GASTROENTEROLOGY AND HEPATOLOGY

HEMATOLOGY AND ONCOLOGY

INFECTIOUS DISEASES AND HIV/AIDS

NEPHROLOGY

NEUROLOGY AND PSYCHIATRY

18th Edition

HARRISON'S™
PRINCIPLES OF
INTERNAL
MEDICINE

EDITORS OF PREVIOUS EDITIONS

18th Edition

HARRISON'S™
PRINCIPLES OF
INTERNAL
MEDICINE

EDITORS

Dan L. Longo, MD

Professor of Medicine, Harvard Medical School;
Senior Physician, Brigham and Women's Hospital; Deputy Editor,
New England Journal of Medicine, Boston, Massachusetts

Dennis L. Kasper, MD

William Ellery Channing Professor of Medicine, Professor of
Microbiology and Molecular Genetics, Harvard Medical School;
Director, Channing Laboratory, Department of Medicine,
Brigham and Women's Hospital, Boston, Massachusetts

J. Larry Jameson, MD, PhD

Robert G. Dunlop Professor of Medicine; Dean, University of
Pennsylvania School of Medicine; Executive Vice-President of the
University of Pennsylvania for the Health System,
Philadelphia, Pennsylvania

Anthony S. Fauci, MD

Chief, Laboratory of Immunoregulation; Director, National
Institute of Allergy and Infectious Diseases, National Institutes of
Health, Bethesda, Maryland

Stephen L. Hauser, MD

Robert A. Fishman Distinguished Professor and Chairman,
Department of Neurology, University of California, San Francisco,
San Francisco, California

Joseph Loscalzo, MD, PhD

Hersey Professor of the Theory and Practice of Medicine,
Harvard Medical School; Chairman, Department of Medicine;
Physician-in-Chief, Brigham and Women's Hospital,
Boston, Massachusetts

VOLUME I

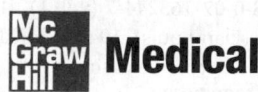

New York   Chicago   San Francisco   Lisbon   London   Madrid   Mexico City
Milan   New Delhi   San Juan   Seoul   Singapore   Sydney   Toronto

Note: Dr. Fauci's work as editor and author was performed outside the scope of his employment as a U.S. government employee. This work represents his personal and professional views and not necessarily those of the U.S. government.

Harrison's ™
PRINCIPLES OF INTERNAL MEDICINE
Eighteenth Edition

2 3 4 5 6 7 8 9 10   DOW/DOW   15 14 13 12

Two Volume Set ISBN 978-0-07174889-6; MHID 0-07-174889-X
Volume 1 ISBN 978-0-07-163244-7; MHID 0-07-163244-1
Volume 2 ISBN 978-0-07-174887-2; MHID 0-07-174887-3
DVD ISBN 978-0-07-174888-9; MHID 0-07-174888-1

FOREIGN LANGUAGE EDITIONS

Arabic (13e): McGraw-Hill Libri Italia srl (1996)
Albanian(17e): Tabernakul Publishing, Skopje, Macedonia
Chinese Long Form (15e): McGraw-Hill International Enterprises, Inc., Taiwan
Chinese Short Form (15e): McGraw-Hill Education (Asia), Singapore
Croatian (16e): Placebo, Split, Croatia
French (16e): Medecine-Sciences Flammarion, Paris, France
German (17e): ABW Wissenschaftsverlagsgesellschaft GmbH, Berlin, Germany
Greek (17e): Parissianos, S.A., Athens, Greece
Italian (17e): The McGraw-Hill Companies, Srl, Milan, Italy
Japanese (17e): MEDSI-Medical Sciences International Ltd, Tokyo, Japan

Korean (17e): McGraw-Hill Korea, Inc., Seoul, Korea
Macedonian (17e): Tabernakul Publishing, Skopje, Macedonia
Polish (17e): Czelej Publishing Company, Lubin, Poland
Portuguese (17e): McGraw-Hill Interamericana Editores, SA de C.V. Mexico City, Mexico
Romanian (17e): Editura All, Bucharest, Romania
Serbian (15e): Publishing House Romanov, Bosnia & Herzegovina, Republic of Serbska
Spanish (17e): McGraw-Hill Interamericana Editores, SA de C.V. Mexico City, Mexico
Turkish (17e): Nobel Tip Kitabevleri, Ltd., Istanbul, Turkey
Vietnamese (15e): McGraw-Hill Education (Asia), Singapore

This book was set in Minion Pro by Cenveo Publisher Services. The editors were James F. Shanahan and Kim J. Davis. The production managers were Phil Galea and John Williams; production assistance was provided by Rajni Pisharody at Cenveo Publisher Services. The index was prepared by Susan Hunter and Ann Blum. The text designer was Alan Barnett; cover design was by Anthony Landi. RR Donnelley was printer and binder.

Library of Congress Cataloging-in-Publication Data

Harrison's principles of internal medicine.—18th ed. / editors, Dan L. Longo ... [et al.]. p. ; cm.
  Includes bibliographical references and index.
    ISBN 978-0-07-174889-6 (set)—ISBN 978-0-07-163244-7 (vol. 1)—ISBN 978-0-07-174887-2 (vol. 2)
      1. Internal medicine. I. Longo, Dan L. (Dan Louis), 1949- II. Harrison, Tinsley
Randolph, 1900-1978. III. Title: Principles of internal medicine.
  [DNLM: 1. Internal Medicine. WB 115 H322 2011]
  RC46.H333 2008
  616—dc22   2008053547

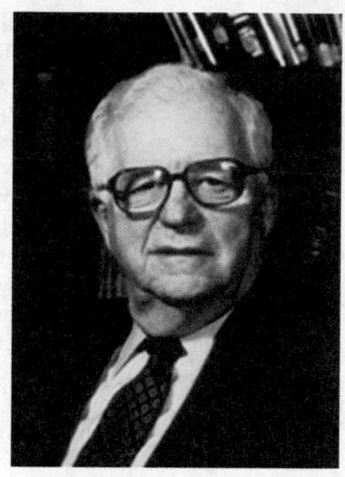

Dedication: Eugene Braunwald

This edition of *Harrison's Principles of Internal Medicine*, the 18th edition, is respectfully and warmly dedicated to our colleague, teacher, mentor, and friend, Eugene Braunwald. Dr. Braunwald has been a fixture on the editorial board of this book since 1967, when the 6th edition was being planned—a period of more than 40 years. No one has served the book so long or with as much distinction. He was an inexhaustible source of ideas and innovations throughout his period of service, for which we and the former editors are most grateful.

Of course, his work on this book was only a small fraction of his prodigious intellectual output. He graduated first in his class from New York University (NYU) School of Medicine, spent two years in internal medicine training at Mount Sinai Hospital, returned to NYU for a year as a research fellow with Andre Cournand (who would later win the Nobel Prize for inventing cardiac catheterization), spent two years as a Clinical Associate at the National Heart Institute, and then completed his final year of internal medicine training on the Osler service at Johns Hopkins. After completing his training, he returned to the National Heart Institute as a tenured senior investigator in 1958 at 29 years of age, becoming Chief of the Cardiology Branch in 1959 and Clinical Director of the institute in 1966. He published about 370 papers during his 10 years at the National Institutes of Health, many of which were seminal findings that became an essential part of the fabric of our cardiovascular knowledge base. In 1968, he was enticed into becoming the founding Chairman of the Department of Medicine at a new medical school, University of California, San Diego (UCSD). During his four years there, he demonstrated that he was not only a creative scientist but an innovative medical educator, administrator, and academic leader. In 1972, he was recruited to be the Hersey Professor of the Theory and Practice of Medicine (the oldest endowed chair in medicine) at Harvard Medical School and Chairman of the Department of Medicine at the Peter Bent Brigham Hospital, a position he held for 24 years. He is now the Distinguished Hersey Professor and the Chairman of the Thrombolysis in Myocardial Infarction (TIMI) Study Group, a cooperative research organization that has completed nearly 60 (and counting) prospective randomized trials that have defined the elements of the optimal care of patients with acute coronary syndromes.

His research has spanned many dimensions of cardiology, in scope and over time. In the earliest phase, he focused on valvular heart disease, which was much more prevalent than it is today because of the late effects of poorly treated rheumatic fever in the preantibiotic era. Among his accomplishments were the very first recordings in humans of the pressure gradient across a stenotic mitral valve and the effects of valvulotomy on hemodynamics; the development of transseptal left heart catheterization, then a breakthrough in the measurement of left heart function in vivo, and now used to treat mitral valve disease, to perform electrophysiology and ablation procedures in the left atrium and to provide access for assist devices; demonstration of the reversibility of high pulmonary vascular resistance by mitral valve replacement in patients with mitral stenosis (high pulmonary vascular resistance had been used to disqualify patients from the operation); and demonstration of the dire prognosis of patients with aortic stenosis when they develop symptoms of heart failure, syncope, or angina (which led to earlier surgical intervention).

Working closely with his surgical colleague at the National Institutes of Health, Glenn Andrew Morrow, he identified a previously unknown disease entity: hypertrophic cardiomyopathy. Based on pressure recordings that showed an unexplained dynamic pressure gradient between the left ventricle and the aorta in the presence of a normal aortic valve, they proposed that the obstruction to left ventricular outflow was caused by left ventricle contraction itself; hypertrophic heart muscle during contraction blocked the flow of blood from the ventricle to the aorta. Hypertrophic cardiomyopathy is now known to be the most common Mendelian inherited heart disease (1 in 500 births). The Braunwald team described the fascinating physiologic changes associated with the condition in detail, including the diagnostic sign of the *reduction* in pulse pressure following a premature contraction instead of the expected potentiation of pulse pressure. They developed treatments (beta blockers and myotomy/myectomy) that are still the cornerstones of therapy 40 years later.

Dr. Braunwald defined fundamental features of the pathophysiology and treatment of heart failure. He and his colleagues documented that normal human heart muscle follows Starling's law (the greater the tension on the muscle, the stronger its contraction) and that left ventricular end-diastolic pressure was a key determinant of stroke volume, stroke work, and stroke power. They showed that these properties were seriously altered in the failing heart, with the length-tension curves shifting dramatically to the left (that is, for any particular amount of stretch on the muscle, contraction extent and velocity were reduced). They also demonstrated the improvement in cardiac function caused by drugs that reduce afterload, including beta blockers and angiotensin-converting enzyme inhibitors or receptor antagonists—treatments that extend the lives of patients with failing hearts. We measure left ventricular ejection fraction today as a method of assessing cardiac function based on concepts and techniques the Braunwald team pioneered.

His work on myocardial ischemia and infarction has formed the basis for current (and likely future) management strategies of this most common disease. It was his work that defined the basic determinants of myocardial oxygen consumption: tension development, contractility, and heart rate account for 92% of consumed oxygen. This finding led directly to the observation that the size of an infarct could be profoundly altered by a number of physiologic and pharmacologic interventions that modify myocardial oxygen consumption and interventions that restore coronary perfusion, especially if implemented within three hours of occlusion. The formation of the Thrombolysis in Myocardial Infarction (TIMI) study group has led to widespread changes in practice and has saved untold numbers of lives. In addition to exploring thrombolytic therapy in its early days, the group has proved the value of early invasive intervention for unstable angina, aggressive lipid-lowering strategies after a heart attack to prevent recurrence and death, and the use of antiplatelet agents and other anticoagulants as adjuncts to coronary artery stenting to prevent restenosis, among others.

His administrative accomplishments are legion. He has served as head of major organizations since he was 31 years old. As the first Chairman of Medicine at UCSD, he took the department from a concept to a leading center in four years, recruiting 75 faculty members and establishing a first-rate training program. Under his leadership, the Brigham and Women's Hospital Department of Medicine grew dramatically, recruited outstanding physician/scientists whose work has influenced every corner of internal medicine, and trained two generations of academic researchers who either stayed on at one or more of the Harvard hospitals or went to other universities and exerted a major influence in academic medicine.

His educational impact extends well beyond the worldwide influence of his mentorship to hundreds of physician scientists and medical educators and his enormous contributions to the cardiology, pulmonology, and renal sections of twelve editions of *Harrison's Principles of Internal Medicine*. Teaching has always been a high priority for him. At UCSD, he helped to establish an educational program in which physicians taught the basic sciences so that the clinical relevance of the information would always be at hand. He created the cardiology textbook *Heart Disease* (now known as *Braunwald's Heart Disease*), wrote a major fraction of its chapters, and has shepherded the book through seven editions.

He has been elected President of nearly every organization to which he belongs. He has published nearly 1300 papers. He is a member of the United States National Academy of Sciences and its Institute of Medicine. A list of his awards and honorary degrees would exceed the length of this dedication. Eugene Braunwald is one of the leading lights in the history of medicine. His indelible impact on the institutions he has led, the practice of cardiology, medical education, this textbook, and the many individuals whom he has trained will continue to be felt in future generations. We therefore dedicate this edition of *Harrison's Principles of Internal Medicine* to him with respect, admiration, and heartfelt gratitude.

THE EDITORS

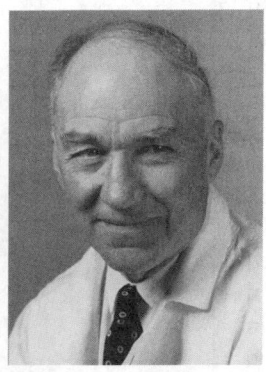

In Memoriam: Raymond D. Adams (1911–2008)

Ray Adams's tenure as editor of *Harrison's Principles of Internal Medicine* began with the second edition, published in 1954; he then remained on the editorial board for more than three decades. Dr. Adams was born in Portland, Oregon and graduated from the University of Oregon and Duke University Medical School. After a discouraging foray into a psycho-analytic career, he found his calling when appointed to the Neurology and Neuropathology Service at Boston City Hospital and then, in 1951, as Chief of the Neurology Service at Massachusetts General Hospital. His contributions to neurology and medicine were prodigious, grounded in a fastidious approach to clinicopathologic correlation. There are few areas of neurology in which he did not have an impact. He identified immune mechanisms and the cause of disability in multiple sclerosis and Guillain-Barré syndrome; clarified nutritional, alcoholic, syphilitic, and metabolic disorders of the nervous system; performed careful studies of embolic stroke and anoxic brain disease; focused attention on mental retardation and language disability as core problems in neurology; and described many muscle diseases. Ray Adams was also an extraordinary clinician and teacher who trained generations of physician-scientists. Today they represent an important part of his legacy. The excellence of *Harrison's* owes much to Dr. Adams, and his commitment to education continues to be reflected in the pages of each new edition.

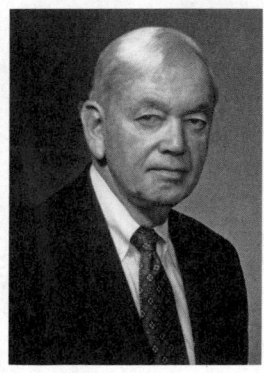

In Memoriam: Robert G. Petersdorf (1926–2006)

An editor of *Harrison's Principles of Internal Medicine* from 1968 through 1990, Robert G. Petersdorf was for many years one of the most powerful figures in American medicine and an internationally recognized expert and educator in infectious diseases. He gained prominence in 1961 through his classic study of fever of unknown origin, conducted at Yale in collaboration with Paul Beeson. During his distinguished career, Dr. Petersdorf held key positions at several institutions, including Chair of the Department of Medicine at the University of Washington in Seattle, President of Brigham and Women's Hospital in Boston, and Vice Chancellor for Health Sciences and Dean of the School of Medicine at the University of California, San Diego. He served from 1986 to 1994 as President of the Association of American Medical Colleges, where he advocated for better communication between the medical community and Congress, for increased enrollment of underrepresented minorities in medical schools, and for greater numbers of primary care doctors in general internal medicine and family practice. As a central figure in the training of many leaders in American medicine, Dr. Petersdorf was described as blunt and demanding but also very kind; a colleague recalled that he constantly reminded students to listen to the patient, who, he maintained, "was always right." Dr. Petersdorf's efforts through seven editions of *Harrison's* were instrumental in establishing the book's pivotal role in the education of students, residents, and practitioners of medicine.

THE EDITORS

NOTICE

Medicine is an ever-changing science. As new research and clinical experience broaden our knowledge, changes in treatment and drug therapy are required. The authors and the publisher of this work have checked with sources believed to be reliable in their efforts to provide information that is complete and generally in accord with the standards accepted at the time of publication. However, in view of the possibility of human error or changes in medical sciences, neither the authors nor the publisher nor any other party who has been involved in the preparation or publication of this work warrants that the information contained herein is in every respect accurate or complete, and they disclaim all responsibility for any errors or omissions or for the results obtained from use of the information contained in this work. Readers are encouraged to confirm the information contained herein with other sources. For example and in particular, readers are advised to check the product information sheet included in the package of each drug they plan to administer to be certain that the information contained in this work is accurate and that changes have not been made in the recommended dose or in the contraindications for administration. This recommendation is of particular importance in connection with new or infrequently used drugs.

COVER ILLUSTRATIONS (VOLUME I)

Background Image: A stylized scanning electron microscopic image of *Mycobacterium tuberculosis*. This bacterium causes most cases of tuberculosis. *(Credit: MedicalRF.com)*

Top Panel: Oxygen-starved cancer cells, microscopic view. Oxygen starvation is something which tumor cells are often exposed to in the center of a solid tumor; those cancer cells that can survive in a low oxygen environment are harder to treat and kill, making the study of cell growth in low oxygen conditions useful. Here, osteocarcoma cells respond to a drug that blocks oxygen use and turn off much of their protein synthesis. Regulatory proteins (green and blue) turn the machinery on and off. Immunofluorescent photomicrograph. *(Credit: Nancy Kedersha, photographer; Science Faction Collection)*

Center Panel: Activated platelet with human red blood cells. *(Credit: David Scharf, photographer; Science Faction Collection.)*

Bottom Panel: X-ray of the lungs. *(Credit: BSIP/Photo Researchers, Inc.)*

CONTENTS

✦ PART 1: Introduction to Clinical Medicine

✦ PART 2: Cardinal Manifestations and Presentation of Diseases

SECTION 1 — Pain

SECTION 2 — Alterations in Body Temperature

SECTION 3 — Nervous System Dysfunction

SECTION 4 — Disorders of Eyes, Ears, Nose, and Throat

CONTENTS

CONTENTS

PART 9: Terrorism and Clinical Medicine

PART 10: Disorders of the Cardiovascular System

CONTENTS

CONTENTS

CONTENTS

CONTENTS

xix

SUMMARIES OF CHAPTERS e1 TO e57

Chapter e1 ◆ Primary Care in Low- and Middle-Income Countries

This chapter looks first at the nature of the health challenges in low- and middle-income countries that underlie the health divide. It then outlines the values and principles of a primary health care approach with a focus on primary care services. Next, the chapter reviews the experience of low- and middle-income countries in addressing health challenges through primary care and a primary health care approach. Finally, the chapter identifies how current challenges and global context provide an agenda and opportunities for the renewal of primary health care and primary care.

Chapter e2 ◆ Complementary, Alternative, and Integrative Medicine

Complementary and alternative medicine (CAM) refers to a group of diverse medical and health care systems, practices, and products that are not considered part of conventional or allopathic medicine or that have historic origins outside mainstream medicine. Most of these practices are used together with conventional therapies and therefore have been called *complementary* to distinguish them from *alternative* practices, which are those used instead of standard care. *Integrative medicine* refers to a style of practice that places strong emphasis on a holistic approach to patient care, focusing on reduced use of technology and preventive strategies for maintenance of health.

Chapter e3 ◆ The Economics of Medical Care

This chapter attempts to explain to physicians how economists think about physicians and medical care. Economists' mode of thinking has shaped health care policy and institutions and, thus, the environment for in which physicians practice. As a result, it may be useful physicians to understand some aspects of this way of thinking even if at times it may seem foreign or uncongenial.

Chapter e4 ◆ Racial and Ethnic Disparities in Health Care

This chapter provides an overview of racial and ethnic disparities in health and health care, identifies root causes, and provides key recommendations to address them at both the clinical and health system level.

Chapter e5 ◆ Ethical Issues in Clinical Medicine

This chapter discusses fundamental and ethical guidelines, patients who lack decision-making capacity, decisions and life-sustaining interventions, conflicts of interest, and just allocation of resources. The chapter helps the physician to follow two fundamental but frequently conflicting ethical principles: respecting patient autonomy and acting in the patient's best interest.

Chapter e6 ◆ Neoplasia During Pregnancy

This chapter looks at the complex problem of cancer in a pregnant woman, covering topics such as cervical cancer, breast cancer, and melanoma during pregnancy. The chapter examines the possible influence of the pregnancy on the natural history of the cancer, the effects of the diagnostic and staging procedures, and the treatments of the cancer on both the mother and the developing fetus. These issues may lead to dilemmas: what is best for the mother may be harmful to the fetus, and what is best for the fetus may be harmful to the mother.

Chapter e7 ◆ Atlas of Rashes Associated With Fever

Given the extremely broad differential diagnosis, the presentation of a patient with fever and rash often poses a thorny diagnostic challenge for even the most astute and experienced clinician. Rapid narrowing of the differential by prompt recognition of a rash's key features can result in appropriate and sometimes life-saving therapy. This atlas presents high-quality images of a variety of rashes that have an infectious etiology and are commonly associated with fever.

Chapter e8 ◆ Video Library of Gait Disorders

Problems with gait and balance are major causes of falls, accidents, and resulting disability, especially in later life, and are often harbingers of neurologic disease. Early diagnosis is essential, especially for treatable conditions, as it may permit the institution of prophylactic measures to prevent dangerous falls, and also to reverse or ameliorate the underlying cause. In this video, examples of gait disorders due to Parkinson's disease, other extrapyramidal disorders, and ataxias, as well as other common gait disorders, are presented.

Chapter e9 ◆ Memory Loss

This chapter discusses the formation of both long- and short-term memories. Long-term memory is divided into declarative and nondeclarative memory; the former is further subdivided into episodic and semantic memories. Short-term, or working, memory relies on different regions of the brain and lesions that disrupt their structure or function can be devastating.

Chapter e10 ◆ Primary Progressive Aphasia, Memory Loss, and Other Focal Cerebral Disorders

Language and memory are essential human functions. For the experienced clinician, the recognition of different types of language and memory disturbances often provides essential clues to the anatomic localization and diagnosis of neurologic disorders. This video illustrates classic disorders of language and speech (including the aphasias), memory (the amnesias), and other disorders of cognition that are commonly encountered in clinical practice.

Chapter e11 ◆ Video Library of Neuro-Ophthalmology

The proper control of eye movements requires the coordinated activity of many different anatomic structures in the peripheral and central nervous system, and in turn manifestations of a diverse array of neurologic and medical disorders are revealed as disorders of eye movement. In this remarkable video collection, an introduction to distinctive eye movement disorders encountered in the context of neuromuscular, paraneoplastic, demyelinating, neurovascular and neurodegenerative disorders is presented.

Chapter e12 ⊘ Atlas of Oral Manifestations of Disease

The health status of the oral cavity is linked to cardiovascular disease, diabetes, and other systemic illnesses. Thus, examining the oral cavity for signs of disease is a key part of the physical exam. This atlas presents numerous outstanding clinical photographs illustrating many of the conditions affecting the teeth, periodontal tissues, and oral mucosa.

Chapter e13 ⊘ Approach to the Patient With a Heart Murmur

This chapter provides comprehensive coverage of heart murmurs (systolic, diastolic, and continuous), their major attributes, and their response to bedside maneuvers, detected by auscultation.

Chapter e14 ⊘ Atlas of Urinary Sediments and Renal Biopsies

This chapter illustrates key diagnostic features of selected diseases in renal biopsy using light microscopy, immunofluorescence, and electron microscopy. Common urinalysis findings are also documented.

Chapter e15 ⊘ Fluid and Electrolyte Imbalances and Acid-Base Disturbances: Case Examples

Acid-base, fluid, and electrolyte disorders can be intimidating to trainees and practicing physicians alike. The real-life clinical vignettes in this chapter have been chosen to reinforce selected concepts covered in the relevant chapters. These are short, directed discussions, focused on key issues in diagnosis and/or therapy.

Chapter e16 ⊘ Atlas of Skin Manifestations of Internal Disease

This atlas provides pictures of a selected group of inflammatory skin eruptions and neoplastic conditions illustrating (1) common skin diseases and lesions, (2) nonmelanoma skin cancer, (3) melanoma and pigmented lesions, (4) infectious disease and the skin, (5) immunologically mediated skin disease, and (6) skin manifestations of internal disease.

Chapter e17 ⊘ Atlas of Hematology and Analysis of Peripheral Blood Smears

This atlas gives many examples of both normal and abnormal blood smears and a guide to blood smear interpretation. A normal peripheral blood smear is shown, as are normal granulocytes, monocytes, eosinophils, basophils, plasma cells, and bone marrow.

Chapter e18 ⊘ Mitochondrial DNA and Heritable Traits and Diseases

The structure and function of mitochondrial DNA (mtDNA) are discussed in depth in this chapter, which includes the proposition that the total cumulative burden of somatic mtDNA mutations acquired with age may contribute to aging and common age-related disturbances.

Chapter e19 ⊘ Systems Biology in Health and Disease

This chapter presents new concepts related to the complex molecular and genetic systems that underlie all human disease. Using the evolving approaches of systems biology, interaction models of human disease that include the molecular networks specific to the disease, as well as those molecular networks that define generic mechanisms common to all disease (e.g., fibrosis and inflammation), are presented. Environmental factors that influence the behavior of these networks and their effects on the patho-phenotype (e.g., epigenesis or posttranslational modification of the proteome) are included in this new disease paradigm.

Chapter e20 ⊘ Thymoma

This chapter begins with a brief overview of the composition and function of the thymus and lists the various abnormalities that can occur and discusses the clinical presentation and differential diagnosis of thymoma as well as staging, pathology and etiology, and treatment.

Chapter e21 ⊘ Less Common Hematologic Malignancies

This chapter focuses on the more unusual forms of hematologic malignancy, covering diseases such as hairy cell leukemia, mediastinal large B cell lymphoma, and Langerhans' cell histiocytosis.

Chapter e22 ⊘ Laboratory Diagnosis of Infectious Diseases

This chapter documents the evolution of methods used in the clinical microbiology laboratory to detect and identify viral, bacterial, fungal, and parasitic agents and to determine the antibiotic susceptibility of bacterial and fungal pathogens.

Chapter e23 ⊘ Infectious Complications of Burns

This chapter details the consequences of breaches in the skin barrier from burns, which may cause massive destruction of the integument as well as derangements in humoral and cellular immunity, permitting the development of infection caused by environmental opportunists and components of the host's skin flora.

Chapter e24 ⊘ Infectious Complications of Bites

This chapter discusses breaches in the skin from bites and scratches that represent a form of immunocompromise and predispose the patient to infection. The treatment section covers wound management, antibiotic therapy for established infection and for prophylactic purposes, and rabies and tetanus prophylaxis.

Chapter e25 ⊘ Laboratory Diagnosis of Parasitic Infections

This chapter emphasizes the importance of the history and epidemiology of a patient's illness. Tables provide clear information on the geographic distribution, transmission, anatomic locations, and methods employed for the diagnosis of flatworm, roundworm, and protozoal infections.

Chapter e26 ⊘ Pharmacology of Agents Used to Treat Parasitic Infections

This chapter deals exclusively with the pharmacologic properties of the agents used to treat infections due to parasites. Specific treatment recommendations for the parasitic diseases of humans are listed in the chapters on those diseases. Information on these agents' major toxicities, spectrum of activity, and safety for use during pregnancy and lactation is presented in Chapter 208.

Chapter e27 ⊘ Atlas of Blood Smears of Malaria and Babesiosis

This chapter provides both thin and thick blood films for *Plasmodium falciparum*, *P. vivax*, *P. ovale*, and *P. malariae*. The thick film allows detection of densities as low as 50 parasites per microliter, with great sensitivity; the thin film is better for speciation and provides useful prognostic information in severe falciparum malaria. One thin blood film showing trophozoites of *Babesia* is included.

Chapter e28 ⊘ Atlas of Electrocardiography

The electrocardiograms in this atlas supplement those illustrated in Chapter 228. The interpretations emphasize findings of specific teaching value.

Chapter e29 ⊘ Atlas of Noninvasive Cardiac Imaging

This chapter provides "real-time" image clips as they are viewed in clinical practice, as well as additional static images. Noninvasive cardiac imaging is essential to the diagnosis and management of patients with known or suspected cardiovascular disease. This atlas supplements Chapter 229, which describes the principles and clinical applications of these important techniques.

Chapter e30 ⊘ Atlas of Cardiac Arrhythmias

The electrocardiograms in this atlas supplement those illustrated in Chapters 232 and 233. The interpretations emphasize findings of specific teaching value.

Chapter e31 ⊘ Cardiac Manifestations of Systemic Disease

This chapter covers the common systemic disorders that have associated cardiac manifestations, such as diabetes mellitus, hyper- and hypothyroidism, and systemic lupus erythematosus.

Chapter e32 ⊘ Atlas of Atherosclerosis

This atlas consists of six videos that highlight some of the current understanding of atherosclerosis. Topics include pulse pressure, plaque instability, rudiments of the clinically important lipoproteins, formation and complications of atherosclerotic plaques, mechanisms of atherogenesis, and metabolic derangements that underlie the metabolic syndrome.

Chapter e33 ⊘ Atlas of Percutaneous Revascularization

This atlas presents seven case studies illustrating the use of percutaneous coronary intervention in a variety of commonly encountered clinical and anatomic situations, such as chronic total occlusion of a coronary artery, bifurcation disease, acute STEMI, saphenous vein graft disease, left main coronary artery disease, multivessel disease, and stent thrombosis.

Chapter e34 ⊘ Atlas of Chest Imaging

This atlas is a collection of interesting chest radiographs and CT scans illustrative of specific major findings that are categorized by those of volume loss, loss of parenchyma, interstitial processes, alveolar processes, bronchiectasis, pleural abnormalities, nodules and masses, and pulmonary vascular abnormalities.

⊘ Chapter e35 Interstitial Cystitis/Painful Bladder Syndrome

This chapter covers interstitial cystitis/painful bladder syndrome, a chronic condition that occurs primarily in women and is characterized by pain perceived to be from the urinary bladder, urinary urgency and frequency, and nocturia.

Chapter e36 ⊘ Video Atlas of Gastrointestinal Endoscopy

Gastrointestinal endoscopy is an increasingly important method for diagnosis and treatment of disease. This atlas demonstrates endoscopic findings in a variety of gastrointestinal infectious, inflammatory, vascular, and neoplastic conditions. Cancer screening and prevention are common indications for gastrointestinal endoscopy, and the premalignant conditions of Barrett's esophagus and colonic polyps are illustrated. Endoscopic treatment modalities for gastrointestinal bleeding, polyps, and biliary stones are demonstrated in video clips.

Chapter e37 ⊘ The Schilling Test

While not available commercially in the United States for the last few years, the Schilling test is performed to determine the cause for cobalamin malabsorption. Since understanding the physiology and pathophysiology of cobalamin absorption is very valuable for enhancing one's understanding of aspects of gastric, pancreatic, and ileal function, discussion of the Schilling test is provided as supplemental information to Chapter 294.

Chapter e38 ⊘ Atlas of Liver Biopsies

Included in this atlas of liver biopsies are examples of common morphologic features of acute and chronic liver disorders, some involving the lobular areas (e.g., the lobular inflammatory changes of acute hepatitis, apoptotic hepatocyte degeneration in acute and chronic hepatitis, virus antigen localization in hepatocyte cytoplasm and/or nuclei, viral inclusion bodies, copper or iron deposition, other inclusion bodies), and others involving the portal tracts (e.g., the portal mononuclear infiltrate that expands and spills over beyond the border of periportal hepatocytes in chronic hepatitis C, autoimmune hepatitis, and liver allograft rejection) or centrizonal areas (e.g., acute acetaminophen hepatotoxicity).

Chapter e39 ⊘ Primary Immunodeficiencies Associated With (or Secondary to) Other Diseases

There are an increasing number of conditions in which a primary immunodeficiency (PID) has been described as one facet of a more complex disease setting. It is essential to consider associated diseases when a PID is identified as the primary manifestation and, conversely, not neglect the potentially harmful consequences of a PID that could be masked by other manifestations of a particular syndrome. This chapter provides descriptions of these syndromes in which the PID is classified according to the arm of the immune system that is affected.

Chapter e40 ⊘ Atlas of the Vasculitic Syndromes

Diagnosis of the vasculitic syndromes is usually based upon characteristic histologic or arteriographic findings in a patient who has clinically compatible features. The images provided in this atlas highlight some of the characteristic histologic and radiographic findings that may be seen in the vasculitic diseases. These images demonstrate the importance that tissue histology may have in securing the diagnosis of vasculitis, the utility of diagnostic imaging in the vasculitic diseases, and the improvements in the care of vasculitis patients that have resulted from radiologic innovations.

Chapter e41 ⊘ Atlas of Clinical Manifestations of Metabolic Diseases

This atlas provides a visual survey of selected metabolic disorders with references to the topics elsewhere in the text. The emerging field of *metabolomics* is based on the premise that the identification and measurement of metabolic products will enhance our understanding of physiology and disease. Over the years, the classification of metabolic diseases has extended beyond traditional pathways involved in fuel metabolism to include disorders such as lysosomal storage diseases or connective tissue diseases.

🔘 Chapter e42 The Neurologic Screening Exam

Knowledge of the basic neurologic examination is an essential clinical skill. A simple neurologic screening examination—assessment of mental status, cranial nerves, motor system, sensory system, coordination, and gait—can be reliably performed in 3-5 minutes. Although the components of the examination may appear daunting at first, skills usually improve rapidly with repetition and practice. In this video, the technique of performing a simple and efficient screening examination is presented.

🔘 Chapter e43 Video Atlas of the Detailed Neurologic Examination

The comprehensive neurologic examination is an irreplaceable tool for the efficient diagnosis of neurologic disorders. Mastery of its details requires knowledge of normal nervous system anatomy and physiology, combined with personal experience performing orderly and systematic examinations on large numbers of patients and healthy individuals. In the hands of a great clinician, the neurologic examination also becomes a thing of beauty—the pinnacle of the art of medicine. In this video, the most commonly used components of the examination are presented in detail, with a particular emphasis on those elements that are most helpful for assessment of common neurologic problems.

🔘 Chapter e44 Atlas of Neuroimaging

This atlas comprises 29 cases to assist the clinician caring for patients with neurologic symptoms. The majority of the images are MRIs; other techniques used are MR and conventional angiography and CT scans. Many neurologic diseases are illustrated, such as tuberculosis of the central nervous system (CNS), neurosyphilis, CNS aspergillosis, neurosarcoid, middle cerebral artery stenosis, CNS vasculitis, Huntington's disease, and acute transverse myelitis.

🔘 Chapter e45 Electrodiagnostic Studies of Nervous System Disorders: EEG, Evoked Potentials, and EMG

This chapter covers the two main techniques for electrodiagnosis of neurologic symptoms: electroencephalogram (EEG) and the electromyogram (EMG). Evoked potentials (sensory, cognitive, and motor) are also covered.

🔘 Chapter e46 Technique of Lumbar Puncture

This chapter covers the procedure of lumbar puncture (LP) in detail (with illustrations), from indications for imaging and laboratory studies prior to LP, analgesia, positioning, and the procedure itself (including dealing with complications that may arise during LP). Also included is a section on the main complication of LP—the post-LP headache—and its causes and therapy and strategies to avoid it.

🔘 Chapter e47 Special Issues in Inpatient Neurologic Consultation

Inpatient neurologic consultations usually involve questions about specific disease processes or prognostication after various cerebral injuries. Common reasons for neurologic consultation include stroke, seizures, altered mental status, headache, and management of coma and other neurocritical care conditions. This chapter focuses on additional common reasons for consultation that are not addressed elsewhere in the text.

🔘 Chapter e48 Neuropsychiatric Illnesses in War Veterans

Neuropsychiatric sequelae are common in combat veterans. Although psychiatric and neurologic problems have been well documented in veterans of prior wars, the conflicts in Iraq and Afghanistan have been unique in terms of the level of commitment by the U.S. Department of Defense, Department of Veterans Affairs, and Veterans Health Administration to support research as the wars have unfolded, and to utilize that knowledge to guide population-level screening, evaluation, and treatment initiatives.

These conflicts, like previous ones, have produced hundreds of thousands of combat veterans, many of whom have received or will need care in government and civilian medical facilities. Two conditions in particular have been labeled the signature injuries related to these wars: post-traumatic stress disorder (PTSD) and mild traumatic brain injury (mTBI)—also known as concussion. Although particular emphasis will be given in this chapter to PTSD and concussion/mTBI, it is important to understand that service in all wars is associated with a number of health concerns that coexist and overlap, and a multidisciplinary patient-centered approach to care is necessary.

🔘 Chapter e49 Heavy Metal Poisoning

This chapter provides specific information about the four main heavy metals that pose a significant threat to health via occupational and environmental exposures: lead, mercury, arsenic, and cadmium. A table clearly details the main sources, metabolism, toxic effects produced, diagnosis, and appropriate therapy for poisoning from these metals.

🔘 Chapter e50 Poisoning and Drug Overdosage

This chapter provides comprehensive coverage of the dose-related adverse effects following exposure to chemicals, drugs, or other xenobiotics. The section on diagnosis gives thorough coverage of the physical examination, laboratory assessment, electrocardiographic and radiologic studies, and *toxicologic analysis*. The treatment section gives detailed coverage of the general principles of care, supportive care, prevention of poison absorption, enhancement of poison elimination, administration of antidotes, and prevention of reexposure.

Chapter e51 🔘 Altitude Illness

Altitude illness can be benign, occurring as acute mountain sickness, or life-threatening, manifesting as high-altitude pulmonary edema or high-altitude cerebral edema. This chapter details the clinical presentation and pathophysiology of altitude illness, providing strategies for its prevention and treatment. The chapter also discusses other problems unrelated to altitude illness (especially neurologic abnormalities) that may be caused by hypoxia at high altitudes. Finally, in line with the increasing popularity of travel to high-altitude locations, the chapter considers the special issues that must be taken into account when travelers have common preexisting conditions, such as hypertension, asthma, and coronary artery disease.

Chapter e52 🔘 Hyperbaric and Diving Medicine

This chapter describes the physical and pharmacologic mechanisms by which hyperbaric oxygen may modulate certain disease processes, and reviews the evidence in support of its use for specific clinical indications. Particular examples include selected problem wounds, delayed tissue injury after radiotherapy, and carbon monoxide poisoning. There is an overview of the highly specialized field of diving medicine, which includes a brief summary of key elements in pathophysiology, diagnosis, and treatment of decompression sickness.

Chapter e53 🔘 The Clinical Laboratory in Modern Health Care

The clinical laboratory plays a critical role in modern health care. This chapter describes the rationale for ordering laboratory tests, the use of critical values, the principles of laboratory-based diagnosis and reference range establishment, sources of error in the testing process, specific issues related to genetic testing, and the regulatory environment in which clinical laboratories operate in the United States.

Clinical procedures are an important component of medical student and resident training, and some are required for board and hospital certification. In these new *Harrison's* e-chapters, video tutorials are presented for performing abdominal paracentesis, thoracentesis, endotracheal intubation, and central venous catheter placement. These videos have been created specifically for *Harrison's*. Each includes the indications, contraindications, equipment, potential complications, and related patient safety considerations. Additional video tutorials covering clinical procedures such as breast biopsy, IV line insertion, phlebotomy, arterial line insertion, arthrocentesis, bone marrow biopsy, lumbar puncture, pelvic examination, thyroid aspiration, basic suturing, and urethral catheterization are available to subscribers of *Harrison's Online* and AccessMedicine (available at *www.accessmedicine.com*).

eCHAPTERS

CONTRIBUTORS

James L. Abbruzzese, MD
Professor and Chair, Department of GI Medical Oncology; M.G. and Lillie Johnson Chair for Cancer Treatment and Research, University of Texas, MD Anderson Cancer Center, Houston, Texas [99]

Jamil Aboulhosn, MD
Assistant Professor, Departments of Medicine and Pediatrics, David Geffen School of Medicine, University of California, Los Angeles, Los Angeles, California [236]

John C. Achermann, MD, PhD
Wellcome Trust Senior Fellow, UCL Institute of Child Health, University College London, London, United Kingdom [349]

John W. Adamson, MD
Clinical Professor of Medicine, Department of Hematology/Oncology, University of California, San Diego, San Diego, California [57, 103]

Anthony A. Amato, MD
Professor of Neurology, Harvard Medical School; Department of Neurology, Brigham and Women's Hospital, Boston, Massachusetts [384, 385, 387]

Michael J. Aminoff, MD, DSc
Professor of Neurology, University of California, San Francisco School of Medicine, San Francisco, California [22, 23, e45]

Neil M. Ampel, MD
Professor of Medicine, University of Arizona, Tucson, Arizona [200]

Kenneth C. Anderson, MD
Kraft Family Professor of Medicine, Harvard Medical School; Chief, Jerome Lipper Multiple Myeloma Center, Dana-Farber Cancer Institute, Boston, Massachusetts [111, 113]

Elliott M. Antman, MD
Professor of Medicine, Harvard Medical School; Brigham and Women's Hospital; Boston, Massachusetts [243, 245]

Frederick R. Appelbaum, MD
Director, Division of Clinical Research, Fred Hutchinson Cancer Research Center, Seattle, Washington [114]

Gordon L. Archer, MD
Professor of Medicine and Microbiology/Immunology; Senior Associate Dean for Research and Research Training, Virginia Commonwealth University School of Medicine, Richmond, Virginia [133]

Cesar A. Arias, MD, PhD
Assistant Professor, University of Texas Medical School, Houston, Texas; Director, Molecular Genetics and Antimicrobial Resistance Unit, Universidad El Bosque, Bogotá, Colombia [137]

Wiebke Arlt, MD, DSc, FRCP, FMedSci
Professor of Medicine, Centre for Endocrinology, Diabetes and Metabolism, School of Clinical and Experimental Medicine, University of Birmingham; Consultant Endocrinologist, University Hospital Birmingham, Birmingham, United Kingdom [342]

Valder R. Arruda, MD, PhD
Associate Professor of Pediatrics, University of Pennsylvania School of Medicine; Division of Hematology, The Children's Hospital of Philadelphia, Philadelphia, Pennsylvania [116]

Arthur K. Asbury, MD, FRCP
Van Meter Professor Emeritus of Neurology, University of Pennsylvania School of Medicine, Philadelphia, Pennsylvania [23]

John R. Asplin, MD
Medical Director, Litholink Corporation; Chicago, Illinois [287]

John C. Atherton, MD, FRCP
Nottingham Digestive Diseases Centre Biomedical Research Unit (NDDC BRU), University of Nottingham and Nottingham University Hospitals NHS Trust, Nottingham, United Kingdom [151]

Evelyn Attia, MD
Professor of Clinical Psychiatry, Columbia College of Physicians and Surgeons; Weill Cornell Medical College, New York, New York [79]

Paul S. Auerbach, MD, MS
Redlich Family Professor, Department of Surgery, Division of Emergency Medicine, Stanford University School of Medicine, Palo Alto, California [396]

K. Frank Austen, MD
AstraZeneca Professor of Respiratory and Inflammatory Diseases; Director, Inflammation and Allergic Diseases Research Section, Harvard Medical School; Brigham and Women's Hospital, Boston, Massachusetts [317]

Eric H. Awtry, MD
Assistant Professor of Medicine, Boston University School of Medicine; Inpatient Clinical Director, Section of Cardiology, Boston Medical Center Boston, Massachusetts [240, e31]

Bruce R. Bacon, MD
James F. King, MD Endowed Chair in Gastroenterology; Professor of Internal Medicine, St. Louis University Liver Center, St. Louis University School of Medicine, St. Louis, Missouri [308, 309]

Lindsey R. Baden, MD
Associate Professor of Medicine, Harvard Medical School; Dana-Farber Cancer Institute, Brigham and Women's Hospital, Boston, Massachusetts [178]

John R. Balmes, MD
Professor of Medicine, San Francisco General Hospital, San Francisco, California [256]

Manisha Balwani, MD, MS
Assistant Professor, Department of Genetics and Genomic Sciences, Mount Sinai School of Medicine of New York University, New York, New York [358]

Peter A. Banks, MD
Professor of Medicine, Harvard Medical School; Senior Physician, Division of Gastroenterology, Brigham and Women's Hospital, Boston, Massachusetts [312, 313]

Robert L. Barbieri, MD
Kate Macy Ladd Professor of Obstetrics, Gynecology and Reproductive Biology, Harvard Medical School; Chairperson, Department of Obstetrics and Gynecology, Brigham and Women's Hospital, Boston, Massachusetts [7]

Joanne M. Bargman, MD, FRCPC
Professor of Medicine, University of Toronto; Staff Nephrologist, University Health Network; Director, Home Peritoneal Dialysis Unit and Co-Director, Renal Rheumatology Lupus Clinic, University Health Network, Toronto, Ontario, Canada [280]

Tamar F. Barlam, MD
Associate Professor of Medicine, Boston University School of Medicine, Boston, Massachusetts [121, 146]

Peter J. Barnes, DM, DSc, FMedSci, FRS
Head of Respiratory Medicine, Imperial College, London, United Kingdom [254]

Richard J. Barohn, MD
Chairman, Department of Neurology; Gertrude and Dewey Ziegler Professor of Neurology, University of Kansas Medical Center, Kansas City, Kansas [384]

Miriam J. Baron, MD
Assistant Professor of Medicine, Harvard Medical School; Associate Physician, Brigham and Women's Hospital, Boston, Massachusetts [127]

Rebecca M. Baron, MD
Assistant Professor, Harvard Medical School; Associate Physician, Department of Pulmonary and Critical Care Medicine, Brigham and Women's Hospital, Boston, Massachusetts [258]

John G. Bartlett, MD
Professor of Medicine and Chief, Division of Infectious Diseases, Department of Medicine, Johns Hopkins School of Medicine, Baltimore, Maryland [258]

Robert C. Basner, MD
Professor of Clinical Medicine, Division of Pulmonary, Allergy, and Critical Care Medicine, Columbia University College of Physicians and Surgeons, New York, New York [Appendix]

Buddha Basnyat, MD, MSc, FACP, FRCP(E)
Principal Investigator, Oxford University Clinical Research Unit-Patan Academy of Health Sciences; Medical Director, Nepal International Clinic, Kathmandu, Nepal [e51]

Shari S. Bassuk, ScD
Epidemiologist, Division of Preventive Medicine, Brigham and Women's Hospital, Boston, Massachusetts [348]

John F. Bateman, PhD
Director, Cell Biology, Development and Disease, Murdoch Childrens Research Institute, Parkville, Victoria, Australia [363]

David W. Bates, MD, MSc
Professor of Medicine, Harvard Medical School; Chief, General Internal Medicine and Primary Care Division, Brigham and Women's Hospital; Medical Director, Clinical and Quality Analysis, Partners HealthCare System, Inc., Boston, Massachusetts [10]

Robert P. Baughman, MD
Department of Internal Medicine, University of Cincinnati Medical Center, Cincinnati, Ohio [329]

M. Flint Beal, MD
Chairman of Neurology and Neuroscience; Neurologist-in-Chief, New York Presbyterian Hospital; Weill Cornell Medical College, New York, New York [366, 376]

Laurence H. Beck, Jr., MD, PhD
Assistant Professor of Medicine, Boston University School of Medicine, Boston, Massachusetts [285]

Nicholas J. Beeching, MA, BM BCh, FRCP, FRACP, FFTM RCPS (Glasg), DCH, DTM&H
Senior Lecturer (Clinical) in Infectious Diseases, Liverpool School of Tropical Medicine; Clinical Lead, Tropical and Infectious Disease Unit, Royal Liverpool University Hospital; Honorary Consultant, Health Protection Agency; Honorary Civilian Consultant in Infectious Diseases, Army Medical Directorate, Liverpool, United Kingdom [157]

Robert S. Benjamin, MD
P.H. and Fay E. Robinson Distinguished Professor and Chair, Department of Sarcoma Medical Oncology, University of Texas MD Anderson Cancer Center, Houston, Texas [98]

Michael H. Bennett, MD, MBBS
Conjoint Associate Professor in Anesthesia and Hyperbaric Medicine; Faculty of Medicine, University of New South Wales; Senior Staff Specialist, Department of Diving and Hyperbaric Medicine, Prince of Wales Hospital, Sydney, Australia [e52]

Edward J. Benz, Jr., MD
Richard and Susan Smith Professor of Medicine, Professor of Pediatrics, Professor of Genetics, Harvard Medical School; President and CEO, Dana-Farber Cancer Institute; Director, Dana-Farber/Harvard Cancer Center (DF/HCC), Boston, Massachusetts [104]

Jean Bergounioux, MD, PhD
Pediatric Intensive Care Unit, Hôpital Necker-Enfants Malades, Paris, France [154]

Joseph R. Betancourt, MD, MPH
Associate Professor of Medicine, Harvard Medical School; Director, The Disparities Solutions Center, Massachusetts General Hospital, Boston, Massachusetts [e4]

Atul K. Bhan, MBBS, MD
Professor of Pathology, Harvard Medical School; Director of Immunopathology, Department of Pathology, Massachusetts General Hospital, Boston, Massachusetts [e38]

Shalender Bhasin, MD
Professor of Medicine; Section Chief, Division of Endocrinology, Diabetes and Nutrition, Boston University School of Medicine, Boston, Massachusetts [346]

Deepak L. Bhatt, MD, MPH
Associate Professor of Medicine, Harvard Medical School; Chief of Cardiology, VA Boston Healthcare System; Director, Integrated Interventional Cardiovascular Program, Brigham and Women's Hospital and VA Boston Healthcare System; Senior Investigator, TIMI Study Group, Boston, Massachusetts [246, e33]

David R. Bickers, MD
Carl Truman Nelson Professor and Chair, Department of Dermatology, College of Physicians and Surgeons, Columbia University Medical Center; Dermatologist-in-Chief, New York Presbyterian Hospital, New York, New York [56]

Henry J. Binder, MD
Professor Emeritus of Medicine; Senior Research Scientist, Yale University, New Haven, Connecticut [294, e37]

William R. Bishai, MD, PhD
Professor and Co-Director, Center for Tuberculosis Research, Department of Medicine, Division of Infectious Diseases, Johns Hopkins University School of Medicine, Baltimore, Maryland [138]

Bruce R. Bistrian, MD, PhD
Professor of Medicine, Harvard Medical School; Chief, Clinical Nutrition, Beth Israel Deaconess Medical Center, Boston, Massachusetts [76]

Martin J. Blaser, MD
Frederick H. King Professor of Internal Medicine; Chair, Department of Medicine; Professor of Microbiology, New York University School of Medicine, New York, New York [151, 155]

Gijs Bleijenberg, PhD
Professor; Head, Expert Centre for Chronic Fatigue, Radboud University Nijmegen Medical Centre, Nijmegen, Netherlands [389]

Clara D. Bloomfield, MD
Distinguished University Professor; William G. Pace, III Professor of Cancer Research; Cancer Scholar and Senior Advisor, The Ohio State University Comprehensive Cancer Center; Arthur G. James Cancer Hospital and Richard J. Solove Research Institute, Columbus, Ohio [109]

Richard S. Blumberg, MD
Chief, Division of Gastroenterology, Brigham and Women's Hospital, Boston, Massachusetts [295]

Jean L. Bolognia, MD
Professor of Dermatology, Yale University School of Medicine, New Haven, Connecticut [53]

Joseph V. Bonventre, MD, PhD
Samuel A. Levine Professor of Medicine, Harvard Medical School; Chief, Renal Division; Chief, BWH HST Division of Bioengineering, Brigham and Women's Hospital, Boston, Massachusetts [279]

George J. Bosl, MD
Professor of Medicine, Weill Cornell Medical College; Chair, Department of Medicine; Patrick M. Byrne Chair in Clinical Oncology, Memorial Sloan-Kettering Cancer Center, New York, New York [96]

Richard C. Boucher, MD
Kenan Professor of Medicine, Pulmonary and Critical Care Medicine; Director, Cystic Fibrosis/Pulmonary Reseach and Treatment Center, University of North Carolina at Chapel Hill, Chapel Hill, North Carolina [259]

Eugene Braunwald, MD, MA (Hon), ScD (Hon) FRCP
Distinguished Hersey Professor of Medicine, Harvard Medical School; Founding Chairman, TIMI Study Group, Brigham and Women's Hospital, Boston, Massachusetts [36, 239, 244]

Irwin M. Braverman, MD
Professor of Dermatology, Yale University School of Medicine, New Haven, Connecticut [53]

Otis W. Brawley, MD
Chief Medical Officer, American Cancer Society Professor of Hematology, Oncology, Medicine, and Epidemiology, Emory University, Atlanta, Georgia [82]

Joel G. Breman, MD, DTPH
Scientist Emeritus, Fogarty International Center, National Institutes of Health, Bethesda, Maryland [210, e27]

George J. Brewer, MD
Morton S. and Henrietta K. Sellner Professor Emeritus of Human Genetics; Emeritus Professor of Internal Medicine, University of Michigan Medical School, Senior Vice President for Research and Development, Adeona Pharmaceuticals, Inc., Ann Arbor, Michigan [360]

Josephine P. Briggs, MD
Director, National Center for Complementary and Alternative Medicine, National Institutes of Health, Bethesda, Maryland [e2]

F. Richard Bringhurst, MD
Associate Professor of Medicine, Harvard Medical School; Physician, Massachusetts General Hospital, Boston, Massachusetts [352]

Steven M. Bromley, MD
Clinical Assistant Professor of Neurology, Department of Medicine, New Jersey School of Medicine and Dentistry–Robert Wood Johnson Medical School, Camden, New Jersey [29]

Kevin E. Brown, MD, MRCP, FRCPath
Consultant Medical Virologist, Virus Reference Department, Health Protection Agency, London, United Kingdom [184]

Robert H. Brown, Jr., MD, PhD
Chairman, Department of Neurology, University of Massachusetts Medical School, Worcester, Massachusetts [374, 387]

Amy E. Bryant, PhD
Research Scientist, Veterans Affairs Medical Center, Boise, Idaho; Affiliate Assistant Professor, University of Washington School of Medicine, Seattle, Washington [142]

Christopher M. Burns, MD
Assistant Professor, Department of Medicine, Section of Rheumatology, Dartmouth Medical School; Dartmouth Hitchcock Medical Center, Lebanon, New Hampshire [359]

David M. Burns, MD
Professor Emeritus, Department of Family and Preventive Medicine, University of California, San Diego School of Medicine, San Diego, California [395]

Stephen B. Calderwood, MD
Morton Swartz MD Academy Professor of Medicine (Microbiology and Molecular Genetics), Harvard Medical School; Chief, Division of Infectious Diseases, Massachusetts General Hospital, Boston, Massachusetts [128]

Michael V. Callahan, MD, DTM&H (UK), MSPH
Clinical Associate Physician, Division of Infectious Diseases, Massachusetts General Hospital, Boston, Massachusetts; Program Manager, Biodefense, Defense Advanced Research Project Agency (DARPA), United States Department of Defense, Washington, DC [18]

Michael Camilleri, MD
Atherton and Winifred W. Bean Professor; Professor of Medicine and Physiology, Mayo Clinic College of Medicine, Rochester, Minnesota [40]

Christopher P. Cannon, MD
Associate Professor of Medicine, Harvard Medical School; Senior Investigator, TIMI Study Group, Brigham and Women's Hospital, Boston, Massachusetts [244]

Jonathan Carapetis, PhD, MBBS, FRACP, FAFPHM
Director, Menzies School of Health Research, Charles Darwin University, Darwin, Australia [322]

Kathryn M. Carbone, MD
Deputy Scientific Director, Division of Intramural Research, National Institute of Dental and Craniofacial Research, Bethesda, Maryland [194]

Brian I. Carr, MD, PhD, FRCP
Professor of Oncology and Hepatology, IRCCS De Bellis Medical Research Institute, Castellana Grotte, Italy [92]

Arturo Casadevall, MD, PhD
Chair, Department of Microbiology and Immunology, Albert Einstein College of Medicine, Bronx, New York [202]

Agustin Castellanos, MD
Professor of Medicine, and Director, Clinical Electrophysiology, Division of Cardiology, University of Miami Miller School of Medicine, Miami, Florida [273]

Bartolome R. Celli, MD
Lecturer on Medicine, Harvard Medical School; Staff Physician, Division of Pulmonary and Critical Care Medicine, Brigham and Women's Hospital, Boston, Massachusetts [269]

Murali Chakinala, MD
Associate Professor of Medicine, Division of Pulmonary and Critical Care Medicine, Washington University School of Medicine, St. Louis, Missouri [234]

Anil Chandraker, MD, FASN, FRCP
Associate Professor of Medicine, Harvard Medical School; Medical Director of Kidney and Pancreas Transplantation; Assistant Director, Schuster Family Transplantation Research Center, Brigham and Women's Hospital; Children's Hospital, Boston, Massachusetts [282]

Stanley W. Chapman, MD
Professor of Medicine, University of Mississippi Medical Center, Jackson, Mississippi [201]

Panithaya Chareonthaitawee, MD
Associate Professor of Medicine, Mayo Clinic College of Medicine, Rochester, Minnesota [229, e29]

Lan X. Chen, MD, PhD
Penn Presbyterian Medical Center, Philadelphia, Pennsylvania [333]

Yuan-Tsong Chen, MD, PhD
Distinguished Research Fellow, Institute of Biomedical Sciences, Academia Sinica, Taiwan [362]

Glenn M. Chertow, MD, MPH
Norman S. Coplon/Satellite Healthcare Professor of Medicine; Chief, Division of Nephrology, Stanford University School of Medicine, Palo Alto, California [281]

John S. Child, MD, FACC, FAHA, FASE
Streisand Professor of Medicine and Cardiology, Geffen School of Medicine, University of California, Los Angeles (UCLA); Director, Ahmanson-UCLA Adult Congenital Heart Disease Center; Director, UCLA Adult Noninvasive Cardiodiagnostics Laboratory, Ronald Reagan-UCLA Medical Center; Los Angeles, California [236]

Augustine M. K. Choi, MD
Parker B. Francis Professor of Medicine, Harvard Medical School; Chief, Division of Pulmonary and Critical Care Medicine, Brigham and Women's Hospital, Boston, Massachusetts [251, 253, 268]

Irene Chong, MRCP, FRCR
Clinical Research Fellow, Royal Marsden NHS Foundation Trust, London and Sutton, United Kingdom [93]

Raymond T. Chung, MD
Associate Professor of Medicine, Harvard Medical School; Director of Hepatology; Vice Chief, Gastrointestinal Unit, Massachusetts General Hospital, Boston, Massachusetts [310]

Fredric L. Coe, MD
Professor of Medicine, University of Chicago, Chicago, Illinois [287]

Jeffrey I. Cohen, MD
Chief, Medical Virology Section, Laboratory of Clinical Infectious Diseases, National Institutes of Health, Bethesda, Maryland [181, 191]

Ronit Cohen-Poradosu, MD
Senior Physician, Department of Clinical Microbiology and Infectious Diseases, Hadassah Hebrew Medical Center, Jerusalem, Israel [164]

Francis S. Collins, MD, PhD
Director, National Institutes of Health, Bethesda, Maryland [83]

Wilson S. Colucci, MD
Thomas J. Ryan Professor of Medicine, Boston University School of Medicine; Chief of Cardiovascular Medicine, Boston Medical Center, Boston, Massachusetts [240, e31]

Darwin L. Conwell, MD
Associate Professor of Medicine, Harvard Medical School; Associate Physician, Division of Gastroenterology, Brigham and Women's Hospital, Boston, Massachusetts [312, 313]

CONTRIBUTORS

Michael J. Corbel, PhD, DSc, FRCPath
Head, Division of Bacteriology, National Institute for Biological Standards and Control, Hertfordshire, United Kingdom [157]

William Edward Corcoran, V, MD
Clinical Instructor, Harvard Medical School; Cardiothoracic Fellow, Department of Anesthesiology, Perioperative, and Pain Medicine, Brigham and Women's Hospital, Boston, Massachusetts [e54]

Kathleen E. Corey, MD, MPH
Clinical and Research Fellow, Harvard Medical School; Fellow, Gastrointestinal Unit, Massachusetts General Hospital, Boston, Massachusetts [43]

Lawrence Corey, MD
Professor of Medicine and Laboratory Medicine and Head, Virology Division, Department of Laboratory Medicine, University of Washington; Head, Program in Infectious Diseases, Fred Hutchinson Cancer Research Center, Seattle, Washington [179]

Felicia Cosman, MD
Professor of Clinical Medicine, Columbia University College of Physicians and Surgeons, New York [354]

Mark A. Creager, MD
Professor of Medicine, Harvard Medical School; Simon C. Fireman Scholar in Cardiovascular Medicine; Director, Vascular Center, Brigham and Women's Hospital, Boston, Massachusetts [248, 249]

Leslie J. Crofford, MD
Gloria W. Singletary Professor of Internal Medicine; Chief, Division of Rheumatology, University of Kentucky, Lexington, Kentucky [335]

Jennifer M. Croswell, MD, MPH
Acting Director, Office of Medical Applications of Research, National Institutes of Health, Bethesda, Maryland [82]

Philip E. Cryer, MD
Irene E. and Michael M. Karl Professor of Endocrinology and Metabolism in Medicine, Washington University School of Medicine; Physician, Barnes-Jewish Hospital, St. Louis, Missouri [345]

David Cunningham, MD, FRCP
Professor of Cancer Medicine, Royal Marsden NHS Foundation Trust, London and Sutton, United Kingdom [93]

John J. Cush, MD
Director of Clinical Rheumatology, Baylor Research Institute, Dallas, Texas [331]

Charles A. Czeisler, MD, PhD, FRCP
Baldino Professor of Sleep Medicine; Director, Division of Sleep Medicine, Harvard Medical School; Chief, Division of Sleep Medicine, Department of Medicine, Brigham and Women's Hospital, Boston, Massachusetts [27]

Marinos C. Dalakas, MD, FAAN
Professor of Neurology, Department of Pathophysiology, National University of Athens Medical School, Athens, Greece [388]

Josep Dalmau, MD, PhD
ICREA Research Professor, Institute for Biomedical Investigations, August Pi i Sunyer (IDIBAPS)/Hospital Clinic, Department of Neurology, University of Barcelona, Barcelona, Spain; Adjunct Professor of Neurology University of Pennsylvania, Philadelphia, Pennsylvania [101]

Daniel F. Danzl, MD
University of Louisville, Department of Emergency Medicine, Louisville, Kentucky [19]

Robert B. Daroff, MD
Professor and Chair Emeritus, Department of Neurology, Case Western Reserve University School of Medicine; University Hospitals–Case Medical Center, Cleveland, Ohio [21]

Charles E. Davis, MD
Professor of Pathology and Medicine, Emeritus, University of California, San Diego School of Medicine; Director Emeritus, Microbiology, University of California, San Diego Medical Center, San Diego, California [e25]

Stephen N. Davis, MBBS, FRCP
Theodore E. Woodward Professor and Chairman, Department of Medicine, University of Maryland School of Medicine; Physician-in-Chief, University of Maryland Medical Center, Baltimore, Maryland [345]

Lisa M. DeAngelis, MD
Professor of Neurology, Weill Cornell Medical College; Chair, Department of Neurology, Memorial Sloan-Kettering Cancer Center, New York, New York [379]

John Del Valle, MD
Professor and Senior Associate Chair of Medicine, Department of Internal Medicine, University of Michigan School of Medicine, Ann Arbor, Michigan [293]

Marie B. Demay, MD
Professor of Medicine, Harvard Medical School; Physician, Massachusetts General Hospital, Boston, Massachusetts [352]

Bradley M. Denker, MD
Associate Professor, Harvard Medical School; Physician, Department of Medicine, Brigham and Women's Hospital; Chief of Nephrology, Harvard Vanguard Medical Associates, Boston, Massachusetts [44]

David W. Denning, MB BS, FRCP, FRCPath
Professor of Medicine and Medical Mycology; Director, National Aspergillosis Centre, The University of Manchester and Wythenshawe Hospital, Manchester, United Kingdom [204]

Robert J. Desnick, MD, PhD
Dean for Genetics and Genomics; Professor and Chairman, Department of Genetics and Genomic Sciences, Mount Sinai School of Medicine of New York University, New York, New York [358]

Richard A. Deyo, MD, MPH
Kaiser Permanente Professor of Evidence-Based Family Medicine, Department of Family Medicine, Department of Medicine, Department of Public Health and Preventive Medicine, Center for Research in Occupational and Environmental Toxicology, Oregon Health and Science University; Clinical Investigator, Kaiser Permanente Center for Health Research, Portland, Oregon [15]

Betty Diamond, MD
The Feinstein Institute for Medical Research, North Shore LIJ Health System; Center for Autoimmunity and Musculoskeletal Diseases, Manhasset, New York [318]

Jules L. Dienstag, MD
Carl W. Walter Professor of Medicine and Dean for Medical Education, Harvard Medical School; Physician, Gastrointestinal Unit, Department of Medicine, Massachusetts General Hospital, Boston, Massachusetts [304, 305, 306, 310, e38]

William P. Dillon, MD
Elizabeth Guillaumin Professor of Radiology, Neurology and Neurosurgery; Executive Vice-Chair, Department of Radiology and Biomedical Imaging, University of California, San Francisco, San Francisco, California [368, e44]

Charles A. Dinarello, MD
Professor of Medicine, Division of Infectious Diseases, University of Colorado School of Medicine, Aurora, Colorado [16]

Raphael Dolin, MD
Maxwell Finland Professor of Medicine (Microbiology and Molecular Genetics), Harvard Medical School; Beth Israel Deaconess Medical Center; Brigham and Women's Hospital, Boston, Massachusetts [178, 186, 187]

Richard L. Doty, PhD
Professor, Department of Otorhinolaryngology: Head and Neck Surgery; Director, Smell and Taste Center, University of Pennsylvania School of Medicine, Philadelphia, Pennsylvania [29]

Neil J. Douglas, MD, MB ChB, DSc, Hon MD, FRCPE
Professor of Respiratory and Sleep Medicine, University of Edinburgh, Edinburgh, Scotland, United Kingdom [265]

Daniel B. Drachman, MD
Professor of Neurology and Neuroscience, W. W. Smith Charitable Trust Professor of Neuroimmunology, Department of Neurology, Johns Hopkins School of Medicine, Baltimore, Maryland [386]

David F. Driscoll, PhD
Associate Professor of Medicine, University of Massachusetts Medical School, Worcester, Massachusetts [76]

Thomas D. DuBose, Jr., MD, MACP
Tinsley R. Harrison Professor and Chair, Internal Medicine; Professor of Physiology and Pharmacology, Department of Internal Medicine, Wake Forest University School of Medicine, Winston-Salem, North Carolina [47, e15]

J. Stephen Dumler, MD
Professor, Division of Medical Microbiology, Department of Pathology, Johns Hopkins University School of Medicine, Baltimore, Maryland [174]

Andrea Dunaif, MD
Charles F. Kettering Professor of Endocrinology and Metabolism; Vice-Chair for Research, Department of Medicine, Northwestern University Feinberg School of Medicine, Chicago, Illinois [6]

Samuel C. Durso, MD, MBA
Mason F. Lord Professor of Medicine; Director, Division of Geriatric Medicine and Gerontology, Johns Hopkins University School of Medicine, Baltimore, Maryland [32, e12]

Janice Dutcher, MD
Department of Oncology, New York Medical College, Montefiore, Bronx, New York [276]

Mark S. Dworkin, MD, MPH&TM
Associate Professor, Division of Epidemiology and Biostatistics, University of Illinois at Chicago School of Public Health, Chicago, Illinois [172]

Johanna Dwyer, DSc, RD
Professor of Medicine (Nutrition), Friedman School of Nutrition Science and Policy, Tufts University School of Medicine; Director, Frances Stern Nutrition Center, Tufts Medical Center, Boston, Massachusetts [73]

Jeffery S. Dzieczkowski, MD
Physician, St. Alphonsus Regional Medical Center; Medical Director, Coagulation Clinic, Saint Alphonsus Medical Group, International Medicine and Travel Medicine, Boise, Idaho [113]

Kim A. Eagle, MD
Albion Walter Hewlett Professor of Internal Medicine; Director, Cardiovascular Center, University of Michigan Health System, Ann Arbor, Michigan [8]

Robert H. Eckel, MD
Professor of Medicine, Division of Endocrinology, Metabolism and Diabetes, Division of Cardiology; Professor of Physiology and Biophysics, Charles A. Boettcher, II Chair in Atherosclerosis, University of Colorado School of Medicine, Anschutz Medical Campus, Director Lipid Clinic, University of Colorado Hospital, Aurora, Colorado [242]

John E. Edwards, Jr., MD
Chief, Division of Infectious Diseases, Harbor/University of California, Los Angeles (UCLA) Medical Center, Torrance, California; Professor of Medicine, David Geffen School of Medicine at UCLA, Los Angeles, California [198, 203]

David A. Ehrmann, MD
Professor of Medicine, The University of Chicago, Chicago, Illinois [49]

Andrew J. Einstein, MD, PhD
Assistant Professor of Clinical Medicine, Columbia University College of Physicians and Surgeons; Department of Medicine, Division of Cardiology, Department of Radiology, Columbia University Medical Center and New York-Presbyterian Hospital, New York, New York [Appendix]

Ezekiel J. Emanuel, MD, PhD
Chief, Department of Clinical Bioethics, National Institutes of Health, Bethesda, Maryland [9]

Joey D. English, MD
Assistant Clinical Professor, Department of Neurology, Univeristy of California, San Francisco, San Francisco, California [370]

John W. Engstrom, MD
Betty Anker Fife Distinguished Professor of Neurology; Neurology Residency Program Director; Clinical Chief of Service, University of California, San Francisco, San Francisco, California [15, 375]

Moshe Ephros, MD
Senior Lecturer, Faculty of Medicine, Technion—Israel Institute of Technology; Pediatric Infectious Disease Unit, Carmel Medical Center; Haifa, Israel [160]

Jonathan A. Epstein, MD, DTMH
William Wikoff Smith Professor of Medicine; Chairman, Department of Cell and Developmental Biology; Scientific Director, Cardiovascular Institute, University of Pennsylvania, Philadelphia, Pennsylvania [224]

Tim Evans, MD, PhD
Assistant Director-General, Information, Evidence, and Research, World Health Organization, Geneva, Switzerland [e1]

Christopher Fanta, MD
Associate Professor of Medicine, Harvard Medical School; Member, Pulmonary and Critical Care Division, Brigham and Women's Hospital, Boston, Massachusetts [34]

Paul Farmer, MD, PhD
Kolokotrones University Professor, Harvard University; Chair, Department of Global Health and Social Medicine, Harvard Medical School; Chief, Division of Global Health Equity, Brigham and Women's Hospital; Co-Founder, Partners in Health, Boston, Massachusetts [2]

Anthony S. Fauci, MD, DSc (Hon), DM&S (Hon), DHL (Hon), DPS (Hon), DLM (Hon), DMS (Hon)
Chief, Laboratory of Immunoregulation; Director, National Institute of Allergy and Infectious Diseases, National Institutes of Health, Bethesda, Maryland [1, 188, 189, 221, 314, 326, e40]

Murray J. Favus, MD
Professor, Department of Medicine, Section of Endocrinology, Diabetes and Metabolism, Director Bone Program, University of Chicago Pritzker School of Medicine, Chicago, Illinois [287, 355]

David P. Faxon, MD
Senior Lecturer, Harvard Medical School; Vice Chair of Medicine for Strategic Planning, Department of Medicine, Brigham and Women's Hospital, Boston, Massachusetts [230, 246, e33]

David T. Felson, MD, MPH
Professor of Medicine and Epidemiology; Chair, Clinical Epidemiology Unit, Boston University School of Medicine, Boston, Massachusetts [332]

Luigi Ferrucci, MD, PhD
Director, Baltimore Longitudinal Study of Aging National Institute of Health, Baltimore, Maryland [72]

Howard L. Fields, MD, PhD
Professor of Neurology, University of California, San Francisco, San Francisco, California [11]

Gregory A. Filice, MD
Professor of Medicine, University of Minnesota; Chief, Infectious Disease Section, Veterans Affairs Medical Center, Minneapolis, Minnesota [162]

Robert Finberg, MD
Chair, Department of Medicine, University of Massachusetts Medical School, Worcester, Massachusetts [86, 132]

Joyce Fingeroth, MD
Associate Professor of Medicine, Harvard Medical School, Boston, Massachusetts [132]

Kurt Fink, MD
Instructor in Anaesthesia, Harvard Medical School; Brigham and Women's Hospital, Boston, Massachusetts [e54]

Alain Fischer, MD, PhD
University Paris Descartes, Inserm Unit 768; Immunology and Pediatric Hematology Unit, Necker Children's Hospital, Paris, France [316, e39]

Jeffrey S. Flier, MD
Caroline Shields Walker Professor of Medicine and Dean, Harvard Medical School, Boston, Massachusetts [77]

Agnes B. Fogo, MD
John L. Shapiro Professor of Pathology; Professor of Medicine and Pediatrics, Vanderbilt University Medical Center, Nashville, Tennessee [e14]

Larry C. Ford, MD
Associate Researcher, Divisions of Clinical Epidemiology and Infectious Diseases, University of Utah, Salt Lake City, Utah [31]

Jane E. Freedman, MD
Professor, Department of Medicine, University of Massachusetts Medical School, Worcester, Massachusetts [117]

Roy Freeman, MBCHB
Professor of Neurology, Harvard Medical School, Boston, Massachusetts [20]

Gyorgy Frendl, MD, PhD
Assistant Professor of Anesthesia and Critical Care, Harvard Medical School; Director of Research, Surgical Critical Care, Brigham and Women's Hospital, Boston, Massachusetts [e54]

Carl E. Freter, MD, PhD
Professor, Department of Internal Medicine, Division of Hematology/Medical Oncology, University of Missouri; Ellis Fischel Cancer Center, Columbia, Missouri [102]

Lawrence S. Friedman, MD
Professor of Medicine, Harvard Medical School; Professor of Medicine, Tufts University School of Medicine; Assistant Chief of Medicine, Massachusetts General Hospital, Boston, Massachusetts; Chair, Department of Medicine, Newton-Wellesley Hospital, Newton, Massachusetts [43]

Sonia Friedman, MD
Assistant Professor of Medicine, Harvard Medical School, Boston, Massachusetts [295]

Anne L. Fuhlbrigge, MD, MS
Assistant Professor, Harvard Medical School; Pulmonary and Critical Care Division, Brigham and Women's Hospital, Boston, Massachusetts [253]

Andre Furtado, MD
Associate Specialist at the Department of Radiology, Neuroradiology Section, University of California, San Francisco, San Francisco, California [e44]

Robert F. Gagel, MD
Professor of Medicine and Head, Division of Internal Medicine, University of Texas MD Anderson Cancer Center, Houston, Texas [351]

Nicholas B. Galifianakis, MD, MPH
Assistant Clinical Professor, Surgical Movement Disorders Center, Department of Neurology, University of California, San Francisco, San Francisco, California [e8]

John I. Gallin, MD
Director, Clinical Center, National Institutes of Health, Bethesda, Maryland [60]

Charlotte A. Gaydos, DrPh, MPH, MS
Professor of Medicine, Johns Hopkins University School of Medicine, Baltimore, Maryland [176]

J. Michael Gaziano, MD, MPH
Professor of Medicine, Harvard Medical School; Chief, Division of Aging, Brigham and Women's Hospital; Director, Massachusetts Veterans Epidemiology Center, Boston VA Healthcare System, Boston, Massachusetts [225]

Thomas A. Gaziano, MD, MSc
Assistant Professor, Harvard Medical School; Assistant Professor, Health Policy and Management, Center for Health Decision Sciences, Harvard School of Public Health; Associate Physician in Cardiovascular Medicine, Department of Cardiology, Brigham and Women's Hospital, Boston, Massachusetts [225]

Susan L. Gearhart, MD
Assistant Professor of Colorectal Surgery and Oncology, The Johns Hopkins University School of Medicine, Baltimore, Maryland [297, 298]

Robert H. Gelber, MD
Clinical Professor of Medicine and Dermatology, University of California, San Francisco, San Francisco, California [166]

Jeffrey A. Gelfand, MD
Clinical Professor of Medicine, Harvard Medical School; Physician, Massachusetts General Hospital, Boston, Massachusetts [18, 211]

Alfred L. George, Jr., MD
Professor of Medicine and Pharmacology; Chief, Division of Genetic Medicine, Vanderbilt University School of Medicine, Nashville, Tennessee [277]

Dale N. Gerding, MD
Professor of Medicine, Loyola University Chicago Stritch School of Medicine; Associate Chief of Staff for Research and Development, Edward Hines, Jr. VA Hospital, Hines, Illinois [129]

Alicia K. Gerke, MD
Associate, Division of Pulmonary and Critical Care Medicine, University of Iowa, Iowa City, Iowa [255]

Michael Geschwind, MD, PhD
Associate Professor of Neurology, Memory and Aging Center, University of California, San Francisco, School of Medicine, San Francisco, California [e8]

Marc G. Ghany, MD, MHSc
Staff Physician, Liver Diseases Branch, National Institute of Diabetes and Digestive and Kidney Diseases, National Institutes of Health, Bethesda, Maryland [301]

Michael Giladi, MD, MSc
Associate Professor of Medicine, Faculty of Medicine, Tel Aviv University, Tel Aviv, Israel [160]

Bruce C. Gilliland,† MD
Professor of Medicine and Laboratory Medicine, University of Washington School of Medicine, Seattle, Washington [337]

Roger I. Glass, MD, PhD
Director, Fogarty International Center, Bethesda, Maryland [190]

Eli Glatstein, MD
Professor and Vice Chairman, Department of Radiation Oncology, Hospital of the University of Pennsylvania, Philadelphia, Pennsylvania [223]

Peter J. Goadsby, MD, PhD, DSc, FRACP FRCP
Professor of Neurology, University of California, San Francisco, California; Honorary Consultant Neurologist, Hospital for Sick Children, London, United Kingdom [14]

Ary L. Goldberger, MD
Professor of Medicine, Harvard Medical School; Wyss Institute for Biologically Inspired Engineering, Harvard University; Beth Israel Deaconess Medical Center, Boston, Massachusetts [228, e28, e30]

David Goldblatt, PhD, MBChB, FRCP, FRCPCH
Professor of Vaccinology and Immunology; Consultant in Paediatric Immunology; Director of Clinical Research and Development; Director, NIHR Biomedical Research Centre, Institute of Child Health; University College London; Great Ormond Street Hospital for Children NHS Trust, London, United Kingdom [134]

Samuel Z. Goldhaber, MD
Professor of Medicine, Harvard Medical School; Director, Venous Thromboembolism Research Group, Cardiovascular Division, Brigham and Women's Hospital, Boston, Massachusetts [262]

Ralph Gonzales, MD, MSPH
Professor of Medicine, University of California, San Francisco, San Francisco, California [31]

Douglas S. Goodin, MD
Professor of Neurology, University of California, San Francisco School of Medicine, San Francisco, California [380]

Craig E. Gordon, MD, MS
Assistant Professor of Medicine, Boston University School of Medicine; Attending, Section of Nephrology, Boston Medical Center, Boston, Massachusetts [284]

Jeffrey I. Gordon, MD
Dr. Robert J. Glaser Distinguished University Professor; Director, Center for Genome Sciences, Washington University School of Medicine, St. Louis, Missouri [64]

Maria Luisa Gorno-Tempini, MD, PhD
Associate Professor of Neurology, Memory and Aging Center, University of California, San Francisco, San Francisco, California [e10]

Gregory A. Grabowski, MD
Professor, Departments of Pediatrics, and Molecular Genetics, Biochemistry, and Microbiology; University of Cincinnati College of Medicine, A. Graeme Mitchell Chair in Human Genetics; Director, Division of Human Genetics, Cincinnati Children's Hosptial Medical Center, Cincinnati, Ohio [361]

Alexander R. Green, MD, MPH
Assistant Professor of Medicine, Harvard Medical School; Associate Director, The Disparities Solutions Center, Massachusetts General Hospital, Boston, Massachusetts [e4]

Norton J. Greenberger, MD
Clinical Professor of Medicine, Harvard Medical School; Senior Physician, Division of Gastroenterology, Brigham and Women's Hospital, Boston, Massachusetts [311, 312, 313]

†Deceased

Daryl R. Gress, MD, FAAN, FCCM
Professor of Neurocritical Care and Stroke; Professor of Neurology, University of California, San Francisco, San Francisco, California [275]

Rasim Gucalp, MD
Professor of Clinical Medicine, Albert Einstein College of Medicine; Associate Chairman for Educational Programs, Department of Oncology; Director, Hematology/Oncology Fellowship, Montefiore Medical Center, Bronx, New York [276]

Kalpana Gupta, MD, MPH
Associate Professor, Department of Medicine, Boston University School of Medicine; Chief, Section of Infectious Diseases, VA Boston Healthcare System, Boston, Massachusetts [288]

John G. Haaga, MD
Deputy Associate Director, Behavioral and Social Research Program, National Institute on Aging, National Institutes of Health, Bethesda, Maryland [70]

Chadi A. Hage, MD
Assistant Professor of Medicine, Pulmonary–Critical Care and Infectious Diseases, Roudebush VA Medical Center; Indiana University, Indianapolis, Indiana [199]

Bevra Hannahs Hahn, MD
Professor of Medicine, University of California, Los Angeles, David Geffen School of Medicine, Los Angeles, California [319]

Janet E. Hall, MD, MSc
Professor of Medicine, Harvard Medical School; Associate Physician, Massachusetts General Hospital, Boston, Massachusetts [50, 347]

Jesse B. Hall, MD, FCCP
Professor of Medicine, Anesthesia and Critical Care; Chief, Section of Pulmonary and Critical Care Medicine, University of Chicago, Chicago, Illinois [267]

Scott A. Halperin, MD
Professor of Pediatrics and Microbiology and Immunology; CIHR/Wyeth Chair in Clinical Vaccine Research; Head, Pediatric Infectious Diseases; Director, Canadian Center for Vaccinology, Dalhousie University, Halifax, Nova Scotia, Canada [148]

R. Doug Hardy, MD
Associate Professor of Internal Medicine and Pediatrics, University of Texas Southwestern Medical Center, Dallas, Texas [175]

Raymond C. Harris, MD
Ann and Roscoe R. Robinson Professor of Medicine; Chief, Division of Nephrology, Vanderbilt University School of Medicine, Nashville, Tennessee [278]

William L. Hasler, MD
Professor of Internal Medicine, Division of Gastroenterology, University of Michigan Health System, Ann Arbor, Michigan [39, 290]

Terry Hassold, PhD
Eastlick Distinguished Professor; Director, Center for Reproductive Biology, Washington State University School of Molecular Biosciences, Pullman, Washington [62]

Stephen L. Hauser, MD
Robert A. Fishman Distinguished Professor and Chairman, Department of Neurology, University of California, San Francisco, San Francisco, California [1, 366, 367, 376, 377, 380, 385, e46]

Barton F. Haynes, MD
Frederic M. Hanes Professor of Medicine and Immunology, Departments of Medicine and Immunology; Director, Duke Human
Vaccine Institute, Duke University School of Medicine, Durham, North Carolina [314]

Douglas C. Heimburger, MD, MS
Professor of Medicine; Associate Director for Education and Training, Vanderbilt Institute for Global Health, Vanderbilt University School of Medicine, Nashville, Tennessee [75]

J. Claude Hemphill, III, MD, MAS
Professor of Clinical Neurology and Neurological Surgery, Department of Neurology, University of California, San Francisco; Director of Neurocritical Care, San Francisco General Hospital, San Francisco, California [275]

Patrick H. Henry, MD
Clinical Adjunct Professor of Medicine, University of Iowa, Iowa City, Iowa [59]

Katherine A. High, MD
Investigator, Howard Hughes Medical Institute; William H. Bennett Professor of Pediatrics, University of Pennsylvania School of Medicine; Director, Center for Cellular and Molecular Therapeutics, Children's Hospital of Philadelphia, Philadelphia, Pennsylvania [68, 116]

Ikuo Hirano, MD
Professor of Medicine, Division of Gastroenterology and Hepatology, Department of Medicine, Northwestern University Feinberg School of Medicine, Chicago, Illinois [38, 292]

Martin S. Hirsch, MD
Professor of Medicine, Harvard Medical School; Professor of Immunology and Infectious Diseases, Harvard School of Public Health; Physician, Massachusetts General Hospital, Cambridge, Massachusetts [182]

Helen H. Hobbs, MD
Professor of Internal Medicine and Molecular Genetics, University of Texas Southwestern Medical Center, Dallas, Texas; Investigator, Howard Hughes Medical Institute, Chevy Chase, Maryland [356]

Judith S. Hochman, MD
Harold Snyder Family Professor of Cardiology; Clinical Chief, Leon Charney Division of Cardiology; Co-Director, NYU-HHC Clinical and Translational Science Institute; Director, Cardiovascular Clinical Research Center, New York University School of Medicine, New York, New York [272]

A. Victor Hoffbrand, DM
Professor Emeritus of Haematology, University College, London; Honorary Consultant Haematologist, Royal Free Hospital, London, United Kingdom [105]

David M. Hoganson, MD
Laboratory for Tissue Engineering and Organ Fabrication Center for Regenerative Medicine, Department of Surgery, Massachusetts General Hospital, Boston, Massachusetts [69]

Charles W. Hoge, MD
Senior Scientist and Staff Psychiatrist, Center for Psychiatry and Neuroscience, Walter Reed Army Institute of Research and Water Reed Army Medical Center, Silver Spring, Maryland [e48]

Elizabeth L. Hohmann, MD
Associate Professor of Medicine and Infectious Diseases, Harvard Medical School; Massachusetts General Hospital, Boston, Massachusetts [139]

Steven M. Holland, MD
Chief, Laboratory of Clinical Infectious Diseases, National Institute of Allergy and Infectious Diseases, National Institutes of Health, Bethesda, Maryland [60, 167]

King K. Holmes, MD, PhD
Chair, Global Health; Professor of Medicine and Global Health; Adjunct Professor, Epidemiology; Director, Center for AIDS and STD; University of Washington School of Medicine; Head, Infectious Diseases Section, Harborview Medical Center, Seattle, Washington [130]

Jay H. Hoofnagle, MD
Director, Liver Diseases Research Branch, National Institute of Diabetes, Digestive and Kidney Diseases, National Institutes of Health, Bethesda, Maryland [301]

Robert Hopkin, MD
Associate Professor of Clinical Pediatrics, University of Cincinnati College of Medicine; Division of Human Genetics, Cincinnati Children's Hospital Medical Center, Cincinnati, Ohio [361]

Leora Horn, MD, MSc
Division of Hematology and Medical Oncology, Vanderbilt University School of Medicine, Nashville, Tennessee [89]

Jonathan C. Horton, MD, PhD
William F. Hoyt Professor of Neuro-ophthalmology, Professor of Ophthalmology, Neurology and Physiology, University of California, San Francisco School of Medicine, San Francisco, California [28]

Howard Hu, MD
Environmental Health Sciences, University of Michigan Schools of Public Health and Medicine, Ann Arbor, Michigan [e49]

Gary W. Hunninghake, MD
Professor, Division of Pulmonary and Critical Care Medicine, University of Iowa, Iowa City, Iowa [255]

Sharon A. Hunt, MD, FACC
Professor, Division of Cardiovascular Medicine, Stanford University, Palo Alto, California [235]

Charles G. Hurst, MD
Chief, Chemical Casualty Care Division, United States Medical Research Institute of Chemical Defense, APG-Edgewood Area, Maryland [222]

Ashraf S. Ibrahim, PhD
Associate Professor of Medicine, Geffen School of Medicine, University of California, Los Angeles (UCLA); Division of Infectious Diseases, Los Angeles Biomedical Research Institute at Harbor–UCLA Medical Center, Torrance, California [205]

David H. Ingbar, MD
Professor of Medicine, Pediatrics, and Physiology; Director, Pulmonary Allergy, Critical Care and Sleep Division, University of Minnesota School of Medicine, Minneapolis, Minnesota [272]

Alan C. Jackson, MD, FRCPC
Professor of Medicine (Neurology) and Medical Microbiology, University of Manitoba; Section Head of Neurology, Winnipeg Regional Health Authority, Winnipeg, Manitoba, Canada [195]

Lisa A. Jackson, MD, MPH
Senior Investigator, Group Health Research Institute; Research Professor, Department of Epidemiology; Adjunct Professor, Department of Medicine, University of Washington, Seattle, Washington [122]

Richard F. Jacobs, MD
Robert H. Fiser, Jr., MD Endowed Chair in Pediatrics; Professor and Chairman, Department of Pediatrics, University of Arkansas for Medical Sciences; President, Arkansas Children's Hospital Research Institute, Little Rock, Arkansas [158]

J. Larry Jameson, MD, PhD
Robert G. Dunlop Professor of Medicine; Dean, University of Pennsylvania School of Medicine; Executive Vice President of the University of Pennsylvania for the Health System, Philadelphia, Pennsylvania [1, 61, 63, 80, 100, 338, 339, 341, 346, 349, e41]

Robert T. Jensen, MD
Digestive Diseases Branch, National Institute of Diabetes; Digestive and Kidney Diseases, National Institutes of Health, Bethesda, Maryland [350]

David H. Johnson, MD, FACP
Donald W. Seldin Distinguished Chair in Internal Medicine; Professor and Chairman, Department of Internal Medicine, University of Texas Southwestern Medical School, Dallas, Texas [89]

James R. Johnson, MD
Professor of Medicine, University of Minnesota, Minneapolis, Minnesota [149]

Stuart Johnson, MD
Associate Professor of Medicine, Loyola University Chicago Stritch School of Medicine; Staff Physician, Edward Hines, Jr. VA Hospital, Hines, Illinois [129]

S. Claiborne Johnston, MD, PhD
Professor of Neurology and Epidemiology, University of California, San Francisco School of Medicine, San Francisco, California [370]

S. Andrew Josephson, MD
Associate Professor, Department of Neurology; Director, Neurohospitalist Program, University of California, San Francisco, San Francisco, California [25, e47]

Harald Jüppner, MD
Professor of Pediatrics, Endocrine Unit and Pediatric Nephrology Unit, Massachusetts General Hospital, Boston, Massachusetts [353]

Peter J. Kahrilas, MD
Gilbert H. Marquardt Professor in Medicine, Division of Gastroenterology, Department of Medicine, Northwestern University Feinberg School of Medicine, Chicago, Illinois [38, 292]

Gail Kang, MD
Assistant Clinical Professor of Neurology, Memory and Aging Center, University of California, San Francisco, San Francisco, California [e8]

Marshall M. Kaplan, MD
Professor of Medicine, Tufts University School of Medicine, Boston, Massachusetts [42, 302]

Adolf W. Karchmer, MD
Professor of Medicine, Harvard Medical School; Division of Infectious Diseases, Beth Israel Deaconess Medical Center, Boston, Massachusetts [124]

Dennis L. Kasper, MD, MA (Hon)
William Ellery Channing Professor of Medicine and Professor of Microbiology and Molecular Genetics, Harvard Medical School; Director, Channing Laboratory, Department of Medicine, Brigham and Women's Hospital, Boston, Massachusetts [1, 119, 121, 127, 146, 164]

Lloyd H. Kasper, MD
Professor of Medicine (Neurology) and Microbiology and Immunology, Dartmouth Medical School, Lebanon, New Hampshire [214]

Daniel L. Kastner, MD, PhD
Scientific Director, National Human Genome Research Institute, National Institutes of Health, Bethesda, Maryland [330]

Carol A. Kauffman, MD
Professor of Internal Medicine, University of Michigan Medical School; Chief, Infectious Diseases Section, Veterans Affairs Ann Arbor Healthcare System, Ann Arbor, Michigan [206]

Elaine T. Kaye, MD
Assistant Clinical Professor of Dermatology, Harvard Medical School, Boston, Massachusetts [17, e7]

Kenneth M. Kaye, MD
Associate Professor of Medicine, Harvard Medical School, Boston, Massachusetts [17, e7]

John A. Kessler, MD
Professor and Chair, Department of Neurology, Northwestern University Feinberg School of Medicine, Chicago, Illinois [67]

Jay S. Keystone, MD, FRCPC, MSc (CTM)
Professor of Medicine, University of Toronto, Toronto, Ontario, Canada [123]

Sundeep Khosla, MD
Professor of Medicine and Physiology, College of Medicine, Mayo Clinic, Rochester, Minnesota [46]

Elliott Kieff, MD, PhD
Harriet Ryan Albee Professor, Harvard Medical School; Chief, Infectious Diseases Division, Brigham and Women's Hospital, Boston, Massachusetts [177]

Anthony A. Killeen, MD, PhD
Associate Professor; Director of Clinical Laboratories, University of Minnesota Medical Center, Minneapolis, Minnesota [e53]

Jim Yong Kim, MD, PhD
Chair, Department of Global Health and Social Medicine, Harvard Medical School; Director, François-Xavier Bagnoud Center for Health and Human Rights, Harvard School of Public Health; Chief, Division of Global Health Equity, Brigham and Women's Hospital, Boston, Massachusetts [2]

Kami Kim, MD
Professor of Medicine (Infectious Diseases) and of Microbiology and Immunology, Albert Einstein College of Medicine, Bronx, New York [214]

Lindsay King, MD
Clinical and Research Fellow, Department of Medicine, Gastrointestinal Unit, Massachusetts General Hospital, Boston, Massachusetts [e56]

Talmadge E. King, Jr., MD
Julius R. Krevans Distinguished Professor in Internal Medicine; Chair, Department of Medicine, University of California, San Francisco, San Francisco, California [261]

Louis V. Kirchhoff, MD, MPH
Professor of Internal Medicine (Infectious Diseases) and Epidemiology, Department of Internal Medicine, The University of Iowa, Iowa City, Iowa [213]

CONTRIBUTORS

Priya S. Kishnani, MD
Professor of Pediatrics, Duke University Medical Center, Durham, North Carolina [362]

Rob Knight, PhD
Assistant Professor, Department of Chemistry and Biochemistry, University of Colorado, Boulder, Colorado [64]

Minoru S. H. Ko, MD, PhD
Senior Investigator and Chief, Developmental Genomics and Aging Section, Laboratory of Genetics, National Institute on Aging, National Institutes of Health, Baltimore, Maryland [65]

Barbara Konkle, MD
Professor of Medicine, Hematology, University of Washington; Director, Translational Research, Puget Sound Blood Center, Seattle, Washington [58, 115]

Peter Kopp, MD
Associate Professor, Division of Endocrinology, Metabolism and Molecular Science, Northwestern University Feinberg School of Medicine, Chicago, Illinois [61]

Walter J. Koroshetz, MD
National Institute of Neurological Disorders and Stroke, National Institutes of Health, Bethesda, Maryland [382]

Thomas R. Kosten, MD
Baylor College of Medicine; Veteran's Administration Medical Center, Houston, Texas [393]

Theodore A. Kotchen, MD
Professor Emeritus, Department of Medicine; Associate Dean for Clinical Research, Medical College of Wisconsin, Milwaukee, Wisconsin [247]

Phyllis E. Kozarsky, MD
Professor of Medicine and Infectious Diseases, Emory University School of Medicine, Atlanta, Georgia [123]

Barnett S. Kramer, MD, MPH
Associate Director for Disease Prevention, Office of Disease Prevention, National Institutes of Health, Bethesda, Maryland [82]

Joel Kramer, PsyD
Clinical Professor of Neuropsychology in Neurology; Director of Neuropsychology, Memory and Aging Center, University of California, San Francisco, San Francisco, California [e10]

Stephen M. Krane, MD
Persis, Cyrus and Marlow B. Harrison Distinguished Professor of Medicine, Harvard Medical School; Massachusetts General Hospital, Boston, Massachusetts [352]

Alexander Kratz, MD, PhD, MPH
Associate Professor of Pathology and Cell Biology, Columbia University College of Physicians and Surgeons; Director, Core Laboratory, Columbia University Medical Center, New York, New York [Appendix]

John P. Kress, MD
Associate Professor of Medicine, Section of Pulmonary and Critical Care, University of Chicago, Chicago, Illinois [267]

Patricia Kritek, MD, EdM
Associate Professor, Division of Pulmonary and Critical Care Medicine, University of Washington, Seattle, Washington [34, 251, e34]

Henry M. Kronenberg, MD
Professor of Medicine, Harvard Medical School; Chief, Endocrine Unit, Massachusetts General Hospital, Boston, Massachusetts [352]

Robert F. Kushner, MD, MS
Professor of Medicine, Northwestern University Feinberg School of Medicine, Chicago, Illinois [78]

Loren Laine, MD
Professor of Medicine, University of Southern California Keck School of Medicine, Los Angeles, California [41]

Anil K. Lalwani, MD
Professor, Departments of Otolaryngology, Pediatrics, and Physiology and Neuroscience, New York University School of Medicine, New York, New York [30]

H. Clifford Lane, MD
Clinical Director; Director, Division of Clinical Research; Deputy Director, Clinical Research and Special Projects; Chief, Clinical and Molecular Retrovirology Section, Laboratory of Immunoregulation, National Institute of Allergy and Infectious Diseases, National Institutes of Health, Bethesda, Maryland [189, 221]

Carol A. Langford, MD, MHS
Director, Center for Vasculitis Care and Research, Department of Rheumatic and Immunologic Diseases, Cleveland Clinic, Cleveland, Ohio [326, 328, 336, 337, e40]

Regina C. LaRocque, MD
Assistant Professor of Medicine, Harvard Medical School; Assistant Physician, Massachusetts General Hospital, Boston, Massachusetts [128]

Wei C. Lau, MD
Associate Professor, Medical Director, Cardiovascular Center Operating Rooms; Director, Adult Cardiovascular and Thoracic Anesthesiology, University of Michigan Health System, Ann Arbor, Michigan [8]

Leslie P. Lawley, MD
Assistant Professor, Department of Dermatology, School of Medicine, Emory University, Atlanta, Georgia [52]

Thomas J. Lawley, MD
William P. Timmie Professor of Dermatology, Dean, Emory University School of Medicine, Atlanta, Georgia [51, 52, 54, e16]

Thomas H. Lee, MD, MSc
Professor of Medicine, Harvard Medical School; Network President, Partners Healthcare System, Boston, Massachusetts [12]

Jane A. Leopold, MD
Associate Professor of Medicine, Harvard Medical School; Brigham and Women's Hospital, Boston, Massachusetts [230, e33]

Nelson Leung, MD
Associate Professor of Medicine, Department of Nephrology and Hypertension, Division of Hematology, Mayo Clinic, Rochester, Minnesota [286]

Bruce D. Levy, MD
Associate Professor of Medicine, Harvard Medical School; Pulmonary and Critical Care Medicine, Brigham and Women's Hospital, Boston, Massachusetts [268]

Julia B. Lewis, MD
Professor, Department of Medicine, Division of Nephrology, Vanderbilt University Medical Center, Nashville, Tennessee [283]

Peter Libby, MD
Mallinckrodt Professor of Medicine, Harvard Medical School; Chief, Cardiovascular Medicine, Brigham and Women's Hospital, Boston, Massachusetts [224, 241, e32]

Richard W. Light, MD
Professor of Medicine, Division of Allergy, Pulmonary, and Critical Care Medicine, Vanderbilt University, Nashville, Tennessee [263]

Julie Lin, MD, MPH
Assistant Professor of Medicine, Harvard Medical School, Boston, Massachusetts [44]

Robert Lindsay, MD, PhD
Chief, Internal Medicine; Professor of Clinical Medicine, Helen Hayes Hospital, West Haverstraw, New York [354]

Marc E. Lippman, MD, MACP
Kathleen and Stanley Glaser Professor; Chairman, Department of Medicine, Deputy Director, Sylvester Comprehensive Cancer Center, University of Miami Miller School of Medicine, Miami, Florida [90]

Peter E. Lipsky, MD
Charlottesville, Virginia [318, 331]

Kathleen D. Liu, MD, PhD, MAS
Assistant Professor, Divisions of Nephrology and Critical Care Medicine, Departments of Medicine and Anesthesia, University of California, San Francisco, San Francisco, California [281]

Bernard Lo, MD
Professor of Medicine; Director, Program in Medical Ethics, University of California, San Francisco, San Francisco, California [e5]

Dan L. Longo, MD
Professor of Medicine, Harvard Medical School; Senior Physician, Brigham and Women's Hospital; Deputy Editor, New England Journal of Medicine, Boston, Massachusetts
[1, 57, 59, 66, 81, 84, 85, 100, 102, 110, 111, 188, e6, e17, e20, e21]

Nicola Longo, MD, PhD, MACP
Professor of Pediatrics; Chief, Division of Medical Genetics, Department of Pediatrics, University of Utah, Salt Lake City, Utah [364, 365]

Joseph Loscalzo, MD, PhD
Hersey Professor of the Theory and Practice of Medicine, Harvard Medical School; Chairman, Department of Medicine; Physician-in-Chief, Brigham and Women's Hospital, Boston, Massachusetts [1, 35, 36, 37, 117, 224, 226, 227, 237, 238, 243, 245, 248, 249, e13, e19]

Phillip A. Low, MD
Robert D. and Patricia E. Kern Professor of Neurology, Mayo Clinic College of Medicine, Rochester, Minnesota [375]

Daniel H. Lowenstein, MD
Dr. Robert B. and Mrs. Ellinor Aird Professor of Neurology; Director, Epilepsy Center, University of California, San Francisco, San Francisco, California [367, 369, e42]

Elyse E. Lower, MD
Medical Oncology and Hematology, University of Cincinnati; Oncology Hematology Care, Inc., Cincinnati, Ohio [329]

Franklin D. Lowy, MD
Professor of Medicine and Pathology, Columbia University College of Physicians and Surgeons, New York, New York [135]

Sheila A. Lukehart, PhD
Professor, Departments of Medicine and Global Health, University of Washington, Seattle, Washington [169, 170]

Lucio Luzzatto, MD, FRCP, FRCPath
Professor of Haematology, University of Genova, Scientific Director Istituto Toscano Tumori, Italy [106]

Lawrence C. Madoff, MD
Professor of Medicine, University of Massachusetts Medical School, Worcester, Massachusetts; Director, Division of Epidemiology and Immunization, Massachusetts Department of Public Health, Jamaica Plain, Massachusetts [119, 334, e23, e24]

Emily Nelson Maher, MD
Clinical Instructor, Department of Anesthesiology, Harvard Medical School; Brigham and Women's Hospital, Boston, Massachusetts [e57]

Adel A. F. Mahmoud, MD, PhD
Professor, Department of Molecular Biology and the Woodrow Wilson School of Public and International Affairs, Princeton University, Princeton, New Jersey [219]

Ronald V. Maier, MD
Jane and Donald D. Trunkey Professor and Vice-Chair, Surgery, University of Washington; Surgeon-in-Chief, Harborview Medical Center, Seattle, Washington [270]

Mark E. Mailliard, MD
Frederick F. Paustian Professor; Chief, Division of Gastroenterology and Hepatology, Department of Internal Medicine, University of Nebraska College of Medicine, Omaha, Nebraska [307]

Hari R. Mallidi, MD
Assistant Professor of Cardiothoracic Surgery; Director of Mechanical Circulatory Support, Stanford University Medical Center, Stanford, California [235]

Hanna Mandel, MD
Director, Pediatric Metabolic Disorders, Rambam Health Care Campus, Haifa, Israel [e18]

Brian F. Mandell, MD, PhD, MACP, FACR
Professor and Chairman of Medicine, Cleveland Clinic Lerner College of Medicine; Department of Rheumatic and Immunologic Disease, Cleveland Clinic, Cleveland, Ohio [336]

Lionel A. Mandell, MD, FRCP(C), FRCP(LOND)
Professor of Medicine, McMaster University, Hamilton, Ontario, Canada [257]

Douglas L. Mann, MD
Lewin Chair and Chief, Cardiovascular Division; Professor of Medicine, Cell Biology and Physiology, Washington University School of Medicine, St. Louis, Missouri [234]

JoAnn E. Manson, MD, DrPH
Professor of Medicine and the Michael and Lee Bell Professor of Women's Health, Harvard Medical School; Chief, Division of Preventive Medicine, Brigham and Women's Hospital, Boston, Massachusetts [348]

Eleftheria Maratos-Flier, MD
Associate Professor of Medicine, Harvard Medical School; Division of Endocrinology, Beth Israel Deaconess Medical Center, Boston, Massachusetts [77]

Francis Marchlinski, MD
Professor of Medicine; Director, Cardiac Electrophysiology, University of Pennsylvania Health System, Philadelphia, Pennsylvania [233]

Guido Marcucci, MD
Professor of Medicine; John B. and Jane T. McCoy Chair in Cancer Research; Associate Director of Translational Research, Comprehensive Cancer Center, The Ohio State University College of Medicine, Columbus, Ohio [109]

Daniel B. Mark, MD, MPH
Professor of Medicine, Duke University Medical Center; Director, Outcomes Research, Duke Clinical Research Institute, Durham, North Carolina [3]

Alexander G. Marneros, MD, PhD
Assistant Professor, Department of Dermatology, Harvard Medical School Boston, Massachusetts; Cutaneous Biology Research Center, Massachusetts General Hospital, Charlestown, Massachusetts [56]

Jeanne M. Marrazzo, MD, MPH
Associate Professor of Medicine, Division of Infectious Diseases, Harborview Medical Center, Seattle, Washington [130]

Thomas Marrie, MD
Dean, Faculty of Medicine, Dalhousie University, Halifax, Nova Scotia, Canada [174]

Gary J. Martin, MD
Raymond J. Langenbach, MD Professor of Medicine; Vice Chairman for Faculty Affairs, Department of Medicine, Northwestern University Feinberg School of Medicine, Chicago, Illinois [4]

George M. Martin, MD
Professor of Pathology Emeritus, Adjunct Professor of Genome Sciences (Retired), University of Washington, Seattle, Washington; Visiting Scholar, Molecular Biology Institute, University of California at Los Angeles, Los Angeles, California [71]

Joseph B. Martin, MD, PhD
Edward R. and Anne G. Lefler Professor, Department of Neurobiology, Harvard Medical School, Boston, Massachusetts [367]

Matthew Martinez, MD
Lehigh Valley Physician Group, Lehigh Valley Heart Specialists, Allentown, Pennsylvania [229, e29]

Susan Maslanka, PhD
Enteric Diseases Laboratory Branch, Centers for Disease Control and Prevention, Atlanta, Georgia [141]

Robert J. Mayer, MD
Stephen B. Kay Family Professor of Medicine, Harvard Medical School, Boston, Massachusetts [91]

Alexander J. McAdam, MD, PhD
Assistant Professor of Pathology, Harvard Medical School, Children's Hospital, Boston, Massachusetts [e22]

Calvin O. McCall, MD
Associate Professor, Department of Dermatology, Virginia Commonwealth University Medical Center; Chief, Dermatology Section, Hunter Holmes McGuire Veterans Affairs Medical Center, Richmond, Virginia [52]

John F. McConville, MD
Assistant Professor of Medicine, University of Chicago, Chicago, Illinois [264]

Kevin T. McVary, MD, FACS
Professor of Urology, Department of Urology, Northwestern University Feinberg School of Medicine, Chicago, Illinois [48]

Nancy K. Mello, PhD
Professor of Psychology (Neuroscience), Harvard Medical School, Boston, Massachusetts; Director, Alcohol and Drug Abuse Research Center, McLean Hospital, Belmont, Massachusetts [394]

Shlomo Melmed, MD
Senior Vice President and Dean of the Medical Faculty, Cedars-Sinai Medical Center, Los Angeles, California [339]

Jack H. Mendelson,† MD
Professor of Psychiatry (Neuroscience), Harvard Medical School, Belmont, Massachusetts [394]

Robert O. Messing, MD
Professor, Department of Neurology; Senior Associate Director, Ernest Gallo Clinic and Research Center, University of California, San Francisco, San Francisco, California [390]

M.-Marsel Mesulam, MD
Professor of Neurology, Psychiatry and Psychology, Cognitive Neurology and Alzheimer's Disease Center, Northwestern University Feinberg School of Medicine, Chicago, Illinois [26]

Susan Miesfeldt, MD
Mercy Hospital, Maine Centers for Cancer Medicine, Scarbrough, Maine [63]

Edgar L. Milford, MD
Associate Professor of Medicine, Harvard Medical School; Director, Tissue Typing Laboratory, Brigham and Women's Hospital, Boston, Massachusetts [282]

Bruce L. Miller, MD
AW and Mary Margaret Clausen Distinguished Professor of Neurology, University of California, San Francisco School of Medicine, San Francisco, California [25, 371, 383, e9, e10]

Samuel I. Miller, MD
Professor of Genome Sciences, Medicine, and Microbiology, University of Washington, Seattle, Washington [153]

Simon J. Mitchell, MB ChB, PhD
Associate Professor in Anesthesiology, Diving and Hyperbaric Medicine, Faculty of Medical and Health Sciences, University of Auckland; Consultant Anesthetist, Auckland City Hospital, Auckland, New Zealand [e52]

Thomas A. Moore, MD, FACP, FIDSA
Chairman, Department of Infectious Diseases, Ochsner Health System, New Orleans, Louisiana [208, e26]

Pat J. Morin, PhD
Senior Investigator, Laboratory of Molecular Biology and Immunology, National Institute on Aging, National Institutes of Health, Baltimore, Maryland [83]

Charles A. Morris, MD, MPH
Instructor in Medicine, Harvard Medical School; Associate Physician, Brigham and Women's Hospital, Boston, Massachusetts [e55, e57]

William J. Moss, MD, MPH
Associate Professor, Departments of Epidemiology, International Health, and Molecular Microbiology and Immunology, Johns Hopkins Bloomberg School of Public Health, Baltimore, Maryland [192]

Robert J. Motzer, MD
Professor of Medicine, Weill Cornell Medical College; Attending Physician, Genitourinary Oncology Service, Memorial Sloan-Kettering Cancer Center, New York, New York [94, 96]

David B. Mount, MD, FRCPC
Assistant Professor of Medicine, Harvard Medical School, Renal Division, VA Boston Healthcare System; Brigham and Women's Hospital, Boston, Massachusetts [45, e15]

Haralampos M. Moutsopoulos, MD, FACP, FRCP, Master ACR
Professor and Director, Department of Pathophysiology, Medical School, National University of Athens, Athens, Greece [320, 324, 327]

†Deceased

Robert S. Munford, MD
Bethesda, Maryland [271]

Nikhil C. Munshi, MD
Associate Professor of Medicine, Harvard Medical School; Associate Director, Jerome Lipper Multiple Myeloma Center, Dana Farber Cancer Institute, Boston, Massachusetts [111]

John R. Murphy, PhD
Professor of Medicine and Microbiology, Boston University School of Medicine, Boston, Massachusetts [138]

Timothy F. Murphy, MD
UB Distinguished Professor of Medicine and Microbiology, University of Buffalo, State University of New York, Buffalo, New York [145]

Barbara E. Murray, MD
J. Ralph Meadows Professor and Director, Division of Infectious Diseases, University of Texas Medical School, Houston, Texas [137]

Joseph A. Murray, MD
Professor of Medicine, Departments of Internal Medicine and Immunology, Mayo Clinic, Rochester, Minnesota [40]

Mark B. Mycyk, MD
Associate Professor, Department of Emergency Medicine, Boston University School of Medicine; Associate Professor, Department of Emergency Medicine; Rush University School of Medicine, Research Director, Division of Toxicology, Cook County Hospital, Chicago, Illinois [e50]

Robert J. Myerburg, MD
Professor, Departments of Medicine and Physiology, Division of Cardiology; AHA Chair in Cardiovascular Research, University of Miami Miller School of Medicine, Miami, Florida [273]

Hari Nadiminti, MD
Clinical Instructor, Department of Dermatology, Emory University School of Medicine, Atlanta, Georgia [87]

Edward T. Naureckas, MD
Associate Professor of Medicine, Section of Pulmonary and Critical Care Medicine, University of Chicago, Chicago, Illinois [252]

Eric G. Neilson, MD
Thomas Fearn Frist Senior Professor of Medicine and Cell and Developmental Biology, Vanderbilt University School of Medicine, Nashville, Tennessee [277, 278, 283, e14]

Gerald T. Nepom, MD, PhD
Director, Benaroya Research Institute at Virginia Mason; Director, Immune Tolerance Network; Professor, University of Washington School of Medicine, Seattle, Washington [315]

Eric J. Nestler, MD, PhD
Nash Family Professor and Chair, Department of Neuroscience; Director, Friedman Brain Institute, Mount Sinai School of Medicine, New York, New York [390]

Hartmut P. H. Neumann, MD
Head, Section Preventative Medicine, Department of Nephrology and General Medicine, Albert-Ludwigs-University of Freiburg, Germany [343]

Joseph P. Newhouse, PhD
John D. MacArthur Professor of Health Policy and Management, Department of Health Care Policy, Harvard Medical School; Department of Health Policy and Management, Harvard School of Public Health, Harvard Kennedy School; Faculty of Arts and Sciences, Harvard University, Boston, Massachusetts [e3]

Jonathan Newmark, MD
Colonel, Medical Corps, US Army; Deputy Joint Program Executive Officer, Medical Systems, Joint Program Executive Office for Chemical/Biological Defense, US Department of Defense, Falls Church, Virginia; Chemical Casualty Care Consultant to the US Army Surgeon General; Adjunct Professor of Neurology, F. Edward Hebert School of Medicine, Uniformed Services University of the Health Sciences, Bethesda, Maryland [222]

Rick A. Nishimura, MD, FACC, FACP
Judd and Mary Morris Leighton Professor of Cardiovascular Diseases; Professor of Medicine; Consultant, Division of Cardiovascular Diseases and Internal Medicine, Mayo Clinic College of Medicine, Rochester, Minnesota [229, e29]

...rt L. Norris, MD
...ssor, Department of Surgery, Division of Emergency Medicine, ...anford University School of Medicine, Palo Alto, California [396]

Thomas B. Nutman, MD
Head, Helminth Immunology Section; Head, Clinical Parasitology Unit, Laboratory of Parasitic Diseases, National Institutes of Health, Bethesda, Maryland [217, 218]

Katherine L. O'Brien, MDCM, MPH, FRCPC
Associate Professor, Center for American Indian Health; Departments of International Health and Epidemiology, Johns Hopkins Bloomberg School of Public Health, Baltimore, Maryland [134]

Richard J. O'Brien, MD
Head, Product Evaluation and Demonstration, Foundation for Innovative and New Diagnostics (FIND), Geneva, Switzerland [165]

Max R. O'Donnell, MD
Assistant Professor of Medicine, Albert Einstein College of Medicine, Bronx, New York [168]

Nigel O'Farrell, MSc, MD, FRCP
Ealing Hospital, London, United Kingdom [161]

Jennifer Ogar, MS
Speech Pathologist, Memory and Aging Center, University of California, San Francisco, San Francisco, California; Acting Chief of Speech Pathology at the Department of Veterans Affairs, Martinez, California [e10]

Patrick T. O'Gara, MD
Professor of Medicine, Harvard Medical School; Director, Clinical Cardiology, Brigham and Women's Hospital, Boston, Massachusetts [227, 237, e13]

C. Warren Olanow MD, FRCPC
Department of Neurology and Neuroscience, Mount Sinai School of Medicine, New York, New York [372]

Andrew B. Onderdonk, PhD
Professor of Pathology, Harvard Medical School; Brigham and Women's Hospital, Boston, Massachusetts [e22]

Chung Owyang, MD
H. Marvin Pollard Professor of Internal Medicine; Chief, Division of Gastroenterology, University of Michigan Health System, Ann Arbor, Michigan [290, 296]

William Pao, MD, PhD
Associate Professor of Medicine, Cancer Biology, and Pathology, Division of Hematology and Medical Oncology, Vanderbilt University School of Medicine, Nashville, Tennessee [89]

Umesh D. Parashar, MBBS, MPH
Lead, Viral Gastroenteritis Epidemiology Team, Division of Viral Diseases, National Center for Immunization and Respiratory Diseases, Centers for Disease Control and Prevention, Atlanta, Georgia [190]

Shreyaskumar R. Patel, MD
Center Medical Director, Sarcoma Center; Professor of Medicine; Deputy Chairman, Department of Sarcoma Medical Oncology, MD Anderson Cancer Center, Houston, Texas [98]

David L. Paterson, MD, PhD
Professor of Medicine, University of Queensland Centre for Clinical Research; Royal Brisbane and Women's Hospital, Brisbane, Australia [150]

Gustav Paumgartner, MD
Professor Emeritus of Medicine, University of Munich, Munich, Germany [311]

David A. Pegues, MD
Hospital Epidemiologist, David Geffen School of Medicine, University of California, Los Angeles, Los Angeles, California [153]

Anton Y. Peleg, MBBS, PhD, MPH, FRACP
Infectious Diseases Physician, Senior Lecturer, and NHMRC Biomedical Fellow, Department of Infectious Diseases and Microbiology, The Alfred Hospital and Monash University, Melbourne, Victoria, Australia [150]

Florencia Pereyra, MD
Assistant Professor of Medicine, Harvard Medical School; Associate Physician, Infectious Disease Division, Brigham and Women's Hospital, Boston, Massachusetts [e23, e24]

Michael A. Pesce, PhD
Professor Emeritus of Pathology and Cell Biology, Columbia University College of Physicians and Surgeons; Columbia University Medical Center, New York, New York [Appendix]

Clarence J. Peters, MD
John Sealy Distinguished University Chair in Tropical and Emerging Virology; Professor, Department of Mirobiology and Immunology; Department of Pathology; Director for Biodefense, Center for Biodefense and Emerging Infectious Diseases, University of Texas Medical Branch, Galveston, Texas [196, 197]

Gerald B. Pier, PhD
Professor of Medicine (Microbiology and Molecular Genetics), Harvard Medical School; Microbiologist, Brigham and Women's Hospital, Boston, Massachusetts [120]

Ronald E. Polk, PharmD
Professor of Pharmacy and Medicine; Chairman, Department of Pharmacy, School of Pharmacy, Virginia Commonwealth University/ Medical College of Virginia Campus, Richmond, Virginia [133]

Richard J. Pollack, PhD
Research Associate Professor, Department of Biology, Boston University; Research Associate, Department of Immunology and Infectious Diseases, Harvard School of Public Health, Boston, Massachusetts [397]

Andrew J. Pollard, PhD, FRCPCH
Professor of Pediatric Infection and Immunity; Director of the Oxford Vaccine Group, Department of Pediatrics, University of Oxford, Oxford, United Kingdom [143]

Reuven Porat, MD
Internal Medicine Department, Tel-Aviv Sourasky Medical Centre; Sackler Faculty of Medicine, Tel-Aviv University, Tel-Aviv, Israel [16]

Daniel A. Portnoy, PhD
Professor of Biochemistry and Molecular Biology, Department of Molecular and Cell Biology, The School of Public Health, University of California, Berkeley, Berkeley, California [139]

John T. Potts, Jr., MD
Director of Research, Massachusetts General Hospital, Boston, Massachusetts [353]

Lawrie W. Powell, MD, PhD
Professor of Medicine; Director, Centre for the Advancement of Clinical Research, Royal Brisbane and Women's Hospital, Brisbane, Australia [357]

Alvin C. Powers, MD
Joe C. Davis Chair in Biomedical Science; Professor of Medicine, Molecular Physiology, and Biophysics; Director, Vanderbilt Diabetes Center; Chief, Division of Diabetes, Endocrinology, and Metabolism, Vanderbilt University School of Medicine, Nashville, Tennessee [344]

Daniel S. Pratt, MD
Assistant Professor of Medicine, Harvard Medical School; Massachusetts General Hospital, Boston, Massachusetts [42, 302]

Michael B. Prentice, MB ChB, PhD, MRCP(UK), FRCPath, FFPRCPI
Professor of Medical Microbiology, Department of Microbiology, University College Cork, Cork, Ireland [159]

Darwin J. Prockop, MD, PhD
Director and Professor, Institute for Regenerative Medicine, Texas A&M Health Science Center College of Medicine at Scott & White, Temple, Texas [363]

Stanley B. Prusiner, MD
Director, Institute for Neurodegenerative Diseases; Professor, Department of Neurology, University of California, San Francisco, San Francisco, California [383]

Howard I. Pryor, II, MD
Laboratory for Tissue Engineering and Organ Fabrication, Center for Regenerative Medicine, Department of Surgery, Massachusetts General Hospital, Boston, Massachusetts [69]

Thomas C. Quinn, MD
Professor of Medicine, Johns Hopkins University, Baltimore, Maryland; Senior Investigator, National Institute of Allergy and Infectious Diseases, National Institutes of Health, Bethesda, Maryland [176]

Gil Rabinovici, MD
Attending Neurologist, Memory and Aging Center, University of California, San Francisco, San Francisco, California [e10]

Daniel J. Rader, MD
Cooper-McClure Professor of Medicine and Pharmacology, University of Pennsylvania School of Medicine, Philadelphia, Pennsylvania [356]

Sanjay Ram, MD
Associate Professor of Medicine, Division of Infectious Diseases and Immunology, University of Massachusetts Medical School, Worcester, Massachusetts [144]

Reuben Ramphal, MD
Professor of Medicine, Molecular Genetics and Microbiology, University of Florida College of Medicine, Gainesville, Florida [152]

Kumanan Rasanathan, MBChB, MPH, FAFPHM
Technical Officer, Department of Ethics, Equity, Trade, and Human Rights, World Health Organization, Geneva, Switzerland [e1]

Neil H. Raskin, MD
Department of Neurology, University of California, San Francisco, San Francisco, San Francisco, California [14]

Anis Rassi, Jr., MD, PhD, FACC, FACP, FAHA
Scientific Director, Anis Rassi Hospital, Goiânia, Brazil [213]

James P. Rathmell, MD
Associate Professor of Anesthesia, Harvard Medical School; Chief, Division of Pain Medicine, Massachusetts General Hospital, Boston, Massachusetts [11]

Mario C. Raviglione, MD
Director, Stop TB Department, World Health Organization, Geneva, Switzerland [165]

Sharon L. Reed, MD
Professor of Pathology and Medicine; Director, Microbiology and Virology Laboratories, University of California, San Diego Medical Center, San Diego, California [e25]

Susan E. Reef, MD
Medical Epidemiologist, Centers for Disease Control and Prevention, Atlanta, Georgia [193]

Richard C. Reichman, MD
Professor of Medicine and of Microbiology and Immunology, University of Rochester School of Medicine and Dentistry, Rochester, New York [185]

John J. Reilly, Jr., MD
Executive Vice Chairman; Department of Medicine; Professor of Medicine, University of Pittsburgh, Pittsburgh, Pennsylvania [260, e34]

John T. Repke, MD
University Professor and Chairman, Department of Obstetrics and Gynecology, Pennsylvania State University College of Medicine, Obstetrician-Gynecologist-in-Chief, The Milton S. Hershey Medical Center, Hershey, Pennsylvania [7]

Victor I. Reus, MD, DFAPA, FACP
Department of Psychiatry, University of California, San Francisco School of Medicine; Langley Porter Neuropsychiatric Institute, San Francisco, San Francisco, California [391]

Joseph Rhatigan, MD
Assistant Professor of Medicine, Harvard Medical School; Assistant Professor, Harvard School of Public Health; Brigham and Women's Hospital, Boston, Massachusetts [2]

Peter A. Rice, MD
Professor of Medicine, Division of Infectious Diseases and Immunology, University of Massachusetts Medical School, Worcester, Massachusetts [144]

Stuart Rich, MD
Professor of Medicine, Department of Medicine, Section of Cardiology, University of Chicago, Chicago, Illinois [250]

Gary S. Richardson, MD
Senior Research Scientist and Staff Physician, Henry Ford Hospital, Detroit, Michigan [27]

Elizabeth Robbins, MD
Clinical Professor of Pediatrics, University of California, San Francisco, San Francisco, California [e46]

Gary L. Robertson, MD
Emeritus Professor of Medicine, Northwestern University Feinberg School of Medicine, Chicago, Illinois [340]

Russell G. Robertson, MD
Vice President for Medical Affairs, Rosalind Franklin University of Medicine and Science; Dean, Chicago Medical School, Chicago, Illinois [80]

Dan M. Roden, MD
William Stokes Professor of Experimental Therapeutics; Assistant Vice-Chancellor for Personalized Medicine, Vanderbilt University School of Medicine, Nashville, Tennessee [5]

James A. Romano, Jr., PhD, DABT
Senior Principal Life Scientist and Technical Fellow, Science Applications International Corporation, Frederick, Maryland [222]

Karen L. Roos, MD
John and Nancy Nelson Professor of Neurology and Professor of Neurological Surgery, Indiana University School of Medicine, Indianapolis, Indiana [381]

Allan H. Ropper, MD
Professor of Neurology, Harvard Medical School; Executive Vice Chair of Neurology, Raymond D. Adams Distinguished Clinician, Brigham and Women's Hospital, Boston, Massachusetts [274, 377, 378]

Roger N. Rosenberg, MD
Zale Distinguished Chair and Professor of Neurology, Department of Neurology, University of Texas Southwestern Medical Center, Dallas, Texas [373]

Myrna R. Rosenfeld, MD, PhD
Professor of Neurology and Chief, Division of Neuro-oncology, University of Pennsylvania, Philadelphia, Pennsylvania [101]

John H. Rubenstein, MD, PhD
Nina Ireland Distinguished Professor in Child Psychiatry, Center for Neurobiology and Psychiatry, Department of Psychiatry, University of California, San Francisco, San Francisco, California [390]

Michael A. Rubin, MD, PhD
Assistant Professor of Medicine, University of Utah School of Medicine, Salt Lake City, Utah [31]

Steven Rubin, MS
Acting Principal Investigator, Center for Biologics Evaluation and Research, Food and Drug Administration, Bethesda, Maryland [194]

Robert M. Russell, MD
Professor Emeritus of Medicine and Nutrition, Tufts University, Boston, Massachusetts; Office of Dietary Supplements, National Institutes of Health, Bethesda, Maryland [74]

Thomas A. Russo, MD, CM, FIDSA
Professor of Medicine and Microbiology and Immunology; Chief, Division of Infectious Diseases, University at Buffalo, State University of New York, Buffalo, New York [149, 163]

Anna Rutherford, MD, MPH
Instructor in Medicine, Harvard Medical School; Associate Physician, Division of Gastroenterology, Hepatology and Endoscopy, Brigham and Women's Hospital, Boston, Massachusetts [e56]

Edward T. Ryan, MD, DTM&H
Associate Professor of Medicine, Harvard Medical School; Associate Professor of Immunology and Infectious Diseases, Harvard School of Public Health; Director, Tropical and Geographic Medicine, Massachusetts General Hospital, Boston, Massachusetts [128, 156]

Miguel Sabria, MD
Professor of Medicine, Autonomous University of Barcelona; Chief, Infectious Diseases Section, Germans Trias I Pujl Hospital, Barcelona, Spain [147]

David J. Salant, MD
Professor of Medicine, Boston University School of Medicine; Chief, Section of Nephrology, Boston Medical Center, Boston, Massachusetts [284, 285]

Martin A. Samuels, MD, DSc(hon), FAAN, MACP, FRCP
Professor of Neurology, Harvard Medical School; Chairman, Department of Neurology, Brigham and Women's Hospital, Boston, Massachusetts [e43, e47]

Philippe Sansonetti, MD, MS
Professor, Collège de France; Institut Pasteur, Paris, France [154]

Jussi J. Saukkonen, MD
Associate Professor of Medicine, Section of Pulmonary, Allergy, and Critical Care Medicine, Boston University School of Medicine, Boston, Massachusetts [168]

Edward A. Sausville, MD, PhD
Professor, Department of Medicine, University of Maryland School of Medicine; Deputy Director and Associate Director for Clinical Research, University of Maryland Marlene and Stewart Greenebaum Cancer Center, Baltimore, Maryland [85]

Mohamed H. Sayegh, MD
Raja N. Khuri Dean, Faculty of Medicine; Professor of Medicine and Immunology; Vice President of Medical Affairs, American University of Beirut, Beirut, Lebanon; Visiting Professor of Medicine and Pediatrics, Harvard Medical School; Director, Schuster Family Transplantation Research Center, Brigham and Women's Hospital; Children's Hospital, Boston, Massachusetts [282]

David T. Scadden, MD
Gerald and Darlene Jordan Professor of Medicine, Harvard Stem Cell Institute, Harvard Medical School; Department of Stem Cell and Regenerative Biology, Massachusetts General Hospital, Boston, Massachusetts [66]

Anthony H. V. Schapira, DSc, MD, FRCP, FMedSci
University Department of Clinical Neurosciences, University College London; National Hospital for Neurology and Neurosurgery, Queen's Square, London, United Kingdom [372]

Howard I. Scher, MD
Professor of Medicine, Weill Cornell Medical College; D. Wayne Calloway Chair in Urologic Oncology; Chief, Genitourinary Oncology Service, Department of Medicine, Memorial Sloan-Kettering Cancer Center, New York, New York [94, 95]

Anne Schuchat, MD
Director, National Center for Immunization and Respiratory Diseases, Centers for Disease Control and Prevention, Atlanta, Georgia [122]

Marc A. Schuckit, MD
Distinguished Professor of Psychiatry, University of California, San Diego School of Medicine, La Jolla, California [392]

H. Ralph Schumacher, MD
Professor of Medicine, Division of Rheumatology, University of Pennsylvania, School of Medicine, Philadelphia, Pennsylvania [333]

Gordon E. Schutze, MD
Professor of Pediatrics, Section of Retrovirology; Vice President, Baylor International Pediatric AIDS Initiative at Texas Children's Hospital, Baylor College of Medicine, Houston, Texas [158]

Stuart Schwartz, PhD
Professor of Human Genetics, Medicine and Pathology, University of Chicago, Chicago, Illinois [62]

Richard M. Schwartzstein, MD
Ellen and Melvin Gordon Professor of Medicine and Medical Education; Associate Chief, Division of Pulmonary, Critical Care, and Sleep Medicine, Beth Israel Deaconess Medical Center, Harvard Medical School, Boston, Massachusetts [33]

William W. Seeley, MD
Associate Professor of Neurology, Memory and Aging Center, University of California, San Francisco, San Francisco, California [371]

Michael V. Seiden, MD, PhD
Professor of Medicine; President and CEO, Fox Chase Cancer Center, Philadelphia, Pennsylvania [97]

Julian L. Seifter, MD
Associate Professor of Medicine, Harvard Medical School; Brigham and Women's Hospital, Boston, Massachusetts [289]

David C. Seldin, MD, PhD
Chief, Section of Hematology-Oncology, Department of Medicine; Director, Amyloid Treatment and Research Program, Boston University School of Medicine; Boston Medical Center, Boston, Massachusetts [112]

Andrew P. Selwyn, MD, MBCHB
Professor of Medicine Brigham and Women's Hospital, Boston, Massachusetts [243]

Ankoor Shah, MD
Department of Medicine, Division of Rheumatology and Immunology, Duke University Medical Center, Durham, North Carolina [321]

Steven D. Shapiro, MD
Jack D. Myers Professor and Chair, Department of Medicine, University of Pittsburgh, Pittsburgh, Pennsylvania [260]

Kanade Shinkai, MD, PhD
Assistant Professor, Department of Dermatology, University of California, San Francisco, San Francisco, California [55]

William Silen, MD
Johnson and Johnson Professor Emeritus of Surgery, Harvard Medical School, Auburndale, Massachusetts [13, 299, 300]

Edwin K. Silverman, MD, PhD
Associate Professor of Medicine, Harvard Medical School; Channing Laboratory, Pulmonary and Critical Care Division, Department of Medicine, Brigham and Women's Hospital, Boston, Massachusetts [260]

Martha Skinner, MD
Professor, Department of Medicine, Boston University School of Medicine, Boston, Massachusetts [112]

Karl Skorecki, MD, FRCP(C), FASN
Annie Chutick Professor in Medicine (Nephrology); Director, Rappaport Research Institute, Technion – Israel Institute of Technology; Director, Medical and Research Development, Rambam Health Care Campus, Haifa, Israel [280, e18]

Wade S. Smith, MD, PhD
Professor of Neurology, Daryl R. Gress Endowed Chair of Neurocritical Care and Stroke; Director, University of California, San Francisco Neurovascular Service, San Francisco, San Francisco, California [275, 370]

A. George Smulian, MBBCh
Associate Professor of Medicine, University of Cincinnati College of Medicine; Chief, Infectious Disease Section, Cincinnati VA Medical Center, Cincinnati, Ohio [207]

Jeremy Sobel, MD, MPH
Medical Officer, Office of Global Health, Centers for Disease Control and Prevention, Atlanta, Georgia [141]

Kelly A. Soderberg, PhD, MPH
Director, Program Management, Duke Human Vaccine Institute, Duke University School of Medicine, Durham, North Carolina [314]

Julian Solway, MD
Walter L. Palmer Distinguished Service Professor of Medicine and Pediatrics; Associate Dean for Translational Medicine, Biological Sciences Division; Vice Chair for Research, Department of Medicine; Chair, Committee on Molecular Medicine, University of Chicago, Chicago, Illinois [252, 264]

Michael F. Sorrell, MD
Robert L. Grissom Professor of Medicine, University of Nebraska Medical Center, Omaha, Nebraska [307]

Frank E. Speizer, MD
E. H. Kass Distinguished Professor of Medicine, Channing Laboratory, Harvard Medical School; Professor of Environmental Science, Harvard School of Public Health, Boston, Massachusetts [256]

Brad Spellberg, MD
Associate Professor of Medicine, Geffen School of Medicine, University of California, Los Angeles (UCLA); Divisions of General Internal Medicine and Infectious Diseases, Los Angeles Biomedical Research Institute at Harbor–UCLA Medical Center, Torrance, California [205]

Jerry L. Spivak, MD
Professor of Medicine and Oncology, Hematology Division, Johns Hopkins University School of Medicine, Baltimore, Maryland [108]

David D. Spragg, MD
Assistant Professor of Medicine, Johns Hopkins University, Baltimore, Maryland [231, 232]

Samuel L. Stanley, Jr., MD
President, Stony Brook University, Stony Brook, New York [209]

E. William St. Clair, MD
Department of Medicine, Division of Rheumatology and Immunology, Duke University Medical Center, Durham, North Carolina [321]

Allen C. Steere, MD
Professor of Medicine, Harvard Medical School; Massachusetts General Hospital, Boston, Massachusetts [173]

Robert S. Stern, MD
Carl J. Herzog Professor of Dermatology, Harvard Medical School; Chair, Department of Dermatology, Beth Israel Deaconess Medical Center, Boston, Massachusetts [55]

Dennis L. Stevens, MD, PhD
Professor of Medicine, University of Washington School of Medicine, Seattle, Washington; Chief, Infectious Disease Section, Veterans Affairs Medical Center, Boise, Idaho [125, 142]

Lynne Warner Stevenson, MD
Professor of Medicine, Harvard Medical School; Director, Heart Failure Program, Brigham and Women's Hospital, Boston, Massachusetts [238]

Stephen E. Straus,† MD
National Institute of Allergy and Infectious Diseases, Bethesda, Maryland [e2]

Stephanie Studenski, MD, MPH
Professor of Geriatric Medicine, Department of Medicine, University of Pittsburgh School of Medicine; Staff Physician, VA Pittsburgh Geriatric Research Education and Clinical Center, Pittsburgh, Pennsylvania [72]

Lewis Sudarsky, MD
Associate Professor of Neurology, Harvard Medical School; Director of Movement Disorders, Brigham and Women's Hospital, Boston, Massachusetts [24]

Donna C. Sullivan, PhD
Professor, Department of Medicine, Division of Infectious Diseases, University of Mississippi Medical School, Jackson, Mississippi [201]

Shyam Sundar, MD
Professor of Medicine, Institute of Medical Sciences, Banaras Hindu University, Varanasi, India [212]

Paolo M. Suter, MD, MS
Professor, Clinic and Policlinic of Internal Medicine, University Hospital, Zurich, Switzerland [74]

Richard Suzman, PhD
Director, Behavioral and Social Research Program, National Institute on Aging, National Institutes of Health, Chevy Chase, Maryland [70]

Morton N. Swartz, MD
Professor of Medicine, Harvard Medical School; Chief, Jackson Firm Medical Service and Infectious Disease Unit, Massachusetts General Hospital, Boston, Massachusetts [382]

Robert A. Swerlick, MD
Alicia Leizman Stonecipher Professor and Chair of Dermatology, Emory University School of Medicine, Atlanta, Georgia [e16]

Geoffrey Tabin, MD
Professor of Ophthalmology and Visual Sciences, University of Utah School of Medicine; Director, International Ophthalmology Division, John A. Moran Eye Center; Director, Himalayan Cataract Project, Salt Lake City, Utah [e51]

Maria Carmela Tartaglia, MD, FRCPC
Clinical Instructor of Neurology, Memory and Aging Center, University of California, San Francisco, San Francisco, California [e10]

Joel D. Taurog, MD
Professor of Internal Medicine, Rheumatic Diseases Division, University of Texas Southwestern Medical Center, Dallas, Texas [325]

Stephen C. Textor, MD
Professor of Medicine, Division of Nephrology and Hypertension, Mayo Clinic, Rochester, Minnesota [286]

†Deceased

C. Louise Thwaites, MD, MBBS
Musculoskeletal Physician, Horsham, West Sussex; Oxford University Clinical Research Unit, Hospital for Tropical Diseases, Ho Chi Minh City, Vietnam [140]

Alan D. Tice, MD, FACP
Infections Limited Hawaii; John A. Burns School of Medicine, University of Hawaii, Honolulu, Hawaii [126]

Zelig A. Tochner, MD
Professor of Radiation Oncology, University of Pennsylvania School of Medicine; Medical Director, Proton Therapy Center, Philadelphia, Pennsylvania [223]

Gordon F. Tomaselli, MD
Michel Mirowski, MD Professor of Cardiology; Professor of Medicine and Cellular and Molecular Medicine; Chief, Division of Cardiology, Johns Hopkins University, Baltimore, Maryland [231, 232]

Mark Topazian, MD
Professor of Medicine, Mayo Clinic, Rochester, Minnesota [291, e36]

Barbara W. Trautner, MD, PhD
Assistant Professor, Section of Infectious Diseases, Baylor College of Medicine; The Michael E. DeBakey Veterans Affairs Medical Center, Houston VA Health Services Research and Development Center of Excellence, Houston, Texas [288]

Jeffrey M. Trent, PhD, FACMG
President and Research Director, Translational Genomics Research Institute, Phoenix, Arizona; Van Andel Research Institute, Grand Rapids, Michigan [83]

Elbert P. Trulock, MD
Rosemary and I. Jerome Flance Professor in Pulmonary Medicine, Washington University School of Medicine, St. Louis, Missouri [266]

Kenneth L. Tyler, MD
Reuler-Lewin Family Professor and Chair, Department of Neurology; Professor of Medicine and Microbiology, University of Colorado School of Medicine, Denver, Colorado; Chief of Neurology, University of Colorado Hospital, Aurora, Colorado [381]

Athanasios G. Tzioufas, MD
Professor, Department of Pathophysiology, National University of Athens School of Medicine, Athens, Greece [324]

Walter J. Urba, MD, PhD
Director of Cancer Research, Robert W. Franz Cancer Research Center, Providence Portland Medical Center, Portland, Oregon [87]

Joseph P. Vacanti, MD
John Homans Professor of Surgery, Harvard Medical School; Surgeon-in-Chief, Massachusetts General Hospital for Children; Deputy Director, Center for Regenerative Medicine, Massachusetts General Hospital, Boston, Massachusetts [69]

Jos W. M. van der Meer, MD, PhD
Professor of Medicine; Head, Department of General Internal Medicine, Radboud University, Nijmegen Medical Centre, Nijmegen, Netherlands [389]

Edouard Vannier, PhD, PharmD
Assistant Professor, Division of Geographic Medicine and Infectious Diseases, Tufts University School of Medicine; Tufts Medical Center, Boston, Massachusetts [211]

Gauri R. Varadhachary, MD
Associate Professor, Department of Gastrointestinal Medical Oncology, University of Texas MD Anderson Cancer Center, Houston, Texas [99]

John Varga, MD
John Hughes Professor of Medicine, Northwestern University Feinberg School of Medicine, Chicago, Illinois [323]

Camilo Jimenez Vasquez, MD
Assistant Professor, Department of Endocrine Neoplasia and Hormonal Disorders, Division of Internal Medicine, University of Texas MD Anderson Cancer Center, Houston, Texas [351]

Joseph M. Vinetz, MD
Professor of Medicine, Division of Infectious Diseases, Department of Medicine, University of California, San Diego, San Diego, California [171]

Indre V. Viskontas, PhD
Visiting Scholar, Memory and Aging Center, University of California, San Francisco, San Francisco, California [e9]

Panayiotis G. Vlachoyiannopoulos, MD
Associate Professor of Medicine-Immunology, Department of Pathophysiology, Medical School, National University of Athens, Athens, Greece [320]

Bert Vogelstein, MD
Professor of Oncology and Pathology; Investigator, Howard Hughes Medical Institute; Sidney Kimmel Comprehensive Cancer Center; Johns Hopkins University School of Medicine, Baltimore, Maryland [83]

Everett E. Vokes, MD
John E. Ultmann Professor and Chairman, Department of Medicine; Physician-in-Chief, University of Chicago Medical Center, Chicago, Illinois [88]

Tamara J. Vokes, MD, FACP
Professor, Department of Medicine, Section of Endocrinology, University of Chicago, Chicago, Illinois [355]

Sushrut S. Waikar, MD, MPH
Assistant Professor of Medicine, Harvard Medical School; Brigham and Women's Hospital, Boston, Massachusetts [279]

Matthew K. Waldor, MD, PhD
Edward H. Kass Professor of Medicine, Channing Laboratory, Brigham and Women's Hospital; Harvard Medical School and Howard Hughes Medical Institute, Boston, Massachusetts [156]

David H. Walker, MD
The Carmage and Martha Walls Distinguished University Chair in Tropical Diseases; Professor and Chairman, Department of Pathology; Executive Director, Center for Biodefense and Emerging Infectious Diseases, University of Texas Medical Branch, Galveston, Texas [174]

Mark F. Walker, MD
Associate Professor, Department of Neurology, Case Western Reserve University School of Medicine; Daroff-Dell'Osso Ocular Motility Laboratory, Louis Stokes Cleveland Department of Veterans Affairs Medical Center, Cleveland, Ohio [21]

B. Timothy Walsh, MD
Professor, Department of Psychiatry, College of Physicians and Surgeons, Columbia University; New York State Psychiatric Institute, New York, New York [79]

Peter D. Walzer, MD, MSc
Professor of Medicine, University of Cincinnati College of Medicine; Associate Chief of Staff for Research, Cincinnati VA Medical Center, Cincinnati, Ohio [207]

Fred Wang, MD
Professor of Medicine, Harvard Medical School; Brigham and Women's Hospital, Boston, Massachusetts [177, 183]

John W. Warren, MD
Professor of Medicine, University of Maryland School of Medicine, Baltimore, Maryland [e35]

Carl V. Washington, MD
Associate Professor of Dermatology, Winship Cancer Center, Emory University School of Medicine, Atlanta, Georgia [87]

Anthony P. Weetman, MD
University of Sheffield School of Medicine, Sheffield, United Kingdom [341]

Robert A. Weinstein, MD
The C Anderson Hedberg MD Professor of Internal Medicine, Rush Medical College; Interim Chairman, Department of Medicine, John Stroger Hospital, Chicago, Illinois [131]

Jeffrey I. Weitz, MD, FRCP(C), FACP
Professor of Medicine and Biochemistry; Executive Director, Thrombosis and Atherosclerosis Research Institute; HSFO/J. F. Mustard Chair in Cardiovascular Research, Canada Research Chair (Tier 1) in Thrombosis, McMaster University, Hamilton, Ontario, Canada [118]

Peter F. Weller, MD
Chief, Infectious Disease Division; Chief, Allergy and Inflammation Division, Beth Israel Deaconess Medical Center, Boston, Massachusetts [215-218, 220]

Patrick Y. Wen, MD
Professor of Neurology, Harvard Medical School; Dana-Farber Cancer Institute, Boston, Massachusetts [379]

Michael R. Wessels, MD
John F. Enders Professor of Pediatrics; Professor of Medicine, Harvard Medical School; Chief, Division of Infectious Diseases, Children's Hospital, Boston, Massachusetts [136]

Meir Wetzler, MD, FACP
Professor of Medicine, Roswell Park Cancer Institute, Buffalo, New York [109]

L. Joseph Wheat, MD
MiraVista Diagnostics and MiraBella Technologies, Indianapolis, Indiana [199]

A. Clinton White, Jr., MD
Director, Infectious Disease Division, Department of Internal Medicine, University of Texas Medical Branch, Galveston, Texas [220]

Nicholas J. White, MD, DSc, FRCP, F Med Sci, FRS
Professor of Tropical Medicine, Faculty of Tropical Medicine, Mahidol University, Bangkok, Thailand [210, e27]

Richard J. Whitley, MD
Distinguished Professor of Pediatrics, Loeb Eminent Scholar Chair in Pediatrics; Professor of Pediatrics, Microbiology, Medicine, and Neurosurgery, University of Alabama at Birmingham, Birmingham, Alabama [180]

John W. Winkelman, MD, PhD
Associate Professor of Psychiatry, Harvard Medical School; Medical Director, Sleep Health Centers, Brigham and Women's Hospital, Boston, Massachusetts [27]

Bruce U. Wintroub, MD
Professor and Chair, Department of Dermatology, University of California, San Francisco, San Francisco, California [55]

Andrea Wolf, MD, MPH
Instructor in Surgery, Harvard Medical School; Chief Resident in Cardiothoracic Surgery, Division of Thoracic Surgery, Brigham and Women's Hospital, Boston, Massachusetts [e55]

Allan W. Wolkoff, MD
Professor of Medicine and Anatomy and Structural Biology; Associate Chair of Medicine for Research; Chief, Division of Gastroenterology and Liver Diseases, Albert Einstein College of Medicine and Montefiore Medical Center, Bronx, New York [303]

John B. Wong, MD
Professor of Medicine, Tufts University School of Medicine; Chief, Division of Clinical Decision Making, Department of Medicine, Tufts Medical Center, Boston, Massachusetts [3]

Louis Michel Wong Kee Song, MD
Associate Professor, Division of Gastroenterology and Hepatology, Mayo Clinic, Rochester, Minnesota [291, e36]

Robert L. Wortmann, MD, FACP, MACR
Professor, Department of Medicine, Dartmouth Medical School and Dartmouth Hitchcock Medical Center, Lebanon, New Hampshire [359]

Shirley H. Wray, MB, ChB, PhD, FRCP
Professor of Neurology, Harvard Medical School; Department of Neurology, Massachusetts General Hospital, Boston, Massachusetts [e11]

Bechien U. Wu, MD
Instructor of Medicine, Harvard Medical School; Associate Physician, Division of Gastroenterology, Brigham and Women's Hospital, Boston, Massachusetts [313]

Richard Wunderink, MD
Professor of Medicine, Division of Pulmonary and Critical Care, Northwestern University Feinberg School of Medicine, Chicago, Illinois [257]

Kim B. Yancey, MD
Professor and Chair, Department of Dermatology, University of Texas Southwestern Medical Center, Dallas, Texas [51, 54]

Janet A. Yellowitz, DMD, MPH
Associate Professor; Director, Geriatric Dentistry, University of Maryland Dental School, Baltimore, Maryland [e12]

CONTRIBUTORS

Lam Minh Yen, MD
Director, Tetanus Intensive Care Unit, Hospital for Tropical Diseases, Ho Chi Minh City, Vietnam [140]

Maria A. Yialamas, MD
Instructor, Harvard Medical School; Associate Program Director, Internal Medicine Residency, Brigham and Women's Hospital, Boston, Massachusetts [e54, e56]

Neal S. Young, MD
Chief, Hematology Branch, National Heart, Lung and Blood Institute, National Institutes of Health, Bethesda, Maryland [107]

Victor L. Yu, MD
Professor of Medicine, Department of Medicine, University of Pittsburgh Medical Center, Pittsburgh, Pennsylvania [147]

Laura A. Zimmerman, MPH
Epidemiologist, Centers for Disease Control and Prevention, Atlanta, Georgia [193]

PREFACE

Welcome to the 18th edition of *Harrison's Principles of Internal Medicine*. In the 62 years since the first edition of this textbook was published, virtually every area of medicine has evolved substantially and many new areas have emerged. In 1949, when the first edition appeared, peptic ulcer disease was thought to be caused by stress, nearly every tumor that was not resected resulted in death, rheumatic heart disease was widely prevalent, and hepatitis B and HIV infection were unknown. In the intervening years, both the infectious cause of and the cure for peptic ulcer disease were identified; advances in diagnosis and treatment made it possible to cure two-thirds of cancers; rheumatic heart disease virtually disappeared; atherosclerotic coronary artery disease waxed and then—at least in part through management of modifiable risk factors—began to wane; hepatitis B and its consequences, cirrhosis and hepatocellular carcinoma, became preventable by a vaccine; and HIV, first viewed as a uniformly fatal worldwide scourge, became a treatable chronic disease. During this same period, the amount of information required for the effective practice of medicine grew unabated, and learning options for students, residents, and practicing physicians also burgeoned to include multiple sources of information in print and electronic formats.

While retaining the founding goals of *Harrison's*, this edition has been modified extensively in light of the varied needs of the book's readers and the diverse methods and formats by which information is now acquired. The print version of the 18th edition is more reader-friendly in several respects: the book is printed in type that is easier to read than prior editions, the graphics and tables have been enhanced for ease of interpretation, and more than 300 new figures are included. This improved format requires publication of the print edition in two volumes conveniently divided by subject matter. A DVD accompanies the book and contains additional e-chapters, videos, and atlases; its image bank includes figures and photographs from the book that can be incorporated into slide presentations. All chapters have been extensively updated by experts in the field. In addition, this edition includes 25 new chapters and more than 100 new authors. The pathophysiologic approach to evaluating patients on the basis of their presentation continues to receive emphasis in an enriched section on the cardinal manifestations of disease. A new section focuses on aging, its demographics and biology, and distinctive clinical issues affecting older patients. The e-chapters have increased in number from 39 to 57 and include a new video atlas of neuro-ophthalmology, an audio-enhanced chapter on the approach to a patient with a heart murmur, a case-based teaching exercise in fluid and electrolyte imbalances and acid-base disturbances, and explorations of infectious complications of burns and bites. New videos demonstrate the neurologic examination and several commonly performed medical procedures. A new chapter focuses on neuropsychiatric problems among war veterans. E-chapters on altitude sickness and hyperbaric and diving medicine form a new section on medical effects of changes in environmental pressure.

For readers who wish to continue using *Harrison's* in a single-volume format, we are pleased to offer two new eBook versions of the 18th edition: a traditional eBook, with text and illustrations from the new edition included for reading on a portable e-reader or on a desktop, and an enhanced eBook developed especially for new tablet devices (e.g., iPad, Galaxy, Playbook, Nook) that offer high-definition resolution of multimedia content and interactive features. The *Harrison's* 18th edition enhanced eBook will contain extensive embedded video footage, including all of the new clinical procedural videos; the wonderful neurologic examination videos from Samuels and Lowenstein; examples of cardiovascular imaging and assessment; and high-resolution versions of more than 2000 color images from the book and the *Harrison's* atlases on the companion DVD. Along with other social media features, the enhanced eBook offers users the opportunity to take and share notes from lectures and their own reading. Additional resources include *Harrison's Online*, a continuously updated electronic resource that highlights and summarizes newly published articles on significant medical findings and advances. *Harrison's Self-Assessment and Board Review*, a useful study guide for board review based on information in the 18th edition, will soon be produced. *Harrison's Manual of Medicine*, a pocket version of *Harrison's Principles of Internal Medicine*, is available in both print and electronic formats.

We have many people to thank for their efforts in producing this book. First, the authors have done a superb job of producing authoritative chapters that synthesize vast amounts of scientific and clinical data to create state-of-the-art descriptions of medical disorders encompassed by internal medicine. In today's information-rich, rapidly evolving environment, they have ensured that this information is current. Helpful suggestions and critical input have been provided by a number of colleagues; particularly notable was the advice of Chung Owyang on the Gastroenterology Section. We are most grateful to our colleagues in each of our editorial offices who have kept track of the work in its various phases and facilitated communication with the authors, with the McGraw-Hill staff, and among the editors: Patricia Conrad, Emily Cowan, Patricia L. Duffey, Gregory K. Folkers, Julie B. McCoy, Elizabeth Robbins, Kristine Shontz, and Stephanie Tribuna.

The staff at McGraw-Hill has been a constant source of support and expertise. James Shanahan, Editor-in-Chief, Internal Medicine, for McGraw-Hill's Professional Publishing Division, has been a superb and insightful partner to the editors, guiding the development of the book and its related products in new formats. Kim Davis seamlessly stepped into the position of Associate Managing Editor, ensuring that the complex production of this multi-authored textbook proceeded in an efficient fashion. Paula Torres, Dominik Pucek, and Michael Crumsho oversaw the production of the new procedural and neurology videos. Phil Galea again served as Production Director on this, his final edition, and did so with a peak performance. Mary A. Murray, Director, International Rights, is retiring from McGraw Hill in 2012, after 50 years with the company. Mary joined the Blakiston Division of McGraw Hill in 1961, when Tinsley Harrison was still the editor of the book. Her first assignment was to distribute reprints of *Harrison's* chapters to the editors and contributors. For the next 23 years, Mary continued to be involved in the editorial process of *Harrison's*. In the early 1990s, she was given responsibility for licensing McGraw-Hill's medical titles; making use of her many cordial connections in global medical publishing, she licensed translations of *Harrison's* into 19 languages. We are extremely grateful to Mary for her many accomplishments in support of the book through 13 editions.

We are privileged to have compiled this 18th edition and are enthusiastic about all that it offers our readers. We learned much in the process of editing *Harrison's* and hope that you will find this edition a uniquely valuable educational resource.

THE EDITORS

PART 1

Introduction to Clinical Medicine

CHAPTER 1

The Practice of Medicine

The Editors

■ THE MODERN-DAY PHYSICIAN

No greater opportunity, responsibility, or obligation can fall to the lot of a human being than to become a physician. In the care of the suffering, [the physician] needs technical skill, scientific knowledge, and human understanding…. Tact, sympathy, and understanding are expected of the physician, for the patient is no mere collection of symptoms, signs, disordered functions, damaged organs, and disturbed emotions. [The patient] is human, fearful, and hopeful, seeking relief, help, and reassurance.

—*Harrison's Principles of Internal Medicine,* 1950

The practice of medicine has changed in significant ways since the first edition of this book appeared more than 60 years ago. The advent of molecular genetics, molecular biology, and molecular pathophysiology, sophisticated new imaging techniques, and advances in bioinformatics and information technology have contributed to an explosion of scientific information that has fundamentally changed the way physicians define, diagnose, treat, and prevent disease. This growth of scientific knowledge is ongoing and accelerating.

The widespread use of electronic medical records and the Internet have altered the way doctors practice medicine and exchange information. As today's physician struggles to integrate copious amounts of scientific knowledge into everyday practice, it is important to remember that the ultimate goal of medicine is to prevent disease and treat sick patients. Despite more than 60 years of scientific advances since the first edition of this text, it is critical to underscore that cultivating the intimate relationship between physician and patient still lies at the heart of successful patient care.

The science and art of medicine

Deductive reasoning and applied technology form the foundation for the solution to many clinical problems. Spectacular advances in biochemistry, cell biology, and genomics, coupled with newly developed imaging techniques, allow access to the innermost parts of the cell and provide a window to the most remote recesses of the body. Revelations about the nature of genes and single cells have opened the portal for formulating a new molecular basis for the physiology of systems. Increasingly, physicians are learning how subtle changes in many different genes can affect the function of cells and organisms. Researchers are beginning to decipher the complex mechanisms by which genes are regulated. Doctors have developed a new appreciation of the role of stem cells in normal tissue function and in the development of cancer, degenerative disease, and other disorders, as well as their emerging role in the treatment of certain diseases. The knowledge gleaned from the science of medicine has already improved and undoubtedly will further improve physicians' understanding of complex disease processes and provide new approaches to disease treatment and prevention. Yet, skill in the most sophisticated application of laboratory technology and in the use of the latest therapeutic modality alone does not make a good physician.

When a patient poses challenging clinical problems, an effective physician must be able to identify the crucial elements in a complex history and physical examination; order the appropriate laboratory, imaging, and diagnostic tests; and extract the key results from the crowded computer printouts of data to determine whether to "treat" or to "watch." Deciding whether a clinical clue is worth pursuing or should be dismissed as a "red herring" and weighing whether a proposed test, preventive measure, or treatment entails a greater risk than the disease itself are essential judgments that a skilled clinician must make many times each day. This combination of medical knowledge, intuition, experience, and judgment defines the *art of medicine,* which is as necessary to the practice of medicine as is a sound scientific base.

■ CLINICAL SKILLS

History-taking

The written history of an illness should include all the facts of medical significance in the life of the patient. Recent events should be given the most attention. The patient should, at some early point, have the opportunity to tell his or her own story of the illness without frequent interruption and, when appropriate, receive expressions of interest, encouragement, and empathy from the physician. Any event related by the patient, however trivial or seemingly irrelevant, may provide the key to solving the medical problem. In general, only patients who feel comfortable with the physician will offer complete information, and thus putting the patient at ease to the greatest extent possible contributes substantially to obtaining an adequate history.

An informative history is more than an orderly listing of symptoms; by listening to patients and noting the way in which they describe their symptoms, physicians can gain valuable insight into the problem. Inflections of voice, facial expression, gestures, and attitude, i.e., "body language," may reveal important clues to the meaning of the symptoms to the patient. Because patients vary in their medical sophistication and ability to recall facts, the reported medical history should be corroborated whenever possible. The social history also can provide important insights into the types of diseases that should be considered. The family history not only identifies rare Mendelian disorders within a family but often reveals risk factors for common disorders, such as coronary heart disease, hypertension, and asthma. A thorough family history may require input from multiple relatives to ensure completeness and accuracy, and once recorded, it can be updated readily. The process of history-taking provides an opportunity to observe the patient's behavior and watch for features to be pursued more thoroughly during the physical examination.

The very act of eliciting the history provides the physician with an opportunity to establish or enhance the unique bond that forms the basis for the ideal patient-physician relationship. This process helps the physician develop an appreciation of the patient's perception of the illness, the patient's expectations of the physician and the health care system, and the financial and social implications of the illness to the patient. Although current health care settings may impose time constraints on patient visits, it is important not to rush the history-taking since this may lead the patient to believe that what he or she is relating is not of importance to the physician and, therefore, may withhold relevant information. The confidentiality of the patient-physician relationship cannot be overemphasized.

Physical examination

The purpose of the physical examination is to identify the physical signs of disease. The significance of these objective indications of disease is enhanced when they confirm a functional or structural change already suggested by the patient's history. At times, however, the physical signs may be the only evidence of disease.

The physical examination should be performed methodically and thoroughly, with consideration for the patient's comfort and modesty. Although attention is often directed by the history to the diseased organ or part of the body, the examination of a new patient must extend from head to toe in an objective search for abnormalities. Unless the physical examination is systematic and is performed in a consistent manner from patient to patient, important segments may be omitted inadvertently. The results of the examination, like the details of the history, should be recorded at the time they are elicited, not hours later, when they are subject to the distortions of memory. Skill in physical diagnosis is acquired with experience, but it is not merely technique that determines success in eliciting signs of disease. The detection of a few scattered petechiae, a faint diastolic murmur, or a small mass in the abdomen is not a question of keener eyes and ears or more sensitive fingers but of a mind alert to those findings. Because physical findings can change with time, the physical examination should be repeated as frequently as the clinical situation warrants. Because a large number of highly sensitive diagnostic tests are available, particularly imaging techniques, it may be tempting to put less emphasis on the physical examination. Indeed, many patients are seen for the first time after a series of diagnostic tests have been performed and the results are known. This fact should not deter the physician from performing a thorough physical examination since clinical findings are often present that have "escaped" the barrage of preexamination diagnostic tests. The act of examining (touching) the patient also offers an opportunity for communication and may have reassuring effects that foster the patient-physician relationship.

Diagnostic studies

Physicians have become increasingly reliant on a wide array of laboratory tests to solve clinical problems. However, accumulated laboratory data do not relieve the physician from the responsibility of carefully observing, examining, and studying the patient. It is also essential to appreciate the limitations of diagnostic tests. By virtue of their impersonal quality, complexity, and apparent precision, they often gain an aura of authority regardless of the fallibility of the tests, the instruments used in the tests, and the individuals performing or interpreting them. Physicians must weigh the expense involved in the laboratory procedures against the value of the information they are likely to provide.

Single laboratory tests are rarely ordered. Instead, physicians generally request "batteries" of multiple tests, which often prove useful. For example, abnormalities of hepatic function may provide the clue to nonspecific symptoms such as generalized weakness and increased fatigability, suggesting the diagnosis of chronic liver disease. Sometimes a single abnormality, such as an elevated serum calcium level, points to a particular disease, such as hyperparathyroidism or an underlying malignancy.

The thoughtful use of screening tests such as low-density lipoprotein cholesterol may be quite useful. A group of laboratory determinations can be carried out conveniently on a single specimen at relatively low cost. Screening tests are most informative when directed toward common diseases or disorders and when their results indicate the need for other useful tests or interventions that may be costly to perform. On the one hand, biochemical measurements, together with simple laboratory examinations such as blood count, urinalysis, and sedimentation rate, often provide a major clue to the presence of a pathologic process. On the other hand, the physician must learn to evaluate occasional abnormalities among the screening tests that may not necessarily connote significant disease. An in-depth workup after a report of an isolated laboratory abnormality in a person who is otherwise well is almost invariably wasteful and unproductive. Because so many tests are performed routinely as screening, it would not be unusual for one or two of them to be slightly abnormal. If there is no suspicion of an underlying illness, these tests ordinarily are repeated to ensure that the abnormality does not represent a laboratory error. If an abnormality is confirmed, it is important to consider its potential significance in the context of the patient's condition and other test results.

The development of technically improved imaging studies with greater sensitivity and specificity is one of the most rapidly advancing areas of medicine. These tests provide remarkably detailed anatomic information that can be a pivotal factor in medical decision-making. Ultrasonography, a variety of isotopic scans, CT, MRI, and positron emission tomography have benefited patients by supplanting older, more invasive approaches and opening new diagnostic vistas. In light of their capabilities and the rapidity with which they can lead to a diagnosis, it is tempting to order a battery of imaging studies. All physicians have had experiences in which imaging studies turned up findings that led to an unexpected diagnosis. Nonetheless, patients must endure each of these tests, and the added cost of unnecessary testing is substantial. Furthermore, investigation of an unexpected abnormal finding may be associated with risk and/or expense and may lead to the diagnosis of an irrelevant or incidental problem. A skilled physician must learn to use these powerful diagnostic tools judiciously, always considering whether the results will alter management and benefit the patient.

■ PRINCIPLES OF PATIENT CARE

Evidence-based medicine

Evidence-based medicine refers to the concept that clinical decisions are formally supported by data, preferably data that are derived from prospectively designed, randomized, controlled clinical trials. This approach is in sharp contrast to anecdotal experience, which often may be biased. Unless they are attuned to the importance of using larger, more objective studies for making decisions, even the most experienced physicians can be influenced by recent encounters with selected patients. Evidence-based medicine has become an increasingly important part of the routine practice of medicine and has led to the publication of a number of practice guidelines.

Practice guidelines

Professional organizations and government agencies are developing formal clinical-practice guidelines to aid physicians and other caregivers in making diagnostic and therapeutic decisions that are evidence-based, cost-effective, and most appropriate to a particular patient and clinical situation. As the evidence base of medicine increases, guidelines can provide a useful framework for managing patients with particular diagnoses or symptoms. They can protect patients—particularly those with inadequate health care benefits—from receiving substandard care. Guidelines also can protect conscientious caregivers from inappropriate charges of malpractice and society from the excessive costs associated with the overuse of medical resources. There are, however, caveats associated with clinical-practice guidelines since they tend to oversimplify the complexities of medicine. Furthermore, groups with differing perspectives may develop divergent recommendations regarding issues as basic as the need for mammographic screening of women in their forties or a prostate-specific antigen (PSA) assay in the serum of men over age 50. Finally, guidelines do not—and cannot be expected to—account for the uniqueness of each individual and his or her illness. The physician's challenge is to integrate into clinical practice the useful recommendations offered by experts without accepting them blindly or being inappropriately constrained by them.

Medical decision-making

Medical decision-making is an important responsibility of the physician and occurs at each stage of the diagnostic and treatment process. It involves the ordering of additional tests, requests for consults, and decisions regarding treatment and prognosis. This process requires an in-depth understanding of the pathophysiology and natural history of disease. As described above, medical decision-making should be evidence-based so that patients derive the full benefit of the scientific knowledge available to physicians. Formulating a differential diagnosis requires not only a broad knowledge base but also the ability to assess the relative probabilities of various diseases. Application of the scientific method, including hypothesis formation and data collection, is essential to the process of accepting or rejecting a particular diagnosis. Analysis of the differential diagnosis is an iterative process. As new information or test results are acquired, the group of disease processes being considered can be contracted or expanded appropriately.

Despite the importance of evidence-based medicine, much of medical decision-making relies on good clinical judgment, a process that is difficult to quantify or even to assess qualitatively. Physicians must use their knowledge and experience as a basis for weighing known factors along with the inevitable uncertainties and the need to use sound judgment; this synthesis of information is particularly important when a relevant evidence base is not available. Several quantitative tools may be invaluable in synthesizing the available information, including diagnostic tests, Bayes' theorem, and multivariate statistical models. *Diagnostic tests* serve to reduce uncertainty about a diagnosis or prognosis in a particular individual and help the physician decide how best to manage that individual's condition. The battery of diagnostic tests complements the history and the physical examination. The accuracy of a particular test is ascertained by determining its sensitivity (true-positive rate) and specificity (true-negative rate) as well as the predictive value of a positive and a negative result. *Bayes' theorem* uses information on a test's sensitivity and specificity, in conjunction with the pretest probability of a diagnosis, to determine mathematically the posttest probability of the diagnosis. More complex clinical problems can be approached with *multivariable statistical models*, which generate highly accurate information even when multiple factors are acting individually or together to affect disease risk, progression, or response to treatment. Studies comparing the performance of statistical models with that of expert clinicians have documented equivalent accuracy, although the models tend to be more consistent. Thus, multivariate statistical models may be particularly helpful to less experienced clinicians. See Chap. 3 for a more thorough discussion of decision-making in clinical medicine.

Electronic medical records

Growing reliance on computers and the strength of information technology are playing an increasingly important role in medicine. Laboratory data are accessed almost universally through computers. Many medical centers now have electronic medical records, computerized order entry, and bar-coded tracking of medications. Some of these systems are interactive and provide reminders or warn of potential medical errors. In many ways, the health care system has lagged behind other industries in the adoption of information technology. Electronic medical records have extraordinary potential for providing rapid access to clinical information, imaging studies, laboratory results, and medications. This type of information is invaluable for ongoing efforts to enhance quality and improve patient safety. Ideally, patient records should be easily transferred across the health care system, providing reliable access to relevant data and historic information. However, technology limitations and concerns about privacy and cost continue to limit a broad-based utilization of electronic health records in most clinical settings. It

also should be emphasized that information technology is merely a tool and can never replace the clinical decisions that are best made by the physician. In this regard, clinical knowledge and an understanding of the patient's needs, supplemented by quantitative tools, still seem to represent the best approach to decision-making in the practice of medicine.

Evaluation of outcomes

Clinicians generally use *objective* and readily measurable parameters to judge the outcome of a therapeutic intervention. For example, findings on physical or laboratory examination—such as the blood pressure level, the patency of a coronary artery on an angiogram, or the size of a mass on a radiologic examination—can provide critically important information. However, patients usually seek medical attention for *subjective* reasons; they wish to obtain relief from pain, preserve or regain function, and enjoy life. The components of a patient's health status or quality of life can include bodily comfort, capacity for physical activity, personal and professional function, sexual function, cognitive function, and overall perception of health. Each of these important areas can be assessed by means of structured interviews or specially designed questionnaires. Such assessments also provide useful parameters by which the physician can judge the patient's subjective view of his or her disability and the response to treatment, particularly in chronic illness. The practice of medicine requires consideration and integration of both objective and subjective outcomes.

Women's health and disease

Although past epidemiologic studies and clinical trials often focused predominantly on men, more recent studies have included more women, and some, like the Women's Health Initiative, have exclusively addressed women's health issues. Significant gender differences exist in diseases that afflict both men and women. Much is still to be learned in this arena, and ongoing studies should enhance physicians' understanding of the mechanisms of gender differences in the course and outcome of certain diseases. For a more complete discussion of women's health, see Chap. 6.

Care of the elderly

The relative proportion of elderly individuals in the populations of developed nations has been growing considerably over the last few decades and will continue to grow. In this regard, the practice of medicine will continue to be greatly influenced by the health care needs of this growing elderly population. The physician must understand and appreciate the decline in physiologic reserve associated with aging; the diminished responses of the elderly to vaccinations such as those against influenza; the different responses of the elderly to common diseases; and disorders that occur commonly with aging, such as depression, dementia, frailty, urinary incontinence, and fractures. For a more complete discussion of medical care for the elderly, see Part 5, Chaps. 70, 71, and 72.

Errors in the delivery of health care

A report from the Institute of Medicine called for an ambitious agenda to reduce medical error rates and improve patient safety by designing and implementing fundamental changes in health care systems. Adverse drug reactions occur in at least 5% of hospitalized patients, and the incidence increases with the use of a large number of drugs. No matter what the clinical situation is, it is the responsibility of the physician to use powerful therapeutic measures wisely, with due regard for their beneficial action, potential dangers, and cost. It is also the responsibility of hospitals and health care organizations to develop systems to reduce risk and ensure patient safety. Medication errors can be reduced through the use of ordering systems that eliminate misreading of handwriting. Implementation of infection control systems, enforcement of hand washing protocols, and careful oversight of antibiotic use can minimize the complications of nosocomial infections.

The role of the physician in the informed consent of the patient

The fundamental principles of medical ethics require physicians to act in the patient's best interest and respect the patient's autonomy. This is particularly relevant to the issue of informed consent. Most patients possess only limited medical knowledge and must rely on their physicians for advice. Physicians must respect their patients' autonomy, fully discussing the alternatives for care and the risks, benefits, and likely consequences of each alternative. Special care should be taken to ensure that a physician seeking a patient's informed consent does not have a real or apparent conflict of interest involving personal gain.

Patients are required to sign a consent form for essentially any diagnostic or therapeutic procedure. In such cases, it is particularly important for the patient to understand clearly the risks and benefits of these procedures; this is the definition of *informed consent*. It is incumbent on the physician to explain the procedures in a clear and understandable manner and to ascertain that the patient comprehends both the nature of the procedure and the attendant risks and benefits. The dread of the unknown, inherent in hospitalization, can be mitigated by such explanations.

The approach to grave prognoses and death

No problem is more distressing than the diagnosis of an incurable disease, particularly when premature death is inevitable. What should the patient and family be told? What measures should be taken to maintain life? What can be done to maintain the quality of life?

Although some would argue otherwise, there is no ironclad rule that the patient must immediately be told "everything" even if the patient is an adult with substantial family responsibilities. Nevertheless, openness and honesty with the patient is a must. A patient must know the expected course of disease to make appropriate plans and preparations. The patient should participate in decision-making with an understanding of the treatment goals (cure or palliation), the disease effects, and the likely treatment effects. A wise and insightful physician often is guided by an understanding of what a patient wants to know and when he or she wants to know it. The patient's religious beliefs also may be taken into consideration. The patient must be given an opportunity to talk with the physician and ask questions. Patients may find it easier to share their feelings about death with their physician, who is likely to be more objective and less emotional, than with family members. As William Osler wrote, "One thing is certain; it is not for you to don the black cap and, assuming the judicial function, take hope away from any patient." Even when the patient directly inquires, "Am I dying?" the physician must attempt to determine whether this is a request for information or for reassurance. Only open communication between the patient and the physician can resolve this question and guide the physician in what to say and how to say it.

The physician should provide or arrange for emotional, physical, and spiritual support and must be compassionate, unhurried, and open. There is much to be gained by the laying on of hands. Pain should be controlled adequately, human dignity maintained, and isolation from family and close friends avoided. These aspects of care tend to be overlooked in hospitals, where the intrusion of life-sustaining apparatus can detract from attention to the whole person and encourage concentration instead on the life-threatening disease, against which the battle ultimately will be lost in any case. In the face of terminal illness, the goal of medicine must shift from *cure* to *care* in the broadest sense of the term. *Primum succurrere*, first hasten to provide help, is a guiding principle. In offering care to a dying patient, a physician must be prepared to provide information to family members and deal with their grief and sometimes their feelings of guilt. It is important for the doctor to assure the family that everything possible has been done. For a more complete discussion of end-of-life care, see Chap. 9.

■ THE PATIENT-PHYSICIAN RELATIONSHIP

The significance of the intimate personal relationship between physician and patient cannot be too strongly emphasized, for in an extraordinarily large number of cases both the diagnosis and treatment are directly dependent on it. One of the essential qualities of the clinician is interest in humanity, **for the secret of the care of the patient is in caring for the patient.**

—Francis W. Peabody, 1881–1927

Physicians must never forget that patients are individual human beings with problems that all too often transcend their physical complaints. They are not "cases" or "admissions" or "diseases." Patients do not fail treatments; treatments fail to benefit patients. This point is particularly important in this era of high technology in clinical medicine. Most patients are anxious and fearful. Physicians should instill confidence and should be reassuring but should never be arrogant. A professional attitude, coupled with warmth and openness, can do much to alleviate anxiety and to encourage patients to share all aspects of their medical history. Empathy and compassion are the essential features of a caring physician. Whatever the patient's attitude is, the physician needs to consider the setting in which an illness occurs—in terms not only of the patients themselves but also of their familial, social, and cultural backgrounds. The ideal patient-physician relationship is based on thorough knowledge of the patient, mutual trust, and the ability to communicate.

The dichotomy of inpatient and outpatient internal medicine

The hospital environment has changed dramatically over the last few decades. In more recent times, emergency departments and critical care units have evolved to identify and manage critically ill patients, allowing them to survive formerly fatal diseases. There is increasing pressure to reduce the length of stay in the hospital and to manage complex disorders in the outpatient setting. This transition has been driven not only by efforts to reduce costs but also by the availability of new outpatient technologies, such as imaging and percutaneous infusion catheters for long-term antibiotics or nutrition, minimally invasive surgical procedures, and evidence that outcomes often are improved by minimizing inpatient hospitalization. Hospitals now consist of multiple distinct levels of care, such as the emergency department, procedure rooms, overnight observation units, critical care units, and palliative care units, in addition to traditional medical beds. A consequence of this differentiation has been the emergence of new specialties such as emergency medicine, intensivists, hospitalists, and end-of-life care. Moreover, these systems frequently involve "handoffs" from the outpatient to the inpatient environment, from the critical care unit to a general medicine floor, and from the hospital to the outpatient environment. Clearly, one of the important challenges in internal medicine is to maintain continuity of care and information flow during these transitions, which threaten the traditional one-to-one relationship between patient and physician. In the current environment, teams of physicians, specialists, and other health care professionals often replace the personal interaction between doctor and patient. The patient can benefit greatly from effective collaboration among a number of health care professionals; however, *it is the duty of the patient's principal or primary physician to provide cohesive guidance through an illness*. To meet this challenge, the primary physician must be familiar with the techniques, skills, and objectives of specialist physicians and allied health professionals. The primary physician must ensure that the patient will benefit from scientific advances and from the expertise of specialists when they are needed while retaining responsibility for the major decisions concerning diagnosis and treatment.

Appreciation of the patient's hospital experience

The hospital is an intimidating environment for most individuals. Hospitalized patients find themselves surrounded by air jets, buttons, and glaring lights; invaded by tubes and wires; and beset by the numerous members of the health care team—nurses, nurses' aides, physicians' assistants, social workers, technologists, physical therapists, medical students, house officers, attending and consulting physicians, and many others. They may be transported to special laboratories and imaging facilities replete with blinking lights, strange sounds, and unfamiliar personnel; they may be left unattended for periods of time; they may be obliged to share a room with other patients, who have their own health problems. It is little wonder that patients may lose their sense of reality. Physicians who can appreciate the hospital experience from the patient's perspective and make an effort to develop a strong personal relationship with the patient in which they may guide the patient through this experience can make a stressful situation more tolerable.

Trends in the delivery of health care: a challenge to the humane physician

Many trends in the delivery of health care tend to make medical care impersonal. These trends, some of which have been mentioned already, include (1) vigorous efforts to reduce the escalating costs of health care; (2) the growing number of managed-care programs, which are intended to reduce costs but in which the patient may have little choice in selecting a physician or in seeing that physician consistently; (3) increasing reliance on technological advances and computerization for many aspects of diagnosis and treatment; (4) the need for numerous physicians to be involved in the care of most patients who are seriously ill; and (5) an increased number of malpractice suits, some of which are justifiable because of medical errors but others of which reflect an unrealistic expectation on the part of many patients that their disease will be cured or that complications will not occur during the course of complex illnesses or procedures.

In light of these changes in the medical care system, it is a major challenge for physicians to maintain the *humane* aspects of medical care. The American Board of Internal Medicine, working together with the American College of Physicians–American Society of Internal Medicine and the European Federation of Internal Medicine, has published a *Charter on Medical Professionalism* that underscores three main principles in physicians' contract with society: (1) the primacy of patient welfare, (2) patient autonomy, and (3) social justice. Medical schools appropriately place substantial emphasis on physician professionalism (Fig. 1-1). The humanistic qualities of a physician must encompass integrity, respect, and compassion. Availability, the expression of sincere concern, the willingness to take the time to explain all aspects of the illness, and a nonjudgmental attitude when dealing with patients whose cultures, lifestyles, attitudes, and values differ from those of the physician are just a

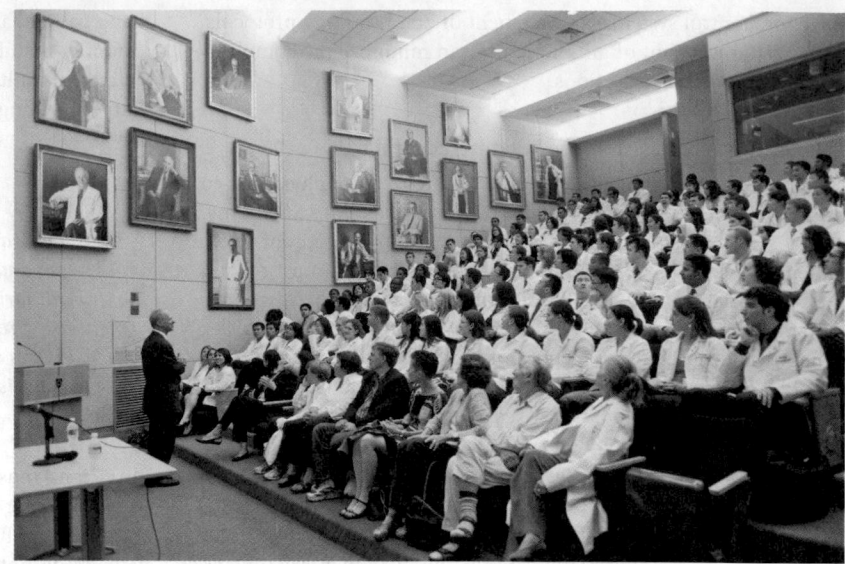

Figure 1-1   A typical "white coat" ceremony in medical school in which students are introduced to the responsibilities of patient care. *(Photo courtesy of Suzanne Camarata Photography; used with permission.)*

few of the characteristics of a humane physician. Every physician will, at times, be challenged by patients who evoke strongly negative or positive emotional responses. Physicians should be alert to their own reactions to such patients and situations and consciously monitor and control their behavior so that the patient's best interest remains the principal motivation for their actions at all times.

An important aspect of patient care involves an appreciation of the patient's "quality of life," a subjective assessment of what each patient values most. This assessment requires detailed, sometimes intimate knowledge of the patient, which usually can be obtained only through deliberate, unhurried, and often repeated conversations. Time pressures will always threaten these interactions, but they should not diminish the importance of understanding and seeking to fulfill the priorities of the patient.

■ THE TWENTY-FIRST-CENTURY PHYSICIAN: EXPANDING FRONTIERS

The era of "omics": genomics, epigenomics, proteomics, microbiomics, metagenomics, metabolomics . . .

In the spring of 2003, the complete sequencing of the human genome was announced, officially ushering in the genomic era. However, even before that landmark accomplishment, the practice of medicine had been evolving as a result of the insights gained from an understanding of the human genome as well as the genomes of a wide variety of microbes, whose genetic sequences were becoming widely available as a result of breathtaking advances in sequencing techniques and informatics. An example is the rapid identification of H1N1 influenza as a potentially fatal pandemic illness and the rapid development and dissemination of an effective protective vaccine. Today, gene expression profiles are being used to guide therapy and inform prognosis for a number of diseases, the use of genotyping is providing a new means to assess the risk of certain diseases as well as variation in response to a number of drugs, and physicians are beginning to understand better the role of certain genes in the causality of common conditions such as obesity and allergies. Despite these advances, scientists are still in the infancy of understanding and utilizing the complexities of genomics in the diagnosis, prevention, and treatment of disease. The task of physicians is complicated by the fact that phenotypes generally are determined not by genes alone but by the interplay of genetic and environmental factors. Indeed, researchers have just begun to scratch the surface of possibilities that the era of genomics will provide to the practice of medicine.

Rapid progress also is being made in other areas of molecular medicine. *Epigenomics* is the study of alterations in chromatin and histone proteins and methylation of DNA sequences that influence gene expression. Epigenetic alterations are associated with a number of cancers and other diseases. The study of the entire library of proteins made in a cell or organ and its relationship to disease is called *proteomics*. Proteomics is now recognized as far more complex than originally considered, enhancing the repertoire of the 30,000 genes in the human genome by alternate splicing and posttranslational processing as well as by an increasing number of posttranslational modifications, many with unique functional consequences. The presence or absence of particular proteins in the circulation or in cells is being explored for diagnostic and disease-screening uses. *Microbiomics* is the study of the bacterial flora of a person. Interesting research is suggesting that the composition of colonic flora may play a role in obesity and in other diseases. *Metagenomics*, of which microbiomics is a part, is the genomic study of environmental species that have the potential to influence human biology directly or indirectly. An example is the study of exposures to microorganisms in farm environments that might be responsible for the lower incidence of asthma among farm-raised children. *Metabolomics* is the study of the range of metabolites in cells or organs and the ways they are altered in disease states. The aging process itself may leave telltale metabolic footprints that allow the prediction (and possibly the prevention) of dysfunction and disease. It seems likely that disease-associated patterns will be sought in lipids, carbohydrates, membranes, mitochondria, and other vital components of cells and tissues. All this new information represents a challenge to the traditional reductionist approach to medical thinking. The variability of results in different patients, together with the large number of variables that can be assessed, creates difficulties in identifying preclinical disease and defining disease states unequivocally. Accordingly, the tools of systems biology are being applied to the myriad information now obtainable from every patient and may provide new approaches to classifying disease. For a more complete discussion of a complex systems approach to human disease, see Chap. e19.

The rapidity of these advances may seem overwhelming to the practicing physician. However, he or she has an important role to play in ensuring that these powerful technologies and sources of new information are applied with sensitivity and intelligence to the patient. Since "omics" is such a rapidly evolving field, physicians and other health care professionals must continue to educate themselves so that they can apply this new knowledge to the benefit of their patients' health and well-being. Genetic testing requires wise counsel based on an understanding of the value and limitations of the tests as well as the implications of their results for specific individuals. For a more complete discussion of genetic testing, see Chap. 63.

The globalization of medicine

Physicians should be cognizant of diseases and health care services beyond local boundaries. Global travel has implications for disease spread, and it is not uncommon for diseases endemic to certain regions to be seen in other regions after a patient has traveled to and returned from those regions. Patients have broader access to unique expertise or clinical trials at distant medical centers, and the cost of travel may be offset by the quality of care at those distant locations. As much as any other factor influencing global aspects of medicine, the Internet has transformed the transfer of medical information throughout the world. This change has been accompanied by the transfer of technological skills through telemedicine and international consultation for radiologic images and pathologic specimens. For a complete discussion of global issues, see Chap. 2.

Medicine on the Internet

On the whole, the Internet has had a very positive effect on the practice of medicine; a wide range of information is available to physicians and patients through personal computers almost instantaneously at any time and from anywhere in the world. This medium holds enormous potential for delivering current information, practice guidelines, state-of-the-art conferences, journal contents, textbooks (including this text), and direct communications with other physicians and specialists, expanding the depth and breadth of information available to the physician about the diagnosis and care of patients. Medical journals are now accessible online, providing rapid sources of new information. This medium also serves to lessen the information gap felt by physicians and health care providers in remote areas by bringing them into direct and timely contact with the latest developments in medical care.

Patients, too, are turning to the Internet in increasing numbers to acquire information about their illnesses and therapies and to join Internet-based support groups. Physicians increasingly are faced with the prospect of dealing with patients who arrive with sophisticated information about their illnesses. In this regard, physicians are challenged in a positive way to keep abreast of the latest relevant information while serving as an "editor" for the patients as they navigate this seemingly endless source of information, the accuracy and validity of which are not uniform.

A critically important caveat is that virtually anything can be published on the Internet, with easy circumvention of the peer-review process that is an essential feature of academic publications. Physicians or patients who search the Internet for medical information must be aware of this danger. Notwithstanding this limitation, appropriate use of the Internet is revolutionizing information access for physicians and patients and in this regard is a great benefit that was not available to earlier practitioners.

Public expectations and accountability

The level of knowledge and sophistication regarding health issues on the part of the general public has grown rapidly over the last few decades. As a result, expectations of the health care system in general and of physicians in particular have risen. Physicians are expected to master rapidly advancing fields (the *science* of medicine) while considering their patients' unique needs (the *art* of medicine). Thus, physicians are held accountable not only for the technical aspects of the care that they provide but also for their patients' satisfaction with the delivery and costs of care.

In many parts of the world, physicians increasingly are expected to account for the way in which they practice medicine by meeting certain standards prescribed by federal and local governments. The hospitalization of patients whose health care costs are reimbursed by the government and other third parties is subjected to utilization review. Thus, a physician must defend the cause for and duration of a patient's hospitalization if it falls outside certain "average" standards. Authorization for reimbursement increasingly is based on documentation of the nature and complexity of an illness, as reflected by recorded elements of the history and physical examination. There is a growing "pay for performance" movement that seeks to link reimbursement to quality of care. The goal of this movement is to improve standards of health care and contain spiraling health care costs. Physicians also are expected to give evidence of their continuing competence through mandatory continuing education, patient record audits, maintenance of certification, and relicensing.

Medical ethics and new technologies

The rapid pace of technological advances has profound implications for medical applications far beyond their traditional roles to prevent, treat, and cure disease. Cloning, genetic engineering, gene therapy, human-computer interfaces, nanotechnology, and designer drugs have the potential to modify inherited predispositions to disease, select desired characteristics in embryos, augment "normal" human performance, replace failing tissues, and substantially prolong life span. Because of their unique training, physicians have a responsibility to help shape the debate concerning the appropriate uses of and limits that should be placed on these new techniques.

The physician as perpetual student

It becomes all too apparent from the time doctors graduate from medical school that as physicians their lot is that of the "perpetual student" and the mosaic of their knowledge and experiences is eternally unfinished. This concept can be at the same time exhilarating and anxiety-provoking. It is exhilarating because doctors will continue to expand knowledge that can be applied to their patients; it is anxiety-provoking because doctors realize that they will never know as much as they want or need to know. At best, doctors will translate this latter feeling into energy to continue to improve themselves and realize their potential as physicians. In this regard, it is the responsibility of a physician to pursue new knowledge continually by reading, attending conferences and courses, and consulting colleagues and the Internet. This is often a difficult task for a busy practitioner; however, such a commitment to continued learning is an integral part of being a physician and must be given the highest priority.

The physician as citizen

Being a physician is a privilege. The capacity to apply one's skills for the benefit of one's fellow human beings is a noble calling. The doctor-patient relationship is inherently unbalanced in the distribution of power. In light of a doctor's influence, he or she must always be aware of the potential impact of what he or she does and says and must always strive to strip away individual biases and preferences to find what is best for the patient. To the extent possible, a physician also should try to act within his or her community to promote health and alleviate suffering. Meeting these goals begins by setting a healthy example and continues in actions that may be taken to deliver needed care even when personal financial compensation may not be available.

G. H. T. Kimble wrote: "It is bad enough that a [person] should be ignorant, for this cuts him [or her] off from the commerce of [people's] minds. It is perhaps worse that a [person] should be poor, for this condemns him [or her] to a life of stint and scheming in which there is no time for dreams and no respite from weariness. But what surely is worse is that a [person] should be unwell, for this prevents his [or her] doing anything much about either his [or her] poverty or his [or her] ignorance." A goal for medicine and its practitioners is to strive to provide the means by which the poor can cease to be unwell.

Learning medicine

It has been about 100 years since the publication of the Flexner Report, a seminal study that transformed medical education and emphasized the scientific foundations of medicine as well as the acquisition of clinical skills. In an era of burgeoning information and access to medical simulation and informatics, many schools are implementing new curricula that emphasize lifelong learning and the acquisition of competencies in teamwork, communication skills, system-based practice, and professionalism. These and other features of the medical school curriculum provide the foundation for many of the themes highlighted in this chapter and are expected to allow physicians to progress from competency to proficiency to mastery with progressive experience and learning.

At a time when the amount of information that one must master to practice medicine continues to expand, increasing pressures both within and outside of medicine have produced strict restrictions on the amount of time a physician in training can spend in the hospital. It was felt that the benefits associated with the continuity of medical care and observation of the patient's progress over time were outstripped by the stresses of long hours on the trainees and the fatigue-related errors they made in caring for patients. Accordingly, physicians in training had limits set on the number of patients they could carry at a time, the number of new patients they could evaluate in a day on call, and the number of hours they could spend in the hospital. In 1980, residents in medicine worked in the hospital more than 90 hours a week on average. In 1989, their hours were restricted to no more than 80 a week. Resident physicians' hours further decreased by about 10% between 1996 and 2008, and in 2010, the Accreditation Council for Graduate Medical Education (ACGME) placed further restrictions on continuing in-hospital duty hours for first year residents (16 hours/shift). The impact of these changes is continuing to be assessed, but the evidence that medical errors have decreased as a consequence is sparse. An unavoidable by-product of fewer hours at work is an increase in the number of "handoffs" of patient responsibility from one physician to another. These transfers often involve a transition from a physician who knows the patient well, having evaluated the patient on admission, to a physician who knows the patient less well. It is imperative that these transitions of responsibility be handled with care and thoroughness with all the relevant information exchanged and acknowledged. The issue of coverage is not limited to physicians in graduate training. The average practicing physician worked 54 hours per week in 1996–1998 and 51 hours per week in 2006–2008.

Research, teaching, and the practice of medicine

The title *doctor* is derived from the Latin *docere*, "to teach," and physicians should share information and medical knowledge with colleagues, students of medicine and related professions, and their patients. The practice of medicine is dependent on the sum total of medical knowledge, which in turn is based on an unending chain of scientific discovery, clinical observation, analysis, and interpretation. Advances in medicine depend on the acquisition of new information through research, and improved medical care requires the transmission of that information. As part of broader societal responsibilities, the physician should encourage patients to participate in ethical and properly approved clinical investigations if they do not impose undue hazard, discomfort, or inconvenience. However, physicians engaged in clinical research must be alert to potential conflicts of interest between their research goals and their obligations to individual patients; the best interests of the patient must always take priority.

To wrest from nature the secrets which have perplexed philosophers in all ages, to track to their sources the causes of disease, to correlate the vast stores of knowledge, that they may be quickly available for the prevention and cure of disease—these are our ambitions.

—William Osler, 1849–1919

FURTHER READINGS

CHARAP MH et al: Internal medicine residency training in the 21st century: Aligning requirements with professional needs. Am J Med 118:1042, 2005

COOKE M et al: American medical education 100 years after the Flexner Report. N Engl J Med 355:1339, 2006

COUNCIL ON GRADUATE MEDICAL EDUCATION: *Thirteenth Report: Physician Education for a Changing Health Care Environment.* U.S. Department of Health and Human Services, Washington, DC

HUNTER DJ et al: From Darwin's finches to canaries in the coal mine—mining the genome for new biology. N Engl J Med 358:2760, 2008

KINGHORN WA: Medical education as moral formation: An Aristotelian account of medical professionalism. Perspect Biol Med 53:87, 2009

LOSCALZO J et al: Human disease classification in the postgenomic era: A complex systems approach. Mol Syst Biol 3:124, 2007

STAIGER DO et al: Trends in the hours of physicians in the United States. JAMA 303:747, 2010

STRAUS SE et al: Teaching evidence-based medicine skills can change practice in a community hospital. J Gen Intern Med 20:340, 2005

CHAPTER **2**

Global Issues in Medicine

Jim Yong Kim
Paul Farmer
Joseph Rhatigan

WHY GLOBAL HEALTH?

Global health, it has been noted, is not a discipline; it is, rather, a collection of problems. A leading group of scholars have defined global health as the study and practice concerned with improving the health of all people and achieving health equity worldwide, with an emphasis on addressing problems that are transnational. No single review can do much more than identify the leading problems in applying evidence-based medicine in settings of great poverty or across national boundaries. This chapter introduces the major international bodies that address these problems; identifies the more significant barriers to improving the health of people who to date have not, by and large, had access to modern medicines; and summarizes population-based data on the most common health problems faced by people living in poverty. Examining specific problems—notably AIDS (Chap. 189) but also tuberculosis (TB, Chap. 165), malaria (Chap. 210), and key noncommunicable diseases—helps sharpen the discussion of barriers to prevention, diagnosis, and care as well as the means of overcoming them. The chapter then discusses the role of health systems and the problem of "brain drain" on those systems. It closes by discussing global health equity, drawing on notions of social justice that once were central to international public health but have fallen out of favor over the last several decades.

BRIEF HISTORY OF GLOBAL HEALTH INSTITUTIONS

Concern about health across national boundaries dates back many centuries, predating the Black Plague and other pandemics. The first organization founded explicitly to tackle cross-border health issues was the Pan American Sanitary Bureau, which was formed by 11 countries in the Americas in 1902. The primary goal of what later became the Pan American Health Organization was the control of infectious diseases across the Americas. Of special concern was yellow fever, which had been running a deadly course through much of South and Central America and posed a threat to the construction of the Panama Canal. In 1948, the United Nations formed the first truly global health institution: the World Health Organization (WHO). In 1958, under the aegis of the WHO and in line with a long-standing focus on communicable diseases that cross borders, leaders in global health initiated the effort that led to what some see as the greatest success in international health: the

eradication of smallpox. Naysayers were surprised when the smallpox eradication campaign, which engaged public health officials throughout the world, proved successful in 1979 during the Cold War. The influence of the WHO waned during the 1980s. In the early 1990s, many observers argued that with its vastly superior financial resources and close if unequal relationships with the governments of poor countries, the World Bank had eclipsed the WHO as the most important multilateral institution working in the area of health. One of the stated goals of the World Bank was to help poor countries identify "cost-effective" interventions worthy of international public support. At the same time, the World Bank encouraged many of those nations to reduce public expenditures in health and education as part of later discredited structural adjustment programs that were imposed as a condition for access to credit and assistance through international financial institutions such as the World Bank and the International Monetary Fund (IMF). At the same time, there was a resurgence of many diseases, including malaria, trypanosomiasis, are schistosomiasis, in Africa. Tuberculosis, an eminently curable disease, remained the world's leading infectious killer of adults. Half a million women per year died in childbirth during the last decade of the twentieth century, and few of the world's largest philanthropic or funding institutions focused on global health.

AIDS, first described in 1981, precipitated a change. In the United States, the advent of this newly described infectious killer marked the culmination of a series of events that discredited talk of "closing the book" on infectious diseases. In Africa, which would emerge as the global epicenter of the pandemic, HIV disease strained TB control programs, and malaria continued to take as many lives as ever. At the dawn of the twenty-first century, these three diseases alone killed an estimated 6 million people each year. New research, new policies, and new funding mechanisms were called for. The last decade has seen the rise of important multilateral global health institutions such as the Global Fund to Fight AIDS, Tuberculosis, and Malaria (GFATM) and the Joint United Nations Programme on HIV/AIDS (UNAIDS); bilateral efforts such as the U.S. President's Emergency Plan for AIDS Relief (PEPFAR); and private philanthropic organizations such as the Bill & Melinda Gates Foundation. Yet with its 193 member states and 147 country offices, the WHO remains preeminent in matters relating to the cross-border spread of infectious diseases and other health threats. In the aftermath of the severe acute respiratory syndrome (SARS) epidemic of 2003, the International Health Regulations—which provide a legal foundation for the WHO's direct investigation of a wide range of global health problems, including pandemic influenza, in any member state—were strengthened and brought into force in May 2007.

Even as attention to and resources for health problems in poor countries grow, the lack of coherence in and among global health institutions may undermine efforts to forge a more comprehensive and effective response. The WHO is still woefully underfunded despite the ever-growing need to engage a wider and more complex range of health issues. In another instance of the paradoxical impact of success, the rapid growth of the Gates Foundation, which is clearly one of the most important developments in the history of global health, has led other foundations to question the wisdom of continuing to invest their more modest resources in this field. This indeed may be what some have called "the golden age of global health," but leaders of major organizations such as the WHO, the GFATM, the United Nations Children's Fund (UNICEF), UNAIDS, PEPFAR, and the Gates Foundation must work together to design an effective architecture that will make the most of the opportunities that now exist. To this end, new and old players in global health must invest heavily in *discovery* (relevant basic science), the *development* of new tools (preventive, diagnostic, and therapeutic), and *delivery* to ensure the equitable provision of health products and services to all who need them.

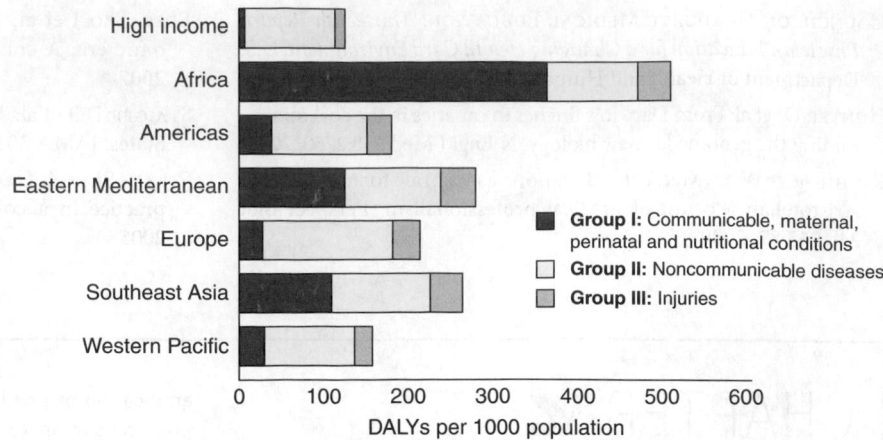

Figure 2-1 Burden of disease, by broad cause and region, 2004. *[Source: World Health Organization. Reprinted with permission (http://www.who.int/healthinfo/global_burden_disease/GBD_report_2004update_full.pdf; accessed January 10, 2010).]*

THE ECONOMICS OF GLOBAL HEALTH

Political and economic concerns have often guided global health interventions. As mentioned, early efforts to control yellow fever were tied to the completion of the Panama Canal. However, the precise nature of the link between economics and health remains a matter for debate. Some economists and demographers argue that improving the health status of populations must begin with economic development; others maintain that addressing ill health is the starting point for development in poor countries. In either case, investment in health care, especially the control of communicable diseases, should lead to increased productivity. The question is where to find the necessary resources to start the predicted "virtuous cycle."

Since 1999, spurred by the leadership of the Gates Foundation and the growing interest in addressing novel and persistent challenges such as AIDS, spending on health in poor countries has increased, with over $80 billion in new funds earmarked for the discovery and development of drugs and diagnostics targeting diseases of the poor; comprehensive responses to the AIDS, TB, and malaria epidemics; vaccine development and delivery; and even improved methods of data collection in resource-poor settings. Nevertheless, to reach the United Nations Millennium Development Goals, that include targets for poverty reduction, universal primary education, and gender equality, spending in the health sector must be increased further. To determine by how much and for how long, it is imperative to improve the ability to assess the global burden of disease (GBD) and plan interventions that more precisely match the need. Refining metrics is an important task for global health: only recently have there been solid assessments of the GBD.

MORTALITY AND THE GLOBAL BURDEN OF DISEASE

Since the late 1980s, serious efforts have been made to calculate the GBD. The first GBD study, conducted in 1990, laid the foundation for the first report on *Disease Control Priorities in Developing Countries* (DCP1) and for the World Bank's 1993 World Development Report *Investing in Health*. Those efforts represented a major advance in the understanding of health status in developing countries. *Investing in Health* has been especially influential: it familiarized a broad audience with cost-effectiveness analysis for specific health interventions and with the notion of disability-adjusted life years

(DALYs). The DALY, which has become a standard measure of the impact of a specific health condition on a population, combines in a single measure both absolute years of life lost and years lost due to disability for incident cases of a condition. (See Fig. 2-1 and Table 2-1 for an analysis of the GBD by DALYs.)

The most recent WHO analysis of the GBD was based on health data from 2004. This report reflects growth in the available data on health in the poorest countries and in the capacity to measure the impact of specific conditions on a population. Yet even in 2004, only 112 of 192 nations surveyed had reliable information on the causes of deaths within their borders. It is essential to expand efforts to collect the most basic health data; this task falls to the WHO, national governments, and certain academic institutions. The lack of complete data has led to considerable uncertainty in estimates of overall mortality rates. The level of uncertainty ranges from as low as ± 1% for estimates of all-cause mortality in developed countries to ± 20% for all-cause mortality in the WHO's African Region. The level of uncertainty in regional prevalence estimates ranges from ± 10% to ± 90%, with a median value of ± 41%. As analytic methods and data quality have improved, however, important trends can be identified in a comparison of GBD estimates from 1990 and 2004.

Of the 58.8 million deaths worldwide in 2004, 30% were due to communicable diseases, maternal and perinatal conditions, and nutritional deficiencies. Although the proportion of all deaths attributable to these causes has decreased marginally since 1990, the share of all deaths due to HIV/AIDS grew from just 2% to >3.5%. Among the fraction of all deaths related to communicable diseases, maternal and perinatal conditions, and nutritional deficiencies, 97% occurred in middle- and low-income countries. The leading cause of death among adults in 2004 was ischemic heart disease, accounting for 16.3% of all deaths in high-income countries, 13.9% in middle-income countries, and 9.4% in low-income countries (Table 2-2). In second place was cerebrovascular disease, that accounted for 9.3% of deaths in high-income countries, 14.2% in middle-income countries, and 5.6% in low-income countries. Although the third leading cause of death in high-income countries was tracheal, bronchial, and lung cancers (that accounted for 5.9% of all deaths), those conditions did not even register in the top 10 places in low-income countries. Among the 10 leading causes of death in low-income countries, 6 were communicable diseases; in high-income countries, however, only one communicable disease—lower respiratory infection—ranked among the top 10 causes of death.

A recent study found that the worldwide mortality figure among children <5 years of age dropped from 11.9 million deaths in 1990 to 7.7 million in 2010. Of the deaths in 2010, 3.1 million (40%) occurred

TABLE 2-1 Leading Causes of Burden of Disease (DALYs), With Countries Grouped by Income, 2004

Disease or Injury	DALYs (millions)	Percent of total DALYs	Disease or Injury	DALYs (millions)	Percent of total DALYs
World			**Middle-income countries**		
1 Lower respiratory infections	94.5	6.2	1 Unipolar depressive disorders	29.0	5.1
2 Diarrheal diseases	72.8	4.8	2 Ischemic heart disease	28.9	5.0
3 Unipolar depressive disorders	65.5	4.3	3 Cerebrovascular disease	27.5	4.8
4 Ischemic heart disease	62.6	4.1	4 Road traffic accidents	21.4	3.7
5 HIV/AIDS	58.5	3.8	5 Lower respiratory infections	16.3	2.8
6 Cerebrovascular disease	46.6	3.1	6 COPD	16.1	2.8
7 Prematurity and low birth weight	44.3	2.9	7 HIV/AIDS	15.0	2.6
8 Birth asphyxia and birth trauma	41.7	2.7	8 Alcohol use disorders	14.9	2.6
9 Road traffic accidents	41.2	2.7	9 Refractive errors	13.7	2.4
10 Neonatal infections and other[b]	40.4	2.7	10 Diarrheal diseases	13.1	2.3
High-income countries			**Low-income countries[a]**		
1 Unipolar depressive disorders	10.0	8.2	1 Lower respiratory infections	76.9	9.3
2 Ischemic heart disease	7.7	6.3	2 Diarrheal diseases	59.2	7.2
3 Cerebrovascular disease	4.8	3.9	3 HIV/AIDS	42.9	5.2
4 Alzheimer's and other dementias	4.4	3.6	4 Malaria	32.8	4.0
5 Alcohol use disorders	4.2	3.4	5 Prematurity and low birth weight	32.1	3.9
6 Hearing loss, adult onset	4.2	3.4	6 Neonatal infections and other[b]	31.4	3.8
7 COPD	3.7	3.0	7 Birth asphyxia and birth trauma	29.8	3.6
8 Diabetes mellitus	3.6	3.0	8 Unipolar depressive disorders	26.5	3.2
9 Trachea, bronchus, lung cancers	3.6	3.0	9 Ischemic heart disease	26.0	3.1
10 Road traffic accidents	3.1	2.6	10 Tuberculosis	22.4	2.7

[a]Countries grouped by gross national income per capita.

[b]This category also includes other noninfectious causes arising in the perinatal period apart from prematurity, low birth weight, birth trauma, and asphyxia. These noninfectious causes are responsible for about 20% of the DALYs shown in this category.

Abbreviation: COPD, chronic obstructive pulmonary disease.

Source: World Health Organization. Reprinted with permission. http://www.who.int/healthinfo/global_burden_disease/GBD_report_2004update_full.pdf.

in the neonatal period. About one-third of these deaths among children <5 years old occurred in southern Asia and almost one-half in sub-Saharan Africa; <1% occurred in high-income countries.

Among persons 15–59 years of age, noncommunicable diseases accounted for more than one-half of all deaths in all regions except sub-Saharan Africa, where communicable diseases, maternal and perinatal conditions, and nutritional deficiencies together accounted for two-thirds of all deaths. Indeed, the HIV mortality rate among 15- to 59-year-olds in sub-Saharan Africa was higher than the mortality rate due to all causes among adults in high-income countries. In this age group, injuries accounted for 23% of all deaths worldwide. Overall, death rates in this age group declined between 1990 and 2004 in all areas except Europe and Central Asia, where cardiovascular diseases and injuries caused increased mortality rates, and sub-Saharan Africa, where the impact of HIV/AIDS in this age cohort was particularly devastating.

There is greater uncertainty in calculating years of life lived with disability for specific conditions than in calculating years of life lost. Best estimates from 2004 reveal that although the prevalence of diseases common in older populations (e.g., dementia and musculoskeletal disease) was higher in high-income countries, the disability experienced as a result of cardiovascular diseases, chronic respiratory diseases, and the long-term impact of communicable diseases was greater in low- and middle-income countries. In most low- and middle-income countries, people lived shorter lives and experienced disability and poor health for a greater proportion of their lives. Indeed, >50% of the GBD occurred in southern Asia and sub-Saharan Africa, which together account for only one-third of the world's population.

Noncommunicable diseases accounted for almost 60% of all deaths in 2004 but, because of the later onset of those diseases, accounted for only 48% of years of life lost. In contrast, because they more often involve younger people, injuries accounted for 12% of years of life lost but for only 10% of deaths. Notably, 45% of the disease burden in middle-income countries in 2004 resulted from noncommunicable conditions; in 1990, the figure was 35%.

Poverty remains one of the most important root causes of poor health worldwide, and the global burden of poverty continues to be high. Among the 6.8 billion people alive today, 43% (~2.7 billion) live on <$2 per day and 17% (~1.1 billion) live on <$1 per day. Comparison of national health indicators with gross domestic product per capita among nations shows a clear relationship between higher gross domestic product and better health, with only a few outliers. Numerous studies also have documented the link between poverty and health within countries.

TABLE 2-2 Leading Causes of Death Worldwide, by Income Group, 2004

Disease or Injury	Deaths (millions)	Percent of Total Deaths	Disease or Injury	Deaths (millions)	Percent of Total Deaths
World			**Middle-income countries**		
1 Ischemic heart disease	7.2	12.2	1 Cerebrovascular disease	3.5	14.2
2 Cerebrovascular disease	5.7	9.7	2 Ischemic heart disease	3.4	13.9
3 Lower respiratory infections	4.2	7.1	3 COPD	1.8	7.4
4 COPD	3.0	5.1	4 Lower respiratory infections	0.9	3.8
5 Diarrheal diseases	2.2	3.7	5 Trachea, bronchus, lung cancers	0.7	2.9
6 HIV/AIDS	2.0	3.5	6 Road traffic accidents	0.7	2.8
7 Tuberculosis	1.5	2.5	7 Hypertensive heart disease	0.6	2.5
8 Trachea, bronchus, lung cancers	1.3	2.3	8 Stomach cancer	0.5	2.2
9 Road traffic accidents	1.3	2.2	9 Tuberculosis	0.5	2.2
10 Prematurity and low birth weight	1.2	2.0	10 Diabetes mellitus	0.5	2.1
High-income countries			**Low-income countries**[a]		
1 Ischemic heart disease	1.3	16.3	1 Lower respiratory infections	2.9	11.2
2 Cerebrovascular disease	0.8	9.3	2 Ischemic heart disease	2.5	9.4
3 Trachea, bronchus, lung cancers	0.5	5.9	3 Diarrheal diseases	1.8	6.9
4 Lower respiratory infections	0.3	3.8	4 HIV/AIDS	1.5	5.7
5 COPD	0.3	3.5	5 Cerebrovascular disease	1.5	5.6
6 Alzheimer's and other dementias	0.3	3.4	6 COPD	0.9	3.6
7 Colon and rectum cancers	0.3	3.3	7 Tuberculosis	0.9	3.5
8 Diabetes mellitus	0.2	2.8	8 Neonatal infections[b]	0.9	3.4
9 Breast cancer	0.2	2.0	9 Malaria	0.9	3.3
10 Stomach cancer	0.1	1.8	10 Prematurity and low birth weight	0.8	3.2

[a]Countries grouped by gross national income per capita: low income ($825 or less), high income ($10,066 or more). Note that these high-income groups differ slightly from those used in the Disease Control Priorities Project.

[b]This category also includes other noninfectious causes arising in the perinatal period, that are responsible for about 20% of the deaths shown in this category.

Abbreviation: COPD, chronic obstructive pulmonary disease.

Source: World Health Organization. Reprinted with permission. *http://www.who.int/healthinfo/global_burden_disease/GBD_report_2004update_full.pdf.*

The Global Burden of Disease Study found that undernutrition was the leading risk factor for poor health. In an era that has seen obesity become a major health concern in many developed countries, the persistence of undernutrition is surely cause for great consternation. Inability to feed the hungry provides evidence of many years of failed development projects and must be addressed as a problem of the highest priority. Indeed, no health care initiative, however generously funded and scientifically justified, will be effective without adequate nutrition.

The second edition of *Disease Control Priorities in Developing Countries* (DCP2), published in 2006, is a document of stunning breadth and ambition, providing cost-effectiveness analyses for >100 interventions and including 21 chapters focused on strategies for strengthening health systems. Cost-effectiveness analyses that compare two relatively equal interventions and facilitate the best choices under constraint are important; however, as both resources and ambitions for global health grow, cost-effectiveness analyses (particularly those based on past conditions) must not hobble the increased worldwide commitment to provide resources and accessible services to all who need them. To illustrate this point, it is instructive to look to AIDS, that in the course of the last three decades has become the world's leading infectious cause of adult death.

■ AIDS

Chapter 189 provides an overview of the AIDS epidemic in the world today. Here the discussion will be limited to AIDS in the developing world. Lessons learned in tackling AIDS in resource-constrained settings are highly relevant to discussions of other chronic diseases, including noncommunicable diseases, for which effective therapies have been developed. Several of these lessons are highlighted below.

In the United States, the availability of highly active antiretroviral therapy (ART) for AIDS has transformed this disease from an inescapably fatal destruction of cell-mediated immunity into a manageable chronic illness. In developing countries, treatment has been offered more broadly only since 2003, and only in the fall of 2008 did the number of patients receiving treatment exceed 40% of the number who need it. (It remains to be seen how many of these fortunate few are receiving ART regularly and with the requisite social support.) Before 2003, many arguments were raised to justify not moving forward rapidly with ART programs for people living with HIV/AIDS in resource-limited settings. The standard litany included the price of therapy compared with the poverty of the patient, the complexity of the intervention, the lack of infrastructure for laboratory monitoring, and the lack of trained health care providers. Narrow cost-effectiveness arguments that created false dichotomies—prevention *or* treatment rather than both—too often went unchallenged. The greatest obstacle at the time was the ambivalence, if not outright silence, of political leaders and experts in public health. The cumulative effect of these factors was to condemn to death tens of millions of poor people in developing countries who had become ill as a result of HIV infection.

The inequity between rich and poor countries in access to HIV treatment has given rise to widespread moral indignation. In several middle-income countries, including Brazil, visionary programs have bridged the access gap. Other innovative projects pioneered by international nongovernmental organizations (NGOs) in diverse settings have clearly established that a very simple approach to ART that is based on intensive community engagement and support can achieve remarkable results. In 2000, the United Nations Accelerating Access Initiative finally brought the research-based and generic pharmaceutical industries into play, and prices of AIDS drugs have fallen significantly. At the same time, fixed-dose combination drugs that are easier to administer have become more widely available.

Building on these lessons, the WHO advocated a public health approach to the treatment of people with AIDS in resource-limited settings. This approach, derived from models of care pioneered by the NGO Partners In Health and other groups, proposed standard first-line treatment regimens based on a simple five-drug formulary, with a more complex (and far more expensive) set of second-line options in reserve. Common clinical protocols were standardized, and intensive training packages for health and community health workers were developed and implemented in many countries. Those efforts were supported by new funding from the World Bank, the GFATM, and PEPFAR. In 2003, the lack of access to ART was declared a global public health emergency by the WHO and UNAIDS, and those two agencies launched the "3 by 5 initiative," setting an ambitious target: to have 3 million people in developing countries in treatment by the end of 2005. Many countries have since set corresponding national targets and have worked to integrate ART into their national AIDS programs and health systems and to harness the synergies between HIV/AIDS treatment and prevention activities. The efficacy of ART is well documented: in the United States, such therapy has prolonged life by an estimated average of 13 years per patient—a better success rate than that obtained with almost any treatment for cancer or for complications of coronary artery disease. Further lessons with implications for policy and action have come from efforts now underway in the developing world. During the last decade, through experiences in >50 countries thus far, the world has seen that ambitious policy goals, adequate funding, and knowledge about implementation can dramatically transform the prospects of people living with HIV infection in developing nations.

■ TUBERCULOSIS

Chapter 165 provides a concise overview of the pathophysiology and treatment of TB, which is closely linked to HIV infection in much of the world. Indeed, a substantial proportion of the resurgence of TB registered in southern Africa may be attributed to HIV co-infection. Even before the advent of HIV, however, it was estimated that fewer than one-half of all cases of TB in developing countries were ever diagnosed, much less treated.

Primarily because of the common failure to diagnose and treat TB, international authorities devised a single strategy to reduce the burden of disease. The DOTS strategy (*d*irectly *o*bserved *t*herapy using *s*hort-course isoniazid- and rifampin-based regimens) was promoted in the early 1990s as highly cost-effective by

the World Bank, the WHO, and other international bodies. Passive case finding of smear-positive patients was central to the strategy, and an uninterrupted drug supply was, of course, deemed necessary for cure. DOTS was clearly effective for most uncomplicated cases of drug-susceptible TB, but a number of shortcomings soon were identified. First, the diagnosis of TB based solely on smear microscopy—a method dating from the late nineteenth century—is not sensitive. Many patients with pulmonary TB and all patients with exclusively extrapulmonary TB are missed by smear microscopy, as are most children with active disease. Second, passive case finding relies on the availability of health care services, that is uneven in the settings where TB is most prevalent. Third, patients with multidrug-resistant TB (MDR-TB) are by definition infected with strains of *Mycobacterium tuberculosis* resistant to isoniazid and rifampin; thus, exclusive reliance on these drugs is ineffective in settings in which drug resistance is an established problem.

The crisis of antibiotic resistance registered in U.S. hospitals is not confined to the industrialized world or to bacterial infections. In some settings, a substantial minority of patients with TB are infected with strains resistant to at least one first-line anti-TB drug. As an effective DOTS-based response to MDR-TB, global health authorities adopted DOTS-Plus, that adds the diagnostics and drugs necessary to manage drug-resistant disease. Even before DOTS-Plus could be brought to scale in resource-constrained settings, however, new strains of extensively drug-resistant (XDR) *M. tuberculosis* began to threaten the success of TB control programs in already beleaguered South Africa, for example, where high rates of HIV infection have led to a doubling of TB incidence over the last decade.

■ TUBERCULOSIS AND AIDS AS CHRONIC DISEASES: LESSONS LEARNED

Strategies effective against MDR-TB have implications for the management of drug-resistant HIV infection and even drug-resistant malaria, which, through repeated infections and a lack of effective therapy, has become a chronic disease in parts of Africa. Indeed, examining AIDS and TB together as chronic diseases makes it possible to draw a number of conclusions, many of them pertinent to global health in general (Fig. 2-2).

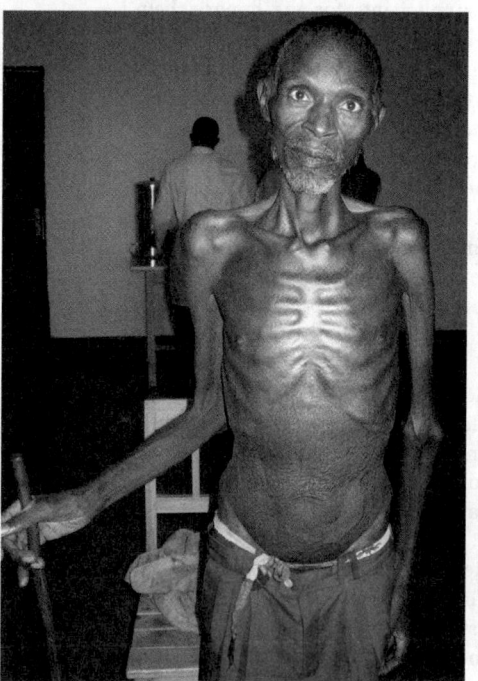
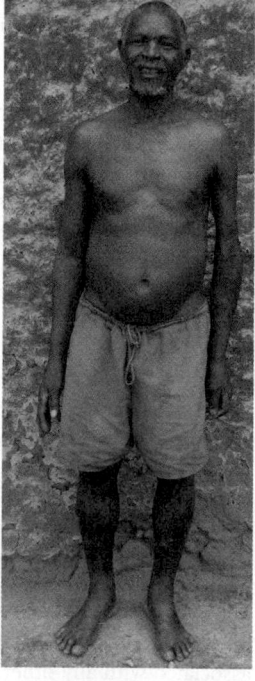

Figure 2-2 An HIV/TB co-infected patient in Rwanda, before (*left*) and after (*right*) 6 months of treatment.

First, charging fees for AIDS prevention and care will pose insurmountable problems for people living in poverty, many of whom will always be unable to pay even modest amounts for services or medications. Like efforts to battle airborne TB, such services might best be seen as a public good for public health. Initially, this approach will require sustained donor contributions, but many African countries have set targets for increased national investments in health, a pledge that could render ambitious programs sustainable in the long run. Meanwhile, as local investments increase, the price of AIDS care is decreasing. The development of generic medications means that ART can now cost <$0.25 per day, and costs continue to decrease to affordable levels in developing countries.

Second, the effective scale-up of pilot projects will require strengthening and sometimes rebuilding health care systems, including those charged with delivering primary care. In the past, the lack of health care infrastructure has been cited as a barrier to providing ART in the world's poorest regions; however, AIDS resources, which are at last considerable, may be marshaled to rebuild public health systems in sub-Saharan Africa and other HIV-burdened regions—precisely the settings in which TB is resurgent.

Third, a lack of trained health care personnel, most notably doctors, is invoked as a reason for the failure to treat AIDS in poor countries. The lack is real, and the brain drain (discussed below) continues. However, one reason doctors leave Africa is that they lack the tools to practice their trade there. AIDS funding provides an opportunity not only to recruit physicians and nurses to underserved regions but also to strengthen health systems by building infrastructure, providing diagnostic and therapeutic resources, and training community health workers to supervise care for AIDS and many other diseases within their communities. Such training should be undertaken even in places where physicians are abundant, since community-based, closely supervised care represents the highest standard of care for chronic disease, whether in the First World or the Third.

Fourth, extreme poverty makes it difficult for many patients to comply with therapy for chronic diseases, whether communicable or not. Indeed, poverty in its many dimensions is far and away the greatest barrier to the scale-up of treatment and prevention programs. It is possible to remove many of the social and economic barriers to adherence, but only with what sometimes are termed "wrap-around services": food supplements for the hungry, help with transportation to clinics, child care, and housing. In many rural regions of Africa, hunger is the major coexisting condition in patients with AIDS or TB, and those consumptive diseases cannot be treated effectively without adequate caloric intake.

Finally, there is a need for a renewed basic-science commitment to the discovery and development of vaccines; more reliable, less expensive diagnostic tools; and new classes of therapeutic agents. This need applies not only to the three leading infectious killers—against none of which is there an effective vaccine—but also to many other neglected diseases of poverty.

■ MALARIA

Chapter 210 reviews the etiology, pathogenesis, and clinical treatment of malaria, the world's third-ranking infectious killer. Malaria's human cost is enormous, with the greatest toll among children, especially African children, living in poverty. An estimated 250 million people have malarial disease each year, and the disease annually kills 1 million people, mostly children under age 5. The poor disproportionately experience the consequences of malaria: 58% of malaria deaths occur in the poorest 20% of the world's population, and 90% are registered in sub-Saharan Africa. The differential magnitude of this mortality burden is greater than that associated with any other disease. Likewise, the morbidity differential is greater for malaria than for diseases caused by other pathogens, as documented in a study from Zambia that revealed a 40% greater

prevalence of parasitemia among children under age 5 in the poorest quintile than in the richest.

Despite experiencing the greatest consequences of malaria, the poor are those least able to access effective prevention and treatment tools. Economists describe the complex interactions between malaria and poverty from an opposite but complementary perspective: they delineate ways in which malaria arrests economic development both for individuals and for whole nations. Microeconomic analyses focusing on direct and indirect costs estimate that malaria may consume up to 10% of a household's annual income. A Ghanaian study that categorized the population by income group highlighted the regressive nature of this cost: the burden of malaria represents only 1% of a wealthy family's income but 34% of a poor household's income.

At the national level, macroeconomic analyses estimate that malaria may reduce the per capita gross national product of a disease-endemic country by 50% relative to that of a nonmalarial country. The causes of this drag include high fertility rates, impaired cognitive development of children, decreased schooling, decreased saving, decreased foreign investment, and restriction of worker mobility. In light of this enormous cost, it is little wonder that an important review by the economists Sachs and Malaney concludes that "where malaria prospers most, human societies have prospered least."

Rolling back malaria

In part because of differences in vector distribution and climate, resource-rich countries offer few blueprints for malaria control and treatment that are applicable in tropical (and resource-poor) settings. In 2001, African heads of state endorsed the WHO Roll Back Malaria (RBM) campaign, which prescribes strategies appropriate for sub-Saharan African countries. In 2008, the RBM partnership launched the Global Malaria Action Plan (GMAP). This global strategy has set out a coordinated approach to control and eliminate the disease and to ensure that gains in one nation are not lost because of failed control measures in neighboring countries. The GMAP recommends a number of key tools to reduce malaria-related morbidity and mortality rates: the use of insecticide-treated bed nets (ITNs), indoor residual spraying (IRS), and artemisinin-based combination therapy (ACT) as well as intermittent preventive treatment during pregnancy, prompt diagnosis, and other vector control measures such as larviciding and environmental management.

Insecticide-treated bed nets ITNs are an efficacious and cost-effective public health intervention. A meta-analysis of controlled trials indicates that malaria incidence is reduced by 50% among persons who sleep under ITNs compared with the incidence among those who do not use nets at all. Even untreated nets reduce malaria incidence by one-quarter. On an individual level, the utility of ITNs extends beyond protection from malaria. Several studies suggest that all-cause mortality is reduced among children under age 5 to a greater degree than can be attributed to the reduction in malarial disease alone. Morbidity (specifically that due to anemia), which predisposes children to diarrheal and respiratory illnesses and pregnant women to the delivery of low-birth-weight infants, is also reduced in populations using ITNs. In some areas, ITNs offer a supplemental benefit by preventing transmission of lymphatic filariasis, cutaneous leishmaniasis, Chagas' disease, and tick-borne relapsing fever. At the community level, investigators suggest that the use of an ITN in just one household may reduce the number of mosquito bites in households up to several hundred meters away. The cost of ITNs per DALY saved is estimated at $10–$38, which qualifies ITNs as a "very efficient use of resources and [a] good candidate for public subsidy."[1]

The WHO recommends that all individuals living in malaria-endemic areas sleep under protective ITNs. About 140 million

---

[1] Nuwaha F: The challenge of chloroquine-resistant malaria in sub-Saharan Africa. Health Policy Plan 16:1, 2001.

long-lasting ITNs were distributed in high-burden African countries in 2006–2008, and rates of household ownership of ITNs in high-burden countries increased to 31%. Although the RBM partnership has seen modest success, the WHO's 2009 World Malaria Report states that the percentage of children <5 years of age using an ITN (24%) remains well below the World Health Assembly's target of 80%. Limited success in scaling up ITN coverage reflects the inadequately acknowledged economic barriers that prevent the destitute sick from accessing critical preventive technologies and the challenges in designing and implementing effective delivery platforms for these products.

Indoor residual spraying IRS is one of the most common interventions for preventing the transmission of malaria in endemic areas. Vector control using insecticides approved by the WHO, including DDT, can effectively reduce or even interrupt malaria transmission. However, studies have indicated that spraying is effective in controlling malaria transmission only if most (~80%) of the structures in the targeted community are treated. Moreover, since a successful program is dependent on well-trained spraying teams as well as on effective monitoring and planning, IRS is difficult to employ and is often reliant on health systems with a strong infrastructure that renders the approach feasible. Regardless of the limitations of IRS, the WHO recommends its use in combination with ITNs. Neither intervention alone is sufficient to prevent transmission of malaria entirely.

Artemisinin-based combination therapy The emergence and spread of chloroquine resistance have increased the necessity for antimalarial combination therapy. To limit the spread of resistance, the WHO now recommends only the use of ACT for uncomplicated falciparum malaria. Like that of other antimalarial interventions, the use of ACT has increased in the last few years, but coverage remains very low in several countries in sub-Saharan Africa. In a 2007–2008 study, fewer than 15% of children under the age of 5 with a fever were receiving ACT in 11 of 13 countries surveyed, although the World Health Assembly's target is 80%. In response, the RBM partnership has focused significant investment on enhancing access to ACT by facilitating its delivery through the public-health sector and developing innovative funding mechanisms (e.g., the Affordable Medicines Facility—malaria) through which consumer prices for ACT can be reduced significantly and ineffective artemisinin monotherapies can be eliminated from the market.

In the last several years, resistance to antimalarial medicines and insecticides has become an even larger problem. In 2009, confirmation of artemisinin resistance was reported. Although the WHO has called for an end to the use of artemisinin monotherapy, the marketing of such therapies continues in many countries. Ongoing use of artemisinin monotherapy increases the likelihood of drug resistance, a deadly prospect that will make malaria far more difficult to treat.

Meeting the challenge of malaria control will continue to require careful study of appropriate preventive and therapeutic strategies in the context of an increasingly sophisticated molecular understanding of the pathogen, vector, and host. However, an appreciation of the economic and structural devastation wrought by malaria—like that inflicted by diarrhea, AIDS, and TB—on the most vulnerable populations should heighten the commitment to the critical analysis of ways to implement proven strategies for the prevention and treatment of these diseases.

■ NONCOMMUNICABLE CHRONIC DISEASES

Although the burden of communicable diseases—especially HIV infection, tuberculosis, and malaria—still accounts for the majority of deaths in resource-poor regions such as sub-Saharan Africa, 60% of all deaths worldwide in 2004 were due to noncommunicable chronic diseases (NCDs). Moreover, 80% of deaths attributable to

NCDs occurred in low- and middle-income countries, where 86% of the global population lives. In 2005, 8.5 million people in the world died of an NCD before their 60th birthday, a figure exceeding the total number of deaths due to AIDS, TB, and malaria combined. By 2020, NCDs will account for 80% of the GBD and for 7 out of every 10 deaths in developing countries. The recent rise in resources for and attention to communicable diseases is both welcome and long overdue, but developing countries already are carrying a "double burden" of communicable and noncommunicable diseases.

Cardiovascular disease

Unlike TB, HIV infection, and malaria—diseases caused by single pathogens that damage multiple organs—cardiovascular diseases reflect injury to a single organ system downstream of a variety of insults. The burden of chronic cardiovascular disease in low-income countries represents one consequence of decades of health system neglect; furthermore, cardiovascular research and investment have long focused on the ischemic conditions that are increasingly common in high- and middle-income countries. Meanwhile, despite awareness of its health impact during the early twentieth century, cardiovascular damage in response to infection and malnutrition has fallen out of view until recently.

The perception of cardiovascular diseases as a problem of elderly populations in middle- and high-income countries has contributed to their neglect by global health institutions. Even in Eastern Europe and Central Asia, where the collapse of the Soviet Union was followed by a catastrophic surge in cardiovascular disease deaths (mortality rates from ischemic heart disease nearly doubled between 1991 and 1994 in Russia, for example), the modest flow of overseas development assistance to the health sector focused on the communicable causes that accounted for <1 in 20 excess deaths during that period.

Predictions of an imminent rise in the share of deaths and disabilities due to NCDs in developing countries have led to calls for preventive policies to restrict tobacco use, improve diet, and increase exercise along with the prescription of multidrug regimens for persons with high levels of vascular risk. Although this agenda could do much to prevent pandemic NCD, it will do little to help those with established heart disease stemming from nonatherogenic pathologies.

The epidemiology of heart failure reflects inequalities in risk factor prevalence and treatment. Heart failure as a consequence of pericardial, myocardial, endocardial, or valvular injury accounts for as many as 1 in 10 admissions to hospitals around the world. Countries have reported a remarkably similar burden of this condition at the health system level since the 1950s, but the causes of heart failure and the age of the people affected vary with resources and ecology. In populations with a high human-development index, coronary artery disease and hypertension among the elderly account for most cases of heart failure. Among the world's poorest billion people, however, heart failure reflects poverty-driven exposure of children and young adults to rheumatogenic strains of streptococci and cardiotropic microorganisms (e.g., HIV, *Trypanosoma cruzi*, enteroviruses, *M. tuberculosis*), untreated high blood pressure, and nutrient deficiencies. The mechanisms of other causes of heart failure common in these populations—such as idiopathic dilated cardiomyopathy, peripartum cardiomyopathy, and endomyocardial fibrosis—remain unclear.

Among the 2.4 million annual cases of pediatric rheumatic heart disease, more than 40% occur in sub-Saharan Africa. This disease leads to more than 33,000 cases of endocarditis, 252,000 strokes, and 680,000 deaths per year—almost all in developing countries. Researchers in Ethiopia have reported annual death rates as high as 12.5% in rural areas. In part because the prevention of rheumatic heart disease has not advanced since the disappearance of this disease in wealthy countries, no part of sub-Saharan Africa has eradicated rheumatic heart disease despite examples of success in Costa Rica, Cuba, and some Caribbean nations.

Strategies to eliminate rheumatic heart disease may depend on active case finding confirmed by echocardiography among high-risk groups as well as efforts to extend access to surgical interventions among children with advanced valvular damage. Partnerships between established surgical programs and areas with limited or nonexistent facilities may help develop capacity and provide care to patients who otherwise would have an early and painful death. A long-term goal is the establishment of regional centers of excellence equipped to provide consistent, accessible, high-quality services.

In stark contrast to the extraordinary lengths to which patients in wealthy countries will go to treat ischemic cardiomyopathy, young patients with nonischemic cardiomyopathies in resource-poor settings have received little attention. These conditions account for as many as 25–30% of admissions for heart failure in sub-Saharan Africa and include poorly understood entities such as peripartum cardiomyopathy (which has an incidence in rural Haiti of 1 per 300 live births) and HIV cardiomyopathy. Multidrug regimens that include beta blockers, angiotensin-converting enzyme (ACE) inhibitors, and other neurohormonal antagonists can dramatically reduce mortality risk and improve quality of life for these patients. Lessons learned in the scale-up of chronic care for HIV infection and TB may be illustrative as progress is made in establishing means to deliver heart failure therapies.

Because systemic investigation of the causes of stroke and heart failure in sub-Saharan Africa has begun only recently, little is known about the impact of elevated blood pressure in this portion of the continent. Modestly elevated blood pressure in the absence of tobacco use in populations with low rates of obesity may confer little risk of adverse events in the short run. In contrast, persistently elevated blood pressure above 180/110 goes largely undetected, untreated, and uncontrolled in this setting. In the Framingham cohort of men 45–74 years old, the prevalence of blood pressures above 210/120 declined from 1.8% in the 1950s to 0.1% in the 1990s with the introduction of effective antihypertensive agents. Although debate continues about appropriate screening strategies and treatment thresholds, rural health centers staffed by nonphysicians must quickly gain access to essential antihypertensive medications.

In 1960, Paul Dudley White and colleagues reported on the prevalence of cardiovascular disease in the region near the Albert Schweitzer Hospital in Lambaréné, Gabon. Although the group found little evidence of myocardial infarction, they concluded that "*the high prevalence of mitral stenosis* [sic] is astonishing. . . . We believe strongly that it is a duty to help bring to these sufferers the benefits of better penicillin prophylaxis and of cardiac surgery when indicated. The same responsibility exists for those with correctable congenital cardiovascular defects."[2] Leaders from tertiary centers in sub-Saharan Africa and elsewhere have continued to call for prevention and treatment of the cardiovascular conditions of the poor. The reconstruction of health services in response to pandemic infectious disease offers an opportunity to identify and treat patients with organ damage and to undertake the prevention of cardiovascular and other chronic conditions of poverty.

Cancer

Low- and middle-income countries accounted for 54% and 60%, respectively, of the 12.4 million cases and 7.6 million deaths due to cancer in 2008. By 2020, the total number of new cancer cases will rise by 29% in developed countries and by 73%

in developing countries. Also by 2020, overall mortality from cancer will increase by 104%, and the increase will be fivefold higher in developing than in developed countries. "Western" lifestyle changes will be responsible for the increased incidence of cancers of the breast, colon, and prostate, but historic realities, sociocultural and behavioral factors, genetics, and poverty itself also will have a profound impact on cancer-related mortality and morbidity rates. Whereas infectious causes are responsible for <10% of cancers in developed countries, they account for 25% of all malignancies in low- and middle-income countries. Infectious causes of cancer such as human papillomavirus (cervical cancer), hepatitis B virus (liver cancer), and *Helicobacter pylori* (stomach cancer) will continue to have a much larger impact in developing countries. Environmental and dietary factors such as indoor air pollution and high-salt diets also help account for increased rates of certain cancers (e.g., lung and stomach cancers). Tobacco use (both smoking and chewing) is the most important source of increased mortality from lung and oral cancers. In contrast to decreasing tobacco use in many developed countries, the number of smokers is growing in developing countries, especially among women and young people.

For many reasons, outcomes of malignancies are far worse in developing countries than in developed nations. Overstretched health systems in poor countries simply are not capable of early detection; 80% of patients already have incurable malignancies at diagnosis. Treatment of cancers is available for only a very small number of mostly wealthy citizens in the majority of poor countries, and even when treatment is available, the range and quality of services are often substandard. Yet this need not be the future. Only a decade ago, MDR-TB and HIV infection were considered untreatable for all but the wealthiest among the world's population. The last decade has made clear the feasibility of creating innovative programs that reduce technical and financial barriers to the provision of care for complex diseases for the world's poorest populations.

Diabetes

The International Diabetes Federation reports that the number of diabetic patients in the world is expected to increase from 285 million in 2010 to 438 million by 2030. Already, more than 70% of diabetic patients live in developing countries where, because those affected are far more frequently under age 65, the complications of micro- and macrovascular disease take a far greater toll. In 2009, the Federation projected an estimated 4 million deaths from diabetes-related illnesses in 2010, with almost 80% of those deaths occurring in low- and middle-income countries.

Obesity and tobacco use

In 2004, the WHO released its Global Strategy on Diet, Physical Activity and Health, which focused on the populationwide promotion of healthy diet and regular physical activity in an effort to reduce the growing global problem of overweight and obesity. Passing this strategy at the World Health Assembly proved difficult because of strong opposition from the food industry and from a number of WHO member states, including the United States. Although globalization has had many positive effects, one negative aspect has been the growth in both developed and developing countries of well-financed lobbies that have aggressively promoted unhealthy dietary changes and increased consumption of alcohol and tobacco. Foreign direct investment in tobacco, beverage, and food products in developing countries reached $327 million in 2002—a figure nearly five times greater than the amount spent during that year to address NCDs by bilateral funding agencies, the WHO, and the World Bank combined.

---

[2] Miller DC et al: Survey of cardiovascular disease among Africans in the vicinity of the Albert Schweitzer Hospital in 1960. Am J Cardiol 19:432, 1962.

The three pillars of prevention

The WHO estimates that 80% of all cases of cardiovascular disease and type 2 diabetes as well as 40% of all cancers can be prevented through the three pillars of healthy diet, physical activity, and avoidance of tobacco. Although there is some evidence that population-based measures can have some impact on these behaviors, it is sobering to note that increasing obesity levels have not been reversed in any population, including the populations of high-income countries with robust diet industries. Nonetheless, in Mauritius, for example, a single policy measure that changed the type of cooking oil available to the population led to a fall in mean serum cholesterol levels. Tobacco avoidance may be the most important and most difficult behavioral modification of all. In the twentieth century, 100 million people worldwide died of tobacco-related diseases; it is projected that >1 billion people will die of these diseases in the twenty-first century, with the vast majority of those deaths in developing countries. Today, 80% of the world's 1.2 billion smokers live in low- and middle-income countries, and although tobacco consumption is falling in most developed countries, it continues to rise at a rate of ~3.4% per year in developing countries. The WHO's 2003 Framework Convention on Tobacco Control represented a major advance, committing all of its signatories to a set of policy measures that have been shown to reduce tobacco consumption. However, most developing countries have continued to take a passive approach to the control of smoking.

■ ENVIRONMENTAL HEALTH

In a recent publication that examined how specific diseases and injuries are affected by environmental risk, the WHO determined that ~24% of the total GBD, one-third of the GBD among children, and 23% of all deaths are due to modifiable environmental factors. Many of these factors lead to deaths from infectious diseases; others lead to deaths from malignancies. Increasingly, etiology and nosology are difficult to parse. As much as 94% of diarrheal disease, which is linked to unsafe drinking water and poor sanitation, can be attributed to environmental factors. Risk factors such as indoor air pollution due to use of solid fuels, exposure to secondhand tobacco smoke, and outdoor air pollution account for 20% of lower respiratory infections in developed countries and as many as 42% of such infections in developing countries. Various forms of unintentional injury and malaria top the list of health problems to which environmental factors contribute. Some 4 million children die every year from causes related to unhealthy environments, and the number of infant deaths due to environmental factors in developing countries is 12 times that in developed countries.

■ MENTAL HEALTH

The WHO reports that some 450 million people worldwide are affected by mental, neurologic, or behavioral problems at any given time and that ~873,000 people die by suicide every year. Major depression is the leading cause of years lost to disability in the world today. One in four patients visiting a health service has at least one mental, neurologic, or behavioral disorder, but most of these disorders are neither diagnosed nor treated. Most low- and middle-income countries devote <1% of their health expenditures to mental health.

Increasingly effective therapies exist for many of the major causes of mental disorders. Effective treatments for many neurologic diseases, including seizure disorders, have long been available. One of the greatest barriers to delivery of such therapies is the paucity of skilled personnel. Most sub-Saharan African countries have only a handful of psychiatrists, for example; most practice in cities and are unavailable within the public sector or to patients living in poverty. Among the few patients who are fortunate enough to see a psychiatrist or neurologist, fewer still are able to adhere to treatment regimens: several surveys of already diagnosed patients ostensibly receiving daily therapy have revealed that among the poor, few can take their medications as prescribed. The same barriers that prevent the poor from having reliable access to insulin or ART prevent them from benefiting from antidepressant, antipsychotic, and antiepileptic agents. To alleviate this problem, some authorities are proposing the training of health workers to provide community-based adherence support, counseling services, and referrals for patients in need of mental health services.

World Mental Health: Problems and Priorities in Low-Income Countries offers a comprehensive analysis of the burden of mental, behavioral, and social problems in low-income countries and relates the mental health consequences of social forces such as violence, dislocation, poverty, and disenfranchisement of women to current economic, political, and environmental concerns.

■ PRIMARY CARE

At the International Conference on Primary Health Care in Alma-Ata (in what is now Kazakhstan) in 1978, public health officials from around the world agreed on a commitment to "Health for All by 2000," a goal to be achieved by providing universal access to primary health care worldwide. Critics argued that the attainment of this goal by the proposed date was impossible. In the ensuing years, a strategy of selective primary health care emerged that included four inexpensive interventions collectively known as GOBI: *g*rowth monitoring, *o*ral rehydration, *b*reast-feeding, and *i*mmunizations for diphtheria, whooping cough, tetanus, polio, TB, and measles. GOBI later was expanded to GOBI-FFF, which also included *f*emale education, *f*ood, and *f*amily planning. Some public health figures saw this as an interim strategy to achieve "health for all," but others criticized it as a retreat from the commitments of Alma-Ata. Similar debates still rage, with "vertical" disease-specific programs for HIV, TB, and malaria often seen as competing with primary health care efforts for critical economic, human, and political resources. Global primary care is examined in detail in Chap. e1.

HEALTH SYSTEMS AND THE BRAIN DRAIN

A significant and frequently invoked barrier to effective health care in resource-poor settings is the lack of medical personnel. In what is termed the *brain drain*, many physicians and nurses emigrate from their home countries to pursue opportunities abroad, leaving behind health systems that are understaffed and ill equipped to deal with the epidemic diseases that ravage local populations. The WHO recommends a minimum of 20 physicians and 100 nurses per 100,000 persons, but recent reports from that organization and others confirm that many countries, especially in sub-Saharan Africa, fall far short of those target numbers. More than one-half of those countries register fewer than 10 physicians per 100,000 population. In contrast, the United States and Cuba register 279 and 596 doctors per 100,000 population, respectively. Similarly, the majority of sub-Saharan African countries do not have even half of the WHO-recommended minimum number of nurses. In addition to these appalling national aggregates, further inequalities in health care staffing exist *within* countries. Rural-urban disparities in health care personnel mirror disparities of both wealth and health. For instance, nearly 90% of Malawi's population is rural, but more than 95% of clinical officers work at urban facilities, and 47% of nurses work at tertiary care facilities. Even community health workers trained to provide first-line services to rural populations often transfer to urban districts. In addition to inter- and intranational transfer of personnel, the AIDS epidemic contributes to personnel shortages across Africa. Although data on the prevalence of HIV infection among health professionals are scarce, the available numbers suggest substantial and adverse impacts on an already overburdened health sector. A study that examined the fates of a small cohort of Ugandan physicians found that at least 22 of the 77 doctors who graduated from Makerere University Medical School in 1984 had died by 2004—most, presumably, of AIDS. The shortage of medical personnel in the areas hardest hit by HIV has profound implications for prevention and treatment efforts in those regions. The cycle of health-sector impoverishment, brain drain, and lack of personnel to fill positions when they are available conspires against ambitious programs to bring ART to persons living with both AIDS and poverty. Furthermore, the education of medical trainees is jeopardized as the ranks of the health and academic communities continue to shrink as a result of migration or disease. The long-term implications are sobering.

A proper biosocial analysis of the brain drain confirms that the flight of health personnel—almost always, as most reviews suggest, from poor to less poor regions—is not simply a question of desire for more equitable remuneration. Epidemiologic trends and access to the tools of the trade are also relevant, as are working conditions in general. In many settings now losing skilled health personnel, the advent of HIV has led to a sharp rise in TB incidence; in the eyes of health care providers, other opportunistic infections also have become insuperable challenges. Together, these forces have conspired to render the provision of proper care almost impossible. One Kenyan medical resident noted, "Before training we thought of doctors as supermen. . . . [Now] we are only mortuary attendants."[3]

In light of the difficult conditions under which these health care personnel work, is it any surprise that the U.S. government's Global AIDS Coordinator remarked in 2004 that there were more Ethiopian physicians practicing in Chicago than in all of Ethiopia? When providing care for the sick becomes a nightmare for those at the beginning of clinical training, physician burnout soon follows among those who carry on in settings of impoverishment. In the public-sector institutions put in place to care for the poorest people, the confluence of epidemic disease, lack of resources with which to respond, and unrealistically high user fees has led to widespread burnout among health workers. Patients and their families are those who pay most dearly for provider burnout, just as they bear the burden of disease and—with the introduction of user fees—much of the cost of responding, however inadequately, to new epidemics and persistent plagues.

CONCLUSION: TOWARD A SCIENCE OF IMPLEMENTATION

Public-health strategies draw largely on quantitative methods—epidemiology, biostatistics, and economics. Clinical practice, including internal medicine, draws on a rapidly expanding knowledge base but remains focused on individual patient care; clinical interventions are rarely population-based. In fact, neither public health nor clinical approaches alone will prove adequate in addressing the problems of global health. There is a long way to go before evidence-based internal medicine is applied effectively among the world's poor. Complex infectious diseases such as AIDS and TB have proved difficult but not impossible to manage; drug resistance and a lack of effective health systems have complicated such work. Beyond communicable disease, in the arena of chronic diseases (e.g., cardiovascular disease), global health is a nascent endeavor. Efforts to address any one of these problems in settings of great scarcity need to be integrated into broader efforts to strengthen failing health systems and alleviate the growing personnel crisis within these systems.

For these reasons, scholarly work and practice in the field once known as international health and now often designated *global health equity* are changing rapidly. That work is still informed by the tension between clinical practice and population-based interventions, between analysis and action. Once metrics are refined, how might they inform efforts to lessen premature morbidity and mortality rates among the world's poor? As in the nineteenth century, human rights perspectives have proved helpful in turning attention to the problems of the destitute sick; such perspectives also may inform strategies of delivering care equitably. A number of university hospitals are developing training programs for physicians with an interest in global health. In medical schools across the United States and in other wealthy countries, interest in global health has been exploding. An informal survey at Harvard Medical School in 2006 revealed that nearly one-quarter of the 160 entering students either had significant global health experience or were planning a career in global health. A similar sea change among trainees has been reported at other medical schools. Half a century or even a decade ago, such high levels of interest would have been unimaginable.

Persistent epidemics, improved metrics, and growing interest have only recently been matched by an unprecedented investment in addressing the health problems of poor people in the developing world. This is a moment of opportunity. To ensure that the opportunity is not wasted, the facts need to be laid out for specialists and laypeople alike. More than 12 million people die each year simply because they live in poverty. An absolute majority of these premature deaths occur in Africa, with the poorer regions of Asia not far behind. Most of these deaths occur because the world's poorest do not have access to the fruits of science. They include deaths from vaccine-preventable illness, deaths during childbirth, deaths from infectious diseases that might be cured with access to antibiotics and other essential medicines, deaths from malaria that would have been prevented by bed nets and access to therapy, and deaths from waterborne illnesses. Other excess mortality is attributable to the inadequacy of efforts to develop new preventive, diagnostic, and therapeutic tools. Those funding the discovery and development of new tools typically neglect the concurrent need for strategies to make them available to the poor. Indeed, some would argue that the biggest challenge facing those who seek to address this outcome gap is the lack of practical means of distribution in the most heavily affected regions.

The development of tools must be followed quickly by their equitable distribution. When new preventive and therapeutic tools are developed without concurrent attention to delivery or implementation, one encounters what sometimes are termed *perverse effects:* even as new tools are developed, inequalities of outcome—lower morbidity and mortality rates among those who can afford access, with sustained high morbidity and mortality among those who cannot—will grow in the absence of an equity plan to deliver the tools to those most at risk. Preventing such a future is the most important goal of global health.

FURTHER READINGS

COHEN J: The new world of global health. Science 311:162, 2006

DESJARLAIS R et al (eds): *World Mental Health: Problems and Priorities in Low-Income Countries.* New York, Oxford University Press, 1995

FARMER PE: *Infections and Inequalities: The Modern Plagues,* 2nd ed. Berkeley, University of California Press, 2001

FAUCI AS et al: Emerging infectious diseases: A 10-year perspective from the National Institute of Allergy and Infectious Diseases. Emerg Infect Dis 11:519, 2005

---

[3] Raviola G et al: HIV, disease plague, demoralization, and "burnout": Resident experience of the medical profession in Nairobi, Kenya. Cult Med Psychiatry 26:55, 2002.

FRENK J: Reinventing primary health care: The need for systems integration. Lancet 374:170, 2009

GAZIANO TA et al: Scaling up interventions for chronic disease prevention: The evidence. Lancet 370:1939, 2007

JAMISON DT et al (eds): *Disease Control Priorities in Developing Countries*, 2nd ed. Washington, DC, Oxford University Press and The World Bank, 2006

MAXIMIZING POSITIVE SYNERGIES COLLABORATIVE GROUP: An assessment of interactions between global health initiatives and country health systems. Lancet 373:2137, 2009

SACHS J, MALANEY O: The economic and social burden of malaria. Nature 415:680, 2002

WORLD HEALTH ORGANIZATION: *The Global Burden of Disease: 2004 Update*. Geneva, World Health Organization, 2008

CHAPTER 3

Decision-Making in Clinical Medicine

Daniel B. Mark
John B. Wong

INTRODUCTION

To a medical student who requires 2 hours to collect a patient's history and perform a physical examination and several additional hours to organize that information into a coherent presentation, an experienced clinician's ability to decide on a diagnosis and management plan in a fraction of the time seems extraordinary. What separates the experienced clinician's performance from that of the novice is an elusive quality called "expertise." The first part of this chapter will provide a brief introduction to what is known about the development of expertise in clinical reasoning.

Equally bewildering to the student are the proper use of diagnostic tests and the integration of the results into the patient's clinical assessment. A novice medical practitioner typically uses a "shotgun" approach to testing, hoping to hit a target without knowing exactly what that target is. The expert, in contrast, usually has a specific target in mind and adjusts the testing strategy to it. The second part of the chapter will review briefly some of the crucial basic statistical concepts useful in the interpretation of diagnostic tests. Quantitative tools available to assist in clinical decision-making also will be discussed.

Evidence-based medicine (EBM) is the term used to describe the integration of the best available research evidence with clinical judgment and experience as applied to the care of individual patients. The third part of the chapter will provide a brief overview of some of the tools of EBM.

■ BRIEF INTRODUCTION TO CLINICAL REASONING

Clinical expertise

It is surprisingly difficult to define clearly what is meant by "clinical expertise." Chess has its masters, music its virtuoso performers, and athletics its Olympians. But in medicine, once training is complete and the boards are passed, there are no further tests or benchmarks of performance or ability that can be used to identify those who have attained the highest level of abilities in their clinical roles. Of course, there are always a few clinicians who are believed by their colleagues to have special problem-solving abilities: the "elite" who are consulted when particularly difficult or obscure cases have baffled everyone else. But for all their expertise, such doctors typically cannot explain what processes and methods they use to achieve their impressive results. Furthermore, it is not clear that their diagnostic virtuosity can be generalized. In other words, an expert on hypertrophic cardiomyopathy may be no better (and possibly worse) than a first-year resident at diagnosing and managing a patient with neutropenia, fever, and hypotension.

Broadly construed, clinical expertise includes not only cognitive dimensions and the integration of verbal and visual cues or information but also complex motor skills that are required in the performance of various invasive and noninvasive procedures and tests. In addition, the ability to communicate effectively with patients and work effectively with members of the medical team could be included as important aspects of "the complete package" of expertise in medicine. In this chapter, however, the focus will be on the cognitive elements (clinical reasoning), particularly as they relate to diagnosis. This focus is driven by two factors. First, the most important "actions" in clinical medicine are not procedures or prescriptions but the judgments (both diagnoses and treatment choices) from which all other aspects of medical care flow. Second, although the research on medical expertise is relatively sparse overall, it is best developed in the area of diagnostic decision-making. Much less work has been done on treatment decisions or the technical skills involved in the performance of procedures.

The obvious difficulty involved in the study of clinical reasoning is that it takes place in the heads of doctors and is therefore not readily observable. Further, doctors may not even be aware of how they reason in many cases, and so they may be unable to describe the processes they use. To overcome this difficulty, one line of research has focused on how doctors *should* reason diagnostically rather than on how they actually *do* reason. In addition, because of the difficulties of empirical research in this area, much of what is known about clinical reasoning comes from empirical studies of nonmedical problem-solving behavior. The field has been influenced by important work from cognitive psychology, sociology, medical education, economics, informatics, and decision sciences. However, because of this diversity of perspectives, no single integrated model of clinical reasoning exists, and not infrequently, different terms and models are proposed for similar phenomena.

Intuitive versus analytic reasoning

One useful contemporary model of reasoning (dual-process theory) distinguishes two general systems of cognitive processes. *Intuition* (System 1) provides rapid effortless judgments from memorized associations—for example, African-American women and hilar adenopathy equals sarcoid—or from the reduction of complex data by means of pattern recognition and other heuristics. Typically, the clinician is unable to say how those judgments were formulated. *Analysis* (System 2), the other form of reasoning in the dual-process model, is slow, methodical, and effortful. These are, of course, idealized extremes of the cognitive continuum. The way these systems interact in different decision problems and the way they differ between experts and novices remain the subject of considerable debate. Much work has also been done to identify how each of these systems can lead to errors in judgment.

Pattern recognition is a complex cognitive process that appears largely intuitive. One can recognize people's faces, the breed of a dog, or the model of an automobile without necessarily being able to say what specific features prompted the recognition. Analogously, an experienced clinician often can recognize the pattern of a diagnosis she or he is very familiar with after a very short amount of time with the patient. The student, who does not have that stored repertoire of diagnostic patterns, must use a more laborious analytic approach along with much more intensive data collection to reach the diagnosis.

The following three brief scenarios of a patient with hemoptysis present three distinct patterns:

- A 46-year-old man presents to his internist with a chief complaint of hemoptysis. He is otherwise healthy, is a nonsmoker, and is recovering from an apparent viral bronchitis. For this patient, the pattern would suggest that the acute bronchitis is responsible for the small amount of blood-streaked sputum the patient has observed. In this case, a chest x-ray may provide sufficient reassurance that a more serious disorder is not present.
- In the second scenario, a 46-year-old patient with the same chief complaint who has a 100-pack-year smoking history, a productive morning cough, and episodes of blood-streaked sputum fits the pattern of carcinoma of the lung. Consequently, along with the chest x-ray, the physician obtains a sputum cytology examination and refers this patient for a chest CT scan.
- In the third scenario, a 46-year-old patient with hemoptysis who is from a developing country is evaluated with an echocardiogram as well, because the physician thinks she hears a soft diastolic rumbling murmur at the apex on cardiac auscultation, suggesting rheumatic mitral stenosis.

The primary mistake that can result from relying on the free use of pattern recognition in diagnosis is *premature closure*: concluding that one already knows the correct diagnosis and therefore failing to complete the data collection that would demonstrate the lack of fit of the initial pattern selected. Consider the following hypothetical example. A 45-year-old male patient with a 3-week history of a "flulike" upper respiratory infection (URI) presented to his physician with symptoms of dyspnea and a productive cough. On the basis of the presenting complaint, the clinician pulled out a "URI assessment form" to obtain patient information that could be beneficial in improving the quality and efficiency of care. The physician quickly completed the examination components outlined on this structured form, noting in particular the absence of fever and a clear chest examination. He then prescribed an antibiotic for presumed bronchitis, showed the patient how to breathe into a paper bag to relieve his "hyperventilation," and sent him home with the reassurance that his illness was not serious. After a sleepless night with significant dyspnea unrelieved by breathing into a bag, the patient developed nausea and vomiting and collapsed. He was brought into the emergency department in cardiac arrest and could not be resuscitated. Autopsy showed a posterior wall myocardial infarction (MI) and a fresh thrombus in an atherosclerotic right coronary artery. What went wrong? The clinician decided, on the basis of the patient's appearance, even before starting the history, that the patient's complaints were not serious. He therefore felt confident that he could perform an abbreviated and focused examination by using the URI assessment protocol rather than considering the broader range of possibilities and performing appropriate tests to confirm or refute his initial hypotheses. In particular, by concentrating on the URI, the clinician failed to elicit the full dyspnea history, which would have suggested a far more serious disorder, and he neglected to search for other symptoms that could have directed him to the correct diagnosis.

Cognitive shortcuts or rules of thumb, sometimes referred to as *heuristics*, are another type of intuitive mental process that can be invoked to understand how experts solve complex problems of the sort encountered daily in clinical medicine with great efficiency. The original work on the use of heuristics in problem solving was done largely in laboratory experiments on psychology undergraduates. The objective of the research program was to test the statistical intuition of those subjects against the rules of statistics to understand how such intuitions could be biased. Hence, discussions of the use of heuristics in decision-making tend to focus more on ways in which their use can lead to errors in judgment than on their successes. Although there are many heuristics of possible relevance to clinical reasoning, only four will be mentioned here.

When assessing a particular patient, clinicians often weigh the probability that the patient's clinical features match those of the class of patients with the leading diagnostic hypotheses being considered. In other words, the clinician is searching for the diagnosis for which the patient appears to be a representative example; this cognitive shortcut is called the *representativeness heuristic*. This heuristic is analogous to pattern recognition. However, if there are two (or more) competing diagnoses that could explain the patient's symptoms, physicians who use the representativeness heuristic can reach erroneous conclusions if they fail to consider the underlying prevalence of the two competing diagnoses (i.e., the prior, or pretest, probabilities). Consider a patient with pleuritic chest pain, dyspnea, and a low-grade fever. A clinician might consider acute pneumonia and acute pulmonary embolism to be the two leading diagnostic alternatives. Using the representativeness heuristic, the clinician might judge both diagnostic candidates to be equally likely, although doing so would be wrong if pneumonia was much more prevalent in the underlying population. Mistakes also may result from a failure to consider that a pattern based on experience with a small number of prior cases probably will be less reliable than one based on greater experience.

A second commonly used cognitive shortcut, the *availability heuristic*, involves judgments made on the basis of how easily prior similar cases or outcomes can be brought to mind. For example, an experienced clinician may recall 20 elderly patients seen over the last few years who presented with painless dyspnea of acute onset and were found to have acute MI. A novice clinician may spend valuable time seeking a pulmonary cause for the symptoms before considering and then confirming the cardiac diagnosis. In this situation, the patient's clinical pattern does not fit the expected pattern of acute MI, but experience with this atypical presentation, along with the ability to recall it, can help direct the physician to the diagnosis.

Errors with the availability heuristic can come from several sources of recall bias. For example, rare catastrophes are likely to be remembered with a clarity and force out of proportion to their value—for example, a patient with a sore throat eventually found to have leukemia or a young athlete with leg pain eventually found to have a sarcoma—and recent experience is, of course, easier to recall and therefore more influential on clinical judgments.

The third commonly used cognitive shortcut, the *anchoring heuristic*, involves estimating a probability by starting from a familiar point (the anchor) and adjusting to the new case from that perspective. Anchoring can be a powerful tool for diagnosis but may be used incorrectly. For example, a clinician may judge the probability of coronary artery disease (CAD) to be very high after a positive exercise thallium test because the prediction has been anchored to the test result ("positive test = high probability of CAD"). Yet, as discussed below, this prediction would be inaccurate if the clinical (pretest) picture of the patient being tested indicated a low probability of disease (e.g., a 30-year-old woman with no risk factors). As illustrated in this example, anchors are not necessarily the same as the pretest probability (see "Measures of Disease Probability and Bayes' Theorem," below).

The fourth heuristic, which might be termed the *simplicity heuristic*, states that clinicians should use the simplest explanation possible that will account adequately for the patient's symptoms or findings (Occam's razor). Although this is an attractive and often useful principle, it is important to remember that there is no biologic basis for it.

Experienced physicians use analytic reasoning processes (System 2) much more often when the problem they face is recognized to be complex or to involve important unfamiliar elements or features. In such situations, the clinician proceeds much more methodically in what has been referred to as the hypothetico-deductive model of reasoning. From the outset, the expert clinician is generating, refining, and discarding diagnostic hypotheses. The questions she asks in the history are driven by the hypotheses she is working with at the moment. Even the physical examination is focused on specific questions. Is the spleen enlarged? How big is the liver? Is it tender? Does it have any palpable masses or nodules? Each question focuses the attention of the examiner on the exclusion of all other inputs until it is answered, allowing the examiner to move on to the next specific question. Each diagnostic hypothesis sets a context for the diagnostic steps to follow and provides testable predictions. For example, if the enlarged and quite tender liver felt on physical examination is due to acute hepatitis (the hypothesis), certain specific liver function tests should be markedly elevated (the prediction). If the tests come back normal, the hypothesis may have to be discarded or substantially modified.

Negative findings often are neglected but are as important as positive ones in establishing and refining diagnostic hypotheses. Chest discomfort that is not provoked or worsened by exertion in an active patient reduces the likelihood that chronic ischemic heart disease is the underlying cause. The absence of a resting tachycardia and thyroid gland enlargement reduces the likelihood of hyperthyroidism in a patient with paroxysmal atrial fibrillation.

The acuity of a patient's illness can play an important role in overriding considerations of prevalence and the other issues described above. For example, clinicians are taught to consider aortic dissection routinely as a possible cause of acute severe chest discomfort along with MI, even though the typical history of dissection is different from that of MI and dissection is far less prevalent (Chap. 248). This recommendation is based on the recognition that a relatively rare but catastrophic diagnosis such as aortic dissection is very difficult to make unless it is explicitly considered as a diagnostic imperative. If the clinician fails to elicit any of the characteristic features of dissection by history and finds equivalent blood pressures in both arms and no pulse deficits, he may feel comfortable discarding the aortic dissection hypothesis. If, however, the chest x-ray shows a possible widened mediastinum, the hypothesis may be reinstated and a diagnostic test ordered [e.g., thoracic computed tomography (CT) scan, transesophageal echocardiogram] to evaluate it more fully. In nonacute situations, the prevalence of potential alternative diagnoses should play a much more prominent role in diagnostic hypothesis generation.

Cognitive scientists studying the thought processes of expert clinicians have observed that clinicians group data into packets, or "chunks," that are stored in their memories and manipulated to generate diagnostic hypotheses. Because short-term memory typically can hold only 7–10 items at a time, the number of packets that can be actively integrated into hypothesis-generating activities is similarly limited. For this reason, the cognitive shortcuts discussed above can play a key role in the generation of diagnostic hypotheses, many of which are discarded as rapidly as they are formed (thus demonstrating that the distinction between analytic and intuitive reasoning is arbitrary and simplistic but useful nonetheless).

Research into the hypothetico-deductive model of reasoning has had surprising difficulty identifying the elements that distinguish experts from novices. This has led to a shift from examining the problem-solving process of experts to analyzing the organization of their knowledge. For example, diagnosis may be based on the resemblance of a new case to prior individual instances (exemplars). Experts have a larger store of recalled cases, for example, visual memory in radiology. In the more abstract prototype model of knowledge, clinicians do not simply rely on specific cases but have constructed elaborate conceptual networks or models of disease to arrive at their conclusions. That is, expertise involves an increased ability to connect symptoms, signs, and risk factors to one another; relate those

findings to possible diagnoses; and identify the additional information necessary to confirm the diagnosis. More recently, fuzzy trace theory has placed greater emphasis on intuitionism in which expertise involves the ability to distill the "gist" or essence of diagnosis by processing less information and discarding extraneous data with an emphasis on memory and meaning or recognition and retrieval.

Although no single theory has emerged to account for the key features of expertise in medical diagnosis, experts have more knowledge about more things and a larger repertoire of cognitive tools to employ in problem solving than do novices. One definition of expertise highlights the ability to make powerful distinctions. Memorization alone is insufficient; instead, expertise involves a working knowledge of the diagnostic possibilities and what features distinguish one from another. What remains less clear is whether there is any didactic program that would allow the accelerated development of a novice into an expert or ensure the same high level of expertise among more experienced physicians. Some current recommendations include using a combined approach to clinical reasoning, that is, emphasizing to students the importance of both conscious deliberative analytic and intuitive pattern recognition nonanalytic reasoning strategies and thus giving students flexibility in applying any particular reasoning strategy to overcome case-specific weaknesses.

■ IMPORTANT MODIFIERS OF CLINICAL DECISION-MAKING

More than a decade of research on variations in clinician practice patterns has shed much light on the forces that shape clinical decisions. These factors can be grouped conceptually into three overlapping categories: (1) factors related to physicians' personal characteristics and practice style, (2) factors related to the practice setting, and (3) factors related to economic incentives.

Factors related to practice style

One of the key roles of the physician in medical care is to serve as the patient's agent to ensure that necessary care is provided at a high level of quality. Factors that influence this role include the physician's knowledge, training, and experience. It is obvious that physicians cannot practice evidence-based medicine (described later in the chapter) if they are unfamiliar with the evidence. As would be expected, specialists generally know the evidence in their field better than do generalists. Surgeons may be more enthusiastic about recommending surgery than are medical doctors because their belief in the beneficial effects of surgery is stronger. For the same reason, invasive cardiologists are much more likely to refer chest pain patients for diagnostic catheterization than are noninvasive cardiologists or generalists. The physician beliefs that drive these different practice styles are based on personal experience, recollection, and interpretation of the available medical evidence. For example, heart failure specialists are much more likely than generalists to achieve target angiotensin-converting enzyme (ACE) inhibitor therapy in their heart failure patients because they are more familiar with what the targets are (as defined by large clinical trials), have more familiarity with the specific drugs (including doses and side effects), and are less likely to overreact to foreseeable problems in therapy such as a rise in creatinine levels or symptomatic hypotension. Other intriguing research has shown a wide distribution of acceptance times of antibiotic therapy for peptic ulcer disease after widespread dissemination of the "evidence" in the medical literature. Some gastroenterologists accepted this new therapy before the evidence was clear (reflecting, perhaps, an aggressive practice style), and some lagged behind (a conservative practice style, associated in this case with older physicians). As a group, internists lagged several years behind gastroenterologists.

An example of the mixed effects on patient outcomes associated with rapid acceptance of new evidence involves the case of adding spironolactone (an aldosterone receptor antagonist) to the drug regimen for patients with systolic heart failure. In a large, well-done clinical trial (Randomized Aldactone Evaluation Study, RALES) published in 1999, this therapy produced a significant reduction in all-cause mortality rates. Over the next 2 years the use of spironolactone increased fivefold in the province of Ontario, Canada. That rapid uptake was associated with a significant increase in the rates of hospital admission for both hyperkalemia- and hyperkalemia-associated deaths. At least some of these adverse effects of using this "evidence-based medicine" appeared to be related to treatment of patients who would not have been eligible for the RALES trial and who had contraindications to the use of the drug.

The opinion of influential leaders also can have an important effect on practice patterns. That influence can occur at both the national level (e.g., expert physicians teaching at national meetings) and the local level (e.g., local educational programs, "curbside consultations"). Opinion leaders do not have to be physicians. When conducting rounds with clinical pharmacists, physicians are less likely to make medication errors and more likely to use target levels of evidence-based therapies.

The patient's welfare is not the only concern that drives clinical decisions. The physician's perception about the risk of a malpractice suit resulting from either an erroneous decision or a bad outcome creates a style of practice referred to as *defensive medicine*. This practice involves using tests and therapies with very small marginal returns to preclude future criticism if there is an adverse outcome. For example, a 40-year-old woman who presents with a long-standing history of intermittent headache and a new severe headache along with a normal neurologic examination has a very low likelihood of having structural intracranial pathology. Performance of a head CT or magnetic resonance imaging (MRI) scan in this situation would constitute defensive medicine. However, the results of the test could provide reassurance to an anxious patient.

Practice setting factors

Factors in this category relate to the physical resources available to the physician's practice and the practice environment. *Physician-induced demand* is a term that refers to the repeated observation that physicians have a remarkable ability to accommodate to and employ the medical facilities available to them. One of the foundational studies in outcomes research showed that physicians in Boston, where the ratio of hospital beds to patients was higher, had an almost 50% higher hospital admission rate than did physicians in New Haven, despite there being no obvious differences in the resulting health or mortality rate of the cities' inhabitants. The physicians in New Haven were not aware of using fewer hospital beds for their patients, nor were the Boston physicians aware of using less stringent criteria to admit patients. In both cities, physicians unconsciously adopted their practice styles to the available level of hospital beds.

Other environmental factors that can influence decision-making include the local availability of specialists for consultations and procedures; "high-tech" facilities such as angiography suites, a heart surgery program, and MRI machines; and fragmentation of care.

Economic incentives

Economic incentives are closely related to the other two categories of practice-modifying factors. Financial issues can exert both stimulatory and inhibitory influences on clinical practice. In general, physicians are paid on a fee-for-service, capitation, or salary basis. In fee-for-service, the more the physician does, the more he gets paid. The economic incentive in this case is to do more. When fees are reduced (discounted fee-for-service), doctors tend to increase the number of services provided. Capitation, in contrast, provides a fixed payment per patient per year, encouraging physicians to take on more patients but to provide each patient with fewer services. Expensive services are more likely to be affected by this type of incentive than are inexpensive preventive services.

Salary compensation plans pay physicians the same regardless of the amount of clinical work performed. The incentive here is to see fewer patients.

In summary, expert clinical decision-making can be appreciated as a complex interplay between cognitive processes used to simplify and organize large amounts of complex information and physician biases reflecting education, training, and experience, all of which are shaped by powerful, sometimes perverse, external forces. In the next section, we will review a set of statistical tools and concepts that can be useful in making clinical decisions in the presence of uncertainty.

INTERPRETATION OF DIAGNOSTIC TESTS IN THE CONTEXT OF DECISION-MAKING

Despite the great technological advances in medicine over the last century, uncertainty remains a key challenge in all aspects of medical decision-making. Compounding this challenge is the massive information overload that characterizes modern medicine. Today's experienced clinician needs access to close to 2 million pieces of information to practice medicine. According to one estimate, doctors subscribe to an average of seven journals, representing over 2500 new articles each year. Of course, to be useful, this information must be integrated with the specific data collected on each patient being cared for. Although computers appear to offer the obvious solution both for management of information and for better quantitation and management of the daily uncertainties of medical care, many practical problems must be solved before computers can be integrated into the clinician's reasoning process in a way that demonstrably improves the quality of care.

Although a fully-integrated computed-based system of diagnosis and management remains a distant possibility, there are tools available now that can assist in aspects of patient management. In addition, understanding the nature of diagnostic test information can help make a clinician a more efficient user of such data. This section of the chapter will review some important concepts related to diagnostic testing.

■ DIAGNOSTIC TESTING: MEASURES OF TEST ACCURACY

The purpose of performing a test on a patient is to reduce uncertainty about the patient's diagnosis or prognosis and to aid the clinician in making management decisions. Although diagnostic tests commonly are thought of as laboratory tests (e.g., measurement of serum amylase level) or procedures (e.g., colonoscopy or bronchoscopy), any technology that changes a physician's understanding of the patient's problem qualifies as a diagnostic test. Thus, even the history and physical examination can be considered a form of diagnostic test. In clinical medicine, it is common to reduce the results of a test to a dichotomous outcome, such as positive or negative, normal or abnormal. In many cases, this simplification results in the waste of useful information. However, such simplification makes it easier to demonstrate some of the quantitative ways in which test results data can be used.

The accuracy of diagnostic tests is defined in relation to an accepted "gold standard," which is presumed to reflect the true state of the patient (Table 3-1). To define the diagnostic performance of a new test, an appropriate population must be identified (ideally, patients on whom the new test would be used), and both the new and the gold standard tests are applied to all subjects (use of an inappropriate population or incomplete application of the gold standard test may lead to biased estimates of test performance). The results of the two tests are then compared. The *sensitivity*, or *true-positive, rate* of the new test is the proportion of patients with disease (defined by the gold standard) who have a positive (new) test. This measure reflects how well the test identifies patients with

TABLE 3-1 Measures of Diagnostic Test Accuracy

	Disease Status	
Test Result	Present	Absent
Positive	True-positive (TP)	False-positive (FP)
negative	false-negative (fn)	true-negative (tn)

Identification of Patients with Disease

True-positive rate (sensitivity) = TP/(TP + FN)
False-negative rate = FN/(TP + FN)
True-positive rate = 1 – false-negative rate

Identification of Patients without Disease

True-negative rate (specificity) = TN/(TN + FP)
False-positive rate = FP/(TN + FP)
True-negative rate = 1 – false-positive rate

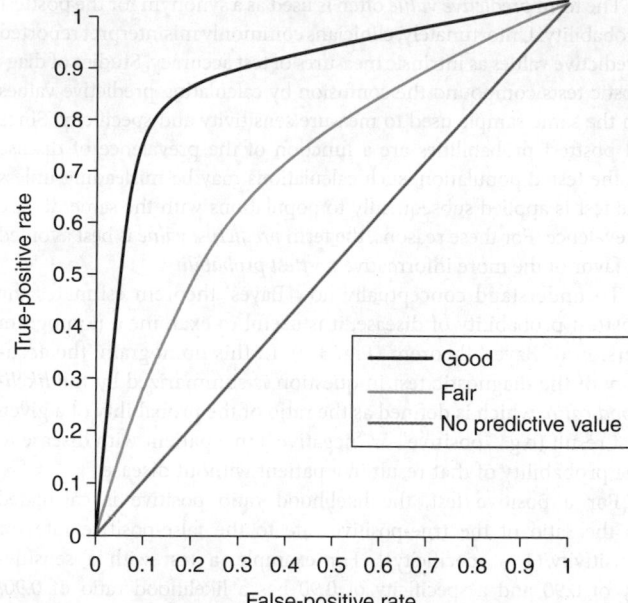

Figure 3-1 Each ROC curve illustrates a trade-off that occurs between improved test sensitivity (accurate detection of patients with disease) and improved test specificity (accurate detection of patients without disease), as the test value defining when the test turns from "negative" to "positive" is varied. A 45° line would indicate a test with no predictive value (sensitivity = specificity at every test value). The area under each ROC curve is a measure of the information content of the test. Thus, a larger ROC area signifies increased diagnostic accuracy.

disease. The proportion of patients with disease who have a negative test is the *false-negative rate* and is calculated as 1 – sensitivity. The proportion of patients without disease who have a negative test is the *specificity,* or *true-negative, rate*. This measure reflects how well the test correctly identifies patients without disease. The proportion of patients without disease who have a positive test is the *false-positive rate*, calculated as 1 – specificity. A perfect test would have a sensitivity of 100% and a specificity of 100% and would completely separate patients with disease from those without it.

Calculating sensitivity and specificity requires selection of a threshold value or cut point at or above which the test is considered "positive." For any specific test, as this cut point is moved to improve sensitivity, specificity falls and vice versa. This dynamic trade-off between more accurate identification of subjects with disease versus those without disease is often displayed graphically as a receiver operating characteristic (ROC) curve (Fig. 3-1). An ROC curve plots sensitivity (*y* axis) versus 1 – specificity (*x* axis). Each point on the curve represents a potential cut point with an associated sensitivity and specificity value. The area under the ROC curve often is used as a quantitative measure of the information content of a test. Values range from 0.5 (no diagnostic information from testing at all; the test is equivalent to flipping a coin) to 1.0 (perfect test).

In the testing literature, ROC areas often are used to compare alternative tests that can be employed for a particular diagnostic problem. The test with the highest area (i.e., closest to 1.0) is presumed to be the most accurate. However, ROC curves are not a panacea for evaluation of diagnostic test utility. Like Bayes' theorem (discussed below), they typically are focused on only one possible test parameter (e.g., ST-segment response in a treadmill exercise test) to the exclusion of other potentially relevant data. In addition, ROC area comparisons do not simulate the way test information actually is used in clinical practice. Finally, biases in the underlying population used to generate the ROC curves (e.g., related to assessment of the test in individuals unrepresentative of those in whom the test will be used clinically) can bias the ROC area and the validity of a comparison among tests.

■ MEASURES OF DISEASE PROBABILITY AND BAYES' THEOREM

Unfortunately, there are no perfect tests. After every test is completed, the true disease state of the patient remains uncertain. Quantifying this residual uncertainty can be done with Bayes' theorem. This theorem provides a simple mathematical way to calculate the posttest probability of disease from three parameters: the pretest probability of disease, the test sensitivity, and the test specificity (Table 3-2). The pretest probability is a quantitative

expression of the confidence in a diagnosis before the test is performed. In the absence of more relevant information, it is usually estimated from the prevalence of the disease in the underlying population. For some common conditions, such as CAD, nomograms and statistical models have been created to generate better estimates of pretest probability from elements of the history and physical examination. The posttest probability, then, is a revised statement of the confidence in the diagnosis, taking into account what was known both before and after the test.

TABLE 3-2 Measures of Disease Probability

Pretest probability of disease = probability of disease before test is performed. May use population prevalence of disease or more patient-specific data to generate this probability estimate.

Posttest probability of disease = probability of disease accounting for both pretest probability and test results. Also called predictive value of the test.

Bayes' theorem computational version:

$$\text{Posttest probability} = \frac{\text{Pretest probability} \times \text{test sensitivity}}{\begin{array}{c}\text{Pretest probability} \times \text{test sensitivity} + \\ (1 - \text{pretest probability}) \times \text{test} \\ \text{false-positive rate}\end{array}}$$

Bayes' theorem example: With a pretest probability of 0.50 and a "positive" diagnostic test result (test sensitivity = 0.90, test specificity = 0.90):

$$\text{Posttest probability} = \frac{(0.50)(0.90)}{(0.50)(0.90) + (0.50)(0.10)}$$

$$= 0.90$$

The term *predictive value* often is used as a synonym for the posttest probability. Unfortunately, clinicians commonly misinterpret reported predictive values as intrinsic measures of test accuracy. Studies of diagnostic tests compound the confusion by calculating predictive values on the same sample used to measure sensitivity and specificity. Since all posttest probabilities are a function of the prevalence of disease in the tested population, such calculations may be misleading unless the test is applied subsequently to populations with the same disease prevalence. For these reasons, the term *predictive value* is best avoided in favor of the more informative *posttest probability*.

To understand conceptually how Bayes' theorem estimates the posttest probability of disease, it is useful to examine a nomogram version of Bayes' theorem (Fig. 3-2). In this nomogram, the accuracy of the diagnostic test in question is summarized by the *likelihood ratio*, which is defined as the ratio of the probability of a given test result (e.g., "positive" or "negative") in a patient with disease to the probability of that result in a patient without disease.

For a positive test, the likelihood ratio positive is calculated as the ratio of the true-positive rate to the false-positive rate [or sensitivity/(1 − specificity)]. For example, a test with a sensitivity of 0.90 and a specificity of 0.90 has a likelihood ratio of 0.90/(1 − 0.90), or 9. Thus, for this hypothetical test, a "positive" result

is 9 times more likely in a patient with the disease than in a patient without it. Most tests in medicine have likelihood ratios for a positive result between 1.5 and 20. Higher values are associated with tests that are more accurate at identifying patients with disease, with values of 10 or greater are of particular note. If sensitivity is excellent but specificity is less so, the likelihood ratio will be reduced substantially (e.g., with a 90% sensitivity but a 60% specificity, the likelihood ratio is 2.25).

For a negative test, the corresponding likelihood ratio negative is the ratio of the false-negative rate to the true-negative rate [or (1 − sensitivity)/specificity]. The smaller the likelihood ratio (i.e., the closer to 0) is, the better the test performs at ruling out disease. The hypothetical test considered above with a sensitivity of 0.9 and a specificity of 0.9 would have a likelihood ratio for a negative test result of (1 − 0.9)/0.9, or 0.11, meaning that a negative result is almost 10 times more likely if the patient is disease-free than if the patient has disease.

■ APPLICATIONS TO DIAGNOSTIC TESTING IN CAD

Consider two tests commonly used in the diagnosis of CAD: an exercise treadmill and an exercise single-photon emission CT (SPECT) myocardial perfusion imaging test (Chap. 229). Meta-analysis has shown that a positive treadmill ST-segment response

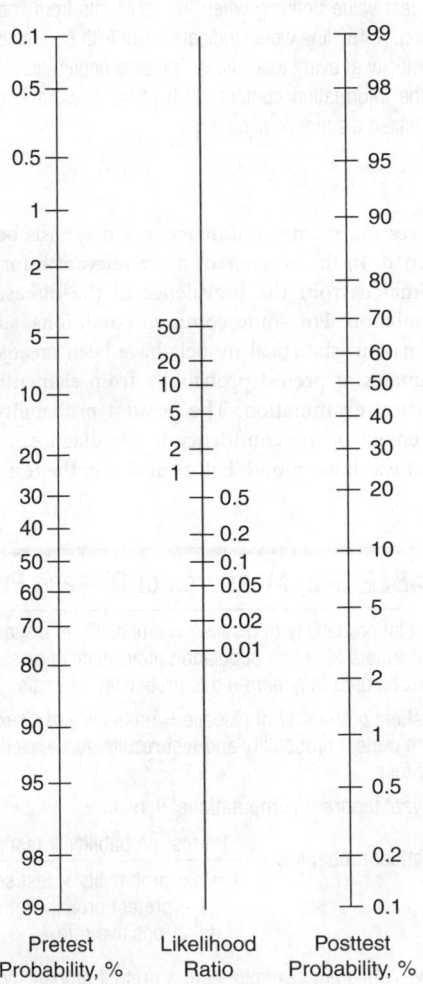

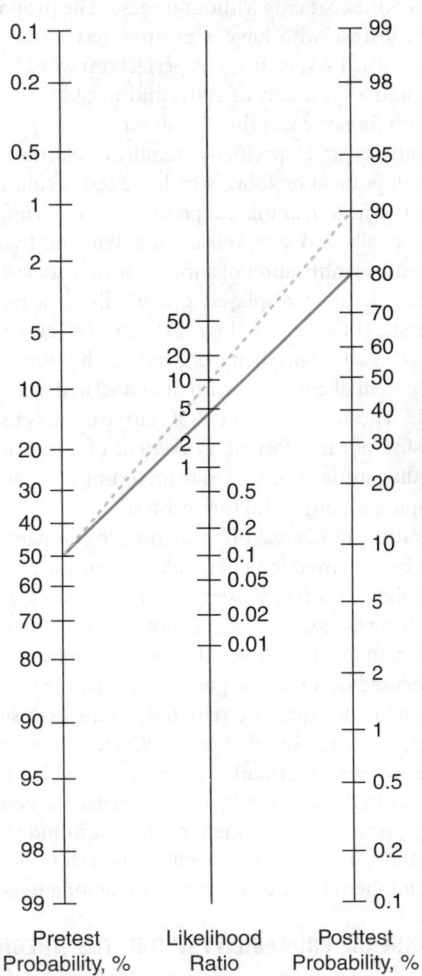

Pretest Probability, %	Likelihood Ratio	Posttest Probability, %

Figure 3-2 Nomogram version of Bayes' theorem used to predict the posttest probability of disease (right-hand scale) using the pretest probability of disease (left-hand scale) and the likelihood ratio for a positive test (middle scale). See text for information on calculation of likelihood ratios. To use, place a straightedge connecting the pretest probability and the likelihood ratio and read off the posttest probability. The right-hand part of the figure

illustrates the value of a positive exercise treadmill test (likelihood ratio 4, green line) and a positive exercise thallium single-photon emission CT perfusion study (likelihood ratio 9, broken yellow line) in a patient with a pretest probability of coronary artery disease of 50%. *(Adapted from Centre for Evidence-Based Medicine: Likelihood ratios. Available at http://www.cebm. net/index.aspx?o=1043.)*

has an average sensitivity of 66% and an average specificity of 84%, yielding a likelihood ratio of 4.1 [0.66/(1 − 0.84)]. If this test is used on a patient with a pretest probability of CAD of 10%, the posttest probability of disease after a positive result rises to only about 30%. If a patient with a pretest probability of CAD of 80% has a positive test result, the posttest probability of disease is about 95%.

The exercise SPECT myocardial perfusion test is a more accurate test for the diagnosis of CAD. For our purposes, assume that the finding of a reversible exercise-induced perfusion defect has both a sensitivity and a specificity of 90%, yielding a likelihood ratio for a positive test of 9.0 [0.90/(1 − 0.90)]. If we again test the low pretest probability patient and that patient has a positive test, by using Fig. 3-2 it can be demonstrated that the posttest probability of CAD rises from 10 to 50%. However, from a decision-making point of view, the more accurate test may not improve diagnostic confidence enough to change management. In fact, the test has moved the physician from being fairly certain that the patient did not have CAD to being completely undecided (a 50:50 chance of disease). In a patient with a pretest probability of 80%, using the more accurate exercise SPECT test raises the posttest probability to 97% (compared with 95% for the exercise treadmill). Again, the more accurate test does not provide enough improvement in posttest confidence to alter management, and neither test has improved much on what was known from clinical data alone.

Although it depends on the sensitivity and specificity, in general, if the pretest probability is low (e.g., 20%), even a positive result on a very accurate test will not move the posttest probability to a range high enough to rule in disease (e.g., 80%). Pretest probabilities are often particularly low in screening situations in which patients are asymptomatic. In such cases, specificity becomes particularly important. For example, in screening first-time female blood donors without risk factors for HIV, a positive test raised the likelihood of HIV to only 67% despite a specificity of 99.995% because the prevalence was 0.01%. One useful mnemonic is *positive SpPin*: a positive test with high specificity rules in disease (keeping in mind the caveats just noted about pretest probability). Conversely, with a high pretest probability, a negative test may not rule out disease adequately if it is not sufficiently sensitive. The other mnemonic is *negative SnNout*: a negative test with high sensitivity rules out disease. Thus, the largest gain in diagnostic confidence from a test occurs when the clinician is most uncertain before performing it (e.g., pretest probability between 30% and 70%). For example, if a patient has a pretest probability for CAD of 50%, a positive exercise treadmill test will move the posttest probability to 80% and a positive exercise SPECT perfusion test will move it to 90% (Fig. 3-2).

Bayes' theorem, as presented above, employs a number of important simplifications that should be considered. First, few tests have only two useful outcomes, positive and negative, and many tests provide numerous pieces of data about the patient. Even if these data can be integrated into a summary result, multiple levels of useful information may be present (e.g., strongly positive, positive, indeterminate, negative, strongly negative). Although Bayes' theorem can be adapted to this more detailed test result format, it is computationally complex to do so. Similarly, when multiple tests are performed, the posttest probability may be used as the pretest probability to interpret the second test. However, this simplification assumes conditional independence—that is, that the results of the first test do not affect the likelihood of the second test result—and this is often not true.

Finally, it has long been asserted that sensitivity and specificity are prevalence-independent parameters of test accuracy, and many texts still make this statement. This statistically useful assumption, however, is clinically simplistic. A treadmill exercise test, for example, has a sensitivity in a population of patients with one-vessel CAD of around 30%, whereas its sensitivity in patients with severe three-vessel CAD approaches 80%. Thus, the best estimate of sensitivity to use in a particular decision often varies, depending on the distribution of disease stages present in the tested population. A hospitalized, symptomatic, or referral population typically has a higher prevalence of disease and, in particular, a higher prevalence of more advanced disease than does an outpatient population. As a consequence, test sensitivity will tend to be higher in hospitalized patients, whereas test specificity will be higher in outpatients.

STATISTICAL PREDICTION MODELS

Bayes' theorem, as presented above, deals with a clinical prediction problem that is unrealistically simple relative to most problems a clinician faces. Prediction models that are based on multivariable statistical models can handle much more complex problems and substantially enhance predictive accuracy for specific situations. Their particular advantage is the ability to take into account many overlapping pieces of information and assign a relative weight to each on the basis of its unique contribution to the prediction in question. For example, a logistic regression model to predict the probability of CAD considers all the relevant independent factors from the clinical examination and diagnostic testing and their significance instead of the small handful of data that clinicians can manage in their heads or with Bayes' theorem. However, despite this strength, the models are too complex computationally to use without a calculator or computer (although this limitation may be overcome once medicine is practiced from a fully computerized platform).

To date, only a handful of prediction models have been validated properly. The importance of independent validation in a population separate from the one used to develop the model cannot be overstated. An unvalidated prediction model should be viewed with the skepticism appropriate for a new drug or medical device that has not been through rigorous clinical trial testing.

When statistical models have been compared directly with expert clinicians, they have been found to be more consistent, as would be expected, but not significantly more accurate. Their biggest promise, then, would seem to be to help less-experienced clinicians become more accurate in their predictions.

FORMAL DECISION SUPPORT TOOLS

DECISION SUPPORT SYSTEMS

Over the last 40 years, many attempts have been made to develop computer systems to aid clinical decision-making and patient management. Conceptually, computers offer a very attractive way to handle the vast information load that today's physicians face. The computer can help by making accurate predictions of outcome, simulating the whole decision process, or providing algorithmic guidance. Computer-based predictions using Bayesian or statistical regression models inform a clinical decision but do not actually reach a "conclusion" or "recommendation." Artificial intelligence systems attempt to simulate or replace human reasoning with a computer-based analogue. To date, such approaches have achieved only limited success. Reminder or protocol-directed systems do not make predictions but use existing algorithms, such as guidelines, to guide clinical practice. In general, however, decision support systems have had little impact on practice. Reminder systems, although not yet in widespread use, have shown the most promise, particularly in correcting drug dosing and promoting adherence to guidelines. The full impact of these approaches will be evaluable only when computers are fully integrated into medical practice.

DECISION ANALYSIS

Compared with the methods discussed above, decision analysis represents a completely different approach to decision support. Its principal application is in decision problems that are complex and involve a substantial risk, a high degree of uncertainty in some key area, or an idiosyncratic feature that does not "fit" the available

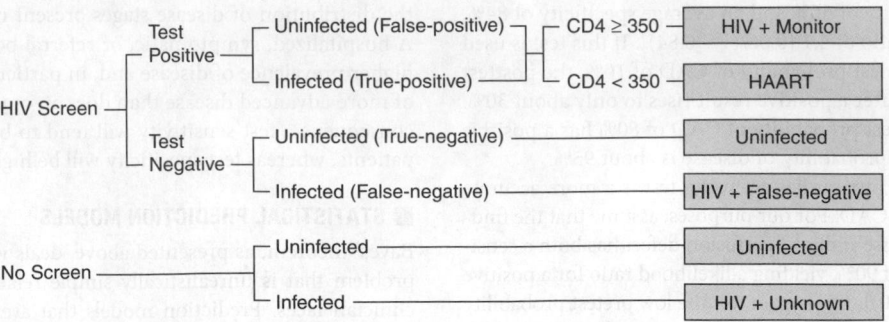

Figure 3-3 Basic structure of decision model used to evaluate strategies for screening for HIV in the general population. HIV, human immunodeficiency virus; HAART, highly active antiretroviral therapy. *(Provided courtesy of G. Sanders, with permission.)*

evidence. An example decision tree created to evaluate strategies for screening for HIV infection is shown in Fig. 3-3. Infected individuals who are unaware of their illness may cause up to 20,000 new cases of HIV infection annually in the United States. In addition, because of delayed diagnosis, about 40% of HIV-positive patients progress to AIDS within a year of the initial diagnosis. Early identification offers the opportunity both to prevent progression to AIDS through the use of serial CD4 counts and measurements of viral load linked to selective use of combination antiretroviral therapy and to encourage reduction of risky sexual behavior.

The Centers for Disease Control and Prevention (CDC) proposed in 2003 that routine HIV testing should be a part of standard medical care. In a decision-model exploration of this proposed strategy compared with usual care, assuming a 1% prevalence of unidentified HIV infection in the population, routine screening of a cohort of 43-year-old men and women increased life expectancy by 5.5 days and cost $194 per subject screened. The cost-effectiveness ratio for screening relative to usual care was $15,078 per quality-adjusted life year (the additional cost to society to increase population health by 1 year of perfect health). Results were sensitive to assumptions about the effectiveness of behavior modification on subsequent sexual behavior, the benefits of early therapy for HIV infection, and the prevalence and incidence of HIV infection in the population targeted. This model, which required over 75 separate data points, provides novel insights into a clinical management problem that has not been subjected to a randomized clinical trial.

Although such models have been developed and used to estimate short- and long-term survival for alternative choices, the process of building and evaluating decision models is generally too complex for use in real-time clinical management. The potential for this tool therefore lies in the development of a set of published or online models addressing a particular decision or policy area that can serve to highlight key pressure points in the problem.

EVIDENCE-BASED MEDICINE

The "art of medicine" is defined traditionally as a practice combining medical knowledge (including scientific evidence), intuition, and judgment in the care of patients (Chap. 1). EBM updates this construct by placing much greater emphasis on the processes by which clinicians gain knowledge of the most up-to-date and relevant clinical research to determine for themselves whether medical interventions alter the disease course and improve the length or quality of life. The meaning of practicing EBM becomes clearer through an examination of its four key steps:

1. Formulating the management question to be answered
2. Searching the literature and online databases for applicable research data

3. Appraising the evidence gathered with regard to its validity and relevance
4. Integrating this appraisal with knowledge about the unique aspects of the patient (including the patient's preferences about the possible outcomes)

Step 1 involves generating well-formulated questions that involve four or five components—PICOD: patient or population, intervention, comparator, outcome, and, sometimes, D for study design, (e.g., does routine percutaneous coronary intervention improve survival compared with initial medical management in 60-year-old men with stable angina and known CAD?) Steps 2 and 3 are the heart of EBM as it is currently used in practice and relate to the underlying fundamental principle that the strength of medical evidence supporting a therapy or strategy is hierarchical. The process of searching the world's research literature and appraising the quality and relevance of studies thus identified can be quite time-consuming and requires skills and training that most clinicians do not possess. Thus, the best starting point for most EBM searches is the identification of recent systematic overviews of the problem in question (Table 3-3).

Generally, the EBM tools listed in Table 3-3 provide access to research information in one of two forms. The first, primary research reports, is the original peer-reviewed research work that is published in medical journals. Initial access to this information in an EBM search may be gained through MEDLINE, which provides access to a huge amount of data in abstract form. However, in using MEDLINE it is often difficult to locate reports that are on point in a sea of irrelevant or unhelpful information and be reasonably certain that important reports have not been overlooked. The second form, systematic reviews, comprehensively summarizes the available evidence on a particular topic up to a certain date and provides the interpretation of the reviewer and thus is the highest level of evidence in the hierarchy. Explicit criteria are used to find all the relevant scientific research and grade its quality. The prototype for this kind of resource is the Cochrane Database of Systematic Reviews. One of the key components of a systematic review is a meta-analysis. The next two sections will review some of the major types of clinical research reports available in the literature and the process of aggregating those data into meta-analyses.

■ SOURCES OF EVIDENCE: CLINICAL TRIALS AND REGISTRIES

The notion of learning from observation of patients is as old as medicine itself. Over the last 50 years, physicians' understanding of how best to turn raw observation into useful evidence has evolved considerably. Case reports, personal anecdotal experience, and small single-center case series are now recognized as having severe limitations in validity and generalizability, and although they may generate hypotheses or be the first reports of adverse events, they

TABLE 3-3 Selected Tools for Finding the Evidence in Evidence-Based Medicine

Name	Description	Web Address	Availability
Evidence-Based Medicine Reviews	Comprehensive electronic database that combines and integrates: 1. The Cochrane Database of Systematic Reviews 2. ACP Journal Club 3. The Database of Abstracts of Reviews of Effectiveness	www.ovid.com	Subscription required. Available through medical center libraries and other institutions.
Cochrane Library	Collection of EBM databases, including The Cochrane Database of Systematic Reviews—full text articles reviewing specific health care topics.	www.cochrane.org	Subscription required. Abstracts of systematic reviews available free online. Some countries have funding to provide free access to all residents.
ACP Journal Club	Collection of summaries of original studies and systematic reviews. Published bimonthly. All data since 1991 available on Web site, updated yearly.	www.acpjc.org	Subscription required.
Clinical Evidence	Monthly updated directory of concise overviews of common clinical interventions.	www.clinicalevidence.com	Subscription required. Free access for United Kingdom and developing countries.
MEDLINE	National Library of Medicine database with citations back to 1966.	www.nlm.nih.gov	Free via Internet.

have no role in formulating modern standards of practice. The major tools used to develop reliable evidence consist of the randomized clinical trial and the large observational registry. A registry or database typically is focused on a disease or syndrome (e.g., cancer, CAD, heart failure), a clinical procedure (e.g., bone marrow transplantation, coronary revascularization), or an administrative process (e.g., claims data used for billing and reimbursement).

By definition, in observational data, the care of the patient is not controlled by the investigator. Carefully collected *prospective* observational data can achieve a level of quality approaching that of major clinical trial data. At the other end of the spectrum, data collected retrospectively (e.g., chart review) are limited in form and content to what previous observers thought was important to record, which may not serve the research question under study particularly well. Data not specifically collected for research (e.g., claims data) often have important limitations that cannot be overcome in the analysis phase of the research. Advantages of observational data include the ability to capture a broader population than is typically represented in clinical trials because of inclusion and exclusion criteria. In addition, observational data are the primary source of evidence for questions for which a randomized trial cannot or will not be performed. For example, it may be difficult or unethical to randomize patients to test diagnostic or therapeutic strategies that are unproven but widely accepted in practice. In addition, patients cannot be randomized to a sex, racial/ethnic group, socioeconomic status, or country of residence. Physicians are also not willing to randomize patients to a potentially harmful intervention, such as smoking or overeating to develop obesity.

The major difference between a well-done randomized clinical trial and a well-done prospective observational study of a particular management strategy is the lack of protection from treatment selection bias in the latter. The use of observational data to compare diagnostic or therapeutic strategies assumes that there is sufficient uncertainty in practice to ensure that similar patients will be managed differently by different physicians. In short, the analysis assumes that there is an element of randomness (in the sense of disorder rather than in the formal statistical sense) to clinical management. In such cases, statistical models attempt to adjust for important imbalances and "level the playing field" so that a fair comparison among treatment options can be made. When management is clearly not random (e.g., all eligible left main coronary artery disease patients are referred for coronary bypass surgery), the problem may be too confounded (biased) for statistical correction, and observational data may not provide reliable evidence.

In general, the use of concurrent controls is vastly preferable to that of historical controls. For example, comparison of current surgical management of left main CAD with left main CAD patients treated medically during the 1970s (the last time these patients were routinely treated with medicine alone) would be extremely misleading since the quality of "medical therapy" has made substantial improvements in the interval.

Randomized controlled clinical trials include the careful prospective design features of the best observational data studies but also include the use of random allocation of treatment. This design provides the best protection against confounding due to treatment selection bias (a major aspect of internal validity). However, the randomized trial may not have good external validity (generalizability) if the process of recruitment into the trial resulted in the exclusion of many potentially eligible subjects.

Consumers of medical evidence need to be aware that randomized trials vary widely in their quality and applicability to practice. The process of designing such a trial often involves a great many compromises. For example, trials designed to gain U.S. Food and Drug Administration (FDA) approval for an investigational drug or device have to address certain regulatory requirements that may result in a trial design different from what practicing clinicians would find useful.

■ META-ANALYSIS

The Greek prefix *meta* signifies something at a later or higher stage of development. Meta-analysis is research done on research data for the purpose of combining and summarizing the available evidence quantitatively. Although it can be used to combine nonrandomized studies, meta-analysis is used most typically to summarize all the randomized trials on a particular therapeutic problem. Ideally, unpublished trials should be identified and included to avoid publication bias (i.e., "negative" trials may not be published). Furthermore, some of the best meta-analyses obtain and analyze the raw individual patient-level data from all trials rather than working only with what is available in the published reports of each trial. Not all published meta-analyses are reliable sources of evidence on a particular problem. Their methodology must be scrutinized carefully to ensure proper study design and analysis. The results of a well-done meta-analysis are likely to be most persuasive if they include at least several large-scale, properly performed randomized trials. Although meta-analysis can help detect benefits when individual trials are inadequately powered (e.g., the benefits of streptokinase thrombolytic therapy in acute MI demonstrated by ISIS-2 in 1988 were evident by the early 1970s through meta-analysis), in cases in which the available trials are small or poorly done, meta-analysis should not be viewed as a remedy for the deficiency in primary trial data.

Meta-analyses typically focus on summary measures of relative treatment benefit, such as odds ratios or relative risks. Clinicians also should examine what absolute risk reduction (ARR) can be expected from the therapy. A useful summary metric of absolute treatment benefit is the number needed to treat (NNT) to prevent one adverse outcome event (e.g., death, stroke). NNT is simply 1/ARR. For example, if a hypothetical therapy reduced mortality rates over a 5-year follow-up by 33% (the relative treatment benefit) from 12% (control arm) to 8% (treatment arm), the absolute risk reduction would be 12% − 8% = 4% and the NNT would be 1/.04, or 25. Thus, it would be necessary to treat 25 patients for 5 years to prevent 1 death. If the hypothetical treatment was applied to a lower-risk population, say, with a 6% 5-year mortality, the 33% relative treatment benefit would reduce absolute mortality by 2% (from 6 to 4%), and the NNT for the same therapy in this lower-risk group of patients would be 50. Although not always made explicit, comparisons of NNT estimates from different studies should account for the duration of follow-up used to create each estimate.

■ CLINICAL PRACTICE GUIDELINES

According to the 1990 Institute of Medicine definition, clinical practice guidelines are "systematically developed statements to assist practitioner and patient decisions about appropriate health care for specific clinical circumstances." This definition emphasizes several crucial features of modern guideline development. First, guidelines are created by using the tools of EBM. In particular, the core of the development process is a systematic literature search followed by a review of the relevant peer-reviewed literature. Second, guidelines usually are focused on a clinical disorder (e.g., adult diabetes, stable angina pectoris) or a health care intervention (e.g., cancer screening). Third, the primary objective of guidelines is to improve the quality of medical care by identifying areas where care should be standardized, based on compelling evidence. Guidelines are intended to "assist" decision-making, not to define explicitly what decisions should be made in a particular situation, in part because evidence alone is never enough for clinical decision-making (e.g., deciding whether to intubate and administer antibiotics for pneumonia in a terminally ill individual, in an individual with dementia, or in an otherwise healthy 30-year-old mother).

Guidelines are narrative documents constructed by an expert panel whose composition often is determined by interested professional organizations. These panels vary in the degree to which they represent all relevant stakeholders. The guideline documents consist of a series of specific management recommendations, a summary indication of the quantity and quality of evidence supporting each recommendation, and a narrative discussion of the recommendations. Many recommendations have little or no supporting evidence and thus reflect the expert consensus of the guideline panel. In part to protect against errors by individual panels, the final step in guideline construction is peer review, followed by a final revision in response to the critiques provided.

Guidelines are closely tied to the process of quality improvement in medicine through their identification of evidence-based best practices. Such practices can be used as quality indicators. Examples include the proportion of acute MI patients who receive aspirin upon admission to a hospital and the proportion of heart failure patients with a depressed ejection fraction treated with an ACE inhibitor. Routine measurement and reporting of such quality indicators can produce selective improvements in quality, since many physicians prefer not to be outliers.

CONCLUSIONS

In this era of EBM, it is tempting to think that all the difficult decisions practitioners face have been or soon will be solved and digested into practice guidelines and computerized reminders. However, EBM provides practitioners with an ideal rather than a finished set of tools with which to manage patients. The significant contribution of EBM has been to promote the development of more powerful and user-friendly EBM tools that can be accessed by busy practitioners. This is an enormously important contribution that is slowly changing the way medicine is practiced. One of the repeated admonitions of EBM pioneers has been to replace reliance on the local "gray-haired expert" (who may be wrong but is rarely in doubt) with a systematic search for and evaluation of the evidence. But EBM has not eliminated the need for subjective judgments. Each systematic review or clinical practice guideline presents the interpretation of "experts" whose biases remain largely invisible to the review's consumers. Moreover, even with such evidence, it is always worth remembering that the response to therapy of the "average" patient represented by the summary clinical trial outcomes may not be what can be expected for the patient sitting in front of a physician in the clinic or hospital. In addition, meta-analyses cannot generate evidence when there are no adequate randomized trials, and most of what clinicians confront in practice will never be thoroughly tested in a randomized trial. For the foreseeable future, excellent clinical reasoning skills and experience supplemented by well-designed quantitative tools and a keen appreciation for individual patient preferences will continue to be of paramount importance in the professional life of medical practitioners.

FURTHER READINGS

DEL MAR C et al: *Clinical Thinking: Evidence, Communication and Decision Making*, Malden, MA, Blackwell, 2006

GRABER ML et al: Diagnostic error in internal medicine. Arch Intern Med 65:1493, 2005

GRIMES DA et al: Refining clinical diagnosis with likelihood ratios. Lancet 365:1500, 2005

KASSIRER JP et al. *Learning Clinical Reasoning*. Baltimore, Lippincott Williams & Wilkins, 2009

NORMAN G et al: Non-analytical models of clinical reasoning: The role of experience. Med Educ 41:1140, 2007

PETERSON ED et al: Association between hospital process performance and outcomes among patients with acute coronary syndromes. JAMA 295:1912, 2006

REILLY BM et al: Translating clinical research into clinical practice: Impact of using prediction rules to make decisions. Ann Intern Med 144:201, 2006

SANDERS GD et al: Cost-effectiveness of screening for HIV in the era of highly active antiretroviral therapy. N Engl J Med 352:570, 2005

TRICOCI P et al: Scientific evidence underlying the AHA/ACC clinical practice guidelines. JAMA 301:831, 2009; erratum in JAMA 301:1544, 2009

CHAPTER 4

Screening and Prevention of Disease

Gary J. Martin

A primary goal of health care is to prevent disease or detect it early enough that intervention will be more effective. Strategies for disease screening and prevention are driven by evidence that testing and intervention are practical and effective. Currently, most screening tests are readily available and inexpensive. Examples include tests that are biochemical (e.g., cholesterol, glucose), physiologic (e.g., blood pressure, growth curves), or radiologic (e.g., mammogram, bone densitometry) or that involve tissue specimens (e.g., Pap smear). In the future, it is anticipated that genetic testing will play an increasingly important role in predicting disease risk (Chap. 63). However, such tests are not widely used except for individuals at risk for high-penetrance genes on the basis of family or ethnic history (e.g., *BRCA1*, *BRCA2*). The identification of low-penetrance but high-frequency genes that cause common disorders such as diabetes, hypertension, and macular degeneration offers the possibility of new genetic tests. However, any new screening test, whether based on genetic or other methods, must be subjected to rigorous evaluation of its sensitivity, specificity, impact on disease, and cost-effectiveness. Physicians and patients are introduced continually to new screening tests, often in advance of complete evaluation. For example, the use of whole-body CT imaging has been advocated as a means to screen for a variety of disorders. Though it is appealing in concept, there is currently no evidence to justify this approach, which is associated with high cost and a substantial risk of false-positive results.

This chapter will review the basic principles of screening and prevention in the primary care setting. Recommendations for specific disorders such as cardiovascular disease, diabetes, and cancer are provided in the chapters dedicated to those topics.

■ BASIC PRINCIPLES OF SCREENING

In general, screening is most effective when applied to relatively common disorders that carry a large disease burden (Table 4-1). The five leading causes of mortality in the United States are heart diseases, malignant neoplasms, accidents, cerebrovascular diseases, and chronic obstructive pulmonary disease. Thus, many prevention strategies are targeted at these conditions. From a global health perspective, these conditions are priorities, but malaria, malnutrition, AIDS, tuberculosis, and violence also carry a heavy disease burden (Chap. 2).

A primary goal of screening is the early detection of a risk factor or disease at a stage at which it can be corrected or cured. For

TABLE 4-1 Lifetime Cumulative Risk

Breast cancer for women	10%
Colon cancer	6%
Cancer of the cervix for women[a]	2%
Domestic violence for women	Up to 15%
Hip fracture for white women	16%

[a]Assuming an unscreened population.

example, most cancers have a better prognosis when identified as premalignant lesions or when they are still resectable. Similarly, early identification of hypertension or hyperlipidemia allows therapeutic interventions that reduce the long-term risk of cardiovascular or cerebrovascular events. However, early detection does not necessarily influence survival. For example, in some studies of lung cancer screening, tumors are identified at an earlier stage but the overall mortality rate does not differ between screened and unscreened populations. The apparent improvement in 5-year survival rates can be attributed to the detection of smaller tumors rather than to a real change in clinical course after diagnosis. Similarly, the detection of prostate cancer may not lead to a difference in the mortality rate because the disease is often indolent and competing morbidities, such as coronary artery disease, may ultimately cause mortality (Chap. 82).

Disorders with a long latency period increase the potential gains associated with detection. For example, cancer of the cervix has a long latency between dysplasia and invasive carcinoma, providing an opportunity for detection by routine screening. It is hoped that the introduction of new papillomavirus vaccines will provide additional disease prevention, ultimately reducing reliance on screening for cervical cancer. For colon cancer, an adenomatous polyp progresses to invasive cancer over 4–12 years, providing an opportunity to detect early lesions by fecal occult blood testing (FOBT) or endoscopy. In contrast, breast cancer screening in premenopausal women is more challenging—and controversial—because of the relatively short interval between development of a localized breast cancer and metastasis to regional nodes (estimated to be ~12 months).

■ METHODS OF MEASURING HEALTH BENEFITS

It is not practical to perform all possible screening procedures. For example, screening for laryngeal cancer in smokers is not currently recommended. It is necessary to examine the strength of evidence in favor of screening measures relative to the cost and risk of false-positive tests. For example, should ultrasound be used to screen for ovarian cancer in average-risk women? It is currently estimated that the unnecessary laparotomies triggered by finding benign ovarian masses would cause more harm than the benefit derived from detecting the occasional curable ovarian cancer.

A variety of endpoints are used to assess the potential gain from screening and prevention interventions:

1. *The number of subjects screened to alter the outcome in one individual.* It is estimated, for example, that 731 women ages 65–69 would need to be screened by dual-energy x-ray absorptiometry (DEXA) and then treated appropriately to prevent one hip fracture from osteoporosis.
2. *The absolute and relative impact of screening on disease outcome.* A meta-analysis of Swedish mammography trials (ages 40–70) found that ~1.2 fewer women per thousand would die from breast cancer if they were screened over a 12-year period. By comparison, ~3 lives per 1000 might be saved from colon cancer in a population (ages 50–75) screened with annual FOBT over a 13-year period. Based on this analysis, colon cancer screening may actually save more women's lives than does mammography. The impact of FOBT (8.8/1000 versus 5.9/1000) might be stated either as 3 lives per 1000 or as a 30% reduction in colon cancer death; thus, it is important to consider both the relative impact and absolute impact on numbers of lives saved.
3. *The cost per year of life saved* is used to assess the effectiveness of many screening and prevention strategies. Typically, strategies that cost <$30,000–50,000 per year of life saved are considered

"cost-effective" (Chap. 3). For example, using alendronate to treat 65-year-old women with osteoporosis approaches this threshold of approximately $30,000 per year of life saved.

4. *Increase in average life expectancy for a population.* Predicted increases in life expectancy for various screening procedures are listed in Table 4-2. It should be noted, however, that the increase in life expectancy is an average that applies to a population, not to an individual. In reality, the vast majority of the screened population does not derive any benefit and possibly incurs a slight risk from false-positive results. A small subset of patients, however, will benefit greatly from being screened. For example, Pap smears do not benefit the 98% of women who never develop cancer of the cervix. However, for the 2% who would develop localized cervical cancer, Pap smears may add as much as 25 years to their lives. Some studies suggest that a 1-month gain of life expectancy is a reasonable goal for a population-based preventive strategy.

The U.S. Preventive Services Task Force (USPSTF) provides recommendations for evidence-based screening (Table 4-3).

TABLE 4-2 Estimated Average Increase in Life Expectancy for a Population

Screening Procedure	Average Increase
Mammography:	
Women, 40–50 years	0–5 days
Women, 50–70 years	1 month
Pap smears, age 18–65	2–3 months
Screening treadmill for a 50-year-old (asymptomatic) man	8 days
PSA and digital rectal exam for a man >50 years	Up to 2 weeks
Getting a 35-year-old smoker to quit	3–5 years
Beginning regular exercise for a 40-year-old man (30 min 3 times a week)	9 months–2 years

Abbreviation: PSA, prostate-specific antigen.

TABLE 4-3 Clinical Preventive Services for Normal-Risk Adults Recommended by the U.S. Preventive Services Task Force

Test or Disorder	Population,[a] Years	Frequency	Chapter Reference
Blood pressure, height and weight	>18	Periodically	77
Cholesterol	Men >35	Every 5 years	241
	Women >45	Every 5 years	
Depression	>18	Periodically[b]	
Diabetes	>45 or earlier, if there are additional risk factors	Every 3 years	344
Pap smear[c]	Within 3 years of onset of sexual activity or 21–65	Every 1–3 years	82
Chlamydia	Women 18–24	Every 1–2 years	176
Mammography[a]	Women >50	Every 2 years	82, 90
Colorectal cancer[a]	>50		82, 91
fecal occult blood and/or		Every year	
sigmoidoscopy or		Every 5 years	
colonoscopy		Every 10 years	
Osteoporosis	Women >65; >60 at risk	Periodically	354
Abdominal aortic aneurysm (ultrasound)	Men 65–75 who have ever smoked	Once	
Alcohol use	>18	Periodically	392
Vision, hearing	>65	Periodically	28, 30
Adult immunization			122, 123
Tetanus-diphtheria (Td)	>18	Every 10 years	
Varicella (VZV)	Susceptibles only, >18	Two doses	
Measles mumps rubella (MMR)	Women, childbearing age	One dose	
Pneumococcal	>65	One dose	
Influenza	>50	Yearly	
Human papillomavirus (HPV)	Up to age 26	If not done prior	

[a]Screening is performed earlier and more frequently when there is a strong family history. Randomized, controlled trials have documented that fecal occult blood testing (FOBT) confers a 15–30% reduction in colon cancer mortality. Although large randomized trials have not been performed for sigmoidoscopy or colonoscopy, well-designed case-control studies suggest similar or greater efficacy relative to FOBT.

[b]If staff support are available.

[c]In the future, Pap smear frequency may be influenced by HPV testing and the HPV vaccine.

Note: Prostate-specific antigen (PSA) testing is capable of enhancing the detection of early-stage prostate cancer, but evidence is inconclusive that it improves health outcomes. PSA testing is recommended by several professional organizations and is widely used in clinical practice, but it is not currently recommended by the U.S. Preventive Services Task Force (Chap. 85).

Source: Adapted from the U.S. Preventive Services Task Force, *Guide to Clinical Prevention Services*, 2009. *http://www.ahrq.gov/clinic/uspstfix.htm.*

In addition to these population-based guidelines, it is reasonable to consider family and social history to identify individuals with special risk (*www.ahrq.gov/clinic/uspstfix.htm*). For example, when there is a significant family history of breast, colon, or prostate cancer, it is prudent to initiate screening about 10 years before the age at which the youngest family member developed cancer. Screening also should be considered for many other common disorders pending the development of further evidence. Three examples are screening for diabetes (using fasting blood glucose), domestic violence, and coronary artery disease in intermediate-risk asymptomatic individuals.

Cost-effectiveness

Screening techniques must be cost-effective if they are to be applied to large populations. Costs include not only the expense of testing but also time away from work, downstream costs from false-positive results, and other potential risks. When the risk-versus-benefit ratio is less favorable, it is useful to provide information to patients and factor their perspectives into the decision-making process. For example, many expert groups, including the USPSTF, recommend an individualized discussion about prostate cancer screening, as the decision-making process is complex and relies heavily on personal issues. Although the early detection of prostate cancer may seem desirable intuitively, risks include false-positive results that can lead to anxiety and unnecessary surgery. Randomized trials for prostate cancer screening have yielded mixed and relatively modest results. Potential complications from surgery and radiation treatment include erectile dysfunction, urinary incontinence, and bowel dysfunction. Some men may decline screening, whereas others may be more willing to accept the risks of an early-detection strategy. Another example of shared decision-making involves the choice of techniques for colon cancer screening (Chap. 82). In controlled studies, the use of annual FOBT reduces colon cancer deaths by 15–30%. Flexible sigmoidoscopy reduces colon cancer deaths by ~60%. Colonoscopy offers the same benefit as or greater benefit than flexible sigmoidoscopy, but its use incurs additional costs and risks. These screening procedures have not been compared directly in the same population, but the estimated cost to society is similar: $10,000–25,000 per year of life saved. Thus, although one patient may prefer the ease of preparation, less time disruption, and the lower risk of flexible sigmoidoscopy, others may prefer the sedation and thoroughness of colonoscopy.

In considering the impact of screening tests, it is important to recognize that tobacco and alcohol use, diet, and exercise constitute the vast majority of factors that influence preventable deaths in developed countries. Perhaps the single greatest preventive health care measure is to help patients quit smoking (Chap. 395).

■ COMMONLY ENCOUNTERED ISSUES

Despite compelling evidence that prevention strategies can have major health care benefits, implementation of these services is challenging because of competing demands on physician and patient time and because of gaps in health care reimbursement. Moreover, efforts to reduce disease risk frequently involve behavior changes (e.g., weight loss, exercise, seat belts) or the management of addictive conditions (e.g., tobacco and alcohol use) that are often recalcitrant to intervention. Public education and economic incentives are often useful, in addition to counseling by health care providers (Table 4-4).

A number of techniques can assist physicians with the growing number of recommended screening tests. An appropriately configured electronic health record can provide reminder systems that make it easier for physicians to track and meet guidelines. Some systems give patients secure access to their medical records, providing an additional means to enhance adherence to routine

TABLE 4-4 Counseling to Prevent Disease

Topic	Chapter Reference
Tobacco cessation	395
Drug and alcohol use	392, 393
Nutrition to maintain caloric balance and vitamin intake	73
Calcium intake in women >18 years	354
Folic acid: Women of childbearing age	74
Oral health	32
Aspirin use to prevent cardiovascular disease in selected men >45 years and women >55 years	241
Chemoprevention of breast cancer in women at high risk	90
STDs and HIV prevention	130, 189
Physical activity	
Sun exposure	56
Injury prevention (loaded handgun, seat belts, bicycle helmet)	
Issues in the elderly	9
Polypharmacy	
Fall prevention	
Hot water heater <120°	
Vision, hearing, dental evaluations	
Immunizations (pneumococcal, influenza)	

Abbreviation: STDs, sexually transmitted diseases.

screening. Systems that provide nurses and other staff with standing orders are effective for smoking prevention and immunizations. The Agency for Healthcare Research and Quality and the Centers for Disease Control and Prevention have developed flow sheets and electronic tools as part of their "Put Prevention into Practice" program (*http://www.ahcpr.gov/clinic/ppipix.htm*). Age-specific recommendations for screening and counseling are summarized in Table 4-5.

A routine health care examination should be performed every 1–3 years before age 50 and every year thereafter. History should include medication use (prescription and nonprescription), allergies, dietary history, use of alcohol and tobacco, sexual practices, and a thorough family history, if not obtained previously. Routine measurements should include assessments of height, weight (body mass index), and blood pressure, in addition to the relevant physical examination. The increasing incidence of skin cancer underscores the importance of screening for suspicious skin lesions. Hearing and vision should be tested after age 65, or earlier if the patient describes difficulties. Other sex- and age-specific examinations are listed in Table 4-3. Counseling and instruction about self-examination (e.g., skin, breast "awareness") can be provided during the routine examination.

Many patients see a physician for ongoing care of chronic illnesses, and this visit provides an opportunity to include a "measure of prevention" for other health problems. For example, a patient seen for management of hypertension or diabetes can have breast cancer screening incorporated into one visit and a discussion about colon cancer screening at the next visit. Other patients may respond more favorably to a clearly defined visit that addresses all relevant screening and prevention interventions. Because of age or comorbidities, it may be appropriate with some patients

TABLE 4-5 Age-Specific Causes of Mortality and Corresponding Preventive Options

Age Group	Leading Causes of Age-Specific Mortality	Screening Prevention Interventions to Consider for Each Specific Population
15–24	1. Accident 2. Homicide 3. Suicide 4. Malignancy 5. Heart disease	• Counseling on routine seat belt use, bicycle/motorcycle/ATV helmets (1) • Counseling on diet and exercise (5) • Discuss dangers of alcohol use while driving, swimming, boating (1) • Ask about vaccination status (tetanus, diphtheria, hepatitis B, MMR, rubella, varicella, meningitis, HPV) • Ask about gun use and/or gun possession (2,3) • Assess for substance abuse history including alcohol (2,3) • Screen for domestic violence (2,3) • Screen for depression and/or suicidal/homicidal ideation (2,3) • Pap smear for cervical cancer screening, discuss STD prevention (4) • Discuss skin, breast awareness, and testicular self-exams (4) • Recommend UV light avoidance and regular sunscreen use (4) • Measurement of blood pressure, height, weight, and body mass index (5) • Discuss health risks of tobacco use, consider emphasis on cosmetic and economic issues to improve quit rates for younger smokers (4,5) • *Chlamydia* screening and contraceptive counseling for sexually active females • HIV, hepatitis B, and syphilis testing if there is high-risk sexual behavior(s) or any prior history of sexually transmitted disease
25–44	1. Accident 2. Malignancy 3. Heart disease 4. Suicide 5. Homicide 6. HIV	*As above plus consider the following:* • Readdress smoking status, encourage cessation at every visit (2,3) • Obtain detailed family history of malignancies and begin early screening/prevention program if patient is at significant increased risk (2) • Assess all cardiac risk factors (including screening for diabetes and hyperlipidemia) and consider primary prevention with aspirin for patients at >3% 5-year risk of a vascular event (3) • Assess for chronic alcohol abuse, risk factors for viral hepatitis, or other risks for development of chronic liver disease • Consider individualized breast cancer screening with mammography at age 40 (2)
45–64	1. Malignancy 2. Heart disease 3. Accident 4. Diabetes mellitus 5. Cerebrovascular disease 6. Chronic lower respiratory disease 7. Chronic liver disease and cirrhosis 8. Suicide	• Consider prostate cancer screen with annual PSA and digital rectal exam at age 50 (or possibly earlier in African Americans or patients with family history) (1) • Begin colorectal cancer screening at age 50 with fecal occult blood testing, flexible sigmoidoscopy, or colonoscopy (1) • Reassess vaccination status at age 50 and give special consideration to vaccines against *Streptococcus pneumoniae*, influenza, tetanus, and viral hepatitis • Consider screening for coronary disease in higher-risk patients (2,5)
≥65	1. Heart disease 2. Malignancy 3. Cerebrovascular disease 4. Chronic lower respiratory disease 5. Alzheimer's disease 6. Influenza and pneumonia 7. Diabetes mellitus 8. Kidney disease 9. Accidents 10. Septicemia	*As above plus consider the following:* • Readdress smoking status, encourage cessation at every visit (1,2,3,4) • One-time ultrasound for AAA in men 65–75 who have ever smoked • Consider pulmonary function testing for all long-term smokers to assess for development of chronic obstructive pulmonary disease (4,6) • Vaccinate all smokers against influenza and *S. pneumoniae* at age 50 (6) • Screen all postmenopausal women (and all men with risk factors) for osteoporosis • Reassess vaccination status at age 65, emphasis on influenza and *S. pneumoniae* (4,6) • Screen for dementia and depression (5) • Screen for visual and hearing problems, home safety issues, and elder abuse (9)

Note: The numbers in parentheses refer to areas of risk in the mortality column affected by the specified intervention.

Abbreviations: AAA, abdominal aortic aneurysm. ATV, all-terrain vehicle; HPV, human papillomavirus; MMR, measles-mumps-rubella; PSA, prostate-specific antigen; STD, sexually transmitted disease; UV, ultraviolet.

to abandon certain screening and prevention activities, although there are fewer data about when to "sunset" these services. The risk of certain cancers, such as cancer of the cervix, ultimately declines, and it is reasonable to cease Pap smears after about age 65 if recent Pap smears have been negative. For breast, colon, and prostate cancer, it is reasonable to reevaluate the need for screening after about age 75. For some older patients with advanced diseases such as severe chronic obstructive pulmonary disease and congestive heart failure and for those who are immobile, the benefit of some screening procedures is low, and other priorities emerge when life expectancy is <10 years. This shift in focus needs to be done tactfully and allows greater focus on the conditions likely to affect quality and length of life.

ACKNOWLEDGMENTS

The author is grateful to Dan Evans, MD, for contributions to this topic in Harrison's Manual of Medicine.

FURTHER READINGS

BARRY MJ: Screening for prostate cancer—the controversy that refuses to die. N Engl J Med 360:1351, 2009

FENTON JJ et al: Delivery of cancer screening: How important is the preventive health examination? Arch Intern Med 167:580, 2007

GREENLAND P et al: Coronary artery calcium score combined with Framingham score for risk prediction in asymptomatic individuals. JAMA 291:210, 2004

KERLIKOWSKE K: Evidence-based breast cancer prevention: The importance of individualized risk. Ann Intern Med 151:750, 2009

RANSOHOFF DF, SANDLER RS: Clinical practice: Screening for colorectal cancer. N Engl J Med 346:40, 2002

U.S. PREVENTIVE SERVICES TASK FORCE: The guide to clinical preventive services, 2009. Agency for Healthcare Research and Quality, Rockville, MD, March 2009. Available at *http://www. ahrq.gov/clinic/pocketgd.htm*

CHAPTER 5

Principles of Clinical Pharmacology

Dan M. Roden

Drugs are the cornerstone of modern therapeutics. Nevertheless, it is well recognized among physicians and in the lay community that the outcome of drug therapy varies widely among individuals. While this variability has been perceived as an unpredictable, and therefore inevitable, accompaniment of drug therapy, this is not the case. The goal of this chapter is to describe the principles of clinical pharmacology that can be used for the safe and optimal use of available and new drugs.

Drugs interact with specific target molecules to produce their beneficial and adverse effects. The chain of events between administration of a drug and production of these effects in the body can be divided into two components, both of which contribute to variability in drug actions. The first component comprises the processes that determine drug delivery to, and removal from, molecular targets. The resulting description of the relationship between drug concentration and time is termed *pharmacokinetics*. The second component of variability in drug action comprises the processes that determine variability in drug actions despite equivalent drug delivery to effector drug sites. This description of the relationship between drug concentration and effect is termed *pharmacodynamics*. As discussed further below, pharmacodynamic variability can arise as a result of variability in function of the target molecule itself or of variability in the broad biologic context in which the drug-target interaction occurs to achieve drug effects.

Two important goals of the discipline of clinical pharmacology are (1) to provide a description of conditions under which drug actions vary among human subjects; and (2) to determine mechanisms underlying this variability, with the goal of improving therapy with available drugs as well as pointing to new drug mechanisms that may be effective in the treatment of human disease. The first steps in the discipline were empirical descriptions of the influence of disease X on drug action Y or of individuals or families with unusual sensitivities to adverse drug effects. These important descriptive findings are now being replaced by an understanding of the molecular mechanisms underlying variability in drug actions. Thus, the effects of disease, drug coadministration, or familial factors in modulating drug action can now be reinterpreted as variability in expression or function of specific genes whose products determine pharmacokinetics and pharmacodynamics. Nevertheless, it is often the personal interaction of the patient with the physician or other health care provider that first identifies unusual variability in drug actions; maintained alertness to unusual drug responses continues to be a key component of improving drug safety.

Unusual drug responses, segregating in families, have been recognized for decades and initially defined the field of *pharmacogenetics*. Now, with an increasing appreciation of common polymorphisms across the human genome, comes the opportunity to reinterpret descriptive mechanisms of variability in drug action as a consequence of specific DNA variants, or sets of variants, among individuals. This approach defines the field of *pharmacogenomics*, which may hold the opportunity of allowing practitioners to integrate a molecular understanding of the basis of disease with an individual's genomic makeup to prescribe personalized, highly effective, and safe therapies.

■ INDICATIONS FOR DRUG THERAPY: RISK VERSUS BENEFIT

It is self-evident that the benefits of drug therapy should outweigh the risks. Benefits fall into two broad categories: those designed to alleviate a symptom and those designed to prolong useful life. An increasing emphasis on the principles of evidence-based medicine and techniques such as large clinical trials and meta-analyses have defined benefits of drug therapy in broad patient populations. Establishing the balance between risk and benefit is not always simple. An increasing body of evidence supports the idea, with which practitioners are very familiar, that individual patients may display responses that are not expected from large population studies and often have comorbidities that typically exclude them from large clinical trials. In addition, therapies that provide symptomatic benefits but shorten life may be entertained in patients with serious and highly symptomatic diseases such as heart failure or cancer. These considerations illustrate the continuing, highly personal nature of the relationship between the prescriber and the patient.

Some adverse effects are so common and so readily associated with drug therapy that they are identified very early during clinical use of a drug. By contrast, serious adverse effects may be sufficiently uncommon that they escape detection for many years after a drug begins to be widely used. The issue of how to identify rare but serious

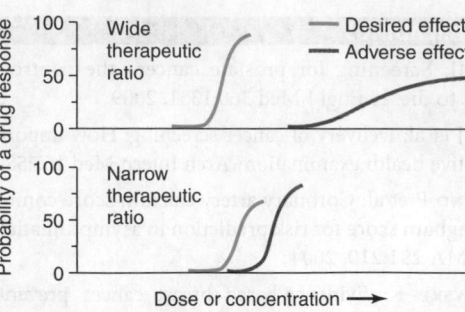

Figure 5-1 The concept of a therapeutic ratio. Each panel illustrates the relationship between increasing dose and cumulative probability of a desired or adverse drug effect. *Top.* A drug with a wide therapeutic ratio, i.e., a wide separation of the two curves. *Bottom.* A drug with a narrow therapeutic ratio; here, the likelihood of adverse effects at therapeutic doses is increased because the curves are not well separated. Further, a steep dose-response curve for adverse effects is especially undesirable, as it implies that even small dosage increments may sharply increase the likelihood of toxicity. When there is a definable relationship between drug concentration (usually measured in plasma) and desirable and adverse effect curves, concentration may be substituted on the abscissa. Note that not all patients necessarily demonstrate a therapeutic response (or adverse effect) at any dose, and that some effects (notably some adverse effects) may occur in a dose-independent fashion.

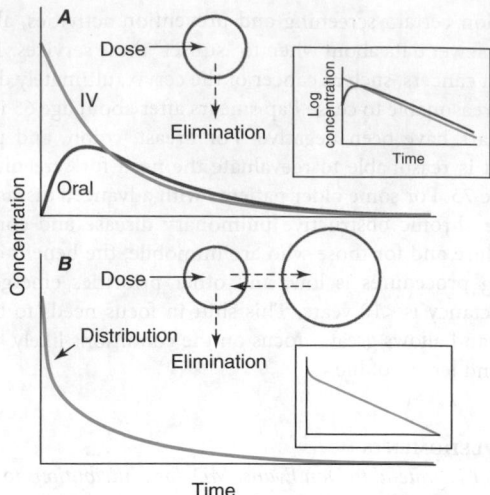

Figure 5-2 Idealized time-plasma concentration curves after a single dose of drug. A. The time course of drug concentration after an instantaneous IV bolus or an oral dose in the one-compartment model shown. The area under the time-concentration curve is clearly less with the oral drug than the IV, indicating incomplete bioavailability. Note that despite this incomplete bioavailability, concentration after the oral dose can be higher than after the IV dose at some time points. The inset shows that the decline of concentrations over time is linear on a log-linear plot, characteristic of first-order elimination, and that oral and IV drug have the same elimination (parallel) time course. **B.** The decline of central compartment concentration when drug is distributed both to and from a peripheral compartment and eliminated from the central compartment. The rapid initial decline of concentration reflects not drug elimination but distribution.

adverse effects (that can profoundly affect the benefit-risk perception in an individual patient) has not been satisfactorily resolved. Potential approaches range from an increased understanding of the molecular and genetic basis of variability in drug actions to expanded postmarketing surveillance mechanisms. None of these have been completely effective, so practitioners must be continuously vigilant to the possibility that unusual symptoms may be related to specific drugs, or combinations of drugs, that their patients receive.

Beneficial and adverse reactions to drug therapy can be described by a series of dose-response relations (Fig. 5-1). Well-tolerated drugs demonstrate a wide margin, termed the *therapeutic ratio*, *therapeutic index*, or *therapeutic window*, between the doses required to produce a therapeutic effect and those producing toxicity. In cases where there is a similar relationship between plasma drug concentration and effects, monitoring plasma concentrations can be a highly effective aid in managing drug therapy by enabling concentrations to be maintained above the minimum required to produce an effect and below the concentration range likely to produce toxicity. Such monitoring has been widely used to guide therapy with specific agents, such as certain antiarrhythmics, anticonvulsants, and antibiotics. Many of the principles in clinical pharmacology and examples outlined below, which can be applied broadly to therapeutics, have been developed in these arenas.

PRINCIPLES OF PHARMACOKINETICS

The processes of absorption, distribution, metabolism, and excretion—collectively termed *drug disposition*—determine the concentration of drug delivered to target effector molecules.

■ ABSORPTION

Bioavailability

When a drug is administered orally, subcutaneously, intramuscularly, rectally, sublingually, or directly into desired sites of action, the amount of drug actually entering the systemic circulation may be less than with the intravenous route (Fig. 5-2A). The fraction of drug available to the systemic circulation by other routes is termed *bioavailability*. Bioavailability may be <100% for two reasons:

(1) absorption is reduced, or (2) the drug undergoes metabolism or elimination prior to entering the systemic circulation.

When a drug is administered by a nonintravenous route, the peak concentration occurs later and is lower than after the same dose given by rapid intravenous injection, reflecting absorption from the site of administration (Fig. 5-2). The extent of absorption may be reduced because a drug is incompletely released from its dosage form, undergoes destruction at its site of administration, or has physicochemical properties such as insolubility that prevent complete absorption from its site of administration. Slow absorption rates are deliberately designed into "slow-release" or "sustained-release" drug formulations in order to minimize variation in plasma concentrations during the interval between doses.

"First-pass" effect

When a drug is administered orally, it must traverse the intestinal epithelium, the portal venous system, and the liver prior to entering the systemic circulation (Fig. 5-3). Once a drug enters the enterocyte, it may undergo metabolism, be transported into the portal vein, or undergo excretion back into the intestinal lumen. Both excretion into the intestinal lumen and metabolism decrease systemic bioavailability. Once a drug passes this enterocyte barrier, it may also be taken up into the hepatocyte, where bioavailability can be further limited by metabolism or excretion into the bile. This elimination in intestine and liver, which reduces the amount of drug delivered to the systemic circulation, is termed *presystemic elimination*, *presystemic extraction*, or *first-pass elimination*.

Drug movement across the membrane of any cell, including enterocytes and hepatocytes, is a combination of passive diffusion and active transport, mediated by specific drug uptake and efflux molecules. The drug transport molecule that has been most widely studied is P-glycoprotein, the product of the normal expression of the *MDR1* gene. P-glycoprotein is expressed on the apical aspect of the enterocyte

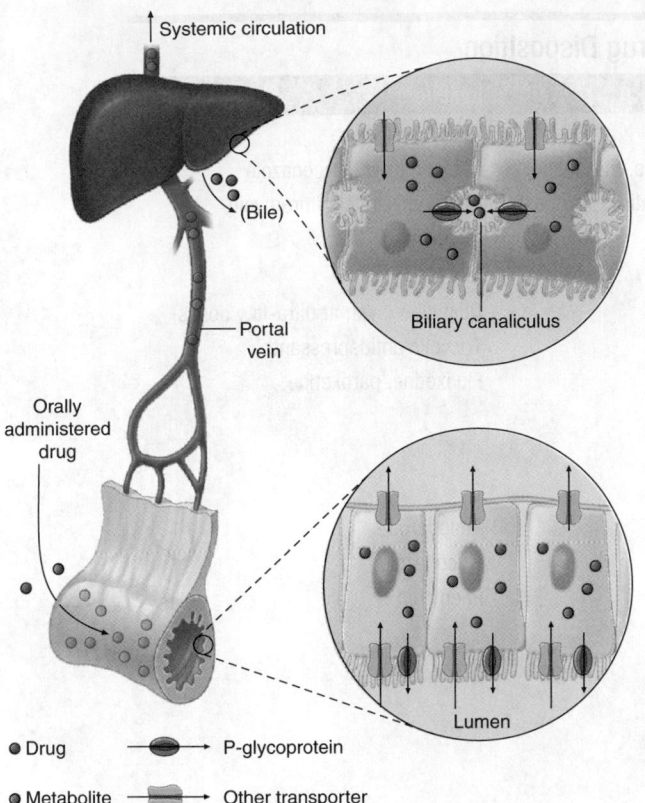

● Drug ⬭➞ P-glycoprotein

● Metabolite ➞ Other transporter

Figure 5-3 Mechanism of presystemic clearance. After drug enters the enterocyte, it can undergo metabolism, excretion into the intestinal lumen, or transport into the portal vein. Similarly, the hepatocyte may accomplish metabolism and biliary excretion prior to the entry of drug and metabolites to the systemic circulation. *[Adapted by permission from DM Roden, in DP Zipes, J Jalife (eds): Cardiac Electrophysiology: From Cell to Bedside, 4th ed. Philadelphia, Saunders, 2003. Copyright 2003 with permission from Elsevier.]*

and on the canalicular aspect of the hepatocyte (Fig. 5-3); in both locations, it serves as an efflux pump, thus limiting availability of drug to the systemic circulation. P-glycoprotein is also an important component of the blood-brain barrier, discussed further below.

Drug metabolism generates compounds that are usually more polar and, hence, more readily excreted than parent drug. Metabolism takes place predominantly in the liver but can occur at other sites such as kidney, intestinal epithelium, lung, and plasma. "Phase I" metabolism involves chemical modification, most often oxidation accomplished by members of the cytochrome P450 (CYP) monooxygenase superfamily. CYPs that are especially important for drug metabolism (Table 5-1) include CYP3A4, CYP3A5, CYP2D6, CYP2C9, CYP2C19, CYP1A2, and CYP2E1, and each drug may be a substrate for one or more of these enzymes. "Phase II" metabolism involves conjugation of specific endogenous compounds to drugs or their metabolites. The enzymes that accomplish phase II reactions include glucuronyl-, acetyl-, sulfo-, and methyltransferases. Drug metabolites may exert important pharmacologic activity, as discussed further below.

Clinical implications of altered bioavailability

Some drugs undergo near-complete presystemic metabolism and, thus, cannot be administered orally. Nitroglycerin cannot be used orally because it is completely extracted prior to reaching the systemic circulation. The drug is, therefore, used by the sublingual or transdermal routes, which bypass presystemic metabolism.

Some drugs with very extensive presystemic metabolism can still be administered by the oral route, using much higher doses than those required intravenously. Thus, a typical intravenous dose of verapamil

is 1–5 mg, compared to the usual single oral dose of 40–120 mg. Administration of low-dose aspirin can result in exposure of cyclooxygenase in platelets in the portal vein to the drug, but systemic sparing because of first-pass aspirin deacylation in the liver. This is an example of presystemic metabolism being exploited to therapeutic advantage.

■ DISTRIBUTION AND ELIMINATION

Most pharmacokinetic processes are first-order; that is, the rate of the process depends on the amount of drug present. Clinically important exceptions are discussed below (see "Principles of Dose Selection"). In the simplest pharmacokinetic model (Fig. 5-2*A*), a drug bolus (D) is administered instantaneously to a central compartment, from which drug elimination occurs as a first-order process. Occasionally, central and other compartments correspond to physiologic spaces (e.g., plasma volume), whereas in others they are simply mathematical functions used to describe drug disposition. The first-order nature of drug elimination leads directly to the relationship describing drug concentration (*C*) at any time (*t*) following the bolus:

$$C = \frac{D}{V_c} \cdot e^{(-0.69t/t_{1/2})}$$

where V_c is the volume of the compartment into which drug is delivered and $t_{1/2}$ is elimination half-life. As a consequence of this relationship, a plot of the logarithm of concentration vs time is a straight line (Fig. 5-2*A*, inset). *Half-life* is the time required for 50% of a first-order process to be complete. Thus, 50% of drug elimination is achieved after one drug-elimination half-life, 75% after two, 87.5% after three, etc. In practice, first-order processes such as elimination are near-complete after four–five half-lives.

In some cases, drug is removed from the central compartment not only by elimination but also by distribution into peripheral compartments. In this case, the plot of plasma concentration vs time after a bolus may demonstrate two (or more) exponential components (Fig. 5-2*B*). In general, the initial rapid drop in drug concentration represents not elimination but drug distribution into and out of peripheral tissues (also first-order processes), while the slower component represents drug elimination; the initial precipitous decline is usually evident with administration by intravenous but not other routes. Drug concentrations at peripheral sites are determined by a balance between drug distribution to and redistribution from those sites, as well as by elimination. Once distribution is near-complete (four–five distribution half-lives), plasma and tissue concentrations decline in parallel.

Clinical implications of half-life measurements

The elimination half-life not only determines the time required for drug concentrations to fall to near-immeasurable levels after a single bolus, it is also the key determinant of the time required for steady-state plasma concentrations to be achieved after any change in drug dosing (Fig. 5-4). This applies to the initiation of chronic drug therapy (whether by multiple oral doses or by continuous intravenous infusion), a change in chronic drug dose or dosing interval, or discontinuation of drug.

Steady state describes the situation during chronic drug administration when the amount of drug administered per unit time equals drug eliminated per unit time. With a continuous intravenous infusion, plasma concentrations at steady state are stable, while with chronic oral drug administration, plasma concentrations vary during the dosing interval but the time-concentration profile between dosing intervals is stable (Fig. 5-4).

■ DRUG DISTRIBUTION

In a typical 70-kg human, plasma volume is ~3 L, blood volume is ~5.5 L, and extracellular water outside the vasculature is ~20 L.

TABLE 5-1 Molecular Pathways Mediating Drug Disposition

Molecule	Substrates[a]	Inhibitors[a]
CYP3A	Calcium channel blockers	Amiodarone
	Antiarrhythmics (lidocaine, quinidine, mexiletine)	Ketoconazole, itraconazole
	HMG-CoA reductase inhibitors ("statins"; see text)	Erythromycin, clarithromycin
	Cyclosporine, tacrolimus	Ritonavir
	Indinavir, saquinavir, ritonavir	
CYP2D6[b]	Timolol, metoprolol, carvedilol	Quinidine (even at ultra-low doses)
	Phenformin	Tricyclic antidepressants
	Codeine	Fluoxetine, paroxetine
	Propafenone, flecainide	
	Tricyclic antidepressants	
	Fluoxetine, paroxetine	
CYP2C9[b]	Warfarin	Amiodarone
	Phenytoin	Fluconazole
	Glipizide	Phenytoin
	Losartan	
CYP2C19[b]	Omeprazole	Omeprazole
	Mephenytoin	
	Clopidogrel	
Thiopurine S-methyltransferase[b]	6-Mercaptopurine, azathioprine	
N-acetyltransferase[b]	Isoniazid	
	Procainamide	
	Hydralazine	
	Some sulfonamides	
UGT1A1[b]	Irinotecan	
Pseudocholinesterase[b]	Succinylcholine	
P-glycoprotein	Digoxin	Quinidine
	HIV protease inhibitors	Amiodarone
	Many CYP3A substrates	Verapamil
		Cyclosporine
		Itraconazole
		Erythromycin

[a]Inhibitors affect the molecular pathway, and thus may affect substrate.

[b]Clinically important genetic variants described; see Table 5-2.

Note: A listing of CYP substrates, inhibitors, and inducers is maintained at *http://medicine.iupui.edu/flockhart/table.htm.*

The volume of distribution of drugs extensively bound to plasma proteins but not to tissue components approaches plasma volume; warfarin is one such example. By contrast, for drugs highly bound to tissues, the volume of distribution can be far greater than any physiologic space. For example, the volume of distribution of digoxin and tricyclic antidepressants is hundreds of liters, obviously exceeding total-body volume. Such drugs are not readily removed by dialysis, an important consideration in overdose.

Clinical implications of drug distribution

In some cases, pharmacologic effects require drug distribution to peripheral sites. In this instance, the time course of drug delivery to and removal from these sites determines the time course of drug effects. Digoxin accesses its cardiac site of action slowly, over a distribution phase of several hours. Thus, after an intravenous dose, plasma levels fall, but those at the site of action increase over hours. Only when

distribution is near-complete does the concentration of digoxin in plasma reflect the pharmacologic effect. For this reason, there should be a 6–8 h wait after administration before plasma levels of digoxin are measured as a guide to therapy. Similarly, anesthetic drug penetration into and removal from the central nervous system (CNS) determines the time course of anesthesia.

Animal models have suggested, and clinical studies are confirming, that limited drug penetration into the brain, the "blood-brain barrier," often represents a robust P-glycoprotein–mediated efflux process from capillary endothelial cells in the cerebral circulation. Thus, drug distribution into the brain may be modulated by changes in P-glycoprotein function.

Loading doses For some drugs, the indication may be so urgent that administration of "loading" dosages is required to achieve rapid elevations of drug concentration and therapeutic effects earlier than with chronic maintenance therapy (Fig. 5-4). Nevertheless, the time

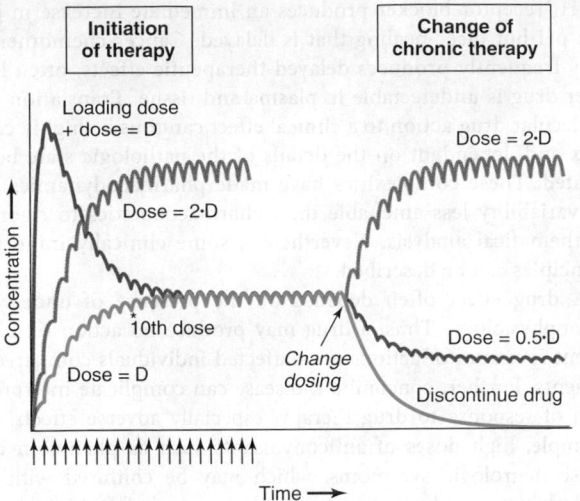

Figure 5-4 Drug accumulation to steady state. In this simulation, drug was administered (arrows) at intervals = 50% of the elimination half-life. Steady state is achieved during initiation of therapy after ~5 elimination half-lives, or 10 doses. A loading dose did not alter the eventual steady state achieved. A doubling of the dose resulted in a doubling of the steady state but the same time course of accumulation. Once steady state is achieved, a change in dose (increase, decrease, or drug discontinuation) results in a new steady state in ~5 elimination half-lives. *[Adapted by permission from DM Roden, in DP Zipes, J Jalife (eds): Cardiac Electrophysiology: From Cell to Bedside, 4th ed. Philadelphia, Saunders, 2003. Copyright 2003 with permission from Elsevier.]*

required for true steady state to be achieved is still determined only by the elimination half-life.

Disease can alter loading requirements: in congestive heart failure, the central volume of distribution of lidocaine is reduced. Therefore, lower-than-normal loading regimens are required to achieve equivalent plasma drug concentrations and to avoid toxicity.

Rate of intravenous administration Although the simulations in Fig. 5-2 use a single intravenous bolus, this is very rarely appropriate in practice because side effects related to transiently very high concentrations can result. Rather, drugs are more usually administered orally or as a slower intravenous infusion. Some drugs are so predictably lethal when infused too rapidly that special precautions should be taken to prevent accidental boluses. For example, solutions of potassium for intravenous administration >20 meq/L should be avoided in all but the most exceptional and carefully monitored circumstances. This minimizes the possibility of cardiac arrest due to accidental increases in infusion rates of more concentrated solutions.

While excessively rapid intravenous drug administration can lead to catastrophic consequences, transiently high drug concentrations after intravenous administration can occasionally be used to advantage. The use of midazolam for intravenous sedation, for example, depends upon its rapid uptake by the brain during the distribution phase to produce sedation quickly, with subsequent egress from the brain during the redistribution of the drug as equilibrium is achieved.

Similarly, adenosine must be administered as a rapid bolus in the treatment of reentrant supraventricular tachycardias (Chap. 233) to prevent elimination by very rapid ($t_{1/2}$ of seconds) uptake into erythrocytes and endothelial cells before the drug can reach its clinical site of action, the atrioventricular node.

■ PLASMA PROTEIN BINDING

Many drugs circulate in the plasma partly bound to plasma proteins. Since only unbound (free) drug can distribute to sites of

pharmacologic action, drug response is related to the free rather than the total circulating plasma drug concentration.

Clinical implications of altered protein binding

For drugs that are normally highly bound to plasma proteins (>90%), small changes in the extent of binding (e.g., due to disease) can produce a large change in the amount of unbound drug, and hence drug effect. The acute-phase reactant α_1-acid glycoprotein binds to basic drugs, such as lidocaine or quinidine, and is increased in a range of common conditions, including myocardial infarction, surgery, neoplastic disease, rheumatoid arthritis, and burns. This increased binding can lead to reduced pharmacologic effects at therapeutic concentrations of total drug. Conversely, conditions such as hypoalbuminemia, liver disease, and renal disease can decrease the extent of drug binding, particularly of acidic and neutral drugs, such as phenytoin. Here, plasma concentration of free drug is increased, so drug efficacy and toxicity are enhanced if total (free + bound) drug concentration is used to monitor therapy.

■ CLEARANCE

Drug elimination reduces the amount of drug in the body over time. An important approach to quantifying this reduction is to consider that drug concentration at the beginning and end of a time period are unchanged and that a specific volume of the body has been "cleared" of the drug during that time period. This defines clearance as volume/time. Clearance includes both drug metabolism and excretion.

Clinical implications of altered clearance

While elimination half-life determines the time required to achieve steady-state plasma concentrations (C_{ss}), the *magnitude* of that steady state is determined by clearance (Cl) and dose alone. For a drug administered as an intravenous infusion, this relationship is:

$$C_{ss} = \text{dosing rate}/Cl \qquad \text{or} \qquad \text{dosing rate} = Cl \cdot C_{ss}$$

When drug is administered orally, the average plasma concentration within a dosing interval ($C_{avg,ss}$) replaces C_{ss}, and the dosage (dose per unit time) must be increased if bioavailability (F) is less than 1:

$$\text{Dose/time} = Cl \cdot C_{avg,ss} / F$$

Genetic variants, drug interactions, or diseases that reduce the activity of drug-metabolizing enzymes or excretory mechanisms may lead to decreased clearance and, hence, a requirement for downward dose adjustment to avoid toxicity. Conversely, some drug interactions and genetic variants increase the function of drug elimination pathways, and, hence, increased drug dosage may be necessary to maintain a therapeutic effect.

■ ACTIVE DRUG METABOLITES

From an evolutionary point of view, drug metabolism may have developed as a defense against noxious xenobiotics (foreign substances, e.g., from plants) to which our ancestors inadvertently exposed themselves. The organization of the drug uptake and efflux pumps and the location of drug metabolism in the intestine and liver prior to drug entry to the systemic circulation (Fig. 5-3) support this idea of a primitive protective function.

However, drug metabolites are not necessarily pharmacologically inactive. Metabolites may produce effects similar to, overlapping with, or distinct from those of the parent drug. For example, *N*-acetylprocainamide (NAPA) is a major metabolite of the antiarrhythmic procainamide. While it exerts antiarrhythmic effects, its electrophysiologic properties differ from those of the parent drug. Indeed, NAPA accumulation is the usual explanation for marked QT prolongation and torsades des pointes ventricular tachycardia (Chap. 233) during therapy with procainamide. Thus, the common laboratory practice of adding procainamide to NAPA concentrations to estimate a total therapeutic effect is inappropriate.

Prodrugs are inactive compounds that require metabolism to generate active metabolites that mediate the drug effects. Examples include many angiotensin-converting enzyme (ACE) inhibitors, the angiotensin receptor blocker losartan, the antineoplastic irinotecan, the anti-estrogen tamoxifen, the analgesic codeine (whose active metabolite morphine probably underlies the opioid effect during codeine administration), and the antiplatelet drug clopidogrel. Drug metabolism has also been implicated in bioactivation of procarcinogens and in generation of reactive metabolites that mediate certain adverse drug effects (e.g., acetaminophen hepatotoxicity, discussed below).

■ THE CONCEPT OF HIGH-RISK PHARMACOKINETICS

When plasma concentrations of active drug depend exclusively on a single metabolic pathway, any condition that inhibits that pathway (be it disease-related, genetic, or due to a drug interaction) can lead to dramatic changes in drug concentrations and marked variability in drug action. This problem of high-risk pharmacokinetics is especially pronounced in two settings. *First*, variability in bioactivation of a prodrug can lead to striking variability in drug action; examples include decreased CYP2D6 activity, which prevents analgesia by codeine, and decreased CYP2C19 activity, which reduces the antiplatelet effects of clopidogrel. The *second* setting is drug elimination that relies on a single pathway. In this case, inhibition of the elimination pathway leads to striking elevation of drug concentration. For drugs with a narrow therapeutic window, this leads to an increased likelihood of dose-related toxicity. An example is digoxin, whose elimination is dependent on P-glycoprotein; many drugs inhibit P-glycoprotein activity (amiodarone, quinidine, erythromycin, cyclosporine, itraconazole) and coadministration of these with digoxin reduces digoxin clearance, and increases toxicity unless maintenance doses are lowered. When drugs undergo elimination by multiple-drug metabolizing or excretory pathways, absence of one pathway (due to a genetic variant or drug interaction) is much less likely to have a large impact on drug concentrations or drug actions.

PRINCIPLES OF PHARMACODYNAMICS

Once a drug accesses a molecular site of action, it alters the function of that molecular target, with the ultimate result of a drug effect that the patient or health care provider can perceive. For drugs used in the urgent treatment of acute symptoms, little or no delay is anticipated (or desired) between the drug-target interaction and the development of a clinical effect. Examples of such acute situations include vascular thrombosis, shock, malignant hypertension, or status epilepticus.

For many conditions, however, the indication for therapy is less urgent, and a delay between the interaction of a drug with its pharmacologic target(s) and a clinical effect is clinically acceptable. Pharmacokinetic mechanisms that can contribute to such a delay include slow elimination (resulting in slow accumulation to steady state), uptake into peripheral compartments, or accumulation of active metabolites. Another common explanation for such a delay is that the clinical effect develops as a downstream consequence of the initial molecular effect the drug produces. Thus, administration of a proton-pump inhibitor or

an H_2-receptor blocker produces an immediate increase in gastric pH but ulcer healing that is delayed. Cancer chemotherapy very frequently produces delayed therapeutic effects, often long after drug is undetectable in plasma and tissue. Translation of a molecular drug action to a clinical effect can thus be highly complex and dependent on the details of the pathologic state being treated. These complexities have made pharmacodynamics and its variability less amenable than pharmacokinetics to rigorous mathematical analysis. Nevertheless, some clinically important principles can be described.

A drug effect often depends on the presence of underlying pathophysiology. Thus, a drug may produce no action or a different spectrum of actions in unaffected individuals compared to patients. Further, concomitant disease can complicate interpretation of response to drug therapy, especially adverse effects. For example, high doses of anticonvulsants such as phenytoin may cause neurologic symptoms, which may be confused with the underlying neurologic disease. Similarly, increasing dyspnea in a patient with chronic lung disease receiving amiodarone therapy could be due to drug, underlying disease, or an intercurrent cardiopulmonary problem. Thus, the presence of chronic lung disease may alter the risk-benefit ratio in a specific patient to argue against the use of amiodarone.

While drugs interact with specific molecular receptors, drug effects may vary over time, even if stable drug and metabolite concentrations are maintained. The drug-receptor interaction occurs in a complex biologic milieu that can vary to modulate the drug effect. For example, ion channel blockade by drugs, an important anticonvulsant and antiarrhythmic effect, is often modulated by membrane potential, itself a function of factors such as extracellular potassium or local ischemia. Receptors may be up- or downregulated by disease or by the drug itself. For example, β-adrenergic blockers upregulate β-receptor density during chronic therapy. While this effect does not usually result in resistance to the therapeutic effect of the drugs, it may produce severe agonist–mediated effects (such as hypertension or tachycardia) if the blocking drug is abruptly withdrawn.

PRINCIPLES OF DOSE SELECTION

The desired goal of therapy with any drug is to maximize the likelihood of a beneficial effect while minimizing the risk of adverse effects. Previous experience with the drug, in controlled clinical trials or in postmarketing use, defines the relationships between dose (or plasma concentration) and these dual effects and provides a starting point for initiation of drug therapy.

Figure 5-1 illustrates the relationships among dose, plasma concentrations, efficacy, and adverse effects and carries with it several important implications:

1. *The target drug effect should be defined when drug treatment is started.* With some drugs, the desired effect may be difficult to measure objectively, or the onset of efficacy can be delayed for weeks or months; drugs used in the treatment of cancer and psychiatric disease are examples. Sometimes a drug is used to treat a symptom, such as pain or palpitations, and here it is the patient who will report whether the selected dose is effective. In yet other settings, such as anticoagulation or hypertension, the desired response can be repeatedly and objectively assessed by simple clinical or laboratory tests.

2. *The nature of anticipated toxicity often dictates the starting dose.* If side effects are minor, it may be acceptable to start at a dose highly likely to achieve efficacy and downtitrate if side effects occur. However, this approach is rarely, if ever, justified if the anticipated toxicity is serious or life-threatening; in this

circumstance, it is more appropriate to initiate therapy with the lowest dose that may produce a desired effect.

3. *The above considerations do not apply if these relationships between dose and effects cannot be defined.* This is especially relevant to some adverse drug effects (discussed in further detail below) whose development are not readily related to drug dose.

4. *If a drug dose does not achieve its desired effect, a dosage increase is justified only if toxicity is absent and the likelihood of serious toxicity is small.* For example, some patients with seizures require plasma levels of phenytoin >20 μg/mL for optimal anticonvulsant activity. Dosages to achieve this effect may be appropriate, if tolerated. Conversely, clinical experience with flecainide suggests that high dosages (e.g., >400 mg/d) may be associated with an increased risk of sudden death; thus dosage increases beyond this limit are ordinarily not appropriate, even if a higher dosage might seem tolerated.

Other mechanisms that can lead to failure of drug effect should also be considered; drug interactions and noncompliance are common examples. These are situations in which measurement of plasma drug concentrations, if available, can be especially useful. Noncompliance is an especially frequent problem in the long-term treatment of diseases such as hypertension and epilepsy, occurring in ≥25% of patients in therapeutic environments in which no special effort is made to involve patients in the responsibility for their own health. Multidrug regimens with multiple doses per day are especially prone to noncompliance.

Monitoring response to therapy, by physiologic measures or by plasma concentration measurements, requires an understanding of the relationships between plasma concentration and anticipated effects. For example, measurement of QT interval is used during treatment with sotalol or dofetilide to avoid marked QT prolongation that can herald serious arrhythmias. In this setting, evaluating the electrocardiogram at the time of anticipated peak plasma concentration and effect (e.g., 1–2 h postdose at steady state) is most appropriate. Maintained high aminoglycoside levels carry a risk of nephrotoxicity, so dosages should be adjusted on the basis of plasma concentrations measured at trough (predose). On the other hand, ensuring aminoglycoside efficacy is accomplished by adjusting dosage so that peak drug concentrations are above a minimal antibacterial concentration. For dose adjustment of other drugs (e.g., anticonvulsants), concentration should be measured at its lowest during the dosing interval, just prior to a dose at steady state (Fig. 5-4), to ensure a maintained therapeutic effect.

■ **CONCENTRATION OF DRUGS IN PLASMA AS A GUIDE TO THERAPY**

Factors such as interactions with other drugs, disease-induced alterations in elimination and distribution, and genetic variation in drug

disposition combine to yield a wide range of plasma levels in patients given the same dose. Hence, if a predictable relationship can be established between plasma drug concentration and beneficial or adverse drug effect, measurement of plasma levels can provide a valuable tool to guide selection of an optimal dose. This is particularly true when there is a narrow range between the plasma levels yielding therapeutic and adverse effects, as with digoxin, theophylline, some antiarrhythmics, aminoglycosides, cyclosporine, and anticonvulsants. By contrast, if no such relationship can be established (e.g., if drug access to important sites of action outside plasma is highly variable), monitoring plasma concentration may not provide an accurate guide to therapy (Fig. 5-5A).

The common situation of first-order elimination implies that average, maximum, and minimum steady-state concentrations are related linearly to the dosing rate. Accordingly, the maintenance dose may be adjusted on the basis of the ratio between the

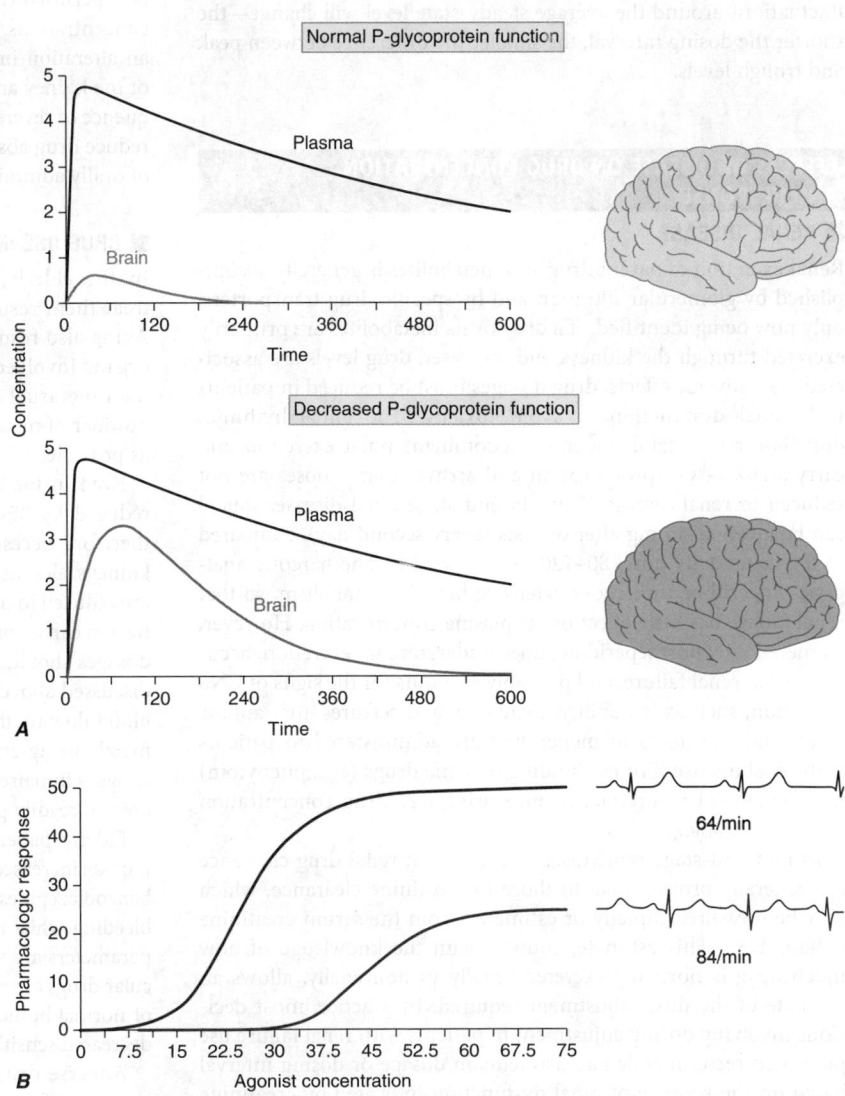

Figure 5-5 *A.* The efflux pump P-glycoprotein excludes drugs from the endothelium of capillaries in the brain, and so constitutes a key element of the blood-brain barrier. Thus, reduced P-glycoprotein function (e.g., due to drug interactions or genetically determined variability in gene transcription) increases penetration of substrate drugs into the brain, even when plasma concentrations are unchanged. *B.* The graph shows an effect of a β₁-receptor polymorphism on receptor function in vitro. Patients with the hypofunctional variant (red) may display lesser heart-rate slowing or blood pressure lowering on exposure to a receptor blocking agent.

desired and measured concentrations *at steady state*; for example, if a doubling of the steady-state plasma concentration is desired, the dose should be doubled. In some cases, elimination becomes saturated at high doses, and the process then occurs at a fixed amount per unit time (zero order). For drugs with this property (e.g., phenytoin and theophylline), plasma concentrations change disproportionately more than the alteration in the dosing rate. In this situation, changes in dose should be small to minimize the degree of unpredictability, and plasma concentration monitoring should be used when available to ensure that dose modification achieves the desired level.

An increase in dosage is usually best achieved by changing the drug dose but not the dosing interval, e.g., by giving 200 mg every 8 h instead of 100 mg every 8 h. However, this approach is acceptable only if the resulting maximum concentration is not toxic and the trough value does not fall below the minimum effective concentration for an undesirable period of time. Alternatively, the steady state may be changed by altering the frequency of intermittent dosing but not the size of each dose. In this case, the magnitude of the fluctuations around the average steady-state level will change—the shorter the dosing interval, the smaller the difference between peak and trough levels.

EFFECTS OF DISEASE ON DRUG CONCENTRATION AND RESPONSE

■ RENAL DISEASE

Renal excretion of parent drug and metabolites is generally accomplished by glomerular filtration and by specific drug transporters, only now being identified. If a drug or its metabolites are primarily excreted through the kidneys and increased drug levels are associated with adverse effects, drug dosages must be reduced in patients with renal dysfunction to avoid toxicity. The antiarrhythmics dofetilide and sotalol undergo predominant renal excretion and carry a risk of QT prolongation and arrhythmias if doses are not reduced in renal disease. Thus, in end-stage renal disease, sotalol can be given as 40 mg after dialysis (every second day), compared to the usual daily dose, 80–120 mg every 12 h. The narcotic analgesic meperidine undergoes extensive hepatic metabolism, so that renal failure has little effect on its plasma concentration. However, its metabolite, normeperidine, does undergo renal excretion, accumulates in renal failure, and probably accounts for the signs of CNS excitation, such as irritability, twitching, and seizures, that appear when multiple doses of meperidine are administered to patients with renal disease. Protein binding of some drugs (e.g., phenytoin) may be altered in uremia, so measuring free drug concentration may be desirable.

In non-end-stage renal disease, changes in renal drug clearance are generally proportional to those in creatinine clearance, which may be measured directly or estimated from the serum creatinine (Chap. 278). This estimate, coupled with the knowledge of how much drug is normally excreted renally vs nonrenally, allows an estimate of the dose adjustment required. In practice, most decisions involving dosing adjustment in patients with renal failure use published recommended adjustments in dosage or dosing interval based on the severity of renal dysfunction indicated by creatinine clearance. Any such modification of dose is a first approximation and should be followed by plasma concentration data (if available) and clinical observation to further optimize therapy for the individual patient.

■ LIVER DISEASE

In contrast to the predictable decline in renal clearance of drugs in renal insufficiency, the effects of diseases like hepatitis or cirrhosis on drug disposition range from impaired to increased drug clearance in an unpredictable fashion. Standard tests of liver function are not useful in adjusting doses. First-pass metabolism may decrease, leading to increased oral bioavailability as a consequence of disrupted hepatocyte function, altered liver architecture, and portacaval shunts. The oral bioavailability for high first-pass drugs such as morphine, meperidine, midazolam, and nifedipine is almost doubled in patients with cirrhosis, compared to those with normal liver function. Therefore, the size of the oral dose of such drugs should be reduced in this setting.

■ HEART FAILURE AND SHOCK

Under conditions of decreased tissue perfusion, the cardiac output is redistributed to preserve blood flow to the heart and brain at the expense of other tissues (Chap. 234). As a result, drugs may be distributed into a smaller volume of distribution, higher drug concentrations will be present in the plasma, and the tissues that are best perfused (the brain and heart) will be exposed to these higher concentrations. If either the brain or heart is sensitive to the drug, an alteration in response will occur. As well, decreased perfusion of the kidney and liver may impair drug clearance. Another consequence of severe heart failure is decreased gut perfusion, which may reduce drug absorption and, thus, lead to reduced or absent effects of orally administered therapies.

■ DRUG USE IN THE ELDERLY

In the elderly, multiple pathologies and medications used to treat them result in more drug interactions and adverse effects. Aging also results in changes in organ function, especially of the organs involved in drug disposition. Initial doses should be less than the usual adult dosage and should be increased slowly. The number of medications, and doses per day, should be kept as low as possible.

Even in the absence of kidney disease, renal clearance may be reduced by 35–50% in elderly patients. Dosage adjustments are therefore necessary for drugs that are eliminated mainly by the kidneys. Because muscle mass and therefore creatinine production are reduced in older individuals, a normal serum creatinine concentration can be present even though creatinine clearance is impaired; dosages should be adjusted on the basis of creatinine clearance, as discussed above. Aging also results in a decrease in the size of, and blood flow to, the liver and possibly in the activity of hepatic drug-metabolizing enzymes; accordingly, the hepatic clearance of some drugs is impaired in the elderly. As with liver disease, these changes are not readily predicted.

Elderly patients may display altered drug sensitivity. Examples include increased analgesic effects of opioids, increased sedation from benzodiazepines and other CNS depressants, and increased risk of bleeding while receiving anticoagulant therapy, even when clotting parameters are well controlled. Exaggerated responses to cardiovascular drugs are also common because of the impaired responsiveness of normal homeostatic mechanisms. Conversely, the elderly display decreased sensitivity to β-adrenergic receptor blockers.

Adverse drug reactions are especially common in the elderly because of altered pharmacokinetics and pharmacodynamics, the frequent use of multidrug regimens, and concomitant disease. For example, use of long half-life benzodiazepines is linked to the occurrence of hip fractures in elderly patients, perhaps reflecting both a risk of falls from these drugs (due to increased sedation) and the increased incidence of osteoporosis in elderly patients. In population surveys of the noninstitutionalized elderly, as many as 10% had at least one adverse drug reaction in the previous year.

GENETIC DETERMINANTS OF THE RESPONSE TO DRUGS

PRINCIPLES OF GENETIC VARIATION AND HUMAN TRAITS

(See also Chaps. 61 and 63) The concept that genetically determined variations in drug metabolism might be associated with variable drug levels and hence, effect, was advanced at the end of the nineteenth century, and the examples of familial clustering of unusual drug responses were noted in the mid-twentieth century. Variants in the human genome resulting in variation in level of expression or function of molecules important for pharmacokinetics and pharmacodynamics are increasingly recognized. These may be mutations (very rare variants, often associated with disease) or polymorphisms, variants that are much more common in a population. Variants may occur at a single nucleotide [single nucleotide polymorphisms (SNPs)] or involve insertion or deletion of one or more nucleotides, occasionally up to thousands. They may be in the exons (coding regions), introns (noncoding intervening sequences), or intergenic regions. Exonic polymorphisms may or may not alter the encoded protein, and variant proteins may or may not display altered function. Similarly, polymorphisms in noncoding regions may or may not alter gene expression and protein level.

As variation in the human genome is increasingly well documented, associations are being described between polymorphisms and various traits (including response to drug therapy). Some of these rely on well-developed chains of evidence, including in vitro studies demonstrating variant protein function, familial aggregation of the variant allele with the trait, and association studies in large populations. In other cases, the associations are less compelling. Identifying replicated associations with important clinical consequences is a challenge that must be overcome before the concept of genotyping to identify optimal drugs (or dosages) in individual patients prior to prescribing can be considered for widespread clinical practice.

Rates of drug efficacy and adverse effects often vary among ethnic groups. Many explanations for such differences are plausible; genomic approaches have now established one mechanism that functionally important variants determining differences in drug response often display differing distributions among ethnic groups. This finding may have importance for drug use among ethnic groups, as well as in drug development.

Approaches to identifying genetic variants modulating drug action

A goal of traditional Mendelian genetics is to identify DNA variants associated with a distinct phenotype in multiple related family members (Chap. 63). The usual approach, linkage analysis, does not generally lend itself to identifying genetic variants contributing to variable drug actions, because it is unusual for a drug response phenotype to be accurately measured in more than one family member, let alone across a kindred. Thus, alternate approaches are used to identify and validate DNA variants contributing to variable drug actions.

Most studies to date have used an understanding of the molecular mechanisms modulating drug action to identify candidate genes in which variants could explain variable drug responses. One very common scenario is that variable drug actions can be attributed to variability in plasma drug concentrations. When plasma drug concentrations vary widely (e.g., more than an order of magnitude), especially if their distribution is nonunimodal as in Fig. 5-6, variants in single genes controlling drug concentrations often contribute. In this case, the most obvious candidate genes are those responsible for drug metabolism and elimination. Other candidate genes are those encoding the target molecules with which drugs interact to produce their effects or molecules modulating that response, including those involved in disease pathogenesis.

The field has also had some success with "unbiased" approaches such as genome-wide association (GWA) (Chap. 61). GWA makes no a priori assumptions about the genetic loci modulating variable drug response and, instead, searches across the whole genome in an "unbiased fashion" to identify loci linked to variable drug response.

GENETICALLY DETERMINED DRUG DISPOSITION AND VARIABLE EFFECTS

Clinically important genetic variants have been described in multiple molecular pathways of drug disposition (Table 5-2). A distinct multimodal distribution of drug disposition (as shown in Fig. 5-6) argues for a predominant effect of variants in a single gene in the metabolism of that substrate. Individuals with two alleles (variants) encoding for nonfunctional protein make up one group, often termed poor metabolizers (PM phenotype); many variants can produce such a loss of function, complicating the use of genotyping in clinical practice. Individuals with one functional allele make up a second (intermediate metabolizers) and may or may not be distinguishable from those with two functional alleles (extensive metabolizers, EMs). Ultra-rapid metabolizers with especially high enzymatic activity (occasionally due to gene duplication; Fig. 5-6) have also been described for some traits. Many drugs in widespread use can inhibit specific drug disposition pathways (Table 5-1), and so EM individuals receiving such inhibitors can respond like PM patients (phenocopying). Polymorphisms in genes encoding drug uptake or drug efflux transporters may be other contributors to variability in drug delivery to target sites and, hence, in drug effects.

CYP Variants

CYP3A4 is the most abundant hepatic and intestinal CYP and is also the enzyme responsible for metabolism of the greatest number of drugs in therapeutic use. CYP3A4 activity is highly variable (up to an order of magnitude) among individuals, but the underlying mechanisms are not yet well understood. A closely related gene, encoding CYP3A5 (which shares substrates with CYP3A4), does display loss-of-function variants, especially in African populations. CYP3A refers to both enzymes.

CYP2D6 is second to CYP3A4 in the number of commonly used drugs that it metabolizes. CYP2D6 activity is polymorphically distributed, with about 7% of European- and African-derived populations (but very few Asians) displaying the PM phenotype (Fig. 5-6). Dozens of loss-of-function variants in the CYP2D6 gene have been described; the PM phenotype arises in individuals with two such alleles. In addition, ultra-rapid metabolizers with multiple functional copies of the CYP2D6 gene have been identified, particularly in Ethiopian, Eritrean, and Saudi individuals.

Codeine is biotransformed by CYP2D6 to the potent active metabolite morphine, so its effects are blunted in PMs and exaggerated in ultra-rapid metabolizers. In the case of drugs with beta-blocking properties metabolized by CYP2D6, greater signs of beta blockade (e.g., bradycardia) are seen in PM subjects than in EMs. This can be seen not only with orally administered beta blockers such as metoprolol and carvedilol, but also with ophthalmic timolol and with the sodium channel–blocking antiarrhythmic propafenone, a CYP2D6 substrate with beta-blocking properties. Further, in EM subjects, propafenone elimination becomes zero-order at higher doses; so, for example, a tripling of the dose may lead to a tenfold increase in drug concentration. Ultra-rapid metabolizers may require very high dosages of tricyclic antidepressants to achieve a therapeutic effect and, with codeine, may display transient euphoria and nausea due to very rapid generation of morphine. Tamoxifen undergoes CYP2D6-mediated biotransformation to an active metabolite, so its efficacy may be in part related to this polymorphism. In addition, the widespread use of selective serotonin reuptake inhibitors (SSRIs) to treat tamoxifen-related hot flashes may also alter the drug's effects because many SSRIs, notably fluoxetine and paroxetine, are also CYP2D6 inhibitors.

TABLE 5-2 Genetic Variants and Drug Responses

Gene	Drugs	Effect of genetic variants*
Variants in Drug Metabolism Pathways		
CYP2C9	Losartan	Decreased bioactivation and effects (PMs)
	Warfarin	Decreased dose requirements; possible increased bleeding risk (PMs)
CYP2C19	Omeprazole, voriconazole	Decreased effect in extensive metabolizers (EMs)
	Celecoxib	Exaggerated effect in PMs
	Clopidogrel	Decreased effect in PMs
CYP2D6	Codeine, tamoxifen	Decreased bioactivation and drug effects in PMs
	Codeine	Morphine-like adverse effects in UMs
	Tricyclic antidepressants	Increased adverse effects in PMs; decreased therapeutic effects in UMs
	Metoprolol, carvedilol, timolol, propafenone	Increased beta blockade in PMs
Dihydropyrimidine dehydrogenase	Capecitabine, fluorouracil	Possible severe toxicity (PMs)
NAT2	Rifampin, isoniazid, pyrazin-amide, hydralazine, procain-amide	Increased risk of toxicity in PMs
Thiopurine S-methyltransferase (*TPMT*)	Azathioprine, 6-mercaptopurine	*3A/*3A (PMs): increased risk of bone marrow aplasia; wild-type homozygote: possible decreased drug action at usual dosages
Uridine diphosphate glucuronosyl-transferase (*UGT1A1*)	Irinotecan	*28/*28 PM homozygotes: increased risk of severe adverse effects (diarrhea, bone marrow aplasia)
Variants in Other Genes		
Glucose 6-phosphate dehydrogenase (G6PD)	Rasburicase, primaquine, chlo-roquine	Increased risk of hemolytic anemia in G6PD-deficient subjects
HLA-B*1501	Carbamazepine	Carriers (1 or 2 alleles) at increased risk of severe skin toxicity
HLA-B*5701	Abacavir	Carriers (1 or 2 alleles) at increased risk of severe skin toxicity
IL28B	Interferon	Variable response in hepatitis C therapy
IL15	Childhood leukemia therapy	Variability in response
SLCO1B1	Simvastatin	Variant non-synonymous single nucleotide polymorphism increases myopathy risk
VKORC1	Warfarin	Decreased dose requirements with variant promoter haplotype
Variants in Other Genomes (Infectious Agents, Tumors)		
Chemokine C-C motif receptor (CCR5)	Maraviroc	Drug effective only in HIV strains with CCR5 detectible
C-KIT	Imatinib	In gastrointestinal stromal tumors, drug indicated only with c-kit–positive cases
Epidermal Growth Factor Receptor (EGFR)	Cetuximab	Clinical trials conducted in patients with EGFR-positive tumors
Her2/neu overexpression	Trastuzumab, lapatinib	Drugs indicated only with tumor overexpression
K-ras mutation	Panitumumab, cetuximab	Lack of efficacy with KRAS mutation
Philadelphia chromosome	Busulfan, dasatinib, nilotinib, imatinib	Decreased efficacy in Philadelphia chromosome–negative chronic myelogenous leukemia

*Drug effect in homozygotes unless otherwise specified.

Note: PM, poor metabolizer (homozygote for reduced or loss of function allele); EM, extensive metabolizer: normal enzymatic activity; UM, ultra-rapid metabolizer (enzymatic activity much greater than normal, e.g., with gene duplication, Fig. 5-6). Further data at U.S. Food and Drug Administration:

http://www.fda.gov/Drugs/ScienceResearch/ResearchAreas/Pharmacogenetics/ucm083378.htm or Pharmacogenetics Research Network/Knowledge Base:

http://www.pharmgkb.org.

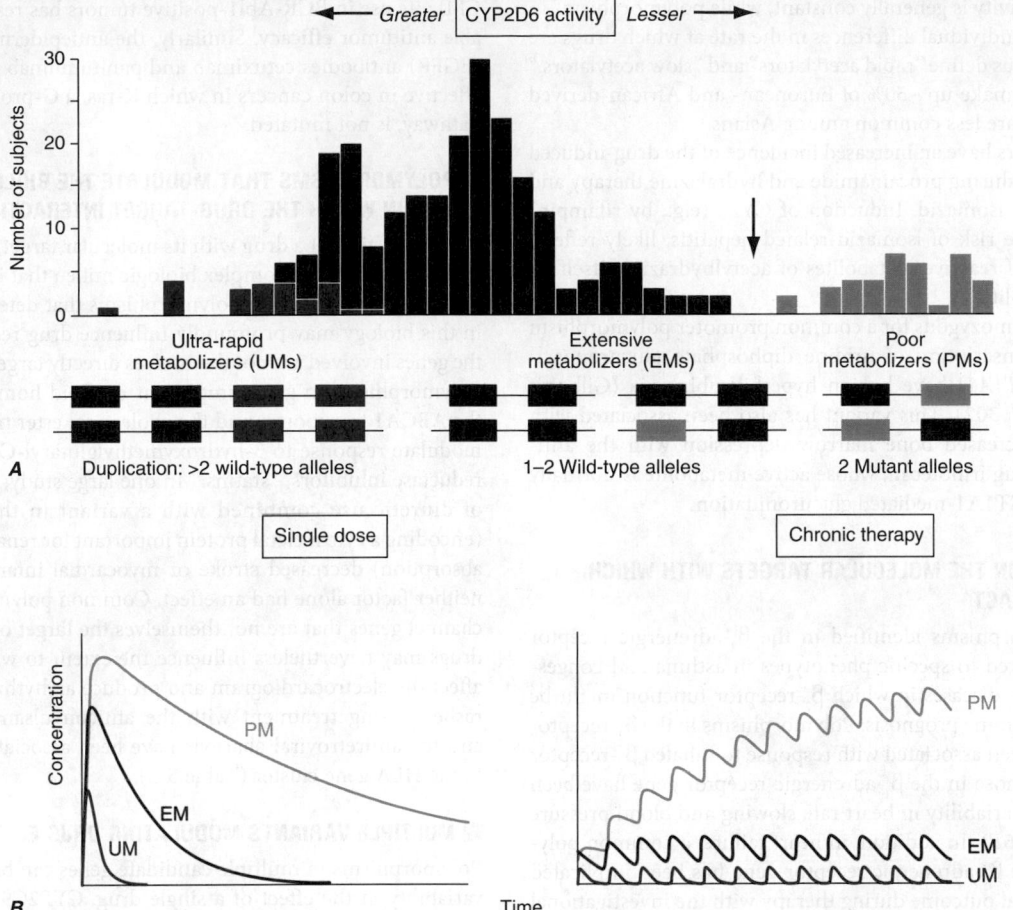

Figure 5-6 **A.** CYP2D6 metabolic activity was assessed in 290 subjects by administration of a test dose of a probe substrate and measurement of urinary formation of the CYP2D6-generated metabolite. The heavy arrow indicates a clear antimode, separating poor metabolizer subjects (PMs, green), with two loss-of-function CYP2D6 alleles, indicated by the intron-exon structures below the bar chart. Individuals with one or two functional alleles are grouped together as extensive metabolizers (EMs, blue). Also shown are ultra-rapid metabolizers (UMs), with 2–12 functional copies of the gene (red), displaying the greatest enzyme activity. *(Adapted by permission from M-L Dahl et al: J Pharmacol Exp Ther 274:516, 1995.)* **B.** These simulations show the predicted effects of CYP2D6 genotype on disposition of a substrate drug. With a single dose (*left*), there is an inverse "gene-dose" relationship between the number of active alleles and the areas under the time-concentration curves (smallest in UM subjects; highest in PM subjects); this indicates that clearance is greatest in UM subjects. In addition, elimination half-life is longest in PM subjects. The right panel shows that these single dose differences are exaggerated during chronic therapy: steady-state concentration is much higher in PM subjects (decreased clearance), as is the time required to achieve steady state (longer elimination half-life).

The PM phenotype for CYP2C19 is common (20%) among Asians and rarer (3–5%) in European-derived populations. The impact of polymorphic CYP2C19-mediated metabolism has been demonstrated with the proton pump inhibitor omeprazole, where ulcer cure rates with "standard" dosages were markedly lower in EM patients (29%) than in PMs (100%). Thus, understanding the importance of this polymorphism would have been important in developing the drug, and knowing a patient's *CYP2C19* genotype should improve therapy. CYP2C19 is responsible for bioactivation of the antiplatelet drug clopidogrel, and several large studies have documented decreased efficacy (e.g., increased myocardial infarction after placement of coronary stents) among Caucasian subjects with reduction of function alleles. In addition, some studies suggest that omeprazole and possibly other proton inhibitors phenocopy this effect.

There are common allelic variants of *CYP2C9* that encode proteins with loss of catalytic function. These variant alleles are associated with increased rates of neurologic complications with phenytoin, hypoglycemia with glipizide, and reduced warfarin dose required

to maintain stable anticoagulation (discussed further below). The angiotensin-receptor blocker losartan is a prodrug that is bioactivated by CYP2C9; as a result, PMs and those receiving inhibitor drugs may display little response to therapy.

Transferase variants

One of the most extensively studied phase II polymorphisms is the PM trait for thiopurine S-methyltransferase (TPMT). TPMT bioinactivates the antileukemic drug 6-mercaptopurine. Further, 6-mercaptopurine is itself an active metabolite of the immunosuppressive azathioprine. Homozygotes for alleles encoding the inactive TPMT (1 in 300 individuals) predictably exhibit severe and potentially fatal pancytopenia on standard doses of azathioprine or 6-mercaptopurine. On the other hand, homozygotes for fully functional alleles may display less anti-inflammatory or antileukemic effect with the drugs.

N-acetylation is catalyzed by hepatic *N*-acetyl transferase (NAT), which represents the activity of two genes, *NAT-1* and *NAT-2*. Both enzymes transfer an acetyl group from acetyl coenzyme A to the drug; NAT-1 activity is generally constant, while polymorphisms in *NAT-2* result in individual differences in the rate at which drugs are acetylated and thus define "rapid acetylators" and "slow acetylators." Slow acetylators make up ~50% of European- and African-derived populations but are less common among Asians.

Slow acetylators have an increased incidence of the drug-induced lupus syndrome during procainamide and hydralazine therapy and of hepatitis with isoniazid. Induction of CYPs (e.g., by rifampin) also increases the risk of isoniazid-related hepatitis, likely reflecting generation of reactive metabolites of acetylhydrazine, itself an isoniazid metabolite.

Individuals homozygous for a common promoter polymorphism that reduces transcription of uridine diphosphate glucuronosyltransferase (*UGT1A1*) have benign hyperbilirubinemia (Gilbert's syndrome; Chap. 302). This variant has also been associated with diarrhea and increased bone marrow depression with the antineoplastic prodrug irinotecan, whose active metabolite is normally detoxified by UGT1A1-mediated glucuronidation.

■ VARIABILITY IN THE MOLECULAR TARGETS WITH WHICH DRUGS INTERACT

Multiple polymorphisms identified in the β_2-adrenergic receptor appear to be linked to specific phenotypes in asthma and congestive heart failure, diseases in which β_2-receptor function might be expected to determine prognosis. Polymorphisms in the β_2-receptor gene have also been associated with response to inhaled β_2-receptor agonists, while those in the β_1-adrenergic receptor gene have been associated with variability in heart rate slowing and blood pressure lowering (Fig. 5-5B). In addition, in heart failure, a common polymorphism in the β_1-adrenergic receptor gene has been implicated in variable clinical outcome during therapy with the investigational beta blocker bucindolol. Response to the 5-lipoxygenase inhibitor zileuton in asthma has been linked to polymorphisms that determine the expression level of the 5-lipoxygenase gene.

Drugs may also interact with genetic pathways of disease to elicit or exacerbate symptoms of the underlying conditions. In the porphyrias, CYP inducers are thought to increase the activity of enzymes proximal to the deficient enzyme, exacerbating or triggering attacks (Chap. 358). Deficiency of glucose-6-phosphate dehydrogenase (G6PD), most often in individuals of African, Mediterranean, or South Asian descent, increases risk of hemolytic anemia in response to primaquine and a number of other drugs that do not cause hemolysis in patients with normal amounts of the enzyme (Chap. 106). Patients with mutations in the ryanodine receptor, which controls intracellular calcium in skeletal muscle and other tissues, may be asymptomatic until exposed to certain general anesthetics, which trigger the syndrome of malignant hyperthermia. Certain antiarrhythmics and other drugs can produce marked QT prolongation and torsades des pointes (Chap. 233), and in some patients this adverse effect represents unmasking of previously subclinical congenital long QT syndrome.

Tumor and infectious agent genomes

The actions of drugs used to treat infectious or neoplastic disease may be modulated by variants in these non-human germline genomes. Genotyping tumors is a rapidly evolving approach to target therapies to underlying mechanisms and to avoid potentially toxic therapy in patients who would derive no benefit (Chap. 83). Trastuzumab, which potentiates anthracycline-related cardiotoxicity, is ineffective in breast cancers that do not express the herceptin receptor. Imatinib targets a specific tyrosine kinase, BCR-Abl1, that is generated by the translocation that creates the Philadelphia chromosome typical of chronic myelogenous leukemia (CML). BCR-Abl1 is not only active but may be central to the pathogenesis of

CML; its use in BCR-Abl1-positive tumors has resulted in remarkable antitumor efficacy. Similarly, the antiepidermal growth factor (EGFR) antibodies cetuximab and panitumumab appear especially effective in colon cancers in which K-ras, a G-protein in the EGFR pathway, is not mutated.

■ POLYMORPHISMS THAT MODULATE THE BIOLOGIC CONTEXT WITHIN WHICH THE DRUG-TARGET INTERACTIONS OCCUR

The interaction of a drug with its molecular target is translated into a clinical action in a complex biologic milieu that is itself often perturbed by disease. Thus, polymorphisms that determine variability in this biology may profoundly influence drug response, although the genes involved are not themselves directly targets of drug action. Polymorphisms in genes important for lipid homeostasis (such as the ABCA1 transporter and the cholesterol ester transport protein) modulate response to 3-hydroxymethylglutaryl-CoA (HMG-CoA) reductase inhibitors, "statins." In one large study, the combination of diuretic use combined with a variant in the adducin gene (encoding a cytoskeletal protein important for renal tubular sodium absorption) decreased stroke or myocardial infarction risk, while neither factor alone had an effect. Common polymorphisms in ion channel genes that are not themselves the target of QT-prolonging drugs may nevertheless influence the extent to which those drugs affect the electrocardiogram and produce arrhythmias. Severe skin rashes during treatment with the anticonvulsant carbamazepine and the antiretroviral abacavir have been associated with variants in the HLA gene cluster (Table 5-2).

■ MULTIPLE VARIANTS MODULATING DRUG EFFECTS

Polymorphisms in multiple candidate genes can be associated with variability in the effect of a single drug. CYP2C9 loss-of-function variants are associated with a requirement for lower maintenance doses of the vitamin K antagonist anticoagulant warfarin. In rarer (<2%) individuals homozygous for these variant alleles, maintenance warfarin dosages may be difficult to establish, and the risk of bleeding complications appears increased. In addition to *CYP2C9*, multiple variants in the promoter region of *VKORC1*, encoding a vitamin K epoxide reductase (the warfarin target), predict warfarin dosages; these promoter variants are in tight *linkage disequilibrium*, i.e., genotyping at one polymorphic site within this *haplotype block* provides reliable information on the identity of genotypes at other linked sites (Chap. 61).

■ GENOME-WIDE ASSOCIATION AND VARIABLE DRUG RESPONSE

A GWA study was used to compare patients with simvastatin-associated myopathy to control tolerating the drugs and identified a single noncoding SNP in *SLCO1B1*, encoding OATP1B1, a drug transporter known to modulate simvastatin uptake into the liver. The SNP was in linkage disequilibrium with a known nonsynonymous SNP modulating OATP1B1 function and was estimated to account for 60% of myopathy risk. GWA approaches have also implicated interferon variants in antileukemic responses and in response to therapy in hepatitis C (Table 5-2).

■ PROSPECTS FOR INCORPORATING PHARMACOGENETIC INFORMATION INTO CLINICAL PRACTICE

The description of genetic variants linked to variable drug responses naturally raises the question of if and how to use this information in practice. Indeed, the U.S. Food and Drug Administration has begun incorporating pharmacogenetic data into information ("package inserts") meant to guide prescribing. A decision to adopt pharmacogenetically guided dosing for a given drug depends on multiple factors. The most important are the magnitude and clinical importance of the genetic effect and the strength of evidence linking genetic variation to variable drug effects (e.g., anecdote versus post-hoc analysis of clinical trial data versus randomized prospective clinical trial). The evidence can be strengthened if statistical arguments from clinical trial data are complemented by an understanding of underlying physiologic mechanisms. Cost versus expected benefit may also be a factor.

When the evidence is compelling and alternate therapies are not available, there is a strong argument for deploying genetic testing as a guide to prescribing. Examples include associations between *UGT1A1* variants and irinotecan toxicity, or between HLA-B*5701 and severe skin toxicity with abacavir. In other situations, the arguments are less compelling: the magnitude of the genetic effect may be smaller, the consequences may be less serious, alternate therapies may be available, or the drug effect may be amenable to monitoring by other approaches. Ongoing clinical trials are addressing the utility of preprescription genotyping in large populations exposed to drugs with known pharmacogenetic variants (e.g., warfarin). Importantly, technological advances are now raising the possibility of inexpensive whole genome sequencing. Incorporating a patient's whole genome sequence into their electronic medical record would allow the information to be accessed as needed for many genetic and pharmacogenetic applications. There are multiple issues (e.g., economic, technological, and ethical) that need to be addressed if such a paradigm is to be adopted (Chap. 61). While barriers to bringing genomic and pharmacogenomic information to the bedside seem daunting, the field is very young and evolving rapidly. Indeed, one major result of understanding the role of genetics in drug action has been improved screening of drugs during the development process to reduce the likelihood of highly variable metabolism or unanticipated toxicity.

INTERACTIONS BETWEEN DRUGS

Drug interactions can complicate therapy by increasing or decreasing the action of a drug; interactions may be based on changes in drug disposition or in drug response in the absence of changes in drug levels. *Interactions must be considered in the differential diagnosis of any unusual response occurring during drug therapy.* Prescribers should recognize that patients often come to them with a legacy of drugs acquired during previous medical experiences, often with multiple physicians who may not be aware of all the patient's medications. A meticulous drug history should include examination of the patient's medications and, if necessary, calls to the pharmacist to identify prescriptions. It should also address the use of agents not often volunteered during questioning, such as over-the-counter (OTC) drugs, health food supplements, and topical agents such as eye drops. Lists of interactions are available from a number of electronic sources. While it is unrealistic to expect the practicing physician to memorize these, certain drugs consistently run the risk of generating interactions, often by inhibiting or inducing specific drug elimination pathways. Examples are presented below and in Table 5-3. Accordingly, when these drugs are started or stopped, prescribers must be especially alert to the possibility of interactions.

■ PHARMACOKINETIC INTERACTIONS CAUSING DECREASED DRUG EFFECTS

Gastrointestinal absorption can be reduced if a drug interaction results in drug binding in the gut, as with aluminum-containing antacids, kaolin-pectin suspensions, or bile acid sequestrants. Drugs such as histamine H_2 receptor antagonists or proton pump inhibitors that alter gastric pH may decrease the solubility and hence absorption of weak bases such as ketoconazole.

Expression of some genes responsible for drug elimination, notably *CYP3A* and *MDR1*, can be markedly increased by "inducing" drugs, such as rifampin, carbamazepine, phenytoin, St. John's

wort, and glutethimide, and by smoking, exposure to chlorinated insecticides such as DDT (CYP1A2), and chronic alcohol ingestion. Administration of inducing agents lowers plasma levels over 2–3 weeks as gene expression is increased. If a drug dose is stabilized in the presence of an inducer that is subsequently stopped, major toxicity can occur as clearance returns to preinduction levels and drug concentrations rise. Individuals vary in the extent to which drug metabolism can be induced, likely through genetic mechanisms.

Interactions that inhibit the bioactivation of prodrugs will similarly decrease drug effects. The analgesic effect of codeine depends on its metabolism to morphine via CYP2D6. Thus, CYP2D6 inhibitors (Table 5-1) are predicted to reduce the analgesic efficacy of codeine in EMs. Similarly, omeprazole, and perhaps other proton pump inhibitors, reduce CYP2C19 activity and have been associated with reduced clopidogrel efficacy.

Interactions that decrease drug delivery to intracellular sites of action can decrease drug effects: tricyclic antidepressants can blunt the antihypertensive effect of clonidine by decreasing its uptake into adrenergic neurons. Reduced CNS penetration of multiple HIV protease inhibitors (with the attendant risk of facilitating viral replication in a sanctuary site) appears attributable to P-glycoprotein-mediated exclusion of the drug from the CNS; indeed, inhibition of P-glycoprotein has been proposed as a therapeutic approach to enhance drug entry to the CNS (Fig. 5-5A).

■ PHARMACOKINETIC INTERACTIONS CAUSING INCREASED DRUG EFFECTS

The most common mechanism here is inhibition of drug elimination. In contrast to induction, new protein synthesis is not involved, and the effect develops as drug and any inhibitor metabolites accumulate (a function of their elimination half-lives). Since shared substrates of a single enzyme can compete for access to the active site of the protein, many CYP substrates can also be considered inhibitors. However, some drugs are especially potent as inhibitors (and occasionally may not even be substrates) of specific drug elimination pathways, and so it is in the use of these agents that clinicians must be most alert to the potential for interactions (Table 5-3). Commonly implicated interacting drugs of this type include amiodarone, cimetidine, erythromycin and some other macrolide antibiotics (clarithromycin but not azithromycin), ketoconazole and other azole antifungals, the antiretroviral agent ritonavir, and high concentrations of grapefruit juice (Table 5-3). The consequences of such interactions will depend on the drug whose elimination is being inhibited; high-risk drugs are those for which alternate pathways of elimination are not available and for which drug accumulation increases the risk of serious toxicity (see "The Concept of High-Risk Pharmacokinetics," above). Examples include CYP3A inhibitors increasing the risk of cyclosporine toxicity or of rhabdomyolysis with some HMG-CoA reductase inhibitors (lovastatin, simvastatin, atorvastatin), and P-glycoprotein inhibitors increasing risk of digoxin toxicity.

These interactions can be exploited to therapeutic benefit. The antiviral ritonavir is a very potent CYP3A4 inhibitor that is sometimes added to anti-HIV regimens, not because of its antiviral effects but because it decreases clearance, and hence increases efficacy, of other anti-HIV agents. Similarly, calcium channel blockers have been deliberately coadministered with cyclosporine to reduce its clearance and thus its maintenance dosage and cost.

Phenytoin, an inducer of many systems, including CYP3A, inhibits CYP2C9. CYP2C9 metabolism of losartan to its active metabolite is inhibited by phenytoin, with potential loss of antihypertensive effect.

Grapefruit (but not orange) juice inhibits CYP3A, especially at high doses; patients receiving drugs where even modest CYP3A inhibition may increase the risk of adverse effects (e.g., cyclosporine,

TABLE 5-3 Drugs With a High Risk of Generating Pharmacokinetic Interactions

Drug	Mechanism	Examples
Antacids Bile acid sequestrants	Reduced absorption	Antacids/tetracyclines Cholestyramine/digoxin
Proton pump inhibitors H_2-receptor blockers	Altered gastric pH	Ketoconazole absorption decreased
Rifampin Carbamazepine Barbiturates Phenytoin St. John's wort Glutethimide	Induction of hepatic metabolism	Decreased concentration and effects of warfarin quinidine cyclosporine losartan oral contraceptives methadone
Tricyclic antidepressants Fluoxetine Quinidine	Inhibitors of CYP2D6	Increased effect of many β blockers Decreased codeine effect
Cimetidine	Inhibitor of multiple CYPs	Increased concentration and effects of warfarin theophylline phenytoin
Ketoconazole, itraconazole Erythromycin, clarithromycin Calcium channel blockers Ritonavir	Inhibitor of CYP3A	Increased concentration and toxicity of some HMG-CoA reductase inhibitors cyclosporine, cisapride, terfenadine (now withdrawn) Increased concentration and effects of indinavir (with ritonavir) Decreased clearance and dose requirement for cyclosporine (with calcium channel blockers)
Allopurinol	Xanthine oxidase inhibitor	Azathioprine and 6-mercaptopurine toxicity
Amiodarone	Inhibitor of many CYPs and of P-glycoprotein	Decreased clearance (risk of toxicity) for warfarin digoxin quinidine
Gemfibrazol (and other fibrates)	CYP3A inhibition	Rhabdomyolysis when co-prescribed with some HMG-CoA reductase inhibitors
Quinidine Amiodarone Verapamil Cyclosporine Itraconazole Erythromycin	P-glycoprotein inhibition	Risk of digoxin toxicity
Phenylbutazone Probenecid Salicylates	Inhibition of renal tubular transport	Increased risk of methotrexate toxicity with salicylates

some HMG-CoA reductase inhibitors) should therefore avoid grapefruit juice.

CYP2D6 is markedly inhibited by quinidine, a number of neuroleptic drugs (chlorpromazine and haloperidol), and the SSRIs fluoxetine and paroxetine. Clinical consequences of fluoxetine's interaction with CYP2D6 substrates may not be apparent for weeks after the drug is started, because of its very long half-life and slow generation of a CYP2D6-inhibiting metabolite.

6-Mercaptopurine is metabolized not only by TPMT but also by xanthine oxidase. When allopurinol, a potent inhibitor of xanthine oxidase, is administered with standard doses of azathioprine or 6-mercaptopurine, life-threatening toxicity (bone marrow suppression) can result.

A number of drugs are secreted by the renal tubular transport systems for organic anions. Inhibition of these systems can cause excessive drug accumulation. Salicylate, for example, reduces the renal clearance of methotrexate, an interaction that may lead to methotrexate toxicity. Renal tubular secretion contributes substantially to the elimination of penicillin, which can be inhibited (to increase its therapeutic effect) by probenecid. Similarly, inhibition of the tubular cation transport system by cimetidine decreases the renal clearance of dofetilide and of procainamide and its active metabolite NAPA.

■ DRUG INTERACTIONS NOT MEDIATED BY CHANGES IN DRUG DISPOSITION

Drugs may act on separate components of a common process to generate effects greater than either has alone. Antithrombotic therapy with combinations of antiplatelet agents (glycoprotein IIb/IIIa inhibitors, aspirin, clopidogrel) and anticoagulants (warfarin, heparins) are often used in the treatment of vascular disease, although such combinations carry an increased risk of bleeding.

Nonsteroidal anti-inflammatory drugs (NSAIDs) cause gastric ulcers, and in patients treated with warfarin, the risk of bleeding from a peptic ulcer is increased almost threefold by concomitant use of an NSAID.

Indomethacin, piroxicam, and probably other NSAIDs antagonize the antihypertensive effects of β-adrenergic receptor blockers, diuretics, ACE inhibitors, and other drugs. The resulting elevation in blood pressure ranges from trivial to severe. This effect is not seen with aspirin and sulindac but has been found with the cyclooxygenase 2 (COX-2) inhibitor celecoxib.

Torsades des pointes ventricular tachycardia during administration of QT-prolonging antiarrhythmics (quinidine, sotalol, dofetilide) occurs much more frequently in patients receiving diuretics, probably reflecting hypokalemia. In vitro, hypokalemia not only prolongs the QT interval in the absence of drug but also potentiates drug block of ion channels that results in QT prolongation. Also, some diuretics have direct electrophysiologic actions that prolong QT.

The administration of supplemental potassium leads to more frequent and more severe hyperkalemia when potassium elimination is reduced by concurrent treatment with ACE inhibitors, spironolactone, amiloride, or triamterene.

The pharmacologic effects of sildenafil result from inhibition of the phosphodiesterase type 5 isoform that inactivates cyclic GMP in the vasculature. Nitroglycerin and related nitrates used to treat angina produce vasodilation by elevating cyclic GMP. Thus, coadministration of these nitrates with sildenafil can cause profound hypotension, which can be catastrophic in patients with coronary disease.

Sometimes, combining drugs can increase overall efficacy and/or reduce drug-specific toxicity. Such therapeutically useful interactions are described in chapters dealing with specific disease entities.

ADVERSE REACTIONS TO DRUGS

The beneficial effects of drugs are coupled with the inescapable risk of untoward effects. The morbidity and mortality from these adverse effects often present diagnostic problems because they can involve every organ and system of the body and may be mistaken for signs of underlying disease. As well, some surveys have suggested that drug therapy for a range of chronic conditions such as psychiatric disease or hypertension does not achieve its desired goal in up to half of treated patients; thus, the most common "adverse" drug effect may be failure of efficacy.

Adverse reactions can be classified in two broad groups. One type results from exaggeration of an intended pharmacologic action of the drug, such as increased bleeding with anticoagulants or bone marrow suppression with antineoplastics. The second type of adverse reaction ensues from toxic effects unrelated to the intended pharmacologic actions. The latter effects are often unanticipated (especially with new drugs) and frequently severe and may result from recognized as well as previously undescribed mechanisms.

Drugs may increase the frequency of an event that is common in a general population, and this may be especially difficult to recognize; an excellent example is the increase in myocardial infarctions with the COX-2 inhibitor rofecoxib. Drugs can also cause rare and serious adverse effects, such as hematologic abnormalities, arrhythmias, severe skin reactions, or hepatic or renal dysfunction. Prior to regulatory approval and marketing, new drugs are tested in relatively few patients who tend to be less sick and to have fewer concomitant diseases than those patients who subsequently receive the drug therapeutically. Because of the relatively small number of patients studied in clinical trials and the selected nature of these patients, rare adverse effects are generally not detected prior to a drug's approval; indeed, if they are detected, the new drugs are generally not approved. Therefore, physicians need to be cautious in the prescription of new drugs and alert for the appearance of previously unrecognized adverse events.

Elucidating mechanisms underlying adverse drug effects can assist development of safer compounds or allow a patient subset at especially high risk to be excluded from drug exposure. National adverse reaction reporting systems, such as those operated by the FDA (suspected adverse reactions can be reported online at *http://www.fda.gov/medwatch/report/hcp.htm*) and the Committee on Safety of Medicines in Great Britain, can prove useful. The publication or reporting of a newly recognized adverse reaction can in a short time stimulate many similar such reports of reactions that previously had gone unrecognized.

Occasionally, "adverse" effects may be exploited to develop an entirely new indication for a drug. Unwanted hair growth during minoxidil treatment of severely hypertensive patients led to development of the drug for hair growth. Sildenafil was initially developed as an antianginal, but its effects to alleviate erectile dysfunction not only led to a new drug indication but also to increased understanding of the role of type 5 phosphodiesterase in erectile tissue. These examples further reinforce the concept that prescribers must remain vigilant to the possibility that unusual symptoms may reflect unappreciated drug effects.

Some 25–50% of patients make errors in self-administration of prescribed medicines, and these errors can be responsible for adverse drug effects. Similarly, patients commit errors in taking OTC drugs by not reading or following the directions on the containers. Physicians must recognize that providing directions with prescriptions does not always guarantee compliance.

In hospitals, drugs are administered in a controlled setting, and patient compliance is, in general, ensured. Errors may occur nevertheless—the wrong drug or dose may be given or the drug may be given to the wrong patient—and improved drug distribution and administration systems are addressing this problem.

■ SCOPE OF THE PROBLEM

Patients receive, on average, 10 different drugs during each hospitalization. The sicker the patient, the more drugs are given, and there is a corresponding increase in the likelihood of adverse drug reactions. When <6 different drugs are given to hospitalized patients, the probability of an adverse reaction is ~5%, but if >15 drugs are given, the probability is >40%. Retrospective analyses of ambulatory patients have revealed adverse drug effects in 20%. Serious adverse reactions are also well-recognized with "herbal" remedies and OTC compounds: examples include kava-associated hepatotoxicity, L-tryptophan-associated eosinophilia-myalgia, and phenylpropanolamine-associated stroke, each of which has caused fatalities.

A small group of widely used drugs accounts for a disproportionate number of reactions. Aspirin and other NSAIDs, analgesics, digoxin, anticoagulants, diuretics, antimicrobials, glucocorticoids, antineoplastics, and hypoglycemic agents account for 90% of reactions, although the drugs involved differ between ambulatory and hospitalized patients.

■ TOXICITY UNRELATED TO A DRUG'S PRIMARY PHARMACOLOGIC ACTIVITY

Cytotoxic reactions

Drugs or more commonly reactive metabolites generated by CYPs can covalently bind to tissue macromolecules (such as proteins or DNA) to cause tissue toxicity. Because of the reactive nature of these metabolites, covalent binding often occurs close to the site of production, typically the liver.

The most common cause of drug-induced hepatotoxicity is acetaminophen overdosage. Normally, reactive metabolites are detoxified by combining with hepatic glutathione. When glutathione becomes depleted, the metabolites bind instead to hepatic protein, with resultant hepatocyte damage. The hepatic necrosis produced by the ingestion of acetaminophen can be prevented or attenuated by the administration of substances such as *N*-acetylcysteine that reduce the binding of electrophilic metabolites to hepatic proteins. The risk of acetaminophen-related hepatic necrosis is increased in patients receiving drugs such as phenobarbital or phenytoin that increase the rate of drug metabolism or ethanol that exhaust glutathione stores. Such toxicity has even occurred with therapeutic dosages, so patients at risk through these mechanisms should be warned.

Immunologic mechanisms

Most pharmacologic agents are small molecules with low molecular weights (<2,000) and thus are poor immunogens. Generation of an immune response to a drug therefore usually requires in vivo activation and covalent linkage to protein, carbohydrate, or nucleic acid.

Drug stimulation of antibody production may mediate tissue injury by several mechanisms. The antibody may attack the drug when the drug is covalently attached to a cell and thereby destroy the cell. This occurs in penicillin-induced hemolytic anemia. Antibody-drug-antigen complexes may be passively adsorbed by a bystander cell, which is then destroyed by activation of complement; this occurs in quinine- and quinidine-induced thrombocytopenia. Heparin-induced thrombocytopenia arises when antibodies against complexes of platelet factor 4 peptide and heparin generate immune complexes that activate platelets; thus, the thrombocytopenia is accompanied by "paradoxical" thrombosis and is treated with thrombin inhibitors. Drugs or their reactive metabolites may alter a host tissue, rendering it antigenic and eliciting autoantibodies. For example, hydralazine and procainamide (or their reactive metabolites) can chemically alter nuclear material, stimulating the formation of antinuclear antibodies and occasionally causing lupus erythematosus. Drug-induced pure red cell aplasia (Chap. 107) is due to an immune-based drug reaction.

Serum sickness (Chap. 317) results from the deposition of circulating drug-antibody complexes on endothelial surfaces. Complement activation occurs, chemotactic factors are generated locally, and an inflammatory response develops at the site of complex entrapment. Arthralgias, urticaria, lymphadenopathy, glomerulonephritis, or cerebritis may result. Foreign proteins (vaccines, streptokinase, therapeutic antibodies) and antibiotics are common causes. Many drugs, particularly antimicrobial agents, ACE inhibitors, and aspirin, can elicit anaphylaxis with production of IgE, which binds to mast cell membranes. Contact with a drug antigen initiates a series of biochemical events in the mast cell and results in the release of mediators that can produce the characteristic urticaria, wheezing, flushing, rhinorrhea, and (occasionally) hypotension.

Drugs may also elicit cell-mediated immune responses. Topically administered substances may interact with sulfhydryl or amino groups in the skin and react with sensitized lymphocytes to produce the rash characteristic of contact dermatitis. Other types of rashes may also result from the interaction of serum factors, drugs, and sensitized lymphocytes.

■ DIAGNOSIS AND TREATMENT OF ADVERSE DRUG REACTIONS

The manifestations of drug-induced diseases frequently resemble those of other diseases, and a given set of manifestations may be produced by different and dissimilar drugs. Recognition of the role of a drug or drugs in an illness depends on appreciation of the possible adverse reactions to drugs in any disease, on identification of the temporal relationship between drug administration and development of the illness, and on familiarity with the common manifestations of the drugs. A suspected adverse drug reaction developing after introduction of a new drug naturally implicates that drug; however, it is also important to remember that a drug interaction may be responsible. Thus, for example, a patient on a chronic stable warfarin dose may develop a bleeding complication after introduction of amiodarone; this does not reflect a direct reaction to amiodarone but rather its effect to inhibit warfarin metabolism. Many associations between particular drugs and specific reactions have been described, but there is always a "first time" for a novel association, and any drug should be suspected of causing an adverse effect if the clinical setting is appropriate.

Illness related to a drug's intended pharmacologic action is often more easily recognized than illness attributable to immune or other mechanisms. For example, side effects such as cardiac arrhythmias in patients receiving digitalis, hypoglycemia in patients given insulin, or bleeding in patients receiving anticoagulants are more readily related to a specific drug than are symptoms such as fever or rash, which may be caused by many drugs or by other factors.

Electronic listings of adverse drug reactions can be useful. However, exhaustive compilations often provide little sense of perspective in terms of frequency and seriousness, which can vary considerably among patients.

Eliciting a drug history from each patient is important for diagnosis. Attention must be directed to OTC drugs and herbal preparations as well as to prescription drugs. Each type can be responsible for adverse drug effects, and adverse interactions may occur between OTC drugs and prescribed drugs. Loss of efficacy of oral contraceptives or cyclosporine by concurrent use of St. John's wort are examples. In addition, it is common for patients to be cared for by several physicians, and duplicative, additive, antagonistic, or synergistic drug combinations may therefore be administered if the physicians are not aware of the patients' drug histories. Every physician should determine what drugs a patient has been taking, for the previous month or two ideally, before prescribing any medications. Medications stopped for inefficacy or adverse effects should be documented to avoid pointless and potentially dangerous reexposure. A frequently overlooked source of additional drug exposure is topical therapy; for example, a patient complaining of bronchospasm may not mention that an ophthalmic beta blocker is being used unless specifically asked. A history of previous adverse drug effects in patients is common. Since these patients have shown a predisposition to drug-induced illnesses, such a history should dictate added caution in prescribing new drugs.

Laboratory studies may include demonstration of serum antibody in some persons with drug allergies involving cellular blood elements, as in agranulocytosis, hemolytic anemia, and thrombocytopenia. For example, both quinine and quinidine can produce platelet agglutination in vitro in the presence of complement and the serum from a patient who has developed thrombocytopenia following use of this drug. Biochemical abnormalities such as G6PD deficiency, serum pseudocholinesterase level, or genotyping may also be useful in diagnosis, often after an adverse effect has occurred in the patient or a family member.

Once an adverse reaction is suspected, discontinuation of the suspected drug followed by disappearance of the reaction is presumptive evidence of a drug-induced illness. Confirming evidence may be sought by cautiously reintroducing the drug and seeing if the reaction reappears. However, that should be done only if confirmation would be useful in the future management of the patient and if the attempt would not entail undue risk. With concentration-dependent adverse reactions, lowering the dosage may cause the reaction to disappear, and raising it may cause the reaction to reappear. When the reaction is thought to be allergic, however, readministration of the drug may be hazardous, since anaphylaxis may develop.

If the patient is receiving many drugs when an adverse reaction is suspected, the drugs likeliest to be responsible can usually be identified; this should include both potential culprit agents as well as drugs that alter their elimination. All drugs may be discontinued at once or, if this is not practical, discontinued one at a time, starting with the ones most suspect, and the patient observed for signs of improvement. The time needed for a concentration-dependent adverse effect to disappear depends on the time required for the concentration to fall below the range associated with the adverse effect; that, in turn, depends on the initial blood level and on the rate of elimination or metabolism of the drug. Adverse effects of drugs with long half-lives or those not directly related to serum concentration may take a considerable time to disappear.

SUMMARY

Modern clinical pharmacology aims to replace empiricism in the use of drugs with therapy based on in-depth understanding of factors that determine an individual's response to drug treatment. Molecular pharmacology, pharmacokinetics, genetics, clinical trials, and the educated prescriber all contribute to this process. No drug response should ever be termed *idiosyncratic*; all responses have a mechanism whose understanding will help guide further therapy with that drug or successors. This rapidly expanding understanding of variability in drug actions makes the process of prescribing drugs increasingly daunting for the practitioner. However, fundamental principles should guide this process:

- The benefits of drug therapy, however defined, should always outweigh the risk.
- The smallest dosage necessary to produce the desired effect should be used.
- The number of medications and doses per day should be minimized.
- Although the literature is rapidly expanding, accessing it is becoming easier; electronic tools to search databases of literature and unbiased opinion will become increasingly commonplace.
- Genetics play a role in determining variability in drug response and may become a part of clinical practice.
- Electronic medical record and pharmacy systems will increasingly incorporate prescribing advice, such as indicated medications not used; unindicated medications being prescribed; and

potential dosing errors, drug interactions, or genetically determined drug responses.

- Prescribers should be particularly wary when adding or stopping specific drugs that are especially liable to provoke interactions and adverse reactions.
- Prescribers should use only a limited number of drugs, with which they are thoroughly familiar.

FURTHER READINGS

COLLET JP et al: Cytochrome P450 2C19 polymorphism in young patients treated with clopidogrel after myocardial infarction: a cohort study. Lancet 373:309, 2009

GE D et al: Genetic variation in IL28B predicts hepatitis C treatment-induced viral clearance. Nature 461:399, 2009

GIACOMINI KM et al: The pharmacogenetics research network: from SNP discovery to clinical drug response. Clin Pharmacol Ther 81:328, 2007

HO PM et al: Risk of adverse outcomes associated with concomitant use of clopidogrel and proton pump inhibitors following acute coronary syndrome. JAMA 301:937, 2009

THE INTERNATIONAL WARFARIN PHARMACOGENETICS CONSORTIUM: Estimation of the warfarin dose with clinical and pharmacogenetic data. N Engl J Med 360:753, 2009

KARAPETIS CS et al: K-ras mutations and benefit from cetuximab in advanced colorectal cancer. N Engl J Med 359:1757, 2008

LIGGETT SB et al: A polymorphism within a conserved β1-adrenergic receptor motif alters cardiac function and β-blocker response in human heart failure. Proc Natl Acad Sci (USA) 103:11288, 2006

LINK E et al: SLCO1B1 variants and statin-induced myopathy—a genomewide study. N Engl J Med 359:789, 2008

MALLAL S et al: HLA-B*5701 Screening for hypersensitivity to abacavir. N Engl J Med 358:568, 2008

MEGA JL et al: Cytochrome P-450 polymorphisms and response to clopidogrel. N Engl J Med 360:354, 2009

RODEN DM, STEIN CM: Clopidogrel and the concept of high risk pharmacokinetics. Circulation 119:2127, 2009

SIMON T et al: Genetic determinants of response to clopidogrel and cardiovascular events. N Engl J Med 360:363, 2009

WEISS ST et al: Creating and evaluating genetic tests predictive of drug response. Nat Rev Drug Discov 7:568, 2008

WILKE RA et al: Identifying genetic risk factors for serious adverse drug reactions: current progress and challenges. Nat Rev Drug Discov 6:904, 2007

WOODCOCK J, LESKO LJ: Pharmacogenetics—tailoring treatment for the outliers. N Engl J Med 360:811, 2009

YANG JJ et al: Genome-wide interrogation of germline genetic variation associated with treatment response in childhood acute lymphoblastic leukemia. JAMA 301:393, 2009

CHAPTER 6

Women's Health

Andrea Dunaif

The study of biologic differences between sexes has emerged as a distinct scientific discipline. A report from the Institute of Medicine (IOM) found that sex has a broad impact on biologic and disease processes and succinctly concluded that sex matters. The National Institutes of Health established the Office of Research on Women's Health in 1990 to develop an agenda for future research in the field. In parallel, women's health has become a distinct clinical discipline with a focus on disorders that occur disproportionately in women. The integration of women's health into internal medicine and other specialties has been accompanied by novel approaches to health care delivery, including greater attention to patient education and involvement in disease prevention and medical decision-making.

The IOM report recommended the term *sex difference* to describe biologic processes that differ between males and females and *gender difference* for features related to social influences. Disorders highlighted here are reviewed in detail in other chapters.

DISEASE RISK: REALITY AND PERCEPTION

The leading causes of death are the same in women and men: (1) heart disease, (2) cancer (Table 6-1; Fig. 6-1). The leading cause of cancer death, lung cancer, is the same in both sexes. Breast cancer is the second leading cause of cancer death in women, but it causes about 60% fewer deaths than does lung cancer. Men are substantially more likely to die from suicide, homicide, and accidents than are women.

Women's risk for many diseases increases at menopause, which occurs at a median age of 51.4 years. In the industrialized world, women spend one-third of their lives in the postmenopausal period. Estrogen levels fall abruptly at menopause, inducing a variety of physiologic and metabolic responses. Rates of cardiovascular disease increase and bone density begins to decrease rapidly after menopause. In the United States, women live on average about 5 years longer than men, with a life expectancy at birth in 2007 of 80.4 years compared with 75.3 years in men. Elderly women outnumber elderly men, so that age-related conditions such as hypertension have a female preponderance. However, the difference in life expectancy between men and women has decreased an average of 0.1 year every year since 1980, and if this convergence in mortality figures continues, it is projected that mortality rates will be similar by 2054.

Women's perception of disease risk is often inaccurate (Fig. 6-2). Public awareness campaigns have resulted in almost 60% of U.S. women knowing that cardiovascular disease is the leading cause of death in women. Nevertheless, the condition they fear most is breast cancer despite the fact that death rates from breast cancer have been falling since the 1990s. In any specific decade of life, a woman's risk for breast cancer never exceeds 1 in 34. Although a woman's lifetime risk of developing breast cancer if she lives past 85 years is about 1 in 9, it is much more likely that she will die from cardiovascular disease than from breast cancer. In other words, many elderly women have breast cancer but die from other causes. Similarly, a minority of women are aware that lung cancer is the leading cause of cancer

TABLE 6-1 Deaths and Percentage of Total Deaths for the Leading Causes of Death by Sex in the United States in 2006

Cause of Death	Female			Male		
	Rank	Deaths	Deaths, %	Rank	Deaths	Deaths, %
Diseases of heart	1	315,930	25.8	1	315,706	26.3
Malignant neoplasms	2	269,819	22.0	2	290,069	24.1
Cerebrovascular diseases	3	82,595	6.7	5	54,524	4.5
Chronic lower respiratory diseases	4	65,323	5.3	4	59,260	4.9
Alzheimer's disease	5	51,281	4.2	9	21,151	1.8
Accidents (unintentional injuries)	6	42,658	3.5	3	78,941	6.6
Diabetes mellitus	7	36,443	3.0	6	36,006	3.0
Pneumonia	8	30,189	2.5	8	25,288	2.1
Renal failure	9	22,229	1.8	10	21,115	1.8
Septicemia	10	18,712	1.5	12	15,522	1.3
Essential hypertension and hypertensive renal disease	11	14,440	1.2	16	9,415	0.8
Other diseases of respiratory system	12	13,916	1.1	14	13,728	1.1
Chronic liver disease and cirrhosis	13	9,689	0.8	11	17,866	1.5
Parkinson's disease	14	8,266	0.7	15	11,300	0.9
Pneumonitis due to solids and liquids	15	7,971	0.7	17	8,916	0.7
Intentional self-harm (suicide)	17	6,992	0.6	7	26,308	2.2
Assault (homicide)	24	3,856	0.3	13	14,717	1.2

Source: Data from Centers for Disease Control and Prevention: National Vital Statistics Reports, Vol. 57, No. 14, April 17, 2009, Table 12, *http://www.cdc.gov/NCHS/data/nvsr/nvsr57/nvsr57_14.pdf.*

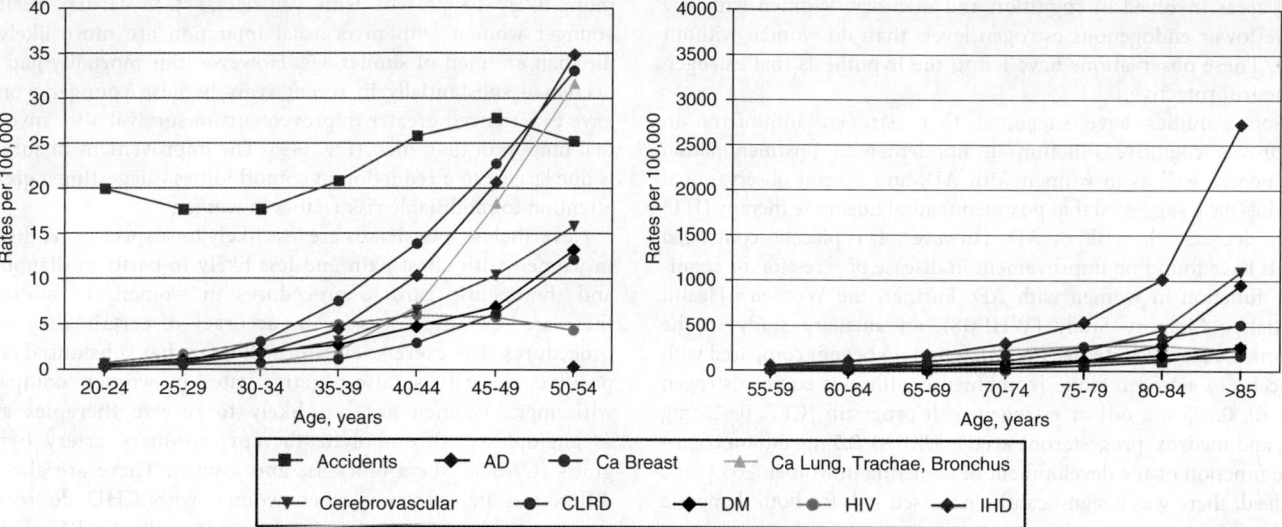

Figure 6-1 **Death rates per 100,000 population for 2006 by 5-year age groups in U.S. women.** Note that the scale of the *y* axis is increased in the graph on the right compared with that on the left. Accidents and HIV/AIDS are the leading causes of death in young women 20–34 years of age. Accidents, breast cancer, and ischemic heart disease (IHD) are the leading causes of death in women 35–49 years of age. IHD becomes the leading cause of death in women beginning at age 50 years. In older women, IHD

remains the leading cause of death, cerebrovascular disease becomes the second leading cause of death, and lung cancer is the leading cause of cancer-related deaths. At age 85 years and beyond, AD becomes the third leading cause of death. AD, Alzheimer's disease; Ca, cancer; CLRD, chronic lower respiratory disease; DM, diabetes mellitus. *(Data adapted from Centers for Disease Control and Prevention, http://www.cdc.gov/nchs/data/dvs/MortFinal2006_WorkTable210R.pdf.)*

death in women. Physicians are also less likely to recognize women's risk for cardiovascular disease. These misconceptions are unfortunate as they perpetuate inadequate attention to modifiable risk factors such as dyslipidemia, hypertension, and cigarette smoking.

SEX DIFFERENCES IN HEALTH AND DISEASE

■ ALZHEIMER'S DISEASE

(See also Chap. 371) Alzheimer's disease (AD) affects approximately twice as many women as men. Because the risk for AD

increases with age, part of this sex difference is accounted for by the fact that women live longer than men. However, additional factors probably contribute to the increased risk for AD in women, including sex differences in brain size, structure, and functional organization. There is emerging evidence for sex-specific differences in gene expression, not only for genes on the X and Y chromosomes but also for some autosomal genes. Estrogens have pleiotropic genomic and nongenomic effects on the central nervous system, including neurotrophic actions in

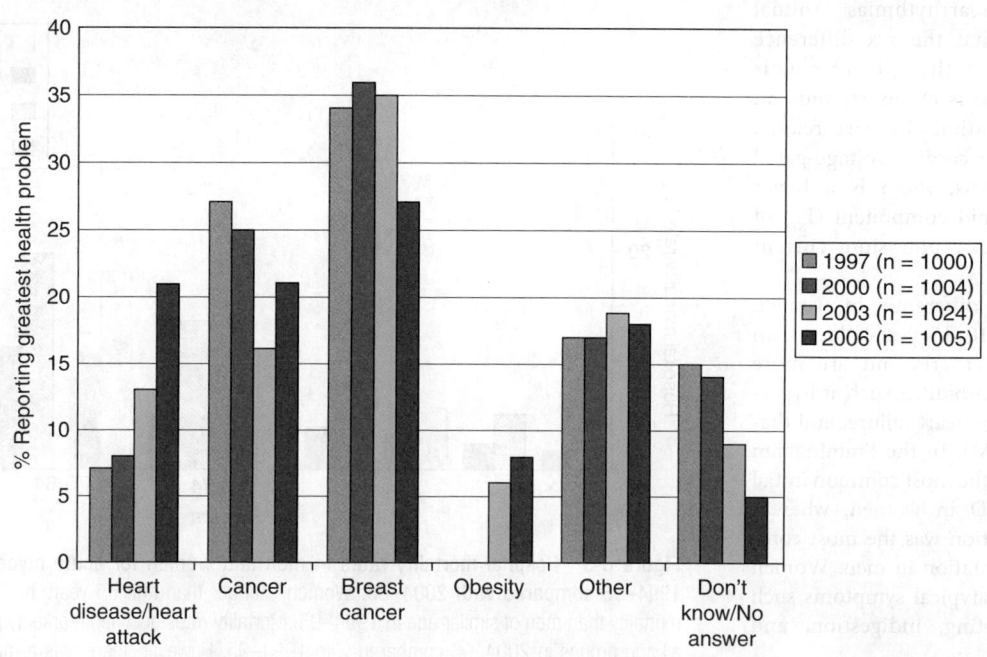

Figure 6-2 **Trends in perceived greatest health problem among women by survey year.** Data for obesity were not available for 1997 and 2000. Significantly more women cited heart disease/heart attack as the

greatest health problem for women in 2006 compared with previous survey years. Breast cancer remained the most commonly identified greatest health risk in all survey years. *(From Christian et al; with permission.)*

key areas involved in cognition and memory. Women with AD have lower endogenous estrogen levels than do women without AD. These observations have led to the hypothesis that estrogen is neuroprotective.

Some studies have suggested that estrogen administration improves cognitive function in nondemented postmenopausal women as well as in women with AD, and several observational studies have suggested that postmenopausal hormone therapy (HT) may decrease the risk of AD. However, HT placebo-controlled trials have found no improvement in disease progression or cognitive function in women with AD. Further, the Women's Health Initiative Memory Study (WHIMS), an ancillary study in the Women's Health Initiative (WHI), found no benefit compared with placebo of estrogen alone [combined continuous equine estrogen (CEE), 0.625 mg qd] or estrogen with progestin [CEE, 0.625 mg qd, and medroxyprogesterone acetate (MPA), 2.5 mg qd] on cognitive function or the development of dementia in women ≥65 years. Indeed, there was a significantly increased risk for both dementia and mild cognitive impairment in women receiving hormone therapy. The possible explanations for the discrepant results between the observational studies and the randomized clinical trials remain unclear (Chap. 348).

■ CARDIOVASCULAR DISEASE

(See also Chap. 243) There are major sex differences in cardiovascular disease, the leading cause of death in men and women in developed countries. Since 1984, more women than men have died of cardiovascular disease. Gonadal steroids have major effects on the cardiovascular system and lipid metabolism. Estrogen increases high-density lipoprotein (HDL) and lowers low-density lipoprotein (LDL), whereas androgens have the opposite effect. Estrogen has direct vasodilatory effects on the vascular endothelium, enhances insulin sensitivity, and has antioxidant as well as anti-inflammatory properties. There is a striking increase in coronary heart disease (CHD) after both natural and surgical menopause, suggesting that endogenous estrogens are cardioprotective. Women also have longer QT intervals on electrocardiograms, and this increases their susceptibility to certain arrhythmias. Animal studies suggest that the sex difference in the duration of the QT interval is caused by the effects of sex steroids on cardiac repolarization, in part related to their effects on cardiac voltage-gated potassium channels; there is a lower density of the rapid component (I_{Kr}) of the delayed rectifier potassium current (I_K) in females.

CHD presents differently in women, who are usually 10–15 years older than their male counterparts and are more likely to have comorbidities such as hypertension, congestive heart failure, and diabetes mellitus (DM). In the Framingham study, angina was the most common initial symptom of CHD in women, whereas myocardial infarction was the most common initial presentation in men. Women more often have atypical symptoms such as nausea, vomiting, indigestion, and upper back pain.

Women with myocardial infarction are more likely to present with cardiac arrest or cardiogenic shock, whereas men are more likely to present with ventricular tachycardia. Further, younger women with myocardial infarction are more likely to die than are men of similar age. However, this mortality gap has decreased substantially in recent years because younger women have experienced greater improvements in survival after myocardial infarction than men (Fig. 6-3). The improvement in survival is due largely to a reduction in comorbidities, suggesting a greater attention to modifiable risk factors in women.

Nevertheless, physicians are less likely to suspect heart disease in women with chest pain and less likely to perform diagnostic and therapeutic cardiac procedures in women. In addition, there are sex differences in the accuracy of certain diagnostic procedures. The exercise electrocardiogram has substantial false-positive as well as false-negative rates in women compared with men. Women are less likely to receive therapies such as angioplasty, thrombolytic therapy, coronary artery bypass grafts (CABGs), beta blockers, and aspirin. There are also sex differences in outcomes when women with CHD do receive therapeutic interventions. Women undergoing CABG surgery have more advanced disease, a higher perioperative mortality rate, less relief of angina, and less graft patency; however, 5- and 10-year survival rates are similar. Women undergoing percutaneous transluminal coronary angioplasty have lower rates of initial angiographic and clinical success than men, but they also have a lower rate of restenosis and a better long-term outcome. Women may benefit less and have more frequent serious bleeding complications from thrombolytic therapy compared with men. Factors such as older age, more comorbid conditions, and more severe CHD in women at the time of events or procedures appear to account in part for the observed sex differences.

Elevated cholesterol levels, hypertension, smoking, obesity, low HDL cholesterol levels, DM, and lack of physical activity are important risk factors for CHD in both men and women. Total triglyceride levels are an independent risk factor for CHD in women but not in men. Low HDL cholesterol and DM are more important risk factors for CHD in women than in men. Smoking is an important

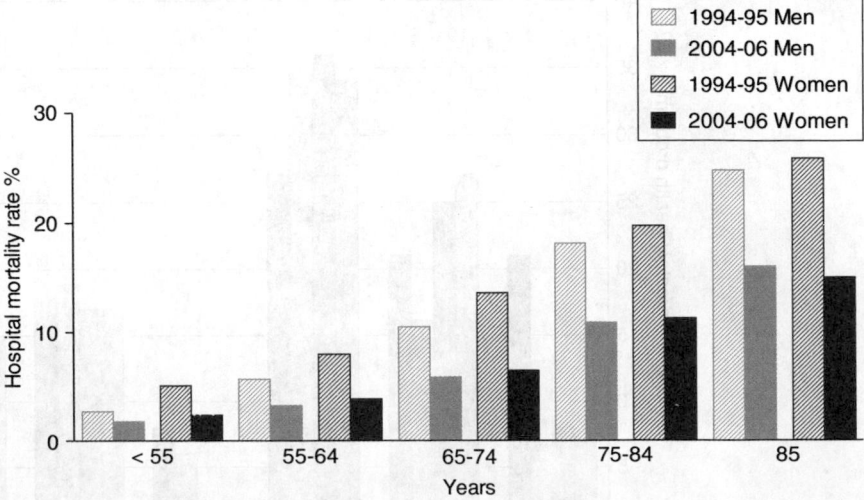

Figure 6-3 Hospital mortality rates in men and women for acute myocardial infarction in 1994–95 compared with 2004–06. Women younger than age 65 years had substantially greater mortality than men of similar age in 1994–95. Mortality rates declined markedly for both sexes across all age groups in 2004–06 compared with 1994–95. However, there was a more striking decrease in mortality in women younger than age 75 years compared with men of similar age. The mortality rate reduction was largest in women less than age 55 years (52.9%) and lowest in men of similar age (33.3%). *(Data adapted from Vaccarino et al.)*

risk factor for CHD in women—it accelerates atherosclerosis, exerts direct negative effects on cardiac function, and is associated with an earlier age of menopause. Cholesterol-lowering drugs are equally effective in men and women for primary and secondary prevention of CHD. However, because of perceptions that women are at lower risk for CHD, they receive fewer interventions for modifiable risk factors than do men.

In contrast to men, randomized trials showed that aspirin was not effective in the primary prevention of CHD in women; it did significantly reduce the risk of ischemic stroke. Secondary prevention in women with known CHD is also suboptimal. At baseline, only about 30% of women enrolled in the Heart and Estrogen/progestin Replacement Study (HERS), a secondary prevention trial in women with established CHD, were taking beta blockers, and only 45% received lipid-lowering medications.

The sex differences in CHD prevalence, beneficial biologic effects of estradiol on the cardiovascular system, and reduced risk for CHD in observational studies of women receiving HT led to the widespread use of HT for the prevention of CHD. However, the WHI, which studied more than 16,000 women on CEE plus MPA or placebo and more than 10,000 women with hysterectomy on CEE alone or placebo, did not demonstrate a benefit of HT for the primary or secondary prevention of CHD. In addition, CEE plus MPA was associated with an increased risk for CHD, particularly in the first year of therapy, whereas CEE alone neither increased nor decreased CHD risk. Both CEE plus MPA and CEE alone were associated with an increased risk for ischemic stroke. There was no evidence for cardioprotective effects of estrogens in smaller randomized trials that used either oral or transdermal estradiol, arguing against the hypothesis that the type of estrogen or its route of administration accounted for the lack of CHD risk reduction.

In the WHI, there was a suggestion of a reduction in CHD risk in women who initiated HT closer to menopause. This finding suggests that the time at which HT is initiated is critical for cardioprotection and is consistent with the "timing hypothesis." According to this hypothesis, HT has differential effects, depending on the stage of atherosclerosis; adverse effects are seen with advanced, unstable lesions. This hypothesis is under investigation in randomized clinical trials, for example, the Kronos Early Estrogen Prevention Study (KEEPS). It is noteworthy that there is no reduction in the risk for ischemic stroke when HT is initiated closer to menopause. HT is discussed further in Chap. 348.

■ DIABETES MELLITUS

(See also Chap. 344) Women are more sensitive to insulin than men are. Despite this, the prevalence of type 2 DM is similar in men and women. There is a sex difference in the relationship between endogenous androgen levels and DM risk: Higher bioavailable testosterone levels are associated with increased risk in women, whereas lower bioavailable testosterone levels are associated with increased risk in men. Polycystic ovary syndrome and gestational DM—common conditions in premenopausal women—are associated with a significantly increased risk for type 2 DM. Premenopausal women with DM lose the cardioprotective effect of female sex and have rates of CHD identical to those in males. These women have impaired endothelial function and reduced coronary vasodilatory responses, which may predispose to cardiovascular complications. Among individuals with DM, women have a greater risk for myocardial infarction than do men. Women with DM are more likely to have left ventricular hypertrophy. In the WHI, CEE plus MPA significantly reduced the incidence of DM, whereas with CEE alone there was only a trend toward decreased DM incidence.

■ HYPERTENSION

(See also Chap. 247) After age 60, hypertension is more common in U.S. women than in men, largely because of the high prevalence of hypertension in older age groups and the longer survival of women. Isolated systolic hypertension is present in 30% of women >60 years. Sex hormones affect blood pressure. Both normotensive and hypertensive women have higher blood pressure levels during the follicular phase than during the luteal phase. In the Nurses Health Study, the relative risk of hypertension was 1.8 in current users of oral contraceptives, but this risk is lower with the newer low-dose contraceptive preparations. HT is not associated with hypertension. Among secondary causes of hypertension, there is a female preponderance of renal artery fibromuscular dysplasia.

The benefits of treatment for hypertension have been dramatic in both women and men. A meta-analysis of the effects of hypertension treatment, the Individual Data Analysis of Antihypertensive Intervention Trial, found a reduction of risk for stroke and for major cardiovascular events in women. The effectiveness of various antihypertensive drugs appears to be comparable in women and men; however, women may experience more side effects. For example, women are more likely to develop cough with angiotensin-converting enzyme inhibitors.

■ AUTOIMMUNE DISORDERS

(See also Chap. 318) Most autoimmune disorders occur more commonly in women than in men; they include autoimmune thyroid and liver diseases, lupus, rheumatoid arthritis (RA), scleroderma, multiple sclerosis (MS), and idiopathic thrombocytopenic purpura. However, there is no sex difference in the incidence of type 1 DM, and ankylosing spondylitis occurs more commonly in men. There are relatively few differences in bacterial disease infection rates between men and women. In general, sex differences in viral diseases can be accounted for by differences in behaviors, such as exposures or rates of immunization. Sex differences in both immune responses and adverse reactions to vaccines have been reported. For example, there is a female preponderance of postvaccination arthritis.

The mechanisms for these sex differences remain obscure. Adaptive immune responses are more robust in women than in men; this may be explained by the stimulatory actions of estrogens and the inhibitory actions of androgens on the cellular mediators of immunity. Consistent with an important role for gonadal hormones, there is variation in immune responses during the menstrual cycle, and the activity of certain autoimmune disorders is altered by castration or pregnancy (e.g., RA and MS may remit during pregnancy). Nevertheless, the majority of studies show that exogenous estrogens and progestins in the form of HT or oral contraceptives do not alter autoimmune disease incidence or activity. Exposure to fetal antigens, including circulating fetal cells that persist in certain tissues, has been speculated to increase the risk of autoimmune responses. There is clearly an important genetic component to autoimmunity, as indicated by the familial clustering and HLA association of many such disorders. However, HLA types are not sexually dimorphic.

■ HIV INFECTION

(See also Chap. 189) Women account for almost 50% of the 40 million persons infected with HIV-1 worldwide. AIDS is an important cause of death in younger women (Fig. 6-1). Heterosexual contact with an at-risk partner is the fastest-growing transmission category, and women are more susceptible to HIV infection than are men. This increased susceptibility is accounted for in part by an increased prevalence of sexually transmitted diseases in women. Some studies have suggested that hormonal contraceptives may increase the risk of HIV transmission. Progesterone has been shown to increase susceptibility to infection in nonhuman primate models of HIV. Women are also more likely to be infected by multiple variants of the virus than are men. Women with HIV have more rapid decreases in their CD4 cell counts than do men. Compared with men, HIV-infected women more frequently develop candidiasis, but Kaposi's sarcoma is less common than it is in men. Women have more adverse reactions, such as lipodystrophy, dyslipidemia, and rash, with antiretroviral therapy than do men. This observation is explained in part by sex differences in the pharmacokinetics of certain antiretroviral drugs, resulting in higher plasma concentrations in women.

■ OBESITY

(See also Chap. 78) The prevalence of obesity is higher in women than in men. Further, >80% of patients who undergo bariatric surgery are women. Pregnancy and menopause are risk factors for obesity. There are major sex differences in body fat distribution. Women characteristically have gluteal and femoral or gynoid pattern of fat distribution, whereas men typically have a central or android pattern. Women have more subcutaneous fat than men. Gonadal steroids appear to be the major regulators of fat distribution through a number of direct effects on adipose tissue. Studies in humans also suggest that gonadal steroids play a role in modulating food intake and energy expenditure.

In men and women, upper-body obesity characterized by increased visceral fat is associated with an increased risk for cardiovascular disease and DM. In women, endogenous androgen levels are positively associated with upper-body obesity, and androgen administration increases visceral fat. In contrast, there is an inverse relationship between endogenous androgen levels and central obesity in men. Further, androgen administration decreases visceral fat in centrally obese men. The reasons for these sex differences in the relationship between visceral fat and androgens are unknown. Obesity increases a woman's risk for certain cancers, in particular postmenopausal breast and endometrial cancer, in part because adipose tissue provides an extragonadal source of estrogen through aromatization of circulating adrenal and ovarian androgens, especially the conversion of androstenedione to estrone. Obesity increases the risk of infertility, miscarriage, and complications of pregnancy.

■ OSTEOPOROSIS

(See also Chap. 354) Osteoporosis is about five times more common in postmenopausal women than in age-matched men, and osteoporotic hip fractures are a major cause of morbidity in elderly women. Men accumulate more bone mass and lose bone more slowly than do women. Sex differences in bone mass are found as early as infancy. Calcium intake, vitamin D, and estrogen all play important roles in bone formation and bone loss. Particularly during adolescence, calcium intake is an important determinant of peak bone mass. Vitamin D deficiency is surprisingly common in elderly women, occurring in >40% of women living in northern latitudes. Receptors for estrogens and androgens have been identified in bone. Estrogen deficiency is associated with increased osteoclast activity and a decreased number of bone-forming units, leading to net bone loss. The aromatase enzyme, which converts androgens to estrogens, is also present in bone. Estrogen is an important determinant of bone mass in men (derived from the aromatization of androgens) as well as in women.

■ PHARMACOLOGY

On average, women have lower body weights, smaller organs, a higher percentage of body fat, and lower total-body water than men.

There are also important sex differences in drug action and metabolism that are not accounted for by these differences in body size and composition. Gonadal steroids alter the binding and metabolism of a number of drugs. Further, menstrual cycle phase and pregnancy can alter drug action. Two-thirds of cases of drug-induced torsades des pointes, a rare, life-threatening ventricular arrhythmia, occur in women because they have a longer, more vulnerable QT interval. These drugs, which include certain antihistamines, antibiotics, antiarrhythmics, and antipsychotics, can prolong cardiac repolarization by blocking cardiac voltage-gated potassium channels, particularly I_{Kr}. Women require lower doses of neuroleptics to control schizophrenia. Women awaken from anesthesia faster than do men given the same doses of anesthetics. Women also take more medications than men, including over-the-counter formulations and supplements. The greater use of medications combined with these biologic differences may account for the reported higher frequency of adverse drug reactions in women than in men.

■ PSYCHOLOGICAL DISORDERS

(See also Chap. 391) Depression, anxiety, and affective and eating disorders (bulimia and anorexia nervosa) are more common in women than in men. Epidemiologic studies from both developed and developing nations consistently find major depression to be twice as common in women as in men, with the sex difference becoming evident in early adolescence. Depression occurs in 10% of women during pregnancy and in 10–15% of women during the postpartum period. There is a high likelihood of recurrence of postpartum depression with subsequent pregnancies. The incidence of major depression diminishes after age 45 years and does not increase with the onset of menopause. Depression in women appears to have a worse prognosis than does depression in men; episodes last longer, and there is a lower rate of spontaneous remission. Schizophrenia and bipolar disorders occur at equal rates in men and women, although there may be sex differences in symptoms.

Both biologic and social factors account for the greater prevalence of depressive disorders in women. Men have higher levels of the neurotransmitter serotonin. Gonadal steroids also affect mood, and fluctuations during the menstrual cycle have been linked to symptoms of premenstrual syndrome. Sex hormones differentially affect the hypothalamic-pituitary-adrenal responses to stress. Testosterone appears to blunt cortisol responses to corticotropin-releasing hormone. Both low and high levels of estrogen can activate the hypothalamic-pituitary-adrenal axis.

■ SLEEP DISORDERS

(See also Chap. 27) There are striking sex differences in sleep and its disorders. During sleep, women have an increased amount of slow-wave activity, differences in timing of delta activity, and an increase in the number of sleep spindles. Testosterone modulates neural control of breathing and upper airway mechanics. Men have a higher prevalence of sleep apnea. Testosterone administration to hypogonadal men as well as to women increases apneic episodes during sleep. Women with the hyperandrogenic disorder polycystic ovary syndrome have an increased prevalence of obstructive sleep apnea, and apneic episodes are positively correlated with their circulating testosterone levels. In contrast, progesterone accelerates breathing, and in the past, progestins were used for treatment of sleep apnea.

■ SUBSTANCE ABUSE AND TOBACCO

(See also Chaps. 392 and 395) Substance abuse is more common in men than in women. However, one-third of Americans who suffer from alcoholism are women. Women alcoholics are less likely to be diagnosed than men. A greater proportion of men than women seek help for alcohol and drug abuse. Men are more likely to go to an alcohol or drug treatment facility, whereas women tend to approach a primary care physician or mental health professional for help under the guise of a psychosocial problem. Late-life alcoholism is more common in women than in men. On average, alcoholic women drink less than alcoholic men but exhibit the same degree of impairment. Blood alcohol levels are higher in women than in men after drinking equivalent amounts of alcohol, adjusted for body weight. This greater bioavailability of alcohol in women is due to both the smaller volume of distribution and the slower gastric metabolism of alcohol secondary to lower activity of gastric alcohol dehydrogenase than is the case in men. In addition, alcoholic women are more likely to abuse tranquilizers, sedatives, and amphetamines. Women alcoholics have a higher mortality rate than do nonalcoholic women and alcoholic men. Women also appear to develop alcoholic liver disease and other alcohol-related diseases with shorter drinking histories and lower levels of alcohol consumption. Alcohol abuse also poses special risks to a woman, adversely affecting fertility and the health of the baby (fetal alcohol syndrome). Even moderate alcohol use increases the risk of breast cancer, hypertension, and stroke in women.

More men than women smoke tobacco, but the prevalence of smoking is declining faster in men than in women. Smoking markedly increases the risk of cardiovascular disease in premenopausal women and is also associated with a decrease in the age of menopause. Women who smoke are more likely to develop chronic obstructive pulmonary disease and lung cancer than men and at lower levels of tobacco exposure.

VIOLENCE AGAINST WOMEN

Domestic violence is the most common cause of physical injury in women, exceeding the combined incidence of all other types of injury (such as from rape, mugging, and auto accidents). Sexual assault is one of the most common crimes against women. One in five adult women in the United States reports having experienced sexual assault during her lifetime. Adult women are much more likely to be raped by a spouse, ex-spouse, or acquaintance than by a stranger. Domestic violence may be an unrecognized feature of certain clinical presentations, such as chronic abdominal pain, headaches, substance abuse, and eating disorders, in addition to more obvious manifestations such as trauma.

SUMMARY

Women's health is now a mature discipline, and the importance of sex differences in biologic processes is well recognized. There has been a striking reduction in the excess mortality rate from myocardial infarction in younger women. Nevertheless, ongoing misperceptions about disease risk not only among women but also among their physicians result in inadequate attention to modifiable risk factors. Research into the fundamental mechanisms of sex differences will provide important biologic insights. Further, those insights will have an impact on both women's and men's health.

FURTHER READINGS

CHRISTIAN AH et al: Nine-year trends and racial and ethnic disparities in women's awareness of heart disease and stroke: An American Heart Association national study. J Womens Health (Larchmt) 16:68, 2007

MOSCA L et al: National study of physician awareness and adherence to cardiovascular disease prevention guidelines. Circulation 111:499, 2005

PRENTICE RL et al: Benefits and risks of postmenopausal hormone therapy when it is initiated soon after menopause. Am J Epidemiol 170:12, 2009

ROSSOUW JE et al: Postmenopausal hormone therapy and risk of cardiovascular disease by age and years since menopause. JAMA 297:1465, 2007

UTIAN WH et al: Estrogen and progestogen use in postmenopausal women: July 2008 position statement of the North American Menopause Society. Menopause 15:584, 2008

VACCARINO V et al: Sex differences in mortality after acute myocardial infarction: Changes from 1994 to 2006. Arch Intern Med 169:1767, 2009

WIZEMANN TM, PARDUE M-L (eds): Exploring the Biological Contributions to Human Health: Does Sex Matter? Washington, DC, National Academy of Sciences, 2001

CHAPTER **7**

Medical Disorders During Pregnancy

Robert L. Barbieri
John T. Repke

Each year, approximately 4 million births occur in the United States, and more than 130 million births occur worldwide. A significant proportion of these are complicated by medical disorders. In the past, many medical disorders were contraindications to pregnancy. Advances in obstetrics, neonatology, obstetric anesthesiology, and medicine have increased the expectation that pregnancy will result in a positive outcome for both mother and fetus despite most of these conditions. Successful pregnancy requires important physiologic adaptations, such as a marked increase in cardiac output.

Medical problems that interfere with the physiologic adaptations of pregnancy increase the risk for poor pregnancy outcome; conversely, in some instances, pregnancy may adversely impact an underlying medical disorder.

HYPERTENSION

(See also Chap. 247) In pregnancy, cardiac output increases by 40%, most of which is due to an increase in stroke volume. Heart rate increases by ~10 beats/min during the third trimester. In the second trimester, systemic vascular resistance decreases and this is associated with a fall in blood pressure. During pregnancy, a blood pressure of 140/90 mmHg is considered to be abnormally elevated and is associated with an increase in perinatal morbidity and mortality. In all pregnant women, the measurement of blood pressure should be performed in the sitting position, because the lateral recumbent position may result in a blood pressure lower than that recorded in the sitting position. The diagnosis of hypertension requires the measurement of two elevated blood pressures, at least 6 h apart. Hypertension during pregnancy is usually caused by preeclampsia, chronic hypertension, gestational hypertension, or renal disease.

■ PREECLAMPSIA

Approximately 5–7% of all pregnant women develop *preeclampsia*, the new onset of hypertension (blood pressure >140/90 mmHg) and proteinuria (>300 mg/24 h) after 20 weeks of gestation. Although the precise pathophysiology of preeclampsia remains unknown, recent studies show excessive placental production of antagonists to both vascular epithelial growth factor (VEGF) (soluble fms-like tyrosine kinase 1 and sflt-1) and transforming growth factor β (TGF-β) (endoglin). These antagonists to VEGF and TGF-β disrupt endothelial and renal glomerular function resulting in edema, hypertension, and proteinuria. The renal histological feature of preeclampsia is glomerular endotheliosis. Glomerular endothelial cells are swollen and encroach on the vascular lumen. Preeclampsia is associated with abnormalities of cerebral circulatory autoregulation, which increase the risk of stroke at near-normal blood pressures. Risk factors for the development of preeclampsia include nulliparity, diabetes mellitus, a history of renal disease or chronic hypertension, a prior history of preeclampsia, extremes of maternal age (>35 years or <15 years), obesity, antiphospholipid antibody syndrome, and multiple gestation.

Severe preeclampsia is the presence of new-onset hypertension and proteinuria accompanied by end organ damage. Features may include marked elevation of blood pressure (>160/110 mmHg), severe proteinuria (>5 g/24 h), or evidence of central nervous system (CNS) dysfunction (headaches, blurred vision, seizures, coma), renal dysfunction (oliguria or creatinine > 1.5 mg/dL), pulmonary edema, hepatocellular injury (ALT > 2-fold the upper limits of normal), hematologic dysfunction (platelet count < 100,000/L or disseminated intravascular coagulation), or placental dysfunction (oligohydramnios or severe intrauterine growth restriction). The HELLP (*h*emolysis, *e*levated *l*iver enzymes, *l*ow *p*latelets) syndrome is a special subgroup of severe preeclampsia and is a major cause of morbidity and mortality in this disease. The presence of platelet dysfunction and coagulation disorders further increases the risk of stroke.

TREATMENT   Preeclampsia

Preeclampsia resolves within a few weeks after delivery. For pregnant women with preeclampsia prior to 37 weeks' gestation, delivery reduces the mother's morbidity but exposes the fetus to the risk of premature birth. The management of preeclampsia is challenging because it requires the clinician to balance the health of the mother and fetus simultaneously. In general, prior to term, women with *mild* preeclampsia may be managed conservatively with bed rest, close monitoring of blood pressure and renal function, and careful fetal surveillance. For women with *severe* preeclampsia, delivery is recommended unless the patient is eligible for expectant management in a tertiary hospital setting. Expectant management of severe preeclampsia remote from term affords some benefits for the fetus but significant risks for the mother.

The definitive treatment of preeclampsia is delivery of the fetus and placenta. For women with severe preeclampsia, aggressive management of blood pressures > 160/110 mmHg reduces the risk of cerebrovascular accidents. Intravenous labetalol or hydralazine are the drugs most commonly used to manage preeclampsia, but labetalol is associated with fewer episodes of maternal hypotension. Nifedipine is also commonly used in pregnancy. Elevated arterial pressure should be reduced slowly to avoid hypotension and a decrease in blood flow to the fetus. Angiotensin-converting enzyme (ACE) inhibitors as well as angiotensin-receptor blockers should be avoided in the second and third trimesters of pregnancy because of their adverse effects on fetal development.

Magnesium sulfate is the treatment of choice for the prevention and treatment of eclamptic seizures. Large, randomized clinical trials have demonstrated the superiority of magnesium sulfate over phenytoin and diazepam, and the efficacy of magnesium sulfate in reducing the risk of seizure and, possibly, the risk of maternal death. Magnesium may prevent seizures by interacting with *N*-methyl-D-aspartate (NMDA) receptors in the CNS. Given the difficulty of predicting eclamptic seizures on the basis of disease severity, once the decision to proceed with delivery is made, most patients carrying a diagnosis of preeclampsia should be treated with magnesium sulfate. Women who have had preeclampsia appear to be at increased risk of cardiovascular and renal disease later in life.

■ CHRONIC ESSENTIAL HYPERTENSION

Pregnancy complicated by chronic essential hypertension is associated with intrauterine growth restriction and increased perinatal mortality. Pregnant women with chronic hypertension are at increased risk for superimposed preeclampsia and abruptio placenta. Women with chronic hypertension should have a thorough prepregnancy evaluation, both to identify remediable causes of hypertension and to ensure that the prescribed antihypertensive agents are not associated with an adverse outcome of pregnancy (e.g., ACE inhibitors, angiotensin-receptor blockers). α-Methyldopa, labetalol, and nifedipine are the most commonly used medications for the treatment of chronic hypertension in pregnancy. α-Methyldopa is a relatively poor antihypertensive drug, but it has a long record of safe use in pregnancy. With the development of newer antihypertensives, also with long records of safe use in pregnancy, and with improved methods of fetal surveillance, we no longer recommend α-methyldopa as first-line therapy for the management of chronic hypertension. Baseline evaluation of renal function is necessary to help differentiate the effects of chronic hypertension versus superimposed preeclampsia, should the hypertension worsen during pregnancy. There are no convincing data that demonstrate that treatment of mild chronic hypertension improves perinatal outcome.

■ GESTATIONAL HYPERTENSION

This is the development of elevated blood pressure during pregnancy or in the first 24 h post-partum in the absence of preexisting chronic hypertension or proteinuria. Mild gestational hypertension that does not progress to preeclampsia has not been associated with adverse pregnancy outcome or adverse long-term prognosis.

RENAL DISEASE

(See also Chaps. 278 and 286) Normal pregnancy is characterized by an increase in glomerular filtration rate and creatinine clearance. This occurs secondary to a rise in renal plasma flow and increased glomerular filtration pressures. Patients with underlying renal disease and hypertension may expect a worsening of hypertension during pregnancy. If superimposed preeclampsia develops, the additional endothelial injury results in a capillary leak syndrome that may make the management challenging. In general, patients with underlying renal disease and hypertension benefit from aggressive management of blood pressure. Preconception counseling is also essential for these patients so that accurate risk assessment and medication changes can occur prior to pregnancy. In general, a prepregnancy serum creatinine level <133 μmol/L (<1.5 mg/dL) is associated with a favorable prognosis. When renal disease worsens during pregnancy, close collaboration between the internist and the maternal-fetal medicine specialist is essential so that decisions regarding delivery can be weighed in the context of sequelae of prematurity for the neonate versus long-term sequelae for the mother with respect to future renal function.

CARDIAC DISEASE

■ VALVULAR HEART DISEASE

(See also Chap. 237) This is the most common cardiac problem complicating pregnancy.

Mitral stenosis

This is the valvular disease most likely to cause death during pregnancy. The pregnancy-induced increase in blood volume, cardiac output, and tachycardia can increase the transmitral pressure gradient and cause pulmonary edema in women with mitral stenosis. Pregnancy associated with long-standing mitral stenosis may result in pulmonary hypertension. Sudden death has been reported when hypovolemia occurs. Careful control of heart rate, especially during labor and delivery, minimizes the impact of tachycardia and reduced ventricular filling times on cardiac function. Pregnant women with mitral stenosis are at increased risk for the development of atrial fibrillation and other tachyarrhythmias. Medical management of severe mitral stenosis and atrial fibrillation with digoxin and beta blockers is recommended. Balloon valvulotomy can be carried out during pregnancy. The immediate postpartum period is a time of particular concern secondary to rapid volume shifts. Careful monitoring of cardiac and fluid status should be observed.

Mitral regurgitation and aortic regurgitation and stenosis

These are generally well tolerated during pregnancy. The pregnancy-induced decrease in systemic vascular resistance reduces the risk of cardiac failure with these conditions. As a rule, mitral valve prolapse does not present problems for the pregnant patient, and aortic stenosis, unless very severe, is well tolerated. In the most severe cases of aortic stenosis, limitation of activity or balloon valvuloplasty may be indicated.

■ CONGENITAL HEART DISEASE

(See also Chap. 236) The presence of a congenital cardiac lesion in the mother increases the risk of congenital cardiac disease in the newborn. Prenatal screening of the fetus for congenital cardiac disease with ultrasound is recommended. Atrial or ventricular septal defect is usually well tolerated during pregnancy in the absence of pulmonary hypertension, provided that the woman's prepregnancy cardiac status is favorable. Use of air filters on IV sets during labor and delivery in patients with intracardiac shunts is recommended.

■ OTHER CARDIAC DISORDERS

Supraventricular tachycardia (Chap. 233) is a common cardiac complication of pregnancy. Treatment is the same as in the nonpregnant patient, and fetal tolerance of medications such as adenosine and calcium channel blockers is acceptable. When necessary, pharmacologic or electric cardioversion may be performed to improve cardiac performance and reduce symptoms. This is generally well tolerated by mother and fetus.

Peripartum cardiomyopathy (Chap. 238) is an uncommon disorder of pregnancy associated with myocarditis, and its etiology remains unknown. Treatment is directed toward symptomatic relief and improvement of cardiac function. Many patients recover completely; others are left with a progressive dilated cardiomyopathy. Recurrence in a subsequent pregnancy has been reported, and women who do not have normal baseline left ventricular function after an episode of peripartum cardiomyopathy should be counseled to avoid pregnancy.

■ SPECIFIC HIGH-RISK CARDIAC LESIONS

Marfan syndrome

(See also Chap. 363) This is an autosomal dominant disease, associated with a high risk of maternal morbidity. Approximately 15% of pregnant women with Marfan syndrome develop a major cardiovascular manifestation during pregnancy, with almost all women surviving. An aortic root diameter <40 mm is considered to be associated with a favorable outcome of pregnancy. Prophylactic therapy with beta blockers has been advocated, although large-scale clinical trials in pregnancy have not been performed. Ehlers-Danlos syndrome (EDS) may be associated with premature labor, and in type IV EDS, there is increased risk of uterine rupture.

Pulmonary hypertension

(See also Chap. 250) Maternal mortality in the setting of severe pulmonary hypertension is high, and primary pulmonary hypertension is a contraindication to pregnancy. Termination of pregnancy may be advisable in these circumstances to preserve the life of the mother. In the Eisenmenger syndrome, i.e., the combination of pulmonary hypertension with right-to-left shunting due to congenital abnormalities (Chap. 236), maternal and fetal death occur frequently. Systemic hypotension may occur after blood loss, prolonged Valsalva maneuver, or regional anesthesia; sudden death secondary to hypotension is a dreaded complication. Management of these patients is challenging, and invasive hemodynamic monitoring during labor and delivery is recommended in severe cases.

In patients with pulmonary hypertension, vaginal delivery is less stressful hemodynamically than cesarean section, which should be reserved for accepted obstetric indications.

DEEP VENOUS THROMBOSIS AND PULMONARY EMBOLISM

(See also Chap. 262) A hypercoagulable state is characteristic of pregnancy, and deep venous thrombosis (DVT) occurs in about 1 in 2000 pregnancies. Pregnancy is associated with an increase in procoagulants such as factors V and VII, and a decrease in anticoagulant activity, including proteins C and S. Pulmonary embolism is one of the most common causes of maternal death in the United States. In pregnant women, DVT occurs much more commonly in the left leg than in the right leg, due to compression of the left iliac vein by the iliac artery and the uterus. Activated protein C resistance caused by the factor V Leiden mutation increases the risk for DVT and pulmonary embolism during pregnancy. Approximately 25% of women with DVT during pregnancy carry the factor V Leiden allele. Additional genetic mutations associated with DVT during pregnancy include the prothrombin G20210A mutation (heterozygotes and homozygotes) and the methylenetetrahydrofolate reductase C677T mutation (homozygotes).

TREATMENT   Deep Venous Thrombosis

Aggressive diagnosis and management of DVT and suspected pulmonary embolism optimize the outcome for mother and fetus. In general, all diagnostic and therapeutic modalities afforded the nonpregnant patient should be utilized in pregnancy. Anticoagulant therapy with low-molecular weight heparin (LMWH) or unfractionated heparin is indicated in pregnant women with DVT. LMWH may be associated with an increased risk of epidural hematoma in women receiving an epidural anesthetic in labor. Four weeks prior to anticipated delivery, LMWH should be switched to unfractionated heparin. Warfarin therapy is contraindicated in the first trimester due to its association with fetal chondrodysplasia punctata. In the second and third trimesters, warfarin may cause fetal optic atrophy and mental retardation. When DVT occurs in the postpartum period, LMWH therapy for 7–10 days may be followed by warfarin therapy for 3–6 months. Warfarin is not contraindicated in breast-feeding women. For women at moderate or high risk of DVT, mechanical or pharmacologic prophylaxis is warranted if they have a cesarean delivery.

ENDOCRINE DISORDERS

◼ DIABETES MELLITUS

(See also Chap. 344) In pregnancy, the fetoplacental unit induces major metabolic changes, the purpose of which is to shunt glucose and amino acids to the fetus while the mother uses ketones and triglycerides to fuel her metabolic needs. These metabolic changes are accompanied by maternal insulin resistance, caused in part by placental production of steroids, a growth hormone variant, and placental lactogen. Although pregnancy has been referred to as a state of "accelerated starvation," it is better characterized as "accelerated ketosis." In pregnancy, after an overnight fast, plasma glucose is lower by 0.8–1.1 mmol/L (15–20 mg/dL) than in the non-pregnant state. This is due to the use of glucose by the fetus. In early pregnancy, fasting may result in circulating glucose concentrations in the range of 2.2 mmol/L (40 mg/dL) and may be associated with symptoms of hypoglycemia. In contrast to the decrease in maternal glucose concentration, plasma hydroxybutyrate and acetoacetate levels rise to two to four times normal after a fast.

TREATMENT   Diabetes Mellitus In Pregnancy

Pregnancy complicated by diabetes mellitus is associated with higher maternal and perinatal morbidity and mortality rates. Preconception counseling and treatment are important for the diabetic patient contemplating pregnancy and can reduce the risk of congenital malformations and improve pregnancy outcome. Folate supplementation reduces the incidence of fetal neural tube defects, which occur with greater frequency in fetuses of diabetic mothers. In addition, optimizing glucose control during key periods of organogenesis reduces other con-genital anomalies including sacral agenesis, caudal dysplasia, renal agenesis, and ventricular septal defect.

Once pregnancy is established, glucose control should be man-aged more aggressively than in the nonpregnant state. In addition to dietary changes, this requires more frequent blood glucose monitoring and often involves additional injections of insulin or conversion to an insulin pump. Fasting blood glucose levels should be maintained at <5.8 mmol/L (<105 mg/dL) with no values >7.8 mmol/L (140 mg/dL). Commencing in the third trimester, regular surveillance of maternal glucose control as well as assessment of fetal growth (obstetric sonography) and fetoplacental oxygenation (fetal heart rate monitoring or biophysical profile) optimizes pregnancy outcome. Pregnant diabetic patients without vascular disease are at greater risk for delivering a macrosomic fetus, and attention to fetal growth via clinical and ultrasound examination is important. Fetal macrosomia is associated with an increased risk of maternal and fetal birth trauma, including permanent newborn Erb's palsy. Pregnant women with diabetes have an increased risk of developing preeclampsia, and those with vascular disease are at greater risk for developing intrauterine growth restriction, which is associated with an increased risk of fetal and neonatal death. Excellent pregnancy outcomes in patients with diabetic nephropathy and proliferative

retinopathy have been reported with aggressive glucose control and intensive maternal and fetal surveillance.

Glycemic control may become more difficult to achieve as preg-nancy progresses due to an increase in insulin resistance. Because of delayed pulmonary maturation of the fetuses of diabetic moth-ers, early delivery should be avoided unless there is biochemical evidence of fetal lung maturity. In general, efforts to control glu-cose and avoid preterm delivery result in the best overall outcome for both mother and newborn. Preterm delivery is generally per-formed only for the usual obstetric indications (e.g., preeclampsia, fetal growth restriction, non-reassuring fetal testing) or for wors-ening maternal renal or active proliferative retinopathy.

◼ GESTATIONAL DIABETES

Gestational diabetes occurs in approximately 4% of pregnancies. All pregnant women should be screened for gestational diabetes unless they are in a low-risk group. Women at low risk for gestational diabetes are those <25 years of age; those with a body mass index < 25 kg/m², no maternal history of macrosomia or gestational diabetes, and no diabetes in a first-degree relative; and those not members of a high-risk ethnic group (African American, Hispanic, Native American). A typical two-step strategy for establishing the diagnosis of gestational diabetes involves administration of a 50-g oral glucose challenge with a single serum glucose measurement at 60 min. If the plasma glucose is <7.8 mmol/L (<140 mg/dL), the test is considered normal. Plasma glucose > 7.8 mmol/L (>140 mg/dL) warrants admin-istration of a 100-g oral glucose challenge with plasma glucose mea-surements obtained in the fasting state and at 1, 2, and 3 h. Normal values are plasma glucose concentrations <5.8 mmol/L (<105 mg/dL), 10.5 mmol/L (190 mg/dL), 9.1 mmol/L (165 mg/dL), and 8.0 mmol/L (145 mg/dL), respectively. Some centers have adopted more sensitive criteria, using <7.5 mmol/L (<130 mg/dL) as the screening threshold and values of <5.3 mmol/L (<95 mg/dL), <10 mmol/L (<180 mg/dL), <8.6 mmol/L (<155 mg/dL), and <7.8 mmol/L (<140 mg/dL) as the upper norms for a 3-h glucose tolerance test. Adverse pregnancy outcomes for mother and fetus appear to increase with glucose as a continuous variable, making it challenging to define the optimal threshold for establishing the diagnosis of gestational diabetes.

Pregnant women with gestational diabetes are at increased risk of stillbirth, preeclampsia, and delivering infants who are large for their gestational age with resulting birth lacerations, shoulder dystocia, and birth trauma including brachial plexus injury. Their fetuses are at risk of hypoglycemia, hyperbilirubinemia, and polycythemia. Tight control of blood sugar during pregnancy and labor can reduce these risks.

TREATMENT   Gestational Diabetes

Treatment of gestational diabetes with a two-step strategy of dietary intervention followed by insulin injections if diet alone does not adequately control blood sugar [fasting glucose < 5.6 mmol/L (<100 mg/dL) and 2-h post-prandial <7.0 mmol/L (<126 mg/dL)] is associated with a decreased risk of birth trauma for the fetus. Oral hypoglycemic agents such as glyburide and metformin have become more commonly utilized for man-aging gestational diabetes refractory to nutritional management. For women with gestational diabetes, within the 10 years after the index pregnancy there is a 40% risk of being diagnosed with diabetes. In women with a history of gestational diabetes, exer-cise, weight loss, and treatment with metformin reduce the risk of developing diabetes. All women with a history of gestational diabetes should be counseled about prevention strategies and evaluated regularly for diabetes.

OBESITY

(See also Chap. 78) Pregnant women who are obese have an increased risk of stillbirth, congenital fetal malformations, gestational diabetes, preeclampsia, urinary tract infections, and post-date deliveries. Women contemplating pregnancy should attempt to achieve a healthy weight prior to conception. For morbidly obese women who have not been able to achieve weight loss with lifestyle changes, bariatric surgery may result in weight loss and improve pregnancy outcomes. Following bariatric surgery, women should delay conception for one year to avoid pregnancy during an interval of rapid metabolic changes.

■ THYROID DISEASE

(See also Chap. 341) In pregnancy, the estrogen-induced increase in thyroxine-binding globulin increases circulating levels of total T_3 and total T_4. The normal range of circulating levels of free T_4, free T_3, and thyroid-stimulating hormone (TSH) remain unaltered by pregnancy.

The thyroid gland normally enlarges during pregnancy. Maternal hyperthyroidism occurs at a rate of ~2 per 1000 pregnancies and is generally well tolerated by pregnant women. Clinical signs and symptoms should alert the physician to the occurrence of this disease. Many of the physiologic adaptations to pregnancy may mimic subtle signs of hyperthyroidism. Although pregnant women are able to tolerate mild hyperthyroidism without adverse sequelae, more severe hyperthyroidism can cause spontaneous abortion or premature labor, and thyroid storm is associated with a significant risk of maternal mortality.

| TREATMENT | Hyperthyroidism In Pregnancy |

Hyperthyroidism in pregnancy should be aggressively evaluated and treated. It is most commonly caused by Graves' disease, but autonomously functioning nodules, gestational trophoblastic disease, thyroiditis, and hyperemesis gravidarum should also be considered. Methimazole crosses the placenta to a greater degree than propylthiouracil and has been associated with fetal aplasia cutis. However, propylthiouracil can be associated with liver failure. Some experts recommend propylthiouracil in the first trimester and methimazole thereafter. Radioiodine should not be used during pregnancy, either for scanning or treatment, because of effects on the fetal thyroid. In emergent circumstances, additional treatment with beta blockers and a saturated solution of potassium iodide may be necessary. Hyperthyroidism is most difficult to control in the first trimester of pregnancy and easiest to control in the third trimester.

Testing for *hypothyroidism* using TSH measurements before or early in pregnancy may be warranted in symptomatic women and women with a personal or family history of thyroid disease. Using this case-finding approach, about 30% of pregnant women with mild hypothyroidism will remain undiagnosed, leading some to recommend universal screening. Children born to women with an elevated serum TSH (and a normal total thyroxine) during pregnancy have impaired performance on neuropsychologic tests. The goal of therapy for hypothyroidism is to maintain the serum TSH in the normal range, and thyroxine is the drug of choice. During pregnancy, the dose of thyroxine required to keep the TSH in the normal range rises. In one study, the mean replacement dose of thyroxine required to maintain the TSH in the normal range was 0.1 mg daily before pregnancy, and it increased to 0.15 mg daily during pregnancy. Since the increased thyroxine requirement occurs as early as the fifth week of pregnancy, one approach is to increase the thyroxine dose by 30% as soon as pregnancy is diagnosed and then adjust the dose by serial measurements of TSH.

HEMATOLOGIC DISORDERS

Pregnancy has been described as a state of physiologic anemia. Part of the reduction in hemoglobin concentration is dilutional, but iron and folate deficiencies are the major causes of correctable anemia during pregnancy.

In populations at high risk for hemoglobinopathies (Chap. 104), hemoglobin electrophoresis should be performed as part of the prenatal screen. Hemoglobinopathies can be associated with increased maternal and fetal morbidity and mortality. Management is tailored to the specific hemoglobinopathy and is generally the same for both pregnant and nonpregnant women. Prenatal diagnosis of hemoglobinopathies in the fetus is readily available and should be discussed with prospective parents either prior to or early in pregnancy.

Thrombocytopenia occurs commonly during pregnancy. The majority of cases are benign gestational thrombocytopenias, but the differential diagnosis should include immune thrombocytopenia (Chap. 115), thrombotic thrombocytopenic purpura, and preeclampsia. Maternal thrombocytopenia may also be caused by disseminated intravascular coagulation (DIC), which is a consumptive coagulopathy characterized by thrombocytopenia, prolonged prothrombin time (PT) and activated partial thromboplastin time (aPTT), elevated fibrin degradation products, and a low fibrinogen concentration. Several catastrophic obstetric events are associated with the development of DIC, including retention of a dead fetus, sepsis, abruptio placenta, and amniotic fluid embolism.

NEUROLOGIC DISORDERS

Headache appearing during pregnancy is usually due to migraine (Chap. 14), a condition that may worsen, improve, or be unaffected by pregnancy. A new or worsening headache, particularly if associated with visual blurring, may signal eclampsia (above) or pseudotumor cerebri (benign intracranial hypertension) (Chap. 28); diplopia due to a sixth-nerve palsy suggests pseudotumor cerebri. The risk of seizures in patients with epilepsy increases in the postpartum period but not consistently during pregnancy; management is discussed in Chap. 369. The risk of stroke is generally thought to increase during pregnancy because of a hypercoagulable state; however, studies suggest that the period of risk occurs primarily in the postpartum period and that both ischemic and hemorrhagic strokes may occur at this time. Guidelines for use of heparin therapy are summarized above (see "Deep Venous Thrombosis and Pulmonary Embolism"); warfarin is teratogenic and should be avoided.

The onset of a new movement disorder during pregnancy suggests chorea gravidarum, a variant of Sydenham's chorea associated with rheumatic fever and streptococcal infection (Chap. 322); the chorea may recur with subsequent pregnancies. Patients with preexisting multiple sclerosis (MS) (Chap. 380) experience a gradual decrease in the risk of relapses as pregnancy progresses and, conversely, an increase in attack risk during the postpartum period. Beta interferons should *not* be administered to pregnant MS patients, but moderate or severe relapses can be safely treated with pulse glucocorticoid therapy. Finally, certain tumors, particularly pituitary adenoma and meningioma (Chap. 379), may manifest during pregnancy because of accelerated growth, possibly driven by hormonal factors.

Peripheral nerve disorders associated with pregnancy include Bell's palsy (idiopathic facial paralysis) (Chap. 384), which is approximately threefold more likely to occur during the third trimester and immediate postpartum period than in the general population. Therapy with glucocorticoids should follow the guidelines established for nonpregnant patients. Entrapment neuropathies are common in the later stages of pregnancy, presumably as a result of fluid retention. Carpal tunnel syndrome (median nerve) presents as pain and paresthesia in the hand, often worse at night, and later with weakness in the thenar muscles. Treatment is generally conservative; wrist splints may be helpful, and glucocorticoid injections or surgical section of the carpal tunnel can usually be postponed. Meralgia paresthetica (lateral femoral cutaneous nerve) consists of pain and numbness in the lateral aspect of the thigh without weakness. Patients are usually reassured to learn that these symptoms are benign and can be expected to remit spontaneously after the pregnancy has been completed. Restless leg syndrome is the most common peripheral nerve and movement disorder in pregnancy. Disordered iron metabolism is the suspected etiology. Management is expectant in most cases.

GASTROINTESTINAL AND LIVER DISEASE

Up to 90% of pregnant women experience nausea and vomiting during the first trimester of pregnancy. Hyperemesis gravidarum is a severe form that prevents adequate fluid and nutritional intake and may require hospitalization to prevent dehydration and malnutrition.

Crohn's disease may be associated with exacerbations in the second and third trimesters. Ulcerative colitis is associated with disease exacerbations in the first trimester and during the early postpartum period. Medical management of these diseases during pregnancy is identical to the management in the nonpregnant state (Chap. 295).

Exacerbation of gall bladder disease is commonly observed during pregnancy. In part, this may be due to pregnancy-induced alteration in the metabolism of bile and fatty acids. Intrahepatic cholestasis of pregnancy is generally a third-trimester event. Profound pruritus may accompany this condition, and it may be associated with increased fetal mortality. Placental bile salt deposition may contribute to progressive uteroplacental insufficiency. Therefore, regular fetal surveillance should be undertaken once the diagnosis of intrahepatic cholestasis is made. Favorable results with ursodiol have been reported.

Acute fatty liver is a rare complication of pregnancy. Frequently confused with the HELLP syndrome (see "Preeclampsia" above) and severe preeclampsia, the diagnosis of acute fatty liver of pregnancy may be facilitated by imaging studies and laboratory evaluation. Acute fatty liver of pregnancy is generally characterized by markedly increased levels of bilirubin and ammonia and by hypoglycemia. Management of acute fatty liver of pregnancy is supportive; recurrence in subsequent pregnancies has been reported.

All pregnant women should be screened for hepatitis B. This information is important for pediatricians after delivery of the infant. All infants receive hepatitis B vaccine. Infants born to mothers who are carriers of hepatitis B surface antigen should also receive hepatitis B immune globulin as soon after birth as possible and preferably within the first 72 h. Screening for hepatitis C is recommended for individuals at high risk for exposure.

INFECTIONS

■ BACTERIAL INFECTIONS

Other than bacterial vaginosis, the most common bacterial infections during pregnancy involve the urinary tract (Chap. 288). Many pregnant women have asymptomatic bacteriuria, most likely due to stasis caused by progestational effects on ureteral and bladder smooth muscle and later in pregnancy due to compression effects of the enlarging uterus. In itself, this condition is not associated with an adverse outcome of pregnancy. However, if asymptomatic bacteriuria is left untreated, symptomatic pyelonephritis may occur. Indeed, ~75% of cases of pregnancy-associated pyelonephritis are the result of untreated asymptomatic bacteriuria. All pregnant women should be screened with a urine culture for asymptomatic bacteriuria at the first prenatal visit. Subsequent screening with nitrite/leukocyte esterase strips is indicated for high-risk women, such as those with sickle cell trait or a history of urinary tract infections. All women

with positive screens should be treated. Pregnant women who develop pyelonephritis need careful monitoring, including inpatient IV antibiotic administration due to the elevated risk of urosepsis and acute respiratory distress syndrome in pregnancy.

Abdominal pain and fever during pregnancy create a clinical dilemma. The diagnosis of greatest concern is intrauterine amniotic infection. While amniotic infection most commonly follows rupture of the membranes, this is not always the case. In general, antibiotic therapy is not recommended as a temporizing measure in these circumstances. If intrauterine infection is suspected, induced delivery with concomitant antibiotic therapy is generally indicated. Intrauterine amniotic infection is most often caused by pathogens such as *Escherichia coli* and group B streptococcus. In high-risk patients at term or in preterm patients, routine intrapartum prophylaxis of group B streptococcal (GBS) disease is recommended. Penicillin G and ampicillin are the drugs of choice. In penicillin-allergic patients, with a low risk of anaphylaxis, cefazolin is recommended. If the patient is at high risk of anaphylaxis, vancomycin is recommended. If the organism is known to be sensitive to clindamycin, this antibiotic may be used. For the reduction of neonatal morbidity due to GBS, universal screening of pregnant women for GBS between 35 and 37 weeks gestation with intrapartum antibiotic treatment of infected women is recommended.

Postpartum infection is a significant cause of maternal morbidity and mortality. Postpartum endomyometritis is more common after cesarean delivery than vaginal delivery and develops in 5% of women after elective repeat cesarean section and in up to 25% after emergency cesarean section, following prolonged labor. Prophylactic antibiotics should be given to all patients undergoing cesarean section, and administration 30–60 minutes prior to skin incision may be preferable to administration at the time of umbilical cord clamping. As most cases of postpartum endomyometritis are polymicrobial, broad-spectrum antibiotic coverage with a penicillin, aminoglycoside, and metronidazole is recommended (Chap. 164). Most cases resolve within 72 h. Women who do not respond to antibiotic treatment for postpartum endomyometritis should be evaluated for septic pelvic thrombophlebitis. Imaging studies may be helpful in establishing the diagnosis, which is primarily a clinical diagnosis of exclusion. Patients with septic pelvic thrombophlebitis generally have tachycardia out of proportion to their fever and respond rapidly to intravenous administration of heparin.

All patients are screened prenatally for gonorrhea and chlamydial infections, and the detection of either should result in prompt treatment. Ceftriaxone and azithromycin are the agents of choice (Chaps. 144 and 176).

■ VIRAL INFECTIONS

Cytomegalovirus infection

Viral infection in pregnancy presents a significant challenge. The most common cause of congenital viral infection in the United States is cytomegalovirus (CMV) (Chap. 182). As many as 50–90% of women of childbearing age have antibodies to CMV, but only rarely does CMV reactivation result in neonatal infection. More commonly, primary CMV infection during pregnancy creates a risk of congenital CMV. No currently accepted treatment of CMV during pregnancy has been demonstrated to protect the fetus effectively. Moreover, it is difficult to predict which fetus will sustain a life-threatening CMV infection. Severe CMV disease in the newborn is characterized most often by petechiae, hepatosplenomegaly, and jaundice. Chorioretinitis, microcephaly, intracranial calcifications, hepatitis, hemolytic anemia, and purpura may also develop. CNS involvement, resulting in the development of psychomotor, ocular, auditory, and dental abnormalities over time, has been described.

Rubella

(See also Chap. 193) Rubella virus is a known teratogen; first-trimester rubella carries a high risk of fetal anomalies, though the risk decreases significantly later in pregnancy. Congenital rubella may be diagnosed by percutaneous umbilical blood sampling with the detection of IgM antibodies in fetal blood. All pregnant women should be screened for their immune status to rubella. Indeed, all women of childbearing age, regardless of pregnancy status, should have their immune status for rubella verified and be immunized if necessary. The incidence of congenital rubella in the United States is extremely low.

Herpesvirus

(See also Chap. 179) The acquisition of genital herpes during pregnancy is associated with spontaneous abortion, prematurity, and congenital and neonatal herpes. A recent cohort study of pregnant women without evidence of previous herpes infection demonstrated that ~2% of the women acquired a new herpes infection during the pregnancy. Approximately 60% of the newly infected women had no clinical symptoms. Infection occurred equally in all three trimesters. If herpes seroconversion occurred early in pregnancy, the risk of transmission to the newborn was very low. In women who acquired genital herpes shortly before delivery, the risk of transmission was high. The risk of active genital herpes lesions at term can be reduced by prescribing acyclovir for the last four weeks of pregnancy to women who have had their first episode of genital herpes during the pregnancy.

Herpesvirus infection in the newborn can be devastating. Disseminated neonatal herpes carries with it high mortality and morbidity rates from CNS involvement. It is recommended that pregnant women with active genital herpes lesions at the time of presentation in labor be delivered by cesarean section.

Parvovirus

(See also Chap. 184) Parvovirus infection (human parvovirus B19) may occur during pregnancy. It rarely causes sequelae, but susceptible women infected during pregnancy may be at risk for fetal hydrops secondary to erythroid aplasia and profound anemia.

HIV infection

(See also Chap. 189) The predominant cause of HIV infection in children is transmission of the virus from the mother to the newborn during the perinatal period. HIV infection with high maternal viral load; low maternal CD4+ T cell count; prolonged labor; prolonged length of membrane rupture; and the presence of other genital tract infections, such as syphilis or herpes, increase the risk of transmission. Advances in antiretroviral therapy now make it possible for many pregnant women to have no detectable viral load as they approach term. These women may elect to attempt a vaginal birth. To reduce the risk of mother-to-newborn transmission, women should be treated during the intrapartum interval with zidovudine and the newborn should also be treated after birth. Breast-feeding may also transmit HIV to the newborn and is therefore contraindicated in most developed countries for HIV-infected mothers.

SUMMARY

Maternal death is defined as the death occurring during pregnancy or within 42 days of completion of the pregnancy from a cause related to or aggravated by the pregnancy, but not from accident or incidental causes. Maternal mortality has decreased steadily during the past 70 years. The maternal death rate has decreased from nearly 600/100,000 live births in 1935 to 13/100,000 live births in 2006. The most common causes of maternal death in the United States today are pulmonary embolism, obstetric hemorrhage, hypertension, sepsis, cardiovascular conditions including peripartum cardiomyopathy, and ectopic pregnancy. With improved diagnostic and therapeutic modalities as well as with advances in the treatment of infertility, more patients with medical complications will be seeking, and be in need of, complex obstetric care. Improving outcome of pregnancy in these women will be best obtained by assembling a team of internists, specialists in maternal-fetal medicine (high-risk obstetrics), and anesthesiologists to counsel these patients about the risks of pregnancy and to plan their treatment prior to conception. The importance of preconception counseling cannot be overstated. It is the responsibility of all physicians caring for women in the reproductive age group to assess their patients' reproductive plans as part of their overall health evaluation.

GLOBAL CONSIDERATIONS

 The maternal mortality ratio in the United States is about 1 in 7500 live births. In some countries in Sub-Saharan Africa and Southeast Asia, the maternal mortality ratio is about 1 in 100 to 1 in 200 live births. The most common cause of maternal mortality in these countries is maternal hemorrhage. The high maternal death rate is due, in part, to inadequate resources, including lack of contraceptive and family-planning services, insufficient number of skilled birth attendants, limited availability of tocolytics, poor nutrition, and a high burden of infectious disease. The high rate of death from peripartum hemorrhage is due, in part, to inadequate access to anesthesia resources, blood-transfusion services, antibiotics, and skilled pelvic surgeons. Maternal death is a global public-health tragedy that could be improved with the application of modest resources.

FURTHER READINGS

Busnell CD et al: Migraines during pregnancy linked to stroke and vascular diseases: US population based case-control study. BMJ 338: b664, 2009

Hogan MC et al: Maternal mortality for 181 countries, 1980-2008: A systematic analysis of progress towards Millennium Development Goal 5. Lancet 375:1609, 2010

Maggard MA et al: Pregnancy and fertility following bariatric surgery. JAMA 300:2286, 2008

Marik PA, Plante LA: Venous thromboembolic disease and pregnancy. N Engl J Med 359:2025, 2008

Ratner RE et al: Prevention of diabetes in women with a history of gestational diabetes: effects of metformin and lifestyle interventions. J Clin Endocrinol Metab 93:4774, 2008

Rowan JA et al: Metformin versus insulin for the treatment of gestational diabetes. N Engl J Med 358:2003, 2009

Schatz M, Dombrowksi MP: Asthma in pregnancy. N Engl J Med 360:1862, 2009

Vaidya B et al: Detection of thyroid dysfunction in early pregnancy: universal screening or targeted high-risk case finding? J Clin Endocrinol Metab 92:203, 2007

Viske BE et al: Preeclampsia and the risk of end-stage renal disease. N Engl J Med 359: 800, 2008

CHAPTER 8

Medical Evaluation of the Surgical Patient

Wei C. Lau

Kim A. Eagle

Cardiovascular and pulmonary complications continue to account for major morbidity and mortality in patients undergoing noncardiac surgery. Emerging evidence-based practices dictate that the internist should perform an individualized evaluation of the surgical patient to provide an accurate preoperative risk assessment and stratification to guide optimum perioperative risk-reduction strategies. This chapter reviews cardiovascular and pulmonary preoperative risk assessment, targeting intermediate- and high-risk patients to strategically guide perioperative therapies to improve outcome. It also reviews perioperative management and prophylaxis of diabetes mellitus, endocarditis, and venous thromboembolism.

ANESTHETICS

Mortality is low with safe delivery of modern anesthesia, especially in low-risk patients undergoing low-risk surgery (Table 8-1). Inhaled anesthetics have predictable circulatory and respiratory effects; all decrease arterial pressure in a dose-dependent manner by reducing sympathetic tone, causing systemic vasodilation, myocardial depression, and decreased cardiac output. Inhaled anesthetics also cause respiratory depression with diminished responses to both hypercapnia and hypoxemia in a dose-dependent manner, and they have a variable effect on heart rate. In combination with neuromuscular blockade, inhaled anesthetic agents also cause reduction in functional residual lung capacity due to loss of diaphragmatic and intercostal muscle function. This decreases lung volume, which may

TABLE 8-1 Surgery: Gradation of Risk of Common Noncardiac Surgical Procedures

Higher	• Emergent major operations, especially elderly
	• Aortic and other noncarotid major vascular surgery (endovascular and nonendovascular)
	• Prolonged surgery associated with large fluid shift and/or blood loss
Intermediate	• Major thoracic surgery
	• Major abdominal surgery
	• Carotid endarterectomy surgery
	• Head/neck surgery
	• Orthopedic surgery
	• Prostate surgery
Lower	• Eye, skin, and superficial surgery
	• Endoscopic procedures

Source: From LA Fleisher et al.

lead to atelectasis in the dependent lung regions and, in turn, may result in arterial hypoxemia from ventilation-perfusion mismatch as well as an increased risk of postoperative pulmonary complications.

Several meta-analyses have shown that overall mortality was lower in patients receiving neuroaxial anesthesia (epidural or spinal) as compared to general (inhaled) anesthesia. Lower rates of venous thrombosis, pulmonary embolism, pneumonia, and respiratory depression were also observed in patients who were provided neuroaxial anesthesia; however, there were no significant differences in cardiac events between the two approaches. A combination of neuroaxial blockade and general anesthesia is useful when it is desired to reduce general anesthesia requirements. Evidence from a meta-analysis of randomized controlled trials also supports postoperative epidural analgesia for the purpose of pain relief for more than 24 h.

EVALUATION OF INTERMEDIATE- TO HIGH-RISK PATIENTS

Simple, standardized preoperative screening questionnaires, such as the one shown in Table 8-2, have been developed for the

TABLE 8-2 Standardized Preoperative Questionnaires[a]

1. Age, weight, height
2. Are you:

   Female and 55 years of age or older or male and 45 years of age of older?

   If yes, are you also 70 years of age or older?
3. Do you take anticoagulant ("blood thinners") medications?
4. Do you have or have you had any of the following heart-related conditions?

   Heart disease

   Heart attack within the last six months

   Angina (chest pain)

   Irregular heartbeat

   Heart failure
5. Do you have or have you ever had any of the following?

   Rheumatoid arthritis

   Kidney disease

   Liver disease

   Diabetes
6. Do you get short of breath when you lie flat?
7. Are you currently on oxygen treatment?
8. Do you have a chronic cough that produces any discharge or fluid?
9. Do you have lung problems or diseases?
10. Have you or any blood member of your family ever had a problem with any anesthesia other than nausea?

    If yes, describe:
11. If female, is it possible that you could be pregnant?

    Pregnancy test:

    Please list date of last menstrual period:

[a]University of Michigan Health System patient information report. Patients who answer yes to any of questions 2–9 should receive a more detailed clinical evaluation.

Source: Adapted from KK Tremper, P Benedict: Anesthesiology 92:1212, 2000; with permission.

purpose of identifying patients at intermediate or high risk who may benefit from a more detailed clinical evaluation. Evaluation of such patients for operation should always begin with a thorough history and physical examination and with a 12-lead resting ECG, in accordance with the American College of Cardiology/ American Heart Association (ACC/AHA) guideline recommendations. The history should focus on symptoms of occult cardiac or pulmonary disease. The urgency of the surgery should be determined, as true emergency procedures are associated with an unavoidably higher morbidity and mortality. Preoperative laboratory testing should be carried out only for specific clinical conditions based on the clinical examination. Thus, healthy patients of any age undergoing elective surgical procedures without coexisting medical conditions should not require any testing unless the degree of surgical stress may result in unusual changes from the baseline state.

■ PREOPERATIVE CARDIAC RISK ASSESSMENT

Assessment of exercise tolerance in the prediction of in-hospital perioperative risk is most helpful in patients who self-report worsening, exercise-induced cardiopulmonary symptoms; those who may benefit from noninvasive or invasive cardiac testing regardless of scheduled surgical procedure; and those with known coronary artery disease (CAD) or with multiple risk factors who are able to exercise. For predicting perioperative events, poor exercise tolerance has been defined as the inability to walk four blocks or climb two flights of stairs at a normal pace or to meet a metabolic equivalent (MET) level of four (e.g., carrying objects of 15–20 lb or playing golf or doubles tennis) because of the development of dyspnea, angina, or excessive fatigue (Table 8-3).

Previous studies have prospectively compared several cardiac risk indices. Given its accuracy and simplicity, the revised cardiac risk index (RCRI) (Table 8-4) is favored. The RCRI relies on the presence or absence of six identifiable predictive factors, which include high-risk surgery, ischemic heart disease, congestive heart failure, cerebrovascular disease, diabetes mellitus, and renal dysfunction. Each of these predictors is assigned one point. The risk of major cardiac events—defined as myocardial infarction, pulmonary edema, ventricular fibrillation or primary cardiac arrest, and complete heart block—can then be predicted. Based on the presence of none, one, two, three, or more of these clinical predictors, the rate of development of one of these major cardiac events is estimated to be 0.5, 1, 5, and 10%, respectively (Fig. 8-1). RCRI 0 has 0.4–0.5% risk of cardiac events; RCRI 1 has 0.9–1.3%; RCRI 2 has 4–6.6%; and RCRI ≥3 has 9–11% risk of cardiac events. The clinical utility of the RCRI is to identify patients with three or more predictors who are at higher risk (≥10%) for cardiac complications and who may benefit from further risk stratification with noninvasive cardiac testing or initiation of preoperative preventive medical management.

TABLE 8-3 Functional Status

Higher	• Difficulty with adult activities of daily living
↑	• Cannot walk four blocks or up two flights of stairs or unable to meet a MET level of four
Risk	• Inactive but no limitation
↓	• Active: easily does vigorous tasks
Lower	• Performs regular vigorous exercises

Source: From LA Fleisher et al.

TABLE 8-4 Revised Cardiac Risk Index Clinical Markers

High-Risk Surgical Procedures

Vascular surgery

Major intraperitoneal or intrathoracic procedures

Ischemic Heart Disease

History of myocardial infarction

Current angina considered to be ischemic

Requiring sublingual nitroglycerin

Positive exercise test

Pathological Q-waves on ECG

History of PTCA and/or CABG with current angina considered to be ischemic

Congestive Heart Failure

Left ventricular failure by physical examination

History of paroxysmal nocturnal dyspnea

History of pulmonary edema

S_3 gallop on cardiac auscultation

Bilateral rales on pulmonary auscultation

Pulmonary edema on chest x-ray

Cerebrovascular Disease

History of transient ischemic attack

History of cerebrovascular accident

Diabetes Mellitus

Treatment with insulin

Chronic Renal Insufficiency

Serum creatinine >2 mg/dL

Abbreviations: CABG, coronary artery bypass grafting; ECG, electrocardiogram; PTCA, percutaneous transluminal coronary angioplasty.

Source: Adapted from TH Lee et al, with permission.

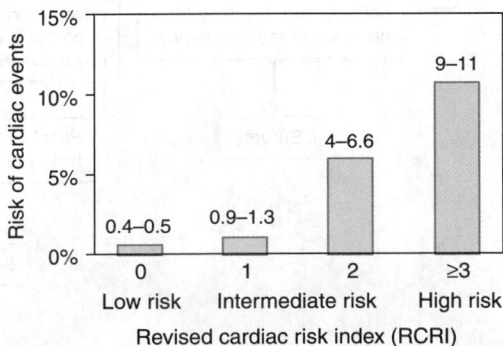

Figure 8-1 Risk stratification based on the RCRI. Derivation and prospective validation of a simple index for prediction of cardiac risk of major noncardiac surgery. Cardiac events include myocardial infarction, pulmonary edema, ventricular fibrillation, cardiac asystole, and complete heart block. *(Adapted from TH Lee et al, with permission.)*

■ PREOPERATIVE NONINVASIVE CARDIAC TESTING FOR RISK STRATIFICATION

There is little evidence to support widespread application of preoperative noninvasive cardiac testing for all patients undergoing major surgery. Rather, a discriminate approach based on clinical risk categorization appears to be both useful clinically and cost-effective. There is potential benefit in identifying asymptomatic but high-risk patients, such as those with left main or left main–equivalent CAD or those with three-vessel CAD with poor left ventricular function who may benefit from coronary revascularization (Chap. 243). However, evidence does not support aggressive attempts to identify patients at intermediate risk with asymptomatic but advanced coronary artery disease, because coronary revascularization appears to offer little advantage over medical therapy.

An RCRI score ≥3 in patients with severe myocardial ischemia on stress testing should lead to consideration of coronary revascularization prior to noncardiac surgery. Noninvasive cardiac testing is most appropriate if it is anticipated that in the event of a strongly positive test a patient will meet guidelines for coronary angiography and coronary revascularization. Pharmacologic stress tests are more useful than exercise testing in patients with functional limitations. Dobutamine echocardiography and persantine, adenosine, or dobutamine nuclear perfusion testing (Chap. 229) have excellent negative predictive values (near 100%) but poor positive predictive values (< 20%) for identification of patients at risk for perioperative myocardial infarction or death. Thus, a negative study is reassuring, but a positive study is a relatively weak predictor of a "hard" perioperative cardiac event. A stepwise approach is illustrated in Fig. 8-2.

■ RISK MODIFICATION USING PREVENTIVE STRATEGIES TO REDUCE CARDIAC RISK

Perioperative coronary revascularization

Currently, potential options for reducing perioperative cardiovascular risk include coronary artery revascularization and/or perioperative medical preventive therapies (Chap. 243). *Prophylactic*

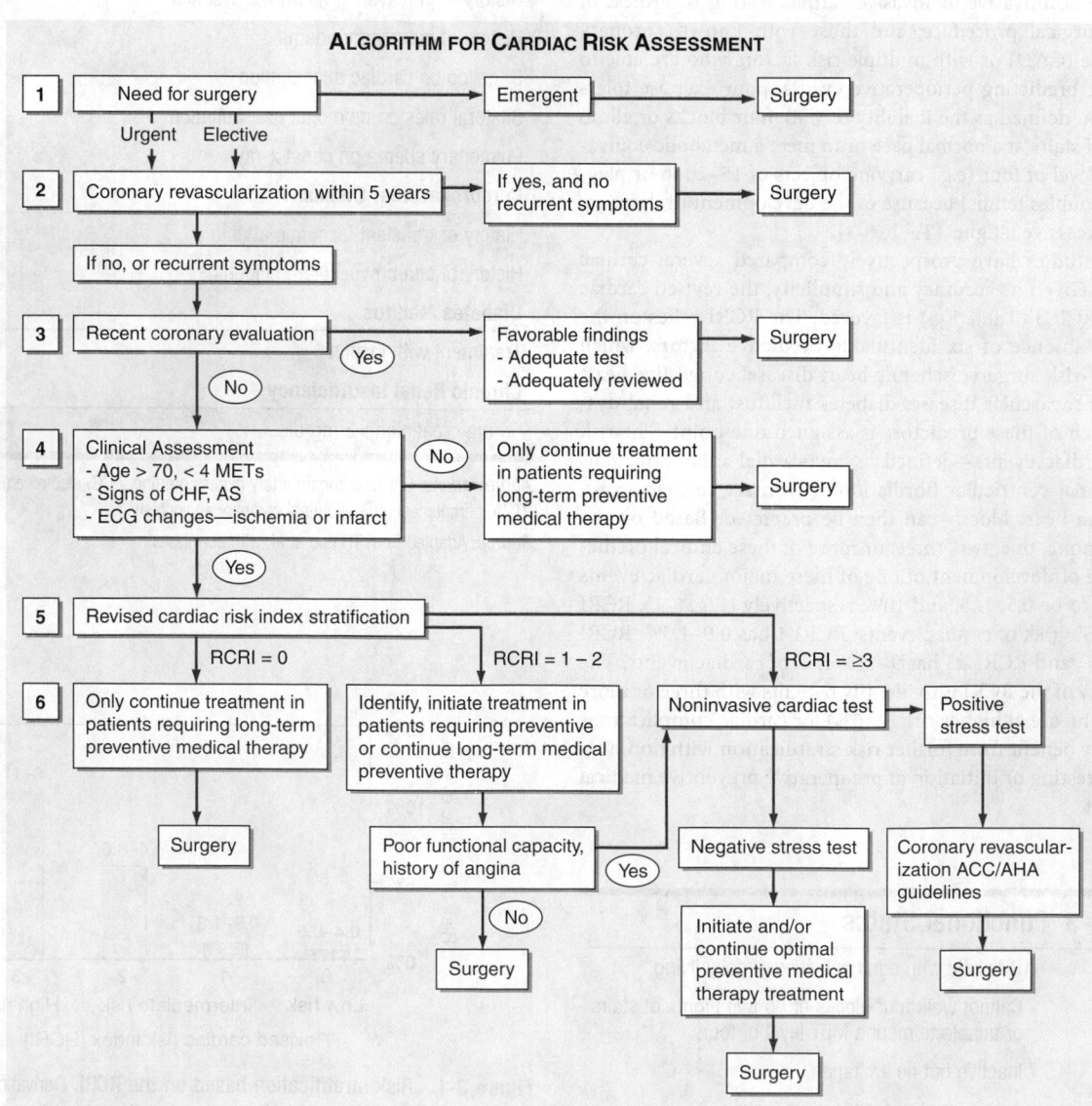

Figure 8-2 Composite algorithm for cardiac risk assessment and stratification in patients undergoing noncardiac surgery. Stepwise clinical evaluation: [1] Emergency surgery; [2] Prior coronary revascularization; [3] Prior coronary evaluation; [4] Clinical assessment; [5] RCRI; [6] Risk modification strategies. Preventative medical therapy = beta blocker and statin therapy. RCRI, revised cardiac risk index. *(Adapted from LA Fleisher et al and TH Lee et al.)*

coronary revascularization with either coronary artery bypass grafting (CABG) or percutaneous coronary intervention (PCI) provides no short- or midterm survival benefit for patients *without* left main CAD or three-vessel CAD in the presence of poor left ventricular systolic function. Although PCI is associated with lower procedural risk than is CABG in the perioperative setting, the placement of a coronary artery stent in a short period of time prior to noncardiac surgery may increase the risk of bleeding during surgery if dual antiplatelet therapy (aspirin and thienopyridine) is administered or it increases the perioperative risk of myocardial infarction and cardiac death due to stent thrombosis if such therapy is withdrawn prematurely (Chap. 246). It is recommended that, if possible, noncardiac surgery be delayed 30–45 days after placement of a bare metal coronary stent and 365 days after a drug-eluting stent. For patients who *must* undergo noncardiac surgery early (> 14 days) after PCI, balloon angioplasty without stent placement appears to be a reasonable alternative because dual antiplatelet therapy is not necessary in such patients.

Perioperative medical preventive therapies Perioperative preventive medical therapy with β-adrenergic antagonists, HMG-CoA reductase inhibitors (statins), and aspirin have the goal of reducing perioperative adrenergic stimulation, ischemia, and inflammation, which are triggered during the perioperative period.

β-adrenergic antagonists The use of perioperative beta blockade should be based on a thorough assessment of a patient's perioperative cardiac risk (RCRI ≥ 2). For patients with or without mild to moderate reactive airway disease, the cardioselective beta blocker of choice should be used and titrated to a target resting heart rate of 60–65 beats/minute. In intermediate- to high-risk patients without a long-term indication for beta blockers, the medications can be administered intravenously as a preoperative medication on the day of surgery, with a targeted heart rate of 60–65 beats/minute and continued for > 7 days (preferably 30 days) postoperatively. Intravenous preparations should be substituted for oral medication if patients are unable to take or absorb pills in the perioperative period. The results from the recent Perioperative Ischemic Evaluation (POISE) trial showed that although cardiac death, nonfatal myocardial infarction, or cardiac arrest was reduced in the patients who received metoprolol as compared to placebo, there was an increased incidence of mortality and stroke in the patients receiving metoprolol because of a high and rapid loading dose of metoprolol. The POISE trial highlights the importance for a clear risk and benefit assessment with careful initiation and titration to therapeutic efficacy of preoperative beta blockers in patients undergoing noncardiac surgery.

The ACC/AHA guidelines recommend the following: (1) Beta blockers *should be continued* in high-risk patients who previously received these drugs and undergo vascular surgery, and they *should be administered* to high-risk patients identified by myocardial ischemia on preoperative assessment who are scheduled to undergo vascular surgery. (2) Beta blockers are *probably recommended* for high-risk patients defined by multiple clinical predictors who undergo intermediate- or high-risk procedures. They *may be considered* for intermediate-risk patients who undergo intermediate- or high-risk procedures and for low-risk patients who undergo vascular surgery.

HMG-CoA reductase inhibitors (statins) A number of prospective and retrospective studies support the perioperative prophylactic use of statins for reduction of cardiac complications in patients with established atherosclerosis. The Dutch Echocardiographic Cardiac Risk Evaluation Applying Stress Echocardiography (DECREASE)-IV study, in addition to confirming the benefit of perioperative bisoprolol in lowering the risk of cardiac death or

myocardial infarction at 30 days, demonstrated a reduced trend in cardiac events in intermediate-risk patients undergoing noncardiac surgery who receive fluvastatin therapy. The use of perioperative statin therapy to reduce perioperative cardiac risk should, therefore, be considered in intermediate- or high-risk patients with atherosclerotic cardiovascular disease who are undergoing major noncardiac surgery.

Angiotensin-converting enzyme (ACE) inhibitors Evidence supports the discontinuation of ACE inhibitors and angiotensin receptor blockers for 24 hours prior to noncardiac surgery due to adverse circulatory effects after induction of anesthesia.

Oral antiplatelet agents Evidence-based recommendations regarding perioperative use of aspirin and/or thienopyridine to reduce cardiac risk currently lack clarity. A substantial increase in perioperative bleeding and transfusion requirement in patients receiving dual antiplatelet therapy has been observed. The discontinuation of thienopyridine and aspirin for 5–7 days prior to major surgery to minimize the risk of perioperative bleeding and transfusion must be balanced with the potential increased risk of an acute coronary syndrome and of subacute stent thrombosis in patients with recent coronary stent implantation. If clinicians elect to withhold antiplatelet agents prior to surgery, they should be restarted as soon as possible postoperatively.

Calcium channel blockers Evidence is lacking to support the use of calcium channel blockers as a prophylactic strategy to decrease perioperative risk in major noncardiac surgery.

■ PREOPERATIVE PULMONARY ASSESSMENT

Perioperative pulmonary complications occur frequently and lead to significant morbidity and mortality. The guidelines from the American College of Physicians recommend the following:

1. All patients undergoing noncardiac surgery should be assessed for risk of pulmonary complications (Table 8-5).
2. Patients undergoing emergency or prolonged (>3 h) surgery; aortic aneurysm repair; vascular surgery; major abdominal, thoracic,

---

TABLE 8-5 Predisposing Risk Factors for Pulmonary Complications

1. Upper respiratory tract infection: cough, dyspnea
2. Age >60 years
3. COPD
4. American Society of Anesthesiologists Class ≥2
5. Functionally dependent
6. Congestive heart failure
7. Serum albumin <3.5 g/dL
8. FEV_1 <2 L
9. MVV <50% of predicted
10. PEF <100 L or 50% predicted value
11. P_{CO_2} ≥45 mmHg
12. P_{O_2} ≤50 mmHg

Abbreviations: COPD, chronic obstructive pulmonary disease; FEV_1, forced expiratory volume in one second; MVV, maximum voluntary ventilation; PEF, peak expiratory flow rate; P_{CO_2}, partial pressure of carbon dioxide; P_{O_2}, partial pressure of oxygen.

Source: Modified from GW Smetana et al and from DN Mohr et al: Postgrad Med 100:247, 1996, with permission.

TABLE 8-6 Risk Modification to Reduce Perioperative Pulmonary Complications

Preoperatively
- Cessation of smoking
- Training in proper breathing (incentive spirometry)
- Inhalation bronchodilator therapy
- Control of infection and secretion, when indicated
- Weight reduction, when appropriate

Intraoperatively
- Limited duration of anesthesia
- Select shorter acting neuromuscular blocking drugs when indicated
- Prevention of aspiration
- Maintenance of optimal bronchodilation

Postoperatively
- Continuation of preoperative measures, with particular attention to

  inspiratory capacity maneuvers

  mobilization of secretions

  early ambulation

  encouragement of coughing

  selective use of a nasogastric tube

  adequate pain control without excessive narcotics

Source: From VA Lawrence et al and from WF Dunn, PD Scanlon, Mayo Clin Proc 68:371, 1993, with permission.

neuro, head, or neck surgery; and general anesthesia should be considered to be at higher risk for postoperative pulmonary complications.

3. Patients at higher risk of pulmonary complications should receive deep breathing exercises and/or incentive spirometry as well as selective use of a nasogastric tube for postoperative nausea, vomiting, or symptomatic abdominal distention to reduce postoperative risk (Table 8-6).

4. Routine preoperative spirometry and chest radiography are less helpful for predicting risk of postoperative pulmonary complications, but may be appropriate for patients with chronic obstructive pulmonary disease (COPD) or asthma.

5. Pulmonary artery catheterization, total parenteral nutrition, and total enteral nutrition are not encouraged for postoperative pulmonary risk reduction.

Other preoperative pulmonary risk-modification strategies

Risk-modification strategies to reduce postoperative pulmonary complications should be implemented, particularly in higher-risk patients. Patients with cough or dyspnea preoperatively should be evaluated to determine the underlying cause of these symptoms. Patients who smoke should be counseled to quit for at least eight weeks prior to elective surgery. Patients with asthma or COPD can be given steroids and bronchodilators pre- and postoperatively to optimize pulmonary function. Bacterial pulmonary infection should be treated preoperatively.

■ DIABETES MELLITUS

(See also Chap. 344) Many patients with diabetes mellitus have significant symptomatic or asymptomatic CAD and may have silent myocardial ischemia due to autonomic dysfunction. Evidence supports intensive perioperative glycemic control to achieve near-normal glucose levels (90–110 mg/dL) versus moderate glycemic control (120–200 mg/dL), using insulin infusion. This practice must be balanced against the risk of hypoglycemic complications. Oral hypoglycemic agonists should be held on the morning of operation. Perioperative hyperglycemia should be treated with intravenous infusion of short-acting insulin or subcutaneous sliding-scale insulin. Patients who are diet-controlled may proceed to surgery with close postoperative monitoring.

■ PROPHYLAXIS FOR INFECTIVE ENDOCARDITIS

(See also Chap. 124) Perioperative prophylactic antibiotics should be administered to patients with congenital or valvular heart disease, prosthetic valves, mitral valve prolapse, or other cardiac abnormalities in accordance with ACC/AHA practice guidelines.

■ PROPHYLAXIS OF VENOUS THROMBOEMBOLISM

(See also Chap. 262) Perioperative prophylaxis of venous thromboembolism should follow established guidelines of the American College of Chest Physicians. Aspirin is not supported as a single agent for thromboprophylaxis. Low-dose unfractionated heparin (≤5000 units subcutaneous bid), low-molecular weight heparin (e.g., enoxaparin 30 mg bid or 40 mg qd) or a pentasaccharide (fondaparinux 2.5 mg qd) for patients at moderate risk, and unfractionated heparin (5000 units subcutaneous tid) for patients at high risk. Graduated compression stockings and pneumatic compression devices are useful supplements to anticoagulant therapy.

FURTHER READINGS

Devereaux PJ et al: Effects of extended-release metoprolol succinate in patients undergoing non-cardiac surgery (POISE trial): A randomized controlled trial. Lancet 371:1839, 2008

Dunkelgruen M et al: Bisoprolol and fluvastatin for the reduction of perioperative cardiac mortality and myocardial infarction in intermediate-risk patients undergoing noncardiovascular surgery: a randomized controlled trial (DECREASE-IV). Ann Surg 249:921, 2009

Fleisher LA et al: ACC/AHA guideline for perioperative cardiovascular evaluation for noncardiac surgery: A report of the American College of Cardiology/American Heart Association Task Force on Practice Guidelines (Writing Committee to Revise the 2002 Guidelines on Perioperative Cardiovascular Evaluation for Noncardiac Surgery). Circulation 116:1971, 2007

Geerts WH et al: Prevention of venous thromboembolism: The Seventh ACCP Conference on Antithrombotic and Thrombolytic Therapy. Chest 126:338S, 2004

Lipshutz AK, Gropper MA: Perioperative glycemic control: An evidence-based review. Anesthesiology 110:408, 2009

Lee TH et al: Derivation and prospective validation of a simple index for prediction of cardiac risk of major noncardiac surgery. Circulation 100:1043, 1999

Lindenauer PK et al: Perioperative beta-blocker therapy and mortality after major noncardiac surgery. N Engl J Med 353:349, 2005

McFalls EO et al: Coronary-artery revascularization before elective major vascular surgery. N Engl J Med 351:2795, 2004

Qaseem A et al: Risk assessment for and strategies to reduce perioperative pulmonary complications for patients undergoing noncardiothoracic surgery: A guideline from the American College of Physicians. Ann Intern Med 144:575, 2006

Smetana GW et al: Preoperative pulmonary risk stratification for noncardiothoracic surgery: Systematic review for the American College of Physicians. Ann Intern Med 144:581, 2006

CHAPTER **9**

Palliative and End-of-Life Care

Ezekiel J. Emanuel

EPIDEMIOLOGY

In 2007, 2,423,712 individuals died in the United States (Table 9-1). Approximately 72% of all deaths occur in those >65 years of age. The epidemiology of mortality is similar in most developed countries; cardiovascular diseases and cancer are the predominant causes of death, a marked change since 1900, when heart disease caused ~8% of all deaths and cancer accounted for <4% of all deaths. In 2006, the year with the most recent available data, AIDS accounted for <1% of all U.S. deaths, although among those age 35–44, it remained one of the top five causes.

It is estimated that in developed countries ~70% of all deaths are preceded by a disease or condition, making it reasonable to plan for dying in the foreseeable future. Cancer has served as the paradigm for terminal care, but it is not the only type of illness with a recognizable and predictable terminal phase. Since heart failure, chronic obstructive pulmonary disease (COPD), chronic liver failure, dementia, and many other conditions have recognizable terminal phases, a systematic approach to end-of-life care should be part of all medical specialties. Many patients with illness-related suffering also can benefit from palliative care regardless of prognosis. Ideally, palliative care should be considered part of comprehensive care for all patients. Reviews of the recent literature have found strong evidence that palliative care can be improved by coordination between caregivers, doctors, and patients for advance care planning, as well as dedicated teams of physicians, nurses, and other providers.

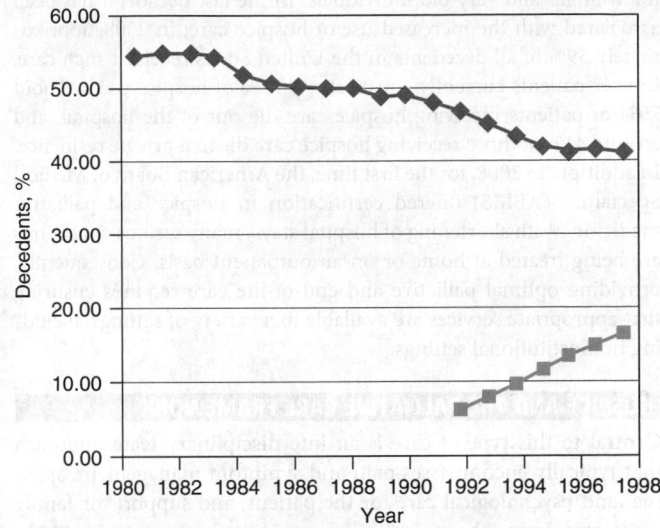

Figure 9-1 **Graph showing trends in the site of death in the last two decades.** ◆, percentage of hospital inpatient deaths; ■, percentage of decedents enrolled in a hospice.

The rapid increases in life expectancy in the United States over the last century have been accompanied by new difficulties facing individuals, families, and society as a whole in addressing the needs of an aging population. These challenges include both more complicated conditions and technologies to address them at the end of life. The development of technologies that can prolong life without restoring full health has led many Americans to seek out alternative end-of-life care settings and approaches that relieve suffering for those with terminal diseases. Over the last few decades in the United States, a significant change in the site of death has occurred that coincides with patient and family preferences. Nearly 60% of Americans died as inpatients in hospitals in 1980. By 2000, the trend was reversing, with ~40% of Americans dying as hospital inpatients (Fig. 9-1). This shift

TABLE 9-1 Ten Leading Causes of Death in the United States and Britain

Cause of Death	United States			Britain	
	Number of Deaths	Percent of Total	Number of Deaths Among People ≥65 Years of Age	Number of Deaths	Percent of Total
All deaths	2,423,712	100	1,759,423	538,254	100
Heart disease	616,067	25.4	510,542	129,009	24
Malignant neoplasms	562,875	23.2	387,515	135,955	25.3
Cerebrovascular diseases	135,952	5.6	117,010	57,808	10.7
Chronic lower respiratory diseases	127,924	5.1	106,845	27,905	5.2
Accidents	123,706	5.1	36,689	10,979	2
Alzheimer's disease	74,632	2.2	71,660	6316	1.2
Diabetes mellitus	71,382	2.9	52,351	34,477	6.4
Influenza and pneumonia	52,717	2.2	49,346	5055	0.9
Nephritis, nephritic syndrome, nephrosis	46,448	1.9	37,377	3287	0.6
Septicemia	34,828	1.4	26,201	2206	0.4

Source: National Center for Health Statistics (data for all age groups from 2007; for age >65, from 2006), *http://www.cdc.gov/nchs;* National Statistics (Great Britain, 2003), *http://www.statistics.gov.uk.*

has been most dramatic for those dying from cancer and COPD and for younger and very old individuals. In the last decade, it has been associated with the increased use of hospice care; in 2008, approximately 39% of all decedents in the United States received such care. Cancer patients currently constitute ~38.3% of hospice users. About 79% of patients receiving hospice care die out of the hospital, and around 41% of those receiving hospice care die in a private residence. In addition, in 2008, for the first time, the American Board of Medical Specialties (ABMS) offered certification in hospice and palliative medicine. With shortening of hospital stays, many serious conditions are being treated at home or on an outpatient basis. Consequently, providing optimal palliative and end-of-life care requires ensuring that appropriate services are available in a variety of settings, including noninstitutional settings.

HOSPICE AND THE PALLIATIVE CARE FRAMEWORK

Central to this type of care is an interdisciplinary team approach that typically encompasses pain and symptom management, spiritual and psychological care for the patient, and support for family caregivers during the patient's illness and the bereavement period.

Terminally ill patients have a wide variety of advanced diseases, often with multiple symptoms that demand relief, and require noninvasive therapeutic regimens to be delivered in flexible care settings. Fundamental to ensuring quality palliative and end-of-life care is a focus on four broad domains: (1) physical symptoms; (2) psychological symptoms; (3) social needs that include interpersonal relationships, caregiving, and economic concerns; and (4) existential or spiritual needs.

A comprehensive assessment screens for and evaluates needs in each of these four domains. Goals for care are established in discussions with the patient and/or family, based on the assessment in each of the domains. Interventions then are aimed at improving or managing symptoms and needs. Although physicians are responsible for certain interventions, especially technical ones, and for coordinating the interventions, they cannot be responsible for providing all of them. Since failing to address any one of the domains is likely to preclude a good death, a well-coordinated, effectively communicating interdisciplinary team takes on special importance in end-of-life care. Depending on the setting, critical members of the interdisciplinary team will include physicians, nurses, social workers, chaplains, nurse's aides, physical therapists, bereavement counselors, and volunteers.

◼ ASSESSMENT AND CARE PLANNING

Comprehensive assessment

Standardized methods for conducting a comprehensive assessment focus on evaluating the patient's condition in all four domains affected by illness: physical, psychological, social, and spiritual. The assessment of physical and mental symptoms should follow a modified version of the traditional medical history and physical examination that emphasizes symptoms. Questions should aim at elucidating symptoms and discerning sources of suffering and gauging how much those symptoms interfere with the patient's quality of life. Standardized assessment is critical. Currently, there are 21 symptom assessment instruments for cancer alone. Further research on and validation of these assessment tools, especially taking into account patient perspectives, could improve their effectiveness. Instruments with good psychometric properties that assess a wide range of symptoms include the Memorial Symptom Assessment Scale (MSAS), the Rotterdam Symptom Checklist, the Worthing Chemotherapy Questionnaire, and the Computerized Symptom Assessment Instrument. These instruments are long and may be useful for initial clinical or for research assessments. Shorter instruments are useful for patients whose performance status does

not permit comprehensive assessments. Suitable shorter instruments include the Condensed Memorial Symptom Assessment Scale, the Edmonton Symptom Assessment System, the M.D. Anderson Symptom Assessment Inventory, and the Symptom Distress Scale. Using such instruments ensures that the assessment is comprehensive and does not focus only on pain and a few other physical symptoms. Invasive tests are best avoided in end-of-life care, and even minimally invasive tests should be evaluated carefully for their benefit-to-burden ratio for the patient. Aspects of the physical examination that are uncomfortable and unlikely to yield useful information can be omitted.

Regarding social needs, health care providers should assess the status of important relationships, financial burdens, caregiving needs, and access to medical care. Relevant questions will include the following: *How often is there someone to feel close to? How has this illness been for your family? How has it affected your relationships? How much help do you need with things like getting meals and getting around? How much trouble do you have getting the medical care you need?* In the area of existential needs, providers should assess distress and the patient's sense of being emotionally and existentially settled and of finding purpose or meaning. Helpful assessment questions can include the following: *How much are you able to find meaning since your illness began? What things are most important to you at this stage?* In addition, it can be helpful to ask how the patient perceives his or her care: *How much do you feel your doctors and nurses respect you? How clear is the information from us about what to expect regarding your illness? How much do you feel that the medical care you are getting fits with your goals?* If concern is detected in any of these areas, deeper evaluative questions are warranted.

Communication

Especially when an illness is life-threatening, there are many emotionally charged and potentially conflict-creating moments, collectively called "bad news" situations, in which empathic and effective communication skills are essential. Those moments include communicating with the patient and/or family about a terminal diagnosis, the patient's prognosis, any treatment failures, deemphasizing efforts to cure and prolong life while focusing more on symptom management and palliation, advance care planning, and the patient's death. Although these conversations can be difficult and lead to tension, research indicates that end-of-life discussions can lead to earlier hospice referrals rather than overly aggressive treatment, benefiting quality of life for patients and improving the bereavement process for families.

Just as surgeons plan and prepare for major operations and investigators rehearse a presentation of research results, physicians and health care providers caring for patients with significant or advanced illness can develop a practiced approach to sharing important information and planning interventions. In addition, families identify as important both how well the physician was prepared to deliver bad news and the setting in which it was delivered. For instance, 27% of families making critical decisions for patients in an intensive care unit (ICU) desired better and more private physical space to communicate with physicians, and 48% found having clergy present reassuring.

An organized and effective seven-step procedure for communicating bad news goes by the acronym P-SPIKES: (1) *p*repare for the discussion, (2) *s*et up a suitable environment, (3) begin the discussion by finding out what the *p*atient and/or family understand, (4) determine how they will comprehend new *i*nformation best and how much they want to know, (5) provide needed new *k*nowledge accordingly, (6) allow for *e*motional responses, and (7) *s*hare plans for the next steps in care. Table 9-2 provides a summary of these steps along with suggested phrases and underlying rationales for

TABLE 9-2 Elements of Communicating Bad News—The P-SPIKES Approach

Acronym	Steps	Aim of the Interaction	Preparations, Questions, or Phrases
P	Preparation	Mentally prepare for the interaction with the patient and/or family.	Review what information needs to be communicated. Plan how you will provide emotional support. Rehearse key steps and phrases in the interaction.
S	Setting of the interaction	Ensure the appropriate setting for a serious and potentially emotionally charged discussion.	Ensure that patient, family, and appropriate social supports are present. Devote sufficient time. Ensure privacy and prevent interruptions by people or beeper. Bring a box of tissues.
P	Patient's perception and preparation	Begin the discussion by establishing the baseline and whether the patient and family can grasp the information. Ease tension by having the patient and family contribute.	Start with open-ended questions to encourage participation. Possible phrases to use: *What do you understand about your illness?* *When you first had symptom X, what did you think it might be?* *What did Dr. X tell you when he or she sent you here?* *What do you think is going to happen?*
I	Invitation and information needs	Discover what information needs the patient and/or family have and what limits they want regarding the bad information.	Possible phrases to use: *If this condition turns out to be something serious, do you want to know?* *Would you like me to tell you all the details of your condition? If not, who would you like me to talk to?*
K	Knowledge of the condition	Provide the bad news or other information to the patient and/or family sensitively.	Do not just dump the information on the patient and family. Check for patient and family understanding. Possible phrases to use: *I feel badly to have to tell you this, but…* *Unfortunately, the tests showed…* *I'm afraid the news is not good…*
E	Empathy and exploration	Identify the cause of the emotions— e.g., poor prognosis. Empathize with the patient and/or family's feelings. Explore by asking open-ended questions.	Strong feelings in reaction to bad news are normal. Acknowledge what the patient and family are feeling. Remind them such feelings are normal, even if frightening. Give them time to respond. Remind patient and family you won't abandon them. Possible phrases to use: *I imagine this is very hard for you to hear.* *You look very upset. Tell me how you are feeling.* *I wish the news were different.* *We'll do whatever we can to help you.*
S	Summary and planning	Delineate for the patient and the family the next steps, including additional tests or interventions.	It is the unknown and uncertain that can increase anxiety. Recommend a schedule with goals and landmarks. Provide your rationale for the patient and/or family to accept (or reject). If the patient and/or family are not ready to discuss the next steps, schedule a follow-up visit.

Source: Adapted from Buckman.

each one. Additional research that further considers the response of patients to systematic methods of delivering bad news could build the evidence base for even more effective communication procedures.

Continuous goal assessment

Major barriers to ensuring quality palliative and end-of-life care include difficulty providing an accurate prognosis and emotional resistance of patients and their families to accepting the implications of a poor prognosis. A practical solution to these barriers is to integrate palliative care with curative care regardless of prognosis.

With this approach, palliative care no longer conveys the message of failure, having no more treatments, or "giving up hope." Fundamental to integrating palliative care with curative therapy is to include continuous goal assessment as part of the routine patient reassessment that occurs at most patient-physician encounters.

Goals for care are numerous, ranging from cure of a specific disease, to prolonging life, to relief of a symptom, to delaying the course of an incurable disease, to adapting to progressive disability without disrupting the family, to finding peace of mind or personal meaning, to dying in a manner that leaves loved ones with positive memories. Discernment of goals for care can be approached through a seven-step protocol: (1) ensure that medical and other information is as complete as reasonably possible and is understood by all relevant parties (see above); (2) explore what the patient and/or family are hoping for while identifying relevant and realistic goals; (3) share all the options with the patient and family; (4) respond with empathy as they adjust to changing expectations; (5) make a plan, emphasizing what can be done toward achieving the realistic goals; (6) follow through with the plan; and (7) review and revise the plan periodically, considering at every encounter whether the goals of care should be reviewed with the patient and/or family. Each of these steps need not be followed in rote order, but together they provide a helpful framework for interactions with patients and their families about goals for care. It can be especially challenging if a patient or family member has difficulty letting go of an unrealistic goal. One strategy is to help them refocus on more realistic goals and also suggest that while hoping for the best, it is still prudent to plan for other outcomes as well.

Advance care planning

Practices Advance care planning is a process of planning for future medical care in case the patient becomes incapable of making medical decisions. A 2010 study of adults 60 or older who died between 2000 and 2006 found that 42% required decision-making about treatment in the final days of life but 70% lacked decision-making capacity. Among those lacking decision-making capacity, around one-third did not have advance planning directives. Ideally, such planning would occur before a health care crisis or the terminal phase of an illness. Unfortunately, diverse barriers prevent this. Although 80% of Americans endorse advance care planning and completing living wills, only 47% have actually done so. Most patients expect physicians to initiate advance care planning and will wait for physicians to broach the subject. Patients also wish to discuss advance care planning with their families. Yet patients with unrealistic expectations are significantly more likely to prefer aggressive treatments. Fewer than one-third of health care providers have completed advance care planning for themselves. Hence, a good first step is for health care providers to complete their own advance care planning. This makes providers aware of the critical choices in the process and the issues that are especially charged and allows them to tell their patients truthfully that they personally have done advance planning.

Steps in effective advance care planning center on (1) introducing the topic, (2) structuring a discussion, (3) reviewing plans that have been discussed by the patient and family, (4) documenting the plans, (5) updating them periodically, and (6) implementing the advance care directives (Table 9-3). Two of the main barriers to advance care planning are problems in raising the topic and difficulty in structuring a succinct discussion. Raising the topic can be done efficiently as a routine matter, noting that it is recommended for all patients, analogous to purchasing insurance or estate planning. Many of the most difficult cases have involved unexpected, acute episodes of brain damage in young individuals.

Structuring a focused discussion is a central communication skill. Identify the health care proxy and recommend his or her involvement in the process of advance care planning. Select a worksheet, preferably one that has been evaluated and demonstrated to produce reliable and valid expressions of patient preferences, and orient the patient and proxy to it. Such worksheets exist for both general and disease-specific situations. Discuss with the patient and proxy one scenario as an example to demonstrate how to think about the issues. It is often helpful to begin with a scenario in which the patient is likely to have settled preferences for care, such as being in a persistent vegetative state. Once the patient's preferences for interventions in this scenario are determined, suggest that the patient and proxy discuss and complete the worksheet for the others. If appropriate, suggest that they involve other family members in the discussion. On a return visit, go over the patient's preferences, checking and resolving any inconsistencies. After having the patient and proxy sign the document, place it in the medical chart and be sure that copies are provided to relevant family members and care sites. Since patients' preferences can change, these documents have to be reviewed periodically.

Types of documents Advance care planning documents are of two broad types. The first includes living wills or instructional directives; these are advisory documents that describe the types of decisions that should direct care. Some are more specific, delineating different scenarios and interventions for the patient to choose from. Among these, some are for general use and others are designed for use by patients with a specific type of disease, such as cancer or HIV. Less specific directives can be general statements of not wanting life-sustaining interventions or forms that describe the values that should guide specific discussions about terminal care. The second type of advance directive allows the designation of a health care proxy (sometimes also referred to as a durable attorney for health care), who is an individual selected by the patient to make decisions. The choice is not either/or; a combined directive that includes a living will and designates a proxy is often used, and the directive should indicate clearly whether the specified patient preferences or the proxy's choice takes precedence if they conflict. Some states have begun to put into practice a "Physician Orders for Life-Sustaining Treatment (POLST)" paradigm, which builds on communication between providers and patients to include guidance for end-of-life care in a color-coordinated form that follows the patient across treatment settings. The procedures for completing advance care planning documents vary according to state law.

A potentially misleading distinction relates to statutory as opposed to advisory documents. Statutory documents are drafted to fulfill relevant state laws. Advisory documents are drafted to reflect the patient's wishes. Both are legal, the first under state law and the latter under common or constitutional law.

Legal aspects As of 2006, 48 states and the District of Columbia had enacted living will legislation. Many states have their own statutory forms. Massachusetts and Michigan do not have living will laws, although both have health care proxy laws. In 25 states, the laws state that the living will is not valid if a woman is pregnant. However, like all other states except Alaska, these states have enacted durable power of attorney for health care laws that permit patients to designate a proxy decision-maker with authority to terminate life-sustaining treatments. Only in Alaska does the law prohibit proxies from terminating life-sustaining treatments. The health reform legislation, the Affordable Care Act of 2010, raised substantial controversy when early versions of the law included Medicare reimbursement for advance care planning consultations. These provisions were withdrawn over accusations that they would lead to the rationing of care for the elderly.

The U.S. Supreme Court has ruled that patients have a constitutional right to decide about refusing and terminating medical interventions, including life-sustaining interventions, and that mentally incompetent patients can exercise this right by providing "clear and convincing evidence" of their preferences. Since advance care directives permit patients to provide such evidence, commentators agree that they are constitutionally protected. Most commentators believe that a state is required to honor any clear advance care directive whether or not it is written on an "official" form. Many states have enacted laws explicitly to honor out-of-state directives. If a patient is not using a statutory form, it may be advisable to attach a statutory form to the advance care directive being used. State-specific forms are readily available free of charge for health care providers and

TABLE 9-3 Steps in Advance Care Planning

Step	Goals to be Achieved and Measures to Cover	Useful Phrases or Points to Make
Introducing advance care planning	Ask the patient what he or she knows about advance care planning and if he or she has already completed an advance care directive. Indicate that you as a physician have completed advance care planning. Indicate that you try to perform advance care planning with all patients regardless of prognosis. Explain the goals of the process as empowering the patient and ensuring that you and the proxy understand the patient's preferences. Provide the patient relevant literature, including the advance care directive that you prefer to use. Recommend the patient identify a proxy decision-maker who should attend the next meeting.	I'd like to talk with you about something I try to discuss with all my patients. It's called advance care planning. In fact, I feel that this is such an important topic that I have done this myself. Are you familiar with advance care planning or living wills? Have you thought about the type of care you would want if you ever became too sick to speak for yourself? That is the purpose of advance care planning. There is no change in health that we have not discussed. I am bringing this up now because it is sensible for everyone, no matter how well or ill, old or young. Have many copies of advance care directives available, including in the waiting room, for patients and families. Know resources for state-specific forms (available at www.nhpco.org).
Structured discussion of scenarios and patient	Affirm that the goal of the process is to follow the patient's wishes if the patient loses decision-making capacity. Elicit the patient's overall goals related to health care. Elicit the patient's preferences for specific interventions in a few salient and common scenarios. Help the patient define the threshold for withdrawing and withholding interventions. Define the patient's preference for the role of the proxy.	Use a structured worksheet with typical scenarios. Begin the discussion with persistent vegetative state and consider other scenarios, such as recovery from an acute event with serious disability, asking the patient about his or her preferences regarding specific interventions, such as ventilators, artificial nutrition, and CPR, and then proceeding to less invasive interventions, such as blood transfusions and antibiotics.
Review the patient's preferences	After the patient has made choices of interventions, review them to ensure they are consistent and the proxy is aware of them.	
Document the patient's preferences	Formally complete the advance care directive and have a witness sign it. Provide a copy for the patient and the proxy. Insert a copy into the patient's medical record and summarize in a progress note.	
Update the directive	Periodically, and with major changes in health status, review the directive with the patient and make any modifications.	
Apply the directive	The directive goes into effect only when the patient becomes unable to make medical decisions for himself or herself. Reread the directive to be sure about its content. Discuss your proposed actions based on the directive with the proxy.	

Abbreviation: CPR, cardiopulmonary resuscitation.

patients and families through the website of the National Hospice and Palliative Care Organization (*http://www.nhpco.org*).

INTERVENTIONS

■ PHYSICAL SYMPTOMS AND THEIR MANAGEMENT

Great emphasis has been placed on addressing dying patients' pain. Some institutions have made pain assessment a fifth vital sign to emphasize its importance. This also has been advocated by large health care systems such as the Veterans' Administration and accrediting bodies such as the Joint Commission on the Accreditation

of Health Care Organizations (JCAHO). Although this embrace of pain as the fifth vital sign has been symbolically important, no data document that it has improved pain management practices. Although good palliative care requires good pain management, it also requires more. The frequency of symptoms varies by disease and other factors. The most common physical and psychological symptoms among all terminally ill patients include pain, fatigue, insomnia, anorexia, dyspnea, depression, anxiety, and nausea and vomiting. In the last days of life, terminal delirium is also common. Assessments of patients with advanced cancer have shown

TABLE 9-4 Common Physical and Psychological Symptoms of Terminally Ill Patients

Physical Symptoms	Psychological Symptoms
Pain	Anxiety
Fatigue and weakness	Depression
Dyspnea	Hopelessness
Insomnia	Meaninglessness
Dry mouth	Irritability
Anorexia	Impaired concentration
Nausea and vomiting	Confusion
Constipation	Delirium
Cough	Loss of libido
Swelling of arms or legs	
Itching	
Diarrhea	
Dysphagia	
Dizziness	
Fecal and urinary incontinence	
Numbness/tingling in hands/feet	

that patients experienced an average of 11.5 different physical and psychological symptoms (Table 9-4).

Evaluations to determine the etiology of these symptoms usually can be limited to the history and physical examination. In some cases, radiologic or other diagnostic examinations will provide sufficient benefit in directing optimal palliative care to warrant the risks, potential discomfort, and inconvenience, especially to a seriously ill patient. Only a few of the common symptoms that present difficult management issues will be addressed in this chapter. Additional information on the management of other symptoms, such as nausea and vomiting, insomnia, and diarrhea, can be found in Chaps. 39 and 81, Chap. 27, and Chap. 40, respectively.

Pain

Frequency The frequency of pain among terminally ill patients varies widely. Substantial pain occurs in 36–90% of patients with advanced cancer. In the SUPPORT study of hospitalized patients with diverse conditions and an estimated survival ≤6 months, 22% reported moderate to severe pain, and caregivers of those patients noted that 50% had similar levels of pain during the last few days of life. A meta-analysis found pain prevalence of 58–69% in studies that included patients characterized as having advanced, metastatic, or terminal cancer; 44–73% in studies that included patients characterized as undergoing cancer treatment; and 21–46% in studies that included posttreatment individuals.

Etiology *Nociceptive pain* is the result of direct mechanical or chemical stimulation of nociceptors and normal neural signaling to the brain. It tends to be localized, aching, throbbing, and cramping. The classic example is bone metastases. *Visceral pain* is caused by nociceptors in gastrointestinal, respiratory, and other organ systems. It is a deep or colicky type of pain classically associated with pancreatitis, myocardial infarction, or tumor invasion of viscera. *Neuropathic pain* arises from disordered nerve signals. It is described by patients as burning, electrical, or shocklike pain. Classic examples are poststroke pain, tumor invasion of the brachial plexus, and herpetic neuralgia.

Assessment Pain is a subjective experience. Depending on the patient's circumstances, perspective, and physiologic condition, the same physical lesion or disease state can produce different levels of reported pain and need for pain relief. Systematic assessment includes eliciting the following: (1) type: throbbing, cramping, burning, etc.; (2) periodicity: continuous, with or without exacerbations, or incident; (3) location; (4) intensity; (5) modifying factors; (6) effects of treatments; (7) functional impact; and (8) impact on patient. Several validated pain assessment measures may be used, such as the Visual Analogue Scale, the Brief Pain Inventory, and the pain component of one of the more comprehensive symptom assessment instruments. Frequent reassessments are essential to assess the effects of interventions.

Interventions Interventions for pain must be tailored to each individual, with the goal of preempting chronic pain and relieving breakthrough pain. At the end of life, there is rarely reason to doubt a patient's report of pain. Pain medications are the cornerstone of management. If they are failing and nonpharmacologic interventions—including radiotherapy and anesthetic or neurosurgical procedures such as peripheral nerve blocks or epidural medications—are required, a pain consultation is appropriate.

Pharmacologic interventions follow the World Health Organization three-step approach involving nonopioid analgesics, mild opioids, and strong opioids, with or without adjuvants (Chap. 11). Nonopioid analgesics, especially nonsteroidal anti-inflammatory drugs (NSAIDs), are the initial treatments for mild pain. They work primarily by inhibiting peripheral prostaglandins and reducing inflammation but also may have central nervous system (CNS) effects. They have a ceiling effect. Ibuprofen, up to 1600 mg/d qid, has a minimal risk of causing bleeding and renal impairment and is a good initial choice. In patients with a history of severe gastrointestinal (GI) or other bleeding, it should be avoided. In patients with a history of mild gastritis or gastroesophageal reflux disease (GERD), acid-lowering therapy such as a proton pump inhibitor should be used. Acetaminophen is an alternative in patients with a history of GI bleeding and can be used safely at up to 4 g/d qid. In patients with liver dysfunction due to metastases or other causes and in patients with heavy alcohol use, doses should be reduced.

If nonopioid analgesics are insufficient, opioids should be introduced. They work by interacting with mu opioid receptors in the CNS to activate pain-inhibitory neurons; most are receptor antagonists. The mixed agonist/antagonist opioids useful for post-acute pain should not be used for the chronic pain in end-of-life care. Weak opioids such as codeine can be used initially. However, if they are escalated and fail to relieve pain, strong opioids such as morphine, 5–10 mg every 4 h, should be used. Nonopioid analgesics should be combined with opioids because they potentiate the effect of opioids.

For continuous pain, opioids should be administered on a regular, around-the-clock basis consistent with their duration of analgesia. They should not be provided only when the patient experiences pain; the goal is to prevent patients from experiencing pain. Patients also should be provided rescue medication, such as liquid morphine, for breakthrough pain, generally at 20% of the baseline dose. Patients should be informed that using the rescue medication does not obviate the need to take the next standard dose of pain medication. If after 24 h the patient's pain remains uncontrolled and recurs before the next dose, requiring the patient to utilize the rescue medication, the daily opioid dose can be increased by the total dose of rescue medications used by the patient, or by 50% for moderate pain and 100% for severe pain of the standing opioid daily dose.

It is inappropriate to start with extended-release preparations. Instead, an initial focus on using short-acting preparations to determine how much is required in the first 24–48 h will allow clinicians to determine opioid needs. Once pain relief is obtained with short-acting preparations, one should switch to extended-release preparations. Even with a stable extended-release preparation regimen, the patient may have incident pain, such as during movement or dressing changes. Short-acting preparations should be taken before such predictable episodes. Although less common, patients may have "end-of-dose failure" with long-acting opioids, meaning that they develop pain after 8 h in the case of an every-12-h medication. In these cases, a trial of giving an every-12-h medication every 8 h is appropriate.

Because of differences in opioid receptors, cross-tolerance among opioids is incomplete, and patients may experience different side effects with different opioids. Therefore, if a patient is not experiencing pain relief or is experiencing too many side effects, a change to another opioid preparation is appropriate. When switching, one should begin with 50–75% of the published equianalgesic dose of the new opioid.

Unlike NSAIDs, opioids have no ceiling effect; therefore, there is no maximum dose no matter how many milligrams the patient is receiving. The appropriate dose is the dose needed to achieve pain relief. This is an important point for clinicians to explain to patients and families. Addiction or excessive respiratory depression is extremely unlikely in the terminally ill; fear of these side effects should neither prevent escalating opioid medications when the patient is experiencing insufficient pain relief nor justify using opioid antagonists.

Opioid side effects should be anticipated and treated preemptively. Nearly all patients experience constipation that can be debilitating (see below). Failure to prevent constipation often results in noncompliance with opioid therapy. Methylnaltrexone is a drug that targets opioid-induced constipation by blocking peripheral opioid receptors but not central receptors for analgesia. In placebo-controlled trials, it has been shown to cause laxation within 24 h of administration. As with the use of opioids, about a third of patients using methylnaltrexone experience nausea and vomiting, but unlike constipation, tolerance develops, usually within a week. Therefore, when one is beginning opioids, an antiemetic such as metoclopramide or a serotonin antagonist often is prescribed prophylactically and stopped after 1 week. Olanzapine also has been shown to have antinausea properties and can be effective in countering delirium or anxiety, with the advantage of some weight gain.

Drowsiness, a common side effect of opioids, also usually abates within a week. During this period, drowsiness can be treated with psychostimulants such as dextroamphetamine, methylphenidate, and modafinil. Modafinil has the advantage of everyday dosing. Pilot reports suggest that donepezil may also be helpful for opiate-induced drowsiness as well as relieving fatigue and anxiety. Metabolites of morphine and most opioids are cleared renally; doses may have to be adjusted for patients with renal failure.

Seriously ill patients who require chronic pain relief rarely if ever become addicted. Suspicion of addiction should not be a reason to withhold pain medications from terminally ill patients. Patients and families may withhold prescribed opioids for fear of addiction or dependence. Physicians and health care providers should reassure patients and families that the patient will not become addicted to opioids if they are used as prescribed for pain relief; this fear should not prevent the patient from taking the medications around the clock. However, diversion of drugs for use by other family members or illicit sale may occur. It may be necessary to advise the patient and caregiver about secure storage of opioids. Contract writing with the patient and family can help. If that fails, transfer to a safe facility may be necessary.

Tolerance is the need to increase medication dosage for the same pain relief without a change in disease. In the case of patients with advanced disease, the need for increasing opioid dosage for pain relief usually is caused by disease progression rather than tolerance.

Physical dependence is indicated by symptoms from the abrupt withdrawal of opioids and should not be confused with addiction.

Adjuvant analgesic medications are nonopioids that potentiate the analgesic effects of opioids. They are especially important in the management of neuropathic pain. Gabapentin, an anticonvulsant initially studied in the setting of herpetic neuralgia, is now the first-line treatment for neuropathic pain from a variety of causes. It is begun at 100–300 mg bid or tid, with 50–100% dose increments every 3 days. Usually 900–3600 mg/d in two or three doses is effective. The combination of gabapentin and nortriptyline may be more effective than gabapentin alone. One potential side effect of gabapentin to be aware of is confusion and drowsiness, especially in the elderly. Other effective adjuvant medications include pregabalin, which has the same mechanism of action as gabapentin but is absorbed more efficiently from the GI tract. Lamotrigine is a novel agent whose mechanism of action is unknown, but it has shown effectiveness. It is recommended to begin at 25–50 mg/d, increasing to 100 mg/d. Carbamazepine, a first-generation agent, has been proved effective in randomized trials for neuropathic pain. Other potentially effective anticonvulsant adjuvants include topiramate (25–50 mg qd or bid, rising to 100–300 mg/d) and oxcarbazepine (75–300 mg bid, rising to 1200 mg bid). Glucocorticoids, preferably dexamethasone given once a day, can be useful in reducing inflammation that causes pain while elevating mood, energy, and appetite. Its main side effects include confusion, sleep difficulties, and fluid retention. Glucocorticoids are especially effective for bone pain and abdominal pain from distention of the GI tract or liver. Other drugs, including clonidine and baclofen, can be effective in pain relief. These drugs are adjuvants and generally should be used in conjunction with—not instead of—opioids. Methadone, carefully dosed because of its unpredictable half-life in many patients, has activity at the N-methyl-D-aspartamate (NMDA) receptor and is useful for complex pain syndromes and neuropathic pain. It generally is reserved for cases in which first-line opioids (morphine, oxycodone, hydromorphone) are either ineffective or unavailable.

Radiation therapy can treat bone pain from single metastatic lesions. Bone pain from multiple metastases can be amenable to radiopharmaceuticals such as strontium 89 and samarium 153. Bisphosphonates [such as pamidronate (90 mg every 4 weeks)] and calcitonin (200 IU intranasally once or twice a day) also provide relief from bone pain but have onset of action of days.

Constipation

Frequency Constipation is reported in up to 87% of patients requiring palliative care.

Etiology Although hypercalcemia and other factors can cause constipation, it is most frequently a predictable consequence of the use of opioids for the relief of pain and dyspnea and of tricyclic antidepressants, from their anticholinergic effects, as well as of the inactivity and poor diet that are common among seriously ill patients. If untreated, constipation can cause substantial pain and vomiting and also is associated with confusion and delirium. Whenever opioids and other medications known to cause constipation are used, preemptive treatment for constipation should be instituted.

Assessment The physician should establish the patient's previous bowel habits, including the frequency, consistency, and volume. Abdominal and rectal examinations should be performed to exclude impaction or acute abdomen. A number of constipation assessment scales are available, although guidelines issued in the *Journal of Palliative Medicine* did not recommend them for routine practice. Four commonly used assessment scales are the Bristol Stool Form Scale, the Constipation Assessment Scale, the Constipation Visual

TABLE 9-5 Medications for the Management of Constipation

Intervention	Dose	Comment
Stimulant laxatives		These agents directly stimulate peristalsis and may reduce colonic absorption of water.
Prune juice	120–240 mL/d	Work in 6–12 h.
Senna (Senokot)	2–8 tablets PO bid	
Bisacodyl	5–15 mg/d PO, PR	
Osmotic laxatives		These agents are not absorbed. They attract and retain water in the gastrointestinal tract.
Lactulose	15–30 mL PO q4–8h	Lactulose may cause flatulence and bloating.
Magnesium hydroxide (Milk of Magnesia)	15–30 mL/d PO	Lactulose works in 1 day, magnesium products in 6 h.
Magnesium citrate	125–250 mL/d PO	
Stool softeners		These agents work by increasing water secretion and as detergents, increasing water penetration into the stool.
Sodium docusate (Colace)	300–600 mg/d PO	Work in 1–3 days.
Calcium docusate	300–600 mg/d PO	
Suppositories and enemas		
Bisacodyl	10–15 PR qd	
Sodium phosphate enema	PR qd	Fixed dose, 4.5 oz, Fleet's.

Analogue Scale, and the Eton Scale Risk Assessment for Constipation. Radiographic assessments beyond a simple flat plate of the abdomen in cases in which obstruction is suspected are rarely necessary.

Intervention Intervention to reestablish comfortable bowel habits and relieve pain and discomfort should be the goals of any measures to address constipation during end-of-life care. Although physical activity, adequate hydration, and dietary treatments with fiber can be helpful, each is limited in its effectiveness for most seriously ill patients, and fiber may exacerbate problems in the setting of dehydration and if impaired motility is the etiology. Fiber is contraindicated in the presence of opioid use. Stimulant and osmotic laxatives, stool softeners, fluids, and enemas are the mainstays of therapy (Table 9-5). In preventing constipation from opioids and other medications, a combination of a laxative and a stool softener (such as senna and docusate) should be used. If after several days of treatment a bowel movement has not occurred, a rectal examination to remove impacted stool and place a suppository is necessary. For patients with impending bowel obstruction or gastric stasis, octreotide to reduce secretions can be helpful. For patients in whom the suspected mechanism is dysmotility, metoclopramide can be helpful.

Nausea

Frequency Up to 70% of patients with advanced cancer have nausea, defined as the subjective sensation of wanting to vomit.

Etiology Nausea and vomiting are both caused by stimulation at one of four sites: the GI tract, the vestibular system, the chemoreceptor trigger zone (CTZ), and the cerebral cortex. Medical treatments for nausea are aimed at receptors at each of these sites: The GI tract contains mechanoreceptors, chemoreceptors, and 5-hydroxytryptamine type 3 (5-HT3) receptors; the vestibular system probably contains histamine and acetylcholine receptors; and the CTZ contains chemoreceptors, dopamine type 2 receptors, and 5-HT3 receptors. An example of nausea that most likely is mediated by the cortex is anticipatory nausea before a dose of chemotherapy or other noxious stimuli.

Specific causes of nausea include metabolic changes (liver failure, uremia from renal failure, hypercalcemia), bowel obstruction, constipation, infection, GERD, vestibular disease, brain metastases, medications (including antibiotics, NSAIDs, proton pump inhibitors, opioids, and chemotherapy), and radiation therapy. Anxiety can also contribute to nausea.

Intervention Medical treatment of nausea is directed at the anatomic and receptor-mediated cause that a careful history and physical examination reveals. When a single specific cause is not found, many advocate beginning treatment with a dopamine antagonist such as haloperidol or prochlorperazine. Prochlorperazine is usually more sedating than haloperidol. When decreased motility is suspected, metoclopramide can be an effective treatment. When inflammation of the GI tract is suspected, glucocorticoids such as dexamethasone are an appropriate treatment. For nausea that follows chemotherapy and radiation therapy, one of the 5-HT3 receptor antagonists (ondansetron, granisetron, dolasetron) is recommended. Clinicians should attempt prevention of postchemotherapy nausea rather than provide treatment after the fact. Current clinical guidelines recommend tailoring the strength of treatments to the specific emetic risk posed by a specific chemotherapy drug. When a vestibular cause (such as "motion sickness" or labyrinthitis) is suspected, antihistamines such as meclizine (whose primary side effect is drowsiness) or anticholinergics such as scopolamine can be effective. In anticipatory nausea, a benzodiazepine such as lorazepam is indicated. As with antihistamines, drowsiness and confusion are the main side effects.

Dyspnea

Frequency Dyspnea is a subjective experience of being short of breath. Nearly 75% of dying patients experience dyspnea at some point in their illness. Dyspnea is among the most distressing physical symptoms and can be even more distressing than pain.

Assessment As with pain, dyspnea is a subjective experience that may not correlate with objective measures of P_{O_2}, P_{CO_2}, or respiratory rate. Consequently, measurements of oxygen saturation through pulse oximetry or blood gases are rarely helpful in guiding therapy. Despite the limitations of existing assessment methods, physicians should regularly assess and document patients' experience of dyspnea and its intensity. Guidelines recommend visual or analogue dyspnea scales to assess the severity of symptoms and the effects of treatment. Potentially reversible or treatable causes of dyspnea include infection, pleural effusions, pulmonary emboli, pulmonary edema, asthma, and tumor encroachment on the airway. However, the risk-versus-benefit ratio of the diagnostic and therapeutic interventions for patients with little time left to live must be considered carefully before one undertakes diagnostic steps. Frequently, the specific etiology cannot be identified, and dyspnea is the consequence of progression of the underlying disease that cannot be treated. The anxiety caused by dyspnea and the choking sensation can significantly exacerbate the underlying dyspnea in a negatively reinforcing cycle.

Interventions When reversible or treatable etiologies are diagnosed, they should be treated as long as the side effects of treatment, such as repeated drainage of effusions or anticoagulants, are less burdensome than the dyspnea itself. More aggressive treatments such as stenting a bronchial lesion may be warranted if it is clear that the dyspnea is due to tumor invasion at that site and if the patient and family understand the risks of such a procedure. Usually, treatment will be symptomatic (Table 9-6). A dyspnea scale and careful monitoring should guide dose adjustment. Low-dose opioids reduce the sensitivity of the central respiratory center and the sensation of dyspnea. If patients are not receiving opioids, weak opioids can be initiated; if patients are already receiving opioids, morphine or other strong opioids should be used. Controlled trials do not support the use of nebulized opioids for dyspnea at the end of life. Phenothiazines and chlorpromazine may be helpful when combined with opioids. Benzodiazepines can be helpful if anxiety is present but should be neither used as first-line therapy nor used alone in the treatment of dyspnea. If the patient has a history of COPD or asthma, inhaled bronchodilators and glucocorticoids may be helpful. If the patient has pulmonary edema due to heart failure, diuresis with a medication such as furosemide is indicated. Excess secretions can be dried with scopolamine, transdermally or intravenously. Oxygen can be used, although it may only be an expensive placebo. For some families and patients, oxygen is distressing; for others, it is reassuring. More general interventions that medical staff can include sitting the patient upright, removing smoke or other irritants such as perfume, ensuring a supply of fresh air with sufficient humidity, and minimizing other factors that can increase anxiety.

Fatigue

Frequency More than 90% of terminally ill patients experience fatigue and/or weakness. Fatigue is one of the most commonly reported symptoms of cancer treatment as well as in the palliative care of multiple sclerosis, COPD, heart failure, and HIV. Fatigue frequently is cited as among the most distressing symptoms.

Etiology The multiple causes of fatigue in the terminally ill can be categorized as resulting from the underlying disease; from disease-induced factors such as tumor necrosis factor and other cytokines; and from secondary factors such as dehydration, anemia, infection, hypothyroidism, and drug side effects. Apart from low caloric intake, loss of muscle mass and changes in muscle enzymes may play an important role in fatigue of terminal illness. The importance of changes in the CNS, especially the reticular activating system, have been hypothesized based on reports of fatigue in patients receiving cranial radiation, experiencing depression, or having chronic pain in the absence of cachexia or other physiologic changes. Finally, depression and other causes of psychological distress can contribute to fatigue.

Assessment Fatigue is subjective; objective changes, even in body mass, may be absent. Consequently, assessment must rely on patient self-reporting. Scales used to measure fatigue, such as the Edmonton Functional Assessment Tool, the Fatigue Self-Report Scales, and the Rhoten Fatigue Scale, are usually appropriate for research rather than clinical purposes. In clinical practice, a simple performance assessment such as the Karnofsky Performance Status or the Eastern Cooperative Oncology Group's question "How much of the day does the patient spend in bed?" may be the best measure. In this 0–4 performance status assessment, 0 = normal activity; 1 = symptomatic without being bedridden; 2 = requiring some, but <50%, bed time; 3 = bedbound more than half the day; and 4 = bedbound all the time. Such a scale allows for assessment over time and correlates with overall disease severity and prognosis. A 2008 review by the European Association of Palliative Care also described several longer assessment tools with 9–20 items, including the Piper Fatigue Inventory, the Multidimensional Fatigue Inventory, and the Brief Fatigue Inventory (BFI).

Interventions At the end of life, fatigue will not be "cured." The goal is to ameliorate it and help patients and families adjust expectations. Behavioral interventions should be utilized to avoid blaming the patient for inactivity and to educate both the family and the patient that the underlying disease causes physiologic changes that produce low energy levels. Understanding that the problem is physiologic and not psychological can help alter expectations regarding the patient's level of physical activity. Practically, this may mean reducing routine activities such as housework and cooking or social events outside the house and making it acceptable to receive guests lying on a couch. At the same time, institution of exercise regimens and physical therapy can raise endorphins, reduce muscle wasting, and reduce the risk of depression. In addition, ensuring good hydration without worsening edema may help reduce fatigue. Discontinuing medications that worsen fatigue may help, including cardiac medications, benzodiazepines, certain antidepressants, or opioids if pain is well-controlled. As end-of-life care proceeds into its final stages, fatigue may protect patients from further suffering, and continued treatment could be detrimental.

Only a few pharmacologic interventions target fatigue and weakness. Glucocorticoids can increase energy and enhance mood. Dexamethasone is preferred for its once-a-day dosing and

TABLE 9-6 Medications for the Management of Dyspnea

Intervention	Dose	Comments
Weak opioids		For patients with mild dyspnea
Codeine (or codeine with 325 mg acetaminophen)	30 mg PO q4h	For opioid-naïve patients
Hydrocodone	5 mg PO q4h	
Strong opioids		For opioid-naïve patients with moderate to severe dyspnea
Morphine	5–10 mg PO q4h	
	30–50% of baseline opioid dose q4h	For patients already taking opioids for pain or other symptoms
Oxycodone	5–10 mg PO q4h	
Hydromorphone	1–2 mg PO q4h	
Anxiolytics		Give a dose every hour until the patient is relaxed, then provide a dose for maintenance
Lorazepam	0.5–2.0 mg PO/SL/IV qh then q4–6h	
Clonazepam	0.25–2.0 mg PO q12h	
Midazolam	0.5 mg IV q15min	

minimal mineralocorticoid activity. Benefit, if any, usually is seen within the first month. Psychostimulants such as dextroamphetamine (5–10 mg PO) and methylphenidate (2.5–5 mg PO) may also enhance energy levels, although a randomized trial did not show methylphenidate beneficial compared with placebo in cancer fatigue. Doses should be given in the morning and at noon to minimize the risk of counterproductive insomnia. Modafinil, developed for narcolepsy, has shown some promise in the treatment of fatigue and has the advantage of once-daily dosing. Its precise role in fatigue at the end of life has not been determined. Anecdotal evidence suggests that L-carnitine may improve fatigue, depression, and sleep disruption.

■ PSYCHOLOGICAL SYMPTOMS AND THEIR MANAGEMENT

Depression

Frequency Depression at the end of life presents an apparently paradoxical situation. Many people believe that depression is normal among seriously ill patients because they are dying. People frequently say, "Wouldn't you be depressed?" However, depression is not a necessary part of terminal illness and can contribute to needless suffering. Although sadness, anxiety, anger, and irritability are normal responses to a serious condition, they are typically of modest intensity and transient. Persistent sadness and anxiety and the physically disabling symptoms that they can lead to are abnormal and suggestive of major depression. Although as many as 75% of terminally ill patients experience depressive symptoms, <25% of terminally ill patients have major depression.

Etiology Previous history of depression, family history of depression or bipolar disorder, and prior suicide attempts are associated with increased risk for depression among terminally ill patients. Other symptoms, such as pain and fatigue, are associated with higher rates of depression; uncontrolled pain can exacerbate depression, and depression can cause patients to be more distressed by pain. Many medications used in the terminal stages, including glucocorticoids, and some anticancer agents, such as tamoxifen, interleukin 2, interferon α, and vincristine, also are associated with depression. Some terminal conditions, such as pancreatic cancer, certain strokes, and heart failure, have been reported to be associated with higher rates of depression, although this is controversial. Finally, depression may be attributable to grief over the loss of a role or function, social isolation, or loneliness.

Assessment Diagnosing depression among seriously ill patients is complicated because many of the vegetative symptoms in the DSM-IV (*Diagnostic and Statistical Manual of Mental Disorders*) criteria for clinical depression—insomnia, anorexia and weight loss, fatigue, decreased libido, and difficulty concentrating—are associated with the dying process itself. The assessment of depression in seriously ill patients therefore should focus on the dysphoric mood, helplessness, hopelessness, and lack of interest and enjoyment and concentration in normal activities. The single questions "How often do you feel downhearted and blue?" (more than a good bit of the time or similar responses) and "Do you feel depressed most of the time?" are appropriate for screening.

Certain conditions may be confused with depression. Endocrinopathies such as hypothyroidism and Cushing's syndrome, electrolyte abnormalities such as hypercalcemia, and akathisia, especially from dopamine-blocking antiemetics such as metoclopramide and prochlorperazine, can mimic depression and should be excluded.

Interventions Physicians must treat any physical symptom, such as pain, that may be causing or exacerbating depression. Fostering adaptation to the many losses that the patient is experiencing can

also be helpful. Nonpharmacologic interventions, including group or individual psychological counseling, and behavioral therapies such as relaxation and imagery can be helpful, especially in combination with drug therapy.

Pharmacologic interventions remain the core of therapy. The same medications are used to treat depression in terminally ill as in non-terminally ill patients. Psychostimulants may be preferred for patients with a poor prognosis or for those with fatigue or opioid-induced somnolence. Psychostimulants are comparatively fast acting, working within a few days instead of the weeks required for selective serotonin reuptake inhibitors (SSRIs). Dextroamphetamine or methylphenidate should be started at 2.5–5.0 mg in the morning and at noon, the same starting doses used for treating fatigue. The dose can be escalated up to 15 mg bid. Modafinil is started at 100 mg qd and can be increased to 200 mg if there is no effect at the lower dose. Pemoline is a nonamphetamine psychostimulant with minimal abuse potential. It is also effective as an antidepressant beginning at 18.75 mg in the morning and at noon. Because it can be absorbed through the buccal mucosa, it is preferred for patients with intestinal obstruction or dysphagia. If it is used for prolonged periods, liver function must be monitored. The psychostimulants can also be combined with more traditional antidepressants while waiting for the antidepressants to become effective and then tapered after a few weeks if necessary. Psychostimulants have side effects, particularly initial anxiety, insomnia, and rarely paranoia, which may necessitate lowering the dose or discontinuing treatment.

Mirtazapine, an antagonist at the postsynaptic serotonin receptors, is a promising psychostimulant. It should be started at 7.5 mg before bed. It has sedating, antiemetic, and anxiolytic properties with few drug interactions. Its side effect of weight gain may be beneficial for seriously ill patients; it is available in orally disintegrating tablets.

For patients with a prognosis of several months or longer, SSRIs, including fluoxetine, sertraline, paroxetine and citalopram, and serotonin-noradrenaline reuptake inhibitors such as venlafaxine, are the preferred treatment because of their efficacy and comparatively few side effects. Because low doses of these medications may be effective for seriously ill patients, one should use half the usual starting dose for healthy adults. The starting dose for fluoxetine is 10 mg once a day. In most cases, once-a-day dosing is possible. The choice of which SSRI to use should be driven by (1) the patient's past success or failure with the specific medication and (2) the most favorable side-effect profile for that specific agent. For instance, for a patient in whom fatigue is a major symptom, a more activating SSRI (fluoxetine) would be appropriate. For a patient in whom anxiety and sleeplessness are major symptoms, a more sedating SSRI (paroxetine) would be appropriate.

Atypical antidepressants are recommended only in selected circumstances, usually with the assistance of a specialty consultation. Trazodone can be an effective antidepressant but is sedating and can cause orthostatic hypotension and, rarely, priapism. Therefore, it should be used only when a sedating effect is desired and is often used for patients with insomnia, at a dose starting at 25 mg. In addition to its antidepressant effects, bupropion is energizing, making it useful for depressed patients who experience fatigue. However, it can cause seizures, preventing its use for patients with a risk of CNS neoplasms or terminal delirium. Finally, alprazolam, a benzodiazepine, starting at 0.25–1.0 mg tid, can be effective in seriously ill patients who have a combination of anxiety and depression. Although it is potent and works quickly, it has many drug interactions and may cause delirium, especially among very ill patients, because of its strong binding to the benzodiazepine–γ-aminobutyric acid (GABA) receptor complex.

Unless used as adjuvants for the treatment of pain, tricyclic antidepressants are not recommended. Similarly, monoamine oxidase (MAO) inhibitors are not recommended because of their side effects and dangerous drug interactions.

Delirium (See Chap. 25)

Frequency In the weeks or months before death, delirium is uncommon, although it may be significantly underdiagnosed. However, delirium becomes relatively common in the hours and days immediately before death. Up to 85% of patients dying from cancer may experience terminal delirium.

Etiology Delirium is a global cerebral dysfunction characterized by alterations in cognition and consciousness. It frequently is preceded by anxiety, changes in sleep patterns (especially reversal of day and night), and decreased attention. In contrast to dementia, delirium has an acute onset, is characterized by fluctuating consciousness and inattention, and is reversible, although reversibility may be more theoretical than real for patients near death. Delirium may occur in a patient with dementia; indeed, patients with dementia are more vulnerable to delirium.

Causes of delirium include metabolic encephalopathy arising from liver or renal failure, hypoxemia, or infection; electrolyte imbalances such as hypercalcemia; paraneoplastic syndromes; dehydration; and primary brain tumors, brain metastases, or leptomeningeal spread of tumor. Commonly, among dying patients, delirium can be caused by side effects of treatments, including radiation for brain metastases, and medications, including opioids, glucocorticoids, anticholinergic drugs, antihistamines, antiemetics, benzodiazepines, and chemotherapeutic agents. The etiology may be multifactorial; e.g., dehydration may exacerbate opioid-induced delirium.

Assessment Delirium should be recognized in any terminally ill patient with new onset of disorientation, impaired cognition, somnolence, fluctuating levels of consciousness, or delusions with or without agitation. Delirium must be distinguished from acute anxiety and depression as well as dementia. The central distinguishing feature is altered consciousness, which usually is not noted in anxiety, depression, and dementia. Although "hyperactive" delirium characterized by overt confusion and agitation is probably more common, patients also should be assessed for "hypoactive" delirium characterized by sleep-wake reversal and decreased alertness.

In some cases, use of formal assessment tools such as the Mini-Mental Status Examination (which does not distinguish delirium from dementia) and the Delirium Rating Scale (which does distinguish delirium from dementia) may be helpful in distinguishing delirium from other processes. The patient's list of medications must be evaluated carefully. Nonetheless, a reversible etiologic factor for delirium is found in fewer than half of terminally ill patients. Because most terminally ill patients experiencing delirium will be very close to death and may be at home, extensive diagnostic evaluations such as lumbar punctures and neuroradiologic examinations are usually inappropriate.

Interventions One of the most important objectives of terminal care is to provide terminally ill patients the lucidity to say goodbye to the people they love. Delirium, especially with agitation during the final days, is distressing to family and caregivers. A strong determinant of bereavement difficulties is witnessing a difficult death. Thus, terminal delirium should be treated aggressively.

At the first sign of delirium, such as day-night reversal with slight changes in mentation, the physician should let the family members know that it is time to be sure that everything they want to say has been said. The family should be informed that delirium is common just before death.

If medications are suspected of being a cause of the delirium, unnecessary agents should be discontinued. Other potentially reversible

TABLE 9-7 Medications for the Management of Delirium

Interventions	Dose
Neuroleptics	
Haloperidol	0.5–5 mg q2–12h, PO/IV/SC/IM
Thioridazine	10–75 mg q4–8h, PO
Chlorpromazine	12.5–50 mg q4–12h, PO/IV/IM
Atypical neuroleptics	
Olanzapine	2.5–5 mg qd or bid, PO
Risperidone	1–3 mg q12h, PO
Anxiolytics	
Lorazepam	0.5–2 mg q1–4h, PO/IV/IM
Midazolam	1–5 mg/h continuous infusion, IV/SC
Anesthetics	
Propofol	0.3–2.0 mg/h continuous infusion, IV

causes, such as constipation, urinary retention, and metabolic abnormalities, should be treated. Supportive measures aimed at providing a familiar environment should be instituted, including restricting visits only to individuals with whom the patient is familiar and eliminating new experiences; orienting the patient, if possible, by providing a clock and calendar; and gently correcting the patient's hallucinations or cognitive mistakes.

Pharmacologic management focuses on the use of neuroleptics and, in the extreme, anesthetics (Table 9-7). Haloperidol remains first-line therapy. Usually, patients can be controlled with a low dose (1–3 mg/d), usually given every 6 h, although some may require as much as 20 mg/d. It can be administered PO, SC, or IV. IM injections should not be used, except when this is the only way to get a patient under control. Olanzapine, an atypical neuroleptic, has shown significant effectiveness in completely resolving delirium in cancer patients. It has other beneficial effects for terminally ill patients, including antinausea, antianxiety, and weight gain. It is useful for patients with longer anticipated life expectancy because it is less likely to cause dysphoria and has a lower risk of dystonic reactions. Also, because it is metabolized through multiple pathways, it can be used in patients with hepatic and renal dysfunction. Olanzapine has the disadvantage that it is available only orally and that it takes a week to reach steady state. The usual dose is 2.5–5 mg PO bid. Chlorpromazine (10–25 mg every 4–6 h) can be useful if sedation is desired and can be administered IV or PR in addition to PO. Dystonic reactions resulting from dopamine blockade are a side effect of neuroleptics, although they are reported to be rare when these drugs are used to treat terminal delirium. If patients develop dystonic reactions, benztropine should be administered. Neuroleptics may be combined with lorazepam to reduce agitation when the delirium is the result of alcohol or sedative withdrawal.

If no response to first-line therapy is seen, a specialty consultation should be obtained with a change to a different medication. If patients fail to improve after a second neuroleptic, sedation with an anesthetic such as propofol or continuous-infusion midazolam may be necessary. By some estimates, at the very end of life as many as 25% of patients experiencing delirium, especially restless delirium with myoclonus or convulsions, may require sedation.

Physical restraints should be used with great reluctance only when the patient's violence is threatening to self or others. If they are used, their appropriateness should be reevaluated frequently.

Insomnia

Frequency Sleep disorders, defined as difficulty initiating sleep or maintaining sleep, sleep difficulty at least 3 nights a week, or sleep difficulty that causes impairment of daytime functioning, occurs in 19–63% of patients with advanced cancer. Some 30–74% of patients with other end-stage conditions, including AIDS, heart disease, COPD, and renal disease, experience insomnia.

Etiology Patients with cancer may have changes in sleep efficiency such as an increase in stage I sleep. Other etiologies of insomnia are coexisting physical illness such as thyroid disease and coexisting psychological illnesses such as depression and anxiety. Medications, including antidepressants, psychostimulants, steroids, and β agonists, are significant contributors to sleep disorders, as are caffeine and alcohol. Multiple over-the-counter medications contain caffeine and antihistamines, which can contribute to sleep disorders.

Assessment Assessment should include specific questions concerning sleep onset, sleep maintenance, and early-morning wakening as these will provide clues to the causative agents and to management. Patients should be asked about previous sleep problems, screened for depression and anxiety, and asked about symptoms of thyroid disease. Caffeine and alcohol are prominent causes of sleep problems, and a careful history of the use of these substances should be obtained. Both excessive use and withdrawal from alcohol can be causes of sleep problems.

Interventions The mainstays of intervention include improvement of sleep hygiene (encouragement of regular time for sleep, decreased nighttime distractions, elimination of caffeine and other stimulants and alcohol), intervention to treat anxiety and depression, and treatment for the insomnia itself. For patients with depression who have insomnia and anxiety, a sedating antidepressant such as mirtazapine can be helpful. In the elderly, trazodone, beginning at 25 mg at nighttime, is an effective sleep aid at doses lower than those which cause its antidepressant effect. Zolpidem may have a decreased incidence of delirium in patients compared with traditional benzodiazepines, but this has not been clearly established. When benzodiazepines are prescribed, short-acting ones (such as lorazepam) are favored over longer-acting (such as diazepam). Patients who receive these medications should be observed for signs of increased confusion and delirium.

■ SOCIAL NEEDS AND THEIR MANAGEMENT

Financial burdens

Frequency Dying can impose substantial economic strains on patients and families, causing distress. In the United States, with one of the least comprehensive health insurance systems among the developed countries, ~20% of terminally ill patients and their families spend >10% of family income on health care costs over and above health insurance premiums. Between 10 and 30% of families sell assets, use savings, or take out a mortgage to pay for the patient's health care costs. Nearly 40% of terminally ill patients in the United States report that the cost of their illness is a moderate or great economic hardship for their family.

The patient is likely to reduce and eventually stop working. In 20% of cases, a family member of the terminally ill patient also stops working to provide care. The major underlying causes of economic burden are related to poor physical functioning and care needs, such as the need for housekeeping, nursing, and personal care. More debilitated patients and poor patients experience greater economic burdens.

Intervention This economic burden should not be ignored as a private matter. It has been associated with a number of adverse health outcomes, including preferring comfort care over life-prolonging care as well as consideration of euthanasia or physician-assisted suicide. Economic burdens increase the psychological distress of families and caregivers of terminally ill patients, and poverty is associated with many adverse health outcomes. Importantly, recent studies found that "patients with advanced cancer who reported having end-of-life conversations with physicians had significantly lower health care costs in their final week of life. Higher costs were associated with worse quality of death." Assistance from a social worker, early on if possible, to ensure access to all available benefits may be helpful. Many patients, families, and health care providers are unaware of options for long-term care insurance, respite care, the Family Medical Leave Act (FMLA), and other sources of assistance. Some of these options (such as respite care) may be part of a formal hospice program but others (such as the FMLA) do not require enrollment in a hospice program.

Relationships

Frequency Settling personal issues and closing the narrative of lived relationships are universal needs. When asked if sudden death or death after an illness is preferable, respondents often initially select the former but soon change to the latter as they reflect on the importance of saying goodbye. Bereaved family members who have not had the chance to say goodbye often have a more difficult grief process.

Interventions Care of seriously ill patients requires efforts to facilitate the types of encounters and time spent with family and friends that are necessary to meet those needs. Family and close friends may need to be accommodated with unrestricted visiting hours, which may include sleeping near the patient even in otherwise regimented institutional settings. Physicians and other health care providers may be able to facilitate and resolve strained interactions between the patient and other family members. Assistance for patients and family members who are unsure about how to create or help preserve memories, whether by providing materials such as a scrapbook or memory box or by offering them suggestions and informational resources, can be deeply appreciated. Taking photographs and creating videos can be especially helpful to terminally ill patients who have younger children or grandchildren.

Family caregivers

Frequency Caring for seriously ill patients places a heavy burden on families. Families frequently are required to provide transportation and homemaking as well as other services. Typically, paid professionals such as home health nurses and hospice workers supplement family care; only about a quarter of all caregiving consists of exclusively paid professional assistance. The trend toward more out-of-hospital deaths will increase reliance on families for end-of-life care. Increasingly, family members are being called upon to provide physical care (such as moving and bathing patients) and medical care (such as assessing symptoms and giving medications) in addition to emotional care and support.

Three-quarters of family caregivers of terminally ill patients are women—wives, daughters, sisters, and even daughters-in-law. Since many are widowed, women tend to be able to rely less on family for caregiving assistance and may need more paid assistance. About 20% of terminally ill patients report substantial unmet needs for nursing and personal care. The impact of caregiving on family caregivers is substantial: both bereaved and current caregivers have a higher mortality rate than that of non-caregiving controls.

Interventions It is imperative to inquire about unmet needs and to try to ensure that those needs are met either through the family or by paid professional services when possible. Community assistance through houses of worship or other community groups often can be mobilized by telephone calls from the medical team to someone the patient or family identifies. Sources of support specifically for family caregivers should be identified through local sources or nationally through groups such as the National Family Caregivers Association (*www.nfcacares.org*), the American Cancer Society (*www.cancer.org*), and the Alzheimer's Association (*www.alz.org*).

■ EXISTENTIAL NEEDS AND THEIR MANAGEMENT

Frequency

Religion and spirituality are often important to dying patients. Nearly 70% of patients report becoming more religious or spiritual when they became terminally ill, and many find comfort in religious or spiritual practices such as prayer. However, ~20% of terminally ill patients become less religious, frequently feeling cheated or betrayed by becoming terminally ill. For other patients, the need is for existential meaning and purpose that is distinct from and may even be antithetical to religion or spirituality. When asked, patients and family caregivers frequently report wanting their professional caregivers to be more attentive to religion and spirituality.

Assessment Health care providers are often hesitant about involving themselves in the religious, spiritual, and existential experiences of their patients because it may seem private or not relevant to the current illness. But physicians and other members of the care team should be able at least to detect spiritual and existential needs. Screening questions have been developed for a physician's spiritual history taking. Spiritual distress can amplify other types of suffering and even masquerade as intractable physical pain, anxiety, or depression. The screening questions in the comprehensive assessment are usually sufficient. Deeper evaluation and intervention are rarely appropriate for the physician unless no other member of a care team is available or suitable. Pastoral care providers may be helpful, whether from the medical institution or from the patient's own community.

Interventions Precisely how religious practices, spirituality, and existential explorations can be facilitated and improve end-of-life care is not well established. What is clear is that for physicians, one main intervention is to inquire about the role and importance of spirituality and religion in a patient's life. This will help a patient feel heard and help physicians identify specific needs. In one study, only 36% of respondents indicated that a clergy member would be comforting. Nevertheless, the increase in religious and spiritual interest among a substantial fraction of dying patients suggests inquiring of individual patients how this need can be addressed. Some evidence supports specific methods of addressing existential needs in patients, ranging from establishing a supportive group environment for terminal patients to individual treatments emphasizing a patient's dignity and sources of meaning.

MANAGING THE LAST STAGES

■ WITHDRAWING AND WITHHOLDING LIFE-SUSTAINING TREATMENT

Legal aspects For centuries, it has been deemed ethical to withhold or withdraw life-sustaining interventions. The current legal consensus in the United States and most developed countries is that patients have a moral as well as constitutional or common law right to refuse medical interventions. American courts also have held that incompetent patients have a right to refuse medical interventions. For patients who are incompetent and terminally ill and who have not completed an advance care directive, next of kin can exercise that right, although this may be restricted in some states, depending how clear and convincing the evidence is of the patient's preferences.

Courts have limited families' ability to terminate life-sustaining treatments in patients who are conscious, incompetent, but not terminally ill. In theory, patients' right to refuse medical therapy can be limited by four countervailing interests: (1) preservation of life, (2) prevention of suicide, (3) protection of third parties such as children, and (4) preservation of the integrity of the medical profession. In practice, these interests almost never override the right of competent patients and incompetent patients who have left explicit and advance care directives.

For incompetent patients who either appointed a proxy without specific indications of their wishes or never completed an advance care directive, three criteria have been suggested to guide the decision to terminate medical interventions. First, some commentators suggest that ordinary care should be administered but extraordinary care could be terminated. Because the ordinary/extraordinary distinction is too vague, courts and commentators widely agree that it should not be used to justify decisions about stopping treatment. Second, many courts have advocated the use of the substituted-judgment criterion, which holds that the proxy decision-makers should try to imagine what the incompetent patient would do if he or she were competent. However, multiple studies indicate that many proxies, even close family members, cannot accurately predict what the patient would have wanted. Therefore, substituted judgment becomes more of a guessing game than a way of fulfilling the patient's wishes. Finally, the best-interests criterion holds that proxies should evaluate treatments by balancing their benefits and risks and select those treatments in which the benefits maximally outweigh the burdens of treatment. Clinicians have a clear and crucial role in this by carefully and dispassionately explaining the known benefits and burdens of specific treatments. Yet even when that information is as clear as possible, different individuals can have very different views of what is in the patient's best interests, and families may have disagreements or even overt conflicts. This criterion has been criticized because there is no single way to determine the balance between benefits and burdens; it depends on a patient's personal values. For instance, for some people being alive even if mentally incapacitated is a benefit, whereas for others it may be the worst possible existence. As a matter of practice, physicians rely on family members to make decisions that they feel are best and object only if those decisions seem to demand treatments that the physicians consider not beneficial.

Practices Withholding and withdrawing acutely life-sustaining medical interventions from terminally ill patients are now standard practice. More than 90% of American patients die without cardiopulmonary resuscitation (CPR), and just as many forgo other potentially life-sustaining interventions. For instance, in ICUs in the period 1987–1988, CPR was performed 49% of the time, but it was performed only 10% of the time in 1992–1993. On average, 3.8 interventions, such as vasopressors and transfusions, were stopped for each dying ICU patient. However, up to 19% of decedents in hospitals received interventions such as extubation, ventilation, and surgery in the 48 h preceding death. However, practices vary widely among hospitals and ICUs, suggesting an important element of physician preferences rather than objective data.

Mechanical ventilation may be the most challenging intervention to withdraw. The two approaches are *terminal extubation*, which is the removal of the endotracheal tube, and *terminal weaning*, which is the gradual reduction of the FI_{O_2} or ventilator rate. One-third of ICU physicians prefer to use the terminal weaning technique, and 13% extubate; the majority of physicians utilize both techniques. The American Thoracic Society's 2008 clinical policy guidelines note that there is no single correct process of ventilator withdrawal and that physicians use and should be proficient in both methods but that the chosen approach should carefully balance benefits and burdens as well as patient and caregiver preferences. Physicians' assessment of patients' likelihood of survival, their prediction of possible cognitive damage, and patients' preferences about the use of life support are primary factors in determining the likelihood of withdrawal of mechanical ventilation. Some recommend terminal weaning because patients do not develop upper airway obstruction and the distress caused by secretions or stridor; however, terminal weaning can prolong the dying process and not allow a patient's family to be with him or her unencumbered by an endotracheal tube. To ensure comfort for conscious or semiconscious patients before withdrawal of the ventilator, neuromuscular blocking agents should be terminated and sedatives and analgesics administered. Removing the neuromuscular blocking agents permits patients to show discomfort, facilitating the titration of sedatives and analgesics; it also permits interactions between patients and their families. A common practice is to inject a bolus of midazolam (2–4 mg) or lorazepam (2–4 mg) before withdrawal, followed by 5–10 mg of morphine and continuous infusion of morphine (50% of the bolus dose per hour) during weaning. In patients who have significant upper airway secretions, IV scopolamine at a rate of 100 μg/h can be administered. Additional boluses of morphine or increases in the infusion rate should be administered for respiratory distress or signs of pain. Higher doses will be needed for patients already receiving sedatives and opioids. Families need to be reassured about treatments for common symptoms after withdrawal of ventilatory support, such as dyspnea and agitation, and warned about the uncertainty of length of survival after withdrawal of ventilatory support: up to 10% of patients unexpectedly survive for 1 day or more after mechanical ventilation is stopped.

◼ FUTILE CARE

Beginning in the late 1980s, some commentators argued that physicians could terminate futile treatments demanded by the families of terminally ill patients. Although no objective definition or standard of futility exists, several categories have been proposed. Physiologic futility means that an intervention will have no physiologic effect. Some have defined qualitative futility as applying to procedures that "fail to end a patient's total dependence on intensive medical care." Quantitative futility occurs "when physicians conclude (through personal experience, experiences shared with colleagues, or consideration of reported empiric data) that in the last 100 cases, a medical treatment has been useless." The term conceals subjective value judgments about when a treatment is "not beneficial." Deciding whether a treatment that obtains an additional 6 weeks of life or a 1% survival advantage confers benefit depends on patients' preferences and goals. Furthermore, physicians' predictions of when treatments were futile deviated markedly from the quantitative definition. When residents thought CPR was quantitatively futile, more than one in five patients had a >10% chance of survival to hospital discharge. Most studies that purport to guide determinations of futility are based on insufficient data to provide statistical confidence for clinical decision-making. Quantitative futility rarely applies in ICU settings. Many commentators reject using futility as a criterion for withdrawing care, preferring instead to consider futility situations as ones that represent conflict that calls for careful negotiation between families and health care providers.

In the wake of a lack of consensus over quantitative measures of futility, many hospitals adopted process-based approaches to resolve disputes over futility and enhance communication with patients and surrogates, including focusing on interests and alternatives rather than opposing positions and generating a wide range of options. Some hospitals have enacted "unilateral DNR" policies to allow clinicians to provide a do-not-resuscitate order in cases in which consensus cannot be reached with families and medical opinion is that resuscitation would be futile if attempted. This type of a policy is not a replacement for careful and patient communication and negotiation but recognizes that agreement cannot always be reached. Over the last 15 years, many states, such as Texas, Virginia, Maryland, and California, have enacted so-called medical futility laws that provide physicians a "safe harbor" from liability if they refuse a patient or family's request for life-sustaining interventions. For instance, in Texas when a disagreement about terminating interventions between the medical team and the family has not been resolved by an ethics consultation, the hospital is supposed to try to facilitate transfer of the patient to an institution willing to provide treatment. If this fails after 10 days, the hospital and physician may unilaterally withdraw treatments determined to be futile. The family may appeal to a state court. Early data suggest that the law increases futility consultations for the ethics committee and that although most families concur with withdrawal, about 10–15% of families refuse to withdraw treatment. Approximately 12 cases have gone to court in Texas in the 7 years since the adoption of the law. As of 2007, there had been 974 ethics committee consultations on medical futility cases and 65 in which committees ruled against families and gave notice that treatment would be terminated. Treatment was withdrawn for 27 of those patients, and the remainder transferred to other facilities or died while awaiting transfer.

◼ EUTHANASIA AND PHYSICIAN-ASSISTED SUICIDE

Euthanasia and physician-assisted suicide are defined in Table 9-8. Terminating life-sustaining care and providing opioid medications to manage symptoms have long been considered ethical by the medical profession and legal by courts and should not be confused with euthanasia or physician-assisted suicide.

Legal aspects Euthanasia is legal in the Netherlands, Belgium, and Luxembourg. It was legalized in the Northern Territory of Australia in 1995, but that legislation was repealed in 1997. Euthanasia is not legal in any state in the United States. With certain conditions, in Switzerland, a layperson can legally assist suicide. In the United States,

TABLE 9-8 Definitions of Assisted Suicide and Euthanasia

Term	Definition	Legal Status
Voluntary active euthanasia	Intentionally administering medications or other interventions to cause the patient's death with the patient's informed consent	Netherlands Belgium
Involuntary active euthanasia	Intentionally administering medications or other interventions to cause the patient's death when the patient was competent to consent but did not—e.g., the patient may not have been asked	Nowhere
Passive euthanasia	Withholding or withdrawing life-sustaining medical treatments from a patient to let him or her die (terminating life-sustaining treatments)	Everywhere
Physician-assisted suicide	A physician provides medications or other interventions to a patient with the understanding that the patient can use them to commit suicide	Oregon Netherlands Belgium Switzerland

physician-assisted suicide is legal in Oregon and Washington State if multiple criteria are met and then only after a process that includes a 15-day waiting period. In 2009, the state supreme court of Montana ruled that state law permits physician-assisted suicide for terminally ill patients. In all other countries and all other states in the United States, physician-assisted suicide and euthanasia are illegal explicitly or by common law.

Practices   Fewer than 10–20% of terminally ill patients actually consider euthanasia and/or physician-assisted suicide for themselves. In the Netherlands and Oregon, >70% of patients utilizing these interventions are dying of cancer; <10% of deaths by euthanasia or physician-assisted suicide involve patients with AIDS or amyotrophic lateral sclerosis. In the Netherlands, the share of deaths attributable to euthanasia or physician-assisted suicide declined from around 2.8% of all deaths in 2001 to around 1.8% in 2005. In 2009, the last year with complete data, around 60 patients in Oregon (~0.2% of all deaths) died by physician-assisted suicide, although this may be an underestimate. In Washington State, between March 2009 (when the law allowing physician-assisted suicide went into force) and December 2009, 36 individuals died from prescribed lethal doses.

Pain is not a primary motivator for patients' requests for or interest in euthanasia and/or physician-assisted suicide. Among the first patients to receive physician-assisted suicide in Oregon, only 1 patient of 15 had inadequate pain control compared with 15 of 43 patients in a control group experiencing inadequate pain relief. Depression, hopelessness, and, more profoundly, concerns about loss of dignity or autonomy or being a burden on family members appear to be primary factors motivating a desire for euthanasia or physician-assisted suicide. In Oregon, fewer than 25% of patients cite pain as the reason for desiring physician-assisted suicide. Most cite losing autonomy, dignity, or enjoyable activities. Over a third note being a burden on family. A study from the Netherlands showed that depressed terminally ill cancer patients were four times more likely to request euthanasia and confirmed that uncontrolled pain was not associated with greater interest in euthanasia.

Euthanasia and physician-assisted suicide are no guarantee of a painless, quick death. Data from the Netherlands indicate that in as many as 20% of cases technical and other problems arose, including patients waking from coma, not becoming comatose, regurgitating medications, and experiencing a prolonged time to death. Data from Oregon indicate that between 1997 and 2009, 20 patients (around 5%) regurgitated after taking prescribed medication, 1 patient awaked, and none experienced seizures. Problems were significantly more common in physician-assisted suicide, sometimes requiring the physician to intervene and provide euthanasia.

Whether practicing in a setting where euthanasia is legal or not, over a career, 12–54% of physicians receive a request for euthanasia or physician-assisted suicide from a patient. Competency in dealing with such a request is crucial. Although challenging, the request can also provide a chance to address intense suffering. After receiving a request for euthanasia and/or physician-assisted suicide, health care providers should carefully clarify the request with empathic, open-ended questions to help elucidate the underlying cause for the request, such as: "What makes you want to consider this option?" Endorsing either moral opposition or moral support for the act tends to be counterproductive, giving an impression of being judgmental or of endorsing the idea that the patient's life is worthless. Health care providers must reassure the patient of continued care and commitment. The patient should be educated about alternative, less controversial options, such as symptom management and withdrawing any unwanted treatments and the reality of euthanasia and/or physician-assisted suicide, since the patient may have misconceptions about their effectiveness as well as the legal implications of the choice. Depression, hopelessness, and other symptoms of psychological distress as well as physical suffering and economic burdens are likely factors motivating the request, and such factors should be assessed and treated aggressively. After these interventions and clarification of options, most patients proceed with another approach, declining life-sustaining interventions, possibly including refusal of nutrition and hydration.

■ CARE DURING THE LAST HOURS

Most laypersons have limited experiences with the actual dying process and death. They frequently do not know what to expect of the final hours and afterward. The family and other caregivers must be prepared, especially if the plan is for the patient to die at home.

Patients in the last days of life typically experience extreme weakness and fatigue and become bedbound; this can lead to pressure sores. The issue of turning patients who are near the end of life, however, must be balanced against the potential discomfort that movement may cause. Patients stop eating and drinking with drying of mucosal membranes and dysphagia. Careful attention to oral swabbing, lubricants for lips, and use of artificial tears can provide a form of care to substitute for attempts at feeding the patient. With loss of the gag reflex and dysphagia, patients may also experience accumulation of oral secretions, producing noises during respiration sometimes called "the death rattle." Scopolamine can reduce the secretions. Patients also experience changes in respiration with periods of apnea or Cheyne-Stokes breathing. Decreased intravascular volume and cardiac output cause tachycardia, hypotension, peripheral coolness, and livedo reticularis (skin mottling). Patients can have urinary and, less frequently, fecal incontinence. Changes in consciousness and neurologic function generally lead to two different paths to death (Fig. 9-2).

Each of these terminal changes can cause patients and families distress, requiring reassurance and targeted interventions (Table 9-9). Informing families that these changes might occur and providing them with an information sheet can help preempt problems and minimize distress. Understanding that patients stop eating because they are dying, not dying because they have stopped eating, can reduce family and caregiver anxiety. Similarly, informing the family and caregivers that the "death rattle" may occur and that it is not indicative of suffocation, choking, or pain can reduce their worry from the breathing sounds.

Families and caregivers may also feel guilty about stopping treatments, fearing that they are "killing" the patient. This may lead to demands for interventions, such as feeding tubes, that may be ineffective. In such cases, the physician should remind the family and caregivers about the inevitability of events and the palliative goals. Interventions may prolong the dying process and cause discomfort. Physicians also should emphasize that withholding treatments is both legal and ethical and that the family members are not the cause of the patient's death. This reassurance may have to be provided multiple times.

Hearing and touch are said to be the last senses to stop functioning. Whether this is the case or not, families and caregivers can be encouraged to communicate with the dying patient. Encouraging them to talk directly to the patient, even if he or she is unconscious, and hold the patient's hand or demonstrate affection in other ways can be an effective way to channel their urge "to do something" for the patient.

When the plan is for the patient to die at home, the physician must inform the family and caregivers how to determine that the patient has died. The cardinal signs are cessation of cardiac function and respiration; the pupils become fixed; the body becomes cool; muscles relax; and incontinence may occur. Remind the family and caregivers that the eyes may remain open even after the patient has

CLINICAL COURSES FOR TERMINALLY ILL PATIENTS

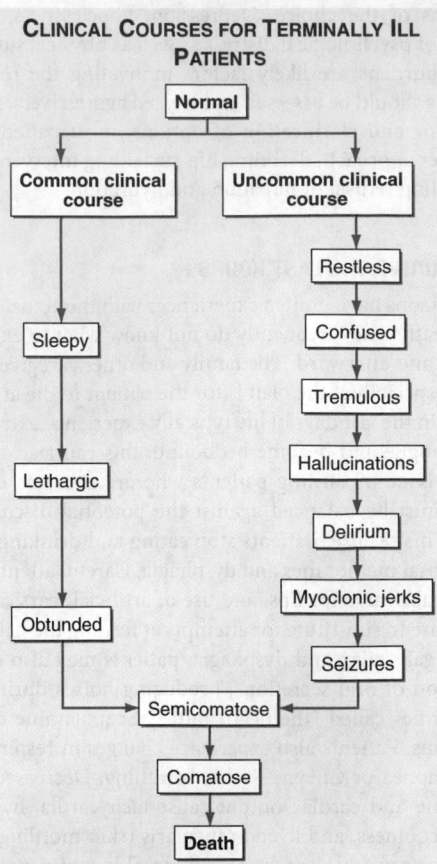

Figure 9-2 Common and uncommon clinical courses in the last days of terminally ill patients. *(Adapted from FD Ferris et al: Module 4: Palliative care, in Comprehensive Guide for the Care of Persons with HIV Disease. Toronto: Mt. Sinai Hospital and Casey Hospice, 1995, http://www.cpsonline. info/content/resources/hivmodule/module4complete.pdf.)*

died because the retroorbital fat pad may be depleted, permitting the orbit to fall posteriorly, which makes it difficult for the eyelids to cover the eyeball.

The physician should establish a plan for who the family or caregivers will contact when the patient is dying or has died. Without a plan, they may panic and call 911, unleashing a cascade of unwanted events, from arrival of emergency personnel and resuscitation to hospital admission. The family and caregivers should be instructed to contact the hospice (if one is involved), the covering physician, or the on-call member of the palliative care team. They should also be told that the medical examiner need not be called unless the state requires it for all deaths. Unless foul play is suspected, the health care team need not contact the medical examiner either.

Just after the patient dies, even the best-prepared family may experience shock and loss and be emotionally distraught. They need time to assimilate the event and be comforted. Health care providers are likely to find it meaningful to write a bereavement card or letter to the family. The purpose is to communicate about the patient, perhaps emphasizing the patient's virtues and the honor it was to care for the patient, and to express concern for the family's hardship. Some physicians attend the funerals of their patients. Although this is beyond any medical obligation, the presence of the physician can be a source of support to the grieving family and provides an opportunity for closure for the physician.

Death of a spouse is a strong predictor of poor health, and even mortality, for the surviving spouse. It may be important to alert the spouse's physician about the death so that he or she is aware of symptoms that might require professional attention.

Determining the best approach to providing palliative care to patients will depend on patient preferences, the availability of caregivers and specialized services in close proximity, institutional resources, and reimbursement. Hospice is a leading, but not the only, model of palliative care services. In the United States, a plurality—40.7%—of hospice care is provided in residential homes. In 2008, just over 20% of hospice care was provided in nursing homes. In the United States, Medicare pays for hospice services under Part A, the hospital insurance part of reimbursement. Two physicians must certify that the patient has a prognosis of ≤6 months if the disease runs its usual course. Prognoses are probabilistic by their nature; patients are not required to die within 6 months but rather to have a condition from which half the individuals with it would not be alive within 6 months. Patients sign a hospice enrollment form that states their intent to forgo curative services related to their terminal illness, but they can still receive medical services for other comorbid conditions. Patients also can withdraw enrollment and reenroll later; the hospice Medicare benefit can be revoked later to secure traditional Medicare benefits. Payments to the hospice are per diem (or capitated), not fee-for-service. Payments are intended to cover physician services for the medical direction of the care team; regular home care visits by registered nurses and licensed practical nurses; home health aid and homemaker services; chaplain services; social work services; bereavement counseling; and medical equipment, supplies, and medications. No specific therapy is excluded, and the goal is for each therapy to be considered for its symptomatic (as opposed to disease-modifying) effect. Additional clinical care, including services of the primary physician, is covered by Medicare Part B even while the hospice Medicare benefit is in place. The health reform legislation signed into law in March 2010—the Affordable Care Act—directs the Secretary of Health and Human Services to gather data on Medicare hospice reimbursement with the goal of reforming payment rates to account for resource use over an entire episode of care. The legislation also requires additional evaluations and reviews of eligibility for hospice care by hospice physicians or nurses. Finally, the legislation establishes a demonstration project for concurrent hospice care in Medicare, which would test and evaluate allowing patients to remain eligible for regular Medicare during hospice care.

By 2008, the mean length of enrollment in a hospice was around 70 days, with the median being 21 days. Such short stays create barriers to establishing high-quality palliative services in patients' homes and also place financial strains on hospice providers since the initial assessments are resource intensive. Physicians should initiate early referrals to the hospice to allow more time for patients to receive palliative care.

Hospice care has been the main method for securing palliative services for terminally ill patients. However, efforts are being made to ensure continuity of palliative care across settings and through time. Palliative care services are becoming available as consultative services and more rarely as palliative care units in hospitals, in day care and other outpatient settings, and in nursing homes. Palliative care consultations for nonhospice patients can be billed as for other consultations under Medicare Part B, the physician reimbursement part. Many believe palliative care should be offered to patients regardless of their prognosis. A patient, his or her family, and physicians should not have to make a "curative vs. palliative care" decision because it is rarely possible to make such a decisive switch to embracing mortality.

Care near the end of life cannot be measured by most of the available validated outcome measures since palliative care does not

TABLE 9-9 Managing Changes in the Patient's Condition During the Final Days and Hours

Changes in the Patient's Condition	Potential Complication	Family's Possible Reaction and Concern	Advice and Intervention
Profound fatigue	Bedbound with development of pressure ulcers that are prone to infection, malodor, and pain, and joint pain	Patient is lazy and giving up.	Reassure family and caregivers that terminal fatigue will not respond to interventions and should not be resisted. Use an air mattress if necessary.
Anorexia	None	Patient is giving up; patient will suffer from hunger and will starve to death.	Reassure family and caregivers that the patient is not eating because he or she is dying; not eating at the end of life does not cause suffering or death. Forced feeding, whether oral, parenteral, or enteral, does not reduce symptoms or prolong life.
Dehydration	Dry mucosal membranes (see below)	Patient will suffer from thirst and die of dehydration.	Reassure family and caregivers that dehydration at the end of life does not cause suffering because patients lose consciousness before any symptom distress. Intravenous hydration can worsen symptoms of dyspnea by pulmonary edema and peripheral edema as well as prolong dying process.
Dysphagia	Inability to swallow oral medications needed for palliative care		Do not force oral intake. Discontinue unnecessary medications that may have been continued, including antibiotics, diuretics, antidepressants, and laxatives. If swallowing pills is difficult, convert essential medications (analgesics, antiemetics, anxiolytics, and psychotropics) to oral solutions, buccal, sublingual, or rectal administration.
"Death rattle"—noisy breathing		Patient is choking and suffocating.	Reassure the family and caregivers that this is caused by secretions in the oropharynx and the patient is not choking. Reduce secretions with scopolamine (0.2–0.4 mg SC q4h or 1–3 patches q3d). Reposition patient to permit drainage of secretions. Do not suction. Suction can cause patient and family discomfort and is usually ineffective.
Apnea, Cheyne-Stokes respirations, dyspnea		Patient is suffocating.	Reassure family and caregivers that unconscious patients do not experience suffocation or air hunger. Apneic episodes are frequently a premorbid change. Opioids or anxiolytics may be used for dyspnea. Oxygen is unlikely to relieve dyspneic symptoms and may prolong the dying process.
Urinary or fecal incontinence	Skin breakdown if days until death Potential transmission of infectious agents to caregivers	Patient is dirty, malodorous, and physically repellent.	Remind family and caregivers to use universal precautions. Frequent changes of bedclothes and bedding. Use diapers, urinary catheter, or rectal tube if diarrhea or high urine output.
Agitation or delirium	Day/night reversal Hurt self or caregivers	Patient is in horrible pain and going to have a horrible death.	Reassure family and caregivers that agitation and delirium do not necessarily connote physical pain. Depending on the prognosis and goals of treatment, consider evaluating for causes of delirium and modify medications. Manage symptoms with haloperidol, chlorpromazine, diazepam, or midazolam.
Dry mucosal membranes	Cracked lips, mouth sores, and candidiasis can also cause pain. Odor	Patient may be malodorous, physically repellent.	Use baking soda mouthwash or saliva preparation q15–30min. Use topical nystatin for candidiasis. Coat lips and nasal mucosa with petroleum jelly q60–90min. Use ophthalmic lubricants q4h or artificial tears q30min.

consider death a bad outcome. Similarly, the family and patients receiving end-of-life care may not desire the elements elicited in current quality-of-life measurements. Symptom control, enhanced family relationships, and quality of bereavement are difficult to measure and are rarely the primary focus of carefully developed or widely used outcome measures. Nevertheless, outcomes are as important in end-of-life care as in any other field of medical care. Specific end-of-life care instruments are being developed both for assessment, such as The Brief Hospice Inventory and NEST (*needs near the end of life screening tool*), and for outcome measures, such as the Palliative Care Outcomes Scale, as well as for prognosis, such as the Palliative Prognostic Index. The field of end-of-life care is entering an era of evidence-based practice and continuous improvement through clinical trials.

FURTHER READINGS

■ WEB SITES

American Academy of Hospice and Palliative Medicine: *www.aahpm.org*

Center to Advance Palliative Care: *http://www.capc.org*

Education in Palliative and End of Life Care (EPEC): *http://www.epec.net*

End of Life—Palliative Education Resource Center: *http://www.eperc.mcw.edu*

Family Caregiver Alliance: *http://www.caregiver.org*

The Medical Directive: *http://www.medicaldirective.org*

National Family Caregivers Association: *http://www.nfcacares.org/*

National Hospice and Palliative Care Organization (including state-specific advance directives): *http://www.nhpco.org*

NCCN: The National Comprehensive Cancer Network palliative care guidelines: *http://www.nccn.org*

■ BOOKS

American Society of Clinical Oncology: *Optimizing Cancer Care—The Importance of Symptom Management,* vols 1 and 2. Alexandria, VA, ASCO, 2001

Buckman R: *How to Break Bad News: A Guide for Health Care Professionals.* Baltimore, Johns Hopkins University Press, 1992

Kuebler KK: *Palliative and End-of-Life Care: Clinical Practice Guide.* Philadelphia, Saunders, 2006

Meier DE et al (eds): *Palliative Care: Transforming the Care of Serious Illness.* San Francisco, Jossey-Bass, 2010

■ ARTICLES

Christakis NA, Allison PD: Mortality after the hospitalization of a spouse. N Engl J Med 354:719, 2006

Emanuel L et al: Integrating palliative care into disease management guidelines. J Palliat Med 7:774, 2004

Gabbay E et al: The empirical basis for determinations of medical futility. J Gen Intern Med 2010

Hugel H et al: The prevalence, key causes and management of insomnia in palliative care patients. J Pain Symptom Manage 27:316, 2004

Kapo J et al: Palliative care for the older adult. J Palliat Med 10:185, 2007

Lanken PN et al: An official American Thoracic Society clinical policy statement: Palliative care for patients with respiratory diseases and critical illnesses. Am J Respir Crit Care Med 177:912 2008

Larken PJ: The management of constipation in palliative care: Clinical practice recommendations. J Palliat Med 22:796, 2008

Lorenz K et al: Evidence for improving palliative care at the end of life: A systematic review. Ann Intern Med 148:147 2008

Lynn J: Serving patients who may die soon and their families: The role of hospice and other services. JAMA 285:925, 2001

Meisel A et al: Seven legal barriers to end-of-life care: Myths, realities, and grains of truth. JAMA 284:2495, 2000

Morrison RS, Meier DE: Palliative care. N Engl J Med 350:2582, 2004

Morrow GR: Guidelines for the treatment of chemotherapy-induced nausea and vomiting. Clin Adv Hematol Oncol 8:4, 2010

Murray SA et al: Illness trajectories and palliative care. BMJ 330:1007, 2005

Qaseem A et al: Evidence-based interventions to improve the palliative care of pain, dyspnea, and depression at the end of life: A clinical practice guideline from the American College of Physicians. Ann Intern Med 148:141, 2008

Radbruch L et al: Fatigue in palliative care patients—an EAPC approach. Palliat Med 22:13, 2008

Silveira M et al: Advance directives and outcomes of surrogate decision making before death. N Engl J Med 362:1211, 2010

Van den Beuken-van Everdingen MH et al: Prevalence of pain in patients with cancer: A systematic review of the past 40 years. Ann Oncol 18:1437, 2007

Wright AA et al: Associations between end-of-life discussions, patient mental health, medical care near death, and caregiver bereavement adjustment. JAMA 300:1665, 2008

Zhang B et al: Health care costs in the last week of life: Associations with end-of-life conversations. Arch Intern Med 169:480, 2009

CHAPTER 10

The Safety and Quality of Health Care

David W. Bates

The safety and quality of care are two of the central dimensions of health care. It is increasingly clear that both could be much better, and in recent years it has become easier to measure safety and quality. In addition, the public is—with good justification—demanding measurement and accountability, and payment for services increasingly will be based on performance in these areas. Thus, physicians must learn about these two domains, how they can be improved, and the relative strengths and limitations of the current ability to measure them.

Safety and quality are closely related but do not completely overlap. The Institute of Medicine has suggested in a seminal series of reports that safety is the first part of quality and that health care first must guarantee that it will deliver safe care, although quality is also pivotal. In the end, it is likely that more net clinical benefit will be derived from improving quality than from improving safety, though both are important and safety is in many ways more tangible to the public. Accordingly, the first section of this chapter will address issues relating to the safety of care and the second will cover quality of care.

■ SAFETY IN HEALTH CARE

Safety theory

Safety theory clearly points out that individuals make errors all the time. Think of driving home from the hospital; you intend to stop and pick up a quart of milk on the way home but find yourself entering your driveway without realizing how you got there. Everybody uses low-level, semiautomatic behavior for many activities in daily life; this kind of error is called a "slip." Slips occur often during care delivery, e.g., when people intend to write an order but forget because they have to complete another action first. "Mistakes," by contrast, are errors of a higher level; they occur in new or nonstereotypic situations in which conscious decisions are being made. An example would be dosing a medication with which a physician is not familiar. The strategies used to prevent slips and mistakes are often different.

Systems theory suggests that most accidents occur as the result of a series of small failures that happen to line up in an individual instance so that an accident can occur (Fig. 10-1). It also suggests that most individuals in an industry such as health care are trying to do the right thing (e.g., deliver safe care), and most accidents thus can be seen as resulting from defects in the systems. Correspondingly, systems should be designed both to make errors less likely and to identify those which do occur, as some inevitably will.

Factors that increase the likelihood of errors

Many factors ubiquitous in health care systems can increase the likelihood of errors, including fatigue, stress, interruptions, complexity, and transitions. The effects of fatigue in other industries are clear, but its effects in health care have been more controversial until recently. For example, the accident rate in truck drivers increases dramatically if they work over a certain number of hours in a week, especially with prolonged shifts. A recent study of house officers in the intensive care unit demonstrated that they were about one-third more likely to make errors when they were on a 24-h shift than when they were on a schedule that allowed them to sleep 8 h the previous night. The American College of Graduate Medical Education (ACGME) has moved to address this issue by putting in place the 80-h workweek. Although this is a step forward, it does not address the most important cause of fatigue-related errors: extended-duty shifts. High levels of stress and workload also can increase error rates. Thus, in extremely high-pressure situations, such as cardiac arrests, errors are more likely to occur. Strategies such as using protocols in these settings can be helpful, as can simply recognizing that the situation is stressful.

Interruptions also increase the likelihood of error and occur frequently in health care delivery. It is common to forget to complete an action when one is interrupted partway through it by a page, for example. Approaches that may be helpful in this area include minimizing the use of interruptions and setting up tools that help define the urgency of an interruption.

In addition, complexity represents a key issue that contributes to errors. Providers are confronted by streams of data, such as laboratory tests and vital signs, many of which provide little useful information but some of which are important and require action or suggest a specific diagnosis. Tools that emphasize specific abnormalities or combinations of abnormalities may be helpful in this area.

Transitions between providers and settings are also common in health care, especially with the advent of the 80-h workweek, and generally represent vulnerabilities. Tools that provide structure in exchanging information, e.g., when transferring care between providers, may be helpful.

The frequency of adverse events in health care

Most large studies focusing on the frequency and consequences of adverse events have been performed in the inpatient setting; some data are available for nursing homes, and much less information is available about the outpatient setting. The Harvard Medical Practice Study, one of the largest studies to address this issue, was performed with hospitalized patients in New York. The primary

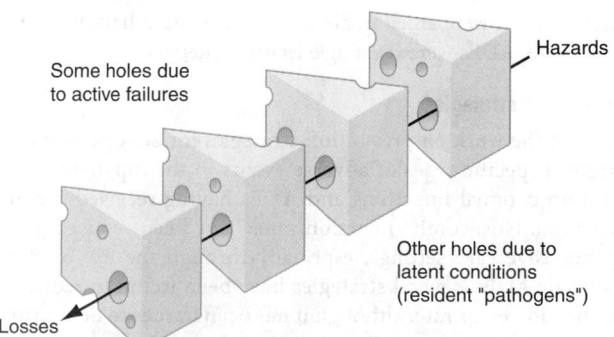

Figure 10-1 **"Swiss cheese" diagram.** Reason has argued that most accidents occur when a series of "latent failures" in a system are present and happen to line up in a given instance, resulting in an accident. Examples of latent failures in the case of a fall might be that the unit was unusually busy that day and that the floor happened to be wet. (*Adapted from J Reason: Human error: Models and management. BMJ 320:768–770, 2000; with permission.*)

outcome was the adverse event, which is an injury caused by medical management rather than the patient's underlying disease. In this study, an event either resulted in death or disability at discharge or prolonged the length of stay by at least 2 days. Key findings were that the adverse event rate was 3.7%, and 58% of the adverse events were considered preventable. Although New York is not representative of the rest of the country, the study was replicated later in Colorado and Utah, where the rates were essentially similar. Since then, other studies have been performed in a variety of developed nations using analogous methodologies, and the rates in developed countries appear to be ~10%. The World Health Organization has focused on this area, forming the World Alliance for Patient Safety, and rates of safety issues in developing and transitional countries appear to be even higher; thus, this is clearly an issue of global proportions.

In the Medical Practice Study, adverse drug events (ADEs) were the most common type, accounting for 19% of adverse events, followed by wound infections (14%) and technical complications (13%). Almost half the adverse events were associated with a surgical procedure. Among nonoperative events, 37% were ADEs, 15% were diagnostic mishaps, 14% were therapeutic mishaps, 13% were procedure-related, and 5% were falls.

ADEs have been studied more than any other category. Studies focusing specifically on ADEs have found that they appear to be much more common than was suggested by the Medical Practice Study, although most other studies use more inclusive criteria. Detection approaches in the research setting include chart review and the use of a computerized ADE monitor, a tool that explores the database and identifies signals that suggest an ADE may have occurred. Studies that use multiple approaches find more ADEs than does any individual approach, suggesting that the true underlying rate in the population is higher than would be identified by an individual approach. About 6–10% of patients admitted to U.S. hospitals experience an ADE.

Injuries caused by drugs are also common in the outpatient setting. One study found a rate of 21 ADEs per every 100 patients per year when patients were called to assess whether they had had a problem with one of their medications. The severity level was lower than in the inpatient setting, but approximately one-third of these ADEs were preventable.

Another area that appears to be very risky is the period immediately after a patient is discharged from the hospital. A recent study of patients hospitalized on a medical service found an adverse event rate of 19%; about a third of those events were preventable, and another third were ameliorable in that they could have been made less severe. ADEs were the single leading category.

Prevention strategies

Most of the work on prevention strategies for adverse events has targeted specific types of adverse events in the inpatient setting, with nosocomial infections and ADEs having received the most attention. Nosocomial infection rates have been reduced greatly in intensive care settings, especially through the use of checklists. For ADEs, several strategies have been found to reduce the medication error rate, although it has been harder to demonstrate that they reduce the ADE rate, and studies with adequate power to demonstrate a clinically meaningful reduction have not been published.

Implementation of checklists to ensure that specific actions are carried out has had a major impact on rates of catheter-associated bloodstream infections and ventilator-associated pneumonia, two of the most serious complications occurring in intensive care. The concept is that there are several specific actions that can reduce the frequency of these issues; when these actions are all carried out for every patient, the result has been an extreme reduction in

the frequency of the associated complication. Furthermore, these practices have been disseminated across wide areas, in particular in the state of Michigan.

Computerized physician order entry (CPOE) linked with clinical decision support has been found to reduce the serious medication error rate; serious medication errors are those which harm someone or have the potential to do so. In one study, CPOE, even with limited decision support, decreased the serious medication error rate by 55%. CPOE can prevent medication errors by suggesting a default dose, ensuring that all orders are complete (e.g., include a dose, route, and frequency), and checking orders for allergies, drug-drug interactions, and drug-laboratory issues. In addition, clinical decision support can suggest the right dose for a patient, tailoring it to the patient's level of renal function and age. In one study, without decision support patients with renal insufficiency received the appropriate dose only one-third of the time, whereas that fraction increased to approximately two-thirds with decision support, and patients with renal insufficiency were discharged from the hospital one-half day earlier. As of 2009, only about 15% of U.S. hospitals had implemented CPOE, but many plan to do so and will receive major financial incentives for achieving this goal.

Another technology that can improve medication safety is bar coding linked with an electronic medication administration record. Bar coding can help ensure that the right patient gets the right medication at the right time. Electronic medication administration records can make it much easier to determine what medications a patient has received. Studies to assess the impact of bar coding on medication safety are under way, and the early results are promising. Another technology that can be used to improve the safety of medication administration is "smart pumps." These are pumps that can be instructed in which medication is being given and at what dose; if the nurse tries to administer too high a dose, he or she will receive a warning.

The national picture around safety

Several organizations, including the National Quality Forum (NQF) and the Joint Commission on Accreditation of Healthcare Organizations (JCAHO), have made recommendations about how to improve safety. In particular, the NQF has released recommendations to the country's hospitals about what practices will most improve the safety of care, which all hospitals are expected to implement (Table 10-1). Many of these practices arise frequently in routine care. One example is "readback," the practice of recording all verbal orders and immediately reading them back to the physician to verify the accuracy of what was heard. Another is to use only standard abbreviations and dose designations, since some abbreviations and dose designations are particularly prone to error; for example, 7U may be read as 70.

Measurement of safety

Measuring the safety of care is quite difficult and expensive, since adverse events are, fortunately, rare. Most hospitals rely on spontaneous reporting to identify errors and adverse events, but this approach has very low sensitivity, with only ~1 in 20 ADEs reported. There are promising research techniques that involve searching the electronic record for signals suggesting that an adverse event has occurred, which probably will be routine in the future but are not yet in wide use. Claims data have been used to identify the frequency of adverse events; this approach works much better for surgical care than for medical care and still requires additional validation. The net result is that except for a few specific types of events, such as falls and nosocomial infections, hospitals have little idea about the true frequency of safety issues.

TABLE 10-1 Safe Practices for Better Health Care[a]

1. Create a health care culture of safety.

2. For designated high-risk, elective surgical procedures or other specified care, patients should be clearly informed of the likely reduced risk of an adverse outcome at treatment facilities that have demonstrated superior outcomes and should be referred to such facilities in accordance with the patient's stated preference.

3. Specify an explicit protocol to be used to ensure an adequate level of nursing based on the institution's usual patient mix and the experience and training of its nursing staff.

4. All patients in general intensive care units (both adult and pediatric) should be managed by physicians who have specific training and certification in critical care medicine ("critical care certified").

5. Pharmacists should participate actively in the medication-use process, including, at a minimum, being available for consultation with prescribers on medication ordering, interpretation and review of medication orders; preparation of medications; dispensing of medications; and administration and monitoring of medications.

6. Verbal orders should be recorded whenever possible and immediately read back to the prescriber; i.e., a health care provider receiving a verbal order should read or repeat back the information that the prescriber conveys to verify the accuracy of what was heard.

7. Use only standardized abbreviations and dose designations.

8. Patient care summaries or other similar records should not be prepared from memory.

9. Ensure that care information, especially changes in orders and new diagnostic information, is transmitted in a timely and clearly understandable form to all of the patient's current health care providers who need that information to provide care.

10. Ask each patient or legal surrogate to recount what he or she has been told during the informed consent discussion.

11. Ensure that written documentation of the patient's preference for life-sustaining treatments is displayed prominently displayed in his or her chart.

12. Implement a computerized prescriber order entry system.

13. Implement a standardized protocol to prevent the mislabeling of radiographs.

14. Implement standardized protocols to prevent the occurrence of wrong-site procedures or wrong-patient procedures.

15. Evaluate each patient undergoing elective surgery for risk of an acute ischemic cardiac event during surgery and provide prophylactic treatment of high-risk patients with beta blockers.

16. Evaluate each patient upon admission, and regularly thereafter, for the risk of developing pressure ulcers. This evaluation should be repeated at regular intervals during care. Clinically appropriate preventive methods should be implemented consequent to the evaluation.

17. Evaluate each patient upon admission, and regularly thereafter, for the risk of developing deep vein thrombosis (DVT)/venous thromboembolism (VTE). Utilize clinically appropriate methods to prevent DVT/VTE.

18. Utilize dedicated antithrombotic (anticoagulation) services that facilitate coordinated care management.

19. Upon admission, and regularly thereafter, evaluate each patient for the risk of aspiration.

20. Adhere to effective methods of preventing central venous catheter–associated bloodstream infections.

21. Evaluate each preoperative patient in light of his or her planned surgical procedure for the risk of surgical site infection and implement appropriate antibiotic prophylaxis and other preventive measures based on that evaluation.

22. Utilize validated protocols to evaluate patients who are at risk for contrast media-induced renal failure and utilize a clinically appropriate method for reducing risk of renal injury based on the patient's kidney function evaluation.

23. Evaluate each patient upon admission, and regularly thereafter, for risk of malnutrition. Employ clinically appropriate strategies to prevent malnutrition.

24. Whenever a pneumatic tourniquet is used, evaluate the patient for the risk of an ischemic and/or thrombotic complication and utilize appropriate prophylactic measures.

25. Decontaminate hands with a hygienic hand rub or by washing with a disinfectant soap before and after direct contact with the patient or objects immediately around the patient.

26. Vaccinate health care workers against influenza to protect both them and patients from influenza.

27. Keep workspaces where medications are prepared clean, orderly, well lit, and free of clutter, distraction, and noise.

28. Standardize the methods for labeling, packaging, and storing medications.

29. Identify all "high alert" drugs (e.g., intravenous adrenergic agonists and antagonists, chemotherapy agents, anticoagulants and antithrombotics, concentrated parenteral electrolytes, general anesthetics, neuromuscular blockers, insulin and oral hypoglycemics, and narcotics and opiates).

30. Dispense medications in unit-dose or, when appropriate, unit-of-use form, whenever possible.

[a] These 30 practices are the recommendations from the National Quality Forum (NQF) for improving the safety of health care; the NQF believes they should be implemented universally in applicable care settings to reduce the risk of patient harm. The practices all have strong supporting evidence and are likely to have a significant benefit.

Nonetheless, all providers have the responsibility to report problems with safety as they are identified. All hospitals have spontaneous reporting systems, and if providers report events as they occur, those events can be used as lessons for subsequent improvement.

Conclusions about safety

It is now abundantly clear that the safety of health care can be improved substantially; as more areas are studied closely, more problems are identified. Compared with the outpatient setting, much more is known about the epidemiology of safety in the inpatient setting, and a number of effective strategies for improving safety have been identified and are being used increasingly. Some effective strategies are also available in the outpatient setting. Transitions appear to be especially risky. The solutions to improving care often will involve systematic techniques such as checklists and often will involve leveraging information technology, but they also will include many other domains, such as use of human factors techniques, team training, and building a culture of safety.

■ QUALITY IN HEALTH CARE

Quality of care has remained somewhat elusive, although the tools for measuring it have increasingly improved. Selecting health care and measuring its quality is a complex process.

Quality theory

Donabedian has suggested that quality of care can be categorized by type of measurement into structure, process, and outcome. *Structure* refers to whether a particular characteristic is present, e.g., whether a hospital has a catheterization laboratory or whether a clinic uses an electronic health record. *Process* refers to the way care is delivered, and examples of process measures are whether a Pap smear was performed at the recommended interval or whether an aspirin was given to a patient with a suspected myocardial infarction. *Outcomes* refer to what actually happens, e.g., the mortality rate in myocardial infarction. It is important to note that good structure and process do not always result in good outcomes. For instance, a patient may present with a suspected myocardial infarction to an institution with a catheterization laboratory and receive recommended care, including aspirin, but still die because of the infarction.

Quality theory also suggests that overall quality will be improved more in the aggregate by raising the level of performance of all providers rather than finding a few poor performers and punishing them. This view suggests that systems changes are especially likely to be helpful in improving quality, since large numbers of providers may be affected simultaneously.

The theory of continuous quality improvement suggests that organizations should be evaluating the care they deliver on an ongoing basis and continually making small changes to improve their individual processes. This approach can be very powerful if embraced over time.

A number of specific tools have been developed to help improve process performance. One of the most important is the Plan-Do-Check-Act cycle (Fig. 10-2). This approach can be used to perform what is called rapid cycle improvement for a process, e.g., the time for a patient with pneumonia to receive antibiotics after diagnosis. Often, specific statistical tools such as control charts are used in conjunction to determine whether progress is being made. Most medical care includes one or many processes, making this tool especially important for improvement.

Factors relating to quality

Many factors can decrease the level of quality, including stress to providers, high or low levels of production pressure, and poor systems, to name but a few examples. Stress can have an adverse effect on quality because it can lead providers to omit important steps, as can a high level of production pressure. Low levels of production pressure sometimes can result in worse quality, as providers may be bored or have little experience with a specific problem. Poor systems can have a tremendous impact on quality, and even extremely dedicated providers typically cannot achieve high levels of performance if they are operating within a poor system.

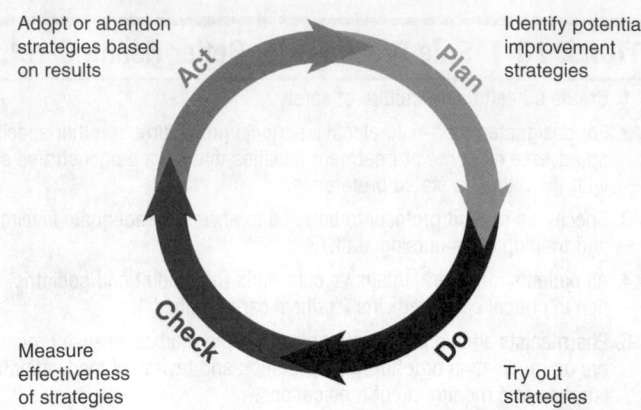

Figure 10-2 Plan-Do-Check-Act (PDCA) cycle. The PDCA cycle approach can be used to improve a specific process rapidly. First, planning is performed, and several potential improvement strategies are identified. Next, these strategies are trialed in small "tests of change." "Checking" entails measuring whether they appeared to make a difference, and "act" refers to acting on the results.

Data about the current state of quality

A recent RAND study has provided the most complete picture of quality of care delivered in the United States to date. The results were sobering. The authors found that across a wide range of quality parameters, patients in the United States received only 55% of recommended care overall; there was little variation by subtype, with scores of 54% for preventive care, 54% for acute care, and 56% for care of chronic conditions, leading the authors to conclude that the chances of getting high-quality care in the United States broadly were little better than those of winning a coin flip.

Work from the Dartmouth Atlas evaluating geographic variation in utilization and quality of care demonstrates that despite large variations in utilization, there is no positive correlation between the two variables at the regional level. An array of data demonstrate, however, that providers with larger volumes for specific conditions, especially for surgical conditions, do have better outcomes.

Strategies for improving quality and performance

A number of specific strategies can be used to improve quality at the individual level, including rationing, education, feedback, incentives, and penalties. *Rationing* has been effective in some specific areas, such as persuading physicians to prescribe within a formulary, but it generally has been resisted. *Education* is effective in the short run and is necessary for changing opinions, but its effect decays fairly rapidly with time. *Feedback* on performance can be given either at the group or the individual level. Feedback is most effective if it is individualized and is given in close temporal proximity to the original events. *Incentives* can be effective, and many believe that this will be a key to improving quality, especially if pay-for-performance with sufficient incentives is broadly implemented (see below). *Penalties* produce provider resentment and rarely are used in health care.

Another set of strategies for improving quality involves changing the systems of care. An example would be introducing reminders about which specific actions need to be taken at a visit for a specific patient, a strategy that has been demonstrated to improve performance in certain situations, e.g., the delivery of preventive services. Another approach that has been effective is the development of "bundles" or groups of quality measures that can be implemented together with a high degree of fidelity. A number of hospitals have implemented a bundle for ventilator-associated pneumonia in the intensive care unit, which includes five measures, including,

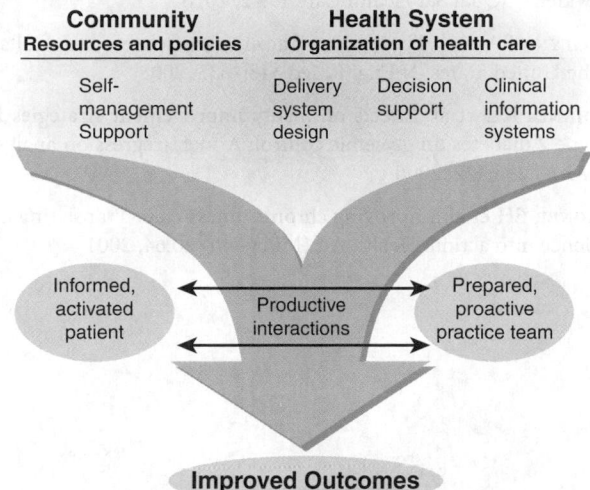

Community
Resources and policies

Health System
Organization of health care

Self-
management
Support

Delivery
system
design

Decision
support

Clinical
information
systems

Informed,
activated
patient

Productive
interactions

Prepared,
proactive
practice team

Improved Outcomes

Figure 10-3   The chronic care model. The chronic care model, which focuses on improving care for chronic diseases, suggests that delivery of high-quality care requires a range of strategies that must closely involve and engage the patient and, in addition, that team care is essential. *(From EH Wagner et al: Eff Clin Pract 1:2, 1998.)*

for example, ensuring that the head of the bed is elevated. The hospitals have found that they were able to improve performance substantially.

Perhaps the most pressing need is to improve the quality of care for chronic diseases. The Chronic Care Model has been developed by Wagner and colleagues (Fig. 10-3); it suggests that a combination of strategies will be necessary, including self-management support, changes in delivery system design, decision support, and information systems, and that these strategies must be delivered by a practice team composed of several providers, not just a physician.

Recent evidence about the relative efficacy of strategies in reducing hemoglobin A_{1c} (HbA_{1c}) in outpatient diabetes care supports this general premise. It is especially notable that the outcome was HbA_{1c}, as it has generally been much more difficult to improve outcome measures than process measures (such as whether an HbA_{1c} was performed). In this meta-analysis, a variety of strategies were effective, but the most effective ones were the use of team changes and the use of a case manager. When cost-effectiveness is considered in addition, it appears likely that an amalgam of strategies will be needed. However, the more expensive strategies, such as the use of case managers, probably will be implemented widely only if pay-for-performance takes hold.

National state of quality measurement

In the inpatient setting, quality measurement is now being performed by a very large proportion of hospitals for several conditions, including myocardial infarction, congestive heart failure, pneumonia, and surgical infection prevention; 20 measures are included in all. This is the result of the Hospital Quality Initiative, which represents a collaboration among many entities, including the Hospital Quality Alliance, the JCAHO, the NQF, and the Agency for Healthcare Research and Quality, among others. The data are housed at the Center for Medicare and Medicaid Services, which publicly releases performance on the measures on a website called *Hospital Compare*. These data are reported voluntarily and are available for a very high proportion of the nation's hospitals. Analyses demonstrate that there is substantial regional variation in quality and that there are important differences among hospitals.

Analyses by the Joint Commission for very similar indicators demonstrate that performance on measures by hospitals did improve over time and that, as might be hoped, lower performers improved more than did higher performers.

Public reporting

Overall, public reporting of quality data is becoming increasingly common. There are now commercial websites that have quality-related data for most regions of the country that can be accessed for a fee. Similarly, national data for hospitals are available. The evidence to date is that patients have not used such data very much but that the data have had an important effect on provider and organization behavior. Instead, patients have relied on provider reputation to make choices. Part of the reason for this choice basis is that until very recently little information was available, and it was not necessarily presented in ways that were easy for patients to access. Many believe that as more information about quality becomes available, it will become increasingly central to patient choices about where to access care.

Pay-for-performance

Currently, providers in the United States get paid exactly the same amount for a specific service regardless of what quality of care is delivered. The theory of pay-for-performance suggests that if providers are paid more for higher-quality care, they will invest in strategies that enable them to deliver that care. The current key issues in the pay-for-performance debate relate to (1) how effective it is, (2) what levels of incentives are needed, and (3) what perverse consequences are produced. The evidence about effectiveness is fairly limited, although a number of studies are ongoing. With respect to levels, most performance incentives around quality have accounted for merely 1–2% of total payment in this country to date, but in the United Kingdom, 40% of general practitioners' salaries have recently been placed at risk based on performance across a wide array of parameters. This has been associated with large improvements in reported quality performance, although it is still unclear to what extent this represents better performance versus better reporting. The potential for perverse consequences exists with any incentive scheme. One problem is that if incentives are tied to outcomes, this introduces the incentive to transfer the sickest patients to other providers and systems. Another concern is that providers will pay too much attention to quality measures with incentives and ignore the rest of the quality picture. The validity of these concerns remains to be determined.

■ CONCLUSIONS

The safety and quality of care in the United States could be improved substantially. A number of interventions are available today that have been demonstrated to improve the safety of care and should be used more widely; others are undergoing evaluation or will be evaluated. Quality also could be dramatically better, and the science of quality improvement is increasingly mature. Implementation of pay-for-performance should make it much easier for organizations to justify investments in improving these parameters, including health information technology; however, many will also require changing the structure of care, e.g., moving to a more team-oriented approach, and ensuring that the patients are more involved in their own care. Measures of safety are still relatively immature and could be made much more robust; it would be particularly useful if organizations had measures they could use in routine operations to assess safety at a reasonable cost. Although the quality measures available are more robust than those for safety, they still cover a relatively small proportion of the entire domain of quality, and more need to be developed. The public and payers are demanding better information about safety and quality as well as better performance in these areas. The clear implication is that these domains will have to be addressed directly by providers.

FURTHER READINGS

BATES DW et al: Effect of computerized physician order entry and a team intervention on prevention of serious medication errors. JAMA 280:1311, 1998

BRENNAN TA et al: Incidence of adverse events and negligence in hospitalized patients: Results from the Harvard Medical Practice Study I. N Engl J Med 324:370, 1991

JHA AK et al: Patient safety research: An overview of the global evidence. Qual Saf Health Care 19:42, 2010

McGLYNN EA et al: The quality of health care delivered to adults in the United States. N Engl J Med 348:2635, 2003

SHOJANIA KG et al: Effects of quality improvement strategies for type 2 diabetes on glycemic control: A meta-regression analysis. JAMA 296:427, 2006

WAGNER EH et al: Improving chronic illness care: Translating evidence into action. Health Aff (Millwood) 20:64, 2001

PART 2

Cardinal Manifestations and Presentation of Diseases

CHAPTER **11**

Pain: Pathophysiology and Management

James P. Rathmell
Howard L. Fields

The task of medicine is to preserve and restore health and to relieve suffering. Understanding pain is essential to both of these goals. Because pain is universally understood as a signal of disease, it is the most common symptom that brings a patient to a physician's attention. The function of the pain sensory system is to protect the body and maintain homeostasis. It does this by detecting, localizing, and identifying potential or actual tissue-damaging processes. Because different diseases produce characteristic patterns of tissue damage, the quality, time course, and location of a patient's pain complaint provide important diagnostic clues. It is the physician's responsibility to provide rapid and effective pain relief.

THE PAIN SENSORY SYSTEM

Pain is an unpleasant sensation localized to a part of the body. It is often described in terms of a penetrating or tissue-destructive process (e.g., stabbing, burning, twisting, tearing, squeezing) and/or of a bodily or emotional reaction (e.g., terrifying, nauseating, sickening). Furthermore, any pain of moderate or higher intensity is accompanied by anxiety and the urge to escape or terminate the feeling. These properties illustrate the duality of pain: it is both sensation and emotion. When it is acute, pain is characteristically associated with behavioral arousal and a stress response consisting of increased blood pressure, heart rate, pupil diameter, and plasma cortisol levels. In addition, local muscle contraction (e.g., limb flexion, abdominal wall rigidity) is often present.

■ PERIPHERAL MECHANISMS

The primary afferent nociceptor

A peripheral nerve consists of the axons of three different types of neurons: primary sensory afferents, motor neurons, and sympathetic postganglionic neurons (Fig. 11-1). The cell bodies of primary sensory afferents are located in the dorsal root ganglia in the vertebral foramina. The primary afferent axon has two branches: one projects centrally into the spinal cord and the other projects peripherally to innervate tissues. Primary afferents are classified by their diameter, degree of myelination, and conduction velocity. The largest-diameter afferent fibers, A-beta (Aβ), respond maximally to light touch and/or moving stimuli; they are present primarily in nerves that innervate the skin. In normal individuals, the activity of these fibers does not produce pain. There are two other classes of primary afferents: the small-diameter myelinated A-delta (Aδ) and the unmyelinated (C fiber) axons (Fig. 11-1). These fibers are present in nerves to the skin and to deep somatic and visceral structures. Some tissues, such as the cornea, are innervated only by Aδ and C fiber afferents. Most Aδ and C fiber afferents respond maximally only to intense (painful) stimuli and produce the subjective experience of pain when they are electrically stimulated; this defines them as *primary afferent nociceptors* (*pain receptors*). The ability to detect painful stimuli is completely abolished when conduction in Aδ and C fiber axons is blocked.

Individual primary afferent nociceptors can respond to several different types of noxious stimuli. For example, most nociceptors respond to heat; intense cold; intense mechanical stimuli, such as a pinch; changes in pH, particularly an acidic environment; and application of chemical irritants including adenosine triphosphate (ATP), serotonin, bradykinin, and histamine.

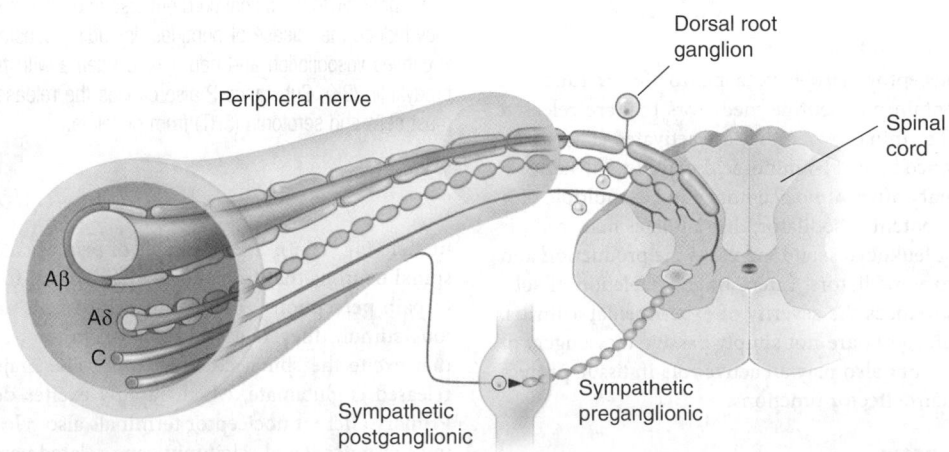

Figure 11-1 Components of a typical cutaneous nerve. There are two distinct functional categories of axons: primary afferents with cell bodies in the dorsal root ganglion, and sympathetic postganglionic fibers with cell bodies in the sympathetic ganglion. Primary afferents include those with large-diameter myelinated (Aβ), small-diameter myelinated (Aδ), and unmyelinated (C) axons. All sympathetic postganglionic fibers are unmyelinated.

Sensitization

When intense, repeated, or prolonged stimuli are applied to damaged or inflamed tissues, the threshold for activating primary afferent nociceptors is lowered, and the frequency of firing is higher for all stimulus intensities. Inflammatory mediators such as bradykinin, nerve-growth factor, some prostaglandins, and leukotrienes contribute to this process, which is called *sensitization*. Sensitization occurs at the level of the peripheral nerve terminal (*peripheral sensitization*) as well as at the level of the dorsal horn of the spinal cord (*central sensitization*). Peripheral sensitization occurs in damaged or inflamed tissues, when inflammatory mediators activate intracellular signal transduction in nociceptors, prompting an increase in the production, transport, and membrane insertion of chemically gated and voltage-gated ion channels. These changes increase the excitability of nociceptor terminals and lower their threshold for activation by mechanical, thermal, and chemical stimuli. Central sensitization occurs when activity, generated by nociceptors during inflammation, enhances the excitability of nerve cells in the dorsal horn of the spinal cord. Following injury and resultant sensitization, normally innocuous stimuli can produce pain. Sensitization is a clinically important process that contributes to tenderness, soreness, and hyperalgesia (increased pain intensity in response to the same noxious stimulus; e.g. moderate pressure causes severe pain). A striking example of sensitization is sunburned skin, in which severe pain can be produced by a gentle slap on the back or a warm shower.

Sensitization is of particular importance for pain and tenderness in deep tissues. Viscera are normally relatively insensitive to noxious mechanical and thermal stimuli, although hollow viscera do generate significant discomfort when distended. In contrast, when affected by a disease process with an inflammatory component, deep structures such as joints or hollow viscera characteristically become exquisitely sensitive to mechanical stimulation.

A large proportion of Aδ and C fiber afferents innervating viscera are completely insensitive in normal noninjured, noninflamed tissue. That is, they cannot be activated by known mechanical or thermal stimuli and are not spontaneously active. However, in the presence of inflammatory mediators, these afferents become sensitive to mechanical stimuli. Such afferents have been termed *silent nociceptors*, and their characteristic properties may explain how, under pathologic conditions, the relatively insensitive deep structures can become the source of severe and debilitating pain and tenderness. Low pH, prostaglandins, leukotrienes, and other inflammatory mediators such as bradykinin play a significant role in sensitization.

Nociceptor-induced inflammation

Primary afferent nociceptors also have a neuroeffector function. Most nociceptors contain polypeptide mediators that are released from their peripheral terminals when they are activated (Fig. 11-2). An example is substance P, an 11-amino-acid peptide. Substance P is released from primary afferent nociceptors and has multiple biologic activities. It is a potent vasodilator, degranulates mast cells, is a chemoattractant for leukocytes, and increases the production and release of inflammatory mediators. Interestingly, depletion of substance P from joints reduces the severity of experimental arthritis. Primary afferent nociceptors are not simply passive messengers of threats to tissue injury but also play an active role in tissue protection through these neuroeffector functions.

■ CENTRAL MECHANISMS

The spinal cord and referred pain

The axons of primary afferent nociceptors enter the spinal cord via the dorsal root. They terminate in the dorsal horn of the spinal gray

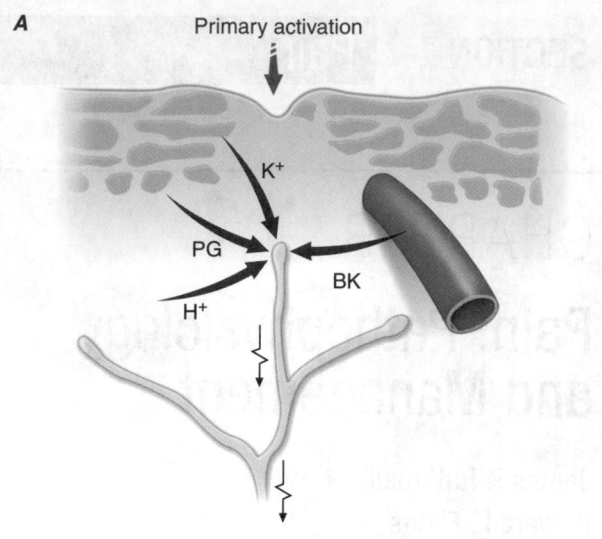

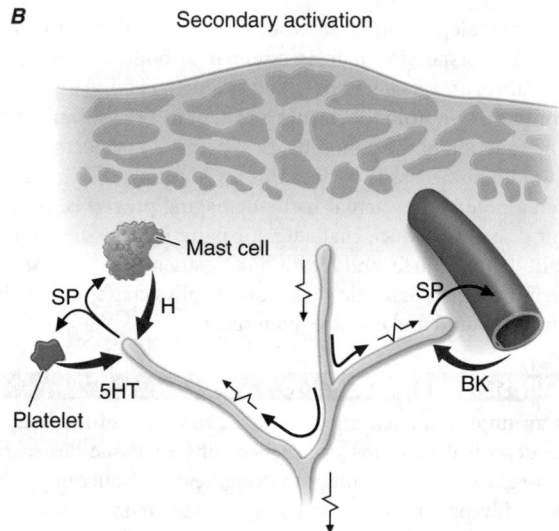

Figure 11-2 **Events leading to activation, sensitization, and spread of sensitization of primary afferent nociceptor terminals.** *A.* Direct activation by intense pressure and consequent cell damage. Cell damage induces lower pH (H^+) and leads to release of potassium (K^+) and to synthesis of prostaglandins (PG) and bradykinin (BK). Prostaglandins increase the sensitivity of the terminal to bradykinin and other pain-producing substances. *B.* Secondary activation. Impulses generated in the stimulated terminal propagate not only to the spinal cord but also into other terminal branches where they induce the release of peptides, including substance P (SP). Substance P causes vasodilation and neurogenic edema with further accumulation of bradykinin (BK). Substance P also causes the release of histamine (H) from mast cells and serotonin (5HT) from platelets.

matter (Fig. 11-3). The terminals of primary afferent axons contact spinal neurons that transmit the pain signal to brain sites involved in pain perception. When primary afferents are activated by noxious stimuli, they release neurotransmitters from their terminals that excite the spinal cord neurons. The major neurotransmitter released is glutamate, which rapidly excites dorsal horn neurons. Primary afferent nociceptor terminals also release peptides, including substance P and calcitonin gene-related peptide, which produce a slower and longer-lasting excitation of the dorsal horn neurons. The axon of each primary afferent contacts many spinal neurons, and each spinal neuron receives convergent inputs from many primary afferents.

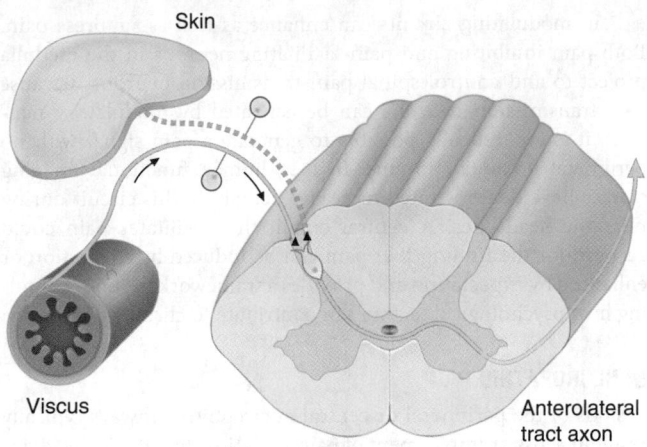

Figure 11-3 The convergence-projection hypothesis of referred pain. According to this hypothesis, visceral afferent nociceptors converge on the same pain-projection neurons as the afferents from the somatic structures in which the pain is perceived. The brain has no way of knowing the actual source of input and mistakenly "projects" the sensation to the somatic structure.

The convergence of sensory inputs to a single spinal pain-transmission neuron is of great importance because it underlies the phenomenon of referred pain. All spinal neurons that receive input from the viscera and deep musculoskeletal structures also receive input from the skin. The convergence patterns are determined by the spinal segment of the dorsal root ganglion that supplies the afferent innervation of a structure. For example, the afferents that supply the central diaphragm are derived from the third and fourth cervical dorsal root ganglia. Primary afferents with cell bodies in these same ganglia supply the skin of the shoulder and lower neck. Thus, sensory inputs from both the shoulder skin and the central diaphragm converge on pain-transmission neurons in the third and fourth cervical spinal segments. *Because of this convergence and the fact that the spinal neurons are most often activated by inputs from the skin, activity evoked in spinal neurons by input from deep structures is mislocalized by the patient to a place that roughly corresponds with the region of skin innervated by the same spinal segment.* Thus, inflammation near the central diaphragm is usually reported as shoulder discomfort. This spatial displacement of pain sensation from the site of the injury that produces it is known as *referred pain*.

Ascending pathways for pain

A majority of spinal neurons contacted by primary afferent nociceptors send their axons to the contralateral thalamus. These axons form the contralateral spinothalamic tract, which lies in the anterolateral white matter of the spinal cord, the lateral edge of the medulla, and the lateral pons and midbrain. The spinothalamic pathway is crucial for pain sensation in humans. Interruption of this pathway produces permanent deficits in pain and temperature discrimination.

Spinothalamic tract axons ascend to several regions of the thalamus. There is tremendous divergence of the pain signal from these thalamic sites to broad areas of the cerebral cortex that subserve different aspects of the pain experience (Fig. 11-4). One of the thalamic projections is to the somatosensory cortex. This projection mediates the purely sensory aspects of pain, i.e., its location, intensity, and quality. Other thalamic neurons project to cortical regions that are linked to emotional responses, such as the cingulate gyrus and other areas of the frontal lobes, including the insular cortex. These pathways to the frontal cortex subserve the affective or unpleasant emotional dimension of pain. This affective dimension

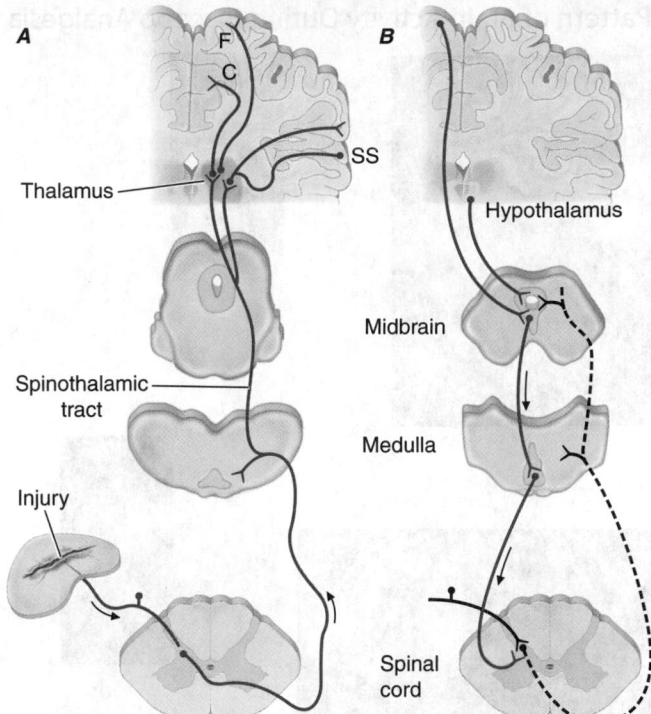

Figure 11-4 Pain transmission and modulatory pathways. *A.* Transmission system for nociceptive messages. Noxious stimuli activate the sensitive peripheral ending of the primary afferent nociceptor by the process of transduction. The message is then transmitted over the peripheral nerve to the spinal cord, where it synapses with cells of origin of the major ascending pain pathway, the spinothalamic tract. The message is relayed in the thalamus to the anterior cingulate (C), frontal insular (F), and somatosensory cortex (SS). *B.* Pain-modulation network. Inputs from frontal cortex and hypothalamus activate cells in the midbrain that control spinal pain-transmission cells via cells in the medulla.

of pain produces suffering and exerts potent control of behavior. Because of this dimension, fear is a constant companion of pain. As a consequence, injury or surgical lesions to areas of the frontal cortex activated by painful stimuli diminish the emotional impact of pain while largely preserving the individual's ability to recognize noxious stimuli as painful.

■ PAIN MODULATION

The pain produced by injuries of similar magnitude is remarkably variable in different situations and in different individuals. For example, athletes have been known to sustain serious fractures with only minor pain, and Beecher's classic World War II survey revealed that many soldiers in battle were unbothered by injuries that would have produced agonizing pain in civilian patients. Furthermore, even the suggestion that a treatment will relieve pain can have a significant analgesic effect (the placebo effect). On the other hand, many patients find even minor injuries (such as venipuncture) frightening and unbearable, and the expectation of pain can induce pain even without a noxious stimulus. The suggestion that pain will worsen following administration of an inert substance can increase its perceived intensity (the nocebo effect).

The powerful effect of expectation and other psychological variables on the perceived intensity of pain is explained by brain circuits that modulate the activity of the pain-transmission pathways. One of these circuits has links to the hypothalamus, midbrain, and medulla, and it selectively controls spinal pain-transmission neurons through a descending pathway (Fig. 11-4).

Pattern of Brain Activity During Placebo Analgesia

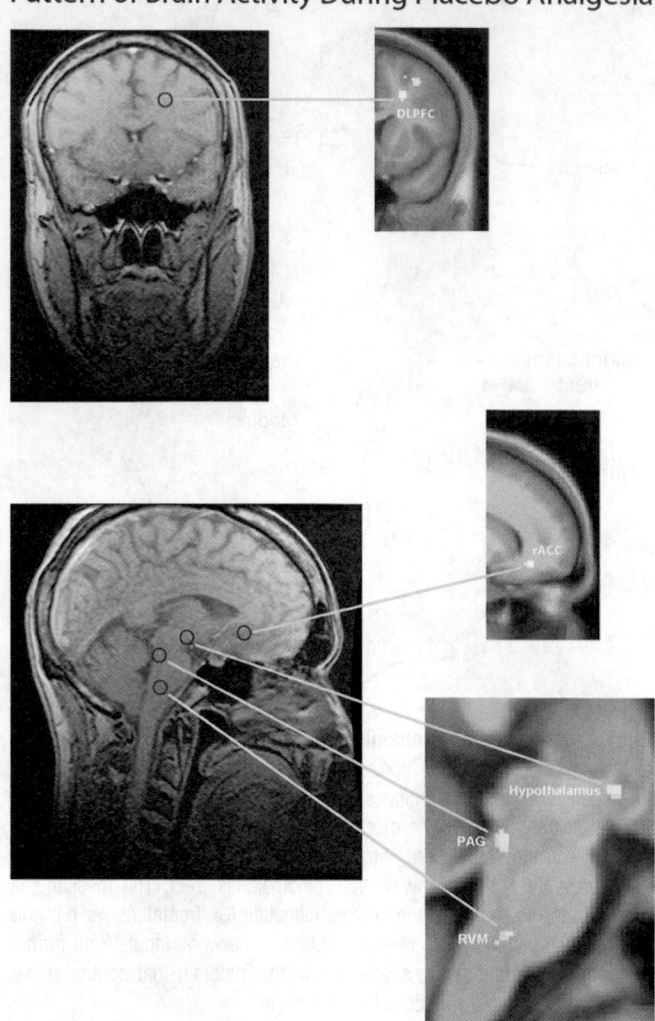

Figure 11-5 Functional magnetic resonance imaging (fMRI) demon-strates placebo-enhanced brain activity in anatomic regions correlating with the opioidergic descending pain control system. Top panel, Frontal fMRI image shows placebo-enhanced brain activity in the dorsal lateral prefrontal cortex (DLPFC). Bottom panel, Sagittal fMRI images show placebo-enhanced responses in the rostral anterior cingulate cortex (rACC), the rostral ventral medullae (RVM), the periaqueductal gray (PAG) area, and the hypothal-amus. The placebo-enhanced activity in all areas was reduced by naloxone, demonstrating the link between the descending opioidergic system and the placebo analgesic response. (*Adapted with permission from Eippert et al.*)

Human brain–imaging studies have implicated this pain-modulating circuit in the pain-relieving effect of attention, sug-gestion, and opioid analgesic medications (Fig. 11-5). Furthermore, each of the component structures of the pathway contains opioid receptors and is sensitive to the direct application of opioid drugs. In animals, lesions of this descending modulatory system reduce the analgesic effect of systemically administered opioids such as mor-phine. Along with the opioid receptor, the component nuclei of this pain-modulating circuit contain endogenous opioid peptides such as the enkephalins and β-endorphin.

The most reliable way to activate this endogenous opioid-mediated modulating system is by suggestion of pain relief or by intense emotion directed away from the pain-causing injury (e.g., during severe threat or an athletic competition). In fact, pain-relieving endogenous opioids are released following surgical procedures and in patients given a placebo for pain relief.

Pain-modulating circuits can enhance as well as suppress pain. Both pain-inhibiting and pain-facilitating neurons in the medulla project to and control spinal pain-transmission neurons. Because pain-transmission neurons can be activated by modulatory neu-rons, it is theoretically possible to generate a pain signal with no peripheral noxious stimulus. In fact, human functional imaging studies have demonstrated increased activity in this circuit during migraine headaches. A central circuit that facilitates pain could account for the finding that pain can be induced by suggestion or enhanced by expectation and provides a framework for understand-ing how psychological factors can contribute to chronic pain.

■ NEUROPATHIC PAIN

Lesions of the peripheral or central nociceptive pathways typically result in a loss or impairment of pain sensation. Paradoxically, dam-age to or dysfunction of these pathways can also produce pain. For example, damage to peripheral nerves, as occurs in diabetic neu-ropathy, or to primary afferents, as in herpes zoster, can result in pain that is referred to the body region innervated by the damaged nerves. Pain may also be produced by damage to the central nervous system (CNS), for example, in some patients following trauma or cerebrovascular injury to spinal cord, brainstem, or thalamic areas that contain central nociceptive pathways. Such neuropathic pains are often severe and are typically resistant to standard treatments for pain.

Neuropathic pain typically has an unusual burning, tingling, or electric shock–like quality and may be triggered by very light touch. These features are rare in other types of pain. On examina-tion, a sensory deficit is characteristically present in the area of the patient's pain. Hyperpathia, a greatly exaggerated pain sensation to innocuous or mild nociceptive stimuli, is also characteristic of neuropathic pain; patients often complain that the very lightest moving stimulus evokes exquisite pain (allodynia). In this regard, it is of clinical interest that a topical preparation of 5% lidocaine in patch form is effective for patients with postherpetic neuralgia who have prominent allodynia.

A variety of mechanisms contribute to neuropathic pain. As with sensitized primary afferent nociceptors, damaged primary affer-ents, including nociceptors, become highly sensitive to mechanical stimulation and may generate impulses in the absence of stimula-tion. Increased sensitivity and spontaneous activity are due, in part, to an increased concentration of sodium channels. Damaged primary afferents may also develop sensitivity to norepinephrine. Interestingly, spinal cord pain-transmission neurons cut off from their normal input may also become spontaneously active. Thus, both CNS and peripheral nervous system hyperactivity contribute to neuropathic pain.

Sympathetically maintained pain

Patients with peripheral nerve injury occasionally develop spon-taneous pain in the region innervated by the nerve. This pain is often described as having a burning quality. The pain typically begins after a delay of hours to days or even weeks and is accom-panied by swelling of the extremity, periarticular bone loss, and arthritic changes in the distal joints. The pain may be relieved by a local anesthetic block of the sympathetic innervation to the affected extremity. Damaged primary afferent nociceptors acquire adrenergic sensitivity and can be activated by stimulation of the sympathetic outflow. This constellation of spontaneous pain and signs of sympathetic dysfunction following injury has been termed *complex regional pain syndrome* (CRPS). When this occurs after an identifiable nerve injury, it is termed CRPS type II (also known as posttraumatic neuralgia or, if severe, *causalgia*). When a similar clinical picture appears without obvious nerve injury, it is termed

CRPS type I (also known as *reflex sympathetic dystrophy*). CRPS can be produced by a variety of injuries, including fractures of bone, soft tissue trauma, myocardial infarction, and stroke (Chap. 375). CRPS type I typically resolves with symptomatic treatment; however, when it persists, detailed examination often reveals evidence of peripheral nerve injury. Although the pathophysiology of CRPS is poorly understood, the pain and the signs of inflammation, when acute, can be rapidly relieved by blocking the sympathetic nervous system. This implies that sympathetic activity can activate undamaged nociceptors when inflammation is present. Signs of sympathetic hyperactivity should be sought in patients with posttraumatic pain and inflammation and no other obvious explanation.

TREATMENT Acute Pain

The ideal treatment for any pain is to remove the cause; thus, while treatment can be initiated immediately, efforts to establish the underlying etiology should always proceed as treatment begins. Sometimes, treating the underlying condition does not immediately relieve pain. Furthermore, some conditions are so painful that rapid and effective analgesia is essential (e.g., the postoperative state, burns, trauma, cancer, or sickle cell crisis). Analgesic medications are a first line of treatment in these cases, and all practitioners should be familiar with their use.

ASPIRIN, ACETAMINOPHEN, AND NONSTEROIDAL ANTI-INFLAMMATORY AGENTS (NSAIDS) These drugs are considered together because they are used for similar problems and may have a similar mechanism of action (Table 11-1). All these compounds inhibit cyclooxygenase (COX), and, except for acetaminophen, all have anti-inflammatory actions, especially at higher dosages. They are particularly effective for mild to moderate headache and for pain of musculoskeletal origin.

Because they are effective for these common types of pain and are available without prescription, COX inhibitors are by far the most commonly used analgesics. They are absorbed well from the gastrointestinal tract and, with occasional use, have only minimal side effects. With chronic use, gastric irritation is a common side effect of aspirin and NSAIDs and is the problem that most frequently limits the dose that can be given. Gastric irritation is most severe with aspirin, which may cause erosion and ulceration of the gastric mucosa leading to bleeding or perforation. Because aspirin irreversibly acetylates platelet cyclooxygenase and thereby interferes with coagulation of the blood, gastrointestinal bleeding is a particular risk. Older age and history of gastrointestinal disease increase the risks of aspirin and NSAIDs. In addition to the well-known gastrointestinal toxicity of NSAIDs, nephrotoxicity is a significant problem for patients using these drugs on a chronic basis. Patients at risk for renal insufficiency, particularly those with significant contraction of their intravascular volume as occurs with chronic diuretic use or acute hypovolemia, should be monitored closely. NSAIDs can also increase blood pressure in some individuals. Long-term treatment with NSAIDs requires regular blood pressure monitoring and treatment if necessary. Although toxic to the liver when taken in high doses, acetaminophen rarely produces gastric irritation and does not interfere with platelet function.

The introduction of a parenteral form of NSAID, ketorolac, extends the usefulness of this class of compounds in the management of acute severe pain. Ketorolac is sufficiently potent and rapid in onset to supplant opioids for many patients with acute severe headache and musculoskeletal pain.

There are two major classes of COX: COX-1 is constitutively expressed, and COX-2 is induced in the inflammatory state.

COX-2–selective drugs have similar analgesic potency and produce less gastric irritation than the nonselective COX inhibitors. The use of COX-2–selective drugs does not appear to lower the risk of nephrotoxicity compared to nonselective NSAIDs. On the other hand, COX-2–selective drugs offer a significant benefit in the management of acute postoperative pain because they do not affect blood coagulation. Nonselective COX inhibitors are usually contraindicated postoperatively because they impair platelet-mediated blood clotting and are thus associated with increased bleeding at the operative site. COX-2 inhibitors, including celecoxib (Celebrex) are associated with increased cardiovascular risk. It is possible that this is a class effect of NSAIDs, excluding aspirin. These drugs are contraindicated in patients in the immediate period after coronary artery bypass surgery and should be used with caution in patients with a history of or significant risk factors for cardiovascular disease.

OPIOID ANALGESICS Opioids are the most potent pain-relieving drugs currently available. Of all analgesics, they have the broadest range of efficacy and provide the most reliable and effective method for rapid pain relief. Although side effects are common, most are reversible: nausea, vomiting, pruritus, and constipation are the most frequent and bothersome side effects. Respiratory depression is uncommon at standard analgesic doses, but can be life-threatening. Opioid-related side effects can be reversed rapidly with the narcotic antagonist naloxone. The physician should not hesitate to use opioid analgesics in patients with acute severe pain. Table 11-1 lists the most commonly used opioid analgesics.

Opioids produce analgesia by actions in the CNS. They activate pain-inhibitory neurons and directly inhibit pain-transmission neurons. Most of the commercially available opioid analgesics act at the same opioid receptor (μ-receptor), differing mainly in potency, speed of onset, duration of action, and optimal route of administration. Some side effects are due to accumulation of nonopioid metabolites that are unique to individual drugs. One striking example of this is normeperidine, a metabolite of meperidine. Normeperidine produces hyperexcitability and seizures that are not reversible with naloxone. Normeperidine accumulation is increased in patients with renal failure.

The most rapid relief with opioids is obtained by intravenous administration; relief with oral administration is significantly slower. Common side effects include nausea, vomiting, constipation, and sedation. The most serious side effect is respiratory depression. Patients with any form of respiratory compromise must be kept under close observation following opioid administration; an oxygen-saturation monitor may be useful. Opioid-induced respiratory depression is typically accompanied by significant sedation and a reduction in respiratory rate. A fall in oxygen saturation represents a critical level of respiratory depression and the need for immediate intervention to prevent life-threatening hypoxemia. Ventilatory assistance should be maintained until the opioid-induced respiratory depression has resolved. The opioid antagonist naloxone should be readily available whenever opioids are used at high doses or in patients with compromised pulmonary function. Opioid effects are dose-related, and there is great variability among patients in the doses that relieve pain and produce side effects. Because of this, initiation of therapy requires titration to optimal dose and interval. The most important principle is to provide adequate pain relief. This requires determining whether the drug has adequately relieved the pain and frequent reassessment to determine the optimal interval for dosing. *The most common error made by physicians in managing severe pain with opioids is to prescribe*

TABLE 11-1 Drugs for Relief of Pain

Generic Name	Dose, mg	Interval	Comments
Nonnarcotic analgesics: usual doses and intervals			
Acetylsalicylic acid	650 PO	q 4 h	Enteric-coated preparations available
Acetaminophen	650 PO	q 4 h	Side effects uncommon
Ibuprofen	400 PO	q 4–6 h	Available without prescription
Naproxen	250–500 PO	q 12 h	Delayed effects may be due to long half-life
Fenoprofen	200 PO	q 4–6 h	Contraindicated in renal disease
Indomethacin	25–50 PO	q 8 h	Gastrointestinal side effects common
Ketorolac	15–60 IM/IV	q 4–6 h	Available for parenteral use
Celecoxib	100–200 PO	q 12–24 h	Useful for arthritis
Valdecoxib	10–20 PO	q12–24 h	Removed from U.S. market in 2005

Generic Name	Parenteral Dose, mg	PO Dose, mg	Comments
Narcotic analgesics: usual doses and intervals			
Codeine	30–60 q 4 h	30–60 q 4 h	Nausea common
Oxycodone	—	5–10 q 4–6 h	Usually available with acetaminophen or aspirin
Morphine	5 q 4 h	30 q 4 h	
Morphine sustained release	—	15–60 bid to tid	Oral slow-release preparation
Hydromorphone	1–2 q 4 h	2–4 q 4 h	Shorter acting than morphine sulfate
Levorphanol	2 q 6–8 h	4 q 6–8 h	Longer acting than morphine sulfate; absorbed well PO
Methadone	5-10 q 6–8 h	5-20 q 6–8 h	Delayed sedation due to long half-life; therapy should not be initiated with greater than 40 mg/day and dose escalation should be made no more frequently than every 3 days
Meperidine	50–100 q 3–4 h	300 q 4 h	Poorly absorbed PO; normeperidine a toxic metabolite; routine use of this agent is not recommended
Butorphanol	—	1–2 q 4 h	Intranasal spray
Fentanyl	25–100 µg/h	—	72-h transdermal patch
Tramadol	—	50–100 q 4–6 h	Mixed opioid/adrenergic action

Generic Name	Uptake Blockade 5-HT	Uptake Blockade NE	Sedative Potency	Anticholinergic Potency	Orthostatic Hypotension	Cardiac Arrhythmia	Ave. Dose, mg/d	Range, mg/d
Antidepressants[a]								
Doxepin	++	+	High	Moderate	Moderate	Less	200	75–400
Amitriptyline	++++	++	High	Highest	Moderate	Yes	150	25–300
Imipramine	++++	++	Moderate	Moderate	High	Yes	200	75–400
Nortriptyline	+++	++	Moderate	Moderate	Low	Yes	100	40–150
Desipramine	+++	++++	Low	Low	Low	Yes	150	50–300
Venlafaxine	+++	++	Low	None	None	No	150	75–400
Duloxetine	+++	+++	Low	None	None	No	40	30–60

Generic Name	PO Dose, mg	Interval	Generic Name	PO Dose, mg	Interval
Anticonvulsants and antiarrhythmics[a]					
Phenytoin	300	daily/qhs	Clonazepam	1	q 6 h
Carbamazepine	200–300	q 6 h	Gabapentin[b]	600–1200	q 8 h
Oxcarbazepine	300	bid	Pregabalin	150–600	bid

[a]Antidepressants, anticonvulsants, and antiarrhythmics have not been approved by the U.S. Food and Drug Administration (FDA) for the treatment of pain.
[b]Gabapentin in doses up to 1800 mg/d is FDA approved for postherpetic neuralgia.
Note: 5-HT, serotonin; NE, norepinephrine.

an inadequate dose. Because many patients are reluctant to complain, this practice leads to needless suffering. In the absence of sedation at the expected time of peak effect, a physician should not hesitate to repeat the initial dose to achieve satisfactory pain relief.

An innovative approach to the problem of achieving adequate pain relief is the use of patient-controlled analgesia (PCA). PCA uses a microprocessor-controlled infusion device that can deliver a baseline continuous dose of an opioid drug as well as preprogrammed additional doses whenever the patient pushes a button. The patient can then titrate the dose to the optimal level. This approach is used most extensively for the management of postoperative pain, but there is no reason why it should not be used for any hospitalized patient with persistent severe pain. PCA is also used for short-term home care of patients with intractable pain, such as that caused by metastatic cancer.

It is important to understand that the PCA device delivers small, repeated doses to maintain pain relief; in patients with severe pain, the pain must first be brought under control with a loading dose before transitioning to the PCA device. The bolus dose of the drug (typically 1 mg morphine, 0.2 mg of hydromorphone, or 10 μg fentanyl) can then be delivered repeatedly as needed. To prevent overdosing, PCA devices are programmed with a lockout period after each demand dose is delivered (5–10 min) and a limit on the total dose delivered per hour. While some have advocated the use of a simultaneous continuous or basal infusion of the PCA drug, this increases the risk of respiratory depression and has not been shown to increase the overall efficacy of the technique.

Many physicians, nurses, and patients have a certain trepidation about using opioids that is based on an exaggerated fear of addiction. In fact, there is a vanishingly small chance of patients becoming addicted to narcotics as a result of their appropriate medical use.

The availability of new routes of administration has extended the usefulness of opioid analgesics. Most important is the availability of spinal administration. Opioids can be infused through a spinal catheter placed either intrathecally or epidurally. By applying opioids directly to the spinal or epidural space adjacent to the spinal cord, regional analgesia can be obtained using relatively low total doses. Indeed, the dose required to produce effective localized analgesia when using morphine intrathecally (0.1–0.3 mg) is a fraction of that required to produce similar analgesia when administered intravenously (5–10 mg). In this way, side effects such as sedation, nausea, and respiratory depression can be minimized. This approach has been used extensively in obstetric procedures and for postoperative pain relief following surgical procedures on the lower extremities. Continuous intrathecal delivery via implanted spinal drug-delivery systems is now commonly used, particularly for the treatment of cancer-related pain that would require sedating doses for adequate pain control if given systemically. Opioids can also be given intranasally (butorphanol), rectally, and transdermally (fentanyl), thus avoiding the discomfort of frequent injections in patients who cannot be given oral medication. The fentanyl transdermal patch has the advantage of providing fairly steady plasma levels, which maximizes patient comfort.

Recent additions to the armamentarium for treating opioid-induced side effects are the peripherally acting opioid antagonists alvimopan (Entereg) and methylnaltrexone (Rellistor). Alvimopan is available as an orally administered agent that is restricted to the intestinal lumen by limited absorption; methylnaltrexone is available in a subcutaneously administered form that has virtually no penetration into the CNS. Both agents act by binding to peripheral μ-receptors, thereby inhibiting or reversing the effects of opioids at these peripheral sites. The action of both agents is restricted to receptor sites outside of the CNS; thus, these drugs can reverse the adverse effects of opioid analgesics that are mediated through their peripheral receptors without reversing their analgesic effects. Both agents are effective for persistent ileus following abdominal surgery to the extent that opioid analgesics used for postoperative pain control contribute to this serious problem. Likewise, both agents have been tested for their effectiveness in treating opioid-induced bowel dysfunction (constipation) in patients taking opioid analgesics on a chronic basis. Although contradictory, the weight of evidence indicates that alvimopan can reduce the incidence and duration of ileus following major abdominal surgery and methylnaltrexone can produce rapid reversal of constipation in many patients receiving opioids on a chronic basis.

Opioid and COX Inhibitor Combinations When used in combination, opioids and COX inhibitors have additive effects. Because a lower dose of each can be used to achieve the same degree of pain relief and their side effects are nonadditive, such combinations are used to lower the severity of dose-related side effects. However, fixed-ratio combinations of an opioid with acetaminophen carry a special risk. Dose escalation as a result of increased severity of pain or decreased opioid effect as a result of tolerance may lead to levels of acetaminophen that are toxic to the liver. Although acetaminophen-related hepatotoxicity is uncommon, it remains a leading cause for liver failure. Thus, many practitioners have moved away from the use of opioid-acetaminophen combination analgesics to avoid the risk of excessive acetaminophen exposure as the dose of the analgesic is escalated.

CHRONIC PAIN

Managing patients with chronic pain is intellectually and emotionally challenging. The patient's problem is often difficult or impossible to diagnose with certainty; such patients are demanding of the physician's time and often appear emotionally distraught. The traditional medical approach of seeking an obscure organic pathology is usually unhelpful. On the other hand, psychological evaluation and behaviorally based treatment paradigms are frequently helpful, particularly in the setting of a multidisciplinary pain-management center. Unfortunately, this approach, while effective, remains largely underused in current medical practice.

There are several factors that can cause, perpetuate, or exacerbate chronic pain. First, of course, the patient may simply have a disease that is characteristically painful for which there is presently no cure. Arthritis, cancer, chronic daily headaches, fibromyalgia, and diabetic neuropathy are examples of this. Second, there may be secondary perpetuating factors that are initiated by disease and persist after that disease has resolved. Examples include damaged sensory nerves, sympathetic efferent activity, and painful reflex muscle contraction. Finally, a variety of psychological conditions can exacerbate or even cause pain.

There are certain areas to which special attention should be paid in a patient's medical history. Because depression is the most common emotional disturbance in patients with chronic pain, patients should be questioned about their mood, appetite, sleep patterns, and daily activity. A simple standardized questionnaire, such as the Beck Depression Inventory, can be a useful screening device. It is important to remember that major depression is a common, treatable, and potentially fatal illness.

Other clues that a significant emotional disturbance is contributing to a patient's chronic pain complaint include pain that occurs in multiple, unrelated sites; a pattern of recurrent, but separate, pain problems beginning in childhood or adolescence; pain beginning at a time of emotional trauma, such as the loss of a parent or spouse; a history of physical or sexual abuse; and past or present substance abuse.

On examination, special attention should be paid to whether the patient guards the painful area and whether certain movements or postures are avoided because of pain. Discovering a mechanical component to the pain can be useful both diagnostically and therapeutically. Painful areas should be examined for deep tenderness, noting whether this is localized to muscle, ligamentous structures, or joints. Chronic myofascial pain is very common, and, in these patients, deep palpation may reveal highly localized trigger points that are firm bands or knots in muscle. Relief of the pain following injection of local anesthetic into these trigger points supports the diagnosis. A neuropathic component to the pain is indicated by evidence of nerve damage, such as sensory impairment, exquisitely sensitive skin, weakness, and muscle atrophy, or loss of deep tendon reflexes. Evidence suggesting sympathetic nervous system involvement includes the presence of diffuse swelling, changes in skin color and temperature, and hypersensitive skin and joint tenderness compared with the normal side. Relief of the pain with a sympathetic block is diagnostic.

A guiding principle in evaluating patients with chronic pain is to assess both emotional and organic factors before initiating therapy. Addressing these issues together, rather than waiting to address emotional issues after organic causes of pain have been ruled out, improves compliance in part because it assures patients that a psychological evaluation does not mean that the physician is questioning the validity of their complaint. Even when an organic cause for a patient's pain can be found, it is still wise to look for other factors. For example, a cancer patient with painful bony metastases may have additional pain due to nerve damage and may also be depressed. Optimal therapy requires that each of these factors be looked for and treated.

TREATMENT   Chronic Pain

Once the evaluation process has been completed and the likely causative and exacerbating factors identified, an explicit treatment plan should be developed. An important part of this process is to identify specific and realistic functional goals for therapy, such as getting a good night's sleep, being able to go shopping, or returning to work. A multidisciplinary approach that uses medications, counseling, physical therapy, nerve blocks, and even surgery may be required to improve the patient's quality of life. There are also some newer, relatively invasive procedures that can be helpful for some patients with intractable pain. These include image-guided interventions such as epidural injection of glucocorticoids for acute radicular pain, radiofrequency treatment of the facet joints for chronic facet-related pain, percutaneous intradiscal treatments for both axial and radicular pain, and placement of implanted intraspinal electrodes and implantation of intrathecal drug-delivery systems for severe and persistent pain that is unresponsive to more conservative treatments. There are no set criteria for predicting which patients will respond to these procedures. They are generally reserved for patients who have not responded to conventional pharmacologic approaches. Referral to a multidisciplinary pain clinic for a full evaluation should precede any invasive procedures. Such referrals are clearly not necessary for all chronic pain patients. For some, pharmacologic management alone can provide adequate relief.

TABLE 11-2   Painful Conditions That Respond to Tricyclic Antidepressants

Postherpetic neuralgia[a]
Diabetic neuropathy[a]
Tension headache[a]
Migraine headache[a]
Rheumatoid arthritis[a,b]
Chronic low back pain[b]
Cancer
Central post-stroke pain

[a]Controlled trials demonstrate analgesia.
[b]Controlled studies indicate benefit but not analgesia.

ANTIDEPRESSANT MEDICATIONS   The tricyclic antidepressants (TCAs), particularly nortriptyline and desipramine (Table 11-1) are useful for the management of chronic pain. Although developed for the treatment of depression, the TCAs have a spectrum of dose-related biologic activities that include analgesia in a variety of chronic clinical conditions. Although the mechanism is unknown, the analgesic effect of TCAs has a more rapid onset and occurs at a lower dose than is typically required for the treatment of depression. Furthermore, patients with chronic pain who are not depressed obtain pain relief with antidepressants. There is evidence that TCAs potentiate opioid analgesia, so they may be useful adjuncts for the treatment of severe persistent pain such as occurs with malignant tumors. Table 11-2 lists some of the painful conditions that respond to TCAs. TCAs are of particular value in the management of neuropathic pain such as occurs in diabetic neuropathy and postherpetic neuralgia, for which there are few other therapeutic options.

The TCAs that have been shown to relieve pain have significant side effects (Table 11-1; Chap. 390). Some of these side effects, such as orthostatic hypotension, drowsiness, cardiac-conduction delay, memory impairment, constipation, and urinary retention, are particularly problematic in elderly patients, and several are additive to the side effects of opioid analgesics. The selective serotonin reuptake inhibitors such as fluoxetine (Prozac) have fewer and less serious side effects than TCAs, but they are much less effective for relieving pain. It is of interest that venlafaxine (Effexor) and duloxetine (Cymbalta), which are nontricyclic antidepressants that block both serotonin and norepinephrine reuptake, appear to retain most of the pain-relieving effect of TCAs with a side-effect profile more like that of the selective serotonin reuptake inhibitors. These drugs may be particularly useful in patients who cannot tolerate the side effects of TCAs.

ANTICONVULSANTS AND ANTIARRHYTHMICS   These drugs are useful primarily for patients with neuropathic pain. Phenytoin (Dilantin) and carbamazepine (Tegretol) were first shown to relieve the pain of trigeminal neuralgia. This pain has a characteristic brief, shooting, electric shock–like quality. In fact, anticonvulsants seem to be particularly helpful for pains that have such a lancinating quality. Newer anticonvulsants, gabapentin (Neurontin) and pregabalin (Lyrica), are effective for a broad range of neuropathic pains. Furthermore, because of their favorable side-effect profile, these newer anticonvulsants are often used as first-line agents.

CHRONIC OPIOID MEDICATION The long-term use of opioids is accepted for patients with pain due to malignant disease. Although opioid use for chronic pain of nonmalignant origin is controversial, it is clear that for many such patients, opioid analgesics are the best available option. This is understandable because opioids are the most potent and have the broadest range of efficacy of any analgesic medications. Although addiction is rare in patients who first use opioids for pain relief, some degree of tolerance and physical dependence is likely with long-term use. Therefore, before embarking on opioid therapy, other options should be explored, and the limitations and risks of opioids should be explained to the patient. It is also important to point out that some opioid analgesic medications have mixed agonist-antagonist properties (e.g., pentazocine and butorphanol). From a practical standpoint, this means that they may worsen pain by inducing an abstinence syndrome in patients who are physically dependent on other opioid analgesics.

With long-term outpatient use of orally administered opioids, it is desirable to use long-acting compounds such as levorphanol, methadone, or sustained-release morphine (Table 11-1). Transdermal fentanyl is another excellent option. The pharmacokinetic profile of these drug preparations enables prolonged pain relief, minimizes side effects such as sedation that are associated with high peak plasma levels, and reduces the likelihood of rebound pain associated with a rapid fall in plasma opioid concentration. While long-acting opioid preparations may provide superior pain relief in patients with a continuous pattern of ongoing pain, others suffer from intermittent severe episodic pain and experience superior pain control and fewer side effects with the periodic use of short-acting opioid analgesics. Constipation is a virtually universal side effect of opioid use and should be treated expectantly. A recent advance for patients with chronic debilitating conditions is the development of methylnaltrexone, a peripherally acting mu opioid antagonist that blocks the constipation and itching associated with chronic opioid use without interfering with analgesia; the usual dose is 0.15 mg/kg of body weight given subcutaneously no more often than once daily.

TREATMENT OF NEUROPATHIC PAIN It is important to individualize treatment for patients with neuropathic pain. Several general principles should guide therapy: the first is to move quickly to provide relief, and the second is to minimize drug side effects. For example, in patients with postherpetic neuralgia and significant cutaneous hypersensitivity, topical lidocaine (Lidoderm patches) can provide immediate relief without side effects. Anticonvulsants (gabapentin or pregabalin, see above) or antidepressants (nortriptyline, desipramine, duloxetine, or venlafaxine) can be used as first-line drugs for patients with neuropathic pain. Systemically administered antiarrhythmic drugs such as lidocaine and mexiletene are less likely to be effective; although intravenous infusion of lidocaine predictably provides analgesia in those with many forms of neuropathic pain, the relief is usually transient, typically lasting just hours after the cessation of the infusion. The oral lidocaine congener mexiletene is poorly tolerated, producing frequent gastrointestinal adverse effects. There is no consensus on which class of drug should be used as a first-line treatment for any chronically painful condition. However, because relatively high doses of anticonvulsants are required for pain relief, sedation is very common. Sedation is also a problem with TCAs but is much less of a problem with serotonin/norepinephrine reuptake inhibitors (SNRIs, e.g., venlafaxine and duloxetine). Thus, in the elderly or in those patients whose daily activities require high-level mental activity, these drugs should be considered the first line. In contrast, opioid medications should be used as a second- or third-line drug class. While highly effective for many painful conditions, opioids are sedating, and their effect tends to lessen over time, leading to dose escalation and, occasionally, a worsening of pain due to physical dependence. Drugs of different classes can be used in combination to optimize pain control.

It is worth emphasizing that many patients, especially those with chronic pain, seek medical attention primarily because they are suffering and because only physicians can provide the medications required for pain relief. A primary responsibility of all physicians is to minimize the physical and emotional discomfort of their patients. Familiarity with pain mechanisms and analgesic medications is an important step toward accomplishing this aim.

FURTHER READINGS

COSTIGAN M: Neuropathic pain: A maladaptive response of the nervous system to damage. Annu Rev Neurosci 32:1, 2009

CRAIG AD: How do you feel? Interoception: The sense of the physiological condition of the body. Nat Rev Neurosci 8:655, 2002

DWORKIN RH: Pharmacologic management of neuropathic pain: Evidence-based recommendations. Pain 123:237, 2007

EIPPERT F et al: Activation of the opioidergic descending pain control system underlies placebo analgesia. Neuron 63:533, 2009

FIELDS HL: Should we be reluctant to prescribe opioids for chronic nonmalignant pain? Pain 129:233, 2007

MACINTYRE PE: Safety and efficacy of patient-controlled analgesia. Br J Anaesth 87:36, 2001

OAKLANDER AL: Is reflex sympathetic dystrophy/complex regional pain syndrome type I a small-fiber neuropathy? Ann Neurol 64:629, 2009

CHAPTER 12

Chest Discomfort

Thomas H. Lee

Chest discomfort is a common challenge for clinicians in the office or emergency department. The differential diagnosis includes conditions affecting organs throughout the thorax and abdomen, with prognostic implications that vary from benign to life-threatening (Table 12-1). Failure to recognize potentially serious conditions such as acute ischemic heart disease, aortic dissection, tension pneumothorax, or pulmonary embolism can lead to serious complications, including death. Conversely, overly conservative management of low-risk patients leads to unnecessary hospital admissions, tests, procedures, and anxiety.

■ CAUSES OF CHEST DISCOMFORT

Myocardial ischemia and injury

Myocardial ischemia occurs when the oxygen supply to the heart is insufficient to meet metabolic needs. This mismatch can result from a decrease in oxygen supply, a rise in demand, or both. The most common underlying cause of myocardial ischemia is obstruction of coronary arteries by atherosclerosis; in the presence of such obstruction, transient ischemic episodes are usually precipitated by an increase in oxygen demand as a result of physical exertion. However, ischemia can also result from psychological stress, fever, or large meals or from compromised oxygen delivery due to anemia, hypoxia, or hypotension. Ventricular hypertrophy due

TABLE 12-1 Diagnoses Among Chest Pain Patients Without Myocardial Infarction

Diagnosis	Percent
Gastroesophageal disease[a]	42
Gastroesophageal reflux	
Esophageal motility disorders	
Peptic ulcer	
Gallstones	
Ischemic heart disease	31
Chest wall syndromes	28
Pericarditis	4
Pleuritis/pneumonia	2
Pulmonary embolism	2
Lung cancer	1.5
Aortic aneurysm	1
Aortic stenosis	1
Herpes zoster	1

[a]In order of frequency.

Source: P Fruergaard et al: Eur Heart J 17:1028, 1996.

to valvular heart disease, hypertrophic cardiomyopathy, or hypertension can predispose the myocardium to ischemia because of impaired penetration of blood flow from epicardial coronary arteries to the endocardium.

Angina pectoris (See also Chap. 243) The chest discomfort of myocardial ischemia is a visceral discomfort that is usually described as a heaviness, pressure, or squeezing (Table 12-2). Other common adjectives for anginal pain are burning and aching. Some patients deny any "pain" but may admit to dyspnea or a vague sense of anxiety. The word "sharp" is sometimes used by patients to describe intensity rather than quality.

The location of angina pectoris is usually retrosternal; most patients do not localize the pain to any small area. The discomfort may radiate to the neck, jaw, teeth, arms, or shoulders, reflecting the common origin in the posterior horn of the spinal cord of sensory neurons supplying the heart and these areas. Some patients present with aching in sites of radiated pain as their only symptoms of ischemia. Occasional patients report epigastric distress with ischemic episodes. Less common is radiation to below the umbilicus or to the back.

Stable angina pectoris usually develops gradually with exertion, emotional excitement, or after heavy meals. Rest or treatment with sublingual nitroglycerin typically leads to relief within several minutes. In contrast, pain that is fleeting (lasting only a few seconds) is rarely ischemic in origin. Similarly, pain that lasts for several hours is unlikely to represent angina, particularly if the patient's electrocardiogram (ECG) does not show evidence of ischemia.

Anginal episodes can be precipitated by any physiologic or psychological stress that induces tachycardia. Most myocardial perfusion occurs during diastole, when there is minimal pressure opposing coronary artery flow from within the left ventricle. Since tachycardia decreases the percentage of the time in which the heart is in diastole, it decreases myocardial perfusion.

Unstable angina and myocardial infarction (See also Chaps. 244 and 245) Patients with these acute ischemic syndromes usually complain of symptoms similar in quality to angina pectoris, but more prolonged and severe. The onset of these syndromes may occur with the patient at rest, or awakened from sleep, and sublingual nitroglycerin may lead to transient or no relief. Accompanying symptoms may include diaphoresis, dyspnea, nausea, and light-headedness.

The physical examination may be completely normal in patients with chest discomfort due to ischemic heart disease. Careful auscultation during ischemic episodes may reveal a third or fourth heart sound, reflecting myocardial systolic or diastolic dysfunction. A transient murmur of mitral regurgitation suggests ischemic papillary muscle dysfunction. Severe episodes of ischemia can lead to pulmonary congestion and even pulmonary edema.

Other cardiac causes Myocardial ischemia caused by hypertrophic cardiomyopathy or aortic stenosis leads to angina pectoris similar to that caused by coronary atherosclerosis. In such cases, a loud systolic murmur or other findings usually suggest that abnormalities other than coronary atherosclerosis may be contributing to the patient's symptoms. Some patients with chest pain and normal coronary angiograms have functional abnormalities of the coronary circulation, ranging from coronary spasm visible on coronary angiography to abnormal vasodilator responses and heightened vasoconstrictor responses. The term "cardiac syndrome X" is used to describe patients with angina-like chest pain and ischemic-appearing ST-segment depression during stress despite normal coronary arteriograms. Some data indicate that many such patients have limited changes in coronary flow in response to pacing stress or coronary vasodilators.

TABLE 12-2 Typical Clinical Features of Major Causes of Acute Chest Discomfort

Condition	Duration	Quality	Location	Associated Features
Angina	More than 2 and less than 10 min	Pressure, tightness, squeezing, heaviness, burning	Retrosternal, often with radiation to or isolated discomfort in neck, jaw, shoulders, or arms—frequently on left	Precipitated by exertion, exposure to cold, psychologic stress S_4 gallop or mitral regurgitation murmur during pain
Unstable angina	10–20 min	Similar to angina but often more severe	Similar to angina	Similar to angina, but occurs with low levels of exertion or even at rest
Acute myocardial infarction	Variable; often more than 30 min	Similar to angina but often more severe	Similar to angina	Unrelieved by nitroglycerin May be associated with evidence of heart failure or arrhythmia
Aortic stenosis	Recurrent episodes as described for angina	As described for angina	As described for angina	Late-peaking systolic murmur radiating to carotid arteries
Pericarditis	Hours to days; may be episodic	Sharp	Retrosternal or toward cardiac apex; may radiate to left shoulder	May be relieved by sitting up and leaning forward Pericardial friction rub
Aortic dissection	Abrupt onset of unrelenting pain	Tearing or ripping sensation; knifelike	Anterior chest, often radiating to back, between shoulder blades	Associated with hypertension and/or underlying connective tissue disorder, e.g., Marfan syndrome Murmur of aortic insufficiency, pericardial rub, pericardial tamponade, or loss of peripheral pulses
Pulmonary embolism	Abrupt onset; several minutes to a few hours	Pleuritic	Often lateral, on the side of the embolism	Dyspnea, tachypnea, tachycardia, and hypotension
Pulmonary hypertension	Variable	Pressure	Substernal	Dyspnea, signs of increased venous pressure including edema and jugular venous distention
Pneumonia or pleuritis	Variable	Pleuritic	Unilateral, often localized	Dyspnea, cough, fever, rales, occasional rub
Spontaneous pneumothorax	Sudden onset; several hours	Pleuritic	Lateral to side of pneumothorax	Dyspnea, decreased breath sounds on side of pneumothorax
Esophageal reflux	10–60 min	Burning	Substernal, epigastric	Worsened by postprandial recumbency Relieved by antacids
Esophageal spasm	2–30 min	Pressure, tightness, burning	Retrosternal	Can closely mimic angina
Peptic ulcer	Prolonged	Burning	Epigastric, substernal	Relieved with food or antacids
Gallbladder disease	Prolonged	Burning, pressure	Epigastric, right upper quadrant, substernal	May follow meal
Musculoskeletal disease	Variable	Aching	Variable	Aggravated by movement May be reproduced by localized pressure on examination
Herpes zoster	Variable	Sharp or burning	Dermatomal distribution	Vesicular rash in area of discomfort
Emotional and psychiatric conditions	Variable; may be fleeting	Variable	Variable; may be retrosternal	Situational factors may precipitate symptoms Anxiety or depression often detectable with careful history

Pericarditis

(See also Chap. 239) The pain in pericarditis is believed to be due to inflammation of the adjacent parietal pleura, since most of the pericardium is believed to be insensitive to pain. Thus, infectious pericarditis, which usually involves adjoining pleural surfaces, tends to be associated with pain, while conditions that cause only local inflammation (e.g., myocardial infarction or uremia) and cardiac tamponade tend to result in mild or no chest pain.

The adjacent parietal pleura receives its sensory supply from several sources, so the pain of pericarditis can be experienced in areas ranging from the shoulder and neck to the abdomen and back. Most typically, the pain is retrosternal and is aggravated by coughing, deep breaths, or changes in position—all of which lead to movements of pleural surfaces. The pain is often worse in the supine position and relieved by sitting upright and leaning forward. Less common is a steady aching discomfort that mimics acute myocardial infarction.

Diseases of the aorta

(See also Chap. 248) *Aortic dissection* is a potentially catastrophic condition that is due to spread of a subintimal hematoma within the wall of the aorta. The hematoma may begin with a tear in the intima of the aorta or with rupture of the vasa vasorum within the aortic media. This syndrome can occur with trauma to the aorta, including motor vehicle accidents or medical procedures in which catheters or intraaortic balloon pumps damage the intima of the aorta. Nontraumatic aortic dissections are rare in the absence of hypertension and/or conditions associated with deterioration of the elastic or muscular components of the media within the aorta's wall. Cystic medial degeneration is a feature of several inherited connective tissue diseases, including Marfan and Ehlers-Danlos syndromes. About half of all aortic dissections in women under 40 years of age occur during pregnancy.

Almost all patients with acute dissections present with severe chest pain, although some patients with chronic dissections are identified without associated symptoms. Unlike the pain of ischemic heart disease, symptoms of aortic dissection tend to reach peak severity immediately, often causing the patient to collapse from its intensity. The classic teaching is that the adjectives used to describe the pain reflect the process occurring within the wall of the aorta—"ripping" and "tearing"—but more recent data suggest that the most common presenting complaint is sudden onset of severe, sharp pain. The location often correlates with the site and extent of the dissection. Thus, dissections that begin in the ascending aorta and extend to the descending aorta tend to cause pain in the front of the chest that extends into the back, between the shoulder blades.

Physical findings may also reflect extension of the aortic dissection that compromises flow into arteries branching off the aorta. Thus, loss of a pulse in one or both arms, cerebrovascular accident, or paraplegia can all be catastrophic consequences of aortic dissection. Hematomas that extend proximally and undermine the coronary arteries or aortic valve apparatus may lead to acute myocardial infarction or acute aortic insufficiency. Rupture of the hematoma into the pericardial space leads to pericardial tamponade.

Another abnormality of the aorta that can cause chest pain is a *thoracic aortic aneurysm*. Aortic aneurysms are frequently asymptomatic but can cause chest pain and other symptoms by compressing adjacent structures. This pain tends to be steady, deep, and sometimes severe.

Pulmonary embolism

(See also Chap. 262) Chest pain due to pulmonary embolism is believed to be due to distention of the pulmonary artery or infarction of a segment of the lung adjacent to the pleura. Massive pulmonary emboli may lead to substernal pain that is suggestive of acute myocardial infarction. More commonly, smaller emboli lead to focal pulmonary infarctions that cause pain that is lateral and pleuritic. Associated symptoms include dyspnea and, occasionally, hemoptysis. Tachycardia is usually present. Although not always present, certain characteristic ECG changes can support the diagnosis.

Pneumothorax

(See also Chap. 263) Sudden onset of pleuritic chest pain and respiratory distress should lead to consideration of spontaneous pneumothorax, as well as pulmonary embolism. Such events may occur without a precipitating event in persons without lung disease, or as a consequence of underlying lung disorders.

Pneumonia or pleuritis

(See also Chaps. 257 and 263) Lung diseases that damage and cause inflammation of the pleura of the lung usually cause a sharp, knife-like pain that is aggravated by inspiration or coughing.

Gastrointestinal conditions

(See also Chap. 292) Esophageal pain from acid reflux from the stomach, spasm, obstruction, or injury can be difficult to differentiate from myocardial syndromes. Acid reflux typically causes a deep burning discomfort that may be exacerbated by alcohol, aspirin, or some foods; this discomfort is often relieved by antacid or other acid-reducing therapies. Acid reflux tends to be exacerbated by lying down and may be worse in early morning when the stomach is empty of food that might otherwise absorb gastric acid.

Esophageal spasm may occur in the presence or absence of acid reflux and leads to a squeezing pain indistinguishable from angina. Prompt relief of esophageal spasm is often provided by antianginal therapies such as sublingual nifedipine, further promoting confusion between these syndromes. Chest pain can also result from injury to the esophagus, such as a Mallory-Weiss tear caused by severe vomiting.

Chest pain can result from diseases of the gastrointestinal tract below the diaphragm, including *peptic ulcer disease*, *biliary disease*, and *pancreatitis*. These conditions usually cause abdominal pain as well as chest discomfort; symptoms are not likely to be associated with exertion. The pain of ulcer disease typically occurs 60 to 90 min after meals, when postprandial acid production is no longer neutralized by food in the stomach. Cholecystitis usually causes a pain that is described as aching, occurring an hour or more after meals.

Neuromusculoskeletal conditions

Cervical disk disease can cause chest pain by compression of nerve roots. Pain in a dermatomal distribution can also be caused by *intercostal muscle cramps* or by *herpes zoster*. Chest pain symptoms due to herpes zoster may occur before skin lesions are apparent.

Costochondral and *chondrosternal syndromes* are the most common causes of anterior chest musculoskeletal pain. Only occasionally are physical signs of costochondritis such as swelling, redness, and warmth (Tietze's syndrome) present. The pain of such syndromes is usually fleeting and sharp, but some patients experience a dull ache that lasts for hours. Direct pressure on the chondrosternal and costochondral junctions may reproduce the pain from these and other musculoskeletal syndromes. Arthritis of the shoulder and spine and bursitis may also cause chest pain. Some patients who have these conditions and myocardial ischemia blur and confuse symptoms of these syndromes.

Emotional and psychiatric conditions

As many as 10% of patients who present to emergency departments with acute chest discomfort have panic disorder or other emotional conditions. The symptoms in these populations are highly variable, but frequently the discomfort is described as visceral tightness or aching that lasts more than 30 min. Some patients offer other atypical descriptions, such as pain that is fleeting, sharp, and/or localized to a small region. The ECG in patients with emotional conditions may be difficult to interpret if hyperventilation causes ST-T-wave abnormalities. A careful history may elicit clues of depression, prior panic attacks, somatization, agoraphobia, or other phobias.

APPROACH TO THE PATIENT   Chest Discomfort

The evaluation of the patient with chest discomfort must accommodate two goals—determining the diagnosis and assessing the safety of the immediate management plan. The latter issue is often dominant when the patient has acute chest discomfort, such as patients seen in the emergency department. In such settings, the clinician must focus first on identifying patients who require aggressive interventions to diagnose or manage potentially life-threatening conditions, including acute ischemic heart disease, acute aortic dissection, pulmonary embolism, and tension pneumothorax. If such conditions are unlikely, the clinician must address questions such as the safety of discharge to home, admission to a non-coronary care unit facility, or immediate exercise testing. Table 12-3 displays a sequence of questions that can be used in the evaluation of the patient with chest discomfort, with the diagnostic entities that are most important for consideration at each stage of the evaluation.

TABLE 12-3 Considerations in the Assessment of the Patient With Chest Discomfort

1. Could the chest discomfort be due to an acute, potentially life-threatening condition that warrants immediate hospitalization and aggressive evaluation?

Acute ischemic heart disease	Pulmonary embolism
Aortic dissection	Spontaneous pneumothorax

2. If not, could the discomfort be due to a chronic condition likely to lead to serious complications?

Stable angina

Aortic stenosis

Pulmonary hypertension

3. If not, could the discomfort be due to an acute condition that warrants specific treatment?

Pericarditis

Pneumonia/pleuritis

Herpes zoster

4. If not, could the discomfort be due to another treatable chronic condition?

Esophageal reflux	Cervical disk disease
Esophageal spasm	Arthritis of the shoulder or spine
Peptic ulcer disease	Costochondritis
Gallbladder disease	Other musculoskeletal disorders
Other gastrointestinal conditions	Anxiety state

ACUTE CHEST DISCOMFORT In patients with acute chest discomfort, the clinician must first assess the patient's respiratory and hemodynamic status. If either is compromised, initial management should focus on stabilizing the patient before the diagnostic evaluation is pursued. If, however, the patient does not require emergent interventions, then a focused history, physical examination, and laboratory evaluation should be performed to assess the patient's risk of life-threatening conditions.

Clinicians who are seeing patients in the office setting should not assume that they do not have acute ischemic heart disease, even if the prevalence may be lower. Malpractice litigation related to myocardial infarctions that were missed during office evaluations is becoming increasingly common, and ECGs were not performed in many such cases. The prevalence of high-risk patients seen in office settings may be increasing due to congestion in emergency departments.

In either setting, the *history* should include questions about the quality and location of the chest discomfort (Table 12-2). The patient should also be asked about the nature of onset of the pain and its duration. Myocardial ischemia is usually associated with a gradual intensification of symptoms over a period of minutes. Pain that is fleeting or that lasts hours without being associated with electrocardiographic changes is not likely to be ischemic in origin. Although the presence of risk factors for coronary artery disease may heighten concern for this diagnosis, the absence of such risk factors does not lower the risk for myocardial ischemia enough to be used to justify a decision to discharge a patient.

Wide radiation of chest pain increases probability that pain is due to myocardial infarction. Radiation of chest pain to the left arm is common with acute ischemic heart disease, but radiation to the right arm is also highly consistent with this diagnosis. Figure 12-1 shows estimates derived from several studies of the impact of various clinical features from the history on the probability that a patient has an acute myocardial infarction.

Right shoulder pain is also common with acute cholecystitis, but this syndrome is usually accompanied by pain that is located in the abdomen rather than chest. Chest pain that radiates between the scapulae raises the question of aortic dissection.

The *physical examination* should include evaluation of blood pressure in both arms and of pulses in both legs. Poor perfusion of a limb may be due to an aortic dissection that has compromised flow to an artery branching from the aorta. Chest auscultation may reveal diminished breath sounds; a pleural rub; or evidence of pneumothorax, pulmonary embolism, pneumonia, or pleurisy. Tension pneumothorax may lead to a shift in the trachea from the midline, away from the side of the pneumothorax. The cardiac examination should seek pericardial rubs, systolic and diastolic murmurs, and third or fourth heart sounds. Pressure on the chest wall may reproduce symptoms in patients with musculoskeletal causes of chest pain; it is important that the clinician ask the patient if the chest pain syndrome is being completely reproduced before drawing too much reassurance that more serious underlying conditions are not present.

An *ECG* is an essential test for adults with chest discomfort that is not due to an obvious traumatic cause. In such patients, the presence of electrocardiographic changes consistent with ischemia or infarction (Chap. 228) is associated with high risks of acute myocardial infarction or unstable angina (Table 12-4); such patients should be admitted to a unit with electrocardiographic monitoring and the capacity to respond to a cardiac arrest. The absence of such changes does not exclude acute ischemic heart disease, but the risk of life-threatening complications is low for patients with normal electrocardiograms or

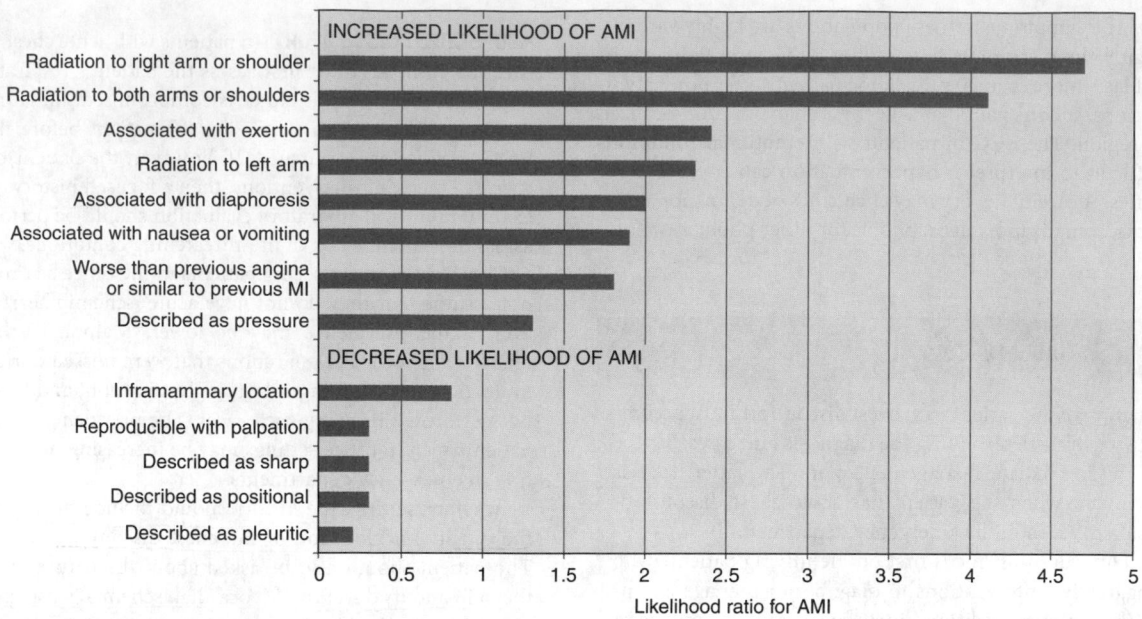

Figure 12-1 Impact of chest pain characteristics on odds of acute myocardial infarction (AMI). *(Figure prepared from data in Swap and Nagurney.)*

only nonspecific ST-T-wave changes. If these patients are not considered appropriate for immediate discharge, they are often candidates for early or immediate exercise testing.

Markers of myocardial injury are often obtained in the emergency department evaluation of acute chest discomfort. In recent years, the cardiac troponins (I and T) have superceded creatine kinase (CK) and CK-MB as the markers of choice for detecting myocardial injury. Some data support the use of other markers, such as myeloperoxidase and B-type natriuretic peptide (BNP), but their roles in routine care have not been established. Single values of any of these markers do not have high sensitivity for acute myocardial infarction or for prediction of complications. Hence, decisions to discharge patients home should not be made on the basis of single negative values of these tests, including the cardiac troponins.

Provocative tests for coronary artery disease are not appropriate for patients with ongoing chest pain. In such patients, rest myocardial perfusion scans can be considered; a normal scan reduces the likelihood of coronary artery disease and can help avoid admission of low-risk patients to the hospital. Computerized tomographic angiography (CTA) is emerging as an alternative diagnostic strategy for patients in whom the likelihood of coronary disease is not clear.

Clinicians frequently employ therapeutic trials with sublingual nitroglycerin or antacids or, in the stable patient seen in the office setting, a proton pump inhibitor. A common error is to assume that a response to any of these interventions clarifies the diagnosis. While such information is often helpful, the patient's response may be due to the placebo effect. Hence, myocardial ischemia should never be considered excluded solely because of a response to antacid therapy. Similarly, failure of nitroglycerin to relieve pain does not exclude the diagnosis of coronary disease.

If the patient's history or examination is consistent with aortic dissection, imaging studies to evaluate the aorta must be pursued promptly because of the high risk of catastrophic complications with this condition. Appropriate tests include a chest CT scan with contrast, MRI, or transesophageal echocardiography. Current data indicate that elevated D-dimer levels should raise clinicians' suspicion of aortic dissection.

Acute pulmonary embolism should be considered in patients with respiratory symptoms, pleuritic chest pain, hemoptysis, or a history of venous thromboembolism or coagulation abnormalities. Initial tests usually include CT angiography or a lung scan, which are sometimes combined with lower extremity venous ultrasound or D-dimer testing.

If patients with acute chest discomfort show no evidence of life-threatening conditions, the clinician should then focus on serious

TABLE 12-4 Prevalence of Acute Ischemic Heart Disease Syndromes Among Subsets of Emergency Department Patients With Chest Pain

Finding	Prevalence Myocardial Infarction, %	Unstable Angina, %
ST elevation (≥1 mm) or Q waves on ECG not known to be old	79	12
Ischemia or strain on ECG not known to be old (ST depression ≥1 mm or ischemic T waves)	20	41
None of the preceding ECG changes but a prior history of angina or myocardial infarction (history of heart attack or nitroglycerin use)	4	51
None of the preceding ECG changes and no prior history of angina or myocardial infarction (history of heart attack or nitroglycerin use)	2	14

Abbreviation: ECG, electrocardiogram.

Unpublished data from Brigham and Women's Hospital Chest Pain Study, 1997–1999.

chronic conditions with the potential to cause major complications, the most common of which is stable angina. Early use of exercise electrocardiography, stress echocardiography, or stress perfusion imaging for such patients, whether in the office or the emergency department, is now an accepted management strategy for low-risk patients. Exercise testing is not appropriate, however, for patients who (1) report pain that is believed to be ischemic occurring at rest or (2) have electrocardiographic changes not known to be old that are consistent with ischemia.

Patients with sustained chest discomfort who do not have evidence for life-threatening conditions should be evaluated for evidence of conditions likely to benefit from acute treatment (Table 12-3). Pericarditis may be suggested by the history, physical examination, and ECG (Table 12-2). Clinicians should carefully assess blood pressure patterns and consider echocardiography in such patients to detect evidence of impending pericardial tamponade. Chest x-rays can be used to evaluate the possibility of pulmonary disease.

■ **GUIDELINES AND CRITICAL PATHWAYS FOR ACUTE CHEST DISCOMFORT**

Guidelines for the initial evaluation for patients with acute chest pain have been developed by the American College of Cardiology, American Heart Association, and other organizations. These guidelines recommend performance of an ECG for virtually all patients with chest pain who do not have an obvious noncardiac cause of their pain, and performance of a chest x-ray for patients with signs or symptoms consistent with congestive heart failure, valvular heart disease, pericardial disease, or aortic dissection or aneurysm.

The American College of Cardiology/American Heart Association guidelines on exercise testing support its use in low-risk patients presenting to the emergency department, as well as in selected intermediate-risk patients. However, these guidelines emphasize that exercise tests should be performed only after patients have been screened for high-risk features or other indicators for hospital admission.

Many medical centers have adopted critical pathways and other forms of guidelines to increase efficiency and to expedite the treatment of patients with high-risk acute ischemic heart disease syndromes. These guidelines emphasize the following strategies:

- Rapid identification and treatment of patients for whom emergent reperfusion therapy, either via percutaneous coronary interventions or thrombolytic agents, is likely to lead to improved outcomes.
- Triage to non-coronary care unit monitored facilities such as intermediate-care units or chest pain units of patients with a low risk for complications, such as patients without new ischemic changes on their ECGs and without ongoing chest pain. Such patients can usually be safely observed in non-coronary care unit settings, undergo early exercise testing, or be discharged home. Risk stratification can be assisted through use of prospectively validated multivariate algorithms that have been published for acute ischemic heart disease and its complications.

- Shortening lengths of stay in the coronary care unit and hospital. Recommendations regarding the minimum length of stay in a monitored bed for a patient who has no further symptoms have decreased in recent years to 12 h or less if exercise testing or other risk stratification technologies are available.

Nonacute chest discomfort

The management of patients who do not require admission to the hospital or who no longer require inpatient observation should seek to identify the cause of the symptoms and the likelihood of major complications. Noninvasive tests for coronary disease serve both to diagnose this condition and to identify patients with high-risk forms of coronary disease who may benefit from revascularization. Gastrointestinal causes of chest pain can be evaluated via endoscopy or radiology studies, or with trials of medical therapy. Emotional and psychiatric conditions warrant appropriate evaluation and treatment; randomized trial data indicate that cognitive therapy and group interventions lead to decreases in symptoms for such patients.

FURTHER READINGS

GIBBONS RJ et al: ACC/AHA 2002 guideline update for exercise testing. A report of the American College of Cardiology/ American Heart Association Task Force on Practice Guidelines (Committee on Exercise Testing). Available at *www.acc.org/ qualityandscience/clinical/guidelines/exercise/dirindex.htm*. Accessed on May 8, 2010

LEBER AW et al: Quantification of obstructive and nonobstructive coronary lesions of 64-slice computed tomography. J Am Coll Cardiol 46:147, 2005

MILLER JM et al: Diagnostic performance of coronary angiography by 64-row CT. N Engl J Med 359:2324, 2008

REICHLIN T et al: Early diagnosis of myocardial infarction with sensitive cardiac troponin assays. N Engl J Med 361:858, 2009

SEQUIST T, LEE TH: Prediction of missed myocardial infarction among symptomatic outpatients without coronary heart disease. Am Heart J 149:74, 2005

SEQUIST TD et al: Missed opportunities in the primary care management of early acute ischemic heart disease. Arch Intern Med 166: 2237, 2006

SUZUKI T et al: Diagnosis of acute aortic dissection by D-dimer. Circulation 119:2702, 2009

SWAP CJ, NAGURNEY JT: Value and limitations of chest pain history in the evaluation of patients with suspected acute coronary syndromes. JAMA 294:2623, 2005

TONG KL et al: Myocardial contrast echocardiography versus Thrombolysis in Myocardial Infarction score in patients presenting to the emergency department with chest pain and a nondiagnostic electrocardiogram. J Am Coll Cardiol 46:928, 2005

TSAI TT et al: Acute aortic syndromes. Circulation 205:3802, 2005

CHAPTER 13

Abdominal Pain

William Silen

The correct interpretation of acute abdominal pain is challenging. Few other clinical situations demand greater judgment, because the most catastrophic of events may be forecast by the subtlest of symptoms and signs. A meticulously executed, detailed history and physical examination are of the greatest importance. The etiologic classification in Table 13-1, although not complete, forms a useful basis for the evaluation of patients with abdominal pain.

The diagnosis of "acute or surgical abdomen" is not an acceptable one because of its often misleading and erroneous connotation. The most obvious of "acute abdomens" may not require operative intervention, and the mildest of abdominal pains may herald an urgently correctable lesion. Any patient with abdominal pain of recent onset requires early and thorough evaluation and accurate diagnosis.

■ SOME MECHANISMS OF PAIN ORIGINATING IN THE ABDOMEN

Inflammation of the parietal peritoneum

The pain of parietal peritoneal inflammation is steady and aching in character and is located directly over the inflamed area, its exact reference being possible because it is transmitted by somatic nerves supplying the parietal peritoneum. The intensity of the pain is dependent on the type and amount of material to which the peritoneal surfaces are exposed in a given time period. For example, the sudden release into the peritoneal cavity of a small quantity of *sterile* acid gastric juice causes much more pain than the same amount of grossly contaminated neutral feces. Enzymatically active pancreatic juice incites more pain and inflammation than does the same amount of sterile bile containing no potent enzymes. Blood and urine are often so bland as to go undetected if their contact with the peritoneum has not been sudden and massive. In the case of bacterial contamination, such as in pelvic inflammatory disease, the pain is frequently of low intensity early in the illness until bacterial multiplication has caused the elaboration of irritating substances.

The rate at which the irritating material is applied to the peritoneum is important. Perforated peptic ulcer may be associated with entirely different clinical pictures dependent only on the rapidity with which the gastric juice enters the peritoneal cavity.

The pain of peritoneal inflammation is invariably accentuated by pressure or changes in tension of the peritoneum, whether produced by palpation or by movement, as in coughing or sneezing. The patient with peritonitis lies quietly in bed, preferring to avoid motion, in contrast to the patient with colic, who may writhe incessantly.

Another characteristic feature of peritoneal irritation is tonic reflex spasm of the abdominal musculature, localized to the involved body segment. The intensity of the tonic muscle spasm accompanying peritoneal inflammation is dependent on the location of the inflammatory process, the rate at which it develops, and the integrity of the nervous system. Spasm over a perforated retrocecal appendix or perforated ulcer into the lesser peritoneal sac may be minimal or absent because of the protective effect of overlying viscera. A slowly developing process often greatly attenuates the degree of muscle spasm. Catastrophic abdominal emergencies such as a perforated ulcer may be associated with minimal or no detectable pain or muscle spasm in obtunded, seriously ill, debilitated elderly patients or in psychotic patients.

Obstruction of hollow viscera

The pain of obstruction of hollow abdominal viscera is classically described as intermittent, or colicky. Yet the lack of a truly cramping character should not be misleading, because distention of a hollow viscus may produce steady pain with only very occasional exacerbations. It is not nearly as well localized as the pain of parietal peritoneal inflammation.

The colicky pain of obstruction of the small intestine is usually periumbilical or supraumbilical and is poorly localized. As the intestine becomes progressively dilated with loss of muscular tone, the colicky nature of the pain may diminish. With superimposed strangulating obstruction, pain may spread to the lower lumbar region if there is traction on the root of the mesentery. The colicky pain of colonic obstruction is of lesser intensity than that of the small intestine and is often located in the infraumbilical area. Lumbar radiation of pain is common in colonic obstruction.

Sudden distention of the biliary tree produces a steady rather than colicky type of pain; hence, the term *biliary colic* is misleading. Acute distention of the gallbladder usually causes pain in the right upper quadrant with radiation to the right posterior region of the thorax or to the tip of the right scapula, but is not uncommonly midline. Distention of the common bile duct is often associated with pain in the epigastrium radiating to the upper part of the lumbar region. Considerable variation is common, however, so that differentiation between these may be impossible. The typical subscapular pain or lumbar radiation is frequently absent. Gradual dilatation of the biliary tree, as in carcinoma of the head of the pancreas, may cause no pain or only a mild aching sensation in the epigastrium or right upper quadrant. The pain of distention of the pancreatic ducts is similar to that described for distention of the common bile duct but, in addition, is very frequently accentuated by recumbency and relieved by the upright position.

Obstruction of the urinary bladder results in dull suprapubic pain, usually low in intensity. Restlessness without specific complaint of pain may be the only sign of a distended bladder in an obtunded patient. In contrast, acute obstruction of the intravesicular portion of the ureter is characterized by severe suprapubic and flank pain that radiates to the penis, scrotum, or inner aspect of the upper thigh. Obstruction of the ureteropelvic junction is felt as pain in the costovertebral angle, whereas obstruction of the remainder of the ureter is associated with flank pain that often extends into the same side of the abdomen.

Vascular disturbances

A frequent misconception, despite abundant experience to the contrary, is that pain associated with intraabdominal vascular disturbances is sudden and catastrophic in nature. The pain of embolism or thrombosis of the superior mesenteric artery or that of impending rupture of an abdominal aortic aneurysm certainly may be severe and diffuse. Yet, just as frequently, the patient with occlusion of the superior mesenteric artery has only mild continuous or cramping diffuse pain for two or three days before vascular collapse or findings of peritoneal inflammation appear. The early, seemingly insignificant discomfort is caused by hyperperistalsis rather than peritoneal inflammation. Indeed, absence of tenderness and rigidity in the presence of continuous, diffuse pain in a patient likely to have vascular disease is quite characteristic of occlusion of the superior mesenteric artery. Abdominal pain with radiation to the sacral region, flank, or genitalia should always signal the possible presence

TABLE 13-1 Some Important Causes of Abdominal Pain

Pain Originating in the Abdomen

Parietal peritoneal inflammation	**Vascular disturbances**
Bacterial contamination	Embolism or thrombosis
Perforated appendix or other perforated viscus	Vascular rupture
Pelvic inflammatory disease	Pressure or torsional occlusion
Chemical irritation	Sickle cell anemia
Perforated ulcer	**Abdominal wall**
Pancreatitis	Distortion or traction of mesentery
Mittelschmerz	Trauma or infection of muscles
Mechanical obstruction of hollow viscera	**Distention of visceral surfaces, e.g., by hemorrhage**
Obstruction of the small or large intestine	Hepatic or renal capsules
Obstruction of the biliary tree	**Inflammation of a viscus**
Obstruction of the ureter	Appendicitis
	Typhoid fever
	Typhlitis

Pain Referred from Extraabdominal Source

Cardiothoracic	Pleurodynia
Acute myocardial infarction	Pneumothorax
Myocarditis, endocarditis, pericarditis	Empyema
Congestive heart failure	Esophageal disease, spasm, rupture, inflammation
Pneumonia	**Genitalia**
Pulmonary embolus	Torsion of the testis

Metabolic Causes

Diabetes	Acute adrenal insufficiency
Uremia	Familial Mediterranean fever
Hyperlipidemia	Porphyria
Hyperparathyroidism	C′1 esterase inhibitor deficiency (angioneurotic edema)

Neurologic/Psychiatric Causes

Herpes zoster	Spinal cord or nerve root compression
Tabes dorsalis	Functional disorders
Causalgia	Psychiatric disorders
Radiculitis from infection or arthritis	

Toxic Causes

Lead poisoning
Insect or animal envenomations
Black widow spiders
Snake bites

Uncertain Mechanisms

Narcotic withdrawal
Heat stroke

of a rupturing abdominal aortic aneurysm. This pain may persist over a period of several days before rupture and collapse occur.

Abdominal wall

Pain arising from the abdominal wall is usually constant and aching. Movement, prolonged standing, and pressure accentuate the discomfort and muscle spasm. In the case of hematoma of the rectus sheath, now most frequently encountered in association with anticoagulant therapy, a mass may be present in the lower quadrants of the abdomen. Simultaneous involvement of muscles in other parts of the body usually serves to differentiate myositis of the abdominal wall from an intraabdominal process that might cause pain in the same region.

■ REFERRED PAIN IN ABDOMINAL DISEASES

Pain referred to the abdomen from the thorax, spine, or genitalia may prove a vexing diagnostic problem, because diseases of the upper part of the abdominal cavity such as acute cholecystitis or perforated ulcer are frequently associated with intrathoracic complications. A most important, yet often forgotten, dictum is that the possibility of intrathoracic disease must be considered in every patient with abdominal pain, especially if the pain is in the upper part of the abdomen. Systematic questioning and examination directed toward detecting myocardial or pulmonary infarction, pneumonia, pericarditis, or esophageal disease (the intrathoracic diseases that most often masquerade as abdominal emergencies) will often provide sufficient clues to establish the proper diagnosis.

Diaphragmatic pleuritis resulting from pneumonia or pulmonary infarction may cause pain in the right upper quadrant and pain in the supraclavicular area, the latter radiation to be distinguished from the referred subscapular pain caused by acute distention of the extrahepatic biliary tree. The ultimate decision as to the origin of abdominal pain may require deliberate and planned observation over a period of several hours, during which repeated questioning and examination will provide the diagnosis or suggest the appropriate studies.

Referred pain of thoracic origin is often accompanied by splinting of the involved hemithorax with respiratory lag and decrease in excursion more marked than that seen in the presence of intraabdominal disease. In addition, apparent abdominal muscle spasm caused by referred pain will diminish during the inspiratory phase of respiration, whereas it is persistent throughout both respiratory phases if it is of abdominal origin. Palpation over the area of referred pain in the abdomen also does not usually accentuate the pain and in many instances actually seems to relieve it. Thoracic disease and abdominal disease frequently coexist and may be difficult or impossible to differentiate. For example, the patient with known biliary tract disease often has epigastric pain during myocardial infarction, or biliary colic may be referred to the precordium or left shoulder in a patient who has suffered previously from angina pectoris. For an explanation of the radiation of pain to a previously diseased area, see Chap. 11.

Referred pain from the spine, which usually involves compression or irritation of nerve roots, is characteristically intensified by certain motions such as cough, sneeze, or strain and is associated with hyperesthesia over the involved dermatomes. Pain referred to the abdomen from the testes or seminal vesicles is generally accentuated by the slightest pressure on either of these organs. The abdominal discomfort is of dull, aching character and is poorly localized.

■ METABOLIC ABDOMINAL CRISES

Pain of metabolic origin may simulate almost any other type of intraabdominal disease. Several mechanisms may be at work. In certain instances, such as hyperlipidemia, the metabolic disease itself may be accompanied by an intraabdominal process such as pancreatitis, which can lead to unnecessary laparotomy unless recognized. $C'1$ esterase deficiency associated with angioneurotic edema is often associated with episodes of severe abdominal pain. Whenever the cause of abdominal pain is obscure, a metabolic origin always must be considered. Abdominal pain is also the hallmark of familial Mediterranean fever (Chap. 330).

The problem of differential diagnosis is often not readily resolved. The pain of porphyria and of lead colic is usually difficult to distinguish from that of intestinal obstruction, because severe hyperperistalsis is a prominent feature of both. The pain of uremia or diabetes is nonspecific, and the pain and tenderness frequently shift in location and intensity. Diabetic acidosis may be precipitated by acute appendicitis or intestinal obstruction, so if prompt resolution of the abdominal pain does not result from correction of the metabolic abnormalities, an underlying organic problem should be suspected. Black widow spider bites produce intense pain and rigidity of the abdominal muscles and back, an area infrequently involved in intraabdominal disease.

■ NEUROGENIC CAUSES

Causalgic pain may occur in diseases that injure sensory nerves. It has a burning character and is usually limited to the distribution of a given peripheral nerve. Normal stimuli such as touch or change in temperature may be transformed into this type of pain, which is frequently present in a patient at rest. The demonstration of irregularly spaced cutaneous pain spots may be the only indication of an old nerve lesion underlying causalgic pain. Even though the pain may be precipitated by gentle palpation, rigidity of the abdominal muscles is absent, and the respirations are not disturbed. Distention of the abdomen is uncommon, and the pain has no relationship to the intake of food.

Pain arising from spinal nerves or roots comes and goes suddenly and is of a lancinating type (Chap. 15). It may be caused by herpes zoster, impingement by arthritis, tumors, herniated nucleus pulposus, diabetes, or syphilis. It is not associated with food intake, abdominal distention, or changes in respiration. Severe muscle spasm, as in the gastric crises of tabes dorsalis, is common but is either relieved or is not accentuated by abdominal palpation. The pain is made worse by movement of the spine and is usually confined to a few dermatomes. Hyperesthesia is very common.

Pain due to functional causes conforms to none of the aforementioned patterns. Mechanism is hard to define. Irritable bowel syndrome (IBS) is a functional gastrointestinal disorder characterized by abdominal pain and altered bowel habits. The diagnosis is made on the basis of clinical criteria (Chap. 296) and after exclusion of demonstrable structural abnormalities. The episodes of abdominal pain are often brought on by stress, and the pain varies considerably in type and location. Nausea and vomiting are rare. Localized tenderness and muscle spasm are inconsistent or absent. The causes of IBS or related functional disorders are not known.

APPROACH TO THE PATIENT Abdominal Pain

Few abdominal conditions require such urgent operative intervention that an orderly approach need be abandoned, no matter how ill the patient. Only those patients with exsanguinating intraabdominal hemorrhage (e.g., ruptured aneurysm) must be rushed to the operating room immediately, but in such instances only a few minutes are required to assess the critical nature of the problem. Under these circumstances, all obstacles must be swept aside, adequate venous access for fluid replacement obtained, and the operation begun. Many patients of this type have died in the radiology department or the emergency room while awaiting such unnecessary examinations as electrocardiograms or CT scans. *There are no contraindications to operation when massive intraabdominal hemorrhage is present.* Fortunately, this situation is relatively rare. These comments do not pertain to gastrointestinal hemorrhage, which can often be managed by other means (Chap. 41).

Nothing will supplant an orderly, painstakingly *detailed history*, which is far more valuable than any laboratory or radiographic examination. This kind of history is laborious and time-consuming, making it not especially popular, even though a reasonably accurate diagnosis can be made on the basis of the history alone in the majority of cases. Computer-aided diagnosis of abdominal pain provides no advantage over clinical assessment alone. In cases of *acute* abdominal pain, a diagnosis is readily established in most instances, whereas success is not so frequent in patients with *chronic* pain. IBS is one of the most common causes of abdominal pain and must always be kept in mind (Chap. 296). The location of the pain can assist in narrowing the differential diagnosis (Table 13-2); however, the *chronological sequence of events* in the patient's history is often more important than emphasis on the location of pain. If the examiner is sufficiently open-minded and unhurried, asks the proper questions, and listens, the patient will usually provide the diagnosis. Careful attention should be paid to the extraabdominal regions that may be responsible for abdominal pain.

TABLE 13-2 Differential Diagnoses of Abdominal Pain by Location

Right Upper Quadrant	Epigastric	Left Upper Quadrant
Cholecystitis	Peptic ulcer disease	Splenic infarct
Cholangitis	Gastritis	Splenic rupture
Pancreatitis	GERD	Splenic abscess
Pneumonia/empyema	Pancreatitis	Gastritis
Pleurisy/pleurodynia	Myocardial infarction	Gastric ulcer
Subdiaphragmatic abscess	Pericarditis	Pancreatitis
Hepatitis	Ruptured aortic aneurysm	Subdiaphragmatic abscess
Budd-Chiari syndrome	Esophagitis	

Right Lower Quadrant	Periumbilical	Left Lower Quadrant
Appendicitis	Early appendicitis	Diverticulitis
Salpingitis	Gastroenteritis	Salpingitis
Inguinal hernia	Bowel obstruction	Inguinal hernia
Ectopic pregnancy	Ruptured aortic aneurysm	Ectopic pregnancy
Nephrolithiasis		Nephrolithiasis
Inflammatory bowel disease		Irritable bowel syndrome
Mesenteric lymphadenitis		Inflammatory bowel disease
Typhlitis		

Diffuse Nonlocalized Pain	
Gastroenteritis	Malaria
Mesenteric ischemia	Familial Mediterranean fever
Bowel obstruction	Metabolic diseases
Irritable bowel syndrome	Psychiatric disease
Peritonitis	
Diabetes	

Abbreviation: GERD, gastroesophageal reflux disease.

An accurate menstrual history in a female patient is essential. Narcotics or analgesics should *not* be withheld until a definitive diagnosis or a definitive plan has been formulated; obfuscation of the diagnosis by adequate analgesia is unlikely.

In the examination, simple critical inspection of the patient, e.g., of facies, position in bed, and respiratory activity, provides valuable clues. The amount of information to be gleaned is directly proportional to the *gentleness* and thoroughness of the examiner. Once a patient with peritoneal inflammation has been examined brusquely, accurate assessment by the next examiner becomes almost impossible. Eliciting rebound tenderness by sudden release of a deeply palpating hand in a patient with suspected peritonitis is cruel and unnecessary. The same information can be obtained by gentle percussion of the abdomen (rebound tenderness on a miniature scale), a maneuver that can be far more precise and localizing. Asking the patient to cough will elicit true rebound tenderness without the need for placing a hand on the abdomen. Furthermore, the forceful demonstration of rebound tenderness will startle and induce protective spasm in a nervous or worried patient in whom true rebound tenderness is not present. A palpable gallbladder will be missed if palpation is so brusque that voluntary muscle spasm becomes superimposed on involuntary muscular rigidity.

As with history taking, sufficient time should be spent in the examination. Abdominal signs may be minimal but nevertheless, if accompanied by consistent symptoms, may be exceptionally meaningful. Abdominal signs may be virtually or totally absent in cases of pelvic peritonitis, so careful *pelvic and rectal examinations are mandatory in every patient with abdominal pain.* Tenderness on pelvic or rectal examination in the absence of other abdominal signs can be caused by operative indications such as perforated appendicitis, diverticulitis, twisted ovarian cyst, and many others.

Much attention has been paid to the presence or absence of peristaltic sounds, their quality, and their frequency. Auscultation of the abdomen is one of the least revealing aspects of the physical examination of a patient with abdominal pain. Catastrophes such as strangulating small intestinal obstruction or perforated appendicitis may occur in the presence of normal peristaltic sounds. Conversely, when the proximal part of the intestine above an obstruction becomes markedly distended and edematous, peristaltic sounds may lose the characteristics of borborygmi and become weak or absent, even when peritonitis is not present. It is usually the severe chemical peritonitis of sudden onset that is associated with the truly silent abdomen. Assessment of the patient's state of hydration is important.

Laboratory examinations may be valuable in assessing the patient with abdominal pain, yet, with few exceptions, they rarely establish a diagnosis. Leukocytosis should never be the single deciding factor as to whether or not operation is indicated. A white blood cell count >20,000/µL may be observed with perforation of a viscus, but pancreatitis, acute cholecystitis, pelvic inflammatory disease, and intestinal infarction may be associated with marked leukocytosis. A normal white blood cell count is not rare in cases of perforation of abdominal viscera. The diagnosis of anemia may be more helpful than the white blood cell count, especially when combined with the history.

The urinalysis may reveal the state of hydration or rule out severe renal disease, diabetes, or urinary infection. Blood urea nitrogen, glucose, and serum bilirubin levels may be helpful. Serum amylase levels may be increased by many diseases other than pancreatitis, e.g., perforated ulcer, strangulating intestinal obstruction, and acute cholecystitis; thus, elevations of serum amylase do not rule out the need for an operation. The determination of the serum lipase may have greater accuracy than that of the serum amylase.

Plain and upright or lateral decubitus radiographs of the abdomen may be of value in cases of intestinal obstruction, perforated ulcer, and a variety of other conditions. They are usually unnecessary in patients with acute appendicitis or strangulated external hernias. In rare instances, barium or water-soluble contrast study of the upper part of the gastrointestinal tract may demonstrate partial intestinal obstruction that may elude diagnosis by other means. If there is any question of obstruction of the colon, oral administration of barium sulfate should be avoided. On the other hand, in cases of suspected colonic obstruction (without perforation), contrast enema may be diagnostic.

In the absence of trauma, peritoneal lavage has been replaced as a diagnostic tool by ultrasound, CT, and laparoscopy. Ultrasonography has proved to be useful in detecting an enlarged gallbladder or pancreas, the presence of gallstones, an enlarged ovary, or a tubal pregnancy. Laparoscopy is especially helpful in diagnosing pelvic conditions, such as ovarian cysts, tubal pregnancies, salpingitis, and acute appendicitis. Radioisotopic hepatobiliary iminodiacetic acid scans (HIDAs) may help differentiate acute cholecystitis from acute pancreatitis. A CT scan may demonstrate an enlarged pancreas, ruptured spleen, or thickened colonic or appendiceal wall and streaking of the mesocolon or mesoappendix characteristic of diverticulitis or appendicitis.

Sometimes, even under the best circumstances with all available aids and with the greatest of clinical skill, a definitive diagnosis cannot be established at the time of the initial examination. Nevertheless, despite lack of a clear anatomic diagnosis, it may be abundantly clear to an experienced and thoughtful physician and surgeon that on clinical grounds alone operation is indicated. Should that decision be questionable, watchful waiting with repeated questioning and examination will often elucidate the true nature of the illness and indicate the proper course of action.

FURTHER READINGS

JONES PF: Suspected acute appendicitis: Trends in management over 30 years. Br J Surg 88:1570, 2001

LYON C, CLARK DC: Diagnosis of acute abdominal pain in older patients. Am Fam Physician 74:1537, 2006

MERLIN MA et al: Evidence-based appendicitis: The initial work-up. Postgrad Med 122:189, 2010

SILEN W: *Cope's Early Diagnosis of the Acute Abdomen*, 21st ed, New York and Oxford: Oxford University Press, 2005

THOMAS SH, SILEN W: Effect on diagnostic efficiency of analgesia for undifferentiated abdominal pain. Br J Surg 90:5, 2003

CHAPTER **14**

Headache

Peter J. Goadsby
Neil H. Raskin

Headache is among the most common reasons patients seek medical attention. Diagnosis and management is based on a careful clinical approach augmented by an understanding of the anatomy, physiology, and pharmacology of the nervous system pathways that mediate the various headache syndromes.

GENERAL PRINCIPLES

A classification system developed by the International Headache Society characterizes headache as primary or secondary (Table 14–1). *Primary headaches* are those in which headache and its associated features are the disorder in itself, whereas *secondary headaches* are those caused by exogenous disorders. Primary headache often results in considerable disability and a decrease in the patient's quality of life. Mild secondary headache, such as that seen in association with upper respiratory tract infections, is common but rarely worrisome. Life-threatening headache is relatively uncommon, but vigilance is required in order to recognize and appropriately treat such patients.

TABLE 14-1 Common Causes of Headache

Primary Headache		Secondary Headache	
Type	%	Type	%
Tension-type	69	Systemic infection	63
Migraine	16	Head injury	4
Idiopathic stabbing	2	Vascular disorders	1
Exertional	1	Subarachnoid hemorrhage	<1
Cluster	0.1	Brain tumor	0.1

Source: After J Olesen et al: *The Headaches.* Philadelphia, Lippincott, Williams & Wilkins, 2005.

■ ANATOMY AND PHYSIOLOGY OF HEADACHE

Pain usually occurs when peripheral nociceptors are stimulated in response to tissue injury, visceral distension, or other factors (Chap. 11). In such situations, pain perception is a normal physiologic response mediated by a healthy nervous system. Pain can also result when pain-producing pathways of the peripheral or central nervous system (CNS) are damaged or activated inappropriately. Headache may originate from either or both mechanisms. Relatively few cranial structures are pain-producing; these include the scalp, middle meningeal artery, dural sinuses, falx cerebri, and proximal segments of the large pial arteries. The ventricular ependyma, choroid plexus, pial veins, and much of the brain parenchyma are not pain-producing.

The key structures involved in primary headache appear to be

- the large intracranial vessels and dura mater and the peripheral terminals of the trigeminal nerve that innervate these structures
- the caudal portion of the trigeminal nucleus, which extends into the dorsal horns of the upper cervical spinal cord and receives input from the first and second cervical nerve roots (the trigeminocervical complex)
- rostral pain-processing regions, such as the ventroposteromedial thalamus and the cortex
- the pain-modulatory systems in the brain that modulate input from trigeminal nociceptors at all levels of the pain-processing pathways

The innervation of the large intracranial vessels and dura mater by the trigeminal nerve is known as the *trigeminovascular system.* Cranial autonomic symptoms, such as *lacrimation* and *nasal congestion,* are prominent in the trigeminal autonomic cephalalgias, including cluster headache and paroxysmal hemicrania, and may also be seen in migraine. These autonomic symptoms reflect activation of cranial parasympathetic pathways, and functional imaging studies indicate that vascular changes in migraine and cluster headache, when present, are similarly driven by these cranial autonomic systems. Migraine and other primary headache types are not "vascular headaches"; these disorders do not reliably manifest vascular changes, and treatment outcomes cannot be predicted by vascular effects. Migraine is a brain disorder, and best understood and managed as such.

■ CLINICAL EVALUATION OF ACUTE, NEW-ONSET HEADACHE

The patient who presents with a new, severe headache has a differential diagnosis that is quite different from the patient with recurrent headaches over many years. In new-onset and severe headache, the probability of finding a potentially serious cause is considerably greater than in recurrent headache. Patients with recent onset of pain require prompt evaluation and appropriate treatment. Serious causes to be considered include meningitis, subarachnoid hemorrhage, epidural or subdural hematoma, glaucoma, tumor, and purulent sinusitis. When worrisome symptoms and signs are present (Table 14–2), rapid diagnosis and management is critical.

TABLE 14-2 Headache Symptoms That Suggest a Serious Underlying Disorder

"Worst" headache ever

First severe headache

Subacute worsening over days or weeks

Abnormal neurologic examination

Fever or unexplained systemic signs

Vomiting that precedes headache

Pain induced by bending, lifting, cough

Pain that disturbs sleep or presents immediately upon awakening

Known systemic illness

Onset after age 55

Pain associated with local tenderness, e.g., region of temporal artery

A complete neurologic examination is an essential first step in the evaluation. In most cases, patients with an abnormal examination or a history of recent-onset headache should be evaluated by a CT or MRI study. As an initial screening procedure for intracranial pathology in this setting, CT and MRI methods appear to be equally sensitive. In some circumstances, a lumbar puncture (LP) is also required, unless a benign etiology can be otherwise established. A general evaluation of acute headache might include the investigation of cardiovascular and renal status by blood pressure monitoring and urine examination; eyes by funduscopy, intraocular pressure measurement, and refraction; cranial arteries by palpation; and cervical spine by the effect of passive movement of the head and by imaging.

The psychological state of the patient should also be evaluated since a relationship exists between head pain and depression. Many patients in chronic daily pain cycles become depressed, although depression itself is rarely a cause of headache. Drugs with antidepressant actions are also effective in the prophylactic treatment of both tension-type headache and migraine.

Underlying recurrent headache disorders may be activated by pain that follows otologic or endodontic surgical procedures. Thus, pain about the head as the result of diseased tissue or trauma may reawaken an otherwise quiescent migrainous syndrome. Treatment of the headache is largely ineffective until the cause of the primary problem is addressed.

Serious underlying conditions that are associated with headache are described below. Brain tumor is a rare cause of headache and even less commonly a cause of severe pain. The vast majority of patients presenting with severe headache have a benign cause.

SECONDARY HEADACHE

The management of secondary headache focuses on diagnosis and treatment of the underlying condition.

■ MENINGITIS

Acute, severe headache with stiff neck and fever suggests meningitis. Lumbar puncture is mandatory. Often there is striking accentuation of pain with eye movement. Meningitis can be easily mistaken for migraine in that the cardinal symptoms of pounding headache, photophobia, nausea, and vomiting are frequently present, perhaps reflecting the underlying biology of some of the patients.

Meningitis is discussed in Chaps. 381 and 382.

■ INTRACRANIAL HEMORRHAGE

Acute, severe headache with stiff neck but without fever suggests subarachnoid hemorrhage. A ruptured aneurysm, arteriovenous malformation, or intraparenchymal hemorrhage may also present with headache alone. Rarely, if the hemorrhage is small or below the foramen magnum, the head CT scan can be normal. Therefore, lumbar puncture may be required to diagnose definitively subarachnoid hemorrhage.

Intracranial hemorrhage is discussed in Chap. 275.

■ BRAIN TUMOR

Approximately 30% of patients with brain tumors consider headache to be their chief complaint. The head pain is usually nondescript—an intermittent deep, dull aching of moderate intensity, which may worsen with exertion or change in position and may be associated with nausea and vomiting. This pattern of symptoms results from migraine far more often than from brain tumor. The headache of brain tumor disturbs sleep in about 10% of patients. Vomiting that precedes the appearance of headache by weeks is highly characteristic of posterior fossa brain tumors. A history of amenorrhea or galactorrhea should lead one to question whether a prolactin-secreting pituitary adenoma (or the polycystic ovary syndrome) is the source of headache. Headache arising de novo in a patient with known malignancy suggests either cerebral metastases or carcinomatous meningitis, or both. Head pain appearing abruptly after bending, lifting, or coughing can be due to a posterior fossa mass, a Chiari malformation, or low CSF volume.

Brain tumors are discussed in Chap. 379.

■ TEMPORAL ARTERITIS

(See also Chaps. 28 and 326) Temporal (giant cell) arteritis is an inflammatory disorder of arteries that frequently involves the extracranial carotid circulation. It is a common disorder of the elderly; its annual incidence is 77 per 100,000 individuals age 50 and older. The average age of onset is 70 years, and women account for 65% of cases. About half of patients with untreated temporal arteritis develop blindness due to involvement of the ophthalmic artery and its branches; indeed, the ischemic optic neuropathy induced by giant cell arteritis is the major cause of rapidly developing bilateral blindness in patients >60 years. Because treatment with glucocorticoids is effective in preventing this complication, prompt recognition of the disorder is important.

Typical presenting symptoms include headache, polymyalgia rheumatica (Chap. 326), jaw claudication, fever, and weight loss. Headache is the dominant symptom and often appears in association with malaise and muscle aches. Head pain may be unilateral or bilateral and is located temporally in 50% of patients but may involve any and all aspects of the cranium. Pain usually appears gradually over a few hours before peak intensity is reached; occasionally, it is explosive in onset. The quality of pain is only seldom throbbing; it is almost invariably described as dull and boring, with superimposed episodic stabbing pains similar to the sharp pains that appear in migraine. Most patients can recognize that the origin of their head pain is superficial, external to the skull, rather than originating deep within the cranium (the pain site for migraineurs). Scalp tenderness is present, often to a marked degree; brushing the hair or resting the head on a pillow may be impossible because of pain. Headache is usually worse at night and often aggravated by exposure to cold. Additional findings may include reddened, tender nodules or red streaking of the skin overlying the temporal arteries, and tenderness of the temporal or, less commonly, the occipital arteries.

The erythrocyte sedimentation rate (ESR) is often, though not always, elevated; a normal ESR does not exclude giant cell arteritis. A temporal artery biopsy followed by immediate treatment with prednisone 80 mg daily for the first 4–6 weeks should be initiated when clinical suspicion is high. The prevalence of migraine among the elderly is substantial, considerably higher than that of giant cell arteritis. Migraineurs often report amelioration of their headaches with prednisone; thus, caution must be used when interpreting the therapeutic response.

■ GLAUCOMA

Glaucoma may present with a prostrating headache associated with nausea and vomiting. The headache often starts with severe eye pain. On physical examination, the eye is often red with a fixed, moderately dilated pupil.

Glaucoma is discussed in Chap. 28.

PRIMARY HEADACHE SYNDROMES

Primary headaches are disorders in which headache and associated features occur in the absence of any exogenous cause (Table 14–1). The most common are migraine, tension-type headache, and cluster headache.

■ MIGRAINE

Migraine, the second most common cause of headache, afflicts approximately 15% of women and 6% of men over a one year period. It is usually an episodic headache associated with certain features such as sensitivity to light, sound, or movement; nausea and vomiting often accompany the headache. A useful description of migraine is a benign and recurring syndrome of headache associated with other symptoms of neurologic dysfunction in varying admixtures (Table 14–3). Migraine can often be recognized by its activators, referred to as *triggers*.

The brain of the migraineur is particularly sensitive to environmental and sensory stimuli; migraine-prone patients do not habituate easily to sensory stimuli. This sensitivity is amplified in females during the menstrual cycle. Headache can be initiated or amplified by various triggers, including glare, bright lights, sounds, or other afferent stimulation; hunger; excess stress; physical exertion; stormy weather or barometric pressure changes; hormonal fluctuations during menses; lack of or excess sleep; and alcohol or other chemical stimulation. Knowledge of a patient's susceptibility to specific triggers can be useful in management strategies involving lifestyle adjustments.

Pathogenesis

The sensory sensitivity that is characteristic of migraine is probably due to dysfunction of monoaminergic sensory control systems located in the brainstem and thalamus (Fig. 14-1).

Activation of cells in the trigeminal nucleus results in the release of vasoactive neuropeptides, particularly calcitonin gene–related peptide (CGRP), at vascular terminations of the trigeminal nerve and within the trigeminal nucleus. CGRP receptor antagonists have now been shown to be effective in the acute treatment of migraine. Centrally, the second-order trigeminal neurons cross the midline and project to ventrobasal and posterior nuclei of the thalamus for further processing. Additionally, there are projections to the

TABLE 14-3 Symptoms Accompanying Severe Migraine Attacks in 500 Patients

Symptom	Patients Affected, %
Nausea	87
Photophobia	82
Lightheadedness	72
Scalp tenderness	65
Vomiting	56
Visual disturbances	36
Paresthesias	33
Vertigo	33
Photopsia	26
Alteration of consciousness	18
Diarrhea	16
Fortification spectra	10
Syncope	10
Seizure	4
Confusional state	4

Source: From NH Raskin, *Headache*, 2nd ed. New York, Churchill Livingston, 1988; with permission.

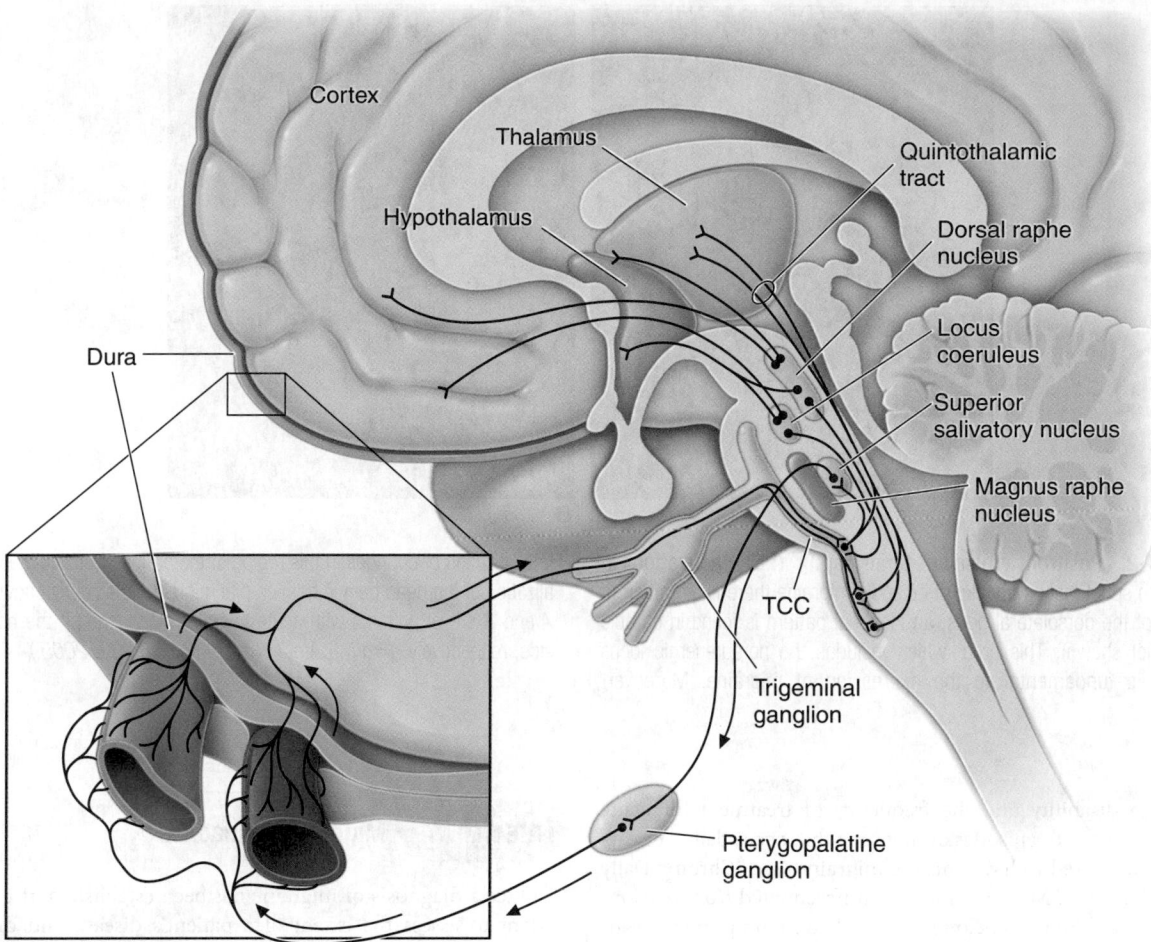

Cortex

Thalamus

Quintothalamic
tract

Hypothalamus

Dorsal raphe
nucleus

Locus
coeruleus

Dura

Superior
salivatory nucleus

Magnus raphe
nucleus

TCC

Trigeminal
ganglion

Pterygopalatine
ganglion

Figure 14-1 Brainstem pathways that modulate sensory input.
The key pathway for pain in migraine is the trigeminovascular input from
the meningeal vessels, which passes through the trigeminal ganglion and
synapses on second-order neurons in the trigeminocervical complex (TCC).
These neurons in turn project in the quintothalamic tract and, after decus-
sating in the brainstem, synapse on neurons in the thalamus. Important
modulation of the trigeminovascular nociceptive input comes from the dorsal
raphe nucleus, locus coeruleus, and nucleus raphe magnus.

periaqueductal gray and hypothalamus, from which reciprocal
descending systems have established antinociceptive effects. Other
brainstem regions likely to be involved in descending modulation of
trigeminal pain include the nucleus locus coeruleus in the pons and
the rostroventromedial medulla.

Pharmacologic and other data point to the involvement of the
neurotransmitter 5-hydroxytryptamine (5-HT; also known as serotonin) in migraine. Approximately 60 years ago, methysergide was
found to antagonize certain peripheral actions of 5-HT and was
introduced as the first drug capable of preventing migraine attacks.
The triptans are designed to selectively stimulate subpopulations
of 5-HT receptors; at least 14 different 5-HT receptors exist in
humans. The triptans are potent agonists of 5-HT_{1B}, 5-HT_{1D}, and
5-HT_{1F} receptors and are less potent at the 5-HT_{1A} receptor. A growing body of data indicates that the antimigraine efficacy of the trip-
tans relates to their ability to stimulate $5\text{-HT}_{1B/1D}$ receptors, which
are located on both blood vessels and nerve terminals. Separately,
it has now been shown that selective 5-HT_{1F} receptor activation,
which has a purely neural effect, can terminate acute migraine.

Data also support a role for dopamine in the pathophysiology of
migraine. Most migraine symptoms can be induced by dopaminergic stimulation. Moreover, there is dopamine receptor hypersensitivity in migraineurs, as demonstrated by the induction of yawning,
nausea, vomiting, hypotension, and other symptoms of a migraine
attack by dopaminergic agonists at doses that do not affect nonmi-
graineurs. Dopamine receptor antagonists are effective therapeutic

agents in migraine, especially when given parenterally or concurrently with other antimigraine agents.

Migraine genes identified by studying families with familial hemiplegic migraine (FHM) reveal involvement of ion
channels, suggesting that alterations in membrane excitability can predispose to migraine. Mutations involving the $\text{Ca}_v2.1$
(P/Q)–type voltage-gated calcium channel *CACNA1A* gene
are now known to cause FHM 1; this mutation is responsi-
ble for about 50% of FHM. Mutations in the $\text{Na}^+\text{-K}^+\text{ATPase}$
ATP1A2 gene, designated FHM 2, are responsible for about 20%
of FHM. Mutations in the neuronal voltage-gated sodium channel *SCN1A* cause FHM 3. Functional neuroimaging has suggested
that brainstem regions in migraine (Fig. 14-2) and the posterior
hypothalamic gray matter region close to the human circadian
pacemaker cells of the suprachiasmatic nucleus in cluster headache
(Fig. 14-3) are good candidates for specific involvement in primary
headache.

Diagnosis and clinical features

Diagnostic criteria for migraine headache are listed in Table 14-4.
A high index of suspicion is required to diagnose migraine: the
migraine aura, consisting of visual disturbances with flashing lights
or zigzag lines moving across the visual field or of other neurologic
symptoms, is reported in only 20–25% of patients. A headache diary
can often be helpful in making the diagnosis; this is also helpful

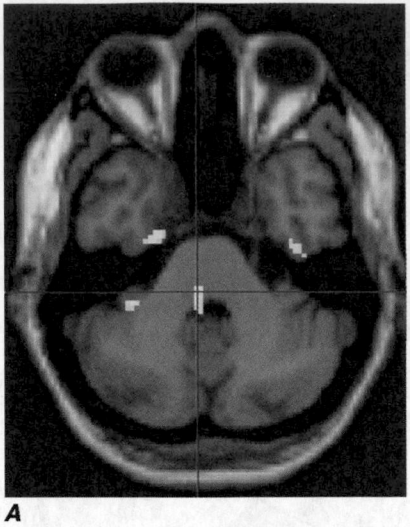
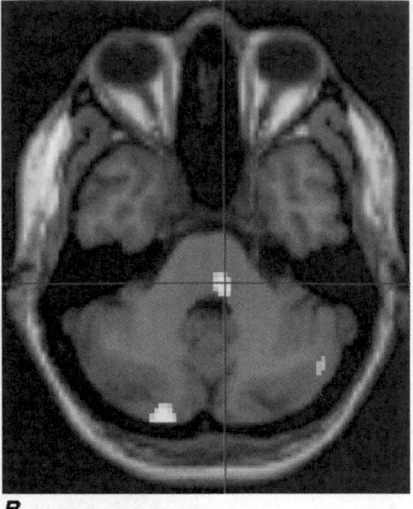

Figure 14-2 Positron emission tomography (PET) activation in migraine. In spontaneous attacks of episodic migraine there is activation of the region of the dorsolateral pons; an identical pattern is found in chronic migraine (not shown). This area, which includes the noradrenergic locus coeruleus, is fundamental to the expression of migraine. Moreover,

lateralization of changes in this region of the brainstem correlates with lateralization of the head pain in hemicranial migraine; the scans shown in panels *A* and *B* are of patients with acute migraine headache on the right and left side, respectively. *(From S Afridi et al: Brain 128:932, 2005.)*

in assessing disability and the frequency of treatment for acute attacks. Patients with episodes of migraine that occur daily or near-daily are considered to have chronic migraine (see "Chronic Daily Headache," below). Migraine must be differentiated from tension-type headache (discussed below), the most common primary headache syndrome seen in clinical practice. *Migraine at its most basic level is headache with associated features, and tension-type headache is headache that is featureless. Most patients with disabling headache probably have migraine.*

Patients with acephalgic migraine experience recurrent neurologic symptoms, often with nausea or vomiting, but with little or no headache. Vertigo can be prominent; it has been estimated that one-third of patients referred for vertigo or dizziness have a primary diagnosis of migraine.

TREATMENT   Migraine Headaches

Once a diagnosis of migraine has been established, it is important to assess the extent of a patient's disease and disability. The Migraine Disability Assessment Score (MIDAS) is a well-validated, easy-to-use tool (Fig. 14-4).

Patient education is an important aspect of migraine management. Information for patients is available at *www.achenet.org*, the website of the American Council for Headache Education (ACHE). It is helpful for patients to understand that migraine is an inherited tendency to headache; that migraine can be modified and controlled by lifestyle adjustments and medications, but it cannot be eradicated; and that, except in some occasions

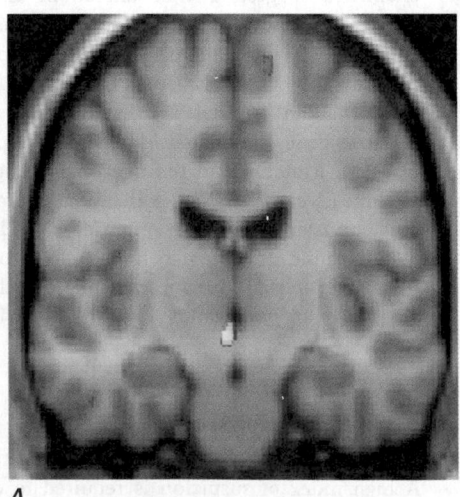
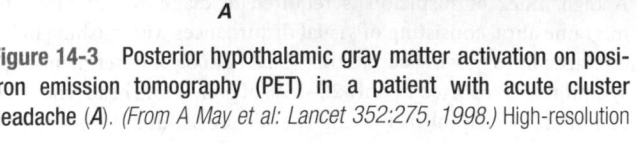
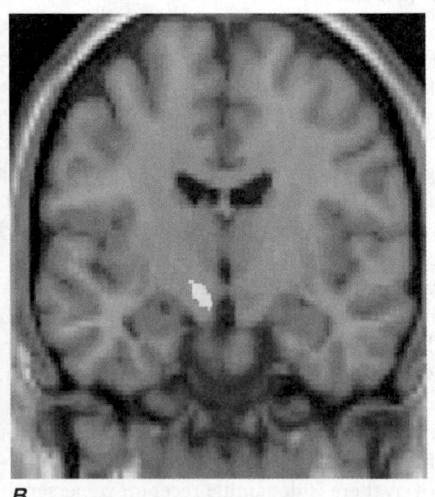

Figure 14-3 Posterior hypothalamic gray matter activation on positron emission tomography (PET) in a patient with acute cluster headache (*A*). *(From A May et al: Lancet 352:275, 1998.)* High-resolution

T1 weighted MRI obtained using voxel-based morphometry demonstrates increased gray matter activity, lateralized to the side of pain in a patient with cluster headache (*B*). *(From A May et al: Nat Med 5:836, 1999.)*

TABLE 14-4 Simplified Diagnostic Criteria for Migraine

Repeated attacks of headache lasting 4–72 h in patients with a normal physical examination, no other reasonable cause for the headache, and:

At Least 2 of the Following Features:	Plus at Least 1 of the Following Features:
Unilateral pain	Nausea/vomiting
Throbbing pain	Photophobia and phonophobia
Aggravation by movement	
Moderate or severe intensity	

Source: Adapted from the International Headache Society Classification (Headache Classification Committee of the International Headache Society, 2004).

in women on oral estrogens or contraceptives, migraine is not associated with serious or life-threatening illnesses.

NONPHARMACOLOGIC MANAGEMENT Migraine can often be managed to some degree by a variety of nonpharmacologic approaches. Most patients benefit by the identification and avoidance of specific headache triggers. A regulated lifestyle is helpful, including a healthful diet, regular exercise, regular sleep patterns, avoidance of excess caffeine and alcohol, and avoidance of acute changes in stress levels.

The measures that benefit a given individual should be used routinely since they provide a simple, cost-effective approach to migraine management. Patients with migraine do not encounter more stress than headache-free individuals; overresponsiveness to stress appears to be the issue. Since the stresses of everyday living cannot be eliminated, lessening one's response to stress by various techniques is helpful for many patients. These may include yoga, transcendental meditation, hypnosis, and conditioning techniques such as biofeedback. For most patients, this approach is, at best, an adjunct to pharmacotherapy. Nonpharmacologic measures are unlikely to prevent all migraine attacks. If these measures fail to prevent an attack, pharmacologic approaches are then needed to abort an attack.

ACUTE ATTACK THERAPIES FOR MIGRAINE The mainstay of pharmacologic therapy is the judicious use of one or more of the many drugs that are effective in migraine (Table 14–5). The selection of the optimal regimen for a given patient depends on a number of factors, the most important of which is the severity of the attack. Mild migraine attacks can usually be managed by oral agents; the average efficacy rate is 50–70%. Severe migraine attacks may require parenteral therapy. Most drugs effective in the treatment of migraine are members of one of three major pharmacologic classes: anti-inflammatory agents, 5-HT$_{1B/1D}$ receptor agonists, and dopamine receptor antagonists.

In general, an adequate dose of whichever agent is chosen should be used as soon as possible after the onset of an attack. If additional medication is required within 60 min because symptoms return or have not abated, the initial dose should be increased for subsequent attacks. Migraine therapy must be individualized; a standard approach for all patients is not possible. A therapeutic

*MIDAS Questionnaire

INSTRUCTIONS: Please answer the following questions about ALL headaches you have had over the last 3 months. Write zero if you did not do the activity in the last 3 months.

1. On how many days in the last 3 months did you miss work or school because of your headaches? .... _____ days

2. How many days in the last 3 months was your productivity at work or school reduced by half or more because of your headaches (*do not include days you counted in question 1 where you missed work or school*)? .... _____ days

3. On how many days in the last 3 months did you **not** do household work because of your headaches? .... _____ days

4. How many days in the last 3 months was your productivity in household work reduced by half or more because of your headaches (*do not include days you counted in question 3 where you did not do household work*)? .... _____ days

5. On how many days in the last 3 months did you miss family, social, or leisure activities because of your headaches? .... _____ days

A. On how many days in the last 3 months did you have a headache? (*If a headache lasted more than one day, count each day.*) .... _____ days

B. On a scale of 0–10, on average how painful were these headaches? (*Where 0 = no pain at all, and 10 = pain as bad as it can be.*) .... _____

*Migraine Disability Assessment Score
(Questions 1–5 are used to calculate the MIDAS score.)
Grade I—Minimal or Infrequent Disability: 0–5
Grade II—Mild or Infrequent Disability: 6–10
Grade III—Moderate Disability: 11–20
Grade IV—Severe Disability: > 20

© Innovative Medical Research 1997

Figure 14-4 MIDAS Questionnaire.

TABLE 14-5 Treatment of Acute Migraine

Drug	Trade Name	Dosage
Simple Analgesics		
Acetaminophen, aspirin, caffeine	Excedrin Migraine	Two tablets or caplets q6h (max 8 per day)
NSAIDs		
Naproxen	Aleve, Anaprox, generic	220–550 mg PO bid
Ibuprofen	Advil, Motrin, Nuprin, generic	400 mg PO q3–4h
Tolfenamic acid	Clotam Rapid	200 mg PO. May repeat ×1 after 1–2 h
5-HT$_1$ Agonists		
Oral		
Ergotamine	Ergomar	One 2 mg sublingual tablet at onset and q^1/$_2$h (max 3 per day, 5 per week)
Ergotamine 1 mg, caffeine 100 mg	Ercaf, Wigraine	One or two tablets at onset, then one tablet q^1/$_2$h (max 6 per day, 10 per week)
Naratriptan	Amerge	2.5 mg tablet at onset; may repeat once after 4 h
Rizatriptan	Maxalt Maxalt-MLT	5–10 mg tablet at onset; may repeat after 2 h (max 30 mg/d)
Sumatriptan	Imitrex	50–100 mg tablet at onset; may repeat after 2 h (max 200 mg/d)
Frovatriptan	Frova	2.5 mg tablet at onset, may repeat after 2 h (max 5 mg/d)
Almotriptan	Axert	12.5 mg tablet at onset, may repeat after 2 h (max 25 mg/d)
Eletriptan	Relpax	40 or 80 mg
Zolmitriptan	Zomig Zomig Rapimelt	2.5 mg tablet at onset; may repeat after 2 h (max 10 mg/d)
Nasal		
Dihydroergotamine	Migranal Nasal Spray	Prior to nasal spray, the pump must be primed 4 times; 1 spray (0.5 mg) is administered, followed in 15 min by a second spray
Sumatriptan	Imitrex Nasal Spray	5–20 mg intranasal spray as 4 sprays of 5 mg or a single 20 mg spray (may repeat once after 2 h, not to exceed a dose of 40 mg/d)
Zolmitriptan	Zomig	5 mg intranasal spray as one spray (may repeat once after 2 h, not to exceed a dose of 10 mg/d)
Parenteral		
Dihydroergotamine	DHE-45	1 mg IV, IM, or SC at onset and q1h (max 3 mg/d, 6 mg per week)
Sumatriptan	Imitrex Injection	6 mg SC at onset (may repeat once after 1 h for max of 2 doses in 24 h)
Dopamine Antagonists		
Oral		
Metoclopramide	Reglan,[a] generic[a]	5–10 mg/d
Prochlorperazine	Compazine,[a] generic[a]	1–25 mg/d
Parenteral		
Chlorpromazine	Generic[a]	0.1 mg/kg IV at 2 mg/min; max 35 mg/d
Metoclopramide	Reglan,[a] generic	10 mg IV
Prochlorperazine	Compazine,[a] generic[a]	10 mg IV
Other		
Oral		
Acetaminophen, 325 mg, *plus* dichloralphenazone, 100 mg, *plus* isometheptene, 65 mg	Midrin, Duradrin, generic	Two capsules at onset followed by 1 capsule q1h (max 5 capsules)
Nasal		
Butorphanol	Stadol[a]	1 mg (1 spray in 1 nostril), may repeat if necessary in 1–2 h
Parenteral		
Narcotics	Generic[a]	Multiple preparations and dosages; see Table 11-1

[a]Not all drugs are specifically indicated by the FDA for migraine. Local regulations and guidelines should be consulted.

Note: Antiemetics (e.g., domperidone 10 mg or ondansetron 4 or 8 mg) or prokinetics (e.g., metoclopramide 10 mg) are sometimes useful adjuncts.

Abbreviations: NSAIDs, nonsteroidal anti-inflammatory drugs; 5-HT, 5-hydroxytryptamine.

TABLE 14-6 Clinical Stratification of Acute Specific Migraine Treatments

Clinical Situation	Treatment Options
Failed NSAIDS/analgesics	**First tier** Sumatriptan 50 mg or 100 mg PO Almotriptan 12.5 mg PO Rizatriptan 10 mg PO Eletriptan 40 mg PO Zolmitriptan 2.5 mg PO **Slower effect/better tolerability** Naratriptan 2.5 mg PO Frovatriptan 2.5 mg PO **Infrequent headache** Ergotamine 1–2 mg PO Dihydroergotamine nasal spray 2 mg
Early nausea or difficulties taking tablets	Zolmitriptan 5 mg nasal spray Sumatriptan 20 mg nasal spray Rizatriptan 10 mg MLT wafer
Headache recurrence	Ergotamine 2 mg (most effective PR/usually with caffeine) Naratriptan 2.5 mg PO Almotriptan 12.5 mg PO Eletriptan 40 mg
Tolerating acute treatments poorly	Naratriptan 2.5 mg Almotriptan 12.5 mg
Early vomiting	Zolmitriptan 5 mg nasal spray Sumatriptan 25 mg PR Sumatriptan 6 mg SC
Menses-related headache	**Prevention** Ergotamine PO at night Estrogen patches **Treatment** Triptans Dihydroergotamine nasal spray
Very rapidly developing symptoms	Zolmitriptan 5 mg nasal spray Sumatriptan 6 mg SC Dihydroergotamine 1 mg IM

regimen may need to be constantly refined until one is identified that provides the patient with rapid, complete, and consistent relief with minimal side effects (Table 14–6).

Nonsteroidal Anti-Inflammatory Drugs (NSAIDs) Both the severity and duration of a migraine attack can be reduced significantly by nonsteroidal anti-inflammatory agents (Table 14–5). Indeed, many undiagnosed migraineurs are self-treated with nonprescription NSAIDs. A general consensus is that NSAIDs are most effective when taken early in the migraine attack. However, the effectiveness of anti-inflammatory agents in migraine is usually less than optimal in moderate or severe migraine attacks. The combination of acetaminophen, aspirin, and caffeine has been approved for use by the U.S. Food and Drug Administration

(FDA) for the treatment of mild to moderate migraine. The combination of aspirin and metoclopramide has been shown to be comparable to a single dose of sumatriptan. Important side effects of NSAIDs include dyspepsia and gastrointestinal irritation.

5-HT₁ RECEPTOR AGONISTS

Oral Stimulation of $5\text{-HT}_{1B/1D}$ receptors can stop an acute migraine attack. Ergotamine and dihydroergotamine are nonselective receptor agonists, while the triptans are selective $5\text{-HT}_{1B/1D}$ receptor agonists. A variety of triptans, $5\text{-HT}_{1B/1D}$ receptor agonists—naratriptan, rizatriptan, eletriptan, sumatriptan, zolmitriptan, almotriptan, and frovatriptan—are now available for the treatment of migraine.

Each drug in the triptan class has similar pharmacologic properties but varies slightly in terms of clinical efficacy. Rizatriptan and eletriptan are the most efficacious of the triptans currently available in the United States. Sumatriptan and zolmitriptan have similar rates of efficacy as well as time to onset, with an advantage of having multiple formulations, whereas almotriptan, frovatriptan, and naratriptan are somewhat slower in onset and are better tolerated. Clinical efficacy appears to be related more to the t_{max} (time to peak plasma level) than to the potency, half-life, or bioavailability. This observation is consistent with a large body of data indicating that faster-acting analgesics are more effective than slower-acting agents.

Unfortunately, monotherapy with a selective oral $5\text{-HT}_{1B/1D}$ agonist does not result in rapid, consistent, and complete relief of migraine in all patients. Triptans are not effective in migraine with aura unless given after the aura is completed and the headache initiated. Side effects are common though often mild and transient. Moreover, $5\text{-HT}_{1B/1D}$ agonists are contraindicated in individuals with a history of cardiovascular and cerebrovascular disease. Recurrence of headache is another important limitation of triptan use and occurs at least occasionally in most patients. Evidence from randomized controlled trials show that coadministration of a longer-acting NSAID, naproxen 500 mg, with sumatriptan will augment the initial effect of sumatriptan and, importantly, reduce rates of headache recurrence.

Ergotamine preparations offer a nonselective means of stimulating 5-HT_1 receptors. A nonnauseating dose of ergotamine should be sought since a dose that provokes nausea is too high and may intensify head pain. Except for a sublingual formulation of ergotamine, oral formulations of ergotamine also contain 100 mg caffeine (theoretically to enhance ergotamine absorption and possibly to add additional analgesic activity). The average oral ergotamine dose for a migraine attack is 2 mg. Since the clinical studies demonstrating the efficacy of ergotamine in migraine predated the clinical trial methodologies used with the triptans, it is difficult to assess the clinical efficacy of ergotamine versus the triptans. In general, ergotamine appears to have a much higher incidence of nausea than triptans, but less headache recurrence.

Nasal The fastest-acting nonparenteral antimigraine therapies that can be self-administered include nasal formulations of dihydroergotamine (Migranal), zolmitriptan (Zomig nasal), or sumatriptan. The nasal sprays result in substantial blood levels within 30–60 min. Although in theory nasal sprays might provide faster and more effective relief of a migraine attack than oral formulations, their reported efficacy is only approximately 50–60%. Studies with an inhalational formulation of dihydroergotamine indicate that its absorption problems can be overcome to produce rapid onset of action with good tolerability.

Parenteral Parenteral administration of drugs such as dihydroergotamine and sumatriptan is approved by the FDA for the rapid relief of a migraine attack. Peak plasma levels of dihydroergotamine are achieved 3 min after IV dosing, 30 min after IM dosing, and 45 min after SC dosing. If an attack has not already peaked, SC or IM administration of 1 mg dihydroergotamine suffices for about 80–90% of patients. Sumatriptan, 6 mg SC, is effective in ~70–80% of patients.

DOPAMINE ANTAGONISTS

Oral Oral dopamine antagonists should be considered as adjunctive therapy in migraine. Drug absorption is impaired during migraine because of reduced gastrointestinal motility. Delayed absorption occurs even in the absence of nausea and is related to the severity of the attack and not its duration. Therefore, when oral NSAIDs and/or triptan agents fail, the addition of a dopamine antagonist such as metoclopramide 10 mg should be considered to enhance gastric absorption. In addition, dopamine antagonists decrease nausea/vomiting and restore normal gastric motility.

Parenteral Parenteral dopamine antagonists (e.g., chlorpromazine, prochlorperazine, metoclopramide) can also provide significant acute relief of migraine; they can be used in combination with parenteral 5-HT$_{1B/1D}$ agonists. A common IV protocol used for the treatment of severe migraine is the administration over 2 min of a mixture of 5 mg of prochlorperazine and 0.5 mg of dihydroergotamine.

OTHER MEDICATIONS FOR ACUTE MIGRAINE

Oral The combination of acetaminophen, dichloralphenazone, and isometheptene, one to two capsules, has been classified by the FDA as "possibly" effective in the treatment of migraine. Since the clinical studies demonstrating the efficacy of this combination analgesic in migraine predated the clinical trial methodologies used with the triptans, it is difficult to compare the efficacy of this sympathomimetic compound to other agents.

Nasal A nasal preparation of butorphanol is available for the treatment of acute pain. As with all narcotics, the use of nasal butorphanol should be limited to a select group of migraineurs, as described below.

Parenteral Narcotics are effective in the acute treatment of migraine. For example, IV meperidine (50–100 mg) is given frequently in the emergency room. This regimen "works" in the sense that the pain of migraine is eliminated. However, this regimen is clearly suboptimal for patients with recurrent headache. Narcotics do not treat the underlying headache mechanism; rather, they act to alter the pain sensation. Moreover, in patients taking oral narcotics such as oxycodone or hydrocodone, narcotic addiction can greatly confuse the treatment of migraine. Narcotic craving and/or withdrawal can aggravate and accentuate migraine. Therefore, it is recommended that narcotic use in migraine be limited to patients with severe, but infrequent, headaches that are unresponsive to other pharmacologic approaches.

MEDICATION-OVERUSE HEADACHE Acute attack medications, particularly codeine or barbiturate-containing compound analgesics, have a propensity to aggravate headache frequency and induce a state of refractory daily or near-daily headache called *medication-overuse headache*. This condition is likely not a separate headache entity but a reaction of the migraine patient to a particular medicine. Migraine patients who have two or more headache days a week should be cautioned about frequent analgesic use (see "Chronic Daily Headache," below).

PREVENTIVE TREATMENTS FOR MIGRAINE Patients with an increasing frequency of migraine attacks, or with attacks that are either unresponsive or poorly responsive to abortive treatments, are good candidates for preventive agents. In general, a preventive medication should be considered in the subset of patients with five or more attacks a month. Significant side effects are associated with the use of many of these agents; furthermore, determination of dose can be difficult since the recommended doses have been derived for conditions other than migraine. The mechanism of action of these drugs is unclear; it seems likely that the brain sensitivity that underlies migraine is modified. Patients are usually started on a low dose of a chosen treatment; the dose is then gradually increased, up to a reasonable maximum to achieve clinical benefit.

Drugs that have the capacity to stabilize migraine are listed in Table 14-7. Drugs must be taken daily, and there is usually a lag of at least 2–12 weeks before an effect is seen. The drugs that have been approved by the FDA for the prophylactic treatment of migraine include propranolol, timolol, sodium valproate, topiramate, and methysergide (not available in the United States). In addition, a number of other drugs appear to display prophylactic efficacy. This group includes amitriptyline, nortriptyline, flunarizine, phenelzine, gabapentin, and cyproheptadine. Placebo-controlled trials of onabotulinum toxin type A in episodic migraine were negative, while, overall, placebo-controlled trials in chronic migraine were positive. Phenelzine and methysergide are usually reserved for recalcitrant cases because of their serious potential side effects. Phenelzine is a monoamine oxidase inhibitor (MAOI); therefore, tyramine-containing foods, decongestants, and meperidine are contraindicated. Methysergide may cause retroperitoneal or cardiac valvular fibrosis when it is used for >6 months, and thus monitoring is required for patients using this drug; the risk of fibrosis is about 1:1500 and is likely to reverse after the drug is stopped.

The probability of success with any one of the antimigraine drugs is 50–75%. Many patients are managed adequately with low-dose amitriptyline, propranolol, topiramate, gabapentin, or valproate. If these agents fail or lead to unacceptable side effects, second-line agents such as methysergide or phenelzine can be used. Once effective stabilization is achieved, the drug is continued for ~6 months and then slowly tapered to assess the continued need. Many patients are able to discontinue medication and experience fewer and milder attacks for long periods, suggesting that these drugs may alter the natural history of migraine.

◼ TENSION-TYPE HEADACHE

Clinical features

The term *tension-type headache* (TTH) is commonly used to describe a chronic head-pain syndrome characterized by bilateral tight, bandlike discomfort. The pain typically builds slowly, fluctuates in severity, and may persist more or less continuously for many days. The headache may be episodic or chronic (present >15 days per month).

A useful clinical approach is to diagnose TTH in patients whose headaches are completely without accompanying features such as nausea, vomiting, photophobia, phonophobia, osmophobia, throbbing, and aggravation with movement. Such an

TABLE 14-7 Preventive Treatments in Migraine[a]

Drug	Dose	Selected Side Effects
Pizotifen[b]	0.5–2 mg qd	Weight gain
		Drowsiness
Beta blocker		
Propranolol	40–120 mg bid	Reduced energy
		Tiredness
		Postural symptoms
		Contraindicated in asthma
Tricyclics		
Amitriptyline	10–75 mg at night	Drowsiness
Dothiepin	25–75 mg at night	
Nortriptyline	25–75 mg at night	**Note:** Some patients may only need a total dose of 10 mg, although generally 1–1.5 mg/kg body weight is required
Anticonvulsants		
Topiramate	25–200 mg/d	Paresthesias
		Cognitive symptoms
		Weight loss
		Glaucoma
		Caution with nephrolithiasis
Valproate	400–600 mg bid	Drowsiness
		Weight gain
		Tremor
		Hair loss
		Fetal abnormalities
		Hematologic or liver abnormalities
Gabapentin	900–3600 mg qd	Dizziness
		Sedation
Serotonergic drugs		
Methysergide	1–4 mg qd	Drowsiness
		Leg cramps
		Hair loss
		Retroperitoneal fibrosis (1-month drug holiday is required every 6 months)
Flunarizine[b]	5–15 mg qd	Drowsiness
		Weight gain
		Depression
		Parkinsonism
No convincing evidence from controlled trials		
Verapamil		
Controlled trials demonstrate *no effect*		
Nimodipine		
Clonidine		
SSRIs: fluoxetine		

[a]Commonly used preventives are listed with typical doses and common side effects. Not all listed medicines are approved by the FDA; local regulations and guidelines should be consulted.
[b]Not available in the United States.

approach neatly separates migraine, which has one or more of these features and is the main differential diagnosis, from TTH. The International Headache Society's main definition of TTH allows an admixture of nausea, photophobia, or phonophobia in various combinations, although the appendix definition does not; this illustrates the difficulty in distinguishing these two clinical entities. In clinical practice, dichotomizing patients on the basis of the presence of associated features (migraine) and the absence of associated features (TTH) is highly recommended. Indeed patients whose headaches fit the TTH phenotype and who have migraine at other times, along with a family history of migraine, migrainous illnesses of childhood, or typical migraine triggers to their migraine attacks, may be biologically different from those who have TTH headache with none of the features.

Pathophysiology

The pathophysiology of TTH is incompletely understood. It seems likely that TTH is due to a primary disorder of CNS pain modulation alone, unlike migraine, which involves a more generalized disturbance of sensory modulation. Data suggest a genetic contribution to TTH, but this may not be a valid finding: given the current diagnostic criteria, the studies undoubtedly included many migraine patients. The name *tension-type headache* implies that pain is a product of *nervous tension*, but there is no clear evidence for tension as an etiology. Muscle contraction has been considered to be a feature that distinguishes TTH from migraine, but there appear to be no differences in contraction between the two headache types.

TREATMENT   Tension-Type Headache

The pain of TTH can generally be managed with simple analgesics such as acetaminophen, aspirin, or NSAIDs. Behavioral approaches including relaxation can also be effective. Clinical studies have demonstrated that triptans in pure TTH are not helpful, although triptans are effective in TTH when the patient also has migraine. For chronic TTH, amitriptyline is the only proven treatment (Table 14–7); other tricyclics, selective serotonin reuptake inhibitors, and the benzodiazepines have not been shown to be effective. There is no evidence for the efficacy of acupuncture. Placebo-controlled trials of onabotulinum toxin type A in chronic TTH have not shown benefit.

■ TRIGEMINAL AUTONOMIC CEPHALALGIAS, INCLUDING CLUSTER HEADACHE

The trigeminal autonomic cephalalgias (TACs) describe a grouping of primary headaches including cluster headache, paroxysmal hemicrania, and SUNCT (*short-lasting unilateral neuralgiform headache attacks with conjunctival injection and tearing*)/SUNA (*short-lasting unilateral neuralgiform headache attacks with cranial autonomic symptoms*). TACs are characterized by relatively short-lasting attacks of head pain associated with cranial autonomic symptoms, such as lacrimation, conjunctival injection, or nasal congestion (Table 14–8). Pain is usually severe and may occur more than once a day. Because of the associated nasal congestion or rhinorrhea, patients are often misdiagnosed with "sinus headache" and treated with decongestants, which are ineffective.

TACs must be differentiated from short-lasting headaches that do not have prominent cranial autonomic syndromes, notably trigeminal neuralgia, primary stabbing headache, and hypnic headache. The cycling pattern and length, frequency, and timing of attacks are useful in classifying patients. Patients with TACs

should undergo pituitary imaging and pituitary function tests as there is an excess of TAC presentations in patients with pituitary tumor–related headache.

Cluster headache

Cluster headache is a rare form of primary headache with a population frequency of approximately 0.1%. The pain is deep, usually retroorbital, often excruciating in intensity, nonfluctuating, and explosive in quality. A core feature of cluster headache is periodicity. At least one of the daily attacks of pain recurs at about the same hour each day for the duration of a cluster bout. The typical cluster headache patient has daily bouts of one to two attacks of relatively short-duration unilateral pain for 8 to 10 weeks a year; this is usually followed by a pain-free interval that averages a little less than 1 year. Cluster headache is characterized as chronic when there is no significant period of sustained remission. Patients are generally perfectly well between episodes. Onset is nocturnal in about 50% of patients, and men are affected three times more often than women. Patients with cluster headache tend to move about during attacks, pacing, rocking, or rubbing their head for relief; some may even become aggressive during attacks. This is in sharp contrast to patients with migraine, who prefer to remain motionless during attacks.

Cluster headache is associated with ipsilateral symptoms of cranial parasympathetic autonomic activation: conjunctival injection or lacrimation, rhinorrhea or nasal congestion, or cranial sympathetic dysfunction such as ptosis. The sympathetic deficit is peripheral and likely to be due to parasympathetic activation with injury to ascending sympathetic fibers surrounding a dilated carotid artery as it passes into the cranial cavity. When present, photophobia and phonophobia are far more likely to be unilateral and on the same side of the pain, rather than bilateral, as is seen in migraine. This phenomenon of unilateral photophobia/phonophobia is characteristic of TACs. Cluster headache is likely to be a disorder involving central pacemaker neurons in the region of the posterior hypothalamus (Fig. 14-3).

TREATMENT   Cluster Headache

The most satisfactory treatment is the administration of drugs to prevent cluster attacks until the bout is over. However, treatment of acute attacks is required for all cluster headache patients at some time.

ACUTE ATTACK TREATMENT   Cluster headache attacks peak rapidly, and thus a treatment with quick onset is required. Many patients with acute cluster headache respond very well to oxygen inhalation. This should be given as 100% oxygen at 10–12 L/min for 15–20 min. It appears that high flow and high oxygen content are important. Sumatriptan 6 mg SC is rapid in onset and will usually shorten an attack to 10–15 min; there is no evidence of tachyphylaxis. Sumatriptan (20 mg) and zolmitriptan (5 mg) nasal sprays are both effective in acute cluster headache, offering a useful option for patients who may not wish to self-inject daily. Oral sumatriptan is not effective for prevention or for acute treatment of cluster headache.

PREVENTIVE TREATMENTS   (Table 14–9) The choice of a preventive treatment in cluster headache depends in part on the length of the bout. Patients with long bouts or those with chronic cluster headache require medicines that are safe when taken for long periods. For patients with relatively short bouts, limited courses of oral glucocorticoids or methysergide (not available in the United States) can be very useful. A 10-day

TABLE 14-8 Clinical Features of the Trigeminal Autonomic Cephalalgias

	Cluster Headache	Paroxysmal Hemicrania	SUNCT
Gender	M > F	F = M	F ~ M
Pain			
Type	Stabbing, boring	Throbbing, boring, stabbing	Burning, stabbing, sharp
Severity	Excruciating	Excruciating	Severe to excruciating
Site	Orbit, temple	Orbit, temple	Periorbital
Attack frequency	1/alternate day–8/d	1–40/d (>5/d for more than half the time)	3–200/d
Duration of attack	15–180 min	2–30 min	5–240 s
Autonomic features	Yes	Yes	Yes (prominent conjunctival injection and lacrimation)[a]
Migrainous features[b]	Yes	Yes	Yes
Alcohol trigger	Yes	No	No
Cutaneous triggers	No	No	Yes
Indomethacin effect	—	Yes[c]	—
Abortive treatment	Sumatriptan injection or nasal spray	No effective treatment	Lidocaine (IV)
	Oxygen		
Prophylactic treatment	Verapamil	Indomethacin	Lamotrigine
	Methysergide		Topiramate
	Lithium		Gabapentin

[a]If conjunctival injection and tearing not present, consider SUNA.
[b]Nausea, photophobia, or phonophobia; photophobia and phonophobia are typically unilateral on the side of the pain.
[c]Indicates complete response to indomethacin.
Abbreviation: SUNCT, short-lasting unilateral neuralgiform headache attacks with conjunctival injection and tearing.

course of prednisone, beginning at 60 mg daily for 7 days and followed by a rapid taper, may interrupt the pain bout for many patients. When ergotamine (1–2 mg) is used, it is most effective when given 1–2 h before an expected attack. Patients who use ergotamine daily must be educated regarding the early symptoms of ergotism, which may include vomiting, numbness, tingling, pain, and cyanosis of the limbs; a weekly limit of 14 mg should be adhered to. Lithium (400–800 mg/d) appears to be particularly useful for the chronic form of the disorder.

TABLE 14-9 Preventive Management of Cluster Headache

Short-Term Prevention	Long-Term Prevention
Episodic Cluster Headache	**Episodic Cluster Headache & Prolonged Chronic Cluster Headache**
Prednisone 1 mg/kg up to 60 mg qd, tapering over 21 days	Verapamil 160–960 mg/d
	Lithium 400–800 mg/d
Methysergide 3–12 mg/d	Methysergide 3–12 mg/d
Verapamil 160–960 mg/d	Topiramate[a] 100–400 mg/d
Greater occipital nerve injection	Gabapentin[a] 1200–3600 mg/d
	Melatonin[a] 9–12 mg/d

[a]Unproven but of potential benefit.

Many experts favor verapamil as the first-line preventive treatment for patients with chronic cluster headache or prolonged bouts. While verapamil compares favorably with lithium in practice, some patients require verapamil doses far in excess of those administered for cardiac disorders. The initial dose range is 40–80 mg twice daily; effective doses may be as high as 960 mg/d. Side effects such as constipation and leg swelling can be problematic. Of paramount concern, however, is the cardiovascular safety of verapamil, particularly at high doses. Verapamil can cause heart block by slowing conduction in the atrioventricular node, a condition that can be monitored by following the PR interval on a standard ECG. Approximately 20% of patients treated with verapamil develop ECG abnormalities, which can be observed with doses as low as 240 mg/d; these abnormalities can worsen over time in patients on stable doses. A baseline ECG is recommended for all patients. The ECG is repeated 10 days after a dose change in those patients whose dose is being increased above 240 mg daily. Dose increases are usually made in 80-mg increments. For patients on long-term verapamil, ECG monitoring every 6 months is advised.

NEUROSTIMULATION THERAPY When medical therapies fail in chronic cluster headache, neurostimulation strategies can be employed. Deep-brain stimulation of the region of the posterior hypothalamic gray matter has proven successful in a substantial proportion of patients. Favorable results have also been reported with the less-invasive approach of occipital nerve stimulation.

■ PAROXYSMAL HEMICRANIA

Paroxysmal hemicrania (PH) is characterized by frequent unilateral, severe, short-lasting episodes of headache. Like cluster headache, the pain tends to be retroorbital but may be experienced all over the head and is associated with autonomic phenomena such as lacrimation and nasal congestion. Patients with remissions are said to have episodic PH, whereas those with the nonremitting form are said to have chronic PH. The essential features of PH are unilateral, very severe pain; short-lasting attacks (2–45 min); very frequent attacks (usually more than five a day); marked autonomic features ipsilateral to the pain; rapid course (<72 h); and excellent response to indomethacin. In contrast to cluster headache, which predominantly affects males, the male:female ratio in PH is close to 1:1.

Indomethacin (25–75 mg tid), which can completely suppress attacks of PH, is the treatment of choice. Although therapy may be complicated by indomethacin-induced gastrointestinal side effects, currently there are no consistently effective alternatives. Topiramate is helpful in some cases. Piroxicam has been used, although it is not as effective as indomethacin. Verapamil, an effective treatment for cluster headache, does not appear to be useful for PH. In occasional patients, PH can coexist with trigeminal neuralgia (PH-tic syndrome); similar to cluster-tic syndrome, each component may require separate treatment.

Secondary PH has been reported with lesions in the region of the sella turcica, including arteriovenous malformation, cavernous sinus meningioma, and epidermoid tumors. Secondary PH is more likely if the patient requires high doses (>200 mg/d) of indomethacin. In patients with apparent bilateral PH, raised CSF pressure should be suspected. It is important to note that indomethacin reduces CSF pressure. When a diagnosis of PH is considered, MRI is indicated to exclude a pituitary lesion.

SUNCT/SUNA

SUNCT (short-lasting unilateral neuralgiform headache attacks with conjunctival injection and tearing) is a rare primary headache syndrome characterized by severe, unilateral orbital or temporal pain that is stabbing or throbbing in quality. Diagnosis requires at least 20 attacks, lasting for 5–240 s; ipsilateral conjunctival injection and lacrimation should be present. In some patients conjunctival injection or lacrimation is missing, and the diagnosis of SUNA (short-lasting unilateral neuralgiform headache attacks with cranial autonomic symptoms) can be made.

Diagnosis The pain of SUNCT/SUNA is unilateral and may be located anywhere in the head. Three basic patterns can be seen: single stabs, which are usually short-lived; groups of stabs; or a longer attack comprising many stabs between which the pain does not completely resolve, thus giving a "saw-tooth" phenomenon with attacks lasting many minutes. Each pattern may be seen in the context of an underlying continuous head pain. Characteristics that lead to a suspected diagnosis of SUNCT are the cutaneous (or other) triggerability of attacks, a lack of refractory period to triggering between attacks, and the lack of a response to indomethacin. Apart from trigeminal sensory disturbance, the neurologic examination is normal in primary SUNCT.

The diagnosis of SUNCT is often confused with trigeminal neuralgia (TN) particularly in first-division TN (Chap. 376). Minimal or no cranial autonomic symptoms and a clear refractory period to triggering indicate a diagnosis of TN.

Secondary (Symptomatic) SUNCT SUNCT can be seen with posterior fossa or pituitary lesions. All patients with SUNCT/SUNA should be evaluated with pituitary function tests and a brain MRI with pituitary views.

ABORTIVE THERAPY Therapy of acute attacks is not a useful concept in SUNCT/SUNA since the attacks are of such short duration. However, IV lidocaine, which arrests the symptoms, can be used in hospitalized patients.

PREVENTIVE THERAPY Long-term prevention to minimize disability and hospitalization is the goal of treatment. The most effective treatment for prevention is lamotrigine, 200–400 mg/d. Topiramate and gabapentin may also be effective. Carbamazepine, 400–500 mg/d, has been reported by patients to offer modest benefit.

Surgical approaches such as microvascular decompression or destructive trigeminal procedures are seldom useful and often produce long-term complications. Greater occipital nerve injection has produced limited benefit in some patients. Occipital nerve stimulation is probably helpful in an important subgroup of these patients. Complete control with deep-brain stimulation of the posterior hypothalamic region was reported in a single patient. For intractable cases, short-term prevention with IV lidocaine can be effective, as can occipital nerve stimulation.

■ CHRONIC DAILY HEADACHE

The broad diagnosis of chronic daily headache (CDH) can be applied when a patient experiences headache on 15 days or more per month. CDH is not a single entity; it encompasses a number of different headache syndromes, including chronic TTH as well as headache secondary to trauma, inflammation, infection, medication overuse, and other causes (Table 14-10). Population-based estimates suggest that about 4% of adults have daily or near-daily headache. Daily headache may be primary or secondary, an important consideration in guiding management of this complaint.

TABLE 14-10 Classification of Chronic Daily Headache

Primary		Secondary
>4 h Daily	**<4 h Daily**	**Secondary**
Chronic migraine[a]	Chronic cluster headache[b]	Posttraumatic
		Head injury
		Iatrogenic
		Postinfectious
Chronic tension-type headache[a]	Chronic paroxysmal hemicrania	Inflammatory, such as
		Giant cell arteritis
		Sarcoidosis
		Behçet's syndrome
Hemicrania continua[a]	SUNCT/SUNA	Chronic CNS infection
New daily persistent headache[a]	Hypnic headache	Medication-overuse headache[a]

[a]May be complicated by analgesic overuse.
[b]Some patients may have headache >4 h/d.
Abbreviations: SUNA, short-lasting unilateral neuralgiform headache attacks with cranial autonomic symptoms; SUNCT, short-lasting unilateral neuralgiform headache attacks with conjunctival injection and tearing.

The first step in the management of patients with CDH is to diagnose any underlying condition (Table 14–10). For patients with primary headaches, diagnosis of the headache type will guide therapy. Preventive treatments such as tricyclics, either amitriptyline or nortriptyline at doses up to 1 mg/kg, are very useful in patients with CDH arising from migraine or tension-type headache. Tricyclics are started in low doses (10–25 mg) daily and may be given 12 h before the expected time of awakening in order to avoid excess morning sleepiness. Anticonvulsants, such as topiramate, valproate, and gabapentin, are also useful in migraineurs. Flunarizine can also be very effective for some patients, as can methysergide or phenelzine.

MANAGEMENT OF MEDICALLY INTRACTABLE DISABLING CHRONIC DAILY HEADACHE   The management of medically intractable headache is difficult. At this time, the only promising approach is occipital nerve stimulation, which appears to modulate thalamic processing in migraine and has also shown promise in chronic cluster headache, SUNCT/SUNA, and hemicrania continua (see below).

MEDICATION-OVERUSE HEADACHE   Overuse of analgesic medication for headache can aggravate headache frequency and induce a state of refractory daily or near-daily headache called *medication-overuse headache*. A proportion of patients who stop taking analgesics will experience substantial improvement in the severity and frequency of their headache. However, even after cessation of analgesic use, many patients continue to have headache, although they may feel clinically improved in some way, especially if they have been using codeine or barbiturates regularly. The residual symptoms probably represent the underlying headache disorder.

Management of Medication Overuse: Outpatients   For patients who overuse medications, it is essential that analgesic use be reduced and eliminated. One approach is to reduce the medication dose by 10% every 1–2 weeks. Immediate cessation of analgesic use is possible for some patients, provided there is no contraindication. Both approaches are facilitated by the use of a medication diary maintained during the month or two before cessation; this helps to identify the scope of the problem. A small dose of an NSAID such as naproxen, 500 mg bid, if tolerated, will help relieve residual pain as analgesic use is reduced. NSAID overuse is not usually a problem for patients with daily headache when the dose is taken once or twice daily; however, overuse problems may develop with more frequent dosing schedules. Once the patient has substantially reduced analgesic use, a preventive medication should be introduced. It must be emphasized that *preventives generally do not work in the presence of analgesic overuse*. The most common cause of unresponsiveness to treatment is the use of a preventive when analgesics continue to be used regularly. For some patients, discontinuing analgesics is very difficult; often the best approach is to directly inform the patient that some degree of pain is inevitable during this initial period.

Management of Medication Overuse: Inpatients   Some patients will require hospitalization for detoxification. Such patients have typically failed efforts at outpatient withdrawal or have a significant medical condition, such as diabetes mellitus, which would complicate withdrawal as an outpatient. Following admission to the hospital, acute medications are withdrawn completely on the first day, in the absence of a contraindication. Antiemetics and fluids are administered as required; clonidine is used for opiate

TABLE 14-11 Differential Diagnosis of New Daily Persistent Headache

Primary	Secondary
Migrainous-type	Subarachnoid hemorrhage
Featureless (tension-type)	Low CSF volume headache
	Raised CSF pressure headache
	Posttraumatic headache[a]
	Chronic meningitis

[a]Includes postinfectious forms.

withdrawal symptoms. For acute intolerable pain during the waking hours aspirin, 1 g IV (not approved in United States), is useful. IM chlorpromazine can be helpful at night; patients must be adequately hydrated. Three to five days into the admission as the effect of the withdrawn substance settles a course of IV dihydroergotamine (DHE) can be employed. DHE, administered every 8 h for 5 consecutive days, can induce a significant remission that allows a preventive treatment to be established. 5-HT$_3$ antagonists, such as ondansetron or granisetron, are often required with DHE to prevent significant nausea, and domperidone (not approved in the United States) orally or by suppository can be very helpful.

NEW DAILY PERSISTENT HEADACHE   New daily persistent headache (NDPH) is a clinically distinct syndrome; its causes are listed in Table 14–11.

Clinical Presentation   The patient with NDPH presents with headache on most if not all days and the patient can clearly, and often vividly, recall the moment of onset. The headache usually begins abruptly, but onset may be more gradual; evolution over 3 days has been proposed as the upper limit for this syndrome. Patients typically recall the exact day and circumstances of the onset of headache; the new, persistent head pain does not remit. The first priority is to distinguish between a primary and a secondary cause of this syndrome. Subarachnoid hemorrhage is the most serious of the secondary causes and must be excluded either by history or appropriate investigation (Chap. 275).

Secondary NDPH

Low CSF Volume Headache   In these syndromes, head pain is positional: it begins when the patient sits or stands upright and resolves upon reclining. The pain, which is occipitofrontal, is usually a dull ache but may be throbbing. Patients with chronic low CSF volume headache typically present with a history of headache from one day to the next that is generally not present on waking but worsens during the day. Recumbency usually improves the headache within minutes, but it takes only minutes to an hour for the pain to return when the patient resumes an upright position.

The most common cause of headache due to persistent low CSF volume is CSF leak following lumbar puncture (LP). Post-LP headache usually begins within 48 h but may be delayed for up to 12 days. Its incidence is between 10 and 30%. Beverages with caffeine may provide temporary relief. Besides LP, index events may include epidural injection or a vigorous Valsalva maneuver, such as from lifting, straining, coughing, clearing the eustachian tubes in an airplane, or multiple orgasms. Spontaneous CSF leaks are well recognized, and the diagnosis should be considered whenever the headache history is typical, even when there is no obvious index event. As time passes from the index event, the

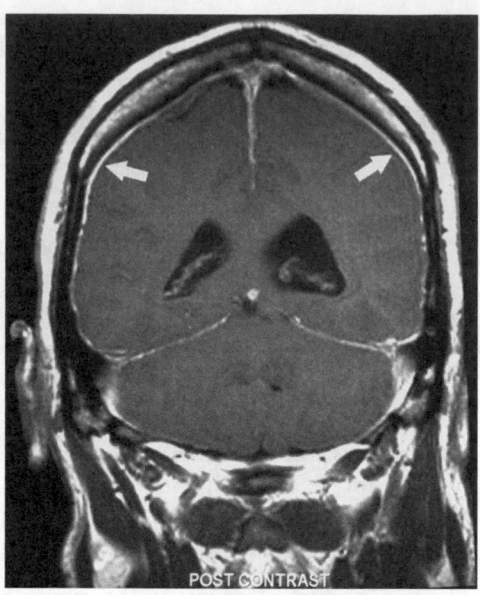

Figure 14-5 Magnetic resonance image showing diffuse meningeal enhancement after gadolinium administration in a patient with low CSF volume headache.

postural nature may become less apparent; cases in which the index event occurred several years before the eventual diagnosis have been recognized. Symptoms appear to result from low volume rather than low pressure: although low CSF pressures, typically 0–50 mmH$_2$O, are usually identified, a pressure as high as 140 mmH$_2$O has been noted with a documented leak.

Postural orthostatic tachycardia syndrome [POTS (Chap. 375)] can present with orthostatic headache similar to low CSF volume headache and is a diagnosis that needs consideration here.

When imaging is indicated to identify the source of a presumed leak, an MRI with gadolinium is the initial study of choice (Fig. 14-5). A striking pattern of diffuse meningeal enhancement is so typical that in the appropriate clinical context the diagnosis is established. Chiari malformations may sometimes be noted on MRI; in such cases, surgery to decompress the posterior fossa usually worsens the headache. Spinal MRI with T2 weighting may reveal a leak and spinal MRI may demonstrate spinal meningeal cysts whose role in these syndromes is yet to be elucidated. The source of CSF leakage may be identified by spinal MRI, by CT, or increasingly with MR myelography, or with ^{111}In-DTPA CSF studies; in the absence of a directly identified site of leakage, early emptying of ^{111}In-DTPA tracer into the bladder or slow progress of tracer across the brain suggests a CSF leak.

Initial treatment for low CSF volume headache is bed rest. For patients with persistent pain, IV caffeine (500 mg in 500 mL saline administered over 2 h) can be very effective. An ECG to screen for arrhythmia should be performed before administration. It is reasonable to administer at least two infusions of caffeine before embarking on additional tests to identify the source of the CSF leak. Since IV caffeine is safe and can be curative, it spares many patients the need for further investigations. If unsuccessful, an abdominal binder may be helpful. If a leak can be identified, an autologous blood patch is usually curative. A blood patch is also effective for post-LP headache; in this setting, the location is empirically determined to be the site of the LP. In patients with intractable pain, oral theophylline is a useful alternative; however, its effect is less rapid than caffeine.

Raised CSF Pressure Headache Raised CSF pressure is well recognized as a cause of headache. Brain imaging can often reveal the cause, such as a space-occupying lesion. NDPH due to raised CSF pressure can be the presenting symptom for patients with idiopathic intracranial hypertension (pseudotumor cerebri) without visual problems, particularly when the fundi are normal. Persistently raised intracranial pressure can trigger chronic migraine. These patients typically present with a history of generalized headache that is present on waking and improves as the day goes on. It is generally worse with recumbency. Visual obscurations are frequent. The diagnosis is relatively straightforward when papilledema is present, but the possibility must be considered even in patients without funduscopic changes. Formal visual field testing should be performed even in the absence of overt ophthalmic involvement. Headache on rising in the morning or nocturnal headache is also characteristic of obstructive sleep apnea or poorly controlled hypertension.

Evaluation of patients suspected to have raised CSF pressure requires brain imaging. It is most efficient to obtain an MRI, including an MR venogram, as the initial study. If there are no contraindications, the CSF pressure should be measured by LP; this should be done when the patient is symptomatic so that both the pressure and the response to removal of 20–30 mL of CSF can be determined. An elevated opening pressure and improvement in headache following removal of CSF is diagnostic.

Initial treatment is with acetazolamide (250–500 mg bid); the headache may improve within weeks. If ineffective, topiramate is the next treatment of choice; it has many actions that may be useful in this setting, including carbonic anhydrase inhibition, weight loss, and neuronal membrane stabilization, likely mediated via effects on phosphorylation pathways. Severely disabled patients who do not respond to medical treatment require intracranial pressure monitoring and may require shunting.

Post-Traumatic Headache A traumatic event can trigger a headache process that lasts for many months or years after the event. The term *trauma* is used in a very broad sense: headache can develop following an injury to the head, but it can also develop after an infectious episode, typically viral meningitis, a flulike illness, or a parasitic infection. Complaints of dizziness, vertigo, and impaired memory can accompany the headache. Symptoms may remit after several weeks or persist for months and even years after the injury. Typically the neurologic examination is normal and CT or MRI studies are unrevealing. Chronic subdural hematoma may on occasion mimic this disorder. In one series, one-third of patients with NDPH reported headache beginning after a transient flulike illness characterized by fever, neck stiffness, photophobia, and marked malaise. Evaluation reveals no apparent cause for the headache. There is no convincing evidence that persistent Epstein-Barr infection plays a role in this syndrome. A complicating factor is that many patients undergo LP during the acute illness; iatrogenic low CSF volume headache must be considered in these cases. Posttraumatic headache may also be seen after carotid dissection and subarachnoid hemorrhage, and following intracranial surgery. The underlying theme appears to be that a traumatic event involving the pain-producing meninges can trigger a headache process that lasts for many years.

Treatment is largely empirical. Tricyclic antidepressants, notably amitriptyline, and anticonvulsants such as topiramate, valproate, and gabapentin, have been used with reported benefit. The MAOI phenelzine may also be useful in carefully selected patients. The headache usually resolves within 3–5 years, but it can be quite disabling.

Primary NDPH   Primary NDPH occurs in both males and females. It can be of the migrainous type, with features of migraine, or it can be featureless, appearing as new-onset TTH (Table 14–11). Migrainous features are common and include unilateral headache and throbbing pain; each feature is present in about one-third of patients. Nausea, photophobia, and/or phonophobia occur in about half of patients. Some patients have a previous history of migraine; however, the proportion of NDPH sufferers with preexisting migraine is no greater than the frequency of migraine in the general population. At 24 months, ~86% of patients are headache-free. Treatment of migrainous-type primary NDPH consists of using the preventive therapies effective in migraine (Table 14–7). Featureless NDPH is one of the primary headache forms most refractory to treatment. Standard preventive therapies can be offered but are often ineffective.

■ OTHER PRIMARY HEADACHES

Hemicrania continua

The essential features of hemicrania continua are moderate and continuous unilateral pain associated with fluctuations of severe pain; complete resolution of pain with indomethacin; and exacerbations that may be associated with autonomic features, including conjunctival injection, lacrimation, and photophobia on the affected side. The age of onset ranges from 11 to 58 years; women are affected twice as often as men. The cause is unknown.

TREATMENT   Hemicrania Continua

Treatment consists of indomethacin; other NSAIDs appear to be of little or no benefit. The IM injection of 100 mg indomethacin has been proposed as a diagnostic tool and administration with a placebo injection in a blinded fashion can be very useful diagnostically. Alternatively, a trial of oral indomethacin, starting with 25 mg tid, then 50 mg tid, and then 75 mg tid, can be given. Up to two weeks at the maximal dose may be necessary to assess whether a dose has a useful effect. Topiramate can be helpful in some patients. Occipital nerve stimulation may have a role in patients with hemicrania continua who are unable to tolerate indomethacin.

Primary stabbing headache

The essential features of primary stabbing headache are stabbing pain confined to the head or, rarely, the face, lasting from 1 to many seconds or minutes and occurring as a single stab or a series of stabs; absence of associated cranial autonomic features; absence of cutaneous triggering of attacks; and a pattern of recurrence at irregular intervals (hours to days). The pains have been variously described as "ice-pick pains" or "jabs and jolts." They are more common in patients with other primary headaches, such as migraine, the TACs, and hemicrania continua.

TREATMENT   Primary Stabbing Headache

The response of primary stabbing headache to indomethacin (25–50 mg two to three times daily) is usually excellent. As a general rule, the symptoms wax and wane, and after a period of control on indomethacin, it is appropriate to withdraw treatment and observe the outcome.

Primary cough headache

Primary cough headache is a generalized headache that begins suddenly, lasts for several minutes, and is precipitated by coughing; it is preventable by avoiding coughing or other precipitating events, which can include sneezing, straining, laughing, or stooping. In all patients with this syndrome, serious etiologies must be excluded before a diagnosis of "benign" primary cough headache can be established. A Chiari malformation or any lesion causing obstruction of CSF pathways or displacing cerebral structures can be the cause of the head pain. Other conditions that can present with cough or exertional headache as the initial symptom include cerebral aneurysm, carotid stenosis, and vertebrobasilar disease. Benign cough headache can resemble benign exertional headache (below), but patients with the former condition are typically older.

TREATMENT   Primary Cough Headache

Indomethacin 25–50 mg two to three times daily is the treatment of choice. Some patients with cough headache obtain pain relief with LP; this is a simple option when compared to prolonged use of indomethacin, and it is effective in about one-third of patients. The mechanism of this response is unclear.

Primary exertional headache

Primary exertional headache has features resembling both cough headache and migraine. It may be precipitated by any form of exercise; it often has the pulsatile quality of migraine. The pain, which can last from 5 min to 24 h, is bilateral and throbbing at onset; migrainous features may develop in patients susceptible to migraine. Primary exertional headache can be prevented by avoiding excessive exertion, particularly in hot weather or at high altitude.

The mechanism of primary exertional headache is unclear. Acute venous distension likely explains one syndrome, the acute onset of headache with straining and breath holding, as in weightlifter's headache. As exertion can result in headache in a number of serious underlying conditions, these must be considered in patients with exertional headache. Pain from angina may be referred to the head, probably by central connections of vagal afferents, and may present as exertional headache (cardiac cephalgia). The link to exercise is the main clinical clue that headache is of cardiac origin. Pheochromocytoma may occasionally cause exertional headache. Intracranial lesions and stenosis of the carotid arteries are other possible etiologies.

TREATMENT   Primary Exertional Headache

Exercise regimens should begin modestly and progress gradually to higher levels of intensity. Indomethacin at daily doses from 25 to 150 mg is generally effective in benign exertional headache. Indomethacin (50 mg), ergotamine (1 mg orally), dihydroergotamine (2 mg by nasal spray), or methysergide (1–2 mg orally given 30–45 min before exercise) are useful prophylactic measures.

Primary sex headache

Sex headache is precipitated by sexual excitement. The pain usually begins as a dull bilateral headache that suddenly becomes intense at orgasm. The headache can be prevented or eased by ceasing sexual activity before orgasm. Three types of sex headache are reported: a dull ache in the head and neck that intensifies as sexual excitement increases; a sudden, severe, explosive headache occurring at orgasm; and a postural headache developing after coitus that resembles the headache of low CSF pressure. The latter arises from vigorous sexual activity and is a form of low CSF pressure headache. Headaches developing at the time of orgasm are not always benign; 5–12% of cases of subarachnoid hemorrhage are precipitated by sexual intercourse. Sex headache is reported by men more often than women and may occur at any time during the years of sexual activity. It may develop on several occasions in succession and then not trouble the patient again, even without an obvious change in sexual activity. In patients who stop sexual activity when headache is first noticed, the pain may subside within a period of 5 min to 2 h. In about half of patients, sex headache will subside within 6 months. About half of patients with sex headache have a history of exertional headaches, but there is no excess of cough headache. Migraine is probably more common in patients with sex headache.

TREATMENT Primary Sex Headache

Benign sex headaches recur irregularly and infrequently. Management can often be limited to reassurance and advice about ceasing sexual activity if a mild, warning headache develops. Propranolol can be used to prevent headache that recurs regularly or frequently, but the dosage required varies from 40 to 200 mg/d. An alternative is the calcium channel–blocking agent diltiazem, 60 mg tid. Ergotamine (1 mg) or indomethacin (25–50 mg) taken about 30–45 min prior to sexual activity can also be helpful.

Primary thunderclap headache

Sudden onset of severe headache may occur in the absence of any known provocation. The differential diagnosis includes the sentinel bleed of an intracranial aneurysm, cervicocephalic arterial dissection, and cerebral venous thrombosis. Headaches of explosive onset may also be caused by the ingestion of sympathomimetic drugs or of tyramine-containing foods in a patient who is taking MAOIs, or they may be a symptom of pheochromocytoma. Whether thunderclap headache can be the presentation of an unruptured cerebral aneurysm is uncertain. When neuroimaging studies and LP exclude subarachnoid hemorrhage, patients with thunderclap headache usually do very well over the long term. In one study of patients whose CT scans and CSF findings were negative, ~15% had recurrent episodes of thunderclap headache, and nearly half subsequently developed migraine or tension-type headache.

The first presentation of any sudden-onset severe headache should be vigorously investigated with neuroimaging (CT or, when possible, MRI with MR angiography) and CSF examination. Formal cerebral angiography should be reserved for those cases in which no primary diagnosis is forthcoming and for clinical situations that are particularly suggestive of intracranial aneurysm. Reversible segmental cerebral vasoconstriction may be seen in primary thunderclap headache without an intracranial aneurysm. In the presence of posterior leukoencephalopathy, the differential diagnosis includes cerebral angiitis, drug toxicity (cyclosporine, intrathecal methotrexate/cytarabine, pseudoephedrine, or cocaine), posttransfusion effects, and postpartum angiopathy. Treatment with nimodipine may be helpful, although by definition the vasoconstriction of primary thunderclap headache resolves spontaneously.

Hypnic headache

This headache syndrome typically begins a few hours after sleep onset. The headaches last from 15 to 30 min and are typically moderately severe and generalized, although they may be unilateral and can be throbbing. Patients may report falling back to sleep only to be awakened by a further attack a few hours later; up to three repetitions of this pattern occur through the night. Daytime naps can also precipitate head pain. Most patients are female, and the onset is usually after age 60 years. Headaches are bilateral in most, but may be unilateral. Photophobia or phonophobia and nausea are usually absent. The major secondary consideration in this headache type is poorly controlled hypertension; 24-h blood pressure monitoring is recommended to detect this treatable condition.

TREATMENT Hypnic Headache

Patients with hypnic headache generally respond to a bedtime dose of lithium carbonate (200–600 mg). For those intolerant of lithium, verapamil (160 mg) or methysergide (1–4 mg at bedtime) may be alternative strategies. One to two cups of coffee or caffeine, 60 mg orally, at bedtime may be effective in approximately one-third of patients. Case reports suggest that flunarizine, 5 mg nightly, can be effective.

FURTHER READINGS

CITTADINI E, GOADSBY PJ: Hemicrania continua: A clinical study of 39 patients with diagnostic implications. Brain 133:1973, 2010

COHEN AS et al: High-flow oxygen for treatment of cluster headache: A randomized trial. JAMA 302:2451, 2009

GOADSBY PJ et al: *Chronic Daily Headache for Clinicians*. Hamilton, Ontario, Canada, BC Decker, 2005

———: Trigeminal autonomic cephalalgias: Paroxysmal hemicrania, SUNCT/SUNA and hemicrania continua. Semin Neurol 30:186, 2010

GOADSBY PJ et al: Trigeminal autonomic cephalalgias: Paroxysmal hemicrania, SUNCT/SUNA and hemicrania continua. Semin Neurol 30:186, 2010

HEADACHE CLASSIFICATION COMMITTEE OF THE INTERNATIONAL HEADACHE SOCIETY: *The International Classification of Headache Disorders*, 2nd ed. Cephalalgia 24:1, 2004

LANCE JW, GOADSBY PJ: *Mechanism and Management of Headache*, 7th ed. Philadelphia, Elsevier, 2005

LIPTON RB, BIGAL M: *Migraine and Other Headache Disorders*. New York, Marcel Dekker, Taylor & Francis, 2006

LODER E: Triptan therapy in migraine. N Engl J Med 363:63, 2010

OLESEN J et al: *The Headaches*. Philadelphia, Lippincott, Williams & Wilkins, 2005

CHAPTER 15

Back and Neck Pain

John W. Engstrom
Richard A. Deyo

The importance of back and neck pain in our society is underscored by the following: (1) the cost of back pain in the United States exceeds $100 billion annually; approximately one-third of these costs are direct health care expenses, and two-thirds are indirect costs resulting from loss of wages and productivity; (2) back symptoms are the most common cause of disability in those <45 years; (3) low back pain is the second most common reason for visiting a physician in the United States; and (4) ~1% of the U.S. population is chronically disabled because of back pain.

ANATOMY OF THE SPINE

The anterior portion of the spine consists of cylindrical vertebral bodies separated by intervertebral disks and held together by the anterior and posterior longitudinal ligaments. The intervertebral disks are composed of a central gelatinous nucleus pulposus surrounded by a tough cartilaginous ring, the annulus fibrosis. Disks are responsible for 25% of spinal column length and allow the bony vertebrae to move easily upon each other (Figs. 15-1 and 15-2). Desiccation of the nucleus pulposus and degeneration of the annulus fibrosus increase with age and results in loss of height. The disks are largest in the cervical and lumbar regions where movements of the spine are greatest. The functions of the anterior spine are to absorb the shock of body movements such as walking and running, and to protect the contents of the spinal canal.

The posterior portion of the spine consists of the vertebral arches and processes. Each arch consists of paired cylindrical pedicles anteriorly and paired laminae posteriorly. The vertebral arch also gives rise to two transverse processes laterally, one spinous process

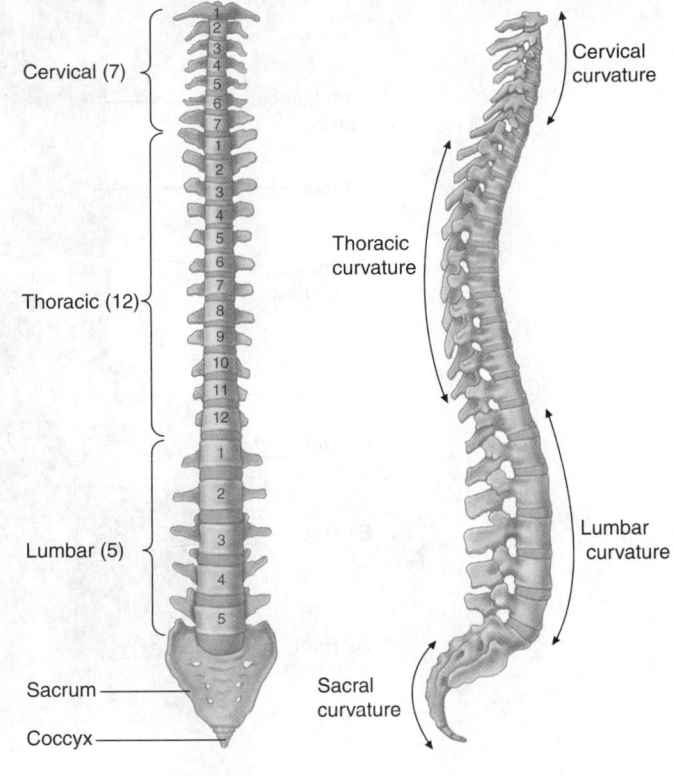

Figure 15-2   Spinal column. *(From A Gauthier Cornuelle, DH Gronefeld: Radiographic Anatomy Positioning. New York, McGraw-Hill, 1998; with permission.)*

posteriorly, plus two superior and two inferior articular facets. The apposition of a superior and inferior facet constitutes a *facet joint*. The functions of the posterior spine are to protect the spinal cord and nerves within the spinal canal and to provide an anchor for the attachment of muscles and ligaments. The contraction of muscles attached to the spinous and transverse processes and laminae works like a system of pulleys and levers that results in flexion, extension, and lateral bending movements of the spine.

Nerve root injury (*radiculopathy*) is a common cause of neck, arm, low back, buttock, and leg pain (Figs. 23-2 and 23-3). The nerve roots exit at a level above their respective vertebral bodies in the cervical region (e.g., the C7 nerve root exits at the C6-C7 level) and below their respective vertebral bodies in the thoracic and lumbar regions (e.g., the T1 nerve root exits at the T1-T2 level). The cervical nerve roots follow a short intraspinal course before exiting. By contrast, because the spinal cord ends at the vertebral L1 or L2 level, the lumbar nerve roots follow a long intraspinal course and can be injured anywhere from the upper lumbar spine to their exit at the intervertebral foramen. For example, disk herniation at the L4-L5 level can produce not only L5 root

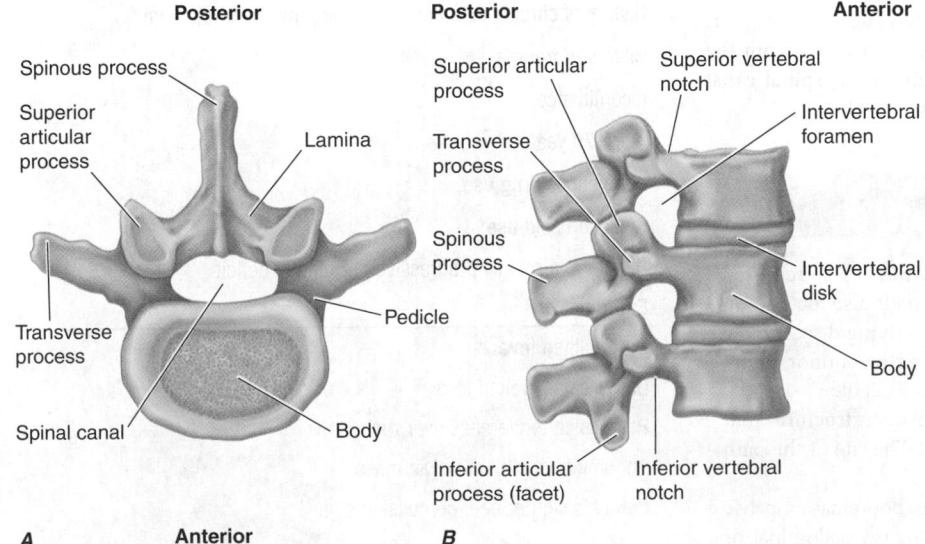

Figure 15-1   Vertebral anatomy. *(From A Gauthier Cornuelle, DH Gronefeld: Radiographic Anatomy Positioning. New York, McGraw-Hill, 1998; with permission.)*

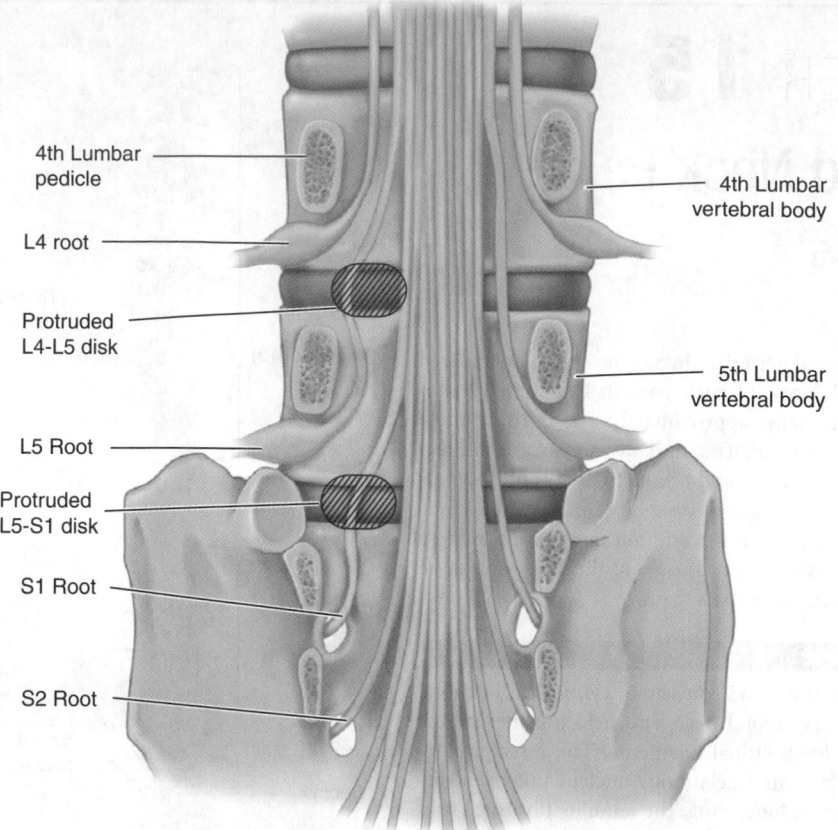

Figure 15-3 **Compression of L5 and S1 roots by herniated disks.** *(From Adams and Victor's Principles of Neurology, 9th ed. New York, McGraw-Hill, 2009; with permission.)*

4th Lumbar pedicle

L4 root

Protruded L4-L5 disk

L5 Root

Protruded L5-S1 disk

S1 Root

S2 Root

4th Lumbar vertebral body

5th Lumbar vertebral body

compression, but also compression of the traversing S1 nerve root (Fig. 15-3).

Pain-sensitive structures of the spine include the periosteum of the vertebrae, dura, facet joints, annulus fibrosus of the intervertebral disk, epidural veins and arteries, and the posterior longitudinal ligament. Disease of these diverse structures may explain many cases of back pain without nerve root compression. The nucleus pulposus of the intervertebral disk is not pain-sensitive under normal circumstances. Pain sensation from within the spinal canal is conveyed partially by the sinuvertebral nerve that arises from the spinal nerve at each spine segment and reenters the spinal canal through the intervertebral foramen at the same level.

APPROACH TO THE PATIENT | **Back Pain**

TYPES OF BACK PAIN Understanding the types of pain reported by patients is the essential first step. Attention is also focused on identification of risk factors for serious underlying diseases; the majority of these are due to radiculopathy, fracture, tumor, infection, or referred pain from visceral structures (Table 15-1).

Local pain is caused by injury to pain-sensitive structures that compress or irritate sensory nerve endings. The site of the pain is near the affected part of the back.

Pain referred to the back may arise from abdominal or pelvic viscera. The pain is usually described as primarily abdominal or pelvic but is accompanied by back pain and usually unaffected by posture. The patient may occasionally complain of back pain only.

TABLE 15-1 Acute Low Back Pain: Risk Factors for an Important Structural Cause

History
Pain worse at rest or at night
Prior history of cancer
History of chronic infection (esp. lung, urinary tract, skin)
History of trauma
Incontinence
Age >70 years
Intravenous drug use
Glucocorticoid use
History of a rapidly progressive neurologic deficit

Examination
Unexplained fever
Unexplained weight loss
Percussion tenderness over the spine
Abdominal, rectal, or pelvic mass
Patrick's sign or heel percussion sign
Straight leg or reverse straight leg–raising signs
Progressive focal neurologic deficit

Pain of spine origin may be located in the back or referred to the buttocks or legs. Diseases affecting the upper lumbar spine tend to refer pain to the lumbar region, groin, or anterior thighs. Diseases affecting the lower lumbar spine tend to produce pain referred to the buttocks, posterior thighs, or rarely the calves or feet. Referred or "sclerotomal" pain may explain instances where the pain crosses multiple dermatomes without evidence of nerve root compression.

Radicular back pain is typically sharp and radiates from the low back to a leg within the territory of a nerve root (see "Lumbar Disk Disease," below). Coughing, sneezing, or voluntary contraction of abdominal muscles (lifting heavy objects or straining at stool) may elicit the radiating pain. The pain may increase in postures that stretch the nerves and nerve roots. Sitting with the leg outstretched places traction on the sciatic nerve and L5 and S1 roots because the nerve passes posterior to the hip. The femoral nerve (L2, L3, and L4 roots) passes anterior to the hip and is not stretched by sitting. The description of the pain alone often fails to distinguish between sclerotomal pain and radiculopathy.

Pain associated with muscle spasm, although of obscure origin, is commonly associated with many spine disorders. The spasms are accompanied by abnormal posture, tense paraspinal muscles, and dull or achy pain in the paraspinal region.

Knowledge of the circumstances associated with the onset of back pain is important when weighing possible serious underlying causes for the pain. Some patients involved in accidents or work-related injuries may exaggerate their pain for the purpose of compensation or for psychological reasons.

EXAMINATION OF THE BACK A physical examination that includes the abdomen and rectum is advisable. Back pain referred from visceral organs may be reproduced during palpation of the abdomen [pancreatitis, abdominal aortic aneurysm (AAA)] or percussion over the costovertebral angles (pyelonephritis).

The normal spine has a cervical and lumbar lordosis, and a thoracic kyphosis. Exaggeration of these normal alignments may result in hyperkyphosis of the thoracic spine or hyperlordosis of the lumbar spine. Inspection may reveal a lateral curvature of the spine (scoliosis) or an asymmetry in the prominence of the paraspinal muscles, suggesting muscle spasm. Back pain of bony spine origin is often reproduced by palpation or percussion over the spinous process of the affected vertebrae.

Forward bending is often limited by paraspinal muscle spasm; the latter may flatten the usual lumbar lordosis. Flexion at the hips is normal in patients with lumbar spine disease, but flexion of the lumbar spine is limited and sometimes painful. Lateral bending to the side opposite the injured spinal element may stretch the damaged tissues, worsen pain, and limit motion. Hyperextension of the spine (with the patient prone or standing) is limited when nerve root compression, facet joint pathology, or other bony spine disease is present.

Pain from hip disease may mimic the pain of lumbar spine disease. Hip pain can be reproduced by internal and external rotation at the hip with the knee and hip in flexion (Patrick's sign) and by tapping the heel with the examiner's palm while the leg is extended (heel percussion sign).

With the patient supine, passive flexion of the extended leg at the hip stretches the L5 and S1 nerve roots and the sciatic nerve (straight leg–raising maneuver). Passive dorsiflexion of the foot during the maneuver adds to the stretch. While flexion to at least 80° is normally possible without causing pain, many patients normally report a tight, stretching sensation in the hamstring muscles unrelated to back pain. The *straight leg–raising (SLR)* test is positive if the maneuver reproduces the patient's usual back or limb pain. Eliciting the SLR sign in the sitting position can help determine if the finding is reproducible. The patient may describe pain in the low back, buttocks, posterior thigh, or lower leg, but the *key feature is reproduction of the patient's usual pain*. The *crossed SLR sign* is positive when flexion of one leg reproduces the usual pain in the opposite leg or buttocks. The crossed SLR sign is less sensitive but more specific for disk herniation than the SLR sign. The nerve or nerve root lesion is always on the side of the pain. The *reverse SLR sign* is elicited by standing the patient next to the examination table and passively extending each leg with the knee fully extended. This maneuver, which stretches the L2-L4 nerve roots, lumbosacral plexus, and femoral nerve, is considered positive if the patient's usual back or limb pain is reproduced.

The neurologic examination includes a search for focal weakness or muscle atrophy, focal reflex changes, diminished sensation in the legs, or signs of spinal cord injury. The examiner should be alert to the possibility of breakaway weakness, defined as fluctuating strength during muscle testing. Breakaway weakness may be due to pain or a combination of pain and underlying true weakness. Breakaway weakness without pain is almost always due to a lack of effort. In uncertain cases, electromyography (EMG) can determine whether or not true weakness due to nerve tissue injury is present. Findings with specific nerve lumbosacral nerve root lesions are shown in Table 15-2 and are discussed below.

LABORATORY, IMAGING, AND EMG STUDIES Routine laboratory studies are rarely needed for the initial evaluation of nonspecific acute (<3 months duration) low back pain (ALBP). If risk factors for a serious underlying cause are present (Table 15-1), then laboratory studies [complete blood count (CBC), erythrocyte sedimentation rate (ESR), urinalysis] are indicated.

CT scanning is superior to routine x-rays for the detection of fractures involving posterior spine structures, craniocervical and craniothoracic junctions, C1 and C2 vertebrae, bone fragments within the spinal canal, or misalignment; CT scans are increasingly used as a primary screening modality for moderate to severe trauma. In the absence of risk factors, these imaging studies are rarely helpful in nonspecific ALBP. MRI and CT-myelography are the radiologic tests of choice for evaluation of most serious diseases involving the spine. MRI is superior for the definition of soft tissue structures, whereas CT-myelography provides optimal imaging of the lateral recess of the spinal canal, and is better tolerated by claustrophobic patients. While the added diagnostic value of modern neuroimaging is significant, there is concern that these studies may be overutilized in patients with benign ALBP.

Electrodiagnostic studies can be used to assess the functional integrity of the peripheral nervous system (Chap. e45). Sensory nerve conduction studies are normal when focal sensory loss is due to nerve root damage because the nerve roots are proximal to the nerve cell bodies in the dorsal root ganglia. Injury to nerve tissue distal to the dorsal root ganglion (e.g., plexus or peripheral nerve) results in reduced sensory nerve signals. Needle EMG complements nerve conduction studies by detecting denervation or reinnervation changes in a myotomal (segmental) distribution. Multiple muscles supplied by different nerve roots and nerves are sampled; the pattern of muscle involvement indicates the nerve root(s) responsible for the injury. Needle EMG provides objective information about motor nerve fiber injury when clinical evaluation of weakness is limited by pain or poor effort. EMG and nerve conduction studies will be normal when sensory nerve root injury or irritation is the source of the pain.

TABLE 15-2 Lumbosacral Radiculopathy—Neurologic Features

Lumbosacral Nerve Roots	Examination Findings			
	Reflex	Sensory	Motor	Pain Distribution
L2[a]	—	Upper anterior thigh	Psoas (hip flexion)	Anterior thigh
L3[a]	—	Lower anterior thigh Anterior knee	Psoas (hip flexion) Quadriceps (knee extension) Thigh adduction	Anterior thigh, knee
L4[a]	Quadriceps (knee)	Medial calf	Quadriceps (knee extension)[b] Thigh adduction Tibialis anterior (foot dorsiflexion)	Knee, medial calf Anterolateral thigh
L5[c]	—	Dorsal surface—foot Lateral calf	Peroneii (foot eversion)[b] Tibialis anterior (foot dorsiflexion) Gluteus medius (hip abduction) Toe dorsiflexors	Lateral calf, dorsal foot, posterolateral thigh, buttocks
S1[c]	Gastrocnemius/soleus (ankle)	Plantar surface—foot Lateral aspect—foot	Gastrocnemius/soleus (foot plantar flexion)[b] Abductor hallucis (toe flexors)[b] Gluteus maximus (hip extension)	Bottom foot, posterior calf, posterior thigh, buttocks

[a]Reverse straight leg–raising sign present—see "Examination of the Back."
[b]These muscles receive the majority of innervation from this root.
[c]Straight leg–raising sign present—see "Examination of the Back."

CAUSES OF BACK PAIN

(Table 15-3)

■ CONGENITAL ANOMALIES OF THE LUMBAR SPINE

Spondylolysis is a bony defect in the vertebral pars interarticularis (a segment near the junction of the pedicle with the lamina); the cause is usually a stress microfracture in a congenitally abnormal segment. It occurs in up to 6% of adolescents. The defect (usually bilateral) is best visualized on plain x-rays, CT scan, or bone scan and is frequently asymptomatic. Symptoms may occur in the setting of a single injury, repeated minor injuries, or growth. Spondylolysis is the most common cause of persistent low back pain in adolescents and is often associated with sports-related activities.

Spondylolisthesis is the anterior slippage of the vertebral body, pedicles, and superior articular facets, leaving the posterior elements behind. Spondylolisthesis can be associated with spondylolysis, congenital anomalies, degenerative spine disease, or other causes of mechanical weakness of the pars (e.g., infection, osteoporosis, tumor, trauma, prior surgery). The slippage may be asymptomatic or may cause low back pain and hamstring tightness, nerve root injury (the L5 root most frequently), symptomatic spinal stenosis, or cauda equina syndrome (CES) in severe cases. Tenderness may be elicited near the segment that has "slipped" forward (most often L4 on L5 or occasionally L5 on S1). A "step" may be present on deep palpation of the posterior elements of the segment above the spondylolisthetic joint. The trunk may be shortened and the abdomen protuberant as a result. Anterolisthesis or retrolisthesis can also occur at other cervical or lumbar levels in adults and be the source of neck or low back pain. Plain x-rays with the neck or low back in flexion and extension will reveal the movement at the abnormal spinal segment. Surgery is considered for pain symptoms that do not respond to conservative measures (e.g., rest, physical therapy), and in cases with progressive neurologic deficit, postural deformity, slippage >50%, or scoliosis.

Spina bifida occulta is a failure of closure of one or several vertebral arches posteriorly; the meninges and spinal cord are normal. A dimple or small lipoma may overlie the defect. Most cases are asymptomatic and discovered incidentally during an evaluation for back pain.

Tethered cord syndrome usually presents as a progressive cauda equina disorder (see below), although myelopathy may also be the initial manifestation. The patient is often a young adult who complains of perineal or perianal pain, sometimes following minor trauma. MRI studies reveal a low-lying conus (below L1-L2) and a short and thickened filum terminale.

■ TRAUMA

A patient complaining of back pain and an inability to move the legs may have a spinal fracture or dislocation, and, with fractures above L1, spinal cord compression. Care must be taken to avoid further damage to the spinal cord or nerve roots by immobilizing the back pending the results of radiologic studies.

Sprains and strains

The terms *low back sprain*, *strain*, and *mechanically induced muscle spasm* refer to minor, self-limited injuries associated with lifting a heavy object, a fall, or a sudden deceleration such as in an automobile accident. These terms are used loosely and do not clearly describe a specific anatomic lesion. The pain is usually confined to the lower back, and there is no radiation to the buttocks or legs. Patients with paraspinal muscle spasm often assume unusual postures.

Traumatic vertebral fractures

Most traumatic fractures of the lumbar vertebral bodies result from injuries producing anterior wedging or compression. With severe trauma, the patient may sustain a fracture-dislocation or a "burst" fracture involving the vertebral body and posterior elements.

TABLE 15-3 Causes of Back or Neck Pain

Congenital/Developmental

Spondylolysis and spondylolisthesis

Kyphoscoliosis

Spina bifida occulta

Tethered spinal cord

Minor Trauma

Strain or sprain

Whiplash injury

Fractures

Trauma—falls, motor vehicle accidents

Atraumatic fractures—osteoporosis, neoplastic infiltration, exogenous steroids, osteomyelitis

Intervertebral Disk Herniation

Degenerative

  Intervertebral foraminal narrowing

  Disk-osteophyte complex

  Internal disk disruption

  LSS with neurogenic claudication

  Uncovertebral joint disease

  Atlantoaxial joint disease (e.g., rheumatoid arthritis)

  Arthritis

  Spondylosis

  Facet or sacroiliac arthropathy

  Neoplasms—metastatic, hematologic, primary bone tumors

Infection/Inflammation

  Vertebral osteomyelitis

  Spinal epidural abscess

  Septic disk (discitis)

  Meningitis

  Lumbar arachnoiditis

  Autoimmune [e.g., ankylosing spondylitis, reactive arthritis (formerly known as Reiter's syndrome)]

Metabolic

  Osteoporosis—hyperparathyroidism, immobility

  Osteosclerosis (e.g., Paget's disease)

Vascular

  Abdominal aortic aneurysm

  Vertebral artery dissection

Other

  Referred pain from visceral disease

  Postural

  Psychiatric, malingering, chronic pain syndromes

Traumatic vertebral fractures are caused by falls from a height (a pars interarticularis fracture of the L5 vertebra is common), sudden deceleration in an automobile accident, or direct injury. Neurologic impairment is common, and early surgical treatment is indicated. In victims of blunt trauma, CT scans of the chest, abdomen, or pelvis can be reformatted to detect associated vertebral fractures.

■ LUMBAR DISK DISEASE

This is a common cause of chronic or recurrent low back and leg pain (Figs. 15-3 and 15-4). Disk disease is most likely to occur at the L4-L5 or L5-S1 levels, but upper lumbar levels are involved occasionally. The cause is often unknown; the risk is increased in overweight individuals. Disk herniation is unusual prior to age 20 years and is rare in the fibrotic disks of the elderly. Genetic factors may play a role in predisposing some patients to disk disease. The pain may be located in the low back only or referred to a leg, buttock, or hip. A sneeze, cough, or trivial movement may cause the nucleus pulposus to prolapse, pushing the frayed and weakened annulus posteriorly. With severe disk disease, the nucleus may protrude through the annulus (herniation) or become extruded to lie as a free fragment in the spinal canal.

The mechanism by which intervertebral disk injury causes back pain is controversial. The inner annulus fibrosus and nucleus pulposus are normally devoid of innervation. Inflammation and production of proinflammatory cytokines within the protruding or ruptured disk may trigger or perpetuate back pain. Ingrowth of nociceptive (pain) nerve fibers into inner portions of a diseased disk may be responsible for chronic "diskogenic" pain. Nerve root injury (radiculopathy) from disk herniation may be due to compression, inflammation, or both; pathologically, demyelination and axonal loss are usually present.

A ruptured disk may be asymptomatic or cause back pain, abnormal posture, limitation of spine motion (particularly flexion), a focal neurologic deficit or radicular pain. A dermatomal pattern of sensory loss or a reduced or absent deep tendon reflex is more suggestive of a specific root lesion than is the pattern of pain. Motor findings (focal weakness, muscle atrophy, or fasciculations) occur less frequently than focal sensory or reflex changes. Symptoms and signs are usually unilateral, but bilateral involvement does occur with large central disk herniations that compress multiple roots or cause inflammation of nerve roots within the spinal canal. Clinical manifestations of specific nerve root lesions are summarized in Table 15-2. There is suggestive evidence that lumbar disk herniation with a nonprogressive nerve root deficit can be managed nonsurgically.

The differential diagnosis covers a variety of serious and treatable conditions, including epidural abscess, hematoma, fracture, or tumor. Fever, constant pain uninfluenced by position, sphincter abnormalities, or signs of spinal cord disease suggest an etiology other than lumbar disk disease. Absence of ankle reflexes can be a normal finding in persons older than age 60 years or a sign of bilateral S1 radiculopathy. An absent deep tendon reflex or focal sensory loss may indicate injury to a nerve root, but other sites of injury along the nerve must also be considered. For example, an absent knee reflex may be due to a femoral neuropathy or an L4 nerve root injury. A loss of sensation over the foot and lateral lower calf may result from a peroneal or lateral sciatic neuropathy or an L5 nerve root injury. Focal muscle atrophy may reflect a nerve root, peripheral nerve, anterior horn cell disease, or disuse.

A lumbar spine MRI scan or CT-myelogram is necessary to establish the location and type of pathology. Spine MRIs yield exquisite views of intraspinal and adjacent soft tissue anatomy. Bony lesions of the lateral recess or intervertebral foramen are optimally visualized by CT-myelography. The correlation of neuroradiologic findings to symptoms, particularly pain, is not simple. Contrast-enhancing

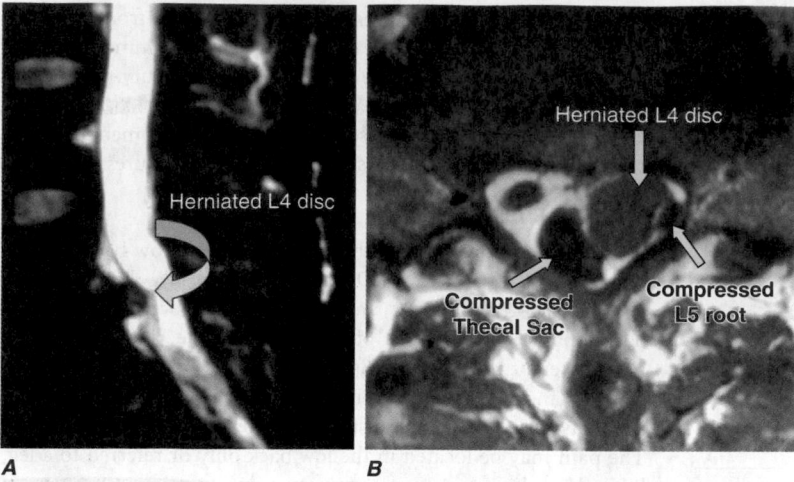

Figure 15-4 Left L5 radiculopathy. *A.* Sagittal T2-weighted image on the left reveals disk herniation at the L4-5 level. *B.* Axial T1-weighted image shows paracentral disk herniation with displacement of the thecal sac medially and the left L5 nerve root posteriorly in the left lateral recess.

tears in the annulus fibrosus or disk protrusions are widely accepted as common sources of back pain; however, studies have found that many asymptomatic adults have similar findings. Asymptomatic disk protrusions are also common and may enhance with contrast. *Furthermore, in patients with known disk herniation treated either medically or surgically, persistence of the herniation 10 years later had no relationship to the clinical outcome.* In summary, MRI findings of disk protrusion, tears in the annulus fibrosus, or contrast enhancement are common incidental findings that, by themselves, should not dictate management decisions for patients with back pain.

The diagnosis of nerve root injury is most secure when the history, examination, results of imaging studies, and the EMG are concordant. The correlation between CT and EMG for localization of nerve root injury is between 65 and 73%. Up to one-third of asymptomatic adults have a lumbar disk protrusion detected by CT or MRI scans.

Management of lumbar disc disease is discussed below.

Cauda equina syndrome (CES) signifies an injury of multiple lumbosacral nerve roots within the spinal canal distal to the termination of the spinal cord at L1-2. Low back pain, weakness and areflexia in the legs, saddle anesthesia, or loss of bladder function may occur. The problem must be distinguished from disorders of the lower spinal cord (conus medullaris syndrome), acute transverse myelitis (Chap. 377), and Guillain-Barré syndrome (Chap. 385). Combined involvement of the conus medullaris and cauda equina can occur. CES is commonly due to a ruptured lumbosacral intervertebral disk, lumbosacral spine fracture, hematoma within the spinal canal (e.g., following lumbar puncture in patients with coagulopathy), compressive tumor, or other mass lesion. Treatment options include surgical decompression, sometimes urgently, in an attempt to restore or preserve motor or sphincter function, or radiotherapy for metastatic tumors (Chap. 379).

■ DEGENERATIVE CONDITIONS

Lumbar spinal stenosis (LSS) describes a narrowed lumbar spinal canal and is frequently asymptomatic. *Neurogenic claudication* is the usual symptom, consisting of back and buttock or leg pain induced by walking or standing and relieved by sitting. Symptoms in the legs are usually bilateral. Lumbar stenosis, by itself, is frequently asymptomatic, and the correlation between the severity of symptoms and degree of stenosis of the spinal canal is poor. Unlike vascular claudication, symptoms are often provoked by standing without walking. Unlike lumbar disk disease, symptoms are usually relieved by sitting. Patients with neurogenic claudication can often walk much farther when leaning over a shopping cart and can pedal a stationary bike while sitting with ease. These flexed positions increase the anteroposterior spinal canal diameter and reduce intraspinal venous hypertension, resulting in pain relief. Focal weakness, sensory loss, or reflex changes may occur when spinal stenosis is associated with neural foraminal narrowing and radiculopathy. Severe neurologic deficits, including paralysis and urinary incontinence, occur only rarely.

LSS can be acquired (75%), congenital, or due to a combination of these factors. Congenital forms (achondroplasia, idiopathic) are characterized by short, thick pedicles that produce both spinal canal and lateral recess stenosis. Acquired factors that contribute to spinal stenosis include degenerative diseases (spondylosis, spondylolisthesis, scoliosis), trauma, spine surgery, metabolic or endocrine disorders (epidural lipomatosis, osteoporosis, acromegaly, renal osteodystrophy, hypoparathyroidism), and Paget's disease. MRI provides the best definition of the abnormal anatomy (Fig. 15-5).

Conservative treatment of symptomatic LSS includes nonsteroidal anti-inflammatory drugs (NSAIDs), acetaminophen, exercise programs, and symptomatic treatment of acute pain episodes. There is insufficient evidence to support the use of epidural glucocorticoid injections. Surgical therapy is considered when medical therapy does not relieve symptoms sufficiently to allow for activities of daily living or when significant focal neurologic signs are present. Most patients with neurogenic claudication treated surgically experience significant relief of back and leg pain within 6 weeks postoperation, and pain relief persists for at least 2 years. Patients treated nonoperatively improve uncommonly. Up to one-quarter develop recurrent stenosis at the same spinal level or an adjacent level 7–10 years after the initial surgery; recurrent symptoms usually respond to a second surgical decompression.

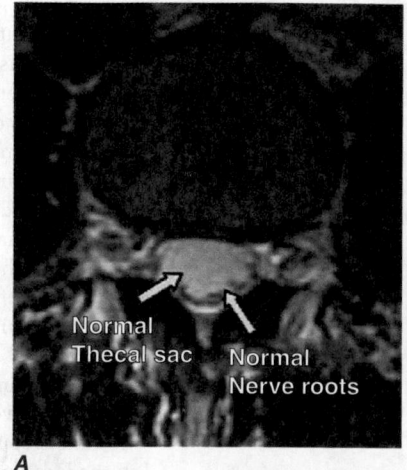
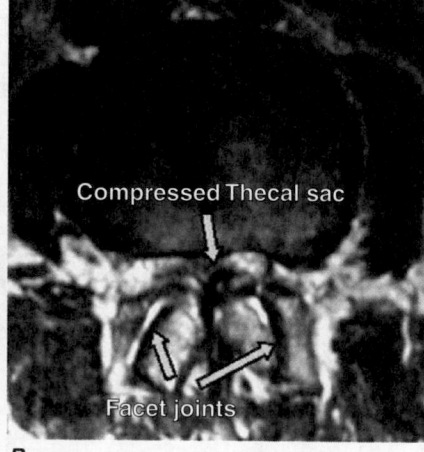

Figure 15-5 Axial T2-weighted images of the lumbar spine. *A.* The image shows a normal thecal sac within the lumbar spinal canal. The thecal sac is bright. The lumbar roots are dark punctuate dots in the posterior thecal sac with the patient supine. *B.* The thecal sac is not well visualized due to severe lumbar spinal canal stenosis, partially the result of hypertrophic facet joints.

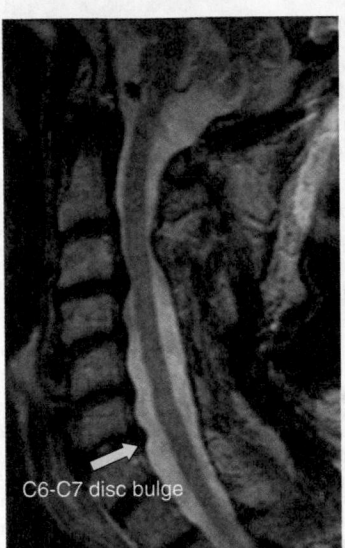

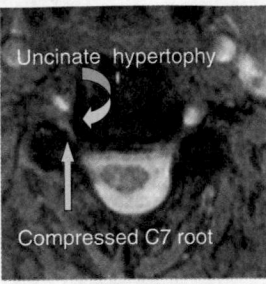

Figure 15-6 Right C7 radiculopathy. A. Sagittal T2-weighted image shows mild disk bulging at C6-C7 and a mildly narrowed spinal canal, but no visible nerve root compression. **B.** Axial T2-weighted image. The combination of uncinate hypertrophy and facet hypertrophy (ovoid dark space just lateral to the C7 root) narrows the right C6-C7 intervertebral foramen resulting in right C7 nerve root compression.

Neural foraminal narrowing with radiculopathy is a common degenerative disorder most often caused by the same processes that cause lumbar spinal stenosis (Figs. 15-1 and 15-6), including osteophytes, lateral disc protrusion, calcified disk-osteophytes, facet joint hypertrophy, uncovertebral joint hypertrophy (cervical spine), congenitally shortened pedicles, or, frequently, a combination of these processes. Neoplasms (primary or metastatic), fractures, infections (epidural abscess), or hematomas are other considerations. These conditions can produce unilateral nerve root symptoms or signs due to bony compression at the intervertebral foramen or lateral recess; symptoms are indistinguishable from disk-related radiculopathy, but treatment may differ depending upon the specific etiology. The history and neurologic examination alone cannot distinguish between these possibilities, and a spinal neuroimaging (CT or MRI) procedure is required to identify the underlying cause. Neurologic findings from the examination and EMG can help direct the attention of the radiologist to specific nerve or root structures that are best visualized on axial images. For *facet joint hypertrophy,* surgical foraminotomy produces long-term relief of leg and back pain in 80–90% of patients. The usefulness of therapeutic facet joint blocks for pain has not been rigorously studied.

ARTHRITIS

Spondylosis, or osteoarthritic spine disease, typically occurs in later life and primarily involves the cervical and lumbosacral spine. Patients often complain of back pain that increases with movement and is associated with stiffness. The relationship between clinical symptoms and radiologic findings is usually not straightforward. Pain may be prominent when x-ray, CT, or MRI findings are minimal, and prominent degenerative spine disease can be seen in asymptomatic patients. Osteophytes or combined disk-osteophytes may cause or contribute to central spinal canal stenosis, lateral recess stenosis, or neural foraminal narrowing.

Ankylosing spondylitis

(See also Chap. 325) This distinctive arthritic spine disease typically presents with the insidious onset of low back and buttock pain.

Patients are often males below age 40. Associated features include morning back stiffness, nocturnal pain, pain unrelieved by rest, an elevated ESR, and the histocompatibility antigen HLA-B27. Onset at a young age and back pain improving with exercise are characteristic. Loss of the normal lumbar lordosis and exaggeration of thoracic kyphosis develop as the disease progresses. Inflammation and erosion of the outer fibers of the annulus fibrosus at the point of contact with the vertebral body are followed by ossification and bony growth that bridges adjacent vertebral bodies and reduces spine mobility in all planes. MRI has been used to assess the presence of inflammation in joints as well as response to treatment and is more sensitive than plain x-rays. In later stages, plain x-rays reveal bridging of vertebral bodies to produce the fused "bamboo spine."

Stress fractures after minimal or no trauma can occur through the spontaneously ankylosed posterior bony elements of the rigid, osteoporotic spine and can produce focal pain, spinal instability, spinal cord compression, or CES. Atlantoaxial subluxation with spinal cord compression can occur in up to 20% of patients over time. Ankylosis of the ribs to the spine and a decrease in the height of the thoracic spine may compromise respiratory function. Therapy with anti–tumor necrosis factor agents is effective in reducing disease activity and improving function. Similar to ankylosing spondylitis, restricted movements may accompany reactive arthritis (formerly known as Reiter's syndrome), psoriatic arthritis, and chronic inflammatory bowel disease.

NEOPLASMS

Back pain is the most common neurologic symptom in patients with systemic cancer and is the presenting symptom in 20%. The cause is usually vertebral body metastasis but can also result from spread of cancer through the intervertebral foramen (especially with lymphoma) or from carcinomatous meningitis. Cancer-related back pain tends to be constant, dull, unrelieved by rest, and worse at night. By contrast, mechanical low back pain usually improves with rest. MRI, CT, and CT-myelography are the studies of choice when spinal metastasis is suspected. Once a metastasis is found, imaging of the entire spine reveals additional tumor deposits in 1/3 of patients. MRI is preferred for soft tissue definition, but the most rapidly available imaging modality is best because the patient's condition may worsen quickly without intervention. Fewer than 5% of patients who are nonambulatory at the time of diagnosis ever regain the ability to walk; thus, early diagnosis is crucial. The management of spinal metastasis is discussed in detail in Chap. 379.

INFECTIONS/INFLAMMATION

Vertebral osteomyelitis is often caused by staphylococci, but other bacteria or tuberculosis (Pott's disease) may be responsible. The primary source of infection is usually the urinary tract, skin, or lungs. Intravenous drug use is a well-recognized risk factor. Whenever pyogenic osteomyelitis is found, the possibility of bacterial endocarditis should be considered. Back pain unrelieved by rest, spine tenderness over the involved spine segment, and an elevated ESR are the most common findings in vertebral osteomyelitis. Fever or an elevated white blood cell count is found in a minority of patients. MRI and CT are sensitive and specific for early detection of osteomyelitis; CT may be more readily available in emergency settings and better tolerated by some patients with severe back pain. The intervertebral disk can also be affected by infection (discitis), and very rarely by tumor.

Spinal epidural abscess (Chap. 377) presents with back pain (aggravated by movement or palpation), fever, radiculopathy, or signs of spinal cord compression. The subacute development of two or more of these findings should increase the index of suspicion for spinal epidural abscess. The abscess may track over multiple spinal levels and is best delineated by spine MRI.

Lumbar adhesive arachnoiditis with radiculopathy is due to fibrosis following inflammation within the subarachnoid space. The fibrosis results in nerve root adhesions, and presents as back and leg pain associated with motor, sensory, or reflex changes. Causes of arachnoiditis include multiple lumbar operations, chronic spinal infections (especially tuberculosis in the developing world), spinal cord injury, intrathecal hemorrhage, myelography (rare), intrathecal injections (glucocorticoids, anesthetics, or other agents), and foreign bodies. The MRI shows clumped nerve roots or loculations of cerebrospinal fluid within the thecal sac. Clumped nerve roots may also occur with demyelinating polyneuropathy or neoplastic infiltration. Treatment is usually unsatisfactory. Microsurgical lysis of adhesions, dorsal rhizotomy, dorsal root ganglionectomy, and epidural steroids have been tried, but outcomes have been poor. Dorsal column stimulation for pain relief has produced varying results.

■ METABOLIC CAUSES

Osteoporosis and osteosclerosis

Immobilization or underlying conditions such as osteomalacia, the postmenopausal state, renal disease, multiple myeloma, hyperparathyroidism, hyperthyroidism, metastatic carcinoma, or glucocorticoid use may accelerate osteoporosis and weaken the vertebral body, leading to compression fractures and pain. Up to two-thirds of compression fractures seen on radiologic imaging are asymptomatic. The most common nontraumatic vertebral body fractures are due to postmenopausal or senile osteoporosis (Chap. 354). The risk of an additional vertebral fracture at 1 year following a first vertebral fracture is 20%. The presence of fever, weight loss, fracture at a level above T4, or other conditions described above should increase the suspicion for a cause other than senile osteoporosis. If tumor is suspected, a bone biopsy or diagnostic search for a primary tumor is indicated. The sole manifestation of a compression fracture may be localized back pain or radicular pain exacerbated by movement and often reproduced by palpation over the spinous process of the affected vertebra. The clinical context, neurologic signs, and radiologic appearance of the spine establish the diagnosis.

Relief of acute pain can often be achieved with acetaminophen or a combination of opioids and acetaminophen. The role of NSAIDs is controversial. Both pain and disability are improved with bracing. Antiresorptive drugs, especially bisphosphonates (e.g., alendronate), have been shown to reduce the risk of osteoporotic fractures and are the preferred treatment to prevent additional fractures. Less than one-third of patients with prior compression fractures are adequately treated for osteoporosis despite the increased risk for future fractures; even fewer at-risk patients without a history of fracture are adequately treated. Interventions [percutaneous vertebroplasty (PVP), kyphoplasty] exist for osteoporotic compression fractures associated with debilitating pain. Controlled studies suggest a benefit for pain reduction acutely, but not at 2 months, when compared with conservative care. Relief of pain following PVP has also been reported in patients with vertebral metastases, myeloma, or hemangiomas.

Osteosclerosis, an abnormally increased bone density often due to Paget's disease, is readily identifiable on routine x-ray studies and can sometimes be a source of back pain. It may be associated with an isolated increase in alkaline phosphatase in an otherwise healthy older person. Spinal cord or nerve root compression can result from bony encroachment. It should not be assumed that Paget's disease is the cause of a patient's back pain until other etiologies have been carefully considered.

For further discussion of these bone disorders, see Chaps. 353–355.

■ REFERRED PAIN FROM VISCERAL DISEASE

Diseases of the thorax, abdomen, or pelvis may refer pain to the posterior portion of the spinal segment that innervates the diseased organ. Occasionally, back pain may be the first and only manifestation. Upper abdominal diseases generally refer pain to the lower thoracic or upper lumbar region (eighth thoracic to the first and second lumbar vertebrae), lower abdominal diseases to the midlumbar region (second to fourth lumbar vertebrae), and pelvic diseases to the sacral region. Local signs (pain with spine palpation, paraspinal muscle spasm) are absent, and little or no pain accompanies routine movements of the spine.

Low Thoracic or Lumbar Pain with Abdominal Disease

Tumors of the posterior wall of the stomach or duodenum typically produce epigastric pain (Chaps. 91 and 293), but midline back or paraspinal pain may occur if retroperitoneal extension is present. Fatty foods occaionally induce back pain associated with biliary disease. Diseases of the pancreas can produce right paraspinal back pain (head of the pancreas involved) or left paraspinal pain (body or tail involved). Pathology in retroperitoneal structures (hemorrhage, tumors, pyelonephritis) can produce paraspinal pain that radiates to the lower abdomen, groin, or anterior thighs. A mass in the iliopsoas region can produce unilateral lumbar pain with radiation toward the groin, labia, or testicle. The sudden appearance of lumbar pain in a patient receiving anticoagulants suggests retroperitoneal hemorrhage.

Isolated low back pain occurs in some patients with a contained rupture of an abdominal aortic aneurysm (AAA). The classic clinical triad of abdominal pain, shock, and back pain occurs in <20% of patients. The typical patient at risk is an elderly male smoker with back pain. Frequently, the diagnosis is initially missed because the symptoms and signs can be nonspecific. Misdiagnoses include nonspecific back pain, diverticulitis, renal colic, sepsis, and myocardial infarction. A careful abdominal examination revealing a pulsatile mass (present in 50–75% of patients) is an important physical finding. Patients with suspected AAA should be evaluated with abdominal ultrasound, CT, or MRI (Chap. 248).

Sacral pain with gynecologic and urologic disease

Pelvic organs rarely cause low back pain, except for gynecologic disorders involving the uterosacral ligaments. The pain is referred to the sacral region. Endometriosis or uterine cancers may invade the uterosacral ligaments. Pain associated with endometriosis is typically premenstrual and often continues until it merges with menstrual pain. Uterine malposition may cause uterosacral ligament traction (retroversion, descensus, and prolapse) or produce sacral pain after prolonged standing.

Menstrual pain may be felt in the sacral region. Poorly localized, cramping pain can radiate down the legs. Pain due to neoplastic infiltration of nerves is typically continuous, progressive in severity, and unrelieved by rest at night. Less commonly, radiation therapy of pelvic tumors may produce sacral pain from late radiation necrosis of tissue. Low back pain that radiates into one or both thighs is common in the last weeks of pregnancy.

Urologic sources of lumbosacral back pain include chronic prostatitis, prostate cancer with spinal metastasis (Chap. 95), and diseases of the kidney or ureter. Lesions of the bladder and testes do not often produce back pain. Infectious, inflammatory, or neoplastic renal diseases may produce ipsilateral lumbosacral pain, as can renal artery or vein thrombosis. Paraspinal lumbar pain may be a symptom of ureteral obstruction due to nephrolithiasis.

OTHER CAUSES OF BACK PAIN

Postural back pain

There is a group of patients with nonspecific chronic low back pain (CLBP) in whom no specific anatomic lesion can be found despite exhaustive investigation. These individuals complain of vague, diffuse back pain with prolonged sitting or standing that is relieved by rest. Exercises to strengthen the paraspinal and abdominal muscles are sometimes helpful.

Psychiatric disease

CLBP may be encountered in patients who seek financial compensation; in malingerers; or in those with concurrent substance abuse. Many patients with CLBP have a history of psychiatric illness (depression, anxiety states), or childhood trauma (physical or sexual abuse) that antedates the onset of back pain. Preoperative psychological assessment has been used to exclude patients with marked psychological impairments that predict a poor surgical outcome from spine surgery.

IDIOPATHIC

The cause of low back pain occasionally remains unclear. Some patients have had multiple operations for disk disease but have persistent pain and disability. The original indications for surgery may have been questionable, with back pain only, no definite neurologic signs, or a minor disk bulge noted on CT or MRI. Scoring systems based upon neurologic signs, psychological factors, physiologic studies, and imaging studies have been devised to minimize the likelihood of unsuccessful surgery.

TREATMENT **Back Pain**

ACUTE LOW BACK PAIN (ALBP) WITHOUT RADICULOPATHY ALBP is defined as pain of <3 months' duration. Full recovery can be expected in 85% of adults with ALBP without leg pain. Most have purely "mechanical" symptoms (i.e., pain that is aggravated by motion and relieved by rest).

The initial assessment excludes serious causes of spine pathology that require urgent intervention, including infection, cancer, or trauma. Risk factors for a serious cause of ALBP are shown in Table 15-1. Laboratory and imaging studies are unnecessary if risk factors are absent. CT or plain spine films are rarely indicated in the first month of symptoms unless a spine fracture is suspected.

The prognosis is generally excellent. Many patients do not seek medical care and apparently improve on their own. Even among those seen in primary care, two-thirds report being substantially improved after seven weeks. This spontaneous improvement can mislead clinicians and researchers about the efficacy of treatment interventions. Perhaps as a result, many ineffective treatments have become widespread in the past, such as bed rest, lumbar traction, sacroiliac fusion, and coccygectomy.

Clinicians should reassure patients that improvement is very likely, and instruct them in self-care. Education is an important part of treatment. Satisfaction and the likelihood of follow-up increase when patients are educated about prognosis, treatment methods, activity modifications, and strategies to prevent future exacerbations. In one study, patients who felt they did not receive an adequate explanation for their symptoms wanted further diagnostic tests. In general, bed rest should be avoided, or kept to a day or two at most, for relief of severe symptoms. Several randomized trials suggest that bed rest does not accelerate the pace of recovery. In general, the best activity

recommendation is for walking and early resumption of normal physical activity, avoiding only strenuous manual labor. Possible advantages of early ambulation for acute back pain include maintenance of cardiovascular conditioning, improved disk and cartilage nutrition, improved bone and muscle strength, and increased endorphin levels. Specific back exercises or early vigorous exercise have not shown benefits for acute back pain, but may be useful for chronic pain. Application of heat by heating pads or heated blankets is sometimes helpful.

Evidence-based guidelines suggest that over-the-counter medicines such as acetaminophen and NSAIDs are first-line options for the treatment of ALBP. Skeletal muscle relaxants, such as cyclobenzaprine or methocarbamol, may be useful, but sedation is a common side effect. Limiting the use of muscle relaxants to nighttime only may be an option for some patients. Because of the risk of abuse of some drugs in this category, including benzodiazepines and carisoprodol, short courses are generally recommended.

It is unclear whether opioid analgesics and tramadol are more effective than NSAIDs or acetaminophen for treating ALBP; most of the available efficacy data are for treatment of chronic back pain. Their use is best reserved for patients who cannot tolerate acetaminophen or NSAIDs, or for those with severe refractory pain. As with muscle relaxants, these drugs are often sedating, so it may be useful to prescribe them at nighttime only. Side effects of short-term opioid use include nausea, constipation and pruritis; risks of long-term opioid use include hypersensitivity to pain, hypogonadism, and dependency.

There is no evidence to support use of oral or injected glucocorticoids for acute low back pain without radiculopathy. Antiepileptic drugs, such as gabapentin, are not FDA approved for treating low back pain, and there is insufficient evidence to support their use in this setting.

Nonpharmacologic treatments for acute low back pain include spinal manipulation, physical therapy, massage, acupuncture, transcutaneous electrical nerve stimulation, ultrasound, diathermy, and magnets. Spinal manipulation appears to be roughly equivalent to conventional medical treatments and may be a useful alternative for patients who wish to avoid or who cannot tolerate drug therapy. There is little evidence to support the use of physical therapy, massage, acupuncture, laser therapy, therapeutic ultrasound, magnets, corsets, or lumbar traction. Though important for chronic pain, back exercises for acute back pain are generally not supported by clinical evidence. There is no useful evidence regarding the value of ice or heat applications for ABLP; many patients report temporary symptomatic relief from ice, and heat may produce a short-term reduction in pain after the first week.

CHRONIC LOW BACK PAIN WITHOUT RADICULOPATHY Chronic low back pain is defined as pain lasting >12 weeks; it accounts for 50% of total back pain costs. Risk factors include obesity, female gender, older age, prior history of back pain, restricted spinal mobility, pain radiating into a leg, high levels of psychological distress, poor self-rated health, minimal physical activity, smoking, job dissatisfaction, and widespread pain. In general, the same treatments that are recommended for acute low back pain can be useful for patients with chronic low back pain. In this setting, however, the benefit of opioid therapy or muscle relaxants is less clear.

Evidence supports the use of exercise therapy, and this can be one of the mainstays of treatment for chronic back pain. Effective regimens have generally included a combination of gradually increasing aerobic exercise, strengthening exercises, and stretching exercises. Motivating patients is sometimes challenging, and supervised exercise is best, for example, with a supportive physical therapist. In general, activity tolerance is the primary goal, while pain relief is secondary. Exercise programs can reverse atrophy in paraspinal muscles and strengthen extensors of the trunk. Supervised intensive physical exercise or "work hardening" regimens have been effective in returning some patients to work, improving walking distance, and reducing pain. In addition, some forms of yoga have been evaluated in randomized trials and may be helpful for patients who are interested.

Medications for chronic low back pain may include acetaminophen, NSAIDs, and tricyclic antidepressants. Trials of the latter suggest some benefit even for patients without evidence of depression. Trials do not support the efficacy of selective serotonin reuptake inhibitors for back pain. However, depression is common among patients with chronic pain and should be appropriately treated.

Cognitive-behavioral therapy is based on evidence that psychological and social factors, as well as somatic pathology, are important in the genesis of chronic pain and disability. The patient's attitudes and beliefs, psychological distress, and patterns of illness behavior may all influence responses to chronic pain. Thus, in addition to addressing pathophysiologic mechanisms, psychological treatments are aimed at reducing disability by modifying cognitive processes and environmental contingencies. Cognitive-behavioral therapy includes efforts to identify and modify patients' thinking about their pain and disability by strategies that may involve imagery, attention diversion, or modifying maladaptive thoughts, feelings, and beliefs. This approach includes educating patients about a multidimensional view of pain, identifying pain-eliciting or pain-aggravating thoughts and feelings, using coping strategies and relaxation techniques, and even hypnosis. A systematic review concluded that such treatments are more effective than a waiting list control group for short-term pain relief; however, long-term results remain unclear. Behavioral treatments may have effects similar in magnitude to exercise therapy.

Back pain is the most common reason for seeking complementary and alternative treatments. The most common of these for back pain are spinal manipulation, acupuncture, and massage. The role of complementary and alternative medicine approaches, aside from spinal manipulation, remains unclear. Biofeedback has not been studied rigorously. As with acute back pain, spinal manipulation may on average offer benefits similar to conventional care. Rigorous recent trials of acupuncture suggest that true acupuncture is not superior to sham acupuncture, but that both may offer an advantage over routine care. Whether this is due entirely to placebo effects or to stimulation provided even by sham acupuncture is uncertain. Some trials of massage therapy have been encouraging, but this has been less well studied than manipulation or acupuncture.

Studies of transcutaneous electrical nerve stimulation (TENS) have reached conflicting conclusions, but a recent evidence-based guideline suggested that there was no convincing evidence for its efficacy in treating chronic back pain.

Various injections, including epidural glucocorticoid injections, facet joint injections, and trigger point injections have been used for treating chronic low back pain. However, in the absence of radiculopathy, there is no evidence that epidural glucocorticoids are effective for treating chronic back pain. Several randomized trials suggest that facet joint injections are not more effective than saline injections, and recent evidence-based guidelines recommend against their use. Similarly, there is little evidence to support the use of trigger point injections. Injection studies are sometimes used diagnostically to help determine the anatomic source of back pain. Reproduction of the patient's typical pain with discography has been used as evidence that a specific disk is the pain generator. Pain relief following a foraminal nerve root block or glucocorticoid injection into a facet has been similarly used as evidence that the facet joint or nerve root is the source. However, the possibility that the injection response was a placebo effect or due to systemic absorption of the glucocorticoids is often not excluded.

Another category of intervention for chronic back pain includes electrothermal and radiofrequency therapies. Intradiscal therapy has been proposed using both types of energy to thermocoagulate and destroy nerves in the intervertebral disc, using specially designed catheters or electrodes. A systematic review has suggested that current evidence does not support the use of these intradiscal therapies.

Radiofrequency denervation is sometimes used to destroy nerves that are thought to mediate pain, and this technique has been used for facet joint pain (with the target nerve being the medial branch of the primary dorsal ramus), for back pain thought to arise from the intervertebral disc (ramus communicans), and radicular back pain (dorsal root ganglia). A few small trials have resulted in conflicting results for facet joint pain. The evidence for presumed discogenic pain and for radicular pain is similarly meager. A trial for patients with chronic radicular pain found no difference between radiofrequency denervation of the dorsal root ganglia and sham treatment. Recent systematic reviews have thus concluded that there is insufficient evidence to reliably evaluate these interventional therapies.

Surgical intervention for chronic low back pain in the absence of radiculopathy has been evaluated in a small number of randomized trials, all conducted in Europe. Each of these studies included patients with back pain and a degenerative disc, but no sciatica. Three of the four trials concluded that lumbar fusion surgery was no more effective than highly structured, rigorous rehabilitation combined with cognitive-behavioral therapy. The fourth trial found an advantage of fusion surgery over haphazard "usual care," which appeared to be less effective than the structured rehabilitation in other trials. Given conflicting evidence, indications for surgery for chronic back pain alone have remained controversial. Both U.S. and British guidelines suggest considering referral for an opinion on spinal fusion for people who have completed an optimal nonsurgical treatment program (including combined physical and psychological treatment) and who have persistent severe back pain for which they would consider surgery.

The newest surgical treatment for degenerated discs with back pain is disc replacement with prosthetic disks. These are generally designed as metal plates with a polyethylene cushion sandwiched in between. The trials that led to approval of these devices compared them to spine fusion, and concluded that the artificial discs were "not inferior." Serious complications appeared to be somewhat more likely with the artificial disc. This treatment remains controversial for low back pain.

Intensive multidisciplinary rehabilitation programs may involve daily or frequent care involving physical therapy, exercise, cognitive-behavioral therapy, a workplace evaluation, and other interventions. For patients who have not responded to other interventions, such programs appear to offer some benefit. Systematic reviews suggest that the evidence is limited and effects are moderate.

Some observers have raised concern that chronic back pain may often be overtreated. The use of opioids, epidural glucocorticoid injections, facet joint injections, and surgical intervention has increased rapidly in the past decade, without corresponding population-level improvements in pain or functioning among patients with back pain. In each case, randomized trials provide only minimal support for these treatments in the setting of chronic back pain without radiculopathy. For low back pain without radiculopathy, new British guidelines explicitly recommend against use of selective serotonin reuptake inhibitors (SSRIs), any type of injection, TENS, lumbar supports, traction, radiofrequency facet joint denervation, intradiscal electrothermal therapy, or intradiscal radio frequency thermocoagulation. Similarly, these treatments are not recommended in guidelines from the American College of Physicians and the American Pain Society. On the other hand, exercise therapy and treatment of depression appear to be underused.

LOW BACK PAIN WITH RADICULOPATHY A common cause of back pain with radiculopathy is a herniated disc with nerve root impingement, resulting in back pain with radiation down the leg. The prognosis for acute low back pain with radiculopathy due to disk herniation (sciatica) is generally favorable, with most patients demonstrating substantial improvement over a matter of months. Serial imaging studies suggest spontaneous regression of the herniated portion of the disc in two-thirds of patients over 6 months. Nonetheless, there are several important treatment options for providing symptom relief while this natural healing process unfolds.

Resumption of normal activity as much as possible is usually the best activity recommendation. Randomized trial evidence suggests that bed rest is ineffective for treating sciatica as well as for back pain alone. Acetaminophen and NSAIDs are appropriate for pain relief, although severe pain may require short courses of opioid analgesics.

Epidural glucocorticoid injections have a role in providing temporary symptom relief for sciatica due to a herniated disc. Although randomized trial evidence is conflicting, there appears to be some overall short-term benefit for pain relief of sciatica. However, there does not appear to be a benefit in terms of reducing subsequent surgical interventions. Diagnostic nerve root blocks have been advocated to determine if pain originates from a specific nerve root. However, improvement may result even when the nerve root is not responsible for the pain; this may occur as a placebo effect, from a pain-generating lesion located distally along the peripheral nerve, or from anesthesia of the sinuvertebral nerve. The utility of diagnostic nerve root blocks remains a subject of debate.

Surgical intervention is indicated for patients who have progressive motor weakness, demonstrated on clinical examination or EMG, as a result of nerve root injury. Urgent surgery is recommended for patients who have evidence of the cauda equina syndrome or spinal cord compression, generally suggested by bowel or bladder dysfunction, diminished sensation in a saddle distribution, a sensory level, bilateral leg weakness, or bilateral leg spasticity.

Surgery is also an important option for patients who have disabling radicular pain despite optimal conservative treatment. Sciatica is perhaps the most common reason for recommending spine surgery. Because patients with a herniated disc and sciatica generally experience rapid improvement over a matter of weeks, most experts do not recommend considering surgery unless the patient has failed to respond to 6–8 weeks of appropriate nonsurgical management. For patients who have not improved, randomized trials indicate that, compared to nonsurgical treatment, surgery results in more rapid pain relief. However, after the first year or two of follow-up, patients with sciatica appear to have much the same level of pain relief and

functional improvement with or without surgery. Thus, both treatment approaches are reasonable, and patient preferences should play a major role in decision making. Some patients will want the fastest possible relief and find surgical risks acceptable. Others will be more risk-averse and more tolerant of symptoms, and will choose watchful waiting if they understand that improvement is likely in the end.

The usual surgical procedure is a partial hemilaminectomy with excision of the prolapsed disk. Fusion of the involved lumbar segments should be considered only if significant spinal instability is present (i.e., degenerative spondylolisthesis). The costs associated with lumbar interbody fusion have increased dramatically in recent years. There are no large prospective, randomized trials comparing fusion to other types of surgical intervention. In one study, patients with persistent low back pain despite an initial diskectomy fared no better with spine fusion than with a conservative regimen of cognitive intervention and exercise. Artificial disks have been in use in Europe for the past decade; their utility remains controversial in the United States.

PAIN IN THE NECK AND SHOULDER

(Table 15-4) Neck pain, which usually arises from diseases of the cervical spine and soft tissues of the neck, is common. Neck pain arising from the cervical spine is typically precipitated by movement and may be accompanied by focal tenderness and limitation of motion. Pain arising from the brachial plexus, shoulder, or peripheral nerves can be confused with cervical spine disease, but the history and examination usually identify a more distal origin for the pain. Cervical spine trauma, disk disease, or spondylosis with intervertebral foraminal narrowing may be asymptomatic or painful and can produce a myelopathy, radiculopathy, or both. The same risk factors for a serious cause of low back pain are thought to apply to neck pain with the addition that neurologic signs of myelopathy (incontinence, sensory level, spastic legs) may also occur. Lhermitte's sign, an electrical shock down the spine with neck flexion, suggests cervical spinal cord involvement from any cause.

■ TRAUMA TO THE CERVICAL SPINE

Trauma to the cervical spine (fractures, subluxation) places the spinal cord at risk for compression. Motor vehicle accidents, violent crimes, or falls account for 87% of cervical spinal cord injuries (Chap. 377). Immediate immobilization of the neck is essential to minimize further spinal cord injury from movement of unstable cervical spine segments. The decision to obtain imaging should be based upon the nature of the injury. The NEXUS low-risk criteria established that normally alert patients without palpation tenderness in the midline; intoxication; neurologic deficits; and painful distracting injuries had a very low likelihood of a clinically significant traumatic injury to the cervical spine. The Canadian C-spine rule recommends that imaging should be obtained following neck region trauma if the patient is >65 years old, has limb paresthesias, or a dangerous mechanism for the injury (e.g., bicycle collision with tree or parked car, fall from height >3 feet or 5 stairs, diving accident). A CT scan is the diagnostic procedure of choice for detection of acute fractures. When traumatic injury to the vertebral arteries or cervical spinal cord is suspected, visualization by MRI with MR angiography is preferred.

Whiplash injury is due to rapid flexion and extension of the neck, usually in automobile accidents, and causes cervical musculoligamental injury. This diagnosis should not be applied to patients with fractures, disk herniation, head injury, focal neurologic findings, or altered consciousness. Up to 50% of persons reporting whiplash injury acutely have persistent neck pain 1 year later.

TABLE 15-4 Cervical Radiculopathy—Neurologic Features

Cervical Nerve Roots	Examination Findings			
	Reflex	Sensory	Motor	Pain Distribution
C5	Biceps	Over lateral deltoid	Supraspinatus* (initial arm abduction) Infraspinatus* (arm external rotation) Deltoid* (arm abduction) Biceps (arm flexion)	Lateral arm, medial scapula
C6	Biceps	Thumb, index fingers Radial hand/forearm	Biceps (arm flexion) Pronator teres (internal forearm rotation)	Lateral forearm, thumb, index finger
C7	Triceps	Middle fingers Dorsum forearm	Triceps* (arm extension) Wrist extensors* Extensor digitorum* (finger extension)	Posterior arm, dorsal forearm, lateral hand
C8	Finger flexors	Little finger Medial hand and forearm	Abductor pollicis brevis (abduction D1) First dorsal interosseous (abduction D2) Abductor digiti minimi (abduction D5)	4th and 5th fingers, medial forearm
T1	Finger flexors	Axilla and medial arm	Abductor pollicis brevis (abduction D1) First dorsal interosseous (abduction D2) Abductor digiti minimi (abduction D5)	Medial arm, axilla

*These muscles receive the majority of innervation from this root.

Once personal compensation for pain and suffering was removed from the Australian health care system, the prognosis for recovery at 1 year from whiplash injury improved also. Imaging of the cervical spine is not cost-effective acutely but is useful to detect disk herniations when symptoms persist for >6 weeks following the injury. Severe initial symptoms have been associated with a poor long-term outcome.

■ CERVICAL DISK DISEASE

Herniation of a lower cervical disk is a common cause of neck, shoulder, arm, or hand pain or tingling. Neck pain, stiffness, and a range of motion limited by pain are the usual manifestations. A herniated cervical disk is responsible for ~25% of cervical radiculopathies. Extension and lateral rotation of the neck narrows the ipsilateral intervertebral foramen and may reproduce radicular symptoms (Spurling's sign). In young persons, acute nerve root compression from a ruptured cervical disk is often due to trauma. Cervical disk herniations are usually posterolateral near the lateral recess. The cervical nerve roots most commonly affected are C7 and C6. Typical patterns of reflex, sensory, and motor changes that accompany specific cervical nerve root lesions are summarized in Table 15-4. While the classic patterns are clinically helpful, there are numerous exceptions because (1) there is overlap in function between adjacent nerve roots, (2) symptoms and signs may be evident in only part of the injured nerve root territory, and (3) the location of pain is the most variable of the clinical features.

■ CERVICAL SPONDYLOSIS

Osteoarthritis of the cervical spine may produce neck pain that radiates into the back of the head, shoulders, or arms, or may be the source of headaches in the posterior occipital region (supplied by the C2-C4 nerve roots). Osteophytes, disk protrusions, or hypertrophic facet or uncovertebral joints may alone or in combination compress one or several nerve roots at the intervertebral foramina (Fig. 15-6);

this compression accounts for 75% of cervical radiculopathies. The roots most commonly affected are C7 and C6. Narrowing of the spinal canal by osteophytes, ossification of the posterior longitudinal ligament (OPLL), or a large central disk may compress the cervical spinal cord. Combinations of radiculopathy and myelopathy may be present. When little or no neck pain accompanies cord compression, the diagnosis may be confused with amyotrophic lateral sclerosis (Chap. 374), multiple sclerosis (Chap. 380), spinal cord tumors, or syringomyelia (Chap. 377). The possibility of cervical spondylosis should be considered even when the patient presents with symptoms or signs in the legs only. MRI is the study of choice to define the anatomic abnormalities, but plain CT is adequate to assess bony spurs, foraminal narrowing, lateral recess stenosis, or OPLL. EMG and nerve conduction studies can localize and assess the severity of the nerve root injury.

■ OTHER CAUSES OF NECK PAIN

Rheumatoid arthritis (RA) (Chap. 321) of the cervical apophyseal joints produces neck pain, stiffness, and limitation of motion. In advanced RA, synovitis of the atlantoaxial joint (C1-C2; Fig. 15-2) may damage the transverse ligament of the atlas, producing forward displacement of the atlas on the axis (atlantoaxial subluxation). Radiologic evidence of atlantoaxial subluxation occurs in 30% of patients with RA. Not surprisingly, the degree of subluxation correlates with the severity of erosive disease. When subluxation is present, careful assessment is important to identify early signs of myelopathy. Occasional patients develop high spinal cord compression leading to quadriparesis, respiratory insufficiency, and death. Surgery should be considered when myelopathy or spinal instability is present. MRI is the imaging modality of choice.

Ankylosing spondylitis can cause neck pain and less commonly atlantoaxial subluxation; surgery may be required to prevent spinal cord compression. Acute *herpes zoster* presents as acute posterior occipital or neck pain prior to the outbreak of vesicles. *Neoplasms* metastatic to the cervical spine, *infections* (osteomyelitis and epidural abscess), and *metabolic bone diseases* may be the cause of neck pain. Neck pain may also be referred from the heart with coronary artery ischemia (cervical angina syndrome).

■ THORACIC OUTLET

The thoracic outlet contains the first rib, the subclavian artery and vein, the brachial plexus, the clavicle, and the lung apex. Injury to these structures may result in postural or movement-induced pain around the shoulder and supraclavicular region. *True neurogenic thoracic outlet syndrome* (TOS) is an uncommon disorder resulting from compression of the lower trunk of the brachial plexus or ventral rami of the C8 or T1 nerve roots most often by an anomalous band of tissue connecting an elongate transverse process at C7 with the first rib. Pain is mild or absent. Signs include weakness and wasting of intrinsic muscles of the hand and diminished sensation on the palmar aspect of the fifth digit. An anteroposterior cervical spine x-ray will show the elongate C7 transverse process, and EMG and nerve conduction studies confirm the diagnosis. Treatment consists of surgical resection of the anomalous band. The weakness and wasting of intrinsic hand muscles typically does not improve, but surgery halts the insidious progression of weakness. *Arterial TOS* results from compression of the subclavian artery by a cervical rib resulting in poststenotic dilatation of the artery and thrombus formation. Blood pressure is reduced in the affected limb, and signs of emboli may be present in the hand. Neurologic signs are absent. Ultrasound can confirm the diagnosis noninvasively. Treatment is with thrombolysis or anticoagulation (with or without embolectomy) and surgical excision of the cervical rib compressing the subclavian artery. *Venous TOS* is due to subclavian vein thrombosis resulting in swelling of the arm and pain. The vein may be compressed by a cervical rib or anomalous scalene muscle. Venography is the diagnostic test of choice. *Disputed TOS* includes a large number of patients with chronic arm and shoulder pain of unclear cause. The lack of sensitive and specific findings on physical examination or laboratory markers for this condition frequently results in diagnostic uncertainty. The role of surgery in disputed TOS is controversial. Multidisciplinary pain management is a conservative approach, although treatment is often unsuccessful.

■ BRACHIAL PLEXUS AND NERVES

Pain from injury to the brachial plexus or peripheral nerves of the arm can occasionally mimic pain of cervical spine origin. Neoplastic infiltration of the lower trunk of the brachial plexus may produce shoulder or supraclavicular pain radiating down the arm, numbness of the fourth and fifth fingers or medial forearm, and weakness of intrinsic hand muscles innervated by the ulnar and median nerves. Delayed radiation injury may produce similar findings, although pain is less often present and almost always less severe. A Pancoast tumor of the lung (Chap. 89) is another cause and should be considered, especially when a Horner's syndrome is present. *Suprascapular neuropathy* may produce severe shoulder pain, weakness, and wasting of the supraspinatus and infraspinatus muscles. *Acute brachial neuritis* is often confused with radiculopathy; the acute onset of severe shoulder or scapular pain is followed typically over days by weakness of the proximal arm and shoulder girdle muscles innervated by the upper brachial plexus. The onset is often preceded by an infection. The long thoracic nerve may be affected; the latter results in a winged scapula. Brachial neuritis may also present as an isolated paralysis of the diaphragm or with involvement of other nerves of the upper limb. Recovery is generally good but may take up to 3 years to be complete.

Occasional cases of carpal tunnel syndrome produce pain and paresthesias extending into the forearm, arm, and shoulder resembling a C5 or C6 root lesion. Lesions of the radial or ulnar nerve can mimic a radiculopathy at C7 or C8, respectively. EMG and nerve conduction studies can accurately localize lesions to the nerve roots, brachial plexus, or peripheral nerves.

For further discussion of peripheral nerve disorders, see Chap. 384.

■ SHOULDER

Pain arising from the shoulder can on occasion mimic pain from the spine. If symptoms and signs of radiculopathy are absent, then the differential diagnosis includes mechanical shoulder pain (tendonitis, bursitis, rotator cuff tear, dislocation, adhesive capsulitis, and cuff impingement under the acromion) and referred pain (subdiaphragmatic irritation, angina, Pancoast tumor). Mechanical pain is often worse at night, associated with local shoulder tenderness and aggravated by abduction, internal rotation, or extension of the arm. Pain from shoulder disease may radiate into the arm or hand, but sensory, motor, and reflex changes are absent.

TREATMENT	Neck Pain Without Radiculopathy

The evidence regarding treatment for neck pain is less complete than that for low back pain. As with low back pain, spontaneous improvement is the norm for acute neck pain, and the usual goal of therapy is to provide symptom relief while natural healing processes proceed.

The evidence in support of nonsurgical treatments for whiplash-associated disorders is generally of poor quality and neither supports nor refutes the effectiveness of common treatments used for symptom relief. Gentle mobilization of the cervical spine combined with exercise programs may be more beneficial than usual care. Evidence is insufficient to recommend for or against the use of cervical traction, neck collars, TENS, ultrasound, diathermy, or massage. The role of acupuncture for neck pain also remains ambiguous, with poor-quality studies and conflicting results.

For patients with neck pain unassociated with trauma, supervised exercise, with or without mobilization, appears to be effective. Exercises often include shoulder rolls and neck stretches. Although there is relatively little evidence about the use of muscle relaxants, analgesics, and NSAIDs in neck pain, many clinicians use these medications in much the same way as for low back pain.

Low-level laser therapy directed at areas of tenderness, local acupuncture points, or a grid of predetermined points is a controversial approach to the treatment of neck pain. The putative benefits might be mediated by anti-inflammatory effects, reduction of skeletal muscle fatigue, or inhibition of transmission at neuromuscular junctions. A 2009 meta-analysis suggested that this treatment may provide greater pain relief than sham therapy for both acute and chronic neck pain. Comparison to other conservative treatment measures is needed.

Although some surgical studies have proposed a role for anterior diskectomy and fusion in patients with neck pain, these studies generally have not been rigorously conducted. A systematic review suggested that there was no valid clinical evidence to support either cervical fusion or cervical disc arthroplasty in patients with neck pain without radiculopathy. Similarly, there is no evidence to support radiofrequency neurotomy or cervical facet injections for neck pain without radiculopathy.

TREATMENT Neck Pain With Radiculopathy

The natural history of neck pain even with radiculopathy is favorable, and many patients will improve without specific therapy. Although there are no randomized trials of NSAIDs for neck pain, a course of NSAIDs, with or without muscle relaxants, may be appropriate initial therapy. Other nonsurgical treatments are commonly used, including opioid analgesics, oral glucocorticoids, cervical traction, and immobilization with a hard or soft cervical collar. However, there are no randomized trials to establish the effectiveness of these treatments in comparison to natural history alone. Soft cervical collars can be modestly helpful by limiting spontaneous and reflex neck movements that exacerbate pain.

As for lumbar radiculopathy, epidural glucocorticoids may provide short-term symptom relief in cervical radiculopathy. If cervical radiculopathy is due to bony compression from cervical spondylosis with foraminal narrowing, then surgical decompression is generally indicated to forestall progression of neurologic signs.

Surgical treatment can produce rapid and substantial symptom relief, although it is unclear whether long-term outcomes are improved over nonsurgical therapy. Reasonable indications for cervical disk surgery include a progressive radicular motor deficit, functionally limiting pain that fails to respond to conservative management, or spinal cord compression.

Surgical treatments include anterior cervical diskectomy alone, laminectomy with discectomy, discectomy with fusion, and disk arthroplasty (implanting an artificial cervical disk). Fusions can be performed with a variety of techniques. The risk of subsequent radiculopathy or myelopathy at cervical segments adjacent to a fusion is ~3% per year and 26% per decade. Although this risk is sometimes portrayed as a late complication of surgery, it may also reflect the natural history of degenerative cervical disk disease. The durability of disk prostheses is uncertain. Available data do not strongly support one surgical technique over another.

FURTHER READINGS

BAGLEY LJ: Imaging of spinal trauma. Radiol Clin North Am 44:1, 2006

BHANGLE SD et al: Back pain made simple: An approach based on principles and evidence. Cleve Clin J Med 76:393, 2009

CASSIDY JD et al: Effect of eliminating compensation for pain and suffering on the outcome of insurance claims for whiplash injury. N Engl J Med 342:1179, 2000

CAVALIER R et al: Spondylolysis and spondylolisthesis in children and adolescents: Diagnosis, natural history, and non-surgical management. J Am Acad Orthop Surg 14:417, 2006

COWAN JA JR et al: Changes in the utilization of spinal fusion in the United States. Neurosurgery 59:1, 2006

DATTA S et al: Systematic assessment of diagnostic accuracy and therapeutic utility of lumbar facet joint interventions. Pain Physician 12:437, 2009

LAMB SE et al: Group cognitive behavioural treatment for low-back pain in primary care: A randomised controlled trial and cost-effectiveness analysis. Lancet 375:916, 2010

MUMMANENI PV et al: Clinical and radiographic analysis of cervical disk arthroplasty compared with allograft fusion: A randomized controlled clinical trial. J Neurosurg Spine 6:198, 2007

PEUL WC et al: Surgery versus prolonged conservative treatment for sciatica. N Engl J Med 356:2245, 2007

WEINSTEIN JN et al: Surgical versus nonsurgical therapy for lumbar spinal stenosis. N Engl J Med 358:794, 2008

WEINSTEIN JN et al: Surgical versus nonsurgical treatment for lumbar degenerative spondylolisthesis. N Engl J Med 356:2257, 2007

WEINSTEIN JN et al: Surgical vs nonoperative treatment for lumbar disc herniation. The spine patient outcomes research trial (SPORT): A randomized trial. JAMA 296:2441, 2006

CHAPTER 16

Fever and Hyperthermia

Charles A. Dinarello
Reuven Porat

Body temperature is controlled by the hypothalamus. Neurons in both the preoptic anterior hypothalamus and the posterior hypothalamus receive two kinds of signals: one from peripheral nerves that transmit information from warmth/cold receptors in the skin and the other from the temperature of the blood bathing the region. These two types of signals are integrated by the thermoregulatory center of the hypothalamus to maintain normal temperature. In a neutral temperature environment, the metabolic rate of humans produces more heat than is necessary to maintain the core body temperature in the range of 36.5–37.5°C (97.7–99.5°F).

A normal body temperature is maintained ordinarily, despite environmental variations, because the hypothalamic thermoregulatory center balances the excess heat production derived from metabolic activity in muscle and the liver with heat dissipation from the skin and lungs. According to studies of healthy individuals 18–40 years of age, the mean oral temperature is 36.8° ± 0.4°C (98.2° ± 0.7°F), with low levels at 6 A.M. and higher levels at 4–6 P.M. The maximum normal oral temperature is 37.2°C (98.9°F) at 6 A.M. and 37.7°C (99.9°F) at 4 P.M.; these values define the 99th percentile for healthy individuals. In light of these studies, an A.M. temperature of >37.2°C (>98.9°F) or a P.M. temperature of >37.7°C (>99.9°F) defines a fever. The normal daily temperature variation is typically 0.5°C (0.9°F). However, in some individuals recovering from a febrile illness, this daily variation can be as great as 1.0°C. During a febrile illness, the diurnal variation usually is maintained, but at higher, febrile levels. The daily temperature variation appears to be fixed in early childhood; in contrast, elderly individuals can exhibit a reduced ability to develop fever, with only a modest fever even in severe infections.

Rectal temperatures are generally 0.4°C (0.7°F) higher than oral readings. The lower oral readings are probably attributable to mouth breathing, which is a factor in patients with respiratory infections and rapid breathing. Lower-esophageal temperatures closely reflect core temperature. Tympanic membrane (TM) thermometers measure radiant heat from the tympanic membrane and nearby ear canal and display that absolute value (unadjusted mode) or a value automatically calculated from the absolute reading on the basis of nomograms relating the radiant temperature measured to actual core temperatures obtained in clinical studies (adjusted mode). These measurements, although convenient, may be more variable than directly determined oral or rectal values. Studies in adults show that readings are lower with unadjusted-mode than with adjusted-mode TM thermometers and that unadjusted-mode TM values are 0.8°C (1.6°F) lower than rectal temperatures.

In women who menstruate, the A.M. temperature is generally lower in the 2 weeks before ovulation; it then rises by ~0.6°C (1°F) with ovulation and remains at that level until menses occur. Body temperature can be elevated in the postprandial state. Pregnancy and endocrinologic dysfunction also affect body temperature.

FEVER VERSUS HYPERTHERMIA

■ FEVER

Fever is an elevation of body temperature that exceeds the normal daily variation and occurs in conjunction with an increase in the hypothalamic set point [e.g., from 37°C to 39°C (98.6°F to 102.2°F)]. This shift of the set point from "normothermic" to febrile levels very much resembles the resetting of the home thermostat to a higher level to raise the ambient temperature in a room. Once the hypothalamic set point is raised, neurons in the vasomotor center are activated and vasoconstriction commences. The individual first notices vasoconstriction in the hands and feet. Shunting of blood away from the periphery to the internal organs essentially decreases heat loss from the skin, and the person feels cold. For most fevers, body temperature increases by 1°–2°C. Shivering, which increases heat production from the muscles, may begin at this time; however, shivering is not required if heat conservation mechanisms raise blood temperature sufficiently. Nonshivering heat production from the liver also contributes to increasing core temperature. In humans, behavioral adjustments (e.g., putting on more clothing or bedding) help raise body temperature by decreasing heat loss.

The processes of heat conservation (vasoconstriction) and heat production (shivering and increased nonshivering thermogenesis) continue until the temperature of the blood bathing the hypothalamic neurons matches the new thermostat setting. Once that point is reached, the hypothalamus maintains the temperature at the febrile level by the same mechanisms of heat balance that function in the afebrile state. When the hypothalamic set point is again reset downward (in response to either a reduction in the concentration of pyrogens or the use of antipyretics), the processes of heat loss through vasodilation and sweating are initiated. Loss of heat by sweating and vasodilation continues until the blood temperature at the hypothalamic level matches the lower setting. Behavioral changes (e.g., removal of clothing) facilitate heat loss.

A fever of >41.5°C (>106.7°F) is called hyperpyrexia. This extraordinarily high fever can develop in patients with severe infections but most commonly occurs in patients with central nervous system (CNS) hemorrhages. In the preantibiotic era, fever due to a variety of infectious diseases rarely exceeded 41.1°C (106°F), and there has been speculation that this natural "thermal ceiling" is mediated by neuropeptides that function as central antipyretics.

In rare cases, the hypothalamic set point is elevated as a result of local trauma, hemorrhage, tumor, or intrinsic hypothalamic malfunction. The term hypothalamic fever sometimes is used to describe elevated temperature caused by abnormal hypothalamic function. However, most patients with hypothalamic damage have subnormal, not supranormal, body temperatures.

■ HYPERTHERMIA

Although most patients with elevated body temperature have fever, there are circumstances in which elevated temperature represents not fever but hyperthermia (also called heat stroke; Table 16-1). Hyperthermia is characterized by an uncontrolled increase in body temperature that exceeds the body's ability to lose heat. The setting of the hypothalamic thermoregulatory center is unchanged. In contrast to fever in infections, hyperthermia does not involve pyrogenic molecules (see "Pyrogens," below). Exogenous heat exposure and endogenous heat production are two mechanisms by which

TABLE 16-1 Causes of Hyperthermia Syndromes

Heat Stroke

Exertional: Exercise in higher than normal heat and/or humidity

Nonexertional: Anticholinergics, including antihistamines; antiparkinsonian drugs; diuretics; phenothiazines

Drug-Induced Hyperthermia

Amphetamines, cocaine, phencyclidine (PCP), methylenedioxymethamphetamine (MDMA; "ecstasy"), lysergic acid diethylamide (LSD), salicylates, lithium, anticholinergics, sympathomimetics

Neuroleptic Malignant Syndrome

Phenothiazines; butyrophenones, including haloperidol and bromperidol; fluoxetine; loxapine; tricyclic dibenzodiazepines; metoclopramide; domperidone; thiothixene; molindone; withdrawal of dopaminergic agents

Serotonin Syndrome

Selective serotonin reuptake inhibitors (SSRIs), monoamine oxidase inhibitors (MAOIs), tricyclic antidepressants

Malignant Hyperthermia

Inhalational anesthetics, succinylcholine

Endocrinopathy

Thyrotoxicosis, pheochromocytoma

Central Nervous System Damage

Cerebral hemorrhage, status epilepticus, hypothalamic injury

Source: After FJ Curley et al (eds): *Intensive Care Medicine*, 3rd ed. Boston, Little, Brown, 1996.

hyperthermia can result in dangerously high internal temperatures. Excessive heat production can easily cause hyperthermia despite physiologic and behavioral control of body temperature. For example, work or exercise in hot environments can produce heat faster than peripheral mechanisms can lose it.

Heat stroke in association with a warm environment may be categorized as exertional or nonexertional. *Exertional heat stroke* typically occurs in individuals exercising at elevated ambient temperatures and/or humidity. In a dry environment and at maximal efficiency, sweating can dissipate ~600 kcal/h, requiring the production of >1 L of sweat. Even in healthy individuals, dehydration or the use of common medications (e.g., over-the-counter antihistamines with anticholinergic side effects) may precipitate exertional heat stroke. *Nonexertional heat stroke* typically occurs in either very young or elderly individuals, particularly during heat waves. According to the Centers for Disease Control and Prevention, there were 7000 deaths attributed to heat injury in the United States from 1979 to 1997. The elderly, the bedridden, persons taking anticholinergic or antiparkinsonian drugs or diuretics, and individuals confined to poorly ventilated and non-air-conditioned environments are most susceptible.

Drug-induced hyperthermia has become increasingly common as a result of the increased use of prescription psychotropic drugs and illicit drugs. Drug-induced hyperthermia may be caused by monoamine oxidase inhibitors (MAOIs), tricyclic antidepressants, and amphetamines and by the illicit use of phencyclidine (PCP), lysergic acid diethylamide (LSD), methylenedioxymethamphetamine (MDMA, "ecstasy"), or cocaine.

Malignant hyperthermia occurs in individuals with an inherited abnormality of skeletal-muscle sarcoplasmic reticulum that causes a rapid increase in intracellular calcium levels in response to

halothane and other inhalational anesthetics or to succinylcholine. Elevated temperature, increased muscle metabolism, muscle rigidity, rhabdomyolysis, acidosis, and cardiovascular instability develop within minutes. This rare condition is often fatal. The *neuroleptic malignant syndrome* occurs in the setting of the use of neuroleptic agents (antipsychotic phenothiazines, haloperidol, prochlorperazine, metoclopramide) or the withdrawal of dopaminergic drugs and is characterized by "lead-pipe" muscle rigidity, extrapyramidal side effects, autonomic dysregulation, and hyperthermia. This disorder appears to be caused by the inhibition of central dopamine receptors in the hypothalamus, which results in increased heat generation and decreased heat dissipation. The *serotonin syndrome*, seen with selective serotonin uptake inhibitors (SSRIs), MAOIs, and other serotonergic medications, has many features that overlap with those of the neuroleptic malignant syndrome (including hyperthermia) but may be distinguished by the presence of diarrhea, tremor, and myoclonus rather than lead-pipe rigidity. Thyrotoxicosis and pheochromocytoma also can cause increased thermogenesis.

It is important to distinguish between fever and hyperthermia since hyperthermia can be rapidly fatal and characteristically does not respond to antipyretics. In an emergency situation, however, making this distinction can be difficult. For example, in systemic sepsis, fever (hyperpyrexia) can be rapid in onset, and temperatures can exceed 40.5°C (104.9°F). Hyperthermia often is diagnosed on the basis of the events immediately preceding the elevation of core temperature—e.g., heat exposure or treatment with drugs that interfere with thermoregulation. In patients with heat stroke syndromes and in those taking drugs that block sweating, the skin is hot but dry, whereas in fever the skin can be cold as a consequence of vasoconstriction. Antipyretics do not reduce the elevated temperature in hyperthermia, whereas in fever—and even in hyperpyrexia—adequate doses of either aspirin or acetaminophen usually result in some decrease in body temperature.

PATHOGENESIS OF FEVER

■ PYROGENS

The term *pyrogen* is used to describe any substance that causes fever. *Exogenous* pyrogens are derived from outside the patient; most are microbial products, microbial toxins, or whole microorganisms. The classic example of an exogenous pyrogen is the lipopolysaccharide (endotoxin) produced by all gram-negative bacteria. Pyrogenic products of gram-positive organisms include the enterotoxins of *Staphylococcus aureus* and the group A and B streptococcal toxins, also called *superantigens*. One staphylococcal toxin of clinical importance is that associated with isolates of *S. aureus* from patients with toxic shock syndrome. These products of staphylococci and streptococci cause fever in experimental animals when injected intravenously at concentrations of 1–10 μg/kg. Endotoxin is a highly pyrogenic molecule in humans: When it is injected intravenously into volunteers, a dose of 2–3 ng/kg produces fever, leukocytosis, acute-phase proteins, and generalized symptoms of malaise.

■ PYROGENIC CYTOKINES

Cytokines are small proteins (molecular mass, 10,000–20,000 Da) that regulate immune, inflammatory, and hematopoietic processes. For example, the elevated leukocytosis seen in several infections with an absolute neutrophilia is the result of the cytokines interleukin (IL) 1 and IL-6. Some cytokines also cause fever; formerly referred to as *endogenous pyrogens*, they are now called *pyrogenic cytokines*. The pyrogenic cytokines include IL-1, IL-6, tumor necrosis factor (TNF), ciliary neurotropic factor (CNTF), and interferon (IFN) α. (IL-18, a member of the IL-1 family, does not appear to be a pyrogenic cytokine.) Other pyrogenic cytokines probably exist. Each cytokine is encoded by a separate gene, and each pyrogenic cytokine has been shown to cause fever in laboratory animals and in humans. When injected into humans, IL-1 and TNF produce fever at low doses (10–100 ng/kg); in contrast, for IL-6, a dose of 1–10 μg/kg is required for fever production.

A wide spectrum of bacterial and fungal products induce the synthesis and release of pyrogenic cytokines, as do viruses. However, fever can be a manifestation of disease in the absence of microbial infection. For example, inflammatory processes, trauma, tissue necrosis, and antigen-antibody complexes can induce the production of IL-1, TNF, and/or IL-6, which—individually or in combination—trigger the hypothalamus to raise the set point to febrile levels.

■ ELEVATION OF THE HYPOTHALAMIC SET POINT BY CYTOKINES

During fever, levels of prostaglandin E_2 (PGE_2) are elevated in hypothalamic tissue and the third cerebral ventricle. The concentrations of PGE_2 are highest near the circumventricular vascular organs (organum vasculosum of lamina terminalis)—networks of enlarged capillaries surrounding the hypothalamic regulatory centers. Destruction of these organs reduces the ability of pyrogens to produce fever. Most studies in animals have failed to show, however, that pyrogenic cytokines pass from the circulation into the brain itself. Thus, it appears that both exogenous and endogenous pyrogens interact with the endothelium of these capillaries and that this interaction is the first step in initiating fever—i.e., in raising the set point to febrile levels.

The key events in the production of fever are illustrated in Fig. 16-1. As has been mentioned, several cell types can produce pyrogenic cytokines. Pyrogenic cytokines such as IL-1, IL-6, and TNF are released from the cells and enter the systemic circulation. Although the systemic effects of these circulating cytokines lead to fever by inducing the synthesis of PGE_2, they also induce PGE_2 in peripheral tissues. The increase in PGE_2 in the periphery accounts for the nonspecific myalgias and arthralgias that often accompany fever. It is thought that some systemic PGE_2 escapes destruction by the lung and gains access to the hypothalamus via the internal carotid. However, it is the elevation of PGE_2 in the brain that starts the process of raising the hypothalamic set point for core temperature.

There are four receptors for PGE_2, and each signals the cell in different ways. Of the four receptors, the third (EP-3) is essential for

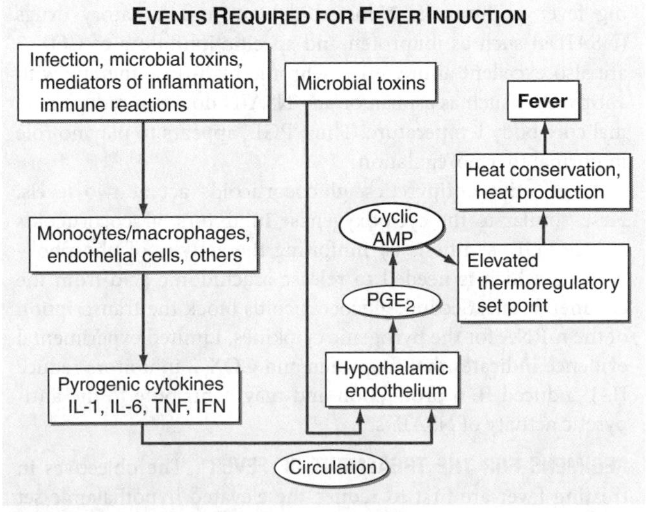

fever: when the gene for this receptor is deleted in mice, no fever follows the injection of IL-1 or endotoxin. Deletion of the other PGE_2 receptor genes leaves the fever mechanism intact. Although PGE_2 is essential for fever, it is not a neurotransmitter. Rather, the release of PGE_2 from the brain side of the hypothalamic endothelium triggers the PGE_2 receptor on glial cells, and this stimulation results in the rapid release of cyclic adenosine 5′-monophosphate (cyclic AMP), which is a neurotransmitter. As shown in Fig. 16-1, the release of cyclic AMP from the glial cells activates neuronal endings from the thermoregulatory center that extend into the area. The elevation of cyclic AMP is thought to account for changes in the hypothalamic set point either directly or indirectly (by inducing the release of neurotransmitters). Distinct receptors for microbial products are located on the hypothalamic endothelium. These receptors are called *Toll-like receptors* and are similar in many ways to IL-1 receptors. The direct activation of Toll-like receptors also results in PGE_2 production and fever.

■ PRODUCTION OF CYTOKINES IN THE CNS

Cytokines produced in the brain may account for the hyperpyrexia of CNS hemorrhage, trauma, or infection. Viral infections of the CNS induce microglial and possibly neuronal production of IL-1, TNF, and IL-6. In experimental animals, the concentration of a cytokine required to cause fever is several orders of magnitude lower with direct injection into the brain substance or brain ventricles than with systemic injection. Therefore, cytokines produced in the CNS can raise the hypothalamic set point, bypassing the circumventricular organs. CNS cytokines probably account for the hyperpyrexia of CNS hemorrhage, trauma, or infection.

APPROACH TO THE PATIENT | **Fever or Hyperthermia**

PHYSICAL EXAMINATION The chronology of events preceding the fever (e.g., exposure to other infected individuals or to vectors of disease) should be ascertained. Electronic devices for measuring oral, tympanic membrane, and rectal temperatures are reliable, but the same site should be used consistently to monitor a febrile disease. Moreover, physicians should be aware that newborns, elderly patients, patients with chronic hepatic or renal failure, and patients taking glucocorticoids may have infections in the absence of fever.

LABORATORY TESTS The workup should include a complete blood count; a differential count should be performed manually or with an instrument sensitive to the identification of juvenile or band forms, toxic granulations, and Döhle bodies, which are suggestive of bacterial infection. Neutropenia may be present with some viral diseases.

Measurement of circulating cytokines in patients with fever is of little use since levels of pyrogenic cytokines in the circulation often are below the detection limit of the assay or do not coincide with fever. In patients with low-grade fevers, the most valuable measurements are C-reactive protein level and erythrocyte sedimentation rate. These markers of inflammatory processes are particularly helpful in detecting the possible presence of occult disease. Acute-phase reactants are discussed in Chap. 271.

FEVER IN RECIPIENTS OF ANTICYTOKINE THERAPY With the increasing use of anticytokines to reduce the activity of IL-1, IL-6, IL-12, or TNF in Crohn's disease, rheumatoid arthritis, or psoriasis, the potential of these therapies to blunt the febrile response must be considered. Chronic administration of anticytokines to block cytokine activity has the distinct clinical drawback of lowering the level of host defenses against both

---

EVENTS REQUIRED FOR FEVER INDUCTION

Figure 16-1 Chronology of events required for the induction of fever. AMP, adenosine 5′-monophosphate; IFN, interferon; IL, interleukin; PGE_2, prostaglandin E_2; TNF, tumor necrosis factor.

routine bacterial and opportunistic infections. The opportunistic infections reported in patients treated with agents that neutralize TNF-α are similar to those reported in the HIV-1-infected population (e.g., new infection with or reactivation of *Mycobacterium tuberculosis*, with dissemination). In nearly all reported cases of infection associated with anticytokine therapy, fever is among the presenting signs. However, the extent to which the febrile response is blunted in these patients remains unknown. This situation is similar to that in patients receiving high-dose glucocorticoid therapy or anti-inflammatory agents such as ibuprofen. Therefore, low-grade fever is of considerable concern in patients receiving anticytokine therapies. The physician must undertake early and rigorous diagnostic evaluation of these patients.

TREATMENT   Fever or Hyperthermia

THE DECISION TO TREAT FEVER   Most fevers are associated with self-limited infections, such as common viral diseases. The use of antipyretics is not contraindicated in these infections: there is no significant clinical evidence that antipyretics delay the resolution of viral or bacterial infections, nor is there evidence that fever facilitates recovery from infection or acts as an adjuvant to the immune system. In short, routine treatment of fever and its symptoms with antipyretics does no harm and does not slow the resolution of common viral and bacterial infections.

However, with bacterial infections, withholding antipyretic therapy can be helpful in evaluating the effectiveness of a particular antibiotic, particularly in the absence of positive cultures of the infecting organism. Therefore, the routine use of antipyretics can mask an inadequately treated bacterial infection. Withholding antipyretics in some cases may facilitate the diagnosis of an unusual febrile disease. Temperature-pulse dissociation (relative bradycardia) occurs in typhoid fever, brucellosis, leptospirosis, some drug-induced fevers, and factitious fever. In newborns, the elderly, patients with chronic hepatic or renal failure, and patients taking glucocorticoids, fever may not be present despite infection. Hypothermia can be observed in patients with septic shock.

Some infections have characteristic patterns in which febrile episodes are separated by intervals of normal temperature. For example, *Plasmodium vivax* causes fever every third day, whereas fever occurs every fourth day with *P. malariae*. Another relapsing fever is related to *Borrelia* infection, with days of fever followed by a several-day afebrile period and then a relapse of days of fever. In the Pel-Ebstein pattern, fever lasting 3–10 days is followed by afebrile periods of 3–10 days; this pattern can be classic for Hodgkin's disease and other lymphomas. In cyclic neutropenia, fevers occur every 21 days and accompany the neutropenia. There is no periodicity of fever in patients with familial Mediterranean fever. However, these patterns have limited or no diagnostic value compared with specific and rapid laboratory tests.

ANTICYTOKINE THERAPY TO REDUCE FEVER IN AUTOIMMUNE AND AUTOINFLAMMATORY DISEASES   Recurrent fever is documented at some point in most autoimmune diseases but in all autoinflammatory diseases. Although fever also can be a manifestation of autoimmune diseases, recurrent fevers are characteristic of autoinflammatory diseases. The autoinflammatory diseases (Table 16-2) include adult and juvenile Still's disease, familial Mediterranean fever, and hyper-IgD syndrome. In addition to recurrent fevers, neutrophilia and serosal inflammation

TABLE 16-2   Autoinflammatory Diseases

Adult and juvenile Still's disease
Cryopyrin-associated periodic syndromes (CAPS)
Familial Mediterranean fever
Hyper-IgD syndrome
Behçet's syndrome
Macrophage activation syndrome
Normocomplementemic urticarial vasculitis
Antisynthetase myositis
PAPA[a] syndrome
Blau syndrome
Gouty arthritis

[a] Pyogenic arthritis, pyoderma gangrenosum, and acne.

characterize autoinflammatory diseases. The fevers associated with these illnesses are reduced dramatically by blocking of IL-1β activity. Anticytokines therefore reduce fever in autoimmune and autoinflammatory diseases. Although fevers in autoinflammatory diseases are mediated by IL-1β, these patients also respond to antipyretics.

MECHANISMS OF ANTIPYRETIC AGENTS   The reduction of fever by lowering of the elevated hypothalamic set point is a direct function of reducing the level of PGE_2 in the thermoregulatory center. The synthesis of PGE_2 depends on the constitutively expressed enzyme cyclooxygenase. The substrate for cyclooxygenase is arachidonic acid released from the cell membrane, and this release is the rate-limiting step in the synthesis of PGE_2. Therefore, inhibitors of cyclooxygenase are potent antipyretics. The antipyretic potency of various drugs is directly correlated with the inhibition of brain cyclooxygenase. Acetaminophen is a poor cyclooxygenase inhibitor in peripheral tissue and lacks noteworthy anti-inflammatory activity; in the brain, however, acetaminophen is oxidized by the p450 cytochrome system, and the oxidized form inhibits cyclooxygenase activity. Moreover, in the brain, the inhibition of another enzyme, COX-3, by acetaminophen may account for the antipyretic effect of this agent. However, COX-3 is not found outside the CNS.

Oral aspirin and acetaminophen are equally effective in reducing fever in humans. Nonsteroidal anti-inflammatory drugs (NSAIDs) such as ibuprofen and specific inhibitors of COX-2 are also excellent antipyretics. Chronic high-dose therapy with antipyretics such as aspirin or any NSAID does not reduce normal core body temperature. Thus, PGE_2 appears to play no role in normal thermoregulation.

As effective antipyretics, glucocorticoids act at two levels. First, similar to the cyclooxygenase inhibitors, glucocorticoids reduce PGE_2 synthesis by inhibiting the activity of phospholipase A_2, which is needed to release arachidonic acid from the cell membrane. Second, glucocorticoids block the transcription of the mRNA for the pyrogenic cytokines. Limited experimental evidence indicates that ibuprofen and COX-2 inhibitors reduce IL-1–induced IL-6 production and may contribute to the antipyretic activity of NSAIDs.

REGIMENS FOR THE TREATMENT OF FEVER   The objectives in treating fever are first to reduce the elevated hypothalamic set point and second to facilitate heat loss. Reducing fever with antipyretics also reduces systemic symptoms of headache, myalgias, and arthralgias.

Oral aspirin and NSAIDs effectively reduce fever but can adversely affect platelets and the gastrointestinal tract. Therefore, use of acetaminophen is preferred as an antipyretic. In children, acetaminophen or oral ibuprofen must be used because aspirin increases the risk of Reye's syndrome. If the patient cannot take oral antipyretics, parenteral preparations of NSAIDs and rectal suppositories of various antipyretics can be used.

Treatment of fever in some patients is highly recommended. Fever increases the demand for oxygen (i.e., for every increase of 1°C over 37°C, there is a 13% increase in oxygen consumption) and can aggravate the condition of patients with preexisting impairment of cardiac, pulmonary, or CNS function. Children with a history of febrile or nonfebrile seizure should be treated aggressively to reduce fever. However, it is unclear what triggers the febrile seizure, and there is no correlation between absolute temperature elevation and onset of a febrile seizure in susceptible children.

In hyperpyrexia, the use of cooling blankets facilitates the reduction of temperature; however, cooling blankets should not be used without oral antipyretics. In hyperpyretic patients with CNS disease or trauma (CNS bleeding), reducing core temperature mitigates the detrimental effects of high temperature on the brain.

TREATING HYPERTHERMIA A high core temperature in a patient with an appropriate history (e.g., environmental heat exposure or treatment with anticholinergic or neuroleptic drugs, tricyclic antidepressants, succinylcholine, or halothane) along with appropriate clinical findings (dry skin, hallucinations, delirium, pupil dilation, muscle rigidity, and/or elevated levels of creatine phosphokinase) suggests hyperthermia. Antipyretics are of no use in treating hyperthermia. Physical cooling with sponging, fans, cooling blankets, and even ice baths should be initiated immediately in conjunction with the administration of IV fluids and appropriate pharmacologic agents (see below). If sufficient cooling is not achieved by external means, internal cooling can be achieved by gastric or peritoneal lavage with iced saline. In extreme circumstances, hemodialysis or even cardiopulmonary bypass with cooling of blood may be performed.

Malignant hyperthermia should be treated immediately with cessation of anesthesia and IV administration of dantrolene sodium. The recommended dose of dantrolene is 1–2.5 mg/kg given intravenously every 6 h for at least 24–48 h—until oral dantrolene can be administered, if needed. Dantrolene at similar doses is indicated in the neuroleptic malignant syndrome and in drug-induced hyperthermia and may even be useful in the hyperthermia of the serotonin syndrome and thyrotoxicosis. The neuroleptic malignant syndrome also may be treated with bromocriptine, levodopa, amantadine, or nifedipine or by induction of muscle paralysis with curare and pancuronium. Tricyclic antidepressant overdose may be treated with physostigmine.

FURTHER READINGS

DE KONING HD et al: Beneficial response to anakinra and thalidomide in Schnitzler's syndrome. Ann Rheum Dis 65:542, 2006

DINARELLO CA: Immunological and inflammatory functions of the interleukin-1 family. Annu Rev Immunol 27:519, 2009

——: Infection, fever, and exogenous and endogenous pyrogens: Some concepts have changed. J Endotoxin Res 10:202, 2004

HAWKINS PN et al: Spectrum of clinical features in Muckle-Wells syndrome and response to anakinra. Arthritis Rheum 50:607, 2004

HOFFMAN HM et al: Prevention of cold-associated acute inflammation in familial cold autoinflammatory syndrome by interleukin-1 receptor antagonist. Lancet 364:1779, 2004

KASTNER DL et al: Autoinflammatory disease reloaded: A clinical perspective. Cell 140:784; 2010

KEANE J et al: Tuberculosis associated with infliximab, a tumor necrosis factor-α-neutralizing agent. N Engl J Med 345:1098, 2001

PASCUAL V et al: Role of interleukin-1 (IL-1) in the pathogenesis of systemic onset juvenile idiopathic arthritis and clinical response to IL-1 blockade. J Exp Med 201:1479, 2005

SIMON A, VAN DER MEER JW: Pathogenesis of familial periodic fever syndromes or hereditary autoinflammatory syndromes. Am J Physiol Regul Integr Comp Physiol 292:R86, 2007

—— et al: Beneficial response to interleukin-1 receptor antagonist in TRAPS. Am J Med 117:208, 2004

WALLIS RS et al: Differential effects of TNF blockers on TB immunity. Ann Rheum Dis 64(Suppl 3):132, 2005

—— et al: Granulomatous infectious diseases associated with tumor necrosis factor antagonists. Clin Infect Dis 38:1261, 2004

CHAPTER 17

Fever and Rash

Elaine T. Kaye
Kenneth M. Kaye

The acutely ill patient with fever and rash often presents a diagnostic challenge for physicians. The distinctive appearance of an eruption in concert with a clinical syndrome may facilitate a prompt diagnosis and the institution of life-saving therapy or critical infection-control interventions. Representative images of many of the rashes discussed in this chapter are included in Chap. e7.

APPROACH TO THE PATIENT   Fever and Rash

A thorough history of patients with fever and rash includes the following relevant information: immune status, medications taken within the previous month, specific travel history, immunization status, exposure to domestic pets and other animals, history of animal (including arthropod) bites, existence of cardiac abnormalities, presence of prosthetic material, recent exposure to ill individuals, and exposure to sexually transmitted diseases. The history should also include the site of the onset of the rash and its direction and rate of spread.

A thorough physical examination entails close attention to the rash, with an assessment and precise definition of its salient features. First, it is critical to determine the *type* of lesions that make up the eruption. *Macules* are flat lesions defined by an area of changed color (i.e., a blanchable erythema). *Papules* are raised, solid lesions <5 mm in diameter; *plaques* are lesions >5 mm in diameter with a flat, plateaulike surface; and *nodules* are lesions >5 mm in diameter with a more rounded configuration. *Wheals* (urticaria, hives) are papules or plaques that are pale pink and may appear annular (ringlike) as they enlarge; classic (nonvasculitic) wheals are transient, lasting only 24 h in any defined area. *Vesicles* (<5 mm) and *bullae* (>5 mm) are circumscribed, elevated lesions containing fluid. *Pustules* are raised lesions containing purulent exudate; vesicular processes such as varicella or herpes simplex may evolve to pustules. *Nonpalpable purpura* is a flat lesion that is due to bleeding into the skin. If <3 mm in diameter, the purpuric lesions are termed *petechiae*; if >3 mm, they are termed *ecchymoses*. *Palpable purpura* is a raised lesion that is due to inflammation of the vessel wall (vasculitis) with subsequent hemorrhage. An *ulcer* is a defect in the skin extending at least into the upper layer of the dermis, and an *eschar* (tâche noire) is a necrotic lesion covered with a black crust.

Other pertinent features of rashes include their *configuration* (i.e., annular or target), the *arrangement* of their lesions, and their *distribution* (i.e., central or peripheral).

For further discussion, see Chaps. 51, 53, and 121.

CLASSIFICATION OF RASH

This chapter reviews rashes that reflect systemic disease, but it does not include localized skin eruptions (i.e., cellulitis, impetigo) that may also be associated with fever (Chap. 125). This chapter does not intend to be all-inclusive, but it covers the most important and most common diseases associated with fever and rash. Rashes are classified herein on the basis of the morphology and distribution of lesions. For practical purposes, this classification system is based on the most typical disease presentations. However, morphology may vary as rashes evolve, and the presentation of diseases with rashes is subject to many variations (Chap. 53). For instance, the classic petechial rash of Rocky Mountain spotted fever (RMSF) (Chap. 174) may initially consist of blanchable erythematous macules distributed peripherally; at times, however, the rash associated with RMSF may not be predominantly acral or no rash may develop at all.

Diseases with fever and rash may be classified by type of eruption: centrally distributed maculopapular, peripheral, confluent desquamative erythematous, vesiculobullous, urticaria-like, nodular, purpuric, ulcerated, or eschar. Diseases are listed by these categories in Table 17-1, and many are highlighted in the text. However, for a more detailed discussion of each disease associated with a rash, the reader is referred to the chapter dealing with that specific disease. (Reference chapters are cited in the text and listed in Table 17-1.)

■ CENTRALLY DISTRIBUTED MACULOPAPULAR ERUPTIONS

Centrally distributed rashes, in which lesions are primarily truncal, are the most common type of eruption. The rash of *rubeola* (measles) starts at the hairline 2–3 days into the illness and moves down the body, sparing the palms and soles (Chap. 192). It begins as discrete erythematous lesions, which become confluent as the rash spreads. Koplik's spots (1- to 2-mm white or bluish lesions with an erythematous halo on the buccal mucosa) are pathognomonic for measles and are generally seen during the first 2 days of symptoms. They should not be confused with Fordyce's spots (ectopic sebaceous glands), which have no erythematous halos and are found in the mouth of healthy individuals. Koplik's spots may briefly overlap with the measles exanthem.

Rubella (German measles) also spreads from the hairline downward; unlike that of measles, however, the rash of rubella tends to clear from originally affected areas as it migrates, and it may be pruritic (Chap. 193). Forchheimer spots (palatal petechiae) may develop but are nonspecific because they also develop in mononucleosis (Chap. 181) and scarlet fever (Chap. 136). Postauricular and suboccipital adenopathy and arthritis are common among adults with rubella. Exposure of pregnant women to ill individuals should be avoided, as rubella causes severe congenital abnormalities. Numerous strains of enteroviruses (Chap. 191), primarily echoviruses and coxsackieviruses, cause nonspecific syndromes of fever and eruptions that may mimic rubella or measles. Patients with infectious mononucleosis caused by Epstein-Barr virus (Chap. 181) or with primary infection caused by HIV (Chap. 189) may exhibit pharyngitis, lymphadenopathy, and a nonspecific maculopapular exanthem.

The rash of *erythema infectiosum* (fifth disease), which is caused by human parvovirus B19, primarily affects children 3–12 years old; it develops after fever has resolved as a bright blanchable erythema on the cheeks ("slapped cheeks") with perioral pallor (Chap. 184). A more diffuse rash (often pruritic) appears the next day on the trunk and extremities and then rapidly develops into a lacy reticular eruption that may wax and wane (especially with temperature change) over 3 weeks. Adults with fifth disease often have arthritis, and fetal hydrops can develop in association with this condition in pregnant women.

Exanthem subitum (roseola) is caused by human herpesvirus 6 and is most common among children <3 years of age (Chap. 182). As in erythema infectiosum, the rash usually appears after fever has subsided. It consists of 2- to 3-mm rose-pink macules and papules that rarely coalesce, which occur initially on the trunk and sometimes on the extremities (sparing the face) and fade within 2 days.

TABLE 17-1 Diseases Associated With Fever and Rash

Disease	Etiology	Description	Group Affected/ Epidemiologic Factors	Clinical Syndrome	Chapter
Centrally Distributed Maculopapular Eruptions					
Acute meningococ-cemia[a]	—	—	—	—	143
Drug-induced hypersensitivity syndrome/drug reaction with eosinophilia and systemic symptoms (DIHS/DRESS)[b]	—	—	—	—	55
Rubeola (measles, first disease)	Paramyxovirus	Discrete lesions that become confluent as rash spreads from hairline downward, sparing palms and soles; lasts ≥3 days; Koplik's spots	Nonimmune individuals	Cough, conjunctivitis, coryza, severe prostration	192
Rubella (German measles, third disease)	Togavirus	Spreads from hairline downward, clearing as it spreads; Forschheimer spots	Nonimmune individuals	Adenopathy, arthritis	193
Erythema infectiosum (fifth disease)	Human parvovirus B19	Bright-red "slapped-cheeks" appearance followed by lacy reticular rash that waxes and wanes over 3 weeks; rarely, papular-purpuric "gloves-and-socks" syndrome on hands and feet	Most common among children 3–12 years old; occurs in winter and spring	Mild fever; arthritis in adults; rash following resolution of fever	184
Exanthem subitum (roseola, sixth disease)	Human herpesvirus 6	Diffuse maculopapular eruption over trunk and neck; resolves within 2 days	Usually affects children <3 years old	Rash following resolution of fever; similar to Boston exanthem (echovirus 16); febrile seizures may occur	182
Primary HIV infection	HIV	Nonspecific diffuse macules and papules; less commonly, urticarial or vesicular oral or genital ulcers	Individuals recently infected with HIV	Pharyngitis, adenopathy, arthralgias	189
Infectious mononucleosis	Epstein-Barr virus	Diffuse maculopapular eruption (5% of cases; 90% if ampicillin is given); urticaria, petechiae in some cases; periorbital edema (50%); palatal petechiae (25%)	Adolescents, young adults	Hepatosplenomegaly, pharyngitis, cervical lymphadenopathy, atypical lymphocytosis, heterophile antibody	181
Other viral exanthems	Echoviruses 2, 4, 9, 11, 16, 19, 25; coxsackieviruses A9, B1, B5; etc.	Wide range of skin findings that may mimic rubella or measles	Affect children more commonly than adults	Nonspecific viral syndromes	191
Exanthematous drug-induced eruption	Drugs (antibiotics, anticonvulsants, diuretics, etc.)	Intensely pruritic, bright-red macules and papules, symmetric on trunk and extremities; may become confluent	Occurs 2–3 days after exposure in previously sensitized individuals; otherwise, after 2–3 weeks (but can occur anytime, even shortly after drug is discontinued)	Variable findings: fever and eosinophilia	55
Epidemic typhus	*Rickettsia prowazekii*	Maculopapular eruption appearing in axillae, spreading to trunk and later to extremities; usually spares face, palms, soles; evolves from blanchable macules to confluent eruption with petechiae; rash evanescent in recrudescent typhus (Brill-Zinsser disease)	Exposure to body lice; occurrence of recrudescent typhus as relapse after 30–50 years	Headache, myalgias; 10–40% mortality if untreated; milder clinical presentation in recrudescent form	174
Endemic (murine) typhus	*Rickettsia typhi*	Maculopapular eruption, usually sparing palms, soles	Exposure to rat or cat fleas	Headache, myalgias	174

(continued)

TABLE 17-1 Diseases Associated With Fever and Rash (*Continued*)

Disease	Etiology	Description	Group Affected/ Epidemiologic Factors	Clinical Syndrome	Chapter
Centrally Distributed Maculopapular Eruptions (*continued*)					
Scrub typhus	*Orientia tsutsugamushi*	Diffuse macular rash starting on trunk; eschar at site of mite bite	Endemic in South Pacific, Australia, Asia; transmitted by mites	Headache, myalgias, regional adenopathy; mortality up to 30% if untreated	174
Rickettsial spotted fevers	*Rickettsia conorii* (boutonneuse fever), *Rickettsia australis* (North Queensland tick typhus), *Rickettsia sibirica* (Siberian tick typhus), and others	Eschar common at bite site; maculopapular (rarely, vesicular and petechial) eruption on proximal extremities, spreading to trunk and face	Exposure to ticks; *R. conorii* in Mediterranean region, India, Africa; *R. australis* in Australia; *R. sibirica* in Siberia, Mongolia	Headache, myalgias, regional adenopathy	174
Human monocytotropic ehrlichiosis[c]	*Ehrlichia chaffeensis*	Maculopapular eruption (40% of cases), involves trunk and extremities; may be petechial	Tick-borne; most common in U.S. Southeast, southern Midwest, and mid-Atlantic regions	Headache, myalgias, leukopenia	174
Leptospirosis	*Leptospira interrogans*	Maculopapular eruption; conjunctivitis; scleral hemorrhage in some cases	Exposure to water contaminated with animal urine	Myalgias; aseptic meningitis; *fulminant form*: icterohemorrhagic fever (Weil's disease)	171
Lyme disease	*Borrelia burgdorferi*	Papule expanding to erythematous annular lesion with central clearing (erythema migrans; average diameter, 15 cm), sometimes with concentric rings, sometimes with indurated or vesicular center; multiple secondary erythema migrans lesions in some cases	Bite of tick vector	Headache, myalgias, chills, photophobia occurring acutely; CNS disease, myocardial disease, arthritis weeks to months later in some cases	173
Southern tick-associated rash illness (STARI, Master's disease)	*Borrelia lonestari*	Similar to erythema migrans of Lyme disease with several differences, including: multiple secondary lesions less likely; lesions tending to be smaller (average diameter, ~8 cm); central clearing more likely	Bite of tick vector *Amblyomma americanum* (Lone Star tick); often found in regions where Lyme disease is uncommon, including southern United States	Compared with Lyme disease: fewer constitutional symptoms, tick bite more likely to be recalled; other Lyme disease sequelae lacking	173
Typhoid fever	*Salmonella typhi*	Transient, blanchable erythematous macules and papules, 2–4 mm, usually on trunk (rose spots)	Ingestion of contaminated food or water (rare in U.S.)	Variable abdominal pain and diarrhea; headache, myalgias, hepatosplenomegaly	153
Dengue fever[d]	Dengue virus (4 serotypes; flaviviruses)	Rash in 50% of cases; initially diffuse flushing; midway through illness, onset of maculopapular rash, which begins on trunk and spreads centrifugally to extremities and face; pruritus, hyperesthesia in some cases; after defervescence, petechiae on extremities in some cases	Occurs in tropics and subtropics; transmitted by mosquito	Headache, musculoskeletal pain ("breakbone fever"); leukopenia; occasionally biphasic ("saddleback") fever	196
Rat-bite fever (sodoku)	*Spirillum minus*	Eschar at bite site; then blotchy violaceous or red-brown rash involving trunk and extremities	Rat bite; primarily found in Asia; rare in U.S.	Regional adenopathy, recurrent fevers if untreated	e24
Relapsing fever	*Borrelia* species	Central rash at end of febrile episode; petechiae in some cases	Exposure to ticks or body lice	Recurrent fever, headache, myalgias, hepatosplenomegaly	172

(*continued*)

TABLE 17-1 Diseases Associated With Fever and Rash (*Continued*)

Disease	Etiology	Description	Group Affected/ Epidemiologic Factors	Clinical Syndrome	Chapter
Centrally Distributed Maculopapular Eruptions (*continued*)					
Erythema marginatum (rheumatic fever)	Group A *Streptococcus*	Erythematous annular papules and plaques occurring as polycyclic lesions in waves over trunk, proximal extremities; evolving and resolving within hours	Patients with rheumatic fever	Pharyngitis preceding polyarthritis, carditis, subcutaneous nodules, chorea	322
Systemic lupus erythematosus	Autoimmune disease	Macular and papular erythema, often in sun-exposed areas; discoid lupus lesions (local atrophy, scale, pigmentary changes); periungual telangiectasis; malar rash; vasculitis sometimes causing urticaria, palpable purpura; oral erosions in some cases	Most common in young to middle-aged women; flares precipitated by sun exposure	Arthritis; cardiac, pulmonary, renal, hematologic, and vasculitic disease	319
Still's disease	Autoimmune disease	Transient 2- to 5-mm erythematous papules appearing at height of fever on trunk, proximal extremities; lesions evanescent	Children and young adults	High spiking fever, polyarthritis, splenomegaly; erythrocyte sedimentation rate, >100 mm/h	337
African trypanosomiasis	*Trypanosoma brucei rhodesiense/ gambiense*	Blotchy or annular erythematous macular and papular rash (trypanid), primarily on trunk; pruritus; chancre at site of tsetse fly bite may precede rash by several weeks	Tsetse fly bite in East (*T. brucei rhodesiense*) or West (*T. brucei gambiense*) Africa	Hemolymphatic disease followed by meningoencephalitis; Winterbottom's sign (posterior cervical lymphadenopathy) (*T. brucei gambiense*)	213
Arcanobacterial pharyngitis	*Arcanobacterium (Corynebacterium) haemolyticum*	Diffuse, erythematous, maculopapular eruption involving trunk and proximal extremities; may desquamate	Children and young adults	Exudative pharyngitis, lymphadenopathy	138
Peripheral Eruptions					
Chronic meningococcemia, disseminated gonococcal infection,[a] human parvovirus B19 infection[e]	—	—	—	—	143, 144, 184
Rocky Mountain spotted fever	*Rickettsia rickettsii*	Rash beginning on wrists and ankles and spreading centripetally; appears on palms and soles later in disease; lesion evolution from blanchable macules to petechiae	Tick vector; widespread but more common in southeastern and southwest-central U.S.	Headache, myalgias, abdominal pain; mortality up to 40% if untreated	174
Secondary syphilis	*Treponema pallidum*	Coincident primary chancre in 10% of cases; copper-colored, scaly papular eruption, diffuse but prominent on palms and soles; rash never vesicular in adults; condyloma latum, mucous patches, and alopecia in some cases	Sexually transmitted	Fever, constitutional symptoms	169
Chikungunya fever	Chikungunya virus	Maculopapular eruption; prominent on upper extremities and face, but can also occur on trunk and lower extremities	*Aedes aegypti* and *A. albopictus* mosquito bites; primarily in Africa and Indian Ocean region	Severe polyarticular, migratory arthralgias, especially involving small joints (e.g., hands, wrists, ankles)	196
Hand-foot-and-mouth disease	Coxsackievirus A16 most common cause	Tender vesicles, erosions in mouth; 0.25-cm papules on hands and feet with rim of erythema evolving into tender vesicles	Summer and fall; primarily children <10 years old; multiple family members	Transient fever	191

(*continued*)

TABLE 17-1 Diseases Associated With Fever and Rash (*Continued*)

Disease	Etiology	Description	Group Affected/ Epidemiologic Factors	Clinical Syndrome	Chapter
Peripheral Eruptions (*continued*)					
Erythema multiforme (EM)	Infection, drugs, idiopathic causes	Target lesions (central erythema surrounded by area of clearing and another rim of erythema) up to 2 cm; symmetric on knees, elbows, palms, soles; spreads centripetally; papular, sometimes vesicular; when extensive and involving mucous membranes, termed *EM major*	Herpes simplex virus or *Mycoplasma pneumoniae* infection; drug intake (i.e., sulfa, phenytoin, penicillin)	50% younger than 20 years old; fever more common in most severe form, EM major, which can be confused with Stevens-Johnson syndrome (but EM major lacks prominent skin sloughing)	—*f*
Rat-bite fever (Haverhill fever)	*Streptobacillus moniliformis*	Maculopapular eruption over palms, soles, and extremities; tends to be more severe at joints; eruption sometimes becoming generalized; may be purpuric; may desquamate	Rat bite, ingestion of contaminated food	Myalgias; arthritis (50%); fever recurrence in some cases	e24
Bacterial endocarditis	*Streptococcus*, *Staphylococcus*, etc.	*Subacute course*: Osler's nodes (tender pink nodules on finger or toe pads); petechiae on skin and mucosa; splinter hemorrhages. *Acute course (Staphylococcus aureus)*: Janeway lesions (painless erythematous or hemorrhagic macules, usually on palms and soles)	Abnormal heart valve (*Streptococcus*), intravenous drug use	New or changing heart murmur	124
Confluent Desquamative Erythemas					
Scarlet fever (second disease)	Group A *Streptococcus* (pyrogenic exotoxins A, B, C)	Diffuse blanchable erythema beginning on face and spreading to trunk and extremities; circumoral pallor; "sandpaper" texture to skin; accentuation of linear erythema in skin folds (Pastia's lines); enanthem of white evolving into red "strawberry" tongue; desquamation in second week	Most common among children 2–10 years old; usually follows group A streptococcal pharyngitis	Fever, pharyngitis, headache	136
Kawasaki disease	Idiopathic causes	Rash similar to scarlet fever (scarlatiniform) or erythema multiforme; fissuring of lips, strawberry tongue; conjunctivitis; edema of hands, feet; desquamation later in disease	Children <8 years old	Cervical adenopathy, pharyngitis, coronary artery vasculitis	53, 326
Streptococcal toxic shock syndrome	Group A *Streptococcus* (associated with pyrogenic exotoxin A and/or B or certain M types)	When present, rash often scarlatiniform	May occur in setting of severe group A streptococcal infections (e.g., necrotizing fasciitis, bacteremia, pneumonia)	Multiorgan failure, hypotension; 30% mortality rate	136
Staphylococcal toxic shock syndrome	*S. aureus* (toxic shock syndrome toxin 1, enterotoxin B or C)	Diffuse erythema involving palms; pronounced erythema of mucosal surfaces; conjunctivitis; desquamation 7–10 days into illness	Colonization with toxin-producing *S. aureus*	Fever >39°C (>102°F), hypotension, multiorgan dysfunction	135
Staphylococcal scalded-skin syndrome	*S. aureus*, phage group II	Diffuse tender erythema, often with bullae and desquamation; Nikolsky's sign	Colonization with toxin-producing *S. aureus*; occurs in children <10 years old (termed "Ritter's disease" in neonates) or adults with renal dysfunction	Irritability; nasal or conjunctival secretions	135

(*continued*)

TABLE 17-1 Diseases Associated With Fever and Rash (*Continued*)

Disease	Etiology	Description	Group Affected/ Epidemiologic Factors	Clinical Syndrome	Chapter
Confluent Desquamative Erythemas (*continued*)					
Exfoliative erythro-derma syndrome	Underlying psoriasis, eczema, drug eruption, mycosis fungoides	Diffuse erythema (often scaling) interspersed with lesions of underlying condition	Usually occurs in adults over age 50; more common among men	Fever, chills (i.e., difficulty with thermoregulation); lymphadenopathy	52, 55
DIHS/DRESS	Aromatic anticonvulsants; other drugs, including sulfonamides, minocycline	Maculopapular eruption (mimicking exanthematous drug rash) sometimes progressing to exfoliative erythroderma; profound edema, especially facial; pustules may occur	Individuals genetically unable to detoxify arene oxides (anticonvulsants), patients with slow *N*-acetylating capacity (sulfonamides)	Lymphadenopathy, multiorgan failure (especially hepatic), eosinophilia, atypical lymphocytes; mimics sepsis	55
Stevens-Johnson syndrome (SJS), toxic epidermal necrolysis (TEN)	Drugs (80% of cases; often allopurinol, anticonvulsants, antibiotics), infection, idiopathic	Erythematous and purpuric macules, sometimes targetoid, or diffuse erythema progressing to bullae, with sloughing and necrosis of entire epidermis; Nikolsky's sign; involves mucosal surfaces; TEN (>30% epidermal necrosis) is maximal form; SJS involves <10%; SJS/TEN overlap involves 10–30% of epidermis	Uncommon among children; more common among patients with HIV infection, SLE, certain HLA types, or slow acetylators	Dehydration, sepsis sometimes resulting from lack of normal skin integrity; up to 30% mortality	55
Vesiculobullous or Pustular Eruptions					
Hand-foot-and-mouth syndrome[g]; staphylo-coccal scalded-skin syndrome; toxic epidermal necrolysis[b]; DIHS/DRESS[b]	—	—	—	—	—[f]
Varicella (chickenpox)	Varicella-zoster virus	Macules (2–3 mm) evolving into papules, then vesicles (sometimes umbilicated), on an erythematous base ("dewdrops on a rose petal"); pustules then forming and crusting; lesions appearing in crops; may involve scalp, mouth; intensely pruritic	Usually affects children; 10% of adults susceptible; most common in late winter and spring	Malaise; generally mild disease in healthy children; more severe disease with complications in adults and immunocompromised children	180
Pseudomonas "hot-tub" folliculitis	*Pseudomonas aeruginosa*	Pruritic erythematous follicular, papular, vesicular, or pustular lesions that may involve axillae, buttocks, abdomen, and especially areas occluded by bathing suits; can manifest as tender isolated nodules on palmar or plantar surfaces (the latter designated "*Pseudomonas* hot-foot syndrome")	Bathers in hot tubs or swimming pools; occurs in outbreaks	Earache, sore eyes and/or throat; generally self-limited	152
Variola (smallpox)	Variola major virus	Red macules on tongue, palate evolving to papules and vesicles; skin macules evolving to papules, then vesicles, then pustules over 1 week, with subsequent lesion crusting; lesions initially appearing on face and spreading centrifugally from trunk to extremities; differs from varicella in that (1) skin lesions in any given area are at same stage of development and (2) there is a prominent distribution of lesions on face and extremities (including palms, soles)	Nonimmune individuals exposed to smallpox	Prodrome of fever, headache, backache, myalgias; vomiting in 50% of cases	221

(*continued*)

TABLE 17-1 Diseases Associated With Fever and Rash (*Continued*)

Disease	Etiology	Description	Group Affected/ Epidemiologic Factors	Clinical Syndrome	Chapter
Vesiculobullous or Pustular Eruptions (*continued*)					
Primary herpes simplex virus (HSV) infection	HSV	Erythema rapidly followed by hallmark painful *grouped vesicles* that may evolve into pustules that ulcerate, especially on mucosal surfaces; lesions at site of inoculation: commonly gingivostomatitis for HSV-1 and genital lesions for HSV-2; recurrent disease milder (e.g., herpes labialis does not involve oral mucosa)	Primary infection most common among children and young adults for HSV-1 and among sexually active young adults for HSV-2; no fever in recurrent infection	Regional lymphadenopathy	179
Disseminated herpesvirus infection	Varicella-zoster virus or HSV	Generalized vesicles that can evolve to pustules and ulcerations; individual lesions similar for varicella-zoster and HSV. *Zoster cutaneous dissemination*: >25 lesions extending outside involved dermatome. *HSV*: extensive, progressive mucocutaneous lesions that may occur in absence of dissemination, sometimes disseminate in eczematous skin (eczema herpeticum); HSV visceral dissemination may occur with only localized mucocutaneous disease; in disseminated neonatal disease, skin lesions diagnostically helpful when present, but rash absent in a substantial minority of cases	Patients with immunosuppression, eczema; neonates	Visceral organ involvement (especially liver) in some cases; neonatal disease particularly severe	179, 180, 381
Rickettsialpox	*Rickettsia akari*	Eschar found at site of mite bite; generalized rash involving face, trunk, extremities; may involve palms and soles; <100 papules and plaques (2–10 mm); tops of lesions developing vesicles that may evolve into pustules	Seen in urban settings; transmitted by mouse mites	Headache, myalgias, regional adenopathy; mild disease	174
Acute generalized eruptive pustulosis (AGEP)	Drugs (mostly anticonvulsants or antimicrobials); also viral	Tiny sterile nonfollicular pustules on erythematous, edematous skin; begins on face and in body folds, then becomes generalized	Appears 2–21 days after start of drug therapy, depending on whether previously sensitized	Acute fever, pruritus, leukocytosis	55
Disseminated *Vibrio vulnificus* infection	*V. vulnificus*	Erythematous lesions evolving into hemorrhagic bullae and then into necrotic ulcers	Patients with cirrhosis, diabetes, renal failure; exposure by ingestion of contaminated saltwater, seafood	Hypotension; 50% mortality	156
Ecthyma gangrenosum	*P. aeruginosa*, other gram-negative rods, fungi	Indurated plaque evolving into hemorrhagic bulla or pustule that sloughs, resulting in eschar formation; erythematous halo; most common in axillary, groin, perianal regions	Usually affects neutropenic patients; occurs in up to 28% of individuals with *Pseudomonas* bacteremia	Clinical signs of sepsis	152
Urticaria-like Eruptions					
Urticarial vasculitis	Serum sickness, often due to infection (including hepatitis B, enteroviral, parasitic), drugs; connective tissue disease	Erythematous, edematous "urticaria-like" plaques, pruritic or burning; unlike urticaria: typical lesion duration >24 h (up to 5 days) and lack of complete lesion blanching with compression due to hemorrhage	Patients with serum sickness (including hepatitis B), connective tissue disease	Fever variable; arthralgias/arthritis	326[f]

(continued)

TABLE 17-1 Diseases Associated With Fever and Rash (*Continued*)

Disease	Etiology	Description	Group Affected/ Epidemiologic Factors	Clinical Syndrome	Chapter
Nodular Eruptions					
Disseminated infection	Fungi (e.g., candidiasis, histoplasmosis, cryptococcosis, sporotrichosis, coccidioidomycosis); mycobacteria	Subcutaneous nodules (up to 3 cm); fluctuance, draining common with mycobacteria; necrotic nodules (extremities, periorbital or nasal regions) common with *Aspergillus, Mucor*	Immunocompromised hosts (i.e., bone marrow transplant recipients, patients undergoing chemotherapy, HIV-infected patients, alcoholics)	Features vary with organism	—[f]
Erythema nodosum (septal panniculitis)	Infections (e.g., streptococcal, fungal, mycobacterial, yersinial); drugs (e.g., sulfas, penicillins, oral contraceptives); sarcoidosis; idiopathic causes	Large, violaceous, nonulcerative, subcutaneous nodules; exquisitely tender; usually on lower legs but also on upper extremities	More common among girls and women 15–30 years old	Arthralgias (50%); features vary with associated condition	—[f]
Sweet's syndrome (acute febrile neutrophilic dermatosis)	Yersinial infection; lymphoproliferative disorders; idiopathic causes	Tender red or blue edematous nodules giving impression of vesiculation; usually on face, neck, upper extremities; when on lower extremities, may mimic erythema nodosum	More common among women and among persons 30–60 years old; 20% of cases associated with malignancy (men and women equally affected in this group)	Headache, arthralgias, leukocytosis	53
Bacillary angiomatosis	*Bartonella henselae, B. quintana*	Many forms, including erythematous, smooth vascular nodules; friable, exophytic lesions; erythematous plaques (may be dry, scaly); subcutaneous nodules (may be erythematous)	Usually patients with HIV infection	Peliosis of liver and spleen in some cases; lesions sometimes involving multiple organs; bacteremia	160
Purpuric Eruptions					
Rocky Mountain spotted fever, rat-bite fever, endocarditis[g]; epidemic typhus[e]; dengue fever[d]; human parvovirus B19 infection[e]	—	—	—	—	—[f]
Acute meningococcemia	*Neisseria meningitidis*	Initially pink maculopapular lesions evolving into petechiae; petechiae rapidly becoming numerous, sometimes enlarging and becoming vesicular; trunk, extremities most commonly involved; may appear on face, hands, feet; may include purpura fulminans (see below) reflecting disseminated intravascular coagulation	Most common among children, individuals with asplenia or terminal complement component deficiency (C5–C8)	Hypotension, meningitis (sometimes preceded by upper respiratory infection)	143
Purpura fulminans	Severe disseminated intravascular coagulation	Large ecchymoses with sharply irregular shapes evolving into hemorrhagic bullae and then into black necrotic lesions	Individuals with sepsis (e.g., involving *N. meningitidis*), malignancy, or massive trauma; asplenic patients at high risk for sepsis	Hypotension	143, 271
Chronic meningococcemia	*N. meningitidis*	Variety of recurrent eruptions, including pink maculopapular; nodular (usually on lower extremities); petechial (sometimes developing vesicular centers); purpuric areas with pale blue-gray centers	Individuals with complement deficiencies	Fevers, sometimes intermittent; arthritis, myalgias, headache	143

(continued)

TABLE 17-1 Diseases Associated With Fever and Rash (*Continued*)

Disease	Etiology	Description	Group Affected/ Epidemiologic Factors	Clinical Syndrome	Chapter
Purpuric Eruptions (*continued*)					
Disseminated gonococcal infection	*Neisseria gonorrhoeae*	Papules (1–5 mm) evolving over 1–2 days into hemorrhagic pustules with gray necrotic centers; hemorrhagic bullae occurring rarely; lesions (usually <40) distributed peripherally near joints (more commonly on upper extremities)	Sexually active individuals (more often females), some with complement deficiency	Low-grade fever, tenosynovitis, arthritis	144
Enteroviral petechial rash	Usually echovirus 9 or coxsackievirus A9	Disseminated petechial lesions (may also be maculopapular, vesicular, or urticarial)	Often occurs in outbreaks	Pharyngitis, headache; aseptic meningitis with echovirus 9	191
Viral hemorrhagic fever	Arboviruses (including dengue) and arenaviruses	Petechial rash	Residence in or travel to endemic areas, other virus exposure	Triad of fever, shock, hemorrhage from mucosa or gastrointestinal tract	196, 197
Thrombotic thrombocytopenic purpura/ hemolytic-uremic syndrome	Idiopathic, *Escherichia coli* 0157:H7 (Shiga toxin), drugs	Petechiae	Individuals with *E. coli* 0157:H7 gastroenteritis (especially children), cancer chemotherapy, HIV infection, autoimmune diseases; pregnant/ postpartum women	Fever (not always present), hemolytic anemia, thrombocytopenia, renal dysfunction, neurologic dysfunction; coagulation studies normal	53, 106, 115, 149, 154
Cutaneous small-vessel vasculitis (leukocytoclastic vasculitis)	Infections (including group A *Streptococcus*, viral hepatitis), drugs, chemicals, food allergens, idiopathic causes	Palpable purpuric lesions appearing in crops on legs or other dependent areas; may become vesicular or ulcerative; usually resolve over 3–4 weeks	Occurs in a wide spectrum of diseases, including connective tissue disease, cryoglobulinemia, malignancy, Henoch-Schönlein purpura (HSP); more common among children	Fever, malaise, arthralgias, myalgias; systemic vasculitis in some cases; renal, joint, and gastrointestinal involvement commonly seen in HSP	53
Eruptions with Ulcers and/or Eschars					
Scrub typhus, rickettsial spotted fevers, rat-bite fever[e]; rickettsialpox, ecthyma gangrenosum[h]	—	—	—	—	—[f]
Tularemia	*Francisella tularensis*	Ulceroglandular form: erythematous, tender papule evolves into necrotic, tender ulcer with raised borders; in 35% of cases, eruptions (maculopapular, vesiculopapular, acneiform, urticarial, erythema nodosum, or erythema multiforme) may occur	Exposure to ticks, biting flies, infected animals	Fever, headache, lymphadenopathy	158
Anthrax	*Bacillus anthracis*	Pruritic papule enlarging and evolving into a 1- by 3-cm painless ulcer surrounded by vesicles and then developing a central eschar with edema; residual scar	Exposure to infected animals or animal products, other exposure to anthrax spores	Lymphadenopathy, headache	221

[a]See "Purpuric eruptions."

[b]See "Confluent desquamative erythemas."

[c]In human granulocytotropic ehrlichiosis or anaplasmosis (caused by *Anaplasma phagocytophila;* most common in the upper midwestern and northeastern regions of the United States), rash is rare.

[d]See "Viral hemorrhagic fever" under "Purpuric eruptions" for dengue hemorrhagic fever/dengue shock syndrome.

[e]See "Centrally distributed maculopapular eruptions."

[f]See etiology-specific chapters.

[g]See "Peripheral eruptions."

[h]See "Vesiculobullous or pustular eruptions."

Although drug reactions have many manifestations, including urticaria, exanthematous *drug-induced eruptions* (Chap. 55) are most common and are often difficult to distinguish from viral exanthems. Eruptions elicited by drugs are usually more intensely erythematous and pruritic than viral exanthems, but this distinction is not reliable. A history of new medications and an absence of prostration may help to distinguish a drug-related rash from an eruption of another etiology. Rashes may persist for up to two weeks after administration of the offending agent is discontinued. Certain populations are more prone than others to drug rashes. Of HIV-infected patients, 50–60% develop a rash in response to sulfa drugs; 90% of patients with mononucleosis due to Epstein-Barr virus develop a rash when given ampicillin.

Rickettsial illnesses (Chap. 174) should be considered in the evaluation of individuals with centrally distributed maculopapular eruptions. The usual setting for *epidemic typhus* is a site of war or natural disaster in which people are exposed to body lice. *Endemic typhus* or *leptospirosis* (the latter caused by a spirochete) (Chap. 171) may be seen in urban environments where rodents proliferate. Outside the United States, other rickettsial diseases cause a spotted-fever syndrome and should be considered in residents of or travelers to endemic areas. Similarly, *typhoid fever*, a nonrickettsial disease caused by *Salmonella typhi* (Chap. 153), is usually acquired during travel outside the United States. Dengue fever, caused by a mosquito-transmitted flavivirus, occurs in tropical and subtropical regions of the world (Chap. 196).

Some centrally distributed maculopapular eruptions have distinctive features. Erythema migrans, the rash of Lyme disease (Chap. 173), typically manifests as singular or multiple annular plaques. Untreated erythema migrans lesions usually fade within a month but may persist for more than a year. Southern tick-associated rash illness (STARI) has an erythema migrans–like rash but is less severe than Lyme disease and often occurs in regions where Lyme is not endemic. *Erythema marginatum*, the rash of acute rheumatic fever (Chap. 322), has a distinctive pattern of enlarging and shifting transient annular lesions.

Collagen vascular diseases may cause fever and rash. Patients with *systemic lupus erythematosus* (Chap. 319) typically develop a sharply defined, erythematous eruption in a butterfly distribution on the cheeks (malar rash) as well as many other skin manifestations. *Still's disease* (Chap. 337) presents as an evanescent, salmon-colored rash on the trunk and proximal extremities that coincides with fever spikes.

■ PERIPHERAL ERUPTIONS

These rashes are alike in that they are most prominent peripherally or begin in peripheral (acral) areas before spreading centripetally. Early diagnosis and therapy are critical in RMSF (Chap. 174) because of its grave prognosis if untreated. Lesions evolve from macular to petechial, start on the wrists and ankles, spread centripetally, and appear on the palms and soles only later in the disease. The rash of *secondary syphilis* (Chap. 169), which may be generalized but is prominent on the palms and soles, should be considered in the differential diagnosis of pityriasis rosea, especially in sexually active patients. Chikungunya fever (Chap. 196), which is transmitted by mosquito bite in Africa and the Indian Ocean region, is associated with a maculopapular eruption and severe polyarticular small-joint arthralgias. *Hand-foot-and-mouth disease* (Chap. 191), most commonly caused by coxsackievirus A16, is distinguished by tender vesicles distributed peripherally and in the mouth; outbreaks commonly occur within families. The classic target lesions of *erythema multiforme* appear symmetrically on the elbows, knees, palms, soles, and face. In severe cases, these lesions spread diffusely and involve mucosal surfaces. Lesions may develop on the hands and feet in *endocarditis* (Chap. 124).

■ CONFLUENT DESQUAMATIVE ERYTHEMAS

These eruptions consist of diffuse erythema frequently followed by desquamation. The eruptions caused by group A *Streptococcus* or *Staphylococcus aureus* are toxin-mediated. *Scarlet fever* (Chap. 136) usually follows pharyngitis; patients have a facial flush, a "strawberry" tongue, and accentuated petechiae in body folds (Pastia's lines). *Kawasaki disease* (Chaps. 53 and 326) presents in the pediatric population as fissuring of the lips, a strawberry tongue, conjunctivitis, adenopathy, and sometimes cardiac abnormalities. *Streptococcal toxic shock syndrome* (Chap. 136) manifests with hypotension, multiorgan failure, and, often, a severe group A streptococcal infection (e.g., necrotizing fasciitis). *Staphylococcal toxic shock syndrome* (Chap. 135) also presents with hypotension, and multiorgan failure, but usually only *S. aureus* colonization—not a severe *S. aureus* infection—is documented. *Staphylococcal scalded-skin syndrome* (Chap. 135) is seen primarily in children and in immunocompromised adults. Generalized erythema is often evident during the prodrome of fever and malaise; profound tenderness of the skin is distinctive. In the exfoliative stage, the skin can be induced to form bullae with light lateral pressure (Nikolsky's sign). In a mild form, a scarlatiniform eruption mimics scarlet fever, but the patient does not exhibit a strawberry tongue or circumoral pallor. In contrast to the staphylococcal scalded-skin syndrome, in which the cleavage plane is superficial in the epidermis, *toxic epidermal necrolysis* (Chap. 55), a maximal variant of Stevens-Johnson syndrome, involves sloughing of the entire epidermis, resulting in severe disease. *Exfoliative erythroderma syndrome* (Chaps. 52 and 55) is a serious reaction associated with systemic toxicity that is often due to eczema, psoriasis, a drug reaction, or mycosis fungoides. Drug-induced hypersensitivity syndrome (DIHS) due to antiepileptic and antibiotic agents (Chap. 55) initially appears similar to an exanthematous drug reaction but may progress to exfoliative erythroderma; it is accompanied by multiorgan failure and has an associated mortality rate of ~10%.

■ VESICULOBULLOUS OR PUSTULAR ERUPTIONS

Varicella (Chap. 180) is highly contagious, often occurring in winter or spring. At any point in time, within a given region of the body, varicella lesions are in different stages of development. In immunocompromised hosts, varicella vesicles may lack the characteristic erythematous base or may appear hemorrhagic. Lesions of *Pseudomonas* "hot-tub" folliculitis (Chap. 152) are also pruritic and may appear similar to those of varicella. However, hot-tub folliculitis generally occurs in outbreaks after bathing in hot tubs or swimming pools, and lesions occur in regions occluded by bathing suits. Lesions of *variola* (smallpox) (Chap. 221) also appear similar to those of varicella but are all at the same stage of development in a given region of the body. Variola lesions are most prominent on the face and extremities, while varicella lesions are most prominent on the trunk. Herpes simplex virus infection (Chap. 179) is characterized by hallmark grouped vesicles on an erythematous base. Primary herpes infection is accompanied by fever and toxicity, while recurrent disease is milder. *Rickettsialpox* (Chap. 174) is often documented in urban settings and is characterized by vesicles followed by pustules. It can be distinguished from varicella by an eschar at the site of the mouse-mite bite and the papule/plaque base of each vesicle. Acute generalized eruptive pustulosis (AGEP) should be considered in individuals who are acutely febrile and are taking new medications, especially anticonvulsant or antimicrobial agents (Chap. 55). Disseminated *Vibrio vulnificus* infection (Chap. 156) or *ecthyma gangrenosum* due to *Pseudomonas aeruginosa* (Chap. 152) should be considered in immunosuppressed individuals with sepsis and hemorrhagic bullae.

URTICARIA-LIKE ERUPTIONS

Individuals with classic urticaria ("hives") usually have a hypersensitivity reaction without associated fever. In the presence of fever, urticaria-like eruptions are usually due to *urticarial vasculitis* (Chap. 326). Unlike individual lesions of classic urticaria, which last up to 24 h, these lesions may last 3–5 days. Etiologies include serum sickness (often induced by drugs such as penicillins, sulfas, salicylates, or barbiturates), connective-tissue disease (e.g., systemic lupus erythematosus or Sjögren's syndrome), and infection (e.g., with hepatitis B virus, enteroviruses, or parasites). Malignancy, especially lymphoma, may be associated with fever and chronic urticaria (Chap. 53).

NODULAR ERUPTIONS

In immunocompromised hosts, nodular lesions often represent disseminated infection. Patients with disseminated *candidiasis* (often due to *Candida tropicalis*) may have a triad of fever, myalgias, and eruptive nodules (Chap. 203). Disseminated *cryptococcosis* lesions (Chap. 202) may resemble molluscum contagiosum (Chap. 183). Necrosis of nodules should raise the suspicion of *aspergillosis* (Chap. 204) or *mucormycosis* (Chap. 205). *Erythema nodosum* presents with exquisitely tender nodules on the lower extremities. *Sweet's syndrome* (Chap. 53) should be considered in individuals with multiple nodules and plaques, often so edematous that they give the appearance of vesicles or bullae. Sweet's syndrome may affect either healthy individuals or persons with lymphoproliferative disease.

PURPURIC ERUPTIONS

Acute meningococcemia (Chap. 143) classically presents in children as a petechial eruption, but initial lesions may appear as blanchable macules or urticaria. RMSF should be considered in the differential diagnosis of acute meningococcemia. *Echovirus 9 infection* (Chap. 191) may mimic acute meningococcemia; patients should be treated as if they have bacterial sepsis because prompt differentiation of these conditions may be impossible. Large ecchymotic areas of *purpura fulminans* (Chaps. 143 and 271) reflect severe underlying disseminated intravascular coagulation, which may be due to infectious or noninfectious causes. The lesions of *chronic meningococcemia* (Chap. 143) may have a variety of morphologies, including petechial. Purpuric nodules may develop on the legs and resemble erythema nodosum but lack its exquisite tenderness. Lesions of *disseminated gonococcemia* (Chap. 144) are distinctive, sparse, countable hemorrhagic pustules, usually located near joints. The lesions of chronic meningococcemia and those of gonococcemia may be indistinguishable in terms of appearance and

distribution. *Viral hemorrhagic fever* (Chaps. 196 and 197) should be considered in patients with an appropriate travel history and a petechial rash. *Thrombotic thrombocytopenic purpura* (Chaps. 53, 106, and 115) and *hemolytic-uremic syndrome* (Chaps. 115, 149, and 154) are closely related and are noninfectious causes of fever and petechiae. *Cutaneous small-vessel vasculitis* (leukocytoclastic vasculitis) typically manifests as palpable purpura and has a wide variety of causes (Chap. 53).

ERUPTIONS WITH ULCERS OR ESCHARS

The presence of an ulcer or eschar in the setting of a more widespread eruption can provide an important diagnostic clue. For example, the presence of an eschar may suggest the diagnosis of scrub typhus or rickettsialpox (Chap. 174) in the appropriate setting. In other illnesses (e.g., anthrax) (Chap. 221), an ulcer or eschar may be the only skin manifestation.

FURTHER READINGS

CHERRY JD: Contemporary infectious exanthems. Clin Infect Dis 16:199, 1993

———: Cutaneous manifestations of systemic infections, in *Textbook of Pediatric Infectious Diseases*, vol. 1, 4th ed, RD Feigin, JD Cherry (eds). Philadelphia, Saunders, 1998, pp 713–737

EICHENFIELD LF et al (eds): *Neonatal Dermatology*, 2nd ed. Philadelphia, Saunders, 2008

LEVIN S, GOODMAN LJ: An approach to acute fever and rash (AFR) in the adult. Curr Clin Top Infect Dis 15:19, 1995

PALLER AS, MANCINI AJ (eds): *Hurwitz Clinical Pediatric Dermatology*, 3rd ed. Philadelphia, Elsevier Saunders, 2006

SCHLOSSBERG D: Fever and rash. Infect Dis Clin North Am 10:101, 1996

WEBER DJ et al: The acutely ill patient with fever and rash, in *Principles and Practice of Infectious Diseases*, vol 1, 7th ed, GL Mandell et al (eds). Philadelphia, Elsevier Churchill Livingstone, 2010, pp 791–807

WENNER HA: Virus diseases associated with cutaneous eruptions. Prog Med Virol 16:269, 1973

WOLFF K, JOHNSON RAJ: *Fitzpatrick's Color Atlas and Synopsis of Clinical Dermatology*, 6th ed. New York, McGraw-Hill, 2009

——— et al (eds): *Fitzpatrick's Dermatology in General Medicine*, 7th ed. New York, McGraw-Hill, 2008

CHAPTER **18**
Fever of Unknown Origin

Jeffrey A. Gelfand
Michael V. Callahan

DEFINITION AND CLASSIFICATION

Fever of unknown origin (FUO) was defined by Petersdorf and Beeson in 1961 as (1) temperatures of >38.3°C (>101°F) on several occasions; (2) a duration of fever of >3 weeks; and (3) failure to reach a diagnosis despite 1 week of inpatient investigation. While

this classification has stood for more than 30 years, Durack and Street have proposed a revised system for classification of FUO that better accounts for nonendemic and emerging diseases, improved diagnostic technologies, and adverse reactions to new therapeutic interventions. This updated classification includes (1) classic FUO, (2) nosocomial FUO, (3) neutropenic FUO, and (4) FUO associated with HIV infection.

Classic FUO corresponds closely to the earlier definition of FUO, differing only with regard to the prior requirement for 1 week's study in the hospital. The newer definition is broader, stipulating three outpatient visits or 3 days in the hospital without elucidation of a cause or 1 week of "intelligent and invasive" ambulatory investigation. In *nosocomial FUO*, a temperature of ≥38.3°C (≥101°F) develops on several occasions in a hospitalized patient who is receiving acute care and in whom infection was not manifest or incubating on admission. Three days of investigation, including at least 2 days' incubation of cultures, is the minimum requirement for this diagnosis. *Neutropenic FUO* is defined as a temperature of ≥38.3°C (≥101°F) on several occasions in a patient whose neutrophil count is <500/μL or is expected to fall to that level in 1–2 days. The diagnosis of neutropenic FUO is invoked if a specific cause is not identified after 3 days of investigation, including at least 2 days' incubation of cultures. *HIV-associated FUO* is defined by a temperature of ≥38.3°C (≥101°F) on several occasions over a period of >4 weeks for outpatients or >3 days for hospitalized patients with HIV infection. This diagnosis is invoked if appropriate investigation over 3 days, including 2 days' incubation of cultures, reveals no source.

Adoption of these categories of FUO in the literature has allowed a more rational compilation of data regarding these disparate groups. In the remainder of this chapter, the discussion will focus on classic FUO in the adult patient unless otherwise specified.

CAUSES OF CLASSIC FUO

Table 18-1 summarizes the findings of several large studies of FUO carried out since the advent of the antibiotic era, including a prospective study of 167 adult patients with FUO encompassing all eight university hospitals in the Netherlands and using a standardized protocol in which the first author reviewed every patient's case. Coincident with the widespread use of antibiotics, increasingly useful diagnostic technologies—both noninvasive and invasive—have been developed. Newer studies reflect not only changing patterns of disease but also the impact of diagnostic techniques that make it possible to eliminate many patients with specific illness from the FUO category. The ubiquitous use of potent broad-spectrum antibiotics may have decreased the number of infections causing FUO. The wide availability of ultrasonography, CT, MRI, radionuclide scanning, and positron emission tomography (PET) scanning has enhanced the detection of localized infections and of occult neoplasms and lymphomas in patients previously thought to have FUO. Likewise, the widespread availability of highly specific and sensitive immunologic testing has reduced the number of undetected cases of adult Still's disease, systemic lupus erythematosus, and polyarteritis nodosa.

Infections such as extrapulmonary tuberculosis and—in endemic areas—typhoid fever and malaria remain a leading diagnosable cause of FUO. Prolonged mononucleosis syndromes caused by Epstein-Barr virus, cytomegalovirus (CMV), or HIV are conditions whose consideration as a cause of FUO are sometimes confounded by delayed antibody responses. Intraabdominal abscesses (sometimes poorly localized) and renal, retroperitoneal, and paraspinal abscesses continue to be difficult to diagnose. Renal malacoplakia,

with submucosal plaques or nodules involving the urinary tract, may cause fatal FUO if untreated; it is associated with intracellular bacterial infection, is seen in patients with defects of intracellular bacterial killing, and is treated with fluoroquinolones or trimethoprim-sulfamethoxazole. Occasionally, other organs may be involved. Osteomyelitis, especially where prosthetic devices have been implanted, must be considered. Although true culture-negative infective endocarditis is rare, one may be misled by cryptic endocarditis caused by indolent, slow-growing microorganisms of the HACEK group (*Haemophilus aphrophilus*, *Aggregatibacter* (formerly *Actinobacillus*) *actinomycetemcomitans*, *Cardiobacterium hominis*, *Eikenella corrodens*, and *Kingella kingae*), *Bartonella* spp. (previously *Rochalimaea*), *Legionella* spp., *Coxiella burnetii*, *Chlamydophila psittaci*, and fungi. Prostatitis, dental abscesses, sinusitis, and cholangitis continue to be sources of occult fever.

Fungal diseases, most notably histoplasmosis involving the reticuloendothelial system, may cause FUO, particularly outside of the endemic regions where these diseases may be more readily recognized. FUO following travel to neotropical regions and the desert southwest of the United States, even for very limited periods, should prompt evaluation for paracoccidioidomycosis and coccidioidomycosis, respectively. The rising popularity of adventure travel among citizens of Western countries has increased the incidence in these nations of presentation for FUO due to otherwise uncommon endemic vector-borne infections, notably Chikungunya fever and scrub typhus. FUO with headache should prompt examination of spinal fluid for *Cryptococcus neoformans*, *Mycobacterium tuberculosis*, and travel-acquired trypanosomes. Malaria (which may result from transfusion, failure to take a prescribed prophylactic agent, or infection with a drug-resistant *Plasmodium* strain) continues to be a cause of FUO, particularly of the asynchronous variety. A related protozoan infection, babesiosis, may cause FUO and is increasing in geographic distribution and in incidence, especially among the elderly and the immunosuppressed.

In most earlier series, neoplasms were the next most common cause of FUO after infections (Table 18-1). In more recent series, a decrease in the percentage of FUO cases due to malignancy was attributed to improvement in diagnostic technologies—in particular, high-resolution tomography, MRI, PET scanning, and tumor antigen assays. This observation does not diminish the importance of considering neoplasia in the initial diagnostic evaluation of a patient with fever. A number of patients in these series had temporal arteritis, adult Still's disease, drug-related fever, and factitious fever. In recent series, ~25–50% of cases of FUO have remained undiagnosed. The general term *noninfectious inflammatory diseases* applies to systemic rheumatologic or vasculitic diseases such as

TABLE 18-1 Classic FUO in Adults

Authors (Year of Publication)	Years of Study	No. of Cases	Infections (%)	Neoplasms (%)	Noninfectious Inflammatory Diseases (%)	Miscellaneous Causes (%)	Undiagnosed Causes (%)
Petersdorf and Beeson (1961)	1952–1957	100	36	19	19[a]	19[a]	7
Larson and Featherstone (1982)	1970–1980	105	30	31	16[a]	11[a]	12
Knockaert and Vanneste (1992)	1980–1989	199	22.5	7	23[a]	21.5[a]	25.5
de Kleijn et al. (1997, Part I)	1992–1994	167	26	12.5	24	8	30
Bleeker-Rovers et al. (2007)	2003–2005	73	16	7	22[b]	4	51

[a]Authors' raw data retabulated to conform to altered diagnostic categories.
[b]Connective tissue diseases.
Source: Modified from de Kleijn et al., 1997 (Part I).

polymyalgia rheumatica, lupus, and adult Still's disease as well as to granulomatous diseases such as sarcoidosis, Crohn's disease, and granulomatous hepatitis.

In the elderly, multisystem disease is the most frequent cause of FUO, giant-cell arteritis being the leading etiologic entity in this category. In patients >50 years of age, this disease accounts for 15–20% of FUO cases. Tuberculosis is the most common infection causing FUO in the elderly, and colon cancer is an important cause of FUO with malignancy in this age group.

Many diseases have been grouped in the various studies as "miscellaneous." On this list are drug fever, pulmonary embolism, factitious fever, the hereditary periodic fever syndromes [familial Mediterranean fever, hyper-IgD syndrome, tumor necrosis factor (TNF) receptor–associated periodic syndrome (also known as TRAPS or familial Hibernian fever), familial cold urticaria, and the Muckle-Wells syndrome)], and congenital lysosomal storage diseases such as Gaucher's and Fabry's disease.

A drug-related etiology must be considered in any case of prolonged fever. Any febrile pattern may be elicited by a drug. Virtually all classes of drugs can cause fever, but antimicrobial agents (especially β-lactam antibiotics), cardiovascular drugs (e.g., quinidine), antineoplastic drugs, and drugs acting on the central nervous system (e.g., phenytoin) are particularly common causes. The use of TNF inhibitors for treatment of inflammatory diseases has led to atypical presentations of tuberculosis, histoplasmosis, coccidioidomycosis, and JC virus infection associated with FUO.

It is axiomatic that, as the duration of fever increases, the likelihood of an infectious cause decreases, even for the more indolent infectious etiologies (e.g., brucellosis, paracoccidioidomycosis, malaria due to *Plasmodium malariae*). In a series of 347 patients referred to the National Institutes of Health from 1961 to 1977, only 6% had an infection (Table 18-2). A significant proportion (9%) had factitious fevers—i.e., fevers due either to false elevations of temperature or to self-induced disease. A substantial number of these factitious cases were in young women in the health professions. It is worth noting that 8% of the patients with prolonged fevers (some of whom had completely normal liver function studies) had granulomatous hepatitis, and 6% had adult Still's disease.

TABLE 18-2 Causes of FUO Lasting >6 Months

Cause	Cases, %
None identified	19
Miscellaneous causes	13
Factitious causes	9
Granulomatous hepatitis	8
Neoplasm	7
Still's disease	6
Infection	6
Collagen vascular disease	4
Familial Mediterranean fever	3
No fever[a]	27

[a]No actual fever observed during 2–3 weeks of inpatient observation. Includes patients with exaggerated circadian rhythm.

Source: From a study of 347 patients referred to the National Institutes of Health from 1961–1977 with a presumptive diagnosis of FUO of >6 months' duration (Data from R Aduan et al: Prolonged fever of unknown origin. Clin Res 26:558A, 1978).

After prolonged investigation, 19% of cases still had no specific diagnosis. A total of 27% of patients had no actual fever during inpatient observation or had an exaggerated circadian temperature rhythm without chills, elevated pulse, or other abnormalities.

■ GLOBAL CONSIDERATIONS

More than 200 conditions may be considered in the differential diagnosis of classic FUO in adults; the most common of these are listed in Table 18-3. This list applies predominantly to Western nations such as the United States. The workup of FUO must take into careful consideration the patient's country of origin, recent and remote travel (including past service in foreign wars), unusual environmental exposures associated with travel or hobbies (e.g., caving, hunting, and safaris), and pets. The increasing number of returning sojourners with exotic travel itineraries underscores the need for a detailed history of travel and associated activities in the setting of undiagnosed fever, as do the changing demographics of the travelers themselves. For example, increasing numbers of travelers are immunosuppressed, are undergoing disease-modifying interventions such as TNF-α suppression, or have recently reconstituted immunity. Immigrants with unexplained fever, including naturalized citizens who have left their countries of origin decades previously, should be carefully interviewed with regard to childhood exposures, including immunization with nonstandard or unidentified live vaccines. In both foreign-born individuals and veterans of foreign wars, subclinical infections may be unmasked decades after exposure by new malignancies or immunosuppressive conditions. The differential diagnosis of FUO must also take into account changes in the range of arthropod vectors or the possibility that local permissive vectors have become infected with previously nonendemic pathogens. Evaluation of FUO in underresourced medical settings requires increased reliance on history and clinical examination. Patients, family members, and close occupational contacts may need to be interviewed. If specialized laboratory and imaging studies cannot be conducted, diagnosis may be facilitated by maximizing the quality and precision of locally available approaches (e.g., culture of lysed, centrifuged blood cultures, and microscopic examination by an experienced technician). Emerging infectious diseases may include FUO first presenting as clusters of cases in remote regions; insight may be gained from contacting local epidemiologists.

The possibility of international and domestic terrorist activity involving the intentional release of infectious agents, many of which cause illnesses presenting with prolonged fever, underscores the need for obtaining an insightful environmental, occupational, and professional history, with early notification of public health authorities in cases of suspicious etiology (Chap. 221). Moreover, the global spread of genetic engineering technologies raises the possibility that traditional agents—including Centers for Disease Control Categories A, B, and C agents; see Table 221-2)—that circumvent vaccine-acquired immunity could be developed or that novel recombinant organisms could be engineered to produce clinical or laboratory responses that defy current diagnostic approaches.

■ SPECIALIZED DIAGNOSTIC STUDIES

Classic FUO

A stepwise flow chart depicting the diagnostic workup and therapeutic management of FUO is provided in Fig. 18-1. In this flow chart, reference is made to "potentially diagnostic clues," as outlined by de Kleijn and colleagues; these clues may be key findings in the history (e.g., travel), localizing signs, or key symptoms. Certain specific diagnostic maneuvers become critical in dealing with prolonged fevers. If

TABLE 18-3 Causes of FUO in Adults in the United States

Infections

Localized pyogenic infections
Appendicitis
Cat-scratch disease
Cholangitis
Cholecystitis
Dental abscess
Diverticulitis/abscess
Lesser sac abscess
Liver abscess
Mesenteric lymphadenitis
Osteomyelitis
Pancreatic abscess
Pelvic inflammatory disease
Perinephric/intrarenal abscess
Prostatic abscess
Renal malacoplakia
Sinusitis
Subphrenic abscess
Suppurative thrombophlebitis
Tuboovarian abscess

Intravascular infections
Bacterial aortitis
Bacterial endocarditis
Vascular catheter infection

Systemic bacterial infections
Bartonellosis
Brucellosis
Campylobacter infection
Cat-scratch disease/bacillary
   angiomatosis (*B. henselae*)
Gonococcemia
Legionnaires' disease
Leptospirosis
Listeriosis
Lyme disease
Melioidosis
Meningococcemia
Rat-bite fever
Relapsing fever
Salmonellosis
Syphilis
Tularemia
Typhoid fever
Vibriosis
Yersinia infection

Mycobacterial infections
M. avium/M. intracellulare infections
Other atypical mycobacterial infections
Tuberculosis

Other bacterial infections
Actinomycosis
Bacillary angiomatosis
Nocardiosis
Whipple's disease

Rickettsial infections
Anaplasmosis
Ehrlichiosis
Murine typhus
Q fever
Rickettsialpox
Rocky Mountain spotted fever
Scrub typhus

Mycoplasmal infections
Chlamydial infections
Lymphogranuloma venereum
Psittacosis
TWAR (*C. pneumoniae*) infection

Viral infections
Chikungunya fever
Colorado tick fever
Coxsackievirus group B infection
Cytomegalovirus infection
Dengue
Epstein-Barr virus infection
Hepatitis A, B, C, D, and E
HIV infection
Human herpesvirus 6 infection
Lymphocytic choriomeningitis
Parvovirus B19 infection
Picornavirus infection

Fungal infections
Aspergillosis
Blastomycosis
Candidiasis
Coccidioidomycosis
Cryptococcosis
Histoplasmosis
Mucormycosis
Paracoccidioidomycosis
Pneumocystis infection
Sporotrichosis

Parasitic infections
Amebiasis
Babesiosis
Chagas' disease
Leishmaniasis
Malaria
Strongyloidiasis
Toxocariasis
Toxoplasmosis
Trichinellosis

Presumed infections, agent undetermined
Kawasaki's disease (mucocutaneous lymph
   node syndrome)
Kikuchi's necrotizing lymphadenitis

Neoplasms

Malignant
Colon cancer
Gall bladder carcinoma
Hepatoma
Hodgkin's lymphoma
Immunoblastic T-cell lymphoma
Leukemia
Lymphomatoid granulomatosis
Malignant histiocytosis
Non-Hodgkin's lymphoma
Pancreatic cancer
Renal cell carcinoma
Sarcoma

Benign
Atrial myxoma
Castleman's disease
Renal angiomyolipoma

Habitual Hyperthermia
(Exaggerated circadian rhythm)

Collagen Vascular/Hypersensitivity Diseases
Adult Still's disease
Behçet's disease
Erythema multiforme
Erythema nodosum
Giant-cell arteritis/polymyalgia rheumatica
Hypersensitivity pneumonitis
Hypersensitivity vasculitis
Mixed connective-tissue disease
Polyarteritis nodosa
Relapsing polychondritis
Rheumatic fever
Rheumatoid arthritis
Schnitzler's syndrome
Systemic lupus erythematosus
Takayasu's aortitis
Weber-Christian disease
Granulomatosis with polyangiitis (Wegener's)

Granulomatous Diseases
Crohn's disease
Granulomatous hepatitis
Midline granuloma
Sarcoidosis

Miscellaneous Conditions
Aortic dissection
Drug fever
Gout
Hematomas
Hemoglobinopathies
Laennec's cirrhosis
PFPA syndrome: periodic fever, adenitis,
   pharyngitis, aphthae
Postmyocardial infarction syndrome
Recurrent pulmonary emboli
Subacute thyroiditis (de Quervain's)
Tissue infarction/necrosis

Inherited and Metabolic Diseases
Adrenal insufficiency
Cyclic neutropenia
Deafness, urticaria, and amyloidosis
Fabry disease
Familial cold urticaria
Familial Mediterranean fever
Hyperimmunoglobulinemia D and periodic fever
Muckle-Wells syndrome
Tumor necrosis factor receptor–associated
   periodic syndrome (familial Hibernian fever)
Type V hypertriglyceridemia

Thermoregulatory Disorders

Central
Brain tumor
Cerebrovascular accident
Encephalitis
Hypothalamic dysfunction

Peripheral
Hyperthyroidism
Pheochromocytoma

Factitious Fevers
"Afebrile" FUO [<38.3°C (100.94°F)]

Source: Modified from RK Root, RG Petersdorf, in JD Wilson et al (eds): *Harrison's Principles of Internal Medicine,* 12th ed. New York, McGraw-Hill, 1991.

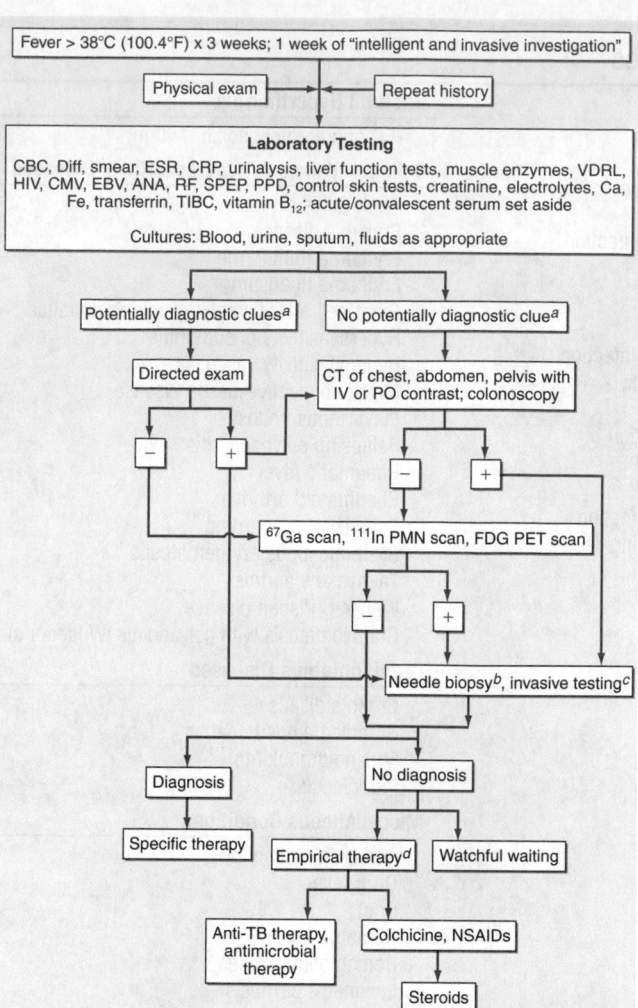

Figure 18-1 Approach to the patient with classic FUO. [a]"Potentially diagnostic clues," as outlined by de Kleijn and colleagues (1997, Part II), may be key findings in the history, localizing signs, or key symptoms. [b]Needle biopsy of liver as well as any other tissue indicated by "potentially diagnostic clues." [c]Invasive testing could involve laparoscopy. [d]Empirical therapy is a last resort, given the good prognosis of most patients with FUO persisting without a diagnosis. *Abbreviations:* ANA, antinuclear antibody; CBC, complete blood count; CMV, cytomegalovirus; CRP, C-reactive protein; CT, computed tomography; Diff, differential; EBV, Epstein-Barr virus; ESR, erythrocyte sedimentation rate; FDG, fluorodeoxyglucose F18; NSAIDs, non-steroidal anti-inflammatory drugs; PET, positron emission tomography; PMN, polymorphonuclear leukocyte; PPD, purified protein derivative; RF, rheumatoid factor; SPEP, serum protein electrophoresis; TB, tuberculosis; TIBC, total iron-binding capacity; VDRL, Venereal Disease Research Laboratory test.

factitious fever is suspected, temperature-taking should be supervised, and simultaneous urine and body temperatures should be measured. Thick blood smears should be examined for *Plasmodium*; thin blood smears, prepared with proper technique and quality stains and subjected to expert microscopy, should be used to speciate *Plasmodium* and to identify *Babesia, Trypanosoma, Leishmania, Leptospira, Rickettsia,* and *Borrelia*. Specialized staining of mononuclear cells and granulocytes can help to identify intracellular bacteria, protozoal amastigotes, and the inclusion bodies of ehrlichiosis and anaplasmosis. Any tissue removed during prior relevant surgery should be reexamined; slides should be requested, and, if necessary, paraffin blocks of fixed pathologic material should be reexamined and additional special studies performed. Relevant x-rays should be reexamined; review of prior

radiologic reports may be insufficient. Serum should be set aside in the laboratory as soon as possible and retained for future examination for rising antibody titers.

Febrile agglutinins is a vague term that, in most laboratories, refers to serologic studies for salmonellosis, brucellosis, and rickettsial diseases. These studies are seldom useful, having low sensitivity and variable specificity. Multiple blood samples (no fewer than three and rarely more than six, including samples for anaerobic culture) should be cultured in the laboratory—with and without increased CO_2—for 2 to 3 weeks to ensure ample growth time for any HACEK organisms (Chap. 146). It is critical to inform the laboratory of the intent to test for unusual organisms. Specialized media should be used if an exposure or travel history suggests uncommon causes of endocarditis, such as *Histoplasma, Chlamydophila, Mycoplasma, Bartonella, Coxiella,* or *Tropheryma whipplei*. Blood culture media should be supplemented with L-cysteine or pyridoxal to assist in the isolation of nutritionally variant streptococci. Lysis-centrifugation blood culture techniques should be employed when prior antimicrobial therapy or fungal or atypical mycobacterial infection is suspected. It should be noted that sequential cultures positive for multiple organisms may reflect self-injection of contaminated substances. Cultures of sinus fluid and pulmonary secretions on multiple permissive cell lines may prove helpful in identifying new respiratory viruses implicated in FUO. Urine cultures, including cultures for mycobacteria, fungi, and CMV, are indicated. In the setting of recurrent fevers with lymphocytic meningitis (Mollaret's meningitis), cerebrospinal fluid can be tested for herpesvirus, with use of the polymerase chain reaction (PCR) to amplify and detect viral nucleic acid (Chap. 179). A highly multiplexed oligonucleotide microarray using PCR amplification and containing probes for all recognized virus species hosted by vertebrates and up to 135 bacterial, 73 fungal, and 63 parasitic genera and species has been developed but has not yet been approved for clinical use. The continued clinical validation of such microarrays will further diminish rates of undiagnosed FUO of infectious etiology.

In any FUO workup, the erythrocyte sedimentation rate (ESR) should be determined. Striking elevation of the ESR and anemia of chronic disease are frequently seen in association with giant cell arteritis or polymyalgia rheumatica—common causes of FUO in patients >50 years of age. Still's disease is suggested by elevations of ESR, leukocytosis, and anemia and is often accompanied by arthralgias, polyserositis (pleuritis, pericarditis), lymphadenopathy, splenomegaly, and rash. The C-reactive protein level may be a useful cross-reference for the ESR and is a more sensitive and specific indicator of an "acute-phase" inflammatory metabolic response. Antinuclear antibody, antineutrophil cytoplasmic antibody, rheumatoid factor, and serum cryoglobulins should be measured to rule out other collagen vascular diseases and vasculitis. Elevated levels of angiotensin-converting enzyme in serum may point to sarcoidosis. With rare exceptions, the intermediate-strength purified protein derivative (PPD) skin test should be used to screen patients with classic FUO for tuberculosis. Concurrent control tests, such as the mumps skin test antigen (Aventis-Pasteur, Swiftwater, PA), should be employed. It should be kept in mind that both the PPD tuberculin skin test (TST) and control tests may yield false-negative results in patients with miliary tuberculosis, sarcoidosis, Hodgkin's disease, malnutrition, or AIDS. Two interferon γ–release assays have been approved by the U.S. Food and Drug Administration for the diagnosis of tuberculosis. These tests—the QuantiFERON-TB Gold In-Tube (QFT-GIT) assay and the T-SPOT TB assay—measure the production of interferon γ by T lymphocytes upon exposure to antigens of *M. tuberculosis*. In direct comparisons, the sensitivity of the QFT-GIT test was statistically similar to that of the TST for detecting infection in persons with untreated, culture-confirmed tuberculosis. The QFT-GIT test is more specific, is less influenced by previous infection with nontuberculous mycobacteria, and is not affected by prior vaccination with bacille Calmette-Guérin (BCG); TSTs are variably affected by these factors. Repeating the QFT-GIT test does not boost the in vitro response, while injection of PPD for the TST can boost subsequent TST responses, primarily in persons who have been infected with nontuberculous mycobacteria or vaccinated with BCG. Negative results in the QFT-GIT test—as in the TST—do not definitively exclude a diagnosis of tuberculosis.

Noninvasive procedures should include an upper gastrointestinal contrast study with small-bowel follow-through and colonoscopy to examine the terminal ileum and cecum for early evidence of lymphoma or subclinical Crohn's disease. Colonoscopy is especially strongly indicated in the elderly. Chest x-rays should be repeated if new symptoms arise. Sputum should be induced with an ultrasonic nebulizer for cultures, cytology, and molecular diagnostic testing. If there are pulmonary signs or symptoms, bronchoscopy with bronchoalveolar lavage for cultures, PCR, and cytology should be considered. High-resolution spiral CT of the chest and abdomen should be performed with both IV and oral contrast. If a spinal or paraspinal lesion is suspected, however, MRI is preferred. MRI may be superior to CT in demonstrating intraabdominal abscesses and aortic dissection, but the comparative utility of MRI and CT in the diagnosis of FUO is unknown. At present, abdominal CT with contrast should be used unless MRI is specifically indicated. Arteriography may be useful for patients in whom systemic necrotizing vasculitis is suspected. Saccular aneurysms may be seen, most commonly in renal or hepatic vessels, and may permit diagnosis of arteritis when biopsy is difficult. Ultrasonography of the abdomen is useful for investigation of the hepatobiliary tract, kidneys, spleen, and pelvis. Echocardiography may be helpful in an evaluation for bacterial endocarditis, pericarditis, nonbacterial thrombotic endocarditis, and atrial myxomas. Transesophageal echocardiography is preferred for these lesions.

Radionuclide scanning procedures using technetium (Tc) 99m sulfur colloid, gallium (Ga) 67 citrate, or indium (In) 111–labeled leukocytes may be useful in identifying and/or localizing inflammatory processes such as aortitis or abscess. In one study, Ga scintigraphy yielded useful diagnostic information in almost one-third of cases, and it was suggested that this procedure might actually be used before other imaging techniques if no specific organ is suspected of being abnormal. It is likely that PET scanning, which provides quicker results (hours vs days), will prove even more sensitive and specific than ^{67}Ga scanning in FUO. ^{99m}Tc bone scan should be undertaken to look for osteomyelitis or bony metastases; ^{67}Ga scan may be used to identify sarcoidosis (Chap. 329) or *Pneumocystis* infection (Chap. 207) in the lungs or Crohn's disease (Chap. 295) in the abdomen. ^{111}In-labeled white blood cell (WBC) scan may be used to locate abscesses. With these scans, false-positive and false-negative findings are common. Fluorodeoxyglucose F18 (FDG) PET scanning appears to be superior to other forms of nuclear imaging. The FDG used in PET scans accumulates in tumors and at sites of inflammation and has even been shown to accumulate reliably at sites of vasculitis. Where available, FDG PET scanning should therefore be chosen over ^{67}Ga scanning in the diagnosis of FUO.

Biopsy of the liver and bone marrow should be considered in the workup of FUO if the studies mentioned above are unrevealing and if fever is prolonged. Granulomatous hepatitis has been diagnosed by liver biopsy, even when liver enzymes are normal and no other diagnostic clues point to liver disease. All biopsy specimens should be cultured for bacteria, mycobacteria, and fungi. Likewise, in the absence of clues pointing to the bone marrow, bone marrow biopsy (not simple aspiration) for histology and culture has yielded diagnoses late in the workup. When possible, a section of the tissue

block should be retained for further sections or stains. At some research centers, PCR technology makes it possible in some cases to identify and speciate mycobacterial DNA in paraffin-embedded, fixed tissues. Thus, a retrospective diagnosis can sometimes be made on the basis of studies of long-fixed pathologic tissues. In a patient over age 50 (or occasionally in a younger patient) with the appropriate symptoms and laboratory findings, "blind biopsy" of one or both temporal arteries may yield a diagnosis of arteritis. Tenderness or decreased pulsation, if noted, should guide the selection of a site for biopsy. Lymph node biopsy may be helpful if nodes are enlarged, but inguinal nodes are often palpable and are seldom diagnostically useful.

Exploratory laparotomy has been performed when all other diagnostic procedures fail but has largely been replaced by imaging and guided-biopsy techniques. Peritoneal lavage may be used as a minimally invasive approach to peritoneal cytology studies. Laparoscopic biopsy may provide more adequate guided sampling of lymph nodes or liver, with less invasive morbidity.

Nosocomial FUO

(See also Chap. 131) The primary considerations in diagnosing nosocomial FUO are the underlying susceptibility of the patient coupled with the potential complications of hospitalization. The original surgical or procedural field is the place to begin a directed physical and laboratory examination for abscesses, hematomas, or infected foreign bodies. More than 50% of patients with nosocomial FUO are infected. Intravascular lines, septic phlebitis, and prostheses are all suspect. In this setting, the best approach is to focus on sites where occult infections may be sequestered, such as the sinuses of intubated patients or a prostatic abscess in a man with a urinary catheter. *Clostridium difficile* colitis may be associated with fever and leukocytosis before the onset of diarrhea. In ~25% of patients with nosocomial FUO, the fever has a noninfectious cause. Among these causes are acalculous cholecystitis, deep-vein thrombophlebitis, and pulmonary embolism. Drug fever, transfusion reactions, alcohol/drug withdrawal, adrenal insufficiency, thyroiditis, pancreatitis, gout, and pseudogout are among the many possible causes to consider. As in classic FUO, repeated meticulous physical examinations, coupled with focused diagnostic techniques, are imperative. Multiple blood, wound, and fluid cultures are mandatory. The pace of diagnostic tests is accelerated, and the threshold for procedures—CT scans, ultrasonography, ^{111}In WBC scans, noninvasive venous studies—is low. Even so, 20% of cases of nosocomial FUO may go undiagnosed.

Like diagnostic measures, therapeutic maneuvers must be swift and decisive, as many patients are already critically ill. IV lines must be changed (and cultured), drugs stopped for 72 hours, and empirical therapy started if bacteremia, fungemia, or persistently high virus loads are a threat. In many hospital settings, empirical antibiotic therapy for nosocomial FUO now includes vancomycin for coverage of methicillin-resistant *Staphylococcus aureus* as well as broad-spectrum gram-negative coverage with piperacillin/tazobactam, ticarcillin/clavulanate, imipenem, or meropenem. Practice guidelines covering many of these issues have been published jointly by the Infectious Diseases Society of America (IDSA) and the American College of Critical Care Medicine and can be accessed on the IDSA website (*www.journals.uchicago.edu/IDSA/guidelines*).

Neutropenic FUO

(See also Chap. 86) Neutropenic patients are susceptible to focal bacterial and fungal infections, to bacteremic infections, to infections involving catheters (including septic thrombophlebitis), and to perianal infections. *Candida* and *Aspergillus* infections are common. Infections due to herpes simplex virus or CMV are sometimes causes of FUO in this group. While the duration of illness may be short in these patients, the consequences of untreated infection may be catastrophic; 50–60% of febrile neutropenic patients are infected, and 20% are bacteremic. The IDSA has published extensive practice guidelines covering these critically ill neutropenic patients (*www.journals.uchicago.edu/IDSA/guidelines*). In these patients, severe mucositis, quinolone prophylaxis, colonization with methicillin-resistant *S. aureus*, obvious catheter-related infection, or hypotension dictates the use of vancomycin plus ceftazidime, cefepime, or a carbapenem with or without an aminoglycoside to provide empirical coverage for bacterial sepsis.

HIV-Associated FUO

HIV infection alone may be a cause of fever. The infectious etiology varies with the extent of immunosuppression and the geographic region. Infection due to *Mycobacterium avium* or *M. intracellulare*, tuberculosis, toxoplasmosis, CMV infection, *Pneumocystis* infection, salmonellosis, cryptococcosis, histoplasmosis, strongyloidiasis, non-Hodgkin's lymphoma, and (of particular importance) drug fever are all possible causes of FUO. Mycobacterial infection can be diagnosed by blood cultures and by liver, bone marrow, and lymph node biopsies. Chest CT should be performed to identify enlarged mediastinal nodes. Serologic studies may reveal cryptococcal antigen, and ^{67}Ga scan may help identify *Pneumocystis* pulmonary infection. FUO has an infectious etiology in >80% of HIV-infected patients, but drug fever and lymphoma remain important considerations. Treatment of HIV-associated FUO depends on many factors and is discussed in Chap. 189.

TREATMENT   Fever of Unknown Origin

The focus here is on classic FUO. Other modifiers of FUO—neutropenia, HIV infection, a nosocomial setting—all vastly affect the risk equation and dictate therapy based on the probability of various causes of fever and on the calculated risks and benefits of a guided empirical approach. The age and physical state of the patient are factors as well: the frail, elderly patient may merit a trial of empirical therapy earlier than the robust young adult.

The emphasis in patients with classic FUO is on continued observation and examination, with the avoidance of "shotgun" empirical therapy. Antibiotic therapy (even that for tuberculosis) may irrevocably alter the ability to culture fastidious bacteria or mycobacteria and delineate ultimate cause. However, vital-sign instability or neutropenia is an indication for empirical therapy with a fluoroquinolone plus piperacillin or the regimen mentioned above (see "Nosocomial FUO"), for example. Cirrhosis, asplenia, disease-modifying biologic therapy, intercurrent immunosuppressive drug use, or exotic travel or environmental exposures (e.g., cave interiors) may all tip the balance toward earlier empirical anti-infective therapy. If the TST is positive or if granulomatous hepatitis or other granulomatous disease is present with anergy (and sarcoid seems unlikely), then a therapeutic trial for tuberculosis should be undertaken, with treatment usually continued for up to 6 weeks. A failure of the fever to respond over this period suggests an alternative diagnosis.

The response of rheumatic fever and Still's disease to aspirin and nonsteroidal anti-inflammatory drugs (NSAIDs) may be dramatic. The effects of glucocorticoids on temporal arteritis, polymyalgia rheumatica, and granulomatous hepatitis are equally dramatic. Colchicine is highly effective in preventing attacks of familial Mediterranean fever but is of little use once an attack is well under way. The ability of glucocorticoids and NSAIDs to mask fever while permitting the spread of infection dictates that their use be avoided unless infection has been largely ruled out and unless inflammatory disease is both probable and debilitating or threatening.

When no underlying source of FUO is identified after prolonged observation (>6 months), the prognosis is generally good, however vexing the fever may be to the patient. Under such circumstances, debilitating symptoms are treated with NSAIDs, and glucocorticoids are the last resort. The initiation of empirical therapy does not mark the end of the diagnostic workup; rather, it commits the physician to continued thoughtful reexamination and evaluation. Patience, compassion, equanimity, vigilance, and intellectual flexibility are indispensable attributes for the clinician in dealing successfully with FUO.

ACKNOWLEDGMENTS

Sheldon M. Wolff, MD, now deceased, was an author of a previous version of this chapter. It is to his memory that the chapter is dedicated. The substantial contributions of Charles A. Dinarello, MD, to this chapter in previous editions are gratefully acknowledged.

FURTHER READINGS

BLEEKER-ROVERS CP et al: A prospective multicenter study on fever of unknown origin: The yield of a structured diagnostic protocol. Medicine 86:26, 2007

——— et al: Fever of unknown origin. Semin Nucl Med 39:81, 2009

DE KLEIJN EM et al: Fever of unknown origin (FUO): I. A prospective multicenter study of 167 patients with FUO, using fixed epidemiologic entry criteria. Medicine 76:392, 1997

——— et al: Fever of unknown origin (FUO): II. Diagnostic procedures in a prospective multicenter study of 167 patients. Medicine 76:401, 1997

GOTO M et al: A retrospective review of 226 hospitalized patients with fever. Intern Med 46:17, 2007

HIGH KP et al: IDSA guidelines: Clinical practice guideline for the evaluation of fever and infection in older adult residents of long-term care facilities: 2008 update by the Infectious Diseases Society of America. Clin Infect Dis 48:149, 2009

HOT A et al: Yield of bone marrow examination in diagnosing the source of fever of unknown origin. Arch Intern Med 169:2018, 2009

KNOCKAERT DC et al: Fever of unknown origin in adults: 40 years on. J Intern Med 253:263, 2003

MOURAD O et al: A comprehensive evidence-based approach to fever of unknown origin. Arch Intern Med 163:545, 2003

O'GRADY NP et al: Guidelines for evaluation of new fever in critically ill adult patients: 2008 update from the American College of Critical Care Medicine and the Infectious Diseases Society of America. Crit Care Med 36:1330, 2008

SIMONS KS et al: F-18-fluorodeoxyglucose positron emission tomography combined with CT in critically ill patients with suspected infection. Intensive Care Med 36:504, 2010

ZENONE T: Fever of unknown origin in adults: Evaluation of 144 cases in a non-university hospital. Scand J Infect Dis 38:632, 2006

CHAPTER 19

Hypothermia and Frostbite

Daniel F. Danzl

HYPOTHERMIA

Accidental hypothermia occurs when there is an unintentional drop in the body's core temperature below 35°C (95°F). At this temperature, many of the compensatory physiologic mechanisms that conserve heat begin to fail. *Primary accidental hypothermia* is a result of the direct exposure of a previously healthy individual to the cold. The mortality rate is much higher for patients who develop *secondary hypothermia* as a complication of a serious systemic disorder.

■ CAUSES

Primary accidental hypothermia is geographically and seasonally pervasive. Although most cases occur in the winter months and in colder climates, it is surprisingly common in warmer regions as well. Multiple variables make individuals at the extremes of age, the elderly and neonates, particularly vulnerable to hypothermia (Table 19-1). The elderly have diminished thermal perception and are more susceptible to immobility, malnutrition, and systemic illnesses that interfere with heat generation or conservation. Dementia, psychiatric illness, and socioeconomic factors often compound these problems by impeding adequate measures

TABLE 19-1 Risk Factors for Hypothermia

Age extremes	Endocrine-related
Elderly	Diabetes mellitus
Neonates	Hypoglycemia
Environmental exposure	Hypothyroidism
Occupational	Adrenal insufficiency
Sports-related	Hypopituitarism
Inadequate clothing	Neurologic-related
Immersion	Cerebrovascular accident
Toxicologic and pharmacologic	Hypothalamic disorders
Ethanol	Parkinson's disease
Phenothiazines	Spinal cord injury
Barbiturates	Multisystem
Carcinomatosis	Trauma
Anesthetics	Sepsis
Neuromuscular blockers	Shock
Antidepressants	Hepatic or renal failure
Insufficient fuel	Burns and exfoliative dermatologic disorders
Malnutrition	Immobility or debilitation
Marasmus	
Kwashiorkor	

to prevent hypothermia. Neonates have high rates of heat loss because of their increased surface-to-mass ratio and their lack of effective shivering and adaptive behavioral responses. At all ages, malnutrition can contribute to heat loss because of diminished subcutaneous fat and as a result of depleted energy stores used for thermogenesis.

Individuals whose occupations or hobbies entail extensive exposure to cold weather are at increased risk for hypothermia. Military history is replete with hypothermic tragedies. Hunters, sailors, skiers, and climbers also are at great risk of exposure, whether it involves injury, changes in weather, or lack of preparedness.

Ethanol causes vasodilation (which increases heat loss), reduces thermogenesis and gluconeogenesis, and may impair judgment or lead to obtundation. Phenothiazines, barbiturates, benzodiazepines, cyclic antidepressants, and many other medications reduce centrally mediated vasoconstriction. Up to 25% of patients admitted to an intensive care unit because of drug overdose are hypothermic. Anesthetics can block the shivering responses; their effects are compounded when patients are not insulated adequately in the operating or recovery rooms.

Several types of endocrine dysfunction can lead to hypothermia. Hypothyroidism—particularly when extreme, as in myxedema coma—reduces the metabolic rate and impairs thermogenesis and behavioral responses. Adrenal insufficiency and hypopituitarism also increase susceptibility to hypothermia. Hypoglycemia, most commonly caused by insulin or oral hypoglycemic drugs, is associated with hypothermia, in part a result of neuroglycopenic effects on hypothalamic function. Increased osmolality and metabolic derangements associated with uremia, diabetic ketoacidosis, and lactic acidosis can lead to altered hypothalamic thermoregulation.

Neurologic injury from trauma, cerebrovascular accident, subarachnoid hemorrhage, and hypothalamic lesion increases susceptibility to hypothermia. Agenesis of the corpus callosum, or Shapiro syndrome, is one cause of episodic hypothermia, characterized by profuse perspiration followed by a rapid fall in temperature. Acute spinal cord injury disrupts the autonomic pathways that lead to shivering and prevents cold-induced reflex vasoconstrictive responses.

Hypothermia associated with sepsis is a poor prognostic sign. Hepatic failure causes decreased glycogen stores and gluconeogenesis, as well as a diminished shivering response. In acute myocardial infarction associated with low cardiac output, hypothermia may be reversed after adequate resuscitation. With extensive burns, psoriasis, erythrodermas, and other skin diseases, increased peripheral blood flow leads to excessive heat loss.

■ THERMOREGULATION

Heat loss occurs through five mechanisms: radiation (55–65% of heat loss), conduction (10–15% of heat loss but much greater in cold water), convection (increased in the wind), respiration, and evaporation (which are affected by the ambient temperature and the relative humidity).

The preoptic anterior hypothalamus normally orchestrates thermoregulation (Chap. 16). The immediate defense of thermoneutrality is via the autonomic nervous system, whereas delayed control is mediated by the endocrine system. Autonomic nervous system responses include the release of norepinephrine, increased muscle tone, and shivering, leading to thermogenesis and an increase in the basal metabolic rate. Cutaneous cold thermoreception causes direct reflex vasoconstriction to conserve heat. Prolonged exposure to cold also stimulates the thyroid axis, leading to an increased metabolic rate.

CLINICAL PRESENTATION

In most cases of hypothermia, the history of exposure to environmental factors, such as prolonged exposure to the outdoors without adequate clothing, makes the diagnosis straightforward. In urban settings, however, the presentation is often more subtle and other disease processes, toxin exposures, or psychiatric diagnoses should be considered.

After initial stimulation by hypothermia, there is progressive depression of all organ systems. The timing of the appearance of these clinical manifestations varies widely (Table 19-2). Without knowing the core temperature, it can be difficult to interpret other vital signs. For example, a tachycardia disproportionate to the core temperature suggests secondary hypothermia resulting from hypoglycemia, hypovolemia, or a toxin overdose. Because carbon dioxide production declines progressively, the respiratory rate should be low; persistent hyperventilation suggests a central nervous system (CNS) lesion or one of the organic acidoses. A markedly depressed level of consciousness in a patient with mild hypothermia should raise suspicion of an overdose or CNS dysfunction due to infection or trauma.

Physical examination findings can also be altered by hypothermia. For instance, the assumption that areflexia is solely attributable to hypothermia can obscure and delay the diagnosis of a spinal cord lesion. Patients with hypothermia may be confused or combative; these symptoms abate more rapidly with rewarming than with chemical or physical restraint. A classic example of maladaptive behavior in patients with hypothermia is paradoxical undressing, which involves the inappropriate removal of clothing in response to a cold stress. The cold-induced ileus and abdominal rectus spasm can mimic, or mask, the presentation of an acute abdomen (Chap. 13).

When a patient in hypothermic cardiac arrest is first discovered, cardiopulmonary resuscitation is indicated unless (1) a do-not-resuscitate status is verified, (2) obviously lethal injuries are identified, or (3) the depression of a frozen chest wall is not possible. As the resuscitation proceeds, the prognosis is grave if there is evidence of widespread cell lysis, as reflected by potassium levels >10 mmol/L (10 meq/L). Other findings that may preclude continuing resuscitation include a core temperature <10–12°C (50–54°F), a pH <6.5, and evidence of intravascular thrombosis with a fibrinogen value <0.5 g/L (<50 mg/dL). The decision to terminate resuscitation before rewarming the patient past 33°C (91°F) should be predicated on the type and severity of the precipitants of hypothermia. There are no validated prognostic indicators for recovery from hypothermia. A history of asphyxia with secondary cooling is the most important negative predictor of survival.

■ DIAGNOSIS AND STABILIZATION

Hypothermia is confirmed by measuring the core temperature, preferably at two sites. Rectal probes should be placed to a depth of 15 cm and not adjacent to cold feces. A simultaneous esophageal probe should be placed 24 cm below the larynx; it may read falsely high during heated inhalation therapy. Relying solely on infrared tympanic thermography is not advisable.

After a diagnosis of hypothermia is established, cardiac monitoring should be instituted, along with attempts to limit further heat loss. If the patient is in ventricular fibrillation, one defibrillation

TABLE 19-2 Physiologic Changes Associated With Accidental Hypothermia

Severity	Body Temperature	Central Nervous System	Cardiovascular	Respiratory	Renal and Endocrine	Neuromuscular
Mild	35°C (95°F)–32.2°C (90°F)	Linear depression of cerebral metabolism; amnesia; apathy; dysarthria; impaired judgment; maladaptive behavior	Tachycardia, then progressive bradycardia; cardiac cycle prolongation; vasoconstriction; increase in cardiac output and blood pressure	Tachypnea, then progressive decrease in respiratory minute volume; declining oxygen consumption; bronchorrhea; bronchospasm	Diuresis; increase in catecholamines, adrenal steroids, triiodothyronine and thyroxine; increase in metabolism with shivering	Increased preshivering muscle tone, then fatiguing
Moderate	<32.2°C (90°F)–28°C (82.4°F)	EEG abnormalities; progressive depression of level of consciousness; pupillary dilation; paradoxical undressing; hallucinations	Progressive decrease in pulse and cardiac output; increased atrial and ventricular arrhythmias; suggestive (J- wave) ECG changes	Hypoventilation; 50% decrease in carbon dioxide production per 8°C (46°F) drop in temperature; absence of protective airway reflexes	50% increase in renal blood flow; renal autoregulation intact; impaired insulin action	Hyporeflexia; diminishing shivering-induced thermogenesis; rigidity
Severe	<28°C (82.4°F)	Loss of cerebrovascular autoregulation; decline in cerebral blood flow; coma; loss of ocular reflexes; progressive decrease in EEG	Progressive decrease in blood pressure, heart rate, and cardiac output; re-entrant dysrhythmias; maximum risk of ventricular fibrillation; asystole	Pulmonic congestion and edema; 75% decrease in oxygen consumption; apnea	Decrease in renal blood flow parallels decrease in cardiac output; extreme oliguria; poikilothermia; 80% decrease in basal metabolism	No motion; decreased nerve-conduction velocity; peripheral areflexia; no corneal or oculocephalic reflexes

Source: Modified from DF Danzl, RS Pozos: N Engl J Med 331:1756, 1994.

attempt (2 J/kg) should be administered. If the rhythm does not convert, the patient should be rewarmed to 30°C (86°F) before defibrillation attempts are repeated. Supplemental oxygenation is always warranted, since tissue oxygenation is affected adversely by the leftward shift of the oxyhemoglobin dissociation curve. Pulse oximetry may be unreliable in patients with vasoconstriction. If protective airway reflexes are absent, gentle endotracheal intubation should be performed. Adequate preoxygenation will prevent ventricular arrhythmias. Although cardiac pacing for hypothermic bradydysrhythmias is rarely indicated, the transthoracic technique is preferable.

Insertion of a gastric tube prevents dilation secondary to decreased bowel motility. Indwelling bladder catheters facilitate monitoring of cold-induced diuresis. Dehydration is encountered commonly with chronic hypothermia, and most patients benefit from a bolus of crystalloid. Normal saline is preferable to lactated Ringer's solution, as the liver in hypothermic patients inefficiently metabolizes lactate. The placement of a pulmonary artery catheter can cause perforation of the less compliant pulmonary artery. Insertion of a central venous catheter into the cold right atrium should be avoided, since this can precipitate arrhythmias.

Arterial blood gases should not be corrected for temperature (Chap. 47). An uncorrected pH of 7.42 and a P_{CO_2} of 40 mmHg reflect appropriate alveolar ventilation and acid-base balance at any core temperature. Acid-base imbalances should be corrected gradually, since the bicarbonate buffering system is inefficient. A common error is overzealous hyperventilation in the setting of depressed CO_2 production. When the P_{CO_2} decreases 10 mmHg at 28°C (82°F), it doubles the pH increase of 0.08 that occurs at 37°C (99°F).

The severity of anemia may be underestimated because the hematocrit increases 2% for each 1°C drop in temperature. White blood cell sequestration and bone marrow suppression are common, potentially masking an infection. Although hypokalemia is more common in chronic hypothermia, hyperkalemia also occurs; the expected electrocardiographic changes can be obscured by hypothermia. Patients with renal insufficiency, metabolic acidoses, or rhabdomyolysis are at greatest risk for electrolyte disturbances.

Coagulopathies are common because cold inhibits the enzymatic reactions required for activation of the intrinsic cascade. In addition, thromboxane B_2 production by platelets is temperature-dependent, and platelet function is impaired. The administration of platelets and fresh frozen plasma is therefore not effective. The prothrombin or partial thromboplastin times or INR (international normalized ratio) can be deceptively normal and contrast with the observed in vivo coagulopathy. This contradiction occurs because all coagulation tests are routinely performed at 37°C (99°F), and the enzymes are thus rewarmed.

▥ REWARMING STRATEGIES

The key initial decision is whether to rewarm the patient passively or actively. *Passive external rewarming* simply involves covering and insulating the patient in a warm environment. With the head also covered, the rate of rewarming is usually 0.5° to 2°C (33° to 36°F) per hour. This technique is ideal for previously healthy patients who develop acute, mild primary accidental hypothermia. The patient must have sufficient glycogen to support endogenous thermogenesis.

The application of heat directly to the extremities of patients with chronic severe hypothermia should be avoided because it can induce peripheral vasodilation and precipitate core temperature "afterdrop," a response characterized by a continual decline in the core temperature after removal of the patient from the cold. Truncal heat application reduces the risk of afterdrop.

Active rewarming is necessary under the following circumstances: core temperature <32°C (90°F) (poikilothermia), cardiovascular instability, age extremes, CNS dysfunction, hormone insufficiency, and suspicion of secondary hypothermia. *Active external rewarming* is best accomplished with forced-air heating blankets. Other options include devices that circulate water through external heat exchange pads, radiant heat sources, and hot packs. Monitoring a patient with hypothermia in a heated tub is extremely difficult. Electric blankets should be avoided because vasoconstricted skin is easily burned.

There are numerous widely available options for *active core rewarming*. Airway rewarming with heated humidified oxygen [40°–45°C (104°–113°F)] is a convenient option via mask or endotracheal tube. Although airway rewarming provides less heat than do some other forms of active core rewarming, it eliminates respiratory heat loss and adds 1°–2°C (34°–36°F) to the overall rewarming rate. Crystalloids should be heated to 40°–42°C (104°–108°F), but the quantity of heat provided is significant only during massive volume resuscitation. The most efficient method for heating and delivering fluid or blood is with a countercurrent in-line heat exchanger. Heated irrigation of the gastrointestinal tract or bladder transfers minimal heat because of the limited available surface area. These methods should be reserved for patients in cardiac arrest and then used in combination with all available active rewarming techniques. Closed thoracic lavage is far more efficient in severely hypothermic patients with cardiac arrest. The hemithoraxes are irrigated through two large-bore thoracostomy tubes that are inserted into the hemithoraxes. Thoracostomy tubes should not be placed in the left chest of a spontaneously perfusing patient for purposes of rewarming. Peritoneal lavage with the dialysate at 40°–45°C (104°–113°F) efficiently transfers heat when delivered through two catheters with outflow suction. Like peritoneal dialysis, standard hemodialysis is especially useful for patients with electrolyte abnormalities, rhabdomyolysis, or toxin ingestions. Another option involves the central venous insertion of a rapid endovascular warming device.

Extracorporeal blood rewarming options (Table 19-3) should be considered in severely hypothermic patients, especially those with *primary accidental hypothermia*. Cardiopulmonary bypass should be considered in nonperfusing patients without documented contraindications to resuscitation. Circulatory support may be the only effective option in patients with completely frozen extremities or those with significant tissue destruction coupled with rhabdomyolysis. There is no evidence that extremely rapid rewarming improves survival in perfusing patients. The best strategy is usually a combination of passive, truncal active, and active core rewarming techniques.

TREATMENT ▸ Hypothermia

When a patient is hypothermic, target organs and the cardiovascular system respond minimally to most medications. Generally, IV medications are withheld below 30°C (86°F). If they are given, an increased interval between doses can prevent cumulative toxicity during rewarming because of increased binding of drugs to proteins as well as impaired metabolism and excretion. As an example, the administration of repeated doses of digoxin or insulin would be ineffective while the patient is hypothermic, and the residual drugs are potentially toxic during rewarming.

Achieving a mean arterial pressure of at least 60 mmHg should be an early objective. If the hypotension does not respond to crystalloid/colloid infusion and rewarming, low-dose dopamine (2–5 μg/kg per min) support should be considered. Perfusion of the vasoconstricted cardiovascular system also may be improved with low-dose IV nitroglycerin.

TABLE 19-3 Options for Extracorporeal Blood Rewarming

Extracorporeal Rewarming (ECR) Technique	Considerations
Continuous venovenous (CVV)	Circuit—CV catheter to CV or dual lumen CV or peripheral catheter
	No oxygenator/circulatory support
	Flow rates 150–400 mL/min
	ROR 2°–3°C (36°–37°F)/h
Hemodialysis (HD)	Circuit—single- or dual-vessel cannulation
	Stabilizes electrolyte or toxicologic abnormalities
	Exchange cycle volumes 200–500 mL/min
	ROR 2°–3°C (36°–37°F)/h
Continuous arteriovenous rewarming (CAVR)	Circuit—percutaneous 8.5 Fr femoral catheters
	Requires BP 60 mmHg systolic
	No perfusionist/pump/anticoagulation
	Flow rates 225–375 mL/min
	ROR 3°–4°C (37°–39°F)/h
Cardiopulmonary bypass (CPB)	Circuit—full circulatory support with pump and oxygenator
	Perfusate-temperature gradient [5°–10°C (41°–50°F)]
	Flow rates 2–7 L/min (ave. 3–4)
	ROR up to 9.5°C (49°F)/h

Abbreviations: BP, blood pressure; CV, central venous; ROR, rate of rewarming.

Atrial arrhythmias should be monitored initially without intervention, as the ventricular response will be slow, and unless preexistent, most will convert spontaneously during rewarming. The role of prophylaxis and treatment of ventricular arrhythmias is problematic. Preexisting ventricular ectopy may be suppressed by hypothermia and reappear during rewarming. None of the class I agents has proved to be safe and efficacious. There is also no evidence that the class III ventricular antiarrhythmic amiodarone is safe. Initiating empirical therapy for adrenal insufficiency usually is not warranted unless there is a history suggesting steroid dependence or hypoadrenalism or a failure to rewarm with standard therapy. The administration of parenteral levothyroxine to euthyroid patients with hypothermia, however, is potentially hazardous. Because laboratory results can be delayed and confounded by the presence of the sick euthyroid syndrome (Chap. 341), historic clues or physical findings suggestive of hypothyroidism should be sought. When myxedema is the cause of hypothermia, the relaxation phase of the Achilles reflex is prolonged more than is the contraction phase.

Hypothermia obscures most of the symptoms and signs of infection, notably fever and leukocytosis. Shaking rigors from infection may be mistaken for shivering. Except in mild cases,

extensive cultures and repeated physical examinations are essential. Unless an infectious source is identified, empirical antibiotic prophylaxis is most warranted in the elderly, neonates, and immunocompromised patients.

Preventive measures should be discussed with high-risk individuals, such as the elderly and people whose work frequently exposes them to extreme cold. The importance of layered clothing and headgear, adequate shelter, increased caloric intake, and the avoidance of ethanol should be emphasized, along with access to rescue services.

FROSTBITE

Peripheral cold injuries include both freezing and nonfreezing injuries to tissue. Tissue freezes quickly when in contact with thermal conductors such as metal and volatile solutions. Other predisposing factors include constrictive clothing or boots, immobility, and vasoconstrictive medications. Frostbite occurs when the tissue temperature drops below 0°C (32°F). Ice crystal formation subsequently distorts and destroys the cellular architecture. Once the vascular endothelium is damaged, stasis progresses rapidly to microvascular thrombosis. After the tissue thaws, there is progressive dermal ischemia. The microvasculature begins to collapse, arteriovenous shunting increases tissue pressures, and edema forms. Finally, thrombosis, ischemia, and superficial necrosis appear. The development of mummification and demarcation may take weeks to months.

■ CLINICAL PRESENTATION

The initial presentation of frostbite can be deceptively benign. The symptoms always include a sensory deficiency affecting light touch, pain, and temperature perception. The acral areas and distal extremities are the most common insensate areas. Some patients complain of a clumsy or "chunk of wood" sensation in the extremity.

Deep frostbitten tissue can appear waxy, mottled, yellow, or violaceous-white. Favorable presenting signs include some warmth or sensation with normal color. The injury is often superficial if the subcutaneous tissue is pliable or if the dermis can be rolled over bony prominences.

Clinically, it is most practical to classify frostbite as superficial or deep. Superficial does not entail tissue loss. Superficial frostbite causes only anesthesia and erythema. The appearance of vesiculation surrounded by edema and erythema implies deeper involvement (Fig. 19-1). Hemorrhagic vesicles reflect a serious injury to the microvasculature and indicate severe frostbite. Damages in subcuticular, muscular, or osseous tissues may result in amputation.

The two most common nonfreezing peripheral cold injuries are *chilblain (pernio)* and *immersion (trench) foot*. Chilblain results from neuronal and endothelial damage induced by repetitive exposure to dry cold. Young females, particularly those with a history of Raynaud's phenomenon, are at greatest risk. Persistent vasospasticity and vasculitis can cause erythema, mild edema, and pruritus. Eventually plaques, blue nodules, and ulcerations develop. These lesions typically involve the dorsa of the hands and feet. In contrast, immersion (trench) foot results from repetitive exposure to wet cold above the freezing point. The feet initially appear cyanotic, cold, and edematous. The subsequent development of bullae is often indistinguishable from frostbite. This vesiculation rapidly progresses to ulceration and liquefaction gangrene. Patients with milder cases complain of hyperhidrosis, cold sensitivity, and painful ambulation for many years.

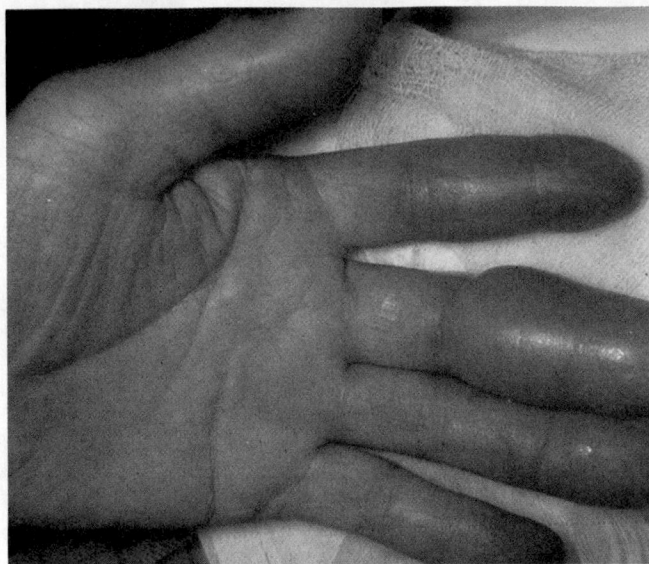

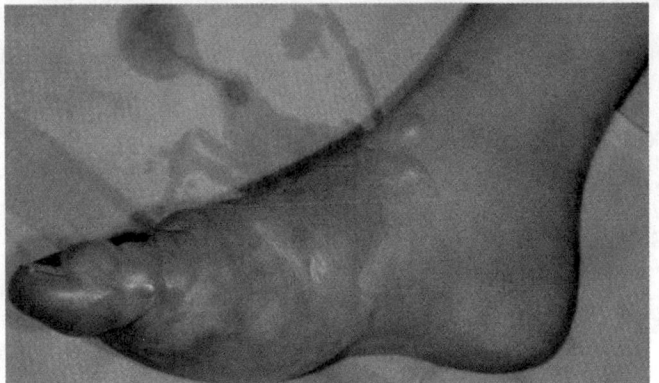

Figure 19-1 **Frostbite with vesiculation,** surrounded by edema and erythema.

Frostbite

Frozen tissue should be thawed rapidly and completely by immersion in circulating water at 37°–40°C (99°–104°F). Rapid rewarming often produces an initial hyperemia. The early formation of large clear distal blebs is more favorable than that of smaller proximal dark hemorrhagic blebs. A common error is the premature termination of thawing, since the reestablishment of perfusion is intensely painful. Parenteral narcotics will be necessary with deep frostbite. If cyanosis persists after rewarming, the tissue compartment pressures should be monitored carefully.

Numerous experimental antithrombotic and vasodilatory treatment regimens have been evaluated. There is no conclusive evidence that dextran, heparin, steroids, calcium channel blockers, hyperbaric oxygen, or prostaglandin inhibitors salvage tissue. Intraarterial thrombolysis may reduce the need for digital and more proximal amputations when administered within 24 h of severe injuries. A treatment protocol for frostbite is summarized in Table 19-4.

Unless infection develops, any decision regarding debridement or amputation should be deferred until there is clear evidence of demarcation, mummification, and sloughing. Magnetic resonance angiography may demonstrate the line of demarcation earlier than does clinical demarcation. The most common symptomatic sequelae reflect neuronal injury and the persistently abnormal sympathetic tone, including paresthesias, thermal misperception, and hyperhidrosis. Delayed findings include nail deformities, cutaneous carcinomas, and epiphyseal damage in children.

Management of the chilblain syndrome is usually supportive. With refractory perniosis, alternatives include nifedipine, steroids, and limaprost, a prostaglandin E_1 analogue.

TABLE 19-4 Treatment for Frostbite

Before Thawing	During Thawing	After Thawing
Remove from environment	Consider parenteral analgesia and ketorolac	Gently dry and protect part; elevate; pledgets between toes, if macerated
Prevent partial thawing and refreezing	Administer ibuprofen, 400 mg PO	If clear vesicles are intact, aspirate sterilely; if broken, debride and dress with antibiotic or sterile aloe vera ointment
Stabilize core temperature and treat hypothermia	Immerse part in 37°–40°C (99°–104°F) (thermometer-monitored) circulating water containing an antiseptic soap until distal flush (10–45 min)	Leave hemorrhagic vesicles intact to prevent dessication and infection
Protect frozen part—no friction or massage	Encourage patient to gently move part	Continue ibuprofen 400 mg PO (12 mg/kg per day) q8–12h
Address medical or surgical conditions	If pain is refractory, reduce water temperature to 35°–37°C (95°–99°F) and administer parenteral narcotics	Consider tetanus and streptococcal prophylaxis; elevate part Hydrotherapy at 37°C (99°F) Consider phenoxybenzamine or thrombolysis in severe cases

FURTHER READINGS

ALFONZO A et al: Survival after 5-h resuscitation attempt for hypothermic cardiac arrest using CVVG for extracorporeal rewarming. Nephrol Dial Transplant 24:1054, 2009

BRUEN KJ et al: Reduction of the incidence of amputation in frostbite injury with thrombolytic therapy. Arch Surg 142:546, 2007

DANZL DF: Accidental hypothermia, in *Rosen's Emergency Medicine: Concepts and Clinical Practice*, 7th ed, J Marx et al (eds). Philadelphia, Mosby, 2010, p. 1861

JURKOVICH GJ: Environmental cold-induced injury. Surg Clin North Am 87:247, 2007

KEMPAINEN RR, BRUNETTE DD: The evaluation and management of accidental hypothermia. Respir Care 49:192, 2004

MULCAHY AR, WATTS MR: Accidental hypothermia: An evidence-based approach. Emerg Med Pract 11:1, 2009

CHAPTER 20

Syncope

Roy Freeman

Syncope is a transient, self-limited loss of consciousness due to acute global impairment of cerebral blood flow. The onset is rapid, duration brief, and recovery spontaneous and complete. Other causes of transient loss of consciousness need to be distinguished from syncope; these include seizures, vertebrobasilar ischemia, hypoxemia, and hypoglycemia. A syncopal prodrome (*presyncope*) is common, although loss of consciousness may occur without any warning symptoms. Typical presyncopal symptoms include dizziness, lightheadedness or faintness, weakness, fatigue, and visual and auditory disturbances. The causes of syncope can be divided into three general categories: (1) neurally mediated syncope (also called *reflex syncope*), (2) orthostatic hypotension, and (3) cardiac syncope.

Neurally mediated syncope comprises a heterogeneous group of functional disorders that are characterized by a transient change in the reflexes responsible for maintaining cardiovascular homeostasis. Episodic vasodilation and bradycardia occur in varying combinations, resulting in temporary failure of blood pressure control. In contrast, in patients with orthostatic hypotension due to autonomic failure, these cardiovascular homeostatic reflexes are chronically impaired. Cardiac syncope may be due to arrhythmias or structural cardiac diseases that cause a decrease in cardiac output. The clinical features, underlying pathophysiologic mechanisms, therapeutic interventions, and prognoses differ markedly among these three causes.

EPIDEMIOLOGY AND NATURAL HISTORY

Syncope is a common presenting problem, accounting for approximately 3% of all emergency room visits and 1% of all hospital admissions. The annual cost for syncope-related hospitalization in the United States is ~ $2 billion. Syncope has a lifetime cumulative incidence of up to 35% in the general population. The peak incidence in the young occurs between ages 10 and 30 years, with a median peak around 15 years. Neurally mediated syncope is the etiology in the vast majority of these cases. In elderly adults, there is a sharp rise in the incidence of syncope after 70 years.

In population-based studies, neurally mediated syncope is the most common cause of syncope. The incidence is slightly higher in females than males. In young subjects there is often a family history in first-degree relatives. Cardiovascular disease due to structural disease or arrhythmias is the next most common cause in most series, particularly in emergency room settings and in older patients. Orthostatic hypotension also increases in prevalence with age because of the reduced baroreflex responsiveness, decreased cardiac compliance, and attenuation of the vestibulosympathetic reflex associated with aging. In the elderly, orthostatic hypotension is substantially more common in institutionalized (54–68%) than community dwelling (6%) individuals, an observation most likely explained by the greater prevalence of predisposing neurologic disorders, physiologic impairment, and vasoactive medication use among institutionalized patients.

TABLE 20-1 High-Risk Features Indicating Hospitalization or Intensive Evaluation of Syncope

Chest pain suggesting coronary ischemia
Features of congestive heart failure
Moderate or severe valvular disease
Moderate or severe structural cardiac disease
Electrocardiographic features of ischemia
History of ventricular arrhythmias
Prolonged QT interval (>500 msec)
Repetitive sinoatrial block or sinus pauses
Persistent sinus bradycardia
Trifascicular block
Atrial fibrillation
Nonsustained ventricular tachycardia
Family history of sudden death
Preexcitation syndromes
Brugada pattern on ECG

The prognosis after a single syncopal event for all age groups is generally benign. In particular, syncope of noncardiac and unexplained origin in younger individuals has an excellent prognosis; life expectancy is unaffected. By contrast, syncope due to a cardiac cause, either structural heart disease or primary arrhythmic disease, is associated with an increased risk of sudden cardiac death and mortality from other causes. Similarly, mortality rate is increased in individuals with syncope due to orthostatic hypotension related to age and the associated comorbid conditions (Table 20-1).

PATHOPHYSIOLOGY

The upright posture imposes a unique physiologic stress upon humans; most, although not all, syncopal episodes occur from a standing position. Standing results in pooling of 500–1000 mL of blood in the lower extremities and splanchnic circulation. There is a decrease in venous return to the heart and reduced ventricular filling that result in diminished cardiac output and blood pressure. These hemodynamic changes provoke a compensatory reflex response, initiated by the baroreceptors in the carotid sinus and aortic arch, resulting in increased sympathetic outflow and decreased vagal nerve activity (Fig. 20-1). The reflex increases peripheral resistance, venous return to the heart, and cardiac output and thus limits the fall in blood pressure. If this response fails, as is the case chronically in orthostatic hypotension and transiently in neurally mediated syncope, cerebral hypoperfusion occurs.

Syncope is a consequence of global cerebral hypoperfusion and thus represents a failure of cerebral blood flow autoregulatory mechanisms. Myogenic factors, local metabolites, and to a lesser extent autonomic neurovascular control are responsible for the

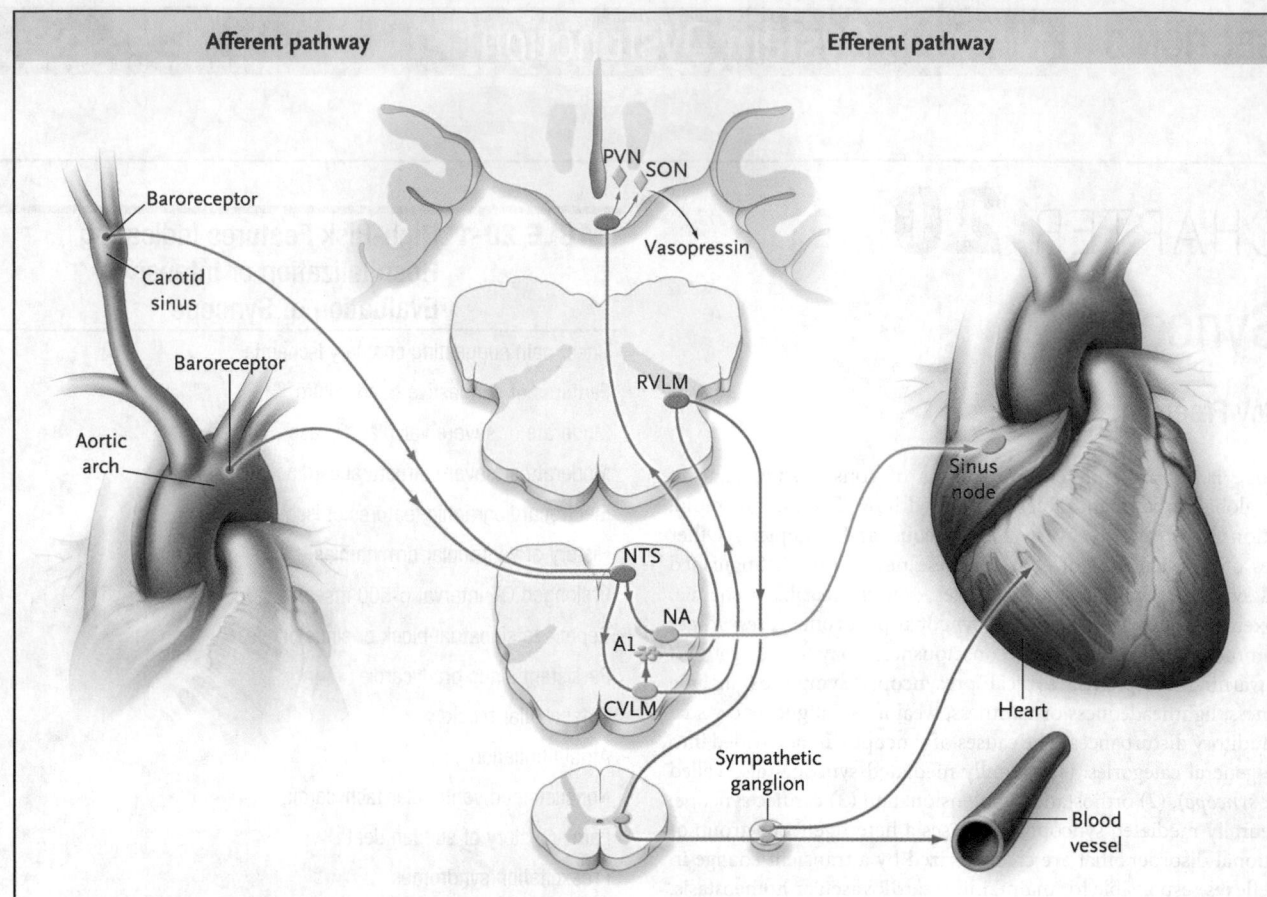

Figure 20-1   The Baroreflex. A decrease in arterial pressure unloads the baroreceptors—the terminals of afferent fibers of the glossopharyngeal and vagus nerves—that are situated in the carotid sinus and aortic arch. This leads to a reduction in the afferent impulses that are relayed from these mechanoreceptors through the glossopharyngeal and vagus nerves to the nucleus of the tractus solitarius (NTS) in the dorsomedial medulla. The reduced baroreceptor afferent activity produces a decrease in vagal nerve input to the sinus node that is mediated by the neuroanatomical connections of the NTS to the nucleus ambiguus (NA). There is an increase in sympathetic efferent activity that is mediated by the NTS projections to the caudal ventrolateral medulla (CVLM) (an excitatory pathway) and from there to the rostral ventrolateral medulla (RVLM) (an inhibitory pathway). The activation of RVLM presympathetic neurons in response to hypotension is thus predominantly due to disinhibition. In response to a sustained fall in blood pressure, vasopressin release is mediated by projections from the A1 noradrenergic cell group in the ventrolateral medulla. This projection activates vasopressin-synthesizing neurons in the magnocellular portion of the paraventricular nucleus (PVN) and the supraoptic nucleus (SON) of the hypothalamus. Blue denotes sympathetic neurons and green parasympathetic neurons.) *(From R Freeman: N Engl J Med 358:615, 2008.)*

autoregulation of cerebral blood flow (Chap. 275). Typically cerebral blood flow ranges from 50 to 60 mL/min per 100 g brain tissue and remains relatively constant over perfusion pressures ranging from 50 to 150 mmHg. Cessation of blood flow for 6–8 seconds will result in loss of consciousness, while impairment of consciousness ensues when blood flow decreases to 25 mL/min per 100 g brain tissue.

From the clinical standpoint, a fall in systemic systolic blood pressure to ~ 50 mmHg or lower will result in syncope. A decrease in cardiac output and/or systemic vascular resistance—the determinants of blood pressure—thus underlies the pathophysiology of syncope. Common causes of impaired cardiac output include decreased effective circulating blood volume; increased thoracic pressure; massive pulmonary embolus; cardiac brady- and tachyarrhythmias; valvular heart disease; and myocardial dysfunction. Systemic vascular resistance may be decreased by central and peripheral autonomic nervous system diseases, sympatholytic medications, and transiently during neurally mediated syncope. Increased cerebral vascular resistance, most frequently due to hypocarbia induced by hyperventilation, may also contribute to the pathophysiology of syncope.

The sequence of changes on the electroencephalogram of syncopal subjects during syncope comprises background slowing (often of high amplitude), followed by attenuation or cessation of cortical activity prior to return of slow waves, and then normal activity. Despite the presence of myoclonic movements and other motor activity, electroencephalographic seizure discharges are not present in syncopal subjects.

CLASSIFICATION

■ NEURALLY MEDIATED SYNCOPE

Neurally mediated syncope is the final pathway of a complex central and peripheral nervous system reflex arc. There is a sudden, transient change in autonomic efferent activity characterized by increased parasympathetic outflow causing bradycardia and sympathoinhibition causing vasodilation. The change in autonomic efferent activity leads to a decrease in blood pressure and a subsequent fall in cerebral blood flow to below the limits of autoregulation (Fig. 20-2). In order to elicit this reflex, a normal or functioning autonomic nervous system is necessary; this is in contrast to the situation in autonomic failure. The triggers of the afferent limb of

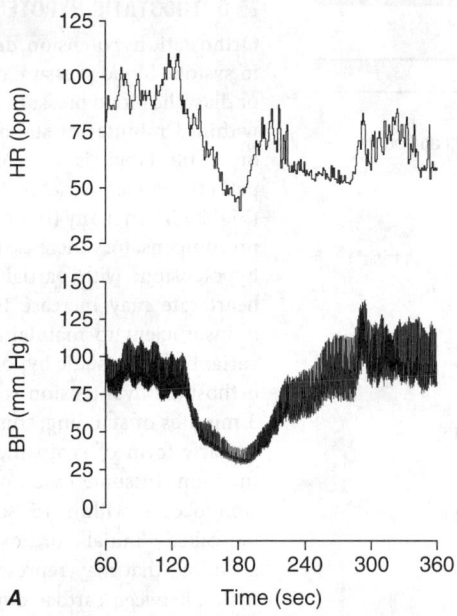
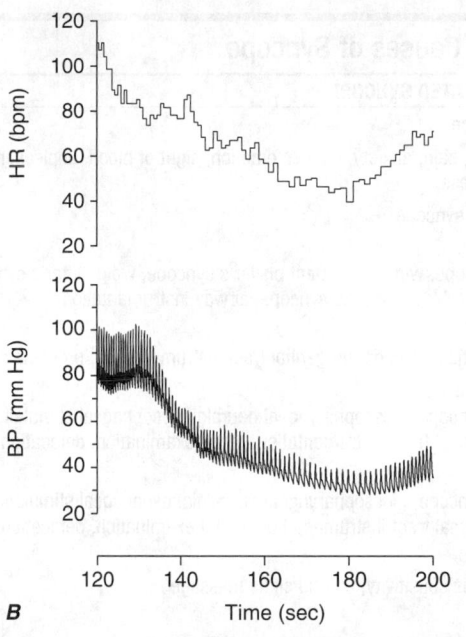

Figure 20-2 *A.* **The paroxysmal hypotensive-bradycardic response** that is characteristic of neurally mediated syncope. Noninvasive beat-to-beat blood pressure and heart rate are shown over 5 minutes (from 60 to 360 seconds) of an upright tilt on a tilt table. *B.* The same tracing expanded to show 80 seconds of the episode (from 80 to 200 seconds). BP, blood pressure; bpm, beats per minute; HR, heart rate.

the reflex arc vary and may be clearly defined, e.g., the carotid sinus, the gastrointestinal tract, or the bladder. In many cases, however, the afferent arc is less easily recognized and, under many circumstances, the cause is multifactorial. Under these circumstances it is likely that multiple afferent pathways converge on the central autonomic network within the medulla that integrates the neural impulses and mediates the vasodepressor-bradycardic response.

Classification of neurally mediated syncope

Neurally mediated syncope may be subdivided based on the afferent pathway and provocative trigger. Vasovagal syncope (the common faint) is provoked by intense emotion, pain, and/or orthostatic stress, whereas the situational reflex syncopes have specific localized stimuli that provoke the reflex vasodilation and bradycardia that leads to syncope. The underlying mechanisms have been identified and pathophysiology delineated for most of these situational reflex syncopes. The afferent trigger may originate in the pulmonary system, gastrointestinal system, urogenital system, heart, and carotid artery (Table 20-2). Hyperventilation leading to hypocarbia and cerebral vasoconstriction, and raised intrathoracic pressure that impairs venous return to the heart, play a central role in many of the situational reflex syncopes. The afferent pathway of the reflex arc differs among these disorders but the efferent response via the vagus and sympathetic pathways is similar.

Alternately, neurally mediated syncope may be subdivided based on the predominant efferent pathway. Vasodepressor syncope describes syncope predominantly due to efferent, sympathetic, vasoconstrictor failure; cardioinhibitory syncope describes syncope predominantly associated with bradycardia or asystole due to increased vagal outflow; while mixed syncope describes syncope in which there are both vagal and sympathetic reflex changes.

Features of neurally mediated syncope

In addition to symptoms of orthostatic intolerance such as dizziness, lightheadedness, and fatigue, premonitory features of autonomic activation may be present in patients with neurally mediated syncope. These include diaphoresis, pallor, palpitations, nausea, hyperventilation, and yawning. During the syncopal event proximal and distal myoclonus (typically arrhythmic and multifocal) may occur, raising the possibility of epilepsy. The eyes typically remain open and usually deviate upward. Urinary but not fecal incontinence may occur. Postictal confusion is rare, although visual and auditory hallucinations are sometimes reported.

While some predisposing factors and provocative stimuli are well established (for example, motionless upright posture, warm ambient temperature, intravascular volume depletion, alcohol ingestion, hypoxemia, anemia, pain, the sight of blood, venipuncture, and intense emotion), the underlying basis for the widely different thresholds for syncope among individuals exposed to the same provocative stimulus is not known. A genetic basis for neurally mediated syncope may exist; several studies have reported an increased incidence of syncope in first-degree relatives of fainters, but no gene or genetic marker has been identified, and environmental, social, and cultural factors have not been excluded by these studies.

TREATMENT Neurally Mediated Syncope

Reassurance, avoidance of provocative stimuli, and plasma volume expansion with fluid and salt are the cornerstones of the management of neurally mediated syncope. Isometric counter-pressure maneuvers of the limbs (leg crossing or handgrip and arm tensing) may raise blood pressure and, by maintaining pressure in the autoregulatory zone, avoid or delay the onset of syncope. Randomized controlled trials support this intervention.

Fludrocortisone, vasoconstricting agents, and beta-adrenoreceptor antagonists are widely used by experts to treat refractory patients, although there is no consistent evidence from randomized, controlled trials for any pharmacotherapy to treat neurally mediated syncope. Because vasodilation is the dominant pathophysiologic syncopal mechanism in most patients, use of a cardiac pacemaker is rarely beneficial. Possible exceptions are older patients in whom syncope is associated with asystole or severe bradycardia, and patients with prominent cardioinhibition due to carotid sinus syndrome. In these patients, dual-chamber pacing may be helpful.

TABLE 20-2 Causes of Syncope

A. NEURALLY MEDIATED SYNCOPE

Vasovagal syncope

Provoked fear, pain, anxiety, intense emotion, sight of blood, unpleasant sights and odors, orthostatic stress

Situational reflex syncope

Pulmonary

Cough syncope, wind instrument player's syncope, weightlifter's syncope, "mess trick"[a] and "fainting lark,"[b] sneeze syncope, airway instrumentation

Urogenital

Postmicturition syncope, urogenital tract instrumentation, prostatic massage

Gastrointestinal

Swallow syncope, glossopharyngeal neuralgia, esophageal stimulation, gastrointestinal tract instrumentation, rectal examination, defecation syncope

Cardiac

Swallow syncope, glossopharyngeal neuralgia, esophageal stimulation, gastrointestinal tract instrumentation, rectal examination, defecation syncope

Carotid sinus

Carotid sinus sensitivity, carotid sinus massage

Ocular

Ocular pressure, ocular examination, ocular surgery

B. ORTHOSTATIC HYPOTENSION

Primary autonomic failure due to idiopathic central and peripheral neurodegenerative diseases—the "synucleinopathies"

Lewy body diseases

Parkinson's disease

Lewy body dementia

Pure autonomic failure

Multiple system atrophy (the Shy-Drager syndrome)

Secondary autonomic failure due to autonomic peripheral neuropathies

Diabetes

Hereditary amyloidosis (familial amyloid polyneuropathy)

Primary amyloidosis (AL amyloidosis; immunoglobulin light chain associated)

Hereditary sensory and autonomic neuropathies (HSAN) (especially type III—familial dysautonomia)

Idiopathic immune-mediated autonomic neuropathy

Autoimmune autonomic ganglionopathy

Sjögren's syndrome

Paraneoplastic autonomic neuropathy

HIV neuropathy

Postprandial hypotension

Iatrogenic (drug-induced)

Volume depletion

C. CARDIAC SYNCOPE

Arrhythmias

Sinus node dysfunction

Atrioventricular dysfunction

Supraventricular tachycardias

Ventricular tachycardias

Inherited channelopathies

Cardiac structural disease

Valvular disease

Myocardial ischemia

Obstructive and other cardiomyopathies

Atrial myxoma

Pericardial effusions and tamponade

[a]Hyperventilation for 1 minute, followed by sudden chest compression.
[b]Hyperventilation (20 breaths) in a squatting position, rapid rise to standing, then Valsalva.

■ ORTHOSTATIC HYPOTENSION

Orthostatic hypotension, defined as a reduction in systolic blood pressure of at least 20 mmHg or diastolic blood pressure of at least 10 mmHg within 3 minutes of standing or head-up tilt on a tilt table, is a manifestation of sympathetic vasoconstrictor (autonomic) failure (Fig. 20-3). In many (but not all) cases, there is no compensatory increase in heart rate despite hypotension; with partial autonomic failure, heart rate may increase to some degree but is insufficient to maintain cardiac output. A variant of orthostatic hypotension is "delayed" orthostatic hypotension which occurs beyond 3 minutes of standing; this may reflect a mild or early form of sympathetic adrenergic dysfunction. In some cases, orthostatic hypotension occurs within 15 seconds of standing (so-called "initial" orthostatic hypotension), a finding that may represent a transient mismatch between cardiac output and peripheral vascular resistance and does not represent autonomic failure.

Characteristic symptoms of orthostatic hypotension include light-headedness, dizziness, and presyncope (near-faintness) occurring in response to sudden postural change. However, symptoms may be absent or nonspecific, such as generalized weakness, fatigue, cognitive slowing, leg buckling, or headache. Visual blurring may occur, likely due to retinal or occipital lobe ischemia. Neck pain—typically in the suboccipital, posterior cervical, and shoulder region (the "coat-hanger headache"), most likely due to neck muscle ischemia, may be the only symptom. Patients may report orthostatic dyspnea (thought to reflect ventilation-perfusion mismatch due to inadequate perfusion of ventilated lung apices) or angina (attributed to impaired myocardial perfusion even with normal coronary arteries). Symptoms may be exacerbated by exertion, prolonged standing, increased ambient temperature, or meals. Syncope is usually preceded by warning symptoms, but may occur suddenly, suggesting the possibility of a seizure or cardiac cause.

Supine hypertension is common in patients with orthostatic hypotension due to autonomic failure, affecting over 50% of patients in some series. Orthostatic hypotension may present after initiation of therapy for hypertension, and supine hypertension may follow treatment of orthostatic hypotension. However, in other cases, the association of the two conditions is unrelated to therapy; it may in part be explained by baroreflex dysfunction in the presence of residual sympathetic outflow, particularly in patients with central autonomic degeneration.

Causes of neurogenic orthostatic hypotension

Causes of neurogenic orthostatic hypotension include central and peripheral autonomic nervous system dysfunction (Chap. 375).

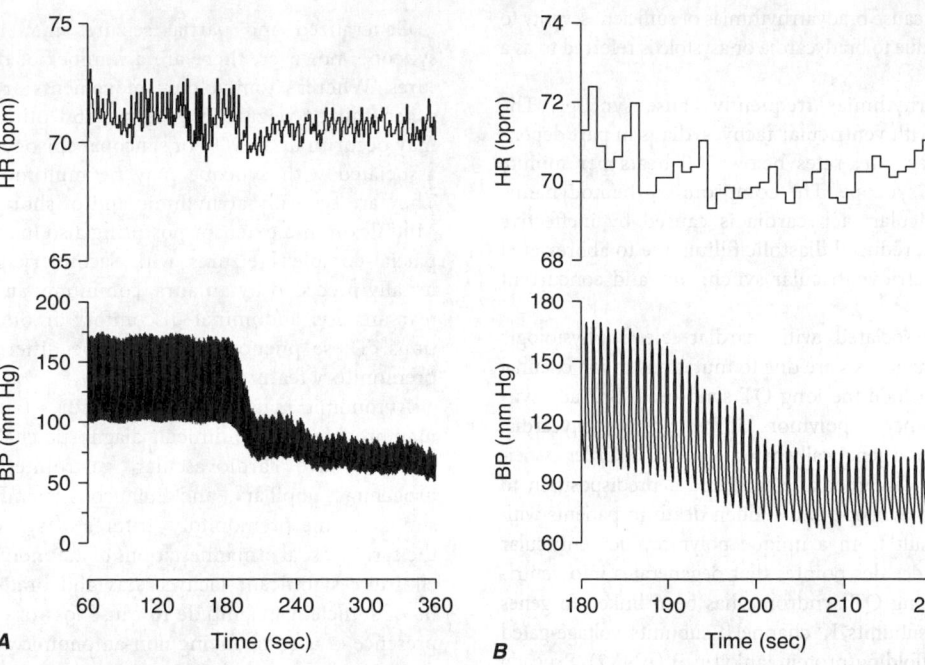

Figure 20-3 **A. The gradual fall in blood pressure** without a compensatory heart rate increase that is characteristic of orthostatic hypotension due to autonomic failure. Blood pressure and heart rate are shown over 5 minutes (from 60 to 360 seconds) of an upright tilt on a tilt table. **B.** The same tracing expanded to show 40 seconds of the episode (from 180 to 220 seconds). BP, blood pressure; bpm, beats per minute; HR, heart rate.

Autonomic dysfunction of other organ systems (including the bladder, bowels, sexual organs, and sudomotor system) of varying severity frequently accompanies orthostatic hypotension in these disorders (Table 20-2).

The primary autonomic degenerative disorders are multiple system atrophy (the Shy-Drager syndrome; Chap. 375), Parkinson's disease (Chap. 372), dementia with Lewy bodies (Chap. 371), and pure autonomic failure (Chap. 375). These are often grouped together as "synucleinopathies" due to the presence of alpha-synuclein, a small protein that precipitates predominantly in the cytoplasm of neurons in the Lewy body disorders (Parkinson's disease, dementia with Lewy bodies, and pure autonomic failure) and in the glia in multiple system atrophy.

Peripheral autonomic dysfunction may also accompany small fiber peripheral neuropathies such as those seen in diabetes, amyloid, immune-mediated neuropathies, hereditary sensory and autonomic neuropathies (HSAN; particularly HSAN type III; familial dysautonomia), and inflammatory neuropathies (Chaps. 385 and 386). Less frequently, orthostatic hypotension is associated with the peripheral neuropathies that accompany vitamin B_{12} deficiency, neurotoxic exposure, HIV and other infections, and porphyria.

Patients with autonomic failure and the elderly are susceptible to falls in blood pressure associated with meals. The magnitude of the blood pressure fall is exacerbated by large meals, meals high in carbohydrate, and alcohol intake. The mechanism of postprandial syncope is not fully elucidated.

Orthostatic hypotension is often iatrogenic. Drugs from several classes may lower peripheral resistance (e.g., alpha-adrenoreceptor antagonists used to treat hypertension and prostatic hypertrophy; antihypertensive agents of several classes; nitrates and other vasodilators; tricyclic agents and phenothiazines). Iatrogenic volume depletion due to diuresis and volume depletion due to medical causes (hemorrhage, vomiting, diarrhea, or decreased fluid intake) may also result in decreased effective circulatory volume, orthostatic hypotension, and syncope.

TREATMENT   Orthostatic Hypotension

The first step is to remove reversible causes—usually vasoactive medications (Table 375-6). Next, nonpharmacologic interventions should be introduced. These interventions include patient education regarding staged moves from supine to upright; warnings about the hypotensive effects of meal ingestion; instructions about the isometric counterpressure maneuvers that increase intravascular pressure (see above); and raising the head of the bed to reduce supine hypertension. Intravascular volume should be expanded by increasing dietary fluid and salt. If these nonpharmacologic measures fail, pharmacologic intervention with fludrocortisone acetate and vasoconstricting agents such as midodrine and pseudoephedrine should be introduced. Some patients with intractable symptoms require additional therapy with supplementary agents that include pyridostigmine, yohimbine, desmopressin acetate (DDAVP), and erythropoietin (Chap. 375).

■ CARDIAC SYNCOPE

Cardiac (or cardiovascular) syncope is caused by arrhythmias and structural heart disease. These may occur in combination because structural disease renders the heart more vulnerable to abnormal electrical activity.

Arrhythmias

Bradyarrhythmias that cause syncope include those due to severe sinus node dysfunction (e.g., sinus arrest or sinoatrial block) and atrioventricular block (e.g., Mobitz type II, high-grade, and complete AV block). The bradyarrhythmias due to sinus node dysfunction are often associated with an atrial tachyarrhythmia, a disorder known as the tachycardia-bradycardia syndrome. A prolonged pause following the termination of a tachycardic episode is a frequent cause of syncope in patients with the tachycardia-bradycardia syndrome. Medications of several classes may also cause bradyarrhythmias of sufficient severity to cause syncope. Syncope due to bradycardia or asystole is referred to as a Stokes-Adams attack.

Ventricular tachyarrhythmias frequently cause syncope. The likelihood of syncope with ventricular tachycardia is in part dependent on the ventricular rate; rates below 200 beats per minute are less likely to cause syncope. The compromised hemodynamic function during ventricular tachycardia is caused by ineffective ventricular contraction, reduced diastolic filling due to abbreviated filling periods, loss of atrioventricular synchrony, and concurrent myocardial ischemia.

Several disorders associated with cardiac electrophysiologic instability and arrhythmogenesis are due to mutations in ion channel subunit genes. These include the long QT syndrome, Brugada syndrome, and catecholaminergic polymorphic ventricular tachycardia. The long QT syndrome is a genetically heterogeneous disorder associated with prolonged cardiac repolarization and a predisposition to ventricular arrhythmias. Syncope and sudden death in patients with long QT syndrome result from a unique polymorphic ventricular tachycardia called torsades des pointes that degenerates into ventricular fibrillation. The long QT syndrome has been linked to genes encoding K^+ channel α-subunits, K^+ channel β-subunits, voltage-gated Na^+ channel, and a scaffolding protein, ankyrin B (ANK2). Brugada syndrome is characterized by idiopathic ventricular fibrillation in association with right ventricular electrocardiogram (ECG) abnormalities without structural heart disease. This disorder is also genetically heterogeneous, although it is most frequently linked to mutations in the Na^+ channel α-subunit, SCN5A. Catecholaminergic polymorphic tachycardia is an inherited, genetically heterogeneous disorder associated with exercise-or stress-induced ventricular arrhythmias, syncope, or sudden death. Acquired QT interval prolongation, most commonly due to drugs, may also result in ventricular arrhythmias and syncope. These disorders are discussed in detail in Chap. 233.

Structural disease

Structural heart disease, (e.g., valvular disease, myocardial ischemia, hypertrophic and other cardiomyopathies, cardiac masses such as atrial myxoma, and pericardial effusions) may lead to syncope by compromising cardiac output. Structural disease may also contribute to other pathophysiologic mechanisms of syncope. For example, cardiac structural disease may predispose to arrhythmogenesis; aggressive treatment of cardiac failure with diuretics and/or vasodilators may lead to orthostatic hypotension; and inappropriate reflex vasodilation may occur with structural disorders such as aortic stenosis and hypertrophic cardiomyopathy, possibly provoked by increased ventricular contractility.

TREATMENT   Cardiac Syncope

Treatment of cardiac disease depends upon the underlying disorder. Therapies for arrhythmias include cardiac pacing for sinus node disease and AV block, and ablation, anti-arrhythmic drugs, and cardioverter-defibrillators for atrial and ventricular tachyarrhythmias. These disorders are best managed by physicians with specialized skills in this area.

APPROACH TO THE PATIENT   Syncope

DIFFERENTIAL DIAGNOSIS   Syncope is easily diagnosed when the characteristic features are present; however, several disorders with transient real or apparent loss of consciousness may create diagnostic confusion.

Generalized and partial seizures may be confused with syncope; however, there are a number of differentiating features. Whereas tonic-clonic movements are the hallmark of a generalized seizure, myoclonic and other movements also may occur in up to 90% of syncopal episodes. Myoclonic jerks associated with syncope may be multifocal or generalized. They are typically arrhythmic and of short duration (<30 s). Mild flexor and extensor posturing also may occur. Partial- or partial-complex seizures with secondary generalization are usually preceded by an aura, commonly an unpleasant smell; fear anxiety; abdominal discomfort or other visceral sensations. These phenomena should be differentiated from the premonitory features of syncope.

Autonomic manifestations of seizures (autonomic epilepsy) may provide a more difficult diagnostic challenge. Autonomic seizures have cardiovascular, gastrointestinal, pulmonary, urogenital, pupillary, and cutaneous manifestations that are similar to the premonitory features of syncope. Furthermore, the cardiovascular manifestations of autonomic epilepsy include clinically significant tachycardias and bradycardias that may be of sufficient magnitude to cause loss of consciousness. The presence of accompanying non-autonomic auras may help differentiate these episodes from syncope.

Loss of consciousness associated with a seizure usually lasts longer than 5 minutes and is associated with prolonged postictal drowsiness and disorientation, whereas reorientation occurs almost immediately after a syncopal event. Muscle aches may occur after both syncope and seizures, although they tend to last longer following a seizure. Seizures, unlike syncope, are rarely provoked by emotions or pain. Incontinence of urine may occur with both seizures and syncope; however, fecal incontinence does not occur with syncope.

Hypoglycemia may cause transient loss of consciousness, typically in individuals with Type 1 or Type 2 diabetes treated with insulin. The clinical features associated with impending or actual hypoglycemia include tremor, palpitations, anxiety, diaphoresis, hunger, and paresthesias. These symptoms are due to autonomic activation to counter the falling blood glucose. Hunger, in particular, is not a typical premonitory feature of syncope. Hypoglycemia also impairs neuronal function, leading to fatigue, weakness, dizziness, and cognitive and behavioral symptoms. Diagnostic difficulties may occur in individuals in strict glycemic control; repeated hypoglycemia impairs the counterregulatory response and leads to a loss of the characteristic warning symptoms that are the hallmark of hypoglycemia.

Patients with cataplexy experience an abrupt partial or complete loss of muscular tone triggered by strong emotions, typically anger or laughter. Unlike syncope, consciousness is maintained throughout the attacks, which typically last between 30 seconds and 2 minutes. There are no premonitory symptoms. Cataplexy occurs in 60–75% of patients with narcolepsy.

The clinical interview and interrogation of eyewitnesses usually allows differentiation of syncope from falls due to vestibular dysfunction, cerebellar disease, extrapyramidal system dysfunction, and other gait disorders. If the fall is accompanied by head trauma, a postconcussive syndrome, amnesia for the precipitating events, and/or the presence of loss of consciousness may contribute to diagnostic difficulty.

Apparent loss of consciousness can be a manifestation of psychiatric disorders such as generalized anxiety, panic disorders, major depression, and somatization disorder. These possibilities should be considered in individuals who faint frequently without prodromal symptoms. Such patients are rarely injured despite numerous falls. There are no clinically significant hemodynamic changes concurrent with these episodes. In contrast, transient loss of consciousness due to vasovagal syncope precipitated by fear, stress, anxiety, and emotional distress is accompanied by hypotension, bradycardia, or both.

INITIAL EVALUATION The goals of the initial evaluation are to determine whether the transient loss of consciousness was due to syncope; to identify the cause; and to assess risk for future episodes and serious harm (Table 20-1). The initial evaluation should include a detailed history, thorough questioning of eyewitnesses, and a complete physical and neurologic examination. Blood pressure and heart rate should be measured in the supine position and after 3 minutes of standing to determine whether orthostatic hypotension is present. An ECG should be performed if there is suspicion of syncope due to an arrhythmia or underlying cardiac disease. Relevant electrocardiographic abnormalities include bradyarrhythmias or tachyarrhythmias, atrioventricular block, ischemia, old myocardial infarction, long QT syndrome, and bundle branch block. This initial assessment will lead to the identification of a cause of syncope in approximately 50% of patients and also allows stratification of patients at risk for cardiac mortality.

Laboratory Tests Baseline laboratory blood tests are rarely helpful in identifying the cause of syncope. Blood tests should be performed when specific disorders, e.g., myocardial infarction, anemia, and secondary autonomic failure are suspected (Table 20-2).

Autonomic Nervous System Testing (Chap. 375) Autonomic testing including tilt table testing can be performed in specialized centers. Autonomic testing is helpful to uncover objective evidence of autonomic failure and also to demonstrate a predisposition to neurally mediated syncope. Autonomic testing includes assessments of parasympathetic autonomic nervous system function (e.g., heart rate variability to deep respiration and a Valsalva maneuver), sympathetic cholinergic function (e.g., thermoregulatory sweat response and quantitative sudomotor axon reflex test), and sympathetic adrenergic function (e.g., blood pressure response to a Valsalva maneuver and a tilt table test with beat-to-beat blood pressure measurement). The hemodynamic abnormalities demonstrated on tilt table test (Figs. 20-2 and 20-3) may be useful in distinguishing orthostatic hypotension due to autonomic failure from the hypotensive bradycardic response of neurally mediated syncope. Similarly, the tilt table test may help identify patients with syncope due to delayed or initial orthostatic hypotension.

Carotid sinus massage should be considered in patients with symptoms suggestive of carotid sinus syncope and in patients over age 50 years with recurrent syncope of unknown etiology. This test should only be carried out under continuous ECG and blood pressure monitoring and should be avoided in patients with carotid bruits, plaques, or stenosis.

Cardiac Evaluation ECG monitoring is indicated for patients with a high pretest probability of arrhythmia causing syncope. Patients should be monitored in hospital if the likelihood of a life-threatening arrhythmia is high, e.g., patients with severe structural or coronary artery disease, nonsustained ventricular tachycardia, trifascicular heart block, prolonged QT interval, Brugada's syndrome ECG pattern, and family history of sudden cardiac death. Outpatient Holter monitoring is recommended for patients who experience frequent syncopal episodes (one

or more per week), whereas loop recorders, which continually record and erase cardiac rhythm, are indicated for patients with suspected arrhythmias with low risk of sudden cardiac death. Loop recorders may be external (recommended for evaluation of episodes that occur at a frequency of greater than one per month) or implantable (if syncope occurs less frequently).

Echocardiography should be performed in patients with a history of cardiac disease or if abnormalities are found on physical examination or the electrocardiogram. Echocardiographic diagnoses that may be responsible for syncope include aortic stenosis, hypertrophic cardiomyopathy, cardiac tumors, aortic dissection, and pericardial tamponade. Echocardiography also has a role in risk stratification based on the left ventricular ejection fraction.

Treadmill exercise testing with ECG and blood pressure monitoring should be performed in patients who have experienced syncope during or shortly after exercise. Treadmill testing may help identify exercise-induced arrhythmias (e.g., tachycardia-related AV block) and exercise-induced exaggerated vasodilation.

Electrophysiologic studies are indicated in patients with structural heart disease and ECG abnormalities in whom noninvasive investigations have failed to yield a diagnosis. Electrophysiologic studies have low sensitivity and specificity and should only be performed when a high pretest probability exists. Currently, this test is rarely performed to evaluate patients with syncope.

Psychiatric Evaluation Screening for psychiatric disorders may be appropriate in patients with recurrent unexplained syncope episodes. Tilt table testing, with demonstration of symptoms in the absence of hemodynamic change, may be useful in reproducing syncope in patients with suspected psychogenic syncope.

FURTHER READINGS

COLEMAN N et al: Syncope, in *Course and Treatment of Neurological Diseases*, 2nd ed, T Brandt et al (eds). San Diego Academic Press, 2003

FREEMAN R: Autonomic peripheral neuropathy. Lancet 365:1259, 2005

——: Clinical practice. Neurogenic orthostatic hypotension. N Engl J Med 358:615, 2008

GANZEBOOM KS et al: Lifetime cumulative incidence of syncope in the general population: A study of 549 Dutch subjects aged 35–60 years. J Cardiovasc Electrophysiol 17:1172, 2006

KAUFMANN H, BIAGGIONI I: Autonomic failure in neurodegenerative disorders. Semin Neurol 23:351, 2003

LEMPERT T: Recognizing syncope: Pitfalls and surprises. J R Soc Med 89:372, 1996

MOYA A et al: Guidelines for the diagnosis and management of syncope (version 2009): The Task Force for the Diagnosis and Management of Syncope of the European Society of Cardiology (ESC). Eur Heart J 30:2631, 2009

SHAH M et al: Molecular basis of arrhythmias. Circulation 112:2517, 2005

SULE S et al: Etiology of syncope in patients hospitalized with syncope and predictors of mortality and rehospitalization for syncope at 27-month follow-up. Clin Cardiol 34:35, 2011

WIELING W et al: Symptoms and signs of syncope: A review of the link between physiology and clinical clues. Brain 132:2630, 2009

CHAPTER 21
Dizziness and Vertigo

Mark F. Walker
Robert B. Daroff

Dizziness is a common, vexing symptom, and epidemiologic data indicate that more than 20% of adults experience dizziness within a given year. The diagnosis is frequently challenging, in part because patients use the term to refer to a variety of different sensations, including feelings of faintness, spinning, and other illusions of motion, imbalance, and anxiety. Other descriptive words, such as *light-headedness*, are equally ambiguous, referring in some cases to a presyncopal sensation due to hypoperfusion of the brain and in others to disequilibrium and imbalance. Patients often have difficulty distinguishing among these various symptoms, and the words they choose do not describe the underlying etiology reliably.

Vascular disorders cause presyncopal dizziness as a result of cardiac dysrhythmia, orthostatic hypotension, medication effects, or another cause. Such presyncopal sensations vary in duration; they may increase in severity until loss of consciousness occurs, or they may resolve before loss of consciousness if the cerebral ischemia is corrected. Faintness and syncope, which are discussed in detail in Chap. 20, should always be considered when one is evaluating patients with brief episodes of dizziness or dizziness that occurs with upright posture.

Vestibular causes of dizziness may be due to peripheral lesions that affect the labyrinths or vestibular nerves or to involvement of the central vestibular pathways. They may be paroxysmal or due to a fixed unilateral or bilateral vestibular deficit. Acute unilateral lesions cause vertigo due to a sudden imbalance in vestibular inputs from the two labyrinths. Bilateral lesions cause imbalance and instability of vision when the head moves (*oscillopsia*). Other causes of dizziness include nonvestibular imbalance and gait disorders (e.g., loss of proprioception from sensory neuropathy, parkinsonism) and anxiety.

In evaluating patients with dizziness, questions to consider include the following: (1) is it dangerous (e.g., arrhythmia, transient ischemic attack/stroke)? (2) is it vestibular? and (3) if vestibular, is it peripheral or central? A careful history and examination often provide enough information to answer these questions and determine whether additional studies or referral to a specialist is necessary.

APPROACH TO THE PATIENT Dizziness

HISTORY   When a patient presents with dizziness, the first step is to delineate more precisely the nature of the symptom. In the case of vestibular disorders, the physical symptoms depend on whether the lesion is unilateral or bilateral and whether it is acute or chronic and progressive. Vertigo, an illusion of self or environmental motion, implies asymmetry of vestibular inputs from the two labyrinths or in their central pathways and is usually acute. Symmetric bilateral vestibular hypofunction causes imbalance but no vertigo. Because of the ambiguity in patients' descriptions of their symptoms, diagnosis based simply on symptom character is typically unreliable. The history should focus closely on other features, including whether dizziness is paroxysmal or has

occurred only once, the duration of each episode, any provoking factors, and the symptoms that accompany the dizziness.

Causes of dizziness can be divided into episodes that last for seconds, minutes, hours, or days. Common causes of brief dizziness (seconds) include benign paroxysmal positional vertigo (BPPV) and orthostatic hypotension, both of which typically are provoked by changes in position. Attacks of migrainous vertigo and Ménière's disease often last hours. When episodes are of intermediate duration (minutes), transient ischemic attacks of the posterior circulation should be considered, although these episodes also could be due to migraine or a number of other causes.

Symptoms that accompany vertigo may be helpful in distinguishing peripheral vestibular lesions from central causes. Unilateral hearing loss and other aural symptoms (ear pain, pressure, fullness) typically point to a peripheral cause. Because the auditory pathways quickly become bilateral upon entering the brainstem, central lesions are unlikely to cause unilateral hearing loss (unless the lesion lies near the root entry zone of the auditory nerve). Symptoms such as double vision, numbness, and limb ataxia suggest a brainstem or cerebellar lesion.

EXAMINATION   Because dizziness and imbalance can be a manifestation of a variety of neurologic disorders, the neurologic examination is important in the evaluation of these patients. Particular focus should be given to assessment of eye movements, vestibular function, and hearing. The range of eye movements and whether they are equal in each eye should be observed. Peripheral eye movement disorders (e.g., cranial neuropathies, eye muscle weakness) are usually *disconjugate* (different in the two eyes). One should check pursuit (the ability to follow a smoothly moving target) and saccades (the ability to look back and forth accurately between two targets). Poor pursuit or inaccurate (*dysmetric*) saccades usually indicates central pathology, often involving the cerebellum. Finally, one should look for spontaneous nystagmus, an involuntary back-and-forth movement of the eyes. Most often nystagmus is of the jerk type, in which a slow drift (*slow phase*) in one direction alternates with a rapid saccadic movement (*quick phase* or *fast phase*) in the opposite direction that resets the position of the eyes in the orbits. Table 21-1 lists features that help distinguish peripheral vestibular nystagmus from central nystagmus. Except in the case of acute vestibulopathy (e.g., vestibular neuritis), if primary position nystagmus is easily seen in the light, it is probably due to a central cause. Two forms of nystagmus that are characteristic of lesions of the cerebellar pathways are vertical nystagmus with downward fast phases (downbeat nystagmus) and horizontal nystagmus that changes direction with gaze (gaze-evoked nystagmus).

Specialists find that the most useful bedside test of peripheral vestibular function is the *head impulse test*, in which the vestibuloocular reflex (VOR) is assessed with small-amplitude (approximately 20 degrees) rapid head rotations; beginning in the primary position, the head is rotated to the left or right while the patient is instructed to fixate on the examiner's face. If the VOR is deficient, a catch-up saccade is seen at the end of the rotation. This test can identify both unilateral (deficient VOR when the head is rotated toward the weak side) and bilateral vestibular hypofunction.

All patients with episodic dizziness, especially if it is provoked by positional change, should be tested with the Dix-Hallpike maneuver. The patient begins in a sitting position with the head turned 45 degrees; holding the back of the head, the examiner then gently lowers the patient into a supine position with the

TABLE 21-1 Features of Peripheral and Central Vertigo

Sign or Symptom	Peripheral (Labyrinth or Vestibular Nerve)	Central (Brainstem or Cerebellum)
Direction of associated nystagmus	Unidirectional; fast phase opposite lesion[a]	Bidirectional (direction-changing) or unidirectional
Purely horizontal nystagmus without torsional component	Uncommon	May be present
Purely vertical or purely torsional nystagmus	Never present[b]	May be present
Visual fixation	Inhibits nystagmus	No inhibition
Tinnitus and/or deafness	Often present	Usually absent
Associated central nervous system abnormalities	None	Extremely common (e.g., diplopia, hiccups, cranial neuropathies, dysarthria)
Common causes	Benign paroxysmal positional vertigo, infection (labyrinthitis), vestibular neuritis, Ménière's disease, labyrinthine ischemia, trauma, toxin	Vascular, demyelinating, neoplasm

[a]In Ménière's disease, the direction of the fast phase is variable.
[b]Combined vertical-torsional nystagmus suggests BPPV.

head extended backward by about 20 degrees, and observes for nystagmus; after 30 s the patient is raised to the sitting position and after a 1-min rest the procedure is repeated with the head turned to the other side. Use of Frenzel eyeglasses (self-illuminated goggles with convex lenses that blur the patient's vision but allow the examiner to see the eyes greatly magnified) can improve the sensitivity of the test. If transient upbeating and torsional nystagmus are elicited in the supine position, posterior canal BPPV can be diagnosed confidently and treated with a repositioning maneuver, and additional testing can be avoided.

Dynamic visual acuity is a functional test that can be useful in assessing vestibular function. Visual acuity is measured with the head still and when the head is rotated back and forth by the examiner (about 1–2 Hz). A drop in visual acuity during head motion of more than one line on a near card or Snellen chart is abnormal.

The choice of ancillary tests should be guided by the history and examination findings. Audiometry should be performed whenever a vestibular disorder is suspected. Unilateral sensorineural hearing loss supports a peripheral disorder (e.g., vestibular schwannoma). Predominantly low-frequency hearing loss is characteristic of Ménière's disease. Electro- or videonystagmography includes recordings of spontaneous nystagmus (if present), pursuit, and saccades; caloric testing to assess the responses of the two horizontal semicircular canals; and measurement of positional nystagmus. Patients with unexplained unilateral hearing loss or vestibular hypofunction should undergo magnetic resonance imaging of the internal auditory canals, including administration of gadolinium, to rule out a schwannoma.

TREATMENT Dizziness

Treatment of vestibular symptoms should be driven by the underlying diagnosis. Simply treating dizziness with vestibular suppressant medications is often not helpful and may make the symptoms worse. The diagnostic and specific treatment approaches for the most commonly encountered vestibular disorders are discussed below.

Acute prolonged vertigo

An acute unilateral vestibular lesion causes constant vertigo, nausea, vomiting, oscillopsia (motion of the visual scene), and imbalance. These symptoms are due to a sudden asymmetry of inputs from the two labyrinths or in their central connections, simulating a continuous rotation of the head. Unlike BPPV, the vertigo persists even when the head is not moving.

When a patient presents with an acute vestibular syndrome, the most important question is whether the lesion is central (e.g., a cerebellar or brainstem infarct or hemorrhage), which may be life-threatening, or peripheral, affecting the vestibular nerve or labyrinth. Attention should be given to any symptoms or signs that point to central dysfunction (diplopia, weakness or numbness, dysarthria). The pattern of spontaneous nystagmus, if present, may be helpful (Table 21-1). If the head impulse test is normal, an acute peripheral vestibular lesion is unlikely. However, a central lesion cannot always be excluded with certainly on the basis of symptoms and examination alone; thus, older patients with vascular risk factors who present with an acute vestibular syndrome generally should be evaluated for the possibility of stroke even when there are no specific findings that indicate a central lesion.

Most patients with vestibular neuritis recover spontaneously, but glucocorticoids can improve outcome if administered within 3 days of symptom onset. Antiviral medications are of no proven benefit unless there is evidence to suggest herpes zoster oticus (Ramsay Hunt syndrome). Vestibular suppressant medications may reduce acute symptoms but should be avoided after the first several days as they may impede central compensation and recovery. Patients should be encouraged to resume a normal level of activity as soon as possible, and directed vestibular rehabilitation therapy may accelerate improvement.

Benign paroxysmal positional vertigo

BPPV is a common cause of recurrent vertigo. Episodes are brief (<1 min and typically 15–20 s) and are always provoked by changes in head position relative to gravity, such as lying down, rolling over in bed, rising from a supine position, and extending the head to look upward. The attacks are caused by free-floating otoconia (calcium carbonate crystals) that have been dislodged from the utricular macula and have moved into one of the semicircular canals, usually the posterior canal. When head position changes, gravity causes the otoconia to move within the canal, producing vertigo and nystagmus. With posterior canal BPPV, the nystagmus beats upward and torsionally (the upper poles of the eyes beat toward the affected ear). Less commonly, the otoconia enter the horizontal canal, resulting in a horizontal nystagmus when the patient is lying with either ear down. Superior (also called anterior) canal involvement is rare. BPPV is treated with repositioning maneuvers that utilize gravity to remove the otoconia from the semicircular canal. For posterior canal BPPV, the Epley maneuver is the most commonly used procedure. For more refractory cases of BPPV, patients can be taught a variant of this maneuver that they can perform alone at home.

Vestibular migraine

Vestibular symptoms occur frequently in migraine, sometimes as a headache aura but often independent of headache. The duration of vertigo may be from minutes to hours, and some patients also experience more prolonged periods of disequilibrium (lasting days to weeks). Motion sensitivity and sensitivity to visual motion (e.g., movies) are common in patients with vestibular migraine. Although data from controlled studies are generally lacking, vestibular migraine typically is treated with medications that are used for prophylaxis of migraine headaches. Antiemetics may be helpful to relieve symptoms at the time of an attack.

Ménière's disease

Attacks of Ménière's disease consist of vertigo, hearing loss, and pain, pressure, or fullness in the affected ear. The hearing loss and aural symptoms are key features that distinguish Ménière's disease from other peripheral vestibulopathies. Audiometry at the time of an attack shows a characteristic asymmetric low-frequency hearing loss; hearing commonly improves between attacks, although permanent hearing loss may occur eventually. Ménière's disease is thought to be due to excess fluid (endolymph) in the inner ear, hence the term *endolymphatic hydrops*. Patients suspected of having Ménière's disease should be referred to an otolaryngologist for further evaluation. Diuretics and sodium restriction are the initial treatments. If attacks persist, injections of gentamicin into the middle ear are typically the next line of therapy. Full ablative procedures (vestibular nerve section, labyrinthectomy) seldom are required.

Vestibular schwannoma

Vestibular schwannomas (sometimes less correctly termed *acoustic neuromas*) and other tumors at the cerebellopontine angle cause slowly progressive unilateral sensorineural hearing loss and vestibular hypofunction. These patients typically do not have vertigo, because the gradual vestibular deficit is compensated centrally as it develops. The diagnosis often is not made until there is sufficient hearing loss to be noticed. The examination will show a deficient Halmagyi-Curthoys head impulse response when the head is rotated toward the affected side. Any patient with unexplained asymmetric vestibular function (e.g., no prior history of vestibular neuritis) or asymmetric sensorineural hearing loss (documented on audiometry) should undergo MRI of the internal auditory canals, including gadolinium administration, to rule out a schwannoma.

Bilateral vestibular hypofunction

Patients with bilateral loss of vestibular function also typically do not have vertigo, since vestibular function is lost on both sides simultaneously, thus there is no asymmetry of vestibular input. Symptoms include loss of balance, particularly in the dark, where vestibular input is most critical, and oscillopsia during head movement, such as while walking or riding in a car. Bilateral vestibular hypofunction may be (1) idiopathic and progressive, (2) part of a neurodegenerative disorder, or (3) iatrogenic, due to medication

ototoxicity (most commonly gentamicin or other aminoglycoside antibiotics). Other causes include bilateral vestibular schwannomas (neurofibromatosis type 2), autoimmune disease, meningeal-based infection or tumor, and other toxins. It also may occur in patients with peripheral polyneuropathy; in these patients, both vestibular loss and impaired proprioception may contribute to poor balance. Finally, unilateral processes such as vestibular neuritis and Ménière's disease may involve both ears sequentially, resulting in bilateral vestibulopathy.

Examination findings include diminished dynamic visual acuity (see above) due to loss of stable vision when the head is moving, abnormal head impulse responses in both directions, and a Romberg sign. In the laboratory, responses to caloric testing are reduced. Patients with bilateral vestibular hypofunction should be referred for vestibular rehabilitation therapy. Vestibular suppressant medications should not be used, as they will increase the imbalance. Evaluation by a neurologist is important not only to confirm the diagnosis but also to consider any other associated neurologic abnormalities that may clarify the etiology.

TABLE 21-2 Treatment of Vertigo

Agent[a]	Dose[b]
Antihistamines	
Meclizine	25–50 mg 3 times daily
Dimenhydrinate	50 mg 1–2 times daily
Promethazine	25 mg 2–3 times daily (also can be given rectally and IM)
Benzodiazepines	
Diazepam	2.5 mg 1–3 times daily
Clonazepam	0.25 mg 1–3 times daily
Anticholinergic	
Scopolamine transdermal[c]	Patch
Physical therapy	
Repositioning maneuvers[d]	
Vestibular rehabilitation	
Other	
Diuretics and/or low-sodium (1 g/d) diet[e]	
Antimigrainous drugs[f]	
Methylprednisolone[g]	100 mg daily days 1–3; 80 mg daily days 4–6; 60 mg daily days 7–9; 40 mg daily days 10–12; 20 mg daily days 13–15; 10 mg daily days 16–18, 20, 22
Selective serotonin reuptake inhibitors[h]	

[a] All listed drugs are approved by the U.S. Food and Drug Administration, but most are not approved for the treatment of vertigo.

[b] Usual oral (unless otherwise stated) starting dose in adults; a higher maintenance dose can be reached by a gradual increase.

[c] For motion sickness only.

[d] For benign paroxysmal positional vertigo.

[e] For Ménière's disease.

[f] For vestibular migraine.

[g] For acute vestibular neuritis (started within three days of onset).

[h] For psychosomatic vertigo.

Psychosomatic dizziness

Psychological factors play an important role in chronic dizziness. First, dizziness may be a somatic manifestation of a psychiatric condition such as major depression, anxiety, or panic disorder. Second, patients may develop anxiety and autonomic symptoms as a consequence or comorbidity of an independent vestibular disorder. One particular form of this has been termed variously *phobic postural vertigo*, *psychophysiologic vertigo*, or *chronic subjective dizziness*. These patients have a chronic feeling (months or longer) of dizziness and disequilibrium, an increased sensitivity to self-motion and visual motion (e.g., movies), and a particular intensification of symptoms when moving through complex visual environments such as supermarkets (*visual vertigo*). Although there may be a past history of an acute vestibular disorder (e.g., vestibular neuritis), the neurootologic examination and vestibular testing are normal or indicative of a compensated vestibular deficit, indicating that the ongoing subjective dizziness cannot be explained by a primary vestibular disorder. Anxiety disorders are common in patients with chronic dizziness and contribute substantially to the morbidity. Thus, treatment with antianxiety medications [selective serotonin reuptake inhibitors (SSRIs)] and cognitive/behavioral therapy may be helpful. Vestibular rehabilitation therapy is also sometimes beneficial. Vestibular suppressant medications generally should be avoided. This condition should be suspected when the patient states, "My dizziness is so bad, I'm afraid to leave my house" (agoraphobia). General treatment of vertigo consists of vestibular suppressant medications and vestibular rehabilitation therapy.

TREATMENT	Vertigo

Table 21-2 provides a list of commonly used medications for suppression of vertigo. As noted, these medications should be reserved for short-term control of active vertigo, such as during the first few days of acute vestibular neuritis, or for acute attacks of Ménière's disease. They are less helpful for chronic dizziness and, as previously stated, may hinder central compensation. An exception is that benzodiazepines may attenuate psychosomatic dizziness and the associated anxiety, although SSRIs are generally preferable in such patients.

Vestibular rehabilitation therapy promotes central adaptation processes that compensate for vestibular loss and also may help habituate motion sensitivity and other symptoms of psychosomatic dizziness. The general approach is to use a graded series of exercises that progressively challenge gaze stabilization and balance.

FURTHER READINGS

BRONSTEIN AM et al: Chronic dizziness: A practical approach. Pract Neurol 10:129, 2010

HALMAGYI GM: Diagnosis and management of vertigo. Clin Med 5:159, 2005

JEN JC: Bilateral vestibulopathy: Clinical, diagnostic, and genetic considerations. Semin Neurol 29:528, 2009

LEMPERT T et al: Vertigo as a symptom of migraine. Ann NY Acad Sci 1164:242, 2009

RUCKENSTEIN MJ, STAAB JP: Chronic subjective dizziness. Otolaryngol Clin North Am 42:71, 2009

STRUPP M, BRANDT T: Vestibular neuritis. Semin Neurol 29:509, 2009

WALKER MF, ZEE DS: Bedside vestibular examination. Otolaryngol Clin North Am 33: 495, 2000

ZINGLER VC et al: Causative factors and epidemiology of bilateral vestibulopathy in 255 patients. Ann Neurol 61:524, 2007

CHAPTER **22**
Weakness and Paralysis

Michael J. Aminoff

Normal motor function involves integrated muscle activity that is modulated by the activity of the cerebral cortex, basal ganglia, cerebellum, and spinal cord. Motor system dysfunction leads to weakness or paralysis, which is discussed in this chapter, or to ataxia (Chap. 373) or abnormal movements (Chap. 372). The mode of onset, distribution, and accompaniments of weakness help suggest its cause.

Weakness is a reduction in the power that can be exerted by one or more muscles. Increased fatigability or limitation in function due to pain or articular stiffness often is confused with weakness by patients. *Increased fatigability* is the inability to sustain the performance of an activity that should be normal for a person of the same age, sex, and size. Increased time is required sometimes for full power to be exerted, and this *bradykinesia* may be misinterpreted as weakness. Severe proprioceptive sensory loss also may lead to complaints of weakness because adequate feedback information about the direction and power of movements is lacking. Finally, *apraxia*, a disorder of planning and initiating a skilled or learned movement unrelated to a significant motor or sensory deficit (Chap. 26), sometimes is mistaken for weakness.

Paralysis indicates weakness that is so severe that a muscle cannot be contracted at all, whereas *paresis* refers to weakness that is mild or moderate. The prefix "hemi-" refers to one-half of the body, "para-" to both legs, and "quadri-" to all four limbs. The suffix "-plegia" signifies severe weakness or paralysis.

The distribution of weakness helps to indicate the site of the underlying lesion. Weakness from involvement of upper motor neurons occurs particularly in the extensors and abductors of the upper limb and the flexors of the lower limb. Lower motor neuron weakness does not have this selectivity but depends on whether involvement is at the level of the anterior horn cells, nerve root, limb plexus, or peripheral nerve—only muscles supplied by the affected structure are weak. Myopathic weakness is generally most marked in proximal muscles, whereas weakness from impaired neuromuscular transmission has no specific pattern of involvement. Weakness often is accompanied by other neurologic abnormalities that help indicate the site of the responsible lesion. These abnormalities include changes in tone, muscle bulk, muscle stretch reflexes, and cutaneous reflexes (Table 22-1).

TABLE 22-1 Signs That Distinguish the Origin of Weakness

Sign	Upper Motor Neuron	Lower Motor Neuron	Myopathic
Atrophy	None	Severe	Mild
Fasciculations	None	Common	None
Tone	Spastic	Decreased	Normal/decreased
Distribution of weakness	Pyramidal/regional	Distal/segmental	Proximal
Tendon reflexes	Hyperactive	Hypoactive/absent	Normal/hypoactive
Babinski sign	Present	Absent	Absent

Tone is the resistance of a muscle to passive stretch. Central nervous system (CNS) abnormalities that cause weakness generally produce *spasticity*, an increase in tone associated with disease of upper motor neurons. Spasticity is velocity-dependent, has a sudden release after reaching a maximum (the "clasp-knife" phenomenon), and predominantly affects the antigravity muscles (i.e., upper-limb flexors and lower-limb extensors). Spasticity is distinct from rigidity and paratonia, two other types of hypertonia. *Rigidity* is increased tone that is present throughout the range of motion (a "lead pipe" or "plastic" stiffness) and affects flexors and extensors equally; it sometimes has a cogwheel quality that is enhanced by voluntary movement of the contralateral limb (reinforcement). Rigidity occurs with certain extrapyramidal disorders, such as Parkinson's disease. *Paratonia* (or *gegenhalten*) is increased tone that varies irregularly in a manner that may seem related to the degree of relaxation, is present throughout the range of motion, and affects flexors and extensors equally; it usually results from disease of the frontal lobes. Weakness with *decreased tone* (*flaccidity*) or normal tone occurs with disorders of *motor units*. A motor unit consists of a single lower motor neuron and all the muscle fibers that it innervates.

Muscle bulk generally is not affected in patients with upper motor neuron lesions, although mild disuse atrophy eventually may occur. By contrast, atrophy is often conspicuous when a lower motor neuron lesion is responsible for weakness and also may occur with advanced muscle disease.

Muscle stretch (tendon) reflexes are usually increased with upper motor neuron lesions, although they may be decreased or absent for a variable period immediately after onset of an acute lesion. This is usually—but not invariably—accompanied by abnormalities of *cutaneous reflexes* (such as superficial abdominals; Chap. 367) and, in particular, by an extensor plantar (Babinski) response. The muscle stretch reflexes are depressed in patients with lower motor neuron lesions when there is direct involvement of specific reflex arcs. The stretch reflexes generally are preserved in patients with myopathic weakness except in advanced stages, when they sometimes are attenuated. In disorders of the neuromuscular junction, the intensity of the reflex responses may be affected by preceding voluntary activity of affected muscles; that activity may lead to enhancement of initially depressed reflexes in Lambert-Eaton myasthenic syndrome and, conversely, to depression of initially normal reflexes in myasthenia gravis (Chap. 386).

The distinction of *neuropathic* (lower motor neuron) from *myopathic* weakness is sometimes difficult clinically, although distal weakness is likely to be neuropathic, and symmetric proximal weakness myopathic. *Fasciculations* (visible or palpable twitch within a muscle due to the spontaneous discharge of a motor unit) and early atrophy indicate that weakness is neuropathic.

■ PATHOGENESIS

Upper motor neuron weakness

This pattern of weakness results from disorders that affect the upper motor neurons or their axons in the cerebral cortex, subcortical white matter, internal capsule, brainstem, or spinal cord (Fig. 22-1). These lesions produce weakness through decreased activation of the lower motor neurons. In general, distal muscle groups are affected more severely than are proximal ones, and axial movements are spared unless the lesion is severe and bilateral. With corticobulbar involvement, weakness usually is observed only in the lower face and tongue; extraocular, upper facial, pharyngeal, and jaw muscles almost always are spared. With bilateral corticobulbar lesions, *pseudobulbar palsy* often develops: dysarthria, dysphagia, dysphonia, and emotional lability accompany bilateral facial weakness and a brisk jaw jerk. Spasticity accompanies upper motor neuron weakness but may not be present in the acute phase. Upper motor neuron lesions also affect the ability to perform rapid repetitive movements. Such movements are slow and coarse, but normal rhythmicity is maintained. Finger-nose-finger and heel-knee-shin maneuvers are performed slowly but adequately.

Lower motor neuron weakness

This pattern results from disorders of cell bodies of lower motor neurons in the brainstem motor nuclei and the anterior horn of the spinal cord or from dysfunction of the axons of these neurons as they pass to skeletal muscle (Fig. 22-2). Weakness is due to a decrease in the number of muscle fibers that can be activated through a loss of α motor neurons or disruption of their connections to muscle. Loss of γ motor neurons does not cause weakness but decreases tension on the muscle spindles, which decreases muscle tone and attenuates the stretch reflexes elicited on examination. An absent stretch reflex suggests involvement of spindle afferent fibers.

When a motor unit becomes diseased, especially in anterior horn cell diseases, it may discharge spontaneously, producing *fasciculations* that may be seen or felt clinically or recorded by electromyography (EMG). When α motor neurons or their axons degenerate, the denervated muscle fibers also may discharge spontaneously. These single muscle fiber discharges, or *fibrillation potentials,* cannot be seen or felt but can be recorded with EMG. If lower motor neuron weakness is present, recruitment of motor units is delayed or reduced, with fewer than normal activated at a particular discharge frequency. This contrasts with weakness of the upper motor neuron type, in which a normal number of motor units is activated at a given frequency but with a diminished maximal discharge frequency.

Myopathic weakness

Myopathic weakness is produced by disorders of the muscle fibers. Disorders of the neuromuscular junctions also produce weakness, but this is variable in degree and distribution and is influenced

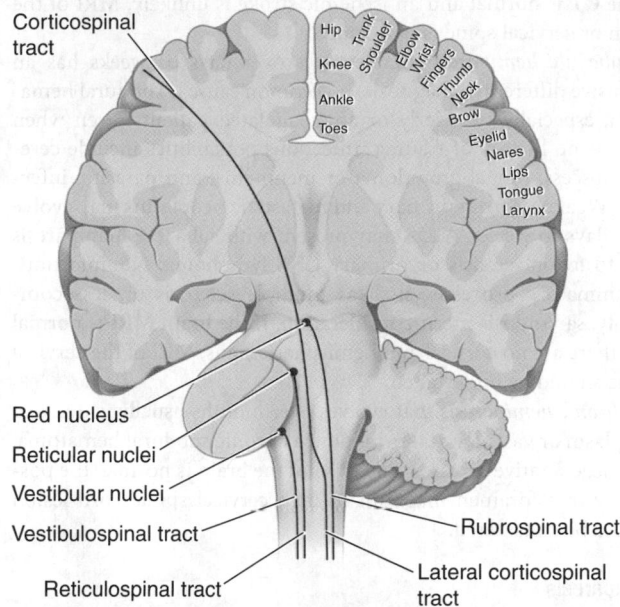

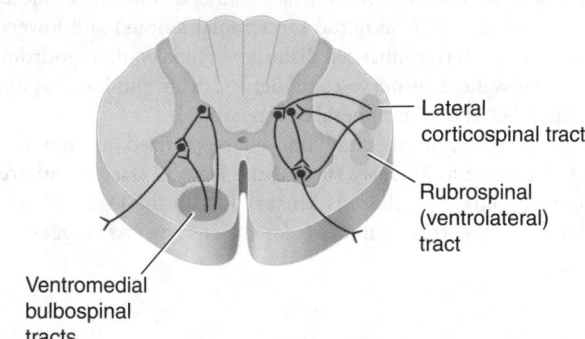

Figure 22-1 The corticospinal and bulbospinal upper motor neuron pathways. Upper motor neurons have their cell bodies in layer V of the primary motor cortex (the precentral gyrus, or Brodmann's area 4) and in the premotor and supplemental motor cortex (area 6). The upper motor neurons in the primary motor cortex are somatotopically organized, as illustrated on the right side of the figure.

Axons of the upper motor neurons descend through the subcortical white matter and the posterior limb of the internal capsule. Axons of the *pyramidal* or *corticospinal system* descend through the brainstem in the cerebral peduncle of the midbrain, the basis pontis, and the medullary pyramids. At the cervicomedullary junction, most pyramidal axons decussate into the contralateral corticospinal tract of the lateral spinal cord, but 10–30% remain ipsilateral in the anterior spinal cord. Pyramidal neurons make direct monosynaptic connections with lower motor neurons. They innervate most densely the lower motor neurons of hand muscles and are involved in the execution of learned, fine movements. Corticobulbar neurons are similar to corticospinal neurons but innervate brainstem motor nuclei.

Bulbospinal upper motor neurons influence strength and tone but are not part of the pyramidal system. The descending *ventromedial bulbospinal pathways* originate in the tectum of the midbrain (tectospinal pathway), the vestibular nuclei (vestibulospinal pathway), and the reticular formation (reticulospinal pathway). These pathways influence axial and proximal muscles and are involved in the maintenance of posture and integrated movements of the limbs and trunk. The descending *ventrolateral bulbospinal pathways*, which originate predominantly in the red nucleus (rubrospinal pathway), facilitate distal limb muscles. The bulbospinal system sometimes is referred to as the *extrapyramidal upper motor neuron system*. In all figures, nerve cell bodies and axon terminals are shown, respectively, as closed circles and forks.

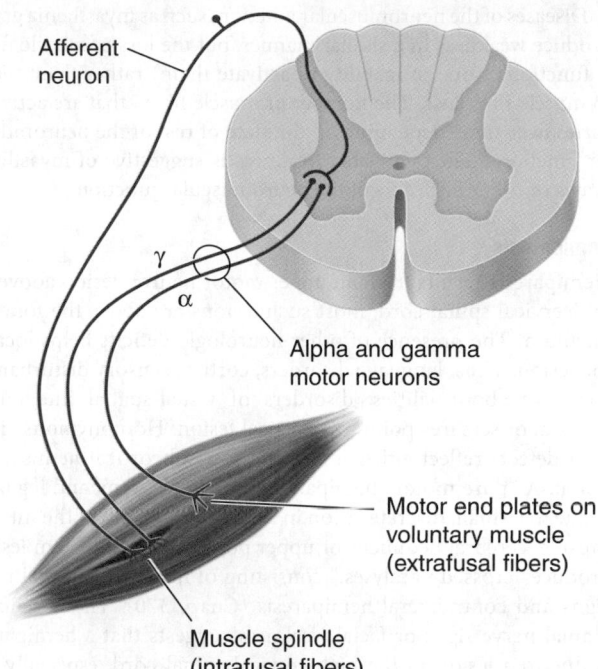

Figure 22-2 Lower motor neurons are divided into α and γ types. The larger α motor neurons are more numerous and innervate the extrafusal muscle fibers of the motor unit. Loss of α motor neurons or disruption of their axons produces lower motor neuron weakness. The smaller, less numerous γ motor neurons innervate the intrafusal muscle fibers of the muscle spindle and contribute to normal tone and stretch reflexes. The α motor neuron receives direct excitatory input from corticomotoneurons and primary muscle spindle afferents. The α and γ motor neurons also receive excitatory input from other descending upper motor neuron pathways, segmental sensory inputs, and interneurons. The α motor neurons receive direct inhibition from Renshaw cell interneurons, and other interneurons indirectly inhibit the α and γ motor neurons.

A tendon reflex requires the function of all the illustrated structures. A tap on a tendon stretches muscle spindles (which are tonically activated by γ motor neurons) and activates the primary spindle afferent neurons. These neurons stimulate the α motor neurons in the spinal cord, producing a brief muscle contraction, which is the familiar tendon reflex.

by preceding activity of the affected muscle. At a muscle fiber, if the nerve terminal releases a normal number of acetylcholine molecules presynaptically and a sufficient number of postsynaptic acetylcholine receptors are opened, the end plate reaches threshold and thereby generates an action potential that spreads across the muscle fiber membrane and into the transverse tubular system. This electrical excitation activates intracellular events that produce an energy-dependent contraction of the muscle fiber (excitation-contraction coupling).

Myopathic weakness is produced by a decrease in the number or contractile force of muscle fibers activated within motor units. With muscular dystrophies, inflammatory myopathies, or myopathies with muscle fiber necrosis, the number of muscle fibers is reduced within many motor units. On EMG, the size of each motor unit action potential is decreased, and motor units must be recruited more rapidly than normal to produce the desired power. Some myopathies produce weakness through loss of contractile force of muscle fibers or through relatively selective involvement of type II (fast) fibers. These myopathies may not affect the size of individual motor unit action potentials and are detected by a discrepancy between the electrical activity and force of a muscle.

Diseases of the neuromuscular junction, such as myasthenia gravis, produce weakness in a similar manner, but the loss of muscle fibers is functional (due to inability to activate them) rather than related to muscle fiber loss. The number of muscle fibers that are activated varies over time, depending on the state of rest of the neuromuscular junctions. Thus, fatigable weakness is suggestive of myasthenia gravis or other disorders of the neuromuscular junction.

Hemiparesis

Hemiparesis results from an upper motor neuron lesion above the midcervical spinal cord; most such lesions are above the foramen magnum. The presence of other neurologic deficits helps localize the lesion. Thus, language disorders, cortical sensory disturbances, cognitive abnormalities, disorders of visual-spatial integration, apraxia, or seizures point to a cortical lesion. Homonymous visual field defects reflect either a cortical or a subcortical hemispheric lesion. A "pure motor" hemiparesis of the face, arm, and leg often is due to a small, discrete lesion in the posterior limb of the internal capsule, cerebral peduncle, or upper pons. Some brainstem lesions produce "crossed paralyses," consisting of ipsilateral cranial nerve signs and contralateral hemiparesis (Chap. 370). The absence of cranial nerve signs or facial weakness suggests that a hemiparesis is due to a lesion in the high cervical spinal cord, especially if it is associated with ipsilateral loss of proprioception and contralateral loss of pain and temperature sense (the Brown-Séquard syndrome).

Acute or episodic hemiparesis usually results from ischemic or hemorrhagic stroke but also may relate to hemorrhage occurring into brain tumors or may be a result of trauma; other causes include a focal structural lesion or an inflammatory process as in multiple sclerosis, abscess, or sarcoidosis. Evaluation (Fig. 22-3) begins immediately with a CT scan of the brain and laboratory studies.

If the CT is normal and an ischemic stroke is unlikely, MRI of the brain or cervical spine is performed.

Subacute hemiparesis that evolves over days or weeks has an extensive differential diagnosis. A common cause is subdural hematoma, especially in elderly or anticoagulated patients, even when there is no history of trauma. Infectious possibilities include cerebral abscess, fungal granuloma or meningitis, and parasitic infection. Weakness from primary and metastatic neoplasms may evolve over days to weeks. AIDS may present with subacute hemiparesis due to toxoplasmosis or primary CNS lymphoma. Noninfectious inflammatory processes such as multiple sclerosis or, less commonly, sarcoidosis merit consideration. If the brain MRI is normal and there are no cortical and hemispheric signs, MRI of the cervical spine should be undertaken.

Chronic hemiparesis that evolves over months usually is due to a neoplasm or vascular malformation, a chronic subdural hematoma, or a degenerative disease. If an MRI of the brain is normal, the possibility of a foramen magnum or high cervical spinal cord lesion should be considered.

Paraparesis

An intraspinal lesion at or below the upper thoracic spinal cord level is most commonly responsible, but a paraparesis also may result from lesions at other locations that disturb upper motor neurons (especially parasagittal intracranial lesions) and lower motor neurons [anterior horn cell disorders, cauda equina syndromes due to involvement of nerve roots derived from the lower spinal cord (Chap. 377), and peripheral neuropathies].

Acute paraparesis may not be recognized as due to spinal cord disease at an early stage if the legs are flaccid and areflexic. Usually, however, there is sensory loss in the legs with an upper level on the trunk, a dissociated sensory loss suggestive of a

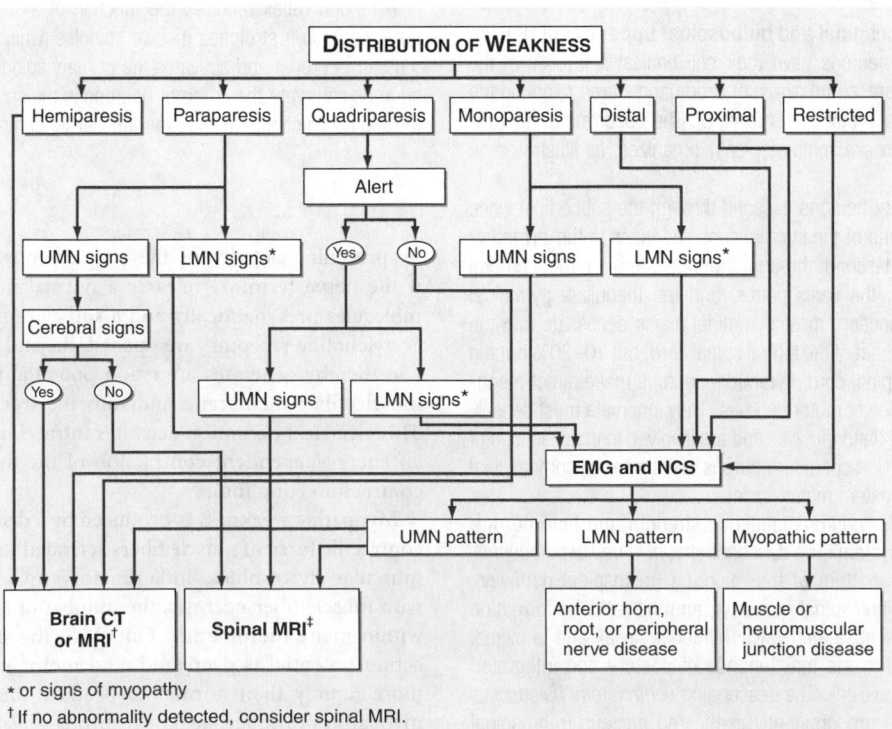

* or signs of myopathy
† If no abnormality detected, consider spinal MRI.
‡ If no abnormality detected, consider myelogram or brain MRI.

Figure 22-3   An algorithm for the initial workup of a patient with weakness. CT, computed tomography; EMG, electromyography; LMN, lower motor neuron; MRI, magnetic resonance imaging; NCS, nerve conduction studies; UMN, upper motor neuron.

central cord syndrome, or exaggerated stretch reflexes in the legs with normal reflexes in the arms. It is important to image the spinal cord (Fig. 22-3). Compressive lesions (particularly epidural tumor, abscess, and hematoma but also a prolapsed intervertebral disk and vertebral involvement by malignancy or infection), spinal cord infarction (proprioception usually is spared), an arteriovenous fistula or other vascular anomaly, and transverse myelitis are among the possible causes (Chap. 377).

Diseases of the cerebral hemispheres that produce acute parapresis include anterior cerebral artery ischemia (shoulder shrug also is affected), superior sagittal sinus or cortical venous thrombosis, and acute hydrocephalus. If upper motor neuron signs are associated with drowsiness, confusion, seizures, or other hemispheric signs, MRI of the brain should be undertaken.

Paraparesis may result from a cauda equina syndrome, for example, after trauma to the low back, a midline disk herniation, or an intraspinal tumor; although sphincters are affected, hip flexion often is spared, as is sensation over the anterolateral thighs. Rarely, paraparesis is caused by a rapidly evolving anterior horn cell disease (such as poliovirus or West Nile virus infection), peripheral neuropathy (such as Guillain-Barré syndrome; Chap. 385), or myopathy (Chap. 387). In such cases, electrophysiologic studies are diagnostically helpful and refocus the subsequent evaluation.

Subacute or chronic paraparesis with spasticity is caused by upper motor neuron disease. When there is associated lower-limb sensory loss and sphincter involvement, a chronic spinal cord disorder is likely (Chap. 377). If an MRI of the spinal cord is normal, MRI of the brain may be indicated. If hemispheric signs are present, a parasagittal meningioma or chronic hydrocephalus is likely and MRI of the brain is the initial test. In the rare situation in which a long-standing paraparesis has a lower motor neuron or myopathic etiology, the localization usually is suspected on clinical grounds by the absence of spasticity and confirmed by EMG and nerve conduction tests.

Quadriparesis or generalized weakness

Generalized weakness may be due to disorders of the CNS or the motor unit. Although the terms *quadriparesis* and *generalized weakness* often are used interchangeably, quadriparesis is commonly used when an upper motor neuron cause is suspected, and generalized weakness when a disease of the motor unit is likely. Weakness from CNS disorders usually is associated with changes in consciousness or cognition, with spasticity and brisk stretch reflexes, and with alterations of sensation. Most neuromuscular causes of generalized weakness are associated with normal mental function, hypotonia, and hypoactive muscle stretch reflexes. The major causes of intermittent weakness are listed in Table 22-2. A patient with generalized fatigability without objective weakness may have the chronic fatigue syndrome (Chap. 389).

Acute quadriparesis Acute quadriparesis with onset over minutes may result from disorders of upper motor neurons (e.g., anoxia, hypotension, brainstem or cervical cord ischemia, trauma, and systemic metabolic abnormalities) or muscle (electrolyte disturbances, certain inborn errors of muscle energy metabolism, toxins, and periodic paralyses). Onset over hours to weeks may, in addition to these disorders, be due to lower motor neuron disorders. Guillain-Barré syndrome (Chap. 385) is the most common lower motor neuron weakness that progresses over days to 4 weeks; the finding of an elevated protein level in the cerebrospinal fluid is helpful but may be absent early in the course.

In obtunded patients, evaluation begins with a CT scan of the brain. If upper motor neuron signs are present but the patient is alert, the initial test is usually an MRI of the cervical cord. If weakness is lower motor neuron, myopathic, or uncertain in origin, the

TABLE 22-2 Causes of Episodic Generalized Weakness

1. Electrolyte disturbances, e.g., hypokalemia, hyperkalemia, hypercalcemia, hypernatremia, hyponatremia, hypophosphatemia, hypermagnesemia
2. Muscle disorders
   a. Channelopathies (periodic paralyses)
   b. Metabolic defects of muscle (impaired carbohydrate or fatty acid utilization; abnormal mitochondrial function)
3. Neuromuscular junction disorders
   a. Myasthenia gravis
   b. Lambert-Eaton myasthenic syndrome
4. Central nervous system disorders
   a. Transient ischemic attacks of the brainstem
   b. Transient global cerebral ischemia
   c. Multiple sclerosis

clinical approach begins with blood studies to determine the level of muscle enzymes and electrolytes and an EMG and nerve conduction study.

Subacute or chronic quadriparesis When quadriparesis due to upper motor neuron disease develops over weeks, months, or years, the distinction between disorders of the cerebral hemispheres, brainstem, and cervical spinal cord is usually possible clinically. An MRI is obtained of the clinically suspected site of pathology. EMG and nerve conduction studies help distinguish lower motor neuron disease (which usually presents with weakness that is most profound distally) from myopathic weakness, which is typically proximal.

Monoparesis

Monoparesis usually is due to lower motor neuron disease, with or without associated sensory involvement. Upper motor neuron weakness occasionally presents as a monoparesis of distal and nonantigravity muscles. Myopathic weakness rarely is limited to one limb.

Acute monoparesis If the weakness is predominantly in distal and nonantigravity muscles and is not associated with sensory impairment or pain, focal cortical ischemia is likely (Chap. 370); diagnostic possibilities are similar to those for acute hemiparesis. Sensory loss and pain usually accompany acute lower motor neuron weakness; the weakness commonly is localized to a single nerve root or peripheral nerve within the limb but occasionally reflects plexus involvement. If lower motor neuron weakness is suspected or the pattern of weakness is uncertain, the clinical approach begins with an EMG and a nerve conduction study.

Subacute or chronic monoparesis Weakness and atrophy that develop over weeks or months are usually of lower motor neuron origin. If they are associated with sensory symptoms, a peripheral cause (nerve, root, or plexus) is likely; in the absence of such symptoms, anterior horn cell disease should be considered. In either case, an electrodiagnostic study is indicated. If weakness is of the upper motor neuron type, a discrete cortical (precentral gyrus) or cord lesion may be responsible, and an imaging study of the appropriate site is performed.

Distal weakness

Involvement of two or more limbs distally suggests lower motor neuron or peripheral nerve disease. Acute distal lower limb weakness results occasionally from an acute toxic polyneuropathy or cauda equina syndrome. Distal symmetric weakness usually develops over weeks, months, or years and, when associated with numbness, is due to diseases of peripheral nerves (Chap. 384). Anterior horn cell disease may begin distally but is typically asymmetric and without accompanying numbness (Chap. 374). Rarely, myopathies present with distal weakness (Chap. 387). Electrodiagnostic studies help localize the disorder (Fig. 22-3).

Proximal weakness

Myopathy often produces symmetric weakness of the pelvic or shoulder girdle muscles (Chap. 387). Diseases of the neuromuscular junction [such as myasthenia gravis (Chap. 386)], may present with symmetric proximal weakness often associated with ptosis, diplopia, or bulbar weakness and fluctuating in severity during the day. The extreme fatigability present in some cases of myasthenia gravis may even suggest episodic weakness, but strength rarely returns fully to normal. In anterior horn cell disease, proximal weakness is usually asymmetric, but it may be symmetric if familial. Numbness does not occur with any of these diseases. The evaluation usually begins with determination of the serum creatine kinase level and electrophysiologic studies.

Weakness in a restricted distribution

Weakness may not fit any of these patterns, being limited, for example, to the extraocular, hemifacial, bulbar, or respiratory muscles. If it is unilateral, restricted weakness usually is due to lower motor neuron or peripheral nerve disease, such as in a facial palsy or an isolated superior oblique muscle paresis. Weakness of part of a limb usually is due to a peripheral nerve lesion such as carpal tunnel syndrome or another entrapment neuropathy. Relatively symmetric weakness of extraocular or bulbar muscles usually is due to a myopathy (Chap. 387) or neuromuscular junction disorder (Chap. 386). Bilateral facial palsy with areflexia suggests Guillain-Barré syndrome (Chap. 385). Worsening of relatively symmetric weakness with fatigue is characteristic of neuromuscular junction disorders. Asymmetric bulbar weakness usually is due to motor neuron disease. Weakness limited to respiratory muscles is uncommon and usually is due to motor neuron disease, myasthenia gravis, or polymyositis/dermatomyositis (Chap. 388).

CHAPTER **23**

Numbness, Tingling, and Sensory Loss

Michael J. Aminoff
Arthur K. Asbury

Normal somatic sensation reflects a continuous monitoring process, little of which reaches consciousness under ordinary conditions. By contrast, disordered sensation, particularly when experienced as painful, is alarming and dominates the patient's attention. Physicians should be able to recognize abnormal sensations by how they are described, know their type and likely site of origin, and understand their implications. Pain is considered separately in Chap. 11.

■ POSITIVE AND NEGATIVE SYMPTOMS

Abnormal sensory symptoms can be divided into two categories: positive and negative. The prototypical positive symptom is tingling (pins and needles); other positive sensory phenomena include altered sensations that are described as pricking, bandlike, lightning-like shooting feelings (lancinations), aching, knifelike, twisting, drawing, pulling, tightening, burning, searing, electrical, or raw feelings. Such symptoms are often painful.

Positive phenomena usually result from trains of impulses generated at sites of lowered threshold or heightened excitability along a peripheral or central sensory pathway. The nature and severity of the abnormal sensation depend on the number, rate, timing, and distribution of ectopic impulses and the type and function of nervous tissue in which they arise. Because positive phenomena represent excessive activity in sensory pathways, they are not necessarily associated with a sensory deficit (loss) on examination.

Negative phenomena represent loss of sensory function and are characterized by diminished or absent feeling that often is experienced as numbness and by abnormal findings on sensory examination. In disorders affecting peripheral sensation, it is estimated that at least one-half the afferent axons innervating a particular site are lost or functionless before a sensory deficit can be demonstrated by clinical examination. This threshold varies in accordance with how rapidly function is lost in sensory nerve fibers. If the rate of loss is slow, lack of cutaneous feeling may be unnoticed by the patient and difficult to demonstrate on examination, even though few sensory fibers are functioning; if it is rapid, both positive and negative phenomena are usually conspicuous. Subclinical degrees of sensory dysfunction may be revealed by sensory nerve conduction studies or somatosensory evoked potentials (Chap. e45).

Whereas sensory symptoms may be either positive or negative, sensory signs on examination are always a measure of negative phenomena.

■ TERMINOLOGY

Words used to characterize sensory disturbance are descriptive and based on convention. Paresthesias and dysesthesias are general terms used to denote positive sensory symptoms. The term *paresthesias* typically refers to tingling or pins-and-needles sensations but may include a wide variety of other abnormal sensations, except pain; it sometimes implies that the abnormal sensations are perceived spontaneously. The more general term *dysesthesias* denotes all types of abnormal sensations, including painful ones, regardless of whether a stimulus is evident.

Another set of terms refers to sensory abnormalities found on examination. *Hypesthesia* or *hypoesthesia* refers to a reduction of cutaneous sensation to a specific type of testing such as pressure, light touch, and warm or cold stimuli; *anesthesia,* to a complete absence of skin sensation to the same stimuli plus pinprick; and *hypalgesia* or *analgesia,* to reduced or absent pain perception (nociception), such as perception of the pricking quality elicited by a pin. *Hyperesthesia* means pain or increased sensitivity in response to touch. Similarly, *allodynia* describes the situation in which a nonpainful stimulus, once perceived, is experienced as painful, even excruciating. An example is elicitation of a painful sensation by application of a vibrating tuning fork. *Hyperalgesia* denotes severe pain in response to a mildly noxious stimulus, and *hyperpathia*, a broad term, encompasses all the phenomena described by hyperesthesia, allodynia, and hyperalgesia. With hyperpathia, the threshold for a sensory stimulus is increased and perception is delayed, but once felt, it is unduly painful.

Disorders of deep sensation arising from muscle spindles, tendons, and joints affect proprioception (position sense). Manifestations include imbalance (particularly with eyes closed or in the dark), clumsiness of precision movements, and unsteadiness of gait, which are referred to collectively as *sensory ataxia*. Other findings on examination usually, but not invariably, include reduced or absent joint position and vibratory sensibility and absent deep tendon reflexes in the affected limbs. The Romberg sign is positive, which means that the patient sways markedly or topples when asked to stand with feet close together and eyes closed. In severe states of deafferentation involving deep sensation, the patient cannot walk or stand unaided or even sit unsupported. Continuous involuntary movements (*pseudoathetosis*) of the outstretched hands and fingers occur, particularly with eyes closed.

■ ANATOMY OF SENSATION

Cutaneous afferent innervation is conveyed by a rich variety of receptors, both naked nerve endings (nociceptors and thermoreceptors) and encapsulated terminals (mechanoreceptors). Each type of receptor has its own set of sensitivities to specific stimuli, size and distinctness of receptive fields, and adaptational qualities. Much of the knowledge about these receptors has come from the development of techniques to study single intact nerve fibers intraneurally in awake, unanesthetized human subjects. It is possible not only to record from but also to stimulate single fibers in isolation. A single impulse, whether elicited by a natural stimulus or evoked by electrical microstimulation in a large myelinated afferent fiber, may be both perceived and localized.

Afferent fibers of all sizes in peripheral nerve trunks traverse the dorsal roots and enter the dorsal horn of the spinal cord (Fig. 23-1). From there the smaller fibers take a route to the parietal cortex different from that of the larger fibers. The polysynaptic projections of the smaller fibers (unmyelinated and small myelinated), which subserve mainly nociception, temperature sensibility, and touch, cross and ascend in the opposite anterior and lateral columns of the spinal cord, through the brainstem, to the ventral posterolateral (VPL) nucleus of the thalamus and ultimately project to the postcentral gyrus of the parietal cortex (Chap. 11). This is the *spinothalamic pathway* or *anterolateral system*. The larger fibers, which subserve tactile and position sense and kinesthesia, project rostrally in the posterior column on the same side of the spinal cord and make their first synapse in the gracile or cuneate nucleus of the lower medulla. Axons of second-order neurons decussate and ascend in the medial lemniscus located medially in the medulla and in the tegmentum of the pons and midbrain and synapse in the VPL nucleus; third-order neurons project to parietal cortex. This large-fiber system is referred to as the *posterior column–medial lemniscal pathway* (lemniscal, for short). Note that although the lemniscal and the anterolateral pathways both project up the spinal cord to the thalamus, it is the (crossed) anterolateral pathway that is referred to as the *spinothalamic tract* by convention.

Although the fiber types and functions that make up the spinothalamic and lemniscal systems are relatively well known, many other fibers, particularly those associated with touch, pressure, and position sense, ascend in a diffusely distributed pattern both ipsilaterally and contralaterally in the anterolateral quadrants of the spinal cord. This explains why a complete lesion of the posterior columns of the spinal cord may be associated with little sensory deficit on examination.

EXAMINATION OF SENSATION

The main components of the sensory examination are tests of primary sensation (pain, touch, vibration, joint position, and thermal sensation; (Table 23-1).

Some general principles pertain. The examiner must depend on patient responses, particularly when testing cutaneous sensation (pin, touch, warm, or cold), and this complicates interpretation. Further, examination may be limited in some patients. In a stuporous patient, for example, sensory examination is reduced to observing the briskness of withdrawal in response to a pinch or another noxious stimulus. Comparison of response on one side of the body to that on the other is essential. In an alert but uncooperative patient, it may not be possible to examine cutaneous sensation, but some idea of proprioceptive function may be gained by noting the patient's best performance of movements requiring balance and precision. Frequently, patients present with sensory symptoms that do not fit an anatomic localization and that are accompanied by either no abnormalities or gross inconsistencies on examination. The examiner should consider whether the sensory symptoms are a disguised request for help with psychological or situational problems. Discretion must be used in pursuing this possibility. Finally, sensory examination of a patient who has no neurologic complaints can be brief and consist of pinprick, touch, and vibration testing in the hands and feet plus evaluation of stance and gait, including the Romberg maneuver. Evaluation of stance and gait also tests the integrity of motor and cerebellar systems.

Primary sensation

(See Table 23-1) The sense of pain usually is tested with a clean pin, with the patient asked to focus on the pricking or unpleasant quality of the stimulus, not just the pressure or touch sensation elicited. Areas of hypalgesia should be mapped by proceeding radially from the most hypalgesic site (Figs. 23-2, 23-3 and 23-4).

Temperature sensation to both hot and cold is best tested with small containers filled with water of the desired temperature. This is impractical in most settings. An alternative way to test cold sensation is to touch a metal object, such as a tuning fork at room temperature, to the skin. For testing warm temperatures, the tuning fork or another metal object may be held under warm water of the desired temperature and then used. The appreciation of both cold and warmth should be tested because different receptors respond to each.

Touch usually is tested with a wisp of cotton or a fine camel hair brush. In general, it is better to avoid testing touch on hairy skin because of the profusion of the sensory endings that surround each hair follicle.

Joint position testing is a measure of proprioception, one of the most important functions of the sensory system. With the patient's eyes closed, joint position is tested in the distal interphalangeal joint of the great toe and fingers. If errors are made in recognizing the direction of passive movements, more proximal joints are tested. A test of proximal joint position sense, primarily at the shoulder, is performed by asking the patient to bring the two index fingers together with arms extended and eyes closed. Normal individuals can do this accurately, with errors of 1 cm or less.

The sense of vibration is tested with a tuning fork that vibrates at 128 Hz. Vibration usually is tested over bony points, beginning distally; in the feet it is tested over the dorsal surface of the distal phalanx of the big toes and at the malleoli of the ankles, and in the hands dorsally at the distal phalanx of the fingers. If abnormalities are found, more proximal sites can be examined. Vibratory thresholds at the same site in the patient and the examiner may be compared for control purposes.

Quantitative sensory testing

Effective sensory testing devices are now available commercially. Quantitative sensory testing is particularly useful for serial evaluation

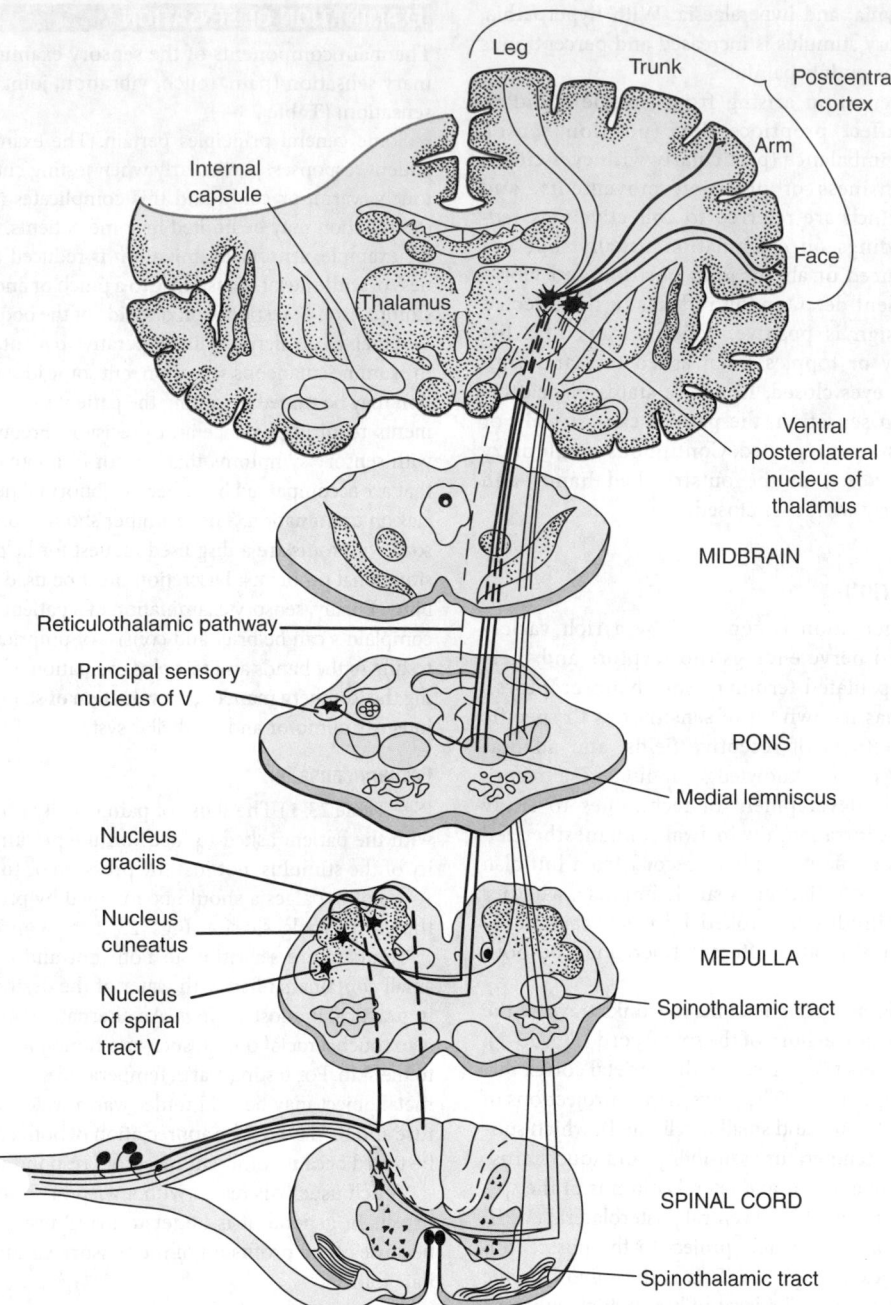

Figure 23-1 The main somatosensory pathways. The spinothalamic tract (pain, thermal sense) and the posterior column–lemniscal system (touch, pressure, joint position) are shown. Offshoots from the ascending anterolateral fasciculus (spinothalamic tract) to nuclei in the medulla, pons, and mesencephalon and nuclear terminations of the tract are indicated. *(From AH Ropper, RH Brown, in Adams and Victor's Principles of Neurology, 9th ed. New York, McGraw-Hill, 2009.)*

of cutaneous sensation in clinical trials. Threshold testing for touch and vibratory and thermal sensation is the most widely used application.

Cortical sensation

The most commonly used tests of cortical function are two-point discrimination, touch localization, and bilateral simultaneous stimulation and tests for graphesthesia and stereognosis. Abnormalities of these sensory tests, in the presence of normal primary sensation in an alert cooperative patient, signify a lesion of the parietal cortex or thalamocortical projections to the parietal lobe. If primary sensation is altered, these cortical discriminative functions usually will be abnormal also. Comparisons should always be made between

analogous sites on the two sides of the body because the deficit with a specific parietal lesion is likely to be unilateral. Interside comparisons are important for all cortical sensory testing.

Two-point discrimination is tested with special calipers, the points of which may be set from 2 mm to several centimeters apart and then applied simultaneously to the site to be tested. The pulp of the fingertips is a common site to test; a normal individual can distinguish about 3-mm separation of points there.

Touch localization is performed by light pressure for an instant with the examiner's fingertip or a wisp of cotton wool; the patient, whose eyes are closed, is required to identify the site of touch with the fingertip. *Bilateral simultaneous stimulation* at analogous sites (e.g.,

TABLE 23-1 Testing Primary Sensation

Sense	Test Device	Endings Activated	Fiber Size Mediating	Central Pathway
Pain	Pinprick	Cutaneous nociceptors	Small	SpTh, also D
Temperature, heat	Warm metal object	Cutaneous thermoreceptors for hot	Small	SpTh
Temperature, cold	Cold metal object	Cutaneous thermoreceptors for cold	Small	SpTh
Touch	Cotton wisp, fine brush	Cutaneous mechanoreceptors, also naked endings	Large and small	Lem, also D and SpTh
Vibration	Tuning fork, 128 Hz	Mechanoreceptors, especially pacinian corpuscles	Large	Lem, also D
Joint position	Passive movement of specific joints	Joint capsule and tendon endings, muscle spindles	Large	Lem, also D

Abbreviations: D, diffuse ascending projections in ipsilateral and contralateral anterolateral columns; SpTh, spinothalamic projection, contralateral; Lem, posterior column and lemniscal projection, ipsilateral.

the dorsum of both hands) can be carried out to determine whether the perception of touch is extinguished consistently on one side or the other. The phenomenon is referred to as *extinction or neglect*. *Graphesthesia* refers to the capacity to recognize with eyes closed letters or numbers drawn by the examiner's fingertip on the palm of the hand. Once again, interside comparison is of prime importance. Inability to recognize numbers or letters is termed *agraphesthesia*.

Stereognosis refers to the ability to identify common objects by palpation, recognizing their shape, texture, and size. Common standard objects such as keys, paper clips, and coins are best used. Patients with normal stereognosis should be able to distinguish a dime from a penny and a nickel from a quarter without looking. Patients should be allowed to feel the object with only one hand at a time. If they are unable to identify it in one hand, it should be placed

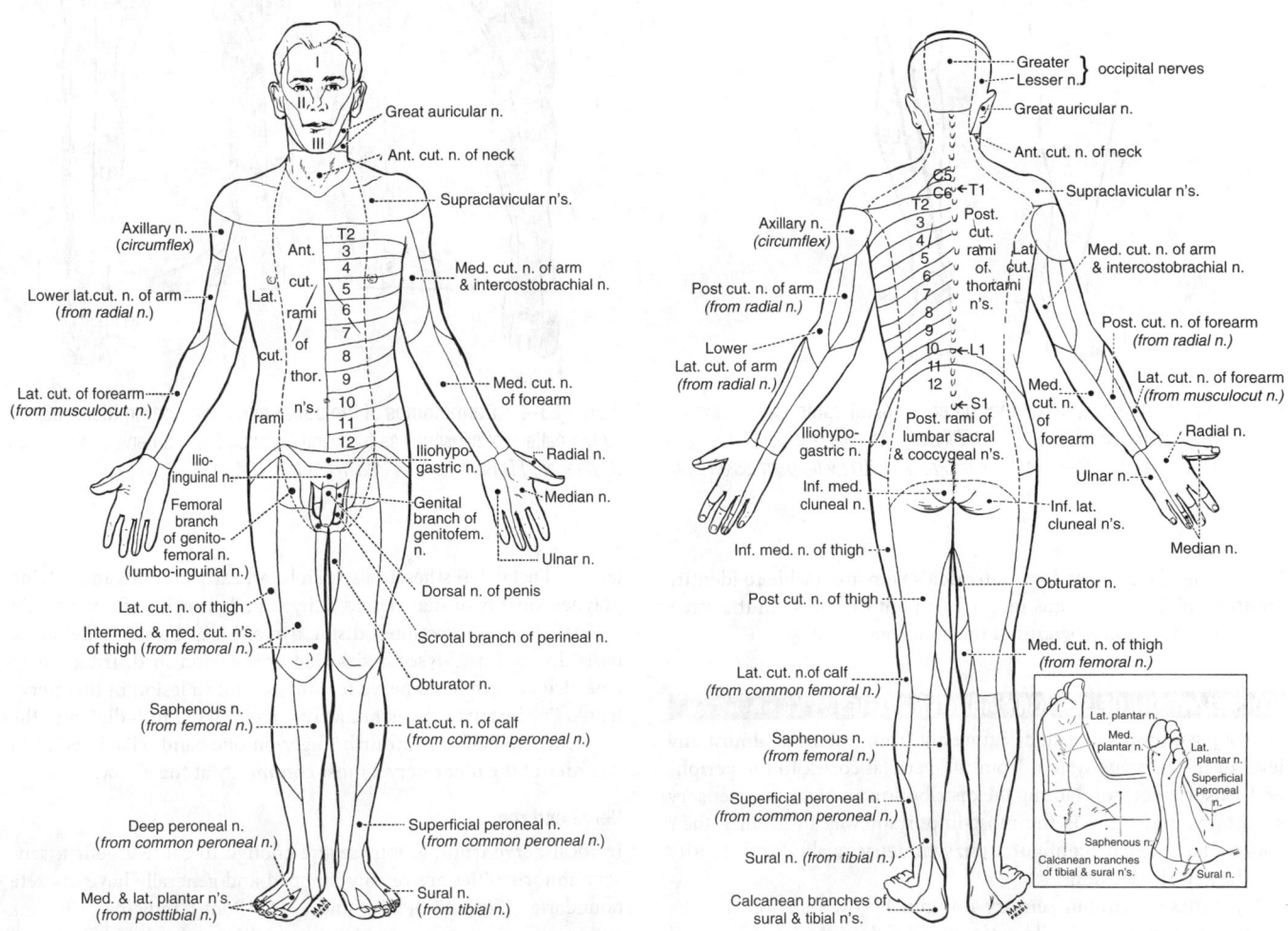

Figure 23-2 **The cutaneous fields of peripheral nerves.** *(Reproduced by permission from W Haymaker, B Woodhall: Peripheral Nerve Injuries, 2nd ed. Philadelphia, Saunders, 1953.)*

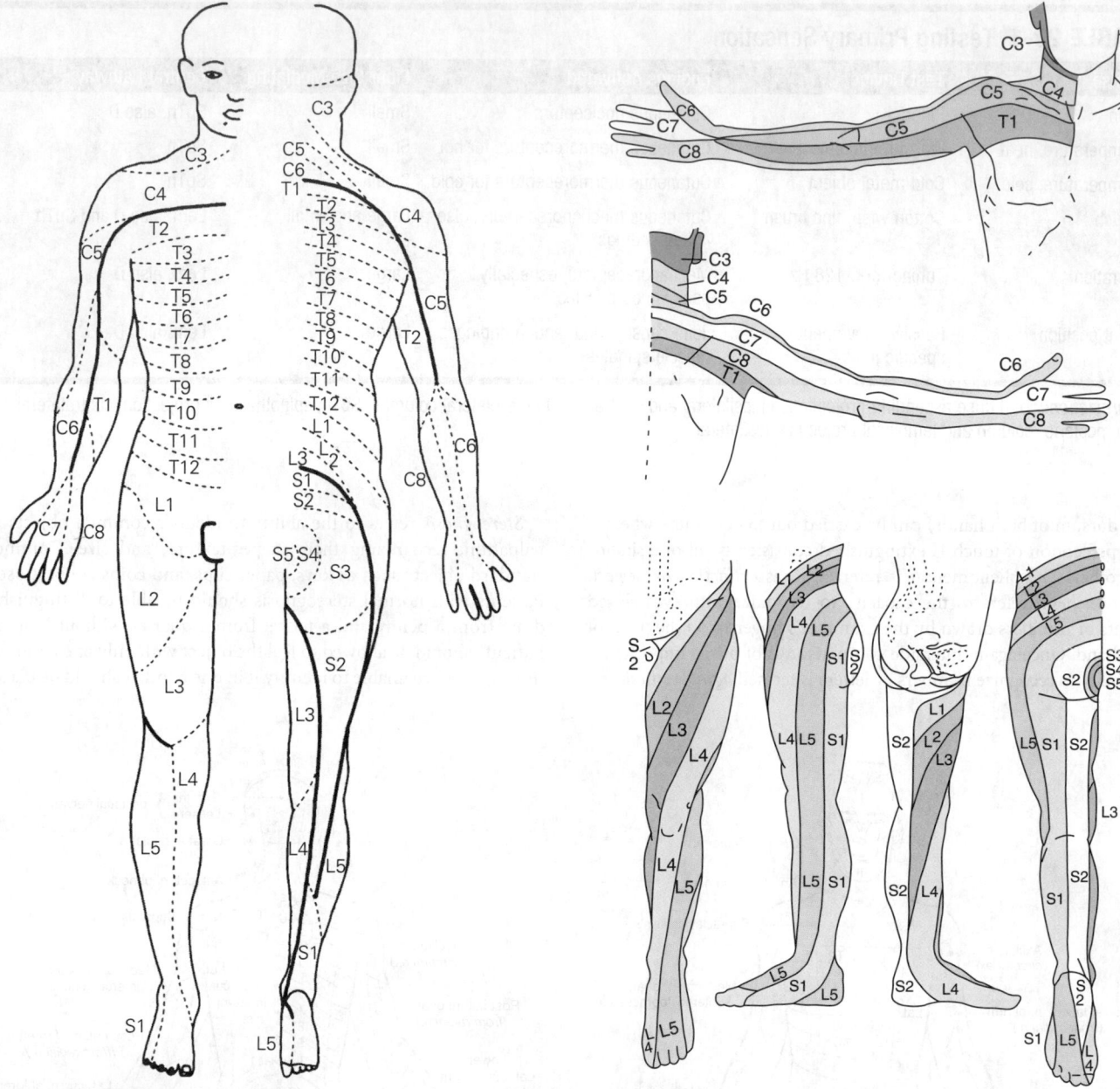

Figure 23-3 **Distribution of the sensory spinal roots** on the surface of the body (dermatomes). *(From D Sinclair: Mechanisms of Cutaneous Sensation. Oxford, UK, Oxford University Press, 1981; with permission from Dr. David Sinclair.)*

Figure 23-4 **Dermatomes of the upper and lower extremities,** outlined by the pattern of sensory loss following lesions of single nerve roots. *(From JJ Keegan, FD Garrett: Anat Rec 102:409, 1948.)*

in the other for comparison. Individuals who are unable to identify common objects and coins in one hand but can do so in the other are said to have *astereognosis* of the abnormal hand.

LOCALIZATION OF SENSORY ABNORMALITIES

Sensory symptoms and signs can result from lesions at almost any level of the nervous system from the parietal cortex to the peripheral sensory receptor. Noting the distribution and nature of sensory symptoms and signs is the most important way to localize their source. Their extent, configuration, symmetry, quality, and severity are the key observations.

Dysesthesias without sensory findings by examination may be difficult to interpret. To illustrate, tingling dysesthesias in an acral distribution (hands and feet) can be systemic in origin, e.g., secondary to hyperventilation, or induced by a medication such as acetazo-

lamide. Distal dysesthesias also can be an early event in an evolving polyneuropathy or may herald a myelopathy, such as from vitamin B_{12} deficiency. Sometimes distal dysesthesias have no definable basis. In contrast, dysesthesias that correspond in distribution to a particular peripheral nerve territory denote a lesion of that nerve trunk. For instance, dysesthesias restricted to the fifth digit and the adjacent one-half of the fourth finger on one hand reliably point to disorder of the ulnar nerve, most commonly at the elbow.

Nerve and root

In focal nerve trunk lesions severe enough to cause a deficit, sensory abnormalities are readily mapped and generally have discrete boundaries (Figs. 23-2, 23-3 and 23-4). Root ("radicular") lesions frequently are accompanied by deep, aching pain along the course of the related nerve trunk. With compression of a fifth lumbar (L5) or first sacral (S1) root, as from a ruptured intervertebral disk, sciatica (radicular pain relating to the sciatic nerve trunk) is a common manifestation (Chap. 15). With a lesion affecting a single root, sensory deficits may be minimal or absent because adjacent root territories overlap extensively.

Isolated mononeuropathies may cause symptoms beyond the territory supplied by the affected nerve, but abnormalities on examination typically are confined to appropriate anatomic boundaries. In multiple mononeuropathies, symptoms and signs occur in discrete territories supplied by different individual nerves and—as more nerves are affected—may simulate a polyneuropathy if deficits become confluent. With polyneuropathies, sensory deficits are generally graded, distal, and symmetric in distribution (Chap. 384). Dysesthesias, followed by numbness, begin in the toes and ascend symmetrically. When dysesthesias reach the knees, they usually also have appeared in the fingertips. The process appears to be nerve length–dependent, and the deficit is often described as "stocking-glove" in type. Involvement of both hands and feet also occurs with lesions of the upper cervical cord or the brainstem, but an upper level of the sensory disturbance may then be found on the trunk and other evidence of a central lesion may be present, such as sphincter involvement or signs of an upper motor neuron lesion (Chap. 22). Although most polyneuropathies are pansensory and affect all modalities of sensation, selective sensory dysfunction according to nerve fiber size may occur. Small-fiber polyneuropathies are characterized by burning, painful dysesthesias with reduced pinprick and thermal sensation but with sparing of proprioception, motor function, and deep tendon reflexes. Touch is involved variably; when it is spared, the sensory pattern is referred to as exhibiting *sensory dissociation*. Sensory dissociation may occur with spinal cord lesions as well as small-fiber neuropathies. Large-fiber polyneuropathies are characterized by vibration and position sense deficits, imbalance, absent tendon reflexes, and variable motor dysfunction but preservation of most cutaneous sensation. Dysesthesias, if present at all, tend to be tingling or bandlike in quality.

Sensory neuronopathy is characterized by widespread but asymmetric sensory loss occurring in a non-length-dependent manner so that it may occur proximally or distally and in the arms, legs, or both. Pain and numbness progress to sensory ataxia and impairment of all sensory modalities with time. This condition is usually paraneoplastic or idiopathic in origin (Chaps. 101 and 384).

Spinal cord

(See also Chap. 377) If the spinal cord is transected, all sensation is lost below the level of transection. Bladder and bowel function also are lost, as is motor function. Hemisection of the spinal cord produces the Brown-Séquard syndrome, with absent pain and temperature sensation contralaterally and loss of proprioceptive sensation and power ipsilaterally below the lesion (see Figs. 23-1 and 377-1).

Numbness or paresthesias in both feet may arise from a spinal cord lesion; this is especially likely when the upper level of the sensory loss extends to the trunk. When all extremities are affected, the lesion is probably in the cervical region or brainstem unless a peripheral neuropathy is responsible. The presence of upper motor neuron signs (Chap. 22) supports a central lesion; a hyperesthetic band on the trunk may suggest the level of involvement.

A dissociated sensory loss can reflect spinothalamic tract involvement in the spinal cord, especially if the deficit is unilateral and has an upper level on the torso. Bilateral spinothalamic tract involvement occurs with lesions affecting the center of the spinal cord, such as in syringomyelia. There is a dissociated sensory loss with impairment of pinprick and temperature appreciation but relative preservation of light touch, position sense, and vibration appreciation.

Dysfunction of the posterior columns in the spinal cord or of the posterior root entry zone may lead to a bandlike sensation around the trunk or a feeling of tight pressure in one or more limbs. Flexion of the neck sometimes leads to an electric shock–like sensation that radiates down the back and into the legs (Lhermitte's sign) in patients with a cervical lesion affecting the posterior columns, such as from multiple sclerosis, cervical spondylosis, or recent irradiation to the cervical region.

Brainstem

Crossed patterns of sensory disturbance, in which one side of the face and the opposite side of the body are affected, localize to the lateral medulla. Here a small lesion may damage both the ipsilateral descending trigeminal tract and the ascending spinothalamic fibers subserving the opposite arm, leg, and hemitorso (see "Lateral medullary syndrome" in Fig. 370-10). A lesion in the tegmentum of the pons and midbrain, where the lemniscal and spinothalamic tracts merge, causes pansensory loss contralaterally.

Thalamus

Hemisensory disturbance with tingling numbness from head to foot is often thalamic in origin but also can arise from the anterior parietal region. If abrupt in onset, the lesion is likely to be due to a small stroke (lacunar infarction), particularly if localized to the thalamus. Occasionally, with lesions affecting the VPL nucleus or adjacent white matter, a syndrome of thalamic pain, also called *Déjerine-Roussy syndrome*, may ensue. The persistent, unrelenting unilateral pain often is described in dramatic terms.

Cortex

With lesions of the parietal lobe involving either the cortex or the subjacent white matter, the most prominent symptoms are contralateral hemineglect, hemi-inattention, and a tendency not to use the affected hand and arm. On cortical sensory testing (e.g., two-point discrimination, graphesthesia), abnormalities are often found but primary sensation is usually intact. Anterior parietal infarction may present as a pseudothalamic syndrome with contralateral loss of primary sensation from head to toe. Dysesthesias or a sense of numbness may also occur and, rarely, a painful state.

Focal sensory seizures

These seizures generally are due to lesions in the area of the postcentral or precentral gyrus. The principal symptom of focal sensory seizures is tingling, but additional, more complex sensations may occur, such as a rushing feeling, a sense of warmth, or a sense of movement without detectable motion. Symptoms typically are unilateral; commonly begin in the arm or hand, face, or foot; and often spread in a manner that reflects the cortical representation of different bodily parts, as in a Jacksonian march. Duration of seizures is variable; seizures may be transient, lasting only for seconds, or persist for an hour or more. Focal motor features may supervene, often becoming generalized with loss of consciousness and tonic-clonic jerking.

CHAPTER **24**

Gait and Balance Disorders

Lewis Sudarsky

■ PREVALENCE, MORBIDITY, AND MORTALITY

Gait and balance problems are common in the elderly and contribute to the risk of falls and injury. Gait disorders have been described in 15% of individuals older than age 65 years. By age 80 years, one person in four will use a mechanical aid to assist ambulation. Among those 85 and older, the prevalence of gait abnormality approaches 40%. In epidemiologic studies, gait disorders are consistently identified as a major risk factor for falls and injury.

A substantial number of older persons report insecure balance and experience falls and fear of falling. Prospective studies indicate that 30% of those age >65 years fall each year; the proportion is even higher in frail elderly and nursing home patients. Each year, 8% of individuals age >75 years suffer a serious fall-related injury. Hip fractures often result in hospitalization and nursing home admission. For each person who is physically disabled, there are others whose functional independence is constrained by anxiety and fear of falling. Nearly one in five elderly individuals voluntarily limits activity because of fear of falling. With loss of ambulation, there is a diminished quality of life and increased morbidity and mortality rates.

■ ANATOMY AND PHYSIOLOGY

Upright bipedal gait depends on the successful integration of postural control and locomotion. These functions are widely distributed in the central nervous system. The biomechanics of bipedal walking are complex, and the performance is easily compromised by neurologic deficit at any level. Command and control centers in the brainstem, cerebellum, and forebrain modify the action of spinal pattern generators to promote stepping. While a form of "fictive locomotion" can be elicited from quadrupedal animals after spinal transection, this capacity is limited in primates. Step generation in primates is dependent on locomotor centers in the pontine tegmentum, midbrain, and subthalamic region. Locomotor synergies are executed through the reticular formation and descending pathways in the ventromedial spinal cord. Cerebral control provides a goal and purpose for walking and is involved in avoidance of obstacles and adaptation of locomotor programs to context and terrain.

Postural control requires the maintenance of the center of mass over the base of support through the gait cycle. Unconscious postural adjustments maintain standing balance: long latency responses are measurable in the leg muscles, beginning 110 milliseconds after a perturbation. Forward motion of the center of mass provides propulsive force for stepping, but failure to maintain the center of mass within stability limits results in falls. The anatomic substrate for dynamic balance has not been well defined, but the vestibular nucleus and midline cerebellum contribute to balance control in animals. Human patients with damage to these structures have impaired balance with standing and walking.

Standing balance depends on good-quality sensory information about the position of the body center with respect to the environment, support surface, and gravitational forces. Sensory information for postural control is primarily generated by the visual system, the vestibular system, and by proprioceptive receptors in the muscle spindles and joints. A healthy redundancy of sensory afferent information is generally available, but loss of two of the three pathways is sufficient to compromise standing balance. Balance disorders in older individuals sometimes result from multiple insults in the peripheral sensory systems (e.g., visual loss, vestibular deficit, peripheral neuropathy), critically degrading the quality of afferent information needed for balance stability.

Older patients with cognitive impairment from neurodegenerative diseases appear to be particularly prone to falls and injury. Frailty, muscle weakness, and deconditioning also contribute to the risk. It has been shown that older people who continue walking while talking are at increased risk for falls. There is a growing literature on the use of attentional resources to manage gait and balance. Walking is generally considered to be unconscious and automatic, but the ability to walk while attending a cognitive task (dual-task walking) may be compromised in frail elderly with a history of falls. Older patients with deficits in executive function may have particular difficulty in managing the attentional resources needed for dynamic balance when distracted.

■ DISORDERS OF GAIT

The heterogeneity of gait disorders observed in clinical practice reflects the large network of neural systems involved in the task. Walking is vulnerable to neurologic disease at every level. Gait disorders have been classified descriptively, based on the abnormal physiology and biomechanics. One problem with this approach is that many failing gaits look fundamentally similar. This overlap reflects common patterns of adaptation to threatened balance stability and declining performance. *The gait disorder observed clinically must be viewed as the product of a neurologic deficit and a functional adaptation.* Unique features of the failing gait are often overwhelmed by the adaptive response. Some of the common patterns of abnormal gait are summarized below. Gait disorders can also be classified by etiology, as listed in Table 24-1.

TABLE 24-1 Etiology of Gait Disorders

	Cases	Percent
Sensory deficits	22	18.3
Myelopathy	20	16.7
Multiple infarcts	18	15.0
Parkinsonism	14	11.7
Cerebellar degeneration	8	6.7
Hydrocephalus	8	6.7
Toxic/metabolic	3	2.5
Psychogenic	4	3.3
Other	6	5.0
Unknown cause	17	14.2
Total	120	100%

Source: Reproduced with permission from J Masdeu et al: *Gait Disorders of Aging: With Special Reference to Falls.* Boston, Little Brown, 1995.

Cautious gait

The term *cautious gait* is used to describe the patient who walks with an abbreviated stride and lowered center of mass, as if walking on a slippery surface. This disorder is both common and nonspecific. It is, in essence, an adaptation to a perceived postural threat. There may be an associated fear of falling. In one study, this disorder was observed in more than one-third of older patients with a higher level gait disturbance. Physical therapy often improves walking to the degree that follow-up observation may reveal a more specific underlying disorder.

Stiff-legged gait

Spastic gait is characterized by stiffness in the legs, an imbalance of muscle tone, and a tendency to circumduct and scuff the feet. The disorder reflects compromise of corticospinal command and overactivity of spinal reflexes. The patient may walk on his or her toes. In extreme instances, the legs cross due to increased tone in the adductors. Upper motor neuron signs are present on physical examination. Shoes often reflect an uneven pattern of wear across the outside. The disorder may be cerebral or spinal in origin.

Myelopathy from cervical spondylosis is a common cause of spastic or spastic-ataxic gait. Demyelinating disease and trauma are the leading causes of myelopathy in younger patients. In a chronic progressive myelopathy of unknown cause, workup with laboratory and imaging tests may establish a diagnosis. A family history should suggest hereditary spastic paraplegia (HSP; Chap. 374). Genetic testing is now available for some of the common HSP mutations. Tropical spastic paraparesis related to the retrovirus HTLV-I is endemic in parts of the Caribbean and South America. A structural lesion, such as tumor or spinal vascular malformation, should be excluded with appropriate testing. Spinal cord disorders are discussed in detail in Chap. 377.

With cerebral spasticity, asymmetry is common, involvement of the upper extremities is usually observed, and dysarthria is often an associated feature. Common causes include vascular disease (stroke), multiple sclerosis, and perinatal injury to the nervous system (cerebral palsy).

Other stiff-legged gaits include dystonia (Chap. 387) and stiff-person syndrome. Dystonia is a disorder characterized by sustained muscle contractions, resulting in repetitive twisting movements and abnormal posture. It often has a genetic basis. Dystonic spasms produce plantar flexion and inversion of the feet, sometimes with torsion of the trunk. In autoimmune stiff-person syndrome (Chap. 101), there is exaggerated lordosis of the lumbar spine and overactivity of antagonist muscles, which restricts trunk and lower limb movement and results in a wooden or fixed posture.

Parkinsonism and freezing gait

Parkinson's disease (Chap. 372) is common, affecting 1% of the population age >55 years. The stooped posture and shuffling gait are characteristic and distinctive features. Patients sometimes accelerate (festinate) with walking or display retropulsion. There may be difficulty with gait initiation (freezing) and a tendency to turn en bloc. Imbalance and falls may develop as the disease progresses over years. Gait freezing is described in 7% of Parkinson's patients within 2 years of onset, 26% by the end of 5 years. Freezing of gait is even more common in some of the Parkinson's-related neurodegenerative disorders, such as progressive supranuclear palsy, multiple-system atrophy, and corticobasal degeneration. These patients frequently present with axial stiffness, postural instability, and a shuffling gait while lacking the characteristic pill-rolling tremor of Parkinson's disease. Falls within the first year suggest the possibility of progressive supranuclear palsy.

Hyperkinetic movement disorders also produce characteristic and recognizable disturbances in gait. In Huntington's disease (Chap. 371), the unpredictable occurrence of choreic movements gives the gait a dancing quality. Tardive dyskinesia is the cause of many odd, stereotypic gait disorders seen in patients chronically exposed to antipsychotics and other drugs that block the D_2 dopamine receptor.

Frontal gait disorder

Frontal gait disorder, sometimes known as "gait apraxia," is common in the elderly and has a variety of causes. The term is used to describe a shuffling, freezing gait with imbalance and other signs of higher cerebral dysfunction. Typical features include a wide base of support, short stride, shuffling along the floor, and difficulty with starts and turns. Many patients exhibit difficulty with gait initiation, descriptively characterized as the "slipping clutch" syndrome. The term *lower body parkinsonism* is also used to describe such patients. Strength is generally preserved, and patients are able to make stepping movements when not standing and maintaining balance at the same time. This disorder is best considered a higher level motor control disorder, as opposed to an apraxia (Chap. 26).

The most common cause of frontal gait disorder is vascular disease, particularly subcortical small-vessel disease. Lesions are frequently found in the deep frontal white matter and centrum ovale. Gait disorder may be the salient feature in hypertensive patients with ischemic lesions of the deep hemisphere white matter (Binswanger's disease). The clinical syndrome includes mental change (variable in degree), dysarthria, pseudobulbar affect (emotional disinhibition), increased tone, and hyperreflexia in the lower limbs.

Communicating hydrocephalus in adults also presents with a gait disorder of this type. Other features of the diagnostic triad (mental change, incontinence) may be absent in the initial stages. MRI demonstrates ventricular enlargement, an enlarged flow void about the aqueduct, and a variable degree of periventricular white matter change. A lumbar puncture or dynamic test is necessary to confirm the presence of hydrocephalus.

Cerebellar gait ataxia

Disorders of the cerebellum have a dramatic impact on gait and balance. Cerebellar gait ataxia is characterized by a wide base of support, lateral instability of the trunk, erratic foot placement, and decompensation of balance when attempting to walk tandem. Difficulty maintaining balance when turning is often an early feature. Patients are unable to walk tandem heel to toe, and display truncal sway in narrow-based or tandem stance. They show considerable variation in their tendency to fall in daily life.

Causes of cerebellar ataxia in older patients include stroke, trauma, tumor, and neurodegenerative disease, including multiple-system atrophy (Chaps. 372 and 375) and various forms of hereditary cerebellar degeneration (Chap. 373). A short expansion at the site of the fragile X mutation (fragile X pre-mutation) has been associated with gait ataxia in older men. Alcoholic cerebellar degeneration can be screened by history and often confirmed by MRI. In patients with ataxia, MRI demonstrates the extent and topography of cerebellar atrophy.

Sensory ataxia

As reviewed above, balance depends on high-quality afferent information from the visual and the vestibular systems and proprioception. When this information is lost or degraded, balance during locomotion is impaired and instability results. The sensory ataxia of tabetic neurosyphilis is a classic example. The contemporary equivalent is the patient with neuropathy affecting large fibers. Vitamin B_{12} deficiency is a treatable cause of large-fiber sensory loss

TABLE 24-2 Features of Cerebellar Ataxia, Sensory Ataxia, and Frontal Gait Disorders

	Cerebellar Ataxia	Sensory Ataxia	Frontal Gait
Base of support	Wide-based	Narrow base, looks down	Wide-based
Velocity	Variable	Slow	Very slow
Stride	Irregular, lurching	Regular with path deviation	Short, shuffling
Romberg	+/−	Unsteady, falls	+/−
Heel → shin	Abnormal	+/−	Normal
Initiation	Normal	Normal	Hesitant
Turns	Unsteady	+/−	Hesitant, multistep
Postural instability	+	+++	++++ Poor postural synergies getting up from a chair
Falls	Late event	Frequent	Frequent

in the spinal cord and peripheral nervous system. Joint position and vibration sense are diminished in the lower limbs. The stance in such patients is destabilized by eye closure; they often look down at their feet when walking and do poorly in the dark. Patients have been described with imbalance from bilateral vestibular loss, caused by disease or by exposure to ototoxic drugs. Table 24-2 compares sensory ataxia with cerebellar ataxia and frontal gait disorder. Some frail older patients exhibit a syndrome of imbalance from the combined effect of multiple sensory deficits. Such patients have disturbances in proprioception, vision, and vestibular sense that impair postural support.

Neuromuscular disease

Patients with neuromuscular disease often have an abnormal gait, occasionally as a presenting feature. With distal weakness (peripheral neuropathy) the step height is increased to compensate for footdrop, and the sole of the foot may slap on the floor during weight acceptance. Neuropathy may be associated with a degree of sensory imbalance, as described above. Patients with myopathy or muscular dystrophy more typically exhibit proximal weakness. Weakness of the hip girdle may result in a degree of excess pelvic sway during locomotion.

Toxic and metabolic disorders

Alcohol intoxication is the most common cause of acute walking difficulty. Chronic toxicity from medications and metabolic disturbances can impair motor function and gait. Mental status changes may be present, and examination may reveal asterixis or myoclonus. Static equilibrium is disturbed, and such patients are easily thrown off balance. Disequilibrium is particularly evident in patients with chronic renal disease and those with hepatic failure, in whom asterixis may impair postural support. Sedative drugs, especially neuroleptics and long-acting benzodiazepines, affect postural control and increase the risk for falls. These disorders are important to recognize because they are often treatable.

Psychogenic gait disorder

Psychogenic disorders are common in neurologic practice, and the presentation often involves gait. Some patients with extreme anxiety or phobia walk with exaggerated caution with abduction of the arms, as if walking on ice. This inappropriately overcautious gait differs in degree from the gait of the patient who is insecure and making adjustments for imbalance. Depressed patients exhibit primarily slowness, a manifestation of psychomotor retardation, and lack of purpose in their stride. Hysterical gait disorders are among the most spectacular encountered. Odd gyrations of posture with wastage of muscular energy (astasia-abasia), extreme slow motion, and dramatic fluctuations over time may be observed in patients with somatoform disorders and conversion reaction.

APPROACH TO THE PATIENT ▶ **Slowly Progressive Disorder of Gait**

When reviewing the history, it is helpful to inquire about the onset and progression of disability. Initial awareness of an unsteady gait often follows a fall. Stepwise evolution or sudden progression suggests vascular disease. Gait disorder may be associated with urinary urgency and incontinence, particularly in patients with cervical spine disease or hydrocephalus. It is always important to review the use of alcohol and medications that affect gait and balance. Information on localization derived from the neurologic examination can be helpful to narrow the list of possible diagnoses.

Gait observation provides an immediate sense of the patient's degree of disability. Characteristic patterns of abnormality are sometimes observed, though failing gaits often look fundamentally similar. Cadence (steps/min), velocity, and stride length can be recorded by timing a patient over a fixed distance. Watching the patient get out of a chair provides a good functional assessment of balance.

Brain imaging studies may be informative in patients with an undiagnosed disorder of gait. MRI is sensitive for cerebral lesions of vascular or demyelinating disease and is a good screening test for occult hydrocephalus. Patients with recurrent falls are at risk for subdural hematoma. Many elderly patients with gait and balance difficulty have white matter abnormalities in the periventricular region and centrum semiovale. While these lesions may be an incidental finding, a substantial burden of white matter disease will ultimately impact cerebral control of locomotion.

■ DISORDERS OF BALANCE

Balance is the ability to maintain equilibrium: a state in which opposing physical forces cancel. In physiology, this is taken to mean the ability to control the center of mass with respect to gravity and the support surface. In reality, we are not consciously aware of what or where our center of mass is, but everyone, including gymnasts, figure skaters, and platform divers, moves so as to manage it. Imbalance implies a disturbance of equilibrium. Disorders of balance present with difficulty maintaining posture standing and walking and with a subjective sense of disequilibrium, a form of dizziness.

The cerebellum and vestibular system organize antigravity responses needed to maintain the upright posture. As reviewed above, these responses are physiologically complex, and the anatomic representation is not well understood. Failure, resulting in disequilibrium, can occur at several levels: cerebellar, vestibular, somatosensory, and higher level disequilibrium. Patients with hereditary ataxia or alcoholic cerebellar degeneration do not generally complain of dizziness, but balance is visibly impaired. Neurologic examination will reveal a variety of cerebellar signs. Postural compensation may prevent falls early on, but falls inevitably occur with disease progression. The progression of a neurodegenerative ataxia is often measured by the number of years to loss of stable ambulation. Vestibular disorders (Chap. 21) have symptoms and signs in three categories: (1) vertigo, the subjective appreciation or illusion of movement; (2) nystagmus, a vestibulo-oculomotor sign; and (3) poor standing balance, an impairment of vestibulospinal function. Not every patient has all manifestations. Patients with vestibular deficits related to ototoxic drugs may lack vertigo or obvious nystagmus, but balance is impaired on standing and walking, and the patient cannot navigate in the dark. Laboratory testing is available to explore vestibulo-oculomotor and vestibulospinal deficits.

Somatosensory deficits also produce imbalance and falls. There is often a subjective sense of insecure balance and fear of falling. Postural control is compromised by eye closure (Romberg's sign); these patients also have difficulty navigating in the dark. A dramatic example is the patient with autoimmune subacute sensory neuropathy, sometimes a paraneoplastic disorder (Chap. 101). Compensatory strategies enable such patients to walk in the virtual absence of proprioception, but the task requires active visual monitoring. Patients with higher level disorders of equilibrium have difficulty maintaining balance in daily life and may present with falls. There may be reduced awareness of balance impairment. Classic examples include patients with progressive supranuclear palsy and normal pressure hydrocephalus. Patients on sedating medications are also in this category. In prospective studies, cognitive impairment and the use of sedative medications substantially increase the risk for falls.

◼ FALLS

Falls are common in the elderly; 30% of people older than age 65 years living in the community fall each year. Modest changes in balance function have been described in fit older subjects as a result of normal aging. Subtle deficits in sensory systems, attention, and motor reaction time contribute to the risk, and environmental hazards abound. Epidemiologic studies have identified a number of risk factors for falls, summarized in Table 24-3. A fall is not a neurologic problem, nor reason for referral to a specialist, but there are circumstances in which neurologic evaluation is appropriate. In a classic study, 90% of fall events occurred among 10% of individuals, a group known as *recurrent fallers*. Some of these are frail older persons with chronic diseases. Recurrent falls sometimes indicate the presence of serious balance impairment. Syncope, seizure, or falls related to loss of consciousness require appropriate evaluation and treatment (Chaps. 20 and 369).

The descriptive classification of falls is as difficult as the classification of gait disorders, for many of the same reasons. Postural control systems are widely distributed, and a number of disease-related abnormalities occur. Unlike gait problems that are apparent on observation, falls are rarely observed in the office. The patient and family may have limited information about what triggered the fall. Injuries can complicate the physical examination. While there is no standard nosology of falls, common patterns can be identified.

Slipping, tripping, and "mechanical falls"

Slipping on icy pavement, tripping on obstacles, and falls related to obvious environmental factors are often termed *mechanical falls*.

TABLE 24-3 Risk Factors for Falls, a Meta-Analysis: Summary of Sixteen Controlled Studies

Risk Factor	Mean RR (OR)	Range
Weakness	4.9	1.9–10.3
Balance deficit	3.2	1.6–5.4
Gait disorder	3.0	1.7–4.8
Visual deficit	2.8	1.1–7.4
Mobility limitation	2.5	1.0–5.3
Cognitive impairment	2.4	2.0–4.7
Impaired functional status	2.0	1.0–3.1
Postural hypotension	1.9	1.0–3.4

Abbreviations: OR, odds ratios from retrospective studies; RR, relative risks from prospective studies.

Source: Reproduced with permission from J Masdeu et al: *Gait Disorders of Aging: With Special Reference to Falls.* Boston, Little Brown, 1995.

They occasionally occur in healthy individuals with good balance compensation. Frequent tripping falls raise suspicion about an underlying neurologic deficit. Patients with spasticity, leg weakness, or footdrop experience tripping falls.

Weakness and frailty

Patients who lack strength in antigravity muscles have difficulty rising from a chair, fatigue easily when walking, and have difficulty maintaining their balance after a perturbation. These patients are often unable to get up after a fall and may be on the floor for an hour or more before help arrives. Deconditioning of this sort is often treatable. Resistance strength training can increase muscle mass and leg strength in people in their eighties and nineties.

Drop attacks and collapsing falls

Drop attacks are sudden collapsing falls without loss of consciousness. Patients who collapse from lack of postural tone present a diagnostic challenge. The patient may report that his or her legs just gave out underneath; the family may describe the patient as "collapsing in a heap." Orthostatic hypotension may be a factor in some such falls. Asterixis or epilepsy may impair postural support. A colloid cyst of the third ventricle can present with intermittent obstruction of the foramen of Monroe, resulting in a drop attack. While collapsing falls are more common in older patients with vascular risk factors, they should not be confused with vertebrobasilar ischemic attacks.

Toppling falls

Some patients maintain tone in antigravity muscles but fall over like a tree trunk, as if postural defenses had disengaged. There may be a consistent direction to such falls. The patient with cerebellar pathology may lean and topple over toward the side of the lesion. Patients with lesions of the vestibular system or its central pathways may experience lateral pulsion and toppling falls. Patients with progressive supranuclear palsy often fall over backward. Falls of this nature occur in patients with advanced Parkinson's disease once postural instability has developed.

Gait freezing

Another fall pattern in Parkinson's disease and related disorders is the fall due to freezing of gait. The feet stick to the floor and the center of mass keeps moving, resulting in a disequilibrium from which the patient has difficulty recovering. This sequence of events can result in a forward fall. Gait freezing can also occur as the patient attempts to turn and change direction. Similarly, the patient with Parkinson's disease and festinating gait may find his feet unable to keep up, resulting in a forward fall.

Falls related to sensory deficit

Patients with somatosensory, visual, or vestibular deficits are prone to falls. These patients have particular difficulty dealing with poor illumination or walking on uneven ground. These patients often express subjective imbalance, apprehension, and fear of falling. Deficits in joint position and vibration sense are apparent on physical examination.

TREATMENT   Interventions to Reduce the Risk of Falls and Injury

Efforts should be made to define the etiology of the gait disorder and mechanism of the falls. Standing blood pressure should be recorded. Specific treatment may be possible, once a diagnosis is established. Therapeutic intervention is often recommended for older patients at substantial risk for falls, even if no neurologic disease is identified. A home visit to look for environmental hazards can be helpful. A variety of modifications may be recommended to improve safety, including improved lighting and the installation of grab bars and nonslip surfaces.

Rehabilitation interventions attempt to improve muscle strength and balance stability and to make the patient more resistant to injury. High-intensity resistance strength training with weights and machines is useful to improve muscle mass, even in frail older patients. Improvements are realized in posture and gait, which should translate to reduced risk of falls and injury. Sensory balance training is another approach to improve

balance stability. Measurable gains can be achieved in a few weeks of training, and benefits can be maintained over 6 months by a 10- to 20-min home exercise program. This strategy is particularly successful in patients with vestibular and somatosensory balance disorders. The Yale Health and Aging study used a strategy of targeted, multiple risk factor abatement to reduce falls in the elderly. Prescription medications were adjusted, and home-based exercise programs were tailored to the patients' needs, based on an initial geriatric assessment. The program realized a 44% reduction in falls, compared with a control group of patients who had periodic social visits.

FURTHER READINGS

BEAUCHET O et al: Stops walking when talking: A predictor of falls in older adults? Eur J Neurol 16:786, 2009

BRONSTEIN A et al: Clinical Disorders of Balance, Posture and Gait. London, Arnold Press, 2003

DE LAAT KF et al: Loss of white matter integrity is associated with gait disorders in cerebral small vessel disease. Brain 134:73, 2011

GILLESPIE LD et al: Interventions for preventing falls in older people living in the community. Cochrane Rev CD007146, 2009

NUTT JG et al: Human walking and higher-level gait disorders. Neurol 43:268, 1993

SNIJDERS AH et al: Neurological gait disorders in elderly people: Clinical approach and classification. Lancet Neurol 6:63, 2007

SPRINGER S et al: Dual-tasking effects on gait variability: The role of aging, falls, and executive function. Mov Disord 21:950, 2006

SUDARSKY L: Gait disorders in the elderly. N Engl J Med 322:1441, 1990

———: Psychogenic gait disorders. Semin Neurol 26:351, 2006

TINETTI ME, KUMAR C: The patient who falls: "It's always a trade-off." JAMA 20:258, 2010

CHAPTER **25**

Confusion and Delirium

S. Andrew Josephson
Bruce L. Miller

Confusion, a mental and behavioral state of reduced comprehension, coherence, and capacity to reason, is one of the most common problems encountered in medicine, accounting for a large number of emergency department visits, hospital admissions, and inpatient consultations. *Delirium*, a term used to describe an acute confusional state, remains a major cause of morbidity and mortality rates, costing billions of dollars yearly in health care costs in the United States alone. Delirium often goes unrecognized despite clear evidence that it is usually the cognitive manifestation of serious underlying medical or neurologic illness.

■ CLINICAL FEATURES OF DELIRIUM

A multitude of terms are used to describe delirium, including *encephalopathy, acute brain failure, acute confusional state,* and

postoperative or intensive care unit (ICU) psychosis. Delirium has many clinical manifestations, but essentially it is defined as a relatively acute decline in cognition that fluctuates over hours or days. The hallmark of delirium is a deficit of attention, although all cognitive domains—including memory, executive function, visuospatial tasks, and language—are variably involved. Associated symptoms may include altered sleep-wake cycles, perceptual disturbances such as hallucinations or delusions, affect changes, and autonomic findings that include heart rate and blood pressure instability.

Delirium is a clinical diagnosis that can be made only at the bedside. Two broad clinical categories have been described—the hyperactive and hypoactive subtypes—that are based on differential psychomotor features. The cognitive syndrome associated with severe alcohol withdrawal remains the classic example of the hyperactive subtype, featuring prominent hallucinations, agitation, and hyperarousal, often accompanied by life-threatening autonomic instability. In striking contrast is the hypoactive subtype, exemplified by opiate intoxication, in which patients are withdrawn and quiet, with prominent apathy and psychomotor slowing.

This dichotomy between subtypes of delirium is a useful construct, but patients often fall somewhere along a spectrum between the hyperactive and hypoactive extremes, sometimes fluctuating from one to the other within minutes. Therefore, clinicians must recognize the broad range of presentations of delirium to identify all patients with this potentially reversible cognitive disturbance.

Hyperactive patients, such as those with delirium tremens, are easily recognized by their characteristic severe agitation, tremor, hallucinations, and autonomic instability. Patients who are quietly disturbed are overlooked more often on the medical wards and in the ICU, yet multiple studies suggest that this underrecognized hypoactive subtype is associated with worse outcomes.

The reversibility of delirium is emphasized because many etiologies, such as systemic infection and medication effects, can be treated easily. However, the long-term cognitive effects of delirium remain largely unknown and understudied. Some episodes of delirium continue for weeks, months, or even years. The persistence of delirium in some patients and its high recurrence rate may be due to inadequate treatment of the underlying etiology of the syndrome. In some instances, delirium does not disappear because there is underlying permanent neuronal damage. Even after an episode of delirium resolves, there may be lingering effects of the disorder. A patient's recall of events after delirium varies widely, ranging from complete amnesia to repeated reexperiencing of the frightening period of confusion in a disturbing manner, similar to what is seen in patients with posttraumatic stress disorder.

■ RISK FACTORS

An effective primary prevention strategy for delirium begins with identification of patients at highest risk, including those preparing for elective surgery or being admitted to the hospital. Although no single validated scoring system has been widely accepted as a screen for asymptomatic patients, there are multiple well-established risk factors for delirium.

The two most consistently identified risks are older age and baseline cognitive dysfunction. Individuals who are over age 65 or exhibit low scores on standardized tests of cognition develop delirium upon hospitalization at a rate approaching 50%. Whether age and baseline cognitive dysfunction are truly independent risk factors is uncertain. Other predisposing factors include sensory deprivation, such as preexisting hearing and visual impairment, as well as indices for poor overall health, including baseline immobility, malnutrition, and underlying medical or neurologic illness.

In-hospital risks for delirium include the use of bladder catheterization, physical restraints, sleep and sensory deprivation, and the addition of three or more new medications. Avoiding such risks remains a key component of delirium prevention as well as treatment. Surgical and anesthetic risk factors for the development of postoperative delirium include specific procedures such as those involving cardiopulmonary bypass and inadequate or excessive treatment of pain in the immediate postoperative period.

The relationship between delirium and dementia (Chap. 371) is complicated by significant overlap between the two conditions, and it is not always simple to distinguish between them. Dementia and preexisting cognitive dysfunction serve as major risk factors for delirium, and at least two-thirds of cases of delirium occur in patients with coexisting underlying dementia. A form of dementia with parkinsonism, termed *dementia with Lewy bodies*, is characterized by a fluctuating course, prominent visual hallucinations, parkinsonism, and an attentional deficit that clinically resembles hyperactive delirium. Delirium in the elderly often reflects an insult to the brain that is vulnerable due to an underlying neurodegenerative condition. Therefore, the development of delirium sometimes heralds the onset of a previously unrecognized brain disorder.

■ EPIDEMIOLOGY

Delirium is a common disease, but its reported incidence has varied widely with the criteria used to define the disorder. Estimates of delirium in hospitalized patients range from 14 to 56%, with higher rates reported for elderly patients and patients undergoing hip surgery. Older patients in the ICU have especially high rates of delirium that range from 70 to 87%. The condition is not recognized in up to one-third of delirious inpatients, and the diagnosis is especially problematic in the ICU environment, where cognitive dysfunction is often difficult to appreciate in the setting of serious systemic illness and sedation. Delirium in the ICU should be viewed as an important manifestation of organ dysfunction not unlike liver, kidney, or heart failure. Outside the acute hospital setting, delirium occurs in nearly two-thirds of patients in nursing homes and in over 80% of those at the end of life. These estimates emphasize the remarkably high frequency of this cognitive syndrome in older patients, a population expected to grow in the upcoming decade with the aging of the "baby boom" generation.

In previous decades an episode of delirium was viewed as a transient condition that carried a benign prognosis. Delirium now has been clearly associated with substantial morbidity rate and increased mortality rate and increasingly is recognized as a sign of serious underlying illness. Recent estimates of in-hospital mortality rates among delirious patients have ranged from 25 to 33%, a rate similar to that of patients with sepsis. Patients with an in-hospital episode of delirium have a higher mortality rate in the months and years after their illness compared with age-matched nondelirious hospitalized patients. Delirious hospitalized patients have a longer length of stay, are more likely to be discharged to a nursing home, and are more likely to experience subsequent episodes of delirium; as a result, this condition has enormous economic implications.

■ PATHOGENESIS

The pathogenesis and anatomy of delirium are incompletely understood. The attentional deficit that serves as the neuropsychological hallmark of delirium appears to have a diffuse localization with the brainstem, thalamus, prefrontal cortex, and parietal lobes. Rarely, focal lesions such as ischemic strokes have led to delirium in otherwise healthy persons; right parietal and medial dorsal thalamic lesions have been reported most commonly, pointing to the relevance of these areas to delirium pathogenesis. In most cases, delirium results from widespread disturbances in cortical and subcortical regions rather than a focal neuroanatomic cause. Electroencephalogram (EEG) data in persons with delirium usually show symmetric slowing, a nonspecific finding that supports diffuse cerebral dysfunction.

Deficiency of acetylcholine often plays a key role in delirium pathogenesis. Medications with anticholinergic properties can precipitate delirium in susceptible individuals, and therapies designed to boost cholinergic tone such as cholinesterase inhibitors have, in small trials, been shown to relieve symptoms of delirium. Dementia patients are susceptible to episodes of delirium, and those with Alzheimer's pathology are known to have a chronic cholinergic deficiency state due to degeneration of acetylcholine-producing neurons in the basal forebrain. Another common dementia associated with decreased acetylcholine levels, dementia with Lewy bodies, clinically mimics delirium in some patients. Other neurotransmitters are also likely to be involved in this diffuse cerebral disorder. For example, increases in dopamine can also lead to delirium. Patients with Parkinson's disease treated with dopaminergic medications can develop a delirium-like state that features visual hallucinations, fluctuations, and confusion. In contrast, reducing dopaminergic tone with dopamine antagonists such as typical and atypical antipsychotic medications has long been recognized as effective symptomatic treatment in patients with delirium.

Not all individuals exposed to the same insult will develop signs of delirium. A low dose of an anticholinergic medication may have no cognitive effects on a healthy young adult but may produce a florid delirium in an elderly person with known underlying dementia. However, an extremely high dose of the same anticholinergic medication may lead to delirium even in healthy young persons. This concept of delirium developing as the result of an insult in predisposed individuals is currently the most widely accepted pathogenic construct. Therefore, if a previously healthy individual with no known history of cognitive illness develops delirium in the setting of a relatively minor insult such as elective surgery or hospitalization, an unrecognized underlying neurologic illness such as a neurodegenerative disease, multiple previous strokes, or another diffuse cerebral cause should be considered. In this context, delirium can be viewed as the symptom resulting from a "stress test for the brain" induced by the insult. Exposure to known inciting factors such as systemic infection and offending drugs can unmask a decreased cerebral reserve and herald a serious underlying and potentially treatable illness.

APPROACH TO THE PATIENT   Delirium

As the diagnosis of delirium is clinical and is made at the bedside, a careful history and physical examination is necessary in evaluating patients with possible confusional states. Screening tools can aid physicians and nurses in identifying patients with delirium, including the Confusion Assessment Method (CAM); the Organic Brain Syndrome Scale; the Delirium Rating Scale; and, in the ICU, the Delirium Detection Score and the ICU version of the CAM. Using the CAM, a diagnosis of delirium is made if there is (1) an acute onset and fluctuating course and (2) inattention accompanied by either (3) disorganized thinking or (4) an altered level of consciousness. These scales are based on criteria from the American Psychiatric Association's *Diagnostic and Statistical Manual of Mental Disorders* (DSM) or the World Health Organization's International Classification of Diseases (ICD). Unfortunately, these scales do not identify the full spectrum of patients with delirium. All patients who are acutely confused should be presumed delirious regardless of their presentation due to the wide variety of possible clinical features. A course that fluctuates over hours or days and may worsen at night (termed *sundowning*) is typical but not essential for the diagnosis. Observation of the patient usually will reveal an altered level of consciousness or a deficit of attention. Other hallmark features that may be present in a delirious patient include alteration of sleep-wake cycles, thought disturbances such as hallucinations or delusions, autonomic instability, and changes in affect.

HISTORY   It may be difficult to elicit an accurate history in delirious patients who have altered levels of consciousness or impaired attention. Information from a collateral source such as a spouse or another family member is therefore invaluable. The three most important pieces of history are the patient's baseline cognitive function, the time course of the present illness, and current medications.

Premorbid cognitive function can be assessed through the collateral source or, if needed, via a review of outpatient records. Delirium by definition represents a change that is relatively acute, usually over hours to days, from a cognitive baseline. As a result, an acute confusional state is nearly impossible to diagnose without some knowledge of baseline cognitive function. Without this information, many patients with dementia or depression may be mistaken as delirious during a single initial evaluation. Patients with a more hypoactive, apathetic presentation with psychomotor slowing may be identified as being different from baseline only through conversations with family members. A number of validated instruments have been shown to diagnose cognitive dysfunction accurately by using a collateral source,

including the modified Blessed Dementia Rating Scale and the Clinical Dementia Rating (CDR). Baseline cognitive impairment is common in patients with delirium. Even when no such history of cognitive impairment is elicited, there should still be a high suspicion for a previously unrecognized underlying neurologic disorder.

Establishing the time course of cognitive change is important not only to make a diagnosis of delirium but also to correlate the onset of the illness with potentially treatable etiologies such as recent medication changes or symptoms of systemic infection.

Medications remain a common cause of delirium, especially compounds with anticholinergic or sedative properties. It is estimated that nearly one-third of all cases of delirium are secondary to medications, especially in the elderly. Medication histories should include all prescription as well as over-the-counter and herbal substances taken by the patient and any recent changes in dosing or formulation, including substitution of generics for brand-name medications.

Other important elements of the history include screening for symptoms of organ failure or systemic infection, which often contributes to delirium in the elderly. A history of illicit drug use, alcoholism, or toxin exposure is common in younger delirious patients. Finally, asking the patient and collateral source about other symptoms that may accompany delirium, such as depression and hallucinations, may help identify potential therapeutic targets.

PHYSICAL EXAMINATION   The general physical examination in a delirious patient should include a careful screening for signs of infection such as fever, tachypnea, pulmonary consolidation, heart murmur, and stiff neck. The patient's fluid status should be assessed; both dehydration and fluid overload with resultant hypoxemia have been associated with delirium, and each is usually easily rectified. The appearance of the skin can be helpful, showing jaundice in hepatic encephalopathy, cyanosis in hypoxemia, or needle tracks in patients using intravenous drugs.

The neurologic examination requires a careful assessment of mental status. Patients with delirium often present with a fluctuating course; therefore, the diagnosis can be missed when one relies on a single time point of evaluation. Some but not all patients exhibit the characteristic pattern of sundowning, a worsening of their condition in the evening. In these cases, assessment only during morning rounds may be falsely reassuring.

An altered level of consciousness ranging from hyperarousal to lethargy to coma is present in most patients with delirium and can be assessed easily at the bedside. In a patient with a relatively normal level of consciousness, a screen for an attentional deficit is in order, as this deficit is the classic neuropsychological hallmark of delirium. Attention can be assessed while taking a history from the patient. Tangential speech, a fragmentary flow of ideas, or inability to follow complex commands often signifies an attentional problem. There are formal neuropsychological tests to assess attention, but a simple bedside test of digit span forward is quick and fairly sensitive. In this task, patients are asked to repeat successively longer random strings of digits beginning with two digits in a row. Average adults can repeat a string of five to seven digits before faltering; a digit span of four or less usually indicates an attentional deficit unless hearing or language barriers are present.

More formal neuropsychological testing can be extraordinarily helpful in assessing a delirious patient, but it is usually too cumbersome and time-consuming in the inpatient setting. A simple Mini Mental Status Examination (MMSE) (see Table 371-5) can provide some information regarding orientation, language, and visuospatial skills; however, performance of some tasks on the MMSE such as spelling "world" backward and serial subtraction of digits will be impaired by delirious patients' attentional deficits alone and are therefore unreliable.

The remainder of the screening neurologic examination should focus on identifying new focal neurologic deficits. Focal strokes or mass lesions in isolation are rarely the cause of delirium, but patients with underlying extensive cerebrovascular disease or neurodegenerative conditions may not be able to cognitively tolerate even relatively small new insults. Patients also should be screened for additional signs of neurodegenerative conditions such as parkinsonism, which is seen not only in idiopathic Parkinson's disease but also in other dementing conditions such as Alzheimer's disease, dementia with Lewy bodies, and progressive supranuclear palsy. The presence of multifocal myoclonus or asterixis on the motor examination is nonspecific but usually indicates a metabolic or toxic etiology of the delirium.

ETIOLOGY Some etiologies can be easily discerned through a careful history and physical examination, whereas others require confirmation with laboratory studies, imaging, or other ancillary tests. A large, diverse group of insults can lead to delirium, and the cause in many patients is often multifactorial. Common etiologies are listed in Table 25-1.

Prescribed, over-the-counter, and herbal medications are common precipitants of delirium. Drugs with anticholinergic properties, narcotics, and benzodiazepines are especially common offenders, but nearly any compound can lead to cognitive dysfunction in a predisposed patient. Whereas an elderly patient with baseline dementia may become delirious upon exposure to a relatively low dose of a medication, less susceptible individuals may become delirious only with very high doses of the same medication. This observation emphasizes the importance of correlating the timing of recent medication changes, including dose and formulation, with the onset of cognitive dysfunction.

In younger patients especially, illicit drugs and toxins are common causes of delirium. In addition to more classic drugs of abuse, the recent rise in availability of so-called club drugs, such as methylenedioxymethamphetamine (MDMA, ecstasy), γ-hydroxybutyrate (GHB), and the phencyclidine (PCP)-like agent ketamine, has led to an increase in delirious young persons presenting to acute care settings. Many common prescription drugs such as oral narcotics and benzodiazepines are often abused and readily available on the street. Alcohol intoxication with high serum levels can cause confusion, but more commonly it is withdrawal from alcohol that leads to a classic hyperactive delirium. Alcohol and benzodiazepine withdrawal should be considered in all cases of delirium as even patients who drink only a few servings of alcohol every day can experience relatively severe withdrawal symptoms upon hospitalization.

Metabolic abnormalities such as electrolyte disturbances of sodium, calcium, magnesium, or glucose can cause delirium, and mild derangements can lead to substantial cognitive disturbances in susceptible individuals. Other common metabolic etiologies include liver and renal failure, hypercarbia and hypoxemia, vitamin deficiencies of thiamine and B_{12}, autoimmune disorders including central nervous system (CNS) vasculitis, and endocrinopathies such as thyroid and adrenal disorders.

Systemic infections often cause delirium, especially in the elderly. A common scenario involves the development of an acute cognitive decline in the setting of a urinary tract infection in a patient with baseline dementia. Pneumonia, skin infections such as cellulitis, and frank sepsis also can lead to delirium.

TABLE 25-1 Common Etiologies of Delirium

Toxins
Prescription medications: especially those with anticholinergic properties, narcotics, and benzodiazepines
Drugs of abuse: alcohol intoxication and alcohol withdrawal, opiates, ecstasy, LSD, GHB, PCP, ketamine, cocaine
Poisons: inhalants, carbon monoxide, ethylene glycol, pesticides

Metabolic conditions
Electrolyte disturbances: hypoglycemia, hyperglycemia, hyponatremia, hypernatremia, hypercalcemia, hypocalcemia, hypomagnesemia
Hypothermia and hyperthermia
Pulmonary failure: hypoxemia and hypercarbia
Liver failure/hepatic encephalopathy
Renal failure/uremia
Cardiac failure
Vitamin deficiencies: B_{12}, thiamine, folate, niacin
Dehydration and malnutrition
Anemia

Infections
Systemic infections: urinary tract infections, pneumonia, skin and soft tissue infections, sepsis
CNS infections: meningitis, encephalitis, brain abscess

Endocrinologic conditions
Hyperthyroidism, hypothyroidism
Hyperparathyroidism
Adrenal insufficiency

Cerebrovascular disorders
Global hypoperfusion states
Hypertensive encephalopathy
Focal ischemic strokes and hemorrhages: especially nondominant parietal and thalamic lesions

Autoimmune disorders
CNS vasculitis
Cerebral lupus

Seizure-related disorders
Nonconvulsive status epilepticus
Intermittent seizures with prolonged postictal states

Neoplastic disorders
Diffuse metastases to the brain
Gliomatosis cerebri
Carcinomatous meningitis

Hospitalization

Terminal end-of-life delirium

Abbreviations: LSD, lysergic acid diethylamide; GHB, γ-hydroxybutyrate; PCP, phencyclidine; CNS, central nervous system.

This so-called septic encephalopathy, often seen in the ICU, is probably due to the release of proinflammatory cytokines and their diffuse cerebral effects. CNS infections such as meningitis, encephalitis, and abscess are less common etiologies of delirium; however, in light of the high mortality rates associated with these conditions when they are not treated quickly, clinicians must always maintain a high index of suspicion.

In some susceptible individuals, exposure to the unfamiliar environment of a hospital can lead to delirium. This etiology usually occurs as part of a multifactorial delirium and should be considered a diagnosis of exclusion after all other causes have been thoroughly investigated. Many primary prevention and treatment strategies for delirium involve relatively simple methods to address the aspects of the inpatient setting that are most confusing.

Cerebrovascular etiologies are usually due to global hypoperfusion in the setting of systemic hypotension from heart failure, septic shock, dehydration, or anemia. Focal strokes in the right parietal lobe and medial dorsal thalamus rarely can lead to a delirious state. A more common scenario involves a new focal stroke or hemorrhage causing confusion in a patient who has decreased cerebral reserve. In these individuals, it is sometimes difficult to distinguish between cognitive dysfunction resulting from the new neurovascular insult itself and delirium due to the infectious, metabolic, and pharmacologic complications that can accompany hospitalization after stroke.

Because a fluctuating course often is seen in delirium, intermittent seizures may be overlooked when one is considering potential etiologies. Both nonconvulsive status epilepticus and recurrent focal or generalized seizures followed by postictal confusion can cause delirium; EEG remains essential for this diagnosis. Seizure activity spreading from an electrical focus in a mass or infarct can explain global cognitive dysfunction caused by relatively small lesions.

It is very common for patients to experience delirium at the end of life in palliative care settings. This condition, sometimes described as *terminal restlessness*, must be identified and treated aggressively as it is an important cause of patient and family discomfort at the end of life. It should be remembered that these patients also may be suffering from more common etiologies of delirium such as systemic infection.

LABORATORY AND DIAGNOSTIC EVALUATION A cost-effective approach to the diagnostic evaluation of delirium allows the history and physical examination to guide tests. No established algorithm for workup will fit all delirious patients due to the staggering number of potential etiologies, but one stepwise approach is detailed in Table 25-2. If a clear precipitant is identified early, such as an offending medication, little further workup is required. If, however, no likely etiology is uncovered with initial evaluation, an aggressive search for an underlying cause should be initiated.

Basic screening labs, including a complete blood count, electrolyte panel, and tests of liver and renal function, should be obtained in all patients with delirium. In elderly patients, screening for systemic infection, including chest radiography, urinalysis and culture, and possibly blood cultures, is important. In younger individuals, serum and urine drug and toxicology screening may be appropriate early in the workup. Additional laboratory tests addressing other autoimmune, endocrinologic, metabolic, and infectious etiologies should be reserved for patients in whom the diagnosis remains unclear after initial testing.

Multiple studies have demonstrated that brain imaging in patients with delirium is often unhelpful. However, if the initial workup is unrevealing, most clinicians quickly move toward imaging of the brain to exclude structural causes. A noncontrast CT scan can identify large masses and hemorrhages but is otherwise relatively insensitive for discovering an etiology of delirium. The ability of MRI to identify most acute ischemic strokes as well as to provide neuroanatomic detail that gives clues to possible infectious, inflammatory, neurodegenerative, and neoplastic conditions makes it the test of choice. Since MRI techniques are

TABLE 25-2 Stepwise Evaluation of a Patient With Delirium

Initial evaluation

  History with special attention to medications (including over-the-counter and herbals)

  General physical examination and neurologic examination

  Complete blood count

  Electrolyte panel including calcium, magnesium, phosphorus

  Liver function tests, including albumin

  Renal function tests

First-tier further evaluation guided by initial evaluation

  Systemic infection screen

    Urinalysis and culture

    Chest radiograph

    Blood cultures

  Electrocardiogram

  Arterial blood gas

  Serum and/or urine toxicology screen (perform earlier in young persons)

  Brain imaging with MRI with diffusion and gadolinium (preferred) or CT

  Suspected CNS infection: lumbar puncture after brain imaging

  Suspected seizure-related etiology: electroencephalogram (EEG) (if high suspicion, should be performed immediately)

Second-tier further evaluation

  Vitamin levels: B$_{12}$, folate, thiamine

  Endocrinologic laboratories: thyroid-stimulating hormone (TSH) and free T$_4$; cortisol

  Serum ammonia

  Sedimentation rate

  Autoimmune serologies: antinuclear antibodies (ANA), complement levels; p-ANCA, c-ANCA

  Infectious serologies: rapid plasmin reagin (RPR); fungal and viral serologies if high suspicion; HIV antibody

  Lumbar puncture (if not already performed)

  Brain MRI with and without gadolinium (if not already performed)

Abbreviations: p-ANCA, perinuclear antineutrophil cytoplasmic antibody; c-ANCA, cytoplasmic antineutrophil cytoplasmic antibody.

limited by availability, speed of imaging, patient cooperation, and contraindications to magnetic exposure, many clinicians begin with CT scanning and proceed to MRI if the etiology of delirium remains elusive.

Lumbar puncture (LP) must be obtained immediately after appropriate neuroimaging in all patients in whom CNS infection is suspected. Spinal fluid examination can also be useful in identifying inflammatory and neoplastic conditions as well as in the diagnosis of hepatic encephalopathy through elevated cerebrospinal fluid (CSF) glutamine levels. As a result, LP should be considered in any delirious patient with a negative workup. EEG does not have a routine role in the workup of delirium, but it remains invaluable if seizure-related etiologies are considered.

TREATMENT   Delirium

Management of delirium begins with treatment of the underlying inciting factor (e.g., patients with systemic infections should be given appropriate antibiotics, and underlying electrolyte disturbances judiciously corrected). These treatments often lead to prompt resolution of delirium. Blindly targeting the symptoms of delirium pharmacologically only serves to prolong the time patients remain in the confused state and may mask important diagnostic information. Recent trials of medications used to boost cholinergic tone in delirious patients have led to mixed results, and this strategy is not currently recommended.

Relatively simple methods of supportive care can be highly effective in treating patients with delirium. Reorientation by the nursing staff and family combined with visible clocks, calendars, and outside-facing windows can reduce confusion. Sensory isolation should be prevented by providing glasses and hearing aids to patients who need them. Sundowning can be addressed to a large extent through vigilance to appropriate sleep-wake cycles. During the day, a well-lit room should be accompanied by activities or exercises to prevent napping. At night, a quiet, dark environment with limited interruptions by staff can assure proper rest. These sleep-wake cycle interventions are especially important in the ICU setting as the usual constant 24-h activity commonly provokes delirium. Attempting to mimic the home environment as much as possible also has been shown to help treat and even prevent delirium. Visits from friends and family throughout the day minimize the anxiety associated with the constant flow of new faces of staff and physicians. Allowing hospitalized patients to have access to home bedding, clothing, and nightstand objects makes the hospital environment less foreign and therefore less confusing. Simple standard nursing practices such as maintaining proper nutrition and volume status as well as managing incontinence and skin breakdown also help alleviate discomfort and resulting confusion.

In some instances, patients pose a threat to their own safety or to the safety of staff members, and acute management is required. Bed alarms and personal sitters are more effective and much less disorienting than physical restraints. Chemical restraints should be avoided, but when necessary, very low dose typical or atypical antipsychotic medications administered on an as-needed basis are effective. The recent association of antipsychotic use in the elderly with increased mortality rates underscores the importance of using these medications judiciously and only as a last resort. Benzodiazepines are not as effective as antipsychotics and often worsen confusion through their sedative properties. Although many clinicians still use benzodiazepines to treat acute confusion, their use should be limited to cases in which delirium is caused by alcohol or benzodiazepine withdrawal.

■ PREVENTION

In light of the high morbidity associated with delirium and the tremendously increased health care costs that accompany it, development of an effective strategy to prevent delirium in hospitalized patients is extremely important. Successful identification of high-risk patients is the first step, followed by initiation of appropriate interventions. One trial randomized more than 850 elderly inpatients to simple standardized protocols used to manage risk factors for delirium, including cognitive impairment, immobility, visual impairment, hearing impairment, sleep deprivation, and dehydration. Significant reductions in the number and duration of episodes of delirium were observed in the treatment group, but unfortunately, delirium recurrence rates were unchanged. Recent trials in the ICU have focused on identifying sedatives, such as dexmedetomidine, that are less likely to lead to delirium in critically ill patients. All hospitals and health care systems should work toward developing standardized protocols to address common risk factors with the goal of decreasing the incidence of delirium.

ACKNOWLEDGMENT

In the 16th edition, Allan H. Ropper contributed to a section on acute confusional states that was incorporated into this current chapter.

FURTHER READINGS

FONG TG et al: Delirium in elderly adults: Diagnosis, prevention, and treatment. Nat Rev Neurol 5:210, 2009

GIRARD TD et al: Delirium as a predictor of long-term cognitive impairment in survivors of critical illness. Crit Care Med 38:1513, 2010

INOUYE SK et al: Clarifying confusion: The confusion assessment method. A new method for detection of delirium. Ann Intern Med 113:941, 1990

———: A multicomponent intervention to prevent delirium in hospitalized older patients. N Engl J Med 340:669, 1999

LAT I et al: The impact of delirium on clinical outcomes in mechanically ventilated surgical and trauma patients. Crit Care Med 37:1898, 2009

RIKER RR et al: Dexmedetomidine vs midazolam for sedation of critically ill patients: A randomized trial. JAMA 301:489, 2009

CHAPTER 26

Aphasia, Memory Loss, and Other Focal Cerebral Disorders

M.-Marsel Mesulam

The cerebral cortex of the human brain contains approximately 20 billion neurons spread over an area of 2.5 m². The *primary sensory* areas provide an obligatory portal for the entry of sensory information into cortical circuitry, and the *primary motor* areas provide a final common pathway for coordinating complex motor acts. The primary sensory and motor areas constitute 10% of the cerebral cortex. The rest is subsumed by modality-selective, heteromodal, paralimbic, and limbic areas collectively known as the *association cortex* (Fig. 26-1). The association cortex mediates the integrative processes that subserve cognition, emotion, and behavior. A systematic testing of these mental functions is necessary for the effective clinical assessment of the association cortex and its diseases.

According to current thinking, there are no centers for "hearing words," "perceiving space," or "storing memories." Cognitive and behavioral functions (domains) are coordinated by intersecting *large-scale neural networks* that contain interconnected cortical and subcortical components. The network approach to higher cerebral function has at least four implications of clinical relevance: (1) A single domain such as language or memory can be disrupted by damage to any one of several areas as long as those areas belong to the same network, (2) damage confined to a single area can give rise to multiple deficits involving the functions of all the networks that intersect in that region, (3) damage to a network component may give rise to minimal or transient deficits if other parts of the network undergo compensatory reorganization, and (4) individual anatomic sites within a network display a relative (but not absolute) specialization for different behavioral aspects of the relevant function. Five anatomically defined large-scale networks are most relevant to clinical practice: (1) a perisylvian network for language, (2) a parietofrontal network for spatial cognition, (3) an occipitotemporal network for face and object recognition, (4) a limbic network for retentive memory, and (5) a prefrontal network for cognitive and behavioral control.

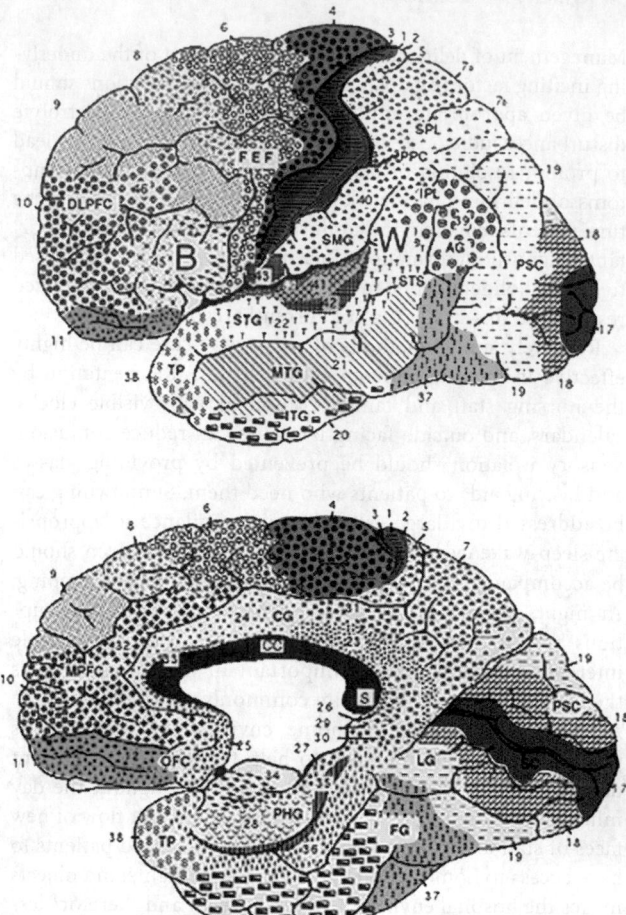

Figure 26-1   Lateral (*top*) and medial (*bottom*) views of the cerebral hemispheres. The numbers refer to the Brodmann cytoarchitectonic designations. Area 17 corresponds to the primary visual cortex, 41–42 to the primary auditory cortex, 1–3 to the primary somatosensory cortex, and 4 to the primary motor cortex. The rest of the cerebral cortex contains association areas. AG, angular gyrus; B, Broca's area; CC, corpus callosum; CG, cingulate gyrus; DLPFC, dorsolateral prefrontal cortex; FEF, frontal eye fields (premotor cortex); FG, fusiform gyrus; IPL, inferior parietal lobule; ITG, inferior temporal gyrus; LG, lingual gyrus; MPFC, medial prefrontal cortex; MTG, middle temporal gyrus; OFC, orbitofrontal cortex; PHG, parahippocampal gyrus; PPC, posterior parietal cortex; PSC, peristriate cortex; SC, striate cortex; SMG, supramarginal gyrus; SPL, superior parietal lobule; STG, superior temporal gyrus; STS, superior temporal sulcus; TP, temporopolar cortex; W, Wernicke's area.

THE LEFT PERISYLVIAN NETWORK FOR LANGUAGE: APHASIAS AND RELATED CONDITIONS

Language allows the communication and elaboration of thoughts and experiences by linking them to arbitrary symbols known as words. The neural substrate of language is composed of a distributed network centered in the perisylvian region of the *left* hemisphere. The posterior pole of this network is located at the temporoparietal junction and includes a region known as *Wernicke's area*. An essential function of Wernicke's area is to transform sensory inputs into their neural word representations so that they can establish the distributed associations that give a word its meaning. The anterior pole of the language network is located in the inferior frontal gyrus and includes a region known as *Broca's area*. An essential function of this area is to transform neural word representations into their articulatory sequences so that the words can be uttered in the form of spoken language. The sequencing function of Broca's area also

appears to involve the ordering of words into sentences that contain a meaning-appropriate *syntax* (grammar). Wernicke's and Broca's areas are interconnected with each other and with additional perisylvian, temporal, prefrontal, and posterior parietal regions, making up a neural network that subserves the various aspects of language function. Damage to any one of these components or to their interconnections can give rise to language disturbances (*aphasia*). Aphasia should be diagnosed only when there are deficits in the formal aspects of language, such as naming, word choice, comprehension, spelling, and syntax. Dysarthria and mutism do not by themselves lead to a diagnosis of aphasia. The language network shows a left hemisphere dominance pattern in the vast majority of the population. In approximately 90% of right-handers and 60% of left-handers, aphasia occurs only after lesions of the left hemisphere. In some individuals no hemispheric dominance for language can be discerned, and in some others (including a small minority of right handers) there is a right hemisphere dominance for language. A language disturbance that occurs after a right hemisphere lesion in a right hander is called *crossed aphasia*.

■ CLINICAL EXAMINATION

The clinical examination of language should include the assessment of naming, spontaneous speech, comprehension, repetition, reading, and writing. A deficit of naming (*anomia*) is the single most common finding in aphasic patients. When asked to name a common object (pencil or wristwatch), the patient may fail to come up with the appropriate word, may provide a circumlocutious description of the object ("the thing for writing"), or may come up with the wrong word (*paraphasia*). If the patient offers an incorrect but related word ("pen" for "pencil"), the naming error is known as a *semantic paraphasia*; if the word approximates the correct answer but is phonetically inaccurate ("plentil" for "pencil"), it is known as a *phonemic paraphasia*. Asking the patient to name body parts, geometric shapes, and component parts of objects (lapel of coat, cap of pen) can elicit mild forms of anomia in patients who otherwise can name common objects. In most anomias, the patient cannot retrieve the appropriate name when shown an object but can point to the appropriate object when the name is provided by the examiner. This is known as a one-way (or retrieval-based) naming deficit. A two-way naming deficit exists if the patient can neither provide nor recognize the correct name, indicating the likely presence of a comprehension impairment for the word. *Spontaneous speech* is described as "fluent" if it maintains appropriate output volume, phrase length, and melody or as "nonfluent" if it is sparse and halting and average utterance length is below four words. The examiner also should note if the speech is paraphasic or circumlocutious; if it shows a relative paucity of substantive nouns and action verbs versus function words (prepositions, conjunctions); and if word order, tenses, suffixes, prefixes, plurals, and possessives are appropriate. *Comprehension* can be tested by assessing the patient's ability to follow conversation, asking yes-no questions ("Can a dog fly?", "Does it snow in summer?") or asking the patient to point to appropriate objects ("Where is the source of illumination in this room?"). Statements with embedded clauses or a passive voice construction ("If a tiger is eaten by a lion, which animal stays alive?") help assess the ability to comprehend complex syntactic structure.

Commands to close or open the eyes, stand up, sit down, or roll over should not be used to assess overall comprehension since appropriate responses aimed at such axial movements can be preserved in patients who otherwise have profound comprehension deficits. *Repetition* is assessed by asking the patient to repeat single words, short sentences, or strings of words such as "No ifs, ands, or buts." The testing of repetition with tongue twisters such as "hippopotamus" and "Irish constabulary" provides a better assessment of dysarthria and pallilalia than of aphasia. Aphasic patients who have little difficulty with tongue twisters may have a particularly hard time repeating a string of function words. It is important to make sure that the number of words does not exceed the patient's attention span. Otherwise, the failure of repetition becomes a reflection of the narrowed attention span rather than an indication of an aphasic deficit. *Reading* should be assessed for deficits in reading aloud as well as comprehension. *Writing* is assessed for spelling errors, word order, and grammar. *Alexia* describes an inability to either read aloud or comprehend single words and simple sentences; *agraphia* (or *dysgraphia*) is used to describe an acquired deficit in the spelling or grammar of written language.

The correspondence between individual deficits of language function and lesion location does not display a rigid one-to-one relationship and should be conceptualized within the context of the distributed network model. Nonetheless, the classification of aphasias into specific clinical syndromes helps determine the most likely anatomic distribution of the underlying neurologic disease and has implications for etiology and prognosis (Table 26-1). The syndromes listed in Table 26-1 are most applicable to aphasias caused by cerebrovascular accidents (CVAs). They can be divided into "central" syndromes, which result from damage to the two epicenters of the language network (Broca's and Wernicke's areas), and "disconnection" syndromes, which arise from lesions that interrupt the functional connectivity of those centers with each other and with the other components of the language network. The syndromes outlined below are idealizations; pure syndromes occur rarely.

Wernicke's aphasia

Comprehension is impaired for spoken and written language, for single words as well as sentences. Language output is fluent but is highly paraphasic and circumlocutious. The tendency for paraphasic errors may be so pronounced that it leads to strings of neologisms, which form the basis of what is known as "jargon

TABLE 26-1 Clinical Features of Aphasias and Related Conditions

	Comprehension	Repetition of Spoken Language	Naming	Fluency
Wernicke's	Impaired	Impaired	Impaired	Preserved or increased
Broca's	Preserved (except grammar)	Impaired	Impaired	Decreased
Global	Impaired	Impaired	Impaired	Decreased
Conduction	Preserved	Impaired	Impaired	Preserved
Nonfluent (motor) transcortical	Preserved	Preserved	Impaired	Impaired
Fluent (sensory) transcortical	Impaired	Preserved	Impaired	Preserved
Isolation	Impaired	Echolalia	Impaired	No purposeful speech
Anomic	Preserved	Preserved	Impaired	Preserved except for word-finding pauses
Pure word deafness	Impaired only for spoken language	Impaired	Preserved	Preserved
Pure alexia	Impaired only for reading	Preserved	Preserved	Preserved

aphasia." Speech contains large numbers of function words (e.g., prepositions, conjunctions) but few substantive nouns or verbs that refer to specific actions. The output is therefore voluminous but uninformative. For example, a patient attempts to describe how his wife accidentally threw away something important, perhaps his dentures: "We don't need it anymore, she says. And with it when that was downstairs was my teeth-tick ... a ... den ... dentith ... my dentist. And they happened to be in that bag ... see? How could this have happened? How could a thing like this happen ... So she says we won't need it anymore ... I didn't think we'd use it. And now if I have any problems anybody coming a month from now, 4 months from now, or 6 months from now, I have a new dentist. Where my two ... two little pieces of dentist that I use ... that I ... all gone. If she throws the whole thing away ... visit some friends of hers and she can't throw them away."

Gestures and pantomime do not improve communication. The patient does not seem to realize that his or her language is incomprehensible and may appear angry and impatient when the examiner fails to decipher the meaning of a severely paraphasic statement. In some patients this type of aphasia can be associated with severe agitation and paranoid behaviors. One area of comprehension that may be preserved is the ability to follow commands aimed at axial musculature. The dissociation between the failure to understand simple questions ("What is your name?") in a patient who rapidly closes his or her eyes, sits up, or rolls over when asked to do so is characteristic of Wernicke's aphasia and helps differentiate it from deafness, psychiatric disease, or malingering. Patients with Wernicke's aphasia cannot express their thoughts in meaning-appropriate words and cannot decode the meaning of words in any modality of input. This aphasia therefore has expressive as well as receptive components. Repetition, naming, reading, and writing also are impaired.

The lesion site most commonly associated with Wernicke's aphasia is the posterior portion of the language network and tends to involve at least parts of Wernicke's area. An embolus to the inferior division of the middle cerebral artery, to the posterior temporal or angular branches in particular, is the most common etiology (Chap. 370). Intracerebral hemorrhage, severe head trauma, and neoplasm are other causes. A coexisting right hemianopia or superior quadrantanopia is common and mild right nasolabial flattening may be found, but otherwise the examination is often unrevealing. The paraphasic, neologistic speech in an agitated patient with an otherwise unremarkable neurologic examination may lead to the suspicion of a primary psychiatric disorder such as schizophrenia or mania, but the other components characteristic of acquired aphasia and the absence of prior psychiatric disease usually settle the issue. Some patients with Wernicke's aphasia due to intracerebral hemorrhage or head trauma may improve as the hemorrhage or the injury heals. In most other patients, prognosis for recovery of language function is guarded.

Broca's aphasia

Speech is nonfluent, labored, interrupted by many word-finding pauses, and usually dysarthric. It is impoverished in function words but enriched in meaning-appropriate nouns and verbs. Abnormal word order and the inappropriate deployment of *bound morphemes* (word endings used to denote tenses, possessives, or plurals) lead to a characteristic agrammatism. Speech is telegraphic and pithy but quite informative. In the following passage, a patient with Broca's aphasia describes his medical history: "I see ... the dotor, dotor sent me ... Bosson. Go to hospital. Dotor ... kept me beside. Two, tee days, doctor send me home."

Output may be reduced to a grunt or single word ("yes" or "no"), which is emitted with different intonations in an attempt to express

approval or disapproval. In addition to fluency, naming and repetition are impaired. Comprehension of spoken language is intact except for syntactically difficult sentences with a passive voice structure or embedded clauses. Reading comprehension also is preserved with the occasional exception of a specific inability to read small grammatical words such as conjunctions and pronouns. The last two features indicate that Broca's aphasia is not just an "expressive" or "motor" disorder and that it also may involve a comprehension deficit for function words and syntax. Patients with Broca's aphasia can be tearful, easily frustrated, and profoundly depressed. Insight into their condition is preserved, in contrast to Wernicke's aphasia. Even when spontaneous speech is severely dysarthric, the patient may be able to display a relatively normal articulation of words when singing. This dissociation has been used to develop specific therapeutic approaches (melodic intonation therapy) for Broca's aphasia. Additional neurologic deficits usually include right facial weakness, hemiparesis or hemiplegia, and a buccofacial apraxia characterized by an inability to carry out motor commands involving oropharyngeal and facial musculature (e.g., patients are unable to demonstrate how to blow out a match or suck through a straw). Visual fields are intact. The cause is most often infarction of Broca's area (the inferior frontal convolution; "B" in Fig. 26-1) and surrounding anterior perisylvian and insular cortex due to occlusion of the superior division of the middle cerebral artery (Chap. 370). Mass lesions, including tumor, intracerebral hemorrhage, and abscess, also may be responsible. Small lesions confined to the posterior part of Broca's area may lead to a nonaphasic and often reversible deficit of speech articulation that usually is accompanied by mild right facial weakness. When the cause of Broca's aphasia is stroke, recovery of language function generally peaks within 2 to 6 months, after which time further progress is limited.

Global aphasia

Speech output is nonfluent, and comprehension of spoken language is severely impaired. Naming, repetition, reading, and writing also are impaired. This syndrome represents the combined dysfunction of Broca's and Wernicke's areas and usually results from strokes that involve the entire middle cerebral artery distribution in the left hemisphere. Most patients are initially mute or say a few words, such as "hi" or "yes." Related signs include right hemiplegia, hemisensory loss, and homonymous hemianopia. Occasionally, a patient with a lesion in Wernicke's area will present with a global aphasia that soon resolves into Wernicke's aphasia.

Conduction aphasia

Speech output is fluent but paraphasic, comprehension of spoken language is intact, and repetition is severely impaired. Naming and writing also are impaired. Reading aloud is impaired, but reading comprehension is preserved. The lesion sites spare Broca's and Wernicke's areas but may induce a functional disconnection between the two so that neural word representations formed in Wernicke's area and adjacent regions cannot be conveyed to Broca's area for assembly into corresponding articulatory patterns. Occasionally, a Wernicke's area lesion gives rise to a transient Wernicke's aphasia that rapidly resolves into a conduction aphasia. The paraphasic output in conduction aphasia interferes with the ability to express meaning, but this deficit is not nearly as severe as the one displayed by patients with Wernicke's aphasia. Associated neurologic signs in conduction aphasia vary according to the primary lesion site.

Nonfluent transcortical aphasia (transcortical motor aphasia)

The features are similar to those of Broca's aphasia, but repetition is intact and agrammatism may be less pronounced. The neurologic examination may be otherwise intact, but a right hemiparesis also can exist. The lesion site disconnects the intact language network from prefrontal areas of the brain and usually involves the anterior watershed zone between anterior and middle cerebral artery territories or the supplementary motor cortex in the territory of the anterior cerebral artery.

Fluent transcortical aphasia (transcortical sensory aphasia)

Clinical features are similar to those of Wernicke's aphasia, but repetition is intact. The lesion site disconnects the intact core of the language network from other temporoparietal association areas. Associated neurologic findings may include hemianopia. Cerebrovascular lesions (e.g., infarctions in the posterior watershed zone) and neoplasms that involve the temporoparietal cortex posterior to Wernicke's area are the most common causes.

Isolation aphasia

This rare syndrome represents a combination of the two transcortical aphasias. Comprehension is severely impaired, and there is no purposeful speech output. The patient may parrot fragments of heard conversations (echolalia), indicating that the neural mechanisms for repetition are at least partially intact. This condition represents the pathologic function of the language network when it is isolated from other regions of the brain. Broca's and Wernicke's areas tend to be spared, but there is damage to the surrounding frontal, parietal, and temporal cortex. Lesions are patchy and can be associated with anoxia, carbon monoxide poisoning, or complete watershed zone infarctions.

Anomic aphasia

This form of aphasia may be considered the "minimal dysfunction" syndrome of the language network. Articulation, comprehension, and repetition are intact, but confrontation naming, word finding, and spelling are impaired. Speech is enriched in function words but impoverished in substantive nouns and verbs denoting specific actions. Language output is fluent but paraphasic, circumlocutious, and uninformative. Fluency may be interrupted by word-finding hesitations. The lesion sites can be anywhere within the left hemisphere language network, including the middle and inferior temporal gyri. *Anomic aphasia is the single most common language disturbance seen in head trauma, metabolic encephalopathy, and Alzheimer's disease.*

Pure word deafness

The most common causes are either bilateral or left-sided middle cerebral artery (MCA) strokes affecting the superior temporal gyrus. The net effect of the underlying lesion is to interrupt the flow of information from the auditory association cortex to Wernicke's area. Patients have no difficulty understanding written language and can express themselves well in spoken or written language. They have no difficulty interpreting and reacting to environmental sounds since primary auditory cortex and subcortical auditory relays are intact. Since auditory information cannot be conveyed to the language network, however, it cannot be decoded into neural word representations, and the patient reacts to speech as if it were in an alien tongue that cannot be deciphered. Patients cannot repeat spoken language but have no difficulty naming objects. In time, patients with pure word deafness teach themselves lipreading and may appear to have improved. There may be no additional neurologic findings, but agitated paranoid reactions are common in the acute stages. Cerebrovascular lesions are the most common cause.

Pure alexia without agraphia

This is the visual equivalent of pure word deafness. The lesions (usually a combination of damage to the left occipital cortex and

to a posterior sector of the corpus callosum—the splenium) interrupt the flow of visual input into the language network. There is usually a right hemianopia, but the core language network remains unaffected. The patient can understand and produce spoken language, name objects in the left visual hemifield, repeat, and write. However, the patient acts as if illiterate when asked to read even the simplest sentence because the visual information from the written words (presented to the intact left visual hemifield) cannot reach the language network. Objects in the left hemifield may be named accurately because they activate nonvisual associations in the right hemisphere, which in turn can access the language network through transcallosal pathways anterior to the splenium. Patients with this syndrome also may lose the ability to name colors, although they can match colors. This is known as a *color anomia*. The most common etiology of pure alexia is a vascular lesion in the territory of the posterior cerebral artery or an infiltrating neoplasm in the left occipital cortex that involves the optic radiations as well as the crossing fibers of the splenium. Since the posterior cerebral artery also supplies medial temporal components of the limbic system, a patient with pure alexia also may experience an amnesia, but this is usually transient because the limbic lesion is unilateral.

Aphemia

There is an acute onset of severely impaired fluency (often mutism), which cannot be accounted for by corticobulbar, cerebellar, or extrapyramidal dysfunction. Recovery is the rule and involves an intermediate stage of hoarse whispering. Writing, reading, and comprehension are intact, and so this is not a true aphasic syndrome. Partial lesions of Broca's area or subcortical lesions that undercut its connections with other parts of the brain may be present. Occasionally, the lesion site is on the medial aspects of the frontal lobes and may involve the supplementary motor cortex of the left hemisphere.

Apraxia

This generic term designates a complex motor deficit that cannot be attributed to pyramidal, extrapyramidal, cerebellar, or sensory dysfunction and that does not arise from the patient's failure to understand the nature of the task. The form that is encountered most frequently in clinical practice is known as *ideomotor apraxia*. Commands to perform a specific motor act ("cough," "blow out a match") or pantomime the use of a common tool (a comb, hammer, straw, or toothbrush) in the absence of the real object cannot be followed. The patient's ability to comprehend the command is ascertained by demonstrating multiple movements and establishing that the correct one can be recognized. Some patients with this type of apraxia can imitate the appropriate movement (when it is demonstrated by the examiner) and show no impairment when handed the real object, indicating that the sensorimotor mechanisms necessary for the movement are intact. Some forms of ideomotor apraxia represent a disconnection of the language network from pyramidal motor systems: commands to execute complex movements are understood but cannot be conveyed to the appropriate motor areas even though the relevant motor mechanisms are intact. *Buccofacial apraxia* involves apraxic deficits in movements of the face and mouth. *Limb apraxia* encompasses apraxic deficits in movements of the arms and legs. Ideomotor apraxia almost always is caused by lesions in the left hemisphere and is commonly associated with aphasic syndromes, especially Broca's aphasia and conduction aphasia. Its presence cannot be ascertained in patients with language comprehension deficits. The ability to follow commands aimed at axial musculature ("close the eyes," "stand up") is subserved by different pathways and may be intact in otherwise severely aphasic and apraxic patients. Since the handling of real objects is not impaired, ideomotor apraxia by itself causes no major limitation of daily living activities. Patients with lesions of the anterior corpus callosum can display ideomotor apraxia confined to the left side of the body, a sign known as *sympathetic dyspraxia*. A severe form of sympathetic dyspraxia known as the *alien hand* syndrome is characterized by additional features of motor disinhibition on the left hand.

Ideational apraxia refers to a deficit in the execution of a goal-directed sequence of movements in patients who have no difficulty executing the individual components of the sequence. For example, when the patient is asked to pick up a pen and write, the sequence of uncapping the pen, placing the cap at the opposite end, turning the point toward the writing surface, and writing may be disrupted, and the patient may be seen trying to write with the wrong end of the pen or even with the removed cap. These motor sequencing problems usually are seen in the context of confusional states and dementias rather than focal lesions associated with aphasic conditions. *Limb-kinetic apraxia* involves a clumsiness in the actual use of tools that cannot be attributed to sensory, pyramidal, extrapyramidal, or cerebellar dysfunction. This condition can emerge in the context of focal premotor cortex lesions or *corticobasal degeneration*.

Gerstmann's syndrome

The combination of *acalculia* (impairment of simple arithmetic), *dysgraphia* (impaired writing), *finger anomia* (an inability to name individual fingers such as the index and thumb), and *right-left confusion* (an inability to tell whether a hand, foot, or arm of the patient or examiner is on the right or left side of the body) is known as Gerstmann's syndrome. In making this diagnosis it is important to establish that the finger and left-right naming deficits are not part of a more generalized anomia and that the patient is not otherwise aphasic. When Gerstmann's syndrome is seen in isolation, it is commonly associated with damage to the inferior parietal lobule (especially the angular gyrus) in the left hemisphere.

Aprosodia

Variations of melodic stress and intonation influence the meaning and impact of spoken language. For example, the two statements "He *is* clever." and "He is *clever*?" contain an identical word choice and syntax but convey vastly different messages because of differences in the intonation and stress with which the statements are uttered. This aspect of language is known as *prosody*. Damage to perisylvian areas in the right hemisphere can interfere with speech prosody and can lead to syndromes of aprosodia. Damage to right hemisphere regions corresponding to Wernicke's area can selectively impair decoding of speech prosody, whereas damage to right hemisphere regions corresponding to Broca's area yields a greater impairment in the ability to introduce meaning-appropriate prosody into spoken language. The latter deficit is the most common type of aprosodia identified in clinical practice; the patient produces grammatically correct language with accurate word choice, but the statements are uttered in a monotone that interferes with the ability to convey the intended stress and affect. Patients with this type of aprosodia give the mistaken impression of being depressed or indifferent.

Subcortical aphasia

Damage to subcortical components of the language network (e.g., the striatum and thalamus of the left hemisphere) also can lead to aphasia. The resulting syndromes contain combinations of deficits in the various aspects of language but rarely fit the specific patterns described in Table 26-1. In a patient with a CVA, an anomic aphasia accompanied by dysarthria or a fluent aphasia with hemiparesis should raise the suspicion of a subcortical lesion site.

Progressive aphasias

Aphasias caused by cerebrovascular accidents start suddenly and display maximal deficits at the onset. The underlying lesion is relatively circumscribed and is associated with a total loss of neural function in at least part of the lesion site. These are the "classic" aphasias described above. Aphasias caused by neurodegenerative diseases have an insidious onset and a relentless progression so that the symptomatology changes over time. Since the neuronal loss within the areas encompassed by the neurodegeneration is partial and since it tends to include multiple components of the language network, the clinico-anatomic patterns are different from those described in Table 26-1.

Clinical presentation and diagnosis of primary progressive aphasia (PPA) When a neurodegenerative disease selectively undermines language function, a clinical diagnosis of PPA is made. A patient with PPA comes to medical attention because of word-finding difficulties, abnormal speech patterns, word-comprehension impairments, or spelling errors of recent onset. PPA is diagnosed when other mental faculties, such as memory for daily events, visuospatial skills (assessed by tests of drawing and face recognition), and comportment (assessed by history obtained from a third party), remain relatively intact; when language is the major area of dysfunction for the first few years of the disease; and when structural brain imaging does not reveal a specific lesion, other than atrophy, that accounts for the language deficit. Impairments in other cognitive functions may emerge eventually, but the language dysfunction remains the most salient feature and deteriorates most rapidly throughout the illness.

Language in PPA The language impairment in PPA varies from patient to patient. Some patients cannot find the right words to express thoughts; others cannot understand the meaning of heard or seen words; still others cannot name objects in the environment. The language impairment can be fluent (that is, with normal articulation, flow, and number of words per utterance) or nonfluent. The single most common sign of primary progressive aphasia is an inability to come up with the right word during conversation and/or an inability to name objects shown by the examiner (anomia). Distinct forms of agrammatism and/or word comprehension deficits also can arise. The agrammatism consists of inappropriate word order and misuse of small grammatical words. Comprehension deficits, if present, start with an occasional inability to understand single low-frequency words and gradually progress to encompass the comprehension of conversational speech.

The impairments of syntax, comprehension, naming, or writing in PPA form slightly different patterns from those seen in CVA-caused aphasias. Three subtypes of PPA can be recognized: an agrammatic variant characterized by poor fluency and impaired grammar, a semantic variant characterized by preserved fluency and syntax but poor single word comprehension, and a logopenic variant characterized by preserved syntax and comprehension but frequent word-finding pauses during spontaneous speech. The agrammatic variant also is known as *progressive nonfluent aphasia* and displays similarities to Broca's aphasia. However, dysarthria is usually absent. The semantic variant of PPA displays similarities to Wernicke's aphasia, but the comprehension difficulty tends to be most profound for single words denoting concrete objects.

Pathophysiology The three variants of PPA display overlapping distributions of neuronal loss, but the agrammatic variant is most closely associated with atrophy in the anterior parts of the language network (where Broca's area is located), the semantic variant with atrophy in the anterior temporal components of the language network, and the logopenic variant with atrophy in the temporoparietal component of the language network. The abnormalities may remain confined to the left hemisphere perisylvian and anterior temporal cortices initially, but gradual deterioration in PPA leads to a loss of syndromic specificity as the disease progresses.

Neuropathology In the majority of PPA cases, the neuropathology falls within the family of frontotemporal lobar degenerations (FTLDs) and displays various combinations of focal neuronal loss, gliosis, tau-positive inclusions including Pick bodies, and tau-negative TDP-43 inclusions. Familial forms of PPA with TDP-43 inclusions recently were linked to mutations of the progranulin gene on chromosome 17. The agrammatic variant most frequently is associated with tauopathy, whereas the semantic variant is most closely associated with TDP-43 inclusions. Alzheimer's pathology is seen most frequently in the logopenic variant. The clinical subtyping of PPA thus may help predict the nature of the underlying neuropathology. The intriguing possibility has been raised that a personal or family history of dyslexia may be a risk factor for primary progressive aphasia, at least in some patients, suggesting that this disease may arise on a background of genetic or developmental vulnerability that affects language-related areas of the brain.

THE PARIETOFRONTAL NETWORK FOR SPATIAL ORIENTATION: NEGLECT AND RELATED CONDITIONS

■ HEMISPATIAL NEGLECT

Adaptive orientation to significant events within the extrapersonal space is subserved by a large-scale network containing three major cortical components. The *cingulate cortex* provides access to a motivational mapping of the extrapersonal space, the *posterior parietal cortex* to a sensorimotor representation of salient extrapersonal events, and the *frontal eye fields* to motor strategies for attentional behaviors (Fig. 26-2). Subcortical components of this network include the striatum and the thalamus. Contralesional hemispatial neglect represents one outcome of damage to any of the cortical or subcortical components of this network. *The traditional view that hemispatial neglect always denotes a parietal lobe lesion is inaccurate.* In keeping with this anatomic organization, the clinical manifestations of neglect display three behavioral components: sensory events (or their mental representations) within the neglected hemispace have a lesser impact on overall awareness, there is a paucity of exploratory and orienting acts directed toward the neglected hemispace, and the patient behaves as if the neglected hemispace were motivationally devalued.

According to one model of spatial cognition, the right hemisphere directs attention within the *entire* extrapersonal space, whereas the left hemisphere directs attention mostly within the contralateral right hemispace. Consequently, unilateral left hemisphere lesions do not give rise to much contralesional neglect since the global attentional mechanisms of the right hemisphere can compensate for the loss of the *contralaterally* directed attentional functions of the left hemisphere. Unilateral right hemisphere lesions, however, give rise to severe contralesional left hemispatial neglect because the unaffected left hemisphere does not contain ipsilateral attentional mechanisms. This model is consistent with clinical experience, which shows that contralesional neglect is more common, severe, and lasting after damage to the right hemisphere than after damage to the left hemisphere. Severe neglect for the right hemispace is rare, even in left-handers with left hemisphere lesions.

Clinical examination

Patients with severe neglect may fail to dress, shave, or groom the left side of the body; fail to eat food placed on the left side of the tray; and fail to read the left half of sentences. When the examiner draws a large circle [12 to 15 cm (5 to 6 in.) in diameter] and asks the patient to place the numbers 1 to 12 as if the circle represented the face of a clock, there is a tendency to crowd the numbers on the right side and leave the left side empty. When asked to copy a simple line drawing, the patient fails to copy detail on the left, and

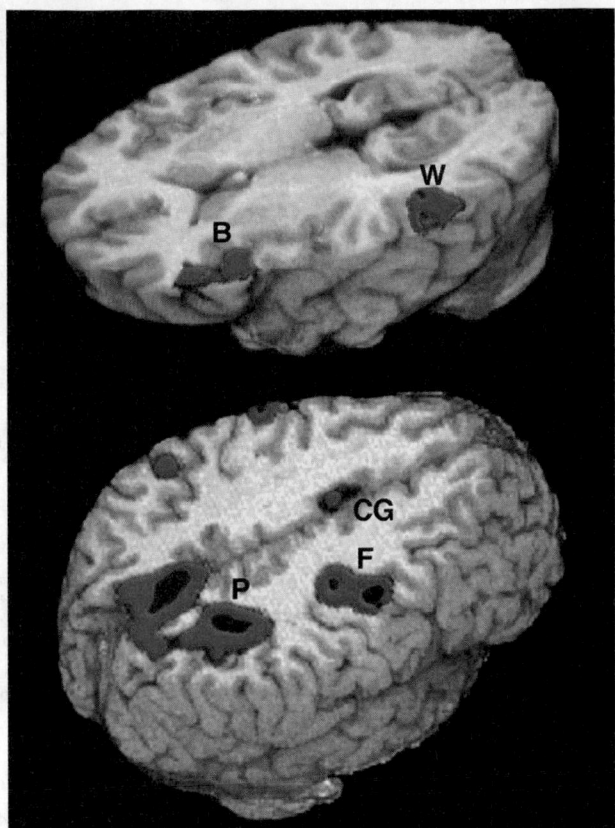

Figure 26-2 **Functional magnetic resonance imaging** of language and spatial attention in neurologically intact subjects. The red and black areas show regions of task-related significant activation. (*Top*) The subjects were asked to determine if two words were synonymous. This language task led to the simultaneous activation of the two epicenters of the language network, Broca's area (B) and Wernicke's area (W). The activations are exclusively in the left hemisphere. (*Bottom*) The subjects were asked to shift spatial attention to a peripheral target. This task led to the simultaneous activation of the three epicenters of the attentional network: the posterior parietal cortex (P), the frontal eye fields (F), and the cingulate gyrus (CG). The activations are predominantly in the right hemisphere. (*Courtesy of Darren Gitelman, MD; with permission.*)

when the patient is asked to write, there is a tendency to leave an unusually wide margin on the left.

Two bedside tests that are useful in assessing neglect are *simultaneous bilateral stimulation* and *visual target cancellation*. In the former, the examiner provides either unilateral or simultaneous bilateral stimulation in the visual, auditory, and tactile modalities. After right hemisphere injury, patients who have no difficulty detecting unilateral stimuli on either side experience the bilaterally presented stimulus as coming only from the right. This phenomenon is known as *extinction* and is a manifestation of the sensory-representational aspect of hemispatial neglect. In the target detection task, targets (e.g., A's) are interspersed with foils (e.g., other letters of the alphabet) on a 21.5- to 28.0-cm (8.5 to 11 in.) sheet of paper, and the patient is asked to circle all the targets. A failure to detect targets on the left is a manifestation of the exploratory deficit in hemispatial neglect (Fig. 26-3A). Hemianopia is not by itself sufficient to cause the target detection failure since the patient is free to turn the head and eyes to the left. Target detection failures therefore reflect a distortion of spatial attention, not just of sensory input. The normal tendency in target detection tasks is to start from the left upper quadrant and move systematically in horizontal or vertical sweeps. Some patients show a tendency to start the process from the

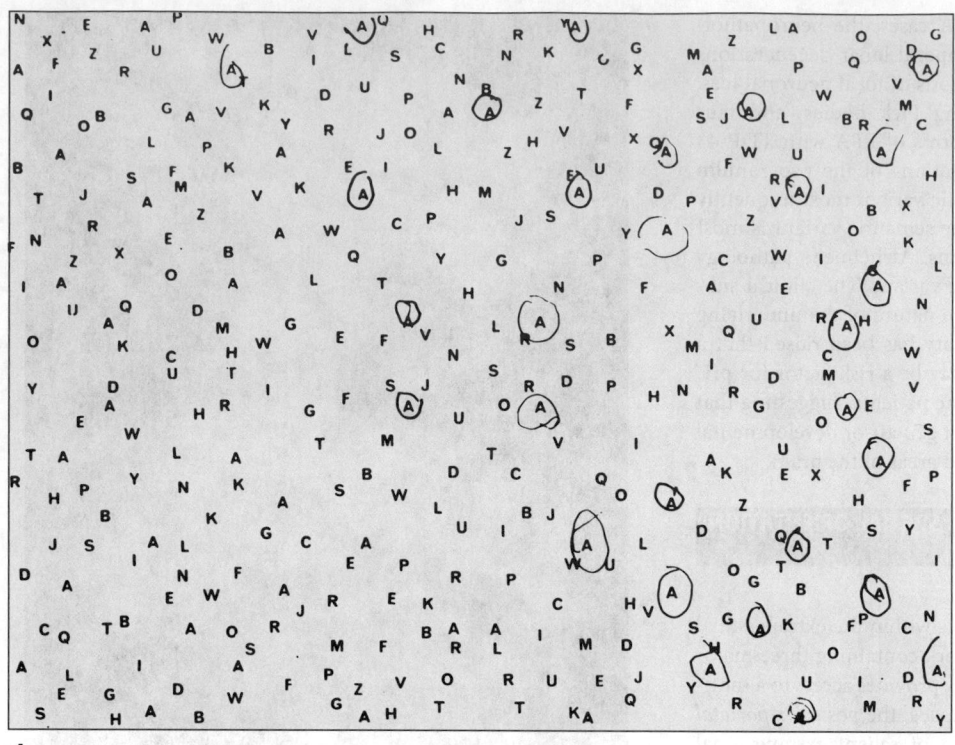

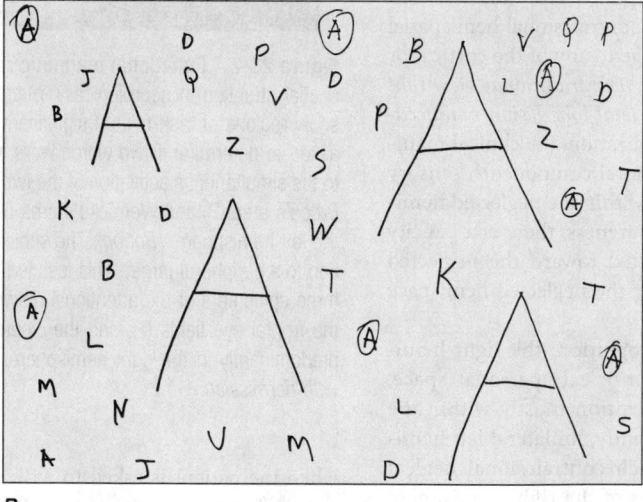

Figure 26-3 **A.** A 47-year-old man with a large frontoparietal lesion in the right hemisphere was asked to circle all the A's. Only targets on the right are circled. This is a manifestation of left hemispatial neglect. **B.** A 70-year-old woman with a 2-year history of degenerative dementia was able to circle most of the small targets but ignored the larger ones. This is a manifestation of simultanagnosia.

for additional information. A patient with simultanagnosia "misses the forest for the trees." Complex visual scenes cannot be grasped in their entirety, leading to severe limitations in the visual identification of objects and scenes. For example, a patient who is shown a table lamp and asked to name the object may look at its circular base and call it an ashtray. Some patients with simultanagnosia report that objects they look at may vanish suddenly, probably indicating an inability to look back at the original point of gaze after brief saccadic displacements. Movement and distracting stimuli greatly exacerbate the difficulties of visual perception. Simultanagnosia sometimes can occur without the other two components of Bálint's syndrome.

A modification of the letter cancellation task described above can be used for the bedside diagnosis of simultanagnosia. In this modification, some of the targets (e.g., A's) are made to be much larger than the others [7.5 to 10 cm vs. 2.5 cm (3 to 4 in. vs. 1 in.) in height], and all targets are embedded among foils. Patients with simultanagnosia display a counterintuitive but characteristic tendency to miss the larger targets (Fig. 26-3B). This occurs because the information needed for the identification of the larger targets cannot be confined to the immediate line of gaze and requires the integration of visual information across a more extensive field of view. The greater difficulty in the detection of the larger targets also indicates that poor acuity is not responsible for the impairment of visual function and that the problem is central rather than peripheral.

Another manifestation of bilateral (or right-sided) dorsal parietal lobe lesions is *dressing apraxia*. A patient with this condition is unable to align the body axis with the axis of the garment and can be seen struggling as he or she holds a coat from its bottom or extends his or her arm into a fold of the garment rather than into its sleeve. Lesions that involve the posterior parietal cortex also lead to severe difficulties in copying simple line drawings. This is known as a *construction apraxia* and is much more severe if the lesion is in the right hemisphere. In some patients with right hemisphere lesions, the drawing difficulties are confined to the left side of the figure and represent a manifestation of hemispatial neglect; in others, there is a more universal deficit in reproducing contours and three-dimensional perspective. Dressing apraxia and construction apraxia represent special instances of a more general disturbance in spatial orientation.

Causes of spatial disorientation

Cerebrovascular lesions and neoplasms in the right hemisphere are the most common causes of hemispatial neglect. Depending on the

right and proceed in a haphazard fashion. This represents a subtle manifestation of left neglect even if the patient eventually manages to detect all the appropriate targets. Some patients with neglect also may deny the existence of hemiparesis and may even deny ownership of the paralyzed limb, a condition known as *anosognosia*.

■ BÁLINT'S SYNDROME, SIMULTANAGNOSIA, DRESSING APRAXIA, AND CONSTRUCTION APRAXIA

Bilateral involvement of the network for spatial attention, especially its parietal components, leads to a state of severe spatial disorientation known as *Bálint's syndrome*. Bálint's syndrome involves deficits in the orderly visuomotor scanning of the environment (*oculomotor apraxia*) and in accurate manual reaching toward visual targets (*optic ataxia*). The third and most dramatic component of Bálint's syndrome is known as *simultanagnosia* and reflects an inability to integrate visual information in the center of gaze with more peripheral information. The patient gets stuck on the detail that falls in the center of gaze without attempting to scan the visual environment site of the lesion, a patient with neglect also may have hemiparesis, hemihypesthesia, and hemianopia on the left, but these are not invariant findings. The majority of these patients display considerable improvement of hemispatial neglect, usually within the first several weeks. Bálint's syndrome results from bilateral dorsal parietal lesions; common settings include watershed infarction between the middle and posterior cerebral artery territories, hypoglycemia, and sagittal sinus thrombosis.

A progressive form of spatial disorientation known as the *posterior cortical atrophy* syndrome most commonly represents a variant of Alzheimer's disease with unusual concentrations of neurofibrillary degeneration in the parieto-occipital cortex and the superior colliculus. The patient displays a progressive Bálint's syndrome, usually accompanied by dressing and construction apraxia. Corticobasal degeneration, a type of FTLD with abnormal tau inclusions, can have an asymmetric distribution. When the atrophy shows a predilection for the right cerebral hemisphere, a progressive left hemineglect syndrome emerges on a background of left-sided extrapyramidal dysfunction.

THE OCCIPITOTEMPORAL NETWORK FOR FACE AND OBJECT RECOGNITION: PROSOPAGNOSIA AND OBJECT AGNOSIA

Perceptual information about faces and objects initially is encoded in primary (striate) visual cortex and adjacent (upstream) peristriate visual association areas. This information subsequently is relayed first to the downstream visual association areas of occipitotemporal cortex and then to other heteromodal and paralimbic areas of the cerebral cortex. Bilateral lesions in the fusiform and lingual gyri of the occipitotemporal cortex disrupt this process and interfere with the ability of otherwise intact perceptual information to activate the distributed multimodal associations that lead to the recognition of faces and objects. The resultant face and object recognition deficits are known as *associative prosopagnosia* and *visual object agnosia*.

A patient with prosopagnosia cannot recognize familiar faces, including, sometimes, the reflection of his or her own face in the mirror. This is not a perceptual deficit since prosopagnosic patients easily can tell whether two faces are identical. Furthermore, a prosopagnosic patient who cannot recognize a familiar face by visual inspection alone can use auditory cues to reach appropriate recognition if allowed to listen to the person's voice. The deficit in prosopagnosia is therefore modality-specific and reflects the existence of a lesion that prevents the activation of otherwise intact multimodal templates by relevant visual input. The deficit in prosopagnosia is not limited to the recognition of faces but also can extend to the recognition of individual members of larger generic object groups. For example, prosopagnosic patients characteristically have no difficulty with the generic identification of a face as a face or a car as a car, but they cannot recognize the identity of an individual face or the make of an individual car. This reflects a visual recognition deficit for proprietary features that characterize individual members of an object class. When recognition problems become more generalized and extend to the generic identification of common objects, the condition is known as *visual object agnosia*. In contrast to prosopagnosic patients, those with object agnosia cannot recognize a face as a face or a car as a car. It is important to distinguish visual object agnosia from anomia. A patient with anomia cannot name the object but can describe its use. In contrast, a patient with visual agnosia is unable either to name a visually presented object or to describe its use. Face and object recognition disorders also can result from the simultanagnosia of Bálint's syndrome, in which case they are known as *apperceptive* agnosias as opposed to the *associative* agnosias that result from inferior temporal lobe lesions.

■ CAUSES

The characteristic lesions in prosopagnosia and visual object agnosia consist of bilateral infarctions in the territory of the posterior cerebral arteries. Associated deficits can include visual field defects (especially superior quadrantanopias) and a centrally based color blindness known as achromatopsia. Rarely, the responsible lesion is unilateral. In such cases, prosopagnosia is associated with lesions in the right hemisphere, and object agnosia with lesions in the left. Degenerative diseases of anterior and inferior temporal cortex can cause progressive associative prosopagnosia and object agnosia. The combination of progressive associative agnosia and a fluent aphasia is known as *semantic dementia* and usually is caused by FTLD with TDP-43 inclusions. Patients with semantic dementia fail to recognize faces and objects and cannot understand the meaning of words denoting objects.

THE LIMBIC NETWORK FOR EPISODIC MEMORY: AMNESIAS

Limbic and paralimbic areas (such as the hippocampus, amygdala, and entorhinal cortex), the anterior and medial nuclei of the thalamus, the medial and basal parts of the striatum, and the hypothalamus collectively constitute a distributed network known as the *limbic system*. The behavioral affiliations of this network include the coordination of emotion, motivation, autonomic tone, and endocrine function. An additional area of specialization for the limbic network and the one that is of most relevance to clinical practice is that of declarative (conscious) memory for recent episodes and experiences. A disturbance in this function is known as an *amnestic state*. In the absence of deficits in motivation, attention, language, or visuospatial function, the clinical diagnosis of a persistent global amnestic state is always associated with bilateral damage to the limbic network, usually within the hippocampo-entorhinal complex or the thalamus.

Although the limbic network is the site of damage for amnestic states, it is almost certainly not the storage site for memories. Memories are stored in widely distributed form throughout the cerebral cortex. The role attributed to the limbic network is to bind these distributed fragments into coherent events and experiences that can sustain conscious recall. Damage to the limbic network does not necessarily destroy memories but interferes with their conscious (declarative) recall in coherent form. The individual fragments of information remain preserved despite the limbic lesions and can sustain what is known as *implicit memory*. For example, patients with amnestic states can acquire new motor or perceptual skills even though they may have no conscious knowledge of the experiences that led to the acquisition of these skills.

The memory disturbance in the amnestic state is multimodal and includes retrograde and anterograde components. The *retrograde amnesia* involves an inability to recall experiences that occurred before the onset of the amnestic state. Relatively recent events are more vulnerable to retrograde amnesia than are more remote and more extensively consolidated events. A patient who comes to the emergency room complaining that he cannot remember his or her identity but can remember the events of the previous day almost certainly does not have a neurologic cause of memory disturbance. The second and most important component of the amnestic state is the *anterograde amnesia*, which indicates an inability to store, retain, and recall new knowledge. Patients with amnestic states cannot remember what they ate a few minutes ago or the details of an important event they may have experienced a few hours ago. In the acute stages, there also may be a tendency to fill in memory gaps with inaccurate, fabricated, and often implausible information. This is known as *confabulation*. Patients with the amnestic syndrome forget that they forget and tend to deny the existence of a memory problem when questioned.

◼ CLINICAL EXAMINATION

A patient with an amnestic state is almost always disoriented, especially to time. Accurate temporal orientation and accurate knowledge of current news rule out a major amnestic state. The anterograde component of an amnestic state can be tested with a list of four to five words read aloud by the examiner up to five times or until the patient can immediately repeat the entire list without an intervening delay. In the next phase of testing, the patient is allowed to concentrate on the words and rehearse them internally for 1 min before being asked to recall them. Accurate performance in this phase indicates that the patient is motivated and sufficiently attentive to hold the words online for at least 1 min. The final phase of the testing involves a retention period of 5 to 10 min during which the patient is engaged in other tasks. Adequate recall at the end of this interval requires offline storage, retention, and retrieval. Amnestic patients fail this phase of the task and may even forget that they were given a list of words to remember. Accurate recognition of the words by multiple choice in a patient who cannot recall them indicates a less severe memory disturbance that affects mostly the retrieval stage of memory. The retrograde component of an amnesia can be assessed with questions related to autobiographical or historic events. The anterograde component of amnestic states is usually much more prominent than the retrograde component. In rare instances, usually associated with temporal lobe epilepsy or benzodiazepine intake, the retrograde component may dominate.

The assessment of memory can be quite challenging. Bedside evaluations may detect only the most severe impairments. Less severe memory impairments, as in the case of patients with temporal lobe epilepsy, mild head injury, or early dementia, require quantitative evaluations by neuropsychologists. Confusional states caused by toxic-metabolic encephalopathies and some types of frontal lobe damage interfere with attentional capacity and lead to secondary memory impairments, even in the absence of any limbic lesions. This sort of memory impairment can be differentiated from the amnestic state by the presence of additional impairments in the attention-related tasks described below in the section on the frontal lobes.

◼ CAUSES, INCLUDING ALZHEIMER'S DISEASE

Many neurologic diseases can give rise to an amnestic state. They include tumors (of the sphenoid wing, posterior corpus callosum, thalamus, or medial temporal lobe), infarctions (in the territories of the anterior or posterior cerebral arteries), head trauma, herpes simplex encephalitis, Wernicke-Korsakoff encephalopathy, paraneoplastic limbic encephalitis, and degenerative dementias such as Alzheimer's disease and Pick's disease. The one common denominator of all these diseases is the presence of bilateral lesions within one or more components in the limbic network. Occasionally, unilateral left-sided hippocampal lesions can give rise to an amnestic state, but the memory disorder tends to be transient. Depending on the nature and distribution of the underlying neurologic disease, the patient also may have visual field deficits, eye movement limitations, or cerebellar findings.

Alzheimer's disease (AD) and its prodromal state of mild cognitive impairment (MCI) are the most common causes of progressive memory impairments. Temporal disorientation and poor recall of recent conversations are early manifestations. The predilection of the entorhinal cortex and hippocampus for early neurofibrillary degeneration in the MCI-AD spectrum is responsible for the initially selective impairment of episodic memory. In time, a full amnestic state emerges, but usually with additional impairments in language, attention, and visuospatial skills as the neurofibrillary degeneration spreads to additional neocortical areas.

Transient global amnesia is a distinctive syndrome usually seen in late middle age. Patients become acutely disoriented and repeatedly ask who they are, where they are, and what they are doing. The spell is characterized by anterograde amnesia (inability to retain new information) and a retrograde amnesia for relatively recent events that occurred before the onset. The syndrome usually resolves within 24 to 48 h and is followed by the filling in of the period affected by the retrograde amnesia, although there is persistent loss of memory for the events that occurred during the ictus. Recurrences are noted in approximately 20% of patients. Migraine, temporal lobe seizures, and perfusion abnormalities in the posterior cerebral territory have been postulated as causes of transient global amnesia. The absence of associated neurologic findings occasionally may lead to the incorrect diagnosis of a psychiatric disorder.

THE PREFRONTAL NETWORK FOR ATTENTION AND BEHAVIOR

Approximately one-third of all the cerebral cortex in the human brain is situated in the frontal lobes. The frontal lobes can be subdivided into motor-premotor, dorsolateral prefrontal, medial prefrontal, and orbitofrontal components. The terms *frontal lobe syndrome* and *prefrontal cortex* refer only to the last three of these four components. These are the parts of the cerebral cortex that show the greatest phylogenetic expansion in primates, especially in humans. The dorsolateral prefrontal, medial prefrontal, and orbitofrontal areas, along with the subcortical structures with which they are interconnected (i.e., the head of the caudate and the dorsomedial nucleus of the thalamus), collectively make up a large-scale network that coordinates exceedingly complex aspects of human cognition and behavior.

The prefrontal network plays an important role in behaviors that require multitasking and the integration of thought with emotion. Its integrity appears important for the simultaneous awareness of context, options, consequences, relevance, and emotional impact that allows the formulation of adaptive inferences, decisions, and actions. Damage to this part of the brain impairs mental flexibility, reasoning, hypothesis formation, abstract thinking, foresight, judgment, the online (attentive) holding of information, and the ability to inhibit inappropriate responses. Cognitive operations impaired by prefrontal cortex lesions often are referred to as "executive functions."

Even very large bilateral prefrontal lesions may leave all sensory, motor, and basic cognitive functions intact while leading to isolated but dramatic alterations of personality and behavior. The most common clinical manifestations of damage to the prefrontal network take the form of two relatively distinct syndromes. In the *frontal abulic syndrome*, the patient shows a loss of initiative, creativity, and curiosity and displays a pervasive emotional blandness and apathy. In the *frontal disinhibition syndrome*, the patient becomes socially disinhibited and shows severe impairments of judgment, insight, and foresight. The dissociation between intact intellectual function and a total lack of even rudimentary common sense is striking. Despite the preservation of all essential memory functions, the patient cannot learn from experience and continues to display inappropriate behaviors without appearing to feel emotional pain, guilt, or regret when those behaviors repeatedly lead to disastrous consequences. The impairments may emerge only in real-life situations when behavior is under minimal external control and may not be apparent within the structured environment of the medical office. Testing judgment by asking patients what they would do if they detected a fire in a theater or found a stamped and addressed envelope on the road is not very informative since patients who answer these questions wisely in the office may still act very foolishly in the more complex real-life setting. The physician must therefore be prepared to make a diagnosis of frontal lobe disease on the basis of historic information alone even when the mental state is quite intact in the office examination.

■ CLINICAL EXAMINATION

The emergence of developmentally primitive reflexes, also known as frontal release signs, such as grasping (elicited by stroking the palm) and sucking (elicited by stroking the lips) are seen primarily in patients with large structural lesions that extend into the premotor components of the frontal lobes or in the context of metabolic encephalopathies. The vast majority of patients with prefrontal lesions and frontal lobe behavioral syndromes do not display these reflexes.

Damage to the frontal lobe disrupts a variety of attention-related functions, including working memory (the transient online holding of information), concentration span, the scanning and retrieval of stored information, the inhibition of immediate but inappropriate responses, and mental flexibility. The capacity for focusing on a trend of thought and the ability to shift the focus of attention voluntarily from one thought or stimulus to another can become impaired. Digit span (which should be seven forward and five reverse) is decreased; the recitation of the months of the year in reverse order (which should take less than 15 s) is slowed; and the fluency in producing words starting with the letter a, f, or s that can be generated in 1 min (normally ≥ 12 per letter) is diminished even in nonaphasic patients. Characteristically, there is a progressive slowing of performance as the task proceeds; e.g., a patient asked to count backward by threes may say "100, 97, 94, ... 91, ... 88," etc., and may not complete the task. In "go–no go" tasks (where the instruction is to raise the finger upon hearing one tap but keep it still upon hearing two taps), the patient shows a characteristic inability to keep still in response to the "no go" stimulus. Mental flexibility (tested by the ability to shift from one criterion to another in sorting or matching tasks) is impoverished; distractibility by irrelevant stimuli is increased; and there is a pronounced tendency for impersistence and perseveration.

These attentional deficits disrupt the orderly registration and retrieval of new information and lead to *secondary* memory deficits. Those memory deficits can be differentiated from the *primary* memory impairments of the amnestic state by showing that they improve when the attentional load of the task is decreased. Working memory (also known as immediate memory) is an attentional function based on the temporary online holding of information. It is closely associated with the integrity of the prefrontal network and the ascending reticular activating system. Retentive memory, in contrast, depends on the stable (offline) storage of information and is associated with the integrity of the limbic network. The distinction of the underlying neural mechanisms is illustrated by the observation that severely amnestic patients who cannot remember events that occurred a few minutes ago may have intact if not superior working memory capacity as shown in tests of digit span.

■ CAUSES: TRAUMA, NEOPLASM, AND FRONTOTEMPORAL DEMENTIA

The abulic syndrome tends to be associated with damage in dorsal prefrontal cortex, and the disinhibition syndrome with damage in ventral prefrontal cortex. These syndromes tend to arise almost exclusively after bilateral lesions. Unilateral lesions confined to the prefrontal cortex may remain silent until the pathology spreads to the other side; this explains why thromboembolic CVA is an unusual cause of the frontal lobe syndrome. Common settings for frontal lobe syndromes include head trauma, ruptured aneurysms, hydrocephalus, tumors (including metastases, glioblastoma, and falx or olfactory groove meningiomas), and focal degenerative diseases.

A major clinical form of FTLD known as the behavioral variant of frontotemporal dementia (bvFTD) causes a progressive frontal lobe syndrome that can start as early as the fifth decade of life. In these patients, the anterior temporal lobe and caudate nucleus are also atrophic. The behavioral changes can include shoplifting, compulsive gambling, sexual indiscretions, and obsessive-compulsive preoccupations, arising on a background of indifference. In many patients with Alzheimer's disease, neurofibrillary degeneration eventually spreads to prefrontal cortex and gives rise to components of the frontal lobe syndrome, but almost always on a background of severe memory impairment.

Lesions in the caudate nucleus or in the dorsomedial nucleus of the thalamus (subcortical components of the prefrontal network) also can produce a frontal lobe syndrome. This is one reason why the changes in mental state associated with degenerative basal ganglia diseases such as Parkinson's disease and Huntington's disease may take the form of a frontal lobe syndrome. Because of its widespread connections with other regions of association cortex, one essential computational role of the prefrontal network is to function as an integrator, or "orchestrator," for other networks. Bilateral multifocal lesions of the cerebral hemispheres, none of which are individually large enough to cause specific cognitive deficits such as aphasia and neglect, can collectively interfere with the connectivity and integrating function of the prefrontal cortex. A frontal lobe syndrome is the single most common behavioral profile associated with a variety of bilateral multifocal brain diseases, including metabolic encephalopathy, multiple sclerosis, and vitamin B_{12} deficiency, among others. Many patients with the clinical diagnosis of a frontal lobe syndrome tend to have lesions that do not involve prefrontal cortex but involve either the subcortical components of the prefrontal network or its connections with other parts of the brain. To avoid making a diagnosis of "frontal lobe syndrome" in a patient with no evidence of frontal cortex disease, it is advisable to use the diagnostic term *frontal network syndrome*, with the understanding that the responsible lesions can lie anywhere within this distributed network.

A patient with frontal lobe disease raises potential dilemmas in differential diagnosis: the abulia and blandness may be misinterpreted as depression, and the disinhibition as idiopathic mania or acting out. Appropriate intervention may be delayed while a treatable tumor keeps expanding. An informed approach to frontal lobe disease and its behavioral manifestations may help prevent such errors.

CARING FOR PATIENTS WITH DEFICITS OF HIGHER CEREBRAL FUNCTION

Some of the deficits described in this chapter are so complex that they may bewilder not only the patient and family but also the physician. It is imperative to carry out a systematic clinical evaluation to characterize the nature of the deficits and explain them in lay terms to the patient and family. Such an explanation can allay at least some of the anxieties, address the mistaken impression that the deficit (e.g., social disinhibition or inability to recognize family members) is psychologically motivated, and lead to practical suggestions for daily living activities. The consultation of a skilled neuropsychologist may aid in the formulation of diagnosis and management. Patients with simultanagnosia, for example, may benefit from the counterintuitive instruction to stand back when they cannot find an item so that a greater search area falls within the immediate field of gaze. Some patients with frontal lobe disease can be extremely irritable and abusive to spouses yet display all the appropriate social graces during a visit to the medical office. In such cases, the history may be more important than the bedside examination in charting a course of treatment.

Reactive depression is common in patients with higher cerebral dysfunction and should be treated. These patients may be overly sensitive to the usual doses of antidepressants or anxiolytics and require a careful titration of dosage. Brain damage may cause a dissociation between feeling states and their expression so that a patient who may superficially appear jocular could still be suffering from an underlying depression that needs to be treated. In many cases, agitation may be controlled with reassurance. In other cases, treatment with benzodiazepines, antiepilectics, or sedating antidepressants may become necessary. If neuroleptics become absolutely necessary for the control of agitation, atypical neuroleptics are preferable because of their lower extrapyramidal side effects. Treatment with neuroleptics in elderly patients with dementia requires weighing the potential benefits against the potentially serious side effects.

Spontaneous improvement of cognitive deficits due to acute neurologic lesions is common. It is most rapid in the first few weeks but may continue for up to 2 years, especially in young individuals with single brain lesions. The mechanisms for this recovery are incompletely understood. Some of the initial deficits appear to arise from remote dysfunction (diaschisis) in parts of the brain that are interconnected with the site of initial injury. Improvement in these patients may reflect, at least in part, a normalization of the remote dysfunction. Other mechanisms may involve functional reorganization in surviving neurons adjacent to the injury or the compensatory use of homologous structures, e.g., the right superior temporal gyrus with recovery from Wernicke's aphasia. In some patients with large lesions involving Broca's and Wernicke's areas, only Wernicke's area may show contralateral compensatory reorganization (or bilateral functionality), giving rise to a situation in which a lesion that should have caused a global aphasia becomes associated with a residual Broca's aphasia. Prognosis for recovery from aphasia is best when Wernicke's area is spared. Cognitive rehabilitation procedures have been used in the treatment of higher cortical deficits. There are few controlled studies, but some show a benefit of rehabilitation in the recovery from hemispatial neglect and aphasia. Some types of deficits may be more prone to recovery than others. For example, patients with CVA and nonfluent aphasias are more likely to benefit from speech therapy than are patients with fluent aphasias and comprehension deficits. In general, lesions that lead to a denial of illness (e.g., anosognosia) are associated with cognitive deficits that are more resistant to rehabilitation. Periodic neuropsychological assessment is necessary for quantifying the pace of the improvement (or of the progression in the case of dementias) and for generating specific recommendations for cognitive rehabilitation, modifications in the home environment, the timetable for returning to work in patients recovering from acute lesions, and the scheduling of retirement or disability status in patients with degenerative diseases. Determining driving competence is challenging, especially in the early stages of dementing diseases. The diagnosis of a neurodegenerative disease is not by itself sufficient for asking the patient to stop driving. An on-the-road driving test and reports from family members may help time decisions related to this very important activity.

There is a mistaken belief that dementias are anatomically diffuse and that they cause global cognitive impairments. This is true only at the terminal stages. During most of the clinical course, dementias are exquisitely selective with respect to anatomy and cognitive pattern. Alzheimer's disease, for example, causes the greatest destruction in medial temporal areas belonging to the memory network and is clinically characterized by a correspondingly severe amnesia. There are other dementias in which memory is intact. Selective degeneration of the frontal lobes in FTLD leads to a gradual dissolution of behavior and executive functions. Primary progressive aphasia is characterized by a gradual atrophy of the left perisylvian language network and a selective dissolution of language that can remain isolated for up to 10 years. An enlightened approach to the differential diagnosis and to the individualized care of patients with acute and progressive damage to the cerebral cortex requires an understanding of the principles that link neural networks to higher cerebral functions.

FURTHER READINGS

BARTSCH T el al: Selective affection of hippocampal CA-1 neurons in patients with transient global amnesia without long-term sequelae. Brain, 129:2874, 2006

CATANI M et al: Perisylvian language networks of the human brain. Ann Neurol 57:8, 2006

DELEON J et al: Neural regions essential for distinct cognitive processes underlying picture naming. Brain, 130:1408, 2007

DORICCI F et al: White matter (dis)connections and gray matter (dys)functions in visual neglect: Gaining insights into the brain networks of spatial awareness. Cortex 44:983, 2008

HEISS W-D et al: Differential capacity of left and right hemispheric areas for compensation of poststroke aphasia. Ann Neurol 45:430, 1999

LEIGUARDA RC, MARSDEN CD: Limb apraxias: Higher-order disorders of sensorimotor integration. Brain 123:860, 2000

MESULAM M: Representation, inference and transcendent encoding in neurocognitive networks of the human brain. Ann Neurol 64:367, 2008

_____ et al: Quantitative template for subtyping primary progressive aphasia. Arch Neurol 66:1545, 2009

RUFF CC et al: Hemispheric differences in frontal and parietal influences on human occipital cortex: Direct confirmation with concurrent TMS-fMRI. J Cogn Neurosci 21:1146, 2008

RUSCONI E et al: A disconnection account of Gerstmann syndrome: Functional neuroanatomy evidence. Ann Neurol 66:654, 2009

SCHMAHMANN JD, PANDYA DN: Disconnection syndromes of basal ganglia, thalamus, and cerebrocerebellar systems. Cortex 44:1037, 2008

SEELEY W et al: Early frontotemporal dementia targets neurons unique to apes and humans. Ann Neurol 60:660, 2006

WEINTRAUB S, MESULAM M: With or without FUS, it is the anatomy that dictates the dementia phenotype. Brain 132:2906, 2009

CHAPTER 27

Sleep Disorders

Charles A. Czeisler
John W. Winkelman
Gary S. Richardson

Disturbed sleep is among the most frequent health complaints physicians encounter. More than one-half of adults in the United States experience at least intermittent sleep disturbance. For most, it is an occasional night of poor sleep or daytime sleepiness. However, the Institute of Medicine has estimated that 50–70 million Americans suffer from a chronic disorder of sleep and wakefulness, which can lead to serious impairment of daytime functioning. In addition, such problems may contribute to or exacerbate medical or psychiatric conditions. Thirty years ago, many such complaints were treated with hypnotic medications without further diagnostic evaluation. Since then, a distinct class of sleep and arousal disorders has been identified.

PHYSIOLOGY OF SLEEP AND WAKEFULNESS

Given the opportunity, most adults will sleep 7–8 h per night, although the timing, duration, and internal structure of sleep vary among healthy individuals and as a function of age. At the extremes, infants and the elderly have frequent interruptions of sleep. In the United States, adults tend to have one consolidated sleep episode per day, although in some cultures sleep may be divided into a mid-afternoon nap and a shortened night sleep. Two principal neural systems govern the expression of the sleep and wakefulness states within the daily cycle. The first potentiates sleep in proportion to the duration of wakefulness (the "sleep homeostat"), while the second rhythmically modulates sleep and wakefulness tendencies at appropriate phases of the 24-h day (the circadian clock). Intrinsic abnormalities in the function of either of these systems, or extrinsic disturbances (environmental, drug- or illness-related) that supersede their normal expression, can lead to clinically recognizable sleep disorders.

STATES AND STAGES OF SLEEP

States and stages of human sleep are defined on the basis of characteristic patterns in the electroencephalogram (EEG), the electrooculogram (EOG—a measure of eye-movement activity), and the surface electromyogram (EMG) measured on the chin and neck. The continuous recording of this array of electrophysiologic parameters to define sleep and wakefulness is termed *polysomnography*.

Polysomnographic profiles define two states of sleep: (1) rapid-eye-movement (REM) sleep and (2) non-rapid-eye-movement (NREM) sleep. NREM sleep is further subdivided into three stages, characterized by increasing arousal threshold and slowing of the cortical EEG. REM sleep is characterized by a low-amplitude, mixed-frequency EEG similar to that of NREM stage N1 sleep. The EOG shows bursts of REM similar to those seen during eyes-open wakefulness. Chin EMG activity is absent, reflecting the brainstem-mediated muscle atonia that is characteristic of that state.

ORGANIZATION OF HUMAN SLEEP

Normal nocturnal sleep in adults displays a consistent organization from night to night (Fig. 27-1). After sleep onset, sleep usually progresses through NREM stages N1–N3 sleep within 45–60 min. Slow-wave sleep (NREM stage N3 sleep) predominates in the first third of the night and comprises 15–25% of total nocturnal sleep time in young adults. The percentage of slow-wave sleep is influenced by several factors, most notably age (see below). Prior sleep deprivation increases the rapidity of sleep onset and both the intensity and amount of slow-wave sleep.

The first REM sleep episode usually occurs in the second hour of sleep. More rapid onset of REM sleep in an adult (particularly if <30 min) may suggest pathology such as endogenous depression, narcolepsy, circadian rhythm disorders, or drug withdrawal. NREM and REM alternate through the night with an average period of 90–110 min (the "ultradian" sleep cycle). Overall, REM sleep constitutes 20–25% of total sleep, and NREM stages N1 and N2 are 50–60%.

Age has a profound impact on sleep state organization (Fig. 27-1). Slow-wave sleep is most intense and prominent during childhood, decreasing sharply coincident with puberty and across the second and third decades of life. After age 30, there is a continued decline in the amount of slow-wave sleep, and the amplitude of delta EEG activity comprising slow-wave sleep is profoundly reduced. The depth of slow-wave sleep, as measured by the arousal threshold to auditory stimulation, also decreases with age. In the otherwise healthy older person, slow-wave sleep may be completely absent, particularly in males. Paradoxically, older people are better able to tolerate acute sleep deprivation than young adults, maintaining reaction time and sustaining vigilance with fewer lapses of attention.

A different age profile exists for REM sleep than for slow-wave sleep. In infancy, REM sleep may comprise 50% of total sleep time, and the percentage is inversely proportional to developmental age. The amount of REM sleep falls off sharply over the first postnatal year as a mature REM-NREM cycle develops; thereafter, REM sleep occupies a relatively constant percentage of total sleep time.

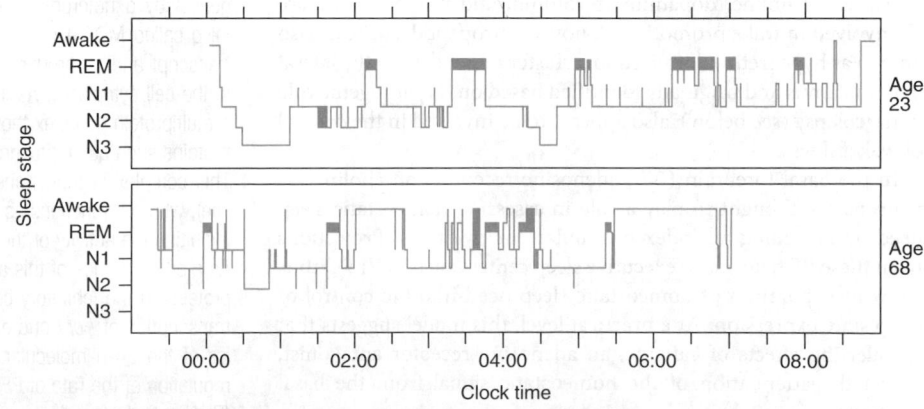

Figure 27-1 **Stages of REM sleep** (solid bars), the three stages of NREM sleep, and wakefulness over the course of the entire night for representative young and older adult men. Characteristic features of sleep in older people include reduction of slow-wave sleep, frequent spontaneous awakenings, early sleep onset, and early morning awakening. *(From the Division of Sleep Medicine, Brigham and Women's Hospital.)*

■ NEUROANATOMY OF SLEEP

Experimental studies in animals have variously implicated the medullary reticular formation, the thalamus, and the basal forebrain in the generation of sleep, while the brainstem reticular formation, the midbrain, the subthalamus, the thalamus, and the basal forebrain have all been suggested to play a role in the generation of wakefulness or EEG arousal.

Current models suggest that the capacity for sleep and wakefulness generation is distributed along an axial "core" of neurons extending from the brainstem rostrally to the basal forebrain. A cluster of γ-aminobutyric acid (GABA) and galaninergic neurons in the ventrolateral preoptic (VLPO) hypothalamus is selectively activated coincident with sleep onset. These neurons project to and inhibit the multiple neural wakefulness centers that comprise the ascending arousal system, and selective cell-specific lesions of VLPO substantially reduce sleep time, indicating that the hypothalamic VLPO neurons play an executive role in sleep regulation. More recent data have identified another sleep center, the median preoptic nucleus (MnPOn) of the hypothalamus with similar activation patterns and projections, suggesting that, like that of wakefulness, executive control of sleep may also be multicentric.

Specific regions in the pons are associated with the neurophysiologic correlates of REM sleep. Small lesions in the dorsal pons result in the loss of the descending muscle inhibition normally associated with REM sleep; microinjections of the cholinergic agonist carbachol into the pontine reticular formation produce a state with all of the features of REM sleep. These experimental manipulations are mimicked by pathologic conditions in humans and animals. A prominent feature of narcolepsy, for example, is abrupt, complete, or partial paralysis (cataplexy) in response to a variety of stimuli, a pathologic activation of neural systems mediating the atonia of normal REM sleep. In narcoleptic dogs, physostigmine, a central cholinesterase inhibitor, increases the frequency of cataplexy episodes, while atropine decreases their frequency. Conversely, in REM sleep behavior disorder (see below), patients suffer from a failure of normal motor inhibition during REM sleep, resulting in involuntary, occasionally violent, movement arising out of dream episodes.

■ NEUROCHEMISTRY OF SLEEP

Early experimental studies that focused on the raphe nuclei of the brainstem appeared to implicate serotonin as the primary sleep-promoting neurotransmitter, while catecholamines were considered to be responsible for wakefulness. Simple neurochemical models have given way to more complex formulations involving multiple parallel waking systems. Pharmacologic studies suggest that histamine, acetylcholine, dopamine, serotonin, and noradrenaline are all involved in wake promotion. A novel neuropeptide, orexin (also known as hypocretin), localized to a cluster of neurons in the lateral hypothalamus and originally identified based on its pathogenic role in narcolepsy (see below), also appears to be involved in the control of wakefulness.

In the basal forebrain (BF), adenosine receptors on cholinergic neurons are thought to play a role in assessing homeostatic sleep need by providing an index of cellular energy status. Projections from these BF neurons to executive sleep centers such as VLPO thus allow incorporation of homeostatic sleep need into the control of sleep state expression. At a practical level, this model suggests that the alerting effects of caffeine, an adenosine receptor antagonist, reflect the attenuation of the homeostatic signal from the basal forebrain.

The prominent hypnotic effects of benzodiazepine receptor agonists suggest that endogenous ligands of this receptor may be involved in normal sleep physiology. While neurosteroids with activity at this receptor have been identified, their role in normal

sleep-wake control remains unclear. In addition, a broad array of endogenous sleep- and wake-promoting substances have been identified, the role of which in normal sleep-wake control remains unclear. These include corticotropin-releasing hormone (CRH), prostaglandin D$_2$, delta sleep–inducing peptide, muramyl dipeptide, interleukin 1, fatty acid primary amides, and melatonin.

■ PHYSIOLOGY OF CIRCADIAN RHYTHMICITY

The sleep-wake cycle is the most evident of the many 24-h rhythms in humans. Prominent daily variations also occur in endocrine, thermoregulatory, cardiac, pulmonary, renal, gastrointestinal, and neurobehavioral functions. At the molecular level, endogenous circadian rhythmicity is driven by self-sustaining transcriptional/translational feedback loops (Fig. 27-2). In evaluating a daily variation in humans, it is important to distinguish between those rhythmic components passively evoked by periodic environmental or behavioral changes (e.g., the increase in blood pressure and heart rate that occurs upon assumption of the upright posture) and those actively driven by an endogenous oscillatory process (e.g., the circadian variation in plasma cortisol that persists under a variety of environmental and behavioral conditions).

While it is now recognized that many peripheral tissues in mammals have circadian clocks that regulate diverse physiologic processes, these independent tissue-specific oscillations are coordinated by a central neural pacemaker located in the suprachiasmatic nuclei (SCN) of the hypothalamus. Bilateral destruction of these nuclei results in a loss of the endogenous circadian rhythm of

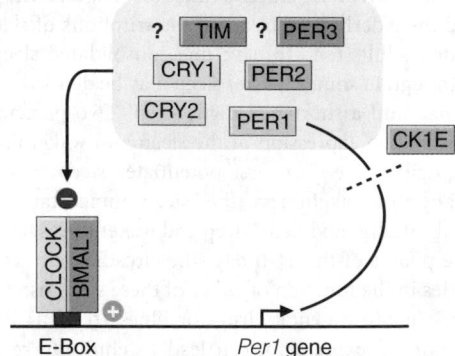

Figure 27-2   Model of the molecular feedback loop at the core of the mammalian circadian clock. The positive element of the feedback loop (+) is the transcriptional activation of the Per1 gene (and probably other clock genes) by a heterodimer of the transcription factors CLOCK and BMAL1 (also called MOP3) bound to an E-box DNA regulatory element. The *Per1* transcript and its product, the clock component PER1 protein, accumulate in the cell cytoplasm. As it accumulates, the PER1 protein is recruited into a multiprotein complex thought to contain other circadian clock component proteins such as cryptochromes (CRYs), Period proteins (PERs), and others. This complex is then transported into the cell nucleus (across the dotted line), where it functions as the negative element in the feedback loop (–) by inhibiting the activity of the CLOCK-BMAL1 transcription factor heterodimer. As a consequence of this action, the concentration of PER1 and other clock proteins in the inhibitory complex falls, allowing CLOCK-BMAL1 to activate transcription of *Per1* and other genes and begin another cycle. The dynamics of the 24-h molecular cycle are controlled at several levels, including regulation of the rate of PER protein degradation by casein kinase-1 epsilon (CK1E). Additional limbs of this genetic regulatory network, omitted for the sake of clarity, are thought to contribute stability. Question marks denote putative clock proteins, such as Timeless (TIM), as yet lacking genetic proof of a role in the mammalian clock mechanism. *(Copyright Charles J. Weitz, PhD, Department of Neurobiology, Harvard Medical School.)*

locomotor activity, which can be restored only by transplantation of the same structure from a donor animal. The genetically determined period of this endogenous neural oscillator, which averages ~24.2 h in humans, is normally synchronized to the 24-h period of the environmental light-dark cycle. Small differences in circadian period underlie variations in diurnal preference, with the circadian period shorter in individuals who typically rise early compared to those who typically go to bed late. Entrainment of mammalian circadian rhythms by the light-dark cycle is mediated via the retino-hypothalamic tract, a monosynaptic pathway that links specialized, photoreceptive retinal ganglion cells directly to the SCN. Humans are exquisitely sensitive to the resetting effects of light, particularly the shorter wavelengths (~460–500 nm) of the visible spectrum.

The timing and internal architecture of sleep are directly coupled to the output of the endogenous circadian pacemaker. Paradoxically, the endogenous circadian rhythms of sleep tendency, sleepiness, and REM sleep propensity all peak near the habitual wake time, just after the nadir of the endogenous circadian temperature cycle, whereas the circadian wake propensity rhythm peaks 1–3 h before the habitual bedtime. These rhythms are thus timed to oppose the homeostatic decline of sleep tendency during the habitual sleep episode and the rise of sleep tendency throughout the usual waking day, respectively. Misalignment of the output of the endogenous circadian pacemaker with the desired sleep-wake cycle can, therefore, induce insomnia, decreased alertness, and impaired performance evident in night-shift workers and airline travelers.

■ BEHAVIORAL CORRELATES OF SLEEP STATES AND STAGES

Polysomnographic staging of sleep correlates with behavioral changes during specific states and stages. During the transitional state between wakefulness and sleep (stage N1 sleep), subjects may respond to faint auditory or visual signals without "awakening." Short-term memory incorporation is inhibited at the onset of NREM stage N1 sleep, which may explain why individuals aroused from that transitional sleep stage frequently deny having been asleep. Such transitions may intrude upon behavioral wakefulness after sleep deprivation, notwithstanding attempts to remain continuously awake (see "Shift-Work Disorder," below).

Awakenings from REM sleep are associated with recall of vivid dream imagery >80% of the time. The reliability of dream recall increases with REM sleep episodes occurring later in the night. Imagery may also be reported after NREM sleep interruptions, though these typically lack the detail and vividness of REM sleep dreams. The incidence of NREM sleep dream recall can be increased by selective REM sleep deprivation, suggesting that REM sleep and dreaming per se are not inexorably linked.

■ PHYSIOLOGIC CORRELATES OF SLEEP STATES AND STAGES

All major physiologic systems are influenced by sleep. Changes in cardiovascular function include a decrease in blood pressure and heart rate during NREM and particularly during slow-wave sleep. During REM sleep, phasic activity (bursts of eye movements) is associated with variability in both blood pressure and heart rate mediated principally by the vagus nerve. Cardiac dysrhythmias may occur selectively during REM sleep. Respiratory function also changes. In comparison to relaxed wakefulness, respiratory rate becomes more regular during NREM sleep (especially slow-wave sleep) and tonic REM sleep and becomes very irregular during phasic REM sleep. Minute ventilation decreases in NREM sleep out of proportion to the decrease in metabolic rate at sleep onset, resulting in a higher PCO_2.

Endocrine function also varies with sleep. Slow-wave sleep is associated with secretion of growth hormone in men, while sleep in general is associated with augmented secretion of prolactin in both men and women. Sleep has a complex effect on the secretion of luteinizing hormone (LH): during puberty, sleep is associated with increased LH secretion, whereas sleep in the postpubertal female inhibits LH secretion in the early follicular phase of the menstrual cycle. Sleep onset (and probably slow-wave sleep) is associated with inhibition of thyroid-stimulating hormone and of the adrenocorticotropic hormone–cortisol axis, an effect that is superimposed on the prominent circadian rhythms in the two systems.

The pineal hormone melatonin is secreted predominantly at night in both day- and night-active species, reflecting the direct modulation of pineal activity by the circadian pacemaker through a circuitous neural pathway from the SCN to the pineal gland. Melatonin secretion is not dependent upon the occurrence of sleep, persisting in individuals kept awake at night. Secretion is inhibited by ambient light, an effect mediated by a neural connection from the retina via the SCN. The role of endogenous melatonin in normal sleep-wake regulation is unclear, but administration of exogenous melatonin can potentiate sleepiness and facilitate sleep onset when administered in the afternoon or evening, at a time when endogenous melatonin levels are low. The efficacy of melatonin as a sleep-promoting therapy for patients with insomnia is currently not known.

Sleep is also accompanied by alterations of thermoregulatory function. NREM sleep is associated with an attenuation of thermoregulatory responses to either heat or cold stress, and animal studies of thermosensitive neurons in the hypothalamus document an NREM-sleep-dependent reduction of the thermoregulatory set-point. REM sleep is associated with complete absence of thermoregulatory responsiveness, resulting in functional poikilothermy. However, the potential adverse impact of this failure of thermoregulation is blunted by inhibition of REM sleep by extreme ambient temperatures.

DISORDERS OF SLEEP AND WAKEFULNESS

APPROACH TO THE PATIENT: Sleep Disorders

Patients may seek help from a physician because of one of several symptoms: (1) an acute or chronic inability to initiate or maintain sleep adequately at night (insomnia); (2) chronic fatigue, sleepiness, or tiredness during the day; or (3) a behavioral manifestation associated with sleep itself. The specific approach to an insomnia complaint will depend on the nature of comorbid medical or psychiatric disease, if present. In general, however, the insomnia complaint should be specifically addressed as soon as it is recognized. This more aggressive approach reflects growing evidence that chronic insomnia may contribute to comorbid disease processes. For example, specific management of symptomatic insomnia at the time of diagnosis of major depressive disorder (MDD) has been shown to positively impact the response to antidepressants. Evidence that insomnia and sleep loss affect the perception of pain suggests that a similar approach is warranted in acute and chronic pain management. In general, at least for chronic insomnia, there is little evidence justifying an expectant approach in which specific insomnia therapy is deferred while comorbid disease is first addressed.

Table 27-1 outlines the diagnostic and therapeutic approach to the patient with a complaint of excessive daytime sleepiness.

A careful history is essential. In particular, the duration, severity, and consistency of the symptoms are important, along with the patient's estimate of the consequences of the sleep disorder on waking function. Information from a friend or family member can be invaluable; some patients may be unaware of, or will underreport, such potentially embarrassing symptoms as heavy snoring or falling asleep while driving.

TABLE 27-1 Evaluation of the Patient With the Complaint of Excessive Daytime Somnolence

Findings on History and Physical Examination	Diagnostic Evaluation	Diagnosis	Therapy
Obesity, snoring, hypertension	Polysomnography with respiratory monitoring	Obstructive sleep apnea	Continuous positive airway pressure; ENT surgery (e.g., uvulopalatopharyngoplasty); dental appliance; pharmacologic therapy (e.g., protriptyline); weight loss
Cataplexy, hypnogogic hallucinations, sleep paralysis, family history	Polysomnography with multiple sleep latency testing	Narcolepsy-cataplexy syndrome	Stimulants (e.g., modafinil, methylphenidate); REM-suppressant antidepressants (e.g., protriptyline); genetic counseling
Restless legs, disturbed sleep, predisposing medical condition (e.g., iron deficiency or renal failure)	Assessment for predisposing medical conditions	Restless legs syndrome	Treatment of predisposing condition, if possible; dopamine agonists (e.g., pramipexole, ropinirole)
Disturbed sleep, predisposing medical conditions (e.g., asthma), and/or predisposing medical therapies (e.g., theophylline)	Sleep-wake diary recording	Insomnias (see text)	Treatment of predisposing condition and/or change in therapy, if possible; behavioral therapy; short-acting benzodiazepine receptor agonist (e.g., zolpidem)

Abbreviations: EMG, electromyogram; ENT, ears, nose, throat; REM, rapid eye movement.

Patients with excessive sleepiness should be advised to avoid all driving until effective therapy has been achieved.

Completion by the patient of a day-by-day sleep-work-drug log for at least 2 weeks can help the physician better understand the nature of the complaint. Work times and sleep times (including daytime naps and nocturnal awakenings) as well as drug and alcohol use, including caffeine and hypnotics, should be noted each day.

Polysomnography is necessary for the diagnosis of specific disorders such as narcolepsy and sleep apnea and may be of utility in other settings as well.

■ EVALUATION OF INSOMNIA

Insomnia is the complaint of inadequate sleep; it can be classified according to the nature of sleep disruption and the duration of the complaint. Insomnia is subdivided into difficulty falling asleep (*sleep onset insomnia*), frequent or sustained awakenings (*sleep maintenance insomnia*), or early morning awakenings (*sleep offset insomnia*), though most insomnia patients present with two or more of these symptoms. Other insomnia patients present with persistent sleepiness/fatigue despite sleep of adequate duration (*nonrestorative sleep*). Similarly, the duration of the symptom influences diagnostic and therapeutic considerations. An insomnia complaint lasting one to several nights (within a single episode) is termed *transient insomnia* and is typically the result of situational stress or a change in sleep schedule or environment (e.g., jet lag disorder). *Short-term insomnia* lasts from a few days to 3 weeks. Disruption of this duration is usually associated with more protracted stress, such as recovery from surgery or short-term illness. *Long-term insomnia*, or *chronic insomnia*, lasts for months or years and, in contrast with short-term insomnia, requires a thorough evaluation of underlying causes (see below). Chronic insomnia is often a waxing and waning disorder, with spontaneous or stressor-induced exacerbations.

An occasional night of poor sleep, typically in the setting of stress or excitement about external events, is both common and without lasting consequences. However, persistent insomnia can lead to impaired daytime function, injury due to accidents, and the development of major depression. In addition, there is emerging evidence that individuals with chronic insomnia have increased utilization of health care resources, even after controlling for comorbid medical and psychiatric disorders.

All insomnias can be exacerbated and perpetuated by behaviors that are not conducive to initiating or maintaining sleep. *Inadequate sleep hygiene* is characterized by a behavior pattern prior to sleep or a bedroom environment that is not conducive to sleep, or irregularity in the timing or duration of the nightly sleep episode. Noise, light, or technology (e.g., television, radio, cell phone, mobile email device or computer) in the bedroom can interfere with sleep, as can a bed partner with periodic limb movements during sleep or one who snores loudly. Clocks can heighten the anxiety about the time it has taken to fall asleep. Drugs that act on the central nervous system, large meals, vigorous exercise, or hot showers just before sleep may all interfere with sleep onset. Many individuals participate in stressful work-related activities in the evening, producing a state incompatible with sleep onset. In preference to hypnotic medications, patients should be counseled to avoid stressful activities before bed, develop a soporific bedtime ritual, and prepare and reserve the bedroom environment for sleeping. Consistent, regular bedtimes and rising times should be maintained daily, including weekends.

■ PRIMARY INSOMNIA

Many patients with chronic insomnia have no clear, single identifiable underlying cause for their difficulties with sleep. Rather, such patients often have multiple etiologies for their insomnia, which may evolve over the years. In addition, the chief sleep complaint may change over time, with initial insomnia predominating at one point, and multiple awakenings or nonrestorative sleep occurring at other times. Subsyndromal psychiatric disorders (e.g., anxiety and mood complaints), negative conditioning to the sleep environment (psychophysiologic insomnia, see below), amplification of the time spent awake (paradoxical insomnia), physiologic hyperarousal, and poor sleep hygiene (see above) may all be present. As these processes may be both causes and consequences of chronic insomnia, many individuals will have a progressive course to their symptoms in which the severity is proportional to the chronicity, and much of the complaint may persist even after effective treatment of the initial inciting etiology. Treatment of insomnia is often directed to each of the putative contributing factors: behavior therapies for anxiety and negative conditioning (see below), pharmacotherapy and/or psychotherapy for mood/anxiety disorders, and an emphasis on maintenance of good sleep hygiene.

If insomnia persists after treatment of these contributing factors, empirical pharmacotherapy is often used on a nightly or intermittent basis. A variety of sedative compounds are used for this purpose. Alcohol and antihistamines are the most commonly used nonprescription sleep aids. The former may help with sleep onset but is associated with sleep disruption during the night and can escalate into abuse, dependence, and withdrawal in the predisposed individual. Antihistamines, which are the primary active ingredient in most over-the-counter sleep aids, may be of benefit when used intermittently but often produce rapid tolerance and may have multiple side effects (especially anticholinergic), which limit their use, particularly in the elderly. Benzodiazepine-receptor agonists are the most effective and well-tolerated class of medications for insomnia. The broad range of half-lives allows flexibility in the duration of sedative action. The most commonly prescribed agents in this family are zaleplon (5–20 mg), with a half-life of 1–2 h; zolpidem (5–10 mg) and triazolam (0.125–0.25 mg), with half-lives of 2–3 h; eszopiclone (1–3 mg), with a half-life of 5.5–8 h; and temazepam (15–30 mg) and lorazepam (0.5–2 mg), with half-lives of 6–12 h. Generally, side effects are minimal when the dose is kept low and the serum concentration is minimized during the waking hours (by using the shortest-acting effective agent). At least one benzodiazepine receptor agonist (eszopiclone) continues to be effective for 6 months of nightly use. However, longer durations of use have not been evaluated, and it is unclear whether this is true of other agents in this class. Moreover, with even brief continuous use of benzodiazepine-receptor agonists, rebound insomnia can occur upon discontinuation. The likelihood of rebound insomnia and tolerance can be minimized by short durations of treatment, intermittent use, or gradual tapering of the dose. For acute insomnia, nightly use of a benzodiazepine receptor agonist for a maximum of 2–4 weeks is advisable. For chronic insomnia, intermittent use is recommended, unless the consequences of untreated insomnia outweigh concerns regarding chronic use. Benzodiazepine receptor agonists should be avoided, or used very judiciously, in patients with a history of substance or alcohol abuse. The heterocyclic antidepressants (trazodone, amitriptyline, and doxepin) are the most commonly prescribed alternatives to benzodiazepine-receptor agonists due to their lack of abuse potential and lower cost. Trazodone (25–100 mg) is used more commonly than the tricyclic antidepressants as it has a much shorter half-life (5–9 h), has much less anticholinergic activity (sparing patients, particularly the elderly, constipation, urinary retention, and tachycardia), is associated with less weight gain, and is much safer in overdose. The risk of priapism is small (~1 in 10,000).

Psychophysiologic insomnia

Persistent *psychophysiologic insomnia* is a behavioral disorder in which patients are preoccupied with a perceived inability to sleep adequately at night. This sleep disorder begins like any other acute insomnia; however, the poor sleep habits and sleep-related anxiety ("insomnia phobia") persist long after the initial incident. Such patients become hyperaroused by their own efforts to sleep or by the sleep environment, and the insomnia becomes a conditioned or learned response. Patients may be able to fall asleep more easily at unscheduled times (when not trying) or outside the home environment. Polysomnographic recording in patients with psychophysiologic insomnia reveals an objective sleep disturbance, often with an abnormally long sleep latency; frequent nocturnal awakenings; and an increased amount of stage N1 transitional sleep. Rigorous attention should be paid to improving sleep hygiene, correction of counterproductive, arousing behaviors before bedtime, and minimizing

exaggerated beliefs regarding the negative consequences of insomnia. Behavioral therapies are the treatment modality of choice, with intermittent use of medications. When patients are awake for >20 min, they should read or perform other relaxing activities to distract themselves from insomnia-related anxiety. In addition, bedtime and wake time should be scheduled to restrict time in bed to be equal to their perceived total sleep time. This will generally produce sleep deprivation, greater sleep drive, and, eventually, better sleep. Time in bed can then be gradually expanded. In addition, methods directed toward producing relaxation in the sleep setting (e.g., meditation, muscle relaxation) are encouraged.

Adjustment insomnia (acute insomnia)

This typically develops after a change in the sleeping environment (e.g., in an unfamiliar hotel or hospital bed) or before or after a significant life event, such as a change of occupation, loss of a loved one, illness, or anxiety over a deadline or examination. Increased sleep latency, frequent awakenings from sleep, and early morning awakening can all occur. Recovery is generally rapid, usually within a few weeks. Treatment is symptomatic, with intermittent use of hypnotics and resolution of the underlying stress. *Altitude insomnia* describes a sleep disturbance that is a common consequence of exposure to high altitude. Periodic breathing of the Cheyne-Stokes type occurs during NREM sleep about half the time at high altitude, with restoration of a regular breathing pattern during REM sleep. Both hypoxia and hypocapnia are thought to be involved in the development of periodic breathing. Frequent awakenings and poor quality sleep characterize altitude insomnia, which is generally worse on the first few nights at high altitude but may persist. Treatment with acetazolamide can decrease time spent in periodic breathing and substantially reduce hypoxia during sleep.

■ COMORBID INSOMNIA

Insomnia associated with mental disorders

Approximately 80% of patients with psychiatric disorders describe sleep complaints. There is considerable heterogeneity, however, in the nature of the sleep disturbance both between conditions and among patients with the same condition. *Depression* can be associated with sleep onset insomnia, sleep maintenance insomnia, or early morning wakefulness. However, hypersomnia occurs in some depressed patients, especially adolescents and those with either bipolar or seasonal (fall/winter) depression (Chap. 391). Indeed, sleep disturbance is an important vegetative sign of depression and may commence before any mood changes are perceived by the patient. Consistent polysomnographic findings in depression include decreased REM sleep latency, lengthened first REM sleep episode, and shortened first NREM sleep episode; however, these findings are not specific for depression, and the extent of these changes varies with age and symptomatology. Depressed patients also show decreased slow-wave sleep and reduced sleep continuity.

In *mania* and *hypomania*, sleep latency is increased and total sleep time can be reduced. Patients with *anxiety disorders* tend not to show the changes in REM sleep and slow-wave sleep seen in endogenously depressed patients. *Chronic alcoholics* lack slow-wave sleep, have decreased amounts of REM sleep (as an acute response to alcohol), and have frequent arousals throughout the night. This is associated with impaired daytime alertness. The sleep of chronic alcoholics may remain disturbed for years after discontinuance of alcohol usage. Sleep architecture and physiology are disturbed in *schizophrenia*, with a decreased amount of slow-wave sleep (NREM stage N3 sleep) and a lack of augmentation of REM sleep following REM sleep deprivation; chronic schizophrenics often show daynight reversal, sleep fragmentation, and insomnia.

Insomnia associated with neurologic disorders

A variety of neurologic diseases result in sleep disruption through both indirect, nonspecific mechanisms (e.g., pain in cervical spondylosis or low back pain) or by impairment of central neural structures involved in the generation and control of sleep itself. For example, *dementia* from any cause has long been associated with disturbances in the timing of the sleep-wake cycle, often characterized by nocturnal wandering and an exacerbation of symptomatology at night (so-called sundowning).

Epilepsy may rarely present as a sleep complaint (Chap. 369). Often the history is of abnormal behavior, at times with convulsive movements during sleep. The differential diagnosis includes REM sleep behavior disorder, sleep apnea syndrome, and periodic movements of sleep (see above). Diagnosis requires nocturnal polysomnography with a full EEG montage. Other neurologic diseases associated with abnormal movements, such as *Parkinson's disease, hemiballismus, Huntington's chorea,* and *Tourette's syndrome* (Chap. 372), are also associated with disrupted sleep, presumably through secondary mechanisms. However, the abnormal movements themselves are greatly reduced during sleep. Headache syndromes (*migraine* or *cluster headache*) may show sleep-associated exacerbations (Chap. 14) by unknown mechanisms.

Fatal familial insomnia is a rare hereditary disorder caused by degeneration of anterior and dorsomedial nuclei of the thalamus. Insomnia is a prominent early symptom. Patients develop progressive autonomic dysfunction, followed by dysarthria, myoclonus, coma, and death. The pathogenesis is a mutation in the prion gene (Chap. 383).

Insomnia associated with other medical disorders

A number of medical conditions are associated with disruptions of sleep. The association is frequently nonspecific, e.g., sleep disruption due to chronic pain from rheumatologic disorders. Attention to this association is important in that sleep-associated symptoms are often the presenting or most bothersome complaint. Treatment of the underlying medical problem is the most useful approach. Sleep disruption can also result from the use of medications such as glucocorticoids (see below).

One prominent association is between sleep disruption and *asthma*. In many asthmatics there is a prominent daily variation in airway resistance that results in marked increases in asthmatic symptoms at night, especially during sleep. In addition, treatment of asthma with theophylline-based compounds, adrenergic agonists, or glucocorticoids can independently disrupt sleep. When sleep disruption is a side effect of asthma treatment, inhaled glucocorticoids (e.g., beclomethasone) that do not disrupt sleep may provide a useful alternative.

Cardiac ischemia may also be associated with sleep disruption. The ischemia itself may result from increases in sympathetic tone as a result of sleep apnea. Patients may present with complaints of nightmares or vivid, disturbing dreams, with or without awareness of the more classic symptoms of angina or of the sleep-disordered breathing. Treatment of the sleep apnea may substantially improve the angina and the nocturnal sleep quality. *Paroxysmal nocturnal dyspnea* can also occur as a consequence of sleep-associated cardiac ischemia that causes pulmonary congestion exacerbated by the recumbent posture.

Chronic obstructive pulmonary disease is also associated with sleep disruption, as is *cystic fibrosis, menopause, hyperthyroidism, gastroesophageal reflux, chronic renal failure,* and *liver failure.*

■ MEDICATION-, DRUG-, OR ALCOHOL-DEPENDENT INSOMNIA

Disturbed sleep can result from ingestion of a wide variety of agents. Caffeine is perhaps the most common pharmacologic cause of insomnia. It produces increased latency to sleep onset, more frequent arousals during sleep, and a reduction in total sleep time for up to 8–14 h after ingestion. Even small amounts of coffee can significantly disturb sleep in some patients; therefore, a 1- to 2-month trial without caffeine should be attempted in patients with these symptoms. Similarly, alcohol and nicotine can interfere with sleep, despite the fact that many patients use them to relax and promote sleep. Although alcohol can increase drowsiness and shorten sleep latency, even moderate amounts of alcohol increase awakenings in the second half of the night. In addition, alcohol ingestion prior to sleep is contraindicated in patients with sleep apnea because of the inhibitory effects of alcohol on upper airway muscle tone. Acutely, amphetamines and cocaine suppress both REM sleep and total sleep time, which return to normal with chronic use. Withdrawal leads to an REM sleep rebound. A number of prescribed medications can produce insomnia. Antidepressants, sympathomimetics, and glucocorticoids are common causes. In addition, severe rebound insomnia can result from the acute withdrawal of hypnotics, especially following the use of high doses of benzodiazepines with a short half-life. For this reason, hypnotic doses should be low to moderate, and prolonged drug tapering is encouraged.

■ RESTLESS LEGS SYNDROME (RLS)

Patients with this sensorimotor disorder report an irresistible urge to move the legs, or sometimes the upper extremities, that is often associated with creepy-crawling or aching dysesthesias deep within the affected limbs. For most patients with RLS, the dysesthesias and restlessness are much worse in the evening or night compared to the daytime and frequently interfere with the ability to fall asleep. The symptoms appear with inactivity and are temporarily relieved by movement. In contrast, paresthesias secondary to peripheral neuropathy persist with activity. The severity of this chronic disorder may wax and wane over time and can be exacerbated by sleep deprivation, caffeine, alcohol, serotonergic antidepressants, and pregnancy. The prevalence is 1–5% of young to middle-age adults and 10–20% of those aged >60 years. There appear to be important differences in RLS prevalence among racial groups, with higher prevalence in those of Northern European ancestry. Roughly one-third of patients (particularly those with an early age of onset) will have multiple affected family members. At least three separate chromosomal loci have been identified in familial RLS, though no gene has been identified to date. Iron deficiency and renal failure may cause RLS, which is then considered secondary RLS. The symptoms of RLS are exquisitely sensitive to dopaminergic drugs (e.g., pramipexole 0.25–0.5 mg q8PM or ropinirole 0.5–4 mg q8PM), which are the treatments of choice. Opioids, benzodiazepines, and gabapentin may also be of therapeutic value. Most patients with restless legs also experience periodic limb movements of sleep, although the reverse is not the case.

■ PERIODIC LIMB MOVEMENT DISORDER (PLMD)

Periodic limb movements of sleep (PLMS), previously known as *nocturnal myoclonus*, consists of stereotyped, 0.5- to 5.0-s extensions of the great toe and dorsiflexion of the foot, which recur every 20–40 s during NREM sleep, in episodes lasting from minutes to hours, as documented by bilateral surface EMG recordings of the anterior tibialis on polysomnography. PLMS is the principal objective polysomnographic finding in 17% of patients with insomnia and 11% of those with excessive daytime somnolence (Fig. 27-3). It is often unclear whether it is an incidental finding or the cause of disturbed sleep. When deemed to be the latter, PLMS is called PLMD. PLMS occurs in a wide variety of sleep disorders (including narcolepsy, sleep apnea, REM sleep behavior disorder, and various forms of insomnia) and may be associated with frequent arousals and an increased number of sleep-stage transitions. The pathophysiology

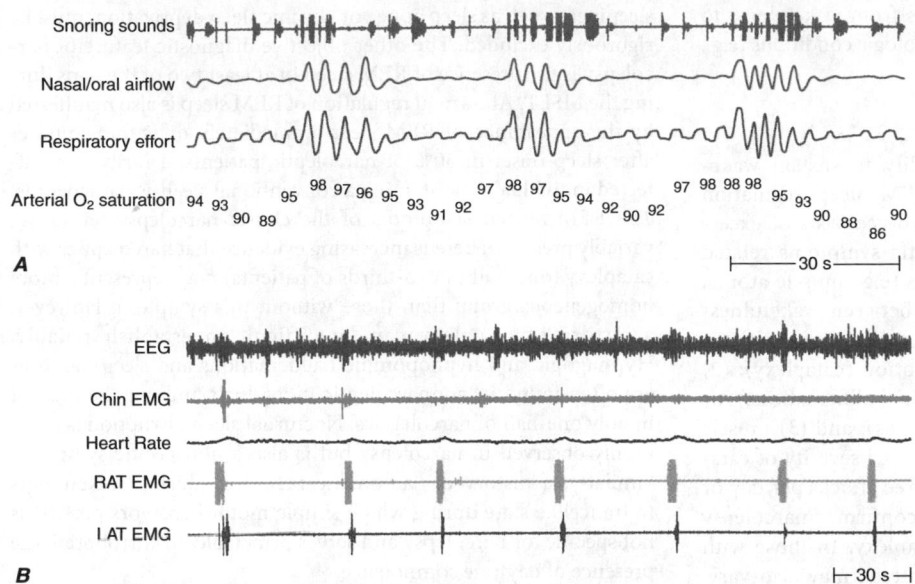

Figure 27-3 Polysomnographic recordings of (A) obstructive sleep apnea and (B) periodic limb movement of sleep. Note the snoring and reduction in air flow in the presence of continued respiratory effort, associated with the subsequent oxygen desaturation (upper panel). Periodic limb movements occur with a relatively constant intermovement interval and are associated with changes in the EEG and heart rate acceleration (lower panel). RAT, right anterior tibialis; LAT, left anterior tibialis. (From the Division of Sleep Medicine, Brigham and Women's Hospital.)

is not well understood, though individuals with high spinal transections can exhibit periodic leg movements during sleep, suggesting the existence of a spinal generator. Treatment options include dopaminergic medications or benzodiazepines.

▓ EVALUATION OF DAYTIME SLEEPINESS

Daytime impairment due to sleep loss may be difficult to quantify for several reasons. First, patients may be unaware of the extent of sleep deprivation. In obstructive sleep apnea, for example, the brief arousals from sleep associated with respiratory recovery after each apneic episode results in daytime sleepiness, despite the fact that the patient may be unaware of the sleep fragmentation. Second, subjective descriptions of waking impairment vary from patient to patient. Patients may describe themselves as "sleepy," "fatigued," or "tired" and may have a clear sense of the meaning of those terms, while others may use the same terms to describe a completely different condition. Third, sleepiness, particularly when profound, may affect judgment in a manner analogous to ethanol, such that subjective awareness of the condition and the consequent cognitive and motor impairment is reduced. Finally, patients may be reluctant to admit that sleepiness is a problem, both because they are generally unaware of what constitutes normal alertness and because sleepiness is generally viewed pejoratively, ascribed more often to a deficit in motivation than to an inadequately addressed physiologic sleep need.

Specific questioning about the occurrence of sleep episodes during normal waking hours, both intentional and unintentional, is necessary to determine the extent of the adverse effects of sleepiness on a patient's daytime function. Specific areas to be addressed include the occurrence of inadvertent sleep episodes while driving or in other safety-related settings, sleepiness while at work or school (and the relationship of sleepiness to work and school performance), and the effect of sleepiness on social and family life. Standardized questionnaires, e.g., the Epworth Sleepiness Scale, are now commonly used in clinical and research settings to quantify daytime sleep tendency and screen for excessive sleepiness.

Driving is particularly hazardous for patients with increased sleepiness. Reaction time is equally impaired by 24 h of sleep loss as by a blood alcohol level of 0.10 g/dL. More than half of Americans admit to having fallen asleep while driving. An estimated 250,000 motor vehicle crashes per year are due to drowsy drivers, causing about 20% of all serious crash injuries and deaths. Drowsy driving legislation, aimed at improving education of all drivers about the hazards of driving drowsy and establishing sanctions comparable to those for drunk driving, has been enacted in New Jersey and is pending in several other states. Screening for sleep disorders, provision of an adequate number of safe highway rest areas, maintenance of unobstructed shoulder rumble strips, and strict enforcement and compliance monitoring of hours-of-service policies are needed to reduce the risk of sleep-related transportation crashes. Evidence for significant daytime impairment in association either with the diagnosis of a primary sleep disorder, such as narcolepsy or sleep apnea, or with imposed or self-selected sleep-wake schedules (see "Shift-Work Disorder," below) raises the issue of the physician's responsibility to notify motor vehicle licensing authorities of the increased risk of sleepiness-related motor vehicle crashes. As with epilepsy, legal requirements vary from state to state, and existing legal precedents do not provide a consistent interpretation of the balance between the physician's responsibility and the patient's right to privacy. At a minimum, physicians should inform patients who report a history of nodding off or falling asleep at the wheel or who have excessive daytime sleepiness about the increased risk of operating a motor vehicle, advise such patients not to drive a motor vehicle until the cause of the excessive sleepiness has been diagnosed and successful treatment has been implemented, and reevaluate the patient to determine when it is safe for the patient to resume driving. Each of those steps should be documented in the patient's medical record.

The distinction between fatigue and sleepiness can be useful in the differentiation of patients with complaints of fatigue or tiredness in the setting of disorders such as fibromyalgia (Chap. 335), chronic fatigue syndrome (Chap. 389), or endocrine deficiencies such as hypothyroidism (Chap. 341) or Addison's disease (Chap. 342). While patients with these disorders can typically distinguish their daytime symptoms from the sleepiness that occurs with sleep deprivation, substantial overlap can occur. This is particularly true when the primary disorder also results in chronic sleep disruption (e.g., sleep apnea in hypothyroidism) or in abnormal sleep (e.g., fibromyalgia).

While clinical evaluation of the complaint of excessive sleepiness is usually adequate, objective quantification is sometimes necessary. Assessment of daytime functioning as an index of the adequacy of sleep can be made with the multiple sleep latency test (MSLT), which utilizes repeated measurement of sleep latency (time to onset of sleep) under standardized conditions during a day following quantified nocturnal sleep. The average latency across four to six tests (administered every 2 h across the waking day) provides an objective measure of daytime sleep tendency. Disorders of sleep that result in pathologic daytime somnolence can be reliably distinguished with the MSLT. In addition, the multiple measurements of sleep onset may identify direct transitions from wakefulness to REM sleep that are suggestive of specific pathologic conditions (e.g., narcolepsy).

■ NARCOLEPSY

Narcolepsy is both a disorder of the ability to sustain wakefulness voluntarily and a disorder of REM sleep regulation (Table 27-2). The classic "narcolepsy tetrad" consists of excessive daytime somnolence plus three specific symptoms related to an intrusion of REM sleep characteristics (e.g., muscle atonia, vivid dream imagery) into the transition between wakefulness and sleep: (1) sudden weakness or loss of muscle tone without loss of consciousness, often elicited by emotion (cataplexy); (2) hallucinations at sleep onset (hypnagogic hallucinations) or upon awakening (hypnopompic hallucinations); and (3) muscle paralysis upon awakening (sleep paralysis). The severity of cataplexy varies, as patients may have two to three attacks per day or per decade. Some patients with objectively confirmed narcolepsy (see below) may show no evidence of cataplexy. In those with cataplexy, the extent and duration of an attack may also vary, from a transient sagging of the jaw lasting a few seconds to rare cases of flaccid paralysis of the entire voluntary musculature for up to 20–30 min. Symptoms of narcolepsy typically begin in the second decade, although the onset ranges from ages 5–50 years. Once established, the disease is chronic without remissions. Secondary forms of narcolepsy have been described (e.g., after head trauma).

Narcolepsy affects about 1 in 4000 people in the United States and appears to have a genetic basis. Recently, several convergent lines of evidence suggest that the hypothalamic neuropeptide hypocretin (orexin) is involved in the pathogenesis of narcolepsy: (1) a mutation in the hypocretin receptor 2 gene has been associated with canine narcolepsy; (2) hypocretin "knockout" mice that are genetically unable to produce this neuropeptide exhibit behavioral and electrophysiologic features resembling human narcolepsy; and (3) cerebrospinal fluid levels of hypocretin are reduced in most patients who have narcolepsy with cataplexy. The inheritance pattern of narcolepsy in humans is more complex than in the canine model. However, almost all narcoleptics with cataplexy are positive for HLA DQB1*0602 (Chap. 315), suggesting that an autoimmune process may be responsible.

Diagnosis

The diagnostic criteria continue to be a matter of debate. Certainly, objective verification of excessive daytime somnolence, typically with MSLT mean sleep latencies <8 min, is an essential if nonspecific diagnostic feature. Other conditions that cause excessive sleepiness, such as sleep apnea or chronic sleep deprivation, must be rigorously excluded. The other objective diagnostic feature of narcolepsy is the presence of REM sleep in at least two of the naps during the MSLT. Abnormal regulation of REM sleep is also manifested by the appearance of REM sleep immediately or within minutes after sleep onset in 50% of narcoleptic patients, a rarity in unaffected individuals maintaining a conventional sleep-wake schedule. The REM-related symptoms of the classic narcolepsy tetrad are variably present. There is increasing evidence that narcoleptics with cataplexy (one-half to two-thirds of patients) may represent a more homogeneous group than those without this symptom. However, a history of cataplexy can be difficult to establish reliably. Hypnagogic and hypnopompic hallucinations and sleep paralysis are often found in nonnarcoleptic individuals and may be present in only one-half of narcoleptics. Nocturnal sleep disruption is commonly observed in narcolepsy but is also a nonspecific symptom. Similarly, a history of "automatic behavior" during wakefulness (a trancelike state during which simple motor behaviors persist) is not specific for narcolepsy and serves principally to corroborate the presence of daytime somnolence.

TREATMENT	Narcolepsy

The treatment of narcolepsy is symptomatic. Somnolence is treated with wake-promoting therapeutics. Modafinil is now the drug of choice, principally because it is associated with fewer side effects than older stimulants and has a long half-life; 200–400 mg is given as a single daily dose. Older drugs such as methylphenidate (10 mg bid to 20 mg qid) or dextroamphetamine (10 mg bid) are still used as alternatives, particularly in refractory patients.

These latter medications are now available in slow-release formulations, extending their duration of action and allowing once-daily dosing.

Treatment of the REM-related phenomena of cataplexy, hypnagogic hallucinations, and sleep paralysis requires the potent REM sleep suppression produced by antidepressant medications. The tricyclic antidepressants [e.g., protriptyline (10–40 mg/d) and clomipramine (25–50 mg/d)] and the selective serotonin reuptake inhibitors (SSRIs) [e.g., fluoxetine (10–20 mg/d)] are commonly used for this purpose. Efficacy of the antidepressants is limited largely by anticholinergic side effects (tricyclics) and by sleep disturbance and sexual dysfunction (SSRIs). Alternately, gamma hydroxybutyrate (GHB), given at bedtime, and 4 h later, is effective in reducing daytime cataplectic episodes. Adequate nocturnal sleep time and planned daytime naps (when possible) are important preventive measures.

■ SLEEP APNEA SYNDROMES

Respiratory dysfunction during sleep is a common, serious cause of excessive daytime somnolence as well as of disturbed nocturnal sleep. An estimated 2–5 million individuals in the United States have a reduction or cessation of breathing for 10–150 s from thirty to several hundred times every night during sleep. These episodes may be due to either an occlusion of the airway (obstructive sleep apnea), absence of respiratory effort (central sleep apnea), or a combination of these factors (mixed sleep apnea) (Fig. 27-3). Failure to recognize and treat these conditions appropriately may lead to impairment of daytime alertness, increased risk of sleep-related motor vehicle accidents, hypertension and other serious cardiovascular complications, and increased mortality. Sleep apnea is particularly prevalent in overweight men and in the elderly, yet it is estimated to remain undiagnosed in 80–90% of affected individuals.

TABLE 27-2 Prevalence of Symptoms in Narcolepsy

Symptom	Prevalence, %
Excessive daytime somnolence	100
Disturbed sleep	87
Cataplexy	76
Hypnagogic hallucinations	68
Sleep paralysis	64
Memory problems	50

Source: Modified from TA Roth, L Merlotti, in SA Burton et al (eds): *Narcolepsy 3rd International Symposium: Selected Symposium Proceedings.* Chicago, Matrix Communications, 1989.

This is unfortunate since effective treatments are available. Readers are referred to Chap. 265 for a comprehensive review of the diagnosis and treatment of patients with these conditions.

■ PARASOMNIAS

The term *parasomnia* refers to abnormal behaviors or experiences that arise from or occur during sleep. A continuum of parasomnias arise from NREM sleep, from brief confusional arousals to sleepwalking and night terrors. The presenting complaint is usually related to the behavior itself, but the parasomnias can disturb sleep continuity or lead to mild impairments in daytime alertness. Two main parasomnias occur in REM sleep: REM sleep behavior disorder (RBD), which will be described below, and nightmare disorder.

Sleepwalking (somnambulism)

Patients affected by this disorder carry out automatic motor activities that range from simple to complex. Individuals may walk, urinate inappropriately, eat, or exit from the house while remaining only partially aware. Full arousal may be difficult, and individuals may rarely respond to attempted awakening with agitation or even violence. Sleepwalking arises from slow-wave sleep (NREM stage N3 sleep), usually in the first 2 h of the night, and is most common in children and adolescents, when these sleep stages are most robust. Episodes are usually isolated but may be recurrent in 1–6% of patients. The cause is unknown, though it has a familial basis in roughly one-third of cases.

Sleep terrors

This disorder, also called *pavor nocturnus*, occurs primarily in young children during the first several hours after sleep onset, in slow-wave sleep (NREM stage N3 sleep). The child suddenly screams, exhibiting autonomic arousal with sweating, tachycardia, and hyperventilation. The individual may be difficult to arouse and rarely recalls the episode on awakening in the morning. Parents are usually reassured to learn that the condition is self-limited and benign and that no specific therapy is indicated. Both sleep terrors and sleepwalking represent abnormalities of arousal. In contrast, *nightmares* occur during REM sleep and cause full arousal, with intact memory for the unpleasant episode.

Sleep bruxism

Bruxism is an involuntary, forceful grinding of teeth during sleep that affects 10–20% of the population. The patient is usually unaware of the problem. The typical age of onset is 17–20 years, and spontaneous remission usually occurs by age 40. Sex distribution appears to be equal. In many cases, the diagnosis is made during dental examination, damage is minor, and no treatment is indicated. In more severe cases, treatment with a rubber tooth guard is necessary to prevent disfiguring tooth injury. Stress management or, in some cases, biofeedback can be useful when bruxism is a manifestation of psychological stress. There are anecdotal reports of benefit using benzodiazepines.

Sleep enuresis

Bedwetting, like sleepwalking and night terrors, is another parasomnia that occurs during sleep in the young. Before age 5 or 6 years, nocturnal enuresis should probably be considered a normal feature of development. The condition usually improves spontaneously by puberty, has a prevalence in late adolescence of 1–3%, and is rare in adulthood. In older patients with enuresis, a distinction must be made between primary and secondary enuresis, the latter being defined as bedwetting in patients who have previously been fully continent for 6–12 months. Treatment of primary enuresis is reserved for patients of appropriate age (>5 or 6 years) and consists of bladder training exercises and behavioral therapy. Urologic abnormalities are more common in primary enuresis and must be assessed by urologic examination. Important causes of secondary enuresis include emotional disturbances, urinary tract infections or malformations, cauda equina lesions, epilepsy, sleep apnea, and certain medications. Symptomatic pharmacotherapy is usually accomplished with desmopressin (0.2 mg qhs), oxybutynin chloride (5–10 mg qhs), or imipramine (10–50 mg qhs).

Miscellaneous parasomnias

Other clinical entities may be characterized as a parasomnia or a sleep-related movement disorder in that they occur selectively during sleep and are associated with some degree of sleep disruption. Examples include *jactatio capitis nocturna* (nocturnal headbanging, rhythmic movement disorder), confusional arousals, sleep-related eating disorder, and nocturnal leg cramps.

REM sleep behavior disorder (RBD)

RBD is a rare condition that is distinct from other parasomnias in that it occurs during REM sleep. It primarily afflicts men of middle age or older, many of whom have an existing, or developing, neurologic disease. Approximately one-half of patients with RBD will develop Parkinson's disease (Chap. 372) within 10–20 years. Presenting symptoms consist of agitated or violent behavior during sleep, as reported by a bed partner. In contrast to typical somnambulism, injury to the patient or bed partner is not uncommon, and, upon awakening, the patient reports vivid, often unpleasant, dream imagery. The principal differential diagnosis is nocturnal seizures, which can be excluded with polysomnography. In RBD, seizure activity is absent on the EEG, and disinhibition of the usual motor atonia is observed in the EMG during REM sleep, at times associated with complex motor behaviors. The pathogenesis is unclear, but damage to brainstem areas mediating descending motor inhibition during REM sleep may be responsible. In support of this hypothesis are the remarkable similarities between RBD and the sleep of animals with bilateral lesions of the pontine tegmentum in areas controlling REM sleep motor inhibition. Treatment with clonazepam (0.5–1.0 mg qhs) provides sustained improvement in almost all reported cases.

CIRCADIAN RHYTHM SLEEP DISORDERS

A subset of patients presenting with either insomnia or hypersomnia may have a disorder of sleep *timing* rather than sleep *generation*. Disorders of sleep timing can be either organic [i.e., due to an abnormality of circadian pacemaker(s) or its input from entraining stimuli] or environmental (i.e., due to a disruption of exposure to entraining stimuli from the environment). Regardless of etiology, the symptoms reflect the influence of the underlying circadian pacemaker on sleep-wake function. Thus, effective therapeutic approaches should aim to entrain the oscillator at an appropriate phase.

Jet lag disorder

More than 60 million persons experience transmeridian air travel annually, which is often associated with excessive daytime sleepiness, sleep onset insomnia, and frequent arousals from sleep, particularly in the latter half of the night. Gastrointestinal discomfort is common. The syndrome is transient, typically lasting 2–14 d depending on the number of time zones crossed, the direction of travel, and the traveler's age and phase-shifting capacity. Travelers who spend more time outdoors reportedly adapt more quickly than those who remain in hotel rooms, presumably due to brighter (outdoor) light exposure. Avoidance of antecedent sleep loss and obtaining nap sleep on the afternoon prior to overnight travel greatly reduce the difficulty of extended wakefulness. Laboratory studies suggest that sub milligram doses of the pineal hormone melatonin can enhance sleep efficiency, but only if taken when endogenous melatonin concentrations are low (i.e., during biologic daytime), and that melatonin may induce phase shifts in human rhythms. A large-scale clinical trial evaluating the safety and efficacy of melatonin as a treatment for jet lag disorder and other circadian sleep disorders is needed.

In addition to jet lag associated with travel across time zones, many patients report a behavioral pattern that has been termed *social jet lag*, in which their bedtimes and wake times on weekends or days off occur 4–8 h later than they do during the week. This recurrent displacement of the timing of the sleep-wake cycle is common in adolescents and young adults and is associated with sleep onset insomnia, poorer academic performance, increased risk of depressive symptoms, and excessive daytime sleepiness.

Shift-work disorder

More than 7 million workers in the United States regularly work at night, either on a permanent or rotating schedule. Many more begin work between 4 A.M. and 7 A.M., requiring them to commute and then work during the time of day that they would otherwise be asleep. In addition, each week millions more elect to remain awake at night to meet deadlines, drive long distances, or participate in recreational activities. This results in both sleep loss and misalignment of the circadian rhythm with respect to the sleep-wake cycle.

Studies of regular night-shift workers indicate that the circadian timing system usually fails to adapt successfully to such inverted schedules. This leads to a misalignment between the desired work-rest schedule and the output of the pacemaker and in disturbed daytime sleep in most individuals. Sleep deprivation, increased length of time awake prior to work, and misalignment of circadian phase produce decreased alertness and performance, increased reaction time, and increased risk of performance lapses, thereby resulting in greater safety hazards among night workers and other sleep-deprived individuals. Sleep disturbance nearly doubles the risk of a fatal work accident. Additional problems include higher rates of breast, colorectal, and prostate cancer and of cardiac, gastrointestinal, and reproductive disorders in long-term night-shift workers. Recently, the World Health Organization has added night-shift work to its list of probable carcinogens.

Sleep onset is associated with marked attenuation in perception of both auditory and visual stimuli and lapses of consciousness. The sleepy individual may thus attempt to perform routine and familiar motor tasks during the transition state between wakefulness and sleep (stage N1 sleep) in the absence of adequate processing of sensory input from the environment. Motor vehicle operators are especially vulnerable to sleep-related accidents since the sleep-deprived driver or operator often fails to heed the warning signs of fatigue. Such attempts to override the powerful biologic drive for sleep by the sheer force of will can yield a catastrophic outcome when sleep processes intrude involuntarily upon the waking brain. Such sleep-related attentional failures typically last only seconds but are known on occasion to persist for longer durations. These frequent brief intrusions of stage N1 sleep into behavioral wakefulness are a major component of the impaired psychomotor performance seen with sleepiness. There is a significant increase in the risk of sleep-related, fatal-to-the-driver highway crashes in the early morning and late afternoon hours, coincident with bimodal peaks in the daily rhythm of sleep tendency.

Resident physicians constitute another group of workers at risk for accidents and other adverse consequences of lack of sleep and misalignment of the circadian rhythm. Recurrent scheduling of resident physicians to work shifts of 24 h or more consecutive hours impairs psychomotor performance to a degree that is comparable to

alcohol intoxication, doubles the risk of attentional failures among intensive care unit interns working at night, and significantly increases the risk of serious medical errors in intensive care units, including a fivefold increase in the risk of serious diagnostic mistakes. Some 20% of hospital interns report making a fatigue-related mistake that injured a patient, and 5% admit making a fatigue-related mistake that results in the death of a patient. Moreover, working for >24 h consecutively increases the risk of percutaneous injuries and more than doubles the risk of motor vehicle crashes on the commute home. For these reasons, in 2008 the Institute of Medicine concluded that the practice of scheduling resident physicians to work for more than 16 consecutive hours without sleep is hazardous for both resident physicians and their patients.

From 5 to 10% of individuals scheduled to work at night or in the early morning hours have much greater than average difficulties remaining awake during night work and sleeping during the day; these individuals are diagnosed with chronic and severe shift-work disorder (SWD). Patients with this disorder have a level of excessive sleepiness during night work and insomnia during day sleep that the physician judges to be clinically significant; the condition is associated with an increased risk of sleep-related accidents and with some of the illnesses associated with night-shift work. Patients with chronic and severe SWD are profoundly sleepy at night. In fact, their sleep latencies during night work average just 2 min, comparable to mean sleep latency durations of patients with narcolepsy or severe daytime sleep apnea.

TREATMENT   Shift-Work Disorder

Caffeine is frequently used to promote wakefulness. However, it cannot forestall sleep indefinitely, and it does not shield users from sleep-related performance lapses. Postural changes, exercise, and strategic placement of nap opportunities can sometimes temporarily reduce the risk of fatigue-related performance lapses. Properly timed exposure to bright light can facilitate rapid adaptation to night-shift work.

While many techniques (e.g., light treatment) used to facilitate adaptation to night-shift work may help patients with this disorder, modafinil is the only therapeutic intervention that has ever been evaluated as a treatment for this specific patient population. Modafinil (200 mg, taken 30–60 min before the start of each night shift) is approved by the U.S. Food and Drug Administration as a treatment for the excessive sleepiness during night work in patients with SWD. Although treatment with modafinil significantly increases sleep latency and reduces the risk of lapses of attention during night work, SWD patients remain excessively sleepy at night, even while being treated with modafinil.

Safety programs should promote education about sleep and increase awareness of the hazards associated with night work. The goal should be to minimize both sleep deprivation and circadian disruption. Work schedules should be designed to minimize (1) exposure to night work, (2) the frequency of shift rotation so that shifts do not rotate more than once every 2–3 weeks, (3) the number of consecutive night shifts, and (4) the duration of night shifts. Shift durations of >16 h should be universally recognized as increasing the risk of sleep-related errors and performance lapses to a level that is unacceptable in nonemergency circumstances. At least 11 h off duty should be provided between work shifts, with at least one day off every week and two consecutive days off every month. Additional off duty time should be allocated after night work, since sleep efficiency is much lower during daytime hours.

Delayed sleep phase disorder

Delayed sleep phase disorder is characterized by (1) reported sleep onset and wake times intractably later than desired, (2) actual sleep times at nearly the same clock hours daily, and (3) essentially normal all-night polysomnography except for delayed sleep onset. Patients exhibit an abnormally delayed endogenous circadian phase, with the temperature minimum during the constant routine occurring later than normal. This delayed phase could be due to (1) an abnormally long, genetically determined intrinsic period of the endogenous circadian pacemaker; (2) an abnormally reduced phase-advancing capacity of the pacemaker; (3) a slower rate of buildup of homeostatic sleep drive during wakefulness; or (4) an irregular prior sleep-wake schedule, characterized by frequent nights when the patient chooses to remain awake well past midnight (for social, school, or work reasons). In most cases, it is difficult to distinguish among these factors, since patients with an abnormally long intrinsic period are more likely to "choose" such late-night activities because they are unable to sleep at that time. Patients tend to be young adults. This self-perpetuating condition can persist for years and does not usually respond to attempts to reestablish normal bedtime hours. Treatment methods involving bright-light phototherapy during the morning hours or melatonin administration in the evening hours show promise in these patients, although the relapse rate is high.

Advanced sleep phase disorder

Advanced sleep phase disorder (ASPD) is the converse of the delayed sleep phase syndrome. Most commonly, this syndrome occurs in older people, 15% of whom report that they cannot sleep past 5 A.M., with twice that number complaining that they wake up too early at least several times per week. Patients with ASPD experience excessive daytime sleepiness during the evening hours, when they have great difficulty remaining awake, even in social settings. Typically, patients awaken from 3 to 5 A.M. each day, often several hours before their desired wake times. In addition to age-related ASPD, an early-onset familial variant of this condition has also been reported. In one such family, autosomal dominant ASPD was due to a missense mutation in a circadian clock component (PER2, as shown in Fig. 27-2) that altered the circadian period. Patients with ASPD may benefit from bright-light phototherapy during the evening hours, designed to reset the circadian pacemaker to a later hour.

Non-24-h sleep-wake disorder

This condition can occur when the synchronizing input (i.e., the light-dark cycle) from the environment to the circadian pacemaker is compromised (as in many blind people with no light perception) or when the maximal phase-advancing capacity of the circadian pacemaker is not adequate to accommodate the difference between the 24-h geophysical day and the intrinsic period of the pacemaker in the patient. Alternatively, patients' self-selected exposure to artificial light may drive the circadian pacemaker to a >24-h schedule. Affected patients are not able to maintain a stable phase relationship between the output of the pacemaker and the 24-h day. Such patients typically present with an incremental pattern of successive delays in sleep propensity, progressing in and out of phase with local time. When the patient's endogenous circadian rhythms are out of phase with the local environment, insomnia coexists with excessive daytime sleepiness. Conversely, when the endogenous circadian rhythms are in phase with the local environment, symptoms remit. The intervals between symptomatic periods may last several weeks to several months. Blind individuals unable to perceive light are particularly susceptible to this disorder, although it can occur in sighted patients. Nightly low-dose (0.5 mg) melatonin administration has been reported to improve sleep and, in some cases, to induce synchronization of the circadian pacemaker.

■ MEDICAL IMPLICATIONS OF CIRCADIAN RHYTHMICITY

Prominent circadian variations have been reported in the incidence of acute myocardial infarction, sudden cardiac death, and stroke, the leading causes of death in the United States. Platelet aggregability is increased in the early morning hours, coincident with the peak incidence of these cardiovascular events. Misalignment of circadian phase, such as occurs during night-shift work, induces insulin resistance and higher glucose levels in response to a standard meal. Blood pressure of night workers with sleep apnea is higher than that of day workers. A better understanding of the possible role of circadian rhythmicity in the acute destabilization of a chronic condition such as atherosclerotic disease could improve the understanding of its pathophysiology.

Diagnostic and therapeutic procedures may also be affected by the time of day at which data are collected. Examples include blood pressure, body temperature, the dexamethasone suppression test, and plasma cortisol levels. The timing of chemotherapy administration has been reported to have an effect on the outcome of treatment. In addition, both the toxicity and effectiveness of drugs can vary during the day. For example, more than a fivefold difference has been observed in mortality rates following administration of toxic agents to experimental animals at different times of day. Anesthetic agents are particularly sensitive to time-of-day effects. Finally, the physician must be increasingly aware of the public health risks associated with the ever-increasing demands made by the duty-rest-recreation schedules in our round-the-clock society.

FURTHER READINGS

AHMED I, THORPY M: Clinical features, diagnosis and treatment of narcolepsy. Clin Chest Med 31:371, 2010

CZEISLER CA: Medical and genetic differences in the adverse impact of sleep loss on performance: Ethical considerations for the medical profession. Trans Am Clin Climatol Assoc 120:249, 2009

DODSON ER et al: Therapeutics for circadian rhythm sleep disorder. Sleep Med Clin 5:701, 2010

DOGHRAMJI K: The evaluation and management of insomnia. Clin Chest Med 31:327, 2010

GAY PC: Sleep and sleep-disordered breathing in the hospitalized patient. Respir Care 55:1240, 2010

MONJAN AA: Perspective on sleep and aging. Front Neurol 1:124, 2010

ROMERO-CORRAL A et al: Interactions between obesity and obstructive sleep apnea: Implications for treatment. Chest 137:711, 2010

CHAPTER **28**

Disorders of the Eye

Jonathan C. Horton

THE HUMAN VISUAL SYSTEM

The visual system provides a supremely efficient means for the rapid assimilation of information from the environment to aid in the guidance of behavior. The act of seeing begins with the capture of images focused by the cornea and lens on a light-sensitive membrane in the back of the eye called the *retina*. The retina is actually part of the brain, banished to the periphery to serve as a transducer for the conversion of patterns of light energy into neuronal signals. Light is absorbed by photopigment in two types of receptors: rods and cones. In the human retina there are 100 million rods and 5 million cones. The rods operate in dim (scotopic) illumination. The cones function under daylight (photopic) conditions. The cone system is specialized for color perception and high spatial resolution. The majority of cones are within the macula, the portion of the retina that serves the central 10° of vision. In the middle of the macula a small pit termed the *fovea*, packed exclusively with cones, provides the best visual acuity.

Photoreceptors hyperpolarize in response to light, activating bipolar, amacrine, and horizontal cells in the inner nuclear layer. After processing of photoreceptor responses by this complex retinal circuit, the flow of sensory information ultimately converges on a final common pathway: the ganglion cells. These cells translate the visual image impinging on the retina into a continuously varying barrage of action potentials that propagates along the primary optic pathway to visual centers within the brain. There are a million ganglion cells in each retina and hence a million fibers in each optic nerve.

Ganglion cell axons sweep along the inner surface of the retina in the nerve fiber layer, exit the eye at the optic disc, and travel through the optic nerve, optic chiasm, and optic tract to reach targets in the brain. The majority of fibers synapse on cells in the lateral geniculate body, a thalamic relay station. Cells in the lateral geniculate body project in turn to the primary visual cortex. This massive afferent retinogeniculocortical sensory pathway provides the neural substrate for visual perception. Although the lateral geniculate body is the main target of the retina, separate classes of ganglion cells project to other subcortical visual nuclei involved in different functions. Ganglion cells that mediate pupillary constriction and circadian rhythms are light sensitive owing to a novel visual pigment, melanopsin. Pupil responses are mediated by input to the pretectal olivary nuclei in the midbrain. The pretectal nuclei send their output to the Edinger-Westphal nuclei, which in turn provide parasympathetic innervation to the iris sphincter via an interneuron in the ciliary ganglion. Circadian rhythms are timed by a retinal projection to the suprachiasmatic nucleus. Visual orientation and eye movements are served by retinal input to the superior colliculus. Gaze stabilization and optokinetic reflexes are governed by a group of small retinal targets known collectively as the *brainstem accessory optic system.*

The eyes must be rotated constantly within their orbits to place and maintain targets of visual interest on the fovea. This activity, called *foveation*, or looking, is governed by an elaborate efferent motor system. Each eye is moved by six extraocular muscles that are supplied by cranial nerves from the oculomotor (III), trochlear (IV), and abducens (VI) nuclei. Activity in these ocular motor nuclei is coordinated by pontine and midbrain mechanisms for smooth pursuit, saccades, and gaze stabilization during head and body movements. Large regions of the frontal and parietooccipital cortex control these brainstem eye movement centers by providing descending supranuclear input.

CLINICAL ASSESSMENT OF VISUAL FUNCTION

■ REFRACTIVE STATE

In approaching a patient with reduced vision, the first step is to decide whether refractive error is responsible. In *emmetropia*, parallel rays from infinity are focused perfectly on the retina. Sadly, this condition is enjoyed by only a minority of the population. In *myopia*, the globe is too long, and light rays come to a focal point in front of the retina. Near objects can be seen clearly, but distant objects require a diverging lens in front of the eye. In *hyperopia*, the globe is too short, and hence a converging lens is used to supplement the refractive power of the eye. In *astigmatism*, the corneal surface is not perfectly spherical, necessitating a cylindrical corrective lens. In recent years it has become possible to correct refractive error with the excimer laser by performing LASIK (laser in situ keratomileusis) to alter the curvature of the cornea.

With the onset of middle age, *presbyopia* develops as the lens within the eye becomes unable to increase its refractive power to accommodate on near objects. To compensate for presbyopia, an emmetropic patient must use reading glasses. A patient already wearing glasses for distance correction usually switches to bifocals. The only exception is a myopic patient, who may achieve clear vision at near simply by removing glasses containing the distance prescription.

Refractive errors usually develop slowly and remain stable after adolescence, except in unusual circumstances. For example, the acute onset of diabetes mellitus can produce sudden myopia because of lens edema induced by hyperglycemia. Testing vision through a pinhole aperture is a useful way to screen quickly for refractive error. If visual acuity is better through a pinhole than it is with the unaided eye, the patient needs refraction to obtain best corrected visual acuity.

■ VISUAL ACUITY

The Snellen chart is used to test acuity at a distance of 6 m (20 ft). For convenience, a scale version of the Snellen chart called the Rosenbaum card is held at 36 cm (14 in.) from the patient (Fig. 28-1). All subjects should be able to read the 6/6 m (20/20 ft) line with each eye using their refractive correction, if any. Patients who need reading glasses because of presbyopia must wear them for accurate testing with the Rosenbaum card. If 6/6 (20/20) acuity is not present in each eye, the deficiency in vision must be explained. If it is worse than 6/240 (20/800), acuity should be recorded in terms of counting fingers, hand motions, light perception, or no light perception. Legal blindness is defined by the Internal Revenue Service as a best corrected acuity of 6/60 (20/200) or less in the better eye or a binocular visual field subtending 20° or less. For driving the laws vary by state, but most states require a corrected acuity of 6/12 (20/40) in at least one eye for unrestricted privileges. Patients with a homonymous hemianopia should not drive.

ROSENBAUM POCKET VISION SCREENER

95

874

2843

		Point	Jaeger	distance equivalent
				$\frac{20}{800}$
				$\frac{20}{400}$
		26	16	$\frac{20}{200}$
638 EШƎ XOO		14	10	$\frac{20}{100}$
8745 ƎMШ OXO		10	7	$\frac{20}{70}$
63925 MEƎ XOX		8	5	$\frac{20}{50}$
428365 ШEM OXO		6	3	$\frac{20}{40}$
374258 ƎШƎ XXO		5	2	$\frac{20}{30}$
937826 ШME XOO		4	1	$\frac{20}{25}$
428739 EШM OOX		3	1+	$\frac{20}{20}$

Card is held in good light 14 inches from eye. Record vision for each eye separately with and without glasses. Presbyopic patients should read thru bifocal segment. Check myopes with glasses only.

DESIGN COURTESY J. G. ROSENBAUM, M.D.

PUPIL GAUGE (mm.)

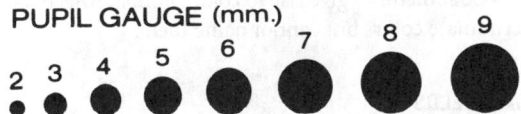

2 3 4 5 6 7 8 9

Figure 28-1 **The Rosenbaum card is a miniature, scale version of the Snellen chart for testing visual acuity at near.** When the visual acuity is recorded, the Snellen distance equivalent should bear a notation indicating that vision was tested at near, not at 6 m (20 ft), or else the Jaeger number system should be used to report the acuity.

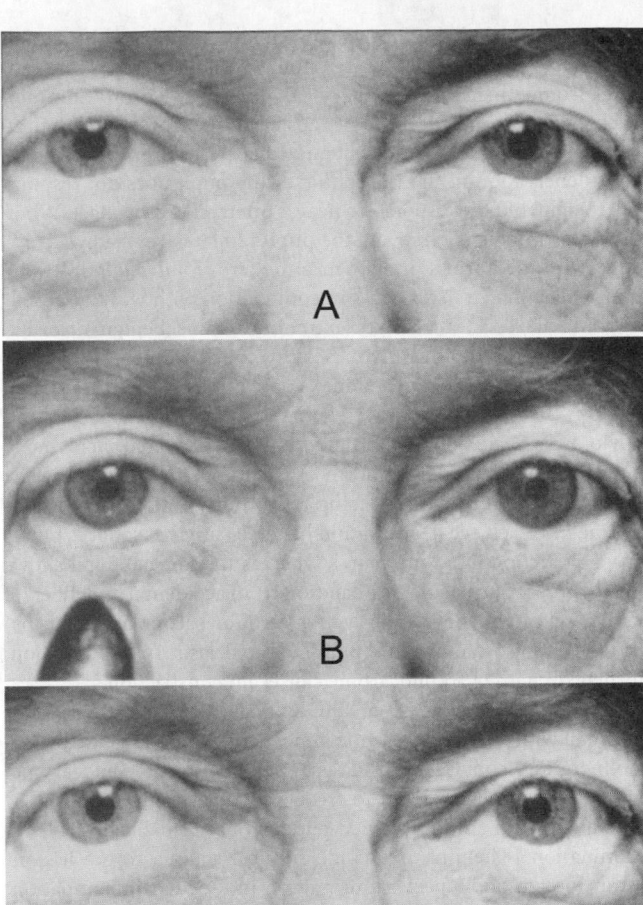

Figure 28-2 Demonstration of a relative afferent pupil defect (Marcus Gunn pupil) in the left eye, done with the patient fixating on a distant target. **A.** With dim background lighting, the pupils are equal and relatively large. **B.** Shining a flashlight into the right eye evokes equal, strong constriction of both pupils. **C.** Swinging the flashlight over to the damaged left eye causes dilation of both pupils, although they remain smaller than in **A.** Swinging the flashlight back over to the healthy right eye would result in symmetric constriction back to the appearance shown in **B.** Note that the pupils always remain equal; the damage to the left retina/optic nerve is revealed by weaker bilateral pupil constriction to a flashlight in the left eye compared with the right eye. *(From P Levatin: Arch Ophthalmol 62:768, 1959. Copyright © 1959 American Medical Association. All rights reserved.)*

■ PUPILS

The pupils should be tested individually in dim light with the patient fixating on a distant target. If the pupils respond briskly to light, there is no need to check the near response, because isolated loss of constriction (miosis) to accommodation does not occur. For this reason, the ubiquitous abbreviation PERRLA (pupils equal, round, and reactive to light and accommodation) implies a wasted effort with the last step. However, it is important to test the near response if the light response is poor or absent. Light-near dissociation occurs with neurosyphilis (Argyll Robertson pupil), with lesions of the dorsal midbrain (obstructive hydrocephalus, pineal region tumors), and after aberrant regeneration (oculomotor nerve palsy, Adie's tonic pupil).

An eye with no light perception has no pupillary response to direct light stimulation. If the retina or optic nerve is only partially injured, the direct pupillary response will be weaker than the consensual pupillary response evoked by shining a light into the other eye. This *relative afferent pupillary defect* (Marcus Gunn pupil) can be elicited with the swinging flashlight test (Fig. 28-2). It is an extremely useful sign in retrobulbar optic neuritis and other optic nerve diseases, in which it may be the sole objective evidence for disease.

Subtle inequality in pupil size, up to 0.5 mm, is a fairly common finding in normal persons. The diagnosis of essential or physiologic anisocoria is secure as long as the relative pupil asymmetry remains constant as ambient lighting varies. Anisocoria that increases in dim light indicates a sympathetic paresis of the iris dilator muscle. The triad of miosis with ipsilateral ptosis and anhidrosis constitutes *Horner's syndrome*, although anhidrosis is an inconstant feature. Brainstem stroke, carotid dissection, and neoplasm impinging on the sympathetic chain occasionally are identified as the cause of Horner's syndrome, but most cases are idiopathic.

Anisocoria that increases in bright light suggests a parasympathetic palsy. The first concern is an oculomotor nerve paresis. This possibility is excluded if the eye movements are full and the patient has no ptosis or diplopia. Acute pupillary dilation (mydriasis) can result from damage to the ciliary ganglion in the orbit. Common mechanisms are infection (herpes zoster, influenza), trauma (blunt, penetrating, surgical), and ischemia (diabetes, temporal arteritis). After denervation of the iris sphincter the pupil does not respond well to light, but the response to near is often relatively intact. When the near stimulus is removed, the pupil redilates very slowly compared with the normal pupil, hence the term *tonic pupil*. In *Adie's syndrome*, a tonic pupil occurs in conjunction with weak or absent tendon reflexes in the lower extremities. This benign disorder, which occurs predominantly in healthy young women, is assumed to represent a mild dysautonomia. Tonic pupils are also associated with Shy-Drager syndrome, segmental hypohidrosis, diabetes, and amyloidosis. Occasionally, a tonic pupil is discovered incidentally in an otherwise completely normal, asymptomatic individual. The diagnosis is confirmed by placing a drop of dilute (0.125%) pilocarpine into each eye. Denervation hypersensitivity produces pupillary constriction in a tonic pupil, whereas the normal pupil shows no response. Pharmacologic dilatation from accidental or deliberate instillation of anticholinergic agents (atropine, scopolamine drops) into the eye also can produce pupillary mydriasis. In this situation, normal strength (1%) pilocarpine causes no constriction.

Both pupils are affected equally by systemic medications. They are small with narcotic use (morphine, heroin) and large with anticholinergics (scopolamine). Parasympathetic agents (pilocarpine, demecarium bromide) used to treat glaucoma produce miosis. In any patient with an unexplained pupillary abnormality, a slit-lamp examination is helpful to exclude surgical trauma to the iris, an occult foreign body, perforating injury, intraocular inflammation, adhesions (synechia), angle-closure glaucoma, and iris sphincter rupture from blunt trauma.

◼ EYE MOVEMENTS AND ALIGNMENT

Eye movements are tested by asking the patient, with both eyes open, to pursue a small target such as a penlight into the cardinal fields of gaze. Normal ocular versions are smooth, symmetric, full, and maintained in all directions without nystagmus. Saccades, or quick refixation eye movements, are assessed by having the patient look back and forth between two stationary targets. The eyes should move rapidly and accurately in a single jump to their target. Ocular alignment can be judged by holding a penlight directly in front of the patient at about 1 m. If the eyes are straight, the corneal light reflex will be centered in the middle of each pupil. To test eye alignment more precisely, the cover test is useful. The patient is instructed to gaze upon a small fixation target in the distance. One eye is covered suddenly while the second eye is observed. If the second eye shifts to fixate on the target, it was misaligned. If it does not move, the first eye is uncovered and the test is repeated on the second eye. If neither eye moves, the eyes are aligned orthotropically. If the eyes are orthotropic in primary gaze but the patient complains of diplopia, the cover test should be performed with the head tilted or turned in whatever direction elicits diplopia. With practice the examiner can detect an ocular deviation (heterotropia) as small as 1–2° with the cover test. Deviations can be measured by placing prisms in front of the misaligned eye to determine the power required to neutralize the fixation shift evoked by covering the other eye.

◼ STEREOPSIS

Stereoacuity is determined by presenting targets with retinal disparity separately to each eye by using polarized images. The most popular office tests measure a range of thresholds from 800–40 seconds of arc. Normal stereoacuity is 40 seconds of arc. If a patient achieves this level of stereoacuity, one is assured that the eyes are aligned orthotropically and that vision is intact in each eye. Random dot stereograms have no monocular depth cues and provide an excellent screening test for strabismus and amblyopia in children.

◼ COLOR VISION

The retina contains three classes of cones, with visual pigments of differing peak spectral sensitivity: red (560 nm), green (530 nm), and blue (430 nm). The red and green cone pigments are encoded on the X chromosome, and the blue cone pigment on chromosome 7. Mutations of the blue cone pigment are exceedingly rare. Mutations of the red and green pigments cause congenital X-linked color blindness in 8% of males. Affected individuals are not truly color blind; rather, they differ from normal subjects in the way they perceive color and the way they combine primary monochromatic lights to match a particular color. Anomalous trichromats have three cone types, but a mutation in one cone pigment (usually red or green) causes a shift in peak spectral sensitivity, altering the proportion of primary colors required to achieve a color match. Dichromats have only two cone types and therefore will accept a color match based on only two primary colors. Anomalous trichromats and dichromats have 6/6 (20/20) visual acuity, but their hue discrimination is impaired. Ishihara color plates can be used to detect red-green color blindness. The test plates contain a hidden number that is visible only to subjects with color confusion from red-green color blindness. Because color blindness is almost exclusively X-linked, it is worth screening only male children.

The Ishihara plates often are used to detect acquired defects in color vision, although they are intended as a screening test for congenital color blindness. Acquired defects in color vision frequently result from disease of the macula or optic nerve. For example, patients with a history of optic neuritis often complain of color desaturation long after their visual acuity has returned to normal. Color blindness also can result from bilateral strokes involving the ventral portion of the occipital lobe (cerebral achromatopsia). Such patients can perceive only shades of gray and also may have difficulty recognizing faces (prosopagnosia). Infarcts of the dominant occipital lobe sometimes give rise to color anomia. Affected patients can discriminate colors but cannot name them.

◼ VISUAL FIELDS

Vision can be impaired by damage to the visual system anywhere from the eyes to the occipital lobes. One can localize the site of the lesion with considerable accuracy by mapping the visual field deficit by finger confrontation and then correlating it with the topographic anatomy of the visual pathway (Fig. 28-3). Quantitative visual field mapping is performed by computer-driven perimeters (Humphrey, Octopus) that present a target of variable intensity at fixed positions in the visual field (Fig. 28-3*A*). By generating an automated printout of light thresholds, these static perimeters provide a sensitive means of detecting scotomas in the visual field. They are exceedingly useful for serial assessment of visual function in chronic diseases such as glaucoma and pseudotumor cerebri.

The crux of visual field analysis is to decide whether a lesion is before, at, or behind the optic chiasm. If a scotoma is confined to one eye, it must be due to a lesion anterior to the chiasm, involving either the optic nerve or the retina. Retinal lesions produce scotomas that correspond optically to their location in the fundus. For example, a superior-nasal retinal detachment results in an inferior-temporal field cut. Damage to the macula causes a central scotoma (Fig. 28-3*B*).

Optic nerve disease produces characteristic patterns of visual field loss. Glaucoma selectively destroys axons that enter the superotemporal or inferotemporal poles of the optic disc, resulting in arcuate scotomas shaped like a Turkish scimitar, which

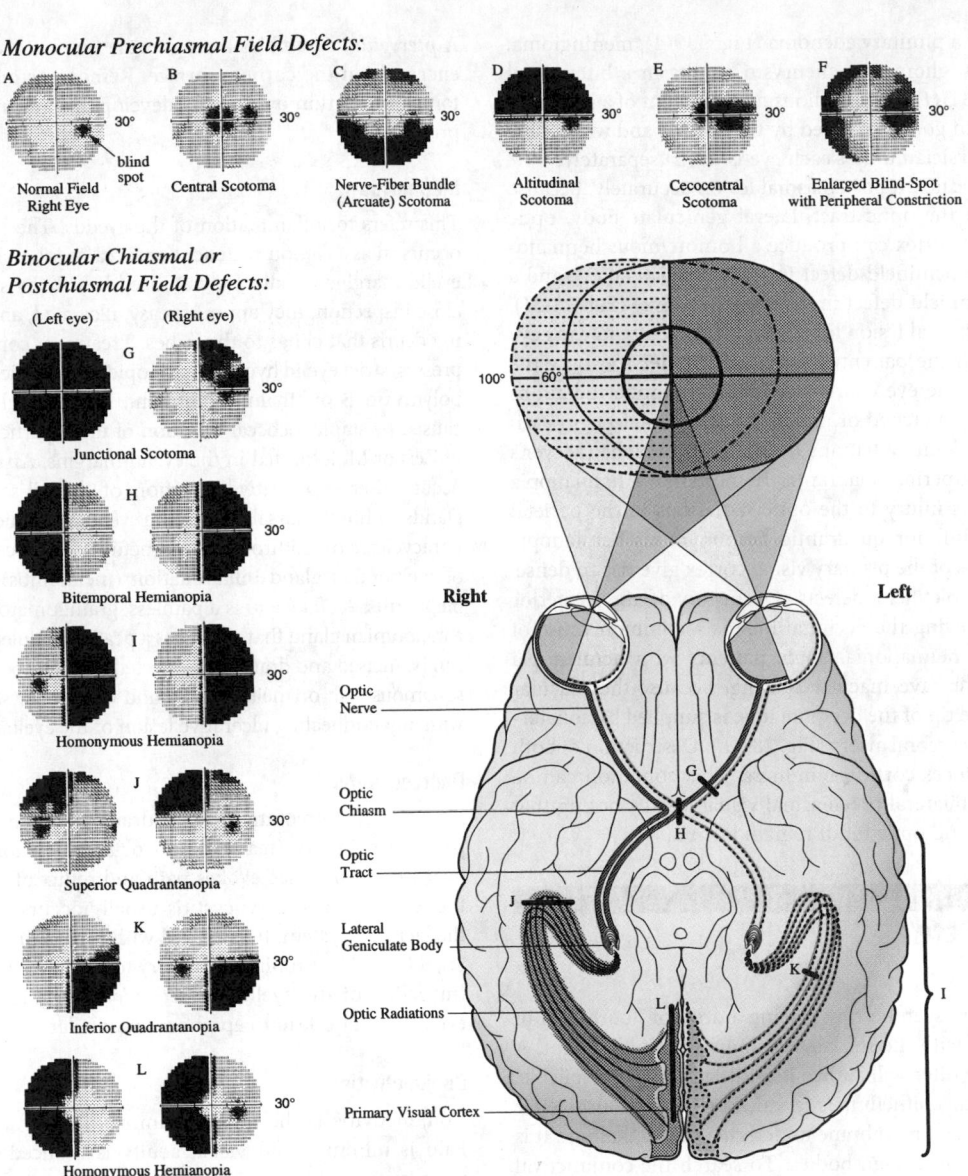

Figure 28-3 Ventral view of the brain, correlating patterns of visual field loss with the sites of lesions in the visual pathway. The visual fields overlap partially, creating 120° of central binocular field flanked by a 40° monocular crescent on either side. The visual field maps in this figure were done with a computer-driven perimeter (Humphrey Instruments, Carl Zeiss, Inc.). It plots the retinal sensitivity to light in the central 30° by using a gray scale format. Areas of visual field loss are shown in black. The examples of common monocular, prechiasmal field defects are all shown for the right eye. By convention, the visual fields are always recorded with the left eye's field on the left and the right eye's field on the right, just as the patient sees the world.

emanate from the blind spot and curve around fixation to end flat against the horizontal meridian (Fig. 28-3*C*). This type of field defect mirrors the arrangement of the nerve fiber layer in the temporal retina. Arcuate or nerve fiber layer scotomas also result from optic neuritis, ischemic optic neuropathy, optic disc drusen, and branch retinal artery or vein occlusion.

Damage to the entire upper or lower pole of the optic disc causes an altitudinal field cut that follows the horizontal meridian (Fig. 28-3*D*). This pattern of visual field loss is typical of ischemic optic neuropathy but also results from retinal vascular occlusion, advanced glaucoma, and optic neuritis.

About half the fibers in the optic nerve originate from ganglion cells serving the macula. Damage to papillomacular fibers causes a cecocentral scotoma that encompasses the blind spot and macula (Fig. 28-3*E*). If the damage is irreversible, pallor eventually appears in the temporal portion of the optic disc. Temporal pallor from a

cecocentral scotoma may develop in optic neuritis, nutritional optic neuropathy, toxic optic neuropathy, Leber's hereditary optic neuropathy, and compressive optic neuropathy. It is worth mentioning that the temporal side of the optic disc is slightly more pale than the nasal side in most normal individuals. Therefore, it sometimes can be difficult to decide whether the temporal pallor visible on fundus examination represents a pathologic change. Pallor of the nasal rim of the optic disc is a less equivocal sign of optic atrophy.

At the optic chiasm, fibers from nasal ganglion cells decussate into the contralateral optic tract. Crossed fibers are damaged more by compression than are uncrossed fibers. As a result, mass lesions of the sellar region cause a temporal hemianopia in each eye. Tumors anterior to the optic chiasm, such as meningiomas of the tuberculum sella, produce a junctional scotoma characterized by an optic neuropathy in one eye and a superior-temporal field cut in the other eye (Fig. 28-3*G*). More symmetric compression of the optic chiasm by a pituitary adenoma (Fig. 339-4), meningioma, craniopharyngioma, glioma, or aneurysm results in a bitemporal hemianopia (Fig. 28-3H). The insidious development of a bitemporal hemianopia often goes unnoticed by the patient and will escape detection by the physician unless each eye is tested separately.

It is difficult to localize a postchiasmal lesion accurately, because injury anywhere in the optic tract, lateral geniculate body, optic radiations, or visual cortex can produce a homonymous hemianopia (i.e., a temporal hemifield defect in the contralateral eye and a matching nasal hemifield defect in the ipsilateral eye) (Fig. 28-3I). A unilateral postchiasmal lesion leaves the visual acuity in each eye unaffected, although the patient may read the letters on only the left or right half of the eye chart. Lesions of the optic radiations tend to cause poorly matched or incongruous field defects in each eye. Damage to the optic radiations in the temporal lobe (Meyer's loop) produces a superior quadrantic homonymous hemianopia (Fig. 28-3J), whereas injury to the optic radiations in the parietal lobe results in an inferior quadrantic homonymous hemianopia (Fig. 28-3K). Lesions of the primary visual cortex give rise to dense, congruous hemianopic field defects. Occlusion of the posterior cerebral artery supplying the occipital lobe is a common cause of total homonymous hemianopia. Some patients with hemianopia after occipital stroke have macular sparing, because the macular representation at the tip of the occipital lobe is supplied by collaterals from the middle cerebral artery (Fig. 28-3L). Destruction of both occipital lobes produces cortical blindness. This condition can be distinguished from bilateral prechiasmal visual loss by noting that the pupil responses and optic fundi remain normal.

DISORDERS

■ RED OR PAINFUL EYE

Corneal abrasions

Corneal abrasions are seen best by placing a drop of fluorescein in the eye and looking with the slit lamp, using a cobalt-blue light. A penlight with a blue filter will suffice if a slit lamp is not available. Damage to the corneal epithelium is revealed by yellow fluorescence of the exposed basement membrane underlying the epithelium. It is important to check for foreign bodies. To search the conjunctival fornices, the lower lid should be pulled down and the upper lid everted. A foreign body can be removed with a moistened cotton-tipped applicator after a drop of a topical anesthetic such as proparacaine has been placed in the eye. Alternatively, it may be possible to flush the foreign body from the eye by irrigating copiously with saline or artificial tears. If the corneal epithelium has been abraded, antibiotic ointment and a patch should be applied to the eye. A drop of an intermediate-acting cycloplegic such as cyclopentolate hydrochloride 1% helps reduce pain by relaxing the ciliary body. The eye should be reexamined the next day. Minor abrasions may not require patching and cycloplegia.

Subconjunctival hemorrhage

This results from rupture of small vessels bridging the potential space between the episclera and the conjunctiva. Blood dissecting into this space can produce a spectacular red eye, but vision is not affected and the hemorrhage resolves without treatment. Subconjunctival hemorrhage is usually spontaneous but can result from blunt trauma, eye rubbing, or vigorous coughing. Occasionally it is a clue to an underlying bleeding disorder.

Pinguecula

Pinguecula is a small, raised conjunctival nodule at the temporal or nasal limbus. In adults such lesions are extremely common and have little significance unless they become inflamed (pingueculitis).

A *pterygium* resembles a pinguecula but has crossed the limbus to encroach on the corneal surface. Removal is justified when symptoms of irritation or blurring develop, but recurrence is a common problem.

Blepharitis

This refers to inflammation of the eyelids. The most common form occurs in association with acne rosacea or seborrheic dermatitis. The eyelid margins usually are colonized heavily by staphylococci. Upon close inspection, they appear greasy, ulcerated, and crusted with scaling debris that clings to the lashes. Treatment consists of warm compresses, strict eyelid hygiene, and topical antibiotics such as bacitracin/polymyxin B ophthalmic ointment. An external *hordeolum* (sty) is caused by staphylococcal infection of the superficial accessory glands of Zeis or Moll located in the eyelid margins. An internal hordeolum occurs after suppurative infection of the oil-secreting meibomian glands within the tarsal plate of the eyelid. Systemic antibiotics, usually tetracyclines or azithromycin, sometimes are necessary for treatment of meibomian gland inflammation (meibomitis) or chronic, severe blepharitis. A *chalazion* is a painless, granulomatous inflammation of a meibomian gland that produces a pealike nodule within the eyelid. It can be incised and drained or injected with glucocorticoids. Basal cell, squamous cell, or meibomian gland carcinoma should be suspected with any nonhealing ulcerative lesion of the eyelids.

Dacryocystitis

An inflammation of the lacrimal drainage system, dacryocystitis can produce epiphora (tearing) and ocular injection. Gentle pressure over the lacrimal sac evokes pain and reflux of mucus or pus from the tear puncta. Dacryocystitis usually occurs after obstruction of the lacrimal system. It is treated with topical and systemic antibiotics, followed by probing or surgery to reestablish patency. *Entropion* (inversion of the eyelid) or *ectropion* (sagging or eversion of the eyelid) can also lead to epiphora and ocular irritation.

Conjunctivitis

Conjunctivitis is the most common cause of a red, irritated eye. Pain is minimal, and visual acuity is reduced only slightly. The most common viral etiology is adenovirus infection. It causes a watery discharge, a mild foreign-body sensation, and photophobia. Bacterial infection tends to produce a more mucopurulent exudate. Mild cases of infectious conjunctivitis usually are treated empirically with broad-spectrum topical ocular antibiotics such as sulfacetamide 10%, polymyxin-bacitracin, or a trimethoprim-polymyxin combination. Smears and cultures usually are reserved for severe, resistant, or recurrent cases of conjunctivitis. To prevent contagion, patients should be admonished to wash their hands frequently, not to touch their eyes, and to avoid direct contact with others.

Allergic conjunctivitis

This condition is extremely common and often is mistaken for infectious conjunctivitis. Itching, redness, and epiphora are typical. The palpebral conjunctiva may become hypertropic with giant excrescences called cobblestone papillae. Irritation from contact lenses or any chronic foreign body also can induce formation of cobblestone papillae. *Atopic conjunctivitis* occurs in subjects with atopic dermatitis or asthma. Symptoms caused by allergic conjunctivitis can be alleviated with cold compresses, topical vasoconstrictors, antihistamines, and mast cell stabilizers such as cromolyn sodium. Topical glucocorticoid solutions provide dramatic relief of immune-mediated forms of conjunctivitis, but their long-term use is ill advised because of the complications of glaucoma, cataract, and secondary infection. Topical nonsteroidal anti-inflammatory drugs (NSAIDs) (e.g., ketorolac tromethamine) are better alternatives.

Keratoconjunctivitis sicca

Also known as dry eye, this produces a burning foreign-body sensation, injection, and photophobia. In mild cases the eye appears surprisingly normal, but tear production measured by wetting of a filter paper (Schirmer strip) is deficient. A variety of systemic drugs, including antihistaminic, anticholinergic, and psychotropic medications, result in dry eye by reducing lacrimal secretion. Disorders that involve the lacrimal gland directly, such as sarcoidosis and Sjögren's syndrome, also cause dry eye. Patients may develop dry eye after radiation therapy if the treatment field includes the orbits. Problems with ocular drying are also common after lesions affecting cranial nerve V or VII. Corneal anesthesia is particularly dangerous, because the absence of a normal blink reflex exposes the cornea to injury without pain to warn the patient. Dry eye is managed by frequent and liberal application of artificial tears and ocular lubricants. In severe cases the tear puncta can be plugged or cauterized to reduce lacrimal outflow.

Keratitis

Keratitis is a threat to vision because of the risk of corneal clouding, scarring, and perforation. Worldwide, the two leading causes of blindness from keratitis are trachoma from chlamydial infection and vitamin A deficiency related to malnutrition. In the United States, contact lenses play a major role in corneal infection and ulceration. They should not be worn by anyone with an active eye infection. In evaluating the cornea, it is important to differentiate between a superficial infection (*keratoconjunctivitis*) and a deeper, more serious ulcerative process. The latter is accompanied by greater visual loss, pain, photophobia, redness, and discharge. Slit-lamp examination shows disruption of the corneal epithelium, a cloudy infiltrate or abscess in the stroma, and an inflammatory cellular reaction in the anterior chamber. In severe cases, pus settles at the bottom of the anterior chamber, giving rise to a hypopyon. Immediate empirical antibiotic therapy should be initiated after corneal scrapings are obtained for Gram's stain, Giemsa stain, and cultures. Fortified topical antibiotics are most effective, supplemented with subconjunctival antibiotics as required. A fungal etiology should always be considered in a patient with keratitis. Fungal infection is common in warm humid climates, especially after penetration of the cornea by plant or vegetable material.

Herpes simplex

The *herpesviruses* are a major cause of blindness from keratitis. Most adults in the United States have serum antibodies to herpes simplex, indicating prior viral infection (Chap. 179). Primary ocular infection generally is caused by herpes simplex type 1 rather than type 2. It manifests as a unilateral follicular blepharoconjunctivitis that is easily confused with adenoviral conjunctivitis unless telltale vesicles appear on the periocular skin or conjunctiva. A dendritic pattern of corneal epithelial ulceration revealed by fluorescein staining is pathognomonic for herpes infection but is seen in only a minority of primary infections. Recurrent ocular infection arises from reactivation of the latent herpesvirus. Viral eruption in the corneal epithelium may result in the characteristic herpes dendrite. Involvement of the corneal stroma produces edema, vascularization, and iridocyclitis. Herpes keratitis is treated with topical antiviral agents, cycloplegics, and oral acyclovir. Topical glucocorticoids are effective in mitigating corneal scarring but must be used with extreme caution because of the danger of corneal melting and perforation. Topical glucocorticoids also carry the risk of prolonging infection and inducing glaucoma.

Herpes zoster

Herpes zoster from reactivation of latent varicella (chickenpox) virus causes a dermatomal pattern of painful vesicular dermatitis. Ocular symptoms can occur after zoster eruption in any branch of the trigeminal nerve but are particularly common when vesicles form on the nose, reflecting nasociliary (V1) nerve involvement (Hutchinson's sign). Herpes zoster ophthalmicus produces corneal dendrites, which can be difficult to distinguish from those seen in herpes simplex. Stromal keratitis, anterior uveitis, raised intraocular pressure, ocular motor nerve palsies, acute retinal necrosis, and postherpetic scarring and neuralgia are other common sequelae. Herpes zoster ophthalmicus is treated with antiviral agents and cycloplegics. In severe cases, glucocorticoids may be added to prevent permanent visual loss from corneal scarring.

Episcleritis

This is an inflammation of the episclera, a thin layer of connective tissue between the conjunctiva and the sclera. Episcleritis resembles conjunctivitis, but it is a more localized process and discharge is absent. Most cases of episcleritis are idiopathic, but some occur in the setting of an autoimmune disease. *Scleritis* refers to a deeper, more severe inflammatory process that frequently is associated with a connective tissue disease such as rheumatoid arthritis, lupus erythematosus, polyarteritis nodosa, granulomatosis with polyangiitis (Wegener's) or relapsing polychondritis. The inflammation and thickening of the sclera can be diffuse or nodular. In anterior forms of scleritis, the globe assumes a violet hue and the patient complains of severe ocular tenderness and pain. With posterior scleritis the pain and redness may be less marked, but there is often proptosis, choroidal effusion, reduced motility, and visual loss. Episcleritis and scleritis should be treated with NSAIDs. If these agents fail, topical or even systemic glucocorticoid therapy may be necessary, especially if an underlying autoimmune process is active.

Uveitis

Involving the anterior structures of the eye, uveitis also is called *iritis* or *iridocyclitis*. The diagnosis requires slit-lamp examination to identify inflammatory cells floating in the aqueous humor or deposited on the corneal endothelium (keratic precipitates). Anterior uveitis develops in sarcoidosis, ankylosing spondylitis, juvenile rheumatoid arthritis, inflammatory bowel disease, psoriasis, reactive arthritis (formerly known as Reiter's syndrome), and Behçet's disease. It also is associated with herpes infections, syphilis, Lyme disease, onchocerciasis, tuberculosis, and leprosy. Although anterior uveitis can occur in conjunction with many diseases, no cause is found to explain the majority of cases. For this reason, laboratory evaluation usually is reserved for patients with recurrent or severe anterior uveitis. Treatment is aimed at reducing inflammation and scarring by judicious use of topical glucocorticoids. Dilatation of the pupil reduces pain and prevents the formation of synechiae.

Posterior uveitis

This is diagnosed by observing inflammation of the vitreous, retina, or choroid on fundus examination. It is more likely than anterior uveitis to be associated with an identifiable systemic disease. Some patients have panuveitis, or inflammation of both the anterior and posterior segments of the eye. Posterior uveitis is a manifestation of autoimmune diseases such as sarcoidosis, Behçet's disease, Vogt-Koyanagi-Harada syndrome, and inflammatory bowel disease (Fig. 28-4). It also accompanies diseases such as toxoplasmosis, onchocerciasis, cysticercosis, coccidioidomycosis, toxocariasis, and histoplasmosis; infections caused by organisms such as *Candida*, *Pneumocystis carinii*, *Cryptococcus*, *Aspergillus*, herpes, and cytomegalovirus (see Fig. 182-1); and other diseases, such as syphilis, Lyme disease, tuberculosis, cat-scratch disease, Whipple's disease, and brucellosis. In multiple sclerosis, chronic inflammatory changes can develop in the extreme periphery of the retina (pars planitis or intermediate uveitis).

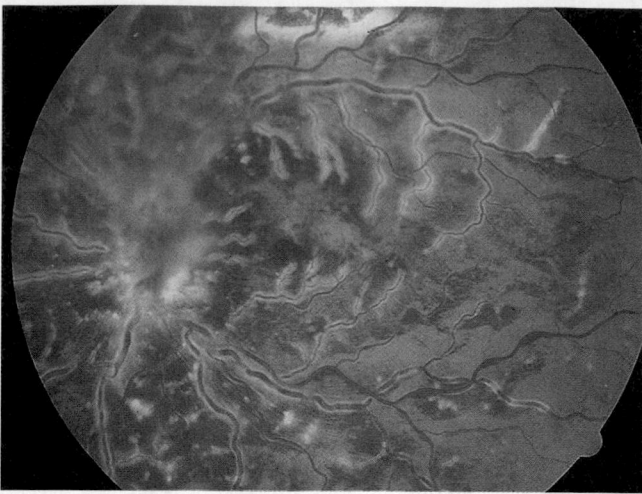

Figure 28-4   Retinal vasculitis, uveitis, and hemorrhage in a 32-year-old woman with Crohn's disease. Note that the veins are frosted with a white exudate. Visual acuity improved from 20/400 to 20/20 after treatment with intravenous methylprednisolone.

Acute angle-closure glaucoma

This is a rare and frequently misdiagnosed cause of a red, painful eye. Susceptible eyes have a shallow anterior chamber because the eye has either a short axial length (hyperopia) or a lens enlarged by the gradual development of cataract. When the pupil becomes mid-dilated, the peripheral iris blocks aqueous outflow via the anterior chamber angle and the intraocular pressure rises abruptly, producing pain, injection, corneal edema, obscurations, and blurred vision. In some patients, ocular symptoms are overshadowed by nausea, vomiting, or headache, prompting a fruitless workup for abdominal or neurologic disease. The diagnosis is made by measuring the intraocular pressure during an acute attack or by observing a narrow chamber angle by means of a specially mirrored contact lens. Acute angle closure is treated with acetazolamide (PO or IV), topical beta blockers, prostaglandin analogues, α_2-adrenergic agonists, and pilocarpine to induce miosis. If these measures fail, a laser can be used to create a hole in the peripheral iris to relieve pupillary block. Many physicians are reluctant to dilate patients routinely for fundus examination because they fear precipitating an angle-closure glaucoma. The risk is actually remote and more than outweighed by the potential benefit to patients of discovering a hidden fundus lesion visible only through a fully dilated pupil. Moreover, a single attack of angle closure after pharmacologic dilatation rarely causes any permanent damage to the eye and serves as an inadvertent provocative test to identify patients with narrow angles who would benefit from prophylactic laser iridectomy.

Endophthalmitis

This results from bacterial, viral, fungal, or parasitic infection of the internal structures of the eye. It usually is acquired by hematogenous seeding from a remote site. Chronically ill, diabetic, or immunosuppressed patients, especially those with a history of indwelling IV catheters or positive blood cultures, are at greatest risk for endogenous endophthalmitis. Although most patients have ocular pain and injection, visual loss is sometimes the only symptom. Septic emboli from a diseased heart valve or a dental abscess that lodge in the retinal circulation can give rise to endophthalmitis. White-centered retinal hemorrhages (Roth's spots) are considered pathognomonic for subacute bacterial endocarditis, but they also appear in leukemia, diabetes, and many other conditions. Endophthalmitis also occurs as a complication of ocular surgery, occasionally months or even years after the operation. An occult

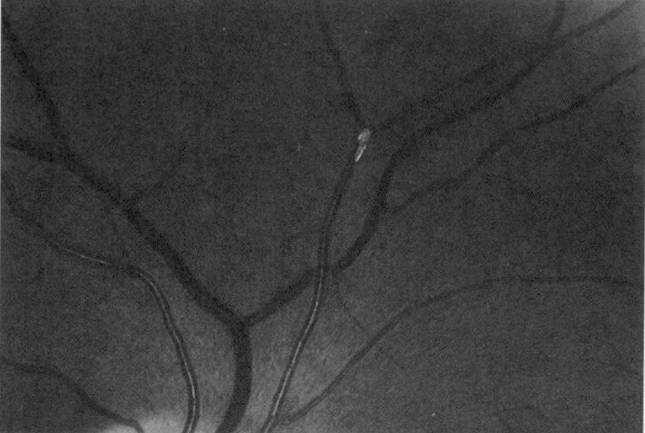

Figure 28-5   Hollenhorst plaque lodged at the bifurcation of a retinal arteriole proves that a patient is shedding emboli from the carotid artery, great vessels, or heart.

penetrating foreign body or unrecognized trauma to the globe should be considered in any patient with unexplained intraocular infection or inflammation.

■ TRANSIENT OR SUDDEN VISUAL LOSS

Amaurosis fugax

This term refers to a transient ischemic attack of the retina (Chap. 370). Because neural tissue has a high rate of metabolism, interruption of blood flow to the retina for more than a few seconds results in *transient monocular blindness*, a term used interchangeably with amaurosis fugax. Patients describe a rapid fading of vision like a curtain descending, sometimes affecting only a portion of the visual field. Amaurosis fugax usually results from an embolus that becomes stuck within a retinal arteriole (Fig. 28-5). If the embolus breaks up or passes, flow is restored and vision returns quickly to normal without permanent damage. With prolonged interruption of blood flow, the inner retina suffers infarction. Ophthalmoscopy reveals zones of whitened, edematous retina following the distribution of branch retinal arterioles. Complete occlusion of the central retinal artery produces arrest of blood flow and a milky retina with a cherry-red fovea (Fig. 28-6). Emboli are composed of cholesterol

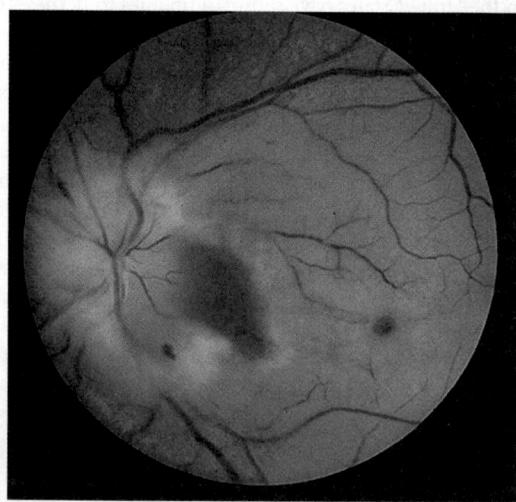

Figure 28-6   Central retinal artery occlusion combined with ischemic optic neuropathy in a 19-year-old woman with an elevated titer of anticardiolipin antibodies. Note the orange dot (rather than cherry red) corresponding to the fovea and the spared patch of retina just temporal to the optic disc.

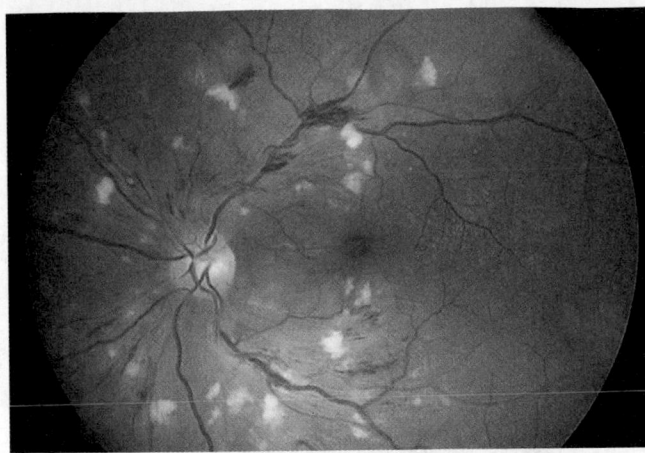

Figure 28-7 Hypertensive retinopathy with scattered flame (splinter) hemorrhages and cotton-wool spots (nerve fiber layer infarcts) in a patient with headache and a blood pressure of 234/120.

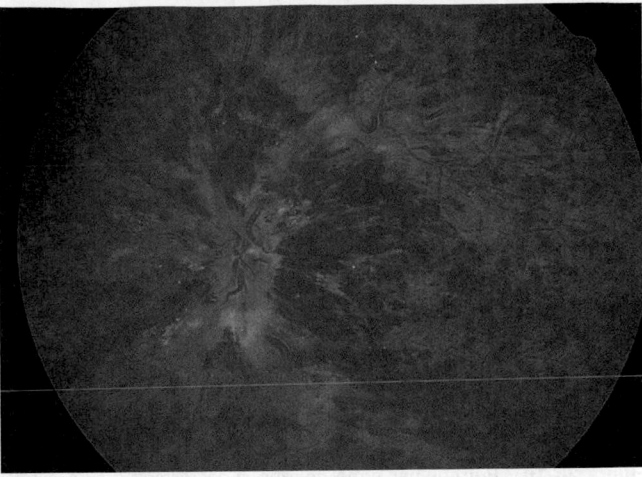

Figure 28-8 Central retinal vein occlusion can produce massive retinal hemorrhage ("blood and thunder"), ischemia, and vision loss.

(Hollenhorst plaque), calcium, or platelet-fibrin debris. The most common source is an atherosclerotic plaque in the carotid artery or aorta, although emboli also can arise from the heart, especially in patients with diseased valves, atrial fibrillation, or wall motion abnormalities.

In rare instances, amaurosis fugax results from low central retinal artery perfusion pressure in a patient with a critical stenosis of the ipsilateral carotid artery and poor collateral flow via the circle of Willis. In this situation, amaurosis fugax develops when there is a dip in systemic blood pressure or a slight worsening of the carotid stenosis. Sometimes there is contralateral motor or sensory loss, indicating concomitant hemispheric cerebral ischemia.

Retinal arterial occlusion also occurs rarely in association with retinal migraine, lupus erythematosus, anticardiolipin antibodies (Fig. 28-6), anticoagulant deficiency states (protein S, protein C, and antithrombin deficiency), pregnancy, IV drug abuse, blood dyscrasias, dysproteinemias, and temporal arteritis.

Marked *systemic hypertension* causes sclerosis of retinal arterioles, splinter hemorrhages, focal infarcts of the nerve fiber layer (cotton-wool spots), and leakage of lipid and fluid (hard exudate) into the macula (Fig. 28-7). In hypertensive crisis, sudden visual loss can result from vasospasm of retinal arterioles and retinal ischemia. In addition, acute hypertension may produce visual loss from ischemic swelling of the optic disc. Patients with acute hypertensive retinopathy should be treated by lowering the blood pressure. However, the blood pressure should not be reduced precipitously, because there is a danger of optic disc infarction from sudden hypoperfusion.

Impending *branch* or *central retinal vein occlusion* can produce prolonged visual obscurations that resemble those described by patients with amaurosis fugax. The veins appear engorged and phlebitic, with numerous retinal hemorrhages (Fig. 28-8). In some patients venous blood flow recovers spontaneously, whereas others evolve a frank obstruction with extensive retinal bleeding ("blood and thunder" appearance), infarction, and visual loss. Venous occlusion of the retina is often idiopathic, but hypertension, diabetes, and glaucoma are prominent risk factors. Polycythemia, thrombocythemia, or other factors leading to an underlying hypercoagulable state should be corrected; aspirin treatment may be beneficial.

Anterior ischemic optic neuropathy (AION)

This is caused by insufficient blood flow through the posterior ciliary arteries that supply the optic disc. It produces painless, monocular visual loss that is usually sudden, although some patients have progressive worsening. The optic disc appears swollen and surrounded by nerve fiber layer splinter hemorrhages (Fig. 28-9). AION is divided into two forms: arteritic and nonarteritic. The nonarteritic form is most common. No specific cause can be identified, although diabetes and hypertension are common risk factors. No treatment is available. About 5% of patients, especially those >age 60, develop the arteritic form of AION in conjunction with giant cell (temporal) arteritis (Chap. 326). It is urgent to recognize arteritic AION so that high doses of glucocorticoids can be instituted immediately to prevent blindness in the second eye. Symptoms of polymyalgia rheumatica may be present; the sedimentation rate and C-reactive protein level are usually elevated. In a patient with visual loss from suspected arteritic AION, temporal artery biopsy is mandatory to confirm the diagnosis. Glucocorticoids should be started immediately, without waiting for the biopsy to be completed. The diagnosis of arteritic AION is difficult to sustain in the face of a negative temporal artery biopsy, but such cases do occur rarely.

Posterior ischemic optic neuropathy

This is an uncommon cause of acute visual loss, induced by the combination of severe anemia and hypotension. Cases have been reported after major blood loss during surgery, exsanguinating

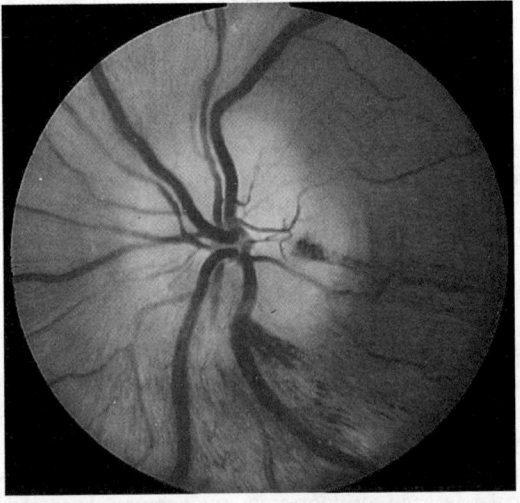

Figure 28-9 Anterior ischemic optic neuropathy from temporal arteritis in a 78-year-old woman with pallid disc swelling, hemorrhage, visual loss, myalgia, and an erythrocyte sedimentation rate of 86 mm/h.

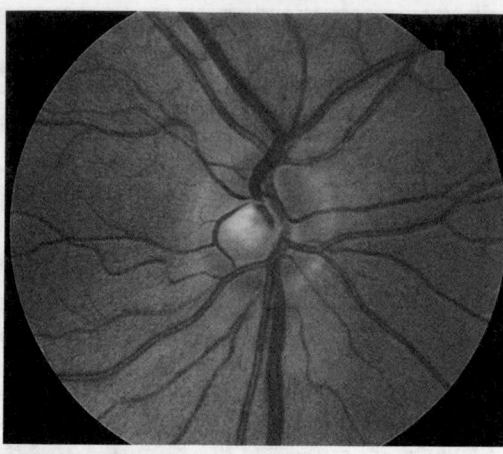

Figure 28-10 Retrobulbar optic neuritis is characterized by a normal fundus examination initially, hence the rubric "the doctor sees nothing, and the patient sees nothing." Optic atrophy develops after severe or repeated attacks.

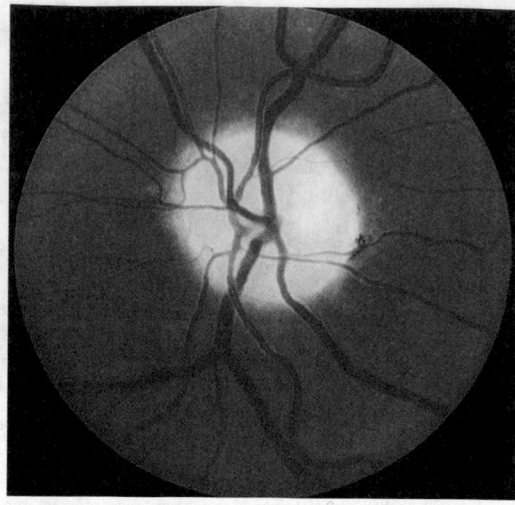

Figure 28-11 Optic atrophy is not a specific diagnosis but refers to the combination of optic disc pallor, arteriolar narrowing, and nerve fiber layer destruction produced by a host of eye diseases, especially optic neuropathies.

trauma, gastrointestinal bleeding, and renal dialysis. The fundus usually appears normal, although optic disc swelling develops if the process extends far enough anteriorly. Vision can be salvaged in some patients by prompt blood transfusion and reversal of hypotension.

Optic neuritis

This is a common inflammatory disease of the optic nerve. In the Optic Neuritis Treatment Trial (ONTT), the mean age of patients was 32 years, 77% were female, 92% had ocular pain (especially with eye movements), and 35% had optic disc swelling. In most patients, the demyelinating event was retrobulbar and the ocular fundus appeared normal on initial examination (Fig. 28-10), although optic disc pallor slowly developed over subsequent months.

Virtually all patients experience a gradual recovery of vision after a single episode of optic neuritis, even without treatment. This rule is so reliable that failure of vision to improve after a first attack of optic neuritis casts doubt on the original diagnosis. Treatment with high-dose IV methylprednisolone (250 mg every 6 h for 3 days) followed by oral prednisone (1 mg/kg per d for 11 days) makes no difference in final acuity (measured 6 months after the attack), but the recovery of visual function occurs more rapidly.

For some patients, optic neuritis remains an isolated event. However, the ONTT showed that the 15-year cumulative probability of developing clinically definite multiple sclerosis after optic neuritis is 50%. In patients with two or more demyelinating plaques on brain magnetic resonance (MR) imaging, treatment with interferon β-1a can retard the development of more lesions. In summary, an MR scan is recommended in every patient with a first attack of optic neuritis. When visual loss is severe (worse than 20/100), treatment with IV followed by oral glucocorticoids hastens recovery. If multiple lesions are present on the MR scan, treatment with interferon β-1a should be considered.

Leber's hereditary optic neuropathy

This disease usually affects young men, causing gradual, painless, severe central visual loss in one eye, followed weeks or months later by the same process in the other eye. Acutely, the optic disc appears mildly plethoric with surface capillary telangiectases but no vascular leakage on fluorescein angiography. Eventually optic atrophy ensues. Leber's optic neuropathy is caused by a point mutation at codon 11778 in the mitochondrial gene encoding nicotinamide adenine dinucleotide dehydrogenase (NADH) subunit 4.

Additional mutations responsible for the disease have been identified, most in mitochondrial genes that encode proteins involved in electron transport. Mitochondrial mutations that cause Leber's neuropathy are inherited from the mother by all her children, but usually only sons develop symptoms.

Toxic optic neuropathy

This can result in acute visual loss with bilateral optic disc swelling and central or cecocentral scotomas. Such cases have been reported to result from exposure to ethambutol, methyl alcohol (moonshine), ethylene glycol (antifreeze), or carbon monoxide. In toxic optic neuropathy, visual loss also can develop gradually and produce optic atrophy (Fig. 28-11) without a phase of acute optic disc edema. Many agents have been implicated as a cause of toxic optic neuropathy, but the evidence supporting the association for many is weak. The following is a partial list of potential offending drugs or toxins: disulfiram, ethchlorvynol, chloramphenicol, amiodarone, monoclonal anti-CD3 antibody, ciprofloxacin, digitalis, streptomycin, lead, arsenic, thallium, D-penicillamine, isoniazid, emetine, and sulfonamides. Deficiency states induced by starvation, malabsorption, or alcoholism can lead to insidious visual loss. Thiamine, vitamin B_{12}, and folate levels should be checked in any patient with unexplained bilateral central scotomas and optic pallor.

Papilledema

This connotes bilateral optic disc swelling from raised intracranial pressure (Fig. 28-12). Headache is a common but not invariable accompaniment. All other forms of optic disc swelling (e.g., from optic neuritis or ischemic optic neuropathy, should be called "optic disc edema"). This convention is arbitrary but serves to avoid confusion. Often it is difficult to differentiate papilledema from other forms of optic disc edema by fundus examination alone. Transient visual obscurations are a classic symptom of papilledema. They can occur in only one eye or simultaneously in both eyes. They usually last seconds but can persist longer. Obscurations follow abrupt shifts in posture or happen spontaneously. When obscurations are prolonged or spontaneous, the papilledema is more threatening. Visual acuity is not affected by papilledema unless the papilledema is severe, long-standing, or accompanied by macular edema and hemorrhage. Visual field testing shows enlarged blind spots and peripheral constriction (Fig. 28-3*F*). With unremitting papilledema, peripheral visual field loss progresses in an insidious fashion

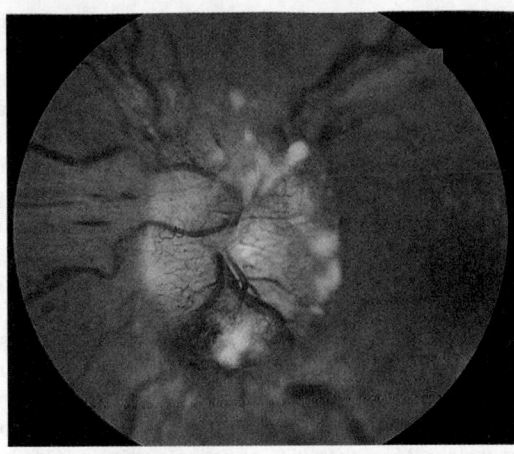

Figure 28-12 Papilledema means optic disc edema from raised intracranial pressure. This obese young woman with pseudotumor cerebri was misdiagnosed as a migraineur until fundus examination was performed, showing optic disc elevation, hemorrhages, and cotton-wool spots.

while the optic nerve develops atrophy. In this setting, reduction of optic disc swelling is an ominous sign of a dying nerve rather than an encouraging indication of resolving papilledema.

Evaluation of papilledema requires neuroimaging to exclude an intracranial lesion. MR angiography is appropriate in selected cases to search for a dural venous sinus occlusion or an arteriovenous shunt. If neuroradiologic studies are negative, the subarachnoid opening pressure should be measured by lumbar puncture. An elevated pressure, with normal cerebrospinal fluid, points by exclusion to the diagnosis of *pseudotumor cerebri* (idiopathic intracranial hypertension). The majority of patients are young, female, and obese. Treatment with a carbonic anhydrase inhibitor such as acetazolamide lowers intracranial pressure by reducing the production of cerebrospinal fluid. Weight reduction is vital but often unsuccessful. If acetazolamide and weight loss fail and visual field loss is progressive, a shunt should be performed without delay to prevent blindness. Occasionally, emergency surgery is required for sudden blindness caused by fulminant papilledema.

Optic disc drusen

These are refractile deposits within the substance of the optic nerve head (Fig. 28-13). They are unrelated to drusen of the retina, which occur in age-related macular degeneration. Optic disc drusen are most common in people of northern European descent. Their diagnosis

is obvious when they are visible as glittering particles on the surface of the optic disc. However, in many patients they are hidden beneath the surface, producing pseudopapilledema. It is important to recognize optic disc drusen to avoid an unnecessary evaluation for papilledema. Ultrasound or CT scanning is sensitive for detection of buried optic disc drusen because they contain calcium. In most patients, optic disc drusen are an incidental, innocuous finding, but they can produce visual obscurations. On perimetry they give rise to enlarged blind spots and arcuate scotomas from damage to the optic disc. With increasing age, drusen tend to become more exposed on the disc surface as optic atrophy develops. Hemorrhage, choroidal neovascular membrane, and AION are more likely to occur in patients with optic disc drusen. No treatment is available.

Vitreous degeneration

This occurs in all individuals with advancing age, leading to visual symptoms. Opacities develop in the vitreous, casting annoying shadows on the retina. As the eye moves, these distracting "floaters" move synchronously, with a slight lag caused by inertia of the vitreous gel. Vitreous traction on the retina causes mechanical stimulation, resulting in perception of flashing lights. This photopsia is brief and is confined to one eye, in contrast to the bilateral, prolonged scintillations of cortical migraine. Contraction of the vitreous can result in sudden separation from the retina, heralded by an alarming shower of floaters and photopsia. This process, known as *vitreous detachment*, is a common involutional event in the elderly. It is not harmful unless it damages the retina. A careful examination of the dilated fundus is important in any patient complaining of floaters or photopsia to search for peripheral tears or holes. If such a lesion is found, laser application can forestall a retinal detachment. Occasionally a tear ruptures a retinal blood vessel, causing vitreous hemorrhage and sudden loss of vision. On attempted ophthalmoscopy the fundus is hidden by a dark red haze of blood. Ultrasound is required to examine the interior of the eye for a retinal tear or detachment. If the hemorrhage does not resolve spontaneously, the vitreous can be removed surgically. Vitreous hemorrhage also results from the fragile neovascular vessels that proliferate on the surface of the retina in diabetes, sickle cell anemia, and other ischemic ocular diseases.

Retinal detachment

This produces symptoms of floaters, flashing lights, and a scotoma in the peripheral visual field corresponding to the detachment (Fig. 28-14). If the detachment includes the fovea, there is an

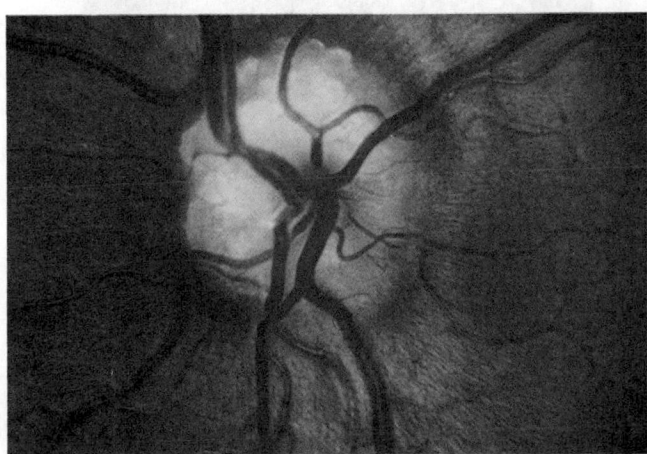

Figure 28-13 Optic disc drusen are calcified deposits of unknown etiology within the optic disc. They sometimes are confused with papilledema.

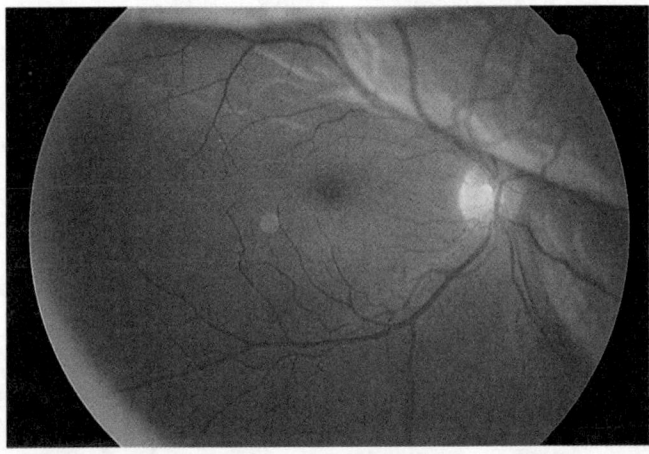

Figure 28-14 Retinal detachment appears as an elevated sheet of retinal tissue with folds. In this patient the fovea was spared, so acuity was normal, but a superior detachment produced an inferior scotoma.

afferent pupil defect and the visual acuity is reduced. In most eyes, retinal detachment starts with a hole, flap, or tear in the peripheral retina (rhegmatogenous retinal detachment). Patients with peripheral retinal thinning (lattice degeneration) are particularly vulnerable to this process. Once a break has developed in the retina, liquefied vitreous is free to enter the subretinal space, separating the retina from the pigment epithelium. The combination of vitreous traction on the retinal surface and passage of fluid behind the retina leads inexorably to detachment. Patients with a history of myopia, trauma, or prior cataract extraction are at greatest risk for retinal detachment. The diagnosis is confirmed by ophthalmoscopic examination of the dilated eye.

Classic migraine

(See also Chap. 14) This usually occurs with a visual aura lasting about 20 min. In a typical attack, a small central disturbance in the field of vision marches toward the periphery, leaving a transient scotoma in its wake. The expanding border of migraine scotoma has a scintillating, dancing, or zigzag edge, resembling the bastions of a fortified city, hence the term *fortification spectra*. Patients' descriptions of fortification spectra vary widely and can be confused with amaurosis fugax. Migraine patterns usually last longer and are perceived in both eyes, whereas amaurosis fugax is briefer and occurs in only one eye. Migraine phenomena also remain visible in the dark or with the eyes closed. Generally they are confined to either the right or the left visual hemifield, but sometimes both fields are involved simultaneously. Patients often have a long history of stereotypic attacks. After the visual symptoms recede, headache develops in most patients.

Transient ischemic attacks

Vertebrobasilar insufficiency may result in acute homonymous visual symptoms. Many patients mistakenly describe symptoms in the left or right eye when in fact the symptoms are occurring in the left or right hemifield of both eyes. Interruption of blood supply to the visual cortex causes a sudden fogging or graying of vision, occasionally with flashing lights or other positive phenomena that mimic migraine. Cortical ischemic attacks are briefer in duration than migraine, occur in older patients, and are not followed by headache. There may be associated signs of brainstem ischemia, such as diplopia, vertigo, numbness, weakness, and dysarthria.

Stroke

Stroke occurs when interruption of blood supply from the posterior cerebral artery to the visual cortex is prolonged. The only finding on examination is a homonymous visual field defect that stops abruptly at the vertical meridian. Occipital lobe stroke usually is due to thrombotic occlusion of the vertebrobasilar system, embolus, or dissection. Lobar hemorrhage, tumor, abscess, and arteriovenous malformation are other common causes of hemianopic cortical visual loss.

Factitious (functional, nonorganic) visual loss

This is claimed by hysterics or malingerers. The latter account for the vast majority, seeking sympathy, special treatment, or financial gain by feigning loss of sight. The diagnosis is suspected when the history is atypical, physical findings are lacking or contradictory, inconsistencies emerge on testing, and a secondary motive can be identified. In our litigious society, the fraudulent pursuit of recompense has spawned an epidemic of factitious visual loss.

■ CHRONIC VISUAL LOSS

Cataract

Cataract is a clouding of the lens sufficient to reduce vision. Most cataracts develop slowly as a result of aging, leading to gradual impairment of vision. The formation of cataract occurs more rapidly in patients with a history of ocular trauma, uveitis, or diabetes mellitus. Cataracts are acquired in a variety of genetic diseases, such as myotonic dystrophy, neurofibromatosis type 2, and galactosemia. Radiation therapy and glucocorticoid treatment can induce cataract as a side effect. The cataracts associated with radiation or glucocorticoids have a typical posterior subcapsular location. Cataract can be detected by noting an impaired red reflex when viewing light reflected from the fundus with an ophthalmoscope or by examining the dilated eye with the slit lamp.

The only treatment for cataract is surgical extraction of the opacified lens. Over a million cataract operations are performed each year in the United States. The operation generally is done under local anesthesia on an outpatient basis. A plastic or silicone intraocular lens is placed within the empty lens capsule in the posterior chamber, substituting for the natural lens and leading to rapid recovery of sight. More than 95% of patients who undergo cataract extraction can expect an improvement in vision. In some patients, the lens capsule remaining in the eye after cataract extraction eventually turns cloudy, causing secondary loss of vision. A small opening is made in the lens capsule with a laser to restore clarity.

Glaucoma

Glaucoma is a slowly progressive, insidious optic neuropathy that usually is associated with chronic elevation of intraocular pressure. In African Americans it is the leading cause of blindness. The mechanism by which raised intraocular pressure injures the optic nerve is not understood. Axons entering the inferotemporal and superotemporal aspects of the optic disc are damaged first, producing typical nerve fiber bundle or arcuate scotomas on perimetric testing. As fibers are destroyed, the neural rim of the optic disc shrinks and the physiologic cup within the optic disc enlarges (Fig. 28-15). This process is referred to as pathologic "cupping." The cup-to-disc diameter is expressed as a ratio (e.g., 0.2/1). The cup-to-disc ratio ranges widely in normal individuals, making it difficult to diagnose glaucoma reliably simply by observing an unusually large or deep optic cup. Careful documentation of serial examinations is helpful. In a patient with physiologic cupping the large cup remains stable, whereas in a patient with glaucoma it expands relentlessly over the years. Detection of visual field loss by computerized perimetry also contributes to the diagnosis. Finally, most patients with glaucoma have raised intraocular pressure. However, many patients with typical glaucomatous cupping and visual field loss have intraocular pressures that apparently never exceed the normal limit of 20 mmHg (so-called low-tension glaucoma).

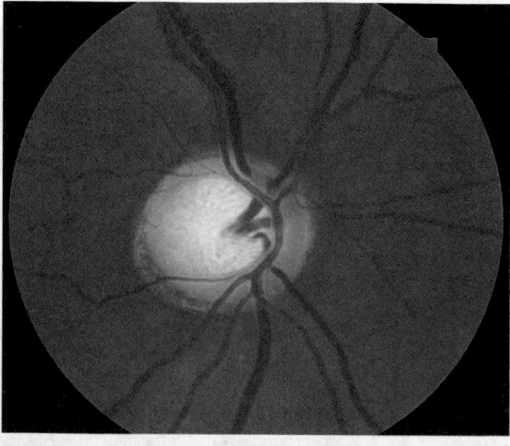

Figure 28-15 Glaucoma results in "cupping" as the neural rim is destroyed and the central cup becomes enlarged and excavated. The cup-to-disc ratio is about 0.7/1.0 in this patient.

In acute angle-closure glaucoma, the eye is red and painful due to abrupt, severe elevation of intraocular pressure. Such cases account for only a minority of glaucoma cases: most patients have open, anterior chamber angles. The cause of raised intraocular pressure in open angle glaucoma is unknown, but it is associated with gene mutations in the heritable forms.

Glaucoma is usually painless (except in angle-closure glaucoma). Foveal acuity is spared until end-stage disease is reached. For these reasons, severe and irreversible damage can occur before either the patient or the physician recognizes the diagnosis. Screening of patients for glaucoma by noting the cup-to-disc ratio on ophthalmoscopy and by measuring intraocular pressure is vital. Glaucoma is treated with topical adrenergic agonists, cholinergic agonists, beta blockers, and prostaglandin analogues. Occasionally, systemic absorption of beta blocker from eyedrops can be sufficient to cause side effects of bradycardia, hypotension, heart block, bronchospasm, or depression. Topical or oral carbonic anhydrase inhibitors are used to lower intraocular pressure by reducing aqueous production. Laser treatment of the trabecular meshwork in the anterior chamber angle improves aqueous outflow from the eye. If medical or laser treatments fail to halt optic nerve damage from glaucoma, a filter must be constructed surgically (trabeculectomy) or a valve placed to release aqueous from the eye in a controlled fashion.

Macular degeneration

This is a major cause of gradual, painless, bilateral central visual loss in the elderly. The old term, "senile macular degeneration," misinterpreted by many patients as an unflattering reference, has been replaced with "age-related macular degeneration." It occurs in a nonexudative (dry) form and an exudative (wet) form. Inflammation may be important in both forms of macular degeneration; recent genetic data indicate that susceptibility is associated with variants in the gene for complement factor H, an inhibitor of the alternative complement pathway. The nonexudative process begins with the accumulation of extracellular deposits called drusen underneath the retinal pigment epithelium. On ophthalmoscopy, they are pleomorphic but generally appear as small discrete yellow lesions clustered in the macula (Fig. 28-16). With time they become larger, more numerous, and confluent. The retinal pigment epithelium becomes focally detached and atrophic, causing visual loss by interfering with photoreceptor function. Treatment with vitamins C and E, betacarotene, and zinc may retard dry macular degeneration.

Exudative macular degeneration, which develops in only a minority of patients, occurs when neovascular vessels from the choroid grow through defects in Bruch's membrane and proliferate underneath the retinal pigment epithelium or the retina. Leakage from these vessels produces elevation of the retina, with distortion (metamorphopsia) and blurring of vision. Although the onset of these symptoms is usually gradual, bleeding from a subretinal choroidal neovascular membrane sometimes causes acute visual loss. Neovascular membranes can be difficult to see on fundus examination because they are located beneath the retina. Fluorescein angiography and optical coherence tomography, a new technique for acquiring images of the retina in cross-section, are extremely useful for their detection. Major or repeated hemorrhage under the retina from neovascular membranes results in fibrosis, development of a round (disciform) macular scar, and permanent loss of central vision.

A major therapeutic advance has occurred recently with the discovery that exudative macular degeneration can be treated with intraocular injection of a vascular endothelial growth factor antagonist. Either bevacizumab or ranibizumab is administered by direct injection into the vitreous cavity, beginning on a monthly basis. These antibodies cause the regression of neovascular membranes by blocking the action of vascular endothelial growth factor, thereby improving visual acuity.

Central serous chorioretinopathy

This primarily affects males between the ages of 20 and 50. Leakage of serous fluid from the choroid causes small, localized detachment of the retinal pigment epithelium and the neurosensory retina. These detachments produce acute or chronic symptoms of metamorphopsia and blurred vision when the macula is involved. They are difficult to visualize with a direct ophthalmoscope because the detached retina is transparent and only slightly elevated. Diagnosis of central serous chorioretinopathy is made easily by fluorescein angiography, which shows dye streaming into the subretinal space. The cause of central serous chorioretinopathy is unknown. Symptoms may resolve spontaneously if the retina reattaches, but recurrent detachment is common. Laser photocoagulation has benefited some patients with this condition.

Diabetic retinopathy

A rare disease until 1921, when the discovery of insulin resulted in a dramatic improvement in life expectancy for patients with diabetes mellitus, diabetic retinopathy is now a leading cause of blindness in the United States. The retinopathy takes years to develop but eventually appears in nearly all cases. Regular surveillance of the dilated fundus is crucial for any patient with diabetes. In advanced diabetic retinopathy, the proliferation of neovascular vessels leads to blindness from vitreous hemorrhage, retinal detachment, and glaucoma (see Fig. 344-9). These complications can be avoided in most patients by administration of panretinal laser photocoagulation at the appropriate point in the evolution of the disease. For further discussion of the manifestations and management of diabetic retinopathy, see Chap. 344.

Retinitis pigmentosa

This is a general term for a disparate group of rod-cone dystrophies characterized by progressive night blindness, visual field constriction with a ring scotoma, loss of acuity, and an abnormal electroretinogram (ERG). It occurs sporadically or in an autosomal recessive, dominant, or X-linked pattern. Irregular black deposits of clumped pigment in the peripheral retina, called *bone spicules* because of their vague resemblance to the spicules of cancellous bone, give the disease its name (Fig. 28-17). The name is actually a misnomer because retinitis pigmentosa is not an inflammatory process. Most cases are due to a mutation in the gene for rhodopsin,

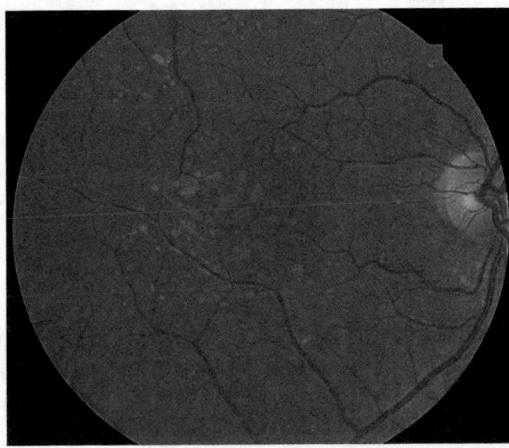

Figure 28-16 Age-related macular degeneration begins with the accumulation of drusen within the macula. They appear as scattered yellow subretinal deposits.

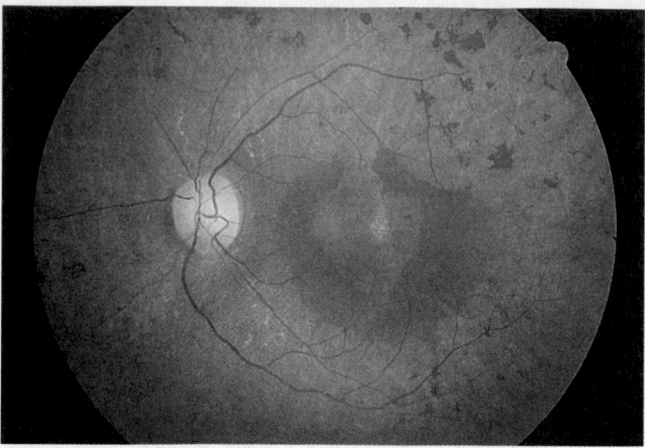

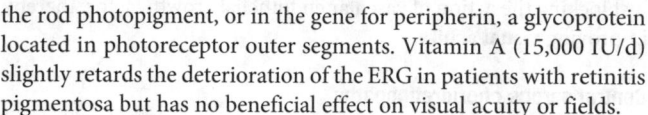

Figure 28-17 Retinitis pigmentosa with black clumps of pigment in the retinal periphery known as "bone spicules." There is also atrophy of the retinal pigment epithelium, making the vasculature of the choroid easily visible.

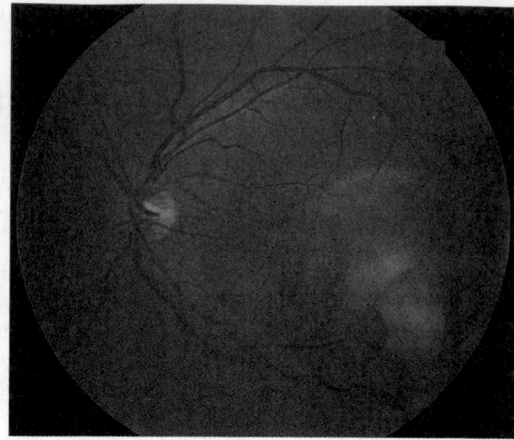

Figure 28-18 Melanoma of the choroid, appearing as an elevated dark mass in the inferior temporal fundus, just encroaching upon the fovea.

the rod photopigment, or in the gene for peripherin, a glycoprotein located in photoreceptor outer segments. Vitamin A (15,000 IU/d) slightly retards the deterioration of the ERG in patients with retinitis pigmentosa but has no beneficial effect on visual acuity or fields.

Leber's congenital amaurosis, a rare cone dystrophy, has been treated by replacement of the missing RPE65 protein through gene therapy, resulting in modest improvement in visual function. Some forms of retinitis pigmentosa occur in association with rare, hereditary systemic diseases (olivopontocerebellar degeneration, Bassen-Kornzweig disease, Kearns-Sayre syndrome, Refsum's disease). Chronic treatment with chloroquine, hydroxychloroquine, and phenothiazines (especially thioridazine) can produce visual loss from a toxic retinopathy that resembles retinitis pigmentosa.

Epiretinal membrane

This is a fibrocellular tissue that grows across the inner surface of the retina, causing metamorphopsia and reduced visual acuity from distortion of the macula. A crinkled, cellophane-like membrane is visible on the retinal examination. Epiretinal membrane is most common in patients over 50 years of age and is usually unilateral. Most cases are idiopathic, but some occur as a result of hypertensive retinopathy, diabetes, retinal detachment, or trauma. When visual acuity is reduced to the level of about 6/24 (20/80), vitrectomy and surgical peeling of the membrane to relieve macular puckering are recommended. Contraction of an epiretinal membrane sometimes gives rise to a *macular hole*. Most macular holes, however, are caused by local vitreous traction within the fovea. Vitrectomy can improve acuity in selected cases.

Melanoma and other tumors

Melanoma is the most common primary tumor of the eye (Fig. 28-18). It causes photopsia, an enlarging scotoma, and loss of vision. A small melanoma is often difficult to differentiate from a benign choroidal nevus. Serial examinations are required to document a malignant pattern of growth. Treatment of melanoma is controversial. Options include enucleation, local resection, and irradiation. *Metastatic tumors* to the eye outnumber primary tumors. Breast and lung carcinomas have a special propensity to spread to the choroid or iris. Leukemia and lymphoma also commonly invade ocular tissues. Sometimes their only sign on eye examination is cellular debris in the vitreous, which can masquerade as a chronic posterior uveitis. *Retrobulbar tumor* of the optic nerve (meningioma, glioma) or *chiasmal tumor* (pituitary adenoma, meningioma) produces gradual visual loss with few objective findings except for optic

disc pallor. Rarely, sudden expansion of a pituitary adenoma from infarction and bleeding (*pituitary apoplexy*) causes acute retrobulbar visual loss, with headache, nausea, and ocular motor nerve palsies. In any patient with visual field loss or optic atrophy, CT or MR scanning should be considered if the cause remains unknown after careful review of the history and thorough examination of the eye.

■ PROPTOSIS

When the globes appear asymmetric, the clinician must first decide which eye is abnormal. Is one eye recessed within the orbit (*enophthalmos*), or is the other eye protuberant (*exophthalmos*, or *proptosis*)? A small globe or a Horner's syndrome can give the appearance of enophthalmos. True enophthalmos occurs commonly after trauma, from atrophy of retrobulbar fat, or from fracture of the orbital floor. The position of the eyes within the orbits is measured by using a Hertel exophthalmometer, a handheld instrument that records the position of the anterior corneal surface relative to the lateral orbital rim. If this instrument is not available, relative eye position can be judged by bending the patient's head forward and looking down upon the orbits. A proptosis of only 2 mm in one eye is detectable from this perspective. The development of proptosis implies a space-occupying lesion in the orbit and usually warrants CT or MR imaging.

Graves' ophthalmopathy

This is the leading cause of proptosis in adults (Chap. 341). The proptosis is often asymmetric and can even appear to be unilateral. Orbital inflammation and engorgement of the extraocular muscles, particularly the medial rectus and the inferior rectus, account for the protrusion of the globe. Corneal exposure, lid retraction, conjunctival injection, restriction of gaze, diplopia, and visual loss from optic nerve compression are cardinal symptoms. Graves' ophthalmopathy is treated with oral prednisone (60 mg/d) for 1 month, followed by a taper over several months, topical lubricants, eyelid surgery, eye muscle surgery, or orbital decompression. Radiation therapy is not effective.

Orbital pseudotumor

This is an idiopathic, inflammatory orbital syndrome that frequently is confused with Graves' ophthalmopathy. Symptoms are pain, limited eye movements, proptosis, and congestion. Evaluation for sarcoidosis, granulomatosis with polyangiitis (Wegener's), and other types of orbital vasculitis or collagen-vascular disease is negative. Imaging often shows swollen eye muscles (orbital myositis) with enlarged tendons. By contrast, in Graves' ophthalmopathy the tendons of the eye muscles usually are spared. The Tolosa-Hunt syndrome may be regarded as an extension of orbital pseudotumor through the superior orbital fissure into the cavernous sinus. The diagnosis of orbital pseudotumor is difficult. Biopsy of the orbit frequently yields nonspecific evidence of fat infiltration by lymphocytes, plasma cells, and eosinophils. A dramatic response to a therapeutic trial of systemic glucocorticoids indirectly provides the best confirmation of the diagnosis.

Orbital cellulitis

This causes pain, lid erythema, proptosis, conjunctival chemosis, restricted motility, decreased acuity, afferent pupillary defect, fever, and leukocytosis. It often arises from the paranasal sinuses, especially by contiguous spread of infection from the ethmoid sinus through the lamina papyracea of the medial orbit. A history of recent upper respiratory tract infection, chronic sinusitis, thick mucus secretions, or dental disease is significant in any patient with suspected orbital cellulitis. Blood cultures should be obtained, but they are usually negative. Most patients respond to empirical therapy with broad-spectrum IV antibiotics. Occasionally, orbital cellulitis follows an overwhelming course, with massive proptosis, blindness, septic cavernous sinus thrombosis, and meningitis. To avert this disaster, orbital cellulitis should be managed aggressively in the early stages, with immediate imaging of the orbits and antibiotic therapy that includes coverage of methicillin-resistant *Staphylococcus aureus* (MRSA). Prompt surgical drainage of an orbital abscess or paranasal sinusitis is indicated if optic nerve function deteriorates despite antibiotics.

Tumors

Tumors of the orbit cause painless, progressive proptosis. The most common primary tumors are hemangioma, lymphangioma, neurofibroma, dermoid cyst, adenoid cystic carcinoma, optic nerve glioma, optic nerve meningioma, and benign mixed tumor of the lacrimal gland. Metastatic tumor to the orbit occurs frequently in breast carcinoma, lung carcinoma, and lymphoma. Diagnosis by fine-needle aspiration followed by urgent radiation therapy sometimes can preserve vision.

Carotid cavernous fistulas

With anterior drainage through the orbit these fistulas produce proptosis, diplopia, glaucoma, and corkscrew, arterialized conjunctival vessels. Direct fistulas usually result from trauma. They are easily diagnosed because of the prominent signs produced by high-flow, high-pressure shunting. Indirect fistulas, or dural arteriovenous malformations, are more likely to occur spontaneously, especially in older women. The signs are more subtle, and the diagnosis frequently is missed. The combination of slight proptosis, diplopia, enlarged muscles, and an injected eye often is mistaken for thyroid ophthalmopathy. A bruit heard upon auscultation of the head or reported by the patient is a valuable diagnostic clue. Imaging shows an enlarged superior ophthalmic vein in the orbits. Carotid cavernous shunts can be eliminated by intravascular embolization.

■ PTOSIS

Blepharoptosis

This is an abnormal drooping of the eyelid. Unilateral or bilateral ptosis can be congenital, from dysgenesis of the levator palpebrae superioris, or from abnormal insertion of its aponeurosis into the eyelid. Acquired ptosis can develop so gradually that the patient is unaware of the problem. Inspection of old photographs is helpful in dating the onset. A history of prior trauma, eye surgery, contact lens use, diplopia, systemic symptoms (e.g., dysphagia or peripheral muscle weakness), or a family history of ptosis should be sought.

Fluctuating ptosis that worsens late in the day is typical of myasthenia gravis. Examination should focus on evidence for proptosis, eyelid masses or deformities, inflammation, pupil inequality, or limitation of motility. The width of the palpebral fissures is measured in primary gaze to quantitate the degree of ptosis. The ptosis will be underestimated if the patient compensates by lifting the brow with the frontalis muscle.

Mechanical ptosis

This occurs in many elderly patients from stretching and redundancy of eyelid skin and subcutaneous fat (dermatochalasis). The extra weight of these sagging tissues causes the lid to droop. Enlargement or deformation of the eyelid from infection, tumor, trauma, or inflammation also results in ptosis on a purely mechanical basis.

Aponeurotic ptosis

This is an acquired dehiscence or stretching of the aponeurotic tendon, which connects the levator muscle to the tarsal plate of the eyelid. It occurs commonly in older patients, presumably from loss of connective tissue elasticity. Aponeurotic ptosis is also a common sequela of eyelid swelling from infection or blunt trauma to the orbit, cataract surgery, or hard contact lens use.

Myogenic ptosis

The causes of *myogenic ptosis* include myasthenia gravis (Chap. 386) and a number of rare myopathies that manifest with ptosis. The term *chronic progressive external ophthalmoplegia* refers to a spectrum of systemic diseases caused by mutations of mitochondrial DNA. As the name implies, the most prominent findings are symmetric, slowly progressive ptosis and limitation of eye movements. In general, diplopia is a late symptom because all eye movements are reduced equally. In the *Kearns-Sayre* variant, retinal pigmentary changes and abnormalities of cardiac conduction develop. Peripheral muscle biopsy shows characteristic "ragged-red fibers." *Oculopharyngeal dystrophy* is a distinct autosomal dominant disease with onset in middle age, characterized by ptosis, limited eye movements, and trouble swallowing. *Myotonic dystrophy*, another autosomal dominant disorder, causes ptosis, ophthalmoparesis, cataract, and pigmentary retinopathy. Patients have muscle wasting, myotonia, frontal balding, and cardiac abnormalities.

Neurogenic ptosis

This results from a lesion affecting the innervation to either of the two muscles that open the eyelid: Müller's muscle or the levator palpebrae superioris. Examination of the pupil helps distinguish between these two possibilities. In Horner's syndrome, the eye with ptosis has a smaller pupil and the eye movements are full. In an oculomotor nerve palsy, the eye with the ptosis has a larger or a normal pupil. If the pupil is normal but there is limitation of adduction, elevation, and depression, a pupil-sparing oculomotor nerve palsy is likely (see next section). Rarely, a lesion affecting the small, central subnucleus of the oculomotor complex will cause bilateral ptosis with normal eye movements and pupils.

■ DOUBLE VISION (DIPLOPIA)

The first point to clarify is whether diplopia persists in either eye after the opposite eye is covered. If it does, the diagnosis is monocular diplopia. The cause is usually intrinsic to the eye and therefore has no dire implications for the patient. Corneal aberrations (e.g., keratoconus, pterygium), uncorrected refractive error, cataract, or foveal traction may give rise to monocular diplopia. Occasionally it is a symptom of malingering or psychiatric disease. Diplopia alleviated by covering one eye is binocular diplopia and is caused by disruption of ocular alignment. Inquiry should be made into the nature of the double vision (purely side-by-side versus partial vertical displacement of images), mode of onset, duration, intermittency, diurnal variation, and associated neurologic or systemic symptoms. If the patient has diplopia while being examined, motility testing should reveal a deficiency corresponding to the patient's symptoms. However, subtle limitation of ocular excursions is often difficult to detect. For example, a patient with a slight left abducens nerve paresis may appear to have full eye movements despite a complaint of horizontal diplopia upon looking to the left. In this situation, the cover test provides a more sensitive method for demonstrating the ocular misalignment. It should be conducted in primary gaze and then with the head turned and tilted in each direction. In the above example, a cover test with the head turned to the right will maximize the fixation shift evoked by the cover test.

Occasionally, a cover test performed in an asymptomatic patient during a routine examination will reveal an ocular deviation. If the eye movements are full and the ocular misalignment is equal in all directions of gaze (concomitant deviation), the diagnosis is strabismus. In this condition, which affects about 1% of the population, fusion is disrupted in infancy or early childhood. To avoid diplopia, vision is suppressed from the nonfixating eye. In some children, this leads to impaired vision (amblyopia, or "lazy" eye) in the deviated eye.

Binocular diplopia results from a wide range of processes: infectious, neoplastic, metabolic, degenerative, inflammatory, and vascular. One must decide whether the diplopia is neurogenic in origin or is due to restriction of globe rotation by local disease in the orbit. Orbital pseudotumor, myositis, infection, tumor, thyroid disease, and muscle entrapment (e.g., from a blowout fracture) cause restrictive diplopia. The diagnosis of restriction is usually made by recognizing other associated signs and symptoms of local orbital disease in conjunction with imaging.

Myasthenia gravis

(See also Chap. 386) This is a major cause of diplopia. The diplopia is often intermittent, variable, and not confined to any single ocular motor nerve distribution. The pupils are always normal. Fluctuating ptosis may be present. Many patients have a purely ocular form of the disease, with no evidence of systemic muscular weakness. The diagnosis can be confirmed by an IV edrophonium injection or by an assay for antiacetylcholine receptor antibodies. Negative results from these tests do not exclude the diagnosis. *Botulism* from food or wound poisoning can mimic ocular myasthenia.

After restrictive orbital disease and myasthenia gravis are excluded, a lesion of a cranial nerve supplying innervation to the extraocular muscles is the most likely cause of binocular diplopia.

Oculomotor nerve

The third cranial nerve innervates the medial, inferior, and superior recti; inferior oblique; levator palpebrae superioris; and the iris sphincter. Total palsy of the oculomotor nerve causes ptosis, results in a dilated pupil, and leaves the eye "down and out" because of the unopposed action of the lateral rectus and superior oblique. This combination of findings is obvious. More challenging is the diagnosis of early or partial oculomotor nerve palsy. In this setting, any combination of ptosis, pupil dilation, and weakness of the eye muscles supplied by the oculomotor nerve may be encountered. Frequent serial examinations during the evolving phase of the palsy help ensure that the diagnosis is not missed. The advent of an oculomotor nerve palsy with a pupil involvement, especially when accompanied by pain, suggests a compressive lesion, such as a tumor or circle of Willis aneurysm. Neuroimaging should be obtained, along with a CT or MR angiogram. Occasionally, a catheter arteriogram must be done to exclude an aneurysm.

A lesion of the oculomotor nucleus in the rostral midbrain produces signs that differ from those caused by a lesion of the nerve itself. There is bilateral ptosis because the levator muscle is innervated by a single central subnucleus. There is also weakness of the contralateral superior rectus, because it is supplied by the oculomotor nucleus on the other side. Occasionally both superior recti are weak. Isolated nuclear oculomotor palsy is rare. Usually neurologic examination reveals additional signs that suggest brainstem damage from infarction, hemorrhage, tumor, or infection.

Injury to structures surrounding fascicles of the oculomotor nerve descending through the midbrain has given rise to a number of classic eponymic designations. In *Nothnagel's syndrome*, injury to the superior cerebellar peduncle causes ipsilateral oculomotor palsy and contralateral cerebellar ataxia. In *Benedikt's syndrome*, injury to the red nucleus results in ipsilateral oculomotor palsy and contralateral tremor, chorea, and athetosis. *Claude's syndrome* incorporates features of both of these syndromes, by injury to both the red nucleus and the superior cerebellar peduncle. Finally, in *Weber's syndrome*, injury to the cerebral peduncle causes ipsilateral oculomotor palsy with contralateral hemiparesis.

In the subarachnoid space the oculomotor nerve is vulnerable to aneurysm, meningitis, tumor, infarction, and compression. In cerebral herniation the nerve becomes trapped between the edge of the tentorium and the uncus of the temporal lobe. Oculomotor palsy also can result from midbrain torsion and hemorrhages during herniation. In the cavernous sinus, oculomotor palsy arises from carotid aneurysm, carotid cavernous fistula, cavernous sinus thrombosis, tumor (pituitary adenoma, meningioma, metastasis), herpes zoster infection, and the Tolosa-Hunt syndrome.

The etiology of an isolated, pupil-sparing oculomotor palsy often remains an enigma even after neuroimaging and extensive laboratory testing. Most cases are thought to result from microvascular infarction of the nerve somewhere along its course from the brainstem to the orbit. Usually the patient complains of pain. Diabetes, hypertension, and vascular disease are major risk factors. Spontaneous recovery over a period of months is the rule. If this fails to occur or if new findings develop, the diagnosis of microvascular oculomotor nerve palsy should be reconsidered. Aberrant regeneration is common when the oculomotor nerve is injured by trauma or compression (tumor, aneurysm). Miswiring of sprouting fibers to the levator muscle and the rectus muscles results in elevation of the eyelid upon downgaze or adduction. The pupil also constricts upon attempted adduction, elevation, or depression of the globe. Aberrant regeneration is not seen after oculomotor palsy from microvascular infarct and hence vitiates that diagnosis.

Trochlear nerve

The fourth cranial nerve originates in the midbrain, just caudal to the oculomotor nerve complex. Fibers exit the brainstem dorsally and cross to innervate the contralateral superior oblique. The principal actions of this muscle are to depress and intort the globe. A palsy therefore results in hypertropia and excyclotorsion. The cyclotorsion seldom is noticed by patients. Instead, they complain of vertical diplopia, especially upon reading or looking down. The vertical diplopia also is exacerbated by tilting the head toward the side with the muscle palsy and alleviated by tilting it away. This "head tilt test" is a cardinal diagnostic feature.

Isolated trochlear nerve palsy results from all the causes listed above for the oculomotor nerve except aneurysm. The trochlear nerve is particularly apt to suffer injury after closed head trauma. The free edge of the tentorium is thought to impinge on the nerve during a concussive blow. Most isolated trochlear nerve palsies are idiopathic and hence are diagnosed by exclusion as "microvascular."

Spontaneous improvement occurs over a period of months in most patients. A base-down prism (conveniently applied to the patient's glasses as a stick-on Fresnel lens) may serve as a temporary measure to alleviate diplopia. If the palsy does not resolve, the eyes can be realigned by weakening the inferior oblique muscle.

Abducens nerve

The sixth cranial nerve innervates the lateral rectus muscle. A palsy produces horizontal diplopia, worse on gaze to the side of the lesion. A nuclear lesion has different consequences, because the abducens nucleus contains interneurons that project via the medial longitudinal fasciculus to the medial rectus subnucleus of the contralateral oculomotor complex. Therefore, an abducens nuclear lesion produces a complete lateral gaze palsy from weakness of both the ipsilateral lateral rectus and the contralateral medial rectus. *Foville's syndrome* after dorsal pontine injury includes lateral gaze palsy, ipsilateral facial palsy, and contralateral hemiparesis incurred by damage to descending corticospinal fibers. *Millard-Gubler syndrome* from ventral pontine injury is similar except for the eye findings. There is lateral rectus weakness only, instead of gaze palsy, because the abducens fascicle is injured rather than the nucleus. Infarct, tumor, hemorrhage, vascular malformation, and multiple sclerosis are the most common etiologies of brainstem abducens palsy.

After leaving the ventral pons, the abducens nerve runs forward along the clivus to pierce the dura at the petrous apex, where it enters the cavernous sinus. Along its subarachnoid course it is susceptible to meningitis, tumor (meningioma, chordoma, carcinomatous meningitis), subarachnoid hemorrhage, trauma, and compression by aneurysm or dolichoectatic vessels. At the petrous apex, mastoiditis can produce deafness, pain, and ipsilateral abducens palsy (*Gradenigo's syndrome*). In the cavernous sinus, the nerve can be affected by carotid aneurysm, carotid cavernous fistula, tumor (pituitary adenoma, meningioma, nasopharyngeal carcinoma), herpes infection, and Tolosa-Hunt syndrome.

Unilateral or bilateral abducens palsy is a classic sign of raised intracranial pressure. The diagnosis can be confirmed if papilledema is observed on fundus examination. The mechanism is still debated but probably is related to rostral-caudal displacement of the brainstem. The same phenomenon accounts for abducens palsy from low intracranial pressure (e.g., after lumbar puncture, spinal anesthesia, or spontaneous dural cerebrospinal fluid leak).

Treatment of abducens palsy is aimed at prompt correction of the underlying cause. However, the cause remains obscure in many instances despite diligent evaluation. As was mentioned above for isolated trochlear or oculomotor palsy, most cases are assumed to represent microvascular infarcts because they often occur in the setting of diabetes or other vascular risk factors. Some cases may develop as a postinfectious mononeuritis (e.g., after a viral flu). Patching one eye or applying a temporary prism will provide relief of diplopia until the palsy resolves. If recovery is incomplete, eye muscle surgery nearly always can realign the eyes, at least in primary position. A patient with an abducens palsy that fails to improve should be reevaluated for an occult etiology (e.g., chordoma, carcinomatous meningitis, carotid cavernous fistula, myasthenia gravis). Skull base tumors are easily missed even on contrast-enhanced neuroimaging studies.

Multiple ocular motor nerve palsies

These should not be attributed to spontaneous microvascular events affecting more than one cranial nerve at a time. This remarkable coincidence does occur, especially in diabetic patients, but the diagnosis is made only in retrospect after all other diagnostic alternatives have been exhausted. Neuroimaging should focus on the cavernous sinus, superior orbital fissure, and orbital apex, where all three ocular motor nerves are in close proximity. In a diabetic or immunocompromised host, fungal infection (*Aspergillus*, Mucorales, *Cryptococcus*) is a common cause of multiple nerve palsies. In a patient with systemic malignancy, carcinomatous meningitis is a likely diagnosis. Cytologic examination may be negative despite repeated sampling of the cerebrospinal fluid. The cancer-associated Lambert-Eaton myasthenic syndrome also can produce ophthalmoplegia. Giant cell (temporal) arteritis occasionally manifests as diplopia from ischemic palsies of extraocular muscles. Fisher's syndrome, an ocular variant of Guillain-Barré, produces ophthalmoplegia with areflexia and ataxia. Often the ataxia is mild, and the reflexes are normal. Antiganglioside antibodies (GQ1b) can be detected in about 50% of cases.

Supranuclear disorders of gaze

These are often mistaken for multiple ocular motor nerve palsies. For example, Wernicke's encephalopathy can produce nystagmus and a partial deficit of horizontal and vertical gaze that mimics a combined abducens and oculomotor nerve palsy. The disorder occurs in malnourished or alcoholic patients and can be reversed by thiamine. Infarct, hemorrhage, tumor, multiple sclerosis, encephalitis, vasculitis, and Whipple's disease are other important causes of supranuclear gaze palsy. Disorders of vertical gaze, especially downward saccades, are an early feature of progressive supranuclear palsy. Smooth pursuit is affected later in the course of the disease. Parkinson's disease, Huntington's disease, and olivopontocerebellar degeneration also can affect vertical gaze.

The *frontal eye field* of the cerebral cortex is involved in generation of saccades to the contralateral side. After hemispheric stroke, the eyes usually deviate toward the lesioned side because of the unopposed action of the frontal eye field in the normal hemisphere. With time, this deficit resolves. Seizures generally have the opposite effect: the eyes deviate conjugately away from the irritative focus. *Parietal lesions* disrupt smooth pursuit of targets moving toward the side of the lesion. Bilateral parietal lesions produce *Bálint's syndrome*, which is characterized by impaired eye-hand coordination (optic ataxia), difficulty initiating voluntary eye movements (ocular apraxia), and visuospatial disorientation (simultanagnosia).

Horizontal gaze

Descending cortical inputs mediating horizontal gaze ultimately converge at the level of the pons. Neurons in the paramedian pontine reticular formation are responsible for controlling conjugate gaze toward the same side. They project directly to the ipsilateral abducens nucleus. A lesion of either the paramedian pontine reticular formation or the abducens nucleus causes an ipsilateral conjugate gaze palsy. Lesions at either locus produce nearly identical clinical syndromes, with the following exception: vestibular stimulation (oculocephalic maneuver or caloric irrigation) will succeed in driving the eyes conjugately to the side in a patient with a lesion of the paramedian pontine reticular formation but not in a patient with a lesion of the abducens nucleus.

Internuclear ophthalmoplegia This results from damage to the medial longitudinal fasciculus ascending from the abducens nucleus in the pons to the oculomotor nucleus in the midbrain (hence, "internuclear"). Damage to fibers carrying the conjugate signal from abducens interneurons to the contralateral medial rectus motoneurons results in a failure of adduction on attempted lateral gaze. For example, a patient with a left internuclear ophthalmoplegia (INO) will have slowed or absent adducting movements of the left eye (Fig. 28-19). A patient with bilateral injury to the medial

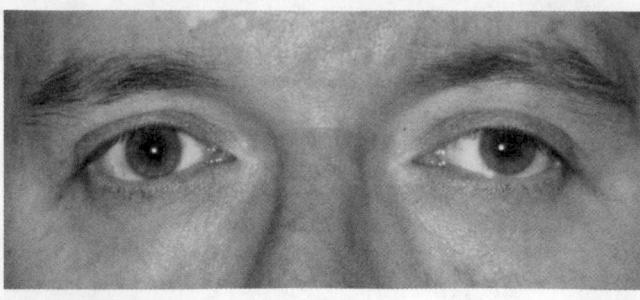

A

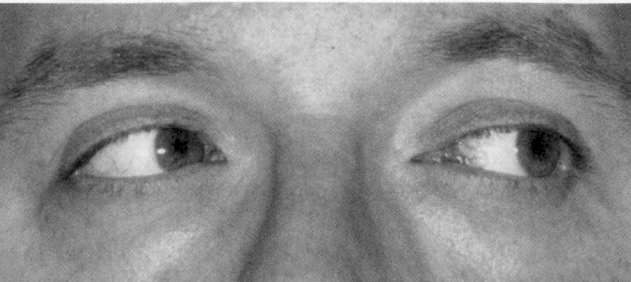

B

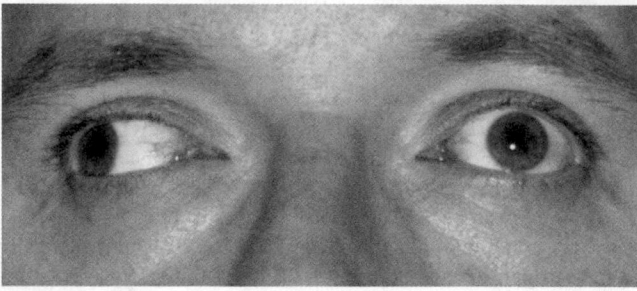

C

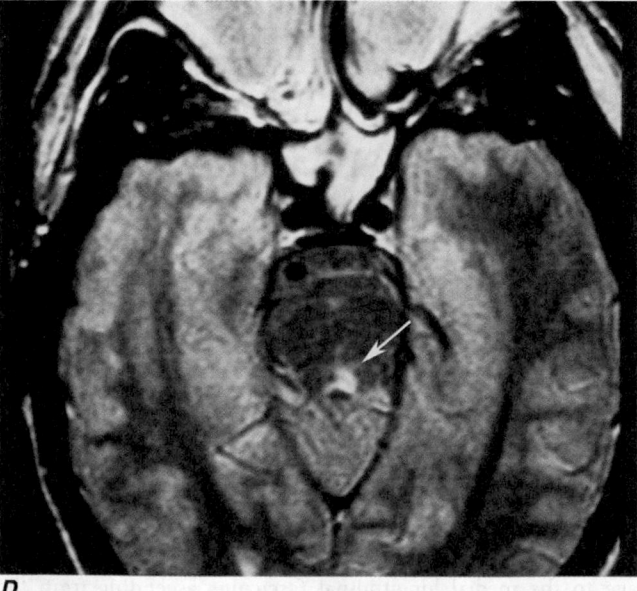

D

Figure 28-19   Left internuclear ophthalmoplegia (INO). *A.* In primary position of gaze the eyes appear normal. ***B.*** Horizontal gaze to the left is intact. ***C.*** On attempted horizontal gaze to the right, the left eye fails to adduct. In mildly affected patients the eye may adduct partially or more slowly than normal. Nystagmus is usually present in the abducted eye. ***D.*** T2-weighted axial MRI image through the pons showing a demyelinating plaque in the left medial longitudinal fasciculus (*arrow*).

longitudinal fasciculus will have bilateral INO. Multiple sclerosis is the most common cause, although tumor, stroke, trauma, or any brainstem process may be responsible. *One-and-a-half syndrome* is due to a combined lesion of the medial longitudinal fasciculus and the abducens nucleus on the same side. The patient's only horizontal eye movement is abduction of the eye on the other side.

Vertical gaze

This is controlled at the level of the midbrain. The neuronal circuits affected in disorders of vertical gaze are not fully elucidated, but lesions of the rostral interstitial nucleus of the medial longitudinal fasciculus and the interstitial nucleus of Cajal cause supranuclear paresis of upgaze, downgaze, or all vertical eye movements. Distal basilar artery ischemia is the most common etiology. *Skew deviation* refers to a vertical misalignment of the eyes, usually constant in all positions of gaze. The finding has poor localizing value because skew deviation has been reported after lesions in widespread regions of the brainstem and cerebellum.

Parinaud's syndrome   Also known as dorsal midbrain syndrome, this is a distinct supranuclear vertical gaze disorder caused by damage to the posterior commissure. It is a classic sign of hydrocephalus from aqueductal stenosis. Pineal region tumors, cysticercosis, and stroke also cause Parinaud's syndrome. Features include loss of upgaze (and sometimes downgaze), convergence-retraction nystagmus on attempted upgaze, downward ocular deviation ("setting sun" sign), lid retraction (Collier's sign), skew deviation, pseudoabducens palsy, and light-near dissociation of the pupils.

Nystagmus

This is a rhythmic oscillation of the eyes, occurring physiologically from vestibular and optokinetic stimulation or pathologically in a wide variety of diseases (Chap. 21). Abnormalities of the eyes or optic nerves, present at birth or acquired in childhood, can produce a complex, searching nystagmus with irregular pendular (sinusoidal) and jerk features. This nystagmus is commonly referred to as *congenital sensory nystagmus.* This is a poor term because even in children with congenital lesions, the nystagmus does not appear until several months of age. *Congenital motor nystagmus,* which looks similar to congenital sensory nystagmus, develops in the absence of any abnormality of the sensory visual system. Visual acuity also is reduced in congenital motor nystagmus, probably by the nystagmus itself, but seldom below a level of 20/200.

Jerk nystagmus   This is characterized by a slow drift off the target, followed by a fast corrective saccade. By convention, the nystagmus is named after the quick phase. Jerk nystagmus can be downbeat, upbeat, horizontal (left or right), and torsional. The pattern of nystagmus may vary with gaze position. Some patients will be oblivious to their nystagmus. Others will complain of blurred vision or a subjective to-and-fro movement of the environment (oscillopsia) corresponding to the nystagmus. Fine nystagmus may be difficult to see on gross examination of the eyes. Observation of nystagmoid movements of the optic disc on ophthalmoscopy is a sensitive way to detect subtle nystagmus.

Gaze-evoked nystagmus   This is the most common form of jerk nystagmus. When the eyes are held eccentrically in the orbits, they have a natural tendency to drift back to primary position. The subject compensates by making a corrective saccade to maintain the deviated eye position. Many normal patients have mild gaze-evoked nystagmus. Exaggerated gaze-evoked nystagmus can be induced by drugs (sedatives, anticonvulsants, alcohol); muscle paresis; myasthenia gravis; demyelinating disease; and cerebellopontine angle, brainstem, and cerebellar lesions.

Vestibular nystagmus *Vestibular nystagmus* results from dysfunction of the labyrinth (Ménière's disease), vestibular nerve, or vestibular nucleus in the brainstem. Peripheral vestibular nystagmus often occurs in discrete attacks, with symptoms of nausea and vertigo. There may be associated tinnitus and hearing loss. Sudden shifts in head position may provoke or exacerbate symptoms.

Downbeat nystagmus *Downbeat nystagmus* results from lesions near the craniocervical junction (Chiari malformation, basilar invagination). It also has been reported in brainstem or cerebellar stroke, lithium or anticonvulsant intoxication, alcoholism, and multiple sclerosis. *Upbeat nystagmus* is associated with damage to the pontine tegmentum from stroke, demyelination, or tumor.

Opsoclonus

This rare, dramatic disorder of eye movements consists of bursts of consecutive saccades (saccadomania). When the saccades are confined to the horizontal plane, the term *ocular flutter* is preferred. It can result from viral encephalitis, trauma, or a paraneoplastic effect of neuroblastoma, breast carcinoma, and other malignancies. It has also been reported as a benign, transient phenomenon in otherwise healthy patients.

FURTHER READINGS

ALBERT DM et al (eds): *Albert and Jakobiec's Principles and Practice of Ophthalmology*, 3rd ed. Philadelphia, Saunders, 2008

CHEUNG N et al: Diabetic retinopathy. Lancet 376:124, 2010

D'AMICO DJ: Clinical practice: Primary retinal detachment. N Engl J Med 359:2346, 2008

JAGER RD et al: Age-related macular degeneration. N Engl J Med 358:2606, 2008

MAGUIRE AM et al: Safety and efficacy of gene transfer for Leber's congenital amaurosis. N Engl J Med 358:2240, 2008

MANCUSO K et al: Gene therapy for red-green colour blindness in adult primates. Nature 461:784, 2009

OPTIC NEURITIS STUDY GROUP: Multiple sclerosis risk after optic neuritis: Final optic neuritis treatment trial follow-up. Arch Neurol 65:1545, 2008

CHAPTER **29**

Disorders of Smell and Taste

Richard L. Doty
Steven M. Bromley

All environmental chemicals necessary for life enter the body by the nose and mouth. The senses of smell (olfaction) and taste (gustation) monitor those chemicals, determine the flavor and palatability of foods and beverages, and warn of dangerous environmental conditions, including fire, air pollution, leaking natural gas, and bacteria-laden foodstuffs. These senses contribute significantly to quality of life and, when dysfunctional, can have untoward physical and psychological consequences. A basic understanding of these senses in health and disease is critical for the physician, since thousands of patients present to doctors' offices each year with complaints of chemosensory dysfunction. Among the more important developments in neurology has been the discovery that decreased smell function is perhaps the first sign of neurodegenerative diseases such as Alzheimer's disease (AD) and Parkinson's disease (PD), signifying their "presymptomatic" phase.

■ ANATOMY AND PHYSIOLOGY

Olfactory system

Odorous chemicals enter the nose during inhalation and active sniffing as well as during deglutition. After reaching the highest recesses of the nasal cavity, they dissolve in the olfactory mucus and diffuse or are actively transported to receptors on the cilia of olfactory receptor cells. The cilia, dendrites, cell bodies, and proximal axonal segments of these bipolar cells are situated within a specialized neuroepithelium that covers the cribriform plate, the superior nasal septum, the superior turbinate, and sectors of the middle turbinate (Fig. 29-1). Each of the ~6 million bipolar receptor cells expresses only one of ~450 receptor protein types, most of which respond to more than a single chemical. When damaged, the receptor cells can be replaced by stem cells near the basement membrane. Unfortunately, such replacement is often incomplete.

After coalescing into bundles surrounded by glia-like ensheathing cells (termed fila), the receptor cell axons pass through the cribriform plate to the olfactory bulbs, where they synapse with dendrites of other cell types within the glomeruli (Fig. 29-2). These spherical structures, which make up a distinct layer of the olfactory bulb, are a site of convergence of information, since many more fibers enter than leave them. Receptor cells that express the same type of receptor project to the same glomeruli, effectively making each glomerulus a functional unit. The major projection neurons of the olfactory system—the mitral and tufted cells—send primary dendrites into the glomeruli, connecting not only with the incoming receptor cell axons but with dendrites of periglomerular cells. The activity of the mitral/tufted cells is modulated by the periglomerular cells, secondary dendrites from other mitral/tufted cells, and granule cells, the most numerous cells of the bulb. The latter cells, which are largely GABAergic, receive inputs from central brain structures and modulate the output of the mitral/tufted cells. Interestingly, like the olfactory receptor cells, some cells within the bulb undergo replacement. Thus, neuroblasts formed within the anterior subventricular zone of the brain migrate along the rostral migratory stream, ultimately becoming granule and periglomerular cells.

The axons of the mitral and tufted cells synapse within the primary olfactory cortex (POC) (Fig. 29-3). The POC is defined as the cortical structures that receive direct projections from the olfactory bulb, most notably the piriform and entorhinal cortices. Although olfaction is unique in that its initial afferent projections bypass the thalamus, persons with damage to the thalamus can exhibit olfactory deficits, particularly ones of odor identification. Those deficits probably reflect the involvement of thalamic connections between the primary olfactory cortex and the orbitofrontal cortex (OFC), where odor identification occurs. The close anatomic ties

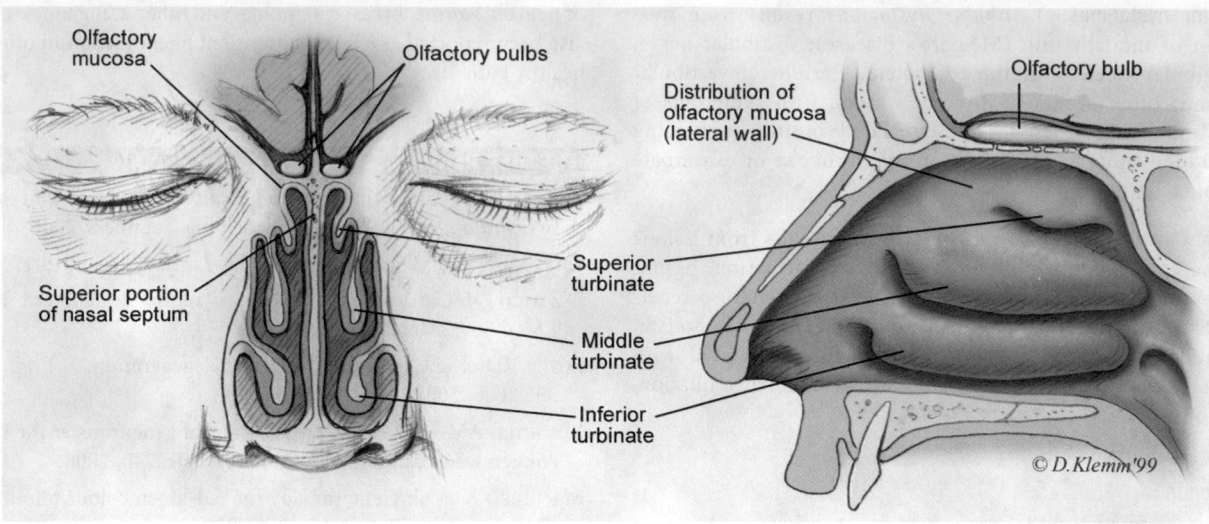

Figure 29-1 **Anatomy of the olfactory neural pathways**, showing the distribution of olfactory receptors in the roof of the nasal cavity. *[Copyright David Klemm, Faculty and Curriculum Support (FACS), Georgetown University Medical Center; used with permission.]*

between the olfactory system and the amygdala, hippocampus, and hypothalamus help explain the intimate associations between odor perception and cognitive functions such as memory, motivation, arousal, autonomic activity, digestion, and sex.

Taste system

Tastants are sensed by specialized receptor cells present within taste buds: small grapefruit-like segmented structures on the lateral margins and dorsum of the tongue, the roof of the mouth, the pharynx, the larynx, and the superior esophagus (Fig. 29-4). Lingual taste

buds are embedded in well-defined protuberances termed fungiform, foliate, and circumvallate papillae. After dissolving in a liquid, tastants enter the opening of the taste bud—the taste pore—and bind to receptors on microvilli, small extensions of receptor cells within each taste bud. Such binding changes the electrical potential across the taste cell, resulting in neurotransmitter release onto the first-order taste neurons. Although humans have ~7500 taste buds, not all harbor taste-sensitive cells; some contain only one class of receptor (e.g., cells responsive only to sugars), whereas others contain cells sensitive to more than one class. The number of taste

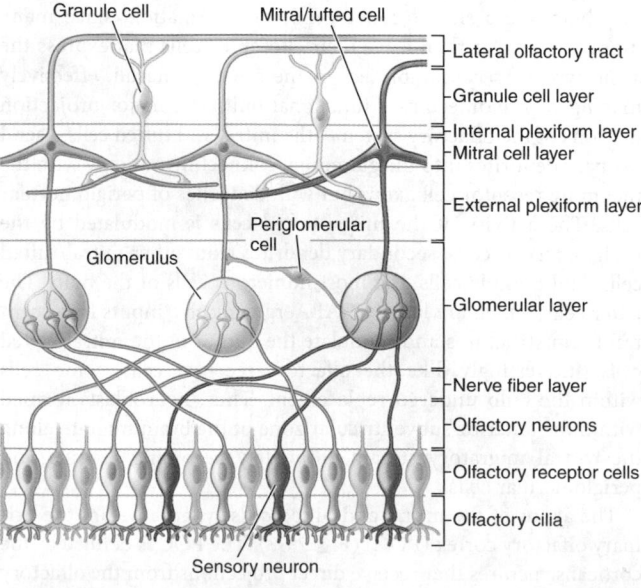

Figure 29-2 **Schematic of the layers and wiring of the olfactory bulb.** Each receptor type (red, green, blue) projects to a common glomerulus. The neural activity within each glomerulus is modulated by periglomerular cells. The activity of the primary projection cells, the mitral and tufted cells, is modulated by granule cells, periglomerular cells, and secondary dendrites from other mitral and tufted cells. *(From www.med.yale.edu/neurosurg/ treloar/index.html.)*

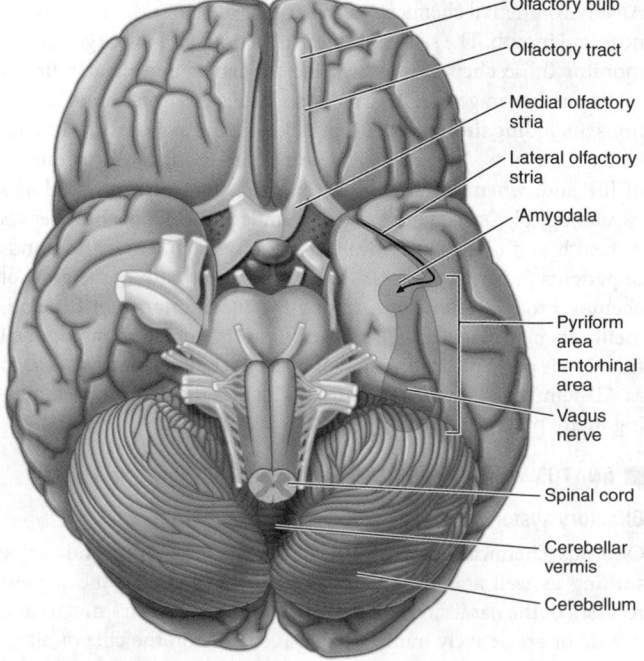

Figure 29-3 **Anatomy of the base of the brain** showing the primary olfactory cortex.

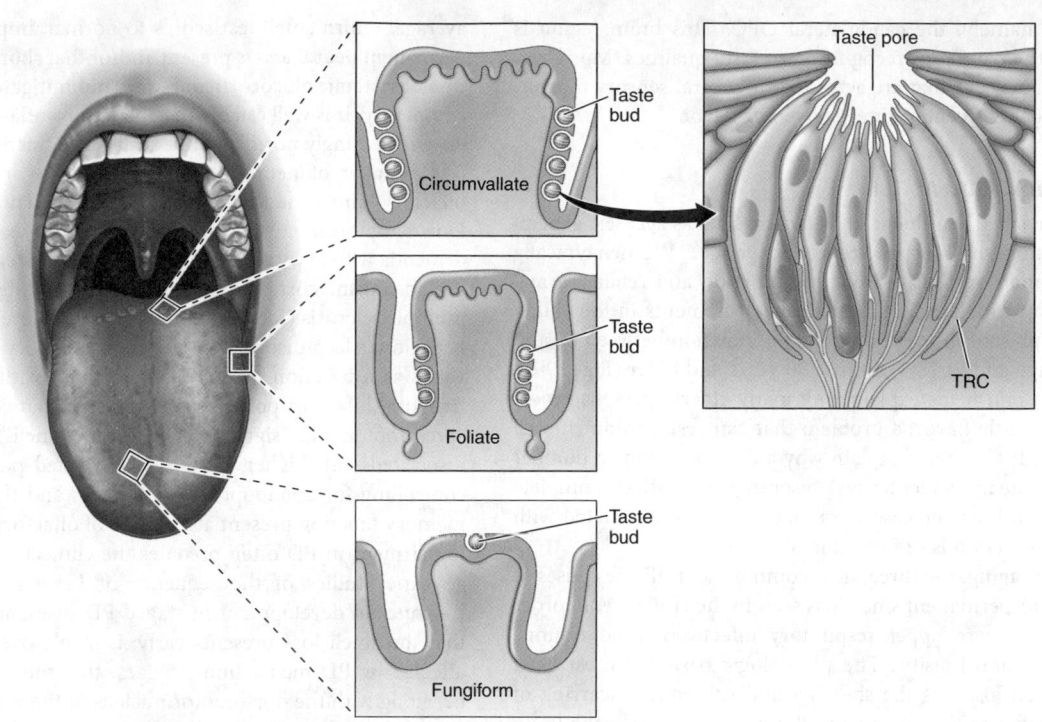

Figure 29-4 **Schematic of the taste bud** and its opening (pore), as well as the location of buds on the three major types of papillae: fungiform (anterior), foliate (lateral), and circumvallate (posterior). TRC, taste receptor cell.

receptor cells per taste bud ranges from zero to well over 100. A small family of three G-protein-coupled receptors (GPCRs)—T1R1, T1R2, and T1R3—mediate sweet and umami taste sensations. Umami ("savory") refers to the flavors of meat, cheese, and broth due to glutamate and related compounds. Bitter sensations, in contrast, depend on T2R receptors, a family of ~30 GPCRs expressed on cells different from those which express the sweet and umami receptors. T2Rs sense a wide range of bitter substances but do not distinguish among them. Sour tastants are sensed by the PKD2L1 receptor, a member of the transient receptor potential protein (TRP) family. Perception of salty sensations, such as those induced by sodium chloride, arises from the entry of Na^+ ions into the cells via specialized membrane channels such as the amiloride-sensitive Na^+ channel.

Taste information is sent to the brain via three cranial nerves (CNs): CN VII (the *facial nerve,* which involves the intermediate nerve with its branches, the greater petrosal and chorda tympani nerves); CN IX (the *glossopharyngeal nerve*); and CN X (the *vagus nerve*) (Fig. 29-5). CN VII innervates the anterior tongue and all of the soft palate, CN IX innervates the posterior tongue, and CN X innervates the laryngeal surface of the epiglottis, the larynx, and the proximal portion of the esophagus. The mandibular branch of CN V (V_3) conveys somatosensory information (e.g., touch, burning, cooling, irritation) to the brain. Although not technically a gustatory nerve, CN V shares primary nerve routes with many of the gustatory nerve fibers and adds temperature, texture, pungency, and spiciness to the taste experience. The chorda tympani nerve is notable for taking a recurrent course through the facial canal in the petrosal portion of the temporal bone, passing through the middle ear, then exiting the skull via the petrotympanic fissure, where it joins the lingual nerve (a division of CN V) near the tongue. This nerve also carries parasympathetic fibers to the submandibular and sublingual glands, whereas the greater petrosal nerve supplies the palatine glands, thereby influencing saliva production.

The axons of the projection cells that synapse with taste buds enter the rostral portion of the nucleus of the solitary tract (NTS)

within the medulla of the brainstem (Fig. 29-5). From the NTS, neurons then project to a division of the ventroposteromedial thalamic nucleus (VPM) via the medial lemniscus. From there projections are made to the rostral part of the frontal operculum and adjoining insula, a brain region considered the *primary taste cortex* (PTC). Projections from the primary taste cortex then go to the *secondary*

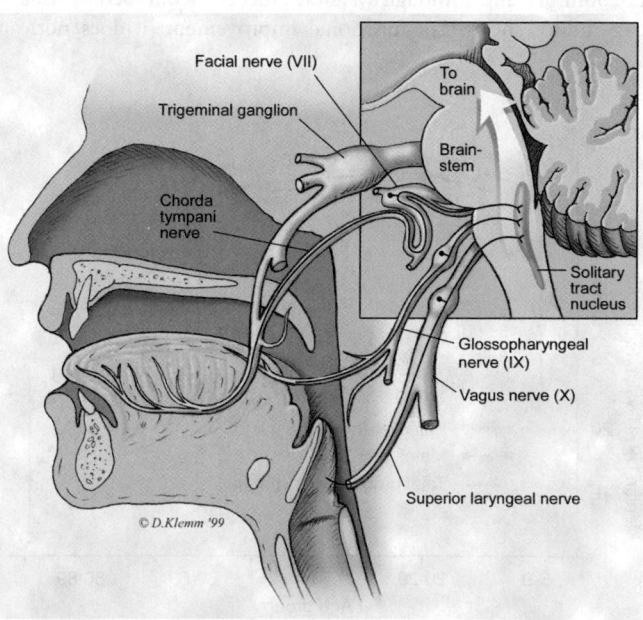

Figure 29-5 **Schematic of the cranial nerves** that mediate taste function, including the chorda tympani nerve (CN VII), the glossopharyngeal nerve (CN IX), and the vagus nerve (CN X). *[Copyright David Klemm, Faculty and Curriculum Support (FACS), Georgetown University Medical Center; used with permission.]*

taste cortex, namely, the caudolateral OFC. This brain region is involved in the conscious recognition of taste qualities. Moreover, since it contains cells that are activated by several sensory modalities, it is probably a center for establishing "flavor."

■ DISORDERS OF OLFACTION

The ability to smell is influenced by factors such as age, sex, general health, nutrition, smoking, and reproductive state. Women typically outperform men on tests of olfactory function and retain normal smell function to a later age. Significant decrements in the ability to smell are present in over 50% of the population between 65 and 80 years of age and in 75% of those 80 years and older (Fig. 29-6). Such *presbyosmia* helps explain why many elderly persons report that food has little flavor, a problem that can result in nutritional disturbances. It also helps explain why a disproportionate number of the elderly die in accidental gas poisonings. A relatively complete listing of conditions and disorders that have been associated with olfactory dysfunction is presented in Table 29-1.

Aside from aging, the three most common identifiable causes of long-lasting or permanent smell loss seen in the clinic are, in order of frequency, severe upper respiratory infections, head trauma, and chronic rhinosinusitis. The physiologic basis for most head trauma–related losses is the shearing and subsequent scarring of the olfactory fila as they pass from the nasal cavity into the brain cavity. The cribriform plate does not have to be fractured or show pathology for smell loss to be present. Severity of trauma, as indexed by a poor Glasgow Coma Rating on presentation and the length of posttraumatic amnesia, is associated with higher risk of olfactory impairment. Fewer than 10% of posttraumatic anosmic patients recover age-related normal function over time. Upper respiratory infections, such as those associated with the common cold, influenza, pneumonia, or HIV, can directly and permanently harm the olfactory epithelium by decreasing receptor cell numbers, damaging cilia on remaining receptor cells, and inducing the replacement of sensory epithelium with respiratory epithelium. The smell loss associated with chronic rhinosinusitis is related to disease severity, with most loss occurring in cases in which rhinosinusitis and polyposis are both present. Although systemic glucocorticoid therapy usually can induce short-term functional improvement, it does not, on

average, return smell test scores to normal, implying that chronic permanent neural loss is present and/or that short-term administration of systemic glucocorticoids does not mitigate the inflammation completely. It is well established that microinflammation in an otherwise seemingly normal epithelium can influence smell function.

A number of neurodegenerative diseases are accompanied by olfactory impairment, including AD, PD, Huntington's disease, Down syndrome, parkinsonism-dementia complex of Guam, dementia with Lewy bodies (DLB), multiple system atrophy, vascular parkinsonism, corticobasal syndrome, frontotemporal dementia, multiple sclerosis (MS), and idiopathic rapid eye movement (REM) behavioral sleep disorder (iRBD). The olfactory disturbance of MS varies as a function of the plaque activity within the frontal and temporal lobes. In postmortem studies of patients with very mild "presymptomatic" signs of AD, poorer smell function has been associated with higher levels of AD-related pathology even after controlling for apolipoprotein E4 alleles and the level of episodic memory function present at the time of olfactory testing. Olfactory impairment in PD often predates the clinical diagnosis by at least 4 years. Studies of the sequence of Lewy body and abnormal α-synuclein development in staged PD cases, along with evidence that the smell loss presents early, is stable over time, and is not affected by PD medications, suggest that the olfactory bulbs may be, along with the dorsomotor nucleus of the vagus, the site of first neural damage in PD. Smell loss is more marked in patients with early clinical manifestations of DLB than in those with mild AD. Interestingly, smell loss is minimal or nonexistent in progressive supranuclear palsy and 1-methyl-4-phenyl-1,2,3,6-tetrahydropyridine (MPTP)-induced parkinsonism.

The smell loss seen in iRBD is of the same magnitude as that found in PD. This is of particular interest to clinicians since patients with iRBD frequently develop PD and hyposmia. iRBD may actually represent an early associated condition of PD. REM behavior disorder not only is seen in its idiopathic form but also can be associated with narcolepsy. This led to a study of narcoleptic patients with and without REM behavior disorder that demonstrated that narcolepsy, independent of REM behavior disorder, was associated with significant impairments in olfactory function. Orexin A, also known as hypocretin-1, is dramatically diminished or undetectable in the cerebrospinal fluid of patients with narcolepsy and cataplexy. The orexin-containing neurons in the hypothalamus project throughout the olfactory system (from the olfactory epithelium to the olfactory cortex), and damage to these orexin-containing projections may be one underlying mechanism for impaired olfactory performance in narcoleptic patients. The administration of intranasal orexin A (hypocretin-1) appears to result in improved olfactory function relative to a placebo, supporting the notion that mild olfactory impairment is not only a primary feature of narcolepsy with cataplexies but that CNS orexin deficiency may be a fundamental part of the mechanism for this loss.

■ DISORDERS OF TASTE

The majority of patients who present with complaints of taste dysfunction exhibit olfactory, not taste, loss. This is the case because most flavors attributed to taste actually depend on retronasal stimulation of the olfactory receptors during deglutition. As noted earlier, taste buds only mediate basic tastes such as sweet, sour, bitter, salty, and umami. Significant impairment of whole-mouth gustatory function is rare outside of generalized metabolic disturbances or systemic use of some medications, since taste bud regeneration occurs and peripheral damage alone would require the involvement of multiple cranial nerve pathways. Nonetheless, taste can be influenced by (1) the release of foul-tasting materials from the oral cavity from oral medical conditions and appliances (e.g. gingivitis, purulent

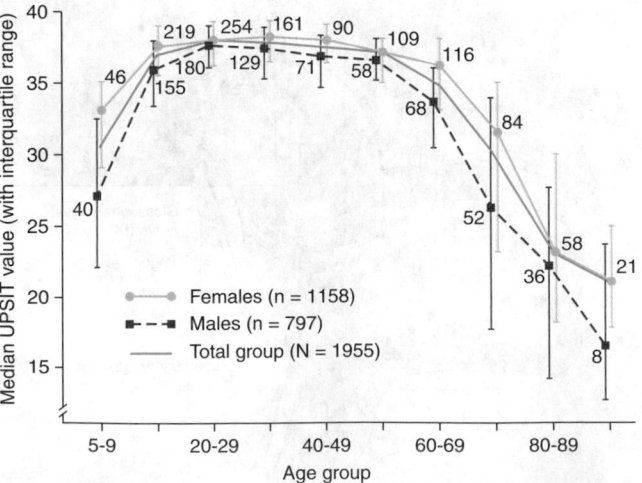

Figure 29-6 Scores on the University of Pennsylvania Smell Identification Test (UPSIT) as a function of subject age and sex. Numbers by each data point indicate sample sizes. Note that women identify odorants better than men at all ages. *(From Doty et al: Science 226:1421, 1984. Copyright 1984 American Association for the Advancement of Science.)*

TABLE 29-1 Disorders and Conditions Associated With Compromised Olfactory Function as Measured by Olfactory Testing

22q11 deletion syndrome	Liver disease
AIDS/HIV infection	Lubag disease
Adenoid hypertrophy	Medications
Adrenal cortical insufficiency	Migraine
Age	Multiple sclerosis
Alcoholism	Multi-infarct dementia
Allergies	Narcolepsy with cataplexy
Alzheimer's disease	Neoplasms, cranial/nasal
Amyotrophic lateral sclerosis	Nutritional deficiencies
Anorexia nervosa	Obstructive pulmonary disease
Asperger's syndrome	Obesity
Ataxias	Obsessive-compulsive disorder
Attention deficit/hyperactivity disorder	Orthostatic tremor
Bardet-Biedl syndrome	Panic disorder
Chemical exposure	Parkinson's disease
Chronic obstructive pulmonary disease	Pick's disease
Congenital	Posttraumatic stress disorder
Cushing's syndrome	Pregnancy
Cystic fibrosis	Pseudohypoparathyroidism
Degenerative ataxias	Psychopathy
Diabetes	Radiation (therapeutic, cranial)
Down syndrome	REM behavior disorder
Epilepsy	Refsum disease
Facial paralysis	Renal failure/end-stage kidney disease
Frontotemporal lobe degeneration	Restless leg syndrome
Gonadal dysgenesis (Turner syndrome)	Rhinosinusitis/polyposis
Guamanian ALS/PD/dementia syndrome	Schizophrenia
Head trauma	Seasonal affective disorder
Herpes simplex encephalitis	Sjögren's syndrome
Hypothyroidism	Stroke
Huntington's disease	Tobacco smoking
Iatrogenesis	Toxic chemical exposure
Kallmann's syndrome	Upper respiratory infections
Korsakoff's psychosis	Usher syndrome
Leprosy	Vitamin B$_{12}$ deficiency

sialadenitis), (2) transport problems of tastants to the taste buds (e.g., drying of the orolingual mucosa, infections, inflammatory conditions), (3) damage to the taste buds themselves (e.g., local trauma, invasive carcinomas), (4) damage to the neural pathways innervating the taste buds (e.g., middle ear infections), (5) damage to central structures (e.g., multiple sclerosis, tumor, epilepsy, stroke), and (6) systemic disturbances of metabolism (e.g., diabetes, thyroid disease, medications). Bell's palsy is among the most common causes of CN VII injury that results in taste disturbance. Unlike CN VII, CN IX is relatively protected along its path, although iatrogenic interventions

such as tonsillectomy, bronchoscopy, laryngoscopy, and radiation therapy can result in selective injury. Migraine is associated on rare occasions with a gustatory prodrome or aura, and certain tastes may trigger a migraine. Although a number of disorders can affect CN IX, including tumors, trauma, vascular lesions, and infection, it remains unclear if noticeable taste disturbance can result from such factors.

Although both taste and smell can be adversely influenced by pharmacologic agents, drug-related taste alterations are more common. Indeed, over 250 medications have been reported to alter the ability to taste. Major offenders include antineoplastic agents, antirheumatic drugs, antibiotics, and blood pressure medications. Terbinafine, a commonly used antifungal, has been linked to taste disturbance lasting up to 3 years. In a controlled trial, nearly two-thirds of individuals taking eszopiclone (Lunesta) experienced a bitter dysgeusia which was stronger in women, systematically related to the time since drug administration, and positively correlated with both blood and saliva levels of the drug. Intranasal use of nasal gels and sprays containing zinc—common over-the-counter prophylactics for upper respiratory viral infections—has been implicated in loss of smell function. Whether their efficacy in preventing such infections, which are the most common cause of anosmia and hyposmia, outweighs their potential detriment to smell function requires study.

As with olfaction, a number of systemic disorders can affect taste. They include chronic renal failure, end-stage liver disease, vitamin and mineral deficiencies, diabetes, and hypothyroidism, to name a few. Psychiatric conditions can be associated with chemosensory alterations (e.g., depression, schizophrenia, bulimia). A review of tactile, gustatory, and olfactory hallucinations demonstrated that no one type of hallucinatory experience is pathognomonic to any specific diagnosis.

■ CLINICAL EVALUATION

In most cases, a careful clinical history will establish the probable etiology of a chemosensory problem, including questions about its nature, onset, duration, and pattern of fluctuations. *Sudden loss* suggests the possibility of head trauma, ischemia, infection, or a psychiatric condition. *Gradual loss* can reflect the development of a progressive obstructive lesion. *Intermittent loss* suggests the likelihood of an inflammatory process. The patient should be asked about potential precipitating events, such as cold or flu infections before symptom onset, as they often are underappreciated. Information regarding head trauma, smoking habits, drug and alcohol abuse (e.g., intranasal cocaine, chronic alcoholism in the context of Wernicke's and Korsakoff's syndromes), exposures to pesticides and other toxic agents, and medical interventions are also informative. A determination of all the medications the patient was taking before and at the time of symptom onset is important, since many can cause chemosensory disturbances. Comorbid medical conditions associated with smell impairment, such as renal failure, liver disease, hypothyroidism, diabetes, and dementia, should be assessed. Delayed puberty in association with anosmia (with or without midline craniofacial abnormalities, deafness, and renal anomalies) suggests the possibility of Kallmann syndrome. Recollection of epistaxis, discharge (clear, purulent, or bloody), nasal obstruction, allergies, and somatic symptoms, including headache or irritation, may have localizing value. Questions related to memory, parkinsonian signs, and seizure activity (e.g., automatisms, occurrence of blackouts, auras, and déjà vu) should be posed. Pending litigation and the possibility of malingering should be considered.

Neurologic and otorhinolaryngologic (ORL) examinations, along with appropriate brain and nasosinus imaging, aid in the evaluation of patients with olfactory or gustatory complaints. The neural evaluation should focus on cranial nerve function, with particular attention to possible skull base and intracranial lesions. Visual acuity, field, and optic disc examinations aid in the detection of intracranial mass lesions that induce elevations in intracranial pressure (papilledema) and optic atrophy, especially when one is considering Foster Kennedy syndrome (ipsilateral optic nerve atrophy and contralateral papilledema usually due to a meningioma near the olfactory bulb or tract). The ORL examination should thoroughly assess the intranasal architecture and mucosal surfaces. Polyps, masses, and adhesions of the turbinates to the septum may compromise the flow of air to the olfactory receptors, since less than a fifth of the inspired air traverses the olfactory cleft in the unobstructed state. Blood serum tests may be helpful to identify conditions such as diabetes, infection, heavy metal exposure, nutritional deficiency (e.g., vitamins B_6 and B_{12}), allergy, and thyroid, liver, and kidney disease.

As with other sensory disorders, quantitative sensory testing is advised. Self-reports of patients can be misleading, and a number who complain of chemosensory dysfunction have normal function for their age and sex. Quantitative smell and taste testing provides valid information for worker's compensation and other legal claims as well as a way to assess treatment interventions accurately. A number of standardized olfactory and taste tests are commercially available. Most evaluate the ability of patients to detect and identify odors or tastes. For example, the most widely used of these tests, the 40-item University of Pennsylvania Smell Identification Test (UPSIT), employs norms based on nearly 4000 normal subjects. A determination is made of both absolute dysfunction (i.e., mild loss, moderate loss, severe loss, total loss, probable malingering) and relative dysfunction (percentile rank for age and sex). Although electrophysiologic testing is available at some smell and taste centers (e.g., odor event-related potentials), such tests require complex stimulus presentation and recording equipment and rarely provide additional diagnostic information. In addition to electrogustometers, commercial chemical taste tests are now available. Most employ filter paper strips impregnated with tastants, so no stimulus preparation is required. Like the UPSIT, these tests have published norms for establishing the degree of dysfunction.

■ TREATMENT AND MANAGEMENT

Because of the various mechanisms by which olfactory and gustatory disturbance can occur, management of patients tends to be condition-specific. For example, patients with hypothyroidism, diabetes, or infections need to be given specific treatments to correct the underlying process adversely influencing chemoreception. For most patients who present primarily with obstructive/transport loss affecting the nasal and paranasal regions (e.g., allergic rhinitis, polyposis, intranasal neoplasms, nasal deviations), medical and/or surgical intervention is often beneficial. Antifungal and antibiotic treatments may reverse taste problems secondary to candidiasis or other oral infections. Chlorohexidine mouthwash mitigates some salty or bitter dysgeusias, conceivably as a result of its strong positive charge. Excessive dryness of the oral mucosa is a problem with many medications and conditions, and artificial saliva (e.g., Xerolube) or oral pilocarpine treatments may prove beneficial. Other methods to improve salivary flow include the use of mints, lozenges, or sugarless gum. Flavor enhancers may make food more palatable (e.g., monosodium glutamate), but caution is advised to avoid overusing ingredients containing sodium or sugar, particularly in circumstances in which a patient also has underlying hypertension or diabetes. Medications that induce distortions of taste often can be discontinued and replaced with other types of medications or modes of therapy. As mentioned earlier, pharmacologic agents result in taste disturbances much more frequently than smell disturbances, and over 250 medications have been reported to alter the sense of taste. Many drug-related effects are long-lasting and are not reversed by short-term drug discontinuance.

A study of endoscopic sinus surgery in patients with chronic rhinosinusitis and hyposmia revealed that patients with severe olfactory dysfunction before the surgery had a more dramatic and sustained improvement over time compared with patients with more mild olfactory dysfunction before intervention. In the case of intranasal and sinus-related inflammatory conditions such as those seen with allergy, viruses, and traumas, the use of intranasal or systemic glucocorticoids may be helpful. One common approach is a short course of oral prednisone, typically 60 mg daily for 4 days and then tapered by 10 mg daily. The utility of restoring olfaction with either topical or systemic glucocorticoids has been studied. Topical intranasal glucocorticoids were less effective in general than systemic glucocorticoids; however, nasal steroid administration techniques were not analyzed. Intranasal glucocorticoids are more effective if administered in Moffett's position (head in the inverted position such as over the edge of the bed with the bridge of the nose perpendicular to the floor). After head trauma, an initial trial of glucocorticoids may help reduce local edema and the potential deleterious deposition of scar tissue around olfactory fila at the level of the cribriform plate.

Treatments are limited for patients with chemosensory loss or primary injury to neural pathways. Nonetheless, spontaneous recovery can occur. In a follow-up study of 542 patients presenting with smell loss from a variety of causes, modest improvement occurred over an average period of 4 years in about half the participants. However, only 11% of the anosmic and 23% of the hyposmic patients regained normal age-related function. Interestingly, the amount of dysfunction present at the time of presentation, not etiology, was the best predictor of prognosis. Other predictors were the patient's age and the time between the onset of dysfunction and initial testing.

A nonblinded study reported that patients with hyposmia may benefit from smelling strong odors (e.g., eucalyptol, citronella, eugenol, and phenyl ethyl alcohol) before going to bed and immediately upon awaking each day over the course of several months. The rationale for this approach comes from animal studies demonstrating that prolonged exposure to odorants can induce increased neural activity within the olfactory bulb. α-Lipoic acid (200 mg two or three times daily), an essential cofactor for many enzyme complexes with possible antioxidant effects, has been reported to be beneficial in mitigating smell loss after viral infection of the upper respiratory tract, although double-blind studies are needed to confirm this observation. This agent has also been suggested to be useful in some cases of hypogeusia and burning mouth syndrome.

The use of zinc and vitamin A in treating olfactory disturbances is controversial; not much benefit is obtained beyond replenishing established deficiencies. However, zinc improves taste function secondary to hepatic deficiencies, and retinoids (bioactive vitamin A derivatives) are known to play an essential role in the survival of olfactory neurons. One protocol in which zinc was infused with chemotherapy treatments suggested a possible protective effect against developing taste impairment. Diseases of the alimentary tract can not only influence chemoreceptive function but occasionally influence B_{12} absorption. This can result in a relative deficiency of B_{12}, theoretically contributing to olfactory nerve disturbance. B_2 (riboflavin) and magnesium supplements are reported in the alternative medicine literature to aid in the management of migraine headaches that may be associated with smell dysfunction.

A number of medicines have been reported to ameliorate olfactory symptoms, although strong scientific evidence for efficacy is generally lacking. A report that theophylline improved smell function was not double-blinded and lacked a control group, failing to take into account that some meaningful improvement occurs without treatment. Indeed, the percentage of patients reported to be responsive to the treatment was about the same as that noted by others to show spontaneous improvement over a similar time period (~50%). Antiepileptics and some antidepressants (e.g. amitriptyline) have been used to treat dysosmias and smell distortions, particularly after head trauma. Ironically, amitriptyline is also frequently on the list of medications that can ultimately distort smell and taste function, possibly from its anticholinergic effects. The use of donepezil (an acetylcholinesterase inhibitor) in AD may result in improvements in smell identification measures that correlate with overall clinician-based impressions of change scales [Clinician Interview Based Impression of Severity (CIBIC)-plus]. Smell identification function could become a useful measure to assess overall treatment response with this medication.

A major and often overlooked element of therapy comes from chemosensory testing itself. Confirmation or lack of confirmation of loss is beneficial to patients who come to believe, in light of unsupportive family members and medical providers, that they may be "crazy." In cases in which the loss is minor, patients can be informed of the likelihood of a more positive prognosis. Importantly, quantitative testing places the patient's problem into overall perspective. Thus, it is often therapeutic for an older person to know that although his or her smell function is not what it used to be, it still falls above the average of his or her peer group. Without testing, many such patients are simply told they are getting old and nothing can be done for them, leading in some cases to depression and decreased self-esteem.

FURTHER READINGS

Bromley SM, Doty RL: Olfaction in dentistry. Oral Dis 16:221, 2010

Calderón-Garcidueñas L et al: Urban air pollution: Influences on olfactory function and pathology in exposed children and young adults. Exp Toxicol Pathol 62:91, 2010

Deems DA et al: Smell and taste disorders: A study of 750 patients from the University of Pennsylvania Smell and Taste Center. Arch Otolaryngol Head Neck Surg 117:519, 1991

Doty RL: The olfactory vector hypothesis of neurodegenerative disease: Is it viable? Ann Neurol 63:7, 2008

—— (ed): Handbook of Olfaction and Gustation. New York, Marcel Dekker, 2003

—— et al: Drug-induced taste disorders: Incidence, prevention and management. Drug Safety 31:199, 2008

Gottfried JA: Function follows form: Ecological constraints on odor codes and olfactory percepts. Curr Opin Neurobiol 19:422, 2009

Hawkes CH, Doty RL. Neurology of Olfaction. Cambridge, Cambridge University Press, 2009

Kern RC: Chronic sinusitis and anosmia: Pathologic changes in the olfactory mucosa. Laryngoscope 110:1071, 2000

London B et al: Predictors of prognosis in patients with olfactory disturbance. Ann Neurol 63:159, 2008

CHAPTER **30**

Disorders of Hearing

Anil K. Lalwani

Hearing loss is one of the most common sensory disorders in humans and can present at any age. Nearly 10% of the adult population has some hearing loss, and one-third of individuals age >65 years have a hearing loss of sufficient magnitude to require a hearing aid.

■ PHYSIOLOGY OF HEARING

The function of the external and middle ear is to amplify sound to facilitate conversion of the mechanical energy of the sound wave into an electrical signal by the inner ear hair cells, a process called mechanotransduction (Fig. 30-1). Sound waves enter the external auditory canal and set the tympanic membrane in motion, which in turn moves the malleus, incus, and stapes of the middle ear. Movement of the footplate of the stapes causes pressure changes in the fluid-filled inner ear, eliciting a traveling wave in the basilar membrane of the cochlea. The tympanic membrane and the ossicular chain in the middle ear serve as an impedance-matching mechanism, improving the efficiency of energy transfer from air to the fluid-filled inner ear.

Stereocilia of the hair cells of the organ of Corti, which rests on the basilar membrane, are in contact with the tectorial membrane and are deformed by the traveling wave. A point of maximal displacement of the basilar membrane is determined by the frequency of the stimulating tone. High-frequency tones cause maximal displacement of the basilar membrane near the base of the cochlea, whereas for low-frequency sounds, the point of maximal displacement is toward the apex of the cochlea.

The inner and outer hair cells of the organ of Corti have different innervation patterns, but both are mechanoreceptors. The afferent innervation relates principally to the inner hair cells, and the efferent innervation relates principally to outer hair cells. The motil-ity of the outer hair cells alters the micromechanics of the inner hair cells, creating a cochlear amplifier, which explains the exquisite sensitivity and frequency selectivity of the cochlea.

Beginning in the cochlea, the frequency specificity is maintained at each point of the central auditory pathway: dorsal and ventral cochlear nuclei, trapezoid body, superior olivary complex, lateral lemniscus, inferior colliculus, medial geniculate body, and auditory cortex. At low frequencies, individual auditory nerve fibers can respond more or less synchronously with the stimulating tone. At higher frequencies, phase-locking occurs so that neurons alternate in response to particular phases of the cycle of the sound wave. Intensity is encoded by the amount of neural activity in individual neurons, the number of neurons that are active, and the specific neurons that are activated.

■ DISORDERS OF THE SENSE OF HEARING

Hearing loss can result from disorders of the auricle, external auditory canal, middle ear, inner ear, or central auditory pathways (Fig. 30-2). *In general, lesions in the auricle, external auditory canal, or middle ear that impede the transmission of sound from the external environment to the inner ear cause conductive hearing loss, whereas lesions that impair mechanotransduction in the inner ear or transmission of the electrical signal along the eighth nerve to the brain cause sensorineural hearing loss.*

Conductive hearing loss

The external ear, the external auditory canal, and the middle ear apparatus is designed to collect and amplify sound and efficiently transfer the mechanical energy of the sound wave to the fluid-filled cochlea. Factors that obstruct the transmission of sound or serve to dampen the acoustical energy result in conductive hearing loss. Conductive hearing loss can occur from obstruction of the external auditory canal by cerumen, debris, and foreign bodies; swelling of the lining of the canal; atresia or neoplasms of the canal; perforations of the tympanic membrane; disruption of the ossicular chain, as occurs with necrosis of the long process of the incus in trauma or infection; otosclerosis; or fluid, scarring, or neoplasms in the middle ear. Rarely, inner ear malformations or pathologies may also be associated with conductive hearing loss.

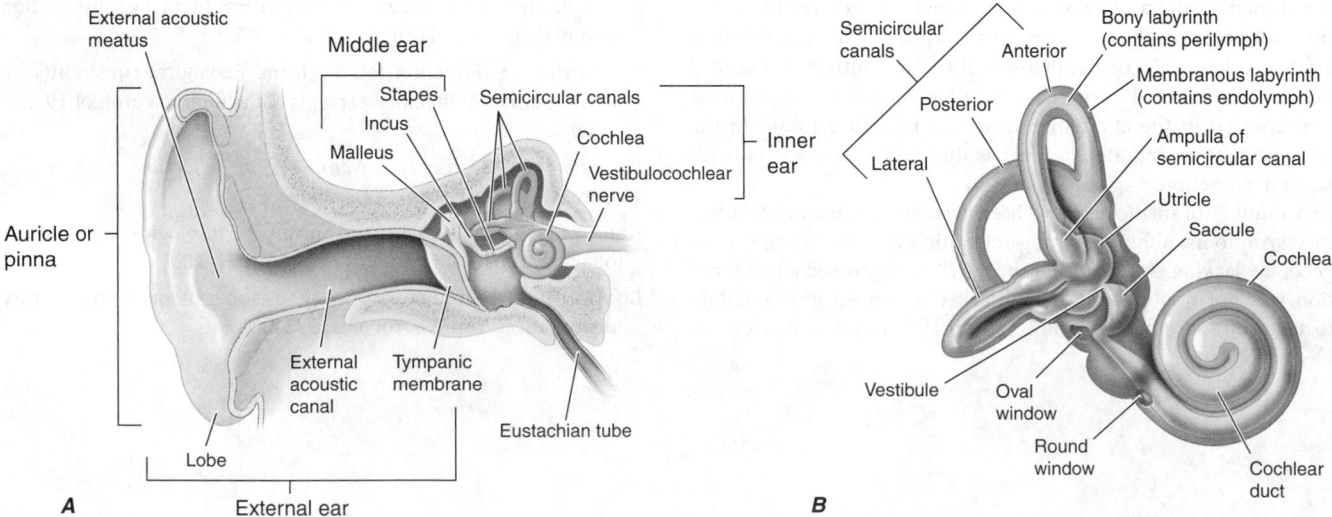

Figure 30-1 Ear anatomy. *A.* Drawing of modified coronal section through external ear and temporal bone, with structures of the middle and inner ear demonstrated. ***B.*** High-resolution view of inner ear.

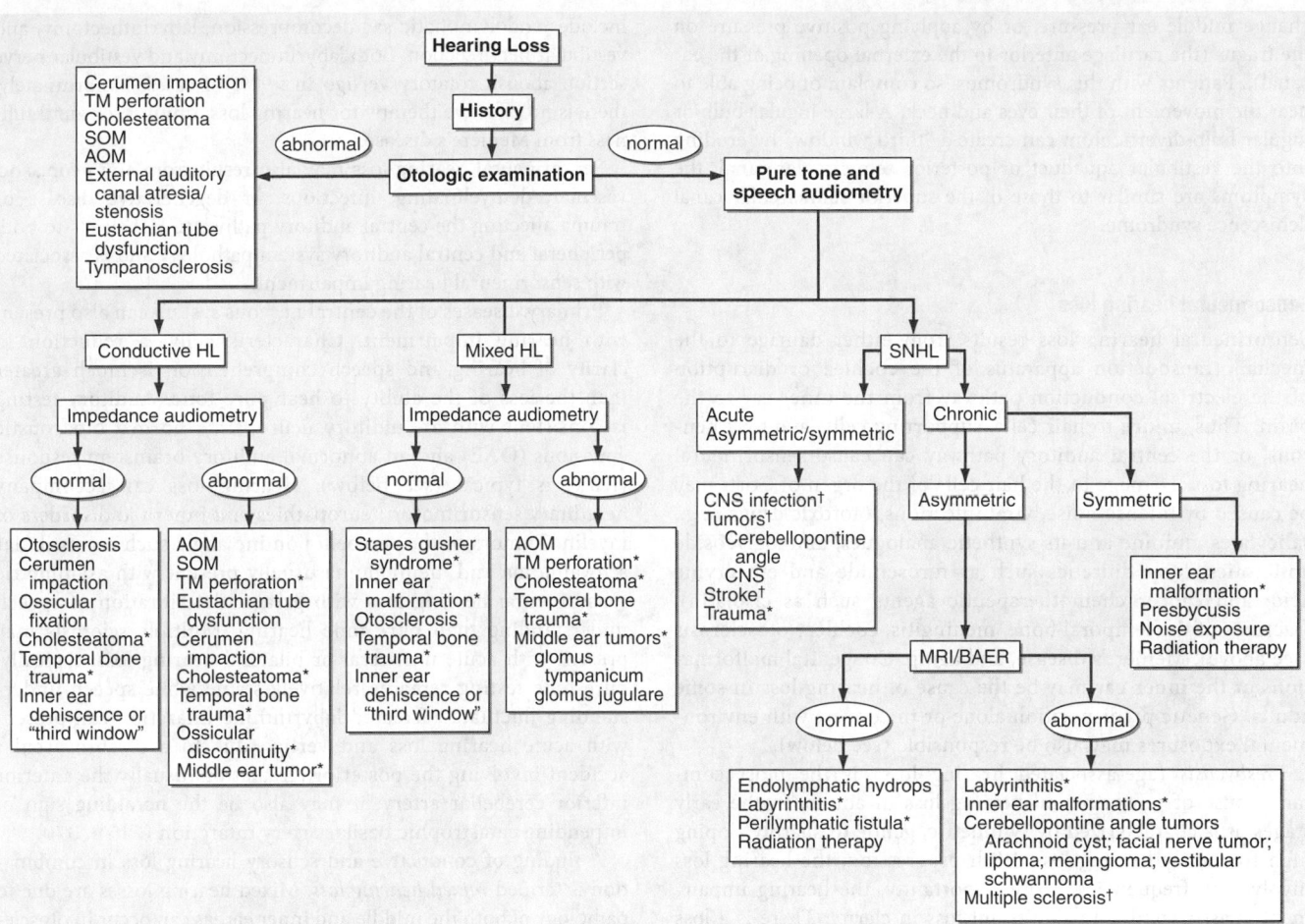

Figure 30-2 An algorithm for the approach to hearing loss. HL, hearing loss; SNHL, sensorineural hearing loss; TM, tympanic membrane; SOM, serous otitis media; AOM, acute otitis media; BAER, brainstem auditory evoked response; *, CT scan of temporal bone; †, MRI scan.

Eustachian tube dysfunction is extremely common in adults and may predispose to acute otitis media (AOM) or serous otitis media (SOM). Trauma, AOM, or chronic otitis media are the usual factors responsible for tympanic membrane perforation. While small perforations often heal spontaneously, larger defects usually require surgical intervention. Tympanoplasty is highly effective (>90%) in the repair of tympanic membrane perforations. Otoscopy is usually sufficient to diagnose AOM, SOM, chronic otitis media, cerumen impaction, tympanic membrane perforation, and eustachian tube dysfunction; tympanometry can be useful to confirm the clinical suspicion of these conditions.

Cholesteatoma, a benign tumor composed of stratified squamous epithelium in the middle ear or mastoid, occurs frequently in adults. This is a slowly growing lesion that destroys bone and normal ear tissue. Theories of pathogenesis include traumatic immigration and invasion of squamous epithelium through a retraction pocket, implantation of squamous epithelia in the middle ear through a perforation or surgery, and metaplasia following chronic infection and irritation. On examination, there is often a perforation of the tympanic membrane filled with cheesy white squamous debris. A chronically draining ear that fails to respond to appropriate antibiotic therapy should raise suspicion of a cholesteatoma. Conductive hearing loss secondary to ossicular erosion is common. Surgery is required to remove this destructive process.

Conductive hearing loss with a normal ear canal and intact tympanic membrane suggests either ossicular pathology or the presence of "third window" in the inner ear (see below).

Fixation of the stapes from *otosclerosis* is a common cause of low-frequency conductive hearing loss. It occurs equally in men and women and is inherited as an autosomal dominant trait with incomplete penetrance; in some cases, it may be a manifestation of osteogenesis imperfecta. Hearing impairment usually presents between the late teens and the forties. In women, the otosclerotic process is accelerated during pregnancy, and the hearing loss is often first noticeable at this time. A hearing aid or a simple outpatient surgical procedure (stapedectomy) can provide adequate auditory rehabilitation. Extension of otosclerosis beyond the stapes footplate to involve the cochlea (cochlear otosclerosis) can lead to mixed or sensorineural hearing loss. Fluoride therapy to prevent hearing loss from cochlear otosclerosis is of uncertain value.

Disorders that lead to the formation of a pathologic "third window" in the inner ear can be associated with conductive hearing loss. There are normally two major openings, or windows, that connect the inner ear with the middle ear and serve as conduits for transmission of sound; these are, respectively, the oval and round windows. A third window is formed where the normally hard otic bone surrounding the inner ear is eroded; dissipation of the acoustic energy at the third window is responsible for the "inner ear conductive hearing loss." The superior semicircular canal dehiscence syndrome resulting from erosion of the otic bone over the superior circular canal can present with conductive hearing loss that mimics otosclerosis. A common symptom is vertigo evoked by loud sounds (Tullio phenomenon), by Valsalva maneuvers that change middle ear pressure, or by applying positive pressure on the tragus (the cartilage anterior to the external opening of the ear canal). Patients with this syndrome also complain of being able to hear the movement of their eyes and neck. A large jugular bulb or jugular bulb diverticulum can create a "third window" by eroding into the vestibular aqueduct or posterior semicircular canal; the symptoms are similar to those of the superior semicircular canal dehiscence syndrome.

Sensorineural hearing loss

Sensorineural hearing loss results from either damage to the mechanotransduction apparatus of the cochlea or disruption of the electrical conduction pathway from the inner ear to the brain. Thus, injury to hair cells, supporting cells, auditory neurons, or the central auditory pathway can cause sensorineural hearing loss. Damage to the hair cells of the organ of Corti may be caused by intense noise, viral infections, ototoxic drugs (e.g., salicylates, quinine and its synthetic analogues, aminoglycoside antibiotics, loop diuretics such as furosemide and ethacrynic acid, and cancer chemotherapeutic agents such as cisplatin), fractures of the temporal bone, meningitis, cochlear otosclerosis (see above), Ménière's disease, and aging. Congenital malformations of the inner ear may be the cause of hearing loss in some adults. Genetic predisposition alone or in concert with environmental exposures may also be responsible (see below).

Presbycusis (age-associated hearing loss) is the most common cause of sensorineural hearing loss in adults. In the early stages, it is characterized by symmetric, gentle to sharply sloping high-frequency hearing loss. With progression, the hearing loss involves all frequencies. More importantly, the hearing impairment is associated with significant loss in clarity. There is a loss of discrimination for phonemes, recruitment (abnormal growth of loudness), and particular difficulty in understanding speech in noisy environments such as at restaurants and social events. Hearing aids are helpful in enhancing the signal-to-noise ratio by amplifying sounds that are close to the listener. *Although hearing aids are able to amplify sounds, they cannot restore the clarity of hearing.* Thus, amplification with hearing aids may provide only limited rehabilitation once the word recognition score deteriorates below 50%. Cochlear implants are the treatment of choice when hearing aids prove inadequate, even when hearing loss is incomplete (see below).

Ménière's disease is characterized by episodic vertigo, fluctuating sensorineural hearing loss, tinnitus, and aural fullness. Tinnitus and/or deafness may be absent during the initial attacks of vertigo, but it invariably appears as the disease progresses and increases in severity during acute attacks. The annual incidence of Ménière's disease is 0.5–7.5 per 1000; onset is most frequently in the fifth decade of life but may also occur in young adults or the elderly. Histologically, there is distention of the endolymphatic system (endolymphatic hydrops) leading to degeneration of vestibular and cochlear hair cells. This may result from endolymphatic sac dysfunction secondary to infection, trauma, autoimmune disease, inflammatory causes, or tumor; an idiopathic etiology constitutes the largest category and is most accurately referred to as Ménière's disease. Although any pattern of hearing loss can be observed, typically, low-frequency, unilateral sensorineural hearing impairment is present. MRI should be obtained to exclude retrocochlear pathology such as a cerebellopontine angle tumor or demyelinating disorder. Therapy is directed toward the control of vertigo. A 2-g/d low-salt diet is the mainstay of treatment for control of rotatory vertigo. Diuretics, a short course of glucocorticoids, and intratympanic gentamicin may also be useful adjuncts in recalcitrant cases. Surgical therapy of vertigo is reserved for unresponsive cases and includes endolymphatic sac decompression, labyrinthectomy, and vestibular nerve section. Both labyrinthectomy and vestibular nerve section abolish rotatory vertigo in >90% of cases. Unfortunately, there is no effective therapy for hearing loss, tinnitus, or aural fullness from Ménière's disease.

Sensorineural hearing loss may also result from any neoplastic, vascular, demyelinating, infectious, or degenerative disease or trauma affecting the central auditory pathways. HIV leads to both peripheral and central auditory system pathology and is associated with sensorineural hearing impairment.

Primary diseases of the central nervous system can also present with hearing impairment. Characteristically, a reduction in clarity of hearing and speech comprehension is much greater than the loss of the ability to hear pure tone. Auditory testing is consistent with an auditory neuropathy; normal otoacoustic emissions (OAE) and an abnormal auditory brainstem response (ABR) is typical (see below). Hearing loss can accompany hereditary sensorimotor neuropathies and inherited disorders of myelin. Tumors of the cerebellopontine angle such as vestibular schwannoma and meningioma usually present with asymmetric sensorineural hearing loss with greater deterioration of speech understanding than pure tone hearing. Multiple sclerosis may present with acute unilateral or bilateral hearing loss; typically, pure tone testing remains relatively stable while speech understanding fluctuates. Isolated labyrinthine infarction can present with acute hearing loss and vertigo due to a cerebrovascular accident involving the posterior circulation, usually the anterior inferior cerebellar artery; it may also be the heralding sign of impending catastrophic basilar artery infarction (Chap. 370).

A finding of conductive and sensory hearing loss in combination is termed *mixed hearing loss*. Mixed hearing losses are due to pathology of both the middle and inner ear, as can occur in otosclerosis involving the ossicles and the cochlea, head trauma, chronic otitis media, cholesteatoma, middle ear tumors, and some inner ear malformations.

Trauma resulting in temporal bone fractures may be associated with conductive, sensorineural, or mixed hearing loss. If the fracture spares the inner ear, there may simply be conductive hearing loss due to rupture of the tympanic membrane or disruption of the ossicular chain. These abnormalities can be surgically corrected. Profound hearing loss and severe vertigo are associated with temporal bone fractures involving the inner ear. A perilymphatic fistula associated with leakage of inner ear fluid into the middle ear can occur and may require surgical repair. An associated facial nerve injury is not uncommon. CT is best suited to assess fracture of the traumatized temporal bone, evaluate the ear canal, and determine the integrity of the ossicular chain and the involvement of the inner ear. CSF leaks that accompany temporal bone fractures are usually self-limited; the value of prophylactic antibiotics is uncertain.

Tinnitus is defined as the perception of a sound when there is no sound in the environment. It may have a buzzing, roaring, or ringing quality and may be pulsatile (synchronous with the heartbeat). Tinnitus is often associated with either a conductive or sensorineural hearing loss. The pathophysiology of tinnitus is not well understood. The cause of the tinnitus can usually be determined by finding the cause of the associated hearing loss. Tinnitus may be the first symptom of a serious condition such as a vestibular schwannoma. Pulsatile tinnitus requires evaluation of the vascular system of the head to exclude vascular tumors such as glomus jugulare tumors, aneurysms, dural arteriovenous fistulas, and stenotic arterial lesions; it may also occur with SOM. It is most commonly associated with some abnormality of the jugular bulb such as a large jugular bulb or jugular bulb diverticulum.

GENETIC CAUSES OF HEARING LOSS

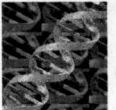

More than half of childhood hearing impairment is thought to be hereditary; hereditary hearing impairment (HHI) can also manifest later in life. HHI may be classified as either nonsyndromic, when hearing loss is the only clinical abnormality, or syndromic, when hearing loss is associated with anomalies in other organ systems. Nearly two-thirds of HHIs are nonsyndromic, and the remaining one-third are syndromic. Between 70 and 80% of nonsyndromic HHI is inherited in an autosomal recessive manner and designated DFNB; another 15–20% is autosomal dominant (DFNA). Less than 5% is X-linked or maternally inherited via the mitochondria.

Nearly 100 loci harboring genes for nonsyndromic HHI have been mapped, with equal numbers of dominant and recessive modes of inheritance; numerous genes have now been cloned (Table 30-1). The hearing genes fall into the categories of structural proteins (MYH9, MYO7A, MYO15, TECTA, DIAPH1), transcription factors (POU3F4, POU4F3), ion channels (KCNQ4, SLC26A4), and gap junction proteins (GJB2, GJB3, GJB6). Several of these genes, including GJB2, TECTA, and TMC1, cause both autosomal dominant and recessive forms of nonsyndromic HHI. In general, the hearing loss associated with dominant genes has its onset in adolescence or adulthood and varies in severity, whereas the hearing loss associated with recessive inheritance is congenital and profound. Connexin 26, product of the GJB2 gene, is particularly important because it is responsible for nearly 20% of all cases of childhood deafness; half of genetic deafness in children is GJB2-related. Two frameshift mutations, 35delG and 167delT, account for >50% of the cases; however, screening for these two mutations alone is insufficient and sequencing of the entire gene is required to diagnose GJB2-related recessive deafness. The 167delT mutation is highly prevalent in Ashkenazi Jews; ~1 in 1765 individuals in this population are homozygous and affected. The hearing loss can also vary among the members of the same family, suggesting that other genes or factors influence the auditory phenotype.

In addition to GJB2, several other nonsyndromic genes are associated with hearing loss that progresses with age. The contribution of genetics to presbycusis is also becoming better

TABLE 30-1 Hereditary Hearing Impairment Genes

Designation	Gene	Function
Autosomal Dominant		
	CRYM	Thyroid hormone–binding protein
DFNA1	DIAPH1	Cytoskeletal protein
DFNA2A	KCNQ4	Potassium channel
DFNA2B	GJB3 (Cx31)	Gap junction
DFNA3A	GJB2 (Cx26)	Gap junction
DFNA3B	GJB6 (Cx30)	Gap junction
DFNA4	MYH14	Class II nonmuscle myosin
DFNA5	DFNA5	Unknown
DFNA6/14/38	WFS1	Transmembrane protein
DFNA8/12	TECTA	Tectorial membrane protein
DFNA9	COCH	Unknown
DFNA10	EYA4	Developmental gene
DFNA11	MYO7A	Cytoskeletal protein
DFNA13	COL11A2	Cytoskeletal protein
DFNA15	POU4F3	Transcription factor
DFNA17	MYH9	Cytoskeletal protein
DFNA20/26	ACTG1	Cytoskeletal protein
DFNA22	MYO6	Unconventional myosin
DFNA28	TFCP2L3	Transcription factor
DFNA36	TMC1	Transmembrane protein
DFNA44	CCDC50	Effector of EGF-mediated signaling
DFNA48	MYO1A	Unconventional myosin
DFNA50	MIRN96	MicroRNA
DFNA51	TJP2	Tight junction protein
Autosomal Recessive		
DFNB1A	GJB2 (CX26)	Gap junction
DFNB1B	GJB6 (CX30)	Gap junction
DFNB2	MYO7A	Cytoskeletal protein
DFNB3	MYO15	Cytoskeletal protein
DFNB4	PDS(SLC26A4)	Chloride/iodide transporter
DFNB6	TMIE	Transmembrane protein
DFNB7/B11	TMC1	Transmembrane protein
DFNB9	OTOF	Trafficking of membrane vesicles
DFNB8/10	TMPRSS3	Transmembrane serine protease
DFNB12	CDH23	Intercellular adherence protein
DFNB16	STRC	Stereocilia protein
DFNB18	USH1C	Unknown
DFNB21	TECTA	Tectorial membrane protein
DFNB22	OTOA	Gel attachment to nonsensory cell
DFNB23	PCDH15	Morphogenesis and cohesion
DFNB24	RDX	Cytoskeletal protein
DFNB25	GRXCR1	Reversible S-glutathionylation of proteins
DFNB28	TRIOBP	Cytoskeletal-organizing protein
DFNB29	CLDN14	Tight junctions
DFNB30	MYO3A	Hybrid motor-signaling myosin
DFNB31	WHRN	PDZ domain–containing protein
DFNB35	ESRRB	Estrogen-related receptor beta protein
DFNB36	ESPN	Ca-insensitive actin-bundling protein
DFNB37	MYO6	Unconventional myosin
DFNB39	HFG	Hepatocyte growth factor
DFNB49	MARVELD2	Tight junction protein
DFNB53	COL11A2	Collagen protein
DFNB59	PJVK	Zn-binding protein
DFNB61	SLC26A5	Motor protein
DFNB63	LRTOMT/COMT2	Putative methyltransferase
DFNB66/67	LHFPL5	Tetraspan protein
DFNB77	LOXHD1	Stereociliary protein
DFNB79	TPRN	Unknown
DFNB82	GPSM2	G protein signaling modulator
DFNB84	PTPRQ	Type III receptor-like protein-tyrosine phosphatase family

TABLE 30-2 Syndromic Hereditary Hearing Impairment Genes

Syndrome	Gene	Function
Alport syndrome	COL4A3-5	Cytoskeletal protein
BOR syndrome	EYA1	Developmental gene
	SIX5	Developmental gene
	SIX1	Developmental gene
Jervell and Lange-Nielsen syndrome	KCNQ1	Delayed rectifier K+ channel
	KCNE1	Delayed rectifier K+ channel
Norrie disease	NDP	Cell-cell interactions
Pendred syndrome	SLC26A4	Chloride/iodide transporter
	FOXI1	Transcriptional activator of SLC26A4
Treacher Collins	TCOF1	Nucleolar-cytoplasmic transport
Usher syndrome	MYO7A	Cytoskeletal protein
	USH1C	Unknown
	CDH23	Intercellular adherence protein
	PCDH15	Cell adhesion molecule
	SANS	Harmonin-associated protein
	USH2A	Cell adhesion molecule
	VLGR1	G protein–coupled receptor
	USH3	Unknown
	WHRN	PDZ domain–containing protein
WS type I, III	PAX3	Transcription factor
WS type II	MITF	Transcription factor
	SNAI2	Transcription factor
WS type IV	EDNRB	Endothelin B receptor
	EDN3	Endothelin B receptor ligand
	SOX10	Transcription factor

Abbreviations: BOR, branchio-oto-renal syndrome; WS, Waardenburg syndrome.

understood. Sensitivity to aminoglycoside ototoxicity can be maternally transmitted through a mitochondrial mutation. Susceptibility to noise-induced hearing loss may also be genetically determined.

There are >400 syndromic forms of hearing loss. These include Usher syndrome (retinitis pigmentosa and hearing loss), Waardenburg syndrome (pigmentary abnormality and hearing loss), Pendred syndrome (thyroid organification defect and hearing loss), Alport syndrome (renal disease and hearing loss), Jervell and Lange-Nielsen syndrome (prolonged QT interval and hearing loss), neurofibromatosis type 2 (bilateral acoustic schwannoma), and mitochondrial disorders [mitochondrial encephalopathy, lactic acidosis, and stroke-like episodes (MELAS); myoclonic epilepsy and ragged red fibers (MERRF); progressive external ophthalmoplegia (PEO)] (Table 30-2).

APPROACH TO THE PATIENT: Disorders of the Sense of Hearing

The goal in the evaluation of a patient with auditory complaints is to determine (1) the nature of the hearing impairment (conductive vs. sensorineural vs. mixed), (2) the severity of the impairment (mild, moderate, severe, profound), (3) the anatomy of the impairment (external ear, middle ear, inner ear, or central auditory pathway), and (4) the etiology. The history should elicit characteristics of the hearing loss, including the duration of deafness, unilateral vs. bilateral involvement, nature of onset (sudden vs. insidious), and rate of progression (rapid vs. slow). Symptoms of tinnitus, vertigo, imbalance, aural fullness, otorrhea, headache, facial nerve dysfunction, and head and neck paresthesias should be noted. Information regarding head trauma, exposure to ototoxins, occupational or recreational noise exposure, and family history of hearing impairment may also be important. A sudden onset of unilateral hearing loss, with or without tinnitus, may represent a viral infection of the inner ear or a stroke. Patients with unilateral hearing loss (sensory or conductive) usually complain of reduced hearing, poor sound localization, and difficulty hearing clearly with background noise. Gradual progression of a hearing deficit is common with otosclerosis, noise-induced hearing loss, vestibular schwannoma, or Ménière's disease. Small vestibular schwannomas typically present with asymmetric hearing impairment, tinnitus, and imbalance (rarely vertigo); cranial neuropathy, in particular of the trigeminal or facial nerve, may accompany larger tumors. In addition to hearing loss, Ménière's disease may be associated with episodic vertigo, tinnitus, and aural fullness. Hearing loss with otorrhea is most likely due to chronic otitis media or cholesteatoma.

Examination should include the auricle, external ear canal, and tympanic membrane. The external ear canal of the elderly is often dry and fragile; it is preferable to clean cerumen with wall-mounted suction or cerumen loops and to avoid irrigation. In examining the eardrum, the topography of the tympanic membrane is more important than the presence or absence of the light reflex. In addition to the pars tensa (the lower two-thirds of the eardrum), the pars flaccida above the short process of the malleus should also be examined for retraction pockets that may be evidence of chronic eustachian tube dysfunction or cholesteatoma. Insufflation of the ear canal is necessary to assess tympanic membrane mobility and compliance. Careful inspection of the nose, nasopharynx, and upper respiratory tract is indicated. Unilateral serous effusion should prompt a fiberoptic examination of the nasopharynx to exclude neoplasms. Cranial nerves should be evaluated with special attention to facial and trigeminal nerves, which are commonly affected with tumors involving the cerebellopontine angle.

The Rinne and Weber tuning fork tests, with a 512-Hz tuning fork, are used to screen for hearing loss, differentiate conductive from sensorineural hearing losses, and to confirm the findings of audiologic evaluation. Rinne's test compares the ability to hear by air conduction with the ability to hear by bone conduction. The tines of a vibrating tuning fork are held near the opening of the external auditory canal, and then the stem is placed on the mastoid process; for direct contact, it may be placed on teeth or dentures. The patient is asked to indicate whether the tone is louder by air conduction or bone conduction. Normally, and in the presence of sensorineural hearing loss, a tone is heard louder by air conduction than by bone conduction; however, with conductive hearing loss of ≥30 dB (see "Audiologic Assessment," below), the bone-conduction stimulus is perceived as louder than the air-conduction stimulus. For the Weber test, the stem of a vibrating tuning fork is placed on the head in the midline and the patient asked whether the tone is heard in both ears or better in one ear than in the other. With a unilateral conductive hearing loss, the tone is perceived in the affected ear. With a unilateral sensorineural hearing loss, the tone is perceived in the unaffected ear. A 5-dB difference in hearing between the two ears is required for lateralization.

LABORATORY ASSESSMENT OF HEARING

Audiologic assessment

The minimum audiologic assessment for hearing loss should include the measurement of pure tone air-conduction and bone-conduction thresholds, speech reception threshold, word recognition score, tympanometry, acoustic reflexes, and acoustic-reflex decay. This test battery provides a screening evaluation of the entire auditory system and allows one to determine whether further differentiation of a sensory (cochlear) from a neural (retrocochlear) hearing loss is indicated.

Pure tone audiometry assesses hearing acuity for pure tones. The test is administered by an audiologist and is performed in a sound-attenuated chamber. The pure tone stimulus is delivered with an audiometer, an electronic device that allows the presentation of specific frequencies (generally between 250 and 8000 Hz) at specific intensities. Air- and bone-conduction thresholds are established for each ear. Air-conduction thresholds are determined by presenting the stimulus in air with the use of headphones. Bone-conduction thresholds are determined by placing the stem of a vibrating tuning fork or an oscillator of an audiometer in contact with the head. In the presence of a hearing loss, broad-spectrum noise is presented to the nontest ear for *masking* purposes so that responses are based on perception from the ear under test.

The responses are measured in decibels. An *audiogram* is a plot of intensity in decibels of hearing threshold versus frequency. A decibel (dB) is equal to 20 times the logarithm of the ratio of the sound pressure required to achieve threshold in the patient to the sound pressure required to achieve threshold in a normal hearing person. Therefore, a change of 6 dB represents doubling of sound pressure, and a change of 20 dB represents a tenfold change in sound pressure. Loudness, which depends on the frequency, intensity, and duration of a sound, doubles with approximately each 10-dB increase in sound pressure level. Pitch, on the other hand, does not directly correlate with frequency. The perception of pitch changes slowly in the low and high frequencies. In the middle tones, which are important for human speech, pitch varies more rapidly with changes in frequency.

Pure tone audiometry establishes the presence and severity of hearing impairment, unilateral vs. bilateral involvement, and the type of hearing loss. Conductive hearing losses with a large mass component, as is often seen in middle ear effusions, produce elevation of thresholds that predominate in the higher frequencies. Conductive hearing losses with a large stiffness component, as in fixation of the footplate of the stapes in early otosclerosis, produce threshold elevations in the lower frequencies. Often, the conductive hearing loss involves all frequencies, suggesting involvement of both stiffness and mass. In general, sensorineural hearing losses such as presbycusis affect higher frequencies more than lower frequencies. An exception is Ménière's disease, which is characteristically associated with low-frequency sensorineural hearing loss. Noise-induced hearing loss has an unusual pattern of hearing impairment in which the loss at 4000 Hz is greater than at higher frequencies. Vestibular schwannomas characteristically affect the higher frequencies, but any pattern of hearing loss can be observed.

Speech recognition requires greater synchronous neural firing than is necessary for appreciation of pure tones. *Speech audiometry* tests the clarity with which one hears. The *speech reception threshold* (SRT) is defined as the intensity at which speech is recognized as a meaningful symbol and is obtained by presenting two-syllable words with an equal accent on each syllable. The intensity at which the patient can repeat 50% of the words correctly is the SRT. Once the SRT is determined, discrimination or word recognition ability is tested by presenting one-syllable words at 25–40 dB above the SRT.

The words are phonetically balanced in that the phonemes (speech sounds) occur in the list of words at the same frequency that they occur in ordinary conversational English. An individual with normal hearing or conductive hearing loss can repeat 88–100% of the phonetically balanced words correctly. Patients with a sensorineural hearing loss have variable loss of discrimination. As a general rule, neural lesions produce greater deficits in discrimination than do cochlear lesions. For example, in a patient with mild asymmetric sensorineural hearing loss, a clue to the diagnosis of vestibular schwannoma is the presence of greater than expected deterioration in discrimination ability. Deterioration in discrimination ability at higher intensities above the SRT also suggests a lesion in the eighth nerve or central auditory pathways.

Tympanometry measures the impedance of the middle ear to sound and is useful in diagnosis of middle-ear effusions. A *tympanogram* is the graphic representation of change in impedance or compliance as the pressure in the ear canal is changed. Normally, the middle ear is most compliant at atmospheric pressure, and the compliance decreases as the pressure is increased or decreased (type A); this pattern is seen with normal hearing or in the presence of sensorineural hearing loss. Compliance that does not change with change in pressure suggests middle-ear effusion (type B). With a negative pressure in the middle ear, as with eustachian tube obstruction, the point of maximal compliance occurs with negative pressure in the ear canal (type C). A tympanogram in which no point of maximal compliance can be obtained is most commonly seen with discontinuity of the ossicular chain (type A_d). A reduction in the maximal compliance peak can be seen in otosclerosis (type A_s).

During tympanometry, an intense tone elicits contraction of the stapedius muscle. The change in compliance of the middle ear with contraction of the stapedius muscle can be detected. The presence or absence of this *acoustic reflex* is important in determining the etiology of hearing loss as well as in the anatomic localization of facial nerve paralysis. The acoustic reflex can help differentiate between conductive hearing loss due to otosclerosis and that caused by an inner ear "third window": it is absent in otosclerosis and present in inner ear conductive hearing loss. Normal or elevated acoustic reflex thresholds in an individual with sensorineural hearing impairment suggests a cochlear hearing loss. An absent acoustic reflex in the setting of sensorineural hearing loss is not helpful in localizing the site of lesion. Assessment of *acoustic reflex decay* helps differentiate sensory from neural hearing losses. In neural hearing loss, the reflex adapts or decays with time.

Otoacoustic emissions (OAE) generated by outer hair cells only can be measured with microphones inserted into the external auditory canal. The emissions may be spontaneous or evoked with sound stimulation. The presence of OAEs indicates that the outer hair cells of the organ of Corti are intact and can be used to assess auditory thresholds and to distinguish sensory from neural hearing losses.

Evoked responses

Electrocochleography measures the earliest evoked potentials generated in the cochlea and the auditory nerve. Receptor potentials recorded include the cochlear microphonic, generated by the outer hair cells of the organ of Corti, and the summating potential, generated by the inner hair cells in response to sound. The whole nerve action potential representing the composite firing of the first-order neurons can also be recorded during electrocochleography. Clinically, the test is useful in the diagnosis of Ménière's disease, where an elevation of the ratio of summating potential to action potential is seen.

Brainstem auditory evoked responses (BAERs), also known as *auditory brainstem responses* (ABRs), are useful in differentiating the site of sensorineural hearing loss. In response to sound, five distinct electrical potentials arising from different stations along the peripheral and central auditory pathway can be identified using computer averaging from scalp surface electrodes. BAERs are valuable in situations in which patients cannot or will not give reliable voluntary thresholds. They are also used to assess the integrity of the auditory nerve and brainstem in various clinical situations, including intraoperative monitoring and in determination of brain death.

The *vestibular-evoked myogenic potential (VEMP) test* elicits a vestibulocollic reflex whose afferent limb arises from acoustically sensitive cells in the saccule, with signals conducted via the inferior vestibular nerve. VEMP is a biphasic, short-latency response recorded from the tonically contracted sternocleidomastoid muscle in response to loud auditory clicks or tones. VEMPs may be diminished or absent in patients with early and late Ménière's disease, vestibular neuritis, benign paroxysmal positional vertigo, and vestibular schwannoma. On the other hand, the threshold for VEMPs may be lower in cases of superior canal dehiscence, other inner ear dehiscence, and perilymphatic fistula.

Imaging studies

The choice of radiologic tests is largely determined by whether the goal is to evaluate the bony anatomy of the external, middle, and inner ear or to image the auditory nerve and brain. Axial and coronal CT of the temporal bone with fine 0.3- to 0.6-mm cuts is ideal for determining the caliber of the external auditory canal, integrity of the ossicular chain, and presence of middle-ear or mastoid disease; it can also detect inner ear malformations. CT is also ideal for the detection of bone erosion with chronic otitis media and cholesteatoma. MRI is superior to CT for imaging of retrocochlear pathology such as vestibular schwannoma, meningioma, other lesions of the cerebellopontine angle, demyelinating lesions of the brainstem, and brain tumors. Both CT and MRI are equally capable of identifying inner ear malformations and assessing cochlear patency for preoperative evaluation of patients for cochlear implantation.

TREATMENT   Disorders of the Sense of Hearing

In general, conductive hearing losses are amenable to surgical correction, while sensorineural hearing losses are more difficult to manage. Atresia of the ear canal can be surgically repaired, often with significant improvement in hearing. Tympanic membrane perforations due to chronic otitis media or trauma can be repaired with an outpatient tympanoplasty. Likewise, conductive hearing loss associated with otosclerosis can be treated by stapedectomy, which is successful in 90–95% of cases. Tympanostomy tubes allow the prompt return of normal hearing in individuals with middle ear effusions. Hearing aids are effective and well tolerated in patients with conductive hearing losses.

Patients with mild, moderate, and severe sensorineural hearing losses are regularly rehabilitated with hearing aids of varying configuration and strength. Hearing aids have been improved to provide greater fidelity and have been miniaturized. The current generation of hearing aids can be placed entirely within the ear canal, thus reducing any stigma associated with their use. In general, the more severe the hearing impairment, the larger the hearing aid required for auditory rehabilitation. Digital hearing aids lend themselves to individual programming, and multiple and directional microphones at the ear level may be helpful in noisy surroundings. Since all hearing aids amplify noise as well as speech, the only absolute solution to the problem of noise is to place the microphone closer to the speaker than the noise source. This arrangement is not possible with a self-contained, cosmetically acceptable device. A significant limitation of rehabilitation with a hearing aid is that while it is able to enhance detection of sound with amplification, it cannot restore clarity of hearing that is lost with presbycusis.

Patients with unilateral deafness have difficulty with sound localization and reduced clarity of hearing in background noise. They may benefit from a CROS (contralateral routing of signal) hearing aid in which a microphone is placed on the hearing-impaired side and the sound is transmitted to the receiver placed on the contralateral ear. The same result may be obtained with a bone-anchored hearing aid (BAHA), in which a hearing aid clamps to a screw osseointegrated into the skull on the hearing-impaired side. Like the CROS hearing aid, the BAHA transfers the acoustic signal to the contralateral hearing ear, but it does so by vibrating the skull. Patients with profound deafness on one side and some hearing loss in the better ear are candidates for a BICROS hearing aid; it differs from the CROS hearing aid in that the patient wears a hearing aid, and not simply a receiver, in the better ear. Unfortunately, CROS and BAHA devices are often judged by patients to be unsatisfactory.

In many situations, including lectures and the theater, hearing-impaired persons benefit from assistive devices that are based on the principle of having the speaker closer to the microphone than any source of noise. Assistive devices include infrared and frequency-modulated (FM) transmission as well as an electromagnetic loop around the room for transmission to the individual's hearing aid. Hearing aids with telecoils can also be used with properly equipped telephones in the same way.

In the event that the hearing aid provides inadequate rehabilitation, cochlear implants may be appropriate. Criteria for implantation include severe to profound hearing loss with open-set sentence cognition of ≤40% under best aided conditions. Worldwide, nearly 200,000 hearing impaired children and adults have received cochlear implants. Cochlear implants are neural prostheses that convert sound energy to electrical energy and can be used to stimulate the auditory division of the eighth nerve directly. In most cases of profound hearing impairment, the auditory hair cells are lost but the ganglionic cells of the auditory division of the eighth nerve are preserved. Cochlear implants consist of electrodes that are inserted into the cochlea through the round window, speech processors that extract acoustical elements of speech for conversion to electrical currents, and a means of transmitting the electrical energy through the skin. Patients with implants experience sound that helps with speech reading, allows open-set word recognition, and helps in modulating the person's own voice. Usually, within the first 3–6 months after implantation, adult patients can understand speech without visual cues. With the current generation of multichannel cochlear implants, nearly 75% of patients are able to converse on the telephone. For individuals who have had both eighth nerves destroyed by trauma or bilateral vestibular schwannomas (e.g., neurofibromatosis type 2), brainstem auditory implants placed near the cochlear nucleus may provide auditory rehabilitation.

Tinnitus often accompanies hearing loss. As for background noise, tinnitus can degrade speech comprehension in individuals with hearing impairment. Therapy for tinnitus is usually directed toward minimizing the appreciation of tinnitus. Relief of the tinnitus may be obtained by masking it with background music. Hearing aids are also helpful in tinnitus suppression, as are tinnitus maskers, devices that present a sound to the affected ear that is more pleasant to listen to than the tinnitus. The use of a tinnitus masker is often followed by several hours of inhibition of the tinnitus. Antidepressants have been shown to be beneficial in helping patients cope with tinnitus.

Hard-of-hearing individuals often benefit from a reduction in unnecessary noise in the environment (e.g., radio or television) to enhance the signal-to-noise ratio. Speech comprehension is aided by lip reading; therefore, the impaired listener should be seated so that the face of the speaker is well illuminated and easily seen. Although speech should be in a loud, clear voice, one should be aware that in sensorineural hearing losses in general and in hard-of-hearing elderly in particular, recruitment (abnormal perception of loud sounds) may be troublesome. Above all, optimal communication cannot take place without both parties giving it their full and undivided attention.

■ PREVENTION

Conductive hearing losses may be prevented by prompt antibiotic therapy of adequate duration for AOM and by ventilation of the middle ear with tympanostomy tubes in middle-ear effusions lasting ≥12 weeks. Loss of vestibular function and deafness due to aminoglycoside antibiotics can largely be prevented by careful monitoring of serum peak and trough levels.

Some 10 million Americans have noise-induced hearing loss, and 20 million are exposed to hazardous noise in their employment. Noise-induced hearing loss can be prevented by avoidance of exposure to loud noise or by regular use of ear plugs or fluid-filled ear muffs to attenuate intense sound. High-risk activities for noise-induced hearing loss include wood and metal working with electrical equipment and target practice and hunting with small firearms. All internal-combustion and electric engines, including snow and leaf blowers, snowmobiles, outboard motors, and chain saws, require protection of the user with hearing protectors. Virtually all noise-induced hearing loss is preventable through education, which should begin before the teenage years. Programs of industrial conservation of hearing are required by Occupational Safety and Health Administration (OSHA) when the exposure over an 8-h period averages 85 dB. OSHA mandates that workers in such noisy environments have hearing monitoring and protection programs that include a pre-employment screen, annual audiologic assessment, as well as the mandatory use of hearing protectors. Exposure to loud sounds above 85 dB in the work environment is restricted by OSHA, with halving of allowed exposure time for each increment of 5 dB above this threshold: for example 90 dB exposure is permitted for 8 h; 95 dB for 4 h, and 100 dB for 2 h.

FURTHER READINGS

Bishop CE, Eby TL: The current status of audiologic rehabilitation for profound unilateral sensorineural hearing loss. Laryngoscope 120:552, 2010

Hilgert N et al: Function and expression pattern of nonsyndromic deafness genes. Curr Mol Med 9:546, 2009

Lalwani AK (ed): *Current Diagnosis and Treatment in Otolaryngology—Head & Neck Surgery*, 3rd ed. New York, McGraw-Hill, 2011

Merchant SN, Rosowski JJ: Conductive hearing loss caused by third-window lesions of the inner ear. Otol Neurotol 29:282, 2008

Sprinzl GM, Riechelmann H: Current trends in treating hearing loss in elderly people: A review of the technology and treatment options—a mini-review. Gerontology 56:351, 2010

CHAPTER 31

Pharyngitis, Sinusitis, Otitis, and Other Upper Respiratory Tract Infections

Michael A. Rubin

Larry C. Ford

Ralph Gonzales

Infections of the upper respiratory tract (URIs) have a tremendous impact on public health. They are among the most common reasons for visits to primary care providers, and although the illnesses are typically mild, their high incidence and transmission rates place them among the leading causes of time lost from work or school. Even though a minority (~25%) of cases are caused by bacteria, URIs are the leading diagnoses for which antibiotics are prescribed on an outpatient basis in the United States. The enormous consumption of antibiotics for these illnesses has contributed to the rise in antibiotic resistance among common community-acquired pathogens such as *Streptococcus pneumoniae*—a trend that in itself has had an enormous influence on public health.

Although most URIs are caused by viruses, distinguishing patients with primary viral infection from those with primary bacterial infection is difficult. Signs and symptoms of bacterial and viral URIs are typically indistinguishable. Until consistent, inexpensive, and rapid testing becomes available and is used widely, acute infections will be diagnosed largely on clinical grounds. The judicious use and potential for misuse of antibiotics in this setting pose definite challenges.

NONSPECIFIC INFECTIONS OF THE UPPER RESPIRATORY TRACT

Nonspecific URIs are a broadly defined group of disorders that collectively constitute the leading cause of ambulatory care visits in the United States. By definition, nonspecific URIs have no prominent localizing features. They are identified by a variety of descriptive names, including *acute infective rhinitis*, *acute rhinopharyngitis/ nasopharyngitis*, *acute coryza*, and *acute nasal catarrh*, as well as by the inclusive label *common cold*.

Etiology

The large assortment of URI classifications reflects the wide variety of causative infectious agents and the varied manifestations of common pathogens. Nearly all nonspecific URIs are caused by viruses spanning multiple virus families and many antigenic types. For instance, there are at least 100 immunotypes of rhinovirus

(Chap. 186), the most common cause of URI (~30–40% of cases); other causes include influenza virus (three immuno-types; Chap. 187) as well as parainfluenza virus (four immuno-types), coronavirus (at least three immunotypes), and adenovirus (47 immunotypes) (Chap. 186). Respiratory syncytial virus (RSV), a well-established pathogen in pediatric populations, is also a recognized cause of significant disease in elderly and immuno-compromised individuals. A host of additional viruses, including some viruses not typically associated with URIs (e.g., enterovi-ruses, rubella virus, and varicella-zoster virus), account for a small percentage of cases in adults each year. Although new diagnostic modalities [e.g., nasopharyngeal swab for polymerase chain reac-tion (PCR)] can assign a viral etiology, there are few specific treatment options, and no pathogen is identified in a substantial proportion of cases. A specific diagnostic workup beyond a clinical diagnosis is generally unnecessary in an otherwise healthy adult.

Clinical manifestations

The signs and symptoms of nonspecific URI are similar to those of other URIs but lack a pronounced localization to one particular anatomic location, such as the sinuses, pharynx, or lower airway. Nonspecific URI commonly presents as an acute, mild, and self-limited catarrhal syndrome with a median dura-tion of ~1 week (range, 2–10 days). Signs and symptoms are diverse and frequently variable across patients. The principal signs and symptoms of nonspecific URI include rhinorrhea (with or without purulence), nasal congestion, cough, and sore throat. Other manifestations, such as fever, malaise, sneezing, lymphadenopathy, and hoarseness, are more variable, with fever more common among infants and young children. This vary-ing presentation may reflect differences in host response as well as in infecting organisms; myalgias and fatigue, for example, sometimes are seen with influenza and parainfluenza infections, whereas conjunctivitis may suggest infection with adenovirus or enterovirus. Findings on physical examination are frequently nonspecific and unimpressive. Between 0.5% and 2% of colds are complicated by secondary bacterial infections (e.g., rhino-sinusitis, otitis media, and pneumonia), particularly in higher-risk populations such as infants, elderly persons, and chronically ill individuals. Secondary bacterial infections usually are associated with a prolonged course of illness, increased severity of illness, and localization of signs and symptoms, often as a rebound after initial clinical improvement. Purulent secretions from the nares or throat often are misinterpreted as an indication of bacterial sinusitis or pharyngitis. These secretions, however, are also seen in nonspecific URI and, in the absence of other clinical features, are poor predictors of bacterial infection.

TREATMENT   Upper Respiratory Infections

Antibiotics have no role in the treatment of uncomplicated nonspecific URI, and their misuse probably facilitates the emer-gence of antimicrobial resistance; even in healthy volunteers, a single course of azithromycin or clarithromycin can lead to macrolide resistance among oral streptococci months later. In the absence of clinical evidence of bacterial infection, treatment remains entirely symptom-based, with use of decongestants and nonsteroidal anti-inflammatory drugs. Other therapies directed at specific symptoms are often useful, including dextromethorphan for cough and lozenges with topical anesthetic for sore throat. Clinical trials of zinc, vitamin C, echinacea, and other alternative remedies have revealed no consistent benefit for the treatment of nonspecific URI.

INFECTIONS OF THE SINUS

Rhinosinusitis refers to an inflammatory condition involving the four paired structures surrounding the nasal cavities. Although most cases of sinusitis involve more than one sinus, the maxillary sinus is most commonly involved; next, in order of frequency, are the ethmoid, frontal, and sphenoid sinuses. Each sinus is lined with a respiratory epithelium that produces mucus, which is transported out by ciliary action through the sinus ostium and into the nasal cavity. Normally, mucus does not accumulate in the sinuses, which remain mostly sterile despite their adjacency to the bacterium-filled nasal passages. When the sinus ostia are obstructed, however, or when ciliary clearance is impaired or absent, the secretions can be retained, producing the typical signs and symptoms of sinusitis. As these secretions accumulate with obstruction, they become more susceptible to infection with a variety of pathogens, including viruses, bacteria, and fungi. Sinusitis affects a tremendous propor-tion of the population, accounts for millions of visits to primary care physicians each year, and is the fifth leading diagnosis for which antibiotics are prescribed. It typically is classified by duration of illness (acute vs. chronic); by etiology (infectious vs. noninfectious); and, when infectious, by the offending pathogen type (viral, bacterial, or fungal).

■ ACUTE RHINOSINUSITIS

Acute rhinosinusitis—defined as sinusitis of <4 weeks' duration—constitutes the vast majority of sinusitis cases. Most cases are diagnosed in the ambulatory care setting and occur primarily as a consequence of a preceding viral URI. Differentiating acute bacte-rial from viral sinusitis on clinical grounds is difficult. Therefore, it is perhaps not surprising that antibiotics are prescribed frequently (in 85–98% of all cases) for this condition.

Etiology

The ostial obstruction that results in rhinosinusitis can arise from both infectious and noninfectious causes. Noninfectious causes include allergic rhinitis (with either mucosal edema or polyp obstruction), barotrauma (e.g., from deep-sea diving or air travel), and exposure to chemical irritants. Obstruction also can occur with nasal and sinus tumors (e.g., squamous cell carcinoma) or granu-lomatous diseases (e.g., granulomatosis with polyangiitis (Wegener's) or rhinoscleroma), and conditions leading to altered mucus content (e.g., cystic fibrosis) can cause sinusitis through impaired mucus clearance. In ICUs, nasotracheal intubation and nasogastric tubes are major risk factors for nosocomial sinusitis.

Viral rhinosinusitis is far more common than bacterial sinusitis, although relatively few studies have sampled sinus aspirates for the presence of different viruses. In the studies that have done so, the viruses most commonly isolated—both alone and with bacteria—have been rhinovirus, parainfluenza virus, and influ-enza virus. Bacterial causes of sinusitis have been better described. Among community-acquired cases, *S. pneumoniae* and nontypable *Haemophilus influenzae* are the most common pathogens, account-ing for 50–60% of cases. *Moraxella catarrhalis* causes disease in a significant percentage (20%) of children but a lesser percentage in adults. Other streptococcal species and *Staphylococcus aureus* cause only a small percentage of cases, although there is increasing concern about community-acquired methicillin-resistant *S. aureus* (MRSA) as an emerging cause. It is difficult to assess whether a cultured bacterium represents a true infecting organism, an insufficiently deep sample (which would not be expected to be sterile), or—especially in the case of previous sinus surgeries—a colonizing organism. Anaerobes occasionally are found in asso-ciation with infections of the roots of premolar teeth that spread into the adjacent maxillary sinuses. The role of *Chlamydophila pneumoniae* and *Mycoplasma pneumoniae* in the pathogenesis of acute sinusitis is unclear. Nosocomial cases commonly are associated with bacteria found in the hospital environment, including *S. aureus, Pseudomonas aeruginosa, Serratia marcescens, Klebsiella pneumoniae*, and *Enterobacter* species. Often, these infections are polymicrobial and involve organisms that are highly resistant to numerous antibiotics. Fungi are also established causes of sinusitis, although most acute cases are in immunocompromised patients and represent invasive, life-threatening infections. The best-known example is rhinocerebral mucormycosis caused by fungi of the order Mucorales, which includes *Rhizopus, Rhizomucor, Mucor, Mycocladus* (*formerly Absidia*), and *Cunninghamella* (Chap. 205). These infections classically occur in diabetic patients with ketoacidosis but also can develop in transplant recipients, patients with hematologic malignancies, and patients receiving chronic glucocorticoid or deferoxamine therapy. Other hyaline molds, such as *Aspergillus* and *Fusarium* species, are also occasional causes of this disease.

Clinical manifestations

Most cases of acute sinusitis present after or in conjunction with a viral URI, and it can be difficult to discriminate the clinical features of one from the other. A large proportion of patients with colds have sinus inflammation, although, as previously stated, true bacterial sinusitis complicates only 0.2–2% of these viral infections. Common presenting symptoms of sinusitis include nasal drainage and congestion, facial pain or pressure, and headache. Thick, purulent or discolored nasal discharge is often thought to indicate bacterial sinusitis but also occurs early in viral infections such as the common cold and is not specific to bacterial infection. Other nonspecific manifestations include cough, sneezing, and fever. Tooth pain, most often involving the upper molars, as well as halitosis can be associated with bacterial sinusitis.

In acute sinusitis, sinus pain or pressure often localizes to the involved sinus (particularly the maxillary sinus) and can be worse when the patient bends over or is supine. Although rare, manifestations of advanced sphenoid or ethmoid sinus infection can be profound, including severe frontal or retroorbital pain radiating to the occiput, thrombosis of the cavernous sinus, and signs of orbital cellulitis. Acute focal sinusitis is uncommon but should be considered over the maxillary sinus and fever in patients with severe symptoms, regardless of illness duration. Similarly, patients with advanced frontal sinusitis can present with a condition known as *Pott's puffy tumor*, with soft tissue swelling and pitting edema over the frontal bone from a communicating subperiosteal abscess. Life-threatening complications of sinusitis include meningitis, epidural abscess, and cerebral abscess.

Patients with acute fungal rhinosinusitis (such as mucormycosis; Chap. 205) often present with symptoms related to pressure effects, particularly when the infection has spread to the orbits and cavernous sinus. Signs such as orbital swelling and cellulitis, proptosis, ptosis, and decreased extraocular movement are common, as is retroorbital or periorbital pain. Nasopharyngeal ulcerations, epistaxis, and headaches are also common, and involvement of cranial nerves V and VII has been described in more advanced cases. Bony erosion may be evident on examination. Often the patient does not appear seriously ill despite the rapidly progressive nature of these infections.

Patients with acute nosocomial sinusitis are often critically ill and thus do not manifest the typical clinical features of sinus disease. This diagnosis should be suspected, however, when hospitalized patients who have appropriate risk factors (e.g., nasotracheal intubation) develop fever without another apparent cause.

Diagnosis

Distinguishing viral from bacterial rhinosinusitis in the ambulatory setting is usually difficult because of the relatively low sensitivity and specificity of the common clinical features. One clinical feature that has been used to help guide diagnostic and therapeutic decision making is illness duration. Because acute bacterial sinusitis is uncommon in patients whose symptoms have lasted <10 days, expert panels now recommend reserving this diagnosis for patients with "persistent" symptoms (i.e., symptoms lasting >10 days in adults or >10–14 days in children) accompanied by the three cardinal signs of purulent nasal discharge, nasal obstruction, and facial pain (Table 31-1). Even among patients who meet these criteria, only 40–50% have true bacterial sinusitis. The use of CT or sinus radiography is not recommended for acute disease, particularly early in the course of illness (i.e., at <10 days) in light of the high prevalence of similar abnormalities among patients with acute viral rhinosinusitis. In the evaluation of persistent, recurrent, or chronic sinusitis, CT of the sinuses is the radiographic study of choice.

The clinical history and/or setting often can identify cases of acute anaerobic bacterial sinusitis, acute fungal sinusitis, or sinusitis from noninfectious causes (e.g., allergic rhinosinusitis). In the case of an immunocompromised patient with acute fungal sinus infection, immediate examination by an otolaryngologist is required. Biopsy specimens from involved areas should be examined by a pathologist for evidence of fungal hyphal elements and tissue invasion. Cases of suspected acute nosocomial sinusitis should be confirmed by sinus CT. Because therapy should target the offending organism, a sinus aspirate for culture and susceptibility testing should be obtained, if possible, before the initiation of antimicrobial therapy.

TREATMENT Acute Sinusitis

Most patients with a clinical diagnosis of acute rhinosinusitis improve without antibiotic therapy. The preferred initial approach in patients with mild to moderate symptoms of short duration is therapy aimed at symptom relief and facilitation of sinus drainage, such as with oral and topical decongestants, nasal saline lavage, and—at least in patients with a history of chronic sinusitis or allergies—nasal glucocorticoids. Newer studies have cast doubt on the role of antibiotics and inhaled glucocorticoids in acute rhinosinusitis. In one notable double-blind, randomized, placebo-controlled trial, neither antibiotics nor topical glucocorticoids had a significant impact on cure in the study population of patients, the majority of whom had had symptoms for <7 days. Adult patients whose condition does not improve after 7 days, children whose condition does not improve after 10–14 days, and patients with more severe symptoms (regardless of duration) should be treated with antibiotics (Table 31-1). Empirical therapy for adults with community-acquired sinusitis should consist of the narrowest-spectrum agent active against the most common bacterial pathogens, including *S. pneumoniae* and *H. influenzae*, e.g., amoxicillin. No clinical trials support the use of broad-spectrum agents for routine cases of bacterial sinusitis, even in the current era of drug-resistant *S. pneumoniae*. Up to 10% of patients do not respond to initial antimicrobial therapy; sinus aspiration and/or lavage by an otolaryngologist should be considered in these cases. Antibiotic prophylaxis to prevent episodes of recurrent acute bacterial sinusitis is not recommended.

Surgical intervention and IV antibiotic administration usually are reserved for patients with severe disease or those with

TABLE 31-1 Guidelines for the Diagnosis and Treatment of Acute Sinusitis

Age Group	Diagnostic Criteria	Treatment Recommendations[a]
Adults	Moderate symptoms (e.g., nasal purulence/congestion or cough) for >10 d *or* Severe symptoms of any duration, including unilateral/focal facial swelling or tooth pain	*Initial therapy:* Amoxicillin, 500 mg PO tid or 875 mg PO bid *Penicillin allergy:* TMP-SMX, 1 DS tablet PO bid for 10–14 d *Exposure to antibiotics within 30 d or >30% prevalence of penicillin-resistant Streptococcus pneumoniae:* Amoxicillin/clavulanate (extended release), 2000 mg PO bid; *or* Antipneumococcal fluoroquinolone (e.g., levofloxacin, 500 mg PO qd) *Recent treatment failure:* Amoxicillin/clavulanate (extended release), 2000 mg PO bid; *or* Amoxicillin, 1500 mg bid, plus clindamycin, 300 mg PO qid; *or* Antipneumococcal fluoroquinolone (e.g., levofloxacin, 500 mg PO qd)
Children	Moderate symptoms (e.g., nasal purulence/congestion or cough) for >10–14 d *or* Severe symptoms of any duration, including fever (>102°F), unilateral/focal facial swelling or pain	*Initial therapy:* Amoxicillin, 45–90 mg/kg qd (up to 2 g) PO in divided doses (bid or tid); *or* Cefuroxime axetil, 30 mg/kg qd PO in divided doses (bid); *or* Cefdinir, 14 mg/kg PO qd *Exposure to antibiotics within 30 d, recent treatment failure, or >30% prevalence of penicillin-resistant S. pneumoniae:* Amoxicillin, 90 mg/kg qd (up to 2 g) PO in divided doses (bid), plus clavulanate, 6.4 mg/kg qd PO in divided doses (bid) (extra-strength suspension); *or* Cefuroxime axetil, 30 mg/kg qd PO in divided doses (bid); *or* Cefdinir, 14 mg/kg PO qd

[a]Unless otherwise specified, the duration of therapy is generally 10 days, with appropriate follow-up.

Abbreviations: DS, double-strength; TMP-SMX, trimethoprim-sulfamethoxazole.

Sources: American Academy of Pediatrics Subcommittee on Management of Sinusitis and Committee on Quality Improvement, 2001; Rosenfeld et al., 2007.

intracranial complications such as abscess and orbital involvement. Immunocompromised patients with acute invasive fungal sinusitis usually require extensive surgical debridement and treatment with IV antifungal agents active against fungal hyphal forms, such as amphotericin B. Specific therapy should be individualized according to the fungal species and its susceptibilities as well as the individual patient's characteristics.

Treatment of nosocomial sinusitis should begin with broad-spectrum antibiotics to cover common and often resistant pathogens such as *S. aureus* and gram-negative bacilli. Therapy then should be tailored to the results of culture and susceptibility testing of sinus aspirates.

■ CHRONIC SINUSITIS

Chronic sinusitis is characterized by symptoms of sinus inflammation lasting >12 weeks. This illness is most commonly associated with either bacteria or fungi, and clinical cure in most cases is very difficult. Many patients have undergone treatment with repeated courses of antibacterial agents and multiple sinus surgeries, increasing their risk of colonization with antibiotic-resistant pathogens and of surgical complications. These patients often have high rates of morbidity, sometimes over many years.

In *chronic bacterial sinusitis*, infection is thought to be due to the impairment of mucociliary clearance from repeated infections rather than to persistent bacterial infection. The pathogenesis of this condition, however, is poorly understood. Although certain conditions (e.g., cystic fibrosis) can predispose patients to chronic

bacterial sinusitis, most patients with chronic rhinosinusitis do not have obvious underlying conditions that result in the obstruction of sinus drainage, the impairment of ciliary action, or immune dysfunction. Patients experience constant nasal congestion and sinus pressure, with intermittent periods of greater severity, which may persist for years. CT can be helpful in determining the extent of disease, detecting an underlying anatomic defect or obstructing process (e.g., a polyp), and assessing the response to therapy. The management team should include an otolaryngologist to conduct endoscopic examinations and obtain tissue samples for histologic examination and culture. An endoscopy-derived culture not only has a higher yield but also allows direct visualization for abnormal anatomy.

Chronic fungal sinusitis is a disease of immunocompetent hosts and is usually noninvasive, although slowly progressive invasive disease sometimes is seen. Noninvasive disease, which typically is associated with hyaline molds such as *Aspergillus* species and dematiaceous molds such as *Curvularia* or *Bipolaris* species, can present as a number of different scenarios. In mild, indolent disease, which usually occurs in the setting of repeated failures of antibacterial therapy, only nonspecific mucosal changes may be seen on sinus CT. Although there is some controversy on this point, endoscopic surgery is usually curative in these cases, with no need for antifungal therapy. Another form of disease presents as long-standing, often unilateral symptoms and opacification of a single sinus on imaging studies as a result of a mycetoma (fungus ball) within the sinus. Treatment for this condition is also surgical, although systemic antifungal therapy may be warranted in the rare case in which bony erosion occurs. A third form of disease, known as *allergic fungal sinusitis*, is seen in patients with a history of nasal polyposis and asthma, who often have had multiple sinus surgeries. Patients with this condition produce a thick, eosinophil-laden mucus with the consistency of peanut butter that contains sparse fungal hyphae on histologic examination. These patients often present with pansinusitis.

TREATMENT   Chronic Sinusitis

Treatment of chronic bacterial sinusitis can be challenging and consists primarily of repeated culture-guided courses of antibiotics, sometimes for 3–4 weeks at a time; administration of intranasal glucocorticoids; and mechanical irrigation of the sinus with sterile saline solution. When this management approach fails, sinus surgery may be indicated and sometimes provides significant, albeit short-term, alleviation. Treatment of chronic fungal sinusitis consists of surgical removal of impacted mucus. Recurrence, unfortunately, is common.

INFECTIONS OF THE EAR AND MASTOID

Infections of the ear and associated structures can involve both the middle and the external ear, including the skin, cartilage, periosteum, ear canal, and tympanic and mastoid cavities. Both viruses and bacteria are known causes of these infections, some of which result in significant morbidity if not treated appropriately.

■ INFECTIONS OF THE EXTERNAL EAR STRUCTURES

Infections involving the structures of the external ear are often difficult to differentiate from noninfectious inflammatory conditions with similar clinical manifestations. Clinicians should consider inflammatory disorders as possible causes of external ear irritation, particularly in the absence of local or regional adenopathy. Aside from the more salient causes of inflammation, such as trauma, insect bite, and overexposure to sunlight or extreme cold, the differential diagnosis should include less common conditions such as autoimmune disorders (e.g., lupus or relapsing polychondritis) and vasculitides (e.g., granulomatosis with polyangiitis [Wegener's]).

Auricular cellulitis

Auricular cellulitis is an infection of the skin overlying the external ear and typically follows minor local trauma. It presents as the typical signs and symptoms of cellulitis, with tenderness, erythema, swelling, and warmth of the external ear (particularly the lobule) but without apparent involvement of the ear canal or inner structures. Treatment consists of warm compresses and oral antibiotics such as dicloxacillin that are active against typical skin and soft tissue pathogens (specifically, *S. aureus* and streptococci). IV antibiotics such as a first-generation cephalosporin (e.g., cefazolin) or a penicillinase-resistant penicillin (e.g., nafcillin) occasionally are needed for more severe cases, with consideration of MRSA if either risk factors or failure of therapy point to this organism.

Perichondritis

Perichondritis, an infection of the perichondrium of the auricular cartilage, typically follows local trauma (e.g., ear piercing, burns, or lacerations). Occasionally, when the infection spreads down to the cartilage of the pinna itself, patients may develop chondritis. The infection may closely resemble auricular cellulitis, with erythema, swelling, and extreme tenderness of the pinna, although the lobule is less often involved in perichondritis. The most common patho-gens are *P. aeruginosa* and *S. aureus*, although other gram-negative and gram-positive organisms occasionally are involved. Treatment consists of systemic antibiotics active against both *P. aeruginosa* and *S. aureus*. An antipseudomonal penicillin (e.g., piperacillin) or a combination of a penicillinase-resistant penicillin and an antipseudomonal quinolone (e.g., nafcillin plus ciprofloxacin) is typically used. Incision and drainage may be helpful for culture and for resolution of infection, which often takes weeks. When perichondritis fails to respond to adequate antimicrobial therapy, clinicians should consider a noninfectious inflammatory etiology such as relapsing polychondritis.

Otitis externa

The term *otitis externa* refers to a collection of diseases involving primarily the auditory meatus. Otitis externa usually results from a combination of heat and retained moisture, with desquamation and maceration of the epithelium of the outer ear canal. The disease exists in several forms: localized, diffuse, chronic, and invasive. All forms are predominantly bacterial in origin, with *P. aeruginosa* and *S. aureus* the most common pathogens.

Acute localized otitis externa (*furunculosis*) can develop in the outer third of the ear canal, where skin overlies cartilage and hair follicles are numerous. As in furunculosis elsewhere on the body, *S. aureus* is the usual pathogen, and treatment typically consists of an oral antistaphylococcal penicillin (e.g., dicloxacillin), with incision and drainage in cases of abscess formation.

Acute diffuse otitis externa is also known as *swimmer's ear*, although it can develop in patients who have not recently been swimming. Heat, humidity, and the loss of protective cerumen lead to excessive moisture and elevation of the pH in the ear canal, which in turn lead to skin maceration and irritation. Infection may then occur; the predominant pathogen is *P. aeruginosa*, although other gram-negative and gram-positive organisms—and rarely yeasts—have been recovered from patients with this condition. The illness often starts with itching and progresses to severe pain, which usually is elicited by manipulation of the pinna or tragus. The onset of pain generally is accompanied by the development of an erythematous, swollen ear canal, often with scant white, clumpy discharge. Treatment consists of cleansing the canal to remove debris and enhance the activity of topical therapeutic agents—usually hypertonic saline or mixtures of alcohol and acetic acid. Inflammation also can be decreased by adding glucocorticoids to the treatment regimen or by using Burow's solution (aluminum acetate in water). Antibiotics are most effective when given topically. Otic mixtures provide adequate pathogen coverage; these preparations usually combine neomycin with polymyxin, with or without glucocorticoids. Systemic antimicrobial agents typically are reserved for severe disease or infections in immunocompromised hosts.

Chronic otitis externa is caused primarily by repeated local irritation, most commonly arising from persistent drainage from a chronic middle-ear infection. Other causes of repeated irritation, such as insertion of cotton swabs or other foreign objects into the ear canal, can lead to this condition, as can rare chronic infections such as syphilis, tuberculosis, and leprosy. Chronic otitis externa typically presents as erythematous, scaling dermatitis in which the predominant symptom is pruritus rather than pain; this condition must be differentiated from several others that produce a similar clinical picture, such as atopic dermatitis, seborrheic dermatitis, psoriasis, and dermatomycosis. Therapy consists of identifying and treating or removing the offending process, although successful resolution is frequently difficult.

Invasive otitis externa, also known as *malignant* or *necrotizing* otitis externa, is an aggressive and potentially life-threatening disease that occurs predominantly in elderly diabetic patients and other immunocompromised persons. The disease begins in the external canal as a soft tissue infection that progresses slowly over weeks to months and often is difficult to distinguish from a severe case of chronic otitis externa because of the presence of purulent otorrhea and an erythematous swollen ear and external canal. Severe, deep-seated otalgia, frequently out of proportion to findings on examination, is often noted and can help differentiate invasive from chronic otitis externa. The characteristic finding on examination is granulation tissue in the posteroinferior wall of the external canal, near the junction of bone and cartilage. If left unchecked, the infection can migrate to the base of the skull (resulting in skull-base osteomyelitis) and onto the meninges and brain, with a high-associated mortality rate. Cranial nerve involvement is seen occasionally, with the facial nerve usually affected first and most often. Thrombosis of the sigmoid sinus can occur if the infection extends to that area. CT, which can reveal osseous erosion of the temporal bone and skull base, can be used to help determine the extent of disease, as can gallium and technetium-99 scintigraphy studies. *P. aeruginosa* is by far the most common pathogen, although *S. aureus*, *S. epidermidis*, *Aspergillus*, *Actinomyces*, and some gram-negative bacteria have also been associated with this disease. In all cases, the external ear canal should be cleansed and a biopsy specimen of the granulation tissue within the canal (or of deeper tissues) obtained for culture of the offending organism. IV antibiotic therapy should be given for a prolonged course (6–8 weeks) and directed specifically toward the recovered pathogen. For *P. aeruginosa*, the regimen typically includes an antipseudomonal penicillin or cephalosporin (e.g., piperacillin or ceftazidime) with an aminoglycoside. A fluoroquinolone antibiotic is frequently used in place of the aminoglycoside and can even be administered orally because of the excellent bioavailability of this drug class. In addition, antibiotic drops containing an agent active against *Pseudomonas* (e.g., ciprofloxacin) usually are prescribed and are combined with glucocorticoids to reduce inflammation. Cases of invasive *Pseudomonas* otitis externa recognized in the early stages sometimes can be treated with oral and otic fluoroquinolones alone, albeit with close follow-up. Extensive surgical debridement, once an important component of the treatment approach, is now rarely indicated.

In necrotizing otitis externa, recurrence is documented up to 20% of the time. Aggressive glycemic control in diabetics is important not only for effective treatment but also for prevention of recurrence. The role of hyperbaric oxygen has not been clearly established.

■ INFECTIONS OF MIDDLE-EAR STRUCTURES

Otitis media is an inflammatory condition of the middle ear that results from dysfunction of the eustachian tube in association with a number of illnesses, including URIs and chronic rhinosinusitis. The inflammatory response to these conditions leads to the development of a sterile transudate within the middle ear and mastoid cavities. Infection may occur if bacteria or viruses from the nasopharynx contaminate this fluid, producing an acute (or sometimes chronic) illness.

Acute otitis media

Acute otitis media results when pathogens from the nasopharynx are introduced into the inflammatory fluid collected in the middle ear (e.g., by nose blowing during a URI). The proliferation of these pathogens in this space leads to the development of the typical signs and symptoms of acute middle-ear infection. The diagnosis of acute otitis media requires the demonstration of fluid in the middle ear [with tympanic membrane (TM) immobility] and the accompanying signs or symptoms of local or systemic illness (Table 31-2).

Etiology Acute otitis media typically follows a viral URI. The causative viruses (most commonly RSV, influenza virus, rhinovirus,

and enterovirus) can themselves cause subsequent acute otitis media; more often, they predispose the patient to bacterial otitis media. Studies using tympanocentesis have consistently found *S. pneumoniae* to be the most important bacterial cause, isolated in up to 35% of cases. *H. influenzae* (nontypable strains) and *M. catarrhalis* are also common bacterial causes of acute otitis media, and concern is increasing about community strains of MRSA as an emerging etiologic agent. Viruses, such as those mentioned above, have been recovered either alone or with bacteria in 17–40% of cases.

Clinical manifestations Fluid in the middle ear is typically demonstrated or confirmed with pneumatic otoscopy. In the absence of fluid, the tympanic membrane moves visibly with the application of positive and negative pressure, but this movement is dampened when fluid is present. With bacterial infection, the tympanic membrane can also be erythematous, bulging, or retracted and occasionally can perforate spontaneously. The signs and symptoms accompanying infection can be local or systemic, including otalgia, otorrhea, diminished hearing, fever, and irritability. Erythema of the tympanic membrane is often evident but is nonspecific as it frequently is seen in association with inflammation of the upper respiratory mucosa (e.g., during examination of young children). Other signs and symptoms that are occasionally reported include vertigo, nystagmus, and tinnitus.

TREATMENT   Acute Otitis Media

There has been considerable debate on the usefulness of antibiotics for the treatment of acute otitis media. A higher proportion of treated than untreated patients are free of illness 3–5 days after diagnosis. The difficulty of predicting which patients will benefit from antibiotic therapy has led to different approaches. In the Netherlands, for instance, physicians typically manage acute otitis media with initial observation, administering anti-inflammatory agents for aggressive pain management and reserving antibiotics for high-risk patients, patients with complicated disease, or patients whose condition does not improve after 48–72 h. In contrast, many experts in the United States continue to recommend antibiotic therapy for children <6 months old in light of the higher frequency of secondary complications in this young and functionally immunocompromised population. However, observation without antimicrobial therapy is now the recommended option in the United States for acute otitis media in children ≥2 years of age and for mild to moderate disease without middle-ear effusion in children 6 months to 2 years of age. Treatment is typically indicated for patients <6 months old; for children 6 months to 2 years old who have middle-ear effusion and signs/symptoms of middle-ear inflammation; for all patients >2 years old who have bilateral disease, tympanic membrane perforation, immunocompromise, or emesis; and for any patient who has severe symptoms, including a fever ≥39°C or moderate to severe otalgia (Table 31-2).

Because most studies of the etiologic agents of acute otitis media consistently document similar pathogen profiles, therapy is generally empirical except in those few cases in which tympanocentesis is warranted—e.g., cases in newborns, cases refractory to therapy, and cases in patients who are severely ill or immunodeficient. Despite resistance to penicillin and amoxicillin in roughly one-quarter of *S. pneumoniae* isolates, one-third of *H. influenzae* isolates, and nearly all *M. catarrhalis* isolates, outcome studies continue to find that amoxicillin is as successful as any other agent, and it remains the drug of first choice in

TABLE 31-2 Guidelines for the Diagnosis and Treatment of Acute Otitis Media

Illness Severity	Diagnostic Criteria	Treatment Recommendations
Mild to moderate	>2 yrs *or* 6 mo to 2 yrs without middle-ear effusion	*Observation alone* (deferring antibiotic therapy for 48–72 h and limiting management to symptom relief)
	<6 mo; *or* 6 mo to 2 yrs with middle-ear effusion (fluid in the middle ear, evidenced by decreased TM mobility, air/fluid level behind TM, bulging TM, purulent otorrhea) *and* acute onset of signs and symptoms of middle-ear inflammation, including fever, otalgia, decreased hearing, tinnitus, vertigo, erythematous TM; *or* >2 yrs with bilateral disease, TM perforation, high fever, immunocompromise, emesis	*Initial therapy*[a] Amoxicillin, 80–90 mg/kg qd (up to 2 g) PO in divided doses (bid or tid); *or* Cefdinir, 14 mg/kg qd PO in 1 dose or divided doses (bid); *or* Cefuroxime, 30 mg/kg qd PO in divided doses (bid); *or* Azithromycin, 10 mg/kg qd PO on day 1 followed by 5 mg/kg qd PO for 4 d *Exposure to antibiotics within 30 d or recent treatment failure*[a,b]: Amoxicillin, 90 mg/kg qd (up to 2 g) PO in divided doses (bid), plus clavulanate, 6.4 mg/kg qd PO in divided doses (bid); *or* Ceftriaxone, 50 mg/kg IV/IM qd for 3 d; *or* Clindamycin, 30–40 mg/kg qd PO in divided doses (tid)
Severe	As above, with temperature ≥39.0°C (102°F) *or* Moderate to severe otalgia	*Initial therapy*[a] Amoxicillin, 90 mg/kg qd (up to 2 g) PO in divided doses (bid), plus clavulanate, 6.4 mg/kg qd PO in divided doses (bid); *or* Ceftriaxone, 50 mg/kg IV/IM qd for 3 d *Exposure to antibiotics within 30 d or recent treatment failure*[a,b] Ceftriaxone, 50 mg/kg IV/IM qd for 3 d; *or* Clindamycin, 30–40 mg/kg qd PO in divided doses (tid); *or* Consider tympanocentesis with culture

[a]Duration (unless otherwise specified): 10 days for patients <6 years old and patients with severe disease; 5–7 days (with consideration of observation only in previously healthy individuals with mild disease) for patients ≥6 years old.

[b]Failure to improve and/or clinical worsening after 48–72 h of observation or treatment.

Abbreviation: TM, tympanic membrane.

Source: American Academy of Pediatrics Subcommittee on Management of Acute Otitis Media, 2004.

recommendations from multiple sources (Table 31-2). Therapy for uncomplicated acute otitis media typically is administered for 5–7 days to patients ≥6 years old; longer courses (e.g., 10 days) should be reserved for children <6 years old and patients with severe disease, in whom short-course therapy may be inadequate.

A switch in regimen is recommended if there is no clinical improvement by the third day of therapy in light of the possibility of infection with a β-lactamase-producing strain of *H. influenzae* or *M. catarrhalis* or with a strain of penicillin-resistant *S. pneumoniae*. Decongestants and antihistamines are frequently used as adjunctive agents to reduce congestion and relieve obstruction of the eustachian tube, but clinical trials have yielded no significant evidence of benefit with either class of agents.

Recurrent acute otitis media

Recurrent acute otitis media (more than three episodes within 6 months or four episodes within 12 months) generally is due to relapse or reinfection, although data indicate that the majority of early recurrences are new infections. In general, the same pathogens responsible for acute otitis media cause recurrent disease; even so, the recommended treatment consists of antibiotics active against β-lactamase-producing organisms. Antibiotic prophylaxis [e.g., with trimethoprim sulfamethoxazole (TMP-SMX) or amoxicillin]

can reduce recurrences in patients with recurrent acute otitis media by an average of one episode per year, but this benefit is small compared with the cost of the drug and the high likelihood of colonization with antibiotic-resistant pathogens. Other approaches, including placement of tympanostomy tubes, adenoidectomy, and tonsillectomy plus adenoidectomy, are of questionable overall value in light of the relatively small benefit compared with the potential for complications.

Serous otitis media

In serous otitis media (otitis media with effusion), fluid is present in the middle ear for an extended period in the absence of signs and symptoms of infection. In general, acute effusions are self-limited; most resolve in 2–4 weeks. In some cases, however (in particular after an episode of acute otitis media), effusions can persist for months. These chronic effusions are often associated with significant hearing loss in the affected ear. In younger children, persistent effusions and decreased hearing can be associated with impairment of language acquisition skills. The great majority of cases of otitis media with effusion resolve spontaneously within 3 months without antibiotic therapy. Antibiotic therapy or myringotomy with insertion of tympanostomy tubes typically is reserved for patients in whom bilateral effusion (1) has persisted for at least 3 months and (2) is associated with significant bilateral hearing loss. With this conservative approach and the application of strict diagnostic criteria for acute otitis media and otitis media with effusion, it is estimated that 6–8 million courses of antibiotics could be avoided each year in the United States.

Chronic otitis media

Chronic suppurative otitis media is characterized by persistent or recurrent purulent otorrhea in the setting of tympanic membrane perforation. Usually, there is also some degree of conductive hearing loss. This condition can be categorized as active or inactive. Inactive disease is characterized by a central perforation of the tympanic membrane, which allows drainage of purulent fluid from the middle ear. When the perforation is more peripheral, squamous epithelium from the auditory canal may invade the middle ear through the perforation, forming a mass of keratinaceous debris (*cholesteatoma*) at the site of invasion. This mass can enlarge and has the potential to erode bone and promote further infection, which can lead to meningitis, brain abscess, or paralysis of cranial nerve VII. Treatment of chronic active otitis media is surgical; mastoidectomy, myringoplasty, and tympanoplasty can be performed as outpatient surgical procedures, with an overall success rate of ~80%. Chronic inactive otitis media is more difficult to cure, usually requiring repeated courses of topical antibiotic drops during periods of drainage. Systemic antibiotics may offer better cure rates, but their role in the treatment of this condition remains unclear.

Mastoiditis

Acute mastoiditis was relatively common among children before the introduction of antibiotics. Because the mastoid air cells connect with the middle ear, the process of fluid collection and infection is usually the same in the mastoid as in the middle ear. Early and frequent treatment of acute otitis media is most likely the reason that the incidence of acute mastoiditis has declined to only 1.2–2.0 cases per 100,000 person-years in countries with high prescribing rates for acute otitis media.

In countries such as the Netherlands, where antibiotics are used sparingly for acute otitis media, the incidence rate of acute mastoiditis is roughly twice that in countries like the United States. However, neighboring Denmark has a rate of acute mastoiditis similar to that in the Netherlands but an antibiotic-prescribing rate for acute otitis media more similar to that in the United States.

In typical acute mastoiditis, purulent exudate collects in the mastoid air cells (Fig. 31-1), producing pressure that may result in erosion of the surrounding bone and formation of abscess-like cavities that are usually evident on CT. Patients typically present with pain, erythema, and swelling of the mastoid process along with displacement of the pinna, usually in conjunction with the typical signs and symptoms of acute middle-ear infection. Rarely, patients can develop severe complications if the infection tracks under the periosteum of the temporal bone to cause a subperiosteal abscess, erodes through the mastoid tip to cause a deep neck abscess, or extends posteriorly to cause septic thrombosis of the lateral sinus.

Purulent fluid should be cultured whenever possible to help guide antimicrobial therapy. Initial empirical therapy usually is directed against the typical organisms associated with acute otitis media, such as *S. pneumoniae*, *H. influenzae*, and *M. catarrhalis*. Some patients with more severe or prolonged courses of illness should be treated for infection with *S. aureus* and gram-negative bacilli (including *Pseudomonas*). Broad empirical therapy is usually narrowed once culture results become available. Most patients can be treated conservatively with IV antibiotics; surgery (cortical mastoidectomy) can be reserved for complicated cases and those in which conservative treatment has failed.

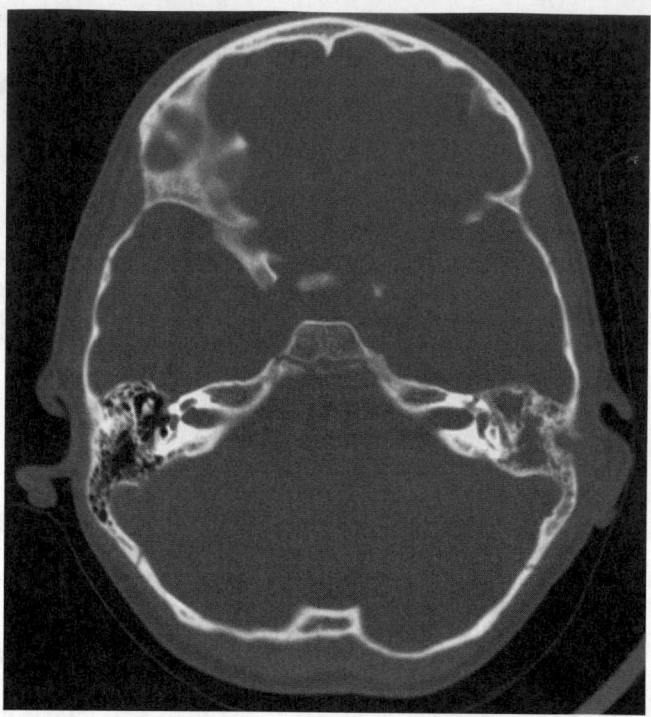

Figure 31-1 Acute mastoiditis. Axial CT image shows an acute fluid collection within the mastoid air cells on the left.

INFECTIONS OF THE PHARYNX AND ORAL CAVITY

Oropharyngeal infections range from mild, self-limited viral illnesses to serious, life-threatening bacterial infections. The most common presenting symptom is sore throat—one of the most common reasons for ambulatory care visits by both adults and children. Although sore throat is a symptom in many noninfectious illnesses as well, the overwhelming majority of patients with a new sore throat have acute pharyngitis of viral or bacterial etiology.

■ ACUTE PHARYNGITIS

Millions of visits to primary care providers each year are for sore throat; the majority of cases of acute pharyngitis are caused by typical respiratory viruses. The most important source of concern is infection with group A β-hemolytic *Streptococcus* (*S. pyogenes*) that is associated with acute glomerulonephritis and acute rheumatic fever. The risk of rheumatic fever can be reduced by timely penicillin therapy.

Etiology

A wide variety of organisms cause acute pharyngitis. The relative importance of the different pathogens can only be estimated, since a significant proportion of cases (~30%) have no identified cause. Together, respiratory viruses are the most common identifiable cause of acute pharyngitis, with rhinoviruses and coronaviruses accounting for large proportions of cases (~20% and at least 5%, respectively). Influenza virus, parainfluenza virus, and adenovirus also account for a measurable share of cases, the latter as part of the more clinically severe syndrome of pharyngoconjunctival fever. Other important but less common viral causes include herpes simplex virus (HSV) types 1 and 2, coxsackievirus A, cytomegalovirus (CMV), and Epstein-Barr virus (EBV). Acute HIV infection can present as acute pharyngitis and should be considered in at-risk populations.

Acute bacterial pharyngitis is typically caused by *S. pyogenes*, which accounts for ~5–15% of all cases of acute pharyngitis in adults; rates vary with the season and with utilization of the health care system. Group A streptococcal pharyngitis is primarily a disease of children 5–15 years of age; it is uncommon among children <3 years old, as is rheumatic fever. Streptococci of groups C and G account for a minority of cases, although these serogroups are nonrheumatogenic. *Fusobacterium necrophorum* has been increasingly recognized as a cause of pharyngitis in adolescents and young adults and is isolated nearly as often as group A streptococci. This information is important because of the rare but life-threatening Lemierre's disease, which is generally associated with *F. necrophorum* and is usually preceded by pharyngitis (see "Oral Infections," below). The remaining bacterial causes of acute pharyngitis are seen infrequently (<1% of cases each) but should be considered in appropriate exposure groups because of the severity of illness if left untreated; these etiologic agents include *Neisseria gonorrhoeae*, *Corynebacterium diphtheriae*, *Corynebacterium ulcerans*, *Yersinia enterocolitica*, and *Treponema pallidum* (in secondary syphilis). Anaerobic bacteria can also cause acute pharyngitis (*Vincent's angina*) and can contribute to more serious polymicrobial infections, such as peritonsillar or retropharyngeal abscess (see below). Atypical organisms such as *M. pneumoniae* and *C. pneumoniae* have been recovered from patients with acute pharyngitis; whether these agents are commensals or causes of acute infection is debatable.

Clinical manifestations

Although the signs and symptoms accompanying acute pharyngitis are not reliable predictors of the etiologic agent, the clinical presentation occasionally suggests that one etiology is more likely than another. Acute pharyngitis due to respiratory viruses such as rhinovirus or coronavirus is usually not severe and typically is associated with a constellation of coryzal symptoms better characterized as nonspecific URI. Findings on physical examination are uncommon; fever is rare, and tender cervical adenopathy and pharyngeal exudates are not seen. In contrast, acute pharyngitis from influenza virus can be severe and is much more likely to be associated with fever as well as with myalgias, headache, and cough. The presentation of pharyngoconjunctival fever due to adenovirus infection is similar. Since pharyngeal exudate may be present on examination, this condition can be difficult to differentiate from streptococcal pharyngitis. However, adenoviral pharyngitis is distinguished by the presence of conjunctivitis in one-third to one-half of patients. Acute pharyngitis from primary HSV infection can also mimic streptococcal pharyngitis in some cases, with pharyngeal inflammation and exudate, but the presence of vesicles and shallow ulcers on the palate can help differentiate the two diseases. This HSV syndrome is distinct from pharyngitis caused by coxsackievirus (*herpangina*), which is associated with small vesicles that develop on the soft palate and uvula and then rupture to form shallow white ulcers. Acute exudative pharyngitis coupled with fever, fatigue, generalized lymphadenopathy, and (on occasion) splenomegaly is characteristic of infectious mononucleosis due to EBV or CMV. Acute primary infection with HIV is frequently associated with fever and acute pharyngitis as well as with myalgias, arthralgias, malaise, and occasionally a nonpruritic maculopapular rash, which may be followed by lymphadenopathy and mucosal ulcerations without exudate.

The clinical features of acute pharyngitis caused by streptococci of groups A, C, and G are all similar, ranging from a relatively mild illness without many accompanying symptoms to clinically severe cases with profound pharyngeal pain, fever, chills, and abdominal pain. A hyperemic pharyngeal membrane with tonsillar hypertrophy and exudate is usually seen, along with tender anterior cervical adenopathy. Coryzal manifestations, including cough, are typically absent; when present, they suggest a viral etiology. Strains of *S. pyogenes* that generate erythrogenic toxin can also produce scarlet fever characterized by an erythematous rash and strawberry tongue.

The other types of acute bacterial pharyngitis (e.g., gonococcal, diphtherial, and yersinial) often present as exudative pharyngitis with or without other clinical features. Their etiologies are often suggested only by the clinical history.

Diagnosis

The primary goal of diagnostic testing is to separate acute streptococcal pharyngitis from pharyngitis of other etiologies (particularly viral) so that antibiotics can be prescribed more efficiently for patients to whom they may be beneficial. The most appropriate standard for the diagnosis of streptococcal pharyngitis, however, has not been established definitively. Throat swab culture is generally regarded as the most appropriate but cannot distinguish between infection and colonization and requires 24–48 h to yield results that vary with technique and culture conditions. Rapid antigen-detection tests offer good specificity (>90%) but lower sensitivity when implemented in routine practice. The sensitivity has also been shown to vary across the clinical spectrum of disease (65–90%). Several clinical prediction systems (Table 31-3) can increase the sensitivity of rapid antigen-detection tests to >90% in controlled settings. Since the sensitivities achieved in routine clinical practice are often lower, several medical and professional societies continue to recommend that all negative rapid antigen-detection tests in children be confirmed by a throat culture to limit transmission and complications of illness caused by group A streptococci. The Centers for Disease Control and Prevention, the Infectious Diseases Society of America, and the American Academy of Family Physicians do not recommend backup culture when adults have negative results in a highly sensitive rapid antigen-detection test, however, because of the lower prevalence and smaller benefit in this age group.

Cultures and rapid diagnostic tests for other causes of acute pharyngitis, such as influenza virus, adenovirus, HSV, EBV, CMV, and *M. pneumoniae*, are available in some locations and can be used when these infections are suspected. The diagnosis of acute EBV infection depends primarily on the detection of antibodies to the virus with a heterophile agglutination assay (monospot slide test) or enzyme-linked immunosorbent assay. Testing for HIV RNA or antigen (p24) should be performed when acute primary HIV infection is suspected. If other bacterial causes are suspected (particularly *N. gonorrhoeae*, *C. diphtheriae*, or *Y. enterocolitica*), specific cultures should be requested since these organisms may be missed on routine throat swab culture.

TREATMENT   Pharyngitis

Antibiotic treatment of pharyngitis due to *S. pyogenes* confers numerous benefits, including a decrease in the risk of rheumatic fever. The magnitude of this benefit is fairly small, since rheumatic fever is now a rare disease, even among untreated patients. Nevertheless, when therapy is started within 48 h of illness onset, symptom duration is decreased. An additional benefit of therapy is the potential to reduce the transmission of streptococcal pharyngitis, particularly in areas of overcrowding or close contact. Antibiotic therapy for acute pharyngitis is therefore recommended in cases in which *S. pyogenes* is confirmed as the etiologic agent by rapid antigen-detection test or throat swab culture. Otherwise, antibiotics should be given in routine cases only when another bacterial cause has been identified. Effective therapy for streptococcal pharyngitis consists of either a single dose of IM benzathine penicillin or a full 10-day course of oral penicillin (Table 31-3).

 Erythromycin can be used in place of penicillin, although resistance to erythromycin among *S. pyogenes* strains in some parts of the world (particularly Europe) can

TABLE 31-3 Guidelines for the Diagnosis and Treatment of Acute Pharyngitis

Age Group	Diagnostic Criteria	Treatment Recommendations[a]
Adults	Clinical suspicion of streptococcal pharyngitis (e.g., fever, tonsillar swelling, exudate, enlarged/tender anterior cervical lymph nodes, absence of cough or coryza)[b] with: History of rheumatic fever *or* Documented household exposure *or* Positive rapid strep screen	Penicillin VK, 500 mg PO tid; *or* Amoxicillin, 500 mg PO bid; *or* Erythromycin, 250 mg PO qid; *or* Benzathine penicillin G, single dose of 1.2 million units IM
Children	Clinical suspicion of streptococcal pharyngitis (e.g., tonsillar swelling, exudate, enlarged/tender anterior cervical lymph nodes, absence of coryza) with: History of rheumatic fever *or* Documented household exposure *or* Positive rapid strep screen *or* Positive throat culture (for patients with negative rapid strep screen)	Amoxicillin, 45 mg/kg qd PO in divided doses (bid or tid); *or* Penicillin VK, 50 mg/kg qd PO in divided doses (bid); *or* Cephalexin, 50 mg/kg qd PO in divided doses (qid); *or* Benzathine penicillin G, single dose of 25,000 units/kg IM

[a]Unless otherwise specified, the duration of therapy is generally 10 days, with appropriate follow-up.

[b]Some organizations support treating adults who have these symptoms and signs without administering a rapid streptococcal antigen test.

Sources: Cooper et al, 2001; Schwartz et al, 1998.

prohibit the use of this drug. Newer (and more expensive) antibiotics are also active against streptococci but offer no greater efficacy than the agents mentioned above. Testing for cure is unnecessary and may reveal only chronic colonization. There is no evidence to support antibiotic treatment of group C or G streptococcal pharyngitis or pharyngitis in which mycoplasmas or chlamydiae have been recovered. Penicillin prophylaxis (benzathine penicillin G, 1.2 million units IM every 3–4 weeks) is indicated for patients at risk of recurrent rheumatic fever.

Treatment of viral pharyngitis is entirely symptom-based except in infection with influenza virus or HSV. For influenza, the repertoire of therapeutic agents includes the adamantanes amantadine and rimantadine and the neuraminidase inhibitors oseltamivir and zanamivir. Administration of all these agents needs to be started within 36–48 h of symptom onset to reduce illness duration meaningfully. Among these agents, only oseltamivir and zanamivir are active against both influenza A and influenza B and therefore can be used when local patterns of infection and antiviral resistance are unknown. Oropharyngeal HSV infection sometimes responds to treatment with antiviral agents such as acyclovir, although these drugs are often reserved for immunosuppressed patients.

Complications

Although rheumatic fever is the best-known complication of acute streptococcal pharyngitis, the risk of its following acute infection remains quite low. Other complications include acute glomerulonephritis and numerous suppurative conditions, such as peritonsillar abscess (*quinsy*), otitis media, mastoiditis, sinusitis, bacteremia, and pneumonia—all of which occur at low rates. Although antibiotic treatment of acute streptococcal pharyngitis can prevent the development of rheumatic fever, there is no evidence that it can prevent acute glomerulonephritis. Some evidence supports antibiotic use to prevent the suppurative complications of streptococcal pharyngitis, particularly peritonsillar abscess, which can also involve oral anaerobes such as *Fusobacterium*. Abscesses usually are accompanied by severe pharyngeal pain, dysphagia, fever, and dehydration; in addition, medial displacement of the tonsil and lateral displacement of

the uvula are often evident on examination. Although early use of IV antibiotics (e.g., clindamycin, penicillin G with metronidazole) may obviate the need for surgical drainage in some cases, treatment typically involves needle aspiration or incision and drainage.

ORAL INFECTIONS

Aside from periodontal disease such as gingivitis, infections of the oral cavity most commonly involve HSV or *Candida* species. In addition to causing painful cold sores on the lips, HSV can infect the tongue and buccal mucosa, causing the formation of irritating vesicles. Although topical antiviral agents (e.g., acyclovir and penciclovir) can be used externally for cold sores, oral or IV acyclovir is often needed for primary infections, extensive oral infections, and infections in immunocompromised patients. Oropharyngeal candidiasis (*thrush*) is caused by a variety of *Candida* species, most often *C. albicans*. Thrush occurs predominantly in neonates, immunocompromised patients (especially those with AIDS), and recipients of prolonged antibiotic or glucocorticoid therapy. In addition to sore throat, patients often report a burning tongue, and physical examination reveals friable white or gray plaques on the gingiva, tongue, and oral mucosa. Treatment that usually consists of an oral antifungal suspension (nystatin or clotrimazole) or oral fluconazole, is frequently successful. In the uncommon cases of fluconazole-refractory thrush that are seen in some patients with AIDS, other therapeutic options include oral formulations of itraconazole, amphotericin B, posaconazole, or voriconazole as well as an IV echinocandin (caspofungin, micafungin, or anidulafungin) or amphotericin B deoxycholate, if needed. In these cases, therapy based on culture and susceptibility test results is ideal.

Vincent's angina, also known as *acute necrotizing ulcerative gingivitis* or *trench mouth*, is a unique and dramatic form of gingivitis characterized by painful, inflamed gingiva with ulcerations of the interdental papillae that bleed easily. Since oral anaerobes are the cause, patients typically have halitosis and frequently present with fever, malaise, and lymphadenopathy. Treatment consists of debridement and oral administration of penicillin plus metronidazole, with clindamycin alone as an alternative.

Ludwig's angina is a rapidly progressive, potentially fulminant form of cellulitis that involves the bilateral sublingual and submandibular spaces and that typically originates from an infected or recently extracted tooth, most commonly the lower second and third molars. Improved dental care has reduced the incidence of this disorder substantially. Infection in these areas leads to dysphagia, odynophagia, and "woody" edema in the sublingual region, forcing the tongue up and back with the potential for airway obstruction. Fever, dysarthria, and drooling also may be noted, and patients may speak in a "hot potato" voice. Intubation or tracheostomy may be necessary to secure the airway, as asphyxiation is the most common cause of death. Patients should be monitored closely and treated promptly with IV antibiotics directed against streptococci and oral anaerobes. Recommended agents include ampicillin/sulbactam and high-dose penicillin plus metronidazole.

Postanginal septicemia (Lemierre's disease) is a rare anaerobic oropharyngeal infection caused predominantly by *F. necrophorum*. The illness typically starts as a sore throat (most commonly in adolescents and young adults), which may present as exudative tonsillitis or peritonsillar abscess. Infection of the deep pharyngeal tissue allows organisms to drain into the lateral pharyngeal space, which contains the carotid artery and internal jugular vein. Septic thrombophlebitis of the internal jugular vein can result, with associated pain, dysphagia, and neck swelling and stiffness. Sepsis usually occurs 3–10 days after the onset of sore throat and is often coupled with metastatic infection to the lung and other distant sites. Occasionally, the infection can extend along the carotid sheath and into the posterior mediastinum, resulting in mediastinitis, or it can erode into the carotid artery, with the early sign of repeated small bleeds into the mouth. The mortality rate from these invasive infections can be as high as 50%. Treatment consists of IV antibiotics (penicillin G or clindamycin) and surgical drainage of any purulent collections. The concomitant use of anticoagulants to prevent embolization remains controversial but is often advised, with careful consideration of both the risks and the benefits.

INFECTIONS OF THE LARYNX AND EPIGLOTTIS

■ LARYNGITIS

Laryngitis is defined as any inflammatory process involving the larynx and can be caused by a variety of infectious and noninfectious processes. The vast majority of laryngitis cases seen in clinical practice in developed countries are acute. Acute laryngitis is a common syndrome caused predominantly by the same viruses responsible for many other URIs. In fact, most cases of acute laryngitis occur in the setting of a viral URI.

Etiology

Nearly all major respiratory viruses have been implicated in acute viral laryngitis, including rhinovirus, influenza virus, parainfluenza virus, adenovirus, coxsackievirus, coronavirus, and RSV. Acute laryngitis can also be associated with acute bacterial respiratory infections such as those caused by group A *Streptococcus* or *C. diphtheriae* (although diphtheria has been virtually eliminated in the United States). Another bacterial pathogen thought to play a role (albeit unclear) in the pathogenesis of acute laryngitis is *M. catarrhalis*, which has been recovered on nasopharyngeal culture in a significant percentage of cases.

Chronic laryngitis of infectious etiology is much less common in developed than in developing countries. Laryngitis due to *Mycobacterium tuberculosis* is often difficult to distinguish from laryngeal cancer, in part because of the frequent absence of signs, symptoms, and radiographic findings typical of pulmonary disease. *Histoplasma* and *Blastomyces* may cause laryngitis, often as a complication of systemic infection. *Candida* species can cause laryngitis as well, often in association with thrush or esophagitis and particularly in immunosuppressed patients. Rare cases of chronic laryngitis are due to *Coccidioides* and *Cryptococcus*.

Clinical manifestations

Laryngitis is characterized by hoarseness and also can be associated with reduced vocal pitch or aphonia. As acute laryngitis is caused predominantly by respiratory viruses, these symptoms usually occur in association with other symptoms and signs of URI, including rhinorrhea, nasal congestion, cough, and sore throat. Direct laryngoscopy often reveals diffuse laryngeal erythema and edema, along with vascular engorgement of the vocal folds. In addition, chronic disease (e.g., tuberculous laryngitis) often includes mucosal nodules and ulcerations visible on laryngoscopy; these lesions sometimes are mistaken for laryngeal cancer.

> **TREATMENT**   Laryngitis

Acute laryngitis usually is treated with humidification and voice rest alone. Antibiotics are not recommended except when group A *Streptococcus* is cultured, in which case penicillin is the drug of choice. The choice of therapy for chronic laryngitis depends on the pathogen, whose identification usually requires biopsy with culture. Patients with laryngeal tuberculosis are highly contagious because of the large number of organisms that are easily aerosolized. These patients should be managed in the same way as patients with active pulmonary disease.

■ CROUP

The term *croup* actually denotes a group of diseases collectively referred to as "croup syndrome," all of which are acute and predominantly viral respiratory illnesses characterized by marked swelling of the subglottic region of the larynx. Croup primarily affects children <6 years old. For a detailed discussion of this entity, the reader should consult a textbook of pediatric medicine.

■ EPIGLOTTITIS

Acute epiglottitis (supraglottitis) is an acute, rapidly progressive form of cellulitis of the epiglottis and adjacent structures that can result in complete—and potentially fatal—airway obstruction in both children and adults. Before the widespread use of *H. influenzae* type b (Hib) vaccine, this entity was much more common among children, with a peak incidence at ~3.5 years of age. In some countries, mass vaccination against Hib has reduced the annual incidence of acute epiglottitis in children by >90%; in contrast, the annual incidence in adults has changed little since the introduction of Hib vaccine. Because of the danger of airway obstruction, acute epiglottitis constitutes a medical emergency, particularly in children, and prompt diagnosis and airway protection are of the utmost importance.

Etiology

After the introduction of the Hib vaccine in the mid-1980s, disease incidence among children in the United States declined dramatically. Nevertheless, lack of vaccination or vaccine failure has meant that many pediatric cases seen today are still due to Hib. In adults and (more recently) in children, a variety of other bacterial pathogens have been associated with epiglottitis, the most common being group A *Streptococcus*. Other pathogens seen less frequently include *S. pneumoniae*, *Haemophilus parainfluenzae*, and *S. aureus* (including MRSA). Viruses have not been established as causes of acute epiglottitis.

Clinical manifestations and diagnosis

Epiglottitis typically presents more acutely in young children than in adolescents or adults. On presentation, most children have had symptoms for <24 h, including high fever, severe sore throat, tachycardia, systemic toxicity, and (in many cases) drooling while sitting forward. Symptoms and signs of respiratory obstruction may also be present and may progress rapidly. The somewhat milder illness in adolescents and adults often follows 1–2 days of severe sore throat and is commonly accompanied by dyspnea, drooling, and stridor. Physical examination of patients with acute epiglottitis may reveal moderate or severe respiratory distress, with inspiratory stridor and retractions of the chest wall. These findings *diminish* as the disease progresses and the patient tires. Conversely, oropharyngeal examination reveals infection that is much less severe than would be predicted from the symptoms—a finding that should alert the clinician to a cause of symptoms and obstruction that lies beyond the tonsils. The diagnosis often is made on clinical grounds, although direct fiberoptic laryngoscopy is frequently performed in a controlled environment (e.g., an operating room) to visualize and culture the typical edematous "cherry-red" epiglottis and facilitate placement of an endotracheal tube. Direct visualization in an examination room (i.e., with a tongue blade and indirect laryngoscopy) is not recommended because of the risk of immediate laryngospasm and complete airway obstruction. Lateral neck radiographs and laboratory tests can assist in the diagnosis but may delay the critical securing of the airway and cause the patient to be moved or repositioned more than is necessary, thereby increasing the risk of further airway compromise. Neck radiographs typically reveal an enlarged edematous epiglottis (the "thumbprint sign," Fig. 31-2), usually with a dilated hypopharynx and normal subglottic structures. Laboratory tests characteristically document mild to moderate leukocytosis with a predominance of neutrophils. Blood cultures are positive in a significant proportion of cases.

TREATMENT Epiglottitis

Security of the airway is always of primary concern in acute epiglottitis, even if the diagnosis is only suspected. Mere observation for signs of impending airway obstruction is not routinely

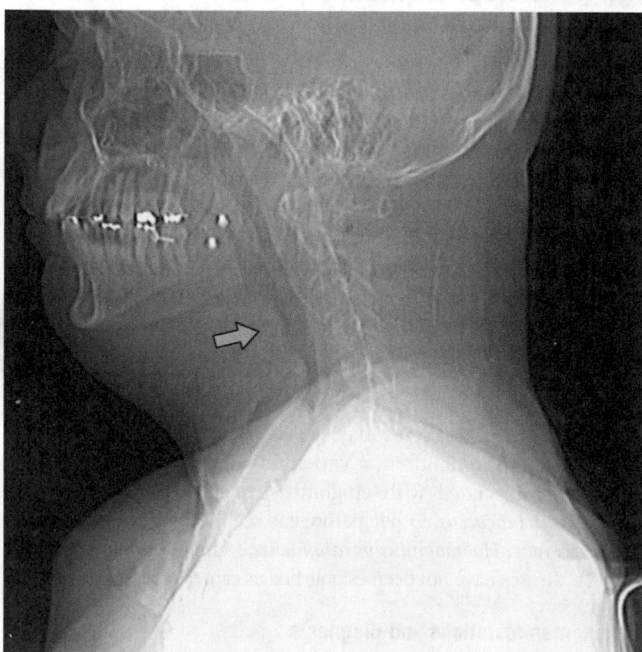

Figure 31-2 Acute epiglottitis. In this lateral soft tissue radiograph of the neck, the arrow indicates the enlarged edematous epiglottis (the "thumbprint sign").

recommended, particularly in children. Many adults have been managed with observation only since the illness is perceived to be milder in this age group, but some data suggest that this approach may be risky and probably should be reserved only for adult patients who have yet to develop dyspnea or stridor. Once the airway has been secured and specimens of blood and epiglottis tissue have been obtained for culture, treatment with IV antibiotics should be given to cover the most likely organisms, particularly *H. influenzae*. Because rates of ampicillin resistance in this organism have risen significantly in recent years, therapy with a β-lactam/β-lactamase inhibitor combination or a second- or third-generation cephalosporin is recommended. Typically, ampicillin/sulbactam, cefuroxime, cefotaxime, or ceftriaxone is given, with clindamycin and TMP-SMX reserved for patients allergic to β-lactams. Antibiotic therapy should be continued for 7–10 days and should be tailored to the organism recovered in culture. If the household contacts of a patient with *H. influenzae* epiglottitis include an unvaccinated child under age 4, all members of the household (including the patient) should receive prophylactic rifampin for 4 days to eradicate carriage of *H. influenzae*.

INFECTIONS OF THE DEEP NECK STRUCTURES

Deep neck infections are usually extensions of infection from other primary sites, most often within the pharynx or oral cavity. Many of these infections are life threatening but are difficult to detect at early stages, when they may be more easily managed. Three of the most clinically relevant spaces in the neck are the submandibular (and sublingual) space, the lateral pharyngeal (or parapharyngeal) space, and the retropharyngeal space. These spaces communicate with one another and with other important structures in the head, neck, and thorax, providing pathogens with easy access to areas that include the mediastinum, carotid sheath, skull base, and meninges. Once infection reaches these sensitive areas, mortality rates can be as high as 20–50%.

Infection of the submandibular and/or sublingual space typically originates from an infected or recently extracted lower tooth. The result is the severe, life-threatening infection referred to as Ludwig's angina (see "Oral Infections," above). Infection of the lateral pharyngeal (or parapharyngeal) space is most often a complication of common infections of the oral cavity and upper respiratory tract, including tonsillitis, peritonsillar abscess, pharyngitis, mastoiditis, and periodontal infection. This space, situated deep in the lateral wall of the pharynx, contains a number of sensitive structures, including the carotid artery, internal jugular vein, cervical sympathetic chain, and portions of cranial nerves IX through XII; at its distal end, it opens into the posterior mediastinum. Involvement of this space with infection can therefore be rapidly fatal. Examination may reveal some tonsillar displacement, trismus, and neck rigidity, but swelling of the lateral pharyngeal wall can easily be missed. The diagnosis can be confirmed by CT. Treatment consists of airway management, operative drainage of fluid collections, and at least 10 days of IV therapy with an antibiotic active against streptococci and oral anaerobes (e.g., ampicillin/sulbactam). A particularly severe form of this infection involving the components of the carotid sheath (postanginal septicemia, Lemierre's disease) is described above (see "Oral Infections"). Infection of the retropharyngeal space can also be extremely dangerous, as this space runs posterior to the pharynx from the skull base to the superior mediastinum. Infections in this space are more common among children <5 years old because of the presence of several small retropharyngeal lymph nodes that typically atrophy by age 4 years. Infection is usually a consequence of extension from another site of infection, most commonly, acute pharyngitis. Other sources include otitis media, tonsillitis, dental infections, Ludwig's angina, and anterior extension of vertebral osteomyelitis. Retropharyngeal space infection also can follow penetrating trauma to the posterior pharynx (e.g., from an endoscopic procedure). Infections are commonly polymicrobial, involving a mixture of aerobes and anaerobes; group A β-hemolytic streptococci and *S. aureus* are the most common pathogens. *M. tuberculosis* was a common cause in the past but now is rarely involved in the United States.

Patients with retropharyngeal abscess typically present with sore throat, fever, dysphagia, and neck pain and are often drooling because of difficulty and pain with swallowing. Examination may reveal tender cervical adenopathy, neck swelling, and diffuse erythema and edema of the posterior pharynx as well as a bulge in the posterior pharyngeal wall that may not be obvious on routine inspection. A soft tissue mass is usually demonstrable by lateral neck radiography or CT. Because of the risk of airway obstruction, treatment begins with securing of the airway, followed by a combination of surgical drainage and IV antibiotic administration. Initial empirical therapy should cover streptococci, oral anaerobes, and *S. aureus*; ampicillin/sulbactam, clindamycin alone, or clindamycin plus ceftriaxone is usually effective. Complications result primarily from extension to other areas (e.g., rupture into the posterior pharynx may lead to aspiration pneumonia and empyema). Extension may also occur to the lateral pharyngeal space and mediastinum, resulting in mediastinitis and pericarditis, or into nearby major blood vessels. All these events are associated with a high mortality rate.

FURTHER READINGS

AMERICAN ACADEMY OF PEDIATRICS SUBCOMMITTEE ON MANAGEMENT OF ACUTE OTITIS MEDIA: Diagnosis and management of acute otitis media. Pediatrics 113:1451, 2004

AMERICAN ACADEMY OF PEDIATRICS SUBCOMMITTEE ON MANAGEMENT OF SINUSITIS AND COMMITTEE ON QUALITY IMPROVEMENT: Clinical practice guideline: Management of sinusitis. Pediatrics 108:798, 2001

CENTOR RM: Expand the pharyngitis paradigm for adolescents and young adults. Ann Intern Med 151:812, 2009

COOPER RJ et al: Principles of appropriate antibiotic use for acute pharyngitis in adults: Background. Ann Intern Med 134:509, 2001

GONZALES R et al: Principles of appropriate antibiotic use for treatment of nonspecific upper respiratory tract infections in adults: Background. Ann Intern Med 134:490, 2001

GRIJALVA CG et al: Antibiotic prescription rates for acute respiratory tract infections in US ambulatory settings. JAMA 302:758, 2009

MEROPOL SB: Valuing reduced antibiotic use for pediatric acute otitis media. Pediatrics 122:669, 2008

RAFEI K et al: Airway infectious disease emergencies. Pediatr Clin North Am 53:215, 2006

ROSENFELD RM et al: Clinical practice guideline: Adult sinusitis. Otolaryngol Head Neck Surg 137(3 Suppl):S1, 2007

SCHWARTZ B et al: Pharyngitis—principles of judicious use of antimicrobial agents. Pediatrics 101:171, 1998

THOMPSON P et al: Effect of antibiotics for otitis media on mastoiditis in children: A retrospective cohort study using the United Kingdom general practice research database. Pediatrics 123:424, 2009

WILLIAMSON IG et al: Antibiotics and topical nasal steroid for treatment of acute maxillary sinusitis. JAMA 298:2487, 2007

YOUNG J et al: Antibiotics for adults with clinically diagnosed acute rhinosinusitis: A meta-analysis of individual patient data. Lancet 371:908, 2008

CHAPTER **32**

Oral Manifestations of Disease

Samuel C. Durso

As primary care physicians and consultants, internists are often asked to evaluate patients with disease of the oral soft tissues, teeth, and pharynx. Knowledge of the oral milieu and its unique structures is necessary to guide preventive services and recognize oral manifestations of local or systemic disease (Chap. e12). Furthermore, internists frequently collaborate with dentists in the care of patients who have a variety of medical conditions that affect oral health or who undergo dental procedures that increase their risk of medical complications.

DISEASES OF THE TEETH AND PERIODONTAL STRUCTURES

■ TOOTH AND PERIODONTAL STRUCTURE

Tooth formation begins during the sixth week of embryonic life and continues through the first 17 years of age. Tooth development begins in utero and continues until after the tooth erupts. Normally, all 20 deciduous teeth have erupted by age 3 and have been shed by age 13. Permanent teeth, eventually totaling 32, begin to erupt by age 6 and have completely erupted by age 14, though third molars (wisdom teeth) may erupt later.

The erupted tooth consists of the visible crown covered with enamel and the root submerged below the gum line and covered with bonelike cementum. *Dentin*, a material that is denser than bone and exquisitely sensitive to pain, forms the majority of the tooth substance. Dentin surrounds a core of myxomatous *pulp* containing the vascular and nerve supply. The tooth is held firmly in the alveolar socket by the *periodontium*, supporting structures that consist of the gingivae, alveolar bone, cementum, and periodontal ligament. The periodontal ligament tenaciously binds the tooth's cementum to the alveolar bone. Above this ligament is a collar of attached gingiva just below the crown. A few millimeters of unattached or free gingiva (1–3 mm) overlap the base of the crown, forming a shallow sulcus along the gum-tooth margin.

Dental caries, pulpal and periapical disease, and complications

Dental caries begin asymptomatically as a destructive process of the hard surface of the tooth. *Streptococcus mutans*, principally, along with other bacteria colonize the organic buffering film on the tooth surface to produce *plaque*. If not removed by brushing or the natural cleaning action of saliva and oral soft tissues, bacterial acids demineralize the enamel. Fissures and pits on the occlusion surfaces are the most frequent sites of decay. Surfaces adjacent to tooth restorations and exposed roots are also vulnerable, particularly as teeth are retained in an aging population. Over time, dental caries extend to the underlying dentin, leading to cavitation of the enamel and, ultimately, penetration to the tooth pulp, producing *acute pulpitis*. At this early stage, when the pulp infection is limited, the tooth becomes sensitive to percussion and hot or cold, and pain resolves immediately when the irritating stimulus is removed. Should the infection spread throughout the pulp, *irreversible pulpitis* occurs, leading to pulp necrosis. At this late stage, pain is severe and has a sharp or throbbing visceral quality that may be worse when the patient lies down. Once pulp necrosis is complete, pain may be constant or intermittent, but cold sensitivity is lost.

Treatment of caries involves removal of the softened and infected hard tissue; sealing the exposed dentin; and restoration of the tooth structure with silver amalgam, composite resin, gold, or porcelain. Once irreversible pulpitis occurs, root canal therapy is necessary, and the contents of the pulp chamber and root canals are removed, followed by thorough cleaning, antisepsis, and filling with an inert material. Alternatively, the tooth may be extracted.

Pulpal infection, if it does not egress through the decayed enamel, leads to *periapical abscess* formation, which produces pain on chewing. If the infection is mild and chronic, a *periapical granuloma* or eventually a *periapical cyst* forms, either of which produces radiolucency at the root apex. When unchecked, a periapical abscess can erode into the alveolar bone producing osteomyelitis, penetrate and drain through the gingivae (parulis or gumboil), or track along deep fascial planes, producing a virulent cellulitis (Ludwig's angina) involving the submandibular space and floor of the mouth (Chap. 164). Elderly patients, those with diabetes mellitus, and patients taking glucocorticoids may experience little or no pain and fever as these complications develop.

Periodontal disease

Periodontal disease accounts for more tooth loss than caries, particularly in the elderly. Like dental caries, chronic infection of the gingiva and anchoring structures of the tooth begins with formation of bacterial plaque. The process begins invisibly above the gum line and in the gingival sulcus. Plaque, including mineralized plaque (calculus), is preventable by appropriate dental hygiene, including periodic professional cleaning. Left undisturbed, chronic inflammation ensues and produces a painless hyperemia of the free and attached gingivae (*gingivitis*) that typically bleeds with brushing. If ignored, severe *periodontitis* occurs, leading to deepening of the physiologic sulcus and destruction of the periodontal ligament. Pockets develop around the teeth and become filled with pus and debris. As the periodontium is destroyed, teeth loosen and exfoliate. Eventually, there is resorption of the alveolar bone. A role for the chronic inflammation resulting from chronic periodontal disease in promoting coronary heart disease and stroke has been proposed. Epidemiologic studies demonstrate a moderate but significant association between chronic periodontal inflammation and atherogenesis, though a causal role remains unproven.

Acute and aggressive forms of periodontal disease are less common than the chronic forms described above. However, if the host is stressed or exposed to a new pathogen, rapidly progressive and destructive disease of the periodontal tissue can occur. A virulent example is *acute necrotizing ulcerative gingivitis* (ANUG) or *Vincent's infection*. Stress, poor oral hygiene, and tobacco and alcohol use are risk factors. The presentation includes sudden gingival inflammation, ulceration, bleeding, interdental gingival necrosis, and fetid halitosis. *Localized juvenile periodontitis*, seen in adolescents, is particularly destructive and appears to be associated with impaired neutrophil chemotaxis. *AIDS-related periodontitis* resembles ANUG in some patients or a more destructive form of adult chronic periodontitis in others. It may also produce a gangrene-like destructive process of the oral soft tissues and bone that resembles *noma*, seen in severely malnourished children in developing nations.

Prevention of tooth decay and periodontal infection

Despite the reduced prevalence of dental caries and periodontal disease in the United States due in large part to water fluoridation and improved dental care, respectively, both diseases constitute a major public health problem worldwide and for certain groups. The internist should promote preventive dental care and hygiene as part of health maintenance. Special populations at high risk for dental caries and periodontal disease include those with xerostomia, diabetics, alcoholics, tobacco users, those with Down's syndrome, and those with gingival hyperplasia. Furthermore, patients lacking dental-care access (low socioeconomic status) and those with reduced ability to provide self-care (e.g., nursing home residents and those with dementia or upper-extremity disability) suffer at a disproportionate rate. It is important to provide counseling regarding regular dental hygiene and professional cleaning, use of fluoride-containing toothpaste, professional fluoride treatments, and use of electric toothbrushes for patients with limited dexterity and to give instruction to caregivers for those unable to perform self-care. Internists caring for international students studying in the United States should be aware of the high prevalence of dental decay in this population. Cost, fear of dental care, and language and cultural differences may create barriers that prevent some from seeking preventive dental services.

Developmental and systemic disease affecting the teeth and periodontium

Malocclusion is the most common developmental problem, which, in addition to a problem with cosmesis, can interfere with mastication unless corrected through orthodontic techniques. Impacted third molars are common and occasionally become infected. Acquired prognathism due to *acromegaly* may also lead to malocclusion, as may deformity of the maxilla and mandible due to *Paget's disease* of the bone. Delayed tooth eruption, receding chin, and a protruding tongue are occasional features of *cretinism* and *hypopituitarism*. Congenital syphilis produces tapering, notched (Hutchinson's) incisors and finely nodular (mulberry) molar crowns.

Enamel hypoplasia results in crown defects ranging from pits to deep fissures of primary or permanent teeth. Intrauterine infection (syphilis, rubella), vitamin deficiency (A, C, or D), disorders of calcium metabolism (malabsorption, vitamin D–resistant rickets, hypoparathyroidism), prematurity, high fever, or rare inherited defects (*amelogenesis imperfecta*) are all causes. Tetracycline, given in sufficiently high doses during the first eight years, may produce enamel hypoplasia and discoloration. Exposure to endogenous pigments can discolor developing teeth: *erythroblastosis fetalis* (green or bluish-black), congenital liver disease (green or yellow-brown), and porphyria (red or brown that fluoresces with ultraviolet light). *Mottled enamel* occurs if excessive fluoride is ingested during development. Worn enamel is seen with age, bruxism, or excessive acid exposure (e.g., chronic gastric reflux or bulimia).

Premature tooth loss resulting from periodontitis is seen with cyclic neutropenia, Papillon-Lefèvre syndrome, Chédiak-Higashi syndrome, and leukemia. Rapid focal tooth loosening is most often due to infection, but rarer causes include Langerhans cell histiocytosis, Ewing's sarcoma, osteosarcoma, or Burkitt's lymphoma. Early loss of primary teeth is a feature of *hypophosphatasia*, a rare inborn error of metabolism.

Pregnancy may produce severe gingivitis and localized *pyogenic granulomas*. Severe periodontal disease occurs with Down's syndrome and diabetes mellitus. *Gingival hyperplasia* may be caused by phenytoin, calcium channel blockers (e.g., nifedipine), and cyclosporine. *Idiopathic familial gingival fibromatosis* and several syndrome-related disorders appear similar. Removal of the medication often reverses the drug-induced form, though surgery may be needed to control both. *Linear gingival erythema* is variably seen in patients with advanced HIV infection and probably represents immune deficiency and decreased neutrophil activity. Diffuse or focal gingival swelling may be a feature of early or late acute myelomonocytic leukemia (AMML) as well as of other lymphoproliferative disorders. A rare, but pathognomonic, sign of Wegener's granulomatosis is a red-purplish, granular gingivitis (strawberry gums).

DISEASES OF THE ORAL MUCOSA

Infection

Most oral mucosal diseases involve microorganisms (Table 32-1).

Pigmented lesions

See Table 32-2.

Dermatologic diseases

See Tables 32-1, 32-2, and 32-3 and Chaps. 51–55.

Diseases of the tongue

See Table 32-4.

HIV disease and AIDS

See Tables 32-1, 32-2, 32-3, and 32-5; Chap. 189; and Figures 181-1 and 203-1.

Ulcers

Ulceration is the most common oral mucosal lesion. Although there are many causes, the host and pattern of lesions, including the presence of systemic features, narrow the differential diagnosis (Table 32-1). Most acute ulcers are painful and self-limited. Recurrent aphthous ulcers and herpes simplex infection constitute the majority. Persistent and deep aphthous ulcers can be idiopathic or seen with HIV/AIDS. Aphthous lesions are often the presenting symptom in *Behçet's syndrome* (Chap. 327). Similar-appearing, though less painful, lesions may occur with reactive arthritis (formerly known as Reiter's syndrome), and aphthous ulcers are occasionally present during phases of discoid or *systemic lupus erythematosus* (Chap. 323). Aphthous-like ulcers are seen in Crohn's disease (Chap. 295), but unlike the common aphthous variety, they may exhibit granulomatous inflammation histologically. Recurrent aphthae in some patients with *celiac disease* have been reported to remit with elimination of gluten.

Of major concern are chronic, relatively painless ulcers and mixed red/white patches (erythroplakia and leukoplakia) of more than two weeks' duration. Squamous cell carcinoma and premalignant dysplasia should be considered early and a diagnostic biopsy obtained. The importance is underscored because early-stage malignancy is vastly more treatable than late-stage disease. High-risk sites include the lower lip, floor of the mouth, ventral and lateral tongue, and soft palate–tonsillar pillar complex. Significant risk factors for oral cancer in Western countries include sun exposure (lower lip) and tobacco and alcohol use. In India and some other Asian countries, smokeless tobacco mixed with betel nut, slaked lime, and spices is a common cause of oral cancer. Less common etiologies include syphilis and Plummer-Vinson syndrome (iron deficiency).

Rarer causes of chronic oral ulcer such as tuberculosis, fungal infection, granulomatosis with polyangiitis (Wegener's), and midline granuloma may look identical to carcinoma. Making the correct diagnosis depends on recognizing other clinical features and biopsy of the lesion. The syphilitic chancre is typically painless and therefore easily missed. Regional lymphadenopathy is invariably present. Confirmation is achieved using appropriate bacterial and serologic tests.

Disorders of mucosal fragility often produce painful oral ulcers that fail to heal within two weeks. *Mucous membrane pemphigoid*

and *pemphigus vulgaris* are the major acquired disorders. While clinical features are often distinctive, immunohistochemical examination should be performed for diagnosis and to distinguish these entities from *lichen planus* and drug reactions.

Hematologic and nutritional disease

Internists are more likely to encounter patients with acquired, rather than congenital, bleeding disorders. Bleeding after minor trauma should stop after 15 min and within an hour of tooth extraction if local pressure is applied. More prolonged bleeding, if not due to continued injury or rupture of a large vessel, should lead to investigation for a clotting abnormality. In addition to bleeding, petechiae and ecchymoses are prone to occur at the line of vibration between the soft and hard palates in patients with platelet dysfunction or thrombocytopenia.

All forms of leukemia, but particularly acute myelomonocytic leukemia, can produce gingival bleeding, ulcers, and gingival enlargement. Oral ulcers are a feature of agranulocytosis, and ulcers and mucositis are often severe complications of chemotherapy and radiation therapy for hematologic and other malignancies. Plummer-Vinson syndrome (iron deficiency, angular stomatitis, glossitis, and dysphagia) raises the risk of oral squamous cell cancer and esophageal cancer at the postcricoidal tissue web. Atrophic papillae and a red, burning tongue may occur with pernicious anemia. B-group vitamin deficiencies produce many of these same symptoms as well as oral ulceration and cheilosis. Swollen, bleeding gums, ulcers, and loosening of the teeth are a consequence of scurvy.

NONDENTAL CAUSES OF ORAL PAIN

Most, but not all, oral pain emanates from inflamed or injured tooth pulp or periodontal tissues. Nonodontogenic causes may be overlooked. In most instances, toothache is predictable and proportional to the stimulus applied, and an identifiable condition (e.g., caries, abscess) is found. Local anesthesia eliminates pain originating from dental or periodontal structures, but not referred pains. The most common nondental origin is myofascial pain referred from muscles of mastication, which become tender and ache with increased use. Many sufferers exhibit bruxism (the grinding of teeth, often during sleep) that is secondary to stress and anxiety. *Temporomandibular disorder* is closely related. It affects both sexes with a higher prevalence in women. Features include pain, limited mandibular movement, and temporomandibular joint sounds. The etiologies are complex, and malocclusion does not play the primary role once attributed to it. *Osteoarthritis* is a common cause of masticatory pain. Anti-inflammatory medication, jaw rest, soft foods, and heat provide relief. The temporomandibular joint is involved in 50% of patients with *rheumatoid arthritis* and is usually a late feature of severe disease. Bilateral preauricular pain, particularly in the morning, limits range of motion.

Migrainous neuralgia may be localized to the mouth. Episodes of pain and remission without identifiable cause and absence of relief with local anesthesia are important clues. *Trigeminal neuralgia (tic douloureux)* may involve the entire branch or part of the mandibular or maxillary branches of the fifth cranial nerve and produce pain in one or a few teeth. Pain may occur spontaneously or may be triggered by touching the lip or gingiva, brushing the teeth, or chewing. *Glossopharyngeal neuralgia* produces similar acute neuropathic symptoms in the distribution of the ninth cranial nerve. Swallowing, sneezing, coughing, or pressure on the tragus of the ear triggers pain that is felt in the base of the tongue, pharynx, and soft palate and may be referred to the temporomandibular joint. *Neuritis* involving the maxillary and mandibular divisions of the trigeminal nerve (e.g., maxillary sinusitis, neuroma, and leukemic infiltrate) is distinguished from ordinary toothache by the neuropathic

TABLE 32-1 Vesicular, Bullous, or Ulcerative Lesions of the Oral Mucosa

Condition	Usual Location	Clinical Features	Course
Viral Diseases			
Primary acute herpetic gingivostomatitis [herpes simplex virus (HSV) type 1, rarely type 2]	Lip and oral mucosa (buccal, gingival, lingual mucosa)	Labial vesicles that rupture and crust, and intraoral vesicles that quickly ulcerate; extremely painful; acute gingivitis, fever, malaise, foul odor, and cervical lymphadenopathy; occurs primarily in infants, children, and young adults	Heals spontaneously in 10–14 days. Unless secondarily infected, lesions lasting >3 weeks are not due to primary HSV infection
Recurrent herpes labialis	Mucocutaneous junction of lip, perioral skin	Eruption of groups of vesicles that may coalesce, then rupture and crust; painful to pressure or spicy foods	Lasts about 1 week, but condition may be prolonged if secondarily infected. If severe, topical or oral antiviral may reduce healing time
Recurrent intraoral herpes simplex	Palate and gingiva	Small vesicles on keratinized epithelium that rupture and coalesce; painful	Heals spontaneously in about 1 week. If severe, topical or oral antiviral may reduce healing time.
Chickenpox (varicella-zoster virus)	Gingiva and oral mucosa	Skin lesions may be accompanied by small vesicles on oral mucosa that rupture to form shallow ulcers; may coalesce to form large bullous lesions that ulcerate; mucosa may have generalized erythema	Lesions heal spontaneously within 2 weeks
Herpes zoster (reactivation of varicella-zoster virus)	Cheek, tongue, gingiva, or palate	Unilateral vesicular eruptions and ulceration in linear pattern following sensory distribution of trigeminal nerve or one of its branches	Gradual healing without scarring unless secondarily infected; postherpetic neuralgia is common. Oral acyclovir, famciclovir, or valacyclovir reduce healing time and postherpetic neuralgia
Infectious mononucleosis (Epstein-Barr virus)	Oral mucosa	Fatigue, sore throat, malaise, fever, and cervical lymphadenopathy; numerous small ulcers usually appear several days before lymphadenopathy; gingival bleeding and multiple petechiae at junction of hard and soft palates	Oral lesions disappear during convalescence; no treatment though glucocorticoids indicated if tonsillar swelling compromises airway
Herpangina (coxsackievirus A; also possibly coxsackie B and echovirus)	Oral mucosa, pharynx, tongue	Sudden onset of fever, sore throat, and oropharyngeal vesicles, usually in children under 4 years, during summer months; diffuse pharyngeal congestion and vesicles (1–2 mm), grayish-white surrounded by red areola; vesicles enlarge and ulcerate	Incubation period 2–9 days; fever for 1–4 days; recovery uneventful
Hand, foot, and mouth disease (coxsackievirus A16 most common)	Oral mucosa, pharynx, palms, and soles	Fever, malaise, headache with oropharyngeal vesicles that become painful, shallow ulcers; highly infectious; usually affects children under age 10	Incubation period 2–18 days; lesions heal spontaneously in 2–4 weeks
Primary HIV infection	Gingiva, palate, and pharynx	Acute gingivitis and oropharyngeal ulceration, associated with febrile illness resembling mononucleosis and including lymphadenopathy	Followed by HIV seroconversion, asymptomatic HIV infection, and usually ultimately by HIV disease
Bacterial or Fungal Diseases			
Acute necrotizing ulcerative gingivitis ("trench mouth," Vincent's infection)	Gingiva	Painful, bleeding gingiva characterized by necrosis and ulceration of gingival papillae and margins plus lymphadenopathy and foul odor	Debridement and diluted (1:3) peroxide lavage provide relief within 24 h; antibiotics in acutely ill patients; relapse may occur
Prenatal (congenital) syphilis	Palate, jaws, tongue, and teeth	Gummatous involvement of palate, jaws, and facial bones; Hutchinson's incisors, mulberry molars, glossitis, mucous patches, and fissures on corner of mouth	Tooth deformities in permanent dentition irreversible
Primary syphilis (chancre)	Lesion appears where organism enters body; may occur on lips, tongue, or tonsillar area	Small papule developing rapidly into a large, painless ulcer with indurated border; unilateral lymphadenopathy; chancre and lymph nodes containing spirochetes; serologic tests positive by third to fourth weeks	Healing of chancre in 1–2 months, followed by secondary syphilis in 6–8 weeks
Secondary syphilis	Oral mucosa frequently involved with mucous patches, primarily on palate, also at commissures of mouth	Maculopapular lesions of oral mucosa, 5–10 mm in diameter with central ulceration covered by grayish membrane; eruptions occurring on various mucosal surfaces and skin accompanied by fever, malaise, and sore throat	Lesions may persist from several weeks to a year

(continued)

Condition	Usual Location	Clinical Features	Course
Tertiary syphilis	Palate and tongue	Gummatous infiltration of palate or tongue followed by ulceration and fibrosis; atrophy of tongue papillae produces characteristic bald tongue and glossitis	Gumma may destroy palate, causing complete perforation
Gonorrhea	Lesions may occur in mouth at site of inoculation or secondarily by hematogenous spread from a primary focus elsewhere	Most pharyngeal infection is asymptomatic; may produce burning or itching sensation; oropharynx and tonsils may be ulcerated and erythematous; saliva viscous and fetid	More difficult to eradicate than urogenital infection, though pharyngitis usually resolves with appropriate antimicrobial treatment
Tuberculosis	Tongue, tonsillar area, soft palate	A painless, solitary, 1–5 cm, irregular ulcer covered with a persistent exudate; ulcer has a firm undermined border	Autoinoculation from pulmonary infection usual; lesions resolve with appropriate antimicrobial therapy
Cervicofacial actinomycosis	Swellings in region of face, neck, and floor of mouth	Infection may be associated with an extraction, jaw fracture, or eruption of molar tooth; in acute form resembles an acute pyogenic abscess, but contains yellow "sulfur granules" (gram-positive mycelia and their hyphae)	Typically, swelling is hard and grows painlessly; multiple abscesses with draining tracts develop; penicillin first choice; surgery usually necessary
Histoplasmosis	Any area of the mouth, particularly tongue, gingiva, or palate	Nodular, verrucous, or granulomatous lesions; ulcers are indurated and painful; usual source hematogenous or pulmonary, but may be primary	Systemic antifungal therapy necessary to treat
Candidiasis (Table 32-3)			

Dermatologic Diseases

Condition	Usual Location	Clinical Features	Course
Mucous membrane pemphigoid	Typically produces marked gingival erythema and ulceration; other areas of oral cavity, esophagus, and vagina may be affected	Painful, grayish-white collapsed vesicles or bullae of full-thickness epithelium with peripheral erythematous zone; gingival lesions desquamate, leaving ulcerated area	Protracted course with remissions and exacerbations; involvement of different sites occurs slowly; glucocorticoids may temporarily reduce symptoms but do not control the disease
Erythema multiforme minor and major (Stevens-Johnson syndrome)	Primarily the oral mucosa and the skin of hands and feet	Intraoral ruptured bullae surrounded by an inflammatory area; lips may show hemorrhagic crusts; the "iris," or "target," lesion on the skin is pathognomonic; patient may have severe signs of toxicity	Onset very rapid; usually idiopathic, but may be associated with trigger such as drug reaction; condition may last 3–6 weeks; mortality with EM major 5–15% if untreated
Pemphigus vulgaris	Oral mucosa and skin; sites of mechanical trauma (soft/hard palate, frenulum, lips, buccal mucosa)	Usually (>70%) presents with oral lesions; fragile, ruptured bullae and ulcerated oral areas; mostly in older adults	With repeated occurrence of bullae, toxicity may lead to cachexia, infection, and death within 2 years; often controllable with oral glucocorticoids
Lichen planus	Oral mucosa and skin	White striae in mouth; purplish nodules on skin at sites of friction; occasionally causes oral mucosal ulcers and erosive gingivitis	White striae alone usually asymptomatic; erosive lesions often difficult to treat, but may respond to glucocorticoids

Other Conditions

Condition	Usual Location	Clinical Features	Course
Recurrent aphthous ulcers	Usually on nonkeratinized oral mucosa (buccal and labial mucosa, floor of mouth, soft palate, lateral and ventral tongue)	Single or clusters of painful ulcers with surrounding erythematous border; lesions may be 1–2 mm in diameter in crops (herpetiform), 1–5 mm (minor), or 5–15 mm (major)	Lesions heal in 1–2 weeks but may recur monthly or several times a year; protective barrier with orabase and topical steroids give symptomatic relief; systemic glucocorticoids may be needed in severe cases
Behçet's syndrome	Oral mucosa, eyes, genitalia, gut, and CNS	Multiple aphthous ulcers in mouth; inflammatory ocular changes, ulcerative lesions on genitalia; inflammatory bowel disease and CNS disease	Oral lesions often first manifestation; persist several weeks and heal without scarring
Traumatic ulcers	Anywhere on oral mucosa; dentures frequently responsible for ulcers in vestibule	Localized, discrete ulcerated lesions with red border; produced by accidental biting of mucosa, penetration by a foreign object, or chronic irritation by a denture	Lesions usually heal in 7–10 days when irritant is removed, unless secondarily infected

(continued)

TABLE 32-1 Vesicular, Bullous, or Ulcerative Lesions of the Oral Mucosa (*Continued*)

Condition	Usual Location	Clinical Features	Course
Squamous cell carcinoma	Any area in the mouth, most commonly on lower lip, tongue, and floor of mouth	Ulcer with elevated, indurated border; failure to heal, pain not prominent; lesions tend to arise in areas of erythro/leukoplakia or in smooth atrophic tongue	Invades and destroys underlying tissues; frequently metastasizes to regional lymph nodes
Acute myeloid leukemia (usually monocytic)	Gingiva	Gingival swelling and superficial ulceration followed by hyperplasia of gingiva with extensive necrosis and hemorrhage; deep ulcers may occur elsewhere on the mucosa complicated by secondary infection	Usually responds to systemic treatment of leukemia; occasionally requires local radiation therapy
Lymphoma	Gingiva, tongue, palate and tonsillar area	Elevated, ulcerated area that may proliferate rapidly, giving the appearance of traumatic inflammation	Fatal if untreated; may indicate underlying HIV infection
Chemical or thermal burns	Any area in mouth	White slough due to contact with corrosive agents (e.g., aspirin, hot cheese) applied locally; removal of slough leaves raw, painful surface	Lesion heals in several weeks if not secondarily infected

Note: CNS, central nervous system.

TABLE 32-2 Pigmented Lesions of the Oral Mucosa

Condition	Usual Location	Clinical Features	Course
Oral melanotic macule	Any area of the mouth	Discrete or diffuse localized, brown to black macule	Remains indefinitely; no growth
Diffuse melanin pigmentation	Any area of the mouth	Diffuse pale to dark-brown pigmentation; may be physiologic ("racial") or due to smoking	Remains indefinitely
Nevi	Any area of the mouth	Discrete, localized, brown to black pigmentation	Remains indefinitely
Malignant melanoma	Any area of the mouth	Can be flat and diffuse, painless, brown to black, or can be raised and nodular	Expands and invades early; metastasis leads to death
Addison's disease	Any area of the mouth, but mostly buccal mucosa	Blotches or spots of bluish-black to dark-brown pigmentation occurring early in the disease, accompanied by diffuse pigmentation of skin; other symptoms of adrenal insufficiency	Condition controlled by adrenal steroid replacement
Peutz-Jeghers syndrome	Any area of the mouth	Dark-brown spots on lips, buccal mucosa, with characteristic distribution of pigment around lips, nose, eyes, and on hands; concomitant intestinal polyposis	Oral pigmented lesions remain indefinitely; gastrointestinal polyps may become malignant
Drug ingestion (neuroleptics, oral contraceptives, minocycline, zidovudine, quinine derivatives)	Any area of the mouth	Brown, black, or gray areas of pigmentation	Gradually disappears following cessation of drug
Amalgam tattoo	Gingiva and alveolar mucosa	Small blue-black pigmented areas associated with embedded amalgam particles in soft tissues; these may show up on radiographs as radiopaque particles in some cases	Remains indefinitely
Heavy metal pigmentation (bismuth, mercury, lead)	Gingival margin	Thin blue-black pigmented line along gingival margin; rarely seen except for children exposed to lead-based paint	Indicative of systemic absorption; no significance for oral health
Black hairy tongue	Dorsum of tongue	Elongation of filiform papillae of tongue, which become stained by coffee, tea, tobacco, or pigmented bacteria	Improves within 1–2 weeks with gentle brushing of tongue or discontinuation of antibiotic if due to bacterial overgrowth
Fordyce "spots"	Buccal and labial mucosa	Numerous small yellowish spots just beneath mucosal surface; no symptoms; due to hyperplasia of sebaceous glands	Benign; remains without apparent change
Kaposi's sarcoma	Palate most common, but may occur in any other site	Red or blue plaques of variable size and shape; often enlarge, become nodular and may ulcerate	Usually indicative of HIV infection or non-Hodgkin's lymphoma; rarely fatal, but may require treatment for comfort or cosmesis
Mucous retention cysts	Buccal and labial mucosa	Bluish-clear fluid-filled cyst due to extravasated mucous from injured minor salivary gland	Benign; painless unless traumatized; may be removed surgically

TABLE 32-3 White Lesions of Oral Mucosa

Condition	Usual Location	Clinical Features	Course
Lichen planus	Buccal mucosa, tongue, gingiva, and lips; skin	Striae, white plaques, red areas, ulcers in mouth; purplish papules on skin; may be asymptomatic, sore, or painful; lichenoid drug reactions may look similar	Protracted; responds to topical glucocorticoids
White sponge nevus	Oral mucosa, vagina, anal mucosa	Painless white thickening of epithelium; adolescent/early adult onset; familial	Benign and permanent
Smoker's leukoplakia and smokeless tobacco lesions	Any area of oral mucosa, sometimes related to location of habit	White patch that may become firm, rough, or red-fissured and ulcerated; may become sore and painful but usually painless	May or may not resolve with cessation of habit; 2% develop squamous cell carcinoma; early biopsy essential
Erythroplakia with or without white patches	Floor of mouth common in men; tongue and buccal mucosa in women	Velvety, reddish plaque; occasionally mixed with white patches or smooth red areas	High risk of squamous cell cancer; early biopsy essential
Candidiasis	Any area in mouth	*Pseudomembranous type* ("thrush"): creamy white curdlike patches that reveal a raw, bleeding surface when scraped; found in sick infants, debilitated elderly patients receiving high doses of glucocorticoids or broad-spectrum antibiotics, or in patients with AIDS	Responds favorably to antifungal therapy and correction of predisposing causes where possible
		Erythematous type: flat, red, sometimes sore areas in same groups of patients	Course same as for pseudomembranous type
		Candidal leukoplakia: nonremovable white thickening of epithelium due to *Candida*	Responds to prolonged antifungal therapy
		Angular cheilitis: sore fissures at corner of mouth	Responds to topical antifungal therapy
Hairy leukoplakia	Usually lateral tongue, rarely elsewhere on oral mucosa	White areas ranging from small and flat to extensive accentuation of vertical folds; found in HIV carriers in all risk groups for AIDS	Due to EBV; responds to high-dose acyclovir but recurs; rarely causes discomfort unless secondarily infected with *Candida*
Warts (papillomavirus)	Anywhere on skin and oral mucosa	Single or multiple papillary lesions, with thick, white keratinized surfaces containing many pointed projections; cauliflower lesions covered with normal-colored mucosa or multiple pink or pale bumps (focal epithelial hyperplasia)	Lesions grow rapidly and spread; consider squamous cell carcinoma and rule out with biopsy; excision or laser therapy; may regress in HIV infected patients on antiretroviral therapy

Note: EBV, Epstein-Barr virus.

TABLE 32-4 Alterations of the Tongue

Type of Change	Clinical Features
Size or Morphology Changes	
Macroglossia	Enlarged tongue that may be part of a syndrome found in developmental conditions such as Down syndrome, Simpson-Golabi-Behmel syndrome, or Beckwith-Wiedemann syndrome may be due to tumor (hemangioma or lymphangioma), metabolic disease (such as primary amyloidosis), or endocrine disturbance (such as acromegaly or cretinism)
Fissured ("scrotal") tongue	Dorsal surface and sides of tongue covered by painless shallow or deep fissures that may collect debris and become irritated
Median rhomboid glossitis	Congenital abnormality of tongue with ovoid, denuded area in median posterior portion of the tongue; may be associated with candidiasis and may respond to antifungals
Color Changes	
"Geographic" tongue (benign migratory glossitis)	Asymptomatic inflammatory condition of the tongue, with rapid loss and regrowth of filiform papillae, leading to appearance of denuded red patches "wandering" across the surface of the tongue
Hairy tongue	Elongation of filiform papillae of the medial dorsal surface area due to failure of keratin layer of the papillae to desquamate normally; brownish-black coloration may be due to staining by tobacco, food, or chromogenic organisms
"Strawberry" and "raspberry" tongue	Appearance of tongue during scarlet fever due to the hypertrophy of fungiform papillae plus changes in the filiform papillae
"Bald" tongue	Atrophy may be associated with xerostomia, pernicious anemia, iron-deficiency anemia, pellagra, or syphilis; may be accompanied by painful burning sensation; may be an expression of erythematous candidiasis and respond to antifungals

TABLE 32-5 Oral Lesions Associated With HIV Infection

Lesion Morphology	Etiologies
Papules, nodules, plaques	Candidiasis (hyperplastic and pseudomembranous)[a]
	Condyloma acuminatum (human papillomavirus infection)
	Squamous cell carcinoma (preinvasive and invasive)
	Non-Hodgkin's lymphoma[a]
	Hairy leukoplakia[a]
Ulcers	Recurrent aphthous ulcers[a]
	Angular cheilitis
	Squamous cell carcinoma
	Acute necrotizing ulcerative gingivitis[a]
	Necrotizing ulcerative periodontitis[a]
	Necrotizing ulcerative stomatitis
	Non-Hodgkin's lymphoma[a]
	Viral infection (herpes simplex, herpes zoster, cytomegalovirus)
	Mycobacterium tuberculosis, Mycobacterium avium-intracellulare
	Fungal infection (histoplasmosis, cryptococcosis, candidiasis, geotrichosis, aspergillosis)
	Bacterial infection (*Escherichia coli, Enterobacter cloacae, Klebsiella pneumoniae, Pseudomonas aeruginosa*)
	Drug reactions (single or multiple ulcers)
Pigmented lesions	Kaposi's sarcoma[a]
	Bacillary angiomatosis (skin and visceral lesions more common than oral)
	Zidovudine pigmentation (skin, nails, and occasionally oral mucosa)
	Addison's disease
Miscellaneous	Linear gingival erythema[a]

[a]Strongly associated with HIV infection.

quality of the pain. Occasionally, *phantom pain* follows tooth extraction. Often the earliest symptom of Bell's palsy in the day or so before facial weakness develops is pain and hyperalgesia behind the ear and side of the face. Likewise, similar symptoms may precede visible lesions of herpes zoster infecting the seventh nerve (Ramsey-Hunt syndrome) or trigeminal nerve. *Postherpetic neuralgia* may follow either condition. *Coronary ischemia* may produce pain exclusively in the face and jaw and, like typical angina pectoris, is usually reproducible with increased myocardial demand. Aching in several upper molar or premolar teeth that is unrelieved by anesthetizing the teeth may point to *maxillary sinusitis.*

Giant cell arteritis is notorious for producing headache, but it may also produce facial pain or sore throat without headache. Jaw and tongue claudication with chewing or talking is relatively common. Tongue infarction is rare. Patients with subacute thyroiditis often experience pain referred to the face or jaw before the tender thyroid gland and transient hyperthyroidism are appreciated.

Burning mouth syndrome (glossodynia) is present in the absence of an identifiable cause (e.g., vitamin B_{12} deficiency, iron deficiency, diabetes mellitus, low-grade *Candida* infection, food sensitivity, or subtle xerostomia) and predominantly affects postmenopausal women. The etiology may be neuropathic. Clonazepam, alpha-lipoic acid, and cognitive behavioral therapy have benefited some. Some cases associated with ACE inhibitors have remitted when the drug was discontinued.

DISEASES OF THE SALIVARY GLANDS

Saliva is essential to oral health. Its absence leads to tooth decay and loss. Its major components, water and mucin, serve as a cleansing solvent and lubricating fluid. In addition, it contains antimicrobial factors (e.g., lysozyme, lactoperoxidase, secretory IgA), epidermal growth factor, minerals, and buffering systems. The major salivary glands secrete intermittently in response to autonomic stimulation, which is high during a meal but low otherwise. Hundreds of minor glands in the lips and cheeks secrete mucus continuously. Consequently, oral function becomes impaired when salivary function is reduced. Dry mouth (*xerostomia*) is perceived when salivary flow is reduced by 50%. The most common etiology is medication, especially drugs with anticholinergic properties, but also alpha and beta blockers, calcium channel blockers, and diuretics. Other causes include Sjögren's syndrome, chronic parotitis, salivary duct obstruction, diabetes mellitus, HIV/AIDS, and radiation therapy that includes the salivary glands in the field (Hodgkin's disease and head and neck cancer). Management involves eliminating or limiting drying medications, preventive dental care, and supplementing oral liquid. Sugarless mints or chewing gum may stimulate salivary secretion if dysfunction is mild. When sufficient exocrine tissue remains, pilocarpine or cevimeline has been shown to increase secretions. Commercial saliva substitutes or gels relieve dryness but must be supplemented with fluoride applications to prevent caries.

Sialolithiasis presents most often as painful swelling but in some instances as just swelling or pain. Conservative therapy consists of local heat, massage, and hydration. Promotion of salivary secretion with mints or lemon drops may flush out small stones. Antibiotic treatment is necessary when bacterial infection in suspected. In adults, *acute bacterial parotitis* is typically unilateral and most commonly affects postoperative, dehydrated, and debilitated patients. *Staphylococcus aureus* including methicillin-resistant forms and anaerobic bacteria are the most common pathogens. Chronic bacterial sialadenitis results from lowered salivary secretion and recurrent bacterial infection. When suspected bacterial infection is not responsive to therapy, the differential diagnosis should be expanded to include benign and malignant neoplasms, lymphoproliferative disorders, Sjögren's syndrome, sarcoidosis, tuberculosis, lymphadenitis, actinomycosis, and granulomatosis with polyangiitis (Wegener's). Bilateral nontender parotid enlargement occurs with diabetes mellitus, cirrhosis, bulimia, HIV/AIDS, and drugs (e.g., iodide, propylthiouracil).

Pleomorphic adenoma comprises two-thirds of all salivary neoplasms. The parotid is the principal salivary gland affected, and the tumor presents as a firm, slow-growing mass. Though benign, recurrence is common if resection is incomplete. Malignant tumors such as mucoepidermoid carcinoma, adenoid cystic carcinoma, and adenocarcinoma tend to grow relatively fast, depending upon grade. They may ulcerate and invade nerves, producing numbness and facial paralysis. Surgical resection is the primary treatment. Radiation therapy (particularly neutron-beam therapy) is used when surgery is not feasible and it is used post-resection for certain histological types with a high risk of recurrence. Malignant salivary gland tumors have a 5-year survival rate of about 68%.

DENTAL CARE OF MEDICALLY COMPLEX PATIENTS

Routine dental care (e.g., extraction, scaling and cleaning, tooth restoration, and root canal) is remarkably safe. The most common concerns regarding care of dental patients with medical disease are fear of excessive bleeding for patients on anticoagulants, infection of the heart valves and prosthetic devices from hematogenous seeding of oral flora, and cardiovascular complications resulting from vasopressors used with local anesthetics during dental treatment. Experience confirms that the risks of any of these complications are very low.

Patients undergoing tooth extraction or alveolar and gingival surgery rarely experience uncontrolled bleeding when warfarin anticoagulation is maintained within the therapeutic range currently recommended for prevention of venous thrombosis, atrial fibrillation, or mechanical heart valve. Embolic complications and death, however, have been reported during subtherapeutic anticoagulation. Therapeutic anticoagulation should be confirmed before and continued through the procedure. Likewise, low-dose aspirin (e.g., 81–325 mg) can be safely continued. For patients on aspirin and another antiplatelet medication (e.g., clopidogrel), the decision to continue the second antiplatelet medication should be based on individual consideration of the risks of thrombosis and bleeding.

Patients at risk for bacterial endocarditis (Chap. 124) should maintain optimal oral hygiene, including flossing, and have regular professional cleaning. Currently, guidelines recommend that prophylactic antibiotics be restricted to those patients at high risk of bacterial endocarditis who undergo dental and oral procedures that involve significant manipulation of gingival or periapical tissue or penetration of the oral mucosa. If unexpected bleeding occurs, antibiotics given within 2 h following the procedure provide effective prophylaxis.

Hematogenous bacterial seeding from oral infection can undoubtedly produce late prosthetic joint infection and therefore requires removal of the infected tissue (e.g., drainage, extraction, root canal) and appropriate antibiotic therapy. However, evidence that late prosthetic joint infection occurs following routine dental procedures is lacking. For this reason, antibiotic prophylaxis is not recommended before dental surgery in patients with orthopedic pins, screws, and plates. It is, however, advised within the first 2 years after joint replacement for patients who have inflammatory arthropathies, immunosuppression, type 1 diabetes mellitus, previous prosthetic joint infection, hemophilia, or malnourishment.

Concern often arises regarding the use of vasoconstrictors in patients with hypertension and heart disease. Vasoconstrictors enhance the depth and duration of local anesthesia, thus reducing the anesthetic dose and potential toxicity. If intravascular injection is avoided, 2% lidocaine with 1:100,000 epinephrine (limited to a total of 0.036 mg epinephrine) can be used safely in those with controlled hypertension and stable coronary heart disease, arrhythmia, or congestive heart failure. Precaution should be taken with patients taking tricyclic antidepressants and nonselective beta blockers because these drugs may potentiate the effect of epinephrine.

Elective dental treatments should be postponed for at least one month after myocardial infarction, after which the risk of reinfarction is low provided the patient is medically stable (e.g., stable rhythm, stable angina, and free of heart failure). Patients who have suffered a stroke should have elective dental care deferred for six months. In both situations, effective stress reduction requires good pain control, including the use of the minimal amount of vasoconstrictor necessary to provide good hemostasis and local anesthesia.

Bisphosphonate therapy is associated with *osteonecrosis* of the jaw. However, the risk with oral bisphosphonate therapy is very low. Most patients affected have received high-dose aminobisphosphonate therapy for multiple myeloma or metastatic breast cancer and have undergone tooth extraction or dental surgery. Intra-oral lesions appear as exposed yellow-white hard bone involving the mandible or maxilla. Two-thirds are painful. Screening tests for determining risk of osteonecrosis are unreliable. Patients slated for aminobisphosphonate therapy should receive preventive dental care that reduces the risk of infection and need for future dentoalveolar surgery.

HALITOSIS

Halitosis typically emanates from the oral cavity or nasal passages. Volatile sulfur compounds resulting from bacterial decay of food and cellular debris account for the malodor. Periodontal disease, caries, acute forms of gingivitis, poorly fitting dentures, oral abscess, and tongue coating are usual causes. Treatment includes correcting poor hygiene, treating infection, and tongue brushing. Xerostomia can produce and exacerbate halitosis. Pockets of decay in the tonsillar crypts, esophageal diverticulum, esophageal stasis (e.g., achalasia, stricture), sinusitis, and lung abscess account for some instances. A few systemic diseases produce distinctive odors: renal failure (ammoniacal), hepatic (fishy), and ketoacidosis (fruity). *Helicobacter pylori* gastritis can also produce ammoniac breath. If no odor is detectable, then pseudohalitosis or even halitophobia must be considered. These conditions represent varying degrees of psychiatric illness.

AGING AND ORAL HEALTH

While tooth loss and dental disease are not normal consequences of aging, a complex array of structural and functional changes occurs with age that can affect oral health. Subtle changes in tooth structure (e.g., diminished pulp space and volume, sclerosis of dentinal tubules, and altered proportions of nerve and vascular pulp content) result in diminished or altered pain sensitivity, reduced reparative capacity, and increased tooth brittleness. In addition, age-associated fatty replacement of salivary acini may reduce physiologic reserve, thus increasing the risk of xerostomia.

Poor oral hygiene often results when vision fails or when patients lose manual dexterity and upper-extremity flexibility. This is particularly common for nursing home residents and must be emphasized because regular oral cleaning and dental care have been shown to reduce the incidence of pneumonia and mortality in this population. Other risks for dental decay include limited lifetime fluoride exposure and preference by some older adults for intensely sweet foods when taste and olfaction wane. These factors occur in an increasing proportion of persons over age 75 who retain teeth that have extensive restorations and exposed roots. Without assiduous care, decay can become quite advanced yet remain asymptomatic. Consequently, much or the entire tooth can be destroyed before the process is detected.

Periodontal disease, a leading cause of tooth loss, is indicated by loss of alveolar bone height. Over 90% of Americans have some degree of periodontal disease by age 50. Healthy adults who have not experienced significant alveolar bone loss by the sixth decade do not typically develop significant worsening with advancing age.

Complete edentulousness with advanced age, though less common than in previous decades, is still present in approximately 50% of Americans age ≥85. Speech, mastication, and facial contours are dramatically affected. Edentulousness may also worsen obstructive sleep apnea, particularly in those without symptoms while wearing dentures. Dentures can improve speech articulation and restore diminished facial contours. Mastication is restored less predictably, and those expecting dentures to improve oral intake are often disappointed. Dentures require periodic adjustment to accommodate inevitable remodeling that leads to a diminished volume of the alveolar ridge. Pain can result from friction or traumatic lesions produced by loose dentures. Poor fit and poor oral hygiene may permit candidiasis to develop. This may be asymptomatic or painful and is indicated by erythematous smooth or granular tissue conforming to an area covered by the appliance.

FURTHER READINGS

Durso SC: Interaction with other health team members in caring for elderly patients. Dent Clin N Am 49:377, 2005

Edwards EJ et al: Updated recommendations for managing the care of patients receiving oral bisphosphonate therapy: an advisory statement from the American Dental Association Council on Scientific Affairs. J Am Dent Assoc 139 :1674, 2008

Little JW. Periodontal disease and heart disease: Are they related? Gen Dent. 56:733, 2008

—— et al (eds): *Dental Management of the Medically Compromised Patient*, 7th ed. St. Louis, Mosby, 2008

Logan RM: Links between oral and gastrointestinal health. Curr Opin Support Palliat Care 4:31, 2010

CHAPTER **33**

Dyspnea

Richard M. Schwartzstein

DYSPNEA

The American Thoracic Society defines *dyspnea* as a "subjective experience of breathing discomfort that consists of qualitatively distinct sensations that vary in intensity. The experience derives from interactions among multiple physiological, psychological, social, and environmental factors and may induce secondary physiological and behavioral responses." Dyspnea, a symptom, must be distinguished from the signs of increased work of breathing.

■ MECHANISMS OF DYSPNEA

Respiratory sensations are the consequence of interactions between the *efferent*, or outgoing, motor output from the brain to the ventilatory muscles (feed-forward) and the *afferent*, or incoming, sensory input from receptors throughout the body (feedback), as well as the integrative processing of this information that we infer must be occurring in the brain (Fig. 33-1). In contrast to painful sensations, which can often be attributed to the stimulation of a single nerve ending, dyspnea sensations are more commonly viewed as holistic, more akin to hunger or thirst. A given disease state may lead to dyspnea by one or more mechanisms, some of which may be operative under some circumstances, e.g., exercise, but not others, e.g., a change in position.

Motor efferents

Disorders of the ventilatory pump, most commonly increase airway resistance or stiffness (decreased compliance) of the respiratory system, are associated with increased work of breathing or a sense of an increased effort to breathe. When the muscles are weak or fatigued, greater effort is required, even though the mechanics of the system are normal. The increased neural output from the motor cortex is sensed via a corollary discharge, a neural signal that is sent to the sensory cortex at the same time that motor output is directed to the ventilatory muscles.

Sensory afferents

Chemoreceptors in the carotid bodies and medulla are activated by hypoxemia, acute hypercapnia, and acidemia. Stimulation of these receptors, as well as others that lead to an increase in ventilation, produce a sensation of air hunger. Mechanoreceptors in the lungs, when stimulated by bronchospasm, lead to a sensation of chest tightness. J-receptors, sensitive to interstitial edema, and pulmonary vascular receptors, activated by acute changes in pulmonary artery pressure, appear to contribute to air hunger. Hyperinflation is associated with the sensation of increased work of breathing and an inability to get a deep breath or of an unsatisfying breath. Metaboreceptors, located in skeletal muscle, are believed to be activated by changes in the local biochemical milieu of the tissue active during exercise and, when stimulated, contribute to the breathing discomfort.

Integration: Efferent-reafferent mismatch

A discrepancy or mismatch between the feed-forward message to the ventilatory muscles and the feedback from receptors that monitor the response of the ventilatory pump increases the intensity of dyspnea. This is particularly important when there is a mechanical derangement of the ventilatory pump, such as in asthma or chronic obstructive pulmonary disease (COPD).

Anxiety

Acute anxiety may increase the severity of dyspnea either by altering the interpretation of sensory data or by leading to patterns of breathing that heighten physiologic abnormalities in the respiratory system. In patients with expiratory flow limitation, for example, the increased respiratory rate that accompanies acute anxiety leads to hyperinflation, increased work and effort of breathing, and a sense of an unsatisfying breath.

■ ASSESSING DYSPNEA

Quality of sensation

As with pain, dyspnea assessment begins with a determination of the quality of the discomfort (Table 33-1). Dyspnea questionnaires, or lists of phrases commonly used by patients, assist those who have difficulty describing their breathing sensations.

Sensory intensity

A modified Borg scale or visual analogue scale can be utilized to measure dyspnea at rest, immediately following exercise, or on recall

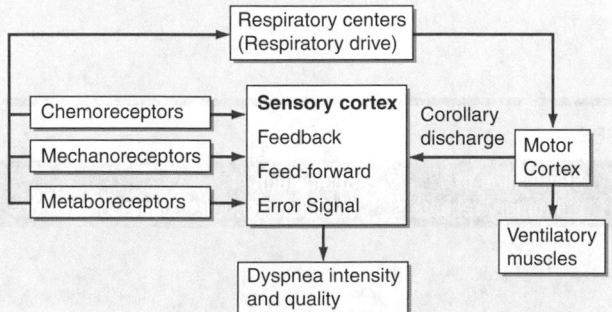

ALGORITHM FOR THE INPUTS IN DYSPNEA PRODUCTION

Figure 33-1 Hypothetical model for integration of sensory inputs in the production of dyspnea. Afferent information from the receptors throughout the respiratory system projects directly to the sensory cortex to contribute to primary qualitative sensory experiences and provide feedback on the action of the ventilatory pump. Afferents also project to the areas of the brain responsible for control of ventilation. The motor cortex, responding to input from the control centers, sends neural messages to the ventilatory muscles and a corollary discharge to the sensory cortex (feed-forward with respect to the instructions sent to the muscles). If the feed-forward and feedback messages do not match, an error signal is generated and the intensity of dyspnea increases. *(Adapted from Gillette and Schwartzstein, 2005.)*

TABLE 33-1 Association of Qualitative Descriptors and Pathophysiologic Mechanisms of Shortness of Breath

Descriptor	Pathophysiology
Chest tightness or constriction	Bronchoconstriction, interstitial edema (asthma, myocardial ischemia)
Increased work or effort of breathing	Airway obstruction, neuromuscular disease (COPD, moderate to severe asthma, myopathy, kyphoscoliosis)
Air hunger, need to breathe, urge to breathe	Increased drive to breathe (CHF, pulmonary embolism, moderate to severe airflow obstruction)
Cannot get a deep breath, unsatisfying breath	Hyperinflation (asthma, COPD) and restricted tidal volume (pulmonary fibrosis, chest wall restriction)
Heavy breathing, rapid breathing, breathing more	Deconditioning

Abbreviations: CHF, congestive heart failure; COPD, chronic obstructive pulmonary disease.

Source: From Schwartzstein and Feller-Kopman.

of a reproducible physical task, e.g., climbing the stairs at home. An alternative approach is to inquire about the activities a patient can do, i.e., to gain a sense of the patient's disability. The Baseline Dyspnea Index and the Chronic Respiratory Disease Questionnaire are commonly used tools for this purpose.

Affective dimension

For a sensation to be reported as a symptom, it must be perceived as unpleasant and interpreted as abnormal. Laboratory studies have demonstrated that air hunger evokes a stronger affective response than does increased effort or work of breathing. Some therapies for dyspnea, such as pulmonary rehabilitation, may reduce breathing discomfort, in part, by altering this dimension.

■ DIFFERENTIAL DIAGNOSIS

Dyspnea is the consequence of deviations from normal function in the cardiopulmonary systems. These deviations produce breathlessness as a consequence of increased drive to breathe; increased effort or work of breathing; and/or stimulation of receptors in the heart, lungs, or vascular system. Most diseases of the respiratory system are associated with alterations in the mechanical properties of the lungs and/or chest wall, frequently as a consequence of disease of the airways or lung parenchyma. In contrast, disorders of the cardiovascular system more commonly lead to dyspnea by causing gas exchange abnormalities or stimulating pulmonary and/or vascular receptors (Table 33-2).

Respiratory system dyspnea

Diseases of the airways Asthma and COPD, the most common obstructive lung diseases, are characterized by expiratory airflow obstruction, which typically leads to dynamic hyperinflation of the lungs and chest wall. Patients with moderate to severe disease have increased resistive and elastic loads (a term that relates to the stiffness of the system) on the ventilatory muscles and increased work of breathing. Patients with acute bronchoconstriction also complain of a sense of tightness, which can exist even when lung function is still within the normal range. These patients commonly hyperventilate. Both the chest tightness and hyperventilation are probably due to stimulation of pulmonary receptors. Both asthma and COPD may lead to hypoxemia and hypercapnia from ventilation-perfusion (V̇/Q̇) mismatch (and diffusion limitation during exercise with emphysema); hypoxemia is much more common than hypercapnia as a consequence of the different ways in which oxygen and carbon dioxide bind to hemoglobin.

Diseases of the chest wall Conditions that stiffen the chest wall, such as kyphoscoliosis, or that weaken ventilatory muscles, such as myasthenia gravis or the Guillain-Barré syndrome, are also associated with an increased effort to breathe. Large pleural effusions may contribute to dyspnea, both by increasing the work of breathing and by stimulating pulmonary receptors if there is associated atelectasis.

Diseases of the lung parenchyma Interstitial lung diseases, which may arise from infections, occupational exposures, or autoimmune

TABLE 33-2 Mechanisms of Dyspnea in Common Diseases

Disease	↑ Work of breathing	↑ Drive to breathe	Hypoxemia[a]	Acute Hypercapnia[a]	Stimulation of pulmonary receptors	Stimulation of vascular receptors	Metaboreceptors
COPD	•		•	•			
Asthma	•	•	•	•	•		
ILD	•	•	•		•		
PVD		•	•			•	
CPE	•	•	•		•	•	•
NCPE	•	•	•		•		
Anemia							•
Decond							•

[a]Hypoxemia and hypercapnia are not always present in these conditions. When hypoxemia is present, dyspnea usually persists, albeit at a reduced intensity, with correction of hypoxemia by the administration of supplemental oxygen.

Abbreviations: COPD, chronic obstructive pulmonary disease; CPE, cardiogenic pulmonary edema; Decond, deconditioning; ILD, interstitial lung disease; NCPE, noncardiogenic pulmonary edema; PVD, pulmonary vascular disease.

disorders, are associated with increased stiffness (decreased compliance) of the lungs and increased work of breathing. In addition, $\dot{V}/\dot{Q}$ mismatch, and destruction and/or thickening of the alveolar-capillary interface may lead to hypoxemia and an increased drive to breathe. Stimulation of pulmonary receptors may further enhance the hyperventilation characteristic of mild to moderate interstitial disease.

Cardiovascular system dyspnea

Diseases of the left heart Diseases of the myocardium resulting from coronary artery disease and nonischemic cardiomyopathies result in a greater left-ventricular end-diastolic volume and an elevation of the left-ventricular end-diastolic, as well as pulmonary capillary pressures. These elevated pressures lead to interstitial edema and stimulation of pulmonary receptors, thereby causing dyspnea; hypoxemia due to $\dot{V}/\dot{Q}$ mismatch may also contribute to breathlessness. Diastolic dysfunction, characterized by a very stiff left ventricle, may lead to severe dyspnea with relatively mild degrees of physical activity, particularly if it is associated with mitral regurgitation.

Diseases of the pulmonary vasculature Pulmonary thromboembolic disease and primary diseases of the pulmonary circulation (primary pulmonary hypertension, pulmonary vasculitis) cause dyspnea via increased pulmonary-artery pressure and stimulation of pulmonary receptors. Hyperventilation is common, and hypoxemia may be present. However, in most cases, use of supplemental oxygen has minimal effect on the severity of dyspnea and hyperventilation.

Diseases of the pericardium Constrictive pericarditis and cardiac tamponade are both associated with increased intracardiac and pulmonary vascular pressures, which are the likely cause of dyspnea in these conditions. To the extent that cardiac output is limited, at rest or with exercise, stimulation of metaboreceptors and chemoreceptors (if lactic acidosis develops) contribute as well.

Dyspnea with normal respiratory and cardiovascular systems

Mild to moderate anemia is associated with breathing discomfort during exercise. This is thought to be related to stimulation of metaboreceptors; oxygen saturation is normal in patients with anemia. The breathlessness associated with obesity is probably due to multiple mechanisms, including high cardiac output and impaired ventilatory pump function (decreased compliance of the chest wall). Cardiovascular deconditioning (poor fitness) is characterized by the early development of anaerobic metabolism and the stimulation of chemoreceptors and metaboreceptors.

APPROACH TO THE PATIENT ▶ **Dyspnea**

(Fig. 33-2) In obtaining a *history*, the patient should be asked to describe in his/her own words what the discomfort feels like, as well as the effect of position, infections, and environmental stimuli on the dyspnea. Orthopnea is a common indicator of congestive heart failure (CHF), mechanical impairment of the diaphragm associated with obesity, or asthma triggered by esophageal reflux. Nocturnal dyspnea suggests CHF or asthma. Acute, intermittent episodes of dyspnea are more likely to reflect episodes of myocardial ischemia, bronchospasm, or pulmonary embolism, while chronic persistent dyspnea is typical of COPD, interstitial lung disease, and chronic thromboembolic

disease. Risk factors for occupational lung disease and for coronary artery disease should be elicited. Left atrial myxoma or hepatopulmonary syndrome should be considered when the patient complains of *platypnea*, defined as dyspnea in the upright position with relief in the supine position.

The *physical examination* should begin during the interview of the patient. Inability of the patient to speak in full sentences before stopping to get a deep breath suggests a condition that leads to stimulation of the controller or an impairment of the ventilatory pump with reduced vital capacity. Evidence for increased work of breathing (supraclavicular retractions, use of accessory muscles of ventilation, and the tripod position, characterized by sitting with one's hands braced on the knees) is indicative of increased airway resistance or stiff lungs and chest wall. When measuring the vital signs, one should accurately assess the respiratory rate and measure the pulsus paradoxus (Chap. 239); if it is >10 mmHg, consider the presence of COPD or acute asthma. During the general examination, signs of anemia (pale conjunctivae), cyanosis, and cirrhosis (spider angiomata, gynecomastia) should be sought. Examination of the chest should focus on symmetry of movement; percussion (dullness indicative of pleural effusion, hyperresonance a sign of emphysema); and auscultation (wheezes, rales, rhonchi, prolonged expiratory phase, diminished breath sounds, which are clues to disorders of the airways, and interstitial edema or fibrosis). The cardiac examination should focus on signs of elevated right heart pressures (jugular venous distention, edema, accentuated pulmonic component to the second heart sound); left ventricular dysfunction (S3 and S4 gallops); and valvular disease (murmurs). When examining the abdomen with the patient in the supine position, it should be noted whether there is paradoxical movement of the abdomen (inward motion during inspiration), a sign of diaphragmatic weakness; rounding of the abdomen during exhalation is suggestive of pulmonary edema. Clubbing of the digits may be an indication of interstitial pulmonary fibrosis, and the presence of joint swelling or deformation as well as changes consistent with Raynaud's disease may be indicative of a collagen-vascular process that can be associated with pulmonary disease.

Patients with exertional dyspnea should be asked to walk under observation in order to reproduce the symptoms. The patient should be examined for new findings that were not present at rest and for oxygen saturation.

Following the history and physical examination, a *chest radiograph* should be obtained. The lung volumes should be assessed (hyperinflation indicates obstructive lung disease; low lung volumes suggest interstitial edema or fibrosis, diaphragmatic dysfunction, or impaired chest wall motion). The pulmonary parenchyma should be examined for evidence of interstitial disease and emphysema. Prominent pulmonary vasculature in the upper zones indicates pulmonary venous hypertension, while enlarged central pulmonary arteries suggest pulmonary artery hypertension. An enlarged cardiac silhouette suggests a dilated cardiomyopathy or valvular disease. Bilateral pleural effusions are typical of CHF and some forms of collagen vascular disease. Unilateral effusions raise the specter of carcinoma and pulmonary embolism but may also occur in heart failure. *Computed tomography* (CT) *of the chest* is generally reserved for further evaluation of the lung parenchyma (interstitial lung disease) and possible pulmonary embolism.

Laboratory studies should include an electrocardiogram to look for evidence of ventricular hypertrophy and prior myocardial infarction. Echocardiography is indicated in patients in whom systolic dysfunction, pulmonary hypertension, or valvular heart disease is suspected. Bronchoprovocation testing is useful in patients with intermittent symptoms suggestive of asthma but normal physical examination and lung function; up to one-third of patients with the clinical diagnosis of asthma do not have reactive airways disease when formally tested.

DISTINGUISHING CARDIOVASCULAR FROM RESPIRATORY SYSTEM DYSPNEA

If a patient has evidence of both pulmonary and cardiac disease, a cardiopulmonary exercise test should be carried out to determine which system is responsible for the exercise limitation. If, at peak exercise, the patient achieves predicted maximal ventilation, demonstrates an increase in dead space or hypoxemia, or develops bronchospasm, the respiratory system is probably the cause of the problem. Alternatively, if the heart rate is >85% of the predicted maximum, if anaerobic threshold occurs early, if the blood pressure becomes excessively high or decreases during exercise, if the O_2 pulse (O_2 consumption/heart rate, an indicator of stroke volume) falls, or if there are ischemic changes on the electrocardiogram, an abnormality of the cardiovascular system is likely the explanation for the breathing discomfort.

TREATMENT Dyspnea

The first goal is to correct the underlying problem responsible for the symptom. If this is not possible, one attempts to lessen the intensity of the symptom and its effect on the patient's quality of life. Supplemental O_2 should be administered if the resting O_2 saturation is ≤89% or if the patient's saturation drops to these levels with activity. For patients with COPD, pulmonary rehabilitation programs have demonstrated positive effects on dyspnea, exercise capacity, and rates of hospitalization. Studies of anxiolytics and antidepressants have not demonstrated consistent benefit. Experimental interventions—e.g., cold air on the face, chest-wall vibration, and inhaled furosemide—to modulate the afferent information from receptors throughout the respiratory system are being studied.

PULMONARY EDEMA

■ MECHANISMS OF FLUID ACCUMULATION

The extent to which fluid accumulates in the interstitium of the lung depends on the balance of hydrostatic and oncotic forces within the pulmonary capillaries and in the surrounding tissue. Hydrostatic pressure favors movement of fluid from the capillary into the interstitium. The oncotic pressure, which is determined by the protein concentration in the blood, favors movement of fluid into the vessel. Albumin, the primary protein in the plasma, may be low in conditions such as cirrhosis and nephrotic syndrome. While hypoalbuminemia favors movement of fluid into the tissue for any given hydrostatic pressure in the capillary, it is usually not sufficient by itself to cause interstitial edema. In a healthy individual, the tight junctions of the capillary endothelium are impermeable to proteins, and the lymphatics in the tissue carry away the small amounts of protein that may leak out; together, these factors result in an oncotic force that maintains fluid in the capillary. Disruption of the endothelial barrier, however, allows protein to escape the capillary bed and enhances the movement of fluid into the tissue of the lung.

Cardiogenic pulmonary edema

(See also Chap. 272) Cardiac abnormalities that lead to an increase in pulmonary venous pressure shift the balance of forces between the capillary and the interstitium. Hydrostatic pressure is increased and fluid exits the capillary at an increased rate, resulting in interstitial and, in more severe cases, alveolar edema. The development of pleural effusions may further compromise respiratory system function and contribute to breathing discomfort.

Early signs of pulmonary edema include exertional dyspnea and orthopnea. Chest radiographs show peribronchial thickening, prominent vascular markings in the upper lung zones, and Kerley B lines. As the pulmonary edema worsens, alveoli fill with fluid; the

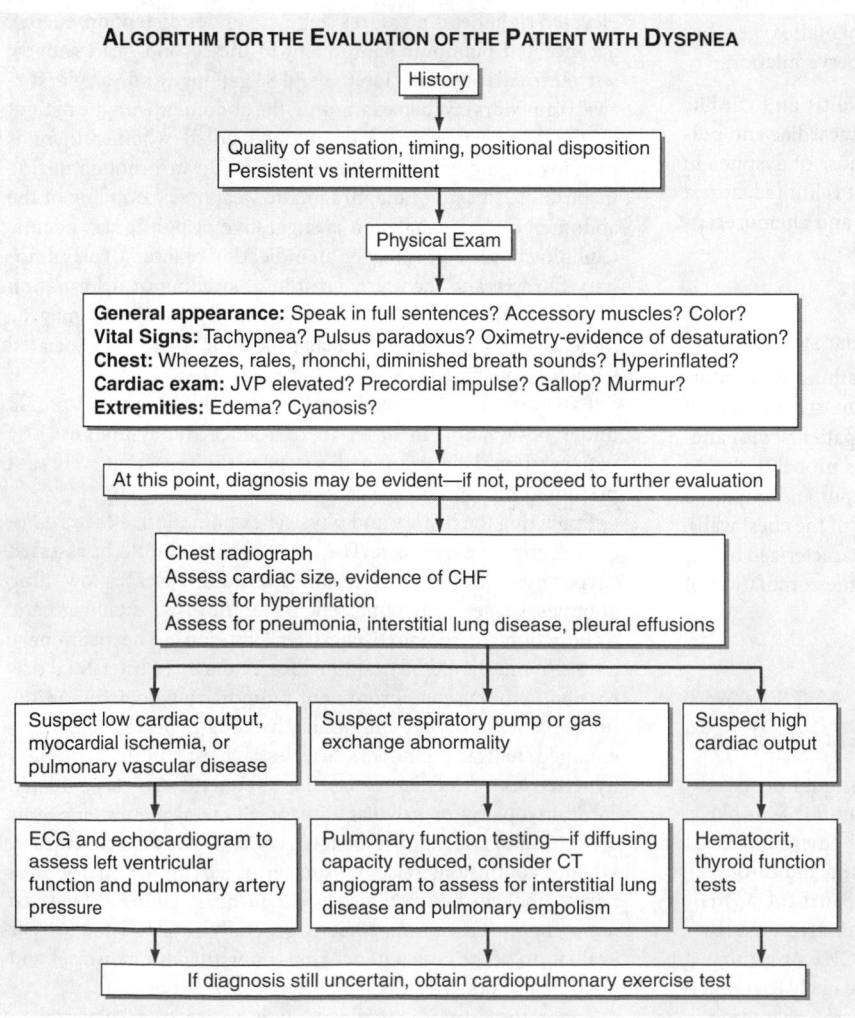

ALGORITHM FOR THE EVALUATION OF THE PATIENT WITH DYSPNEA

History
↓
Quality of sensation, timing, positional disposition
Persistent vs intermittent
↓
Physical Exam
↓
General appearance: Speak in full sentences? Accessory muscles? Color?
Vital Signs: Tachypnea? Pulsus paradoxus? Oximetry-evidence of desaturation?
Chest: Wheezes, rales, rhonchi, diminished breath sounds? Hyperinflated?
Cardiac exam: JVP elevated? Precordial impulse? Gallop? Murmur?
Extremities: Edema? Cyanosis?
↓
At this point, diagnosis may be evident—if not, proceed to further evaluation
↓
Chest radiograph
Assess cardiac size, evidence of CHF
Assess for hyperinflation
Assess for pneumonia, interstitial lung disease, pleural effusions

Suspect low cardiac output, myocardial ischemia, or pulmonary vascular disease	Suspect respiratory pump or gas exchange abnormality	Suspect high cardiac output
ECG and echocardiogram to assess left ventricular function and pulmonary artery pressure	Pulmonary function testing—if diffusing capacity reduced, consider CT angiogram to assess for interstitial lung disease and pulmonary embolism	Hematocrit, thyroid function tests

↓
If diagnosis still uncertain, obtain cardiopulmonary exercise test

Figure 33-2 An algorithm for the evaluation of the patient with dyspnea. JVP, jugular venous pulse; CHF, congestive heart failure; ECG, electrocardiogram; CT, computed tomography. *(Adapted from Schwartzstein and Feller-Kopman, 2003.)*

chest radiograph shows patchy alveolar filling, typically in a perihilar distribution, which then progresses to diffuse alveolar infiltrates. Increasing airway edema is associated with rhonchi and wheezes.

Noncardiogenic pulmonary edema

In noncardiogenic pulmonary edema, lung water increases due to damage of the pulmonary capillary lining with leakage of proteins and other macromolecules into the tissue; fluid follows the protein as oncotic forces are shifted from the vessel to the surrounding lung tissue. This process is associated with dysfunction of the surfactant lining the alveoli, increased surface forces, and a propensity for the alveoli to collapse at low lung volumes. Physiologically, noncardiogenic pulmonary edema is characterized by intrapulmonary shunt with hypoxemia and decreased pulmonary compliance. Pathologically, hyaline membranes are evident in the alveoli, and inflammation leading to pulmonary fibrosis may be seen. Clinically, the picture ranges from mild dyspnea to respiratory failure. Auscultation of the lungs may be relatively normal despite chest radiographs that show diffuse alveolar infiltrates. CT scans demonstrate that the distribution of alveolar edema is more heterogeneous than was once thought. Although normal intracardiac pressures are considered by many to be part of the definition of noncardiogenic pulmonary edema, the pathology of the process, as described above, is distinctly different, and one can observe a combination of cardiogenic and noncardiogenic pulmonary edema in some patients.

It is useful to categorize the causes of noncardiogenic pulmonary edema in terms of whether the injury to the lung is likely to result from direct, indirect, or pulmonary vascular causes (Table 33-3). Direct injuries are mediated via the airways (e.g., aspiration) or as the consequence of blunt chest trauma. Indirect injury is the consequence of mediators that reach the lung via the blood stream. The third category includes conditions that may be the consequence of acute changes in pulmonary vascular pressures, possibly the result of sudden autonomic discharge in the case of neurogenic and high-altitude pulmonary edema, or sudden swings of pleural pressure, as well as transient damage to the pulmonary capillaries in the case of reexpansion pulmonary edema.

Distinguishing cardiogenic from noncardiogenic pulmonary edema

The *history* is essential for assessing the likelihood of underlying cardiac disease as well as for identification of one of the conditions associated with noncardiogenic pulmonary edema. The *physical examination* in cardiogenic pulmonary edema is notable for evidence of increased intracardiac pressures (S3 gallop, elevated jugular venous pulse, peripheral edema), and rales and/or wheezes on auscultation of the chest. In contrast, the physical examination in noncardiogenic pulmonary edema is dominated by the findings of the precipitating condition; pulmonary findings may be relatively normal in the early stages. The *chest radiograph* in cardiogenic pulmonary edema typically shows an enlarged cardiac silhouette, vascular redistribution, interstitial thickening, and perihilar alveolar infiltrates; pleural effusions are common. In noncardiogenic pulmonary edema, heart size is normal, alveolar infiltrates are distributed more uniformly throughout the lungs, and pleural effusions are uncommon. Finally, the *hypoxemia* of cardiogenic pulmonary edema is due largely to $\dot{V}/Q$ mismatch and responds to the administration of supplemental oxygen. In contrast, hypoxemia in noncardiogenic pulmonary edema is due primarily to intrapulmonary shunting and typically persists despite high concentrations of inhaled O_2.

FURTHER READINGS

AARON SD et al: Overdiagnosis of asthma in obese and nonobese adults. CMAJ 179:1121, 2008

ABIDOV A et al: Prognostic significance of dyspnea in patients referred for cardiac stress testing. N Engl J Med 353:1889, 2005

BANZETT RB et al: The affective dimension of laboratory dyspnea: Air hunger is more unpleasant than work/effort. Am J Respir Crit Care Med 177:1384, 2008

Dyspnea mechanisms, assessment, and management: A consensus statement. Am J Respir Crit Care Med 159:321, 1999

GILLETTE MA, SCHWARTZSTEIN RM: Mechanisms of dyspnea, in *Supportive Care in Respiratory Disease*, SH Ahmedzai and MF Muer (eds). Oxford, U.K., Oxford University Press, 2005

MAHLER DA et al: Descriptors of breathlessness in cardiorespiratory diseases. Am J Respir Crit Care Med 154:1357, 1996

——, O'DONNELL DE (eds): *Dyspnea: Mechanisms, Measurement, and Management.* New York, Marcel Dekker, 2005

SCHWARTZSTEIN RM: The language of dyspnea, in *Dyspnea: Mechanisms, Measurement, and Management*, DA Mahler and DE O'Donnell (eds). New York, Marcel Dekker, 2005

——, FELLER-KOPMAN D: Shortness of breath, in *Primary Cardiology*, 2nd ed, E Braunwald and L Goldman (eds). Philadelphia: WB Saunders, 2003

TABLE 33-3 Common Causes of Noncardiogenic Pulmonary Edema

Direct Injury to Lung

Chest trauma, pulmonary contusion
Aspiration
Smoke inhalation
Pneumonia
Oxygen toxicity
Pulmonary embolism, reperfusion

Hematogenous Injury to Lung

Sepsis
Pancreatitis
Nonthoracic trauma
Leukoagglutination reactions
Multiple transfusions
Intravenous drug use, e.g., heroin
Cardiopulmonary bypass

Possible Lung Injury Plus Elevated Hydrostatic Pressures

High-altitude pulmonary edema
Neurogenic pulmonary edema
Reexpansion pulmonary edema

CHAPTER 34
Cough and Hemoptysis

Patricia Kritek

Christopher Fanta

COUGH

Cough provides an essential protective function for human airways and lungs. Without an effective cough reflex, we are at risk for retained airway secretions and aspirated material, predisposing to infection, atelectasis, and respiratory compromise. At the other extreme, excessive coughing can be exhausting; can be complicated by emesis, syncope, muscular pain, or rib fractures; and can aggravate abdominal or inguinal hernias and urinary incontinence. Cough is often a clue to the presence of respiratory disease. In many instances, cough is an expected and accepted manifestation of disease, such as during an acute respiratory tract infection. However, persistent cough in the absence of other respiratory symptoms commonly causes patients to seek medical attention, accounting for as many as 10–30% of referrals to pulmonary specialists.

◼ COUGH MECHANISM

Spontaneous cough is triggered by stimulation of sensory nerve endings that are thought to be primarily rapidly adapting receptors and C-fibers. Both chemical (e.g., capsaicin) and mechanical (e.g., particulates in air pollution) stimuli may initiate the cough reflex. A cationic ion channel, called the type-1 vanilloid receptor, is found on rapidly adapting receptors and C-fibers; it is the receptor for capsaicin, and its expression is increased in patients with chronic cough. Afferent nerve endings richly innervate the pharynx, larynx, and airways to the level of terminal bronchioles and into the lung parenchyma. They may also be found in the external auditory meatus (the auricular branch of the vagus nerve, called the Arnold nerve) and in the esophagus. Sensory signals travel via the vagus and superior laryngeal nerves to a region of the brainstem in the nucleus tractus solitarius, vaguely identified as the "cough center." Mechanical stimulation of bronchial mucosa in a transplanted lung (in which the vagus nerve has been severed) does not produce cough.

The cough reflex involves a highly orchestrated series of involuntary muscular actions, with the potential for input from cortical pathways as well. The vocal cords adduct, leading to transient upper-airway occlusion. Expiratory muscles contract, generating positive intrathoracic pressures as high as 300 mm Hg. With sudden release of the laryngeal contraction, rapid expiratory flows are generated, exceeding the normal "envelope" of maximal expiratory flow seen on the flow-volume curve (Fig. 34-1). Bronchial smooth muscle contraction together with dynamic compression of airways narrows airway lumens and maximizes the velocity of exhalation (as fast as 50 miles per hour). The kinetic energy available to dislodge mucus from the inside of airway walls is directly proportional to the square of the velocity of expiratory airflow. A deep breath preceding a cough optimizes the function of the expiratory muscles; a series of repetitive coughs at successively lower lung volumes sweeps the point of maximal expiratory velocity progressively further into the lung periphery.

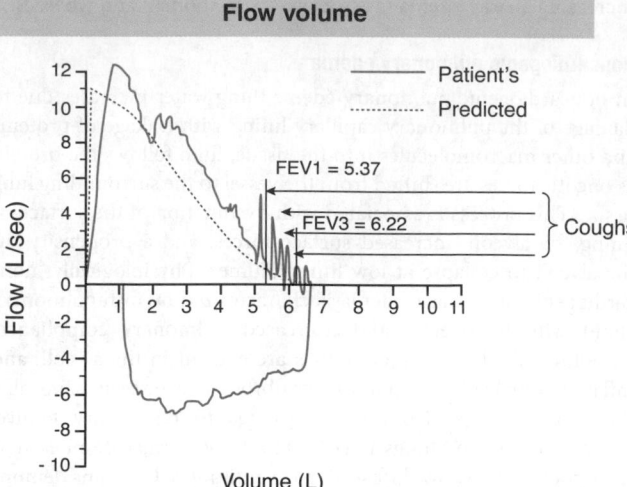

Figure 34-1   Flow-Volume Loop. Flow-volume curve with spikes of high expiratory flow achieved with cough.

◼ IMPAIRED COUGH

Weak or ineffective cough compromises the ability to clear lower respiratory tract infections, predisposing to more serious infections and their sequelae. Weakness, paralysis, or pain of the expiratory (abdominal and intercostal) muscles is foremost on the list of causes of impaired cough (Table 34-1). Cough strength is generally assessed qualitatively; peak expiratory flow or maximal expiratory pressure at the mouth can be used as a surrogate marker for cough strength. A variety of assistive devices and techniques have been developed to improve cough strength, spanning the gamut from simple (splinting the abdominal muscles with a tightly-held pillow to reduce post-operative pain while coughing) to complex (a mechanical cough-assist device applied via face mask or tracheal tube that applies a cycle of positive pressure followed rapidly by negative pressure). Cough may fail to clear secretions despite a preserved ability to generate normal expiratory velocities, either due to abnormal airway secretions (e.g., bronchiectasis due to cystic fibrosis) or structural abnormalities of the airways (e.g., tracheomalacia with expiratory collapse during cough).

◼ SYMPTOMATIC COUGH

The cough of chronic bronchitis in long-term cigarette smokers rarely leads the patient to seek medical advice. It lasts only seconds to a few minutes, is productive of benign-appearing mucoid sputum,

TABLE 34-1 Causes of Impaired Cough

Decreased expiratory-muscle strength

Decreased inspiratory-muscle strength

Chest-wall deformity

Impaired glottic closure or tracheostomy

Tracheomalacia

Abnormal airway secretions

Central respiratory depression (e.g., anesthesia, sedation, or coma)

and is not discomforting. Similarly, cough may occur in the context of other respiratory symptoms that, together, point to a diagnosis, such as when cough is accompanied by wheezing, shortness of breath, and chest tightness after exposure to a cat or other sources of allergens. At times, however, cough is the dominant or sole symptom of disease, and it may be of sufficient duration and severity that relief is sought. The duration of cough is a clue to its etiology. Acute cough (<3 weeks) is most commonly due to a respiratory tract infection, aspiration event, or inhalation of noxious chemicals or smoke. Subacute cough (3–8 weeks duration) is frequently the residuum from a tracheobronchitis, such as in pertussis or "postviral tussive syndrome." Chronic cough (>8 weeks) may be caused by a wide variety of cardiopulmonary diseases, including those of inflammatory, infectious, neoplastic, and cardiovascular etiologies. When initial assessment with chest examination and radiograph is normal, cough-variant asthma, gastroesophageal reflux, nasopharyngeal drainage, and medications (angiotensin converting enzyme [ACE] inhibitors) are the most common causes of chronic cough. Cough of less than 8 weeks' duration may be the early manifestation of a disease causing chronic cough.

■ ASSESSMENT OF CHRONIC COUGH

Details as to the sound, time of occurrence during the day, and pattern of coughing infrequently provide useful etiology clues. Regardless of cause, cough often worsens when one first lies down at night or with talking or in association with the hyperpnea of exercise; it frequently improves with sleep. Exceptions might include the characteristic inspiratory whoop after a paroxysm of coughing that suggests pertussis or the cough that occurs only with certain allergic exposures or exercise in cold air, as in asthma. Useful historical questions include the circumstances surrounding the onset of cough, what makes the cough better or worse, and whether or not the cough produces sputum.

The physical examination seeks clues to the presence of cardiopulmonary disease, including findings such as wheezing or crackles on chest examination. Examination of the auditory canals and tympanic membranes (for irritation of the tympanic membrane resulting in stimulation of Arnold's nerve), the nasal passageways (for rhinitis), and nails (for clubbing) may also provide etiologic clues. Because cough can be a manifestation of a systemic disease, such as sarcoidosis or vasculitis, a thorough general examination is equally important.

In virtually all instances, evaluation of chronic cough merits a chest radiograph. The list of diseases that can cause persistent coughing without other symptoms and without detectable abnormality on physical examination is long. It includes serious illnesses such as Hodgkin's disease in young adults and lung cancer in an older population. An abnormal chest film leads to evaluation of the radiographic abnormality to explain the symptom of cough. A normal chest image provides valuable reassurance to the patient and the patient's family, who may have imagined the direst explanation for the cough.

In a patient with chronic productive cough, examination of expectorated sputum is warranted. Purulent-appearing sputum should be sent for routine bacterial culture and, in certain circumstances, mycobacterial culture as well. Cytologic examination of mucoid sputum may be useful to assess for malignancy and to distinguish neutrophilic from eosinophilic bronchitis. Expectoration of blood—whether streaks of blood, blood mixed with airway secretions, or pure blood—deserves a special approach to assessment and management, as discussed below.

■ CHRONIC COUGH WITH A NORMAL CHEST RADIOGRAPH

It is commonly held that use of an angiotensin-converting enzyme inhibitor; post-nasal drainage; gastroesophageal reflux; and asthma, alone or in combination, account for more than 90% of patients who have chronic cough and a normal or noncontributory chest radiograph. However, clinical experience does not support this contention, and strict adherence to this concept discourages the search for alternative explanations by both clinicians and researchers. On the one hand, chronic idiopathic cough is common and its management deserves study and discussion. On the other hand, serious pulmonary diseases, including inflammatory lung diseases, chronic infections, and neoplasms, may remain occult on plain chest imaging and require additional testing for detection.

ACE inhibitor-induced cough occurs in 5–30% of patients taking ACE inhibitors and is not dose-dependent. Any patient with chronic unexplained cough who is taking an ACE inhibitor should be given a trial period off the medication, regardless of the timing of the onset of cough relative to the initiation of ACE inhibitor therapy. In most instances, a safe alternative is available; angiotensin-receptor blockers do not cause cough. Failure to observe a decrease in cough after one month off medication argues strongly against this diagnosis. ACE metabolizes bradykinin and other tachykinins, such as substance P. The mechanism of ACE inhibitor cough may involve sensitization of sensory nerve endings due to accumulation of bradykinin. In support of this hypothesis, polymorphisms in the neurokinin-2 receptor gene are associated with ACE inhibitor–induced cough.

Post-nasal drainage of any etiology can cause cough as a response to stimulation of sensory receptors of the cough-reflex pathway in the hypopharynx or aspiration of draining secretions into the trachea. Clues to this etiology include symptoms of post-nasal drip, frequent throat clearing, and sneezing and rhinorrhea. On speculum examination of the nose, one may see excess mucoid or purulent secretions, inflamed and edematous nasal mucosa, and/or nasal polyps; in addition, one might visualize secretions or a cobblestoned appearance of the mucosa along the posterior pharyngeal wall. Unfortunately, there is no means by which to quantitate post-nasal drainage. In many instances, one is left to rely on a qualitative judgment based on subjective information provided by the patient. This assessment must also be counterbalanced by the fact that many people who have chronic post-nasal drainage do not experience cough.

Linking gastroesophageal reflux to chronic cough poses similar challenges. It is thought that reflux of gastric contents into the lower esophagus may trigger cough via reflex pathways initiated in the esophageal mucosa. Reflux to the level of the pharynx with consequent aspiration of gastric contents causes a chemical bronchitis and possible pneumonitis that can elicit cough for days after the aspiration event. Retrosternal burning after meals or on recumbency, frequent eructation, hoarseness, and throat pain are potential clues to gastroesophageal reflux. Reflux may also elicit no or minimal symptoms. Glottic inflammation may be a clue to recurrent reflux to the level of the throat, but it is a nonspecific finding and requires direct or indirect laryngoscopy for detection. Quantification of the frequency and level of reflux requires a somewhat invasive procedure to measure esophageal pH directly (a catheter with pH probe placed nasopharyngeally in the esophagus for 24 h, or pH monitoring using a radiotransmitter capsule placed endoscopically into the esophagus). Precise interpretation of test results enabling one to link reflux and cough in a causative way remains debated. Again, assigning the cause of cough to gastroesophageal reflux must be weighed against the observation that many people with chronic reflux (such as frequently occurs during pregnancy) do not experience chronic cough.

Cough alone as a manifestation of asthma is common in children but not in adults. Cough due to asthma in the absence of wheezing, shortness of breath, and chest tightness is referred to as "cough-variant asthma." A history suggestive of cough-variant asthma ties the onset of cough to typical triggers for asthma and resolution of cough upon withdrawal from exposure to them. Objective testing can establish the diagnosis of asthma (airflow obstruction on spirometry that varies over time or reverses in response to bronchodilator) or exclude it with certainty (negative response to bronchoprovocation challenge, such as with methacholine). In a patient capable of making reliable measurements, home expiratory peak flow monitoring can be used as a cost-effective method to support or discount a diagnosis of asthma.

Chronic eosinophilic bronchitis causes chronic cough with a normal chest radiograph. This condition is characterized by sputum eosinophilia in excess of 3% without airflow obstruction or bronchial hyperresponsiveness and is successfully treated with inhaled glucocorticoids.

Treatment of chronic cough in a patient with a normal chest radiograph is often empiric and is targeted at the most likely cause or causes of cough as determined by history, physical examination, and possibly pulmonary-function testing. Therapy for post-nasal drainage depends on the presumed etiology (infection, allergy, or vasomotor rhinitis) and may include systemic antihistamines; antibiotics; nasal saline irrigation; and nasal pump sprays with corticosteroids, antihistamines, or anticholinergics. Antacids, histamine type-2 (H2) receptor antagonists, and proton-pump inhibitors are used to neutralize or decrease production of gastric acid in gastroesophageal reflux disease; dietary changes, elevation of the head and torso during sleep, and medications to improve gastric emptying are additional therapies. Cough-variant asthma typically responds well to inhaled glucocorticoids and intermittent use of inhaled beta-agonist bronchodilators.

Patients who fail to respond to treatment of the common causes of cough or who have had these causes excluded by appropriate diagnostic testing should undergo chest CT. Examples of diseases causing cough that may be missed on chest x-ray include carcinoid tumor, early interstitial lung disease, bronchiectasis, and atypical mycobacterial pulmonary infection. On the other hand, patients with chronic cough who have normal chest examination, lung function, oxygenation, and chest CT imaging can be reassured as to the absence of serious pulmonary pathology.

■ SYMPTOMATIC TREATMENT OF COUGH

Chronic idiopathic cough is distressingly common. It is often experienced as a tickle or sensitivity in the throat area, occurs more often in women, and is typically "dry" or at most productive of scant amounts of mucoid sputum. It can be exhausting, interfere with work, and cause social embarrassment. Once serious underlying cardiopulmonary pathology has been excluded, an attempt at cough suppression is appropriate. Most effective are narcotic cough suppressants, such as codeine or hydrocodone, which are thought to act in the "cough center" in the brainstem. The tendency of narcotic cough suppressants to cause drowsiness and constipation and their potential for addictive dependence limit their appeal for long-term use. Dextromethorphan is an over-the-counter, centrally acting cough suppressant with fewer side effects and less efficacy compared to the narcotic cough suppressants. It is thought to have a different site of action than narcotic cough suppressants and can be used in combination with them if necessary. Benzonatate is thought to inhibit neural activity of sensory nerves in the cough-reflex pathway. It is generally free of side effects; however, its effectiveness in suppressing cough is variable and unpredictable. Novel cough suppressants without the limitations of currently available therapies are greatly needed. Approaches that are being explored include development of neurokinin receptor antagonists, type-1 vanilloid receptor antagonists, and novel opioid and opioidlike receptor agonists.

HEMOPTYSIS

Hemoptysis is the expectoration of blood from the respiratory tract. It can arise from any part of the respiratory tract, from the alveoli to the glottis. It is important, however, to distinguish hemoptysis from epistaxis (i.e., bleeding from the nasopharynx) and hematemesis (i.e., bleeding from the upper gastrointestinal tract). Hemoptysis can range from blood-tinged sputum to life-threatening large volumes of bright red blood. For most patients, any degree of hemoptysis can be anxiety-producing and often prompts medical evaluation.

While precise epidemiologic data are lacking, the most common etiology of hemoptysis is infection of the medium-sized airways. In the United States, this is usually due to a viral or bacterial bronchitis. Hemoptysis can arise in the setting of either acute bronchitis or during an exacerbation of chronic bronchitis. Worldwide, the most common cause of hemoptysis is tuberculous infection presumably owing to the high prevalence of the disease and its predilection for cavity formation. While these are the most common causes, there is an extensive differential diagnosis for hemoptysis, and a step-wise approach to the evaluation of this symptom is appropriate.

■ ETIOLOGY

One way to approach the source of hemoptysis is systematically to assess for potential sites of bleeding from the alveolus to the mouth. Diffuse bleeding in the alveolar space, often referred to as diffuse alveolar hemorrhage (DAH), may present with hemoptysis, although this is not always the case. Causes of DAH can be divided into inflammatory and noninflammatory types. Inflammatory DAH is due to small vessel vasculitis/capillaritis from a variety of diseases, including granulomatosis with polyangiitis (Wegener's) and microscopic polyangiitis. Similarly, systemic autoimmune disease, such as systemic lupus erythematosus (SLE), can manifest as pulmonary capillaritis and result in DAH. Antibodies to the alveolar basement membrane, as are seen in Goodpasture's disease, can also result in alveolar hemorrhage. In the early time period after a bone marrow transplant (BMT), patients can also develop a form of inflammatory DAH, which can be catastrophic and life-threatening. The exact pathophysiology of this process is not well understood, but DAH should be suspected in patients with sudden-onset dyspnea and hypoxemia in the first 100 days after a BMT.

Alveoli can also bleed due to noninflammatory causes, most commonly due to direct inhalational injury. This category includes thermal injury from fires, inhalation of illicit substances (e.g., cocaine), and inhalation of toxic chemicals. If alveoli are irritated from any process, patients with thrombocytopenia, coagulopathy, or antiplatelet or anticoagulant use will have an increased risk of developing hemoptysis.

As already noted, the most common site of hemoptysis is bleeding from the small- to medium-sized airways. Irritation and injury of the bronchial mucosal can lead to small-volume bleeding. More significant hemoptysis can also occur because of the proximity of the bronchial artery and vein to the airway, running together in what is often referred to as the "bronchovascular bundle." In the smaller airways, these blood vessels are close to the airspace and, therefore, lesser degrees of inflammation or injury can result in rupture of these vessels into the airways. Of note, while alveolar hemorrhage arises from capillaries that are part of the low-pressure pulmonary circulation, bronchial bleeding is generally from bronchial arteries, which are under systemic pressure and, therefore, predisposed to larger-volume bleeding.

Any infection of the airways can result in hemoptysis, although, most commonly, acute bronchitis is caused by viral infection. In patients with a history of chronic bronchitis, bacterial super infection with organisms such as *Streptococcus pneumoniae*, *Hemophilus* influenzae, or *Moraxella catarrhalis* can also result in hemoptysis. Patients with bronchiectasis, a permanent dilation and irregularity of the airways, are particularly prone to hemoptysis due to anatomic abnormalities that bring the bronchial arteries closer to the mucosal surface and the associated chronic inflammatory state. One common presentation of patients with advanced cystic fibrosis, the prototypical bronchiectatic lung disease, is hemoptysis, which, at times, can be life-threatening.

Pneumonias of any sort can cause hemoptysis. Tuberculous infection, which can lead to bronchiectasis or cavitary pneumonia, is a very common cause of hemoptysis worldwide. Community-acquired pneumonia and lung abscess can also result in bleeding. Once again, if the infection results in cavitation, there is a greater likelihood of bleeding due to erosion into blood vessels. Infections with *Staphylococcus aureus* and gram-negative rods (e.g., *Klebsiella pneumoniae*) are more likely to cause necrotizing lung infections and, thus, are more often associated with hemoptysis. Previous severe pneumonias can cause scarring and abnormal lung architecture, which may predispose a patient to hemoptysis with subsequent infections.

While it is not commonly seen in North America, pulmonary paragonimiasis (i.e., infection with the lung fluke *Paragonimus westermani*) often presents with fever, cough, and hemoptysis. This infection is a public health issue in Southeast Asia and China and is commonly confused with active tuberculosis, because the clinical pictures can be similar. Paragonimiasis should be considered in recent immigrants from endemic areas with new or recurrent hemoptysis. In addition, there are reports of pulmonary paragonimiasis in the United States secondary to ingestion of crayfish or small crabs.

Other causes of irritation of the airways resulting in hemoptysis include inhalation of toxic chemicals, thermal injury, direct trauma from suctioning of the airways (particularly in intubated patients), and irritation from inhalation of foreign bodies. All of these etiologies should be suggested by the individual patient's history and exposures.

Perhaps the most feared cause of hemoptysis is bronchogenic lung cancer, although hemoptysis is not a particularly common presenting symptom of this disease with only approximately 10% of patients having frank hemoptysis on initial assessment. Cancers arising in the proximal airways are much more likely to cause hemoptysis, although any malignancy in the chest can do so. Because both squamous cell carcinoma and small cell carcinoma are more commonly central and large at presentation, they are more often a cause of hemoptysis. These cancers can present with large-volume and life-threatening hemoptysis because of erosion into the hilar vessels. Carcinoid tumors, which are almost exclusively found as endobronchial lesions with friable mucosa, can also present with hemoptysis.

In addition to cancers arising in the lung, metastatic disease in the pulmonary parenchyma can also bleed. Malignancies that commonly metastasize to the lungs include renal cell, breast, colon, testicular, and thyroid cancers as well as melanoma. While they are not a common way for metastatic disease to present, multiple pulmonary nodules and hemoptysis should raise the suspicion for this etiology.

Finally, disease of the pulmonary vasculature can cause hemoptysis. Perhaps most commonly, congestive heart failure with transmission of elevated left atrial pressures, if severe enough, can lead to rupture of small alveolar capillaries. These patients rarely present with bright red blood but more commonly have pink, frothy sputum or blood-tinged secretions. Patients with a focal jet of mitral regurgitation can present with an upper-lobe infiltrate on chest radiograph together with hemoptysis. This is thought to be due to focal increases in pulmonary capillary pressure due to the regurgitant jet. Pulmonary arterio-venous malformations are prone to bleeding. Pulmonary embolism can also lead to the development of hemoptysis, which is generally associated with pulmonary infarction. Pulmonary arterial hypertension from other causes rarely results in hemoptysis.

EVALUATION

As with most symptoms, the initial step in the evaluation of hemoptysis is a thorough history and physical examination (Fig. 34-2). As already mentioned, questioning should begin with determining if the bleeding is truly from the respiratory tract and not the nasopharynx or gastrointestinal tract, because these sources of bleeding require different evaluation and treatment approaches.

■ HISTORY AND PHYSICAL EXAM

The nature of the hemoptysis, whether they are blood-tinged, purulent secretions; pink, frothy sputum; or frank blood, may be helpful in determining an etiology. Specific triggers of the bleeding, such as recent inhalation exposures as well as any previous episodes of hemoptysis, should be elicited during history-taking. Monthly hemoptysis in a woman suggests catamenial hemoptysis from pulmonary endometriosis. The volume of the hemoptysis is also important not only in determining the cause, but in gauging the urgency for further diagnostic and therapeutic maneuvers. Patients rarely exsanguinate from hemoptysis but can effectively "drown" in aspirated blood. Large-volume hemoptysis, referred to as *massive hemoptysis*, is variably defined as hemoptysis of greater than 200–600 cc in 24 h. Massive hemoptysis should be considered a medical emergency. The medical urgency related to hemoptysis depends on both the amount of bleeding and the severity of underlying pulmonary disease.

All patients should be asked about current or former cigarette smoking; this behavior predisposes to both chronic bronchitis and increases the likelihood of bronchogenic cancer. Symptoms suggestive of respiratory tract infection— including fever, chills, and dyspnea—should be elicited. The practitioner should inquire about recent inhalation exposures or use of illicit substances as well as risk factors for venous thromboembolism.

Past medical history of malignancy or treatment thereof, rheumatologic disease, vascular disease, or underlying lung disease such as bronchiectasis may be relevant to the cause of hemoptysis. Because many of the causes of DAH can be part of a pulmonary-renal syndrome, specific inquiry into a history of renal insufficiency also is important.

The physical examination begins with an assessment of vital signs and oxygen saturation to gauge whether there is evidence of life-threatening bleeding. Tachycardia, hypotension, and decreased oxygen saturation should dictate a more expedited evaluation of hemoptysis. Specific focus on respiratory and cardiac examinations are important and should include inspection of the nares, auscultation of the lungs and heart, assessment of the lower extremities for symmetric or asymmetric edema, and evaluation for jugular venous distention. Clubbing of the digits may suggest underlying lung diseases such as bronchogenic carcinoma or bronchiectasis, which predispose to hemoptysis. Similarly, mucocutaneous telangiectasias should raise the specter of pulmonary arterial-venous malformations.

■ DIAGNOSTIC EVALUATION

For most patients, the next step in evaluation of hemoptysis should be a standard chest radiograph. If a source of bleeding is not identified on plain film, a CT of the chest should be obtained. CT allows better delineation of bronchiectasis, alveolar filling, cavitary infiltrates, and masses than does chest x-ray; it also gives further information on mediastinal lymphadenopathy, which may support a diagnosis of thoracic malignancy. The practitioner should consider a CT protocol to assess for pulmonary embolism if the history or examination suggests venous thromboembolism as a cause of the bleeding.

Laboratory studies should include a complete blood count to assess both the hematocrit as well as platelet count and coagulation studies. Renal function and urinalysis should be assessed because of the possibility of pulmonary-renal syndromes presenting with

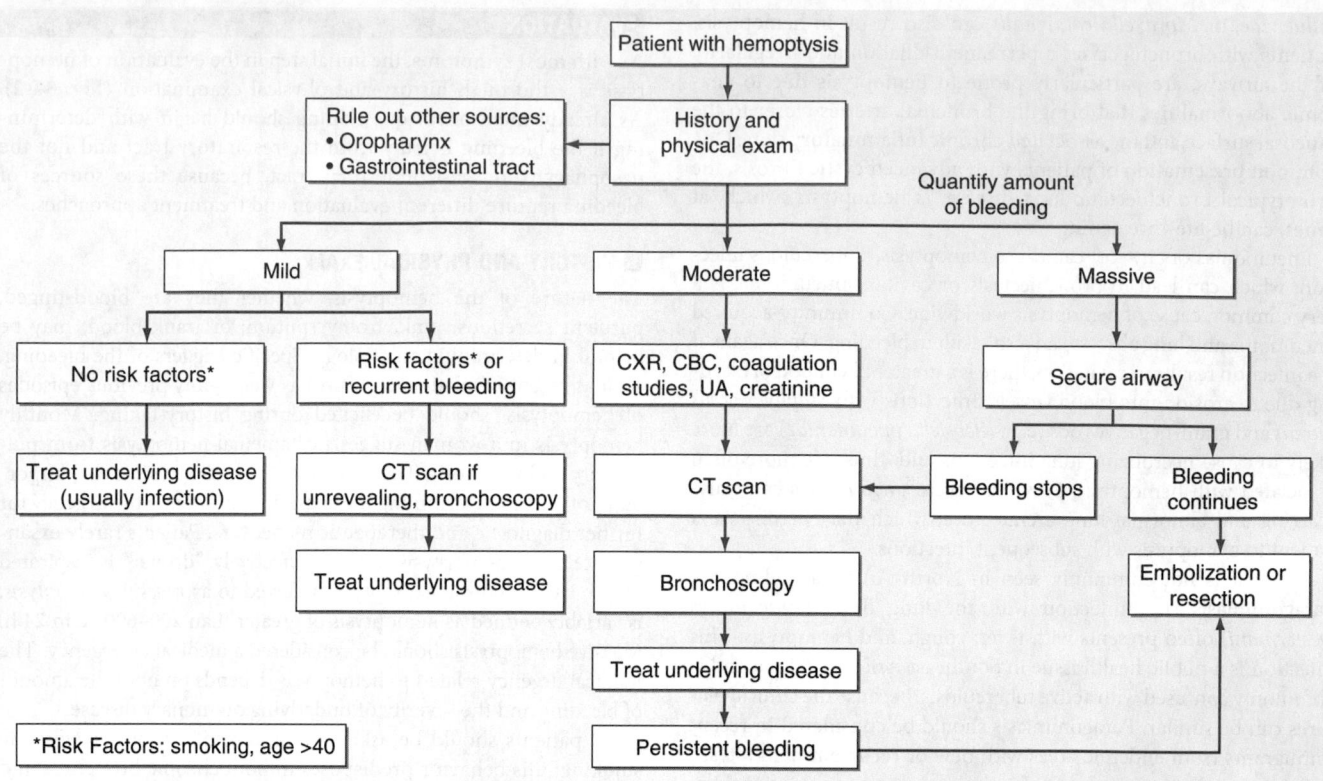

Figure 34-2 Flowchart—evaluation of hemoptysis. Decision tree for evaluation of hemoptysis. CBC, complete blood count; CT, computed tomography; CXR, chest x-ray; UA, urinalysis.

hemoptysis. Acute renal insufficiency, or red blood cells or red blood cell casts on urinalysis should increase suspicion for small-vessel vasculitis, and studies such as antineutrophil cytoplasmic antibody (ANCA), antiglomerular basement membrane antibody (anti-GBM), and antinuclear antibody (ANA), should be considered. If a patient is producing sputum, Gram and acid-fast stains as well as culture should be obtained.

If all of these studies are unrevealing, bronchoscopy should be considered. In any patient with a history of cigarette smoking, airway inspection should be part of the evaluation of new hemoptysis. Because these patients are at increased risk of bronchogenic carcinoma, and endobronchial lesions are often not reliably visualized on computed tomogram, bronchoscopy should be seriously considered to add to the completeness of the evaluation.

TREATMENT   Hemoptysis

For the most part, the treatment of hemoptysis will vary based on its etiology. However, large-volume, life-threatening hemoptysis generally requires immediate intervention regardless of the cause. The first step is to establish a patent airway usually by endotracheal intubation and subsequent mechanical ventilation. As most large-volume hemoptysis arises from an airway lesion, it is ideal if the site of the bleeding can be identified either by chest imaging or bronchoscopy (more commonly rigid than flexible). The goal is then to isolate the bleeding to one lung and not allow the preserved airspaces in the other lung to be filled with blood, further impairing gas exchange. Patients should be placed with the bleeding lung in a dependent position (i.e., bleeding-side down) and, if possible, dual lumen endotracheal tubes or an airway blocker should be placed in the proximal airway of the bleeding lung. These interventions generally require

the assistance of anesthesiologists, interventional pulmonologists, or thoracic surgeons.

If the bleeding does not stop with therapies of the underlying cause and passage of time, severe hemoptysis from bronchial arteries can be treated with angiographic embolization of the culprit bronchial artery. This intervention should only be entertained in the most severe and life-threatening cases of hemoptysis because there is a risk of unintentional spinal-artery embolization and consequent paraplegia with this procedure. Endobronchial lesions can be treated with a variety of bronchoscopically directed interventions, including cauterization and laser therapy. In extreme conditions, surgical resection of the affected region of lung is considered. Most cases of hemoptysis will resolve with treatment of the infection or inflammatory process or with removal of the offending stimulus.

FURTHER READINGS

BIDWELL JL, PACHNER RW: Hemoptysis: diagnosis and management. Am Fam Physician 72:1253, 2005

CHUNG KF, PAVORD ID: Prevalence, pathogenesis, and causes of chronic cough. Lancet 37: 1364, 2008

IRWIN RS et al: Diagnosis and management of cough executive summary: ACCP evidence-based clinical practice guidelines. Chest 129:1S, 2006

JEAN-BAPTISTE E: Clinical assessment and management of massive hemoptysis. Crit Care Med 28:1642, 2000

LARA AR, SCHWARZ MI: Diffuse alveolar hemorrhage. Chest 137:1164, 2010

PAVORD ID, CHUNG KF: Management of chronic cough. Lancet 371: 1375, 2008

CHAPTER **35**

Hypoxia and Cyanosis

Joseph Loscalzo

HYPOXIA

The fundamental purpose of the cardiorespiratory system is to deliver O_2 and nutrients to cells and to remove CO_2 and other metabolic products from them. Proper maintenance of this function depends not only on intact cardiovascular and respiratory systems but also on an adequate number of red blood cells and hemoglobin and a supply of inspired gas containing adequate O_2.

■ RESPONSES TO HYPOXIA

Decreased O_2 availability to cells results in an inhibition of oxidative phosphorylation and increased anaerobic glycolysis. This switch from aerobic to anaerobic metabolism, the Pasteur effect, maintains some, albeit reduced, adenosine 5'-triphosphate (ATP) production. In severe hypoxia, when ATP production is inadequate to meet the energy requirements of ionic and osmotic equilibrium, cell membrane depolarization leads to uncontrolled Ca^{2+} influx and activation of Ca^{2+}-dependent phospholipases and proteases. These events, in turn, cause cell swelling and, ultimately, cell death.

The adaptations to hypoxia are mediated, in part, by the upregulation of genes encoding a variety of proteins, including glycolytic enzymes such as phosphoglycerate kinase and phosphofructokinase, as well as the glucose transporters Glut-1 and Glut-2; and by growth factors, such as vascular endothelial growth factor (VEGF) and erythropoietin, which enhance erythrocyte production. The hypoxia-induced increase in expression of these key proteins is governed by the hypoxia-sensitive transcription factor, hypoxia-inducible factor-1 (HIF-1).

During hypoxia, systemic arterioles dilate, at least in part, by opening of K_{ATP} channels in vascular smooth-muscle cells due to the hypoxia-induced reduction in ATP concentration. By contrast, in pulmonary vascular smooth-muscle cells, inhibition of K^+ channels causes depolarization which, in turn, activates voltage-gated Ca^{2+} channels raising the cytosolic $[Ca^{2+}]$ and causing smooth-muscle cell contraction. Hypoxia-induced pulmonary arterial constriction shunts blood away from poorly ventilated portions toward better ventilated portions of the lung; however, it also increases pulmonary vascular resistance and right ventricular afterload.

Effects on the central nervous system

Changes in the central nervous system (CNS), particularly the higher centers, are especially important consequences of hypoxia. Acute hypoxia causes impaired judgment, motor incoordination, and a clinical picture resembling acute alcohol intoxication. High-altitude illness is characterized by headache secondary to cerebral vasodilation, gastrointestinal symptoms, dizziness, insomnia, fatigue, or somnolence. Pulmonary arterial and sometimes venous constriction cause capillary leakage and high-altitude pulmonary edema (HAPE) (Chap. 33), which intensifies hypoxia, further promoting vasoconstriction. Rarely, high-altitude cerebral edema (HACE) develops, which is manifest by severe headache and papilledema and can cause coma. As hypoxia becomes more severe, the regulatory centers of the brainstem are affected, and death usually results from respiratory failure.

■ CAUSES OF HYPOXIA

Respiratory hypoxia

When hypoxia occurs from respiratory failure, PaO_2 declines, and when respiratory failure is persistent, the hemoglobin-oxygen (Hb-O_2) dissociation curve (Fig. 104-2) is displaced to the right, with greater quantities of O_2 released at any level of tissue PO_2. Arterial hypoxemia, i.e., a reduction of O_2 saturation of arterial blood (SaO_2), and consequent cyanosis are likely to be more marked when such depression of PaO_2 results from pulmonary disease than when the depression occurs as the result of a decline in the fraction of oxygen in inspired air (FIO_2). In this latter situation, $PaCO_2$ falls secondary to anoxia-induced hyperventilation and the Hb-O_2 dissociation curve is displaced to the left, limiting the decline in SaO_2 at any level of PaO_2.

The most common cause of respiratory hypoxia is *ventilation-perfusion mismatch* resulting from perfusion of poorly ventilated alveoli. Respiratory hypoxemia may also be caused by *hypoventilation*, in which case it is then associated with an elevation of $PaCO_2$ (Chap. 252). These two forms of respiratory hypoxia are usually correctable by inspiring 100% O_2 for several minutes. A third cause of respiratory hypoxia is shunting of blood across the lung from the pulmonary arterial to the venous bed (*intrapulmonary right-to-left shunting*) by perfusion of nonventilated portions of the lung, as in pulmonary atelectasis or through pulmonary arteriovenous connections. The low PaO_2 in this situation is only partially corrected by an FIO_2 of 100%.

Hypoxia secondary to high altitude

As one ascends rapidly to 3000 m (~10,000 ft), the reduction of the O_2 content of inspired air (FIO_2) leads to a decrease in alveolar PO_2 to approximately 60 mmHg, and a condition termed *high-altitude illness* develops (see above). At higher altitudes, arterial saturation declines rapidly and symptoms become more serious; and at 5000 m, unacclimated individuals usually cease to be able to function normally owing to the changes in CNS function described above.

Hypoxia secondary to right-to-left extrapulmonary shunting

From a physiologic viewpoint, this cause of hypoxia resembles intrapulmonary right-to-left shunting but is caused by congenital cardiac malformations, such as tetralogy of Fallot, transposition of the great arteries, and Eisenmenger's syndrome (Chap. 236). As in pulmonary right-to-left shunting, the PaO_2 cannot be restored to normal with inspiration of 100% O_2.

Anemic hypoxia

A reduction in hemoglobin concentration of the blood is accompanied by a corresponding decline in the O_2-carrying capacity of the blood. Although the PaO_2 is normal in anemic hypoxia, the absolute quantity of O_2 transported per unit volume of blood is diminished. As the anemic blood passes through the capillaries and the usual quantity of O_2 is removed from it, the PO_2 and saturation in the venous blood decline to a greater extent than normal.

Carbon monoxide (CO) intoxication

(See also Chap. e49) Hemoglobin that binds with CO (carboxyhemoglobin, COHb) is unavailable for O_2 transport. In addition, the presence of COHb shifts the Hb-O_2 dissociation curve to the left (Fig. 104-2) so that O_2 is unloaded only at lower tensions, contributing further to tissue hypoxia.

Circulatory hypoxia

As in anemic hypoxia, the PaO_2 is usually normal, but venous and tissue PO_2 values are reduced as a consequence of reduced tissue perfusion and greater tissue O_2 extraction. This pathophysiology leads to an increased arterial-mixed venous O_2 difference (a-v-O_2 difference), or gradient. Generalized circulatory hypoxia occurs in heart failure (Chap. 234) and in most forms of shock (Chap. 270).

Specific organ hypoxia

Localized circulatory hypoxia may occur as a result of decreased perfusion secondary to arterial obstruction, as in localized athero-sclerosis in any vascular bed, or as a consequence of vasoconstriction, as observed in Raynaud's phenomenon (Chap. 249). Localized hypoxia may also result from venous obstruction and the resultant expansion of interstitial fluid causing arteriolar compression and, thereby, reduction of arterial inflow. Edema, which increases the distance through which O_2 must diffuse before it reaches cells, can also cause localized hypoxia. In an attempt to maintain adequate perfusion to more vital organs in patients with reduced cardiac output secondary to heart failure or hypovolemic shock, vasoconstriction may reduce perfusion in the limbs and skin, causing hypoxia of these regions.

Increased O_2 requirements

If the O_2 consumption of tissues is elevated without a corresponding increase in perfusion, tissue hypoxia ensues and the Po_2 in venous blood declines. Ordinarily, the clinical picture of patients with hypoxia due to an elevated metabolic rate, as in fever or thyro-toxicosis, is quite different from that in other types of hypoxia: the skin is warm and flushed owing to increased cutaneous blood flow that dissipates the excessive heat produced, and cyanosis is usually absent.

Exercise is a classic example of increased tissue O_2 requirements. These increased demands are normally met by several mechanisms operating simultaneously: (1) increase in the cardiac output and ventilation and, thus, O_2 delivery to the tissues; (2) a preferential shift in blood flow to the exercising muscles by changing vascular resistances in the circulatory beds of exercising tissues, directly and/or reflexly; (3) an increase in O_2 extraction from the delivered blood and a widening of the arteriovenous O_2 difference; and (4) a reduction in the pH of the tissues and capillary blood, shifting the Hb-O_2 curve to the right (Fig. 104-2), and unloading more O_2 from hemoglobin. If the capacity of these mechanisms is exceeded, then hypoxia, especially of the exercising muscles, will result.

Improper oxygen utilization

Cyanide (Chap. e50) and several other similarly acting poisons cause cellular hypoxia. The tissues are unable to utilize O_2, and, as a consequence, the venous blood tends to have a high O_2 tension. This condition has been termed *histotoxic hypoxia*.

■ ADAPTATION TO HYPOXIA

An important component of the respiratory response to hypoxia originates in special chemosensitive cells in the carotid and aortic bodies and in the respiratory center in the brainstem. The stimulation of these cells by hypoxia increases ventilation, with a loss of CO_2, and can lead to respiratory alkalosis. When combined with the metabolic acidosis resulting from the production of lactic acid, the serum bicarbonate level declines (Chap. 47).

With the reduction of Pao_2, cerebrovascular resistance decreases and cerebral blood flow increases in an attempt to maintain O_2 delivery to the brain. However, when the reduction of Pao_2 is accompanied by hyperventilation and a reduction of $Paco_2$, cerebrovascular resistance rises, cerebral blood flow falls, and tissue hypoxia intensifies.

The diffuse, systemic vasodilation that occurs in generalized hypoxia increases the cardiac output. In patients with underlying heart disease, the requirements of peripheral tissues for an increase of cardiac output with hypoxia may precipitate congestive heart failure. In patients with ischemic heart disease, a reduced Pao_2 may intensify myocardial ischemia and further impair left ventricular function.

One of the important compensatory mechanisms for chronic hypoxia is an increase in the hemoglobin concentration and in the number of red blood cells in the circulating blood, i.e., the development of polycythemia secondary to erythropoietin production (Chap. 108). In persons with chronic hypoxemia secondary to prolonged residence at a high altitude (>13,000 ft, 4200 m), a condition termed *chronic mountain sickness* develops. This disorder is characterized by a blunted respiratory drive, reduced ventilation, erythrocytosis, cyanosis, weakness, right ventricular enlargement secondary to pulmonary hypertension, and even stupor.

CYANOSIS

Cyanosis refers to a bluish color of the skin and mucous membranes resulting from an increased quantity of reduced hemoglobin (i.e., deoxygenated hemoglobin) or of hemoglobin derivatives (e.g., methemoglobin or sulfhemoglobin) in the small blood vessels of those tissues. It is usually most marked in the lips, nail beds, ears, and malar eminences. Cyanosis, especially if developed recently, is more commonly detected by a family member than the patient. The florid skin characteristic of polycythemia vera (Chap. 108) must be distinguished from the true cyanosis discussed here. A cherry-colored flush, rather than cyanosis, is caused by COHb (Chap. e50).

The degree of cyanosis is modified by the color of the cutaneous pigment and the thickness of the skin, as well as by the state of the cutaneous capillaries. The accurate clinical detection of the presence and degree of cyanosis is difficult, as proved by oximetric studies. In some instances, central cyanosis can be detected reliably when the Sao_2 has fallen to 85%; in others, particularly in dark-skinned persons, it may not be detected until it has declined to 75%. In the latter case, examination of the mucous membranes in the oral cavity and the conjunctivae rather than examination of the skin is more helpful in the detection of cyanosis.

The increase in the quantity of reduced hemoglobin in the mucocutaneous vessels that produces cyanosis may be brought about either by an increase in the quantity of venous blood as a result of dilation of the venules and venous ends of the capillaries or by a reduction in the Sao_2 in the capillary blood. In general, cyanosis becomes apparent when the concentration of reduced hemoglobin in capillary blood exceeds 40 g/L (4 g/dL).

It is the *absolute*, rather than the *relative*, quantity of reduced hemoglobin that is important in producing cyanosis. Thus, in a patient with severe anemia, the *relative* quantity of reduced hemoglobin in the venous blood may be very large when considered in relation to the total quantity of hemoglobin in the blood. However, since the concentration of the latter is markedly reduced, the *absolute* quantity of reduced hemoglobin may still be small, and, therefore, patients with severe anemia and even *marked* arterial desaturation may not display cyanosis. Conversely, the higher the total hemoglobin content, the greater the tendency toward cyanosis; thus, patients with marked polycythemia tend to be cyanotic at higher levels of Sao_2 than patients with normal hematocrit values. Likewise, local passive congestion, which causes an increase in the total quantity of reduced hemoglobin in the vessels in a given area, may cause cyanosis. Cyanosis is also observed when nonfunctional hemoglobin, such as methemoglobin or sulfhemoglobin (Chap. 104), is present in blood.

Cyanosis may be subdivided into central and peripheral types. In *central* cyanosis, the Sao_2 is reduced or an abnormal hemoglobin derivative is present, and the mucous membranes and skin are both affected. *Peripheral* cyanosis is due to a slowing of blood flow and abnormally great extraction of O_2 from normally saturated arterial blood; it results from vasoconstriction and diminished peripheral blood flow, such as occurs in cold exposure, shock, congestive failure, and peripheral vascular disease. Often in these conditions, the mucous membranes of the oral cavity or those beneath the tongue may be spared. Clinical differentiation between central and peripheral cyanosis may not always be simple, and in conditions such as cardiogenic shock with pulmonary edema there may be a mixture of both types.

■ DIFFERENTIAL DIAGNOSIS

Central cyanosis

(Table 35-1) Decreased Sao_2 results from a marked reduction in the Pao_2. This reduction may be brought about by a decline in the Fio_2 without sufficient compensatory alveolar hyperventilation to maintain alveolar Po_2. Cyanosis usually becomes manifest in an ascent to an altitude of 4000 m (13,000 ft).

Seriously *impaired pulmonary function*, through perfusion of unventilated or poorly ventilated areas of the lung or alveolar hypoventilation, is a common cause of central cyanosis (Chap. 252). This condition may occur acutely, as in extensive pneumonia or pulmonary edema, or chronically, with chronic pulmonary diseases (e.g., emphysema). In the latter situation, secondary polycythemia is generally present and clubbing of the fingers (see below) may occur. Another cause of reduced Sao_2 is *shunting of systemic venous blood into the arterial circuit*. Certain forms of congenital heart disease are associated with cyanosis on this basis (see above and Chap. 236).

Pulmonary arteriovenous fistulae may be congenital or acquired, solitary or multiple, microscopic or massive. The severity of cyanosis produced by these fistulae depends on their size and number. They occur with some frequency in hereditary hemorrhagic telangiectasia. Sao_2 reduction and cyanosis may also occur in some patients with cirrhosis, presumably as a consequence of pulmonary arteriovenous fistulae or portal vein–pulmonary vein anastomoses.

TABLE 35-1 Causes of Cyanosis

Central Cyanosis

Decreased arterial oxygen saturation
  Decreased atmospheric pressure—high altitude
  Impaired pulmonary function
    Alveolar hypoventilation
    Uneven relationships between pulmonary ventilation and
      perfusion (perfusion of hypoventilated alveoli)
    Impaired oxygen diffusion
  Anatomic shunts
    Certain types of congenital heart disease
    Pulmonary arteriovenous fistulas
    Multiple small intrapulmonary shunts
  Hemoglobin with low affinity for oxygen
Hemoglobin abnormalities
  Methemoglobinemia—hereditary, acquired
  Sulfhemoglobinemia—acquired
  Carboxyhemoglobinemia (not true cyanosis)

Peripheral Cyanosis

Reduced cardiac output
Cold exposure
Redistribution of blood flow from extremities
Arterial obstruction
Venous obstruction

In patients with cardiac or pulmonary right-to-left shunts, the presence and severity of cyanosis depend on the size of the shunt relative to the systemic flow as well as on the Hb-O_2 saturation of the venous blood. With increased extraction of O_2 from the blood by the exercising muscles, the venous blood returning to the right side of the heart is more unsaturated than at rest, and shunting of this blood intensifies the cyanosis. Secondary polycythemia occurs frequently in patients in this setting and contributes to the cyanosis.

Cyanosis can be caused by small quantities of circulating methemoglobin (Hb Fe^{3+}) and by even smaller quantities of sulfhemoglobin (Chap. 104); both of these hemoglobin derivatives are unable to bind oxygen. Although they are uncommon causes of cyanosis, these abnormal hemoglobin species should be sought by spectroscopy when cyanosis is not readily explained by malfunction of the circulatory or respiratory systems. Generally, digital clubbing does not occur with them.

Peripheral cyanosis

Probably the most common cause of peripheral cyanosis is the normal vasoconstriction resulting from exposure to cold air or water. When cardiac output is reduced, cutaneous vasoconstriction occurs as a compensatory mechanism so that blood is diverted from the skin to more vital areas such as the CNS and heart, and cyanosis of the extremities may result even though the arterial blood is normally saturated.

Arterial obstruction to an extremity, as with an embolus, or arteriolar constriction, as in cold-induced vasospasm (Raynaud's phenomenon) (Chap. 249), generally results in pallor and coldness, and there may be associated cyanosis. Venous obstruction, as in thrombophlebitis or deep venous thrombosis, dilates the subpapillary venous plexuses and thereby intensifies cyanosis.

APPROACH TO THE PATIENT ▶ **Cyanosis**

Certain features are important in arriving at the cause of cyanosis:

1. It is important to ascertain the time of onset of cyanosis. Cyanosis present since birth or infancy is usually due to congenital heart disease.
2. Central and peripheral cyanosis must be differentiated. Evidence of disorders of the respiratory or cardiovascular systems are helpful. Massage or gentle warming of a cyanotic extremity will increase peripheral blood flow and abolish peripheral, but not central, cyanosis.
3. The presence or absence of clubbing of the digits (see below) should be ascertained. The combination of cyanosis and clubbing is frequent in patients with congenital heart disease and right-to-left shunting and is seen occasionally in patients with pulmonary disease, such as lung abscess or pulmonary arteriovenous fistulae. In contrast, peripheral cyanosis or acutely developing central cyanosis is *not* associated with clubbed digits.
4. Pao_2 and Sao_2 should be determined, and, in patients with cyanosis in whom the mechanism is obscure, spectroscopic examination of the blood performed to look for abnormal types of hemoglobin (critical in the differential diagnosis of cyanosis).

CLUBBING

The selective bulbous enlargement of the distal segments of the fingers and toes due to proliferation of connective tissue, particularly on the dorsal surface, is termed *clubbing*; there is also increased sponginess of the soft tissue at the base of the clubbed nail. Clubbing may be hereditary, idiopathic, or acquired and associated with a variety of disorders, including cyanotic congenital heart disease (see above), infective endocarditis, and a variety of pulmonary conditions (among them primary and metastatic lung cancer, bronchiectasis, asbestosis, sarcoidosis, lung abscess, cystic fibrosis, tuberculosis, and mesothelioma), as well as with some gastrointestinal diseases (including inflammatory bowel disease and hepatic cirrhosis). In some instances, it is occupational, e.g., in jackhammer operators.

Clubbing in patients with primary and metastatic lung cancer, mesothelioma, bronchiectasis, or hepatic cirrhosis may be associated with *hypertrophic osteoarthropathy*. In this condition, the subperiosteal formation of new bone in the distal diaphyses of the long bones of the extremities causes pain and symmetric arthritis-like changes in the shoulders, knees, ankles, wrists, and elbows. The diagnosis of hypertrophic osteoarthropathy may be confirmed by bone radiograph or MRI. Although the mechanism of clubbing is unclear, it appears to be secondary to humoral substances that cause dilation of the vessels of the distal digits as well as growth factors released from unfragmented platelet precursors in the digital circulation.

ACKNOWLEDGEMENTS

Dr. Eugene Braunwald authored this chapter in the previous edition. Some of the material from the 17th edition has been carried forward.

FURTHER READINGS

FAWCETT RS et al: Nail abnormalities: Clues to systemic disease. Am Fam Physician 69:1417, 2004

GIORDANO FJ: Oxygen, oxidative stress, hypoxia, and heart failure. J Clin Invest 115:500, 2005

GRIFFEY RT et al: Cyanosis. J Emerg Med 18:369, 2000

HACKETT PH, ROACH RC: Current concepts: High altitude illness. N Engl J Med 345:107, 2001

LEÓN-VELARDE F et al: Chronic mountain sickness and the heart. Prog Cardiovasc Dis 52:540, 2010

LEVY MM: Pathophysiology of oxygen delivery in respiratory failure. Chest 128:547S, 2005

MICHIELS C: Physiological and pathological responses to hypoxia. Am J Pathol 164:1875, 2004

SCHERRER U et al: New insights in the pathogenesis of high-altitude pulmonary edema. Prog Cardiovasc Dis 52:485, 2010

SEMENZA GL: Involvement of oxygen-sensing pathways in physiological and pathological erythropoiesis. Blood 114:2015, 2009

SPICKNALL KE et al: Clubbing: an update on diagnosis, differential diagnosis, pathophysiology, and clinical relevance. J Am Acad Dermatol 52:1020, 2005

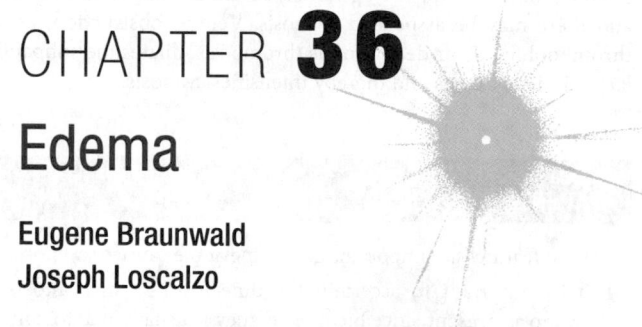

CHAPTER 36

Edema

Eugene Braunwald
Joseph Loscalzo

Edema is defined as a clinically apparent increase in the interstitial fluid volume, which may expand by several liters before the abnormality is evident. Therefore, a weight gain of several kilograms usually precedes overt manifestations of edema, and a similar weight loss from diuresis can be induced in a slightly edematous patient before "dry weight" is achieved. *Anasarca* refers to gross, generalized edema. *Ascites* (Chap. 43) and *hydrothorax* refer to accumulation of excess fluid in the peritoneal and pleural cavities, respectively, and are considered special forms of edema.

Depending on its cause and mechanism, edema may be localized or have a generalized distribution. Edema is recognized in its generalized form by puffiness of the face, which is most readily apparent in the periorbital areas, and by the persistence of an indentation of the skin after pressure; this is known as "pitting" edema. In its more subtle form, edema may be detected by noting that after the stethoscope is removed from the chest wall, the rim of the bell leaves an indentation on the skin of the chest for a few minutes. When the ring on a finger fits more snugly than in the past or when a patient complains of difficulty putting on shoes, particularly in the evening, edema may be present.

■ PATHOGENESIS

About one-third of total-body water is confined to the extracellular space. Approximately 75% of the latter is interstitial fluid, and the remainder is in the plasma compartment.

Starling forces

The forces that regulate the disposition of fluid between these two components of the extracellular compartment frequently are referred to as the *Starling forces*. The hydrostatic pressure within the vascular system and the colloid oncotic pressure in the interstitial fluid tend to promote movement of fluid from the vascular to the extravascular space. By contrast, the colloid oncotic pressure contributed by plasma proteins and the hydrostatic pressure within the interstitial fluid promote the movement of fluid into the vascular compartment.

As a consequence of these forces, there is movement of water and diffusible solutes from the vascular space at the arteriolar end of the capillaries. Fluid is returned from the interstitial space into the vascular system at the venous end of the capillaries and by way of the lymphatics. Unless these channels are obstructed, lymph flow rises with increases in net movement of fluid from the vascular compartment to the interstitium. These flows are usually balanced so that there is a steady state in the sizes of the intravascular and interstitial compartments, yet a large exchange between them occurs. However, if either the hydrostatic or the oncotic pressure gradient is altered significantly, a further net movement of fluid between the two components of the extracellular space will take place. The development of edema then depends on one or more alterations in the Starling forces so that there is increased flow of fluid from the vascular system into the interstitium or into a body cavity.

Edema due to an increase in capillary pressure may result from an elevation of venous pressure caused by obstruction to venous and/or lymphatic drainage. An increase in capillary pressure may be generalized, as occurs in congestive heart failure (see below). The Starling forces also may be imbalanced when the colloid oncotic pressure of the plasma is reduced owing to any factor that may induce hypoalbuminemia, such as severe malnutrition, liver disease, loss of protein into the urine or into the gastrointestinal tract, or a severe catabolic state. Edema may be localized to one extremity when venous pressure is elevated due to unilateral thrombophlebitis (see below).

Capillary damage

Edema may also result from damage to the capillary endothelium, which increases its permeability and permits the transfer of proteins into the interstitial compartment. Injury to the capillary wall can result from drugs, viral or bacterial agents, and thermal or mechanical trauma. Increased capillary permeability also may be a consequence of a hypersensitivity reaction and is characteristic of immune injury. Damage to the capillary endothelium is presumably responsible for inflammatory edema, which is usually nonpitting, localized, and accompanied by other signs of inflammation—i.e., erythema, heat, and tenderness.

Reduction of effective arterial volume

In many forms of edema, the effective arterial blood volume, a parameter that represents the filling of the arterial tree, is reduced. Underfilling of the arterial tree may be caused by a reduction of cardiac output and/or systemic vascular resistance. As a consequence of underfilling, a series of physiologic responses designed to restore the effective arterial volume to normal are set into motion. A key element of these responses is the retention of salt and, therefore, of water, ultimately leading to edema.

Renal factors and the renin-angiotensin-aldosterone (RAA) system

(See also Chap. 342) In the final analysis, renal retention of Na^+ is central to the development of generalized edema (Fig. 36-1). The diminished renal blood flow characteristic of states in which the effective arterial blood volume is reduced is translated by the renal juxtaglomerular cells (specialized myoepithelial cells surrounding the afferent arteriole) into a signal for increased renin release. Renin is an enzyme with a molecular mass of about 40,000 Da that acts on its substrate, angiotensinogen, an α_2-globulin synthesized by the liver, to release angiotensin I, a decapeptide, which in turn is converted to angiotensin II (AII), an octapeptide. AII has generalized vasoconstrictor properties; it is especially active on the renal efferent arterioles. This action reduces the hydrostatic pressure in the peritubular capillaries, whereas the increased filtration fraction raises the colloid osmotic pressure in these vessels, thereby enhancing salt and water reabsorption in the proximal tubule as well as in the ascending limb of the loop of Henle.

The renin-angiotensin-aldosterone (RAA) system has long been recognized as a hormonal system; however, it also operates locally. Intrarenally produced AII contributes to glomerular efferent arteriolar constriction, and this "tubuloglomerular feedback" causes salt and water retention and thereby contributes to the formation of edema.

AII that enters the systemic circulation stimulates the production of aldosterone by the zona glomerulosa of the adrenal cortex. Aldosterone in turn enhances Na^+ reabsorption (and K^+ excretion) by the collecting tubule. In patients with heart failure, not only is aldosterone secretion elevated but the biologic

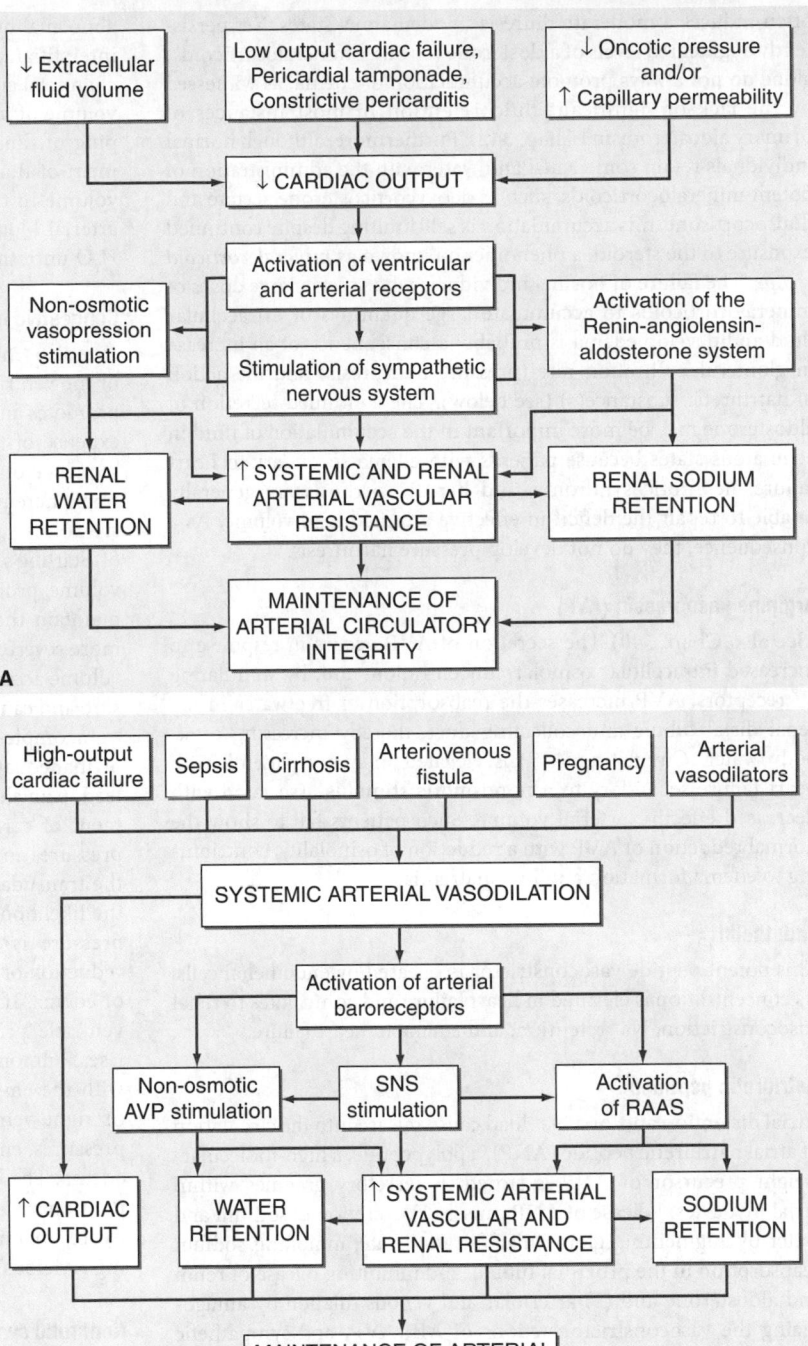

Figure 36-1 Clinical conditions in which a decrease in cardiac output (*A*) and systemic arterial vasodilation (*B*) cause arterial underfilling with resulting neurohumoral activation and renal sodium and water retention. In addition to activating the neurohumoral axis, adrenergic stimulation causes renal vasoconstriction and enhances sodium and fluid transport by the proximal tubule epithelium. SNS, sympathetic nervous system; RAAS, renin-angiotensin aldosterone system. (*Reprinted from RW Schrier: Ann Intern Med 113:155, 1990.*)

half-life of aldosterone is prolonged, which increases further the plasma level of the hormone. A depression of hepatic blood flow, especially during exercise, is responsible for reduced hepatic catabolism of aldosterone.

Increased quantities of aldosterone are secreted in heart failure and in other edematous states, and blockade of the action of aldosterone by spironolactone or eplerenone (aldosterone antagonists) or by amiloride (a blocker of epithelial Na^+ channels) often induces a moderate diuresis in edematous states. Yet persistently augmented levels of aldosterone (or other mineralocorticoids) alone do not always promote accumulation of edema, as witnessed by the lack of significant fluid retention in most instances of primary aldosteronism (Chap. 342). Furthermore, although normal individuals retain some NaCl and water with the administration of potent mineralocorticoids, such as deoxycorticosterone acetate and fludrocortisone, this accumulation is self-limiting despite continued exposure to the steroid, a phenomenon known as *mineralocorticoid escape*. The failure of normal individuals who receive large doses of mineralocorticoids to accumulate large quantities of extracellular fluid and develop edema is probably a consequence of an increase in glomerular filtration rate (pressure natriuresis) and the action of natriuretic substance(s) (see below). The continued secretion of aldosterone may be more important in the accumulation of fluid in edematous states because patients with edema secondary to heart failure, nephrotic syndrome, and hepatic cirrhosis are generally unable to repair the deficit in effective arterial blood volume. As a consequence, they do not develop pressure natriuresis.

Arginine vasopressin (AVP)

(See also Chap. 340) The secretion of AVP occurs in response to increased intracellular osmolar concentration, and, by stimulating V_2 receptors, AVP increases the reabsorption of free water in the renal distal tubule and collecting duct, thereby increasing total-body water. Circulating AVP is elevated in many patients with heart failure secondary to a nonosmotic stimulus associated with decreased effective arterial volume. Such patients fail to show the normal reduction of AVP with a reduction of osmolality, contributing to edema formation and hyponatremia.

Endothelin

This potent peptide vasoconstrictor is released by endothelial cells. Its concentration is elevated in heart failure and contributes to renal vasoconstriction, Na$^+$ retention, and edema in heart failure.

Natriuretic peptides

Atrial distention and/or a Na$^+$ load cause release into the circulation of atrial natriuretic peptide (ANP), a polypeptide; a high-molecular-weight precursor of ANP is stored in secretory granules within atrial myocytes. Release of ANP causes (1) excretion of sodium and water by augmenting glomerular filtration rate, inhibiting sodium reabsorption in the proximal tubule, and inhibiting release of renin and aldosterone and (2) arteriolar and venous dilation by antagonizing the vasoconstrictor actions of AII, AVP, and sympathetic stimulation. Thus, ANP has the capacity to oppose Na$^+$ retention and arterial pressure elevation in hypervolemic states.

The closely related brain natriuretic peptide (BNP) is stored primarily in ventricular myocardium and is released when ventricular diastolic pressure rises. Its actions are similar to those of ANP, and both BNP and ANP bind to the natriuretic receptor-A, which is found in the myocardium. Yet another natriuretic peptide, C-type (CNP), is of endothelial and renal origin. CNP binds preferentially to the natriuretic peptide receptor-B, which is expressed principally in veins. Circulating levels of ANP and BNP are elevated in congestive heart failure and in cirrhosis with ascites, but obviously not sufficiently to prevent edema formation. In addition, in edematous states there is abnormal resistance to the actions of natriuretic peptides.

■ CLINICAL CAUSES OF EDEMA

Obstruction of venous (and lymphatic) drainage of a limb

In this condition the hydrostatic pressure in the capillary bed upstream (proximal) to the obstruction increases so that an abnormal quantity of fluid is transferred from the vascular to the interstitial space. Since the alternative route (i.e., the lymphatic channels) also may be obstructed or maximally filled, an increased volume of interstitial fluid in the limb develops (i.e., there is trapping of fluid in the interstitium of the extremity). The displacement of fluid into a limb may occur at the expense of the blood volume in the remainder of the body, thereby reducing effective arterial blood volume and leading to the retention of NaCl and H$_2$O until the deficit in plasma volume has been corrected.

Congestive heart failure

(See also Chap. 234) In this disorder the impaired systolic emptying of the ventricle(s) and/or the impairment of ventricular relaxation promotes an accumulation of blood in the venous circulation at the expense of the effective arterial volume, and the aforementioned sequence of events (Fig. 36-1) is initiated. In mild heart failure, a small increment of total blood volume may repair the deficit of arterial volume and establish a new steady state. Through the operation of Starling's law of the heart, an increase in ventricular diastolic volume promotes a more forceful contraction and may thereby maintain the cardiac output. However, if the cardiac disorder is more severe, fluid retention continues, and the increment in blood volume accumulates in the venous circulation, raising venous pressure and causing edema.

Incomplete ventricular emptying (systolic heart failure) and/or inadequate ventricular relaxation (diastolic heart failure) both lead to an elevation of ventricular diastolic pressure. If the impairment of cardiac function primarily involves the right ventricle, pressures in the systemic veins and capillaries rise, augmenting the transudation of fluid into the interstitial space and enhancing the likelihood of peripheral edema. The elevated systemic venous pressure is transmitted to the thoracic duct with consequent reduction of lymph drainage, further increasing the accumulation of edema. If the impairment of cardiac function involves the left ventricle primarily, pulmonary venous and capillary pressures rise. Pulmonary artery pressure rises, and this in turn interferes with the emptying of the right ventricle, leading to an elevation of right ventricular diastolic and central and systemic venous pressures, enhancing the likelihood of the formation of peripheral edema. The elevation of pulmonary capillary pressure may cause pulmonary edema, which impairs gas exchange. The resulting hypoxemia may impair cardiac function further, sometimes causing a vicious circle.

Nephrotic syndrome and other hypoalbuminemic states

(See also Chap. 283) The primary alteration in this disorder is a diminished colloid oncotic pressure due to losses of large quantities of protein into the urine. With severe hypoalbuminemia and the consequent reduced colloid osmotic pressure, the NaCl and H$_2$O that are retained cannot be restrained within the vascular compartment, and total and effective arterial blood volumes decline. This process initiates the edema-forming sequence of events described above, including activation of the RAA system. Impaired renal function contributes further to the formation of edema. A similar sequence of events occurs in other conditions that lead to *severe* hypoalbuminemia, including (1) severe nutritional deficiency states, (2) severe, chronic liver disease (see below), and (3) protein-losing enteropathy.

Cirrhosis

(See also Chaps. 43 and 308) This condition is characterized in part by hepatic venous outflow blockade, which in turn expands the splanchnic blood volume and increases hepatic lymph formation. Intrahepatic hypertension acts as a stimulus for renal

TABLE 36-1 Drugs Associated With Edema Formation

Nonsteroidal anti-inflammatory drugs
Antihypertensive agents
    Direct arterial/arteriolar vasodilators
        Hydralazine
        Clonidine
        Methyldopa
        Guanethidine
        Minoxidil
    Calcium channel antagonists
    α-Adrenergic antagonists
    Thiazolidinediones
Steroid hormones
    Glucocorticoids
    Anabolic steroids
    Estrogens
    Progestins
Cyclosporine
Growth hormone
Immunotherapies
    Interleukin 2
    OKT3 monoclonal antibody

Source: From Chertow.

Na^+ retention and a reduction of effective arterial blood volume. These alterations frequently are complicated by hypoalbuminemia secondary to reduced hepatic synthesis, as well as systemic vasodilation. These effects reduce the effective arterial blood volume further, leading to activation of the RAA system, renal sympathetic nerves, and other $NaCl$- and H_2O-retaining mechanisms. The concentration of circulating aldosterone often is elevated by the failure of the liver to metabolize this hormone. Initially, the excess interstitial fluid is localized preferentially proximal (upstream) to the congested portal venous system and obstructed hepatic lymphatics, i.e., in the peritoneal cavity (ascites, Chap. 43). In later stages, particularly when there is severe hypoalbuminemia, peripheral edema may develop. The excess production of prostaglandins (PGE_2 and PGI_2) in cirrhosis attenuates renal Na^+ retention. When the synthesis of these substances is inhibited by nonsteroidal anti-inflammatory drugs (NSAIDs), renal function deteriorates and Na^+ retention increases.

Drug-induced edema

A large number of widely used drugs can cause edema (Table 36-1). Mechanisms include renal vasoconstriction (NSAIDs and cyclosporine), arteriolar dilation (vasodilators), augmented renal Na^+ reabsorption (steroid hormones), and capillary damage (interleukin 2).

DIFFERENTIAL DIAGNOSIS

■ LOCALIZED EDEMA

(See also Chap. 249) Localized edema due to venous or lymphatic obstruction may be caused by thrombophlebitis, chronic lymphangitis, resection of regional lymph nodes, filariasis, etc. Lymphedema is particularly intractable because restriction of lymphatic flow results in increased protein concentration in the interstitial fluid, a circumstance that aggravates retention of fluid.

■ GENERALIZED EDEMA

The differences among the major causes of generalized edema are shown in Table 36-2.

A majority of patients with generalized edema develop cardiac, renal, hepatic, or nutritional disorders. Consequently, the differential diagnosis of generalized edema should be directed toward identifying or excluding these several conditions.

Edema of heart failure

(See also Chap. 234) The presence of heart disease, as manifested by cardiac enlargement and a gallop rhythm, together with evidence of cardiac failure, such as dyspnea, basilar rales, venous distention, and hepatomegaly, usually indicates that edema results from heart failure. Noninvasive tests such as echocardiography may be helpful in establishing the diagnosis of heart disease. The edema of heart failure typically occurs in the dependent portions of the body.

Edema of acute glomerulonephritis and other forms of renal failure

(See also Chap. 283) The edema that occurs during the acute phases of glomerulonephritis is characteristically associated with hematuria, proteinuria, and hypertension. Although some evidence supports the view that the fluid retention is due to increased capillary permeability, in most instances, the edema results from primary retention of $NaCl$ and H_2O by the kidneys owing to renal insufficiency. This state differs from congestive heart failure in that it is characterized by a normal (or sometimes even increased) cardiac output and a normal arterial–mixed venous oxygen difference. Patients with edema due to renal failure commonly have evidence of arterial hypertension as well as pulmonary congestion on chest roentgenogram even without cardiac enlargement, but they may not develop orthopnea. Patients with *chronic* renal failure may also develop edema due to primary renal retention of $NaCl$ and H_2O.

Edema of the nephrotic syndrome

(See also Chap. 283) Marked proteinuria (>3.5 g/d), hypoalbuminemia (<35 g/L), and, in some instances, hypercholesterolemia are present. This syndrome may occur during the course of a variety of kidney diseases, which include glomerulonephritis, diabetic glomerulosclerosis, and hypersensitivity reactions. A history of previous renal disease may or may not be elicited.

Edema of cirrhosis

(See also Chap. 308) Ascites and biochemical and clinical evidence of hepatic disease (collateral venous channels, jaundice, and spider angiomata) characterize edema of hepatic origin. The ascites (Chap. 43) is frequently refractory to treatment because it collects as a result of a combination of obstruction of hepatic lymphatic drainage, portal hypertension, and hypoalbuminemia. A sizable accumulation of ascitic fluid may increase intra-abdominal pressure and impede venous return from the lower extremities; hence, it tends to promote accumulation of edema in this region as well.

Edema of nutritional origin

A diet grossly deficient in protein over a prolonged period may produce hypoproteinemia and edema. The latter may be intensified by the development of beriberi heart disease, which also is of nutritional origin, in which multiple peripheral arteriovenous

TABLE 36-2 Principal Causes of Generalized Edema: History, Physical Examination, and Laboratory Findings

Organ System	History	Physical Examination	Laboratory Findings
Cardiac	Dyspnea with exertion prominent—often associated with orthopnea—or paroxysmal nocturnal dyspnea	Elevated jugular venous pressure, ventricular (S_3) gallop; occasionally with displaced or dyskinetic apical pulse; peripheral cyanosis, cool extremities, small pulse pressure when severe	Elevated urea nitrogen-to-creatinine ratio common; elevated uric acid; serum sodium often diminished; liver enzymes occasionally elevated with hepatic congestion
Hepatic	Dyspnea uncommon, except if associated with significant degree of ascites; most often a history of ethanol abuse	Frequently associated with ascites; jugular venous pressure normal or low; blood pressure lower than in renal or cardiac disease; one or more additional signs of chronic liver disease (jaundice, palmar erythema, Dupuytren's contracture, spider angiomata, male gynecomastia; asterixis and other signs of encephalopathy) may be present	If severe, reductions in serum albumin, cholesterol, other hepatic proteins (transferrin, fibrinogen); liver enzymes elevated, depending on the cause and acuity of liver injury; tendency toward hypokalemia, respiratory alkalosis; macrocytosis from folate deficiency
Renal (CRF)	Usually chronic: may be associated with uremic signs and symptoms, including decreased appetite, altered (metallic or fishy) taste, altered sleep pattern, difficulty concentrating, restless legs or myoclonus; dyspnea can be present, but generally less prominent than in heart failure	Elevated blood pressure; hypertensive retinopathy; nitrogenous fetor; pericardial friction rub in advanced cases with uremia	Albuminuria, hypoalbuminemia; sometimes, elevation of serum creatinine and urea nitrogen; hyperkalemia, metabolic acidosis, hyperphosphatemia, hypocalcemia, anemia (usually normocytic)
Renal (NS)	Childhood diabetes mellitus; plasma cell dyscrasias	Periorbital edema; hypertension	Proteinuria (3.5 g/d); hypoalbuminemia; hypercholesterolemia; microscopic hematuria

Abbreviations: CRF, chronic renal failure; NS, nephrotic syndrome.

Source: Modified from Chertow.

fistulas result in reduced effective systemic perfusion and effective arterial blood volume, thereby enhancing edema formation (Chap. 74). Edema may actually become intensified when famished subjects are first provided with an adequate diet. The ingestion of more food may increase the quantity of NaCl ingested, which is then retained along with H_2O. So-called refeeding edema also may be linked to increased release of insulin, which directly increases tubular Na^+ reabsorption. In addition to hypoalbuminemia, hypokalemia and caloric deficits may be involved in the edema of starvation.

Other causes of edema

These causes include hypothyroidism (myxedema) and hyperthyroidism (pretibial myxedema secondary to Graves' disease), the edema in which is typically nonpitting and due to deposition of hyaluronic acid and, in Graves' disease, lymphocytic infiltration and inflammation; exogenous hyperadrenocortism; pregnancy; and administration of estrogens and vasodilators, particularly dihydropyridines such as nifedipine.

◼ DISTRIBUTION OF EDEMA

The distribution of edema is an important guide to its cause. Thus, edema limited to one leg or to one or both arms is usually the result of venous and/or lymphatic obstruction. Edema resulting from hypoproteinemia characteristically is generalized, but it is especially evident in the very soft tissues of the eyelids and face and tends to be most pronounced in the morning because of the recumbent posture assumed during the night. Less common causes of facial edema include trichinosis, allergic reactions, and myxedema. Edema associated with heart failure, by contrast, tends to be more extensive in the legs and to be accentuated in the evening, a feature also determined largely by posture. When patients with heart failure have been confined to bed, edema may be most prominent in the presacral region. Paralysis reduces lymphatic and venous drainage on the affected side and may be responsible for unilateral edema.

◼ ADDITIONAL FACTORS IN DIAGNOSIS

The color, thickness, and sensitivity of the skin are significant. Local tenderness and warmth suggest inflammation. Local cyanosis may signify venous obstruction. In individuals who have had repeated episodes of prolonged edema, the skin over the involved areas may be thickened, indurated, and often red.

Estimation of the venous pressure is of importance in evaluating edema. Ordinarily, a significant generalized increase in venous pressure can be recognized by the level at which cervical veins collapse (Chap. 227). In patients with obstruction of the superior vena cava, edema is confined to the face, neck, and upper extremities, in which the venous pressure is elevated compared with that in the lower extremities. Severe heart failure may cause ascites that may be distinguished from the ascites caused by hepatic cirrhosis by the jugular venous pressure, which is usually elevated in heart failure and normal in cirrhosis.

Determination of the concentration of serum albumin aids importantly in identifying those patients in whom edema is due, at least in part, to diminished intravascular colloid oncotic pressure. The presence of proteinuria also affords useful clues. The absence of proteinuria excludes nephrotic syndrome but cannot exclude nonproteinuric causes of renal failure. Slight to moderate proteinuria is the rule in patients with heart failure.

APPROACH TO THE
PATIENT | Edema

An important first question is whether the edema is localized or generalized. If it is localized, the local phenomena that may be responsible should be considered. If the edema is generalized, one should first determine if there is serious hypoalbuminemia, e.g., serum albumin <25 g/L. If so, the history, physical examination, urinalysis, and other laboratory data will help evaluate the question of cirrhosis, severe malnutrition, or the nephrotic syndrome as the underlying disorder. If hypoalbuminemia is not present, one should determine if there is evidence of congestive heart failure severe enough to promote generalized edema. Finally, one should determine whether the patient has an adequate urine output or if there is significant oliguria or anuria. These abnormalities are discussed in Chaps. 44, 279, and 280.

FURTHER READINGS

BANSAL S et al: Sodium retention in heart failure and cirrhosis: Potential role of natriuretic doses of mineralocorticoid antagonist? Circ Heart Fail 2:370, 2009

CHERTOW GM: Approach to the patient with edema, in *Primary Cardiology*, 2nd ed, E Braunwald, L Goldman (eds). Philadelphia, Saunders, 2003, pp 117–128

LEE CYW, BURNETT JC Jr: Natriuretic peptides and therapeutic application. Heart Fail Rev 12:131, 2007

MCCULLOUGH JC: Renal disorders and heart disease, in *Braunwald's Heart Disease*, 8th ed, P Libby et al (eds). Philadelphia, Saunders, 2008

SCHRIER RW: Decreased effective blood volume in edematous disorders: What does this mean? J Am Soc Nephrol 18:2028, 2007

SKORECKI KL et al: Extracellular fluid and edema formation, in *Brenner and Rector's The Kidney*, 8th ed. Philadelphia, Elsevier, 2008

STREETEN DH: Idiopathic edema: Pathogenesis, clinical features, and treatment. Endocrinol Metab Clin North Am 24:531, 1995

CHAPTER **37**

Palpitations

Joseph Loscalzo

Palpitations are extremely common among patients who present to their internist and can best be defined as an intermittent "thumping," "pounding," or "fluttering" sensation in the chest. This sensation can be either intermittent or sustained and either regular or irregular. Most patients interpret palpitations as an unusual awareness of the heartbeat, and become especially concerned when they sense that they have had "skipped" or "missing" heartbeats. Palpitations are often noted when the patient is quietly resting, during which time other stimuli are minimal. Palpitations that are positional generally reflect a structural process within (e.g., atrial myxoma) or adjacent to (e.g., mediastinal mass) the heart.

Palpitations are brought about by cardiac (43%), psychiatric (31%), miscellaneous (10%), and unknown (16%) causes, according to one large series. Among the cardiovascular causes are premature atrial and ventricular contractions, supraventricular and ventricular arrhythmias, mitral valve prolapse (with or without associated arrhythmias), aortic insufficiency, atrial myxoma, and pulmonary embolism. Intermittent palpitations are commonly caused by premature atrial or ventricular contractions: the post-extrasystolic beat is sensed by the patient owing to the increase in ventricular end-diastolic dimension following the pause in the cardiac cycle and the increased strength of contraction (post-extrasystolic potentiation) of that beat. Regular, sustained palpitations can be caused by regular supraventricular and ventricular tachycardias. Irregular, sustained palpitations can be caused by atrial fibrillation. It is important to note that most arrhythmias are not associated with palpitations. In those that are, it is often useful either to ask the patient to "tap out" the rhythm of the palpitations or to take his/her pulse while experiencing palpitations. In general, hyperdynamic cardiovascular states caused by catecholaminergic stimulation from exercise, stress, or pheochromocytoma can lead to palpitations. Palpitations

are common among athletes, especially older endurance athletes. In addition, the enlarged ventricle of aortic regurgitation and accompanying hyperdynamic precordium frequently lead to the sensation of palpitations. Other factors that enhance the strength of myocardial contraction, including tobacco, caffeine, aminophylline, atropine, thyroxine, cocaine, and amphetamines, can cause palpitations.

Psychiatric causes of palpitations include panic attacks or disorders, anxiety states, and somatization, alone or in combination. Patients with psychiatric causes for palpitations more commonly report a longer duration of the sensation (>15 min) and other accompanying symptoms than do patients with other causes. Among the miscellaneous causes of palpitations included are thyrotoxicosis, drugs (see above) and ethanol, spontaneous skeletal muscle contractions of the chest wall, pheochromocytoma, and systemic mastocytosis.

APPROACH TO THE
PATIENT | Palpitations

The principal goal in assessing patients with palpitations is to determine if the symptom is caused by a life-threatening arrhythmia. Patients with preexisting coronary artery disease (CAD) or risk factors for CAD are at greatest risk for ventricular arrhythmias as a cause for palpitations. In addition, the association of palpitations with other symptoms suggesting hemodynamic compromise, including syncope or lightheadedness, supports this diagnosis. Palpitations caused by sustained tachyarrhythmias in patients with CAD can be accompanied by angina pectoris or dyspnea, and in patients with ventricular dysfunction (systolic or diastolic), aortic stenosis, hypertrophic cardiomyopathy, or mitral stenosis, with or without CAD, can be accompanied by dyspnea from increased left atrial and pulmonary venous pressure.

Key features of the physical examination that will help confirm or refute the presence of an arrhythmia as a cause for the palpitations and its adverse hemodynamic consequences include measurement of the vital signs, assessment of the jugular venous pressure and pulse, and auscultation of the chest and precordium. A resting electrocardiogram can be used to document the arrhythmia. If exertion is known to induce the arrhythmia and accompanying palpitations, exercise electrocardiography can be used to make the diagnosis. If the arrhythmia is sufficiently infrequent, other methods must be used, including continuous electrocardiographic (Holter) monitoring; telephonic monitoring, through which the patient can transmit an electrocardiographic tracing during a sensed episode; loop recordings (external or implantable), which can capture the electrocardiographic event for later review; and mobile cardiac outpatient telemetry. Recent data suggest that Holter monitoring is of limited clinical utility, while the implantable loop recorder and mobile cardiac outpatient telemetry are safe and possibly more cost-effective in the assessment of patients with recurrent, unexplained palpitations.

Most patients with palpitations do not have serious arrhythmias or underlying structural heart disease. Occasional benign atrial or ventricular premature contractions can often be managed with beta-blocker therapy if sufficiently troubling to the patient. Palpitations incited by alcohol, tobacco, or illicit drugs need to be managed by abstention, while those caused by pharmacologic agents should be addressed by considering alternate therapies when appropriate or possible. Psychiatric causes of palpitations may benefit from cognitive or pharmacotherapies. The physician should note that palpitations are at the very least bothersome and, on occasion, frightening to the patient. Once

serious causes for the symptom have been excluded, the patient should be reassured that the palpitations will not adversely affect prognosis.

FURTHER READINGS

ABBOTT AV: Diagnostic approach to palpitations. Am Fam Phys 71:743, 2005

GIADA F et al: Recurrent unexplained palpitations (RUP) study. J Am Coll Cardiol 49:1951, 2007

LAWLESS CE, BRINER W: Palpitations in athletes. Sports Med 38:687, 2008

OLSON JA et al: Utility of mobile cardiac outpatient telemetry for the diagnosis of palpitations, presyncope, syncope, and the assessment of therapy efficacy. J Cardiovasc Electrophysiol 18:473, 2007

SULFI S et al: Limited clinical utility of Holter monitoring in patients with palpitations or altered consciousness: analysis of 8973 recordings in 7394 patients. Ann Noninvasive Electrocardiol 13:39, 2008

WEBER BE, KAPOOR WN: Evaluation and outcomes of patients with palpitations. Am J Med 100:138, 1996

CHAPTER **38**

Dysphagia

Ikuo Hirano

Peter J. Kahrilas

Dysphagia—difficulty with swallowing—refers to problems with the transit of food or liquid from the mouth to the hypopharynx or through the esophagus. Severe dysphagia can compromise nutrition, cause aspiration, and reduce quality of life. Additional terminology pertaining to swallowing dysfunction is as follows. *Aphagia* denotes complete esophageal obstruction, most commonly encountered in the acute setting of a food bolus or foreign body impaction. *Odynophagia* refers to painful swallowing, typically resulting from mucosal ulceration within the oropharynx or esophagus. It commonly is accompanied by dysphagia, but the converse is not true. *Globus pharyngeus* is a foreign body sensation localized in the neck that does not interfere with swallowing and sometimes is relieved by swallowing. *Transfer dysphagia* frequently results in nasal regurgitation and pulmonary aspiration during swallowing and is characteristic of oropharyngeal dysphagia. *Phagophobia* (fear of swallowing) and *refusal to swallow* may be psychogenic or related to anticipatory anxiety about food bolus obstruction, odynophagia, or aspiration.

■ PHYSIOLOGY OF SWALLOWING

Swallowing begins with a voluntary (oral) phase that includes preparation during which food is masticated and mixed with saliva. This is followed by a transfer phase during which the bolus is pushed into the pharynx by the tongue. Bolus entry into the hypopharynx initiates the pharyngeal swallow response, which is centrally mediated and involves a complex series of actions, the net result of which is to propel food through the pharynx into the esophagus while preventing its entry into the airway. To accomplish this, the larynx is elevated and pulled forward, actions that also facilitate upper esophageal sphincter (UES) opening. Tongue pulsion then propels the bolus through the UES, followed by a peristaltic contraction that clears residue from the pharynx and through the esophagus. The lower esophageal sphincter (LES) relaxes as the food enters the esophagus and remains relaxed until the peristaltic contraction has delivered the bolus into the stomach. Peristaltic contractions elicited in response to a swallow are called *primary peristalsis* and involve sequenced inhibition followed by contraction of the musculature along the entire length of the esophagus. The inhibition that precedes the peristaltic contraction is called *deglutitive inhibition*. Local distention of the esophagus anywhere along its length, as may occur with gastroesophageal reflux, activates *secondary peristalsis* that begins at the point of distention and proceeds distally. Tertiary esophageal contractions are nonperistaltic, disordered esophageal contractions that may be observed to occur spontaneously during fluoroscopic observation.

The musculature of the oral cavity, pharynx, UES, and cervical esophagus is striated and directly innervated by lower motor neurons carried in cranial nerves (Fig. 38-1). Oral cavity muscles are innervated by the fifth (trigeminal) and seventh (facial) cranial nerves;

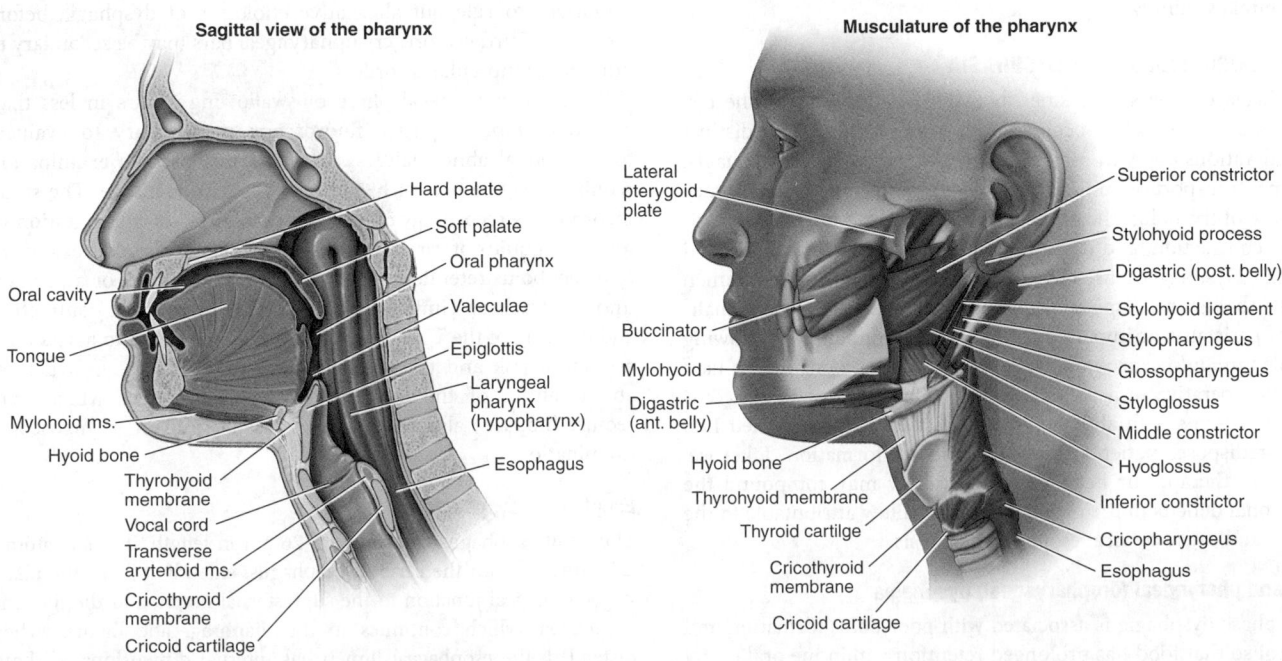

Sagittal view of the pharynx

Hard palate
Soft palate
Oral pharynx
Valeculae
Epiglottis
Laryngeal pharynx (hypopharynx)
Esophagus

Oral cavity
Tongue
Mylohoid ms.
Hyoid bone
Thyrohyoid membrane
Vocal cord
Transverse arytenoid ms.
Cricothyroid membrane
Cricoid cartilage

Musculature of the pharynx

Lateral pterygoid plate
Buccinator
Mylohyoid
Digastric (ant. belly)
Hyoid bone
Thyrohyoid membrane
Thyroid cartilge
Cricothyroid membrane
Cricoid cartilage

Superior constrictor
Stylohyoid process
Digastric (post. belly)
Stylohyoid ligament
Stylopharyngeus
Glossopharyngeus
Styloglossus
Middle constrictor
Hyoglossus
Inferior constrictor
Cricopharyngeus
Esophagus

Figure 38-1 Sagittal and diagrammatic views of the musculature involved in enacting oropharyngeal swallowing. Note the dominance of the tongue in the sagittal view and the intimate relationship between the entrance to the larynx (airway) and the esophagus. In the resting configuration illustrated, the esophageal inlet is closed. This is transiently reconfigured such that the esophageal inlet is open and the laryngeal inlet closed during swallowing. [Adapted from PJ Kahrilas, in DW Gelfand and JE Richter (eds): Dysphagia: Diagnosis and Treatment. New York: Igaku-Shoin Medical Publishers, 1989, pp. 11–28.]

the tongue, by the twelfth (hypoglossal) cranial nerve. Pharyngeal muscles are innervated by the ninth (glossopharyngeal) and tenth (vagus) cranial nerves.

Physiologically, the UES consists of the cricopharyngeus muscle, the adjacent inferior pharyngeal constrictor, and the proximal portion of the cervical esophagus. UES innervation is derived from the vagus nerve, whereas the innervation to the musculature acting on the UES to facilitate its opening during swallowing comes from the fifth, seventh, and twelfth cranial nerves. The UES remains closed at rest owing to both its inherent elastic properties and neurogenically mediated contraction of the cricopharyngeus muscle. UES opening during swallowing involves both cessation of vagal excitation to the cricopharyngeus and simultaneous contraction of the suprahyoid and geniohyoid muscles that pull open the UES in conjunction with the upward and forward displacement of the larynx.

The neuromuscular apparatus for peristalsis is distinct in proximal and distal parts of the esophagus. The cervical esophagus, like the pharyngeal musculature, consists of striated muscle and is directly innervated by lower motor neurons of the vagus nerve. Peristalsis in the proximal esophagus is governed by the sequential activation of the vagal motor neurons in the nucleus ambiguus. In contrast, the distal esophagus and LES are composed of smooth muscle and are controlled by excitatory and inhibitory neurons within the esophageal myenteric plexus. Medullary preganglionic neurons from the dorsal motor nucleus of the vagus trigger peristalsis via these ganglionic neurons during primary peristalsis. Neurotransmitters of the excitatory ganglionic neurons are acetylcholine and substance P; those of the inhibitory neurons are vasoactive intestinal peptide and nitric oxide. Peristalsis results from the patterned activation of inhibitory followed by excitatory ganglionic neurons, with progressive dominance of the inhibitory neurons distally. Similarly, LES relaxation occurs with the onset of deglutitive inhibition and persists until the peristaltic sequence is complete. At rest, the LES is contracted because of excitatory ganglionic stimulation and its intrinsic myogenic tone, a property that distinguishes it from the adjacent esophagus. The function of the LES is supplemented by the surrounding muscle of the right diaphragmatic crus, which acts as an external sphincter during inspiration, cough, or abdominal straining.

■ PATHOPHYSIOLOGY OF DYSPHAGIA

Dysphagia can be subclassified both by location and by the circumstances in which it occurs. With respect to location, distinct considerations apply to oral, pharyngeal, or esophageal dysphagia. Normal transport of an ingested bolus depends on the consistency and size of the bolus, the caliber of the lumen, the integrity of peristaltic contraction, and deglutitive inhibition of both the UES and the LES. Dysphagia caused by an oversized bolus or a narrow lumen is called *structural dysphagia*, whereas dysphagia due to abnormalities of peristalsis or impaired sphincter relaxation after swallowing is called *propulsive* or *motor dysphagia*. More than one mechanism may be operative in a patient with dysphagia. Scleroderma commonly presents with absent peristalsis as well as a weakened LES that predisposes patients to peptic stricture formation. Likewise, radiation therapy for head and neck cancer may compound the functional deficits in the oropharyngeal swallow attributable to the tumor and cause cervical esophageal stenosis.

Oral and pharyngeal (oropharyngeal) dysphagia

Oral-phase dysphagia is associated with poor bolus formation and control so that food has prolonged retention within the oral cavity and may seep out of the mouth. Drooling and difficulty in initiating swallowing are other characteristic signs. Poor bolus control also may lead to premature spillage of food into the hypopharynx with resultant aspiration into the trachea or regurgitation into the nasal

cavity. Pharyngeal-phase dysphagia is associated with retention of food in the pharynx due to poor tongue or pharyngeal propulsion or obstruction at the UES. Signs and symptoms of concomitant hoarseness or cranial nerve dysfunction may be associated with oropharyngeal dysphagia.

Oropharyngeal dysphagia may be due to neurologic, muscular, structural, iatrogenic, infectious, and metabolic causes. Iatrogenic, neurologic, and structural pathologies are most common. Iatrogenic causes include surgery and radiation, often in the setting of head and neck cancer. Neurogenic dysphagia resulting from cerebrovascular accidents, Parkinson's disease, and amyotrophic lateral sclerosis is a major source of morbidity related to aspiration and malnutrition. Medullary nuclei directly innervate the oropharynx. Lateralization of pharyngeal dysphagia implies either a structural pharyngeal lesion or a neurologic process that selectively targeted the ipsilateral brainstem nuclei or cranial nerve. Advances in functional brain imaging have elucidated an important role of the cerebral cortex in swallow function and dysphagia. Asymmetry in the cortical representation of the pharynx provides an explanation for the dysphagia that occurs as a consequence of unilateral cortical cerebrovascular accidents.

Oropharyngeal structural lesions causing dysphagia include Zenker's diverticulum, cricopharyngeal bar, and neoplasia. Zenker's diverticulum typically is encountered in elderly patients, with an estimated prevalence between 1:1000 and 1:10,000. In addition to dysphagia, patients may present with regurgitation of particulate food debris, aspiration, and halitosis. The pathogenesis is related to stenosis of the cricopharyngeus that causes diminished opening of the UES and results in increased hypopharyngeal pressure during swallowing with development of a pulsion diverticulum immediately above the cricopharyngeus in a region of potential weakness known as Killian's dehiscence. A cricopharyngeal bar, appearing as a prominent indentation behind the lower third of the cricoid cartilage, is related to Zenker's diverticulum in that it involves limited distensibility of the cricopharyngeus and can lead to the formation of a Zenker's diverticulum. However, a cricopharyngeal bar is a common radiographic finding, and most patients with transient cricopharyngeal bars are asymptomatic, making it important to rule out alternative etiologies of dysphagia before treatment. Furthermore, cricopharyngeal bars may be secondary to other neuromuscular disorders.

Since the pharyngeal phase of swallowing occurs in less than a second, rapid-sequence fluoroscopy is necessary to evaluate for functional abnormalities. Adequate fluoroscopic examination requires that the patient be conscious and cooperative. The study incorporates recordings of swallow sequences during ingestion of food and liquids of varying consistencies. The pharynx is examined to detect bolus retention, regurgitation into the nose, or aspiration into the trachea. Timing and integrity of pharyngeal contraction and opening of the UES with a swallow are analyzed to assess both aspiration risk and the potential for swallow therapy. Structural abnormalities of the oropharynx, especially those which may require biopsies, also should be assessed by direct laryngoscopic examination.

Esophageal dysphagia

The adult esophagus measures 18–26 cm in length and is anatomically divided into the cervical esophagus, extending from the pharyngoesophageal junction to the suprasternal notch, and the thoracic esophagus, which continues to the diaphragmatic hiatus. When distended, the esophageal lumen has internal dimensions of about 2 cm in the anteroposterior plane and 3 cm in the lateral plane. Solid food dysphagia becomes common when the lumen is narrowed to <13 mm but also can occur with larger diameters in the setting of poorly masticated food or motor dysfunction. Circumferential lesions are more likely to cause dysphagia than are lesions that involve only a partial circumference of the esophageal wall. The most common structural causes of dysphagia are Schatzki's rings, eosinophilic esophagitis, and peptic strictures. Dysphagia also occurs in the setting of gastroesophageal reflux disease without a stricture, perhaps on the basis of altered esophageal sensation, distensibility, or motor function.

Propulsive disorders leading to esophageal dysphagia result from abnormalities of peristalsis and/or deglutitive inhibition, potentially affecting the cervical or thoracic esophagus. Since striated muscle pathology usually involves both the oropharynx and the cervical esophagus, the clinical manifestations usually are dominated by oropharyngeal dysphagia. Diseases affecting smooth muscle involve both the thoracic esophagus and the LES. A dominant manifestation of this, absent peristalsis, refers to either the complete absence of swallow-induced contraction or the presence of nonperistaltic, disordered contractions. Absent peristalsis and failure of deglutitive LES relaxation are the defining features of achalasia. In diffuse esophageal spasm (DES), LES function is normal, with the disordered motility restricted to the esophageal body. Absent peristalsis combined with severe weakness of the LES is a nonspecific pattern commonly found in patients with scleroderma.

| APPROACH TO THE PATIENT | Dysphagia |

Figure 38-2 shows an algorithm for the approach to a patient with dysphagia.

HISTORY The patient history is extremely valuable in making a presumptive diagnosis or at least substantially restricting the differential diagnoses in most patients. Key elements of the history are the localization of dysphagia, the circumstances in which dysphagia is experienced, other symptoms associated with dysphagia, and progression. Dysphagia that localizes to the suprasternal notch may indicate either an oropharyngeal or an esophageal etiology as distal dysphagia is referred proximally about 30% of the time. Dysphagia that localizes to the chest is esophageal in origin. Nasal regurgitation and tracheobronchial aspiration with swallowing are hallmarks of oropharyngeal dysphagia or a tracheoesophageal fistula. The presence of hoarseness may be another important diagnostic clue. When hoarseness precedes dysphagia, the primary lesion is usually laryngeal; hoarseness that occurs after the development of dysphagia may result from compromise of the recurrent laryngeal nerve by a malignancy. The type of food causing dysphagia is a crucial detail. Intermittent dysphagia that occurs only with solid food implies structural dysphagia, whereas constant dysphagia with both liquids and solids strongly suggests a motor abnormality. Two caveats to this pattern are that despite having a motor abnormality, patients with scleroderma generally develop mild dysphagia for solids only and, somewhat paradoxically, that patients with oropharyngeal dysphagia often have greater difficulty managing liquids than solids. Dysphagia that is progressive over the course of weeks to months raises concern for neoplasia. Episodic dysphagia to solids that is unchanged over years indicates a benign disease process such as a Schatzki's ring or eosinophilic esophagitis. Food impaction with a prolonged inability to pass an ingested bolus even with ingestion of liquid is typical of a structural dysphagia. Chest pain frequently accompanies dysphagia whether it is related to motor disorders, structural disorders, or reflux disease. A prolonged history of heartburn preceding the onset of dysphagia is suggestive of peptic stricture

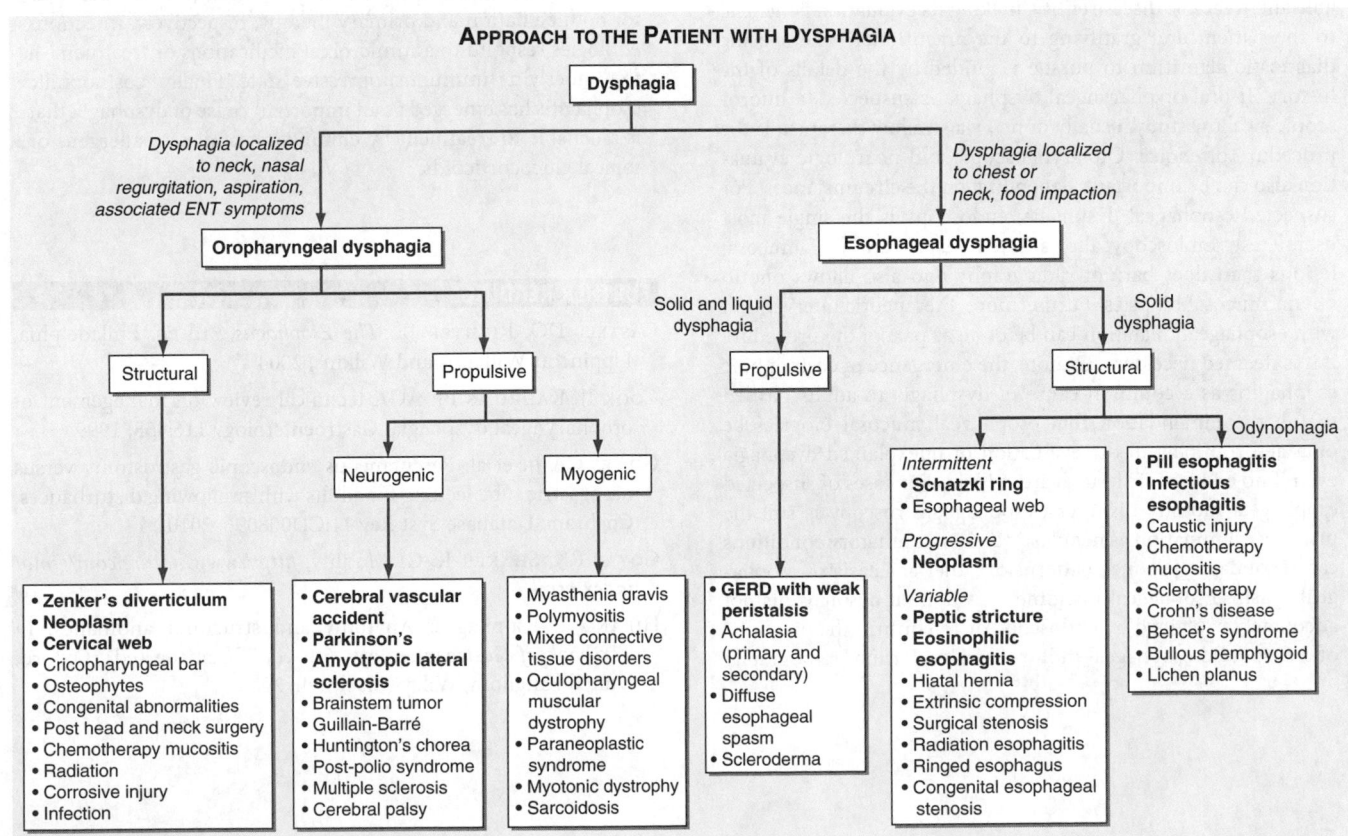

Figure 38-2 Approach to the patient with dysphagia. Etiologies in bold print are the most common. ENT, ear, nose, and throat; GERD, gastroesophageal reflux disease.

and, less commonly, esophageal adenocarcinoma. A history of prolonged nasogastric intubation, esophageal or head and neck surgery, ingestion of caustic agents or pills, previous radiation or chemotherapy, or associated mucocutaneous diseases may help isolate the cause of dysphagia. With accompanying odynophagia, which usually is indicative of ulceration, infectious or pill-induced esophagitis should be suspected. In patients with AIDS or other immunocompromised states, esophagitis due to opportunistic infections such as *Candida*, herpes simplex virus, or cytomegalovirus and to tumors such as Kaposi's sarcoma and lymphoma should be considered. A strong history of atopy increases concerns for eosinophilic esophagitis.

PHYSICAL EXAMINATION Physical examination is important in the evaluation of oral and pharyngeal dysphagia because dysphagia is usually only one of many manifestations of a more global disease process. Signs of bulbar or pseudobulbar palsy, including dysarthria, dysphonia, ptosis, tongue atrophy, and hyperactive jaw jerk, in addition to evidence of generalized neuromuscular disease, should be elicited. The neck should be examined for thyromegaly. A careful inspection of the mouth and pharynx should disclose lesions that may interfere with passage of food. Physical examination is less helpful in the evaluation of esophageal dysphagia as most relevant pathology is restricted to the esophagus. The notable exception is skin disease. Changes in the skin may suggest a diagnosis of scleroderma or mucocutaneous diseases such as pemphigoid and epidermolysis bullosa, all of which can involve the esophagus.

DIAGNOSTIC PROCEDURES Although most instances of dysphagia are attributable to benign disease processes, dysphagia is also a cardinal symptom of several malignancies, making it an important symptom to evaluate. Even when not attributable to malignancy, dysphagia is usually a manifestation of an identifiable and treatable disease entity, making its evaluation beneficial to the patient and gratifying to the practitioner. The specific diagnostic algorithm to pursue is guided by the details of the history. If oral or pharyngeal dysphagia is suspected, a fluoroscopic swallow study, usually done by a swallow therapist, is the procedure of choice. Otolaryngoscopic and neurologic evaluation also can be important, depending on the circumstances. For suspected esophageal dysphagia, endoscopy is the single most useful test. Endoscopy allows better visualization of mucosal lesions than does barium radiography and also allows one to obtain mucosal biopsies. Furthermore, therapeutic intervention with esophageal dilatation can be done as part of the procedure if it is deemed necessary. Of note, the emergence of eosinophilic esophagitis as a common cause of dysphagia in adults has led to the recommendation that esophageal mucosal biopsies be obtained routinely in the evaluation of unexplained dysphagia even if no endoscopic lesions are evident. For cases of suspected esophageal motility disorders, esophagogastroscopy is still the primary examination as neoplastic and inflammatory conditions can secondarily produce patterns of either achalasia or esophageal spasm. Esophageal manometry is done if dysphagia is not adequately explained by endoscopy or to confirm the diagnosis of a suspected esophageal motor disorder. Barium radiography can provide useful adjunctive information in cases of subtle or complex esophageal strictures, esophageal diverticula, or paraesophageal herniation. In specific cases, CT examination and endoscopic ultrasonography may be useful.

TREATMENT Treatment of dysphagia depends on both the locus and the specific etiology. Oropharyngeal dysphagia most commonly results from functional deficits caused by neurologic disorders. In such circumstances, the treatment focuses on utilizing postures or maneuvers devised to reduce pharyngeal residue and enhance airway protection learned under the direction of a trained swallow therapist. Aspiration risk may be reduced by altering the consistency of ingested food and liquid. Dysphagia resulting from a cerebrovascular accident usually, but not always, spontaneously improves within the first few weeks after the event. More severe and persistent cases may require gastrostomy and enteral feeding. Patients with myasthenia gravis (Chap. 386) and polymyositis (Chap. 388) may respond to medical treatment of the primary neuromuscular disease. Surgical intervention with cricopharyngeal myotomy is usually not helpful, with the exception of specific disorders such as the idiopathic cricopharyngeal bar, Zenker's diverticulum, and oculopharyngeal muscular dystrophy. Chronic neurologic disorders such as Parkinson's disease and amyotrophic lateral sclerosis may manifest with severe oropharyngeal dysphagia. Feeding by a nasogastric tube or an endoscopically placed gastrostomy tube may be considered for nutritional support; however, these maneuvers do not provide protection against aspiration of salivary secretions or refluxed gastric contents.

Treatment of esophageal dysphagia is covered in detail in Chap. 292. The majority of causes of esophageal dysphagia are effectively managed by means of esophageal dilatation using bougie or balloon dilators. Cancer and achalasia are often managed surgically, although endoscopic techniques are available for both palliation and primary therapy, respectively. Infectious etiologies respond to antimicrobial medications or treatment of the underlying immunosuppressive state. Finally, eosinophilic esophagitis has emerged as an important cause of dysphagia that is amenable to treatment by elimination of dietary allergens or topical glucocorticoids.

FURTHER READINGS

CASTELL DO, RICHTER JE: *The Esophagus*, 3rd ed. Philadelphia, Lippincott Williams and Wilkins, 2004

COOK IJ, KAHRILAS PJ: AGA technical review on management of oropharyngeal dysphagia. Gastroenterology 116:455, 1999

GOMES CA JR et al: Percutaneous endoscopic gastrostomy versus nasogastric tube feeding for adults with swallowing disturbances. Cochrane Database Syst Rev 11:CD008096, 2010

GOYAL RK, SHAKER R: GI Motility. *http://www.nature.com/gimo/index.html*

HIRANO I: Esophagus: Anatomy and structural anomalies, in *Textbook of Gastroenterology*, 5th ed, T Yamada (ed). Oxford, United Kingdom, Wiley-Blackwell, 2008

CHAPTER 39

Nausea, Vomiting, and Indigestion

William L. Hasler

Nausea is the subjective feeling of a need to vomit. *Vomiting* (emesis) is the oral expulsion of gastrointestinal contents resulting from contractions of gut and thoracoabdominal wall musculature. Vomiting is contrasted with *regurgitation*, the effortless passage of gastric contents into the mouth. *Rumination* is the repeated regurgitation of stomach contents, which may be rechewed and reswallowed. In contrast to vomiting, these phenomena often exhibit volitional control. *Indigestion* is a nonspecific term that encompasses a variety of upper abdominal complaints including nausea, vomiting, heartburn, regurgitation, and dyspepsia (the presence of symptoms thought to originate in the gastroduodenal region). Some individuals with dyspepsia report predominantly epigastric burning, gnawing discomfort, or pain. Others with dyspepsia experience a constellation of symptoms including postprandial fullness, early satiety (an inability to complete a meal due to premature fullness), bloating, eructation (belching), and anorexia.

NAUSEA AND VOMITING

■ MECHANISMS

Vomiting is coordinated by the brainstem and is effected by responses in the gut, pharynx, and thoracoabdominal wall. The mechanisms underlying nausea are poorly understood but likely involve the cerebral cortex, because nausea requires conscious perception. This is supported by electroencephalographic studies showing activation of temporofrontal regions during nausea.

Coordination of emesis

Brain stem nuclei—including the nucleus tractus solitarius; dorsal vagal and phrenic nuclei; medullary nuclei that regulate respiration; and nuclei that control pharyngeal, facial, and tongue movements—coordinate the initiation of emesis. Neurotransmitters involved in this coordination are uncertain, but neurokinin NK_1, serotonin 5-HT_3, and vasopressin pathways may participate.

Somatic and visceral muscles exhibit stereotypic responses during emesis. Inspiratory thoracic and abdominal wall muscles contract, producing high intrathoracic and intraabdominal pressures that facilitate expulsion of gastric contents. The gastric cardia herniates across the diaphragm and the larynx moves upward to promote oral propulsion of the vomitus. Under normal conditions, distally migrating gut contractions are regulated by an electrical phenomenon, the slow wave, which cycles at 3 cycles/min in the stomach and 11 cycles/min in the duodenum. With emesis, there is slow-wave abolition and initiation of orally propagating spikes that evoke retrograde contractions that assist in oral expulsion of intestinal contents.

Activators of emesis

Emetic stimuli act at several sites. Emesis provoked by unpleasant thoughts or smells originates in the cerebral cortex, whereas cranial nerves mediate vomiting after gag reflex activation. Motion sickness and inner ear disorders act on the labyrinthine apparatus, whereas gastric irritants and cytotoxic agents such as cisplatin stimulate gastroduodenal vagal afferent nerves. Nongastric visceral afferents are activated by intestinal and colonic obstruction and mesenteric ischemia. The area postrema, a medullary nucleus, responds to bloodborne emetic stimuli and is termed the *chemoreceptor trigger zone*. Many emetogenic drugs act on the area postrema, as do bacterial toxins and metabolic factors produced during uremia, hypoxia, and ketoacidosis.

Neurotransmitters that mediate induction of vomiting are selective for these anatomic sites. Labyrinthine disorders stimulate vestibular muscarinic M_1 and histaminergic H_1 receptors, whereas vagal afferent stimuli activate serotonin 5-HT_3 receptors. The area postrema is richly served by nerves acting on 5-HT_3, M_1, H_1, and dopamine D_2 subtypes. Transmitters in the cerebral cortex are poorly understood, although cannabinoid CB_1 pathways may participate. Optimal pharmacologic therapy of vomiting requires understanding of these pathways.

■ DIFFERENTIAL DIAGNOSIS

Nausea and vomiting are caused by conditions within and outside the gut as well as by drugs and circulating toxins (Table 39-1).

Intraperitoneal disorders

Visceral obstruction and inflammation of hollow and solid viscera may produce vomiting. Gastric obstruction results from ulcer disease and malignancy, while small-bowel and colonic obstruction occur because of adhesions, benign or malignant tumors, volvulus, intussusception, or inflammatory diseases such as Crohn's disease. The superior mesenteric artery syndrome, occurring after weight loss or prolonged bed rest, results when the duodenum is compressed by the overlying superior mesenteric artery. Abdominal irradiation impairs intestinal motor function and induces strictures. Biliary colic causes nausea via action on visceral afferent nerves. Vomiting with pancreatitis, cholecystitis, and appendicitis is due to visceral irritation and induction of ileus. Enteric infections with viruses or bacteria such as *Staphylococcus aureus* and *Bacillus cereus* commonly cause vomiting, especially in children. Opportunistic infections such as cytomegalovirus or herpes simplex virus induce emesis in immunocompromised individuals.

Disordered gut sensorimotor function commonly causes nausea and vomiting. *Gastroparesis* is defined as a delay in gastric emptying of food and occurs after vagotomy, with pancreatic adenocarcinoma, with mesenteric vascular insufficiency, or in systemic diseases such as diabetes, scleroderma, and amyloidosis. The most common form of disease, idiopathic gastroparesis, occurs in the absence of systemic illness and may follow a viral prodrome, suggesting an infectious etiology. Intestinal pseudoobstruction is characterized by disrupted intestinal and colonic motor activity and leads to retention of food residue and secretions; bacterial overgrowth; nutrient malabsorption; and symptoms of nausea, vomiting, bloating, pain, and altered defecation. *Intestinal pseudoobstruction* may be idiopathic or inherited as a familial visceral myopathy or neuropathy, or it may result from systemic disease or as a paraneoplastic complication of a malignancy such as small cell lung carcinoma. Patients with gastroesophageal reflux may report nausea and vomiting, as do some individuals with irritable bowel syndrome (IBS).

Other functional disorders without organic abnormalities have been characterized in adults. *Chronic idiopathic nausea* is defined as nausea without vomiting occurring several times weekly, whereas *functional vomiting* is defined as one or more vomiting episodes weekly in the absence of an eating disorder or psychiatric disease. *Cyclic vomiting syndrome* is a rare disorder of unknown etiology

TABLE 39-1 Causes of Nausea and Vomiting

Intraperitoneal	Extraperitoneal	Medications/Metabolic Disorders

Obstructing disorders
  Pyloric obstruction
  Small bowel obstruction
  Colonic obstruction
  Superior mesenteric artery syndrome
	Cardiopulmonary disease
	  Cardiomyopathy
	  Myocardial infarction
		Drugs
		  Cancer chemotherapy
		  Antibiotics
		  Cardiac antiarrhythmics
		  Digoxin
		  Oral hypoglycemics
		  Oral contraceptives

Enteric infections
  Viral
  Bacterial
	Labyrinthine disease
	  Motion sickness
	  Labyrinthitis
	  Malignancy	

Inflammatory diseases
  Cholecystitis
  Pancreatitis
  Appendicitis
  Hepatitis
	Intracerebral disorders
	  Malignancy
	  Hemorrhage
	  Abscess
	  Hydrocephalus
		Endocrine/metabolic disease
		  Pregnancy
		  Uremia
		  Ketoacidosis
		  Thyroid and parathyroid disease
		  Adrenal insufficiency

Altered sensorimotor function
  Gastroparesis
  Intestinal pseudoobstruction
  Gastroesophageal reflux
  Chronic idiopathic nausea
  Functional vomiting
  Cyclic vomiting syndrome
	Psychiatric illness
	  Anorexia and bulimia nervosa
	  Depression
		Toxins
		  Liver failure
		  Ethanol

Biliary colic	Postoperative vomiting	
Abdominal irradiation		

that produces periodic discrete episodes of relentless nausea and vomiting. The syndrome shows a strong association with migraine headaches, suggesting that some cases may be migraine variants. Cyclic vomiting is most common in children, although adult cases have been described in association with rapid gastric emptying and with chronic cannabis use.

Extraperitoneal disorders

Myocardial infarction and congestive heart failure may cause nausea and vomiting. Postoperative emesis occurs after 25% of surgeries, most commonly laparotomy and orthopedic surgery, and is more prevalent in women. Increased intracranial pressure from tumors, bleeding, abscess, or obstruction to cerebrospinal fluid outflow produces prominent vomiting with or without nausea. Motion sickness, labyrinthitis, and Ménière's disease evoke emesis via labyrinthine pathways. Patients with psychiatric illnesses including anorexia nervosa, bulimia nervosa, anxiety, and depression may report significant nausea that may be associated with delayed gastric emptying.

Medications and metabolic disorders

Drugs evoke vomiting by action on the stomach (analgesics, erythromycin) or area postrema (digoxin, opiates, anti-Parkinsonian drugs). Emetogenic agents include antibiotics, cardiac antiarrhythmics, antihypertensives, oral hypoglycemics, and contraceptives. Cancer chemotherapy causes vomiting that is acute (within hours of administration), delayed (after one or more days), or anticipatory. Acute emesis resulting from highly emetogenic agents such as cisplatin is mediated by 5-HT$_3$ pathways, whereas delayed emesis is 5-HT$_3$-independent. Anticipatory nausea often responds better to anxiolytic therapy than to antiemetics.

Several metabolic disorders elicit nausea and vomiting. Pregnancy is the most prevalent endocrinologic cause of nausea, which affects 70% of women in the first trimester. Hyperemesis gravidarum is a severe form of nausea of pregnancy that can produce significant fluid loss and electrolyte disturbances. Uremia, ketoacidosis, and

adrenal insufficiency, as well as parathyroid and thyroid disease, are other metabolic causes of emesis.

Circulating toxins evoke emesis via effects on the area postrema. Endogenous toxins are generated in fulminant liver failure, whereas exogenous enterotoxins may be produced by enteric bacterial infection. Ethanol intoxication is a common toxic etiology of nausea and vomiting.

APPROACH TO THE PATIENT   **Nausea and Vomiting**

HISTORY AND PHYSICAL EXAMINATION The history helps define the etiology of unexplained nausea and vomiting. Drugs, toxins, and gastrointestinal infections commonly cause acute symptoms, whereas established illnesses evoke chronic complaints. Pyloric obstruction and gastroparesis produce vomiting within one hour of eating, whereas emesis from intestinal obstruction occurs later. In severe cases of gastroparesis, the vomitus may contain food residue ingested hours or days previously. Hematemesis raises suspicion of an ulcer, malignancy, or Mallory-Weiss tear, whereas feculent emesis is noted with distal intestinal or colonic obstruction. Bilious vomiting excludes gastric obstruction, while emesis of undigested food is consistent with a Zenker's diverticulum or achalasia. Relief of abdominal pain by emesis characterizes intestinal obstruction, whereas vomiting has no effect on pancreatitis or cholecystitis pain. Pronounced weight loss raises concern about malignancy or obstruction. Fevers suggest inflammation; an intracranial source is considered if there are headaches or visual field changes. Vertigo or tinnitus indicates labyrinthine disease.

The physical examination complements information from the history. Orthostatic hypotension and reduced skin turgor indicate intravascular fluid loss. Pulmonary abnormalities raise concern for aspiration of vomitus. Abdominal auscultation may reveal absent bowel sounds with ileus. High-pitched rushes suggest bowel obstruction, while a succussion splash upon abrupt lateral movement of the patient is found with gastroparesis or pyloric obstruction. Tenderness or involuntary guarding raises suspicion of inflammation, whereas fecal blood suggests mucosal injury from ulcer, ischemia, or tumor. Neurologic disease presents with papilledema, visual field loss, or focal neural abnormalities. Neoplasm is suggested by palpation of masses or adenopathy.

DIAGNOSTIC TESTING For intractable symptoms or an elusive diagnosis, selected screening tests can direct clinical care. Electrolyte replacement is indicated for hypokalemia or metabolic alkalosis. Detection of iron-deficiency anemia mandates a search for mucosal injury. Pancreaticobiliary disease is indicated by abnormal pancreatic or liver biochemistries, whereas endocrinologic, rheumatologic, or paraneoplastic etiologies are suggested by hormone or serologic abnormalities. If bowel obstruction is suspected, supine and upright abdominal radiographs may show intestinal air-fluid levels with reduced colonic air. Ileus is characterized by diffusely dilated air-filled bowel loops.

Anatomic studies may be indicated if initial testing is nondiagnostic. Upper endoscopy detects ulcers or malignancy, while small-bowel barium radiography diagnoses partial intestinal obstruction. Colonoscopy or contrast enema radiography can detect colonic obstruction. Ultrasound or CT defines intraperitoneal inflammatory processes, while CT or MRI of the head can delineate intracranial disease. Advances in CT and MRI enterography have improved definition of bowel inflammation, as in Crohn's disease. Mesenteric angiography, CT, or MRI is useful for suspected ischemia.

Gastrointestinal motility testing may detect a motor disorder that contributes to symptoms when anatomic abnormalities are absent. Gastroparesis commonly is diagnosed using gastric scintigraphy, by which emptying of a radiolabeled meal is measured. Isotopic breath tests and wireless motility capsule methods have been validated and may become important alternatives to scintigraphy to define gastroparesis. The diagnosis of intestinal pseudoobstruction often is suggested by abnormal barium transit and luminal dilation on small-bowel contrast radiography. Delayed small-bowel transit also may be detected by wireless capsule techniques. Small-intestinal manometry can confirm the diagnosis and further characterize the motor abnormality as neuropathic or myopathic based on contractile patterns. Such investigation can obviate the need for open intestinal biopsy to evaluate for smooth muscle or neuronal degeneration.

TREATMENT Nausea and Vomiting

GENERAL PRINCIPLES Therapy of vomiting is tailored to correcting medically or surgically remediable abnormalities if possible. Hospitalization is considered for severe dehydration, especially if oral fluid replenishment cannot be sustained. Once oral intake is tolerated, nutrients are restarted with liquids that are low in fat, as lipids delay gastric emptying. Foods high in indigestible residues are avoided because these also prolong gastric retention.

ANTIEMETIC MEDICATIONS The most commonly used antiemetic agents act on sites in the central nervous system (Table 39-2). Antihistamines such as meclizine and dimenhydrinate and anticholinergic drugs like scopolamine act on labyrinthine pathways and are useful in motion sickness and inner ear disorders. Dopamine D_2 antagonists treat emesis evoked by area postrema stimuli and are useful for medication, toxic, and metabolic etiologies. Dopamine antagonists freely cross the blood-brain barrier and cause anxiety, dystonic reactions, hyperprolactinemic effects (galactorrhea

TABLE 39-2 Treatment of Nausea and Vomiting

Treatment	Mechanism	Examples	Clinical Indications
Antiemetic agents	Antihistaminergic	Dimenhydrinate, meclizine	Motion sickness, inner ear disease
	Anticholinergic	Scopolamine	Motion sickness, inner ear disease
	Antidopaminergic	Prochlorperazine, thiethylperazine	Medication-, toxin-, or metabolic-induced emesis
	5-HT₃ antagonist	Ondansetron, granisetron	Chemotherapy- and radiation-induced emesis, postoperative emesis
	NK₁ antagonist	Aprepitant	Chemotherapy-induced nausea and vomiting
	Tricyclic antidepressant	Amitriptyline, nortriptyline	Chronic idiopathic nausea, functional vomiting, cyclic vomiting syndrome, ?gastroparesis
	Other antidepressant	Mirtazapine	?Functional vomiting, ?gastroparesis
Prokinetic agents	5-HT₄ agonist and antidopaminergic	Metoclopramide	Gastroparesis
	Motilin agonist	Erythromycin	Gastroparesis, ?intestinal pseudoobstruction
	Peripheral antidopaminergic	Domperidone	Gastroparesis
	Somatostatin analogue	Octreotide	Intestinal pseudoobstruction
	Acetylcholinesterase inhibitor	Pyridostigmine	?Small intestinal dysmotility/pseudoobstruction
Special settings	Benzodiazepines	Lorazepam	Anticipatory nausea and vomiting with chemotherapy
	Glucocorticoids	Methylprednisolone, dexamethasone	Chemotherapy-induced emesis
	Cannabinoids	Tetrahydrocannabinol	?Chemotherapy-induced emesis

Note: ?, indication is uncertain.

and sexual dysfunction), and irreversible tardive dyskinesia.

Other drug classes exhibit antiemetic properties. Serotonin 5-HT$_3$ antagonists such as ondansetron and granisetron exhibit utility in postoperative vomiting, after radiation therapy, and for preventing cancer chemotherapy–induced emesis. The usefulness of 5-HT$_3$ antagonists for other causes of emesis is less well established. Low-dose tricyclic antidepressant agents provide symptomatic benefit in patients with chronic idiopathic nausea and functional vomiting as well as in diabetic patients with nausea and vomiting whose disease is of long standing. Other antidepressants such as mirtazapine also may exhibit antiemetic effects.

GASTROINTESTINAL MOTOR STIMULANTS   Drugs that stimulate gastric emptying are indicated for gastroparesis (Table 39-2). Metoclopramide, a combined 5-HT$_4$ agonist and D$_2$ antagonist, exhibits efficacy in gastroparesis, but antidopaminergic side effects, particularly tardive dyskinesia, limit its use in <25% of patients. Erythromycin, a macrolide antibiotic, increases gastroduodenal motility by action on receptors for motilin, an endogenous stimulant of fasting motor activity. Intravenous erythromycin is useful for inpatients with refractory gastroparesis; however, oral forms also have some utility. Domperidone, a D$_2$ antagonist not available in the United States, exhibits prokinetic and antiemetic effects but does not cross into most other brain regions; thus, anxiety and dystonic reactions are rare. The main side effects of domperidone relate to induction of hyperprolactinemia via effects on pituitary regions served by a porous blood-brain barrier.

Refractory upper gut motility disorders pose significant challenges. Liquid suspensions of prokinetic drugs may be beneficial, because liquids empty from the stomach more rapidly than pills do. Metoclopramide can be administered subcutaneously in patients unresponsive to oral drugs. Intestinal pseudoobstruction may respond to the somatostatin analogue octreotide, which induces propagative small intestinal motor complexes. Acetylcholinesterase inhibitors such as pyridostigmine are anecdotally observed to benefit some patients with small bowel dysmotility. Pyloric injections of botulinum toxin are reported in uncontrolled studies to benefit patients with gastroparesis. Placement of a feeding jejunostomy reduces hospitalizations and improves overall health in some patients with drug-refractory gastroparesis. Surgical options are limited for unresponsive cases, but postvagotomy gastroparesis may improve with near-total resection of the stomach. Implanted gastric electrical stimulators may reduce symptoms, enhance nutrition, improve quality of life, and decrease health care expenditures in medication-refractory gastroparesis, although small controlled trials report only modest benefits with this method.

SELECTED CLINICAL SETTINGS   Some cancer chemotherapeutic agents such as cisplatin are intensely emetogenic (Chap. 85). Given prophylactically, 5-HT$_3$ antagonists prevent chemotherapy-induced acute vomiting in most cases (Table 39-2). Optimal antiemetic effects often are obtained with a 5-HT$_3$ antagonist combined with a glucocorticoid. Benzodiazepines such as lorazepam are useful to reduce anticipatory nausea and vomiting. Therapy of delayed emesis 1–5 days after chemotherapy is less successful. Neurokinin NK$_1$ antagonists (e.g., aprepitant) exhibit antiemetic and antinausea effects during both the acute and delayed periods after chemotherapy. Cannabinoids such as tetrahydrocannabinol, long advocated for cancer-associated emesis, produce significant side effects and exhibit no more efficacy than antidopaminergic agents. Most antiemetic regimens produce greater reductions in vomiting than in nausea.

The clinician should exercise caution in managing the pregnant patient with nausea. Studies of the teratogenic effects of available antiemetic agents provide conflicting results. Few controlled trials have been performed in nausea of pregnancy, although antihistamines such as meclizine and antidopaminergics such as prochlorperazine demonstrate efficacy greater than placebo. Some obstetricians offer alternative therapies such as pyridoxine, acupressure, or ginger.

Controlling emesis in cyclic vomiting syndrome is a challenge. In many patients, prophylaxis with tricyclic antidepressants, cyproheptadine, or β-adrenoceptor antagonists can reduce the frequency of attacks. Intravenous 5-HT$_3$ antagonists combined with the sedating effects of a benzodiazepine such as lorazepam are a mainstay of treatment of acute symptom flares. Small studies report benefits with antimigraine therapies, including the serotonin 5-HT$_1$ agonist sumatriptan, as well as selected anticonvulsant drugs such as zonisamide and levetiracetam.

INDIGESTION

■ MECHANISMS

The most common causes of indigestion are gastroesophageal reflux and functional dyspepsia. Other cases are a consequence of a more serious organic illness.

Gastroesophageal reflux

Gastroesophageal reflux can result from a variety of physiologic defects. Reduced lower esophageal sphincter (LES) tone is an important cause of reflux in scleroderma and pregnancy; it may also be a factor in patients without other systemic conditions. Many individuals exhibit frequent transient LES relaxations during which acid or nonacidic fluid bathes the esophagus. Overeating and aerophagia can transiently override the barrier function of the LES, whereas impaired esophageal body motility and reduced salivary secretion prolong fluid exposure. The role of hiatal hernias is controversial—although most reflux patients exhibit hiatal hernias, most individuals with hiatal hernias do not have excess heartburn.

Gastric motor dysfunction

Disturbed gastric motility is purported to cause gastroesophageal reflux in some cases of indigestion. Delayed gastric emptying is also found in 25–50% of functional dyspeptics. The relation of these defects to symptom induction is uncertain; studies show poor correlation between symptom severity and degrees of motor dysfunction. Impaired gastric fundus relaxation after eating may underlie selected dyspeptic symptoms like bloating, nausea, and early satiety.

Visceral afferent hypersensitivity

Disturbed gastric sensory function is proposed as a pathogenic factor in functional dyspepsia. Visceral afferent hypersensitivity was first demonstrated in patients with IBS who had heightened perception of rectal balloon inflation without changes in rectal compliance. Similarly, dyspeptic patients experience discomfort with fundic distention to lower pressures than healthy controls. Some patients with heartburn exhibit no increase in reflux of acid or nonacidic fluid. These individuals with functional heartburn are believed to have heightened perception of normal esophageal pH and volume.

Other factors

Helicobacter pylori has a clear etiologic role in peptic ulcer disease, but ulcers cause a minority of cases of dyspepsia. *H. pylori* is considered to be a minor factor in the genesis of functional dyspepsia.

In contrast, functional dyspepsia is associated with a reduced sense of physical and mental well-being and is exacerbated by stress, suggesting important roles for psychological factors. Analgesics cause dyspepsia, while nitrates, calcium channel blockers, theophylline, and progesterone promote gastroesophageal reflux. Other stimuli that induce reflux include ethanol, tobacco, and caffeine via LES relaxation. Genetic factors may promote development of reflux.

◼ DIFFERENTIAL DIAGNOSIS

Gastroesophageal reflux disease

Gastroesophageal reflux disease (GERD) is prevalent in Western society. Heartburn is reported once monthly by 40% of Americans and daily by 7–10%. Most cases of heartburn occur because of excess acid reflux, although reflux of non-acidic fluid may produce similar symptoms. Alkaline reflux esophagitis produces GERD-like symptoms most often in patients who have had surgery for peptic ulcer disease. Approximately 10% of patients with heartburn of a functional nature exhibit normal degrees of esophageal acid exposure and no increase in nonacidic reflux.

Functional dyspepsia

Nearly 25% of the populace has dyspepsia at least 6 times yearly, but only 10–20% of these individuals present to physicians. Functional dyspepsia, the cause of symptoms in 60% of dyspeptic patients, is defined as ≥3 months of bothersome postprandial fullness, early satiety, or epigastric pain or burning with symptom onset at least 6 months before diagnosis in the absence of organic cause. Most cases follow a benign course, but some patients with *H. pylori* infection or on nonsteroidal anti-inflammatory drugs (NSAIDs) develop ulcers. As with idiopathic gastroparesis, some cases of functional dyspepsia result from prior gastrointestinal infection.

Ulcer disease

In most cases of GERD, there is no destruction of the esophagus. However, 5% of patients develop esophageal ulcers, and some form strictures. Symptoms do not reliably distinguish nonerosive from erosive or ulcerative esophagitis. Some 15–25% of cases of dyspepsia stem from ulcers of the stomach or duodenum. The most common causes of ulcer disease are gastric infection with *H. pylori* and use of NSAIDs. Other rare causes of gastroduodenal ulcer include Crohn's disease (Chap. 295) and Zollinger-Ellison syndrome (Chap. 293), a condition resulting from gastrin overproduction by an endocrine tumor.

Malignancy

Dyspeptic patients often seek care because of fear of cancer. However, <2% of cases result from gastroesophageal malignancy. Esophageal squamous cell carcinoma occurs most often in those with histories of tobacco or ethanol intake. Other risk factors include prior caustic ingestion, achalasia, and the hereditary disorder tylosis. Esophageal adenocarcinoma usually complicates long-standing acid reflux. Between 8 and 20% of GERD patients exhibit intestinal metaplasia of the esophagus, termed *Barrett's metaplasia*. This condition predisposes to esophageal adenocarcinoma (Chap. 91). Gastric malignancies include adenocarcinoma, which is prevalent in certain Asian societies, and lymphoma.

Other causes

Opportunistic fungal or viral esophageal infections may produce heartburn or chest discomfort but more often cause odynophagia. Other causes of esophageal inflammation include eosinophilic esophagitis and pill esophagitis. Biliary colic is in the differential diagnosis of dyspepsia, but most patients with true biliary colic report discrete episodes of right upper quadrant or epigastric pain rather than chronic burning discomfort, nausea, and bloating. Intestinal lactase deficiency produces gas, bloating, discomfort, and diarrhea after lactose ingestion. Lactase deficiency occurs in 15–25% of whites of northern European descent but is more common in blacks and Asians. Intolerance of other carbohydrates (e.g., fructose, sorbitol) produces similar symptoms. Small-intestinal bacterial overgrowth may produce dyspepsia, often with bowel dysfunction, distention, and malabsorption. Eosinophilic infiltration of the duodenal mucosa is described in some cases of dyspepsia. Pancreatic disease (chronic pancreatitis and malignancy), hepatocellular carcinoma, celiac disease, Ménétrier's disease, infiltrative diseases (sarcoidosis and eosinophilic gastroenteritis), mesenteric ischemia, thyroid and parathyroid disease, and abdominal wall strain cause dyspepsia. Extraperitoneal etiologies of indigestion include congestive heart failure and tuberculosis. Investigation is ongoing into genetic markers that predispose to developing functional dyspepsia.

APPROACH TO THE PATIENT | **Indigestion**

HISTORY AND PHYSICAL EXAMINATION   Care of the patient with indigestion requires a thorough interview. GERD classically produces heartburn, a substernal warmth in the epigastrium that moves toward the neck. Heartburn often is exacerbated by meals and may awaken the patient. Associated symptoms include regurgitation of acid or nonacidic fluid and water brash, the reflex release of salty salivary secretions into the mouth. Atypical symptoms include pharyngitis, asthma, cough, bronchitis, hoarseness, and chest pain that mimics angina. Some patients with acid reflux on esophageal pH testing do not report heartburn, but note abdominal pain or other symptoms.

Some patients with dyspepsia report a predominance of epigastric pain or burning that is intermittent and not generalized or localized to other regions. Others experience a postprandial distress syndrome characterized by fullness occurring after normal-sized meals and early satiety that prevents completion of regular meals, with associated bloating, belching, or nausea. Functional dyspepsia overlaps with other functional disorders such as IBS.

The physical exam with GERD and functional dyspepsia usually is normal. In atypical GERD, pharyngeal erythema and wheezing may be noted. Recurrent acid regurgitation may cause poor dentition. Functional dyspeptics may report epigastric tenderness or distention.

Discrimination between functional and organic causes of indigestion mandates exclusion of selected historic and examination features. Odynophagia suggests esophageal infection, while dysphagia is worrisome for a benign or malignant esophageal blockage. Other alarming features include unexplained weight loss, recurrent vomiting, occult or gross gastrointestinal bleeding, jaundice, a palpable mass or adenopathy, and a family history of gastrointestinal malignancy.

DIAGNOSTIC TESTING   Because indigestion is prevalent and most cases result from GERD or functional dyspepsia, a general principle is to perform only limited and directed diagnostic testing of selected individuals.

Once alarm factors are excluded (Table 39-3), patients with typical GERD do not need further evaluation and are treated empirically. Upper endoscopy is indicated to exclude mucosal injury in cases with atypical symptoms, symptoms unresponsive to acid suppressing drugs, or alarm factors. For heartburn >5 years in duration, especially in patients >50 years old, endoscopy is

TABLE 39-3 Alarm Symptoms in GERD

Odynophagia

Unexplained weight loss

Recurrent vomiting

Occult or gross gastrointestinal bleeding

Jaundice

Palpable mass or adenopathy

Family history of gastrointestinal malignancy

recommended to screen for Barrett's metaplasia. However, the clinical benefits and cost-effectiveness of this approach have not been validated in controlled studies. Ambulatory esophageal pH testing using a catheter method or an implanted esophageal capsule device is considered for drug-refractory symptoms and atypical symptoms like unexplained chest pain. Esophageal manometry most commonly is ordered when surgical treatment of GERD is considered. A low LES pressure may predict failure of drug therapy and helps select patients who may require surgery. Demonstration of disordered esophageal body peristalsis may affect the decision to operate or modify the type of operation chosen. High-resolution manometric methods improve characterization of ineffective esophageal propulsion, which may contribute to impaired esophageal acid clearance in some GERD patients. Manometry with provocative testing may clarify the diagnosis in patients with atypical symptoms. Blind perfusion of saline and then acid into the esophagus, known as the *Bernstein test*, can delineate whether unexplained chest discomfort results from acid reflux. Nonacidic reflux may be suggested by nuclear medicine reflux scanning or detected by combined esophageal impedance-pH testing, which increases the diagnostic yield by 15% versus pH testing alone. Ambulatory measurement of esophageal bilirubin levels facilitates diagnosis of alkaline reflux.

Upper endoscopy is performed as the initial diagnostic test in patients with unexplained dyspepsia who are >55 years old or who have alarm factors because of the elevated risks of malignancy and ulcer in these groups. The management approach to patients <55 years old without alarm factors is dependent on the local prevalence of *H. pylori* infection. For individuals in regions with low *H. pylori* prevalence (<10%), a 4-week trial of an acid-suppressing medication such as a proton pump inhibitor is recommended. If this fails, a "test and treat" approach is most commonly applied. *H. pylori* status is determined with urea breath testing, stool antigen measurement, or blood serology testing. Those who are *H. pylori* positive are given therapy to eradicate the infection. If symptoms resolve on either regimen, no further intervention is required. For patients in areas with high *H. pylori* prevalence (>10%), an initial test and treat approach is advocated, with a subsequent trial of an acid-suppressing regimen offered for those in whom *H. pylori* treatment fails or for those who are negative for the infection. In each of these patient subsets, upper endoscopy is reserved for those whose symptoms fail to respond to therapy.

Further testing is indicated if other factors are present. If bleeding is reported, a blood count is obtained to exclude anemia. Thyroid chemistries or calcium levels screen for metabolic disease, whereas serologies may suggest celiac disease. For possible pancreaticobiliary causes, pancreatic and liver chemistries are obtained. If abnormalities are found, ultrasound or CT may

give important information. Gastric emptying measurement is considered to exclude gastroparesis in patients whose dyspeptic symptoms resemble postprandial distress when drug therapy fails. Gastric scintigraphy also assesses for gastroparesis in patients with GERD, especially if surgical intervention is being considered. Breath testing after carbohydrate ingestion may detect lactase deficiency, intolerance to other carbohydrates, or small-intestinal bacterial overgrowth.

TREATMENT General Principles

For mild indigestion, reassurance that a careful evaluation revealed no serious organic disease may be the only intervention needed. Drugs that cause gastroesophageal reflux or dyspepsia should be stopped, if possible. Patients with GERD should limit ethanol, caffeine, chocolate, and tobacco use because of their effects on the LES. Other measures in GERD include ingesting a low-fat diet, avoiding snacks before bedtime, and elevating the head of the bed.

Specific therapies for organic disease should be offered when possible. Surgery is appropriate in disorders like biliary colic, while diet changes are indicated for lactase deficiency or celiac disease. Some illnesses such as peptic ulcer disease may be cured by specific medical regimens. However, because most indigestion is caused by GERD or functional dyspepsia, medications that reduce gastric acid, modulate motility, or blunt gastric sensitivity are indicated.

ACID-SUPPRESSING OR NEUTRALIZING MEDICATIONS Drugs that reduce or neutralize gastric acid are often prescribed for GERD. Histamine H_2 antagonists such as cimetidine, ranitidine, famotidine, and nizatidine are useful in mild to moderate GERD. For severe symptoms or for many cases of erosive or ulcerative esophagitis, proton pump inhibitors such as omeprazole, lansoprazole, rabeprazole, pantoprazole, esomeprazole, or dexlansoprazole are needed. These drugs, which inhibit gastric H^+, K^+-ATPase, are more potent than H_2 antagonists. Up to one third of GERD patients do not respond to proton pump inhibitors; one third of these patients have nonacidic reflux while 10% have persistent acid-related disease. Acid suppressants may be taken continuously or on demand depending on symptom severity. Infrequent potential complications of long-term proton pump inhibitors may include infection, small intestinal bacterial overgrowth, nutrient deficiency (vitamin B_{12}, iron, calcium), bone demineralization, and impaired medication absorption (e.g. clopidogrel). Many patients started on a proton pump inhibitor can be stepped down to an H_2 antagonist. Combining a proton pump inhibitor with an H_2 antagonist is provided for some refractory cases.

Acid-suppressing drugs are also effective in appropriately selected patients with functional dyspepsia. Meta-analysis of eight controlled trials calculated a risk ratio of 0.86, with a 95% confidence interval of 0.78–0.95, favoring proton pump inhibitor therapy over placebo. The benefits of less potent acid reducing therapies such as H_2 antagonists are unproven.

Liquid antacids are useful for short-term control of mild GERD but are less effective for severe disease unless given at high doses that elicit side effects (diarrhea and constipation with magnesium- and aluminum-containing agents, respectively). Alginic acid in combination with antacids may form a floating barrier to acid reflux in individuals with upright symptoms. Sucralfate is a salt of aluminum hydroxide and sucrose octasulfate that buffers acid and binds pepsin and bile salts. Its efficacy in GERD is felt to be comparable to that of H₂ antagonists.

HELICOBACTER PYLORI ERADICATION *H. pylori* eradication is clearly indicated only for peptic ulcer and mucosa-associated lymphoid tissue gastric lymphoma. The utility of eradication therapy in functional dyspepsia is less well established, but <15% of cases relate to this infection. Meta-analysis of 13 controlled trials calculated a risk ratio of 0.91, with a 95% confidence interval of 0.87–0.96, favoring *H. pylori* eradication therapy over placebo. Several drug combinations show efficacy in eliminating the infection (Chap. 293); most include 10–14 days of a proton pump inhibitor or bismuth subsalicylate in concert with two antibiotics. *H. pylori* infection is associated with reduced prevalence of GERD, especially in the elderly. However, eradication of the infection does not worsen GERD symptoms. To date, no consensus recommendations regarding *H. pylori* eradication in GERD patients have been offered.

AGENTS THAT MODIFY GASTROINTESTINAL MOTOR ACTIVITY Motor stimulants (also known as prokinetics) such as metoclopramide, erythromycin, and domperidone have limited utility in GERD. Several studies have evaluated the effectiveness of motor-stimulating drugs in functional dyspepsia; however, convincing evidence of their benefits has not been found. Some clinicians suggest that patients with symptoms resembling postprandial distress may respond preferentially to prokinetic drugs. The γ-aminobutyric acid B (GABA-B) agonist baclofen reduces esophageal exposure to acid and non-acidic fluids by inhibiting transient LES relaxations; this drug is proposed for refractory acid and non-acid reflux.

OTHER OPTIONS Antireflux surgery (fundoplication) is most often offered to GERD patients who are young and may require lifelong therapy, have typical heartburn and regurgitation, and are responsive to proton pump inhibitors. Surgery also is effective for some cases of non-acidic reflux. Individuals who may respond less well to operative therapy include those with atypical symptoms and those who have esophageal body motor disturbances. Fundoplications are performed laparoscopically when possible and include the Nissen and Toupet procedures in which the proximal stomach is partly or completely wrapped around the distal esophagus to increase LES pressure. Dysphagia, gas-bloat syndrome, and gastroparesis may be long-term complications of these procedures. The utility and safety of endoscopic therapies for increasing the barrier function of the gastroesophageal junction, including radiofrequency energy delivery and gastroplication, have not been fully investigated for patients with refractory GERD.

Some patients with functional heartburn and functional dyspepsia refractory to standard therapies may respond to low-dose antidepressants in tricyclic and other classes. Their mechanism of action is unknown but may involve blunting of visceral pain processing in the brain. Gas and bloating are among the most troubling symptoms in some patients with indigestion and can be difficult to treat. Dietary exclusion of gas-producing foods such as legumes and use of simethicone or activated charcoal provide benefits in some cases. Therapies that modify gut flora, including antibiotics and probiotic preparations containing active bacterial cultures, are useful for cases of bacterial overgrowth and functional lower gastrointestinal disorders, but their utility in functional dyspepsia is unproven. Psychological treatments may be offered for refractory functional dyspepsia, but no convincing data suggest their efficacy.

FURTHER READINGS

CAMILLERI M, TACK JF: Current medical treatments of dyspepsia and irritable bowel syndrome. Gastroenterol Clin North Am 39:481, 2010

DEVAULT KR, TALLEY NJ: Insights into the future of gastric acid suppression. Nature Rev Gastroenterol Hepatol 6: 524, 2009

HASLER WL: Methods of gastric electrical stimulation and pacing: a review of their benefits and mechanisms of action in gastroparesis and obesity. Neurogastroenterol Motil 21: 229, 2009

HESKETH PJ: Chemotherapy-induced nausea and vomiting. N Engl J Med 358: 2482, 2008

KAHRILAS PJ, SIFRIM D: High-resolution manometry and impedance-pH/manometry: valuable tools in clinical and investigational esophagology. Gastroenterology 135: 756, 2008

—— et al: American Gastroenterological Association Institute technical review on the management of gastroesophageal reflux disease. Gastroenterology 135: 1392, 2008

OLDEN KW, CHEPYALA P: Functional nausea and vomiting. Nature Clin Pract Gastroenterol Hepatol 5: 202, 2008

PARKMAN HP, JONES MP: Tests of gastric neuromuscular function. Gastroenterology 136: 1526, 2009

SHAFI MA, BRESALIER RS: The gastrointestinal complications of oncologic therapy. Gastroenterol Clin North Am 39:629, 2010

STAPLETON J, WO JM: Current treatment of nausea and vomiting associated with gastroparesis: antiemetics, prokinetics, tricyclics. Gastroenterol Clin North Am 19: 57, 2009

CHAPTER **40**

Diarrhea and Constipation

Michael Camilleri
Joseph A. Murray

Diarrhea and constipation are exceedingly common and, together, exact an enormous toll in terms of mortality, morbidity, social inconvenience, loss of work productivity, and consumption of medical resources. Worldwide, >1 billion individuals suffer one or more episodes of acute diarrhea each year. Among the 100 million persons affected annually by acute diarrhea in the United States, nearly half must restrict activities, 10% consult physicians, ~250,000 require hospitalization, and ~5000 die (primarily the elderly). The annual economic burden to society may exceed $20 billion. Acute infectious diarrhea remains one of the most common causes of mortality in developing countries, particularly among children, accounting for 2–3 million deaths per year. Constipation, by contrast, is rarely associated with mortality and is exceedingly common in developed countries, leading to frequent self-medication and, in a third of those, to medical consultation. Population statistics on chronic diarrhea and constipation are more uncertain, perhaps due to variable definitions and reporting, but the frequency of these conditions is also high. United States population surveys put prevalence rates for chronic diarrhea at 2–7% and for chronic constipation at 12–19%, with women being affected twice as often as men. Diarrhea and constipation are among the most common patient complaints faced by internists and primary care physicians, and they account for nearly 50% of referrals to gastroenterologists.

Although diarrhea and constipation may present as mere nuisance symptoms at one extreme, they can be severe or life-threatening at the other. Even mild symptoms may signal a serious underlying gastrointestinal lesion, such as colorectal cancer, or systemic disorder, such as thyroid disease. Given the heterogeneous causes and potential severity of these common complaints, it is imperative for clinicians to appreciate the pathophysiology, etiologic classification, diagnostic strategies, and principles of management of diarrhea and constipation, so that rational and cost-effective care can be delivered.

NORMAL PHYSIOLOGY

While the primary function of the small intestine is the digestion and assimilation of nutrients from food, the small intestine and colon together perform important functions that regulate the secretion and absorption of water and electrolytes, the storage and subsequent transport of intraluminal contents aborally, and the salvage of some nutrients after bacterial metabolism of carbohydrate that are not absorbed in the small intestine. The main motor functions are summarized in Table 40-1. Alterations in fluid and electrolyte handling contribute significantly to diarrhea. Alterations in motor and sensory functions of the colon result in highly prevalent syndromes such as irritable bowel syndrome (IBS), chronic diarrhea, and chronic constipation.

■ NEURAL CONTROL

The small intestine and colon have intrinsic and extrinsic innervation. The *intrinsic innervation*, also called the enteric nervous system, comprises myenteric, submucosal, and mucosal neuronal

TABLE 40-1 Normal Gastrointestinal Motility: Functions at Different Anatomic Levels

Stomach and small bowel
Synchronized MMC in fasting
Accommodation, trituration, mixing, transit
Stomach ~3 h
Small bowel ~3 h
Ileal reservoir empties boluses
Colon: irregular mixing, fermentation, absorption, transit
Ascending, transverse: reservoirs
Descending: conduit
Sigmoid/rectum: volitional reservoir

Note: MMC, migrating motor complex.

layers. The function of these layers is modulated by interneurons through the actions of neurotransmitter amines or peptides, including acetylcholine, vasoactive intestinal peptide (VIP), opioids, norepinephrine, serotonin, Adenosine triphosphate (ATP), and nitric oxide (NO). The myenteric plexus regulates smooth-muscle function, and the submucosal plexus affects secretion, absorption, and mucosal blood flow.

The *extrinsic innervations* of the small intestine and colon are part of the autonomic nervous system and also modulate motor and secretory functions. The parasympathetic nerves convey visceral sensory and excitatory pathways to the colon. Parasympathetic fibers via the vagus nerve reach the small intestine and proximal colon along the branches of the superior mesenteric artery. The distal colon is supplied by sacral parasympathetic nerves (S_{2-4}) via the pelvic plexus; these fibers course through the wall of the colon as ascending intracolonic fibers as far as, and in some instances including, the proximal colon. The chief excitatory neurotransmitters controlling motor function are acetylcholine and the tachykinins, such as substance P. The sympathetic nerve supply modulates motor functions and reaches the small intestine and colon alongside their arterial vessels. Sympathetic input to the gut is generally excitatory to sphincters and inhibitory to nonsphincteric muscle. Visceral afferents convey sensation from the gut to the central nervous system (CNS); initially, they course along sympathetic fibers, but as they approach the spinal cord they separate, have cell bodies in the dorsal root ganglion, and enter the dorsal horn of the spinal cord. Afferent signals are conveyed to the brain along the lateral spinothalamic tract and the nociceptive dorsal column pathway and are then projected beyond the thalamus and brainstem to the insula and cerebral cortex to be perceived. Other afferent fibers synapse in the prevertebral ganglia and reflexly modulate intestinal motility.

■ INTESTINAL FLUID ABSORPTION AND SECRETION

On an average day, 9 L of fluid enter the gastrointestinal (GI) tract, ~1 L of residual fluid reaches the colon, and the stool excretion of fluid constitutes about 0.2 L/d. The colon has a large capacitance and functional reserve and may recover up to four times its usual volume of 0.8 L/d, provided the rate of flow permits reabsorption to occur. Thus, the colon can partially compensate for excess fluid delivery to the colon because of intestinal absorptive or secretory disorders.

In the colon, sodium absorption is predominantly electrogenic, and uptake takes place at the apical membrane; it is compensated for by the export functions of the basolateral sodium pump. A variety of neural and non-neural mediators regulate colonic fluid and electrolyte balance, including cholinergic, adrenergic, and serotonergic mediators. Angiotensin and aldosterone also influence colonic absorption, reflecting the common embryologic development of the distal colonic epithelium and the renal tubules.

■ SMALL-INTESTINAL MOTILITY

During fasting, the motility of the small intestine is characterized by a cyclical event called the migrating motor complex (MMC), which serves to clear nondigestible residue from the small intestine (the intestinal "housekeeper"). This organized, propagated series of contractions last, on average, 4 min, occurs every 60–90 min, and usually involve the entire small intestine. After food ingestion, the small intestine produces irregular, mixing contractions of relatively low amplitude, except in the distal ileum where more powerful contractions occur intermittently and empty the ileum by bolus transfers.

■ ILEOCOLONIC STORAGE AND SALVAGE

The distal ileum acts as a reservoir, emptying intermittently by bolus movements. This action allows time for salvage of fluids, electrolytes, and nutrients. Segmentation by haustra compartmentalizes the colon and facilitates mixing, retention of residue, and formation of solid stools. There is increased appreciation of the intimate interaction between the colonic function and the luminal ecology. The resident bacteria in the colon are necessary for the digestion of unabsorbed carbohydrates that reach the colon even in health, thereby providing a vital source of nutrients to the mucosa. Normal colonic flora also keeps pathogens at bay by a variety of mechanisms. In health, the ascending and transverse regions of colon function as reservoirs (average transit, 15 h), and the descending colon acts as a conduit (average transit, 3 h). The colon is efficient at conserving sodium and water, a function that is particularly important in sodium-depleted patients in whom the small intestine alone is unable to maintain sodium balance. Diarrhea or constipation may result from alteration in the reservoir function of the proximal colon or the propulsive function of the left colon. Constipation may also result from disturbances of the rectal or sigmoid reservoir, typically as a result of dysfunction of the pelvic floor, the anal sphincters, or the coordination of defecation.

■ COLONIC MOTILITY AND TONE

The small intestinal MMC only rarely continues into the colon. However, short duration or phasic contractions mix colonic contents, and high-amplitude (>75 mmHg) propagated contractions (HAPCs) are sometimes associated with mass movements through the colon and normally occur approximately five times per day, usually on awakening in the morning and postprandially. Increased frequency of HAPCs may result in diarrhea or urgency. The predominant phasic contractions in the colon are irregular and non-propagated and serve a "mixing" function.

Colonic tone refers to the background contractility upon which phasic contractile activity (typically contractions lasting <15 s) is superimposed. It is an important cofactor in the colon's capacitance (volume accommodation) and sensation.

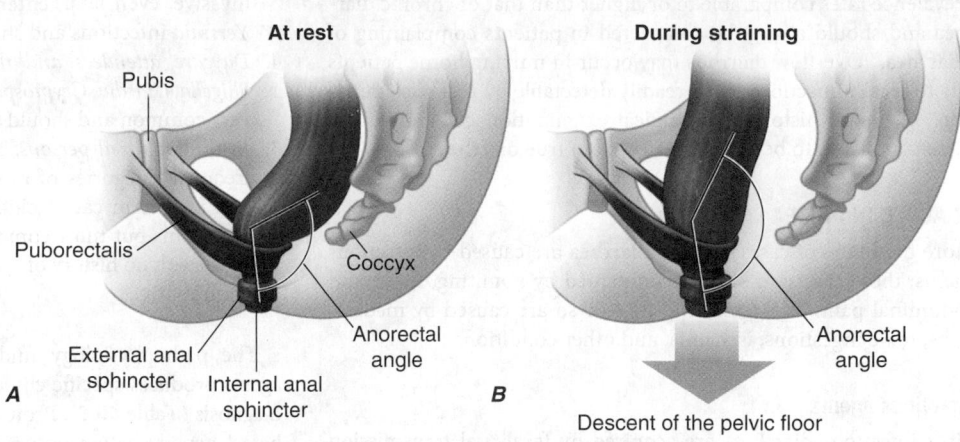

Figure 40-1 Sagittal view of the anorectum (A) at rest and (B) during straining to defecate. Continence is maintained by normal rectal sensation and tonic contraction of the internal anal sphincter and the puborectalis muscle, which wraps around the anorectum, maintaining an anorectal angle between 80° and 110°. During defecation, the pelvic floor muscles (including the puborectalis) relax, allowing the anorectal angle to straighten by at least 15°, and the perineum descends by 1–3.5 cm. The external anal sphincter also relaxes and reduces pressure on the anal canal. *(Reproduced with permission from Lembo and Camilleri.)*

■ COLONIC MOTILITY AFTER MEAL INGESTION

After meal ingestion, colonic phasic and tonic contractility increase for a period of ~2 h. The initial phase (~10 min) is mediated by the vagus nerve in response to mechanical distention of the stomach. The subsequent response of the colon requires caloric stimulation and is mediated at least in part by hormones (e.g., gastrin and serotonin).

■ DEFECATION

Tonic contraction of the puborectalis muscle, which forms a sling around the rectoanal junction, is important to maintain continence; during defecation, sacral parasympathetic nerves relax this muscle, facilitating the straightening of the rectoanal angle (Fig. 40-1). Distention of the rectum results in transient relaxation of the internal anal sphincter via intrinsic and reflex sympathetic innervation. As sigmoid and rectal contractions increase the pressure within the rectum, the rectosigmoid angle opens by >15°. Voluntary relaxation of the external anal sphincter (striated muscle innervated by the pudendal nerve) in response to the sensation produced by distention permits the evacuation of feces; this evacuation process can be augmented by an increase in intraabdominal pressure created by the Valsalva maneuver. Defecation can also be delayed voluntarily by contraction of the external anal sphincter.

DIARRHEA

■ DEFINITION

Diarrhea is loosely defined as passage of abnormally liquid or unformed stools at an increased frequency. For adults on a typical Western diet, stool weight >200 g/d can generally be considered diarrheal. Diarrhea may be further defined as *acute* if <2 weeks, *persistent* if 2–4 weeks, and *chronic* if >4 weeks in duration.

Two common conditions, usually associated with the passage of stool totaling <200 g/d, must be distinguished from diarrhea, because diagnostic and therapeutic algorithms differ. *Pseudodiarrhea*, or the frequent passage of small volumes of stool, is often associated with rectal urgency and accompanies IBS or proctitis. *Fecal incontinence* is the involuntary discharge of rectal contents and is most often caused by neuromuscular disorders or structural anorectal problems. Diarrhea and urgency, especially if severe, may aggravate or cause incontinence. Pseudodiarrhea and fecal incontinence occur at prevalence rates comparable to or higher than that of chronic diarrhea and should always be considered in patients complaining of "diarrhea." Overflow diarrhea may occur in nursing home patients due to fecal impaction that is readily detectable by rectal examination. A careful history and physical examination generally allow these conditions to be discriminated from true diarrhea.

■ ACUTE DIARRHEA

More than 90% of cases of acute diarrhea are caused by infectious agents; these cases are often accompanied by vomiting, fever, and abdominal pain. The remaining 10% or so are caused by medications, toxic ingestions, ischemia, and other conditions.

Infectious agents

Most infectious diarrheas are acquired by fecal-oral transmission or, more commonly, via ingestion of food or water contaminated with pathogens from human or animal feces. In the immunocompetent person, the resident fecal microflora, containing >500 taxonomically distinct species, are rarely the source of diarrhea and may actually play a role in suppressing the growth of ingested pathogens. Disturbances of flora by antibiotics can lead to diarrhea by reducing the digestive function or by allowing the overgrowth of pathogens, such as *Clostridium difficile* (Chap. 129). Acute infection or injury occurs when the ingested agent overwhelms or bypasses the host's mucosal immune and nonimmune (gastric acid, digestive enzymes, mucus secretion, peristalsis, and suppressive resident flora) defenses. Established clinical associations with specific enteropathogens may offer diagnostic clues.

In the United States, five high-risk groups are recognized:

1. *Travelers.* Nearly 40% of tourists to endemic regions of Latin America, Africa, and Asia develop so-called traveler's diarrhea, most commonly due to enterotoxigenic or enteroaggregative *Escherichia coli* as well as to *Campylobacter, Shigella, Aeromonas,* norovirus, *Coronavirus,* and *Salmonella.* Visitors to Russia (especially St. Petersburg) may have increased risk of *Giardia*-associated diarrhea; visitors to Nepal may acquire *Cyclospora.* Campers, backpackers, and swimmers in wilderness areas may become infected with *Giardia.* Cruise ships may be affected by outbreaks of gastroenteritis caused by agents such as norovirus.

2. *Consumers of certain foods.* Diarrhea closely following food consumption at a picnic, banquet, or restaurant may suggest infection with *Salmonella, Campylobacter,* or *Shigella* from chicken; enterohemorrhagic *E. coli* (O157:H7) from undercooked hamburger; *Bacillus cereus* from fried rice or other reheated food; *Staphylococcus aureus* or *Salmonella* from mayonnaise or creams; *Salmonella* from eggs; *Listeria* from uncooked foods or soft cheeses; and *Vibrio* species, *Salmonella,* or acute hepatitis A from seafood, especially if raw.

3. *Immunodeficient persons.* Individuals at risk for diarrhea include those with either primary immunodeficiency (e.g., IgA deficiency, common variable hypogammaglobulinemia, chronic granulomatous disease) or the much more common secondary immunodeficiency states (e.g., AIDS, senescence, pharmacologic suppression). Common enteric pathogens often cause a more severe and protracted diarrheal illness, and, particularly in persons with AIDS, opportunistic infections, such as by *Mycobacterium* species, certain viruses (cytomegalovirus, adenovirus, and herpes simplex), and protozoa (*Cryptosporidium, Isospora belli,* Microsporida, and *Blastocystis hominis*) may also play a role (Chap. 189). In patients with AIDS, agents transmitted venereally per rectum (e.g., *Neisseria gonorrhoeae, Treponema pallidum, Chlamydia*) may contribute to proctocolitis. Persons with hemochromatosis are especially prone to

invasive, even fatal, enteric infections with *Vibrio* species and *Yersinia* infections and should avoid raw fish.

4. *Daycare attendees and their family members.* Infections with *Shigella, Giardia, Cryptosporidium,* rotavirus, and other agents are very common and should be considered.

5. *Institutionalized persons.* Infectious diarrhea is one of the most frequent categories of nosocomial infections in many hospitals and long-term care facilities; the causes are a variety of microorganisms but most commonly *C. difficile. C. difficile* can affect those with no history of antibiotic use and may be acquired in the community.

The pathophysiology underlying acute diarrhea by infectious agents produces specific clinical features that may also be helpful in diagnosis (Table 40-2). Profuse, watery diarrhea secondary to small-bowel hypersecretion occurs with ingestion of preformed bacterial toxins, enterotoxin-producing bacteria, and enteroadherent pathogens. Diarrhea associated with marked vomiting and minimal or no fever may occur abruptly within a few hours after ingestion of the former two types; vomiting is usually less, abdominal cramping or bloating is greater, and fever is higher with the latter. Cytotoxin-producing and invasive microorganisms all cause high fever and abdominal pain. Invasive bacteria and *Entamoeba histolytica* often cause bloody diarrhea (referred to as *dysentery*). *Yersinia* invades the terminal ileal and proximal colon mucosa and may cause especially severe abdominal pain with tenderness mimicking acute appendicitis.

Finally, infectious diarrhea may be associated with systemic manifestations. Reactive arthritis (formerly known as Reiter's syndrome), arthritis, urethritis, and conjunctivitis may accompany or follow infections by *Salmonella, Campylobacter, Shigella,* and *Yersinia.* Yersiniosis may also lead to an autoimmune-type thyroiditis, pericarditis, and glomerulonephritis. Both enterohemorrhagic *E. coli* (O157:H7) and *Shigella* can lead to the *hemolytic-uremic syndrome* with an attendant high mortality rate. The syndrome of postinfectious IBS has now been recognized as a complication of infectious diarrhea. Acute diarrhea can also be a major symptom of several systemic infections including *viral hepatitis, listeriosis, legionellosis,* and *toxic shock syndrome.*

Other causes

Side effects from medications are probably the most common noninfectious causes of acute diarrhea, and etiology may be suggested by a temporal association between use and symptom onset. Although innumerable medications may produce diarrhea, some of the more frequently incriminated include antibiotics, cardiac antidysrhythmics, antihypertensives, nonsteroidal anti-inflammatory drugs (NSAIDs), certain antidepressants, chemotherapeutic agents, bronchodilators, antacids, and laxatives. Occlusive or nonocclusive *ischemic colitis* typically occurs in persons >50 years; often presents as acute lower abdominal pain preceding watery, then bloody diarrhea; and generally results in acute inflammatory changes in the sigmoid or left colon while sparing the rectum. Acute diarrhea may accompany colonic *diverticulitis* and *graft-versus-host disease.* Acute diarrhea, often associated with systemic compromise, can follow ingestion of toxins including organophosphate insecticides; amanita and other mushrooms; arsenic; and preformed environmental toxins in seafood, such as ciguatera and scombroid. Acute anaphylaxis to food ingestion can have a similar presentation. Conditions causing chronic diarrhea can also be confused with acute diarrhea early in their course. This confusion may occur with inflammatory bowel disease (IBD) and some of the other inflammatory chronic diarrheas that may have an abrupt rather than insidious onset and exhibit features that mimic infection.

TABLE 40-2 Association Between Pathobiology of Causative Agents and Clinical Features in Acute Infectious Diarrhea

Pathobiology/Agents	Incubation Period	Vomiting	Abdominal Pain	Fever	Diarrhea
Toxin producers					
Preformed toxin					
Bacillus cereus, Staphylococcus aureus, Clostridium perfringens	1–8 h 8–24 h	3–4+	1–2+	0–1+	3–4+, watery
Enterotoxin					
Vibrio cholerae, enterotoxigenic *Escherichia coli, Klebsiella pneumoniae, Aeromonas* species	8–72 h	2–4+	1–2+	0–1+	3–4+, watery
Enteroadherent					
Enteropathogenic and enteroadherent *E. coli, Giardia* organisms, cryptosporidiosis, helminths	1–8 d	0–1+	1–3+	0–2+	1–2+, watery, mushy
Cytotoxin producers					
C. difficile	1–3 d	0–1+	3–4+	1–2+	1–3+, usually watery, occasionally bloody
Hemorrhagic *E. coli*	12–72 h	0–1+	3–4+	1–2+	1–3+, initially watery, quickly bloody
Invasive organisms					
Minimal inflammation					
Rotavirus and norovirus	1–3 d	1–3+	2–3+	3–4+	1–3+, watery
Variable inflammation					
Salmonella, Campylobacter, and *Aeromonas* species, *Vibrio parahaemolyticus, Yersinia*	12 h–11 d	0–3+	2–4+	3–4+	1–4+, watery or bloody
Severe inflammation					
Shigella species, enteroinvasive *E. coli, Entamoeba histolytica*	12 h–8 d	0–1+	3–4+	3–4+	1–2+, bloody

Source: Adapted from DW Powell, in T Yamada (ed): *Textbook of Gastroenterology and Hepatology*, 4th ed. Philadelphia, Lippincott Williams & Wilkins, 2003.

APPROACH TO THE PATIENT | Acute Diarrhea

The decision to evaluate acute diarrhea depends on its severity and duration and on various host factors (Fig. 40-2). Most episodes of acute diarrhea are mild and self-limited and do not justify the cost and potential morbidity rate of diagnostic or pharmacologic interventions. Indications for evaluation include profuse diarrhea with dehydration, grossly bloody stools, fever ≥38.5°C (≥101°F), duration >48 h without improvement, recent antibiotic use, new community outbreaks, associated severe abdominal pain in patients >50 years, and elderly (≥70 years) or immunocompromised patients. In some cases of moderately severe febrile diarrhea associated with fecal leukocytes (or increased fecal levels of the leukocyte proteins) or with gross blood, a diagnostic evaluation might be avoided in favor of an empirical antibiotic trial (see below).

The cornerstone of diagnosis in those suspected of severe acute infectious diarrhea is microbiologic analysis of the stool. Workup includes cultures for bacterial and viral pathogens, direct inspection for ova and parasites, and immunoassays for certain bacterial toxins (*C. difficile*), viral antigens (rotavirus), and protozoal antigens (*Giardia, E. histolytica*). The aforementioned clinical and epidemiologic associations may assist in focusing the evaluation. If a particular pathogen or set of possible pathogens is so implicated, then either the whole panel of routine studies may not be necessary or, in some instances, special cultures may be appropriate as for enterohemorrhagic and other types of *E. coli*, *Vibrio* species, and *Yersinia*. Molecular diagnosis of pathogens in stool can be made by identification of unique DNA sequences; and evolving microarray technologies could lead to a more rapid, sensitive, specific, and cost-effective diagnostic approach in the future.

Persistent diarrhea is commonly due to *Giardia* (Chap. 209), but additional causative organisms that should be considered include *C. difficile* (especially if antibiotics had been administered), *E. histolytica*, *Cryptosporidium*, *Campylobacter*, and others. If stool studies are unrevealing, flexible sigmoidoscopy with biopsies and upper endoscopy with duodenal aspirates and biopsies may be indicated. Brainerd diarrhea is an increasingly recognized entity characterized by an abrupt-onset diarrhea that persists for at least 4 weeks, but may last 1–3 years, and is thought to be of infectious origin. It may be associated with subtle inflammation of the distal small intestine or proximal colon.

Structural examination by sigmoidoscopy, colonoscopy, or abdominal CT scanning (or other imaging approaches) may be appropriate in patients with uncharacterized persistent diarrhea to exclude IBD or as an initial approach in patients with suspected noninfectious acute diarrhea such as might be caused by ischemic colitis, diverticulitis, or partial bowel obstruction.

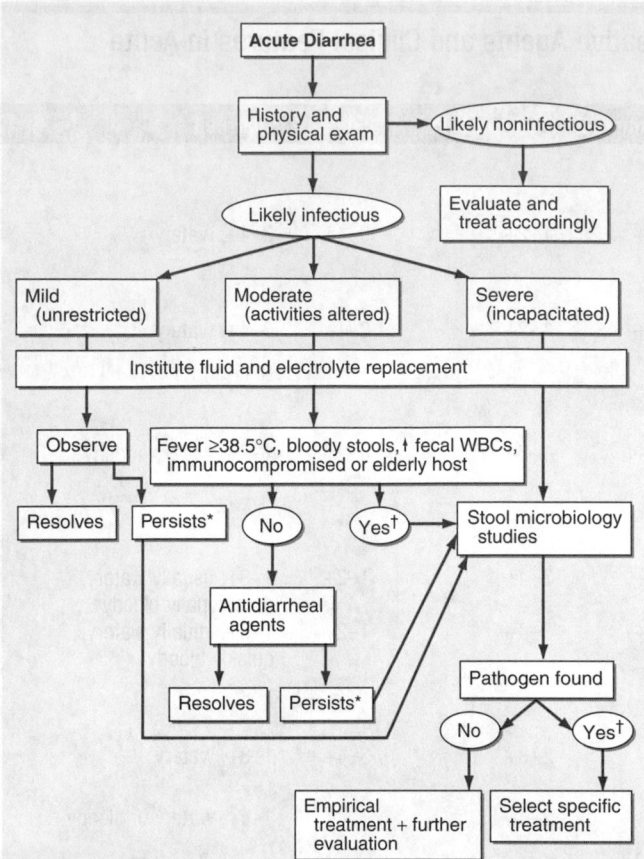

Figure 40-2 Algorithm for the management of acute diarrhea. Consider empirical Rx before evaluation with (*) metronidazole and with (†) quinolone. WBCs, white blood cells.

TREATMENT   Acute Diarrhea

Fluid and electrolyte replacement are of central importance to all forms of acute diarrhea. Fluid replacement alone may suffice for mild cases. Oral sugar-electrolyte solutions (sport drinks or designed formulations) should be instituted promptly with severe diarrhea to limit dehydration, which is the major cause of death. Profoundly dehydrated patients, especially infants and the elderly, require IV rehydration.

In moderately severe nonfebrile and nonbloody diarrhea, antimotility and antisecretory agents such as loperamide can be useful adjuncts to control symptoms. Such agents should be avoided with febrile dysentery, which may be exacerbated or prolonged by them. Bismuth subsalicylate may reduce symptoms of vomiting and diarrhea but should not be used to treat immunocompromised patients or those with renal impairment because of the risk of bismuth encephalopathy.

Judicious use of antibiotics is appropriate in selected instances of acute diarrhea and may reduce its severity and duration (Fig. 40-2). Many physicians treat moderately to severely ill patients with febrile dysentery empirically without diagnostic evaluation using a quinolone, such as ciprofloxacin (500 mg bid for 3–5 d). Empirical treatment can also be considered for suspected giardiasis with metronidazole (250 mg qid for 7 d). Selection of antibiotics and dosage regimens are otherwise dictated by specific pathogens, geographic patterns of resistance, and conditions found (Chaps. 128, 149, and 153–159). Antibiotic coverage is indicated, whether or not a causative organism is discovered, in patients who are immunocompromised, have mechanical heart valves or recent vascular grafts, or are elderly. Bismuth subsalicylate may reduce the frequency of traveler's diarrhea. Antibiotic prophylaxis is only indicated for certain patients traveling to high-risk countries in whom the likelihood or seriousness of acquired diarrhea would be especially high, including those with immunocompromise, IBD, hemochromatosis, or gastric achlorhydria. Use of ciprofloxacin or rifaximin may reduce bacterial diarrhea in such travelers by 90%, though rifaximin is not suitable for invasive disease, but rather as treatment for uncomplicated traveler's diarrhea. Finally, physicians should be vigilant to identify if an outbreak of diarrheal illness is occurring and to alert the public health authorities promptly. This may reduce the ultimate size of the affected population.

◼ CHRONIC DIARRHEA

Diarrhea lasting >4 weeks warrants evaluation to exclude serious underlying pathology. In contrast to acute diarrhea, most of the causes of chronic diarrhea are noninfectious. The classification of chronic diarrhea by pathophysiologic mechanism facilitates a rational approach to management, though many diseases cause diarrhea by more than one mechanism (Table 40-3).

Secretory causes

Secretory diarrheas are due to derangements in fluid and electrolyte transport across the enterocolonic mucosa. They are characterized clinically by watery, large-volume fecal outputs that are typically painless and persist with fasting. Because there is no malabsorbed solute, stool osmolality is accounted for by normal endogenous electrolytes with no fecal osmotic gap.

Medications   Side effects from regular ingestion of drugs and toxins are the most common secretory causes of chronic diarrhea. Hundreds of prescription and over-the-counter medications (see "Acute Diarrhea, Other Causes," above) may produce diarrhea. Surreptitious or habitual use of stimulant laxatives [e.g., senna, cascara, bisacodyl, ricinoleic acid (castor oil)] must also be considered. Chronic ethanol consumption may cause a secretory-type diarrhea due to enterocyte injury with impaired sodium and water absorption as well as rapid transit and other alterations. Inadvertent ingestion of certain environmental toxins (e.g., arsenic) may lead to chronic rather than acute forms of diarrhea. Certain bacterial infections may occasionally persist and be associated with a secretory-type diarrhea.

Bowel resection, mucosal disease, or enterocolic fistula   These conditions may result in a secretory-type diarrhea because of inadequate surface for reabsorption of secreted fluids and electrolytes. Unlike other secretory diarrheas, this subset of conditions tends to worsen with eating. With disease (e.g., Crohn's ileitis) or resection of <100 cm of terminal ileum, dihydroxy bile acids may escape absorption and stimulate colonic secretion (cholorrheic diarrhea). This mechanism may contribute to so-called *idiopathic secretory diarrhea*, in which bile acids are functionally malabsorbed from a normal-appearing terminal ileum. This *idiopathic bile acid malabsorption* may account for an average of 40% of unexplained chronic diarrhea. Reduced negative feedback regulation of bile acid synthesis by fibroblast growth factor 19 produced by enterocytes results in a degree of bile-acid synthesis that exceeds the normal capacity for ileal reabsorption, producing bile acid diarrhea.

Partial bowel obstruction, ostomy stricture, or fecal impaction may paradoxically lead to increased fecal output due to fluid hypersecretion.

TABLE 40-3 Major Causes of Chronic Diarrhea According to Predominant Pathophysiologic Mechanism

Secretory causes

Exogenous stimulant laxatives

Chronic ethanol ingestion

Other drugs and toxins

Endogenous laxatives (dihydroxy bile acids)

Idiopathic secretory diarrhea

Certain bacterial infections

Bowel resection, disease, or fistula (↓ absorption)

Partial bowel obstruction or fecal impaction

Hormone-producing tumors (carcinoid, VIPoma, medullary cancer of thyroid, mastocytosis, gastrinoma, colorectal villous adenoma)

Addison's disease

Congenital electrolyte absorption defects

Osmotic causes

Osmotic laxatives (Mg^{2+}, PO_4^{-3}, SO_4^{-2})

Lactase and other disaccharide deficiencies

Nonabsorbable carbohydrates (sorbitol, lactulose, polyethylene glycol)

Steatorrheal causes

Intraluminal maldigestion (pancreatic exocrine insufficiency, bacterial overgrowth, bariatric surgery, liver disease)

Mucosal malabsorption (celiac sprue, Whipple's disease, infections, abetalipoproteinemia, ischemia)

Postmucosal obstruction (1° or 2° lymphatic obstruction)

Inflammatory causes

Idiopathic inflammatory bowel disease (Crohn's, chronic ulcerative colitis)

Lymphocytic and collagenous colitis

Immune-related mucosal disease (1° or 2° immuno-deficiencies, food allergy, eosinophilic gastroenteritis, graft-vs-host disease)

Infections (invasive bacteria, viruses, and parasites, Brainerd diarrhea)

Radiation injury

Gastrointestinal malignancies

Dysmotile causes

Irritable bowel syndrome (including postinfectious IBS)

Visceral neuromyopathies

Hyperthyroidism

Drugs (prokinetic agents)

Postvagotomy

Factitial causes

Munchausen

Eating disorders

Iatrogenic causes

Cholecystectomy

Ileal resection

Bariatric surgery

Vagotomy, fundoplication

Hormones Although uncommon, the classic examples of secretory diarrhea are those mediated by hormones. *Metastatic gastrointestinal carcinoid tumors* or, rarely, *primary bronchial carcinoids* may produce watery diarrhea alone or as part of the carcinoid syndrome that comprises episodic flushing, wheezing, dyspnea, and right-sided valvular heart disease. Diarrhea is due to the release into the circulation of potent intestinal secretagogues including serotonin, histamine, prostaglandins, and various kinins. Pellagra-like skin lesions may rarely occur as the result of serotonin overproduction with niacin depletion. *Gastrinoma*, one of the most common neuroendocrine tumors, most typically presents with refractory peptic ulcers, but diarrhea occurs in up to one-third of cases and may be the only clinical manifestation in 10%. While other secretagogues released with gastrin may play a role, the diarrhea most often results from fat maldigestion owing to pancreatic enzyme inactivation by

low intraduodenal pH. The watery diarrhea hypokalemia achlorhydria syndrome, also called *pancreatic cholera*, is due to a non-β cell pancreatic adenoma, referred to as a *VIPoma*, that secretes VIP and a host of other peptide hormones including pancreatic polypeptide, secretin, gastrin, gastrin-inhibitory polypeptide (also called glucose-dependent insulinotropic peptide), neurotensin, calcitonin, and prostaglandins. The secretory diarrhea is often massive with stool volumes >3 L/d; daily volumes as high as 20 L have been reported. Life-threatening dehydration; neuromuscular dysfunction from associated hypokalemia, hypomagnesemia, or hypercalcemia; flushing; and hyperglycemia may accompany a VIPoma. *Medullary carcinoma of the thyroid* may present with watery diarrhea caused by calcitonin, other secretory peptides, or prostaglandins. Prominent diarrhea is often associated with metastatic disease and poor prognosis. *Systemic mastocytosis*, which may be associated with the skin lesion urticaria pigmentosa, may cause diarrhea that is either secretory and mediated by histamine or inflammatory due to intestinal infiltration by mast cells. Large *colorectal villous adenomas* may rarely be associated with a secretory diarrhea that may cause hypokalemia, can be inhibited by NSAIDs, and are apparently mediated by prostaglandins.

Congenital defects in ion absorption Rarely, defects in specific carriers associated with ion absorption cause watery diarrhea from birth. These disorders include defective Cl^-/HCO_3^- exchange (*congenital chloridorrhea*) with alkalosis (which results from a mutated *DRA* [down-regulated in adenoma] gene) and defective Na^+/H^+ exchange (*congential sodium diarrhea*), which results from a mutation in the *NHE3* (sodium-hydrogen exchanger) gene and results in acidosis.

Some hormone deficiencies may be associated with watery diarrhea, such as occurs with adrenocortical insufficiency (Addison's disease) that may be accompanied by skin hyperpigmentation.

Osmotic causes

Osmotic diarrhea occurs when ingested, poorly absorbable, osmotically active solutes draw enough fluid into the lumen to exceed the reabsorptive capacity of the colon. Fecal water output increases in proportion to such a solute load. Osmotic diarrhea characteristically ceases with fasting or with discontinuation of the causative agent.

Osmotic laxatives Ingestion of magnesium-containing antacids, health supplements, or laxatives may induce osmotic diarrhea typified by a stool osmotic gap (>50 mosmol/L): serum osmolarity (typically 290 mosmol/kg)-[2 x (fecal sodium + potassium concentration)]. Measurement of fecal osmolarity is no longer recommended because, even when measured immediately after evacuation, it may be erroneous because carbohydrates are metabolized by colonic bacteria, causing an increase in osmolarity.

Carbohydrate malabsorption Carbohydrate malabsorption due to acquired or congenital defects in brush-border disaccharidases and other enzymes leads to osmotic diarrhea with a low pH. One of the most common causes of chronic diarrhea in adults is *lactase deficiency*, which affects three-fourths of non-whites worldwide and 5–30% of persons in the United States; the total lactose load at any one time influences the symptoms experienced. Most patients learn to avoid milk products without requiring treatment with enzyme supplements. Some sugars, such as sorbitol, lactulose, or fructose, are frequently malabsorbed, and diarrhea ensues with ingestion of medications, gum, or candies sweetened with these poorly or incompletely absorbed sugars.

Steatorrheal causes

Fat malabsorption may lead to greasy, foul-smelling, difficult-to-flush diarrhea often associated with weight loss and nutritional deficiencies due to concomitant malabsorption of amino acids and vitamins. Increased fecal output is caused by the osmotic effects of fatty acids, especially after bacterial hydroxylation, and, to a lesser extent, by the neutral fat. Quantitatively, steatorrhea is defined as stool fat exceeding the normal 7 g/d; rapid-transit diarrhea may result in fecal fat up to 14 g/d; daily fecal fat averages 15–25 g with small intestinal diseases and is often >32 g with pancreatic exocrine insufficiency. Intraluminal maldigestion, mucosal malabsorption, or lymphatic obstruction may produce steatorrhea.

Intraluminal maldigestion This condition most commonly results from pancreatic exocrine insufficiency, which occurs when >90% of pancreatic secretory function is lost. *Chronic pancreatitis*, usually a sequel of ethanol abuse, most frequently causes pancreatic insufficiency. Other causes include *cystic fibrosis*; *pancreatic duct obstruction*; and, rarely, *somatostatinoma*. Bacterial overgrowth in the small intestine may deconjugate bile acids and alter micelle formation, impairing fat digestion; it occurs with stasis from a blind-loop, small-bowel diverticulum or dysmotility and is especially likely in the elderly. Finally, cirrhosis or biliary obstruction may lead to mild steatorrhea due to deficient intraluminal bile acid concentration.

Mucosal malabsorption Mucosal malabsorption occurs from a variety of enteropathies, but it most commonly occurs from *celiac disease*. This gluten-sensitive enteropathy affects all ages and is characterized by villous atrophy and crypt hyperplasia in the proximal small bowel and can present with fatty diarrhea associated with multiple nutritional deficiencies of varying severity. Celiac disease is much more frequent than previously thought; it affects ~1% of the population, frequently presents without steatorrhea, can mimic IBS, and has many other GI and extraintestinal manifestations. *Tropical sprue* may produce a similar histologic and clinical syndrome but occurs in residents of or travelers to tropical climates; abrupt onset and response to antibiotics suggest an infectious etiology. *Whipple's disease*, due to the bacillus *Tropheryma whipplei* and histiocytic infiltration of the small-bowel mucosa, is a less common cause of steatorrhea that most typically occurs in young or middle-aged men; it is frequently associated with arthralgias, fever, lymphadenopathy, and extreme fatigue, and it may affect the CNS and endocardium. A similar clinical and histologic picture results from *Mycobacterium avium-intracellulare* infection in patients with AIDS. *Abetalipoproteinemia* is a rare defect of chylomicron formation and fat malabsorption in children, associated with acanthocytic erythrocytes, ataxia, and retinitis pigmentosa. Several other conditions may cause mucosal malabsorption including infections, especially with protozoa such as *Giardia*; numerous medications (e.g., colchicine, cholestyramine, neomycin); amyloidosis; and chronic ischemia.

Postmucosal lymphatic obstruction The pathophysiology of this condition, which is due to the rare *congenital intestinal lymphangiectasia* or to *acquired lymphatic obstruction* secondary to trauma, tumor, cardiac disease or infection, leads to the unique constellation of fat malabsorption with enteric losses of protein (often causing edema) and lymphocytopenia. Carbohydrate and amino acid absorption are preserved.

Inflammatory causes

Inflammatory diarrheas are generally accompanied by pain, fever, bleeding, or other manifestations of inflammation. The mechanism of diarrhea may not only be exudation but, depending on lesion site, may include fat malabsorption, disrupted fluid/electrolyte absorption, and hypersecretion or hypermotility from release of cytokines and other inflammatory mediators. The unifying feature on stool analysis is the presence of leukocytes or leukocyte-derived proteins such as calprotectin. With severe inflammation, exudative protein loss can lead to anasarca (generalized edema). Any middle-aged or older person with chronic inflammatory-type diarrhea, especially with blood, should be carefully evaluated to exclude a colorectal tumor.

Idiopathic inflammatory bowel disease The illnesses in this category, which include *Crohn's disease* and *chronic ulcerative colitis*, are among the most common organic causes of chronic diarrhea in adults and range in severity from mild to fulminant and life-threatening. They may be associated with uveitis, polyarthralgias, cholestatic liver disease (primary sclerosing cholangitis), and skin lesions (erythema nodosum, pyoderma gangrenosum). *Microscopic colitis*, including both lymphocytic and *collagenous colitis*, is an increasingly recognized cause of chronic watery diarrhea, especially in middle-aged women and those on NSAIDs, statins, proton pump inhibitors (PPIs), and selective serotonin reuptake inhibitors (SSRIs); biopsy of a normal-appearing colon is required for histologic diagnosis. It may coexist with symptoms suggesting IBS or with celiac sprue. It typically responds well to anti-inflammatory drugs (e.g., bismuth), to the opioid agonist loperamide, or to budesonide.

Primary or secondary forms of immunodeficiency Immunodeficiency may lead to prolonged infectious diarrhea. With selective IgA deficiency or common variable *hypogammaglobulinemia*, diarrhea is particularly prevalent and often the result of giardiasis, bacterial overgrowth, or sprue.

Eosinophilic gastroenteritis Eosinophil infiltration of the mucosa, muscularis, or serosa at any level of the GI tract may cause diarrhea, pain, vomiting, or ascites. Affected patients often have an atopic history, Charcot-Leyden crystals due to extruded eosinophil contents may be seen on microscopic inspection of stool, and peripheral eosinophilia is present in 50–75% of patients. While hypersensitivity to certain foods occurs in adults, true food allergy causing chronic diarrhea is rare.

Other causes Chronic inflammatory diarrhea may be caused by *radiation enterocolitis*, *chronic graft-versus-host disease*, *Behçet's syndrome*, and *Cronkhite-Canada syndrome*, among others.

Dysmotility causes

Rapid transit may accompany many diarrheas as a secondary or contributing phenomenon, but primary dysmotility is an unusual etiology of true diarrhea. Stool features often suggest a secretory diarrhea, but mild steatorrhea of up to 14 g of fat per day can be produced by maldigestion from rapid transit alone. *Hyperthyroidism*, *carcinoid syndrome*, and certain drugs (e.g., prostaglandins, prokinetic agents) may produce hypermotility with resultant diarrhea. Primary visceral neuromyopathies or idiopathic acquired intestinal pseudoobstruction may lead to stasis with secondary bacterial overgrowth causing diarrhea. *Diabetic diarrhea*, often accompanied by peripheral and generalized autonomic neuropathies, may occur in part because of intestinal dysmotility.

The exceedingly common IBS (10% point prevalence, 1–2% per year incidence) is characterized by disturbed intestinal and colonic motor and sensory responses to various stimuli. Symptoms of stool frequency typically cease at night, alternate with periods of constipation, are accompanied by abdominal pain relieved with defecation, and rarely result in weight loss.

Factitial causes

Factitial diarrhea accounts for up to 15% of unexplained diarrheas referred to tertiary care centers. Either as a form of *Munchausen syndrome* (deception or self-injury for secondary gain) or *eating disorders*, some patients covertly self-administer laxatives alone or in combination with other medications (e.g., diuretics) or surreptitiously add water or urine to stool sent for analysis. Such patients are typically women, often with histories of psychiatric illness, and disproportionately from careers in health care. Hypotension and hypokalemia are common co-presenting features. The evaluation of such patients may be difficult: contamination of the stool with water or urine is suggested by very low or high stool osmolarity, respectively. Such patients often deny this possibility when confronted, but they do benefit from psychiatric counseling when they acknowledge their behavior.

Chronic Diarrhea

The laboratory tools available to evaluate the very common problem of chronic diarrhea are extensive, and many are costly and invasive. As such, the diagnostic evaluation must be rationally directed by a careful history and physical examination (Fig. 40-3A). When this strategy is unrevealing, simple triage tests are often warranted to direct the choice of more complex investigations (Fig. 40-3B). The history, physical examination (Table 40-4), and routine blood studies should attempt to characterize the mechanism of diarrhea, identify diagnostically helpful associations, and assess the patient's fluid/electrolyte and nutritional status. Patients should be questioned about the onset, duration, pattern, aggravating (especially diet) and relieving factors, and stool characteristics of their diarrhea. The presence or absence of fecal incontinence, fever, weight loss, pain, certain exposures (travel, medications, contacts with diarrhea), and common extraintestinal manifestations (skin changes, arthralgias, oral aphthous ulcers) should be noted. A family history of IBD or sprue may indicate those possibilities.

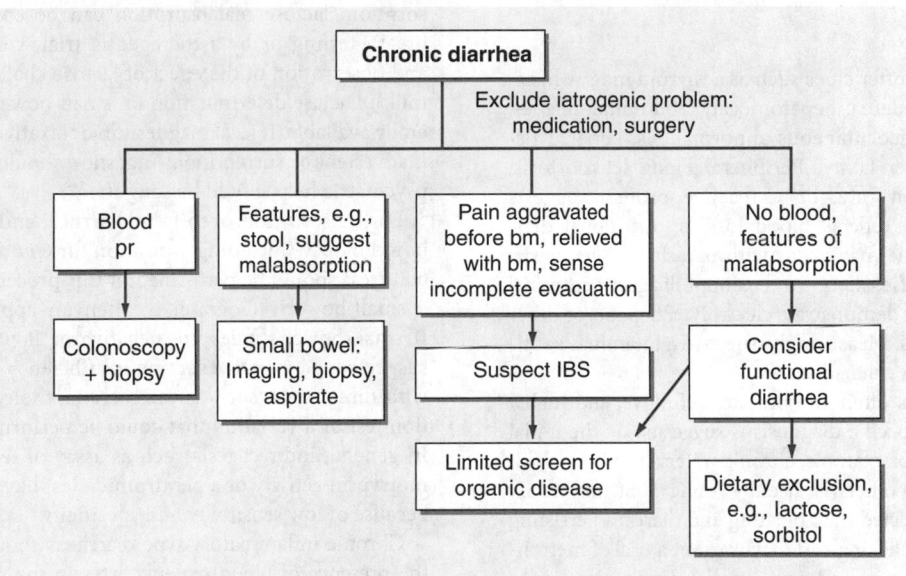

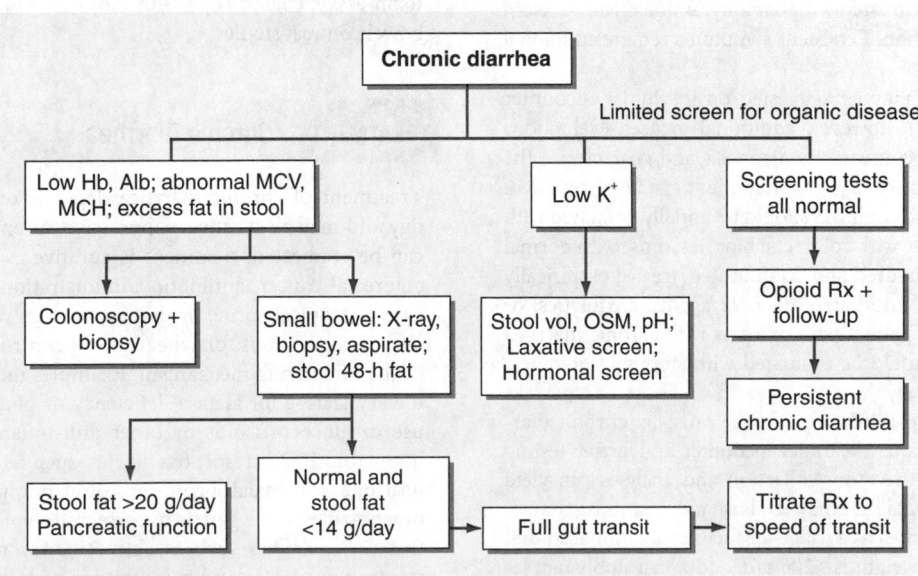

Figure 40-3   Chronic diarrhea. A. Initial management based on accompanying symptoms or features. **B.** Evaluation based on findings from a limited age-appropriate screen for organic disease. pr, per rectum; bm, bowel movement; IBS, irritable bowel syndrome; Hb, hemoglobin; Alb, albumin; MCV, mean corpuscular volume; MCH, mean corpuscular hemoglobin; OSM, osmolality. *(Reprinted from M Camilleri: Clin Gastroenterol Hepatol. 2:198, 2004.)*

TABLE 40-4 Physical Examination in Patients With Chronic Diarrhea

1. Are there general features to suggest malabsorption or inflammatory bowel disease (IBD) such as anemia, dermatitis herpetiformis, edema, or clubbing?

2. Are there features to suggest underlying autonomic neuropathy or collagen-vascular disease in the pupils, orthostasis, skin, hands, or joints?

3. Is there an abdominal mass or tenderness?

4. Are there any abnormalities of rectal mucosa, rectal defects, or altered anal sphincter functions?

5. Are there any mucocutaneous manifestations of systemic disease such as dermatitis herpetiformis (celiac disease), erythema nodosum (ulcerative colitis), flushing (carcinoid), or oral ulcers for IBD or celiac disease?

Physical findings may offer clues such as a thyroid mass, wheezing, heart murmurs, edema, hepatomegaly, abdominal masses, lymphadenopathy, mucocutaneous abnormalities, perianal fistulas, or anal sphincter laxity. Peripheral blood leukocytosis, elevated sedimentation rate, or C-reactive protein suggests inflammation; anemia reflects blood loss or nutritional deficiencies; or eosinophilia may occur with parasitoses, neoplasia, collagen-vascular disease, allergy, or eosinophilic gastroenteritis. Blood chemistries may demonstrate electrolyte, hepatic, or other metabolic disturbances. Measuring tissue transglutaminase antibodies may help detect celiac disease.

A therapeutic trial is often appropriate, definitive, and highly cost effective when a specific diagnosis is suggested on the initial physician encounter. For example, chronic watery diarrhea, which ceases with fasting in an otherwise healthy young adult, may justify a trial of a lactose-restricted diet; bloating and diarrhea persisting since a mountain backpacking trip may warrant a trial of metronidazole for likely giardiasis; and postprandial diarrhea persisting following resection of terminal ileum might be due to bile acid malabsorption and be treated with cholestyramine or colesevelam before further evaluation. Persistent symptoms require additional investigation.

Certain diagnoses may be suggested on the initial encounter (e.g., idiopathic IBD); however, additional focused evaluations may be necessary to confirm the diagnosis and characterize the severity or extent of disease so that treatment can be best guided. Patients suspected of having IBS should be initially evaluated with flexible sigmoidoscopy with colorectal biopsies; those with normal findings might be reassured and, as indicated, treated empirically with antispasmodics, antidiarrheals, bulk agents, anxiolytics, or antidepressants. Any patient who presents with chronic diarrhea and hematochezia should be evaluated with stool microbiologic studies and colonoscopy.

In an estimated two-thirds of cases, the cause for chronic diarrhea remains unclear after the initial encounter, and further testing is required. Quantitative stool collection and analyses can yield important objective data that may establish a diagnosis or characterize the type of diarrhea as a triage for focused additional studies (Fig. 40-3B). If stool weight is >200 g/d, additional stool analyses should be performed that might include electrolyte concentration, pH, occult blood testing, leukocyte inspection (or leukocyte protein assay), fat quantitation, and laxative screens.

For secretory diarrheas (watery, normal osmotic gap), possible medication-related side effects or surreptitious laxative use

should be reconsidered. Microbiologic studies should be done including fecal bacterial cultures (including media for *Aeromonas* and *Pleisiomonas*), inspection for ova and parasites, and *Giardia* antigen assay (the most sensitive test for giardiasis). Small-bowel bacterial overgrowth can be excluded by intestinal aspirates with quantitative cultures or with glucose or lactulose breath tests involving measurement of breath hydrogen, methane, or other metabolite (e.g., $^{14}CO_2$). However, interpretation of these breath tests may be confounded by disturbances of intestinal transit. Upper endoscopy and colonoscopy with biopsies and small-bowel barium x-rays are helpful to rule out structural or occult inflammatory disease. When suggested by history or other findings, screens for peptide hormones should be pursued (e.g., serum gastrin, VIP, calcitonin, and thyroid hormone/thyroid-stimulating hormone, or urinary 5-hydroxyindolacetic acid, and histamine).

Further evaluation of osmotic diarrhea should include tests for lactose intolerance and magnesium ingestion, the two most common causes. Low fecal pH suggests carbohydrate malabsorption; lactose malabsorption can be confirmed by lactose breath testing or by a therapeutic trial with lactose exclusion and observation of the effect of lactose challenge (e.g., a liter of milk). Lactase determination on small-bowel biopsy is not generally available. If fecal magnesium or laxative levels are elevated, inadvertent or surreptitious ingestion should be considered and psychiatric help should be sought.

For those with proven fatty diarrhea, endoscopy with small-bowel biopsy (including aspiration for *Giardia* and quantitative cultures) should be performed; if this procedure is unrevealing, a small-bowel radiograph is often an appropriate next step. If small-bowel studies are negative or if pancreatic disease is suspected, pancreatic exocrine insufficiency should be excluded with direct tests, such as the secretin-cholecystokinin stimulation test or a variation that could be performed endoscopically. In general, indirect tests such as assay of fecal elastase or chymotrypsin activity or a bentiromide test have fallen out of favor because of low sensitivity and specificity.

Chronic inflammatory-type diarrheas should be suspected by the presence of blood or leukocytes in the stool. Such findings warrant stool cultures; inspection for ova and parasites; *C. difficile* toxin assay; colonoscopy with biopsies; and, if indicated, small-bowel contrast studies.

TREATMENT   Chronic Diarrhea

Treatment of chronic diarrhea depends on the specific etiology and may be curative, suppressive, or empirical. If the cause can be eradicated, treatment is curative as with resection of a colorectal cancer, antibiotic administration for Whipple's disease or tropical sprue, or discontinuation of a drug. For many chronic conditions, diarrhea can be controlled by suppression of the underlying mechanism. Examples include elimination of dietary lactose for lactase deficiency or gluten for celiac sprue, use of glucocorticoids or other anti-inflammatory agents for idiopathic IBDs, adsorptive agents such as cholestyramine for ileal bile acid malabsorption, proton pump inhibitors such as omeprazole for the gastric hypersecretion of gastrinomas, somatostatin analogues such as octreotide for malignant carcinoid syndrome, prostaglandin inhibitors such as indomethacin for medullary carcinoma of the thyroid, and pancreatic enzyme replacement for pancreatic insufficiency. When the specific cause or mechanism of chronic diarrhea evades diagnosis, empirical therapy may be beneficial. Mild opiates, such as diphenoxylate or loperamide, are often helpful in mild or moderate watery diarrhea. For those with more severe diarrhea, codeine or tincture of opium may be beneficial. Such antimotility agents should be avoided with severe IBD, because toxic megacolon may be precipitated. Clonidine, an α_2-adrenergic agonist, may allow control of diabetic diarrhea. For all patients with chronic diarrhea, fluid and electrolyte repletion is an important component of management (see "Acute Diarrhea," above). Replacement of fat-soluble vitamins may also be necessary in patients with chronic steatorrhea.

CONSTIPATION

■ DEFINITION

Constipation is a common complaint in clinical practice and usually refers to persistent, difficult, infrequent, or seemingly incomplete defecation. Because of the wide range of normal bowel habits, constipation is difficult to define precisely. Most persons have at least three bowel movements per week; however, low stool frequency alone is not the sole criterion for the diagnosis of constipation. Many constipated patients have a normal frequency of defecation but complain of excessive straining, hard stools, lower abdominal fullness, or a sense of incomplete evacuation. The individual patient's symptoms must be analyzed in detail to ascertain what is meant by "constipation" or "difficulty" with defecation.

Stool form and consistency are well correlated with the time elapsed from the preceding defecation. Hard, pellety stools occur with slow transit, while loose, watery stools are associated with rapid transit. Both small pellety or very large stools are more difficult to expel than normal stools.

The perception of hard stools or excessive straining is more difficult to assess objectively, and the need for enemas or digital disimpaction is a clinically useful way to corroborate the patient's perceptions of difficult defecation.

Psychosocial or cultural factors may also be important. A person whose parents attached great importance to daily defecation will become greatly concerned when he or she misses a daily bowel movement; some children withhold stool to gain attention or because of fear of pain from anal irritation; and some adults habitually ignore or delay the call to have a bowel movement.

■ CAUSES

Pathophysiologically, chronic constipation generally results from inadequate fiber or fluid intake or from disordered colonic transit or anorectal function. These result from neurogastroenterologic disturbance, certain drugs, advancing age, or in association with a large number of systemic diseases that affect the GI tract (Table 40-5). Constipation of recent onset may be a symptom of significant organic disease such as tumor or stricture. In *idiopathic constipation*, a subset of patients exhibit delayed emptying of the ascending and transverse colon with prolongation of transit (often in the proximal colon) and a reduced frequency of propulsive HAPCs. *Outlet obstruction to defecation* (also called *evacuation disorders*) may cause delayed colonic transit, which is usually corrected by biofeedback retraining of the disordered defecation. Constipation of any cause may be exacerbated by hospitalization or chronic illnesses that lead to physical or mental impairment and result in inactivity or physical immobility.

APPROACH TO THE PATIENT ▶ Constipation

A careful history should explore the patient's symptoms and confirm whether he or she is indeed constipated based on frequency (e.g., fewer than three bowel movements per week),

TABLE 40-5 Causes of Constipation in Adults

Types of Constipation and Causes	Examples
Recent onset	
Colonic obstruction	Neoplasm; stricture: ischemic, diverticular, inflammatory
Anal sphincter spasm	Anal fissure, painful hemorrhoids
Medications	
Chronic	
Irritable bowel syndrome	Constipation-predominant, alternating
Medications	Ca^{2+} blockers, antidepressants
Colonic pseudoobstruction	Slow-transit constipation, megacolon (rare Hirschsprung's, Chagas' diseases)
Disorders of rectal evacuation	Pelvic floor dysfunction; anismus; descending perineum syndrome; rectal mucosal prolapse; rectocele
Endocrinopathies	Hypothyroidism, hypercalcemia, pregnancy
Psychiatric disorders	Depression, eating disorders, drugs
Neurologic disease	Parkinsonism, multiple sclerosis, spinal cord injury
Generalized muscle disease	Progressive systemic sclerosis

consistency (lumpy/hard), excessive straining, prolonged defecation time, or need to support the perineum or digitate the anorectum. In the vast majority of cases (probably >90%), there is no underlying cause (e.g., cancer, depression, or hypothyroidism), and constipation responds to ample hydration, exercise, and supplementation of dietary fiber (15–25 g/d). A good diet and medication history and attention to psychosocial issues are key. Physical examination and, particularly, a rectal examination should exclude fecal impaction and most of the important diseases that present with constipation and possibly indicate features suggesting an evacuation disorder (e.g., high anal sphincter tone).

The presence of weight loss, rectal bleeding, or anemia with constipation mandates either flexible sigmoidoscopy plus barium enema or colonoscopy alone, particularly in patients >40 years, to exclude structural diseases such as cancer or strictures. Colonoscopy alone is most cost-effective in this setting because it provides an opportunity to biopsy mucosal lesions, perform polypectomy, or dilate strictures. Barium enema has advantages over colonoscopy in the patient with isolated constipation because it is less costly and identifies colonic dilation and all significant mucosal lesions or strictures that are likely to present with constipation. Melanosis coli, or pigmentation of the colon mucosa, indicates the use of anthraquinone laxatives such as cascara or senna; however, this is usually apparent from a careful history. An unexpected disorder such as megacolon or cathartic colon may also be detected by colonic radiographs. Measurement of serum calcium, potassium, and thyroid-stimulating hormone levels will identify rare patients with metabolic disorders.

Patients with more troublesome constipation may not respond to fiber alone and may be helped by a bowel-training regimen: taking an osmotic laxative (lactulose, sorbitol, polyethylene glycol) and evacuating with enema or glycerine suppository as needed. After breakfast, a distraction-free 15–20 min on the toilet without straining is encouraged. Excessive straining may lead to development of hemorrhoids, and, if there is weakness of the pelvic floor or injury to the pudendal nerve, may result in obstructed defecation from descending perineum syndrome several years later. Those few who do not benefit from the simple measures delineated above or require long-term treatment with potent laxatives, with the attendant risk of developing laxative abuse syndrome, are assumed to have severe or intractable constipation and should have further investigation (Fig. 40-4). Novel agents that induce secretion (e.g., lubiprostone, a chloride channel activator) are also available.

■ INVESTIGATION OF SEVERE CONSTIPATION

A small minority (probably <5%) of patients have severe or "intractable" constipation. These are the patients most likely to be seen by gastroenterologists or in referral centers. Further observation of the patient may occasionally reveal a previously unrecognized cause, such as an evacuation disorder, laxative abuse, malingering, or psychological disorder. In these patients, evaluations of the physiologic function of the colon and pelvic floor and of psychological status aid in the rational choice of treatment. Even among these highly selected patients with severe constipation, a cause can be identified in only about two-thirds of tertiary referral patients (see below).

Measurement of colonic transit

Radiopaque marker transit tests are easy, repeatable, generally safe, inexpensive, reliable, and highly applicable in evaluating constipated patients in clinical practice. Several validated methods are very simple. For example, radiopaque markers are ingested; an abdominal flat film taken 5 days later should indicate passage of 80% of the markers out of the colon without the use of laxatives or enemas. This test does not provide useful information about the transit profile of the stomach and small bowel.

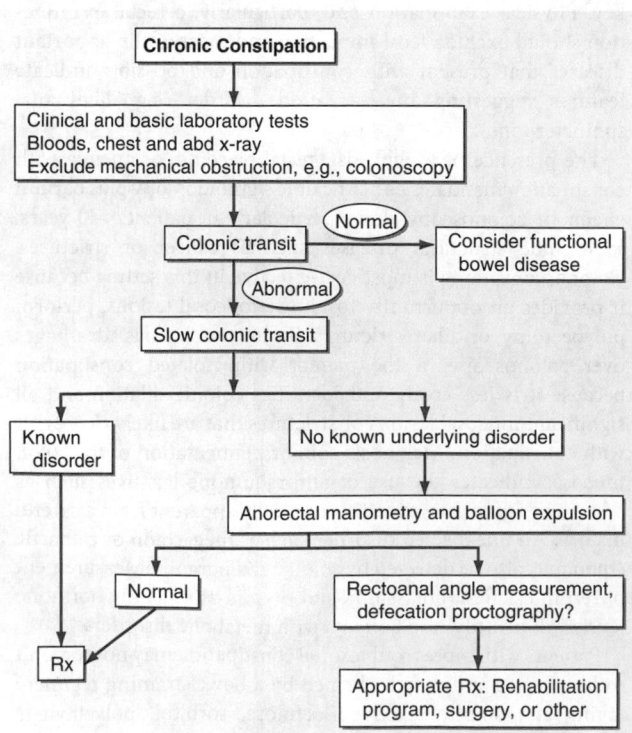

Figure 40-4 Algorithm for the management of constipation.

Radioscintigraphy with a delayed-release capsule containing radiolabeled particles has been used to noninvasively characterize normal, accelerated, or delayed colonic function over 24–48 h with low radiation exposure. This approach simultaneously assesses gastric, small bowel (which may be important in ~20% of patients with delayed colonic transit because they reflect a more generalized GI motility disorder), and colonic transit. The disadvantages are the greater cost and the need for specific materials prepared in a nuclear medicine laboratory.

Anorectal and pelvic floor tests

Pelvic floor dysfunction is suggested by the inability to evacuate the rectum, a feeling of persistent rectal fullness, rectal pain, the need to extract stool from the rectum digitally, application of pressure on the posterior wall of the vagina, support of the perineum during straining, and excessive straining. These significant symptoms should be contrasted with the sense of incomplete rectal evacuation, which is common in IBS.

Formal psychological evaluation may identify eating disorders, "control issues," depression, or post-traumatic stress disorders that may respond to cognitive or other intervention and may be important in restoring quality of life to patients who might present with chronic constipation.

A simple clinical test in the office to document a nonrelaxing puborectalis muscle is to have the patient strain to expel the index finger during a digital rectal examination. Motion of the puborectalis posteriorly during straining indicates proper coordination of the pelvic floor muscles.

Measurement of perineal descent is relatively easy to gauge clinically by placing the patient in the left decubitus position and watching the perineum to detect inadequate descent (<1.5 cm, a sign of pelvic floor dysfunction) or perineal ballooning during straining relative to bony landmarks (>4 cm, suggesting excessive perineal descent).

A useful overall test of evacuation is the balloon expulsion test. A balloon-tipped urinary catheter is placed and inflated with 50 mL of water. Normally, a patient can expel it while seated on a toilet or in the left lateral decubitus position. In the lateral position, the weight needed to facilitate expulsion of the balloon is determined; normally, expulsion occurs with <200 g added.

Anorectal manometry, when used in the evaluation of patients with severe constipation, may find an excessively high resting (>80 mmHg) or squeeze anal sphincter tone, suggesting anismus (anal sphincter spasm). This test also identifies rare syndromes, such as adult Hirschsprung's disease, by the absence of the rectoanal inhibitory reflex.

Defecography (a dynamic barium enema including lateral views obtained during barium expulsion) reveals "soft abnormalities" in many patients; the most relevant findings are the measured changes in rectoanal angle, anatomic defects of the rectum such as internal mucosal prolapse, and enteroceles or rectoceles. Surgically remediable conditions are identified in only a few patients. These include severe, whole-thickness intussusception with complete outlet obstruction due to funnel-shaped plugging at the anal canal or an extremely large rectocele that fills preferentially during attempts at defecation instead of expulsion of the barium through the anus. In summary, defecography requires an interested and experienced radiologist, and abnormalities are not pathognomonic for pelvic floor dysfunction. The most common cause of outlet obstruction is failure of the puborectalis muscle to relax; this is not identified by defecography but requires a dynamic study such as proctography. MRI is being developed as an alternative and provides more information about the structure and function of the pelvic floor, distal colorectum, and anal sphincters.

Dynamic imaging studies such as proctography during defecation or scintigraphic expulsion of artificial stool help measure perineal descent and the rectoanal angle during rest, squeezing, and straining, and scintigraphic expulsion quantitates the amount of "artificial stool" emptied. Lack of straightening of the rectoanal angle by at least 15° during defecation confirms pelvic floor dysfunction.

Neurologic testing (electromyography) is more helpful in the evaluation of patients with incontinence than of those with symptoms suggesting obstructed defecation. The absence of neurologic signs in the lower extremities suggests that any documented denervation of the puborectalis results from pelvic (e.g., obstetric) injury or from stretching of the pudendal nerve by chronic, long-standing straining. Constipation is common among patients with spinal cord injuries, neurologic diseases such as Parkinson's disease, multiple sclerosis, and diabetic neuropathy.

Spinal-evoked responses during electrical rectal stimulation or stimulation of external anal sphincter contraction by applying magnetic stimulation over the lumbosacral cord identify patients with limited sacral neuropathies with sufficient residual nerve conduction to attempt biofeedback training.

In summary, a balloon expulsion test is an important screening test for anorectal dysfunction. If positive, an anatomic evaluation of the rectum or anal sphincters and an assessment of pelvic floor relaxation are the tools for evaluating patients in whom obstructed defecation is suspected.

TREATMENT Constipation

After the cause of constipation is characterized, a treatment decision can be made. Slow-transit constipation requires aggressive medical or surgical treatment; anismus or pelvic floor dysfunction usually responds to biofeedback management (Fig. 40-4). However, only ~60% of patients with severe constipation are found to have such a physiologic disorder (half with colonic transit delay and half with evacuation disorder). Patients with spinal cord injuries or other neurologic disorders require a dedicated bowel regimen that often includes rectal stimulation, enema therapy, and carefully timed laxative therapy.

Patients with slow-transit constipation are treated with bulk, osmotic, prokinetic, secretory, and stimulant laxatives including fiber, psyllium, milk of magnesia, lactulose, polyethylene glycol (colonic lavage solution), lubiprostone, and bisacodyl. Newer treatment aimed at enhancing motility and secretion may have application in circumstances such as constipation-predominant IBS in females or severe constipation. If a three- to six-month trial of medical therapy fails and patients continue to have documented slow-transit constipation unassociated with obstructed defecation, the patients should be considered for laparoscopic colectomy with ileorectostomy; however, this should not be undertaken if there is continued evidence of an evacuation disorder or a generalized GI dysmotility. Referral to a specialized center for further tests of colonic motor function

is warranted. The decision to resort to surgery is facilitated in the presence of megacolon and megarectum. The complications after surgery include small-bowel obstruction (11%) and fecal soiling, particularly at night during the first postoperative year. Frequency of defecation is 3–8 per day during the first year, dropping to 1–3 per day from the second year after surgery.

Patients who have a combined (evacuation and transit/motility) disorder should pursue pelvic floor retraining (biofeedback and muscle relaxation), psychological counseling, and dietetic advice first, followed by colectomy and ileorectostomy if colonic transit studies do not normalize and symptoms are intractable despite biofeedback and optimized medical therapy. In patients with pelvic floor dysfunction alone, biofeedback training has a 70–80% success rate, measured by the acquisition of comfortable stool habits. Attempts to manage pelvic floor dysfunction with operations (internal anal sphincter or puborectalis muscle division) have achieved only mediocre success and have been largely abandoned.

FURTHER READINGS

BARTLETT JG: Narrative review: The new epidemic of *Clostridium difficile*–associated enteric disease. Ann Intern Med 145:758, 2006

BINDER HJ: Causes of chronic diarrhea. N Engl J Med 355:236, 2006

CAMILLERI M: Chronic diarrhea: A review on pathophysiology and management for the clinical gastroenterologist. Clin Gastroenterol Hepatol 2:198, 2004

DUPONT HL: Clinical practice. Bacterial diarrhea. N Engl J Med 361:1560, 2009

LEMBO A, CAMILLERI M: Chronic constipation. N Engl J Med 349:1360, 2003

MUSHER DM, MUSHER BL: Contagious acute gastrointestinal infections. N Engl J Med 351:2417, 2004

NAVANEETHAN U, GIANNELLA RA: Mechanisms of infectious diarrhea. Nat Clin Pract Gastroenterol Hepatol 5:637, 2008

RIDDLE MS, et al: Effect of adjunctive loperamide in combination with antibiotics on treatment outcomes in traveler's diarrhea: a systematic review and meta-analysis. Clin Infect Dis 47:1007, 2008

ROSTOM A, et al: American Gastroenterological Association (AGA) Institute technical review on the diagnosis and management of celiac disease. Gastroenterology 131:1981, 2006

WALD A: Clinical practice. Fecal incontinence in adults. N Engl J Med 356:1648, 2007

WALTERS JR, et al: A new mechanism for bile acid diarrhea: defective feedback inhibition of bile acid biosynthesis. Clin Gastroenterol Hepatol 7:1189, 2009

WHITEHEAD WE, BHARUCHA AE: Diagnosis and treatment of pelvic floor disorders: What's new and what to do. Gastroenterology 138:1231, 2010

CHAPTER **41**

Gastrointestinal Bleeding

Loren Laine

Bleeding from the gastrointestinal (GI) tract may present in five ways. *Hematemesis* is vomitus of red blood or "coffee-grounds" material. *Melena* is black, tarry, foul-smelling stool. *Hematochezia* is the passage of bright red or maroon blood from the rectum. *Occult GI bleeding* (GIB) may be identified in the absence of overt bleeding by a fecal occult blood test or the presence of iron deficiency. Finally, patients may present only with *symptoms of blood loss or anemia* such as lightheadedness, syncope, angina, or dyspnea.

■ SOURCES OF GASTROINTESTINAL BLEEDING

Upper gastrointestinal sources of bleeding

(Table 41-1) The annual incidence of hospital admissions for upper GIB (UGIB) in the United States and Europe is ~0.1%, with a mortality rate of ~5–10%. Patients rarely die from exsanguination; rather, they die due to decompensation from other underlying illnesses. The mortality rate for patients <60 years in the absence of major concurrent illness is <1%. Independent predictors of rebleeding and death in patients hospitalized with UGIB include increasing age, comorbidities, and hemodynamic compromise (tachycardia or hypotension).

Peptic ulcers are the most common cause of UGIB, accounting for up to ~50% of cases; an increasing proportion is due to nonsteroidal anti-inflammatory drugs (NSAIDs), with the prevalence of *Helicobacter pylori* decreasing. Mallory-Weiss tears account for ~5–10% of cases. The proportion of patients bleeding from varices varies widely from ~5 to 40%, depending on the population. Hemorrhagic or erosive gastropathy (e.g., due to NSAIDs or alcohol) and erosive esophagitis often cause mild UGIB, but major bleeding is rare.

Peptic ulcers In addition to clinical features, characteristics of an ulcer at endoscopy provide important prognostic information. One-third of patients with active bleeding or a nonbleeding visible vessel

TABLE 41-1 Sources of Bleeding in Patients Hospitalized for Upper GI Bleeding

Sources of Bleeding	Proportion of Patients, %
Ulcers	31–67
Varices	6–39
Mallory-Weiss tears	2–8
Gastroduodenal erosions	2–18
Erosive esophagitis	1–13
Neoplasm	2–8
Vascular ectasias	0–6
No source identified	5–14

Source: Data on hospitalizations from year 2000 onward from Am J Gastroenterol 98:1494, 2003; Gastrointest Endosc 57:AB147, 2003; 60;875, 2004; Eur J Gastroenterol Hepatol 16:177, 2004; 17:641, 2005; J Clin Gastroenterol 42:128, 2008; World J Gastroenterol 14:5046, 2008; Dig Dis Sci 54:333, 2009.

have further bleeding that requires urgent surgery if they are treated conservatively. These patients clearly benefit from endoscopic therapy with bipolar electrocoagulation; heater probe; injection therapy (e.g., absolute alcohol, 1:10,000 epinephrine); and/or clips with reductions in bleeding, hospital stay, mortality rate, and costs. In contrast, patients with clean-based ulcers have rates of recurrent bleeding approaching zero. If there is no other reason for hospitalization, such patients may be discharged on the first hospital day, following stabilization. Patients without clean-based ulcers should usually remain in the hospital for three days because most episodes of recurrent bleeding occur within three days.

Randomized controlled trials document that a high-dose, constant-infusion IV proton pump inhibitor (PPI) (e.g., omeprazole 80-mg bolus and 8-mg/h infusion), designed to sustain intragastric pH > 6 and enhance clot stability, decreases further bleeding and mortality in patients with high-risk ulcers (active bleeding, nonbleeding visible vessel, adherent clot) when given after endoscopic therapy. Institution of PPI therapy at presentation in all patients with UGIB decreases high-risk ulcer characteristics (e.g., active bleeding) but does not significantly improve outcomes such as further bleeding, transfusions, or mortality as compared to initiating therapy only when high-risk ulcers are identified at the time of endoscopy.

Approximately one-third of patients with bleeding ulcers will rebleed within the next 1–2 years if no preventive strategies are employed. Prevention of recurrent bleeding focuses on the three main factors in ulcer pathogenesis, *H. pylori*, NSAIDs, and acid. Eradication of *H. pylori* in patients with bleeding ulcers decreases rates of rebleeding to <5%. If a bleeding ulcer develops in a patient taking NSAIDs, the NSAIDs should be discontinued, if possible. If NSAIDs must be continued or reinstituted, a cyclooxygenase 2 (COX-2) selective inhibitor (coxib) plus a PPI should be used. PPI co-therapy alone or a coxib alone is associated with an annual rebleeding rate of ~10% in patients with a recent bleeding ulcer, while combination of a coxib and PPI provides a further significant decrease in recurrent ulcer bleeding. Patients with cardiovascular disease who develop bleeding ulcers while taking low-dose aspirin should restart aspirin as soon as possible after their bleeding episode (e.g., ≤ 7 days). A randomized trial showed that failure to restart aspirin was associated with a nonsignificant difference in rebleeding (5% vs. 10% at 30 days), but a significant increase in mortality at 30 days (9% vs. 1%) and 8 weeks (13% vs. 1%) as compared to immediate reinstitution of aspirin. Patients with bleeding ulcers unrelated to *H. pylori* or NSAIDs should remain on full-dose antisecretory therapy indefinitely. Peptic ulcers are discussed in Chap. 293.

Mallory-Weiss tears The classic history is vomiting, retching, or coughing preceding hematemesis, especially in an alcoholic patient. Bleeding from these tears, which are usually on the gastric side of the gastroesophageal junction, stops spontaneously in 80–90% of patients and recurs in only 0–7%. Endoscopic therapy is indicated for actively bleeding Mallory-Weiss tears. Angiographic therapy with embolization and operative therapy with oversewing of the tear are rarely required. Mallory-Weiss tears are discussed in Chap. 292.

Esophageal varices Patients with variceal hemorrhage have poorer outcomes than patients with other sources of UGIB. Endoscopic therapy for acute bleeding and repeated sessions of endoscopic therapy to eradicate esophageal varices significantly reduce rebleeding and mortality. Ligation is the endoscopic therapy of choice for esophageal varices because it has less rebleeding, a lower mortality rate, fewer local complications, and it requires fewer treatment sessions to achieve variceal eradication than sclerotherapy.

Octreotide (50-μg bolus and 50-μg/h IV infusion for 2–5 days) further helps in the control of acute bleeding when used in combination with endoscopic therapy. Other vasoactive agents such as somatostatin and terlipressin, available outside the United States, are also effective. Antibiotic therapy (e.g., ceftriaxone) is also recommended for patients with cirrhosis presenting with UGIB because antibiotics decrease bacterial infections and mortality in this population. Over the long term, treatment with nonselective beta blockers decreases recurrent bleeding from esophageal varices. Chronic therapy with beta blockers plus endoscopic ligation is recommended for prevention of recurrent esophageal variceal bleeding.

In patients who have persistent or recurrent bleeding despite endoscopic and medical therapy, more invasive therapy with transjugular intrahepatic portosystemic shunt (TIPS) is recommended. Older studies indicate that most patients with TIPS developed shunt stenosis within 1–2 years and required reintervention to maintain shunt patency. The use of coated stents appears to decrease shunt dysfunction by ~50% in the first 2 years. A randomized comparison of TIPS (with uncoated stents) and distal splenorenal shunt in Child-Pugh class A or B cirrhotic patients with refractory variceal bleeding revealed no significant difference in rebleeding, encephalopathy, or survival, but had a much higher rate of reintervention with TIPS (82% vs. 11%). Therefore, decompressive surgery may be an option in patients with milder, well-compensated cirrhosis.

Portal hypertension is also responsible for bleeding from gastric varices, varices in the small and large intestine, and portal hypertensive gastropathy and enterocolopathy.

Hemorrhagic and erosive gastropathy ("gastritis") Hemorrhagic and erosive gastropathy, often labeled gastritis, refers to endoscopically visualized subepithelial hemorrhages and erosions. These are mucosal lesions and, thus, do not cause major bleeding. They develop in various clinical settings, the most important of which are NSAID use, alcohol intake, and stress. Half of patients who chronically ingest NSAIDs have erosions (15–30% have ulcers), while up to 20% of actively drinking alcoholic patients with symptoms of UGIB have evidence of subepithelial hemorrhages or erosions.

Stress-related gastric mucosal injury occurs only in extremely sick patients: those who have experienced serious trauma, major surgery, burns covering more than one-third of the body surface area, major intracranial disease, or severe medical illness (i.e., ventilator dependence, coagulopathy). Significant bleeding probably does not develop unless ulceration occurs. The mortality rate in these patients is quite high because of their serious underlying illnesses.

The incidence of bleeding from stress-related gastric mucosal injury or ulceration has decreased dramatically in recent years, most likely due to better care of critically ill patients. Pharmacologic prophylaxis for bleeding may be considered in the high-risk patients mentioned above. Multiple trials document the efficacy of intravenous H_2-receptor antagonist therapy, which is more effective than sucralfate but not superior to a PPI immediate-release suspension given via nasogastric tube. Prophylactic therapy decreases bleeding but does not lower the mortality rate.

Other causes Other less frequent causes of UGIB include erosive duodenitis, neoplasms, aortoenteric fistulas, vascular lesions [including hereditary hemorrhagic telangiectasias (Osler-Weber-Rendu) and gastric antral vascular ectasia ("watermelon stomach")], Dieulafoy's lesion (in which an aberrant vessel in the mucosa bleeds from a pinpoint mucosal defect), prolapse gastropathy (prolapse of proximal stomach into esophagus with retching, especially in alcoholics), and hemobilia or hemosuccus pancreaticus (bleeding from the bile duct or pancreatic duct).

Small-intestinal sources of bleeding

Small-intestinal sources of bleeding (bleeding from sites beyond the reach of the standard upper endoscope) are difficult to diagnose and are responsible for the majority of cases of obscure GIB. Fortunately, small-intestinal bleeding is uncommon. The most common causes in adults are vascular ectasias, tumors (e.g., adenocarcinoma, leiomyoma, lymphoma, benign polyps, carcinoid, metastases, and lipoma), and NSAID-induced erosions and ulcers. Other less common causes in adults include Crohn's disease, infection, ischemia, vasculitis, small-bowel varices, diverticula, Meckel's diverticulum, duplication cysts, and intussusception.

Meckel's diverticulum is the most common cause of significant lower GIB (LGIB) in children, decreasing in frequency as a cause of bleeding with age. In adults <40–50 years, small-bowel tumors often account for obscure GIB; in patients >50–60 years, vascular ectasias and NSAID-induced lesions are more commonly responsible.

Vascular ectasias should be treated with endoscopic therapy if possible. Surgical therapy can be used for vascular ectasias isolated to a segment of the small intestine when endoscopic therapy is unsuccessful. Although estrogen/progesterone compounds have been used for vascular ectasias, a double-blind trial found no benefit in prevention of recurrent bleeding. Isolated lesions, such as tumors, diverticula, or duplications, are generally treated with surgical resection.

Colonic sources of bleeding

The incidence of hospitalizations for LGIB is ≥20% that for UGIB. Hemorrhoids are probably the most common cause of LGIB; anal fissures also cause minor bleeding and pain. If these local anal processes, which rarely require hospitalization, are excluded, the most common causes of LGIB in adults are diverticula, vascular ectasias (especially in the proximal colon of patients >70 years), neoplasms (primarily adenocarcinoma), and colitis—most commonly infectious or idiopathic inflammatory bowel disease, but occasionally ischemic or radiation-induced. Uncommon causes include post-polypectomy bleeding, solitary rectal ulcer syndrome, NSAID-induced ulcers or colitis, trauma, varices (most commonly rectal), lymphoid nodular hyperplasia, vasculitis, and aortocolic fistulas. In children and adolescents, the most common colonic causes of significant GIB are inflammatory bowel disease and juvenile polyps.

Diverticular bleeding is abrupt in onset, usually painless, sometimes massive, and often from the right colon; minor and occult bleeding is not characteristic. Clinical reports suggest that bleeding colonic diverticula stop bleeding spontaneously in ~80% of patients and rebleed in about 20–25% of patients. Intraarterial vasopressin or embolization by superselective technique should stop bleeding in a majority of patients. If bleeding persists or recurs, segmental surgical resection is indicated.

Bleeding from right colonic vascular ectasias in the elderly may be overt or occult; it tends to be chronic and only occasionally is hemodynamically significant. Endoscopic hemostatic therapy may be useful in the treatment of vascular ectasias, as well as discrete bleeding ulcers and post-polypectomy bleeding, while endoscopic polypectomy, if possible, is used for bleeding colonic polyps. Surgical therapy is generally required for major, persistent, or recurrent bleeding from the wide variety of colonic sources of GIB that cannot be treated medically, angiographically, or endoscopically.

| APPROACH TO THE PATIENT | **Gastrointestinal Bleeding** |

Measurement of the heart rate and blood pressure is the best way to initially assess a patient with GIB. Clinically significant bleeding leads to postural changes in heart rate or blood pressure, tachycardia, and, finally, recumbent hypotension. In contrast, the hemoglobin does not fall immediately with acute GIB, due to proportionate reductions in plasma and red cell volumes (i.e., "people bleed whole blood"). Thus, hemoglobin may be normal

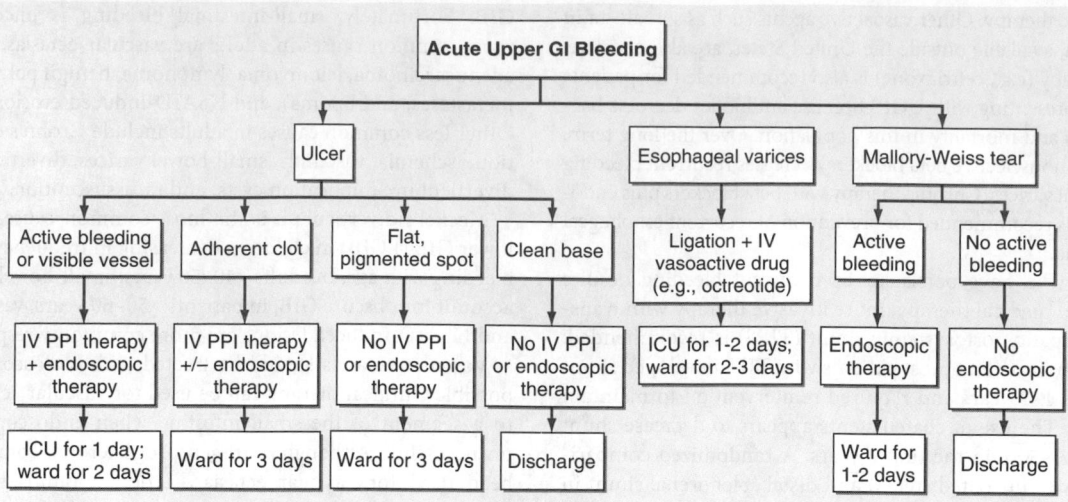

Figure 41-1 Suggested algorithm for patients with acute upper gastrointestinal bleeding. Recommendations on level of care and time of discharge assume patient is stabilized without further bleeding or other concomitant medical problems. ICU, intensive care unit; PPI, proton pump inhibitor.

or only minimally decreased at the initial presentation of a severe bleeding episode. As extravascular fluid enters the vascular space to restore volume, the hemoglobin falls, but this process may take up to 72 h. Patients with slow, chronic GIB may have very low hemoglobin values despite normal blood pressure and heart rate. With the development of iron-deficiency anemia, the mean corpuscular volume will be low and red blood cell distribution width will increase.

DIFFERENTIATION OF UPPER FROM LOWER GIB Hematemesis indicates an upper GI source of bleeding (above the ligament of Treitz). Melena indicates that blood has been present in the GI tract for at least 14 h (and as long as 3–5 days). The more proximal the bleeding site, the more likely melena will occur. Hematochezia usually represents a lower GI source of bleeding, although an upper GI lesion may bleed so briskly that blood does not remain in the bowel long enough for melena to develop. When hematochezia is the presenting symptom of UGIB, it is associated with hemodynamic instability and dropping hemoglobin. Bleeding lesions of the small bowel may present as melena or hematochezia. Other clues to UGIB include hyperactive bowel sounds and an elevated blood urea nitrogen level (due to volume depletion and blood proteins absorbed in the small intestine).

A nonbloody nasogastric aspirate may be seen in up to 18% of patients with UGIB—usually from a duodenal source. Even a bile-stained appearance does not exclude a bleeding postpyloric lesion because reports of bile in the aspirate are incorrect in ~50% of cases. Testing of aspirates that are not grossly bloody for occult blood is not useful.

DIAGNOSTIC EVALUATION OF THE PATIENT WITH GIB
Upper GIB (Fig. 41-1) History and physical examination are not usually diagnostic of the source of GIB. Upper endoscopy is the test of choice in patients with UGIB and should be performed urgently in patients who present with hemodynamic instability (hypotension, tachycardia, or postural changes in heart rate or blood pressure). Early endoscopy is also beneficial in cases of milder bleeding for management decisions. Patients with major bleeding and high-risk endoscopic findings (e.g., varices, ulcers with active bleeding or a visible vessel) benefit from endoscopic

hemostatic therapy, while patients with low-risk lesions (e.g., clean-based ulcers, nonbleeding Mallory-Weiss tears, erosive or hemorrhagic gastropathy) who have stable vital signs and hemoglobin, and no other medical problems, can be discharged home.

Lower GIB (Fig. 41-2) Patients with hematochezia and hemodynamic instability should have upper endoscopy to rule out an upper GI source before evaluation of the lower GI tract. Patients with

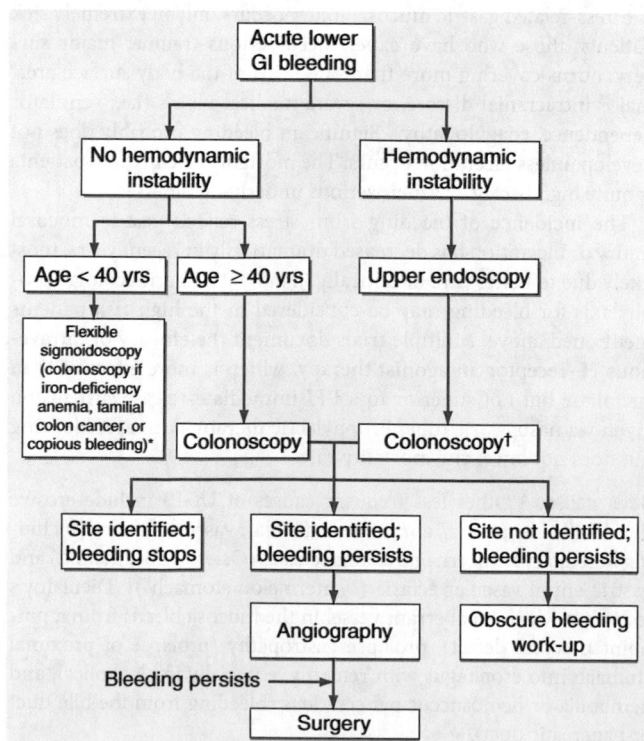

Figure 41-2 Suggested algorithm for patients with acute lower gastrointestinal bleeding. *Some suggest colonoscopy for any degree of rectal bleeding in patients <40 years as well. †If massive bleeding does not allow time for colonic lavage, proceed to angiography.

presumed LGIB may undergo early sigmoidoscopy for the detection of obvious, low-lying lesions. However, the procedure is difficult with brisk bleeding, and it is usually not possible to identify the area of bleeding. Sigmoidoscopy is useful primarily in patients <40 years with minor bleeding.

Colonoscopy after an oral lavage solution is the procedure of choice in patients admitted with LGIB unless bleeding is too massive or unless sigmoidoscopy has disclosed an obvious actively bleeding lesion. ^{99m}Tc-labeled red cell scan allows repeated imaging for up to 24 h and may identify the general location of bleeding. However, radionuclide scans should be interpreted with caution because results, especially from later images, are highly variable. In active LGIB, angiography can detect the site of bleeding (extravasation of contrast into the gut) and permits treatment with embolization or intraarterial infusion of vasopressin. Even after bleeding has stopped, angiography may identify lesions with abnormal vasculature, such as vascular ectasias or tumors.

GIB of Obscure Origin Obscure GIB is defined as persistent or recurrent bleeding for which no source has been identified by routine endoscopic and contrast x-ray studies; it may be overt (melena, hematochezia) or occult (iron-deficiency anemia). Current guidelines suggest angiography as the initial test for massive obscure bleeding, and video capsule endoscopy, which allows examination of the entire small intestine, for all others. Push enteroscopy, with a specially designed enteroscope or a pediatric colonoscope to inspect the entire duodenum and part of the jejunum, also may be considered as an initial evaluation. A systematic review of 14 trials comparing push enteroscopy to capsule revealed "clinically significant findings" in 26% and 56% of patients, respectively. However, in contrast to enteroscopy, lack of control of the capsule prevents its manipulation and full visualization of the intestine; in addition, tissue cannot be sampled and therapy cannot be applied.

If capsule endoscopy is positive, management (e.g., enteroscopy, laparoscopy) is dictated by the finding. If capsule is negative, current recommendations suggest patients may be either observed, or if their clinical course mandates (e.g., recurrent bleeding, need for transfusions or hospitalization), undergo further testing. Newer endoscopic techniques (e.g., double-balloon, single-balloon, and spiral enteroscopy) allow the endoscopist to examine, obtain specimens from, and provide therapy to much or all of the small intestine. Newer imaging techniques (CT and MR enterography) are now frequently being used in place of older specialized small-bowel radiographic exams (e.g., enteroclysis). Other tests include ^{99m}Tc-labeled red blood cell scintigraphy; angiography, which may be useful even if bleeding has subsided because it may disclose vascular anomalies or tumor vessels; and ^{99m}Tc-pertechnetate scintigraphy for diagnosis of Meckel's diverticulum (especially in young patients). When all tests are unrevealing, intraoperative endoscopy is indicated in patients with severe recurrent or persistent bleeding requiring repeated transfusions.

Positive Fecal Occult Blood Test Fecal occult blood testing is recommended only for colorectal cancer screening and may be used in average-risk adults (beginning at age 50) and in adults with a first-degree relative with colorectal neoplasm at ≥60 years or two second-degree relatives with colorectal cancer (beginning at age 40). A positive test necessitates colonoscopy. If evaluation of the colon is negative, further workup is not recommended unless iron-deficiency anemia or GI symptoms are present.

FURTHER READINGS

BARKUN AN et al: International consensus recommendations on the management of patients with nonvariceal upper gastrointestinal bleeding. Ann Intern Med 152:101, 2010

CONRAD SA et al: Randomized, double-blind comparison of immediate-release omeprazole oral suspension versus intravenous cimetidine for the prevention of upper gastrointestinal bleeding in critically ill patients. Crit Care Med 33:760, 2005

GARCIA-TSAO G et al: Prevention and management of gastroesophageal varices and variceal hemorrhage in cirrhosis. Am J Gastroenterol 102:2086, 2007

HENDERSON JM et al: Distal splenorenal shunt versus transjugular intrahepatic portal systematic shunt for variceal bleeding: A randomized trial. Gastroenterology 130:1643, 2006

LAINE L, McQUAID KR: Endoscopic therapy for bleeding ulcers: an evidence-based approach based on meta-analyses of randomized controlled trials. Clin Gastroenterol Hepatol 7:33, 2009

RAJU GS et al: American Gastroenterological Association (AGA) Institute technical review on obscure gastrointestinal bleeding. Gastroenterology 133:1697, 2007

ROCKALL TA et al: Risk assessment after acute upper gastrointestinal haemorrhage. Gut 38:316, 1996

SUNG JJY et al: Continuation of low-dose aspirin in peptic ulcer bleeding. A randomized trial. Ann Intern Med 152:1, 2010

TRIESTER SL et al: A meta-analysis of the yield of capsule endoscopy compared to other diagnostic modalities in patients with obscure gastrointestinal bleeding. Am J Gastroenterol 100:2407, 2005

CHAPTER **42**

Jaundice

Daniel S. Pratt
Marshall M. Kaplan

Jaundice, or icterus, is a yellowish discoloration of tissue resulting from the deposition of bilirubin. Tissue deposition of bilirubin occurs only in the presence of serum hyperbilirubinemia and is a sign of either liver disease or, less often, a hemolytic disorder. The degree of serum bilirubin elevation can be estimated by physical examination. Slight increases in serum bilirubin are best detected by examining the sclerae, which have a particular affinity for bilirubin due to their high elastin content. The presence of scleral icterus indicates a serum bilirubin of at least 51 μmol/L (3 mg/dL). The ability to detect scleral icterus is made more difficult if the examining room has fluorescent lighting. If the examiner suspects scleral icterus, a second place to examine is underneath the tongue. As serum bilirubin levels rise, the skin will eventually become yellow in light-skinned patients and even green if the process is long-standing; the green color is produced by oxidation of bilirubin to biliverdin.

The differential diagnosis for yellowing of the skin is limited. In addition to jaundice, it includes carotenoderma, the use of the drug quinacrine, and excessive exposure to phenols. Carotenoderma is the yellow color imparted to the skin by the presence of carotene; it occurs in healthy individuals who ingest excessive amounts of vegetables and fruits that contain carotene, such as carrots, leafy vegetables, squash, peaches, and oranges. Unlike jaundice, where the yellow coloration of the skin is uniformly distributed over the body, in carotenoderma, the pigment is concentrated on the palms, soles, forehead, and nasolabial folds. Carotenoderma can be distinguished from jaundice by the sparing of the sclerae. Quinacrine causes a yellow discoloration of the skin in 4–37% of patients treated with it. Unlike carotene, quinacrine can cause discoloration of the sclerae.

Another sensitive indicator of increased serum bilirubin is darkening of the urine, which is due to the renal excretion of conjugated bilirubin. Patients often describe their urine as tea- or cola-colored. Bilirubinuria indicates an elevation of the direct serum bilirubin fraction and, therefore, the presence of liver disease.

Increased serum bilirubin levels occur when an imbalance exists between bilirubin production and clearance. A logical evaluation of the patient who is jaundiced requires an understanding of bilirubin production and metabolism.

■ PRODUCTION AND METABOLISM OF BILIRUBIN

(See also Chap. 303) Bilirubin, a tetrapyrrole pigment, is a breakdown product of heme (ferroprotoporphyrin IX). About 70–80% of the 250–300 mg of bilirubin produced each day is derived from the breakdown of hemoglobin in senescent red blood cells. The remainder comes from prematurely destroyed erythroid cells in bone marrow and from the turnover of hemoproteins such as myoglobin and cytochromes found in tissues throughout the body.

The formation of bilirubin occurs in reticuloendothelial cells, primarily in the spleen and liver. The first reaction, catalyzed by the microsomal enzyme heme oxygenase, oxidatively cleaves the α bridge of the porphyrin group and opens the heme ring. The end products of this reaction are biliverdin, carbon monoxide, and iron. The second reaction, catalyzed by the cytosolic enzyme biliverdin reductase, reduces the central methylene bridge of biliverdin and

converts it to bilirubin. Bilirubin formed in the reticuloendothelial cells is virtually insoluble in water. This is due to tight internal hydrogen bonding between the water-soluble moieties of bilirubin, proprionic acid carboxyl groups of one dipyrrolic half of the molecule with the imino and lactam groups of the opposite half. This configuration blocks solvent access to the polar residues of bilirubin and places the hydrophobic residues on the outside. To be transported in blood, bilirubin must be solubilized. This is accomplished by its reversible, noncovalent binding to albumin. Unconjugated bilirubin bound to albumin is transported to the liver, where it, but not the albumin, is taken up by hepatocytes via a process that at least partly involves carrier-mediated membrane transport. No specific bilirubin transporter has yet been identified (Chap. 303, Fig. 303-1).

After entering the hepatocyte, unconjugated bilirubin is bound in the cytosol to a number of proteins including proteins in the glutathione-S-transferase superfamily. These proteins serve both to reduce efflux of bilirubin back into the serum and to present the bilirubin for conjugation. In the endoplasmic reticulum, bilirubin is solubilized by conjugation to glucuronic acid, a process that disrupts the internal hydrogen bonds and yields bilirubin monoglucuronide and diglucuronide. The conjugation of glucuronic acid to bilirubin is catalyzed by bilirubin uridine diphosphate-glucuronosyl transferase (UDPGT). The now hydrophilic bilirubin conjugates diffuse from the endoplasmic reticulum to the canalicular membrane, where bilirubin monoglucuronide and diglucuronide are actively transported into canalicular bile by an energy-dependent mechanism involving the multiple drug resistance protein 2.

The conjugated bilirubin excreted into bile drains into the duodenum and passes unchanged through the proximal small bowel. Conjugated bilirubin is not taken up by the intestinal mucosa. When the conjugated bilirubin reaches the distal ileum and colon, it is hydrolyzed to unconjugated bilirubin by bacterial β-glucuronidases. The unconjugated bilirubin is reduced by normal gut bacteria to form a group of colorless tetrapyrroles called urobilinogens. About 80–90% of these products are excreted in feces, either unchanged or oxidized to orange derivatives called urobilins. The remaining 10–20% of the urobilinogens are passively absorbed, enter the portal venous blood, and are reexcreted by the liver. A small fraction (usually <3 mg/dL) escapes hepatic uptake, filters across the renal glomerulus, and is excreted in urine.

■ MEASUREMENT OF SERUM BILIRUBIN

The terms direct and indirect bilirubin, conjugated and unconjugated bilirubin, respectively, are based on the original van den Bergh reaction. This assay, or a variation of it, is still used in most clinical chemistry laboratories to determine the serum bilirubin level. In this assay, bilirubin is exposed to diazotized sulfanilic acid, splitting into two relatively stable dipyrrylmethene azopigments that absorb maximally at 540 nm, allowing for photometric analysis. The direct fraction is that which reacts with diazotized sulfanilic acid in the absence of an accelerator substance such as alcohol. The direct fraction provides an approximate determination of the conjugated bilirubin in serum. The total serum bilirubin is the amount that reacts after the addition of alcohol. The indirect fraction is the difference between the total and the direct bilirubin and provides an estimate of the unconjugated bilirubin in serum.

With the van den Bergh method, the normal serum bilirubin concentration usually is 17 μmol/L (<1 mg/dL). Up to 30%, or 5.1 μmol/L (0.3 mg/dL), of the total may be direct-reacting (conjugated) bilirubin. Total serum bilirubin concentrations are between 3.4 and 15.4 μmol/L (0.2 and 0.9 mg/dL) in 95% of a normal population.

Several new techniques, although less convenient to perform, have added considerably to our understanding of bilirubin metabolism.

First, they demonstrate that in normal persons or those with Gilbert's syndrome, almost 100% of the serum bilirubin is unconjugated; <3% is monoconjugated bilirubin. Second, in jaundiced patients with hepatobiliary disease, the total serum bilirubin concentration measured by these new, more accurate methods is lower than the values found with diazo methods. This suggests that there are diazo-positive compounds distinct from bilirubin in the serum of patients with hepatobiliary disease. Third, these studies indicate that, in jaundiced patients with hepatobiliary disease, monoglucuronides of bilirubin predominate over the diglucuronides. Fourth, part of the direct-reacting bilirubin fraction includes conjugated bilirubin that is covalently linked to albumin. This albumin-linked bilirubin fraction (*delta fraction,* or *biliprotein*) represents an important fraction of total serum bilirubin in patients with cholestasis and hepatobiliary disorders. Albumin-bound conjugated bilirubin is formed in serum when hepatic excretion of bilirubin glucuronides is impaired and the glucuronides are present in serum in increasing amounts. By virtue of its tight binding to albumin, the clearance rate of albumin-bound bilirubin from serum approximates the half-life of albumin, 12–14 days, rather than the short half-life of bilirubin, about 4 hours.

The prolonged half-life of albumin-bound conjugated bilirubin explains two previously unexplained enigmas in jaundiced patients with liver disease: (1) that some patients with conjugated hyperbilirubinemia do not exhibit bilirubinuria during the recovery phase of their disease because the bilirubin is covalently bound to albumin and therefore not filtered by the renal glomeruli, and (2) that the elevated serum bilirubin level declines more slowly than expected in some patients who otherwise appear to be recovering satisfactorily. Late in the recovery phase of hepatobiliary disorders, all the conjugated bilirubin may be in the albumin-linked form. Its value in serum falls slowly because of the long half-life of albumin.

■ MEASUREMENT OF URINE BILIRUBIN

Unconjugated bilirubin is always bound to albumin in the serum, is not filtered by the kidney, and is not found in the urine. Conjugated bilirubin is filtered at the glomerulus and the majority is reabsorbed by the proximal tubules; a small fraction is excreted in the urine. Any bilirubin found in the urine is conjugated bilirubin. The presence of bilirubinuria implies the presence of liver disease. A urine dipstick test (Ictotest) gives the same information as fractionation of the serum bilirubin. This test is very accurate. A false-negative test is possible in patients with prolonged cholestasis due to the predominance of conjugated bilirubin covalently bound to albumin.

APPROACH TO THE PATIENT ▶ Bilirubin

The bilirubin present in serum represents a balance between input from production of bilirubin and hepatic/biliary removal of the pigment. Hyperbilirubinemia may result from (1) overproduction of bilirubin; (2) impaired uptake, conjugation, or excretion of bilirubin; or (3) regurgitation of unconjugated or conjugated bilirubin from damaged hepatocytes or bile ducts. An increase in unconjugated bilirubin in serum results from either overproduction, impairment of uptake, or conjugation of bilirubin. An increase in conjugated bilirubin is due to decreased excretion into the bile ductules or backward leakage of the pigment. The initial steps in evaluating the patient with jaundice are to determine (1) whether the hyperbilirubinemia is predominantly conjugated or unconjugated in nature, and (2) whether other biochemical liver tests are abnormal. The thoughtful interpretation of limited data will allow for a rational evaluation of the patient (Fig. 42-1).

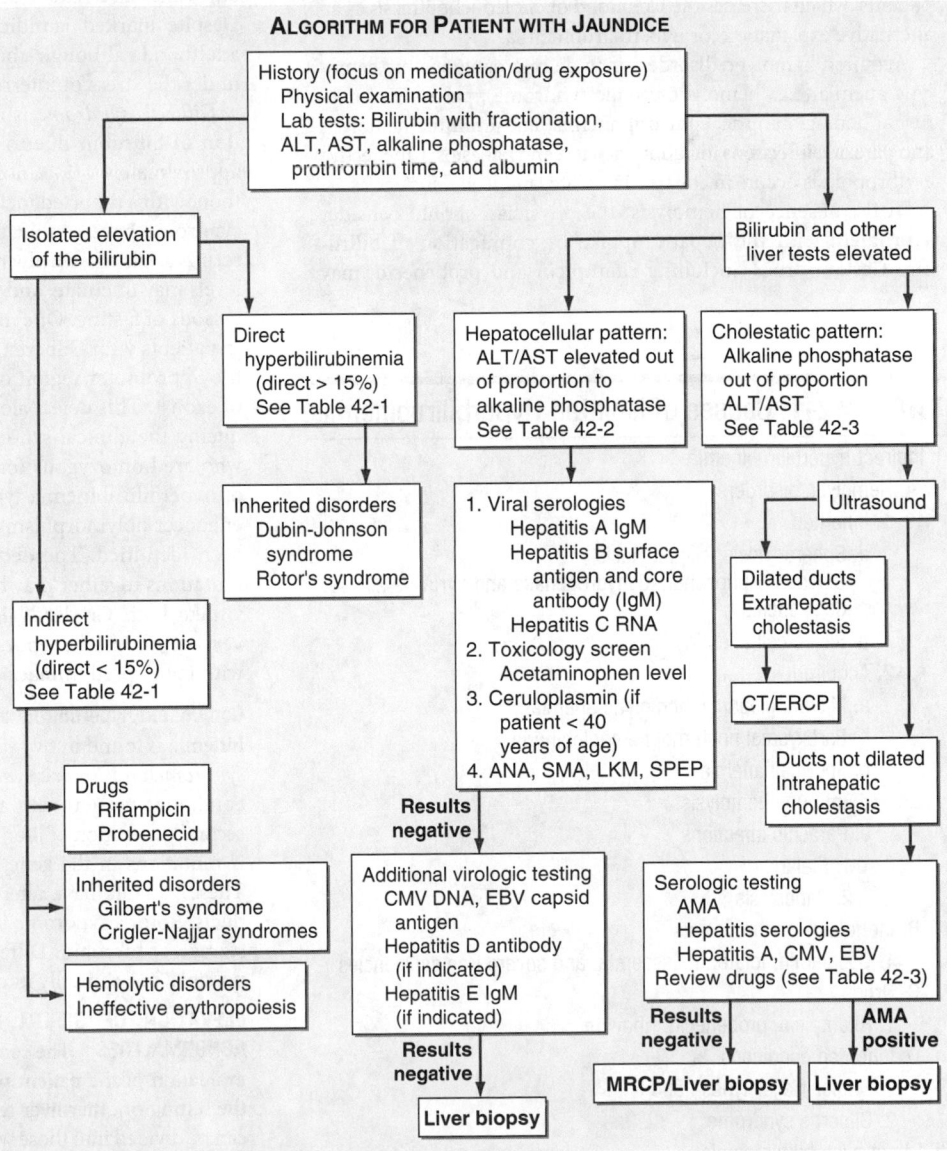

Figure 42-1 Evaluation of the patient with jaundice. ALT, alanine aminotransferase; AMA, antimitochondrial antibody; ANA, antinuclear antibody; AST, aspartate aminotransferase; CMV, cytomegalovirus; EBV, Epstein-Barr virus; LKM, liver-kidney microsomal antibody; MRCP, magnetic resonance cholangiopancreatography; SMA, smooth-muscle antibody; SPEP, serum protein electrophoresis.

This discussion will focus solely on the evaluation of the adult patient with jaundice.

ISOLATED ELEVATION OF SERUM BILIRUBIN

Unconjugated Hyperbilirubinemia The differential diagnosis of an isolated unconjugated hyperbilirubinemia is limited (Table 42-1). The critical determination is whether the patient is suffering from a hemolytic process resulting in an overproduction of bilirubin (hemolytic disorders and ineffective erythropoiesis) or from impaired hepatic uptake/conjugation of bilirubin (drug effect or genetic disorders).

Hemolytic disorders that cause excessive heme production may be either inherited or acquired. Inherited disorders include spherocytosis, sickle cell anemia, thalassemia, and deficiency of red cell enzymes such as pyruvate kinase and glucose-6-phosphate dehydrogenase. In these conditions, the serum bilirubin rarely exceeds 86 μmol/L (5 mg/dL). Higher levels may occur when there is coexistent renal or hepatocellular dysfunction or in acute hemolysis such as a sickle cell crisis. In evaluating jaundice in patients with chronic hemolysis, it is important to remember the high incidence of pigmented (calcium bilirubinate) gallstones found in these patients, which increases the likelihood of choledocholithiasis as an alternative explanation for hyperbilirubinemia.

Acquired hemolytic disorders include microangiopathic hemolytic anemia (e.g., hemolytic-uremic syndrome), paroxysmal nocturnal hemoglobinuria, spur cell anemia, and immune hemolysis and parasitic infections including malaria and babesiosis. Ineffective erythropoiesis occurs in cobalamin, folate, and iron deficiencies.

In the absence of hemolysis, the physician should consider a problem with the hepatic uptake or conjugation of bilirubin. Certain drugs, including rifampicin and probenecid, may cause unconjugated hyperbilirubinemia by diminishing hepatic uptake of bilirubin. Impaired bilirubin conjugation occurs in three genetic conditions: Crigler-Najjar syndrome, types I and II, and Gilbert's syndrome. *Crigler-Najjar type I* is an exceptionally rare condition found in neonates and characterized by severe jaundice [bilirubin > 342 μmol/L (>20 mg/dL)] and neurologic impairment due to kernicterus, frequently leading to death in infancy or childhood. These patients have a complete absence of bilirubin UDPGT activity, usually due to mutations in the critical 3′ domain of the *UDPGT* gene, and are totally unable to conjugate, hence cannot excrete, bilirubin. The only effective treatment is orthotopic liver transplantation. Use of gene therapy and allogeneic hepatocyte infusion are experimental approaches of future promise for this devastating disease.

Crigler-Najjar type II is somewhat more common than type I. Patients live into adulthood with serum bilirubin levels that range from 103–428 μmol/L (6–25 mg/dL). In these patients, mutations in the bilirubin *UDPGT* gene cause reduced but not completely absent activity of the enzyme. Bilirubin UDPGT activity can be induced by the administration of phenobarbital, which can reduce serum bilirubin levels in these patients. Despite marked jaundice, these patients usually survive into adulthood, although they may be susceptible to kernicterus under the stress of intercurrent illness or surgery.

Gilbert's syndrome is also marked by the impaired conjugation of bilirubin due to reduced bilirubin UDPGT activity to approximately 1/3 of normal. Gilbert's syndrome is very common, with a reported incidence of 3–12%. Patients with Gilbert's syndrome have a mild unconjugated hyperbilirubinemia with serum levels almost always <103 μmol/L (6 mg/dL). The serum levels may fluctuate, and jaundice is often identified only during periods of fasting. One molecular defect that has been identified in patients with Gilbert's syndrome is in the TATAA element in the 5′ promoter region of the bilirubin *UDPGT* gene upstream of exon 1. This defect alone is not necessarily sufficient for producing the clinical syndrome of Gilbert's as there are patients who are homozygous for this defect yet do not have the levels of hyperbilirubinemia typically seen in Gilbert's syndrome. An enhancer polymorphism that lowers transcriptional activity has been identified. The decrease in transcription caused by both mutations together may be critical for producing the syndrome. Unlike both Crigler-Najjar syndromes, Gilbert's syndrome is very common. The reported incidence is 3–7% of the population with males predominating over females by a ratio of 2–7:1.

Conjugated Hyperbilirubinemia Elevated conjugated hyperbilirubinemia is found in two rare inherited conditions: *Dubin-Johnson syndrome* and *Rotor's syndrome* (Table 42-1). Patients with both conditions present with asymptomatic jaundice, typically in the second generation of life. The defect in Dubin-Johnson syndrome is mutations in the gene for multiple drug resistance protein 2. These patients have altered excretion of bilirubin into the bile ducts. Rotor's syndrome seems to be a problem with the hepatic storage of bilirubin. Differentiating between these syndromes is possible, but clinically unnecessary, due to their benign nature.

ELEVATION OF SERUM BILIRUBIN WITH OTHER LIVER TEST ABNORMALITIES

The remainder of this chapter will focus on the evaluation of the patient with a conjugated hyperbilirubinemia in the setting of other liver test abnormalities. This group of patients can be divided into those with a primary hepatocellular process and those with intra- or extrahepatic cholestasis. Being able to make this differentiation will guide the physician's evaluation (Fig. 42-1). This differentiation is made on the basis of the history and physical examination as well as the pattern of liver test abnormalities.

TABLE 42-1 Causes of Isolated Hyperbilirubinemia

I. Indirect hyperbilirubinemia
  A. Hemolytic disorders
    1. Inherited
      a. Spherocytosis, elliptocytosis
        Glucose-6-phosphate dehydrogenase and pyruvate kinase deficiencies
      b. Sickle cell anemia
    2. Acquired
      a. Microangiopathic hemolytic anemias
      b. Paroxysmal nocturnal hemoglobinuria
      c. Spur cell anemia
      d. Immune hemolysis
      e. Parasitic infections
        1. Malaria
        2. Babesiosis
  B. Ineffective erythropoiesis
    1. Cobalamin, folate, thalassemia, and severe iron deficiencies
  C. Drugs
    1. Rifampicin, probenecid, ribavirin
  D. Inherited conditions
    1. Crigler-Najjar types I and II
    2. Gilbert's syndrome
II. Direct hyperbilirubinemia
  A. Inherited conditions
    1. Dubin-Johnson syndrome
    2. Rotor's syndrome

History A complete medical history is perhaps the single most important part of the evaluation of the patient with unexplained jaundice. Important considerations include the use of or exposure to any chemical or medication, either physician-prescribed, over-the-counter, complementary or alternative medicines such as herbal and vitamin preparations, or other drugs such as anabolic steroids. The patient should be carefully questioned about possible parenteral exposures, including transfusions, intravenous and intranasal drug use, tattoos, and sexual activity. Other important questions include recent travel history; exposure to people with jaundice; exposure to possibly contaminated foods; occupational exposure to hepatotoxins; alcohol consumption; the duration of jaundice; and the presence of any accompanying symptoms such as arthralgias, myalgias, rash, anorexia, weight loss, abdominal pain, fever, pruritus, and changes in the urine and stool. While none of these latter symptoms are specific for any one condition, they can suggest a particular diagnosis. A history of arthralgias and myalgias predating jaundice suggests hepatitis, either viral or drug-related. Jaundice associated with the sudden onset of severe right upper quadrant pain and shaking chills suggests choledocholithiasis and ascending cholangitis.

Physical Examination The general assessment should include assessment of the patient's nutritional status. Temporal and proximal muscle wasting suggests long-standing diseases such as pancreatic cancer or cirrhosis. Stigmata of chronic liver disease, including spider nevi, palmar erythema, gynecomastia, caput medusae, Dupuytren's contractures, parotid gland enlargement, and testicular atrophy are commonly seen in advanced alcoholic (Laennec's) cirrhosis and occasionally in other types of cirrhosis. An enlarged left supraclavicular node (Virchow's node) or periumbilical nodule (Sister Mary Joseph's nodule) suggests an abdominal malignancy. Jugular venous distention, a sign of right-sided heart failure, suggests hepatic congestion. Right pleural effusion, in the absence of clinically apparent ascites, may be seen in advanced cirrhosis.

The abdominal examination should focus on the size and consistency of the liver, whether the spleen is palpable and hence enlarged, and whether there is ascites present. Patients with cirrhosis may have an enlarged left lobe of the liver, which is felt below the xiphoid, and an enlarged spleen. A grossly enlarged nodular liver or an obvious abdominal mass suggests malignancy. An enlarged tender liver could be viral or alcoholic hepatitis; an infiltrative process such as amyloid; or, less often, an acutely congested liver secondary to right-sided heart failure. Severe right upper quadrant tenderness with respiratory arrest on inspiration (Murphy's sign) suggests cholecystitis or, occasionally, ascending cholangitis. Ascites in the presence of jaundice suggests either cirrhosis or malignancy with peritoneal spread.

Laboratory Tests When the physician encounters a patient with unexplained jaundice, there is a battery of tests that are helpful in the initial evaluation. These include total and direct serum bilirubin with fractionation, aminotransferases, alkaline phosphatase, albumin, and prothrombin time tests. Enzyme tests [alanine aminotransferase (ALT), aspartate aminotransferase (AST), and alkaline phosphatase (ALP)] are helpful in differentiating between a hepatocellular process and a cholestatic process (Table 302-1; Fig. 42-1), a critical step in determining what additional workup is indicated. Patients with a hepatocellular process generally have a disproportionate rise in the aminotransferases compared to the ALP. Patients with a cholestatic process have a disproportionate rise in the ALP compared to the aminotransferases. The bilirubin can be prominently elevated in both hepatocellular and cholestatic conditions and, therefore, is not necessarily helpful in differentiating between the two.

In addition to the enzyme tests, all jaundiced patients should have additional blood tests, specifically an albumin level and a prothrombin time, to assess liver function. A low albumin level suggests a chronic process such as cirrhosis or cancer. A normal albumin level is suggestive of a more acute process such as viral hepatitis or choledocholithiasis. An elevated prothrombin time indicates either vitamin K deficiency due to prolonged jaundice and malabsorption of vitamin K or significant hepatocellular dysfunction. The failure of the prothrombin time to correct with parenteral administration of vitamin K indicates severe hepatocellular injury.

The results of the bilirubin, enzyme tests, albumin, and prothrombin time tests will usually indicate whether a jaundiced patient has a hepatocellular or a cholestatic disease, as well as some indication of the duration and severity of the disease. The causes and evaluation of hepatocellular and cholestatic diseases are quite different.

Hepatocellular Conditions Hepatocellular diseases that can cause jaundice include viral hepatitis, drug or environmental toxicity, alcohol, and end-stage cirrhosis from any cause (Table 42-2). Wilson's disease, once believed to occur primarily in young adults, should be considered in all adults if no other cause of jaundice is found. Autoimmune hepatitis is typically seen in young to middle-aged women but may affect men and women of any age. Alcoholic hepatitis can be differentiated from viral and toxin-related hepatitis by the pattern of the aminotransferases. Patients with alcoholic hepatitis typically have an AST:ALT ratio of at least 2:1. The AST rarely exceeds 300 U/L. Patients with acute viral hepatitis and toxin-related injury severe enough to produce jaundice typically have aminotransferases > 500 U/L, with the ALT greater than or equal to the AST. The degree of aminotransferase elevation can occasionally help in differentiating between hepatocellular and cholestatic processes. While ALT and AST values less than 8 times normal may be seen in either hepatocellular or cholestatic liver disease, values 25 times normal or higher are seen primarily in acute hepatocellular diseases. Patients with

TABLE 42-2 Hepatocellular Conditions That May Produce Jaundice

Viral hepatitis
  Hepatitis A, B, C, D, and E
  Epstein-Barr virus
  Cytomegalovirus
  Herpes simplex
Alcohol
Drug toxicity
  Predictable, dose-dependent (e.g., acetaminophen)
  Unpredictable, idiosyncratic (e.g., isoniazid)
Environmental toxins
  Vinyl chloride
  Jamaica bush tea—pyrrolizidine alkaloids
  Kava Kava
  Wild mushrooms—*Amanita phalloides* or *A. verna*
Wilson's disease
Autoimmune hepatitis

jaundice from cirrhosis can have normal or only slight elevations of the aminotransferases.

When the physician determines that the patient has a hepatocellular disease, appropriate testing for acute viral hepatitis includes a hepatitis A IgM antibody, a hepatitis B surface antigen and core IgM antibody, and a hepatitis C viral RNA test. It can take many weeks for the hepatitis C antibody to become detectable, making it an unreliable test if acute hepatitis C is suspected. Depending on circumstances, studies for hepatitis D and E, Epstein-Barr virus (EBV), and cytomegalovirus (CMV) may be indicated. Ceruloplasmin is the initial screening test for Wilson's disease. Testing for autoimmune hepatitis usually includes an antinuclear antibody and measurement of specific immunoglobulins.

Drug-induced hepatocellular injury can be classified either as predictable or unpredictable. Predictable drug reactions are dose-dependent and affect all patients who ingest a toxic dose of the drug in question. The classic example is acetaminophen hepatotoxicity. Unpredictable or idiosyncratic drug reactions are not dose-dependent and occur in a minority of patients. A great number of drugs can cause idiosyncratic hepatic injury. Environmental toxins are also an important cause of hepatocellular injury. Examples include industrial chemicals such as vinyl chloride, herbal preparations containing pyrrolizidine alkaloids (Jamaica bush tea) and Kava Kava, and the mushrooms *Amanita phalloides* or *A. verna* that contain highly hepatotoxic amatoxins.

Cholestatic Conditions   When the pattern of the liver tests suggests a cholestatic disorder, the next step is to determine whether it is intra- or extrahepatic cholestasis (Fig. 42-1). Distinguishing intrahepatic from extrahepatic cholestasis may be difficult. History, physical examination, and laboratory tests are often not helpful. The next appropriate test is an ultrasound. The ultrasound is inexpensive, does not expose the patient to ionizing radiation, and can detect dilation of the intra- and extrahepatic biliary tree with a high degree of sensitivity and specificity. The absence of biliary dilatation suggests intrahepatic cholestasis, while the presence of biliary dilatation indicates extrahepatic cholestasis. False-negative results occur in patients with partial obstruction of the common bile duct or in patients with cirrhosis or primary sclerosing cholangitis (PSC) where scarring prevents the intrahepatic ducts from dilating.

Although ultrasonography may indicate extrahepatic cholestasis, it rarely identifies the site or cause of obstruction. The distal common bile duct is a particularly difficult area to visualize by ultrasound because of overlying bowel gas. Appropriate next tests include CT, magnetic resonance cholangiography (MRCP), and endoscopic retrograde cholangiopancreatography (ERCP). CT scanning and MRCP are better than ultrasonography for assessing the head of the pancreas and for identifying choledocholithiasis in the distal common bile duct, particularly when the ducts are not dilated. ERCP is the "gold standard" for identifying choledocholithiasis. It is performed by introducing a side-viewing endoscope perorally into the duodenum. The ampulla of Vater is visualized, and a catheter is advanced through the ampulla. Injection of dye allows for the visualization of the common bile duct and the pancreatic duct. Beyond its diagnostic capabilities, ERCP allows for therapeutic interventions, including the removal of common bile duct stones and the placement of stents. In patients in whom ERCP is unsuccessful and there is a high likelihood of the need for a therapeutic intervention, transhepatic cholangiography can provide the same information and allow for intervention. MRCP has replaced ERCP as the initial diagnostic test in cases where the need for intervention is felt to be small.

In patients with apparent *intrahepatic cholestasis*, the diagnosis is often made by serologic testing in combination with percutaneous liver biopsy. The list of possible causes of intrahepatic cholestasis is long and varied (Table 42-3). A number of conditions that typically cause a hepatocellular pattern of injury can also present as a cholestatic variant. Both hepatitis B and C can cause a cholestatic hepatitis (fibrosing cholestatic hepatitis). This disease variant has been reported in patients who have undergone solid organ transplantation. Hepatitis A, alcoholic hepatitis, EBV, and CMV may also present as cholestatic liver disease.

TABLE 42-3 Cholestatic Conditions That May Produce Jaundice

I. Intrahepatic
 A. Viral hepatitis
  1. Fibrosing cholestatic hepatitis—hepatitis B and C
  2. Hepatitis A, Epstein-Barr virus, cytomegalovirus
 B. Alcoholic hepatitis
 C. Drug toxicity
  1. Pure cholestasis—anabolic and contraceptive steroids
  2. Cholestatic hepatitis—chlorpromazine, erythromycin estolate
  3. Chronic cholestasis—chlorpromazine and prochlorperazine
 D. Primary biliary cirrhosis
 E. Primary sclerosing cholangitis
 F. Vanishing bile duct syndrome
  1. Chronic rejection of liver transplants
  2. Sarcoidosis
  3. Drugs
 G. Inherited
  1. Progressive familial intrahepatic cholestasis
  2. Benign recurrent cholestasis
 H. Cholestasis of pregnancy
 I. Total parenteral nutrition
 J. Nonhepatobiliary sepsis
 K. Benign postoperative cholestasis
 L. Paraneoplastic syndrome
 M. Venoocclusive disease
 N. Graft-versus-host disease
 O. Infiltrative disease
  1. TB
  2. Lymphoma
  3. Amyloid
 P. Infections
  1. Malaria
  2. Leptospirosis
II. Extrahepatic
 A. Malignant
  1. Cholangiocarcinoma
  2. Pancreatic cancer
  3. Gallbladder cancer
  4. Ampullary cancer
  5. Malignant involvement of the porta hepatis lymph nodes
 B. Benign
  1. Choledocholithiasis
  2. Postoperative biliary structures
  3. Primary sclerosing cholangitis
  4. Chronic pancreatitis
  5. AIDS cholangiopathy
  6. Mirizzi's syndrome
  7. Parasitic disease (ascariasis)

Drugs may cause intrahepatic cholestasis, a variant of drug-induced hepatitis. Drug-induced cholestasis is usually reversible after eliminating the offending drug, although it may take many months for cholestasis to resolve. Drugs most commonly associated with cholestasis are the anabolic and contraceptive steroids. Cholestatic hepatitis has been reported with chlorpromazine, imipramine, tolbutamide, sulindac, cimetidine, and erythromycin estolate. It also occurs in patients taking trimethoprim; sulfamethoxazole; and penicillin-based antibiotics such as ampicillin, dicloxacillin, and clavulinic acid. Rarely, cholestasis may be chronic and associated with progressive fibrosis despite early discontinuation of the drug. Chronic cholestasis has been associated with chlorpromazine and prochlorperazine.

Primary biliary cirrhosis is an autoimmune disease predominantly of middle-aged women in which there is a progressive destruction of interlobular bile ducts. The diagnosis is made by the presence of the antimitochondrial antibody that is found in 95% of patients. *Primary sclerosing cholangitis* is characterized by the destruction and fibrosis of larger bile ducts. The disease may involve only the intrahepatic ducts and present as intrahepatic cholestasis. However, in 95% of patients with PSC, both intra- and extrahepatic ducts are involved. The diagnosis of PSC is made by imaging the biliary tree. The pathognomonic findings are multiple strictures of bile ducts with dilatations proximal to the strictures. Approximately 75% of patients with PSC have inflammatory bowel disease.

The *vanishing bile duct syndrome* and *adult bile ductopenia* are rare conditions in which there are a decreased number of bile ducts seen in liver biopsy specimens. The histologic picture is similar to that found in primary biliary cirrhosis. This picture is seen in patients who develop chronic rejection after liver transplantation and in those who develop graft-versus-host disease after bone marrow transplantation. Vanishing bile duct syndrome also occurs in rare cases of sarcoidosis, in patients taking certain drugs including chlorpromazine, and idiopathically.

There are also familial forms of intrahepatic cholestasis. The familial intrahepatic cholestatic syndromes include *progressive familial intrahepatic cholestasis* (PFIC) *types 1–3,* and *benign recurrent cholestasis* (BRC). PFIC1 and BRC are autosomal recessive diseases that result from mutations in the *ATP8B1* gene that encodes a protein belonging to the subfamily of P-type ATPases; the exact function of this protein remains poorly defined. While PFIC1 is a progressive condition that manifests in childhood, BRC presents later than PFIC1 and is marked by recurrent episodes of jaundice and pruritus; the episodes are self-limited but can be debilitating. PFIC2 is caused by mutations in the *ABCB11* gene, which encodes the bile salt export pump, and PFIC3 is caused by mutations in the multidrug-resistant P-glycoprotein 3. *Cholestasis of pregnancy* occurs in the second and third trimesters and resolves after delivery. Its cause is unknown, but the condition is probably inherited and cholestasis can be triggered by estrogen administration.

Other causes of intrahepatic cholestasis include total parenteral nutrition (TPN); nonhepatobiliary sepsis; benign postoperative cholestasis; and a paraneoplastic syndrome associated with a number of different malignancies, including Hodgkin's disease, medullary thyroid cancer, renal cell cancer, renal sarcoma, T cell lymphoma, prostate cancer, and several gastrointestinal malignancies. The term *Stauffer's syndrome* has been used for intrahepatic cholestasis specifically associated with renal cell cancer. In patients developing cholestasis in the intensive care unit, the major considerations should be sepsis, shock liver, and TPN jaundice. Jaundice occurring after bone marrow transplantation is most likely due to venoocclusive disease or graft-versus-host disease.

Jaundice with associated liver dysfunction can be seen in severe cases of *Plasmodium falciparum*. The jaundice in these cases is a combination of indirect hyperbilirubinemia from hemolysis and both cholestatic and hepatocellular jaundice. Poor outcomes are seen in these cases when the jaundice is accompanied by encephalopathy and renal failure. Weil's disease, a severe presentation of leptospirosis, is marked by jaundice with renal failure, fever, headache, and muscle pain.

Causes of *extrahepatic cholestasis* can be split into malignant and benign (Table 42-3). Malignant causes include pancreatic, gallbladder, ampullary, and cholangiocarcinoma. The latter is most commonly associated with PSC and is exceptionally difficult to diagnose because its appearance is often identical to that of PSC. Pancreatic and gallbladder tumors, as well as cholangiocarcinoma, are rarely resectable and have poor prognoses. Ampullary carcinoma has the highest surgical cure rate of all the tumors that present as painless jaundice. Hilar lymphadenopathy due to metastases from other cancers may cause obstruction of the extrahepatic biliary tree.

Choledocholithiasis is the most common cause of extrahepatic cholestasis. The clinical presentation can range from mild right upper quadrant discomfort with only minimal elevations of the enzyme tests to ascending cholangitis with jaundice, sepsis, and circulatory collapse. PSC may occur with clinically important strictures limited to the extrahepatic biliary tree. In cases where there is a dominant stricture, patients can be effectively managed with serial endoscopic dilatations. Chronic pancreatitis rarely causes strictures of the distal common bile duct, where it passes through the head of the pancreas. AIDS cholangiopathy is a condition, usually due to infection of the bile duct epithelium with CMV or cryptosporidia, which has a cholangiographic appearance similar to that of PSC. These patients usually present with greatly elevated serum alkaline phosphatase levels (mean, 800 IU/L), but the bilirubin is often near normal. These patients do not typically present with jaundice.

■ SUMMARY

The goal of this chapter is not to provide an encyclopedic review of all of the conditions that can cause jaundice. Rather, it is intended to provide a framework that helps a physician to evaluate the patient with jaundice in a logical way (Fig. 42-1).

Simply stated, the initial step is to obtain appropriate blood tests to determine if the patient has an isolated elevation of serum bilirubin. If so, is the bilirubin elevation due to an increased unconjugated or conjugated fraction? If the hyperbilirubinemia is accompanied by other liver test abnormalities, is the disorder hepatocellular or cholestatic? If cholestatic, is it intra- or extrahepatic? All of these questions can be answered with a thoughtful history, physical examination, and interpretation of laboratory and radiologic tests and procedures.

FURTHER READINGS

Bosma PJ: Inherited disorders of bilirubin metabolism. J Hepatol 38:107, 2003

Ferenci P: Wilson's disease. Clin Gastroenterol Hepatol 3:726, 2005

Glasova H, Beuers U: Extrahepatic manifestations of cholestasis. J Gastroenterol Hepatol 9:938, 2002

Pratt DS, Kaplan MM: Laboratory tests, in *Schiff's Diseases of the Liver*, 10th ed, ER Schiff et al (eds). Philadelphia, Lippincott Williams & Wilkins, 2006

Trauner M et al: Molecular pathogenesis of cholestasis. N Engl J Med 339:1217, 1998

CHAPTER 43

Abdominal Swelling and Ascites

Kathleen E. Corey

Lawrence S. Friedman

ABDOMINAL SWELLING

Abdominal swelling is a manifestation of numerous diseases. Patients may complain of bloating or abdominal fullness and may note increasing abdominal girth on the basis of increased clothing or belt size. Abdominal discomfort is often reported, but pain is less frequent. When abdominal pain does accompany swelling, it is frequently the result of an intraabdominal infection, peritonitis, or pancreatitis. Patients with abdominal distention from ascites (fluid in the abdomen) may report the new onset of an inguinal or umbilical hernia. Dyspnea may result from pressure against the diaphragm and the inability to expand the lungs fully.

The causes of abdominal swelling can be remembered conveniently by the *six Fs*: flatus, fat, fluid, fetus, feces, or a "fatal growth" (often a neoplasm).

FLATUS

Abdominal swelling may be the result of increased intestinal gas. The normal small intestine contains approximately 200 mL of gas made up of nitrogen, oxygen, carbon dioxide, hydrogen, and methane. Nitrogen and oxygen are consumed (swallowed), whereas carbon dioxide, hydrogen, and methane are produced intraluminally by bacterial fermentation. Increased intestinal gas can occur in a number of conditions. Aerophagia, the swallowing of air, can result in increased amounts of oxygen and nitrogen in the small intestine and lead to abdominal swelling. Aerophagia typically results from gulping food; chewing gum; smoking; or as a response to anxiety, which leads to repetitive belching. In some cases, increased intestinal gas is the result of bacterial metabolism of excess fermentable substances such as lactose and other oligosaccharides that can lead to production of hydrogen, carbon dioxide, or methane. In many cases, the precise cause of abdominal distention cannot be determined. In some persons, particularly those with irritable bowel syndrome and bloating, the subjective sense of abdominal pressure is attributable to impaired intestinal transit of gas rather than increased gas volume. Abdominal distention, an objective increase in girth, is the result of a lack of coordination between diaphragmatic contraction and anterior abdominal wall relaxation in response to an increase in intraabdominal volume loads. Occasionally, increased lumbar lordosis accounts for apparent abdominal distention.

FAT

Weight gain with an increase in abdominal fat can result in an increase in abdominal girth and can be perceived as abdominal swelling. Abdominal fat may be the result of an imbalance between calorie intake and energy expenditure associated with a poor diet and sedentary lifestyle and also can be a manifestation of certain diseases such as Cushing's syndrome. Excess abdominal fat has been associated with an increased risk of insulin resistance and cardiovascular disease.

FLUID

Fluid within the abdominal cavity, or ascites, often results in abdominal distention and is discussed in detail below.

FETUS

Pregnancy results in increased abdominal girth. Typically, an increase in abdominal size is first noted at 12 to 14 weeks of gestation, when the uterus moves from the pelvis into the abdomen. Abdominal distention may be seen before this point as a result of fluid retention and relaxation of the abdominal muscles.

FECES

Increased stool in the colon, in the setting of severe constipation or intestinal obstruction, also leads to increased abdominal girth. These conditions often are accompanied by abdominal pain, nausea, and vomiting and can be diagnosed by imaging studies.

FATAL GROWTH

An abdominal mass can result in abdominal swelling. Enlargement of the intraabdominal organs, specifically the liver (hepatomegaly) or spleen (splenomegaly) or an abdominal aortic aneurysm, can result in abdominal distention. Bladder distention also may result in abdominal swelling. In addition, malignancies, abscesses, or cysts can grow to sizes that lead to increased abdominal girth.

HISTORY AND PHYSICAL EXAMINATION

Determining the etiology of abdominal swelling begins with history-taking and a physical examination. Patients should be questioned regarding symptoms suggestive of malignancy, including weight loss, night sweats, and anorexia. Inability to pass stool or flatus together with nausea or vomiting suggest bowel obstruction, severe constipation, or an ileus (lack of peristalsis). Increased eructation and flatus may point toward aerophagia or increased intestinal production of gas. Patients should be questioned about risk factors for or symptoms of chronic liver disease, including excessive alcohol use and jaundice, which suggest ascites. Patients should also be asked about other symptoms of medical conditions, including heart failure and tuberculosis, which may cause ascites.

Physical examination should assess for signs of systemic disease. The presence of lymphadenopathy, especially supraclavicular lymphadenopathy (Virchow's node), suggests metastatic abdominal malignancy. Care also should be taken during the cardiac examination to evaluate for elevation of jugular venous pressure (JVP); Kussmaul's sign (elevation of the JVP during inspiration); or a pericardial knock, which may be seen in heart failure or constrictive pericarditis, as well as a murmur of tricuspid regurgitation. Spider angiomas, palmar erythema, dilated superficial veins around the umbilicus (caput medusae), and gynecomastia suggest chronic liver disease.

The abdominal examination should begin with inspection for the presence of uneven distention or an obvious mass. Auscultation should follow. The absence of bowel sounds or the presence of high-pitched localized bowel sounds point toward an ileus or intestinal obstruction. An umbilical venous hum may suggest the presence of portal hypertension, and a harsh bruit over the liver is heard rarely in patients with hepatocellular carcinoma or alcoholic hepatitis. Abdominal swelling caused by intestinal gas can be differentiated from swelling caused by fluid or a solid mass by percussion; an abdomen filled with gas is tympanic, whereas an abdomen containing a mass or fluid is dull to percussion. The absence of abdominal dullness, however, does not exclude ascites, because a minimum of 1500 mL of ascites is required for detection on physical

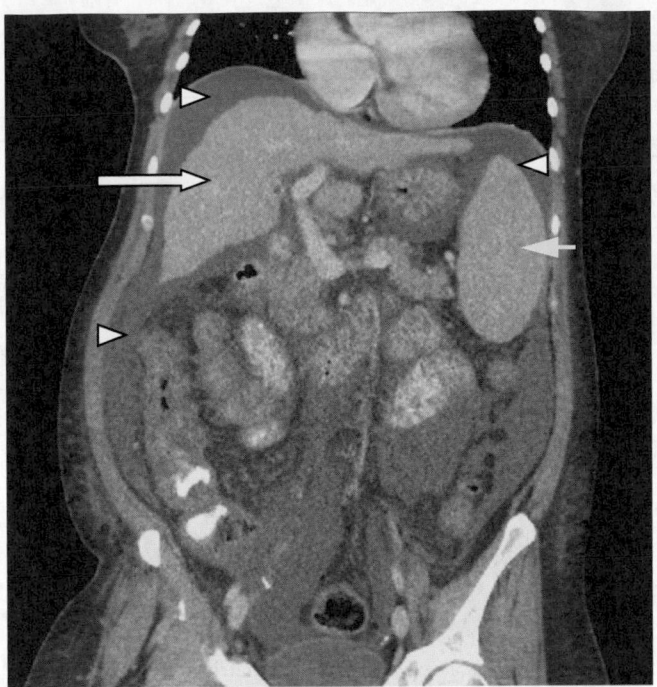

Figure 43-1 CT of a patient with a cirrhotic, nodular liver (white arrow), splenomegaly (yellow arrow), and ascites (arrowheads).

examination. Finally, the abdomen should be palpated to assess for tenderness, a mass, enlargement of the spleen or liver, or presence of a nodular liver suggesting cirrhosis or tumor. Light palpation of the liver may detect pulsations suggesting retrograde vascular flow from the heart in patients with right-sided heart failure, particularly tricuspid regurgitation.

IMAGING AND LABORATORY EVALUATION

Abdominal x-rays can be used to detect dilated loops of bowel, suggesting intestinal obstruction or ileus. An abdominal ultrasound can detect as little as 100 mL of ascites, hepatosplenomegaly, a nodular liver, or a mass. Ultrasound is often inadequate to detect retroperitoneal lymphadenopathy or a pancreatic lesion because of overlying bowel gas. If malignancy or pancreatic disease is suspected, CT can be performed. CT may also detect changes associated with advanced cirrhosis and portal hypertension (Fig. 43-1).

Laboratory evaluation should include liver biochemical testing, a serum albumin level, a prothrombin time (international normalized ratio) to assess hepatic function, and a complete blood count to evaluate for the presence of cytopenias that may result from portal hypertension or leukocytosis, anemia, and thrombocytosis that may result from systemic infection. Serum amylase and lipase levels should be checked to evaluate the patient for acute pancreatitis. Urinary protein quantitation is indicated when nephrotic syndrome, which may cause ascites, is suspected.

In selected cases, measurement of the hepatic venous pressure gradient (pressure across the liver between the portal and hepatic veins) can be obtained via cannulation of the hepatic vein to confirm that ascites is caused by cirrhosis (see Chapter 308). In some cases, a liver biopsy may be necessary to confirm cirrhosis.

ASCITES

PATHOGENESIS IN CIRRHOSIS

Ascites in patients with cirrhosis is the result of portal hypertension and renal salt and water retention. Portal hypertension signifies elevation of the pressure within the portal vein. According to

Ohm's law, pressure is the product of resistance and flow. Increased hepatic resistance occurs by several mechanisms. First, the development of hepatic fibrosis, which defines cirrhosis, disrupts the normal architecture of the hepatic sinusoids and impedes normal blood flow through the liver. Second, activation of hepatic stellate cells, which mediate fibrogenesis, leads to smooth muscle contraction and fibrosis. Finally, cirrhosis is associated with a decrease in endothelial nitric oxide synthetase (eNOS) production, which results in decreased nitric oxide production and increased intrahepatic vasoconstriction.

The development of cirrhosis is also associated with increased systemic circulating levels of nitric oxide (contrary to the decrease seen intrahepatically) as well as increased levels of vascular endothelial growth factor and tumor necrosis factor that result in splanchnic arterial vasodilatation. Vasodilatation of the splanchnic circulation results in pooling of blood and a decrease in the effective circulating volume, which is perceived by the kidneys as hypovolemia. Compensatory vasoconstriction via release of antidiuretic hormone ensues, thereby leading to free water retention and activation of the sympathetic nervous system and renin angiotensin aldosterone system, leading in turn to renal sodium and water retention.

PATHOGENESIS IN THE ABSENCE OF CIRRHOSIS

Ascites in the absence of cirrhosis generally results from peritoneal carcinomatosis, peritoneal infection, or pancreatic disease. Peritoneal carcinomatosis can result from primary peritoneal malignancies such as mesothelioma or sarcoma, abdominal malignancies such as gastric or colonic adenocarcinoma, or metastatic disease from breast or lung carcinoma or melanoma (Fig. 43-2). The tumor cells lining the peritoneum produce a protein-rich fluid that contributes to the development of ascites. Fluid from the extracellular space is drawn into the peritoneum, further contributing to the development of ascites. Tuberculous peritonitis causes ascites via a similar mechanism; tubercles deposited on the peritoneum exude a proteinaceous fluid. Pancreatic ascites results from leakage of pancreatic enzymes into the peritoneum.

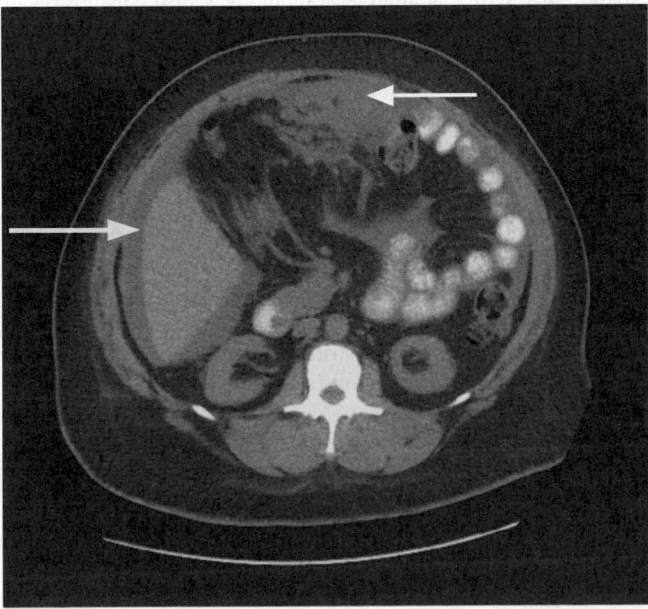

Figure 43-2 CT of a patient with peritoneal carcinomatosis (white arrow) and ascites (yellow arrow).

■ CAUSES

Cirrhosis accounts for 84% of cases of ascites. Cardiac ascites, peritoneal carcinomatosis, and "mixed" ascites resulting from cirrhosis and a second disease account for 10 to 15% of cases. Less common causes of ascites include massive hepatic metastasis, infection (tuberculosis, *Chlamydia*), pancreatitis, and renal disease (nephrotic syndrome). Rare causes of ascites include hypothyroidism and familial Mediterranean fever.

■ EVALUATION

Once the presence of ascites has been confirmed, the etiology of the ascites is best determined by *paracentesis*. Paracentesis is a bedside procedure in which a needle or small catheter is passed transcutaneously to extract ascitic fluid from the peritoneum. The lower quadrants are the most frequent sites for paracentesis. Occasionally, an infraumbilical approach is used. The left lower quadrant is preferred because of the greater depth of ascites and thinner abdominal wall. Paracentesis is a safe procedure even in patients with coagulopathy; complications, including abdominal wall hematomas, hypotension, hepatorenal syndrome, and infection, are infrequent.

Once ascitic fluid has been extracted, its gross appearance should be examined. Turbid fluid can result from infection or tumor cells within the fluid. White, milky fluid indicates the presence of triglycerides in levels > 200 mg/dL (and often > 1000 mg/dL), which is the hallmark of *chylous ascites*. Chylous ascites results from lymphatic disruption that may occur with trauma, cirrhosis, tumor, tuberculosis, or certain congenital abnormalities. Dark brown fluid can reflect a high bilirubin concentration and indicates biliary tract perforation. Black fluid may indicate the presence of pancreatic necrosis or metastatic melanoma.

The ascitic fluid should be sent for measurement of the albumin and total protein levels, cell and differential counts, and, if infection is suspected, Gram's stain and culture, with inoculation of the fluid into blood culture bottles at the patient's bedside to maximize the yield. In addition, a serum albumin level should be sent simultaneously to permit calculation of the *serum-ascites albumin gradient* (SAAG).

The SAAG is useful for distinguishing ascites caused by portal hypertension from nonportal hypertensive ascites (Fig. 43-3). The SAAG reflects the pressure within the hepatic sinusoids and correlates with the hepatic venous pressure gradient. The SAAG is calculated by subtracting the ascitic albumin from the serum albumin and does not change with diuresis. A SAAG ≥ 1.1 g/dL reflects the presence of portal hypertension and indicates that the ascites is from an increased pressure in the hepatic sinusoids. According to Starling's law, a high SAAG reflects the oncotic pressure that counterbalances the portal pressure. Possible causes include cirrhosis, cardiac ascites, sinusoidal obstruction syndrome (venoocclusive disease), massive liver metastasis, or hepatic vein thrombosis (Budd-Chiari syndrome). A SAAG < 1.1 g/dL indicates that the ascites is not related to portal hypertension as in tuberculous peritonitis, peritoneal carcinomatosis, or pancreatic ascites.

For high-SAAG (≥ 1.1) ascites, the ascitic protein level can provide further clues to the etiology (see Fig. 43-3). An ascitic protein level of ≥ 2.5 g/dL indicates that the hepatic sinusoids are normal and allows passage of protein into the ascites, as occurs in cardiac ascites, sinusoidal obstruction syndrome, or early Budd-Chiari syndrome. An ascitic protein level < 2.5 g/dL indicates that the hepatic sinusoids have been damaged and scarred and no longer allow passage

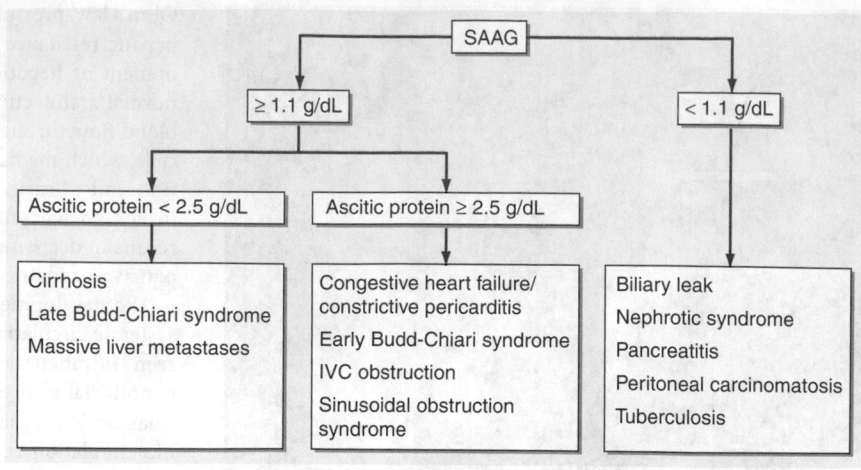

Figure 43-3 Algorithm for the diagnosis of ascites according to the serum-ascites albumin gradient (SAAG). IVC, inferior vena cava.

of protein, as occurs with cirrhosis, late Budd-Chiari syndrome, or massive liver metastases. Pro-brain-type natriuretic peptide (BNP) is a natriuretic hormone released by the heart as a result of increased volume and ventricular wall stretch. High levels of BNP in serum occur in heart failure and may be useful in identifying congestive heart failure as the cause of high-SAAG ascites.

Further tests are indicated only in specific clinical circumstances. When secondary peritonitis resulting from a perforated hollow viscus is suspected, ascitic glucose and lactate dehydrogenase (LDH) levels can be sent. In contrast to "spontaneous" bacterial peritonitis (SBP), which may complicate cirrhotic ascites, secondary peritonitis is suggested by an ascitic glucose level <50 mg/dL, an ascitic LDH greater than the serum LDH level, and multiple pathogens on ascitic fluid culture. When pancreatic ascites is suspected, an ascitic amylase should be measured and is typically >1000 mg/dL. Cytology can be useful in the diagnosis of peritoneal carcinomatosis. At least 50 mL of fluid should be obtained and sent for immediate processing. Tuberculous peritonitis can be difficult to diagnose by paracentesis. A smear for acid-fast bacilli has a sensitivity of only 0 to 3%, and a culture increases the sensitivity for diagnosis to 35 to 50%. In patients without cirrhosis, an elevated ascitic adenosine deaminase level has a sensitivity of more than 90% when a cut-off value of 30 to 45 U/L is used. When the cause of ascites remains uncertain, laparotomy or laparoscopy with peritoneal biopsies for histology and culture remains the gold standard.

TREATMENT   Ascites

The initial treatment of cirrhotic ascites is restriction of sodium intake to 2 g/d. When sodium restriction alone is inadequate to control ascites, oral diuretics, typically the combination of spironolactone and furosemide, are used. Spironolactone is an aldosterone antagonist that inhibits Na⁺ resorption in the distal convoluted tubule of the kidney. Use of spironolactone may be limited by hyponatremia, hyperkalemia, and painful gynecomastia. If the gynecomastia is distressing, amiloride, 5–40 mg/d, may be substituted for spironolactone. Furosemide is a loop diuretic that is generally combined with spironolactone in a ratio of 40:100; maximal daily doses of spironolactone and furosemide are generally 400 mg and 160 mg, respectively.

Refractory cirrhotic ascites is defined by the persistence of ascites despite sodium restriction and maximal (or maximally tolerated) diuretic use. Refractory ascites can be managed by serial large volume paracentesis (LVP) or a transjugular intrahepatic peritoneal shunt (TIPS), a radiologically placed portosystemic shunt to decompress the hepatic sinusoids. TIPS is superior to LVP in reducing the reaccumulation of ascites but is associated with an increased frequency of hepatic encephalopathy with no difference in mortality rates.

Malignant ascites does not respond to sodium restriction or diuretics. Patients must undergo serial LVPs, transcutaneous drainage catheter placement, or, rarely, creation of a peritovenous shunt (a shunt from the abdominal cavity to the vena cava).

Ascites caused by tuberculous peritonitis is treated with standard antituberculosis therapy. Noncirrhotic ascites of other causes is treated by correction of the precipitating condition.

◼ COMPLICATIONS

Spontaneous bacterial peritonitis (SBP) is a common and potentially lethal complication of cirrhotic ascites. SBP also can occasionally complicate ascites caused by nephrotic syndrome, heart failure, acute hepatitis, and acute liver failure but is rare in malignant ascites. Patients with SBP generally note an increase in abdominal girth; however, abdominal tenderness is found in only 40% of patients, and rebound tenderness is rare. Patients may present with fever, nausea, vomiting, or the new onset of or exacerbation of preexisting hepatic encephalopathy.

SBP is defined by a polymorphonuclear neutrophil (PMN) count of ≥250/mm³ in the ascitic fluid. Ascitic fluid cultures typically reveal one bacterial pathogen. The presence of multiple pathogens in the setting of an elevated ascitic PMN count suggests secondary peritonitis from a ruptured viscus or abscess. The presence of multiple pathogens without an elevated PMN count suggests bowel perforation from the paracentesis needle. SBP is generally the result of enteric bacteria that have translocated across an edematous bowel wall. The most common pathogens are Gram-negative rods, including *Escherichia coli* and *Klebsiella*, as well as streptococci and enterococci.

Treatment of SBP with an antibiotic such as intravenous cefotaxime is effective against gram-negative and Gram-positive aerobes. Five days of treatment are sufficient if the patient improves clinically.

Cirrhotic patients with a history of SBP, an ascitic fluid total protein concentration <1 g/dL, or active gastrointestinal bleeding should receive prophylactic antibiotics to prevent SBP; oral norfloxacin is commonly used. Diuresis increases the activity of ascitic fluid protein opsonins and may decrease the risk of SBP.

Hepatic hydrothorax occurs when ascites, often caused by cirrhosis, migrates via fenestrae in the diaphragm into the pleural space and can result in shortness of breath, hypoxia, and infection. Treatment is similar to that of cirrhotic ascites and includes sodium restriction, diuretics, and, if needed, thoracentesis or TIPS placement. Chest tube placement should be avoided.

FURTHER READINGS

HOEFS JC: Serum protein concentration and portal pressure determine the ascitic fluid protein concentration in patients with chronic liver disease. J Lab Clin Med 102:260, 1983

RUNYON BA: Cardiac ascites: A characterization. J Clin Gastroenterol 10:410, 1988

——: Management of adult patients with ascites due to cirrhosis: An update. Hepatology 49:2087, 2009

——, et al: Diuresis increases ascitic fluid opsonic activity in patients who survive spontaneous bacterial peritonitis. J Hepatol 14:249, 1992

——, et al: Ascitic fluid analysis in malignancy-related ascites. Hepatology 8:1104, 1988

SHEER TA, et al: Usefulness of serum N-terminal-ProBNP in distinguishing ascites due to cirrhosis from ascites due to heart failure. J Clin Gastroenterol 44:e23, 2010

SIMRÉN M: Bloating and abdominal distention: Not so poorly understood anymore! Gastroenterology 136:1487, 2009

CHAPTER 44

Azotemia and Urinary Abnormalities

Julie Lin

Bradley M. Denker

Normal kidney functions occur through numerous cellular processes to maintain body homeostasis. Disturbances in any of those functions can lead to a constellation of abnormalities that may be detrimental to survival. The clinical manifestations of those disorders depend on the pathophysiology of the renal injury and often are identified initially as a complex of symptoms, abnormal physical findings, and laboratory changes that together make possible the identification of specific syndromes. These renal syndromes (Table 44-1) may arise as a consequence of a systemic illness or can occur as a primary renal disease. Nephrologic syndromes usually consist of several elements that reflect the underlying pathologic processes. The duration and severity of the disease affect those findings and typically include one or more of the following: (1) reduction in glomerular filtration rate (GFR) (azotemia), (2) abnormalities of urine sediment [red blood cells (RBC), white blood cells, casts, and crystals], (3) abnormal excretion of serum proteins (proteinuria), (4) disturbances in urine volume (oliguria, anuria, polyuria), (5) presence of hypertension and/or expanded total body fluid volume (edema), (6) electrolyte abnormalities, (7) in some syndromes, fever/pain. The combination of these findings should permit identification of one of the major nephrologic syndromes (Table 44-1) and will allow differential diagnoses to be narrowed and the appropriate diagnostic evaluation and therapeutic course to be determined. All these syndromes and their associated diseases are discussed in more detail in subsequent chapters. This chapter focuses on several aspects of renal abnormalities that are critically important for distinguishing among those processes: (1) reduction in GFR leading to azotemia, (2) alterations of the urinary sediment and/or protein excretion, and (3) abnormalities of urinary volume.

AZOTEMIA

■ ASSESSMENT OF GLOMERULAR FILTRATION RATE (GFR)

Monitoring the GFR is important in both the hospital and outpatient settings, and several different methodologies are available. GFR is the primary metric for kidney "function," and its direct measurement involves administration of a radioactive isotope (such as inulin or iothalamate) that is filtered at the glomerulus but neither reabsorbed nor secreted throughout the tubule. Clearance of inulin or iothalamate in milliliters per minute equals the GFR and is calculated from the rate of removal from the blood and appearance in the urine over several hours. Direct GFR measurements are frequently available through nuclear radiology departments. In most clinical circumstances direct measurement of GFR is not available, and the serum creatinine level is used as a surrogate to estimate GFR. Serum creatinine is the most widely used marker for GFR, and the GFR is related directly to the urine creatinine excretion and inversely to the serum creatinine (U_{Cr}/P_{Cr}). Based on this relationship and some important caveats (discussed below), the GFR will fall in roughly inverse proportion to the rise in P_{Cr}. Failure to account for GFR reductions in drug dosing can lead to significant morbidity and mortality from drug toxicities (e.g., digoxin, aminoglycosides). In the outpatient setting, the serum creatinine serves as an estimate for GFR (although much less accurate; see below). In patients with chronic progressive renal disease, there is an approximately linear relationship between $1/P_{Cr}$ (y axis) and time (x axis). The slope of that line will remain constant for an individual patient, and when values are obtained that do not fall on the line, an investigation for a superimposed acute process (e.g., volume depletion, drug reaction) should be initiated. Signs and symptoms of uremia develop at significantly different levels of serum creatinine, depending on the patient (size, age, and sex), the underlying renal disease, the existence of concurrent diseases, and true GFR. In general, patients do not develop symptomatic uremia until renal insufficiency is quite severe (GFR <15 mL/min).

A significantly reduced GFR (either acute or chronic) usually is reflected in a rise in serum creatinine and leads to retention of nitrogenous waste products (azotemia) such as urea. Azotemia may result from reduced renal perfusion, intrinsic renal disease, or postrenal processes (ureteral obstruction; see below and Fig. 44-1). Precise determination of GFR is problematic as both commonly measured indices (urea and creatinine) have characteristics that affect their accuracy as markers of clearance. Urea clearance may underestimate GFR significantly because of urea reabsorption by the tubule. In contrast, creatinine is derived from muscle metabolism of creatine, and its generation varies little from day to day.

Creatinine clearance, an approximation of GFR, is measured from plasma and urinary creatinine excretion rates for a defined time period (usually 24 h) and is expressed in milliliters per minute: $CrCl = (U_{vol} \times U_{Cr})/(P_{Cr} \times T_{min})$. Creatinine is useful for estimating GFR because it is a small, freely filtered solute that is not reabsorbed by the tubules. Serum creatinine levels can increase acutely from dietary ingestion of cooked meat, however, and creatinine can be secreted into the proximal tubule through an organic cation pathway (especially in advanced progressive chronic kidney disease), leading to overestimation of GFR. When a timed collection for creatinine clearance is not available, decisions about drug dosing must be based on serum creatinine alone. Two formulas are used widely to estimate kidney function from serum creatinine: (1) Cockcroft-Gault and (2) four-variable MDRD (Modification of Diet in Renal Disease).

Cockcroft-Gault: CrCl (mL/min) = (140 − age (years) × weight (kg)
$$\times [0.85 \text{ if female}])/(72 \times sCr \text{ (mg/dL)})$$

MDRD: eGFR (mL/min per 1.73 m²) = 186.3 × P_{Cr} ($e^{-1.154}$) × age ($e^{-0.203}$)
$$\times (0.742 \text{ if female}) \times (1.21 \text{ if black}).$$

Numerous websites are available for making these calculations (*www.kidney.org/professionals/kdoqi/gfr_calculator.cfm*). A newer CKD-EPI eGFR was developed by pooling several cohorts with and without kidney disease who had data on directly measured GFR and appears to be more accurate:

CKD-EPI: eGFR = 141 × min (Scr/k, 1)[a] × max (Scr/k, 1)$^{-1.209}$
$$\times 0.993^{Age} \times 1.018 \text{ [if female]} \times 1.159 \text{ [if black]}$$

where Scr is serum creatinine, k is 0.7 for females and 0.9 for males, a is −0.329 for females and −0.411 for males, min indicates the

TABLE 44-1 Initial Clinical and Laboratory Data Base for Defining Major Syndromes in Nephrology

Syndromes	Important Clues to Diagnosis	Findings That Are Common	Location of Discussion of Disease-Causing Syndrome
Acute or rapidly progressive renal failure	Anuria Oliguria Documented recent decline in GFR	Hypertension, hematuria Proteinuria, pyuria Casts, edema	Chaps. 279, 283, 285, 289
Acute nephritis	Hematuria, RBC casts Azotemia, oliguria Edema, hypertension	Proteinuria Pyuria Circulatory congestion	Chap. 283
Chronic renal failure	Azotemia for >3 months Prolonged symptoms or signs of uremia Symptoms or signs of renal osteodystrophy Kidneys reduced in size bilaterally Broad casts in urinary sediment	Proteinuria Casts Polyuria, nocturia Edema, hypertension Electrolyte disorders	Chaps. 278, 280
Nephrotic syndrome	Proteinuria >3.5 g per 1.73 m² per 24 h Hypoalbuminemia Edema Hyperlipidemia	Casts Lipiduria	Chap. 283
Asymptomatic urinary abnormalities	Hematuria Proteinuria (below nephrotic range) Sterile pyuria, casts		Chap. 283
Urinary tract infection/pyelonephritis	Bacteriuria >10⁵ colonies per milliliter Other infectious agent documented in urine Pyuria, leukocyte casts Frequency, urgency Bladder tenderness, flank tenderness	Hematuria Mild azotemia Mild proteinuria Fever	Chap. 288
Renal tubule defects	Electrolyte disorders Polyuria, nocturia Renal calcification Large kidneys Renal transport defects	Hematuria "Tubular" proteinuria (<1 g/24 h) Enuresis	Chaps. 284, 285
Hypertension	Systolic/diastolic hypertension	Proteinuria Casts Azotemia	Chaps. 247, 286
Nephrolithiasis	Previous history of stone passage or removal Previous history of stone seen by x-ray Renal colic	Hematuria Pyuria Frequency, urgency	Chap. 287
Urinary tract obstruction	Azotemia, oliguria, anuria Polyuria, nocturia, urinary retention Slowing of urinary stream Large prostate, large kidneys Flank tenderness, full bladder after voiding	Hematuria Pyuria Enuresis, dysuria	Chap. 289

Abbreviations: GFR; glomerular filtration rate; RBC, red blood cell.

minimum of Scr/k or 1, and max indicates the maximum of Scr/k or 1 (*http://www.qxmd.com/renal/Calculate-CKD-EPI-GFR.php*).

Several limitations of using serum creatinine–based estimating equations must be acknowledged. Each equation, along with the 24-h urine collection for measurement of creatinine clearance, is based on the assumption that the patient is in steady state, without daily increases or decreases in serum creatinine levels as a result of rapidly changing GFR. The MDRD equation has poorer accuracy when GFR >60 mL/min per 1.73 m². The gradual loss of muscle from chronic illness, chronic use of glucocorticoids, or malnutrition can mask significant changes in GFR with small or imperceptible changes in serum creatinine concentration. Cystatin C is a member of the cystatin superfamily of cysteine protease inhibitors and is produced at a relatively constant rate from all nucleated cells. Serum cystatin C has been proposed to be a more sensitive marker of early GFR decline than is plasma creatinine; however, like serum creatinine, cystatin C is influenced by age, race, and sex and additionally is associated with diabetes, smoking, and markers of inflammation.

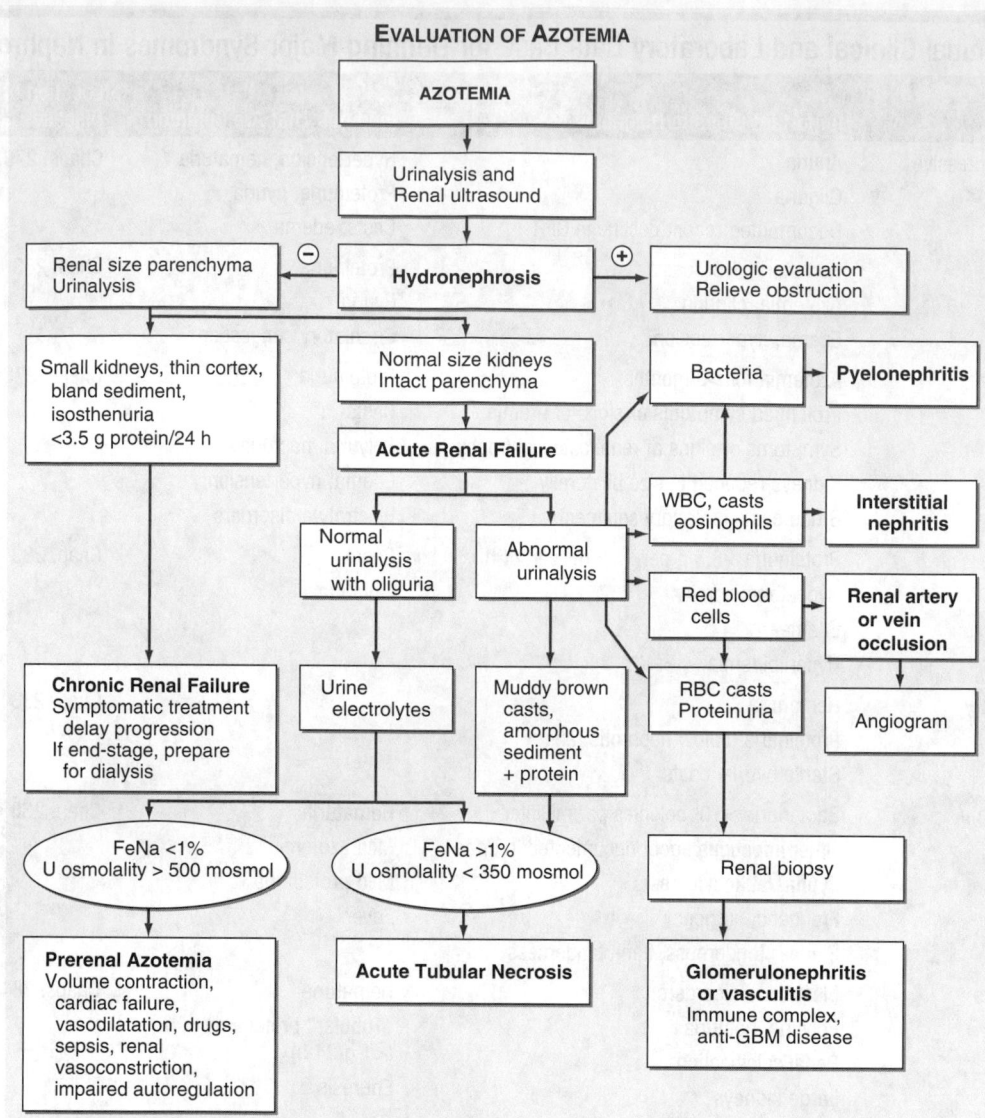

EVALUATION OF AZOTEMIA

Figure 44-1 Approach to the patient with azotemia. FeNa, fractional excretion of sodium; GBM, glomerular basement membrane; RBC, red blood cell; WBC, white blood cell.

APPROACH TO THE
PATIENT ▶ Azotemia

Once it has been established that GFR is reduced, the physician must decide if this represents acute or chronic renal injury. The clinical situation, history, and laboratory data often make this an easy distinction. However, the laboratory abnormalities characteristic of chronic renal failure, including anemia, hypocalcemia, and hyperphosphatemia, often are also present in patients presenting with acute renal failure. Radiographic evidence of renal osteodystrophy (Chap. 280) can be seen only in chronic renal failure but is a very late finding, and these patients are usually on dialysis. The urinalysis and renal ultrasound occasionally can facilitate distinguishing acute from chronic renal failure. An approach to the evaluation of azotemic patients is shown in Fig. 44-1. Patients with advanced chronic renal insufficiency often have some proteinuria, nonconcentrated urine (isosthenuria; isoosmotic with plasma), and small kidneys on ultrasound, characterized by increased echogenicity and cortical thinning. Treatment should be directed toward slowing the progression of renal disease and providing symptomatic relief for edema, acidosis, anemia, and hyperphosphatemia, as discussed in Chap. 280. Acute

renal failure (Chap. 279) can result from processes that affect renal blood flow (prerenal azotemia), intrinsic renal diseases (affecting small vessels, glomeruli, or tubules), or postrenal processes (obstruction to urine flow in ureters, bladder, or urethra) (Chap. 289).

Prerenal Failure Decreased renal perfusion accounts for 40–80% of acute renal failure and, if appropriately treated, is readily reversible. The etiologies of prerenal azotemia include any cause of decreased circulating blood volume (gastrointestinal hemorrhage, burns, diarrhea, diuretics), volume sequestration (pancreatitis, peritonitis, rhabdomyolysis), or decreased effective arterial volume (cardiogenic shock, sepsis). Renal perfusion also can be affected by reductions in cardiac output from peripheral vasodilation (sepsis, drugs) or profound renal vasoconstriction [severe heart failure, hepatorenal syndrome, drugs such as nonsteroidal anti-inflammatory drugs (NSAIDs)]. True or "effective" arterial hypovolemia leads to a fall in mean arterial pressure, which in turn triggers a series of neural and humoral responses that include activation of the sympathetic nervous and renin-angiotensin-aldosterone systems and antidiuretic hormone (ADH) release. GFR is maintained by prostaglandin-mediated

TABLE 44-2 Laboratory Findings in Acute Renal Failure

Index	Prerenal Azotemia	Oliguric Acute Renal Failure
BUN/P_{Cr} ratio	>20:1	10-15:1
Urine sodium (U_{Na}), meq/L	<20	>40
Urine osmolality, mosmol/L H_2O	>500	<350
Fractional excretion of sodium	<1%	>2%
$$FE_{Na} = \frac{U_{Na} \times P_{Cr} \times 100}{P_{Na} \times U_{Cr}}$$		
Urine/plasma creatinine (U_{Cr}/P_{Cr})	>40	<20

Abbreviations: BUN, blood urea nitrogen; P_{Cr}, plasma creatinine; P_{Na}, plasma sodium concentration; U_{Cr}, urine creatinine concentration; U_{Na}, urine sodium concentration.

relaxation of afferent arterioles and angiotensin II–mediated constriction of efferent arterioles. Once the mean arterial pressure falls below 80 mmHg, there is a steep decline in GFR.

Blockade of prostaglandin production by NSAIDs can result in severe vasoconstriction and acute renal failure. Blocking angiotensin action with angiotensin-converting enzyme (ACE) inhibitors or angiotensin receptor blockers (ARBs) decreases efferent arteriolar tone and in turn decreases glomerular capillary perfusion pressure. Patients on NSAIDs and/or ACE inhibitors/ARBs are most susceptible to hemodynamically mediated acute renal failure when blood volume is reduced for any reason. Patients with bilateral renal artery stenosis (or stenosis in a solitary kidney) are dependent on efferent arteriolar vasoconstriction for maintenance of glomerular filtration pressure and are particularly susceptible to a precipitous decline in GFR when given ACE inhibitors or ARBs.

Prolonged renal hypoperfusion may lead to acute tubular necrosis (ATN), an intrinsic renal disease that is discussed below. The urinalysis and urinary electrolytes can be useful in distinguishing prerenal azotemia from ATN (Table 44-2). The urine of patients with prerenal azotemia can be predicted from the stimulatory actions of norepinephrine, angiotensin II, ADH, and low tubule fluid flow rate on salt and water reabsorption. In prerenal conditions, the tubules are intact, leading to a concentrated urine (>500 mosmol), avid Na retention (urine Na concentration <20 mM/L, fractional excretion of Na <1%), and U_{Cr}/P_{Cr} >40 (Table 44-2). The prerenal urine sediment is usually normal or has occasional hyaline and granular casts, whereas the sediment of ATN usually is filled with cellular debris and dark (muddy brown) granular casts.

Postrenal Azotemia Urinary tract obstruction accounts for <5% of cases of acute renal failure, but it is usually reversible and must be ruled out early in the evaluation (Fig. 44-1). Since a single kidney is capable of adequate clearance, obstructive acute renal failure requires obstruction at the urethra or bladder outlet, bilateral ureteral obstruction, or unilateral obstruction in a patient with a single functioning kidney. Obstruction usually is diagnosed by the presence of ureteral and renal pelvic dilation on renal ultrasound. However, early in the course of obstruction or if the ureters are unable to dilate (e.g., encasement by pelvic tumors or periureteral), the ultrasound examination may be negative. The specific urologic conditions that cause obstruction are discussed in Chap. 289.

Intrinsic Renal Disease When prerenal and postrenal azotemia have been excluded as etiologies of renal failure, an intrinsic parenchymal renal disease is present. Intrinsic renal disease can arise from processes involving large renal vessels, intrarenal microvasculature and glomeruli, or the tubulointerstitium. Ischemic and toxic ATN account for ~90% of cases of acute intrinsic renal failure. As outlined in Fig. 44-1, the clinical setting and urinalysis are helpful in separating the possible etiologies of acute intrinsic renal failure. Prerenal azotemia and ATN are part of a spectrum of renal hypoperfusion; evidence of structural tubule injury is present in ATN, whereas prompt reversibility occurs with prerenal azotemia upon restoration of adequate renal perfusion. Thus, ATN often can be distinguished from prerenal azotemia by urinalysis and urine electrolyte composition (Table 44-2 and Fig. 44-1). Ischemic ATN is observed most frequently in patients who have undergone major surgery, trauma, severe hypovolemia, overwhelming sepsis, or extensive burns. Nephrotoxic ATN complicates the administration of many common medications, usually by inducing a combination of intrarenal vasoconstriction, direct tubule toxicity, and/or tubule obstruction. The kidney is vulnerable to toxic injury by virtue of its rich blood supply (25% of cardiac output) and its ability to concentrate and metabolize toxins. A diligent search for hypotension and nephrotoxins usually will uncover the specific etiology of ATN. Discontinuation of nephrotoxins and stabilization of blood pressure often will suffice without the need for dialysis while the tubules recover. An extensive list of potential drugs and toxins implicated in ATN can be found in Chap. 279.

Processes that involve the tubules and interstitium can lead to acute kidney injury (AKI), a subtype of acute renal failure. These processes include drug-induced interstitial nephritis (especially antibiotics, NSAIDs, and diuretics), severe infections (both bacterial and viral), systemic diseases (e.g., systemic lupus erythematosus), and infiltrative disorders (e.g., sarcoid, lymphoma, or leukemia). A list of drugs associated with allergic interstitial nephritis can be found in Chap. 285. The urinalysis usually shows mild to moderate proteinuria, hematuria, and pyuria (~75% of cases) and occasionally shows white blood cell casts. The finding of RBC casts in interstitial nephritis has been reported but should prompt a search for glomerular diseases (Fig. 44-1). Occasionally, renal biopsy will be needed to distinguish among these possibilities. The finding of eosinophils in the urine is suggestive of allergic interstitial nephritis or atheroembolic renal disease and is optimally observed by using a Hansel stain. The absence of eosinophiluria, however, does not exclude these etiologies.

Occlusion of large renal vessels including arteries and veins is an uncommon cause of acute renal failure. A significant reduction in GFR by this mechanism suggests bilateral processes or a unilateral process in a patient with a single functioning kidney. Renal arteries can be occluded with atheroemboli, thromboemboli, in situ thrombosis, aortic dissection, or vasculitis. Atheroembolic renal failure can occur spontaneously but most often is associated with recent aortic instrumentation. The emboli are cholesterol-rich and lodge in medium and small renal arteries, leading to an eosinophil-rich inflammatory reaction. Patients with atheroembolic acute renal failure often have a normal urinalysis, but the urine may contain eosinophils and casts. The diagnosis can be confirmed by renal biopsy, but this is often unnecessary when other stigmata of atheroemboli are present (livedo reticularis, distal peripheral infarcts, eosinophilia). Renal artery thrombosis may lead to mild proteinuria and hematuria, whereas renal vein thrombosis typically induces heavy proteinuria and hematuria. These vascular complications often require angiography for confirmation and are discussed in Chap. 286.

EVALUATION OF HEMATURIA

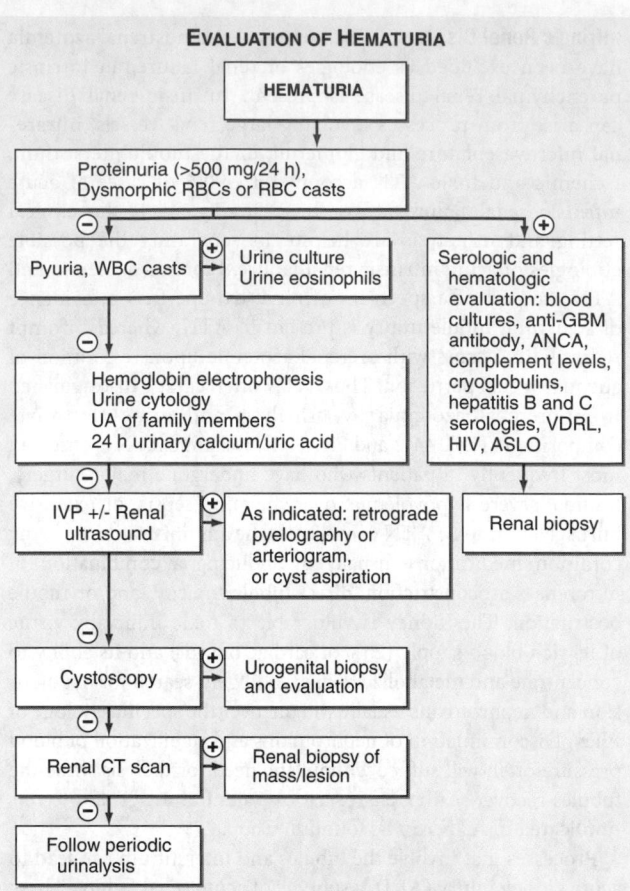

Figure 44-2 Approach to the patient with hematuria. ANCA, antineutrophil cytoplasmic antibody; ASLO, antistreptolysin O; CT, computed tomography; GBM, glomerular basement membrane; IVP, intravenous pyelography; RBC, red blood cell; UA, urinalysis; VDRL, Venereal Disease Research Laboratory; WBC, white blood cell.

Diseases of the glomeruli (glomerulonephritis and vasculitis) and the renal microvasculature (hemolytic-uremic syndromes, thrombotic thrombocytopenic purpura, and malignant hypertension) usually present with various combinations of glomerular injury: proteinuria, hematuria, reduced GFR, and alterations of sodium excretion that lead to hypertension, edema, and circulatory congestion (acute nephritic syndrome). These findings may occur as primary renal diseases or as renal manifestations of systemic diseases. The clinical setting and other laboratory data help distinguish primary renal diseases from systemic diseases. The finding of RBC casts in the urine is an indication for early renal biopsy (Fig. 44-1) as the pathologic pattern has important implications for diagnosis, prognosis, and treatment. Hematuria without RBC casts also can be an indication of glomerular disease; this evaluation is summarized in Fig. 44-2. A detailed discussion of glomerulonephritis and diseases of the microvasculature can be found in Chap. 285.

Oliguria and Anuria *Oliguria* refers to a 24-h urine output <400 mL, and *anuria* is the complete absence of urine formation (<100 mL). Anuria can be caused by total urinary tract obstruction, total renal artery or vein occlusion, and shock (manifested by severe hypotension and intense renal vasoconstriction). Cortical necrosis, ATN, and rapidly progressive glomerulonephritis occasionally cause anuria. Oliguria can accompany any cause of acute renal failure and carries a more serious prognosis for renal recovery in all conditions except prerenal azotemia. *Nonoliguria* refers to urine output >400 mL/d in patients with acute or chronic azotemia.

With nonoliguric ATN, disturbances of potassium and hydrogen balance are less severe than in oliguric patients, and recovery to normal renal function is usually more rapid.

ABNORMALITIES OF THE URINE

■ PROTEINURIA

The evaluation of proteinuria is shown schematically in Fig. 44-3 and typically is initiated after detection of proteinuria by dipstick examination. The dipstick measurement detects only albumin and gives false-positive results when pH >7.0 and the urine is very concentrated or contaminated with blood. Because the dipstick relies on urinary albumin concentration, a very dilute urine may obscure significant proteinuria on dipstick examination. Quantification of urinary albumin on a spot urine sample (ideally from a first morning void) by measuring an albumin-to-creatinine ratio (ACR) is helpful in approximating a 24-h albumin excretion rate (AER) where ACR (mg/g) ≈AER (mg/24 h). Furthermore, proteinuria that is not predominantly albumin will be missed by dipstick screening. This is particularly important for the detection of Bence Jones proteins in the urine of patients with multiple myeloma. Tests to measure total urine protein concentration accurately rely on precipitation with sulfosalicylic or trichloracetic acid (Fig. 44-3).

The magnitude of proteinuria and the protein composition of the urine depend on the mechanism of renal injury that leads to protein losses. Both charge and size selectivity normally prevent virtually all plasma albumin, globulins, and other high-molecular-weight proteins from crossing the glomerular wall; however, if this barrier is disrupted, plasma proteins may leak into the urine (glomerular proteinuria; Fig. 44-3). Smaller proteins (<20 kDa) are freely filtered but are readily reabsorbed by the proximal tubule. Traditionally, healthy individuals excrete <150 mg/d of total protein and <30 mg/d of albumin. However, even at albuminuria levels <30 mg/d, risk for progression to overt nephropathy or subsequent cardiovascular disease is increased. The remainder of the protein in the urine is secreted by the tubules (Tamm-Horsfall, IgA, and urokinase) or represents small amounts of filtered β_2-microglobulin, apoproteins, enzymes, and peptide hormones. Another mechanism of proteinuria occurs when there is excessive production of an abnormal protein that exceeds the capacity of the tubule for reabsorption. This most commonly occurs with plasma cell dyscrasias, such as multiple myeloma, amyloidosis, and lymphomas that are associated with monoclonal production of immunoglobulin light chains.

The normal glomerular endothelial cell forms a barrier composed of pores of ~100 nm that retain blood cells but offer little impediment to passage of most proteins. The glomerular basement membrane traps most large proteins (>100 kDa), and the foot processes of epithelial cells (podocytes) cover the urinary side of the glomerular basement membrane and produce a series of narrow channels (slit diaphragms) to allow molecular passage of small solutes and water but not proteins. Some glomerular diseases, such as minimal change disease, cause fusion of glomerular epithelial cell foot processes, resulting in predominantly "selective" (Fig. 44-3) loss of albumin. Other glomerular diseases can present with disruption of the basement membrane and slit diaphragms (e.g., by immune complex deposition), resulting in losses of albumin and other plasma proteins. The fusion of foot processes causes increased pressure across the capillary basement membrane, resulting in areas with larger pore sizes. The combination of increased pressure and larger pores results in significant proteinuria ("nonselective"; Fig. 44-3).

When the total daily excretion of protein is >3.5 g, hypoalbuminemia, hyperlipidemia, and edema (nephrotic syndrome; Fig. 44-3) are often present as well. However, total daily urinary protein excretion >3.5 g can occur without the other features of the nephrotic syndrome in a variety of other renal diseases (Fig. 44-3). Plasma cell dyscrasias (multiple myeloma) can be associated with large

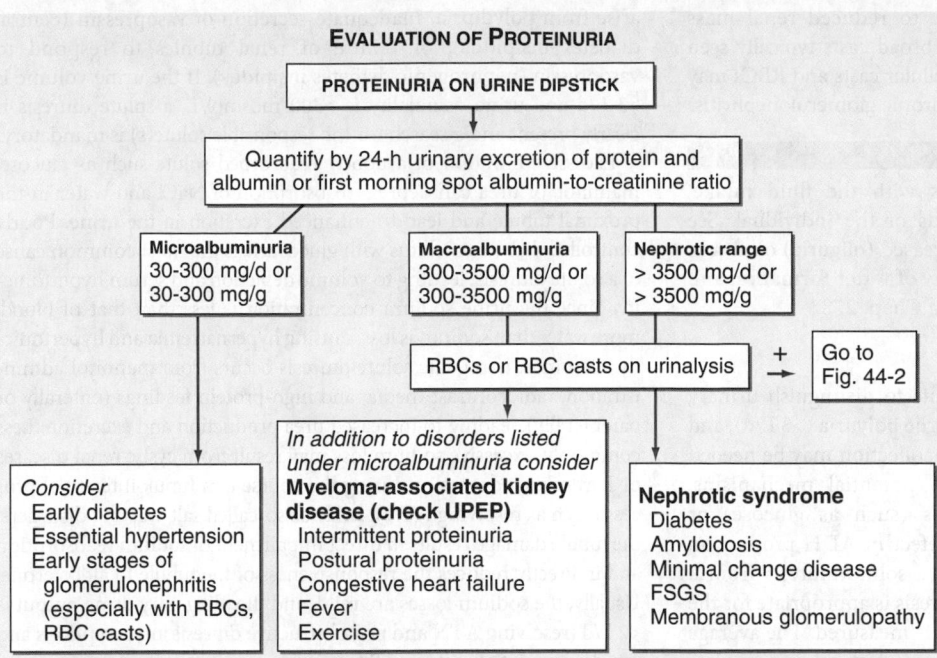

EVALUATION OF PROTEINURIA

PROTEINURIA ON URINE DIPSTICK

↓

Quantify by 24-h urinary excretion of protein and albumin or first morning spot albumin-to-creatinine ratio

| Microalbuminuria 30-300 mg/d or 30-300 mg/g | Macroalbuminuria 300-3500 mg/d or 300-3500 mg/g | Nephrotic range > 3500 mg/d or > 3500 mg/g |

RBCs or RBC casts on urinalysis + → Go to Fig. 44-2

Consider
Early diabetes
Essential hypertension
Early stages of glomerulonephritis (especially with RBCs, RBC casts)

In addition to disorders listed under microalbuminuria consider
Myeloma-associated kidney disease (check UPEP)
Intermittent proteinuria
Postural proteinuria
Congestive heart failure
Fever
Exercise

Nephrotic syndrome
Diabetes
Amyloidosis
Minimal change disease
FSGS
Membranous glomerulopathy

Figure 44-3   Approach to the patient with proteinuria. Investigation of proteinuria is often initiated by a positive dipstick on routine urinalysis. Conventional dipsticks detect predominantly albumin and provide a semi-quantitative assessment (trace, 1+, 2+, or 3+), which is influenced by urinary concentration as reflected by urine specific gravity (minimum <1.005, maximum 1.030). However, more exact determination of proteinuria should employ a spot morning protein/creatinine ratio (mg/g) or a 24-h urine collection (mg/24 h). FSGS, focal segmental glomerulosclerosis; MPGN, membranoproliferative glomerulonephritis; RBC, red blood cell.

amounts of excreted light chains in the urine, which may not be detected by dipstick. The light chains produced from these disorders are filtered by the glomerulus and overwhelm the reabsorptive capacity of the proximal tubule.. Renal failure from these disorders occurs through a variety of mechanisms, including tubule obstruction (cast nephropathy) and light chain deposition.

Hypoalbuminemia in nephrotic syndrome occurs through excessive urinary losses and increased proximal tubule catabolism of filtered albumin. Edema forms from renal sodium retention and reduced plasma oncotic pressure, which favors fluid movement from capillaries to interstitium. To compensate for the perceived decrease in effective intravascular volume, activation of the renin-angiotensin system, stimulation of ADH, and activation of the sympathetic nervous system occur that promote continued renal salt and water reabsorption and progressive edema. The urinary loss of regulatory proteins and changes in hepatic synthesis contribute to the other manifestations of the nephrotic syndrome. A hypercoagulable state may arise from urinary losses of antithrombin III, reduced serum levels of proteins S and C, hyperfibrinogenemia, and enhanced platelet aggregation. Hypercholesterolemia may be severe and results from increased hepatic lipoprotein synthesis. Loss of immunoglobulins contributes to an increased risk of infection. Many diseases (some listed in Fig. 44-3) and drugs can cause the nephrotic syndrome; a complete list can be found in Chap. 283.

■ HEMATURIA, PYURIA, AND CASTS

Isolated hematuria without proteinuria, other cells, or casts is often indicative of bleeding from the urinary tract. Hematuria is defined as two to five RBCs per high-power field (HPF) and can be detected by dipstick. A false-positive dipstick for hematuria (where no RBCs are seen on urine microscopy) may occur when myoglobinuria is present, often in the setting of rhabdomyolysis. Common causes of isolated hematuria include stones, neoplasms, tuberculosis, trauma, and

prostatitis. Gross hematuria with blood clots is usually not an intrinsic renal process; rather, it suggests a postrenal source in the urinary collecting system. Evaluation of patients presenting with microscopic hematuria is outlined in Fig. 44-2. A single urinalysis with hematuria is common and can result from menstruation, viral illness, allergy, exercise, or mild trauma. Persistent or significant hematuria (>3 RBCs/HPF on three urinalyses, a single urinalysis with >100 RBCs, or gross hematuria) is associated with significant renal or urologic lesions in 9.1% of cases. Even patients who are chronically anticoagulated should be investigated as outlined in Fig. 44-2. The suspicion for urogenital neoplasms in patients with isolated painless hematuria and nondysmorphic RBCs increases with age. Neoplasms are rare in the pediatric population, and isolated hematuria is more likely to be "idiopathic" or associated with a congenital anomaly. Hematuria with pyuria and bacteriuria is typical of infection and should be treated with antibiotics after appropriate cultures. Acute cystitis or urethritis in women can cause gross hematuria. Hypercalciuria and hyperuricosuria are also risk factors for unexplained isolated hematuria in both children and adults. In some of these patients (50–60%), reducing calcium and uric acid excretion through dietary interventions can eliminate the microscopic hematuria.

Isolated microscopic hematuria can be a manifestation of glomerular diseases. The RBCs of glomerular origin are often dysmorphic when examined by phase-contrast microscopy. Irregular shapes of RBCs may also result from pH and osmolarity changes produced along the distal nephron. Observer variability in detecting dysmorphic RBCs is common. The most common etiologies of isolated glomerular hematuria are IgA nephropathy, hereditary nephritis, and thin basement membrane disease. IgA nephropathy and hereditary nephritis can lead to episodic gross hematuria. A family history of renal failure is often present in patients with hereditary nephritis, and patients with thin basement membrane disease often have other family members with microscopic hematuria. A renal biopsy is needed for the definitive diagnosis of these disorders, which are discussed in more detail in Chap. 283. Hematuria with dysmorphic RBCs, RBC casts, and protein excretion >500 mg/d is virtually diagnostic of glomerulonephritis. RBC casts form as RBCs that enter the tubule fluid become trapped in a cylindrical mold of gelled Tamm-Horsfall protein. Even in the absence of azotemia, these patients should undergo serologic evaluation and renal biopsy as outlined in Fig. 44-2.

Isolated pyuria is unusual since inflammatory reactions in the kidney or collecting system also are associated with hematuria. The presence of bacteria suggests infection, and white blood cell casts with bacteria are indicative of pyelonephritis. White blood cells and/or white blood cell casts also may be seen in acute glomerulonephritis as well as in tubulointerstitial processes such as interstitial nephritis and transplant rejection. In chronic renal diseases, degenerated cellular casts called *waxy casts* can be seen in the urine. *Broad casts* are thought to arise in the dilated tubules of enlarged nephrons that have undergone compensatory hypertrophy in response to reduced renal mass (i.e., chronic renal failure). A mixture of broad casts typically seen with chronic renal failure together with cellular casts and RBCs may be seen in smoldering processes such as chronic glomerulonephritis.

ABNORMALITIES OF URINE VOLUME

The volume of urine produced varies with the fluid intake, renal function, and physiologic demands of the individual. See "Azotemia," above, for discussion of decreased (oliguria) or absent urine production (anuria). The physiology of water formation and renal water conservation are discussed in Chap. 278.

◼ POLYURIA

By history, it is often difficult for patients to distinguish urinary frequency (often of small volumes) from true polyuria (>3 L/d), and a quantification of volume by 24-h urine collection may be needed (Fig. 44-4). Polyuria results from two potential mechanisms: (1) excretion of nonabsorbable solutes (such as glucose) or (2) excretion of water (usually from a defect in ADH production or renal responsiveness). To distinguish a solute diuresis from a water diuresis and to determine if the diuresis is appropriate for the clinical circumstances, a urine osmolality is measured. The average person excretes between 600 and 800 mosmol of solutes per day, primarily as urea and electrolytes. If the urine output is >3 L/d and the urine is dilute (<250 mosmol/L), total mosmol excretion is normal and a water diuresis is present. This circumstance could arise from polydipsia, inadequate secretion of vasopressin (central diabetes insipidus), or failure of renal tubules to respond to vasopressin (nephrogenic diabetes insipidus). If the urine volume is >3 L/d and urine osmolality is >300 mosmol/L, a solute diuresis is clearly present and a search for the responsible solute(s) is mandatory.

Excessive filtration of a poorly reabsorbed solute such as glucose, mannitol, or urea can depress reabsorption of NaCl and water in the proximal tubule and lead to enhanced excretion in the urine. Poorly controlled diabetes mellitus with glucosuria is the most common cause of a solute diuresis, leading to volume depletion and serum hypertonicity. Since the urine sodium concentration is less than that of blood, more water than sodium is lost, causing hypernatremia and hypertonicity. Common iatrogenic solute diuresis occurs from mannitol administration, radiocontrast media, and high-protein feedings (enterally or parenterally), leading to increased urea production and excretion. Less commonly, excessive sodium loss may result from cystic renal diseases or Bartter's syndrome or during the course of a tubulointerstitial process (such as resolving ATN). In these so-called salt-wasting disorders, the tubule damage results in direct impairment of sodium reabsorption and indirectly reduces the responsiveness of the tubule to aldosterone. Usually, the sodium losses are mild, and the obligatory urine output is <2 L/d (resolving ATN and postobstructive diuresis are exceptions and may be associated with significant natriuresis and polyuria).

Formation of large volumes of dilute urine is usually due to polydipsic states or diabetes insipidus. Primary polydipsia can result from habit, psychiatric disorders, neurologic lesions, or medications. During deliberate polydipsia, extracellular fluid volume is normal or expanded and plasma vasopressin levels are reduced because serum osmolality tends to be near the lower limits of normal. Urine osmolality should also be maximally dilute at 50 mosmol/L.

Central diabetes insipidus may be idiopathic in origin or secondary to a variety of hypothalamic conditions, including posthypophysectomy or trauma or neoplastic, inflammatory, vascular, or infectious hypothalamic diseases. Idiopathic central diabetes insipidus is associated with selective destruction of the vasopressin-secreting neurons in the supraoptic and paraventricular nuclei and can be inherited as an autosomal dominant trait or occur spontaneously. Nephrogenic diabetes insipidus can occur in a variety of clinical situations, as summarized in Fig. 44-4.

A plasma vasopressin level is recommended as the best method for distinguishing between central and nephrogenic diabetes insipidus. Alternatively, a water deprivation test plus exogenous vasopressin may distinguish primary polydipsia from central and nephrogenic diabetes insipidus. For a detailed discussion, see Chap. 340.

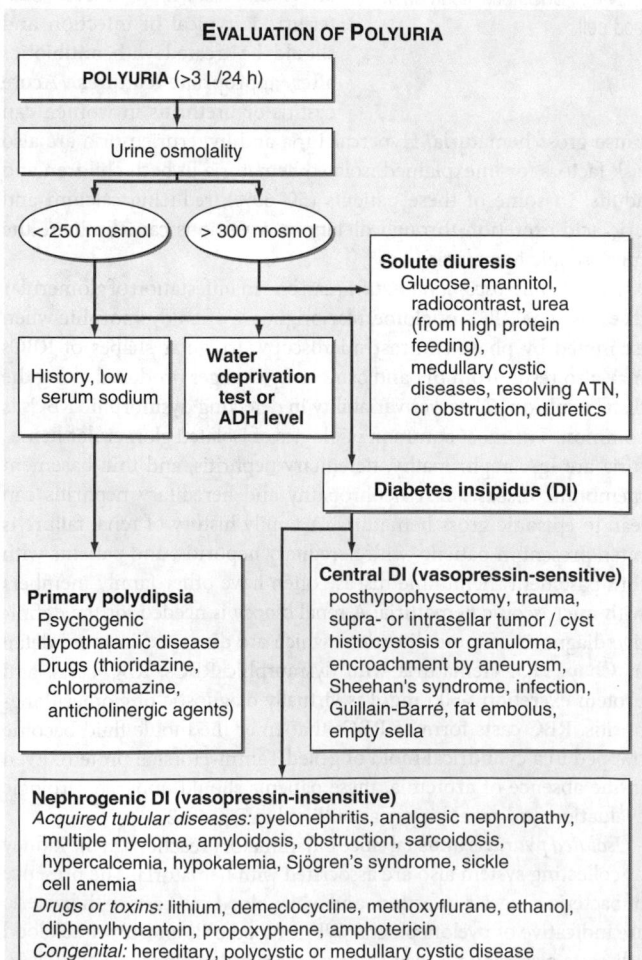

Figure 44-4 Approach to the patient with polyuria. ADH, antidiuretic hormone; ATN, acute tubular necrosis.

FURTHER READINGS

ANDERSON S et al: Renal and systemic manifestations of glomerular disease, in *Brenner & Rector's The Kidney*, 8th ed, BM Brenner (ed). Philadelphia, Saunders, 2008, pp. 820–838

ISRANI AK, KASISKE BL: Laboratory assessment of renal disease: Clearance, urinalysis and renal biopsy, in *Brenner & Rector's The Kidney*, 8th ed, BM Brenner (ed). Philadelphia, Saunders, 2008, pp 724–756

RODRIGO E et al: Measurement of renal function in pre-ESRD patients. Kidney Int Suppl 80:11, 2002

SASAKI S: Nephrogenic diabetes insipidus: Update of genetic and clinical aspects. Nephrol Dial Transplant 19:1351, 2004

SHRIER RW et al: Acute renal failure: Definitions, diagnosis, pathogenesis and therapy. J Clin Invest 114:5, 2004

VERBALIS JG, BERL T: Disorders of water balance, in *Brenner & Rector's The Kidney*, 8th ed, BM Brenner (ed). Philadelphia, Saunders, 2008, pp 459–504

CHAPTER 45

Fluid and Electrolyte Disturbances

David B. Mount

SODIUM AND WATER

■ COMPOSITION OF BODY FLUIDS

Water is the most abundant constituent in the body, accounting for ~50% of body weight in women and 60% in men. Total body water is distributed in two major compartments: 55–75% is intracellular [intracellular fluid (ICF)], and 25–45% is extracellular [extracellular fluid (ECF)]. ECF is subdivided into intravascular (plasma water) and extravascular (interstitial) spaces in a ratio of 1:3. Fluid movement between the intravascular and interstitial spaces occurs across the capillary wall and is determined by Starling forces, i.e., capillary hydraulic pressure and colloid osmotic pressure. The transcapillary hydraulic pressure gradient exceeds the corresponding oncotic pressure gradient, thus favoring the movement of plasma ultrafiltrate into the extravascular space. The return of fluid into the intravascular compartment occurs via lymphatic flow.

The solute or particle concentration of a fluid is known as its osmolality and is expressed as milliosmoles per kilogram of water (mosmol/kg). Water easily diffuses across most cell membranes to achieve osmotic equilibrium (ECF osmolality = ICF osmolality). Notably, the extracellular and intracellular solute compositions differ considerably owing to the activity of various transporters, channels, and ATP-driven membrane pumps. The major ECF particles are Na^+ and its accompanying anions Cl^- and HCO_3^-, whereas K^+ and organic phosphate esters (ATP, creatine phosphate, and phospholipids) are the predominant ICF osmoles. Solutes that are restricted to the ECF or the ICF determine the tonicity or effective osmolality of that compartment. Certain solutes, particularly urea, do not contribute to water shifts across most membranes and are thus known as *ineffective osmoles*.

Water balance

Vasopressin secretion, water ingestion, and renal water transport collaborate to maintain human body fluid osmolality between 280 and 295 mosmol/kg. Vasopressin (AVP) is synthesized in magnocellular neurons within the hypothalamus; the distal axons of those neurons project to the posterior pituitary or neurohypophysis, from which AVP is released into the circulation. A network of central osmoreceptor neurons that includes the AVP-expressing magnocellular neurons themselves sense circulating osmolality via nonselective, stretch-activated cation channels. These osmoreceptor neurons are activated or inhibited by modest increases and decreases in circulating osmolality, respectively; activation leads to AVP release and thirst.

AVP secretion is stimulated as systemic osmolality increases above a threshold level of ~285 mosmol/kg, above which there is a linear relationship between osmolality and circulating AVP (Fig. 45-1). Thirst and thus water ingestion also are activated at ~285 mosmol/kg, beyond which there is an equivalent linear increase in the perceived intensity of thirst as a function of circulating osmolality. Changes in blood volume and blood pressure

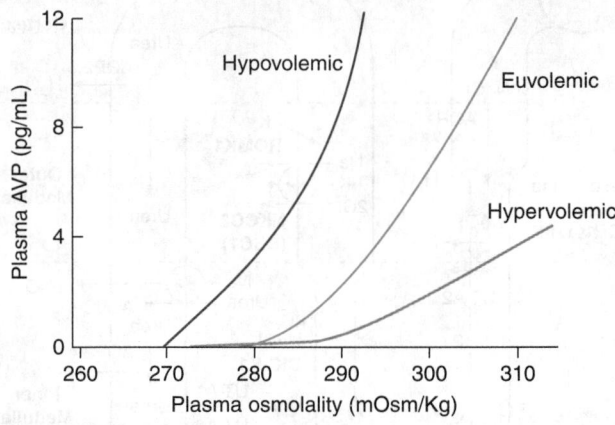

Figure 45-1 Circulating levels of vasopressin (AVP) in response to changes in osmolality. Plasma vasopressin becomes detectable in euvolemic, healthy individuals at a threshold of ~285 mOsm/Kg, above which there is a linear relationship between osmolality and circulating AVP. The vasopressin response to osmolality is modulated strongly by volume status. The osmotic threshold is thus slightly lower in hypovolemia, with a steeper response curve; hypervolemia reduces the sensitivity of circulating AVP levels to osmolality.

are also direct stimuli for AVP release and thirst, albeit with a less sensitive response profile. Of perhaps greater clinical relevance to the pathophysiology of water homeostasis, ECF volume strongly modulates the relationship between circulating osmolality and AVP release so that *hypovolemia* reduces the osmotic threshold and increases the slope of the response curve to osmolality; *hypervolemia* has the opposite effect, increasing the osmotic threshold and reducing the slope of the response curve (Fig. 45-1). Notably, AVP has a half-life in the circulation of only 10–20 min; thus, changes in extracellular fluid volume and/or circulating osmolality can affect water homeostasis rapidly. In addition to volume status, a number of nonosmotic stimuli have potent activating effects on osmosensitive neurons and AVP release, including nausea, intracerebral angiotensin II, serotonin, and multiple drugs.

The excretion or retention of electrolyte-free water by the kidney is modulated by circulating AVP. AVP acts on renal V_2-type receptors in the thick ascending limb of Henle and principal cells of the collecting duct (CD), increasing cyclic adenosine monophosphate (AMP) and activating protein kinase A (PKA)–dependent phosphorylation of multiple transport proteins. The AVP- and PKA-dependent activation of Na^+-Cl^- and K^+ transport by the thick ascending limb of the loop of Henle (TALH) is a key participant in the countercurrent mechanism (Fig. 45-2). The countercurrent mechanism ultimately increases the interstitial osmolality in the inner medulla of the kidney, driving water absorption across the renal collecting duct. However, water, salt, and solute transport by both proximal and distal nephron segments participates in the renal concentrating mechanism (Fig. 45-2). Water transport across apical and basolateral aquaporin-1 water channels in the descending thin limb of the loop of Henle is thus involved, as is passive absorption of Na^+-Cl^- by the thin ascending limb, via apical and basolateral CLC-K1 chloride channels and paracellular Na^+ transport. Renal urea transport in turn plays important roles in the generation of the medullary osmotic gradient and the ability to excrete solute-free water under conditions of both high and low protein intake (Fig. 45-2).

AVP-induced, PKA-dependent phosphorylation of the aquaporin-2 water channel in principal cells stimulates the insertion of active water channels into the lumen of the collecting duct, resulting in

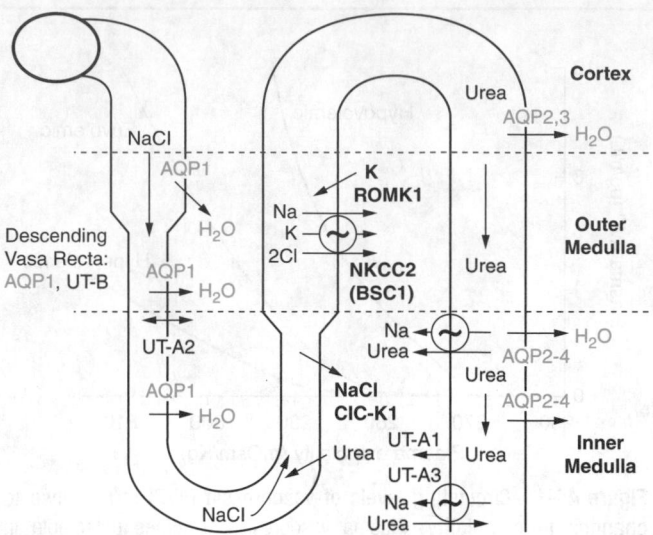

Figure 45-2 The renal concentrating mechanism. Water, salt, and solute transport by both proximal and distal nephron segments participates in the renal concentrating mechanism (see text for details). Diagram showing the location of the major transport proteins involved; a loop of Henle is depicted on the left, a collecting duct on the right. UT, urea transporter; AQP, aquaporin; NKCC2, Na-K-2Cl cotransporter; ROMK, renal outer medullary K+ channel; CLC-K1, chloride channel. *(From JM Sands: J Am Soc Nephrol 13:2795, 2002; with permission.)*

transepithelial water absorption down the medullary osmotic gradient (Fig. 45-3). Under antidiuretic conditions, with increased circulating AVP, the kidney reabsorbs water filtered by the glomerulus, equilibrating the osmolality across the collecting duct epithelium

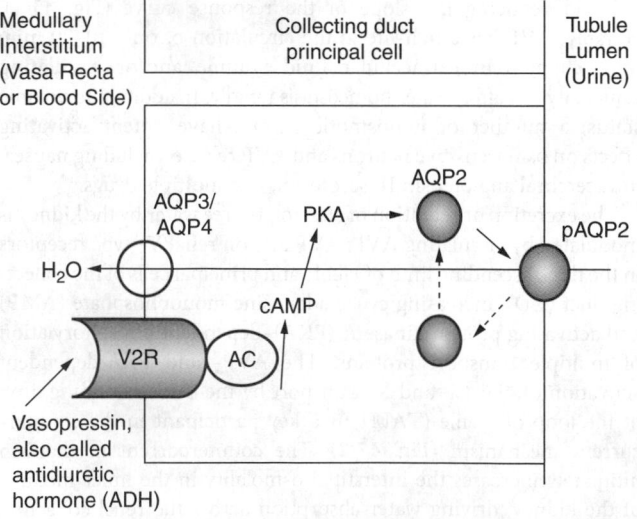

Figure 45-3 Vasopressin and the regulation of water permeability in the renal collecting duct. Vasopressin binds to the type 2 vasopressin receptor (V2R) on the basolateral membrane of principal cells, activates adenylyl cyclase (AC), increases intracellular cyclic adenosine monophosphatase (cAMP), and stimulates protein kinase A (PKA) activity. Cytoplasmic vesicles carrying aquaporin-2 (AQP) water channel proteins are inserted into the luminal membrane in response to vasopressin, increasing the water permeability of this membrane. When vasopressin stimulation ends, water channels are retrieved by an endocytic process and water permeability returns to its low basal rate. The AQP3 and AQP4 water channels are expressed on the basolateral membrane and complete the transcellular pathway for water reabsorption. pAQP2 = phosphorylated aquaporin-2. *(From JM Sands, DG Bichet: Ann Intern Med 144:186, 2006; with permission.)*

to excrete a hypertonic, concentrated urine (osmolality of up to 1200 mosmol/kg). In the absence of circulating AVP, insertion of aquaporin-2 channels and water absorption across the collecting duct are essentially abolished, resulting in secretion of a hypotonic, dilute urine (osmolality as low as 30–50 mosmol/kg). Abnormalities in this final common pathway are involved in most disorders of water homeostasis, e.g., a reduced or absent insertion of active aquaporin-2 water channels into the membrane of principal cells in diabetes insipidus.

Maintenance of arterial circulatory integrity

Sodium is actively pumped out of cells by the Na+, K+-ATPase membrane pump. In consequence, 85–90% of body Na+ is extracellular, and the extracellular fluid volume (ECFV) is a function of total-body Na+ content. Arterial perfusion and circulatory integrity are, in turn, determined by renal Na+ retention or excretion, in addition to the modulation of systemic arterial resistance. Within the kidney, Na+ is filtered by the glomeruli and then sequentially reabsorbed by the renal tubules. The Na+ cation typically is reabsorbed with the chloride anion (Cl−); thus, chloride homeostasis also affects the ECFV. On a quantitative level, at a glomerular filtration rate (GFR) of 180 L/d and serum Na+ of ~140 mM, the kidney filters some 25,200 mmol/d of Na+. This is equivalent to ~1.5 kg of salt, which would occupy roughly 10 times the extracellular space; 99.6% of filtered Na+-Cl− must be reabsorbed to excrete 100 mM per day. Minute changes in renal Na+-Cl− excretion will thus have significant effects on the ECFV, leading to edema syndromes or hypovolemia.

Approximately two-thirds of filtered Na+-Cl− is reabsorbed by the renal proximal tubule via both paracellular and transcellular mechanisms. The TALH subsequently reabsorbs another 25–30% of filtered Na+-Cl− via the apical, furosemide-sensitive Na+-K+-2Cl− cotransporter. The adjacent aldosterone-sensitive distal nephron, which encompasses the distal convoluted tubule (DCT), connecting tubule (CNT), and collecting duct, accomplishes the "fine-tuning" of renal Na+-Cl− excretion. The thiazide-sensitive apical Na+-Cl− cotransporter (NCC) reabsorbs 5–10% of filtered Na+-Cl− in the DCT. Principal cells in the CNT and CD reabsorb Na+ via electrogenic, amiloride-sensitive epithelial Na+ channels (ENaC); Cl− ions are reabsorbed primarily by adjacent intercalated cells via apical Cl− exchange (Cl−-OH− and Cl−-HCO3− exchange, mediated by the SLC26A4 anion exchanger) (Fig. 45-4).

Renal tubular reabsorption of filtered Na+-Cl− is regulated by multiple circulating and paracrine hormones in addition to the activity of renal nerves. Angiotensin II activates proximal Na+-Cl− reabsorption, as do adrenergic receptors under the influence of renal sympathetic innervation; locally generated dopamine, in contrast, has a *natriuretic* effect. Aldosterone primarily activates Na+-Cl− reabsorption within the aldosterone-sensitive distal nephron. In particular, aldosterone activates the ENaC channel in principal cells, inducing Na+ absorption and promoting K+ excretion (see Fig. 45-4).

Circulatory integrity is critical for the perfusion and function of vital organs. Underfilling of the arterial circulation is sensed by ventricular and vascular pressure receptors, resulting in a neurohumoral activation (increased sympathetic tone, activation of the renin-angiotensin-aldosterone axis, and increased circulating AVP) that synergistically increases renal Na+-Cl− reabsorption, vascular resistance, and renal water reabsorption. This occurs in the context of decreased cardiac output, as occurs in hypovolemic states, low-output cardiac failure, decreased oncotic pressure, and/or increased capillary permeability. Alternatively, excessive arterial vasodilation results in *relative* arterial underfilling, leading to neurohumoral activation in the defense of tissue perfusion. These physiologic responses play important roles in many of the disorders discussed

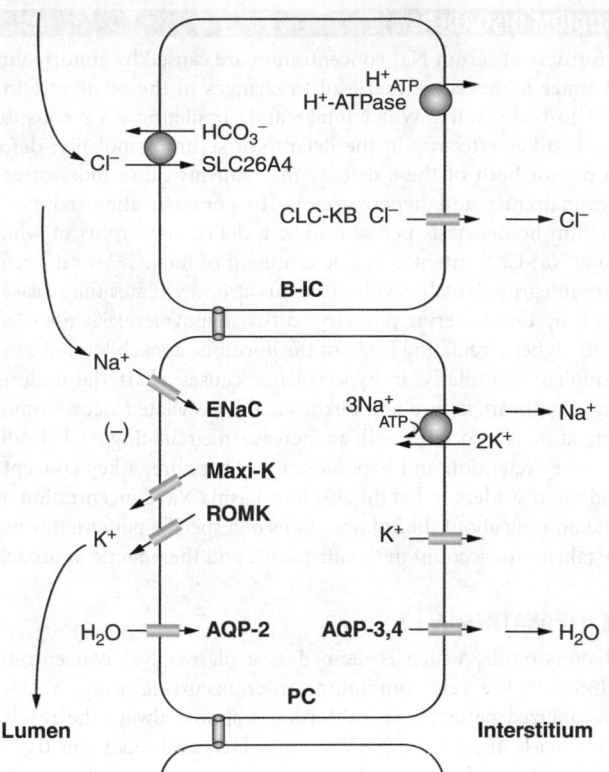

Figure 45-4 Sodium, water, and potassium transport in principal cells (PC) and adjacent β-intercalated cells (B-IC). The absorption of Na+ via the amiloride-sensitive epithelial sodium channel (ENaC) generates a lumen-negative potential difference that drives K+ excretion through the apical secretory K+ channel ROMK (renal outer medullary K+ channel) and/ or the flow-dependent maxi-K channel. Transepithelial Cl– transport occurs in adjacent β-intercalated cells via apical Cl–-HCO₃– and Cl–-OH– exchange (SLC26A4 anion exchanger, also known as pendrin) basolateral CLC chloride channels. Water is absorbed down the osmotic gradient by principal cells, through the apical aquaporin-2 (AQP-2) and basolateral aquaporin-3 and aquaporin-4 (Fig. 45-3).

to increased urinary Na+-Cl– excretion. Other drugs can induce natriuresis as a side effect. For example, acetazolamide can inhibit proximal tubular Na+-Cl– absorption through its inhibition of carbonic anhydrase; other drugs, such as the antibiotics trimethroprim and pentamidine, inhibit distal tubular Na+ reabsorption through the amiloride-sensitive ENaC channel, leading to urinary Na+-Cl– loss. Hereditary defects in renal transport proteins also are associated with reduced reabsorption of filtered Na+-Cl– and/or water. Alternatively, mineralocorticoid deficiency, mineralocorticoid resistance, or inhibition of the mineralocorticoid receptor (MLR) can reduce Na+-Cl– reabsorption by the aldosterone-sensitive distal nephron. Finally, tubulointerstitial injury, as occurs in interstitial nephritis, acute tubular injury, or obstructive uropathy, can reduce distal tubular Na+-Cl– and/or water absorption.

Excessive excretion of free water, i.e., water without electrolytes, also can lead to hypovolemia. However, the effect on ECFV is usually less marked in light of the fact that two-thirds of the water volume is lost from the ICF. Excessive renal water excretion occurs in the setting of decreased circulating AVP or renal resistance to AVP (central and nephrogenic diabetes insipidus, respectively).

Extrarenal causes Nonrenal causes of hypovolemia include fluid loss from the gastrointestinal tract, skin, and respiratory system. Accumulations of fluid within specific tissue compartments—typically the interstitium, peritoneum, or gastrointestinal tract—also can cause hypovolemia.

Approximately 9 L of fluid enters the gastrointestinal tract daily, 2 L by ingestion and 7 L by secretion; almost 98% of this volume is absorbed so that daily fecal fluid loss is only 100–200 mL. Impaired gastrointestinal reabsorption or enhanced secretion of fluid can cause hypovolemia. Since gastric secretions have a low pH (high H+ concentration), whereas biliary, pancreatic, and intestinal secretions are alkaline (high HCO₃– concentration), vomiting and diarrhea often are accompanied by metabolic alkalosis and acidosis, respectively.

Evaporation of water from the skin and respiratory tract (so-called insensible losses) is the major route for loss of solute-free water, which is typically 500–650 mL/d in healthy adults. This evaporative loss can increase during febrile illness or prolonged heat exposure. Hyperventilation also can increase insensible losses via the respiratory tract, particularly in ventilated patients; the humidity of inspired air is another determining factor. In addition, increased exertion and/or ambient temperature will increase insensible losses via sweat, which is hypotonic to plasma. Profuse sweating without adequate repletion of water and Na+-Cl– thus can lead to both hypovolemia and hypertonicity. Alternatively, replacement of these insensible losses with a surfeit of free water without adequate replacement of electrolytes may lead to hypovolemic hyponatremia.

Excessive fluid accumulation in interstitial and/or peritoneal spaces also can cause intravascular hypovolemia. Increases in vascular permeability and/or a reduction in oncotic pressure (hypoalbuminemia) alter Starling forces, resulting in excessive "third spacing" of the ECFV. This occurs in sepsis syndrome, burns, pancreatitis, nutritional hypoalbuminemia, and peritonitis. Alternatively, distributive hypovolemia can result from accumulation of fluid within specific compartments, for example, within the bowel lumen in gastrointestinal obstruction or ileus. Hypovolemia also can occur after extracorporeal hemorrhage or after significant hemorrhage into an expandable space, for example, the retroperitoneum.

Diagnostic evaluation

A careful history usually determines the etiologic cause of hypovolemia. Symptoms of hypovolemia are nonspecific and include fatigue, weakness, thirst, and postural dizziness; more severe symptoms and signs include oliguria, cyanosis, abdominal and chest

in this chapter. In particular, it is important to appreciate that AVP functions in the defense of circulatory integrity, inducing vasoconstriction, increasing sympathetic nervous system tone, increasing renal retention of both water and Na+-Cl–, and modulating the arterial baroreceptor reflex. Most of these responses involve activation of systemic V₁A AVP receptors, but concomitant activation of V₂ receptors in the kidney can result in renal water retention and hyponatremia.

▣ HYPOVOLEMIA

Etiology

True volume depletion, or hypovolemia, generally refers to a state of combined salt and water loss that leads to contraction of the ECFV. The loss of salt and water may be renal or nonrenal in origin.

Renal causes Excessive urinary Na+-Cl– and water loss is a feature of several conditions. A high filtered load of endogenous solutes, such as glucose and urea, can impair tubular reabsorption of Na+-Cl– and water, leading to an osmotic diuresis. Exogenous mannitol, which often is used to decrease intracerebral pressure, is filtered by glomeruli but not reabsorbed by the proximal tubule, thus causing an osmotic diuresis. Pharmacologic diuretics selectively impair Na+-Cl– reabsorption at specific sites along the nephron, leading pain, and confusion or obtundation. Associated electrolyte disorders may cause additional symptoms, for example, muscle weakness in patients with hypokalemia. On examination, diminished skin turgor and dry oral mucous membranes are less than ideal markers of a decreased ECFV in adult patients; reliable signs of hypovolemia include a decreased jugular venous pressure (JVP), orthostatic tachycardia (an increase of >15–20 beats per minute upon standing), and orthostatic hypotension (a >10–20-mmHg drop in blood pressure on standing). More severe fluid loss leads to hypovolemic shock, with hypotension, tachycardia, peripheral vasoconstriction, and peripheral hypoperfusion; these patients may exhibit peripheral cyanosis, cold extremities, oliguria, and altered mental status.

Routine chemistries may reveal an increase in blood urea nitrogen (BUN) and creatinine, reflecting a decrease in GFR. Creatinine is the more dependable measure of GFR, since BUN levels may be influenced by an increase in tubular reabsorption (prerenal azotemia), an increase in urea generation in catabolic states, hyperalimentation, or gastrointestinal bleeding and/or a decreased urea generation in decreased protein intake. In hypovolemic shock, liver function tests and cardiac biomarkers may show evidence of hepatic and cardiac ischemia, respectively. Routine chemistries and/or blood gases may reveal evidence of acid-base disorders. For example, bicarbonate loss due to diarrheal illness is a very common cause of metabolic acidosis; alternatively, patients with severe hypovolemic shock may develop lactic acidosis with an elevated anion gap.

The neurohumoral response to hypovolemia stimulates an increase in renal tubular Na^+ and water reabsorption. Therefore, the urine Na^+ concentration is typically <20 mM in nonrenal causes of hypovolemia, with a urine osmolality of >450 mosmol/kg. The reduction in both GFR and distal tubular Na^+ delivery may cause a defect in renal potassium excretion, with an increase in plasma K^+ concentration. Of note, patients with hypovolemia and a hypochloremic alkalosis due to vomiting, diarrhea, or diuretics typically have a urine Na^+ concentration >20 mM and urine pH >7.0 due to the increase in filtered HCO_3^-; the urine Cl^- concentration in this setting is a more accurate indicator of volume status, with a level <25 mM suggestive of hypovolemia. The urine Na^+ concentration is often >20 mM in patients with *renal* causes of hypovolemia, such as acute tubular necrosis; similarly, patients with diabetes insipidus will have an inappropriately dilute urine.

TREATMENT   Hypovolemia

The therapeutic goals in hypovolemia are to restore normovolemia and replace ongoing fluid losses. Mild hypovolemia usually can be treated with oral hydration and resumption of a normal maintenance diet. More severe hypovolemia requires intravenous hydration, with the choice of solution tailored to the underlying pathophysiology. Isotonic, "normal" saline (0.9% NaCl, 154 mM Na^+) is the most appropriate resuscitation fluid for normonatremic or hyponatremic patients with severe hypovolemia; colloid solutions such as intravenous albumin are not demonstrably superior for this purpose. Hypernatremic patients should receive a hypotonic solution: 5% dextrose if there has been only water loss (as in diabetes insipidus) or hypotonic saline (1/2 or 1/4 normal saline) if there has been water and Na^+-Cl^- loss. Patients with bicarbonate loss and metabolic acidosis, as occurs frequently in diarrhea, should receive intravenous bicarbonate, either an isotonic solution (150 meq of Na^+-HCO_3^- in 5% dextrose) or a more hypotonic bicarbonate solution in dextrose or dilute saline. Patients with severe hemorrhage or anemia should receive red cell transfusions without increasing the hematocrit beyond 35%.

Disorders of serum Na^+ concentration are caused by abnormalities in water homeostasis that lead to changes in the relative ratio of Na^+ to body water. Water intake and circulating AVP constitute the two key effectors in the defense of serum osmolality; defects in one or both of these defense mechanisms cause most cases of hyponatremia and hypernatremia. In contrast, abnormalities in sodium homeostasis per se lead to a deficit or surplus of whole-body Na^+-Cl^- content, a key determinant of the ECFV and circulatory integrity. Notably, volume status also modulates the release of AVP by the posterior pituitary so that hypovolemia is associated with higher circulating levels of the hormone at each level of serum osmolality. Similarly, in hypervolemic causes of arterial underfilling, e.g., heart failure and cirrhosis, the associated neurohumoral activation is associated with an increase in circulating AVP, leading to water retention and hyponatremia. Therefore, a key concept in sodium disorders is that the absolute plasma Na^+ concentration tells one nothing about the volume status of a specific patient; this must be taken into account in the diagnostic and therapeutic approach.

■ HYPONATREMIA

Hyponatremia, which is defined as a plasma Na^+ concentration <135 mM, is a very common disorder, occurring in up to 22% of hospitalized patients. This disorder is almost always the result of an increase in circulating AVP and/or increased renal sensitivity to AVP, combined with any intake of free water; a notable exception is hyponatremia due to low solute intake (see below). The underlying pathophysiology for the exaggerated or inappropriate AVP response differs in patients with hyponatremia as a function of their ECFV. Hyponatremia thus is subdivided diagnostically into three groups, depending on clinical history and volume status: hypovolemic, euvolemic, and hypervolemic (Fig. 45-5).

Hypovolemic hyponatremia

Hypovolemia causes a marked neurohumoral activation, increasing circulating levels of AVP. The increase in circulating AVP helps preserve blood pressure via vascular and baroreceptor V_{1A} receptors and increases water reabsorption via renal V_2 receptors; activation of V_2 receptors can lead to hyponatremia in the setting of increased free-water intake. Nonrenal causes of hypovolemic hyponatremia include gastrointestinal (GI) loss (vomiting, diarrhea, tube drainage, etc.) and insensible loss (sweating, burns) of Na^+-Cl^- and water in the absence of adequate oral replacement; urine Na^+ concentration is typically <20 mM. Notably, these patients may be clinically classified as euvolemic, with only the reduced urinary Na^+ concentration to indicate the cause of their hyponatremia. Indeed, a urine Na^+ concentration <20 mM in the absence of a cause of hypervolemic hyponatremia predicts a rapid increase in plasma Na^+ concentration in response to intravenous normal saline; saline induces a water diuresis in this setting, as circulating AVP levels plummet.

The *renal* causes of hypovolemic hyponatremia share an inappropriate loss of Na^+-Cl^- in the urine, leading to volume depletion and an increase in circulating AVP; urine Na^+ concentration is typically >20 mM (Fig. 45-5). A deficiency in circulating aldosterone and/or its renal effects can lead to hyponatremia in primary adrenal insufficiency and other causes of hypoaldosteronism; hyperkalemia and hyponatremia in a hypotensive and/or hypovolemic patient with high urine Na^+ concentration (much >20 mM) should strongly suggest this diagnosis. Salt-losing nephropathies may lead to hyponatremia when sodium intake is reduced due to impaired renal tubular function; typical causes include reflux nephropathy, interstitial nephropathies, post-obstructive uropathy, medullary cystic disease, and the recovery phase of acute tubular necrosis. Thiazide diuretics cause hyponatremia via a number of mechanisms, including

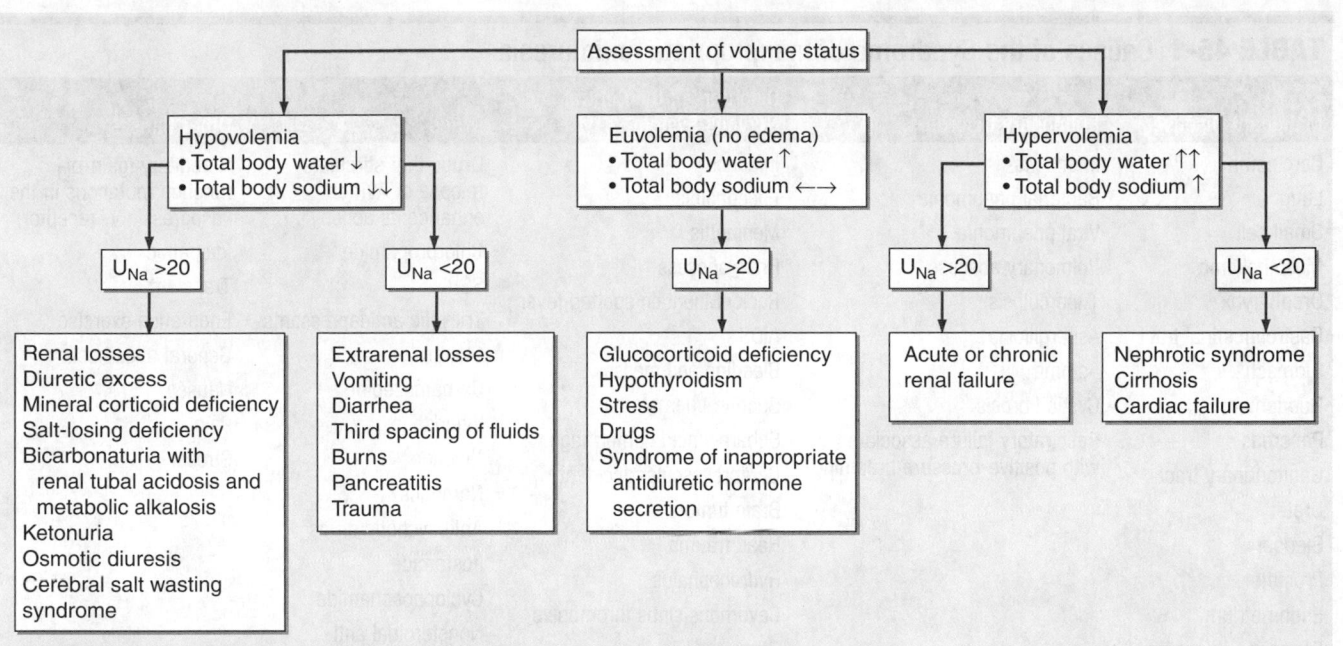

Figure 45-5 The diagnostic approach to hyponatremia. *[From S Kumar, T Berl: Diseases of water metabolism, in Atlas of Diseases of the Kidney, RW Schrier (ed). Philadelphia, Current Medicine, Inc, 1999; with permission.]*

polydipsia and diuretic-induced volume depletion. Notably, thiazides do not inhibit the renal concentrating mechanism so that circulating AVP has a maximal effect on renal water retention. In contrast, loop diuretics, which are associated less frequently with hyponatremia, inhibit Na+-Cl− and K+ absorption by the TALH, blunting the countercurrent mechanism and reducing the ability to concentrate the urine. Increased excretion of an osmotically active nonreabsorbable or poorly reabsorbable solute also can lead to volume depletion and hyponatremia; important causes include glycosuria, ketonuria (e.g., in starvation or in diabetic or alcoholic ketoacidosis), and bicarbonaturia (e.g., in renal tubular acidosis or metabolic alkalosis, in which the associated bicarbonaturia leads to loss of Na+).

Finally, the syndrome of "cerebral salt wasting" is a rare cause of hypovolemic hyponatremia, encompassing hyponatremia with clinical hypovolemia and inappropriate natriuresis in association with intracranial disease; associated disorders include subarachnoid hemorrhage, traumatic brain injury, craniotomy, encephalitis, and meningitis. Distinction from the more common syndrome of inappropriate antidiuresis (SIAD) is critical, since cerebral salt wasting typically responds to aggressive Na+-Cl− repletion.

Hypervolemic hyponatremia

Patients with hypervolemic hyponatremia develop an increase in total body Na+-Cl− that is accompanied by a proportionately *greater* increase in total body water, leading to a reduced plasma Na+ concentration. As in hypovolemic hyponatremia, the causative disorders can be separated by the effect on urine Na+ concentration, with acute or chronic renal failure uniquely associated with an increase in urine Na+ concentration (Fig. 45-5). The pathophysiology of hyponatremia in the sodium-avid edematous disorders [congestive heart failure (CHF), cirrhosis, and nephrotic syndrome] is similar to that in hypovolemic hyponatremia except that arterial filling and circulatory integrity are decreased due to the specific etiologic factors, e.g., cardiac dysfunction in CHF and peripheral vasodilation in cirrhosis. Urine Na+ concentration is typically very low, i.e., <10 m*M*, even

after hydration with normal saline; this Na+-avid state may be obscured by diuretic therapy. The degree of hyponatremia provides an indirect index of the associated neurohumoral activation and is an important prognostic indicator in hypervolemic hyponatremia.

Euvolemic hyponatremia

Euvolemic hyponatremia can occur in moderate to severe hypothyroidism, with correction after the achievement of a euthyroid state. Severe hyponatremia also can be a consequence of secondary adrenal insufficiency due to pituitary disease; whereas the deficit in circulating aldosterone in primary adrenal insufficiency causes *hypovolemic* hyponatremia, the predominant glucocorticoid deficiency in secondary adrenal failure is associated with *euvolemic* hyponatremia. Glucocorticoids exert a negative feedback on AVP release by the posterior pituitary so that hydrocortisone replacement in these patients will rapidly normalize the AVP response to osmolality, reducing circulating AVP.

The syndrome of inappropriate antidiuresis is the most common cause of euvolemic hyponatremia (Table 45-1). The generation of hyponatremia in SIAD requires an intake of free water, with persistent intake at serum osmolalities that are lower than the usual threshold for thirst; as one would expect, the osmotic threshold and osmotic response curves for the sensation of thirst are shifted downward in patients with SIAD. Four distinct patterns of AVP secretion have been recognized in patients with SIAD, independent for the most part of the underlying cause. Unregulated, erratic AVP secretion is seen in about a third of patients, with no obvious correlation between serum osmolality and circulating AVP levels. Other patients fail to suppress AVP secretion at lower serum osmolalities, with a normal response curve to hyperosmolar conditions; others have a reset osmostat, with a lower threshold osmolality and a left-shifted osmotic response curve. The fourth subset consists of patients who have essentially no detectable circulating AVP, suggesting either a gain in function in renal water reabsorption or a circulating antidiuretic substance that is distinct from AVP.

TABLE 45-1 Causes of the Syndrome of Inappropriate Antidiuresis

Malignant Diseases	Pulmonary Disorders	Disorders of the Central Nervous System	Drugs	Other Causes
Carcinoma	Infections	Infection	Drugs that stimulate release of AVP or enhance its action	Hereditary (gain-of-function mutations in the vasopressin V_2 receptor)
Lung	Bacterial pneumonia	Encephalitis	Chlorpropamide	Idiopathic
Small cell	Viral pneumonia	Meningitis	SSRIs	Transient
Mesothelioma	Pulmonary abscess	Brain abscess	Tricyclic antidepressants	Endurance exercise
Oropharynx	Tuberculosis	Rocky Mountain spotted fever	Clofibrate	General anesthesia
Gastrointestinal tract	Aspergillosis	AIDS	Carbamazepine	Nausea
Stomach	Asthma	Bleeding and masses	Vincristine	Pain
Duodenum	Cystic fibrosis	Subdural hematoma	Nicotine	Stress
Pancreas	Respiratory failure associated with positive-pressure breathing	Subarachnoid hemorrhage	Narcotics	
Genitourinary tract		Cerebrovascular accident	Antipsychotic drugs	
Ureter		Brain tumors	Ifosfamide	
Bladder		Head trauma	Cyclophosphamide	
Prostate		Hydrocephalus	Nonsteroidal anti-inflammatory drugs	
Endometrium		Cavernous sinus thrombosis	MDMA (ecstasy)	
Endocrine thymoma		Other	AVP analogues	
Lymphomas		Multiple sclerosis	Desmopressin	
Sarcomas		Guillain-Barré syndrome	Oxytocin	
Ewing's sarcoma		Shy-Drager syndrome	Vasopressin	
		Delerium tremens		
		Acute intermittent polyphyria		

Abbreviations: AIDS, acquired immunodeficiency syndrome; AVP, vasopressin; MDMA, 3,4-methylenedioxymethamphetamine (ecstasy); SSRI, selective serotonin reuptake inhibitor.

Source: From Ellison and Berl.

Gain-in-function mutations of a single specific residue in the V_2 vasopressin receptor have been described in some of these patients, leading to constitutive activation of the receptor in the absence of AVP and a nephrogenic subset of SIAD.

Strictly speaking, patients with SIAD are not euvolemic but are subclinically volume expanded due to AVP-induced water and Na^+-Cl^- retention; vasopressin escape mechanisms invoked by sustained increases in AVP serve to limit distal renal tubular transport, preserving a modestly hypervolemic steady state. Serum uric acid is often low (<4 mg/dL) in patients with SIAD, consistent with suppressed proximal tubular transport in the setting of increased distal tubular Na^+-Cl^- and water transport; in contrast, patients with hypovolemic hyponatremia are often hyperuricemic due to a shared activation of proximal tubular Na^+-Cl^- and urate transport.

Common causes of SIAD include pulmonary disease (pneumonia, tuberculosis, pleural effusion, etc.) and central nervous system (CNS) diseases (tumor, subarachnoid hemorrhage, meningitis, etc.). SIAD also occurs with malignancies, most commonly with small cell lung carcinoma (75% of cases of malignancy-associated SIAD); ~10% of patients with this tumor will have a plasma Na^+ concentration <130 mM at presentation. SIAD is also a common complication of certain drugs, most commonly the selective serotonin reuptake inhibitors (SSRIs). Other drugs can potentiate the renal effect of AVP without exerting direct effects on circulating AVP levels (Table 45-1).

Low solute intake and hyponatremia

Hyponatremia occasionally can occur in patients with a very low intake of dietary solutes. Classically, this occurs in alcoholics whose sole nutrient is beer, hence the diagnostic label "beer potomania";

beer is very low in protein and salt content, containing only 1–2 millimole per liter of Na^+. The syndrome also has been described in nonalcoholic patients with highly restricted solute intake due to nutrient-restricted diets, e.g., extreme vegetarian diets. Patients with hyponatremia due to low solute intake typically present with a very low urine osmolality, <100–200 mosmol/kg, with a urine Na^+ concentration that is <10–20 mM. The fundamental abnormality is the inadequate dietary intake of solutes; the reduced urinary solute excretion limits water excretion so that hyponatremia ensues after relatively modest polydipsia. The ability to excrete a free-water load is thus a function of urinary solute excretion; at a urine osmolality of 80 mosmol/kg, free-water clearance is 2.7 L daily for a solute excretion of 300 mosmol/d, 5.4 L daily at 600 mosmol/d, and 8.1 L at 900 mosmol/d. AVP levels have not been reported in patients with beer potomania but are expected to be suppressed or rapidly suppressible with saline hydration; this fits with the overly rapid correction in plasma Na^+ concentration that can be seen with saline hydration. Resumption of a normal diet and/or saline hydration also will correct the causative deficit in urinary solute excretion so that patients with beer potomania typically correct their plasma Na^+ concentration promptly after admission to the hospital.

Clinical features of hyponatremia

Hyponatremia induces generalized cellular swelling, a consequence of water movement down the osmotic gradient from the hypotonic ECF to the ICF. The symptoms of hyponatremia are primarily neurologic, reflecting the development of cerebral edema within a rigid skull. The initial CNS response to acute hyponatremia is an increase in interstitial pressure, leading to shunting of ECF and solutes from the interstitial space into the cerebrospinal fluid and then into the

TABLE 45-2 Causes of Acute Hyponatremia

Iatrogenic

   Postoperative: premenopausal women

   Hypotonic fluids with cause of ↑ vasopressin

   Glycine irrigation: TURP, uterine surgery

   Colonoscopy preparation

   Recent institution of thiazides

Polydipsia

MDMA ingestion

Exercise-induced

Multifactorial, e.g., thiazide and polydipsia

Abbreviations: MDMA, 3,4-methylenedioxymethamphetamine (ecstasy); TURP, transurethral resection of the prostate.

systemic circulation. This is accompanied by an efflux of the major intracellular ions, Na^+, K^+, and Cl^-, from brain cells. Acute hyponatremic encephalopathy ensues when these volume regulatory mechanisms are overwhelmed by a rapid decrease in tonicity, resulting in acute cerebral edema. Early symptoms can include nausea, headache, and vomiting. However, severe complications can evolve rapidly, including seizure activity, brainstem herniation, coma, and death. A key complication of acute hyponatremia is normocapnic or hypercapnic respiratory failure; the associated hypoxemia may amplify the neurologic injury. Normocapnic respiratory failure in this setting typically is due to noncardiogenic, neurogenic pulmonary edema, with a normal pulmonary capillary wedge pressure.

Acute symptomatic hyponatremia is a medical emergency that occurs in a number of specific settings (Table 45-2). Women, particularly before menopause, are much more likely to develop encephalopathy and severe neurologic sequelae. Acute hyponatremia often has an iatrogenic component, e.g., when hypotonic intravenous fluids are given to postoperative patients with an increase in circulating AVP. Exercise-associated hyponatremia, an important clinical issue at marathons and other endurance events, similarly has been linked to both a nonosmotic increase in circulating AVP and excessive free-water intake. The recreational drug ecstasy (MDMA, 3,4-methylenedioxymethamphetamine) causes a rapid and potent induction of both thirst and AVP, leading to severe acute hyponatremia.

Persistent, chronic hyponatremia results in an efflux of organic osmolytes (creatine, betaine, glutamate, *myo*-inositol, and taurine) from brain cells; this response reduces intracellular osmolality and the osmotic gradient, favoring water entry. This reduction in intracellular osmolytes is largely complete within 48 h, the time period that clinically defines chronic hyponatremia; this temporal definition has considerable relevance for the treatment of hyponatremia (see below). The cellular response to chronic hyponatremia does not fully protect patients from symptoms, which can include vomiting, nausea, confusion, and seizures, usually at a plasma Na^+ concentration <125 m*M*. Even patients who are judged asymptomatic can manifest subtle gait and cognitive defects that reverse with correction of hyponatremia; notably, chronic asymptomatic hyponatremia increases the risk of falls. Chronic hyponatremia also increases the risk of bony fractures owing to the associated neurologic dysfunction and to a hyponatremia-associated reduction in bone density. Therefore, every attempt should be made to correct plasma Na^+ concentration safely in patients with chronic hyponatremia,

even in the absence of overt symptoms (see the section on treatment of hyponatremia, below).

The management of chronic hyponatremia is complicated significantly by the asymmetry of the cellular response to correction of plasma Na^+ concentration. Specifically, the *reaccumulation* of organic osmolytes by brain cells is attenuated and delayed as osmolality increases after correction of hyponatremia, sometimes resulting in degenerative loss of oligodendrocytes and an osmotic demyelination syndrome (ODS). Overly rapid correction of hyponatremia (>8–10 m*M* in 24 h or 18 m*M* in 48 h) also is associated with a disruption in integrity of the blood-brain barrier, allowing the entry of immune mediators that may contribute to demyelination. The lesions of ODS classically affect the pons, a structure in which the delay in the reaccumulation of osmotic osmolytes is particularly pronounced; clinically, patients with central pontine myelinolysis can present one or more days after overcorrection of hyponatremia with para- or quadraparesis, dysphagia, dysarthria, diplopia, a "locked-in syndrome," and/or loss of consciousness. Other regions of the brain also can be involved in ODS, most commonly in association with lesions of the pons but occasionally in isolation; in order of frequency, the lesions of extrapontine myelinolysis can occur in the cerebellum, lateral geniculate body, thalamus, putamen, and cerebral cortex or subcortex. The clinical presentation of ODS therefore can vary as a function of the extent and localization of extrapontine myelinolysis, with the reported development of ataxia, mutism, parkinsonism, dystonia, and catatonia. Relowering of plasma Na^+ concentration after overly rapid correction can prevent or attenuate ODS (see the section on treatment of hyponatremia, below). However, even appropriately slow correction can be associated with ODS, particularly in patients with additional risk factors; these factors include alcoholism, malnutrition, hypokalemia, and liver transplantation.

Diagnostic evaluation of hyponatremia

Clinical assessment of hyponatremic patients should focus on the underlying cause; a detailed drug history is particularly crucial (Table 45-1). A careful clinical assessment of volume status is obligatory for the classical diagnostic approach to hyponatremia (Fig. 45-5). Hyponatremia is frequently multifactorial, particularly when severe; clinical evaluation should consider *all* the possible causes for excessive circulating AVP, including volume status, drugs, and the presence of nausea and/or pain. Radiologic imaging also may be appropriate to assess whether patients have a pulmonary or CNS cause for hyponatremia. A screening chest x-ray may fail to detect a small cell carcinoma of the lung; CT scanning of the thorax should be considered in patients at high risk for this tumor, e.g., patients with a history of smoking.

Laboratory investigation should include a measurement of serum osmolality to exclude pseudohyponatremia, which is defined as the coexistence of hyponatremia with a normal or increased plasma tonicity. Most clinical laboratories measure plasma Na^+ concentration by testing diluted samples with automated ion-sensitive electrodes, correcting for this dilution by assuming that plasma is 93% water; this correction factor can be inaccurate in patients with pseudohyponatremia due to extreme hyperlipidemia and/or hyperproteinemia, in whom serum lipid or protein makes up a greater percentage of plasma volume. The measured osmolality also should be converted to the effective osmolality (tonicity) by subtracting the measured concentration of urea (divided by 2.8 if in mg/dL); patients with hyponatremia have an effective osmolality <275 mosmol/kg.

Elevated BUN and creatinine in routine chemistries also can indicate renal dysfunction as a potential cause of hyponatremia, whereas hyperkalemia may suggest adrenal insufficiency or hypoaldosteronism. Serum glucose also should be measured; plasma Na^+

347

concentration falls by ~1.6 to 2.4 mM for every 100-mg/dL increase in glucose due to glucose-induced water efflux from cells; this "true" hyponatremia resolves after correction of hyperglycemia. Measurement of serum uric acid also should be performed; whereas patients with SIAD-type physiology typically will be hypouricemic (serum uric acid <4 mg/dL), volume-depleted patients often will be hyperuricemic. In the appropriate clinical setting, thyroid, adrenal, and pituitary function should also be tested; hypothyroidism and secondary adrenal failure due to pituitary insufficiency are important causes of euvolemic hyponatremia, whereas primary adrenal failure causes hypovolemic hyponatremia. A cosyntropin stimulation test is necessary to assess for primary adrenal insufficiency.

Urine electrolytes and osmolality are crucial tests in the initial evaluation of hyponatremia. A urine Na$^+$ concentration <20–30 mM is consistent with hypovolemic hyponatremia in the clinical absence of a hypervolemic, Na$^+$-avid syndrome such as CHF (Fig. 45-5). In contrast, patients with SIAD typically excrete urine with a Na$^+$ concentration that is >30 mM. However, there can be substantial overlap in urine Na$^+$ concentration values in patients with SIAD and hypovolemic hyponatremia, particularly in the elderly; the ultimate "gold standard" for the diagnosis of hypovolemic hyponatremia is the demonstration that plasma Na$^+$ concentration corrects after hydration with normal saline. Patients with thiazide-associated hyponatremia also may present with a higher than expected urine Na$^+$ concentration and other findings suggestive of SIAD; one should defer making a diagnosis of SIAD in these patients until 1–2 weeks after discontinuation of the thiazide. A urine osmolality <100 mosmol/kg is suggestive of polydipsia; urine osmolality >400 mosmol/kg indicates that AVP excess is playing a more dominant role, whereas intermediate values are more consistent with multifactorial pathophysiology (e.g., AVP excess with a significant component of polydipsia). Patients with hyponatremia due to decreased solute intake (beer potomania) typically have urine Na$^+$ concentration <20 mM and urine osmolality in the range of <100 to the low 200's. Finally, the measurement of urine K$^+$ concentration is required to calculate the urine:plasma electrolyte ratio, which is useful to predict the response to fluid restriction (see the section on treatment of hyponatremia, below).

TREATMENT   Hyponatremia

Three major considerations guide therapy for hyponatremia. First, the presence and/or severity of symptoms determine the urgency and goals of therapy. Patients with acute hyponatremia (Table 45-2) present with symptoms that can range from headache, nausea, and/or vomiting to seizures, obtundation, and central herniation; patients with chronic hyponatremia that is present for >48 h are less likely to have severe symptoms. Second, patients with chronic hyponatremia are at risk for ODS if plasma Na$^+$ concentration is corrected by >8–10 mM within the first 24 h and/or by >18 mM within the first 48 h. Third, the response to interventions such as hypertonic saline, isotonic saline, and vasopressin antagonists can be highly unpredictable, and so frequent monitoring of plasma Na$^+$ concentration during corrective therapy is imperative.

Once the urgency in correcting the plasma Na$^+$ concentration has been established and appropriate therapy instituted, the focus should be on treatment or withdrawal of the underlying cause. Patients with euvolemic hyponatremia due to SIAD, hypothyroidism, or secondary adrenal failure will respond to successful treatment of the underlying cause, with an increase in plasma Na$^+$ concentration. However, not all causes of SIAD are immediately reversible, necessitating pharmacologic

therapy to increase the plasma Na$^+$ concentration (see below). Hypovolemic hyponatremia will respond to intravenous hydration with isotonic normal saline, with a rapid reduction in circulating AVP and a brisk water diuresis; it may be necessary to reduce the rate of correction if the history suggests that hyponatremia has been chronic, i.e., present for more than 48 h (see below). Hypervolemic hyponatremia due to congestive heart failure often responds to improved therapy of the underlying cardiomyopathy, e.g., after the institution or intensification of angiotensin-converting enzyme (ACE) inhibition. Finally, patients with hyponatremia due to beer potomania and low solute intake respond very rapidly to intravenous saline and the resumption of a normal diet. Notably, patients with beer potomania have a very high risk of developing ODS due to the associated hypokalemia, alcoholism, and malnutrition and the high risk of overcorrecting the plasma Na$^+$ concentration.

Water deprivation has long been a cornerstone of therapy for chronic hyponatremia. However, patients who are excreting minimal electrolyte-free water will require aggressive fluid restriction; this can be very difficult for patients with SIAD to tolerate because their thirst is also inappropriately stimulated. The urine:plasma electrolyte ratio (urinary [Na$^+$]+[K$^+$]/plasma [Na$^+$]) can be exploited as a quick indicator of electrolyte-free water excretion (Table 45-3); patients with a ratio >1 should be restricted more aggressively (<500 mL/d), those with a ratio ~1 should be restricted to 500–700 mL/d, and those with a ratio <1 should be restricted to <1 L/d. In hypokalemic patients, potassium replacement will serve to increase plasma Na$^+$ concentration in light of the fact that the plasma Na$^+$ concentration is a function of both exchangeable Na$^+$ and exchangeable K$^+$ divided by total body water; a corollary is that aggressive repletion of K$^+$ has the potential to overcorrect the plasma Na$^+$ concentration even in the absence of hypertonic saline. Plasma Na$^+$ concentration also tends to respond to an increase in dietary solute intake, which increases the ability to excrete free water; however, the use of oral urea and/or salt tablets for this purpose is generally not practical or well tolerated.

TABLE 45-3   Management of Hypernatremia

Water Deficit

1. Estimate total-body water (TBW): 50% of body weight in women and 60% in men

2. Calculate free-water deficit: $\{([Na^+]{-}140)/140\} \times TBW$

3. Administer deficit over 48–72 h, without increasing the plasma Na$^+$ concentration by >10 mM/24 h

Ongoing Water Losses

4. Calculate electrolyte-free water clearance, C_eH_2O:

$$C_eH_2O = \frac{V\,(1 - U_{Na} + U_K)}{P_{Na}}$$

where V is urinary volume, U_{Na} is urinary [Na$^+$], U_K is urinary [K$^+$], and P_{Na} is plasma [Na$^+$]

Insensible Losses

5. ~10 mL/kg per day: less if ventilated, more if febrile

Total

6. Add components to determine water deficit and ongoing water loss; correct the water deficit over 48–72 h and replace daily water loss. Avoid correction of plasma [Na$^+$] by >10 mM/d

Patients in whom therapy with fluid restriction, potassium replacement, and/or increased solute intake fails may require pharmacologic therapy to increase their plasma Na^+ concentration. Many patients with SIAD respond to combined therapy with oral furosemide, 20 mg twice a day (higher doses may be necessary in renal insufficiency), and oral salt tablets; furosemide serves to inhibit the renal countercurrent mechanism and blunt urinary concentrating ability, whereas the salt tablets counteract diuretic-associated natriuresis. Demeclocycline is a potent inhibitor of principal cells and can be utilized in patients whose Na^+ levels do not increase in response to furosemide and salt tablets. However, this agent can be associated with a reduction in GFR due to excessive natriuresis and/or direct renal toxicity; it should be avoided in cirrhotic patients in particular, who are at higher risk of nephrotoxicity due to drug accumulation.

Vasopressin antagonists (vaptans) are highly effective in treating SIAD and hypervolemic hyponatremia due to heart failure or cirrhosis, reliably increasing plasma Na^+ concentration as a result of their aquaretic effects (augmentation of free-water clearance). Most of these agents specifically antagonize the V_2 vasopressin receptor; tolvaptan is currently the only oral V_2 antagonist approved by the U.S. Food and Drug Administration. Conivaptan, the only available intravenous vaptan, is a mixed V_{1A}/V_2 antagonist with a modest risk of hypotension due to V_{1A} receptor inhibition. Therapy with vaptans must be initiated in a hospital setting, with a liberalization of fluid restriction (>2 L/d) and close monitoring of plasma Na^+ concentration. Although these agents are approved for the management of all but hypovolemic hyponatremia and acute hyponatremia, the clinical indications for them are not completely clear. Oral tolvaptan is perhaps most appropriate for the management of significant and persistent SIAD (e.g., in small cell lung carcinoma) that has not responded to water restriction and/or oral furosemide and salt tablets.

Treatment of acute symptomatic hyponatremia should include hypertonic 3% saline (513 mM) to acutely increase plasma Na^+ concentration by 1–2 mM/h to a total of 4–6 mM; this modest increase is typically sufficient to alleviate severe acute symptoms, after which corrective guidelines for "chronic" hyponatremia are appropriate (see below). A number of equations have been developed to estimate the required rate of hypertonic saline. The traditional approach is to calculate a Na^+ deficit, in which the Na^+ deficit = 0.6 × body weight × (target plasma Na^+ concentration – starting plasma Na^+ concentration), followed by a calculation of the required rate. Regardless of the method used to determine the rate of administration, the increase in plasma Na^+ concentration can be highly unpredictable during treatment with hypertonic saline due to rapid changes in the underlying physiology; plasma Na^+ concentration should be monitored every 2–4 h during treatment, with appropriate changes in therapy based on the observed rate of change. The administration of supplemental oxygen and ventilatory support is also critical in the management of patients with acute hyponatremia who develop acute pulmonary edema or hypercapnic respiratory failure. Intravenous loop diuretics will help treat acute pulmonary edema and also increase free-water excretion by interfering with the renal countercurrent multiplication system. Vasopressin antagonists do *not* have an approved role in the management of acute hyponatremia.

The rate of correction should be comparatively slow in *chronic* hyponatremia (<8–10 mM in the first 24 h and <18 mM in the first 48 h) to avoid ODS. Overcorrection of the plasma Na^+ concentration can occur when AVP levels rapidly normalize, for example, after treatment of patients with chronic hypovolemic

hyponatremia with intravenous saline or after glucocorticoid replacement in patients with hypopituitarism and secondary adrenal failure. Approximately 10% of patients treated with vaptans will overcorrect; the risk is increased if water intake is not liberalized. If the plasma Na^+ concentration overcorrects after therapy—whether with hypertonic saline, isotonic saline, or a vaptan—hyponatremia can be reinduced safely or stabilized by the administration of the vasopressin *agonist* desmopressin acetate (DDAVP) and/or the administration of free water, typically intravenous D5W; the goal is to prevent or reverse the development of ODS.

■ HYPERNATREMIA

Etiology

Hypernatremia is defined as an increase in the plasma Na^+ concentration to >145 mM. Considerably less common than hyponatremia, hypernatremia nonetheless is associated with mortality rates as high as 40–60%, mostly due to the severity of the associated underlying disease processes. Hypernatremia is usually the result of a combined water and electrolyte deficit, with losses of H_2O in excess of those of Na^+. Less frequently, the ingestion or iatrogenic administration of excess Na^+ can be causative, for example, after IV administration of excessive hypertonic Na^+-Cl^- or Na^+-HCO_3^- (Fig. 45-6).

Elderly individuals with reduced thirst and/or diminished access to fluids are at the highest risk of developing hypernatremia. Patients with hypernatremia may rarely have a central defect in hypothalamic osmoreceptor function, with a mixture of both decreased thirst and reduced AVP secretion. Causes of this adipsic diabetes insipidus include primary or metastatic tumor, occlusion or ligation of the anterior communicating artery, trauma, hydrocephalus, and inflammation.

Hypernatremia can develop after the loss of water via both renal and nonrenal routes. Insensible losses of water may increase in the setting of fever, exercise, heat exposure, severe burns, or mechanical

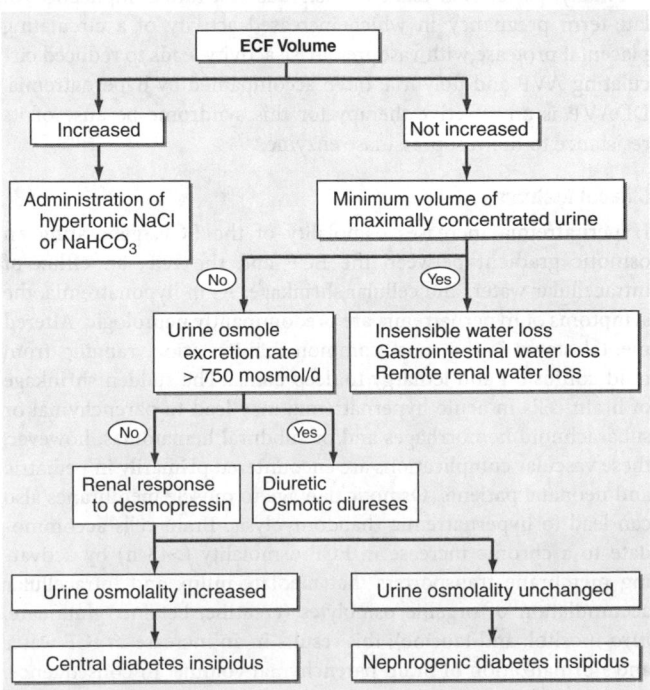

Figure 45-6 **The diagnostic approach to hypernatremia.** ECF, extracellular fluid.

ventilation. Diarrhea is the most common gastrointestinal cause of hypernatremia. Notably, osmotic diarrhea and viral gastroenteritis typically generate stools with Na^+ and K^+ <100 mM, thus leading to water loss and hypernatremia; in contrast, secretory diarrhea typically results in isotonic stool and thus hypovolemia with or without hypovolemic hyponatremia.

Common causes of renal water loss include osmotic diuresis secondary to hyperglycemia, excess urea, postobstructive diuresis, and mannitol; these disorders share an increase in urinary solute excretion and urinary osmolality (see "Diagnostic Approach," below). Hypernatremia due to a water diuresis occurs in central or nephrogenic diabetes insipidus (DI).

Nephrogenic DI (NDI) is characterized by renal resistance to AVP, which can be partial or complete (see "Diagnostic Approach," below). Genetic causes include loss-of-function mutations in the X-linked V_2 receptor; mutations in the AVP-responsive aquaporin-2 water channel can cause autosomal recessive and autosomal dominant nephrogenic DI, whereas recessive deficiency of the aquaporin-1 water channel causes a more modest concentrating defect (Fig. 45-2). Hypercalcemia also can cause polyuria and NDI; calcium signals directly through the calcium-sensing receptor to downregulate Na^+, K^+, and Cl^- transport by the TALH and water transport in principal cells, thus reducing renal concentrating ability in hypercalcemia. Another common acquired cause of NDI is hypokalemia, which inhibits the renal response to AVP and downregulates aquaporin-2 expression. Several drugs can cause acquired NDI, in particular lithium, ifosfamide, and several antiviral agents. Lithium causes NDI by multiple mechanisms, including direct inhibition of renal glycogen synthase kinase-3 (GSK3), a kinase thought to be the pharmacologic target of lithium in bipolar disease; GSK3 is required for the response of principal cells to AVP. The entry of lithium through the amiloride-sensitive Na^+ channel ENaC (Fig. 45-4) is required for the effect of the drug on principal cells; thus, combined therapy with lithium and amiloride can mitigate lithium-associated NDI. However, lithium causes chronic tubulointerstitial scarring and chronic kidney disease after prolonged therapy so that patients may have a persistent NDI long after stopping the drug, with a reduced therapeutic benefit from amiloride.

Finally, gestational diabetes insipidus is a rare complication of late-term pregnancy in which increased activity of a circulating placental protease with vasopressinase activity leads to reduced circulating AVP and polyuria, often accompanied by hypernatremia. DDAVP is an effective therapy for this syndrome because of its resistance to the vasopressinase enzyme.

Clinical features

Hypernatremia increases osmolality of the ECF, generating an osmotic gradient between the ECF and the ICF, an efflux of intracellular water, and cellular shrinkage. As in hyponatremia, the symptoms of hypernatremia are predominantly neurologic. Altered mental status is the most common manifestation, ranging from mild confusion and lethargy to deep coma. The sudden shrinkage of brain cells in acute hypernatremia may lead to parenchymal or subarachnoid hemorrhages and/or subdural hematomas; however, these vascular complications are encountered primarily in pediatric and neonatal patients. Osmotic damage to muscle membranes also can lead to hypernatremic rhabdomyolysis. Brain cells accommodate to a chronic increase in ECF osmolality (>48 h) by activating membrane transporters that mediate influx and intracellular accumulation of organic osmolytes (creatine, betaine, glutamate, *myo*-inositol, and taurine); this results in an increase in ICF water and normalization of brain parenchymal volume. In consequence, patients with *chronic* hypernatremia are less likely to develop severe neurologic compromise. However, the cellular response to chronic hypernatremia predisposes these patients to the development of

cerebral edema and seizures during overly rapid hydration (overcorrection of plasma Na^+ concentration by >10 mM/d).

Diagnostic approach

The history should focus on the presence or absence of thirst, polyuria, and/or an extrarenal source for water loss, such as diarrhea. The physical examination should include a detailed neurologic exam and an assessment of the ECFV; patients with a particularly large water deficit and/or a combined deficit in electrolytes and water may be hypovolemic, with reduced JVP and orthostasis. Accurate documentation of daily fluid intake and daily urine output is also critical for the diagnosis and management of hypernatremia.

Laboratory investigation should include a measurement of serum and urine osmolality in addition to urine electrolytes. The appropriate response to hypernatremia and a serum osmolality >295 mosmol/kg is an increase in circulating AVP and the excretion of low volumes (<500 mL/d) of maximally concentrated urine, i.e., urine with osmolality >800 mosmol/kg; if this is the case, an extrarenal source of water loss is primarily responsible for the generation of hypernatremia. Many patients with hypernatremia are polyuric; if an osmotic diuresis is responsible, with excessive excretion of Na^+-Cl^-, glucose, and/or urea, solute excretion will be >750–1000 mosmol/d (>15 mosmol/kg body water per day) (Fig. 45-6). More commonly, patients with hypernatremia and polyuria will have a predominant water diuresis, with excessive excretion of hypotonic, dilute urine.

Adequate differentiation between nephrogenic and central causes of DI requires the measurement of the response in urinary osmolality to DDAVP, combined with measurement of circulating AVP in the setting of hypertonicity. By definition, patients with baseline hypernatremia are hypertonic, with an adequate stimulus for AVP by the posterior pituitary. Therefore, in contrast to polyuric patients with a normal or reduced baseline plasma Na^+ concentration and osmolality, a water deprivation test (Chap. 44) is unnecessary in hypernatremia; indeed, water deprivation is absolutely contraindicated in this setting because of the risk for worsening the hypernatremia. Patients with NDI will fail to respond to DDAVP, with a urine osmolality that increases by <50% or <150 mosmol/kg from baseline, in combination with a normal or high circulating AVP level; patients with central DI will respond to DDAVP, with a reduced circulating AVP. Patients may exhibit a partial response to DDAVP, with a >50% rise in urine osmolality that nonetheless fails to reach 800 mosmol/kg; the level of circulating AVP will help differentiate the underlying cause, i.e., nephrogenic versus central DI. In pregnant patients, AVP assays should be drawn in tubes containing the protease inhibitor 1,10-phenanthroline to prevent in vitro degradation of AVP by placental vasopressinase.

For patients with hypernatremia due to renal loss of water it is critical to quantify *ongoing* daily losses using the calculated electrolyte-free water clearance in addition to calculation of the baseline water deficit (the relevant formulas are discussed in Table 45-3). This requires daily measurement of urine electrolytes, combined with accurate measurement of daily urine volume.

TREATMENT   Hypernatremia

The underlying cause of hypernatremia should be withdrawn or corrected, whether it is drugs, hyperglycemia, hypercalcemia, hypokalemia, or diarrhea. The approach to the correction of hypernatremia is outlined in Table 45-3. It is imperative to correct hypernatremia slowly to avoid cerebral edema, typically replacing the calculated free-water deficit over 48 h. Notably, the plasma Na^+ concentration should be corrected by no more than 10 mM/d, which may take longer than 48 h in patients with severe hypernatremia (>160 mM). A rare exception is patients with acute hypernatremia (<48 h) due to sodium loading, who can safely be corrected rapidly at a rate of 1 mM/h.

Water ideally should be administered by mouth or by nasogastric tube as the most direct way to provide free water, i.e., water without electrolytes. Alternatively, patients can receive free water in dextrose-containing IV solutions such as 5% dextrose (D5W); blood glucose should be monitored to avoid hyperglycemia. Depending on the history, blood pressure, or clinical volume status, it may be appropriate to treat initially with hypotonic saline solutions (1/4 or 1/2 normal saline); normal saline is usually inappropriate in the absence of very severe hypernatremia, in which normal saline is proportionally more hypotonic relative to plasma, or frank hypotension. Calculation of urinary electrolyte-free water clearance (see Table 45-3) is required to estimate daily, ongoing loss of free water in patients with nephrogenic or central DI, which should be replenished daily.

Additional therapy may be feasible in specific cases. Patients with central DI should respond to the administration of intravenous, intranasal, or oral DDAVP. Patients with NDI due to lithium may reduce their polyuria with amiloride (2.5–10 mg/d), which decreases entry of lithium into principal cells by inhibiting ENaC (see above); in practice, however, most patients with lithium-associated DI are able to compensate for their polyuria simply by increasing their daily water intake. Thiazides may reduce polyuria due to NDI, ostensibly by inducing hypovolemia and increasing proximal tubular water reabsorption. Occasionally, nonsteroidal anti-inflammatory drugs (NSAIDs) have been used to treat polyuria associated with NDI, reducing the negative effect of intrarenal prostaglandins on urinary concentrating mechanisms; however, this creates the risk of NSAID-associated gastric and/or renal toxicity. Furthermore, it must be emphasized that thiazides, amiloride, and NSAIDs are appropriate only for *chronic* management of polyuria from NDI and have *no* role in the acute management of associated hypernatremia, in which the focus is on replacing free-water deficits and ongoing free-water loss.

POTASSIUM DISORDERS

Homeostatic mechanisms maintain plasma K$^+$ concentration between 3.5 and 5.0 mM despite marked variation in dietary K$^+$ intake. In a healthy individual at steady state, the entire daily intake of potassium is excreted, approximately 90% in the urine and 10% in the stool; the kidney thus plays a dominant role in potassium homeostasis. However, more than 98% of total-body potassium is intracellular, chiefly in muscle; buffering of extracellular K$^+$ by this large intracellular pool plays a crucial role in the regulation of plasma K$^+$ concentration. Changes in the exchange and distribution of intra- and extracellular K$^+$ thus can lead to marked hypo- or hyperkalemia. A corollary is that massive necrosis and the attendant release of tissue K$^+$ can cause severe hyperkalemia, particularly in the setting of acute kidney injury and reduced excretion of K$^+$.

Changes in whole-body K$^+$ content are mediated primarily by the kidney, which *reabsorbs* filtered K$^+$ in hypokalemic, K$^+$-deficient states and *secretes* K$^+$ in hyperkalemic, K$^+$-replete states. Although K$^+$ is transported along the entire nephron, it is the principal cells of the connecting tubule (CNT) and cortical collecting duct (CD) that play a dominant role in renal K$^+$ secretion, whereas alpha-intercalated cells of the outer medullary CD function in renal tubular reabsorption of filtered K$^+$ in K$^+$-deficient states. In principal cells, apical Na$^+$ entry via the amiloride-sensitive ENaC generates a lumen-negative

potential difference that drives passive K$^+$ exit through apical K$^+$ channels (Fig. 45-4). Two major K$^+$ channels mediate distal tubular K$^+$ secretion: the secretory K$^+$ channel ROMK (the renal outer medullary K$^+$ channel, also known as Kir1.1 or KcnJ1) and the flow-sensitive maxi-K K$^+$ channel (also known as the BK K$^+$ channel). ROMK is thought to mediate the bulk of constitutive K$^+$ secretion, whereas increases in distal flow rate and/or genetic absence of ROMK activate K$^+$ secretion via the maxi-K channel.

An appreciation of the relationship between ENaC-dependent Na$^+$ entry and distal K$^+$ secretion (Fig. 45-4) is required for the bedside interpretation of potassium disorders. For example, decreased distal delivery of Na$^+$, as occurs in hypovolemic, prerenal states, tends to blunt the ability to excrete K$^+$, leading to hyperkalemia; in contrast, an *increase* in distal delivery of Na$^+$ and distal flow rate, as occurs after treatment with thiazide and loop diuretics, can enhance K$^+$ secretion and lead to hypokalemia. Hyperkalemia is also a predictable consequence of drugs that directly inhibit ENaC due to the role of this Na$^+$ channel in generating a lumen-negative potential difference. Aldosterone in turn has a major influence on potassium excretion, increasing the activity of ENaC channels and thus amplifying the driving force for K$^+$ secretion across the luminal membrane of principal cells. Abnormalities in the renin-angiotensin-aldosterone system thus can cause both hypokalemia and hyperkalemia. Notably, however, potassium excess and potassium restriction have opposing, aldosterone-independent effects on the density and activity of apical K$^+$ channels in the distal nephron; i.e., other factors modulate the renal capacity to secrete K$^+$. In addition, potassium restriction and hypokalemia activate aldosterone-independent distal *reabsorption* of filtered K$^+$, activating apical H$^+$/K$^+$-ATPase activity in intercalated cells within the outer medullary CD. Reflective perhaps of this physiology, changes in plasma K$^+$ concentration are not universal in disorders associated with changes in aldosterone activity.

■ HYPOKALEMIA

Hypokalemia, defined as a plasma K$^+$ concentration <3.6 mM, occurs in up to 20% of hospitalized patients. Hypokalemia is associated with a tenfold increase in in-hospital mortality rates due to adverse effects on cardiac rhythm, blood pressure, and cardiovascular morbidity rate. Mechanistically, hypokalemia can be caused by redistribution of K$^+$ between tissues and the ECF or by renal and nonrenal loss of K$^+$ (Table 45-4). Systemic hypomagnesemia also can cause treatment-resistant hypokalemia due to a combination of reduced cellular uptake of K$^+$ and exaggerated renal secretion. Spurious hypokalemia or pseudohypokalemia occasionally can result from in vitro cellular uptake of K$^+$ after venipuncture, for example, due to profound leukocytosis in acute leukemia.

Redistribution and hypokalemia

Insulin, β_2-adrenergic activity, and thyroid hormone promote Na$^+$,K$^+$-ATPase-mediated cellular uptake of K$^+$, leading to hypokalemia. Inhibition of passive *efflux* of K$^+$ also can cause hypokalemia, albeit rarely; this typically occurs in the setting of systemic inhibition of K$^+$ channels by toxic barium ions. Exogenous insulin can cause iatrogenic hypokalemia, particularly during the management of K$^+$-deficient states such as diabetic ketoacidosis. Alternatively, the stimulation of *endogenous* insulin can provoke hypokalemia, hypomagnesemia, and/or hypophosphatemia in malnourished patients who are given a carbohydrate load. Alterations in the activity of the endogenous sympathetic nervous system can cause hypokalemia in several settings, including alcohol withdrawal, hyperthyroidism, acute myocardial infarction, and severe head injury. β_2 agonists, including both bronchodilators and tocolytics (ritodrine), are powerful activators of cellular K$^+$ uptake;

TABLE 45-4 Causes of Hypokalemia

I. Decreased intake
   A. Starvation
   B. Clay ingestion
II. Redistribution into cells
   A. Acid-base
      1. Metabolic alkalosis
   B. Hormonal
      1. Insulin
      2. Increased β_2-adrenergic sympathetic activity: post-myocardial infarction, head injury
      3. β_2-Adrenergic agonists: bronchodilators, tocolytics
      4. α-Adrenergic antagonists
      5. Thyrotoxic periodic paralysis
      6. Downstream stimulation of Na^+/K^+-ATPase: theophylline, caffeine
   C. Anabolic state
      1. Vitamin B_{12} or folic acid administration (red blood cell production)
      2. Granulocyte-macrophage colony-stimulating factor (white blood cell production)
      3. Total parenteral nutrition
   D. Other
      1. Pseudohypokalemia
      2. Hypothermia
      3. Familial hypokalemic periodic paralysis
      4. Barium toxicity: systemic inhibition of "leak" K^+ channels
III. Increased loss
   A. Nonrenal
      1. Gastrointestinal loss (diarrhea)
      2. Integumentary loss (sweat)
   B. Renal
      1. Increased distal flow and distal Na^+ delivery: diuretics, osmotic diuresis, salt-wasting nephropathies
      2. Increased secretion of potassium
         a. Mineralocorticoid excess: primary hyperaldosteronism [aldosterone-producing adenomas (APAs)], primary or unilateral adrenal hyperplasia (PAH), idiopathic hyperaldosteronism (IHA) due to bilateral adrenal hyperplasia, and adrenal carcinoma], familial hyperaldosteronism (FH-I, FH-II, congenital adrenal hyperplasias), secondary hyperaldosteronism (malignant hypertension, renin-secreting tumors, renal artery stenosis, hypovolemia), Cushing's syndrome, Bartter's syndrome, Gitelman's syndrome
         b. Apparent mineralocorticoid excess: genetic deficiency of 11β-dehydrogenase-2 (syndrome of apparent mineralocorticoid excess), inhibition of 11β-dehydrogenase-2 (glycyrrhetinic/glycyrrhizinic acid and/or carbenoxolone; licorice, food products, drugs), Liddle's syndrome [genetic activation of epithelial Na^+ channels (ENaC)]
         c. Distal delivery of nonreabsorbed anions: vomiting, nasogastric suction, proximal renal tubular acidosis, diabetic ketoacidosis, glue sniffing (toluene abuse), penicillin derivatives (penicillin, nafcillin, dicloxacillin, ticarcillin, oxacillin, and carbenicillin)
      3. Magnesium deficiency

"hidden" sympathomimetics such as pseudoephedrine and ephedrine in cough syrup or dieting agents also may cause unexpected hypokalemia. Finally, xanthine-dependent activation of cyclic AMP–dependent signaling downstream of the β_2 receptor can lead to hypokalemia, usually in the setting of overdose (theophylline) or marked overingestion (dietary caffeine).

Redistributive hypokalemia also can occur in the setting of hyperthyroidism, with periodic attacks of hypokalemic paralysis [thyrotoxic periodic paralysis (TPP)]. Similar episodes of hypokalemic weakness in the absence of thyroid abnormalities occur in *familial* hypokalemic periodic paralysis, usually caused by missense mutations of voltage sensor domains within the α_1 subunit of L-type calcium channels or the skeletal Na^+ channel; these mutations generate an abnormal gating pore current activated by hyperpolarization. TPP develops more frequently in patients of Asian or Hispanic origin; this shared predisposition has been linked to genetic variation in Kir2.6, a muscle-specific, thyroid hormone–responsive K^+ channel. Patients typically present with weakness of the extremities and limb girdles, with paralytic episodes that occur most frequently between 1 and 6 A.M. Signs and symptoms of hyperthyroidism are not invariably present. Hypokalemia is usually profound and almost invariably is accompanied by hypophosphatemia and hypomagnesemia. The hypokalemia in TPP is attributed to both direct and indirect activation of Na^+,K^+-ATPase, resulting in increased uptake of K^+ by muscle and other tissues. Increases in β-adrenergic activity play an important role in that high-dose propranolol (3 mg/kg) rapidly reverses the associated hypokalemia, hypophosphatemia, and paralysis.

Nonrenal loss of potassium

The loss of K^+ in sweat is typically low except under extremes of physical exertion. Direct gastric losses of K^+ due to vomiting or nasogastric suctioning are also minimal; however, the ensuing hypochloremic alkalosis results in persistent kaliuresis due to secondary hyperaldosteronism and bicarbonaturia, i.e., a *renal* loss of K^+. Intestinal loss of K^+ due to diarrhea is a globally important cause of hypokalemia in light of the worldwide prevalence of diarrheal disease. Noninfectious gastrointestinal processes such as celiac disease, ileostomy, villous adenomas, VIPomas, and chronic laxative abuse also can cause significant hypokalemia. Colonic pseudo-obstruction (Ogilvie's syndrome) can lead to hypokalemia from secretory diarrhea with an abnormally high potassium content caused by a marked activation of colonic K^+ secretion.

Renal loss of potassium

Drugs can increase renal K^+ excretion by a variety of different mechanisms. Diuretics are a particularly common cause due to associated increases in distal tubular Na^+ delivery and distal tubular flow rate in addition to secondary hyperaldosteronism. Thiazides have an effect on plasma K^+ concentration greater than that of loop diuretics despite their lesser natriuretic effect. The higher propensity of thiazides to cause hypokalemia may be secondary to thiazide-associated hypocalciuria versus the *hypercalciuria* seen with loop diuretics; increases in downstream luminal calcium in response to loop diuretics will inhibit ENaC in principal cells, thus reducing the lumen-negative potential difference and attenuating distal K^+ excretion. High doses of penicillin-related antibiotics (nafcillin, dicloxacillin, ticarcillin, oxacillin, and carbenicillin) can increase obligatory K^+ excretion by acting as nonreabsorbable anions in the distal nephron. Finally, several renal tubular toxins cause renal K^+ and magnesium wasting, leading to hypokalemia and hypomagnesemia; these drugs include aminoglycosides, amphotericin, foscarnet, cisplatin, and ifosfamide (see also "Magnesium Deficiency and Hypokalemia," below).

Aldosterone activates the ENaC channel in principal cells via multiple synergistic mechanisms, thus increasing the driving force for K$^+$ excretion. In consequence, increases in aldosterone bioactivity and/or gains in function of aldosterone-dependent signaling pathways are associated with hypokalemia. Increases in circulating aldosterone (hyperaldosteronism) may be primary or secondary. Increased levels of circulating renin in secondary forms of hyperaldosteronism lead to increased angiotensin II (AT-II) and thus aldosterone; renal artery stenosis is perhaps the most common cause (Table 45-4). Primary hyperaldosteronism may be genetic or acquired. Hypertension and hypokalemia due to increases in circulating 11-deoxycorticosterone occur in patients with congenital adrenal hyperplasia caused by defects in either steroid 11β-hydroxylase or steroid 17α-hydroxylase; deficient 11β-hydroxylase results in associated virilization and other signs of androgen excess, whereas reduced sex steroids in 17α-hydroxylase deficiency lead to hypogonadism. The two major forms of *isolated* primary hyperaldosteronism are familial hyperaldosteronism type I [FH-I, also known as glucocorticoid-remediable hyperaldosteronism (GRA)] and familial hyperaldosteronism type II (FH-II), in which aldosterone production is not repressible by exogenous glucocorticoids. FH-I is caused by a chimeric gene duplication between the homologous 11β-hydroxylase (*CYP11B1*) and aldosterone synthase (*CYP11B2*) genes, fusing the adrenocorticotropic hormone (ACTH)-responsive 11β-hydroxylase promoter to the coding region of aldosterone synthase; this chimeric gene is under the control of ACTH and thus is repressible by glucocorticoids.

Acquired causes of primary hyperaldosteronism include aldosterone-producing adenomas (APAs), primary or unilateral adrenal hyperplasia (PAH), idiopathic hyperaldosteronism (IHA) due to bilateral adrenal hyperplasia, and adrenal carcinoma; APA and IHA account for close to 60% and 40%, respectively, of diagnosed cases of hyperaldosteronism. Random testing of plasma renin activity (PRA) and aldosterone is a helpful screening tool in hypokalemic and/or hypertensive patients, with an aldosterone:PRA ratio >50 suggestive of primary hyperaldosteronism.

The glucocorticoid cortisol has affinity for the mineralocorticoid receptor (MLR) equal to that of aldosterone, with resultant mineralocorticoid-like activity. However, cells in the aldosterone-sensitive distal nephron are protected from this illicit activation by the enzyme 11β-hydroxysteroid dehydrogenase-2 (11βHSD-2), which converts cortisol to cortisone; cortisone has minimal affinity for the MLR. Recessive loss-of-function mutations in the *11βHSD-2* gene thus are associated with cortisol-dependent activation of the MLR and the syndrome of apparent mineralocorticoid excess (SAME), encompassing hypertension, hypokalemia, hypercalciuria, and metabolic alkalosis, with suppressed PRA and suppressed aldosterone. A similar syndrome is caused by biochemical inhibition of 11βHSD-2 by glycyrrhetinic/glycyrrhizinic acid and/or carbenoxolone. Glycyrrhizinic acid is a natural sweetener found in licorice root, typically encountered in licorice and its many guises or as a flavoring agent in tobacco and food products.

Finally, hypokalemia may occur with systemic increases in glucocorticoids. In Cushing's syndrome caused by increases in pituitary ACTH (Chap. 342) the incidence of hypokalemia is only 10%, whereas it is 60–100% in patients with ectopic secretion of ACTH despite a similar incidence of hypertension. Indirect evidence suggests that the activity of renal 11βHSD-2 is reduced in patients with ectopic ACTH compared with Cushing's syndrome, resulting in a syndrome of apparent mineralocorticoid excess.

Finally, defects in multiple renal tubular transport pathways are associated with hypokalemia. For example, loss-of-function mutations in subunits of the acidifying H$^+$-ATPase in alpha-intercalated cells cause hypokalemic distal renal tubular acidosis, as do many acquired disorders of the distal nephron. Liddle's syndrome is caused by autosomal dominant gain-in-function mutations of ENaC subunits. Disease-associated mutations either activate the channel directly or abrogate aldosterone-inhibited retrieval of ENaC subunits from the plasma membrane; the end result is increased expression of activated ENaC channels at the plasma membrane of principal cells. Patients classically manifest severe hypertension with hypokalemia that is unresponsive to spironolactone yet sensitive to amiloride. Hypertension and hypokalemia are, however, variable aspects of the Liddle's phenotype; more consistent features include a blunted aldosterone response to ACTH and reduced urinary aldosterone excretion.

Loss of the transport functions of the TALH and DCT nephron segments causes two distinct subtypes of hereditary hypokalemic alkalosis, with TALH dysfunction causing Bartter's syndrome (BS) and DCT dysfunction causing Gitelman's syndrome (GS). Patients with "classic" BS typically have polyuria and polydipsia due to the reduction in renal concentrating ability. They may have an increase in urinary calcium excretion, and 20% are hypomagnesemic. Other features include marked activation of the renin-angiotensin-aldosterone axis. Patients with "antenatal" BS have a severe systemic disorder characterized by marked electrolyte wasting, polyhydramnios, and hypercalciuria with nephrocalcinosis; renal prostaglandin synthesis and excretion are increased significantly, accounting for many of the systemic symptoms. There are five disease genes for BS, all of which function in some aspect of regulated Na$^+$, K$^+$, and Cl$^-$ transport by the TALH. Gitelman's syndrome is, in contrast, genetically homogeneous, caused almost exclusively by loss-of-function mutations in the thiazide-sensitive Na$^+$-Cl$^-$ cotransporter of the DCT. Patients with GS are uniformly hypomagnesemic and exhibit marked hypocalciuria rather than the hypercalciuria typically seen in BS; urinary calcium excretion is thus a critical diagnostic test in GS. GS has a milder phenotype than BS; however, patients with GS may suffer from chondrocalcinosis, an abnormal deposition of calcium pyrophosphate dihydrate (CPPD) in joint cartilage (Chap. 284).

Magnesium deficiency and hypokalemia

Magnesium depletion has inhibitory effects on muscle Na$^+$,K$^+$-ATPase activity, reducing influx into muscle cells and causing a secondary kaliuresis. In addition, magnesium depletion causes exaggerated K$^+$ secretion by the distal nephron; this is attributed to a reduction in the magnesium-dependent, intracellular block of K$^+$ efflux through the secretory K$^+$ channel of principal cells (ROMK; Fig. 45-4). Regardless of the dominant mechanism(s), hypomagnesemic patients are clinically refractory to K$^+$ replacement in the absence of Mg^{2+} repletion. Notably, magnesium deficiency is also a common concomitant of hypokalemia, since many disorders of the distal nephron may cause both potassium and magnesium wasting (Chap. 284).

Clinical features

Hypokalemia has prominent effects on cardiac, skeletal, and intestinal muscle cells. In particular, it is a major risk factor for both ventricular and atrial arrhythmias. Hypokalemia predisposes to digoxin toxicity by a number of mechanisms, including reduced competition between K$^+$ and digoxin for shared binding sites on cardiac Na$^+$,K$^+$-ATPase subunits. Electrocardiographic changes in hypokalemia include broad flat T waves, ST depression, and QT prolongation; these are most marked when serum K$^+$ is <2.7 mmol/L. Hypokalemia also results in hyperpolarization of skeletal muscle, thus impairing the capacity to depolarize and contract; weakness and even paralysis may ensue. It also causes a skeletal myopathy and predisposes to rhabdomyolysis. Finally, the paralytic effects of hypokalemia on intestinal smooth muscle may cause intestinal ileus.

The functional effects of hypokalemia on the kidney include Na^+-Cl^- and HCO_3^- retention, polyuria, phosphaturia, hypocitraturia, and an activation of renal ammoniagenesis. Bicarbonate retention and other acid-base effects of hypokalemia can contribute to the generation of metabolic alkalosis. Hypokalemic polyuria is due to a combination of polydipsia and an AVP-resistant renal concentrating defect. Structural changes in the kidney due to hypokalemia include a relatively specific vacuolizing injury to proximal tubular cells, interstitial nephritis, and renal cysts. Hypokalemia also predisposes to acute kidney injury and can lead to end-stage renal disease in patients with long-standing hypokalemia due to eating disorders and/or laxative abuse.

Hypokalemia and/or reduced dietary K^+ are implicated in the pathophysiology and progression of hypertension, heart failure, and stroke. For example, short-term K^+ restriction in healthy humans and patients with essential hypertension induces Na^+-Cl^- retention and hypertension. Correction of hypokalemia is particularly important in hypertensive patients treated with diuretics, in whom blood pressure improves with the establishment of normokalemia.

Diagnostic approach

The cause of hypokalemia is usually evident from history, physical examination, and/or basic laboratory tests. The history should focus on medications (e.g., laxatives, diuretics, antibiotics), diet and dietary habits (e.g., licorice), and/or symptoms that suggest a particular cause (e.g., periodic weakness, diarrhea). The physical examination should pay particular attention to blood pressure, volume status, and signs suggestive of specific hypokalemic disorders, e.g., hyperthyroidism and Cushing's syndrome. Initial laboratory evaluation should include electrolytes, BUN, creatinine, serum osmolality, Mg^{2+}, Ca^{2+}, a complete blood count, and urinary pH (Fig. 45-7). The presence of a non-anion-gap acidosis suggests a distal, hypokalemic renal tubular acidosis or diarrhea; calculation of the urinary anion gap can help differentiate these two diagnoses. Renal K^+ excretion can be assessed with a 24-h urine collection; a 24-h K^+ excretion of <15 mM is indicative of an extrarenal cause of hypokalemia (Fig. 45-7). Alternatively, serum and urine osmolality can be used to calculate the transtubular K^+ gradient (TTKG), which should be <3-4 in the presence of hypokalemia (see the section on hyperkalemia in this chapter). Urine Cl^- is usually decreased in patients with hypokalemia from a nonreabsorbable anion, such as antibiotics or HCO_3^-. Other causes of chronic, hypokalemic alkalosis are surreptitious vomiting, diuretic abuse, and GS. Hypokalemic patients with bulimia thus have a urinary Cl^- <10 mmol/L; urine Na^+, K^+, and Cl^- are persistently elevated in GS due to loss of function in the thiazide-sensitive Na^+-Cl^- cotransporter but less elevated in diuretic abuse and with greater variability. Urine diuretic screens for loop diuretics and thiazides may be necessary to further exclude diuretic abuse.

Other tests, such as urinary Ca^{2+}, thyroid function tests, and/or PRA and aldosterone levels, may be appropriate in specific cases. A plasma aldosterone:PRA ratio >50 is suggestive of hyperaldosteronism. Patients with hyperaldosteronism or apparent mineralocorticoid excess may require further testing, for example, adrenal vein sampling (Chap. 342) or the clinically available tests for specific genetic causes (FH-I, SAME, Liddle's syndrome, etc.). Patients with primary aldosteronism thus should be tested for the chimeric FH-I/GRA gene (see above) if they are younger than 20 years of age or have a family history of primary aldosteronism or stroke at a young age (<40 years). Preliminary differentiation of Liddle's syndrome due to mutant ENaC channels from SAME due to mutant 11βHSD-2 (see above)—both of which cause hypokalemia and hypertension with aldosterone suppression—can be made on a clinical basis; patients with Liddle's syndrome should respond to amiloride (ENaC inhibition) but not spironolactone, whereas patients with SAME will respond to spironolactone.

TREATMENT   Hypokalemia

The goals of therapy for hypokalemia are to prevent life-threatening and/or chronic consequences, replace the associated K^+ deficit, and correct the underlying cause and/or mitigate future hypokalemia. The urgency of therapy depends on the severity of hypokalemia, associated clinical factors (cardiac disease, digoxin therapy, etc.), and the rate of decline in serum K^+. Urgent but cautious K^+ replacement should be considered in patients with severe redistributive hypokalemia (plasma K^+ concentration <2.5 mM) and/or when serious complications ensue; however, this creates a risk of rebound hyperkalemia after resolution of the underlying cause. When excessive activity of the sympathetic nervous system is thought to play a dominant role in redistributive hypokalemia, as in thyrotoxic periodic paralysis, high-dose propranolol (3 mg/kg) should be considered; this nonspecific β-adrenergic blocker will correct hypokalemia without the risk of rebound hyperkalemia.

Oral replacement with K^+-Cl^- is the mainstay of therapy for hypokalemia. Potassium phosphate, oral or IV, may be appropriate in patients with combined hypokalemia and hypophosphatemia. Potassium bicarbonate or potassium citrate should be considered in patients with concomitant metabolic acidosis. Notably, hypomagnesemic patients are refractory to K^+ replacement alone, and so concomitant Mg^{2+} deficiency should *always* be corrected with oral or intravenous repletion. The deficit of K^+ and the rate of correction should be estimated as accurately as possible; renal function, medications, and comorbid conditions such as diabetes should be considered to gauge the risk of overcorrection. In the absence of abnormal K^+ redistribution, the total deficit correlates with serum K^+ so that serum K^+ drops by approximately 0.27 mM for every 100-mmol reduction in total-body stores; loss of 400 to 800 mmol of total-body K^+ results in a reduction in serum K^+ of approximately 2.0 mM. However, because of the difficulty in assessing the deficit accurately, plasma K^+ concentration must be monitored carefully during repletion.

The use of intravenous administration should be limited to patients unable to utilize the enteral route or in the setting of severe complications (paralysis, arrhythmia, etc.). Intravenous K^+-Cl^- should always be administered in saline solutions rather than dextrose since the dextrose-induced increase in insulin can acutely exacerbate hypokalemia. The peripheral intravenous dose is usually 20–40 mmol of K^+-Cl^- per liter; higher concentrations can cause localized pain from chemical phlebitis, irritation, and sclerosis. If hypokalemia is severe (<2.5 mmol/L) and/or critically symptomatic, intravenous K^+-Cl^- can be administered through a central vein with cardiac monitoring in an intensive care setting at rates of 10–20 mmol/h; higher rates should be reserved for acutely life-threatening complications. The absolute amount of administered K^+ should be restricted (e.g., 20 mmol in 100 mL of saline solution) to prevent inadvertent infusion of a large dose. Femoral veins are preferable, since infusion through internal jugular or subclavian central lines can acutely increase the local concentration of K^+ and affect cardiac conduction.

Strategies to minimize K^+ losses also should be considered. These measures may include minimizing the dose of non-K^+-sparing diuretics, restricting Na^+ intake, and using clinically appropriate combinations of non-K^+-sparing and K^+-sparing medications (e.g., loop diuretics with ACE inhibitors).

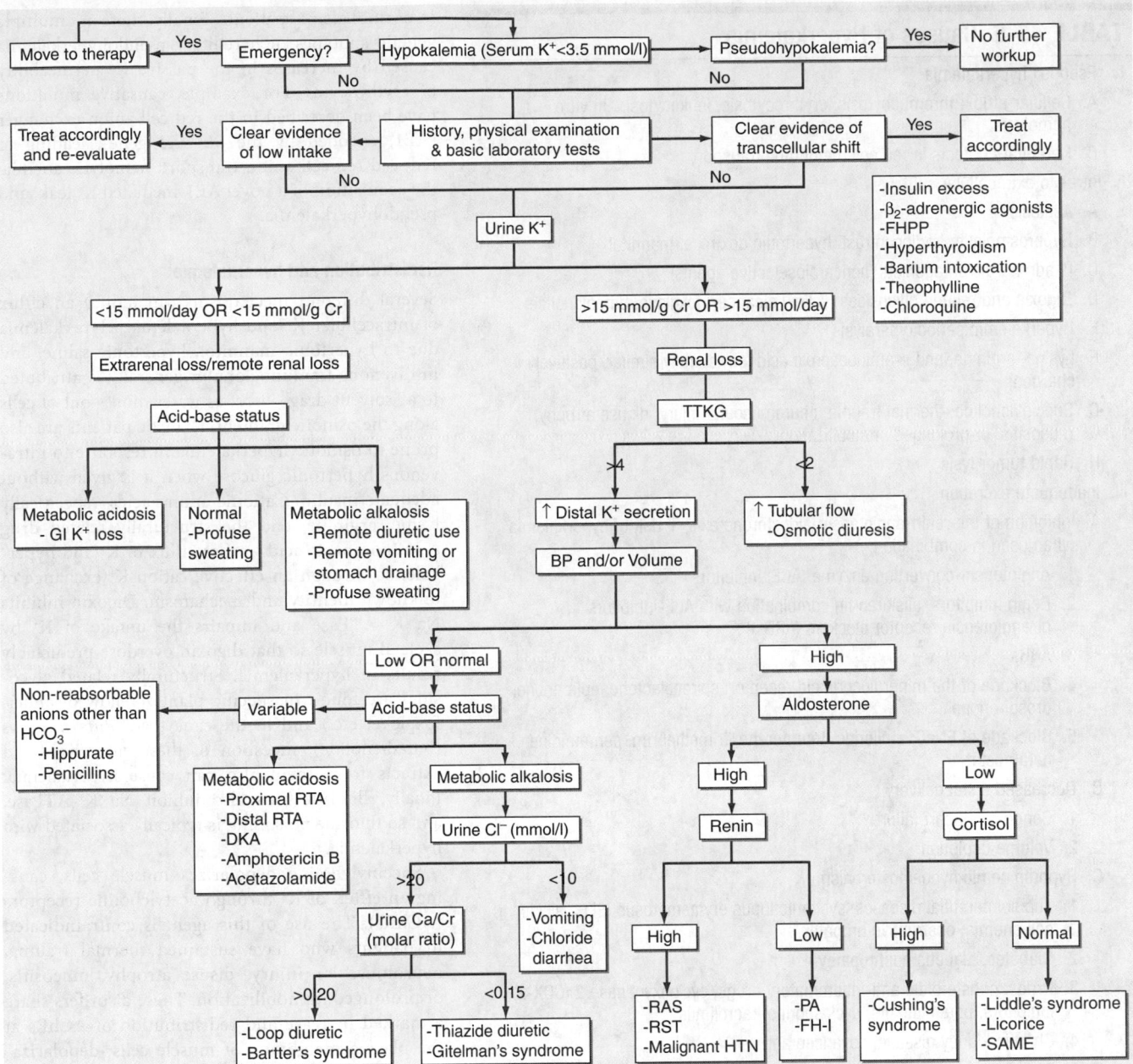

Figure 45-7 The diagnostic approach to hypokalemia. See text for details. BP, blood pressure; DKA, diabetic ketoacidosis; FHPP, familial hypokalemic periodic paralysis; FH-I, familial hyperaldosteronism type I; GI, gastrointestinal; HTN, hypertension; PA, primary aldosteronism; RAS, renal artery stenosis; RST, renin-secreting tumor; RTA, renal tubular acidosis; SAME, syndrome of apparent mineralocorticoid excess; TTKG, transtubular potassium gradient. *(From Mount and Zandi-Nejad; with permission.)*

■ HYPERKALEMIA

Hyperkalemia is defined as a plasma potassium level of 5.5 m*M*. It occurs in up to 10% of hospitalized patients; severe hyperkalemia (>6.0 m*M*) occurs in approximately 1%, with a significantly increased risk of mortality. Although redistribution and reduced tissue uptake can acutely cause hyperkalemia, a decrease in renal K$^+$ excretion is the most common underlying cause (Table 45-5). Excessive intake of K$^+$ is a rare cause because of the adaptive capacity to increase renal secretion; however, dietary intake can have a major effect in susceptible patients, e.g., diabetic patients with hyporeninemic hypoaldosteronism and chronic kidney disease. Drugs that have an impact on the renin-angiotensin-aldosterone axis are also a major cause of hyperkalemia.

Pseudohyperkalemia

Hyperkalemia should be distinguished from factitious hyperkalemia or pseudohyperkalemia, an artifactual increase in serum K$^+$ due to the release of K$^+$ during or after venipuncture. Pseudohyperkalemia can occur in the setting of excessive muscle activity during venipuncture (fist clenching, etc.), a marked increase in cellular elements (thrombocytosis, leukocytosis, and/or erythrocytosis) with in vitro efflux of K$^+$, and acute anxiety during venipuncture with respiratory alkalosis and redistributive hyperkalemia. Cooling of blood after venipuncture is another cause, due to reduced cellular uptake; the converse is the increased uptake of K$^+$ by cells at high ambient temperatures, leading to normal values for hyperkalemic patients and/or to spurious hypokalemia

TABLE 45-5 Causes of Hyperkalemia

I. "Pseudo" hyperkalemia

  A. Cellular efflux: thrombocytosis, erythrocytosis, leukocytosis, in vitro hemolysis

  B. Hereditary defects in red cell membrane transport

II. Intra- to extracellular shift

  A. Acidosis

  B. Hyperosmolality; radiocontrast, hypertonic dextrose, mannitol

  C. β-adrenergic antagonists (noncardioselective agents)

  D. Digoxin and related glycosides (yellow oleander, foxglove, bufadienolide)

  E. Hyperkalemic periodic paralysis

  F. Lysine, arginine, and ε-aminocaproic acid (structurally similar, positively charged)

  G. Succinylcholine; thermal trauma, neuromuscular injury, disuse atrophy, mucositis, or prolonged immobilization

  H. Rapid tumor lysis

III. Inadequate excretion

  A. Inhibition of the renin-angiotensin-aldosterone axis; ↑ risk of hyperkalemia when used in combination

    1. Angiotensin-converting enzyme (ACE) inhibitors

    2. Renin inhibitors: aliskiren [in combination with ACE-inhibitors or angiotensin receptor blockers (ARBs)]

    3. ARBs

    4. Blockade of the mineralocorticoid receptor: spironolactone, eplerenone, drospirenone

    5. Blockade of ENaC: amiloride, triamterene, trimethoprim, pentamidine, nafamostat

  B. Decreased distal delivery

    1. Congestive heart failure

    2. Volume depletion

  C. Hyporeninemic hypoaldosteronism

    1. Tubulointerstitial diseases: systemic lupus erythematosus (SLE), sickle cell anemia, obstructive uropathy

    2. Diabetes, diabetic nephropathy

    3. Drugs: nonsteroidal anti-inflammatory drugs, cyclooxygenase 2 (COX-2) inhibitors, beta blockers, cyclosporine, tacrolimus

    4. Chronic kidney disease, advanced age

    5. Pseudohypoaldosteronism type II: defects in WNK1 or WNK4 kinases

  D. Renal resistance to mineralocorticoid

    1. Tubulointerstitial diseases: SLE, amyloidosis, sickle cell anemia, obstructive uropathy, post-acute tubular necrosis

    2. Hereditary: pseudohypoaldosteronism type I: defects in the mineralocorticoid receptor *or* ENaC

  E. Advanced renal insufficiency

    1. Chronic kidney disease

    2. End-stage renal disease

    3. Acute oliguric kidney injury

  F. Primary adrenal insufficiency

    1. Autoimmune: Addison's disease, polyglandular endocrinopathy

    2. Infectious: HIV, cytomegalovirus, tuberculosis, disseminated fungal infection

    3. Infiltrative: amyloidosis, malignancy, metastatic cancer

    4. Drug-associated: heparin, low-molecular-weight heparin

    5. Hereditary: adrenal hypoplasia congenita, congenital lipoid adrenal hyperplasia, aldosterone synthase deficiency

    6. Adrenal hemorrhage or infarction, including in antiphospholipid syndrome

in normokalemic patients. Finally, there are multiple genetic subtypes of hereditary pseudohyperkalemia caused by increases in the passive K^+ permeability of erythrocytes. For example, causative mutations have been described in the red cell anion exchanger (AE1, encoded by the *SLC4A1* gene), leading to reduced red cell anion transport, hemolytic anemia, the acquisition of a novel AE1-mediated K^+ leak, and pseudohyperkalemia.

Redistribution and hyperkalemia

Several different mechanisms can induce an efflux of intracellular K^+ and hyperkalemia. Hyperkalemia due to hypertonic mannitol, hypertonic saline, and intravenous immunoglobulin generally is attributed to a "solvent drag" effect as water moves out of cells along the osmotic gradient. Diabetic patients are also prone to osmotic hyperkalemia in response to intravenous hypertonic glucose when it is given without adequate insulin. Cationic amino acids—specifically lysine, arginine, and the structurally related drug ε-aminocaproic acid—cause efflux of K^+ and hyperkalemia through an effective cation-K^+ exchange of unknown identity and mechanism. Digoxin inhibits Na^+,K^+-ATPase and impairs the uptake of K^+ by skeletal muscle so that digoxin overdose predictably results in hyperkalemia. Structurally related glycosides are found in specific plants (yellow oleander, foxglove, etc.) and in the cane toad, *Bufo marinus* (bufadienolide); ingestion of these substances and extracts from them also can cause hyperkalemia. Finally, fluoride ions also inhibit Na^+,K^+-ATPase, and so fluoride poisoning is typically associated with hyperkalemia.

Succinylcholine depolarizes muscle cells, causing an efflux of K^+ through acetylcholine receptors (AChRs). The use of this agent is contraindicated in patients who have sustained thermal trauma, neuromuscular injury, disuse atrophy, mucositis, or prolonged immobilization. These disorders share a marked increase and redistribution of AChRs at the plasma membrane of muscle cells; depolarization of these upregulated AChRs by succinylcholine leads to an exaggerated efflux of K^+ through the receptor-associated cation channels, resulting in acute hyperkalemia.

Hyperkalemia due to excess intake or tissue necrosis

Increased intake of even small amounts of K^+ may provoke severe hyperkalemia in patients with predisposing factors; hence, an assessment of dietary intake is crucial. Foods rich in potassium include tomatoes, bananas, and citrus fruits; occult sources of K^+, particularly K^+-containing salt substitutes, also may contribute significantly. Iatrogenic causes include simple overreplacement with K^+-Cl^- and the administration of a potassium-containing medication (e.g., K^+-penicillin) to a susceptible patient. Red cell transfusion is a well-described cause of hyperkalemia, typically in the setting of massive transfusions. Finally, tissue necrosis, as in acute tumor lysis syndrome and rhabdomyolysis, predictably causes hyperkalemia from the release of intracellular K^+.

Hypoaldosteronism and hyperkalemia

Aldosterone release from the adrenal gland may be reduced by hyporeninemic hypoaldosteronism, medications, or primary hypoaldosteronism or by isolated deficiency of ACTH (secondary hypoaldosteronism). Primary hypoaldosteronism may be genetic or acquired (Chap. 342) but is commonly caused by autoimmunity either in Addison's disease or in the context of a polyglandular endocrinopathy. HIV has surpassed tuberculosis as the most important infectious cause of adrenal insufficiency. The adrenal involvement in HIV disease is usually subclinical; however, adrenal insufficiency may be precipitated by stress, drugs such as ketoconazole that inhibit steroidogenesis, or the acute withdrawal of steroid agents such as megestrol.

Hyporeninemic hypoaldosteronism is a very common predisposing factor in several overlapping subsets of hyperkalemic patients: diabetic patients, the elderly, and patients with renal insufficiency. Classically, these patients should have suppressed PRA and aldosterone; approximately 50% have an associated acidosis with a reduced renal excretion of NH_4^+, a positive urinary anion gap, and urine pH <5.5. Most patients are volume expanded, with secondary increases in circulating atrial natriuretic peptide (ANP) that inhibit both renal renin release and adrenal aldosterone release.

Renal disease and hyperkalemia

Chronic kidney disease and end-stage kidney disease are very common causes of hyperkalemia because of the associated deficit or absence of functioning nephrons. Hyperkalemia is more common in oliguric acute kidney injury; distal tubular flow rate and Na^+ delivery is less of a limiting factor in nonoliguric patients. Hyperkalemia out of proportion to GFR can also be seen in the context of tubulointerstitial disease that affects the distal nephron, such as amyloidosis, sickle cell anemia, interstitial nephritis, and obstructive uropathy.

Hereditary renal causes of hyperkalemia have overlapping clinical features with hypoaldosteronism, hence the diagnostic label *pseudohypoaldosteronism* (PHA). PHA-I has both an autosomal recessive and an autosomal dominant form. The autosomal dominant form is due to loss-of-function mutations in MLR; the recessive form is caused by various combinations of mutations in the three subunits of ENaC, resulting in impaired Na^+ channel activity in principal cells and other tissues. Patients with recessive PHA-I experience lifelong salt wasting, hypotension, and hyperkalemia, whereas the phenotype of autosomal dominant PHA-I due to MLR dysfunction improves in adulthood. Pseudohypoaldosteronism type II (PHA-II, also known as hereditary hypertension with hyperkalemia) is in every respect the mirror image of GS caused by loss of function in NCC, the thiazide-sensitive Na^+-Cl^- cotransporter (see above); the clinical phenotype includes hypertension, hyperkalemia, hyperchloremic metabolic acidosis, suppressed PRA and aldosterone, hypercalciuria, and reduced bone density. PHA-II thus behaves like a gain of function in NCC, and treatment with thiazides results in resolution of the entire clinical phenotype; however, PHA-II is caused by mutations in the WNK1 and WNK4 serine-threonine kinases, which regulate NCC activity.

Medication-associated hyperkalemia

Most medications associated with hyperkalemia cause inhibition of some component of the renin-angiotensin-aldosterone axis. ACE inhibitors, angiotensin-receptor blockers, renin inhibitors, and mineralocorticoid receptors are predictable and common causes of hyperkalemia, particularly when prescribed in combination. The oral contraceptive agent Yasmin-28 contains the progestin drospirenone, which inhibits the MLR and can cause hyperkalemia in susceptible patients. Cyclosporine, tacrolimus, NSAIDs,

and cyclooxygenase 2 (COX-2) inhibitors cause hyperkalemia by multiple mechanisms but share the ability to cause hyporeninemic hypoaldosteronism. Notably, most drugs that affect the renin-angiotensin-aldosterone axis also block the local adrenal response to hyperkalemia, thus attenuating the *direct* stimulation of aldosterone release by increased plasma K^+ concentration.

Inhibition of apical ENaC activity in the distal nephron by amiloride and other K^+-sparing diuretics results in hyperkalemia, often with a voltage-dependent hyperchloremic acidosis and/or hypovolemic hyponatremia. Amiloride is structurally similar to the antibiotics trimethoprim (TMP) and pentamidine, which also block ENaC; risk factors for TMP-associated hyperkalemia include the administered dose, renal insufficiency, and hyporeninemic hypoaldosteronism. Indirect inhibition of ENaC at the plasma membrane is also a cause of hyperkalemia; nafamostat, a protease inhibitor utilized in the management of pancreatitis, inhibits aldosterone-induced proteases that activate ENaC by proteolytic cleavage.

Clinical features

Hyperkalemia is a medical emergency because of its effects on the heart. Cardiac arrhythmias associated with hyperkalemia include sinus bradycardia, sinus arrest, slow idioventricular rhythms, ventricular tachycardia, ventricular fibrillation, and asystole. Mild increases in extracellular K^+ affect the repolarization phase of the cardiac action potential, resulting in changes in T-wave morphology; further increase in plasma K^+ concentration depresses intracardiac conduction, with progressive prolongation of the PR and QRS intervals. Severe hyperkalemia results in loss of the P wave and a progressive widening of the QRS complex; development of a sine-wave sinoventricular rhythm suggests impending ventricular fibrillation or asystole. Classically, the electrocardiographic manifestations in hyperkalemia progress from tall peaked T waves (5.5–6.5 mM), to a loss of P waves (6.5–7.5 mM), to a widened QRS complex (7–8 mM), and ultimately to a sine wave pattern (8 mM). However, these changes are notoriously insensitive, particularly in patients with chronic kidney disease or end-stage renal disease.

Hyperkalemia from a variety of causes can also present with ascending paralysis; this is denoted secondary hyperkalemic paralysis to differentiate it from familial hyperkalemic periodic paralysis (HYPP). The presentation may include diaphragmatic paralysis and respiratory failure. Patients with familial HYPP develop myopathic weakness during hyperkalemia induced by increased K^+ intake or rest after heavy exercise. Depolarization of skeletal muscle by hyperkalemia unmasks an inactivation defect in skeletal Na^+ channels; autosomal dominant mutations in the *SCN4A* gene encoding this channel are the predominant cause.

Within the kidney, hyperkalemia has negative effects on the ability to excrete an acid load, and so hyperkalemia per se can contribute to metabolic acidosis. This defect appears to be due in part to competition between K^+ and NH_4^+ for reabsorption by the TALH and subsequent countercurrent multiplication, ultimately reducing the medullary gradient for NH_3/NH_4 excretion by the distal nephron. Regardless of the underlying mechanism, restoration of normokalemia can in many instances correct hyperkalemic metabolic acidosis.

Diagnostic approach

The first priority in the management of hyperkalemia is to assess the need for emergency treatment, followed by a comprehensive workup to determine the cause (Fig. 45-8). History and physical examination should focus on medications, diet and dietary supplements, risk factors for kidney failure, reduction in urine output, blood pressure, and volume status. Initial laboratory tests should include electrolytes, BUN, creatinine, serum osmolality, Mg^{2+} and

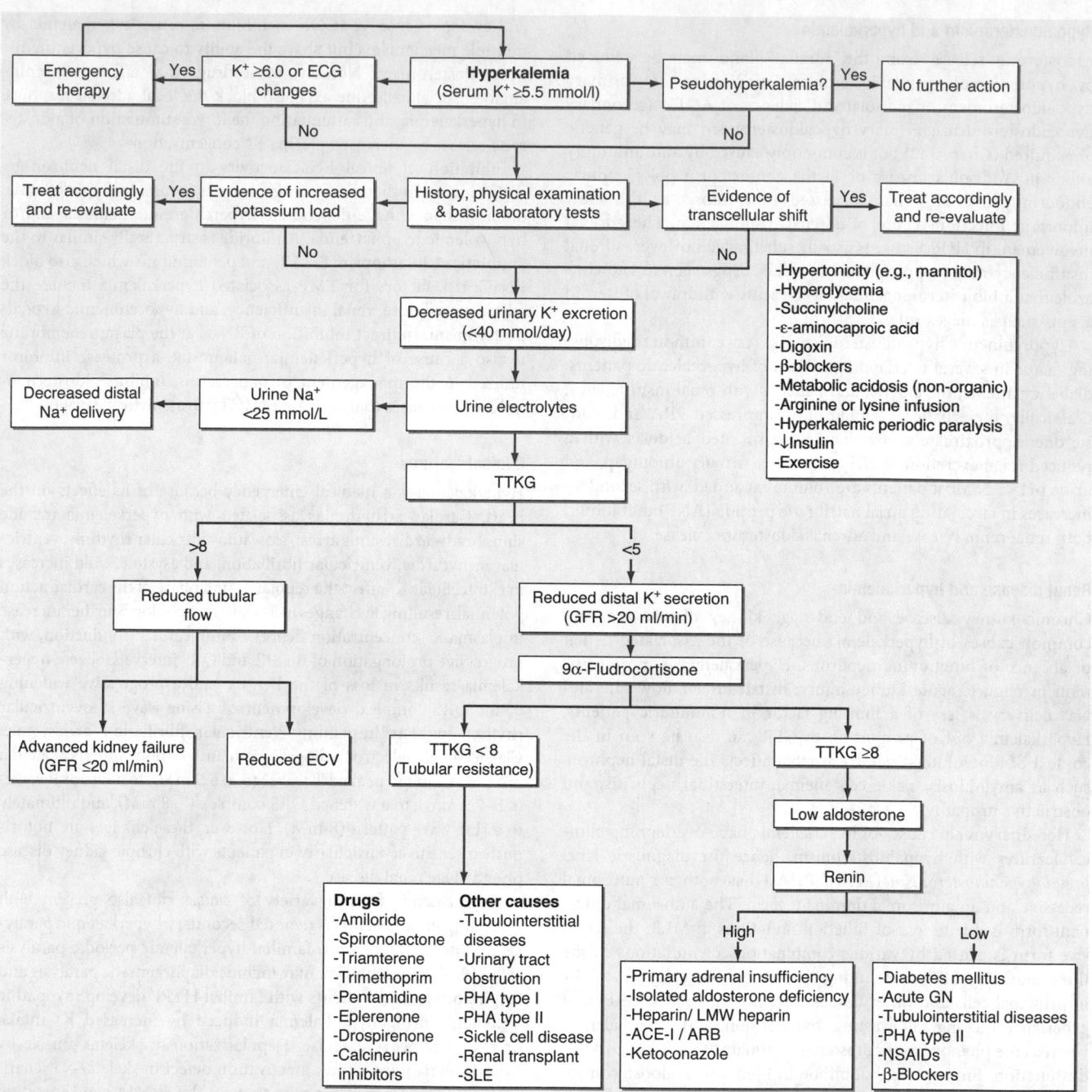

Figure 45-8 The diagnostic approach to hyperkalemia. See text for details. ACE-I, angiotensin converting enzyme inhibitor; acute GN, acute glomerulonephritis; ARB, angiotensin II receptor blocker; ECG, electrocardiogram; ECV, effective circulatory volume; GFR, glomerular filtration rate; LMW heparin, low-molecular-weight heparin; NSAIDs, nonsteroidal anti-inflammatory drugs; PHA, pseudohypoaldosteronism; SLE, systemic lupus erythematosus; TTKG, transtubular potassium gradient. *(From Mount and Zandi-Nejad; with permission.)*

Ca^{2+}, a complete blood count, and urinary pH. A urine Na^+ concentration <20 mM indicates that distal Na^+ delivery is a limiting factor in K^+ excretion; volume repletion with 0.9% saline or treatment with furosemide may be effective in reducing plasma K^+ concentration. Serum and urine osmolality is required for calculation of the TTKG (Fig. 45-8). The expected values of the TTKG are largely based on historic data and are <3-4 in the presence of hypokalemia and >6-7 in the presence of hyperkalemia. TTKG is measured as follows:

$$TTKG = \frac{[K^+]_{urine} \times osmol_{serum}}{[K^+]_{serum} \times osmol_{urine}}$$

TREATMENT Hyperkalemia

Electrocardiographic manifestations of hyperkalemia should be considered a medical emergency and treated urgently. However, patients with significant hyperkalemia (plasma K^+ concentration ≥6.5–7 mM) in the absence of ECG changes should be aggressively managed because of the limitations of ECG changes as a predictor of cardiac toxicity. Urgent management of hyperkalemia includes admission to the hospital, continuous cardiac monitoring, and immediate treatment. The treatment of hyperkalemia is divided into three stages:

1. *Immediate antagonism of the cardiac effects of hyperkalemia.* Intravenous calcium serves to protect the heart while measures are taken to correct hyperkalemia. Calcium raises the action potential threshold and reduces excitability without changing the resting membrane potential. By restoring the difference between the resting and threshold potentials, calcium reverses the depolarization blockade caused by hyperkalemia. The recommended dose is 10 mL of 10% calcium gluconate (3–4 mL of calcium chloride), infused intravenously over 2 to 3 min with cardiac monitoring. The effect of the infusion starts in 1–3 min and lasts 30–60 min; the dose should be repeated if there is no change in ECG findings or if they recur after initial improvement. Hypercalcemia potentiates the cardiac toxicity of digoxin; hence, intravenous calcium should be used with extreme caution in patients taking this medication. If judged necessary, 10 mL of 10% calcium gluconate can be added to 100 mL of 5% dextrose in water and infused over 20–30 min to avoid acute hypercalcemia.

2. *Rapid reduction in plasma K^+ concentration by redistribution into cells.* Insulin lowers plasma K^+ concentration by shifting K^+ into cells. The recommended dose is 10 units of IV regular insulin followed immediately by 50 mL of 50% dextrose (D50W, 25 g of glucose total); the effect begins in 10–20 min, peaks at 30–60 min, and lasts 4 to 6 h. Bolus D50W without insulin is *never* appropriate because of the risk of acutely worsening hyperkalemia due to the osmotic effect of hypertonic glucose. Hypoglycemia is common with insulin plus glucose; hence, this should be followed by an infusion of 10% dextrose at 50 to 75 mL/h, with close monitoring of plasma glucose concentration. In hyperkalemic patients with glucose concentrations ≥200–250 mg/dL, insulin should be administered *without* glucose, again with close monitoring of glucose concentrations.

3. β_2-agonists, most commonly albuterol, are effective but underutilized agents for the acute management of hyperkalemia. Albuterol and insulin with glucose have an additive effect on plasma K^+ concentration; however, ~20% of patients with end-stage renal disease are resistant to the effect of β_2-agonists; hence, these drugs should not be used without insulin. The recommended dose for inhaled albuterol is 10–20 mg of nebulized albuterol in 4 mL of normal saline, inhaled over 10 min; the effect starts at about 30 min, reaches its peak at about 90 min, and lasts 2–6 h. Hyperglycemia is a side effect, along with tachycardia; β_2-agonists should be used with caution in hyperkalemic patients with known cardiac disease.

Intravenous bicarbonate has no role in the routine treatment of hyperkalemia. It should be reserved for patients with hyperkalemia and concomitant metabolic acidosis, and only if judged appropriate for management of the acidosis. It should not be given as a hypertonic intravenous bolus in light of the risk of hypernatremia but should be infused in an isotonic or hypotonic fluid (e.g., 150 meq in 1 L of D5W).

Removal of potassium. This typically is accomplished by using cation exchange resins, diuretics, and/or dialysis. Sodium polystyrene sulfonate (SPS) exchanges Na^+ for K^+ in the gastrointestinal tract and increases the fecal excretion of K^+. The recommended dose of SPS is 15-30 g, typically given in a premade suspension with 33% sorbitol to avoid constipation. The effect of SPS on plasma K^+ concentration is slow; the full effect may take up to 24 hours and usually requires repeated doses every 4–6 hours. Intestinal necrosis is the most serious complication of SPS. Studies in experimental animals suggest that sorbitol is required for the intestinal injury; however, SPS crystals can often be detected in the injured human intestine, suggesting a direct role for SPS crystals in this complication. Regardless, in light of the risk of intestinal necrosis, the U.S. Food and Drug Administration has recently stated that the administration of sorbitol with SPS is no longer recommended; however, administering SPS without sorbitol might not eliminate the risk of intestinal necrosis, given the evident role for the SPS resin. Therefore, clinicians must carefully consider whether emergency treatment with SPS is necessary and appropriate for the treatment of hyperkalemia; for example, SPS is unnecessary if acute dialysis is appropriate and immediately available. If SPS is administered, the preparation should ideally not contain sorbitol. Reasonable substitutes for the laxative effect of sorbitol include lactulose and some preparations of polyethylene glycol 3350; however, data demonstrating the efficacy and safety of these laxatives with SPS are not available. SPS should not be administered in patients at higher risk for intestinal necrosis, including postoperative patients, patients with a history of bowel obstruction, patients with slow intestinal transit, patients with ischemic bowel disease, and renal transplant patients. Loop and thiazide diuretics can be utilized to reduce plasma K^+ concentration in volume-replete or hypervolemic patients with sufficient renal function for a diuretic response. Finally, hemodialysis is the most effective and reliable method to reduce plasma K^+ concentration; peritoneal dialysis is considerably less effective. The amount of K^+ removed during hemodialysis depends on the relative distribution of K^+ between ICF and ECF (potentially affected by prior therapy for hyperkalemia), the type and surface area of the dialyzer used, dialysate and blood flow rates, the dialysate flow rate, dialysis duration, and the plasma to dialysate K^+ gradient.

FURTHER READINGS

ADROGUE HJ, MADIAS NE: Hypernatremia. N Engl J Med 342:1493, 2000

ELLISON DH, BERL T: Clinical practice: The syndrome of inappropriate antidiuresis. N Engl J Med 356:2064, 2007

MOHMAND HK et al: Hypertonic saline for hyponatremia: Risk of inadvertent overcorrection. Clin J Am Soc Nephrol 2:1110, 2007

MOUNT DB, ZANDI-NEJAD K: Disorders of potassium balance, in *Brenner and Rector's The Kidney*, 8th ed, BM Brenner (ed). Philadelphia, W.B. Saunders, 2008, pp 547–587

PERIANAYAGAM A et al: DDAVP is effective in preventing and reversing inadvertent overcorrection of hyponatremia. Clin J Am Soc Nephrol 3:331, 2008

SCHRIER RW: Decreased effective blood volume in edematous disorders: What does this mean? J Am Soc Nephrol 18:2028, 2007

―――― et al: Tolvaptan, a selective oral vasopressin V2-receptor antagonist, for hyponatremia. N Engl J Med 355:2099, 2006

STERNS RH et al: Ion-exchange resins for the treatment of hyperkalemia: Are they safe and effective? J Am Soc Nephrol 21:733, 2010

CHAPTER 46

Hypercalcemia and Hypocalcemia

Sundeep Khosla

The calcium ion plays a critical role in normal cellular function and signaling, regulating diverse physiologic processes such as neuromuscular signaling, cardiac contractility, hormone secretion, and blood coagulation. Thus, extracellular calcium concentrations are maintained within an exquisitely narrow range through a series of feedback mechanisms that involve parathyroid hormone (PTH) and the active vitamin D metabolite 1,25-dihydroxyvitamin D [1,25(OH)$_2$D]. These feedback mechanisms are orchestrated by integrating signals between the parathyroid glands, kidney, intestine, and bone (Fig. 46-1; Chap. 352).

Disorders of serum calcium concentration are relatively common and often serve as a harbinger of underlying disease. This chapter provides a brief summary of the approach to patients with altered serum calcium levels. See Chap. 353 for a detailed discussion of this topic.

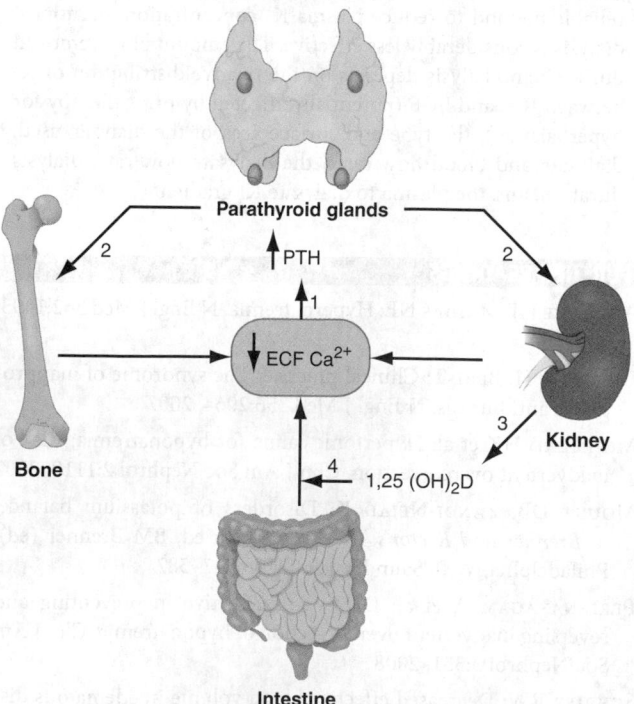

Figure 46-1   Feedback mechanisms maintaining extracellular calcium concentrations within a narrow, physiologic range [8.9–10.1 mg/dL (2.2–2.5 mM)]. A decrease in extracellular (ECF) calcium (Ca^{2+}) triggers an increase in parathyroid hormone (PTH) secretion (1) via the calcium sensor receptor on parathyroid cells. PTH, in turn, results in increased tubular reabsorption of calcium by the kidney (2) and resorption of calcium from bone (2) and also stimulates renal 1,25(OH)$_2$D production (3). 1,25(OH)$_2$D, in turn, acts principally on the intestine to increase calcium absorption (4). Collectively, these homeostatic mechanisms serve to restore serum calcium levels to normal.

HYPERCALCEMIA

ETIOLOGY

The causes of hypercalcemia can be understood and classified based on derangements in the normal feedback mechanisms that regulate serum calcium (Table 46-1). Excess PTH production, which is not appropriately suppressed by increased serum calcium concentrations, occurs in primary neoplastic disorders of the parathyroid glands (parathyroid adenomas; hyperplasia; or, rarely, carcinoma) that are associated with increased parathyroid cell mass and impaired feedback inhibition by calcium. Inappropriate PTH secretion for the ambient level of serum calcium also occurs with heterozygous inactivating calcium sensor receptor (CaSR) mutations, which impair extracellular calcium sensing by the parathyroid glands and the kidneys, resulting in familial hypocalciuric hypercalcemia (FHH). Although PTH secretion by tumors is extremely rare, many solid tumors produce PTH-related peptide (PTHrP), which shares homology with PTH in the first 13 amino acids and binds the PTH receptor, thus mimicking effects of PTH on bone and the kidney. In PTHrP-mediated hypercalcemia of malignancy, PTH levels are suppressed by the high serum calcium levels. Hypercalcemia associated with granulomatous disease (e.g., sarcoidosis) or lymphomas is caused by enhanced conversion of 25(OH)D to the potent 1,25(OH)$_2$D. In these disorders, 1,25(OH)$_2$D enhances intestinal calcium absorption, resulting in hypercalcemia and suppressed PTH. Disorders that directly increase calcium mobilization from bone, such as hyperthyroidism or osteolytic metastases, also lead to hypercalcemia with suppressed PTH secretion as does exogenous calcium overload, as in milk-alkali syndrome, or total parenteral nutrition with excessive calcium supplementation.

TABLE 46-1   Causes of Hypercalcemia

Excessive PTH production

Primary hyperparathyroidism (adenoma, hyperplasia, rarely carcinoma)

Tertiary hyperparathyroidism (long-term stimulation of PTH secretion in renal insufficiency)

Ectopic PTH secretion (very rare)

Inactivating mutations in the CaSR (FHH)

Alterations in CaSR function (lithium therapy)

Hypercalcemia of malignancy

Overproduction of PTHrP (many solid tumors)

Lytic skeletal metastases (breast, myeloma)

Excessive 1,25(OH)$_2$D production

Granulomatous diseases (sarcoidosis, tuberculosis, silicosis)

Lymphomas

Vitamin D intoxication

Primary increase in bone resorption

Hyperthyroidism

Immobilization

Excessive calcium intake

Milk-alkali syndrome

Total parenteral nutrition

Other causes

Endocrine disorders (adrenal insufficiency, pheochromocytoma, VIPoma)

Medications (thiazides, vitamin A, antiestrogens)

Abbreviations: CaSR, calcium sensor receptor; FHH, familial hypocalciuric hypercalcemia; PTH, parathyroid hormone; PTHrP, PTH-related peptide.

■ CLINICAL MANIFESTATIONS

Mild hypercalcemia (up to 11–11.5 mg/dL) is usually asymptomatic and recognized only on routine calcium measurements. Some patients may complain of vague neuropsychiatric symptoms, including trouble concentrating, personality changes, or depression. Other presenting symptoms may include peptic ulcer disease or nephrolithiasis, and fracture risk may be increased. More severe hypercalcemia (>12–13 mg/dL), particularly if it develops acutely, may result in lethargy, stupor, or coma, as well as gastrointestinal symptoms (nausea, anorexia, constipation, or pancreatitis). Hypercalcemia decreases renal concentrating ability, which may cause polyuria and polydipsia. With long-standing hyperparathyroidism, patients may present with bone pain or pathologic fractures. Finally, hypercalcemia can result in significant electrocardiographic changes, including bradycardia, AV block, and short QT interval; changes in serum calcium can be monitored by following the QT interval (Fig. 228-16).

■ DIAGNOSTIC APPROACH

The first step in the diagnostic evaluation of hyper- or hypocalcemia is to ensure that the alteration in serum calcium levels is not due to abnormal albumin concentrations. About 50% of total calcium is ionized, and the rest is bound principally to albumin. Although direct measurements of ionized calcium are possible, they are easily influenced by collection methods and other artifacts; thus, it is generally preferable to measure total calcium and albumin to "correct" the serum calcium. When serum albumin concentrations are reduced, a corrected calcium concentration is calculated by adding 0.2 mM (0.8 mg/dL) to the total calcium level for every decrement in serum albumin of 1.0 g/dL below the reference value of 4.1 g/dL for albumin, and, conversely, for elevations in serum albumin.

A detailed history may provide important clues regarding the etiology of the hypercalcemia (Table 46-1). Chronic hypercalcemia is most commonly caused by primary hyperparathyroidism, as opposed to the second most common etiology of hypercalcemia, an underlying malignancy. The history should include medication use, previous neck surgery, and systemic symptoms suggestive of sarcoidosis or lymphoma.

Once true hypercalcemia is established, the second most important laboratory test in the diagnostic evaluation is a PTH level using a two-site assay for the intact hormone. Increases in PTH are often accompanied by hypophosphatemia. In addition, serum creatinine should be measured to assess renal function; hypercalcemia may impair renal function, and renal clearance of PTH may be altered depending on the fragments detected by the assay. If the PTH level is increased (or "inappropriately normal") in the setting of elevated calcium and low phosphorus, the diagnosis is almost always primary hyperparathyroidism. Because individuals with familial hypocalciuric hypercalcemia (FHH) may also present with mildly elevated PTH levels and hypercalcemia, this diagnosis should be considered and excluded because parathyroid surgery is ineffective in this condition. A calcium/creatinine clearance ratio (calculated as urine calcium/serum calcium divided by urine creatinine/serum creatinine) of <0.01 is suggestive of FHH, particularly when there is a family history of mild, asymptomatic hypercalcemia. In addition, a number of laboratories are now offering sequence analysis of the CaSR gene for the definitive diagnosis of FHH. Ectopic PTH secretion is extremely rare.

A suppressed PTH level in the face of hypercalcemia is consistent with non-parathyroid-mediated hypercalcemia, most often due to underlying malignancy. Although a tumor that causes hypercalcemia is generally overt, a PTHrP level may be needed to establish the diagnosis of hypercalcemia of malignancy. Serum 1,25(OH)$_2$D levels are increased in granulomatous disorders, and clinical evaluation in combination with laboratory testing will generally provide a diagnosis for the various disorders listed in Table 46-1.

TREATMENT Hypercalcemia

Mild, asymptomatic hypercalcemia does not require immediate therapy, and management should be dictated by the underlying diagnosis. By contrast, significant, symptomatic hypercalcemia usually requires therapeutic intervention independent of the etiology of hypercalcemia. Initial therapy of significant hypercalcemia begins with volume expansion because hypercalcemia invariably leads to dehydration; 4–6 L of intravenous saline may be required over the first 24 h, keeping in mind that underlying comorbidities (e.g., congestive heart failure) may require the use of loop diuretics to enhance sodium and calcium excretion. However, loop diuretics should not be initiated until the volume status has been restored to normal. If there is increased calcium mobilization from bone (as in malignancy or severe hyperparathyroidism), drugs that inhibit bone resorption should be considered. Zoledronic acid (e.g., 4 mg intravenously over ~30 min), pamidronate (e.g., 60–90 mg intravenously over 2–4 h), and etidronate (e.g., 7.5 mg/kg per day for 3–7 consecutive days) are approved by the U.S. Food and Drug Administration for the treatment of hypercalcemia of malignancy in adults. Onset of action is within 1–3 days, with normalization of serum calcium levels occurring in 60–90% of patients. Bisphosphonate infusions may need to be repeated if hypercalcemia relapses. Because of their effectiveness, bisphosphonates have replaced calcitonin or plicamycin, which are rarely used in current practice for the management of hypercalcemia. In rare instances, dialysis may be necessary. Finally, while intravenous phosphate chelates calcium and decreases serum calcium levels, this therapy can be toxic because calcium-phosphate complexes may deposit in tissues and cause extensive organ damage.

In patients with 1,25(OH)$_2$D-mediated hypercalcemia, glucocorticoids are the preferred therapy, as they decrease 1,25(OH)$_2$D production. Intravenous hydrocortisone (100–300 mg daily) or oral prednisone (40–60 mg daily) for 3–7 days are used most often. Other drugs, such as ketoconazole, chloroquine, and hydroxychloroquine, may also decrease 1,25(OH)$_2$D production and are used occasionally.

HYPOCALCEMIA

■ ETIOLOGY

The causes of hypocalcemia can be differentiated according to whether serum PTH levels are low (hypoparathyroidism) or high (secondary hyperparathyroidism). Although there are many potential causes of hypocalcemia, impaired PTH or vitamin D production are the most common etiologies (Table 46-2) (Chap. 353). Because PTH is the main defense against hypocalcemia, disorders associated with deficient PTH production or secretion may be associated with profound, life-threatening hypocalcemia. In adults, hypoparathyroidism most commonly results from inadvertent damage to all four glands during thyroid or parathyroid gland surgery. Hypoparathyroidism is a cardinal feature of autoimmune endocrinopathies (Chap. 351); rarely, it may be associated with infiltrative diseases such as sarcoidosis. Impaired PTH secretion may be secondary to magnesium deficiency or to activating mutations in the CaSR, which suppress PTH, leading to effects that are opposite to those that occur in FHH.

Vitamin D deficiency, impaired 1,25(OH)$_2$D production (primarily secondary to renal insufficiency), or vitamin D resistance also cause hypocalcemia. However, the degree of hypocalcemia in these disorders is generally not as severe as that seen with hypoparathyroidism because the parathyroids are capable of mounting a compensatory increase in PTH secretion. Hypocalcemia may also

TABLE 46-2 Causes of Hypocalcemia

Low Parathyroid Hormone Levels (Hypoparathyroidism)

Parathyroid agenesis
  Isolated
  DiGeorge syndrome
Parathyroid destruction
  Surgical
  Radiation
  Infiltration by metastases or systemic diseases
  Autoimmune
Reduced parathyroid function
  Hypomagnesemia
  Activating CaSR mutations

High Parathyroid Hormone Levels (Secondary Hyperparathyroidism)

Vitamin D deficiency or impaired $1,25(OH)_2D$ production/action
  Nutritional vitamin D deficiency (poor intake or absorption)
  Renal insufficiency with impaired $1,25(OH)_2D$ production
  Vitamin D resistance, including receptor defects
Parathyroid hormone resistance syndromes
  PTH receptor mutations
  Pseudohypoparathyroidism (G protein mutations)
Drugs
  Calcium chelators
  Inhibitors of bone resorption (bisphosphonates, plicamycin)
  Altered vitamin D metabolism (phenytoin, ketoconazole)
Miscellaneous causes
  Acute pancreatitis
  Acute rhabdomyolysis
  Hungry bone syndrome after parathyroidectomy
  Osteoblastic metastases with marked stimulation of bone formation (prostate cancer)

Abbreviations: CaSR, calcium sensor receptor; PTH, parathyroid hormone.

occur in conditions associated with severe tissue injury such as burns, rhabdomyolysis, tumor lysis, or pancreatitis. The cause of hypocalcemia in these settings may include a combination of low albumin, hyperphosphatemia, tissue deposition of calcium, and impaired PTH secretion.

■ CLINICAL MANIFESTATIONS

Patients with hypocalcemia may be asymptomatic if the decreases in serum calcium are relatively mild and chronic, or they may present with life-threatening complications. Moderate to severe hypocalcemia is associated with paresthesias, usually of the fingers, toes, and circumoral regions, and is caused by increased neuromuscular irritability. On physical examination, a Chvostek's sign (twitching of the circumoral muscles in response to gentle tapping of the facial nerve just anterior to the ear) may be elicited, although it is also present in ~10% of normal individuals. Carpal spasm may be induced by inflation of a blood pressure cuff to 20 mmHg above the patient's systolic blood pressure for 3 min (Trousseau's sign). Severe hypocalcemia can induce seizures, carpopedal spasm, bronchospasm, laryngospasm, and prolongation of the QT interval.

■ DIAGNOSTIC APPROACH

In addition to measuring serum calcium, it is useful to determine albumin, phosphorus, and magnesium levels. As for the evaluation of hypercalcemia, determining the PTH level is central to the evaluation of hypocalcemia. A suppressed (or "inappropriately low") PTH level in the setting of hypocalcemia establishes absent or reduced PTH secretion (hypoparathyroidism) as the cause of the hypocalcemia. Further history will often elicit the underlying cause (i.e., parathyroid agenesis vs. destruction). By contrast, an elevated PTH level (secondary hyperparathyroidism) should direct attention to the vitamin D axis as the cause of the hypocalcemia. Nutritional vitamin D deficiency is best assessed by obtaining serum 25-hydroxyvitamin D levels, which reflect vitamin D stores. In the setting of renal insufficiency or suspected vitamin D resistance, serum $1,25(OH)_2D$ levels are informative.

TREATMENT   Hypocalcemia

The approach to treatment depends on the severity of the hypocalcemia, the rapidity with which it develops, and the accompanying complications (e.g., seizures, laryngospasm). Acute, symptomatic hypocalcemia is initially managed with calcium gluconate, 10 mL 10% wt/vol (90 mg or 2.2 mmol) intravenously, diluted in 50 mL of 5% dextrose or 0.9% sodium chloride, given intravenously over 5 min. Continuing hypocalcemia often requires a constant intravenous infusion (typically 10 ampuls of calcium gluconate or 900 mg of calcium in 1 L of 5% dextrose or 0.9% sodium chloride administered over 24 h). Accompanying hypomagnesemia, if present, should be treated with appropriate magnesium supplementation.

Chronic hypocalcemia due to hypoparathyroidism is treated with calcium supplements (1000–1500 mg/d elemental calcium in divided doses) and either vitamin D_2 or D_3 (25,000–100,000 U daily) or calcitriol [$1,25(OH)_2D$, 0.25–2 μg/d]. Other vitamin D metabolites (dihydrotachysterol, alfacalcidiol) are now used less frequently. Vitamin D deficiency, however, is best treated using vitamin D supplementation, with the dose depending on the severity of the deficit and the underlying cause. Thus, nutritional vitamin D deficiency generally responds to relatively low doses of vitamin D (50,000 U, 2–3 times per week for several months), while vitamin D deficiency due to malabsorption may require much higher doses (100,000 U/d or more). The treatment goal is to bring serum calcium into the low normal range and to avoid hypercalciuria, which may lead to nephrolithiasis.

FURTHER READINGS

Bilezikian JP: Primary hyperparathyroidism and hypoparathyroidism, in *Conn's Current Therapy*, RE Rakel, ET Bope (eds), Philadelphia, Elsevier, 2009

Bilezikian JP, Khan AA et al: Guidelines for the management of asymptomatic primary hyperparathyroidism: Summary statement from the third international workship. J Clin Endocrinol Metab 94:335, 2009

Egbuna OI, Brown EM: Hypercalcaemic and hypocalcaemic conditions due to calcium-sensing receptor mutations. Best Pract Clin Rheumatol 22:129, 2008

Shoback D: Clinical practice. Hypoparathyroidism. N Engl J Med 359:391, 2008

Stewart AF: Hypercalcemia associated with cancer. N Engl J Med 352:373, 2005

CHAPTER **47**

Acidosis and Alkalosis

Thomas D. DuBose, Jr.

NORMAL ACID-BASE HOMEOSTASIS

Systemic arterial pH is maintained between 7.35 and 7.45 by extracellular and intracellular chemical buffering together with respiratory and renal regulatory mechanisms. The control of arterial CO_2 tension (Pa_{CO_2}) by the central nervous system (CNS) and respiratory systems and the control of the plasma bicarbonate by the kidneys stabilize the arterial pH by excretion or retention of acid or alkali. The metabolic and respiratory components that regulate systemic pH are described by the Henderson-Hasselbalch equation:

$$pH = 6.1 + \log \frac{HCO_3^-}{Pa_{CO_2} \times 0.0301}$$

Under most circumstances, CO_2 production and excretion are matched, and the usual steady-state Pa_{CO_2} is maintained at 40 mmHg. Underexcretion of CO_2 produces hypercapnia, and overexcretion causes hypocapnia. Nevertheless, production and excretion are again matched at a new steady-state Pa_{CO_2}. Therefore, the Pa_{CO_2} is regulated primarily by neural respiratory factors and is not subject to regulation by the rate of CO_2 production. Hypercapnia is usually the result of hypoventilation rather than of increased CO_2 production. Increases or decreases in Pa_{CO_2} represent derangements of neural respiratory control or are due to compensatory changes in response to a primary alteration in the plasma $[HCO_3^-]$.

The kidneys regulate plasma $[HCO_3^-]$ through three main processes: (1) "reabsorption" of filtered HCO_3^-, (2) formation of titratable acid, and (3) excretion of NH_4^+ in the urine. The kidney filters ~4000 mmol of HCO_3^- per day. To reabsorb the filtered load of HCO_3^-, the renal tubules must therefore secrete 4000 mmol of hydrogen ions. Between 80 and 90% of HCO_3^- is reabsorbed in the proximal tubule. The distal nephron reabsorbs the remainder and secretes H^+ to defend systemic pH. While this quantity of protons, 40–60 mmol/d, is small, it must be secreted to prevent chronic positive H^+ balance and metabolic acidosis. This quantity of secreted protons is represented in the urine as titratable acid and NH_4^+. Metabolic acidosis in the face of normal renal function increases NH_4^+ production and excretion. NH_4^+ production and excretion are impaired in chronic renal failure, hyperkalemia, and renal tubular acidosis.

DIAGNOSIS OF GENERAL TYPES OF DISTURBANCES

The most common clinical disturbances are simple acid-base disorders; i.e., metabolic acidosis or alkalosis or respiratory acidosis or alkalosis. Because compensation is not complete, the pH is abnormal in simple disturbances. More complicated clinical situations can give rise to mixed acid-base disturbances.

■ SIMPLE ACID-BASE DISORDERS

Primary respiratory disturbances (primary changes in Pa_{CO_2}) invoke compensatory metabolic responses (secondary changes in $[HCO_3^-]$), and primary metabolic disturbances elicit predictable compensatory respiratory responses (secondary changes in Pa_{CO_2}). Physiologic compensation can be predicted from the relationships displayed in Table 47-1. Metabolic acidosis due to an increase in

TABLE 47-1 Prediction of Compensatory Responses on Simple Acid-Base Disturbances and Pattern of Changes

Disorder	Prediction of Compensation	Range of Values		
		pH	HCO_3^-	Pa_{CO_2}
Metabolic acidosis	$Pa_{CO_2} = (1.5 \times HCO_3^-) + 8 \pm 2$ or Pa_{CO_2} will ↓ 1.25 mmHg per mmol/L ↓ in $[HCO_3^-]$ or $Pa_{CO_2} = [HCO_3^-] + 15$	Low	Low	Low
Metabolic alkalosis	Pa_{CO_2} will ↑ 0.75 mmHg per mmol/L ↑ in $[HCO_3^-]$ or Pa_{CO_2} will ↑ 6 mmHg per 10 mmol/L ↑ in $[HCO_3^-]$ or $Pa_{CO_2} = [HCO_3^-] + 15$	High	High	High
Respiratory alkalosis		High	Low	Low
Acute	$[HCO_3^-]$ will ↓ 0.2 mmol/L per mmHg ↓ in Pa_{CO_2}			
Chronic	$[HCO_3^-]$ will ↓ 0.4 mmol/L per mmHg ↓ in Pa_{CO_2}			
Respiratory acidosis		Low	High	High
Acute	$[HCO_3^-]$ will ↑ 0.1 mmol/L per mmHg ↑ in Pa_{CO_2}			
Chronic	$[HCO_3^-]$ will ↑ 0.4 mmol/L per mmHg ↑ in Pa_{CO_2}			

endogenous acids (e.g., ketoacidosis) lowers extracellular fluid $[HCO_3^-]$ and decreases extracellular pH. This stimulates the medullary chemoreceptors to increase ventilation and to return the ratio of $[HCO_3^-]$ to Pa_{CO_2}, and thus pH, toward, but not to, normal. The degree of respiratory compensation expected in a simple form of metabolic acidosis can be predicted from the relationship: $Pa_{CO_2} = (1.5 \times [HCO_3^-]) + 8 \pm 2$. Thus, a patient with metabolic acidosis and $[HCO_3^-]$ of 12 mmol/L would be expected to have a Pa_{CO_2} between 24 and 28 mmHg. Values for Pa_{CO_2} <24 or >28 mmHg define a mixed disturbance (metabolic acidosis and respiratory alkalosis or metabolic alkalosis and respiratory acidosis, respectively). Another way to judge the appropriateness of the response in $[HCO_3^-]$

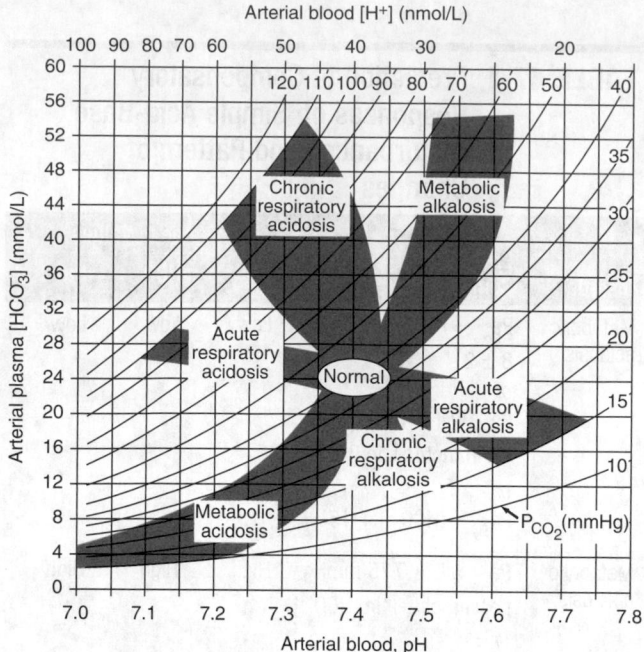

Figure 47-1   Acid-base nomogram. Shown are the 90% confidence limits (range of values) of the normal respiratory and metabolic compensations for primary acid-base disturbances. *(From DuBose, used with permission.)*

or Pa_{CO_2} is to use an acid-base nomogram (Fig. 47-1). While the shaded areas of the nomogram show the 95% confidence limits for normal compensation in simple disturbances, finding acid-base values within the shaded area does not necessarily rule out a mixed disturbance. Imposition of one disorder over another may result in values lying within the area of a third. Thus, the nomogram, while convenient, is not a substitute for the equations in Table 47-1.

■ MIXED ACID-BASE DISORDERS

Mixed acid-base disorders—defined as independently coexisting disorders, not merely compensatory responses—are often seen in patients in critical care units and can lead to dangerous extremes of pH (Table 47-2). A patient with diabetic ketoacidosis (metabolic acidosis) may develop an independent respiratory problem (e.g., pneumonia) leading to respiratory acidosis or alkalosis. Patients with underlying pulmonary disease (e.g., COPD) may not respond to metabolic acidosis with an appropriate ventilatory response because of insufficient respiratory reserve. Such imposition of respiratory acidosis on metabolic acidosis can lead to severe acidemia. When metabolic acidosis and metabolic alkalosis coexist in the same patient, the pH may be normal or near normal. When the pH is normal, an elevated anion gap (AG; see below) reliably denotes the presence of an AG metabolic acidosis. A discrepancy in the ΔAG (prevailing minus normal AG) and the ΔHCO$_3^-$ (normal minus prevailing HCO$_3^-$) indicates the presence of a mixed high-gap acidosis—metabolic alkalosis (see example below). A diabetic patient with ketoacidosis may have renal dysfunction resulting in simultaneous metabolic acidosis. Patients who have ingested an overdose of drug combinations such as sedatives and salicylates may have mixed disturbances as a result of the acid-base response to the individual drugs (metabolic acidosis mixed with respiratory acidosis or respiratory alkalosis, respectively). Triple acid-base disturbances are more complex. For example, patients with metabolic acidosis due to alcoholic ketoacidosis may develop metabolic alkalosis due to vomiting and superimposed respiratory alkalosis due to the hyperventilation of hepatic dysfunction or alcohol withdrawal.

TABLE 47-2   Examples of Mixed Acid-Base Disorders

Mixed Metabolic and Respiratory

Metabolic acidosis—respiratory alkalosis

Key: High- or normal-AG metabolic acidosis; prevailing Pa_{CO_2} *below* predicted value (Table 47-1)

Example: Na$^+$, 140; K$^+$, 4.0; Cl$^-$, 106; HCO$_3^-$, 14; AG, 20; Pa_{CO_2}, 24; pH, 7.39 (lactic acidosis, sepsis in ICU)

Metabolic acidosis—respiratory acidosis

Key: High- or normal-AG metabolic acidosis; prevailing Pa_{CO_2} *above* predicted value (Table 47-1)

Example: Na$^+$, 140; K$^+$, 4.0; Cl$^-$, 102; HCO$_3^-$, 18; AG, 20; Pa_{CO_2}, 38; pH, 7.30 (severe pneumonia, pulmonary edema)

Metabolic alkalosis—respiratory alkalosis

Key: Pa_{CO_2} does not increase as predicted; pH higher than expected

Example: Na$^+$, 140; K$^+$, 4.0; Cl$^-$, 91; HCO$_3^-$, 33; AG, 16; Pa_{CO_2}, 38; pH, 7.55 (liver disease and diuretics)

Metabolic alkalosis—respiratory acidosis

Key: Pa_{CO_2} higher than predicted; pH normal

Example: Na$^+$, 140; K$^+$, 3.5; Cl$^-$, 88; HCO$_3^-$, 42; AG, 10; Pa_{CO_2}, 67; pH, 7.42 (COPD on diuretics)

Mixed Metabolic Disorders

Metabolic acidosis—metabolic alkalosis

Key: Only detectable with high-AG acidosis; ΔAG >> ΔHCO$_3^-$

Example: Na$^+$, 140; K$^+$, 3.0; Cl$^-$, 95; HCO$_3^-$, 25; AG, 20; Pa_{CO_2}, 40; pH, 7.42 (uremia with vomiting)

Metabolic acidosis—metabolic acidosis

Key: Mixed high-AG—normal-AG acidosis; ΔHCO$_3^-$ accounted for by combined change in ΔAG and ΔCl$^-$

Example: Na$^+$, 135; K$^+$, 3.0; Cl$^-$, 110; HCO$_3^-$, 10; AG, 15; Pa_{CO_2}, 25; pH, 7.20 (diarrhea and lactic acidosis, toluene toxicity, treatment of diabetic ketoacidosis)

Abbreviations: AG, anion gap; COPD, chronic obstructive pulmonary disease; ICU, intensive care unit.

> **APPROACH TO THE PATIENT**   **Acid-Base Disorders**

A stepwise approach to the diagnosis of acid-base disorders follows (Table 47-3). Care should be taken when measuring blood gases to obtain the arterial blood sample without using excessive heparin. Blood for electrolytes and arterial blood gases should be drawn simultaneously prior to therapy, because an increase in [HCO$_3^-$] occurs with metabolic alkalosis and respiratory acidosis. Conversely, a decrease in [HCO$_3^-$] occurs in metabolic acidosis and respiratory alkalosis. In the determination of arterial blood gases by the clinical laboratory, both pH and Pa_{CO_2} are measured, and the [HCO$_3^-$] is calculated from the Henderson-Hasselbalch equation. This calculated value should be compared with the measured [HCO$_3^-$] (total CO$_2$) on the electrolyte panel. These two values should agree within 2 mmol/L. If they do not, the values may not have been drawn simultaneously, a laboratory error may be present, or an error could have been made in calculating the [HCO$_3^-$]. After verifying the blood acid-base values, the precise acid-base disorder can then be identified.

TABLE 47-3 Steps in Acid-Base Diagnosis

1. Obtain arterial blood gas (ABG) and electrolytes simultaneously.
2. Compare [HCO_3^-] on ABG and electrolytes to verify accuracy.
3. Calculate anion gap (AG).
4. Know four causes of high-AG acidosis (ketoacidosis, lactic acid acidosis, renal failure, and toxins).
5. Know two causes of hyperchloremic or nongap acidosis (bicarbonate loss from GI tract, renal tubular acidosis).
6. Estimate compensatory response (Table 47-1).
7. Compare ΔAG and ΔHCO_3^-.
8. Compare change in [Cl^-] with change in [Na^+].

CALCULATE THE ANION GAP All evaluations of acid-base disorders should include a simple calculation of the AG; it represents those unmeasured anions in plasma (normally 10 to 12 mmol/L) and is calculated as follows: $AG = Na^+ - (Cl^- + HCO_3^-)$. The unmeasured anions include anionic proteins, (e.g., albumin), phosphate, sulfate, and organic anions. When acid anions, such as acetoacetate and lactate, accumulate in extracellular fluid, the AG increases, causing a high-AG acidosis. An increase in the AG is most often due to an increase in unmeasured anions and, less commonly, is due to a decrease in unmeasured cations (calcium, magnesium, potassium). In addition, the AG may increase with an increase in anionic albumin, because of either increased albumin concentration or alkalosis, which alters albumin charge. A decrease in the AG can be due to (1) an increase in unmeasured cations; (2) the addition to the blood of abnormal cations, such as lithium (lithium intoxication) or cationic immunoglobulins (plasma cell dyscrasias); (3) a reduction in the major plasma anion albumin concentration (nephrotic syndrome); (4) a decrease in the effective anionic charge on albumin by acidosis; or (5) hyperviscosity and severe hyperlipidemia, which can lead to an underestimation of sodium and chloride concentrations. A fall in serum albumin by 1 g/dL from the normal value (4.5 g/dL) decreases the AG by 2.5 meq/L. Know the common causes of a high-AG acidosis (Table 47-3).

In the face of a normal serum albumin, a high AG is usually due to non-chloride containing acids that contain inorganic (phosphate, sulfate), organic (ketoacids, lactate, uremic organic anions), exogenous (salicylate or ingested toxins with organic acid production), or unidentified anions. The high AG is significant even if an additional acid-base disorder is superimposed to modify the [HCO_3^-] independently. Simultaneous metabolic acidosis of the high-AG variety plus either chronic respiratory acidosis or metabolic alkalosis represents such a situation in which [HCO_3^-] may be normal or even high (Table 47-3). Compare the change in [HCO_3^-] (ΔHCO_3^-) and the change in the AG (ΔAG).

Similarly, normal values for [HCO_3^-], Pa_{CO_2}, and pH do not ensure the absence of an acid-base disturbance. For instance, an alcoholic who has been vomiting may develop a metabolic alkalosis with a pH of 7.55, Pa_{CO_2} of 47 mmHg, [HCO_3^-] of 40 mmol/L, [Na^+] of 135, [Cl^-] of 80, and [K^+] of 2.8. If such a patient were then to develop a superimposed alcoholic ketoacidosis with a β-hydroxybutyrate concentration of 15 mM, arterial pH would fall to 7.40, [HCO_3^-] to 25 mmol/L, and the Pa_{CO_2} to 40 mmHg. Although these blood gases are normal, the AG is elevated at 30 mmol/L, indicating a mixed metabolic alkalosis and metabolic acidosis. A mixture of high-gap acidosis and metabolic

alkalosis is recognized easily by comparing the differences (Δ values) in the normal to prevailing patient values. In this example, the ΔHCO_3^- is 0 (25 – 25 mmol/L) but the ΔAG is 20 (30 – 10 mmol/L). Therefore, 20 mmol/L is unaccounted for in the Δ/Δ value (ΔAG to ΔHCO_3^-).

METABOLIC ACIDOSIS

Metabolic acidosis can occur because of an increase in endogenous acid production (such as lactate and ketoacids), loss of bicarbonate (as in diarrhea), or accumulation of endogenous acids (as in renal failure). Metabolic acidosis has profound effects on the respiratory, cardiac, and nervous systems. The fall in blood pH is accompanied by a characteristic increase in ventilation, especially the tidal volume (Kussmaul respiration). Intrinsic cardiac contractility may be depressed, but inotropic function can be normal because of catecholamine release. Both peripheral arterial vasodilation and central venoconstriction can be present; the decrease in central and pulmonary vascular compliance predisposes to pulmonary edema with even minimal volume overload. CNS function is depressed, with headache, lethargy, stupor, and, in some cases, even coma. Glucose intolerance may also occur.

There are two major categories of clinical metabolic acidosis: high-AG and normal-AG, or hyperchloremic acidosis (Table 47-3 and Table 47-4).

TREATMENT Metabolic Acidosis

Treatment of metabolic acidosis with alkali should be reserved for severe acidemia except when the patient has no "potential HCO_3^-" in plasma. Potential [HCO_3^-] can be estimated from the increment (Δ) in the AG (ΔAG = patient's AG – 10). It must be determined if the acid anion in plasma is metabolizable (i.e., β-hydroxybutyrate, acetoacetate, and lactate) or nonmetabolizable (anions that accumulate in chronic renal failure and after toxin ingestion). The latter requires return of renal function to replenish the [HCO_3^-] deficit, a slow and often unpredictable process. Consequently, patients with a normal AG acidosis (hyperchloremic acidosis), a slightly elevated AG (mixed hyperchloremic and AG acidosis), or an AG attributable to a nonmetabolizable anion in the face of renal failure should receive alkali therapy, either PO ($NaHCO_3$ or Shohl's solution) or IV ($NaHCO_3$), in an amount necessary to slowly increase the plasma [HCO_3^-] into the 20–22 mmol/L range.

Controversy exists, however, in regard to the use of alkali in patients with a pure AG acidosis owing to accumulation of a metabolizable organic acid anion (ketoacidosis or lactic

TABLE 47-4 Causes of High–Anion Gap Metabolic Acidosis

Lactic acidosis	Toxins
Ketoacidosis	Ethylene glycol
Diabetic	Methanol
Alcoholic	Salicylates
Starvation	Propylene glycol
	Pyroglutamic acid
	Renal failure (acute and chronic)

acidosis). In general, severe acidosis (pH < 7.10) warrants the IV administration of 50–100 meq of NaHCO₃, over 30–45 min, during the initial 1–2 h of therapy. Provision of such modest quantities of alkali in this situation seems to provide an added measure of safety, but it is essential to monitor plasma electrolytes during the course of therapy, because the [K⁺] may decline as pH rises. The goal is to increase the [HCO₃⁻] to 10 meq/L and the pH to 7.20, not to increase these values to normal.

HIGH–ANION GAP ACIDOSES

APPROACH TO THE PATIENT | **High–Anion Gap Acidoses**

There are four principal causes of a high-AG acidosis: (1) lactic acidosis, (2) ketoacidosis, (3) ingested toxins, and (4) acute and chronic renal failure (Table 47-4). Initial screening to differentiate the high-AG acidoses should include (1) a probe of the history for evidence of drug and toxin ingestion and measurement of arterial blood gas to detect coexistent respiratory alkalosis (salicylates); (2) determination of whether diabetes mellitus is present (diabetic ketoacidosis); (3) a search for evidence of alcoholism or increased levels of β-hydroxybutyrate (alcoholic ketoacidosis); (4) observation for clinical signs of uremia and determination of the blood urea nitrogen (BUN) and creatinine (uremic acidosis); (5) inspection of the urine for oxalate crystals (ethylene glycol); and (6) recognition of the numerous clinical settings in which lactate levels may be increased (hypotension, shock, cardiac failure, leukemia, cancer, and drug or toxin ingestion).

Lactic acidosis

An increase in plasma L-lactate may be secondary to poor tissue perfusion (type A)—circulatory insufficiency (shock, cardiac failure), severe anemia, mitochondrial enzyme defects, and inhibitors (carbon monoxide, cyanide)—or to aerobic disorders (type B)—malignancies, nucleoside analogue reverse transcriptase inhibitors in HIV, diabetes mellitus, renal or hepatic failure, thiamine deficiency, severe infections (cholera, malaria), seizures, or drugs/toxins (biguanides, ethanol, methanol, propylene glycol, isoniazid, and fructose). Propylene glycol may be used as a vehicle for IV medications including lorazepam, and toxicity has been reported in several settings. Unrecognized bowel ischemia or infarction in a patient with severe atherosclerosis or cardiac decompensation receiving vasopressors is a common cause of lactic acidosis. Pyroglutamic acidemia has been reported in critically ill patients receiving acetaminophen, which is associated with depletion of glutathione. D-Lactic acid acidosis, which may be associated with jejunoileal bypass, short bowel syndrome, or intestinal obstruction, is due to formation of D-lactate by gut bacteria.

APPROACH TO THE PATIENT | **Lactic Acid Acidosis**

The underlying condition that disrupts lactate metabolism must first be corrected; tissue perfusion must be restored when inadequate. Vasoconstrictors should be avoided, if possible, because they may worsen tissue perfusion. Alkali therapy is generally advocated for acute, severe acidemia (pH < 7.15) to improve cardiac function and lactate use. However, NaHCO₃ therapy may paradoxically depress cardiac performance and exacerbate acidosis by enhancing lactate production (HCO₃⁻ stimulates phosphofructokinase). While the use of alkali in moderate lactic acidosis is controversial, it is generally agreed that attempts to return the pH or [HCO₃⁻] to normal by administration of

exogenous NaHCO₃ are deleterious. A reasonable approach is to infuse sufficient NaHCO₃ to raise the arterial pH to no more than 7.2 over 30–40 min.

NaHCO₃ therapy can cause fluid overload and hypertension because the amount required can be massive when accumulation of lactic acid is relentless. Fluid administration is poorly tolerated because of central venoconstriction, especially in the oliguric patient. When the underlying cause of the lactic acidosis can be remedied, blood lactate will be converted to HCO₃⁻ and may result in an overshoot alkalosis.

Ketoacidosis

Diabetic ketoacidosis (DKA) This condition is caused by increased fatty acid metabolism and the accumulation of ketoacids (acetoacetate and β-hydroxybutyrate). DKA usually occurs in insulin-dependent diabetes mellitus in association with cessation of insulin or an intercurrent illness such as an infection, gastroenteritis, pancreatitis, or myocardial infarction, which increases insulin requirements temporarily and acutely. The accumulation of ketoacids accounts for the increment in the AG and is accompanied most often by hyperglycemia [glucose > 17 mmol/L (300 mg/dL)]. The relationship between the ΔAG and ΔHCO₃⁻ is typically ~1:1 in DKA. It should be noted that, because insulin prevents production of ketones, bicarbonate therapy is rarely needed except with extreme acidemia (pH < 7.1), and then in only limited amounts. Patients with DKA are typically volume depleted and require fluid resuscitation with isotonic saline. Volume overexpansion with IV-fluid administration is not uncommon, however, and contributes to the development of a hyperchloremic acidosis during treatment of DKA. The mainstay for treatment of this condition is IV regular insulin and is described in Chap. 344 in more detail.

Alcoholic ketoacidosis (AKA) Chronic alcoholics can develop ketoacidosis when alcohol consumption is abruptly curtailed and nutrition is poor. AKA is usually associated with binge drinking, vomiting, abdominal pain, starvation, and volume depletion. The glucose concentration is variable, and acidosis may be severe because of elevated ketones, predominantly β-hydroxybutyrate. Hypoperfusion may enhance lactic acid production, chronic respiratory alkalosis may accompany liver disease, and metabolic alkalosis can result from vomiting (refer to the relationship between ΔAG and ΔHCO₃⁻). Thus, mixed acid-base disorders are common in AKA. As the circulation is restored by administration of isotonic saline, the preferential accumulation of β-hydroxybutyrate is then shifted to acetoacetate. This explains the common clinical observation of an increasingly positive nitroprusside reaction as the patient improves. The nitroprusside ketone reaction (Acetest) can detect acetoacetic acid but not β-hydroxybutyrate, so that the degree of ketosis and ketonuria can not only change with therapy, but can be underestimated initially. Patients with AKA usually present with relatively normal renal function, as opposed to DKA, where renal function is often compromised because of volume depletion (osmotic diuresis) or diabetic nephropathy. The AKA patient with normal renal function may excrete relatively large quantities of ketoacids in the urine, therefore, and may have a relatively normal AG and a discrepancy in the ΔAG/ΔHCO₃⁻ relationship.

TREATMENT | **Alcoholic Ketoacidosis**

Extracellular fluid deficits almost always accompany AKA and should be repleted by IV administration of saline and glucose (5% dextrose in 0.9% NaCl). Hypophosphatemia, hypokalemia, and hypomagnesemia may coexist and should be corrected. Hypophosphatemia usually emerges 12–24 h after admission, may be exacerbated by glucose infusion, and, if severe, may induce rhabdomyolysis. Upper gastrointestinal hemorrhage, pancreatitis, and pneumonia may accompany this disorder.

Drug- and toxin-induced acidosis

Salicylates (See also Chap. e49) Salicylate intoxication in adults usually causes respiratory alkalosis or a mixture of high-AG metabolic acidosis and respiratory alkalosis. Only a portion of the AG is due to salicylates. Lactic acid production is also often increased.

TREATMENT   Salicylate-Induced Acidosis

Vigorous gastric lavage with isotonic saline (not $NaHCO_3$) should be initiated immediately, followed by administration of activated charcoal per NG tube. In the acidotic patient, to facilitate removal of salicylate, intravenous $NaHCO_3$ is administered in amounts adequate to alkalinize the urine and to maintain urine output (urine pH > 7.5). While this form of therapy is straightforward in acidotic patients, a coexisting respiratory alkalosis may make this approach hazardous. Alkalemic patients should not receive $NaHCO_3$. Acetazolamide may be administered in the face of alkalemia, when an alkaline diuresis cannot be achieved, or to ameliorate volume overload associated with $NaHCO_3$ administration, but this drug can cause systemic metabolic acidosis if HCO_3^- is not replaced. Hypokalemia should be anticipated with an alkaline diuresis and should be treated promptly and aggressively. Glucose-containing fluids should be administered because of the danger of hypoglycemia. Excessive insensible fluid losses may cause severe volume depletion and hypernatremia. If renal failure prevents rapid clearance of salicylate, hemodialysis can be performed against a bicarbonate dialysate.

Alcohols Under most physiologic conditions, sodium, urea, and glucose generate the osmotic pressure of blood. Plasma osmolality is calculated according to the following expression: $P_{osm} = 2Na^+ + Glu + BUN$ (all in mmol/L), or, using conventional laboratory values in which glucose and BUN are expressed in milligrams per deciliter: $P_{osm} = 2Na^+ + Glu/18 + BUN/2.8$. The calculated and determined osmolality should agree within 10–15 mmol/kg H_2O. When the measured osmolality exceeds the calculated osmolality by >15–20 mmol/kg H_2O, one of two circumstances prevails. Either the serum sodium is spuriously low, as with hyperlipidemia or hyperproteinemia (pseudohyponatremia), or osmolytes other than sodium salts, glucose, or urea have accumulated in plasma. Examples of such osmolytes include mannitol, radiocontrast media, ethanol, isopropyl alcohol, ethylene glycol, propylene glycol, methanol, and acetone. In this situation, the difference between the calculated osmolality and the measured osmolality (*osmolar gap*) is proportional to the concentration of the unmeasured solute. With an appropriate clinical history and index of suspicion, identification of an osmolar gap is helpful in identifying the presence of poison-associated AG acidosis. Three alcohols may cause fatal intoxications: ethylene glycol, methanol, and isopropyl alcohol. All cause an elevated osmolal gap, but only the first two cause a high-AG acidosis.

Ethylene glycol (See also Chap. e49) Ingestion of ethylene glycol (commonly used in antifreeze) leads to a metabolic acidosis and severe damage to the CNS, heart, lungs, and kidneys. The increased AG and osmolar gap are attributable to ethylene glycol

and its metabolites, oxalic acid, glycolic acid, and other organic acids. Lactic acid production increases secondary to inhibition of the tricarboxylic acid cycle and altered intracellular redox state. Diagnosis is facilitated by recognizing oxalate crystals in the urine, the presence of an osmolar gap in serum, and a high-AG acidosis. Treatment should not be delayed while awaiting measurement of ethylene glycol levels in this setting.

TREATMENT   Ethylene Glycol–Induced Acidosis

This includes the prompt institution of a saline or osmotic diuresis, thiamine and pyridoxine supplements, fomepizole or ethanol, and hemodialysis. The IV administration of the alcohol dehydrogenase inhibitor fomepizole (4-methylpyrazole; 15 mg/kg as a loading dose) or ethanol IV to achieve a level of 22 mmol/L (100 mg/dL) serves to lessen toxicity because they compete with ethylene glycol for metabolism by alcohol dehydrogenase. Fomepizole, although expensive, is the agent of choice and offers the advantages of a predictable decline in ethylene glycol levels without excessive obtundation during ethyl alcohol infusion. Hemodialysis is indicated when the arterial pH is <7.3, or the osmolar gap exceeds 20 mOsm/kg.

Methanol (See also Chap. e49) The ingestion of methanol (wood alcohol) causes metabolic acidosis, and its metabolites formaldehyde and formic acid cause severe optic nerve and CNS damage. Lactic acid, ketoacids, and other unidentified organic acids may contribute to the acidosis. Due to its low molecular mass (32 Da), an osmolar gap is usually present.

TREATMENT   Methanol-Induced Acidosis

This is similar to that for ethylene glycol intoxication, including general supportive measures, fomepizole, and hemodialysis (as above).

Isopropyl alcohol Ingested isopropanol is absorbed rapidly and may be fatal when as little as 150 mL of rubbing alcohol, solvent, or de-icer is consumed. A plasma level >400 mg/dL is life-threatening. Isopropyl alcohol differs from ethylene glycol and methanol in that the parent compound, not the metabolites, causes toxicity, and an AG acidosis is not present because acetone is rapidly excreted.

TREATMENT   Isopropyl Alcohol Toxicity

Isopropanol alcohol toxicity is treated by watchful waiting and supportive therapy; IV fluids, pressors, ventilatory support if needed, and occasionally hemodialysis for prolonged coma or levels >400 mg/dL.

Renal failure

(See also Chap. 280) The hyperchloremic acidosis of moderate renal insufficiency is eventually converted to the high-AG acidosis of advanced renal failure. Poor filtration and reabsorption of organic anions contribute to the pathogenesis. As renal disease progresses, the number of functioning nephrons eventually becomes insufficient to keep pace with net acid production. Uremic acidosis is characterized, therefore, by a reduced rate of NH_4^+ production and excretion. The acid retained in chronic renal disease is buffered by alkaline salts from bone. Despite significant retention of acid (up to 20 mmol/d), the serum $[HCO_3^-]$ does not decrease further, indicating participation of buffers outside the extracellular compartment. Chronic metabolic acidosis results in significant loss of bone mass due to reduction in bone calcium carbonate. Chronic acidosis also increases urinary calcium excretion, proportional to cumulative acid retention.

TREATMENT   Renal Failure

Because of the association of renal failure acidosis with muscle catabolism and bone disease, both uremic acidosis and the hyperchloremic acidosis of renal failure require oral alkali replacement to maintain the $[HCO_3^-]$ between 20 and 24 mmol/L. This can be accomplished with relatively modest amounts of alkali (1.0–1.5 mmol/kg body weight per day). Sodium citrate (Shohl's solution) or $NaHCO_3$ tablets (650-mg tablets contain 7.8 meq) are equally effective alkalinizing salts. Citrate enhances the absorption of aluminum from the gastrointestinal tract and should never be given together with aluminum-containing antacids because of the risk of aluminum intoxication. When hyperkalemia is present, furosemide (60–80 mg/d) should be added.

■ NON–ANION GAP METABOLIC ACIDOSES

Alkali can be lost from the gastrointestinal tract in diarrhea or from the kidneys (renal tubular acidosis, RTA). In these disorders (Table 47-5), reciprocal changes in $[Cl^-]$ and $[HCO_3^-]$ result in a normal AG. In pure non–AG acidosis, therefore, the increase in $[Cl^-]$ above the normal value approximates the decrease in $[HCO_3^-]$. The absence of such a relationship suggests a mixed disturbance.

TREATMENT   Non–Anion Gap Metabolic Acidoses

In diarrhea, stools contain a higher $[HCO_3^-]$ and decomposed HCO_3^- than plasma so that metabolic acidosis develops along with volume depletion. Instead of an acid urine pH (as anticipated with systemic acidosis), urine pH is usually around 6 because metabolic acidosis and hypokalemia increase renal synthesis and excretion of NH_4^+, thus providing a urinary buffer that increases urine pH. Metabolic acidosis due to gastrointestinal losses with a high urine pH can be differentiated from RTA because urinary NH_4^+ excretion is typically low in RTA and high with diarrhea. Urinary NH_4^+ levels can be estimated by calculating the urine anion gap (UAG): UAG = $[Na^+ + K^+]_u - [Cl^-]_u$. When $[Cl^-]_u > [Na^+ + K^+]_u$, the UAG is negative by definition. This indicates that the urine ammonium level is appropriately increased, suggesting an extrarenal cause of the acidosis. Conversely, when the UAG is positive, the urine ammonium level is low, suggesting a renal cause of the acidosis.

Loss of functioning renal parenchyma by progressive renal disease leads to hyperchloremic acidosis when the glomerular filtration rate (GFR) is between 20 and 50 mL/min and to uremic acidosis with a high AG when the GFR falls to <20 mL/min. In advanced renal failure, ammoniagenesis is reduced in proportion to the loss of functional renal mass, and ammonium accumulation and trapping in the outer medullary collecting tubule may also be impaired. Because of adaptive increases in K^+ secretion by the collecting duct

TABLE 47-5 Causes of Non–Anion Gap Acidosis

I. Gastrointestinal bicarbonate loss
   A. Diarrhea
   B. External pancreatic or small-bowel drainage
   C. Ureterosigmoidostomy, jejunal loop, ileal loop
   D. Drugs
      1. Calcium chloride (acidifying agent)
      2. Magnesium sulfate (diarrhea)
      3. Cholestyramine (bile acid diarrhea)
II. Renal acidosis
   A. Hypokalemia
      1. Proximal RTA (type 2)
         Drug-induced: acetazolamide, topiramate
      2. Distal (classic) RTA (type 1)
         Drug induced: amphotericin B, ifosfamide
   B. Hyperkalemia
      1. Generalized distal nephron dysfunction (type 4 RTA)
         a. Mineralocorticoid deficiency
         b. Mineralocorticoid resistance (autosomal dominant PHA I)
         c. Voltage defect (autosomal dominant PHA I and PHA II)
         d. Tubulointerstitial disease
III. Drug-induced hyperkalemia (with renal insufficiency)
   A. Potassium-sparing diuretics (amiloride, triamterene, spironolactone)
   B. Trimethoprim
   C. Pentamidine
   D. ACE-Is and ARBs
   E. Nonsteroidal anti-inflammatory drugs
   F. Cyclosporine and tacrolimus
IV. Other
   A. Acid loads (ammonium chloride, hyperalimentation)
   B. Loss of potential bicarbonate: ketosis with ketone excretion
   C. Expansion acidosis (rapid saline administration)
   D. Hippurate
   E. Cation exchange resins

Abbreviations: ACE-I, angiotensin-converting enzyme inhibitor; ARB, angiotensin receptor blocker; PHA, pseudohypoaldosteronism; RTA, renal tubular acidosis.

and colon, the acidosis of chronic renal insufficiency is typically normokalemic.

Proximal RTA (type 2 RTA) (Chap. 284) is most often due to generalized proximal tubular dysfunction manifested by glycosuria, generalized aminoaciduria, and phosphaturia (Fanconi syndrome). With a low plasma $[HCO_3^-]$, the urine pH is acid (pH < 5.5). The fractional excretion of $[HCO_3^-]$ may exceed 10–15% when the serum $HCO_3^- > 20$ mmol/L. Because HCO_3^- is not reabsorbed normally in the proximal tubule, therapy with $NaHCO_3$ will enhance renal potassium wasting and hypokalemia.

The typical findings in acquired or inherited forms of classic distal RTA (type 1 RTA) include hypokalemia, non-AG metabolic acidosis, low urinary NH_4^+ excretion (positive UAG, low urine $[NH_4^+]$), and inappropriately high urine pH (pH > 5.5). Most patients have hypocitraturia and hypercalciuria, so nephrolithiasis, nephrocalcinosis, and bone disease are common. In generalized distal nephron dysfunction (type 4 RTA), hyperkalemia is disproportionate to the reduction in GFR because of coexisting dysfunction of potassium and acid secretion. Urinary ammonium excretion is invariably depressed, and renal function may be compromised, for example, due to diabetic nephropathy, obstructive uropathy, or chronic tubulointerstitial disease.

Hyporeninemic hypoaldosteronism typically causes non-AG metabolic acidosis, most commonly in older adults with diabetes mellitus or tubulointerstitial disease and renal insufficiency. Patients usually have mild to moderate CKD (GFR, 20–50 mL/min) and acidosis, with elevation in serum [K+] (5.2–6.0 mmol/L), concurrent hypertension, and congestive heart failure. Both the metabolic acidosis and the hyperkalemia are out of proportion to impairment in GFR. Nonsteroidal anti-inflammatory drugs, trimethoprim, pentamidine, and angiotensin-converting enzyme (ACE) inhibitors can also cause non-AG metabolic acidosis in patients with renal insufficiency (Table 47-5).

METABOLIC ALKALOSIS

Metabolic alkalosis is manifested by an elevated arterial pH, an increase in the serum $[HCO_3^-]$, and an increase in Pa_{CO_2} as a result of compensatory alveolar hypoventilation (Table 47-1). It is often accompanied by hypochloremia and hypokalemia. The arterial pH establishes the diagnosis, because it is increased in metabolic alkalosis and decreased or normal in respiratory acidosis. Metabolic alkalosis frequently occurs in association with other disorders such as respiratory acidosis or alkalosis or metabolic acidosis.

■ PATHOGENESIS

Metabolic alkalosis occurs as a result of net gain of $[HCO_3^-]$ or loss of nonvolatile acid (usually HCl by vomiting) from the extracellular fluid. For HCO_3^- to be added to the extracellular fluid, it must be administered exogenously or synthesized endogenously, in part or entirely by the kidneys. Because it is unusual for alkali to be added to the body, the disorder involves a generative stage, in which the loss of acid usually causes alkalosis, and a maintenance stage, in which the kidneys fail to compensate by excreting HCO_3^-.

Under normal circumstances, the kidneys have an impressive capacity to excrete HCO_3^-. Continuation of metabolic alkalosis represents a failure of the kidneys to eliminate HCO_3^- in the usual manner. The kidneys will retain, rather than excrete, the excess alkali and maintain the alkalosis if (1) volume deficiency, chloride deficiency, and K+ deficiency exist in combination with a reduced GFR, which augments distal tubule H+ secretion; or (2) hypokalemia exists because of autonomous hyperaldosteronism. In the first example, alkalosis is corrected by administration of NaCl and KCl, whereas, in the latter, it is necessary to repair the alkalosis by pharmacologic or surgical intervention, not with saline administration.

■ DIFFERENTIAL DIAGNOSIS

To establish the cause of metabolic alkalosis (Table 47-6), it is necessary to assess the status of the extracellular fluid volume (ECFV), the recumbent and upright blood pressure, the serum [K+], and the renin-aldosterone system. For example, the presence of chronic hypertension and chronic hypokalemia in an alkalotic patient suggests either mineralocorticoid excess or that the hypertensive patient is receiving diuretics. Low plasma renin activity and normal urine

TABLE 47-6 Causes of Metabolic Alkalosis

I. Exogenous HCO_3^- loads
   A. Acute alkali administration
   B. Milk-alkali syndrome

II. Effective ECFV contraction, normotension, K+ deficiency, and secondary hyperreninemic hyperaldosteronism
   A. Gastrointestinal origin
      1. Vomiting
      2. Gastric aspiration
      3. Congenital chloridorrhea
      4. Villous adenoma
   B. Renal origin
      1. Diuretics
      2. Posthypercapnic state
      3. Hypercalcemia/hypoparathyroidism
      4. Recovery from lactic acidosis or ketoacidosis
      5. Nonreabsorbable anions including penicillin, carbenicillin
      6. Mg^{2+} deficiency
      7. K+ depletion
      8. Bartter's syndrome (loss of function mutations in TALH)
      9. Gitelman's syndrome (loss of function mutation in Na^+-Cl^- cotransporter in DCT)

III. ECFV expansion, hypertension, K+ deficiency, and mineralocorticoid excess
   A. High renin
      1. Renal artery stenosis
      2. Accelerated hypertension
      3. Renin-secreting tumor
      4. Estrogen therapy
   B. Low renin
      1. Primary aldosteronism
         a. Adenoma
         b. Hyperplasia
         c. Carcinoma
      2. Adrenal enzyme defects
         a. 11 β-Hydroxylase deficiency
         b. 17 α-Hydroxylase deficiency
      3. Cushing's syndrome or disease
      4. Other
         a. Licorice
         b. Carbenoxolone
         c. Chewer's tobacco

IV. Gain-of-function mutation of renal sodium channel with ECFV expansion, hypertension, K+ deficiency, and hyporeninemic-hypoaldosteronism
   A. Liddle's syndrome

Abbreviations: DCT, distal convoluted tubule; ECFV, extracellular fluid volume; TALH, thick ascending limb of Henle's loop.

[Na$^+$] and [Cl$^-$] in a patient who is not taking diuretics indicate a primary mineralocorticoid excess syndrome. The combination of hypokalemia and alkalosis in a normotensive, nonedematous patient can be due to Bartter's or Gitelman's syndrome, magnesium deficiency, vomiting, exogenous alkali, or diuretic ingestion. Determination of urine electrolytes (especially the urine [Cl$^-$]) and screening of the urine for diuretics may be helpful. If the urine is alkaline, with an elevated [Na$^+$] and [K$^+$] but low [Cl$^-$], the diagnosis is usually either vomiting (overt or surreptitious) or alkali ingestion. If the urine is relatively acid and has low concentrations of Na$^+$, K$^+$, and Cl$^-$, the most likely possibilities are prior vomiting, the posthypercapnic state, or prior diuretic ingestion. If, on the other hand, neither the urine sodium, potassium, nor chloride concentrations are depressed, magnesium deficiency, Bartter's or Gitelman's syndrome, or current diuretic ingestion should be considered. Bartter's syndrome is distinguished from Gitelman's syndrome because of hypocalciuria and hypomagnesemia in the latter disorder.

Alkali administration

Chronic administration of alkali to individuals with normal renal function rarely causes alkalosis. However, in patients with coexistent hemodynamic disturbances, alkalosis can develop because the normal capacity to excrete HCO$_3^-$ may be exceeded or there may be enhanced reabsorption of HCO$_3^-$. Such patients include those who receive HCO$_3^-$ (PO or IV), acetate loads (parenteral hyperalimentation solutions), citrate loads (transfusions), or antacids plus cation-exchange resins (aluminum hydroxide and sodium polystyrene sulfonate). Nursing-home patients receiving tube feedings have a higher incidence of metabolic alkalosis than nursing-home patients receiving oral feedings.

▣ METABOLIC ALKALOSIS ASSOCIATED WITH ECFV CONTRACTION, K$^+$ DEPLETION, AND SECONDARY HYPERRENINEMIC HYPERALDOSTERONISM

Gastrointestinal origin

Gastrointestinal loss of H$^+$ from vomiting or gastric aspiration results in retention of HCO$_3^-$. The loss of fluid and NaCl in vomitus or nasogastric suction results in contraction of the ECFV and an increase in the secretion of renin and aldosterone. Volume contraction through a reduction in GFR results in an enhanced capacity of the renal tubule to reabsorb HCO$_3^-$. During active vomiting, however, the filtered load of bicarbonate is acutely increased to the point that the reabsorptive capacity of the proximal tubule for HCO$_3^-$ is exceeded. The excess NaHCO$_3$ issuing out of the proximal tubule reaches the distal tubule, where H$^+$ secretion is enhanced by an aldosterone and the delivery of the poorly reabsorbed anion, HCO$_3^-$. Correction of the contracted ECFV with NaCl and repair of K$^+$ deficits corrects the acid-base disorder, and chloride deficiency.

Renal origin

Diuretics (See also Chap. 234) Drugs that induce chloruresis, such as thiazides and loop diuretics (furosemide, bumetanide, torsemide, and ethacrynic acid), acutely diminish the ECFV without altering the total body bicarbonate content. The serum [HCO$_3^-$] increases because the reduced ECFV "contracts" the [HCO$_3^-$] in the plasma (contraction alkalosis). The chronic administration of diuretics tends to generate an alkalosis by increasing distal salt delivery, so that K$^+$ and H$^+$ secretion are stimulated. The alkalosis is maintained by persistence of the contraction of the ECFV, secondary hyperaldosteronism, K$^+$ deficiency, and the direct effect of the diuretic (as long as diuretic administration continues). Repair of the alkalosis is achieved by providing isotonic saline to correct the ECFV deficit.

Solute losing disorders: Bartter's syndrome and Gitelman's syndrome See Chap. 284.

Nonreabsorbable anions and magnesium deficiency Administration of large quantities of nonreabsorbable anions, such as penicillin or carbenicillin, can enhance distal acidification and K$^+$ secretion by increasing the transepithelial potential difference. Mg^{2+} deficiency results in hypokalemic alkalosis by enhancing distal acidification through stimulation of renin and hence aldosterone secretion.

Potassium depletion Chronic K$^+$ depletion may cause metabolic alkalosis by increasing urinary acid excretion. Both NH$_4^+$ production and absorption are enhanced and HCO$_3^-$ reabsorption is stimulated. Chronic K$^+$ deficiency upregulates the renal H$^+$, K$^+$-ATPase to increase K$^+$ absorption at the expense of enhanced H$^+$ secretion. Alkalosis associated with severe K$^+$ depletion is resistant to salt administration, but repair of the K$^+$ deficiency corrects the alkalosis.

After treatment of lactic acidosis or ketoacidosis When an underlying stimulus for the generation of lactic acid or ketoacid is removed rapidly, as with repair of circulatory insufficiency or with insulin therapy, the lactate or ketones are metabolized to yield an equivalent amount of HCO$_3^-$. Other sources of new HCO$_3^-$ are additive with the original amount generated by organic anion metabolism to create a surfeit of HCO$_3^-$. Such sources include (1) new HCO$_3^-$ added to the blood by the kidneys as a result of enhanced acid excretion during the preexisting period of acidosis, and (2) alkali therapy during the treatment phase of the acidosis. Acidosis-induced contraction of the ECFV and K$^+$ deficiency act to sustain the alkalosis.

Posthypercapnia Prolonged CO$_2$ retention with chronic respiratory acidosis enhances renal HCO$_3^-$ absorption and the generation of new HCO$_3^-$ (increased net acid excretion). If the Pa$_{CO_2}$ is returned to normal, metabolic alkalosis results from the persistently elevated [HCO$_3^-$]. Alkalosis develops if the elevated Pa$_{CO_2}$ is abruptly returned toward normal by a change in mechanically controlled ventilation. Associated ECFV contraction does not allow complete repair of the alkalosis by correction of the Pa$_{CO_2}$ alone, and alkalosis persists until Cl$^-$ supplementation is provided.

▣ METABOLIC ALKALOSIS ASSOCIATED WITH ECFV EXPANSION, HYPERTENSION, AND HYPERALDOSTERONISM

Increased aldosterone levels may be the result of autonomous primary adrenal overproduction or of secondary aldosterone release due to renal overproduction of renin. Mineralocorticoid excess increases net acid excretion and may result in metabolic alkalosis, which may be worsened by associated K$^+$ deficiency. ECFV expansion from salt retention causes hypertension. The kaliuresis persists because of mineralocorticoid excess and distal Na$^+$ absorption causing enhanced K$^+$ excretion, continued K$^+$ depletion with polydipsia, inability to concentrate the urine, and polyuria.

Liddle's syndrome (Chap. 284) results from increased activity of the collecting duct Na$^+$ channel (ENaC) and is a rare monogenic form of hypertension due to volume expansion manifested as hypokalemic alkalosis and normal aldosterone levels.

Symptoms

With metabolic alkalosis, changes in CNS and peripheral nervous system function are similar to those of hypocalcemia (Chap. 352); symptoms include mental confusion; obtundation; and a predisposition to seizures, paresthesia, muscular cramping, tetany, aggravation of arrhythmias, and hypoxemia in chronic obstructive pulmonary disease. Related electrolyte abnormalities include hypokalemia and hypophosphatemia.

TREATMENT Metabolic Alkalosis

This is primarily directed at correcting the underlying stimulus for HCO_3^- generation. If primary aldosteronism, renal artery stenosis, or Cushing's syndrome is present, correction of the underlying cause will reverse the alkalosis. [H^+] loss by the stomach or kidneys can be mitigated by the use of proton pump inhibitors or the discontinuation of diuretics. The second aspect of treatment is to remove the factors that sustain the inappropriate increase in HCO_3^- reabsorption, such as ECFV contraction or K^+ deficiency. K^+ deficits should always be repaired. Isotonic saline is usually sufficient to reverse the alkalosis if ECFV contraction is present.

If associated conditions preclude infusion of saline, renal HCO_3^- loss can be accelerated by administration of acetazolamide, a carbonic anhydrase inhibitor, which is usually effective in patients with adequate renal function but can worsen K^+ losses. Dilute hydrochloric acid (0.1 N HCl) is also effective but can cause hemolysis, and must be delivered centrally and slowly. Hemodialysis against a dialysate low in [HCO_3^-] and high in [Cl^-] can be effective when renal function is impaired.

RESPIRATORY ACIDOSIS

Respiratory acidosis can be due to severe pulmonary disease, respiratory muscle fatigue, or abnormalities in ventilatory control and is recognized by an increase in Pa_{CO_2} and decrease in pH (Table 47-7). In acute respiratory acidosis, there is an immediate compensatory elevation (due to cellular buffering mechanisms) in HCO_3^-, which increases 1 mmol/L for every 10-mmHg increase in Pa_{CO_2}. In chronic respiratory acidosis (>24 h), renal adaptation increases the [HCO_3^-] by 4 mmol/L for every 10-mmHg increase in Pa_{CO_2}. The serum HCO_3^- usually does not increase above 38 mmol/L.

The clinical features vary according to the severity and duration of the respiratory acidosis, the underlying disease, and whether there is accompanying hypoxemia. A rapid increase in Pa_{CO_2} may cause anxiety, dyspnea, confusion, psychosis, and hallucinations and may progress to coma. Lesser degrees of dysfunction in chronic hypercapnia include sleep disturbances; loss of memory; daytime somnolence; personality changes; impairment of coordination; and motor disturbances such as tremor, myoclonic jerks, and asterixis. Headaches and other signs that mimic raised intracranial pressure, such as papilledema, abnormal reflexes, and focal muscle weakness, are due to vasoconstriction secondary to loss of the vasodilator effects of CO_2.

Depression of the respiratory center by a variety of drugs, injury, or disease can produce respiratory acidosis. This may occur acutely with general anesthetics, sedatives, and head trauma or chronically with sedatives, alcohol, intracranial tumors, and the syndromes of sleep-disordered breathing including the primary alveolar and obesity-hypoventilation syndromes (Chaps. 264 and 265). Abnormalities or disease in the motor neurons, neuromuscular junction, and skeletal muscle can cause hypoventilation via respiratory muscle fatigue. Mechanical ventilation, when not properly adjusted and supervised, may result in respiratory acidosis, particularly if CO_2 production suddenly rises (because of fever, agitation, sepsis, or overfeeding) or alveolar ventilation falls because of worsening pulmonary function. High levels of positive end-expiratory pressure in the presence of reduced cardiac output may cause hypercapnia as a result of large increases in alveolar dead space (Chap. 252). Permissive hypercapnia is being used with increasing frequency because of studies suggesting lower mortality rates than with conventional mechanical ventilation, especially

TABLE 47-7 Respiratory Acid-Base Disorders

I. Alkalosis
  A. Central nervous system stimulation
    1. Pain
    2. Anxiety, psychosis
    3. Fever
    4. Cerebrovascular accident
    5. Meningitis, encephalitis
    6. Tumor
    7. Trauma
  B. Hypoxemia or tissue hypoxia
    1. High altitude
    2. Pneumonia, pulmonary edema
    3. Aspiration
    4. Severe anemia
  C. Drugs or hormones
    1. Pregnancy, progesterone
    2. Salicylates
    3. Cardiac failure
  D. Stimulation of chest receptors
    1. Hemothorax
    2. Flail chest
    3. Cardiac failure
    4. Pulmonary embolism
  E. Miscellaneous
    1. Septicemia
    2. Hepatic failure
    3. Mechanical hyperventilation
    4. Heat exposure
    5. Recovery from metabolic acidosis

II. Acidosis
  A. Central
    1. Drugs (anesthetics, morphine, sedatives)
    2. Stroke
    3. Infection
  B. Airway
    1. Obstruction
    2. Asthma
  C. Parenchyma
    1. Emphysema
    2. Pneumoconiosis
    3. Bronchitis
    4. Adult respiratory distress syndrome
    5. Barotrauma
  D. Neuromuscular
    1. Poliomyelitis
    2. Kyphoscoliosis
    3. Myasthenia
    4. Muscular dystrophies
  E. Miscellaneous
    1. Obesity
    2. Hypoventilation
    3. Permissive hypercapnia

with severe CNS or heart disease. The respiratory acidosis associated with permissive hypercapnia may require administration of $NaHCO_3$ to increase the arterial pH to 7.25 but overcorrection of the acidemia may be deleterious.

Acute hypercapnia follows sudden occlusion of the upper airway or generalized bronchospasm as in severe asthma, anaphylaxis, inhalational burn, or toxin injury. Chronic hypercapnia and respiratory acidosis occur in end-stage obstructive lung disease. Restrictive disorders involving both the chest wall and the lungs can cause respiratory acidosis because the high metabolic cost of respiration causes ventilatory muscle fatigue. Advanced stages of intrapulmonary and extrapulmonary restrictive defects present as chronic respiratory acidosis.

The diagnosis of respiratory acidosis requires the measurement of Pa_{CO_2} and arterial pH. A detailed history and physical examination often indicate the cause. Pulmonary function studies (Chap. 252), including spirometry, diffusion capacity for carbon monoxide, lung volumes, and arterial Pa_{CO_2} and O_2 saturation, usually make it possible to determine if respiratory acidosis is secondary to lung disease. The workup for nonpulmonary causes should include a detailed drug history, measurement of hematocrit, and assessment of upper airway, chest wall, pleura, and neuromuscular function.

TREATMENT   Respiratory Acidosis

The management of respiratory acidosis depends on its severity and rate of onset. Acute respiratory acidosis can be life-threatening, and measures to reverse the underlying cause should be undertaken simultaneously with restoration of adequate alveolar ventilation. This may necessitate tracheal intubation and assisted mechanical ventilation. Oxygen administration should be titrated carefully in patients with severe obstructive pulmonary disease and chronic CO_2 retention who are breathing spontaneously (Chap. 260). When oxygen is used injudiciously, these patients may experience progression of the respiratory acidosis. Aggressive and rapid correction of hypercapnia should be avoided, because the falling Pa_{CO_2} may provoke the same complications noted with acute respiratory alkalosis (i.e., cardiac arrhythmias, reduced cerebral perfusion, and seizures). The Pa_{CO_2} should be lowered gradually in chronic respiratory acidosis, aiming to restore the Pa_{CO_2} to baseline levels and to provide sufficient Cl^- and K^+ to enhance the renal excretion of HCO_3^-.

Chronic respiratory acidosis is frequently difficult to correct, but measures aimed at improving lung function (Chap. 260) can help some patients and forestall further deterioration in most.

RESPIRATORY ALKALOSIS

Alveolar hyperventilation decreases Pa_{CO_2} and increases the HCO_3^-/Pa_{CO_2} ratio, thus increasing pH (Table 47-7). Nonbicarbonate cellular buffers respond by consuming HCO_3^-. Hypocapnia develops when a sufficiently strong ventilatory stimulus causes CO_2 output in the lungs to exceed its metabolic production by tissues. Plasma pH and $[HCO_3^-]$ appear to vary proportionately with Pa_{CO_2} over a range from 40–15 mmHg. The relationship between arterial $[H^+]$ concentration and Pa_{CO_2} is ~0.7 mmol/L per mmHg (or 0.01 pH unit/mmHg), and that for plasma $[HCO_3^-]$ is 0.2 mmol/L per mmHg. Hypocapnia sustained for >2–6 h is further compensated by a decrease in renal ammonium and titratable acid excretion and a reduction in filtered HCO_3^- reabsorption. Full renal adaptation to respiratory alkalosis may take several days and requires normal volume status and renal function. The kidneys appear to respond

directly to the lowered Pa_{CO_2} rather than to alkalosis per se. In chronic respiratory alkalosis a 1-mmHg fall in Pa_{CO_2} causes a 0.4- to 0.5-mmol/L drop in $[HCO_3^-]$ and a 0.3-mmol/L fall (or 0.003 rise in pH) in $[H^+]$.

The effects of respiratory alkalosis vary according to duration and severity but are primarily those of the underlying disease. Reduced cerebral blood flow as a consequence of a rapid decline in Pa_{CO_2} may cause dizziness, mental confusion, and seizures, even in the absence of hypoxemia. The cardiovascular effects of acute hypocapnia in the conscious human are generally minimal, but in the anesthetized or mechanically ventilated patient, cardiac output and blood pressure may fall because of the depressant effects of anesthesia and positive-pressure ventilation on heart rate, systemic resistance, and venous return. Cardiac arrhythmias may occur in patients with heart disease as a result of changes in oxygen unloading by blood from a left shift in the hemoglobin-oxygen dissociation curve (Bohr effect). Acute respiratory alkalosis causes intracellular shifts of Na^+, K^+, and PO_4^{2-} and reduces free $[Ca^{2+}]$ by increasing the protein-bound fraction. Hypocapnia-induced hypokalemia is usually minor.

Chronic respiratory alkalosis is the most common acid-base disturbance in critically ill patients and, when severe, portends a poor prognosis. Many cardiopulmonary disorders manifest respiratory alkalosis in their early to intermediate stages, and the finding of normocapnia and hypoxemia in a patient with hyperventilation may herald the onset of rapid respiratory failure and should prompt an assessment to determine if the patient is becoming fatigued. Respiratory alkalosis is common during mechanical ventilation.

The hyperventilation syndrome may be disabling. Paresthesia; circumoral numbness; chest wall tightness or pain; dizziness; inability to take an adequate breath; and, rarely, tetany may be sufficiently stressful to perpetuate the disorder. Arterial blood-gas analysis demonstrates an acute or chronic respiratory alkalosis, often with hypocapnia in the range of 15–30 mmHg and no hypoxemia. CNS diseases or injury can produce several patterns of hyperventilation and sustained Pa_{CO_2} levels of 20–30 mmHg. Hyperthyroidism, high caloric loads, and exercise raise the basal metabolic rate, but ventilation usually rises in proportion so that arterial blood gases are unchanged and respiratory alkalosis does not develop. Salicylates are the most common cause of drug-induced respiratory alkalosis as a result of direct stimulation of the medullary chemoreceptor (Chap. e49). The methylxanthines, theophylline, and aminophylline stimulate ventilation and increase the ventilatory response to CO_2. Progesterone increases ventilation and lowers arterial Pa_{CO_2} by as much as 5–10 mmHg. Therefore, chronic respiratory alkalosis is a common feature of pregnancy. Respiratory alkalosis is also prominent in liver failure, and the severity correlates with the degree of hepatic insufficiency. Respiratory alkalosis is often an early finding in gram-negative septicemia, before fever, hypoxemia, or hypotension develops.

The diagnosis of respiratory alkalosis depends on measurement of arterial pH and Pa_{CO_2}. The plasma $[K^+]$ is often reduced and the $[Cl^-]$ increased. In the acute phase, respiratory alkalosis is not associated with increased renal HCO_3^- excretion, but within hours net acid excretion is reduced. In general, the HCO_3^- concentration falls by 2.0 mmol/L for each 10-mmHg decrease in Pa_{CO_2}. Chronic hypocapnia reduces the serum $[HCO_3^-]$ by 4.0 mmol/L for each 10-mmHg decrease in Pa_{CO_2}. It is unusual to observe a plasma $HCO_3^- < 12$ mmol/L as a result of a pure respiratory alkalosis.

When a diagnosis of respiratory alkalosis is made, its cause should be investigated. The diagnosis of hyperventilation syndrome is made by exclusion. In difficult cases, it may be important to rule out other conditions such as pulmonary embolism, coronary artery disease, and hyperthyroidism.

TREATMENT Respiratory Alkalosis

The management of respiratory alkalosis is directed toward alleviation of the underlying disorder. If respiratory alkalosis complicates ventilator management, changes in dead space, tidal volume, and frequency can minimize the hypocapnia. Patients with the hyperventilation syndrome may benefit from reassurance, rebreathing from a paper bag during symptomatic attacks, and attention to underlying psychological stress. Antidepressants and sedatives are not recommended. β-Adrenergic blockers may ameliorate peripheral manifestations of the hyperadrenergic state.

FURTHER READINGS

DuBose TD: Metabolic alkalosis, in *Primer on Kidney Diseases,* 5th ed, A Greenberg (ed). Saunders Elsevier, 2009, pp 84-90

DuBose TD Jr: Acid-base disorders, in *Brenner and Rector's The Kidney,* 8th ed, BM Brenner (ed). Philadelphia, Saunders, 2008, pp 505-546

———, Alpern RJ: Renal tubular acidosis, in *The Metabolic and Molecular Bases of Inherited Disease,* 8th ed, CR Scriver et al (eds). New York, McGraw-Hill, 2001

Kraut JA, Madias NE: Metabolic acidosis: Pathophysiology, diagnosis and management. Nat Rev Nephrol. 6:274, 2010

Laski ME, Wesson DE: Lactic acidosis, in *Acid-Base and Electrolyte Disorders—A Companion to Brenner and Rector's The Kidney,* TD DuBose, LL Hamm (eds). Philadelphia, Saunders, 2002, pp 83–107

Madias NE: Respiratory alkalosis, in *Acid-Base and Electrolyte Disorders—A Companion to Brenner and Rector's The Kidney,* TD DuBose, LL Hamm (eds). Philadelphia, Saunders, 2002, pp 147–164

CHAPTER **48**

Sexual Dysfunction

Kevin T. McVary

Male sexual dysfunction affects 10–25% of middle-aged and elderly men, and female sexual dysfunction occurs with a similar frequency. Demographic changes, the popularity of newer treatments, and greater awareness of sexual dysfunction by patients and society have led to increased diagnosis and associated health care expenditures for the management of this common disorder. Because many patients are reluctant to initiate discussion of their sex lives, physicians should address this topic directly to elicit a history of sexual dysfunction.

MALE SEXUAL DYSFUNCTION

▇ PHYSIOLOGY OF MALE SEXUAL RESPONSE

Normal male sexual function requires (1) an intact libido, (2) the ability to achieve and maintain penile erection, (3) ejaculation, and (4) detumescence. *Libido* refers to sexual desire and is influenced by a variety of visual, olfactory, tactile, auditory, imaginative, and hormonal stimuli. Sex steroids, particularly testosterone, act to increase libido. Libido can be diminished by hormonal or psychiatric disorders and by medications.

Penile tumescence leading to erection depends on an increased flow of blood into the lacunar network accompanied by complete relaxation of the arteries and corporal smooth muscle. The microarchitecture of the corpora is composed of a mass of smooth muscle (trabecula) that contains a network of endothelial-lined vessels (lacunar spaces). Subsequent compression of the trabecular smooth muscle against the fibroelastic tunica albuginea causes a passive closure of the emissary veins and accumulation of blood in the corpora. In the presence of a full erection and a competent valve mechanism, the corpora become noncompressible cylinders from which blood does not escape.

The central nervous system (CNS) exerts an important influence by either stimulating or antagonizing spinal pathways that mediate erectile function and ejaculation. The erectile response is mediated by a combination of central (psychogenic) innervation and peripheral (reflexogenic) innervation. Sensory nerves that originate from receptors in the penile skin and glans converge to form the dorsal nerve of the penis, which travels to the S2-S4 dorsal root ganglia via the pudendal nerve. Parasympathetic nerve fibers to the penis arise from neurons in the intermediolateral columns of the S2-S4 sacral spinal segments. Sympathetic innervation originates from the T-11 to the L-2 spinal segments and descends through the hypogastric plexus.

Neural input to smooth-muscle tone is crucial to the initiation and maintenance of an erection. There is also an intricate interaction between the corporal smooth-muscle cell and its overlying endothelial cell lining (Fig. 48-1A). Nitric oxide, which induces vascular relaxation, promotes erection and is opposed by endothelin 1 (ET-1) and Rho kinase, which mediate vascular contraction.

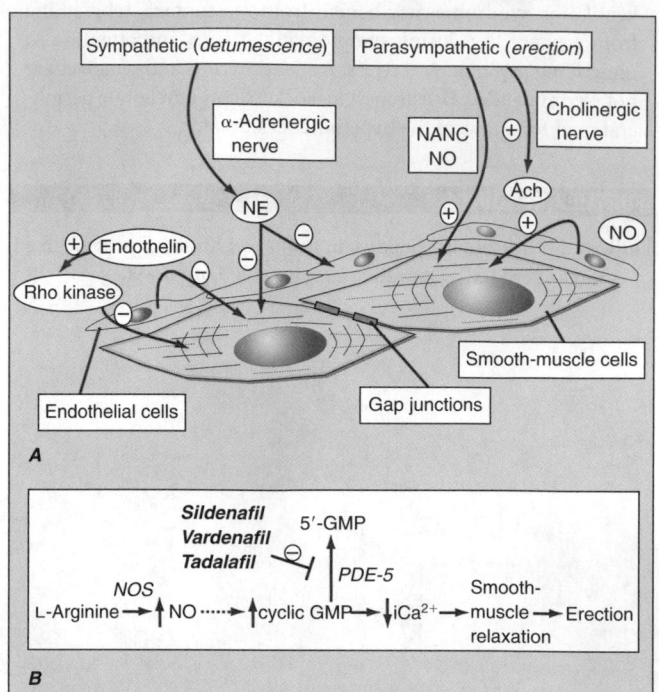

Figure 48-1 Pathways that control erection and detumescence. *A.* Erection is mediated by cholinergic parasympathetic pathways and nonadrenergic, noncholinergic (NANC) pathways, which release nitric oxide (NO). Endothelial cells also release NO, which induces vascular smooth-muscle cell relaxation, allowing enhanced blood flow and leading to erection. Detumescence is mediated by sympathetic pathways that release norepinephrine and stimulate α-adrenergic pathways, leading to contraction of vascular smooth-muscle cells. Endothelin, released from endothelial cells, also induces contraction. Rho kinase activation via endothelin activity (among others) also contributes to detumescence by alteration of calcium signaling. *B.* Biochemical pathways of NO synthesis and action. Sildenafil, vardenafil, and tadalafil enhance erectile function by inhibiting phosphodiesterase type 5 (PDE-5), thereby maintaining high levels of cyclic 3′,5′-guanosine monophosphate (cyclic GMP). NOS, nitric oxide synthase; iCa^{2+}, intracellular calcium.

Nitric oxide is synthesized from L-arginine by nitric oxide synthase and is released from the nonadrenergic, noncholinergic (NANC) autonomic nerve supply to act postjunctionally on smooth-muscle cells. Nitric oxide increases the production of cyclic 3′,5′-guanosine monophosphate (cyclic GMP), which induces relaxation of smooth muscle (Fig. 48-1B). Cyclic GMP is gradually broken down by phosphodiesterase type 5 (PDE-5). Inhibitors of PDE-5 such as the oral medications sildenafil, vardenafil, and tadalafil maintain erections by reducing the breakdown of cyclic GMP. However, if nitric oxide is not produced at some level, PDE-5 inhibitors are ineffective, as these drugs facilitate, but do not initiate, the initial enzyme cascade. In addition to nitric oxide, vasoactive prostaglandins (PGE_1, $PGF_{2\alpha}$) are synthesized within the cavernosal tissue and increase cyclic AMP levels, also leading to relaxation of cavernosal smooth-muscle cells.

Ejaculation is stimulated by the sympathetic nervous system; this results in contraction of the epididymis, vas deferens, seminal vesicles, and prostate, causing seminal fluid to enter the urethra. Seminal fluid emission is followed by rhythmic contractions of the bulbocavernosus and ischiocavernosus muscles, leading to ejaculation. *Premature ejaculation* usually is related to anxiety or a learned behavior and is amenable to behavioral therapy or treatment with medications such as selective serotonin reuptake inhibitors (SSRIs). *Retrograde ejaculation* results when the internal urethral sphincter does not close; it may occur in men with diabetes or after surgery involving the bladder neck.

Detumescence is mediated by norepinephrine from the sympathetic nerves, endothelin from the vascular surface, and smooth-muscle contraction induced by postsynaptic α-adrenergic receptors and activation of Rho kinase. These events increase venous outflow and restore the flaccid state. Venous leak can cause premature detumescence and is caused by insufficient relaxation of the corporal smooth muscle rather than a specific anatomic defect. *Priapism* refers to a persistent and painful erection and may be associated with sickle cell anemia, hypercoagulable states, spinal cord injury, or injection of vasodilator agents into the penis.

■ ERECTILE DYSFUNCTION

Epidemiology

Erectile dysfunction (ED) is not considered a normal part of the aging process. Nonetheless, it is associated with certain physiologic and psychological changes related to age. In the Massachusetts Male Aging Study (MMAS), a community-based survey of men age 40–70, 52% of responders reported some degree of ED. Complete ED occurred in 10% of respondents, moderate ED in 25%, and minimal ED in 17%. The incidence of moderate or severe ED more than doubled between the ages of 40 and 70. In the National Health and Social Life Survey (NHSLS), which included a sample of men and women age 18–59, 10% of men reported being unable to maintain an erection (corresponding to the proportion of men in the MMAS reporting severe ED). Incidence was highest among men in the age group 50–59 (21%) and men who were poor (14%), divorced (14%), and less educated (13%).

The incidence of ED is also higher among men with certain medical disorders, such as diabetes mellitus, obesity, lower urinary tract symptoms secondary to benign prostatic hyperplasia (BPH), heart disease, hypertension, and decreased high-density lipoprotein (HDL) levels. Cardiovascular disease and ED share etiologies as well as pathophysiology (e.g., endothelial dysfunction), and the degree of ED appears to correlate with the severity of cardiovascular disease. Consequently, ED represents a "sentinel symptom" in patients with occult cardiovascular and peripheral vascular disease.

Smoking is also a significant risk factor in the development of ED. Medications used in treating diabetes or cardiovascular disease are additional risk factors (see below). There is a higher incidence of ED among men who have undergone radiation or surgery for prostate cancer and in those with a lower spinal cord injury. Psychological causes of ED include depression, anger, stress from unemployment, and other stress-related causes.

Pathophysiology

ED may result from three basic mechanisms: (1) failure to initiate (psychogenic, endocrinologic, or neurogenic), (2) failure to fill (arteriogenic), and (3) failure to store adequate blood volume within the lacunar network (venoocclusive dysfunction). These categories are not mutually exclusive, and multiple factors contribute to ED in many patients. For example, diminished filling pressure can lead secondarily to venous leak. Psychogenic factors frequently coexist with other etiologic factors and should be considered in all cases. Diabetic, atherosclerotic, and drug-related causes account for >80% of cases of ED in older men.

Vasculogenic The most common organic cause of ED is a disturbance of blood flow to and from the penis. Atherosclerotic or traumatic arterial disease can decrease flow to the lacunar spaces, resulting in decreased rigidity and an increased time to full erection. Excessive outflow through the veins despite adequate inflow also may contribute to ED. Structural alterations to the fibroelastic components of the corpora may cause a loss of compliance and inability to compress the tunical veins. This condition may result from aging, increased cross-linking of collagen fibers induced by nonenzymatic glycosylation, hypoxemia, or altered synthesis of collagen associated with hypercholesterolemia.

Neurogenic Disorders that affect the sacral spinal cord or the autonomic fibers to the penis preclude nervous system relaxation of penile smooth muscle, thus leading to ED. In patients with spinal cord injury, the degree of ED depends on the completeness and level of the lesion. Patients with incomplete lesions or injuries to the upper part of the spinal cord are more likely to retain erectile capabilities than are those with complete lesions or injuries to the lower part. Although 75% of patients with spinal cord injuries have some erectile capability, only 25% have erections sufficient for penetration. Other neurologic disorders commonly associated with ED include multiple sclerosis and peripheral neuropathy. The latter is often due to either diabetes or alcoholism. Pelvic surgery may cause ED through disruption of the autonomic nerve supply.

Endocrinologic Androgens increase libido, but their exact role in erectile function is unclear. Individuals with castrate levels of testosterone can achieve erections from visual or sexual stimuli. Nonetheless, normal levels of testosterone appear to be important for erectile function, particularly in older males. Androgen replacement therapy can improve depressed erectile function when it is secondary to hypogonadism; however, it is not useful for ED when endogenous testosterone levels are normal. Increased prolactin may decrease libido by suppressing gonadotropin-releasing hormone (GnRH), and it also leads to decreased testosterone levels. Treatment of hyperprolactinemia with dopamine agonists can restore libido and testosterone.

Diabetic ED occurs in 35–75% of men with diabetes mellitus. Pathologic mechanisms are related primarily to diabetes-associated vascular and neurologic complications. Diabetic macrovascular complications are related mainly to age, whereas microvascular complications correlate with the duration of diabetes and the degree of glycemic control (Chap. 344). Individuals with diabetes also have reduced amounts of nitric oxide synthase in both endothelial and neural tissues.

Psychogenic Two mechanisms contribute to the inhibition of erections in psychogenic ED. First, psychogenic stimuli to the sacral cord may inhibit reflexogenic responses, thereby blocking activation of vasodilator outflow to the penis. Second, excess sympathetic stimulation in an anxious man may increase penile smooth-muscle tone. The most common causes of psychogenic ED are performance anxiety, depression, relationship conflict, loss of attraction, sexual inhibition, conflicts over sexual preference, sexual abuse in childhood, and fear of pregnancy or sexually transmitted disease. Almost all patients with ED, even when it has a clear-cut organic basis, develop a psychogenic component as a reaction to ED.

Medication-related Medication-induced ED (Table 48-1) is estimated to occur in 25% of men seen in general medical outpatient clinics. The adverse effects related to drug therapy are additive, especially in older men. In addition to the drug itself, the disease being treated is likely to contribute to sexual dysfunction. Among the antihypertensive agents, the thiazide diuretics and beta blockers have been implicated most frequently. Calcium channel blockers and

TABLE 48-1 Drugs Associated With Erectile Dysfunction

Classification	Drugs
Diuretics	Thiazides
	Spironolactone
Antihypertensives	Calcium channel blockers
	Methyldopa
	Clonidine
	Reserpine
	Beta blockers
	Guanethidine
Cardiac/antihyperlipidemics	Digoxin
	Gemfibrozil
	Clofibrate
Antidepressants	Selective serotonin reuptake inhibitors
	Tricyclic antidepressants
	Lithium
	Monoamine oxidase inhibitors
Tranquilizers	Butyrophenones
	Phenothiazines
H$_2$ antagonists	Ranitidine
	Cimetidine
Hormones	Progesterone
	Estrogens
	Corticosteroids
	GnRH agonists
	5α-Reductase inhibitors
	Cyproterone acetate
Cytotoxic agents	Cyclophosphamide
	Methotrexate
	Roferon-A
Anticholinergics	Disopyramide
	Anticonvulsants
Recreational	Ethanol
	Cocaine
	Marijuana

Abbreviation: GnRH, gonadotropin-releasing hormone.

angiotensin converting-enzyme inhibitors are cited less frequently. These drugs may act directly at the corporal level (e.g., calcium channel blockers) or indirectly by reducing pelvic blood pressure, which is important in the development of penile rigidity. α-Adrenergic blockers are less likely to cause ED. Estrogens, GnRH agonists, H$_2$ antagonists, and spironolactone cause ED by suppressing gonadotropin production or by blocking androgen action. Antidepressant and antipsychotic agents—particularly neuroleptics, tricyclics, and SSRIs—are associated with erectile, ejaculatory, orgasmic, and sexual desire difficulties.

If there is a strong association between the institution of a drug and the onset of ED, alternative medications should be considered. Otherwise, it is often practical to treat the ED without attempting multiple changes in medications, as it may be difficult to establish a causal role for a drug.

A good physician-patient relationship helps unravel the possible causes of ED, many of which require discussion of personal and sometimes embarrassing topics. For this reason, a primary care provider is often ideally suited to initiate the evaluation. However, a significant percentage of men experience ED and remain undiagnosed unless specifically questioned about this issue. By far the most common reason for underreporting of ED is patient embarrassment. Once the topic is initiated by the physician, patients are more willing to discuss their potency issues. A complete medical and sexual history should be taken in an effort to assess whether the cause of ED is organic, psychogenic, or multifactorial (Fig. 48-2).

Both the patient and his sexual partner should be interviewed regarding sexual history. ED should be distinguished from other sexual problems, such as premature ejaculation. Lifestyle factors such as sexual orientation, the patient's distress from ED, performance anxiety, and details of sexual techniques should be addressed. Standardized questionnaires are available to assess ED, including the International Index of Erectile Function (IIEF) and the more easily administered Sexual Health Inventory for Men (SHIM), a validated abridged version of the IIEF.

The initial evaluation of ED begins with a review of the patient's medical, surgical, sexual, and psychosocial histories. The history should note whether the patient has experienced pelvic trauma, surgery, or radiation. In light of the increasing recognition of the relationship between lower urinary tract symptoms and ED, it is advisable to evaluate for the presence of symptoms of bladder outlet obstruction. Questions should focus on the onset of symptoms, the presence and duration of partial erections, and the progression of ED. A history of nocturnal or early morning erections is useful for distinguishing physiologic ED from psychogenic ED. Nocturnal erections occur during rapid eye movement (REM) sleep and require intact neurologic and circulatory systems. Organic causes of ED generally are characterized by a gradual and persistent change in rigidity or the inability to sustain nocturnal, coital, or self-stimulated erections. The patient should be questioned about the presence of penile curvature or pain with coitus. It is also important to address libido, as decreased sexual drive and ED are sometimes

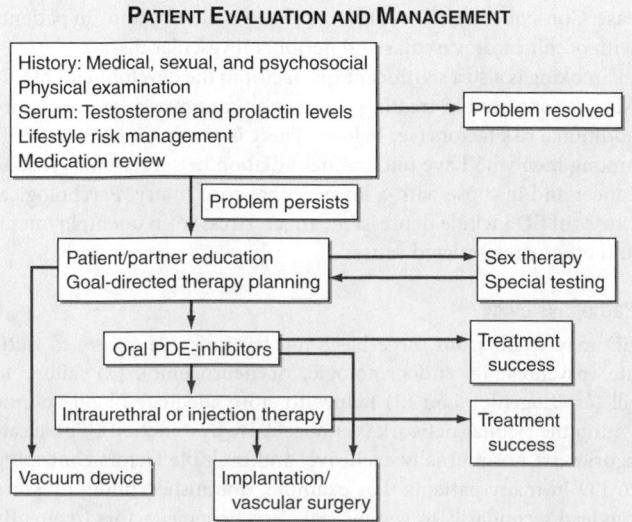

PATIENT EVALUATION AND MANAGEMENT

Figure 48-2 Algorithm for the evaluation and management of patients with ED. PDE, phosphodiesterase.

the earliest signs of endocrine abnormalities (e.g., increased prolactin, decreased testosterone levels). It is useful to ask whether the problem is confined to coitus with one partner or also involves other partners; ED not uncommonly arises in association with new or extramarital sexual relationships. Situational ED, as opposed to consistent ED, suggests psychogenic causes. Ejaculation is much less commonly affected than erection, but questions should be asked about whether ejaculation is normal, premature, delayed, or absent. Relevant risk factors should be identified, such as diabetes mellitus, coronary artery disease (CAD), and neurologic disorders. The patient's surgical history should be explored with an emphasis on bowel, bladder, prostate, and vascular procedures. A complete drug history is also important. Social changes that may precipitate ED are also crucial to the evaluation, including health worries, spousal death, divorce, relationship difficulties, and financial concerns.

Because ED commonly involves a host of endothelial cell risk factors, men with ED report higher rates of overt and silent myocardial infarction. Therefore, ED in an otherwise asymptomatic male warrants consideration of other vascular disorders, including CAD.

The physical examination is an essential element in the assessment of ED. Signs of hypertension as well as evidence of thyroid, hepatic, hematologic, cardiovascular, or renal diseases should be sought. An assessment should be made of the endocrine and vascular systems, the external genitalia, and the prostate gland. The penis should be palpated carefully along the corpora to detect fibrotic plaques. Reduced testicular size and loss of secondary sexual characteristics are suggestive of hypogonadism. Neurologic examination should include assessment of anal sphincter tone, investigation of the bulbocavernosus reflex, and testing for peripheral neuropathy.

Although hyperprolactinemia is uncommon, a serum prolactin level should be measured, as decreased libido and/or ED may be the presenting symptoms of a prolactinoma or another mass lesion of the sella (Chap. 339). The serum testosterone level should be measured, and if it is low, gonadotropins should be measured to determine whether hypogonadism is primary (testicular) or secondary (hypothalamic-pituitary) in origin (Chap. 346). If not performed recently, serum chemistries, complete blood count (CBC), and lipid profiles may be of value, as they can yield evidence of anemia, diabetes, hyperlipidemia, or other systemic diseases associated with ED. Determination of serum prostate-specific antigen (PSA) should be conducted according to recommended clinical guidelines (Chap. 95).

Additional diagnostic testing is rarely necessary in the evaluation of ED. However, in selected patients, specialized testing may provide insight into pathologic mechanisms of ED and aid in the selection of treatment options. Optional specialized testing includes (1) studies of nocturnal penile tumescence and rigidity, (2) vascular testing (in-office injection of vasoactive substances, penile Doppler ultrasound, penile angiography, dynamic infusion cavernosography/cavernosometry), (3) neurologic testing (biothesiometry-graded vibratory perception, somatosensory evoked potentials), and (4) psychological diagnostic tests. The information potentially gained from these procedures must be balanced against their invasiveness and cost.

TREATMENT   Male Sexual Dysfunction

PATIENT EDUCATION   Patient and partner education is essential in the treatment of ED. In goal-directed therapy, education facilitates understanding of the disease, the results of the tests, and the selection of treatment. Discussion of treatment options helps clarify how treatment is best offered and stratify first- and second-line therapies. Patients with high-risk lifestyle issues such as obesity, smoking, alcohol abuse, and recreational drug use should be counseled on the role those factors play in the development of ED.

Therapies currently employed for the treatment of ED include oral phosphodiesterase type 5 inhibitor therapy (most commonly used), injection therapies, testosterone therapy, penile devices, and psychological therapy. In addition, limited data suggest that treatments for underlying risk factors and comorbidities—for example, weight loss, exercise, stress reduction, and smoking cessation—may improve erectile function. Decisions regarding therapy should take into account the preferences and expectations of patients and their partners.

ORAL AGENTS   Sildenafil, tadalafil, and vardenafil are the only approved and effective oral agents for the treatment of ED. These three medications have markedly improved the management of ED because they are effective for the treatment of a broad range of causes, including psychogenic, diabetic, vasculogenic, postradical prostatectomy (nerve-sparing procedures), and spinal cord injury. They belong to a class of medications that are selective and potent inhibitors of PDE-5, the predominant phosphodiesterase isoform found in the penis. They are administered in graduated doses and enhance erections after sexual stimulation. The onset of action is approximately 60–120 min, depending on the medication used and other factors, such as recent food intake. Reduced initial doses should be considered for patients who are elderly, are taking concomitant alpha blockers, have renal insufficiency, or are taking medications that inhibit the CYP3A4 metabolic pathway in the liver (e.g., erythromycin, cimetidine, ketoconazole, and possibly itraconazole and mibefradil), as they may increase the serum concentration of the PDE-5 inhibitors (PDE-5i) or promote hypotension.

Several randomized trials have demonstrated the efficacy of this class of medications. There are no compelling data to support the superiority of one PDE-5i over another.

Patients may fail to respond to a PDE-5i for several reasons (Table 48-2). Some patients may not tolerate PDE-5i secondary to adverse events from vasodilation in nonpenile tissues expressing PDE-5 or from the inhibition of homologous nonpenile isozymes (i.e., PDE-6 found in the retina). Abnormal vision attributed to the effects of PDE-5i on retinal PDE-6 is of short duration, reported only with sildenafil and not thought to be clinically significant. A more serious concern is the possibility that PDE-5i may cause nonarteritic anterior ischemic optic neuropathy; although data to support that association are limited, it is prudent to avoid the use of these agents in men with a prior history of nonarteritic anterior ischemic optic neuropathy.

TABLE 48-2 Issues to Consider If Patients Report Failure of PDE-5i to Improve Erectile Dysfunction

➤ A trial of medication on at least six different days at the maximal dose should be made before declaring patient nonresponsive to PDE-5i use

➤ Taking medication after a high-fat meal

➤ Failure to include physical and psychic stimulation at the time of foreplay to induce endogenous NO

➤ Unrecognized hypogonadism

Abbreviations: NO, nitric oxide; PDE 5i, phosphodiesterase type 5 inhibitor.

Testosterone supplementation combined with a PDE-5i may be beneficial in improving erectile function in hypogonadal men with ED who are unresponsive to PDE-5i alone. These drugs do not affect ejaculation, orgasm, or sexual drive. Side effects associated with PDE-5i include headaches (19%), facial flushing (9%), dyspepsia (6%), and nasal congestion (4%). Approximately 7% of men using sildenafil may experience transient altered color vision (blue halo effect), and 6% of men taking tadalafil may experience loin pain. PDE-5i is contraindicated in men receiving nitrate therapy for cardiovascular disease, including agents delivered by the oral, sublingual, transnasal, and topical routes. These agents can potentiate its hypotensive effect and may result in profound shock. Likewise, amyl/butyl nitrate "poppers" may have a fatal synergistic effect on blood pressure. PDE-5i also should be avoided in patients with congestive heart failure and cardiomyopathy because of the risk of vascular collapse. Because sexual activity leads to an increase in physiologic expenditure [5–6 metabolic equivalents (METS)], physicians have been advised to exercise caution in prescribing any drug for sexual activity to those with active coronary disease, heart failure, borderline hypotension, or hypovolemia and to those on complex antihypertensive regimens.

Although the various forms of PDE-5i have a common mechanism of action, there are a few differences among the three agents. Tadalafil is unique in its longer half-life. All three drugs are effective for patients with ED of all ages, severities, and etiologies. Although there are pharmacokinetic and pharmacodynamic differences among these agents, clinically relevant differences are not clear.

ANDROGEN THERAPY Testosterone replacement is used to treat both primary and secondary causes of hypogonadism (Chap. 346). Androgen supplementation in the setting of normal testosterone is rarely efficacious in the treatment of ED and is discouraged. Methods of androgen replacement include transdermal patches and gels, parenteral administration of long-acting testosterone esters (enanthate and cypionate), and oral preparations (17 α-alkylated derivatives) (Chap. 346). Oral androgen preparations have the potential for hepatotoxicity and should be avoided.

Men who receive testosterone should be reevaluated after 1–3 months and at least annually thereafter for testosterone levels, erectile function, and adverse effects, which may include gynecomastia, sleep apnea, development or exacerbation of lower urinary tract symptoms or benign prostatic hyperplasia, prostate cancer, lowering of HDL, erythrocytosis, elevations of liver function tests, and reduced fertility. Periodic reevaluation should include measurement of CBC and PSA and digital rectal exam. Therapy should be discontinued in patients who do not respond within 3 months.

VACUUM CONSTRICTION DEVICES Vacuum constriction devices (VCDs) are a well-established noninvasive therapy. They are a reasonable treatment alternative for select patients who cannot take sildenafil or do not desire other interventions. VCDs draw venous blood into the penis and use a constriction ring to restrict venous return and maintain tumescence. Adverse events with VCD include pain, numbness, bruising, and altered ejaculation. Additionally, many patients complain that the devices are cumbersome and that the induced erections have a nonphysiologic appearance and feel.

INTRAURETHRAL ALPROSTADIL If a patient fails to respond to oral agents, a reasonable next choice is intraurethral or self-injection of vasoactive substances. Intraurethral prostaglandin E₁ (alprostadil), in the form of a semisolid pellet (doses of 125–1000 μg), is delivered with an applicator. Approximately 65% of men receiving intraurethral alprostadil respond with an erection when tested in the office, but only 50% achieve successful coitus at home. Intraurethral insertion is associated with a markedly reduced incidence of priapism in comparison to intracavernosal injection.

INTRACAVERNOSAL SELF-INJECTION Injection of synthetic formulations of alprostadil is effective in 70–80% of patients with ED, but discontinuation rates are high because of the invasive nature of administration. Doses range between 1 and 40 μg. Injection therapy is contraindicated in men with a history of hypersensitivity to the drug and men at risk for priapism (hypercoagulable states, sickle cell disease). Side effects include local adverse events, prolonged erections, pain, and fibrosis with chronic use. Various combinations of alprostadil, phentolamine, and/or papaverine sometimes are used.

SURGERY A less frequently used form of therapy for ED involves the surgical implantation of a semirigid or inflatable penile prosthesis. The choice of prosthesis is dependent on patient preference and should take into account body habitus and manual dexterity, which may affect the ability of the patient to manipulate the device. Because of the permanence of prosthetic devices, patients should be advised to first consider less invasive options for treatment. These surgical treatments are invasive, are associated with potential complications, and generally are reserved for treatment of refractory ED. Despite their high cost and invasiveness, penile prostheses are associated with high rates of patient and partner satisfaction.

SEX THERAPY A course of sex therapy may be useful for addressing specific interpersonal factors that may affect sexual functioning. Sex therapy generally consists of in-session discussion and at-home exercises specific to the person and the relationship. Psychosexual therapy involves techniques such as sensate focus (nongenital massage), sensory awareness exercises, correction of misconceptions about sexuality, and interpersonal difficulties therapy (e.g., open communication about sexual issues, physical intimacy scheduling, and behavioral interventions). These approaches may be useful in patients who have psychogenic or social components to their ED, although data from randomized trials are scanty and inconsistent. It is preferable if therapy includes both partners if the patient is involved in an ongoing relationship.

FEMALE SEXUAL DYSFUNCTION

Female sexual dysfunction (FSD) has traditionally included disorders of desire, arousal, pain, and muted orgasm. The associated risk factors for FSD are similar to those in males: cardiovascular disease, endocrine disorders, hypertension, neurologic disorders, and smoking (Table 48-3).

■ EPIDEMIOLOGY

Epidemiologic data are limited, but the available estimates suggest that as many as 43% of women complain of at least one sexual problem. Despite the recent interest in organic causes of FSD, desire and arousal phase disorders (including lubrication complaints) remain the most common presenting problems when surveyed in a community-based population.

■ PHYSIOLOGY OF THE FEMALE SEXUAL RESPONSE

The female sexual response requires the presence of estrogens. A role for androgens is also likely but less well established. In the CNS, estrogens and androgens work synergistically to enhance sexual arousal and response. A number of studies report enhanced libido in women during preovulatory phases of the menstrual cycle, suggesting that hormones involved in the ovulatory surge (e.g., estrogens) increase desire.

TABLE 48-3 Risk Factors for Female Sexual Dysfunction

Neurologic disease: stroke, spinal cord injury, parkinsonism

Trauma, genital surgery, radiation

Endocrinopathies: diabetes, hyperprolactinemia

Liver and/or renal failure

Cardiovascular disease

Psychological factors and interpersonal relationship disorders: sexual abuse, life stressors

Medications

    Antiandrogens: cimetidine, spironolactone

    Antidepressants, alcohol, hypnotics, sedatives

    Antiestrogens or GnRH antagonists

    Antihistamines, sympathomimetic amines

    Antihypertensives: diuretics, calcium channel blockers

    Alkylating agents

    Anticholinergics

Abbreviation: GnRH, gonadotropin-releasing hormone.

Sexual motivation is heavily influenced by context, including the environment and partner factors. Once sufficient sexual desire is reached, sexual arousal is mediated by the central and autonomic nervous systems. Cerebral sympathetic outflow is thought to increase desire, and peripheral parasympathetic activity results in clitoral vasocongestion and vaginal secretion (lubrication).

The neurotransmitters for clitoral corporal engorgement are similar to those in the male, with a prominent role for neural, smooth-muscle, and endothelial released nitric oxide (NO). A fine network of vaginal nerves and arterioles promotes a vaginal transudate. The major transmitters of this complex vaginal response are not certain, but roles for NO and vasointestinal polypeptide (VIP) are suspected. Investigators studying the normal female sexual response have challenged the long-held construct of a linear and unmitigated relationship between initial desire, arousal, vasocongestion, lubrication, and eventual orgasm. Caregivers should consider a paradigm of a positive emotional and physical outcome with one, many, or no orgasmic peak and release.

Although there are anatomic differences as well as variation in the density of vascular and neural beds in males and females, the primary effectors of sexual response are strikingly similar. Intact sensation is important for arousal. Thus, reduced levels of sexual functioning are more common in women with peripheral neuropathies (e.g., diabetes). Vaginal lubrication is a transudate of serum that results from the increased pelvic blood flow associated with arousal. Vascular insufficiency from a variety of causes may compromise adequate lubrication and result in dyspareunia. Cavernosal and arteriole smooth-muscle relaxation occurs via increased nitric oxide synthase (NOS) activity and produces engorgement in the clitoris and the surrounding vestibule. Orgasm requires an intact sympathetic outflow tract; hence, orgasmic disorders are common in female patients with spinal cord injuries.

APPROACH TO THE PATIENT: Female Sexual Dysfunction

Many women do not volunteer information about their sexual response. Open-ended questions in a supportive atmosphere are helpful in initiating a discussion of sexual fitness in women who are reluctant to discuss such issues. Once a complaint has been voiced, a comprehensive evaluation should be performed, including a medical history, a psychosocial history, a physical examination, and limited laboratory testing.

The history should include the usual medical, surgical, obstetric, psychological, gynecologic, sexual, and social information. Past experiences, intimacy, knowledge, and partner availability should also be ascertained. Medical disorders that may affect sexual health should be delineated. They include diabetes, cardiovascular disease, gynecologic conditions, obstetric history, depression, anxiety disorders, and neurologic disease. Medications should be reviewed as they may affect arousal, libido, and orgasm. The need for counseling and recognizing life stresses should be identified. The physical examination should assess the genitalia, including the clitoris. Pelvic floor examination may identify prolapse or other disorders. Laboratory studies are needed, especially if menopausal status is uncertain. Estradiol, follicle-stimulating hormone (FSH), and luteinizing hormone (LH) are usually obtained, and dehydroepiandrosterone (DHEA) should be considered as it reflects adrenal androgen secretion. A CBC, liver function assessment, and lipid studies may be useful, if not otherwise obtained. Complicated diagnostic evaluation such as clitoral Doppler ultrasonography and biothesiometry require expensive equipment and are of uncertain utility. It is important for the patient to identify which symptoms are most distressing.

The evaluation of FSD previously occurred mainly in a psychosocial context. However, inconsistencies between diagnostic categories based only on psychosocial considerations and the emerging recognition of organic etiologies have led to a new classification of FSD. This diagnostic scheme is based on four components that are not mutually exclusive: (1) *Hypoactive sexual desire*—the persistent or recurrent lack of sexual thoughts and/or receptivity to sexual activity, which causes personal distress. Hypoactive sexual desire may result from endocrine failure or may be associated with psychological or emotional disorders, (2) *Sexual arousal disorder*—the persistent or recurrent inability to attain or maintain sexual excitement, which causes personal distress, (3) *Orgasmic disorder*—the persistent or recurrent loss of orgasmic potential after sufficient sexual stimulation and arousal, which causes personal distress, and (4) *Sexual pain disorder*—persistent or recurrent genital pain associated with noncoital sexual stimulation, which causes personal distress. This newer classification emphasizes "personal distress" as a requirement for dysfunction and provides clinicians with an organized framework for evaluation before or in conjunction with more traditional counseling methods.

TREATMENT: Female Sexual Dysfunction

GENERAL An open discussion with the patient is important as couples may need to be educated about normal anatomy and physiologic responses, including the role of orgasm, in sexual encounters. Physiologic changes associated with aging and/or disease should be explained. Couples may need to be reminded that clitoral stimulation rather than coital intromission may be more beneficial.

Behavioral modification and nonpharmacologic therapies should be a first step. Patient and partner counseling may improve communication and relationship strains. Lifestyle changes involving known risk factors can be an important part of the treatment process. Emphasis on maximizing physical health and avoiding lifestyles (e.g., smoking, alcohol abuse) and medications likely to produce FSD is important (Table 48-3). The use of topical lubricants may address complaints of dyspareunia and dryness. Contributing medications such as antidepressants may need to be altered, including the use of medications with less impact on sexual function, dose reduction, medication switching, or drug holidays.

HORMONAL THERAPY In postmenopausal women, estrogen replacement therapy may be helpful in treating vaginal atrophy, decreasing coital pain, and improving clitoral sensitivity (Chap. 348). Estrogen replacement in the form of local cream is the preferred method, as it avoids systemic side effects. Androgen levels in women decline substantially before menopause. However, low levels of testosterone or DHEA are not effective predictors of a positive therapeutic outcome with androgen therapy. The widespread use of exogenous androgens is not supported by the literature except in select circumstances (premature ovarian failure or menopausal states) and in secondary arousal disorders.

ORAL AGENTS The efficacy of PDE-5i in FDS has been a marked disappointment in light of the proposed role of nitric oxide–dependent physiology in the normal female sexual response. The use of PDE-5i for FSD should be discouraged pending proof that it is effective.

CLITORAL VACUUM DEVICE In patients with arousal and orgasmic difficulties, the option of using a clitoral vacuum device may be explored. This handheld battery-operated device has a small soft plastic cup that applies a vacuum over the stimulated clitoris. This causes increased cavernosal blood flow, engorgement, and vaginal lubrication.

FURTHER READINGS

ARAUJO AB et al: Changes in sexual function in middle-aged and older men: Longitudinal data from the Massachusetts male aging study. J Am Geriatr Soc 52:1502, 2004

BHASIN S et al: Sexual dysfunction in men and women with endocrine disorders. Lancet 369:597, 2007

BURNETT AL: Erectile dysfunction. J Urol 175:S25, 2006

CAPPELLERI JC et al: A 5-year review of research and clinical experience. Int J Impot Res 17:307, 2005

DAVIS SR et al: Endocrine aspects of female sexual dysfunction. J Sex Med 1:82, 2004

DOGGRELL SA: Comparison of clinical trials with sildenafil, vardenafil, and tadalafil in erectile dysfunction. Expert Opin Pharmacother 6:75, 2005

ESPOSITO K et al: Effect of lifestyle changes on erectile dysfunction in obese men: A randomized controlled trial. JAMA 291:2978, 2004

INMAN BA et al. A population-based, longitudinal study of erectile dysfunction and future coronary artery disease. Mayo Clin Proc 84:108, 2009

PAULS RN et al: Female sexual dysfunction: Principles of diagnosis and therapy. Obstet Gynecol Surv 60:196, 2005

REES PM et al: Sexual function in men and women with neurological disorders. Lancet 369(9560):512, 2007

THOMPSON IM et al: Erectile dysfunction and subsequent cardiovascular disease. JAMA 294:2996, 2005

CHAPTER **49**

Hirsutism and Virilization

David A. Ehrmann

Hirsutism, which is defined as androgen-dependent excessive male-pattern hair growth, affects approximately 10% of women. Hirsutism is most often idiopathic or the consequence of androgen excess associated with the polycystic ovarian syndrome (PCOS). Less frequently, it may result from adrenal androgen overproduction as occurs in nonclassic congenital adrenal hyperplasia (CAH) (Table 49-1). Rarely, it is a harbinger of a serious underlying condition. Cutaneous manifestations commonly associated with hirsutism include acne and male-pattern balding (androgenic alopecia). *Virilization* refers to a condition in which androgen levels are sufficiently high to cause additional signs and symptoms, such as deepening of the voice, breast atrophy, increased muscle bulk, clitoromegaly, and increased libido; virilization is an ominous sign that suggests the possibility of an ovarian or adrenal neoplasm.

■ HAIR FOLLICLE GROWTH AND DIFFERENTIATION

Hair can be categorized as either *vellus* (fine, soft, and not pigmented) or *terminal* (long, coarse, and pigmented). The number of hair follicles does not change over an individual's lifetime, but the follicle size and type of hair can change in response to numerous factors, particularly androgens. Androgens are necessary for terminal hair and sebaceous gland development and mediate differentiation of pilosebaceous units (PSUs) into either a terminal hair follicle or a sebaceous gland. In the former case, androgens transform the vellus hair into a terminal hair; in the latter case, the sebaceous component proliferates and the hair remains vellus.

There are three phases in the cycle of hair growth: (1) *anagen* (growth phase), (2) *catagen* (involution phase), and (3) *telogen* (rest phase). Depending on the body site, hormonal regulation may play an important role in the hair growth cycle. For example, the eyebrows, eyelashes, and vellus hairs are androgen-insensitive, whereas the axillary and pubic areas are sensitive to low levels of androgens. Hair growth on the face, chest, upper abdomen, and back requires higher levels of androgens and is therefore more characteristic of the pattern typically seen in men. Androgen excess in women leads to increased hair growth in most androgen-sensitive sites except in the scalp region, where hair loss occurs because androgens cause scalp hairs to spend less time in the anagen phase.

Although androgen excess underlies most cases of hirsutism, there is only a modest correlation between androgen levels and the quantity of hair growth. This is due to the fact that hair growth from the follicle also depends on local growth factors, and there is variability in end organ (PSU) sensitivity. Genetic factors and ethnic background also influence hair growth. In general, dark-haired individuals tend to be more hirsute than blond or fair individuals. Asians and Native Americans have relatively sparse hair in regions sensitive to high androgen levels, whereas people of Mediterranean descent are more hirsute.

■ CLINICAL ASSESSMENT

Historic elements relevant to the assessment of hirsutism include the age at onset and rate of progression of hair growth and associated symptoms or signs (e.g., acne). Depending on the cause, excess

TABLE 49-1 Causes of Hirsutism

Gonadal hyperandrogenism
  Ovarian hyperandrogenism
  Polycystic ovary syndrome/functional ovarian hyperandrogenism
  Ovarian steroidogenic blocks
  Syndromes of extreme insulin resistance
  Ovarian neoplasms
Adrenal hyperandrogenism
  Premature adrenarche
  Functional adrenal hyperandrogenism
  Congenital adrenal hyperplasia (nonclassic and classic)
  Abnormal cortisol action/metabolism
  Adrenal neoplasms
Other endocrine disorders
  Cushing's syndrome
  Hyperprolactinemia
  Acromegaly
Peripheral androgen overproduction
  Obesity
  Idiopathic
Pregnancy-related hyperandrogenism
  Hyperreactio luteinalis
  Thecoma of pregnancy
Drugs
  Androgens
  Oral contraceptives containing androgenic progestins
  Minoxidil
  Phenytoin
  Diazoxide
  Cyclosporine
True hermaphroditism

hair growth typically is first noted during the second and third decades of life. The growth is usually slow but progressive. Sudden development and rapid progression of hirsutism suggest the possibility of an androgen-secreting neoplasm, in which case virilization also may be present.

The age at onset of menstrual cycles (menarche) and the pattern of the menstrual cycle should be ascertained; irregular cycles from the time of menarche onward are more likely to result from ovarian rather than adrenal androgen excess. Associated symptoms such as galactorrhea should prompt evaluation for hyperprolactinemia (Chap. 339) and possibly hypothyroidism (Chap. 341). Hypertension, striae, easy bruising, centripetal weight gain, and weakness suggest hypercortisolism (Cushing's syndrome; Chap. 342). Rarely, patients with growth hormone excess (i.e., acromegaly) present with hirsutism. Use of medications such as phenytoin, minoxidil, and cyclosporine may be associated with androgen-independent excess hair growth (i.e., hypertrichosis). A family history of infertility and/or hirsutism may indicate disorders such as nonclassic CAH (Chap. 342).

Physical examination should include measurement of height and weight and calculation of body mass index (BMI). A BMI >25 kg/m^2 is indicative of excess weight for height, and values >30 kg/m^2 are often seen in association with hirsutism, probably the result of increased conversion of androgen precursors to testosterone.

Notation should be made of blood pressure, as adrenal causes may be associated with hypertension. Cutaneous signs sometimes associated with androgen excess and insulin resistance include acanthosis nigricans and skin tags.

An objective clinical assessment of hair distribution and quantity is central to the evaluation in any woman presenting with hirsutism. This assessment permits the distinction between hirsutism and hypertrichosis and provides a baseline reference point to gauge the response to treatment. A simple and commonly used method to grade hair growth is the modified scale of Ferriman and Gallwey (Fig. 49-1), in which each of nine androgen-sensitive sites is graded from 0 to 4. Approximately 95% of white women have a score below 8 on this scale; thus, it is normal for most women to have some hair growth in androgen-sensitive sites. Scores above 8 suggest excess androgen-mediated hair growth, a finding that should be assessed further by means of hormonal evaluation (see below). In racial/ethnic groups that are less likely to manifest hirsutism (e.g., Asian women), additional cutaneous evidence of androgen excess should be sought, including pustular acne and thinning scalp hair.

■ HORMONAL EVALUATION

Androgens are secreted by the ovaries and adrenal glands in response to their respective tropic hormones: luteinizing hormone (LH) and adrenocorticotropic hormone (ACTH). The principal circulating steroids involved in the etiology of hirsutism are testosterone, androstenedione, and dehydroepiandrosterone (DHEA) and its sulfated form (DHEAS). The ovaries and adrenal glands normally contribute about equally to testosterone production. Approximately half of the total testosterone originates from direct glandular secretion, and the remainder is derived from the peripheral conversion of androstenedione and DHEA (Chap. 346).

Although it is the most important circulating androgen, testosterone is in effect the penultimate androgen in mediating hirsutism; it is converted to the more potent dihydrotestosterone (DHT) by the enzyme 5α-reductase, which is located in the PSU. DHT has a higher affinity for, and slower dissociation from, the androgen receptor. The local production of DHT allows it to serve as the primary mediator of androgen action at the level of the pilosebaceous unit. There are two isoenzymes of 5α-reductase: Type 2 is found in the prostate gland and in hair follicles, and type 1 is found primarily in sebaceous glands.

One approach to testing for hyperandrogenemia is depicted in Fig. 49-2. In addition to measuring blood levels of testosterone and DHEAS, it is important to measure the level of free (or unbound) testosterone. The fraction of testosterone that is not bound to its carrier protein, sex hormone–binding globulin (SHBG), is biologically available for conversion to DHT and binding to androgen receptors. Hyperinsulinemia and/or androgen excess decrease hepatic production of SHBG, resulting in levels of total testosterone within the high-normal range, whereas the unbound hormone is elevated more substantially. Although there is a decline in ovarian testosterone production after menopause, ovarian estrogen production decreases to an even greater extent, and the concentration of SHBG is reduced. Consequently, there is an increase in the relative proportion of unbound testosterone, and it may exacerbate hirsutism after menopause.

A baseline plasma total testosterone level >12 nmol/L (>3.5 ng/mL) usually indicates a virilizing tumor, whereas a level >7 nmol/L (>2 ng/mL) is suggestive. A basal DHEAS level >18.5 μmol/L (>7000 μg/L) suggests an adrenal tumor. Although DHEAS has been proposed as a "marker" of predominant adrenal androgen excess, it is not unusual to find modest elevations in DHEAS among women with PCOS. Computed tomography (CT) or magnetic resonance imaging (MRI) should be used to localize an adrenal mass,

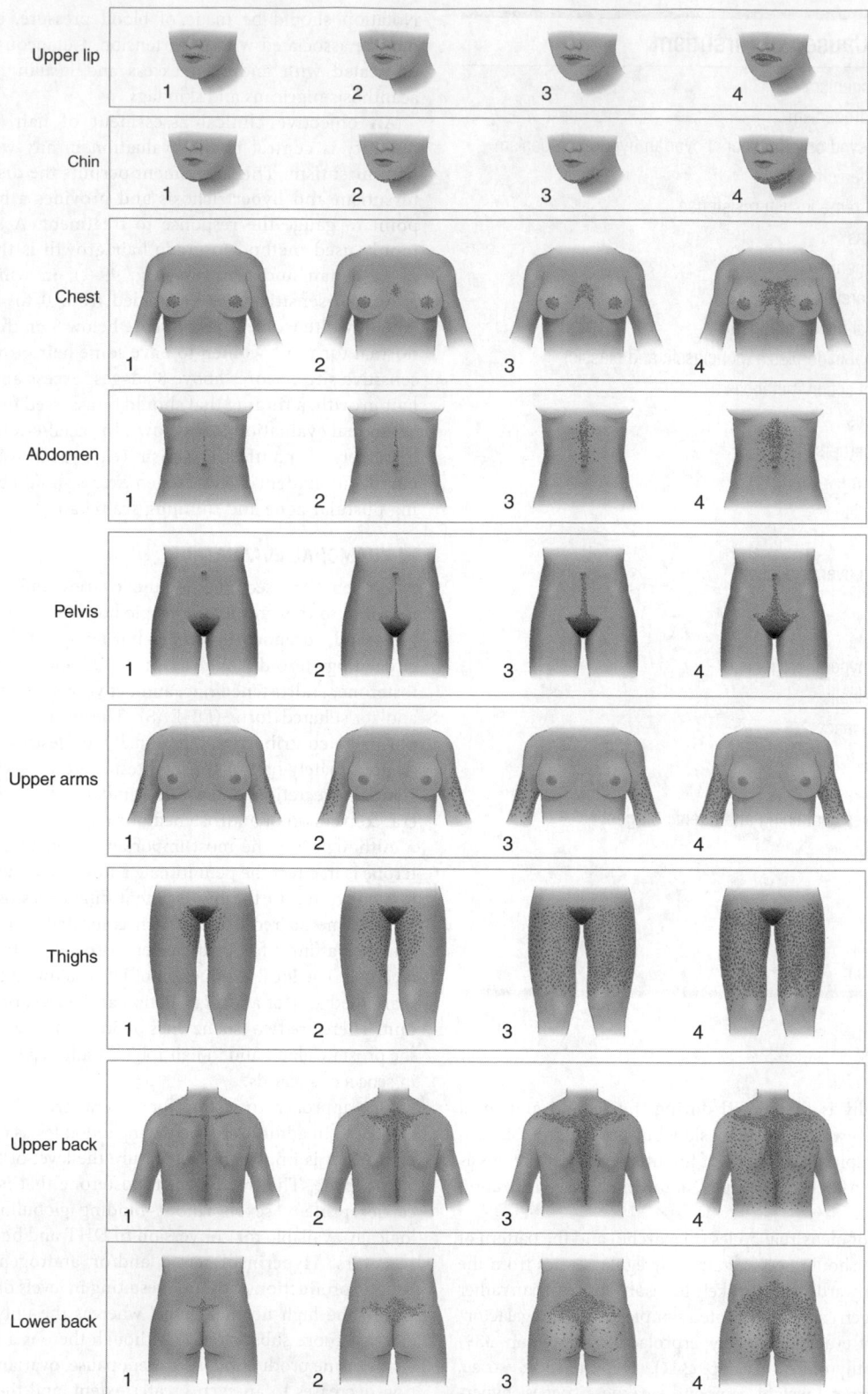

Figure 49-1   Hirsutism scoring scale of Ferriman and Gallwey. The nine body areas that have androgen-sensitive areas are graded from 0 (no terminal hair) to 4 (frankly virile) to obtain a total score. A normal hirsutism score is <8. *[Modified from DA Ehrmann et al: Hyperandrogenism, hirsutism, and polycystic ovary syndrome, in LJ DeGroot and JL Jameson (eds), Endocrinology, 5th ed. Philadelphia, Saunders, 2006; with permission.]*

and ultrasound usually suffices to identify an ovarian mass if clinical evaluation and hormonal levels suggest these possibilities.

PCOS is the most common cause of ovarian androgen excess (Chap. 347). An increased ratio of LH to follicle-stimulating

hormone is characteristic in carefully studied patients with PCOS. However, because of the pulsatile nature of gonadotropin secretion, this finding may be absent in up to half of women with PCOS. Transvaginal ultrasound classically shows enlarged ovaries and increased stroma in women with PCOS. However, cystic ovaries also may be found in women without clinical or laboratory features of PCOS. Although usually limited to a research setting, a gonadotropin-releasing hormone agonist test can be used to make a specific diagnosis of ovarian hyperandrogenism. A peak 17-hydroxyprogesterone level ≥7.8 nmol/L (≥2.6 µg/L) after the administration of 100 µg nafarelin (or 10 µg/kg leuprolide) subcutaneously is virtually diagnostic of ovarian hyperandrogenism.

Because adrenal androgens are readily suppressed by low doses of glucocorticoids, the dexamethasone androgen-suppression test may broadly distinguish ovarian from adrenal androgen overproduction. A blood sample is obtained before and after the administration of dexa-methasone (0.5 mg orally every 6 h for 4 days). An adrenal source is suggested by suppression of unbound testosterone into the normal range; incomplete suppression suggests ovarian androgen excess. An overnight 1-mg dexamethasone suppression test, with measurement of 8:00 A.M. serum cortisol, is useful when there is clinical suspicion of Cushing's syndrome (Chap. 342).

Nonclassic CAH is most commonly due to 21-hydroxylase deficiency but also can be caused by autosomal recessive defects in other steroidogenic enzymes necessary for adrenal corticosteroid synthesis (Chap. 342). Because of the enzyme defect, the adrenal gland cannot secrete glucocorticoids (especially cortisol) efficiently. This results in diminished negative feedback inhibition of ACTH, leading to compensatory adrenal hyperplasia and the accumulation of steroid precursors that subsequently are converted to androgen. Deficiency of 21-hydroxylase can be reliably excluded by determining a morning 17-hydroxyprogesterone level <6 nmol/L (<2 µg/L) (drawn in the follicular phase). Alternatively, 21-hydroxylase deficiency can be diagnosed by measurement of 17-hydroxyprogesterone 1 h after the administration of 250 µg of synthetic ACTH (cosyntropin) intravenously.

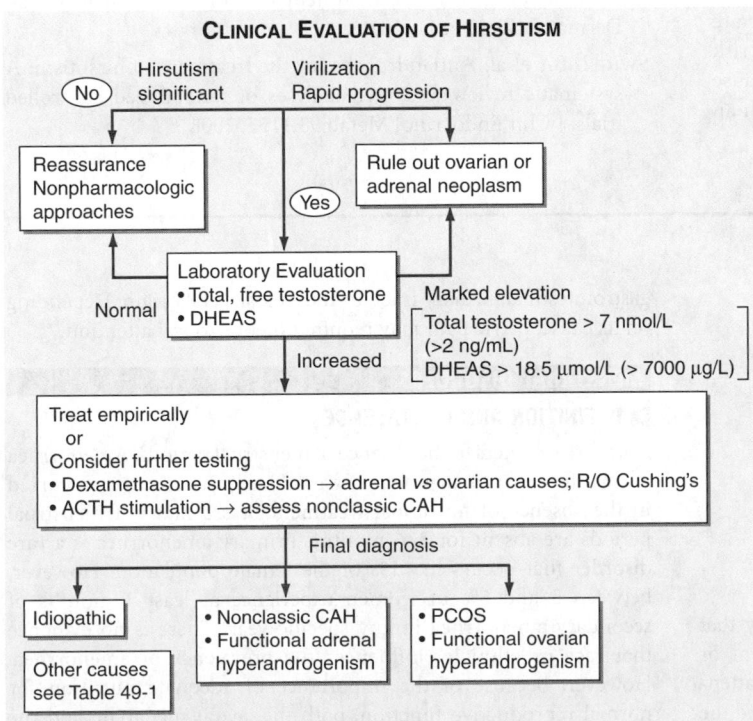

CLINICAL EVALUATION OF HIRSUTISM

Figure 49-2 Algorithm for the evaluation and differential diagnosis of hirsutism. ACTH, adrenocorticotropic hormone; CAH, congenital adrenal hyperplasia; DHEAS, sulfated form of dehydroepiandrosterone; PCOS, polycystic ovarian syndrome.

TREATMENT ▶ Hirsutism

Treatment of hirsutism may be accomplished pharmacologically or by mechanical means of hair removal. Nonpharmacologic treatments should be considered in all patients either as the only treatment or as an adjunct to drug therapy.

Nonpharmacologic treatments include (1) bleaching, (2) depilatory (removal from the skin surface) such as shaving and chemical treatments, and (3) epilatory (removal of the hair including the root) such as plucking, waxing, electrolysis, and laser therapy. Despite perceptions to the contrary, shaving does not increase the rate or density of hair growth. Chemical depilatory treatments may be useful for mild hirsutism that affects only limited skin areas, though they can cause skin irritation. Wax treatment removes hair temporarily but is uncomfortable. Electrolysis is effective for more permanent hair removal, particularly in the hands of a skilled electrologist. Laser phototherapy appears to be efficacious for hair removal. It delays hair regrowth and causes permanent hair removal in most patients. The long-term effects and complications associated with laser treatment are being evaluated.

Pharmacologic therapy is directed at interrupting one or more of the steps in the pathway of androgen synthesis and action: (1) suppression of adrenal and/or ovarian androgen production, (2) enhancement of androgen-binding to plasma-binding proteins, particularly SHBG, (3) impairment of the peripheral conversion of androgen precursors to active androgen, and (4) inhibition of androgen action at the target tissue level. Attenuation of hair growth is typically not evident until 4–6 months after initiation of medical treatment and in most cases leads to only a modest reduction in hair growth.

Combination estrogen-progestin therapy in the form of an oral contraceptive is usually the first-line endocrine treatment for hirsutism and acne, after cosmetic and dermatologic management. The estrogenic component of most oral contraceptives currently in use is either ethinyl estradiol or mestranol. The suppression of LH leads to reduced production of ovarian androgens. The reduced androgen levels also result in a dose-related increase in SHBG, thus lowering the fraction of unbound plasma testosterone. Combination therapy also has been demonstrated to decrease DHEAS, perhaps by reducing ACTH levels. Estrogens also have a direct, dose-dependent suppressive effect on sebaceous cell function.

The choice of a specific oral contraceptive should be predicated on the progestational component, as progestins vary in their suppressive effect on SHBG levels and in their androgenic potential. Ethynodiol diacetate has relatively low androgenic potential, whereas progestins such as norgestrel and levonorgestrel are particularly androgenic, as judged from their attenuation of the estrogen-induced increase in SHBG. Norgestimate exemplifies the newer generation of progestins that are virtually nonandrogenic. Drospirenone, an analogue of spironolactone that has both antimineralocorticoid and antiandrogenic activities, has been approved for use as a progestational agent in combination with ethinyl estradiol.

Oral contraceptives are contraindicated in women with a history of thromboembolic disease and women with increased risk of breast or other estrogen-dependent cancers (Chap. 348). There is a relative contraindication to the use of oral contraceptives in smokers and those with hypertension or a history of migraine headaches. In most trials, estrogen-progestin therapy alone improves the extent of acne by a maximum of 50–70%. The effect on hair growth may not be evident for 6 months, and the maximum effect may require 9–12 months owing to the length of the hair growth cycle. Improvements in hirsutism are typically in the range of 20%, but there may be an arrest of further progression of hair growth.

Adrenal androgens are more sensitive than cortisol to the suppressive effects of glucocorticoids. Therefore, glucocorticoids are the mainstay of treatment in patients with CAH. Although glucocorticoids have been reported to restore ovulatory function in some women with PCOS, this effect is highly variable. Because of side effects from excessive glucocorticoids, low doses should be used. Dexamethasone (0.2–0.5 mg) or prednisone (5–10 mg) should be taken at bedtime to achieve maximal suppression by inhibiting the nocturnal surge of ACTH.

Cyproterone acetate is the prototypic antiandrogen. It acts mainly by competitive inhibition of the binding of testosterone and DHT to the androgen receptor. In addition, it may enhance the metabolic clearance of testosterone by inducing hepatic enzymes. Although not available for use in the United States, cyproterone acetate is widely used in Canada, Mexico, and Europe. Cyproterone (50–100 mg) is given on days 1–15 and ethinyl estradiol (50 μg) is given on days 5–26 of the menstrual cycle. Side effects include irregular uterine bleeding, nausea, headache, fatigue, weight gain, and decreased libido.

Spironolactone, which usually is used as a mineralocorticoid antagonist, is also a weak antiandrogen. It is almost as effective as cyproterone acetate when used at high enough doses (100–200 mg daily). Patients should be monitored intermittently for hyperkalemia or hypotension, though these side effects are uncommon. Pregnancy should be avoided because of the risk of feminization of a male fetus. Spironolactone can also cause menstrual irregularity. It often is used in combination with an oral contraceptive, which suppresses ovarian androgen production and helps prevent pregnancy.

Flutamide is a potent nonsteroidal antiandrogen that is effective in treating hirsutism, but concerns about the induction of hepatocellular dysfunction have limited its use. Finasteride is a competitive inhibitor of 5α-reductase type 2. Beneficial effects on hirsutism have been reported, but the predominance of 5α-reductase type 1 in the PSU appears to account for its limited efficacy. Finasteride would also be expected to impair sexual differentiation in a male fetus, and it should not be used in women who may become pregnant.

Eflornithine cream (Vaniqa) has been approved as a novel treatment for unwanted facial hair in women, but long-term efficacy remains to be established. It can cause skin irritation under exaggerated conditions of use. Ultimately, the choice of any specific agent(s) must be tailored to the unique needs of the patient being treated. As noted previously, pharmacologic treatments for hirsutism should be used in conjunction with nonpharmacologic approaches. It is also helpful to review the pattern of female hair distribution in the normal population to dispel unrealistic expectations.

FURTHER READINGS

EHRMANN DA: Polycystic ovary syndrome. N Engl J Med 352:1223, 2005

MARTIN KA et al: Evaluation and treatment of hirsutism in premenopausal women: An Endocrine Society clinical practice guideline. J Clin Endocrinol Metab 93:1105, 2008

PALL M et al: The phenotype of hirsute women: A comparison of polycystic ovary syndrome and 21-hydroxylase–deficient nonclassic adrenal hyperplasia. Fertil Steril 94:684, 2010

RATHNAYAKE D, SINCLAIR: Innovative use of spironolactone as an antiandrogen in the treatment of female pattern hair loss. Dermatol Clin 28:611, 2010

SWIGLO BA et al: Antiandrogens for the treatment of hirsutism: A systematic review and metaanalyses of randomized controlled trials. J Clin Endocrinol Metab 93:1153, 2008

CHAPTER 50

Menstrual Disorders and Pelvic Pain

Janet E. Hall

Menstrual dysfunction can signal an underlying abnormality that may have long-term health consequences. Although frequent or prolonged bleeding usually prompts a woman to seek medical attention, infrequent or absent bleeding may seem less troubling and the patient may not bring it to the attention of the physician. Thus, a focused menstrual history is a critical part of every encounter with a female patient. Pelvic pain is a common complaint that may relate to an abnormality of the reproductive organs but also may be of gastrointestinal, urinary tract, or musculoskeletal origin. Depending on its cause, pelvic pain may require urgent surgical attention.

MENSTRUAL DISORDERS

DEFINITION AND PREVALENCE

Amenorrhea refers to the absence of menstrual periods. Amenorrhea is classified as *primary* if menstrual bleeding has never occurred in the absence of hormonal treatment or *secondary* if menstrual periods are absent for 3–6 months. Primary amenorrhea is a rare disorder that occurs in <1% of the female population. However, between 3 and 5% of women experience at least 3 months of secondary amenorrhea in any specific year. There is no evidence that race or ethnicity influences the prevalence of amenorrhea. However, because of the importance of adequate nutrition for normal reproductive function, both the age at menarche and the prevalence of secondary amenorrhea vary significantly in different parts of the world.

Oligomenorrhea is defined as a cycle length >35 days or <10 menses per year. Both the frequency and the amount of vaginal bleeding are irregular in oligomenorrhea. It is often associated with anovulation, which also can occur with intermenstrual intervals <24 days or vaginal bleeding for >7 days. Frequent or heavy irregular bleeding is termed *dysfunctional uterine bleeding* if anatomic uterine lesions or a bleeding diathesis has been excluded.

Primary amenorrhea

The absence of menses by age 16 has been used traditionally to define primary amenorrhea. However, other factors, such as growth, secondary sexual characteristics, the presence of cyclic pelvic pain, and the secular trend toward an earlier age of menarche, particularly in African-American girls, also influence the age at which primary amenorrhea should be investigated. Thus, an evaluation for amenorrhea should be initiated by age 15 or 16 in the presence of normal growth and secondary sexual characteristics; age 13 in the absence of secondary sexual characteristics or if height is less than the third percentile; age 12 or 13 in the presence of breast development and cyclic pelvic pain; or within 2 years of breast development if menarche, defined by the first menstrual period, has not occurred.

Secondary amenorrhea or oligomenorrhea

Anovulation and irregular cycles are relatively common for up to 2 years after menarche and for 1–2 years before the final menstrual period. In the intervening years, menstrual cycle length is ~28 days, with an intermenstrual interval normally ranging between 25 and 35 days. Cycle-to-cycle variability in an individual woman who is ovulating consistently is generally +/– 2 days. Pregnancy is the most common cause of amenorrhea and should be excluded early in any evaluation of menstrual irregularity. However, many women occasionally miss a single period. Three or more months of secondary amenorrhea should prompt an evaluation, as should a history of intermenstrual intervals >35 or <21 days or bleeding that persists for >7 days.

■ DIAGNOSIS

Evaluation of menstrual dysfunction depends on understanding the interrelationships between the four critical components of the reproductive tract: (1) the hypothalamus, (2) the pituitary, (3) the ovaries, and (4) the uterus and outflow tract (Fig. 50-1; Chap. 347). This system is maintained by complex negative and positive feedback loops involving the ovarian steroids (estradiol and progesterone) and peptides (inhibin B and inhibin A) and the hypothalamic [gonadotropin-releasing hormone (GnRH)] and pituitary [follicle-stimulating hormone (FSH) and luteinizing hormone (LH)] components of this system (Fig. 50-1).

Disorders of menstrual function can be thought of in two main categories: disorders of the uterus and outflow tract and disorders of ovulation. Many of the conditions that cause primary amenorrhea are congenital but go unrecognized until the time of normal puberty (e.g., genetic, chromosomal, and anatomic abnormalities). All causes of secondary amenorrhea also can cause primary amenorrhea.

Disorders of the uterus or outflow tract

Abnormalities of the uterus and outflow tract typically present as primary amenorrhea. In patients with normal pubertal development and a blind vagina, the differential diagnosis includes *obstruction* by a transverse vaginal septum or imperforate hymen; *müllerian agenesis* (Mayer-Rokitansky-Kuster-Hauser syndrome), which has been associated with mutations in the *WNT4* gene; and *androgen insensitivity syndrome* (AIS), which is an X-linked recessive disorder that accounts for ~10% of all cases of primary amenorrhea (Chap. 346). Patients with AIS have a 46,XY karyotype, but because of the lack of androgen receptor responsiveness, they have severe underandrogenization and female external genitalia. The absence of pubic and axillary hair distinguishes them clinically from patients with müllerian agenesis. *Asherman syndrome* presents as secondary amenorrhea or hypomenorrhea and results from partial or complete obliteration of the uterine cavity by adhesions that prevent normal growth and shedding of the endometrium. Curettage performed for pregnancy complications accounts for >90% of cases; genital tuberculosis is an important cause in regions where it is endemic.

TREATMENT	Disorders of the Uterus or Outflow Tract

Obstruction of the outflow tract requires surgical correction. The risk of endometriosis is increased with this condition, perhaps because of retrograde menstrual flow. *Müllerian agenesis* also may require surgical intervention, although vaginal dilatation is

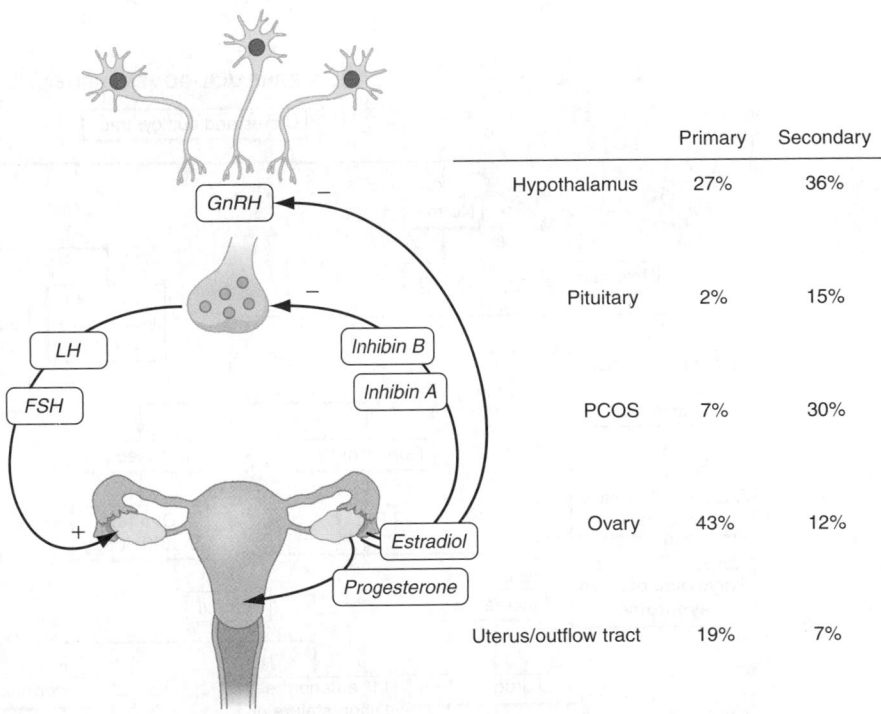

	Primary	Secondary
Hypothalamus	27%	36%
Pituitary	2%	15%
PCOS	7%	30%
Ovary	43%	12%
Uterus/outflow tract	19%	7%

Figure 50-1 Role of the hypothalamic-pituitary-gonadal axis in the etiology of amenorrhea. Gonadotropin-releasing hormone (GnRH) secretion from the hypothalamus stimulates follicle-stimulating hormone (FSH) and luteinizing hormone (LH) secretion from the pituitary to induce ovarian folliculogenesis and steroidogenesis. Ovarian secretion of estradiol and progesterone controls the shedding of the endometrium, resulting in menses, and, in combination with the inhibins, provides feedback regulation of the hypothalamus and pituitary to control secretion of FSH and LH. The prevalence of amenorrhea resulting from abnormalities at each level of the reproductive system (hypothalamus, pituitary, ovary, uterus and outflow tract) varies depending on whether amenorrhea is primary or secondary. PCOS, polycystic ovarian syndrome.

adequate in some patients. Because ovarian function is normal, assisted reproductive techniques can be used with a surrogate carrier. *Androgen resistance syndrome* requires gonadectomy because there is risk of gonadoblastoma in the dysgenetic gonads. Whether this should be performed in early childhood or after completion of breast development is controversial. Estrogen replacement is indicated after gonadectomy, and vaginal dilatation may be required to allow sexual intercourse.

Disorders of ovulation

Once uterus and outflow tract abnormalities have been excluded, other causes of amenorrhea involve disorders of ovulation. The differential diagnosis is based on the results of initial tests, including a pregnancy test, gonadotropins (to determine whether the cause is likely to be ovarian or central), and assessment of hyperandrogenism (Fig. 50-2).

Hypogonadotropic hypogonadism Low estrogen levels in combination with normal or low levels of LH and FSH are seen with anatomic, genetic, or functional abnormalities that interfere with hypothalamic GnRH secretion or normal pituitary responsiveness to GnRH. Although relatively uncommon, tumors and infiltrative diseases should be considered in the differential diagnosis of hypogonadotropic hypogonadism (Chap. 339). These disorders may present with primary or secondary amenorrhea. They may occur in association with other features suggestive of hypothalamic or pituitary dysfunction, such as short stature, diabetes insipidus, galactorrhea, and headache. Hypogonadotropic hypogonadism also may be seen after cranial irradiation. In the postpartum period, it

may be caused by pituitary necrosis (Sheehan's syndrome) or lymphocytic hypophysitis. Because reproductive dysfunction is commonly associated with hyperprolactinemia from neuroanatomic lesions or medications, prolactin should be measured in all patients with hypogonadotropic hypogonadism (Chap. 339).

Isolated hypogonadotropic hypogonadism (IHH) occurs in women, although it is more common in men. IHH generally presents with primary amenorrhea and is associated with anosmia in about 50% of women (termed Kallmann syndrome). Genetic causes of IHH have been identified in approximately 35% of patients (Chaps. 346 and 347).

Functional hypothalamic amenorrhea (HA) is caused by a mismatch between energy expenditure and energy intake. Recent studies suggest that variants in genes associated with IHH may increase susceptibility to these environmental inputs, accounting in part for the clinical variability in this disorder. Leptin secretion may play a key role in transducing the signals from the periphery to the hypothalamus in HA. The hypothalamic-pituitary-adrenal axis also may play a role. The diagnosis of HA generally can be made on the basis of a careful history, a physical examination, and the demonstration of low levels of gonadotropins and normal prolactin levels. Eating disorders and chronic disease must be specifically excluded (Chap. 79). An atypical history, headache, signs of other hypothalamic dysfunction, or hyperprolactinemia, even if mild, necessitates cranial imaging with CT or MRI to exclude a neuroanatomic cause.

Hypergonadotropic hypogonadism Ovarian failure is considered premature when it occurs in women <40 years old and accounts for ~10% of secondary amenorrhea. *Primary ovarian insufficiency*

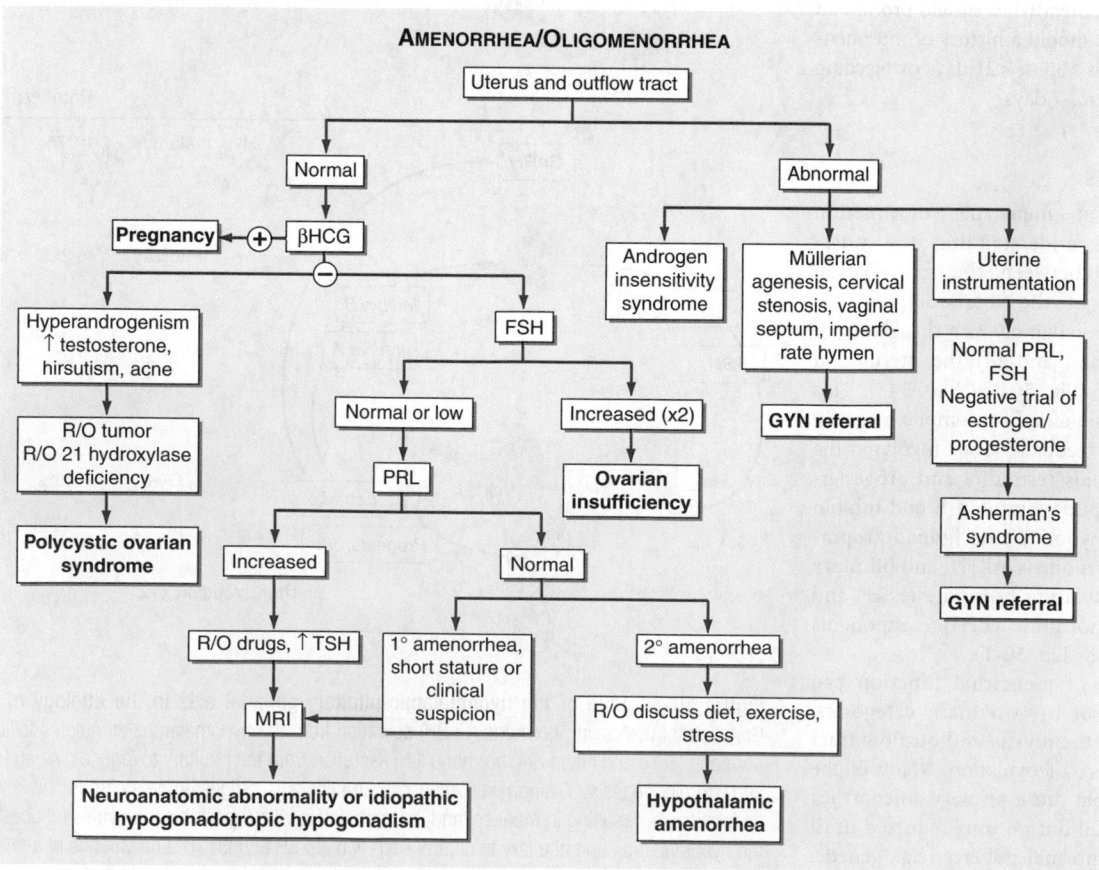

Figure 50-2 Algorithm for evaluation of amenorrhea. β-hCG, human chorionic gonadotropin; FSH, follicle-stimulating hormone; PRL, prolactin; TSH, thyroid-stimulating hormone.

(POI) has generally replaced the terms *premature menopause* and *premature ovarian failure* in recognition that this disorder represents a continuum of impaired ovarian function. Ovarian insufficiency is associated with the loss of negative-feedback restraint on the hypothalamus and pituitary, resulting in increased FSH and LH levels. FSH is a better marker of ovarian failure as its levels are less variable than those of LH. As with natural menopause, POI may wax and wane, and serial measurements may be necessary to establish the diagnosis.

Once the diagnosis of POI has been established, further evaluation is indicated because of other health problems that may be associated with POI. For example, POI occurs in association with a variety of chromosomal abnormalities, including Turner syndrome, autoimmune polyglandular failure syndromes, radio- and chemotherapy, and galactosemia. The recognition that early ovarian failure occurs in premutation carriers of the fragile X syndrome is important because of the increased risk of severe mental retardation in male children with *FMR1* mutations. In the majority of cases, however, a cause for POI is not determined.

Hypergonadotropic hypogonadism occurs rarely in other disorders, such as mutations in the FSH or LH receptors. Aromatase deficiency and 17α-hydroxylase deficiency are associated with elevated gonadotropins with hyperandrogenism and hypertension, respectively. Gonadotropin-secreting tumors in women of reproductive age generally present with high, rather than low, estrogen levels and cause ovarian hyperstimulation or dysfunctional bleeding.

TREATMENT   Hypo- and Hypergonadotropic Causes of Amenorrhea

Amenorrhea almost always is associated with chronically low levels of estrogen, whether it is caused by hypogonadotropic hypogonadism or ovarian insufficiency. Development of secondary sexual characteristics requires gradual titration of estradiol replacement with eventual addition of progestin. Symptoms of hypoestrogenism can be treated with hormone replacement therapy or oral contraceptive pills. Patients with hypogonadotropic hypogonadism who are interested in fertility require treatment with pulsatile GnRH or exogenous FSH and LH, whereas patients with ovarian failure can consider oocyte donation, which has a high chance of success in this population.

Polycystic ovarian syndrome (PCOS)   PCOS is diagnosed on the basis of a combination of clinical or biochemical evidence of hyperandrogenism, amenorrhea or oligomenorrhea, and the ultrasound appearance of polycystic ovaries. Approximately half of patients with PCOS are obese, and abnormalities in insulin dynamics are common, as is metabolic syndrome. Symptoms generally begin shortly after menarche and are slowly progressive. Lean patients with PCOS generally have high LH levels in the presence of normal to low levels of FSH and estradiol. The LH/FSH ratio is less pronounced in obese patients in whom insulin resistance is a more prominent feature.

TREATMENT   Polycystic Ovarian Syndrome

A major abnormality in patients with PCOS is the failure of regular, predictable ovulation. Thus, these patients are at risk for the development of dysfunctional bleeding and endometrial hyperplasia associated with unopposed estrogen exposure. Endometrial protection can be achieved with the use of oral contraceptives or progestins (medroxyprogesterone acetate, 5–10 mg, or prometrium, 200 mg daily for 10–14 days of each

month). Oral contraceptives are also useful for management of hyperandrogenic symptoms, as is spironolactone, which functions as a weak androgen receptor antagonist. Management of the associated metabolic syndrome may be appropriate for some patients (Chap. 242). For patients interested in fertility, weight control is a critical first step. Clomiphene citrate is highly effective as a first-line treatment, with or without the addition of metformin. Exogenous gonadotropins can be used by experienced practitioners.

PELVIC PAIN

The mechanisms that cause pelvic pain are similar to those which cause abdominal pain (Chap. 13) and include inflammation of the parietal peritoneum, obstruction of hollow viscera, vascular disturbances, and pain originating in the abdominal wall. Pelvic pain may reflect pelvic disease per se but also may reflect extrapelvic disorders that refer pain to the pelvis. In up to 60% of cases, pelvic pain can be attributed to gastrointestinal problems, including appendicitis, cholecystitis, infections, intestinal obstruction, diverticulitis, and inflammatory bowel disease. Urinary tract and musculoskeletal disorders are also common causes of pelvic pain.

APPROACH TO THE PATIENT   Pelvic Pain

A thorough history that includes the type, location, radiation, and status with respect to increasing or decreasing severity can help identify the cause of acute pelvic pain. Specific associations with vaginal bleeding, sexual activity, defecation, urination, movement, or eating should be specifically sought. A careful menstrual history is essential to assess the possibility of pregnancy. Determination of whether the pain is acute versus chronic and cyclic versus noncyclic will direct further investigation (Table 50-1). However, disorders that cause cyclic pain occasionally may cause noncyclic pain, and the converse is also true.

■ ACUTE PELVIC PAIN

Pelvic inflammatory disease most commonly presents with bilateral lower abdominal pain. It is generally of recent onset and is exacerbated by intercourse or jarring movements. Fever is present in about

TABLE 50-1 Causes of Pelvic Pain

	Acute	Chronic
Cyclic pelvic pain		Premenstrual symptoms
		Mittelschmerz
		Dysmenorrhea
		Endometriosis
Noncyclic pelvic pain	Pelvic inflammatory disease	Pelvic congestion syndrome
	Ruptured or hemorrhagic ovarian cyst or ovarian torsion	Adhesions and retroversion of the uterus
	Ectopic pregnancy	Pelvic malignancy
	Endometritis	Vulvodynia
	Acute growth or degeneration of uterine myoma	History of sexual abuse

half of these patients; abnormal uterine bleeding occurs in about one-third. New vaginal discharge, urethritis, and chills may be present but are less specific signs. *Adnexal pathology* can present acutely and may be due to rupture, bleeding or torsion of cysts, or, much less commonly, neoplasms of the ovary, fallopian tubes, or paraovarian areas. Fever may be present with ovarian torsion. *Ectopic pregnancy* is associated with right- or left-sided lower abdominal pain and vaginal bleeding, with clinical signs generally appearing 6–8 weeks after the last normal menstrual period. Orthostatic signs and fever may be present. Risk factors include the presence of known tubal disease, previous ectopic pregnancies, a history of infertility, diethyl-stilbestrol (DES) exposure of the mother in utero, or a history of pelvic infections. *Uterine pathology* includes endometritis and, less frequently, degenerating leiomyomas (fibroids). Endometritis often is associated with vaginal bleeding and systemic signs of infection. It occurs in the setting of sexually transmitted infections, uterine instrumentation, or postpartum infection.

A sensitive pregnancy test, complete blood count with differential, urinalysis, tests for chlamydial and gonococcal infections, and abdominal ultrasound aid in making the diagnosis and directing further management.

TREATMENT   Acute Pelvic Pain

Treatment of acute pelvic pain depends on the suspected etiology but may require surgical or gynecologic intervention. Conservative management is an important consideration for ovarian cysts, if torsion is not suspected, to avoid unnecessary pelvic surgery and the subsequent risk of infertility due to adhesions. The majority of unruptured ectopic pregnancies are now treated with methotrexate, which is effective in 84–96% of cases. However, surgical treatment may be required.

■ CHRONIC PELVIC PAIN

Some women experience discomfort at the time of ovulation (*mittelschmerz*). The pain can be quite intense but is generally of short duration. The mechanism is thought to involve rapid expansion of the dominant follicle, although it also may be caused by peritoneal irritation by follicular fluid released at the time of ovulation. Many women experience premenstrual symptoms such as breast discomfort, food cravings, and abdominal bloating or discomfort. These moliminal symptoms are a good predictor of ovulation, although their absence is less helpful.

Dysmenorrhea

Dysmenorrhea refers to the crampy lower abdominal discomfort that begins with the onset of menstrual bleeding and gradually decreases over the next 12–72 h. It may be associated with nausea, diarrhea, fatigue, and headache and occurs in 60–93% of adolescents, beginning with the establishment of regular ovulatory cycles. Its prevalence decreases after pregnancy and with the use of oral contraceptives.

Primary dysmenorrhea results from increased stores of prostaglandin precursors, which are generated by sequential stimulation of the uterus by estrogen and progesterone. During menstruation these precursors are converted to prostaglandins, which cause intense uterine contractions, decreased blood flow, and increased peripheral nerve hypersensitivity, resulting in pain.

Secondary dysmenorrhea is caused by underlying pelvic pathology. *Endometriosis* results from the presence of endometrial glands and stroma outside the uterus. These deposits of ectopic endometrium respond to hormonal stimulation and cause dysmenorrhea, which generally precedes menstruation by several days. Endometriosis also may be associated with painful intercourse, painful bowel movements, and tender nodules in the uterosacral ligament. Fibrosis and adhesions can produce lateral displacement of the cervix. The CA125 level may be increased, but it has low negative predictive value. Definitive diagnosis requires laparoscopy. Symptomatology does not always predict the extent of endometriosis. Other secondary causes of dysmenorrhea include adenomyosis, a condition caused by the presence of ectopic endometrial glands and stroma within the myometrium. Cervical stenosis may result from trauma, infection, or surgery.

TREATMENT   Dysmenorrhea

Local application of heat; use of vitamins B_1, B_6, and E and magnesium; acupuncture; yoga; and exercise are of some benefit for the treatment of dysmenorrhea. However, non-steroidal anti-inflammatory drugs (NSAIDs) are the most effective treatment and provide >80% sustained response rates. Ibuprofen, naproxen, ketoprofen, mefanamic acid, and nimesulide are all superior to placebo. Treatment should be started a day before expected menses and generally is continued for 2–3 days. Oral contraceptives also reduce symptoms of dysmenorrhea. Failure of response to NSAIDs and oral contraceptives is suggestive of a pelvic disorder such as endometriosis, and diagnostic laparoscopy should be considered to guide further treatment.

FURTHER READINGS

GORDON CM: Clinical practice: Functional hypothalamic amenorrhea. N Engl J Med 33:365, 2010

HALL JE: Neuroendocrine control of the menstrual cycle, in *Yen and Jaffe's Reproductive Endocrinology*, 6th ed, JF Strauss III, RL Barbieri (eds). Philadelphia, Elsevier, 2009, pp 139–154

HOWARD FM: Endometriosis and mechanisms of pelvic pain. J Minim Invasive Gynecol 16:540, 2009

NELSON LM: Clinical practice: Primary ovarian insufficiency. N Engl J Med 360:606, 2009

PALLAIS JC et al: Kallmann syndrome, in *GeneReviews,* RA Pagon et al (eds). Seattle, University of Washington, 1993–2007 [updated April 8, 2010]. *http://www.ncbi.nlm.nih.gov/bookshelf/br.fcgi?book=gene*

SULTAN C et al: Mayer-Rokitansky-Kuster-Hauser syndrome: Recent clinical and genetic findings. Gynecol Endocrinol 25:88, 2009

WITTENBERGER MD et al: The FMR1 premutation and reproduction. Fertil Steril 87:456, 2007

ZAHRADNIK HP et al: Nonsteroidal anti-inflammatory drugs and hormonal contraceptives for pain relief from dysmenorrhea: A review. Contraception 81:185, 2010

CHAPTER **51**

Approach to the Patient With a Skin Disorder

Thomas J. Lawley

Kim B. Yancey

The challenge of examining the skin lies in distinguishing normal from abnormal, significant findings from trivial ones, and in integrating pertinent signs and symptoms into an appropriate differential diagnosis. The fact that the largest organ in the body is visible is both an advantage and a disadvantage to those who examine it. It is advantageous because no special instrumentation is necessary and because the skin can be biopsied with little morbidity. However, the casual observer can be misled by a variety of stimuli and overlook important, subtle signs of skin or systemic disease. For instance, the sometimes minor differences in color and shape that distinguish a melanoma (Fig. 51-1) from a benign nevomelanocytic nevus (Fig. 51-2) can be difficult to recognize. To aid in the interpretation of skin lesions, a variety of descriptive terms have been developed to characterize cutaneous lesions (Tables 51-1, 51-2, and 51-3 as well as Fig. 51-3) and to formulate a differential diagnosis (Table 51-4). For instance, the finding of scaling papules (present in patients with psoriasis or atopic dermatitis) places the patient in a different diagnostic category than would hemorrhagic papules, which may indicate vasculitis or sepsis (Figs. 51-4 and 51-5, respectively). It is also important to differentiate primary from secondary skin lesions. If the examiner focuses on linear erosions overlying an area of erythema and scaling, he or she may incorrectly assume that the

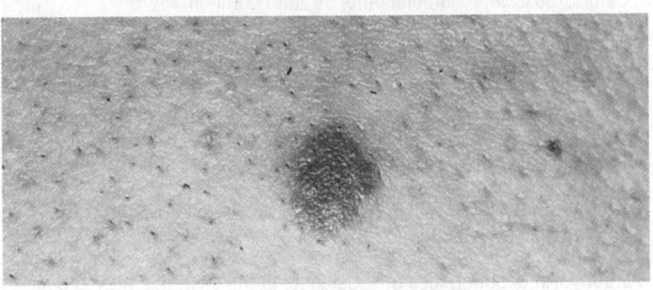

Figure 51-2 Nevomelanocytic nevus. Nevi are benign proliferations of nevomelanocytes characterized by regularly shaped hyperpigmented macules or papules of a uniform color.

erosion is the primary lesion and the redness and scale are secondary, while the correct interpretation would be that the patient has a pruritic eczematous dermatitis with erosions caused by scratching.

APPROACH TO THE PATIENT ▶ Skin Disorder

In examining the skin it is usually advisable to assess the patient before taking an extensive history. This way, the entire cutaneous surface is sure to be evaluated, and objective findings can be integrated with relevant historic data. Four basic features

TABLE 51-1 Description of Primary Skin Lesions

Macule: A flat, colored lesion, <2 cm in diameter, not raised above the surface of the surrounding skin. A "freckle," or ephelid, is a prototype pigmented macule.

Patch: A large (>2 cm) flat lesion with a color different from the surrounding skin. This differs from a macule only in size.

Papule: A small, solid lesion, <0.5 cm in diameter, raised above the surface of the surrounding skin and, hence, palpable (e.g., a closed comedone, or whitehead, in acne).

Nodule: A larger (0.5–5.0 cm), firm lesion raised above the surface of the surrounding skin. This differs from a papule only in size (e.g., a dermal nevomelanocytic nevus).

Tumor: A solid, raised growth >5 cm in diameter.

Plaque: A large (>1 cm), flat-topped, raised lesion; edges may either be distinct (e.g., in psoriasis) or gradually blend with surrounding skin (e.g., in eczematous dermatitis).

Vesicle: A small, fluid-filled lesion, <0.5 cm in diameter, raised above the plane of surrounding skin. Fluid is often visible, and the lesions are translucent [e.g., vesicles in allergic contact dermatitis caused by *Toxicodendron* (poison ivy)].

Pustule: A vesicle filled with leukocytes. Note: The presence of pustules does not necessarily signify the existence of an infection.

Bulla: A fluid-filled, raised, often translucent lesion >0.5 cm in diameter.

Wheal: A raised, erythematous, edematous papule or plaque, usually representing short-lived vasodilatation and vasopermeability.

Telangiectasia: A dilated, superficial blood vessel.

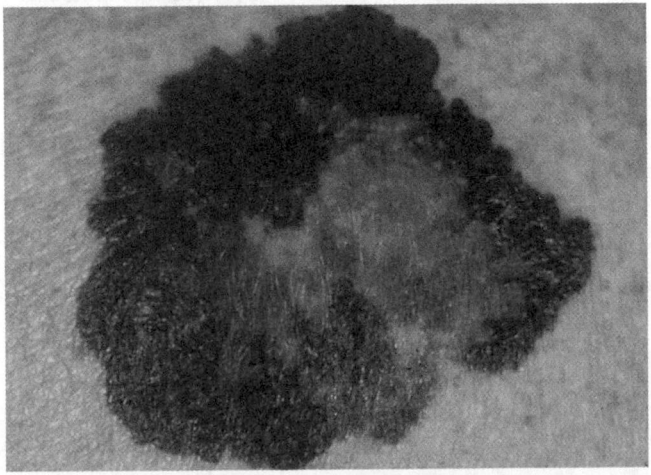

Figure 51-1 Superficial spreading melanoma. This is the most common type of melanoma. Such lesions usually demonstrate asymmetry, border irregularity, color variegation (black, blue, brown, pink, and white), a diameter >6 mm, and a history of change (e.g., an increase in size or development of associated symptoms such as pruritus or pain).

TABLE 51-2 Description of Secondary Skin Lesions

Lichenification: A distinctive thickening of the skin that is characterized by accentuated skin-fold markings.

Scale: Excessive accumulation of stratum corneum.

Crust: Dried exudate of body fluids that may be either yellow (i.e., serous crust) or red (i.e., hemorrhagic crust).

Erosion: Loss of epidermis without an associated loss of dermis.

Ulcer: Loss of epidermis and at least a portion of the underlying dermis.

Excoriation: Linear, angular erosions that may be covered by crust and are caused by scratching.

Atrophy: An acquired loss of substance. In the skin, this may appear as a depression with intact epidermis (i.e., loss of dermal or subcutaneous tissue) or as sites of shiny, delicate, wrinkled lesions (i.e., epidermal atrophy).

Scar: A change in the skin secondary to trauma or inflammation. Sites may be erythematous, hypopigmented, or hyperpigmented depending on their age or character. Sites on hair-bearing areas may be characterized by destruction of hair follicles.

of a skin lesion must be noted and considered during a physical examination: the distribution of the eruption, the types of primary and secondary lesions, the shape of individual lesions, and the arrangement of the lesions. An ideal skin examination includes evaluation of the skin, hair, and nails as well as the mucous membranes of the mouth, eyes, nose, nasopharynx, and anogenital region. In the initial examination it is important

TABLE 51-3 Common Dermatologic Terms

Alopecia: Hair loss; it may be partial or complete.

Annular: Ring-shaped lesions.

Cyst: A soft, raised, encapsulated lesion filled with semisolid or liquid contents.

Herpetiform: Grouped lesions.

Lichenoid: Violaceous to purple, polygonal lesions that resemble those seen in lichen planus.

Milia: Small, firm, white papules filled with keratin.

Morbilliform: Generalized, small erythematous macules and/or papules that resemble lesions seen in measles.

Nummular: Coin-shaped lesions.

Poikiloderma: Skin that displays variegated pigmentation, atrophy, and telangiectases.

Polycyclic: A configuration of skin lesions formed from coalescing rings or incomplete rings.

Pruritus: A sensation that elicits the desire to scratch. Pruritus is often the predominant symptom of inflammatory skin diseases (e.g., atopic dermatitis, allergic contact dermatitis); it is also commonly associated with xerosis and aged skin. Systemic conditions that can be associated with pruritus include chronic renal disease, cholestasis, pregnancy, malignancy, thyroid disease, polycythemia vera, and delusions of parasitosis.

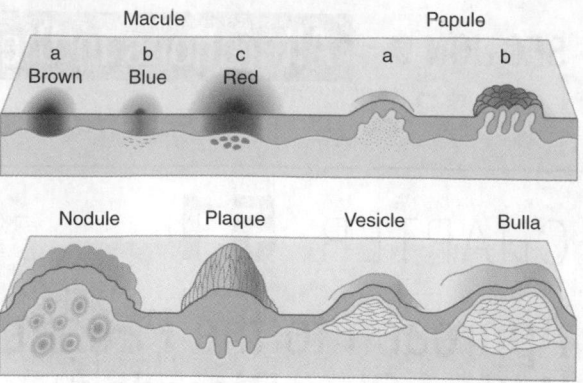

Figure 51-3   A schematic representation of several common primary skin lesions (see Table 51-1).

that the patient be disrobed as completely as possible. This will minimize chances of missing important individual skin lesions and make it possible to assess the distribution of the eruption accurately. The patient should first be viewed from a distance of about 1.5–2 m (4–6 ft) so that the general character of the skin and the distribution of lesions can be evaluated. Indeed, the distribution of lesions often correlates highly with diagnosis (Fig. 51-6). For example, a hospitalized patient with a generalized erythematous exanthem is more likely to have a drug eruption than is a patient with a similar rash limited to the sun-exposed portions of the face. Once the distribution of the lesions has been established, the nature of the primary lesion must be determined. Thus, when lesions are distributed on elbows, knees, and scalp, the most likely possibility based solely on distribution is psoriasis or dermatitis herpetiformis (Figs. 51-7 and 51-8, respectively). The primary lesion in psoriasis is a scaly papule that soon forms erythematous plaques covered with a white scale, whereas that of dermatitis herpetiformis is an urticarial papule that quickly becomes a small vesicle. In this manner, identification of the primary lesion directs the examiner toward the proper diagnosis. Secondary changes in skin can also be quite helpful. For example, scale represents excessive epidermis, while crust is the result of a discontinuous epithelial cell layer. Palpation of skin lesions can also yield insight into the character of an eruption. Thus, red papules on the lower extremities that blanch with pressure can be a manifestation of many different diseases, but hemorrhagic red papules that do not blanch with pressure indicate palpable purpura characteristic of necrotizing vasculitis (Fig. 51-4).

The shape of lesions is also an important feature. Flat, round, erythematous papules and plaques are common in many cutaneous diseases. However, target-shaped lesions that consist in part of erythematous plaques are specific for erythema multiforme (Fig. 51-9). In the same way, the arrangement of individual lesions is important. Erythematous papules and vesicles can occur in many conditions, but their arrangement in a specific linear array suggests an external etiology such as allergic contact (Fig. 51-10) or primary irritant dermatitis. In contrast, lesions with a generalized arrangement are common and suggest a systemic etiology.

As in other branches of medicine, a complete history should be obtained to emphasize the following features:

1. Evolution of lesions
   a. Site of onset
   b. Manner in which the eruption progressed or spread

TABLE 51-4 Selected Common Dermatologic Conditions

Diagnosis	Common Distribution	Usual Morphology	Diagnosis	Common Distribution	Usual Morphology
Acne vulgaris	Face, upper back, chest	Open and closed comedones, erythematous papules, pustules, cysts	Seborrheic keratosis	Trunk, face	Brown plaques with adherent, greasy scale; "stuck on" appearance
Rosacea	Blush area of cheeks, nose, forehead, chin	Erythema, telangiectases, papules, pustules	Folliculitis	Any hair-bearing area	Follicular pustules
			Impetigo	Anywhere	Papules, vesicles, pustules, often with honey-colored crusts
Seborrheic dermatitis	Scalp, eyebrows, perinasal areas	Erythema with greasy yellow-brown scale	Herpes simplex	Lips, genitalia	Grouped vesicles progressing to crusted erosions
Atopic dermatitis	Antecubital and popliteal fossae; may be widespread	Patches and plaques of erythema, scaling, and lichenification; pruritus	Herpes zoster	Dermatomal, usually trunk but may be anywhere	Vesicles limited to a dermatome (often painful)
Stasis dermatitis	Ankles, lower legs over medial malleoli	Patches of erythema and scaling on background of hyperpigmentation associated with signs of venous insufficiency	Varicella	Face, trunk, relative sparing of extremities	Lesions arise in crops and quickly progress from erythematous macules, to papules, to vesicles, to pustules, to crusted sites
Dyshidrotic eczema	Palms, soles, sides of fingers and toes	Deep vesicles	Pityriasis rosea	Trunk (Christmas tree pattern); herald patch followed by multiple smaller lesions	Symmetric erythematous patches with a collarette of scale
Allergic contact dermatitis	Anywhere	Localized erythema, vesicles, scale, and pruritus (e.g., fingers, earlobes—nickel; dorsal aspect of foot—shoe; exposed surfaces—poison ivy)	Tinea versicolor	Chest, back, abdomen, proximal extremities	Scaly hyper- or hypopigmented macules
Psoriasis	Elbows, knees, scalp, lower back, fingernails (may be generalized)	Papules and plaques covered with silvery scale; nails have pits	Candidiasis	Groin, beneath breasts, vagina, oral cavity	Erythematous macerated areas with satellite pustules; white, friable patches on mucous membranes
Lichen planus	Wrists, ankles, mouth (may be widespread)	Violaceous flat-topped papules and plaques	Dermatophytosis	Feet, groin, beard, or scalp	Varies with site, (e.g., tinea corporis—scaly annular patch)
Keratosis pilaris	Extensor surfaces of arms and thighs, buttocks	Keratotic follicular papules with surrounding erythema	Scabies	Groin, axillae, between fingers and toes, beneath breasts	Excoriated papules, burrows, pruritus
Melasma	Forehead, cheeks, temples, upper lip	Tan to brown patches	Insect bites	Anywhere	Erythematous papules with central puncta
Vitiligo	Periorificial, trunk, extensor surfaces of extremities, flexor wrists, axillae	Chalk-white macules	Cherry angioma	Trunk	Red, blood-filled papules
			Keloid	Anywhere (site of previous injury)	Firm tumor, pink, purple, or brown
			Dermatofibroma	Anywhere	Firm red to brown nodule that shows dimpling of overlying skin with lateral compression
Actinic keratosis	Sun-exposed areas	Skin-colored or red-brown macule or papule with dry, rough, adherent scale	Acrochordons (skin tags)	Groin, axilla, neck	Fleshy papules
Basal cell carcinoma	Face	Papule with pearly, telangiectatic border on sun-damaged skin	Urticaria	Anywhere	Wheals, sometimes with surrounding flare; pruritus
Squamous cell carcinoma	Face, especially lower lip, ears	Indurated and possibly hyperkeratotic lesions often showing ulceration and/or crusting	Transient acantholytic dermatosis	Trunk, especially anterior chest	Erythematous papules
			Xerosis	Extensor extremities, especially legs	Dry, erythematous, scaling patches; pruritus

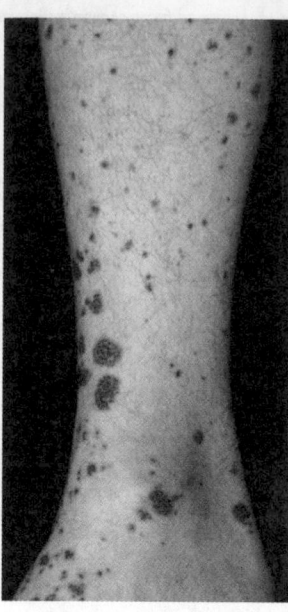

Figure 51-4 Necrotizing vasculitis. Palpable purpuric papules on the lower legs are seen in this patient with cutaneous small vessel vasculitis. *(Courtesy of Robert Swerlick, MD; with permission.)*

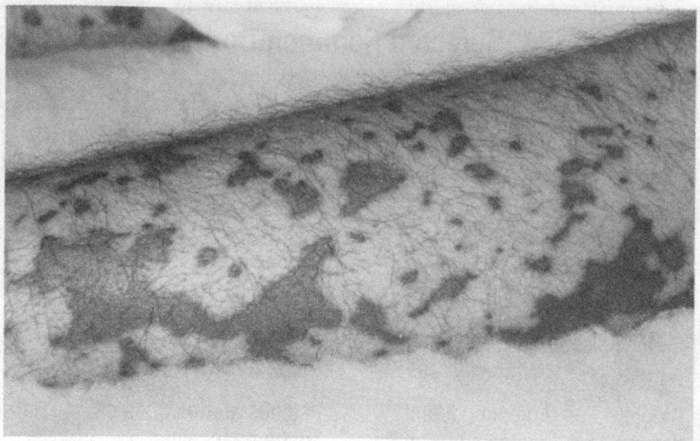

Figure 51-5 Meningococcemia. An example of fulminant meningococcemia with extensive angular purpuric patches. *(Courtesy of Stephen E. Gellis, MD; with permission.)*

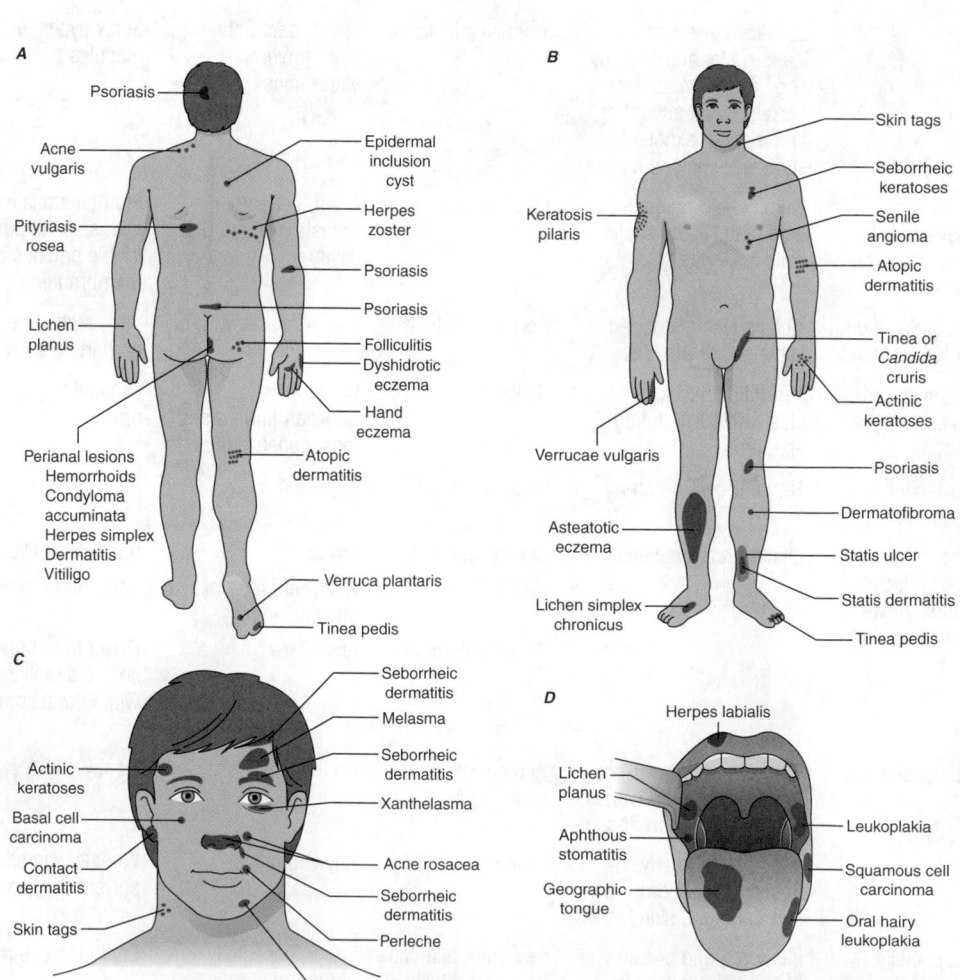

Figure 51-6 *A–D.* The distribution of some common dermatologic diseases and lesions.

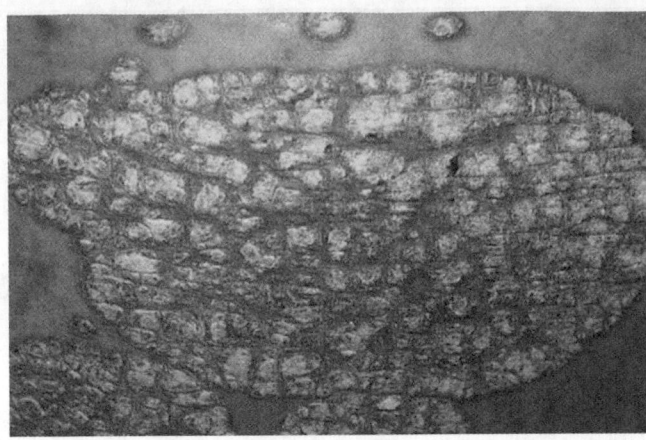

Figure 51-7 Psoriasis. This papulosquamous skin disease is characterized by small and large erythematous papules and plaques with overlying adherent silvery scale.

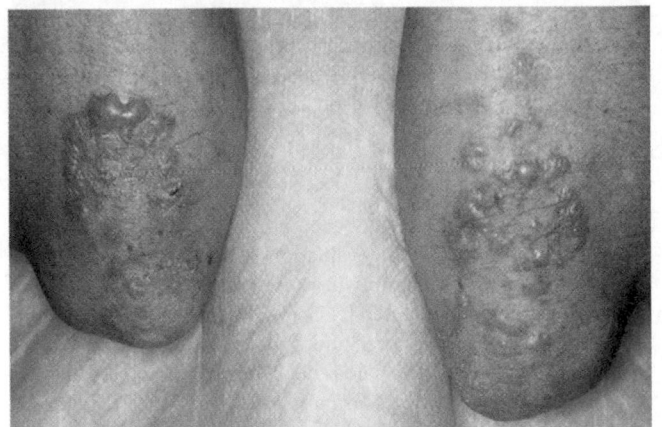

Figure 51-8 Dermatitis herpetiformis. This disorder typically displays pruritic, grouped papulovesicles on elbows, knees, buttocks, and posterior scalp. Vesicles are often excoriated due to associated pruritus.

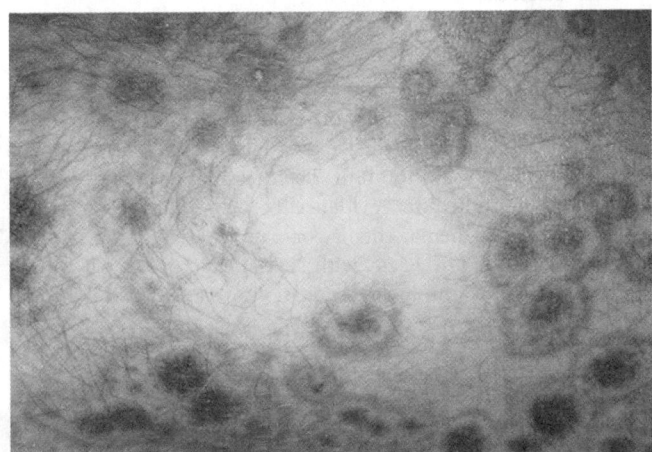

Figure 51-9 Erythema multiforme. This eruption is characterized by multiple erythematous plaques with a target or iris morphology. It usually represents a hypersensitivity reaction to drugs (e.g., sulfonylamides) or infections (e.g., HSV). *(Courtesy of the Yale Resident's Slide Collection; with permission.)*

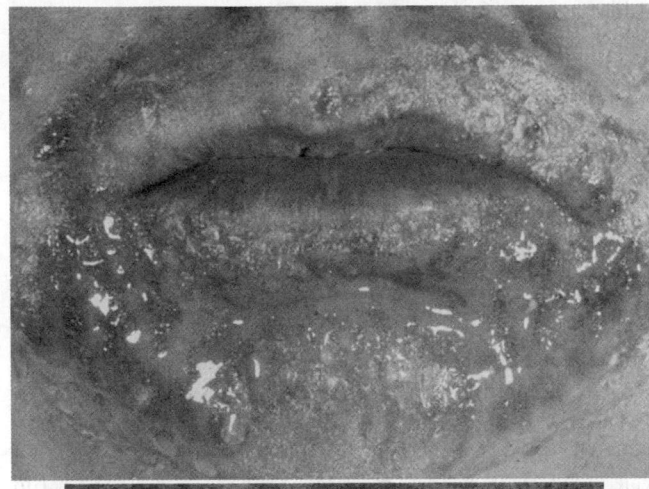

A

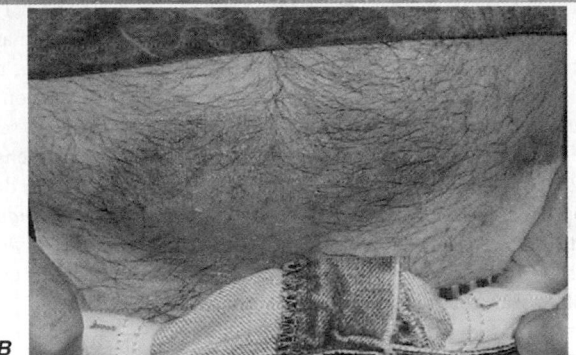

B

Figure 51-10 Allergic contact dermatitis (ACD). *A.* An example of ACD in its acute phase, with sharply demarcated, weeping, eczematous plaques in a perioral distribution. *B.* ACD in its chronic phase demonstrating an erythematous, lichenified, weeping plaque on skin chronically exposed to nickel in a metal snap. *(B, Courtesy of Robert Swerlick, MD; with permission.)*

  c. Duration
  d. Periods of resolution or improvement in chronic eruptions
 2. Symptoms associated with the eruption
  a. Itching, burning, pain, numbness
  b. What, if anything, has relieved symptoms
  c. Time of day when symptoms are most severe
 3. Current or recent medications (prescribed as well as over-the-counter)
 4. Associated systemic symptoms (e.g., malaise, fever, arthralgias)
 5. Ongoing or previous illnesses
 6. History of allergies
 7. Presence of photosensitivity
 8. Review of systems
 9. Family history (particularly relevant for patients with melanoma, atopy, psoriasis, or acne)
 10. Social, sexual, or travel history as relevant to the patient

■ DIAGNOSTIC TECHNIQUES

Many skin diseases can be diagnosed on gross clinical appearance, but sometimes relatively simple diagnostic procedures can yield valuable information. In most instances, they can be performed at the bedside with a minimum of equipment.

Skin biopsy

A skin biopsy is a straightforward minor surgical procedure; however, it is important to biopsy a lesion that is most likely to yield diagnostic findings. This decision may require expertise in skin diseases and knowledge of superficial anatomic structures in selected areas of the body. In this procedure, a small area of skin is anesthetized with 1% lidocaine with or without epinephrine. The skin lesion in question can be excised or saucerized with a scalpel or removed by punch biopsy. In the latter technique, a punch is pressed against the surface of the skin and rotated with downward pressure until it penetrates to the subcutaneous tissue. The circular biopsy is then lifted with forceps, and the bottom is cut with iris scissors. Biopsy sites may or may not need suture closure, depending on size and location.

KOH preparation

A potassium hydroxide (KOH) preparation is performed on scaling skin lesions where a fungal infection is suspected. The edge of such a lesion is scraped gently with a no. 15 scalpel blade, and the removed scale is collected on a glass microscope slide then treated with 1 to 2 drops of a solution of 10–20% KOH. KOH dissolves keratin and allows easier visualization of fungal elements. Brief heating of the slide accelerates dissolution of keratin. When the preparation is viewed under the microscope, the refractile hyphae will be seen more easily when the light intensity is reduced and the condenser is lowered. This technique can be used to identify hyphae in dermatophyte infections, pseudohyphae and budding yeast in *Candida* infections (see Fig. 203-1), and "spaghetti and meatballs" yeast forms in tinea versicolor. The same sampling technique can be used to obtain scale for culture of selected pathogenic organisms.

Tzanck smear

A Tzanck smear is a cytologic technique most often used in the diagnosis of herpesvirus infections [herpes simplex virus (HSV) or varicella zoster virus (VZV)] (see Figs. 180-1 and 180-3). An early vesicle, not a pustule or crusted lesion, is unroofed, and the base of the lesion is scraped gently with a scalpel blade. The material is placed on a glass slide, air-dried, and stained with Giemsa or Wright's stain. Multinucleated epithelial giant cells suggest the presence of HSV or VZV; culture or immunofluorescence, or genetic testing must be performed to identify the specific virus.

Diascopy

Diascopy is designed to assess whether a skin lesion will blanch with pressure as, for example, in determining whether a red lesion is hemorrhagic or simply blood-filled. Urticaria (Fig. 51-11) will

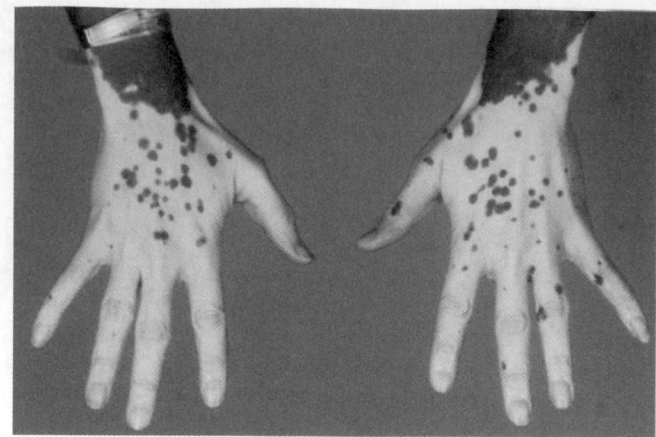

Figure 51-12 **Vitiligo.** Characteristic lesions display an acral distribution and striking depigmentation as a result of loss of melanocytes.

blanch with pressure, whereas a purpuric lesion caused by necrotizing vasculitis (Fig. 51-4) will not. Diascopy is performed by pressing a microscope slide or magnifying lens against a lesion and noting the amount of blanching that occurs. Granulomas often have an opaque to transparent, brown-pink "apple jelly" appearance on diascopy.

Wood's light

A Wood's lamp generates 360-nm ultraviolet (or "black") light that can be used to aid the evaluation of certain skin disorders. For example, a Wood's lamp will cause erythrasma (a superficial, intertriginous infection caused by *Corynebacterium minutissimum*) to show a characteristic coral pink color, and wounds colonized by *Pseudomonas* to appear pale blue. Tinea capitis caused by certain dermatophytes such as *Microsporum canis* or *M. audouini* exhibits a yellow fluorescence. Pigmented lesions of the epidermis such as freckles are accentuated, while dermal pigment such as postinflammatory hyperpigmentation fades under a Wood's light. Vitiligo (Fig. 51-12) appears totally white under a Wood's lamp, and previously unsuspected areas of involvement often become apparent. A Wood's lamp may also aid in the demonstration of tinea versicolor and in recognition of ash leaf spots in patients with tuberous sclerosis.

Patch tests

Patch testing is designed to document sensitivity to a specific antigen. In this procedure, a battery of suspected allergens is applied to the patient's back under occlusive dressings and allowed to remain in contact with the skin for 48 h. The dressings are removed, and the area is examined for evidence of delayed hypersensitivity reactions (e.g., erythema, edema, or papulovesicles). This test is best performed by physicians with special expertise in patch testing and is often helpful in the evaluation of patients with chronic dermatitis.

FURTHER READINGS

HABIF TP: *Clinical Dermatology: A Color Guide to Diagnosis and Therapy,* 4th ed. Philadelphia, Mosby, 2004

JAMES WD et al: *Andrews' Diseases of the Skin: Clinical Dermatology,* 10th ed. Philadelphia, Elsevier, 2006

WOLFF K et al (eds): *Fitzpatrick's Dermatology in General Medicine,* 7th ed. New York, McGraw-Hill, 2008

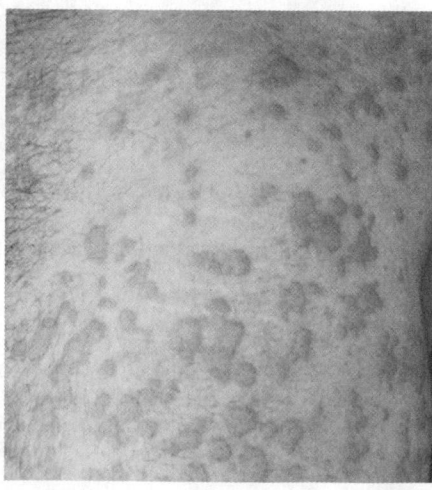

Figure 51-11 **Urticaria.** Discrete and confluent, edematous, erythematous papules and plaques are characteristic of this whealing eruption.

CHAPTER 52

Eczema, Psoriasis, Cutaneous Infections, Acne, and Other Common Skin Disorders

Leslie P. Lawley

Calvin O. McCall

Thomas J. Lawley

ECZEMA AND DERMATITIS

Eczema is a type of dermatitis and these terms are often used synonymously (atopic eczema or atopic dermatitis). Eczema is a reaction pattern that presents with variable clinical findings and the common histologic finding of spongiosis (intercellular edema of the epidermis). Eczema is the final common expression for a number of disorders, including those discussed in the following sections. Primary lesions may include erythematous macules, papules, and vesicles, which can coalesce to form patches and plaques. In severe eczema, secondary lesions from infection or excoriation, marked by weeping and crusting, may predominate. In chronic eczematous conditions, lichenification (cutaneous hypertrophy and accentuation of normal skin markings) may alter the characteristic appearance of eczema.

■ ATOPIC DERMATITIS

Atopic dermatitis (AD) is the cutaneous expression of the atopic state, characterized by a family history of asthma, allergic rhinitis, or eczema. The prevalence of AD is increasing worldwide. Some of its features are shown in Table 52-1.

The etiology of AD is only partially defined, but there is a clear genetic predisposition. When both parents are affected by AD, >80% of their children manifest the disease. When only one parent is affected, the prevalence drops to slightly over 50%. Patients with AD may display a variety of immunoregulatory abnormalities including increased IgE synthesis; increased serum IgE; and impaired, delayed-type hypersensitivity reactions.

The clinical presentation often varies with age. Half of patients with AD present within the first year of life, and 80% present by 5 years of age. About 80% ultimately coexpress allergic rhinitis or asthma. The infantile pattern is characterized by weeping inflammatory patches and crusted plaques on the face, neck, and extensor surfaces. The childhood and adolescent pattern is marked by dermatitis of flexural skin, particularly in the antecubital and popliteal fossae (Fig. 52-1). AD may resolve spontaneously, but approximately 40% of all individuals affected as children will have dermatitis in adult life. The distribution of lesions may be similar to those seen in childhood; however, adults frequently have localized disease, manifesting as lichen simplex chronicus or hand eczema (see below). In patients with localized disease, AD may be suspected because of a typical personal history, family history, or the presence of cutaneous stigmata of AD such as perioral pallor, an extra fold of skin beneath the lower eyelid (Dennie-Morgan folds), increased palmar skin markings, and an increased incidence of cutaneous

TABLE 52-1 Clinical Features of Atopic Dermatitis

1. Pruritus and scratching
2. Course marked by exacerbations and remissions
3. Lesions typical of eczematous dermatitis
4. Personal or family history of atopy (asthma, allergic rhinitis, food allergies, or eczema)
5. Clinical course lasting longer than 6 weeks
6. Lichenification of skin

infections, particularly with *Staphylococcus aureus*. Regardless of other manifestations, pruritus is a prominent characteristic of AD in all age groups and is exacerbated by dry skin. Many of the cutaneous findings in affected patients, such as lichenification, are secondary to rubbing and scratching.

TREATMENT   Atopic Dermatitis

Therapy of AD should include avoidance of cutaneous irritants, adequate moisturizing through the application of emollients, judicious use of topical anti-inflammatory agents, and prompt treatment of secondary infection. Patients should be instructed to bathe no more often than daily, using warm or cool water, and to use only mild bath soap. Immediately after bathing, while the skin is still moist, a topical anti-inflammatory agent in a cream or ointment base should be applied to areas of dermatitis, and all other skin areas should be lubricated with a moisturizer. Approximately 30 g of a topical agent is required to cover the entire body surface of an average adult.

Low- to midpotency topical glucocorticoids are employed in most treatment regimens for AD. Skin atrophy and the potential for systemic absorption are constant concerns, especially with more potent agents. Low-potency topical glucocorticoids or nonglucocorticoid anti-inflammatory agents should be selected for use on the face and intertriginous areas to minimize the risk of skin atrophy. Two nonglucocorticoid anti-inflammatory agents are available: tacrolimus ointment and pimecrolimus

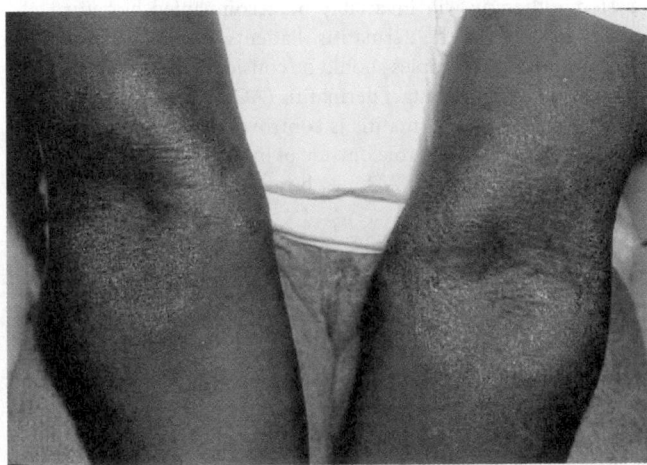

Figure 52-1 Atopic dermatitis. Hyperpigmentation, lichenification, and scaling in the antecubital fossae are seen in this patient with atopic dermatitis. (*Courtesy of Robert Swerlick, MD; with permission.*)

cream. These agents are macrolide immunosuppressants that are approved by the U.S. Food and Drug Administration (FDA) for topical use in AD. Reports of broader effectiveness appear in the literature. These agents do not cause skin atrophy, nor do they suppress the hypothalamic-pituitary-adrenal axis. Recently, however, concerns have emerged regarding the potential for lymphomas in patients treated with these agents. Thus, caution should be exercised when considering these agents. Currently, they are also more costly than topical glucocorticoids. Barrier-repair products are also nonglucocorticoid agents and are gaining popularity in treating AD.

Secondary infection of eczematous skin may lead to exacerbation of AD. Crusted and weeping skin lesions may be infected with *S. aureus*. When secondary infection is suspected, eczematous lesions should be cultured and patients treated with systemic antibiotics active against *S. aureus*. The initial use of penicillinase-resistant penicillins or cephalosporins is preferable. Dicloxacillin or cephalexin (250 mg qid for 7–10 days) is generally adequate for adults; however, antibiotic selection must be directed by culture results and clinical response. More than 50% of *S. aureus* (SA) isolates are now methacillin resistant (MR) in some communities—community-acquired MRSA (CA-MRSA). Current recommendations for the treatment of CA-MRSA infection in adults include trimethoprim/sulfamethoxazole (1 double strength bid), minocycline (100 mg bid), doxycycline (100 mg bid), or clindamycin (300–450 mg qid). Duration of therapy should be 7–10 days. Inducible resistance may limit clindamycin's usefulness. The latter can be detected by the double-disk diffusion test, which should be ordered if the isolate is erythromycin-resistant and clindamycin-sensitive. As an adjunct, the use of antibacterial washes or dilute sodium hypochlorite baths (0.005% bleach) and intermittent nasal mupirocin may be useful.

Control of pruritus is essential for treatment, because AD often represents "an itch that rashes." Antihistamines are most often used to control pruritus, and mild sedation may be responsible for their antipruritic action. Sedation may also limit their usefulness; however, when used at bedtime, sedating antihistamines may improve the patient's sleep. Unlike their effects in urticaria, nonsedating antihistamines and selective H_2 blockers are of little use in controlling the pruritus of AD.

Treatment with systemic glucocorticoids should be limited to severe exacerbations unresponsive to topical therapy. In the patient with chronic AD, therapy with systemic glucocorticoids will generally clear the skin only briefly, and cessation of the systemic therapy will invariably be accompanied by return, if not worsening, of the dermatitis. Patients who do not respond to conventional therapies should be considered for patch testing to rule out allergic contact dermatitis (ACD). The role of dietary allergens in atopic dermatitis is controversial, and there is little evidence they play any role outside of infancy where a small percentage of patients with AD may be affected by food allergens.

■ LICHEN SIMPLEX CHRONICUS

Lichen simplex chronicus may represent the end stage of a variety of pruritic and eczematous disorders, including atopic dermatitis. It consists of a circumscribed plaque or plaques of lichenified skin due to chronic scratching or rubbing. Common areas involved include the posterior nuchal region, dorsum of the feet, and ankles. Treatment of lichen simplex chronicus centers on breaking the cycle of chronic itching and scratching. High-potency topical glucocorticoids are helpful in most cases, but in recalcitrant cases, application of topical glucocorticoids under occlusion, or intralesional injection of glucocorticoids may be required. Oral antihistamines such as

hydroxyzine (10–25 mg every 6 h) or tricyclic antidepressants with antihistaminic activity, such as doxepin (10–25 mg at bedtime), are useful primarily due to their sedating action. Higher doses of these agents may be required, but sedation can become bothersome. Patients need to be counseled regarding driving or operating heavy equipment after taking these medications.

■ CONTACT DERMATITIS

Contact dermatitis is an inflammatory process in skin caused by an exogenous agent or agents that directly or indirectly injure the skin. This injury may be caused by an inherent characteristic of a compound—irritant contact dermatitis (ICD). An example of ICD would be dermatitis induced by a concentrated acid or base. Agents that cause ACD induce an antigen-specific immune response (poison ivy dermatitis). The clinical lesions of contact dermatitis may be acute (wet and edematous) or chronic (dry, thickened, and scaly), depending on the persistence of the insult (see Fig. 51-10).

Irritant contact dermatitis

ICD is generally well demarcated and often localized to areas of thin skin (eyelids, intertriginous areas) or to areas where the irritant was occluded. Lesions may range from minimal skin erythema to areas of marked edema, vesicles, and ulcers. Chronic low-grade irritant dermatitis is the most common type of ICD, and the most common area of involvement is the hands (see below). The most common irritants encountered are chronic wet work, soaps, and detergents. Treatment should be directed to avoidance of irritants and use of protective gloves or clothing.

Allergic contact dermatitis

ACD is a manifestation of delayed-type hypersensitivity mediated by memory T lymphocytes in the skin. The most common cause of ACD is exposure to plants, especially to members of the family Anacardiaceae, including the genus *Toxicodendron*. Poison ivy, poison oak, and poison sumac are members of this genus and cause an allergic reaction marked by erythema, vesiculation, and severe pruritus. The eruption is often linear or angular, corresponding to areas where plants have touched the skin. The sensitizing antigen common to these plants is urushiol, an oleoresin containing the active ingredient pentadecylcatechol. The oleoresin may adhere to skin, clothing, tools, and pets, and contaminated articles may cause dermatitis even after prolonged storage. Blister fluid does not contain urushiol and is not capable of inducing skin eruption in exposed subjects.

TREATMENT	Contact Dermatitis

If contact dermatitis is suspected and an offending agent is identified and removed, the eruption will resolve. Usually, treatment with high-potency topical glucocorticoids is enough to relieve symptoms while the dermatitis runs its course. For those patients who require systemic therapy, daily oral prednisone beginning at 1 mg/kg, but usually ≤60 mg/d, is sufficient. It should be tapered over 2 to 3 weeks, and each daily dose given in the morning with food.

Identification of a contact allergen can be a difficult and time-consuming task. Patients with dermatitis unresponsive to conventional therapy or with an unusual and patterned distribution should be suspected of having ACD. They should be questioned carefully regarding occupational exposures and topical medications. Common sensitizers include preservatives in topical preparations, nickel sulfate, potassium dichromate, thimerosal, neomycin sulfate, fragrances, formaldehyde, and rubber-curing agents. Patch testing is helpful in identifying these agents but should not be attempted on patients with widespread active dermatitis or on those taking systemic glucocorticoids.

HAND ECZEMA

Hand eczema is a very common, chronic skin disorder in which both exogenous and endogenous factors play important roles. It may be associated with other cutaneous disorders such as atopic dermatitis, and contact with various agents may be involved. It represents a large proportion of occupation-associated skin disease. Chronic, excessive exposure to water and detergents, harsh chemicals, or allergens may initiate or aggravate this disorder. It may present with dryness and cracking of the skin of the hands as well as with variable amounts of erythema and edema. Often, the dermatitis will begin under rings where water and irritants are trapped. Dyshidrotic eczema, a variant of hand eczema, presents with multiple, intensely pruritic, small papules and vesicles occurring on the thenar and hypothenar eminences and the sides of the fingers (Fig. 52-2). Lesions tend to occur in crops that slowly form crusts and then heal.

The evaluation of a patient with hand eczema should include an assessment of potential occupation-associated exposures. The history should be directed to identifying possible irritant or allergen exposures.

TREATMENT Hand Eczema

Therapy of hand eczema is directed toward avoidance of irritants, identification of possible contact allergens, treatment of coexistent infection, and application of topical glucocorticoids. Whenever possible, the hands should be protected by gloves, preferably vinyl. The use of rubber gloves (latex) to protect dermatitic skin is sometimes associated with the development of hypersensitivity reactions to components of the gloves. Patients can be treated with cool moist compresses, followed by application of a mid- to high-potency topical glucocorticoid in a cream or ointment base. As with atopic dermatitis, treatment of secondary infection is essential for good control. In addition, patients with hand eczema should be examined for dermatophyte infection by KOH preparation and culture (see below).

NUMMULAR ECZEMA

Nummular eczema is characterized by circular or oval "coinlike" lesions, beginning as small edematous papules that become crusted and scaly. The etiology of nummular eczema is unknown, but dry skin is a contributing factor. Common locations are the trunk or the extensor surfaces of the extremities, particularly on the pretibial areas or dorsum of the hands. It occurs more frequently in men and is most commonly seen in middle age. The treatment of nummular eczema is similar to that for atopic dermatitis.

ASTEATOTIC ECZEMA

Asteatotic eczema, also known as *xerotic eczema* or *"winter itch,"* is a mildly inflammatory dermatitis that develops in areas of extremely dry skin, especially during the dry winter months. Clinically, there may be considerable overlap with nummular eczema. This form of eczema accounts for a large number of physician visits because of the associated pruritus. Fine cracks and scale, with or without erythema, characteristically develop in areas of dry skin, especially on the anterior surfaces of the lower extremities in elderly patients. Asteatotic eczema responds well to topical moisturizers and the avoidance of cutaneous irritants. Overbathing and the use of harsh soaps exacerbate asteatotic eczema.

STASIS DERMATITIS AND STASIS ULCERATION

Stasis dermatitis develops on the lower extremities secondary to venous incompetence and chronic edema. Patients may give a history of deep venous thrombosis, have evidence of vein removal, or varicose veins. Early findings in stasis dermatitis consist of mild erythema and scaling associated with pruritus. The typical initial site of involvement is the medial aspect of the ankle, often over a distended vein (Fig. 52-3).

Stasis dermatitis may become acutely inflamed, with crusting and exudate. In this state, it is easily confused with cellulitis. Chronic stasis dermatitis is often associated with dermal fibrosis that is recognized clinically as brawny edema of the skin. As the disorder progresses, the dermatitis becomes progressively pigmented, due to chronic erythrocyte extravasation leading to cutaneous hemosiderin deposition. Stasis dermatitis may be complicated by secondary infection and contact dermatitis. Severe stasis dermatitis may precede the development of stasis ulcers.

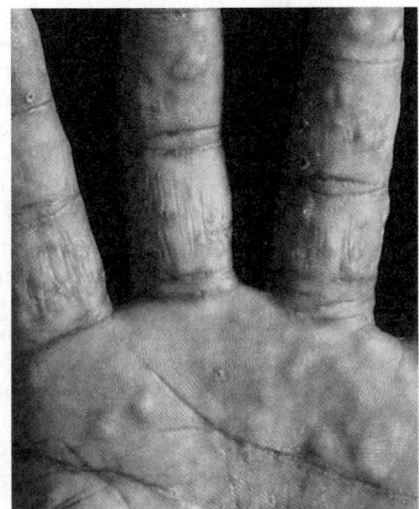

Figure 52-2 Dyshidrotic eczema. This example is characterized by deep-seated vesicles and scaling on palms and lateral fingers, and the disease is often associated with an atopic diathesis.

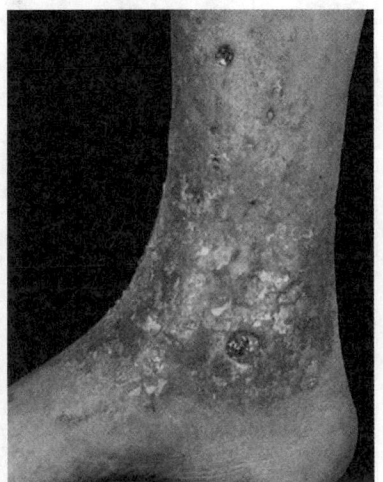

Figure 52-3 Stasis dermatitis. An example of stasis dermatitis showing erythematous, scaly, and oozing patches over the lower leg. Several stasis ulcers are also seen in this patient.

TREATMENT Stasis Dermatitis and Stasis Ulceration

Patients with stasis dermatitis and stasis ulceration benefit greatly from leg elevation and the routine use of compression stockings with a gradient of at least 30–40 mmHg. Stockings providing less compression, such as antiembolism hose, are poor substitutes. Use of emollients and/or midpotency topical glucocorticoids and avoidance of irritants are also helpful in treating stasis dermatitis. Protecting the legs from injury, including scratching, and control of chronic edema are essential to prevent ulcers. Diuretics may be required to adequately control chronic edema.

Stasis ulcers are difficult to treat, and resolution is slow. It is extremely important to elevate the affected limb as much as possible. The ulcer should be kept clear of necrotic material by gentle debridement and covered with a semipermeable dressing and a compression dressing or compression stocking. Glucocorticoids should not be applied to ulcers, because they may retard healing; however, they may be applied to the surrounding skin to control itching, scratching, and additional trauma. Secondarily infected lesions should be treated with appropriate oral antibiotics, but it should be noted that all ulcers will become colonized with bacteria, and the purpose of antibiotic therapy should not be to clear all bacterial growth. Care must be taken to exclude treatable causes of leg ulcers (hypercoagulation, vasculitis) before beginning the chronic management outlined above.

■ SEBORRHEIC DERMATITIS

Seborrheic dermatitis is a common, chronic disorder, characterized by greasy scales overlying erythematous patches or plaques. Induration and scale are generally less prominent than in psoriasis, but clinical overlap exists between these diseases—"sebopsoriasis." The most common location is in the scalp, where it may be recognized as severe dandruff. On the face, seborrheic dermatitis affects the eyebrows, eyelids, glabella, and nasolabial folds (Fig. 52-4). Scaling of the external auditory canal is common in seborrheic dermatitis. In addition, the postauricular areas often become macerated and tender. Seborrheic dermatitis may also develop in the central chest, axilla, groin, submammary folds, and gluteal cleft. Rarely, it may cause a widespread generalized dermatitis. Pruritus is variable.

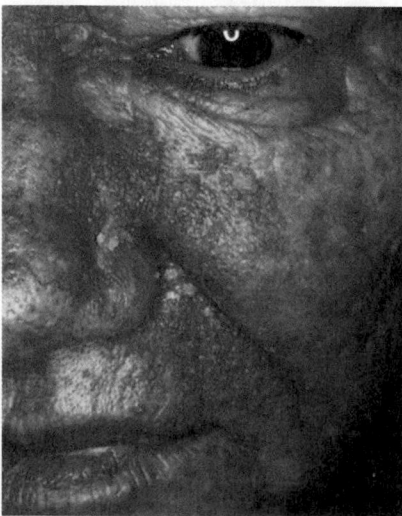

Figure 52-4 Seborrheic dermatitis. Central facial erythema with overlying greasy, yellowish scale is seen in this patient. (*Courtesy of Jean Bolognia, MD; with permission.*)

Seborrheic dermatitis may be evident within the first few weeks of life, and within this context it typically occurs in the scalp ("cradle cap"), face, or groin. It is rarely seen in children beyond infancy but becomes evident again during adult life. Although it is frequently seen in patients with Parkinson's disease, in those who have had cerebrovascular accidents, and in those with HIV infection, the overwhelming majority of individuals with seborrheic dermatitis have no underlying disorder.

TREATMENT Seborrheic Dermatitis

Treatment with low-potency topical glucocorticoids in conjunction with a topical antifungal agent, such as ketoconazole cream or ciclopirox cream, is often effective. The scalp and beard areas may benefit from antidandruff shampoos, which should be left in place 3–5 min before rinsing. High-potency topical glucocorticoid solutions (betamethasone or clobetasol) are effective for control of severe scalp involvement. High-potency glucocorticoids should not be used on the face because this is often associated with steroid-induced rosacea or atrophy.

PAPULOSQUAMOUS DISORDERS (TABLE 52-2)

■ PSORIASIS

Psoriasis is one of the most common dermatologic diseases, affecting up to 1% of the world's population. It is a chronic inflammatory skin disorder clinically characterized by erythematous, sharply demarcated papules and rounded plaques, covered by silvery micaceous scale. The skin lesions of psoriasis are variably pruritic. Traumatized areas often develop lesions of psoriasis (Koebner's or isomorphic phenomenon). In addition, other external factors may exacerbate psoriasis including infections, stress, and medications (lithium, beta blockers, and antimalarials).

The most common variety of psoriasis is called *plaque-type*. Patients with plaque-type psoriasis will have stable, slowly enlarging plaques, which remain basically unchanged for long periods of time. The most commonly involved areas are the elbows, knees, gluteal cleft, and the scalp. Involvement tends to be symmetric. Plaque psoriasis generally develops slowly and runs an indolent course. It rarely remits spontaneously. *Inverse psoriasis* affects the intertriginous regions including the axilla, groin, submammary region, and navel; it also tends to affect the scalp, palms, and soles. The individual lesions are sharply demarcated plaques (see Fig. 51-7), but they may be moist and without scale due to their locations.

Guttate psoriasis (eruptive psoriasis) is most common in children and young adults. It develops acutely in individuals without psoriasis or in those with chronic plaque psoriasis. Patients present with many small erythematous, scaling papules, frequently after upper respiratory tract infection with β-hemolytic streptococci. The differential diagnosis should include pityriasis rosea and secondary syphilis.

Pustular psoriasis is another variant. Patients may have disease localized to the palms and soles, or the disease may be generalized. Regardless of the extent of disease, the skin is erythematous with pustules and variable scale. Localized to the palms and soles, it is easily confused with eczema. When generalized, episodes are characterized by fever [39°–40°C (102.2°–104.0°F)] lasting several days, an accompanying generalized eruption of sterile pustules, and a background of intense erythema; patients may become erythrodermic. Episodes of fever and pustules are recurrent. Local irritants, pregnancy, medications, infections, and systemic glucocorticoid withdrawal can precipitate this form of psoriasis. Oral retinoids are the treatment of choice in nonpregnant patients.

Fingernail involvement, appearing as punctate pitting, onycholysis, nail thickening, or subungual hyperkeratosis may be a clue to the diagnosis of psoriasis when the clinical presentation is not classic.

TABLE 52-2 Papulosquamous Disorders

	Clinical Features	Other Notable Features	Histologic Features
Psoriasis	Sharply demarcated, erythematous plaques with mica-like scale; predominantly elbows, knees, and scalp; atypical forms may localize to intertriginous areas; eruptive forms may be associated with infection	May be aggravated by certain drugs, infection; severe forms seen associated with HIV	Acanthosis, vascular proliferation
Lichen planus	Purple polygonal papules marked by severe pruritus; lacy white markings, especially associated with mucous membrane lesions	Certain drugs may induce: thiazides, antimalarial drugs	Interface dermatitis
Pityriasis rosea	Rash often preceded by herald patch; oval to round plaques with trailing scale; most often affects the trunk, and eruption lines up in skinfolds giving a "fir treelike" appearance; generally spares palms and soles	Variable pruritus; self-limited resolving in 2–8 weeks; may be imitated by secondary syphilis	Pathologic features often nonspecific
Dermatophytosis	Polymorphous appearance depending on dermatophyte, body site, and host response; sharply defined to ill-demarcated scaly plaques with or without inflammation; may be associated with hair loss	KOH preparation may show branching hyphae; culture helpful	Hyphae and neutrophils in stratum corneum

According to the National Psoriasis Foundation, up to 30% of patients with psoriasis have psoriatic arthritis (PsA). There are five subtypes of PsA: symmetric, asymmetric, distal interphalangeal predominant (DIP), spondylitis, and arthritis mutilans. Symmetric arthritis resembles rheumatoid arthritis, but is usually milder. Asymmetric arthritis can involve any joint and may present as "sausage digits." DIP is the classic form, but occurs in only about 5% of patients with PsA. It may involve fingers and toes. Spondylitis also occurs in about 5% of patients with PsA. Arthritis mutilans is severe and deforming. It affects primarily the small joints of the hands and feet. It accounts for less than 5% of PsA.

The etiology of psoriasis is still poorly understood, but there is clearly a genetic component to the disease. Over 50% of patients with psoriasis report a positive family history. Psoriatic lesions demonstrate infiltrates of activated T cells that are thought to elaborate cytokines responsible for keratinocyte hyperproliferation, which results in the characteristic clinical findings. Agents inhibiting T cell activation, clonal expansion, or release of proinflammatory cytokines are often effective for the treatment of severe psoriasis (see below).

TREATMENT   Psoriasis

Treatment of psoriasis depends on the type, location, and extent of disease. All patients should be instructed to avoid excess drying or irritation of their skin and to maintain adequate cutaneous hydration. Most patients with localized, plaque-type psoriasis can be managed with midpotency topical glucocorticoids, although their long-term use is often accompanied by loss of effectiveness (tachyphylaxis) and atrophy of the skin. A topical vitamin D analogue (calcipotriene) and a retinoid (tazarotene) are also efficacious in the treatment of limited psoriasis and have largely replaced other topical agents such as coal tar, salicylic acid, and anthralin.

Ultraviolet light, natural or artificial, is an effective therapy for many patients with widespread psoriasis. Ultraviolet B (UV-B) light, narrowband UV-B, and ultraviolet A (UV-A) spectrum with either oral or topical psoralens (PUVA) are also extremely effective. The long-term use of UV light may be associated with an increased incidence of nonmelanoma and melanoma skin cancer. UV-light therapy is contraindicated in patients receiving cyclosporine and should be used with great care in all immunocompromised patients due to an increased risk of developing skin cancers.

Various systemic agents can be used for severe, widespread psoriatic disease (Table 52-3). Oral glucocorticoids should not be used for the treatment of psoriasis due to the potential for developing life-threatening pustular psoriasis when therapy is discontinued. Methotrexate is an effective agent, especially in patients with psoriatic arthritis. The synthetic retinoid acitretin is useful, especially when immunosuppression must be avoided; however, teratogenicity limits its use.

The evidence implicating psoriasis as a T cell–mediated disorder has directed therapeutic efforts to immunoregulation. Cyclosporine and other immunosuppressive agents can be very effective in the treatment of psoriasis, and much attention is currently directed toward the development of biologic agents with more selective immunosuppressive properties and better safety profiles (Table 52-4). Experience with these agents is limited, and information regarding combination therapy and adverse events continues to emerge. Use of tumor necrosis factor (TNF-α) inhibitors may worsen congestive heart failure (CHF), and they should be used with caution in those at risk for or known to have CHF. Further, none of the immunosuppressive agents used in the treatment of psoriasis should be initiated if the patient has a severe infection; patients on such therapy should be routinely screened for tuberculosis. There have been reports of progressive multifocal leukoencephalopathy in association with treatment with the TNF-α inhibitors. Malignancies, including a risk or history of certain malignancies, may limit the use of these systemic agents.

■ LICHEN PLANUS

Lichen planus (LP) is a papulosquamous disorder that may affect the skin, scalp, nails, and mucous membranes. The primary cutaneous lesions are pruritic, polygonal, flat-topped, violaceous papules. Close examination of the surface of these papules often reveals a network of gray lines (Wickham's striae). The skin lesions may occur anywhere but have a predilection for the wrists, shins, lower back, and genitalia (Fig. 52-5). Involvement of the scalp, lichen planopilaris, may lead to scarring alopecia, and nail involvement may lead to permanent deformity or loss of fingernails and toenails. LP commonly involves mucous membranes, particularly the buccal mucosa, where it can present a spectrum of disease from a mild, white, reticulate eruption of the mucosa to a severe, erosive stomatitis. Erosive stomatitis may persist for years and may be linked to an increased risk of oral

TABLE 52-3 FDA-Approved Systemic Therapy for Psoriasis

Agent	Medication Class	Administration Route	Administration Frequency	Adverse Events (Selected)
Methotrexate	Antimetabolite	Oral	Weekly	Hepatotoxicity, pulmonary toxicity, pancytopenia, potential for increased malignancies, ulcerative stomatitis, nausea, diarrhea, teratogenicity
Acitretin	Retinoid	Oral	Daily	Teratogenicity, osteophyte formation, hyperlipidemia, flare of inflammatory bowel disease, hepatoxicity, depression
Cyclosporine	Calcineurin inhibitor	Oral	Twice daily	Renal dysfunction, hypertension, hyperkalemia, hyperuricemia, hypomagnesemia, hyperlipidemia, increased risk of malignancies

squamous cell carcinoma. Cutaneous eruptions clinically resembling LP have been observed after administration of numerous drugs, including thiazide diuretics, gold, antimalarials, penicillamine, and phenothiazines, and in patients with skin lesions of chronic graft-versus-host disease. In addition, LP may be associated with hepatitis C infection. The course of LP is variable, but most patients have spontaneous remissions 6 months to 2 years after the onset of disease. Topical glucocorticoids are the mainstay of therapy.

■ PITYRIASIS ROSEA

Pityriasis rosea (PR) is a papulosquamous eruption of unknown etiology occurring more commonly in the spring and fall. Its first manifestation is the development of a 2- to 6-cm annular lesion (the herald patch). This is followed in a few days to a few weeks by the appearance of many smaller annular or papular lesions with a predilection to occur on the trunk (Fig. 52-6). The lesions are generally oval, with their long axis parallel to the skinfold lines. Individual lesions may range in color from red to brown and have a trailing scale. PR shares many clinical features with the eruption of secondary syphilis, but palm and sole lesions are extremely rare in PR and common in secondary syphilis. The eruption tends to be moderately pruritic and lasts 3 to 8 weeks. Treatment is directed at alleviating pruritus and consists of oral antihistamines; midpotency topical glucocorticoids; and, in some cases, the use of UV-B phototherapy.

CUTANEOUS INFECTIONS (TABLE 52-5)

■ IMPETIGO, ECTHYMA, AND FURUNCULOSIS

Impetigo is a common superficial bacterial infection of skin caused most often by *S. aureus* (Chap. 135), and in some cases by group

A β-hemolytic streptococci (Chap. 136). The primary lesion is a superficial pustule that ruptures and forms a characteristic yellow-brown honey-colored crust (Chap. 136). Lesions may occur on normal skin—primary infection—or in areas already affected by another skin disease—secondary infection. Lesions caused by staphylococci may be tense, clear bullae, and this less common form of the disease is called *bullous impetigo*. Blisters are caused by the production of exfoliative toxin by *S. aureus* phage type II. This is the same toxin responsible for staphylococcal scalded-skin syndrome (SSSS), often resulting in dramatic loss of the superficial epidermis due to blistering. SSSS is much more common in children than in adults; however, it should be considered along with toxic epidermal necrolysis and severe drug eruptions in patients with widespread blistering of the skin. *Ecthyma* is a variant of impetigo that causes punched-out ulcerative lesions. It may result from neglected or inadequately treated impetigo. Treatment of both ecthyma and impetigo involves gentle debridement of adherent crusts, which is facilitated by the use of soaks and topical antibiotics, in conjunction with appropriate oral antibiotics. *Furunculosis* is also caused by *S. aureus*, and this disorder has gained prominence in the last decade because of CA-MRSA. A furuncle, or boil, is a painful, erythematous, nodule that can occur on any cutaneous surface. The lesions may be solitary but are most often multiple. Patients frequently believe they have been bitten by spiders or insects. Family members or close contacts may also be affected. Furuncles can rupture and drain spontaneously or may need incision and drainage, which may be adequate therapy for small solitary furuncles without cellulitis or systemic symptoms. Whenever possible, lesional material should be sent for culture. Current recommendations for methicillin-sensitive infections are β-lactam antibiotics. Therapy for CA-MRSA was

TABLE 52-4 Biologics Approved for Psoriasis or Psoriatic Arthritis

Agent	Mechanism of Action	Indication	Administration Route	Administration Frequency	Warnings
Alefacept	Anti-CD-2	Ps	IM	Once weekly × 12 weeks; may repeat	Lymphopenia, potential for increased malignancies, serious infections
Etanercept	Anti TNF-α	Ps, PsA	SC	Once or twice weekly	Serious infections, neurologic events, hematologic events, potential for increased malignancies
Adalimumab	Anti TNF-α	PsA	SC	Every other week	Serious infections, neurologic events, potential for increased malignancies, hypersensitivity reactions, hematologic events
Infliximab	Anti TNF-α	PsA	IV	Initial infusion followed by infusions at week 2, 6, then every 8 weeks	Serious infections, hepatotoxicity, hematologic events, hypersensitivity reactions, neurologic events, potential for increased malignancies

Abbreviations: IM, intramuscular; Ps, psoriasis; PsA, psoriatic arthritis; SC, subcutaneous; TNF, tumor necrosis factor.

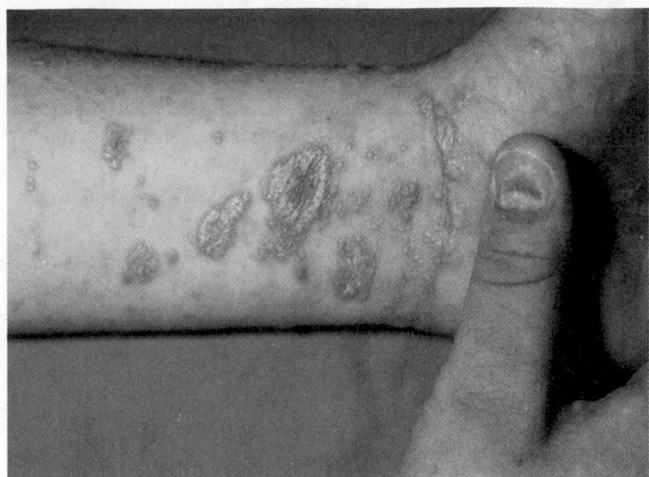

Figure 52-5 Lichen planus. An example of lichen planus showing multiple flat-topped, violaceous papules and plaques. Nail dystrophy as seen in this patient's thumbnail may also be a feature. (*Courtesy of Robert Swerlick, MD; with permission.*)

discussed previously (see "Atopic Dermatitis"). Warm compresses and nasal mupirocin are helpful therapeutic additions. Severe infections may require IV antibiotics.

■ ERYSIPELAS AND CELLULITIS

See Chap. 125.

■ DERMATOPHYTOSIS

Dermatophytes are fungi that infect skin, hair, and nails and include members of the genera *Trichophyton, Microsporum*, and *Epidermophyton*. Tinea corporis, or infection of the relatively hairless skin of the body (glabrous skin), may have a variable appearance depending on the extent of the associated inflammatory reaction. Typical infections have an annular appearance that patients refer to as "ringworm." Deep inflammatory nodules or granulomas occur in some infections—especially in those infections inappropriately treated with mid- to high-potency topical glucocorticoids. Involvement of the groin (tinea cruris) is more common in males than females. It presents as a scaling, erythematous eruption sparing the scrotum.

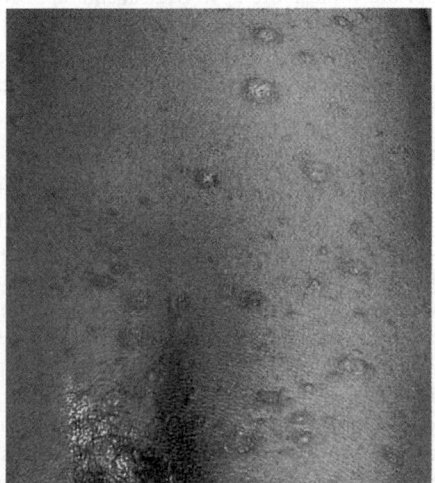

Figure 52-6 Pityriasis rosea. In this patient with pityriasis rosea, multiple round to oval erythematous patches with fine central scale are distributed along the skin tension lines on the trunk.

Infection of the foot (tinea pedis) is the most common dermatophyte infection and is often chronic; it is characterized by variable erythema, edema, scaling, pruritus, and, occasionally, vesiculation. Involvement may be widespread or localized but generally involves the web space between the fourth and fifth toes. Infection of the nails (tinea unguium or onychomycosis) occurs in many patients with tinea pedis and is characterized by opacified, thickened nails and subungual debris. The distal-lateral variant is most common. Proximal subungual onychomycosis may be a marker for HIV infection or other immunocompromised states. Dermatophyte infection of the scalp (tinea capitis) continues to be common, particularly affecting inner-city children, but it also affects adults. The predominant organism is *T. tonsurans*, which can produce a relatively noninflammatory infection with mild scale and hair loss that is diffuse or localized. *T. tonsurans* can also cause a markedly inflammatory dermatosis with edema and nodules. This latter presentation is a kerion.

The diagnosis of tinea can be made from skin scrapings, nail scrapings, or hair by culture or direct microscopic examination with potassium hydroxide (KOH). Nail clippings may be sent for histologic examination with periodic acid-Schiff (PAS) stain.

TREATMENT **Dermatophytosis**

Both topical and systemic therapies may be used to treat dermatophyte infections. Treatment depends on the site involved and the type of infection. Topical therapy is generally effective for uncomplicated tinea corporis, tinea cruris, and limited tinea pedis. It is not effective as a monotherapy for tinea capitis or onychomycosis. Topical imidazoles, triazoles, and allylamines may be effective therapies for dermatophyte infections, but nystatin is not active against dermatophytes. Topicals are generally applied twice daily, and treatment should continue 1 week beyond clinical resolution of the infection. Tinea pedis often requires longer treatment courses and it frequently relapses. Oral antifungal agents may be required for recalcitrant tinea pedis or tinea corporis.

Oral antifungal agents are required for dermatophyte infections involving the hair and nails and for other infections unresponsive to topical therapy. A fungal etiology should be confirmed by direct microscopic examination or by culture prior to prescribing oral antifungal agents. All of the oral agents may cause hepatotoxicity and should not be used in women who are pregnant or breast-feeding.

Griseofulvin is the only oral agent approved in the United States for dermatophyte infections involving the skin, hair, or nails. When griseofulvin is used, a daily dose of 500 mg microsized or 375 mg ultramicrosized griseofulvin administered with a fatty meal is an adequate dose for most dermatophyte infections. Higher doses are required for some cases of tinea pedis and tinea capitis. Markedly inflammatory tinea capitis may result in scarring and hair loss, and systemic or topical glucocorticoids may be helpful in preventing these sequelae. The duration of antifungal therapy may be 2 weeks for uncomplicated tinea corporis, 8–12 weeks for tinea capitis, or as long as 6–18 months for nail infections. Due to high relapse rates, griseofulvin is seldom used for nail infections. Common side effects of griseofulvin include gastrointestinal distress, headache, and urticaria.

Oral itraconazole and terbinafine are approved for onychomycosis. Itraconazole is given as either continuous daily therapy (200 mg/d) or pulses (200 mg bid for 1 week per month) administered with food. Fingernails require 2 months of continuous therapy or two pulses. Toenails require 3 months of continuous therapy or three pulses. Itraconazole has the potential for serious interactions with other drugs requiring the P450 enzyme system for metabolism. Terbinafine (250 mg/d) is also effective

TABLE 52-5 Common Skin Infections

	Clinical Features	Etiologic Agent	Treatment
Impetigo	Honey-colored crusted papules, plaques, or bullae	Group A streptococcus and *Staphylococcus aureus*	Systemic or topical antistaphylococcal antibiotics
Dermatophytosis	Inflammatory or noninflammatory annular scaly plaques; may have hair loss; groin involvement spares scrotum; hyphae on KOH preparation	*Trichophyton, Epidermophyton,* or *Microsporum* sp.	Topical azoles, systemic griseofulvin, terbinafine, or azoles
Candidiasis	Inflammatory papules and plaques with satellite pustules, frequently in intertriginous areas; may involve scrotum; pseudohyphae on KOH preparation	*Candida albicans* and other *Candida* sp.	Topical nystatin or azoles; systemic azoles for resistant disease
Tinea versicolor	Hyper- or hypopigmented scaly patches on the trunk; characteristic mixture of hyphae and spores ("spaghetti and meatballs") on KOH preparation	*Malassezia furfur*	Topical selenium sulfide lotion or azoles

for onychomycosis. Therapy with terbinafine is continued for 6 weeks for fingernail infections and 12 weeks for toenail infections. Terbinafine has fewer drug-drug interactions, but caution should be used with patients who are on multiple medications.

■ TINEA VERSICOLOR

Tinea versicolor is caused by a nondermatophyte, dimorphic fungus, *Malassezia furfur*, a normal inhabitant of the skin. The expression of infection is promoted by heat and humidity. The typical lesions consist of oval scaly macules, papules, and patches concentrated on the chest, shoulders, and back, but only rarely on the face or distal extremities. On dark skin, they often appear as hypopigmented areas, while on light skin, they are slightly erythematous or hyperpigmented. A KOH preparation from scaling lesions will demonstrate a confluence of short hyphae and round spores ("spaghetti and meatballs"). Lotions or shampoos containing sulfur, salicylic acid, or selenium sulfide will clear the infection if used daily for 1 to 2 weeks and then weekly thereafter. These preparations are irritating if left on the skin for more than 10 minutes; thus, they should be washed off completely. Treatment with some oral antifungal agents is also effective, but they do not provide lasting results and they are not FDA-approved for this indication. Ketoconazole has been used as have itraconazole and fluconazole. Griseofulvin is not effective, and terbinafine is not reliably effective for tinea versicolor.

■ CANDIDIASIS

Candidiasis is a fungal infection caused by a related group of yeasts, whose manifestations may be localized to the skin, or, rarely, may be systemic and life-threatening. The causative organism is usually *Candida albicans*, but may also be *C. tropicalis, C. parapsilosis,* or *C. krusei*. These organisms are normal saprophytic inhabitants of the gastrointestinal tract but may overgrow (usually due to broad-spectrum antibiotic therapy) and cause disease at a number of cutaneous sites. Other predisposing factors include diabetes mellitus, chronic intertrigo, oral contraceptive use, and cellular immune deficiency. Candidiasis is a very common infection in HIV-infected individuals (Chap. 189). The oral cavity is commonly involved. Lesions may occur on the tongue or buccal mucosa (thrush) and appear as white plaques. Microscopic examination of scrapings demonstrates both pseudohyphae and yeast forms. Fissured, macerated lesions at the corners of the mouth (perlèche) are often seen in individuals with poorly fitting dentures and may also be associated with candidal

infection. In addition, candidal infections have an affinity for sites that are chronically wet and macerated, including the skin around nails (onycholysis and paronychia) and in intertriginous areas. Intertriginous lesions are characteristically edematous, erythematous, and scaly, with scattered "satellite pustules." In males, there is often involvement of the penis and scrotum as well as the inner aspect of the thighs. In contrast to dermatophyte infections, candidal infections are frequently painful and accompanied by a marked inflammatory response. Diagnosis of candidal infection is based upon the clinical pattern and demonstration of yeast on KOH preparation or culture.

TREATMENT ▶ Candidiasis

Treatment involves removing any predisposing factors such as antibiotic therapy or chronic wetness and the use of appropriate topical or systemic antifungal agents. Effective topicals include nystatin or azoles (miconazole, clotrimazole, econazole, or ketoconazole). The associated inflammatory response accompanying candidal infection on glabrous skin can be treated with a mild glucocorticoid lotion or cream (2.5% hydrocortisone). Systemic therapy is usually reserved for immunosuppressed patients or individuals with chronic or recurrent disease who fail to respond to appropriate topical therapy. Oral agents approved for the treatment of candidiasis include itraconazole and fluconazole. Oral nystatin is only effective for candidiasis of the gastrointestinal tract. Griseofulvin and terbinafine are not effective.

■ WARTS

Warts are cutaneous neoplasms caused by papilloma viruses. More than 100 different human papilloma viruses (HPV) have been described. A typical wart, verruca vulgaris, is sessile, dome-shaped, and usually about a centimeter in diameter. Its surface is hyperkeratotic consisting of many small filamentous projections. The HPV that cause typical verruca vulgaris also cause typical plantar warts, flat warts (or verruca plana), and filiform warts. Plantar warts are endophytic and are covered by thick keratin. Paring of the wart will generally demonstrate a central core of keratinized debris and punctate bleeding points. Filiform warts are most commonly seen on the face, neck, and skinfolds and present as papillomatous lesions on a narrow base. Flat warts are only slightly elevated and have a velvety, nonverrucous surface. They have a propensity for the face, arms, and legs and are often spread by shaving.

Genital warts begin as small papillomas that may grow to form large, fungating lesions. In women, they may involve either the labia, perineum, or perianal skin. In addition, the mucosa of the vagina, urethra, and anus can be involved as well as the cervical epithelium. In men, the lesions often occur initially in the coronal sulcus but may be seen on the shaft of the penis, the scrotum, perianal skin, or in the urethra.

Appreciable evidence has accumulated that suggests HPV plays a role in the development of neoplasia of the uterine cervix and anogenital skin (Chap. 97). HPV types 16 and 18 have been most intensely studied and are the major risk factors for intraepithelial neoplasia and squamous cell carcinoma of the cervix, anus, vulva, and penis. The risk is higher in patients immunosuppressed after solid organ transplantation and in those infected with HIV. Recent evidence also implicates other types. Histologic examination of biopsies from affected sites may reveal changes associated with typical warts and/or features typical of intraepidermal carcinoma (Bowen's disease). Squamous cell carcinomas associated with HPV infections have also been observed in extragenital skin (Chap. 87). This is most commonly seen in patients immunosuppressed after organ transplantation. Patients on long-term immunosuppression should be monitored for the development of squamous cell carcinoma and other cutaneous malignancies.

TREATMENT ▶ Warts

Treatment of warts, other than anogenital warts, should be tempered by the observation that a majority of warts in normal individuals resolve spontaneously within 1 to 2 years. There are many modalities available to treat warts, but no single therapy is universally effective. Factors that influence the choice of therapy include the location of the wart, the extent of disease, the age and immunologic status of the patient, and the patient's desire for therapy. Perhaps the most useful and convenient method for treating warts in almost any location is cryotherapy with liquid nitrogen. Equally effective for nongenital warts, but requiring much more patient compliance, is the use of keratolytic agents such as salicylic acid plasters or solutions. For genital warts, in-office application of a podophyllin solution is moderately effective but may be associated with marked local reactions. Prescription preparations of dilute, purified podophyllin are available for home use. Topical imiquimod, a potent inducer of local cytokine release, has also been approved for use in genital warts. Conventional and laser surgical procedures may be required for recalcitrant warts. Recurrence of warts appears to be common to all these modalities. A highly effective vaccine for selected types of HPV has been recently approved by the FDA, and its use will likely reduce the incidence of anogenital and cervical carcinoma.

■ HERPES SIMPLEX
See Chap. 179.

■ HERPES ZOSTER
See Chap. 180.

ACNE

■ ACNE VULGARIS

Acne vulgaris is a self-limited disorder primarily of teenagers and young adults, although perhaps 10–20% of adults may continue to experience some form of the disorder. The permissive factor for the expression of the disease in adolescence is the increase in sebum production by sebaceous glands after puberty. Small cysts, called *comedones*, form in hair follicles due to blockage of the follicular orifice by retention of keratinous material and sebum. The activity of bacteria (*Propionibacterium*

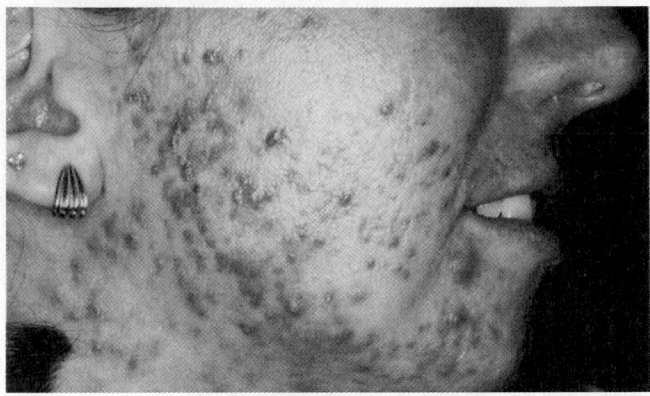

Figure 52-7   Acne vulgaris. An example of acne vulgaris with inflammatory papules, pustules, and comedones. (*Courtesy of Kalman Watsky, MD; with permission.*)

acnes) within the comedones releases free fatty acids from sebum, causes inflammation within the cyst, and results in rupture of the cyst wall. An inflammatory foreign-body reaction develops as result of extrusion of oily and keratinous debris from the cyst.

The clinical hallmark of acne vulgaris is the comedone, which may be closed (whitehead) or open (blackhead). Closed comedones appear as 1- to 2-mm pebbly white papules, which are accentuated when the skin is stretched. They are the precursors of inflammatory lesions of acne vulgaris. The contents of closed comedones are not easily expressed. Open comedones, which rarely result in inflammatory acne lesions, have a large dilated follicular orifice and are filled with easily expressible oxidized, darkened, oily debris. Comedones are usually accompanied by inflammatory lesions: papules, pustules, or nodules.

The earliest lesions seen in adolescence are generally mildly inflamed or noninflammatory comedones on the forehead. Subsequently, more typical inflammatory lesions develop on the cheeks, nose, and chin (Fig. 52-7). The most common location for acne is the face, but involvement of the chest and back is common. Most disease remains mild and does not lead to scarring. A small number of patients develop large inflammatory cysts and nodules, which may drain and result in significant scarring. Regardless of the severity, acne may affect a patient's quality of life. If adequately treated, this may be a transient effect. In the case of severe, scarring acne, the effects can be permanent and profound. Early therapeutic intervention in severe acne is essential.

Exogenous and endogenous factors can alter the expression of acne vulgaris. Friction and trauma (from headbands or chin straps of athletic helmets), application of comedogenic topical agents (cosmetics or hair preparations), or chronic topical exposure to certain industrial compounds may elicit or aggravate acne. Glucocorticoids, topical or systemic, may also elicit acne. Other systemic medications such as oral contraceptive pills, lithium, isoniazid, androgenic steroids, halogens, phenytoin, and phenobarbital may produce acneiform eruptions or aggravate preexisting acne. Genetic factors and polycystic ovary disease may also play a role.

TREATMENT ▶ Acne Vulgaris

Treatment of acne vulgaris is directed toward elimination of comedones by normalization of follicular keratinization, decreasing sebaceous gland activity, decreasing the population of *P. acnes*, and decreasing inflammation. Minimal to moderate pauci-inflammatory disease may respond adequately to local therapy alone. Although areas affected with acne should be kept clean, overly vigorous scrubbing may aggravate acne due to mechanical rupture of comedones. Topical agents such as retinoic acid, benzoyl peroxide, or salicylic acid may alter the pattern of epidermal desquamation, preventing the formation of comedones and aiding in the resolution of preexisting cysts. Topical antibacterial agents such as azelaic acid, topical erythromycin, or clindamycin are also useful adjuncts to therapy.

Patients with moderate to severe acne with a prominent inflammatory component will benefit from the addition of systemic therapy, such as tetracycline in doses of 250–500 mg bid or doxycycline, 100 mg bid. Minocycline is also useful. Such antibiotics appear to have anti-inflammatory effects independent of their antibacterial effects. Female patients who do not respond to oral antibiotics may benefit from hormonal therapy. Several oral contraceptives are now approved by the FDA for use in the treatment of acne vulgaris.

Patients with severe nodulocystic acne unresponsive to the therapies discussed above may benefit from treatment with the synthetic retinoid isotretinoin. Its dose is based on the patient's weight, and it is given once daily for 5 months. Results are excellent in appropriately selected patients. Its use is highly regulated due to its potential for severe adverse events, primarily teratogenicity. In addition, patients receiving this medication develop extremely dry skin, cheilitis, and must be followed for development of hypertriglyceridemia.

Recently, there have also been concerns that isotretinoin is associated with severe depression in some patients. At present, prescribers must enroll in a program designed to prevent pregnancy and adverse events while patients are taking isotretinoin. These measures are imposed to ensure that all prescribers are familiar with the risks of isotretinoin; that all female patients have two negative pregnancy tests prior to initiating therapy and a negative pregnancy test prior to each refill; and that all patients have been warned about the risks associated with isotretinoin.

ACNE ROSACEA

Acne rosacea, commonly referred to as rosacea, is an inflammatory disorder predominantly affecting the central face. Those most often affected are Caucasians of northern European background, but it is seen in patients with dark skin also. It is seen almost exclusively in adults, only rarely affecting patients <30 years. Rosacea is more common in women, but those most severely affected are men. It is characterized by the presence of erythema, telangiectases, and superficial pustules (Fig. 52-8), but is not associated with the presence of comedones. Rosacea rarely involves the chest or back.

There is a relationship between the tendency for facial flushing and the subsequent development of acne rosacea. Often, individuals with rosacea initially demonstrate a pronounced flushing reaction. This may be in response to heat, emotional stimuli, alcohol, hot drinks, or spicy foods. As the disease progresses, the flush persists longer and longer and may eventually become permanent. Papules, pustules, and telangiectases can become superimposed on the persistent flush. Rosacea of very long standing may lead to connective tissue overgrowth, particularly of the nose (rhinophyma). Rosacea may also be complicated by various inflammatory disorders of the eye, including keratitis, blepharitis, iritis, and recurrent chalazion. These ocular problems are potentially sight-threatening and warrant ophthalmologic evaluation.

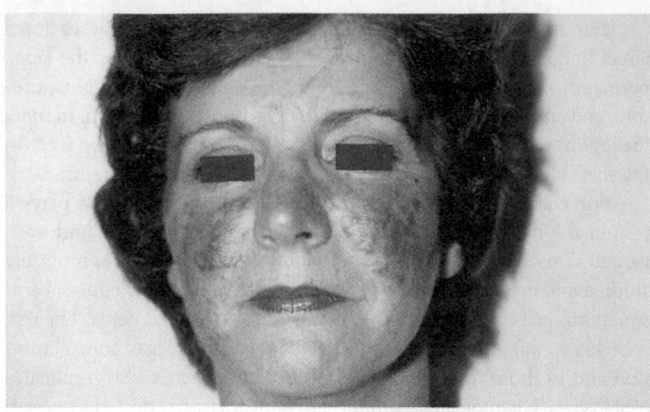

Figure 52-8 Acne rosacea. Prominent facial erythema, telangiectasia, scattered papules, and small pustules are seen in this patient with acne rosacea. (*Courtesy of Robert Swerlick, MD; with permission.*)

TREATMENT Acne Rosacea

Acne rosacea can be treated topically or systemically. Mild disease often responds to topical metronidazole or sodium sulfacetamide. More severe disease requires oral tetracyclines: tetracycline 250–500 mg bid, doxycycline 100 mg bid, or minocycline 50–100 mg bid. Residual telangiectasia may respond to laser therapy. Topical glucocorticoids, especially potent agents, should be avoided because chronic use of these preparations may elicit rosacea. Topical therapy of the skin is not effective treatment for ocular disease.

SKIN DISEASES AND SMALLPOX VACCINATION

Because of a higher incidence of adverse events associated with smallpox vaccination in patients with a history of certain skin diseases, including atopic dermatitis, eczema, and psoriasis, such vaccination is contraindicated in patients with these conditions in the absence of a bioterrorism attack and a real or potential exposure to smallpox. In the case of such exposure, the risk of smallpox infection outweighs the risk of adverse events from the vaccine (Chap. 221).

FURTHER READINGS

BOLOGNIA JL, JORIZZO JL, RAPINI RP (eds): *Dermatology*, 2nd ed. Philadelphia, Mosby, 2009

JAMES WD et al: *Andrews' Diseases of the Skin Clinical Dermatology*, 10th ed. Philadelphia, Saunders-Elsevier, 2006

WOLFF K, GOLDSMITH LA, KATZ SI, et al (eds): *Fitzpatrick's Dermatology in General Medicine*, 7th ed. New York, McGraw Hill, 2008

WOLFF K, JOHNSON RA: *Fitzpatrick's Color Atlas and Synopsis of Clinical Dermatology*, 6th ed. New York, McGraw-Hill, 2009

WOLVERTON SE (ed): *Comprehensive Dermatologic Drug Therapy* 2nd ed. Philadelphia, Saunders, 2007

CHAPTER 53

Skin Manifestations of Internal Disease

Jean L. Bolognia
Irwin M. Braverman

It is a generally accepted concept in medicine that the skin can develop signs of internal disease. Therefore, in textbooks of medicine, one finds a chapter describing in detail the major systemic disorders that can be identified by cutaneous signs. The underlying assumption of such a chapter is that the clinician has been able to identify the specific disorder in the patient and needs only to read about it in the textbook. In reality, concise differential diagnoses and the identification of these disorders are actually difficult for the nondermatologist because he or she is not well-versed in the recognition of cutaneous lesions or their spectrum of presentations. Therefore, this chapter covers this particular topic of cutaneous medicine not by discussing individual disorders, but by describing and discussing the various presenting clinical signs and symptoms that indicate the presence of these disorders. Concise differential diagnoses will be generated in which the significant diseases will be briefly discussed and distinguished from the more common disorders that have minimal or no significance for internal diseases. The latter disorders are reviewed in table form and always need to be excluded when considering the former. For a detailed description of individual diseases, the reader should consult a dermatologic text.

PAPULOSQUAMOUS SKIN LESIONS

(Table 53-1) When an eruption is characterized by elevated lesions, papules (<1 cm), or plaques (>1 cm), in association with scale, it is referred to as a *papulosquamous lesion*. The most common papulosquamous diseases—*psoriasis, tinea, pityriasis rosea*, and *lichen planus*—are primary cutaneous disorders (Chap. 52). When psoriatic lesions are accompanied by arthritis, the possibility of psoriatic arthritis or reactive arthritis (formerly known as Reiter's syndrome) should be considered. A history of oral ulcers, conjunctivitis, uveitis, and/or urethritis points to the latter diagnosis. Lithium, beta blockers, HIV or streptococcal infections, and a rapid taper of systemic glucocorticoids are known to exacerbate psoriasis. Emerging comorbidities in psoriasis include cardiovascular disease and metabolic syndrome.

Whenever the diagnosis of pityriasis rosea or lichen planus is made, it is important to review the patient's medications because the eruption can be treated by simply discontinuing the offending agent. Pityriasis rosea–like drug eruptions are seen most commonly with beta blockers, angiotensin-converting enzyme (ACE) inhibitors, and metronidazole, while the drugs that can produce a lichenoid eruption include thiazides, antimalarials, quinidine, beta blockers, and ACE inhibitors. In some populations, there is a higher prevalence of hepatitis C viral infection in patients with lichen planus. Lichen planus–like lesions are also observed in chronic graft-versus-host disease.

In its early stages, the mycosis fungoides (MF) form of *cutaneous T cell lymphoma* (CTCL) may be confused with eczema or psoriasis, but it often fails to respond to the appropriate therapy for those inflammatory diseases. MF can develop within lesions of large-plaque parapsoriasis and is suggested by an increase in the thickness of

TABLE 53-1 Selected Causes of Papulosquamous Skin Lesions

1. Primary cutaneous disorders
   a. Psoriasis[a]
   b. Tinea[a]
   c. Pityriasis rosea[a]
   d. Lichen planus[a]
   e. Parapsoriasis
   f. Bowen's disease (squamous cell carcinoma in situ)[b]
2. Drugs
3. Systemic diseases
   a. Lupus erythematosus[c]
   b. Cutaneous T cell lymphoma; in particular, mycosis fungoides[d]
   c. Secondary syphilis
   d. Reactive arthritis (formerly known as Reiter's syndrome)
   e. Sarcoidosis[e]

[a]Discussed in detail in Chap. 52; cardiovascular disease and metabolic syndrome are emerging comorbidities in psoriasis; primarily in Europe, hepatitis C virus is associated with oral lichen planus.
[b]Associated with chronic sun exposure and exposure to arsenic.
[c]See also Red Lesions in "Papulonodular Skin Lesions."
[d]Also cutaneous lesions of HTLV-1-associated adult T cell leukemia/lymphoma.
[e]See also Red-Brown Lesions in "Papulonodular Skin Lesions."

the lesions. The diagnosis of MF is established by skin biopsy in which collections of atypical T lymphocytes are found in the epidermis and dermis. As the disease progresses, cutaneous tumors and lymph node involvement may appear.

In *secondary syphilis*, there are scattered red-brown papules with thin scale. The eruption often involves the palms and soles and can resemble pityriasis rosea. Associated findings are helpful in making the diagnosis and include annular plaques on the face, nonscarring alopecia, condyloma lata (broad-based and moist), and mucous patches as well as lymphadenopathy, malaise, fever, headache, and myalgias. The interval between the primary chancre and the secondary stage is usually 4–8 weeks, and spontaneous resolution without appropriate therapy is seen.

ERYTHRODERMA

(Table 53-2) *Erythroderma* is the term used when the majority of the skin surface is erythematous (red in color). There may be

TABLE 53-2 Causes of Erythroderma

1. Primary cutaneous disorders
   a. Psoriasis[a]
   b. Dermatitis [atopic, contact >> stasis (with autosensitization) or seborrheic][a]
   c. Pityriasis rubra pilaris
2. Drugs
3. Systemic diseases
   a. Cutaneous T cell lymphoma
   b. Lymphoma
4. Idiopathic

[a]Discussed in detail in Chap. 52.

associated scale, erosions, or pustules as well as shedding of the hair and nails. Potential systemic manifestations include fever, chills, hypothermia, reactive lymphadenopathy, peripheral edema, hypoalbuminemia, and high-output cardiac failure. The major etiologies of erythroderma are (1) cutaneous diseases such as psoriasis and dermatitis (Table 53-3); (2) drugs; (3) systemic diseases, most commonly CTCL; and (4) idiopathic. In the first three groups, the location and description of the initial lesions, prior to the development of the erythroderma, aid in the diagnosis. For example, a history of red scaly plaques on the elbows and knees would point to psoriasis. It is also important to examine the skin carefully for a migration of the erythema and associated secondary changes such as pustules or erosions. Migratory waves of erythema studded with superficial pustules are seen in *pustular psoriasis.*

Drug-induced erythroderma (exfoliative dermatitis) may begin as an exanthematous (morbilliform) eruption (Chap. 55) or may arise as diffuse erythema. A number of drugs can produce an erythroderma, including penicillins, sulfonamides, carbamazepine, phenytoin, and allopurinol. Fever and peripheral eosinophilia often accompany the eruption, and there may also be facial swelling, hepatitis, myocarditis, and allergic interstitial nephritis; this constellation is frequently referred to as *drug reaction with eosinophilia and systemic symptoms* (DRESS). In addition, these reactions, especially to anticonvulsants, can lead to a pseudolymphoma syndrome (with adenopathy and circulating atypical lymphocytes), while reactions to allopurinol may be accompanied by gastrointestinal bleeding.

The most common malignancy that is associated with erythroderma is CTCL; in some series, up to 25% of the cases of

TABLE 53-3 Erythroderma (Primary Cutaneous Disorders)

	Initial Lesions	Location of Initial Lesions	Other Findings	Diagnostic Aids	Treatment
Psoriasis[a]	Pink-red, silvery scale, sharply demarcated	Elbows, knees, scalp, presacral area	Nail dystrophy, arthritis, pustules; SAPHO syndrome, especially with palmoplantar pustulosis	Skin biopsy	Topical glucocorticoids, vitamin D; UV-B (narrowband); oral retinoid and/or PUVA; MTX, cyclosporine, anti-TNF agents, anti-IL-12/23 Ab
Dermatitis[a]					
Atopic	Acute: Erythema, fine scale, crust, indistinct borders	Antecubital and popliteal fossae, neck, hands, eyelids	Pruritus	Skin biopsy	Topical glucocorticoids, tacrolimus, pimecrolimus, tar, and antipruritics; oral antihistamines; open wet dressings; UV-B ± UV-A; PUVA; oral/IM glucocorticoids; MTX; mycophenolate mofetil; cyclosporine
			Personal and/or family history of atopy, including asthma, allergic rhinitis or conjunctivitis, and atopic dermatitis		
	Chronic: Lichenification (increased skin markings)		Exclude secondary infection with *S. aureus* or HSV		
			Exclude superimposed irritant or allergic contact dermatitis		Topical or oral antibiotics
Contact	Local: Erythema, crusting, vesicles, and bullae	Depends on offending agent	Irritant—onset often within hours	Patch testing; open use test	Remove irritant or allergen; topical glucocorticoids; oral antihistamines; oral/IM glucocorticoids
			Allergic—delayed-type hypersensitivity; lag time of 48 h		
	Systemic: Erythema, fine scale, crust	Generalized vs major intertriginous zones (especially groin)	Patient has history of allergic contact dermatitis to topical agent and then receives systemic medication that is structurally related, e.g., ethylenediamine (topical), aminophylline (IV)	Patch testing	Same as local
Seborrheic (rare) in adults	Pink-red, greasy scale	Scalp, nasolabial folds, eyebrows, intertriginous zones	Flares with stress, HIV infection	Skin biopsy	Topical glucocorticoids and imidazoles
			Associated with Parkinson's disease		
Stasis (with autosensitization)	Erythema, crusting, excoriations	Lower extremities	Pruritus, lower extremity edema, varicosities, hemosiderin deposits	Skin biopsy	Topical glucocorticoids; open wet dressings; leg elevation; pressure stockings
			History of venous ulcers, thrombophlebitis, and/or cellulitis		
			Exclude cellulitis		
			Exclude superimposed contact dermatitis, e.g., topical neomycin		
Pityriasis rubra pilaris	Orange-red, perifollicular papules	Generalized, but characteristic "skip" areas of normal skin	Wax-like palmoplantar keratoderma	Skin biopsy	Isotretinoin or acitretin; MTX
			Exclude cutaneous T cell lymphoma		

[a]Discussed in detail in Chap. 52.

Note: Ab, antibody; HSV, herpes simplex virus; IL, interleukin; IM, intramuscular; MTX, methotrexate; PUVA, *p*soralens + *u*ltraviolet A irradiation; SAPHO, *s*ynovitis, *a*cne, *p*ustulosis, *h*yperostosis and *o*steitis (also referred to as chronic recurrent multifocal osteomyelitis); TNF, tumor necrosis factor; UV-A, *u*ltraviolet A irradiation; UV-B, *u*ltraviolet B irradiation.

erythroderma were due to CTCL. The patient may progress from isolated plaques and tumors, but, more commonly, the erythroderma is present throughout the course of the disease (Sézary syndrome). In the Sézary syndrome, there are circulating atypical T lymphocytes, pruritus, and lymphadenopathy. In cases of erythroderma where there is no apparent cause (idiopathic), longitudinal evaluation is mandatory to monitor for the possible development of CTCL. There have been isolated case reports of erythroderma secondary to some solid tumors—lung, liver, prostate, thyroid, and colon—but it is primarily during a late stage of the disease.

ALOPECIA

(Table 53-4) The two major forms of alopecia are scarring and nonscarring. In *scarring alopecia*, there are associated fibrosis, inflammation, and loss of hair follicles. A smooth scalp with a decreased number of follicular openings is usually observed clinically, but in some cases, the changes are seen only in biopsy specimens from affected areas. In *nonscarring alopecia*, the hair shafts are gone, but the hair follicles are preserved, explaining the reversible nature of nonscarring alopecia.

The most common causes of nonscarring alopecia include *telogen effluvium, androgenetic alopecia, alopecia areata, tinea capitis*, and the early phase of *traumatic alopecia* (Table 53-5). In women with

TABLE 53-4 Causes of Alopecia

I. Nonscarring alopecia
  A. Primary cutaneous disorders
    1. Telogen effluvium
    2. Androgenetic alopecia
    3. Alopecia areata
    4. Tinea capitis
    5. Traumatic alopecia[a]
  B. Drugs
  C. Systemic diseases
    I. Systemic lupus erythematosus
    2. Secondary syphilis
    3. Hypothyroidism
    4. Hyperthyroidism
    5. Hypopituitarism
    6. Deficiencies of protein, iron, biotin, and zinc
II. Scarring alopecia
  A. Primary cutaneous disorders
    1. Cutaneous lupus (chronic discoid lesions)[b]
    2. Lichen planus
    3. Central centrifugal cicatricial alopecia
    4. Folliculitis decalvans
    5. Linear scleroderma (morphea)
  B. Systemic diseases
    1. Discoid lesions in the setting of systemic lupus erythematosus[b]
    2. Sarcoidosis
    3. Cutaneous metastases

[a]Most patients with trichotillomania, pressure-induced alopecia, early stages of traction alopecia.

[b]While the majority of patients with discoid lesions have only cutaneous disease, these lesions do represent one of the 11 American College of Rheumatology criteria (1982) for systemic lupus erythematosus.

androgenetic alopecia, an elevation in circulating levels of androgens may be seen as a result of ovarian or adrenal gland dysfunction. When there are signs of virilization, such as a deepened voice and enlarged clitoris, the possibility of an ovarian or adrenal gland tumor should be considered.

Exposure to various drugs can also cause diffuse hair loss, usually by inducing a telogen effluvium. An exception is the anagen effluvium observed with antimitotic agents such as daunorubicin. Alopecia is a side effect of the following drugs: warfarin, heparin, propylthiouracil, carbimazole, vitamin A, isotretinoin, acitretin, lithium, beta blockers, colchicine, and amphetamines. Fortunately, spontaneous regrowth usually follows discontinuation of the offending agent.

Less commonly, nonscarring alopecia is associated with *lupus erythematosus* and *secondary syphilis*. In systemic lupus there are two forms of alopecia—one is scarring secondary to discoid lesions (see below), and the other is nonscarring. The latter form may be diffuse and involve the entire scalp or it may be localized to the frontal scalp, with the appearance of multiple short hairs ("lupus hairs") as a sign of initial regrowth. Scattered, poorly circumscribed patches of alopecia with a "moth-eaten" appearance are a manifestation of the secondary stage of syphilis. Diffuse thinning of the hair is also associated with hypothyroidism and hyperthyroidism (Table 53-4).

Scarring alopecia is more frequently the result of a primary cutaneous disorder such as *lichen planus, folliculitis decalvans, chronic cutaneous (discoid) lupus*, or *linear scleroderma (morphea)* than it is a sign of systemic disease. Although the scarring lesions of *discoid lupus* can be seen in patients with systemic lupus, in the majority of cases, the disease process is limited to the skin. Less common causes of scarring alopecia include *sarcoidosis* (see "Papulonodular Skin Lesions," below) and *cutaneous metastases*.

In the early phases of discoid lupus, lichen planus, and folliculitis decalvans, there are circumscribed areas of alopecia. Fibrosis and subsequent loss of hair follicles are observed primarily in the center of the individual lesions; the inflammatory process is most prominent at the periphery. The areas of active inflammation in discoid lupus are erythematous with scale, whereas the areas of previous inflammation are often hypopigmented with a rim of hyperpigmentation. In lichen planus, the peripheral perifollicular macules are usually violet-colored. A complete examination of the skin and oral mucosa combined with a biopsy and direct immunofluorescence microscopy will aid in distinguishing these two entities. The peripheral active lesions in folliculitis decalvans are follicular pustules; these patients can develop a reactive arthritis.

FIGURATE SKIN LESIONS

(Table 53-6) In *figurate eruptions*, the lesions form rings and arcs that are usually erythematous but can be skin-colored to brown. Most commonly, they are due to primary cutaneous diseases such as *tinea, urticaria, erythema annulare centrifugum*, and *granuloma annulare* (Chaps. 52 and 54). An underlying systemic illness is found in a second, less common group of migratory annular erythemas. It includes *erythema gyratum repens, erythema migrans, erythema marginatum*, and *necrolytic migratory erythema*.

In erythema gyratum repens, one sees numerous mobile concentric arcs and wavefronts that resemble the grain in wood. A search for an underlying malignancy is mandatory in a patient with this eruption. Erythema migrans is the cutaneous manifestation of Lyme disease, which is caused by the spirochete *Borrelia burgdorferi*. In the initial stage (3–30 days after tick bite), a single annular lesion is usually seen, which can expand to ≥10 cm in diameter. Within several days, approximately half the patients develop multiple smaller erythematous lesions at sites distant from the bite. Associated symptoms include fever, headache, photophobia,

TABLE 53-5 Nonscarring Alopecia (Primary Cutaneous Disorders)

	Clinical Characteristics	Pathogenesis	Treatment
Telogen effluvium	Diffuse shedding of normal hairs Follows major stress (high fever, severe infection) or change in hormones (postpartum) Reversible without treatment	Stress causes more of the asynchronous growth cycles of individual hairs to become synchronous; therefore, larger numbers of growing (anagen) hairs simultaneously enter the dying (telogen) phase	Observation; discontinue any drugs that have alopecia as a side effect; must exclude underlying metabolic causes, e.g., hypothyroidism, hyperthyroidism
Androgenetic alopecia (male pattern; female pattern)	Miniaturization of hairs along the midline of the scalp Recession of the anterior scalp line in men and some women	Increased sensitivity of affected hairs to the effects of androgens Increased levels of circulating androgens (ovarian or adrenal source in women)	If no evidence of hyperandrogen state, then topical minoxidil; finasteride[a]; spironolactone (women); hair transplant
Alopecia areata	Well-circumscribed, circular areas of hair loss, 2–5 cm in diameter In extensive cases, coalescence of lesions and/or involvement of other hair-bearing surfaces of the body Pitting of the nails	The germinative zones of the hair follicles are surrounded by T lymphocytes Occasional associated diseases: hyperthyroidism, hypothyroidism, vitiligo, Down syndrome	Topical anthralin or tazarotene; intralesional glucocorticoids; topical contact sensitizers
Tinea capitis	Varies from scaling with minimal hair loss to discrete patches with "black dots" (broken hairs) to boggy plaque with pustules (kerion)[b]	Invasion of hairs by dermatophytes, most commonly *Trichophyton tonsurans*	Oral griseofulvin or terbinafine plus 2.5% selenium sulfide or ketoconazole shampoo; examine family members
Traumatic alopecia[c]	Broken hairs Irregular outline	Traction with curlers, rubber bands, braiding Exposure to heat or chemicals (e.g., hair straighteners) Mechanical pulling (trichotillomania)	Discontinuation of offending hair style or chemical treatments; trichotillomania may require hair clipping and observation of shaved hairs or biopsy for diagnosis, possibly followed by psychotherapy

[a] To date, FDA-approved for men.

[b] Scarring alopecia can occur at sites of kerions.

[c] May also be scarring, especially late-stage traction alopecia.

myalgias, arthralgias, and malar rash. Erythema marginatum is seen in patients with rheumatic fever, primarily on the trunk. Lesions are pink-red in color, flat to mildly elevated, and transient.

TABLE 53-6 Causes of Figurate Skin Lesions

I. Primary cutaneous disorders

  A. Tinea

  B. Urticaria (primary in ≥90% of patients)

  C. Erythema annulare centrifugum

  D. Granuloma annulare

  E. Psoriasis

II. Systemic diseases

  A. Migratory

    1. Erythema migrans

    2. Urticaria (≤10% of patients)

    3. Erythema gyratum repens

    4. Erythema marginatum

    5. Pustular psoriasis (generalized)

    6. Necrolytic migratory erythema (glucagonoma syndrome)[a]

  B. Nonmigratory

    1. Sarcoidosis

    2. Subacute cutaneous lupus erythematosus

    3. Secondary syphilis

    4. Cutaneous T cell lymphoma (especially mycosis fungoides)

[a] Migratory erythema with erosions; favors lower extremities and girdle area.

There are additional cutaneous diseases that present as annular eruptions but lack an obvious migratory component. Examples include *CTCL, subacute cutaneous lupus, secondary syphilis,* and *sarcoidosis* (see "Papulonodular Skin Lesions," below).

ACNE

(Table 53-7) In addition to *acne vulgaris* and *acne rosacea,* the two major forms of acne (Chap. 52), there are drugs and systemic diseases that can lead to acneiform eruptions.

TABLE 53-7 Causes of Acneiform Eruptions

I. Primary cutaneous disorders

  A. Acne vulgaris

  B. Acne rosacea

II. Drugs, e.g., anabolic steroids, glucocorticoids, lithium, EGFR[a] inhibitors, iodides

III. Systemic diseases

  A. Increased androgen production

    1. Adrenal origin, e.g., Cushing's disease, 21-hydroxylase deficiency

    2. Ovarian origin, e.g., polycystic ovary syndrome

  B. Cryptococcosis, disseminated

  C. Dimorphic fungi

  D. Behçet's disease

[a] EGFR, epidermal growth factor receptor.

Patients with the *carcinoid syndrome* have episodes of flushing of the head, neck, and sometimes the trunk. Resultant skin changes of the face, in particular telangiectasias, may mimic the clinical appearance of acne rosacea.

PUSTULAR LESIONS

Acneiform eruptions (see "Acne," above) and *folliculitis* represent the most common pustular dermatoses. An important consideration in the evaluation of follicular pustules is a determination of the associated pathogen, e.g., normal flora, *Staphylococcus aureus*, *Pseudomonas aeruginosa* ("hot tub" folliculitis), *Malassezia*, and dermatophytes (Majocchi's granuloma). Noninfectious forms of folliculitis include HIV-associated eosinophilic folliculitis and folliculitis secondary to drugs such as glucocorticoids, lithium, and epidermal growth factor receptor (EGFR) inhibitors. Administration of high-dose systemic glucocorticoids can result in a widespread eruption of follicular pustules on the trunk, characterized by lesions in the same stage of development. With regard to underlying systemic diseases, nonfollicular-based pustules are a characteristic component of pustular psoriasis (sterile) and can be seen in septic emboli of bacterial or fungal origin (see "Purpura," below). In patients with acute generalized exanthematous pustulosis (AGEP) due primarily to medications (e.g., cephalosporins), there are large areas of erythema studded with multiple sterile pustules in addition to neutrophilia.

TELANGIECTASIAS

(Table 53-8) To distinguish the various types of telangiectasias, it is important to examine the shape and configuration of the dilated blood vessels. *Linear telangiectasias* are seen on the face of patients with *actinically damaged skin* and *acne rosacea,* and they are found on the legs of patients with *venous hypertension* and *essential telangiectasia.* Patients with an unusual form of *mastocytosis* (telangiectasia macularis eruptiva perstans) and the *carcinoid syndrome* (see "Acne," above) also have linear telangiectasias. Lastly, linear telangiectasias are found in areas of cutaneous inflammation.

TABLE 53-8 Causes of Telangiectasias

I. Primary cutaneous disorders

A. Linear
1. Acne rosacea
2. Actinically damaged skin
3. Venous hypertension
4. Essential telangiectasia
5. Within basal cell carcinomas

B. Poikiloderma
1. Ionizing radiation[a]
2. Poikiloderma vasculare atrophicans

C. Spider angioma
1. Idiopathic
2. Pregnancy

II. Systemic diseases

A. Linear
1. Carcinoid
2. Ataxia-telangiectasia
3. Mastocytosis

B. Poikiloderma
1. Dermatomyositis
2. Cutaneous T cell lymphoma
3. Xeroderma pigmentosum

C. Mat
1. Scleroderma

D. Periungual
1. Lupus erythematosus
2. Scleroderma
3. Dermatomyositis
4. Hereditary hemorrhagic telangiectasia

E. Papular
1. Hereditary hemorrhagic telangiectasia

F. Spider angioma
1. Cirrhosis

[a]Becoming less common.

For example, lesions of discoid lupus frequently have telangiectasias within them.

Poikiloderma is a term used to describe a patch of skin with: (1) reticulated hypo- and hyperpigmentation, (2) wrinkling secondary to epidermal atrophy, and (3) telangiectasias. Poikiloderma does not imply a single disease entity—although it is becoming less common, it is seen in skin damaged by *ionizing radiation* as well as in patients with autoimmune connective tissue diseases, primarily *dermatomyositis* (DM), and rare genodermatoses (e.g., Kindler syndrome).

In *systemic sclerosis (scleroderma)* the dilated blood vessels have a unique configuration and are known as *mat telangiectasias.* The lesions are broad macules that usually measure 2–7 mm in diameter but occasionally are larger. Mats have a polygonal or oval shape and their erythematous color may appear uniform, but, upon closer inspection, the erythema is the result of delicate telangiectasias. The most common locations for mat telangiectasias are the face, oral mucosa, and hands—peripheral sites that are prone to intermittent ischemia. The CREST (*c*alcinosis cutis, *R*aynaud's phenomenon, *e*sophageal dysmotility, *s*clerodactyly, and *t*elangiectasia) variant of scleroderma (Chap. 323) is associated with a chronic course and anticentromere antibodies. Mat telangiectasias are an important clue to the diagnosis of the CREST syndrome as well as systemic scleroderma because they may be the only cutaneous finding.

Periungual telangiectasias are pathognomonic signs of the three major autoimmune connective tissue diseases: *lupus erythematosus*, *scleroderma*, and *DM*. They are easily visualized by the naked eye and occur in at least two-thirds of these patients. In both DM and lupus, there is associated nailfold erythema, and in DM, the erythema is often accompanied by "ragged" cuticles and fingertip tenderness. Under 10× magnification, the blood vessels in the nailfolds of lupus patients are tortuous and resemble "glomeruli," whereas in scleroderma and DM, there is a loss of capillary loops and those that remain are markedly dilated.

In *hereditary hemorrhagic telangiectasia* (Osler-Rendu-Weber disease), the lesions usually appear during adulthood and are most commonly seen on the mucous membranes, face, and distal extremities, including under the nails. They represent arteriovenous (AV) malformations of the dermal microvasculature, are dark red in color, and are usually slightly elevated. When the skin is stretched over an individual lesion, an eccentric punctum with radiating legs is seen. Although the degree of systemic involvement varies in this autosomal dominant disease (due primarily to mutations in either the endoglin or activin receptor–like kinase gene), the major symptoms are recurrent epistaxis and gastrointestinal bleeding. The fact that these mucosal telangiectasias are actually AV communications helps to explain their tendency to bleed.

HYPOPIGMENTATION

(Table 53-9) Disorders of hypopigmentation are often classified as either diffuse or localized. The classic example of *diffuse hypopigmentation* is *oculocutaneous albinism* (OCA). The most common forms are due to mutations in the tyrosinase gene (type I) or the *P* gene (type II); patients with type IA OCA have a total lack of enzyme activity. At birth, different forms of OCA can appear similar—white hair, gray-blue eyes, and pink-white skin. However, the patients with no tyrosinase activity maintain this phenotype, whereas those with decreased activity will acquire some pigmentation of the eyes, hair, and skin as they age. The degree of pigment formation is also a function of racial background, and the pigmentary dilution is more readily apparent when patients are compared to their first-degree relatives. The ocular findings in OCA correlate with the degree of hypopigmentation and include decreased visual acuity, nystagmus, photophobia, and a lack of normal binocular vision.

TABLE 53-9 Causes of Hypopigmentation

I. Primary cutaneous disorders
   A. Diffuse
      1. Generalized vitiligo[a]
   B. Localized
      1. Idiopathic guttate hypomelanosis
      2. Postinflammatory
      3. Tinea (pityriasis) versicolor
      4. Vitiligo[a]
      5. Chemical- or drug-enduced leukoderma
      6. Nevus depigmentosus
      7. Piebaldism
II. Systemic diseases
   A. Diffuse
      1. Oculocutaneous albinism[b]
      2. Hermansky-Pudlak syndrome[b,c]
      3. Chédiak-Higashi syndrome[b,d]
      4. Phenylketonuria
      5. Homocystinuria
   B. Localized
      1. Scleroderma
      2. Melanoma-associated leukoderma
      3. Sarcoidosis
      4. Cutaneous T cell lymphoma (especially mycosis fungoides)
      5. Tuberculoid and indeterminate leprosy
      6. Onchocerciasis
      7. Tuberous sclerosis
      8. Hypomelanosis of Ito/mosaicism/linear nevoid hypopigmentation
      9. Incontinentia pigmenti (stage IV)
      10. Vogt-Koyanagi-Harada syndrome
      11. Waardenburg syndrome

[a]Absence of melanocytes.

[b]Normal number of melanocytes.

[c]Platelet storage defect and restrictive lung disease secondary to deposits of ceroid-like material; due to mutations in β subunit of adaptor protein 3 as well as subunits of *b*iogenesis of *l*ysosome-related *o*rganelles *c*omplex (BLOC)-1, -2, and -3.

[d]Giant lysosomal granules and recurrent infections.

The differential diagnosis of *localized hypomelanosis* includes the following primary cutaneous disorders: *idiopathic guttate hypomelanosis, postinflammatory hypopigmentation, tinea (pityriasis) versicolor, vitiligo, chemical- or drug-induced leukoderma, nevus depigmentosus* (see below), and *piebaldism* (Table 53-9). In this group of diseases, the areas of involvement are macules or patches with a decrease or absence of pigmentation. Patients with vitiligo also have an increased incidence of several autoimmune disorders, including Hashimoto's thyroiditis, Graves' disease, pernicious anemia, Addison's disease, uveitis, alopecia areata, chronic mucocutaneous candidiasis, and the polyglandular autoimmune syndromes (types I and II). Diseases of the thyroid gland are the most frequently associated disorders, occurring in up to 30% of patients with vitiligo. Circulating autoantibodies are often found, and the most common ones are antithyroglobulin, antimicrosomal, and antithyroid-stimulating hormone receptor antibodies.

There are four systemic diseases that should be considered in a patient with skin findings suggestive of vitiligo—*Vogt-Koyanagi-Harada syndrome, scleroderma, onchocerciasis,* and *melanoma-associated leukoderma.* A history of aseptic meningitis, nontraumatic uveitis, tinnitus, hearing loss, and/or dysacousia points to the diagnosis of the Vogt-Koyanagi-Harada syndrome. In these patients, the face and scalp are the most common locations of pigment loss. The vitiligo-like leukoderma seen in patients with scleroderma has a clinical resemblance to idiopathic vitiligo that has begun to repigment as a result of treatment; that is, perifollicular macules of normal pigmentation are seen within areas of depigmentation. The basis of this leukoderma is unknown; there is no evidence of inflammation in areas of involvement, but it can resolve if the underlying connective tissue disease becomes inactive. In contrast to idiopathic vitiligo, melanoma-associated leukoderma often begins on the trunk, and its appearance should prompt a search for metastatic disease. It is also seen in patients undergoing immunotherapy for melanoma, with cytotoxic T lymphocytes presumably recognizing cell surface antigens common to melanoma cells and melanocytes, and is associated with a greater likelihood of a clinical response.

There are two systemic disorders (neurocristopathies) that may have the cutaneous findings of piebaldism (Table 53-10). They are *Shah-Waardenburg syndrome* and *Waardenburg syndrome.* A possible explanation for both disorders is an abnormal embryonic migration or survival of two neural crest–derived elements, one of them being melanocytes and the other myenteric ganglion cells (leading to Hirschsprung disease in Shah-Waardenburg syndrome) or auditory nerve cells (Waardenburg syndrome). The latter syndrome is characterized by congenital sensorineural hearing loss, dystopia canthorum (lateral displacement of the inner canthi but normal interpupillary distance), heterochromic irises, and a broad nasal root, in addition to the piebaldism. Patients with Waardenburg syndrome have been shown to have mutations in three genes, including two (*PAX-3* and *MITF*) that encode DNA-binding proteins, while patients with Hirschsprung disease plus white spotting have mutations in one of three genes—endothelin 3, endothelin B receptor, and *SOX-10.*

In *tuberous sclerosis,* the earliest cutaneous sign is an ash leaf spot. These lesions are often present at birth and are usually multiple; however, detection may require Wood's lamp examination, especially in fair-skinned individuals. The pigment within them is reduced, but not absent. The average size is 1–3 cm, and the common shapes are polygonal and lance-ovate. Examination of the patient for additional cutaneous signs such as multiple angiofibromas of the face (adenoma sebaceum), ungual and gingival fibromas, fibrous plaques of the forehead, and connective tissue nevi (shagreen patches) is recommended. It is important to remember that an ash leaf spot on the scalp will result in a circumscribed patch of lightly pigmented hair. Internal manifestations include seizures, mental retardation, central nervous system (CNS) and retinal hamartomas, pulmonary lymphangioleiomyomatosis (women), renal angiomyolipomas, and cardiac rhabdomyomas. The latter can be detected in up to 60% of children (<18 years) with tuberous sclerosis by echocardiography.

Nevus depigmentosus is a stable, well-circumscribed hypomelanosis that is present at birth. There is usually a single oval or rectangular lesion, but when there are multiple lesions, the possibility of tuberous sclerosis needs to be considered. In *linear nevoid hypopigmentation* or *pigmentary mosaicism,* terms that are replacing hypomelanosis of Ito and segmental or systematized nevus depigmentosus, streaks and swirls of hypopigmentation are observed. Up to a third of patients in a referral population had associated abnormalities involving the musculoskeletal system (asymmetry), the CNS (seizures and mental retardation), and the eyes (strabismus and hypertelorism). Chromosomal mosaicism has been detected in

TABLE 53-10 Hypopigmentation (Primary Cutaneous Disorders, Localized)

	Clinical Characteristics	Wood's Lamp Examination (UV-A; Peak = 365 nm)	Skin Biopsy Specimen	Pathogenesis	Treatment
Idiopathic guttate hypomelanosis	Common; acquired; 1–4 mm in diameter Shins and extensor forearms	Less enhancement than vitiligo	Abrupt decrease in epidermal melanin content	Possible somatic mutations as a reflection of aging; UV exposure	None
Postinflammatory hypopigmentation	Can develop within active lesions, as in subacute cutaneous lupus, or after the lesion fades, as in dermatitis	Depends on particular disease Usually less enhancement than in vitiligo	Type of inflammatory infiltrate depends on specific disease	Block in transfer of melanin from melanocytes to keratinocytes could be secondary to edema or decrease in contact time Destruction of melanocytes if inflammatory cells attack basal layer of epidermis	Treat underlying inflammatory disease
Pityriasis (tinea) versicolor	Common disorder Upper trunk and neck (shawl-like distribution), groin Young adults Macules have fine white scale when scratched	Golden fluorescence	Hyphal forms and budding yeast in stratum corneum	Invasion of stratum corneum by the yeast *Malassezia* Yeast is lipophilic and produces C_9 and C_{11} dicarboxylic acids, which in vitro inhibit tyrosinase	Selenium sulfide 2.5%; topical imidazoles; oral imidazoles or triazoles
Vitiligo	Acquired; progressive Symmetric areas of complete pigment loss Periorificial—around mouth, nose, eyes, nipples, umbilicus, anus Other areas—flexor wrists, extensor distal extremities Segmental form is less common—unilateral, dermatomal-like	More apparent Chalk-white	Absence of melanocytes Mild inflammation	Autoimmune phenomenon that results in destruction of melanocytes—primarily cellular (circulating skin-homing autoreactive T cells)	Topical glucocorticoids; topical calcineurin inhibitors; NBUV-B; PUVA; transplants, if stable; depigmentation (topical MBEH), if widespread
Chemical- or drug-induced leukoderma	Similar appearance to vitiligo Often begins on hands when associated with chemical exposure Satellite lesions in areas not exposed to chemicals	More apparent Chalk-white	Decreased number or absence of melanocytes	Exposure to chemicals that selectively destroy melanocytes, in particular phenols and catechols (germicides; adhesives) or ingestion of drugs such as imatinib Release of cellular antigens and activation of circulating lymphocytes may explain satellite phenomenon Possible inhibition of KIT receptor	Avoid exposure to offending agent, then treat as vitiligo Drug-induced variant may undergo repigmentation when medication is discontinued
Piebaldism	Autosomal dominant Congenital, stable White forelock Areas of hypomelanosis contain normally pigmented and hyperpigmented macules of various sizes Symmetric involvement of central forehead, ventral trunk, and mid regions of upper and lower extremities	Enhancement of leukoderma and hyperpigmented macules	Hypomelanotic areas—few to no melanocytes	Defect in migration of melanoblasts from neural crest to involved skin or failure of melanoblasts to survive or differentiate in these areas Mutations within the c-*kit* protooncogene that encodes the tyrosine kinase receptor for stem cell growth factor (kit ligand)	None; occasionally transplants

Abbreviations: MBEH, monobenzylether of hydroquinone; NBUV-B, *narrow*b and *u*ltraviolet B; PUVA, *p*soralens +*u*ltraviolet A irradiation.

these patients, lending support to the hypothesis that the pattern is the result of the migration of two clones of primordial melanocytes, each with a different pigment potential.

Localized areas of decreased pigmentation are commonly seen as a result of cutaneous inflammation (Table 53-10) and have been observed in the skin overlying active lesions of sarcoidosis (see "Papulonodular Skin Lesions," below) as well as in CTCL. Cutaneous infections also present as disorders of hypopigmentation, and in *tuberculoid leprosy*, there are a few asymmetric patches of hypomelanosis that have associated anesthesia, anhidrosis, and alopecia. Biopsy specimens of the palpable border show dermal granulomas that contain rare, if any, *Mycobacterium leprae* organisms.

HYPERPIGMENTATION

(Table 53-11) Disorders of hyperpigmentation are also divided into two groups—localized and diffuse. The localized forms are due to an epidermal alteration, a proliferation of melanocytes, or an increase in pigment production. Both seborrheic keratoses and acanthosis nigricans belong to the first group. *Seborrheic keratoses* are common lesions, but in one rare clinical setting, they are a sign of systemic disease, and that setting is the sudden appearance of multiple lesions, often with an inflammatory base and in association with acrochordons (skin tags) and acanthosis nigricans. This is termed the *sign of Leser-Trélat* and alerts the clinician to search for an internal malignancy. *Acanthosis nigricans* can also be a reflection of an internal malignancy, most commonly of the gastrointestinal tract, and it appears as velvety hyperpigmentation, primarily in flexural areas. However, in the majority of patients, acanthosis nigricans is associated with obesity and insulin resistance, but it may be a reflection of an endocrinopathy such as acromegaly, Cushing's syndrome, polycystic ovary syndrome, or insulin-resistant diabetes mellitus (type A, type B, and lipoatrophic forms).

A proliferation of melanocytes results in the following pigmented lesions: *lentigo*, *melanocytic nevus*, and *melanoma* (Chap. 87). In an adult, the majority of lentigines are related to sun exposure, which explains their distribution. However, in the Peutz-Jeghers and LEOPARD [*l*entigines; *E*CG abnormalities, primarily conduction defects; *o*cular hypertelorism; *p*ulmonary stenosis and subaortic valvular stenosis; *a*bnormal genitalia (cryptorchidism, hypospadias); *r*etardation of growth; and *d*eafness (sensorineural)] syndromes, lentigines do serve as a clue to systemic disease. In *LEOPARD syndrome*, hundreds of lentigines develop during childhood and are scattered over the entire surface of the body. The lentigines in patients with *Peutz-Jeghers syndrome* are located primarily around the nose and mouth, on the hands and feet, and within the oral cavity. While the pigmented macules on the face may fade with age, the oral lesions persist. However, similar intraoral lesions are also seen in Addison's disease, Laugier-Hunziker syndrome (no internal manifestations), and as a normal finding in darkly pigmented individuals. Patients with this autosomal dominant syndrome (due to mutations in a novel serine threonine kinase gene) have multiple benign polyps of the gastrointestinal tract, testicular or ovarian tumors, and an increased risk of developing gastrointestinal (primarily colon) and pancreatic cancers.

In the Carney complex, numerous lentigines are also seen but they are in association with cardiac myxomas. This autosomal dominant disorder is also known as the *LAMB* (*l*entigines, *a*trial myxomas, *m*ucocutaneous myxomas, and *b*lue nevi) *syndrome* or *NAME* [*n*evi, *a*trial myxoma, *m*yxoid neurofibroma, and *e*phelides (freckles)] *syndrome*. These patients can also have evidence of endocrine overactivity in the form of Cushing's syndrome (pigmented nodular adrenocortical disease) and acromegaly.

The third type of localized hyperpigmentation is due to a local increase in pigment production, and it includes *ephelides* and

TABLE 53-11 Causes of Hyperpigmentation

I. Primary cutaneous disorders
  A. Localized
    1. Epidermal alteration
      a. Seborrheic keratosis
      b. Pigmented actinic keratosis
    2. Proliferation of melanocytes
      a. Lentigo
      b. Melanocytic nevus (mole)
      c. Melanoma
    3. Increased pigment production
      a. Ephelide (freckle)
      b. Café au lait macule
      c. Postinflammatory hyperpigmentation
  B. Localized and diffuse
    1. Drugs
II. Systemic diseases
  A. Localized
    1. Epidermal alteration
      a. Seborrheic keratoses (sign of Leser-Trélat)
      b. Acanthosis nigricans (insulin resistance, other endocrine disorders, paraneoplastic)
    2. Proliferation of melanocytes
      a. Lentigines (Peutz-Jeghers and LEOPARD syndromes; xeroderma pigmentosum)
      b. Melanocytic nevi [Carney complex (LAMB and NAME syndromes)][a]
    3. Increased pigment production
      a. Café au lait macules (neurofibromatosis, McCune-Albright syndrome[b])
      b. Urticaria pigmentosa[c]
    4. Dermal pigmentation
      a. Incontinentia pigmenti (stage III)
      b. Dyskeratosis congenita
  B. Diffuse
    1. Endocrinopathies
      a. Addison's disease
      b. Nelson syndrome
      c. Ectopic ACTH syndrome
    2. Metabolic
      a. Porphyria cutanea tarda
      b. Hemochromatosis
      c. Vitamin B_{12}, folate deficiency
      d. Pellagra
      e. Malabsorption, including Whipple's disease
    3. Melanosis secondary to metastatic melanoma
    4. Autoimmune
      a. Biliary cirrhosis
      b. Scleroderma
      c. POEMS syndrome
      d. Eosinophilia-myalgia syndrome[d]
    5. Drugs and metals

[a]Also lentigines.

[b]Polyostotic fibrous dysplasia.

[c]See also "Papulonodular Skin Lesions."

[d]Late 1980s.

Abbreviations: LAMB, *l*entigines, *a*trial myxomas, *m*ucocutaneous myxomas, and *b*lue nevi; LEOPARD, *l*entigines, *E*CG abnormalities, *o*cular hypertelorism, *p*ulmonary stenosis and subaortic valvular stenosis, *a*bnormal genitalia, *r*etardation of growth, and *d*eafness (sensorineural); NAME, *n*evi, *a*trial myxoma, *m*yxoid neurofibroma, and *e*phelides (freckles); POEMS, *p*olyneuropathy, *o*rganomegaly, *e*ndocrinopathies, *M*-protein, and *s*kin changes.

café au lait macules (CALM). While a single CALM can be seen in up to 10% of the normal population, the presence of multiple or large-sized CALM raises the possibility of an associated genodermatosis, e.g., neurofibromatosis (NF) or McCune-Albright syndrome. CALM are flat, uniformly brown in color (usually two shades darker than uninvolved skin), and can- vary in size from 0.5–12 cm. Approximately 80–90% of adult patients with *type I NF* will have six or more CALM measuring ≥1.5 cm in diameter. Additional findings are discussed in the section on neurofibromas (see "Papulonodular Skin Lesions," below). In comparison with NF, the CALM in patients with *McCune-Albright syndrome* [polyostotic fibrous dysplasia with precocious puberty in females due to mosaicism for an activating mutation in a G protein ($G_s\alpha$) gene] are usually larger, more irregular in outline, and tend to respect the midline.

In incontinentia pigmenti, dyskeratosis congenita, and bleomycin pigmentation, the areas of localized hyperpigmentation form a pattern—swirled in the first, reticulated in the second, and flagellate in the third. In *dyskeratosis congenita*, atrophic reticulated hyperpigmentation is seen on the neck, trunk, and thighs and is accompanied by nail dystrophy, pancytopenia, and leukoplakia of the oral and anal mucosae. The latter often develops into squamous cell carcinoma. In addition to the flagellate pigmentation (linear streaks) on the trunk, patients receiving bleomycin often have hyperpigmentation overlying the elbows, knees, and small joints of the hand.

Localized hyperpigmentation is seen as a side effect of several other *systemic medications*, including those that produce fixed drug reactions [nonsteroidal anti-inflammatory drugs (NSAIDs), sulfonamides, barbiturates, and tetracyclines] and those that can complex with melanin (antimalarials) or iron (minocycline). Fixed drug eruptions recur in the exact same location as circular areas of erythema that can become bullous and then resolve as brown macules. The eruption usually appears within hours of administration of the offending agent, and common locations include the genitalia, extremities, and perioral region. Chloroquine and hydroxychloroquine produce gray-brown to blue-black discoloration of the shins, hard palate, and face, while blue macules (often misdiagnosed as bruises) can be seen on the lower extremities and in sites of inflammation with prolonged minocycline administration. Estrogen in oral contraceptives can induce melasma—symmetric brown patches on the face, especially the cheeks, upper lip, and forehead. Similar changes are seen in pregnancy and in patients receiving phenytoin.

In the diffuse forms of hyperpigmentation, the darkening of the skin may be of equal intensity over the entire body or may be accentuated in sun-exposed areas. The causes of diffuse hyperpigmentation can be divided into four major groups—endocrine, metabolic, autoimmune, and drugs. The endocrinopathies that frequently have associated hyperpigmentation include *Addison's disease*, *Nelson syndrome*, and *ectopic ACTH syndrome*. In these diseases, the increased pigmentation is diffuse but is accentuated in sun-exposed areas, the palmar creases, sites of friction, and scars. An overproduction of the pituitary hormones α-MSH (melanocyte-stimulating hormone) and ACTH can lead to an increase in melanocyte activity. These peptides are products of the proopiomelanocortin gene and exhibit homology; e.g., α-MSH and ACTH share 13 amino acids. A minority of the patients with Cushing's disease or hyperthyroidism have generalized hyperpigmentation.

The metabolic causes of hyperpigmentation include *porphyria cutanea tarda* (PCT), *hemochromatosis, vitamin B_{12} deficiency, folic acid deficiency, pellagra,* and *malabsorption,* including *Whipple's disease.* In patients with PCT (see "Vesicles/Bullae," below), the skin darkening is seen in sun-exposed areas and is a reflection of the photoreactive properties of porphyrins. The increased level of iron

in the skin of patients with hemochromatosis stimulates melanin pigment production and leads to the classic bronze color. Patients with pellagra have a brown discoloration of the skin, especially in sun-exposed areas, as a result of nicotinic acid (niacin) deficiency. In the areas of increased pigmentation, there is a thin, varnish-like scale. These changes are also seen in patients who are vitamin B_6 deficient, have functioning carcinoid tumors (increased consumption of niacin), or take isoniazid. Approximately 50% of the patients with Whipple's disease have an associated generalized hyperpigmentation in association with diarrhea, weight loss, arthritis, and lymphadenopathy. A diffuse, slate-blue color is seen in patients with *melanosis secondary to metastatic melanoma.* Although there is a debate as to whether the color is due to single-cell metastases in the dermis or to a widespread deposition of melanin resulting from the high concentration of circulating melanin precursors, there is more evidence to support the latter.

Of the autoimmune diseases associated with diffuse hyperpigmentation, *biliary cirrhosis* and *scleroderma* are the most common, and occasionally, both disorders are seen in the same patient. The skin is dark brown in color, especially in sun-exposed areas. In biliary cirrhosis, the hyperpigmentation is accompanied by pruritus, jaundice, and xanthomas, whereas in scleroderma, it is accompanied by sclerosis of the extremities, face, and, less commonly, the trunk. Additional clues to the diagnosis of scleroderma are mat and periungual telangiectasias, calcinosis cutis, Raynaud's phenomenon, and distal ulcerations (see "Telangiectasias," above). The differential diagnosis of cutaneous sclerosis with hyperpigmentation includes the POEMS [*p*olyneuropathy; *o*rganomegaly (liver, spleen, lymph nodes); *e*ndocrinopathies (impotence, gynecomastia); *M*-protein; and *s*kin changes] syndrome. The skin changes include hyperpigmentation, induration, hypertrichosis, and angiomas.

Diffuse hyperpigmentation that is due to drugs or metals can result from one of several mechanisms—induction of melanin pigment formation, complexing of the drug or its metabolites to melanin, and deposits of the drug in the dermis. Busulfan, cyclophosphamide, 5-fluorouracil, and inorganic arsenic induce pigment production. Complexes containing melanin or iron plus the drug or its metabolites are seen in patients receiving minocycline, and a diffuse, blue-gray, muddy appearance within sun-exposed areas may develop, in addition to pigmentation of the mucous membranes, teeth, nails, bones, and thyroid. Administration of amiodarone can result in both a phototoxic eruption (exaggerated sunburn) and/or a slate-gray to violaceous discoloration of sun-exposed skin. Biopsy specimens of the latter show yellow-brown granules in dermal macrophages, which represent intralysosomal accumulations of lipids, amiodarone, and its metabolites. Actual deposits of a particular drug or metal in the skin are seen with silver (argyria), where the skin appears blue-gray in color; gold (chrysiasis), where the skin has a brown to blue-gray color; and clofazimine, where the skin appears reddish brown. The associated hyperpigmentation is accentuated in sun-exposed areas, and discoloration of the eye is seen with gold (sclerae) and clofazimine (conjunctivae).

VESICLES/BULLAE

(Table 53-12) Depending on their size, cutaneous blisters are referred to as *vesicles* (<0.5 cm) or *bullae* (>0.5 cm). The primary autoimmune blistering disorders include *pemphigus vulgaris, pemphigus foliaceus, pemphigus erythematosus, paraneoplastic pemphigus, bullous pemphigoid, gestational pemphigoid, cicatricial pemphigoid, epidermolysis bullosa acquisita, linear IgA bullous dermatosis (LABD),* and *dermatitis herpetiformis* (Chap. 54).

Vesicles and bullae are also seen in *contact dermatitis*, both allergic and irritant forms (Chap. 52). When there is a linear arrangement of vesicular lesions, an exogenous cause should be suspected. Bullous disease secondary to the ingestion of drugs can take one

TABLE 53-12 Causes of Vesicles/Bullae

I. Primary mucocutaneous diseases
  A. Primary blistering diseases (autoimmune)
    1. Pemphigus[a]
    2. Bullous pemphigoid[b]
    3. Gestational pemphigoid[b]
    4. Cicatricial pemphigoid[b]
    5. Dermatitis herpetiformis[b,c]
    6. Linear IgA bullous dermatosis[b]
    7. Epidermolysis bullosa acquisita[b,d]
  B. Secondary blistering diseases
    1. Contact dermatitis[a]
    2. Erythema multiforme[e]
    3. Stevens-Johnson syndrome[e]
    4. Toxic epidermal necrolysis[e]
  C. Infections
    1. Varicella/zoster virus[a,f]
    2. Herpes simplex virus[a,f]
    3. Enteroviruses, e.g., hand-foot-and-mouth disease
    4. Staphylococcal scalded-skin syndrome[a,g]
    5. Bullous impetigo[a]
II. Systemic diseases
  A. Autoimmune
    1. Paraneoplastic pemphigus[a]
  B. Infections
    1. Cutaneous emboli[b]
  C. Metabolic
    1. Diabetic bullae[a,b]
    2. Porphyria cutanea tarda[b]
    3. Porphyria variegata[b]
    4. Pseudoporphyria[b]
    5. Bullous dermatosis of hemodialysis[b]
  D. Ischemia
    1. Coma bullae

[a]Intraepidermal.

[b]Subepidermal.

[c]Associated with gluten enteropathy.

[d]Associated with inflammatory bowel disease.

[e]Degeneration of cells within the basal layer of the epidermis can give impression split is subepidermal.

[f]Also systemic.

[g]In adults, associated with renal failure and immunocompromised state.

of several forms, including phototoxic eruptions, isolated bullae, Stevens-Johnson syndrome (SJS), and toxic epidermal necrolysis (TEN) (Chap. 55). Clinically, phototoxic eruptions resemble an exaggerated sunburn with diffuse erythema and bullae in sun-exposed areas. The most commonly associated drugs are doxycycline, quinolones, thiazides, NSAIDs, voriconazole, and psoralens. The development of a phototoxic eruption is dependent on the doses of both the drug and ultraviolet (UV)-A irradiation.

Toxic epidermal necrolysis is characterized by bullae that arise on widespread areas of erythema and then slough. This results in large areas of denuded skin. The associated morbidity, such as sepsis, and mortality rates are relatively high and are a function of the extent of epidermal necrosis. In addition, these patients may also have involvement of the mucous membranes and respiratory and intestinal tracts. Drugs are the primary cause of TEN, and the most common offenders are phenytoin, barbiturates, carbamazepine, sulfonamides, aminopenicillins, allopurinol, and NSAIDs. Severe acute graft-versus-host disease (grade 4), drug-induced LABD, and the acute syndrome of apoptotic pan-epidermolysis (ASAP) in patients with lupus can also resemble TEN.

In *erythema multiforme* (EM), the primary lesions are pink-red macules and edematous papules, the centers of which may become vesicular. In contrast to a morbilliform exanthem, the clue to the diagnosis of EM, and especially SJS, is the development of a "dusky" violet color in the center of the lesions. Target or iris lesions are also characteristic of EM and arise as a result of active centers and borders in combination with centrifugal spread. However, iris lesions need not be present to make the diagnosis of EM.

EM has been subdivided into two major groups: (1) EM minor due to herpes simplex virus (HSV) and (2) EM major due to HSV; *Mycoplasma pneumoniae*; or, occasionally, drugs. Involvement of the mucous membranes (oral, nasal, ocular, and genital) is seen more commonly in the latter form. Hemorrhagic crusts of the lips are characteristic of EM major and SJS as well as herpes simplex, pemphigus vulgaris, and paraneoplastic pemphigus. Fever, malaise, myalgias, sore throat, and cough may precede or accompany the eruption. The lesions of EM usually resolve over 2–4 weeks but may be recurrent, especially when due to HSV. In addition to HSV (in which lesions usually appear 7–12 days after the viral eruption), EM can also follow vaccinations, radiation therapy, and exposure to environmental toxins, including the oleoresin in poison ivy.

Induction of SJS is most often due to drugs, especially sulfonamides, phenytoin, barbiturates, aminopenicillins, non-nucleoside reverse transcriptase inhibitors, and carbamazepine. Widespread dusky macules and significant mucosal involvement are characteristic of SJS, and the cutaneous lesions may or may not develop epidermal detachment. If the latter occurs, by definition, it is limited to <10% of the body surface area (BSA). Greater involvement leads to the diagnosis of SJS/TEN overlap (10–30% BSA) or TEN (>30% BSA).

In addition to primary blistering disorders and hypersensitivity reactions, bacterial and viral infections can lead to vesicles and bullae. The most common infectious agents are HSV (Chap. 179), varicella-zoster virus (Chap. 180), and *S. aureus* (Chap. 135).

Staphylococcal scalded-skin syndrome (SSSS) and *bullous impetigo* are two blistering disorders associated with staphylococcal (phage group II) infection. In SSSS, the initial findings are redness and tenderness of the central face, neck, trunk, and intertriginous zones. This is followed by short-lived flaccid bullae and a slough or exfoliation of the superficial epidermis. Crusted areas then develop, characteristically around the mouth. SSSS is distinguished from TEN by the following features: younger age group (primarily infants), more superficial site of blister formation, no oral lesions, shorter course, lower morbidity and mortality rates, and an association with staphylococcal exfoliative toxin ("exfoliatin"), not drugs. A rapid diagnosis of SSSS versus TEN can be made by a frozen section of the blister roof or exfoliative cytology of the blister contents. In SSSS the site of staphylococcal infection is usually extracutaneous (conjunctivitis, rhinorrhea, otitis media, pharyngitis, tonsillitis), and the cutaneous lesions are sterile, whereas in bullous impetigo, the skin lesions are the site of infection. Impetigo is more localized than SSSS and usually presents with honey-colored crusts. Occasionally, superficial purulent blisters also form. *Cutaneous emboli* from gram-negative infections may present as isolated bullae, but the base of the lesion is purpuric or necrotic, and it may develop into an ulcer (see "Purpura," below).

Several metabolic disorders are associated with blister formation, including diabetes mellitus, renal failure, and porphyria. Local hypoxemia secondary to decreased cutaneous blood flow can also produce blisters, which explains the presence of bullae over pressure points in comatose patients (coma bullae). In *diabetes mellitus*, tense bullae with clear viscous fluid arise on normal skin. The lesions can be as large as 6 cm in diameter and are located on the distal extremities. There are several types of porphyria, but the most common form with cutaneous findings is *porphyria cutanea tarda* (PCT). In sun-exposed areas (primarily the face and hands), the skin is very fragile, with trauma leading to erosions mixed with tense vesicles. These lesions then heal with scarring and formation of milia; the latter are firm, 1- to 2-mm white or yellow papules that represent epidermoid inclusion cysts. Associated findings can include hypertrichosis of the lateral malar region (men) or face (women) and, in sun-exposed areas, hyperpigmentation and firm sclerotic plaques. An elevated level of urinary uroporphyrins confirms the diagnosis and is due to a decrease in uroporphyrinogen decarboxylase activity. Precipitating agents include alcohol, iron, chlorinated hydrocarbons, hepatitis C infection, and hepatomas.

The differential diagnosis of PCT includes (1) *porphyria variegata*—the skin signs of PCT plus the systemic findings of acute intermittent porphyria; it has a diagnostic plasma porphyrin fluorescence emission at 626 nm; (2) *drug-induced* pseudoporphyria—the clinical and histologic findings are similar to PCT, but porphyrins are normal; etiologic agents include naproxen and other NSAIDs, furosemide, tetracycline, and retinoids; (3) *bullous dermatosis of hemodialysis*—the same appearance as PCT, but porphyrins are usually normal or occasionally borderline elevated; patients have chronic renal failure and are on hemodialysis; (4) PCT associated with hepatomas and hemodialysis; and (5) *epidermolysis bullosa acquisita* (Chap. 54).

EXANTHEMS

(Table 53-13) Exanthems are characterized by an acute generalized eruption. The most common presentation is erythematous macules

TABLE 53-13 Causes of Exanthems

I. Morbilliform
  A. Drugs
  B. Viral
    1. Rubeola (measles)
    2. Rubella
    3. Erythema infectiosum (reticulated on extremities)
    4. Epstein-Barr virus, echovirus, coxsackievirus, CMV, and adenovirus infections
    5. Early HIV infection (plus mucosal ulcerations)
  C. Bacterial
    1. Typhoid fever
    2. Early secondary syphilis
    3. Early *Rickettsia* infections
    4. Early meningococcemia
  D. Acute graft-versus-host disease
  E. Kawasaki's disease
II. Scarlatiniform
  A. Scarlet fever
  B. Toxic shock syndrome
  C. Kawasaki's disease
  D. Early staphylococcal scalded-skin syndrome

Abbreviations: CMV, cytomegalovirus; HIV, human immunodeficiency virus.

and papules (morbilliform) and less often confluent blanching erythema (scarlatiniform). *Morbilliform* eruptions are usually due to either drugs or viral infections. For example, up to 5% of patients receiving penicillins, sulfonamides, phenytoin, or nevirapine will develop a maculopapular eruption. Accompanying signs may include pruritus, fever, eosinophilia, and transient lymphadenopathy. Similar maculopapular eruptions are seen in the classic childhood viral exanthems, including (1) *rubeola* (measles)—a prodrome of coryza, cough, and conjunctivitis followed by Koplik's spots on the buccal mucosa; the eruption begins behind the ears, at the hairline, and on the forehead and then spreads down the body, often becoming confluent; (2) *rubella*—the eruption begins on the forehead and face and then spreads down the body; it resolves in the same order and is associated with retroauricular and suboccipital lymphadenopathy; and (3) *erythema infectiosum* (fifth disease)—erythema of the cheeks is followed by a reticulated pattern on the extremities; it is secondary to a parvovirus B19 infection, and an associated arthritis is seen in adults.

Both measles and rubella can occur in unvaccinated adults, and an atypical form of measles is seen in adults immunized with either killed measles vaccine or killed vaccine followed in time by live vaccine. In contrast to classic measles, the eruption of atypical measles begins on the palms, soles, wrists, and knuckles, and the lesions may become purpuric. The patient with atypical measles can have pulmonary involvement and be quite ill. Rubelliform and roseoliform eruptions are also associated with *Epstein-Barr virus* (5–15% of patients), *echovirus, coxsackievirus, cytomegalovirus, adenovirus, dengue virus,* and *West Nile virus* infections. Detection of specific IgM antibodies or fourfold elevations in IgG antibodies allows the proper diagnosis. Occasionally, a maculopapular drug eruption is a reflection of an underlying viral infection. For example, about 95% of the patients with infectious mononucleosis who are given ampicillin will develop a rash.

Of note, early in the course of infections with *Rickettsia* and meningococcus, prior to the development of purpura, the lesions may be erythematous macules and papules. This is also the case in chickenpox prior to the development of vesicles. Maculopapular eruptions are associated with early *HIV infection*, early secondary *syphilis, typhoid fever,* and *acute graft-versus-host disease.* In the last, lesions frequently begin on the dorsal hands and forearms; the macular rose spots of typhoid fever involve primarily the anterior trunk.

The prototypic *scarlatiniform* eruption is seen in *scarlet fever* and is due to an erythrotoxin produced by group A β-hemolytic streptococcal infections, most commonly pharyngitis. This eruption is characterized by diffuse erythema, which begins on the neck and upper trunk, and red follicular puncta. Additional findings include a white strawberry tongue (white coating with red papillae) followed by a red strawberry tongue (red tongue with red papillae); petechiae of the palate; a facial flush with circumoral pallor; linear petechiae in the antecubital fossae; and desquamation of the involved skin, palms, and soles 5–20 days after onset of the eruption. A similar desquamation of the palms and soles is seen in toxic shock syndrome (TSS), Kawasaki's disease, and after severe febrile illnesses. Certain strains of staphylococci also produce an erythrotoxin that leads to the same clinical findings as in streptococcal scarlet fever, except that the anti-streptolysin O or -DNase B titers are not elevated.

In *toxic shock syndrome*, staphylococcal (phage group I) infections produce an exotoxin (TSST-1) that causes the fever and rash as well as enterotoxins. Initially, the majority of cases were reported in menstruating women who were using tampons. However, other sites of infection, including wounds and nasal packing, can lead to TSS. The diagnosis of TSS is based on clinical criteria (Chap. 135), and three of these involve mucocutaneous sites (diffuse erythema of the skin, desquamation of the palms and soles 1–2 weeks after onset of illness, and involvement of the mucous membranes). The latter is characterized as hyperemia of the vagina, oropharynx, or conjunctivae. Similar systemic findings have been described in *streptococcal toxic shock syndrome* (Chap. 136), and although an exanthem is seen less often than in TSS due to a staphylococcal infection, the underlying infection is often in the soft tissue.

The cutaneous eruption in *Kawasaki's disease* (mucocutaneous lymph node syndrome) (Chap. 326) is polymorphous, but the two most common forms are morbilliform and scarlatiniform. Additional mucocutaneous findings include bilateral conjunctival injection; erythema and edema of the hands and feet followed by desquamation; and diffuse erythema of the oropharynx, red strawberry tongue, and dry fissured lips. This clinical picture can resemble TSS and scarlet fever, but clues to the diagnosis of Kawasaki's disease are cervical lymphadenopathy, cheilitis, and thrombocytosis. The most serious associated systemic finding in this disease is coronary aneurysms secondary to arteritis. Aneurysms may lead to sudden death, primarily within the first 30 days of the illness. Scarlatiniform eruptions are also seen in the early phase of SSSS (see "Vesicles/Bullae," above) and as reactions to drugs.

URTICARIA

(Table 53-14) *Urticaria* (hives) are transient lesions that are composed of a central wheal surrounded by an erythematous halo. Individual lesions are round, oval, or figurate and are often pruritic. Acute and chronic urticaria have a wide variety of allergic etiologies and reflect edema in the dermis. Urticarial lesions can also be seen in patients with mastocytosis (urticaria pigmentosa), hypo- or hyperthyroidism, and systemic-onset juvenile idiopathic arthritis (Still's disease). In both juvenile- and adult-onset Still's disease, the lesions coincide with the fever spike, are transient, and are due to dermal infiltrates of neutrophils.

The common *physical urticarias* include dermatographism, solar urticaria, cold urticaria, and cholinergic urticaria. Patients with *dermatographism* exhibit linear wheals following minor pressure or scratching of the skin. It is a common disorder, affecting ~5% of the population. *Solar urticaria* characteristically occurs within minutes of sun exposure and is a skin sign of one systemic disease—erythropoietic protoporphyria. In addition to the urticaria, these patients have subtle pitted scarring of the nose and hands.

TABLE 53-14 Causes of Urticaria and Angioedema

I. Primary cutaneous disorders
  A. Acute and chronic urticaria[a]
  B. Physical urticaria
    1. Dermatographism
    2. Solar urticaria[b]
    3. Cold urticaria[b]
    4. Cholinergic urticaria[b]
  C. Angioedema (hereditary and acquired)[b]
II. Systemic diseases
  A. Urticarial vasculitis
  B. Hepatitis B or C infection
  C. Serum sickness
  D. Angioedema (hereditary and acquired)

[a] A small minority develop anaphylaxis.
[b] Also systemic.

Cold urticaria is precipitated by exposure to the cold, and therefore exposed areas are usually affected. In occasional patients, the disease is associated with abnormal circulating proteins—more commonly cryoglobulins and less commonly cryofibrinogens. Additional systemic symptoms include wheezing and syncope, thus explaining the need for these patients to avoid swimming in cold water. *Cholinergic urticaria* is precipitated by heat, exercise, or emotion and is characterized by small wheals with relatively large flares. It is occasionally associated with wheezing.

Whereas urticarias are the result of dermal edema, subcutaneous edema leads to the clinical picture of *angioedema*. Sites of involvement include the eyelids, lips, tongue, larynx, and gastrointestinal tract as well as the subcutaneous tissue. Angioedema occurs alone or in combination with urticaria, including urticarial vasculitis and the physical urticarias. Both acquired and hereditary (autosomal dominant) forms of angioedema occur (Chap. 317), and in the latter, urticaria is rarely, if ever, seen.

Urticarial vasculitis is an immune complex disease that may be confused with simple urticaria. In contrast to simple urticaria, individual lesions tend to last longer than 24 h and usually develop central petechiae that can be observed even after the urticarial phase has resolved. The patient may also complain of burning rather than pruritus. On biopsy, there is a leukocytoclastic vasculitis of the small blood vessels. Although many cases of urticarial vasculitis are idiopathic in origin, it can be a reflection of an underlying systemic illness such as lupus erythematosus, Sjögren's syndrome, or hereditary complement deficiency. There is a spectrum of urticarial vasculitis that ranges from purely cutaneous to multisystem involvement. The most common systemic signs and symptoms are arthralgias and/or arthritis, nephritis, and crampy abdominal pain, with asthma and chronic obstructive lung disease seen less often. Hypocomplementemia occurs in one- to two-thirds of patients, even in the idiopathic cases. Urticarial vasculitis can also be seen in patients with *hepatitis B* and *hepatitis C* infections, *serum sickness*, and *serum sickness–like illnesses* (e.g., due to cefaclor, minocycline).

PAPULONODULAR SKIN LESIONS

(Table 53-15) In the *papulonodular diseases*, the lesions are elevated above the surface of the skin and may coalesce to form plaques. The location, consistency, and color of the lesions are the keys to their diagnosis; this section is organized on the basis of color.

■ WHITE LESIONS

In *calcinosis cutis* there are firm white to white-yellow papules with an irregular surface. When the contents are expressed, a chalky white material is seen. *Dystrophic calcification* is seen at sites of previous inflammation or damage to the skin. It develops in acne scars as well as on the distal extremities of patients with scleroderma and in the subcutaneous tissue and intermuscular fascial planes in DM. The latter is more extensive and is more commonly seen in children. An elevated calcium phosphate product, most commonly due to secondary hyperparathyroidism in the setting of renal failure, can lead to nodules of *metastatic calcinosis cutis*, which tend to be subcutaneous and periarticular. These patients can also develop calcification of muscular arteries and subsequent ischemic necrosis (calciphylaxis).

■ SKIN-COLORED LESIONS

There are several types of skin-colored lesions, including epidermoid inclusion cysts, lipomas, rheumatoid nodules, neurofibromas, angiofibromas, neuromas, and adnexal tumors such as tricholemmomas. Both *epidermoid inclusion cysts* and *lipomas* are very common mobile subcutaneous nodules—the former are

TABLE 53-15 Papulonodular Skin Lesions According to Color Groups

I. White
   A. Calcinosis cutis

II. Skin-colored
   A. Rheumatoid nodules
   B. Neurofibromas (von Recklinghausen's disease)
   C. Angiofibromas (tuberous sclerosis, MEN syndrome, type 1)
   D. Neuromas (MEN syndrome, type 2b)
   E. Adnexal tumors
      1. Basal cell carcinomas (nevoid basal cell carcinoma syndrome)
      2. Tricholemmomas (Cowden disease)
   F. Osteomas (Gardner syndrome)
   G. Primary cutaneous disorders
      1. Epidermal inclusion cysts[a]
      2. Lipomas

III. Pink/translucent[b]
   A. Amyloidosis
   B. Papular mucinosis

IV. Yellow
   A. Xanthomas
   B. Tophi
   C. Necrobiosis lipoidica
   D. Pseudoxanthoma elasticum
   E. Sebaceous adenomas (Torre syndrome)

V. Red[b]
   A. Papules
      1. Angiokeratomas (Fabry disease)
      2. Bacillary angiomatosis (primarily in AIDS)
   B. Papules/plaques
      1. Cutaneous lupus
      2. Lymphoma cutis
      3. Leukemia cutis
      4. Sweet syndrome
   C. Nodules
      1. Panniculitis
      2. Cutaneous polyarteritis nodosa
      3. Systemic vasculitis
   D. Primary cutaneous disorders
      1. Arthropod bites
      2. Cherry hemangiomas
      3. Infections, e.g., erysipelas, sporotrichosis
      4. Polymorphous light eruption
      5. Lymphocytoma cutis (pseudolymphoma)

VI. Red-brown[b]
   A. Sarcoidosis
   B. Sweet's syndrome
   C. Urticaria pigmentosa
   D. Erythema elevatum diutinum (chronic leukocytoclastic vasculitis)
   E. Lupus vulgaris

VII. Blue[b]
   A. Venous malformations (e.g., blue rubber bleb syndrome)
   B. Primary cutaneous disorders
      1. Venous lake
      2. Blue nevus

VIII. Violaceous
   A. Lupus pernio (sarcoidosis)
   B. Lymphoma cutis
   C. Cutaneous lupus

IX. Purple
   A. Kaposi's sarcoma
   B. Angiosarcoma
   C. Palpable purpura (see Table 53-16)

X. Brown-black[c]

XI. Any color
   A. Metastases

[a]If multiple with childhood onset, consider Gardner syndrome.

[b]May have darker hue in more darkly pigmented individuals.

[c]See also "Hyperpigmentation."

Abbreviation: MEN, multiple endocrine neoplasia.

rubbery and drain cheeselike material (sebum and keratin) if incised. Lipomas are firm and somewhat lobulated on palpation. When extensive facial epidermoid inclusion cysts develop during childhood or there is a family history of such lesions, the patient should be examined for other signs of Gardner syndrome, including osteomas and desmoid tumors. *Rheumatoid nodules* are firm 0.5- to 4-cm nodules that favor the extensor aspect of joints, especially the elbows. They are seen in ~20% of patients with rheumatoid arthritis and 6% of patients with Still's disease. Biopsies of the nodules show palisading granulomas. Similar lesions that are smaller and shorter-lived are seen in rheumatic fever.

Neurofibromas (benign Schwann cell tumors) are soft papules or nodules that exhibit the "button-hole" sign; that is, they invaginate into the skin with pressure in a manner similar to a hernia. Single lesions are seen in normal individuals, but multiple neurofibromas, usually in combination with six or more CALM measuring >1.5 cm (see "Hyperpigmentation," above), axillary freckling, and multiple Lisch nodules, are seen in von Recklinghausen's disease (NF type I;

Chap. 379). In some patients, the neurofibromas are localized and unilateral due to somatic mosaicism.

Angiofibromas are firm pink to skin-colored papules that measure from 3 mm to a few centimeters in diameter. When multiple lesions are located on the central cheeks (adenoma sebaceum), the patient has tuberous sclerosis or multiple endocrine neoplasia (MEN) syndrome, type 1. The former is an autosomal disorder due to mutations in two different genes, and the associated findings are discussed in the section on ash leaf spots as well as in Chap. 379.

Neuromas (benign proliferations of nerve fibers) are also firm, skin-colored papules. They are more commonly found at sites of amputation and as rudimentary supernumerary digits. However, when there are multiple neuromas on the eyelids, lips, distal tongue, and/or oral mucosa, the patient should be investigated for other signs of the MEN syndrome, type 2b. Associated findings include marfanoid habitus, protuberant lips, intestinal ganglioneuromas, and medullary thyroid carcinoma (>75% of patients; Chap. 351).

Adnexal tumors are derived from pluripotent cells of the epidermis that can differentiate toward hair, sebaceous, apocrine, or eccrine glands or remain undifferentiated. *Basal cell carcinomas* (BCCs) are examples of adnexal tumors that have little or no evidence of differentiation. Clinically, they are translucent papules with rolled borders, telangiectasias, and central erosion. BCCs commonly arise in sun-damaged skin of the head and neck as well as the upper trunk. When a patient has multiple BCCs, especially prior to age 30, the possibility of the nevoid basal cell carcinoma syndrome should be raised. It is inherited as an autosomal dominant trait and is associated with jaw cysts, palmar and plantar pits, frontal bossing, medulloblastomas, and calcification of the falx cerebri and diaphragma sellae. *Tricholemmomas* are also skin-colored adnexal tumors but differentiate toward hair follicles and can have a wartlike appearance. The presence of multiple tricholemmomas on the face and cobblestoning of the oral mucosa points to the diagnosis of Cowden disease (multiple hamartoma syndrome) due to mutations in the phosphatase and tensin homolog (*PTEN*) gene. Internal organ involvement (in decreasing order of frequency) includes fibrocystic disease and carcinoma of the breast, adenomas and carcinomas of the thyroid, and gastrointestinal polyposis. Keratoses of the palms, soles, and dorsal aspect of the hands are also seen.

■ PINK LESIONS

The cutaneous lesions associated with primary systemic *amyloidosis* are often pink in color and translucent. Common locations are the face, especially the periorbital and perioral regions, and flexural areas. On biopsy, homogeneous deposits of amyloid are seen in the dermis and in the walls of blood vessels; the latter lead to an increase in vessel wall fragility. As a result, petechiae and purpura develop in clinically normal skin as well as in lesional skin following minor trauma, hence the term *pinch purpura*. Amyloid deposits are also seen in the striated muscle of the tongue and result in macroglossia.

Even though specific mucocutaneous lesions are rarely seen in secondary amyloidosis and are present in only ~30% of the patients with primary amyloidosis, a rapid diagnosis of systemic amyloidosis can be made by an examination of abdominal subcutaneous fat. By special staining, deposits are seen around blood vessels or individual fat cells in 40–50% of patients. There are also three forms of amyloidosis that are limited to the skin and that should not be construed as cutaneous lesions of systemic amyloidosis. They are macular amyloidosis (upper back), lichenoid amyloidosis (usually lower extremities), and nodular amyloidosis. In macular and lichenoid amyloidosis, the deposits are composed of altered epidermal keratin. Early-onset macular and lichenoid amyloidosis have been associated with MEN syndrome, type 2a.

Patients with *multicentric reticulohistiocytosis* also have pink-colored papules and nodules on the face and mucous membranes as well as on the extensor surface of the hands and forearms. They have a polyarthritis that can mimic rheumatoid arthritis clinically. On histologic examination, the papules have characteristic giant cells that are not seen in biopsies of rheumatoid nodules. Pink to skin-colored papules that are firm, 2–5 mm in diameter, and often in a linear arrangement are seen in patients with *papular mucinosis*. This disease is also referred to as *generalized lichen myxedematosus* or *scleromyxedema*. The latter name comes from the induration of the face and extremities that may accompany the papular eruption. Biopsy specimens of the papules show localized mucin deposition, and serum protein electrophoresis and/or immunofixation electrophoresis demonstrates a monoclonal spike of IgG, usually with a λ light chain.

■ YELLOW LESIONS

Several systemic disorders are characterized by yellow-colored cutaneous papules or plaques—hyperlipidemia (xanthomas), gout (tophi), diabetes (necrobiosis lipoidica), pseudoxanthoma elasticum, and Torre syndrome (sebaceous tumors). Eruptive xanthomas are the most common form of *xanthomas* and are associated with hypertriglyceridemia (types I, III, IV, and V). Crops of yellow papules with erythematous halos occur primarily on the extensor surfaces of the extremities and the buttocks, and they spontaneously involute with a fall in serum triglycerides. Increased β-lipoproteins (primarily types II and III) result in one or more of the following types of xanthoma: xanthelasma, tendon xanthomas, and plane xanthomas. Xanthelasma are found on the eyelids, whereas tendon xanthomas are frequently associated with the Achilles and extensor finger tendons; plane xanthomas are flat and favor the palmar creases, face, upper trunk, and scars. Tuberous xanthomas are frequently associated with hypertriglyceridemia, but they are also seen in patients with hypercholesterolemia (type II) and are found most frequently over the large joints or hand. Biopsy specimens of xanthomas show collections of lipid-containing macrophages (foam cells).

Patients with several disorders, including biliary cirrhosis, can have a secondary form of hyperlipidemia with associated tuberous and planar xanthomas. However, patients with plasma cell dyscrasias have *normolipemic flat xanthomas*. This latter form of xanthoma may be ≥12 cm in diameter and is most frequently seen on the upper trunk or side of the neck. It is important to note that the most common setting for eruptive xanthomas is uncontrolled diabetes mellitus. The least specific sign for hyperlipidemia is xanthelasma, because at least 50% of the patients with this finding have normal lipid profiles.

In *tophaceous gout*, there are deposits of monosodium urate in the skin around the joints, particularly those of the hands and feet. Additional sites of *tophi* formation include the helix of the ear and the olecranon and prepatellar bursae. The lesions are firm, yellow in color, and occasionally discharge a chalky material. Their size varies from 1 mm to 7 cm, and the diagnosis can be established by polarization of the aspirated contents of a lesion. Lesions of *necrobiosis lipoidica* are found primarily on the shins (90%), and patients can have diabetes mellitus or develop it subsequently. Characteristic findings include a central yellow color, atrophy (transparency), telangiectasias, and a red to red-brown border. Ulcerations can also develop within the plaques. Biopsy specimens show necrobiosis of collagen and granulomatous inflammation.

In *pseudoxanthoma elasticum* (PXE), due to mutations in the gene *ABCC6*, there is an abnormal deposition of calcium on the elastic fibers of the skin, eye, and blood vessels. In the skin, the flexural areas such as the neck, axillae, antecubital fossae, and inguinal area are the primary sites of involvement. Yellow papules coalesce to form reticulated plaques that have an appearance similar to that of plucked chicken skin. In severely affected skin, hanging, redundant folds develop. Biopsy specimens of involved skin show swollen and irregularly clumped elastic fibers with deposits of calcium. In the eye, the calcium deposits in Bruch's membrane lead to angioid streaks and choroiditis; in the arteries of the heart, kidney, gastrointestinal tract, and extremities, the deposits lead to angina, hypertension, gastrointestinal bleeding, and claudication, respectively. Long-term administration of D-penicillamine can lead to PXE-like skin changes as well as elastic fiber alterations in internal organs.

Adnexal tumors that have differentiated toward sebaceous glands include sebaceous adenoma, sebaceous carcinoma, and sebaceous hyperplasia. Except for sebaceous hyperplasia, which is commonly seen on the face, these tumors are fairly rare. Patients with Torre syndrome have one or more *sebaceous adenoma(s)*, and they can also have sebaceous carcinomas and sebaceous hyperplasia as well as keratoacanthomas. The internal manifestations of Torre syndrome include *multiple* carcinomas of the gastrointestinal tract (primarily colon) as well as cancers of the larynx, genitourinary tract, and breast.

RED LESIONS

Cutaneous lesions that are red in color have a wide variety of etiologies; in an attempt to simplify their identification, they will be subdivided into papules, papules/plaques, and subcutaneous nodules. Common red papules include *arthropod bites* and *cherry hemangiomas*; the latter are small, bright-red, dome-shaped papules that represent benign proliferation of capillaries. In patients with AIDS (see Chapter 189), the development of multiple red hemangioma-like lesions points to bacillary angiomatosis, and biopsy specimens show clusters of bacilli that stain positive with the Warthin-Starry stain; the pathogens have been identified as *Bartonella henselae* and *B. quintana*. Disseminated visceral disease is seen primarily in immunocompromised hosts but can occur in immunocompetent individuals.

Multiple *angiokeratomas* are seen in Fabry disease, an X-linked recessive lysosomal storage disease that is due to a deficiency of α-galactosidase A. The lesions are red to red-blue in color and can be quite small in size (1–3 mm), with the most common location being the lower trunk. Associated findings include chronic renal failure, peripheral neuropathy, and corneal opacities (cornea verticillata). Electron photomicrographs of angiokeratomas and clinically normal skin demonstrate lamellar lipid deposits in fibroblasts, pericytes, and endothelial cells that are diagnostic of this disease. Widespread acute eruptions of erythematous papules are discussed in the section on exanthems.

There are several infectious diseases that present as erythematous papules or nodules in a lymphocutaneous or sporotrichoid pattern, i.e., in a linear arrangement along the lymphatic channels. The two most common etiologies are *Sporothrix schenckii* (sporotrichosis) and the atypical mycobacterium *M. marinum*. The organisms are introduced as a result of trauma, and a primary inoculation site is often seen in addition to the lymphatic nodules. Additional causes include *Nocardia*, *Leishmania*, and other dimorphic fungi; culture of lesional tissue will aid in the diagnosis.

The diseases that are characterized by erythematous plaques with scale are reviewed in the papulosquamous section, and the various forms of dermatitis are discussed in the section on erythroderma. Additional disorders in the differential diagnosis of red papules/plaques include *erysipelas*, *polymorphous light eruption* (PMLE), *cutaneous lymphoid hyperplasia* (lymphocytoma cutis), *cutaneous lupus*, *lymphoma cutis*, and *leukemia cutis*. The first three diseases represent primary cutaneous disorders. PMLE is characterized by erythematous papules and plaques in a primarily sun-exposed distribution—dorsum of the hand, extensor forearm, and upper trunk. Lesions follow exposure to UV-B and/or UV-A, and in higher latitudes, PMLE is most severe in the late spring and early summer. A process referred to as "hardening" occurs with continued UV exposure, and the eruption fades, but in temperate climates, it will recur in the spring. PMLE must be differentiated from cutaneous lupus, and this is accomplished by observation of the natural history, histologic examination, and direct immunofluorescence of the lesions. Cutaneous lymphoid hyperplasia (pseudolymphoma) is a *benign* polyclonal proliferation of lymphocytes in the skin that presents as infiltrated pink-red to red-purple papules and plaques; it must be distinguished from lymphoma cutis.

Several types of red plaques are seen in patients with systemic *lupus*, including (1) erythematous urticarial plaques across the cheeks and nose in the classic butterfly rash; (2) erythematous discoid lesions with fine or "carpet-tack" scale, telangiectasias, central hypopigmentation, peripheral hyperpigmentation, follicular plugging, and atrophy located on the face, scalp, external ears, arms, and upper trunk; and (3) psoriasiform or annular lesions of subacute cutaneous lupus with hypopigmented centers located primarily on the extensor arms and upper trunk. Additional mucocutaneous findings include (1) a violaceous flush on the face and V of the neck; (2) photosensitivity; (3) urticarial vasculitis (see "Urticaria," above); (4) lupus panniculitis (see below); (5) diffuse alopecia; (6) alopecia secondary to discoid lesions; (7) periungual telangiectasias and erythema; (8) EM-like lesions that may become bullous; (9) oral ulcers; and (10) distal ulcerations secondary to Raynaud's phenomenon, vasculitis, or livedoid vasculopathy. Patients with only discoid lesions usually have the form of lupus that is limited to the skin. However, 2–10% of these patients eventually develop systemic lupus. Direct immunofluorescence of involved skin shows deposits of IgG or IgM and C3 in a granular distribution along the dermal-epidermal junction.

In *lymphoma cutis*, there is a proliferation of malignant lymphocytes in the skin, and the clinical appearance resembles that of cutaneous lymphoid hyperplasia—infiltrated pink-red to red-purple papules and plaques. Lymphoma cutis can occur anywhere on the surface of the skin, whereas the sites of predilection for lymphocytomas include the malar ridge, tip of the nose, and earlobes. Patients with non-Hodgkin's lymphomas have specific cutaneous lesions more often than those with Hodgkin's disease, and, occasionally, the skin nodules precede the development of extracutaneous non-Hodgkin's lymphoma or represent the only site of involvement (e.g., primary cutaneous B cell lymphoma). Arcuate lesions are sometimes seen in lymphoma and lymphocytoma cutis as well as in CTCL. *Adult T cell leukemia/lymphoma* that develops in association with HTLV-1 infection is characterized by cutaneous plaques, hypercalcemia, and circulating CD25+ lymphocytes. *Leukemia cutis* has the same appearance as lymphoma cutis, and specific lesions are seen more commonly in monocytic leukemias than in lymphocytic or granulocytic leukemias. Cutaneous chloromas (granulocytic sarcomas) may precede the appearance of circulating blasts in acute myelogenous leukemia and, as such, represent a form of aleukemic leukemia cutis.

Common causes of erythematous subcutaneous nodules include inflamed epidermoid inclusion cysts, acne cysts, and furuncles. *Panniculitis*, an inflammation of the fat, also presents as subcutaneous nodules and is frequently a sign of systemic disease. There are several forms of panniculitis, including erythema nodosum, erythema induratum/nodular vasculitis, lupus profundus, lipodermatosclerosis, α₁-antitrypsin deficiency, factitial, and fat necrosis secondary to pancreatic disease. Except for erythema nodosum, these lesions may break down and ulcerate or heal with a scar. The shin is the most common location for the nodules of erythema nodosum, whereas the calf is the most common location for lesions of erythema induratum. In erythema nodosum, the nodules are initially red but then develop a blue color as they resolve. Patients with erythema nodosum but no underlying systemic illness can still have fever, malaise, leukocytosis, arthralgias, and/or arthritis. However, the possibility of an underlying illness should be excluded, and the most common associations are streptococcal infections, upper respiratory viral infections, sarcoidosis, and inflammatory bowel disease in addition to drugs (oral contraceptives, sulfonamides, penicillins, bromides, iodides). Less common associations include bacterial gastroenteritis (*Yersinia*, *Salmonella*) and coccidioidomycosis followed by tuberculosis, histoplasmosis, brucellosis, and infections with *Chlamydophila pneumoniae* or *Chlamydia trachomatis*, *Mycoplasma pneumoniae*, or hepatitis B virus.

Erythema induratum and nodular vasculitis have overlapping features clinically and histologically, and whether they represent two separate entities or the ends of a single disease spectrum is a point of debate; in general, the latter is usually idiopathic and the former is associated with the presence of *M. tuberculosis* DNA by polymerase chain reaction (PCR) within skin lesions. The lesions of lupus panniculitis are found primarily on the cheeks, upper arms, and buttocks (sites of abundant fat) and are seen in both the cutaneous and systemic forms of lupus. The overlying skin may be normal, erythematous, or have the changes of discoid lupus. The subcutaneous fat necrosis that is associated with pancreatic disease is presumably secondary to circulating lipases and is seen in patients with pancreatic carcinoma as well as in patients with acute and chronic pancreatitis. In this disorder, there may be an associated arthritis, fever, and inflammation of visceral fat. Histologic examination of deep incisional biopsy specimens will aid in the diagnosis of the particular type of panniculitis.

Subcutaneous erythematous nodules are also seen in *cutaneous polyarteritis nodosa* (PAN) and as a manifestation of *systemic vasculitis*, e.g., systemic PAN, allergic granulomatosis, or granulomatosis with polyangiitis (Wegener's) (Chap. 326). Cutaneous PAN presents with painful subcutaneous nodules and ulcers within a red-purple, netlike pattern of livedo reticularis. The latter is due to slowed blood flow through the superficial horizontal venous plexus. The majority of lesions are found on the lower extremity, and while arthralgias and myalgias may accompany cutaneous PAN, there is no evidence of systemic involvement. In both the cutaneous and systemic forms of vasculitis, skin biopsy specimens of the associated nodules will show the changes characteristic of a vasculitis; the size of the vessel involved will depend on the particular disease.

RED-BROWN LESIONS

The cutaneous lesions in *sarcoidosis* (Chap. 329) are classically red to red-brown in color, and with diascopy (pressure with a glass slide), a yellow-brown residual color is observed that is secondary to the granulomatous infiltrate. The waxy papules and plaques may be found anywhere on the skin, but the face is the most common location. Usually there are no surface changes, but occasionally the lesions will have scale. Biopsy specimens of the papules show "naked" granulomas in the dermis, i.e., granulomas surrounded by a minimal number of lymphocytes. Other cutaneous findings in sarcoidosis include annular lesions with an atrophic or scaly center, papules within scars, hypopigmented macules and papules, alopecia, acquired ichthyosis, erythema nodosum, and lupus pernio (see below).

The differential diagnosis of sarcoidosis includes foreign-body granulomas produced by chemicals such as beryllium and zirconium, late secondary syphilis, and *lupus vulgaris*. Lupus vulgaris is a form of cutaneous tuberculosis that is seen in previously infected and sensitized individuals. There is often underlying active tuberculosis elsewhere, usually in the lungs or lymph nodes. Lesions occur primarily in the head and neck region and are red-brown plaques with a yellow-brown color on diascopy. Secondary scarring and squamous cell carcinomas can develop within the plaques. Cultures or PCR analysis of the lesions should be performed because it is rare for the acid-fast stain to show bacilli within the dermal granulomas.

Sweet's syndrome is characterized by red to red-brown plaques and nodules that are frequently painful and occur primarily on the head, neck, and upper (and, less often, lower) extremities. The patients also have fever, neutrophilia, and a dense dermal infiltrate of neutrophils in the lesions. In ~10% of the patients, there is an associated malignancy, most commonly acute myelogenous leukemia. Sweet's syndrome has also been reported with inflammatory bowel disease, systemic lupus, and solid tumors (primarily of the genitourinary tract) as well as drugs [e.g., *all-trans*-retinoic acid, granulocyte colony-stimulating factor (G-CSF)]. The differential diagnosis includes neutrophilic eccrine hidradenitis; atypical forms of pyoderma gangrenosum; and, occasionally, cellulitis. Extracutaneous sites of involvement include joints, muscles, eye, kidney (proteinuria, occasionally glomerulonephritis), and lung (neutrophilic infiltrates). The idiopathic form of Sweet's syndrome is seen more often in women, following a respiratory tract infection.

A generalized distribution of red-brown macules and papules is seen in the form of mastocytosis known as *urticaria pigmentosa* (Chap. 317). Each lesion represents a collection of mast cells in the dermis, with hyperpigmentation of the overlying epidermis. Stimuli such as rubbing cause these mast cells to degranulate, and this leads to the formation of localized urticaria (Darier's sign). Additional symptoms can result from mast cell degranulation and include headache, flushing, diarrhea, and pruritus. Mast cells also infiltrate various organs such as the liver, spleen, and gastrointestinal tract, and accumulations of mast cells in the bones may produce either osteosclerotic or osteolytic lesions on radiographs. In the majority of these patients, however, the internal involvement remains indolent. A subtype of chronic cutaneous small-vessel vasculitis, *erythema elevatum diutinum* (EED), also presents with papules that are red-brown in color. The papules coalesce into plaques on the extensor surfaces of knees, elbows, and the small joints of the hand. Flares of EED have been associated with streptococcal infections.

BLUE LESIONS

Lesions that are blue in color are the result of either vascular ectasias and tumors or melanin pigment in the dermis. *Venous lakes* (ectasias) are compressible dark-blue lesions that are found commonly in the head and neck region. *Venous malformations* are also compressible blue papulonodules and plaques that can occur anywhere on the body, including the oral mucosa. When there are multiple rather than single congenital lesions, the patient may have the blue rubber bleb syndrome or Maffucci's syndrome. Patients with the blue rubber bleb syndrome also have vascular anomalies of the gastrointestinal tract that may bleed, whereas patients with Maffucci's syndrome have associated dyschondroplasia and osteochondromas. *Blue nevi* (moles) are seen when there are collections of pigment-producing nevus cells in the dermis. These benign papular lesions are dome-shaped and occur most commonly on the dorsum of the hand or foot or in the head and neck region.

VIOLACEOUS LESIONS

Violaceous papules and plaques are seen in *lupus pernio, lymphoma cutis,* and *cutaneous lupus.* Lupus pernio is a particular type of sarcoidosis that involves the tip and alar rim of the nose as well as the earlobes, with lesions that are violaceous in color rather than red-brown. This form of sarcoidosis is associated with involvement of the upper respiratory tract. The plaques of lymphoma cutis and cutaneous lupus may be red or violaceous in color and were discussed above.

PURPLE LESIONS

Purple-colored papules and plaques are seen in vascular tumors, such as *Kaposi's sarcoma* (Chap. 189) and *angiosarcoma*, and when there is extravasation of red blood cells into the skin in association with inflammation, as in *palpable purpura* (see "Purpura," below). Patients with congenital or acquired AV fistulas and venous hypertension can develop purple papules on the lower extremities that can resemble Kaposi's sarcoma clinically and histologically; this condition is referred to as pseudo-Kaposi sarcoma (acral angiodermatitis). Angiosarcoma is found most commonly on the scalp and face of elderly patients or within areas of chronic lymphedema and presents as purple papules and plaques. In the head and neck region, the tumor often extends beyond the clinically defined borders and may be accompanied by facial edema.

BROWN AND BLACK LESIONS

Brown- and black-colored papules are reviewed in "Hyperpigmentation," above.

■ **CUTANEOUS METASTASES**

These are discussed last because they can have a wide range of colors. Most commonly, they present as either firm, skin-colored subcutaneous nodules or firm, red to red-brown papulonodules. The lesions of lymphoma cutis range from pink-red to plum in color, whereas metastatic melanoma can be pink, blue, or black in color. Cutaneous metastases develop from hematogenous or lymphatic spread and are most often due to the following primary carcinomas: in men, melanoma, oropharynx, lung, and colon; and in women, breast, melanoma, and ovary. These metastatic lesions may be the initial presentation of the carcinoma, especially when the primary site is the lung.

PURPURA

(Table 53-16) *Purpura* are seen when there is an extravasation of red blood cells into the dermis and, as a result, the lesions do not blanch with pressure. This is in contrast to those erythematous or violet-colored lesions that are due to localized vasodilatation—they do blanch with pressure. Purpura (≥3 mm) and petechiae (≤2 mm) are divided into two major groups: palpable and nonpalpable. The most frequent causes of *nonpalpable* petechiae and purpura are primary cutaneous disorders such as *trauma, solar (actinic) purpura,* and *capillaritis.* Less common causes are *steroid purpura* and *livedoid vasculopathy* (see "Ulcers," below). Solar purpura are seen primarily on the extensor forearms, while steroid purpura secondary to potent topical glucocorticoids or endogenous or exogenous Cushing's syndrome can be more widespread. In both cases, there is alteration of the supporting connective tissue that surrounds the dermal blood vessels. In contrast, the petechiae that result from capillaritis are found primarily on the lower extremities. In capillaritis, there is an extravasation of erythrocytes as a result of perivascular lymphocytic inflammation. The petechiae are bright red, 1–2 mm in size, and scattered within annular or coin-shaped yellow-brown macules. The yellow-brown color is caused by hemosiderin deposits within the dermis.

Systemic causes of nonpalpable purpura fall into several categories, and those secondary to clotting disturbances and vascular fragility will be discussed first. The former group includes *thrombocytopenia* (Chap. 115), *abnormal platelet function* as is seen in uremia, and *clotting factor defects.* The initial site of presentation for thrombocytopenia-induced petechiae is the distal lower extremity. Capillary fragility leads to nonpalpable purpura in patients with systemic *amyloidosis* (see "Papulonodular Skin Lesions," above), disorders of collagen production such as *Ehlers-Danlos syndrome,* and *scurvy.* In scurvy, there are flattened corkscrew hairs with surrounding hemorrhage on the lower extremities, in addition to gingivitis. Vitamin C is a cofactor for lysyl hydroxylase, an enzyme involved in the posttranslational modification of procollagen that is necessary for cross-link formation.

In contrast to the previous group of disorders, the purpura (noninflammatory with a retiform outline) seen in the following group of diseases are associated with thrombi formation within vessels. It is important to note that these thrombi are demonstrable in skin biopsy specimens. This group of disorders includes disseminated intravascular coagulation (DIC), monoclonal cryoglobulinemia, thrombocytosis, thrombotic thrombocytopenic purpura, antiphospholipid antibody syndrome, and reactions to warfarin and heparin (heparin-induced thrombocytopenia and thrombosis). DIC is triggered by several types of infection (gram-negative, gram-positive, viral, and rickettsial) as well as by tissue injury and neoplasms. Widespread purpura and hemorrhagic infarcts of the distal extremities are seen. Similar lesions are found in purpura fulminans, which is a form of DIC associated with fever and hypotension that occurs more commonly in children following

TABLE 53-16 Causes of Purpura

I. Primary cutaneous disorders
  A. Nonpalpable
    1. Trauma
    2. Solar (actinic, senile) purpura
    3. Steroid purpura
    4. Capillaritis
    5. Livedoid vasculopathy in the setting of venous hypertension[a]
II. Systemic diseases
  A. Nonpalpable
    1. Clotting disturbances
      a. Thrombocytopenia (including ITP)
      b. Abnormal platelet function
      c. Clotting factor defects
    2. Vascular fragility
      a. Amyloidosis
      b. Ehlers-Danlos syndrome
      c. Scurvy
    3. Thrombi
      a. Disseminated intravascular coagulation
      b. Monoclonal cryoglobulinemia
      c. Heparin-induced thrombocytopenia and thrombosis
      d. Thrombocytosis
      e. Thrombotic thrombocytopenic purpura
      f. Antiphospholipid antibody syndrome
      g. Warfarin reaction
      h. Homozygous protein C or protein S deficiency
    4. Emboli
      a. Cholesterol
      b. Fat
    5. Possible immune complex
      a. Gardner-Diamond syndrome (autoerythrocyte sensitivity)
      b. Waldenström's hypergammaglobulinemic purpura
  B. Palpable
    1. Vasculitis
      a. Cutaneous small-vessel vasculitis
      b. Polyarteritis nodosa
    2. Emboli[b]
      a. Acute meningococcemia
      b. Disseminated gonococcal infection
      c. Rocky Mountain spotted fever
      d. Ecthyma gangrenosum

[a]Also associated with underlying disorders that lead to hypercoagulability, e.g. factor V Leiden, protein C dysfunction/deficiency.

[b]Bacterial, fungal, or parasitic.

Abbreviation: ITP, idiopathic thrombocytopenic purpura.

an infectious illness such as varicella, scarlet fever, or an upper respiratory tract infection. In both disorders, hemorrhagic bullae can develop in involved skin.

Monoclonal cryoglobulinemia is associated with multiple myeloma, Waldenström's macroglobulinemia, chronic lymphocytic leukemia, and lymphoma. Purpura, primarily of the lower extremities, and hemorrhagic infarcts of the fingers and toes are seen in these patients. Exacerbations of disease activity can follow cold exposure or an increase in serum viscosity. Biopsy specimens show precipitates of the cryoglobulin within dermal vessels. Similar deposits have been found in the lung, brain, and renal glomeruli. Patients with *thrombotic thrombocytopenic purpura* can also have hemorrhagic infarcts as a result of intravascular thromboses. Additional signs include thrombocytopenic purpura, fever, and microangiopathic hemolytic anemia.

Administration of *warfarin* can result in painful areas of erythema that become purpuric and then necrotic with an adherent black eschar; the condition is referred to as warfarin-induced necrosis. This reaction is seen more often in women and in areas with abundant subcutaneous fat—breasts, abdomen, buttocks, thighs, and calves. The erythema and purpura develop between the third and tenth day of therapy, most likely as a result of a transient imbalance in the levels of anticoagulant and procoagulant vitamin K–dependent factors. Continued therapy does not exacerbate preexisting lesions, and patients with an inherited or acquired deficiency of protein C are at increased risk for this particular reaction as well as for purpura fulminans.

Purpura secondary to *cholesterol emboli* are usually seen on the lower extremities of patients with atherosclerotic vascular disease. They often follow anticoagulant therapy or an invasive vascular procedure such as an arteriogram but also occur spontaneously from disintegration of atheromatous plaques. Associated findings include livedo reticularis, gangrene, cyanosis, and ischemic ulcerations. Multiple step sections of the biopsy specimen may be necessary to demonstrate the cholesterol clefts within the vessels. Petechiae are also an important sign of *fat embolism* and occur primarily on the upper body 2–3 days after a major injury. By using special fixatives, the emboli can be demonstrated in biopsy specimens of the petechiae. Emboli of tumor or thrombus are seen in patients with atrial myxomas and marantic endocarditis.

In the *Gardner-Diamond syndrome* (autoerythrocyte sensitivity), female patients develop large ecchymoses within areas of painful, warm erythema. Intradermal injections of autologous erythrocytes or phosphatidyl serine derived from the red cell membrane can reproduce the lesions in some patients; however, there are instances where a reaction is seen at an injection site of the forearm but not in the midback region. The latter has led some observers to view Gardner-Diamond syndrome as a cutaneous manifestation of severe emotional stress. More recently, the possibility of platelet dysfunction (as assessed via aggregation studies) has been raised. *Waldenström's hypergammaglobulinemic purpura* is a chronic disorder characterized by petechiae on the lower extremities. There are circulating complexes of IgG–anti-IgG molecules, and exacerbations are associated with prolonged standing or walking.

Palpable purpura are further subdivided into vasculitic and embolic. In the group of vasculitic disorders, cutaneous small-vessel vasculitis, also known as *leukocytoclastic vasculitis* (LCV), is the one most commonly associated with palpable purpura (Chap. 326). Underlying etiologies include drugs (e.g., antibiotics), infections (e.g., hepatitis C virus), and autoimmune connective tissue diseases (e.g. rheumatoid arthritis, Sjögren syndrome, lupus). *Henoch-Schönlein purpura* (HSP) is a subtype of acute LCV that is seen primarily in children and adolescents following an upper respiratory infection. The majority of lesions are found on the lower extremities and buttocks. Systemic manifestations include fever, arthralgias (primarily of the knees and ankles), abdominal pain, gastrointestinal bleeding, and nephritis. Direct immunofluorescence examination shows deposits of IgA within dermal blood vessel walls. Renal disease is of particular concern in adults with HSP. In *polyarteritis nodosa*, specific cutaneous lesions result from a vasculitis of arterial vessels (arteritis) or there may be an associated LCV. Arteritis leads to an infarct of the skin, and this explains the irregular outline of the purpura (see below).

Several types of infectious emboli can give rise to palpable purpura. These embolic lesions are usually *irregular* in outline as opposed to the lesions of LCV, which are *circular* in outline. The irregular outline is indicative of a cutaneous infarct, and the size corresponds to the area of skin that received its blood supply from that particular arteriole or artery. The palpable purpura in LCV are circular because the erythrocytes simply diffuse out evenly from the postcapillary venules as a result of inflammation. Infectious emboli are most commonly due to gram-negative cocci (meningococcus, gonococcus), gram-negative rods (Enterobacteriaceae), and gram-positive cocci (*Staphylococcus*). Additional causes include *Rickettsia* and, in immunocompromised patients, *Candida* and other opportunistic fungi.

The embolic lesions in *acute meningococcemia* are found primarily on the trunk, lower extremities, and sites of pressure, and a gunmetal-gray color often develops within them. Their size varies from a few millimeters to several centimeters, and the organisms can be cultured from the lesions. Associated findings include a preceding upper respiratory tract infection; fever; meningitis; DIC; and, in some patients, a deficiency of the terminal components of complement. In *disseminated gonococcal infection* (arthritis-dermatitis syndrome), a small number of papules and vesicopustules with central purpura or hemorrhagic necrosis are found on the distal extremities. Additional symptoms include arthralgias, tenosynovitis, and fever. To establish the diagnosis, a Gram stain of these lesions should be performed. *Rocky Mountain spotted fever* is a tick-borne disease that is caused by *R. rickettsii*. A several-day history of fever, chills, severe headache, and photophobia precedes the onset of the cutaneous eruption. The initial lesions are erythematous macules and papules on the wrists, ankles, palms, and soles. With time, the lesions spread centripetally and become purpuric.

Lesions of *ecthyma gangrenosum* begin as edematous, erythematous papules or plaques and then develop central purpura and necrosis. Bullae formation also occurs in these lesions, and they are frequently found in the girdle region. The organism that is classically associated with ecthyma gangrenosum is *Pseudomonas aeruginosa*, but other gram-negative rods such as *Klebsiella*, *Escherichia coli*, and *Serratia* can produce similar lesions. In immunocompromised hosts, the list of potential pathogens is expanded to include *Candida* and other opportunistic fungi (e.g., *Aspergillus*, *Fusarium*).

ULCERS

The approach to the patient with a cutaneous ulcer is outlined in Table 53-17. Peripheral vascular diseases of the extremities are reviewed in Chap. 249, as is Raynaud's phenomenon.

Livedoid vasculopathy (livedoid vasculitis; atrophie blanche) represents a combination of a vasculopathy plus intravascular thrombosis. Purpuric lesions and livedo reticularis are found in association with *painful* ulcerations of the lower extremities. These ulcers are often slow to heal, but when they do, irregularly shaped white scars form. The majority of cases are secondary to venous hypertension, but possible underlying illnesses include cryofibrinogenemia and disorders of hypercoagulability, e.g., the antiphospholipid antibody syndrome (Chaps. 117 and 320).

In *pyoderma gangrenosum*, the border of untreated ulcers has a characteristic appearance consisting of an undermined necrotic violaceous edge and a peripheral erythematous halo. The ulcers often begin as pustules that then expand rather rapidly to a size as large as 20 cm. Although these lesions are most commonly found on the lower extremities, they can arise anywhere on the surface of the body, including sites of trauma (pathergy). An estimated 30–50% of cases are idiopathic, and the most common associated disorders are ulcerative colitis and Crohn's disease. Less commonly, pyoderma

TABLE 53-17 Causes of Mucocutaneous Ulcers

I. Primary cutaneous disorders
  A. Peripheral vascular disease (Chap. 249)
    1. Venous
    2. Arterial[a]
  B. Livedoid vasculopathy in the setting of venous hypertension[b]
  C. Squamous cell carcinoma, e.g., within scars, basal cell carcinomas
  D. Infections, e.g., ecthyma caused by *Streptococcus* (Chap. 136)
  E. Physical, e.g., trauma, pressure
  F. Drugs, e.g., hydroxyurea
II. Systemic diseases
  A. Lower legs
    1. Small-vessel and medium-vessel vasculitis[c]
    2. Hemoglobinopathies (Chap. 104)
    3. Cryoglobulinemia,[c] cryofibrinogenemia
    4. Cholesterol emboli[c]
    5. Necrobiosis lipoidica[d]
    6. Antiphospholipid syndrome (Chap. 116)
    7. Neuropathic[e] (Chap. 344)
    8. Panniculitis
    9. Kaposi's sarcoma, acral angiodermatitis
  B. Hands and feet
    1. Raynaud's phenomenon (Chap. 249)
    2. Buerger disease
  C. Generalized
    1. Pyoderma gangrenosum, but most commonly legs
    2. Calciphylaxis (Chap. 353)
    3. Infections, e.g., dimorphic fungi, leishmaniasis
    4. Lymphoma
  D. Face, especially perioral, and anogenital
    1. Chronic herpes simplex[f]
III. Mucosal
  A. Behçet's syndrome (Chap. 327)
  B. Erythema multiforme major, Stevens-Johnson syndrome, TEN
  C. Primary blistering disorders (Chap. 54)
  D. Lupus erythematosus, lichen planus
  E. Inflammatory bowel disease
  F. Acute HIV infection
  G. Reactive arthritis (formerly known as Reiter's syndrome)

[a]Underlying atherosclerosis.

[b]Also associated with underlying disorders that lead to hypercoagulability, e.g., factor V Leiden, protein C dysfunction/deficiency, anti-phospholipid antibodies.

[c]Reviewed in section on Purpura.

[d]Reviewed in section on Papulonodular Skin Lesions.

[e]Favors plantar surface of the foot.

[f]Sign of immunosuppression.

Abbreviation: TEN, toxic epidermal necrolysis.

gangrenosum is associated with seropositive rheumatoid arthritis, acute and chronic myelogenous leukemia, hairy cell leukemia, and myelofibrosis. Additional findings in these patients, even those with idiopathic disease, are cutaneous anergy and a monoclonal gammopathy, usually IgA. Because the histology of pyoderma gangrenosum may be nonspecific (dermal infiltrate of neutrophils when in untreated state), the diagnosis requires clinicopathologic correlation, in particular, the exclusion of similar-appearing ulcers such as necrotizing vasculitis, Meleney's ulcer (synergistic infection at a site of trauma or surgery), dimorphic fungi, cutaneous amebiasis, spider bites, and factitial. In the myeloproliferative disorders, the ulcers may be more superficial with a pustulobullous border, and these lesions provide a connection between classic pyoderma gangrenosum and acute febrile neutrophilic dermatosis (Sweet's syndrome).

FEVER AND RASH

The major considerations in a patient with a fever and a rash are inflammatory diseases versus infectious diseases. In the hospital setting, the most common scenario is a patient who has a drug rash plus a fever secondary to an underlying infection. However, it should be emphasized that a drug reaction can lead to both a cutaneous eruption and a fever ("drug fever"), especially in the setting of DRESS or AGEP. Additional inflammatory diseases that are often associated with a fever include pustular psoriasis, erythroderma, and Sweet's syndrome. Lyme disease, secondary syphilis, and viral and bacterial exanthems (see "Exanthems," above) are examples of infectious diseases that produce a rash and a fever. Lastly, it is important to determine whether or not the cutaneous lesions represent septic emboli (see "Purpura," above). Such lesions usually have evidence of ischemia in the form of purpura, necrosis, or impending necrosis (gunmetal-gray color). In the patient with thrombocytopenia, however, purpura can be seen in inflammatory reactions such as morbilliform drug eruptions and infectious lesions.

FURTHER READINGS

Bolognia JL et al: *Dermatology*, 2nd ed. Philadelphia, Mosby, 2008

Braverman IM: *Skin Signs of Systemic Disease*, 3rd ed. Philadelphia, Saunders, 1998

Callen JP et al: *Dermatological Signs of Internal Disease*, 4th ed. Philadelphia, Saunders, 2009

Mckee PH et al: *Pathology of the Skin*, 3rd ed. London, Elsevier, 2005

Spitz JL: *Genodermatoses: A Clinical Guide to Genetic Skin Disorders*, 2nd ed. Philadelphia, Lippincott Williams & Wilkins, 2004

CHAPTER 54

Immunologically Mediated Skin Diseases

Kim B. Yancey

Thomas J. Lawley

A number of immunologically mediated skin diseases and immunologically mediated systemic disorders with cutaneous manifestations are now recognized as distinct entities with consistent clinical, histologic, and immunopathologic findings. Clinically, these disorders are characterized by morbidity (pain, pruritus, disfigurement) and, in some instances, by mortality (largely due to loss of epidermal barrier function and/or secondary infection). The major features of the more common immunologically mediated skin diseases are summarized in this chapter (Table 54-1) as are the systemic disorders with cutaneous manifestations.

AUTOIMMUNE CUTANEOUS DISEASES

■ PEMPHIGUS VULGARIS

Pemphigus refers to a group of autoantibody-mediated intraepidermal blistering diseases characterized by loss of cohesion between epidermal cells (a process termed *acantholysis*). Manual pressure to the skin of these patients may elicit the separation of the epidermis (Nikolsky's sign). This finding, while characteristic of pemphigus, is not specific to this group of disorders and is also seen in toxic epidermal necrolysis, Stevens-Johnson syndrome, and a few other skin diseases.

Pemphigus vulgaris (PV) is a mucocutaneous blistering disease that predominates in patients >40 years. PV typically begins on mucosal surfaces and often progresses to involve the skin. PV is characterized by fragile, flaccid blisters that rupture to produce extensive denudation of mucous membranes and skin (Fig. 54-1). PV typically involves the mouth, scalp, face, neck, axilla, groin, and trunk. PV may be associated with severe skin pain; some patients

TABLE 54-1 Immunologically Mediated Blistering Diseases

Disease	Clinical	Histology	Immunopathology	Autoantigens[a]
Pemphigus foliaceus	Crusts and shallow erosions on scalp, central face, upper chest, and back	Acantholytic blister formed in superficial layer of epidermis	Cell surface deposits of IgG on keratinocytes	Dsg1
Pemphigus vulgaris	Flaccid blisters, denuded skin, oromucosal lesions	Acantholytic blister formed in suprabasal layer of epidermis	Cell surface deposits of IgG on keratinocytes	Dsg3 (plus Dsg1 in patients with skin involvement)
Paraneoplastic pemphigus	Painful stomatitis with papulosquamous or lichenoid eruptions that progress to blisters	Acantholysis, keratinocyte necrosis and vacuolar interface dermatitis	Cell surface deposits of IgG and C3 on keratinocytes and (variably) similar immunoreactants in epidermal BMZ	Plakin protein family members and desmosomal cadherins (see text for details)
Bullous pemphigoid	Large tense blisters on flexor surfaces and trunk	Subepidermal blister with eosinophil-rich infiltrate	Linear band of IgG and/or C3 in epidermal BMZ	BPAG1, BPAG2
Pemphigoid gestationis	Pruritic, urticarial plaques, rimmed by vesicles and bullae on the trunk and extremities	Teardrop-shaped, subepidermal blisters in dermal papillae; eosinophil-rich infiltrate	Linear band of C3 in epidermal BMZ	BPAG2 (plus BPAG1 in some patients)
Linear IgA disease	Pruritic small papules on extensor surfaces; occasionally larger, arciform blisters	Subepidermal blister with neutrophil-rich infiltrate	Linear band of IgA in epidermal BMZ	BPAG2 (see text for specific details)
Cicatricial pemphigoid	Erosive and/or blistering lesions of mucous membranes and possibly the skin; scarring of some sites	Subepidermal blister that may or may not include a leukocytic infiltrate	Linear band of IgG, IgA, and/or C3 in epidermal BMZ	BPAG2, laminin-332, or others
Epidermolysis bullosa acquisita	Blisters, erosions, scars, and milia on sites exposed to trauma; widespread, inflammatory, tense blisters may be seen initially	Subepidermal blister that may or may not include a leukocytic infiltrate	Linear band of IgG and/or C3 in epidermal BMZ	Type VII collagen
Dermatitis herpetiformis	Extremely pruritic small papules and vesicles on elbows, knees, buttocks, and posterior neck	Subepidermal blister with neutrophils in dermal papillae	Granular deposits of IgA in dermal papillae	Epidermal transglutaminase

[a]Autoantigens bound by these patients' autoantibodies are defined as follows: Dsg1, desmoglein 1; Dsg3, desmoglein 3; BPAG1, bullous pemphigoid antigen 1; BPAG2, bullous pemphigoid antigen 2.

Abbreviation: BMZ, basement membrane zone.

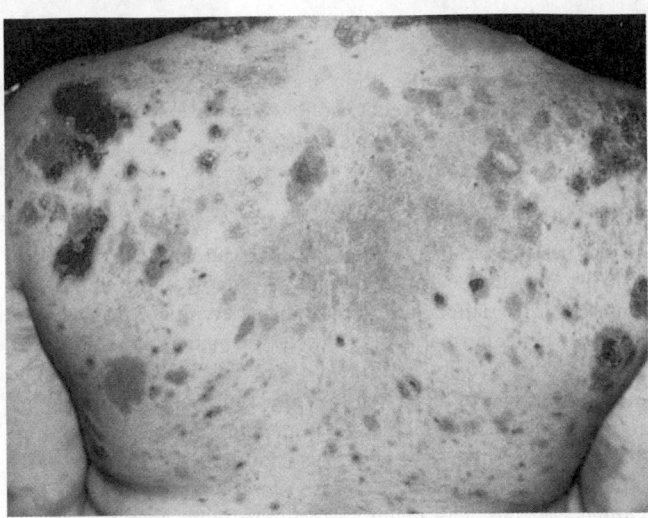

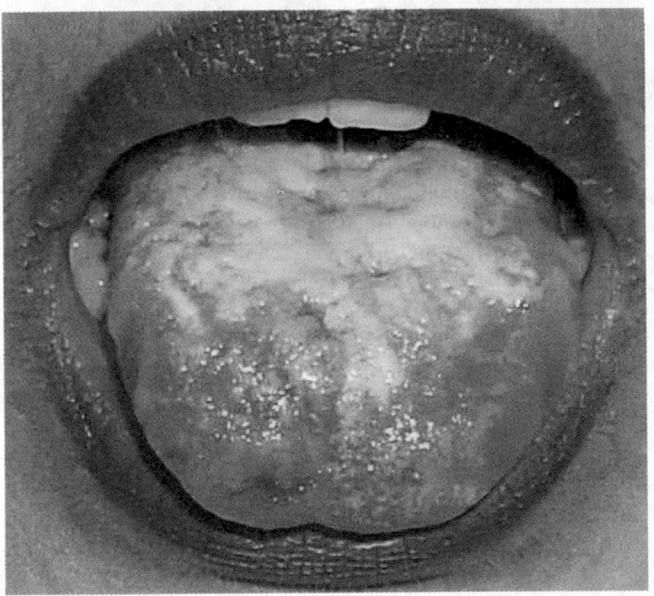

Figure 54-1 Pemphigus vulgaris. *A.* Pemphigus vulgaris demonstrating flaccid bullae that are easily ruptured, resulting in multiple erosions and crusted plaques. ***B.*** Pemphigus vulgaris almost invariably involves the oral mucosa and may present with erosions involving the gingiva, buccal mucosa, palate, posterior pharynx, or the tongue. (***B,*** *Courtesy of Robert Swerlick, MD; with permission.)*

microscopy of lesional or intact patient skin shows deposits of IgG on the surface of keratinocytes; deposits of complement components are typically found in lesional but not uninvolved skin. Deposits of IgG on keratinocytes are derived from circulating autoantibodies directed against cell-surface autoantigens. Such circulating autoantibodies can be demonstrated in 80–90% of PV patients by indirect immunofluorescence microscopy; monkey esophagus is the optimal substrate for these studies. Patients with PV have IgG autoantibodies directed against *desmogleins* (Dsgs), transmembrane desmosomal glycoproteins that belong to the cadherin family of calcium-dependent adhesion molecules. Such autoantibodies can be precisely quantitated by enzyme-linked immunosorbent assay (ELISA). Patients with early PV (i.e., mucosal disease) have IgG autoantibodies directed against Dsg3; patients with advanced PV (i.e., mucocutaneous disease) have IgG autoantibodies directed against both Dsg3 and Dsg1. Experimental studies have shown that autoantibodies from patients with PV are pathogenic (i.e., responsible for blister formation) and that their titer correlates with disease activity. Recent studies have shown that the anti-Dsg autoantibody profile in these patients' sera as well as the tissue distribution of Dsg3 and Dsg1 determine the site of blister formation in patients with pemphigus. Coexpression of Dsg3 and Dsg1 by epidermal cells protects against pathogenic IgG directed against either cadherin but not pathogenic autoantibodies directed against both.

PV can be life threatening. Prior to the availability of glucocorticoids, the mortality ranged from 60–90%; the current mortality is ~5%. Common causes of morbidity and mortality are infection and complications of treatment with glucocorticoids. Bad prognostic factors include advanced age, widespread involvement, and the requirement for high doses of glucocorticoids (with or without other immunosuppressive agents) for control of disease. The course of PV in individual patients is variable and difficult to predict. Some patients achieve remission, while others may require long-term treatment or succumb to complications of their disease or its treatment. The mainstay of treatment is systemic glucocorticoids. Patients with moderate to severe PV are usually started on prednisone, 1 mg/kg per day. If new lesions continue to appear after 1–2 weeks of treatment, the dose may need to be increased and/or combined with other immunosuppressive agents such as azathioprine (2–2.5 mg/kg per d), mycophenolate mofetil (20–35 mg/kg per d), or cyclophosphamide (1–2 mg/kg per d). Patients with severe, treatment-resistant disease may derive benefit from plasmapheresis [six high-volume exchanges (i.e., 2–3 L per exchange) over ~2 weeks], IV immunoglobulin (IVIg) (2 g/kg over 3–5 days every 6–8 weeks), or rituximab (375 mg/m^2 per week × 4, or 1,000 mg on days 1 and 15). It is important to bring severe or progressive disease under control quickly to lessen the severity and/or duration of this disorder. Accordingly, some have suggested that rituximab and daily glucocorticoids should be used early in PV patients to avert the development of treatment-resistant disease.

■ PEMPHIGUS FOLIACEUS

Pemphigus foliaceus (PF) is distinguished from PV by several features. In PF, acantholytic blisters are located high within the epidermis, usually just beneath the stratum corneum. Hence, PF is a more superficial blistering disease than PV. The distribution of lesions in the two disorders is much the same, except that in PF, mucous membranes are almost always spared. Patients with PF rarely demonstrate intact blisters but rather exhibit shallow erosions associated with erythema, scale, and crust formation. Mild cases of PF resemble severe seborrheic dermatitis; severe PF may cause extensive exfoliation. Sun exposure (ultraviolet irradiation) may be an aggravating factor. *Fogo selvagem* (FS), an endemic form of PF thought to develop as a consequence of environmental stimuli

experience pruritus as well. Lesions usually heal without scarring, except at sites complicated by secondary infection or mechanically induced dermal wounds. Postinflammatory hyperpigmentation is usually present at sites of healed lesions for some time.

Biopsies of early lesions demonstrate intraepidermal vesicle formation secondary to loss of cohesion between epidermal cells (i.e., acantholytic blisters). Blister cavities contain acantholytic epidermal cells, which appear as round homogeneous cells containing hyperchromatic nuclei. Basal keratinocytes remain attached to the epidermal basement membrane; hence, blister formation is within the suprabasal portion of the epidermis. Lesional skin may contain focal collections of intraepidermal eosinophils within blister cavities; dermal alterations are slight, often limited to an eosinophil-predominant leukocytic infiltrate. Direct immunofluorescence (e.g., insect bites), is found in south central rural Brazil as well as selected sites in Latin America and Tunisia.

Patients with PF have immunopathologic features in common with PV. Specifically, direct immunofluorescence microscopy of perilesional skin demonstrates IgG on the surface of keratinocytes. Similarly, patients with PF have circulating IgG autoantibodies directed against the surface of keratinocytes. In PF, autoantibodies are directed against Dsg1, a 160-kDa desmosomal cadherin. These autoantibodies can be quantitated by ELISA. As noted for PV, the autoantibody profile in patients with PF (i.e., anti-Dsg1 IgG) and the tissue distribution of this autoantigen (i.e., expression in oral mucosa that is compensated by coexpression of Dsg3) are thought to account for the distribution of lesions in this disease.

Although pemphigus has been associated with several autoimmune diseases, its association with thymoma and/or myasthenia gravis is particularly notable. To date, >30 cases of thymoma and/or myasthenia gravis have been reported in association with pemphigus, usually with PF. Patients may also develop pemphigus as a consequence of drug exposure; drug-induced pemphigus usually resembles PF rather than PV. Drugs containing a thiol group in their chemical structure (e.g., penicillamine, captopril, enalapril) are most commonly associated with drug-induced pemphigus. Nonthiol drugs linked to pemphigus include penicillins, cephalosporins, and piroxicam. It has been suggested that thiol- and nonthiol-containing drugs induce pemphigus via biochemical and immunologic mechanisms, respectively. Hence, the better prognosis upon drug withdrawal in cases of pemphigus induced by thiol-containing medications. Some cases of drug-induced pemphigus are durable and require treatment with systemic glucocorticoids and/or immunosuppressive agents.

PF is generally a less severe disease than PV and carries a better prognosis. Localized disease can sometimes be treated with topical or intralesional glucocorticoids; more active cases can usually be controlled with systemic glucocorticoids. Patients with severe, treatment-resistant disease may require more aggressive interventions as described above for patients with PV.

■ PARANEOPLASTIC PEMPHIGUS

Paraneoplastic pemphigus (PNP) is an autoimmune acantholytic mucocutaneous disease associated with an occult or confirmed neoplasm. Patients with PNP typically show painful mucosal erosive lesions in association with papulosquamous and/or lichenoid eruptions that often progress to blisters. Palm and sole involvement are common in these patients and raise the possibility that prior reports of neoplasia-associated erythema multiforme actually may have represented unrecognized cases of PNP. Biopsies of lesional skin from these patients show varying combinations of acantholysis, keratinocyte necrosis, and vacuolar-interface dermatitis. Direct immunofluorescence microscopy of patient's skin shows deposits of IgG and complement on the surface of keratinocytes and (variably) similar immunoreactants in the epidermal basement membrane zone. Patients with PNP have IgG autoantibodies against cytoplasmic proteins that are members of the plakin family (e.g., desmoplakins I and II, bullous pemphigoid antigen 1, envoplakin, periplakin, and plectin) and cell-surface proteins that are members of the cadherin family (e.g., Dsg1 and Dsg3). Passive transfer studies have shown that autoantibodies from patients with PNP are pathogenic.

The predominant neoplasms associated with PNP are non-Hodgkin's lymphoma, chronic lymphocytic leukemia, thymoma, spindle cell tumors, Waldenström's macroglobulinemia, and Castleman's disease; the latter is particularly common among children with PNP. Rare cases of seronegative PNP have been reported in patients with B cell malignancies previously treated with rituximab. In addition to severe skin lesions, many patients with PNP develop life-threatening bronchiolitis obliterans. PNP is generally resistant to conventional therapies (i.e., those used to treat PV); rarely patients may improve (or even remit) following ablation or removal of underlying neoplasms.

■ BULLOUS PEMPHIGOID

Bullous pemphigoid (BP) is a polymorphic autoimmune subepidermal blistering disease usually seen in the elderly. Initial lesions may consist of urticarial plaques; most patients eventually display tense blisters on either normal-appearing or erythematous skin (Fig. 54-2). The lesions are usually distributed over the lower abdomen, groin, and flexor surface of the extremities; oral mucosal lesions are found in some patients. Pruritus may be nonexistent or severe. As lesions evolve, tense blisters tend to rupture and be replaced by erosions with or without surmounting crust. Nontraumatized blisters heal without scarring. The major histocompatibility complex class II allele HLA-DQβ1*0301 is prevalent in patients with BP. Despite isolated reports, several studies have shown that patients with BP do not have an increased incidence of malignancy in comparison with appropriately age- and gender-matched controls.

Biopsies of early lesional skin demonstrate subepidermal blisters and histologic features that roughly correlate with the clinical character of the particular lesion under study. Lesions on normal-appearing skin generally show a sparse perivascular leukocytic infiltrate with some eosinophils; conversely, biopsies of inflammatory lesions typically show an eosinophil-rich infiltrate at sites of vesicle formation and in perivascular areas. In addition to eosinophils, cell-rich lesions also contain mononuclear cells and neutrophils. It is not possible to distinguish BP from other subepidermal blistering diseases by routine histologic studies alone.

Direct immunofluorescence microscopy of normal-appearing perilesional skin from patients with BP shows linear deposits of IgG and/or C3 in the epidermal basement membrane. The sera of ~70% of these patients contain circulating IgG autoantibodies that bind the epidermal basement membrane of normal human skin in indirect immunofluorescence microscopy. IgG from an even higher

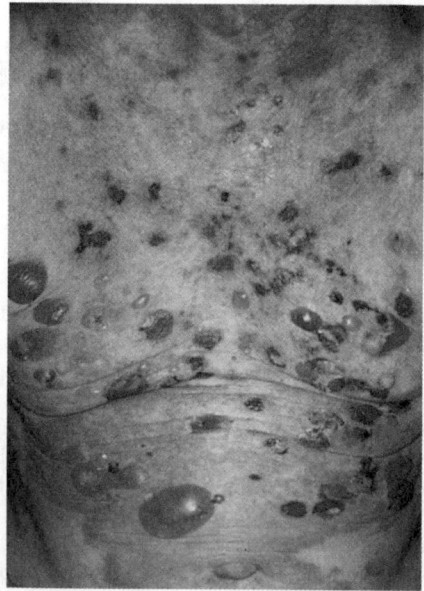

Figure 54-2 Bullous pemphigoid with tense vesicles and bullae on erythematous, urticarial bases. *(Courtesy of the Yale Resident's Slide Collection; with permission).*

percentage of patients shows reactivity to the epidermal side of 1 *M* NaCl split skin [an alternative immunofluorescence microscopy test substrate used to distinguish circulating IgG anti-basement membrane autoantibodies in patients with BP from those in patients with similar, yet different, subepidermal blistering diseases (see below)]. In BP, circulating autoantibodies recognize 230- and 180-kDa hemidesmosome-associated proteins in basal keratinocytes [i.e., bullous pemphigoid antigen (BPAG)1 and BPAG2, respectively]. Autoantibodies against BPAG2 are thought to deposit in situ, activate complement, produce dermal mast cell degranulation, and generate granulocyte-rich infiltrates that cause tissue damage and blister formation.

BP may persist for months to years, with exacerbations or remissions. Extensive involvement may result in widespread erosions and compromise cutaneous integrity; deaths may occur in elderly and/or debilitated patients. The mainstay of treatment is systemic glucocorticoids. Patients with local or minimal disease can sometimes be controlled with topical glucocorticoids alone; patients with more extensive lesions generally respond to systemic glucocorticoids either alone or in combination with immunosuppressive agents. Patients will usually respond to prednisone, 0.75–1 mg/kg per d. In some instances, azathioprine (2–2.5 mg/kg per d), mycophenolate mofetil (20–35 mg/kg per d), or cyclophosphamide (1–2 mg/kg per d) are necessary adjuncts.

■ PEMPHIGOID GESTATIONIS

Pemphigoid gestationis (PG), also known as *herpes gestationis*, is a rare, nonviral, subepidermal blistering disease of pregnancy and the puerperium. PG may begin during any trimester of pregnancy or present shortly after delivery. Lesions are usually distributed over the abdomen, trunk, and extremities; mucous membrane lesions are rare. Skin lesions in these patients may be quite polymorphic and consist of erythematous urticarial papules and plaques, vesiculopapules, and/or frank bullae. Lesions are almost always very pruritic. Severe exacerbations of PG frequently occur after delivery, typically within 24–48 hours. PG tends to recur in subsequent pregnancies, often beginning earlier during such gestations. Brief flare-ups of disease may occur with resumption of menses and may develop in patients later exposed to oral contraceptives. Occasionally, infants of affected mothers demonstrate transient skin lesions.

Biopsies of early lesional skin show teardrop-shaped subepidermal vesicles forming in dermal papillae in association with an eosinophil-rich leukocytic infiltrate. Differentiation of PG from other subepidermal bullous diseases by light microscopy is difficult. However, direct immunofluorescence microscopy of perilesional skin from PG patients reveals the immunopathologic hallmark of this disorder—linear deposits of C3 in epidermal basement membrane. These deposits develop as a consequence of complement activation produced by low titer IgG anti-basement membrane autoantibodies directed against BPAG2, the same hemidesmosome-associated protein that is targeted by autoantibodies in patients with BP—a subepidermal bullous disease that resembles PG clinically, histologically, and immunopathologically.

The goals of therapy in patients with PG are to prevent the development of new lesions, relieve intense pruritus, and care for erosions at sites of blister formation. Many patients require treatment with moderate doses of daily glucocorticoids (i.e., 20–40 mg prednisone) at some point in their course. Mild cases (or brief flare-ups) may be controlled by vigorous use of potent topical glucocorticoids. Infants born of mothers with PG appear to be at increased risk of being slightly premature or "small for dates." Current evidence suggests that there is no difference in the incidence of uncomplicated live births in PG patients treated with systemic glucocorticoids and in those managed more conservatively. If systemic glucocorticoids are administered, newborns are at risk for development of reversible adrenal insufficiency.

■ DERMATITIS HERPETIFORMIS

Dermatitis herpetiformis (DH) is an intensely pruritic, papulovesicular skin disease characterized by lesions symmetrically distributed over extensor surfaces (i.e., elbows, knees, buttocks, back, scalp, and posterior neck) (see Fig. 51-8). Primary lesions in this disorder consist of papules, papulovesicles, or urticarial plaques. Because pruritus is prominent, patients may present with excoriations and crusted papules but no observable primary lesions. Patients sometimes report that their pruritus has a distinctive burning or stinging component; the onset of such local symptoms reliably heralds the development of distinct clinical lesions 12–24 hours later. Almost all DH patients have an associated, usually subclinical, gluten-sensitive enteropathy (Chap. 294), and >90% express the HLA-B8/DRw3 and HLA-DQw2 haplotypes. DH may present at any age, including childhood; onset in the second to fourth decades is most common. The disease is typically chronic.

Biopsy of early lesional skin reveals neutrophil-rich infiltrates within dermal papillae. Neutrophils, fibrin, edema, and microvesicle formation at these sites are characteristic of early disease. Older lesions may demonstrate nonspecific features of a subepidermal bulla or an excoriated papule. Because the clinical and histologic features of this disease can be variable and resemble other subepidermal blistering disorders, the diagnosis is confirmed by direct immunofluorescence microscopy of normal-appearing perilesional skin. Such studies demonstrate granular deposits of IgA (with or without complement components) in the papillary dermis and along the epidermal basement membrane zone. IgA deposits in the skin are unaffected by control of disease with medication; however, these immunoreactants diminish in intensity or disappear in patients maintained for long periods on a strict gluten-free diet (see below). Patients with DH have granular deposits of IgA in their epidermal basement membrane zone and should be distinguished from individuals with linear IgA deposits at this site (see below).

Although most DH patients do not report overt gastrointestinal symptoms or have laboratory evidence of malabsorption, biopsies of the small bowel usually reveal blunting of intestinal villi and a lymphocytic infiltrate in the lamina propria. As is true for patients with celiac disease, this gastrointestinal abnormality can be reversed by a gluten-free diet. Moreover, if maintained, this diet alone may control the skin disease and eventuate in clearance of IgA deposits from these patients' epidermal basement membrane zones. Subsequent gluten exposure in such patients alters the morphology of their small bowel, elicits a flare-up of their skin disease, and is associated with the reappearance of IgA in their epidermal basement membrane zones. As in patients with celiac disease, dietary gluten sensitivity in patients with DH is associated with IgA antiendomysial autoantibodies that target tissue transglutaminase. Recent studies indicate that patients with DH also have high-avidity IgA autoantibodies against epidermal transglutaminase 3 and that the latter is co-localized with granular deposits of IgA in the papillary dermis of DH patients. Patients with DH also have an increased incidence of thyroid abnormalities, achlorhydria, atrophic gastritis, and anti-gastric parietal cell autoantibodies. These associations likely relate to the high frequency of the HLA-B8/DRw3 haplotype in these patients, because this marker is commonly linked to autoimmune disorders. The mainstay of treatment of DH is dapsone, a sulfone. Patients respond rapidly (24–48 hours) to dapsone (50–200 mg/d), but require careful pretreatment evaluation and close follow-up to ensure that complications are avoided or controlled. All patients on >100 mg/d dapsone will have some hemolysis and methemoglobinemia, which are expected pharmacologic side effects of this agent. Gluten restriction can control DH and lessen dapsone requirements; this diet must rigidly exclude gluten to be of maximal benefit. Many months of dietary restriction may be necessary before a beneficial result is achieved. Good dietary counseling by a trained dietitian is essential.

■ LINEAR IgA DISEASE

Linear IgA disease, once considered a variant form of dermatitis herpetiformis, is actually a separate and distinct entity. Clinically, these patients may resemble individuals with DH, BP, or other subepidermal blistering diseases. Lesions typically consist of papulovesicles, bullae, and/or urticarial plaques predominantly on central or flexural sites. Oral mucosal involvement occurs in some patients. Severe pruritus resembles that seen in patients with DH. Patients with linear IgA disease do not have an increased frequency of the HLA-B8/DRw3 haplotype or an associated enteropathy and, hence, are not candidates for treatment with a gluten-free diet.

Histologic alterations in early lesions may be virtually indistinguishable from those in DH. However, direct immunofluorescence microscopy of normal-appearing perilesional skin reveals linear deposits of IgA (and often C3) in the epidermal basement membrane zone. Most patients with linear IgA disease demonstrate circulating IgA anti-basement membrane autoantibodies directed against neoepitopes in the proteolytically processed extracellular domain of BPAG2. These patients generally respond to treatment with dapsone, 50–200 mg/d.

■ EPIDERMOLYSIS BULLOSA ACQUISITA

Epidermolysis bullosa acquisita (EBA) is a rare, noninherited, polymorphic, chronic, subepidermal blistering disease. (The inherited form is discussed in Chap. 363.) Patients with classic or noninflammatory EBA have blisters on noninflamed skin, atrophic scars, milia, nail dystrophy, and oral lesions. Because lesions generally occur at sites exposed to minor trauma, classic EBA is considered to be a mechanobullous disease. Other patients with EBA have widespread inflammatory scarring and bullous lesions that resemble severe BP. Inflammatory EBA may evolve into the classic, noninflammatory form of this disease. Rarely patients present with lesions that predominate on mucous membranes. The HLA-DR2 haplotype is found with increased frequency in EBA patients. Recent studies suggest that EBA is sometimes associated with inflammatory bowel disease (especially Crohn's disease).

The histology of lesional skin varies depending on the character of the lesion being studied. Noninflammatory bullae show subepidermal blisters with a sparse leukocytic infiltrate and resemble those in patients with porphyria cutanea tarda. Inflammatory lesions consist of neutrophil-rich subepidermal blisters. EBA patients have continuous deposits of IgG (and frequently C3) in a linear pattern within the epidermal basement membrane zone. Ultrastructurally, these immunoreactants are found in the sublamina densa region in association with anchoring fibrils. Approximately 50% of EBA patients have demonstrable circulating IgG anti-basement membrane autoantibodies directed against type VII collagen—the collagen species that comprises anchoring fibrils. Such IgG autoantibodies bind the dermal side of 1 M NaCl split skin (in contrast to IgG autoantibodies in patients with BP). Studies have shown that passive transfer of experimental or patient IgG directed against type VII collagen can produce lesions in mice that clinically, histologically, and immunopathologically resemble those seen in patients with inflammatory EBA.

Treatment of EBA is generally unsatisfactory. Some patients with inflammatory EBA may respond to systemic glucocorticoids, either alone or in combination with immunosuppressive agents. Other patients (especially those with neutrophil-rich inflammatory

lesions) may respond to dapsone. The chronic, noninflammatory form of this disease is largely resistant to treatment, although some patients may respond to cyclosporine, azathioprine, or IVIg.

■ CICATRICIAL PEMPHIGOID

Cicatricial pemphigoid (CP) is a rare, acquired, subepithelial immunobullous disease characterized by erosive lesions of mucous membranes and skin that result in scarring of at least some sites of involvement. Common sites of involvement include the oral mucosa (especially the gingiva) and conjunctiva; other sites that may be affected include the nasopharyngeal, laryngeal, esophageal, and anogenital mucosa. Skin lesions (present in about one-third of patients) tend to predominate on the scalp, face, and upper trunk and generally consist of a few scattered erosions or tense blisters on an erythematous or urticarial base. CP is typically a chronic and progressive disorder. Serious complications may arise as a consequence of ocular, laryngeal, esophageal, or anogenital lesions. Erosive conjunctivitis may result in shortened fornices, symblephara, ankyloblepharon, entropion, corneal opacities, and (in severe cases) blindness. Similarly, erosive lesions of the larynx may cause hoarseness, pain, and tissue loss that, if unrecognized and untreated, may eventuate in complete destruction of the airway. Esophageal lesions may result in stenosis and/or strictures that could place patients at risk for aspiration. Strictures might also complicate anogenital involvement.

Biopsies of lesional tissue generally demonstrate subepithelial vesiculobullae and a mononuclear leukocytic infiltrate. Neutrophils and eosinophils may be seen in biopsies of early lesions; older lesions may demonstrate a scant leukocytic infiltrate and fibrosis. Direct immunofluorescence microscopy of perilesional tissue typically demonstrates deposits of IgG, IgA, and/or C3 in the epidermal basement membrane of these patients. Because many of these patients show no evidence of circulating anti-basement membrane autoantibodies, testing of perilesional skin is important diagnostically. Although CP was once thought to be a single nosologic entity, it is now largely regarded as a disease phenotype that may develop as a consequence of an autoimmune reaction against a variety of different molecules in epidermal basement membrane (e.g., BPAG2, laminin-332, type VII collagen, and other antigens yet to be completely defined). Recent studies suggest that CP patients with anti-laminin-332 autoantibodies have an increased relative risk for cancer. Treatment of CP is largely dependent upon sites of involvement. Due to potentially severe complications, patients with ocular, laryngeal, esophageal, and/or anogenital involvement require aggressive systemic treatment with dapsone, prednisone, or the latter in combination with another immunosuppressive agent (e.g., azathioprine, mycophenolate mofetil, or cyclophosphamide) or IVIg. Less threatening forms of the disease may be managed with topical or intralesional glucocorticoids.

AUTOIMMUNE SYSTEMIC DISEASES WITH PROMINENT CUTANEOUS FEATURES

■ DERMATOMYOSITIS

The cutaneous manifestations of dermatomyositis (Chap. 388) are often distinctive, but, at times, they may resemble those of systemic lupus erythematosus (SLE) (Chap. 319), scleroderma (Chap. 323), or other overlapping connective tissue diseases (Chap. 323). The extent and severity of cutaneous disease may or may not correlate with the extent and severity of the myositis. The cutaneous manifestations of dermatomyositis are similar, whether the disease appears in children or the elderly, except that calcification of subcutaneous tissue is a common late sequela in childhood dermatomyositis.

The cutaneous signs of dermatomyositis may precede or follow the development of myositis by weeks to years. Cases lacking

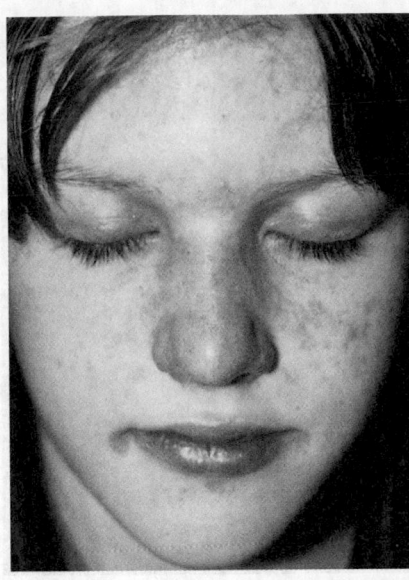

Figure 54-3 Dermatomyositis. Periorbital violaceous erythema characterizes the classic heliotrope rash. *(Courtesy of James Krell, MD; with permission.)*

muscle involvement (i.e., dermatomyositis sine myositis) have also been reported. The most common manifestation is a purple-red discoloration of the upper eyelids, sometimes associated with scaling ("heliotrope" erythema; Fig. 54-3) and periorbital edema. Erythema on the cheeks and nose in a "butterfly" distribution may resemble the malar eruption of SLE. Erythematous or violaceous scaling patches are common on the upper anterior chest; posterior neck; scalp; and the extensor surfaces of the arms, legs, and hands. Erythema and scaling may be particularly prominent over the elbows, knees, and the dorsal interphalangeal joints. Approximately one-third of patients have violaceous, flat-topped papules over the dorsal interphalangeal joints that are pathognomonic of dermatomyositis (Gottron's sign or Gottron's papules; Fig. 54-4). These lesions can be contrasted with the erythema and scaling on the dorsum of the fingers that spares the skin over the interphalangeal joints of some SLE patients. Periungual telangiectasia may be prominent. Lacy or reticulated erythema may be associated

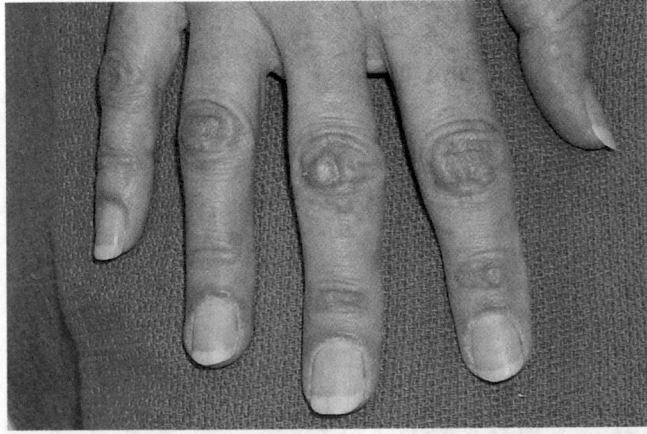

Figure 54-4 Gottron's sign. Dermatomyositis often involves the hands as erythematous flat-topped papules over the knuckles (Gottron's sign). Periungual telangiectases are also evident.

with fine scaling on the extensor surfaces of the thighs and upper arms. Other patients, particularly those with long-standing disease, develop areas of hypopigmentation, hyperpigmentation, mild atrophy, and telangiectasia known as *poikiloderma*. Poikiloderma is rare in both SLE and scleroderma and, thus, can serve as a clinical sign that distinguishes dermatomyositis from these two diseases. Cutaneous changes may be similar in scleroderma and dermatomyositis and may include thickening and binding down of the skin of the hands (sclerodactyly) as well as Raynaud's phenomenon. However, the presence of severe muscle disease, Gottron's papules, heliotrope erythema, and poikiloderma serve to distinguish patients with dermatomyositis. Skin biopsy of erythematous, scaling lesions of dermatomyositis may reveal only mild nonspecific inflammation but sometimes may show changes indistinguishable from those found in SLE, including epidermal atrophy, hydropic degeneration of basal keratinocytes, edema of the upper dermis, and a mild mononuclear cell infiltrate. Direct immunofluorescence microscopy of lesional skin is usually negative, although granular deposits of immunoglobulin(s) and complement in the epidermal basement membrane zone have been described in some patients. Treatment should be directed at the systemic disease. Topical glucocorticoids are sometimes useful; patients should avoid exposure to ultraviolet irradiation and aggressively use photoprotective measures including use of broad-spectrum sunscreens.

■ LUPUS ERYTHEMATOSUS

The cutaneous manifestations of lupus erythematosus (LE) (Chap. 319) can be divided into acute, subacute, and chronic types. *Acute cutaneous LE* is characterized by erythema of the nose and malar eminences in a "butterfly" distribution (Fig. 54-5). The erythema is often sudden in onset, accompanied by edema and fine scale, and correlated with systemic involvement. Patients may have widespread involvement of the face as well as erythema and scaling of the extensor surfaces of the extremities and upper chest. These acute lesions, while sometimes evanescent, usually last for days and are often associated with exacerbations of systemic disease. Skin biopsy of acute lesions may show only a sparse dermal infiltrate of mononuclear cells and dermal edema. In some instances, cellular infiltrates around blood vessels and hair follicles are notable, as is hydropic degeneration of basal cells of the epidermis. Direct immunofluorescence microscopy of lesional skin frequently reveals deposits of immunoglobulin(s) and complement in the epidermal basement membrane zone. Treatment is aimed at control of systemic disease; photoprotection in this as well as in other forms of LE is very important.

Subacute cutaneous lupus erythematosus (SCLE) is characterized by a widespread photosensitive, nonscarring eruption. Most of these patients have SLE in which renal and CNS involvement is mild or absent. SCLE may present as a papulosquamous eruption that resembles psoriasis or annular lesions that resemble those seen in erythema multiforme. In the papulosquamous form, discrete erythematous papules arise on the back, chest, shoulders, extensor surfaces of the arms, and the dorsum of the hands; lesions are uncommon on the face, flexor surfaces of the arms, and below the waist. These slightly scaling papules tend to merge into large plaques, some with a reticulate appearance. The annular form involves the same areas and presents with erythematous papules that evolve into oval, circular, or polycyclic lesions. The lesions of SCLE are more widespread but have less tendency for scarring than do lesions of discoid LE. Skin biopsy reveals a dense mononuclear cell infiltrate around hair follicles and blood vessels in the superficial dermis, combined with hydropic degeneration of basal cells in the epidermis. Direct immunofluorescence microscopy of lesional skin reveals deposits of immunoglobulin(s) in the epidermal basement

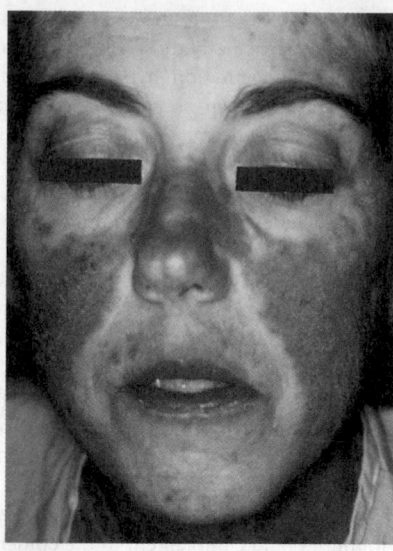

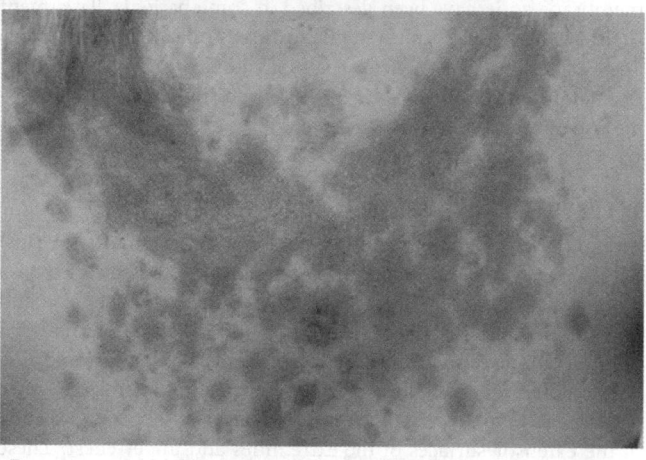

Figure 54-5 ***A.* Acute cutaneous lupus erythematosus** showing prominent, scaly, malar erythema. Involvement of other sun-exposed sites is also common. ***B.* Acute cutaneous LE** on the upper chest demonstrating brightly erythematous and slightly edematous papules and plaques. (***B****, Courtesy of Robert Swerlick, MD; with permission.*)

membrane zone in about one-half of these cases. A particulate pattern of IgG deposition throughout the epidermis has been associated with SCLE. Most SCLE patients have anti-Ro autoantibodies. Local therapy alone is usually unsuccessful. Most patients require treatment with aminoquinoline antimalarials. Low-dose therapy with oral glucocorticoids is sometimes necessary. Photoprotective measures against both ultraviolet B and A wavelengths are very important.

Discoid lupus erythematosus (DLE, also called *chronic cutaneous LE*) is characterized by discrete lesions, most often found on the face, scalp, and/or external ears. The lesions are erythematous papules or plaques with a thick, adherent scale that occludes hair follicles (follicular plugging). When the scale is removed, its underside shows small excrescences that correlate with the openings of hair follicles (so-called "carpet tacking"), a finding relatively specific for DLE. Long-standing lesions develop central atrophy, scarring, and hypopigmentation but frequently have erythematous, sometimes raised borders (Fig. 54-6). These lesions persist for years and tend to expand slowly. Only 5–10% of patients with DLE meet the American Rheumatism Association criteria for SLE. However, typical discoid lesions are frequently seen in patients with SLE. Biopsy of DLE lesions shows hyperkeratosis, follicular plugging, atrophy

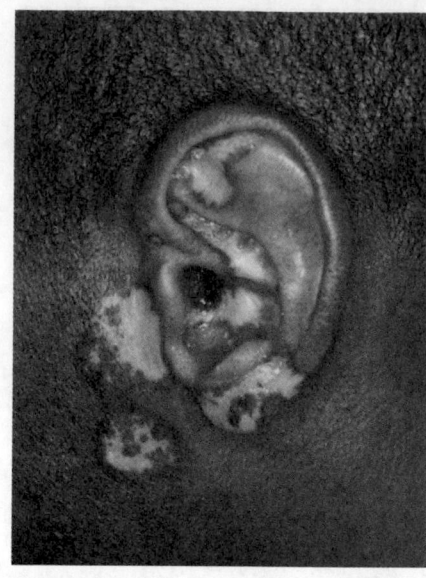

Figure 54-6 Discoid lupus erythematosus. Violaceous, hyperpigmented, atrophic plaques, often with evidence of follicular plugging, which may result in scarring, are characteristic of discoid lupus erythematosus (also called chronic cutaneous lupus erythematosus).

of the epidermis, hydropic degeneration of basal keratinocytes, and a mononuclear cell infiltrate adjacent to epidermal, adnexal, and microvascular basement membranes. Direct immunofluorescence microscopy demonstrates immunoglobulin(s) and complement deposits at the basement membrane zone in ~90% of cases. Treatment is focused on control of local cutaneous disease and consists mainly of photoprotection and topical or intralesional glucocorticoids. If local therapy is ineffective, use of aminoquinoline antimalarials may be indicated.

■ SCLERODERMA AND MORPHEA

The skin changes of scleroderma (Chap. 323) usually begin on the hands, feet, and face, with episodes of recurrent nonpitting edema. Sclerosis of the skin begins distally on the fingers (sclerodactyly) and spreads proximally, usually accompanied by resorption of bone of the fingertips, which may have punched out ulcers, stellate scars, or areas of hemorrhage (Fig. 54-7). The fingers may

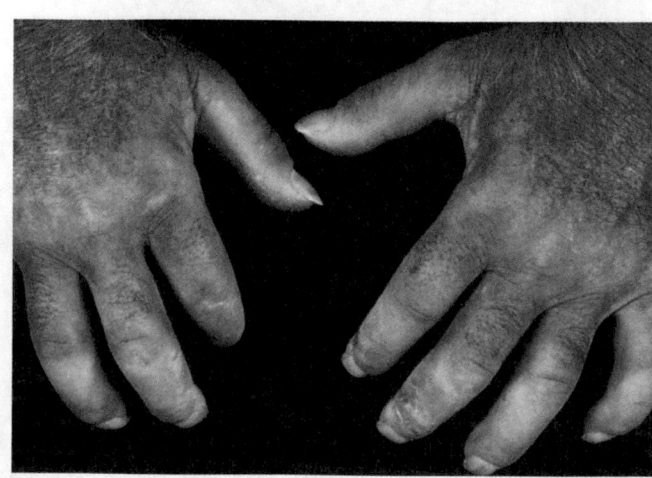

Figure 54-7 Scleroderma showing acral sclerosis and focal digital ulcers.

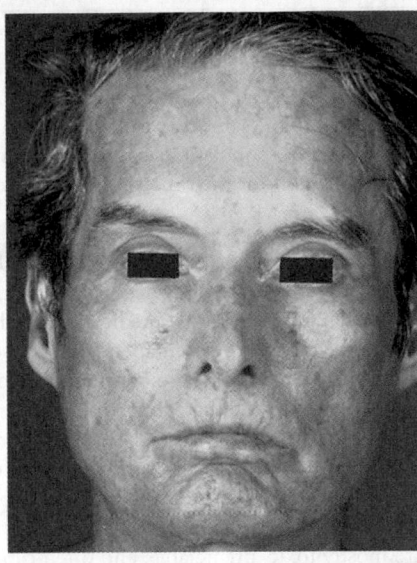

Figure 54-8 **Scleroderma** often eventuates in development of an expressionless, masklike facies.

actually shrink in size and become sausage-shaped, and because the fingernails are usually unaffected, the nails may curve over the end of the fingertips. Periungual telangiectases are usually present, but periungual erythema is rare. In advanced cases, the extremities show contractures and calcinosis cutis. Facial involvement includes a smooth, unwrinkled brow, taut skin over the nose, shrinkage of tissue around the mouth, and perioral radial furrowing (Fig. 54-8). Matlike telangiectases are often present, particularly on the face and hands. Involved skin feels indurated, smooth, and bound to underlying structures; hyper- and hypopigmentation are also often present. Raynaud's phenomenon (i.e., cold-induced blanching, cyanosis, and reactive hyperemia) is present in almost all patients and can precede development of scleroderma by many years. Linear scleroderma is a limited form of disease that presents in a linear, bandlike distribution and tends to involve deep as well as superficial layers of skin. The combination of calcinosis cutis, Raynaud's phenomenon, esophageal dysmotility, sclerodactyly, and telangiectasia has been termed the *CREST syndrome*. Anticentromere antibodies have been reported in a very high percentage of patients with the CREST syndrome but in only a small minority of patients with scleroderma. Skin biopsy reveals thickening of the dermis and homogenization of collagen bundles. Direct immunofluorescence microscopy of lesional skin is usually negative.

Morphea is characterized by localized thickening and sclerosis of skin; it dominates on the trunk. This disorder may affect children or adults. Morphea begins as erythematous or flesh-colored plaques that become sclerotic, develop central hypopigmentation, and demonstrate an erythematous border. In most cases, patients have one or a few lesions, and the disease is termed *localized morphea*. In some patients, widespread cutaneous lesions may occur without systemic involvement. This form is called *generalized morphea*.

Many adults with generalized morphea have concomitant rheumatic or other autoimmune disorders. Skin biopsy of morphea is indistinguishable from that of scleroderma. Scleroderma and morphea are usually quite resistant to therapy. For this reason, physical therapy to prevent joint contractures and to maintain function is employed and is often helpful. Treatment options for early, rapidly progressive disease include phototherapy (UVA1 or PUVA) or methotrexate 15–20 mg per week alone or in combination with daily glucocorticoids.

Diffuse fasciitis with eosinophilia is a clinical entity that can sometimes be confused with scleroderma. There is usually the sudden onset of swelling, induration, and erythema of the extremities frequently following significant physical exertion. The proximal portions of extremities (arms, forearms, thighs, legs) are more often involved than are the hands and feet. While the skin is indurated, it is usually not bound down as in scleroderma; contractures may occur early secondary to fascial involvement. The latter may also cause muscle groups to be separated and veins to appear depressed (i.e., the "groove sign"). These skin findings are accompanied by peripheral blood eosinophilia, increased erythrocyte sedimentation rate, and sometimes hypergammaglobulinemia. Deep biopsy of affected areas of skin reveals inflammation and thickening of the deep fascia overlying muscle. An inflammatory infiltrate composed of eosinophils and mononuclear cells is usually found. Patients with eosinophilic fasciitis appear to be at increased risk to develop bone marrow failure or other hematologic abnormalities. While the ultimate course of eosinophilic fasciitis is uncertain, many patients respond favorably to treatment with prednisone in doses ranging from 40–60 mg/d.

The *eosinophilia-myalgia syndrome*, a disorder reported in epidemic numbers in 1989 and linked to ingestion of L-tryptophan manufactured by a single company in Japan, is a multisystem disorder characterized by debilitating myalgias and absolute eosinophilia in association with varying combinations of arthralgias, pulmonary symptoms, and peripheral edema. In a later phase (3–6 months after initial symptoms), these patients often develop localized sclerodermatous skin changes, weight loss, and/or neuropathy (Chap. 323). The precise cause of this syndrome, which may resemble other sclerotic skin conditions, is unknown. However, the implicated lots of L-tryptophan contained the contaminant 1,1-ethylidene bis[tryptophan]. This contaminant may be pathogenic or a marker for another substance that provokes the disorder.

FURTHER READINGS

ANHALT GJ: Paraneoplastic pemphigus. J Investig Dermatol Symp Proc 9:29, 2004

OLASZ EB, YANCEY KB: Bullous pemphigoid and related subepidermal autoimmune blistering diseases, in *Current Directions in Autoimmunity: Dermatologic Immunity*, BJ Nickoloff, FO Nestle (eds). Basel, Karger Press, 2008, pp 141-166

PAYNE AS et al: Desmosomes and disease: Pemphigus and bullous impetigo. Curr Opin Cell Biol 16:536, 2004

SONTHEIMER RD: Skin manifestations of systemic autoimmune connective tissue disease: Diagnostics and therapeutics. Best Pract Res Clin Rheumatol 18:429, 2004

CHAPTER **55**

Cutaneous Drug Reactions

Kanade Shinkai

Robert S. Stern

Bruce U. Wintroub

Cutaneous reactions are among the most frequent adverse reactions to drugs. Most are benign, but a few can be life threatening. Prompt recognition of severe reactions, drug withdrawal, and appropriate therapeutic interventions can minimize toxicity. This chapter focuses on adverse cutaneous reactions to systemic medications; it covers their incidence, patterns, and pathogenesis and provides some practical guidelines on treatment, assessment of causality, and future use of drugs.

USE OF PRESCRIPTION DRUGS IN THE UNITED STATES

In the United States, more than 3 billion prescriptions for over 60,000 drug products, which include more than 2000 different active agents, are dispensed annually. Hospital inpatients alone annually receive about 120 million courses of drug therapy, and half of adult Americans receive prescription drugs on a regular outpatient basis. Many patients use over-the-counter medicines that may cause adverse cutaneous reactions.

INCIDENCE OF CUTANEOUS REACTIONS

Several large cohort studies established that acute cutaneous reaction to drugs affected about 3% of hospital inpatients. Reactions usually occur a few days to 4 weeks after initiation of therapy.

Many drugs of common use are associated with a 1–2% rate of "rashes" during premarketing clinical trials. The risk is often higher when medications are used in general, unselected populations. The rate may reach 3–7% for amoxicillin, sulfamethoxazole, and many anticonvulsants. It may be even higher with anti-HIV agents.

In addition to acute eruptions, a variety of skin diseases can be induced or exacerbated by prolonged use of drugs (e.g., pruritus, pigmentation, nail or hair disorders, psoriasis, pemphigoid, and pemphigus). These drug reactions are not frequent, but neither their incidence nor their impact on public health has been evaluated.

In a series of 48,005 inpatients over a 20-year period, morbilliform rash (91%) and urticaria (6%) were the most frequent skin reactions. Severe reactions are actually too rare to be detected in such cohorts. Although rare, severe cutaneous reactions to drugs have an important impact on health and on the risk-versus-benefit evaluation of medicines because of significant sequelae, including mortality. In one prospective study in the hospital setting, adverse drug rash was responsible for hospitalization, increased the duration of hospital stay, or was life threatening. Some populations are at increased risk of drug reactions: patients with collagen vascular diseases, bone marrow graft recipients, and those with acute Epstein-Barr virus infection. The pathophysiology underlying this association is unknown. It has also been established that HIV infection increases the risk of drug allergy, including severe hypersensitivity reactions (Chap. 189). This was true for many drugs but has been evaluated mainly with sulfamethoxazole. Up to 40% of HIV-infected patients had skin reactions when treated with high doses, and about 15% reacted to the same dosage that induced eruption in 3–5% of non-HIV-infected populations. How HIV promotes sensitivity to certain medications or their metabolites remains unclear.

PATHOGENESIS OF DRUG REACTIONS

The skin is commonly affected by adverse drug reactions. The list of conditions that can be triggered by medications includes nearly all dermatologic diseases. Adverse cutaneous responses to drugs can arise as a result of immunologic or nonimmunologic mechanisms. Examples of responses that arise from nonimmunologic mechanisms are pigmentary changes related to accumulation in the dermis of amiodarone, antimalarials, minocycline, quinolones, alteration of hair follicles by antimetabolites, and lipodystrophy associated with metabolic effects of anti-HIV medications. These side effects are mostly toxic, predictable, and often can be avoided in part by simple preventive measures.

■ IMMUNOLOGIC DRUG REACTIONS

Evidence suggests an immunologic basis for most acute drug eruptions, benign or severe. Drug-specific T cell clones can be derived from the blood or from skin lesions of patients with a variety of drug allergies, strongly suggesting that drugs can be recognized as antigens by human T cells and that these T cells play a role in drug allergy. Specific clones were obtained with penicillin G, amoxicillin, cephalosporins, sulfamethoxazole, phenobarbital, carbamazepine, lamotrigine (i.e., many of the medications that are frequently a cause of drug eruptions). Both CD4 and CD8 clones have been obtained; however, their specific roles in the manifestations of allergy have not been elucidated. Drug presentation to T cells was MHC-restricted and may involve hapten-peptide complexes formed between drugs or reactive metabolites and endogenous cell-surface proteins.

Once a drug has induced an immune response, the final phenotype of the reaction probably depends on the nature of effectors: cytotoxic (CD8+) T cells in blistering and certain hypersensitivity reactions, chemokines for reactions mediated by neutrophils or eosinophils, and collaboration with B cells for production of specific antibodies for urticarial reactions.

Immediate reactions

Immediate reactions depend on the release of mediators of inflammation by tissue mast cells or circulating basophilic leukocytes. These mediators include histamine, leukotrienes, prostaglandins, platelet-activating factor, enzymes, and proteoglycans. Drugs can trigger mediator release either directly ("anaphylactoid" reaction) or through IgE-specific antibodies. These reactions usually manifest in the skin and gastrointestinal, respiratory, and cardiovascular systems (Chap. 317). Primary symptoms and signs include pruritus, urticaria, nausea, vomiting, abdominal cramps, bronchospasm, laryngeal edema, and, occasionally, anaphylactic shock with hypotension and death. They occur within minutes of drug exposure. Nonsteroidal anti-inflammatory drugs (NSAIDs), including aspirin, and radiocontrast media are frequent causes of direct mast cell degranulation or anaphylactoid reactions, which can occur on first exposure. Penicillins and muscle relaxants used in general anesthesia are the most frequent causes of IgE-dependent reactions to drugs, which require prior sensitization. Release of mediators is triggered when polyvalent drug protein conjugates cross-link IgE molecules fixed to sensitized cells. Certain routes of administration favor different clinical patterns (e.g., gastrointestinal effects from oral route, circulatory effects from intravenous route).

Immune complex–dependent reactions

Serum sickness is produced by tissue deposition of circulating immune complexes with consumption of complement. It is characterized by fever, arthritis, nephritis, neuritis, edema, and an urticarial, papular, or purpuric rash (Chap. 326). First described following administration of nonhuman sera, it currently occurs in the setting of monoclonal antibodies and other similar medications. In classic serum sickness, symptoms develop 6 days or more after exposure to a drug, the latent period representing the time needed to synthesize antibody. Cephalosporin administration may be associated with a clinically similar "serum sickness-like" reaction in children. The mechanism of this reaction is unknown but is unrelated to complement activation and lacks immune complex formation, vasculitis, or renal disease.

Cutaneous or systemic vasculitis, a relatively rare cutaneous complication of drugs, may also be a result of immune complex deposition (Chap. 326).

Delayed hypersensitivity

Delayed hypersensitivity directed by drug-specific T cells is probably the most important mechanism in the etiology of the most common drug eruptions—morbilliform eruptions—and also of rare and severe forms such as hypersensitivity syndrome, acute generalized exanthematous pustulosis (AGEP), Stevens-Johnson syndrome (SJS), and toxic epidermal necrolysis (TEN). Drug-specific T cells have been detected in these types of drug eruptions. It remains unknown why T cell stimulation by medications leads to reactions that are clinically so diverse.

Contrary to what has been believed for years, the antigen is more often the native drug itself than its metabolites. Drug-specific cytotoxic T cells have been detected in the skin lesions of fixed drug eruptions and of TEN. In TEN, blisters that result from accumulation of interstitial fluid under the necrotic epidermis contain T lymphocytes reactive to autologous lymphocytes and keratinocytes in a drug-specific, HLA-restricted, and perforin/granzyme-mediated pathway.

Drug-specific clones producing CXCL8, a neutrophil-attracting chemokine, were obtained from skin biopsies of patients with AGEP, a neutrophil-mediated drug reaction.

Genetic factors and cutaneous drug reactions

Genetic determinants may predispose individuals to severe drug reactions by affecting either drug metabolism or immune responses to drugs. Polymorphisms in cytochrome P450 enzymes may increase susceptibility to drug toxicity, highlighting a role for differential pharmacokinetic or pharmacodynamic effects. It has also been suspected that a slow acetylator phenotype increases the risk of rash from sulfonamides. However, in two large prospective cohorts of HIV-infected patients treated with sulfonamides, no association of drug eruption with acetylation genotype was found.

Associations between drug hypersensitivities and HLA haplotypes also suggest a key role for immune mechanisms. Hypersensitivity to the anti-HIV medication abacavir is strongly associated with HLA B*5701. In Taiwan, within a homogeneous Han Chinese population, a 100% association was observed between SJS or TEN related to carbamazepine and HLA B*1502. In the same population, another 100% association was found between SJS, TEN, or hypersensitivity syndrome/drug reaction with eosinophilia and systemic symptoms (DRESS) related to allopurinol and HLA B*5801. Additional adverse cutaneous drug reactions have been linked to other HLA haplotypes. However, the strong associations found in Taiwan have not been observed in other countries with more heterogeneous populations. Development of molecular screening tests for abacavir hypersensitivity is under way as a model for implementing individualized pharmacogenetic screening in clinical practice.

CLINICAL PRESENTATION OF CUTANEOUS DRUG REACTIONS

■ NONIMMUNE CUTANEOUS REACTIONS

Exacerbation or induction of dermatologic diseases

A variety of drugs can exacerbate preexisting diseases or sometimes induce a disease that may or may not disappear after withdrawal of the inducing medication. For example, NSAIDs, lithium, beta blockers, TNF-α cytokine antagonists, and angiotensin-converting enzyme (ACE) inhibitors can exacerbate plaque psoriasis, while antimalarials and withdrawal of systemic glucocorticoids can worsen pustular psoriasis. Acne may be induced by glucocorticoids, androgens, lithium, and antidepressants. Minocycline and thiazide diuretics may exacerbate subacute systemic lupus erythematosus; and pemphigus can be induced by D-penicillamine, captopril, and other ACE inhibitors. Furosemide is associated with drug-induced bullous pemphigoid. The hypothesis that a drug may be responsible should always be considered, especially in cases with atypical clinical presentation.

Photosensitivity eruptions

Photosensitivity eruptions are usually most marked in sun-exposed areas but may extend to sun-protected areas. The mechanism is almost always phototoxicity. Phototoxic reactions resemble sunburn and can occur with first exposure to a drug. Blistering may occur in drug-related pseudoporphyria. The severity of the reactions depends on the tissue level of the drug, its efficiency as a photosensitizer, and the extent of exposure to the activating wavelengths of ultraviolet light (Chap. 56).

Common orally administered photosensitizing drugs include many fluoroquinolones and tetracycline antibiotics. Other drugs less frequently encountered are chlorpromazine, thiazides, and several NSAIDs (ibuprofen, naproxen, piroxicam). Voriconazole may result in severe photosensitivity and accelerated photo-induced aging in certain organ transplant recipients.

Because UV-A and visible light, which trigger these reactions, are not easily absorbed by nonopaque sunscreens and are transmitted through window glass, photosensitivity reactions may be difficult to block. Photosensitivity reactions abate with removal of either the drug or ultraviolet radiation, use of high-potency sunscreens that block UV-A light, and treating the reaction as one would a sunburn. Rarely, individuals develop persistent reactivity to light, necessitating long-term avoidance of sun exposure.

Pigmentation changes

Drugs, either systemic or topical, may cause a variety of pigmentary changes in the skin. Oral contraceptives may induce melasma. Long-term minocycline, pefloxacin, and amiodarone may cause blue-gray pigmentation. Long-term, high-dose phenothiazine results in gray-brown pigmentation of sun-exposed areas. Numerous cancer chemotherapeutic agents may be associated with characteristic patterns of pigmentation (e.g., bleomycin, busulfan, daunorubicin, cyclophosphamide, hydroxyurea, and methotrexate). Pigmentation changes may also occur in mucous membranes (busulfan), nails (zidovudine), hair, and teeth.

Warfarin necrosis of skin

This rare reaction usually occurs between the third and tenth days of therapy with warfarin, usually in women. Common sites are breasts, thighs, and buttocks (Fig. 55-1). Lesions are sharply demarcated, erythematous, indurated, and purpuric and may progress to form large, irregular, hemorrhagic bullae with eventual necrosis and slow-healing eschar formation. These lesions can be life threatening.

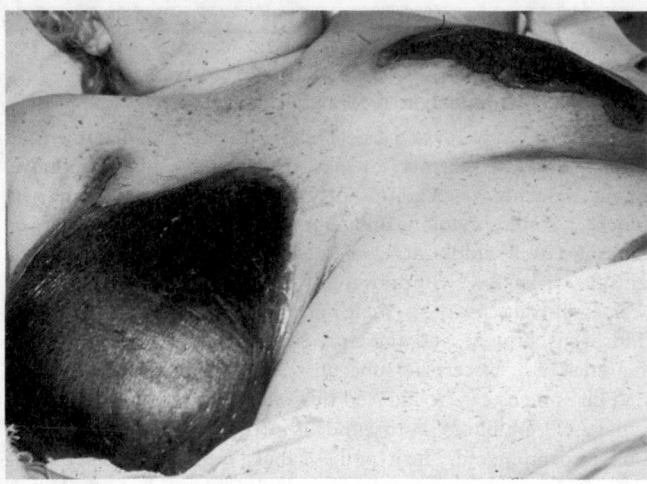

Figure 55-1 Warfarin necrosis.

Development of the syndrome is unrelated to drug dose, and the course is not altered by discontinuation of the drug after onset of the eruption. Warfarin reactions are associated with protein C deficiency. Warfarin anticoagulation in heterozygotes for protein C deficiency causes a precipitous fall in circulating levels of protein C, permitting hypercoagulability and thrombosis in the cutaneous microvasculature, with consequent areas of necrosis. Similar reactions have been associated with heparin. Heparin-induced necrosis may have clinically similar features but is probably due to heparin-induced platelet aggregation with subsequent occlusion of blood vessels; it can affect areas adjacent to the injection site or more distant sites if infused.

Warfarin-induced cutaneous necrosis is treated with vitamin K, heparin, and intensive wound care. Treatment with protein C concentrates may also be helpful.

Drug-induced hair disorders

Drug-induced hair loss Medications may affect hair follicles at two different phases of their growth cycle: anagen (growth) or telogen (resting). *Anagen effluvium* occurs within days of drug administration, especially with antimetabolite or other chemotherapeutic drugs. In contrast, in *telogen effluvium*, the delay is 2 to 4 months following initiation of a new medication, or after childbirth, acute illness, or severe stress. In drug-related cases, both present as diffuse nonscarring alopecia most often reversible after discontinuation of the responsible agent.

The prevalence and severity of alopecia depend on the drug as well as on an individual's predisposition. A considerable number of drugs have been reported to induce hair loss. These include antineoplastic agents (alkylating agents, bleomycin, vinca alkaloids, platinum compounds), anticonvulsants (carbamazepine, valproate), antihypertensive drugs (beta blockers), antidepressants, antithyroid drugs, interferons (IFNs), oral contraceptives, and cholesterol-lowering agents.

Hirsutism Hirsutism is an excessive growth of terminal hair with masculine hair growth pattern in a female, most often on the face and trunk. Hirsutism results from androgenic stimulation of hormone-sensitive hair follicles.

Anabolic steroids, oral contraceptives of the nonsteroid progesterone type, testosterone, and corticotropin can induce hirsutism.

Hypertrichosis Hypertrichosis differs from hirsutism by being located mainly on the forehead and temporal regions of the face. It

is usually reversible. Drugs responsible for hypertrichosis include anti-inflammatory drugs, glucocorticoids, vasodilators (diazoxide, minoxidil), diuretics (acetazolamide), anticonvulsants (phenytoin), immunosuppressive agents, psoralens, and zidovudine.

Changes in hair color or structure are uncommon adverse effects from medications. Hair discoloration may occur with chloroquine, IFN-α, chemotherapeutic agents, and tyrosine kinase inhibitors. Changes in hair structure have been observed in patients given epidermal growth factor receptor (EGFR) inhibitors.

Drug-induced nail disorders

Drug-related nail disorders usually involve several or all 20 nails and need months to resolve after withdrawal of the offending agent. The pathogenesis is most often toxic. Drug-induced nail changes include Beau's line (transverse depression of the nail plate), onycholysis (detachment of the distal part of the nail plate), onychomadesis (detachment of the proximal part of the nail plate), pigmentation, and paronychia (inflammation of periungual skin).

Onycholysis Onycholysis occurs with tetracyclines, fluoroquinolones, phenothiazines, and psoralens, as well as in persons taking NSAIDs, captopril, retinoids, sodium valproate, and many chemotherapeutic agents such as anthracyclines or taxanes including paclitaxel and docetaxel. The risk of onycholysis in patients receiving cytotoxic drugs can be increased by exposure to sunlight.

Onychomadesis Onychomadesis is caused by temporary arrest of nail matrix mitotic activity. Common drugs reported to induce onychomadesis include carbamazepine, lithium, retinoids, and chemotherapeutic agents such as cyclophosphamide and vincristine.

Paronychia Paronychia and multiple pyogenic granuloma with progressive and painful periungual abscess of fingers and toes are a side effect of systemic retinoids, lamivudine, indinavir, and anti-EGFR monoclonal antibodies (cetuximab, gefitinib).

Nail discoloration Some drugs—including anthracyclines, taxanes, fluorouracil, and zidovudine—may induce nail bed hyperpigmentation through melanocyte stimulation. It appears to be reversible and dose-dependent.

Pruritus

Pruritus is a common symptom of most drug eruptions, but it may also occur without skin lesions as the only manifestation of drug intolerance. Severe pruritus may occur in up to 50% of African patients treated with antimalarials and leads to poor compliance. It is much rarer in Caucasians.

■ IMMUNE CUTANEOUS REACTIONS: BENIGN

Maculopapular eruptions

Morbilliform or maculopapular eruptions (Fig. 55-2) are the most common of all drug-induced reactions, often start on the trunk or intertriginous areas, and consist of erythematous macules and papules that are frequently symmetric and may become confluent. Involvement of mucous membranes is unusual, with the exception of scaly lips; the eruption may be associated with moderate to severe pruritus and fever. Diagnosis is rarely assisted by laboratory testing. Skin biopsy is useless because it shows normal skin or very mild and nonspecific changes. A viral exanthem is the principal differential diagnostic consideration, especially in children, and graft-versus-host-disease in the proper clinical setting. Absence of enanthems; absence of symptoms in ears, nose, throat, and upper respiratory tract; and polymorphism of the skin lesions support a drug rather than a viral eruption.

Maculopapular reactions usually develop within 1 week of initiation of therapy and last less than 2 weeks. Occasionally, these

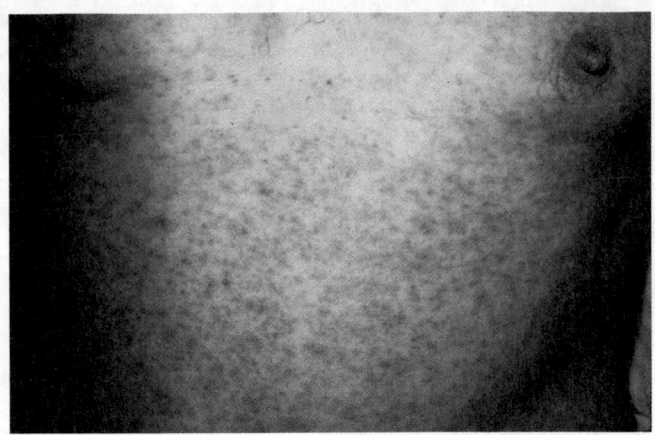

Figure 55-2 Morbilliform drug eruption.

eruptions decrease with continued use of the responsible drug. Because the eruption may also worsen, the suspect drug should be discontinued unless it is essential. Oral antihistamines, emollients, and soothing baths may help relieve pruritus. Short courses of potent topical glucocorticoids can reduce inflammation and symptoms. Systemic glucocorticoid treatment is rarely indicated.

Urticaria/angioedema

Urticaria is the second most frequent type of cutaneous reaction to drugs. However, "drug allergy" explains no more than 10–20% of acute urticaria cases. It is a skin reaction characterized by pruritic, red wheals of varying size. Individual lesions rarely last more than 24 hours. Deep edema within dermal and subcutaneous tissues is known as *angioedema*. Angioedema may involve respiratory and gastrointestinal mucous membranes. Urticaria and angioedema may be part of a life-threatening anaphylactic reaction.

Drug-induced urticaria may be caused by three mechanisms: an IgE-dependent mechanism, circulating immune complexes (serum sickness), and nonimmunologic activation of effector pathways. IgE-dependent urticarial reactions usually occur within 36 hours of drug exposure but can occur within minutes. Immune complex–induced urticaria associated with serum sickness usually occurs 6–12 days after first exposure. In this syndrome, the urticarial eruption may be accompanied by fever, hematuria, arthralgias, hepatic dysfunction, and neurologic symptoms. Certain drugs, such as NSAIDs, ACE inhibitors, angiotensin II antagonists, and radiographic dyes, may induce urticarial reactions, angioedema, and anaphylaxis in the absence of drug-specific antibody through direct mast-cell degranulation.

Although ACE inhibitors, aspirin, penicillin, and blood products are the most frequent causes of urticarial eruptions, urticaria has been observed in association with nearly all drugs. Drugs may also cause chronic urticaria, which lasts more than 6 weeks. Aspirin frequently exacerbates this problem.

The treatment of urticaria or angioedema depends on the severity of the reaction and the rate at which it is evolving. In severe cases with respiratory or cardiovascular compromise, epinephrine is the mainstay of therapy, but its effect is reduced in patients using beta blockers. Treatment with systemic glucocorticoids, sometimes administered IV, is helpful. In addition to drug withdrawal, for patients with only cutaneous symptoms and without symptoms of angioedema or anaphylaxis, oral antihistamines are usually sufficient.

Fixed drug eruptions

These reactions are characterized by one or more sharply demarcated, erythematous lesions, sometimes leading to a blister. Hyperpigmentation often results after resolution of the acute inflammation. With rechallenge, the lesion recurs in the same (i.e., fixed) location. Lesions often involve the lips, hands, legs, face, genitalia, and oral mucosa and cause a burning sensation. Most patients have multiple lesions. Fixed drug eruptions have been associated with pseudoephedrine (frequently a nonpigmented reaction), phenolphthalein (in laxatives), sulfonamides, tetracyclines, NSAIDs, and barbiturates. Patch testing has been used in Europe to help establish the etiology.

◼ IMMUNE CUTANEOUS REACTIONS: SEVERE

Vasculitis

Cutaneous small-vessel vasculitis often presents as palpable purpuric lesions that may be generalized or limited to the lower extremities or other dependent areas (Chap. 326). Urticarial lesions, ulcers, and hemorrhagic blisters also occur. Vasculitis may involve other organs, including the liver, kidney, brain, and joints. Drugs are implicated as a cause of 10–15% of all cases of vasculitides. Infection, malignancy, and collagen vascular disease are responsible for the majority non-drug related cases.

Propylthiouracil induces a cutaneous vasculitis that is accompanied by leukopenia and splenomegaly. Direct immunofluorescent changes in these lesions suggest immune-complex deposition. Drugs implicated in vasculitis include allopurinol, thiazides, sulfonamides, other antimicrobials, and several NSAIDs. The presence of eosinophils in the perivascular infiltrate of skin biopsy suggests a drug etiology.

Pustular eruptions

AGEP is a rare reaction pattern that is often associated with exposure to drugs. Usually beginning on the face or intertriginous areas, small nonfollicular pustules overlying erythematous and edematous skin may coalesce and lead to superficial ulceration. Differentiating this eruption from TEN in its initial stages may be difficult. A skin biopsy is important and shows scattered pustules in the upper part of the epidermis instead of the full-thickness necrosis that characterizes TEN. Fever is present with elevated neutrophil counts, and sepsis is often suspected. Acute pustular psoriasis is the principal differential diagnostic consideration. AGEP often begins within a few days of initiating drug treatment, most notably antibiotics. For other associated drugs (e.g., diltiazem, chloroquine, hydroxychloroquine, or terbinafine), AGEP begins later: 7–14 days after initiation of treatment.

Hypersensitivity syndrome

Initially described with phenytoin, hypersensitivity syndrome—a multiorgan drug-induced reaction—is also known as *DRESS (drug reaction with eosinophilia and systemic symptoms)* and *drug-induced hypersensitivity syndrome (DIHS)*. It presents as a widespread erythematous eruption that may become purpuric or lichenoid and is accompanied by many of the following features: fever, facial and periorbital edema, tender and generalized lymphadenopathy, leukocytosis (often with atypical lymphocytes and eosinophilia), hepatitis, and sometimes nephritis or pneumonitis. The cutaneous reaction usually begins 2 to 8 weeks after the drug is started and lasts longer than mild eruptions after drug cessation. Signs and symptoms may persist for several weeks, especially those associated with hepatitis. The eruption recurs with rechallenge, and cross-reactions among aromatic anticonvulsants, including phenytoin, carbamazepine, and barbiturates, are frequent. Other drugs causing this syndrome include lamotrigine, minocycline, dapsone, allopurinol, and sulfonamides, as well as abacavir and zalcitabine in HIV-infected patients. Hypersensitivity to reactive drug metabolites, hydroxylamine for sulfamethoxazole, and arene oxide for aromatic anticonvulsants may be involved in the pathogenesis of DRESS. Reactivation of herpes viruses, especially of herpes virus 6, has been reported to be frequent in this syndrome. The role of virus infection is still unclear; it may contribute to long-lasting manifestations such as hepatitis or encephalitis. Mortality rates as high as 10% have been reported; mortality is highest in association with hepatitis. Systemic glucocorticoids (prednisone, 1.5–2 mg/kg per d) should be started with slow taper over 8–12 weeks. Topical, high-potency glucocorticoids may also be helpful. In all cases, rapid withdrawal of the suspected drug is required. Patients should be closely monitored for resolution of organ dysfunction and for development of late-onset autoimmune thyroiditis (up to 6 months).

Stevens-Johnson syndrome and toxic epidermal necrolysis

SJS and *TEN* are characterized by blisters and epidermal detachment resulting from epidermal necrosis in the absence of substantial dermal inflammation. The term *Stevens-Johnson syndrome* is now used to describe cases with blisters developing on target lesions, dusky or purpuric macules in which mucosal involvement is significant, and total body surface area blistering and eventual detachment is <10%. The term *Stevens-Johnson syndrome/toxic epidermal necrolysis overlap* is used to describe cases with 10–30% detachment, and TEN is used to describe cases with >30% detachment. Erythema multiforme major is now considered by most to be different from SJS. Erythema multiforme (EM) is characterized by mucosal involvement and true "target" lesions or atypical raised target lesions often more acrally distributed and with limited extent of skin detachment. EM is most often triggered by infection, particularly herpes simplex virus or *mycoplasma pneumoniae*.

Patients with SJS, SJS/TEN, or TEN initially present with acute symptoms, painful skin lesions, fever >39°C (102.2°F), sore throat, and conjunctivitis resulting from mucosal membrane and ocular lesions. Intestinal and pulmonary involvements are associated with a poor prognosis, as are a greater extent of epidermal detachment and older age. About 10% and 30% of SJS- and TEN-affected persons die from their disease, respectively. Drugs that most commonly cause SJS or TEN are sulfonamides, nevirapine, allopurinol, lamotrigine, aromatic anticonvulsants, and the oxicam NSAIDs. At this time, SJS or TEN have no treatment of proven efficacy. The best results come from early diagnosis, immediate discontinuation of any suspected drug, supportive therapy, and paying close attention to ocular complications and infection. Frozen-section skin biopsy may aid in rapid diagnosis. Systemic glucocorticoid therapy (prednisone 1 to 2 mg/kg) may be useful early in the evolution of the disease, but long-term systemic glucocorticoid use has been associated with higher mortality. After initial enthusiasm for the use of intravenous immunoglobulin (IVIG) in the treatment of SJS/TEN, some recent data suggest IVIG is unlikely to benefit these patients. Randomized studies to more definitively assess the potential benefit of systemic glucocorticoids and IVIG are lacking and difficult to perform but are necessary.

DRUGS OF SPECIAL INTEREST

◼ ALLOPURINOL

Together with sulfonamides and antiepileptics, allopurinol is a frequent cause of mild maculopapular eruptions (in at least 3% of users) and may also cause more severe reactions including hypersensitivity/DRESS and SJS/TEN; patients with HLA B*5801 are highly susceptible to these severe reactions.

◼ ANTI-HIV MEDICATIONS

In clinical trials, combinations of highly active antiretroviral treatments were frequently associated with ≥10% "drug eruptions." Two drugs, nevirapine and abacavir, have been associated with specific risks.

Nevirapine has both a high risk of maculopapular eruptions and a very high risk (about 1 in 1000) of SJS or TEN. Progressive escalation of daily doses has been shown to decrease the risk of mild eruption but does not abrogate the risk of severe reactions.

Abacavir is associated with a 4–8% risk of a hypersensitivity reaction, which is remarkable because of the association of symptoms suggesting a type I hypersensitivity reaction (dyspnea, diarrhea, low blood pressure, shock on rechallenge) as well as signs of delayed hypersensitivity (rash, late onset hepatitis). The risk is lower in patients of African ancestry and strongly correlated with HLA B*5701. Evidence supports patch testing for abacavir hypersensitivity, and additional molecular screening methods are being developed to identify susceptible individuals.

◼ PENICILLIN

Incidence of cutaneous reactions due to penicillin is about 1%. About 85% of cutaneous reactions are morbilliform, and about 10% are urticaria or angioedema. Anaphylaxis and serum sickness appear to be due to IgE antibodies in serum.

Delayed reactions, mainly maculopapular eruptions, are much more common with aminopenicillins, involving 4–7% of users. The question of cross-reactivity between β-lactam antibiotics and preventing the risk of anaphylaxis is discussed below ("Management of a Patient with a Drug Eruption"). Approximately 10% of patients with penicillin allergies will also develop allergic reactions to cephalosporin class antibiotics.

◼ NONSTEROIDAL ANTI-INFLAMMATORY DRUGS

Most NSAIDs, including aspirin, cause immediate, allergy-like symptoms in susceptible individuals. Approximately 1% of persons experience urticaria or angioedema, and rare individuals (0.5%) experience rhinosinusitis and asthma.

Urticaria/angioedema may be delayed up to 24 hours and may occur at any age. The rhinosinusitis-asthma syndrome generally develops within 1 hour of drug administration. Recurrences are frequent and can be complicated by nasal and sinus infection, polyposis, bloody discharge, and nasal eosinophilia. In many individuals with this syndrome, potentially life-threatening asthma may ensue whenever NSAIDs are subsequently ingested. Proof of the association of symptoms and NSAID use requires either clear-cut history of symptoms following drug ingestion or an oral challenge. That procedure must be conducted only in a hospital setting by experienced personnel. Cross-reactivity between NSAIDs that inhibit cyclooxygenase (COX) 1 is common, while reactivity to COX-2 inhibitors is less frequent. The reaction is pharmacologic, and patients who are sensitive to NSAIDs cannot be identified by assessment of IgE antibody to aspirin, lymphocyte sensitization, or in vitro immunologic testing.

Other reactions can also occur with NSAIDs, including phototoxicity with many agents, a pattern of pseudoporphyria being often related to naproxen, hypersensitivity/DRESS (oxicam derivatives, COX-2 inhibitors), and SJS or TEN (phenylbutazone, oxicam derivatives).

◼ RADIOCONTRAST MEDIA

Many patients are exposed to radiocontrast agents, which can be a cause of adverse drug reactions. High-osmolality radiocontrast media were about five times more likely to induce urticaria (1%) or anaphylaxis than were newer low-osmolality media. Severe reactions are rare with either type of contrast media. About one-third of those with mild reactions to previous exposure react on re-exposure. Pretreatment with prednisone and diphenhydramine reduces reaction rates. Persons with a reaction to a high-osmolality contrast media should be given low-osmolality media if later contrast studies are required.

A new association between certain types of gadolinium contrast and nephrogenic systemic fibrosis, a condition of sclerosing skin with rare internal organ involvement, has been reported; advanced renal compromise may be an important risk factor.

ANTICONVULSANTS

Phenobarbital, phenytoin, carbamazepine, and lamotrigine are associated with many types of severe reactions in adults and a high incidence of less-severe reactions in children. These drugs carry the highest risk of SJS, TEN, and hypersensitivity syndrome in immunologically normal patients. There are strong HLA associations with anticonvulsant-induced toxicity in Han Chinese (see above). Aromatic anticonvulsants can induce a pseudolymphoma syndrome and induce gingival hyperplasia.

The overall rate of lamotrigine associated rash is lower in patients whose doses are slowly increased, but whether or not the risk of more severe reactions is reduced by slow dose escalation is less clear. Patients who also use valproate, which increases lamotrigine levels and half life, have a higher risk of skin reactions.

SULFONAMIDES

Antibacterial sulfonamides cause cutaneous eruptions at a high rate and are among the drugs most frequently implicated in SJS and TEN. The combination of sulfamethoxazole and trimethoprim frequently induces adverse cutaneous reactions in patients with AIDS (Chap. 182). Desensitization is often successful in AIDS patients with morbilliform eruptions but is not recommended in AIDS patients who manifested erythroderma or a bullous reaction in response to their earlier sulfonamide exposure.

Reaction rates are much lower with nonantibiotic sulfonamides, including diuretics or antidiabetic agents. Cross-reactivity between antibiotic and nonantibiotic sulfonamides is at most infrequent.

VANCOMYCIN

Vancomycin causes two unusual but recognizable cutaneous reactions: linear IgA bullous dermatosis (a transient, blistering eruption) and *red man syndrome*. Red man syndrome occurs during rapid IV infusion of vancomycin. This is thought to be a histamine-related anaphylactoid reaction characterized by flushing, diffuse maculopapular eruption, hypotension, and, in rare cases, cardiac arrest.

AGENTS USED IN CANCER CHEMOTHERAPY

Because many agents used in cancer chemotherapy inhibit cell division, rapidly proliferating elements of the skin, including hair, mucous membranes, and appendages, are sensitive to their effects. As a result, stomatitis and alopecia are among the most frequent dose-dependent side effects of chemotherapy. Various nail abnormalities have been described: onycholysis, dystrophy, Beau's lines, white lines, and pigmentation. Sterile cellulitis and phlebitis and ulceration of pressure areas occur with many of these agents. Also reported is acral erythema, which begins with dysesthesia followed by redness and a painful edematous eruption of the palms and soles, and is caused by cytarabine, doxorubicin, methotrexate, hydroxyurea, and 5-fluorouracil. Pyridoxine alleviates symptoms of acral erythema. Urticaria, angioedema, and exfoliative dermatitis also have been seen, as has local and diffuse hyperpigmentation.

Hypersensitivity to carboplatin or cisplatin is not rare (with an incidence of 10–20%) among patients receiving multiple treatments with these drugs. It is probably IgE mediated. Moderate to severe reactions, including respiratory distress and hypotension, are also observed in 10–20% of patients receiving paclitaxel regardless of premedication with glucocorticoids and histamine H(1) and H(2) antagonists.

Cetuximab and other EGF receptor antagonists induce follicular eruptions and nail toxicity after a mean interval of 10 days in a majority of patients. Xerosis, eczematous eruptions, and pruritus also frequently occur with EGF receptor antagonists. The severity of the eruption correlates with a better anticancer effect. Systemic antibiotics, topical antiacne treatments, and supportive care are helpful. Sorafenib, a tyrosine kinase inhibitor, may result in follicular eruptions and bullous palmoplantar eruptions with dysesthesia.

GLUCOCORTICOIDS

Both systemic and topical glucocorticoids cause a variety of skin changes, including acneiform eruptions, atrophy, striae, and other stigmata of Cushing's syndrome. And, in sufficiently high doses, glucocorticoids can retard wound healing. Patients using glucocorticoids are at higher risk for bacterial, yeast, and fungal skin infections that may be misinterpreted as drug eruptions but are instead drug side effects. Allergy to glucocorticoids may also occur either as contact dermatitis to topical formulations or as systemic reactions, including anaphylaxis.

BIOLOGIC THERAPIES

These include cytokines, cytokine antagonists, and monoclonal antibodies.

Injection-site reactions are the most frequent adverse events. The severity varies from mild redness to deep inflammation and necrosis. In most cases, the treatment can be continued and the severity of reactions will decrease with time.

Like all foreign proteins, monoclonal antibodies may induce urticaria, angioedema, anaphylactic reactions, and serum sickness. Production of inactivating antibodies to the drug may occur, classically with infliximab, and may be prevented by concomitant administration of low-dose methotrexate.

Alopecia is a common complication of IFN-α. A nonspecific, highly pruritic "dermatitis" is frequent in patients receiving IFN and ribavirin for hepatitis C.

Induction or exacerbation of various immune-mediated disorders, especially lupus erythematosus, has been reported with interleukin 2, IFN-α, and antitumor necrosis factor α.

Granulocyte colony-stimulating factor may induce various neutrophilic dermatoses, including Sweet's syndrome and pyoderma gangrenosum, and can exacerbate psoriasis.

ANTIMALARIAL AGENTS

Antimalarial agents are used as therapy for several skin diseases, including the skin manifestations of lupus and polymorphous light eruption, but they can also induce cutaneous reactions. The most frequent is pruritus, which occurs in up to 50% of African patients receiving chloroquine and may be severe enough to lead to discontinuation of treatment.

Pigmentation disturbances, including black pigmentation of the face, mucous membranes, and pretibial and subungual areas, occur with antimalarials. Quinacrine (mepacrine) causes generalized, cutaneous yellow discoloration. Less frequent reactions include pustular eruptions (AGEP) and hypersensitivity/DRESS.

MANAGEMENT OF A PATIENT WITH A DRUG ERUPTION

There are four main questions to answer regarding an eruption:

1. Is it a drug reaction?
2. Is it a severe eruption or the onset of a form that may become severe?
3. Which drug(s) are suspected, and which drug(s) should be withdrawn?
4. What is recommended for future use of drugs?

EARLY DIAGNOSIS OF SEVERE ERUPTIONS

Rapid recognition of adverse drug reactions that may become serious or life threatening is paramount. Table 55-1 lists clinical and laboratory features that, if present, suggest that the reaction may be serious. Table 55-2 provides key features of the most serious adverse cutaneous reactions. Intensity of symptoms and rapid progression of signs should raise the suspicion of a severe eruption. Any doubt should lead to prompt consultation with a dermatologist and/or referral of the patient to a specialized center.

CONFIRMATION OF DRUG REACTION

The probability of drug etiology varies with the pattern of the reaction. Only fixed drug eruptions are always drug-induced. Morbilliform eruptions are usually viral in children and drug-induced in adults. Among severe reactions, drugs account for 10–20% for anaphylaxis and vasculitis and between 70–90% for AGEP, DRESS, SJS, or TEN. Skin biopsy helps in characterizing the reaction but does not indicate drug causality. Blood counts and liver and renal function tests are important for evaluating organ involvement. The association of mild elevation of liver enzymes and high eosinophil count is frequent but not specific for a drug reaction. Blood tests that could identify an alternative cause, antihistone antibody tests, and serology or polymerase chain reaction for infections may be of great importance for final assessment of etiology.

WHAT DRUG(S) TO SUSPECT AND WITHDRAW

Most cases of drug eruptions occur during the first course of treatment with a new medication. A notable exception is IgE-mediated urticaria and anaphylaxis that need presensitization and develop a few minutes to a few hours after rechallenge. Characteristic time of onset to drug reaction: 4–14 days for morbilliform eruptions, 5–28 days for SJS/TEN, and 14–48 days for DRESS. Medications introduced for the first time in the relevant time frame are prime suspects. Two other important elements to suspect causality at this stage are (1) previous experience with the drug in the population and (2) alternative etiologic candidates.

The decision to continue or discontinue any medication will depend on the severity of the reaction, the severity of the primary disease, the degree of suspicion of causality, and the feasibility of an alternative safer treatment. In severe drug reactions, elimination of all possible suspect drugs or unnecessary medications should be attempted. Some rashes may disappear when "treating through" a benign drug-related eruption as seen in patients with AIDS treated for opportunistic infections with antibacterial sulfonamides. The decision to treat through an eruption should, however, remain the exception and withdrawal of every suspect drug the general rule. On the other hand, drugs that are not suspected and are important for the patient, (e.g., antihypertensive agents) generally should not be quickly withdrawn. This approach prevents reluctance to future use of these agents.

RECOMMENDATION FOR FUTURE USE OF DRUGS

The aims are (1) to prevent the recurrence of the drug eruption and (2) not to compromise future treatments by contraindicating otherwise useful medications.

Begin with thorough assessment of drug causality. Drug causality is evaluated based on timing of the reaction, evaluation of other possible causes, effect of drug withdrawal or continuation, and knowledge of medications that have been associated with the observed reaction. Combination of these criteria leads to considering the causality as definite, probable, possible, or unlikely.

A drug with "unlikely" causality or that has been continued when the reaction improved or was reintroduced without a reaction can be administered safely.

A drug with a "definite" or "probable" causality should be contraindicated, and a warning card or medical alert tag (e.g., wristband) given to the patient.

A drug with a "possible" causality may be submitted to further investigations depending on the expected need for future treatment.

The usefulness of drug tests is still debated. Many in vitro immunologic assays have been developed, but the predictive value of these tests has not been validated in any large series of affected patients; these tests exist primarily for research and not clinical purposes.

In patients with history suggesting immediate IgE-mediated reactions to penicillin, skin testing with major and minor determinants of penicillins or cephalosporins has proved useful for identifying patients at risk of anaphylactic reactions to these agents. However, skin tests themselves carry a small risk of anaphylaxis. Negative skin tests do not totally rule out IgE-mediated reactivity, but the risk of anaphylaxis in response to penicillin administration in patients with negative skin tests is about 1% while about two-thirds of patients with a positive skin test experience an allergic response on rechallenge.

For patients with late drug reactions, the clinical usefulness of skin tests is more questionable. At least one of a combination of several tests (prick, patch, and intradermal) is positive in 50–70% of patients with a reaction "definitely" attributed to a single medication. This low sensitivity probably contributes to the fact that readministration of drugs that had been tested negative resulted in up to 17% eruptions.

CROSS-SENSITIVITY

Because of the possibility of cross-sensitivity among chemically related drugs, many physicians recommend avoidance of not only the medication that induced the reaction but also all drugs of the same pharmacologic class.

TABLE 55-1 Clinical and Laboratory Findings Associated With More Serious Drug-Induced Cutaneous Clinical Findings

Cutaneous
  Generalized erythema
  Facial edema or central facial involvement
  Skin pain
  Palpable purpura
  Target lesions
  Skin necrosis
  Blisters or epidermal detachment
  Positive Nikolsky's sign
  Mucous membrane erosions
  Urticaria
  Swelling of tongue

General
  High fever [temperature >40°C (>104°F)]
  Enlarged lymph nodes
  Arthralgias or arthritis
  Shortness of breath, wheezing, hypotension

Laboratory results
  Eosinophil count >1000/μL
  Lymphocytosis with atypical lymphocytes
  Abnormal liver or kidney function tests

Source: Adapted from Roujeau and Stern.

TABLE 55-2 Clinical Features of Severe Cutaneous Drug Reactions

Diagnosis	Mucosal Lesions	Typical Skin Lesions	Frequent Signs and Symptoms	Alternative Causes Not Related to Drugs
Stevens-Johnson syndrome	Erosions usually at two or more sites	Small blisters on dusky purpuric macules or atypical targets; rare areas of confluence; detachment ≤10% of body surface area	Most cases involve fever	10-20% cause not determined
Toxic epidermal necrolysis[a]	Erosions usually at two or more sites	Individual lesions like those seen in Stevens-Johnson syndrome; confluent erythema; outer layer of epidermis separates readily from basal layer with lateral pressure; large sheet of necrotic epidermis; total detachment of >30% of body surface area	Nearly all cases involve fever, "acute skin failure," leukopenia	10–20% cause not determined
Hypersensitivity syndrome	Infrequent	Severe exanthematous rash (may become purpuric), exfoliative dermatitis, facial edema	30–50% of cases involve fever, lymphadenopathy, hepatitis, nephritis, carditis, eosinophilia, atypical lymphocytes	Cutaneous lymphoma
Acute generalized exanthematous pustulosis	About 20% erosions mouth, tongue	Initially nonfollicular small pustules overlying edematous erythema, sometimes leading to superficial erosions	Fever, burning, pruritus, facial swelling, leukocytosis, hypocalcemia	Infection
Serum sickness or reactions resembling serum sickness	Absent	Morbilliform lesions, sometimes with urticaria	Fever, arthralgias	Infection
Anticoagulant-induced necrosis	Infrequent	Erythema then purpura and necrosis, especially of fatty areas	Pain in affected areas	Disseminated intravascular coagulopathy, septicemia
Angioedema	Often involved	Urticaria or swelling of central part of face	Respiratory distress, cardiovascular collapse	Insect stings, foods

[a]Overlap of Stevens-Johnson syndrome and toxic epidermal necrolysis with features of both and attachment of 10–30% of body surface area may occur.

Source: Adapted from Roujeau and Stern.

There are two types of cross-sensitivity. Reactions that depend on a pharmacologic interaction may recur with all drugs that target the same pathway, whether they are structurally similar or not. This is the case with angioedema caused by NSAIDs and ACE inhibitors. In this situation, the risk of recurrence varies from drug to drug in a particular class; however, avoidance of all drugs in the class is usually recommended. Immune recognition of structurally related drugs is the second mechanism by which cross-sensitivity occurs. A classic example is hypersensitivity to aromatic antiepileptics (barbiturates, phenytoin, carbamazepine) with up to 50% reaction to a second drug in patients who reacted to one. For other drugs, in vitro as well as in vivo data have suggested that cross-reactivity existed only between compounds with very similar chemical structures. Sulfamethoxazole-specific lymphocytes may occasionally recognize a few other antibacterial sulfonamides but not diuretics, antidiabetic drugs, or anti-COX2 NSAIDs with a sulfonamide group.

Recent data suggest that although the risk of a drug eruption to another drug was increased in persons with a prior reaction, "cross-sensitivity" was probably not the explanation. As an example, persons with a history of an allergic-like reaction to penicillin were at higher risk to develop a reaction to antibacterial sulfonamides than to cephalosporin.

These data suggest that the list of drugs to avoid after a drug reaction should be limited to the causative one(s) and to a few very similar medications.

Because of growing evidence that some severe cutaneous reactions to drugs are associated with HLA genes, it is probably wise to recommend that first-degree family members of patients with severe cutaneous reactions also should avoid these causative medications.

Desensitization can be considered in those with a history of reaction to a medication that must be used again. Efficacy of such procedures has been demonstrated in cases of immediate reaction to penicillin and positive skin tests, anaphylactic reactions to platinum chemotherapy, and delayed reactions to sulfonamides in patients with AIDS. Various protocols are available, including oral and parenteral approaches. Oral desensitization appears to have a lower risk of serious anaphylactic reactions. However, desensitization carries the risk of anaphylaxis regardless of how it is performed and should be performed in monitored clinical settings such as an intensive care unit. After desensitization, many patients experience non-life-threatening reactions during therapy with the culprit drug.

▇ REPORTING

Any severe reaction to drugs should be reported to a regulatory agency or to pharmaceutical companies (e.g., MedWatch, *http://www.fda.gov/Safety/MedWatch/default.htm*). Because severe reactions are too rare to be detected in premarketing clinical trials, spontaneous reports are of critical importance for early detection of unexpected life-threatening events. To be useful, the report should contain enough details to permit ascertainment of severity and drug causality. This permits recognition of similar cases that may be reported from several different sources.

ACKNOWLEDGMENTS

We acknowledge the contribution of Dr. Jean-Claude Roujeau to this chapter in the previous edition.

FURTHER READINGS

AUQUIER-DUNANT A et al: Severe cutaneous adverse reactions. Correlations between clinical patterns and causes of erythema multiforme majus, Stevens-Johnson syndrome, and toxic epidermal necrolysis: Results of an international prospective study. Arch Dermatol 138:1019, 2002

BACHOT N, ROUJEAU JC: Differential diagnosis of severe cutaneous drug eruptions. Am J Clin Dermatol 4:561, 2003

BIGBY M: Rates of cutaneous reactions to drugs. Arch Dermatol 137:765, 2001

ELIASZEWICZ M et al: Prospective evaluation of risk factors of cutaneous drug reactions to sulfonamides in patients with AIDS. J Am Acad Dermatol 47:40, 2002

HIRSCH LJ et al: Predictors of lamotrigine-associated rash. Epilepsia 47:318, 2006

HUNG SI et al: HLA B*5801 allele as a genetic marker for severe cutaneous reactions caused by allopurinol. Proc Natl Acad Sci USA 102:4134, 2005

LANGE-ASSCHENFELDT C et al: Cutaneous adverse reactions to psychotropic drugs: data from a multicenter surveillance program. J Clin Psychiatry 70:1258, 2009

LIN D, TUCKER MJ, RIEDER MJ: Increased adverse drug reactions to antimicrobials and anticonvulsants in patients with HIV infection. Ann Pharm 40:1594, 2006

MOCKENHAUPT M et al: Stevens-Johnson syndrome and toxic epidermal necrolysis: Assessment of medication risks with emphasis on recently marketed drugs. The EuroSCAR-Study. J Invest Dermatol 128:35, 2008

PERAZELLA MA: Advanced kidney disease, gadolinium and nephrogenic systemic fibrosis: The perfect storm. Curr Opin Nephrol Hypertens 18:519, 2009

PHILLIPS EJ, MALLAL SA: HLA and drug-induced toxicity. Curr Opin Mol Therap 11:231, 2009

ROUJEAU JC, STERN RS: Severe adverse cutaneous reactions to drugs. N Engl J Med 331:1272, 1994

CHAPTER **56**

Photosensitivity and Other Reactions to Light

Alexander G. Marneros

David R. Bickers

SOLAR RADIATION

Sunlight is the most visible and obvious source of comfort in the environment. The sun provides the beneficial effects of warmth and vitamin D synthesis; however, acute and chronic sun exposure also have pathologic consequences. Few effects of sun exposure beyond those affecting the skin have been identified, but cutaneous exposure to sunlight is the major cause of human skin cancer and can have immunosuppressive effects as well.

The sun's energy reaching the earth's surface is limited to components of the ultraviolet (UV), the visible, and portions of the infrared spectra. The cutoff at the short end of the UV is at ~290 nm; this is due primarily to stratospheric ozone formed by highly energetic ionizing radiation, preventing penetration to the earth's surface of the shorter, more energetic, potentially more harmful wavelengths of solar radiation. Indeed, concern about destruction of the ozone layer by chlorofluorocarbons released into the atmosphere has led to international agreements to reduce production of those chemicals.

Measurements of solar flux indicate that there is a twentyfold regional variation in the amount of energy at 300 nm that reaches the earth's surface. This variability relates to seasonal effects, the path that sunlight traverses through ozone and air, the altitude (4% increase for each 300 m of elevation), the latitude (increasing intensity with decreasing latitude), and the amount of cloud cover, fog, and pollution.

The major components of the photobiologic action spectrum capable of affecting human skin include the UV and visible wavelengths between 290 and 700 nm. In addition, the wavelengths beyond 700 nm in the infrared spectrum primarily emit heat and in certain circumstances may exacerbate the pathologic effects of energy in the UV and visible spectra.

The UV spectrum reaching the earth represents <10% of total incident solar energy and is arbitrarily divided into two major segments, UV-B and UV-A, constituting the wavelengths from 290–400 nm. UV-B consists of wavelengths between 290 and 320 nm. This portion of the photobiologic action spectrum is the most efficient in producing redness or erythema in human skin and hence sometimes is known as the "sunburn spectrum." UV-A includes wavelengths between 320 and 400 nm and is ~1000-fold less efficient in producing skin redness than is UV-B.

The wavelengths between 400 and 700 nm are visible to the human eye. The photon energy in the visible spectrum is not capable of damaging human skin in the absence of a photosensitizing chemical. Without the absorption of energy by a molecule, there can be no photosensitivity. Thus, the *absorption spectrum* of a molecule is defined as the range of wavelengths absorbed by it, whereas the *action spectrum* for an effect of incident radiation is defined as the range of wavelengths that evoke the response.

Photosensitivity occurs when a photon-absorbing chemical (chromophore) present in the skin absorbs incident energy, becomes excited, and transfers the absorbed energy to various structures or to oxygen.

■ UV RADIATION (UVR) AND SKIN STRUCTURE AND FUNCTION

Skin consists of two major compartments: the outer epidermis, which is a stratified squamous epithelium, and the underlying dermis, which is rich in matrix proteins such as collagens and elastin. Both compartments are susceptible to damage from sun exposure.

Cardinal Manifestations and Presentation of Diseases

PART 2

The epidermis and the dermis contain several chromophores capable of absorbing incident solar energy, including nucleic acids, proteins, and lipids. The outermost epidermal layer, the stratum corneum, is a major absorber of UV-B, and <10% of incident UV-B wavelengths penetrate through the epidermis to the dermis. Approximately 3% of radiation below 300 nm, 20% of radiation below 360 nm, and 33% of short visible radiation reaches the basal cell layer in untanned human skin. In contrast, UV-A readily penetrates to the dermis and is capable of altering structural and matrix proteins that contribute to photoaging of chronically sun-exposed skin, particularly in individuals of light complexion. Thus, longer wavelengths can penetrate more deeply into the skin.

Molecular targets for UVR-induced skin effects

Epidermal DNA, predominantly in keratinocytes and in Langerhans cells (LCs), which are dendritic antigen-presenting cells, absorbs UV-B and undergoes structural changes between adjacent pyrimidine bases (thymine or cytosine), including the formation of cyclobutane dimers and 6,4-photoproducts. These structural changes are potentially mutagenic and are found in most basal cell and squamous cell skin cancers. They can be repaired by cellular mechanisms that result in their recognition and excision and the restoration of normal base sequences. The efficient repair of these structural aberrations is crucial, since individuals with defective DNA repair are at high risk for the development of cutaneous cancer. For example, patients with xeroderma pigmentosum (XP), an autosomal recessive disorder, are characterized by variably deficient repair of UV-induced photoproducts, and their skin phenotype often manifests the dry, leathery appearance of prematurely photoaged skin as well as basal cell and squamous cell carcinomas and melanoma in the first two decades of life. Studies in mice using knockout gene technology have verified the importance of functional genes regulating these repair pathways in preventing the development of UV-induced cancer. Furthermore, incorporation of a bacterial DNA repair enzyme, T4 endonuclease V, into liposomes in a product applied to the skin of patients with XP selectively removes cyclobutane pyrimidine dimers and reduces the degree of solar damage and skin cancer. This approach also may benefit other patients who are susceptible to skin cancer, such as organ transplant recipients receiving chronic immunosuppressive drug therapy. DNA damage in LCs may contribute to the known immunosuppressive effects of UV-B (see "Immunologic Effects," below).

In addition to DNA, molecular oxygen is a target for incident solar UVR, leading to the generation of reactive oxygen species (ROS). These ROS can damage skin components, such as epidermal lipids, either free lipids in the stratum corneum or cell membrane lipids. UVR also can target proteins, leading to increased cross-linking and degradation of matrix proteins in the dermis and thus to photoaging changes known as solar elastosis.

Cutaneous optics and chromophores

Chromophores are endogenous or exogenous chemical components that can absorb physical energy. Endogenous chromophores are of two types: (1) normal components of skin, including nucleic acids, proteins, lipids, and 7-dehydrocholesterol, the precursor of vitamin D, and (2) components that are synthesized elsewhere in the body that circulate in the bloodstream and diffuse into the skin, such as porphyrins. Normally, only trace amounts of porphyrins are present in the skin, but in selected diseases known as the porphyrias (Chap. 358), increased amounts are released into the circulation from the bone marrow and the liver and are transported to the skin, where they absorb incident energy both in the Soret band, around 400 nm (short visible), and to a lesser extent in the red portion of the visible spectrum (580–660 nm). This results in the generation of

ROS that can mediate structural damage to the skin, manifested as erythema, edema, urticaria, or blister formation. It is of interest that photoexcited porphyrins are currently used therapeutically in treating nonmelanoma skin cancers and their precursor lesions, actinic keratoses. Known as photodynamic therapy (PDT), this modality generates ROS in the skin, leading to cell death. Topical photosensitizers used in PDT are the porphyrin precursors 5-aminolevulinic acid (ALA) and methyl aminolevulinate (MAL), which are converted to porphyrins in the skin. It is believed that PDT targets tumor cells for destruction more selectively than it targets adjacent nonneoplastic cells. The efficacy of PDT requires appropriate timing of the application of MAL and ALA to the affected skin followed by exposure to artificial sources of visible light. High-intensity blue light has been used successfully for the treatment of thin actinic keratoses. Red light has a longer wavelength and penetrates more deeply into the skin and is more beneficial in the treatment of superficial basal cell carcinomas.

Acute effects of sun exposure

The acute effects of skin exposure to sunlight include sunburn and vitamin D synthesis.

Sunburn This painful skin condition is an acute inflammatory response of the skin predominantly to UV-B. Generally, an individual's ability to tolerate sunlight is inversely proportional to that individual's degree of melanin pigmentation. Melanin, a complex polymer of tyrosine derivatives, is synthesized in specialized epidermal dendritic cells known as melanocytes and is packaged into melanosomes that are transferred via dendritic process into keratinocytes, thereby providing photoprotection and simultaneously darkening the skin. Sun-induced melanogenesis is a consequence of increased tyrosinase activity in melanocytes. Central to the suntan response is the melanocortin-1 receptor (MC1R), and mutations in this gene account for the wide variation in human skin and hair color. The human MC1R gene encodes a 317-amino-acid G protein-coupled receptor (melanocortin receptor) that binds α-melanocyte-stimulating hormone (α-MSH), which is secreted in the skin mainly by keratinocytes in response to UVR. This UV-induced expression of α-MSH is controlled by the tumor suppressor p53, and absence of functional p53 is known to ablate the tanning response in a mouse model. Activation of the melanocortin receptor leads to increased intracellular cyclic adenosine 5′-monophosphate (cyclic AMP) and protein kinase A activation, followed by increased transcription of microphthalmia transcription factor (MITF), which stimulates melanogenesis. Since the precursor of α-MSH, proopiomelanocortin (POMC), is also the precursor of β-endorphin, UVR results in increased pigmentation and β-endorphin production, probably promoting sun-seeking behaviors.

The Fitzpatrick classification of human skin is a function of the efficiency of the epidermal-melanin unit and usually can be ascertained by asking an individual two questions: (1) Do you burn after sun exposure? and (2) Do you tan after sun exposure? The answers to these questions permit division of the population into six skin types varying from type I (always burn, never tan) to type VI (never burn, always tan) (Table 56-1).

Sunburn erythema is due to vasodilation of dermal blood vessels. There is a lag in time between skin exposure to sunlight and the development of visible redness (usually 4–12 h), suggesting that an epidermal chromophore causes delayed production and/or release of vasoactive mediator(s), or cytokines, that diffuse to the dermal vasculature to evoke vasodilation.

The action spectrum for sunburn erythema includes UV-B and UV-A. Photons in the UV-B are at least 1000-fold more efficient than photons in the UV-A in evoking the response. However, UV-A may contribute to sunburn erythema at midday, when

TABLE 56-1 Skin Type and Sunburn Sensitivity (Fitzpatrick Classification)

Type	Description
I	Always burn, never tan
II	Always burn, sometimes tan
III	Sometimes burn, sometimes tan
IV	Sometimes burn, always tan
V	Never burn, sometimes tan
VI	Never burn, always tan

much more UV-A than UV-B is present in the solar spectrum. The erythema that accompanies the inflammatory response induced by UVR results from the orchestrated release of cytokines, along with growth factors or lipid mediators, and the generation of ROS. Furthermore, it is known that UV-induced activation of nuclear factor-κB (NF-κB)-dependent gene transcription can augment release of several proinflammatory cytokines and vasoactive mediators, including interleukin 1 (IL-1), IL-6, IL-8, IL-12, vascular endothelial growth factor, prostaglandin E_2, and tumor necrosis factor α. Local accumulation of these cytokines occurs in sunburned skin, providing chemotactic factors that attract neutrophils and macrophages, which can cause cell damage through generation of ROS. UVR also promotes infiltration of inflammatory cells through induced expression of adhesion molecules such as E-selectin and intercellular adhesion molecule-1 (ICAM-1) on endothelial cells and ICAM-1 on keratinocytes. It is of interest that nonsteroidal anti-inflammatory drugs (NSAIDs) can reduce sunburn erythema. UVR also has been shown to activate phospholipase A_2, resulting in increased eicosanoids, such as prostaglandin E_2, which is known to be a potent inducer of sunburn erythema, thereby explaining how cyclooxygenase inhibitors can reduce sunburn erythema.

Epidermal changes in sunburn include the induction of "sunburn cells," which are keratinocytes undergoing p53-dependent apoptosis as a defense for the elimination of cells that harbor UV-B-induced structural DNA damage.

Vitamin D photochemistry Cutaneous exposure to UV-B causes photolysis of epidermal 7-dehydrocholesterol, converting it to pre-vitamin D_3, which then undergoes a temperature-dependent isomerization to form the stable hormone vitamin D_3. This compound then diffuses to the dermal vasculature and circulates to the liver and kidney, where it is converted to the dihydroxylated functional hormone 1,25-dihydroxyvitamin D_3[1,25$(OH)_2D_3$]. Vitamin D metabolites from the circulation and those produced in the skin itself can augment epidermal differentiation signaling and inhibit keratinocyte proliferation. These effects on keratinocytes are used therapeutically in psoriasis with the topical application of synthetic vitamin D analogues. In addition, vitamin D is increasingly recognized to have beneficial effects in several other inflammatory conditions, and there is some evidence to suggest that it is associated with a reduced risk for various internal malignancies, aside from its classic physiologic effects on calcium metabolism and bone homeostasis. There is controversy regarding the risk/benefit of sun exposure in vitamin D homeostasis. At present, it is important to emphasize that there is no clear-cut evidence to suggest that the use of sunscreens substantially diminishes vitamin D levels. Since aging also substantially decreases the ability of human skin to photocatalytically produce vitamin D_3, the widespread use of sunscreens that filter out UV-B has led to the concern that vitamin D deficiency may become a significant clinical problem in the elderly. However, the amount of sunlight needed to produce sufficient

vitamin D is small and does not justify increased sun exposure or tanning behavior. Increased nutritional supplementation of vitamin D is advocated in patients with vitamin D deficiency rather than increasing UV exposure that is associated with carcinogenic and other types of photodamage.

Chronic effects of sun exposure: nonmalignant

The clinical features of photodamaged sun-exposed skin consist of wrinkling, blotchiness, and telangiectasia and a roughened, irregular, "weather-beaten" leathery appearance. Whether this photoaging represents accelerated chronologic aging or a separate and distinct process is not clear.

Within chronically sun-exposed epidermis, there is thickening (acanthosis) and morphologic heterogeneity within the basal cell layer. Higher but irregular melanosome content may be present in some keratinocytes, indicating prolonged residence of the cells in the basal cell layer. These structural changes may help explain the leathery texture and the blotchy discoloration of sun-damaged skin.

UV-A is important in the pathogenesis of photoaging in human skin, and ROS probably are involved. The dermis and its connective tissue matrix are the major site for sun-associated chronic damage, manifest as solar elastosis, a massive increase in thickened irregular masses of abnormal-appearing elastic fibers. Collagen fibers are also abnormally clumped in the deeper dermis of sun-damaged skin. The chromophore(s), the action spectra, and the specific biochemical events orchestrating these changes are only partially understood, although UV-A seems to be primarily involved. This could be due to the predominance of UV-A in the solar energy reaching the earth's surface as well as the fact that UV-A penetrates more deeply into the dermis. Chronologically aged sun-protected skin and photoaged skin share important molecular features, including connective tissue damage and elevated matrix metalloproteinases (MMPs). MMPs are enzymes involved in the degradation of the extracellular matrix, and UV-A induces expression of MMPs, including MMP-1 and MMP-3, leading to increased collagen breakdown. In addition, UV-A reduces type I procollagen mRNA expression. Thus, chronic UVR reduces functional collagen content in the dermis. Based on these observations, it is not surprising that high-dose UV-A phototherapy may have beneficial effects in some patients with localized fibrotic diseases of the skin, such as localized scleroderma.

Chronic effects of sun exposure: malignant

One of the major known consequences of chronic skin exposure to sunlight is nonmelanoma skin cancer. The two most common types of nonmelanoma skin cancer are *basal cell carcinoma* (BCC) and *squamous cell carcinoma* (SCC; Chap. 87). A model for skin cancer induction involves three major steps: initiation, promotion, and progression. Exposure of human skin to sunlight results in *initiation*, a step by which structural (mutagenic) changes in DNA evoke an irreversible alteration in the target cell (*keratinocyte*) that begins the tumorigenic process. Exposure to a tumor initiator such as UV-B is believed to be a necessary but not sufficient step in the malignant process, since initiated skin cells not exposed to tumor promoters generally do not develop tumors. The second stage in tumor development is *promotion*, a multistep process by which chronic exposure to sunlight evokes further changes that culminate in the clonal expansion of initiated cells and cause the development, over many years, of premalignant growths known as *actinic keratoses*, a minority of which may progress to form SCCs. Based on extensive studies, it seems clear that UV-B is a *complete carcinogen*, meaning that it can act as both a tumor initiator and a promoter.

The third and final step in the malignant process is *malignant conversion* of benign precursors into malignant lesions, a process thought to require additional genetic alterations.

On a molecular level skin carcinogenesis is thought to be caused by the accumulation of gene mutations that result in inactivation of tumor suppressors, activation of oncogenes, or reactivation of cellular signaling pathways that normally are expressed only during embryologic development of the epidermis.

Accumulation of mutations in the tumor-suppressor gene *p53* as a result of UV-induced DNA damage has been found in both SCCs and BCCs and is probably important in promoting skin carcinogenesis. Indeed, both human and murine UV-induced skin cancers have characteristic *p53* mutations (C → T and CC → TT transitions) that are present in the majority of these lesions. Studies in mice have shown that sunscreens can substantially reduce the frequency of these signature mutations in *p53* and dramatically inhibit the induction of tumors.

BCCs also manifest inactivating mutations in the tumor-suppressor gene known as *patched*, which results in activation of hedgehog signaling, and enhanced activity of *smoothened*, which in turn causes downstream activation of transcription factors that augment cell proliferation. Thus, these tumors can manifest mutations in both *p53* and *patched* or *smothered*. New evidence links alterations in the Wnt/β-catenin signaling pathway known to be critical for hair follicle development, to skin cancer as well. Thus interactions between this pathway and the hedgehog signaling pathway appear to be involved in both skin carcinogenesis and the embryologic development of the skin and hair follicles.

Studies in mouse models have strengthened the hypothesis that SCCs and BCCs are derived from cells in the epidermis with properties of stem cells, and the cells of origin for these skin cancers may be derived from the hair bulge region. The transcription factor Myc is important for stem cell maintenance in the skin, and oncogenic activation of Myc has been implicated in the development of BCCs and SCCs. Thus, nonmelanoma skin cancer involves mutations and alterations in multiple genes and pathways that occur as a result of the chronic accumulation of such changes promoted by exposure to environmental factors such as solar radiation.

Sun exposure causes nonmelanoma cancers and melanoma of the skin, although the evidence is far more direct for its role in nonmelanoma skin cancer (BCC and SCC) than its role in melanoma. Approximately 80% of nonmelanoma skin cancers develop on sun-exposed body areas, including the face, neck, and hands. Major risk factors include male sex, childhood sun exposures, older age, fair skin, and residence at latitudes closer to the equator. Whites of darker complexions (e.g., Hispanics) have one-tenth the risk of developing such cancers compared with fair-skinned individuals. Blacks are at substantially reduced risk for skin cancer. More than 1.3 million individuals in the United States develop nonmelanoma skin cancer annually, and the lifetime risk for a fair-skinned individual to develop such a neoplasm is estimated at ~15%. A consensus exists that the incidence of nonmelanoma skin cancer in the population is increasing at a rate of 2–3% per year for unknown reasons. One potential explanation is the widespread use of indoor tanning. It is estimated that 30 million people tan indoors in the United States annually, including >2 million adolescents.

The relationship of sun exposure to melanoma development is less clear-cut, but suggestive evidence supports an association. The strongest risk factors for melanoma include positive family history for melanoma, multiple dysplastic nevi, and prior melanoma. Melanomas occasionally develop by the teenage years, indicating that the latent period for tumor growth is less than that for nonmelanoma skin cancer. Melanomas are among the most rapidly increasing among all human malignancies (Chap. 87). Epidemiologic studies of immigrant populations of similar ethnic background indicate that individuals who are born in one area or who migrate to the same locale before age 10 have higher age-specific melanoma

rates than do individuals arriving later. It is thus reasonable to conclude that life in a sunny climate from birth or early childhood increases the risk of melanoma. In general, risk does not correlate with cumulative sun exposure but may be related to the duration and extent of exposure in childhood. Epidemiologic studies have shown that indoor tanning is a risk factor for melanoma.

Meta-analysis of 17 case-control studies in patients with melanoma concluded that the protective effect of sunscreens against this type of tumor could not be substantiated, but this probably is due to failure to control for confounding factors such as sunscreen stability and frequency of application. Since no prospective studies are available to address this issue, it seems reasonable to recommend that patients at risk for melanoma utilize photoprotection such as sun avoidance, high sun protective factor (SPF) sunscreens, and protective clothing.

Immunologic effects

Exposure to solar radiation causes local (inhibition of immune responses to antigens applied at the irradiated site) and systemic (inhibition of immune responses to antigens applied at remote unirradiated sites) immunosuppression. For example, administration of modest doses of UV-B to human skin reduces the degree of allergic sensitization to the potent contact allergen dinitrochlorobenzene. This is associated with depletion of epidermal LCs.

An example of the systemic immunosuppressive effects of higher doses of UVR is the diminished immunologic response to antigens introduced either epicutaneously or intracutaneously at sites distant from the irradiated site.

The major chromophores in the upper epidermis that initiate UV-mediated immunosuppression include DNA, *trans*-urocanic acid, and membrane components. The action spectrum for UV-induced immunosuppression closely mimics the absorption spectrum of DNA. Pyrimidine dimers in LCs may inhibit antigen presentation. The absorption spectrum of epidermal urocanic acid closely mimics the action spectrum for UV-B-induced immunosuppression as well. Urocanic acid is a metabolic product of the essential amino acid histidine and accumulates in the upper epidermis through breakdown of the histidine-rich protein filaggrin due to the absence of its catabolizing enzyme in keratinocytes. It is synthesized as a *trans*-isomer, and UV-induced *trans-cis* isomerization of urocanic acid in the stratum corneum leads to its immunosuppressive effects. *Cis*-urocanic acid has been proposed to exert its immunosuppressive effects through a variety of mechanisms, including inhibition of antigen presentation by LCs.

One important consequence of chronic sun exposure and the concomitant immunosuppression is enhanced risk of skin cancer. The molecular mechanisms of photocarcinogenesis are complex and only partially understood. In part, UV-B activates regulatory T cells that suppress antitumor immune responses via IL-10 expression, whereas in the absence of high UV-B exposure, epidermal antigen-presenting cells present tumor-associated antigens and induce protective immunity, thereby inhibiting skin tumorigenesis. UV-induced DNA damage is a major molecular trigger of this immunosuppressive effect.

Perhaps the most graphic demonstration of the role of immunosuppression in enhancing the risk of nonmelanoma skin cancer has come from studies of patients who are organ transplant recipients who are chronically treated with immunosuppressive antirejection drug regimens. More than 50% of transplant patients develop BCCs and SCCs, and these cancers are the most common malignancies arising in immunosuppressed solid-organ transplant recipients. Rates of BCCs and SCCs increase with the duration and the degree of immunosuppression. These patients require close periodic monitoring and rigorous photoprotection through the use of sunscreens, protective clothing, and sun avoidance.

■ PHOTOSENSITIVITY DISEASES

The diagnosis of photosensitivity requires a careful history to define the duration of the signs and symptoms, the length of time between exposure to sunlight and the development of subjective complaints, and visible changes in the skin. The age of onset can also be a helpful clue; for example, the acute photosensitivity of erythropoietic protoporphyria almost always begins in childhood, whereas the chronic photosensitivity of porphyria cutanea tarda (PCT) typically begins in the fourth and fifth decades. A history of exposure to topical and systemic drugs and chemicals may provide important clues. Many classes of drugs can cause photosensitivity on the basis of either phototoxicity or photoallergy. Fragrances such as musk ambrette that were previously present in numerous cosmetic products are also potent photosensitizers.

Examination of the skin also may offer important clues. Anatomic areas that are naturally protected from direct sunlight, such as the hairy scalp, the upper eyelids, the retroauricular areas, and the infranasal and submental regions, may be spared, whereas exposed areas show characteristic features of the pathologic process. These anatomic localization patterns are often helpful but not infallible in making the diagnosis. For example, airborne contact sensitizers that are blown onto the skin may produce a dermatitis that can be difficult to distinguish from photosensitivity despite the fact that such material may trigger skin reactivity in areas shielded from direct sunlight.

Many dermatologic conditions may be caused or aggravated by sunlight (Table 56-2). The role of light in evoking these responses may be dependent on genetic abnormalities ranging from well-described defects in DNA repair that occur in XP to the inherited abnormalities in heme synthesis that characterize the porphyrias. In certain photosensitivity diseases the chromophore has been identified, whereas in the majority, the energy-absorbing agent is unknown.

Polymorphous light eruption

After sunburn, the most common type of photosensitivity disease is *polymorphous light eruption* (PLE). Many affected individuals never seek medical attention because the condition is often transient, becoming manifest each spring with initial sun exposure but then subsiding spontaneously with continuing exposure, a phenomenon known as "hardening." The major manifestations of PLE include pruritic (often intensely so) erythematous papules that may coalesce into plaques in a patchy distribution on exposed areas of the trunk and forearms. The face is usually less seriously involved. Whereas the morphologic skin findings remain similar for each patient with subsequent recurrences, significant interindividual variations in skin findings are characteristic (hence the term "polymorphous").

The diagnosis can be confirmed by skin biopsy and by performing phototest procedures in which skin is exposed to multiple erythema doses of UV-A and UV-B. The action spectrum for PLE is usually within these portions of the solar spectrum.

Whereas the treatment of an acute flare of PLE may require topical or systemic glucocorticoids, approaches to prevent PLE are important and include the use of broad-spectrum sunscreens and the induction of hardening by the cautious administration of artificial UV-B (broad-band or narrow-band) and/or UV-A radiation or the use of psoralen plus UV-A (PUVA) photochemotherapy for 2–4 weeks before initial sun exposure. Such prophylactic phototherapy or photochemotherapy at the beginning of spring may prevent the occurrence of PLE throughout the summer.

Phototoxicity and photoallergy

These photosensitivity disorders are related to the topical or systemic administration of drugs and other chemicals. Both reactions

TABLE 56-2 Classification of Photosensitivity Diseases

Type	Disease
Genetic	Erythropoietic porphyria
	Erythropoietic protoporphyria
	Porphyria cutanea tarda—familial
	Variegate porphyria
	Hepatoerythropoietic porphyria
	Albinism
	Xeroderma pigmentosum
	Rothmund-Thomson syndrome
	Bloom syndrome
	Cockayne's disease
	Kindler syndrome
	Phenylketonuria
Metabolic	Porphyria cutanea tarda—sporadic
	Hartnup disease
	Kwashiorkor
	Pellagra
	Carcinoid syndrome
Phototoxic	
Internal	Drugs
External	Drugs, plants, food
Photoallergic	
Immediate	Solar urticaria
Delayed	Drug photoallergy
	Persistent light reaction/chronic actinic dermatitis
Neoplastic and degenerative	Photoaging
	Actinic keratosis
	Melanoma and nonmelanoma skin cancer
Idiopathic	Polymorphous light eruption
	Hydroa aestivale
	Actinic prurigo
Photoaggravated	Lupus erythematosus
	Systemic
	Subacute cutaneous
	Discoid
	Dermatomyositis
	Herpes simplex
	Lichen planus actinicus
	Acne vulgaris (aestivale)

require the absorption of energy by a drug or chemical resulting in the production of an excited-state photosensitizer that can transfer its absorbed energy to a bystander molecule or to molecular oxygen, thereby generating tissue-destructive chemical species, including ROS.

Phototoxicity is a nonimmunologic reaction caused by drugs and chemicals, a few of which are listed in Table 56-3. The usual clinical manifestations include erythema resembling a sunburn reaction that quickly desquamates, or "peels," within several days. In addition, edema, vesicles, and bullae may occur.

TABLE 56-3 Phototoxic Drugs

	Topical	Systemic
Amiodarone		+
Dacarbazine		+
Fluoroquinolones		+
5-Fluorouracil	+	+
Furosemide		+
Nalidixic acid		+
Phenothiazines		+
Psoralens	+	+
Retinoids	+/−	+
Sulfonamides		+
Sulfonylureas		+
Tetracyclines		+
Thiazides		+
Vinblastine		+

Photoallergy is much less common and is distinct in that it is an immunopathologic process. The excited-state photosensitizer may create highly unstable haptenic free radicals that bind covalently to macromolecules to form a functional antigen capable of evoking a delayed hypersensitivity response. Some of the drugs and chemicals that produce photoallergy are listed in Table 56-4. The clinical manifestations typically differ from those of phototoxicity in that an intensely pruritic eczematous dermatitis tends to predominate and evolves into lichenified, thickened, "leathery" changes in sun-exposed areas. A small subset (perhaps 5–10%) of patients with photoallergy may develop a persistent exquisite hypersensitivity to light even when the offending drug or chemical is identified and eliminated, a condition known as *persistent light reaction*.

TABLE 56-4 Photoallergic Drugs

	Topical	Systemic
6-Methylcoumarin	+	
Aminobenzoic acid and esters	+	
Bithionol	+	
Chlorpromazine		+
Diclofenac		+
Fluoroquinolones		+
Halogenated salicylanilides	+	
Hypericin (St John's wort)	+	+
Musk ambrette	+	
Piroxicam		+
Promethazine		+
Sulfonamides		+
Sulfonylureas		+

A very uncommon type of persistent photosensitivity is known as *chronic actinic dermatitis*. These patients are typically elderly men with a long history of preexisting allergic contact dermatitis or photosensitivity. They are usually exquisitely sensitive to UV-B, UV-A, and visible wavelengths.

Diagnostic confirmation of phototoxicity and photoallergy often can be obtained by using phototest procedures. In patients with suspected phototoxicity, determining the minimal erythema dose (MED) while the patient is exposed to a suspected agent and then repeating the MED after discontinuation of the agent may provide a clue to the causative drug or chemical. Photopatch testing can be performed to confirm the diagnosis of photoallergy. This is a simple variant of ordinary patch testing in which a series of known photoallergens is applied to the skin in duplicate and one set is irradiated with a suberythema dose of UV-A. Development of eczematous changes at sites exposed to sensitizer and light is a positive result. The characteristic abnormality in patients with persistent light reaction is a diminished threshold to erythema evoked by UV-B. Patients with chronic actinic dermatitis usually manifest a broad spectrum of UV hyperresponsiveness and require meticulous photoprotection, including avoiding sun exposure, high (>30) SPF sunscreens, and in severe cases systemic immunosuppression, preferably with azathioprine (1–2 mg/kg per day).

The management of drug photosensitivity involves first and foremost the elimination of exposure to the chemical agents responsible for the reaction and minimization of sun exposure. The acute symptoms of phototoxicity may be ameliorated by cool moist compresses, topical glucocorticoids, and systemically administered NSAIDs. In severely affected individuals, a rapidly tapered course of systemic glucocorticoids may be useful. Judicious use of analgesics may be necessary.

Photoallergic reactions require a similar management approach. Furthermore, patients with persistent light reaction and chronic actinic dermatitis must be meticulously protected against light exposure. In selected patients in whom chronic systemic high-dose glucocorticoids pose unacceptable risks, it may be necessary to employ an immunosuppressive drug such as azathioprine, cyclophosphamide, cyclosporine, or mycophenolate mofetil.

Porphyria

The porphyrias (Chap. 358) are a group of diseases that have in common inherited or acquired derangements in the synthesis of heme. Heme is an iron-chelated tetrapyrrole or porphyrin, and the nonmetal chelated porphyrins are potent photosensitizers that absorb light intensely in both the short (400–410 nm) and the long (580–650 nm) portions of the visible spectrum.

Heme cannot be reutilized and must be synthesized continuously, and the two body compartments with the largest capacity for its production are the bone marrow and the liver. Accordingly, the porphyrias originate in one or the other of these organs, with the end result of excessive endogenous production of potent photosensitizing porphyrins. The porphyrins circulate in the bloodstream and diffuse into the skin, where they absorb solar energy, become photoexcited, generate ROS, and evoke cutaneous photosensitivity. The mechanism of porphyrin photosensitization is known to be photodynamic, or oxygen-dependent, and is mediated by ROS such as singlet oxygen and superoxide anions.

Porphyria cutanea tarda (PCT) is the most common type of human porphyria and is associated with decreased activity of the enzyme uroporphyrinogen decarboxylase. There are two basic types of PCT: (1) the sporadic or acquired type, generally seen in individuals ingesting ethanol or receiving estrogens, and (2) the inherited type, in which there is autosomal dominant transmission of deficient enzyme activity. Both forms are associated with increased hepatic iron stores.

In both types of PCT, the predominant feature is a chronic photosensitivity characterized by increased fragility of sun-exposed skin, particularly areas subject to repeated trauma, such as the dorsa of the hands, the forearms, the face, and the ears. The predominant skin lesions are vesicles and bullae that rupture, producing moist erosions, often with a hemorrhagic base, that heal slowly with crusting and purplish discoloration of the affected skin. Hypertrichosis, mottled pigmentary change, and scleroderma-like induration are associated features. Biochemical confirmation of the diagnosis can be obtained by measurement of urinary porphyrin excretion, plasma porphyrin assay, and assay of erythrocyte and/or hepatic uroporphyrinogen decarboxylase. Multiple mutations of the uroporphyrinogen decarboxylase gene have been identified in human populations. Some patients with PCT have associated mutations in the *HFE* gene, which is linked to hemochromatosis. This could contribute to the iron overload seen in PCT, although iron status as measured by serum ferritin, iron levels, and transferrin saturation is no different from that in PCT patients without *HFE* mutations. Prior hepatitis C virus infection appears to be an independent risk factor for PCT.

Treatment of PCT consists of repeated phlebotomies to diminish the excessive hepatic iron stores and/or intermittent low doses of the antimalarial drugs chloroquine and hydroxychloroquine. Long-term remission of the disease can be achieved if the patient eliminates exposure to porphyrinogenic agents.

Erythropoietic protoporphyria originates in the bone marrow and is due to a decrease in the mitochondrial enzyme ferrochelatase secondary to numerous gene mutations. The major clinical features include an acute photosensitivity characterized by subjective burning and stinging of exposed skin that often develops during or just after sun exposure. There may be associated skin swelling and, after repeated episodes, a waxlike scarring.

The diagnosis is confirmed by demonstration of elevated levels of free erythrocyte protoporphyrin. Detection of increased plasma protoporphyrin helps differentiate lead poisoning and iron-deficiency anemia, in both of which elevated erythrocyte protoporphyrin levels occur in the absence of cutaneous photosensitivity and elevated plasma protoporphyrin levels.

Treatment consists of reducing sun exposure and the oral administration of the carotenoid β-carotene, which is an effective scavenger of free radicals. This drug increases tolerance to sun exposure in many affected individuals, although it has no effect on deficient ferrochelatase.

An algorithm for managing patients with photosensitivity is illustrated in Fig. 56-1.

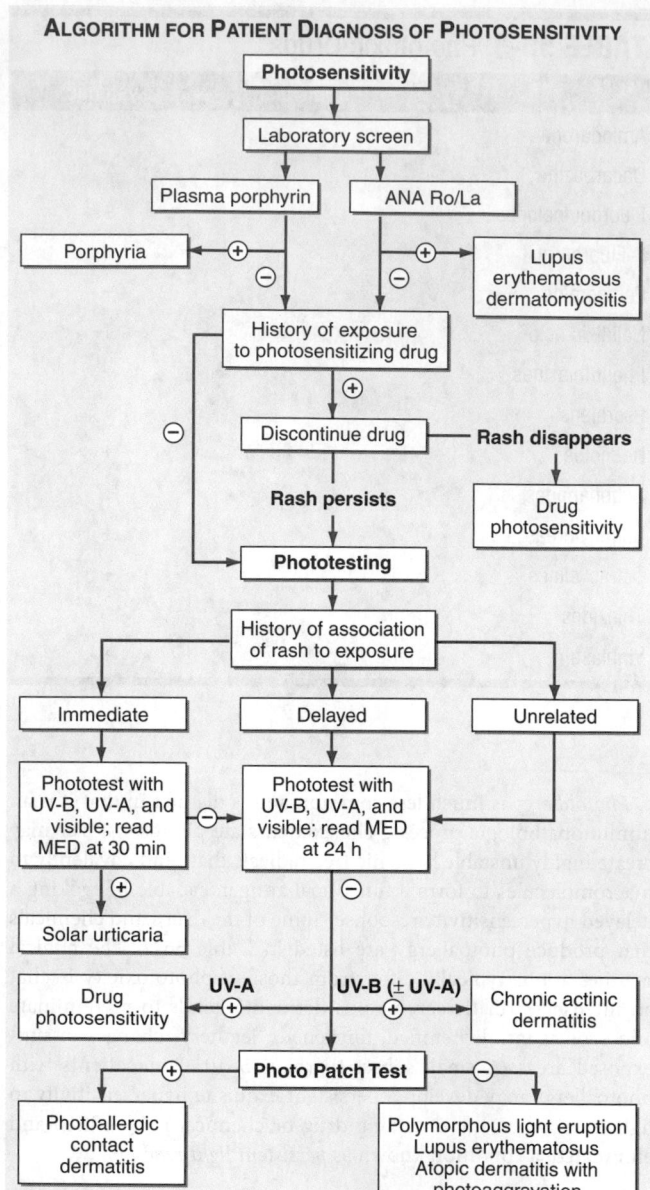

Figure 56-1 An algorithm for the diagnosis of a patient with photosensitivity.

PHOTOPROTECTION

Since photosensitivity of the skin results from exposure to sunlight, it follows that absolute avoidance of the sun will eliminate these disorders. Unfortunately, contemporary lifestyles make this an impractical alternative for most individuals, and this has led to a search for better approaches to photoprotection.

Natural photoprotection is provided by structural proteins in the epidermis, particularly keratins and melanin. The amount of melanin and its distribution in cells are genetically regulated, and individuals of darker complexion (skin types IV–VI) are at decreased risk for the development of acute sunburn and cutaneous malignancy.

Other forms of photoprotection include clothing and sunscreens. Clothing constructed of tightly woven sun-protective fabrics, irrespective of color, affords substantial protection. Wide-brimmed hats, long sleeves, and trousers all reduce direct exposure. Sunscreens are now considered over-the-counter drugs, and category I ingredients are recognized by the U.S. Food and Drug Administration (FDA)

as monographed and safe and effective. Those ingredients are listed in Table 56-5. Sunscreens are rated for their photoprotective effect by their sun protection factor. The SPF is simply a ratio of the time required to produce sunburn erythema with and without sunscreen application. Thus, the SPF of sunscreens reflects mainly protection from UV-B and does not reflect protection from UV-A. The monograph stipulates that sunscreens must be rated on a scale ranging from minimal (SPF ≥2 and <12) to moderate (SPF ≥12 and <30) to high (SPF ≥30, labeled as 30+).

Broad-spectrum sunscreens contain in addition to UV-B-absorbing chemicals UV-A-absorbing chemicals, such as avobenzone and ecamsule (terephthalylidene dicamphor sulfonic acid). These chemicals absorb UVR and transfer the absorbed energy to surrounding cells either as heat or by emission of fluorescence or phosphorescence. In contrast, physical UV blockers (zinc oxide and titanium dioxide) scatter or reflect UVR.

In addition to light absorption, a critical determinant of the sustained photoprotective effect of sunscreens is their water resistance.

TABLE 56-5 FDA Category 1 Monographed Sunscreen Ingredients[a]

Ingredients	Maximum Concentration, %
p-Aminobenzoic acid (PABA)	15
Avobenzone	3
Cinoxate	3
Dioxybenzone (benzophenone-8)	3
Ecamsule[b]	15
Homosalate	15
Menthyl anthranilate	5
Octocrylene	10
Octyl methoxycinnamate	7.5
Octyl salicylate	5
Oxybenzone (benzophenone-3)	6
Padimate O (octyl dimethyl PABA)	8
Phenylbenzimidazole sulfonic acid	4
Sulisobenzone (benzophenone-4)	10
Titanium dioxide	25
Trolamine salicylate	12
Zinc oxide	25

[a]FDA, U.S. Food and Drug Administration.
[b]Recently approved by the FDA.

The FDA monograph has defined strict testing criteria for sunscreens making this claim.

Some degree of photoprotection can be achieved by limiting the time of exposure during the day. Since a large part of an individual's total lifetime sun exposure may occur by age 18, it is important to educate parents and young children about the hazards of sunlight. Simply eliminating exposure at midday will substantially reduce lifetime UV-B exposure.

PHOTOTHERAPY AND PHOTOCHEMOTHERAPY

UVR also can be used therapeutically. The administration of UV-B alone or in combination with topically applied agents can induce remissions of many dermatologic diseases, including psoriasis and atopic dermatitis. In particular, narrow-band UV-B treatments (with fluorescent bulbs emitting radiation at ~311 nm) have enhanced efficacy compared with broad-band UV-B in the treatment of psoriasis.

Photochemotherapy in which topically applied or systemically administered psoralens are combined with UV-A (PUVA) is also effective in treating psoriasis and the early stages of cutaneous T cell lymphoma and vitiligo. Psoralens are tricyclic furocoumarins that, when intercalated into DNA and exposed to UV-A, form adducts with pyrimidine bases and eventually form DNA cross-links. These structural changes are thought to decrease DNA synthesis and relate

to the improvement that occurs in psoriasis. The reason why PUVA photochemotherapy is effective in cutaneous T cell lymphoma is not clear, but it has been shown to induce apoptosis of atypical T-lymphocyte populations in the skin. Consequently, direct treatment of circulating atypical lymphocytes by extracorporeal photochemotherapy (photopheresis) has been used in Sézary syndrome as well as in other severe systemic diseases with circulating atypical lymphocytes, such as graft-versus-host disease.

In addition to its effects on DNA, PUVA photochemotherapy stimulates epidermal thickening and melanin synthesis; the latter provides the rationale for its use in the depigmenting disease vitiligo, together with its anti-inflammatory effects. Oral 8-methoxypsoralen and UV-A appear to be most effective in this regard, but as many as 100 treatments extending over 12–18 months may be required to promote satisfactory repigmentation.

Not surprisingly the major side effects of long-term UV-B phototherapy and PUVA photochemotherapy mimic those seen in individuals with chronic sun exposure and include skin dryness, actinic keratoses, and an increased risk of skin cancer. Despite these risks, the therapeutic index of these modalities continues to be excellent. It is important to choose the most appropriate phototherapy treatment approach for a specific dermatologic disease. For example, narrow-band UV-B has been reported in several studies to be as effective as PUVA photochemotherapy in the treatment of psoriasis but to have a lower risk of skin cancer development than PUVA.

FURTHER READING

Benjamin CL, Ananthaswamy HN: p53 and the pathogenesis of skin cancer. Toxicol Appl Pharmacol 224:221, 2007

Cui R et al: Central role of p53 in the suntan response and pathologic hyperpigmentation. Cell 128:853, 2007

Deeb KK et al: Vitamin D signaling pathways in cancer: Potential for anticancer therapeutics. Nat Rev Cancer 7:684, 2007

Epstein EH: Basal cell carcinomas: Attack of the hedgehog. Nat Rev Cancer 8(10):1275, 2008

Laga AC, Murphy GF: The translational basis of human cutaneous photoaging. Am J Pathol 174:357, 2009

Malanchi I et al: Cutaneous cancer stem cell maintenance is dependent on beta-catenin signalling. Nature 452:650, 2008

Miller AJ, Mihm MC Jr: Melanoma. N Engl J Med 355:51, 2006

Morison WL: Photosensitivity. N Engl J Med 350:111, 2004

Sage RJ, Lim HW: Therapeutic Hotline: Recommendations on photoprotection and vitamin D. Dermatol Ther 23:82, 2010

Schade N et al: Ultraviolet B radiation–induced immunosuppression: Molecular mechanisms and cellular alterations. Photochem Photobiol Sci 3:699, 2005

Wong TH, Rees JL: The relation between melanocortin I receptor variation and generation of phenotypic diversity in the cutaneous response to ultraviolet radiation. Peptides 26:1965, 2005

Yaar M, Gilchrest BA: Photoageing: Mechanism, prevention and therapy. Br J Dermatol 157: 874, 2007

Yang SH et al: Pathological responses to oncogenic Hedgehog signaling in skin are dependent on canonical Wnt/β-catenin signaling. Nat Genet 40: 1130, 2008

CHAPTER **57**

Anemia and Polycythemia

John W. Adamson

Dan L. Longo

HEMATOPOIESIS AND THE PHYSIOLOGIC BASIS OF RED CELL PRODUCTION

Hematopoiesis is the process by which the formed elements of blood are produced. The process is regulated through a series of steps beginning with the hematopoietic stem cell. Stem cells are capable of producing red cells, all classes of granulocytes, monocytes, platelets, and the cells of the immune system. The precise molecular mechanism—either intrinsic to the stem cell itself or through the action of extrinsic factors—by which the stem cell becomes committed to a given lineage is not fully defined. However, experiments in mice suggest that erythroid cells come from a common erythroid/megakaryocyte progenitor that does not develop in the absence of expression of the GATA-1 and FOG-1 (friend of GATA-1) transcription factors (Chap. 66). Following lineage commitment, hematopoietic progenitor and precursor cells come increasingly under the regulatory influence of growth factors and hormones. For red cell production, erythropoietin (EPO) is the regulatory hormone. EPO is required for the maintenance of committed erythroid progenitor cells that, in the absence of the hormone, undergo programmed cell death (*apoptosis*). The regulated process of red cell production is *erythropoiesis*, and its key elements are illustrated in Fig. 57-1.

In the bone marrow, the first morphologically recognizable erythroid precursor is the pronormoblast. This cell can undergo four to five cell divisions, which result in the production of 16–32 mature red cells. With increased EPO production, or the administration of EPO as a drug, early progenitor cell numbers are amplified and, in turn, give rise to increased numbers of erythrocytes. The regulation of EPO production itself is linked to tissue oxygenation.

In mammals, O_2 is transported to tissues bound to the hemoglobin contained within circulating red cells. The mature red cell is 8 μm in diameter, anucleate, discoid in shape, and extremely pliable in order to traverse the microcirculation successfully; its membrane integrity is maintained by the intracellular generation of ATP. Normal red cell production results in the daily replacement of 0.8–1% of all circulating red cells in the body, since the average red cell lives 100–120 days. The organ responsible for red cell production is called the *erythron*. The erythron is a dynamic organ made up of a rapidly proliferating pool of marrow erythroid precursor cells and a large mass of mature circulating red blood cells. The size of the red cell mass reflects the balance of red cell production and destruction. The physiologic basis of red cell production and destruction provides an understanding of the mechanisms that can lead to anemia.

The physiologic regulator of red cell production, the glycoprotein hormone EPO, is produced and released by peritubular capillary lining cells within the kidney. These cells are highly specialized epithelial-like cells. A small amount of EPO is produced by hepatocytes. The fundamental stimulus for EPO production is the availability of O_2 for tissue metabolic needs. Key to EPO gene regulation is hypoxia-inducible factor (HIF)-1α. In the presence of O_2, HIF-1α is hydroxylated at a key proline, allowing HIF-1α to be ubiquitinylated and degraded via the proteasome pathway. If O_2 becomes limiting, this critical hydroxylation step does not occur, allowing HIF-1α to partner with other proteins, translocate to the nucleus, and upregulate the EPO gene, among others.

Impaired O_2 delivery to the kidney can result from a decreased red cell mass (*anemia*), impaired O_2 loading of the hemoglobin molecule or a high O_2 affinity mutant hemoglobin (*hypoxemia*), or, rarely, impaired blood flow to the kidney (renal artery stenosis). EPO governs the day-to-day production of red cells, and ambient levels of the hormone can be measured in the plasma by sensitive immunoassays—the normal level being 10–25 U/L. When the hemoglobin concentration falls below 100–120 g/L (10–12 g/dL), plasma EPO levels increase in proportion to the severity of the anemia (Fig. 57-2). In circulation, EPO has a half-clearance time of 6–9 h. EPO acts by binding to specific receptors on the surface of marrow erythroid precursors, inducing them to proliferate and to mature. With EPO stimulation, red cell production can increase four- to fivefold within a 1- to 2-week period, but only in the presence of adequate nutrients, especially iron. The functional capacity of the erythron, therefore, requires normal renal production of EPO, a functioning erythroid marrow, and an adequate supply of substrates for hemoglobin synthesis. A defect in any of these key components can lead to anemia. Generally, anemia is recognized in the laboratory when a patient's hemoglobin level or hematocrit is reduced below an expected value (the normal range). The likelihood and severity of anemia are defined based on the deviation of the patient's hemoglobin/hematocrit from values expected for age- and sex-matched normal subjects. The hemoglobin concentration in adults has a Gaussian distribution. The mean hematocrit value for adult males is 47% (± SD 7) and that for adult females is 42% (± 5). Any single hematocrit or hemoglobin value carries with it a likelihood of associated anemia. Thus, a hematocrit of ≤39% in an adult male or <35% in an adult female has only about a 25% chance of

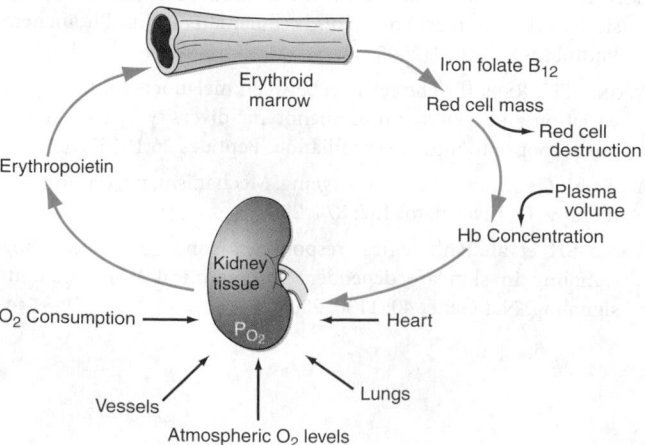

Figure 57-1 The physiologic regulation of red cell production by tissue oxygen tension. Hb, hemoglobin.

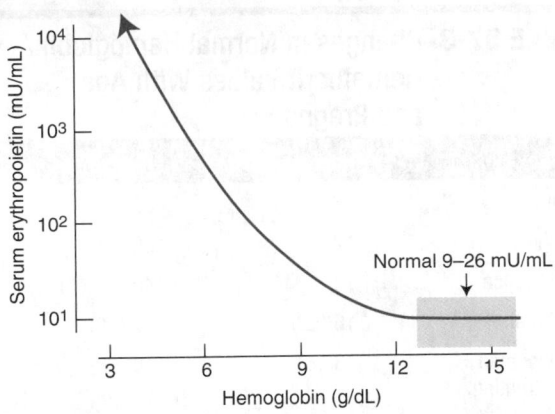

Figure 57-2 Erythropoietin (EPO) levels in response to anemia. When the hemoglobin level falls to 120 g/L (12 g/dL), plasma EPO levels increase logarithmically. In the presence of chronic kidney disease or chronic inflammation, EPO levels are typically lower than expected for the degree of anemia. As individuals age, the level of EPO needed to sustain normal hemoglobin levels appears to increase. *(From Hillman et al.)*

being normal. Suspected low hemoglobin or hematocrit values are more easily interpreted if previous values for the same patient are known for comparison. The World Health Organization (WHO) defines anemia as a hemoglobin level <130 g/L (13 g/dL) in men and <120 g/L (12 g/dL) in women.

The critical elements of erythropoiesis—EPO production, iron availability, the proliferative capacity of the bone marrow, and effective maturation of red cell precursors—are used for the initial classification of anemia (see below).

ANEMIA

CLINICAL PRESENTATION OF ANEMIA

Signs and symptoms

Anemia is most often recognized by abnormal screening laboratory tests. Patients less commonly present with advanced anemia and its attendant signs and symptoms. Acute anemia is due to blood loss or hemolysis. If blood loss is mild, enhanced O_2 delivery is achieved through changes in the O_2–hemoglobin dissociation curve mediated by a decreased pH or increased CO_2 (*Bohr effect*). With acute blood loss, hypovolemia dominates the clinical picture and the hematocrit and hemoglobin levels do not reflect the volume of blood lost. Signs of vascular instability appear with acute losses of 10–15% of the total blood volume. In such patients, the issue is not anemia but hypotension and decreased organ perfusion. When >30% of the blood volume is lost suddenly, patients are unable to compensate with the usual mechanisms of vascular contraction and changes in regional blood flow. The patient prefers to remain supine and will show postural hypotension and tachycardia. If the volume of blood lost is >40% (i.e., >2 L in the average-sized adult), signs of hypovolemic shock including confusion, dyspnea, diaphoresis, hypotension, and tachycardia appear (Chap. 106). Such patients have significant deficits in vital organ perfusion and require immediate volume replacement.

With acute hemolysis, the signs and symptoms depend on the mechanism that leads to red cell destruction. Intravascular hemolysis with release of free hemoglobin may be associated with acute back pain, free hemoglobin in the plasma and urine, and renal failure. Symptoms associated with more chronic or progressive anemia depend on the age of the patient and the adequacy of blood supply to critical organs. Symptoms associated with moderate anemia include fatigue, loss of stamina, breathlessness,

and tachycardia (particularly with physical exertion). However, because of the intrinsic compensatory mechanisms that govern the O_2–hemoglobin dissociation curve, the gradual onset of anemia—particularly in young patients—may not be associated with signs or symptoms until the anemia is severe [hemoglobin <70–80 g/L (7–8 g/dL)]. When anemia develops over a period of days or weeks, the total blood volume is normal to slightly increased, and changes in cardiac output and regional blood flow help compensate for the overall loss in O_2-carrying capacity. Changes in the position of the O_2–hemoglobin dissociation curve account for some of the compensatory response to anemia. With chronic anemia, intracellular levels of 2,3-bisphosphoglycerate rise, shifting the dissociation curve to the right and facilitating O_2 unloading. This compensatory mechanism can only maintain normal tissue O_2 delivery in the face of a 20–30 g/L (2–3 g/dL) deficit in hemoglobin concentration. Finally, further protection of O_2 delivery to vital organs is achieved by the shunting of blood away from organs that are relatively rich in blood supply, particularly the kidney, gut, and skin.

Certain disorders are commonly associated with anemia. Chronic inflammatory states (e.g., infection, rheumatoid arthritis, cancer) are associated with mild to moderate anemia, whereas lymphoproliferative disorders, such as chronic lymphocytic leukemia and certain other B cell neoplasms, may be associated with autoimmune hemolysis.

APPROACH TO THE PATIENT: Anemia

The evaluation of the patient with anemia requires a careful history and physical examination. Nutritional history related to drugs or alcohol intake and family history of anemia should always be assessed. Certain geographic backgrounds and ethnic origins are associated with an increased likelihood of an inherited disorder of the hemoglobin molecule or intermediary metabolism. Glucose-6-phosphate dehydrogenase (G6PD) deficiency and certain hemoglobinopathies are seen more commonly in those of Middle Eastern or African origin, including African Americans who have a high frequency of G6PD deficiency. Other information that may be useful includes exposure to certain toxic agents or drugs and symptoms related to other disorders commonly associated with anemia. These include symptoms and signs such as bleeding, fatigue, malaise, fever, weight loss, night sweats, and other systemic symptoms. Clues to the mechanisms of anemia may be provided on physical examination by findings of infection, blood in the stool, lymphadenopathy, splenomegaly, or petechiae. Splenomegaly and lymphadenopathy suggest an underlying lymphoproliferative disease, while petechiae suggest platelet dysfunction. Past laboratory measurements are helpful to determine a time of onset.

In the anemic patient, physical examination may demonstrate a forceful heartbeat, strong peripheral pulses, and a systolic "flow" murmur. The skin and mucous membranes may be pale if the hemoglobin is <80–100 g/L (8–10 g/dL). This part of the physical examination should focus on areas where vessels are close to the surface such as the mucous membranes, nail beds, and palmar creases. If the palmar creases are lighter in color than the surrounding skin when the hand is hyperextended, the hemoglobin level is usually <80 g/L (8 g/dL).

LABORATORY EVALUATION Table 57-1 lists the tests used in the initial workup of anemia. A routine complete blood count (CBC) is required as part of the evaluation and includes the hemoglobin, hematocrit, and red cell indices: the mean cell volume (MCV) in femtoliters, mean cell hemoglobin (MCH) in picograms per cell, and mean concentration of hemoglobin per

TABLE 57-1 Laboratory Tests in Anemia Diagnosis

I. Complete blood count (CBC)
   A. Red blood cell count
      1. Hemoglobin
      2. Hematocrit
      3. Reticulocyte count
   B. Red blood cell indices
      1. Mean cell volume (MCV)
      2. Mean cell hemoglobin (MCH)
      3. Mean cell hemoglobin concentration (MCHC)
      4. Red cell distribution width (RDW)
   C. White blood cell count
      1. Cell differential
      2. Nuclear segmentation of neutrophils
   D. Platelet count
   E. Cell morphology
      1. Cell size
      2. Hemoglobin content
      3. Anisocytosis
      4. Poikilocytosis
      5. Polychromasia

II. Iron supply studies
   A. Serum iron
   B. Total iron-binding capacity
   C. Serum ferritin
III. Marrow examination
   A. Aspirate
      1. M/E ratio[a]
      2. Cell morphology
      3. Iron stain
   B. Biopsy
      1. Cellularity
      2. Morphology

[a]M/E ratio, ratio of myeloid to erythroid precursors.

TABLE 57-3 Changes in Normal Hemoglobin/Hematocrit Values With Age and Pregnancy

Age/Sex	Hemoglobin g/dL	Hematocrit %
At birth	17	52
Childhood	12	36
Adolescence	13	40
Adult man	16 (±2)	47 (±6)
Adult woman (menstruating)	13 (±2)	40 (±6)
Adult woman (postmenopausal)	14 (±2)	42 (±6)
During pregnancy	12 (±2)	37 (±6)

Source: From Hillman et al.

volume of red cells (MCHC) in grams per liter (non-SI: grams per deciliter). The red cell indices are calculated as shown in Table 57-2, and the normal variations in the hemoglobin and hematocrit with age are shown in Table 57-3. A number of physiologic factors affect the CBC, including age, sex, pregnancy, smoking, and altitude. High-normal hemoglobin values may be seen in men and women who live at altitude or smoke heavily. Hemoglobin elevations due to smoking reflect normal compensation due to the displacement of O_2 by CO in hemoglobin binding. Other important information is provided by the reticulocyte count and measurements of iron supply including *serum iron*, *total iron-binding capacity* (TIBC; an indirect measure of the transferrin level), and *serum ferritin*. Marked alterations in the red cell indices usually reflect disorders of maturation or iron deficiency. A careful evaluation of the peripheral blood smear is important, and clinical laboratories often provide a description of both the red and white cells, a white cell differential count, and the platelet count. In patients with severe anemia

TABLE 57-2 Red Blood Cell Indices

Index	Normal Value
Mean cell volume (MCV) = (hematocrit × 10)/(red cell count × 10⁶)	90 ± 8 fL
Mean cell hemoglobin (MCH) = (hemoglobin × 10)/(red cell count × 10⁶)	30 ± 3 pg
Mean cell hemoglobin concentration = (hemoglobin × 10)/hematocrit, or MCH/MCV	33 ± 2%

and abnormalities in red blood cell morphology and/or low reticulocyte counts, a bone marrow aspirate or biopsy can assist in the diagnosis. Other tests of value in the diagnosis of specific anemias are discussed in chapters on specific disease states.

The components of the CBC also help in the classification of anemia. *Microcytosis* is reflected by a lower than normal MCV (<80), whereas high values (>100) reflect *macrocytosis*. The MCH and MCHC reflect defects in hemoglobin synthesis (*hypochromia*). Automated cell counters describe the red cell volume distribution width (RDW). The MCV (representing the peak of the distribution curve) is insensitive to the appearance of small populations of macrocytes or microcytes. An experienced laboratory technician will be able to identify minor populations of large or small cells or hypochromic cells before the red cell indices change.

Peripheral Blood Smear The peripheral blood smear provides important information about defects in red cell production (Chap. e17). As a complement to the red cell indices, the blood smear also reveals variations in cell size (*anisocytosis*) and shape (*poikilocytosis*). The degree of anisocytosis usually correlates with increases in the RDW or the range of cell sizes. Poikilocytosis suggests a defect in the maturation of red cell precursors in the bone marrow or fragmentation of circulating red cells. The blood smear may also reveal *polychromasia*—red cells that are slightly larger than normal and grayish blue in color on the Wright-Giemsa stain. These cells are reticulocytes that have been prematurely released from the bone marrow, and their color represents residual amounts of ribosomal RNA. These cells appear in circulation in response to EPO stimulation or to architectural damage of the bone marrow (fibrosis, infiltration of the marrow by malignant cells, etc.) that results in their disordered release from the marrow. The appearance of nucleated red cells, Howell-Jolly bodies, target cells, sickle cells, and others may provide clues to specific disorders (Figs. 57-3 to 57-11).

Reticulocyte Count An accurate reticulocyte count is key to the initial classification of anemia. Normally, reticulocytes are red cells that have been recently released from the bone marrow. They are identified by staining with a supravital dye that precipitates the ribosomal RNA (Fig. 57-12). These precipitates appear as blue or black punctate spots. This residual RNA is metabolized over the first 24–36 h of the reticulocyte's life span in circulation. Normally, the reticulocyte count ranges from 1 to

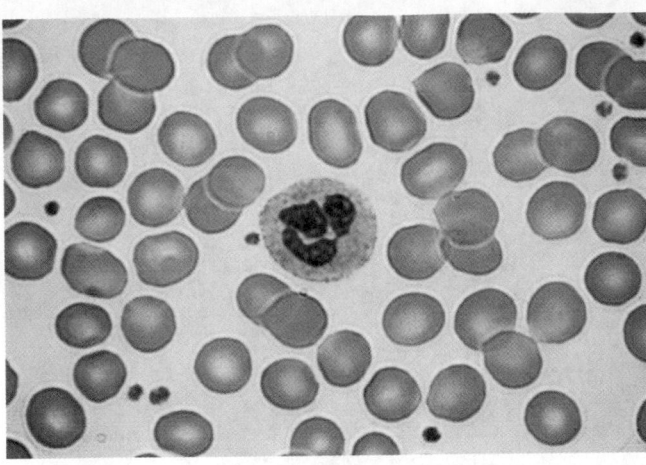

Figure 57-3 Normal blood smear (Wright stain). High-power field showing normal red cells, a neutrophil, and a few platelets. *(From Hillman et al.)*

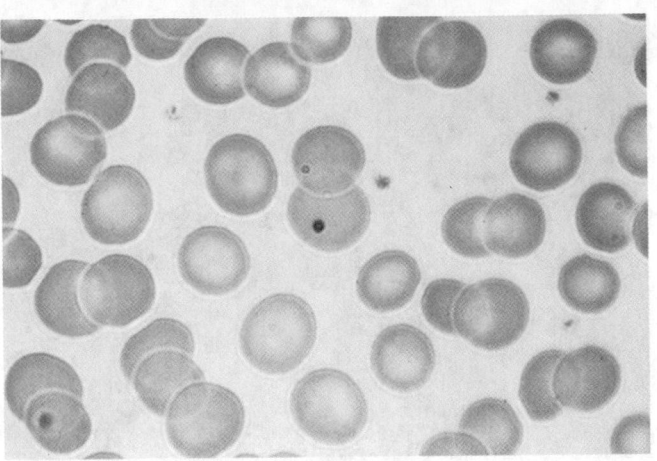

Figure 57-6 Howell-Jolly bodies. In the absence of a functional spleen, nuclear remnants are not culled from the red cells and remain as small homogeneously staining blue inclusions on Wright stain. *(From Hillman et al.)*

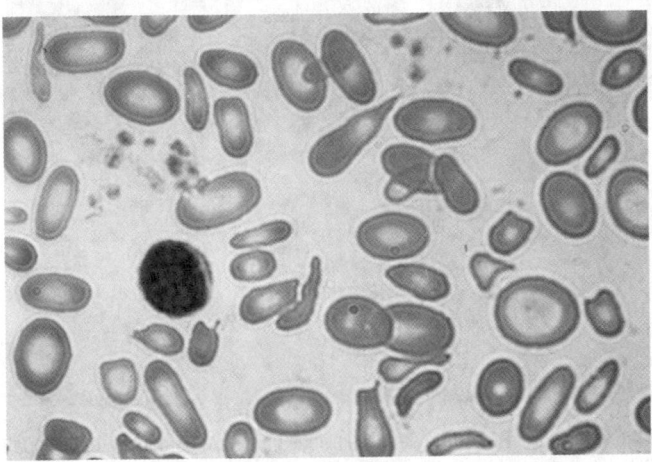

Figure 57-4 Severe iron-deficiency anemia. Microcytic and hypochromic red cells smaller than the nucleus of a lymphocyte associated with marked variation in size (anisocytosis) and shape (poikilocytosis). *(From Hillman et al.)*

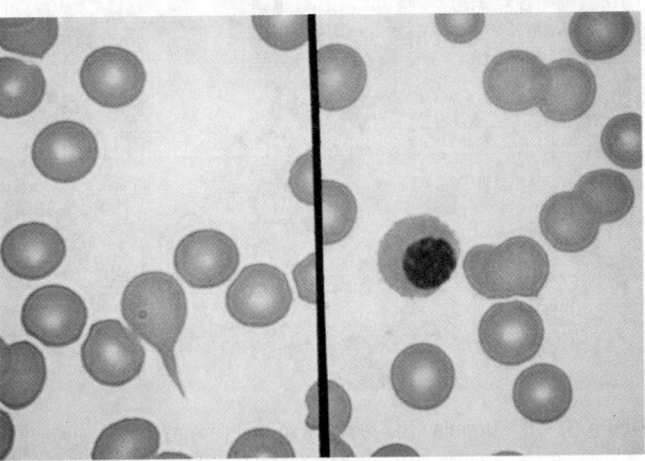

Figure 57-7 Red cell changes in myelofibrosis. The left panel shows a teardrop-shaped cell. The right panel shows a nucleated red cell. These forms are seen in myelofibrosis.

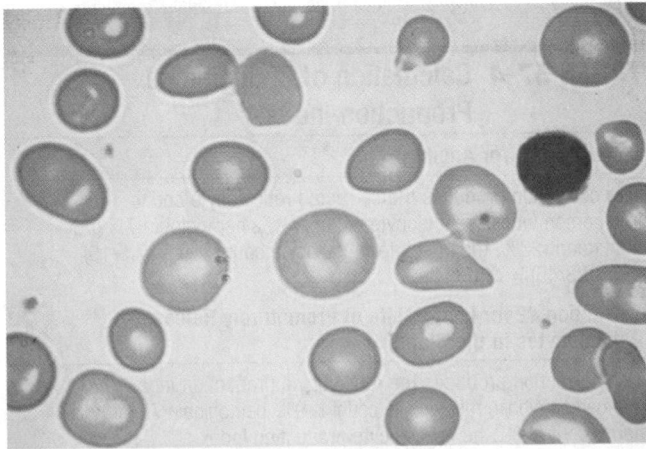

Figure 57-5 Macrocytosis. Red cells are larger than a small lymphocyte and well hemoglobinized. Often macrocytes are oval shaped (macro-ovalocytes).

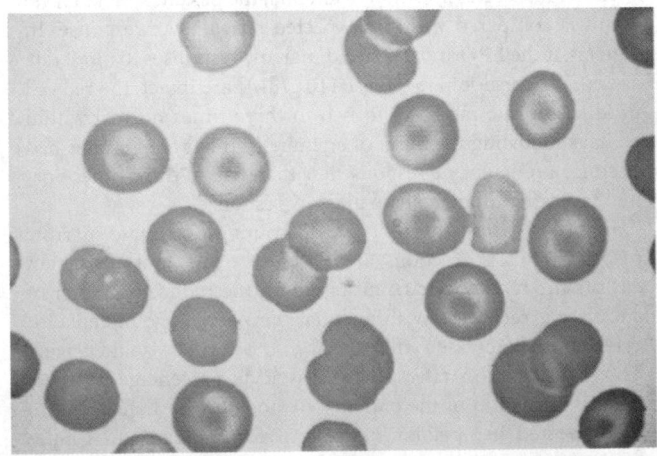

Figure 57-8 Target cells. Target cells have a bull's-eye appearance and are seen in thalassemia and in liver disease. *(From Hillman et al.)*

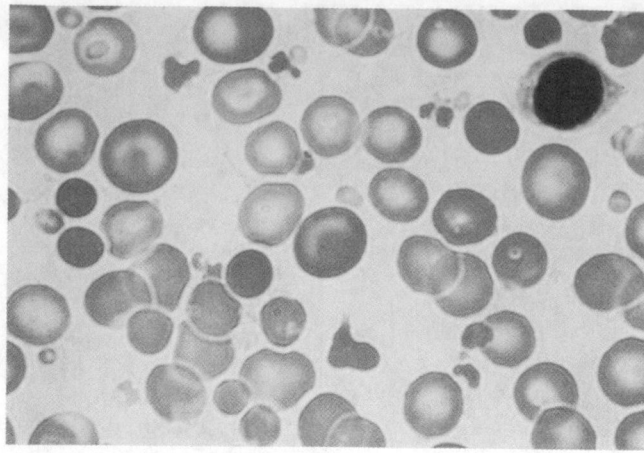

Figure 57-9 **Red cell fragmentation.** Red cells may become fragmented in the presence of foreign bodies in the circulation, such as mechanical heart valves, or in the setting of thermal injury. *(From Hillman et al.)*

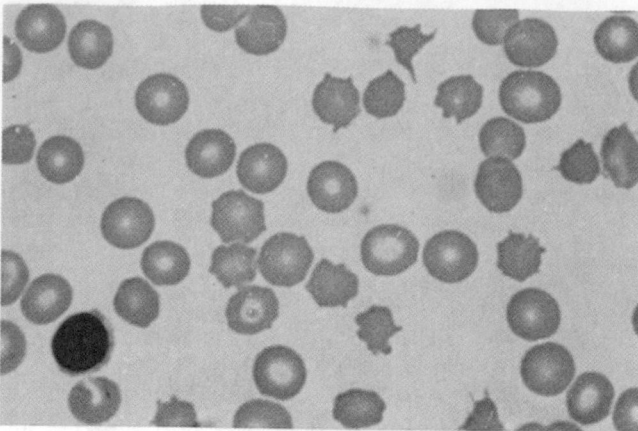

Figure 57-11 **Spur cells.** Spur cells are recognized as distorted red cells containing several irregularly distributed thornlike projections. Cells with this morphologic abnormality are also called acanthocytes. *(From Hillman et al.)*

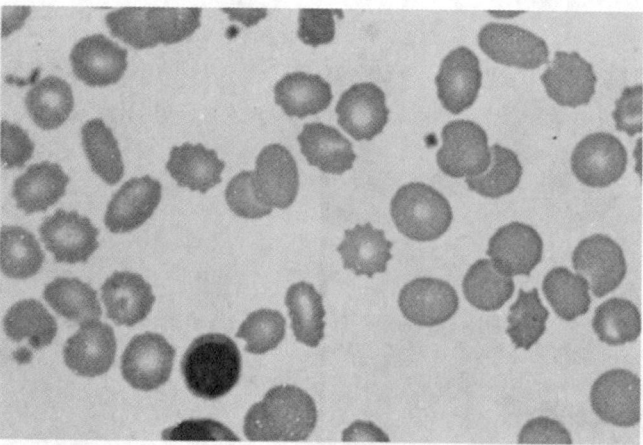

Figure 57-10 **Uremia.** The red cells in uremia may acquire numerous regularly spaced, small, spiny projections. Such cells, called burr cells or echinocytes, are readily distinguishable from irregularly spiculated acanthocytes shown in Fig. 57-11.

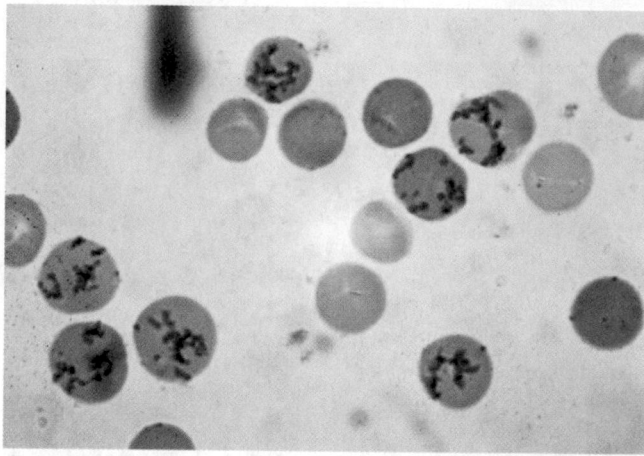

Figure 57-12 **Reticulocytes.** Methylene blue stain demonstrates residual RNA in newly made red cells. *(From Hillman et al.)*

2% and reflects the daily replacement of 0.8–1.0% of the circulating red cell population. A corrected reticulocyte count provides a reliable measure of red cell production.

In the initial classification of anemia, the patient's reticulocyte count is compared with the expected reticulocyte response. In general, if the EPO and erythroid marrow responses to moderate anemia [hemoglobin < 100 g/L (10 g/dL)] are intact, the red cell production rate increases to two to three times normal within 10 days following the onset of anemia. In the face of established anemia, a reticulocyte response less than two to three times normal indicates an inadequate marrow response.

In order to use the reticulocyte count to estimate marrow response, two corrections are necessary. The first correction adjusts the reticulocyte count based on the reduced number of circulating red cells. With anemia, the percentage of reticulocytes may be increased while the absolute number is unchanged. To correct for this effect, the reticulocyte percentage is multiplied by the ratio of the patient's hemoglobin or hematocrit to the expected hemoglobin/hematocrit for the age and gender of the patient (Table 57-4). This provides an estimate of the reticulocyte count corrected for anemia. In order to convert the corrected reticulocyte count to an index of marrow production, a further correction is required, depending on whether some

of the reticulocytes in circulation have been released from the marrow prematurely. For this second correction, the peripheral blood smear is examined to see if there are polychromatophilic macrocytes present.

TABLE 57-4 Calculation of Reticulocyte Production Index

Correction #1 for Anemia:

This correction produces the corrected reticulocyte count
In a person whose reticulocyte count is 9%, hemoglobin 7.5 g/dL, hematocrit 23%, the absolute reticulocyte count = 9 × (7.5/15) [or × (23/45)]= 4.5%

Correction #2 for Longer Life of Prematurely Released Reticulocytes in the Blood:

This correction produces the reticulocyte production index
In a person whose reticulocyte count is 9%, hemoglobin 7.5 gm/dL, hematocrit 23%, the reticulocyte production index

$$= 9 \times \frac{(7.5 / 15)(\text{hemoglobin correction})}{2(\text{maturation time correction})} = 2.25$$

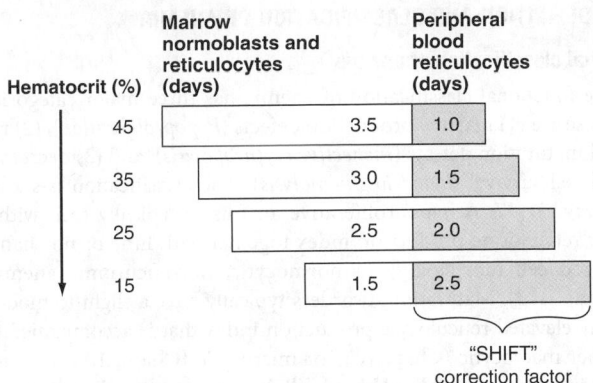

Figure 57-13   **Correction of the reticulocyte count.** In order to use the reticulocyte count as an indicator of effective red cell production, the reticulocyte percentage must be corrected based on the level of anemia and the circulating life span of the reticulocytes. Erythroid cells take ~4.5 days to mature. At a normal hemoglobin, reticulocytes are released to the circulation with ~1 day left as reticulocytes. However, with different levels of anemia, reticulocytes (and even earlier erythroid cells) may be released from the marrow prematurely. Most patients come to clinical attention with hematocrits in the mid-20s, and thus a correction factor of 2 is commonly used because the observed reticulocytes will live for 2 days in the circulation before losing their RNA.

These cells, representing prematurely released reticulocytes, are referred to as "shift" cells, and the relationship between the degree of shift and the necessary shift correction factor is shown in Fig. 57-13. The correction is necessary because these prematurely released cells survive as reticulocytes in circulation for >1 day, thereby providing a falsely high estimate of daily red cell production. If polychromasia is increased, the reticulocyte count, already corrected for anemia, should be divided again by 2 to account for the prolonged reticulocyte maturation time. The second correction factor varies from 1 to 3 depending on the severity of anemia. In general, a correction of 2 is commonly used. An appropriate correction is shown in Table 57-4. If polychromatophilic cells are not seen on the blood smear, the second correction is not required. The now doubly corrected reticulocyte count is the *reticulocyte production index*, and it provides an estimate of marrow production relative to normal.

Premature release of reticulocytes is normally due to increased EPO stimulation. However, if the integrity of the bone marrow release process is lost through tumor infiltration, fibrosis, or other disorders, the appearance of nucleated red cells or polychromatophilic macrocytes should still invoke the second reticulocyte correction. The shift correction should always be applied to a patient with anemia and a very high reticulocyte count to provide a true index of effective red cell production. Patients with severe chronic hemolytic anemia may increase red cell production as much as six- to sevenfold. This measure alone, therefore, confirms the fact that the patient has an appropriate EPO response, a normally functioning bone marrow, and sufficient iron available to meet the demands for new red cell formation. Table 57-5 demonstrates the normal marrow response to anemia. If the reticulocyte production index is <2 in the face of established anemia, a defect in erythroid marrow proliferation or maturation must be present.

TABLE 57-5   Normal Marrow Response to Anemia

Hematocrit	Production Index	Reticulocytes (incl corrections)	Marrow M/E Ratio
45	1	1	3:1
35	2.0–3.0	4.8%/3.8/2.5	2:1–1:1
25	3.0–5.0	14%/8/4.0	1:1–1:2
15	3.0–5.0	30%/10/4.0	1:1–1:2

Tests of Iron Supply and Storage   The laboratory measurements that reflect the availability of iron for hemoglobin synthesis include the serum iron, the TIBC, and the percent transferrin saturation. The percent transferrin saturation is derived by dividing the serum iron level (× 100) by the TIBC. The normal serum iron ranges from 9 to 27 μmol/L (50–150 μg/dL), while the normal TIBC is 54–64 μmol/L (300–360 μg/dL); the normal transferrin saturation ranges from 25 to 50%. A diurnal variation in the serum iron leads to a variation in the percent transferrin saturation. The serum ferritin is used to evaluate total body iron stores. Adult males have serum ferritin levels that average ~100 μg/L, corresponding to iron stores of ~1 g. Adult females have lower serum ferritin levels averaging 30 μg/L, reflecting lower iron stores (~300 mg). A serum ferritin level of 10–15 μg/L represents depletion of body iron stores. However, ferritin is also an acute-phase reactant and, in the presence of acute or chronic inflammation, may rise several-fold above baseline levels. As a rule, a serum ferritin >200 μg/L means there is at least some iron in tissue stores.

Bone Marrow Examination   A bone marrow aspirate and smear or a needle biopsy can be useful in the evaluation of some patients with anemia. In patients with hypoproliferative anemia and normal iron status, a bone marrow is indicated. Marrow examination can diagnose primary marrow disorders such as myelofibrosis, a red cell maturation defect, or an infiltrative disease (Figs. 57-14 to 57-16). The increase or decrease of one cell lineage (myeloid vs. erythroid) compared to another is obtained by a differential count of nucleated cells in a bone

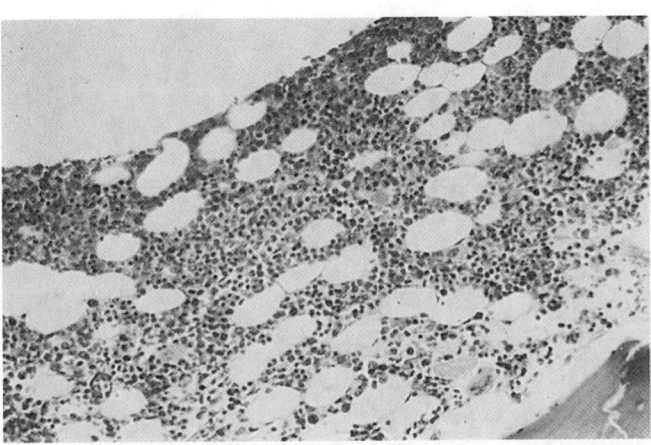

Figure 57-14   **Normal bone marrow.** This is a low-power view of a section of a normal bone marrow biopsy stained with hematoxylin and eosin (H&E). Note that the nucleated cellular elements account for ~40–50% and the fat (clear areas) accounts for ~50–60% of the area. *(From Hillman et al.)*

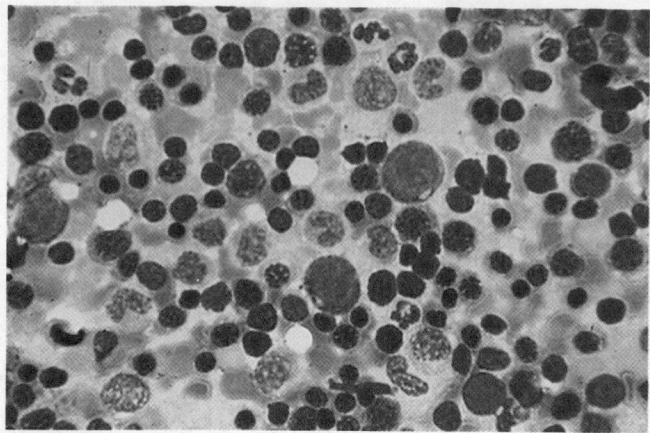

Figure 57-15 Erythroid hyperplasia. This marrow shows an increase in the fraction of cells in the erythroid lineage as might be seen when a normal marrow compensates for acute blood loss or hemolysis. The M/E ratio is about 1:1. M/E, myeloid/erythroid. *(From Hillman et al.)*

marrow smear [the myeloid/erythroid (M/E) ratio]. A patient with a hypoproliferative anemia (see below) and a reticulocyte production index <2 will demonstrate an M/E ratio of 2 or 3:1. In contrast, patients with hemolytic disease and a production index >3 will have an M/E ratio of at least 1:1. Maturation disorders are identified from the discrepancy between the M/E ratio and the reticulocyte production index (see below). Either the marrow smear or biopsy can be stained for the presence of iron stores or iron in developing red cells. The storage iron is in the form of ferritin or *hemosiderin*. On carefully prepared bone marrow smears, small ferritin granules can normally be seen under oil immersion in 20–40% of developing erythroblasts. Such cells are called *sideroblasts*.

OTHER LABORATORY MEASUREMENTS Additional laboratory tests may be of value in confirming specific diagnoses. For details of these tests and how they are applied in individual disorders, see Chaps. 103 to 107.

■ DEFINITION AND CLASSIFICATION OF ANEMIA

Initial classification of anemia

The functional classification of anemia has three major categories. These are (1) marrow production defects (*hypoproliferation*), (2) red cell maturation defects (*ineffective erythropoiesis*), and (3) decreased red cell survival (*blood loss/hemolysis*). The classification is shown in Fig. 57-17. A hypoproliferative anemia is typically seen with a low reticulocyte production index together with little or no change in red cell morphology (a normocytic, normochromic anemia) (Chap. 103). Maturation disorders typically have a slight to moderately elevated reticulocyte production index that is accompanied by either macrocytic (Chap. 105) or microcytic (Chaps. 103, 104) red cell indices. Increased red blood cell destruction secondary to hemolysis results in an increase in the reticulocyte production index to at least three times normal (Chap. 106), provided sufficient iron is available. Hemorrhagic anemia does not typically result in production indices of more than 2.0–2.5 times normal because of the limitations placed on expansion of the erythroid marrow by iron availability.

In the first branch point of the classification of anemia, a reticulocyte production index >2.5 indicates that hemolysis is most likely. A reticulocyte production index <2 indicates either a hypoproliferative anemia or maturation disorder. The latter two possibilities can often be distinguished by the red cell indices, by examination of the peripheral blood smear, or by a marrow examination. If the red cell indices are normal, the anemia is almost certainly hypoproliferative in nature. Maturation disorders are characterized by ineffective red cell production and a low reticulocyte production index. Bizarre red cell shapes—macrocytes or hypochromic microcytes—are seen on the peripheral blood smear. With a hypoproliferative anemia, no erythroid hyperplasia is noted in the marrow, whereas patients with ineffective red cell production have erythroid hyperplasia and an M/E ratio <1:1.

ALGORITHM OF THE PHYSIOLOGIC CLASSIFICATION OF ANEMIA

```
                    Anemia
                      │
             CBC, reticulocyte
                  count
                 ┌────┴──────────────┐
           Index < 2.5          Index ≥ 2.5
                │                     │
          Red cell              Hemolysis/
         morphology             hemorrhage
          ┌────┴─────┐               │
    Normocytic    Micro or      ─ Blood loss
   normochromic   macrocytic
        │             │         ─ Intravascular
  Hypoproliferative  Maturation    hemolysis
                     disorder
                               ─ Metabolic defect
 ─ Marrow damage   ─ Cytoplasmic defects
   • Infiltration/   • Iron deficiency   ─ Membrane
     fibrosis        • Thalassemia         abnormality
   • Aplasia         • Sideroblastic
 ─ Iron deficiency     anemia          ─ Hemoglobinopathy

 ─ ↓ Stimulation   ─ Nuclear defects   ─ Immune destruction
   • Inflammation    • Folate deficiency
   • Metabolic defect • Vitamin B₁₂ deficiency ─ Fragmentation
   • Renal disease   • Drug toxicity      hemolysis
                     • Refractory anemia
```

Figure 57-17 The physiologic classification of anemia. CBC, complete blood count.

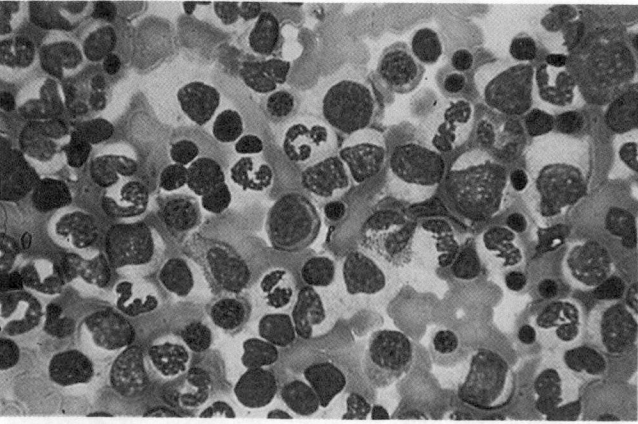

Figure 57-16 Myeloid hyperplasia. This marrow shows an increase in the fraction of cells in the myeloid or granulocytic lineage as might be seen in a normal marrow responding to infection. The M/E ratio is >3:1. M/E, myeloid/erythroid. *(From Hillman et al.)*

Hypoproliferative anemias

At least 75% of all cases of anemia are hypoproliferative in nature. A hypoproliferative anemia reflects absolute or relative marrow failure in which the erythroid marrow has not proliferated appropriately for the degree of anemia. The majority of hypoproliferative anemias are due to mild to moderate iron deficiency or inflammation. A hypoproliferative anemia can result from marrow damage, iron deficiency, or inadequate EPO stimulation. The last may reflect impaired renal function, suppression of EPO production by inflammatory cytokines such as interleukin 1, or reduced tissue needs for O_2 from metabolic disease such as hypothyroidism. Only occasionally is the marrow unable to produce red cells at a normal rate, and this is most prevalent in patients with renal failure. With diabetes mellitus or myeloma, the EPO deficiency may be more marked than would be predicted by the degree of renal insufficiency. In general, hypoproliferative anemias are characterized by normocytic, normochromic red cells, although microcytic, hypochromic cells may be observed with mild iron deficiency or long-standing chronic inflammatory disease. The key laboratory tests in distinguishing between the various forms of hypoproliferative anemia include the serum iron and iron-binding capacity, evaluation of renal and thyroid function, a marrow biopsy or aspirate to detect marrow damage or infiltrative disease, and serum ferritin to assess iron stores. An iron stain of the marrow will determine the pattern of iron distribution. Patients with the anemia of acute or chronic inflammation show a distinctive pattern of serum iron (low), TIBC (normal or low), percent transferrin saturation (low), and serum ferritin (normal or high). These changes in iron values are brought about by hepcidin, the iron regulatory hormone that is increased in inflammation (Chap. 103). A distinct pattern of results is noted in mild to moderate iron deficiency (low serum iron, high TIBC, low percent transferrin saturation, low serum ferritin) (Chap. 103). Marrow damage by drugs, infiltrative disease such as leukemia or lymphoma, or marrow aplasia are diagnosed from the peripheral blood and bone marrow morphology. With infiltrative disease or fibrosis, a marrow biopsy is required.

Maturation disorders

The presence of anemia with an inappropriately low reticulocyte production index, macro- or microcytosis on smear, and abnormal red cell indices suggests a maturation disorder. Maturation disorders are divided into two categories: nuclear maturation defects, associated with macrocytosis, and cytoplasmic maturation defects, associated with microcytosis and hypochromia usually from defects in hemoglobin synthesis. The inappropriately low reticulocyte production index is a reflection of the ineffective erythropoiesis that results from the destruction within the marrow of developing erythroblasts. Bone marrow examination shows erythroid hyperplasia.

Nuclear maturation defects result from vitamin B_{12} or folic acid deficiency, drug damage, or myelodysplasia. Drugs that interfere with cellular DNA synthesis, such as methotrexate or alkylating agents, can produce a nuclear maturation defect. Alcohol, alone, is also capable of producing macrocytosis and a variable degree of anemia, but this is usually associated with folic acid deficiency. Measurements of folic acid and vitamin B_{12} are critical not only in identifying the specific vitamin deficiency but also because they reflect different pathogenetic mechanisms (Chap. 105).

Cytoplasmic maturation defects result from severe iron deficiency or abnormalities in globin or heme synthesis. Iron deficiency occupies an unusual position in the classification of anemia. If the iron-deficiency anemia is mild to moderate, erythroid marrow proliferation is blunted and the anemia is classified as hypoproliferative. However, if the anemia is severe and prolonged, the erythroid marrow will become hyperplastic despite the inadequate iron supply, and the anemia will be classified as ineffective erythropoiesis with a cytoplasmic maturation defect. In either case, an inappropriately low reticulocyte production index, microcytosis, and a classic pattern of iron values make the diagnosis clear and easily distinguish iron deficiency from other cytoplasmic maturation defects such as the thalassemias. Defects in heme synthesis, in contrast to globin synthesis, are less common and may be acquired or inherited (Chap. 358). Acquired abnormalities are usually associated with myelodysplasia, may lead to either a macro- or microcytic anemia, and are frequently associated with mitochondrial iron loading. In these cases, iron is taken up by the mitochondria of the developing erythroid cell but not incorporated into heme. The iron-encrusted mitochondria surround the nucleus of the erythroid cell, forming a ring. Based on the distinctive finding of so-called ringed sideroblasts on the marrow iron stain, patients are diagnosed as having a sideroblastic anemia—almost always reflecting myelodysplasia. Again, studies of iron parameters are helpful in the differential diagnosis of these patients.

Blood loss/hemolytic anemia

In contrast to anemias associated with an inappropriately low reticulocyte production index, hemolysis is associated with red cell production indices ≥2.5 times normal. The stimulated erythropoiesis is reflected in the blood smear by the appearance of increased numbers of polychromatophilic macrocytes. A marrow examination is rarely indicated if the reticulocyte production index is increased appropriately. The red cell indices are typically normocytic or slightly macrocytic, reflecting the increased number of reticulocytes. Acute blood loss is not associated with an increased reticulocyte production index because of the time required to increase EPO production and, subsequently, marrow proliferation. Subacute blood loss may be associated with modest reticulocytosis. Anemia from chronic blood loss presents more often as iron deficiency than with the picture of increased red cell production.

The evaluation of blood loss anemia is usually not difficult. Most problems arise when a patient presents with an increased red cell production index from an episode of acute blood loss that went unrecognized. The cause of the anemia and increased red cell production may not be obvious. The confirmation of a recovering state may require observations over a period of 2–3 weeks, during which the hemoglobin concentration will be seen to rise and the reticulocyte production index fall (Chap. 106).

Hemolytic disease, while dramatic, is among the least common forms of anemia. The ability to sustain a high reticulocyte production index reflects the ability of the erythroid marrow to compensate for hemolysis and, in the case of extravascular hemolysis, the efficient recycling of iron from the destroyed red cells to support red cell production. With intravascular hemolysis, such as paroxysmal nocturnal hemoglobinuria, the loss of iron may limit the marrow response. The level of response depends on the severity of the anemia and the nature of the underlying disease process.

Hemoglobinopathies, such as sickle cell disease and the thalassemias, present a mixed picture. The reticulocyte index may be high but is inappropriately low for the degree of marrow erythroid hyperplasia (Chap. 104).

Hemolytic anemias present in different ways. Some appear suddenly as an acute, self-limited episode of intravascular or extravascular hemolysis, a presentation pattern often seen in patients with autoimmune hemolysis or with inherited defects of the Embden-Meyerhof pathway or the glutathione reductase pathway. Patients with inherited disorders of the hemoglobin molecule or red cell membrane generally have a lifelong clinical history typical of the disease process. Those with chronic hemolytic disease, such as hereditary spherocytosis, may actually present not with anemia but with a complication stemming from the prolonged increase in red cell destruction such as symptomatic bilirubin gallstones or splenomegaly. Patients with chronic hemolysis are also susceptible to aplastic crises if an infectious process interrupts red cell production.

The differential diagnosis of an acute or chronic hemolytic event requires the careful integration of family history, the pattern of clinical presentation and—whether the disease is congenital or acquired—by a careful examination of the peripheral blood smear. Precise diagnosis may require more specialized laboratory tests, such as hemoglobin electrophoresis or a screen for red cell enzymes. Acquired defects in red cell survival are often immunologically mediated and require a direct or indirect antiglobulin test or a cold agglutinin titer to detect the presence of hemolytic antibodies or complement-mediated red cell destruction (Chap. 106).

TREATMENT   Anemia

An overriding principle is to initiate treatment of mild to moderate anemia only when a specific diagnosis is made. Rarely, in the acute setting, anemia may be so severe that red cell transfusions are required before a specific diagnosis is made. Whether the anemia is of acute or gradual onset, the selection of the appropriate treatment is determined by the documented cause(s) of the anemia. Often, the cause of the anemia is multifactorial. For example, a patient with severe rheumatoid arthritis who has been taking anti-inflammatory drugs may have a hypoproliferative anemia associated with chronic inflammation as well as chronic blood loss associated with intermittent gastrointestinal bleeding. In every circumstance, it is important to evaluate the patient's iron status fully before and during the treatment of any anemia. Transfusion is discussed in Chap. 113; iron therapy is discussed in Chap. 103; treatment of megaloblastic anemia is discussed in Chap. 105; treatment of other entities is discussed in their respective chapters (sickle cell anemia, Chap. 104; hemolytic anemias, Chap. 106; aplastic anemia and myelodysplasia, Chap. 107).

Therapeutic options for the treatment of anemias have expanded dramatically during the past 25 years. Blood component therapy is available and safe. Recombinant EPO as an adjunct to anemia management has transformed the lives of patients with chronic renal failure on dialysis and reduced transfusion needs of anemic cancer patients receiving chemotherapy. Eventually, patients with inherited disorders of globin synthesis or mutations in the globin gene, such as sickle cell disease, may benefit from the successful introduction of targeted genetic therapy (Chap. 68).

POLYCYTHEMIA

Polycythemia is defined as an increase in the hemoglobin above normal. This increase may be real or only apparent because of a decrease in plasma volume (spurious or relative polycythemia). The term *erythrocytosis* may be used interchangeably with polycythemia, but some draw a distinction between them: erythrocytosis implies documentation of increased red cell mass, whereas polycythemia refers to any increase in red cells. Often patients with polycythemia are detected through an incidental finding of elevated hemoglobin or hematocrit levels. Concern that the hemoglobin level may be abnormally high is usually triggered at 170 g/L (17 g/dL) for men and 150 g/L (15 g/dL) for women. Hematocrit levels >50% in men or >45% in women may be abnormal.

Hematocrits >60% in men and >55% in women are almost invariably associated with an increased red cell mass. Given that the machine that quantitates red cell parameters actually measures hemoglobin concentrations and calculates hematocrits, hemoglobin levels may be a better index.

Features of the clinical history that are useful in the differential diagnosis include smoking history; current living at high altitude; or a history of congenital heart disease, sleep apnea, or chronic lung disease.

Patients with polycythemia may be asymptomatic or experience symptoms related to the increased red cell mass or the underlying disease process that leads to the increased red cell mass. The dominant symptoms from an increased red cell mass are related to hyperviscosity and thrombosis (both venous and arterial), because the blood viscosity increases logarithmically at hematocrits >55%. Manifestations range from digital ischemia to Budd-Chiari syndrome with hepatic vein thrombosis. Abdominal vessel thromboses are particularly common. Neurologic symptoms such as vertigo, tinnitus, headache, and visual disturbances may occur. Hypertension is often present. Patients with *polycythemia vera* may have aquagenic pruritus and symptoms related to hepatosplenomegaly. Patients may have easy bruising, epistaxis, or bleeding from the gastrointestinal tract. Peptic ulcer disease is common. Patients with hypoxemia may develop cyanosis on minimal exertion or have headache, impaired mental acuity, and fatigue.

The physical examination usually reveals a ruddy complexion. Splenomegaly favors polycythemia vera as the diagnosis (Chap. 108). The presence of cyanosis or evidence of a right-to-left shunt suggests congenital heart disease presenting in the adult, particularly tetralogy of Fallot's or Eisenmenger's syndrome (Chap. 236). Increased blood viscosity raises pulmonary artery pressure; hypoxemia can lead to increased pulmonary vascular resistance. Together, these factors can produce cor pulmonale.

Polycythemia can be spurious (related to a decrease in plasma volume; Gaisbock's syndrome), primary, or secondary in origin. The secondary causes are all associated with increases in EPO levels: either a physiologically adapted appropriate elevation based on tissue hypoxia (lung disease, high altitude, CO poisoning, high-affinity hemoglobinopathy) or an abnormal overproduction (renal cysts, renal artery stenosis, tumors with ectopic EPO production). A rare familial form of polycythemia is associated with normal EPO levels but hyperresponsive EPO receptors due to mutations.

APPROACH TO THE PATIENT   Polycythemia

As shown in Fig. 57-18, the first step is to document the presence of an increased red cell mass using the principle of isotope dilution by administering ^{51}Cr-labeled autologous red blood cells to the patient and sampling blood radioactivity over a 2-h period. If the red cell mass is normal (<36 mL/kg in men, <32 mL/kg in women), the patient has spurious or relative polycythemia. If the red cell mass is increased (>36 mL/kg in men, >32 mL/kg in women), serum EPO levels should be measured. If EPO levels are low or unmeasurable, the patient most likely has polycythemia vera. Tests that support this diagnosis include elevated white blood cell count, increased absolute basophil count, and thrombocytosis. A mutation in *JAK-2* (Val617Phe), a key member of the cytokine intracellular signaling pathway, can be found in 70–95% of patients with polycythemia vera.

If serum EPO levels are elevated, one needs to distinguish whether the elevation is a physiologic response to hypoxia or is related to autonomous EPO production. Patients with low

AN APPROACH TO DIAGNOSING PATIENTS WITH POLYCYTHEMIA

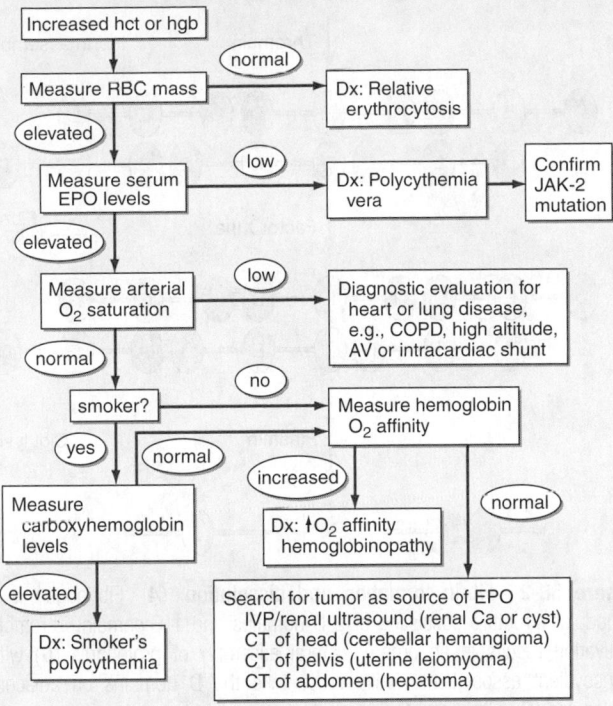

Figure 57-18   An approach to the differential diagnosis of patients with an elevated hemoglobin (possible polycythemia). AV, atrioventricular; COPD, chronic obstructive pulmonary disease; EPO, erythropoietin; hct, hematocrit; IVP, intravenous pyelogram; RBC, red blood cell.

arterial O_2 saturation (<92%) should be further evaluated for the presence of heart or lung disease, if they are not living at high altitude. Patients with normal O_2 saturation who are smokers may have elevated EPO levels because of CO displacement of O_2. If carboxyhemoglobin (COHb) levels are high, the diagnosis is "smoker's polycythemia." Such patients should be urged to stop smoking. Those who cannot stop smoking require phlebotomy to control their polycythemia. Patients with normal O_2 saturation who do not smoke either have an abnormal hemoglobin that does not deliver O_2 to the tissues (evaluated by finding elevated O_2–hemoglobin affinity) or have a source of EPO production that is not responding to the normal feedback inhibition. Further workup is dictated by the differential diagnosis of EPO-producing neoplasms. Hepatoma, uterine leiomyoma, and renal cancer or cysts are all detectable with abdominopelvic CT scans. Cerebellar hemangiomas may produce EPO, but they present with localizing neurologic signs and symptoms rather than polycythemia-related symptoms.

FURTHER READINGS

HILLMAN RS et al: *Hematology in Clinical Practice*, 5th ed. New York, McGraw-Hill, 2010

McMULLIN MF: The classification and diagnosis of erythrocytosis. Int J Lab Hematol 30:447, 2008

RIZZO JD et al: American Society of Hematology/American Society of Clinical Oncology clinical practice guideline update on the use of epoetin and darbepoetin in adult patients with cancer. Blood 116:4045, 2010

CHAPTER **58**

Bleeding and Thrombosis

Barbara Konkle

The human hemostatic system provides a natural balance between procoagulant and anticoagulant forces. The procoagulant forces include platelet adhesion and aggregation and fibrin clot formation; anticoagulant forces include the natural inhibitors of coagulation and fibrinolysis. Under normal circumstances, hemostasis is regulated to promote blood flow; however, it is also prepared to clot blood rapidly to arrest blood flow and prevent exsanguination. After bleeding is successfully halted, the system remodels the damaged vessel to restore normal blood flow. The major components of the hemostatic system, which function in concert, are (1) platelets and other formed elements of blood, such as monocytes and red cells; (2) plasma proteins (the coagulation and fibrinolytic factors and inhibitors); and (3) the vessel wall.

STEPS OF NORMAL HEMOSTASIS

■ PLATELET PLUG FORMATION

On vascular injury, platelets adhere to the site of injury, usually the denuded vascular intimal surface. Platelet adhesion is mediated primarily by von Willebrand factor (VWF), a large multimeric

protein present in both plasma and the extracellular matrix of the subendothelial vessel wall, which serves as the primary "molecular glue," providing sufficient strength to withstand the high levels of shear stress that would tend to detach them with the flow of blood. Platelet adhesion is also facilitated by direct binding to subendothelial collagen through specific platelet membrane collagen receptors.

Platelet adhesion results in subsequent platelet activation and aggregation. This process is enhanced and amplified by humoral mediators in plasma (e.g., epinephrine, thrombin); mediators released from activated platelets (e.g., adenosine diphosphate, serotonin); and vessel wall extracellular matrix constituents that come in contact with adherent platelets (e.g., collagen, VWF). Activated platelets undergo the release reaction, during which they secrete contents that further promote aggregation and inhibit the naturally anticoagulant endothelial cell factors. During platelet aggregation (platelet-platelet interaction), additional platelets are recruited from the circulation to the site of vascular injury, leading to the formation of an occlusive platelet thrombus. The platelet plug is anchored and stabilized by the developing fibrin mesh.

The platelet glycoprotein (Gp) IIb/IIIa ($\alpha_{IIb}\beta_3$) complex is the most abundant receptor on the platelet surface. Platelet activation converts the normally inactive Gp IIb/IIIa receptor into an active receptor, enabling binding to fibrinogen and VWF. Because the surface of each platelet has about 50,000 Gp IIb/IIIa-binding sites, numerous activated platelets recruited to the site of vascular injury can rapidly form an occlusive aggregate by means of a dense network of intercellular fibrinogen bridges. Since this receptor is the key mediator of platelet aggregation, it has become an effective target for antiplatelet therapy.

■ FIBRIN CLOT FORMATION

Plasma coagulation proteins (*clotting factors*) normally circulate in plasma in their inactive forms. The sequence of coagulation protein reactions that culminate in the formation of fibrin was originally described as a *waterfall* or a *cascade*. Two pathways of blood coagulation have been described in the past: the so-called extrinsic, or tissue factor, pathway and the so-called intrinsic, or contact activation, pathway. We now know that coagulation is normally initiated through tissue factor (TF) exposure and activation through the classic *extrinsic pathway* but with critically important amplification through elements of the classic *intrinsic pathway*, as illustrated in Fig. 58-1. These reactions take place on phospholipid surfaces, usually the activated platelet surface. Coagulation testing in the laboratory can reflect other influences due to the artificial nature of the in vitro systems used (see below).

The immediate trigger for coagulation is vascular damage that exposes blood to TF that is constitutively expressed on the surfaces of subendothelial cellular components of the vessel wall, such as smooth muscle cells and fibroblasts. TF is also present in circulating microparticles, presumably shed from cells including monocytes and platelets. TF binds the serine protease factor VIIa; the complex activates factor X to factor Xa. Alternatively, the complex can indirectly activate factor X by initially converting factor IX to factor IXa, which then activates factor X. The participation of factor XI in hemostasis is not dependent on its activation by factor XIIa but rather on its positive feedback activation by thrombin. Thus, factor XIa functions in the propagation and amplification, rather than in the initiation, of the coagulation cascade.

Factor Xa can be formed through the actions of either the tissue factor/factor VIIa complex or factor IXa (with factor VIIIa as a cofactor) and converts prothrombin to thrombin, the pivotal protease of the coagulation system. The essential cofactor for this reaction is factor Va. Like the homologous factor VIIIa, factor Va is produced by thrombin-induced limited proteolysis of factor V. Thrombin is a multifunctional enzyme that converts soluble plasma fibrinogen to an insoluble fibrin matrix. Fibrin polymerization involves an orderly process of intermolecular associations

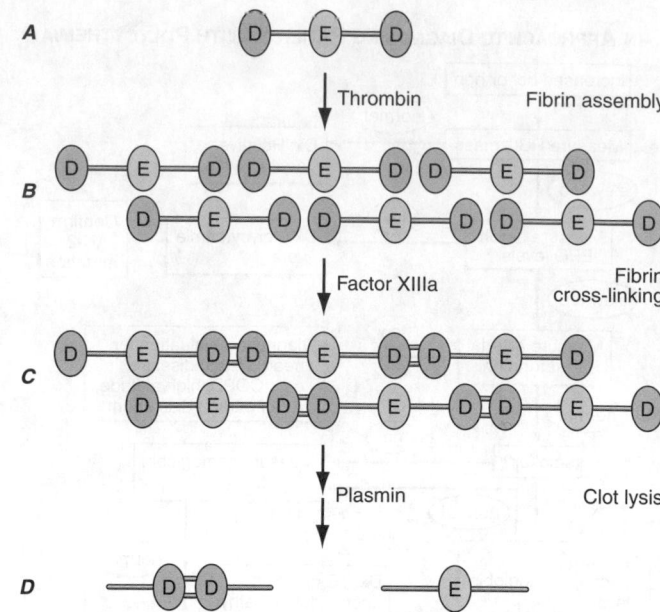

Figure 58-2   Fibrin formation and dissolution. (*A*). Fibrinogen is a trinodular structure consisting of 2 D domains and 1 E domain. Thrombin activation results in an ordered lateral assembly of protofibrils (*B*) with noncovalent associations. FXIIIa cross-links the D domains on adjacent molecules (*C*). Fibrin and fibrinogen (not shown) lysis by plasmin occurs at discrete sites and results in intermediary fibrin(ogen) degradation products (not shown). D-Dimers are the product of complete lysis of fibrin (*D*), maintaining the cross-linked D domains.

(Fig. 58-2). Thrombin also activates factor XIII (fibrin-stabilizing factor) to factor XIIIa, which covalently cross-links and thereby stabilizes the fibrin clot.

The assembly of the clotting factors on activated cell membrane surfaces greatly accelerates their reaction rates and also serves to localize blood clotting to sites of vascular injury. The critical cell membrane components, acidic phospholipids, are not normally exposed on resting cell membrane surfaces. However, when platelets, monocytes, and endothelial cells are activated by vascular injury or inflammatory stimuli, the procoagulant head groups of the membrane anionic phospholipids become translocated to the surfaces of these cells or released as part of microparticles, making them available to support and promote the plasma coagulation reactions.

ANTITHROMBOTIC MECHANISMS

Several physiologic antithrombotic mechanisms act in concert to prevent clotting under normal circumstances. These mechanisms operate to preserve blood fluidity and to limit blood clotting to specific focal sites of vascular injury. Endothelial cells have many antithrombotic effects. They produce prostacyclin, nitric oxide, and ectoADPase/CD39, which act to inhibit platelet binding, secretion, and aggregation. Endothelial cells produce anticoagulant factors including heparan proteoglycans, antithrombin, TF pathway inhibitor, and thrombomodulin. They also activate fibrinolytic mechanisms through the

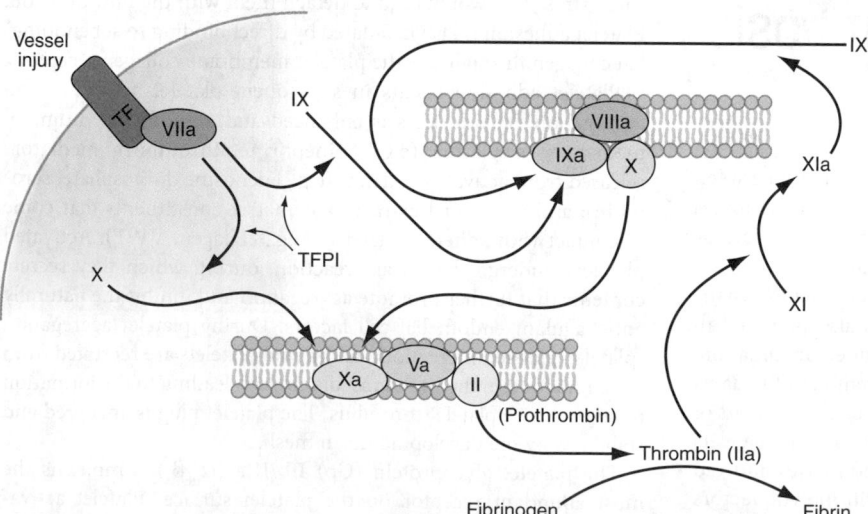

Figure 58-1   Coagulation is initiated by tissue factor (TF) exposure, which, with factor (F)VIIa, activates FIX and FX, which in turn, with FVIII and FV as cofactors, respectively, results in thrombin formation and subsequent conversion of fibrinogen to fibrin. Thrombin activates FXI, FVIII, and FV, amplifying the coagulation signal. Once the TF/FVIIa/FXa complex is formed, tissue factor pathway inhibitor (TFPI) inhibits the TF/FVIIa pathway, making coagulation dependent on the amplification loop through FIX/FVIII. Coagulation requires calcium (not shown) and takes place on phospholipid surfaces, usually the activated platelet membrane.

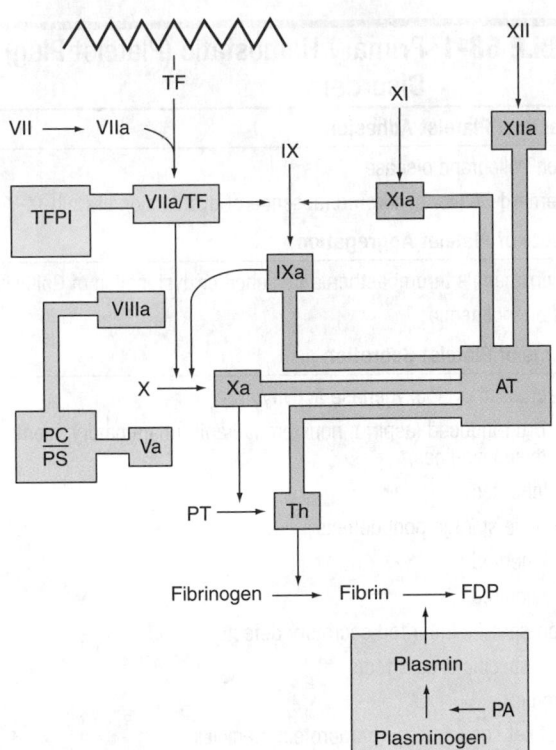

Figure 58-3 **Sites of action of the four major physiologic antithrombotic pathways:** antithrombin (AT); protein C/S (PC/PS); tissue factor pathway inhibitor (TFPI); and the fibrinolytic system, consisting of plasminogen, plasminogen activator (PA), and plasmin. PT, prothrombin; Th, thrombin; FDP, fibrin(ogen) degradation products. *[Modified from BA Konkle, AI Schafer, in DP Zipes et al (eds): Braunwald's Heart Disease, 7th ed. Philadelphia, Saunders, 2005.]*

production of tissue plasminogen activator 1, urokinase, plasminogen activator inhibitor, and annexin-2. The sites of action of the major physiologic antithrombotic pathways are shown in Fig. 58-3.

Antithrombin (or antithrombin III) is the major plasma protease inhibitor of thrombin and the other clotting factors in coagulation. Antithrombin neutralizes thrombin and other activated coagulation factors by forming a complex between the active site of the enzyme and the reactive center of antithrombin. The rate of formation of these inactivating complexes increases by a factor of several thousand in the presence of heparin. Antithrombin inactivation of thrombin and other activated clotting factors occurs physiologically on vascular surfaces, where glycosoaminoglycans, including heparan sulfates, are present to catalyze these reactions. Inherited quantitative or qualitative deficiencies of antithrombin lead to a lifelong predisposition to venous thromboembolism.

Protein C is a plasma glycoprotein that becomes an anticoagulant when it is activated by thrombin. The thrombin-induced activation of protein C occurs physiologically on thrombomodulin, a transmembrane proteoglycan-binding site for thrombin on endothelial cell surfaces. The binding of protein C to its receptor on endothelial cells places it in proximity to the thrombin-thrombomodulin complex, thereby enhancing its activation efficiency. Activated protein C acts as an anticoagulant by cleaving and inactivating activated factors V and VIII. This reaction is accelerated by a cofactor, protein S, which, like protein C, is a glycoprotein that undergoes vitamin K–dependent posttranslational modification. Quantitative or qualitative deficiencies of protein C or protein S, or resistance to the action of activated protein C by a specific mutation at its target cleavage site in factor Va (factor V Leiden), lead to hypercoagulable states.

Tissue factor pathway inhibitor (TFPI) is a plasma protease inhibitor that regulates the TF–induced extrinsic pathway of coagulation. TFPI inhibits the TF/FVIIa/FXa complex, essentially turning off the TF/FVIIa initiation of coagulation, which then becomes dependent on the "amplification loop" via FXI and FVIII activation by thrombin. TFPI is bound to lipoprotein and can also be released by heparin from endothelial cells, where it is bound to glycosoaminoglycans, and from platelets. The heparin-mediated release of TFPI may play a role in the anticoagulant effects of unfractionated and low-molecular-weight heparins.

■ THE FIBRINOLYTIC SYSTEM

Any thrombin that escapes the inhibitory effects of the physiologic anticoagulant systems is available to convert fibrinogen to fibrin. In response, the endogenous fibrinolytic system is then activated to dispose of intravascular fibrin and thereby maintain or reestablish the patency of the circulation. Just as thrombin is the key protease enzyme of the coagulation system, plasmin is the major protease enzyme of the fibrinolytic system, acting to digest fibrin to fibrin degradation products. The general scheme of fibrinolysis and its control is shown in Fig. 58-4.

The plasminogen activators, tissue type plasminogen activator (tPA) and the urokinase type plasminogen activator cleave (uPA), cleave the Arg560-Val561 bond of plasminogen to generate the active enzyme plasmin. The lysine-binding sites of plasmin (and plasminogen) permit it to bind to fibrin, so that physiologic fibrinolysis is "fibrin specific." Both plasminogen (through its lysine-binding sites) and tPA possess specific affinity for fibrin and thereby bind selectively to clots. The assembly of a ternary complex, consisting of fibrin, plasminogen, and tPA, promotes the localized interaction between plasminogen and tPA and greatly accelerates the rate of plasminogen activation to plasmin. Moreover, partial degradation of fibrin by plasmin exposes new plasminogen and tPA-binding sites in carboxy-terminus lysine residues of fibrin fragments to enhance these reactions further. This creates a highly efficient mechanism to generate plasmin focally on the fibrin clot, which then becomes plasmin's substrate for digestion to fibrin degradation products. Plasmin cleaves fibrin at distinct sites of the fibrin molecule leading to the generation of characteristic fibrin fragments during the process of fibrinolysis (Fig. 58-2). The sites of plasmin cleavage of fibrin are the same as those in fibrinogen. However, when plasmin acts on covalently cross-linked fibrin, D-dimers are released; hence, D-dimers can be measured in plasma

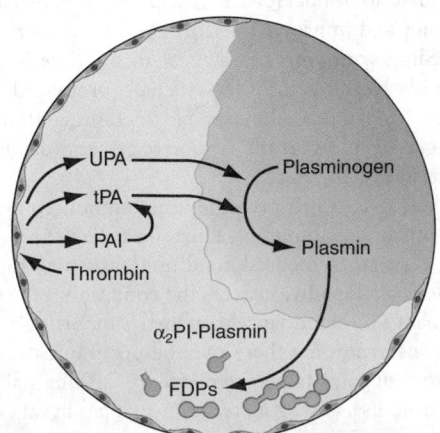

Figure 58-4 **A schematic diagram of the fibrinolytic system.** Tissue plasminogen activator (tPA) is released from endothelial cells, binds the fibrin clot, and activates plasminogen to plasmin. Excess fibrin is degraded by plasmin to distinct degradation products (FDPs). Any free plasmin is complexed with α_2-antiplasmin (α_2PI).

as a relatively specific test of fibrin (rather than fibrinogen) degradation. D-dimer assays can be used as sensitive markers of blood clot formation, and some have been validated for clinical use to exclude the diagnosis of deep-venous thrombosis (DVT) and pulmonary embolism in selected populations.

Physiologic regulation of fibrinolysis occurs primarily at three levels: (1) plasminogen activator inhibitors (PAIs), specifically PAI-1 and PAI-2, inhibit the physiologic plasminogen activators; (2) the thrombin-activatable fibrinolysis inhibitor (TAFI) limits fibrinolysis; and (3) α_2-antiplasmin inhibits plasmin. PAI1 is the primary inhibitor of tPA and uPA in plasma. TAFI cleaves the N-terminal lysine residues of fibrin, which aid in localization of plasmin activity. α_2-Antiplasmin is the main inhibitor of plasmin in human plasma, inactivating any non-fibrin clot-associated plasmin.

APPROACH TO THE PATIENT: Bleeding and Thrombosis

CLINICAL PRESENTATION Disorders of hemostasis may be either inherited or acquired. A detailed personal and family history is key in determining the chronicity of symptoms and the likelihood of the disorder being inherited, and it provides clues to underlying conditions that have contributed to the bleeding or thrombotic state. In addition, the history can give clues as to the etiology by determining (1) the bleeding (mucosal and/or joint) or thrombosis (arterial and/or venous) site and (2) whether an underlying bleeding or clotting tendency was enhanced by another medical condition or the introduction of medications or dietary supplements.

History of Bleeding   A history of bleeding is the most important predictor of bleeding risk. In evaluating a patient for a bleeding disorder, a history of at-risk situations, including the response to past surgeries, should be assessed. Does the patient have a history of spontaneous or trauma/surgery-induced bleeding? Spontaneous hemarthroses are a hallmark of moderate and severe factor VIII and IX deficiency and, in rare circumstances, of other clotting factor deficiencies. Mucosal bleeding symptoms are more suggestive of underlying platelet disorders or von Willebrand disease (VWD), termed *disorders of primary hemostasis or platelet plug formation*. Disorders affecting primary hemostasis are shown in Table 58-1.

A bleeding score has been validated as a tool to predict patients more likely to have Type 1 VWD. Studies are under way to validate additional formats, including ones that are easier to administer and improving performance in pediatric populations. Bleeding symptoms that appear to be more common in patients with bleeding disorders include prolonged bleeding with surgery, dental procedures and extractions, and/or trauma, menorrhagia or postpartum hemorrhage, and large bruises (often described with lumps).

Easy bruising and menorrhagia are common complaints in patients with and without bleeding disorders. Easy bruising can also be a sign of medical conditions in which there is no identifiable coagulopathy; instead, the conditions are caused by an abnormality of blood vessels or their supporting tissues. In Ehlers-Danlos syndrome there may be posttraumatic bleeding and a history of joint hyperextensibility. Cushing's syndrome, chronic steroid use, and aging result in changes in skin and subcutaneous tissue, and subcutaneous bleeding occurs in response to minor trauma. The latter has been termed *senile purpura*.

Epistaxis is a common symptom, particularly in children and in dry climates, and may not reflect an underlying bleeding disorder. However it is the most common symptom in hereditary hemorrhagic telangiectasia and in boys with VWD. Clues that

TABLE 58-1 Primary Hemostatic (Platelet Plug) Disorders

Defects of Platelet Adhesion

Von Willebrand disease

Bernard-Soulier syndrome (absence of dysfunction of GpIb-IX-V)

Defects of Platelet Aggregation

Glanzmann's thrombasthenia (absence or dysfunction of GpIIbIIIa)

Afibrinogenemia

Defects of Platelet Secretion

Decreased cyclooxygenase activity

   Drug-induced (aspirin, nonsteroidal anti-inflammatory agents, thienopyridines)

   Inherited

Granule storage pool defects

   Inherited

   Acquired

Non-specific inherited secretory defects

Non-specific drug effects

Uremia

Platelet coating (e.g., paraprotein, penicillin)

Defect of Platelet Coagulant Activity

Scott's syndrome

epistaxis is a symptom of an underlying bleeding disorder include lack of seasonal variation and bleeding that requires medical evaluation or treatment, including cauterization. Bleeding with eruption of primary teeth is seen in children with more severe bleeding disorders, such as moderate and severe hemophilia. It is uncommon in children with mild bleeding disorders. Patients with disorders of primary hemostasis (platelet adhesion) may have increased bleeding after dental cleanings and other procedures that involve gum manipulation.

Menorrhagia is defined quantitatively as a loss of >80 mL of blood per cycle, based on blood loss required to produce iron-deficiency anemia. A complaint of heavy menses is subjective and has a poor correlation with excessive blood loss. Predictors of menorrhagia include bleeding resulting in iron-deficiency anemia or a need for blood transfusion, passage of clots >1 inch in diameter and changing a pad or tampon more than hourly. Menorrhagia is a common symptom in women with underlying bleeding disorders and is reported in the majority of women with VWD and factor XI deficiency and in symptomatic carriers of hemophilia A. Women with underlying bleeding disorders are more likely to have other bleeding symptoms, including bleeding after dental extractions, postoperative bleeding, and postpartum bleeding, and are much more likely to have menorrhagia beginning at menarche than women with menorrhagia due to other causes.

Postpartum hemorrhage (PPH) is a common symptom in women with underlying bleeding disorders. In women with Type 1 VWD and symptomatic carriers of hemophilia in whom levels of VWF and FVIII usually normalize during pregnancy, PPH may be delayed. Women with a history of postpartum hemorrhage have a high risk of recurrence with subsequent pregnancies. Rupture of ovarian cysts with intraabdominal hemorrhage has also been reported in women with underlying bleeding disorders.

Tonsillectomy is a major hemostatic challenge, as intact hemostatic mechanisms are essential to prevent excessive bleeding from the tonsillar bed. Bleeding may occur early after surgery or after approximately 7 days postoperatively, with loss of the eschar at the operative site. Similar delayed bleeding is seen after colonic polyp resection. Gastrointestinal (GI) bleeding and hematuria are usually due to underlying pathology, and procedures to identify and treat the bleeding site should be undertaken, even in patients with known bleeding disorders. VWD, particularly types 2 and 3, has been associated with angiodysplasia of the bowel and GI bleeding.

Hemarthroses and spontaneous muscle hematomas are characteristic of moderate or severe congenital factor VIII or IX deficiency. They can also be seen in moderate and severe deficiencies of fibrinogen, prothrombin, and of factors V, VII, and X. Spontaneous hemarthroses occur rarely in other bleeding disorders except for severe VWD, with associated FVIII levels <5%. Muscle and soft tissue bleeds are also common in acquired FVIII deficiency. Bleeding into a joint results in severe pain and swelling, as well as loss of function, but is rarely associated with discoloration from bruising around the joint. Life-threatening sites of bleeding include bleeding into the oropharynx, where bleeding can obstruct the airway, into the central nervous system, and into the retroperitoneum. Central nervous system bleeding is the major cause of bleeding-related deaths in patients with severe congenital factor deficiencies.

Prohemorrhagic Effects of Medications and Dietary Supplements
Aspirin and other nonsteroidal inflammatory drugs (NSAIDs) that inhibit cyclooxygenase 1 impair primary hemostasis and may exacerbate bleeding from another cause or even unmask a previously occult mild bleeding disorder such as VWD. All NSAIDs, however, can precipitate gastrointestinal bleeding, which may be more severe in patients with underlying bleeding disorders. The aspirin effect on platelet function as assessed by aggregometry can persist for up to 7 days, although it has frequently returned to normal by 3 days after the last dose. The effect of other NSAIDs is shorter, as the inhibitor effect is reversed when the drug is removed. Thienopyridines (clopidogrel and prasugrel) inhibit ADP-mediated platelet aggregation and like NSAIDs can precipitate or exacerbate bleeding symptoms.

Many herbal supplements can impair hemostatic function (Table 58-2). Some are more convincingly associated with a bleeding risk than others. Fish oil or concentrated omega 3 fatty acid supplements impair platelet function. They alter platelet biochemistry to produce more PGI3, a more potent platelet inhibitor than prostacyclin (PGI2), and more thromboxane A3, a less potent platelet activator than thromboxane A2. In fact, diets naturally rich in omega 3 fatty acids can result in a prolonged bleeding time and abnormal platelet aggregation studies, but the actual associated bleeding risk is unclear. Vitamin E appears to inhibit protein kinase C–mediated platelet aggregation and nitric oxide production. In patients with unexplained bruising or bleeding, it is prudent to review any new medications or supplements and discontinue those that may be associated with bleeding.

Underlying Systemic Diseases That Cause or Exacerbate a Bleeding Tendency
Acquired bleeding disorders are commonly secondary to, or associated with, systemic disease. The clinical evaluation of a patient with a bleeding tendency must therefore include a thorough assessment for evidence of underlying disease. Bruising or mucosal bleeding may be the presenting complaint in liver disease, severe renal impairment, hypothyroidism, paraproteinemias or amyloidosis, and conditions causing bone marrow failure. All coagulation factors are synthesized in the liver, and hepatic failure results in combined factor deficiencies. This is often compounded by thrombocytopenia from splenomegaly due to portal hypertension. Coagulation factors II, VII, IX, X and proteins C, S,

TABLE 58-2 Herbal Supplements Associated With Increased Bleeding

Herbs With Potential Anti-Platelet Activity

Ginkgo (*Ginkgo biloba L.*)
Garlic (*Allium sativum*)
Bilberry (*Vaccinium myrtillus*)
Ginger (*Gingiber officinale*)
Dong quai (*Angelica sinensis*)
Feverfew (*Tanacetum parthenium*)
Asian ginseng (*Panax ginseng*)
American ginseng (*Panax quinquefolius*)
Siberian ginseng/eleuthero (*Eleuterococcus senticosus*)
Turmeric (*Circuma longa*)
Meadowsweet (*Filipendula ulmaria*)
Willow (*Salix* spp.)

Coumarin-Containing Herbs

Motherworth (*Leonurus cardiaca*)
Chamomile (*Matricaria recutita, Chamaemelum mobile*)
Horse chestnut (*Aesculus hippocastanum*)
Red clover (*Trifolium pratense*)
Fenugreek (*Trigonella foenum-graecum*)

and Z are dependent on vitamin K for posttranslational modification. Although vitamin K is required in both procoagulant and anticoagulant processes, the phenotype of vitamin K deficiency or the warfarin effect on coagulation is bleeding.

The normal blood platelet count is 150,000–450,000/μL. Thrombocytopenia results from decreased production, increased destruction, and/or sequestration. Although the bleeding risk varies somewhat by the reason for the thrombocytopenia, bleeding rarely occurs in isolated thrombocytopenia at counts <50,000/μL and usually not until <10,000–20,000/μL. Coexisting coagulopathies, as is seen in liver failure or disseminated coagulation; infection, platelet-inhibitory drugs; and underlying medical conditions can all increase the risk of bleeding in the thrombocytopenic patient. Most procedures can be performed in patients with a platelet count of 50,000/μL. The level needed for major surgery will depend on the type of surgery and the patients' underlying medical state, although a count of approximately 80,000/μL is likely sufficient.

HISTORY OF THROMBOSIS The risk of thrombosis, like that of bleeding, is influenced by both genetic and environmental influences. The major risk factor for arterial thrombosis is atherosclerosis, while for venous thrombosis the risk factors are immobility, surgery, underlying medical conditions such as malignancy, medications such as hormonal therapy, obesity, and genetic predispositions. Factors that increase risks for venous and for both venous and arterial thromboses are shown in Table 58-3.

The most important point in a history related to venous thrombosis is determining whether the thrombotic event was idiopathic (meaning there was no clear precipitating factor) or was a precipitated event. In patients without underlying malignancy, having an idiopathic event is the strongest predictor of recurrence of venous thromboembolism. In patients who have a vague history of thrombosis, a history of being treated with warfarin suggests a past DVT. Age is an important risk factor for venous thrombosis—the risk of DVT increasing per decade, with an approximate incidence of 1/100,000 per year in early childhood to 200 per year among

TABLE 58-3 Risk Factors for Thrombosis

Venous	Venous and Arterial
Inherited	**Inherited**
Factor V Leiden	Homocystinuria
Prothrombin G20210A	Dysfibrinogenemia
Antithrombin deficiency	
Protein C deficiency	**Mixed (inherited and acquired)**
Protein S deficiency	Hyperhomocysteinemia
Elevated FVIII	
	Acquired
Acquired	Malignancy
Age	Antiphospholipid antibody syndrome
Previous thrombosis	Hormonal therapy
Immobilization	Polycythemia vera
Major surgery	Essential thrombocythemia
Pregnancy and puerperium	Paroxysmal nocturnal hemoglobinuria
Hospitalization	Thrombotic thrombocytopenic purpura
Obesity	Heparin-induced thrombocytopenia
Infection	Disseminated intravascular coagulation
APC resistance, nongenetic	
Smoking	
Unknown*	
Elevated factor II, IX, XI	
Elevated TAFI levels	
Low levels of TFPI	

*Unknown whether risk is inherited or acquired.

Abbreviations: APC, activated protein C; TAFI, thrombin-activatable fibrinolysis inhibitor; TFPI, tissue factor pathway inhibitor.

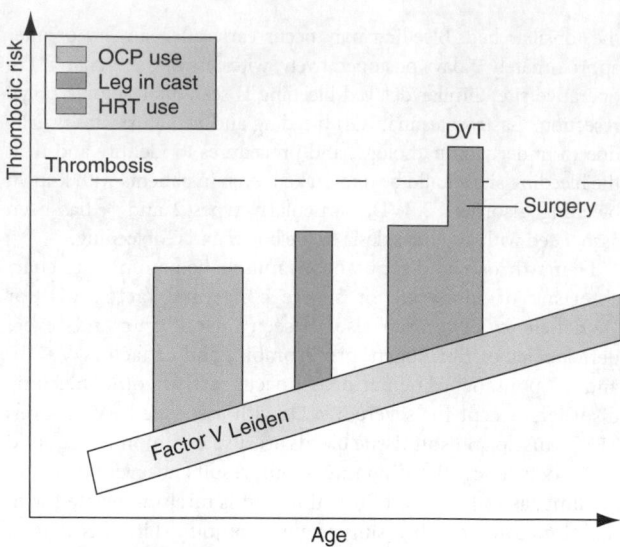

Figure 58-5 Thrombotic risk over time. Shown schematically is an individual's thrombotic risk over time. An underlying factor V Leiden mutation provides a "theoretically" constant increased risk. The thrombotic risk increases with age and, intermittently, with oral contraceptive (OCP) or hormone replacement (HRT) use; other events may increase the risk further. At some point the cumulative risk may increase to the threshold for thrombosis and result in deep-venous thrombosis (DVT). Note: The magnitude and duration of risk portrayed in the figure is meant for example only and may not precisely reflect the relative risk determined by clinical study. *[From BA Konkle, A Schafer, in DP Zipes et al (eds): Braunwald's Heart Disease, 7th ed. Philadelphia, Saunders, 2005; modified with permission from FR Rosendaal: Venous thrombosis: A multicausal disease. Lancet 353:1167, 1999.]*

octogenarians. Family history is helpful in determining if there is a genetic predisposition and how strong that predisposition appears to be. A genetic thrombophilia that confers a relatively small increased risk, such as being a heterozygote for the prothrombin G20210A or factor V Leiden mutation, may be a minor determinant of risk in an elderly individual undergoing a high-risk surgical procedure. As illustrated in Fig. 58-5, a thrombotic event usually has more than one contributing factor. Predisposing factors must be carefully assessed to determine the risk of recurrent thrombosis and, with consideration of the patient's bleeding risk, determine the length of anticoagulation. Similar consideration should be given in determining the need to test the patient and family members for thrombophilias.

LABORATORY EVALUATION Careful history taking and clinical examination are essential components in the assessment of bleeding and thrombotic risk. The use of laboratory tests of coagulation complement, but cannot substitute for, clinical assessment. No test exists that provides a global assessment of hemostasis. The bleeding time has been used to assess bleeding risk; however, it does not predict bleeding risk with surgery and it is not recommended for this indication. The PFA-100, an instrument that measures platelet-dependent coagulation under flow conditions, is more sensitive and specific for platelet disorders and VWD than the bleeding time; however it is not sensitive enough to rule out underlying mild bleeding disorders. Also, its utility in predicting bleeding risk has not been determined.

For routine preoperative and preprocedure testing, an abnormal prothrombin time (PT) may detect liver disease or vitamin K deficiency that had not been previously appreciated. Studies have not confirmed the usefulness of an activated partial thromboplastin time (aPTT) in preoperative evaluations in patients with a negative bleeding history. The primary use of coagulation testing should be to confirm the presence and type of bleeding disorder in a patient with a suspicious clinical history.

Because of the nature of coagulation assays, proper sample acquisition and handling is critical to obtaining valid results. In patients with abnormal coagulation assays who have no bleeding history, repeat studies with attention to these factors frequently results in normal values. Most coagulation assays are performed in sodium citrate anticoagulated plasma that is recalcified for the assay. Because the anticoagulant is in liquid solution and needs to be added to blood in proportion to the plasma volume, incorrectly filled or inadequately mixed blood collection tubes will give erroneous results. Vacutainer tubes should be filled to >90% of the recommended fill, which is usually denoted by a line on the tube. An elevated hematocrit (>55%) can result in a false value due to a decreased plasma to anticoagulant ratio.

Screening Assays The most commonly used screening tests are the PT, aPTT, and platelet count. The PT assesses the factors I (fibrinogen), II (prothrombin), V, VII, and X (Fig. 58-6). The PT measures the time for clot formation of the citrated plasma after recalcification and addition of thromboplastin, a mixture of TF and phospholipids. The sensitivity of the assay varies by the source of thromboplastin. The relationship between defects in secondary hemostasis (fibrin formation) and coagulation test abnormalities is shown in Table 58-4. To adjust for this variability, the overall sensitivity of different thromboplastins to reduction of the vitamin K–dependent clotting factors II, VII, IX, and X in anticoagulation patients is now expressed as the International Sensitivity Index (ISI). An inverse relationship exists between ISI and thromboplastin sensitivity. The international normalized ratio (INR) is then determined based on the formula: $INR = (PT_{patient}/PT_{normal\ mean})^{ISI}$.

The INR was developed to assess anticoagulation due to reduction of vitamin K–dependent coagulation factors; it is

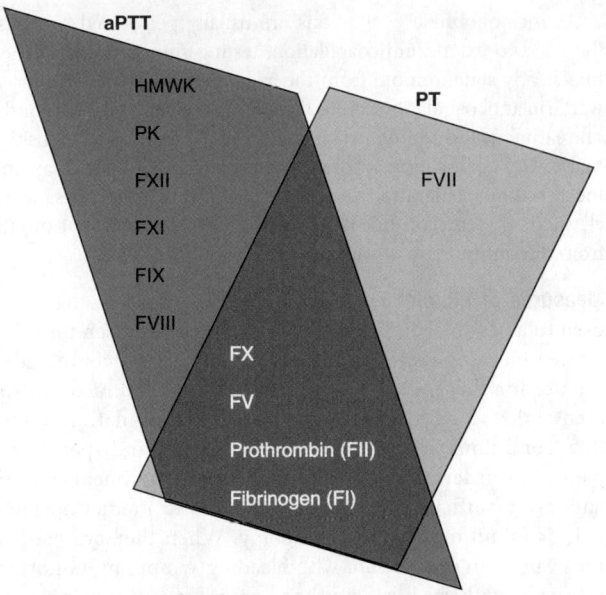

Figure 58-6 **Coagulation factor activity** tested in the activated partial thromboplastin time (aPTT) in red and prothrombin time (PT) in green, or both. F, factor; HMWK, high-molecular-weight kininogen; PK, prekallikrein.

TABLE 58-4 Hemostatic Disorders and Coagulation Test Abnormalities

Prolonged Activated Partial Thromboplastin Time (aPTT)

No clinical bleeding—↓ factors XII, high-molecular-weight kininogen, prekallikrein

Variable, but usually mild, bleeding—↓ factor XI, mild↓ FVIII and FIX

Frequent, severe bleeding—severe deficiencies of FVIII and FIX

Heparin

Prolonged Prothrombin Time (PT)

Factor VII deficiency

Vitamin K deficiency—early

Warfarin anticoagulation

Prolonged aPTT and PT

Factor II, V, X, or fibrinogen deficiency

Vitamin K deficiency—late

Direct thrombin inhibitors

Prolonged Thrombin Time

Heparin or heparin-like inhibitors

Mild or no bleeding—dysfibrinogenemia

Frequent, severe bleeding—afibrinogenemia

Prolonged PT and/or aPTT Not Corrected with Mixing with Normal Plasma

Bleeding—specific factor inhibitor

No symptoms, or clotting and/or pregnancy loss—lupus anticoagulant

Disseminated intravascular coagulation

Heparin or direct thrombin inhibitor

Abnormal Clot Solubility

Factor XIII deficiency

Inhibitors or defective cross-linking

Rapid Clot Lysis

Deficiency of α_2-antiplasmin or plasminogen activator inhibitor 1

Treatment with fibrinolytic therapy

---

commonly used in the evaluation of patients with liver disease. While it does allow comparison between laboratories, reagent sensitivity as used to determine the ISI is not the same in liver disease as with warfarin anticoagulation. In addition, progressive liver failure is associated with variable changes in coagulation factors; the degree of prolongation of either the PT or the INR only roughly predicts the bleeding risk. Thrombin generation has been shown to be normal in many patients with mild to moderate liver dysfunction. As the PT only measures one aspect of hemostasis affected by liver dysfunction, we likely overestimate the bleeding risk of a mildly elevated INR in this setting.

The aPTT assesses the intrinsic and common coagulation pathways, factors XI, IX, VIII, X, V, II, fibrinogen, and also prekallikrein, high-molecular-weight kininogen and factor XII (Fig. 58-6). The aPTT reagent contains phospholipids derived from either animal or vegetable sources that function as a platelet substitute in the coagulation pathways and includes an activator of the intrinsic coagulation system, such as nonparticulate ellagic acid or the particulate activators kaolin, celite, or micronized silica.

The phospholipid composition of aPTT reagents varies, which influences the sensitivity of individual reagents to clotting factor deficiencies and to inhibitors such as heparin and lupus anticoagulants. Thus, aPTT results will vary from one laboratory to another and the normal range in the laboratory where the testing occurs should be used in the interpretation. Local laboratories cam relate their aPTT values to the therapeutic heparin anticoagulation by correlating aPTT values with direct measurements of heparin activity (anti-Xa or protamine titration assays) in samples from heparinized patients, although correlation between these assays is often poor. The aPTT reagent will vary in sensitivity to individual factor deficiencies and usually becomes prolonged with individual factor deficiencies of 30–50%.

Mixing Studies Mixing studies are used to evaluate a prolonged aPTT or, less commonly PT, to distinguish between a factor deficiency and an inhibitor. In this assay, normal plasma and patient plasma are mixed in a 1:1 ratio, and the aPTT or PT is determined immediately and after incubation at 37°C for varying times, typically 30, 60, and/or 120 min. With isolated factor deficiencies, the aPTT will correct with mixing and stay corrected with incubation. With aPTT prolongation due to a lupus anticoagulant, the mixing and incubation will show no correction. In acquired neutralizing factor antibodies, such as an acquired factor VIII inhibitor, the initial assay may or may not correct immediately after mixing but will prolong or remain prolonged with incubation at 37°C. Failure to correct with mixing can also be due to the presence of other inhibitors or interfering substances such as heparin, fibrin split products, and paraproteins.

Specific Factor Assays Decisions to proceed with specific clotting factor assays will be influenced by the clinical situation and the results of coagulation screening tests. Precise diagnosis and effective management of inherited and acquired coagulation deficiencies necessitate quantitation of the relevant factors.

When bleeding is severe, specific assays are often urgently required to guide appropriate therapy. Individual factor assays are usually performed as modifications of the mixing study, where the patient's plasma is mixed with plasma deficient in the factor being studied. This will correct all factor deficiencies to >50%, thus making prolongation of clot formation due to a factor deficiency dependent on the factor missing from the added plasma.

Testing for Antiphospholipid Antibodies Antibodies to phospholipids (cardiolipin) or phospholipid-binding proteins (β_2-microglobulin and others) are detected by ELISA. When these antibodies interfere with phospholipid-dependent coagulation tests, they are termed *lupus anticoagulants*. The aPTT has variability sensitivity to lupus anticoagulants, depending in part on the aPTT reagents used. An assay utilizing a sensitive reagent has been termed an *LA-PTT*. The dilute Russell viper venom test (dRVVT) and the tissue thromboplastin inhibition (TTI) test are modifications of standard tests with the phospholipid reagent decreased, thus increasing the sensitivity to antibodies that interfere with the phospholipid component. The tests, however, are not specific for lupus anticoagulants, as factor deficiencies or other inhibitors will also result in prolongation. Documentation of a lupus anticoagulant requires not only prolongation of a phospholipid-dependent coagulation test but also lack of correction when mixed with normal plasma and correction with the addition of activated platelet membranes or certain phospholipids, e.g. hexagonal phase.

Other Coagulation Tests The thrombin time and the reptilase time measure fibrinogen conversion to fibrin and are prolonged when the fibrinogen level is low (usually <80–100 mg/dL), qualitatively abnormal, as seen in inherited or acquired dysfibrinogenemias, or when fibrin/fibrinogen degradation products interfere. The thrombin time, but not the reptilase time, is prolonged in the presence of heparin. Measurement of anti–factor Xa plasma inhibitory activity is a test frequently used to assess low-molecular-weight heparin (LMWH) levels or as a direct measurement of unfractionated heparin (UFH) activity. Heparin in the patient sample inhibits the enzymatic conversion of a Xa-specific chromogenic substrate to colored product by factor Xa. Standard curves are created using multiple concentrations of UFH and LMWH and are used to calculate the concentration of anti-Xa activity in the patient plasma.

Laboratory Testing for Thrombophilia. Laboratory assays to detect thrombophilic states include molecular diagnostics and immunologic and functional assays. These assays vary in their sensitivity and specificity for the condition being tested. Furthermore, acute thrombosis, acute illnesses, inflammatory conditions, pregnancy, and medications affect levels of many coagulation factors and their inhibitors. Antithrombin is decreased by heparin and in the setting of acute thrombosis. Protein C and S levels may be increased in the setting of acute thrombosis and are decreased by warfarin. Antiphospholipid antibodies are frequently transiently positive in acute illness. Testing for genetic thrombophilias should, in general, only be performed when there is a strong family history of thrombosis and results would affect clinical decision making.

As thrombophilia evaluations are usually performed to assess the need to extend anticoagulation, testing should be performed in a steady state, remote from the acute event. In most instances, warfarin anticoagulation can be stopped after the initial 3–6 months of treatment, and testing performed at least 3 weeks later. Sensitive markers of coagulation activation, notably the D-dimer assay and the thrombin generation test, hold promise as predictors, when elevated, of recurrent thrombosis when measured at least 1 month from discontinuation of warfarin.

Measures of Platelet Function. The bleeding time has been used to assess bleeding risk; however, it has not been found to predict bleeding risk with surgery, and it is not recommended for use for this indication. The PFA-100 and similar instruments that measure platelet-dependent coagulation under flow conditions are generally more sensitive and specific for platelet disorders and VWD than the bleeding time; however, data are insufficient to support their use to predict bleeding risk or monitor response to therapy. When they are used in the evaluation of a patient with bleeding symptoms, abnormal results, as with the bleeding time, require specific testing, such as VWF assays and/or platelet aggregation studies. Since all of these "screening" assays may miss patients with mild bleeding disorders, further studies are needed to define their role in hemostasis testing.

For classic platelet aggregometry, various agonists are added to the patient's platelet-rich plasma and platelet aggregation is observed. Tests of platelet secretion in response to agonists can also be measured. These tests are affected by many factors, including numerous medications, and the association between minor defects in aggregation or secretion in these assays and bleeding risk is not clearly established.

ACKNOWLEDGMENT
Robert I. Handin, MD, contributed this chapter in the 16th edition and some material from that chapter has been retained here.

FURTHER READINGS

BAGLIN T et al: Clinical guidelines for testing for heritable thrombophilia. Br J Haematol 149:209, 2010

COSMI B et al: Usefulness of repeated D-dimer testing after stopping anticoagulation for a first episode of unprovoked venous thromboembolism: The PROLONG II prospective study. Blood 115:481, 2010

GALLI M: The antiphospholipid triangle. J Thromb Haemost 8:234, 2010

LIJFERING WM et al: Risk factors for venous thrombosis—current understanding from an epidemiological point of view. Br J Haematol 149:824, 2010

PENGO V et al: Antiphospholipid syndrome: Critical analysis of the diagnostic path. Lupus 19:428, 2010

WAGENMAN BL et al: The laboratory approach to inherited and acquired coagulation factor deficiencies. Clin Lab Med 29:229, 2009

WHEELER AP, RICE TW: Coagulopathy in critically ill patients: Soluble clotting factors and hemostatic testing. Chest 137:185, 2010

CHAPTER 59

Enlargement of Lymph Nodes and Spleen

Patrick H. Henry
Dan L. Longo

This chapter is intended to serve as a guide to the evaluation of patients who present with enlargement of the lymph nodes (*lymphadenopathy*) or the spleen (*splenomegaly*). Lymphadenopathy is a rather common clinical finding in primary care settings, whereas palpable splenomegaly is less so.

LYMPHADENOPATHY

Lymphadenopathy may be an incidental finding in patients being examined for various reasons, or it may be a presenting sign or symptom of the patient's illness. The physician must eventually decide whether the lymphadenopathy is a normal finding or one that requires further study, up to and including biopsy. Soft, flat, submandibular nodes (<1 cm) are often palpable in healthy children and young adults; healthy adults may have palpable inguinal nodes of up to 2 cm, which are considered normal. Further evaluation of these normal nodes is not warranted. In contrast, if the physician believes the node(s) to be abnormal, then pursuit of a more precise diagnosis is needed.

APPROACH TO THE PATIENT Lymphadenopathy

Lymphadenopathy may be a primary or secondary manifestation of numerous disorders, as shown in Table 59-1. Many of these disorders are infrequent causes of lymphadenopathy. In primary care practice, more than two-thirds of patients with lymphadenopathy have nonspecific causes or upper respiratory illnesses (viral or bacterial) and <1% have a malignancy. In one study, 84% of patients referred for evaluation of lymphadenopathy had a "benign" diagnosis. The remaining 16% had a malignancy (lymphoma or metastatic adenocarcinoma). Of the patients with benign lymphadenopathy, 63% had a nonspecific or reactive etiology (no causative agent found), and the remainder had a specific cause demonstrated, most commonly infectious mononucleosis, toxoplasmosis, or tuberculosis. Thus, the vast majority of patients with lymphadenopathy will have a nonspecific etiology requiring few diagnostic tests.

CLINICAL ASSESSMENT The physician will be aided in the pursuit of an explanation for the lymphadenopathy by a careful medical history, physical examination, selected laboratory tests, and perhaps an excisional lymph node biopsy.

The *medical history* should reveal the setting in which lymphadenopathy is occurring. Symptoms such as sore throat, cough, fever, night sweats, fatigue, weight loss, or pain in the nodes should be sought. The patient's age, sex, occupation, exposure to pets, sexual behavior, and use of drugs such as diphenylhydantoin are other important historic points. For example, children and young adults usually have benign (i.e., nonmalignant) disorders that account for the observed lymphadenopathy such as

TABLE 59-1 Diseases Associated With Lymphadenopathy

1. Infectious diseases
    a. Viral—infectious mononucleosis syndromes (EBV, CMV), infectious hepatitis, herpes simplex, herpesvirus-6, varicella-zoster virus, rubella, measles, adenovirus, HIV, epidemic keratoconjunctivitis, vaccinia, herpesvirus-8
    b. Bacterial—streptococci, staphylococci, cat-scratch disease, brucellosis, tularemia, plague, chancroid, melioidosis, glanders, tuberculosis, atypical mycobacterial infection, primary and secondary syphilis, diphtheria, leprosy
    c. Fungal—histoplasmosis, coccidioidomycosis, paracoccidioidomycosis
    d. Chlamydial—lymphogranuloma venereum, trachoma
    e. Parasitic—toxoplasmosis, leishmaniasis, trypanosomiasis, filariasis
    f. Rickettsial—scrub typhus, rickettsialpox, Q fever

2. Immunologic diseases
    a. Rheumatoid arthritis
    b. Juvenile rheumatoid arthritis
    c. Mixed connective tissue disease
    d. Systemic lupus erythematosus
    e. Dermatomyositis
    f. Sjögren's syndrome
    g. Serum sickness
    h. Drug hypersensitivity—diphenylhydantoin, hydralazine, allopurinol, primidone, gold, carbamazepine, etc.
    i. Angioimmunoblastic lymphadenopathy
    j. Primary biliary cirrhosis
    k. Graft-vs.-host disease
    l. Silicone-associated
    m. Autoimmune lymphoproliferative syndrome

3. Malignant diseases
    a. Hematologic—Hodgkin's disease, non-Hodgkin's lymphomas, acute or chronic lymphocytic leukemia, hairy cell leukemia, malignant histiocytosis, amyloidosis
    b. Metastatic—from numerous primary sites

4. Lipid storage diseases—Gaucher's, Niemann-Pick, Fabry, Tangier

5. Endocrine diseases—hyperthyroidism

6. Other disorders
    a. Castleman's disease (giant lymph node hyperplasia)
    b. Sarcoidosis
    c. Dermatopathic lymphadenitis
    d. Lymphomatoid granulomatosis
    e. Histiocytic necrotizing lymphadenitis (Kikuchi's disease)
    f. Sinus histiocytosis with massive lymphadenopathy (Rosai-Dorfman disease)
    g. Mucocutaneous lymph node syndrome (Kawasaki's disease)
    h. Histiocytosis X
    i. Familial Mediterranean fever
    j. Severe hypertriglyceridemia
    k. Vascular transformation of sinuses
    l. Inflammatory pseudotumor of lymph node
    m. Congestive heart failure

Abbreviations: CMV, cytomegalovirus; EBV, Epstein-Barr virus.

viral or bacterial upper respiratory infections; infectious mononucleosis; toxoplasmosis; and, in some countries, tuberculosis. In contrast, after age 50, the incidence of malignant disorders increases and that of benign disorders decreases.

The *physical examination* can provide useful clues such as the extent of lymphadenopathy (localized or generalized), size of nodes, texture, presence or absence of nodal tenderness, signs of inflammation over the node, skin lesions, and splenomegaly. A thorough ear, nose, and throat (ENT) examination is indicated in adult patients with cervical adenopathy and a history of tobacco use. Localized or regional adenopathy implies involvement of a single anatomic area. Generalized adenopathy has been defined as involvement of three or more noncontiguous lymph node areas. Many of the causes of lymphadenopathy (Table 59-1) can produce localized *or* generalized adenopathy, so this distinction is of limited utility in the differential diagnosis. Nevertheless, generalized lymphadenopathy is frequently associated with nonmalignant disorders such as infectious mononucleosis [Epstein-Barr virus (EBV) or cytomegalovirus (CMV)], toxoplasmosis, AIDS, other viral infections, systemic lupus erythematosus (SLE), and mixed connective tissue disease. Acute and chronic lymphocytic leukemias and malignant lymphomas also produce generalized adenopathy in adults.

The site of localized or regional adenopathy may provide a useful clue about the cause. Occipital adenopathy often reflects an infection of the scalp, and preauricular adenopathy accompanies conjunctival infections and cat-scratch disease. The most frequent site of regional adenopathy is the neck, and most of the causes are benign—upper respiratory infections, oral and dental lesions, infectious mononucleosis, or other viral illnesses. The chief malignant causes include metastatic cancer from head and neck, breast, lung, and thyroid primaries. Enlargement of supraclavicular and scalene nodes is always abnormal. Because these nodes drain regions of the lung and retroperitoneal space, they can reflect lymphomas, other cancers, or infectious processes arising in these areas. Virchow's node is an enlarged left supraclavicular node infiltrated with metastatic cancer from a gastrointestinal primary. Metastases to supraclavicular nodes also occur from lung, breast, testis, or ovarian cancers. Tuberculosis, sarcoidosis, and toxoplasmosis are nonneoplastic causes of supraclavicular adenopathy. Axillary adenopathy is usually due to injuries or localized infections of the ipsilateral upper extremity. Malignant causes include melanoma or lymphoma and, in women, breast cancer. Inguinal lymphadenopathy is usually secondary to infections or trauma of the lower extremities and may accompany sexually transmitted diseases such as lymphogranuloma venereum, primary syphilis, genital herpes, or chancroid. These nodes may also be involved by lymphomas and metastatic cancer from primary lesions of the rectum, genitalia, or lower extremities (melanoma).

The size and texture of the lymph node(s) and the presence of pain are useful parameters in evaluating a patient with lymphadenopathy. Nodes <1.0 cm² in area (1.0 cm × 1.0 cm or less) are almost always secondary to benign, nonspecific reactive causes. In one retrospective analysis of younger patients (9–25 years) who had a lymph node biopsy, a maximum diameter of >2 cm served as one discriminant for predicting that the biopsy would reveal malignant or granulomatous disease. Another study showed that a lymph node size of 2.25 cm² (1.5 cm × 1.5 cm) was the best size limit for distinguishing malignant or granulomatous lymphadenopathy from other causes of lymphadenopathy. Patients with node(s) ≤1.0 cm² should be observed after excluding infectious mononucleosis and/or toxoplasmosis unless there are symptoms and signs of an underlying systemic illness.

The texture of lymph nodes may be described as soft, firm, rubbery, hard, discrete, matted, tender, movable, or fixed. Tenderness is found when the capsule is stretched during rapid enlargement, usually secondary to an inflammatory process. Some malignant diseases such as acute leukemia may produce rapid enlargement and pain in the nodes. Nodes involved by lymphoma tend to be large, discrete, symmetric, rubbery, firm, mobile, and nontender. Nodes containing metastatic cancer are often hard, nontender, and nonmovable because of fixation to surrounding tissues. The coexistence of splenomegaly in the patient with lymphadenopathy implies a systemic illness such as infectious mononucleosis, lymphoma, acute or chronic leukemia, SLE, sarcoidosis, toxoplasmosis, cat-scratch disease, or other less common hematologic disorders. The patient's story should provide helpful clues about the underlying systemic illness.

Nonsuperficial presentations (thoracic or abdominal) of adenopathy are usually detected as the result of a symptom-directed diagnostic workup. Thoracic adenopathy may be detected by routine chest radiography or during the workup for superficial adenopathy. It may also be found because the patient complains of a cough or wheezing from airway compression; hoarseness from recurrent laryngeal nerve involvement; dysphagia from esophageal compression; or swelling of the neck, face, or arms secondary to compression of the superior vena cava or subclavian vein. The differential diagnosis of mediastinal and hilar adenopathy includes primary lung disorders and systemic illnesses that characteristically involve mediastinal or hilar nodes. In the young, mediastinal adenopathy is associated with infectious mononucleosis and sarcoidosis. In endemic regions, histoplasmosis can cause unilateral paratracheal lymph node involvement that mimics lymphoma. Tuberculosis can also cause unilateral adenopathy. In older patients, the differential diagnosis includes primary lung cancer (especially among smokers), lymphomas, metastatic carcinoma (usually lung), tuberculosis, fungal infection, and sarcoidosis.

Enlarged intraabdominal or retroperitoneal nodes are usually malignant. Although tuberculosis may present as mesenteric lymphadenitis, these masses usually contain lymphomas or, in young men, germ cell tumors.

LABORATORY INVESTIGATION The laboratory investigation of patients with lymphadenopathy must be tailored to elucidate the etiology suspected from the patient's history and physical findings. One study from a family practice clinic evaluated 249 younger patients with "enlarged lymph nodes, not infected" or "lymphadenitis." No laboratory studies were obtained in 51%. When studies were performed, the most common were a complete blood count (CBC) (33%), throat culture (16%), chest x-ray (12%), or monospot test (10%). Only eight patients (3%) had a node biopsy, and half of those were normal or reactive. The CBC can provide useful data for the diagnosis of acute or chronic leukemias, EBV or CMV mononucleosis, lymphoma with a leukemic component, pyogenic infections, or immune cytopenias in illnesses such as SLE. Serologic studies may demonstrate antibodies specific to components of EBV, CMV, HIV, and other viruses; *Toxoplasma gondii*; *Brucella*; etc. If SLE is suspected, antinuclear and anti-DNA antibody studies are warranted.

The chest x-ray is usually negative, but the presence of a pulmonary infiltrate or mediastinal lymphadenopathy would suggest tuberculosis, histoplasmosis, sarcoidosis, lymphoma, primary lung cancer, or metastatic cancer and demands further investigation.

A variety of imaging techniques (CT, MRI, ultrasound, color Doppler ultrasonography) have been employed to differentiate benign from malignant lymph nodes, especially in patients with head and neck cancer. CT and MRI are comparably accurate (65–90%) in the diagnosis of metastases to cervical lymph nodes. Ultrasonography has been used to determine the long (L) axis, short (S) axis, and a ratio of long to short axis in cervical nodes. An L/S ratio of <2.0 has a sensitivity and a specificity of 95% for distinguishing benign and malignant nodes in patients with head and neck cancer. This ratio has greater specificity and sensitivity than palpation or measurement of either the long or the short axis alone.

The indications for lymph node biopsy are imprecise, yet it is a valuable diagnostic tool. The decision to biopsy may be made early in a patient's evaluation or delayed for up to two weeks. Prompt biopsy should occur if the patient's history and physical findings suggest a malignancy; examples include a solitary, hard, nontender cervical node in an older patient who is a chronic user of tobacco; supraclavicular adenopathy; and solitary or generalized adenopathy that is firm, movable, and suggestive of lymphoma. If a primary head and neck cancer is suspected as the basis of a solitary, hard cervical node, then a careful ENT examination should be performed. Any mucosal lesion that is suspicious for a primary neoplastic process should be biopsied first. If no mucosal lesion is detected, an excisional biopsy of the largest node should be performed. Fine-needle aspiration should not be performed as the first diagnostic procedure. Most diagnoses require more tissue than such aspiration can provide, and it often delays a definitive diagnosis. Fine-needle aspiration should be reserved for thyroid nodules and for confirmation of relapse in patients whose primary diagnosis is known. If the primary physician is uncertain about whether to proceed to biopsy, consultation with a hematologist or medical oncologist should be helpful. In primary care practices, <5% of lymphadenopathy patients will require a biopsy. That percentage will be considerably larger in referral practices, i.e., hematology, oncology, or ENT.

Two groups have reported algorithms that they claim will identify more precisely those lymphadenopathy patients who should have a biopsy. Both reports were retrospective analyses in referral practices. The first study involved patients 9–25 years of age who had a node biopsy performed. Three variables were identified that predicted those young patients with peripheral lymphadenopathy who should undergo biopsy; lymph node size >2 cm in diameter and abnormal chest x-ray had positive predictive values, whereas recent ENT symptoms had negative predictive values. The second study evaluated 220 lymphadenopathy patients in a hematology unit and identified five variables [lymph node size, location (supraclavicular or non-supraclavicular), age (>40 years or <40 years), texture (nonhard or hard), and tenderness] that were used in a mathematical model to identify those patients requiring a biopsy. Positive predictive value was found for age >40 years, supraclavicular location, node size >2.25 cm², hard texture, and lack of pain or tenderness. Negative predictive value was evident for age <40 years, node size <1.0 cm², nonhard texture, and tender or painful nodes. Ninety-one percent of those who required biopsy were correctly classified by this model. Because both of these studies were retrospective analyses and one was limited to young patients, it is not known how useful these models would be if applied prospectively in a primary care setting.

Most lymphadenopathy patients do not require a biopsy, and at least half require no laboratory studies. If the patient's history and physical findings point to a benign cause for lymphadenopathy,

careful follow-up at a 2- to 4-week interval can be employed. The patient should be instructed to return for reevaluation if there is an increase in the size of the nodels). Antibiotics are not indicated for lymphadenopathy unless strong evidence of a bacterial infection is present. Glucocorticoids should not be used to treat lymphadenopathy because their lympholytic effect obscures some diagnoses (lymphoma, leukemia, Castleman's disease) and they contribute to delayed healing or activation of underlying infections. An exception to this statement is the life-threatening pharyngeal obstruction by enlarged lymphoid tissue in Waldeyer's ring that is occasionally seen in infectious mononucleosis.

SPLENOMEGALY

■ STRUCTURE AND FUNCTION OF THE SPLEEN

The spleen is a reticuloendothelial organ that has its embryologic origin in the dorsal mesogastrium at about five weeks' gestation. It arises in a series of hillocks, migrates to its normal adult location in the left upper quadrant (LUQ), and is attached to the stomach via the gastrolienal ligament and to the kidney via the lienorenal ligament. When the hillocks fail to unify into a single tissue mass, accessory spleens may develop in around 20% of persons. The function of the spleen has been elusive. Galen believed it was the source of "black bile" or melancholia, and the word *hypochondria* (literally, beneath the ribs) and the idiom "to vent one's spleen" attest to the beliefs that the spleen had an important influence on the psyche and emotions. In humans, its normal physiologic roles seem to be the following:

1. Maintenance of quality control over erythrocytes in the red pulp by removal of senescent and defective red blood cells. The spleen accomplishes this function through a unique organization of its parenchyma and vasculature (Fig. 59-1).

2. Synthesis of antibodies in the white pulp.

3. The removal of antibody-coated bacteria and antibody-coated blood cells from the circulation.

An increase in these normal functions may result in splenomegaly.

The spleen is composed of *red pulp* and *white pulp*, which are Malpighi's terms for the red blood–filled sinuses and reticuloendothelial cell–lined cords and the white lymphoid follicles arrayed within the red pulp matrix. The spleen is in the portal circulation. The reason for this is unknown but may relate to the fact that lower blood pressure allows less rapid flow and minimizes damage to normal erythrocytes. Blood flows into the spleen at a rate of about 150 mL/min through the splenic artery, which ultimately ramifies into central arterioles. Some blood goes from the arterioles to capillaries and then to splenic veins and out of the spleen, but the majority of blood from central arterioles flows into the macrophage-lined sinuses and cords. The blood entering the sinuses reenters the circulation through the splenic venules, but the blood entering the cords is subjected to an inspection of sorts. To return to the circulation, the blood cells in the cords must squeeze through slits in the cord lining to enter the sinuses that lead to the venules. Old and damaged erythrocytes are less deformable and are retained in the cords, where they are destroyed and their components recycled. Red cell–inclusion bodies such as parasites (Chaps. 210 and e27), nuclear residua (Howell-Jolly bodies, see Fig. 57-6), or denatured hemoglobin (Heinz bodies) are pinched off in the process of passing through the slits, a process called *pitting*. The culling of dead and damaged cells and the pitting of cells with inclusions appear to occur without significant delay because the blood transit time through the spleen is only slightly slower than in other organs.

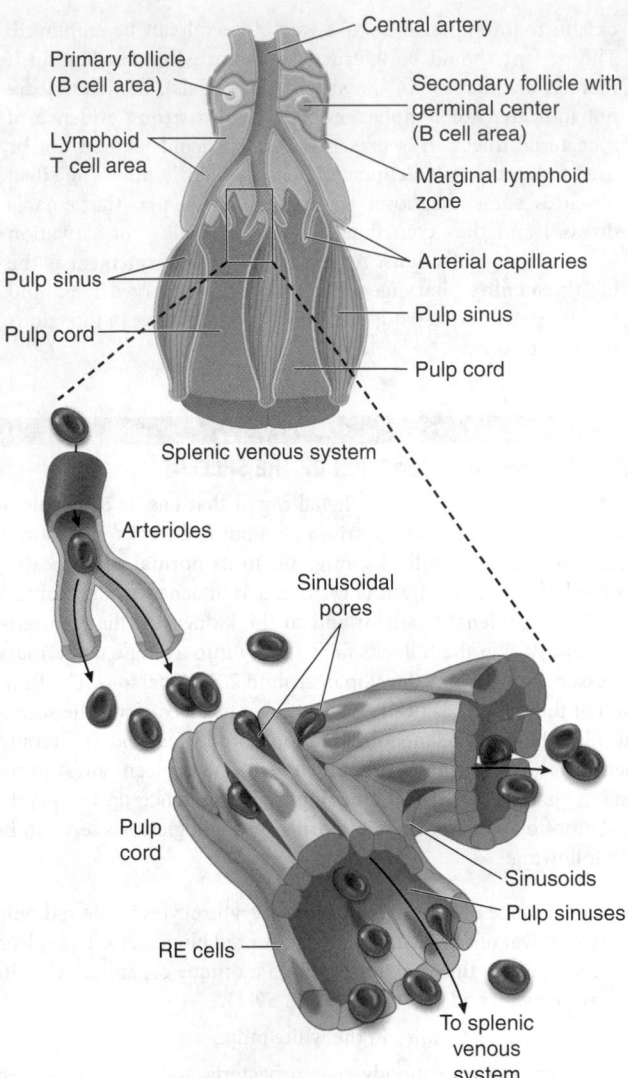

Figure 59-1 Schematic spleen structure. The spleen comprises many units of red and white pulp centered around small branches of the splenic artery, called *central arteries*. White pulp is lymphoid in nature and contains B cell follicles, a marginal zone around the follicles, and T cell–rich areas sheathing arterioles. The red pulp areas include pulp sinuses and pulp cords. The cords are dead ends. In order to regain access to the circulation, red blood cells must traverse tiny openings in the sinusoidal lining. Stiff, damaged, or old red cells cannot enter the sinuses. RE, reticuloendthelial. *(Bottom portion of figure from RS Hillman, KA Ault: Hematology in Clinical Practice, 4th ed. New York, McGraw-Hill, 2005.)*

The spleen is also capable of assisting the host in adapting to its hostile environment. It has at least three adaptive functions: (1) clearance of bacteria and particulates from the blood, (2) the generation of immune responses to certain pathogens, and (3) the generation of cellular components of the blood under circumstances in which the marrow is unable to meet the needs (i.e., extramedullary hematopoiesis). The latter adaptation is a recapitulation of the blood-forming function the spleen plays during gestation. In some animals, the spleen also serves a role in the vascular adaptation to stress because it stores red blood cells (often hemoconcentrated to higher hematocrits than normal) under normal circumstances and contracts under the influence of β-adrenergic stimulation to provide the animal with an autotransfusion and improved oxygen-carrying capacity. However, the normal human spleen does not sequester or store red blood cells and does not contract in response to

sympathetic stimuli. The normal human spleen contains approximately one-third of the total body platelets and a significant number of marginated neutrophils. These sequestered cells are available when needed to respond to bleeding or infection.

APPROACH TO THE PATIENT: Splenomegaly

CLINICAL ASSESSMENT The most common *symptoms* produced by diseases involving the spleen are pain and a heavy sensation in the LUQ. Massive splenomegaly may cause early satiety. Pain may result from acute swelling of the spleen with stretching of the capsule, infarction, or inflammation of the capsule. For many years, it was believed that splenic infarction was clinically silent, which, at times, is true. However, Soma Weiss, in his classic 1942 report of the self-observations by a Harvard medical student on the clinical course of subacute bacterial endocarditis, documented that severe LUQ and pleuritic chest pain may accompany thromboembolic occlusion of splenic blood flow. Vascular occlusion, with infarction and pain, is commonly seen in children with sickle cell crises. Rupture of the spleen, from either trauma or infiltrative disease that breaks the capsule, may result in intraperitoneal bleeding, shock, and death. The rupture itself may be painless.

A palpable spleen is the major *physical sign* produced by diseases affecting the spleen and suggests enlargement of the organ. The normal spleen weighs <250 g, decreases in size with age, normally lies entirely within the rib cage, has a maximum cephalocaudad diameter of 13 cm by ultrasonography or maximum length of 12 cm and/or width of 7 cm by radionuclide scan, and is usually not palpable. However, a palpable spleen was found in 3% of 2200 asymptomatic, male, freshman college students. Follow-up at 3 years revealed that 30% of those students still had a palpable spleen without any increase in disease prevalence. Ten-year follow-up found no evidence for lymphoid malignancies. Furthermore, in some tropical countries (e.g., New Guinea), the incidence of splenomegaly may reach 60%. Thus, the presence of a palpable spleen does not always equate with presence of disease. Even when disease is present, splenomegaly may not reflect the primary disease but rather a reaction to it. For example, in patients with Hodgkin's disease, only two-thirds of the palpable spleens show involvement by the cancer.

Physical examination of the spleen uses primarily the techniques of palpation and percussion. Inspection may reveal fullness in the LUQ that descends on inspiration, a finding associated with a massively enlarged spleen. Auscultation may reveal a venous hum or friction rub.

Palpation can be accomplished by bimanual palpation, ballotment, and palpation from above (Middleton maneuver). For bimanual palpation, which is at least as reliable as the other techniques, the patient is supine with flexed knees. The examiner's left hand is placed on the lower rib cage and pulls the skin toward the costal margin, allowing the fingertips of the right hand to feel the tip of the spleen as it descends while the patient inspires slowly, smoothly, and deeply. Palpation is begun with the right hand in the left lower quadrant with gradual movement toward the left costal margin, thereby identifying the lower edge of a massively enlarged spleen. When the spleen tip is felt, the finding is recorded as centimeters below the left costal margin at some arbitrary point, i.e., 10–15 cm, from the midpoint of the umbilicus or the xiphisternal junction. This allows other examiners to compare findings or the initial examiner to determine changes in size over time. Bimanual palpation in the right lateral decubitus position adds nothing to the supine examination.

Percussion for splenic dullness is accomplished with any of three techniques described by Nixon, Castell, or Barkun:

1. *Nixon's method*: The patient is placed on the right side so that the spleen lies above the colon and stomach. Percussion begins at the lower level of pulmonary resonance in the posterior axillary line and proceeds diagonally along a perpendicular line toward the lower midanterior costal margin. The upper border of dullness is normally 6–8 cm above the costal margin. Dullness >8 cm in an adult is presumed to indicate splenic enlargement.

2. *Castell's method*: With the patient supine, percussion in the lowest intercostal space in the anterior axillary line (8th or 9th) produces a resonant note if the spleen is normal in size. This is true during expiration or full inspiration. A dull percussion note on full inspiration suggests splenomegaly.

3. *Percussion of Traube's semilunar space*: The borders of Traube's space are the sixth rib superiorly, the left midaxillary line laterally, and the left costal margin inferiorly. The patient is supine with the left arm slightly abducted. During normal breathing, this space is percussed from medial to lateral margins, yielding a normal resonant sound. A dull percussion note suggests splenomegaly.

Studies comparing methods of percussion and palpation with a standard of ultrasonography or scintigraphy have revealed sensitivity of 56–71% for palpation and 59–82% for percussion. Reproducibility among examiners is better for palpation than percussion. Both techniques are less reliable in obese patients or patients who have just eaten. Thus, the physical examination techniques of palpation and percussion are imprecise at best. It has been suggested that the examiner perform percussion first and, if positive, proceed to palpation; if the spleen is palpable, then one can be reasonably confident that splenomegaly exists. However, not all LUQ masses are enlarged spleens; gastric or colon tumors and pancreatic or renal cysts or tumors can mimic splenomegaly.

The presence of an enlarged spleen can be more precisely determined, if necessary, by liver-spleen radionuclide scan, CT, MRI, or ultrasonography. The latter technique is the current procedure of choice for routine assessment of spleen size (normal = a maximum cephalocaudad diameter of 13 cm) because it has high sensitivity and specificity and is safe, noninvasive, quick, mobile, and less costly. Nuclear medicine scans are accurate, sensitive, and reliable but are costly, require greater time to generate data, and use immobile equipment. They have the advantage of demonstrating accessory splenic tissue. CT and MRI provide accurate determination of spleen size, but the equipment is immobile and the procedures are expensive. MRI appears to offer no advantage over CT. Changes in spleen structure such as mass lesions, infarcts, inhomogeneous infiltrates, and cysts are more readily assessed by CT, MRI, or ultrasonography. None of these techniques is very reliable in the detection of patchy infiltration (e.g., Hodgkin's disease).

DIFFERENTIAL DIAGNOSIS Many of the diseases associated with splenomegaly are listed in Table 59-2. They are grouped according to the presumed basic mechanisms responsible for organ enlargement:

1. Hyperplasia or hypertrophy related to a particular splenic function such as reticuloendothelial hyperplasia (work hypertrophy) in diseases such as hereditary spherocytosis or thalassemia syndromes that require removal of large numbers of defective red blood cells; immune hyperplasia in response

to systemic infection (infectious mononucleosis, subacute bacterial endocarditis) or to immunologic diseases (immune thrombocytopenia, SLE, Felty's syndrome).

2. Passive congestion due to decreased blood flow from the spleen in conditions that produce portal hypertension (cirrhosis, Budd-Chiari syndrome, congestive heart failure).

3. Infiltrative diseases of the spleen (lymphomas, metastatic cancer, amyloidosis, Gaucher's disease, myeloproliferative disorders with extramedullary hematopoiesis).

The differential diagnostic possibilities are much fewer when the spleen is "massively enlarged," palpable more than 8 cm below the left costal margin or its drained weight is ≥1000 g (Table 59-3). The vast majority of such patients will have non-Hodgkin's lymphoma, chronic lymphocytic leukemia, hairy cell leukemia, chronic myeloid leukemia, myelofibrosis with myeloid metaplasia, or polycythemia vera.

LABORATORY ASSESSMENT The major laboratory abnormalities accompanying splenomegaly are determined by the underlying systemic illness. Erythrocyte counts may be normal, decreased (thalassemia major syndromes, SLE, cirrhosis with portal hypertension), or increased (polycythemia vera). Granulocyte counts may be normal, decreased (Felty's syndrome, congestive splenomegaly, leukemias), or increased (infections or inflammatory disease, myeloproliferative disorders). Similarly, the platelet count may be normal, decreased when there is enhanced sequestration or destruction of platelets in an enlarged spleen (congestive splenomegaly, Gaucher's disease, immune thrombocytopenia), or increased in the myeloproliferative disorders such as polycythemia vera.

The CBC may reveal cytopenia of one or more blood cell types, which should suggest *hypersplenism*. This condition is characterized by splenomegaly, cytopenia(s), normal or hyperplastic bone marrow, and a response to splenectomy. The latter characteristic is less precise because reversal of cytopenia, particularly granulocytopenia, is sometimes not sustained after splenectomy. The cytopenias result from increased destruction of the cellular elements secondary to reduced flow of blood through enlarged and congested cords (congestive splenomegaly) or to immune-mediated mechanisms. In hypersplenism, various cell types usually have normal morphology on the peripheral blood smear, although the red cells may be spherocytic due to loss of surface area during their longer transit through the enlarged spleen. The increased marrow production of red cells should be reflected as an increased reticulocyte production index, although the value may be less than expected due to increased sequestration of reticulocytes in the spleen.

The need for additional laboratory studies is dictated by the differential diagnosis of the underlying illness of which splenomegaly is a manifestation.

■ **SPLENECTOMY**

Splenectomy is infrequently performed for diagnostic purposes, especially in the absence of clinical illness or other diagnostic tests that suggest underlying disease. More often, splenectomy is performed for symptom control in patients with massive splenomegaly, for disease control in patients with traumatic splenic rupture, or for correction of cytopenias in patients with hypersplenism or immune-mediated destruction of one or more cellular blood elements. Splenectomy is necessary for staging of patients with Hodgkin's disease only in those with clinical stage I or II disease in whom radiation therapy alone is contemplated as the treatment. Noninvasive staging of the spleen in Hodgkin's disease is not a

TABLE 59-2 Diseases Associated With Splenomegaly Grouped by Pathogenic Mechanism

Enlargement Due to Increased Demand for Splenic Function

Reticuloendothelial system hyperplasia (for removal of defective erythrocytes)	Malaria
Spherocytosis	Leishmaniasis
Early sickle cell anemia	Trypanosomiasis
Ovalocytosis	Ehrlichiosis
Thalassemia major	Disordered immunoregulation
Hemoglobinopathies	Rheumatoid arthritis (Felty's syndrome)
Paroxysmal nocturnal hemoglobinuria	Systemic lupus erythematosus
Pernicious anemia	Collagen vascular diseases
Immune hyperplasia	Serum sickness
Response to infection (viral, bacterial, fungal, parasitic)	Immune hemolytic anemias
Infectious mononucleosis	Immune thrombocytopenias
AIDS	Immune neutropenias
Viral hepatitis	Drug reactions
Cytomegalovirus	Angioimmunoblastic lymphadenopathy
Subacute bacterial endocarditis	Sarcoidosis
Bacterial septicemia	Thyrotoxicosis (benign lymphoid hypertrophy)
Congenital syphilis	Interleukin 2 therapy
Splenic abscess	Extramedullary hematopoiesis
Tuberculosis	Myelofibrosis
Histoplasmosis	Marrow damage by toxins, radiation, strontium
	Marrow infiltration by tumors, leukemias, Gaucher's disease

Enlargement Due to Abnormal Splenic or Portal Blood Flow

Cirrhosis	Splenic artery aneurysm
Hepatic vein obstruction	Hepatic schistosomiasis
Portal vein obstruction, intrahepatic or extrahepatic	Congestive heart failure
Cavernous transformation of the portal vein	Hepatic echinococcosis
Splenic vein obstruction	Portal hypertension (any cause including the above): "Banti's disease"

Infiltration of the Spleen

Intracellular or extracellular depositions	Hodgkin's disease
Amyloidosis	Myeloproliferative syndromes (e.g., polycythemia vera, essential thrombocytosis)
Gaucher's disease	
Niemann-Pick disease	Angiosarcomas
Tangier disease	Metastatic tumors (melanoma is most common)
Hurler's syndrome and other mucopolysaccharidoses	Eosinophilic granuloma
Hyperlipidemias	Histiocytosis X
Benign and malignant cellular infiltrations	Hamartomas
Leukemias (acute, chronic, lymphoid, myeloid, monocytic)	Hemangiomas, fibromas, lymphangiomas
Lymphomas	Splenic cysts

Unknown Etiology

Idiopathic splenomegaly	Iron-deficiency anemia
Berylliosis	

sufficiently reliable basis for treatment decisions because one-third of normal-sized spleens will be involved with Hodgkin's disease and one-third of enlarged spleens will be tumor-free. The widespread use of systemic therapy to test all stages of Hodgkin's disease has made staging laparotomy with splenectomy unnecessary. Although splenectomy in chronic myeloid leukemia (CMC) does not affect the natural history of disease, removal of the massive spleen usually makes patients significantly more comfortable and simplifies their management by significantly reducing transfusion requirements.

The improvements in therapy of CML have reduced the need for splenectomy for symptom control. Splenectomy is an effective secondary or tertiary treatment for two chronic B cell leukemias, hairy cell leukemia and prolymphocytic leukemia, and for the very rare splenic mantle cell or marginal zone lymphoma. Splenectomy in these diseases may be associated with significant tumor regression in bone marrow and other sites of disease. Similar regressions of systemic disease have been noted after splenic irradiation in some types of lymphoid tumors, especially chronic lymphocytic leukemia

TABLE 59-3 Diseases Associated With Massive Splenomegaly*

Chronic myeloid leukemia	Gaucher's disease
Lymphomas	Chronic lymphocytic leukemia
Hairy cell leukemia	Sarcoidosis
Myelofibrosis with myeloid metaplasia	Autoimmune hemolytic anemia
Polycythemia vera	Diffuse splenic hemangiomatosis

*The spleen extends greater than 8 cm below left costal margin and/or weighs more than 1000 g.

and prolymphocytic leukemia. This has been termed the *abscopal effect*. Such systemic tumor responses to local therapy directed at the spleen suggest that some hormone or growth factor produced by the spleen may affect tumor cell proliferation, but this conjecture is not yet substantiated. A common therapeutic indication for splenectomy is traumatic or iatrogenic splenic rupture. In a fraction of patients with splenic rupture, peritoneal seeding of splenic fragments can lead to *splenosis*—the presence of multiple rests of spleen tissue not connected to the portal circulation. This ectopic spleen tissue may cause pain or gastrointestinal obstruction, as in endometriosis. A large number of hematologic, immunologic, and congestive causes of splenomegaly can lead to destruction of one or more cellular blood elements. In the majority of such cases, splenectomy can correct the cytopenias, particularly anemia and thrombocytopenia. In a large series of patients seen in two tertiary care centers, the indication for splenectomy was diagnostic in 10% of patients, therapeutic in 44%, staging for Hodgkin's disease in 20%, and incidental to another procedure in 26%. Perhaps the only contraindication to splenectomy is the presence of marrow failure, in which the enlarged spleen is the only source of hematopoietic tissue.

The absence of the spleen has minimal long-term effects on the hematologic profile. In the immediate postsplenectomy period, leukocytosis (up to 25,000/μL) and thrombocytosis (up to 1×10^6/μL) may develop, but within 2–3 weeks, blood cell counts and survival of each cell lineage are usually normal. The chronic manifestations of splenectomy are marked variation in size and shape of erythrocytes (anisocytosis, poikilocytosis) and the presence of Howell-Jolly bodies (nuclear remnants), Heinz bodies (denatured hemoglobin), basophilic stippling, and an occasional nucleated erythrocyte in the peripheral blood. When such erythrocyte abnormalities appear in a patient whose spleen has not been removed, one should suspect splenic infiltration by tumor that has interfered with its normal culling and pitting function.

The most serious consequence of splenectomy is increased susceptibility to bacterial infections, particularly those with capsules such as *Streptococcus pneumoniae*, *Haemophilus influenzae*, and some gram-negative enteric organisms. Patients under age 20 years are particularly susceptible to overwhelming sepsis with *S. pneumoniae*, and the overall actuarial risk of sepsis in patients who have had their spleens removed is about 7% in 10 years. The case-fatality rate for pneumococcal sepsis in splenectomized patients is 50–80%. About 25% of patients without spleens will develop a serious infection at some time in their life. The frequency is highest within the first three years after splenectomy. About 15% of the infections are polymicrobial, and lung, skin, and blood are the most common sites. No increased risk of viral infection has been noted in patients who have no spleen. The susceptibility to bacterial infections relates to the inability to remove opsonized bacteria from the bloodstream and a defect in making antibodies to T cell–independent antigens such as the polysaccharide components of bacterial capsules. Pneumococcal

vaccine should be administered to all patients two weeks before elective splenectomy. The Advisory Committee on Immunization Practices recommends that these patients receive repeat vaccination five years post-splenectomy. Efficacy has not been proven for this group, and the recommendation discounts the possibility that administration of the vaccine may actually lower the titer of specific pneumococcal antibodies. A more effective pneumococcal conjugate vaccine that involves T cells in the response is now available (Prevenar, 7-valent). The vaccine to *Neisseria meningitidis* should also be given to patients in whom elective splenectomy is planned. Although efficacy data for *Haemophilus influenzae* type b vaccine are not available for older children or adults, it may be given to patients who have had a splenectomy.

Splenectomized patients should be educated to consider any unexplained fever as a medical emergency. Prompt medical attention with evaluation and treatment of suspected bacteremia may be life-saving. Routine chemoprophylaxis with oral penicillin can result in the emergence of drug-resistant strains and is not recommended.

In addition to an increased susceptibility to bacterial infections, splenectomized patients are also more susceptible to the parasitic disease babesiosis. The splenectomized patient should avoid areas where the parasite *Babesia* is endemic (e.g., Cape Cod, MA).

Surgical removal of the spleen is an obvious cause of hyposplenism. Patients with sickle cell disease often suffer from autosplenectomy as a result of splenic destruction by the numerous infarcts associated with sickle cell crises during childhood. Indeed, the presence of a palpable spleen in a patient with sickle cell disease after age five suggests a coexisting hemoglobinopathy, e.g., thalassemia or hemoglobin C. In addition, patients who receive splenic irradiation for a neoplastic or autoimmune disease are also functionally hyposplenic. The term *hyposplenism* is preferred to *asplenism* in referring to the physiologic consequences of splenectomy because asplenia is a rare, specific, and fatal congenital abnormality in which there is a failure of the left side of the coelomic cavity (which includes the splenic anlagen) to develop normally. Infants with asplenia have no spleens, but that is the least of their problems. The right side of the developing embryo is duplicated on the left so there is liver where the spleen should be, there are two right lungs, and the heart comprises two right atria and two right ventricles.

FURTHER READINGS

Barkun AN et al: The bedside assessment of splenic enlargement. Am J Med 91:512, 1991

Center for Disease Control and Prevention: Recommended adult immunization schedule—United States, 2009. MMWR 57:Q-1, 2009

Facchetti F: Tumors of the spleen. Int J Surg Pathol 18:136S, 2010

Graves SA et al: Does this patient have splenomegaly? JAMA 270:2218, 1993

Kraus MD et al: The spleen as a diagnostic specimen: A review of ten years' experience at two tertiary care institutions. Cancer 91:2001, 2001

McIntyre OR, Ebaugh FG Jr: Palpable spleens: Ten year follow-up. Ann Intern Med 90:130, 1979

Mikocka-Walus A et al: Management of spleen injuries: The current profile. ANZ J Surg 80:157, 2010

Pangalis GA et al: Clinical approach to lymphadenopathy. Semin Oncol 20:570, 1993

Williamson HA Jr: Lymphadenopathy in a family practice: A descriptive study of 240 cases. J Fam Pract 20:449, 1985

CHAPTER 60

Disorders of Granulocytes and Monocytes

Steven M. Holland
John I. Gallin

Leukocytes, the major cells comprising inflammatory and immune responses, include neutrophils, T and B lymphocytes, natural killer (NK) cells, monocytes, eosinophils, and basophils. These cells have specific functions, such as antibody production by B lymphocytes or destruction of bacteria by neutrophils, but in no single infectious disease is the exact role of the cell types completely established. Thus, whereas neutrophils are classically thought to be critical to host defense against bacteria, they may also play important roles in defense against viral infections.

The blood delivers leukocytes to the various tissues from the bone marrow, where they are produced. Normal blood leukocyte counts are 4.3–10.8 × 10⁹/L, with neutrophils representing 45–74% of the cells, bands 0–4%, lymphocytes 16–45%, monocytes 4–10%, eosinophils 0–7%, and basophils 0–2%. Variation among individuals and among different ethnic groups can be substantial, with lower leukocyte numbers for certain African-American ethnic groups. The various leukocytes are derived from a common stem cell in the bone marrow. Three-fourths of the nucleated cells of bone marrow are committed to the production of leukocytes. Leukocyte maturation in the marrow is under the regulatory control of a number of different factors, known as colony-stimulating factors (CSFs) and interleukins (ILs). Because an alteration in the number and type of leukocytes is often associated with disease processes, total white blood cell (WBC) count (cells per μL) and differential counts are informative. This chapter focuses on neutrophils, monocytes, and eosinophils. Lymphocytes and basophils are discussed in Chaps. 314 and 317, respectively.

NEUTROPHILS

■ MATURATION

Important events in neutrophil life are summarized in Fig. 60-1. In normal humans, neutrophils are produced only in the bone marrow. The minimum number of stem cells necessary to support hematopoiesis is estimated to be 400–500 at any one time. Human blood monocytes, tissue macrophages, and stromal cells produce CSFs, hormones required for the growth of monocytes and neutrophils in the bone marrow. The hematopoietic system not only

produces enough neutrophils (~1.3 × 10¹¹ cells per 80-kg person per day) to carry out physiologic functions but also has a large reserve stored in the marrow, which can be mobilized in response to inflammation or infection. An increase in the number of blood neutrophils is called *neutrophilia*, and the presence of immature cells is termed a *shift to the left*. A decrease in the number of blood neutrophils is called *neutropenia*.

Neutrophils and monocytes evolve from pluripotent stem cells under the influence of cytokines and CSFs (Fig. 60-2). The proliferation phase through the metamyelocyte takes about 1 week, while the maturation phase from metamyelocyte to mature neutrophil takes another week. The myeloblast is the first recognizable precursor cell and is followed by the *promyelocyte*. The promyelocyte evolves when the classic lysosomal granules, called the *primary*, or *azurophil, granules* are produced. The primary granules contain hydrolases, elastase, myeloperoxidase, cathepsin G, cationic proteins, and bactericidal/permeability-increasing protein, which is important for killing gram-negative bacteria. Azurophil granules also contain *defensins*, a family of cysteine-rich polypeptides with broad antimicrobial activity against bacteria, fungi, and certain enveloped viruses. The promyelocyte divides to produce the *myelocyte*, a cell responsible for the synthesis of the *specific*, or *secondary, granules*, which contain unique (specific) constituents such as lactoferrin, vitamin B₁₂–binding protein, membrane components of the reduced nicotinamide-adenine dinucleotide phosphate (NADPH) oxidase required for hydrogen peroxide production, histaminase, and receptors for certain chemoattractants and adherence-promoting factors (CR3) as well as receptors for the basement membrane component, laminin. The secondary granules do not contain acid hydrolases and therefore are not classic lysosomes. Packaging of secondary granule contents during myelopoiesis is controlled by CCAAT/enhancer binding protein-ε. Secondary granule contents

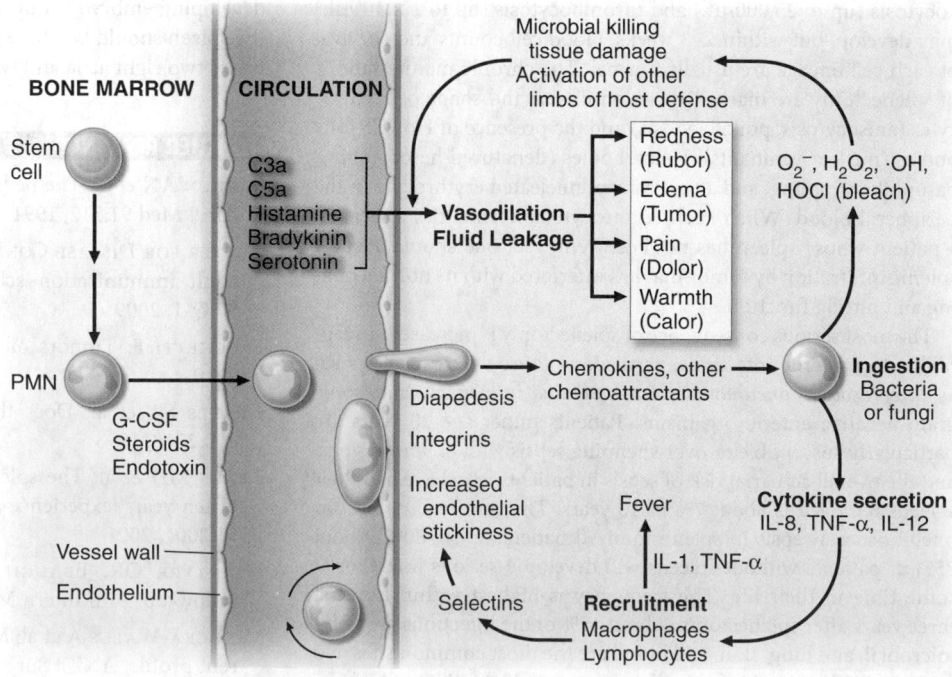

Figure 60-1   Schematic events in neutrophil production, recruitment, and inflammation. The four cardinal signs of inflammation (rubor, tumor, calor, dolor) are indicated, as are the interactions of neutrophils with other cells and cytokines. PMN, polymorphonuclear leukocyte; G-CSF, granulocyte colony-stimulating factor; IL, interleukin; TNF-α, tumor necrosis factor α.

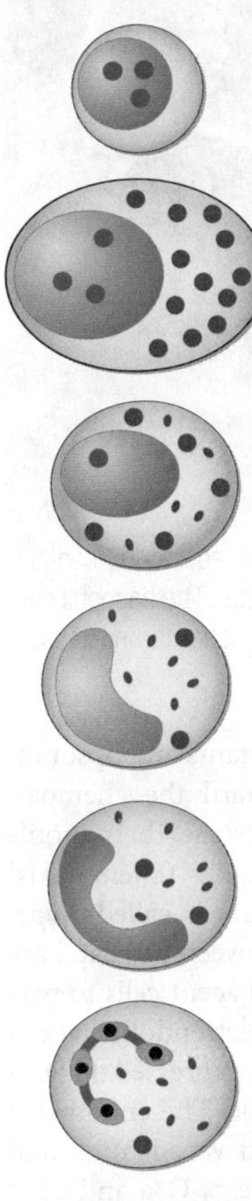

Cell	Stage	Surface Markers[a]	Characteristics
	MYELOBLAST	CD33, CD13, CD15	Prominent nucleoli
	PROMYELOCYTE	CD33, CD13, CD15	Large cell Primary granules appear
	MYELOCYTE	CD33, CD13, CD15, CD14, CD11b	Secondary granules appear
	METAMYELOCYTE	CD33, CD13, CD15, CD14, CD11b	Kidney bean–shaped nucleus
	BAND FORM	CD33, CD13, CD15, CD14, CD11b CD10, CD16	Condensed, band–shaped nucleus
	NEUTROPHIL	CD33, CD13, CD15, CD14, CD11b CD10, CD16	Condensed, multilobed nucleus

[a]CD= Cluster Determinant; ● Nucleolus; ● Primary granule; ◦ Secondary granule.

Figure 60-2 Stages of neutrophil development shown schematically. G-CSF (granulocyte colony-stimulating factor) and GM-CSF (granulocyte-macrophage colony-stimulating factor) are critical to this process. Identifying cellular characteristics and specific cell-surface markers are listed for each maturational stage.

are readily released extracellularly, and their mobilization is important in modulating inflammation. During the final stages of maturation, no cell division occurs, and the cell passes through the metamyelocyte stage and then to the band neutrophil with a sausage-shaped nucleus (Fig. 60-3). As the band cell matures, the nucleus assumes a lobulated configuration. The nucleus of neutrophils normally contains up to four segments (Fig. 60-4). Excessive segmentation (more than five nuclear lobes) may be a manifestation of folate or vitamin B₁₂ deficiency or the congenital neutropenia syndrome of warts, hypogammaglobulinemia, infections, and myelokathexis (WHIM) described below. The Pelger-Hüet anomaly (Fig. 60-5), an infrequent dominant benign inherited trait, results in neutrophils with distinctive bilobed nuclei that must be distinguished from band forms. Acquired bilobed nuclei, pseudo Pelger-Hüet anomaly, can occur with acute infections or in myelodysplastic syndromes. The physiologic role of the normal multilobed nucleus of neutrophils is unknown, but it may allow great deformation of neutrophils during migration into tissues at sites of inflammation.

In severe acute bacterial infection, prominent neutrophil cytoplasmic granules, called *toxic granulations*, are occasionally seen. Toxic granulations are immature or abnormally staining azurophil granules. Cytoplasmic inclusions, also called *Döhle bodies* (Fig. 60-3), can be seen during infection and are fragments of ribosome-rich endoplasmic reticulum. Large neutrophil vacuoles are often present

in acute bacterial infection and probably represent pinocytosed (internalized) membrane.

Neutrophils are heterogeneous in function. Monoclonal antibodies have been developed that recognize only a subset of mature neutrophils. The meaning of neutrophil heterogeneity is not known.

The morphology of eosinophils and basophils is shown in Fig. 60-6.

■ MARROW RELEASE AND CIRCULATING COMPARTMENTS

Specific signals, including IL-1, tumor necrosis factor α (TNF-α), the CSFs, complement fragments, and chemokines, mobilize leukocytes from the bone marrow and deliver them to the blood in an unstimulated state. Under normal conditions, ~90% of the neutrophil pool is in the bone marrow, 2–3% in the circulation, and the remainder in the tissues (Fig. 60-7).

The circulating pool exists in two dynamic compartments: one freely flowing and one marginated. The freely flowing pool is about one-half the neutrophils in the basal state and is composed of those cells that are in the blood and not in contact with the endothelium. Marginated leukocytes are those that are in close physical contact with the endothelium (Fig. 60-8). In the pulmonary circulation, where an extensive capillary bed (~1000 capillaries per alveolus) exists, margination occurs because the capillaries are about the same size as a mature neutrophil. Therefore, neutrophil fluidity and deformability are necessary to make the transit through the pulmonary bed. Increased neutrophil rigidity and decreased deformability lead to augmented neutrophil trapping and margination in the lung. In contrast, in the systemic postcapillary venules, margination is mediated by the interaction of specific cell-surface molecules called *selectins*. Selectins are glycoproteins expressed on neutrophils and endothelial cells, among others, that cause a low-affinity interaction, resulting in "rolling" of the neutrophil along the endothelial surface. On neutrophils, the

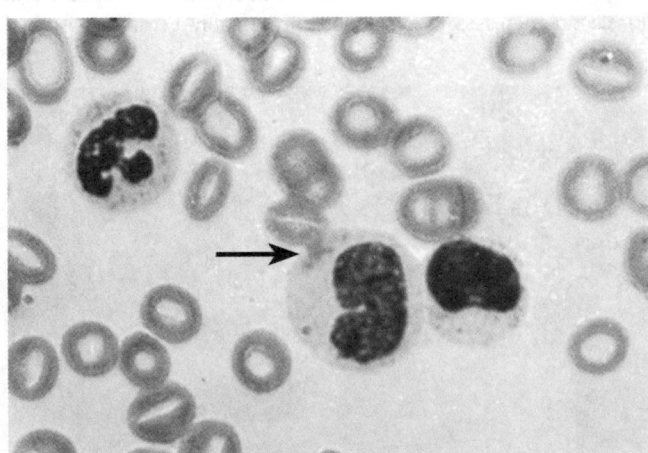

Figure 60-3 Neutrophil band with Döhle body. The neutrophil with a sausage-shaped nucleus in the center of the field is a band form. Döhle bodies are discrete, blue-staining nongranular areas found in the periphery of the cytoplasm of the neutrophil in infections and other toxic states. They represent aggregates of rough endoplasmic reticulum.

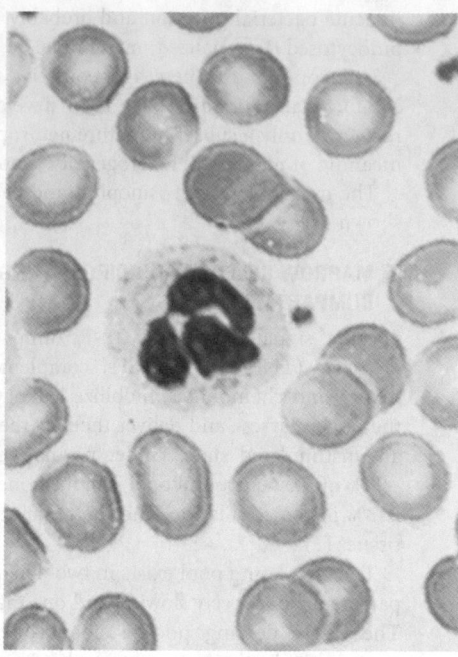

Figure 60-4   Normal granulocyte. The normal granulocyte has a segmented nucleus with heavy, clumped chromatin; fine neutrophilic granules are dispersed throughout the cytoplasm.

molecule L-selectin [cluster determinant (CD) 62L] binds to glycosylated proteins on endothelial cells [e.g., glycosylation-dependent cell adhesion molecule (GlyCAM1) and CD34]. Glycoproteins on neutrophils, most importantly sialyl-Lewis^x (SLe^x, CD15s), are targets for binding of selectins expressed on endothelial cells [E-selectin (CD62E) and P-selectin (CD62P)] and other leukocytes. In response to chemotactic stimuli from injured tissues (e.g., complement product C5a, leukotriene B$_4$, IL-8) or bacterial products [e.g., *N*-formylmethionylleucylphenylalanine (f-metleuphe)], neutrophil adhesiveness increases, and the cells "stick" to the endothelium through *integrins*. The integrins are leukocyte glycoproteins that exist as complexes of a common CD18 β chain with CD11a (LFA-1), CD11b (called Mac-1, CR3, or the C3bi receptor), and CD11c (called p150,95 or CR4). CD11a/CD18 and CD11b/CD18 bind to specific endothelial receptors [intercellular adhesion molecules (ICAM) 1 and 2].

On cell stimulation, L-selectin is shed from neutrophils, and E-selectin increases in the blood, presumably because it is shed

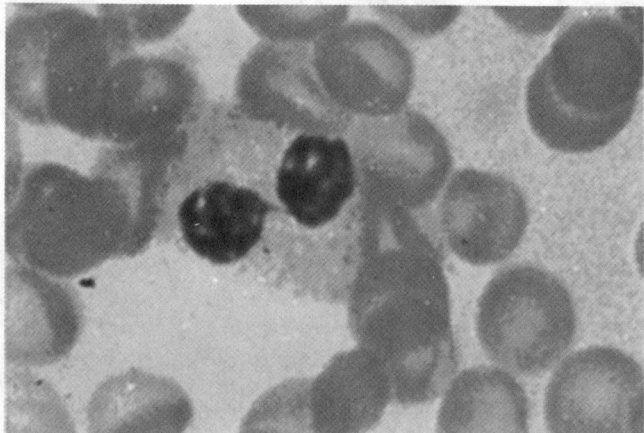

Figure 60-5   Pelger-Hüet anomaly. In this benign disorder, the majority of granulocytes are bilobed. The nucleus frequently has a spectacle-like, or "pince-nez," configuration.

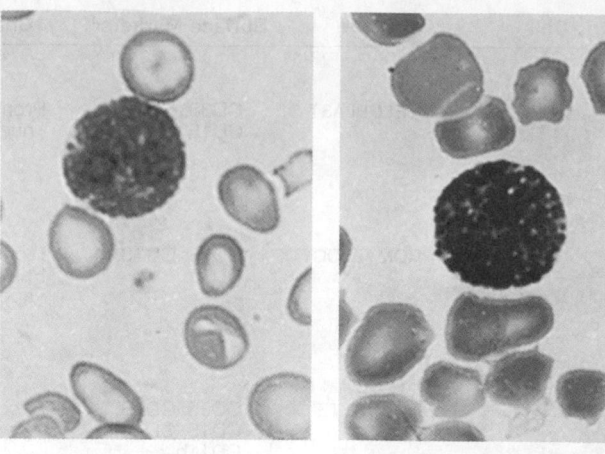

Figure 60-6   Normal eosinophil and basophil. The eosinophil contains large, bright orange granules and usually a bilobed nucleus. The basophil contains large purple-black granules that fill the cell and obscure the nucleus.

from endothelial cells; receptors for chemoattractants and opsonins are mobilized; and the phagocytes orient toward the chemoattractant source in the extravascular space, increase their motile activity (chemokinesis), and migrate directionally (chemotaxis) into tissues. The process of migration into tissues is called *diapedesis* and involves the crawling of neutrophils between postcapillary endothelial cells that open junctions between adjacent cells to permit leukocyte passage. Diapedesis involves platelet/endothelial cell adhesion molecule (PECAM) 1 (CD31), which is expressed on both the emigrating leukocyte and the endothelial cells. The endothelial responses (increased blood flow from increased vasodilation and permeability) are mediated by anaphylatoxins (e.g., C3a and C5a) as well as vasodilators such as histamine, bradykinin, serotonin, nitric oxide, vascular endothelial growth factor (VEGF), and prostaglandins E and I. Cytokines regulate some of these processes

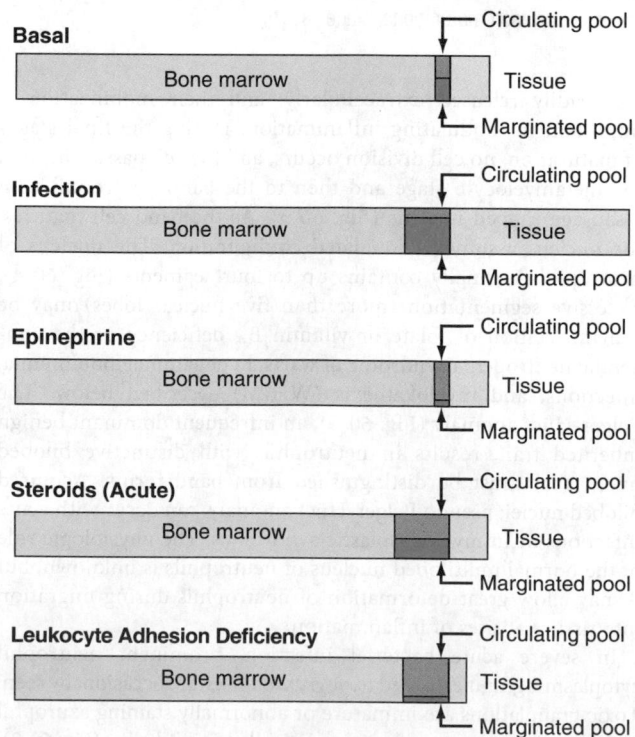

Figure 60-7   Schematic neutrophil distribution and kinetics between the different anatomic and functional pools.

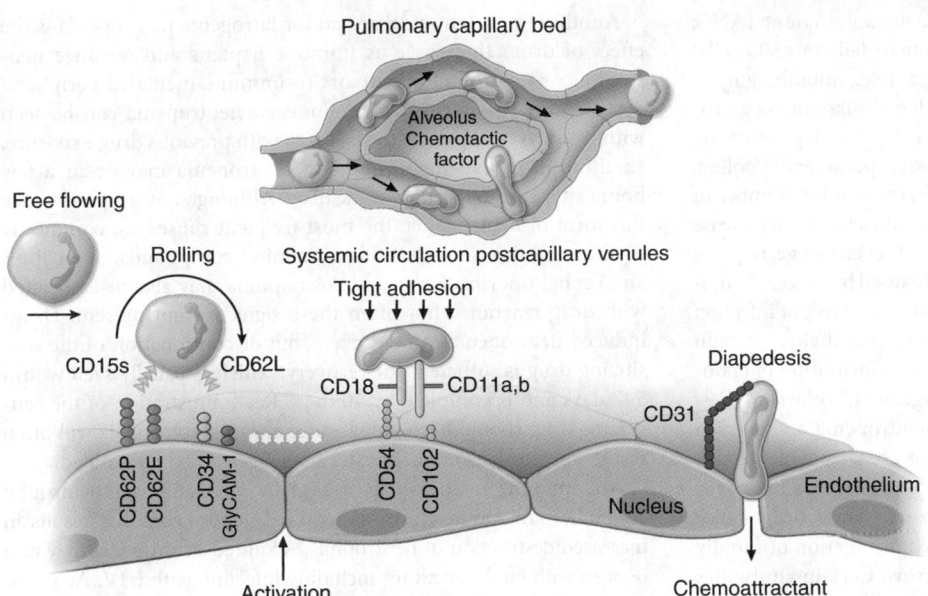

Figure 60-8 Neutrophil travel through the pulmonary capillaries is dependent on neutrophil deformability. Neutrophil rigidity (e.g., caused by C5a) enhances pulmonary trapping and response to pulmonary pathogens in a way that is not so dependent on cell-surface receptors. Intraalveolar chemotactic factors, such as those caused by certain bacteria (e.g., *Streptococcus pneumoniae*), lead to diapedesis of neutrophils from the pulmonary capillaries into the alveolar space. Neutrophil interaction with the endothelium of the systemic postcapillary venules is dependent on molecules of attachment. The neutrophil "rolls" along the endothelium using selectins: neutrophil CD15s (sialyl-Lewis^x) binds to CD62E (E-selectin) and CD62P (P-selectin) on endothelial cells; CD62L (L-selectin) on neutrophils binds to CD34 and other molecules (e.g., GlyCAM-1) expressed on endothelium. Chemokines or other activation factors stimulate integrin-mediated "tight adhesion": CD11a/CD18 (LFA-1) and CD11b/CD18 (Mac-1, CR3) bind to CD54 (ICAM-1) and CD102 (ICAM-2) on the endothelium. Diapedesis occurs between endothelial cells: CD31 (PECAM-1) expressed by the emigrating neutrophil interacts with CD31 expressed at the endothelial cell-cell junction. CD, cluster determinant; GlyCAM, glycosylation-dependent cell adhesion molecule; ICAM, intercellular adhesion molecule; PECAM, platelet/endothelial cell adhesion molecule.

[e.g., TNF-α induction of VEGF, interferon (IFN) γ inhibition of prostaglandin E].

In the healthy adult, most neutrophils leave the body by migration through the mucous membrane of the gastrointestinal tract. Normally, neutrophils spend a short time in the circulation (half-life, 6–7 h). Senescent neutrophils are cleared from the circulation by macrophages in the lung and spleen. Once in the tissues, neutrophils release enzymes, such as collagenase and elastase, which may help establish abscess cavities. Neutrophils ingest pathogenic materials that have been opsonized by IgG and C3b. Fibronectin and the tetrapeptide tuftsin also facilitate phagocytosis.

With phagocytosis comes a burst of oxygen consumption and activation of the hexose-monophosphate shunt. A membrane-associated NADPH oxidase, consisting of membrane and cytosolic components, is assembled and catalyzes the reduction of oxygen to superoxide anion, which is then converted to hydrogen peroxide and other toxic oxygen products (e.g., hydroxyl radical). Hydrogen peroxide + chloride + neutrophil myeloperoxidase generate hypochlorous acid (bleach), hypochlorite, and chlorine. These products oxidize and halogenate microorganisms and tumor cells and, when uncontrolled, can damage host tissue. Strongly cationic proteins, defensins, elastase, cathepsins, and probably nitric oxide also participate in microbial killing. Lactoferrin chelates iron, an important growth factor for microorganisms, especially fungi. Other enzymes, such as lysozyme and acid proteases, help digest microbial debris. After 1–4 days in tissues, neutrophils die. The apoptosis of neutrophils is also cytokine-regulated; granulocyte colony-stimulating factor (G-CSF) and IFN-γ prolong their life span. Under certain conditions, such as in delayed-type hypersensitivity, monocyte accumulation occurs within 6–12 h of initiation of inflammation. Neutrophils,

monocytes, microorganisms in various states of digestion, and altered local tissue cells make up the inflammatory exudate, pus. Myeloperoxidase confers the characteristic green color to pus and may participate in turning off the inflammatory process by inactivating chemoattractants and immobilizing phagocytic cells.

Neutrophils respond to certain cytokines [IFN-γ, granulocyte-macrophage colony-stimulating factor (GM-CSF), IL-8] and produce cytokines and chemotactic signals [TNF-α, IL-8, macrophage inflammatory protein (MIP) 1] that modulate the inflammatory response. In the presence of fibrinogen, f-metleuphe or leukotriene B$_4$ induces IL-8 production by neutrophils, providing autocrine amplification of inflammation. *Chemokines* (*chemo*attractant *cytokines*) are small proteins produced by many different cell types, including endothelial cells, fibroblasts, epithelial cells, neutrophils, and monocytes, that regulate neutrophil, monocyte, eosinophil, and lymphocyte recruitment and activation. Chemokines transduce their signals through heterotrimeric G protein–linked receptors that have seven cell membrane–spanning domains, the same type of cell-surface receptor that mediates the response to the classic chemoattractants f-metleuphe and C5a. Four major groups of chemokines are recognized based on the cysteine structure near the N terminus: C, CC, CXC, and CXXXC. The CXC cytokines such as IL-8 mainly attract neutrophils; CC chemokines such as MIP-1 attract lymphocytes, monocytes, eosinophils, and basophils; the C chemokine lymphotactin is T cell tropic; the CXXXC chemokine fractalkine attracts neutrophils, monocytes, and T cells. These molecules and their receptors not only regulate the trafficking and activation of inflammatory cells, but specific chemokine receptors serve as co-receptors for HIV infection (Chap. 189) and have a role in other viral infections such as West Nile infection and atherogenesis.

■ NEUTROPHIL ABNORMALITIES

Defects in the neutrophil life cycle can lead to dysfunction and compromised host defenses. Inflammation is often depressed, and the clinical result is often recurrent, with severe bacterial and fungal infections. Aphthous ulcers of mucous membranes (gray ulcers without pus) and gingivitis and periodontal disease suggest a phagocytic cell disorder. Patients with congenital phagocyte defects can have infections within the first few days of life. Skin, ear, upper and lower respiratory tract, and bone infections are common. Sepsis and meningitis are rare. In some disorders, the frequency of infection is variable, and patients can go for months or even years without major infection. Aggressive management of these congenital diseases has extended the life span of patients well beyond 30 years.

Neutropenia

The consequences of absent neutrophils are dramatic. Susceptibility to infectious diseases increases sharply when neutrophil counts fall below 1000 cells/μL. When the absolute neutrophil count (ANC; band forms and mature neutrophils combined) falls to <500 cells/μL, control of endogenous microbial flora (e.g., mouth, gut) is impaired; when the ANC is <200/μL, the local inflammatory process is absent. Neutropenia can be due to depressed production, increased peripheral destruction, or excessive peripheral pooling. A falling neutrophil count or a significant decrease in the number of neutrophils below steady-state levels, together with a failure to increase neutrophil counts in the setting of infection or other challenge, requires investigation. Acute neutropenia, such as that caused by cancer chemotherapy, is more likely to be associated with increased risk of infection than neutropenia of long duration (months to years) that reverses in response to infection or carefully controlled administration of endotoxin (see "Laboratory Diagnosis and Management," below).

Some causes of inherited and acquired neutropenia are listed in Table 60-1. The most common neutropenias are iatrogenic, resulting from the use of cytotoxic or immunosuppressive therapies for malignancy or control of autoimmune disorders. These drugs cause neutropenia because they result in decreased production of rapidly growing progenitor (stem) cells of the marrow. Certain antibiotics such as chloramphenicol, trimethoprim-sulfamethoxazole, flucytosine, vidarabine, and the antiretroviral drug zidovudine may cause neutropenia by inhibiting proliferation of myeloid precursors. Azathioprine and 6-mercaptopurine are metabolized by the enzyme thiopurine methyltransferase (TMPT), hypofunctional polymorphisms in which can lead to accumulation of 6-thioguanine and profound marrow toxicity. The marrow suppression is generally dose-related and dependent on continued administration of the drug. Cessation of the offending agent and recombinant human G-CSF usually reverse these forms of neutropenia.

TABLE 60-1 Causes of Neutropenia

Decreased Production

Drug-induced—alkylating agents (nitrogen mustard, busulfan, chlorambucil, cyclophosphamide); antimetabolites (methotrexate, 6-mercaptopurine, 5-flucytosine); noncytotoxic agents [antibiotics (chloramphenicol, penicillins, sulfonamides), phenothiazines, tranquilizers (meprobamate), anticonvulsants (carbamazepine), antipsychotics (clozapine), certain diuretics, anti-inflammatory agents, antithyroid drugs, many others]

Hematologic diseases—idiopathic, cyclic neutropenia, Chédiak-Higashi syndrome, aplastic anemia, infantile genetic disorders (see text)

Tumor invasion, myelofibrosis

Nutritional deficiency—vitamin B_{12}, folate (especially alcoholics)

Infection—tuberculosis, typhoid fever, brucellosis, tularemia, measles, infectious mononucleosis, malaria, viral hepatitis, leishmaniasis, AIDS

Peripheral Destruction

Antineutrophil antibodies and/or splenic or lung trapping

Autoimmune disorders—Felty's syndrome, rheumatoid arthritis, lupus erythematosus

Drugs as haptens—aminopyrine, α-methyldopa, phenylbutazone, mercurial diuretics, some phenothiazines

Granulomatosis with polyangiitis (Wegener's)

Peripheral Pooling (Transient Neutropenia)

Overwhelming bacterial infection (acute endotoxemia)

Hemodialysis

Cardiopulmonary bypass

Another important mechanism for iatrogenic neutropenia is the effect of drugs that serve as immune haptens and sensitize neutrophils or neutrophil precursors to immune-mediated peripheral destruction. This form of drug-induced neutropenia can be seen within 7 days of exposure to the drug; with previous drug exposure, resulting in preexisting antibodies, neutropenia may occur a few hours after administration of the drug. Although any drug can cause this form of neutropenia, the most frequent causes are commonly used antibiotics, such as sulfa-containing compounds, penicillins, and cephalosporins. Fever and eosinophilia may also be associated with drug reactions, but often these signs are not present. Drug-induced neutropenia can be severe, but discontinuation of the sensitizing drug is sufficient for recovery, which is usually seen within 5–7 days and is complete by 10 days. Readministration of the sensitizing drug should be avoided, since abrupt neutropenia will often result. For this reason, diagnostic challenge should be avoided.

Autoimmune neutropenias caused by circulating antineutrophil antibodies are another form of acquired neutropenia that results in increased destruction of neutrophils. Acquired neutropenia may also be seen with viral infections, including infection with HIV. Acquired neutropenia may be cyclic in nature, occurring at intervals of several weeks. Acquired cyclic or stable neutropenia may be associated with an expansion of large granular lymphocytes (LGLs), which may be T cells, NK cells, or NK-like cells. Patients with large granular lymphocytosis may have moderate blood and bone marrow lymphocytosis, neutropenia, polyclonal hypergammaglobulinemia, splenomegaly, rheumatoid arthritis, and absence of lymphadenopathy. Such patients may have a chronic and relatively stable course. Recurrent bacterial infections are frequent. Benign and malignant forms of this syndrome occur. In some patients, a spontaneous regression has occurred even after 11 years, suggesting an immunoregulatory defect as the basis for at least one form of the disorder. Glucocorticoids, cyclosporine, and methotrexate are commonly used to manage these cytopenias.

Hereditary neutropenias

Hereditary neutropenias are rare and may manifest in early childhood as a profound constant neutropenia or agranulocytosis. Congenital forms of neutropenia include Kostmann's syndrome (neutrophil count <100/μL), which is often fatal and due to mutations in the anti-apoptosis gene *HAX-1*; severe chronic neutropenia (neutrophil count of 300–1500/μL) due to mutations in neutrophil elastase (ELA-2); hereditary cyclic neutropenia, or, more appropriately, cyclic hematopoiesis, also due to mutations in neutrophil elastase (ELA-2); the cartilage-hair hypoplasia syndrome due to mutations in the mitochondrial RNA-processing endoribonuclease RMRP; Shwachman-Diamond syndrome associated with pancreatic insufficiency due to mutations in the Shwachman-Bodian-Diamond syndrome gene *SBDS*; the WHIM [*w*arts, *h*ypogammaglobulinemia, *i*nfections, *m*yelokathexis (retention of WBCs in the marrow)] syndrome, characterized by neutrophil hypersegmentation and bone marrow myeloid arrest due to mutations in the chemokine receptor CXCR4; and neutropenias associated with other immune defects, such as X-linked agammaglobulinemia, Wiskott-Aldrich syndrome, and CD40 ligand deficiency. Mutations in the G-CSF receptor can develop in severe congenital neutropenia and are linked to leukemia. Absence of both myeloid and lymphoid cells is seen in reticular dysgenesis, due to mutations in the nuclear genome-encoded mitochondrial enzyme adenylate kinase-2 (AK2).

Maternal factors can be associated with neutropenia in the newborn. Transplacental transfer of IgG directed against antigens on fetal neutrophils can result in peripheral destruction. Drugs (e.g., thiazides) ingested during pregnancy can cause neutropenia in the newborn by either depressed production or peripheral destruction.

In Felty's syndrome—the triad of rheumatoid arthritis, splenomegaly, and neutropenia (Chap. 321)—spleen-produced antibodies can shorten neutrophil life span, while LGLs can attack marrow

TABLE 60-2 Causes of Neutrophilia

Increased Production

Idiopathic

Drug-induced—glucocorticoids, G-CSF

Infection—bacterial, fungal, sometimes viral

Inflammation—thermal injury, tissue necrosis, myocardial and pulmonary infarction, hypersensitivity states, collagen vascular diseases

Myeloproliferative diseases—myelocytic leukemia, myeloid metaplasia, polycythemia vera

Increased Marrow Release

Glucocorticoids

Acute infection (endotoxin)

Inflammation—thermal injury

Decreased or Defective Margination

Drugs—epinephrine, glucocorticoids, nonsteroidal anti-inflammatory agents

Stress, excitement, vigorous exercise

Leukocyte adhesion deficiency type 1 (CD18); leukocyte adhesion deficiency type 2 (selectin ligand, CD15s); leukocyte adhesion deficiency type 3 (Kindlin-3)

Miscellaneous

Metabolic disorders—ketoacidosis, acute renal failure, eclampsia, acute poisoning

Drugs—lithium

Other—metastatic carcinoma, acute hemorrhage or hemolysis

Abbreviation: G-CSF, granulocyte colony-stimulating factor.

neutrophil precursors. Splenectomy may increase the neutrophil count in Felty's syndrome and lower serum neutrophil-binding IgG. Some Felty's syndrome patients also have neutropenia associated with an increased number of LGLs. Splenomegaly with peripheral trapping and destruction of neutrophils is also seen in lysosomal storage diseases and in portal hypertension.

Neutrophilia

Neutrophilia results from increased neutrophil production, increased marrow release, or defective margination (Table 60-2). The most important acute cause of neutrophilia is infection. Neutrophilia from acute infection represents both increased production and increased marrow release. Increased production is also associated with chronic inflammation and certain myeloproliferative diseases. Increased marrow release and mobilization of the marginated leukocyte pool are induced by glucocorticoids. Release of epinephrine, as with vigorous exercise, excitement, or stress, will demarginate neutrophils in the spleen and lungs and double the neutrophil count in minutes. Cigarette smoking can elevate neutrophil counts above the normal range. Leukocytosis with cell counts of 10,000–25,000/μL occurs in response to infection and other forms of acute inflammation and results from both release of the marginated pool and mobilization of marrow reserves. Persistent neutrophilia with cell counts of ≥30,000–50,000/μL is called a *leukemoid reaction*, a term often used to distinguish this degree of neutrophilia from leukemia. In a leukemoid reaction, the circulating neutrophils are usually mature and not clonally derived.

Abnormal neutrophil function

Inherited and acquired abnormalities of phagocyte function are listed in Table 60-3. The resulting diseases are best considered in terms of the functional defects of adherence, chemotaxis, and microbicidal activity. The distinguishing features of the important inherited disorders of phagocyte function are shown in Table 60-4.

Disorders of adhesion Three main types of leukocyte adhesion deficiency (LAD) have been described. All are autosomal recessive and result in the inability of neutrophils to exit the circulation to sites of infection, leading to leukocytosis and increased susceptibility to infection (Fig. 60-8). Patients with LAD 1 have mutations in CD18, the common component of the integrins LFA-1, Mac-1, and p150,95, leading to a defect in tight adhesion between neutrophils and the endothelium. The heterodimer formed by CD18/CD11b (Mac-1) is also the receptor for the complement-derived opsonin C3bi (CR3). The *CD18* gene is located on distal chromosome 21q. The severity of the defect determines the severity of clinical disease. Complete lack of expression of the leukocyte integrins results in a severe phenotype in which inflammatory stimuli do not increase the expression of leukocyte integrins on neutrophils or activated T and B cells. Neutrophils (and monocytes) from patients with LAD 1 adhere poorly to endothelial cells and protein-coated surfaces and exhibit defective spreading, aggregation, and chemotaxis. Patients with LAD 1 have recurrent bacterial infections involving the skin, oral and genital mucosa, and respiratory and intestinal tracts;

TABLE 60-3 Types of Granulocyte and Monocyte Disorders

Function	Cause of Indicated Dysfunction		
	Drug-Induced	Acquired	Inherited
Adherence-aggregation	Aspirin, colchicine, alcohol, glucocorticoids, ibuprofen, piroxicam	Neonatal state, hemodialysis	Leukocyte adhesion deficiency types 1, 2, and 3
Deformability		Leukemia, neonatal state, diabetes mellitus, immature neutrophils	
Chemokinesis-chemotaxis	Glucocorticoids (high dose), auranofin, colchicine (weak effect), phenylbutazone, naproxen, indomethacin, interleukin 2	Thermal injury, malignancy, malnutrition, periodontal disease, neonatal state, systemic lupus erythematosus, rheumatoid arthritis, diabetes mellitus, sepsis, influenza virus infection, herpes simplex virus infection, acrodermatitis enteropathica, AIDS	Chédiak-Higashi syndrome, neutrophil-specific granule deficiency, hyper IgE–recurrent infection (Job's) syndrome (in some patients), Down syndrome, α-mannosidase deficiency, leukocyte adhesion deficiencies, Wiskott-Aldrich syndrome
Microbicidal activity	Colchicine, cyclophosphamide, glucocorticoids (high dose), TNF-α blocking antibodies	Leukemia, aplastic anemia, certain neutropenias, tuftsin deficiency, thermal injury, sepsis, neonatal state, diabetes mellitus, malnutrition, AIDS	Chédiak-Higashi syndrome, neutrophil-specific granule deficiency, chronic granulomatous disease, defects in IFN- /IL-12 axis

Abbreviations: IFN, interferon; IL, interleukin; TNF-α, tumor necrosis factor alpha.

TABLE 60-4 Inherited Disorders of Phagocyte Function: Differential Features

Clinical Manifestations	Cellular or Molecular Defects	Diagnosis
Chronic Granulomatous Diseases (70% X-linked, 30% Autosomal Recessive)		
Severe infections of skin, ears, lungs, liver, and bone with catalase-positive micro-organisms such as *Staphylococcus aureus*, *Burkholderia cepacia*, *Aspergillus* spp., *Chromobacterium violaceum*; often hard to culture organism; excessive inflammation with granulomas, frequent lymph node suppuration; granulomas can obstruct GI or GU tracts; gingivitis, aphthous ulcers, seborrheic dermatitis	No respiratory burst due to the lack of one of five NADPH oxidase subunits in neutrophils, monocytes, and eosinophils	DHR or NBT test; no superoxide and H_2O_2 production by neutrophils; immunoblot for NADPH oxidase components; genetic detection
Chédiak-Higashi Syndrome (Autosomal Recessive)		
Recurrent pyogenic infections, especially with *S. aureus;* many patients get lymphoma-like illness during adolescence; periodontal disease; partial oculocutaneous albinism, nystagmus, progressive peripheral neuropathy, mental retardation in some patients	Reduced chemotaxis and phagolysosome fusion, increased respiratory burst activity, defective egress from marrow, abnormal skin window; defect in *CHS1*	Giant primary granules in neutrophils and other granule-bearing cells (Wright's stain); genetic detection
Specific Granule Deficiency (Autosomal Recessive)		
Recurrent infections of skin, ears, and sinopulmonary tract; delayed wound healing; decreased inflammation; bleeding diathesis	Abnormal chemotaxis, impaired respiratory burst and bacterial killing, failure to upregulate chemotactic and adhesion receptors with stimulation, defect in transcription of granule proteins; defect in C/EBPε	Lack of secondary (specific) granules in neutrophils (Wright's stain), no neutrophil-specific granule contents (i.e., lactoferrin), no defensins, platelet α granule abnormality; genetic detection
Myeloperoxidase Deficiency (Autosomal Recessive)		
Clinically normal except in patients with underlying disease such as diabetes mellitus; then candidiasis or other fungal infections	No myeloperoxidase due to pre- and posttranslational defects in myeloperoxidase deficiency	No peroxidase in neutrophils; genetic detection
Leukocyte Adhesion Deficiency		
Type 1: Delayed separation of umbilical cord, sustained neutrophilia, recurrent infections of skin and mucosa, gingivitis, periodontal disease	Impaired phagocyte adherence, aggregation, spreading, chemotaxis, phagocytosis of C3bi-coated particles; defective production of CD18 subunit common to leukocyte integrins	Reduced phagocyte surface expression of the CD18-containing integrins with monoclonal antibodies against LFA-1 (CD18/CD11a), Mac-1 or CR3 (CD18/CD11b), p150,95 (CD18/CD11c); genetic detection
Type 2: Mental retardation, short stature, Bombay (hh) blood phenotype, recurrent infections, neutrophilia	Impaired phagocyte rolling along endothelium due to defects in fucose transporter	Reduced phagocyte surface expression of Sialyl-Lewis^x, with monoclonal antibodies against CD15s; genetic detection
Type 3: Petechial hemorrhage, recurrent infections	Impaired signaling for integrin activation resulting in impaired adhesion due to mutation in *FERMT3*	Reduced signaling for adhesion through integrins; genetic detection
Phagocyte Activation Defects (X-linked and Autosomal Recessive)		
NEMO deficiency: mild hypohidrotic ectodermal dysplasia; broad-based immune defect: pyogenic and encapsulated bacteria, viruses, *Pneumocystis*, mycobacteria; X-linked	Impaired phagocyte activation by IL-1, IL-18, TLR, CD40L, TNF-α leading to problems with inflammation and antibody production	Poor in vitro response to endotoxin; lack of NF-κB activation; genetic detection
IRAK4 and MyD88 deficiency: susceptibility to pyogenic bacteria such as staphylococci, streptococci, clostridia; resistant to candida; autosomal recessive	Impaired phagocyte activation by endotoxin through TLR and other pathways; TNF-α signaling preserved	Poor in vitro response to endotoxin; lack of NF-κB activation by endotoxin; genetic detection
Hyper IgE–Recurrent Infection Syndrome (Autosomal Dominant) (Job's Syndrome)		
Eczematoid or pruritic dermatitis, "cold" skin abscesses, recurrent pneumonias with *S. aureus* with bronchopleural fistulas and cyst formation, mild eosinophilia, mucocutaneous candidiasis, characteristic facies, restrictive lung disease, scoliosis, delayed primary dental deciduation	Reduced chemotaxis in some patients, reduced suppressor T cell activity. Mutation in *STAT3*	Somatic and immune features involving lungs, skeleton, and immune system; serum IgE > 2000 IU/mL; genetic testing
DOCK8 deficiency (autosomal recessive) Severe eczema, atopic dermatitis, cutaneous abscesses, HSV, HPV, and molluscum infections, severe allergies, cancer	Impaired T cell proliferation to mitogens	Severe allergies, viral infections, high IgE, eosinophilia, low IgM, progressive lymphopenia, genetic detection

(continued)

TABLE 60-4 Inherited Disorders of Phagocyte Function: Differential Features (*Continued*)

Clinical Manifestations	Cellular or Molecular Defects	Diagnosis
Mycobacteria Susceptibility (Autosomal Dominant and Recessive Forms)		
Severe extrapulmonary or disseminated infections with bacille Calmette-Guérin (BCG), nontuberculous mycobacteria, salmonella, histoplasmosis, coccidioidomycosis, poor granuloma formation	Inability to kill intracellular organisms due to low IFN-γ production or response; mutations in IFN-γ receptors, IL-12 receptor, IL-12 p40, STAT1, NEMO	Low or very high levels of IFN-γ receptor 1; functional assays of cytokine production and response; genetic detection

Abbreviations: C/EBPε, CCAAT/enhancer binding protein-ε; DHR, dihydrorhodamine (oxidation test); DOCK8, dedicator of cytokinesis 8; GI, gastrointestinal; GU, genitourinary; HPV, human papilloma virus; HSV, herpes simplex virus; IFN, interferon; IL, interleukin; IRAK4, IL-1 receptor–associated kinase 4; LFA-1, leukocyte function–associated antigen 1; MyD88, myeloid differentiation primary response gene 88; NADPH, nicotinamide–adenine dinueleotide phosphate; NBT, nitroblue tetrazolium (dye test); NEMO, NF-κB essential modulator; NF-κB, nuclear factor κB; STAT1, –3, signal transducer and activator of transcription 1, –3; TLR, Toll-like receptor; TNF, tumor necrosis factor.

persistent leukocytosis (resting neutrophil counts of 15,000–20,000/ µL) because cells do not marginate; and, in severe cases, a history of delayed separation of the umbilical stump. Infections, especially of the skin, may become necrotic with progressively enlarging borders, slow healing, and development of dysplastic scars. The most common bacteria are *Staphylococcus aureus* and enteric gram-negative bacteria. LAD 2 is caused by an abnormality of fucosylation of SLeˣ (CD15s), the ligand on neutrophils that interacts with selectins on endothelial cells and is responsible for neutrophil rolling along the endothelium. Infection susceptibility in LAD 2 appears to be less severe than in LAD 1. LAD 2 is also known as *congenital disorder of glycosylation IIc* (CDGIIc) due to mutation in a GDP-fucose transporter (SLC35C1). LAD 3 is characterized by infection susceptibility, leukocytosis, and petechial hemorrhage due to impaired integrin activation caused by mutations in the gene *FERMT3*.

Disorders of neutrophil granules The most common neutrophil defect is myeloperoxidase deficiency, a primary granule defect inherited as an autosomal recessive trait; the incidence is ~1 in 2000 persons. Isolated myeloperoxidase deficiency is not associated with clinically compromised defenses, presumably because other defense systems such as hydrogen peroxide generation are amplified. Microbicidal activity of neutrophils is delayed but not absent. Myeloperoxidase deficiency may make other acquired host defense defects more serious. An acquired form of myeloperoxidase deficiency occurs in myelomonocytic leukemia and acute myeloid leukemia.

Chédiak-Higashi syndrome (CHS) is a rare disease with autosomal recessive inheritance due to defects in the lysosomal transport protein LYST, encoded by the gene *CHS1* at 1q42. This protein is required for normal packaging and disbursement of granules. Neutrophils (and all cells containing lysosomes) from patients with CHS characteristically have large granules (Fig. 60-9), making it a systemic disease. Patients with CHS have nystagmus, partial oculocutaneous albinism, and an increased number of infections resulting from many bacterial agents. Some CHS patients develop an "accelerated phase" in childhood with a hemophagocytic syndrome and an aggressive lymphoma requiring bone marrow transplantation. CHS neutrophils and monocytes have impaired chemotaxis and abnormal rates of microbial killing due to slow rates of fusion of the lysosomal granules with phagosomes. NK cell function is also impaired. CHS patients may develop a severe disabling peripheral neuropathy in adulthood that can lead to bed confinement.

Specific granule deficiency is a rare autosomal recessive disease in which the production of secondary granules and their contents, as well as the primary granule component defensins, is defective. The defect in bacterial killing leads to severe bacterial infections. One type of specific granule deficiency is due to a mutation in the CCAAT/enhancer binding protein-ε, a regulator of expression of granule components.

Chronic granulomatous disease Chronic granulomatous disease (CGD) is a group of disorders of granulocyte and monocyte oxidative metabolism. Although CGD is rare, with an incidence of 1 in 200,000 individuals, it is an important model of defective neutrophil oxidative metabolism. Most often CGD is inherited as an X-linked recessive trait; 30% of patients inherit the disease in an autosomal recessive pattern. Mutations in the genes for the five proteins that assemble at the plasma membrane account for all patients with CGD. Two proteins (a 91-kDa protein, abnormal in X-linked CGD, and a 22-kDa protein, absent in one form of autosomal recessive CGD) form the heterodimer cytochrome b-558 in the plasma membrane. Three other proteins (40-, 47-, and 67-kDa, abnormal in the other autosomal recessive forms of CGD) are cytoplasmic in origin and interact with the cytochrome after cell activation to form NADPH oxidase, required for hydrogen peroxide production. Leukocytes from patients with CGD have severely diminished hydrogen peroxide production. The genes involved in each of the defects have been cloned and sequenced and the chromosome locations identified. Patients with CGD characteristically have increased numbers of infections due to catalase-positive microorganisms (organisms that destroy their

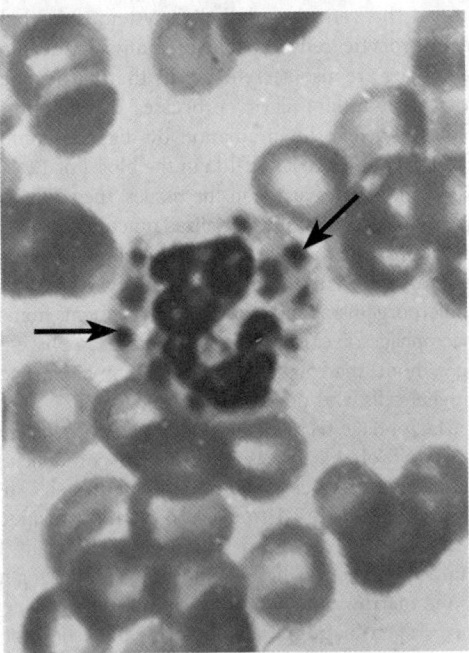

Figure 60-9 Chédiak-Higashi syndrome. The granulocytes contain huge cytoplasmic granules formed from aggregation and fusion of azurophilic and specific granules. Large abnormal granules are found in other granule-containing cells throughout the body.

own hydrogen peroxide). When patients with CGD become infected, they often have extensive inflammatory reactions, and lymph node suppuration is common despite the administration of appropriate antibiotics. Aphthous ulcers and chronic inflammation of the nares are often present. Granulomas are frequent and can obstruct the gastrointestinal or genitourinary tracts. The excessive inflammation reflects failure to downregulate inflammation, reflecting failure to inhibit the synthesis, degradation of or response to chemoattractants or residual antigens, leading to persistent neutrophil accumulation. Impaired killing of intracellular microorganisms by macrophages may lead to persistent cell-mediated immune activation and granuloma formation. Autoimmune complications such as immune thrombocytopenic purpura and juvenile rheumatoid arthritis are also increased in CGD. In addition, discoid lupus is more common in X-linked carriers. Late complications including nodular regenerative hyperplasia and portal hypertension are increasingly recognized in long-term survivors of severe CGD.

Disorders of phagocyte activation Phagocytes depend on cell-surface stimulation to induce signals that evoke multiple levels of the inflammatory response, including cytokine synthesis, chemotaxis, and antigen presentation. Mutations affecting the major pathway that signals through NF-κB have been noted in patients with a variety of infection susceptibility syndromes. If the defects are at a very late stage of signal transduction, in the protein critical for NF-κB activation known as the NF-κB essential modulator (NEMO), then affected males develop ectodermal dysplasia and severe immune deficiency with susceptibility to bacteria, fungi, mycobacteria, and viruses. If the defects in NF-κB activation are closer to the cell-surface receptors, in the proteins transducing Toll-like receptor signals, IL-1 receptor–associated kinase 4 (IRAK4), and myeloid differentiation primary response gene 88 (MyD88), then children have a marked susceptibility to pyogenic infections early in life but develop resistance to infection later.

MONONUCLEAR PHAGOCYTES

The mononuclear phagocyte system is composed of monoblasts, promonocytes, and monocytes, in addition to the structurally diverse tissue macrophages that make up what was previously referred to as the reticuloendothelial system. Macrophages are long-lived phagocytic cells capable of many of the functions of neutrophils. They are also secretory cells that participate in many immunologic and inflammatory processes distinct from neutrophils. Monocytes leave the circulation by diapedesis more slowly than neutrophils and have a half-life in the blood of 12–24 h.

After blood monocytes arrive in the tissues, they differentiate into macrophages ("big eaters") with specialized functions suited for specific anatomic locations. Macrophages are particularly abundant in capillary walls of the lung, spleen, liver, and bone marrow, where they function to remove microorganisms and other noxious elements from the blood. Alveolar macrophages, liver Kupffer cells, splenic macrophages, peritoneal macrophages, bone marrow macrophages, lymphatic macrophages, brain microglial cells, and dendritic macrophages all have specialized functions. Macrophage-secreted products include lysozyme, neutral proteases, acid hydrolases, arginase, complement components, enzyme inhibitors (plasmin, α_2-macroglobulin), binding proteins (transferrin, fibronectin, transcobalamin II), nucleosides, and cytokines (TNF-α; IL-1, -8, -12, -18). IL-1 (Chaps. 16 and 314) has many functions, including initiating fever in the hypothalamus, mobilizing leukocytes from the bone marrow, and activating lymphocytes and neutrophils. TNF-α is a pyrogen that duplicates many of the actions of IL-1 and plays an important role in the pathogenesis of gram-negative shock (Chap. 271). TNF-α stimulates production of hydrogen peroxide and related toxic oxygen species by macrophages and neutrophils. In addition, TNF-α induces catabolic changes that contribute to the profound wasting (cachexia) associated with many chronic diseases.

Other macrophage-secreted products include reactive oxygen and nitrogen metabolites, bioactive lipids (arachidonic acid metabolites and platelet-activating factors), chemokines, CSFs, and factors stimulating fibroblast and vessel proliferation. Macrophages help regulate the replication of lymphocytes and participate in the killing of tumors, viruses, and certain bacteria (*Mycobacterium tuberculosis* and *Listeria monocytogenes*). Macrophages are key effector cells in the elimination of intracellular microorganisms. Their ability to fuse to form giant cells that coalesce into granulomas in response to some inflammatory stimuli is important in the elimination of intracellular microbes and is under the control of IFN-γ. Nitric oxide induced by IFN-γ is an important effector against intracellular parasites, including tuberculosis and *Leishmania*.

Macrophages play an important role in the immune response (Chap. 314). They process and present antigen to lymphocytes and secrete cytokines that modulate and direct lymphocyte development and function. Macrophages participate in autoimmune phenomena by removing immune complexes and other substances from the circulation. Polymorphisms in macrophage receptors for immunoglobulin (FcγRII) determine susceptibility to some infections and autoimmune diseases. In wound healing, they dispose of senescent cells, and they contribute to atheroma development. Macrophage elastase mediates development of emphysema from cigarette smoking.

■ DISORDERS OF THE MONONUCLEAR PHAGOCYTE SYSTEM

Many disorders of neutrophils extend to mononuclear phagocytes. Thus, drugs that suppress neutrophil production in the bone marrow can cause monocytopenia. Transient monocytopenia occurs after stress or glucocorticoid administration. Monocytosis is associated with tuberculosis, brucellosis, subacute bacterial endocarditis, Rocky Mountain spotted fever, malaria, and visceral leishmaniasis (kala azar). Monocytosis also occurs with malignancies, leukemias, myeloproliferative syndromes, hemolytic anemias, chronic idiopathic neutropenias, and granulomatous diseases such as sarcoidosis, regional enteritis, and some collagen vascular diseases. Patients with LAD, hyperimmunoglobulin E–recurrent infection (Job's) syndrome, CHS, and CGD all have defects in the mononuclear phagocyte system.

Monocyte cytokine production or response is impaired in some patients with disseminated nontuberculous mycobacterial infection who are not infected with HIV. Genetic defects in the pathways regulated by IFN-γ and IL-12 lead to impaired killing of intracellular bacteria, mycobacteria, salmonellae, and certain viruses (Fig. 60-10).

Certain viral infections impair mononuclear phagocyte function. For example, influenza virus infection causes abnormal monocyte chemotaxis. Mononuclear phagocytes can be infected by HIV using CCR5, the chemokine receptor that acts as a co-receptor with CD4 for HIV. T lymphocytes produce IFN-γ, which induces FcR expression and phagocytosis and stimulates hydrogen peroxide production by mononuclear phagocytes and neutrophils. In certain diseases, such as AIDS, IFN-γ production may be deficient, whereas in other diseases, such as T cell lymphomas, excessive release of IFN-γ may be associated with erythrophagocytosis by splenic macrophages.

Autoinflammatory diseases are characterized by abnormal cytokine regulation, leading to excess inflammation in the absence of infection. These diseases can mimic infectious or immunodeficient syndromes. Gain-of-function mutations in the TNF-α receptor cause TNF-α receptor–associated periodic syndrome (TRAPS), which is characterized by recurrent fever in the absence of infection, due to persistent stimulation of the TNF-α receptor (Chap. 330). Diseases with abnormal IL-1 regulation leading to fever include familial Mediterranean fever due to mutations in *PYRIN*. Mutations in *cold-induced autoinflammatory syndrome 1* (*CIAS1*) lead to neonatal-onset multisystem autoinflammatory disease, familial cold urticaria, and Muckle-Wells syndrome. The syndrome of *pyoderma*

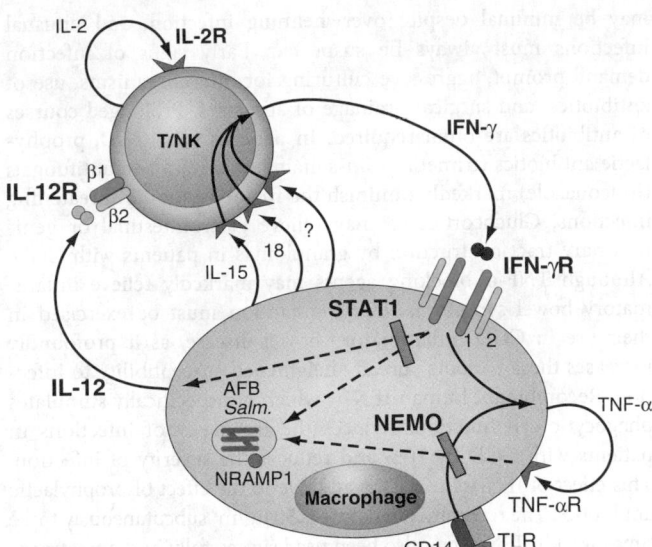

Figure 60-10 Lymphocyte-macrophage interactions underlying resistance to mycobacteria and other intracellular parasites such as *Salmonella*. Mycobacteria infect macrophages, leading to the production of IL-12, which activates T or NK cells through its receptor, leading to production of IL-2 and IFN-γ. IFN-γ acts through its receptor on macrophages to upregulate TNF-γ and IL-12 and kill intracellular parasites. Mutant forms of the cytokines and receptors shown in large type have been found in severe cases of nontuberculous mycobacterial infection and salmonellosis. AFB, acid fast bacilli; IFN, interferon; IL, interleukin; NEMO, NF-κB essential modulator; NK, natural killer; STAT1, signal transducer and activator of transcription 1; TLR, Toll-like receptor; TNF, tumor necrosis factor.

gangrenosum, *a*cne, and sterile *p*yogenic *a*rthritis (PAPA syndrome) is caused by mutations in *CD2BP1*. In contrast to these syndromes of overexpression of proinflammatory cytokines, blockade of TNF-α by the antagonists infliximab, adalimumab, certolizumab, or etanercept has been associated with severe infections due to tuberculosis, nontuberculous mycobacteria, and fungi (Chap. 330).

Monocytopenia occurs with acute infections, with stress, and after treatment with glucocorticoids. Monocytopenia also occurs in aplastic anemia, hairy cell leukemia, acute myeloid leukemia, and as a direct result of myelotoxic drugs.

EOSINOPHILS

Eosinophils and neutrophils share similar morphology, many lysosomal constituents, phagocytic capacity, and oxidative metabolism. Eosinophils express a specific chemoattractant receptor and respond to a specific chemokine, eotaxin, but little is known about their required role. Eosinophils are much longer lived than neutrophils, and unlike neutrophils, tissue eosinophils can recirculate. During most infections, eosinophils appear unimportant. However, in invasive helminthic infections, such as hookworm, schistosomiasis, strongyloidiasis, toxocariasis, trichinosis, filariasis, echinococcosis, and cysticercosis, the eosinophil plays a central role in host defense. Eosinophils are associated with bronchial asthma, cutaneous allergic reactions, and other hypersensitivity states.

The distinctive feature of the red-staining (Wright's stain) eosinophil granule is its crystalline core consisting of an arginine-rich protein (major basic protein) with histaminase activity, important in host defense against parasites. Eosinophil granules also contain a unique eosinophil peroxidase that catalyzes the oxidation of many substances by hydrogen peroxide and may facilitate killing of microorganisms.

Eosinophil peroxidase, in the presence of hydrogen peroxide and halide, initiates mast cell secretion in vitro and thereby promotes inflammation. Eosinophils contain cationic proteins, some of which bind to heparin and reduce its anticoagulant activity. Eosinophil-derived neurotoxin and eosinophil cationic protein are ribonucleases that can kill respiratory syncytial virus. Eosinophil cytoplasm contains Charcot-Leyden crystal protein, a hexagonal bipyramidal crystal first observed in a patient with leukemia and then in sputum of patients with asthma; this protein is lysophospholipase and may function to detoxify certain lysophospholipids.

Several factors enhance the eosinophil's function in host defense. T cell–derived factors enhance the ability of eosinophils to kill parasites. Mast cell–derived eosinophil chemotactic factor of anaphylaxis (ECFa) increases the number of eosinophil complement receptors and enhances eosinophil killing of parasites. Eosinophil CSFs (e.g., IL-5) produced by macrophages increase eosinophil production in the bone marrow and activate eosinophils to kill parasites.

EOSINOPHILIA

Eosinophilia is the presence of >500 eosinophils per μL of blood and is common in many settings besides parasite infection. Significant tissue eosinophilia can occur without an elevated blood count. A common cause of eosinophilia is allergic reaction to drugs (iodides, aspirin, sulfonamides, nitrofurantoin, penicillins, and cephalosporins). Allergies such as hay fever, asthma, eczema, serum sickness, allergic vasculitis, and pemphigus are associated with eosinophilia. Eosinophilia also occurs in collagen vascular diseases (e.g., rheumatoid arthritis, eosinophilic fasciitis, allergic angiitis, and periarteritis nodosa) and malignancies (e.g., Hodgkin disease; mycosis fungoides; chronic myeloid leukemia; and cancer of the lung, stomach, pancreas, ovary, or uterus), as well as in Job's syndrome, DOCK8 deficiency (see below), and CGD. Eosinophilia is commonly present in helminthic infections. IL-5 is the dominant eosinophil growth factor. Therapeutic administration of the cytokines IL-2 and GM-CSF frequently leads to transient eosinophilia. The most dramatic hypereosinophilic syndromes are Loeffler's syndrome, tropical pulmonary eosinophilia, Loeffler's endocarditis, eosinophilic leukemia, and idiopathic hypereosinophilic syndrome (50,000–100,000/μL). IL-5 is the dominant eosinophil growth factor, and can be specifically inhibited with the monoclonal antibody mepolizumab.

The idiopathic hypereosinophilic syndrome represents a heterogeneous group of disorders with the common feature of prolonged eosinophilia of unknown cause and organ system dysfunction, including the heart, central nervous system, kidneys, lungs, gastrointestinal tract, and skin. The bone marrow is involved in all affected individuals, but the most severe complications involve the heart and central nervous system. Clinical manifestations and organ dysfunction are highly variable. Eosinophils are found in the involved tissues and likely cause tissue damage by local deposition of toxic eosinophil proteins such as eosinophil cationic protein and major basic protein. In the heart, the pathologic changes lead to thrombosis, endocardial fibrosis, and restrictive endomyocardiopathy. The damage to tissues in other organ systems is similar. Some cases are due to mutations involving the platelet-derived growth factor receptor, and these are extremely sensitive to the tyrosine kinase inhibitor imatinib. Glucocorticoids, hydroxyurea, and IFN-α each have been used successfully, as have therapeutic antibodies against IL-5. Cardiovascular complications are managed aggressively.

The *eosinophilia-myalgia syndrome* is a multisystem disease, with prominent cutaneous, hematologic, and visceral manifestations, that frequently evolves into a chronic course and can occasionally be fatal. The syndrome is characterized by eosinophilia (eosinophil count >1000/μL) and generalized disabling myalgias without other recognized causes. Eosinophilic fasciitis, pneumonitis, and myocarditis; neuropathy culminating in respiratory failure; and encephalopathy may occur. The disease is caused by ingesting contaminants in L-tryptophan–containing products. Eosinophils, lymphocytes, macrophages, and fibroblasts accumulate in the affected tissues, but their role in pathogenesis is unclear. Activation of eosinophils and fibroblasts and the deposition of eosinophil-derived toxic proteins in affected tissues may contribute. IL-5 and transforming growth factor β have been implicated as potential mediators. Treatment is withdrawal of products containing L-tryptophan and the administration of glucocorticoids. Most patients recover fully, remain stable, or show slow recovery, but the disease can be fatal in up to 5% of patients.

■ EOSINOPENIA

Eosinopenia occurs with stress, such as acute bacterial infection, and after treatment with glucocorticoids. The mechanism of eosinopenia of acute bacterial infection is unknown but is independent of endogenous glucocorticoids, since it occurs in animals after total adrenalectomy. There is no known adverse effect of eosinopenia.

HYPERIMMUNOGLOBULIN E–RECURRENT INFECTION SYNDROME

The hyperimmunoglobulin E–recurrent infection syndrome, or Job's syndrome, is a rare multisystem disease in which the immune and somatic systems are affected, including neutrophils, monocytes, T cells, B cells, and osteoclasts. Autosomal dominant mutations in signal transducer and activator of transcription 3 (STAT3) lead to inhibition of normal STAT signaling with broad and profound effects. Patients have characteristic facies with broad nose, kyphoscoliosis and osteoporosis, and eczema. The primary teeth erupt normally but do not deciduate, often requiring extraction. Patients develop recurrent sinopulmonary and cutaneous infections that tend to be much less inflamed than appropriate for the degree of infection and have been referred to as "cold abscesses." Characteristically, pneumonias cavitate, leading to pneumatoceles. Coronary artery aneurysms are common, as are cerebral demyelinated plaques that accumulate with age. Importantly, IL-17–producing cells, which are thought responsible for protection against extracellular and mucosal infections, are profoundly reduced in Job's syndrome. Despite very high IgE levels, these patients do not have elevated levels of allergy. An important syndrome with clinical overlap with STAT3 deficiency is due to autosomal recessive defects in dedicator of cytokinesis 8 (DOCK8). In DOCK8 deficiency, IgE elevation is joined to severe allergy, viral susceptibility, and increased rates of cancer.

LABORATORY DIAGNOSIS AND MANAGEMENT

Initial studies of WBC and differential and often a bone marrow examination may be followed by assessment of bone marrow reserves (steroid challenge test), marginated circulating pool of cells (epinephrine challenge test), and marginating ability (endotoxin challenge test) (Fig. 60-7). In vivo assessment of inflammation is possible with a Rebuck skin window test or an in vivo skin blister assay, which measures the ability of leukocytes and inflammatory mediators to accumulate locally in the skin. In vitro tests of phagocyte aggregation, adherence, chemotaxis, phagocytosis, degranulation, and microbicidal activity (for *S. aureus*) may help pinpoint cellular or humoral lesions. Deficiencies of oxidative metabolism are detected with either the nitroblue tetrazolium (NBT) dye test or the dihydrorhodamine (DHR) oxidation test. These tests are based on the ability of products of oxidative metabolism to alter the oxidation states of reporter molecules so that they can be detected microscopically (NBT) or by flow cytometry (DHR). Qualitative studies of superoxide and hydrogen peroxide production may further define neutrophil oxidative function.

Patients with leukopenias or leukocyte dysfunction often have delayed inflammatory responses. Therefore, clinical manifestations may be minimal despite overwhelming infection, and unusual infections must always be suspected. Early signs of infection demand prompt, aggressive culturing for microorganisms, use of antibiotics, and surgical drainage of abscesses. Prolonged courses of antibiotics are often required. In patients with CGD, prophylactic antibiotics (trimethoprim-sulfamethoxazole) and antifungals (itraconazole) markedly diminish the frequency of life-threatening infections. Glucocorticoids may relieve gastrointestinal or genitourinary tract obstruction by granulomas in patients with CGD. Although TNF-α blocking agents may markedly relieve inflammatory bowel symptoms, extreme caution must be exercised in their use in CGD inflammatory bowel disease, as it profoundly increases these patients' already heightened susceptibility to infection. Recombinant human IFN-γ, which nonspecifically stimulates phagocytic cell function, reduces the frequency of infections in patients with CGD by 70% and reduces the severity of infection. This effect of IFN-γ in CGD is additive to the effect of prophylactic antibiotics. The recommended dose is 50 μg/m² subcutaneously three times weekly. IFN-γ has also been used successfully in the treatment of leprosy, nontuberculous mycobacteria, and visceral leishmaniasis.

Rigorous oral hygiene reduces but does not eliminate the discomfort of gingivitis, periodontal disease, and aphthous ulcers; chlorhexidine mouthwash and tooth brushing with a hydrogen peroxide–sodium bicarbonate paste helps many patients. Oral antifungal agents (fluconazole, itraconazole, voriconazole, posaconazole) have reduced mucocutaneous candidiasis in patients with Job's syndrome. Androgens, glucocorticoids, lithium, and immunosuppressive therapy have been used to restore myelopoiesis in patients with neutropenia due to impaired production. Recombinant G-CSF is useful in the management of certain forms of neutropenia due to depressed neutrophil production, especially those related to cancer chemotherapy. Patients with chronic neutropenia with evidence of a good bone marrow reserve need not receive prophylactic antibiotics. Patients with chronic or cyclic neutrophil counts <500/μL may benefit from prophylactic antibiotics and G-CSF during periods of neutropenia. Oral trimethoprim-sulfamethoxazole (160/800 mg) twice daily can prevent infection. Increased numbers of fungal infections are not seen in patients with CGD on this regimen. Oral quinolones such as levofloxacin and ciprofloxacin are alternatives.

In the setting of cytotoxic chemotherapy with severe, persistent neutropenia, trimethoprim-sulfamethoxazole prevents *Pneumocystis jirovecii* pneumonia. These patients, and patients with phagocytic cell dysfunction, should avoid heavy exposure to airborne soil, dust, or decaying matter (mulch, manure), which are often rich in *Nocardia* and the spores of *Aspergillus* and other fungi. Restriction of activities or social contact has no proven role in reducing risk of infection.

Although aggressive medical care for many patients with phagocytic disorders can allow them to go for years without a life-threatening infection, there may still be delayed effects of prolonged antimicrobials and other inflammatory complications. Cure of most congenital phagocyte defects is possible by bone marrow transplantation, and rates of success are improving (Chap. 114). The identification of specific gene defects in patients with LAD 1, CGD, and other immunodeficiencies has led to gene therapy trials in a number of genetic white cell disorders.

FURTHER READINGS

HEIMALL J et al: Pathogenesis of hyper IgE syndrome. Clin Rev Allergy Immunol 38:32, 2010

HOLLAND SM: Chronic granulomatous disease. Clin Rev Allergy Immunol 38:3, 2010

International Union of Immunological Societies Expert Committee on Primary Immunodeficiencies: Primary immunodeficiencies: 2009 update. J Allergy Clin Immunol 124:1161, 2009

Klein C, Welte K: Genetic insights into congenital neutropenia. Clin Rev Allergy Immunol 38:68, 2010

Kuhns DB, et al: Residual NADPH opidase and survival in chronic granulomatous disease. N Engl J Med 363:2600, 2010

Notarangelo LD: Primary immunodeficiencies. J Allergy Clin Immunol 125:S182, 2010.

Ogbogu PU et al: Hypereosinophilic syndrome: A multicenter, retrospective analysis of clinical characteristics and response to therapy. J Allergy Clin Immunol 124:1319, 2009

van de Vosse E et al: Genetic deficiencies of innate immune signalling in human infectious disease. Lancet Infect Dis 9:688, 2009

PART 3

Genes, the Environment, and Disease

CHAPTER **61**

Principles of Human Genetics

J. Larry Jameson
Peter Kopp

IMPACT OF GENETICS ON MEDICAL PRACTICE

The beginning of the new millennium was marked by the announcement that the vast majority of the human genome had been sequenced. This milestone in the exploration of the human genome was preceded by numerous conceptual and technologic advances. They include, among others, the elucidation of the DNA double-helix structure, the discovery of restriction enzymes and the polymerase chain reaction (PCR), the development and automatization of DNA sequencing, and the generation of genetic and physical maps by the Human Genome Project (HGP). The consequences of this wealth of knowledge for the practice of medicine are profound. First, the most significant impact of genetics has been to enhance our understanding of disease etiology and pathogenesis. However, genetics is playing an increasingly prominent role in the diagnosis, prevention, and treatment of disease (Chap. 63). Genetic approaches have proven invaluable for the detection of infectious pathogens and are used clinically to identify agents that are difficult to culture such as mycobacteria, viruses, and parasites. In many cases, molecular genetics has improved the feasibility and accuracy of diagnostic testing and is beginning to open new avenues for therapy, including gene and cellular therapy (Chaps. 68 and 67). Molecular genetics has significantly changed the treatment of human disease. Peptide hormones, growth factors, cytokines, and vaccines can now be produced in large amounts using recombinant DNA technology. Targeted modifications of these peptides provide the practitioner with improved therapeutic tools, as illustrated by genetically modified insulin analogues with more favorable kinetics. There is hope that a better understanding of the genetic basis of human disease will also have an increasing impact on disease prevention.

Genetics has traditionally been viewed through the window of relatively rare single-gene diseases. Taken together, these disorders account for ~10% of pediatric admissions and childhood mortality. It is, however, increasingly apparent that virtually every medical condition has a genetic component. As is often evident from a patient's family history, many common disorders such as hypertension, heart disease, asthma, diabetes mellitus, and mental illnesses are significantly influenced by the genetic background. These polygenic or multifactorial (complex) disorders involve the contributions of many different genes, as well as environmental factors that can modify disease risk (Chap. 63). Genome-wide association studies (GWAS) have elucidated numerous disease-associated loci and are providing novel insights into the allelic architecture of complex traits. These studies have been facilitated by the availability of comprehensive catalogues of human single-nucleotide polymorphism (SNP) haplotypes generated through the HapMap Project.

Cancer has a genetic basis since it results from acquired somatic mutations in genes controlling growth, apoptosis, and cellular differentiation (Chap. 83). In addition, the development of many cancers is associated with a hereditary predisposition. The prevalence of genetic diseases, combined with their severity and chronic nature, imposes great financial, social, and emotional burdens on society.

Genetics has historically focused predominantly on chromosomal and metabolic disorders, reflecting the long-standing availability of techniques to diagnose these conditions. For example, conditions such as trisomy 21 (Down syndrome) or monosomy X (Turner's syndrome) can be diagnosed using cytogenetics (Chap. 62). Likewise, many metabolic disorders (e.g., phenylketonuria, familial hypercholesterolemia) are diagnosed using biochemical analyses. Recent advances in DNA diagnostics have extended the field of genetics to include virtually all medical specialties. In cardiology, for example, the molecular basis of inherited cardiomyopathies and ion channel defects that predispose to arrhythmias is being defined (Chaps. 233 and 238). In neurology, genetics has unmasked the pathophysiology of a startling number of neurodegenerative disorders (Chap. 366). Hematology has evolved dramatically, from its incipient genetic descriptions of hemoglobinopathies to the current understanding of the molecular basis of red cell membrane defects, clotting disorders, and thrombotic disorders (Chaps. 104 and 116).

New concepts derived from genetic studies can sometimes clarify the pathogenesis of disorders that were previously opaque. For example, although many different genetic defects can cause peripheral neuropathies, disruption of the normal folding of the myelin sheaths is frequently a common final pathway (Chap. 384). Several genetic causes of obesity appear to converge on a physiologic pathway that involves products of the proopiomelanocortin polypeptide and the MC4R receptor, thus identifying a key mechanism for appetite control (Chap. 77). A similar phenomenon is emerging for genetically distinct forms of Alzheimer's disease, several of which lead to the formation of neurofibrillary tangles (Chap. 371). The identification of defective genes often leads to the detection of cellular pathways involved in key physiologic processes. Examples include identification of the cystic fibrosis conductance regulator (*CFTR*) gene; the Duchenne's muscular dystrophy (*DMD*) gene, which encodes dystrophin; and the fibroblast growth factor receptor-3 (*FGFR3*) gene, which is responsible for achondroplastic dwarfism. Similarly, transgenic (over)expression, and targeted gene "knock-out" and "knock-in" models help to unravel the physiologic function of genes.

The astounding rate at which new genetic information is being generated creates a major challenge for physicians, health care providers, and basic investigators. The terminology and techniques used for discovery evolve continuously. Much genetic information resides in databases or is being published in basic science journals. Databases provide easy access to the expanding information about the human genome, genetic disease, and genetic testing (Table 61-1). For example, several thousand monogenic disorders are summarized in a large, continuously evolving compendium, referred to as the *Online Mendelian Inheritance in Man* (OMIM) catalogue (Table 61-1). The ongoing refinement of bioinformatics is simplifying the access to this daunting onslaught of new information.

■ CHROMOSOMES AND DNA REPLICATION

Organization of DNA into chromosomes

Size of the human genome The human genome is divided into 23 different chromosomes, including 22 autosomes (numbered 1–22) and the X and Y sex chromosomes. Adult cells are *diploid*, meaning they contain two homologous sets of 22 autosomes and a pair of sex chromosomes. Females have two X chromosomes (XX), whereas males have one X and one Y chromosome (XY). As a consequence of meiosis, germ cells (sperm or oocytes) are haploid and contain one set of 22 autosomes and one of the sex chromosomes. At the

TABLE 61-1 Selected Databases Relevant for Genomics and Genetic Disorders

Site	URL	Comment
National Center for Biotechnology Information (NCBI)	http://www.ncbi.nlm.nih.gov/	Broad access to biomedical and genomic information, literature (PubMed), sequence databases, software for analyses of nucleotides and proteins
		Extensive links to other databases, genome resources, and tutorials
National Human Genome Research Institute	http://www.genome.gov/	Web links providing information about the human genome sequence, genomes of other organisms, and genomic research
Ensembl Genome browser	http://www.ensembl.org	Maps and sequence information of eukaryotic genomes
Online Mendelian Inheritance in Man	http://www.ncbi.nlm.nih.gov/omim	Online compendium of Mendelian disorders and human genes causing genetic disorders
Office of Biotechnology Activities National Institutes of Health	http://oba.od.nih.gov/oba	Information about recombinant DNA and gene transfer
		Medical, ethical, legal, and social issues raised by genetic testing
		Medical, ethical, legal, and social issues raised by xenotransplantation
American College of Medical Genetics	http://www.acmg.net/	Extensive links to other databases relevant for the diagnosis, treatment, and prevention of genetic disease
Cancer Genome Anatomy Project (CGAP)	http://cgap.nci.nih.gov/	Information about gene expression profiles of normal, precancer, and cancer cells
GeneTests	http://www.genetests.org/	International directory of genetic testing laboratories and prenatal diagnosis clinics
		Reviews and educational materials
Genomes Online Database (GOLD)	http://www.genomesonline.org/	Information on published and unpublished genomes
HUGO Gene Nomenclature	http://www.genenames.org/	Gene names and symbols
MITOMAP, a human mitochondrial genome database	http://www.mitomap.org/	A compendium of polymorphisms and mutations of the human mitochondrial DNA
Mitochondrial disorders	http://www.neuro.wustl.edu/neuromuscular/mitosyn.html	Overview on clinical syndromes associated with mtDNA mutations
DNA repeat sequences & disease	http://www.neuro.wustl.edu/neuromuscular/mother/dnarep.htm	Overview on clinical syndromes associated with DNA repeats
Online Mendelian Inheritance in Animals (OMIA)	http://omia.angis.org.au/	Online compendium of Mendelian disorders in animals
The Jackson Laboratory	http://www.jax.org/	Information about murine models and the mouse genome
International HapMap Project	http://www.hapmap.org/	Catalogue of haplotypes in different ethnic groups relevant for association studies and pharmacogenomics
Nuclear Receptor Signaling Atlas	http://nursa.org	Atlas of nuclear receptors, coregulators, and ligands
Dolan DNA Learning Center, Cold Spring Harbor Laboratories	http://www.dnalc.org/	Educational material about selected genetic disorders, DNA, eugenics, and genetic origin
The Online Metabolic and Molecular Bases of Inherited Disease (OMMBID)	http://www.ommbid.com/	Online version of the comprehensive text on The Metabolic and Molecular Bases of Inherited Disease

Note: Databases are evolving constantly. Pertinent information may be found by using links listed in the few selected databases. Instructions for the use of genome-related databases have been published [Nat Genet 32(Suppl):1–79, 2002].

time of fertilization, the diploid genome is reconstituted by pairing of the homologous chromosomes from the mother and father. With each cell division (mitosis), chromosomes are replicated, paired, segregated, and divided into two daughter cells (Chap. 62).

Although the exact number of genes encoded by the human genome is still unknown, current estimates predict about 23,000 to 25,000 protein-coding genes, a number that is substantially smaller than initially predicted. A *gene* is a functional unit that is regulated by transcription (see below) and encodes an RNA product, which is most commonly, but not always, translated into a protein that exerts activity within or outside the cell. Historically, genes were identified because they conferred specific traits that are transmitted from one generation to the next. Increasingly, they are characterized based on expression in various tissues (transcriptome). The number of genes greatly underestimates the complexity of genetic expression, as single genes can generate multiple spliced messenger RNA (mRNA) products, which are translated into proteins that are subject to complex posttranslational modification such as phosphorylation. *Proteomics,* the study of the proteome using technologies of large-scale protein separation and identification, is focused on protein variation and function. Similarly, the field of *metabolomics* aims at determining the composition and modifications of the *metabolome*, the complement of low-molecular-weight molecules, many of which participate in various metabolic functions. The human *microbiome* refers to the constellation of viruses, bacteria, and fungi that colonize various human tissues (Chap. 64). Comprehensive characterization of the microbiome has been made feasible by the availability of high-throughput DNA-sequencing methods. Analyses of genomics, proteomics, metabolomics, and the microbiome are heavily dependent on bioinformatics, and they are beginning to reveal how physiologic or pathologic alterations affect *modular networks* rather than *linear pathways* (Chap. e19).

Human DNA consists of ~3 billion base pairs (bp) of DNA per haploid genome. DNA length is normally measured in units of 1000 bp (kilobases, kb) or 1,000,000 bp (megabases, Mb). Not all DNA encodes genes. In fact, genes account for only ~10–15% of DNA. Much of the remaining DNA consists of highly repetitive sequences, the function of which is poorly understood. These repetitive DNA regions, along with nonrepetitive sequences that do not encode genes, may serve a structural role in the packaging of DNA into chromatin [i.e., DNA bound to histone proteins, and chromosomes (Fig. 61-1)]. If only 10% of DNA is expressed and there are 25,000 genes, the average gene would be ~12 kb in length. Although many genes are about this size, the range is quite broad. For example, some genes are only a few hundred bp, whereas others such as the *DMD* gene, are extraordinarily large (2 Mb).

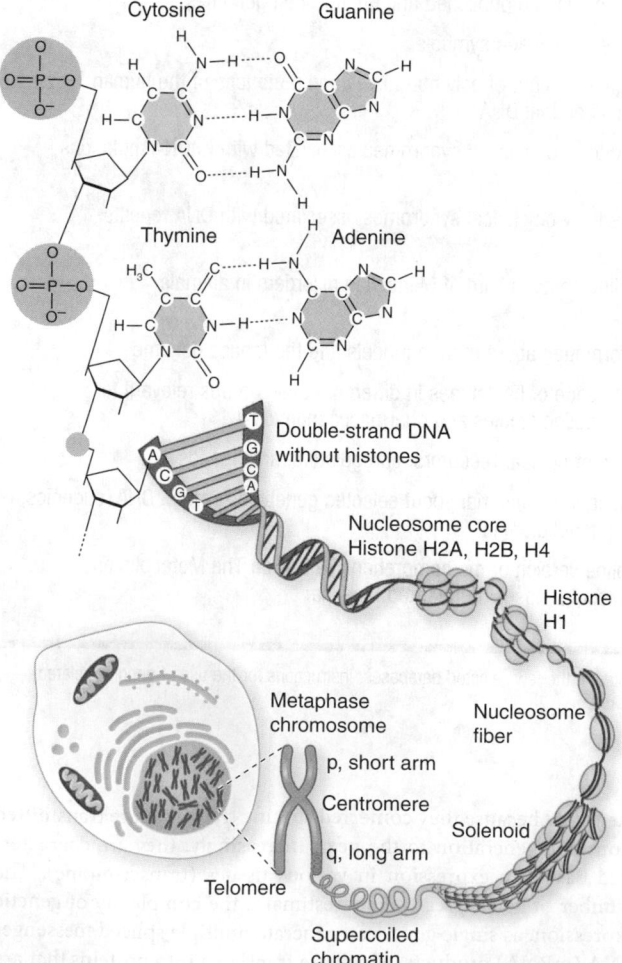

Figure 61-1 Structure of chromatin and chromosomes. Chromatin is composed of double-strand DNA that is wrapped around histone and non-histone proteins forming nucleosomes. The nucleosomes are further organized into solenoid structures. Chromosomes assume their characteristic structure, with short (p) and long (q) arms at the metaphase stage of the cell cycle.

Structure of DNA Each gene is composed of a linear polymer of DNA. DNA is a double-stranded helix composed of four different bases: adenine (A), thymidine (T), guanine (G), and cytosine (C). Adenine is paired to thymidine, and guanine is paired to cytosine, by hydrogen bond interactions that span the double helix. DNA has several remarkable features that make it ideal for the transmission of genetic information. It is relatively stable, at least in comparison to RNA or proteins. The double-stranded nature of DNA and its feature of strict base-pair complementarity permit faithful replication during cell division. As described below, complementarity also allows the transmission of genetic information from DNA → RNA → protein (Fig. 61-2). mRNA is encoded by the so-called sense or coding strand of the DNA double helix and is translated into proteins by ribosomes.

The presence of four different bases provides surprising genetic diversity. In the protein-coding regions of genes, the DNA bases are arranged into codons, a triplet of bases that specifies a particular amino acid. It is possible to arrange the four bases into 64 different triplet codons (4^3). Each codon specifies 1 of the 20 different amino acids, or a regulatory signal such as initiation and stop of translation. Because there are more codons than amino acids, the genetic code is degenerate; that is, most amino acids can be specified by several different codons. By arranging the codons in different combinations and in various lengths, it is possible to generate the tremendous diversity of primary protein structure.

Replication of DNA and mitosis

Genetic information in DNA is transmitted to daughter cells under two different circumstances: (1) somatic cells divide by mitosis, allowing the diploid (2n) genome to replicate itself completely in conjunction with cell division; and (2) germ cells (sperm and ova) undergo meiosis, a process that enables the reduction of the diploid (2n) set of chromosomes to the haploid state (1n) (Chap. 62).

Prior to mitosis, cells exit the resting, or G_0 state, and enter the cell cycle (Chap. 84). After traversing a critical checkpoint in G_1, cells undergo DNA synthesis (S phase), during which the DNA in each chromosome is replicated, yielding two pairs of sister chromatids (2n → 4n). The process of DNA synthesis requires stringent fidelity in order to avoid transmitting errors to subsequent generations of cells. Genetic abnormalities of DNA mismatch/repair include xeroderma pigmentosum, Bloom's syndrome, ataxia telangiectasia, and hereditary nonpolyposis colon cancer (HNPCC), among others. Many of these disorders strongly predispose to neoplasia because of the rapid acquisition of additional mutations (Chap. 83). After completion of DNA synthesis, cells enter G_2 and progress through a second checkpoint before entering mitosis. At this stage, the chromosomes condense and are aligned along the equatorial plate at metaphase. The two identical sister chromatids, held together at the centromere, divide and migrate to opposite poles of the cell (Fig. 63-3). After formation of a nuclear membrane around the two separated sets of chromatids, the cell divides and two daughter cells are formed, thus restoring the diploid (2n) state.

Assortment and segregation of genes during meiosis

Meiosis occurs only in germ cells of the gonads. It shares certain features with mitosis but involves two distinct steps of cell division that reduce the chromosome number to the haploid state. In addition, there is active recombination that generates genetic diversity. During the first cell division, two sister chromatids (2n → 4n) are formed for each chromosome pair and there is an exchange of DNA between homologous paternal and maternal chromosomes. This process involves the formation of *chiasmata*, structures that correspond to the DNA segments that cross over between the maternal and paternal homologues (Fig. 61-3). Usually there is at least one crossover on

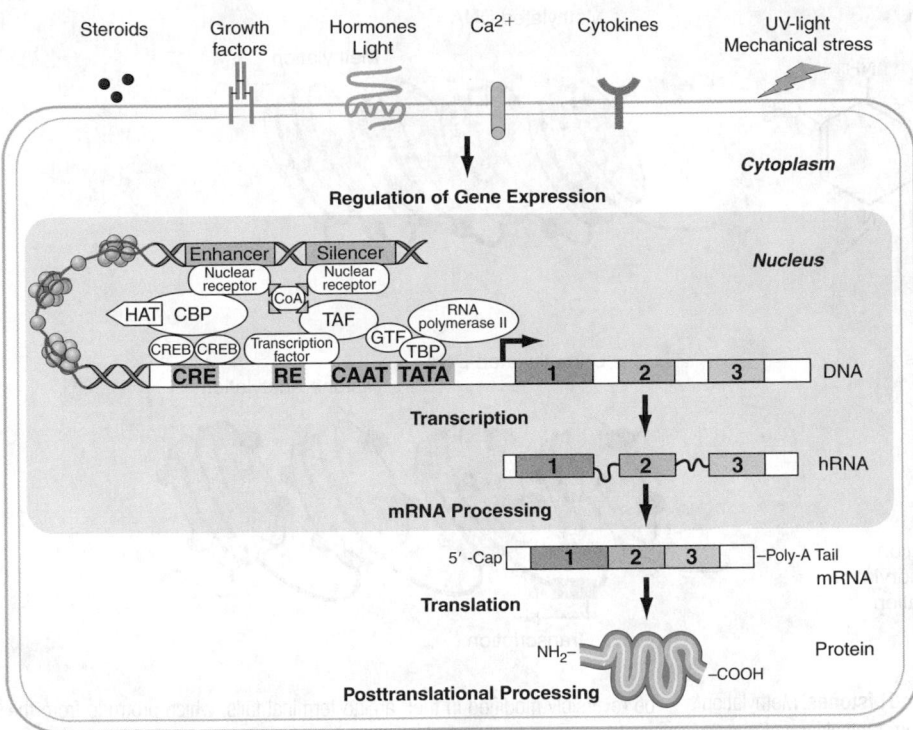

Figure 61-2 Flow of genetic information. Multiple extracellular signals activate intracellular signal cascades that result in altered regulation of gene expression through the interaction of transcription factors with regulatory regions of genes. RNA polymerase transcribes DNA into RNA that is processed to mRNA by excision of intronic sequences. The mRNA is translated into a polypeptide chain to form the mature protein after undergoing posttranslational processing. HAT, histone acetyl transferase; CBP, CREB-binding protein; CREB, cyclic AMP response element–binding protein; CRE, cyclic AMP responsive element; CoA, Co activator; TAF, TBP-associated factors; GTF, general transcription factors; TBP, TATA-binding protein; TATA, TATA box; RE, response element; NH₂, aminoterminus; COOH, carboxyterminus.

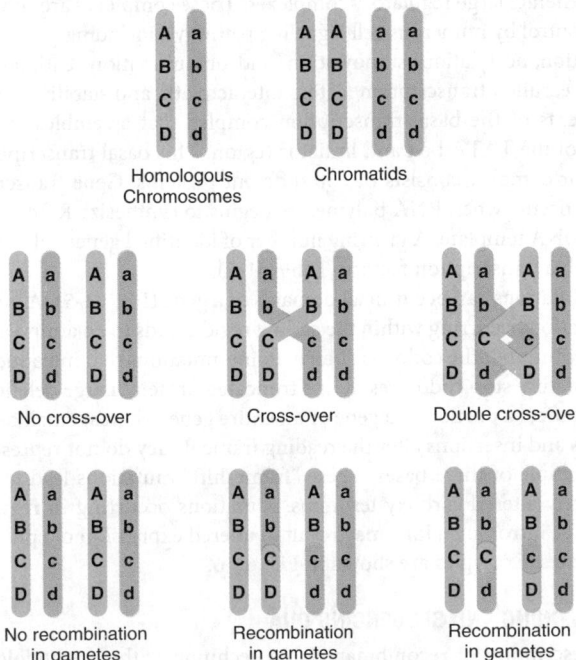

Figure 61-3 Crossing-over and genetic recombination. During chiasma formation, either of the two sister chromatids on one chromosome pairs with one of the chromatids of the homologous chromosome. Genetic recombination occurs through crossing-over and results in recombinant and nonrecombinant chromosome segments in the gametes. Together with the random segregation of the maternal and paternal chromosomes, recombination contributes to genetic diversity and forms the basis of the concept of linkage.

each chromosomal arm; recombination occurs more frequently in female meiosis than in male meiosis. Subsequently, the chromosomes segregate randomly. Because there are 23 chromosomes, there exist 2^{23} (>8 million) possible combinations of chromosomes. Together with the genetic exchanges that occur during recombination, chromosomal segregation generates tremendous diversity, and each gamete is genetically unique. The process of recombination, and the independent segregation of chromosomes, provide the foundation for performing linkage analyses, whereby one attempts to correlate the inheritance of certain chromosomal regions (or linked genes) with the presence of a disease or genetic trait (see below).

After the first meiotic division, which results in two daughter cells ($2n$), the two chromatids of each chromosome separate during a second meiotic division to yield four gametes with a haploid state ($1n$). When the egg is fertilized by sperm, the two haploid sets are combined, thereby restoring the diploid state ($2n$) in the zygote.

■ REGULATION OF GENE EXPRESSION

Mechanisms that regulate gene expression play a critical role in the function of genes. The transcription of genes is controlled primarily by *transcription factors* that bind to DNA sequences in the regulatory regions of genes. As described below, mutations in transcription factors cause a significant number of genetic disorders. Gene expression is also influenced by *epigenetic events (epigenetics)*. DNA and histone modifications can result in the activation or silencing of gene expression (Fig. 61-4). They include heritable changes such as X-inactivation and imprinting, and dynamic alterations in response to environmental influences such as diet, age, or drugs. *Epigenomics* addresses epigenetic changes across the whole genome in a cell or organism. Several genetic disorders such as Prader-Willi syndrome (neonatal hypotonia, developmental delay, obesity, short stature, and hypogonadism) and Albright's hereditary osteodystrophy (resistance to parathyroid hormone, short stature, brachydactyly, resistance to other hormones in certain subtypes), exhibit the consequences of genomic imprinting. Acquired modifications in DNA methylation occur during development and are found in cancer cells, likely contributing to cancer development and progression. Most studies of gene expression have focused on the regulatory DNA elements of genes that control transcription. However, it should be emphasized that gene expression requires a series of steps, including mRNA processing, protein translation, and posttranslational modifications, all of which are actively regulated (Fig. 61-2).

The field of *functional genomics* is based on the concept that understanding alterations of gene expression under various physiologic and pathologic conditions provides insight into the underlying processes, and by revealing certain gene expression profiles, this knowledge may be of diagnostic and therapeutic relevance. The large-scale study of expression profiles, which takes advantage of microarray and bead array technologies, is also referred to as *transcriptomics* because the complement of mRNAs transcribed by the cellular genome is called the *transcriptome*.

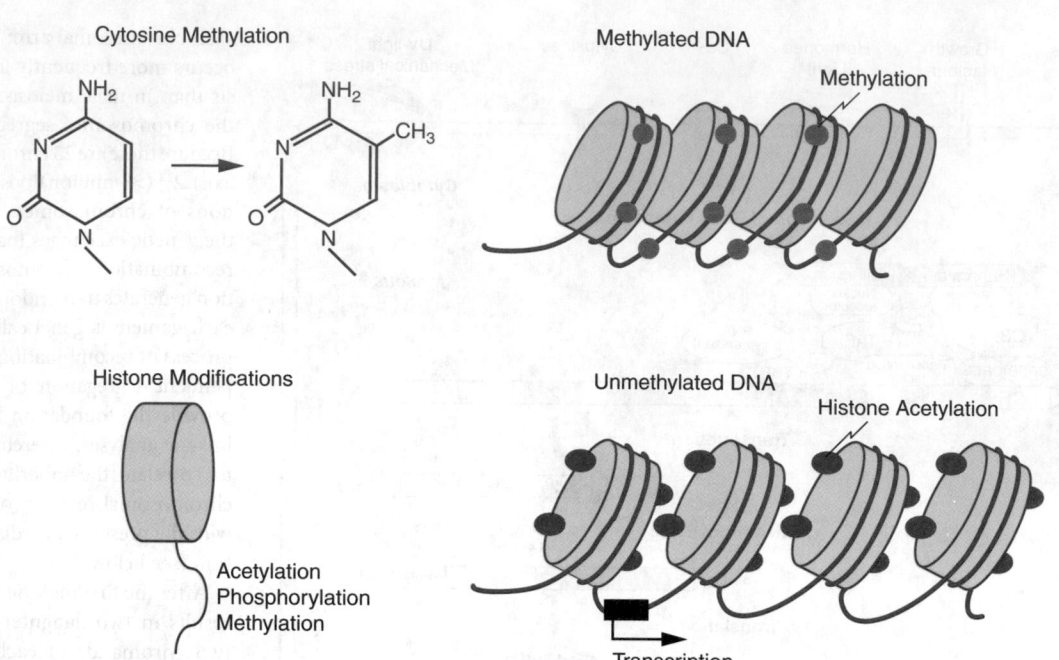

Cytosine Methylation

Histone Modifications

Acetylation
Phosphorylation
Methylation

Methylated DNA

Methylation

Unmethylated DNA

Histone Acetylation

Transcription

Figure 61-4   Epigenetic modifications of DNA and histones. Methylation of cytosine residues is associated with gene silencing. Methylation of certain genomic regions is inherited (imprinting) and is involved in the silencing of one of the two X chromosomes in females (X-inactivation). Alterations in methylation can also be acquired (e.g. in cancer cells). Covalent post-translational modifications of histones and other proteins play an important role in altering chromatin structure and, hence, transcription. Histones can be reversibly modified in their amino-terminal tails, which protrude from the nucleosome core particle, by acetylation of lysine, phosphorylation of serine, or methylation of lysine and arginine residues. Acetylation of histones by histone acetylases (HATs), for example, leads to unwinding of chromatin and accessibility to transcription factors. Conversely, deacetylation by histone deacetylases (HDACs) results in a compact chromatin structure and silencing of transcription.

Structure of genes

A gene product is usually a protein but can occasionally consist of RNA that is not translated (e.g., microRNAs). *Exons* refer to the portion of genes that are eventually spliced together to form mRNA. *Introns* refer to the spacing regions between the exons that are spliced out of precursor RNAs during RNA processing. The gene locus also includes regions that are necessary to control its expression (Fig. 61-2).

The number of DNA sequences and transcription factors that regulate transcription is much greater than originally anticipated. Most genes contain at least 15–20 discrete regulatory elements within 300 bp of the transcription start site. This densely packed promoter region often contains binding sites for ubiquitous transcription factors such as CAAT box/enhancer binding protein (C/EBP), cyclic AMP response element–binding (CREB) protein, selective promoter factor 1 (Sp-1), or activator protein 1 (AP-1). However, factors involved in cell-specific expression may also bind to these sequences. For example, basic helix-loop-helix (bHLH) proteins bind to E-boxes in the promoters of myogenic genes, and steroidogenic factor 1 (SF-1) binds to a specific recognition site in the regulatory region of multiple steroidogenic enzyme genes. Key regulatory elements may also reside at a large distance from the proximal promoter. The globin and the immunoglobulin genes, (e.g., contain *locus control regions* that are several kilobases away from the structural sequences of the gene). Specific groups of transcription factors that bind to these promoter and enhancer sequences provide a combinatorial code for regulating transcription. In this manner, relatively ubiquitous factors interact with more restricted factors to allow each gene to be expressed and regulated in a unique manner that is dependent on developmental state, cell type, and numerous extracellular stimuli. The transcription factors that bind to DNA actually represent only the first level of regulatory control. Other proteins—*co-activators* and *co-repressors*—interact with the DNA-binding transcription factors to generate large regulatory complexes. These complexes are subject to control by numerous cell-signaling pathways, including phosphorylation, acetylation, sumoylation, and ubiquitination. Ultimately, the recruited transcription factors interact with, and stabilize, components of the basal transcription complex that assembles at the site of the TATA box and initiator region. This basal transcription factor complex consists of >30 different proteins. Gene transcription occurs when RNA polymerase begins to synthesize RNA from the DNA template. A growing number of identified genetic diseases involve transcription factors (Table 61-2).

Mutations can occur in all domains of a gene (Fig. 61-5). A point mutation occurring within the coding region leads to an amino acid substitution if the codon is altered. Point mutations that introduce a premature stop codon result in a truncated protein. Large deletions may affect a portion of a gene or an entire gene, whereas small deletions and insertions alter the reading frame if they do not represent a multiple of three bases. These "frameshift" mutations lead to an entirely altered carboxy terminus. Mutations occurring in regulatory or intronic regions may result in altered expression or splicing of genes. Examples are shown in Fig. 61-6.

■ CLONING AND SEQUENCING DNA

A description of recombinant DNA techniques, the methodology used for the manipulation, analysis, and characterization of DNA segments, is beyond the scope of this chapter. These methods are now widely used in genetics and molecular diagnostics.

■ TRANSGENIC MICE AS MODELS OF GENETIC DISEASE

Several organisms have been studied extensively as genetic models, including *Mus musculus* (mouse), *Drosophila melanogaster* (fruit fly),

TABLE 61-2 Selected Examples of Diseases Caused by Mutations and Rearrangements in Transcription Factor Classes

Transcription Factor Class	Example	Associated Disorder
Nuclear receptors	Androgen receptor	Complete or partial androgen insensitivity (recessive missense mutations)
		Spinobulbar muscular atrophy (CAG repeat expansion)
Zinc finger proteins	WT1	WAGR syndrome: Wilms' tumor, aniridia, genitourinary malformations, mental retardation
Basic helix-loop-helix	MITF	Waardenburg's syndrome type 2A
Homeobox	IPF1	Maturity onset of diabetes mellitus type 4 (heterozygous mutation/haploinsufficiency) Pancreatic agenesis (homozygous mutation)
Leucine zipper	Retina leucine zipper (NRL)	Autosomal dominant retinitis pigmentosa
High mobility group (HMG) proteins	SRY	Sex-reversal
Forkhead	HNF4α, HNF1α, HNF1β	Maturity-onset of diabetes mellitus types 1, 3, 5
Paired box	PAX3	Waardenburg's syndrome types 1 and 3
T-box	TBX5	Holt-Oram syndrome (thumb anomalies, atrial or ventricular septum defects, phocomelia)
Cell cycle control proteins	P53	Li-Fraumeni syndrome, other cancers
Coactivators	CREB binding protein (CBP)	Rubinstein-Taybi syndrome
General transcription factors	TATA-binding protein (TBP)	Spinocerebellar ataxia 17 (CAG expansion)
Transcription elongation factor	VHL	von Hippel–Lindau syndrome (renal cell carcinoma, pheochromocytoma, pancreatic tumors, hemangioblastomas)
		Autosomal dominant inheritance, somatic inactivation of second allele (Knudson two-hit model)
Runt	CBFA2	Familial thrombocytopenia with propensity to acute myelogenous leukemia
Chimeric proteins due to translocations	PML–RAR	Acute promyelocytic leukemia t(15;17)(q22;q11.2-q12) translocation

Abbreviations: CREB, cAMP responsive element–binding protein; HNF, hepatocyte nuclear factor; PML, promyelocytic leukemia; RAR, retinoic acid receptor; SRY, sex-determining region Y; VHL, von Hippel–Lindau.

Caenorhabditis elegans (nematode), *Saccharomyces cerevisiae* (baker's yeast), and *Escherichia coli* (colonic bacterium). The ability to use these evolutionarily distant organisms as genetic models that are relevant to human physiology reflects a surprising conservation of genetic pathways and gene function. Transgenic mouse models have been particularly valuable, because many human and mouse genes exhibit similar structure and function, and because manipulation of the mouse genome is relatively straightforward compared to those of other mammalian species.

Transgenic strategies in mice can be divided into two main approaches: (1) expression of a gene by random insertion into the genome, and (2) deletion or targeted mutagenesis of a gene by homologous recombination with the native endogenous gene (knock-out, knock-in) (Table 61-3).

Transgenic expression of genes can be useful for studying disorders that are sensitive to gene dosage. Overexpression of *PMP22*, for example, mimics a common duplication of this gene in type IA Charcot-Marie-Tooth disease (Chap. 384). Duplication of the *PMP22* gene results in high levels of expression of peripheral myelin protein 22, and this dosage effect is responsible for the demyelinating neuropathy. Expression of the Y chromosome–specific gene, *SRY*, in XX females demonstrates that *SRY* is sufficient to induce the formation of testes. This finding confirms the pathogenic role of *SRY* translocations to the X chromosome in sex-reversed XX females. Huntington's disease is an autosomal dominant disorder caused by expansion of a CAG trinucleotide repeat that encodes a polyglutamine tract. Targeted deletion of the Huntington disease's (*HD*) gene does not induce the neurologic disorder. On the other hand, transgenic expression of the entire gene or of the first exon containing the sequence encoding the expanded polyglutamine repeat is sufficient to cause many features of the neurologic disorder, indicating a gain-of-function property for the expanded polyglutamine-containing protein. Transgenic strategies can also be used as precursors to gene therapy. Expression of dystrophin, the protein that is deleted in Duchenne's muscular dystrophy, partially corrects the disorder in a mouse model of Duchenne's. Targeted expression of oncogenes has been valuable to study mechanisms of neoplasia and to generate immortalized cell lines. For example, expression of the simian virus 40 (SV40) large T antigen under the direction of the insulin promoter induces the formation of islet cell tumors.

The creation of gene knock-out and knock-in models takes advantage of the fact that a segment of DNA can be substituted by another that is identical (homologous), or nearly identical, by recombination. This permits integration of deletions that disrupt the gene (knock-out) or selected mutations (knock-in) into the target gene of choice. Many of these gene knock-outs do not have an apparent phenotype, either because of redundant functions of the other genes or because the phenotype is subtle. For example, deletion of the hypoxanthine phosphoribosyltransferase (HPRT) gene (*Hprt*) does not cause characteristic features of Lesch-Nyhan syndrome in mice because of their reliance on adenine phosphoribosyltransferase (APRT) in the purine salvage pathway. Deletion of the retinoblastoma (*Rb*) gene encoding p105 does not lead to retinoblastoma or other tumors that characterize the human syndrome. However, mice with combinatorial deletion of several Rb-related proteins exhibit features similar to the human disorder. These examples underscore the fact that the functions of genes, and their interactions with genetic background and the environment, are not necessarily identical in mice and humans. On the other hand, the deletion of many genes provides a remarkably faithful model of human disorders. In addition to clarifying

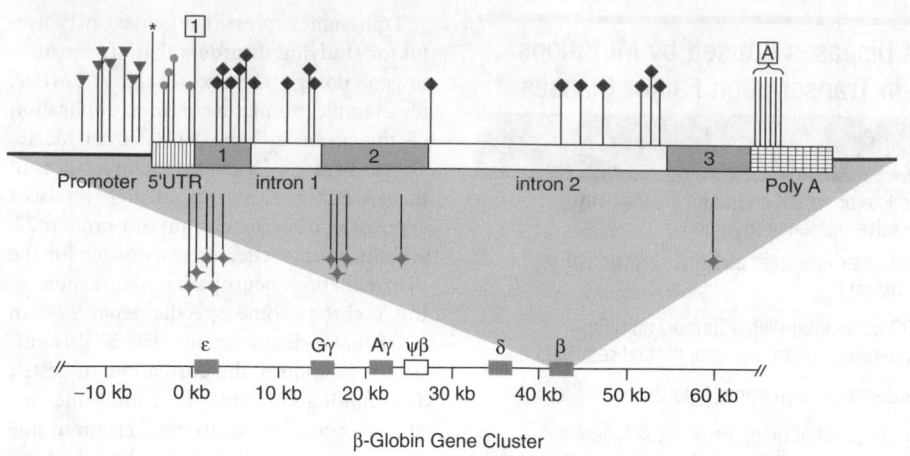

β-Globin Gene Cluster

Figure 61-5 Point mutations causing β-thalassemia as example of allelic heterogeneity. The β-globin gene is located in the globin gene cluster. Point mutations can be located in the promoter, the CAP site, the 5′-untranslated region, the initiation codon, each of the three exons, the introns, or the polyadenylation signal. Many mutations introduce missense or nonsense mutations, whereas others cause defective RNA splicing. Not shown here are deletion mutations of the β-globin gene or larger deletions of the globin locus that can also result in thalassemia. ▼, Promoter mutations; *, CAP site; ●, 5′UTR; ☐1, Initiation codon; ◆, Defective RNA processing; ✦, Missense and nonsense mutations; ☐A, Poly A signal.

pathophysiology, these models facilitate the development of therapies, both genetic and pharmaceutical.

Many variations of these basic approaches now exist that allow genes to be expressed or deleted in specific cell types, at different times during development, or at varying levels. Consequently, transgenic technology has emerged as a powerful strategy for defining the physiologic effects of deleting or overexpressing a gene, as well as providing unique genetic models for dissecting pathophysiology or testing therapies. In addition to transgenic animal models, naturally occurring mutations in mice and other species continue to provide fundamental insights into human disease. A compendium of natural and transgenic animal models is provided in continuously evolving databases (Table 61-1).

IMPLICATIONS OF THE HUMAN GENOME PROJECT

The HGP was initiated in the mid-1980s as an ambitious effort to characterize the human genome, culminating in a complete DNA sequence. The initial main goals were (1) creation of genetic maps, (2) development of physical maps, and (3) determination of the complete human DNA sequence. Some analogies help in appreciating the scope of the HGP. The 23 pairs of human chromosomes encode ~23,000–30,000 genes. The total length of DNA is ~3 billion bp, which is nearly 1000-fold greater than that of the *E. coli* genome. If the human DNA sequence were printed out, it would correspond to about 120 volumes of *Harrison's Principles of Internal Medicine*.

The identification of the ~10 million SNPs estimated to occur in the human genome has generated a catalogue of common genetic variants that occur in human beings from distinct ethnic backgrounds (Fig. 61-7). SNPs that are in close proximity are inherited together (i.e., they are linked) and are referred to as *haplotypes*, hence the name HapMap (Fig. 61-8). The HapMap describes the nature and location of these SNP haplotypes and how they are distributed among individuals within and among populations. The HapMap information is greatly facilitating GWAS designed to elucidate the complex interactions among multiple genes and lifestyle factors in multifactorial disorders (see below). Moreover, haplotype analyses will be useful to assess variations in responses to medications (*pharmacogenomics*) and environmental factors, as well as the prediction of disease predisposition.

The human DNA sequence

The complete DNA sequence of each chromosome provides the highest-resolution physical map. The primary focus of the HGP was to obtain DNA sequence for the entire human genome as well as model organisms. Although the prospect of determining the complete sequence of the human genome seemed daunting several years ago, technical advances in DNA sequencing and bioinformatics led to the completion of a draft human sequence in June 2000, well in advance of the original goal year of 2003. High-quality reference sequences, completed in 2003, further closed gaps and reduced remaining ambiguities, and the HGP announced the completion of the DNA sequence for the last of the human chromosomes in May 2006. The Personal Genome Project (PGP) launched in 2006 aims to completely sequence the genomes from multiple individuals and to associate them with health and physical information to enhance our understanding of

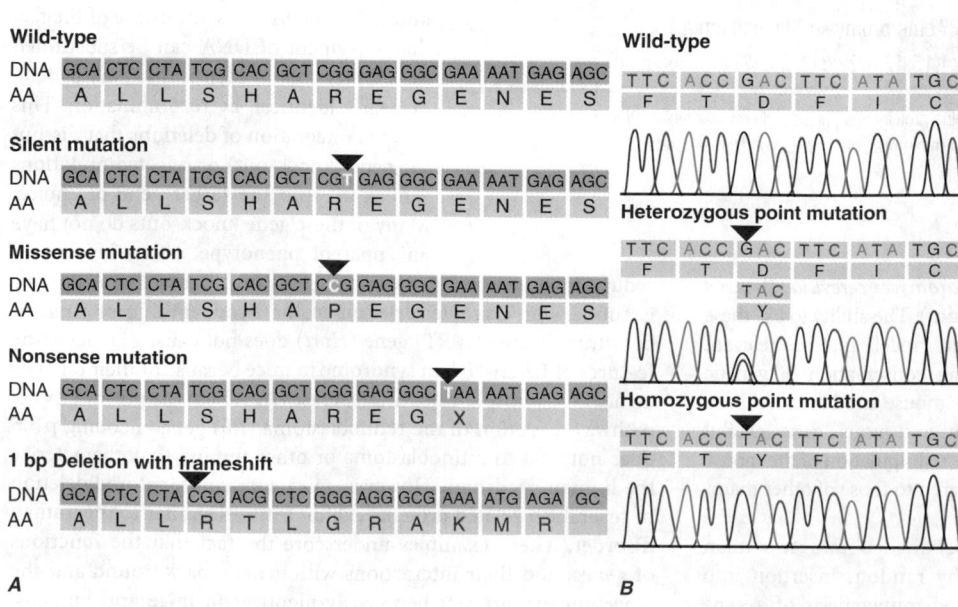

Figure 61-6 A. Examples of mutations. The coding strand is shown with the encoded amino acid sequence. **B.** Chromatograms of sequence analyses after amplification of genomic DNA by polymerase chain reaction.

TABLE 61-3 Genetically Modified Animals

Commonly Used Description	Technical Principle	Remarks
Transgenic	Pronuclear injection of transgene	Commonly used
		Genomic DNA or cDNA constructs
		Random integration of transgene
		Variable copy numbers of transgene
		Variable expression in each individual founder
		Gain-of-function models due to overexpression using tissue-specific promoters
		Loss-of-function models using antisense and dominant negative transgenes
		Inducible expression possible (tetracycline, ecdysone)
		Applicable to several species
(Targeted) Knock-out	Substitution of functional gene with inactive gene by homologous recombination in embryonic stem cells	Predominantly used in mice
		Tissue-specific knock-out possible (Cre/lox)
		Absence of phenotype possible due to redundancy
(Targeted) Knock-in	Introduction of subtle mutation(s) into gene by substitution of endogenous gene with gene carrying a specific mutation. Homologous recombination in embryonic stem cells	Predominantly used in mice
		Can accurately model human disease
Forward genetics	Mutations created randomly by ENU (*N*-ethyl-*N*-nitrourea)	Selection of phenotype followed by genetic characterization
		Useful for identifying novel genes
Congenic strains	Mating of an inbred *donor* strain with a disease phenotype with an inbred *recipient* strain in order to define the genomic region responsible for the disorder	Useful for mapping disease-causing genes
Cloning	Introduction of nucleus into enucleated eggs (nuclear transfer)	Successful in several mammalian species including sheep (Dolly), mice, cows, monkeys
		Cloning of genetically identical individuals
		May affect lifespan
		Ethical concerns

human (patho)physiology. A variety of technical advances in DNA sequencing and computational analyses may soon reduce the cost of obtaining a complete human genome sequence to close to US $1,000. In addition to the human genome, the genomes of numerous organisms have been sequenced completely (~ 1000) or partially (~ 5500) [Genomes Online Database (GOLD); Table 61-1]. They include, among others, eukaryotes such as man and mouse; *S. cerevisiae, C. elegans,* and *D. melanogaster*; bacteria (e.g., *E. coli*); and archeae, viruses, organelles (mitochondriae, chloroplasts), and plants (e.g., *Arabidopsis thaliana*). This information, together with technological advances and refinement of computational bioinformatics, has led to a fast-paced transition from the study of single genes to whole genomes. The current directions arising from the HGP include, among others, (1) the comparison of entire genomes (*comparative genomics*), (2) the study of large-scale expression of RNAs (*functional genomics*) and proteins (*proteomics*) in order to detect differences between various tissues in health and disease, (3) the characterization of the variation among individuals by establishing catalogues of sequence variations and SNPs (HapMap project) and the Personal Genome Project, and (4) the identification of genes that play critical roles in the development of polygenic and multifactorial disorders.

Ethical issues

Implicit in the HGP is the concept that identifying disease-causing genes can lead to improvements in diagnosis, treatment, and prevention. Most individuals can be expected to harbor several serious recessive gene mutations. Completion of the human genome sequence, determination of the association of genetic defects with disease, and studies of genetic variation raise many new issues with implications for the individual and mankind. The controversies concerning the cloning of mammals, the establishment of human ES cells, and the creation of synthetic organisms underscore the relevance of these questions. Moreover, the information gleaned from genotypic results can have quite different impacts, depending on the availability of strategies to modify the course of disease. For example, the identification of mutations that cause multiple endocrine neoplasia (MEN) type 2 or hemochromatosis allows specific interventions for affected family members. On the other hand, at present, the identification of an Alzheimer's or Huntington's disease gene does not alter therapy and outcomes. However, the progress in this area is unpredictable, as underscored by the finding that angiotensin II receptor blockers may slow disease progression in Marfan's syndrome.

Genetic test results can generate anxiety in affected individuals and family members, and there is the possibility of discrimination on the basis of the test results. Most genetic disorders are likely to fall into an intermediate category where the opportunity for prevention or treatment is significant but limited (Chap. 63). For these reasons, the scientific components of the HGP have been paralleled by efforts to examine ethical, social, and legal implications as new issues arise.

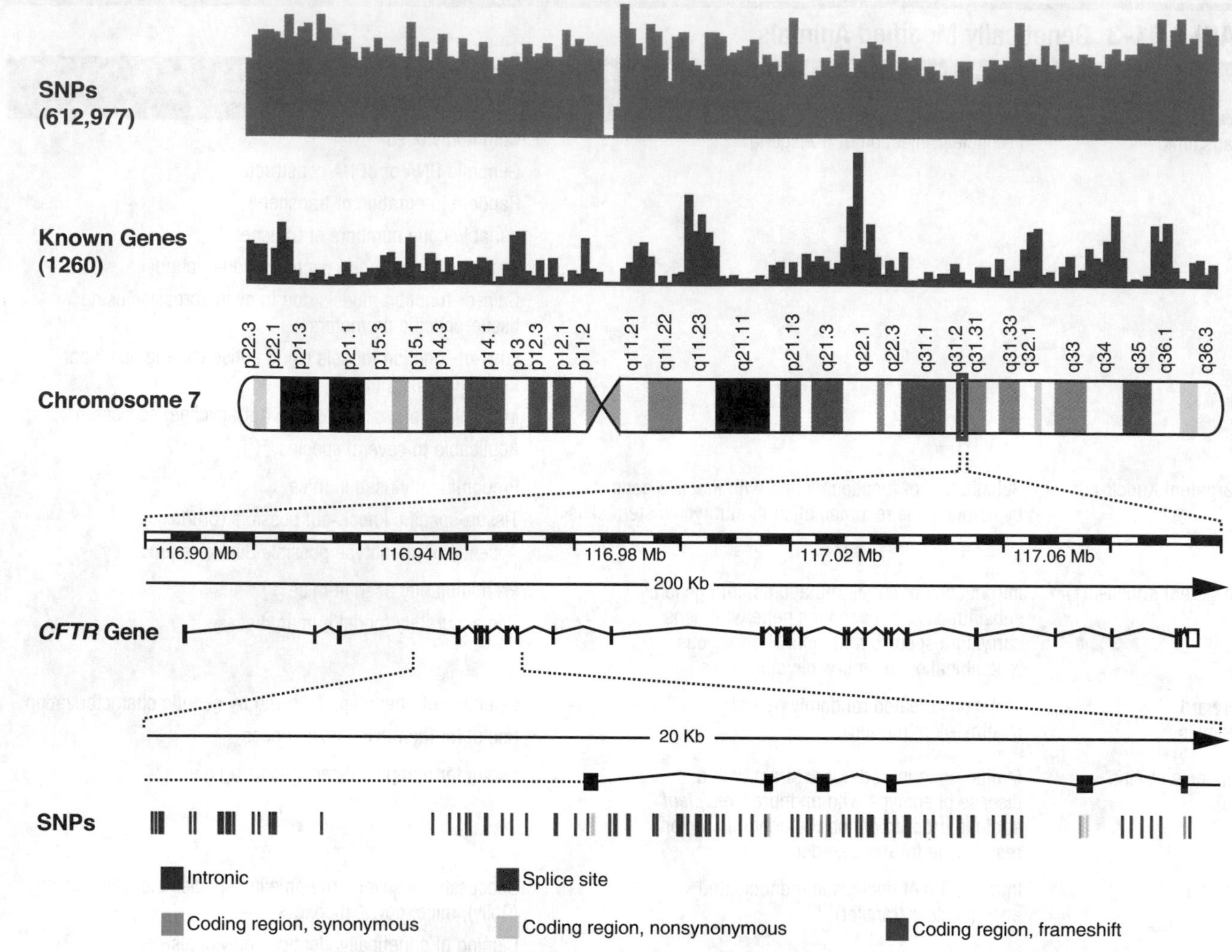

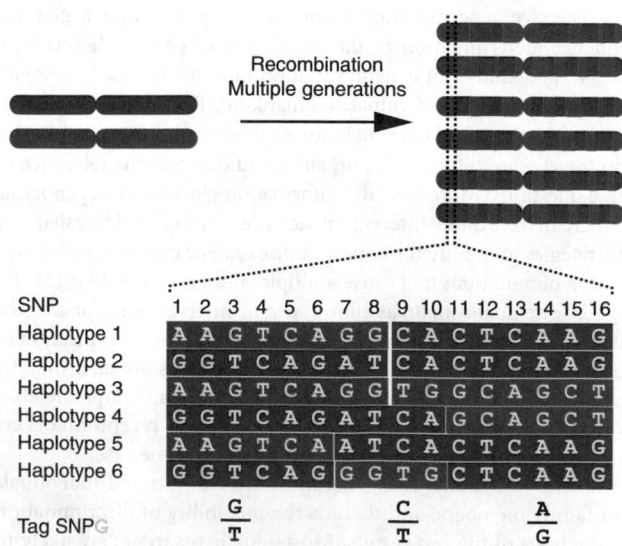

SNPs
(612,977)

Known Genes
(1260)

Chromosome 7

p22.3 p22.1 p21.3 p21.1 p15.3 p15.1 p14.3 p14.1 p13 p12.3 p12.1 p11.2 q11.21 q11.22 q11.23 q21.11 q21.13 q21.3 q22.1 q22.3 q31.1 q31.2 q31.31 q31.33 q32.1 q33 q34 q35 q36.1 q36.3

116.90 Mb   116.94 Mb   116.98 Mb   117.02 Mb   117.06 Mb

← 200 Kb →

CFTR Gene

← 20 Kb →

SNPs

■ Intronic   ■ Splice site

■ Coding region, synonymous   ■ Coding region, nonsynonymous   ■ Coding region, frameshift

Figure 61-7 Chromosome 7 is shown with the density of single nucleotide polymorphisms (SNPs) and genes above. A 200-kb region in 7q31.2 containing the *CFTR* gene is shown below. The *CFTR* gene contains 27 exons. More than 1790 mutations in this gene have been found in patients with cystic fibrosis. A 20-kb region encompassing exons 4–9 is shown further amplified in order to illustrate the SNPs in this region.

Recombination
Multiple generations

SNP	1	2	3	4	5	6	7	8	9	10	11	12	13	14	15	16
Haplotype 1	A	A	G	T	C	A	G	G	C	A	C	T	C	A	A	G
Haplotype 2	G	G	T	C	A	G	A	T	C	A	C	T	C	A	A	G
Haplotype 3	A	A	G	T	C	A	G	G	G	T	G	G	C	A	G	C	T
Haplotype 4	G	G	T	C	A	G	A	T	C	A	G	C	A	G	C	T
Haplotype 5	A	A	G	T	C	A	A	T	C	A	C	T	C	A	A	G
Haplotype 6	G	G	T	C	A	G	G	G	T	G	C	T	C	A	A	G

Tag SNP $\frac{G}{T}$ $\frac{G}{T}$ $\frac{C}{T}$ $\frac{A}{G}$

Figure 61-8 The origin of haplotypes is due to repeated recombination events occurring in multiple generations. Over time, this leads to distinct haplotypes. These haplotype blocks can often be characterized by genotyping selected Tag single-nucleotide polymorphisms, an approach that now facilitates performing genome-wide association studies (GWAS).

The Genetic Information Nondiscrimination Act (GINA), signed into law in 2008, aims to protect individuals against the misuse of genetic information for health insurance and employment. The impact of genetic testing on health care costs is currently unclear. It is likely to vary among disorders and depend on the availability of effective therapeutic modalities. A significant problem arises from the marketing of genetic testing directly to consumers by commercial companies. The validity of these tests has not been defined and there are numerous concerns about the lack of appropriate regulatory oversight, the accuracy and confidentiality of genetic information, the availability of counseling, and the handling of these results.

Many issues raised by the genome project are familiar, in principle, to medical practitioners. For example, an asymptomatic patient with increased low-density lipoprotein (LDL) cholesterol, high blood pressure, or a strong family history of early myocardial infarction is known to be at increased risk of coronary heart disease. In such cases, it is clear that the identification of risk factors and an appropriate intervention are beneficial. Likewise, patients with phenylketonuria, cystic fibrosis, or sickle cell anemia are often identified as having a genetic disease early in life. These precedents can be helpful for adapting policies that relate to genetic information. We can anticipate similar efforts, whether based on genotypes or other markers of genetic predisposition, to be applied to many disorders. One confounding aspect of the rapid expansion of information is that our ability to make clinical decisions often lags behind initial insights into genetic mechanisms of disease. For example, when genes that predispose to breast cancer such as *BRCA1* are described, they generate tremendous public interest in the potential to predict disease, but many years of clinical research are still required to rigorously establish genotype and phenotype correlations.

Whether related to informed consent, participation in research, or the management of a genetic disorder that affects an individual or their families, there is a great need for more information about fundamental principles of genetics. The pervasive nature of the role of genetics in medicine makes it imperative for physicians and other health care professionals to become more informed about genetics and to provide advice and counseling in conjunction with trained genetic counselors (Chap. 63). The application of screening and prevention strategies will therefore require intensive patient and physician education, changes in health care financing, and legislation to protect patient's rights.

Genomics and global health

Genomics may contribute to improvements in global health by providing a better understanding of pathogens and diagnostics, and through contributions to drug development. There is, however, concern about the development of a "genomics divide" because of the costs associated with these developments and uncertainty as to whether these advances will be accessible to the populations of developing countries. The World Health Organization has summarized the current issues and inequities surrounding genomic medicine in a detailed report on *Genomics and World Health*.

■ TRANSMISSION OF GENETIC DISEASE

Origins and types of mutations

A *mutation* can be defined as any change in the primary nucleotide sequence of DNA regardless of its functional consequences. Some mutations may be lethal, others are less deleterious, and some may confer an evolutionary advantage. Mutations can occur in the germline (sperm or oocytes); these can be transmitted to progeny. Alternatively, mutations can occur during embryogenesis or in somatic tissues. Mutations that occur during development lead to *mosaicism*, a situation in which tissues are composed of cells with different genetic constitutions. If the germline is mosaic, a mutation can be transmitted to some progeny but not others, which sometimes leads to confusion in assessing the pattern of inheritance. Somatic mutations that do not affect cell survival can sometimes be detected because of variable phenotypic effects in tissues (e.g., pigmented lesions in McCune-Albright syndrome). Other somatic mutations are associated with neoplasia because they confer a growth advantage to cells. Epigenetic events, heritable changes that do not involve changes in gene sequence (e.g., altered DNA methylation), may influence gene expression or facilitate genetic damage. With the exception of triplet nucleotide repeats, which can expand (see below), mutations are usually stable.

Mutations are structurally diverse—they can involve the entire genome, as in triploidy (one extra set of chromosomes), or gross numerical or structural alterations in chromosomes or individual genes (Chap. 62). Large deletions may affect a portion of a gene or an entire gene, or, if several genes are involved, they may lead to a *contiguous gene syndrome*. Unequal crossing-over between homologous genes can result in fusion gene mutations, as illustrated by color blindness (Chap. 28). Mutations involving single nucleotides are referred to as *point mutations*. Substitutions are called *transitions* if a purine is replaced by another purine base (A ↔ G) or if a pyrimidine is replaced by another pyrimidine (C ↔ T). Changes from a purine to a pyrimidine, or vice versa, are referred to as *transversions*. If the DNA sequence change occurs in a coding region and alters an amino acid, it is called a *missense mutation*. Depending on the functional consequences of such a missense mutation, amino acid substitutions in different regions of the protein can lead to distinct phenotypes. *Polymorphisms* are sequence variations that have a frequency of at least 1%. Usually, they do not result in a perceptible phenotype. Often they consist of single base-pair substitutions that do not alter the protein coding sequence because of the degenerate nature of the genetic code (synonymous polymorphism), although it is possible that some might alter mRNA stability, translation, or the amino acid sequence (nonsynonymous polymorphism) (Fig. 61-7). These types of base substitutions are encountered frequently during genetic testing and must be distinguished from true mutations that alter protein expression or function. Small nucleotide deletions or insertions cause a shift of the codon reading frame (*frameshift*). Most commonly, reading frame alterations result in an abnormal protein segment of variable length before termination of translation occurs at a stop codon (*nonsense mutation*) (Fig. 61-6). Mutations in intronic sequences or in exon junctions may destroy or create splice donor or splice acceptor sites. Mutations may also be found in the regulatory sequences of genes, resulting in reduced gene transcription.

Mutation rates As noted before, mutations represent an important cause of genetic diversity as well as disease. Mutation rates are difficult to determine in humans because many mutations are silent and because testing is often not adequate to detect the phenotypic consequences. Mutation rates vary in different genes but are estimated to occur at a rate of ~10^{-10}/bp per cell division. Germline mutation rates (as opposed to somatic mutations) are relevant in the transmission of genetic disease. Because the population of oocytes is established very early in development, only ~20 cell divisions are required for completed oogenesis, whereas spermatogenesis involves ~30 divisions by the time of puberty and 20 cell divisions each year thereafter. Consequently, the probability of acquiring new point mutations is much greater in the male germline than the female germline, in which rates of aneuploidy are increased (Chap. 62). Thus, the incidence of new point mutations in spermatogonia increases with paternal age (e.g., achondrodysplasia, Marfan's syndrome, neurofibromatosis). It is estimated that about 1 in 10 sperm carries a new deleterious mutation. The rates for new mutations are calculated most readily for autosomal dominant and X-linked disorders and are ~10^{-5}–10^{-6}/locus per generation. Because most monogenic diseases are relatively rare, new mutations account for a significant fraction of cases. This is important in the context of genetic counseling, as a new mutation can be transmitted to the affected individual but does not necessarily imply that the parents are at risk to transmit the disease to other children. An exception to this is when the new mutation occurs early in germline development, leading to *gonadal mosaicism*.

Unequal crossing-over Normally, DNA recombination in germ cells occurs with remarkable fidelity to maintain the precise junction sites for the exchanged DNA sequences (Fig. 61-3). However, mispairing of homologous sequences leads to unequal crossover, with gene duplication on one of the chromosomes and gene deletion on the other chromosome. A significant fraction of growth hormone (*GH*) gene deletions, for example, involve unequal crossing-over (Chap. 339). The *GH* gene is a member of a large gene cluster that includes a GH variant gene as well as several structurally related chorionic somatomammotropin genes and pseudogenes (highly homologous but functionally inactive relatives of a normal gene). Because such gene clusters contain multiple homologous DNA sequences arranged in tandem, they are particularly prone to undergo recombination and, consequently, gene duplication or deletion. On the other hand, duplication of the *PMP22* gene because of unequal crossing-over results in increased gene dosage and type IA Charcot-Marie-Tooth disease. Unequal crossing-over resulting in deletion of *PMP22* causes a distinct neuropathy called *hereditary liability to pressure palsy* (Chap. 384).

Glucocorticoid-remediable aldosteronism (GRA) is caused by a rearrangement involving the genes that encode aldosterone synthase (*CYP11B2*) and steroid 11β-hydroxylase (*CYP11B1*), normally arranged in tandem on chromosome 8q. These two genes are 95% identical, predisposing to gene duplication and deletion by unequal crossing-over. The rearranged gene product contains the regulatory regions of 11β-hydroxylase fused to the coding sequence of aldosterone synthetase. Consequently, the latter enzyme is expressed in the adrenocorticotropic hormone (ACTH)–dependent zona fasciculata of the adrenal gland, resulting in overproduction of mineralocorticoids and hypertension (Chap. 342).

Gene conversion refers to a nonreciprocal exchange of homologous genetic information; it is probably more common than generally recognized. In human genetics, gene conversion has been used to explain how an internal portion of a gene is replaced by a homologous segment copied from another allele or locus; these genetic alterations may range from a few nucleotides to a few thousand nucleotides. As a result of gene conversion, it is possible for short DNA segments of two chromosomes to be identical, even though these sequences are distinct in the parents. A practical consequence of this phenomenon is that nucleotide substitutions can occur during gene conversion between related genes, often altering the function of the gene. In disease states, gene conversion often involves intergenic exchange of DNA between a gene and a related pseudogene. For example, the 21-hydroxylase gene (*CYP21A2*) is adjacent to a nonfunctional pseudogene (*CYP21A1P*). Many of the nucleotide substitutions that are found in the *CYP21A2* gene in patients with congenital adrenal hyperplasia correspond to sequences that are present in the *CYP21A1P* pseudogene, suggesting gene conversion as a mechanism of mutagenesis. In addition, mitotic gene conversion has been suggested as a mechanism to explain revertant mosaicism in which an inherited mutation is "corrected" in certain cells. For example, patients with autosomal recessive generalized atrophic benign epidermolysis bullosa have acquired reverse mutations in one of the two mutated *COL17A1* alleles, leading to clinically unaffected patches of skin.

Insertions and deletions   Although many instances of insertions and deletions occur as a consequence of unequal crossing-over, there is also evidence for internal duplication, inversion, or deletion of DNA sequences. The fact that certain deletions or insertions appear to occur repeatedly as independent events suggests that specific regions within the DNA sequence predispose to these errors. For example, certain regions of the *DMD* gene appear to be hot spots for deletions. Some regions within the human genome are rearrangement hot spots and lead to copy number variations (CNVs).

Errors in DNA repair   Because mutations caused by defects in DNA repair accumulate as somatic cells divide, these types of mutations are particularly important in the context of neoplastic disorders (Chap. 84). Several genetic disorders involving DNA repair enzymes underscore their importance. Patients with xeroderma pigmentosum have defects in DNA damage recognition or in the nucleotide excision and repair pathway (Chap. 87). Exposed skin is dry and pigmented and is extraordinarily sensitive to the mutagenic effects of ultraviolet irradiation. More than 10 different genes have been shown to cause the different forms of xeroderma pigmentosum. This finding is consistent with the earlier classification of this disease into different complementation groups in which normal function is rescued by the fusion of cells derived from two different forms of xeroderma pigmentosum.

Ataxia telangiectasia causes large telangiectatic lesions of the face, cerebellar ataxia, immunologic defects, and hypersensitivity to ionizing radiation (Chap. 373). The discovery of the ataxia telangiectasia mutated (*ATM*) gene reveals that it is homologous to genes involved in DNA repair and control of cell cycle checkpoints. Mutations in the *ATM* gene give rise to defects in meiosis as well as increasing susceptibility to damage from ionizing radiation. Fanconi's anemia is also associated with an increased risk of multiple acquired genetic abnormalities. It is characterized by diverse congenital anomalies and a strong predisposition to develop aplastic anemia and acute myelogenous leukemia (Chap. 109). Cells from these patients are susceptible to chromosomal breaks caused by a defect in genetic recombination. At least 13 different complementation groups have been identified, and several loci and genes associated with Fanconi's anemia have been mapped or cloned. HNPCC (Lynch's syndrome) is characterized by autosomal dominant transmission of colon cancer, young age (<50 years) of presentation, predisposition to lesions in the proximal large bowel, and associated malignancies such as uterine cancer and ovarian cancer. HNPCC is predominantly caused by mutations in one of several different mismatch repair (MMR) genes including MutS homologue 2 (*MSH2*), MutL homologue 1 and 6 (*MLH1, MLH6*), *MSH6*, *PMS1*, and *PMS2* (Chap. 91). These proteins are involved in the detection of nucleotide mismatches and in the recognition of slipped-strand trinucleotide repeats. Germline mutations in these genes lead to microsatellite instability and a high mutation rate in colon cancer. Genetic screening tests for this disorder are now being used for families considered to be at risk (Chap. 63). Recognition of HNPCC allows early screening with colonoscopy and the implementation of prevention strategies using nonsteroidal anti-inflammatory drugs.

Dipyrimidine and CpG sequences   Certain DNA sequences are particularly susceptible to mutagenesis. Successive pyrimidine residues (e.g., T-T or C-C) are subject to the formation of ultraviolet light–induced photoadducts. If these pyrimidine dimers are not repaired by the nucleotide excision repair pathway, mutations will be introduced after DNA synthesis. The dinucleotide C-G, or CpG, is also a hot spot for a specific type of mutation. In this case, methylation of the cytosine is associated with an enhanced rate of deamination to uracil, which is then replaced with thymine. This $C \rightarrow T$ transition (or $G \rightarrow A$ on the opposite strand) accounts for at least one-third of point mutations associated with polymorphisms and mutations. Many of the *MSH2* mutations in HNPCC, for example, involve CpG sequences. In addition to the fact that certain types of mutations ($C \rightarrow T$ or $G \rightarrow A$) are relatively common, the nature of the genetic code also results in overrepresentation of certain amino acid substitutions.

Unstable DNA sequences   *Trinucleotide repeats* may be unstable and expand beyond a critical number. Mechanistically, the expansion is thought to be caused by unequal recombination and slipped mispairing. A premutation represents a small increase in trinucleotide copy number. In subsequent generations, the expanded repeat may increase further in length and result in an increasingly severe phenotype, a process called *dynamic mutation* (see below for discussion of anticipation). Trinucleotide expansion was first recognized as a cause of the fragile X syndrome, one of the most common causes of mental retardation. Other disorders arising from a similar mechanism include Huntington's disease (Chap. 371), X-linked spinobulbar muscular atrophy (Chap. 374), and myotonic dystrophy (Chap. 387). Malignant cells are also characterized by genetic instability, indicating a breakdown in mechanisms that regulate DNA repair and the cell cycle.

Functional consequences of mutations

Functionally, mutations can be broadly classified as gain-of-function and loss-of-function mutations. Gain-of-function mutations are typically dominant (i.e., they result in phenotypic alterations when a single allele is affected). Inactivating mutations are usually recessive, and an affected individual is homozygous or compound heterozygous (e.g., carrying two different mutant alleles of the same gene) for the disease-causing mutations. Alternatively, mutation in a single allele can result in *haploinsufficiency*, a situation in which one normal allele is not sufficient to maintain a normal phenotype. Haploinsufficiency is a commonly observed mechanism in diseases associated with mutations in transcription factors (Table 61-2). Remarkably, the clinical features among patients with an identical mutation in a transcription factor often vary significantly. One mechanism underlying this variability consists in the influence of modifying genes. Haploinsufficiency can also affect the expression of rate-limiting enzymes. For example, haploinsufficiency in enzymes involved in heme synthesis can cause porphyrias (Chap. 358).

An increase in dosage of a gene product may also result in disease, as illustrated by the duplication of the *DAX1* gene in dosage-sensitive sex-reversal (Chap. 349). Mutation in a single allele can also result in loss of function due to a dominant-negative effect. In this case, the mutated allele interferes with the function of the normal gene product by one of several different mechanisms: (1) a mutant protein may interfere with the function of a multimeric protein complex, as illustrated by mutations in type 1 collagen (*COL1A1*, *COL1A2*) genes in osteogenesis imperfecta (Chap. 363); (2) a mutant protein may occupy binding sites on proteins or promoter response elements, as illustrated by thyroid hormone resistance, a disorder in which inactivated thyroid hormone receptor binds to target genes and functions as an antagonist of normal receptors (Chap. 341); or (3) a mutant protein can be cytotoxic as in α_1 antitrypsin deficiency (Chap. 260) or autosomal dominant neurohypophyseal diabetes insipidus (Chap. 340), in which the abnormally folded proteins are trapped within the endoplasmic reticulum and ultimately cause cellular damage.

Genotype and phenotype

Alleles, genotypes, and haplotypes

An observed trait is referred to as a *phenotype*; the genetic information defining the phenotype is called the *genotype*. Alternative forms of a gene or a genetic marker are referred to as *alleles*. Alleles may be polymorphic variants of nucleic acids that have no apparent effect on gene expression or function. In other instances, these variants may have subtle effects on gene expression, thereby conferring the adaptive advantages associated with genetic diversity. On the other hand, allelic variants may reflect mutations in a gene that clearly alter its function. The common Glu6Val (E6V) sickle cell mutation in the β-*globin* gene and the ΔF508 deletion of phenylalanine (F) in the *CFTR* gene are examples of allelic variants of these genes that result in disease. Because each individual has two copies of each chromosome (one inherited from the mother and one inherited from the father), he or she can have only two alleles at a given locus. However, there can be many different alleles in the population. The normal or common allele is usually referred to as *wild type*. When alleles at a given locus are identical, the individual is *homozygous*. Inheriting identical copies of a mutant allele occurs in many autosomal recessive disorders, particularly in circumstances of consanguinity. If the alleles are different on the maternal and the paternal copy of the gene, the individual is *heterozygous* at this locus (Fig. 61-6). If two different mutant alleles are inherited at a given locus, the individual is said to be a *compound heterozygote*. *Hemizygous* is used to describe males with a mutation in an X chromosomal gene or a female with a loss of one X chromosomal locus.

Genotypes describe the specific alleles at a particular locus. For example, there are three common alleles (E2, E3, E4) of the apolipoprotein E (*APOE*) gene. The genotype of an individual can therefore be described as *APOE3/4* or *APOE4/4* or any other variant. These designations indicate which alleles are present on the two chromosomes in the *APOE* gene at locus 19q13.2. In other cases, the genotype might be assigned arbitrary numbers (e.g., 1/2) or letters (e.g., B/b) to distinguish different alleles.

A *haplotype* refers to a group of alleles that are closely linked together at a genomic locus (Fig. 61-8). Haplotypes are useful for tracking the transmission of genomic segments within families and for detecting evidence of genetic recombination, if the crossover event occurs between the alleles (Fig. 61-3). As an example, various alleles at the histocompatibility locus antigen (HLA) on chromosome 6p are used to establish haplotypes associated with certain disease states. For example, 21-hydroxylase deficiency, complement deficiency, and hemochromatosis are each associated with specific HLA haplotypes. It is now recognized that these genes lie in close vicinity to the HLA locus, which explains why HLA associations were identified even before the disease genes were cloned and localized. In other cases, specific HLA associations with diseases such as ankylosing spondylitis (HLA-B27) or type 1 diabetes mellitus (HLA-DR4) reflect the role of specific HLA allelic variants in susceptibility to these autoimmune diseases. The characterization of common SNP haplotypes in numerous populations from different parts of the world through the HapMap project is providing a novel tool for association studies designed to detect genes involved in the pathogenesis of complex disorders (Table 61-1). The presence or absence of certain haplotypes may also become relevant for the customized choice of medical therapies (pharmacogenomics) or for preventive strategies.

Allelic heterogeneity

Allelic heterogeneity refers to the fact that different mutations in the same genetic locus can cause an identical or similar phenotype. For example, many different mutations of the β-globin locus can cause β-thalassemia (Table 61-4) (Fig. 61-5). In essence, allelic heterogeneity reflects the fact that many different mutations are capable of altering protein structure and function. For this reason, maps of inactivating mutations in genes usually show a near-random distribution. Exceptions include (1) a founder effect, in which a particular mutation that does not affect reproductive capacity can be traced to a single individual; (2) "hot spots" for mutations, in which the nature of the DNA sequence predisposes to a recurring mutation; and (3) localization of mutations to certain domains that are particularly critical for protein function. Allelic heterogeneity creates a practical problem for genetic testing because one must often examine the entire genetic locus for mutations, as these can differ in each patient. For example, there are currently 1795 reported mutations in the *CFTR* gene (Fig. 61-7). The mutational analysis initially focuses on a panel of mutations that are particularly frequent (often taking the ethnic background of the patient into account), but a negative result does not exclude the presence of a mutation elsewhere in the gene. One should also be aware that mutational analyses generally focus on the coding region of a gene without considering regulatory and intronic regions. Because disease-causing mutations may be located outside the coding regions, negative results should be interpreted with caution. It is expected that the advent of more comprehensive sequencing technologies will greatly facilitate mutational analyses. It will, however, also introduce challenges because the detection of a sequence alteration alone is not always sufficient to establish that it has a causal role.

Phenotypic heterogeneity

Phenotypic heterogeneity occurs when more than one phenotype is caused by allelic mutations (i.e., different mutations in the same gene) (Table 61-4). For example, laminopathies are monogenic multisystem disorders that result from mutations in the *LMNA* gene, which encodes the nuclear

TABLE 61-4 Selected Examples of Locus Heterogeneity and Phenotypic Heterogeneity

Phenotypic Heterogeneity

Gene, Protein	Phenotype	Inheritance	OMIM
LMNA, Lamin A/C	Emery-Dreifuss muscular dystrophy (AD)	AD	181350
	Familial partial lipodystrophy Dunnigan	AD	151660
	Hutchinson-Gilford progeria	AD	176670
	Atypical Werner's syndrome	AD	150330
	Dilated cardiomyopathy	AD	115200
	Early-onset atrial fibrillation	AD	607554
	Emery-Dreifuss muscular dystrophy (AR)	AR	604929
	Limb-girdle muscular dystrophy type 1B	AR	159001
	Charcot-Marie-Tooth type 2B1	AR	605588
KRAS	Noonan syndrome	AD	163950
	Cardio-facio-cutaneous syndrome	AD	115150

Locus Heterogeneity

Phenotype	Gene	Chromosomal Location	Protein
Familial hypertrophic cardiomyopathy	MYH7	14q12	Myosin heavy chain beta
Genes encoding sarcomeric proteins	TNNT2	1q2	Troponin-T2
	TPM1	15q22.1	Tropomyosin alpha
	MYBPC3	11p11q	Myosin-binding protein C
	TNNI3	19q13.4	Troponin 1
	MYL2	12q23-24.3	Myosin light chain 2
	MYL3	3p	Myosin light chain 3
	TTN	2q24.3	Cardiac titin
	ACTC	15q11	Cardiac alpha actin
	MYH6	14q1	Myosin heavy chain alpha
	MYLK2	20q13.3	Myosin light-peptide kinase
	CAV3	3p25	Caveolin 3
Genes encoding nonsarcomeric proteins	MTT1	Mitochondrial	tRNA isoleucine
	MTTG	Mitochondrial	tRNA glycine
	PRKAG2	7q35-q36	AMP-activated protein kinase γ2 subunit
	DMPK	19q13.2-13.3	Myotonin protein kinase (myotonic dystrophy)
	FRDA	9q13	Frataxin (Friedreich ataxia)
Polycystic kidney disease	PKD1	16p13.3-13.12	Polycystin 1 (AD)
	PKD2	4q21.-23	Polycystin 2 (AD)
	PKHD1	6p21.1-p12	Fibrocystin (AR)
Noonan syndrome	PTPN11	12q24.1	Protein-tyrosine phosphatase 2c
	KRAS	12p12.1	KRAS

Abbreviations: AD, autosomal dominant; AR, autosomal recessive.

lamins A and C. Twelve autosomal dominant and four autosomal recessive disorders are caused by mutations in the *LMNA* gene. They include several forms of lipodystrophies, Emery-Dreifuss muscular dystrophy, progeria syndromes, a form of neuronal Charcot-Marie-Tooth disease (type 2B1), and a group of overlapping syndromes. Remarkably, hierarchical cluster analysis has revealed that the phenotypes vary depending on the position of the mutation. Similarly, identical mutations in the *FGFR2* gene can result in very distinct phenotypes: Crouzon's syndrome (craniofacial synostosis) or Pfeiffer's syndrome (acrocephalopolysyndactyly).

Locus or nonallelic heterogeneity and phenocopies *Nonallelic or locus heterogeneity* refers to the situation in which a similar disease phenotype results from mutations at different genetic loci. This often occurs when more than one gene product produces different subunits of an interacting complex or when different genes are involved in the same genetic cascade or physiologic pathway. For example, osteogenesis imperfecta can arise from mutations in two different procollagen genes (*COL1A1* or *COL1A2*) that are located on different chromosomes (Chap. 363). The effects of inactivating mutations in these two genes are similar because the protein products comprise different subunits of the helical collagen fiber. Similarly, muscular dystrophy syndromes can be caused by mutations in various genes, consistent with the fact that it can be transmitted in an X-linked (Duchenne or Becker), autosomal dominant (limb-girdle muscular dystrophy type 1), or autosomal recessive (limb-girdle muscular dystrophy type 2) manner (Chap. 387). Mutations in the X-linked *DMD* gene, which encodes dystrophin, are the most common cause of muscular dystrophy. This feature reflects the large size of the gene as well as the fact that the phenotype is expressed in hemizygous males because they have only a single copy of the X chromosome. Dystrophin is associated with a large protein complex linked to the membrane-associated cytoskeleton in muscle. Mutations in several different components of this protein complex can also cause muscular dystrophy syndromes. Although the phenotypic features of some of these disorders are distinct, the phenotypic spectrum caused by mutations in different genes overlaps, thereby leading to nonallelic heterogeneity. It should be noted that mutations in dystrophin also cause allelic heterogeneity. For example, mutations in the *DMD* gene can cause either Duchenne's or the less severe Becker's muscular dystrophy, depending on the severity of the protein defect.

Recognition of nonallelic heterogeneity is important for several reasons: (1) the ability to identify disease loci in linkage studies is reduced by including patients with similar phenotypes but different genetic disorders; (2) genetic testing is more complex because several different genes need to be considered along with the possibility of different mutations in each of the candidate genes; and (3) novel information is gained about how genes or proteins interact, providing unique insights into molecular physiology.

Phenocopies refer to circumstances in which nongenetic conditions mimic a genetic disorder. For example, features of toxin- or drug-induced neurologic syndromes can resemble those seen in Huntington's disease, and vascular causes of dementia share phenotypic features with familial forms of Alzheimer's dementia (Chap. 371). Children born with activating mutations of the thyroid-stimulating hormone receptor (TSH-R) exhibit goiter and thyrotoxicosis similar to that seen in neonatal Graves' disease, which is caused by the transfer of maternal autoantibodies to the fetus (Chap. 341). As in nonallelic heterogeneity, the presence of phenocopies has the potential to confound linkage studies and genetic testing. Patient history and subtle differences in phenotype can often provide clues that distinguish these disorders from related genetic conditions.

Variable expressivity and incomplete penetrance   The same genetic mutation may be associated with a phenotypic spectrum in different affected individuals, thereby illustrating the phenomenon of *variable expressivity*. This may include different manifestations of a disorder variably involving different organs (e.g., MEN), the severity of the disorder (e.g., cystic fibrosis), or the age of disease onset (e.g., Alzheimer's dementia). MEN-1 illustrates several of these features. Families with this autosomal dominant disorder develop tumors of the parathyroid gland, endocrine pancreas, and the pituitary gland (Chap. 351). However, the pattern of tumors in the different glands, the age at which tumors develop, and the types of hormones produced vary among affected individuals, even within a given family. In this example, the phenotypic variability arises, in part, because of the requirement for a second mutation in the normal copy of the *MEN1* gene, as well as the large array of different cell types that are susceptible to the effects of *MEN1* gene mutations. In part, variable expression reflects the influence of modifier genes, or genetic background, on the effects of a particular mutation. Even in identical twins, in whom the genetic constitution is essentially the same, one can occasionally see variable expression of a genetic disease.

Interactions with the environment can also influence the course of a disease. For example, the manifestations and severity of hemochromatosis can be influenced by iron intake (Chap. 357), and the course of phenylketonuria is affected by exposure to phenylalanine in the diet (Chap. 364). Other metabolic disorders such as hyperlipidemias and porphyria, also fall into this category. Many mechanisms, including genetic effects and environmental influences, can therefore lead to variable expressivity. In genetic counseling, it is particularly important to recognize this variability, as one cannot always predict the course of disease, even when the mutation is known.

Penetrance refers to the proportion of individuals with a mutant genotype that express the phenotype. If all carriers of a mutant express the phenotype, penetrance is complete, whereas it is said to be *incomplete* or *reduced* if some individuals do not have any features of the phenotype. Dominant conditions with incomplete penetrance are characterized by skipping of generations with unaffected carriers transmitting the mutant gene. For example, hypertrophic obstructive cardiomyopathy (HCM) caused by mutations in the *myosin-binding protein C* gene is a dominant disorder with clinical features in only a subset of patients who carry the mutation (Chap. 237). Patients who have the mutation but no evidence of the disease can still transmit the disorder to subsequent generations. In many conditions with postnatal onset, the proportion of gene carriers who are affected varies with age. Thus, when describing penetrance, one has to specify age. For example, for disorders such as Huntington's disease or familial amyotrophic lateral sclerosis, which present late in life, the rate of penetrance is influenced by the age at which the clinical assessment is performed. *Imprinting* can also modify the penetrance of a disease (see below). For example, in patients with Albright's hereditary osteodystrophy, mutations in the Gsα subunit (*GNAS1* gene) are expressed clinically only in individuals who inherit the mutation from their mother (Chap. 353).

Sex-influenced phenotypes   Certain mutations affect males and females quite differently. In some instances, this is because the gene resides on the X or Y sex chromosomes (X-linked disorders and Y-linked disorders). As a result, the phenotype of mutated X-linked genes will be expressed fully in males but variably in heterozygous females, depending on the degree of X-inactivation and the function of the gene. For example, most heterozygous female carriers of factor VIII deficiency (hemophilia A) are asymptomatic because sufficient factor VIII is produced to prevent a defect in coagulation (Chap. 116). On the other hand, some females heterozygous for the X-linked lipid storage defect caused by α-galactosidase A deficiency (Fabry's disease) experience mild manifestations of painful neuropathy, as well as other features of the disease (Chap. 361). Because only males have a Y chromosome, mutations in genes such as *SRY*, which causes male-to-female sex-reversal, or *DAZ* (deleted in azoospermia), which causes abnormalities of spermatogenesis, are unique to males (Chap. 349).

Other diseases are expressed in a sex-limited manner because of the differential function of the gene product in males and females. Activating mutations in the luteinizing hormone receptor cause dominant male-limited precocious puberty in boys (Chap. 346). The phenotype is unique to males because activation of the receptor induces testosterone production in the testis, whereas it is functionally silent in the immature ovary. Biallelic inactivating mutations of the follicle-stimulating hormone (FSH) receptor cause primary ovarian failure in females because the follicles do not develop in the absence of FSH action. In contrast, affected males have a more subtle phenotype, because testosterone production is preserved (allowing sexual maturation) and spermatogenesis is only partially impaired (Chap. 346). In congenital adrenal hyperplasia, most commonly caused by 21-hydroxylase deficiency, cortisol production is impaired and ACTH stimulation of the adrenal gland leads to increased production of androgenic precursors (Chap. 342). In females, the increased androgen level causes ambiguous genitalia, which can be recognized at the time of birth. In males, the diagnosis may be made on the basis of adrenal insufficiency at birth, because the increased adrenal androgen level does not alter sexual differentiation, or later in childhood, because of the development of precocious puberty. Hemochromatosis is more common in males than in females, presumably because of differences in dietary iron intake and losses associated with menstruation and pregnancy in females (Chap. 357).

Chromosomal disorders

Chromosomal or cytogenetic disorders are caused by numerical or structural aberrations in chromosomes. Deviations in chromosome number are common causes of abortions, developmental disorders, and malformations. *Contiguous gene syndromes* (i.e., large deletions affecting several genes), have been useful for identifying the location of new disease-causing genes. Because of the variable size of gene deletions in different patients, a systematic comparison of phenotypes and locations of deletion breakpoints allows positions of particular genes to be mapped within the critical genomic region.

For discussion of disorders of chromosome number and structure, see Chap. 62.

Monogenic Mendelian disorders

Monogenic human diseases are frequently referred to as *Mendelian disorders* because they obey the principles of genetic transmission originally set forth in Gregor Mendel's classic work. The continuously updated OMIM catalogue lists several thousand of these disorders and provides information about the clinical phenotype,

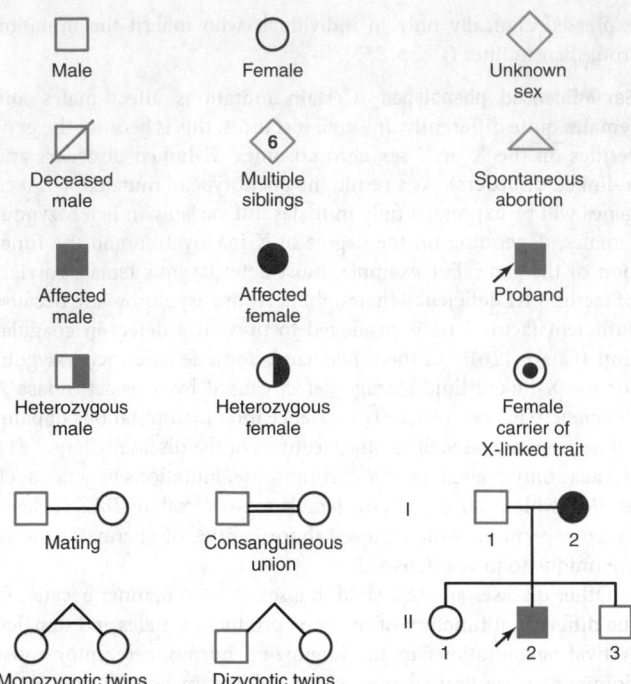

Figure 61-9   Standard pedigree symbols.

molecular basis, allelic variants, and pertinent animal models (Table 61-1). The mode of inheritance for a given phenotypic trait or disease is determined by pedigree analysis. All affected and unaffected individuals in the family are recorded in a pedigree using standard symbols (Fig. 61-9). The principles of allelic segregation, and the transmission of alleles from parents to children, are illustrated in Fig. 61-10. One dominant (A) allele and one recessive (a) allele can display three Mendelian modes of inheritance: autosomal dominant, autosomal recessive, and X-chromosomal. About 65% of human monogenic disorders are autosomal dominant, 25% are autosomal recessive, and 5% are X-linked. Genetic testing is now available for many of these disorders and plays an increasingly important role in clinical medicine (Chap. 63).

Autosomal dominant disorders   Autosomal dominant disorders assume particular relevance because mutations in a single allele are sufficient to cause the disease. In contrast to recessive disorders, in which disease pathogenesis is relatively straightforward because there is loss of gene function, dominant disorders can be caused by various disease mechanisms, many of which are unique to the function of the genetic pathway involved.

In autosomal dominant disorders, individuals are affected in successive generations; the disease does not occur in the offspring

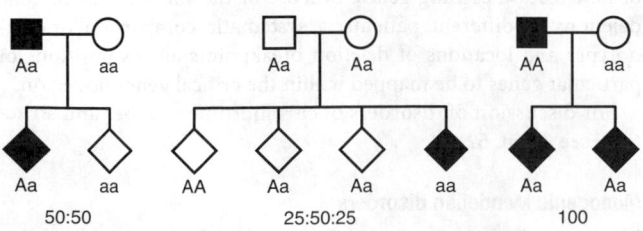

Figure 61-10   Segregation of alleles. Segregation of genotypes in the offspring of parents with one dominant (A) and one recessive (a) allele. The distribution of the parental alleles to their offspring depends on the combination present in the parents. Filled symbols represent affected individuals.

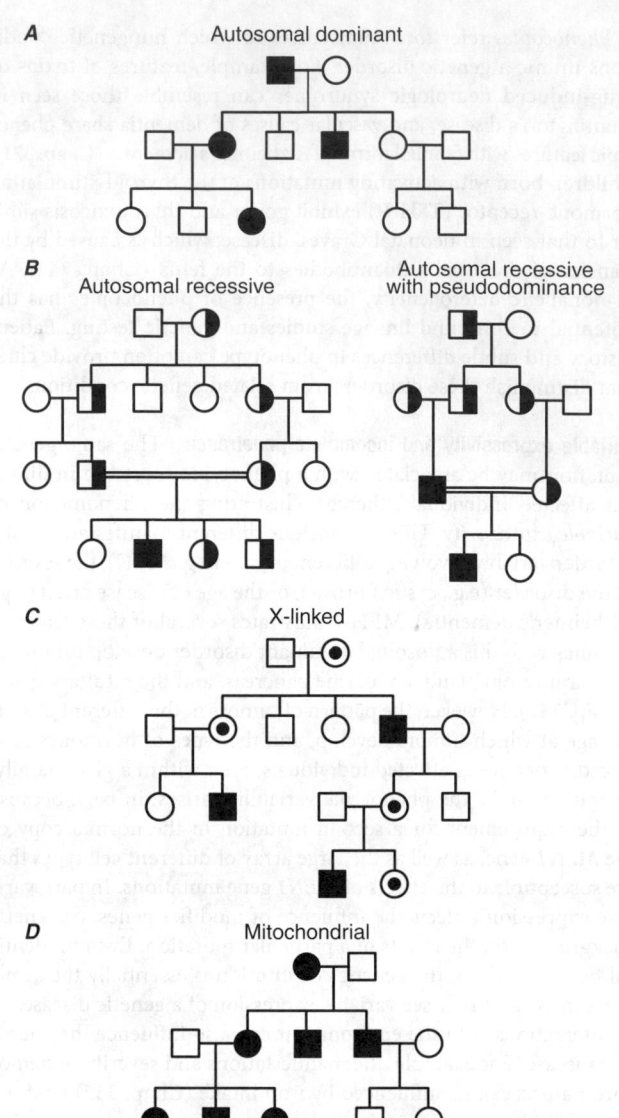

Figure 61-11   Dominant, recessive, X-linked, and mitochondrial (matrilinear) inheritance.

of unaffected individuals. Males and females are affected with equal frequency because the defective gene resides on one of the 22 autosomes (Fig. 61-11A). Autosomal dominant mutations alter one of the two alleles at a given locus. Because the alleles segregate randomly at meiosis, the probability that an offspring will be affected is 50%. Unless there is a new germline mutation, an affected individual has an affected parent. Children with a normal genotype do not transmit the disorder. Due to differences in penetrance or expressivity (see above), the clinical manifestations of autosomal dominant disorders may be variable. Because of these variations, it is sometimes challenging to determine the pattern of inheritance.

It should be recognized, however, that some individuals acquire a mutated gene from an unaffected parent. De novo germline mutations occur more frequently during later cell divisions in gametogenesis, which explains why siblings are rarely affected. As noted before, new germline mutations occur more frequently in fathers of advanced age. For example, the average age of fathers with new germline mutations that cause Marfan's syndrome is ~37 years, whereas fathers who transmit the disease by inheritance have an average age of ~30 years.

Autosomal recessive disorders   In recessive disorders, the mutated alleles result in a complete or partial loss of function. They frequently involve enzymes in metabolic pathways, receptors, or proteins in signaling cascades. In an autosomal recessive disease, the affected individual, who can be of either sex, is a homozygote or compound heterozygote for a single-gene defect. With a few important exceptions, autosomal recessive diseases are rare and often occur in the context of parental consanguinity. The relatively high frequency of certain recessive disorders such as sickle cell anemia, cystic fibrosis, and thalassemia, is partially explained by a selective biologic advantage for the heterozygous state (see below). Though heterozygous carriers of a defective allele are usually clinically normal, they may display subtle differences in phenotype that only become apparent with more precise testing or in the context of certain environmental influences. In sickle cell anemia, for example, heterozygotes are normally asymptomatic. However, in situations of dehydration or diminished oxygen pressure, sickle cell crises can also occur in heterozygotes (Chap. 104).

In most instances, an affected individual is the offspring of heterozygous parents. In this situation, there is a 25% chance that the offspring will have a normal genotype, a 50% probability of a heterozygous state, and a 25% risk of homozygosity for the recessive alleles (Figs. 61-10, 61-11B). In the case of one unaffected heterozygous and one affected homozygous parent, the probability of disease increases to 50% for each child. In this instance, the pedigree analysis mimics an autosomal dominant mode of inheritance (*pseudodominance*). In contrast to autosomal dominant disorders, new mutations in recessive alleles are rarely manifest because they usually result in an asymptomatic carrier state.

X-linked disorders Males have only one X chromosome; consequently, a daughter always inherits her father's X chromosome in addition to one of her mother's two X chromosomes. A son inherits the Y chromosome from his father and one maternal X chromosome. Thus, the characteristic features of X-linked inheritance are (1) the absence of father-to-son transmission, and (2) the fact that all daughters of an affected male are obligate carriers of the mutant allele (Fig. 61-11C). The risk of developing disease due to a mutant X-chromosomal gene differs in the two sexes. Because males have only one X chromosome, they are hemizygous for the mutant allele; thus, they are more likely to develop the mutant phenotype, regardless of whether the mutation is dominant or recessive. A female may be either heterozygous or homozygous for the mutant allele, which may be dominant or recessive. The terms *X-linked dominant* or *X-linked recessive* are therefore only applicable to expression of the mutant phenotype in women. In addition, the expression of X-chromosomal genes is influenced by X chromosome inactivation (see below).

Y-linked disorders The Y chromosome has a relatively small number of genes. One such gene, the sex-region determining Y factor (*SRY*), which encodes the testis-determining factor (*TDF*), is crucial for normal male development. Normally there is infrequent exchange of sequences on the Y chromosome with the X chromosome. The *SRY* region is adjacent to the pseudoautosomal region, a chromosomal segment on the X and Y chromosomes with a high degree of homology. A crossing-over occasionally involves the *SRY* region with the distal tip of the X chromosome during meiosis in the male. Translocations can result in XY females with the Y chromosome lacking the *SRY* gene or XX males harboring the *SRY* gene on one of the X chromosomes (Chap. 349). Point mutations in the *SRY* gene may also result in individuals with an XY genotype and an incomplete female phenotype. Most of these mutations occur de novo. Men with oligospermia/azoospermia frequently have microdeletions on the long arm of the Y chromosome that involve one or more of the azoospermia factor (*AZF*) genes.

Exceptions to simple Mendelian inheritance patterns

Mitochondrial disorders Mendelian inheritance refers to the transmission of genes encoded by DNA contained in the nuclear chromosomes. In addition, each mitochondrion contains several copies of a small circular chromosome. The mitochondrial DNA (mtDNA) is ~16.5 kb and encodes transfer and ribosomal RNAs and 13 proteins that are components of the respiratory chain involved in oxidative phosphorylation and ATP generation. The mitochondrial genome does not recombine and is inherited through the maternal line because sperm does not contribute significant cytoplasmic components to the zygote. A noncoding region of the mitochondrial chromosome, referred to as D-loop, is highly polymorphic. This property, together with the absence of mtDNA recombination, makes it a valuable tool for studies tracing human migration and evolution, and it is also used for specific forensic applications.

Inherited mitochondrial disorders are transmitted in a matrilineal fashion; all children from an affected mother will inherit the disease, but it will not be transmitted from an affected father to his children (Fig. 61-11D). Alterations in the mtDNA affecting enzymes required for oxidative phosphorylation lead to reduction of ATP supply, generation of free radicals, and induction of apoptosis. Several syndromic disorders arising from mutations in the mitochondrial genome are known in humans and they affect both protein-coding and tRNA genes (Tables 61-1 and 61-5). The broad clinical spectrum often involves (cardio)myopathies and encephalopathies because of the high dependence of these tissues on oxidative phosphorylation. The age of onset and the clinical course are highly variable because of the unusual mechanisms of mtDNA transmission, which replicates independently from nuclear DNA. During cell replication, the proportion of wild-type and mutant mitochondria can drift among different cells and tissues. The resulting heterogeneity in the proportion of mitochondria with and without a mutation is referred to as *heteroplasmia* and underlies the phenotypic variability that is characteristic of mitochondrial diseases.

TABLE 61-5 Selected Mitochondrial Diseases

Disease/Syndrome	OMIM #
MELAS syndrome: mitochondrial myopathy with encephalopathy, lactacidosis, and stroke	540000
Leber's optic atrophy: hereditary optical neuropathy	535000
Kearns-Sayre syndrome (KSS): ophthalmoplegia, pigmental degeneration of the retina, cardiomyopathy	530000
MERRF syndrome: myoclonic epilepsy and ragged-red fibers	545000
Neurogenic muscular weakness with ataxia and retinitis pigmentosa (NARP)	551500
Chronic progressive external ophthalmoplegia (CEOP)	258470
Pearson's syndrome (PEAR): bone marrow and pancreatic failure	557000
Autosomal dominant inherited mitochondrial myopathy with mitochondrial deletion (ADMIMY)	157640
Somatic mutations in cytochrome *b* gene: exercise intolerance, lactic acidosis, complex III deficiency, muscle pain, ragged-red fibers	516020

Acquired somatic mutations in mitochondria are thought to be involved in several age-dependent degenerative disorders affecting predominantly muscle and the peripheral and central nervous system (e.g., Alzheimer's and Parkinson's diseases). Establishing that an mtDNA alteration is causal for a clinical phenotype is challenging because of the high degree of polymorphism in mtDNA and the phenotypic variability characteristic of these disorders. Certain pharmacologic treatments may have an impact on mitochondria and/or their function. For example, treatment with the antiretroviral compound azidothymidine (AZT) causes an acquired mitochondrial myopathy through depletion of muscular mtDNA.

Mosaicism Mosaicism refers to the presence of two or more genetically distinct cell lines in the tissues of an individual. It results from a mutation that occurs during embryonic, fetal, or extrauterine development. The developmental stage at which the mutation arises will determine whether germ cells and/or somatic cells are involved. Chromosomal mosaicism results from nondisjunction at an early embryonic mitotic division, leading to the persistence of more than one cell line, as exemplified by some patients with Turner's syndrome (Chap. 349). Somatic mosaicism is characterized by a patchy distribution of genetically altered somatic cells. The McCune-Albright syndrome, for example, is caused by activating mutations in the stimulatory G protein α ($G_s\alpha$) that occur early in development (Chap. 353). The clinical phenotype varies depending on the tissue distribution of the mutation; manifestations include ovarian cysts that secrete sex steroids and cause precocious puberty, polyostotic fibrous dysplasia, café-au-lait skin pigmentation, growth hormone–secreting pituitary adenomas, and hypersecreting autonomous thyroid nodules (Chap. 347).

X-inactivation, imprinting, and uniparental disomy According to traditional Mendelian principles, the parental origin of a mutant gene is irrelevant for the expression of the phenotype. There are, however, important exceptions to this rule. *X-inactivation* prevents the expression of most genes on one of the two X-chromosomes in every cell of a female. Gene inactivation also occurs on selected chromosomal regions of autosomes. This phenomenon, referred to as *genomic imprinting*, leads to inheritable preferential expression of one of the parental alleles. It is of pathophysiologic importance in disorders where the transmission of disease is dependent on the sex of the transmitting parent and, thus, plays an important role in the expression of certain genetic disorders. Two classic examples are the Prader-Willi syndrome and Angelman's syndrome (Chap. 62). Prader-Willi syndrome is characterized by diminished fetal activity, obesity, hypotonia, mental retardation, short stature, and hypogonadotropic hypogonadism. Deletions of the paternal copy of the Prader-Willi locus located on the short arm of chromosome 15 result in a contiguous gene syndrome involving missing paternal copies of the *necdin* and *SNRPN* genes, among others. In contrast, patients with Angelman's syndrome, characterized by mental retardation, seizures, ataxia, and hypotonia, have deletions involving the maternal copy of this region on chromosome 15. These two syndromes may also result from *uniparental disomy*. In this case, the syndromes are not caused by deletions on chromosome 15 but by the inheritance of either two maternal chromosomes (Prader-Willi syndrome) or two paternal chromosomes (Angelman's syndrome).

Imprinting and the related phenomenon of allelic exclusion may be more common than currently documented, as it is difficult to examine levels of mRNA expression from the maternal and paternal alleles in specific tissues or in individual cells. Genomic imprinting, or uniparental disomy, is involved in the pathogenesis of several other disorders and malignancies (Chap. 62). For example, hydatidiform moles contain a normal number of diploid chromosomes, but they are all of paternal origin. The opposite situation occurs in ovarian teratomata, with 46 chromosomes of maternal origin.

Expression of the imprinted gene for insulin-like growth factor II (IGF-II) is involved in the pathogenesis of the cancer-predisposing Beckwith-Wiedemann syndrome (BWS) (Chap. 83). These children show somatic overgrowth with organomegalies and hemihypertrophy, and they have an increased risk of embryonal malignancies such as Wilms' tumor. Normally, only the paternally derived copy of the IGF-II gene is active and the maternal copy is inactive. Imprinting of the *IGF-II* gene is regulated by *H19*, which encodes an RNA transcript that is not translated into protein. Disruption or lack of *H19* methylation leads to a relaxation of *IGF-II* imprinting and expression of both alleles.

Meiotically and mitotically heritable changes in gene expression not associated with DNA sequence alterations are referred to as *epigenetic effects*. These changes involve DNA methylation, histone modifications, and RNA-mediated silencing, resulting in gene repression without a change in the coding sequence. Epigenetic alterations are increasingly recognized to play a role in human diseases such as cancer, mental retardation, hematologic disorders, and possibly in aging. For example, de novo methylation of CpG islands, regions of >500 bp in size with a GC content >55% in promoter regions that are normally unmethylated, is a hallmark of human cancers. Inhibitors of enzymes controlling epigenetic modifications such as histone deacetylases and DNA methyltransferases reverse gene silencing and represent a promising new group of antineoplastic agents.

Somatic mutations Cancer can be defined as a genetic disease at the cellular level (Chap. 83). Cancers are monoclonal in origin, indicating that they have arisen from a single precursor cell with one or several mutations in genes controlling growth (proliferation or apoptosis) and/or differentiation. These acquired somatic mutations are restricted to the tumor and its metastases and are not found in the surrounding normal tissue. The molecular alterations include dominant gain-of-function mutations in oncogenes, recessive loss-of-function mutations in tumor-suppressor genes and DNA repair genes, gene amplification, and chromosome rearrangements. Rarely, a single mutation in certain genes may be sufficient to transform a normal cell into a malignant cell. In most cancers, however, the development of a malignant phenotype requires several genetic alterations for the gradual progression from a normal cell to a cancerous cell, a phenomenon termed *multistep carcinogenesis* (Chaps. 83 and 84). Genomewide analyses of cancers using deep sequencing often reveal somatic rearrangements and mutations in multiple genes. Most human tumors express telomerase, an enzyme formed of a protein and an RNA component, which adds telomere repeats at the ends of chromosomes during replication. This mechanism impedes shortening of the telomeres, which is associated with senescence in normal cells, and is associated with enhanced replicative capacity in cancer cells. Telomerase inhibitors may provide a novel strategy for treating advanced human cancers.

In many cancer syndromes, there is an inherited *predisposition* to tumor formation. In these instances, a germline mutation is inherited in an autosomal dominant fashion inactivating one allele of an autosomal tumor-suppressor gene. If the second allele is inactivated by a somatic mutation or by epigenetic silencing in a given cell, this will lead to neoplastic growth (Knudson two-hit model). Thus, the defective allele in the germline is transmitted in a dominant mode, though tumorigenesis results from a biallelic loss of the tumor-suppressor gene in an affected tissue. The classic example to illustrate this phenomenon is retinoblastoma, which can occur as a sporadic or hereditary tumor. In sporadic retinoblastoma, both copies of the retinoblastoma (RB) gene are inactivated through two somatic events. In hereditary retinoblastoma, one mutated or deleted RB allele is inherited in an autosomal dominant manner and the second allele is inactivated by a subsequent somatic mutation. This two-hit

TABLE 61-6 Selected Trinucleotide Repeat Disorders

Disease	Locus	Repeat	Triplet Length (Normal/Disease)	Inheritance	Gene Product
X-chromosomal spinobulbar muscular atrophy (SBMA)	Xq11-q12	CAG	11–34/40–62	XR	Androgen receptor
Fragile X-syndrome (FRAXA)	Xq27.3	CGG	6–50/200–300	XR	FMR-1 protein
Fragile X-syndrome (FRAXE)	Xq28	GCC	6–25/>200	XR	FMR-2 protein
Dystrophia myotonica (DM)	19q13.2-q13.3	CTG	5–30/200–1000	AD, variable penetrance	Myotonin protein kinase
Huntington's disease (HD)	4p16.3	CAG	6–34/37–180	AD	Huntingtin
Spinocerebellar ataxia type 1 (SCA1)	6p21.3-21.2	CAG	6–39/40–88	AD	Ataxin 1
Spinocerebellar ataxia type 2 (SCA2)	12q24.1	CAG	15–31/34–400	AD	Ataxin 2
Spinocerebellar ataxia type 3 (SCA3); Machado-Joseph disease (MD)	14q21	CAG	13–36/55–86	AD	Ataxin 3
Spinocerebellar ataxia type 6 (SCA6, CACNAIA)	19p13.1-13.2	CAG	4–16/20–33	AD	Alpha 1A voltage-dependent L-type calcium channel
Spinocerebellar ataxia type 7 (SCA7)	3p21.1-p12	CAG	4–19/37 to >300	AD	Ataxin 7
Spinocerebellar ataxia type 12 (SCA12)	5q31	CAG	6–26/66–78	AD	Protein phosphatase 2A
Dentorubral pallidoluysian atrophy (DRPLA)	12p	CAG	7–23/49–75	AD	Atrophin 1
Friedreich ataxia (FRDA1)	9q13-21	GAA	7–22/200–900	AR	Frataxin

Abbreviations: AD, autosomal dominant; AR, autosomal recessive; XR, X-linked recessive.

model applies to other inherited cancer syndromes such as MEN-1 (Chap. 351) and neurofibromatosis type 2 (Chap. 379).

Nucleotide repeat expansion disorders Several diseases are associated with an increase in the number of nucleotide repeats above a certain threshold (Table 61-6). The repeats are sometimes located within the coding region of the genes, as in Huntington's disease or the X-linked form of spinal and bulbar muscular atrophy (SBMA, Kennedy's syndrome). In other instances, the repeats probably alter gene regulatory sequences. If an expansion is present, the DNA fragment is unstable and tends to expand further during cell division. The length of the nucleotide repeat often correlates with the severity of the disease. When repeat length increases from one generation to the next, disease manifestations may worsen or be observed at an earlier age; this phenomenon is referred to as *anticipation*. In Huntington's disease, for example, there is a correlation between age of onset and length of the triplet codon expansion (Chap. 366). Anticipation has also been documented in other diseases caused by dynamic mutations in trinucleotide repeats (Table 61-6). The repeat number may also vary in a tissue-specific manner. In myotonic dystrophy, the CTG repeat may be tenfold greater in muscle tissue than in lymphocytes (Chap. 387).

Complex genetic disorders

The expression of many common diseases such as cardiovascular disease, hypertension, diabetes, asthma, psychiatric disorders, and certain cancers is determined by a combination of genetic background, environmental factors, and lifestyle. A trait is called *polygenic* if multiple genes contribute to the phenotype or *multifactorial* if multiple genes are assumed to interact with environmental factors. Genetic models for these complex traits need to account for genetic heterogeneity and interactions with other genes and the environment. Complex genetic traits may be influenced by modifying genes that

are not linked to the main gene involved in the pathogenesis of the trait. This type of gene-gene interaction, or *epistasis*, plays an important role in polygenic traits that require the simultaneous presence of variations in multiple genes to result in a pathologic phenotype.

Type 2 diabetes mellitus provides a paradigm for considering a multifactorial disorder, as genetic, nutritional, and lifestyle factors are intimately interrelated in disease pathogenesis (Table 61-7) (Chap. 344). The identification of genetic variations and environmental factors that either predispose to or protect against disease is essential for predicting disease risk, designing preventive strategies, and developing novel therapeutic approaches. The study of rare monogenic diseases may provide insight into some of genetic and molecular mechanisms important in the pathogenesis of complex diseases. For example, the identification of the hepatocyte nuclear factor 1α (HNF1α) in maturity-onset of diabetes type 4 defined it as a *candidate gene* in the pathogenesis of diabetes mellitus type 2 (Tables 61-2 and 61-7). Genome scans have identified various loci that may be associated with susceptibility to development of diabetes mellitus in certain populations. Efforts to identify susceptibility genes require very large sample sizes, and positive results may depend on ethnicity, ascertainment criteria, and statistical analysis. Association studies analyzing the potential influence of (biologically functional) SNPs and SNP haplotypes on a particular phenotype are providing new insights into the genes involved in the pathogenesis of these common disorders. Large variants [(micro)deletions, duplications, and inversions] present in the human population also contribute to the pathogenesis of complex disorders, but their contributions remain poorly understood.

Linkage and association studies

There are two primary strategies for mapping genes that cause or increase susceptibility to human disease: (1) classic linkage can be

TABLE 61-7 Genes and Loci Involved in Mono- and Polygenic Forms of Diabetes

Disorder	Genes or Susceptibility Locus	Chromosomal Location	Other Factors
Monogenic forms of diabetes			
MODY 1	HNF4α (hepatocyte nuclear factor 4α)	20q12-q13.1	AD inheritance
MODY 2	GCK (glucokinase)	7p15-p13	
MODY 3	HNF1α (hepatocyte nuclear factor 1α)	12q24.2	
MODY 4	IPF1 (insulin receptor substrate)	13q12.1	
MODY 5 (renal cysts, diabetes)	HNF1β (hepatocyte nuclear factor 1β)	17cen-q21.3	
MODY 6	NeuroD1 (neurogenic differention factor 1)	2q32	
Diabetes mellitus type 2; loci and genes linked and/or associated with susceptibility for diabetes mellitus type 2	*Genes and loci identified by linkage/association studies*		
	CPN10 (Calpain-10)	2q37.3	Diet
	HNF4α (hepatocyte nuclear factor 4α)	20q12-q13.1	Energy expenditure
	PTPN1 (protein-tyrosine phosphatase)	20q13.1-q13.2	Obesity
	PKLR (liver pyruvate kinase)	1q21	
	CASQ1 (calsequestrin 1)	1q21	
	APM1 (adiponectin)	3q27	
	TCF7L2 (transcription factor 7-like 2)	10q25.3	
	1q21-23	1q21-23	
	2q	2q	
	3q22-27	3q22-27	
	8p21-23	8p21-23	
	11q	11q	
	12q24	12q24	
	15	15	
	18p11	18p11	
	20q	20q	
	20p	20p	
	Selected candidate genes with possible contribution		
	PPARγ (Peroxisome proliferator receptor γ)	3p25	
	KCNJ11(ATP-sensitive K channel Kir6.2)	11p15.1	
	ABCC8 (ATP-binding cassette, subfamily c, member 8)	11p15.1	
	Insulin VNTR	11p15	
	IRS-1 (insulin receptor substrate)	2q36	
	PGC1α (PPAR γ coactivator α)	4p15.1	
	ENPP1 (ectonucleotide pyrophosphatase/phosphodiesterase 1)	6q22-23	

Abbreviations: AD, autosomal dominant; MODY, maturity onset diabetes of the young; VNTR, variable number of tandem repeats.

performed based on a known genetic model or, when the model is unknown, by studying pairs of affected relatives; or (2) disease genes can be mapped using allelic association studies (Table 61-8).

Genetic linkage *Genetic linkage* refers to the fact that genes are physically connected, or linked, to one another along the chromosomes. Two fundamental principles are essential for understanding the concept of linkage: (1) when two genes are close together on a chromosome, they are usually transmitted together, unless a recombination event separates them (Figs. 61-3 and 61-7); and (2) the odds of a crossover, or recombination event, between two linked genes is proportional to the distance that separates them. Thus, genes that are farther apart are more likely to undergo a recombination event than genes that are very close together. The detection of chromosomal loci that segregate with a disease by linkage can be used to identify the gene responsible for the disease (*positional cloning*) and to predict the odds of disease gene transmission in genetic counseling.

Polymorphisms are essential for linkage studies because they provide a means to distinguish the maternal and paternal chromosomes in an individual. On average, 1 out of every 1000 bp varies from one person to the next. Although this degree of variation seems

TABLE 61-8 Genetic Approaches for Identifying Disease Genes

Method	Indications and Advantages	Limitations
Linkage Studies		
Classical linkage analysis (parametric methods)	Analysis of monogenic traits Suitable for genome scan Control population not required Useful for multifactorial disorders in isolated populations	Difficult to collect large informative pedigrees Difficult to obtain sufficient statistical power for complex traits
Allele-sharing methods (nonparametric methods) Affected sib and relative pair analyses Sib pair analysis	Suitable for identification of susceptibility genes in polygenic and multifactorial disorders Suitable for genome scan Control population not required if allele frequencies are known Statistical power can be increased by including parents and relatives	Difficult to collect sufficient number of subjects Difficult to obtain sufficient statistical power for complex traits Reduced power compared to classical linkage, but not sensitive to specification of genetic mode
Association Studies		
Case-control studies Linkage disequilibrium Transmission disequilibrium test (TDT) Whole-genome association studies	Suitable for identification of susceptibility genes in polygenic and multifactorial disorders Suitable for testing specific allelic variants of known candidate loci Facilitated by HapMap data, making GWAS more feasible Does not necessarily need relatives	Requires large sample size and matched control population False-positive results in the absence of suitable control population Candidate gene approach does not permit to detect novel genes and pathways Whole-genome association studies very expensive

Abbreviation: GWAS, genome-wide association study

low (99.9% identical), it means that >3 million sequence differences exist between any two unrelated individuals and the probability that the sequence at such loci will differ on the two homologous chromosomes is high (often >70–90%). These sequence variations include variable number of tandem repeats (VNTRs), short tandem repeats (STRs), and SNPs. Most STRs, also called *polymorphic microsatellite markers*, consist of di-, tri-, or tetranucleotide repeats that can be measured readily using PCR (Fig. 61-12). Characterization of SNPs, using DNA chips or beads, permit comprehensive analyses of genetic variation, linkage, and association studies. Although these sequence variations usually have no apparent functional consequences, they provide much of the basis for variation in genetic traits.

In order to identify a chromosomal locus that segregates with a disease, it is necessary to characterize polymorphic DNA markers from affected and unaffected individuals of one or several pedigrees. One can then assess whether certain marker alleles cosegregate with the disease. Markers that are closest to the disease gene are less likely to undergo recombination events and therefore receive a higher linkage score. Linkage is expressed as a lod (logarithm of odds) score—the ratio of the probability that the disease and marker loci are linked rather than unlinked. Lod scores of +3 (1000:1) are generally accepted as supporting linkage, whereas a score of –2 is consistent with the absence of linkage.

An example of the use of linkage analysis is shown in Fig. 61-12. In this case, the gene for the autosomal dominant disorder MEN-1 is known to be located on chromosome 11q13. Using positional cloning, the *MEN1* gene was identified and shown to encode menin, a tumor suppressor. Affected individuals inherit a mutant form of the *MEN1* gene, predisposing them to certain types of tumors (parathyroid, pituitary, pancreatic islet) (Chap. 351). In the tissues that develop a tumor, a "second hit" occurs in the normal copy of the *MEN1* gene. This somatic mutation may be a point mutation, a microdeletion, or loss of a chromosomal fragment (detected as loss of heterozygosity, LOH). Within a given family, linkage to the *MEN1* gene locus can be assessed without necessarily knowing the specific mutation in the *MEN1* gene. Using polymorphic STRs that are close to the *MEN1* gene, one can assess transmission of the different *MEN1* alleles and compare this pattern to development of the disorder to determine which allele is associated with risk of MEN-1. In the pedigree shown, the affected grandfather in generation I carries alleles 3 and 4 on the chromosome with the mutated *MEN1* gene and alleles 2 and 2 on his other chromosome 11. Consistent with linkage of the 3/4 genotype to the *MEN1* locus, his son in generation II is affected, whereas his daughter (who inherits the 2/2 genotype from her father) is unaffected. In the third generation, transmission of the 3/4 genotype indicates risk of developing MEN-1, assuming that no genetic recombination between the 3/4 alleles and the *MEN1* gene has occurred. After a specific mutation in the *MEN1* gene is identified within a family, it is possible to track transmission of the mutation itself, thereby eliminating uncertainty caused by recombination.

Allelic association, linkage disequilibrium, and haplotypes *Allelic association* refers to a situation in which the frequency of an allele is significantly increased or decreased in individuals affected by a particular disease in comparison to controls. Linkage and association differ in several aspects. Genetic linkage is demonstrable in families or sibships. Association studies, on the other hand, compare a population of affected individuals with a control population. Association studies can be performed as case-control studies that include unrelated affected individuals and matched controls, or as family-based studies that compare the frequencies of alleles transmitted or not transmitted to affected children.

Allelic association studies are particularly useful for identifying susceptibility genes in complex diseases. When alleles at two loci

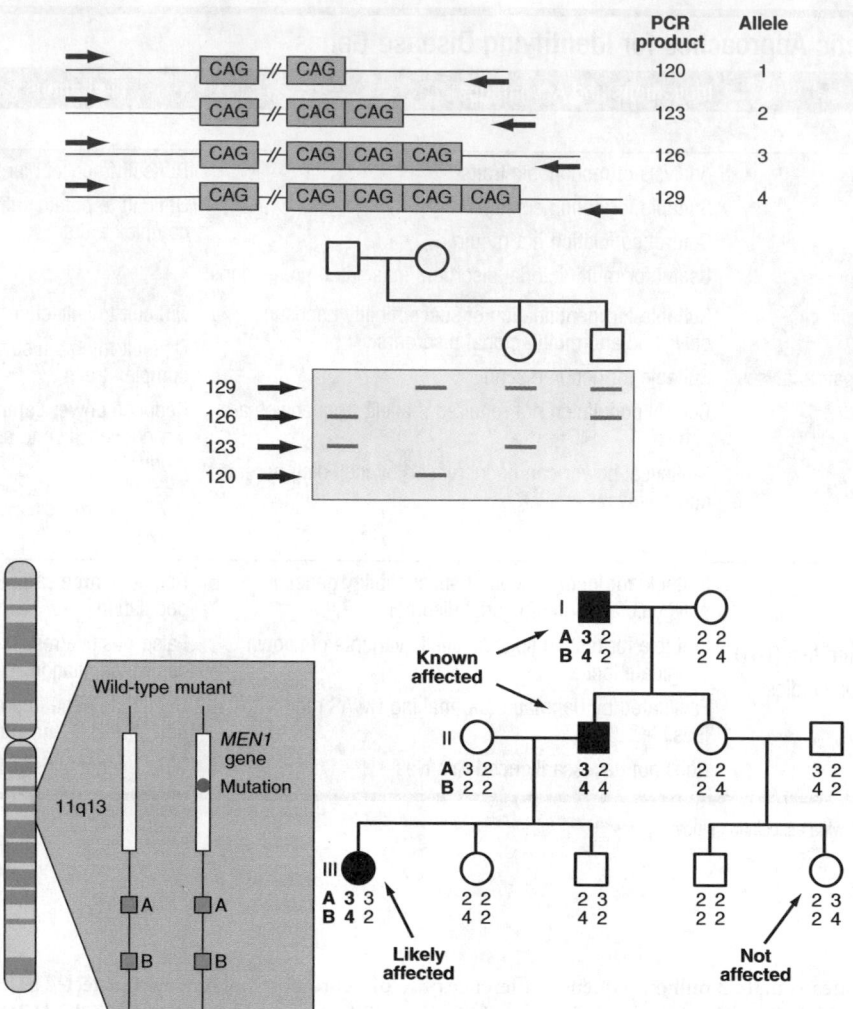

Figure 61-12 CAG repeat length and linkage analysis in multiple endocrine neoplasia (MEN) type 1. *Upper panel.* Detection of different alleles using polymorphic microsatellite markers. The example depicts a CAG trinucleotide repeat. PCR with primers flanking the polymorphic region results in products of variable length, depending on the number of CAG repeats. After characterization of the alleles in the parents, transmission of the paternal and maternal alleles can be determined. ***Lower panel.*** Genotype analysis using microsatellite markers in a family with MEN-1. Two microsatellite markers, A and B, are located in close proximity to the *MEN1* gene on chromosome 11q13. For each individual, the A and B alleles have

been determined. Based on this analysis, the genotype A3,B4 is linked to the disease because it occurs in the two affected individuals I-1 and II-2 but not in unaffected siblings. Because the disease allele is linked to A3,B4 within the affected family, it is likely that the individual III-1 is a carrier of the mutated *MEN1* gene. Although III-5 also has the A3,B4 genotype, she has inherited the allele from her unaffected father (II-4), who is not related to the original family. The A3,B4 genotype is only associated with MEN-1 in the original family, but not in the general population. Therefore, individual III-5 is not at risk for developing the disease.

occur more frequently *in combination* than would be predicted (based on known allele frequencies and recombination fractions), they are said to be in *linkage disequilibrium*. Evidence for linkage disequilibrium can be helpful in mapping disease genes because it suggests that the two loci are tightly linked.

Detecting the genetic factors contributing to the pathogenesis of common complex disorders remains a great challenge. In many instances, these are low-penetrance alleles (i.e., variations that individually only have a subtle effect on disease development, and they can only be identified by unbiased GWAS). Most variants are in noncoding or regulatory sequences but do not alter protein structure. The analysis of complex disorders is further complicated by ethnic differences in disease prevalence, differences in allele frequencies in known susceptibility genes among different populations, locus and allelic heterogeneity, gene-gene and gene-environment interactions, and the possibility of phenocopies. The data generated by the HapMap Project are greatly facilitating GWAS for the characterization of complex disorders. Adjacent SNPs are inherited together as

blocks, and these blocks can be identified by genotyping selected marker SNPs, so-called *Tag SNPs*, thereby reducing cost and workload (Fig. 61-8). The availability of this information permits the characterization of a limited number of SNPs to identify the set of haplotypes present in an individual (e.g., in cases and controls). This, in turn, permits GWAS by searching for associations of certain haplotypes with a disease phenotype of interest, an essential step for unraveling the genetic factors contributing to complex disorders.

Population genetics In population genetics, the focus changes from alterations in an individual's genome to the distribution pattern of different genotypes in the population. In a case where there are only two alleles, A and a, the frequency of the genotypes will be $p^2 + 2pq + q^2 = 1$, with p^2 corresponding to the frequency of AA, $2pq$ to the frequency of Aa, and q^2 to aa. When the frequency of an allele is known, the frequency of the genotype can be calculated. Alternatively, one can determine an allele frequency, if the genotype frequency has been determined.

Allele frequencies vary among ethnic groups and geographic regions. For example, heterozygous mutations in the *CFTR* gene are relatively common in populations of European origin but are rare in the African population. Allele frequencies may vary because certain allelic variants confer a selective advantage. For example, heterozygotes for the sickle cell mutation, which is particularly common in West Africa, are more resistant to malarial infection because the erythrocytes of heterozygotes provide a less favorable environment for *Plasmodium* parasites. Though homozygosity for the sickle cell gene is associated with severe anemia and sickle crises (Chap. 104), heterozygotes have a higher probability of survival because of the reduced morbidity and mortality from malaria; this phenomenon has led to an increased frequency of the mutant allele. Recessive conditions are more prevalent in geographically isolated populations because of the more restricted gene pool.

APPROACH TO THE PATIENT   Inherited Disorders

For the practicing clinician, the family history remains an essential step in recognizing the possibility of a hereditary component. When taking the history, it is useful to draw a detailed pedigree of the first-degree relatives (e.g., parents, siblings, and children), since they share 50% of genes with the patient. Standard symbols for pedigrees are depicted in Fig. 61-9. The family history should include information about ethnic background, age, health status, and (infant) deaths. Next, the physician should explore whether there is a family history of the same or related illnesses to the current problem. An inquiry focused on commonly occurring disorders such as cancers, heart disease, and diabetes mellitus should follow. Because of the possibility of age-dependent expressivity and penetrance, the family history will need intermittent updating. If the findings suggest a genetic disorder, the clinician will have to assess whether some of the patient's relatives may be at risk of carrying or transmitting the disease. In this circumstance, it is useful to confirm and extend the pedigree based on input from several family members. This information may form the basis for carrier detection, genetic counseling, early intervention, and prevention of a disease in relatives of the index patient (Chap. 63).

In instances where a diagnosis at the molecular level may be relevant, the physician will have to identify an appropriate laboratory that can perform the test. Genetic testing is available for a rapidly growing number of monogenic disorders through commercial laboratories. For uncommon disorders, the test may only be performed in a specialized research laboratory. Approved laboratories offering testing for inherited disorders can be identified in continuously updated on-line resources (GeneTests; Table 61-1). If genetic testing is considered, the patient and the family should be informed about the potential implications of positive results, including psychological distress and the possibility of discrimination. The patient or caretakers should be informed about the meaning of a negative result, technical limitations, and the possibility of false-negative and inconclusive results. For these reasons, genetic testing should only be performed after obtaining *informed consent*. Published ethical guidelines address the specific aspects that should be considered when testing children and adolescents. Genetic testing should usually be limited to situations in which the results may have an impact on the medical management.

IDENTIFYING THE DISEASE-CAUSING GENE *Genomic medicine* aims to enhance the quality of medical care through the use of genotypic analysis (DNA testing) to identify genetic predisposition to disease, to select more specific pharmacotherapy, and to design individualized medical care based on genotype. Genotype can be deduced by analysis of protein (e.g., hemoglobin, apoprotein E), mRNA, or DNA. However, technologic advances have made DNA analysis particularly useful because it can be readily applied.

DNA testing is performed by mutational analysis or linkage studies in individuals at risk for a genetic disorder known to be present in a family. Mass screening programs require tests of high sensitivity and specificity to be cost effective. Prerequisites for the success of genetic screening programs include the following: that the disorder is potentially serious; that it can be influenced at a presymptomatic stage by changes in behavior, diet, and/or pharmaceutical manipulations; and that the screening does not result in any harm or discrimination. Screening in Jewish populations for the autosomal recessive neurodegenerative storage disease Tay-Sachs has reduced the number of affected individuals. In contrast, screening for sickle cell trait/disease in African Americans has led to unanticipated problems of discrimination by health insurers and employers. Mass screening programs harbor additional potential problems. For example, screening for the most common genetic alteration in cystic fibrosis, the ΔF508 mutation with a frequency of ~70% in northern Europe is feasible and seems to be effective. One has to keep in mind, however, that there is pronounced allelic heterogeneity and that the disease can be caused by >1700 other mutations. The search for these less common mutations would substantially increase costs but not the effectiveness of the screening program as a whole. Next-generation genome sequencing will permit comprehensive and cost-effective mutational analyses after selective enrichment of candidate genes. For example, tests that sequence all the common genes causing hereditary deafness are already commercially available. Occupational screening programs aim to detect individuals with increased risk for certain professional activities (e.g., α_1 antitrypsin deficiency and smoke or dust exposure).

Mutational Analyses   DNA sequence analysis is now widely used as a diagnostic tool and has significantly enhanced diagnostic accuracy. It is used for determining carrier status and for prenatal testing in monogenic disorders (Chap. 63). Numerous techniques are available for the detection of mutations (Table 61-9). In a very broad sense, one can distinguish between techniques that allow for screening for the absence or presence of known mutations (screening mode) or techniques that definitively characterize mutations. Analyses of large alterations in the genome are possible using classic methods such as cytogenetics, fluorescent in situ hybridization (FISH), and Southern blotting (Chap. 62), as well as more sensitive novel techniques that search for multiple single exon deletions or duplications.

More discrete sequence alterations rely heavily on the use of the PCR, which allows rapid gene amplification and analysis. Moreover, PCR makes it possible to perform genetic testing and mutational analysis with small amounts of DNA extracted from leukocytes or even from single cells, buccal cells, or hair roots. DNA sequencing can be performed directly on PCR products or on fragments cloned into plasmid vectors amplified in bacterial host cells. Sequencing of all exons of the genome or selected chromosomes, or sequencing of numerous candidate genes in a single run, is now possible with next-generation sequencing platforms.

The majority of traditional diagnostic methods were gel-based. Novel technologies for the analysis of mutations, genotyping, large-scale sequencing, and mRNA expression profiles are currently undergoing rapid evolution. DNA chip technologies allow hybridization of DNA or RNA to hundreds of thousands of probes simultaneously. Microarrays are being used clinically for mutational analysis of several human disease genes, as well

TABLE 61-9 Techniques Commonly Used for Mutation Detection

Method	Principle	Type of Mutation Detected
Cytogenetic analysis	Unique visual appearance of various chromosomes	Numerical or structural abnormalities in chromosomes
Fluorescent in situ hybridization (FISH)	Hybridization to chromosomes with fluorescently labeled probes	Numerical or structural abnormalities in chromosomes
Southern blot	Hybridization with genomic probe or cDNA probe after digestion of high-molecular-weight DNA	Large deletion, insertion, rearrangement, expansions of triplet repeat, amplification
Polymerase chain reaction (PCR)	Amplification of DNA segment	Expansion of triplet repeats, variable number of tandem repeats (VNTR), gene rearrangements, translocations; prepare DNA for other mutation methods
Reverse transcriptase PCR (RT-PCR)	Reverse transcription, amplification of DNA segment → absence or reduction of mRNA transcription	Analyze expressed mRNA (cDNA) sequence; detect loss of expression
Traditional DNA sequencing	Direct sequencing of PCR products / Sequencing of DNA segments cloned into plasmid vectors	Point mutations, small deletions and insertions
Next-generation DNA sequencing	Sequencing of large contiguous genomic regions, exome of single or all chromosomes.	Deep sequencing for detection of mutations and SNPs. Sequencing of whole genomes of microorganisms
Microarrays	Hybridization of PCR products to wild-type or mutated oligonucleotides	Point mutations, small deletions and insertions Genotyping of SNPs

as for the identification of viral or bacterial sequence variations. With advances in high-throughput DNA-sequencing technology, complete sequencing of the genome of an individual is expected to cost about $1000 within this decade. Although comprehensive sequencing of large genomic regions or multiple genes is already a reality, the subsequent bioinformatics analysis, assembly of sequence fragments, and comparative alignments remains a significant and commonly underestimated challenge for data handling.

The huge amount of data generated by massive parallel sequencing underscores the need for ongoing attention to ethical and legal concerns. They include, among others, issues related to consent, sequence interpretation, the discovery of incidental findings that are predictors of serious disorders, the ability to link the information to an individual despite the absence of any conventional personal identifier, and data storage.

A general algorithm for the approach to mutational analysis is outlined in Fig. 61-13. The importance of a detailed clinical phenotype cannot be overemphasized. This is the step where one should also consider the possibility of genetic heterogeneity and phenocopies. If obvious candidate genes are suggested by the phenotype, they can be analyzed directly. After identification of a mutation, it is essential to demonstrate that it segregates with the phenotype. The functional characterization of novel mutations is labor intensive and may require analyses in vitro or in transgenic models in order to document the relevance of the genetic alteration.

Prenatal diagnosis of numerous genetic diseases in instances with a high risk for certain disorders is now possible by direct DNA analysis. *Amniocentesis* involves the removal of a small amount of amniotic fluid, usually at 16 weeks of gestation. Cells can be collected and submitted for karyotype analyses, FISH, and mutational analysis of selected genes. The main indications for amniocentesis include advanced maternal age (>35 years), an abnormal serum triple marker test (α-fetoprotein, β human

chorionic gonadotropin, pregnancy-associated plasma protein A, or unconjugated estriol), a family history of chromosomal abnormalities, or a Mendelian disorder amenable to genetic testing. Prenatal diagnosis can also be performed by *chorionic villus sampling* (CVS), in which a small amount of the chorion is removed by a transcervical or transabdominal biopsy. Chromosomes and DNA obtained from these cells can be submitted for cytogenetic and mutational analyses. CVS can be performed earlier in gestation (weeks 9–12) than amniocentesis, an aspect that may be of relevance when termination of pregnancy is a consideration. Later in pregnancy, beginning at about 18 weeks of gestation,

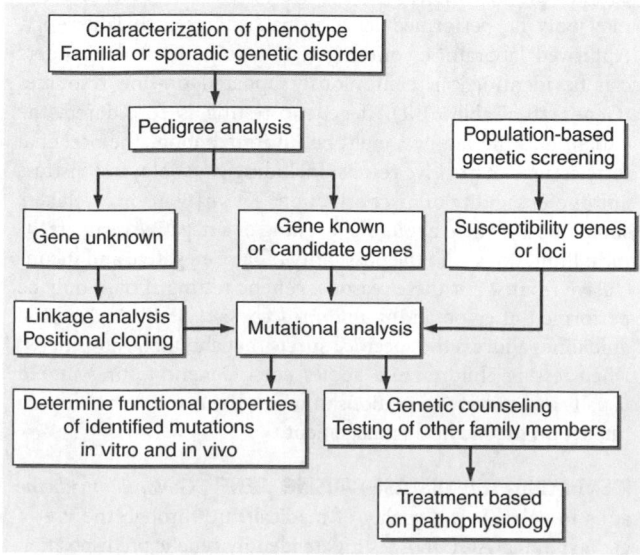

Figure 61-13   Approach to genetic disease.

percutaneous umbilical blood sampling (PUBS) permits collection of fetal blood for lymphocyte culture and analysis. In combination with in vitro fertilization (IVF) techniques, it is even possible to perform genetic diagnoses in a single cell removed from the four- to eight-cell embryo or to analyze the first polar body from an oocyte. Preconceptual diagnosis thereby avoids therapeutic abortions but is extremely costly and labor intensive. Lastly, it has to be emphasized that excluding a specific disorder by any of these approaches is never equivalent to the assurance of having a normal child.

Mutations in certain cancer susceptibility genes such as *BRCA1* and *BRCA2* may identify individuals with an increased risk for the development of malignancies and result in risk-reducing interventions. The detection of mutations is an important diagnostic and prognostic tool in leukemias and lymphomas. The demonstration of the presence or absence of mutations and polymorphisms is also relevant for the rapidly evolving field of pharmacogenomics, including the identification of differences in drug treatment response or metabolism as a function of genetic background. For example, the thiopurine drugs 6-mercaptopurine and azathioprine are commonly used cytotoxic and immunosuppressive agents. They are metabolized by thiopurine methyltransferase (TPMT), an enzyme with variable activity associated with genetic polymorphisms in 10% of whites and complete deficiency in about 1/300 individuals. Patients with intermediate or deficient TPMT activity are at risk for excessive toxicity, including fatal myelosuppression. Characterization of these polymorphisms allows mercaptopurine doses to be modified based on TPMT genotype. Pharmacogenomics may increasingly permit individualized drug therapy, improve drug effectiveness, reduce adverse side effects, and provide cost-effective pharmaceutical care.

FURTHER READINGS

ANTONARAKIS SE et al: Mendelian disorders and multifactorial traits: The big divide or one for all? Nat Rev Genet 11:380, 2010

EICHLER EE et al: Missing heritability and strategies for finding the underlying causes of complex disease. Nat Rev Genet 11:446, 2010

GUTTMACHER AE et al: Personalized genomic information: Preparing for the future of genetic medicine. Nat Rev Genet 11:161, 2010

HAMBURG MA, COLLINS FS: The path to personalized medicine. N Engl J Med 363:301, 2010

HUDSON KL et al: Keeping pace with the times—The Genetic Information Nondiscrimination Act of 2008. N Engl J Med 358:2661, 2008

LA SPADA AR, TAYLOR JP: Repeat expansion disease: Progress and puzzles in disease pathogenesis. Nat Rev Genet 11:247, 2010

METZKER ML: Sequencing technologies—the next generation. Nat Rev Genet 11:31, 2010

PANG T: The impact of genomics on global health. Am J Public Health 92:1077, 2002

SMITH RD et al: Genomics knowledge and equity: A global public goods perspective of the patent system. Bull World Health Organ 82:385, 2004

WAALEN J, BEUTLER E: Genetic screening for low-penetrance variants in protein-coding genes. Annu Rev Genomic Hum Genet 10:431, 2009

ZHANG F et al: Copy number variation in human health, disease, and evolution. Annu Rev Genomic Hum Genet 10:451, 2009

CHAPTER **62**
Chromosome Disorders

Stuart Schwartz

Terry Hassold

In humans, the normal diploid number of chromosomes is 46, consisting of 22 pairs of autosomal chromosomes (numbered 1–22 in decreasing size) and one pair of sex chromosomes (XX in females and XY in males). The genome is estimated to contain approximately 25,000 genes. Even the smallest autosome contains between 200 and 300 genes. Not surprisingly, duplications or deletions of chromosomes, or even small chromosome segments, have profound consequences on normal gene expression, leading to severe developmental and physiologic abnormalities.

Deviations in number or structure of the 46 human chromosomes are astonishingly common, despite severe deleterious consequences. Chromosomal disorders occur in an estimated 10–25% of all pregnancies. They are the leading cause of fetal loss and, among pregnancies surviving to term, the leading known cause of birth defects and mental retardation.

In recent years, the practice of cytogenetics has shifted from conventional cytogenetic methodology to a union of cytogenetic and molecular techniques. Formerly the province of research laboratories, fluorescence in situ hybridization (FISH), genomic array analysis, and related molecular cytogenetic technologies have been incorporated into everyday practice in clinical laboratories. As a result, there is an increased appreciation of the importance of "subtle" constitutional cytogenetic abnormalities such as microdeletions and imprinting disorders, as well as previously recognized translocations and disorders of chromosome number.

VISUALIZING CHROMOSOMES

■ CONVENTIONAL CYTOGENETIC ANALYSIS

In theory, chromosome preparations can be obtained from any actively dividing tissue by causing the cells to arrest in metaphase, the stage of the cell cycle when chromosomes are maximally condensed. In practice, only a small number of tissues are used for routine chromosome analysis: amniocytes or chorionic villi for prenatal testing and blood, bone marrow, or skin fibroblasts for postnatal studies. Samples of blood, bone marrow, and chorionic villi can be processed using short-term culture techniques that yield results in 1–3 days. Analysis of other tissue types typically involves long-term cell culture, requiring 1–3 weeks of processing before cytogenetic analysis is possible.

Cells are isolated at metaphase or prometaphase and treated chemically or enzymatically to reveal chromosome "bands" (Fig. 62-1). Analysis of the number of chromosomes in the cell and the distribution of bands on individual chromosomes allow the identification of numerical or structural abnormalities. This strategy is useful for

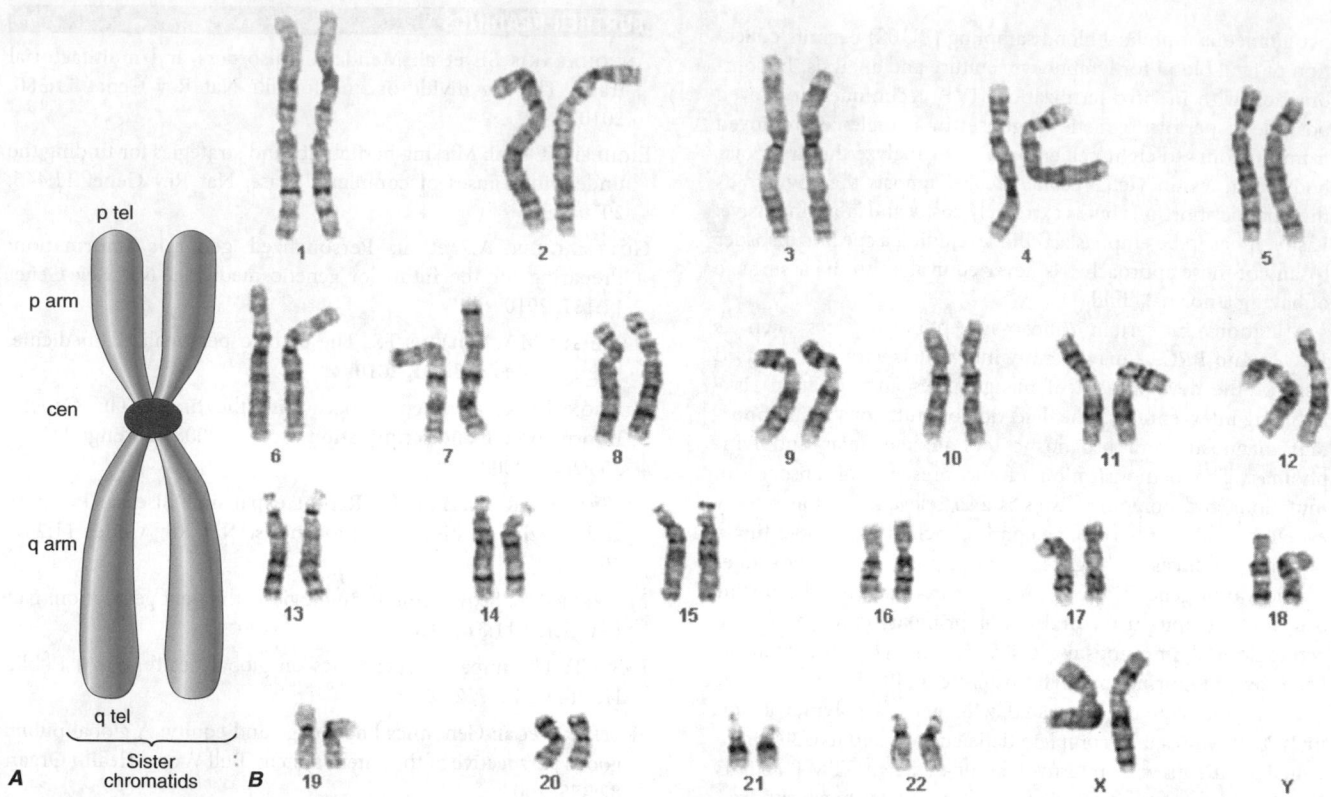

Figure 62-1 *A.* An idealized human chromosome, showing the centromere (cen), long (q) and short (p) arms, and telomeres (tel). *B.* A G-banded human karyotype from a normal (46,XX) female.

characterizing the normal chromosome complement and determining the incidence and types of major chromosome abnormalities.

Each human chromosome contains two specialized structures: a centromere and two telomeres. The centromere, or primary constriction, divides the chromosome into short (p) and long (q) arms and is responsible for the segregation of chromosomes during cell division. The telomeres, or chromosome ends, "cap" the p and q arms and are important for allowing DNA replication at the ends of the chromosomes. Prior to DNA replication, each chromosome consists of a single chromatid copy of the DNA double helix. After DNA replication and continuing until the time of cell division (including metaphase, when chromosomes are typically visualized), each chromosome consists of two identical sister chromatids (Fig. 62-1).

■ MOLECULAR CYTOGENETICS

The introduction of FISH methodologies in the late 1980s revolutionized the field of cytogenetics. In principle, FISH is similar to other DNA–DNA hybridization methodologies. In most instances, the probe is labeled directly with a fluorochrome to allow detection. After the hybridization step, the specimen is counterstained and the preparations are visualized with a fluorescence microscope.

Types of FISH probes

A variety of probes are available for use with FISH, including chromosome-specific paints (chromosome libraries), repetitive probes, and single-copy probes (Fig. 62-2). Chromosome libraries hybridize to sequences that span the entirety of the chromosome from which they are derived and, as a result, they can be used to "paint" individual chromosomes.

Repetitive probes recognize amplified DNA sequences present in chromosomes. The most common are α-satellite DNA probes that

are complementary to DNA sequences found at the centromeric regions of all human chromosomes. A vast number of *single-copy probes* are now available as a result of the human genome project. These probes can be as small as 1 kb, though normally they are much larger and are packaged into fosmids (40 kb), or bacterial artificial chromosomes (BACs) (100–200 kb). The most widely used probes are available commercially, including probes for specific rearrangements identified in a variety of cancers.

Applications of FISH and array technology

The majority of FISH applications involve hybridization of one or two probes of interest as an adjunctive procedure to conventional chromosomal banding techniques. In this regard, FISH can be utilized to identify specific chromosomes, characterize de novo duplications or deletions, and clarify subtle chromosomal rearrangements. Its greatest utilization in constitutional analysis, however, is in the detection of microdeletions (see below). In cancer cytogenetics, it is used extensively in the analysis of structural rearrangements. Though conventional cytogenetic studies can detect some microdeletions, initial detection and/or confirmation with FISH is essential. In fact, since appropriate FISH probes have become available, detection of microdeletion syndromes has increased significantly.

In addition to metaphase FISH, cells can be analyzed at a variety of stages. Interphase analysis, for example, can be used to make a rapid diagnosis in instances when metaphase chromosome preparations are not yet available (e.g., amniotic fluid interphase analysis). Interphase analysis also increases the number of cells available for examination, allows for investigation of nuclear organization, and provides results when cells do not progress to metaphase. One specialized type of interphase analysis involves the application of FISH to paraffin-embedded sections, thereby preserving the architecture of the tissue.

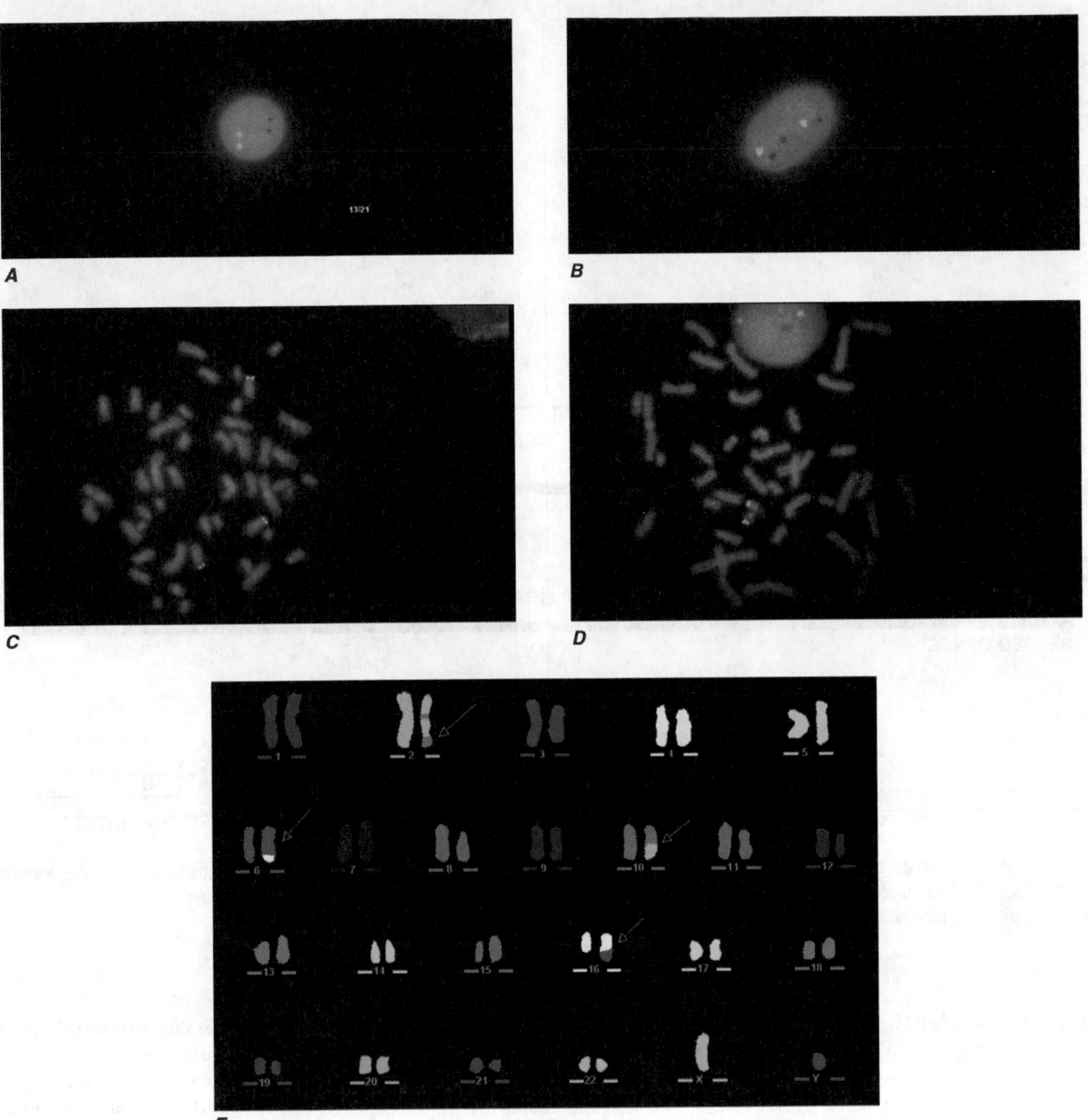

Figure 62-2 **Examples of different applications of fluorescence in situ hybridization (FISH)** to human metaphase and interphase preparations. *A, B.* Aneuploidy detection: Interphase FISH using chromosome 13 (green) and chromosome 21 (red) unique sequence probes on interphase cells from direct amniotic fluid preparations. In "A" (a normal cell), two signals for both chromosomes 13 and 21 are seen; in "B," three signals for chromosome 21 are seen, indicating trisomy 21 in the fetus. *C.* Aneuploidy detection: Two-color FISH with telomere probes from the short arm (green) and the long arm (red) of chromosome 8. Hybridization with these probes shows fluorescence of both probes to three separate chromosomes, indicating the presence of trisomy 8 in this individual. *D.* Microdeletion detection: Two-color FISH is used to detect a microdeletion of chromosome 22 associated with velocardiofacial (VCF) syndrome. A probe for ARSA (a locus on the distal portion of chromosome 22, visualized as a green signal) is observed on both chromosomes 22. However, a probe for TUPLE1 (a locus within the VCF region of chromosome 22, visualized in red) hybridizes to only the normal chromosome. *E.* Characterization of structural rearrangements: M-FISH (multicolor FISH) is used to detect a complex chromosome rearrangement involving a translocation between chromosomes 6 and 16, as well as a translocation and inversion involving chromosomes 2 and 10.

The use of interphase FISH has increased recently, especially for analyses of amniocentesis samples. These studies are performed on uncultured amniotic fluid, typically using DNA probes specific for the chromosomes most commonly identified in trisomies (chromosomes 13, 18, 21, and the X and Y). These studies can be performed rapidly (24–48 hours) and will ascertain about 60% of the abnormalities detected prenatally. Another area in which interphase analysis is routinely utilized is cancer cytogenetics (Chap. 83). Many site-specific translocations are associated with specific types of malignancies. For example, there are probes available for both the Abelson (Abl) oncogene and breakpoint cluster region (bcr) involved in chronic myelogenous leukemia (CML); these probes are labeled in red and green, respectively; the fusion of these genes in CML combines the fluorescent colors and appears as a yellow hybridization signal.

In addition to standard metaphase and interphase FISH analyses, a number of enhanced techniques have been developed for specific types of analysis, including multicolor FISH techniques,

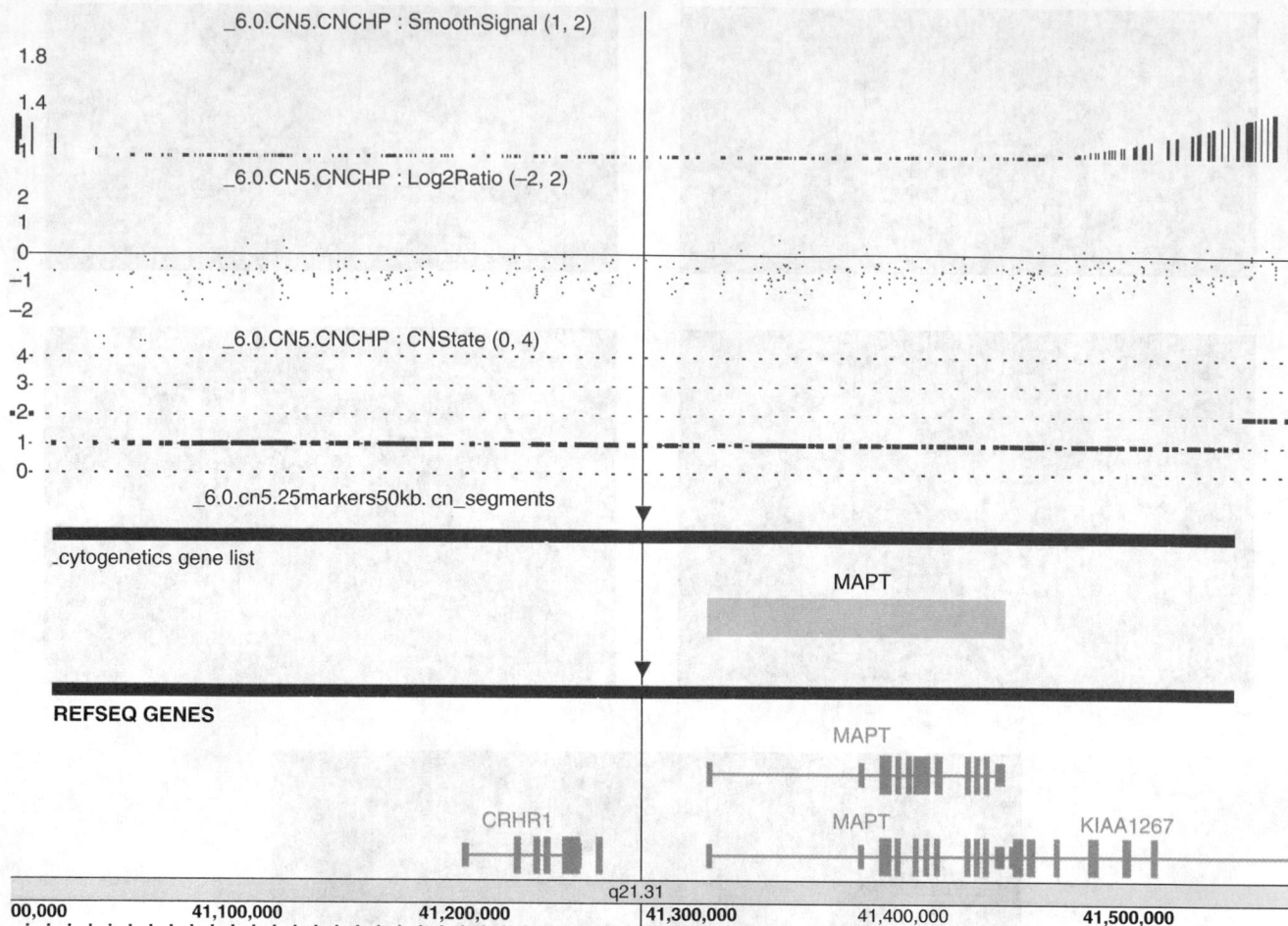

Figure 62-3 **Array analysis to diagnose** human chromosome abnormalities. Detection of a 533-kb deletion in 17q21.31 that includes the *MAPT* gene that is responsible for a newly described microdeletion syndrome. The SNP array illustrates the deletion by changes in the log2 ratio, allele difference, smooth signal, and copy number change.

reverse painting, fiber FISH, and comparative genomic hybridization. *Spectral karyotyping* (SKY) and multicolor FISH (m-FISH) techniques use combinatorially labeled probes that create a unique color for individual chromosomes. This technology is useful in the identification of unknown chromosome material (such as accessory marker chromosomes containing additional material) but has been most commonly used with the complex rearrangements seen in cancer specimens.

Fiber FISH is a technique in which chromosomes are mechanically stretched, using a variety of different methods. It provides a higher resolution of analysis than conventional FISH.

FISH comparative genomic hybridization (CGH) is a method that can be used only when DNA is available from a specimen of interest. The entire DNA specimen from the sample of interest is labeled in one color (e.g., green), and the normal control DNA specimen is indicated by another color (e.g., red). These are mixed in equal amounts and hybridized to normal metaphase chromosomes. The red-to-green ratio is analyzed by a computer program that determines where the DNA of interest may have gains or losses of material. Many of the FISH technologies are now being supplanted by the utilization of array analysis as described below.

The major advance for examining human chromosomes is an extension of the FISH CGH technologies. Specifically, the initial development of CGH arrays used protocols that are similar to standard FISH CGH, except that test DNA is hybridized to DNAs that are spread on arrays, rather than hybridized to normal chromosomes. These arrays are a natural outgrowth of both cytogenetic and FISH analysis, as they can provide a whole-genome analysis (as cytogenetic analysis provides), but at a higher resolution. There are several different types of arrays. CGH arrays utilize either BACs or oligonucleotides, whereas genotyping arrays (SNP arrays) utilize single nucleotide polymorphisms (Fig. 62-3). The resolution of these arrays can be up to 50 kb, far greater than for standard chromosome analysis. This technology has been used to study cryptic chromosomal imbalances in patients with mental retardation and multiple congenital anomalies, as well as in prenatal diagnosis. It has also been used to detect microdeletions and microduplications in cancer and in previously unidentified genomic disorders. This technology is still in development, but it will ultimately be the initial method of study for constitutional abnormalities.

INDICATIONS FOR CYTOGENETIC ANALYSIS

Primary indications for karyotypic analysis vary according to the developmental stage/age of the conceptus/individual under investigation. One especially important application is in prenatal diagnosis (particularly for pregnancies involving older women or women identified at increased risk by screening modalities), assaying for chromosomal abnormalities in either chorionic villi of first-trimester fetuses or amniotic fluid of second-trimester fetuses. Tissue specimens from spontaneously aborted fetuses or stillbirths can also be examined for chromosome abnormalities. Interphase cytogenetics (using FISH) is increasingly being used to study individual blastomeres of preimplantation embryos (with in vitro fertilization-derived pregnancies). This makes it possible to detect aneuploid or structurally unbalanced embryos or, in the case of sex-linked disorders, to identify male conceptuses; such embryos would not be used to initiate pregnancies.

Among infants and children, peripheral blood is examined, most often in individuals with specific phenotypic abnormalities. For example, karyotypic analysis can be used for the confirmation or exclusion of a specific chromosomal syndrome (e.g., trisomy 21); in patients with unexplained psychomotor retardation with or without dysmorphic features; in cases of monogenic disorders associated with mental retardation and/or dysmorphic features; and with abnormalities of sexual differentiation and development. Additionally, the array analysis is being increasingly used in patients with autism.

In adults, peripheral blood can be examined in patients with infertility or recurrent miscarriages, since chromosome abnormalities can lead to meiotic arrest or to genetically unbalanced gametes. An important branch of cytogenetics is concerned with analyses of bone marrow, unstimulated peripheral blood, and lymph nodes of tumors, as chromosomal abnormalities are a common correlate of leukemia, lymphoma, and solid tumors (Chap. 83).

CYTOGENETIC TESTING IN PRENATAL DIAGNOSIS

The vast majority of prenatal diagnostic studies are performed to rule out a chromosomal abnormality, but cells may also be propagated for biochemical studies or molecular analyses of DNA. Three procedures are used to obtain samples for prenatal diagnosis: amniocentesis, chorionic villus sampling (CVS), and fetal blood sampling. Amniocentesis is the most common procedure and is routinely performed at 15–17 weeks of gestation. On some occasions, early amniocentesis at 12–14 weeks is performed to expedite results, although less fluid is obtained at this time. Early amniocentesis carries a greater risk of spontaneous abortion or fetal injury but provides results at an earlier stage of pregnancy.

The vast majority of amniocenteses are performed in the context of advanced maternal age, the best-known correlate of trisomy (see below). Additional reasons for amniocentesis referral include an abnormal "triple- or quad-marker assay" and/or detection of ultrasound abnormalities. In the second trimester, levels of human chorionic gonadotropin (HCG), α-fetoprotein, and unconjugated estriol (and, in the quad assay, inhibin) in the maternal serum are quantified and used to adjust the maternal age–predicted risk of a trisomy 21 or trisomy 18 fetus. More recently, first-trimester screening, involving the measurement of nuchal translucency, and the levels of PAPP-A and HCG are being used to identify women at increased risk. When integrated together, first- and second-trimester testing will identify approximately 93% of trisomy 21 pregnancies. Specific ultrasound abnormalities, when detected at midtrimester, can also be associated with chromosomal defects. When a non-specific ultrasound abnormality is present, the estimated risk of a chromosomal defect is ~16%. Associations of chromosomal abnormalities and specific types of abnormal ultrasound findings are listed in Table 62-1.

CVS is the second most common procedure for genetic prenatal diagnosis. Because this procedure is routinely performed at about 10–12 weeks of gestation, it allows for an earlier detection of abnormalities and a safer pregnancy termination, if desired. CVS is a relatively safe procedure (spontaneous abortions, <0.5–1%). Because there is an increased association of limb defects when the procedure is performed earlier (<10 weeks of gestation), CVS is applicable during a narrow time frame of gestation. CVS involves the use

TABLE 62-1 Frequency of Chromosome Abnormalities, Identified on the Basis of Abnormal Ultrasound Findings

Ultrasound Finding	Chromosomal Abnormalities (Frequency)	
	Average, %	Range in Different Studies, %
Abnormal ultrasound (nonspecific)	16	13–35
Omphalocele	39	26–54
Cystic hygroma	68	46–78
Congenital heart disease	30	8–40
Choroid plexus cyst	5	4–10

of a catheter inserted transvaginally; ~25 mg of villi are aspirated from the chorion frondosum (the fetal portion of the placenta). By adding colchicine directly to the rapidly dividing cytotrophoblasts, results can be obtained within 24–48 hours. Findings from these procedures should be confirmed by analyses of cultured mesenchymal cells, as they are more reliably derived from the fetus.

Percutaneous umbilical blood sampling (PUBS) is a method for obtaining fetal blood during the second and third trimesters of pregnancy. PUBS is usually performed when ultrasound abnormalities are detected late in the second trimester. PUBS is also used when cytogenetic results from amniocentesis need clarification, such as in the detection of mosaicism.

CHROMOSOME ABNORMALITIES

■ CHROMOSOMES IN CELL DIVISION

To understand the etiology of chromosome abnormalities, it is important to review the movement of chromosomes during cell division. In somatic tissues, chromosomes are replicated during the S-phase of the cell cycle, so that each replicated chromosome consists of two identical sister chromatids. When the cell enters mitosis, each of the 46 chromosomes align on the metaphase plate, with the centromeres co-oriented toward opposite spindle poles (Fig. 62-4). At anaphase, the sister chromatids separate, with each of the daughter cells receiving one sister chromatid from each of the 46 chromosomes.

Chromosome segregation is more complicated in germ cell division, since the number of chromosomes must be reduced from 46 to 23 in the mature sperm and eggs. This is accomplished by two rounds of division—meiosis I and meiosis II (Fig. 62-4). In meiosis I, homologous chromosomes pair and exchange genetic material, then align on the metaphase plate, and finally separate from one another. Thus, by the end of meiosis I, only 23 of the original 46 chromosomes are represented in each of the two daughter cells. Meiosis II quickly follows meiosis I and is essentially a "haploid mitosis," involving separation of the sister chromatids in each of the 23 chromosomes.

Although the fundamentals of meiosis are the same in males and females, there are important distinctions, particularly in the timing of meiotic divisions. In males, meiosis begins with puberty and continues throughout the individual's lifetime. In females, meiosis begins prenatally, with oocytes proceeding through the first stages of meiosis I but arresting at mid-prophase. At the time of birth, the first meiotic division is suspended in oocytes. Only after ovulation many years later do oocytes complete meiosis I and proceed

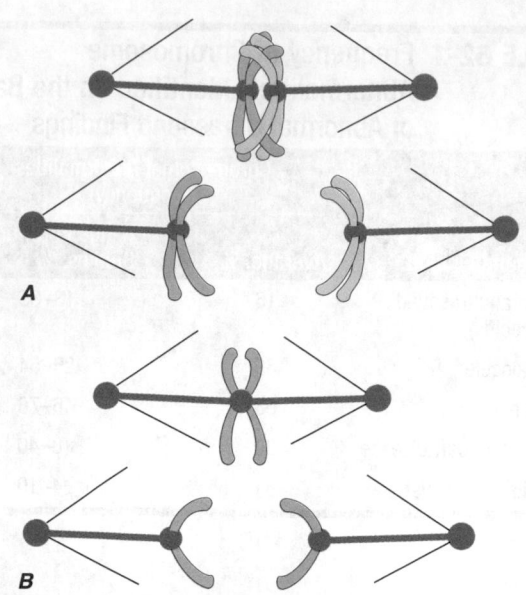

Figure 62-4 Chromosome segregation in meiosis. *A.* In meiosis I, each of the 23 pairs of chromosomes finds its "partner," or homologue, and exchanges genetic material (recombines) with it. At metaphase, each homologous pair aligns on the equatorial plate; at anaphase, each member of the homologous pair segregates from its partner. Thus, at the end of meiosis I, each daughter cell contains 23 chromosomes, with each chromosome consisting of two sister chromatids. ***B.*** In meiosis II, each chromosome aligns on the metaphase plate, and at anaphase, each of the two sister chromatids divides from the other. Thus, at the end of meiosis II, each daughter cell (e.g., the oocyte or spermatocyte) contains 23 chromosomes, with each chromosome consisting of one sister chromatid. In mitosis, the chromosomes behave exactly as they do in meiosis II, except that somatically dividing cells contain 46 chromosomes, not the 23 that are present in the meiosis II cell.

to the metaphase stage of meiosis II; if fertilized, the oocyte then completes the second meiotic division. Thus, in females, the first meiotic division takes at least 10–15 years and as many as 40–45 years to complete. Maternal age-related increases in the incidence of trisomy are likely the consequence of this protracted process of cell division.

■ INCIDENCE AND TYPES OF CHROMOSOME ABNORMALITIES

Errors in meiosis, or in early cleavage divisions, occur with extraordinary frequency. At least 10–25% of all pregnancies, for example, involve chromosomally abnormal conceptions. A large proportion of these terminate in the earliest stages of pregnancy, many of which go unrecognized. Nevertheless, even among clinically recognized pregnancies, nearly 10% of fetuses are chromosomally unbalanced. For the three types of clinically recognized pregnancies—spontaneous abortions, stillbirths, and livebirths—the frequencies of different chromosomal abnormalities are summarized in Table 62-2. The most common abnormalities are numerical, involving fetuses with additional (trisomy) or missing (monosomy) chromosomes, or those with one (triploidy) or two (tetraploidy) additional sets of chromosomes. Structural chromosome abnormalities are much less common, although several of the most important clinical chromosomal disorders involve structural rearrangements (see below).

By far the most common abnormality is trisomy, which is identified in ~25% of spontaneous abortions and 0.3% of newborns. Trisomies for all chromosomes have now been identified in embryos or fetuses, but there is considerable variation in frequency for various chromosomes. For example, trisomy 16 is extraordinarily common, accounting for about one-third of all trisomies in spontaneous abortions, whereas trisomies 1, 5, 11, and 19 have been identified less often. Available evidence suggests two reasons for this variation: (1) some chromosomes (e.g., chromosome 16) are more likely to segregate abnormally or undergo nondisjunction during meiosis than are others; and (2) the potential for development varies widely among different trisomic conditions, with some being eliminated very early in gestation, others surviving to the time of clinical pregnancy recognition, and some (e.g., trisomies 13, 18, and 21 and sex chromosome trisomies) being compatible with survival to term.

CHROMOSOMAL SYNDROMES

While most chromosomally abnormal conceptions perish in utero, several conditions are compatible with survival to term. The best-characterized of these are numerical abnormalities, involving loss or gain of individual chromosomes, and abnormalities resulting from unbalanced translocations. FISH, array analysis, and other molecular studies have led to the identification of two "new" types of chromosome abnormalities, commonly referred to as *microdeletion syndromes* and *imprinting syndromes*.

■ NUMERICAL ABNORMALITIES

Virtually all types of numerical abnormalities are eliminated prenatally, so that only those involving small, gene-poor autosomes or the sex chromosomes are identified with any frequency among liveborns. Clinically, the most important of these is trisomy 21, the most frequent cause of Down syndrome. Depending on the maternal age structure of the population and the utilization of prenatal testing, the incidence of trisomy 21 ranges from 1/600 to 1/1000 livebirths, making it the most common chromosome abnormality in live-born individuals. Like most trisomies, the incidence of trisomy 21 is highly correlated with maternal age, increasing from about 1/1500 livebirths for women 20 years of age to 1/30 for women ≥45 years.

In addition to trisomy 21, only two other autosomal trisomies, 13 and 18,

TABLE 62-2 Frequency and Distribution of Chromosome Abnormalities in Different Types of Clinically Recognizable Pregnancies

Chromosome Abnormality	Frequency of Abnormality			Probability of Surviving to Term, %
	Spontaneous Abortion	Stillbirth	Livebirth	
Trisomy, all	25.1	4.0	0.3	5
+13, 18, 21	4.5	2.7	0.14	15
+16	7.5	—	—	0
Sex chromosome monosomy (45,X)	8.7	0.1	0.01	1
Triploidy	6.4	0.2	—	0
Tetraploidy	2.4	—	—	0
Structural abnormality	2.0	0.8	0.3	45
Total abnormalities	50.0	5.1	0.6	5

occur with any frequency in livebirths. Incidence rates for trisomies 13 and 18 in livebirths are 1/20,000 and 1/10,000, respectively. Unlike trisomy 21 that is associated with near-normal life expectancy, both trisomies 13 and 18 are associated with death in infancy, typically occurring during the first year of life.

Three sex chromosome trisomies—the 47,XXX, 47,XXY (Klinefelter's syndrome), and 47,XYY conditions—are quite common, with each occurring in about 1/2000 newborns. Of all the trisomic conditions, these three have the fewest phenotypic complications. In fact, with the exception of infertility in Klinefelter's syndrome (Chap. 349), it is likely that most individuals with such trisomic conditions would go undetected. The additional Y chromosome in the 47,XYY condition is small and contains only a few genes. Most Y-linked genes are involved in testicular development or spermatogenesis. Thus, dosage imbalance of Y-linked genes has relatively little effect on other developmental processes. The 47,XYY genotype is associated with increased height. Its role in antisocial behavior, postulated initially because of an increased prevalence among some penalized populations, is unclear.

For the 47,XXX and 47,XXY conditions, the situation is different—the X chromosome contains >1000 genes, many of them essential for normal development. How, then, are 47,XXX and 47,XXY individuals spared from the catastrophic consequences of dosage imbalance? The answer lies in the biology of X chromosome gene expression. In normal females, one of the chromosomes undergoes *X inactivation* in somatic cells. The inactivation of the paternal or maternal X chromosome occurs randomly in each somatic cell and thereby serves as a mechanism of dosage compensation, ensuring that males and females have equal expression of most X-linked genes. The inactivation process occurs at the blastocyst stage of development; prior to this, both X chromosomes are active. In addition, not all X-linked genes are inactivated. Some genes on the X chromosome "escape" the inactivating mechanism and are expressed from both X chromosomes. In disorders such as Klinefelter's syndrome, some genes may be expressed from both X chromosomes, resulting in its phenotypic features.

As a rule, monosomic conditions are incompatible with fetal development and, consequently, autosomal monosomies are only rarely identified in spontaneous abortions and are not found among live-born individuals. In fact, the only monosomy compatible with livebirth is the 45,X condition that causes Turner's syndrome. The 45,X chromosome constitution occurs with surprisingly high frequency, present in at least 1–2% of all pregnancies. More than 99% of all 45,X conceptions are spontaneously aborted. Thus, live-born individuals with a 45,X chromosome constitution represent a rare group of survivors. The 45,X phenotype is mild, presumably because the second copy of many X chromosomal genes is normally inactivated. Nonetheless, Turner's syndrome causes gonadal dysgenesis, resulting in infertility and failure to undergo secondary sexual development, along with a number of other phenotypic features (Chap. 349). Several other structural abnormalities of the X chromosome such as deletions, isochromosome X, or ring chromosomes can cause Turner's syndrome. Mosaicism, including 45,X/46,XX, 45,X/47,XXX, 45,X/46,XY, and others, also occurs (see below) and contributes to the phenotypic spectrum in Turner's syndrome.

Because numerical abnormalities originate in meiosis (Table 62-3), affected individuals have missing or extra chromosomes in all cells. In a small proportion of cases, a mitotic nondisjunctional event occurs at an early stage in an individual with an initially normal chromosome constitution. Alternatively, a "normalizing" mitotic nondisjunctional event may result in a normal chromosome complement in some cells of an embryo. In either case, the embryo

TABLE 62-3 Studies of the Parent and Meiotic/Mitotic Stage of Origin of Human Trisomies and Sex Chromosome Monosomy

	Origin, %				
	Paternal		Maternal		
	I	II	I	II	Mitotic
Trisomy					
2	28	—	54	13	6
7	—	—	17	26	57
15	—	15	76	9	—
16	—	1	96	3	—
18	—	—	33	56	11
21	3	5	67	22	2
22	3	—	94	3	—
XXY	46	—	38	14	3
XXX	—	6	60	16	18
Monosomy					
X*	80		20		

*Results pertain to nonmosaic 45,X individuals.

is a mosaic, with some cells bearing a normal chromosome constitution and others an aneuploid number of chromosomes. The phenotypic consequences are difficult to predict because they depend on the timing of nondisjunction and the distribution of normal and abnormal cells in different tissues. Nevertheless, mosaicism may lead to clinical abnormalities indistinguishable from those of nonmosaic individuals (e.g., nearly 5% of all cases of Down syndrome involve individuals with mosaic trisomy 21, and about 15% of individuals with Turner's syndrome are mosaic for various sex chromosomal constitutions as described above).

The origin and etiology of numerical abnormalities

Over the past decade, a number of studies have used DNA polymorphisms to investigate the origin of different types of chromosome abnormalities (Fig. 62-5). The most thoroughly investigated types have been numerical abnormalities (Table 62-4). Sex chromosome monosomy usually results from loss of the paternal sex chromosome, regardless of whether the conception is liveborn or spontaneously aborted.

Trisomies show remarkable variation in parental origin. For example, paternal nondisjunction is responsible for nearly 50% of 47,XXY but only 5–10% of cases of trisomies 13, 14, 15, 21, and 22; it is rarely, if ever, the source of the additional chromosome in trisomy 16. Similarly, there is considerable variability in the meiotic stage of origin. For example, all cases of trisomy 16 may be due to meiosis I errors, whereas for trisomy 21, one-third of cases are associated with meiosis II errors, and for trisomy 18, the majority of cases are apparently due to meiosis II nondisjunction. In spite of this variation in parental and meiotic origin, nondisjunction at maternal meiosis I appears to be the most common source of trisomy.

Maternal age and trisomy

The association between increasing maternal age and trisomy is the most important etiologic factor in congenital chromosomal

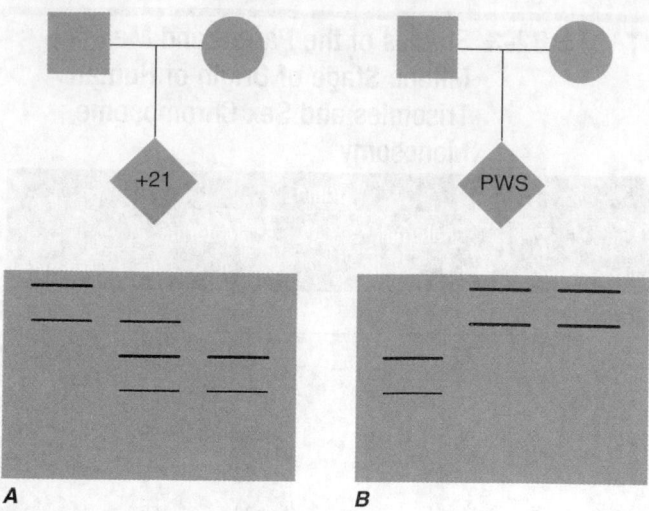

Figure 62-5 Use of DNA technology to determine the origin of chromosome abnormalities. A. Analysis of a chromosome 21–specific DNA polymorphism demonstrates that the trisomic individual received two chromosomes 21 from his mother and one from his father; thus, the extra chromosome 21 resulted from an error in oogenesis. **B.** Inheritance of a chromosome 15–specific DNA polymorphism in an individual with Prader-Willi syndrome (PWS). The affected individual has received two maternal, but no paternal, chromosomes 15; thus, the individual is said to have maternal uniparental disomy 15, a common cause of PWS.

disorders. Among women under the age of 25, ~2% of all clinically recognized pregnancies are trisomic; by the age of 36, however, this figure increases to 10% and by the age of 42, to >33% (Fig. 62-6). This association between maternal age and trisomy is exerted without respect to race, geography, or socioeconomic factors and likely affects segregation of all chromosomes.

Despite the importance of increasing age, little is known about the mechanism by which aging leads to abnormal chromosomal segregation. As noted above, it is thought to originate in maternal meiosis I owing to the protracted time to completion (often ≥40 years) in females, and recent studies suggest that it may be associated with alterations in meiotic crossing-over. In trisomy 21, for example, crossover patterns appear to be similarly abnormal in younger and older mothers of trisomic conceptions. Thus, it has been suggested that two distinct steps, or "hits," may be involved in maternal age-related nondisjunction. The first hit, which is age independent, involves the establishment of a "vulnerable" crossover configuration in the fetal oocyte; the second hit, which is age dependent, involves abnormal processing of the vulnerable bivalent structure at metaphase I. If this model is correct, it suggests that the nondisjunctional process is the same in younger and older women, but it occurs more frequently with aging, possibly because of age-dependent degradation of meiotic proteins.

▪ STRUCTURAL CHROMOSOME ABNORMALITIES

Structural rearrangements involve breakage and reunion of chromosomes. Although less common than numerical abnormalities, they

TABLE 62-4 Some Commonly Identified Microdeletion and Microduplication Syndromes—FISH Analysis

Syndrome	Cytogenetic Location	Principal Features	Imprinting Effects
Langer-Giedion syndrome	8q24.1 (del)	Sparse hair, bulbous nose, variable mental retardation	No
WAGR complex	11p13 (del)	Wilms' tumor, aniridia, genitourinary disorders, mental retardation	No
Beckwith-Wiedemann syndrome	11p15 (dup)	Macrosomia, macroglossia, omphalocele	Yes, occasionally associated with "paternal uniparental disomy" (see text)
Retinoblastoma	13q14.11 (del)	Retinoblastoma due to homozygous loss of functional RB allele	No obvious effect, although abnormal RB allele more likely to be paternal
Prader-Willi syndrome	15q11-13 (del)	Obesity, hypogonadism, mental retardation	Yes, prototypic imprinting disorder (see text)
Angelman syndrome	15q11-13 (del)	Ataxic gait	With Prader-Willi syndrome, prototypic imprinting disorder (see text)
α-Thalassemia and mental retardation	16p13.3 (del)	α-Thalassemia and mental retardation, due to deletion of distal 16p, including α-globin locus	No
Smith-Magenis syndrome	17p11.2 (del)	Brachycephaly, midface hypoplasia, mental retardation	No
Miller-Dieker syndrome	17p13 (del)	Dysmorphic facies, lissencephaly	No
Charcot-Marie-Tooth syndrome type 1A	17p11.2 (dup)	Progressive neuropathy due to microduplication	No
DiGeorge syndrome/ velocardiofacial syndrome	22q11 (del)	Abnormalities of third and fourth branchial arches	No

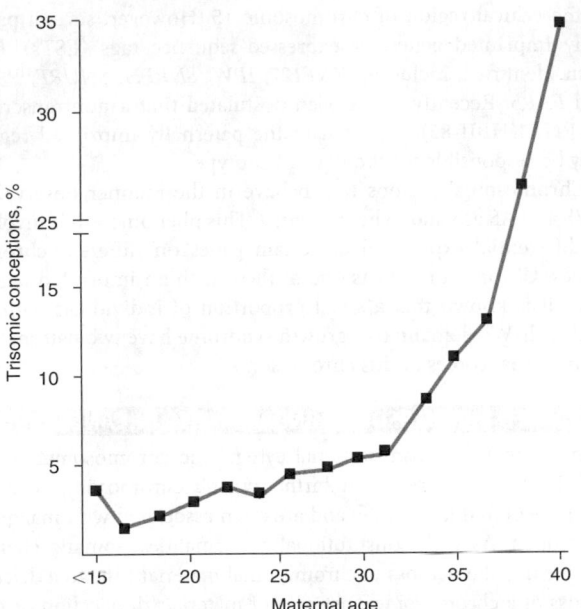

Figure 62-6 Estimated maternal age–adjusted rates of trisomy among all clinically recognized pregnancies (e.g., spontaneous abortions, stillbirths, and livebirths). Among women in their forties, more than 25% of all pregnancies are estimated to involve a trisomic conception; the vast majority of these spontaneously abort, with only trisomies 13, 18, and 21 and sex chromosome trisomies surviving to term with any appreciable frequency.

present additional challenges from a genetic counseling standpoint. This is because structural abnormalities, unlike numerical abnormalities, can be present in "balanced" form in clinically normal individuals but transmitted in "unbalanced" form to progeny, thereby resulting in a hereditary form of chromosome abnormality.

Rearrangements may involve exchanges of material between different chromosomes (translocations) or loss, gain, or rearrangements of individual chromosomes (e.g., deletions, duplications, inversions, rings, or isochromosomes). Of particular clinical importance are *translocations* that involve two basic types: Robertsonian and reciprocal. Robertsonian rearrangements are a special class of translocation, in which the long arms of two acrocentric chromosomes (chromosomes 13, 14, 15, 21, and 22) join together, generating a fusion chromosome that contains virtually all of the genetic material of the original two chromosomes. If the Robertsonian translocation is present in unbalanced form, a monosomic or trisomic conception ensues. For example, ~3% of Down syndrome cases are attributable to unbalanced Robertsonian translocations, most often involving chromosomes 14 and 21. In this instance, the affected individual has 46 chromosomes, including one structurally normal chromosome 14, two structurally normal chromosomes 21, and one fusion 14/21 chromosome. This effect leads to a normal diploid dosage for chromosome 14 and to a triplication of chromosome 21, thus resulting in Down syndrome. Similarly, a small proportion of individuals with trisomy 13 syndrome are clinically affected because of an unbalanced Robertsonian translocation involving chromosome 13.

Reciprocal translocations involve mutual exchanges between any two chromosomes. In this circumstance, the phenotypic consequences associated with unbalanced translocations depend on the location of the breakpoints that dictate the amount of material that has been "exchanged" between the two chromosomes. Because most reciprocal translocations involve unique sets of breakpoints, it is difficult to predict the phenotypic consequences in any one situation. In general, severity is determined by the amount of excess

or missing chromosome material in individuals with unbalanced translocations.

In addition to rearrangements between chromosomes, there are several examples of intrachromosome structural abnormalities. The most common and deleterious of these involve loss of chromosome material due to deletions. The two best-characterized deletion syndromes, Wolf-Hirschhorn syndrome and cri-du-chat syndrome, result from loss of relatively small chromosomal segments on chromosomes 4p and 5p, respectively. Nonetheless, each is associated with multiple congenital anomalies, developmental delays, profound retardation, and reduced lifespan.

Microdeletion syndromes—FISH

The term *contiguous gene syndrome* refers to genetic disorders that mimic a combination of single-gene disorders. They result from the deletion of a small number of tightly clustered genes. Because some are too small to be detected cytogenetically, they are termed *microdeletions*. The application of molecular techniques has led to the identification of at least 18 of these microdeletion syndromes (Table 62-4) that have been diagnosed using a directed FISH analysis. Some of the more common ones include the Wilms' tumor–aniridia complex (WAGR), Miller-Dieker syndrome (MDS), and velocardiofacial (VCF) syndrome. WAGR is characterized by mental retardation and involvement of multiple organs, including kidney (Wilms' tumor), eye (aniridia), and the genitourinary system. The cytogenetic abnormality involves a deletion of a part of the short arm of chromosome 11 (11p13), which typically is detectable on well-banded chromosome preparations. In MDS, a disorder characterized by mental retardation, dysmorphic facies, and lissencephaly, the deletion involves chromosome 17 (17p13.3). Using FISH, 17p deletions have been detected in >90% of patients with MDS as well as in 20% of cases of isolated lissencephaly.

Deletions involving the long arm of chromosome 22 (22q11.21) are the most common microdeletions identified to date, present in ~1/3000 newborns. VCF syndrome, the most commonly associated syndrome, consists of learning disabilities or mild mental retardation, palatal defects, a hypoplastic alae nasi and long nose, and congenital heart defects (conotruncal defect). Some individuals with 22q11.21 deletion are more severely affected and present with DiGeorge syndrome that involves abnormalities in the development of the third and fourth branchial arches leading to thymic hypoplasia, parathyroid hypoplasia, and conotruncal heart defects. In ~30% of these cases, a deletion at 22q11.21 can be detected with high-resolution banding; by combing conventional cytogenetics, FISH, and molecular detection techniques (i.e., Southern blotting or polymerase chain reaction analyses), these rates improve to >90%. Additional studies have demonstrated a surprisingly high frequency of 22q11.21 deletions in individuals with nonsyndromic conotruncal defects. Approximately 10% of individuals with a 22q11.21 deletion inherited it from a parent with a similar deletion.

Smith-Magenis syndrome involves a microdeletion localized to the proximal region of the short arm of chromosome 17 (17p11.2). Affected individuals have mental retardation, dysmorphic facial features, delayed speech, peripheral neuropathy, and behavior abnormalities. Most of these deletions can be detected with cytogenetic analysis, although FISH is available to confirm these findings. In contrast, William syndrome, a chromosome 7 (7q11.23) microdeletion, cannot be diagnosed with standard or high-resolution analysis; it is only detectable utilizing FISH or other molecular methods. Williams' syndrome involves a deletion of the elastin gene and is characterized by mental retardation, dysmorphic features, a gregarious personality, premature aging, and congenital heart disease (usually supravalvular aortic stenosis).

In addition to microdeletion syndromes, there are several well-described microduplication syndromes, one of which is

Charcot-Marie-Tooth type 1A (CMT1A). This is a nerve conduction disease previously thought to be transmitted as a simple autosomal dominant disorder. Recent molecular studies have demonstrated that affected individuals are heterozygous for duplication of a small region of chromosome 17 (17p12). Although it is not yet clear why increased gene dosage would result in CMT1A, the inheritance pattern is explained by the fact that one-half of the offspring of affected individuals inherit the duplication-carrying chromosome.

Microdeletion syndromes—array analysis

All of the above-mentioned microdeletions and microduplications were initially identified clinically because of specific phenotypic features. After these were mapped to specific cytogenetic regions, FISH probes were developed to confirm the clinical diagnosis. With the advent of array analysis, new microdeletion and microduplication syndromes have been identified, often having less specific diagnostic criteria. These microdeletions and microduplications include changes in 16p11.2, 16p13.1, 15q13.3, 1q21.1, and are often ascertained because of autism. Often, the detected genetic changes are familial and parents do not always demonstrate any phenotypic abnormalities. Many of these are believed to be susceptibility genes that might increase an individual's risk for developing a disorder. Other changes such as a microdeletion involving 17q11.21, was not diagnosed before the advent of array analysis, and involves loss of the *MAPT* gene and is seen in patients with mental retardation, dysmorphic features, and hypopigmentation (Fig. 62-3).

■ IMPRINTING DISORDERS

Two microdeletion syndromes, Prader-Willi syndrome (PWS) and Angelman syndrome (AS), exhibit parent-of-origin, or "imprinting," effects. For many years, it has been known that cytogenetically detectable deletions of chromosome 15 occur in a proportion of patients with PWS, as well as in those with AS. This seemed curious, as the clinical manifestations of the two syndromes are very dissimilar, but the deletions appeared identical. PWS is characterized by obesity, hypogonadism, and mild to moderate mental retardation, whereas AS is associated with microcephaly, ataxic gait, seizures, inappropriate laughter, and severe mental retardation. New insight into the pathogenesis of these disorders has been provided by the recognition that parental origin of the deletion determines which phenotype ensues: If the deletion is paternal, the result is PWS, whereas if the deletion is maternal, the result is AS (Fig. 62-5*B*).

This scenario is complicated further by the recognition that not all individuals with PWS or AS carry the chromosome 15 deletion. For such individuals, the parental origin of the chromosome 15 region is again the important determinant. In PWS, for example, nondeletion patients invariably have two maternal and no paternal chromosomes 15 [maternal uniparental disomy (UPD)], whereas for some nondeletion AS patients the reverse is true (paternal UPD). This indicates that at least some genes on chromosome 15 are differently expressed, depending on which parent contributed the chromosome. Additionally, this means that normal fetal development requires the presence of one maternal and one paternal copy of chromosome 15.

Approximately 70% of PWS cases are due to paternal deletions of 15q11-q13, whereas 25% are due to maternal UPD, and about 5% are caused by mutations in a chromosome 15 imprinting center. In AS, 75% of cases are due to maternal deletions, and only 2% are due to paternal UPD. The remaining cases are presumably caused by imprinting mutations (5%), or mutations in the *UBE3A* gene, which is associated with AS. The UPD cases are mostly caused by meiotic nondisjunction resulting in trisomy 15, subsequently followed by a normalizing mitotic nondisjunction event ("trisomy rescue") resulting in two normal chromosomes 15, both from the same parent. *UBE3A* is the only maternally imprinted gene known

in the critical region of chromosome 15. However, several paternally imprinted genes, or expressed-sequence tags (ESTs), have been identified, including *ZNF127, IPW, SNRPN, SNURF, PAR1,* and *PAR5*. Recently it has been postulated that a nontranscribed snoRNA (HBII-85), localized to the paternally imprinted region, may be responsible for the PWS phenotype.

Chromosomal regions that behave in the manner observed in PWS and AS are said to be *imprinted*. This phenomenon is involved in differential expression of certain genes on different chromosomes. Chromosome 11 is one of these with an imprinted region, since it is known that a small proportion of individuals with the Beckwith-Wiedemann overgrowth syndrome have two paternal but no maternal copies of this chromosome.

ACQUIRED CHROMOSOME ABNORMALITIES IN CANCER

In addition to the constitutional cytogenetic chromosomal abnormalities that are present at birth, somatic chromosomal changes can be acquired later in life and are often associated with malignant conditions. As with constitutional abnormalities, somatic changes can include the net loss of chromosomal material (due to a deletion or loss of a chromosome), net gain of material (duplication or gain of a chromosome), and relocation of DNA sequences (translocation). Cytogenetic changes have been particularly well studied in (1) leukemias, e.g., Philadelphia chromosome translocation in CML [t(9;22) (q34.1;q11.2)]; and (2) lymphomas, e.g., translocations of *MYC* in Burkitt's [t(8;14)(q24;q32)]. These and other translocations are useful for diagnosis, classification, and prognosis. Analyses of cytogenetic changes are also useful in certain solid tumors. For example, a complex karyotype with Wilms' tumor, diploidy in medulloblastoma, and Her-2/neu amplification in breast cancer are poor prognostic signs. For detailed discussion of cancer genetics, see Chap. 83.

FURTHER READINGS

Bejjani BA, Shaffer LG: Clinical utility of contemporary molecular cytogenetics. Annu Rev Genomics Hum Genet 9:71, 2008

Ferguson-Smith MA: Cytogenetics and the evolution of cytogenetics. Genet Med 10:553, 2008

Hassold T, Hunt P: Maternal age and chromosomally abnormal pregnancies: What we know and what we wish we knew. Curr Opin Pediatr 21:703, 2009

Lee C et al: Multicolor fluorescence in situ hybridization in clinical cytogenetic diagnostics. Curr Opin Pediatr 13:550, 2002

Maya I et al: Diagnostic utility of array-based comparative genomic hybridization (aCGH) in a prenatal setting. Prenat Diagn 30:1131, 2010

Mefford HC, Eichler EE: Duplication hotspots, rare genomic disorders and common disease. Curr Opin Genet Dev 19:196, 2009

Miller DT et al: Consensus statement: Chromosomal microarray is a first-tier clinical diagnostic test for individuals with developmental disabilities or congenital anomalies. Am J Hum Genet 86:749, 2010

Nasmyth K: Segregating sister genomes: The molecular biology of chromosome separation. Science 297:559, 2002

Rimoin DL et al (eds): *Emery and Rimoin's Principles and Practice of Medical Genetics,* 5th ed. Philadelphia, Churchill Livingstone, 2007

Sharp AJ et al: Discovery of previously unidentified genomic disorders from the duplication architecture of the human genome. Nat Genet 38:1038, 2006

Vorsanova SG et al: Human interphase chromosomes: A review of available molecular cytogenetic technologies. Mol Cytogenet 3:1, 2010

CHAPTER **63**

The Practice of Genetics in Clinical Medicine

Susan Miesfeldt

J. Larry Jameson

APPLICATIONS OF MOLECULAR GENETICS IN CLINICAL MEDICINE

The field of medical genetics has traditionally focused on chromosomal abnormalities (Chap. 62) and Mendelian disorders (Chap. 61). However, there is genetic susceptibility to many common adult-onset diseases, including atherosclerosis, cardiac disorders, asthma, hypertension, autoimmune diseases, diabetes mellitus, macular degeneration, Alzheimer's disease, psychiatric disorders, and many forms of cancer. Genetic contributions to these common disorders involve more than the ultimate expression of the condition; these genes can also influence the severity of illness, progression of disease, and effect of treatment.

The primary care clinician is now faced with the role of recognizing and counseling patients at risk for a number of genetically influenced diseases. Among the greater than 20,000 genes in the human genome, it is estimated that each of us harbors several potentially deleterious mutations. Fortunately, many of these genetic alterations are recessive or clinically silent. An even greater number, however, represent genetic variants that alter disease susceptibility, course, or response to therapy.

Genetic medicine is changing the way diseases are classified, enhancing our understanding of pathophysiology, providing practical information concerning drug metabolism and therapeutic response, and allowing for individualized screening and health care management programs. In view of these changes, the physician must integrate personal medical history, family history, and diagnostic molecular testing into the overall care of individual patients and their families. Patients turn to their primary care providers for guidance about genetic disorders, even though they may also be seeing other specialists. The primary care provider has an important role in educating patients about the indications, benefits, risks, and limitations of genetic testing in the management of a number of diverse diseases. This is a difficult task, because scientific advances in genetic medicine are outpacing the translation of these discoveries into standards of clinical care.

COMMON ADULT-ONSET GENETIC DISORDERS

■ MULTIFACTORIAL INHERITANCE

The risk for many adult-onset disorders reflects the combined effects of genetic factors at multiple loci that may function independently or in combination with other genes or environmental factors. Our understanding of the genetic basis of these disorders is incomplete, despite the clear recognition of genetic susceptibility. In Type 2 diabetes mellitus, for example, the concordance rate in monozygotic twins ranges between 50 and 90%. Diabetes or impaired glucose tolerance occurs in 40% of siblings and in 30% of the offspring of an affected individual. Despite the fact that diabetes affects 5% of the population and exhibits a high degree of heritability, only a few genetic mutations (most of which are rare) that might account for the familial nature of the disease have been identified. They include

certain mitochondrial DNA disorders (Chap. 61), mutations in a cascade of genes that control pancreatic islet cell development and function (*HNF4α, HNF1α, IPF1, TCF7L2, glucokinase*), insulin receptor mutations, and others (Chap. 344). In addition to these known genes, a large number of additional genetic loci that confer disease susceptibility have been identified. Superimposed on this genetic background are environmental or medical influences such as diet, exercise, pregnancy, and medications.

Identifying susceptibility genes associated with multifactorial adult-onset disorders is a formidable task. Nonetheless, a reasonable goal for these types of diseases is to identify genes that increase (or decrease) disease risk by a factor of two or more. For common diseases such as diabetes or heart disease, this level of risk has important implications for health. In much the same way that cholesterol is currently used as a biochemical marker of cardiovascular risk, we can anticipate the development of genetic panels with similar predictive power. The availability of DNA-microarray systems represents an important technology that makes large-scale testing feasible (Chap. 61). Whether to perform a genetic test for a particular inherited adult-onset disorder, such as hemochromatosis, multiple endocrine neoplasia (MEN) type 1, prolonged QT syndrome, or Huntington's disease, is a complex decision; it depends on the clinical features of the disorder, the desires of the patient and family, and whether the results of genetic testing will alter medical decision-making or treatment (see below).

Population screening

Mass genetic screening programs require tests with high enough sensitivity and specificity to be cost-effective. An effective screening program should fulfill the following criteria: the tested disorder is prevalent and serious; it can be influenced presymptomatically through lifestyle changes, screening, medications, or other risk-reducing interventions; and identification of risk does not result in undue discrimination or harm. Screening individuals of Jewish descent for the autosomal recessive neurodegenerative disorder Tay-Sachs disease has resulted in a dramatic decline in the incidence of this syndrome in the United States. On the other hand, screening for sickle cell disease or trait in the African-American population has sometimes resulted in insurance and employment discrimination.

Mass screening for complex genetic disorders can result in potential problems. For example, cystic fibrosis is most commonly associated with the ΔF508 mutation. This variant accounts for 30–80% of mutant alleles, depending on the ethnic group. Nevertheless, cystic fibrosis is associated with pronounced genetic heterogeneity with more than 1000 disease-related mutations. The American College of Medical Genetics recommends a panel of 23 alleles, including the ΔF508 allele, for routine carrier testing. Analysis for the less common cystic fibrosis–associated mutations would greatly impact the cost of testing without significantly influencing the effectiveness of mass screening. Nevertheless, the individual who carries one of the less common cystic fibrosis–associated alterations will not benefit if testing is limited to a routine panel.

Occupational health screening programs hold promise but also raise concerns about employment discrimination. These concerns were brought to light when it was discovered that a railroad company was testing its employees, without consent, for a rare genetic condition that results in susceptibility to carpal tunnel syndrome. The Equal Employment Opportunity Commission argued that the tests were unlawful under the Americans with Disabilities Act.

■ THE FAMILY HISTORY

When two or more first-degree relatives are affected with asthma, cardiovascular disease, Type 2 diabetes, breast cancer, colon cancer, or melanoma, the relative risk ranges from two- to fivefold, underscoring the importance of family history for these prevalent disorders. Pending further advances in genetic testing, in most circumstances, the key to assessing the inherited risk for common adult-onset diseases rests in the collection and interpretation of a detailed personal and family medical history in conjunction with a directed physical examination. For example, a history of multiple family members with early-onset coronary artery disease, glucose intolerance, and hypertension should suggest increased risk for genetic, and perhaps environmental, predisposition to metabolic syndrome (Chap. 242). Individual patients with this family history should be monitored for the possible development of high blood pressure, diabetes, and hyperlipidemia. They should be counseled about the importance of avoiding additional risk factors such as obesity, physical inactivity, and cigarette smoking.

Family history should be recorded in the form of a pedigree. At a minimum, pedigrees should convey health-related data on all first-degree relatives and selected second-degree relatives, including grandparents. When pedigrees appear to suggest an inherited disease, they should be extended to include additional family members. The determination of risk for an asymptomatic individual will vary depending on the size of the pedigree, the number of unaffected relatives, and the types of diagnoses, as well as the age of disease onset. For example, a woman with two first-degree relatives with breast cancer is at greater risk for a Mendelian disorder if she has a total of three female first-degree relatives than if she has a total of ten female first-degree relatives. Additional variables that should be documented in the pedigree include the presence or absence of nonhereditary risk factors among those affected with diseases and the finding of multiple diseases in an individual patient. For instance, a woman with a history of both colon cancer and endometrial cancer is at risk for Lynch syndrome regardless of her family history.

When assessing the personal and family history, the physician should be alert to a younger age of disease onset than is usually seen in the general population. A 30-year-old with acute myocardial infarction should be considered at risk for a hereditary trait, even if there is no family history of premature coronary artery disease (Chap. 241). The absence of the nonhereditary risk factors typically associated with a disease also raises the prospect of genetic causation. A personal or family history of deep vein thrombosis, in the absence of known environmental or medical risk factors, suggests a hereditary thrombotic disorder (Chap. 117). The physical examination also may provide important clues about the risk for a specific inherited disorder. A patient presenting with xanthomas at a young age should prompt consideration of familial hypercholesterolemia. Some adult-onset disease-causing mutations are more prevalent in certain ethnic groups. For instance, >2% of the Ashkenazi population carry one of three specific mutations in the *BRCA1* or *BRCA2* genes. The prevalence of the factor V Leiden allele ranges from 3 to 7% in Caucasians but is much lower in Africans or Asians.

Recall of family history is often inaccurate. This is especially so when the history is remote and families become more dispersed geographically. It can be helpful to ask patients to fill out family history forms before or after their visits, as this provides them with an opportunity to contact relatives. Ideally, this information should be embedded in electronic health records and updated intermittently. Attempts should be made to confirm the illnesses reported in the family history before making important and, in certain circumstances, irreversible management decisions. This process is often labor intensive and ideally involves interviews of additional family members or reviewing medical records, autopsy reports, and death certificates.

Although many inherited disorders will be suggested by the clustering of relatives with the same or related conditions, it is important to note that *disease penetrance* is incomplete for most multifactorial

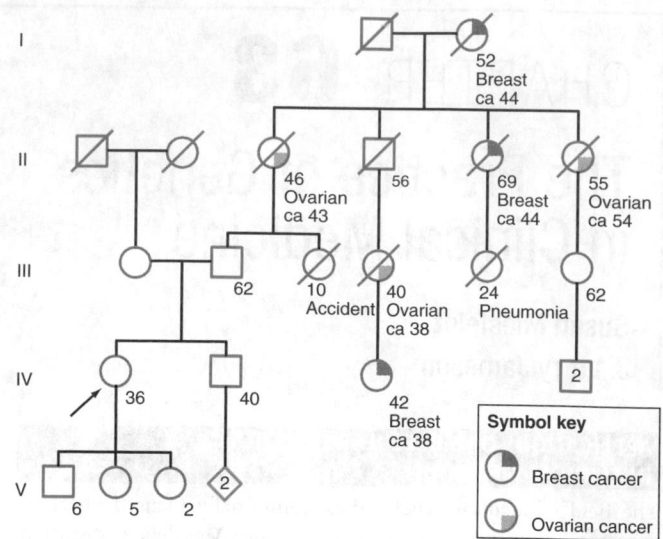

Figure 63-1   A 36-year-old woman (*arrow*) seeks consultation because of her family history of cancer. The patient expresses concern that the multiple cancers in her relatives imply an inherited predisposition to develop cancer. The family history is recorded and records of the patient's relatives confirm the reported diagnoses.

genetic disorders. As a result, the pedigree obtained in such families may not exhibit a clear Mendelian inheritance pattern, as not all family members carrying the disease-associated alleles will manifest a clinical disorder. Furthermore, genes associated with some of these disorders often exhibit *variable expression* of disease. For example, the breast cancer–associated gene *BRCA1* can predispose to several different malignancies in the same family, including cancers of the breast, ovary, and prostate (Chap. 83). For common diseases such as breast cancer, some family members without the disease-causing mutation may also develop breast cancer, representing another confounding variable in the pedigree analysis.

Some of the aforementioned features of the family history are illustrated in Fig. 63-1. In this example, the proband, a 36-year-old woman (IV-1), has a strong history of breast and ovarian cancer on the paternal side of her family. The early age of onset, as well as the co-occurrence of breast and ovarian cancer in this family, suggests the possibility of an inherited mutation in *BRCA1* or *BRCA2*. It is unclear though—without genetic testing—whether her father harbors such a mutation and transmitted it to her. After appropriate genetic counseling of the proband and her family, the most informative approach to DNA analysis in this family is to test the cancer-affected 42-year-old living cousin for the presence of a *BRCA1* or *BRCA2* mutation. If a mutation is found, then it is possible to test for this particular alteration in other family members, if they so desire. In the example shown, if the proband's father has the *BRCA1* mutation, there is a 50:50 probability that the mutation was transmitted to her, and genetic testing can be used to establish the absence or presence of this alteration. In this same example, if a mutation is not detected in the cancer-affected cousin, testing would not be indicated for cancer-unaffected relatives.

GENETIC TESTING FOR ADULT-ONSET DISORDERS

A critical first step before initiating genetic testing is to ensure that the correct clinical diagnosis has been made, whether it is based on family history, characteristic physical findings, or biochemical testing. Careful clinical assessment can define the *phenotype*, thereby preventing unnecessary testing and directing testing toward the most probable candidate genes (Fig. 63-2). For patients identified by population-based screening (e.g., diabetes, hypercholesterolemia),

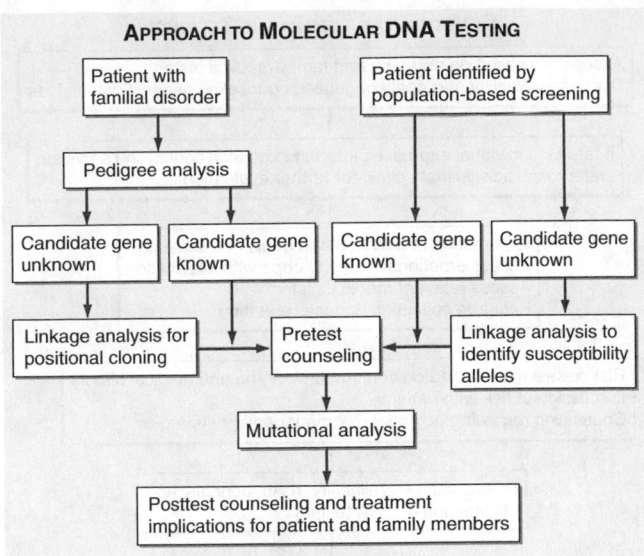

APPROACH TO MOLECULAR DNA TESTING

Figure 63-2 Approach to identifying a disease-causing gene.

testing might involve known candidate genes, or genome-wide linkage studies of the population could be used as part of a research study to identify susceptibility alleles. For patients with a strong family history (e.g., breast cancer, hemochromatosis), testing often includes known candidate genes, or traditional linkage analyses within pedigrees can identify candidate disease-causing genes. Once disease-related genes are known, mutational analyses can be performed after pretest genetic counseling (see below).

Many disorders exhibit the feature of *locus heterogeneity*, which refers to the fact that mutations in different genes can cause phenotypically similar disorders. For example, osteogenesis imperfecta (Chap. 363), long QT syndrome (Chap. 233), muscular dystrophy (Chap. 387), homocystinuria (Chap. 364), retinitis pigmentosa (Chap. 28), and hereditary predisposition to colon cancer (Chap. 91) or breast cancer (Chap. 90) can each be caused by mutations in distinct genes. The pattern of disease transmission, disease risk, clinical course, and treatment may differ significantly, depending on the specific gene affected. In these cases, the choice of which genes to test is often determined by unique clinical and family history features, the relative prevalence of mutations in various genes, or test availability.

■ METHODOLOGIC APPROACHES TO GENETIC TESTING

Genetic testing is performed in much the same way as other specialized laboratory tests. In the United States, genetic testing laboratories are Clinical Laboratory Improvement Act (CLIA) approved to ensure that they meet quality and proficiency standards. A useful information source for various genetic tests is *www.genetests.org*.

DNA testing is most commonly performed by DNA sequence analysis for mutations, although genotype can also be deduced through the study of RNA or protein (e.g., apoprotein E, hemoglobin, immunohistochemistry). For example, immunohistochemical analysis of colorectal cancers for absence of expression of mismatch repair proteins has been proposed as a strategy for universal Lynch syndrome screening. The determination of DNA sequence alterations relies heavily on the use of polymerase chain reaction (PCR), which allows rapid amplification and analysis of the gene of interest. In addition, PCR enables genetic testing on minimal amounts of DNA extracted from a wide range of tissue sources including leukocytes, mucosal epithelial cells, and archival tissues. Amplified DNA can be analyzed directly by DNA sequencing or it can be hybridized to DNA chips or blots to detect the presence of normal and altered

DNA sequences. Direct DNA sequencing is increasingly used for prenatal diagnosis as well as for determination of hereditary disease susceptibility. Analyses of large alterations in the genome are possible using cytogenetics, fluorescent in situ hybridization (FISH), or Southern blotting (Chap. 62).

Protein truncation tests (PTTs) are used to detect mutations that result in the premature termination of a polypeptide occurring during protein synthesis. In this assay, the isolated complementary DNA (cDNA) is transcribed and translated in vitro, and the protein is analyzed by gel electrophoresis. The truncated (mutant) gene product is readily identified as its electrophoretic mobility differs from that of the normal protein. This test has been used most commonly for analyses of large genes with significant genetic heterogeneity such as the *APC* gene.

Like all laboratory analyses, there are limitations to the accuracy and interpretation of genetic tests. In addition to technical errors, genetic tests are sometimes designed to detect only the most common mutations. In this case, a negative result must be qualified by the possibility that the individual may have a mutation that is not included in the test. In addition, a negative result does not mean that there is not a mutation in some other gene that causes a similar inherited disorder. A negative result, in those at risk for the disorder, is typically classified as *uninformative*.

In addition to molecular testing for established disease, genetic testing for susceptibility to chronic disease is being increasingly integrated into the practice of medicine. In most cases, however, the discovery of disease-associated genes has greatly outpaced studies that assess the clinical utility of genetic testing. Until such evidence-based studies are available, predictive molecular testing must be approached with caution and should be offered only to patients who have been adequately counseled and have provided informed consent. In the majority of cases, genetic testing should be offered only to individuals with a suggestive personal or family medical history or in the context of a clinical trial.

Predictive genetic testing falls into two distinct categories. *Presymptomatic testing* applies to diseases where a specific genetic alteration is associated with a near 100% likelihood of developing disease. In contrast, *predisposition testing* predicts a risk for disease that is less than 100%. For example, presymptomatic testing is available for those at risk for Huntington's disease, whereas predisposition testing is considered for those at risk for hereditary breast cancer. It is important to note that, for the majority of adult-onset, multifactorial genetic disorders, testing is only predictive. Test results cannot reveal with confidence whether, when, or how the disease will manifest itself. For example, not everyone with the apolipoprotein E allele (ε4) will develop Alzheimer's disease, and individuals without this genetic marker can still develop the disorder (Chap. 371).

Molecular analysis is generally more informative if testing is initiated in a symptomatic family member because the identification of a mutation can direct the testing of other at-risk family members (whether they are symptomatic or not). In the absence of additional familial or environmental risk factors, individuals who test negative for the mutation found in the affected family member can be informed that they are at general population risk for that particular disease. Furthermore, they can be reassured that they are not at risk for passing the mutation on to their children. On the other hand, asymptomatic family members who test positive for the known mutation must be informed that they are at increased risk for disease development and for transmitting the alteration to their children.

Clinicians providing pretest counseling and education should assess the patient's ability to understand and cope with test results. Individuals who demonstrate signs and symptoms of emotional distress should have their psychosocial needs addressed before proceeding with molecular testing. Generally, genetic testing should not be offered at a time of personal crisis or acute illness within the family. Patients will derive more benefit from test results if they are emotionally able to comprehend and absorb the information. It is important to assess a patient's preconceived notions of their personal likelihood of disease in preparing pretest educational strategies. Often, patients harbor unwarranted fear or denial of their likelihood of genetic risk.

Genetic testing has the potential of affecting the way individual family members relate to one another, both negatively and positively. As a result, patients addressing the option of molecular testing must consider how test results might impact their relationships with relatives, partners, spouses, and friends. In families with a known genetic mutation, those who test positive must consider the impact of their carrier status on their present and future lifestyles; those who test negative may manifest *survivor guilt.* Family members are likely to differ in their emotional and social responses to the same information. Counseling should also address the potential consequences of test results on relationships with a spouse or child. Parents who are found to have a disease-associated mutation often express considerable anxiety and despair as they address the issue of risk to their children.

When a condition does not manifest until adulthood, clinicians will be faced with the question of whether at-risk children should be offered molecular testing and, if so, at what age. Although the matter is debated, several professional organizations have cautioned that genetic testing for adult-onset disorders should not be offered to children. Many of these conditions are not preventable; consequently, such information can pose significant psychosocial risk to the child. In addition, there is concern that testing during childhood violates a child's right to make an informed decision regarding testing upon reaching adulthood. On the other hand, testing should be offered in childhood for disorders that may manifest early in life, especially when management options are available. For example, children at risk for familial adenomatous polyposis (FAP), associated with alterations in the *APC* gene, may develop polyps as early as their teens, and progression to an invasive cancer can occur by their twenties. Likewise, children at risk for MEN type 2, which is caused by mutations in the *RET* protooncogene, may develop medullary thyroid cancer early in childhood, and the issue of prophylactic thyroidectomy should be addressed with the parents of children with documented mutations (Chap. 351).

■ INFORMED CONSENT

When the issue of testing is addressed, patients should be strongly encouraged to involve other relatives in the decision-making process, because molecular diagnostics will likely have an impact on the entire family. Informed consent for molecular testing begins with detailed education and counseling (Fig. 63-3). The patient must fully understand the risks, benefits, and limitations of undergoing the analysis. Informed consent should include a written document, drafted clearly and concisely in a language and format that is comprehensible to the patient, who should be made aware of the disposition of test results. Informed consent should also include a discussion of the mechanics of testing. Most molecular testing for hereditary disease involves DNA-based analysis of peripheral blood. In the majority of circumstances, test results should be given only to the individual, in person, and preferably with a support person in the room.

Because molecular testing of an asymptomatic individual often allows prediction of future risk, the patient should understand any potential long-term medical, psychological, and social implications of this decision. In the United States, legislation affecting health insurance genetic discrimination has evolved through the Genetics Information Nondiscrimination Act. It is important to explore with the patient the potential impact that test results may have on employment and future health as well as disability and life insurance coverage.

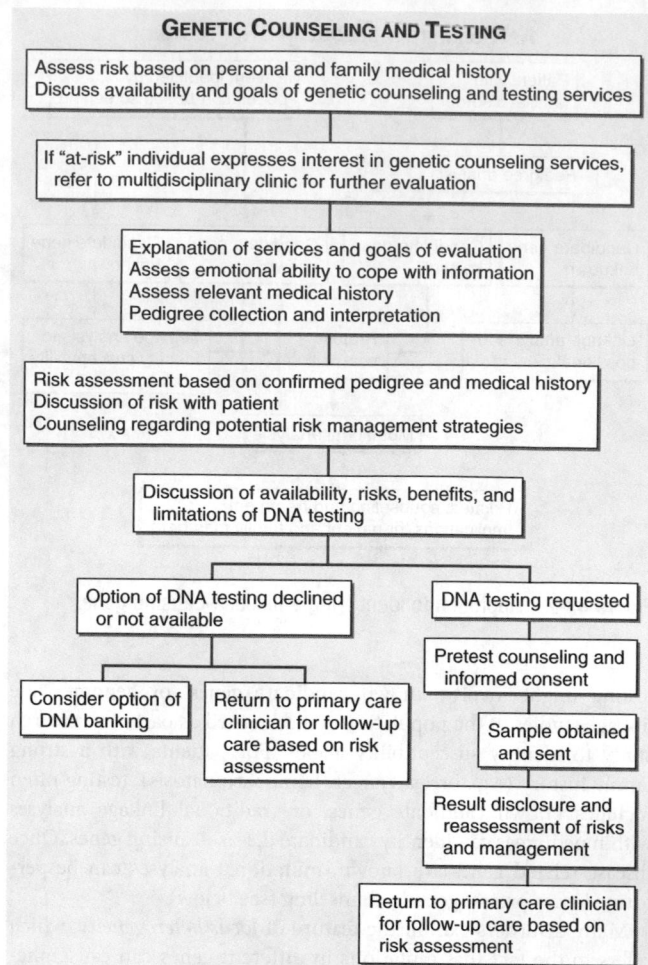

Figure 63-3 Algorithm for genetic counseling in association with genetic testing.

Patients should understand that alternatives to molecular analysis remain available if they decide not to proceed with this option. They should also be notified that testing is available in the future if they are not currently prepared to undergo analysis. The option of DNA banking should be presented so that samples are readily available for future use by family members, if needed.

■ FOLLOW-UP CARE AFTER TESTING

Depending on the nature of the genetic disorder, posttest interventions may include (1) cautious surveillance and appropriate health care screening, (2) specific medical interventions, (3) chemoprevention, (4) risk avoidance, and (5) referral to support services. For example, patients with known pathologic mutations in *BRCA1* or *BRCA2* are strongly encouraged to pursue risk-reducing bilateral salpingo-oophorectomy and are offered intensive screening as well as the option of risk-reducing mastectomy. In addition, such women may be eligible for preventive treatment with tamoxifen or enrollment in a chemoprevention clinical trial. In contrast, those at known risk for Huntington's disease are offered continued follow-up and supportive services, including physical and occupational therapy, and social services or support groups, as indicated. Specific interventions will change as translational research continues to enhance our understanding of these genetic diseases and as more is learned about the functions of the gene products involved.

Individuals who test negative for a mutation in a disease-associated gene identified in an affected family member must be reminded that they may still be at risk for the disease. This is of particular importance for common diseases such as diabetes mellitus, cancer, and coronary artery disease. For example, a woman who finds that she does not carry the disease-associated mutation in *BRCA2* previously discovered in her family must be reminded that she still requires the same breast cancer screening recommended for the general population.

GENETIC COUNSELING AND EDUCATION

Genetic counseling should be distinguished from genetic testing and screening, even though genetic counselors are often involved in issues related to testing. Genetic counseling refers to *a communication process that deals with human problems associated with the occurrence or risk of a genetic disorder in a family.* Genetic risk assessment is complex and often involves elements of uncertainty. Counseling, therefore, includes genetic education as well as psychosocial counseling. Genetic counselors may be called upon by other health care professionals (or by individual patients and families) to address a broad range of issues directly and indirectly related to genetic disease (Table 63-1). The role of the genetic counselor includes the following:

- Gather and document a detailed family history
- Educate patients about general genetic principles related to disease risk, both for themselves and for others in their family
- Assess and enhance the patient's ability to cope with the genetic information offered
- Discuss how nongenetic factors may relate to the ultimate expression of disease
- Address medical management issues
- Assist in determining the role of genetic testing for the individual and family
- Ensure that the patient is aware of the indications, process, risks, benefits, and limitations of the various genetic testing options
- Assist the patient, family, and referring physician in the interpretation of the test results
- Refer the patient and other at-risk family members for additional medical and support services, if necessary

The complexity of genetic counseling and the broad scope of genetic diseases have led to the development of specialized, multidisciplinary clinics designed to provide broad-based support and medical care for those at risk and their family members. Such specialty clinics are well established in the areas of cancer and neurodegenerative disorders and are developing in other areas such as cardiology. The multidisciplinary teams are often composed of medical geneticists, specialist physicians, genetic counselors, nurses, psychologists, social workers, and biomedical ethicists who work together to consider difficult diagnostic, treatment, and testing decisions. Such a format also provides primary care physicians with invaluable support and assistance as they follow and treat at-risk patients.

TABLE 63-1 Indications for Genetic Counseling

Advanced maternal (>35) or paternal (>50) age

Consanguinity

Previous history of a child with birth defects or a genetic disorder

Personal or family history suggestive of a genetic disorder

High-risk ethnic groups; known carriers of genetic alterations

Documented genetic alteration in a family member

Ultrasound or prenatal testing suggesting a genetic disorder

The approach to genetic counseling has important ethical, social, and financial implications. Philosophies related to genetic counseling vary widely by country and center. Counseling is generally offered in a nondirective manner, wherein patients learn to understand how their values factor into a particular medical decision. Nondirective counseling is particularly appropriate when there are no data demonstrating a clear benefit associated with a particular intervention or when an intervention is considered experimental. For example, nondirective genetic counseling is employed when a person is deciding whether to undergo genetic testing for Huntington's disease (Chap. 371). At this time, there is no clear benefit (in terms of medical outcome) to an at-risk individual undergoing genetic testing for this disease, because its course cannot be altered by therapeutic interventions. However, testing can have an important impact on this individual's perception of the future and his or her interpersonal relationships and plans for reproduction. Therefore, the decision to pursue testing rests on the individual's belief system and values. On the other hand, a more directive approach is appropriate when a condition can be treated. In a family with FAP, colon cancer screening and prophylactic colectomy should be recommended for known *APC* mutation carriers. The counselor and clinician following this family must ensure that the at-risk family members have access to the resources necessary to adhere to these recommendations.

Genetic education is central to an individual's ability to make an informed decision regarding testing options and treatment. Although genetic counselors represent one source of genetic education, other health care providers also need to contribute to patient education. Patients at risk for genetic disease should understand fundamental medical genetic principles and terminology relevant to their situation. This includes the concept of genes, how they are transmitted, and how they confer hereditary disease risk. An adequate knowledge of patterns of inheritance will allow patients to understand the probability of disease risk for themselves and other family members. It is also important to impart the concepts of disease penetrance and expression. For most complex adult-onset genetic disorders, asymptomatic patients should be advised that a positive test result does not always translate into future disease development. In addition, the role of nongenetic factors, such as environmental exposures, must be discussed in the context of multifactorial disease risk and disease prevention. Finally, patients should understand the natural history of the disease as well as the potential options for intervention, including screening, prevention, and—in certain circumstances— pharmacologic treatment or prophylactic surgery.

THERAPEUTIC INTERVENTIONS BASED ON GENETIC RISK FOR DISEASE

Specific treatments are now available for an increasing number of genetic disorders, whether identified through population-based screening or directed testing (Table 63-2). Although the strategies for therapeutic interventions are best developed for childhood hereditary metabolic diseases, these principles have made their way into the diagnosis and management of adult-onset disorders. Hereditary hemochromatosis illustrates many of the issues raised by the availability of genetic screening in the adult population. For instance, hemochromatosis is relatively common (approximately 1 in 200 individuals of northern European descent are homozygous), and its complications are potentially preventable through phlebotomy (Chap. 357). The identification of the *HFE* gene, mutations of which are associated with this syndrome, has sparked interest in the use of DNA-based testing for presymptomatic diagnosis of the disorder. However, up to one-third of individuals who are homozygous for the *HFE* mutation do not have evidence of iron overload. Consequently, in the absence of a positive family history, current recommendations include phenotypic screening for evidence of

TABLE 63-2 Examples of Genetic Testing and Possible Interventions

Genetic Disorder	Inheritance	Genes	Interventions
Oncologic			
Lynch syndrome	AD	MSH2, MLH1, MSH6, PMS2,	Early endoscopic screening
Familial adenomatous polyposis	AD	APC	Early endoscopic screening
			Nonsteroidal anti-inflammatory drugs
			Colectomy
Hereditary breast and ovarian cancer	AD	BRCA1, BRCA2	Estrogen receptor antagonists
			Early screening by exams, mammography, and breast MRI
			Risk-reducing surgery
Familial malignant melanoma	AD	CDKN2A, CDK4	Avoidance of UV light
			Screening and biopsies
Basal cell nevus syndrome	AD	PTCH	Avoidance of UV light
			Screening and biopsies
Hematologic			
Factor V Leiden	AD	F5	Avoidance of thrombogenic risk factors and oral contraceptives
Hemophilia A	XL	F8	Factor VIII replacement
Hemophilia B	XL	F9	Factor IX replacement
Glucose 6-PO$_4$ dehydrogenase deficiency	XL	G6PD	Avoidance of oxidant drugs
Cardiovascular			
Hypertrophic cardiomyopathy	AD	MYH7, MYBPC3, TNNT2, TPM1	Echocardiographic screening
			Early pharmacologic intervention
			Myomectomy
Long QT syndrome	AD, AR	KCNQ1, SCN5A, KCNE1, KCNE2	Electrocardiographic screening
			Early pharmacologic intervention
			Implantable cardioverter defibrillator devices
Marfan syndrome	AD	FBN1	Echocardiographic screening
			Prophylactic beta blockers or ACE inhibitors
Gastrointestinal			
Familial Mediterranean fever	AR	MEFV	Colchicine treatment
Hemochromatosis	AR	HFE	Phlebotomy
Pulmonary			
α_1 Antitrypsin deficiency	AR	SERPINA1	Avoidance of smoking
			Avoidance of occupational and environmental toxins
Primary pulmonary hypertension	AD	BMPR2	Pharmacologic intervention
			Lung transplantation
Renal			
Polycystic kidney disease	AD	PKD1, PKD2	Prevention of hypertension
			Prevention of urinary tract infections
			Kidney transplantation
Nephrogenic diabetes insipidus	XL, AR	AVPR2, AQP2	Fluid replacement
			Thiazides with or without amiloride
Endocrine			
Neurohypophyseal diabetes insipidus	AD	AVP	Replace vasopressin
Maturity-onset diabetes of the young	AD	Multiple genes	Screen and treat for diabetes
Familial hypocalciuric hypercalcemia	AD	CASR	Avoidance of parathyroidectomy
Kallmann syndrome	XL	KAL	Induction of puberty with hormone replacement

(continued)

Genetic Disorder	Inheritance	Genes	Interventions
Multiple endocrine neoplasia type 2	AD	*RET*	Prophylactic thyroidectomy
			Screening for pheochromocytoma and hyperparathyroidism
21-hydroxylase deficiency	AR	*CYP21*	Glucocorticoid and mineralocorticoid treatment
Neurologic			
Malignant hyperthermia	AD	*RYR1, CACNA1S*	Avoidance of precipitating anesthetics
Hyperkalemic periodic paralysis	AD	*SCN4A*	Diet rich in carbohydrates and low in potassium
			Avoidance of fasting, strenuous work, or cold temperatures
			Thiazides or acetazolamide
Adrenoleukodystrophy	XL	*ABCD1*	Possible bone marrow transplantation for childhood cerebral form
Duchenne and Becker muscular dystrophy	XL	*DMD*	Corticosteroids
Familial Parkinson disease	AD, AR	*SNCA, PARK2, PINK1, PARK7, LRRK2*	Amantadine, anticholinergics, levodopa, monoamine oxidase B inhibitors
Wilson disease	AR	*ATP7B*	Zinc, trientene

Abbreviations: AD, autosomal dominant; AR, autosomal recessive; CNS, central nervous system; MRI, magnetic resonance imaging; XL, X-linked.

iron overload followed by genetic testing. Whether genetic screening for hemochromatosis will someday be coupled to assessment of phenotypic expression awaits further studies. In contrast to the issue of population screening, it is important to test and counsel other family members when the diagnosis of hemochromatosis has been made in a proband. Testing allows the physician to exclude family members who are not at risk. It also permits presymptomatic detection of iron overload and the institution of treatment (phlebotomy) before the development of organ damage.

Preventive measures and therapeutic interventions are not restricted to metabolic disorders. Identification of familial forms of long QT syndrome, associated with ventricular arrhythmias, allows early electrocardiographic testing and the use of prophylactic antiarrhythmic therapy, overdrive pacemakers, or defibrillators (Chap. 233). Individuals with familial hypertrophic cardiomyopathy can be screened by ultrasound, treated with beta blockers or other drugs, and counseled about the importance of avoiding strenuous exercise and dehydration (Chap. 238). Likewise, individuals with Marfan syndrome can be treated with beta blockers or ACE inhibitors and monitored for the development of aortic aneurysms (Chap. 248). Individuals with α_1 antitrypsin deficiency can be strongly counseled to avoid cigarette smoking and exposure to environmental pulmonary and hepatotoxins. Various host genes influence the pathogenesis of certain infectious diseases in humans, including HIV (Chap. 189). The factor V Leiden allele increases risk of thrombosis (Chap. 58). Approximately 3% of the worldwide population is heterozygous for this mutation. Moreover, it is found in up to 25% of patients with recurrent deep vein thrombosis or pulmonary embolism. Women who are heterozygous or homozygous for this allele should, therefore, avoid the use of oral contraceptives.

The field of pharmacogenomics seeks to identify genes that alter drug metabolism or confer susceptibility to toxic drug reactions. Pharmacogenomics permits individualized drug therapy, resulting in improved treatment outcomes, reduced toxicities, and more cost-effective pharmaceutical care. Examples include succinylcholine sensitivity, thiopurine methyltransferase (TPMT) deficiency, malignant hyperthermia, dihydropyrimidine dehydrogenase deficiency, the porphyrias, and glucose-6-phosphate dehydrogenase (G6PD) deficiency.

As noted above, the identification of genes that increase the risk of specific types of neoplasia is rapidly changing the management of many cancers. Identifying family members with mutations that predispose to FAP or Lynch syndrome can lead to recommendations of early cancer screening or prophylactic surgery (Chap. 91). Similar principles apply to familial forms of melanoma; basal cell carcinoma; and cancers of the breast, ovary, and thyroid gland. It should be recognized, however, that most cancers harbor several distinct genetic abnormalities by the time they acquire invasive or metastatic potential (Chaps. 83 and 84). Consequently, the major impact of genetic testing in these cases is to allow more intensive management, including disease prevention and screening, as it remains very challenging to predict disease penetrance, expression, or clinical course.

Although genetic diagnosis of these and other disorders is still evolving in the clinical setting, predictive testing holds the promise of allowing earlier and more targeted interventions that can reduce morbidity and mortality rates. We can expect the availability of genetic tests to expand, including direct-to-consumer options. A critical challenge for physicians and other health care providers is to keep pace with these advances in genetic medicine and to implement testing judiciously.

FURTHER READINGS

BRAND A et al: The impact of genetics and genomics on public health. Eur J Hum Genet 16:5, 2008

CLAYTON EW: Ethical, legal, and social implications of genomic medicine. N Engl J Med 349:562, 2003

FEERO WG et al: Genomic medicine–an updated primer. N Engl J Med 362:2001, 2010

GREEN NS et al: Newborn screening: Complexities in universal genetic testing. Am J Public Health 96 1955, 2006

HARPER PS: *Practical Genetic Counseling*, 5th ed. Oxford, Butterworth Heinmann, 1998

LUMBRERAS B, et al: Assessing the social meaning, value and implications of research in genomics. J Epidemiol Community Health 61:755, 2007

CHAPTER 64

The Human Microbiome

Jeffrey I. Gordon

Rob Knight

The words *well-being* and *microbes* typically are not spoken in the same breath. Microbes have a strong negative connotation in contemporary societies and are viewed in a warlike context. Disease-producing or pathogenic microbes are indeed serious threats to human health and have received justifiable attention from the inception of the field of microbiology. The list of known and notorious pathogens is long. However, most human encounters with microbes are not hostile but benign or even beneficial. Advances in DNA sequencing and computational biology now permit comprehensive description of the composition of and the roles played by the microbial communities (*microbiota*) associated with the human body.

Like all animals on the planet, humans have had to adapt to a microbe-dominated biosphere. The number of microbes on Earth is staggering. It has been estimated that 10^{30} microbes live in the ocean, in surface and subsurface terrestrial ecosystems, and on and inside animals and plants. Microbes, which are defined here as microscopic living organisms that belong to any of the three known domains of life on Earth (Bacteria, Archaea, and Eukarya), inhabit the exposed exterior and interior surfaces of the human body (e.g., the skin, mouth, airways, gastrointestinal tract, and vagina). The uterus traditionally has been thought to be microbe-free, although new evidence may prompt a reevaluation of the idea that this ecosystem is completely sterile throughout gestation. Colonization with microbes begins no later than during parturition; in the ensuing years, microbes come to outnumber human cells by an estimated tenfold in the human body. Therefore, a comprehensive view of humans as a life form entails consideration of the body's microbial and *Homo sapiens* cells together as a connected network—a coevolved symbiosis ("living together")—in which various body habitats serve as homes to microbial communities. These habitats harbor microbiota composed of members that function as mutualists (both host and microbe benefit from the other's presence), commensals (one partner benefits, and the other is seemingly unaffected), and potential or overt pathogens (one partner benefits, and the other is harmed).

■ HUMAN MICROBIOME PROJECTS

Human microbiome projects (HMPs) reflect this view of the human body as an amalgamation of human and microbial cells as well as human and microbial genes. These projects represent a confluence of ongoing technical and computational advances in the genome sciences. The newest generation of massively parallel DNA sequencers can be used to document—with unprecedented speed and economy—which microbes compose a microbiota and to characterize a microbiota's gene content (its *microbiome*). Key terms relevant to HMPs are defined in Table 64-1.

Computing power and software tools are evolving rapidly to mine the vast amount of data generated by these sequencers. The coevolution of software development and ever-increasing dataset generation is not surprising. In systems ranging from artificial organisms to bacteria to metazoa, coevolution of predators and prey greatly accelerates the evolutionary rate. Dawkins and Krebs

(1979) introduced the concept of an "arms race" in which the predator has a clear advantage in developing better means for consuming its prey and the prey has a clear advantage in developing better means to avoid being eaten. Adaptation to evade a population that is itself adapting proceeds at a far more rapid rate than does adaptation to an environment that can change but cannot evolve in an adaptive way. The same dynamics are apparent in software development: the "consumers" of software produce ever-larger data sets that break the software, in part because the availability of these resources prompts new strategies for exploitation (i.e., the design of experiments that could not have been conceived without the availability of the improved tools). This intimate association between tool users and tool developers is essential for rapid development in terms of what the software can accomplish and what experiments can be conceived and accomplished in HMPs. HMPs also reflect a more ecologic focus of microbiology on the properties and functions of microbial communities; that is, these projects go beyond the properties and functions that individual component species of these communities exhibit when studied in isolation—i.e., outside their native environments.

The ability to characterize the structures and functions of whole microbial communities without culturing their component members has spawned a new field of science known as *metagenomics* (Table 64-1). Metagenomics involves the sequencing of DNA isolated directly from a microbial community residing in a particular environment; the resulting information permits the application of other systems-level techniques, such as profiling of mRNA and protein products expressed by a microbiome and characterization of a community's metabolic activities. The goal of metagenomics (these allied systemwide characterizations) and of HMPs in general is an understanding of the ecologic principles and the various factors that determine how microbial communities are assembled, are maintained, and operate. The results promise to provide a deeper understanding of how habitats and microbial communities coevolve and, in the case of humans, how these communities vary both compositionally and functionally over time at different anatomic sites within an individual and in different groups of people living in different cultural contexts as well as how these communities contribute to human physiologic status, physiologic variation, disease predisposition, and disease pathogenesis.

Furthermore, HMPs address one of the most fundamental questions in genetics: How does environment influence the structure and function of "human genes"? Over a lifetime, each human encounters a unique environment. Part of this personally experienced environment is incorporated into the body habitat–associated microbiota. In this sense, HMPs will expand the conceptualization of "human" genetic potential from a relatively fixed deterministic view in which individuals are seen as inheriting only a defined set of ~20,000 genes from their parents to a view in which each human acquires a microbiome containing a varied assemblage of genes several orders of magnitude larger than the collected *H. sapiens* genes through a process influenced by family, lifestyle, and life experiences as well as by *H. sapiens* genes. International HMPs probably will help determine whether there is a dimension of human evolution that is occurring at the level of the human microbiota and microbiome and—if so—whether, how, and how fast this microbial evolution may be affecting human biology. Finally, these projects probably will raise a number of important questions about personal identity, how to define the origins of health disparities, and issues related to privacy and confidentiality.

TABLE 64-1 Glossary of Terms Used in Discussion of the Human Microbiome

Term	Definition
Culture-independent analysis	A type of analysis that does not require culture of microbes. Information is extracted directly from environmental samples.
Diversity	The distribution of different kinds of organisms in a specific habitat or habitats. *Alpha* diversity is, broadly speaking, the number of kinds of organisms in a single sample; *beta* diversity describes how the types of organisms are partitioned among samples.
Domains of life	The three major branches of life on Earth: the Eukarya (including humans), the Bacteria, and the Archaea
Gnotobiotics	Rearing of animals under sterile (germ-free) conditions. Animals subsequently can be colonized at various stages of their life cycle with defined collections of microbes.
Human microbiome	In ecology, *biome* refers to a habitat and the organisms in it. In this sense, the human *microbiome* would be defined as the collection of microorganisms associated with the human body. However, the term *microbiome* is also used to refer to the collective genomes and genes present in members of a particular microbiota, and the human *metagenome* is the sum of the human genome and microbial genes (microbiome). A *core* human microbiome is defined as everything shared in a particular body habitat among all or the vast majority of human microbiomes. A core microbiome may include a common set of genomes and genes encoding various protein families and/or metabolic capabilities. Microbial genes that are variably represented in different humans may contribute to distinctive physiologic/metabolic phenotypes.
Metagenomics	An emerging field encompassing culture-independent studies of the structures and functions of microbial communities and their interactions with the habitats they occupy. Metagenomics includes (1) shotgun sequencing of microbial DNA isolated directly from a particular environment and (2) high-throughput screening of expression libraries constructed from cloned community DNA to identify specific functions such as antibiotic resistance (*functional* metagenomics). DNA-level analyses provide the foundation for profiling of mRNAs and proteins produced by a microbiome (*meta-transcriptomics* and *meta-proteomics*) and for identification of a community's metabolic network (*meta-metabolomics*).
Microbiota	A microbial community, including Bacteria, Archaea, Eukarya, and viruses, that occupies a specific habitat
Pan-genome	The group of genes found in genomes that make up a particular microbial phylotype, including *core* genes found in all genomes and *dispensable* genes found in a subset of genomes within the phylotype
Phylogenetic analysis	Characterization of the evolutionary relationships between organisms and their gene products
Phylogenetic tree	A "tree" in which organisms are shown according to their relationships to hypothetical common ancestors. When built from molecular sequences, the branch lengths are proportional to the amount of evolutionary change separating each ancestor-descendant pair.
Phylotype	A phylogenetic group of microbes, currently defined by a threshold percentage identity shared among their small subunit rRNA genes (e.g., ≥97% for a species-level phylotype)
Rarefaction	A procedure in which subsampling is used to assess whether all the diversity present in a specific sample or set of samples has been observed at a specific sampling depth and to extrapolate how much additional sampling would be needed to observe all the diversity
Resilience	A community's ability to return to its initial state after a perturbation

■ A TOOLBOX FOR CULTURE-INDEPENDENT METAGENOMIC ANALYSES OF MICROBIAL COMMUNITIES

Most members of complex microbial communities cannot be cultured by conventional laboratory techniques. The vast microbial diversity that exists inside and on the human body cannot be characterized with culture-based approaches, in large part because the metabolic milieu fashioned by these communities in their native habitats cannot be duplicated in vitro at this time. Therefore, investigators have turned to culture-independent methods to identify which organisms are present in a microbiota and in what abundance. The gene widely used to identify microorganisms and classify their evolutionary relationships encodes the major RNA component of the small subunit (SSU) of ribosomes. The SSU rRNA gene has been highly conserved among all known life forms on Earth. This conservation allows SSU rRNA genes from different organisms to be aligned accurately so that regions of nucleotide sequence variation can be identified readily. Pairwise comparisons of SSU rRNA gene sequences from different microbes allow the construction of a phylogenetic tree that represents an evolutionary map; previously unknown organisms can then be assigned a location (coordinate) on that map. This approach, known as *molecular phylogenetics*, allows each organism to be characterized on the basis of its evolutionary distance from other organisms. Different phylogenetic types (phylotypes) can be viewed as branches on an evolutionary tree.

The most straightforward way to define which microbes are present in microbial communities associated with the human body is to amplify SSU rRNA genes by polymerase chain reaction (PCR), using primers directed at regions with nucleotide sequences that are conserved among all bacteria (or archaea or eukaryota) and that flank more variable regions. These variable regions can be used to discriminate among different kinds of organisms belonging to each of the three domains of life. Because bacteria dominate human microbial communities, most efforts have been devoted to defining bacterial diversity in the microbiota.

The coevolution of high-throughput next-generation DNA sequencing with new software tools has led to an SSU rRNA renaissance that allows simultaneous characterization of the diversity present in hundreds to thousands of microbial communities. Sequencing of a small fragment of the 1500-bp (base pair) bacterial 16S rRNA gene has been found to be sufficient for many types of analysis. For example, 250-base reads encompassing a variable region of the gene are suitable for taxonomic assignments and microbial community comparisons provided that the region is chosen carefully. Primer design for PCR of bacterial 16S rRNA genes is a critical factor: differential annealing with different primer pairs designed to amplify different variable regions can lead to over- or underrepresentation of specific taxonomic groups (*taxa*), and different regions within the gene can have somewhat different patterns of evolution. Therefore, caution must be exercised in comparisons of the relative abundance of taxa in samples characterized in different studies using different methods.

A key innovation has been multiplex sequencing with highly parallel DNA sequencers that can generate large numbers of sequences with read lengths of ≥200 nucleotides. Amplicons generated from each microbial-community DNA sample are tagged by incorporation of a unique oligonucleotide barcode into the primer. Amplicons that harbor these sample-specific barcodes can be pooled together so that multiple samples representing multiple communities can be sequenced simultaneously (Fig. 64-1).

One important choice in multiplex barcoded sequencing involves a trade-off between the number of samples that can be processed simultaneously and the number of sequences per sample, which in turn depends on the expected size of the differences between microbial communities. Differences in the microbiota between individuals or between communities occupying different body habitats in the same individual are large; therefore, relatively few (<1000) SSU rRNA reads are required for discrimination among communities. However, the identification of systematic differences in community ecology that correlate with physiologic or pathophysiologic status is confounded by this immense interpersonal variation. For example, 1000 sequences per sample means that species present at 1% abundance can be identified with reasonable confidence, although this

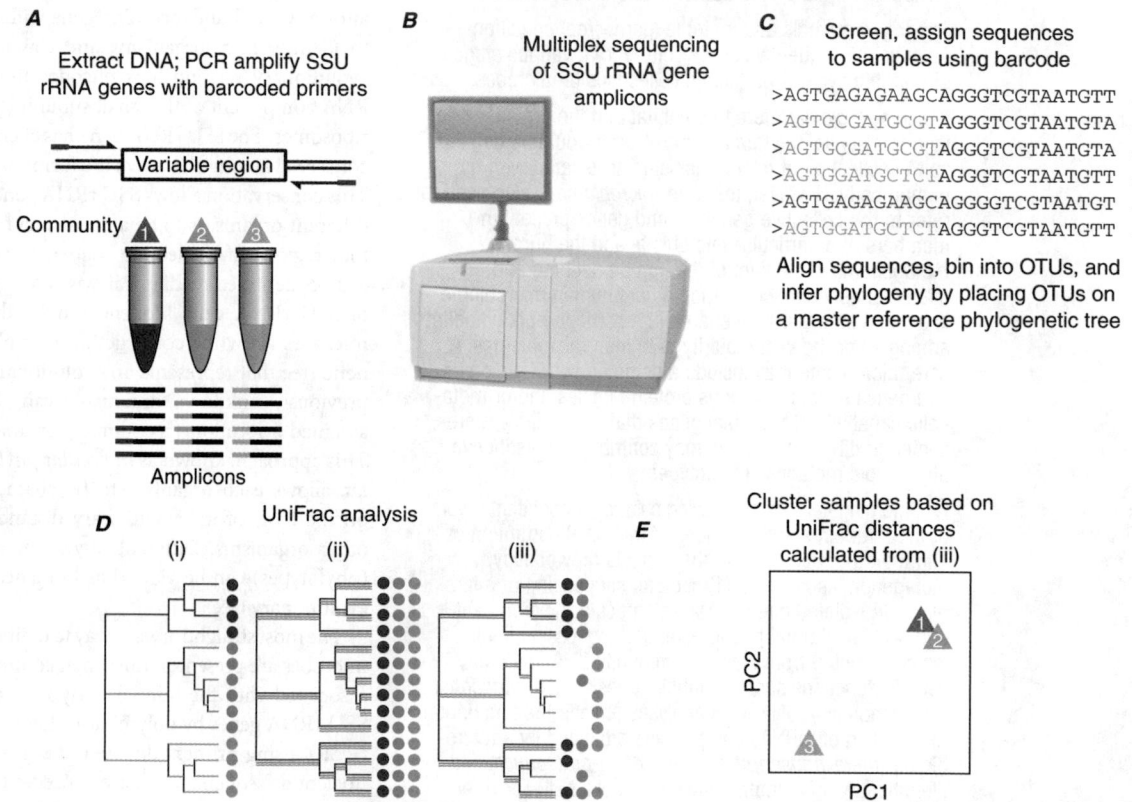

Figure 64-1   Pipeline for culture-independent studies of a microbiota. *(A)* DNA is extracted directly from a sampled human body habitat–associated microbial community. The precise location of the community and relevant patient meta-data are collected. Polymerase chain reaction (PCR) is used to amplify portions of the bacterial 16S rRNA gene containing one or more variable regions. Primers with sample-specific, error-correcting barcodes are designed to recognize the more conserved regions of the 16S rRNA gene that flank the targeted variable region(s). *(B)* Barcoded amplicons from multiple samples (communities 1–3) are pooled and sequenced in batches in a highly parallel next-generation DNA sequencer. *(C)* The resulting reads are processed. Barcodes denote which sample the sequence came from. After barcode sequences are removed in silico, reads are aligned and grouped according to a specified level of shared identity; e.g., sequences that share ≥97% nucleotide sequence identity are regarded as representing a species. Once reads are binned in this fashion, they are placed on a phylogenetic tree of all known bacteria to infer their phylogeny. *(D)* Communities can be compared to one another by either taxon-based methods, in which phylogeny is not considered and the number of shared taxa is simply scored, or phylogenetic methods, in which community similarity is considered in light of the evolutionary relationships of community members. The UniFrac metric is commonly used for phylogenetic-based comparisons. In the three stylized examples here, communities with varying degrees of similarity are shown. Each circle represents an operational taxonomic unit (OTU) which is colored

according to its community of origin and placed on a master phylogenetic tree that includes all lineages from all communities. Branches (*horizontal lines*) are colored with each community that contains members from that branch. Examples (i), (ii), and (iii) vary in the amount of branch length shared between the OTUs from each community. In (i), there is no shared branch length, and the three communities have a similarity score of 0. In (ii), the communities are identical and are assigned a similarity score of 1. In (iii), there is an intermediate level of similarity. Communities represented in red and green share more branch length and thus have a higher similarity score than red versus blue or green versus blue. The amount of shared branch length in each pairwise community comparison provides a distance matrix. *(E)* The results of taxon- or phylogenetic-based distance matrices can be displayed by principal coordinates analysis (PCoA), in which each community is plotted spatially such that the largest component of variance is captured on the x axis (PC1) and the second largest component of variance is displayed on the y axis (PC2). In the example shown, the three communities in (iii) from panel D are compared. Note that for shotgun sequencing of whole-community DNA (microbiome analysis), reads are compared with genes present in the genomes of sequenced cultured microbes and/or with genes that have been annotated by hierarchical classification schemes in various databases, such as KEGG. Communities can then be compared according to the distribution of functional groups in their microbiomes (in a manner analogous to taxon-based methods for 16S rRNA-based comparisons) and the results plotted by PCoA.

level of coverage will fail to identify many of the rarer species-level phylotypes that may provide critical functions for using specific nutrients or for triggering immune responses that greatly affect other components of the microbiota.

The capacity to perform multiplex sequencing of bacterial 16S rRNA genes with highly parallel sequencers creates a problem: traditional tools for aligning sequences and defining taxonomic groups by their sequence similarity [a process known as *picking operational taxonomic units* (OTUs)] and traditional methods for phylogenetic analyses cannot handle the vast data sets involved. Emerging tools for performing large-scale alignments and large-scale taxon-based and phylogenetic analyses are starting to resolve this issue.

Both taxon-based methods (analyses based only on the OTUs present regardless of their evolutionary relationships) and phylogenetic methods (compositional analyses considered in light of the evolutionary relationships of community members) can be useful. The advantages of taxon-based methods are that they reveal directly which taxa contribute to the similarities and differences among samples (communities) and do not rely on possibly inaccurate tree reconstructions. The advantages of phylogenetic methods are that, with the same input data, they use a more accurate picture of evolution to provide clearer results than do taxon-based methods. Unlike taxon-based methods, phylogenetic methods do not assume that all taxa are equally related to one another.

UniFrac, a commonly used phylogenetic method that compares the evolutionary history encompassed within different microbial communities, can be used to compare any two communities by noting the degree to which they share branch length on a master tree of microbial life: the more similar communities are to one another, the more branch length they will share (Fig. 64-1). A matrix of UniFrac-based measurements of distances between each pair of communities can be generated and the results graphed by principal coordinates analysis (PCoA), nonmetric multidimensional scaling (NMDS), or other geometric techniques that project a high-dimensional data set down onto a small number of dimensions that can be visualized and analyzed conveniently. The resulting dimensions show, in descending order, orthogonal contributions to variation in the full data set (Fig. 64-1).

Another level of analysis entails estimation of the richness, or diversity, of a microbial community by plotting the number of different types of SSU rRNA sequences at a specific phylogenetic level (e.g., species, genus) that are identified in a sample as a function of the number of sequences collected. Diversity estimates typically are based on rarefaction procedures, which assess how many species (or genera, etc.) would have been observed in a given sample if only 100, 200, 300, or more sequences had been collected.

■ ASSEMBLING A BACTERIAL 16S rRNA-BASED ATLAS OF THE HUMAN BODY

At several levels, humans are very much alike: their *H. sapiens* genomes are >99% identical, and they have similar collections of human cells. However, microbial communities differ drastically both between people and between habitats within a single human body. The variation is greatest between body sites; for example, the difference between the microbial communities residing in a person's mouth and those residing in that person's gut is comparable to the difference between the communities found in soil and in seawater. Even within a body site, the differences between people are not subtle: both gut and hand communities can differ by 80–90% at the bacterial species level, although the degree of variation in the mouth appears to be somewhat less (see below). The poet John Donne said that "no man is an island"; from a microbial perspective, however, each person consists of not just one isolated island but a whole archipelago of distinct habitats that exchange microbes with one another and with the "outside" at some undetermined level.

As with other ecosystems, human body habitat–associated microbial communities vary over time, and an understanding of this variation is probably essential to a functional understanding of the human microbiota. For example, studies of forests would prove puzzling without an understanding of the succession of events during which plant communities change systematically over time from weedy species colonizing fields to large mature trees. One exciting area opened up by high-throughput sequencing is the potential for tracking multiple body locations in multiple individuals over time, with direct visualization of the flow of microbes among different body habitats and different individuals in the presence or absence of various perturbations, such as antibiotic administration.

International HMPs must address a number of issues during the cataloging of microbial communities that inhabit humans. How many people have to be sampled (breadth) and how extensively (depth) to get a true measure of the extent of microbial diversity in humans? Where and how can investigators consistently sample a defined region of body habitat? In sampling relatively inaccessible microbial communities deep in the interior of the body, how can the risk to the donor be minimized? Defining the spatial features of microbial community structure in the mouth and the skin poses a particularly daunting challenge; for example, there is evidence that each tooth in an individual has a distinctive microbiota and that brushing produces a dramatic, immediate reduction in diversity. How often and over what period should a human being be sampled? What are the effects of gender? What is the impact of a person's relationship to family members who may or may not be sharing living space? What demographic factors should be evaluated (e.g., rural versus urban)? What is the impact of culture, lifestyle, health status, medications, and *H. sapiens* genotype?

Ecologists, who study the macroscopic world of plants and animals, have shown that the composition of a community depends on the order of initial entry of the component species. The same thing is probably true in the microbial world. Studies of bacterial diversity in fecal samples obtained from young adult female mono- and dizygotic twin pairs and their mothers over time have revealed that (1) the communities with the greatest degree of similarity are those derived from the same individual, (2) the similarity in the gut bacterial communities of adult monozygotic twin pairs is not significantly different in degree from the similarity of those of dizygotic twin pairs, and (3) fecal communities are more similar within family members than between members of different families. These results emphasize that early environmental exposures are a critical determinant of adult-gut microbial ecology. In humans, initial exposures depend on the mode of delivery. Babies sampled within 20 min of birth have relatively undifferentiated microbial communities in the mouth, the skin, and the gut. For vaginally delivered babies, these communities resemble the specific microbial communities found in the mother's vagina; for babies delivered by cesarean section, the communities resemble the mother's skin communities. The infant-gut microbiota changes to resemble the adult-gut community over the first 3 years of life and may continue to change throughout life. The stages at which communities in other body habitats reach their highly differentiated adult forms have not been determined.

An initial integrated view of the spatial and temporal distribution of bacteria in the human body has been obtained from a survey of communities of microbiota occupying 27 sites in a few healthy unrelated men and women. The body habitats sampled (on a given day for 2 consecutive days on two occasions separated by 3 months) included the gut (feces), the oral cavity, the external auditory canals, the inside of the nares, and 18 distinct skin locations (Fig. 64-2). Across all body habitats, members of 22 bacterial phyla were detected, but the vast majority of sequences belonged to only four bacterial phyla: Actinobacteria (37%), Firmicutes (34%), Proteobacteria (12%), and Bacteroidetes (10%). UniFrac-based

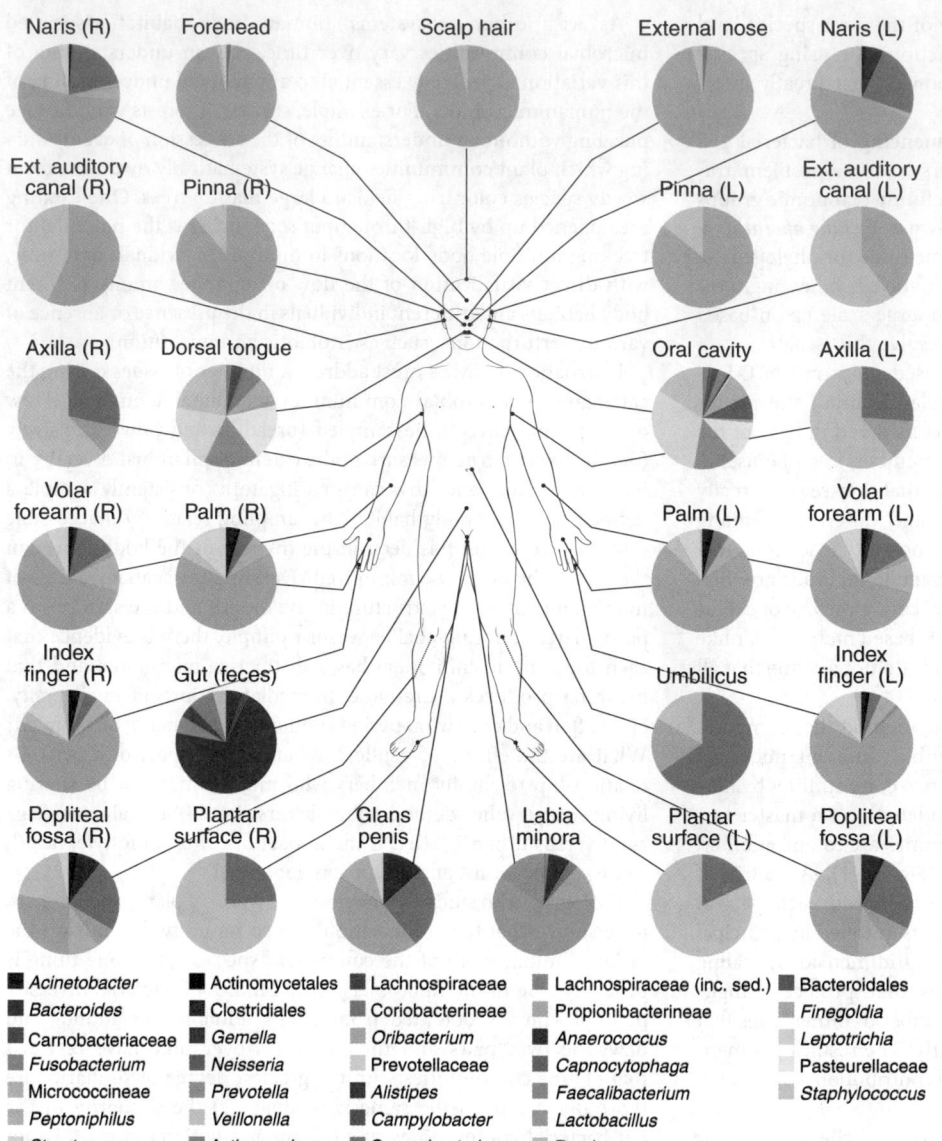

Figure 64-2   Results of a 16S rRNA gene sequence–based study of bacterial diversity in 27 body habitats of nine unrelated healthy human adults. The relative proportions of major phylogenetic groups present in the various microbial communities are shown. Note that skin communities occupying comparable positions on the right and left sides of the body are similar. *(Adapted from Costello et al.)*

PCoA revealed strong primary clustering by body habitat; community composition was significantly less varied within than between habitats. Within habitats, the degree of variation was significantly less within individuals sampled over time than between individuals sampled on a specific day. Finally, after habitat and individual had been taken into account, the degree of variation was significantly less over 1 day than over 3 months. People's daily composite "whole-body" communities revealed perfect grouping by host and month, further emphasizing that the personal microbiota signature remains relatively stable over time.

Several surveys have emphasized that the skin harbors communities with predictable, albeit complex, biogeographic features (Fig. 64-2). To determine whether these differences reflect differences in local environmental factors, the history of the exposure of a specific site to microbes, or both, reciprocal microbiota transplantation has been performed in which microbial communities from one region of the skin are depleted by treatment with germicidal agents and the region (plot) is inoculated with a "foreign" microbiota harvested from different regions of the skin

or from different body habitats from the same person or another individual. Community assembly at the site of transplantation subsequently is tracked over time. Remarkably, assembly proceeds differently at different sites: forearm plots receiving a tongue microbiota remained more similar to tongue communities than to native forearm communities in terms of their composition and diversity. However, forehead plots inoculated with tongue bacteria evolved to become more similar to native forehead communities. Thus, it appears that environmental factors operating at the forehead plot, in addition to the history of exposure to tongue bacteria, shaped community assembly.

These results underscore the need to specify body habitat when conducting microbial surveillance studies designed to examine the flow of normal and pathogenic organisms into and out of different body sites in inpatients and their health care providers. They also tie together several emerging themes from studies of human-associated microbial communities. Notably, there is a high level of *inter*personal variability in every body habitat studied to date. *Intra*personal variation in a specific body habitat is less marked, making longitudinal studies of microbial community ecology in a person before, during, or after a perturbation (e.g., dietary, pharmacologic) an attractive study option.

The resilience of human-associated microbial communities after perturbation has been addressed in several other contexts. One study showed that hand washing led to profound changes in the microbial community, greatly increasing diversity (presumably because of the preferential removal of high-abundance dominant phylotypes such as *Propionibacterium*). Within 6 h, the microbiota had rebounded to resemble the original hand communities. In adults, studies of a few individuals who took a 5-day course of ciprofloxacin showed that restoration of the fecal community after antibiotic administration took several months. Both the nature and the time course of restoration (reconfiguration) varied with the individual. Most previously present taxa returned, although in different proportions. The effects of antibiotics given during the first year of life on the assembly of the microbiota are ill defined. Are these effects transient or persistent? Is the diversity of the adult microbiota affected? Intriguingly, the "hygiene hypothesis" links the development of the human immune system to microbial exposures early in life. Increasing evidence indicates that fewer exposures and less conditioning are associated with an increased risk of allergic disorders such as asthma and various food sensitivities.

Bacterial 16S rRNA–based studies of the midvaginal microbiota in sexually active asymptomatic women have documented significant differences in community configurations among four self-reported ethnic groups (women of white, black, Hispanic, and Asian ancestry). Unlike most other body habitats surveyed, this eco-system is dominated by a single genus, *Lactobacillus*. Four species of this genus together make up more than one-half the bacteria in most of these communities. Five community groups, designated I–V, have been defined. Four groups are dominated by *L. iners, L. crispatus, L. gasseri,* or *L. jensii,* whereas the fifth group includes proportion-ally fewer members of this genus and more anaerobes. The repre-sentation of these community categories was very distinctive within each of the four ethnic groups and correlated with vaginal pH and Nugent scores (a biomarker for bacterial vaginosis). Identification of the factors that determine the assembly of these distinct commu-nities within and between ethnic groups as well as their resistance to or resilience after various physiologic or pathologic perturba-tions will require extensive longitudinal studies within individuals, including assessment of the impact of menstrual cycle, age, preg-nancy, vaginal infections, and antibiotic use.

■ WHO ELSE IS THERE? OTHER BRANCHES OF THE TREE OF LIFE REPRESENTED IN THE HUMAN BODY

Surveys based on SSU rRNA sequencing have focused largely on bacteria, yet the census of "who's there" in human body habitat–associated communities ultimately must take into account the other two domains of life (Archaea and Eukarya) as well as viruses. The representation of the four major Archaea phyla (Euryarchaeota, Crenarchaeota, Nanoarchaeota, and Korarchaeota) in human micro-bial communities and their contributions to community functions are largely ill defined, in part because of the difficulty in optimizing Archaea-directed primer design. Some archaeons are known to play key roles in community metabolism. For example, methane-producing archaeons (methanogens) make up as many as 10% of all anaerobes in the feces of some humans, yet archaeal diversity in the gut microbiota appears to be low, with *Methanobrevibacter smithii* being the dominant species. Gut methanogens improve the effi-ciency of dietary polysaccharide degradation and fermentation by preventing the buildup of hydrogen gas, an end product of fermen-tation. It is not a particularly rewarding job: the task of coupling H_2 oxidation with CO_2 reduction to produce methane (CH_4) is one of the lowest-energy-yielding reactions known in biology.

Culture-independent surveys of eukaryotic diversity in body habitat–associated communities of microbiota have been very limited to date. Information about the representation of members of this domain of life has important implications for defining "normal"; for example, eukaryotic parasites are represented in millions of hosts living in various parts of the world and may be construed as a component of "normal" in these regions. Culture-independent analyses have relied on targeting eukaryotic SSU rRNA genes that encode 18S rRNA as well as the internal transcribed spacer (ITS) regions of fungal rRNA genes. Metagenomic studies of the fecal microbiota of a few healthy human adults indicate that the degree of eukaryotic diversity is lower than that of bacterial diversity, with prominent representation of members of the genus *Blastocystis*—obligate anaerobes with a wide host range whose role as parasites or pathogens in the human gut ecosystem is not clear. The fecal microbiota of these healthy humans also harbored other fungal genera (*Galactomyces, Paecilomyces,* and *Gloeotinia*). As with bacteria, culture-independent and culture-based surveys provide very different pictures of community composition, with *Candida* species appearing dominant among cultivable fecal eukaryotes.

Viruses are *the* major predators on this microbe-dominated planet, determining which microbial strains survive. Most genetic diversity on Earth is viral: viruses move DNA from microbial host to microbial host, harboring host-derived genes as they evolve. The current view is that there are ~10 virus-like particles (VLPs) per microbial cell in virtually all microbial communities. Sequencing of

VLP DNA from purified feces from a group of monozygotic twins and their mothers disclosed that prophages and phages constitute the majority of the virome, with a majority of the phages belonging to the Podoviridae. One survey found that most viral diversity in the distal gut was novel (<20% of VLP sequencing reads exhibited homology to known viruses) and that VLP sequences represented <5% of all fecal microbiome sequences. Time-course studies of the fecal virome revealed that viral populations—like bacterial popu-lations—are most similar within an individual; i.e., interpersonal variation is greater than intrapersonal variation. Unlike bacterial populations, in which community composition is more similar among family members than among unrelated individuals, interper-sonal variations in VLP-associated viral populations are not appre-ciably less pronounced within than between families.

■ THE MICROBIOME: CONVERGENT FUNCTIONS FROM DIFFERENT SPECIES ASSEMBLAGES

Characterization of the microbiome by shotgun sequencing is important because, unlike SSU rRNA analysis, this method provides a direct readout of the genes that are available to perform particular functions in a specific community. The central issues are (1) to what degree variation in species-level assemblages occupying particular body habitats correlates with variation in community gene content and (2) whether groups of genes are represented in a particular body habitat–associated community in most or all individuals. The neu-tral theory of community assembly developed by macroecologists posits that most species in a community will have the same general niche (profession) or will adopt the broadest niche possible, endow-ing the community with functional redundancy. If applicable to the microbial world, neutral community assembly would predict a high level of variation in the types of microbial lineages that occupy a specific body habitat in different individuals (as defined by SSU rRNA sequencing), although the broad functions encoded in the microbiomes of these communities could be quite similar. In addition, chemical food webs are generated when the metabolic product(s) of one type of microbe become the substrate(s) for other microbes. These webs can be incredibly elaborate and can change as microbes adjust their patterns of gene expression and metabolism in response to alterations in nutrient availability. Thus, the sum of all activities of members of a microbial community can be viewed as an emergent rather than a fixed property (Chap. e19).

There are several key challenges in dealing with data obtained from shotgun sequencing of microbiomes. The first challenge is to attain a biomass sufficient for DNA recovery. Most human microbiome characterization has used fecal samples because they can be obtained readily in bulk quantities, 50% of the biomass of stool is microbial, and feces are an excellent proxy for depicting interpersonal differ-ences in gut microbial ecology. At present, microbiome-level analyses typically are based on counts of reads assigned to specific taxa or func-tions. It is challenging to reconstruct metabolic pathways realistically for prediction of symbiotic, syntrophic, or antagonistic relationships among organisms. A number of databases are available for functional assignments; they employ various schemes for hierarchical classifica-tion. Unfortunately, the vast majority of these functional assignments are based on the very limited number of cultured organisms that have been subjected to direct experimental analyses.

Shotgun sequencing of the fecal microbiome has revealed that different microbial communities (species assemblages) converge on the same functional state. In other words, there is a group of microbial genes represented in the guts of unrelated as well as related individuals. This "core" microbiome is enriched in functions related to microbial survival in the gut (e.g., translation; nucleotide, carbo-hydrate, and amino acid metabolism) and in functions that benefit the host (nutrient and energy partitioning from the diet to microbes *and* host). Microbial genes whose proportional representation in gut communities varies among individuals and make up a "variable" microbiome. Pairwise comparisons have shown that family members have functionally more similar gut microbiomes than do unrelated individuals. Thus, intrafamilial transmission of a gut microbiome—which probably contains >100-fold more genes than the human genome—within a specific generation and across multiple generations could shape the biologic features of humans belonging to a kinship. This second dimension of human gene flow (the other occurring at the level of *H. sapiens* genes) could modulate/mediate risks for a variety of pathogenic states.

The generalizability of the observation that vastly different species assemblages converge on similar gene functional repertoires in human body–associated habitats will have profound implications for an understanding of microbial functions in these different environments and the way these functions shape "human" physiologic and metabolic phenotypes. Issues such as the level of intra- and interpersonal variation in the gene content of the microbiome in various body habitats, the sampling depth required to characterize these differences, and the role of the *H. sapiens* genotype in shaping the microbiome genotype will be critical for informing this understanding.

EARLY EXAMPLES OF ASSOCIATIONS BETWEEN THE HUMAN MICROBIOTA AND DISEASE STATES

HMPs probably will expand the scientific view of what constitutes a pathogenic microbe. Pathogens currently are viewed as discrete phylotypes that are able to elicit disease in susceptible hosts; this attribution is, in the best circumstances, based on satisfying Koch's postulates. A more ecologic view is that pathogens do not function in isolation; rather, their invasions and/or emergence as well as their effects on the host reflect interactions with other members of a microbiota. An even more expansive view is that a number of co-occurring organisms can "conspire" to produce pathogenic effects in certain host and environmental contexts, forming a "pathologic community."

The relationships of microbiota and microbiome composition and their function to human diseases are being investigated in many HMPs. The rationale for hypotheses invoking a disease–microbiota/microbiome relationship in many cases emanates from gnotobiotic mouse models (i.e., mice raised in germ-free environments—with no exposure to microbes—and then colonized at specific stages of life with different microbial communities). Germ-free animals are compared with conventionally raised animals of similar genotype or with germ-free mice that have received a microbiota from a conventionally raised mouse donor with a defined phenotype. These comparisons have shown that the gut microbiota plays a key role in the maturation of the innate as well as the adaptive components of the immune system, that the microbiota is a key trigger in the development of inflammatory bowel disease (IBD) in animals that harbor mutations in genes associated with disease risk in humans, and that surface components of certain members of the gut microbiota can specifically modify the activity of the immune system to mitigate or prevent IBD. The risk of development of type 1 diabetes in genetically susceptible mice is modified by the gut microbiota; this fact provides additional evidence for the role of this microbial community in the pathogenesis of certain types of autoimmune disorders.

Gnotobiotic mice provide an excellent system for controlling host genotype, microbial community composition, diet, and housing conditions. Microbial communities harvested from donor mice of defined genotypes and physiologic phenotypes can be used to determine the impact of these communities on formerly germ-free recipients as well as the effect of the recipient on the transplanted microbiota and its microbiome. In this respect, gnotobiotic mice provide an opportunity to combine comparative metagenomic studies of donor communities with functional assays of community properties. Studies of gnotobiotic mice also have revealed that the gut microbiota plays a role in regulating the efficiency of energy and nutrient harvest from the diet; it does so not only by processing otherwise indigestible components of the diet (e.g., polysaccharides) but also by regulating host genes that affect energy storage in adipocytes. The microbiota influences the rate of epithelial turnover in the gut (the rate is slower in germ-free animals), modulates the development of the elaborate microvasculature that underlies the epithelium (capillary network density is markedly reduced in adult germ-free animals but can be restored to normal levels within 2 weeks after gut microbiota transplantation), is a key determinant of whether radiation enteritis follows abdominal or whole-body irradiation (germ-free mice are resistant), and influences gut motility. The impact of the gut microbiota extends beyond the gastrointestinal tract. Heart weight, whether measured echocardiographically or as wet mass and normalized to tibial length or lean body weight, is reduced significantly in germ-free mice; this difference is eliminated within 2 weeks after colonization with a gut microbiota. The presence or absence of a gut microbiota influences certain aspects of behavior, including locomotor activity. This observation raises the question of whether in this coevolved relationship microbes have developed strategies for manipulating certain features of host behavior that are mutually beneficial. For example, it is intriguing that plasma levels of serotonin are several-fold higher in conventionally raised mice than in germ-free mice.

Initial metagenomic studies of relatively small numbers of humans have provided insights into bacterial communities associated with several diseases, offering, for example, new ways to classify bacterial vaginosis, identifying alterations in the cutaneous bacterial communities of patients with psoriatic lesions, demonstrating shifts in the representation of various bacterial taxa in IBD, and revealing differences in the composition of the microbiota and microbiome in obese versus lean individuals as well as before and after bariatric surgery. The challenge provided by such observations is not only to expand the level of sampling to different populations of individuals but also to determine whether these associations are causal or only side effects of other processes.

Ongoing studies are exploring the impact of the microbiota on nutritional status, the development of *Clostridium difficile* colitis and its risk of relapse, the occurrence of necrotizing enterocolitis in premature newborns, the pathogenesis of diabetes, and various other metabolic phenotypes (*metabotypes*). These studies include assessment of the impact of the microbiota on drug metabolism. Comparisons of metabolites in the blood of germ-free and conventionally raised mice by nontargeted mass spectrometry have disclosed hundreds of compounds that are detectable in one but not the other type of animal and whose concentrations are affected markedly by the microbiota. These include compounds that are conjugated with sulfate, glycine, glucuronide, or other charged adducts that also modify xenobiotics, potentially altering the capacity of the host to metabolize these foreign molecules. Analogous events are being observed in humans. For example, metabolism of the analgesic acetaminophen to either sulfonated or glucuronidated forms is associated with predose levels of *p*-cresol, a microbial tyrosine metabolite that competes with acetaminophen for its sulfonate donor and the relevant sulfotransferase enzyme. Higher levels of *p*-cresol correlate with decreased sulfonation and increased glucuronidation of acetaminophen.

An additional series of metagenomic studies is exploring antibiotic resistance reservoirs in human microbial communities. To this end, a recent study of fecal samples used expression cloning: taking random fragments of the microbiome, placing them in expression vectors in a bacterial host, and screening for antibiotic resistance phenotypes. A related study demonstrated that bacteria subsisting on antibiotics are widely distributed in the environment. Capable of degrading a variety of antibiotics, these organisms are extensively drug resistant, phylogenetically diverse, and in many cases related to pathogens; they also harbor many resistance genes identical to those in clinical pathogens.

The role of microbes in therapeutics extends to clinical trials of the impact of probiotics—most recovered from fermented dairy products—on various forms of IBD [pouchitis that occurs in both ileoanal (pull-through) pouches and continent ileostomies or in recurrent *C. difficile* colitis]. A number of questions raised about probiotics typify the issues that surround studies of the role of the microbiota and microbiome in disease pathogenesis and therapeutics. Is there a consistent configuration of the microbiota definable in the study population that is associated with a particular disease state? The answer has diagnostic and mechanistic implications. How is the configuration affected by the intervention? Is there an identifiable reconfiguration? If so, how does it proceed? Are there many routes? Are the pathways related to the initial pretreatment state? If a reconfiguration does occur, is it sustained after cessation of treatment? How is host biology related to the configuration or reconfiguration? As with all studies involving human microbial ecology, the issue of what constitutes a suitable reference control is extremely important: the person himself or herself? family members? age- and sex-matched individuals living in the same locale with similar cultural traditions?

■ IMPACT OF HMPs ON GENETIC DETERMINISM, PERSONAL IDENTITY, CULTURAL TRADITIONS, AND PERSONALIZED MEDICINE

Sets of mono- and dizygotic twins and their family members will be an extremely valuable resource for initially teasing out relationships between environmental exposures, *H. sapiens* genotype, and human microbial ecology. Similarly, monozygotic twins discordant for certain disease states represent a powerful paradigm that enhances the ability to determine whether various diseases (e.g., asthma, IBD, metabolic disorders) can be linked to a person's microbiota and microbiome. It will be important to explore microbial ecology in groups of individuals living in developing countries that are undergoing rapid transformations in lifestyle and experiencing the emergence of a variety of Western diseases. Birth cohort studies (including studies of twins) that are initiated every 10 years in these countries may capture the impact of changes in lifestyle, including diet, on human microbial ecology.

Defining the human metagenome (the genes embedded in the *H. sapiens* genome plus the microbiome) will provide an entirely new level of refinement to the human description of self as well as a potential microbial legacy of personal lifestyle choices. Although this information may promote an appreciation of the origins of certain health disparities, care must be taken to avoid stigmatization of individuals or groups of individuals who have different cultural norms or express different behaviors. Metagenomics is a new field through which to view the influence of cultural traditions on lifestyles and choices that in turn affect human microbial ecology. Cultural anthropologists must examine the impact of this field on the ways in which study volunteers who live in various cultural settings view the natural world that envelops them and the ways this field and their cultural traditions interact to influence their perceptions of forces that affect their lives or their connections to one another within the context of a family or community. The union of metagenomics and cultural anthropology can help reveal how cultural traditions (e.g., the way infants are handled and cared for in early life) influence the flow of microbes between generations of humans, thus shaping the physiologic and genetic features of a kinship.

Finally, although microbiome-directed/related diagnostics and therapeutics would represent a new and different dimension of personalized medicine, sensitivity to the societal impact of this work is essential. This field is changing the human sense of personal identity, relationships with the world, and genetic determinism. Studies of human microbiomes promise to uncover new gene and protein families and probably will reveal novel biotransformations by microbial communities that could have commercial and therapeutic implications. Assessing the microbiome's capacity to metabolize orally administered drugs may be highly instructive for the pharmaceutical industry as it investigates new and more accurate ways to predict drug bioavailability and toxicity. The chemical entities that human microbial communities synthesize to support mutually beneficial relationships with the host may become new classes of drugs; the human genes that these chemical entities target (manipulate) may represent new targets for drug discovery. Microbial strains harvested from the microbiota of people living in various parts of the world with varied diets and lifestyles could expand the repertoire of probiotic strains, including strains that could be added to food to enhance its nutrient value. Microbes, microbial genes, and microbial products may serve as new and valuable biomarkers of physiologic status and distinctive biological properties. Thus, a microbial ecology scan may become a standard component of regular health examinations or a tool for forensic scientists. All these speculations raise questions about how microbial strains and whole microbial communities obtained from volunteers should be archived and distributed as well as about who owns these reagents and discoveries emanating from them.

SUMMARY

HMPs are an important manifestation of progress in the genome sciences, a timely step in the quest to achieve a better understanding of the place of humans in the natural world, and a reflection of the evolving focus of twenty-first-century medicine on disease prevention, new definitions of health, new ways to determine the origins of individual biological differences, and new approaches to elucidate how changes in lifestyle and biosphere affect human biology.

FURTHER READINGS

CLAYTON TA et al: Pharmacometabonomic identification of a significant host-microbiome metabolic interaction affecting human drug metabolism. Proc Natl Acad Sci USA 106:14728, 2009

COSTELLO EK et al: Bacterial community variation in human body habitats across space and time. Science 326:1694, 2009

DANTAS G et al: Bacteria subsisting on antibiotics. Science 320:100, 2008

DAWKINS R, KREBS JR: Arms races between and within species. Proc R Soc Lond B Biol Sci 205:489, 1979

DETHLEFSEN L et al: The pervasive effects of an antibiotic on the human gut microbiota. PLoS Biol 6:e280, 2008

ECKBURG PB et al: Diversity of the human intestinal microbial flora. Science 308:1635, 2005

FIERER N et al: The influence of sex, handedness, and washing on the diversity of hand surface bacteria. Proc Natl Acad Sci USA 105:17994, 2008

GRICE EA et al: Topographical and temporal diversity of the human skin microbiome. Science 324:1190, 2009

HUMAN MICROBIOME JUMPSTART REFERENCE STRAINS CONSORTIUM: A catalog of reference genomes from the human microbiome. Science 328:994, 2010

LEE YK et al: Proinflammatory T-cell responses to gut microbiota promote experimental autoimmune encephalomyeitis. Proc Natl Acad Sci USA 108(Suppl 1):4615, 2011

Mazmanian SI et al: A microbial symbiosis factor prevents inflammatory bowel disease. Nature 453:620, 2008

Qin J et al: A human gut microbial gene catalogue established by metagenomic sequencing. Nature 464:59, 2010

Ravel J et al: Vaginal microbiome of reproductive-age women. Proc Natl Acad Sci USA 108(Suppl 1):4680, 2011

Reyes A et al: Viruses in the fecal microbiota of monozygotic twins and their mothers. Nature 466:334, 2010

Scanlan PD, Marchesi JR: Micro-eukaryotic diversity of the human distal gut microbiota: Qualitative assessment using culture-dependent and -independent analysis of faeces. ISME J 2:1183, 2008

Sommer MOA et al: Functional characterization of the antibiotic reservoir in the human microflora. Science 325:1128, 2009

Turnbaugh PJ et al: A core gut microbiome in obese and lean twins. Nature 457:480, 2009

Volkov I et al: Neutral theory and relative species abundance in ecology. Nature 424:1035, 2003

Wen L et al: Innate immunity and intestinal microbiota in the development of type 1 diabetes. Nature 255:1109, 2008

Wikoff WR et al: Metabolomics analysis reveals large effects of gut microflora on mammalian blood metabolites. Proc Natl Acad Sci USA 106:3698, 2009

PART 4
Regenerative Medicine

CHAPTER **65**
Stem Cell Biology

Minoru S. H. Ko

Stem cell biology is a rapidly expanding field that explores the characteristics and possible clinical applications of a variety of stem cells that serve as the progenitors of more differentiated cell types. In addition to potential therapeutic applications (Chap. 67), patient-derived stem cells can also be used as disease models and a means to test drug effectiveness. Stem cells and their niche are becoming a major focus of medical research because they play central roles in tissue and organ homeostasis and repair, which are important aspects of aging and disease.

■ IDENTIFICATION, ISOLATION, AND DERIVATION OF STEM CELLS

Resident stem cells

The definition of stem cells remains elusive. Stem cells were originally postulated as *unspecified* or *undifferentiated* cells that provide a source of renewal of skin, intestine, and blood cells throughout life. These *resident stem cells* have been identified in a variety of organs (e.g., epithelia of the skin and digestive system, bone marrow, blood vessels, brain, skeletal muscle, liver, testis, and pancreas) based on their specific locations, morphology, and biochemical markers.

Isolated stem cells

Unequivocal identification of stem cells requires their separation and purification, usually based on a combination of specific cell-surface markers. These *isolated stem cells* [e.g., hematopoietic stem (HS) cells] can be studied in detail and used in clinical applications, such as bone marrow transplantation (Chap. 66). However, the lack of specific cell-surface markers for other types of stem cells has made it difficult to isolate them in large quantities. This challenge has been partially addressed in animal models by genetically marking different cell types with green-fluorescence protein driven by cell-specific promoters. Alternatively, putative stem cells have been isolated from a variety of tissues as side population (SP) cells using fluorescence-activated cell sorting after staining with Hoechst 33342 dye.

Cultured stem cells

It is desirable to culture and expand stem cells in vitro to obtain a sufficient quantity for analysis and potential therapeutic use. Although the derivation of stem cells in vitro has been a major obstacle in stem cell biology, the number and types of *cultured stem cells* have increased progressively (Table 65-1). Cultured stem cells derived from resident stem cells are often called *adult stem cells* to distinguish them from *embryonic stem* (ES) and *embryonic germ* (EG) *cells*. However, considering the existence of embryo-derived, tissue-specific stem cells [e.g., trophoblast stem (TS) cells] and the possible derivation of similar cells from an embryo/fetus [e.g., neural stem (NS) cells], it is more appropriate to use the term, *tissue stem cells*.

Successful derivation of cultured stem cells (both embryonic and tissue stem cells) often requires the identification of necessary growth factors and culture conditions, mimicking the microenvironment or *niche* of the resident stem cells. For example, the derivation of mouse TS cells, once considered impossible, became feasible by using FGF4, a ligand expressed by adjacent cells in the developing trophoblast in vivo. Therefore, it may be possible to culture other resident stem cells (e.g., intestinal stem cells) or isolated stem cells (e.g., HS cells) by studying the factors that constitute their normal niche.

■ SELF-RENEWAL AND PROLIFERATION OF STEM CELLS

Symmetric and asymmetric cell division

The most widely accepted stem cell definition is a cell with a unique capacity to produce unaltered daughter cells (*self-renewal*) and to generate specialized cell types (*potency*). Self-renewal can be achieved in two ways. *Asymmetric cell division* produces one daughter cell that is identical to the parental cell and one daughter cell that is different from the parental cell and is a progenitor or differentiated cell. Asymmetric cell division does not increase the number of stem cells. *Symmetric cell division* produces two identical daughter cells. For stem cells to proliferate in vitro, they must divide symmetrically.

Unlimited expansion in vitro

Resident stem cells are often quiescent and divide infrequently. However, once the stem cells are successfully cultured in vitro, they often acquire the capacity to divide continuously and the ability to proliferate beyond the normal passage limit typical of primary cultured cells (sometimes called *immortality*). These features are primarily seen in ES cells but have also been demonstrated for NS cells, MS cells, MAPCs, maGSCs (adult-derived tissue stem cells), and USSCs (newborn-derived tissue stem cells), thereby enhancing the potential of these cells for therapeutic use (Table 65-1).

Stability of genotype and phenotype

The capacity to actively proliferate is often associated with the accumulation of chromosomal abnormalities and mutations. Mouse ES cells appear to be an exception to this rule and tend to maintain their euploid karyotype and genome integrity. By contrast, human ES cells appear to be more susceptible to mutations after long-term culture. However, it is also important to note that even euploid mouse ES cells can form teratomas when injected into immunosuppressed animals, raising concerns about the possible formation of tumors after transplanting actively dividing stem cells.

■ POTENCY AND DIFFERENTIATION OF STEM CELLS

Developmental potency

The term *potency* is used to indicate a cell's ability to differentiate into specialized cell types. The current lack of knowledge about the molecular nature of potency requires the experimental manipulation of stem cells to demonstrate their potency. For example, in vivo testing can be done by injecting stem cells into mouse blastocysts or immunosuppressed adult mice and determining how many different cell types are formed from the injected cells. In vitro testing can be done by differentiating cells in various culture conditions to determine how many different cell types are formed from the cells. However, these in vivo assays are not applicable to human stem cells. The formal test of self-renewal and potency is performed by demonstrating that a single cell possesses such abilities in vitro (*clonality*). Cultured stem cells are tentatively grouped according to their potency (Fig. 65-1).

From totipotency to unipotency

Totipotent cells can form an entire organism autonomously. Only a fertilized egg (zygote) possesses this feature. *Pluripotent cells*

TABLE 65-1 Classification of Cultured Stem Cells

Name	Source	Properties
Embryonic stem cells (ES, ESC)	Blastocysts or immuno-surgically isolated inner cell mass (ICM) from blastocysts.	ES cells grow as tightly adherent multicellular colonies with a population doubling time of ~12 h, maintain a stable euploid karyotype even after extensive culture and manipulation, can differentiate into a variety of cell types *in vitro*, and can contribute to all cell types, including functional sperm and oocytes, when injected into a blastocyst (m). ES cells form relatively flat, compact colonies with a population doubling time of 35–40 h (h).
Embryonic germ cells (EG, EGC)	Primordial germ cells (PGCs) from embryos at E8.5–E12.5 (m). Gonadal tissues from 5–11 week post-fertilization embryo/fetus (h).	EG cells show essentially the same pluripotency as ES cells when injected into mouse blastocysts (m). The only known difference is the imprinting status of some genes (e.g., Igf2r): Imprinting is normally erased during germline development, and thus, the imprinting status of EG cells is different from that of ES cells.
Trophoblast stem cells (TS, TSC)	Trophectoderm of E3.5 blastocysts, extraembryonic ectoderm of E6.5 embryos, and chorionic ectoderm of E7.5 embryos.	TS cells can differentiate into trophoblast giant cells *in vitro* (m). TS can contribute exclusively to all trophoblast subtypes when injected into blastocysts (m).
Extraembryonic endoderm cells (XEN)	ICM from blastocysts	XEN cells can contribute only to the parietal endoderm lineage when injected into a blastocyst (m).
Embryonal carcinoma cells (EC)	Teratocarcinoma—a type of cancer that develops in the testes and ovaries	EC cells rarely show pluripotency *in vitro*, but they can contribute to nearly all cell types when injected into blastocysts (m). EC cells often have an aneuploid karyotype and other genome alterations (m, h).
Mesenchymal stem cells (MS, MSC)	Bone marrow, muscle, adipose tissue, peripheral blood, and umbilical cord blood (m, h)	MS cells can differentiate into mesenchymal cell types, including adipocytes, osteocytes, chondrocytes, and myocytes (m, h).
Multipotent adult stem cells (MAPC)	Bone marrow mononuclear cells (m, h); postnatal muscle and brain (m)	MAPCs are very rare cells that are present within MSC cultures from postnatal bone marrow (m, h). MAPCs can be cultured for >120 population doublings, can differentiate into all tissues *in vivo* when injected into a mouse blastocyst, and can differentiate into various cell lineages of mesodermal, ectodermal, and endodermal origin *in vitro* (m).
Spermatogonial stem cells (SS, SSC)	Newborn testis (m)	SS cells can reconstitute long-term spermatogenesis after transplantation into recipient testes and restore fertility (m).
Germline stem cells (GS, GSC)	Neonatal testis (m)	GS cells can differentiate into three germlayers *in vitro* and contribute to a variety of tissues, including germline, when injected into blastocysts (m).
Multipotent adult germline stem cells (maGSC)	Adult testis (m)	maGSC can differentiate into three germlayers *in vitro* and can contribute to a variety of tissues, including germline, when injected into blastocysts.
Neural stem cells (NS, NSC)	Fetal and adult brain (subventricular zone, ventricular zone, and hippocampus)	NS cells can be cultured as a heterogeneous cell population of monolayer or floating cell clusters called *neurospheres*. NS cells can differentiate into neuron and glia *in vivo* and *in vitro*. Recently, the culture of pure population of symmetrically dividing adherent NS cells became possible.
Unrestricted somatic stem cells (USSC)	Mononuclear fraction of cord blood (h)	USSCs can differentiate into a variety of cell types *in vitro* and can contribute a variety of cells types in *in vivo* transplantation experiments in rat, mouse, and sheep (h). USSCs are CD45⁻ adherent cells and can be expanded to 10^{15} cells without losing pluripotency (h).
Epistem cells (EpiSC)	Early postimplantation epiblast (m)	EpiSCs can differentiate into three germlayers *in vitro* and form teratomas but cannot contribute to normal tissues when injected into blastocysts (m). EpiSCs (m) are shown to be more similar to ESC (h) than ESC (m).
Induced pluripotent stem cells (iPS, iPSC)	Variety of terminally differentiated cells and tissue stem cells (m, h)	ESC-like cells originally derived by introducing four transcription factors (Klf4, Pou5f1/Oct4, Sox2, and Myc) into mouse embryo fibroblasts by retroviral vectors (m). iPS cells are essentially indistinguishable from ES cells. A number of somatic cell types can be converted into iPS cells using different combinations of transcription factors and treatment with small molecules.

Abbreviations: m, mouse; h, human.

(e.g., ES cells) can form almost all of the body's cell lineages (endoderm, mesoderm, and ectoderm), including germ cells. *Multipotent cells* (e.g., HS cells) can form multiple cell lineages but cannot form all of the body's cell lineages. *Oligopotent cells* (e.g., NS cells) can form more than one cell lineage but are more restricted than multipotent cells. Oligopotent cells are sometimes called *progenitor cells* or *precursor cells*; however, these terms are often more strictly used to define partially differentiated or lineage-committed cells (e.g., myeloid progenitor cells) that can divide into different cell types but lack self-renewing capacity. *Unipotent cells* or *monopotent cells*

Stage / Potency	Preimplantation	Embryonic, fetal	Postnatal	Adult
Totipotent	Zygote^{m,h}			
Pluripotent	ES^{m,h}	EG^{m,h} EpiSC^{m}	GS^{m} iPS^{m,h} USSC^{h} MAPC^{m,h}	EC^{m,h} iPS^{m,h} maGSC^{m} MAPC^{m,h}
Multipotent				MS^{m,h}
Oligopotent	TS^{m}			NS^{m,h}
Unipotent	XEN^{m}			SSC^{m}
Terminally differentiated cells				

Figure 65-1 Potency and source developmental stage of cultured stem cells. For abbreviations of stem cells, see Table 65-1. Note that stem cells are often abbreviated with or without "cells," e.g., ES cells or ESCs for embryonic stem cells. m, mouse; h, human.

[e.g., spermatogonial stem (SS) cells] can form a single differentiated cell lineage. Terminally differentiated cells, such as fibroblasts, also have a capacity to proliferate (which may be called self-renewal) but maintain the same cell type (i.e., they have no ability to form another cell type) and are not, therefore, considered unipotent cells.

Nuclear reprogramming

Development naturally progresses from totipotent fertilized eggs to pluripotent epiblast cells to multipotent cells and, finally, to terminally differentiated cells. According to Waddington's epigenetic landscape, this is analogous to a ball moving down a slope. The reversal of the terminally differentiated cells to totipotent or pluripotent cells (called *nuclear reprogramming*) can thus be seen as an uphill gradient that never occurs in normal conditions. However, nuclear reprogramming has been achieved using *nuclear transplantation*, or *nuclear transfer* (NT), procedures (often called "cloning"), where the nucleus of a differentiated cell is transferred into an enucleated oocyte. Although this is an error-prone procedure with a very low success rate, live animals have been produced using adult somatic cells as donors in sheep, mice, and other mammals. In mice, it has been demonstrated that ES cells derived from blastocysts made by somatic cell NT are indistinguishable from normal ES cells. NT can potentially be used to produce *patient-specific ES cells* carrying a genome identical to that of the patient. However, the successful implementation of this procedure has not been reported in humans. Setting aside technical and ethical issues, the limited supply of human oocytes will be a major problem for clinical applications of NT. Alternatively, successful nuclear reprogramming of somatic cells by fusing them with ES cells has been demonstrated in mice and humans. However, it is not yet clear how ES-derived DNA can be removed from hybrid cells.

An approach that has become increasingly successful is the direct conversion of terminally differentiated cells into ES-like cells [called induced pluripotent (iPS) cells] by transiently overexpressing a combination of key transcription factors (TFs). The original method was to infect mouse embryonic fibroblast cells with retrovirus vectors carrying four TFs [*Pou5f1*(*Oct4*), *Sox2*, *Klf4*, and *Myc*] and to identify rare ES-like cells in culture. It was soon adapted to human cells, followed by a more refined procedure (e.g., the use of fewer TFs, different cell types, and different gene-delivery methods). Use of protein cocktails and a variety of small molecules has also been actively pursued, as the goal is to produce patient-specific iPS cells without altering their genetic makeup.

Stem cell plasticity or transdifferentiation

The prevailing paradigm in developmental biology is that once cells are differentiated, their phenotypes are stable. However, a number of reports have shown that tissue stem cells, which have traditionally been thought to be lineage-committed multipotent cells, possessing the capacity to differentiate into cell types outside their lineage restrictions (called *transdifferentiation*). For example, HS cells may be converted into neurons as well as germ cells. This feature may provide a means to use tissue stem cells derived directly from a patient for therapeutic purposes, thereby eliminating the need to use embryonic stem cells or elaborate procedures such as nuclear reprogramming of a patient's somatic cells. However, more strict criteria and rigorous validation are required to establish tissue stem cell plasticity. For example, observations of transdifferentiation may reflect cell fusion, contamination with progenitor cells from other cell lineages, or persistence of pluripotent embryonic cells in adult organs. Therefore, the assignment of potency to each cultured stem cell in Fig. 65-1 should be taken with caution. Whether transdifferentiation exists and can be used for therapeutic purposes remains to be determined conclusively.

Directed differentiation of stem cells

Pluripotent stem cells (e.g., ES and iPS cells) can differentiate into multiple cell types, but in culture, they normally differentiate into heterogeneous cell populations in a stochastic manner. However, for therapeutic uses, it is desirable to direct stem cells into specific cell types (e.g., insulin-secreting beta cells). This is an active area of stem cell research, and protocols are being developed to achieve this goal. In any of these directed cell differentiation systems, the cell phenotype must be evaluated critically.

■ MOLECULAR CHARACTERIZATION OF STEM CELLS

Genomics and proteomics

In addition to standard molecular biological approaches, high-throughput genomics and proteomics have been extensively applied to the analysis of stem cells. For example, DNA microarray analyses have revealed the expression levels of essentially all genes and identified specific markers for some stem cells. Chromatin-immunoprecipitation coupled with next-generation sequencing technologies, capable of producing tens of millions of sequence reads in a single run, have revealed chromatin modifications ("epigenetic marks") relevant to stem cell properties. Similarly, the protein profiles of stem cells have been assessed by using mass spectrometry. These methods are beginning to provide a novel means to characterize and classify various stem cells and the molecular mechanisms that give them their unique characteristics.

ES cell regulation

It is important to identify genes involved in the regulation of stem cell function and to examine the effects of altered gene expression on ES and other stem cells. For example, core networks of TFs such as *Pou5f1* (*Oct4*), *Nanog*, and *Sox2*, govern key gene regulatory pathways/networks for the maintenance of self-renewal and pluripotency of mouse and human ES cells. These TF networks are modulated by specific external factors through signal transduction pathways, such as leukemia inhibitory factor (*Lif*)/*Stat3*, mitogen-activated protein kinase 1/3 (*Mapk1/3*), TGFβ superfamily, and *Wnt*/glycogen synthase kinase 3 beta (*Gsk3b*). Inhibitors of Mapk1/3 and Gsk3b signaling enhance the derivation of ES cells and help to maintain ES cells in a full pluripotency ("ground" or "naive state"). Recent data also indicate that 20–25 nucleotide RNAs, called microRNAs (miRNAs), play an important role in regulating stem cell function by repressing the translation of their target genes. For example, it has been shown that miR-21 regulates cell cycle progression in ES cells and miR-128 prevents the differentiation of hematopoietic progenitor cells. These types of analyses should provide molecular clues about the function of stem cells and lead to a more effective means to manipulate stem cells for future therapeutic use.

FURTHER READINGS

DEPARTMENT OF HEALTH AND HUMAN SERVICES: NIH Stem Cell Information Home Page, 2010. *http://stemcells.nih.gov/index*

GANGARAJU VK, LIN H: MicroRNAs: Key regulators of stem cells. Nat Rev Mol Cell Biol 10:116, 2009

LANZA R et al (eds): *Essentials of Cell Biology*, 2nd ed. San Diego, Academic Press, 2009

NICHOLS J, SMITH A: Naive and primed pluripotent state. Cell Stem Cell 4:487, 2009

NISHIYAMA A et al: Uncovering early response of gene regulatory networks in ESCs by systematic induction of transcription factors. Cell Stem Cell 5:420, 2009

SAHA K, JAENISCH R: Technical challenges in using human induced pluripotent stem cells to Model Disease. Cell Stem Cell 5:584, 2009

YAMANAKA S, BLAU HM: Nuclear reprogramming to a pluripotent state by three approaches. Nature 465:704, 2010

CHAPTER **66**

Hematopoietic Stem Cells

David T. Scadden

Dan L. Longo

All of the cell types in the peripheral blood and some cells in every tissue of the body are derived from hematopoietic (*hemo*: blood; *poiesis*: creation) stem cells. If the hematopoietic stem cell is damaged and can no longer function (e.g., due to a nuclear accident), a person would survive 2–4 weeks in the absence of extraordinary support measures. With the clinical use of hematopoietic stem cells, tens of thousands of lives are saved each year (Chap. 114). Stem cells produce tens of billions of blood cells daily from a stem cell pool that is estimated to be only in the hundreds of thousands. How stem cells do this, how they persist for many decades despite the production demands, and how they may be better used in clinical care are important issues in medicine.

The study of blood cell production has become a paradigm for how other tissues may be organized and regulated. Basic research in hematopoiesis that includes defining stepwise molecular changes accompanying functional changes in maturing cells, aggregating cells into functional subgroups, and demonstrating hematopoietic stem cell regulation by a specialized microenvironment are concepts worked out in hematology, but they offer models for other tissues. Moreover, these concepts may not be restricted to normal tissue function but extend to malignancy. Stem cells are rare cells among a heterogeneous population of cell types, and their behavior is assessed mainly in experimental animal models involving reconstitution of hematopoiesis. Thus, much of what we know about stem cells is imprecise and based on inferences from genetically manipulated animals.

CARDINAL FUNCTIONS OF HEMATOPOIETIC STEM CELLS

All stem cell types have two cardinal functions: self-renewal and differentiation (Fig. 66-1). Stem cells exist to generate, maintain, and repair tissues. They function successfully if they can replace a wide variety of shorter-lived mature cells over prolonged periods. The process of self-renewal (see below) assures that a stem cell population can be sustained over time. Without self-renewal, the stem cell pool would become exhausted and tissue maintenance would not be possible. The process of differentiation leads to production of the effectors of tissue function: mature cells. Without proper differentiation, the integrity of tissue function would be compromised and organ failure would ensue.

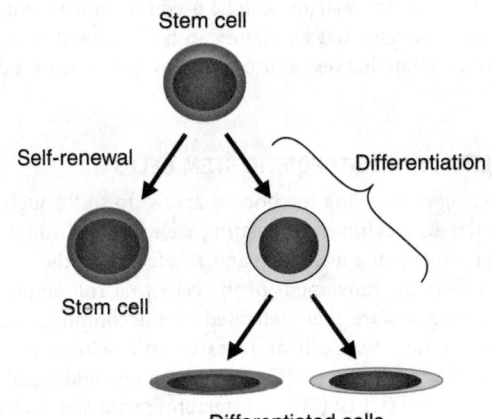

Figure 66-1 Signature characteristics of the stem cell. Stem cells have two essential features: the capacity to differentiate into a variety of mature cell types and the capacity for self-renewal. Intrinsic factors associated with self-renewal include expression of Bmi-1, Gfi-1, PTEN, STAT5, Tel/Atv6, p21, p18, MCL-1, Mel-18, RAE28, and HoxB4. Extrinsic signals for self-renewal include Notch, Wnt, SHH, and Tie2/Ang-1. Based mainly on murine studies, hematopoietic stem cells express the following cell surface molecules: CD34, Thy-1 (CD90), c-Kit receptor (CD117), CD133, CD164, and c-Mpl (CD110, also known as the thrombopoietin receptor).

In the blood, mature cells have variable average life spans, ranging from 7 h for mature neutrophils to a few months for red blood cells to many years for memory lymphocytes. However, the stem cell pool is the central, durable source of all blood and immune cells, maintaining a capacity to produce a broad range of cells from a single cell source, yet keeping itself vigorous over decades of life. As an individual stem cell divides, it has the capacity to accomplish one of three division outcomes: two stem cells, two cells destined for differentiation, or one stem cell and one differentiating cell. The former two outcomes are the result of symmetric cell division, whereas the latter indicates a different outcome for the two daughter cells—an event termed *asymmetric cell division*. The relative balance for these types of outcomes may change during development and under particular kinds of demands on the stem cell pool.

◼ DEVELOPMENTAL BIOLOGY OF HEMATOPOIETIC STEM CELLS

During development, blood cells are produced at different sites. Initially, the yolk sac provides oxygen-carrying red blood cells, and then the placenta and several sites of intraembryonic blood cell production become involved. These intraembryonic sites engage in sequential order, moving from the genital ridge at a site where the aorta, gonadal tissue, and mesonephros are emerging to the fetal liver and then, in the second trimester, to the bone marrow and spleen. As the location of stem cells changes, the cells they produce also change. The yolk sac provides red cells expressing embryonic hemoglobins while intraembryonic sites of hematopoiesis generate red cells, platelets, and the cells of innate immunity. The production of the cells of adaptive immunity occurs when the bone marrow is colonized and the thymus forms. Stem cell proliferation remains high, even in the bone marrow, until shortly after birth, when it appears to dramatically decline. The cells in the bone marrow are thought to arrive by the bloodborne transit of cells from the fetal liver after calcification of the long bones has begun. The presence of stem cells in the circulation is not unique to a time window in development. Rather, hematopoietic stem cells appear to circulate throughout life. The time that cells spend freely circulating appears to be brief (measured in minutes in the mouse), but the cells that do circulate are functional and can be used for transplantation. The number of stem cells that circulate can be increased in a number of ways to facilitate harvest and transfer to the same or a different host.

■ MOBILITY OF HEMATOPOIETIC STEM CELLS

Cells entering and exiting the bone marrow do so through a series of molecular interactions. Circulating stem cells (through CD162 and CD44) engage the lectins P- and E-selectin on the endothelial surface to slow the movement of the cells to a rolling phenotype. Stem cell integrins are then activated and accomplish firm adhesion between the stem cell and vessel wall, with a particularly important role for stem cell VCAM-1 engaging endothelial VLA-4. The chemokine CXCL12 (SDF1) interacting with stem cell CXCR4 receptors also appears to be important in the process of stem cells getting from the circulation to where they engraft in the bone marrow. This is particularly true in the developmental move from fetal liver to bone marrow; however, the role for this molecule in adults appears to be more related to retention of stem cells in the bone marrow rather the process of getting them there. Interrupting that retention process through either specific molecular blockers of the CXCR4/CXCL12 interaction, cleavage of CXCL12, or down-regulation of the receptor can all result in the release of stem cells into the circulation. This process is an increasingly important aspect of recovering stem cells for therapeutic use as it has permitted the harvesting process to be done by leukapheresis rather than bone marrow punctures in the operating room. Refining our knowledge of how stem cells get into and out of the bone marrow may improve our ability to obtain stem cells and make them more efficient at finding their way to the specific sites for blood cell production, the so-called stem cell niche.

■ HEMATOPOIETIC STEM CELL MICROENVIRONMENT

The concept of a specialized microenvironment, or stem cell niche, was first proposed to explain why cells derived from the bone marrow of one animal could be used in transplantation and again be found in the bone marrow of the recipient. This niche is more than just a housing site for stem cells, however. It is an anatomic location where regulatory signals are provided that allow the stem cells to thrive, to expand if needed, and to provide varying amounts of descendant daughter cells. In addition, unregulated growth of stem cells may be problematic based on their undifferentiated state and self-renewal capacity. Thus, the niche must also regulate the number of stem cells produced. In this manner, the niche has the dual function of serving as a site of nurture but imposing limits for stem cells: in effect, acting as both a nutritive and constraining home.

The niche for blood stem cells changes with each of the sites of blood production during development, but for most of human life it is located in the bone marrow. Within the bone marrow, at least two niche sites have been proposed: on trabecular bone surfaces and in the perivascular space. Stem cells may be found in both places by histologic analysis, and functional regulation has been shown at the highly vascular bone surface. Specifically, bone-forming mesenchymal cells, osteoblastic cells, participate in hematopoietic stem cell function, affecting their location, proliferation, and number. The basis for this interaction is through a number of molecules mediating location, such as the chemokine CXCL12 (SDF1), through proliferation signals mediated by angiopoietin 1, and signaling to modulate self-renewal or survival by factors such as Notch ligands, kit ligand, and Wnts. Other bone components, such as the extracellular matrix glycoprotein, osteopontin, and the high ionic calcium found at trabecular surfaces, contribute to the unique microenvironment, or stem cell niche, on trabecular bone. This physiology has practical applications. First, medications altering niche components may have an effect on stem cell function. This has now been shown for a number of compounds, and some are being clinically tested. Second, it is now possible to assess whether the niche participates in disease states and to examine whether targeting the niche with medications may alter the outcome of certain diseases.

■ EXCESS CAPACITY OF HEMATOPOIETIC STEM CELLS

In the absence of disease, one never runs out of hematopoietic stem cells. Indeed, serial transplantation studies in mice suggest that sufficient stem cells are present to reconstitute several animals in succession, with each animal having normal blood cell production. The fact that allogeneic stem cell transplant recipients also never run out of blood cells in their life span, which can extend for decades, argues that even the limiting numbers of stem cells provided to them are sufficient. How stem cells respond to different conditions to increase or decrease their mature cell production remains poorly understood. Clearly, negative feedback mechanisms affect the level of production of most of the cells, leading to the normal tightly regulated blood cell counts. However, many of the regulatory mechanisms that govern production of more mature progenitor cells do not apply or apply differently to stem cells. Similarly, most of the molecules shown to be able to change the size of the stem cell pool have little effect on more mature blood cells. For example, the growth factor erythropoietin, which stimulates red blood cell production from more mature precursor cells, has no effect on stem cells. Similarly, granulocyte colony-stimulating factor drives the rapid proliferation of granulocyte precursors but has little or no effect on the cell cycling of stem cells. Rather, it changes the location of stem cells by indirect means, altering molecules such as CXCL12 that tether stem cells to their niche. Molecules shown to be important for altering the proliferation, self renewal or survival of stem cells, such as cyclin-dependent kinase inhibitors, transcription factors like *Bmi-1*, or microRNAs like miR125a, have little or different effects on progenitor cells. Hematopoietic stem cells have governing mechanisms that are distinct from the cells they generate.

■ HEMATOPOIETIC STEM CELL DIFFERENTIATION

Hematopoietic stem cells sit at the base of a branching hierarchy of cells culminating in the many mature cell types that compose the blood and immune system (Fig. 66-2). The maturation steps leading to terminally differentiated and functional blood cells take place both as a consequence of intrinsic changes in gene expression and niche-directed and cytokine-directed changes in the cells. Our knowledge of the details remains incomplete. As stem cells mature to progenitors, precursors, and, finally, mature effector cells, they undergo a series of functional changes. These include the

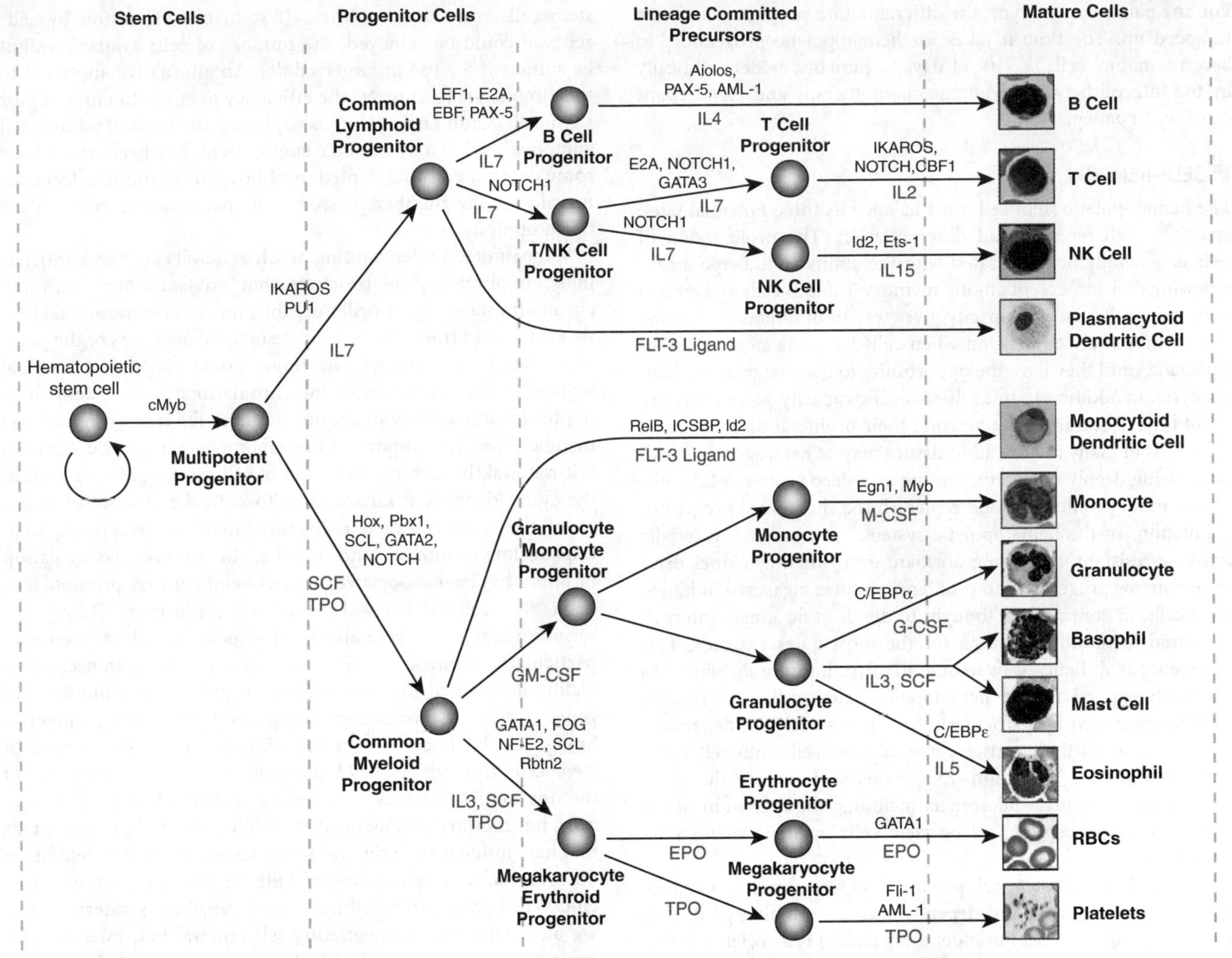

Stem Cells **Progenitor Cells** **Lineage Committed Precursors** **Mature Cells**

Hematopoietic stem cell — cMyb → **Multipotent Progenitor**

IKAROS PU1 / IL7 → **Common Lymphoid Progenitor**

LEF1, E2A, EBF, PAX-5 → **B Cell Progenitor**
Aiolos, PAX-5, AML-1 → **B Cell**
IL4 → **T Cell Progenitor**
IL7 / NOTCH1 → **T/NK Cell Progenitor**
E2A, NOTCH1, GATA3 / IL7 → **T Cell Progenitor**
IKAROS, NOTCH, CBF1 / IL2 → **T Cell**
NOTCH1 / IL7 → **NK Cell Progenitor**
Id2, Ets-1 / IL15 → **NK Cell**
FLT-3 Ligand → **Plasmacytoid Dendritic Cell**

Hox, Pbx1, SCL, GATA2, NOTCH / SCF TPO → **Common Myeloid Progenitor**

GM-CSF → **Granulocyte Monocyte Progenitor**
RelB, ICSBP, Id2 / FLT-3 Ligand → **Monocytoid Dendritic Cell**
→ **Monocyte Progenitor**
Egn1, Myb / M-CSF → **Monocyte**
→ **Granulocyte Progenitor**
C/EBPα / G-CSF → **Granulocyte**
IL3, SCF → **Basophil**
→ **Mast Cell**
C/EBPε / IL5 → **Eosinophil**

GATA1, FOG NF-E2, SCL Rbtn2 / IL3, SCF TPO → **Megakaryocyte Erythroid Progenitor**
EPO → **Erythrocyte Progenitor**
GATA1 / EPO → **RBCs**
TPO → **Megakaryocyte Progenitor**
Fli-1 AML-1 / TPO → **Platelets**

Figure 66-2 Hierarchy of hematopoietic differentiation. *Stem cells* are multipotent cells that are the source of all descendant cells and have the capacity to provide either long-term (measured in years) or short-term (measured in months) cell production. *Progenitor cells* have a more limited spectrum of cells they can produce and are generally a short-lived, highly proliferative population also known as transient amplifying cells. *Precursor cells* are cells committed to a single blood cell lineage but with a continued ability to proliferate; they do not have all the features of a fully mature cell. *Mature cells* are the terminally differentiated product of the differentiation process and are the effector cells of specific activities of the blood and immune system. Progress through the pathways is mediated by alterations in gene expression. The regulation of the differentiation by soluble factors and cell-cell communications within the bone marrow niche are still being defined. The transcription factors that characterize particular cell transitions are illustrated on the arrows; the soluble factors that contribute to the differentiation process are in blue. EPO, erythropoietin; SCF, stem cell factor; TPO, thrombopoietin.

obvious acquisition of functions defining mature blood cells, such as phagocytic capacity or hemoglobin synthesis. They also include the progressive loss of plasticity (i.e., the ability to become other cell types). For example, the myeloid progenitor can make all cells in the myeloid series but none in the lymphoid series. As common myeloid progenitors mature, they become precursors for either monocytes and granulocytes or erythrocytes and megakaryocytes, but not both. Some amount of reversibility of this process may exist early in the differentiation cascade, but that is lost beyond a distinct stage. As cells differentiate, they may also lose proliferative capacity (Fig. 66-3). Mature granulocytes are incapable of proliferation and only increase in number by increased production from precursors. Lymphoid cells retain the capacity to proliferate but have linked their proliferation to the recognition of particular proteins or peptides by specific antigen receptors on their surface. In most tissues the proliferative cell population is a more immature progenitor population. In general, cells within the highly proliferative progenitor cell compartment are also relatively short-lived, making their way through the differentiation process in a defined molecular program involving the sequential activation of particular sets of genes.

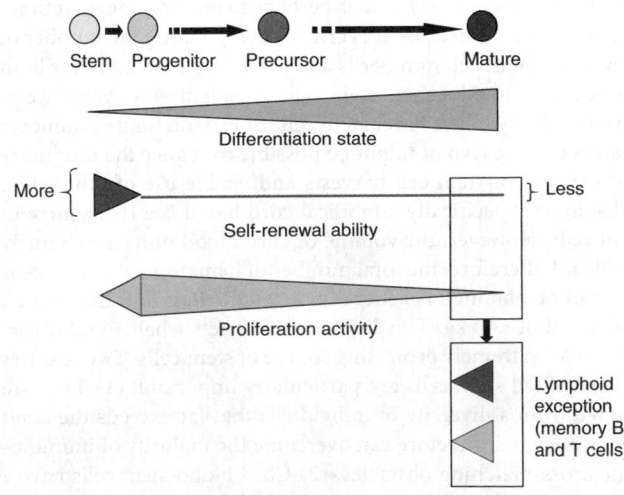

Figure 66-3 Relative function of cells in the hematopoietic hierarchy. The boxes represent distinct functional features of cells in the myeloid (*upper box*) versus lymphoid (*lower box*) lineages.

For any particular cell type, the differentiation program is difficult to speed up. The time it takes for hematopoietic progenitors to become mature cells is ~10–14 days in humans, evident clinically by the interval between cytotoxic chemotherapy and blood count recovery in patients.

■ SELF-RENEWAL

The hematopoietic stem cell must balance its three potential fates: apoptosis, self-renewal, and differentiation. The proliferation of cells is generally not associated with the ability to undergo a self-renewing division except among memory T and B cells and among stem cells. Self-renewal capacity gives way to differentiation as the only option after cell division when cells leave the stem cell compartment, until they have the opportunity to become memory lymphocytes. In addition to this self-renewing capacity, stem cells have an additional feature characterizing their proliferation machinery. Stem cells in many mature adult tissues may be heterogeneous with some being deeply quiescent, serving as a deep reserve, while others are more proliferative and replenish the short-lived progenitor population. In the hematopoietic system, stem cells are generally cytokine-resistant, remaining dormant even when cytokines drive bone marrow progenitors to proliferation rates measured in hours. Stem cells, in contrast, are thought to divide at far longer intervals measured in months to years, for the most quiescent cells. This quiescence is difficult to overcome in vitro, limiting the ability to effectively expand human hematopoietic stem cells. The process may be controlled by particularly high levels of cyclin-dependent kinase inhibitors that restrict entry of stem cells into cell cycle, blocking the G1-S transition. Exogenous signals from the niche also appear to enforce quiescence, including the activation of the tyrosine kinase receptor Tie2 on stem cells by angiopoietin 1 on osteoblasts.

The regulation of stem cell proliferation also appears to change with age. In mice, the cyclin-dependent kinase inhibitor p16INK4a accumulates in stem cells in older animals and is associated with a change in five different stem cell functions, including cell cycling. Lowering expression of p16INK4a in older animals improves stem cell cycling and capacity to reconstitute hematopoiesis in adoptive hosts, making them similar to younger animals. Mature cell numbers are unaffected. Therefore, molecular events governing the specific functions of stem cells are being gradually made clear and offer the potential of new approaches to changing stem cell function for therapy. One critical stem cell function that remains poorly defined is the molecular regulation of self-renewal.

For medicine, self-renewal is perhaps the most important function of stem cells because it is critical in regulating the number of stem cells. Stem cell number is a key limiting parameter for both autologous and allogeneic stem cell transplantation. Were we to have the ability to use fewer stem cells or expand limited numbers of stem cells ex vivo, it might be possible to reduce the morbidity and expense of stem cell harvests and enable use of other stem cell sources. Specifically, umbilical cord blood is a rich source of stem cells. However, the volume of cord blood units is extremely small and, therefore, the total number of hematopoietic stem cells that can be obtained is generally only sufficient to transplant an individual of <40 kg. This limitation restricts what would otherwise be an extremely promising source of stem cells. Two features of cord blood stem cells are particularly important. (1) They are derived from a diversity of individuals that far exceeds the adult donor pool and therefore can overcome the majority of immunologic cross-matching obstacles. (2) Cord blood stem cells have a large number of T cells associated with them, but (paradoxically) they appear to be associated with a lower incidence of graft-versus-host disease when compared with similarly mismatched

stem cells from other sources. If stem cell expansion by self-renewal could be achieved, the number of cells available might be sufficient for use in larger adults. An alternative approach to this problem is to improve the efficiency of engraftment of donor stem cells. Graft engineering is exploring methods of adding cell components that may enhance engraftment. Furthermore, at least some data suggest that depletion of host NK (natural killer) cells may lower the number of stem cells necessary to reconstitute hematopoiesis.

Some limited understanding of self-renewal exists and, intriguingly, implicates gene products that are associated with the chromatin state, a high-order organization of chromosomal DNA that influences transcription. These include members of the polycomb family, a group of zinc finger–containing transcriptional regulators that interact with the chromatin structure, contributing to the accessibility of groups of genes for transcription. One member, *Bmi-1*, is important in enabling hematopoietic stem cell self-renewal through modification of cell cycle regulators such as the cyclin-dependent kinase inhibitors. In the absence of *Bmi-1* or of the transcriptional regulator, Gfi-1, hematopoietic stem cells decline in number and function. In contrast, dysregulation of *Bmi-1* has been associated with leukemia; it may promote leukemic stem cell self-renewal when it is overexpressed. Other transcription regulators have also been associated with self-renewal, particularly homeobox, or "hox," genes. These transcription factors are named for their ability to govern large numbers of genes, including those determining body patterning in invertebrates. HoxB4 is capable of inducing extensive self-renewal of stem cells through its DNA-binding motif. Other members of the hox family of genes have been noted to affect normal stem cells, but they are also associated with leukemia. External signals that may influence the relative self-renewal versus differentiation outcomes of stem cell cycling include the Notch ligands and specific Wnt ligands. Intracellular signal transducing intermediates are also implicated in regulating self-renewal but, interestingly, are not usually associated with the pathways activated by Notch or Wnt receptors. They include PTEN, an inhibitor of the AKT pathway, and STAT5, both of which are usually downstream of activated growth factor receptors and necessary for normal stem cell functions including self-renewal, at least in mouse models. The connections between these molecules remain to be defined, and their role in physiologic regulation of stem cell self-renewal is still poorly understood.

CANCER IS SIMILAR TO AN ORGAN WITH SELF-RENEWING CAPACITY

The relationship of stem cells to cancer is an important evolving dimension of adult stem cell biology. Cancer may share principles of organization with normal tissues. Cancer might have the same hierarchical organization of cells with a base of stem-like cells capable of the signature stem-cell features, self-renewal, and differentiation. These stem-like cells might be the basis for perpetuation of the tumor and represent a slowly dividing, rare population with distinct regulatory mechanisms, including a relationship with a specialized microenvironment. A subpopulation of self-renewing cells has been defined for some, but not all, cancers. A more sophisticated understanding of the stem-cell organization of cancers may lead to improved strategies for developing new therapies for the many common and difficult-to-treat types of malignancies that have been relatively refractory to interventions aimed at dividing cells.

Does the concept of cancer stem cells provide insight into the cellular origin of cancer? The fact that some cells within a cancer have stem cell–like properties does not necessarily mean that the cancer arose in the stem cell itself. Rather, more mature cells could have acquired the self-renewal characteristics of stem cells. Any single genetic event is unlikely to be sufficient to enable full transformation of a normal cell to a frankly malignant one. Rather, cancer is a multistep process, and for the multiple steps to accumulate, the cell of origin must be able to persist for prolonged periods. It must also be able to generate large numbers of daughter cells. The normal stem cell has these properties and, by virtue of its having intrinsic self-renewal capability, may be more readily converted to a malignant phenotype. This hypothesis has been tested experimentally in the hematopoietic system. Taking advantage of the cell-surface markers that distinguish hematopoietic cells of varying maturity, stem cells, progenitors, precursors, and mature cells can be isolated. Powerful transforming gene constructs were placed in these cells, and it was found that the cell with the greatest potential to produce a malignancy was dependent on the transforming gene. In some cases it was the stem cell, but in others, the progenitor cell functioned to initiate and perpetuate the cancer. This shows that cells can acquire stem cell-like properties in malignancy.

WHAT ELSE CAN HEMATOPOIETIC STEM CELLS DO?

Some experimental data have suggested that hematopoietic stem cells or other cells mobilized into the circulation by the same factors that mobilize hematopoietic stem cells are capable of playing a role in healing the vascular and tissue damage associated with stroke and myocardial infarction. These data are controversial, and the applicability of a stem-cell approach to nonhematopoietic conditions remains experimental. However, the application of the evolving knowledge of hematopoietic stem cell biology may lead to wide-ranging clinical uses.

The stem cell, therefore, represents a true dual-edged sword. It has tremendous healing capacity and is essential for life. Uncontrolled, it can threaten the life it maintains. Understanding how stem cells function, the signals that modify their behavior, and the tissue niches that modulate stem cell responses to injury and disease are critical for more effectively developing stem cell–based medicine. That aspect of medicine will include the use of the stem cells and the use of drugs to target stem cells to enhance repair of damaged tissues. It will also include the careful balance of interventions to control stem cells where they may be dysfunctional or malignant.

FURTHER READINGS

DICK JE: Stem cell concepts renew cancer research. Blood 112:4793, 2008

CARLESSO N, CARDOSO AA: Stem cell regulatory niches and their role in normal and malignant hematopoiesis. Curr Opin Hematol 17:281, 2010

LASLO P et al: Gene regulatory networks directing myeloid and lymphoid cell fates with the immune system. Semin Immunol 20:228, 2008

OTTERSBACH K et al: Ontogeny of haematopoiesis: Recent advances and open questions. Br J Haematol 148:343, 2010

SCHULZ C et al: Hematopoietic stem and progenitor cells: Their mobilization and homing to bone marrow and peripheral tissue. Immunol Res 44:160, 2009

CHAPTER 67

Applications of Stem Cell Biology in Clinical Medicine

John A. Kessler

Damage to an organ initiates a series of events that lead to the reconstruction of the damaged tissue, including proliferation, differentiation and migration of various cell types, release of cytokines and chemokines, and remodeling of the extracellular matrix. Endogenous stem and progenitor cells are among the cell populations that are involved in the injury responses. In normal steady-state conditions, an equilibrium is maintained in which endogenous stem cells intrinsic to the tissue replenish dying cells. After tissue injury, stem cells in organs, such as the liver and skin, have a remarkable ability to regenerate the organ, whereas other stem cell populations, such as those in the heart and brain, have a much more limited capability for self-repair. In rare circumstances, circulating stem cells may contribute to regenerative responses by migrating into a tissue and differentiating into organ-specific cell types. The goal of stem cell therapies is to promote cell replacement in organs that are damaged beyond their ability for self-repair.

GENERAL STRATEGIES FOR STEM CELL REPLACEMENT

At least three different therapeutic concepts for cell replacement can be envisaged (Fig. 67-1). One therapeutic approach involves direct administration of stem cells. This may involve injection of the cells directly into the damaged organ, where they can differentiate into the desired cell type. Alternatively, stem cells may be injected systemically since they have the capacity to home in on damaged tissues by following gradients of cytokines and chemokines released by the diseased organ. A second approach involves transplantation of differentiated cells derived from stem cells. For example, pancreatic islet cells would be generated from stem cells before transplantation into diabetic patients and cardiomyocytes would be generated to treat ischemic heart disease. A third approach involves stimulation of endogenous stem cells to facilitate repair. This might be accomplished by administration of appropriate growth factors and drugs that amplify the number of endogenous stem/progenitor cells and/or direct them to differentiate into the desired cell types. Therapeutic stimulation of precursor cells is already a clinical reality in the hematopoietic system, where factors such as erythropoietin, granulocyte colony-stimulating factor (G-CSF), and granulocyte-macrophage colony-stimulating factor (GM-CSF) are used to increase production of specific blood elements. In addition to these strategies for cell replacement, a number of other approaches could involve stem cells for ex vivo or in situ generation of tissues, a process termed tissue engineering (Chap. 69). Stem cells are also excellent candidates as vehicles for cellular gene therapy (Chap. 68). Finally, transplanted stem cells may exert paracrine effects on damaged tissues without differentiating and replacing lost cells.

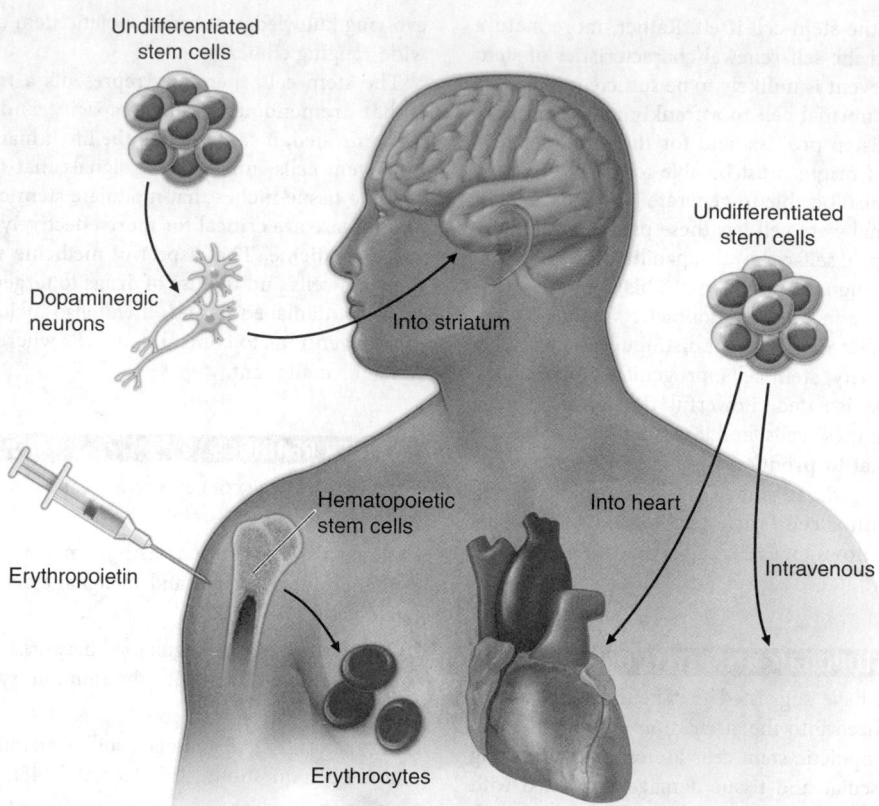

Figure 67-1 Strategies for transplantation of stem cells. 1. Undifferentiated or partially differentiated stem cells may be injected directly into the target organ or intravenously. 2. Stem cells may be differentiated ex vivo before injection into the target organ. 3. Growth factors or other drugs may be injected to stimulate endogenous stem cell populations.

Stem cell transplantation is not a new concept and is already part of established medical practice. Hematopoietic stem cells (Chap. 66) are responsible for the long-term repopulation of all blood elements in recipients of bone marrow transplants, and hematopoietic stem cell transplantation is the gold standard against which other stem cell transplantation therapies will be measured. Transplantation of differentiated cells is also a clinical reality, and donated organs and tissues often are used to replace damaged tissues. However, the need for transplantable tissues and organs far outweighs the available supply, and organ transplantation has limited potential for some tissues, such as the brain. Stem cells offer the possibility of a renewable source of replacement cells for virtually all organs.

SOURCES OF STEM CELLS FOR TISSUE REPAIR

A variety of different types of stem cells (Chap. 65) could be used in regenerative strategies, including embryonic stem (ES) cells, induced pluripotent stem cells (iPS cells), umbilical cord blood stem cells, organ-specific somatic stem cells (e.g., neural stem cells for treatment of the brain), and somatic stem cells that generate cell types specific for the target organ rather than the donor organ (e.g., bone marrow mesenchymal stem cells for cardiac repair). Each cell type has potential advantages and disadvantages, and there are a number of generic problems in developing any of these cell types into a useful and reliable clinical tool.

■ EMBRYONIC STEM CELLS

Embryonic stem cells have the potential to generate all the cell types in the body, and so in theory there are no restrictions on the organs that could be regenerated. They can self-renew endlessly so

that a single cell line with carefully characterized traits potentially could generate almost limitless numbers of cells. In the absence of moral or ethical constraints, unused human blastocysts from fertility clinics could be used to derive new ES cell lines that are matched immunologically with potential transplant recipients. Alternatively, somatic cell nuclear transfer ("therapeutic cloning") could be used to create ES cell lines that are genetically identical to those of the patient. However, human ES cells are difficult to culture and grow slowly. Techniques for differentiating them into specific cell types are just beginning to be developed. Cells tend to develop abnormal karyotypes and other abnormalities with increased time in culture, and ES cells have the potential to form teratomas if all cells are not committed to the desired cell types before transplantation. Further, human ES cells are ethically controversial and, on these grounds, would be unacceptable to some patients and physicians despite their therapeutic potential.

■ INDUCED PLURIPOTENT STEM CELLS

The field of stem cell biology was transformed by the discovery that adult somatic cells can be converted ("reprogrammed") into pluripotent cells by overexpressing four transcription factors normally expressed in pluripotent cells (Chap. 65). These iPS cells share most properties with ES cells, although there are distinct differences in gene expression between ES and iPS cells. Viruses were used initially to insert the transcription factors into somatic cells, making them unsuitable for clinical use. However, a number of strategies have been developed to circumvent this problem, including the insertion of proteins rather than cDNAs; insertion of transposons with the programming factors, followed by their subsequent removal;

and use of floxed viral constructs followed by Cre recombinase to excise the viral constructs. None of these approaches is sufficiently developed for cells to be used clinically, but appropriate techniques are likely to evolve quickly. The potential advantages of such cells are that use of somatic cells from patients would generate iPS cells genetically identical to those of the patient and that the cells do not have the same ethical constraints as ES cells. It is not clear whether the differences in gene expression between ES and iPS cells will have any impact on their potential clinical utility, and studies of both cell types will be essential to resolve this issue.

UMBILICAL CORD STEM CELLS

Umbilical cord blood stem/progenitor cells are widely and easily available, and they appear to be associated with less graft-versus-host disease than are some other cell types, such as marrow stem cells. They have less human leukocyte antigen (HLA) restriction than adult marrow stem cells and are less likely to be contaminated with herpesvirus. However, it is unclear how many different cell types can be generated from umbilical cord blood stem cells, and methods for differentiating these cells into nonhematopoietic phenotypes are largely lacking. Further, the quantity of obtainable cells may be limiting.

ORGAN-SPECIFIC MULTIPOTENT STEM CELLS

Organ-specific multipotent stem cells have the advantage that they are already somewhat specialized and inducement of desired cell types thus may be easier. Cells potentially could be obtained from the patient and amplified in cell culture, circumventing the problems associated with immune rejection. Stem cells are relatively easy to harvest from some tissues, such as bone marrow and blood, but difficult in the case of other tissues, such as heart and brain. However, these populations of cells are more limited in potentiality than are pluripotent ES or iPS cells, and they may be difficult to obtain in large quantities from many organs. Therefore, substantial efforts have been devoted to developing techniques for using more easily obtainable stem cell populations, such as bone marrow mesenchymal stem cells (MSCs) and adipose stem cells, for use in regenerative strategies. Tissue culture evidence suggests that these stem cell populations may be able to generate differentiated cell types unrelated to their organ source, including myocytes, chondrocytes, tendon cells, osteoblasts, cardiomyocytes, adipocytes, hepatocytes, and neurons, a process known as transdifferentiation. However, it is still unclear whether these stem cells are capable of generating differentiated cell types that integrate into organs, survive, and function after transplantation in vivo. A number of early studies of bone marrow–derived stem cells transplanted into heart, liver, and other organs suggested that the cells had differentiated into organ-specific cell types. Subsequent studies, however, revealed that the stem cells had simply fused with cells resident in the organs. Further studies will be necessary to determine whether transdifferentiation of MSCs, adipose stem cells, or other stem cell populations occurs at a high enough frequency to be useful for stem cell replacement therapy.

Regardless of the source of the stem cell used in regenerative strategies, there are a number of generic problems that must be overcome for the development of successful clinical applications. These problems include development of methods for reliably generating large numbers of specific cell types, minimizing the risk of tumor formation or proliferation of inappropriate cell types, ensuring the viability and function of the engrafted cells, overcoming the problems of immune rejection when autografts are not used, and facilitating revascularization of the regenerated tissue. Each organ system will also pose tissue-specific problems for stem cell therapies.

DISEASE-SPECIFIC APPLICATIONS OF STEM CELLS

ISCHEMIC HEART DISEASE AND CARDIOMYOCYTE REGENERATION

Because of the prevalence of ischemic heart disease, extensive efforts have been devoted to the development of strategies for cell replacement of cardiomyocytes. Historically, the adult heart has been viewed as a terminally differentiated organ without the capacity for regeneration. However, recent studies have demonstrated that the heart has the ability to achieve low levels of cardiomyocyte regeneration (Chap. 224). This regeneration appears to be accomplished by cardiac stem cells resident in the heart and possibly by cells originating in the bone marrow. Cardiac stem cells might be an ideal source for therapeutic use, but techniques for isolating, characterizing, and amplifying large numbers of these cells have not been perfected. To effect myocardial repair, stem cell therapy must deliver cells either systemically or locally, and the cells must survive, engraft, and differentiate into functional cardiomyocytes that couple mechanically and electrically with the recipient myocardium. The optimal method for cell delivery is not clear, and various experimental and clinical studies have successfully employed intramyocardial, transendocardial, intravenous, and intracoronary injections. In experimental myocardial infarction, functional improvements have been achieved after transplantation of a variety of different cell types, including ES cells, bone marrow stem cells, endothelial stem cells, and adipose stem cells. Early studies suggested that each of these cell types might have the potential to engraft and generate cardiomyocytes. However, most investigators have found that the generation of new cardiomyocytes by these cells is at best a rare event and that graft survival over long periods is poor. The preponderance of evidence suggests that the beneficial effects of most experimental therapies were not derived from direct stem cell generation of cardiomyocytes but rather from indirect effects of the stem cells on resident cells. It is not clear whether this reflects the release of soluble growth factors, induction of angiogenesis, or another mechanism. The ready availability of bone marrow stem cells facilitated a series of limited clinical trials in human ischemic heart disease. A wide variety of cell delivery methods, cell types, and doses of cells have been used in the various studies, and the fate of the cells and the mechanisms by which they altered cardiac function are open questions. In aggregate, however, these studies have shown a small but measurable improvement in cardiac function and, in some cases, reduction in infarct size. The limited available evidence suggests that the beneficial effects probably reflect an indirect effect of the transplanted cells rather than genuine cell replacement.

DIABETES

Successes with islet cell and pancreas transplantation have provided proof of the concept for cell-based therapies for type 1 diabetes. However, the demand for donor pancreases far exceeds the number available, and maintenance of long-term graft survival is a problem. The search for a renewable source of stem cells capable of regenerating pancreatic islets has therefore been intensive. Pancreatic beta cell turnover occurs even in the normal pancreas, although the source of the new beta cells remains controversial. This suggests that in principle, it should be possible to develop strategies for reconstituting the beta cell population in diabetics. Attempts to devise techniques for promoting endogenous regenerative processes by using combinations of growth factors, drugs, and gene therapy have failed thus far, but this remains a potentially viable approach. A number of different cell types are candidates for use in stem cell replacement strategies, including iPS cells, ES cells, hepatic progenitor cells, pancreatic ductal progenitor cells, and bone marrow stem cells. Successful therapy will depend on the development of a source of cells that can be amplified to produce large numbers of progeny that have the ability to synthesize, store, and release insulin when it is required, primarily in response to changes in the ambient level of glucose. The proliferative capacity of the replacement cells must be tightly regulated to avoid excessive expansion of beta cell numbers with the consequent development of hyperinsulinemia/hypoglycemia, and the cells must withstand immune rejection. Although it has been reported that ES and iPS cells can be differentiated into cells that produce insulin, these cells have a low content of insulin and a high rate of apoptosis and generally lack the capacity to normalize blood glucose in diabetic animals. Thus, ES and iPS cells have not been useful for the large-scale production of differentiated islet cells. During embryogenesis, the pancreas, liver, and gastrointestinal tract are all derived from the anterior endoderm, and transdifferentiation of the pancreas to liver and vice versa has been observed in a number of pathologic conditions. There is also substantial evidence that multipotential stem cells reside within gastric glands and intestinal crypts. These observations suggest that hepatic, pancreatic and/or gastrointestinal precursor cells may be reasonable candidates for cell-based therapy for diabetes, although it is unclear whether insulin-producing cells derived from pancreatic stem cells or liver progenitors can be expanded in vitro to clinically useful numbers. Bone marrow stem cells and neural stem cells both reportedly have the capacity to generate insulin-producing cells, but there is no convincing evidence that either cell type will be clinically useful.

NERVOUS SYSTEM

Substantial progress has been made in developing methodologies for generating neural cells from different stem cell populations. Human ES or iPS cells can be induced to generate cells with the properties of neural stem cells, and these cells in turn give rise to neurons, oligodendroglia, and astrocytes. Reasonably large numbers of these cells can be transplanted into the rodent brain with formation of appropriate cell types and no tumor formation. Multipotent stem cells present in the adult brain also can be easily amplified in number and used to generate all the major neural cell types, but the invasive procedures that would be necessary to obtain autologous cells are a major limitation. Fetal neural stem cells derived from miscarriages or abortions are an alternative but may raise ethical concerns. Nevertheless, a clinical trial of fetal neural stem cells in Batten's disease is in progress. Transdifferentiation of bone marrow and adipose stem cells into neural stem cells, and vice versa, has been reported by numerous investigators, and clinical trials of such cells have begun for a number of neurologic disorders. Clinical trials of a conditionally immortalized human cell line and of human umbilical cord blood cells in stroke are planned. Some evidence suggests that epidermal stem cells also have the potential for neural regeneration. Neurologic disorders that have been targeted for stem cell therapies include spinal cord injury, amyotrophic lateral sclerosis (ALS), stroke, traumatic brain injury, Batten's disease, and Parkinson's disease. In Parkinson's disease the major motor features of the disorder result from the loss of a single cell population—dopaminergic neurons within the substantia nigra—suggesting that cell replacement should be relatively straightforward. However, two clinical trials of fetal nigral transplantation failed to meet their primary endpoint and were complicated by the development of dyskinesia. Transplantation of stem cell–derived dopamine-producing cells offers a number of potential advantages over the fetal transplants, including the ability of stem cells to migrate and disperse within tissue, the potential for engineering regulatable release of dopamine, and the ability to engineer cells to produce factors that will enhance cell survival. Nevertheless, the experience with fetal transplants points out the difficulties that may be encountered.

At least some of the neurologic dysfunction after spinal cord injury reflects demyelination, and both ES cells and marrow-derived stem cells are able to facilitate remyelination after experimental spinal cord injury. Clinical trials of marrow-derived stem cells in this disorder have commenced in a number of countries, and this may be the first disease targeted for the clinical use of ES cells. Marrow-derived stem cells also are being used in the treatment of stroke, traumatic brain injury, and ALS, in which possible benefits are more likely to be due to indirect trophic effects or remyelination than to neuron replacement. At present no population of transplanted stem cells has been shown to have the capacity to generate neurons that extend axons over long distances to form synaptic connections (as would be necessary for replacement of upper motor neurons in ALS, stroke, or other disorders).

LIVER

Liver transplantation is currently the only successful treatment for end-stage liver diseases, but the shortage of liver grafts is a serious problem. Clinical trials of hepatocyte transplantation demonstrate that it potentially can substitute for organ transplantation, but this approach is limited by the paucity of available cells. Potential sources of stem cells for regenerative strategies include endogenous liver stem cells (such as oval cells), ES cells, bone marrow cells, and umbilical cord blood cells. Although a series of studies in humans as well as animals suggested that transplanted bone marrow stem cells can generate hepatocytes, fusion of the transplanted cells with endogenous liver cells, giving the erroneous appearance of new hepatocytes, appears to be the underlying event in most circumstances. The available evidence suggests that transplanted hematopoietic cells can generate hepatocyte-like cells in the liver only at a very low frequency. ES cells can be differentiated into hepatocytes and transplanted in animal models of liver failure without the formation of teratomas.

OTHER ORGAN SYSTEMS AND THE FUTURE

The use of stem cells in regenerative strategies has been studied for many other organ systems and cell types, including skin, eye, cartilage, bone, kidney, lung, endometrium, vascular endothelium, smooth muscle, and striated muscle, among others. In fact, the potential for stem cell regeneration of damaged organs and tissues is virtually limitless. However, there are numerous obstacles to be overcome before stem cell therapies can become a widespread clinical reality. Only hematopoietic stem cells have been adequately characterized by surface markers so that they can be unambiguously identified, a prerequisite for reliable clinical applications. The pathways for differentiating stem cells into specific cellular phenotypes are largely unknown, and there is little ability at present to control the migration of transplanted cells or predict the response of the cells to the environment of diseased organs. Some strategies may employ the coadministration of scaffolding, artificial extracellular matrix, and/or growth factors to orchestrate differentiation of stem cells and their organization into appropriate constituents of the organ. There is currently no way to image stem cells in vivo after transplantation into humans, and it will be necessary to develop techniques to accomplish this. Fortunately, stem cells can be engineered before transplantation to contain a contrast agent that may make this feasible. The potential for tumor formation and the problems associated with immune rejection are impediments, and it will also be necessary to develop techniques for ensuring vascularization of regenerated tissues. There already are many strategies for cell replacement, including vasoactive endothelial growth factor (VEGF) coadministration to foster vascularization of the transplant. Some strategies also include genetically engineering stem cells to have an inducible suicide gene so that the cells can be easily eradicated in the event of tumor formation or another complication. The potential for stem cell therapies to revolutionize medical care is extraordinary, and disorders such as myocardial infarction, diabetes, and Parkinson's disease, among many others, will become potentially curable. However, such stem cell–based therapies are still at a very early stage of development, and perfection of techniques for clinical transplantation of predictable, well-characterized cells is going to be a difficult and lengthy undertaking.

ETHICAL ISSUES

Stem cell therapies raise ethical and socially contentious issues that must be addressed in parallel with the scientific and medical opportunities. This society has great diversity with respect to religious beliefs, concepts of individual rights, tolerance for uncertainty and risk, and boundaries for how scientific interventions should be used to alter the outcome of disease. In the United States, the federal government has authorized research using existing human ES cell lines but still restricts the use of federal funds for developing new human ES cell lines. Ongoing studies of existing lines have indicated that they develop abnormalities with time in culture and that they may be contaminated with mouse proteins. These findings point out the need to develop new human ES cell lines. The development of iPS cell technology may lessen the need for deriving new ES cell lines, but it is still not clear whether the differences in gene expression by ES and iPS cells are important for potential clinical use.

In considering ethical issues associated with the use of stem cells, it is helpful to draw from experience with other scientific advances, such as organ transplantation, recombinant DNA technology, implantation of mechanical devices, neuroscience and cognitive research, in vitro fertilization, and prenatal genetic testing. These and other precedents have pointed to the importance of understanding and testing fundamental biology in the laboratory setting and in animal models before applying new techniques in carefully controlled clinical trials. When these trials occur, they must include full informed consent and provide for careful oversight by external review groups.

Ultimately, there will be medical interventions that are scientifically feasible but ethically or socially unacceptable to some members of a society. Stem cell research raises fundamentally difficult questions about the definition of human life, and it has raised deep fears about the ability to balance issues of justice and safety with the needs of critically ill patients. Health care providers and experts with backgrounds in ethics, law, and sociology, must help guard against the premature or inappropriate application of stem cell therapies and the inappropriate use of vulnerable population groups. However, these therapies offer important new strategies for the treatment of otherwise irreversible disorders. An open dialogue among the scientific community, physicians, patients and their advocates, lawmakers, and the lay population is critically important to raise and address important ethical issues and balance the benefits and risks associated with stem cell transfer.

FURTHER READINGS

Higgs DR: A new dawn for stem-cell therapy. N Engl J Med 358:964, 2008

Kiskinis E, Eggan K: Progress toward the clinical application of patient-specific pluripotent stem cells. J Clin Invest 120:51, 2010

Park IH et al: Disease-specific induced pluripotent stem cells. Cell 134:877, 2008

Parmacek MS, Epstein JA: Cardiomyocyte renewal. N Engl J Med 361:86, 2009

Riazi AM et al: Stem cell sources for regenerative medicine. Methods Mol Biol 482:55, 2009

CHAPTER **68**

Gene Therapy in Clinical Medicine

Katherine A. High

Gene transfer is a novel area of therapeutics in which the active agent is a nucleic acid rather than a protein or small molecule. Because delivery of naked DNA or RNA to a cell is an inefficient process, most gene transfer is carried out using a vector, or gene delivery vehicle. These vehicles have generally been engineered from viruses by deleting some or all of the viral genome and replacing it with the therapeutic gene of interest under the control of a suitable promoter (Table 68-1). Gene transfer strategies can be described in terms of three essential elements: (1) a vector; (2) a gene to be delivered, sometimes called the *transgene*; and (3) a relevant target cell to which the DNA or RNA is delivered. The series of steps in which the donated DNA enters the target cell and expresses the transgene is referred to as *transduction*. Gene delivery can take place in vivo, in which the vector is directly injected into the patient or, in the case of hematopoietic and some other target cells, ex vivo, with removal of the target cells from the patient, followed by return of the modified autologous cells after gene transfer in the laboratory. The latter approach offers opportunities to integrate gene transfer techniques with cellular therapies (Chap. 67).

Gene transfer technology is still under development, although licensing applications for gene therapy products have been filed. Gene therapy is one of the most complex therapeutic modalities yet attempted, and each new disease represents a therapeutic problem for which dosing, safety, and efficacy must be defined. Nonetheless, gene transfer remains one of the most powerful concepts in modern molecular medicine and has the potential to address a host of diseases for which there are currently no cures or, in some cases, no available treatment. More than 5000 subjects have been enrolled in gene transfer studies, and serious adverse events have been rare. Gene therapies are being developed for a wide variety of disease entities (Fig. 68-1).

GENE TRANSFER FOR GENETIC DISEASE

Gene transfer strategies for genetic disease generally involve gene addition therapy. This approach most commonly involves transfer of the missing gene to a physiologically relevant target cell. However, other strategies are possible, including supplying a gene that achieves a similar biologic effect through an alternative pathway (e.g., factor VIIa for hemophilia A), supplying an antisense oligonucleotide to splice out a mutant exon if the sequence is not critical to the function of the protein (as has been done with the dystrophin gene in Duchenne's muscular dystrophy), or downregulating a harmful response through an siRNA. Two distinct strategies are used to achieve long-term gene expression: one is to transduce stem cells with an integrating vector, so that all progeny cells will carry the donated gene; the other is to transduce long-lived cells such as skeletal muscle or neural cells. In the case of long-lived cells, integration into the target cell genome is unnecessary. Instead, because

TABLE 68-1 Characteristics of Gene Delivery Vehicles

Features	Viral Vectors							
	Retroviral	Lentiviral	Adenoviral	AAV	Human Foamy Virus	HSV-1	SV-40	Alphaviruses
Viral genome	RNA	RNA	DNA	DNA	RNA	DNA	DNA	RNA
Cell division requirement	Yes	G1 phase	No	No	No	No	No	No
Packaging limitation	8 kb	8 kb	8–30 kb	5 kb	8.5 kb	40–150 kb	5 kb	5 kb
Immune responses to vector	Few	Few	Extensive	Few	Few	Few in recombinant virus	Few	Few
Genome integration	Yes	Yes	Poor	Poor	Yes	No	Poor	No
Long-term expression	Yes	Yes	No	Yes	Yes	No	No	No
Main advantages	Persistent gene transfer in dividing cells	Persistent gene transfer in transduced tissues	Highly effective in transducing various tissues	Elicits few inflammatory responses, nonpathogenic	Persistent gene expression in both dividing and nondividing cells	Large packaging capacity with persistent gene transfer	Wide host cell range; lack of immunogenicity	Limited immune responses against the vector
Main disadvantages	Theoretical risk of insertional mutagenesis (occurred in three cases)	Might induce oncogenesis in some cases	Viral capsid elicits strong immune responses	Limited packaging capacity	In need of a stable packaging system	Residual cytotoxicity with neuron specificity	Limited packaging capacity	Transduced gene expression is transient

Abbreviations: AAV, adeno-associated virus; HSV, herpes simplex virus; SV, sarcoma virus.

the cells are nondividing, the donated DNA can be stabilized in an episomal form, avoiding problems related to integration and insertional mutagenesis.

Immunodeficiency disorders: proof of principle

Early attempts to effect gene replacement into hematopoietic stem cells (HSCs) were stymied by the relatively low transduction efficiency of retroviral vectors, which require dividing target cells for integration. Because HSCs are normally quiescent, they are a formidable transduction target. However, identification of cytokines that induced cell division without promoting differentiation of stem cells, along with technical improvements in the isolation and transduction of HSCs, led to modest but real gains in transduction efficiency.

The first convincing therapeutic effect from gene transfer occurred with X-linked severe combined immunodeficiency disease (SCID), which results from mutations in the gene (*IL2RG*) encoding the γc subunit of cytokine receptors required for normal development of T and NK cells (Chap. 316). Affected infants present in the first few months of life with overwhelming infections and/or failure to thrive. In this disorder, it was recognized that the transduced cells, even if few in number, would have a proliferative advantage compared to the nontransduced cells, which lack receptors for the cytokines required for lymphocyte development and maturation. Complete reconstitution of the immune system, including documented responses to standard childhood vaccinations, clearing of infections, and remarkable gains in growth occurred in most of the treated children. However, among 20 children

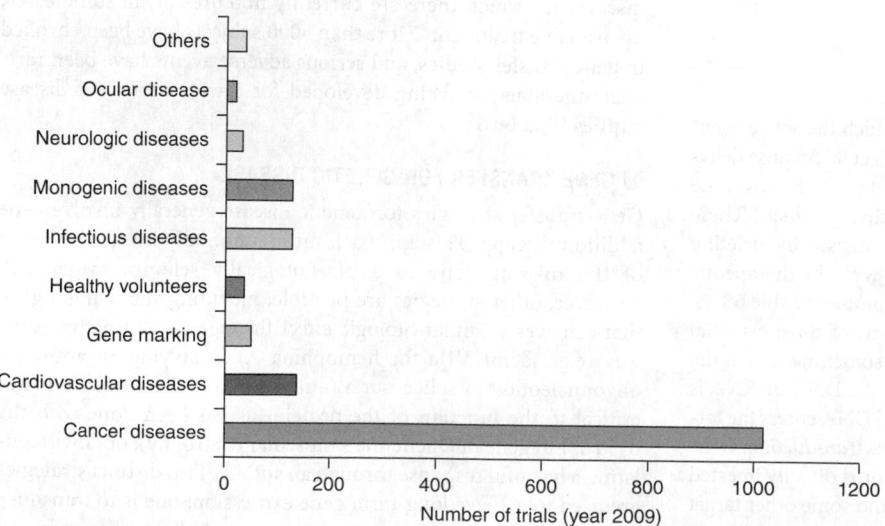

Figure 68-1 Indications in gene therapy clinical trials. The bar graph classifies clinical gene transfer studies by disease. A majority of trials have addressed cancer, with monogenic disorders and cardiovascular diseases the next largest categories. *(Adapted from J Gene Med. New Jersey, Wiley, 2009.)*

TABLE 68-2 Potential Complications of Gene Therapy

Gene silencing: repression of promoter

Genotoxicity: complications arising from insertional mutagenesis

Phenotoxicity: complications arising from overexpression or ectopic expression of the transgene

Immunotoxicity: harmful immune response to either the vector or transgene

Risks of horizontal transmission: shedding of infectious vector into environment

Risks of vertical transmission: germline transmission of donated DNA

---

treated in two separate trials, 5 developed a syndrome similar to T cell acute lymphocytic leukemia, with splenomegaly, rising white blood cell counts, and the emergence of a single clone of T cells. In most of these children, the retroviral vector had integrated within a gene, *LMO-2* (LIM only-2), which encodes a component of a transcription factor complex involved in hematopoietic development. The retroviral long terminal repeat is thought to increase the expression of *LMO-2*.

The X-linked SCID studies were a watershed event in the evolution of gene therapy. They demonstrated conclusively that gene therapy could cure disease; of the 20 children eventually treated in these trials, 18 achieved correction of the immunodeficiency disorder. Unfortunately, 5 later developed a leukemia-like disorder, and 1 died of this complication, but the rest are alive and free of complications for up to 10 years after initial treatment. These studies also demonstrated that insertional mutagenesis leading to cancer was more than a hypothetical possibility (Table 68-2). As a result of the experience in these trials, all protocols using integrating vectors in hematopoietic cells must include a plan for monitoring sites of insertion and clonal proliferation. Strategies to overcome this complication have included employing a "suicide" gene cassette in the vector, so that errant clones can be quickly ablated; or using "insulator" elements in the cassette, which can limit the activation of genes surrounding the insertion site. Lentiviral vectors, which can efficiently transduce nondividing target cells, may prove to be safer than retroviral vectors, based on patterns of integration; the field is thus gradually using these as an alternative to retroviral vectors.

More clear-cut success has been achieved in a gene therapy trial for another form of SCID, adenosine deaminase (ADA) deficiency (Chap. 316). ADA-SCID is clinically similar to X-linked SCID, although it can be treated by enzyme replacement therapy with a pegylated form of the enzyme (PEG-ADA), which leads to immune reconstitution but not always to normal T cell counts. Enzyme replacement therapy is expensive (annual costs: $200,000–$300,000 in U.S. dollars). The initial trials of gene therapy for ADA-SCID were unsuccessful, but modifications of this protocol to include the use of HSCs rather than T cells as the target for transduction; discontinuation of PEG-ADA at the time of vector infusion, so that the transduced cells have a proliferative advantage over the nontransduced; and the use of a mild conditioning regimen to facilitate engraftment of the transduced cells. There have been no complications in the 10 children treated on the Milan protocol, with a median follow-up of >4 years. ADA-SCID, then, is an example where gene therapy has changed therapeutic options for patients. For those with an HLA-identical sibling, bone marrow transplantation is still the best treatment option, but this applies to only a minority of those affected. For those without an HLA-identical match, gene therapy has comparable efficacy to PEG-ADA and does not run the risk of neutralizing antibodies to the bovine enzyme.

Other applications of integrating vectors

More recently, therapeutic success has also been reported in the setting of X-linked adrenoleukodystrophy, a fatal demyelinating disease of the central nervous system (CNS) caused by mutations in the gene encoding an adenosine triphosphate–binding cassette transporter. Deficiency of this protein leads to adrenal insufficiency and accumulation of very-long-chain fatty acids in oligodendrocytes and microglia, disrupting myelin maintenance by these cells. Affected boys present with clinical and neuroradiographic evidence of disease at age 6–8 years and usually die before adolescence. Aubourg and colleagues have shown dramatic stabilization of disease both clinically and radiographically following lentiviral transduction of hematopoietic stem cells in young boys with disease. Other diseases likely to be amenable to transduction of HSCs include Wiskott-Aldrich syndrome, chronic granulomatous disease, thalassemia, and sickle cell disease, with trials under way currently for the first three of these disorders.

Long-term expression in genetic disease: in vivo gene transfer with recombinant adeno-associated viral (AAV) vectors

Recombinant AAV vectors have emerged as attractive gene delivery vehicles for genetic disease. Engineered from a small replication-defective DNA virus, they are devoid of viral coding sequences and trigger very little immune response in experimental animals. They are capable of transducing nondividing target cells, and the donated DNA is stabilized primarily in an episomal form, thus minimizing risks associated with insertional mutagenesis. Because the vector has a tropism for certain long-lived cell types, such as skeletal muscle, the central nervous system, and hepatocytes, long-term expression can be achieved even in the absence of integration.

Clinical trials using recombinant AAV vectors are now ongoing for muscular dystrophies, α_1-antitrypsin deficiency, Parkinson's disease, lipoprotein lipase deficiency, hemophilia B, and a form of congenital blindness called Leber's congenital amaurosis. Hemophilia is often considered a promising disease model for gene transfer, as the gene product does not require precise regulation of expression and biologically active clotting factors can be synthesized in a variety of tissue types, permitting latitude in choice of target tissue. Moreover, raising circulating factor levels from <1% (levels seen in those severely affected) into the range of 5% greatly improves the phenotype of the disease. Preclinical studies with recombinant AAV vectors infused into skeletal muscle or liver have resulted in long-term (>5 years) expression of factor VIII or factor IX in the hemophilic dog model. Administration to skeletal muscle of an AAV vector expressing factor IX in patients with hemophilia was safe and resulted in long-term expression as measured by muscle biopsy, but circulating levels never rose >1% for sustained periods, and a large number of IM injections (>80–100) was required to access a large muscle mass. Intravascular vector delivery has been employed to access large areas of skeletal muscle in animal models of hemophilia and will likely be tested in upcoming trials. Administration of an AAV vector expressing factor IX to the liver in humans with hemophilia resulted in therapeutic circulating levels at the highest dose tested, but expression at these levels (>5%) lasted for only 6–10 weeks before declining to baseline (<1%). A memory T cell response to viral capsid, present in humans but not in other animal species (which are not natural hosts for the virus), may be a contributing factor in the loss of expression (Table 68-2). Trials currently under way are testing two potential strategies to overcome this obstacle—in the first, subjects receive a short course of immunosuppression coadministered with the vector to block the immune response to capsid until the capsid proteins have been degraded and metabolized. In the second, the use of a more efficient expression cassette with a codon-optimized, self-complementary design should allow expression of factor IX at lower doses of vector, which may also elude the immune response.

Early experience with AAV in liver in the hemophilia trial suggested that introduction of small doses of vector into an immuno-privileged site might allow long-term expression, even in humans previously exposed to AAV. This has been most elegantly demonstrated in the setting of the retinal degenerative disease Leber's congenital amaurosis (LCA). LCA, characterized by early-onset blindness, is not currently treatable, and is caused by mutations in several different genes; ~15% of cases of LCA are due to a mutation in a gene, *RPE65*, encoding a retinal pigment epithelial-associated 65 kilodalton protein. In dogs with a null mutation in *RPE65*, sight has been restored after subretinal injection of an AAV vector expressing *RPE65*. Transgene expression appears to be stable, with the first animals treated >10 years ago continuing to manifest electrophysiologic and behavioral evidence of visual function. As is the case for X-linked SCID, gene transfer must occur relatively early in life to achieve optimal correction of the genetic disease, although the exact limitations imposed by age have not yet been defined. AAV-RPE65 trials carried out in both the United States and the United Kingdom have shown restoration of visual and retinal function in more than 20 subjects, with the most marked improvement occurring in the youngest subjects treated (age 8 years). Other inherited retinal degenerative disorders may also be amenable to correction by gene transfer, as are certain complex acquired disorders such as age-related macular degeneration, which affects several million people worldwide. The neovascularization that occurs in age-related macular degeneration can be inhibited by expression of vascular endothelial growth factor (VEGF) inhibitors such as angiostatin, or through the use of RNAi-mediated knockdown of VEGF. Early-phase trials of siRNAs that target VEGF RNA are under way, but these require repeated intravitreal injection of the siRNAs; an AAV vector–mediated approach, which would allow long-term inhibition of the biologic effects of VEGF through a soluble VEGF receptor is now in early-phase clinical testing.

GENE THERAPY FOR CANCER

The majority of clinical gene transfer experience has been in subjects with cancer (Fig. 68-1). As a general rule, a feature that distinguishes gene therapies from conventional cancer therapeutics is that the former are less toxic, in some cases because they are delivered locally (e.g., intratumoral injections), and in other cases because they are targeted specifically to features of the tumor (immunotherapies, antiangiogenic approaches).

Cancer gene therapies can be divided into local and systemic approaches (Table 68-3). Some of the earliest cancer gene therapy trials focused on local delivery of a prodrug or a suicide gene that would increase sensitivity of tumor cells to cytotoxic drugs. A frequently used strategy has been intratumoral injection of an adenoviral vector expressing the thymidine kinase (*TK*) gene. Cells that take up and express the *TK* gene can be killed after the administration of

gancyclovir, which is phosphorylated to a toxic nucleoside by *TK*. Because cell division is required for the toxic nucleoside to affect cell viability, this strategy was initially used in aggressive brain tumors (glioblastoma multiforme) where the cycling tumor cells were affected but the nondividing normal neurons were not. More recently, this approach has been explored for locally recurrent prostate, breast, and colon tumors, among others.

Another local approach uses adenoviral-mediated expression of the tumor suppressor p53, which is mutated in a wide variety of cancers. This strategy has shown complete and partial responses in squamous cell carcinoma of the head and neck, esophageal cancer, and non-small-cell lung cancer after direct intratumoral injection of the vector. Response rates (~15%) are comparable to those of other single agents. The use of oncolytic viruses that selectively replicate in tumor cells but not in normal cells has also shown promise in squamous cell carcinoma of the head and neck and in other solid tumors. This approach is based on the observation that deletion of certain viral genes abolishes their ability to replicate in normal cells but not in tumor cells. An advantage of this strategy is that the replicating vector can proliferate and spread within the tumor, facilitating eventual tumor clearance. However, physical limitations to viral spread, including fibrosis, intermixed normal cells, basement membranes, and necrotic areas within the tumor, may reduce clinical efficacy. Oncolytic viruses are licensed and available in some countries, but not in the United States.

Because metastatic disease rather than uncontrolled growth of the primary tumor is the source of mortality for most cancers, there has been considerable interest in developing systemic gene therapy approaches. One strategy has been to promote more efficient recognition of tumor cells by the immune system. Approaches have included transduction of tumor cells with immune-enhancing genes encoding cytokines, chemokines, or co-stimulatory molecules. Sustained clinical responses provide evidence that the transduced cells can act as a vaccine. In a related approach, patient lymphocytes have been transduced with genes encoding a T cell receptor–like molecule, with a tumor antigen–binding domain fused to an intracellular signaling domain to allow T cell activation, thereby converting normal lymphocytes into cells capable of recognizing and destroying tumor cells. A third immunotherapy approach relies on ex vivo manipulation of dendritic cells to enhance the presentation of tumor antigens. These immunologic approaches may be of particular value in treating minimal residual disease after other anticancer modalities.

Gene transfer strategies have also been developed for inhibiting tumor angiogenesis. These have included constitutive expression of angiogenesis inhibitors such as angiostatin and endostatin; use of siRNA to reduce levels of VEGF or VEGF receptor; and combined approaches in which autologous T cells are genetically modified to recognize antigens specific to tumor vasculature. These studies are still in early-phase testing.

Another novel systemic approach is the use of gene transfer to protect normal cells from the toxicities of chemotherapy. The most extensively studied of these approaches has been transduction of hematopoietic cells with genes encoding resistance to chemotherapeutic agents, including the multidrug resistance gene *MDR1* or the gene encoding O⁶-methylguanine DNA methyltransferase (*MGMT*). Ex vivo transduction of hematopoietic cells, followed by autologous transplantation, is being investigated as a strategy for allowing administration of higher doses of chemotherapy than would otherwise be tolerated.

GENE THERAPY FOR VASCULAR DISEASE

The third major category addressed by gene transfer studies is cardiovascular disease. The most extensive experience has

---

TABLE 68-3 Gene Therapy Strategies in Cancer

Local/regional approaches
    Suicide gene/prodrug
    Suppressor oncogene
    Oncolytic virus
Systemic approaches
    Chemoprotection
    Immunomodulation
    Antiangiogenesis

been in trials designed to increase blood flow to either skeletal (critical limb ischemia) or cardiac muscle (angina/myocardial ischemia). Initial treatment options for both of these groups include mechanical revascularization or medical management, but a subset of patients are not candidates for, or fail, these approaches. These patients have formed the first cohorts for evaluation of gene transfer to achieve therapeutic angiogenesis. The major transgene used has been VEGF, attractive because of its specificity for endothelial cells; other transgenes have included fibroblast growth factor (FGF) and hypoxia-inducible factor 1, α subunit (HIF-1α). The design of most of the trials has included direct IM (or myocardial) injection of either a plasmid or an adenoviral vector expressing the transgene. Both of these vectors are likely to result in only short-term expression of VEGF. This strategy may be adequate, however, as there is no need for continued transgene expression once the new vessels have formed. Direct injection favors local expression, which should help to avoid systemic effects such as retinal neovascularization or new vessel formation in a nascent tumor. Initial trials of adeno-VEGF or plasmid-VEGF injection have resulted in improvement over baseline in terms of frequency of claudication/angina or amounts of nitroglycerin consumption. Study designs including placebo control groups and more objective endpoints (exercise duration at 3 or 6 months, rest and stress cardiac perfusion scans, and regional wall motion assessed by nonfluoroscopic electroanatomic mapping) continue to suggest a beneficial effect of gene transfer, although definitive conclusions will require larger studies. Continuing areas of investigation include choice of the optimal vector (adenoviral vs. plasmid), the optimal transgene (VEGF, HIF-1α, FGF, etc.), the optimal method of delivery in cardiac indications (intracoronary vs. direct myocardial), ideal objective endpoints, and whether concurrent administration of cytokines to mobilize endothelial progenitor cells will augment the therapeutic effect.

◼ OTHER DISEASES

The power and versatility of gene transfer approaches are such that there are few serious disease entities for which gene transfer therapies are *not* under development. Besides those already discussed, other areas of interest include gene therapies for HIV and for neurodegenerative disorders. The latter include studies in patients with Parkinson's disease, where AAV vectors expressing enzymes required for enhanced production of dopamine, or of the inhibitory neurotransmitter γ-aminobutyric acid, have been introduced into affected areas of the brain (striatum, subthalamic nucleus) by stereotactic neurosurgery. In Alzheimer's disease, an ex vivo approach in which autologous fibroblasts are transduced with a retroviral vector expressing nerve growth factor, then reimplanted into the basal forebrain, has slowed the rate of cognitive decline in a small phase I study.

◼ SUMMARY

The development of new classes of therapeutics typically takes two to three decades; monoclonal antibodies and recombinant proteins are recent examples. Gene therapeutics, which entered clinical testing in the early 1990s, are well along in the course of development, and are likely to become increasingly important as a therapeutic modality in the twenty-first century. A central question to be

TABLE 68-4 Taking History From Subjects Enrolled in Gene Transfer Studies

Elements of History for Subjects Enrolled in Gene Transfer Trials

1. What vector was administered? Is it predominantly integrating [retroviral, lentiviral, herpesvirus (latency and reactivation)], or nonintegrating (plasmid, adenoviral, AAV)?

2. What was the route of administration of the vector?

3. What was the target tissue?

4. What gene was transferred in? A disease-related gene? A marker?

5. Were there any adverse events noted after gene transfer?

Screening Questions for Long-Term Follow-Up in Gene Transfer Subjects*

1. Has a new malignancy been diagnosed?

2. Has a new neurologic/ophthalmologic disorder, or exacerbation of a preexisting disorder, been diagnosed?

3. Has a new autoimmune or rheumatologic disorder been diagnosed?

4. Has a new hematologic disorder been diagnosed?

*Factors influencing long-term risk include: integration of the vector into the genome; vector persistence without integration; and transgene-specific effects.

addressed is the long-term safety of gene transfer, and regulatory agencies have mandated a 15-year follow-up for subjects enrolled in gene therapy trials (Table 68-4). Realization of the therapeutic benefits of the Human Genome Project, and of new discoveries such as RNAi, will depend on continued progress in gene transfer technology.

FURTHER READINGS

AIUTI A et al: Gene therapy for immunodeficiency due to adenosine deaminase deficiency. N Engl J Med 360:447, 2009

BREITBACH CJ et al: Navigating the clinical development landscape for oncolytic viruses and other cancer therapeutics: No shortcuts on the road to approval. Cytokine Growth Factor Rev 21:85, 2010

CARTIER N et al: Hematopoietic stem cell gene therapy with a lentiviral vector in X-linked adrenoleukodystrophy. Science 326:818, 2009

Gene Therapy Clinical Trials Worldwide. J Gene Med. John Wiley & Sons, 2009. Accessed at http://www.wiley.co.uk/genetherapy/clinical/

HACEIN-BEY-ABINA S et al: LMO2-associated clonal T cell proliferation in two patients after gene therapy for SCID-X1. Science 302:415, 2003

MAGUIRE AM et al: Age-dependent effects of REP65 gene therapy for Leber's congenital amaurosis: A phase 1 dose escalation trial. Lancet 374:1597, 2009

MANNO CS et al: Successful transduction of liver in hemophilia by AAV-Factor IX and limitations imposed by the host immune response. Nat Med 12:342, 2006

SADELAIN M: T-cell engineering for cancer immunotherapy. Cancer 15:451, 2009

TONGERS GR, Losordo DW: Human studies of angiogenic gene therapy. Circ Res 105:724, 2009

CHAPTER **69**
Tissue Engineering

David M. Hoganson
Howard I. Pryor, II
Joseph P. Vacanti

INTRODUCTION

As medicine therapy advances, we can now realistically set goals for fully functional living replacement of nearly every diseased organ or tissue. In the past several decades, the limitations of nonliving mechanical solutions to organ and tissue dysfunction are now recognized and include dialysis, mechanical heart valves, metallic orthopedic implants, and nonresorbable hernia mesh. Tissue engineering has broad goals including organ development, the elimination of the waiting time for transplants such as the liver and kidney, the creation of living tissue replacements for soft tissue, bone, cartilage, fascia, and virtually every structure in the body.

MATERIALS AND SCAFFOLDS FOR TISSUE ENGINEERING

The principal mechanical supporting structure of any engineered tissue is the scaffold. These three-dimensional constructs are often composed of several materials and support the living cells required to generate a functional tissue (Fig. 69-1). The mechanical properties of the scaffolds, such as strength and elasticity, must correspond to the mechanical properties of the target tissue. Moreover, cells respond to environmental cues such that the scaffold should mimic the target tissue to achieve the desired cell alignment and the three-dimensional arrangement of the cells.

The ideal scaffold materials for engineered tissues are resorbable materials that break down over time. During resorption, the engineered tissue is remodeled by normal healing processes, leaving only living cellular tissue with natural supporting connective tissue. Many implants or organ assist devices are under development utilizing the principles of tissue engineering with nonresorbable materials. These technologies such as lung assist devices, liver assist devices, and even composite implants with resorbable and nonresorbable components for orthopedic and hernia repair represent an important step toward developing fully resorbable scaffolds for all tissues. Current research is focused on resorbable synthetic polymers (e.g., polyglycolic acid, resorbable polyurethanes, polyglycerol sebacic acid); naturally occurring polymers (e.g., collagens, fibrin); and minerals (e.g., calcium triphosphate). Scaffold materials can be supplemented with growth factors or other cytokines to improve cellular incorporation and differentiation. Other surface modifications including surface texturing and protein or antibody coatings may improve cellular adhesion and migration.

Decellularized connective tissue, or organs, represents a rapidly developing area of materials for engineered tissues. Decellularized hearts reseeded with myocardial cells have been demonstrated to function in vitro, and research is focused on expanding this approach to other organs such as the lung and liver as well as soft tissues using material such as decellularized dermis.

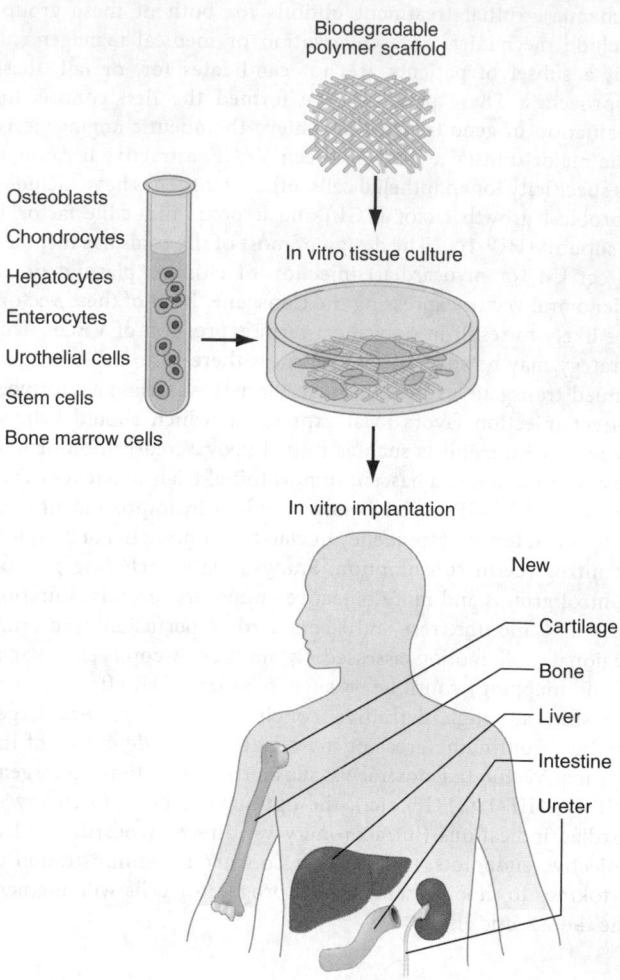

Figure 69-1 Schematic of basic principles of tissue engineering. (*From R Langer, J Vacanti: Science 260:1993; with permission.*)

CELLS FOR TISSUE ENGINEERING

The cellular components of engineered tissues must achieve organ functionality (e.g., hepatocytes), maintain organ structure (e.g., fibroblasts and stromal cells), and deliver blood to the tissue (e.g., endothelial cells and pericytes). The three-dimensional arrangement of the cells is critical for proper function; therefore, coordination of scaffold design and cellular components is essential. Maintenance of appropriate cell-to-cell interactions and cell-to-extracellular matrix interactions establishes the microenvironment that drives the differentiation, proliferation potential, and function of many cell types.

Using autologous cells is a principal goal when developing any engineered tissue. This avoids the tremendous burden of immunosuppression. Induced pluripotent stem cells and adult mesenchymal stem cells (e.g., bone marrow or adipose derived) are two promising autologous progenitor cells sources. Differentiation cues including soluble signals and incorporating genes can drive the progenitor cells into cell lineages and end-organ cells (Chaps. 67 and 68). Finally, achieving an adequate number of cells is important. For example, there are approximately 5×10^{10} hepatocytes in a normal adult liver. Therefore, any cellular differentiation strategy must take into account the number of cells needed to seed the scaffold for appropriate tissue function.

Allogenic cells remain an option for many tissues and have been the principal source of clinically successful engineered tissues to date. Embryonic stem cells continue to hold great promise as an allogenic cell option. Xenogenic cells are important to consider as they are available in large numbers, but their use has been mostly limited to organ support devices (i.e., liver devices) and they are not directly implanted into a patient.

IN VITRO MATURATION OF ENGINEERED TISSUES

Nearly all tissues have baseline mechanical requirements and many tissues such as heart valves, blood vessels, bone, and tendons must have adequate mechanical properties to achieve function. Mechanical forces are important to induce cell alignment and in the production of an extracellular matrix. Bioreactors have been developed to impart the needed mechanical forces to engineered tissues, including shear stress, pusatile flow, and pressure for valves and blood vessels, and axial tension and compression for bone, cartilage, and tendons.

CLINICAL APPLICATIONS

Engineered skin substitutes were the first true clinical success of the principles of tissue engineering (Table 69-1). These clinically available products use autologous fibroblasts grown on a resorbable polymer scaffold for a single-layer product or fibroblasts covered with keratinocytes for a two-layer product. Recent products for promoting the healing of skin and dermal wounds also incorporate autologous fibroblasts delivered into the wound. Autologous chondrocytes are being used to heal damaged joints, and they have shown excellent results. Acellular collagen-based materials derived from human or animal dermis are being implanted for soft tissue reconstruction or hernia repair and become cellularized in vivo with autologous cells. Many engineered tissues are in clinical trials (Table 69-2) or under development, including those for bone, cartilage, nerve, skeletal muscle, small-diameter blood vessels, heart valves, and vital organs, including heart, liver, lung, and kidney.

TABLE 69-1 Examples of FDA-Approved Tissue Engineering Products

Alloderm (LifeCell)	Acellular dermal matrix for tissue repair
Apligraf (Organogenesis)	Living skin equivalent approved for the treatment of venous leg ulcers and diabetic foot ulcers
Carticel (Genzyme Biosurgery)	Autologous chondrocytes approved for cartilage repair
Dermagraft (Smith and Nephew)	Living skin equivalent approved for full-thickness diabetic foot ulcers
Durasis (Cook Surgical Products)	Porcine small-intestine submucosa for replacement of dura mater
Epicel (Genzyme Biosurgery)	Living skin equivalent approved for burn patients
OrCel (Ortec)	Living skin equivalent approved for burn patients
Surgisis (Cook Surgical Products)	Porcine small-intestine submucosa for dermal wounds and reinforcement of weakened tissue
FlexHD (Ethicon)	Acellular dermal matrix for tissue repair
Strattice (LifeCell)	Acellular dermal matrix for tissue repair
DermaMatrix (Synthes)	Acellular dermal matrix for tissue repair

TABLE 69-2 Tissue Engineering Products in Clinical Trials

Dermagen (Laboratoires Genévrier)	Living skin equivalent
Lifeline (Cytograft)	Living small-diameter blood vessel
Hepatocyte Matrix Implant (Baermed)	Resorbable matrix and autologous hepatocytes grafted into omentum to support liver function
TRC (Aastrom)	Autologous adult bone marrow cells for bone grafting
Myocell (Bioheart)	Encapsulated autologous muscle cells for myocardial infarction
MarkII (Excorp)	Extracorporeal liver assist device
HuCNS-SC (Stem Cell Inc)	Human central nervous system stem cells
NT-501 (Neurotech SA)	Encapsulated cell technology for long-term delivery of therapeutic factors to retina
Procord (Proneuron)	Autologous activated macrophage therapy for patients with acute complete spinal cord injury
ChondroCelect (Tigenix)	Autologous chondrocyte implantation
ELAD (Vigagen)	Extracorporeal liver assist device
Neo-Bladder (Tengion)	Living engineered bladder

CHALLENGES AHEAD

Thin tissues such as skin, cartilage, heart valves, and blood vessels are advantageous in that they can survive on diffusion of oxygen and nutrients, while new blood vessels sprout for permanent tissue formation. Thick tissues and solid organs depend on an elaborate network of blood vessels that course within 150–200 μm of each cell in that tissue. The heart requires so much oxygen that often there are blood vessels on both sides of an individual cardiomyocyte. Development of blood vessel networks within tissues is the principal challenge for engineered tissues. Angiogenesis can be used to create capillary networks for musculoskeletal and soft tissues while engineered vascular networks utilizing microfluidic principles are being developed for solid organs such as the liver and lung.

In vitro expansion and differentiation of progenitor cells to tissue-specific cells also remains an important milestone. This includes optimization of the different cell types and ratios for each tissue for long-term tissue function. Conditions necessary for in vitro culture and preimplant logistics such as delivery and storage are just beginning to be addressed for complex tissues.

FURTHER READINGS

BADYLAK SF et al: Extracellular matrix as a biological scaffold material: Structure and function. Acta Biomater 5:1, 2009

GRAYSON WL et al: Biomimetic approach to tissue engineering. Semin Cell Dev Biol 20:665, 2009

HOGANSON DM et al: Tissue engineering and organ structure: A vascularized approach to liver and lung. Pediatr Res 63:520, 2008

KHADEMHOSSEINI A et al: Progress in tissue engineering. Sci Am 300:64, 2009

OTT HC et al: Perfusion-decellularized matrix: Using nature's platform to engineer a bioartificial heart. Nat Med 14:213, 2008

SACKS MS et al: Bioengineering challenges for heart valve tissue engineering. Annu Rev Biomed Eng 11:289, 2009

PART 5
Aging

CHAPTER **70**

World Demography of Aging

Richard Suzman

John G. Haaga

Population aging is transforming the world in dramatic and fundamental ways. The age distributions of populations have changed and will continue to change radically, due to long-term declines in fertility rates and improvements in mortality rates (Table 70-1). This transformation, known as the Demographic Transition, is also accompanied by an epidemiological transition, in which noncommunicable chronic diseases are becoming the major causes of death and contributors to the burden of disease and disability. A concomitant of population aging is the change in key ratios expressing "dependency" of one form or another—the ratio of adults in the workforce to those typically out of the workforce, such as infants, children, retired "young old" (those still active in many ways other than paid work) and the oldest old. Global aging will affect economic growth, migration, patterns of work and retirement, family structures, pension and health systems, and even trade and the relative standing of nations. Both numbers (the size of an age group) and ratios (the ratio of those in the labor force age group to dependants such as the young or retired, or the ratio of children to older people) are important. The size of population age groups might affect the number of hospital beds needed, while the ratio of children to older people, the relative demand for pediatricians and geriatricians.

While the increase in life expectancy, resulting from a series of social, economic, public health, and medical victories over disease, might very well be considered the crowning achievement of the past century and a half, the increased length of life coupled with the shifts in the size of dependent groups relative to the size of the labor force, present formidable long-term challenges.

The pace of the change is accelerating. In countries where the Demographic Transition began earlier, the process was slower: it took France 115 years for the proportion of the age group 65 and older to increase from 7 to 14% of the total population, and the United States will soon have completed this same increase in 69 years. But in countries that started the transition later, the process is occurring much more rapidly: Japan took 26 years to go from 7 to 14% age 65 and older, while China and Brazil are projected to require just 24 years.

Sometime around the year 2020, for the first time ever, the number of people aged 65 and older in the world is expected to exceed that of children under the age of 5. Around the middle of the twentieth century, the under-5 age group constituted almost 15% of the total population and the over-65 age group 5%. It took about 70 years for these two to reach equal proportions. But population forecasts predict it will take only another 30 years for the 65 and older age group to equal about 15% and the younger age group, 5%. By the middle of their careers, medical students in most countries should expect to be practicing in far older populations. Preparations for these changes need to begin decades in advance, and the costs and penalties of waiting can be very high. While some governments have started planning for the long term, many, if not most, have yet to begin.

Population aging around the world in recent decades has followed a broadly similar pattern, starting with a decline in infant and childhood mortality that precedes a decline in fertility; at later stages, mortality at older ages declines as well. Declining fertility began as early as the beginning of the nineteenth century in the United States and France and extended to the rest of Europe and North America and parts of East Asia by the middle of the twentieth century. Since World War II, fertility declines have started in all other world regions. In fact, more than half the world's population now lives in countries or provinces with fertility rates below the replacement level of just over two live births per woman. Mortality rates also began to change, relatively slowly at first, in Western Europe and North America during the nineteenth century. At first, changes were most evident at the youngest ages. Improvements in water supply and sewage handling, as well as in nutrition and housing, accounted for most of the improvement before the 1940s, when antibiotics and vaccines, and increasing education of mothers began to make a major impact. Since the middle of the twentieth century, the "Child Survival Revolution" has spread to all parts of the world. Children almost everywhere in the world are much more likely to reach late middle age now than in previous generations.

Especially since around 1960, mortality at older ages has improved rapidly in most of the developed countries. This improvement has been primarily due to advances in care of heart disease and stroke and in control of conditions like hypertension and hypercholesterolemia that lead to circulatory diseases. In some parts of the world, smoking rates have declined, and these declines have led to lower incidence of many cancers, heart disease, and stroke.

The initial decline in fertility resulted in older age groups becoming a larger fraction of the total population. Declines in adult and old age mortality contributed to the later stages of the process. Life expectancy at birth—the average age to which someone is expected to live, under prevailing mortality conditions—has been calculated at around 28 years in ancient Greece, perhaps 30 years in medieval Britain, and less than 25 years in the colony of Virginia in North America. In the United States, life expectancy climbed slowly during the nineteenth century, reaching 49 years for white women by 1900. White men had a life expectancy 2 years lower than that for white women, and black Americans had life expectancy 14 years lower than did white Americans in 1900. By the early twenty-first century, life expectancy in the United States had improved dramatically for all, with the sex gap wider and the racial gaps narrower than at the beginning of the century: 76 years for white men in 2006; 81 years for white women; and 70 and 76 years for black men and women, respectively.

At later stages of the demographic transition, mortality declines at the oldest ages, leading to increases in the 65 and older population, and the oldest old, those older than age 85 years. Migration can also affect population aging. An influx of young migrants with high birth rates can slow (though not stop) the process, as it has in the United States and Canada; or the out-migration of the young leaving older people behind can accelerate aging at the population level, as it has in many rural areas of the world. Wars and pandemic diseases such as AIDS can also change age composition by decimating particular adult age groups.

Regions of the world are at very different stages of the demographic transition (Fig. 70-1). Of a world population of 6.8 billion in 2009, approximately 11% were older than age 60 years, with Japan (30%)

TABLE 70-1 Selected Indicators of Population Aging, Estimates for 2009 and Projections to 2050; Selected Regions and Countries

	Population Age 60+ (in millions)		Percentage of Population 60+		Life Expectancy at Birth		Life Expectancy at 60		Old Age Support Ratio[a]	
	2009	2050	2009	2050	Male	Female	Male	Female	2009	2050
World	737	2008	11	22	65.4	69.8	18.1	21.2	9	4
More Developed Regions	264	416	21	33	73.6	80.5	19.6	23.7	4	2
Less Developed Regions	473	1592	8	20	63.9	67.4	17.3	19.6	11	4
Least Developed Countries	43	185	5	11	54.7	57.2	15.3	16.8	17	9
Africa	53.8	212.8	5	11	52.9	55.3	15.2	17.1	16	9
Egypt	6.0	24.8	7	19	68.3	71.8	16.2	18.3	14	5
Tanzania	2.1	8.4	5	8	54.6	56.2	16.1	17.6	17	13
Kenya	1.6	7.9	4	9	53.7	54.5	16	17.8	21	11
Nigeria	7.6	27.7	5	10	47.3	48.3	14.5	15.7	17	11
South Africa	3.6	8.1	7	14	49.9	53.2	13.6	17.8	14	7
Asia	399.9	1236.1	10	24	67.1	75.7	17.6	20.3	10	4
China	160.2	440.4	12	31	71.3	74.8	18.2	20.7	9	3
Japan	37.8	44.9	30	44	79	86.2	22.1	27.8	3	1
Rep. of Korea	7.3	18.0	15	41	75.9	82.5	19.7	24.6	7	2
India	88.6	315.6	7	20	62.1	65	16	17.9	13	5
Pakistan	11.1	49.8	6	15	66	66.7	17.6	18.4	15	7
Indonesia	20.2	71.6	9	25	68.7	72.6	16.5	18.5	11	3
Australia	4.1	8.5	19	30	79.1	83.8	22.3	25.8	5	3
New Zealand	0.8	1.6	18	29	78.2	82.2	21.6	24.7	5	3
Europe	158.5	236.4	22	34	71.1[b]	79.1[b]	18.3	22.6	4	2
Russian Federation	25.0	36.8	18	32	60.3	73.1	14.3	19.2	6	3
United Kingdom	13.8	20.9	22	29	77.2	81.6	20.4	24	4	3
Italy	15.8	22.3	26	39	78.1	84.1	21.5	25.9	3	2
Germany	21.1	27.9	26	40	77.1	82.4	20.4	24.6	3	2
France	14.1	22.0	23	33	77.6	84.7	21.6	26.6	4	2
Americas										
United States	56.2	110.5	18	27	76.9	81.4	21.2	24.6	5	3
Canada	6.5	14.1	20	32	78.3	82.9	21.7	25.2	5	2
Mexico	10.0	36.4	9	28	73.8	78.6	20.6	22.9	10	3
Argentina	5.9	12.7	15	25	71.6	79.1	18.1	23	6	3
Brazil	19.1	64.0	10	29	68.7	76	19.5	22.4	10	3

[a]UN Population Division defines Old Age Support Ratio as the number of persons aged 65 or older per one hundred persons aged 15 to 64 years.
[b]The UN includes all European regions in its overall statistics; life expectancy at birth for males ranges from 63.8 years in Eastern Europe to 77.4 years in Western Europe. For women it ranges from 74.8 to 83.1 years in Western Europe.
Source: United Nations Population Division, *World Population Ageing* 2009.

and Europe (22%) being the oldest regions (Germany, Italy, and Sweden have the highest percentages, 25–26%), and the United States and Canada having 21% and 20%, respectively. The percentage of the population older than age 60 years in the United States has remained lower than in Europe, due both to modestly higher fertility rates and to higher rates of immigration. The Caribbean and some Latin American countries average 10% older than age 60 years, with countries such as Uruguay, Cuba, and Argentina in the 15–18% range. Asia has about 10% older than age 60 years, with the population giants close to the average—China (12%), Indonesia (9%), and India (7%). Middle Eastern and African countries have the lowest proportions of older people (5% or lower).

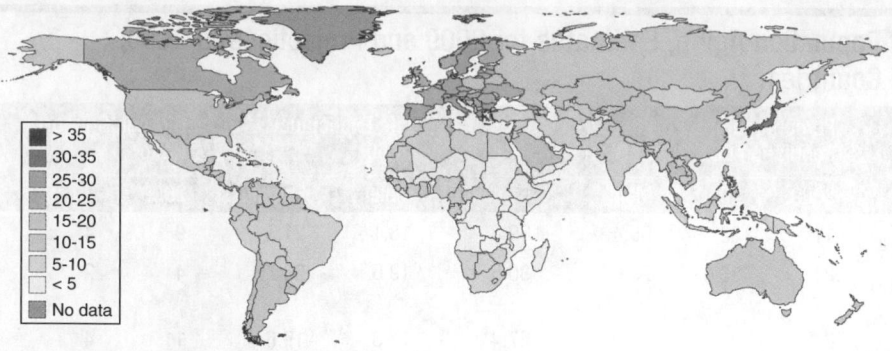

Figure 70-1 Percentages of national populations aged 60+, in 2010. *(From the US Census Bureau, International Database. StatPlanet Mapping Software.)*

Based on estimates from the United Nations Population Division, 737 million people were older than age 60 years in 2009, of whom 264 million lived in more developed countries, 473 million in less developed countries (43 million of the latter living in the least developed countries, as classified by the United Nations). The countries with the largest populations of those aged 60 and older were China (160 million), India (89 million), and the United States (56 million).

NUMBERS–POPULATION SIZE PROJECTIONS

Population projections make use of expected fertility, mortality, and migration rates and should be regarded as uncertain when applied 40 or more years in the future. However, the population that will be aged 60 and older in 2050 have all been born and survived childhood in 2010, so uncertainty about their numbers (as distinct from their proportion of the total population) is not great. Comparing the maps of the world in 2010 (Fig. 70-1) and 2050 (Fig. 70-2), it is apparent that the middle- and low-income countries in Latin America, Asia, and much of Africa will be joining the "oldest" category. In the four decades between 2010 and 2050, the United Nations Population Division projects that the world population aged 60 and older will almost triple to 2.01 billion, with the least developed regions more than quadrupling. China's 60+ population is projected to reach 440 million, India's 316 million, and the United States's 111 million. Over the next 40 years, the median age of the world's population is expected to increase by 10 years.

Current global life expectancy at birth is estimated to be 65.4 for men and 69.8 for women, with the comparable figures for the more developed region being 73.6 and 80.5 years. Life expectancy in the least developed countries averaged only 57.2 for women and 54.7 for men. Life expectancy at birth is heavily influenced by infant and child mortality, which is considerably higher in poor countries. At older ages, the gap between rich and poor nations is narrower; so while women who have reached age 60 in wealthy countries can expect 23.7 more years of life on average, women at age 60 in poor countries live 16.8 years on average—a significant difference but not so stark as the difference in life expectancy at birth. At the lowest levels of per capita GNP, life expectancy shows a powerful positive association with this measure of economic development but then the slope of the relationship flattens out; for countries with average incomes above about $20,000 per years life expectancy is not closely related to income. At each level of economic development, there is significant variation in life expectancy, indicating that many other factors influence life expectancy.

Japan, France, Italy, and Australia currently have life expectancy among the highest in the world, while the United States has lagged behind other high-income countries since about 1980, especially in the case of white women. The causes of this lag are being explored, but the cumulative number of years that people have smoked tobacco by the time they reach older ages appears to play an important role.

GROWTH OF THE OLDEST OLD POPULATION–THOSE OVER AGE 85

A modern feature of population aging has been the almost explosive growth of the age group known as the oldest old, variously defined as those over age 80 or age 85. This is the age group with the highest burden of noncommunicable degenerative disease and related disability. Thirty years ago, this group attracted little attention because they were hidden within the overall older population in most statistical reports; for example, the U.S. Census Bureau merged them into a 65+ category. The reduction of mortality at older ages coupled with larger birth cohorts surviving into old age led to the rapid growth of the oldest old. This age group is predicted to grow at a significantly higher rate than the 60+ population and one estimate has the current 102 million aged 80+ increasing to almost 400 million by 2050 (Table 70-2). Projected increases are astounding: China's 80+ population might increase from 18 to 101 million, India from 8 million to 43 million, the United States from 12 to 32 million, and Japan from 8 to 16 million. The numbers of centenarians are increasing at an even faster rate.

THE FUTURE OF LIFE EXPECTANCY

The members of the population who could potentially become aged 80 and older in 2050 are those aged 40+ who are alive today. The actual numbers who will be age 80 and older in 2050 will therefore depend almost solely on adult and old age mortality rates over the next 40 years. The history of the decline of mortality and increase in life expectancy suggests that improvements in the standard of living including increased and improved education and improved nutrition coupled with improvements in public health stemming from an understanding of the germ theory of disease initially led to the improvements, with medical achievements such as antibiotics and improved understanding of risk factors for cardiovascular and circulatory diseases becoming factors only in the

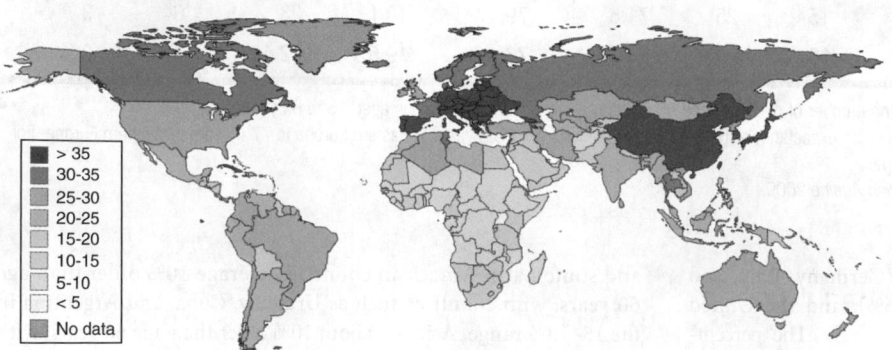

Figure 70-2 Percentages of national populations aged 60 +, in 2050 (projections). *(From the US Census Bureau, International Database. StatPlanet Mapping Software.)*

TABLE 70-2 Estimates (2009) and Projections (2050) for the Population Aged 80 Years and Older: Selected Regions and Countries

	Population Age 80 and Over (in thousands)	
	2009	2050
World	101,873	394,663
More Developed Regions	51,827	120,982
Less Developed Regions	50,046	273,771
Least Developed Countries	3,282	18,221
Africa	4,136	21,042
Kenya	151	686
Congo	20	65
Tanzania	164	810
South Africa	277	1,226
Asia	45,235	227,916
China	18,463	101,354
Japan	7,693	15,864
Rep. of Korea	895	5,618
India	7,754	42,583
Pakistan	1,041	6,156
Indonesia	1,670	11,515
Australia	814	2587
New Zealand	147	472
Europe	29,994	66,147
Russian Federation	3,986	6,984
United Kingdom	2,869	6,235
Italy	3,486	7,670
Germany	4,096	9,926
France	3,324	7,634
Americas		
United States	11,894	31,501
Canada	1,282	4,302
Mexico	1,477	7,944
Argentina	1,030	2,692
Brazil	2,754	14,133

Source: United Nations Population Division, *World Population Ageing* 2009.

post–World War II period with the largest strides for cardiovascular disease coming only in more recent decades. The improvements in educational attainment of succeeding generations have been credited in large part for improvements in child mortality during the past century, since educated mothers are especially likely to understand and take advantage of measures to reduce infection. The effects of continuing progress will likely be seen in coming decades as well, since educational attainment is associated with improved health and survival at older ages. Countries vary in the extent to

which the "future elderly" cohorts will be more educated. China in particular will have a much more educated elderly population in 2050 (with more than two-thirds of the 65+ population having completed secondary school) than it did in 2000 (when only 10% of older people had a secondary education). In the United States and other rich nations, this change has largely taken place already; future changes in educational attainment of the elderly population will be less dramatic.

Holding aside the possibility of new infectious diseases ravaging populations as AIDS did in some African countries, debates about future life expectancy revolve around the balance and influence of risk factors such as obesity, the possibility of reducing the deaths from current killers such as cancer, heart disease, and diabetes, whether there is some natural limit to life expectancy, and the distant though nonzero possibility that science will find a way to slow the basic processes of aging.

While some have posited natural limits to human life expectancy, the limits have been surpassed with some regularity and at the very oldest ages in the leading countries with the highest life expectancy, there appears to be little evidence of any approaching asymptote. Indeed a surprising discovery was that life expectancy in the leading country over the last century and a half, with different countries taking the lead in different epochs, could be represented almost perfectly by a straight line, with the increase for females showing a steady and astonishing increase of three months per year or 2.5 years per decade (Fig. 70-3). No single country kept that pace of improvement the entire time, but this trend does call into question the notion that improvement must slow down, at least in the near future.

There remains a great deal of diversity in health conditions both among and within national populations. There is nothing inevitable about the mortality transition—in several African countries, the prevalence of AIDS has been high enough to cause life expectancy to fall below the levels of 1980. Though none has so far reached a

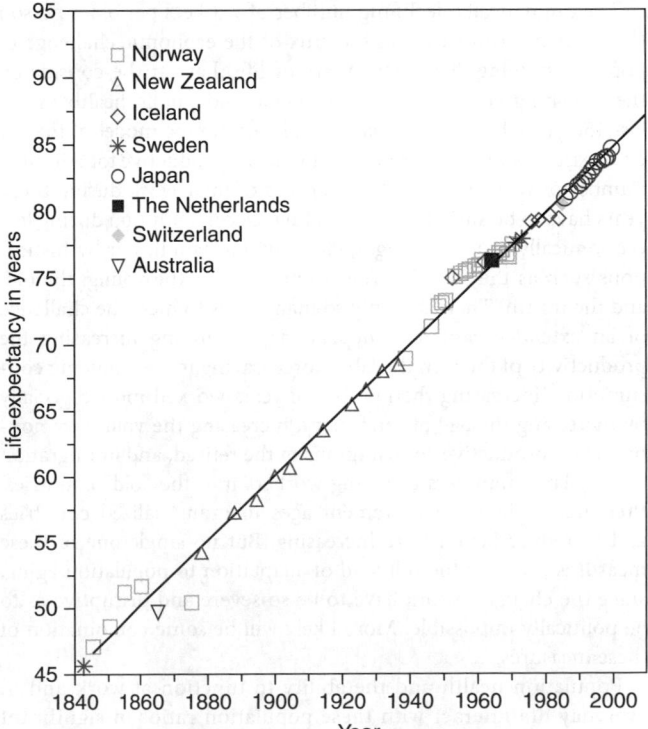

Figure 70-3 Life expectancy in most advanced nations, 1800-2000, females. *(From J Oeppen, JW Vaupel: Science 296:1029, 2002.)*

scale to rival the AIDS epidemic, periodic outbreaks of new influenza viruses or "emerging infectious" agents remind us that infectious diseases could again come to the fore. Progress against chronic disease is also reversible: In Russia and some other countries that formed part of the Soviet Union before 1992, life expectancy for men has been declining, now reaching levels below those of men in South Asia. Much of the gap between Russian and Western European men is explainable by much greater heart disease and injuries among the former.

DEPENDENCY AND CAREGIVING RATIOS

Ratios of different age groups provide useful though crude indicators of potential demands on resources and resource availability. One set of ratios, known variously as dependency or support ratios, compare the age groups who are most likely to be in the labor force with the age groups typically dependent on the productive capacity of those working—the young and the old, or just the old. A commonly used ratio is the number of persons aged 15–64 per persons aged 65 and older. Even though many in some countries do not enter the labor force until significantly older than age 15, retire before age 65 or work past age 65, the ratios do summarize important facts, especially in countries where financial support for the retired comes partially or mainly from those currently in the labor force through either a formal pension system or through the family. While many countries, including China and most African countries do not have formal pension systems except in specialized sectors such as the government sector, in Europe public pensions are quite generous, and face dramatic changes in their dependency ratios. Over the next 40 years, Western Europe faces a drop in the ratio from 4 to 2. In other words, while in crude terms there are today 4 workers supporting the pensions and other costs of each older person, by 2050 there will only be 2. China faces an even steeper drop from 9 of working age to only 3, while Japan declines from 3 to just 1. Even in India, projected to become the most populous country, the decline is quite steep from 13 to 5.

The dramatically declining number of workers per older person (however determined) is at the crux of the economic challenge of population aging. The extra years of life that can be considered the crowning achievement in medicine and public health of the last 150 years have to be financed. The economic model of the life cycle assumes that people are economically productive for a limited number of years and that the proceeds of their work during those years have to be smoothed over to finance consumption during less economically productive ages, either within families or by institutions such as the state in order to provide for the young, the old, and the infirm. There are only so many ways to meet the challenge of an extended period of dependency, including increasing the productivity of those in the labor force, saving more, reducing consumption, increasing the number of years worked most especially by increasing the age of retirement, increasing the voluntary nonmonetary productive contributions of the retired, and immigration of very large numbers of young workers into the "old" countries. Pressures to increase retirement ages in industrialized countries and to reduce benefits are increasing. But no single one of these measures can bear the full load of adaptation to population aging, since the changes would have to be so severe and disruptive as to be politically impossible. More likely will be some combination of these measures.

Population health and the ability to function at work and in everyday life interact with these population ratios in significant ways. The physical and cognitive capacity to continue to work at older ages is crucial if the age of retirement is raised. Similarly, caregiving often requires significant physical and emotional

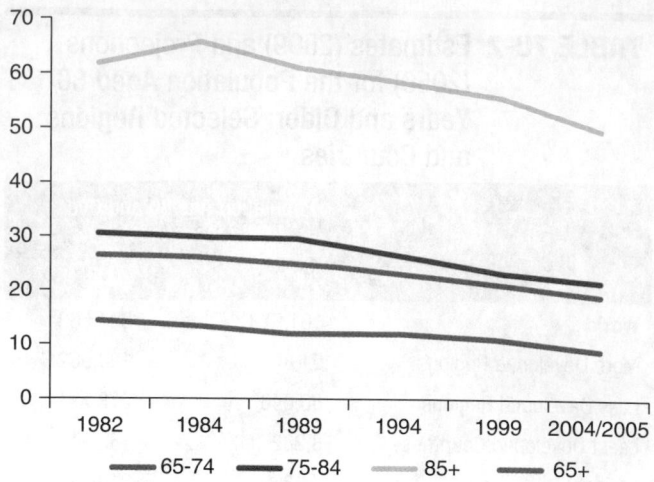

Figure 70-4 Disability prevalence, various years 1982-2005, by age group over 65, United States. *(Adapted from KG Manton et al: Proc Natl Acad Sci U S A. 103:18374, 2006.)*

stamina. Further, healthier older populations require less caregiving and medical services. Just two decades ago, the prevalent view of aging was highly pessimistic. Epidemiologists held that while modern medicine could keep older people alive, nothing much could be done to prevent, delay, or significantly treat the degenerative chronic diseases of aging. The result would be that more and more older people with chronic diseases would be kept from dying, with the consequent piling up of the older people disabled by chronic disease. Surprisingly, between 1984 and about 2000, the prevalence of disability in the 65+ population in the United States declined by about 25%, suggesting that in this respect, aging was more plastic than had been previously believed (Fig. 70-4). All the causes of this significant shift in disability are not yet understood, but rising levels of education, improved treatment of cardiovascular diseases and cataracts, greater availability of assistive devices, and less physically demanding occupations have been found to contribute. One calculation showed that if the rate of improvement could be maintained until 2050, that the numbers of disabled in the older population could be kept constant despite the aging of the baby boomers and the older population itself growing older. Unfortunately, concern is increasing that the rapid increase in obesity rates will negate and perhaps even reverse this most positive trend. Because of the absence of comparable data in other countries, it is uncertain whether the same improvement in disability rates (or recent deceleration) is occurring outside of the United States, but a global network of longitudinal studies on aging, health, and retirement is now providing data to answer the question.

Population aging, and related demographic changes including changes in family structure, could also have powerful though indirect effects through the "supply side" and health care financing. In every country, long-term care of the disabled and the chronically ill relies heavily on informal, typically unpaid caregivers—usually spouses, children, and, increasingly in more developed countries, caregivers for the oldest old are in their 60s and early 70s. Though there are many men who provide care, on the population level, informal caregiving is still mainly done by women. Because both men and women are living longer than in the past, the "young old" in most countries are less likely than in the past to be widows. But because women live longer than men, lack of a spousal caregiver is especially likely to be a problem for older women. Both men and women have fewer children on whom they can call for informal caregiving, because of the worldwide decline in fertility rates. An increasing proportion of older men in Europe and North America have spent much or all of their adult lives apart from their biological children. Lower fertility rates, delayed marriage, and increasing divorce rates among their children mean that people approaching old age may be less likely to have or to have close ties with daughters and daughters-in-law—the adults who have in the past been the most common caregivers apart from spouses. Adult women who in the past have provided uncompensated care (and much other essential volunteer work) are now more likely than in the past to be working for pay, and thus have fewer hours to devote to the unpaid roles.

These broad demographic and economic trends do not dictate particular social adaptations or policy responses, of course. One can imagine many different responses to the challenges of caring for the disabled—increased reliance on home health agencies and assisted living communities, "naturally occurring retirement communities" in which neighbors fulfill many of the roles once reserved for close kin; private or even publicly financed direct payments to compensate formerly unpaid family caregivers (a reform that has proved very popular in Germany)—these and other responses to the challenge of long-term care are being tested in aging countries, and others will no doubt be needed.

THE EPIDEMIOLOGIC TRANSITION—CHANGES IN THE BURDEN OF DISEASE AND RISK FACTORS

The secular improvements in ages at death have been accompanied by changes in causes of death. In the broadest terms, the proportion of deaths due to infectious disease and conditions associated with pregnancy and delivery has fallen, and the proportion due to chronic, noncommunicable diseases, such as heart and cerebrovascular diseases, diabetes, cancers, and age-related neurodegenerative diseases such as Alzheimer's and Parkinson's diseases, has increased steadily and is expected to continue to increase. Figure 70-5 shows results from an international comparative project that drew on a wide variety of data sources to provide estimates of the global burden of disease at the beginning of this century, with projections to future years based on recent trends in disease prevalence and demographic rates. Burden of disease in these pie charts is a composite measure,

one that takes into account both the number of deaths due to a particular disease or condition and the timing of such deaths—an infant death represents a loss of more potential life-years lived than does the death of a very old person. Nor is death the only outcome that matters; most diseases or conditions cause significant disability and suffering even when nonfatal, so this measure of burden captures nonfatal outcomes using statistical weighting. As Table 70-3 shows, the "modern plagues" of chronic noncommunicable diseases are already among the leading causes of premature death and disability

TABLE 70-3 Diseases and Conditions Causing the Greatest Burden of Disease for Low-, Middle-, and High-Income Countries

	Low-Income Countries	Medium-Income Countries	High-Income Countries
1	Lower respiratory infections	Unipolar depressive disorders	Unipolar depressive disorders
2	Diarrheal diseases	Ischemic heart disease	Ischemic heart disease
3	HIV/AIDS	Cerebrovascular disease	Cerebrovascular disease
4	Malaria	Road traffic accidents	Alzheimer's and other dementias
5	Prematurity and low birth weight	Lower respiratory infections	Alcohol use disorders
6	Neonatal infections and other	COPD	Hearing-loss, adult onset
7	Birth asphyxia and birth trauma	HIV/AIDS	COPD
8	Unipolar depressive disorders	Alcohol use disorders	Diabetes mellitus
9	Ischemic heart disease	Refractive errors	Trachea, bronchus, lung cancers
10	Tuberculosis	Diarrheal disease	Road traffic accidents

Note: "Burden of Disease" takes into account years of life lost due to premature death, and also a weighted estimate for years spent with disability, pain, or impairments due to conditions. These estimates are aggregated from many different national reporting systems and special surveys or surveillance systems, with adjustments for incomplete coverage and different reporting schemes. Especially for older people with multiple chronic conditions, it is difficult even for physicians familiar with their case to designate underlying and precipitating causes. For example, Alzheimer's disease and other dementias are treated very differently and cause-of-death data are of little use in studying trends and differences in dementia prevalence.

Abbreviation: COPD, chronic obstructive pulmonary disease.

Source: World Health Organization: *The Global Burden of Disease: 2004 Update.* © World Health Organization 2008. Accessed February 28, 2011 at http://www.who.int/healthinfo/global_burden_disease/2004_report_update/en/index.html.

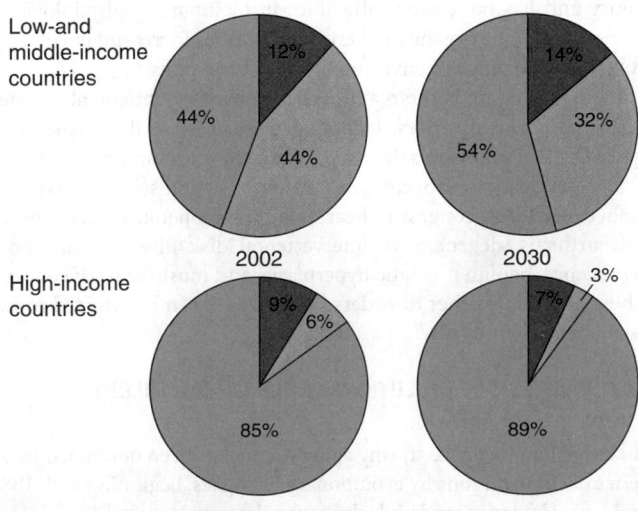

Figure 70-5 Leading causes of burden of illness in world regions 2002 and projected for 2030. *(Adapted from Mathers and Loncar.)*

even in low-income countries. This is due to a mix of factors—lower fertility rates mean fewer infants and children at prime ages of susceptibility to infections; more people reaching older ages when chronic disease incidence is high; and often changing incidence rates due to increased exposure to tobacco, Western diets, and inactivity. Noncommunicable diseases, once thought of as "diseases of affluence"—are projected to account for more than half of the disease burden even in low- and middle-income countries by the year 2030 (Fig. 70-5).

SUMMARY

Population aging is a global phenomenon with profound short- and long-term implications for health and long-term care needs, and indeed for the economic and social wellbeing of nations. The timing and context of aging vary across and within world regions and countries; the industrialized nations became wealthy before they aged significantly, while many of the low resource regions will age before they become significantly industrialized. The variation at both the population level and individual levels indicates that there is a significant degree of flexibility in successful aging, but meeting the challenges will require significant advance planning and preparation. The extent to which research can find solutions that reduce physical and cognitive disability at older ages will be a significant factor in how countries cope with this fundamental transformation of populations and societies.

FURTHER READINGS

CUTLER D et al: The determinants of mortality. J Econ Perspectives 20:97, 2006

KINSELLA K, HE W: US Census Bureau, International Population reports, P95/09-1, in *An Aging World: 2008*. Washington DC, Govt Printing Office 2009

LOPEZ AD et al: The global and regional burden of disease and risk factors in 2001: Health priorities at the beginning of the millennium. Lancet 367:1747, 2006

MATHERS CD, LONCAR D: Projections of global mortality and burden of disease from 2002 to 2030. PLoS Med 3:e442, 2006

SAMIR KC et al: Projection of populations by level of educational attainment, age and sex for 120 countries for 2005-2050. Demographic Research 22:Article 15, 2010 (online at *www.demographic-research.org*)

SCHOENI RF et al: Why is late-life disability declining? Milbank Q 86:47, 2008

United Nations Dept of International Economic and Social Affairs, Population Division (2010). *World Population Ageing 2009*. United Nations, NY, 2010

VAUPEL JW: Biodemography of human ageing. Nature 464:536, 2010

CHAPTER 71

The Biology of Aging

George M. Martin

Thanks largely to the power of genetic analysis in model organisms such as *Caenorhabditis elegans* (a nematode), *Drosophila melanogaster* (a fruit fly), and the laboratory mouse, major advances have been made in the elucidation of what can be termed "public" modulations of intrinsic biological aging—that is to say, commonalities of gene actions across widely diverse phyla that explain, in part, the plasticity of processes of aging. There are hints that at least one such conserved pathway may be operative in our own species. These observations, together with related research on other biochemical pathways, a long history of research on the beneficial effects of dietary restriction (most recently including an initial report of its beneficial effects on healthspan and lifespan in a primate) (Fig. 71-1), and spectacular advances in genomics raise the possibility that we may one day be able to delay the times of onset and decrease the rates of progression of aging processes. Such interventions have the potential to extend the healthspans and, therefore, the functional lifespans of a large proportion of our population. This new knowledge, however, is still very distant from clinical translation. Many remain skeptical of the relevance of these experimental findings. Moreover, we need much more information on the pathophysiology of aging, especially in the invertebrate models that have provided most of our new knowledge concerning genetic modulations of lifespan. We will also require more detailed information on the impact of longevity enhancements upon what can be described as the "terminal decline" of the life course, the stage of life in humans responsible for protracted morbidity, frailty, and the consequent loss of the ability to live independently. These terminal declines account for a very substantial

proportion of all health care costs. Finally, the promising new knowledge needs fuller discussions by ethicists, economists, sociologists, and political scientists, among others, as to the impacts upon society of any large-scale clinical translations.

■ DEFINITIONS OF AGING: SENESCENT PHENOTYPES

Mammalian gerontologists usually define aging in terms of the gradual, insidious, and progressive declines in structure and function (involving molecules, cells, tissues, organs, and organisms) that begin to unfold after the achievement of sexual maturity. These declines affect the germ line as well as the soma. For large populations of individuals, exponential declines in the probability of survival are observed. The aging organism is less successful in its reaction to injury and has increasing difficulties in maintaining physiological homeostasis. The organism, therefore, becomes increasingly vulnerable to a wide range of environmental perturbations.

Biological aging is the major risk factor for essentially all of the major geriatric disorders, including dementias of the Alzheimer type (DAT), Parkinson's disease, age-related macular degeneration, ocular cataracts, presbycusis, all forms of arteriosclerosis, type 2 diabetes mellitus, congestive heart failure, sarcopenia, osteoporosis, osteoarthritis, degenerative intervertebral disk disease, immunosenescence, benign prostatic hyperplasia, and most forms of cancer. These and many other disorders (Table 71-1) can be referred to as "senescent phenotypes."

■ THE CLASSICAL EVOLUTIONARY BIOLOGICAL THEORY OF WHY WE AGE

A compelling theory as to why aging occurs has been developed by a series of contributions by evolutionary biologists, beginning with JBS Haldane. Haldane wondered why certain late-onset disorders, such as Huntington's disease, seemed to be so prevalent in England—perhaps of the order of one per thousand instead of what might have been expected from germ-line mutation rates—perhaps one per million. He concluded that this was because the disease had largely escaped the force of natural selection, because the commonest forms of the

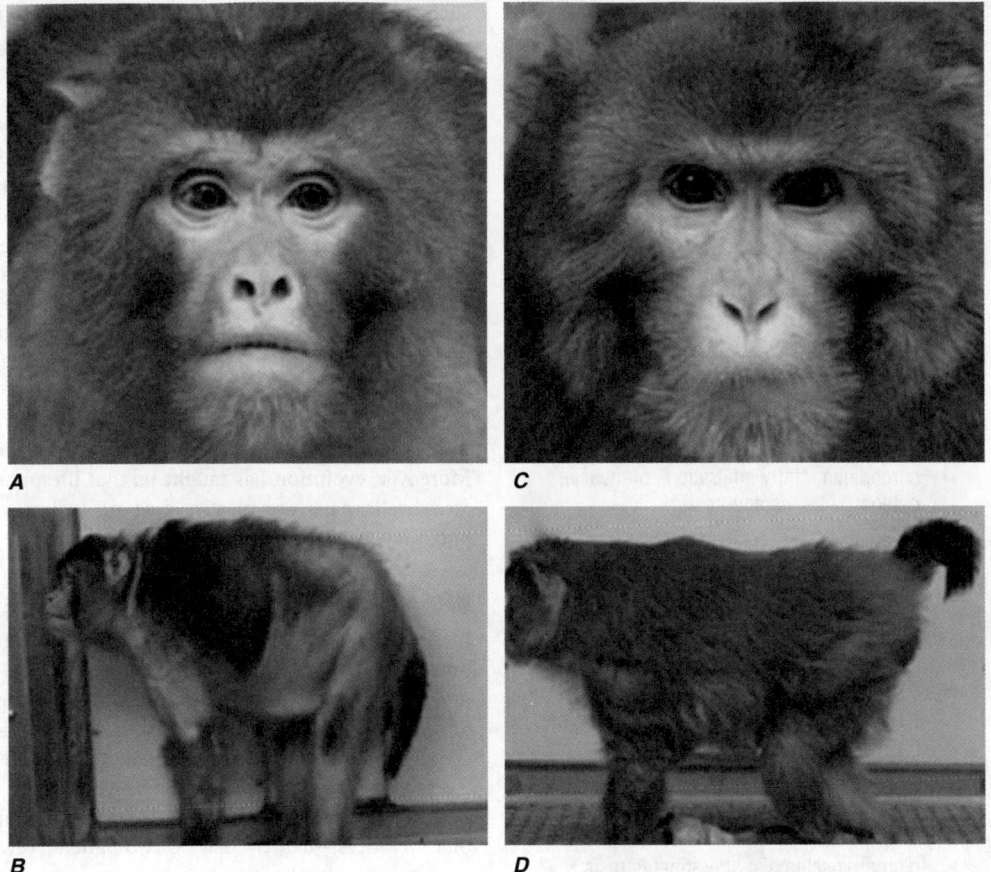

Figure 71-1 *Photographs of an old (age 27.6 years) calorically restricted (CR) Rhesus monkey (A, B) compared to an age-matched control (C, D).* The mean lifespans of control animals in captivity is 27 years and the maximum lifespan is about 40 years. CR (30% of ad libitum fed controls) was initiated as adults (ages 7–14 years). Restricted animals exhibited superior insulin sensitivity, less fat, more muscle mass, and fewer diseases (diabetes, neoplasia, cardiovascular, brain atrophy). Preliminary analyses of survival curves were consistent with enhanced longevity of the CR cohort. *(Reproduced from RJ Colman et al: Science 235:201, 2009; with permission.)*

disease did not manifest until after reproduction had ceased. In age-structured populations (i.e., populations consisting of individuals with a wide range of ages), most of the reproduction is carried out by the younger cohorts. This is because, historically, few individuals living in the wild escaped the effects of infections, predation, nutritional deprivations, and accidents to achieve old age. As such, even late-acting *good* alleles will have only minor contributions to the gene pools of subsequent generations. Peter Medawar extended this idea, arguing that there are numerous such constitutional mutations, an idea that has come to be known as the "mutation accumulation" theory of aging. (These are mutations that one is born with, not somatic mutations.) By this argument, most of us are likely to have been born with some special vulnerability to a late-life disorder or disorders. A second major theory, known as "antagonistic pleiotropy," was developed by George C. Williams. He argued that there are likely to be many genetic alleles that were selected because of their enhancement of reproductive fitness *early* in the life course, but that have negative effects *late* in life, when the force of natural selection will have greatly diminished. A more general conceptualization of tradeoffs between reproduction and lifespan (the "disposable soma" theory) was developed by TBL Kirkwood. The evolutionary theory was quantified by William D. Hamilton and elaborated on by Brian Charlesworth and Michael Rose.

Perhaps the best indication that the field of biogerontology has finally matured as a science is the fact that its most cherished theory, what can now be termed as the "classical" evolutionary theory, has undergone several challenges. First, demographers have noted that at the extremes of old age for organisms as diverse as roundworms, fruit flies, med flies, and humans, rates of *declines* in the force of natural selection diminish. One response to this important challenge (the "cocoon" hypothesis) is that these declines may simply be related to the virtual cessation of locomotor activities at extreme ages. When flies cease flying and worms cease moving, fewer opportunities for serious injuries may result. These "plateaus" in the rates of mortality at very advanced ages are much less striking for people; they might also be related, in part, to diminished motility, as well as to secular trends in the development of central heating, air conditioning, and immunizations. A second challenge comes from geneticists who have discovered that, to our great surprise, many single-gene mutations can substantially increase the lifespans of Baker's yeast, nematodes, and fruit flies This issue has been most systematically explored in *C. elegans*; a meta-analysis of an initial set of unbiased, genome-wide RNAi screens ("knockdowns," but not "knockouts" of gene expression) has tabulated hundreds of single-gene loci capable of enhancing lifespan when they are dialed down. These genes fall into a finite number of pathways and, moreover, many of them fit within the context of antagonistic pleiotropic mechanisms of aging. For example, hypomorphic mutations in genes within the most famous of these pathways, the insulin-like growth factor (IGF)/insulin signaling pathway, may be reporting on an evolutionarily conserved diapause—nature's way of taking time out from the business of development and reproduction during hard times, such as severe shortages of food. The gene actions associated with such diapauses (many of which are still unexplored

TABLE 71-1 Alterations in Proliferative Homeostasis in the Tissues of Aging Humans

Integument	epidermal atrophy, "liver spots", seborrheic keratoses, basal cell ca, squamous cell carcinoma, graying and loss of hair, eccrine sweat gland atrophy, apocrine sweat gland hyperplasia, stasis dermatitis, regional subcutaneous atrophy, hyperplasia
Sensory	lacrimal gland atrophy, corneal degenerations, ocular cataracts, age-related macular degeneration, presbycusis, olfactory loss
Musculoskeletal	sarcopenia, "fatty infiltration" of muscle, osteoarthritis, osteoporosis
Hematopoietic/Immune	anemias, myelodysplastic syndromes, leukemia, lymphoma, monoclonal gammopathy and multiple myeloma, autoimmune disorders (e.g., atrophic gastritis and polycythemia vera), immunosenescence (accelerated in AIDS)
CNS	reactive gliosis, dural and meningeal fibrosis
Cardiovascular	atherosclerosis, arteriolosclerosis, myocardial interstitial fibrosis
Pulmonary	interstitial fibrosis, emphysema
Renal	glomerulosclerosis, interstitial fibrosis
Male Reproductive	benign prostatic hyperplasia (smooth muscle and glands), adenocarcinoma of prostate, testicular atrophy
Female Reproductive	ovarian atrophy and theca cell hyperplasia, endometrial atrophy and hyperplasia, endometrial carcinoma, smooth muscle atrophy, leiomyomas of uterus
Endocrine	parenchymal atrophy with interstitial fibrosis, cell type-specific hyperplasias, adenomas
GI	mucosal and smooth muscle atrophy, hyperplastic polyps, adenomas, adenocarcinomas of colon and rectum

Source: After GM Martin et al: PLoS Genet 3:e125, 2007.

at the biochemical genetic level) understandably result in enhanced resistance to various stresses. A large number of these *C. elegans* "longevity genes" converge upon a single transcription factor, *daf2*, or influence mitochondrial function. Moreover, it is possible that many such genes may be specific for this highly inbred laboratory model. In general, these investigations support, rather than refute, the evolutionary theory of aging.

A third challenge to the theory comes mainly from anthropologists and economists and emphasizes intergenerational transfers of resources. As an oversimplification, this idea is often referred to as "the grandmother hypothesis." Older members of population groups have survived a number of threats to their existence and can pass along to their younger family members information about successful avoidance or adaptation. Field experiments with prides of lions and olive baboons have failed to support this hypothesis. Moreover, while many grandparents are now contributing to the reproductive fitness of their children and grandchildren via transfer of resources, current evidence, while still incomplete, indicates that

such elders were exceedingly rare within populations of our remote ancestors, when the evolution of species-specific gene actions would have evolved. Any such favorable alleles not expressed until those late stages of life would, therefore, have been vastly diluted by the alleles of their progeny.

A final challenge to evolutionary theory comes from a reexamination of the assumptions made by Hamilton in his influential 1966 paper. Baudisch, using different assumptions, demonstrates that, under some conditions, the force of natural selection can *increase* during aging. For example, species of rockfish that continue to grow beyond sexual maturity are much more likely to become predators rather than prey; as such, the force of natural selection would, indeed, become stronger, not weaker, as they age.

The message is that aging is *non-adaptive*. It did not evolve via a program of determinative gene actions that are designed to lead to the death of aging organisms because it is good for the species. Moreover, evolution has taught us that lifespans and their associated healthspans are plastic, thus providing a rationale for the potential effectiveness of future interventions.

■ CLASSES OF GENE ACTION THAT MODULATE RATES OF AGING

If we are ever to intelligently intervene in one or more aging processes, we must be thoroughly familiar with the nature of the underlying gene actions. We must also be aware of the influences of idiosyncratic constitutional mutations, genetic polymorphisms, gene-gene interactions, environmental agents, gene-environmental interactions, and stochastic events. All of these complexities support what most experienced clinicians have learned in the course of their practices—namely that no two patients (even identical twins) age in precisely the same way; they share some commonalities but also have unique subsets of structural and functional impairments. Enhancements in the prevention and treatment of geriatric disorders will, therefore, require a more sophisticated and comprehensive understanding of the cellular, molecular, and integrative physiological underpinnings of these intra-specific variations in the patterns of aging.

The evolutionary biological theory of why we age provides clues as to how we age (i.e., the nature of the underlying gene actions). We can, in fact, outline twelve distinct classes of gene actions suggested by the evolutionary theory.

Class one: good alleles with good effects early and late: *longevity assurance genes*

There are many examples of such genes. For instance, about 150 distinct human genetic loci have already been identified for the repair of DNA. Table 71-2 gives an example of the many different types of genetic loci involved in the oxidative-damage theory of aging. According to that venerable theory, various sources of oxidative damage to macromolecules, notably those produced as byproducts of the oxidative metabolism of mitochondria, are the primary causes of intrinsic biological aging. There is now mounting evidence, however, that this theory is an insufficient explanation for variations in longevity. Nevertheless, increasing evidence also suggests that the modulation of oxidative damage is important for major aspects of healthspan. A cogent example is the evidence that the genetic engineering of mice to provide high concentrations of a human cDNA for catalase directed to the mitochondria greatly ameliorates a form of congestive heart failure responsible for many geriatric hospital admissions. By the criteria of anatomic pathology and echocardiography, the features in aging mice are quite comparable to those observed in aging human subjects. This finding gives support to the proposition that even potentially good novel gene actions can also escape the force of natural selection. Nature has targeted catalase to peroxisomes, but it does not supplement

TABLE 71-2 Categories of Gene Action Relevant to the Oxidative Damage Theory of Aging

Category I	Structural and regulatory genes modulating genesis of free radicals
	Examples: Cytochrome C Oxidase; P450 family
Category II	Structural and regulatory genes for scavenger enzymes
	Examples: SOD-1,2,3; Catalase; γ Glutamyl cysteine synthetase
Category III	Genes regulating flux of nonenzymatic free radical scavengers
	Examples: uric acid synthetic enzymes
Category IV	Genes regulating target copy number
	Examples: Genetic regulation of mitochondrial DNA replication, fusion, fission
Category V	Genes specifying target structure
	Examples: Structural genes for chromatin proteins and membrane lipoproteins
Category VI	Structural and regulatory genes for repair of target macromolecules
	Examples: Specification of machinery for reversal, repair, tolerance of DNA damage
Category VII	Genes specifying the orderly replacement of effete cells
	Examples: Genes modulating DNA replication and cell cycle progression, apoptosis, growth factors, growth factor receptors, and stem cell biology

Source: After GM Martin et al: Nature Genetics 13:25, 1996.

mitochondrial protection by also directing some optimal amount of catalase to the mitochondria to decrease the steady state levels of a dangerous by-product of mitochondrial metabolism, peroxide (H_2O_2). In the presence of iron, H_2O_2 results in the synthesis of the highly reactive hydroxyl radical, with resulting damage to all classes of macromolecules in its immediate vicinity.

The last category (VII) of gene actions listed in Table 71-2 is relevant to a very important aspect of mammalian aging—the maintenance of proliferative homeostasis. As mammals age, there is a puzzling juxtaposition of both atrophy and inappropriate hyperplasia, often side by side. This can involve multiple tissues and is associated with numerous geriatric pathologies (Table 71-1). The hyperplasias may act as tumor promoters, leading to benign and malignant neoplasms.

Tissue atrophy may be attributable, in part, to the accumulating effects of cell apoptosis and necrosis from various causes and the failure of stem cells to compensate for the gradual attenuation of the replicative potentials of somatic cells, a process known as replicative senescence or the "Hayflick limit." It remains controversial as to whether or not an in vivo phenomenon exists that reflects the in vitro phenomenon of replicative senescence. The dominant (but not the only) mechanism responsible for replicative senescence is the loss of telomere repeat units from the ends of chromosomes. The germ line, many stem cells, and most cancers are protected from the erosion of telomeres by an enzyme known as telomerase, but this enzyme is absent from most somatic cells. Scientists shared a 2009 Nobel Prize for research in this field, the first such prize to recognize modern research in biogerontology. Cells that have exited the cell cycle typically do not undergo necrosis or apoptosis. They

have a variety of phenotypes that characterize them as senescent; most notably a senescence-associated secretory phenotype (SASP) that has important consequences for regional pathology. In brief, such cells secrete a range of pro-inflammatory cytokines, metallothioneins, and mitogens. While such cells may be few in number within a given tissue, they can have a "field effect," thus driving the proliferation of neighboring epithelial cells, altering the connective tissue matrix, and contributing to sustained chronic inflammation. The latter is receiving increasing attention as a major concomitant of intrinsic biological aging.

As noted above, Category VII is also highly relevant to the emerging field of regenerative medicine. A possible generalization emerging from research on the interface of stem cell biology with the biology of aging is that a dominant factor in the decline of the success in mobilizing stem cells for the response to injury resides in the microenvironment of stem cells. This has been most effectively demonstrated in the repair of injury to skeletal muscle, in which satellite stem cells are mobilized quite effectively for repair in young mice but not in old mice. A clever parabiotic experiment provided compelling evidence for a non-cellular factor circulating from young to old mice that was capable of markedly ameliorating the deficient repair in the old mice. The satellite stem cell model has also demonstrated a switch, during adult myogenesis, from the Notch pathway—required for stem cell proliferation—to the Wnt pathway—required for effective differentiation. As is the case with so many signal transduction pathways, there is cross-talk between these two pathways. The situation is more complex, however, with evidence of an important role for a member of the transforming growth factor beta family of cytokines. There may also be a role for Klotho, a transmembrane protein with a structure suggestive of certain glycosidases. In any case, the clinical implications of this field of research are clear: as a much less complex and much safer alternative to the transplantation of stem cells, including those derived from the patient's own cells, clinicians might one day be able to inject small molecular weight compounds to "wake up" the patient's endogenous stem cells.

Class two: bad alleles with late-life penetrance: *idiosyncratic constitutional mutations*

There is a national debate concerning health care reform, including the need for legislation for the protection of children with pre-existing genetic disorders. It seems likely, however, that we *all* have pre-existing conditions—namely gene actions that will lead to variable times of onset and variable severities of late-life disorders. Among these gene actions are individually rare but numerically numerous mutations that do not reach some phenotypic level of expression until middle age or beyond, when the effects will have escaped the force of natural selection. A prototypic example is Huntington's disease, one of a number of triplet repeat diseases; those unfortunate enough to have been born with the requisite number of CAG repeats (coding for a run of polyglutamines) in the affected locus will develop the disease after the peak of reproduction. More cogent examples, perhaps, come from rare, but pathogenetically informative, autosomal dominant mutations at three distinct loci resulting in "early" onset DAT. ("Early" here means younger than age 60; most patients are in late middle age when they're diagnosed with these forms of Alzheimer's disease.) To get some estimate of the genetic load of mutations that were known to lead to late-onset dementias of various types, the following is a systematic analysis of several editions of *McKusick's Mendelian Inheritance in Man*. In the 1975 edition, some 55 loci were identified from among 2336 listed at that time. Thirty years ago, the conventional wisdom was that there were ~100,000 protein-coding genes in the human genome. When the results of full genome sequencing were about to appear, geneticists participated in a contest (GeneSweep) to see who got closest to the sequencing results; the low bidder (~26,000 genes) won the event. Assuming that number is, in fact, correct (some new estimates suggest somewhat lower or higher figures), we can conclude that about 2.4% of these protein-coding genes, or a total of 624, have the potential to modulate one's susceptibility to dementing disorders of late life. That has to be an absolutely lower limit of how we can get in trouble with cognition as we age; however, as there are thousands of functionally distinct splice variants and thousands of DNA sequences that code for various families of RNA molecules (the "dark matter" of DNA), most of which seem likely to have a role in the regulation of gene expression. We are also learning about so-called "moonlighting proteins"—single proteins with two distinct functions.

Class three: bad alleles early with good effects late: *paradoxical antagonistic pleiotropy*

In theory, such genes can persist in a population either because of a comparatively recent founder effect, or because the allele participates in a balanced polymorphism. Elevated frequencies of the 4G allele and of the homozygous 4G4G genotype were found in centenarians and were associated with high levels of plasminogen activator inhibitor-1. Such high levels are predictive of recurring myocardial infarction in young men. It is, therefore, paradoxical that these high levels are associated with extreme longevity. Like all such studies with centenarians, however, one requires independent confirmations and more sophisticated controls, such as the use of centenarian progeny and their spouses.

Class four: bad alleles early and late: *segmental progeroid syndromes*

These conditions can be defined as genetic disorders that mimic, to various extents, many, but not all, senescent phenotypes found in the general population. Prototypic examples are the Werner syndrome (WS) ("Progeria of the Adult") and the Hutchinson-Gilford syndrome (HGPS) ("Progeria of Childhood"). WS results from homozygosity for null mutations at the *WRN* locus, which codes for a member of the RecQ family of helicases. To "do business" with DNA, one must first unwind the double helix. The WRN protein appears to have several functions in DNA replication, transcription, recombination, and repair. Telomeres are particularly favored substrates. Almost all HGPS patients suffer from the same C-terminal mutation in the Lamin A gene (*LMNA*), which codes for an intermediate filament that lines the nuclear membrane. The mutation results in the preferential use of a cryptic splice site, resulting in the deletion of a sequence of 50 amino acids. The abnormal gene product (progerin) no longer acts as a substrate for the enzymatic removal of a post-translational modification (farnesylation). This contributes to structurally distorted nuclei and abnormalities in gene expression and has, therefore, led to clinical trials employing farnesylation inhibitors. Other factors are likely to contribute to the pathology, however. Many segmental progeroid syndromes are characterized by genomic instability. For the case of WS, there is a 10–100 fold increase in mutation rates; large deletions are particularly common. There is a striking limitation of the replicative lifespans of somatic cells from such patients, probably related to unrepaired damage of a major product of oxidative damage, 8-oxo-2′-deoxyguanosine, at telomeres. Deficiency of the WRN helicase also results in pro-inflammatory gene actions characteristic of normative aging.

For the case of HGPS, in addition to the genomic instability related to the abnormal structures of nuclei, there are likely to be important aberrations in the regulation of gene expression. Evidence that the study of HGPS can provide insight into normative aging comes from the discovery that small, potentially pathogenetically relevant amounts of progerin can be found in cells from normal individuals and that the effects of this abnormal protein may be particularly relevant for stem cells.

Class five: good alleles early with bad effects late: *antagonistic pleiotropy*

This category of gene action may contribute to three of our most devastating geriatric disorders—cancer, atherosclerosis, and DAT. The evidence that it plays a role in the pathogenesis of cancer comes from research referred to above, largely from the laboratory of Judith Campisi. The underlying hypothesis, as noted above, is that the repression of telomerase in somatic cells and alternative modalities of expediting exit from the mitotic cell cycle (such as DNA damage and oncogenic stimuli), evolved because they were adaptive for young, actively reproducing organisms, where they act as tumor suppressors. Later in life, however, the accumulation of replicative senescent cells may act in tumor promotion, both via mitogenic effects upon neighboring epithelial cells and via degradative actions upon the associated matrix, which may enhance local invasion by neoplastic cells. The arguments for roles in atherosclerosis and in Alzheimer's disease are much more speculative but worthy of more research. For the case of atherosclerosis, an argument can be made that macrophages play a primary pathogenetic role, particularly in the presence of functionally impaired, aged endothelial cells. The primary functions of macrophages are to engulf and destroy pathogens, for which purpose they employ a range of receptors including promiscuous "flypaper" receptors that can also recognize oxidized lipoproteins, which are of relevance to the pathogenesis of atherosclerosis. Given the exposure of modern humans to high-fat diets, late-life deleterious effects of the phagocytosis of oxidized lipoproteins may be an unfortunate tradeoff. Evidence for such a tradeoff has come from experiments with a mouse model of atherosclerosis (APOE knockout mice on a high-fat Western diet). When these mice were crossed with mice deficient in a class-A scavenger receptor (*MSR-A*), there was the expected amelioration of atherosclerosis. These hybrid mice, however, were shown to be highly susceptible to infection with *Listeria monocytogenes* or herpes simplex virus.

The evidence for a role of antagonistic pleiotropic gene action in the pathogenesis of DAT remains modest but is of considerable interest. Most such discussions revolve around polymorphic alleles of the *APOE* gene. The ancestral allele found within primates is the notorious epsilon 4 allele, the single-most important genetic susceptibility factor for common "sporadic" forms of DAT. In populations within the developed world, this has become a minor allele, however. Arguments have been developed that this allele had been (and still is, in some parts of the world) a major allele of *Homo sapiens* because it is under selection for its putative protection against a variety of infectious agents, either because of its enhancement of the immune/inflammatory response or because of its less efficient delivery of lipids to the membranes of infectious agents such as *Trypanosoma brucei*, which must obtain its lipids from its infected host. Yet another antagonistic pleiotropic hypothesis for the existence of DAT in our species comes from studies of polymorphic forms of a locus coding for an adaptor protein of importance in the metabolism of the beta amyloid precursor protein (APP), widely considered to be of central importance in the pathogenesis of DAT. The gene coding for this protein is formally designated as the *APBB1* (Amyloid Beta A4 Precursor Protein-Binding, Family B, Member 1), but is widely referred to as *FE65*. Two laboratories have provided evidence that polymorphic alleles of this locus modulate susceptibility to what has been termed "very-late-onset Alzheimer's disease," that is to say, dementias with onsets after the peak ages of onset of the sporadic late-onset forms of Alzheimer's disease that are associated with the epsilon 4 allele of *APOE* (an association that peaks between 65 and 75 years of age). The *FE65* polymorphism was shown to be independent of the impact of the *APOE* polymorphism. Its minor allele, the dominant allele found in other mammals and primates (species resistant to DAT) was shown to bind with much less avidity to APP. This is likely to significantly alter the modulation of functions of that protein, potentially including the role of the APP/FE65/TIP60 complex in transcription. The authors suggested that the new allele emerged as part of a suite of gene actions to enhance cognitive functions, but that this came with deleterious effects of APP metabolism in late life.

Class six: bad alleles early and late: *nuclear and mitochondrial somatic mutations*

The accumulation of somatic mutations in the tissues of aging mammals has been well-documented and can be surprisingly high. For example, *non-leaky* mutations (i.e., severe loss of function mutations) have been shown to rise exponentially in the renal tubular epithelium of human kidneys, reaching levels—by about age 80—between 10^{-3} and 10^{-4}. If one assumes that, for each such severe mutation, there are of the order of ten "leaky" mutations (i.e., mutations with diminished function), one can conclude that the levels of mutations at the single locus that was investigated could approach one in a hundred cells at advanced ages. In aging mice, the rates of increase and the types of nuclear somatic mutations were found to vary substantially from tissue to tissue. The frequencies of chromosomal mutations from the kidneys of aged F1 hybrid mice were found to be as high as one in three cells, but these remarkable results were likely related, in part, to transient exposures of the cells to ambient oxygen, which is now known to be particularly cytotoxic for murine cells. The late Howard J. Curtis, in an early example of the use of comparative gerontology, demonstrated that the levels of carbon tetrachloride-induced chromosomal mutations in mammals were inversely related to their lifespan potentials.

About 1500 genes (encoded by nuclei and mitochondrial DNA) contribute to the functioning of mitochondria. These targets clearly also contribute to the load of somatic mutations during aging and age-related diseases. The frequency of somatic mutation in mitochondrial DNA is ~500–1000-fold higher than it is in nuclear DNA. The tissues of individuals may, in fact, provide unique and dynamic mosaics of patterns of these mutations, serving as a sort of forensic fingerprint. While we have noted above that there is a waning of support for the idea that lifespan is limited by oxidative damage related to mitochondrial metabolism, arguments are still garnered for a primary role in aging processes. We will require more research on the characterization of the specific types of mitochondrial mutations that might be important actors in normative aging, because certain mutations may be more likely to out-compete wild type molecules within cells. Perhaps mutations with rearrangements of the mitochondrial genome produce more than one origin of replication and may lead to dominance ("homoplasty") of deleterious mutant molecules and thus the death of cells bearing that type of mutation.

In contrast to the present debate on the role of mitochondrial mutations and mitochondrial dysfunctions in the genesis of normative cellular aging, support for the roles of mitochondrial dysfunction in common geriatric diseases is becoming stronger. It is noted above that the evidence for an important role of mitochondrial dysfunction in a common form of geriatric congestive heart failure. The evidence of important roles of dysfunctional mitochondria in the genesis of Parkinson's disease is now quite compelling, given the roles of mutations at the *DJ-1* and *PINK1* loci. There is also great interest in observations of marked increases in the prevalence of mutations in the mitochondrial control region in the brains of patients with DAT. Given the key role of mitochondria in the control of apoptosis, aberrations in this pathway can skew the

balance of cell proliferation and cell death and, therefore, modulate carcinogenesis; there is, in fact, growing interest in targeting mitochondria as treatments for cancer. Mitochondrial deletions appear to be key events in the genesis of sarcopenia. Mitochondrial mutations or dysfunctions may also be involved in the pathogenesis of atherosclerosis. Finally, a novel hypothesis has been proposed implicating changes that occur in utero as influences on diseases of aging. Epidemiologic data show an association of small birth weight with the increased risks of developing type 2 diabetes, metabolic syndrome, and cardiovascular disease in adulthood. Leduc and Levy propose that placental mitochondrial dysfunction is present in cases of placental insufficiency and may be a critical influence on the fetus leading to atherosclerosis in later life.

■ EPIGENETIC SHIFTS IN GENE EXPRESSION

The next six classes of gene action (half of the total) can all be grouped under this heading. The term "epigenetic" refers to covalent chemical alterations in the expressions of DNA that are "on top of" the DNA—that is to say, in contrast to mutations or polymorphisms, they do not change the primary sequence or arrangement of nucleotides. These alterations produce the striking specificities of gene expression that define the numerous functionally distinct mammalian cell types and are essential components in the reactions to various injuries. These chemical changes are of two broad types. One type involves methylations of cytosines, typically at "islands" of CpG runs within domains, such as promoters and enhancers, that regulate gene expression. Such methylations are associated with gene silencing. A second general type involves alterations of specific amino acids within the histone proteins that coat the DNA, such as acetylations (associated with gene activation), deacetylations (associated with gene silencing), phosphorylations, methylations, ubiquitinylations, and ADP ribosylations. Methods for molecular epigenetic analysis are being applied at the single cell level, a key technical development for gerontology, because there are many shifts in the population heterogeneity of tissues during aging. Such studies are of interest in the assessment of yet another antagonistic pleiotropic mechanism of aging (Class Twelve).

Class seven: good alleles downregulated early for good reasons: *adaptive silencing*

Given our evolutionary biological premise that nature does not really "care" much about the impact of gene actions that are going on late in the life course (i.e., when the force of natural selection is very weak), any switches in the degrees of gene expression that are initiated at some earlier stage of life because of their adaptive nature could, in principle, have a life of their own and could, therefore, continue to be downregulated or upregulated to a degree that could eventually become deleterious. The following are two examples of such downregulations, one observed in lab mice and the other in people. The first example occurs at the period of life when the somatic growth of mice is dramatically slowed and when resources are switched toward the business of reproduction. Beginning at around that time, a subset of genes that code for the synthesis of ribosomal proteins is silenced. Consequently, the rates of protein synthesis and protein turnover decline in most tissues. This leads to the accumulation of post-translationally modified proteins, including alterations that lead to diminished functions of those proteins, a process likely to contribute to senescent phenotypes. The second example involves the silencing, probably beginning with human puberty, of the estrogen receptor in human colonic mucosa, including regions of the colon that are particularly susceptible to the development of adenocarcinoma. This silencing continues throughout the adult lifespan and, given other lines of evidence for a role of this locus in the regulation of gene expression, likely plays a role in the development of colon cancer the elderly. Both examples involve gene silencing via methylations of CpG dinucleotides.

Class eight: good alleles upregulated early for good reasons: *adaptive expression*

Here is the counterpoint for the mechanism mentioned above. An example is the enhanced expression of androgenic loci after sexual maturation, a likely contributor to the eventual emergence of benign prostatic hyperplasia later in life.

Class nine: good alleles inappropriately upregulated in late life: *non-adaptive loss of silencing*

The best example of this mechanism comes from research on aging laboratory mice. To cite only one of several examples, a locus (*Atp7a*) on the X-inactivated chromosome (a normal dosage compensation event) increases expression in the spleen with increasing age. While the links to specific pathophysiological effects of this and other aberrant upregulations of genes remains to be elucidated, it seems likely that that there will be contributions to senescent phenotypes, given large number of such alterations.

Class ten: good alleles inappropriately downregulated in late life: *non-adaptive epigenetic loss of expression*

An example comes from studies of monozygotic human twins. Both gains and losses of expression were seen in a large number of loci. While it is possible that a number of these alterations were adaptive responses to age-related changes in physiology ("sageing"), given the very large number of these epigenetic alterations in gene expression, many are likely to have resulted in pathophysiological effects.

Class eleven: good alleles for females, bad effects for males (and vice-versa): *sex-based antagonistic pleiotropy*

It would seem likely that evolution will have optimized gene actions somewhat differently in males versus females to enhance the fitness for these behaviorally, morphologically, and physiologically distinct organisms. Thus, alleles that evolve because of optimization for females may not be optimal for males, and vice versa—a sort of evolutionary battle of the sexes. In fruit flies, a large proportion of the alleles that have been optimized for male fertilization are detrimental for the fecundity of females, and vice versa. Arguments have also been made that, given the exclusive inheritance of mitochondria via the female germ line, mitochondrial structure, and function, including numerous interactions with the nuclear genome, may not work as well in males as they do in females. These effects can translate into differential longevities and patterns of late life dysfunction.

Class twelve: good or bad alleles early with bad effects late: *epigenetic gambling and epigenetic drift*

The histograms of Fig. 71-2 demonstrate a phenomenon that has puzzled gerontologists for generations. Why is it that, despite every effort to control genetics and environment, there are still marked variations in the lifespans of cohorts of experimental animals ranging from worms to mice? By far the best job of controlling for both genetics and environment has been achieved in experiments with *C. elegans* (Fig. 71-2). These organisms are hermaphrodites and, therefore, every diploid locus is driven to homozygosity—in other words, populations of these worms essentially consist of identical twins. They also can be grown in axenic media (devoid of

bacteria) in temperature-controlled suspension cultures, including those with magnetic stirring rods, so that each individual worm "sees" the same food and waste and has equal opportunities for contact with other worms. Nevertheless, lifespans among such genetically defined organisms show considerable variability. This intrinsic variation is sufficient to produce a remarkable degree of overlap in the distributions of lifespans among wild type controls and a long-lived mutant population. These variations in lifespan are not heritable. Therefore, when considering the relative contributions of nature, nurture, and chance to intraspecific variations in lifespan, chance seems to be the dominating factor. Phenotypic evidence for stochastic variations is seen in the differences in the rates of development of aberrations in the ultrastructure of the skeletal muscles of aging worms. Some of these stochastic factors could involve somatic mutations—possibly in mitochondria—but their probable frequencies seem insufficient to explain these striking variations. Therefore, a theory suggests that, based upon the proposition that stochastic variations in gene expression develop in cohorts of all organisms, they enhance survival of the population. In a given environment, some worms may have developed a "lucky" set of gene expressions, while the patterns of gene expression may be quite nonadaptive in some of their identical twins. These individual outcomes could be changed in different environments. It is speculated that such "epigenetic gambling" may have evolved before the development of meiosis as a mechanism to ensure the survival of the species under unpredictable environments. Once initiated, "epigenetic drift" would ensue, eventually leading to departures from physiological homeostasis and senescent phenotypes. Published evidence indicates that epigenetic drift occurs within families of isogenic single cells.

■ THE IDENTIFICATION OF SIGNAL TRANSDUCTION PATHWAYS CAPABLE OF MODULATING LIFESPAN AND THEIR POTENTIAL AS GUIDES TO DRUG TARGETS

Earlier in the chapter evidence was cited for the existence of biochemical genetic pathways (or "signal transduction pathways") that, when appropriately modified, could extend the lifespans of several distantly related species—in other words, there is now evidence for the existence of "public" or shared mechanisms of aging. Because of claims that drugs that act in such pathways may enhance lifespans in model organisms (and, by extrapolation, perhaps in people), we need to review these pathways and the evidence for

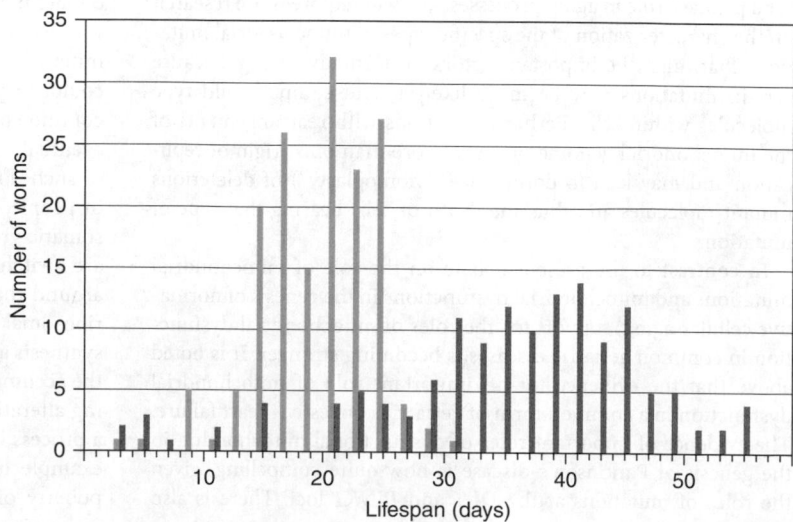

Figure 71-2 Life-span distributions for individual *Caenorhabditis elegans* nematodes in isogenic populations of wild-type (green bars) and age-1 (red bars) strains. *(Reproduced from TB Kirkwood et al: Mech Ageing Dev 126:439, 2005; with permission.)*

pharmacological interventions in more detail. We must keep in mind, however, that there is likely to be extensive cross-talk among these various pathways. Therefore, the "tweaking" of one pathway may have unanticipated effects on distant types of gene actions, especially given the high degree of genetic polymorphism in our species.

The best-documented such longevity-related signaling pathway is the IGF-insulin signaling pathway. The details of this pathway vary somewhat between nematodes, fruit flies, mice, and men, but a key common element is a downstream transcription factor (*daf16* in worms and members of the *FOXO* family in mammals). In response to the regulation of its phosphorylation state, the transcription factors can enter the nucleus and expedite the transcription of a very large suite of genes with diverse activities that serve to enhance the protection of the soma from macromolecular damage. Downregulation of IGF-insulin signaling, as in the case of upstream hypomorphic mutations, releases inhibition of this transcription factor. Such decreased signaling is associated with enhanced longevity. It has also been shown to protect *C. elegans* from the types of proteotoxicity associated with a variety of human neurodegenerative disorders. It is apparent, however, that an optimum level of functioning of this pathway must have evolved to enhance reproductive fitness and survival in both good times and bad times, including the prevention of diabetes mellitus. That such optimization is subject to modulations by genetic polymorphisms in human subjects is suggested by initial findings that exceptionally healthy and exceptionally long-lived subjects (centenarians) exhibit an enrichment of variant hypomorphic alleles for the IGF1 receptor. In that study, it was interesting that the progeny of these centenarians carrying these alleles were more likely to have shorter stature. Such short stature has been associated with a specific haplotype for IGF1 and with longer lifespans of breeds of dogs.

A second pathway (actually two related pathways) involves mTOR signaling. The nomenclature derives from the discovery that this protein, a serine/threonine kinase, is a target of rapamycin, a drug in clinical use as an immunosuppressive agent, for the prevention of coronary artery restenosis and for the treatment of malignant neoplasms. The pathways are involved in a plethora of vital functions, including cell proliferation and survival, the recycling of intracellular materials, aspects of metabolism including nutrient sensing, the generation of ribosomes, and the regulation of protein translation. It has been referred to as the conductor of the cell-signaling symphony. Rapamycin enhances the lifespans and healthspans of mice even when administered at ages roughly comparable to those of 60-year-old humans. While there appeared to be no impact of this treatment upon the numbers of neoplasms, the dominant cause of death of these strains of lab mice, it remains to be seen if the increased lifespan was attributable, at least in part, to a slowing of the rate of growth of these neoplasms.

A third pathway of growing interest to biogerontologists involves a family of histone deacetylases known as sirtuins. Early experiments in yeast demonstrated that such enzymes are associated with the silencing of genes. Their functions are intimately related to the metabolism of nicotinamide adenine dinucleotide (NAD), a coenzyme used as an oxidizing or reducing agent in a variety of essential metabolic processes. Although still controversial, an important member of this family is SIRT1, homologues of which enhance the lifespans of model organisms. SIRT1 is a putative target of resveratrol, which is thought to activate the enzyme and, therefore, might enhance lifespan and, presumably healthspan as well. Health benefits of large doses of resveratrol have been noted in obese, diabetic mice with fatty livers. Resveratrol, a component of red wine, has caught the imagination of the general public and the investment dollars of some pharmaceutical companies. The latter are searching for more potent variants of the molecule; phase IIa clinical trials in patients with type 2 diabetes and other disorders are in progress.

FURTHER READINGS

Austad SN: *Why We Age: What Science Is Discovering About the Body's Journey Through Life.* New York, John Wiley & Sons, 1997

Colman RJ et al: Caloric restriction delays disease onset and mortality in rhesus monkeys. Science 325:201, 2009

Conboy IM et al: Rejuvenation of aged progenitor cells by exposure to a young systemic environment. Nature 433:760, 2005

Coppe JP et al: The senescence-associated secretory phenotype: the dark side of tumor suppression. Annu Rev Pathol 5:99, 2010

Harrison DE et al: Rapamycin fed late in life extends lifespan in genetically heterogeneous mice. Nature 460:392, 2009

Imai SI, Guarente L: Ten years of NAD-dependent SIR2 family deacetylases: implications for metabolic diseases. Trends Pharmacol Sci 31:212, 2010

Kennedy BK: The genetics of ageing: insight from genome-wide approaches in invertebrate model organisms. J Intern Med 263:142, 2008

Kenyon CJ: The genetics of ageing. Nature 464:504, 2010

Leduc L et al: Fetal programming of atherosclerosis: Possible role of the mitochondria. Eur J Obstet Gynecol Reprod Biol 149:127, 2010

Martin GM: *Modalities of Gene Action Predicted by the Classical Evolutionary Theory of Aging*, in VL Bengston et al (Eds). *Handbook of Theories of Aging*, 2nd ed, New York, Springer, 2009, pp 179-191

Partridge L, Gems D: Beyond the evolutionary theory of ageing, from functional genomics to evo-gero. Trends Ecol Evol 21:334, 2006

CHAPTER **72**

Clinical Problems of Aging

Luigi Ferrucci
Stephanie Studenski

While an in-depth understanding of internal medicine serves as a foundation, proper care of older adults should be complemented by insight into the multidimensional effects of aging on disease manifestations, consequences, and response to treatment. In younger adults, individual diseases tend to have a more distinct pathophysiology with well-defined risk factors; the same diseases in older persons may have a less distinct pathophysiology and are often the result of failed homeostatic mechanisms. Causes and clinical manifestations are less specific and can vary widely between individuals. Therefore, the care of older patients demands an understanding of the effects of aging on human physiology and a broader perspective that incorporates geriatric syndromes, disability, social contexts, and goals of care. For example, care planning for the older patient cannot ignore the influence of life expectancy. In fact, the expected remaining years of life can guide recommendations about appropriate preventive and other long-term interventions, and shape discussions about treatment alternatives.

Demography (Chap. 70) Population aging emerged on a worldwide scale for the first time in history within the last century. Since aging influences many facets of life, governments and societies now face new social and economic challenges that impact health care, as well as family and community responsibilities. Figure 72-1 highlights recent and predicted changes in U.S. population structure. The overall number of children has remained relatively stable, but explosive growth has occurred among older populations. The percentage growth is particularly dramatic among the oldest old. For example, the 80–89-year-old group increased more than threefold between

1960 and 2010 and will increase almost tenfold between 1960 and 2050. Women already outlive men by many years and the sex discrepancy in longevity is projected to increase further in the future.

Population aging occurs at different rates in varying geographic regions of the world. Over the last century, Europe, Australia, and North America have had the populations with the greatest proportions of older persons, but Asia and South America are aging rapidly, with a population structure that will resemble the "older" countries by around 2050 (Fig. 72-2). Among older persons, the oldest old (those older than age 80 years) are the fastest growing segment of the population (Fig. 72-3), and the pace of aging is projected to accelerate in most countries in the next 50 years. There is no evidence that the rate of population aging is decreasing.

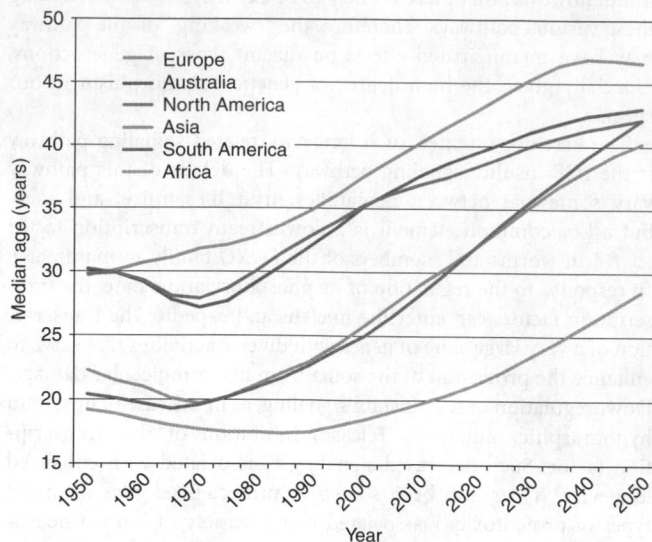

Figure 72-2 Population aging in different geographic regions. *(From United Nations World Population Prospects: The 2008 Revision, http://esa. un.org/unpp.)*

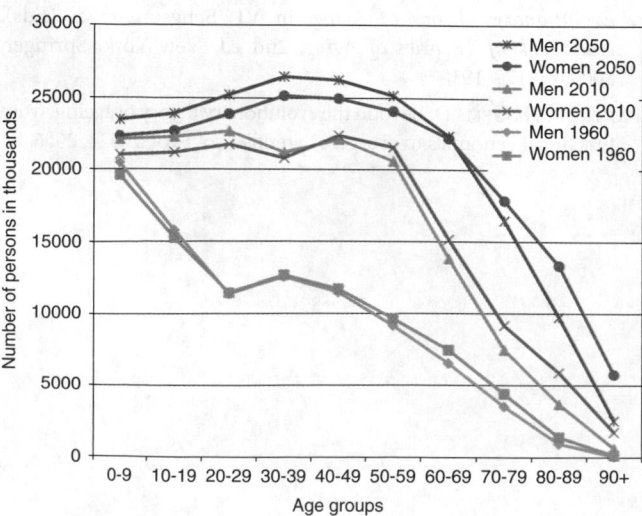

Figure 72-1 Change in the structure of the U.S. population between 1960 and 2050. *(From United Nations World Population Prospects: The 2008 Revision, http://esa.un.org/unpp.)*

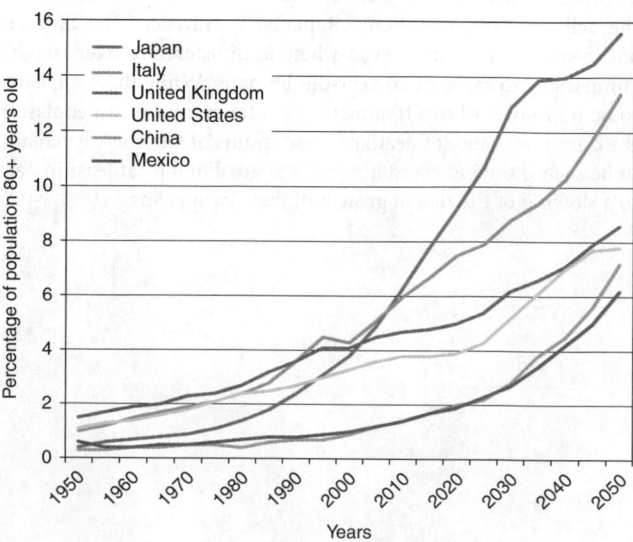

Figure 72-3 Percentage of the population age >80 years from 1950 to 2050 in different representative nations. The pace of aging will accelerate. *(From United Nations World Population Prospects: The 2008 Revision, http:// esa.un.org/unpp.)*

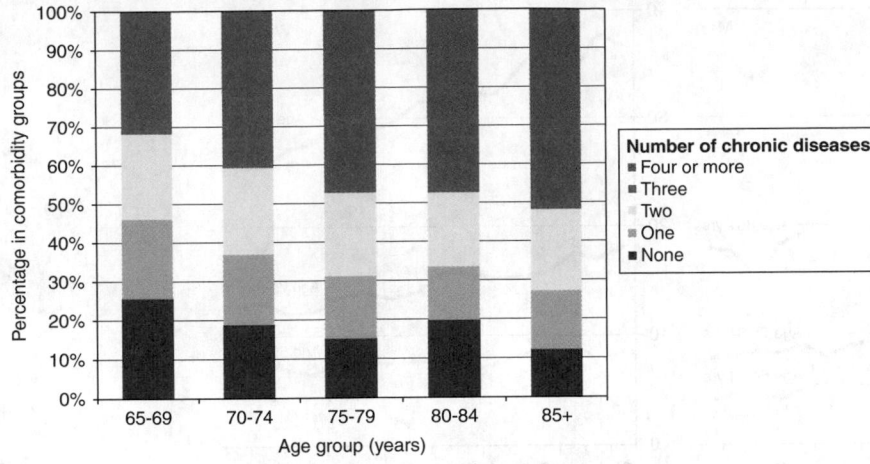

Figure 72-4 Prevalence of comorbidity by age group in persons 65 years and older living in the U.S. and enrolled in Medicare parts A and B in 1999. *(From JL Wolff et al: Arch Intern Med 162:2269, 2002.)*

Population aging and health

Many chronic diseases increase in prevalence with age. It is not unusual for older persons to have multiple chronic diseases (Fig. 72-4) although some seem more susceptible to co-occurring problems compared to others. Functional problems with difficulty or need for help in performing basic activities of daily living (ADLs) (Table 72-1) increase with age and are more common in women than men. In recent decades, the age-specific prevalence of disability has declined, especially in the oldest old. Estimated rates are shown in Fig. 72-5 as the percentage of persons who reported severe difficulty or needed help in bathing, but data on other basic activities of daily living show similar trends. The rate of decline in disability is decreasing, but the magnitude of this decline is small compared to the overwhelming effect of population aging. Thus, the number of people with disability in the United States and other countries is rapidly expanding. Rates of cognitive impairments, such as memory problems, also increase with aging (Fig. 72-6). Chronic disease and disability lead to increased use of health care resources. Health care expenditures increase with age, increase more with disability, and are highest in the last year of life. However, new medical technologies and expensive medications are greater influences on health care costs than population aging alone. General practitioners and internists with little specific training in geriatric medicine provide the bulk of care for older persons.

Systemic effects of aging

Systemic consequences of aging are widespread but can be clustered into four main domains or processes (Fig. 72-7): (1) body composition; (2) balance between energy availability and energy demand; (3) signaling networks that maintain homeostasis; and (4) neurodegeneration. Each domain can be assessed using routine clinical tests, although more detailed research techniques are also available (Table 72-2).

Body composition Profound changes in body composition may be the most evident and inescapable effect of aging (Fig. 72-8). Over the life span, body weight tends to increase through childhood, puberty, and adulthood until late middle age. Weight tends to decline in men between ages 65 and 70 years, and somewhat later in women. Lean body mass, composed predominantly of muscle and visceral organs, decreases steadily after the third decade. In muscle, this atrophy is greater in fast-twitch compared to slow-twitch fibers. Fat mass tends to increase in middle age and then declines in late life, reflecting the trajectory of weight change. Interestingly, waist circumference continues to increase across the life span, suggesting that visceral fat, which is responsible for most of the pathologic consequences of obesity, continues to accumulate. In some individuals, fat also accumulates inside muscle where it affects muscle quality and function. With age, fibro-connective tissue tends to increase in many organ systems. In muscle, fibro-connective tissue buildup also affects muscle quality and function. In combination, the loss of muscle mass and quality result in reduced muscle strength, with ultimate impact on functional capacity and mobility. Muscle strength declines with aging and not only affects functional status but is also a strong independent predictor of mortality (Fig. 72-9). Progressive demineralization and architectural modification occurs in bone, resulting in a decline of bone strength. Loss of bone strength increases the risk of fracture. Sex differences in the effects of aging on bone mass are due to sex differences in peak bone mass and the effects of gonadal hormones on bone. Overall, compared to men, women tend to lose bone at an earlier age and more quickly reach the threshold of low bone strength that increases fracture risk. All of these changes in body composition can be attributed to disruptions in the links between synthesis, degradation, and repair that normally serve to remodel tissues. Body composition can be approximated in clinical practice using weight, height, body mass index (weight in kilograms divided by height in meters squared),

---

TABLE 72-1 Basic and Instrumental Activities of Daily Living

The Basic Activities of Daily Living (ADLs) Consist of These Self-Care Tasks

- Personal hygiene
- Dressing and undressing
- Eating
- Transferring from bed to chair, and back
- Voluntarily controlling urinary and fecal discharge
- Using the toilet
- Moving around (as opposed to being bedridden)

Instrumental Activities of Daily Living (IADLs) Are Not Necessary For Fundamental Functioning, But They Let an Individual Live Independently in a Community

- Doing light housework
- Preparing meals
- Taking medications
- Shopping for groceries or clothes
- Using the telephone
- Managing money
- Using technology (older generations may not be that technologically savvy since they were not as exposed to it during their lifetime.)

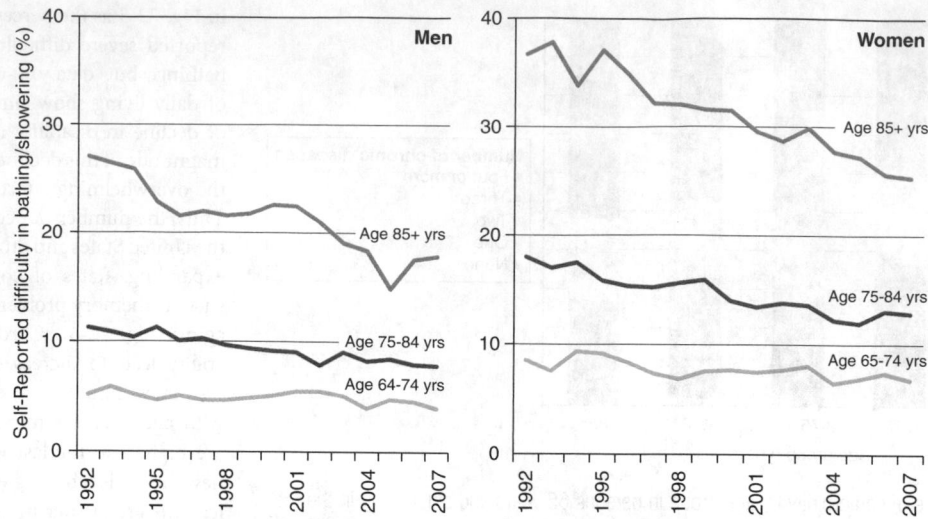

Figure 72-5 Self-reported prevalence of disability (severe difficulty) in bathing/showering between 1992 and 2007, according to age and sex. *(From Medicare Current Beneficiary Survey 1992–2007. Accessed May 26, 2010 at http://205.207.175.93/HDI/TableViewer/.)*

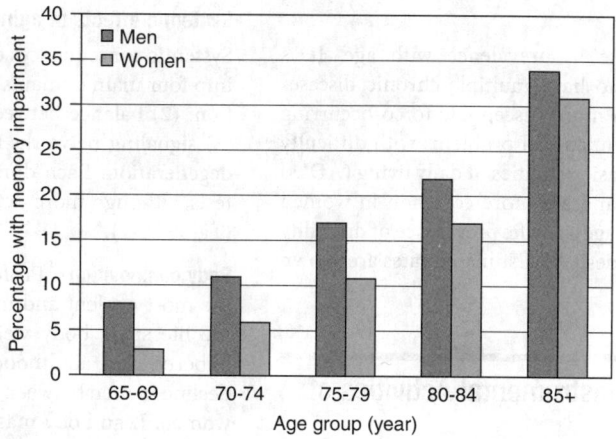

Figure 72-6 Rates of memory impairments in different age groups. The definition of "moderate or severe memory impairment" is 4 or fewer words recalled out of 20. *(Source: Health and Retirement Survey. Accessed February 7, 2011 at http://aoa.gov/agingstatsdotnet/Main_Site/Data/2000_Documents/healthstatus.aspx.)*

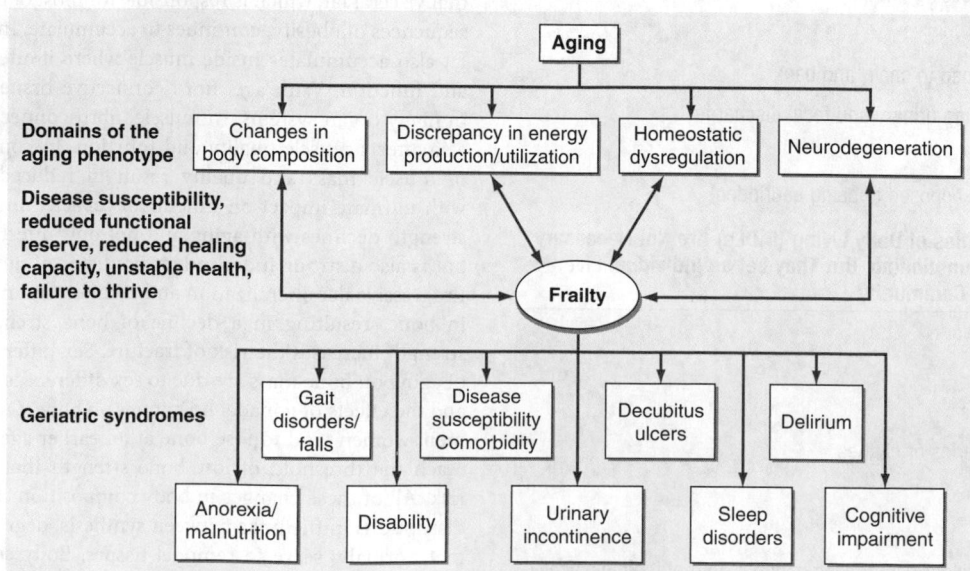

Figure 72-7 A unifying model of aging, frailty, and the geriatric syndromes.

TABLE 72-2 Example of Assessment of the Different Domains of the Aging Phenotype

Body Composition	Energetics	Homeostatic Regulation	Neurodegeneration
Anthropometrics (weight, height, BMI, waist circumference, arm and leg circumference, skin folds)	Self-reported questionnaires investigating physical activity, sense of fatigue/exhaustion, exercise tolerance	Baseline levels of biomarkers and hormone levels	Standard neurologic exam, including assessment of global cognition [Mini Mental State, Montreal Cognitive Assessment (MoCa)]
Muscle strength testing (isometric and isokinetic)	Resting metabolic rate	Inflammatory markers (ESR, CRP, IL-6, TNF-alpha, etc)	Objective assessment of gait, balance, reaction time, coordination
Biomarkers (24-h creatinuria or 3-methyl-histidine)	Performance-based tests of physical function	Nutritional biomarkers (vitamins, antioxidants, etc)	Electroneurography and electromyography
CT and MRI, dual-energy x-ray absorptiometry (DEXA)	Treadmill testing	Response to provocative tests, such as oral glucose tolerance test, dexamethasone test, and others	MRI, fMRI, PET, and other dynamic imaging techniques
Hydrostatic weighing	Objective measures of physical activity (accelerometers, double labeled water)	Stress response	Evoked potentials

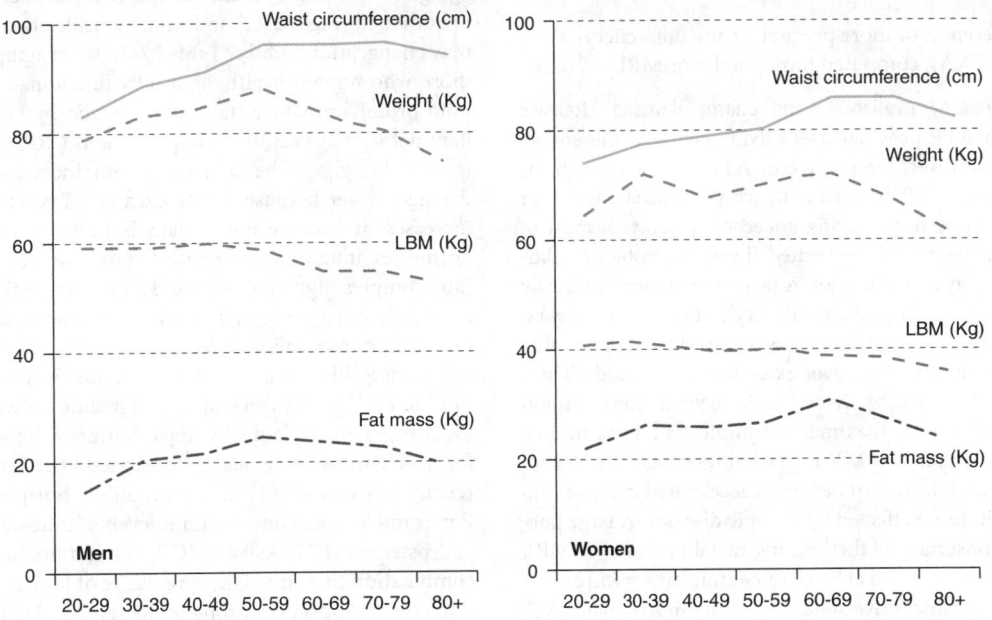

Figure 72-8 Longitudinal changes of weight, body composition, and waist circumference over the life span estimated in 1167 participants of the Baltimore Longitudinal Study of Aging. *Lean Body Mass (LBM) and Fat Mass estimated with DEXA. [Source: The Baltimore Longitudinal study of Aging 2010 (unpublished data).]

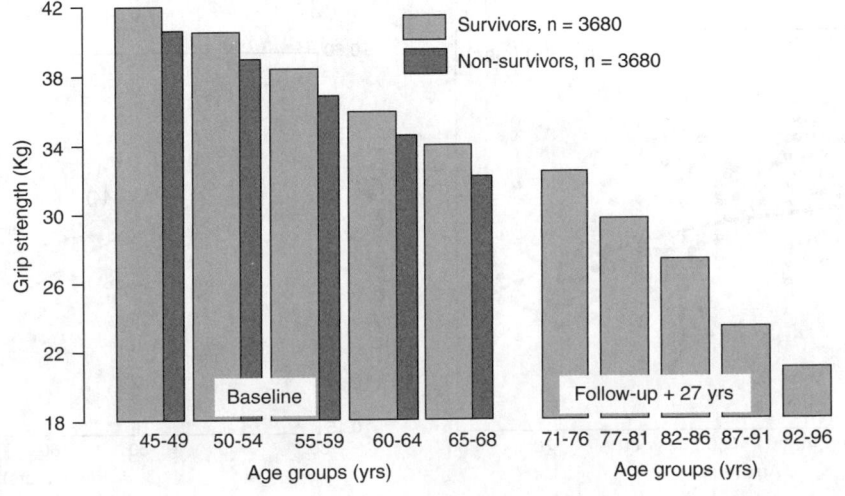

Figure 72-9 Cross-sectional differences and longitudinal changes in muscle strength over a 27-year follow-up. Note that subjects who died during the follow-up had lower baseline muscle strength. (From T Rantanen et al: J Appl Physiol 85:2047, 1998.)

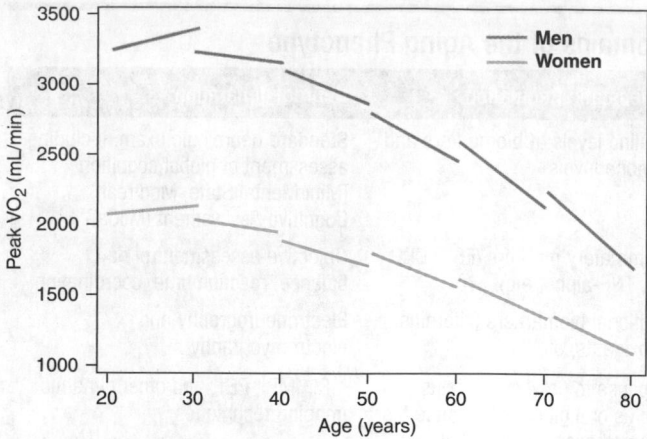

Figure 72-10 Longitudinal changes in aerobic capacity in participants of the Baltimore Longitudinal Study of Aging. *(From JL Fleg: Circulation 112:674, 2005.)*

and waist circumference, or more precisely using dual-energy x-ray absorptiometry (DEXA), computed tomography or MRI.

Balance between energy availability and energy demand Release of phosphate from ATP provides every living cell with the energy required for life. However, the storage of ATP is only enough for 6 seconds; therefore, ATP is constantly resynthesized. Although ATP resynthesis can be done during anaerobic glycolysis, most of the energy used in the body is generated through aerobic metabolism. Therefore, energy comsumption is usually estimated indirectly by oxygen consumption (indirect calorimetry). There is currently no method to measure true "fitness," which is the maximum energy that can be produced by an organism over extended time periods. Thus, fitness is estimated indirectly from peak oxygen consumption (MV_{O_2peak}), often during a maximal treadmill test. Longitudinal studies have demonstrated that MV_{O_2peak} declines progressively with aging (Fig. 72-10), and the rate of decline is accelerated in those who are sedentary and in those affected by chronic diseases. A large portion of energy is consumed as the "resting metabolic rate" (RMR), the amount of energy expended at rest in a neutral temperature environment and in a postabsorptive state. In healthy individuals, RMR declines with aging, mostly due to a decline in the highly metabolically active tissues of lean body mass (Fig. 72-11). However, persons

with unstable homeostasis due to illness require additional energy for compensatory mechanisms. Indeed, an inadequately high RMR is a marker of illness, is an independent risk factor for mortality, and may contribute to the weight loss that often accompanies severe illness. Finally, for reasons that are not yet completely clear, older age, pathology, and physical impairment increase the energy cost of motor activities such as walking. Overall, older individuals with multiple chronic conditions have low available energy levels and require more energy both at rest and during physical activity. Thus, sick older people may consume all their available energy performing the most basic activities of daily living, leading to symptoms of fatigue and restriction to a sedentary existence. Energetic status can be assessed clinically by simply asking the patient about their perceived level of fatigue during daily activities such as walking or dressing. Energy capacity can be assessed more precisely by exercise tolerance during a walking test or a treadmill test coupled with spirometry.

Signaling networks that maintain homeostasis The main signaling pathways that control homeostasis involve hormones, inflammatory mediators, and antioxidants; all are profoundly affected by aging. Sex hormone levels, such as testosterone, decrease with age in both men (Fig. 72-12) and women, while other hormone systems may change more subtly (Table 72-3). Most aging individuals, even those who remain healthy and fully functional, tend to develop a mild proinflammatory state characterized by high levels of proinflammatory markers, including IL-6 and CRP (Fig. 72-13). Aging is also thought to be associated with increased oxidative stress damage, either because the production of reactive oxygen species increases or because antioxidant buffers are less effective. Since hormones, inflammatory markers, and antioxidants are integrated into complex signaling networks, levels of individual biomarkers may well reflect adaptation within homeostatic feedback loops rather than true causative factors. Thus, the therapeutic strategy of single-molecule replacement may be ineffective or even counterproductive. The presence of such signaling networks and feedback loops may help explain why single-hormone "replacement therapy" for problems of aging has demonstrated little benefit. The focus of research in this area is now on multiple-hormonal dysregulation. For example, taken one at a time, levels of testosterone, dehydroepiandrosterone (DHEAs), and IGF-1 do not predict mortality, but in combination they are highly predictive of longevity. This combination effect is especially strong in the setting of congestive heart failure. Similarly, several micronutrients, such as vitamins (especially vitamin D), minerals (selenium and magnesium), and antioxidants

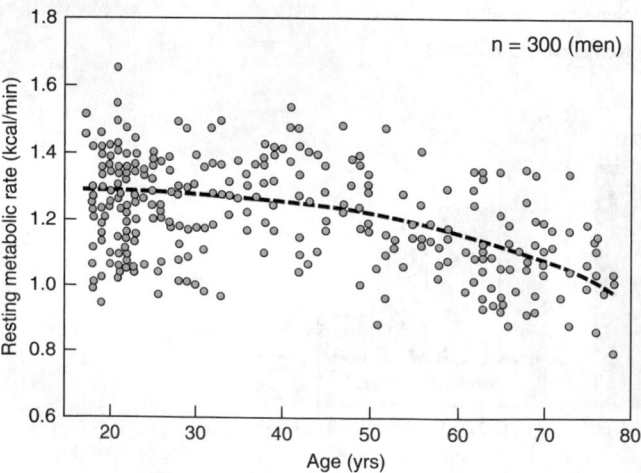

Figure 72-11 Changes in resting metabolic rate with aging. *[Data from the Baltimore Longitudinal Study of Aging (unpublished).]*

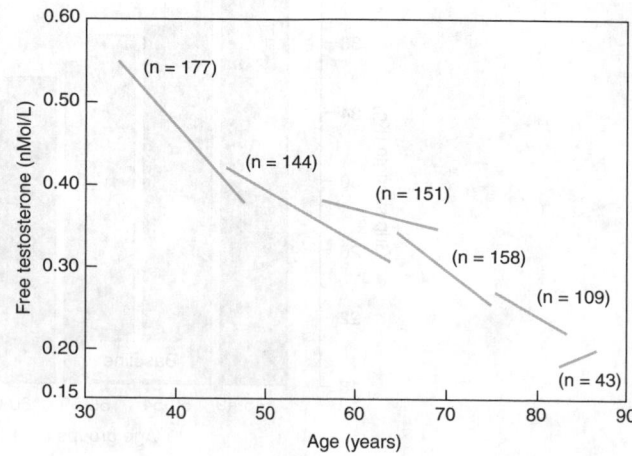

Figure 72-12 Longitudinal changes of free testosterone levels in healthy men. *(From SM Harman et al: J Clin Endocrinol Metab 86:724, 2001.)*

TABLE 72-3 Hormones That Decrease, Remain Stable, and Increase With Aging

Decrease	No Change	Increase
Growth hormone	Prolactin	Cholecystokinin
Luteinizing hormone (men)	Thyrotropin	Luteinizing hormone (women)
Insulin growth factor I	Thyroid hormones	Follicle-stimulating hormone
Testosterone	Epinephrine	Cortisol
Estradiol	Glucagon-like peptide 1	Prolactin
DHEA and DHEAs	Gastric inhibitory polypeptide	Norepinephrine
Pregnenolone		Insulin
25(OH) vitamin D		Parathormone
Aldosterone		
Vasoactive intestinal peptide		
Melatonin		

findings are not specific and their diagnostic utility is unclear (Fig. 72-15). Other neurophysiologic changes in the brain also frequently occur with aging and may contribute to cognitive decline. Functional imaging studies have shown that some older people have diminished coordination between the brain regions responsible for higher-order cognitive functions and that such diminished coordination is correlated with poor cognitive performance. In young healthy individuals, the brain activity associated with executive cognitive functions (e.g., problem solving, decision making) is very well localized while in healthy older individuals, the pattern of cortical activation is more diffuse. Brain pathology has typically been associated with specific diseases; amyloid plaques and neurofibrillary tangles are considered the pathologic hallmarks of Alzheimer's disease. However, these pathologic markers have been found at autopsy in many older individuals who had cognitive testing in the year before death and were found to be normal. Taken together, trends in brain changes with aging suggest that some neurophysiologic manifestations are compensatory adaptations, rather than primary contributors to age-related declines. Because the brain is capable of reorganization and compensation, extensive neurodegeneration may not be clinically evident. Therefore, early detection requires careful testing. Clinically, cortical and subcortical changes are reflected in the high prevalence of "soft," nonspecific neurologic signs, often with slow and unstable gait, poor balance, and slow reaction times. These movement changes can be elicited more overtly using "dual tasks," in which a cognitive and a motor task are performed simultaneously. In a simple version of a dual task, an older adult who has to stop walking in order to talk has been shown to predict increased risk of falls. Poor dual task performance has been interpreted as a marker of reduced overall capacity for central processing, so that simultaneous processing is more constrained. Beyond the brain, the spinal cord also experiences changes after age 60 years, including reduced numbers of motor neurons and damage to myelin. The motor neurons that survive compensate by increased branching complexity, and by serving larger motor units. As motor units become larger, they decline in number at a rate of about 1% per year, starting after the third decade. These larger motor units contribute to reductions in fine-motor control and manual dexterity. Age-related changes also occur in the autonomic nervous system, affecting cardiovascular and splanchnic function.

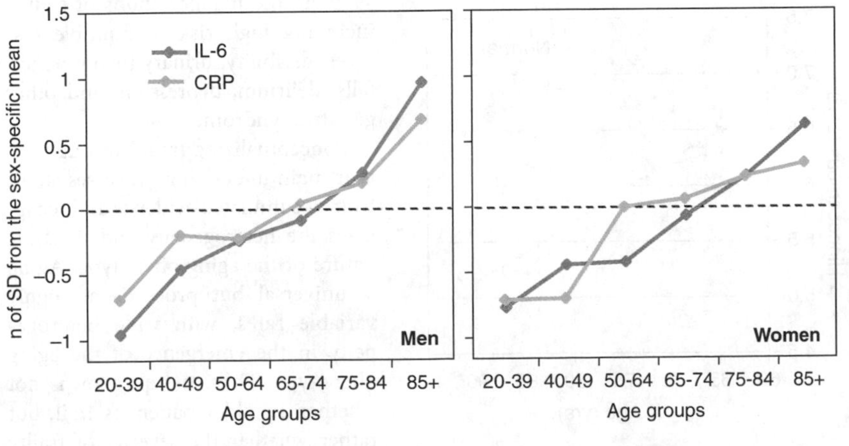

(vitamins D and E), also regulate aspects of metabolism. Low levels of these micronutrients have been associated with accelerated aging and high risk of adverse outcomes. However, except for vitamin D, no clear evidence suggests that supplementation has positive effects on health. Unfortunately, no standard criteria exist that allow the detection and quantification of homeostatic dysregulation.

Neurodegeneration Neurons stop reproducing shortly after birth and their number declines throughout life. Brain atrophy occurs with aging after the age of 60 years. Atrophy proceeds at varying rates in different parts of the brain (Fig. 72-14) and is often accompanied by an inflammatory response and microglial activation. Age-associated brain atrophy may contribute to age-related declines in cognitive and motor function. Atrophy may also be a factor in some brain diseases that may occur with aging, such as mild cognitive impairment (MCI), in which persons have mild but detectable impairments on tests of cognition but no severe disability in daily activities. In MCI, atrophy has been found mostly in the prefrontal cortex and hippocampus, but these

System changes coexist and affect each other: the phenotype of aging is the final common pathway of this interaction While age-related system changes were described individually, in reality, these changes develop in parallel and affect each other through many feed-forward and feedback loops. Some system interactions are well understood, while others are under investigation. For example, body composition interacts with energy balance and signaling. Higher lean body mass increases energy consumption and improves insulin sensitivity and carbohydrate metabolism. Higher fat mass, especially visceral fat mass, is the culprit in the metabolic

Figure 72-13 Change in IL-6 and c-reactive protein with aging. *Values are expressed as Z-Scores to make them comparable. (From L Ferrucci et al: Blood 105:2294, 2005.)

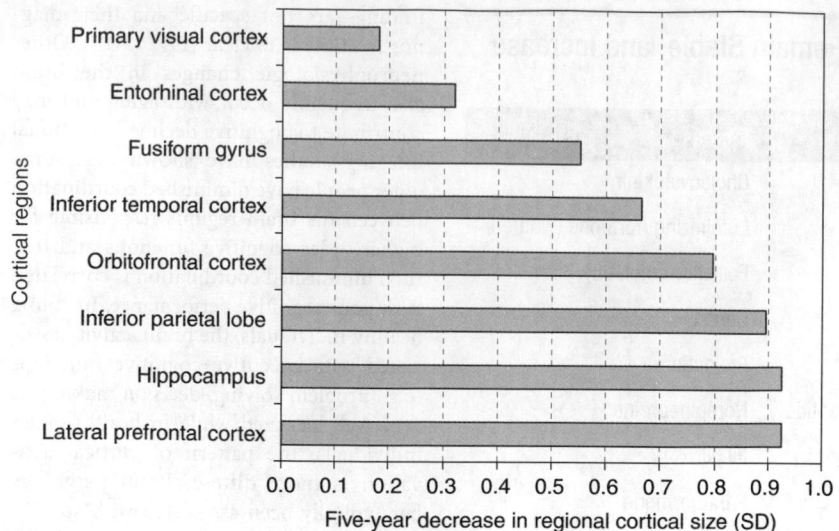

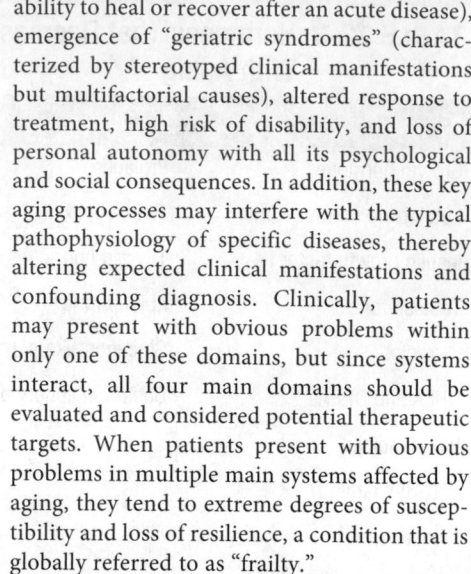

Figure 72-14 Five-year decline in mean volumes measured in standard deviation units (Cohen's *d*) of different brain regions. The primary visual cortex shows the smallest average shrinkage and the prefrontal and inferior parietal cortex and hippocampus showed the highest average shrinkage. *(From N Raz et al: Ann N Y Acad Sci 1097:84, 2007.)*

syndrome and is associated with low testosterone, high SHBG, and increased levels of proinflammatory markers such as C-reactive protein and IL-6. Altered signaling can affect neurodegeneration; insulin resistance and adipokines such as leptin and adiponectin are associated with declines in cognitive function. A state of inflammation, reduced levels of testosterone and IGF-1, combined with loss of motor neurons and dysfunction of the motor unit, have been linked to accelerated decline of muscle mass and strength. Normal intersystem coordination is also affected by aging. The hypothalamus normally functions as a central regulator of metabolism and energy use and coordinates physiologic responses of the entire organism through hormonal signaling; aging-related changes in the hypothalamus alter this control. The central nervous system also controls adaptive sympathetic/parasympathetic activity, so that age-related CNS degeneration may have implications for autonomic function.

The phenotype that results from the aging process is characterized by increased susceptibility to diseases, high risk of multiple coexisting diseases, impaired response to stress (including limited ability to heal or recover after an acute disease), emergence of "geriatric syndromes" (characterized by stereotyped clinical manifestations but multifactorial causes), altered response to treatment, high risk of disability, and loss of personal autonomy with all its psychological and social consequences. In addition, these key aging processes may interfere with the typical pathophysiology of specific diseases, thereby altering expected clinical manifestations and confounding diagnosis. Clinically, patients may present with obvious problems within only one of these domains, but since systems interact, all four main domains should be evaluated and considered potential therapeutic targets. When patients present with obvious problems in multiple main systems affected by aging, they tend to extreme degrees of susceptibility and loss of resilience, a condition that is globally referred to as "frailty."

■ FRAILTY

Frailty has been described as a physiologic syndrome characterized by decreased reserve and diminished resistance to stressors, resulting from cumulative decline across multiple physiologic systems, causing vulnerability to adverse outcomes and high risk of death. A proposed definition characterized by weight loss, fatigue, impaired grip strength, diminished physical activity, and slow gait has shown good internal consistency and strong predictive validity, and has been used in many clinical and epidemiologic studies. However, alternative schools of thought have different diagnostic criteria. For example, frailty has been suggested to be a random accumulation of multiple impairments with aging, and, therefore, no standard criteria for diagnosis can be developed. Regardless of the definition, an extensive literature shows that older persons who are considered frail by any definition have overt changes in the same four main processes—body composition, homeostatic dysregulation, energetic failure, and neurodegeneration, the characteristics of the aging "phenotype." A classic clinical case would be an older woman with sarcopenic obesity characterized by increased body fat and decreased muscle (body composition changes); extremely low exercise tolerance and extreme fatigue (energetic failure); high insulin; low IGF-1; inadequate intake of calories; low vitamin D, E, and carotenoids (signal dysregulation); and memory problems, slow gait, and unstable balance (neurodegeneration). This woman is likely to show all the manifestations of frailty, including high risk of multiple diseases, disability, urinary incontinence, falls, delirium, depression, and other geriatric syndromes.

Conceptualizing frailty through the four main underlying processes stems from accumulated evidence and recognizes the heterogeneity and dynamic nature of the aging phenotype. Aging is universal but proceeds at highly variable rates, with wide heterogeneity in the emergence of the aging phenotype. Thus, the question is not whether an older patient is frail, but rather whether the severity of frailty is beyond the threshold of clinical and behavioral relevance. Understanding

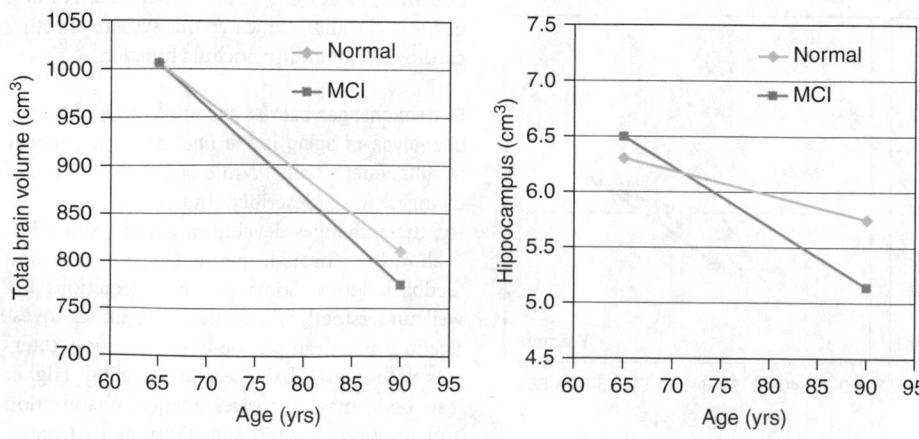

Figure 72-15 Longitudinal changes of regional brain volumes in normal aging and MCI. *(From I Driscoll et al: Neurology 72:1906, 2009.)*

frailty through the lens of four interacting underlying processes also provides an interface with diseases that, like aging itself, affect the "aging phenotype." For example, congestive heart failure is associated with low energy availability, multiple hormonal derangements, and a proinflammatory state, thereby contributing to frailty severity. Parkinson's disease is an example of neurodegeneration that, in an advanced state, affects body composition, energy metabolism, and homeostatic signaling, resulting in a syndrome that closely resembles frailty. Diabetes is especially important to aging and frailty because it harms body composition, energy metabolism, homeostatic dysregulation, and neuronal integrity. Accordingly, a number of studies have found that type 2 diabetes is a strong risk factor for frailty and for many of its consequences. Since disease and aging interact, careful and appropriate treatment of disease is critical to prevent or reduce frailty.

■ CONSEQUENCES OF AGING PROCESSES, THE AGING PHENOTYPE, AND FRAILTY

While the pathophysiology of frailty is still being elucidated, its consequences have been well characterized in prospective studies. Four main consequences are important for clinical practice: (1) ineffective or incomplete homeostatic response to stress, (2) multiple coexisting diseases (multi- or comorbidity) and polypharmacy, (3) physical disability, and (4) the so-called geriatric syndromes. We will briefly address each one of them.

Low resistance to stress Frailty can be considered a progressive loss of reserve in multiple physiologic functions. At an early stage and in the absence of stress, mildly frail older individuals may appear to be normal. However, they have reduced ability to cope with challenges, such as acute diseases, traumas, surgical procedures, or chemotherapy. Acute illness involving a hospital stay is associated with undernutrition and inactivity, which sometimes may be of such magnitude that the residual muscle mass fails to meet the minimal requirement for walking. Even when nutrition is reinstated, energy reserves may be insufficient to adequately rebuild muscle mass. Older persons have a reduced ability to tolerate infections, in part because they are less able to build a dynamic inflammatory response to vaccination or infectious exposure, so that infections are more likely to become severe and systemic and resolve more slowly. In the context of tolerance to stress, assessing aspects of frailty can help estimate ability to withstand the rigors of aggressive treatments, to respond to interventions aimed at infection, to anticipate and prevent complications of hospitalization, and generally to estimate prognosis. Accordingly, treatment plans may be adjusted to improve tolerance and safety; bed rest and hospitalization should be used sparingly; and infections should be prevented, anticipated, and managed assertively.

Comorbidity and polypharmacy Older age is associated with high rates of many chronic diseases (Fig. 72-4). Thus, not unexpectedly, the percentage of individuals affected by multiple medical conditions (co- or multimorbidity) also increases with age. In frail older individuals, comorbidity occurs at higher rates than would be expected from the combined probability of the component conditions. It is likely that frailty and comorbidity affect each other, so that multiple diseases contribute to frailty and frailty increases susceptibility to diseases. Clinically, patients with multiple conditions present unique diagnostic and treatment challenges. Standard diagnostic criteria may not be informative because there are additional confusing signs and symptoms. A classic example is the coexistence of iron and vitamin B_{12} deficiency, creating an apparently normocytic anemia. The risk/benefit ratio for many medical and surgical treatment options may be reduced in the face of other diseases. Drug treatment planning is made more complex because comorbid diseases may affect the absorption, volume of distribution, protein binding, and, especially, elimination of many drugs, leading to fluctuation in therapeutic levels and increased risk of under- or overdosing. Drug excretion is affected by renal and liver changes with aging that may not be detectable with usual clinical tests. Formulas for estimating glomerular filtration rate in older patients are available while estimating changes in hepatic excretion is still a challenge. Patients with many diseases are usually prescribed multiple drugs, especially when they are cared for by multiple specialists who do not communicate. The risk of adverse drug reactions, drug-drug interactions, and poor compliance increases geometrically with the number of drugs prescribed and with the severity of frailty. Some general rules to minimize the chances of adverse drug events are as follows: (a) always ask patients to bring in all medications, including prescription, over-the-counter, vitamins supplements, and herbal preparations (the "brown bag test"); (b) screen for unnecessary drugs—those without a clear indication should be stopped; (c) simplify the regimen in terms of number of agents and schedules, try to avoid frequent changes, and use single daily dose regimens whenever possible; (d) avoid drugs that are expensive or not covered by insurance whenever possible; (e) minimize the number of drugs to those that are absolutely essential and always check for possible interactions; (f) make sure that the patient or an available caregiver understands the administration regimen and provide legible written instructions; and (g) schedule periodic medication reviews.

Disability and impaired recovery from acute-onset disability The prevalence of disability in self-care and home management increases steeply with aging and tends to be higher in women than in men (Fig. 72-5). Physical and cognitive function in older persons reflects overall health status, and predicts health care utilization, institutionalization, and mortality more accurately than any other known biomedical measure. Thus, assessing function and disability and predicting the risk of disability are cornerstones of geriatric medicine. Frailty, regardless of the criteria used for its definition, is a robust and powerful risk factor for disability. Because of this strong relationship, measures of physical function and mobility have been proposed as standard criteria for frailty. However, disability occurs late in the frailty process, after reserve and compensation are exhausted. Early in the development of frailty, body composition change, reduced fitness, homeostatic deregulation, and neurodegeneration can begin without impact on daily function. As opposed to disability in younger persons, where the rule is to look for a clear dominant cause, disability in frail, older persons is almost always multifactorial. Multiple disrupted aging processes are usually involved, even when the precipitating cause seems unique. Excess fat mass, poor muscle strength, reduced lean body mass, poor fitness, reduced energy efficiency, poor nutritional intake, low circulating levels of antioxidant micronutrients, high levels of proinflammatory markers, objective signs of neurologic dysfunction, and cognitive impairment all contribute to disability. The multifactorial nature of disability in frail older persons reduces the capacity for compensation and interferes with functional recovery. For example, a small lacunar stroke that causes problems with balance in a young hypertensive individual can be overcome by standing and walking with the feet further apart, a strategy that requires the brain to adapt, strong muscles, and lots of energy capacity. The same small, lacunar stroke may cause catastrophic disability in an older person already affected by neurodegeneration and weakness who is less able to compensate. As a consequence, interventions aimed at preventing and reducing disability in older persons should have a dual focus on both the precipitating cause and the systems needed for compensation. In the case of the lacunar stroke, interventions to promote mobility function might include stroke prevention, balance rehabilitation, and strength training. As a rule of thumb, the assessment of contributing causes and the design of intervention strategies for disability in older persons should always consider the four main aging processes that contribute to frailty. One of the most popular approaches to disability measurement is a modification of the International Classification of Impairments, Disabilities and Handicaps (World Health Organization, 1980) proposed by the Institute of Medicine (IOM, 1992). This classification infers a causal pathway in four steps: pathology (diseases), impairment (the physical manifestation of diseases), functional limitation (global functions such as walking, grasping, climbing stairs), and disability (ability to fulfill social roles in the environment).

In practice, the assessment of functional limitation and disability is performed either by: 1) self reported questionnaire concerning the degree of ability to perform basic self-care or more complex activities of daily living; 2) performance-based measures of physical function that assess specific domains, such as balance, gait, manual dexterity, coordination, flexibility, and endurance. A concise list of standard tools that can be used to assess physical function in older persons is reported in Table 72-4. In 2001, the WHO officially endorsed a new classification system, the International Classification of Functioning, Disability and Health, known more commonly as ICF. In the ICF, health measures are classified from body, individual, and societal perspectives by means of two lists: a

TABLE 72-4 Tools for Functional Assessment in Older Patients

Measurement Instrument	Evaluation	Activities/ Reference	Notes
Index of independence in Activities of Daily Living (ADLs)	Self-reported	Difficulty/need for help in bathing, dressing, using toilet, transferring, continence, feeding. *Katz S et al: The index of ADL: A standardized measure of biological and psychosocial function. JAMA 1963*	Short and simple but subjective.
Instrumental Activities of Daily Living (IADLs)	Self-reported	Difficulty using the telephone, using car/public transportation, shopping, preparing meals, housework, managing medications, financial management. *Lawton MP et al: Instrumental activities of daily living (IADL) scale: Original observer-rated version. Psychopharmacol Bull 1988*	Short and simple. Gender-biased and cultural-biased items.
Functional Independence Measure (FIM)	Consensus multidisciplinary team	Motor (eating, grooming, bathing, dressing, toileting, bladder/bowel management, transfers, walking, climbing stairs); Cognitive (auditory comprehension, verbal expression, social interaction, problem solving, memory). *Keith RA et al: The functional independence measure: A new tool for rehabilitation. Adv Clin Rehabil 1987*	Administered by trained health professionals.
Barthel Index	Professionally evaluated	Independence and need for help in feeding, transferring from bed to chair and back, grooming, transferring to and from toilet, bathing, walking, stairs, dressing, continence. *Mahoney FI et al: Functional evaluation: The Barthel Index. Md State Med J 1965*	Administered by trained health professionals.
Mobility Questionnaire	Self-reported	Severe difficulty walking 1/4 mile and/or climbing stairs.	Short and simple
Short Physical Performance Battery	Objective performance based	Time to walk 4 m, rise from a chair 5 times, maintain balance for 10 sec in the side-by-side, semi-tandem and tandem positions. *Guralnik JM et al: A short physical performance battery assessing lower extremity function: Association with self-reported disability and prediction of mortality and nursing home admission. J Gerontol 1994*	Some training required.
Berg Balance Scale	Objective and professionally evaluated	Performance in 14 different tasks related to balance. *Berg KO et al: Clinical and laboratory measures of postural balance in an elderly population. Arch Phys Med Rehabil 1992*	Typically used by physical therapists.
Walking Speed	Objective performance	Measure walking speed over a 4 m course. *Studenski S: Bradypedia: Is gait speed ready for clinical use? J Nutr Health Aging 2009*	Simple and powerful but limited to patients who can walk.
6-Minute Walk	Objective performance based	Distance covered in 6 min. *Guyatt GH: The 6-minute walk: A new measure of exercise capacity in patients with chronic heart failure. Can Med Assoc J 1985*	Good measure of fitness, walking capacity/ endurance.
Long Distance Corridor Walk (400 m)	Objective performance based	Time to fast walk 400 m. *Newman AB et al: Association of long-distance corridor walk performance with mortality, cardiovascular disease, mobility limitation, and disability. JAMA 2006*	More challenging than the 6-min walk.

list of body functions and structure and a list of domains of activity and participation. Since an individual's functioning and disability occurs in a context, the ICF also includes a list of environmental factors. A detailed list of codes that allow the classification of body functions, activities, and participation is being developed. The ICF system is widely implemented in Europe and is gaining popularity in the United States.

Impaired cognition is a very important cause of disability but is treated in detail in Chap. 371.

Geriatric syndromes The term *geriatric syndrome* is used to capture clinical conditions that are frequently encountered in older persons, have a deleterious effect on function and quality of life, have multifactorial pathophysiology, often involving systems unrelated to the apparent chief complaint, and are manifested by stereotypical clinical presentations. The list of geriatric syndromes includes incontinence, delirium, falls, pressure ulcers, sleep disorders, problems with eating or feeding, pain, and depressed mood. Dementia and physical disability are also sometimes considered to be geriatric syndromes. Using the term *syndrome* is somewhat misleading since this term is normally used to describe a pattern of symptoms and signs that have a single underlying cause. Geriatric syndromes, by contrast, refer to "multifactorial health conditions that occur when the accumulated effects of impairments in multiple systems render an older person vulnerable to situational challenges." According to this definition, geriatric syndromes reflect the complex interactions between an individual's vulnerabilities and exposure to stressors or challenges. This definition aligns well with the concept that geriatric syndromes should be considered as phenotypic consequences of frailty and that a limited number of shared risk factors contribute to their etiology. Indeed, in various combinations and frequencies, virtually all geriatric syndromes are characterized by body composition changes, energy gaps, signaling disequilibria, and neurodegeneration. For example, detrusor (bladder) underactivity is a multifactorial geriatric condition that contributes to urinary retention in the frail elderly. It is characterized by detrusor muscle loss, fibrosis, and axonal degeneration. A proinflammatory state, and a lack of estrogen signaling, cause bladder muscle loss and detrusor underactivity while a chronic urinary infection may cause detrusor hyperactivity, all factors that may contribute to urinary incontinence.

Due to limited space, only delirium, falls, incontinence, chronic pain, and anorexia are addressed here. Interested readers can consult the references at the end of the chapter for details on other geriatric syndromes.

Delirium (Chap. 25) Delirium is an acute disorder of disturbed attention that fluctuates with time. It affects between 15 and 55% of hospitalized older patients and is associated with high in-hospital mortality and sometimes with permanent brain damage. Figure 72-16 shows brief guidelines for assessment and management of delirium in hospitalized older patients. The clinical presentation of delirium is heterogeneous, but frequent features are (a) rapid decline in level of consciousness with difficulty focusing, shifting, or sustaining attention; (b) cognitive change (rumbling incoherent speech, memory gaps, disorientation, hallucinations) not explained by dementia; and (c) medical history suggestive of preexisting cognitive impairment, frailty, and comorbidity. The strongest predisposing factors for delirium are dementia, any other condition associated with chronic or transient neurologic dysfunction (neurologic diseases, dehydration, alcohol consumption, psychoactive drugs), and sensory (visual and hearing) deprivation, suggesting that delirium is a condition of brain function susceptibility (neurodegeneration or transient neuronal impairment) that cannot avoid decompensation when hit by a stressful event. Many stressful conditions have been implicated as precipitating factors, including surgery, anesthesia, persistent pain, opiates, narcotics, anticholinergics, sleep deprivation, immobilization,

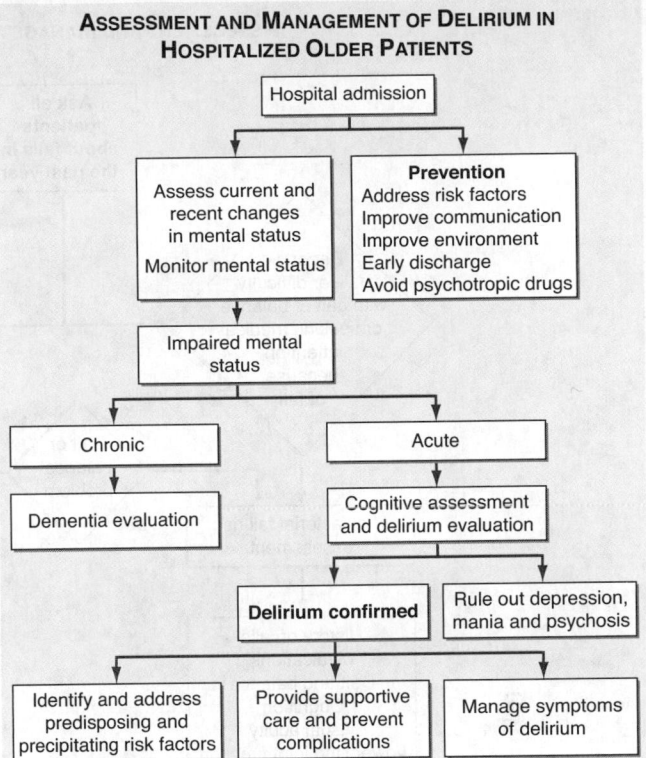

Figure 72-16 Algorithm depicting assessment and management of delirium in hospitalized older patients. *(Modified from SK Inouye: N Engl J Med 354:1157, 2006.)*

hypoxia, malnutrition, and metabolic and electrolyte derangements. Delirium, both onset and severity, can be reduced by anticipatory screening and preventive strategies aimed at reducing precipitating causes. The Confusion Assessment Method (CAM) is a simple, validated tool for screening in the hospital setting. Immediate identification and treatment of precipitating factors, withdrawal of drugs that may have facilitated the insurgence of delirium, and supportive care (management of hypoxia, hydration and nutrition, mobilization, and environmental modifications) are the three pillars of treatment. Whether patients in special Delirium Units have better outcomes is still in question. Physical restraints should be avoided because they tend to increase agitation and injury. Whenever possible, drug treatment should be avoided because it may prolong or aggravate delirium in some cases. The treatment of choice is low-dose haloperidol.

Falls and balance disorders Unstable gait and falls are serious concerns in the older adult because they lead not only to injury but also to restricted activity, increased health care utilization, and even death. Like all geriatric syndromes, problems with balance and falls tend to be multifactorial and are strongly connected with the disrupted aging systems that contribute to frailty. Poor muscle strength, neural damage in the basal ganglia and cerebellum, diabetes, and peripheral neuropathy are all recognized risk factors for falls. Therefore, evaluation and management require a structured multisystem approach that spans the entire frailty spectrum and beyond. Accordingly, interventions to prevent or reduce instability and falls usually require a mix of medical, rehabilitative, and environmental modification approaches. Guidelines for the evaluation and management of falls, released by the American Geriatrics Society, recommend asking all older adults about falls and perceived gait instability (Fig. 72-17). Patients with a positive history of multiple falls, in addition to persons who have sustained one or more injurious falls, should undergo an evaluation of gait and balance

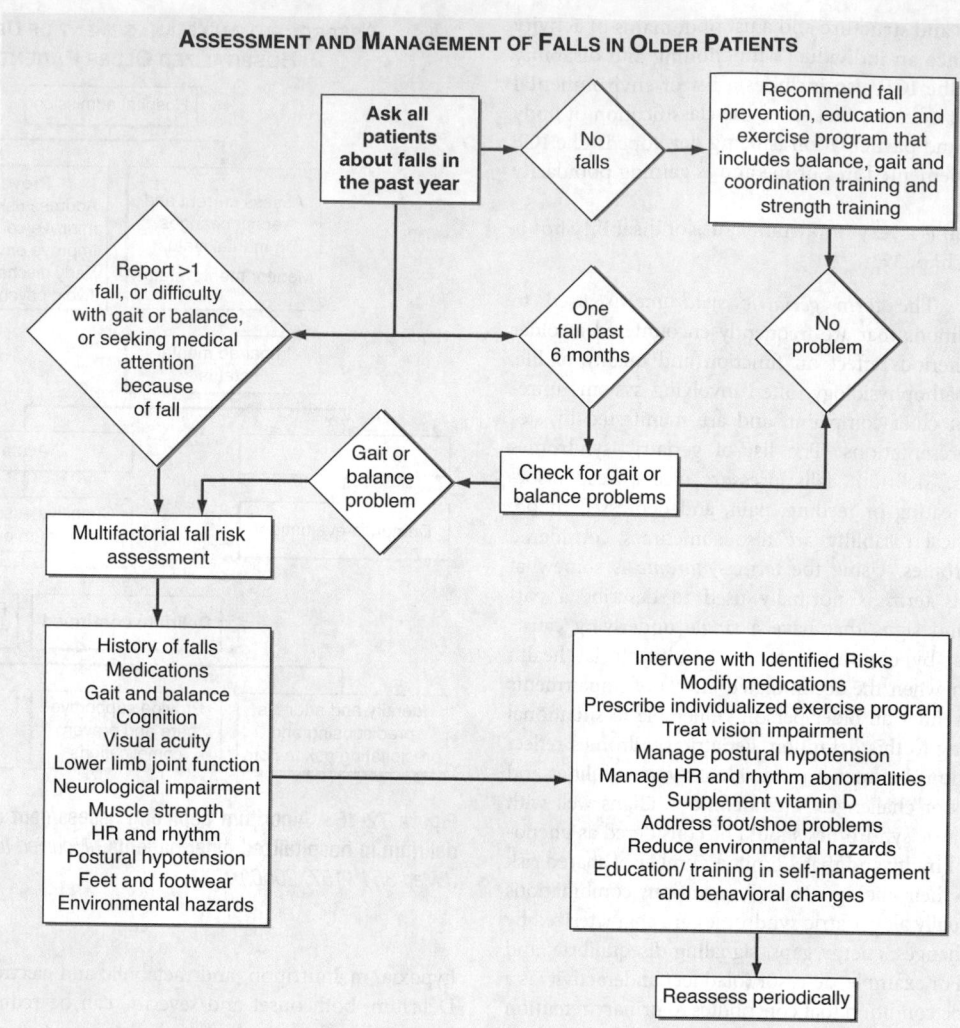

Figure 72-17 Algorithm depicting assessment and management of falls in older patients. *(From American Geriatrics Society and British Geriatrics Society: Clinical Practice Guideline for the Prevention of Falls in Older Persons. New York, American Geriatric Society, 2010.)*

as well as a targeted history and physical examination to detect sensory, nervous system, brain, cardiovascular, and musculoskeletal contributors. Interventions depend on the factors identified but often include medication adjustment, physical therapy, and home modifications. Meta-analyses of falls prevention strategies have found that multifactorial risk assessment and management, as well as individually targeted therapeutic exercise, are effective in reducing falls. Supplementation with vitamin D at 800 IU daily may help reduce falls, especially in older persons with reduced levels.

Persistent pain   Pain from multiple sources is the most common symptom complaint of older adults in primary care settings and is also common in acute care, long-term care, and palliative care settings. Acute pain and cancer pain problems are beyond the scope of this chapter. Persistent pain results in restricted activity, depression, sleep disorders, social isolation, and increases the risk of medication adverse events. The most common causes of persistent pain are musculoskeletal problems, but neuropathic and ischemic pain occur frequently, and multiple concurrent causes are often found. Alterations in mechanical and structural elements of the skeleton commonly lead to secondary problems in other parts of the body, especially to soft tissue or myofascial components. A structured history should obtain information about the quality, severity, and temporal patterns of pain. Physical examination should focus on back and joints as well as trigger points and periarticular areas, as

well as evidence of radicular neurologic patterns and peripheral vascular disease. Pharmacologic management should follow standard progressions as recommended by the World Health Organization (Chap. 11), but side effects to the central nervous system are more likely and must be monitored. For persistent pain, regular analgesic schedules are appropriate and should be combined with nonpharmacologic approaches such as splints, physical exercise, heat, and other modalities. A variety of adjuvant analgesics such as antidepressants and anticonvulsants may be used, but again, effects on reaction time and alertness may be dose limiting, especially in older persons with cognitive impairment. Joint or soft tissue injections may be helpful. Patient education and mutual goal setting are important since pain is usually not fully eliminated, but rather controlled to a tolerable level that maximizes function while minimizing adverse effects.

Urinary incontinence   Urinary incontinence (UI), the involuntary leakage of urine, is highly prevalent in older persons, especially in older women, and has a profound negative impact on quality of life. Approximately 50% of American women will suffer from some form of UI over a lifetime. Increasing age, white race, childbirth, obesity, and medical comorbidity are all risk factors for UI. The three main clinical forms of UI are as follows: (1) *Stress* incontinence is the failure of the sphincteric mechanism to remain closed when there is a sudden increase in intraabdominal pressure, such as a cough or sneeze. In women, this condition is due to insufficient strength of the pelvic floor muscles, while in men it is almost exclusively secondary to prostate surgery. (2) *Urge* incontinence is the loss of urine accompanied by a sudden sensation of need to urinate and is due to detrusor muscle overactivity (lack of inhibition) due to loss of neurologic control or local irritation. (3) *Overflow* incontinence is characterized by urinary dribbling, either constantly or for some period after urination. This condition is due to impaired detrusor contractility (due usually to denervation, for example, in diabetes) or bladder outlet obstruction (prostate hypertrophy in men and cystocele in women). Thus, not surprisingly, the pathogenesis of urinary incontinence is connected to the disrupted aging systems that contribute to frailty, body composition changes (atrophy of the bladder and pelvic floor muscle), and neurodegeneration (both central and peripheral nervous systems). Frailty is a strong risk factor for urinary incontinence. Indeed, older women are more likely to have mixed (urge|stress) incontinence than any pure form (Fig. 72-18). In analogy with the other geriatric syndromes, UI derives from a predisposing condition superimposed on a stressful, precipitating factor. Accordingly, treatment of UI should address both. The first line of treatment is bladder training associated with pelvic muscle exercise (Kegel exercises) that sometimes should be associated with electrical stimulation. Those with possible vaginal or uterine prolapse should be referred to a specialist. Urinary infections should be investigated and eventually treated. A long list of medications can precipitate urinary incontinence, including diuretics, antidepressants, sedative hypnotics, adrenergic agonists or blockers, anticholinergic, and calcium channel blockers. Whenever possible, these medications should be discontinued. Until recently, it was believed that estrogen oral or local treatments improved the UI symptoms in postmenopausal women, but this notion is now controversial. Antimuscarinic drugs such as tolterodine, darifenacin, and fesoterodine are modestly effective for mixed incontinence, but they all can affect cognition and so must be used with caution and careful follow-up monitoring of cognitive status. In some cases, surgical treatment should be considered. Chronic catheterization has many adverse effects and should be limited to chronic urinary retention that cannot be managed in any other way. Bacteriuria always occurs and should be treated only if symptomatic.

Undernutrition and anorexia Normal aging is associated with a decline in food intake that is more marked in men than in women. To some extent, food intake is reduced because energy demand declines as a result of a combination of lower physical activity, decline in lean body mass, and slowed rates of protein turnover. Other contributors to decreased food intake include losses of taste sensation, reduced stomach compliance, higher circulating levels of cholecystokinin, and, in men, low testosterone associated with increased leptin. When food intake decreases to a level below the reduced energy demand, the result is energy malnutrition. Malnutrition in older persons should be considered a geriatric syndrome because it is the result of intrinsic susceptibility due to aging, complicated by multiple superimposed precipitating causes. In addition, many older individuals tend to consume a monotonous diet that lacks sufficient fresh food, fruits, and vegetables, so that intake of important micronutrients is inadequate. Undernutrition in older people is associated with multiple adverse health consequences, including impaired muscle function, decreased bone mass, immune dysfunction, anemia, reduced cognitive function, poor wound healing, delayed recovery from surgery, and increased risk of falls, disability, and mortality. Despite these serious consequences, undernutrition often remains unrecognized until it is very advanced because weight loss tends to be ignored by both patients and physicians. Muscle wasting is a frequent feature of weight loss and malnutrition, often associated with loss of subcutaneous fat. The main causes of weight loss are anorexia, cachexia, sarcopenia, malabsorption, hypermetabolism, and dehydration, almost always in various combinations. Many of these causes can be detected and corrected. Cancer accounts for only 10–15% of cases of weight loss and anorexia in older people. Other important causes include a recent move to a long-term care setting, acute illness (often with inflammation), hospitalization with bed rest for as little as 1–2 days, depression, drugs that cause anorexia and nausea (e.g., digoxin and antibiotics), swallowing problems, oral infections, dental problems, GI pathology, thyroid and other hormonal problems, poverty, and isolation, with reduced access to food. Weight loss may also result from dehydration, possibly related to excess sweating, diarrhea, vomiting, or reduced intake. Early identification is paramount and requires careful weight monitoring. Patients or caregivers should be taught to record weight regularly at home, the patient should be weighed at each clinical encounter, and a record of serial weights should be maintained in the medical record. If malnutrition is suspected, formal assessment should begin with a standardized screening instrument such as the Mini Nutritional Assessment (MNA), the Malnutrition Universal Screening Tool, or the Simplified Nutritional Appetite Questionnaire. The MNA includes questions on appetite, timing of eating, and frequency of meals and taste, and has sensitivity and specificity >75% for future weight loss of ≥5% in older people. Many nutritional supplementations are available and should be initiated early to prevent more severe weight loss and its consequences. When an older patient has malnutrition, the diet should be liberalized and dietary restrictions should be lifted as much as possible. Nutritional supplements should be given between meals to avoid interference with food intake at mealtime. Limited evidence supports the use of any pharmacologic intervention to treat weight loss. The two antianorexic drugs most often prescribed in older persons are megesterol and dronabinol. Both can increase weight, although the gain is mostly fat not muscle, and both have serious side effects. Dronabinol is an excellent drug in the palliative care setting. There is little evidence that intentional weight loss in overweight, older people prolongs life. Weight loss after the age of 70 should probably be limited to those with extreme obesity and should always be medically supervised.

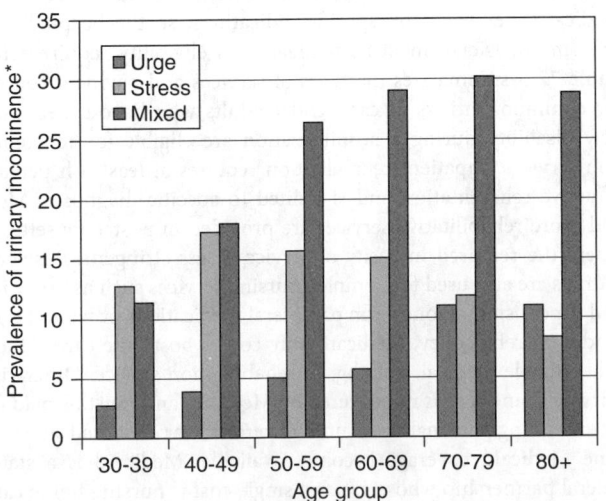

Figure 72-18 Rates of urge, stress and mixed incontinence by age group in a sample of 3552 women. *Based on a sample of 3553 participants. *(From JL Melville et al: Arch Intern Med 165:537, 2005.)*

■ HOW THE PHENOTYPES OF AGING AFFECT DISEASE PRESENTATION

Common diseases in older adults may have unexpected and atypical clinical features. Most age-related changes in clinical presentation, evolution, and response to treatment are due to the interaction between the pathophysiology of disease and the development of age-related system dysregulation. Some diseases directly impact aging systems and, therefore, have a devastating impact on frailty and its consequences. Parkinson's disease (PD) and diabetes are described as examples.

Parkinson's disease (Chap. 372) Most cases of PD begin after age 60 years, and incidence increases up to about age 80 years. Brain aging and PD have long been thought to be related. The nigrostriatal system deteriorates with aging, and many older persons tend to develop a mild form of movement disorder characterized by bradykinesia and stooped posture, that mimics mild PD. Interestingly, in PD, older age at presentation is associated with a more severe and rapid decline in gait, balance, postural problems, and cognition. These age-related motor and cognitive manifestations of PD tend to be poorly responsive to levodopa or dopamine agonist treatments, especially in older persons. Interestingly, age at presentation does not correlate with the severity and progression of other classic PD symptoms such as tremor, rigidity, and bradykinesia, and it does not affect response of these symptoms to levodopa. The pattern of PD features in older persons suggests that late-life PD may reflect a failure of the normal cellular compensatory mechanisms in vulnerable brain regions, and this vulnerability is increased by age-related neurodegeneration, making PD symptoms particularly resistant to levodopa treatment. In addition to the motor symptoms, older PD patients tend to have reduced muscle mass (sarcopenia), eating disorders, and poor levels of fitness. Accordingly, PD is a powerful risk factor for frailty and its consequences, including disability, comorbidity, falls, incontinence, chronic pain, and delirium. Use of levodopa and dopaminergic agonists in older PD patients requires complex dosing schedules and therefore slow-release preparations should be preferred. Both dopaminergic and anticholinergic agents increase the risk of confusion and hallucinations. Use of anticholinergic agents should generally be avoided. For dopaminergic agents, cognitive side effects can be dose-limiting.

Diabetes (Chap. 344) Both the incidence and prevalence of diabetes mellitus increase with aging. Among persons age 65 years and older, the prevalence is about 12%, and is higher in African Americans and Hispanics, reflecting the effects of population aging and the obesity epidemic. Diabetes affects all four main aging systems that contribute to frailty. Obesity, especially visceral obesity, is a strong risk factor for diabetes. Diabetes is associated with both reduced muscle mass and accelerated rates of muscle wasting. Diabetic patients have a higher RMR and poor fitness. Diabetes is associated with multiple hormone dysregulation, a pro-inflammatory state, and excess oxidative stress. Finally, diabetes-induced neurodegeneration involves both the central and peripheral nervous systems. Given these characteristics, not surprisingly, patients with DM are more likely to be frail and to have a very high risk of developing physical disability, depression, delirium, cognitive impairment, urinary incontinence, injurious falls, and persistent pain. Thus, the assessment of older diabetic patients should always include screening and risk factor evaluation for these conditions.

In young and adult patients, the main treatment goal has been strict glycemic control aimed at bringing the hemoglobin A_{1c} level to within normal values. However, the risk/benefit ratio is optimized by using less-aggressive glycemic targets. In fact, in the context of a randomized clinical trial, strict glycemic control was associated with higher mortality. Thus, a more reasonable goal for A_{1c} is 7% or slightly below. Treatment goals are altered further in frail older adults who have a high risk of complications of hypoglycemia and a

life expectancy of less than 5 years. In these cases, an even less stringent target such as 7–8% should be considered, with A_{1c} monitored every 6 or 12 months. Hypoglycemia is particularly difficult to identify in older diabetic patients because autonomic and nervous system symptoms occur at a lower blood sugar level compared to younger diabetics, although the metabolic reactions and neurologic injury effects are similar in young and older diabetics. The autonomic symptoms of hypoglycemia are often masked by beta blockers. Frail older adults are at even higher risk for serious hypoglycemia than are healthier, higher functioning older adults. In older patients with type 2 diabetes, a history of severe hypoglycemic episodes is associated with higher mortality, more severe microvascular complications, and greater risk of dementia. Thus, patients with suspected or documented episodes of hypoglycemia, especially those who are frail or disabled, need more liberal glucose control goals, careful education about hypoglycemia, and close follow-up with the health provider, possibly accompanied by a caregiver. Chlorpropamide has a prolonged half-life, particularly in older adults, and should be avoided because it is associated with high risk for hypoglycemia. Metformin should be use with caution and only in patients free of severe renal insufficiency. Renal insufficiency should be assessed by calculated glomerular filtration rate, or in very old patients who have reduced muscle mass, by a direct measure of creatinine clearance from a 24-h urine collection. Lifestyle changes in diet and exercise and losing a little weight can prevent or delay diabetes in high-risk individuals and is substantially more effective than metformin. Risk of type 2 diabetes decreased by 58% in a study of diet and exercise and this effect was similar in all ages and all ethnic groups. For comparison, the risk reduction with standard care plus metformin was 31 percent.

■ APPROACH TO THE CARE OF OLDER PERSONS

Organization of health care for older adults   The complex underlying physiology of aging leads to multiple coexisting medical problems and functional consequences that are often chronic with recurrent exacerbations and remissions. Combined with social consequences of aging such as widowhood and lack of an available caregiver, older adults must sometimes use nonmedical services to meet functional needs. The end result of these medical, functional, and social factors is that older adults use many health care and social support services and settings. Thus it is incumbent on the internist, whether a generalist or specialist, to be familiar with the scope of settings and services that are used by their patients. For many settings, Medicare reimbursement requires a medical order based on specific indications, so the hospitalist or referring physician must be familiar with eligibility requirements. Table 72-5 summarizes the types of services and payment sources for common settings of care. Older adults who have experienced new disability during a hospitalization are eligible for rehabilitation services. Inpatient rehabilitation requires at least 3 h per day of active rehabilitation and is limited to specific diagnoses. More and more rehabilitative services are provided in postacute settings, where the required intensity of service is less stringent. Postacute settings are also used for complex nursing services such as provision and supervision of long-term parenteral medications or wound care. Under current policy, Medicare only covers postacute care if there is an eligible medical, nursing, or rehabilitation service. Otherwise, nursing home care is not covered by Medicare and must be paid for by expending personal assets until resources are consumed, at which time Medicaid coverage becomes available. Medicaid is a state–federal partnership whose greatest single cost is nursing home care. Thus the need for chronic daily assistance with personal care in a nursing home consumes a large part of most state Medicaid budgets as well as personal assets. Therefore, alternatives to chronic nursing home care are of great interest to states, patients, and families.

TABLE 72-5 Care Setting for Older Patients

Setting	Services	Payment Source
Hospital acute care	Medical, surgical, and psychiatric services that cannot be provided in less complex settings	Medicare, Medicaid, and private insurance
Emergency room	Resuscitation, stabilization, triage, disposition	Medicare, Medicaid, and private insurance
Inpatient rehabilitation	Hospital-based residential program providing team-based, physician-supervised, intensive therapeutic rehabilitation for specific diagnoses	Medicare, Medicaid, and private insurance
Outpatient clinic	Chronic, urgent, and preventive services	Medicare, Medicaid, and private insurance
Postacute care	Medical, nursing, and rehabilitative services after hospitalization, often based in hospitals or nursing homes	Medicare up to 100 days with eligibility requirements
Long-term care	Residential program with daily nursing and aide care for persons who are dependent in self-care	Medicaid, private pay, long-term care insurance
Assisted living	Residential program with daily aide care and housing for persons who are dependent in household management	Private pay
Home health care	Nursing and rehabilitative services for episodes of care provided to persons in the community	Medicare, Medicaid
Day programs	Supervised settings providing nursing and aide care for scheduled hours	Private pay, Medicaid

Some states have developed Medicaid-funded day care programs, sometimes based on the Program for All-inclusive Care of the Elderly (PACE) model. In this situation, older adults who are eligible for both Medicare and Medicaid, and otherwise eligible for chronic nursing home care, can receive coordinated medical and functional services along with a day care setting. For most older adults, a caregiver must be available to provide assistance on weeknights and weekends. Home health services under current policy do not provide chronic functional assistance in the home, but rather are targeted at episodes of care for medical or rehabilitative services for older adults who are considered home bound. Within the past decade, there has been tremendous growth in a broad spectrum of assisted living settings. Such settings do not provide the degree of 24-h nursing supervision or personal aide care that is provided in traditional nursing homes, although distinctions are becoming blurred. Most assisted living settings provide meals, medication supervision, and homemaking services but often require that residents be capable of transporting themselves to a congregate meal site. Most of these settings accept only private pay from residents and their families and thus are hard to access for older adults with limited resources. Some states are exploring coverage for lower-cost residential care services such as family care homes. Some community agencies, whether private or public, can provide homemaker and home aide services to assist the home-bound older adult with functional needs, but there may be income requirements or need for expensive private payment.

Models of care coordination The complexity and fragmentation of care for complex older adults results in both increased costs and increased risk of iatrogenic complications such as missed diagnoses, adverse medication events, further worsening of function, and even death. These serious consequences have led to a strong interest in care coordination through teams of providers, with the goal to reduce unnecessary costs and prevent adverse events. Table 72-6 lists examples of evidence-based models of care coordination that were recommended in a recent Institute of Medicine report. While not mentioned as a specific type of team care, modern information technology has substantial promise to provide consistent readily available information across settings and providers. All such team programs are targeted at prevention and management of chronic and complex problems. Each model has demonstrated evidence for

benefit in clinical trials or quasi-experimental studies, and some have sufficient findings to support meta-analyses. The evidence for benefit is not always consistent between studies or types of care, but includes some support for improved quality of care, quality of life, function, survival, and health care costs and use. Some models of care are disease-specific and focus on common chronic conditions such as diabetes mellitus, congestive heart failure, chronic obstructive pulmonary disease, or stroke. One challenge to these models is that a majority of older adults will have multiple simultaneous conditions, and thus need services from multiple programs that may not communicate among themselves.

Most models of care are difficult to implement in today's health care system because non physician services are not reimbursed, nor is physician effort that is not incorporated into "face to face" time. Thus several models have largely been developed in the Department of Veterans Affairs Health Care system, Medicare Managed Care providers, or other sponsoring agencies. Medicare has developed a series of demonstration projects that can help further build the evidence base and serve policy makers.

■ SCREENING AND PREVENTION IN OLDER PERSONS

In older adults, prevention tests and interventions are less consistently recommended for all asymptomatic patients. The guidelines fail to address the influence of health status and life expectancy on recommendations, although the benefits of prevention are clearly affected by life expectancy. For example, in most types of cancer, screening provides no benefit in patients with a life expectancy of 5 years or less. More research is needed to build an appropriate evidence base for age- and life expectancy–adapted preventive services. Health behavior modification, especially increasing physical activity and improving nutrition, are probably the two interventions with the highest potential to promote healthy aging.

Screening tests

- Osteoporosis: Bone mineral density (BMD) at least once after the age of 65 years. There is little evidence that regular monitoring of BMD improves the prediction of fractures. However, because of limitations in the precision of DEXA the minimal interval between evaluations should be 2–3 years.

TABLE 72-6 Evidence-Based Models of Care Coordination for Older Patients (Institute of Medicine 2009)

Model	Team Members	Services
Interdisciplinary primary care "Medical Home"	Primary care physician plus social worker, nurse, nurse practitioner, or other care coordinators	Coordinate medical and social needs across settings
Case management	Nurse or social worker	Provide education and information to patients and families, may communicate with providers and settings
Disease management	Nurse	Health education and follow-up support for specific chronic diseases
Preventive home visits	Physician, nurse, social worker, and others	Structured assessment of physical, mental, functional, and social status in the home setting, with recommendations for care and prevention
Comprehensive outpatient geriatric assessment and management	Physician, nurse, social worker, plus sometimes others such as pharmacist, rehabilitation therapists, psychologist	Structured assessment of physical, mental, functional, and social status in the outpatient setting, with recommendations for care and prevention. Some programs also take responsibility for implementing the recommendations
Pharmaceutical care management	Pharmacist	Review and recommendations regarding the total medication regimen, provided in any setting
Chronic disease self-management	Nurse, health educator, or other health professional	Health education and coaching for specific chronic conditions
Prevention rehabilitation	Rehabilitation therapist	Anticipatory evaluation, therapeutic exercise, and assistive technology in the home or outpatient setting for older adults with physical disability
Caregiver services	Social worker, psychologist, or other health professional	Education, counseling, and resource referral for caregivers of older adults with chronic functional and mental health problems
Hospital discharge/transition coordination	Nurse, nurse practitioner	Care planning and education for patient and family before and after hospital discharge
Hospital at home	Physician, nurse, pharmacist	Diagnostic testing and medical treatments that can replace hospitalization or reduce length of stay for target conditions
Nursing home care coordination	Nurse practitioner or physician assistant	Scheduled assessment and care planning, as well as education for health workers in chronic care settings
Hospital delirium comprehensive care	Physician, nurse	Prevention, screening, and management of delirium in the hospital setting
Comprehensive inpatient geriatric assessment and management	Physician, nurse, social worker plus sometimes others such as pharmacist, rehabilitation therapists, psychologist	Specialized inpatient settings such as acute care of the elderly (ACE) unit or roving multidisciplinary teams that provide evaluation and recommendations for medical, mental health, functional, and social needs. ACE units and some teams take responsibility for implementation of recommendations

Source: Reproduced with permission from Boult et al.

- Hypertension: Blood pressure at least once a year, more often in patients with hypertension.
- Diabetes: Serum glucose and hemoglobin A_{1c} every 3 years, more often in patients who are obese or hypertensive.
- Lipid disorders: Lipid panel every 5 years, more often in patients with diabetes or any cardiovascular disease.
- Colorectal cancer: Fecal occult blood test, sigmoidoscopy or colonoscopy, regular schedule up to age 75 years. No consensus guidelines after age 75 years.
- Breast cancer: Mammography every 2 years between ages 50 and 74 years. No consensus guidelines after age 75 years.
- Cervical cancer: Pap smear every 3 years up to age 65 years.

Preventive interventions
- Influenza: Immunization annually.
- Shingles: Herpes zoster immunization once after age 50 years.
- Pneumonia: Pneumococcal immunization once at age 65 years.
- Myocardial infarction: Daily aspirin in patients with prevalent cardiovascular disease or with poor cardiovascular risk profile.

- Osteoporosis: Calcium 1200 mg daily and vitamin D at least 800 UI daily.

EXERCISE

Rates of regular physical activity decrease with age and are lowest in older persons. This is unfortunate because physical activity has clear benefits in aging. In older adults, increased physical activity improves physical function, muscle strength, mood, sleep, and metabolic risk profile. Some studies suggest that exercise can improve cognition and prevent dementia, but this is still controversial. Exercise programs, both aerobic and strength training, are feasible and beneficial even in very old and frail individuals. Regular, moderate-intensity exercise can reduce the rate of age-associated decline in physical function. The U.S. Centers for Disease Control and Prevention recommend that older persons should have at least 150 min per week of moderate-intensity aerobic activity (such as brisk walking) and muscle-strengthening activities that work all major muscle groups (legs, hips, back, abdomen, chest, shoulders, and arms) on 2 or more days a week. In the absence of contraindications, more intense and prolonged physical activity provides higher benefits. Frail and sedentary persons may need supervision, at least at the start of the exercise program, to avoid falls and exercise-related injuries.

◼ NUTRITION

Older persons are particularly vulnerable to malnutrition and many problems that affect older patients can be addressed by dietary modification. In spite of this, evidence-based guidelines for individualized dietary modification in the elderly are lacking and older people tend to be poorly compliant with dietary recommendations. Basic principles of a healthy diet that are also valid for older persons are as follows:

- Encourage consumption of fruits and vegetables; they are rich in micronutrients, mineral, and fibers. Whole grains are also a good source of fiber. Keep in mind that some of these foods are costly and thus less accessible to low-income persons.
- Good hydration is essential. Fluid intake should be at least 1000 mL daily.
- Encourage the use of fat-free and low-fat dairy products, legumes, poultry, and lean meats. Encourage consumption of fish at least once a week.
- Match intake of energy (calories) to overall energy needs in order to maintain a healthy weight and body mass index (BMI 20–27). If BMI >27, implement a 5–10% calorie restriction.
- Limit consumption of foods with high caloric density, high sugar, and high salt content (less than 6 g per day).
- Limit the intake of foods with a high content of saturated fatty acids and cholesterol.
- Limit alcohol consumption (1 drink per day or less).
- Older persons who have little exposure to UVB radiation are at risk of vitamin D insufficiency. Thus, vitamin D–fortified foods and/or vitamin D supplements should be introduced in the diet.
- Make sure that the diet includes adequate food-related intake of magnesium, vitamin A, and vitamin B_{12}.
- For constipation: increase dietary fiber to 10–25 g and fluid intake to 1500 mL daily. A bulk laxative (methylcellulose or psyllium) can be added.

◼ NOVEL INTERVENTIONS TO MODIFY AGING PROCESSES

Aging is a complex process with multiple manifestations at the molecular, cellular, organ, and whole organism level. The nature of the aging process is still not fully understood, but aging and its effects may be modulated by appropriate interventions. Dietary and genetic alterations can increase healthy life span and prevent the development of dysregulated systems and the aging phenotype in laboratory model organisms. The mechanisms responsible for life span expansion are "food" sensors typically activated in situations of food shortage, such as IGF (insulin-like growth factor)/insulin and the TOR (target of rapamycin) pathways. Accordingly, a reduction in food intake without malnutrition extends the life span by 10–50% in diverse organisms, from yeast to rhesus monkeys. Mechanisms that mediate the effects of caloric restriction are under intensive study because they are potential targets for interventions aimed at counteracting the emergence of the aging phenotype and its deleterious effects in humans. For example, resveratrol, a natural compound found in grape skin that mimics some of the effects of dietary restriction, increases longevity and improves health when fed to mice on a high-fat diet but has little effect in mice on a standard diet. Other compounds that potentially mimic caloric restriction are currently in development and testing. A high prevalence of IGF-1 receptor gene mutation has been found in Ashkenazi Jewish centenarians and in long-lived individuals, suggesting that the downregulation of IGF-1 signaling may promote human longevity. A 20-year 30% dietary restriction applied to adult rhesus monkeys was shown to be associated with reduced cardiovascular and

cancer morbidity, reduced signs of aging, and higher longevity, though a second such study did not find increased longevity. In humans, dietary restriction is effective against obesity and reduces insulin resistance, inflammation, blood pressure, c-reactive protein, and intima-media thickness of the carotid arteries. However, the beneficial effects of dietary restriction in humans are still controversial, and some potential negative effects have not been sufficiently studied. An interesting effect of caloric restriction in humans is mitochondrial biogenesis. Mitochondrial dysfunction has emerged as a potentially important underlying contributor to aging. Reduced expression of mitochondrial genes is a strongly conserved feature of aging across different species. Interestingly, mitochondria are the machinery for chemical energy production, and brain and muscle are particularly susceptible to defective mitochondrial function. Thus, declining mitochondrial function may be a direct cause of at least three of the main dysregulated systems contributing to the phenotype of aging.

◼ OTHER ASPECTS OF AGING

This chapter touched on some of the fundamental aspects of human aging, focusing mostly on those that are relevant to the care of older patients. Many aspects of geriatric medicine could not be addressed due to space limitations. Valuable topics had to be left out, including details of comprehensive geriatric assessment, depression and anxiety, hypertension, orthostatic hypotension, dementia, vision and hearing impairment, osteoporosis, palliative care, prostate disorders, foot problems, and women's health. Some of these topics are treated extensively elsewhere in this text, sometimes with comments on age-specific issues. The interested reader can find resources for further information at the end of this chapter.

◼ CONCLUSIONS

The universal process of aging is becoming better understood. There appear to be shared underlying cellular and molecular processes that induce widespread dysregulation in key systems. This dysregulation contributes to clinical manifestations of a frailty phenotype and can be used to understand how to evaluate and manage the older patient.

ACKNOWLEDGMENT

We would like to thank our colleagues who provided criticisms and suggestions for improvement of this chapter. We are particularly indebted to Dr. John Morley for his valuable suggestions on the "Anorexia-Malnutrition" section.

FURTHER READINGS

American Geriatrics Society Panel on Pharmacological Management of Persistent Pain in Older Persons. Pharmacological management of persistent pain in older persons. J Am Geriatr Soc 57:1331, 2009

Boult C et al: Successful models of comprehensive care for older adults with chronic conditions: Evidence for the Institute of Medicine's "retooling for an aging America" report. J Am Geriatr Soc 57:2328, 2009

Halter JB et al: *Hazzard's Geriatric Medicine & Gerontology*, 6th ed. New York, McGraw-Hill, 2009

Reuben DB et al: *Geriatrics at Your Fingertips: 2010*, 12th ed. New York, American Geriatric Society, 2010

WEBSITES

The American Geriatric Society *http://www.americangeriatrics.org/*

The Gerontological Society of America *http://www.geron.org/*

World Health Organization Website on Aging *http://www.who.int/topics/ageing/en/*

PART 6
Nutrition

CHAPTER 73

Nutrient Requirements and Dietary Assessment

Johanna Dwyer

Nutrients are substances that are not synthesized in sufficient amounts in the body and therefore must be supplied by the diet. Nutrient requirements for groups of healthy persons have been determined experimentally. For good health, we require energy-providing nutrients (protein, fat, and carbohydrate), vitamins, minerals, and water. Human requirements for organic nutrients include 9 essential amino acids, several fatty acids, glucose, 4 fat-soluble vitamins, 10 water-soluble vitamins, dietary fiber, and choline. Several inorganic substances, including 4 minerals, 7 trace minerals, 3 electrolytes, and the ultra trace elements, must also be supplied by diet.

The required amounts of the essential nutrients differ by age and physiologic state. Conditionally essential nutrients are not required in the diet but must be supplied to individuals who do not synthesize them in adequate amounts, such as those with genetic defects, those having pathologic states with nutritional implications, and developmentally immature infants. Many other organic and inorganic compounds present in foods have health effects. For example, lead and pesticide residues may have toxic effects.

ESSENTIAL NUTRIENT REQUIREMENTS

■ ENERGY

For weight to remain stable, energy intake must match energy output. The major components of energy output are resting energy expenditure (REE) and physical activity; minor sources include the energy cost of metabolizing food (thermic effect of food or specific dynamic action) and shivering thermogenesis (e.g., cold-induced thermogenesis). The average energy intake is about 2600 kcal/d for American men and about 1900 kcal/d for American women, though these estimates vary with body size and activity level. Formulas for estimating REE are useful for assessing the energy needs of an individual whose weight is stable. Thus, for males, REE = 900 + 10m, and for females, REE = 700 + 7m, where m is mass in kilograms. The calculated REE is then adjusted for physical activity level by multiplying by 1.2 for sedentary, 1.4 for moderately active, or 1.8 for very active individuals. The final figure provides an estimate of total caloric needs in a state of energy balance. For further discussion of energy balance in health and disease, see Chap.75.

■ PROTEIN

Dietary protein consists of both essential and nonessential amino acids that are required for protein synthesis. The nine essential amino acids are histidine, isoleucine, leucine, lysine, methionine/cystine, phenylalanine/tyrosine, threonine, tryptophan, and valine. Certain amino acids, such as alanine, can also be used for energy and gluconeogenesis. When energy intake is inadequate, protein intake must be increased, because ingested amino acids are diverted into pathways of glucose synthesis and oxidation. In extreme energy deprivation, protein-calorie malnutrition may ensue (Chap. 75).

For adults, the recommended dietary allowance (RDA) for protein is about 0.6 g/kg desirable body mass per day, assuming that energy needs are met and that the protein is of relatively high biologic value. Current recommendations for a healthy diet call for at least 10 to 14% of calories from protein. Most American diets provide at least those amounts. Biologic value tends to be highest for animal proteins, followed by proteins from legumes (beans), cereals (rice, wheat, corn), and roots. Combinations of plant proteins that complement one another in biologic value, or combinations of animal and plant proteins, can increase biologic value and lower total protein requirements.

Protein needs increase during growth, pregnancy, lactation, and rehabilitation after injury or malnutrition. Tolerance to dietary protein is decreased in renal insufficiency (causing uremia) and in liver failure. Normal protein intake can precipitate encephalopathy in patients with cirrhosis of the liver.

■ FAT AND CARBOHYDRATE

Fats are a concentrated source of energy and constitute, on average, 34% of calories in U.S. diets. However, for optimal health, fat intake should total no more than 30% of calories. Saturated fat and trans-fat should be limited to <10% of calories, and poly-unsaturated fats to <10% of calories, with monounsaturated fats comprising the remainder of fat intake. At least 45–55% of total calories should be derived from carbohydrates. The brain requires about 100 g/d of glucose for fuel; other tissues use about 50 g/d. Some tissues (e.g., brain and red blood cells) rely on glucose supplied either exogenously or from muscle proteolysis. Over time, adaptations in carbohydrate needs are possible during hypocaloric states.

■ WATER

For adults, 1 to 1.5 mL water per kcal of energy expenditure is sufficient under usual conditions to allow for normal variations in physical activity, sweating, and solute load of the diet. Water losses include 50 to 100 mL/d in the feces; 500 to 1000 mL/d by evaporation or exhalation; and, depending on the renal solute load, ≥1000 mL/d in the urine. If external losses increase, intakes must increase accordingly to avoid underhydration. Fever increases water losses by approximately 200 mL/d per °C; diarrheal losses vary, but may be as great as 5 L/d in severe diarrhea. Heavy sweating and vomiting also increase water losses. When renal function is normal and solute intakes are adequate, the kidneys can adjust to increased water intake by excreting up to 18 L/d of excess water (Chap. 340). However, obligatory urine outputs can compromise hydration status when there is inadequate intake or when losses increase in disease or kidney damage.

Infants have high requirements for water because of their large ratio of surface area to volume, the limited capacity of the immature kidney to handle high renal solute loads, and their inability to communicate their thirst. Increased water needs during pregnancy are about 30 mL/d. During lactation, milk production increases water requirements so that approximately 1000 mL/d of additional water is needed, or 1 mL for each mL of milk produced. Special attention must be paid to the water needs of the elderly, who have reduced total body water and blunted thirst sensation, and are more likely to be taking medications such as diuretics.

■ OTHER NUTRIENTS

See Chap. 74 for detailed descriptions of vitamins and trace minerals.

DIETARY REFERENCE INTAKES AND RECOMMENDED DIETARY ALLOWANCES

Fortunately, human life and well-being can be maintained within a fairly wide range for most nutrients. However, the capacity for adaptation is not infinite—too much, as well as too little, intake of a nutrient could have adverse effects or alter the health benefits conferred by another nutrient. Therefore, benchmark recommendations regarding nutrient intakes have been developed to guide clinical practice. These quantitative estimates of nutrient intakes are collectively referred to as the *dietary reference intakes* (DRIs). The DRIs supplant the *recommended daily allowances* (RDAs), the single reference values used in the United States until the early 1990s. DRIs include the *estimated average requirement* (EAR) for nutrients as well as other reference values used for dietary planning for individuals: the RDA, the *adequate intake* (AI), and the tolerable *upper level* (UL). The DRI also include acceptable macronutrient distribution ranges (AMDR) for protein, fat, and carbohydrate. The current DRIs for vitamins and elements are provided in Tables 73-1 and 73-2, respectively.

ESTIMATED AVERAGE REQUIREMENT

When florid manifestations of the classic dietary deficiency diseases such as rickets (deficiency of vitamin D and calcium), scurvy (deficiency of vitamin C), xerophthalmia (deficiency of vitamin A), and protein-calorie malnutrition were common, nutrient adequacy was inferred from the absence of their clinical signs. Later, biochemical and other changes were found to be evident long before the clinical deficiency became apparent. Consequently, criteria of adequacy are now based on biologic markers when they are available. Current efforts focus on the amount of a nutrient that reduces the risk of chronic degenerative diseases. Priority is given to sensitive biochemical, physiologic, or behavioral tests that reflect early changes in regulatory processes; maintenance of body stores of nutrients; or, if available, the amount of a nutrient that minimizes risk of chronic degenerative disease.

The EAR is the amount of a nutrient estimated to be adequate for half of the healthy individuals of a specific age and sex. The types of evidence and criteria used to establish nutrient requirements vary by nutrient, age, and physiologic group. The EAR is not an effective estimate of nutrient adequacy in individuals because it is a median requirement for a group; 50% of individuals in a group fall below the requirement and 50% fall above it. Thus, a person with a usual intake at the EAR has a 50% risk of an inadequate intake. For these reasons, other standards, described below, are more useful for clinical purposes.

RECOMMENDED DIETARY ALLOWANCES

The RDA is the average daily dietary intake level that meets the nutrient requirements of nearly all healthy persons of a specific sex, age, life stage, or physiologic condition (such as pregnancy or lactation). The RDA is the nutrient-intake goal for planning diets of individuals.

The RDA is defined statistically as two standard deviations (SD) above the EAR to ensure that the needs of any given individual are met. Recommendations for individuals of a given age, sex, and weight are easily obtained from a Web-based calculator at *http://fnic.nal.usda.gov/interactiveDRI/*. This online tool allows health professionals to calculate daily nutrient recommendations for dietary planning based on the DRIs for individuals.

The RDAs are used to formulate food guides such as the U.S. Department of Agriculture (USDA) Food Guide Pyramid for individuals, to create food-exchange lists for therapeutic diet planning, and as a standard for describing the nutritional content of processed foods and nutrient-containing dietary supplements. The nutrient content in a food is stated by weight or as a percent of the daily value (DV), a variant of the RDA used in food labeling on the nutrition facts panel that, for an adult, represents the highest RDA for an adult consuming 2000 kcal/d.

The risk of dietary inadequacy increases as intake falls below the RDA. However, the RDA is an overly generous criterion for evaluating nutrient adequacy. For example, by definition the RDA exceeds the actual requirements of all but about 2 to 3% of the population. Therefore, many people whose intake falls below the RDA may still be getting enough of the nutrient.

ADEQUATE INTAKE

It is not possible to set an RDA for some nutrients that do not have an established EAR. In this circumstance, the AI is based on observed, or experimentally determined, approximations of nutrient intakes in healthy people. In the DRIs, AIs rather than RDAs are proposed for infants up to age 1 year, as well as for calcium, chromium, vitamin D, fluoride, manganese, pantothenic acid, biotin, and choline for persons of all ages. Vitamin D and calcium are currently being reevaluated, and more precise values may be available in the near future.

TOLERABLE UPPER LEVELS OF NUTRIENT INTAKE

Excessive nutrient intake can disturb body functions and cause acute, progressive, or permanent disabilities. The tolerable UL is the highest level of chronic nutrient intake (usually daily) that is unlikely to pose a risk of adverse health effects for most of the population. Data on the adverse effects of large amounts of many nutrients are unavailable or too limited to establish a UL. Therefore, the lack of a UL does *not* mean that the risk of adverse effects from high intake is nonexistent. Healthy individuals derive no established benefit from consuming nutrient levels above the RDA or AI. Nutrients in commonly eaten foods rarely exceed the UL. However, highly fortified foods and dietary supplements provide more concentrated amounts of nutrients per serving and, thus, pose a potential risk of toxicity. Nutrient supplements are labeled with supplement facts that express the amount of nutrient in absolute units or as the percent of the DV provided per recommended serving size. Total nutrient consumption, including foods; supplements; and over-the-counter medications, such as antacids, should not exceed RDA levels.

ACCEPTABLE MACRONUTRIENT DISTRIBUTION RANGES

The AMDR is a range of energy providing intakes that the Food and Nutrition Board considers to be healthful for macronutrients. These ranges are 10–35% calories for protein, 20–35% calories for fat, and 45–65% of calories for carbohydrate. Alcohol, which also provides energy, is not a nutrient and recommendations, therefore, are not provided for it.

FACTORS ALTERING NUTRIENT NEEDS

The DRIs are affected by age, sex, rate of growth, pregnancy, lactation, physical activity, concomitant diseases, drugs, and dietary composition. If requirements for nutrient sufficiency are close to levels indicating excess, dietary planning is difficult.

PHYSIOLOGIC FACTORS

Growth, strenuous physical activity, pregnancy, and lactation increase needs for energy and several essential nutrients. Energy needs rise during pregnancy due to the demands of fetal growth and during lactation because of the increased energy required for milk production. Energy needs decrease with loss of lean body mass, the major determinant of REE. Because both health and physical activity tend to decline with age, energy needs of older persons, especially those over 70, tend to be less than those of younger persons.

TABLE 73-1 Dietary Reference Intakes: Recommended Intakes for Individuals—Vitamins

Life-Stage Group	Vitamin, µg/d					Thiamine, mg/d	Riboflavin, mg/d	Niacin, mg/d[e]	Vitamin B₆, mg/d	Folate, µg/d[f]	Vitamin B₁₂, µg/d	Pantothenic Acid, mg/d	Biotin, µg/d	Choline, mg/d[g]
	A[a]	C	D[b,c]	E[d]	K									
Infants														
0–6 mo	400	40	5	4	2.0	0.2	0.3	2	0.1	65	0.4	1.7	5	125
7–12 mo	500	50	5	5	2.5	0.3	0.4	4	0.3	80	0.5	1.8	6	150
Children														
1–3 y	**300**	**15**	5	6	30	**0.5**	**0.5**	**6**	**0.5**	**150**	**0.9**	2	8	200
4–8 y	**400**	**25**	5	7	55	**0.6**	**0.6**	**8**	**0.6**	**200**	**1.2**	3	12	250
Males														
9–13 y	**600**	**45**	5	11	60	**0.9**	**0.9**	**12**	**1.0**	**300**	**1.8**	4	20	375
14–18 y	**900**	**75**	5	15	75	**1.2**	**1.3**	**16**	**1.3**	**400**	**2.4**	5	25	550
19–30 y	**900**	**90**	5	15	120	**1.2**	**1.3**	**16**	**1.3**	**400**	**2.4**	5	30	550
31–50 y	**900**	**90**	5	15	120	**1.2**	**1.3**	**16**	**1.3**	**400**	**2.4**	5	30	550
51–70 y	**900**	**90**	10	15	120	**1.2**	**1.3**	**16**	**1.7**	**400**	**2.4**[h]	5	30	550
>70 y	**900**	**90**	15	15	120	**1.2**	**1.3**	**16**	**1.7**	**400**	**2.4**[h]	5	30	550
Females														
9–13 y	**600**	**45**	5	11	60	**0.9**	**0.9**	**12**	**1.0**	**300**	**1.8**	4	20	375
14–18 y	**700**	**65**	5	15	75	**1.0**	**1.0**	**14**	**1.2**	**400**[i]	**2.4**	5	25	400
19–30 y	**700**	**75**	5	15	90	**1.1**	**1.1**	**14**	**1.3**	**400**[i]	**2.4**	5	30	425
31–50 y	**700**	**75**	5	15	90	**1.1**	**1.1**	**14**	**1.3**	**400**[i]	**2.4**	5	30	425
51–70 y	**700**	**75**	10	15	90	**1.1**	**1.1**	**14**	**1.5**	**400**	**2.4**[h]	5	30	425
>70 y	**700**	**75**	15	15	90	**1.1**	**1.1**	**14**	**1.5**	**400**	**2.4**[h]	5	30	425
Pregnancy														
≤18 y	**750**	**80**	5	15	75	**1.4**	**1.4**	**18**	**1.6**	**600**[j]	**2.6**	6	30	450
19–30 y	**770**	**85**	5	15	90	**1.4**	**1.4**	**18**	**1.9**	**600**[j]	**2.6**	6	30	450
31–50 y	**770**	**85**	5	15	90	**1.4**	**1.4**	**18**	**1.9**	**600**[j]	**2.6**	6	30	450
Lactation														
≤18 y	**1200**	**115**	5	19	75	**1.4**	**1.6**	**17**	**2.0**	**500**	**2.8**	7	35	550
19–30 y	**1300**	**120**	5	19	90	**1.4**	**1.6**	**17**	**2.0**	**500**	**2.8**	7	35	550
31–50 y	**1300**	**120**	5	19	90	**1.4**	**1.6**	**17**	**2.0**	**500**	**2.8**	7	35	550

Note: This table presents recommended dietary allowances (RDAs) in **bold type** and adequate intakes (Als) in ordinary type. RDAs and Als may both be used as goals for individual intake. RDAs are set to meet the needs of almost all individuals (97 to 98%) in a group. For healthy breastfed infants, the AI is the mean intake. The AI for other life stage and gender groups is believed to cover needs of all individuals in the group, but lack of data or uncertainty in the data prevent being able to specify with confidence the percentage of individuals covered by this intake.

[a] As retinol activity equivalents (RAEs). 1 RAE = 1 µg retinol, 12 µg β-carotene, 24 µg α-carotene, or 24 µg β-cryptoxanthin. To calculate RAEs from retinol equivalents (REs) of provitamin A carotenoids in foods, divide the REs by 2. For preformed vitamin A in foods or supplements and for provitamin A carotenoids in supplements, 1 RE = 1 RAE.

[b] As calciferol. 1 µg calciferol = 40 IU vitamin D.

[c] In the absence of adequate exposure to sunlight.

[d] As α-tocopherol. α-Tocopherol includes *RRR*-α-tocopherol, the only form of α-tocopherol that occurs naturally in foods, and the 2*R*-stereoisomeric forms of α-tocopherol (*RRR*-, *RSR*-, *RRS*-, and *RSS*-α-tocopherol) that occur in fortified foods and supplements. It does not include the 2*S*-stereoisomeric forms of -tocopherol (*SRR*-, *SSR*-, *SRS*-, and SSS-α-tocopherol), also found in fortified foods and supplements.

[e] As niacin equivalents (NE). 1 mg of niacin = 60 mg of tryptophan; 0–6 months = preformed niacin (not NE).

[f] As dietary folate equivalents (DFEs). 1 DFE = 1 µg food folate = 0.6 µg of folic acid from fortified food or as a supplement consumed with food = 0.5 µg of a supplement taken on an empty stomach.

[g] Although Als have been set for choline, there are few data to assess whether a dietary supply of choline is needed at all stages of the life cycle, and it may be that the choline requirement can be met by endogenous synthesis at some of these stages.

[h] Because 10 to 30% of older people may malabsorb food-bound B₁₂, it is advisable for those >50 years to meet their RDA mainly by consuming foods fortified with B₁₂ or a supplement containing B₁₂.

[i] In view of evidence linking inadequate folate intake with neural tube defects in the fetus, it is recommended that all women capable of becoming pregnant consume 400 µg from supplements or fortified foods in addition to intake of food folate from a varied diet.

[j] It is assumed that women will continue consuming 400 µg from supplements or fortified food until their pregnancy is confirmed and they enter prenatal care, which ordinarily occurs after the end of the periconceptional period—the critical time for formation of the neural tube.

Source: Food and Nutrition Board, Institute of Medicine—National Academy of Sciences Dietary Reference Intakes, 2000, 2002, reprinted with permission. Courtesy of the National Academy Press, Washington, DC. *http://www.nap.edu.*

TABLE 73-2 Dietary Reference Intakes: Recommended Intakes for Individuals—Elements

Life-Stage Group	Calcium, mg/d	Chromium, μg/d	Copper, μg/d	Fluoride, mg/d	Iodine, μg/d	Iron, mg/d	Magnesium, mg/d	Manganese, mg/d	Molybdenum, μg/d	Phosphorus, mg/d	Selenium, μg/d	Zinc, mg/d
Infants												
0–6 mo	210	0.2	200	0.01	110	0.27	30	0.003	2	100	15	2
7–12 mo	270	5.5	220	0.5	130	**11**	75	0.6	3	275	20	**3**
Children												
1–3 y	500	11	**340**	0.7	**90**	**7**	80	1.2	**17**	**460**	**20**	**3**
4–8 y	800	15	**440**	1	**90**	**10**	130	1.5	**22**	**500**	**30**	**5**
Males												
9–13 y	1300	25	**700**	2	**120**	**8**	240	1.9	**34**	**1250**	**40**	**8**
14–18 y	1300	35	**890**	3	**150**	**11**	410	2.2	**43**	**1250**	**55**	**11**
19–30 y	1000	35	**900**	4	**150**	**8**	400	2.3	**45**	**700**	**55**	**11**
31–50 y	1000	35	**900**	4	**150**	**8**	420	2.3	**45**	**700**	**55**	**11**
51–70 y	1200	30	**900**	4	**150**	**8**	420	2.3	**45**	**700**	**55**	**11**
>70 y	1200	30	**900**	4	**150**	**8**	420	2.3	**45**	**700**	**55**	**11**
Females												
9–13 y	1300	21	**700**	2	**120**	**8**	240	1.6	**34**	**1250**	**40**	**8**
14–18 y	1300	24	**890**	3	**150**	**15**	360	1.6	**43**	**1250**	**55**	**9**
19–30 y	1000	25	**900**	3	**150**	**18**	310	1.8	**45**	**700**	**55**	**8**
31–50 y	1000	25	**900**	3	**150**	**18**	320	1.8	**45**	**700**	**55**	**8**
51–70 y	1200	20	**900**	3	**150**	**8**	320	1.8	**45**	**700**	**55**	**8**
>70 y	1200	20	**900**	3	**150**	**8**	320	1.8	**45**	**700**	**55**	**8**
Pregnancy												
≤18 y	1300	29	**1000**	3	**220**	**27**	400	2.0	**50**	**1250**	**60**	**12**
19–30 y	1000	30	**1000**	3	**220**	**27**	350	2.0	**50**	**700**	**60**	**11**
31–50 y	1000	30	**1000**	3	**220**	**27**	360	2.0	**50**	**700**	**60**	**11**
Lactation												
≤18 y	1300	44	**1300**	3	**290**	**10**	360	2.6	**50**	**1250**	**70**	**13**
19–30 y	1000	45	**1300**	3	**290**	**9**	310	2.6	**50**	**700**	**70**	**12**
31–50 y	1000	45	**1300**	3	**290**	**9**	320	2.6	**50**	**700**	**70**	**12**

Note: This table presents recommended dietary allowances (RDAs) in **bold type** and adequate intakes (AIs) in ordinary type. RDAs and AIs may both be used as goals for individual intake. RDAs are set to meet the needs of almost all individuals (97 to 98%) in a group. For healthy breastfed infants, the AI is the mean intake. The AI for other life stage and gender groups is believed to cover needs of all individuals in the group, but lack of data or uncertainty in the data prevent being able to specify with confidence the percentage of individuals covered by this intake.

Source: Food and Nutrition Board, Institute of Medicine—National Academy of Sciences Dietary Reference Intakes, 2000, 2002, reprinted with permission. Courtesy of the National Academy Press, Washington, DC. *http://www.nap.edu.*

■ DIETARY COMPOSITION

Dietary composition affects the biologic availability and use of nutrients. For example, the absorption of iron may be impaired by high amounts of calcium or lead; also, non-heme iron uptake may be impaired by the lack of ascorbic acid and amino acids in the meal. Protein use by the body may be decreased when essential amino acids are not present in sufficient amounts. Animal foods, such as milk, eggs, and meat, have high biologic values with most of the needed amino acids present in adequate amounts. Plant proteins in corn (maize), soy, and wheat have lower biologic values and must be combined with other plant or animal proteins to achieve optimal use by the body.

■ ROUTE OF ADMINISTRATION

The RDAs apply only to oral intakes. When nutrients are administered parenterally, similar values can sometimes be used for amino acids, carbohydrates, fats, sodium, chloride, potassium, and most of the vitamins, because their intestinal absorption is nearly 100%. However, the oral bioavailability of most mineral elements may be only half that obtained by parenteral administration. For some nutrients that are not readily stored in the body or cannot be stored in large amounts, timing of administration may also be important. For example, amino acids cannot be used for protein synthesis if they are not supplied together; instead, they will be used for energy production.

DISEASE

Specific dietary deficiency diseases include: protein-calorie malnutrition; iron, iodine, and vitamin A deficiency; megaloblastic anemia due to vitamin B$_{12}$ or folic acid deficiency; vitamin D–deficiency rickets and osteomalacia; and scurvy, beriberi, and pellagra (Chaps. 74 and 75). Each deficiency disease is characterized by imbalances at the cellular level between the supply of nutrients or energy and the body's nutritional needs for growth, maintenance, and other functions. Imbalances and excess in nutrient intakes are recognized as risk factors for certain chronic degenerative diseases, such as saturated fat and cholesterol in coronary artery disease; sodium in hypertension; obesity in hormone-dependent endometrial and breast cancers; and ethanol in alcoholism. Because the etiology and pathogenesis of these disorders are multifactorial, diet is only one of many risk factors. Osteoporosis, for example, is associated with calcium deficiency, as well as risk factors related to environment (e.g., smoking, sedentary lifestyle), physiology (e.g., estrogen deficiency), genetic determinants (e.g., defects in collagen metabolism), and drug use (chronic steroids) (Chap. 354).

DIETARY ASSESSMENT

In clinical situations, nutritional assessment is an iterative process that involves: (1) screening for malnutrition, (2) assessing the diet and other data to establish either the absence or presence of malnutrition and its possible causes, (3) planning and implementing the most appropriate nutritional therapy, and (4) reassessing intakes to make sure that they were consumed. Some disease states affect the bioavailability, requirements, use, or excretion of specific nutrients. In these circumstances, specific measurements of various nutrients or their biomarkers may be required to ensure adequate replacement (Chap. 73).

Most health care facilities have nutrition-screening processes in place for identifying possible malnutrition after hospital admission. Nutritional screening is required by the Joint Commission on Accreditation of Healthcare Organizations (JCAHO), but there are no universally recognized or validated standards. The factors that are usually assessed include: abnormal weight for height or body mass index (e.g., BMI <19 or >25); reported weight change (involuntary loss or gain of >5 kg in the past 6 months) (Chap. 80); diagnoses with known nutritional implications (metabolic disease, any disease affecting the gastrointestinal tract, alcoholism, and others); present therapeutic dietary prescription; chronic poor appetite; presence of chewing and swallowing problems or major food intolerances; need for assistance with preparing or shopping for food, eating, or other aspects of self care; and social isolation. Reassessment of nutrition status should occur periodically in hospitalized patients—at least once every week.

A more complete dietary assessment is indicated for patients who exhibit a high risk of or frank malnutrition on nutrition screening. The type of assessment varies based on the clinical setting, severity of the patient's illness, and stability of his or her condition.

ACUTE CARE SETTINGS

In acute-care settings, anorexia, various diseases, test procedures, and medications can compromise dietary intake. Under such circumstances, the goal is to identify and avoid inadequate intake and assure appropriate alimentation. Dietary assessment focuses on what patients are currently eating, whether or not they are able and willing to eat, and whether or not they experience any problems with eating. Dietary intake assessment is based on information from observed intakes; medical record; history; clinical examination; and anthropometric, biochemical, and functional status. The objective is to gather enough information to establish the likelihood of malnutrition due to poor dietary intake or other causes to assess whether nutritional therapy is indicated (Chap. 76).

Simple observations may suffice to suggest inadequate oral intake. These include dietitians' and nurses' notes, the amount of food eaten on trays, frequent tests and procedures that are likely to cause meals to be skipped, nutritionally inadequate diet orders such as clear liquids or full liquids for more than a few days, fever, gastrointestinal distress, vomiting, diarrhea, a comatose state, and diseases or treatments that involve any part of the alimentary tract. Acutely ill patients with diet-related diseases such as diabetes need assessment because an inappropriate diet may exacerbate these conditions and adversely affect other therapies. Abnormal biochemical values [serum albumin levels <35 g/L (<3.5 mg/dL); serum cholesterol levels <3.9 mmol/L (<150 mg/dL)] are nonspecific but may also indicate a need for further nutritional assessment.

Most therapeutic diets offered in hospitals are calculated to meet individual nutrient requirements and the RDA *if they are eaten*. Exceptions include clear liquids, some full-liquid diets, and test diets (such as preparation for gastrointestinal procedures), which are inadequate for several nutrients and should not be used, if possible, for more than 24 h. As much as half of the food served to hospitalized patients is not eaten, and so it cannot be assumed that the intakes of hospitalized patients are adequate. Dietary assessment should compare how much and what food the patient has consumed with the diet that has been provided. Major deviations in intakes of energy, protein, fluids, or other nutrients of special concern for the patient's illness should be noted and corrected.

Nutritional monitoring is especially important for patients who are very ill and who have extended lengths of stay. Patients who are fed by special enteral and parenteral routes also require special nutritional assessment and monitoring by physicians and/or dietitians with certification in nutrition support (Chap. 76).

AMBULATORY SETTINGS

The aim of dietary assessment in the outpatient setting is to determine whether or not the patient's usual diet is a health risk in itself or if it contributes to existing chronic disease-related problems. Dietary assessment also provides the basis for planning a diet that fulfills therapeutic goals while ensuring patient adherence. The outpatient dietary assessment should review the adequacy of present and usual food intakes, including vitamin and mineral supplements, medications, and alcohol, because all of these may affect the patient's nutritional status. The assessment should focus on the dietary constituents that are most likely to be involved or compromised by a specific diagnosis, as well as any co-morbidities that are present. More than one day's intake should be reviewed to provide a better representation of the usual diet.

There are many ways to assess the adequacy of the patient's habitual diet. These include a food guide, a food-exchange list, a diet history, or a food-frequency questionnaire. A commonly used food guide for healthy persons is the USDA's food pyramid, which is useful as a basis for identifying inadequate intakes of essential nutrients, as well as likely excesses in fat, saturated fat, sodium, sugar, and alcohol (Table 73-3). The Web version of the guide provides a calculator that tailors the number of servings suggested for healthy patients of different weights, sexes, ages, and life-cycle stages: *http://www.mypyramidtracker.gov/planner/launchpage.aspx*. Patients who follow ethnic or unusual dietary patterns may need extra instruction on how foods should be categorized, as well as the appropriate portion sizes that constitute a serving. The process of reviewing the guide with patients helps them transition to healthier dietary patterns and identifies food groups eaten in excess of recommendations or in insufficient quantities. For those on therapeutic diets, assessment against food-exchange lists may be useful. These include, for example, the American Diabetes Association food-exchange lists

TABLE 73-3 My Pyramid: The USDA Food Guide Pyramid for Healthy Persons

Servings and Examples of Standard Portion Sizes	Lower: 1600 kcal	Moderate: 2200 kcal	Higher: 2800 kcal
Fruits, cups	1.5	2	2.5
Vegetables, cups	2	3	3.5
Grains, oz eq	5	7	10
(1 slice bread, 1 cup ready to eat cereal, 0.5 cup cooked rice, pasta, cooked cereal)			
Meat and beans, oz eq	5	6	7
(1 oz lean meat, poultry, or fish; 1 egg, 1 Tbsp. peanut butter, 0.25 cup cooked dry beans, or 0.5 oz nuts or seeds)			
Milk, cups	3	3	3
(1 cup milk or yogurt, 1.5 oz natural or 2 oz processed cheese)			
Oils, tsp	5	6	8
Discretionary calorie allowance, kcal (remaining calories after accounting for all of the above)	132	290	426

Abbreviation: oz eq, ounce equivalent.

Source: Data from United States Department of Agriculture. *http://www.MyPyramid.com.*

for diabetes or the American Dietetic Association food-exchange lists for renal disease.

NUTRITIONAL STATUS ASSESSMENT

Full nutritional status assessment is reserved for seriously ill patients and those at very high nutritional risk when the cause of malnutrition is still uncertain after initial clinical evaluation and dietary assessment. It involves multiple dimensions, including documentation of dietary intake, anthropometric measurements, biochemical measurements of blood and urine, clinical examination, health history, and functional status. Therapeutic dietary prescriptions and menu plans for most diseases are available from most hospitals and from the American Dietetic Association. For further discussion of nutritional assessment, see Chap. 75.

GLOBAL CONSIDERATIONS

 The DRI such as the EAR, UL, and energy needs are estimates of physiological requirements based on experimental evidence. Assuming appropriate adjustments are made for age, sex, body size, and physical-activity level, they should be applicable to individuals in most parts of the world. However, the AI are based on customary and adequate intakes in U.S. and Canadian populations, which appear to be compatible with good health, rather than being based on a large body of direct experimental evidence. Similarly, the AMDR represent expert opinion of approximate intakes of energy providing nutrients that are healthful in these North American populations. As such, they should be used with caution in other settings. Nutrient-based standards like the DRI have also been developed by the World Health Organization/Food and Agricultural Organization of the United Nations (WHO/FAO) and are available at their Web site: *http://wwww.who.int/nutrition/topics/nutrecomm/en/index.html.* The different standards have many similarities in their basic concepts, definitions, and nutrient-recommendation levels, but there are some differences from the DRI, due to the functional criteria chosen, environmental differences, the timeliness of the evidence reviewed, and expert judgment.

FURTHER READINGS

KAISER MJ et al: Validation of the mini-nutritional assessment short form (MNA-SF): A practical tool for identification of nutritional status. J Nutr Health Aging 13: 782, 2009

KING JC, GARZA C: Harmonization of nutrient intake values. Food Nutr Bull 28:S1, 2007

GIBSON RS: *Principles of Nutritional Assessment*, 2nd ed, London, Oxford University Press, 2005

MURPHY SP et al: Multivitamin-multimineral supplements' effect on total nutrient intake Am J Clin Nutr 85: 280S, 2007

OTTEN JJ et al (eds): *The Dietary Reference Intakes: The Essential Guide to Nutrient Requirements* Washington Washington, DC, National Academy Press, 2006

SHILS ME et al (eds): *Modern Nutrition in Health and Disease*, 10th ed, Philadelphia, Lippincott, Williams and Wilkins, 2005

CHAPTER 74

Vitamin and Trace Mineral Deficiency and Excess

Robert M. Russell

Paolo M. Suter

Vitamins and trace minerals are required constituents of the human diet since they are inadequately synthesized or not synthesized in the human body. Only small amounts of these substances are needed to carry out essential biochemical reactions (e.g., by acting as coenzymes or prosthetic groups). Overt vitamin or trace mineral deficiencies are rare in Western countries due to a plentiful, varied, and inexpensive food supply; however, multiple nutrient deficiencies may appear together in persons who are chronically ill or alcoholic. After gastric bypass surgery, patients are at high risk for multiple nutrient deficiencies. Moreover, subclinical vitamin and trace mineral deficiencies, as diagnosed by laboratory testing, are quite common in the normal population, especially in the geriatric age group.

Victims of famine, emergency-affected and displaced populations, and refugees are at increased risk for protein-energy malnutrition and classic micronutrient deficiencies (vitamin A, iron, iodine) as well as for thiamine (beriberi), riboflavin, vitamin C (scurvy), and niacin (pellagra) overt deficiencies.

Body stores of vitamins and minerals vary tremendously. For example, vitamin B_{12} and vitamin A stores are large, and an adult may not become deficient for 1 or more years after being on a deficient diet. However, folate and thiamine may become depleted within weeks among those eating a deficient diet. Therapeutic modalities can deplete essential nutrients from the body; for example, hemodialysis removes water-soluble vitamins, which must be replaced by supplementation.

There are several roles for vitamins and trace minerals in diseases: (1) deficiencies of vitamins and minerals may be caused by disease states such as malabsorption; (2) both deficiency and excess of vitamins and minerals can cause disease in and of themselves (e.g., vitamin A intoxication and liver disease); and (3) vitamins and minerals in high doses may be used as drugs (e.g., niacin for hypercholesterolemia). The hematologic-related vitamins and minerals (Chaps. 103, 105) either are not considered or are considered only briefly in this chapter, as are the bone-related vitamins and minerals (vitamin D, calcium, phosphorus; Chap. 352), since they are covered elsewhere (Tables 74-1 and 74-2 and Fig. 74-1).

TABLE 74-1 Principal Clinical Findings of Vitamin Malnutrition

Nutrient	Clinical Finding	Dietary Level per Day Associated with Overt Deficiency in Adults	Contributing Factors to Deficiency
Thiamine	Beriberi: neuropathy, muscle weakness and wasting, cardiomegaly, edema, ophthalmoplegia, confabulation	<0.3 mg/1000 kcal	Alcoholism, chronic diuretic use, hyperemesis
Riboflavin	Magenta tongue, angular stomatitis, seborrhea, cheilosis	<0.6 mg	—
Niacin	Pellagra: pigmented rash of sun-exposed areas, bright red tongue, diarrhea, apathy, memory loss, disorientation	<9.0 niacin equivalents	Alcoholism, vitamin B_6 deficiency, riboflavin deficiency, tryptophan deficiency
Vitamin B_6	Seborrhea, glossitis, convulsions, neuropathy, depression, confusion, microcytic anemia	<0.2 mg	Alcoholism, isoniazid
Folate	Megaloblastic anemia, atrophic glossitis, depression, ↑ homocysteine	<100 µg/d	Alcoholism, sulfasalazine, pyrimethamine, triamterene
Vitamin B_{12}	Megaloblastic anemia, loss of vibratory and position sense, abnormal gait, dementia, impotence, loss of bladder and bowel control, ↑ homocysteine, ↑ methylmalonic acid	<1.0 µg/d	Gastric atrophy (pernicious anemia), terminal ileal disease, strict vegetarianism, acid-reducing drugs (e.g., H_2 blockers)
Vitamin C	Scurvy: petechiae, ecchymosis, coiled hairs, inflamed and bleeding gums, joint effusion, poor wound healing, fatigue	<10 mg/d	Smoking, alcoholism
Vitamin A	Xerophthalmia, night blindness, Bitot's spots, follicular hyperkeratosis, impaired embryonic development, immune dysfunction	<300 µg/d	Fat malabsorption, infection, measles, alcoholism, protein-energy malnutrition
Vitamin D	Rickets: skeletal deformation, rachitic rosary, bowed legs; osteomalacia	<2.0 µg/d	Aging, lack of sunlight exposure, fat malabsorption, deeply pigmented skin
Vitamin E	Peripheral neuropathy, spinocerebellar ataxia, skeletal muscle atrophy, retinopathy	Not described unless underlying contributing factor is present	Occurs only with fat malabsorption or genetic abnormalities of vitamin E metabolism/transport
Vitamin K	Elevated prothrombin time, bleeding	<10 µg/d	Fat malabsorption, liver disease, antibiotic use

TABLE 74-2 Deficiencies and Toxicities of Metals

Element	Deficiency	Toxicity	Tolerable Upper (Dietary) Intake Level
Boron	No biologic function determined	Developmental defects, male sterility, testicular atrophy	20 mg/d (extrapolated from animal data)
Calcium	Reduced bone mass, osteoporosis	Renal insufficiency (milk-alkali syndrome), nephrolithiasis, impaired iron absorption	2500 mg/d (milk-alkali)
Copper	Anemia, growth retardation, defective keratinization and pigmentation of hair, hypothermia, degenerative changes in aortic elastin, osteopenia, mental deterioration	Nausea, vomiting, diarrhea, hepatic failure, tremor, mental deterioration, hemolytic anemia, renal dysfunction	10 mg/d (liver toxicity)
Chromium	Impaired glucose tolerance	Occupational: renal failure, dermatitis, pulmonary cancer	ND
Fluoride	↑ Dental caries	Dental and skeletal fluorosis, osteosclerosis	10 mg/d (fluorosis)
Iodine	Thyroid enlargement, ↓ T$_4$, cretinism	Thyroid dysfunction, acne-like eruptions	1100 µg/d (thyroid dysfunction)
Iron	Muscle abnormalities, koilonychia, pica, anemia, ↓ work performance, impaired cognitive development, premature labor, ↑ perinatal maternal mortality	Gastrointestinal effects (nausea, vomiting, diarrhea, constipation), iron overload with organ damage, acute systemic toxicity	45 mg/d of elemental iron (GI side effects)
Manganese	Impaired growth and skeletal development, reproduction, lipid and carbohydrate metabolism; upper body rash	General: Neurotoxicity, Parkinson-like symptoms Occupational: Encephalitis-like syndrome, Parkinson-like syndrome, psychosis, pneumoconiosis	11 mg/d (neurotoxicity)
Molybdenum	Severe neurologic abnormalities	Reproductive and fetal abnormalities	2 mg/d extrapolated from animal data
Selenium	Cardiomyopathy, heart failure, striated muscle degeneration	General: Alopecia, nausea, vomiting, abnormal nails, emotional lability, peripheral neuropathy, lassitude, garlic odor to breath, dermatitis Occupational: Lung and nasal carcinomas, liver necrosis, pulmonary inflammation	400 µg/d (hair, nail changes)
Phosphorus	Rickets (osteomalacia), proximal muscle weakness, rhabdomyolysis, paresthesia, ataxia, seizure, confusion, heart failure, hemolysis, acidosis	Hyperphosphatemia	4000 mg/d
Zinc	Growth retardation, ↓ taste and smell, alopecia, dermatitis, diarrhea, immune dysfunction, failure to thrive, gonadal atrophy, congenital malformations	General: Reduced copper absorption, gastritis, sweating, fever, nausea, vomiting Occupational: Respiratory distress, pulmonary fibrosis	40 mg/d (impaired copper metabolism)

Abbreviations: GI, gastrointestinal; ND, not determined.

VITAMINS

■ THIAMINE (VITAMIN B$_1$)

Thiamine was the first B vitamin to be identified and therefore is referred to as vitamin B$_1$. Thiamine functions in the decarboxylation of α-ketoacids, such as pyruvate α-ketoglutarate, and branched-chain amino acids and thus is essential for energy generation. In addition, thiamine pyrophosphate acts as a coenzyme for a transketolase reaction that mediates the conversion of hexose and pentose phosphates. It has been postulated that thiamine plays a role in peripheral nerve conduction, although the exact chemical reactions underlying this function are not known.

Food sources

The median intake of thiamine in the United States from food alone is 2 mg/d. Primary food sources for thiamine include yeast, organ meat, pork, legumes, beef, whole grains, and nuts. Milled rice and grains contain little thiamine, if any. Thiamine deficiency is therefore more common in cultures that rely heavily on a rice-based diet. Tea, coffee (regular and decaffeinated), raw fish, and shellfish contain thiaminases, which can destroy the vitamin. Thus, drinking large amounts of tea or coffee can theoretically lower thiamine body stores.

Deficiency

Most dietary deficiency of thiamine worldwide is the result of poor dietary intake. In Western countries, the primary causes of thiamine deficiency are alcoholism and chronic illnesses such as cancer. Alcohol interferes directly with the absorption of thiamine and with the synthesis of thiamine pyrophosphate. Thiamine should always be replenished when a patient with alcoholism is being refed, as carbohydrate repletion without adequate thiamine can precipitate acute thiamine deficiency with lactic acidosis. Other at-risk populations are women with prolonged hyperemesis gravidarum and anorexia, patients with overall poor nutritional status on parenteral glucose, patients after bariatric bypass surgery, and patients on chronic diuretic therapy due to increased urinary thiamine losses.

Maternal thiamine deficiency can lead to infantile beriberi in breast-fed children. Thiamine deficiency should be considered in the setting of motor vehicle accidents associated with head injury.

Thiamine deficiency in its early stage induces anorexia and nonspecific symptoms (e.g., irritability, decrease in short-term

Vitamin	Active derivative or cofactor form	Principal function
Thiamine (B$_1$) 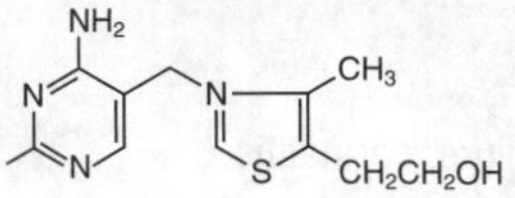	Thiamine pyrophosphate	Coenzyme for cleavage of carbon-carbon bonds; amino acid and carbohydrate metabolism
Riboflavin (B$_2$) 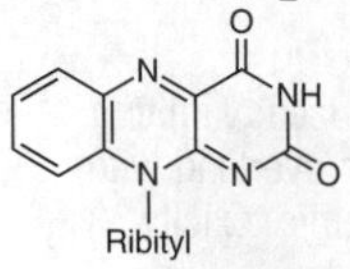	Flavin mononucleotide (FMN) and flavin adenine dinucleotide (FAD)	Cofactor for oxidation, reduction reactions, and covalently attached prosthetic groups for some enzymes
Niacin 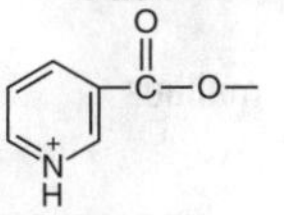	Nicotinamide adenine dinucleotide phosphate (NADP) and nicotinamide adenine dinucleotide (NAD)	Coenzymes for oxidation and reduction reactions
Vitamin B$_6$ 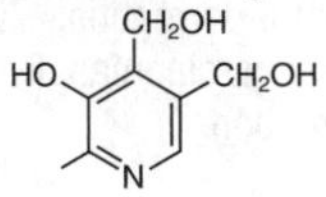	Pyridoxal phosphate	Cofactor for enzymes of amino acid metabolism
Folate 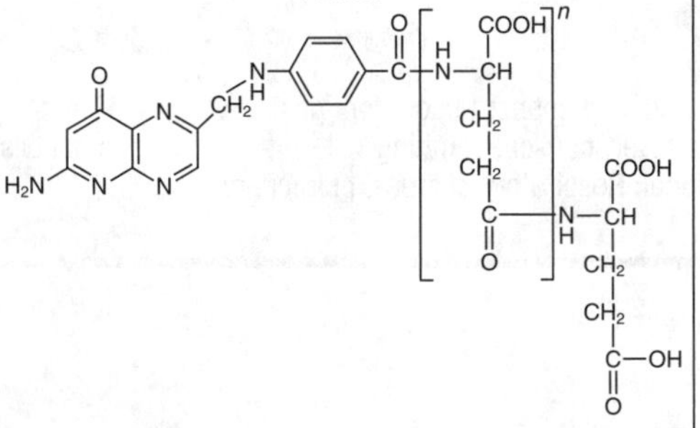	Polyglutamate forms of (5, 6, 7, 8) tetrahydrofolate with carbon unit attachments	Coenzyme for one carbon transfer in nucleic acid and amino acid metabolism
Vitamin B$_{12}$ 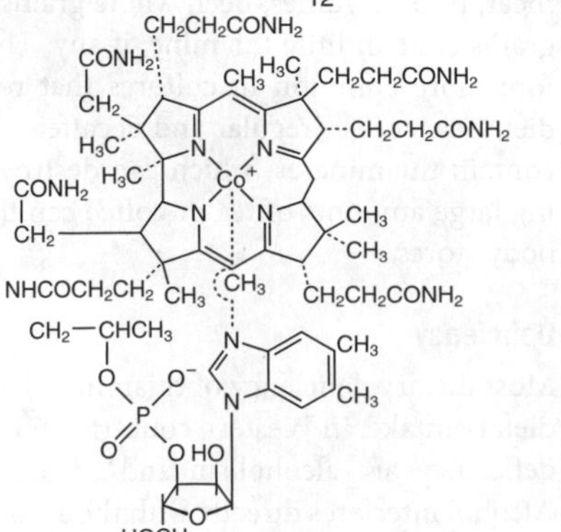	Methylcobalamine Adenosylcobalamin	Coenzyme for methionine synthase and L-methylmalonyl-CoA mutase

Figure 74-1 The structures and principal functions of vitamins associated with human disorders.

Vitamin	Active derivative or cofactor form	Principal function
Vitamin C 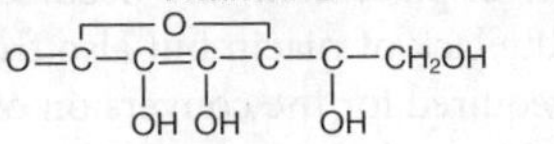	Ascorbic acid and dehydroascorbic acid	Participation as a redox ion in many biologic oxidation and hydrogen transfer reactions
Vitamin A 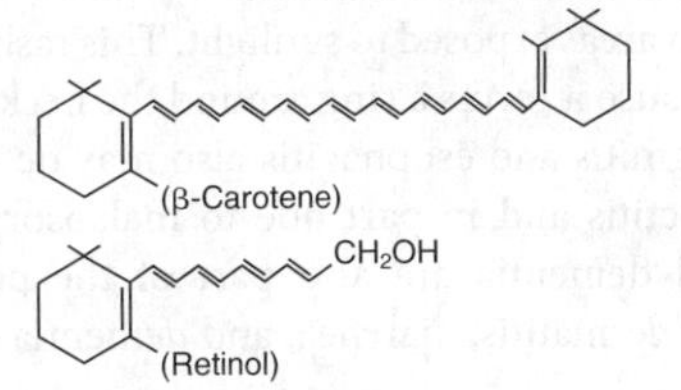 (β-Carotene) (Retinol)	Retinol, retinaldehyde, and retinoic acid	Formation of rhodopsin (vision) and glycoproteins (epithelial cell function); also regulates gene transcription
Vitamin D 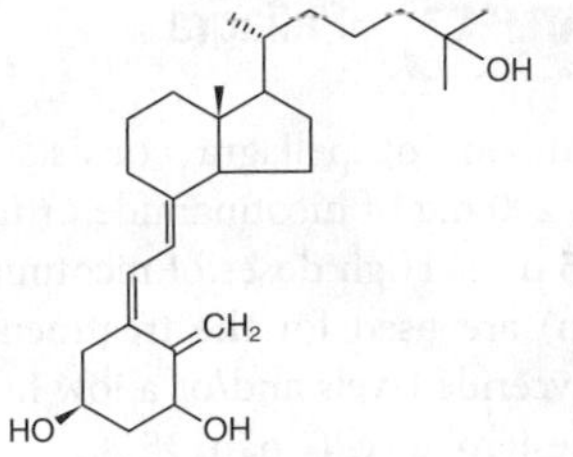	1,25-Dihydroxyvitamin D	Maintenance of blood calcium and phosphorus levels; antiproliferative hormone
Vitamin E 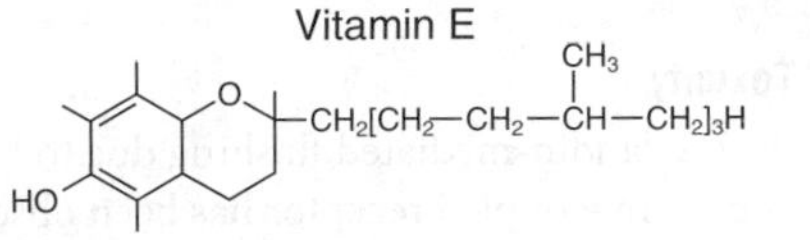	Tocopherols and tocotrienols	Antioxidants
Vitamin K 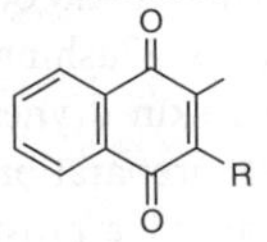	Vitamin K hydroquinone	Cofactor for posttranslation carboxylation of many proteins including essential clotting factors

Figure 74-1 *(Continued)*

memory). Prolonged thiamine deficiency causes beriberi, which is classically categorized as wet or dry, although there is considerable overlap. In either form of beriberi, patients may complain of pain and paresthesia. *Wet beriberi* presents primarily with cardiovascular symptoms, due to impaired myocardial energy metabolism and dysautonomia, and can occur after 3 months of a thiamine-deficient diet. Patients present with an enlarged heart, tachycardia, high-output congestive heart failure, peripheral edema, and peripheral neuritis. Patients with *dry beriberi* present with a symmetric peripheral neuropathy of the motor and sensory systems with diminished reflexes. The neuropathy affects the legs most markedly, and these patients have difficulty rising from a squatting position.

Alcoholic patients with chronic thiamine deficiency also may have central nervous system (CNS) manifestations known as *Wernicke's encephalopathy*, consisting of horizontal nystagmus, ophthalmoplegia (due to weakness of one or more extraocular muscles), cerebellar ataxia, and mental impairment (Chap. 392). When there is an additional loss of memory and a confabulatory psychosis, the syndrome is known as *Wernicke-Korsakoff syndrome*. Despite the typical clinical picture and history, Wernicke-Korsakoff syndrome is underdiagnosed.

The laboratory diagnosis of thiamine deficiency usually is made by a functional enzymatic assay of transketolase activity measured

before and after the addition of thiamine pyrophosphate. A >25% stimulation by the addition of thiamine pyrophosphate (an activity coefficient of 1.25) is interpreted as abnormal. Thiamine or the phosphorylated esters of thiamine in serum or blood also can be measured by high-performance liquid chromatography (HPLC) to detect deficiency.

TREATMENT   Thiamine Deficiency

In acute thiamine deficiency with either cardiovascular or neurologic signs, 100 mg/d of thiamine should be given parenterally for 7 days, followed by 10 mg/d orally until there is complete recovery. Cardiovascular and ophthalmoplegic improvement occurs within 24 h. Other manifestations gradually clear, although psychosis in Wernicke-Korsakoff syndrome may be permanent or persist for several months.

Toxicity

Although anaphylaxis has been reported after high doses of thiamine, no adverse effects have been recorded from either food or supplements at high doses. Thiamine supplements may be bought over the counter in doses of up to 50 mg/d.

■ RIBOFLAVIN (VITAMIN B₂)

Riboflavin is important for the metabolism of fat, carbohydrate, and protein, reflecting its role as a respiratory coenzyme and an electron donor. Enzymes that contain flavin adenine dinucleotide (FAD) or flavin mononucleotide (FMN) as prosthetic groups are known as *flavoenzymes* (e.g., succinic acid dehydrogenase, monoamine oxidase, glutathione reductase). FAD is a cofactor for methyltetrahydrofolate reductase and therefore modulates homocysteine metabolism. The vitamin also plays a role in drug and steroid metabolism, including detoxification reactions.

Although much is known about the chemical and enzymatic reactions of riboflavin, the clinical manifestations of riboflavin deficiency are nonspecific and are similar to those of other deficiencies of B vitamins. Riboflavin deficiency is manifested principally by lesions of the mucocutaneous surfaces of the mouth and skin (Table 74-1). In addition to the mucocutaneous lesions, corneal vascularization, anemia, and personality changes have been described with riboflavin deficiency.

Deficiency and excess

Riboflavin deficiency almost always is due to dietary deficiency. Milk, other dairy products, and enriched breads and cereals are the most important dietary sources of riboflavin in the United States, although lean meat, fish, eggs, broccoli, and legumes are also good sources. Riboflavin is extremely sensitive to light, and milk should be stored in containers that protect against photodegradation. Laboratory diagnosis of riboflavin deficiency can be made by measurement of red blood cell or urinary riboflavin concentrations or by measurement of erythrocyte glutathione reductase activity, with and without added FAD. Because the capacity of the gastrointestinal tract to absorb riboflavin is limited (~20 mg if given in one oral dose), riboflavin toxicity has not been described.

■ NIACIN (VITAMIN B₃)

The term *niacin* refers to nicotinic acid and nicotinamide and their biologically active derivatives. Nicotinic acid and nicotinamide serve as precursors of two coenzymes, nicotinamide adenine dinucleotide (NAD) and NAD phosphate (NADP), which are important in numerous oxidation and reduction reactions in the body. In addition, NAD and NADP are active in adenine diphosphate–ribose transfer reactions involved in DNA repair and calcium mobilization.

Metabolism and requirements

Nicotinic acid and nicotinamide are absorbed well from the stomach and small intestine. Niacin bioavailability is high from beans, milk, meat, and eggs; bioavailability from cereal grains is lower. Since flour is enriched with the "free" niacin (i.e., non-coenzyme form), bioavailability is excellent. Median intakes of niacin in the United States considerably exceed the recommended dietary allowance (RDA).

The amino acid tryptophan can be converted to niacin with an efficiency of 60:1 by weight. Thus, the RDA for niacin is expressed in niacin equivalents. A lower conversion of tryptophan to niacin occurs in vitamin B₆ and/or riboflavin deficiencies and in the presence of isoniazid. The urinary excretion products of niacin include 2-pyridone and 2-methyl nicotinamide, measurements of which are used in the diagnosis of niacin deficiency.

Deficiency

Niacin deficiency causes *pellagra*, which is found mostly among people eating corn-based diets in parts of China, Africa, and India. Pellagra in North America is found mainly among alcoholics; in patients with congenital defects of intestinal and kidney absorption

of tryptophan (Hartnup disease; Chap. 364); and in patients with carcinoid syndrome (Chap. 350), in which there is increased conversion of tryptophan to serotonin. In the setting of famine or population displacement, the occurrence of pellagra results from the absolute lack of niacin but also from the deficiency of micronutrients required for the conversion of tryptophan to niacin (e.g., iron, riboflavin, and pyridoxine). The early symptoms of pellagra include loss of appetite, generalized weakness and irritability, abdominal pain, and vomiting. Bright red glossitis then ensues, followed by a characteristic skin rash that is pigmented and scaling, particularly in skin areas exposed to sunlight. This rash is known as *Casal's necklace* because it forms a ring around the neck; it is seen in advanced cases. Vaginitis and esophagitis also may occur. Diarrhea (in part due to proctitis and in part due to malabsorption), depression, seizures, and dementia are also part of the pellagra syndrome—the four Ds: *d*ermatitis, *d*iarrhea, and *d*ementia leading to *d*eath.

TREATMENT   Pellagra

Treatment of pellagra consists of oral supplementation of 100–200 mg of nicotinamide or nicotinic acid three times daily for 5 days. High doses of nicotinic acid (2 g/d in a time-release form) are used for the treatment of elevated cholesterol and triglyceride levels and/or a low high-density lipoprotein (HDL) cholesterol level (Chap. 356).

Toxicity

Prostaglandin-mediated flushing due to binding of the vitamin to a G protein–coupled receptor has been observed at daily doses as low as 50 mg of niacin when taken as a supplement or as therapy for dyslipidemia. There is no evidence of toxicity from niacin derived from food sources. Flushing always starts in the face and may be accompanied by skin dryness, itching, paresthesia, and headache. Pharmaceutical preparations of nicotinic acid combined with laropiprant, a selective prostaglandin D₂ receptor 1 antagonist, or premedication with aspirin may alleviate these symptoms. Flushing is subject to tachyphylaxis and often improves with time. Nausea, vomiting, and abdominal pain also occur at similar doses of niacin. Hepatic toxicity is the most serious toxic reaction caused by niacin and may present as jaundice with elevated aspartate aminotransferase (AST) and alanine aminotransferase (ALT) levels. A few cases of fulminant hepatitis requiring liver transplantation have been reported at doses of 3–9 g/d. Other toxic reactions include glucose intolerance, hyperuricemia, macular edema, and macular cysts. The combination of nicotinic acid preparations for dyslipidemia with 3-hydroxy-3-methylglutaryl coenzyme A (HMG-CoA) reductase inhibitors may increase the risk of rhabdomyolysis. The upper limit for daily niacin intake has been set at 35 mg. However, this upper limit does not pertain to the therapeutic use of niacin.

■ PYRIDOXINE (VITAMIN B₆)

Vitamin B₆ refers to a family of compounds that include pyridoxine, pyridoxal, pyridoxamine, and their 5′-phosphate derivatives. 5′-Pyridoxal phosphate (PLP) is a cofactor for more than 100 enzymes involved in amino acid metabolism. Vitamin B₆ also is involved in heme and neurotransmitter synthesis and in the metabolism of glycogen, lipids, steroids, sphingoid bases, and several vitamins, including the conversion of tryptophan to niacin.

Dietary sources

Plants contain vitamin B₆ in the form of pyridoxine, whereas animal tissues contain PLP and pyridoxamine phosphate. The vitamin B₆ contained in plants is less bioavailable than that in animal tissues.

Rich food sources of vitamin B_6 include legumes, nuts, wheat bran, and meat, although it is present in all food groups.

Deficiency

Symptoms of vitamin B_6 deficiency include epithelial changes, as seen frequently with other B vitamin deficiencies. In addition, severe vitamin B_6 deficiency can lead to peripheral neuropathy, abnormal electroencephalograms, and personality changes that include depression and confusion. In infants, diarrhea, seizures, and anemia have been reported. Microcytic hypochromic anemia is due to diminished hemoglobin synthesis, since the first enzyme involved in heme biosynthesis (aminolevulinate synthase) requires PLP as a cofactor (Chap. 103). In some case reports, platelet dysfunction has been reported. Since vitamin B_6 is necessary for the conversion of homocysteine to cystathionine, it is possible that chronic low-grade vitamin B_6 deficiency may result in hyperhomocysteinemia and increased risk of cardiovascular disease (Chaps. 241 and 364). Independent of homocysteine, low levels of circulating vitamin B_6 have been associated with inflammation and elevated levels of C-reactive protein.

Certain medications, such as isoniazid, L-dopa, penicillamine, and cycloserine, interact with PLP due to a reaction with carbonyl groups. Pyridoxine should be given concurrently with isoniazid to avoid neuropathy. The increased ratio of AST to ALT seen in alcoholic liver disease reflects the relative vitamin B_6 dependence of ALT. Vitamin B_6 dependency syndromes that require pharmacologic doses of vitamin B_6 are rare; they include cystathionine β-synthase deficiency, pyridoxine-responsive (primarily sideroblastic) anemias, and gyrate atrophy with chorioretinal degeneration due to decreased activity of the mitochondrial enzyme ornithine aminotransferase. In these situations, 100–200 mg/d of oral vitamin B_6 is required for treatment.

High doses of vitamin B_6 have been used to treat carpal tunnel syndrome, premenstrual syndrome, schizophrenia, autism, and diabetic neuropathy but have not been found to be effective.

The laboratory diagnosis of vitamin B_6 deficiency is generally made on the basis of low plasma PLP values (<20 nmol/L). Treatment of vitamin B_6 deficiency is done with 50 mg/d; higher doses of 100–200 mg/d are given if the deficiency is related to medication use. Vitamin B_6 should not be given with L-dopa, since the vitamin interferes with the action of this drug.

Toxicity

The safe upper limit for vitamin B_6 has been set at 100 mg/d, although no adverse effects have been associated with high intakes of vitamin B_6 from food sources only. When toxicity occurs, it causes a severe sensory neuropathy, leaving patients unable to walk. Some cases of photosensitivity and dermatitis have been reported.

■ FOLATE, VITAMIN B_{12}

See Chap. 105.

■ VITAMIN C

Both ascorbic acid and its oxidized product dehydroascorbic acid are biologically active. Actions of vitamin C include antioxidant activity, promotion of nonheme iron absorption, carnitine biosynthesis, the conversion of dopamine to norepinephrine, and the synthesis of many peptide hormones. Vitamin C is also important for connective tissue metabolism and cross-linking (proline hydroxylation), and it is a component of many drug-metabolizing enzyme systems, particularly the mixed-function oxidase systems.

Absorption and dietary sources

Almost complete absorption of vitamin C occurs if <100 mg is administered in a single dose; however, only 50% or less is absorbed at doses >1 g. Enhanced degradation and fecal and urinary excretion of vitamin C occur at higher intake levels.

Good dietary sources of vitamin C include citrus fruits, green vegetables (especially broccoli), tomatoes, and potatoes. Consumption of five servings of fruits and vegetables a day provides vitamin C in excess of the RDA of 90 mg/d for males and 75 mg/d for females. In addition, approximately 40% of the U.S. population consumes vitamin C as a dietary supplement in which "natural forms" of the vitamin are no more bioavailable than synthetic forms. Smoking, hemodialysis, pregnancy, and stress (e.g., infection, trauma) appear to increase vitamin C requirements.

Deficiency

Vitamin C deficiency causes scurvy. In the United States, this is seen primarily among the poor and elderly, in alcoholics who consume <10 mg/d of vitamin C, and in individuals consuming macrobiotic diets. Vitamin C deficiency also can occur in young adults who eat severely unbalanced diets. In addition to generalized fatigue, symptoms of scurvy primarily reflect impaired formation of mature connective tissue and include bleeding into skin (petechiae, ecchymoses, perifollicular hemorrhages); inflamed and bleeding gums; and manifestations of bleeding into joints, the peritoneal cavity, the pericardium, and the adrenal glands. In children, vitamin C deficiency may cause impaired bone growth. Laboratory diagnosis of vitamin C deficiency is made on the basis of low plasma or leukocyte levels.

Administration of vitamin C (200 mg/d) improves the symptoms of scurvy within a matter of several days. High-dose vitamin C supplementation (e.g., 1–2 g/d) may slightly decrease the symptoms and duration of upper respiratory tract infections. Vitamin C supplementation has also been reported to be useful in Chédiak-Higashi syndrome (Chap. 60) and osteogenesis imperfecta (Chap. 363). Diets high in vitamin C have been claimed to lower the incidence of certain cancers, particularly esophageal and gastric cancers. If proved, this effect may be due to the fact that vitamin C can prevent the conversion of nitrites and secondary amines to carcinogenic nitrosamines. However, an intervention study from China did not show vitamin C to be protective. Parenteral ascorbic acid has been suggested to have a potential therapeutic role in the treatment of advanced cancers.

Toxicity

Taking >2 g of vitamin C in a single dose may result in abdominal pain, diarrhea, and nausea. Since vitamin C may be metabolized to oxalate, it is feared that chronic high-dose vitamin C supplementation could result in an increased prevalence of kidney stones. However, this has not been borne out in several trials, except in patients with preexisting renal disease. Thus, it is reasonable to advise patients with a past history of kidney stones not to take large doses of vitamin C. There is also an unproven but possible risk that chronic high doses of vitamin C could promote iron overload in patients taking supplemental iron. High doses of vitamin C can induce hemolysis in patients with glucose-6-phosphate dehydrogenase deficiency, and doses >1 g/d can cause false-negative guaiac reactions as well as interfere with tests for urinary glucose. High doses may interfere with certain drugs (e.g., bortezomib in myeloma patients).

■ BIOTIN

Biotin is a water-soluble vitamin that plays a role in gene expression, gluconeogenesis, and fatty acid synthesis and serves as a CO_2 carrier on the surface of both cytosolic and mitochondrial carboxylase enzymes. The vitamin also functions in the catabolism of specific amino acids (e.g., leucine). Excellent food sources of biotin include organ meat such as liver or kidney, soy, beans, yeast, and egg yolks; however, egg white contains the protein avidin, which strongly binds the vitamin and reduces its bioavailability.

Biotin deficiency due to low dietary intake is rare; rather, deficiency is due to inborn errors of metabolism. Biotin deficiency has been induced by experimental feeding of egg white diets and in patients with short bowels who received biotin-free parenteral nutrition. In adults, biotin deficiency results in mental changes (depression, hallucinations), paresthesia, anorexia, and nausea. A scaling, seborrheic, and erythematous rash may occur around the eyes, nose, and mouth as well as on the extremities. In infants, biotin deficiency presents as hypotonia, lethargy, and apathy. In addition, infants may develop alopecia and a characteristic rash that includes the ears. The laboratory diagnosis of biotin deficiency can be established on the basis of a decreased urinary concentration or an increased urinary excretion of 3-hydroxyisovaleric acid after a leucine challenge. Treatment requires pharmacologic doses of biotin, using up to 10 mg/d. No toxicity is known.

PANTOTHENIC ACID (VITAMIN B$_5$)

Pantothenic acid is a component of coenzyme A and phosphopantetheine, which are involved in fatty acid metabolism and the synthesis of cholesterol, steroid hormones, and all compounds formed from isoprenoid units. In addition, pantothenic acid is involved in the acetylation of proteins. The vitamin is excreted in the urine, and the laboratory diagnosis of deficiency is made on the basis of low urinary vitamin levels.

The vitamin is ubiquitous in the food supply. Liver, yeast, egg yolks, whole grains, and vegetables are particularly good sources. Human pantothenic acid deficiency has been demonstrated only in experimental feeding of diets low in pantothenic acid or by giving a specific pantothenic acid antagonist. The symptoms of pantothenic acid deficiency are nonspecific and include gastrointestinal disturbance, depression, muscle cramps, paresthesia, ataxia, and hypoglycemia. Pantothenic acid deficiency is believed to have caused the burning feet syndrome seen in prisoners of war during World War II. No toxicity of this vitamin has been reported.

CHOLINE

Choline is a precursor for acetylcholine, phospholipids, and betaine. Choline is necessary for the structural integrity of cell membranes, cholinergic neurotransmission, lipid and cholesterol metabolism, methyl-group metabolism, and transmembrane signaling. Recently, a recommended adequate intake was set at 550 mg/d for adult males and 425 mg/d for adult females, although certain genetic polymorphisms can increase an individual's requirement. Choline is thought to be a "conditionally essential" nutrient in that de novo synthesis occurs in the liver and is less than the vitamin's utilization only under certain stress conditions (e.g., alcoholic liver disease). The dietary requirement of choline depends on the status of other methyl-group donors (folate, vitamin B$_{12}$, and methionine) and thus varies widely. Choline is widely distributed in food (e.g., egg yolk, wheat germ, organ meat, milk) in the form of lecithin (phosphatidylcholine). Choline deficiency has occurred in patients receiving parenteral nutrition devoid of choline. Deficiency results in fatty liver, elevated transaminase levels, and skeletal muscle damage with high creatine phosphokinase values. The diagnosis of choline deficiency is currently made on the basis of low plasma levels, although nonspecific conditions (e.g., heavy exercise) may suppress plasma levels.

Toxicity from choline results in hypotension, cholinergic sweating, diarrhea, salivation, and a fishy body odor. The upper limit for choline has been set at 3.5 g/d. Therapeutically, choline has been suggested for patients with dementia and patients at high risk of cardiovascular disease, due to its ability to lower cholesterol and homocysteine levels. However, such benefits have not been firmly documented. Choline- and betaine-restricted diets are of therapeutic value in trimethylaminuria (fish odor syndrome).

FLAVONOIDS

Flavonoids constitute a large family of polyphenols that contribute to the aroma, taste, and color of fruits and vegetables. Major groups of dietary flavonoids include anthocyanidins in berries; catechins in green tea and chocolate; flavonols (e.g., quercitin) in broccoli, kale, leeks, onion, and the skins of grapes and apples; and isoflavones (e.g., genistein) in legumes. Isoflavones have a low bioavailability and are partially metabolized by the intestinal flora. The dietary intake of flavonoids is estimated to be between 10 and 100 mg/d, although this is almost certainly an underestimate due to the lack of knowledge of their concentrations in many foods. Several flavonoids have been shown to have antioxidant activity and to affect cell signaling. From observational epidemiologic studies and limited clinical human and animal studies, flavonoids have been postulated to play a role in the prevention of several chronic diseases, including neurodegenerative disease, diabetes, and osteoporosis. The ultimate importance and usefulness of their compounds against human disease have not been demonstrated.

VITAMIN A

Vitamin A, in the strictest sense, refers to retinol. However, the oxidized metabolites, retinaldehyde and retinoic acid, are also biologically active compounds. The term *retinoids* includes all molecules (including synthetic molecules) that are chemically related to retinol. Retinaldehyde (11-*cis*) is the essential form of vitamin A that is required for normal vision, whereas retinoic acid is necessary for normal morphogenesis, growth, and cell differentiation. Retinoic acid does not function in vision and, in contrast to retinol, is not involved in reproduction. Vitamin A also plays a role in iron utilization, humoral immunity, T cell–mediated immunity, natural killer cell activity, and phagocytosis. Vitamin A is commercially available in esterified forms (e.g., acetate, palmitate) since it is more stable as an ester.

There are more than 600 carotenoids in nature, and approximately 50 of them can be metabolized to vitamin A. β-Carotene is the most prevalent carotenoid in the food supply that has provitamin A activity. In humans, significant fractions of carotenoids are absorbed intact and are stored in liver and fat. It is now estimated that 12 μg or more (range, 4–27 μg) of dietary all-*trans* β-carotene is equivalent to 1 μg of retinol activity, whereas 24 μg or more of other dietary provitamin A carotenoids (e.g., cryptoxanthin, α-carotene) is equivalent to 1 μg of retinol activity. The vitamin A equivalency for a β-carotene supplement in an oily solution is 2:1.

Metabolism

The liver contains approximately 90% of the vitamin A reserves and secretes vitamin A in the form of retinol, which is bound to retinol-binding protein. Once this has occurred, the retinol-binding protein complex interacts with a second protein, transthyretin. This trimolecular complex functions to prevent vitamin A from being filtered by the kidney glomerulus to protect the body against the toxicity of retinol and to allow retinol to be taken up by specific cell-surface receptors that recognize retinol-binding protein. A certain amount of vitamin A enters peripheral cells even if it is not bound to retinol-binding protein. After retinol is internalized by the cell, it becomes bound to a series of cellular retinol-binding proteins, which function as sequestering and transporting agents as well as co-ligands for enzymatic reactions. Certain cells also contain retinoic acid–binding proteins, which have sequestering functions but also shuttle retinoic acid to the nucleus and enable its metabolism.

Retinoic acid is a ligand for certain nuclear receptors that act as transcription factors. Two families of receptors (RAR and RXR receptors) are active in retinoid-mediated gene transcription. Retinoid receptors regulate transcription by binding as dimeric complexes to specific DNA sites, the retinoic acid response elements, in target genes (Chap. 338). The receptors can either stimulate or repress gene expression in response to their ligands. RAR binds all-*trans* retinoic acid and 9-*cis*-retinoic acid, whereas RXR binds only 9-*cis*-retinoic acid.

The retinoid receptors play an important role in controlling cell proliferation and differentiation. Retinoic acid is useful in the treatment of promyelocytic leukemia (Chap. 109) and also is used in the treatment of cystic acne because it inhibits keratinization, decreases sebum secretion, and possibly alters the inflammatory reaction (Chap. 52). RXRs dimerize with other nuclear receptors to function as coregulators of genes responsive to retinoids, thyroid hormone, and calcitriol. RXR agonists induce insulin sensitivity experimentally, perhaps because RXR is a cofactor for the peroxisome-proliferator-activated receptors (PPARs), which are targets for thiazolidinedione drugs such as rosiglitazone and troglitazone (Chap. 344).

Dietary sources

The retinol activity equivalent (RAE) is used to express the vitamin A value of food. One RAE is defined as 1 μg of retinol (0.003491 mmol), 12 μg of β-carotene, and 24 μg of other provitamin A carotenoids. In older literature, vitamin A often was expressed in international units (IU), with 1 μg of retinol being equal to 3.33 IU of retinol and 20 IU of β-carotene, but these units are no longer in scientific use.

Liver, fish, and eggs are excellent food sources for preformed vitamin A; vegetable sources of provitamin A carotenoids include dark green and deeply colored fruits and vegetables. Moderate cooking of vegetables enhances carotenoid release for uptake in the gut. Carotenoid absorption is also aided by some fat in a meal. Infants are particularly susceptible to vitamin A deficiency because neither breast nor cow's milk supplies enough vitamin A to prevent deficiency. In developing countries, chronic dietary deficiency is the main cause of vitamin A deficiency and is exacerbated by infection. In early childhood, low vitamin A status results from inadequate intakes of animal food sources and edible oils, both of which are expensive, coupled with seasonal unavailability of vegetables and fruits and lack of marketed fortified food products. Concurrent zinc deficiency can interfere with the mobilization of vitamin A from liver stores. Alcohol interferes with the conversion of retinol to retinaldehyde in the eye by competing for alcohol (retinol) dehydrogenase. Drugs that interfere with the absorption of vitamin A include mineral oil, neomycin, and cholestyramine.

Deficiency

Vitamin A deficiency is endemic in areas where diets are chronically poor, especially in southern Asia, sub-Saharan Africa, some parts of Latin America, and the western Pacific, including parts of China. Vitamin A status is usually assessed by measuring serum retinol [normal range, 1.05–3.50 μmol/L (30–100 μg/dL)] or blood spot retinol or by tests of dark adaptation. There are stable isotopic or invasive liver biopsy methods to estimate total body stores of vitamin A. Based on deficient serum retinol [<0.70 μmol/L (20 μg/dL)], there are >90 million preschool-age children with vitamin A deficiency, among whom >4 million have an ocular manifestation of deficiency termed *xerophthalmia*. This condition includes milder stages of night blindness and conjunctival xerosis (dryness) with Bitot's spots (white patches of keratinized epithelium appearing on the sclera) as well as rare, potentially blinding corneal ulceration and necrosis. Keratomalacia (softening of the cornea) leads to corneal scarring that blinds at least a quarter of a million children each year and is associated with a fatality rate of 4–25%. However, vitamin A deficiency at any stage poses an increased risk of mortality from diarrhea, dysentery, measles, malaria, and respiratory disease. Vitamin A deficiency can compromise barrier and innate and acquired immune defenses to infection. Vitamin A supplementation can markedly reduce risk of child mortality (23–34%, on average) in areas where deficiency is widely prevalent. About 10% of pregnant women in undernourished settings also develop night blindness, assessed by history, during the latter half of pregnancy, and this moderate vitamin A deficiency is associated with an increased risk of maternal infection and mortality rate.

TREATMENT   Vitamin A Deficiency

Any stage of xerophthalmia should be treated with 60 mg of vitamin A in oily solution, usually contained in a soft-gel capsule. The same dose is repeated 1 and 14 days later. Doses should be reduced by half for patients 6–11 months of age. Mothers with night blindness or Bitot's spots should be given vitamin A orally, either 3 mg daily or 7.5 mg twice a week for 3 months. These regimens are efficacious, and they are less expensive and more widely available than injectable water-miscible vitamin A. A common approach to prevention is to supplement young children in high-risk areas with 60 mg every 4–6 months, with a half dose given to infants 6–11 months of age.

Uncomplicated vitamin A deficiency rarely occurs in industrialized countries. One high-risk group, extremely low-birth-weight infants (<1000 g), is likely to be vitamin A–deficient and should be supplemented with 1500 μg (or RAE) of vitamin A three times a week for 4 weeks. Severe measles in any society can lead to secondary vitamin A deficiency. Children hospitalized with measles should receive two 60-mg doses of vitamin A on two consecutive days. Vitamin A deficiency most often occurs in patients with malabsorptive diseases (e.g., celiac sprue, short-bowel syndrome) who have abnormal dark adaptation or symptoms of night blindness without other ocular changes. Typically, such patients are treated for 1 month with 15 mg/d of a water-miscible preparation of vitamin A. This is followed by a lower maintenance dose, with the exact amount determined by monitoring serum retinol.

There are no specific deficiency signs or symptoms that result from carotenoid deficiency. It was postulated that β-carotene would be an effective chemopreventive agent for cancer because numerous epidemiologic studies had shown that diets high in β-carotene were associated with lower incidences of cancers of the respiratory and digestive systems. However, intervention studies in smokers found that treatment with high doses of β-carotene actually resulted in more lung cancers than did treatment with placebo. Non–provitamin A carotenoids such as lutein and zeaxanthin have been suggested to protect against macular degeneration, and large-scale intervention studies have been undertaken to test this hypothesis. The non–provitamin A carotenoid lycopene has been proposed to protect against prostate cancer. However, the effectiveness of these agents has not been proved by intervention studies, and the mechanisms underlying these purported biologic actions are unknown.

Selective plant breeding techniques that lead to a higher provitamin A content of staple foods may improve vitamin A malnutrition in low-income countries. Moreover, a recently developed genetically modified food (Golden Rice) showed an improved β-carotene to vitamin A conversion ratio of ~3:1.

Toxicity

Acute toxicity of vitamin A was first noted in Arctic explorers who ate polar bear liver and has also been seen after administration of 150 mg in adults or 100 mg in children. Acute toxicity is manifested by increased intracranial pressure, vertigo, diplopia, bulging fontanels in children, seizures, and exfoliative dermatitis; it may result in death. In children being treated for vitamin A deficiency according to the protocols outlined above, transient bulging of fontanels occurs in 2% of infants, and transient nausea, vomiting, and headache occur in 5% of preschoolers. Chronic vitamin A intoxication is largely a concern in industrialized countries and has been seen in normal adults who ingest 15 mg/d and children who ingest 6 mg/d of vitamin A over a period of several months. Manifestations include dry skin, cheilosis, glossitis, vomiting, alopecia, bone demineralization and pain, hypercalcemia, lymph node enlargement, hyperlipidemia, amenorrhea, and features of pseudotumor cerebri with increased intracranial pressure and papilledema. Liver fibrosis with portal hypertension and bone demineralization may result from chronic vitamin A intoxication. When vitamin A is provided in excess to pregnant women, congenital malformations have included spontaneous abortions, craniofacial abnormalities, and valvular heart disease. In pregnancy, the daily dose of vitamin A should not exceed 3 mg. Commercially available retinoid derivatives are also toxic, including 13-*cis*-retinoic acid, which has been associated with birth defects. As a result, contraception should be continued for a least 1 year and possibly longer in women who have taken 13-*cis*-retinoic acid.

In malnourished children, vitamin A supplements (100,000–200,000 IU) as a function of age in several rounds over 2 years are considered to amplify nonspecific effects of vaccines. However, for unclear reasons, there may be a negative effect on mortality rates in incompletely vaccinated girls.

High doses of carotenoids do not result in toxic symptoms but should be avoided in smokers due to an increased risk of lung cancer. Very high doses of β-carotene (~200 mg/d) have been used to treat or prevent the skin rashes of erythropoietic protoporphyria. Carotenemia, which is characterized by a yellowing of the skin (creases of the palms and soles) but not the sclerae, may be present after ingestion of >30 mg of β-carotene daily. Hypothyroid patients are particularly susceptible to the development of carotenemia due to impaired breakdown of carotene to vitamin A. Reduction of carotenes from the diet results in the disappearance of skin yellowing and carotenemia over a period of 30–60 days.

■ VITAMIN D

The metabolism of the fat-soluble vitamin D is described in detail in Chap. 352. The biologic effects of this vitamin are mediated by vitamin D receptors, which are found in most tissues, thus potentially expanding vitamin D actions on nearly all cell systems and organs (e.g., immune cells, brain, breast, colon, and prostate) as well as exerting classic endocrine effects on calcium metabolism and bone health. Vitamin D is thought to be important for maintaining normal function of many nonskeletal tissues such as muscle (including heart muscle), immune function, and inflammation as well as cell proliferation and differentiation. Studies have shown that it may be useful as adjunctive treatment for tuberculosis, psoriasis, and multiple sclerosis or for the prevention of certain cancers. Vitamin D insufficiency may increase the risk of Type 1 diabetes mellitus, cardiovascular disease (insulin resistance, hypertension, or low-grade inflammation), or brain dysfunction (e.g., depression). However, the importance of the exact physiologic role of vitamin D in these non skeletal diseases has not been clarified.

A major source of vitamin D is its synthesis in the skin upon ultraviolet B (UV-B) (wavelength, 290–315 nm) exposure.

Except for fish, food (unless fortified) contains only limited amounts of vitamin D. Vitamin D_2 (ergocalciferol) is obtained from plant sources and is the chemical form found in some supplements.

Deficiency

Vitamin D status has been assessed by measuring serum 25-dihydroxyvitamin D [25(OH)$_2$] vitamin D levels; however, there is no consensus on a uniform assay methodology or on optimal serum levels. The optimal level might, in fact, differ according to the targeted disease entity. Based on epidemiologic and experimental data, a 25(OH)$_2$ vitamin D level >20 ng/mL (≥50 nmol/L; to convert ng/mL to nmol/L, multiply by 2.496) is sufficient for good bone health. Some experts advocate higher serum levels (e.g., >30ng/mL) for other desirable endpoints of vitamin D action.

Risk factors for vitamin D deficiency are old age, lack of sun exposure, dark skin (especially among those living in northern latitudes), fat malabsorption, and obesity. Rickets represents the classic disease of vitamin D deficiency. Signs of deficiency are muscle soreness, weakness, and bone pain. Some of these effects are independent of calcium intake.

The U.S. National Academy of Science recently concluded that the majority of North Americans are receiving adequate amounts of vitamin D (RDA = 15 μg/d or 600 IU/d; Chap. 73). However, for people older than 70 years, the RDA is set at 20 μg/d (800 IU/d). The consumption of fortified or enriched foods as well as suberythemal sun exposure should be encouraged for people at risk for vitamin D deficiency. If an adequate intake cannot be achieved, vitamin D supplements should be taken, especially during the winter months. Vitamin D deficiency can be treated by the oral administration of 50,000 IU/week for 6–8 weeks followed by a maintenance dose of 800 IU/d (100 μg/d) from food and supplements after achievement of normal plasma levels. The physiologic effects of vitamin D_2 and D_3 are identical when ingested over long periods.

Toxicity

The upper limit of intake has been set at 4000 IU/d. Contrary to earlier beliefs, acute vitamin D intoxication is rare and usually is caused by the uncontrolled and excessive ingestion of supplements or faulty food fortification practices. High plasma 1,25(OH)$_2$ vitamin D and high plasma calcium levels are central features of toxicity. Stopping vitamin D and calcium supplements is mandatory, and treatment of hypercalcemia may be required.

■ VITAMIN E

Vitamin E is a collective name for all stereoisomers of tocopherols and tocotrienols, although only the *RR* tocopherols meet human requirements. Vitamin E acts as a chain-breaking antioxidant and is an efficient pyroxyl radical scavenger that protects low-density lipoproteins (LDLs) and polyunsaturated fats in membranes from oxidation. A network of other antioxidants (e.g., vitamin C, glutathione) and enzymes maintains vitamin E in a reduced state. Vitamin E also inhibits prostaglandin synthesis and the activities of protein kinase C and phospholipase A_2.

Absorption and metabolism

After absorption, vitamin E is taken up from chylomicrons by the liver, and a hepatic α-tocopherol transport protein mediates intracellular vitamin E transport and incorporation into very low density lipoprotein (VLDL). The transport protein has particular affinity for the *RRR* isomeric form of α-tocopherol; thus, this natural isomer has the most biologic activity.

Requirement

Vitamin E is widely distributed in the food supply and is particularly high in sunflower oil, safflower oil, and wheat germ oil; γ-tocotrienols are notably present in soybean and corn oils. Vitamin E is also found in meats, nuts, and cereal grains, and small amounts are present in fruits and vegetables. Vitamin E pills containing doses of 50–1000 mg are ingested by about 10% of the U.S. population. The RDA for vitamin E is 15 mg/d (34.9 μmol or 22.5 IU) for all adults. Diets high in polyunsaturated fats may necessitate a slightly higher intake of vitamin E.

Dietary deficiency of vitamin E does not exist. Vitamin E deficiency is seen in only severe and prolonged malabsorptive diseases, such as celiac disease, or after small-intestinal resection. Children with cystic fibrosis or prolonged cholestasis may develop vitamin E deficiency characterized by areflexia and hemolytic anemia. Children with abetalipoproteinemia cannot absorb or transport vitamin E and become deficient quite rapidly. A familial form of isolated vitamin E deficiency also exists; it is due to a defect in the α-tocopherol transport protein. Vitamin E deficiency causes axonal degeneration of the large myelinated axons and results in posterior column and spinocerebellar symptoms. Peripheral neuropathy is initially characterized by areflexia, with progression to an ataxic gait, and by decreased vibration and position sensations. Ophthalmoplegia, skeletal myopathy, and pigmented retinopathy may also be features of vitamin E deficiency. Either vitamin E or selenium deficiency in the host has been shown to increase certain viral mutations and, therefore, virulence. The laboratory diagnosis of vitamin E deficiency is made on the basis of low blood levels of α-tocopherol (<5 μg/mL, or <0.8 mg of α-tocopherol per gram of total lipids).

TREATMENT   Vitamin E Deficiency

Symptomatic vitamin E deficiency should be treated with 800–1200 mg of α-tocopherol per day. Patients with abetalipoproteinemia may need as much as 5000–7000 mg/d. Children with symptomatic vitamin E deficiency should be treated with 400 mg/d orally of water-miscible esters; alternatively, 2 mg/kg per d may be administered intramuscularly. Vitamin E in high doses may protect against oxygen-induced retrolental fibroplasia and bronchopulmonary dysplasia as well as intraventricular hemorrhage of prematurity. Vitamin E has been suggested to increase sexual performance, treat intermittent claudication, and slow the aging process, but evidence for these properties is lacking. When given in combination with other antioxidants, vitamin E may help prevent macular degeneration. High doses (60–800 mg/d) of vitamin E have been shown in controlled trials to improve parameters of immune function and reduce colds in nursing home residents, but intervention studies using vitamin E to prevent cardiovascular disease or cancer have not shown efficacy, and at doses >400 mg/d, vitamin E may even increase all-cause mortality rates.

Toxicity

All forms of vitamin E are absorbed and could contribute to toxicity. *High* doses of vitamin E (>800 mg/d) may reduce platelet aggregation and interfere with vitamin K metabolism and are therefore contraindicated in patients taking warfarin and antiplatelet agents (such as aspirin or clopidogrel). Nausea, flatulence, and diarrhea have been reported at doses >1 g/d.

■ VITAMIN K

There are two natural forms of vitamin K: vitamin K₁, also known as *phylloquinone*, from vegetable and animal sources, and vitamin K₂, or *menaquinone*, which is synthesized by bacterial flora and found in hepatic tissue. Phylloquinone can be converted to menaquinone in some organs.

Vitamin K is required for the posttranslational carboxylation of glutamic acid, which is necessary for calcium binding to γ-carboxylated proteins such as prothrombin (factor II); factors VII, IX, and X; protein C; protein S; and proteins found in bone (osteocalcin) and vascular smooth muscle (e.g., matrix Gla protein). However, the importance of vitamin K for bone mineralization and prevention of vascular calcification is not known. Warfarin-type drugs inhibit γ-carboxylation by preventing the conversion of vitamin K to its active hydroquinone form.

Dietary sources

Vitamin K is found in green leafy vegetables such as kale and spinach, and appreciable amounts are also present in margarine and liver. Vitamin K is present in vegetable oils; olive, canola, and soybean oils are particularly rich sources. The average daily intake by Americans is estimated to be approximately 100 μg/d.

Deficiency

The symptoms of vitamin K deficiency are due to hemorrhage, and newborns are particularly susceptible because of low fat stores, low breast milk levels of vitamin K, sterility of the infantile intestinal tract, liver immaturity, and poor placental transport. Intracranial bleeding, as well as gastrointestinal and skin bleeding, can occur in vitamin K–deficient infants 1–7 days after birth. Thus, vitamin K (1 mg IM) is given prophylactically at the time of delivery.

Vitamin K deficiency in adults may be seen in patients with chronic small-intestinal disease (e.g., celiac disease, Crohn's disease), in those with obstructed biliary tracts, or after small-bowel resection. Broad-spectrum antibiotic treatment can precipitate vitamin K deficiency by reducing gut bacteria, which synthesize menaquinones, and by inhibiting the metabolism of vitamin K. In patients with warfarin therapy, the antiobesity drug orlistat can lead to international normalized ratio (INR) changes due to vitamin K malabsorption. The diagnosis of vitamin K deficiency usually is made on the basis of an elevated prothrombin time or reduced clotting factors, although vitamin K may also be measured directly by HPLC. Vitamin K deficiency is treated by using a parenteral dose of 10 mg. For patients with chronic malabsorption, 1–2 mg/d of vitamin K should be given orally, or 1–2 mg/week can be taken parenterally. Patients with liver disease may have an elevated prothrombin time because of liver cell destruction as well as vitamin K deficiency. If an elevated prothrombin time does not improve on vitamin K therapy, it can be deduced that it is not the result of vitamin K deficiency.

Toxicity

Toxicity from dietary phylloquinones and menaquinones has not been described. High doses of vitamin K can impair the actions of oral anticoagulants.

MINERALS

Table 74-2.

■ CALCIUM

See Chap. 352.

■ ZINC

Zinc is an integral component of many metalloenzymes in the body; it is involved in the synthesis and stabilization of proteins, DNA, and RNA and plays a structural role in ribosomes and membranes.

Zinc is necessary for the binding of steroid hormone receptors and several other transcription factors to DNA. Zinc is absolutely required for normal spermatogenesis, fetal growth, and embryonic development.

Absorption

The absorption of zinc from the diet is inhibited by dietary phytate, fiber, oxalate, iron, and copper, as well as by certain drugs, including penicillamine, sodium valproate, and ethambutol. Meat, shellfish, nuts, and legumes are good sources of bioavailable zinc, whereas zinc in grains and legumes is less available for absorption.

Deficiency

Mild zinc deficiency has been described in many diseases, including diabetes mellitus, HIV/AIDS, cirrhosis, alcoholism, inflammatory bowel disease, malabsorption syndromes, and sickle cell disease. In these diseases, mild chronic zinc deficiency can cause stunted growth in children, decreased taste sensation (hypogeusia), and impaired immune function. Severe chronic zinc deficiency has been described as a cause of hypogonadism and dwarfism in several Middle Eastern countries. In these children, hypopigmented hair is also part of the syndrome. Acrodermatitis enteropathica is a rare autosomal recessive disorder characterized by abnormalities in zinc absorption. Clinical manifestations include diarrhea, alopecia, muscle wasting, depression, irritability, and a rash involving the extremities, face, and perineum. The rash is characterized by vesicular and pustular crusting with scaling and erythema. Occasional patients with Wilson's disease have developed zinc deficiency as a consequence of penicillamine therapy (Chap. 360).

The diagnosis of zinc deficiency is usually made by a serum zinc level <12 µmol/L (<70 µg/dL). Pregnancy and birth control pills may cause a slight depression in serum zinc levels, and hypoalbuminemia from any cause can result in hypozincemia. In acute stress situations, zinc may be redistributed from serum into tissues. Zinc deficiency may be treated with 60 mg elemental zinc, orally twice a day. Zinc gluconate lozenges (13 mg elemental zinc every 2 h while awake) have been reported to reduce the duration and symptoms of the common cold in adults, but studies are conflicting.

Zinc deficiency is prevalent in many developing countries and usually coexists with other micronutrient deficiencies (especially iron). Zinc (20 mg/d) may be an effective adjunctive therapeutic strategy for diarrheal disease and pneumonia in children.

Toxicity

Acute zinc toxicity after oral ingestion causes nausea, vomiting, and fever. Zinc fumes from welding may also be toxic and cause fever, respiratory distress, excessive salivation, sweating, and headache. Chronic large doses of zinc may depress immune function and cause hypochromic anemia as a result of copper deficiency. Intranasal zinc preparations should be avoided because they may lead to irreversible damage of nasal mucosa and anosmia.

■ COPPER

Copper is an integral part of numerous enzyme systemsz, including amine oxidases, ferroxidase (ceruloplasmin), cytochrome-*c* oxidase, superoxide dismutase, and dopamine hydroxylase. Copper is also a component of ferroprotein, a transport protein involved in the basolateral transfer of iron during absorption from the enterocyte. As such, copper plays a role in iron metabolism, melanin synthesis, energy production, neurotransmitter synthesis, and CNS function; the synthesis and cross-linking of elastin and collagen; and the scavenging of superoxide radicals.

Dietary sources of copper include shellfish, liver, nuts, legumes, bran, and organ meats.

Deficiency

Dietary copper deficiency is relatively rare, although it has been described in premature infants who are fed milk diets and in infants with malabsorption (Table 74-2). Copper-deficiency anemia has been reported in patients with malabsorptive diseases and nephrotic syndrome and in patients treated for Wilson's disease with chronic high doses of oral zinc, which can interfere with copper absorption. Menkes' kinky hair syndrome is an X-linked metabolic disturbance of copper metabolism characterized by mental retardation, hypocupremia, and decreased circulating ceruloplasmin (Chap. 363). It is caused by mutations in the copper-transporting *ATP7A* gene. Children with this disease often die within 5 years because of dissecting aneurysms or cardiac rupture. Aceruloplasminemia is a rare autosomal recessive disease characterized by tissue iron overload, mental deterioration, microcytic anemia, and low serum iron and copper concentrations.

The diagnosis of copper deficiency is usually made on the basis of low serum levels of copper (<65 µg/dL) and low ceruloplasmin levels (<20 mg/dL). Serum levels of copper may be elevated in pregnancy or stress conditions since ceruloplasmin is an acute-phase reactant and 90% of circulating copper is bound to ceruloplasmin.

Toxicity

Copper toxicity is usually accidental (Table 74-2). In severe cases, kidney failure, liver failure, and coma may ensue. In Wilson's disease, mutations in the copper-transporting *ATP7B* gene lead to accumulation of copper in the liver and brain, with low blood levels due to decreased ceruloplasmin (Chap. 360).

■ SELENIUM

Selenium, in the form of selenocysteine, is a component of the enzyme glutathione peroxidase, which serves to protect proteins, cell membranes, lipids, and nucleic acids from oxidant molecules. As such, selenium is being actively studied as a chemopreventive agent against certain cancers, such as prostate cancer. Selenocysteine is also found in the deiodinase enzymes, which mediate the deiodination of thyroxine to triiodothyronine (Chap. 341). Rich dietary sources of selenium include seafood, muscle meat, and cereals, although the selenium content of cereal is determined by the soil concentration. Countries with low soil concentrations include parts of Scandinavia, China, and New Zealand. *Keshan disease* is an endemic cardiomyopathy found in children and young women residing in regions of China where dietary intake of selenium is low (<20 µg/d). Concomitant deficiencies of iodine and selenium may worsen the clinical manifestations of cretinism. Chronic ingestion of high amounts of selenium leads to selenosis, characterized by hair and nail brittleness and loss, garlic breath odor, skin rash, myopathy, irritability, and other abnormalities of the nervous system.

■ CHROMIUM

Chromium potentiates the action of insulin in patients with impaired glucose tolerance, presumably by increasing insulin receptor–mediated signaling, although its usefulness in treating Type 2 diabetes is uncertain. In addition, improvement in blood lipid profiles has been reported in some patients. The usefulness of chromium supplements in muscle building has not been substantiated. Rich food sources of chromium include yeast, meat, and grain products. Chromium in the trivalent state is found in supplements and is largely nontoxic; however, chromium-6 is a product of stainless steel welding and is a known pulmonary carcinogen as well as a cause of liver, kidney, and CNS damage.

■ MAGNESIUM

See Chap. 352.

■ FLUORIDE, MANGANESE, AND ULTRATRACE ELEMENTS

An essential function for fluoride in humans has not been described, although it is useful for the maintenance of structure in teeth and bone. Adult fluorosis results in mottled and pitted defects in tooth enamel as well as brittle bone (skeletal fluorosis).

Manganese and molybdenum deficiencies have been reported in patients with rare genetic abnormalities and in a few patients receiving prolonged total parenteral nutrition. Several manganese-specific enzymes have been identified (e.g., manganese superoxide dismutase). Deficiencies of manganese have been reported to result in bone demineralization, poor growth, ataxia, disturbances in carbohydrate and lipid metabolism, and convulsions.

Ultratrace elements are defined as those needed in amounts <1 mg/d. Essentiality has not been established for most ultratrace elements, although selenium, chromium, and iodine are clearly essential (Chap. 341). *Molybdenum* is necessary for the activity of sulfite and xanthine oxidase, and molybdenum deficiency may result in skeletal and brain lesions.

FURTHER READINGS

AASHEIM ET et al: Vitamin status after bariatric surgery: A randomized study of gastric bypass and duodenal switch. Am J Clin Nutr 90:15, 2009

BOOTH SL: Roles for vitamin K beyond coagulation. Annu Rev Nutr 29:89, 2009

HOLICK MF: Deficiency of sunlight and vitamin D. BMJ 336:1318, 2008

LICHTENSTEIN AH, RUSSELL RM: Essential nutrients: Food or supplements? Where should the emphasis be? JAMA 294:351, 2005

NEUHOUSER ML et al. Multivitamin use and risk of cancer and cardiovascular disease in the Women's Health Initiative Cohorts. Arch Intern Med 169:294, 2009

PENNISTON KL, TANUMIHARDJO SA: The acute and chronic toxic effects of vitamin A. Am J Clin Nutr 83:191, 2006

ROSS AC et al (eds): *Dietary Reference Intakes for Calcium and Vitamin D.* Washington, DC, The National Academies Press, 2011

TANG G et al: Golden Rice is an effective source of vitamin A. Am J Clin Nutr 89:1776, 2009

ZEISEL SH, DA COSTA KA: Choline: An essential nutrient for public health. Nutr Rev 67:615, 2009

CHAPTER **75**

Malnutrition and Nutritional Assessment

Douglas C. Heimburger

Malnutrition can arise from primary or secondary causes, with the former resulting from inadequate or poor-quality food intake and the latter from diseases that alter food intake or nutrient requirements, metabolism, or absorption. Primary malnutrition occurs mainly in developing countries and under conditions of political unrest, war, or famine. Secondary malnutrition, the main form encountered in industrialized countries, was largely unrecognized until the early 1970s, when it was appreciated that persons with adequate food supplies can become malnourished as a result of acute or chronic diseases that alter nutrient intake or metabolism, particularly diseases that cause acute or chronic inflammation. Various studies have shown that protein-energy malnutrition (PEM) affects one-third to one-half of patients on general medical and surgical wards in teaching hospitals. The consistent finding that nutritional status influences patient prognosis underscores the importance of preventing, detecting, and treating malnutrition.

PROTEIN-ENERGY MALNUTRITION

Definitions for forms of PEM are in flux. Traditionally, the two major types of PEM have been *marasmus* and *kwashiorkor*. These conditions are compared in Table 75-1. Marasmus has been considered the end result of a long-term deficit of dietary energy, whereas kwashiorkor has been understood to result from a protein-poor diet.

Although the former concept remains essentially correct, evidence is accumulating that PEM syndromes are distinguished by two main features: dietary intake and underlying inflammatory processes. Energy-poor diets with minimal inflammation cause gradual erosion of body mass, resulting in classic marasmus. By contrast, inflammation from acute illnesses such as injury or sepsis and chronic illnesses such as cancer, lung or heart disease, and HIV can erode lean body mass even in the presence of relatively sufficient dietary intake, leading to a kwashiorkor-like state. Quite often, inflammatory illnesses impair appetite and dietary intake, producing combinations of the two.

An international consensus committee has proposed the following revised definitions. *Starvation-related malnutrition* is suggested for instances of chronic starvation without inflammation, *chronic disease–related malnutrition* when inflammation is chronic and of mild to moderate degree, and *acute disease– or injury-related malnutrition* when inflammation is acute and of a severe degree. However, because distinguishing diagnostic criteria for these conditions have not been elaborated, this chapter outlines criteria that have served well and are embedded in the medical literature.

■ MARASMUS OR CACHEXIA

Marasmus is a state in which virtually all available body fat stores have been exhausted due to starvation. Cachexia is a state that involves substantial loss of lean body mass due to chronic systemic inflammation. Conditions that produce cachexia in high-income countries tend to be chronic and indolent, such as cancer and chronic pulmonary disease, whereas marasmus occurs in patients with anorexia nervosa. These conditions are relatively easy to detect because of the patient's starved appearance. The diagnosis is based on fat and muscle wastage resulting from prolonged calorie deficiency and/or inflammation. Diminished skinfold thickness reflects the loss of fat reserves; reduced arm muscle circumference with temporal and interosseous muscle wasting reflects the catabolism of protein throughout the body, including vital organs such as the heart, liver, and kidneys.

TABLE 75-1 Comparison of Marasmus/Cachexia and Kwashiorkor/Protein-Calorie Malnutrition

	Marasmus or Cachexia	Kwashiorkor or Protein-Calorie Malnutrition[a]
Clinical setting	↓ Energy intake	↓ Protein intake during stress state
Time course to develop	Months or years	Weeks
Clinical features	Starved appearance	Well-nourished appearance
	Weight <80% standard for height	Easy hair pluckability[b]
	Triceps skinfold <3 mm	Edema
	Midarm muscle circumference <15 cm	
Laboratory findings	Creatinine-height index <60% standard	Serum albumin <2.8 g/dL
		Total iron-binding capacity <200 μg/dL
		Lymphocytes <1500/μL
		Anergy
Clinical course	Reasonably preserved responsiveness to short-term stress	Infections
		Poor wound healing, decubitus ulcers, skin breakdown
Mortality	Low unless related to underlying disease	High
Diagnostic criteria	Triceps skinfold <3 mm	Serum albumin <2.8 g/dL
	Midarm muscle circumference <15 cm	At least one of the following:
		Poor wound healing, decubitus ulcers, or skin breakdown
		Easy hair pluckability[b]
		Edema

[a]The findings used to diagnose kwashiorkor must be unexplained by other causes.

[b]Tested by *firmly* pulling a lock of hair from the top (not the sides or back), grasping with the thumb and forefinger. An average of three or more hairs removed easily and painlessly is considered abnormal hair pluckability.

Routine laboratory findings in cachexia/marasmus are relatively unremarkable. The creatinine-height index (24-h urinary creatinine excretion compared with normal values based on height) is low, reflecting the loss of muscle mass. Occasionally, the serum albumin level is reduced, but it stays above 2.8 g/dL in uncomplicated cases. Despite a morbid appearance, immunocompetence, wound healing, and the ability to handle short-term stress are reasonably well preserved in most patients.

Pure starvation-related malnutrition is a chronic, fairly well adapted form of starvation rather than an acute illness; it should be treated cautiously in an attempt to reverse the downward trend gradually. Although nutritional support is necessary, overly aggressive repletion can result in severe, even life-threatening metabolic imbalances such as hypophosphatemia and cardiorespiratory failure (refeeding syndrome). When possible, oral or enteral nutritional support is preferred; treatment started slowly allows readaptation of metabolic and intestinal functions (Chap. 76).

■ KWASHIORKOR OR PROTEIN-CALORIE MALNUTRITION (PCM)

By contrast, kwashiorkor or PCM in developed countries occurs mainly in connection with acute, life-threatening illnesses such as trauma and sepsis. The physiologic stress produced by these illnesses increases protein and energy requirements at a time when intake is often limited. A classic scenario for PCM is an acutely stressed patient who receives only 5% dextrose solutions for periods as brief as 2 weeks; this gives rise to the proposed term *acute disease– or injury-related malnutrition*. Although the etiologic mechanisms are not fully known, the protein-sparing response normally seen in starvation is blocked by the stressed state and by carbohydrate infusion.

In its early stages, the physical findings of kwashiorkor/PCM are few and subtle. Fat reserves and muscle mass are initially unaffected, giving the deceptive appearance of adequate nutrition. Signs that support the diagnosis of kwashiorkor/PCM include easy hair pluckability, edema, skin breakdown, and poor wound healing. The major sine qua non is severe reduction of levels of serum proteins such as albumin (<2.8 g/dL) and transferrin (<150 mg/dL) or iron-binding capacity (<200 μg/dL). Cellular immune function is depressed, reflected by lymphopenia (<1500 lymphocytes/μL in adults and older children) and lack of response to skin test antigens (anergy).

The prognosis of adult patients with full-blown kwashiorkor/PCM is not good even with aggressive nutritional support. Surgical wounds often dehisce (fail to heal), pressure sores develop, gastroparesis and diarrhea can occur with enteral feeding, the risk of gastrointestinal bleeding from stress ulcers is increased, host defenses are compromised, and death from overwhelming infection may occur despite antibiotic therapy. Unlike treatment in marasmus, aggressive nutritional support is indicated to restore better metabolic balance rapidly (Chap. 76). Although kwashiorkor in children is less foreboding, perhaps because a lesser degree of stress is required to precipitate the disorder, it is still a serious condition.

■ PHYSIOLOGIC CHARACTERISTICS OF HYPOMETABOLIC AND HYPERMETABOLIC STATES

The metabolic characteristics and nutritional needs of hypermetabolic patients who are stressed from injury, infection, or chronic

TABLE 75-2 Physiologic Characteristics of Hypometabolic and Hypermetabolic States

Physiologic Characteristics	Hypometabolic, Nonstressed Patient (Marasmic)	Hypermetabolic, Stressed Patient (Kwashiorkor Risk*)
Cytokines, catecholamines, glucagon, cortisol, insulin	↓	↑
Metabolic rate, O$_2$ consumption	↓	↑
Proteolysis, gluconeogenesis	↓	↑
Ureagenesis, urea excretion	↓	↑
Fat catabolism, fatty acid utilization	Relative ↑	Absolute ↑
Adaptation to starvation	Normal	Abnormal

*These changes characterize the stressed, kwashiorkor-risk patient seen in developed countries; they differ in some respects from the characteristics of primary kwashiorkor seen in developing countries.

inflammatory illness differ from those of hypometabolic patients who are unstressed but chronically starved. In both cases, nutritional support is important, but misjudgments in selecting the appropriate approach may have serious adverse consequences.

The hypometabolic patient is typified by the relatively less stressed but mildly catabolic and chronically starved individual who, with time, will develop cachexia/marasmus. The hypermetabolic patient stressed from injury or infection is catabolic (experiencing rapid breakdown of body mass) and is at high risk for developing PCM/kwashiorkor if nutritional needs are not met and/or the illness does not resolve quickly. As summarized in Table 75-2, the two states are distinguished by differing perturbations of metabolic rate, rates of protein breakdown (proteolysis), and rates of gluconeogenesis. These differences are mediated by proinflammatory cytokines and counterregulatory hormones—tumor necrosis factor, interleukins 1 and 6, C-reactive protein, catecholamines (epinephrine and norepinephrine), glucagon, and cortisol—that are relatively reduced in hypometabolic patients and increased in hypermetabolic patients. Although insulin levels are also elevated in stressed patients, insulin resistance in the target tissues blocks insulin-mediated anabolic effects.

■ METABOLIC RATE

In starvation and semistarvation, the resting metabolic rate falls between 10 and 30% as an adaptive response to energy restriction, slowing the rate of weight loss. By contrast, resting metabolic rate rises in the presence of physiologic stress in proportion to the degree of the insult. It may increase by about 10% after elective surgery, 20–30% after bone fractures, 30–60% with severe infections such as peritonitis or gram-negative septicemia, and as much as 110% after major burns.

If the metabolic rate (energy requirement) is not matched by energy intake, weight loss results, slowly in hypometabolism and quickly in hypermetabolism. Losses of up to 10% of body mass are unlikely to be detrimental; however, losses greater than this in acutely ill hypermetabolic patients may be associated with rapid deterioration in body function.

■ PROTEIN CATABOLISM

The rate of endogenous protein breakdown (catabolism) to supply energy needs normally falls during uncomplicated energy deprivation. After about 10 days of total starvation, an unstressed individual loses about 12–18 g/d protein (equivalent to approximately 2 oz of muscle tissue or 2–3 g of nitrogen). By contrast, in injury and sepsis, protein breakdown accelerates in proportion to the degree of stress, reaching 30–60 g/d after elective surgery, 60–90 g/d with infection, 100–130 g/d with severe sepsis or skeletal trauma, and >175 g/d with major burns or head injuries. These losses are reflected by proportional increases in the excretion of urea nitrogen, the major by-product of protein breakdown.

■ GLUCONEOGENESIS

The major aim of protein catabolism during a state of starvation is to provide the glucogenic amino acids (especially alanine and glutamine) that serve as substrates for endogenous glucose production (gluconeogenesis) in the liver. In the hypometabolic/starved state, protein breakdown for gluconeogenesis is minimized, especially as ketones derived from fatty acids become the substrate preferred by certain tissues. In the hypermetabolic/stress state, gluconeogenesis increases dramatically and in proportion to the degree of the insult to increase the supply of glucose (the major fuel of reparation). Glucose is the only fuel that can be utilized by hypoxemic tissues (anaerobic glycolysis), white blood cells, and newly generated fibroblasts. Infusions of glucose partially offset a negative energy balance but do not significantly suppress the high rates of gluconeogenesis in catabolic patients. Hence, adequate supplies of protein are needed to replace the amino acids utilized for this metabolic response.

In summary, a hypometabolic patient is adapted to starvation and conserves body mass by reducing the metabolic rate and using fat as the primary fuel (rather than glucose and its precursor amino acids). A hypermetabolic patient also uses fat as a fuel but rapidly breaks down body protein to produce glucose, causing loss of muscle and organ tissue and endangering vital body functions.

MICRONUTRIENT MALNUTRITION

The same illnesses and reductions in nutrient intake that lead to PEM often produce deficiencies of vitamins and minerals as well (Chap. 74). Deficiencies of nutrients that are stored in small amounts (such as the water-soluble vitamins) are lost through external secretions, such as zinc in diarrhea fluid or burn exudate, and are probably more common than generally recognized.

Deficiencies of vitamin C, folic acid, and zinc are reasonably common in sick patients. Signs of scurvy such as corkscrew hairs on the lower extremities are found frequently in chronically ill and/or alcoholic patients. The diagnosis can be confirmed with plasma vitamin C levels. Folic acid intakes and blood levels are often less than optimal, even among healthy persons; when illness, alcoholism, poverty, or poor dentition is present, these deficiencies are common. Low blood zinc levels are prevalent in patients with malabsorption syndromes such as inflammatory bowel disease. Patients with zinc deficiency often exhibit poor wound healing, pressure ulcer formation, and impaired immunity. Thiamine deficiency is a common complication of alcoholism but may be prevented by therapeutic doses of thiamine in patients treated for alcohol abuse.

Patients with low plasma vitamin C levels usually respond to the doses in multivitamin preparations, but patients with deficiencies should be supplemented with 250–500 mg/d. Folic acid is absent from some oral multivitamin preparations; patients with deficiencies should be supplemented with about 1 mg/d. Patients with zinc deficiencies resulting from large external losses sometimes require oral supplementation with 220 mg of zinc sulfate one to three times daily. For these reasons, laboratory assessments of the micronutrient status of patients at high risk are desirable.

Hypophosphatemia develops in hospitalized patients with remarkable frequency and generally results from rapid intracellular shifts of phosphate in cachectic or alcoholic patients receiving intravenous glucose (Chap. 45). The adverse clinical sequelae are numerous; some, such as acute cardiopulmonary failure, are collectively called refeeding syndrome and can be life-threatening.

GLOBAL CONSIDERATIONS

Many developing countries are still faced with high prevalences of the classic forms of PEM: marasmus and kwashiorkor. *Food insecurity*, which characterizes many poor countries, prevents consistent dietary sufficiency and/or quality and leads to endemic or cyclic malnutrition. Factors threatening food security include marked seasonal variations in agricultural productivity (rainy season–dry season cycles), periodic droughts, political unrest or injustice, and disease epidemics, especially HIV/AIDS. The coexistence of malnutrition and disease epidemics exacerbates the latter and increases complications and mortality rates, creating vicious cycles of malnutrition and disease.

As economic prosperity improves, developing countries have been observed to undergo an epidemiologic transition, a component of which has been termed the *nutrition transition*. As improved economic resources make greater dietary diversity possible, middle-income populations (e.g., southern Asia, China, and Latin America) typically begin to adopt lifestyle habits of industrialized nations, with increased consumption of energy and fat and decreased levels of physical activity. This leads to rising levels of obesity, metabolic syndrome, diabetes, cardiovascular disease, and cancer, sometimes coexisting in populations with persistent undernutrition.

Micronutrient deficiencies also remain prevalent in many countries of the world, impairing functional status and productivity and increasing mortality rates. Vitamin A deficiency affects perhaps 20% of the world's population, impairing vision and increasing morbidity and mortality rates from infections, for example, measles. Community vitamin A supplementation programs have significantly reduced measles mortality rates in vulnerable populations. Mild to moderate iron deficiency may be prevalent in up to 50% of the world, resulting from poor dietary diversity coupled with periodic blood loss and pregnancies. Iodine deficiency remains prevalent in about 35% of the world's population, causing goiter, hypothyroidism, and cretinism. Zinc deficiency is endemic in many populations, producing growth retardation, hypogonadism, and dermatoses, and impairing wound healing.

NUTRITIONAL ASSESSMENT

Because interactions between illness and nutrition are complex, many physical and laboratory findings reflect both underlying disease and nutritional status. Therefore, the nutritional evaluation of a patient requires an integration of the history, physical examination, anthropometrics, and laboratory studies. This approach helps both to detect nutritional problems and to prevent concluding that isolated findings indicate nutritional problems when they do not. For example, hypoalbuminemia caused by an underlying illness does not necessarily indicate malnutrition.

■ NUTRITIONAL HISTORY

A nutritional history is directed toward identifying underlying mechanisms that put patients at risk for nutritional depletion or excess. These mechanisms include inadequate intake, impaired absorption, decreased utilization, increased losses, and increased requirements of nutrients.

TABLE 75-3 The High-Risk Patient

Underweight (body mass index <18.5) and/or recent loss of ≥10% of usual body mass

Poor intake: anorexia, food avoidance (e.g., psychiatric condition), or NPO status for more than about 5 days

Protracted nutrient losses: malabsorption, enteric fistulas, draining abscesses or wounds, renal dialysis

Hypermetabolic states: sepsis, protracted fever, extensive trauma or burns

Alcohol abuse or use of drugs with antinutrient or catabolic properties: steroids, antimetabolites (e.g., methotrexate), immunosuppressants, antitumor agents

Impoverishment, isolation, advanced age

Individuals with the characteristics listed in Table 75-3 are at particular risk for nutritional deficiencies.

■ PHYSICAL EXAMINATION

Physical findings that suggest vitamin, mineral, and protein-energy deficiencies and excesses are outlined in Table 75-4. Most of the physical findings are not specific for individual nutrient deficiencies and must be integrated with the historic, anthropometric, and laboratory findings. For example, the finding of follicular hyperkeratosis on the back of the arms is a fairly common, normal finding. However, if it is widespread in a person who consumes little fruit and vegetables and smokes regularly (increasing ascorbic acid requirements), vitamin C deficiency is likely. Similarly, easily pluckable hair may be a consequence of chemotherapy, but in a hospitalized patient who has poorly healing surgical wounds and hypoalbuminemia, it suggests PCM/kwashiorkor.

■ ANTHROPOMETRICS

Anthropometric measurements provide information on body muscle mass and fat reserves. The most practical and commonly used measurements are body weight, height, triceps skinfold (TSF), and midarm muscle circumference (MAMC). Body weight is one of the most useful nutritional parameters to follow in patients who are acutely or chronically ill. Unintentional weight loss during illness often reflects loss of lean body mass (muscle and organ tissue), especially if it is rapid and is not caused by diuresis. This can be an ominous sign since it indicates use of vital body protein stores for metabolic fuel. The reference standard for normal body weight, body mass index (BMI: weight in kilograms divided by height, in meters, squared), is discussed in Chap 78. BMIs <18.5 are considered underweight, 18.5–24.9 are normal, 25–29.9 are overweight, and ≥30 are obese.

Measurement of skinfold thickness is useful for estimating body fat stores, because about 50% of body fat is normally in the subcutaneous region. Skinfold thickness can also permit discrimination of fat mass from muscle mass. The TSF is a convenient site that is generally representative of the body's overall fat level. A thickness <3 mm suggests virtually complete exhaustion of fat stores. The MAMC can be used to estimate skeletal muscle mass, calculated as follows:

$$\text{MAMC (cm)} = \text{upper arm circumference (cm)} - [0.314 \times \text{TSF (mm)}]$$

■ LABORATORY STUDIES

A number of laboratory tests used routinely in clinical medicine can yield valuable information about a patient's nutritional status

TABLE 75-4 Physical Findings of Nutritional Deficiencies

Clinical Findings	Possible Deficiency*	Possible Excess
Hair, Nails		
Corkscrew hairs and unemerged coiled hairs	Vitamin C	
Easily pluckable hair	Protein	
Flag sign (transverse depigmentation of hair)	Protein	
Sparse hair	Protein, biotin, zinc	Vitamin A
Transverse ridging of nails	Protein	
Skin		
Cellophane appearance	Protein	
Cracking (flaky paint or crazy pavement dermatosis)	Protein	
Follicular hyperkeratosis	Vitamins A, C	
Petechiae (especially perifollicular)	Vitamin C	
Purpura	Vitamins C, K	
Pigmentation, scaling of sun-exposed areas	Niacin	
Poor wound healing, decubitus ulcers	Protein, vitamin C, zinc	
Scaling	Vitamin A, essential fatty acids, biotin	Vitamin A
	Zinc (hyperpigmented)	Carotene
Yellow pigmentation sparing sclerae (benign)		
Eyes		
Night blindness	Vitamin A	
Papilledema		Vitamin A
Perioral		
Angular stomatitis	Riboflavin, pyridoxine, niacin	
Cheilosis (dry, cracking, ulcerated lips)	Riboflavin, pyridoxine, niacin	

Clinical Findings	Possible Deficiency*	Possible Excess
Oral		
Atrophic lingual papillae (slick tongue)	Riboflavin, niacin, folate, vitamin B_{12}, protein, iron	
Glossitis (scarlet, raw tongue)	Riboflavin, niacin, pyridoxine, folate, vitamin B_{12}	
Hypogeusesthesia, hyposmia	Zinc	
Swollen, retracted, bleeding gums (if teeth present)	Vitamin C	
Bones, Joints		
Beading of ribs, epiphyseal swelling, bowlegs	Vitamin D	
Tenderness, subperiosteal hemorrhage in children	Vitamin C	
Neurologic		
Confabulation, disorientation	Thiamine (Korsakoff's psychosis)	
Drowsiness, lethargy, vomiting		Vitamin A
Dementia	Niacin, vitamin B_{12}, folate	
Headache		Vitamin A
Ophthalmoplegia	Thiamine, phosphorus	
Peripheral neuropathy (e.g., weakness, paresthesias, ataxia, footdrop, and decreased tendon reflexes, fine tactile sense, vibratory sense, and position sense)	Thiamine, pyridoxine, vitamin B_{12}	Pyridoxine
Tetany	Calcium, magnesium	
Other		
Edema	Protein, thiamine	
Heart failure	Thiamine ("wet" beriberi), phosphorus	
Hepatomegaly	Protein	Vitamin A
Parotid enlargement	Protein (consider also bulimia)	
Sudden heart failure, death	Vitamin C	

*In this table, "protein deficiency" is used to signify kwashiorkor/PCM.

if a slightly different approach to their interpretation is used. For example, abnormally low serum albumin levels, total iron-binding capacity, and anergy may have a distinct explanation, but collectively they may represent kwashiorkor. In the clinical setting of a hypermetabolic, acutely ill patient who is edematous and has easily pluckable hair and inadequate protein intake, the diagnosis of PCM/kwashiorkor is clear-cut. Commonly used laboratory tests for assessing nutritional status are outlined in Table 75-5. The table also provides tips to avoid assigning nutritional significance to tests that may be abnormal for nonnutritional reasons.

Assessment of circulating (visceral) proteins

The serum proteins most commonly used to assess nutritional status include albumin, total iron-binding capacity (or transferrin), thyroxine-binding prealbumin (or transthyretin), and retinol-binding protein. Because they have differing synthesis rates and

TABLE 75-5 Laboratory Tests for Nutritional Assessment

Test (Normal Values)	Nutritional Use	Causes of Normal Value Despite Malnutrition	Other Causes of Abnormal Value
Serum albumin (3.5–5.5 g/dL)	2.8–3.5: Compromised protein status <2.8: Possible kwashiorkor Increasing value reflects positive protein balance	Dehydration Infusion of albumin, fresh-frozen plasma, or whole blood	**Low** Common: Infection and other stress, especially with poor protein intake Burns, trauma Congestive heart failure Fluid overload Severe liver disease Uncommon: Nephrotic syndrome Zinc deficiency Bacterial stasis/overgrowth of small intestine
Serum prealbumin, also called transthyretin (20–40 mg/dL; lower in prepubertal children)	10–15 mg/dL: Mild protein depletion 5–10 mg/dL: Moderate protein depletion <5 mg/dL: Severe protein depletion Increasing value reflects positive protein balance	Chronic renal failure	Similar to serum albumin
Serum total iron-binding capacity (TIBC) 240–450 µg/dL	<200: Compromised protein status, possible kwashiorkor Increasing value reflects positive protein balance More labile than albumin	Iron deficiency	**Low** Similar to serum albumin **High** Iron deficiency
Prothrombin time 12.0–15.5 s	Prolongation: vitamin K deficiency		**Prolonged** Anticoagulant therapy (warfarin) Severe liver disease
Serum creatinine 0.6–1.6 mg/dL	<0.6: Muscle wasting due to prolonged energy deficit Reflects muscle mass		**High** Despite muscle wasting: Renal failure Severe dehydration
24-h urinary creatinine 500–1200 mg/d (standardized for height and sex)	Low value: muscle wasting due to prolonged energy deficit	>24-h collection Decreasing serum creatinine	**Low** Incomplete urine collection Increasing serum creatinine Neuromuscular wasting
24-h urinary urea nitrogen (UUN) <5 g/d (depends on level of protein intake)	Determine level of catabolism (as long as protein intake is ≥10 g below calculated protein loss or <20 g total, but at least 100 g carbohydrate is provided) 5–10 g/d = mild catabolism or normal fed state 10–15 g/d = moderate catabolism >15 g/d = severe catabolism Estimate protein balance Protein balance = protein intake − protein loss where protein loss (protein catabolic rate) = [24-h UUN (g) + 4] × 6.25 Adjustments required in burn patients and others with large nonurinary nitrogen losses and in patients with fluctuating BUN levels (e.g., renal failure)		

(continued)

TABLE 75-5 Laboratory Tests for Nutritional Assessment (*Continued*)

Test (Normal Values)	Nutritional Use	Causes of Normal Value Despite Malnutrition	Other Causes of Abnormal Value
Blood urea nitrogen (BUN) 8–23 mg/dL	<8: Possibly inadequate protein intake 12–23: Possibly adequate protein intake >23: Possibly excessive protein intake If serum creatinine is normal, use BUN If serum creatinine is elevated, use BUN/creatinine ratio (normal range is essentially the same as for BUN)		**Low** Severe liver disease Anabolic state Syndrome of inappropriate antidiuretic hormone **High** Despite poor protein intake: Renal failure (use BUN/creatinine ratio) Congestive heart failure Gastrointestinal hemorrhage

half-lives—the half-life of serum albumin is about 21 days, whereas those of prealbumin and retinol-binding protein are about 2 days and 12 h, respectively—some of these proteins reflect changes in nutritional status more quickly than do others. However, rapid fluctuations can also make shorter-half-life proteins less reliable.

Levels of circulating proteins are influenced by their rates of synthesis and catabolism, "third spacing" (loss into interstitial spaces), and, in some cases, external loss. Although an adequate intake of calories and protein is necessary to achieve optimal circulating protein levels, serum protein levels generally do not reflect protein intake. For example, a drop in the serum level of albumin or transferrin often accompanies significant physiologic stress (e.g., from infection or injury) and is not necessarily an indication of malnutrition or poor intake. A low serum albumin level in a burned patient with both hypermetabolism and increased dermal losses of protein may not indicate malnutrition. However, adequate nutritional support of the patient's calorie and protein needs is critical for returning circulating proteins to normal levels as stress resolves. Thus low values by themselves do not define malnutrition, but they often point to increased risk of malnutrition because of the hypermetabolic stress state. As long as significant physiologic stress persists, serum protein levels remain low, even with aggressive nutritional support. However, if the levels do not rise after the underlying illness improves, the patient's protein and calorie needs should be reassessed to ensure that intake is sufficient.

Assessment of vitamin and mineral status

The use of laboratory tests to confirm suspected micronutrient deficiencies is desirable because the physical findings for those deficiencies are often equivocal or nonspecific. Low blood micronutrient levels can predate more serious clinical manifestations and also may indicate drug-nutrient interactions.

ESTIMATING ENERGY AND PROTEIN REQUIREMENTS

A patient's basal energy expenditures (BEE, measured in kilocalories per day) can be estimated from height, weight, age, and gender by using the Harris-Benedict equations:

$$\text{Men: BEE} = 66.47 + 13.75W + 5.00H - 6.76A$$
$$\text{Women: BEE} = 655.10 + 9.56W + 1.85H - 4.68A$$

where W is weight in kilograms; H is height in centimeters, and A is age in years. After these equations are solved, total energy requirements are estimated by multiplying BEE by a factor that accounts for the stress of illness. Multiplying by 1.1–1.4 yields a range 10–40% above basal that estimates the 24-h energy expenditure of the majority of patients. The lower value (1.1) is used for patients without evidence of significant physiologic stress; the higher value (1.4) is appropriate for patients with marked stress such as sepsis or trauma. The result is used as a 24-h energy goal for feeding.

When it is important to have a more accurate assessment of energy expenditure, it can be measured at the bedside by using indirect calorimetry. This technique is useful in patients who are believed to be hypermetabolic from sepsis or trauma and whose body weights cannot be obtained accurately. Indirect calorimetry can also be useful in patients who have difficulty weaning from a ventilator, as their energy needs should not be exceeded to avoid excessive CO_2 production. Patients at the extremes of weight (e.g., obese persons) and/or age are good candidates as well, because the Harris-Benedict equations were developed from measurements in adults with roughly normal body weights.

Because urea is a major by-product of protein catabolism, the amount of urea nitrogen excreted each day can be used to estimate the rate of protein catabolism and determine whether protein intake is adequate to offset it. Total protein loss and protein balance can be calculated from urinary urea nitrogen (UUN) as follows:

$$\text{Protein catabolic rate (g/d)} = [24\text{-h UUN (g)} + 4]$$
$$\times 6.25 \text{ (g protein/g nitrogen)}$$

The value of 4 g added to the UUN represents a liberal estimate of the unmeasured nitrogen lost in the urine (e.g., creatinine and uric acid), sweat, hair, skin, and feces. When protein intake is low (e.g., less than about 20 g/d), the equation indicates both the patient's protein requirement and the severity of the catabolic state (Table 75-5). More substantial protein intakes can raise the UUN because some of the ingested (or infused) protein is catabolized and converted to UUN. Thus, at lower protein intakes the equation is useful for estimating *requirements*, and at higher protein intakes it is useful for assessing protein *balance*.

$$\text{Protein balance (g/d)} = \text{protein intake} - \text{protein catabolic rate}$$

FURTHER READINGS

BALES CW, RITCHIE CS (eds): *Handbook of Clinical Nutrition and Aging*, 2nd ed. New York, Humana, 2009

GOTTSCHLICH MM (ed): *The A.S.P.E.N. Nutrition Support Core Curriculum: A Case-Based Approach—The Adult Patient.* Silver Spring, MD, A.S.P.E.N., 2007. Available online at *www.nutritioncare.org*

HEIMBURGER DC, ARD JD (eds): *Handbook of Clinical Nutrition*, 4th ed. Philadelphia, Mosby Elsevier, 2006

JENSEN GL et al: Adult starvation and disease-related malnutrition: A proposal for etiology-based diagnosis in the clinical practice setting from the International Consensus Guideline Committee. J Parenter Enteral Nutr 34:156, 2010

SHILS ME et al (eds): *Modern Nutrition in Health and Disease*, 10th ed. Baltimore, Lippincott Williams & Wilkins, 2005

WEST KP et al: Nutrition, in *International Public Health: Diseases, Programs, Systems, and Policies*, 2nd ed, MH Merson et al (eds). Sudbury, MA, Jones and Bartlett, 2006, pp 207–269

CHAPTER 76

Enteral and Parenteral Nutrition Therapy

Bruce R. Bistrian

David F. Driscoll

The ability to provide specialized nutritional support (SNS) represents a major advance in medical therapy. Nutritional support, via either enteral or parenteral routes, is used in two main settings: (1) to provide adequate nutritional intake during the recuperative phase of illness or injury, when the patient's ability to ingest or absorb nutrients is impaired, and (2) to support the patient during the systemic response to inflammation, injury, or infection during an extended critical illness. SNS is also used in patients with permanent loss of intestinal length or function. In addition, an increasing number of elderly patients living in nursing homes and chronic care facilities receive enteral feeding, usually as a consequence of inadequate nutritional intake.

Enteral refers to feeding via a tube placed into the gut to deliver liquid formulas containing all essential nutrients. *Parenteral* refers to the infusion of complete nutrient solutions into the bloodstream via a peripheral vein or, more commonly, by central venous access to meet nutritional needs. Enteral feeding is generally the preferred route because of benefits derived from maintaining the digestive, absorptive, and immunologic barrier functions of the gastrointestinal tract. Small-bore pliable tubes have largely replaced large-bore rubber tubes, making placement easier and more acceptable to patients. Infusion pumps have also improved the delivery of nutrient solutions.

For short-term use, enteral tubes can be placed via the nose into the stomach, duodenum, or jejunum. For long-term use, these sites can be accessed through the abdominal wall using endoscopic, radiologic, or surgical procedures. Intestinal tolerance of tube feeding may be limited during acute illness by gastric retention or diarrhea. Parenteral feeding has greater risk of infection, reflecting the need for venous access, and a greater propensity for inducing hyperglycemia. However, these risks can generally be managed successfully by SNS teams. For the postoperative patient with preexisting malnutrition, or in trauma patients who were previously well nourished, SNS is cost-effective. In the most critically ill patient in the intensive care unit, SNS can enhance survival. Although enteral nutrition (EN) can be provided by most health care teams caring for hospitalized patients, safe and effective parenteral nutrition (PN) usually requires specialized teams.

Requirements for Specialized Nutritional Support

INDICATIONS FOR SPECIALIZED NUTRITIONAL SUPPORT Although at least 15–20% of patients in acute care hospitals have evidence of significant malnutrition, only a small fraction will benefit from SNS. For others, wasting is an inevitable component of a terminal disease and the course of the disease will not be altered by SNS. The decision to use SNS should be based on the likelihood that preventing protein-calorie malnutrition (PCM) will increase the likelihood of recovery, reduce infection rates, improve healing, or otherwise shorten the hospital stay. In the case of the elderly or chronically ill patient for whom full recovery is not anticipated, the decision to feed is usually based on whether SNS will extend the duration or quality of life. The decision-making process used to assess whether to use SNS is depicted in Fig. 76-1.

The first step in deciding to administer SNS is to consider the nutritional implications of the disease process. Is the condition or its treatment likely to impair food intake and absorption for a prolonged period of time? For example, a well-nourished individual can tolerate approximately 7 days of starvation while experiencing a systemic response to inflammation (SRI). The second step is to determine if the patient is already significantly malnourished to the degree that critical functions such as wound healing, immune responses, or ventilatory function are impaired (Chap. 75). An unintentional weight loss of >10% during the previous 6 months or a weight/height <90% of standard, when associated with physiologic impairment, represents significant PCM. Weight loss >20% of usual or <80% of standard reflects severe PCM. The presence or absence of SRI should be noted, since inflammation, injury, and infection increase the rate of lean tissue loss. SRI also has pathophysiologic effects that influence nutritional responses such as fluid retention and hyperglycemia, as well as impairment of anabolic responses to nutritional support.

Once it is determined that a patient is already or at risk of becoming malnourished, the next step is to decide whether SNS will impact positively on the patient's response to disease. In the end stages of many chronic illnesses with accompanying PCM, particularly those due to cancer or terminal neurologic disorders, nutrition may not reverse the PCM or improve quality of life. While the provision of food and water is part of basic medical care, nutrition delivered by tube or catheter, either enterally or parenterally, is associated with risk and discomfort. Thus, SNS should be recommended only when potential benefits exceed risks, and it should be undertaken with the consent of the patient. Like other life support measures, enteral or parenteral therapy is difficult to withdraw once started. Initiating

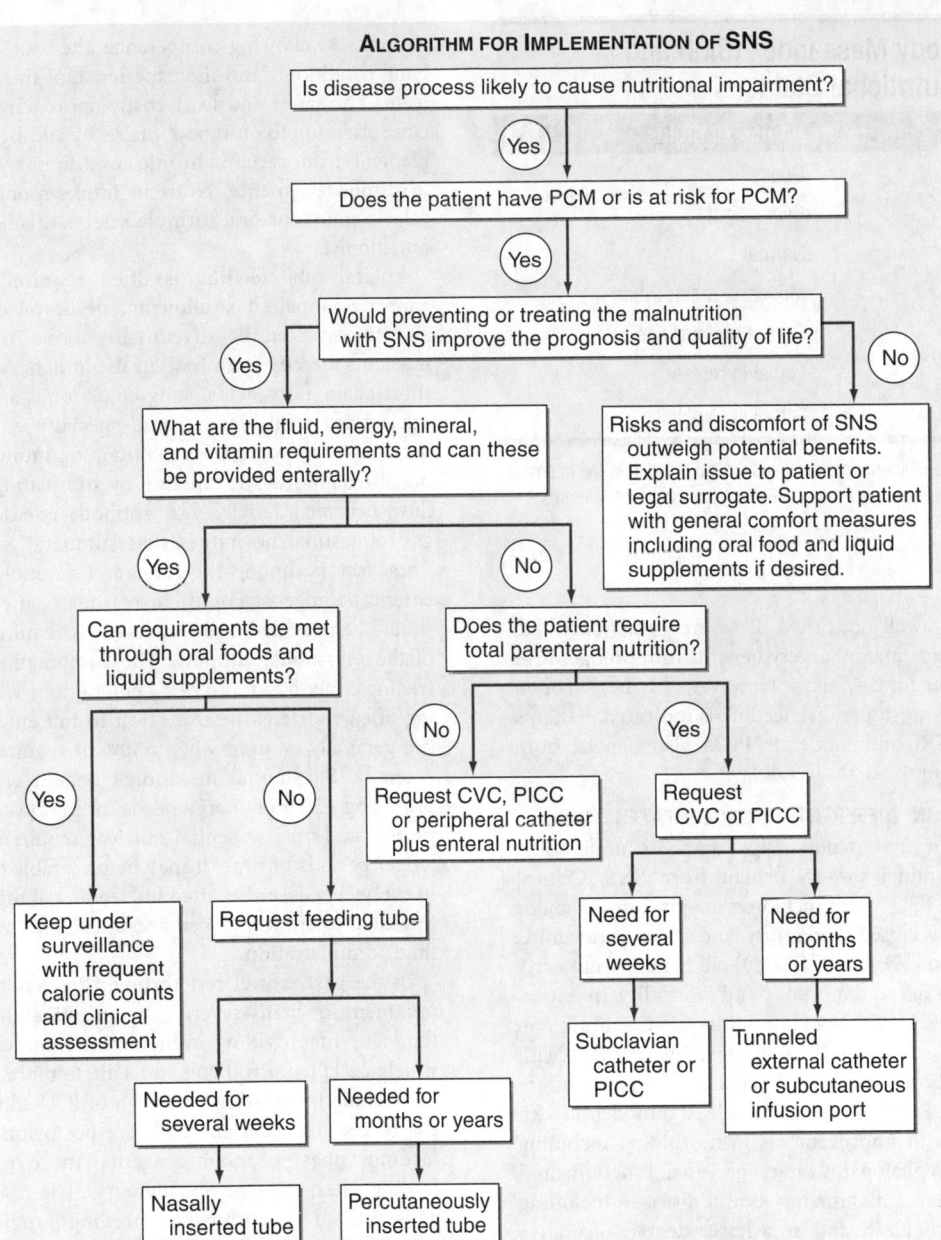

Figure 76-1 Decision-making for the implementation of specialized nutrition support (SNS). CVC, central venous catheter; PICC, peripherally inserted central catheter. *(Adapted from chapter in Harrison's Principles of Internal Medicine, 16e, by Lyn Howard, MD.)*

nutrition support may be appropriate before a final prognosis can be determined, but this should not preclude its subsequent withdrawal. If preventing or treating PCM with SNS is appropriate, nutritional requirements and the method of delivery should be determined. The optimal route depends on the degree of gut function and somewhat on the available technical resources.

The timing of nutritional support is based on evaluation of the preexisting nutritional status, the presence and extent of SRI, and the anticipated clinical course. SRI is identified by the standard clinical signs of leukocytosis, tachycardia, tachypnea, and/or temperature elevation or depression. Although the degree of hypoalbuminemia provides an estimate of SRI severity, normal serum albumin levels will not be restored by adequate nutritional support until the SRI remits, even though nutritional benefits can be achieved by adequate feeding.

The SRI can be graded as severe, moderate, or mild. Examples of severe SRI include sepsis or other inflammatory conditions

like pancreatitis requiring ICU care, multiple trauma with an Injury Severity Score > 20–25 or Acute Physiology and Chronic Health Evaluation II (APACHE II) > 25, closed head injury with a Glasgow Coma Scale < 8, or major third-degree burns of >40% of body surface area. Moderate SRI includes less severe infections, injuries, or inflammatory conditions like pneumonia, major surgery, acute hepatic or renal insufficiency, and exacerbations of ulcerative colitis or regional enteritis requiring hospitalization. PCM should also be defined as severe, moderate, or minimal as assessed by weight/height, percent recent weight loss, and body mass index. The body mass index in relation to nutritional status is listed in Table 76-1. A patient with a severe SRI requires early feeding within the first several days of care because the condition is likely to produce inadequate spontaneous intake over the next 7 days. A moderate SRI, as commonly seen during a postoperative period without oral intake that exceeds 5 days, benefits from adequate feeding by day 5–7 if the

TABLE 76-1 Body Mass Index (BMI) and Nutritional Status

BMI	Nutritional Status
>30 kg/m²	Obese
>25–30 kg/m²	Overweight
20–25 kg/m²	Normal
<18.5 kg/m²	Moderate malnutrition
<16 kg/m²	Severe malnutrition
<13 kg/m²	Lethal in males
<11 kg/m²	Lethal in females

Source: From D Driscoll, B Bistrian: Parenteral and enteral nutrition in the intensive care unit, in *Intensive Care Medicine*, R Irwin, J Rippe (eds). Lippincott Williams & Wilkins, Philadelphia, 2003.

patient was initially well nourished. If severely malnourished, candidates for elective major surgery benefit from preoperative nutritional repletion for 5–7 days. However, this is not often possible. Thus, early postoperative feeding is indicated. Patients with a moderate SRI and moderate PCM also benefit from earlier feeding within the first several days.

EFFICACY OF SNS IN DIFFERENT DISEASE STATES Efficacy studies have shown that malnourished patients undergoing major thoracoabdominal surgery benefit from SNS. Critical illnesses requiring ICU care, including major burns, major trauma, severe sepsis, closed head injury, and severe pancreatitis (positive CT scan and APACHE II > 10), all benefit from early SNS, as indicated by reduced mortality and morbidity. In critical illness, initiation of SNS within 24 h of injury or ICU admission is associated with a ~50% reduction in mortality. Patients with nitrogen accumulation disorders of renal and hepatic failure have a likelihood of PCM of >50% and at least a moderate SRI. SNS is associated with improvements in morbidity, including infection rates, encephalopathy, liver or renal function, and length of hospital stay. Inflammatory bowel disease—including Crohn's disease particularly and, to a lesser degree, ulcerative colitis—often produce PCM. In the outpatient setting, SNS in Crohn's disease can improve nutritional status, quality of life, and the likelihood of remission. With pulmonary disease in the critically ill, SNS improves ventilatory status, and in acute lung injury the use of omega 3 fats as a component of SNS improves gas exchange and respiratory dynamics and reduces the need for mechanical ventilation. Low body mass in chronic obstructive pulmonary disease is associated with diminished pulmonary status and exercise capacity and higher mortality rates. However, there is little convincing evidence that SNS as caloric supplementation improves nutrition or pulmonary function. PCM is also common in the course of cancer and HIV disease, although less so in the latter with the advent of highly active antiretroviral therapy. When PCM develops as a consequence of SRI in these conditions, there is limited likelihood of substantial efficacy or benefit from SNS. However, when PCM develops as a consequence of gastrointestinal dysfunction, SNS can be effective. Although no randomized trials have been performed for SNS provided for hyperemesis gravidarum, there is considerable clinical evidence that it improves pregnancy outcomes.

RISKS AND BENEFITS OF SPECIALIZED NUTRITION SUPPORT The risks are determined primarily by patient factors such as state of alertness, swallowing competence, the route of delivery, underlying conditions, and the experience of the supervising clinical team. The safest and least costly approach is to avoid SNS by close attention to oral food intake, by adding an oral liquid supplement, or in certain chronic conditions by using medications to stimulate appetite. Nutrient intake monitoring by frequent calorie counts or oral formula selection is best performed by a nutritionist.

Enteral tube feeding is often required in patients with anorexia, impaired swallowing, or bowel disease. The bowel and its associated digestive organs derive 70% of their required nutrients directly from food in the lumen. Arginine, glutamine, short-chain fatty acids, long-chain omega 3 fatty acids, and nucleotides available in some specialty enteral formulas are particularly important for maintaining immunity. Enteral feeding also supports gut function by stimulating splanchnic blood flow, neuronal activity, IgA antibody release, and secretion of gastrointestinal hormones that stimulate gut trophic activity. These factors support the gut as an immunologic barrier against enteric pathogens. For these reasons, some luminal nutrition should be provided, even when PN is required to provide most of the nutritional support. The combination of some enteral feeding either by mouth or by enteral tube with parenteral feeding often shortens the transition to full enteral feeding, which can generally be used when >50% of requirements can be met enterally. Substantial nutritional benefit can be achieved by providing ~50% of energy needs for periods of up to 10 days, if protein and other essential nutrient requirements are met. For longer periods of time, it may be preferable to provide 75–80% of energy needs, rather than full feeding, if this improves gastrointestinal tolerance, glycemic control, and avoidance of excess fluid administration.

In the past, bowel rest through PN was the cornerstone of treatment for many severe gastrointestinal disorders. However, the value of providing even minimal amounts of EN is now widely accepted. Protocols to facilitate more widespread use of EN include initiation within 24 h of ICU admission; aggressive use of the head-upright position; postpyloric and nasojejunal feeding tubes; prokinetic agents; more rapid increases in feeding rates; tolerance of higher gastric residuals; and nurse-administered algorithms for feeding progression. PN alone is generally necessary only for severe gut dysfunction due to prolonged ileus, obstruction, or severe hemorrhagic pancreatitis. In the critically ill, feeding adequately by PN beginning within the first 24 h of care improves mortality and is more effective than delayed EN. Early feeding of the critically ill in the ICU is associated with a 50% reduction in mortality, but there is also a 50% increase in infection risk. Much of the increase in morbidity related to PN and EN is due to hyperglycemia, which can be significantly reduced by intensive insulin therapy. The level of glycemia necessary to accomplish this goal, whether <110 mg/dL or only <150 mg/dL, is not yet defined. Surgical patients being adequately fed may benefit from the lower glucose range, but studies of intensive insulin therapy alone without full feeding have shown improved morbidity and mortality outcome with looser control of glucose < 180 mg/dL.

Although PN was initially relatively expensive, its components are now often less expensive than specialty enteral formulas. Percutaneous placement of a central venous catheter into the subclavian or internal jugular vein with advancement into the superior vena cava can be accomplished at the bedside by trained personnel using sterile techniques. Peripherally inserted central catheters (PICCs) can also be placed within the lumen in the central vein, but this technique is usually more appropriate for non-ICU patients. Subclavian or internal jugular catheters carry a greater risk, including pneumothorax or serious vascular damage, but they are well tolerated and can be exchanged over a wire rather than requiring reinsertion when ruling out catheter infection. The peripherally inserted catheters are subject to position-related flow, and the catheter cannot be changed over a wire. Inserting a nasogastric tube is a bedside procedure, but many critically ill patients have impaired gastric emptying that increases the risk of aspiration pneumonia. This risk can be reduced by feeding directly into the jejunum beyond the ligament of Treitz. This usually requires fluoroscopic guidance or endoscopic placement. In patients who have planned laparotomies or other conditions likely to require a prolonged need for SNS, it is advantageous to place a jejunal feeding tube at the time of surgery.

Although most SNS is delivered in hospitals, some patients require it on a long-term basis. If they have a safe environment and a willingness to learn the self-care techniques, SNS can be administered at home. The clinical outcomes of patients with severe intestinal disorders treated with home PN or EN are summarized in Table 76-2. PN infused at home is usually cycled overnight to give greater daytime freedom. Other important considerations in determining the appropriateness of home PN or EN are that the patient's prognosis is longer than several months and that the therapy benefits quality of life. Recent advances in surgical techniques and immunosuppressive therapies have made intestinal transplantation a viable alternative for some patients who require life-long home parenteral nutrition. Although the quality of life can be improved with intestinal transplantation relative to home PN, long-term survival even in the most accomplished centers is still somewhat less with transplantation.

DISEASE-SPECIFIC NUTRITIONAL SUPPORT SNS is basically a support therapy and is primary therapy only for the treatment or prevention of malnutrition. Certain conditions require modification of nutritional support because of organ or system impairment. For instance, in nitrogen accumulation disorders, protein intake may need to be reduced. However, in renal disease, except for brief periods of several days, protein intakes should approach requirement levels of at least 0.8 g/kg or higher up to 1.2 g/kg as long as the blood urea nitrogen does not exceed 100 mg/dL. If this is not possible, then dialysis or other renal replacement therapy should be considered to allow better feeding. In hepatic failure, intakes of 1.2–1.4 g/kg up to the optimal 1.5 g/kg should be attempted, as long as encephalopathy due to protein intolerance is not encountered. In the presence of protein intolerance, formulas containing 33–50% branched-chain amino acids are available and should be provided at the 1.2–1.4-g/kg level. Cardiac patients, and many severely stressed patients, often

TABLE 76-2 Summary of Outcomes for Patients on Home Parenteral and Enteral Nutrition (HPEN)

Diagnosis	Number in Group	Age in Years	Survival[a] on Therapy, %	Therapy Status, % at 1 Year[b]			Rehabilitation[c] Status, % in 1st Year			Complications[d] per Patient-Year	
				Full Oral Nutrition	Continued on HPEN Rx	Died	C	P	M	HPEN	NonHPEN
Home Parenteral Nutrition											
Crohn's disease	562	36	96	70	25	2	60	38	2	0.9	1.1
Ischemic bowel disease	331	49	87	27	48	19	53	41	6	1.4	1.1
Motility disorder	299	45	87	31	44	21	49	39	12	1.3	1.1
Congenital bowel defect	172	5	94	42	47	9	63	27	11	2.1	1.0
Hyperemesis gravidarum	112	28	100	100	0	0	83	16	1	1.5	3.5
Chronic pancreatitis	156	42	90	82	10	5	60	38	2	1.2	2.5
Radiation enteritis	145	58	87	28	49	22	42	49	9	0.8	1.1
Chronic adhesive obstructions	120	53	83	47	34	13	23	68	10	1.7	1.4
Cystic fibrosis	51	17	50	38	13	36	24	66	16	0.8	3.7
Cancer	2122	44	20	26	8	63	29	57	14	1.1	3.3
AIDS	280	33	10	13	6	73	8	63	29	1.6	3.3
Home Enteral Nutrition											
Neurologic disorders of swallowing	1134	65	55	19	25	48	5	24	71	0.3	0.9
Cancer	1644	61	30	30	6	59	21	59	21	0.4	2.7

[a]Survival rates on therapy are values at 1 year, calculated by the life table method. This will differ from the percentage listed as died under Therapy Status, since all patients with known endpoints are considered in this latter measure. The ratio of observed versus expected deaths is equivalent to a Standard Mortality Ratio.

[b]Not shown are those patients who were back in hospital or who had changed therapy type by 12 months.

[c]Rehabilitation is designated complete (C), partial (P), or minimal (M), relative to the patient's ability to sustain normal age-related activity.

[d]Complications refer only to those complications that resulted in rehospitalization.

Source: Derived from North American HPEN Registry. Adapted from chapter in *Harrison's Principles of Internal Medicine*, 16e, by Lyn Howard, MD.

benefit from fluid and sodium restriction to levels of 1000 mL of total parenteral nutrition (TPN) formula and 5–20 meq of sodium per day. In patients with severe chronic PCM characterized by severe weight loss and tissue wasting, TPN must be instituted gradually because of the profound antinatriuresis, antidiuresis, and intracellular accumulation of potassium, magnesium, and phosphorus that develop as a consequence of high insulin levels. This modification of TPN is usually accomplished by limiting fluid intakes initially to about 1000 mL containing modest carbohydrate content of 10–20% dextrose, low sodium, and ample potassium, magnesium, and phosphorus, with careful daily assessment of fluid and electrolyte status. Protein need not be restricted.

THE DESIGN OF INDIVIDUAL REGIMENS

■ FLUID REQUIREMENTS

The normal daily requirement for fluid is 30 mL/kg of body mass from all sources (IV infusions, per tube, or oral intake), plus any replacement of abnormal losses such as from an osmotic diuresis, nasogastric drainage, wound output, or diarrheal/ostomy losses. Electrolyte and mineral losses can be estimated or measured and also need to be replaced (Table 76-3). Fluid restriction may be necessary in patients with fluid overload, and fluid inputs can be limited to 1200 mL/d if urine is the only significant fluid output. When severe fluid overload is present, the optimal TPN solution for central venous administration is a concentrated 1-L solution of 7% crystalline amino acids (70 g) and 21% dextrose (210 g), which provides an amount of nitrogen and glucose that is optimally effective at protein-sparing.

Patients requiring PN or EN in the acute care setting generally have some element of associated hormonal adaptations to their underlying critical illness (e.g., increased secretion of antidiuretic hormone, aldosterone, insulin, glucagon, or cortisol) that cause fluid retention and hyperglycemia. Weight gain in the critically ill, whether receiving SNS or not, is invariably the consequence of fluid retention, since lean tissue accretion, even with feeding, is minimal in the acute phase of illness. Because excess fluid removal can be difficult, limiting fluid intake to allow for balanced intake and output is more effective.

■ ENERGY REQUIREMENTS

Total energy expenditure comprises resting energy expenditure, activity energy expenditure, and the thermal effect of feeding (Chap. 75). Resting energy expenditure (two-thirds) includes the calories necessary for basal metabolism at bed rest. Activity energy expenditure represents one-fourth to one-third of the total, and the thermal effect of feeding is about 10% of the total energy expenditure. For normally nourished healthy individuals, the total energy expenditure is about 30–35 kcal/kg. Although critical illness increases resting energy expenditure, only in initially well-nourished individuals with the highest systemic inflammatory response, such as that from severe multiple trauma, burns, closed head injury, or sepsis, do total energy expenditures reach 40–45 kcal/kg. The chronically ill patient with lean tissue loss has reduced basal energy expenditure, as well as inactivity, which results in a total energy expenditure of about 20–25 kcal/kg. About 95% of such patients need <30 kcal/kg to achieve energy balance. Because providing about 50% of measured energy expenditure as SNS is at least equally efficacious for the first 10 days of critical illness, actual measurement of energy expenditure is not generally necessary in the early period of SNS. However, in patients who remain critically ill beyond several weeks, in the severely malnourished for whom estimates of energy expenditure are unreliable, or in those who are difficult to wean from ventilators, it is reasonable to actually measure energy expenditure and to aim for energy balance to 1.2 times measured expenditure with SNS.

Insulin resistance due to SRI is associated with increased gluconeogenesis and reduced peripheral glucose utilization, predisposing a patient to hyperglycemia. This is aggravated in patients receiving exogenous carbohydrate from SNS. Normalization of blood glucose levels by insulin infusion in critically ill patients receiving SNS reduces morbidity and mortality. In mild or moderately malnourished patients, a reasonable goal is to provide metabolic support to improve protein synthesis and maintain metabolic homeostasis. Hypocaloric nutrition providing only about 1000 kcal/d and 70 g protein for up to 10 days requires less fluid and reduces the likelihood of poor glycemic control. Energy content can be advanced to 20–25 kcal/kg with 1.5 g protein/kg as metabolic conditions permit and definitely during the second week of SNS. Patients with multiple trauma, closed head injury, and severe burns often have much higher energy expenditures, but there is little evidence that providing more than 30 kcal/kg has additional benefit, and it substantially increases the risks of hyperglycemia.

Generally, because glucose is an essential tissue fuel, glucose and amino acids are provided parenterally until the level of resting energy expenditure is reached. At this point, adding fat becomes beneficial, since more parenteral glucose stimulates de novo lipogenesis by the liver—an energy-inefficient process. Polyunsaturated long-chain triglycerides as soybean oil are the chief ingredient in most parenteral fat emulsions and the majority of the fat in enteral feeding formulas. These vegetable oil–based emulsions provide essential fatty acids. Enteral feeding formulas have fat content that ranges from 3% of calories up to as much as 50% of calories, while parenteral fat comes in separate containers as 10%, 20%, and 30% emulsions that can be infused separately or mixed by the pharmacy under controlled conditions as all-in-one or total nutrient admixture with glucose, amino acids, lipid, electrolytes, vitamins, and minerals. Although parenteral fat is required at only about 3% of energy requirements to meet essential fatty acid requirements, when provided as an all-in-one mixture of carbohydrate, fat, and protein, 2–3% fat in the TPN mixtures, representing about 20–30% of calories as fat, is provided to ensure emulsion stability. If given separately, parenteral

TABLE 76-3 Enteric Fluid Volumes and Their Electrolyte Content[a]

	L/d	Na	K	Cl	HCO₃	H
Oral intake	2–3					
Enteric secretions						
Saliva	1–2	15	30	15	50	—
Gastric juice	1.5–2	50–70	5–15	90–120	0	70–100
Bile	0.5–1.5	120–150	5–15	80–120	30–50	—
Pancreatic	0.5–1	100–140	10	70–100	60–110	—
Small intestine	1–2	80–140	10–20	80–120	20–40	—

[a]All in meq/L.

Source: Adapted from chapter in *Harrison's Principles of Internal Medicine*, 16e, by Lyn Howard, MD.

fat should not be provided at rates exceeding 0.11 g/kg body mass per h or about 100 g over 12 h—equivalent to 1 L of 10% parenteral fat and 500 mL of 20% parenteral fat.

Medium-chain triglycerides, which contain saturated fatty acids with chain lengths of 6, 8, 10, or 12 carbons, are provided in a number of enteral feeding formulas because they are absorbed preferentially. Fish oil contains polyunsaturated fatty acids of the omega 3 family, which have been shown to improve immune function and reduce the inflammatory response.

Carbohydrates are provided as hydrous glucose providing 3.4 kcal/g in PN formulas. In enteral formulas, glucose is the carbohydrate source in so-called monomeric diets. These diets provide protein as amino acids and fat in minimal amounts (3%) to meet essential fatty acid requirements. Monomeric formulas are designed to optimize absorption in the seriously compromised gut. These formulas, like the immune-enhancing diets, are quite expensive. In polymeric diets, the carbohydrate source is usually an osmotically less active polysaccharide, protein is usually soy or casein protein, and fat is present in amounts from 25 to 50%. Such formulas are usually well tolerated by patients with normal intestinal length, and some are acceptable for oral consumption.

■ PROTEIN OR AMINO ACID REQUIREMENTS

Although the recommended dietary allowance for protein is 0.8 g/kg per d, maximal rates of repletion occur with 1.5 g/kg in the malnourished. In the severely catabolic patient, this higher level minimizes protein loss. In patients requiring SNS in the acute care setting, at least 1 g/kg is recommended, with greater amounts up to 1.5 g/kg as volume, renal, and hepatic tolerances allow. The standard parenteral and enteral formulas contain protein of high biologic value and meet the requirements for the eight essential amino acids when nitrogen needs are met. In protein-intolerant conditions such as renal and hepatic failure, modified amino acid formulas should be considered. In hepatic failure, higher branched-chain amino acid–enriched formulas appear to improve outcomes. Conditionally essential amino acids like arginine and glutamine may also have some benefit in supplemental amounts.

Protein (nitrogen) balance provides a measure of feeding efficacy of PN or EN. It is calculated as protein intake/6.25 because proteins are on average 16% nitrogen (N), minus the 24-h urine urea N (UUN) plus 4 g N, which reflects other N losses. In the critically ill, a mild negative balance of 2–4 g N/d is usually achievable with a similarly mild positive balance in the recuperating patient. Each g N represents approximately 30 g lean tissue.

■ MINERAL AND VITAMIN REQUIREMENTS

Parenteral electrolyte, vitamin, and trace mineral requirements are summarized in Tables 76-4, 76-5, and 76-6. Electrolyte modifications are necessary with substantial gastrointestinal losses from nasogastric drainage or intestinal losses from fistulas, diarrhea, or ostomy outputs. Such losses also imply extra calcium, magnesium, and zinc losses. Excessive urine or potassium losses with amphotericin, or magnesium losses with cisplatin or in renal failure, necessitate adjustments in sodium, potassium, magnesium, phosphorus, and acid-base balance. Vitamin and trace element requirements are met by the daily provision of a complete parenteral vitamin supplement and trace elements for PN, and with the provision of adequate amounts of enteral feeding formulas that contain these micronutrients.

PARENTERAL NUTRITION

■ INFUSION TECHNIQUE AND PATIENT MONITORING

Parenteral feeding through a peripheral vein is limited by osmolality and volume constraints. Solutions that contain more than 3% amino acids and 5% glucose (290 kcal/L) are poorly tolerated peripherally. Parenteral fat (20%) can be given to increase the calories delivered. The total volume required to provide a marginal protein intake of 60 g and 1680 total kcal is 2.5 L. Moreover, the risk of significant morbidity and mortality from incompatibilities of calcium and phosphate salts is greatest in these low-osmolality, low-glucose regimens. Parenteral feeding via a peripheral vein is generally intended as a supplement to oral feeding and is not optimal for the critically ill. Peripheral parenteral nutrition may benefit from small amounts of heparin at 1000 U/L and co-infusion with parenteral fat to reduce osmolality, but volume constraints still limit the value of this therapy. PICCs can be used for the short term to provide concentrated glucose parenteral solutions of 20–25% dextrose and 4–7% amino acids, while avoiding some of the complications of catheter placement via a large central vein.

TABLE 76-4 Usual Daily Electrolyte Additions to Parenteral Nutrition

Electrolyte	Parenteral Equivalent of RDA	Usual Intake
Sodium		1–2 meq/kg + replacement, but can be as low as 5–40 meq/d
Potassium		40–100 meq/d + replacement of unusual losses
Chloride		As needed for acid-base balance, but usually 2:1 to 1:1 with acetate
Acetate		As needed for acid-base balance
Calcium	10 meq	10–20 meq/d
Magnesium	10 meq	8–16 meq/d
Phosphorus	30 mmol	20–40 mmol

TABLE 76-5 Parenteral Multivitamin Requirements for Adults

Vitamin	Recently Revised Value
Vitamin A	3300 IU
Thiamin (B$_1$)	6 mg
Riboflavin (B$_2$)	3.6 mg
Niacin (B$_3$)	40 mg
Folic acid	600 µg
Pantothenic acid	15 mg
Pyridoxine (B$_6$)	6 mg
Cyanocobalamin (B$_{12}$)	5 µg
Biotin	60 µg
Ascorbic acid (C)	200 mg
Vitamin D	200 IU
Vitamin E	10 IU
Vitamin K[a]	150 µg

[a]A product is available without vitamin K. Vitamin K supplementation is recommended at 2–4 mg/week in patients not receiving oral anticoagulation therapy if using this product.

TABLE 76-6 Parenteral Trace Metal Supplementation for Adults[a]

Trace Mineral	Intake
Zinc	2.5–4 mg/d, an additional 10–15 mg/d per L of stool or ileostomy output
Copper	0.5–1.5 mg/d, possibility of retention in biliary tract obstruction
Manganese	0.1–0.3 mg/d, possibility of retention in biliary tract obstruction
Chromium	10–15 µg/d
Selenium	20–100 µg/d, necessary for long-term PN, optional for short-term TPN
Molybdenum	20–120 µg/d, necessary for long-term PN, optional for short-term PN
Iodine	75–150 µg/d, necessary for long-term PN, optional for short-term PN

[a]Commercial products are available with the first four, first five, and all seven of these metals in recommended amounts.

Note: PN, parenteral nutrition; TPN, total parenteral nutrition.

TABLE 76-7 Monitoring the Patient on Parenteral Nutrition

Clinical Data Monitored Daily

General sense of well-being

Strength as evidenced in getting out of bed, walking, resistance exercise as appropriate

Vital signs including temperature, blood pressure, pulse, and respiratory rate

Fluid balance: weight at least several times weekly, fluid intake (parenteral and enteral) vs. fluid output (urine, stool, gastric drainage, wound, ostomy)

Parenteral nutrition delivery equipment: tubing, pump, filter, catheter, dressing

Nutrient solution composition

Laboratory Daily

Finger-stick glucose	Three times daily until stable
Blood glucose, Na, K, Cl, HCO$_3$, BUN	Daily until stable and fully advanced, then twice weekly
Serum creatinine, albumin, PO$_4$, Ca, Mg, Hb/Hct, WBC	Baseline, then twice weekly
INR	Baseline, then weekly
Micronutrient tests	As indicated

Note: BUN, blood urea nitrogen; Hb, hemoglobin; Hct, hematocrit; INR, international normalized ratio; WBC, white blood cell count.

Source: Adapted from chapter in *Harrison's Principles of Internal Medicine*, 16e, by Lyn Howard, MD.

With PICC lines, however, flow can be position-related, and the lines cannot be exchanged over a wire for infection monitoring. For these reasons, in the critically ill, centrally placed catheters are preferred. The subclavian approach is best tolerated by the patient and is the easiest to dress. The jugular approach is less likely to lead to a pneumothorax. The femoral approach is discouraged because of the greater risk of catheter infection. For long-term feeding in the home, tunneled catheters and implanted ports reduce infection risk and are more acceptable to patients. However, tunneled catheters require placement in the operating room.

Catheters are made of silastic, polyurethane, or polyvinyl chloride. Silastic catheters are less thrombogenic and are best for tunneled catheters. Polyurethane is best for temporary catheters. Dressing changes with dry gauze at regular intervals should be performed by nurses skilled in catheter care to avoid infection. Chlorhexidine solution is more effective than alcohol or iodine compounds. Appropriate monitoring for patients receiving PN is summarized in Table 76-7.

■ COMPLICATIONS

Mechanical

The insertion of a central venous catheter should be performed by trained and experienced personnel using aseptic techniques to limit the major common complications of pneumothorax and inadvertent arterial puncture or injury. Catheter position should be radiographically confirmed to be in the superior vena cava distal to the junction with the jugular or subclavian vein and not directly against the vessel wall. Thrombosis related to the catheter may occur at the site of entry into the vein and extend to encase the catheter. Catheter infection predisposes to thrombosis, as does the SRI. The addition of 6000 U of heparin in the daily parenteral formula in hospitalized patients with temporary catheters reduces the risk of fibrin sheath formation and catheter infection. Temporary catheters that develop a thrombus should be removed and, based on clinical findings, treated with anticoagulants. Thrombolytic therapy can be considered for patients with permanent catheters, depending on the ease of replacement and presence of alternate, reasonably acceptable venous access sites. Low-dose warfarin therapy of 1 mg/d reduces

the risk of thrombosis in permanent catheters used for home PN, but full anticoagulation may be required in patients who have recurrent thrombosis related to permanent catheters. A recent U.S. Food and Drug Administration mandate to reformulate parenteral multivitamins to include vitamin K at a dose of 150 µg daily may affect the efficacy of low-dose warfarin therapy. There is a "no vitamin K" version available for patients receiving this therapy. Catheters can become mechanically occluded and may also become occluded by fibrin at the tip, or by fat, minerals, or drugs intraluminally. These occlusions can be managed with low-dose alteplase for fibrin, with indwelling 70% alcohol for fat, with 0.1 N hydrochloric acid for mineral precipitates, and with either 0.1 N hydrochloric acid or 0.1 N sodium hydroxide for drugs, depending on their pH.

Metabolic

The most common problems related to PN are fluid overload and hyperglycemia (Table 76-8). Hypertonic dextrose stimulates a much higher insulin level than meal feeding. Because insulin is a potent antinatriuretic and antidiuretic hormone, hyperinsulinemia leads to sodium and fluid retention. In the absence of gastrointestinal losses or renal dysfunction, net fluid retention is likely when total fluid intake exceeds 2000 mL/d. Close monitoring of body mass, as well as fluid intake and output, is necessary to prevent this complication. In the absence of significant renal impairment, the sodium content of the urine is likely to be <10 meq/L. Providing sodium in limited amounts of 40 meq/d and the use of both glucose and fat in the PN mixture to lower total glucose and sodium will help reduce fluid retention. The elevated insulin also increases the intracellular transport of potassium, magnesium, and phosphorus, which can

TABLE 76-8 Selected Metabolic Disturbances and Their Correction

Disturbance	Cause	Corrective Action with PN
Hyponatremia	Increased total body water or decreased total body sodium	Decrease free water or increase sodium
Hypernatremia	Occurs commonly with excessive isotonic or hypertonic fluid followed by diuretic administration with free water clearance; can also occur with dehydration and normal total body sodium	Increase free water to produce net positive fluid balance maintaining sodium and chloride balance
Hypokalemia	Inadequate intake relative to need	Use supplements
	Excessive diuresis, tubular dysfunction	Use supplements
	Magnesium deficiency	Increase PN magnesium
	Metabolic alkalosis	Correct alkalosis
	Hyperinsulinemia	Maintain constant PN, increase potassium
Hyperkalemia	Excessive provision	Reduce supplements
	Metabolic acidosis	Evaluate acidosis, treat with PN acetate salt and decrease potassium
	Renal deterioration	Evaluate patient and adjust PN as indicated
Hypocalcemia	Reciprocal response to phosphorus repletion	Increase calcium
	Critical illness effect	Increase calcium
	Severe malabsorption	Supplement calcium
Hypercalcemia	Excessive administration or pathologic (cancer, hyperparathyroidism)	Reduce or eliminate calcium
Hypomagnesemia	Increased requirements due to diuretic use, alcoholism, malabsorption, malnutrition	Supplement magnesium
	Critical illness	Supplement magnesium
Hypophosphatemia	Inadequate intake relative to needs related to malnutrition, alcohol use	Supplement phosphorus
	Increased calcium intake	Use supplements
Hyperphosphatemia	Excessive administration or worsening renal function	Reduce phosphorus
Azotemia	Excessive amino acid infusion or worsening renal function	Reduce amino acid level but consider renal replacement therapy if cannot provide 1 g protein per kg for prolonged periods

Abbreviation: PN, parenteral nutrition.

precipitate a dangerous refeeding syndrome if the total glucose content of the PN solution is advanced too quickly in severely malnourished patients. It is generally best to start PN with <200 g glucose/d to assess glucose tolerance. Regular insulin can be added to the PN formula to establish glycemic control, and the insulin doses can be increased proportionately as the glucose is advanced. As a general rule, patients with insulin-dependent diabetes require about twice their usual home insulin doses when they are receiving TPN at 20–25 kcal/kg, largely as a consequence of parenteral glucose administration and some loss of insulin to the TPN container. As a rough estimate, the amount of insulin can be provided in a similar proportion to the amount of calories provided as TPN relative to full feeding, and the insulin can be placed in the TPN formula. Subcutaneous (SC) regular insulin can be provided to improve glucose control as assessed by measurements of blood glucose every 6 h. About two-thirds of the total 24-h amount can be added to the next day's order, with SC insulin supplements as needed. Advances in TPN concentration should be made when reasonable glucose control is established, and the insulin dose adjusted proportionately to the calories added as glucose and amino acids. These are general rules, and they are conservative. Given the adverse clinical impact of hyperglycemia, it may be necessary to use intensive insulin therapy as a separate infusion with a standard protocol to initially establish control. Once established, this insulin dose can be added to the PN formula. Acid-base imbalance is also common during PN therapy. Amino acid formulas are buffered, but critically ill patients are prone to metabolic acidosis, often due to renal tubular impairment. The use of sodium and potassium acetate salts in the PN formula may address this problem. Bicarbonate salts should not be used because they are incompatible with TPN formulations. Nasogastric drainage produces a hypochloremic alkalosis that can be managed by attention to chloride balance. Occasionally, hydrochloric acid may be required for a more rapid response or when diuretic therapy limits the ability to provide substantial sodium chloride. Up to 100 meq/L and up to 150 meq of hydrochloric acid per day may be placed in a fat-free TPN formula.

Infectious

Infections of the central access catheter rarely occur in the first 72 h. Fever during this period is usually from infection elsewhere or another cause. Fever that develops during PN can be addressed by checking the catheter site and, if the site looks clean, exchanging the catheter over a wire with cultures taken through the catheter and at the catheter tip. If these cultures are negative, as they are most of the time, the new catheter can continue to be used. If a culture is positive for a relatively nonpathogenic bacteria like *Staphylococcus epidermidis*, consider a second exchange over a wire with repeat cultures or replace the catheter depending on the clinical circumstances. If cultures are positive for more pathogenic bacteria, or for fungi like *Candida albicans*, it is generally best to replace the catheter at a new site. Whether antibiotic treatment is required is a clinical decision, but *C. albicans* grown from the blood culture in a patient receiving PN should always be treated because the consequences of failure to treat can be dire.

Catheter infections can be minimized by dedicating the feeding catheter to TPN, without blood sampling or medication administration. Central catheter infections are a serious complication with an attributed mortality of 12–25%. Infections in central venous catheters dedicated to feeding should occur less frequently than 3 per 1000 catheter-days. Home TPN catheters that become infected may be treated through the catheter without removal of the catheter, particularly if the offending organism is *S. epidermidis*. Clearing of the biofilm and fibrin sheath by local treatment of the catheter with indwelling alteplase may increase the likelihood of eradication. Antibiotic lock therapy with high concentrations of antibiotic, with or without heparin in addition to systemic therapy, may improve efficacy. Sepsis with hypotension should precipitate catheter removal in either the temporary or permanent TPN setting.

ENTERAL NUTRITION

■ TUBE PLACEMENT AND PATIENT MONITORING

The types of enteral feeding tubes, methods of insertion, their clinical uses, and potential complications are outlined in Table 76-9.

The different types of enteral formulas are listed in Table 76-10. Patients receiving EN are at risk for many of the same metabolic complications as those who receive PN and should be monitored in the same manner. EN can be a source of similar problems, but not to the same degree, because the insulin response to EN is about half of that seen with PN. Enteral feeding formulas have fixed electrolyte compositions that are generally modest in sodium and somewhat higher in potassium content. Acid-base disturbances can be addressed to a more limited extent with EN. Acetate salts can be added to the formula to treat chronic metabolic acidosis. Calcium chloride can be added to treat mild chronic metabolic alkalosis. Medications and other additives to enteral feeding formulas can clog the tubes (e.g., calcium chloride may interact with casein-based formulas to produce insoluble calcium caseinate products) and may reduce the efficacy of some drugs (e.g., phenytoin). Since small-bore tubes are easily displaced, tube position should be checked at intervals by aspirating and measuring the pH of the gut fluid (<4 in the stomach, >6 in the jejunum).

■ COMPLICATIONS

Aspiration

The debilitated patient with poor gastric emptying and impairment of swallowing and cough is at risk for aspiration; this is particularly true for those who are mechanically ventilated. Tracheal suctioning induces coughing and gastric regurgitation, and cuffs on endotracheal or tracheostomy tubes seldom protect against aspiration. Preventive measures include elevating the head of the

TABLE 76-9 Enteral Feeding Tubes

Type/Insertion Technique	Clinical Uses	Potential Complications
Nasogastric Tube		
External measurement: nostril, ear, xiphisternum; tube stiffened by ice water or stylet; position verified by injecting air and auscultating, or by x-ray	Short-term clinical situation (weeks) or longer periods with intermittent insertion; bolus feeding simpler, but continuous drip with pump better tolerated	Aspiration; ulceration of nasal and esophageal tissues, leading to stricture
Nasoduodenal Tube		
External measurement: nostril, ear, anterior superior iliac spine; tube stiffened by stylet and passed through pylorus under fluoroscopy or with endoscopic loop	Short-term clinical situations where gastric emptying impaired or proximal leak suspected; requires continuous drip with pump	Spontaneous pulling back into stomach (position verified by aspirating content, pH >6); diarrhea common, fiber-containing formulas may help
Gastrostomy Tube		
Percutaneous placement endoscopically, radiologically, or surgically; after tract established, can be converted to a gastric "button"	Long-term clinical situations, swallowing disorders, or impaired small-bowel absorption requiring continuous drip	Aspiration; irritation around tube exit site; peritoneal leak; balloon migration and obstruction of pylorus
Jejunostomy Tube		
Percutaneous placement endoscopically or radiologically via pylorus or endoscopically or surgically directly into the jejunum	Long-term clinical situations where gastric emptying impaired; requires continuous drip with pump; direct endoscopic placement (PEJ) is the most comfortable for patient	Clogging or displacement of tube; jejunal fistula if large-bore tube used; diarrhea from dumping; irritation of surgical anchoring suture
Combined Gastrojejunostomy Tube		
Percutaneous placement endoscopically, radiologically, or surgically; intragastric arm for continuous or intermittent gastric suction; jejunal arm for enteral feeding	Used for patients with impaired gastric emptying and at high risk for aspiration or patients with acute pancreatitis or proximal leaks	Clogging: especially of small-bore jejunal tube

Note: All small tubes are at risk for clogging, especially if used for crushed medications. In long-term enteral patients, gastrostomy and jejunostomy tubes can be exchanged for a low-profile "button" once the tract is established. PEJ, percutaneous endoscopic jejunostomy.

Source: Adapted from chapter in *Harrison's Principles of Internal Medicine*, 16e, by Lyn Howard, MD.

TABLE 76-10 Enteral Formulas

Composition Characteristics	Clinical Indications
Standard Enteral Formula	
1. Complete dietary products (+)[a]	Suitable for most patients requiring tube feeding; some can be used orally
a. Caloric density 1 kcal/mL	
b. Protein ~14% cals, caseinates, soy, lactalbumin	
c. CHO ~60% cals, hydrolyzed corn starch, maltodextrin, sucrose	
d. Fat ~30% cals, corn, soy, safflower oils	
e. Recommended daily intake of all minerals and vitamins in >1500 kcal/d	
f. Osmolality (mosmol/kg): ~300	
Modified Enteral Formulas	
1. Caloric density 1.5–2 kcal/mL (+)	Fluid-restricted patients
2. a. High protein ~20–25% protein (+)	Critically ill patients
b. Hydrolyzed protein to small peptides (+)	Impaired absorption
c. ↑ Arginine, glutamine, nucleotides, ω3 fat (+++)	Immune-enhancing diets
d. ↑ Branched-chain amino acids, ↓ aromatic amino acids (+++)	Liver failure patients intolerant of 0.8 g/kg protein
e. Low protein of high biologic value	Renal failure patient for brief periods if critically ill
3. a. Low-fat partial MCT substitution (+)	Fat malabsorption
b. ↑ Fat >40% cals (++)	Pulmonary failure with CO_2 retention on standard formula, limited utility
c. ↑ Fat from MUFA (++)	Improvement in glycemic index control in diabetes
d. ↑ Fat from ω3 and ↓ ω6 linoleic acid (+++)	Improved ventilation in ARDS
4. Fiber provided as soy polysaccharide (+)	Improved laxation

[a]Cost: + inexpensive; ++ moderately expensive; +++ very expensive.

Note: ARDS, acute respiratory distress syndrome; CHO, carbohydrate; MCT, medium-chain triglyceride; MUFA, monounsaturated fatty acids; ω3 or ω6, polyunsaturated fat with first double bond at carbon 3 (fish oils) or carbon 6 (vegetable oils).

Source: Adapted from chapter in *Harrison's Principles of Internal Medicine*, 16e, by Lyn Howard, MD.

bed to 30 degrees, using nurse-directed algorithms for formula advancement, combining enteral with parenteral feeding, and using post–ligament of Treitz feeding. Tube feeding should not be discontinued for gastric residuals of <300 mL unless there are other signs of gastrointestinal intolerance such as nausea, vomiting, or abdominal distention. Continuous feeding using pumps is better tolerated intragastrically and is essential for feeding into the jejunum. For small-bowel feeding, residuals are not assessed but abdominal pain and distention should be monitored.

Diarrhea

Enteral feeding often leads to diarrhea, especially if bowel function is compromised by disease or drugs, particularly broad-spectrum antibiotics. Diarrhea may be controlled by the use of a continuous drip, with a fiber-containing formula, or by adding an antidiarrheal agent to the formula. However, *Clostridium difficile*, which is a common cause of diarrhea in patients being tube fed, should be ruled out before using antidiarrheal agents. H2 blockers may also assist in reducing the net fluid presented to the colon. Diarrhea associated with enteral feeding does not necessarily imply inadequate absorption of nutrients other than water and electrolytes. Amino acids and glucose are particularly well absorbed in the upper small bowel except in the most diseased or shortest bowel. Since luminal nutrients exert trophic effects on the gut mucosa, it is often appropriate to persist with tube feeding, despite the diarrhea, even when this necessitates supplemental parenteral fluid support.

GLOBAL CONSIDERATIONS

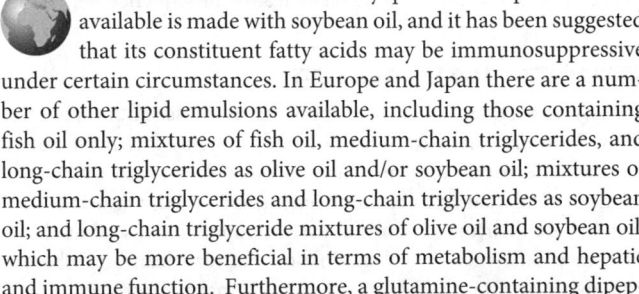 In the United States the only parenteral lipid emulsion available is made with soybean oil, and it has been suggested that its constituent fatty acids may be immunosuppressive under certain circumstances. In Europe and Japan there are a number of other lipid emulsions available, including those containing fish oil only; mixtures of fish oil, medium-chain triglycerides, and long-chain triglycerides as olive oil and/or soybean oil; mixtures of medium-chain triglycerides and long-chain triglycerides as soybean oil; and long-chain triglyceride mixtures of olive oil and soybean oil, which may be more beneficial in terms of metabolism and hepatic and immune function. Furthermore, a glutamine-containing dipeptide for inclusion in TPN formulas is available in Europe and may be helpful in terms of immune function and resistance to infection.

ACKNOWLEDGMENT

The authors acknowledge the contributions of Lyn Howard, MD, the author in earlier editions of HPIM, to material in this chapter.

FURTHER READINGS

Bistrian B, McCowen K: Nutritional support in the adult intensive care unit: Key controversies. Crit Care Med 34:1525, 2006

Centers for Disease Control and Prevention: Reduction in central line–associated bloodstream infections among patients in intensive care units—Pennsylvania, April 2001–March 2005. MMWR Morb Mortal Wkly Rep 54:1013, 2005

FISHBEIN T: Intestinal transplantation. N Engl J Med 361:998, 2009

KORETZ RL et al: Does enteral nutrition affect clinical outcome? A systematic review of the randomized trials. Am J Gastroenterol 102:412, 2007

McCLAVE SA et al: Guidelines for the provision and assessment of nutrition support therapy in the adult critically ill patient: Society of Critical Care Medicine (SCCM) and American Society for Parenteral and Enteral Nutrition (A.S.P.E.N.) JPEN J Parenter Enteral Nutr 33:277, 2009

MILNE A et al: Meta-analysis: Protein and energy supplementation in older people. Ann Intern Med 144:37, 2006

THE NICE-SUGAR STUDY INVESTIGATORS: Intensive versus conventional glucose control in critically ill patients. N Engl J Med 360:1283, 2009

SIMPSON F, DOIG GS: Parenteral vs. enteral nutrition in the critically ill patient: A meta-analysis of trials using the intention to treat principle. Intensive Care Med 31:12, 2005

SINGER P et al: ESPEN guidelines on parenteral nutrition: Intensive care. Clin Nutr 28:387, 2009

VAN DEN BERGHE G et al: Intensive insulin therapy in the critically ill patients. N Engl J Med 345:1359, 2001

ZEIGLER TR: Parenteral nutrition in the critically ill patient. N Engl J Med 361:1088, 2009

CHAPTER **77**

Biology of Obesity

Jeffrey S. Flier
Eleftheria Maratos-Flier

In a world where food supplies are intermittent, the ability to store energy in excess of what is required for immediate use is essential for survival. Fat cells, residing within widely distributed adipose tissue depots, are adapted to store excess energy efficiently as triglyceride and, when needed, to release stored energy as free fatty acids for use at other sites. This physiologic system, orchestrated through endocrine and neural pathways, permits humans to survive starvation for as long as several months. However, in the presence of nutritional abundance and a sedentary lifestyle, and influenced importantly by genetic endowment, this system increases adipose energy stores and produces adverse health consequences.

■ DEFINITION AND MEASUREMENT

Obesity is a state of excess adipose tissue mass. Although often viewed as equivalent to increased body weight, this need not be the case—lean but very muscular individuals may be overweight by numerical standards without having increased adiposity. Body weights are distributed continuously in populations, so that choice of a medically meaningful distinction between lean and obese is somewhat arbitrary. Obesity is therefore more effectively defined by assessing its linkage to morbidity or mortality.

Although not a direct measure of adiposity, the most widely used method to gauge obesity is the *body mass index* (BMI), which is equal to weight/height^2 (in kg/m^2) (Fig. 77-1). Other approaches to quantifying obesity include anthropometry (skinfold thickness), densitometry (underwater weighing), CT or MRI, and electrical impedance. Using data from the Metropolitan Life Tables, BMIs for the midpoint of all heights and frames among both men and women range from 19 to 26 kg/m^2; at a similar BMI, women have more body fat than men. Based on data of substantial morbidity, a BMI of 30 is most commonly used as a threshold for obesity in both men and women. Large-scale epidemiologic studies suggest that all-cause, metabolic, cancer, and cardiovascular morbidity begin to rise (albeit at a slow rate) when BMIs are ≥25, suggesting that the cutoff for obesity should be lowered. Most authorities use the term overweight (rather than obese) to describe individuals with BMIs between 25 and 30. A BMI between 25 and 30 should be viewed as medically significant and worthy of therapeutic intervention, especially in the presence of risk factors that are influenced by adiposity such as hypertension and glucose intolerance.

The distribution of adipose tissue in different anatomic depots also has substantial implications for morbidity. Specifically, intraabdominal and abdominal subcutaneous fat have more significance than subcutaneous fat present in the buttocks and lower extremities. This distinction is most easily made clinically by determining the waist-to-hip ratio, with a ratio >0.9 in women and >1.0 in men being abnormal. Many of the most important complications of obesity such as insulin resistance, diabetes, hypertension, hyperlipidemia, and hyperandrogenism in women, are linked more strongly to intraabdominal and/or upper body fat than to overall adiposity (Chap. 242). The mechanism underlying this association is unknown but may relate to the fact that intraabdominal adipocytes are more lipolytically active than those from other depots. Release of free fatty acids into the portal circulation has adverse metabolic actions, especially on the liver. Whether adipokines and cytokines secreted by visceral adipocytes play an additional role in systemic complications of obesity is an area of active investigation.

■ PREVALENCE

Data from the National Health and Nutrition Examination Surveys (NHANES) show that the percentage of the American adult population with obesity (BMI >30) has increased from 14.5% (between 1976 and 1980) to 33.9% (between 2007 and 2008). As many as 68% of U.S. adults aged ≥20 years were overweight (defined as BMI >25) between the years of 2007 and 2008. Extreme obesity (BMI ≥40) has also increased and affects 5.7% of the population. The increasing prevalence of medically significant obesity raises great concern. Obesity is more common among women and in the poor, and among blacks and Hispanics; the prevalence in children is also rising at a worrisome rate.

■ PHYSIOLOGIC REGULATION OF ENERGY BALANCE

Substantial evidence suggests that body weight is regulated by both endocrine and neural components that ultimately influence the effector arms of energy intake and expenditure. This complex regulatory system is necessary because even small imbalances between energy intake and expenditure will ultimately have large effects on body weight. For example, a 0.3% positive imbalance over 30 years would result in a 9-kg (20-lb) weight gain. This exquisite regulation of energy balance cannot be monitored easily by calorie-counting

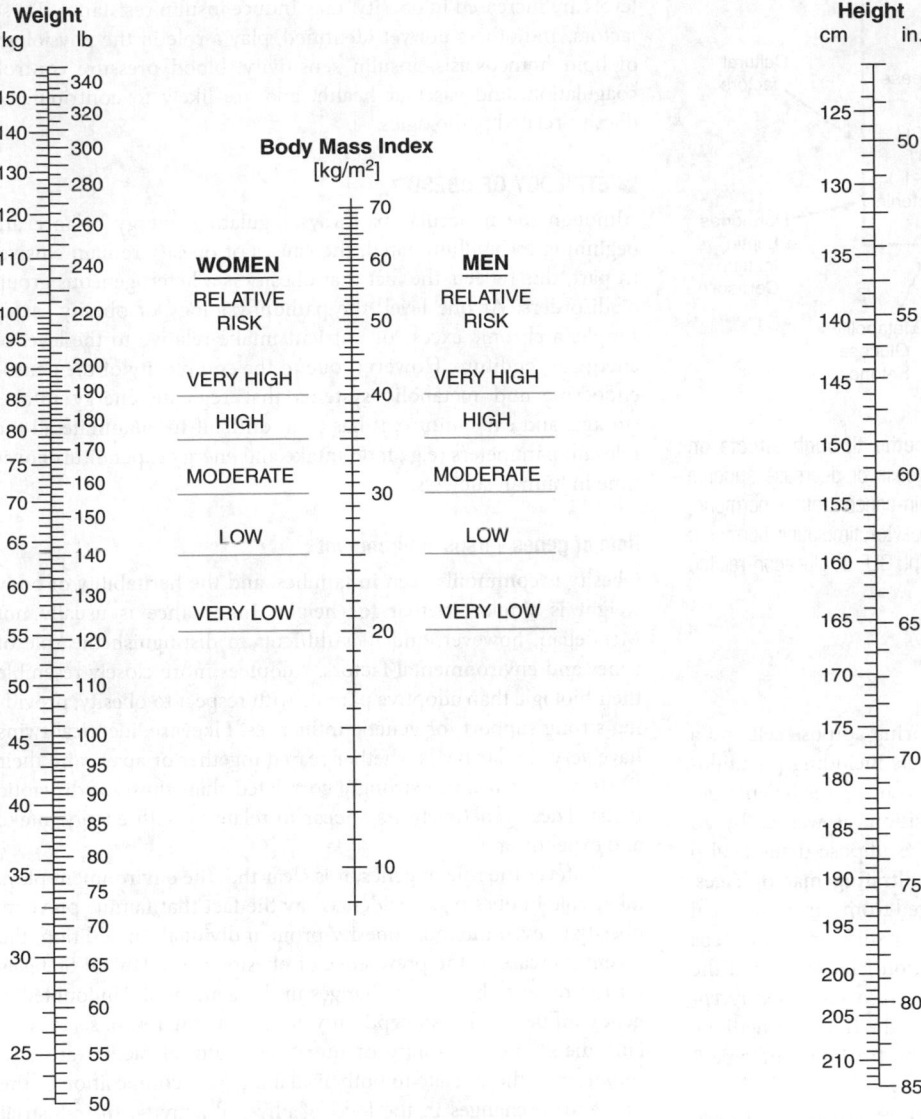

Weight

kg   lb

Body Mass Index
[kg/m²]

WOMEN
RELATIVE
RISK

MEN
RELATIVE
RISK

Height

cm   in.

Figure 77-1   Nomogram for determining body mass index. To use this nomogram, place a ruler or other straight edge between the body weight (without clothes) in kilograms or pounds located on the left-hand line and the height (without shoes) in centimeters or inches located on the right-hand line. The body mass index is read from the middle of the scale and is in metric units. (*Copyright 1979, George A. Bray, MD; used with permission.*)

signals include leptin, insulin, cortisol, and gut peptides. Among the latter is ghrelin, which is made in the stomach and stimulates feeding, and peptide YY (PYY) and cholecystokinin, which is made in the small intestine and signal to the brain through direct action on hypothalamic control centers and/or via the vagus nerve. Metabolites, including glucose, can influence appetite, as seen by the effect of hypoglycemia to induce hunger; however, glucose is not normally a major regulator of appetite. These diverse hormonal, metabolic, and neural signals act by influencing the expression and release of various hypothalamic peptides [e.g., neuropeptide Y (NPY), Agouti-related peptide (AgRP), α-melanocyte-stimulating hormone (α-MSH), and melanin-concentrating hormone (MCH)] that are integrated with serotonergic, catecholaminergic, endocannabinoid, and opioid signaling pathways (see below). Psychological and cultural factors also play a role in the final expression of appetite. Apart from rare genetic syndromes involving leptin, its receptor, and the melanocortin system, specific defects in this complex appetite control network that influence common cases of obesity are not well defined.

Energy expenditure includes the following components: (1) resting or basal metabolic rate; (2) the energy cost of metabolizing and storing food; (3) the thermic effect of exercise; and (4) adaptive thermogenesis, which varies in response to long-term caloric intake (rising with increased intake). Basal metabolic rate accounts for ~70% of daily energy expenditure, whereas active physical activity contributes 5–10%. Thus, a significant component of daily energy consumption is fixed.

Genetic models in mice indicate that mutations in certain genes (e.g., targeted deletion of the insulin receptor in adipose tissue) protect against obesity, apparently by increasing energy expenditure. Adaptive thermogenesis occurs in *brown adipose tissue* (BAT), which plays an important role in energy metabolism in many mammals. In contrast to white adipose tissue, which is used to store energy in the form of lipids, BAT expends stored energy as heat. A mitochondrial *uncoupling protein* (UCP-1) in BAT dissipates the hydrogen ion gradient in the oxidative respiration chain and releases energy as heat. The metabolic activity of BAT is increased by a central action of leptin, acting through the sympathetic nervous system that heavily innervates this tissue. In rodents, BAT deficiency causes obesity and diabetes; stimulation of BAT with a specific adrenergic agonist (β₃ agonist) protects against diabetes and obesity. BAT exists in humans (especially neonates), and although its physiologic role is not yet established, identification of functional BAT in many adults using PET imaging has increased interest in the implications of the tissue for pathogenesis and therapy of obesity.

in relation to physical activity. Rather, body weight regulation or dysregulation depends on a complex interplay of hormonal and neural signals. Alterations in stable weight by forced overfeeding or food deprivation induce physiologic changes that resist these perturbations: with weight loss, appetite increases and energy expenditure falls; with overfeeding, appetite falls and energy expenditure increases. This latter compensatory mechanism frequently fails, however, permitting obesity to develop when food is abundant and physical activity is limited. A major regulator of these adaptive responses is the adipocyte-derived hormone leptin, which acts through brain circuits (predominantly in the hypothalamus) to influence appetite, energy expenditure, and neuroendocrine function (see below).

Appetite is influenced by many factors that are integrated by the brain, most importantly within the hypothalamus (Fig. 77-2). Signals that impinge on the hypothalamic center include neural afferents, hormones, and metabolites. Vagal inputs are particularly important, bringing information from viscera, such as gut distention. Hormonal

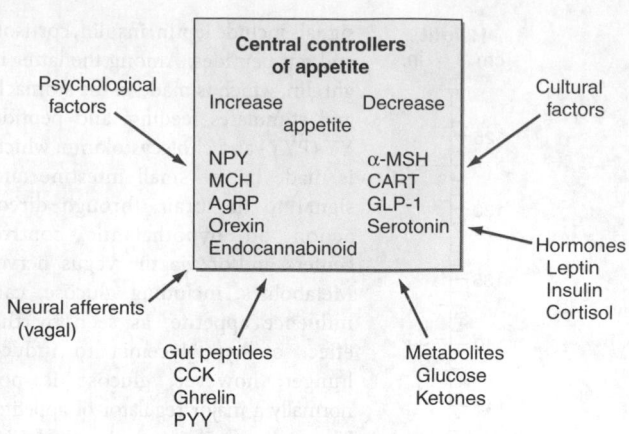

Figure 77-2 **The factors that regulate appetite through effects on central neural circuits.** Some factors that increase or decrease appetite are listed. NPY, neuropeptide Y; MCH, melanin-concentrating hormone; AgRP, Agouti-related peptide; α-MSH, α-melanocyte-stimulating hormone; CART, cocaine- and amphetamine-related transcript; GLP-1, glucagon-related peptide-1; CCK, cholecystokinin.

THE ADIPOCYTE AND ADIPOSE TISSUE

Adipose tissue is composed of the lipid-storing adipose cell and a stromal/vascular compartment in which cells including preadipocytes and macrophages reside. Adipose mass increases by enlargement of adipose cells through lipid deposition, as well as by an increase in the number of adipocytes. Obese adipose tissue is also characterized by increased numbers of infiltrating macrophages. The process by which adipose cells are derived from a mesenchymal preadipocyte involves an orchestrated series of differentiation steps mediated by a cascade of specific transcription factors. One of the key transcription factors is *peroxisome proliferator-activated receptor γ (PPARγ)*, a nuclear receptor that binds the thiazolidinedione class of insulin-sensitizing drugs used in the treatment of type 2 diabetes (Chap. 344).

Although the adipocyte has generally been regarded as a storage depot for fat, it is also an endocrine cell that releases numerous molecules in a regulated fashion (Fig. 77-3). These include the energy balance–regulating hormone leptin, cytokines such as tumor necrosis factor (TNF)-α and interleukin (IL)-6, complement factors such as factor D (also known as *adipsin*), prothrombotic agents such as plasminogen activator inhibitor I, and a component of the blood pressure–regulating system, angiotensinogen. Adiponectin, an abundant adipose-derived protein whose levels are reduced in obesity, enhances insulin sensitivity and lipid oxidation and it has vascular-protective effects, whereas resistin and RBP4, whose

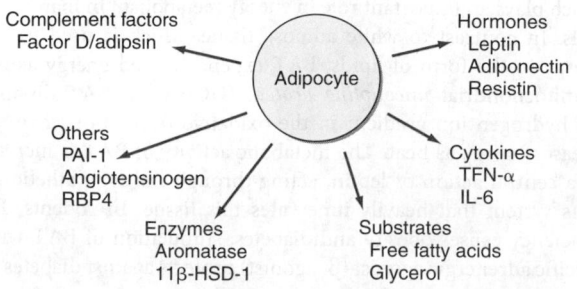

Figure 77-3 **Factors released by the adipocyte that can affect peripheral tissues.** PAI, plasminogen activator inhibitor; TNF, tumor necrosis factor; RBP4, retinal binding protein 4.

levels are increased in obesity, may induce insulin resistance. These factors, and others not yet identified, play a role in the physiology of lipid homeostasis, insulin sensitivity, blood pressure control, coagulation, and vascular health, and are likely to contribute to obesity-related pathologies.

ETIOLOGY OF OBESITY

Although the molecular pathways regulating energy balance are beginning to be illuminated, the causes of obesity remain elusive. In part, this reflects the fact that obesity is a heterogeneous group of disorders. At one level, the pathophysiology of obesity seems simple: a chronic excess of nutrient intake relative to the level of energy expenditure. However, due to the complexity of the neuro-endocrine and metabolic systems that regulate energy intake, storage, and expenditure, it has been difficult to quantitate all the relevant parameters (e.g., food intake and energy expenditure) over time in human subjects.

Role of genes versus environment

Obesity is commonly seen in families, and the heritability of body weight is similar to that for height. Inheritance is usually not Mendelian, however, and it is difficult to distinguish the role of genes and environmental factors. Adoptees more closely resemble their biologic than adoptive parents with respect to obesity, providing strong support for genetic influences. Likewise, identical twins have very similar BMIs whether reared together or apart, and their BMIs are much more strongly correlated than those of dizygotic twins. These genetic effects appear to relate to both energy intake and expenditure.

Whatever the role of genes, it is clear that the environment plays a key role in obesity, as evidenced by the fact that famine prevents obesity in even the most obesity-prone individual. In addition, the recent increase in the prevalence of obesity in the United States is far too rapid to be due to changes in the gene pool. Undoubtedly, genes influence the susceptibility to obesity in response to specific diets and availability of nutrition. Cultural factors are also important—these relate to both availability and composition of the diet and to changes in the level of physical activity. In industrial societies, obesity is more common among poor women, whereas in underdeveloped countries, wealthier women are more often obese. In children, obesity correlates to some degree with time spent watching television. Although the role of diet composition in obesity continues to generate controversy, it appears that high-fat diets may promote obesity when combined with diets rich in simple, rapidly absorbed carbohydrates.

Additional environmental factors may contribute to the increasing obesity prevalence. Both epidemiologic correlations and experimental data suggest that sleep deprivation leads to increased obesity. Changes in gut microbiome with capacity to alter energy balance are receiving experimental support from animal studies, and a possible role for obesigenic viral infections continues to receive sporadic attention.

Specific genetic syndromes

For many years, obesity in rodents has been known to be caused by a number of distinct mutations distributed through the genome. Most of these single-gene mutations cause both hyperphagia and diminished energy expenditure, suggesting a physiologic link between these two parameters of energy homeostasis. Identification of the *ob* gene mutation in genetically obese (ob/ob) mice represented a major breakthrough in the field. The ob/ob mouse develops severe obesity, insulin resistance, and hyperphagia, as well as efficient metabolism (e.g., it gets fat even when ingesting the same number of calories as lean litter mates). The product of the *ob* gene is the peptide leptin,

PART 6 Nutrition

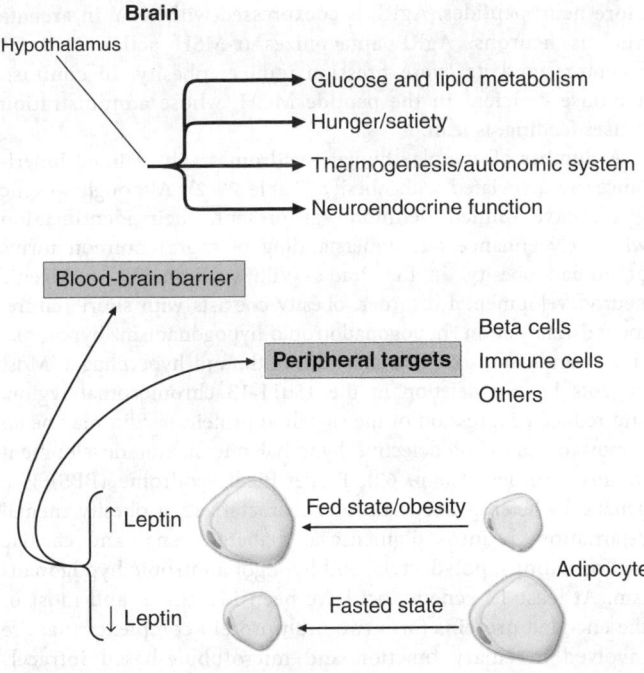

Brain

Hypothalamus

- → Glucose and lipid metabolism
- → Hunger/satiety
- → Thermogenesis/autonomic system
- → Neuroendocrine function

Blood-brain barrier

Peripheral targets

Beta cells
Immune cells
Others

↑ Leptin — Fed state/obesity
↓ Leptin — Fasted state

Adipocyte

Figure 77-4 **The physiologic system regulated by leptin.** Rising or falling leptin levels act through the hypothalamus to influence appetite, energy expenditure, and neuroendocrine function and through peripheral sites to influence systems such as the immune system.

a name derived from the Greek root *leptos*, meaning thin. Leptin is secreted by adipose cells and acts primarily through the hypothalamus. Its level of production provides an index of adipose energy stores (Fig. 77-4). High leptin levels decrease food intake and increase energy expenditure. Another mouse mutant, db/db, which is resistant to leptin, has a mutation in the leptin receptor and develops a similar syndrome. The *ob* gene is present in humans where it is also expressed in fat. Several families with morbid, early-onset obesity caused

by inactivating mutations in either leptin or the leptin receptor have been described, thus demonstrating the biologic relevance of the leptin pathway in humans. Obesity in these individuals begins shortly after birth, is severe, and is accompanied by neuroendocrine abnormalities. The most prominent of these is hypogonadotropic hypogonadism, which is reversed by leptin replacement in the leptin-deficient subset. Central hypothyroidism and growth retardation are seen in the mouse model, but their occurrence in leptin-deficient humans is less clear. To date, there is no evidence that mutations in the leptin or leptin receptor genes play a prominent role in common forms of obesity.

Mutations in several other genes cause severe obesity in humans (Table 77-1); each of these syndromes is rare. Mutations in the gene encoding proopiomelanocortin (POMC) cause severe obesity through failure to synthesize α-MSH, a key neuropeptide that inhibits appetite in the hypothalamus. The absence of POMC also causes secondary adrenal insufficiency due to absence of adrenocorticotropic hormone (ACTH), as well as pale skin and red hair due to absence of α-MSH. Proenzyme convertase 1 (PC-1) mutations are thought to cause obesity by preventing synthesis of α-MSH from its precursor peptide, POMC. α-MSH binds to the type 4 melanocortin receptor (MC4R), a key hypothalamic receptor that inhibits eating. Heterozygous loss-of-function mutations of this receptor account for as much as 5% of severe obesity. These five genetic defects define a pathway through which leptin (by stimulating POMC and increasing α-MSH) restricts food intake and limits weight (Fig. 77-5). The results of genomewide association studies to identify genetic loci responsible for obesity in the general population have so far been disappointing. More than 10 replicated loci linked to obesity have been identified, but together they account for less than 3% of interindividual variation in BMI. The most replicated of these is a gene named *FTO*, which is of unknown function, but like many of the other recently described candidates, is expressed in the brain. Since the heritability of obesity is estimated to be 40–70%, it is likely that many more loci remain to be identified.

In addition to these human obesity genes, studies in rodents reveal several other molecular candidates for hypothalamic mediators of human obesity or leanness. The *tub* gene encodes

TABLE 77-1 **Some Obesity Genes in Humans and Mice**

Gene	Gene Product	Mechanism of Obesity	In Human	In Rodent
Lep (*ob*)	Leptin, a fat-derived hormone	Mutation prevents leptin from delivering satiety signal; brain perceives starvation	Yes	Yes
LepR (*db*)	Leptin receptor	Same as above	Yes	Yes
POMC	Proopiomelanocortin, a precursor of several hormones and neuropeptides	Mutation prevents synthesis of melanocyte-stimulating hormone (MSH), a satiety signal	Yes	Yes
MC4R	Type 4 receptor for MSH	Mutation prevents reception of satiety signal from MSH	Yes	Yes
AgRP	Agouti-related peptide, a neuropeptide expressed in the hypothalamus	Overexpression inhibits signal through *MC4R*	No	Yes
PC-1	Prohormone convertase 1, a processing enzyme	Mutation prevents synthesis of neuropeptide, probably MSH	Yes	No
Fat	Carboxypeptidase E, a processing enzyme	Same as above	No	Yes
Tub	Tub, a hypothalamic protein of unknown function	Hypothalamic dysfunction	No	Yes
TrkB	TrkB, a neurotrophin receptor	Hyperphagia due to uncharacterized hypothalamic defect	Yes	Yes

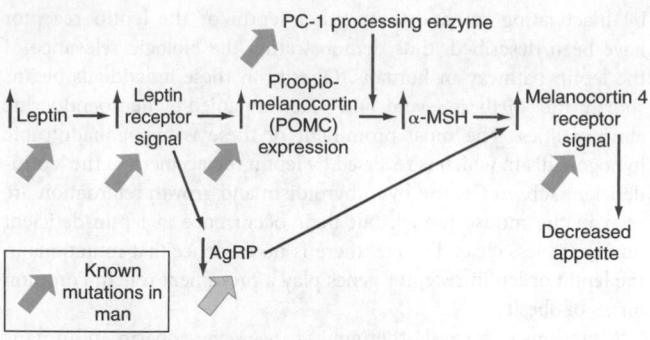

Figure 77-5 **A central pathway through which leptin acts to regulate appetite and body weight.** Leptin signals through proopiomelanocortin (POMC) neurons in the hypothalamus to induce increased production of α-melanocyte-stimulating hormone (α-MSH), requiring the processing enzyme PC-1 (proenzyme convertase 1). α-MSH acts as an agonist on melanocortin-4 receptors to inhibit appetite, and the neuropeptide AgRp (Agouti-related peptide) acts as an antagonist of this receptor. Mutations that cause obesity in humans are indicated by the solid green arrows.

a hypothalamic peptide of unknown function; mutation of this gene causes late-onset obesity. The *fat* gene encodes carboxypeptidase E, a peptide-processing enzyme; mutation of this gene is thought to cause obesity by disrupting production of one or more neuropeptides. AgRP is coexpressed with NPY in arcuate nucleus neurons. AgRP antagonizes α-MSH action at MC4 receptors, and its overexpression induces obesity. In contrast, a mouse deficient in the peptide MCH, whose administration causes feeding, is lean.

A number of complex human syndromes with defined inheritance are associated with obesity (Table 77-2). Although specific genes have limited definition at present, their identification will likely enhance our understanding of more common forms of human obesity. In the Prader-Willi syndrome, a multigenic neurodevelopmental disorder, obesity coexists with short stature, mental retardation, hypogonadotropic hypogonadism, hypotonia, small hands and feet, fish-shaped mouth, and hyperphagia. Most patients have a deletion in the 15q11-13 chromosomal region, and reduced expression of the signaling protein necdin may be an important cause of defective hypothalamic neural development in this disorder (Chap. 62). Bardet-Biedl syndrome (BBS) is a genetically heterogeneous disorder characterized by obesity, mental retardation, retinitis pigmentosa, diabetes, renal and cardiac malformations, polydactyly, and hypogonadotropic hypogonadism. At least 12 genetic loci have been identified, and most of the encoded proteins form two multiprotein complexes that are involved in ciliary function and microtubule-based intracellular transport. Recent evidence suggests that mutations might disrupt leptin receptor trafficking in key hypothalamic neurons, causing leptin resistance.

TABLE 77-2 A Comparison of Syndromes of Obesity—Hypogonadism and Mental Retardation

Feature	Syndrome				
	Prader-Willi	Laurence-Moon-Biedl	Ahlstrom's	Cohen's	Carpenter's
Inheritance	Sporadic; two-thirds have defect	Autosomal recessive	Autosomal recessive	Probably autosomal recessive	Autosomal recessive
Stature	Short	Normal; infrequently short	Normal; infrequently short	Short or tall	Normal
Obesity	Generalized	Generalized	Truncal	Truncal	Truncal, gluteal
	Moderate to severe	Early onset, 1–2 years	Early onset, 2–5 years	Mid-childhood, age 5	
	Onset 1–3 years				
Craniofacies	Narrow bifrontal diameter	Not distinctive	Not distinctive	High nasal bridge	Acrocephaly
	Almond-shaped eyes			Arched palate	Flat nasal bridge
	Strabismus			Open mouth	High-arched palate
	V-shaped mouth			Short philtrum	
	High-arched palate				
Limbs	Small hands and feet	Polydactyly	No abnormalities	Hypotonia	Polydactyly
	Hypotonia			Narrow hands and feet	Syndactyly
					Genu valgum
Reproductive status	1° Hypogonadism	1° Hypogonadism	Hypogonadism in males but not in females	Normal gonadal function or hypogonadotrophic hypogonadism	2° Hypogonadism
Other features	Enamel hypoplasia			Dysplastic ears	
	Hyperphagia			Delayed puberty	
	Temper tantrums				
	Nasal speech				
Mental retardation	Mild to moderate		Normal intelligence	Mild	Slight

Other specific syndromes associated with obesity

Cushing's syndrome Although obese patients commonly have central obesity, hypertension, and glucose intolerance, they lack other specific stigmata of Cushing's syndrome (Chap. 342). Nonetheless, a potential diagnosis of Cushing's syndrome is often entertained. Cortisol production and urinary metabolites (17OH steroids) may be increased in simple obesity. Unlike in Cushing's syndrome, however, cortisol levels in blood and urine in the basal state and in response to corticotropin-releasing hormone (CRH) or ACTH are normal; the overnight 1-mg dexamethasone suppression test is normal in 90%, with the remainder being normal on a standard 2-day low-dose dexamethasone suppression test. Obesity may be associated with excessive local reactivation of cortisol in fat by 11β-hydroxysteroid dehydrogenase 1, an enzyme that converts inactive cortisone to cortisol.

Hypothyroidism The possibility of hypothyroidism should be considered, but it is an uncommon cause of obesity; hypothyroidism is easily ruled out by measuring thyroid-stimulating hormone (TSH). Much of the weight gain that occurs in hypothyroidism is due to myxedema (Chap. 341).

Insulinoma Patients with insulinoma often gain weight as a result of overeating to avoid -hypoglycemic symptoms (Chap. 345). The increased substrate plus high insulin levels promote energy storage in fat. This can be marked in some individuals but is modest in most.

Craniopharyngioma and other disorders involving the hypothalamus Whether through tumors, trauma, or inflammation, hypothalamic dysfunction of systems controlling satiety, hunger, and energy expenditure can cause varying degrees of obesity (Chap. 339). It is uncommon to identify a discrete anatomic basis for these disorders. Subtle hypothalamic dysfunction is probably a more common cause of obesity than can be documented using currently available imaging techniques. Growth hormone (GH), which exerts lipolytic activity, is diminished in obesity and is increased with weight loss. Despite low GH levels, insulin-like growth factor (IGF)-I (somatomedin) production is normal, suggesting that GH suppression is a compensatory response to increased nutritional supply.

Pathogenesis of common obesity

Obesity can result from increased energy intake, decreased energy expenditure, or a combination of the two. Thus, identifying the etiology of obesity should involve measurements of both parameters. However, it is difficult to perform direct and accurate measurements of energy intake in free-living individuals; and the obese, in particular, often underreport intake. Measurements of chronic energy expenditure are possible using doubly labeled water or metabolic chamber/rooms. In subjects at stable weight and body composition, energy intake equals expenditure. Consequently, these techniques allow assessment of energy intake in free-living individuals. The level of energy expenditure differs in established obesity, during periods of weight gain or loss, and in the pre- or postobese state. Studies that fail to take note of this phenomenon are not easily interpreted.

There is continued interest in the concept of a body weight "set point." This idea is supported by physiologic mechanisms centered around a sensing system in adipose tissue that reflects fat stores and a receptor, or "adipostat," that is in the hypothalamic centers. When fat stores are depleted, the adipostat signal is low, and the hypothalamus responds by stimulating hunger and decreasing energy expenditure to conserve energy. Conversely, when fat stores are abundant, the signal is increased, and the hypothalamus responds by decreasing hunger and increasing energy expenditure. The recent discovery of the *ob* gene, and its product leptin, and the *db* gene, whose product is the leptin receptor, provides important elements of a molecular basis for this physiologic concept (see above).

What is the status of food intake in obesity? (Do the obese eat more than the lean?)

This question has stimulated much debate, due in part to the methodologic difficulties inherent in determining food intake. Many obese individuals believe that they eat small quantities of food, and this claim has often been supported by the results of food intake questionnaires. However, it is now established that average energy expenditure increases as individuals get more obese, due primarily to the fact that metabolically active lean tissue mass increases with obesity. Given the laws of thermodynamics, the obese person must therefore eat more than the average lean person to maintain their increased weight. It may be the case, however, that a subset of individuals who are predisposed to obesity have the capacity to become obese initially without an absolute increase in caloric consumption.

What is the state of energy expenditure in obesity?

The average total daily energy expenditure is higher in obese than lean individuals when measured at stable weight. However, energy expenditure falls as weight is lost, due in part to loss of lean body mass and to decreased sympathetic nerve activity. When reduced to near-normal weight and maintained there for awhile, (some) obese individuals have lower energy expenditure than (some) lean individuals. There is also a tendency for those who will develop obesity as infants or children to have lower resting energy expenditure rates than those who remain lean.

The physiologic basis for variable rates of energy expenditure (at a given body weight and level of energy intake) is essentially unknown. A mutation in the human β₃-adrenergic receptor may be associated with increased risk of obesity and/or insulin resistance in certain (but not all) populations.

One recently described component of thermogenesis, called *nonexercise activity thermogenesis* (NEAT), has been linked to obesity. It is the thermogenesis that accompanies physical activities other than volitional exercise such as the activities of daily living, fidgeting, spontaneous muscle contraction, and maintaining posture. NEAT accounts for about two-thirds of the increased daily energy expenditure induced by overfeeding. The wide variation in fat storage seen in overfed individuals is predicted by the degree to which NEAT is induced. The molecular basis for NEAT and its regulation is unknown.

Leptin in typical obesity

The vast majority of obese persons have increased leptin levels but do not have mutations of either leptin or its receptor. They appear, therefore, to have a form of functional "leptin resistance." Data suggesting that some individuals produce less leptin per unit fat mass than others or have a form of relative leptin deficiency that predisposes to obesity are at present contradictory and unsettled. The mechanism for leptin resistance, and whether it can be overcome by raising leptin levels or combining leptin with other treatments in a subset of obese individuals, is not yet established. Some data suggest that leptin may not effectively cross the blood-brain barrier as levels rise. It is also apparent from animal studies that leptin signaling inhibitors, such as SOCS3 and PTP1b, are involved in the leptin-resistant state.

■ PATHOLOGIC CONSEQUENCES OF OBESITY

(See also Chap. 78) Obesity has major adverse effects on health. Obesity is associated with an increase in mortality, with a 50–100% increased risk of death from all causes compared to normal-weight individuals, mostly due to cardiovascular causes. Obesity and over-weight together are the second leading cause of preventable death in the United States, accounting for 300,000 deaths per year. Mortality rates rise as obesity increases, particularly when obesity is associated with increased intraabdominal fat (see above). Life expectancy of a moderately obese individual could be shortened by 2–5 years, and a 20- to 30-year-old male with a BMI >45 may lose 13 years of life. It is also apparent that the degree to which obesity affects particular organ systems is influenced by susceptibility genes that vary in the population.

Insulin resistance and type 2 diabetes mellitus

Hyperinsulinemia and insulin resistance are pervasive features of obesity, increasing with weight gain and diminishing with weight loss (Chap. 242). Insulin resistance is more strongly linked to intraabdominal fat than to fat in other depots. Molecular links between obesity and insulin resistance in fat, muscle, and liver have been sought for many years. Major factors include: (1) insulin itself, by inducing receptor downregulation; (2) free fatty acids that are increased and capable of impairing insulin action; (3) intracellular lipid accumulation; and (4) several circulating peptides produced by adipocytes, including the cytokines TNF-α and IL-6, RBP4, and the "adipokines" adiponectin and resistin that have altered expression in obese adipocytes, and can modify insulin action. Additional mechanisms are obesity-linked inflammation, including infiltration of macrophages into tissues including fat, and induction of the endoplasmic reticulum stress response, that can bring about resistance to insulin action in cells. Despite the prevalence of insulin resistance, most obese individuals do not develop diabetes, suggesting that diabetes requires an interaction between obesity-induced insulin resistance and other factors such as impaired insulin secretion (Chap. 344). Obesity, however, is a major risk factor for diabetes, and as many as 80% of patients with type 2 diabetes mellitus are obese. Weight loss and exercise, even of modest degree, increase insulin sensitivity and often improve glucose control in diabetes.

Reproductive disorders

Disorders that affect the reproductive axis are associated with obesity in both men and women. Male hypogonadism is associated with increased adipose tissue, often distributed in a pattern more typical of females. In men whose weight is >160% ideal body weight (IBW), plasma testosterone and sex hormone–binding globulin (SHBG) are often reduced, and estrogen levels (derived from conversion of adrenal androgens in adipose tissue) are increased (Chap. 346). Gynecomastia may be seen. However, masculinization, libido, potency, and spermatogenesis are preserved in most of these individuals. Free testosterone may be decreased in morbidly obese men whose weight is >200% IBW.

Obesity has long been associated with menstrual abnormalities in women, particularly in women with upper body obesity (Chap. 347). Common findings are increased androgen production, decreased SHBG, and increased peripheral conversion of androgen to estrogen. Most obese women with oligomenorrhea have the polycystic ovarian syndrome (PCOS), with its associated anovulation and ovarian hyperandrogenism; 40% of women with PCOS are obese. Most nonobese women with PCOS are also insulin-resistant, suggesting that insulin resistance, hyperinsulinemia, or the combination of the two are causative or contribute to the ovarian pathophysiology in PCOS in both obese and lean individuals. In obese women with PCOS, weight loss or treatment with insulin-sensitizing drugs often restores normal menses. The increased conversion of androstenedione to estrogen, which occurs to a greater degree in women with lower body obesity, may contribute to the

increased incidence of uterine cancer in postmenopausal women with obesity.

Cardiovascular disease

The Framingham Study revealed that obesity was an independent risk factor for the 26-year incidence of cardiovascular disease in men and women [including coronary disease, stroke, and congestive heart failure (CHF)]. The waist-to-hip ratio may be the best predictor of these risks. When the additional effects of hypertension and glucose intolerance associated with obesity are included, the adverse impact of obesity is even more evident. The effect of obesity on cardiovascular mortality in women may be seen at BMIs as low as 25. Obesity, especially abdominal obesity, is associated with an atherogenic lipid profile; with increased low-density lipoprotein cholesterol, very low density lipoprotein, and triglyceride; and with decreased high density lipoprotein cholesterol and decreased levels of the vascular protective adipokine adiponectin (Chap. 356). Obesity is also associated with hypertension. Measurement of blood pressure in the obese requires use of a larger cuff size to avoid artifactual increases. Obesity-induced hypertension is associated with increased peripheral resistance and cardiac output, increased sympathetic nervous system tone, increased salt sensitivity, and insulin-mediated salt retention; it is often responsive to modest weight loss.

Pulmonary disease

Obesity may be associated with a number of pulmonary abnormalities. These include reduced chest wall compliance, increased work of breathing, increased minute ventilation due to increased metabolic rate, and decreased functional residual capacity and expiratory reserve volume (Chap. 252). Severe obesity may be associated with obstructive sleep apnea and the "obesity hypoventilation syndrome" with attenuated hypoxic and hypercapnic ventilatory responses (Chap. 264). Sleep apnea can be obstructive (most common), central, or mixed and is associated with hypertension. Weight loss (10–20 kg) can bring substantial improvement, as can major weight loss following gastric bypass or restrictive surgery. Continuous positive airway pressure has been used with some success.

Hepatobiliary disease

Obesity is frequently associated with the common disorder nonalcoholic fatty liver disease (NAFLD). This hepatic fatty infiltration of NAFLD can progress in a subset to inflammatory nonalcoholic steatohepatitis (NASH) and more rarely to cirrhosis and hepatocellular carcinoma. Steatosis has been noted to improve following weight loss, secondary to diet or bariatric surgery. The mechanism for the association remains unclear. Obesity is associated with enhanced biliary secretion of cholesterol, supersaturation of bile, and a higher incidence of gallstones, particularly cholesterol gallstones (Chap. 311). A person 50% above IBW has about a sixfold increased incidence of symptomatic gallstones. Paradoxically, fasting increases supersaturation of bile by decreasing the phospholipid component. Fasting-induced cholecystitis is a complication of extreme diets.

Cancer

Obesity in males is associated with higher mortality from cancer, including cancer of the esophagus, colon, rectum, pancreas, liver, and prostate; obesity in females is associated with higher mortality from cancer of the gallbladder, bile ducts, breasts, endometrium, cervix, and ovaries. Some of the latter may be due to increased rates of conversion of androstenedione to estrone in adipose tissue of obese individuals. Other possible mechanistic links are other hormones whose levels are linked to nutritional state, including insulin, leptin, adiponectin, and IGF-1. It has been estimated that obesity accounts for 14% of cancer deaths in men and 20% in women in the United States.

Bone, joint, and cutaneous disease

Obesity is associated with an increased risk of osteoarthritis, no doubt partly due to the trauma of added weight bearing, but potentially linked as well to activation of inflammatory pathways that could promote synovial pathology. The prevalence of gout may also be increased (Chap. 333). Among the skin problems associated with obesity is acanthosis nigricans, manifested by darkening and thickening of the skinfolds on the neck, elbows, and dorsal interphalangeal spaces. Acanthosis reflects the severity of underlying insulin resistance and diminishes with weight loss. Friability of skin may be increased, especially in skinfolds, enhancing the risk of fungal and yeast infections. Finally, venous stasis is increased in the obese.

FURTHER READINGS

BOCHUKOVA EG et al: Large, rare chromosomal deletions associated with severe early-onset obesity. Nature 463:666, 2010

CECIL JE et al: An obesity-associated FTO gene variant and increased energy intake in children. N Engl J Med 359:2558, 2008

FISHER FM et al: Obesity is an FGF21 resistant state. Diabetes 59:2781, 2010

FROY O: Metabolism and circadian rhythms—Implications for obesity. Endocr Rev 31:1, 2010

MISRA A, KHURANA L: Obesity and the metabolic syndrome in developing countries. J Clin Endocrinol Metab 93:S9, 2008

MORTON GJ et al: Central nervous system control of food intake and body weight. Nature 443:289, 2006

VIRTANEN KA et al: Functional brown adipose tissue in healthy adults. N Engl J Med 360:1518, 2009

WALTERS RG et al: A new highly penetrant form of obesity due to deletions on chromosome 16p11.2. Nature 463:671, 2010

ZOBEL DP et al: Variants near MC4R are associated with obesity and influence obesity-related quantitative traits in a population of middle-aged people: Studies of 14,940 Danes. Diabetes 58:757, 2009

CHAPTER 78

Evaluation and Management of Obesity

Robert F. Kushner

Over 66% of U.S. adults are categorized as overweight or obese, and the prevalence of obesity is increasing rapidly in most of the industrialized world. Children and adolescents also are becoming more obese, indicating that the current trends will accelerate over time. Obesity is associated with an increased risk of multiple health problems, including hypertension, Type 2 diabetes, dyslipidemia, degenerative joint disease, and some malignancies. Thus, it is important for physicians to identify, evaluate, and treat patients for obesity and associated comorbid conditions.

■ EVALUATION

Physicians should screen all adult patients for obesity and offer intensive counseling and behavioral interventions to promote sustained weight loss. The five main steps in the evaluation of obesity, as described below, are (1) focused obesity-related history, (2) physical examination to determine the degree and type of obesity, (3) comorbid conditions, (4) fitness level, and (5) the patient's readiness to adopt lifestyle changes.

The obesity-focused history

Information from the history should address the following six questions:

- What factors contribute to the patient's obesity?
- How is the obesity affecting the patient's health?
- What is the patient's level of risk from obesity?
- What are the patient's goals and expectations?
- Is the patient motivated to begin a weight management program?
- What kind of help does the patient need?

Although the vast majority of cases of obesity can be attributed to behavioral features that affect diet and physical activity patterns, the history may suggest secondary causes that merit further evaluation. Disorders to consider include polycystic ovarian syndrome, hypothyroidism, Cushing's syndrome, and hypothalamic disease. Drug-induced weight gain also should be considered. Common causes include medications for diabetes (insulin, sulfonylureas, thiazolidinediones); steroid hormones; psychotropic agents; mood stabilizers (lithium); antidepressants (tricyclics, monoamine oxidase inhibitors, paroxetine, mirtazapine); and antiepileptic drugs (valproate, gabapentin, carbamazepine). Other medications, such as nonsteroidal anti-inflammatory drugs and calcium channel blockers, may cause peripheral edema but do not increase body fat.

The patient's current diet and physical activity patterns may reveal factors that contribute to the development of obesity in addition to identifying behaviors to target for treatment. This type of historic information is best obtained by using a questionnaire in combination with an interview.

BMI and waist circumference

Three key anthropometric measurements are important to evaluate the degree of obesity: weight, height, and waist circumference. The body mass index (BMI), calculated as weight (kg)/height (m)^2, or weight (lbs)/height (inches)^2 × 703, is used to classify weight status and risk of disease (Tables 78-1 and 78-2). BMI is used since it provides an estimate of body fat and is related to risk of disease. Lower BMI thresholds for overweight and obesity have been proposed for the Asia-Pacific region since this population appears to be at risk for glucose and lipid abnormalities at lower body weights.

Excess abdominal fat, assessed by measurement of waist circumference or waist-to-hip ratio, is independently associated with higher risk for diabetes mellitus and cardiovascular disease. Measurement of the waist circumference is a surrogate for visceral

TABLE 78-1 Body Mass Index (BMI) Table

BMI	19	20	21	22	23	24	25	26	27	28	29	30	31	32	33	34	35
Height, inches								Body Weight, pounds									
58	91	96	100	105	110	115	119	124	129	134	138	143	148	153	158	162	167
59	94	99	104	109	114	119	124	128	133	138	143	148	153	158	163	168	173
60	97	102	107	112	118	123	128	133	138	143	148	153	158	163	168	174	179
61	100	106	111	116	122	127	132	137	143	148	153	158	164	169	174	180	185
62	104	109	115	120	126	131	136	142	147	153	158	164	169	175	180	186	191
63	107	113	118	124	130	135	141	146	152	158	163	169	175	180	186	191	197
64	110	116	122	128	134	140	145	151	157	163	169	174	180	186	192	197	204
65	114	120	126	132	138	144	150	156	162	168	174	180	186	192	198	204	210
66	118	124	130	136	142	148	155	161	167	173	179	186	192	198	204	210	216
67	121	127	134	140	146	153	159	166	172	178	185	191	198	204	211	217	223
68	125	131	138	144	151	158	164	171	177	184	190	197	203	210	216	223	230
69	128	135	142	149	155	162	169	176	182	189	196	203	209	216	223	230	236
70	132	139	146	153	160	167	174	181	188	195	202	209	216	222	229	236	243
71	136	143	150	157	165	172	179	186	193	200	208	215	222	229	236	243	250
72	140	147	154	162	169	177	184	191	199	206	213	221	228	235	242	250	258
73	144	151	159	166	174	182	189	197	204	212	219	227	235	242	250	257	265
74	148	155	163	171	179	186	194	202	210	218	225	233	241	249	256	264	272
75	152	160	168	176	184	192	200	208	216	224	232	240	248	256	264	272	279
76	156	164	172	180	189	197	205	213	221	230	238	246	254	263	271	279	287

BMI	36	37	38	39	40	41	42	43	44	45	46	47	48	49	50	51	52	53	54
58	172	177	181	186	191	196	201	205	210	215	220	224	229	234	239	244	248	253	258
59	178	183	188	193	198	203	208	212	217	222	227	232	237	242	247	252	257	262	267
60	184	189	194	199	204	209	215	220	225	230	235	240	245	250	255	261	266	271	276
61	190	195	201	206	211	217	222	227	232	238	243	248	254	259	264	269	275	280	285
62	196	202	207	213	218	224	229	235	240	246	251	256	262	267	273	278	284	289	295
63	203	208	214	220	225	231	237	242	248	254	259	265	270	278	282	287	293	299	304
64	209	215	221	227	232	238	244	250	256	262	267	273	279	285	291	296	302	308	314
65	216	222	228	234	240	246	252	258	264	270	276	282	288	294	300	306	312	318	324
66	223	229	235	241	247	253	260	266	272	278	284	291	297	303	309	315	322	328	334
67	230	236	242	249	255	261	268	274	280	287	293	299	306	312	319	325	331	338	344
68	236	243	249	256	262	269	276	282	289	295	302	308	315	322	328	335	341	348	354
69	243	250	257	263	270	277	284	291	297	304	311	318	324	331	338	345	351	358	365
70	250	257	264	271	278	285	292	299	306	313	320	327	334	341	348	355	362	369	376
71	257	265	272	279	286	293	301	308	315	322	329	338	343	351	358	365	372	379	386
72	265	272	279	287	294	302	309	316	324	331	338	346	353	361	368	375	383	390	397
73	272	280	288	295	302	310	318	325	333	340	348	355	363	371	378	386	393	401	408
74	280	287	295	303	311	319	326	334	342	350	358	365	373	381	389	396	404	412	420
75	287	295	303	311	319	327	335	343	351	359	367	375	383	391	399	407	415	423	431
76	295	304	312	320	328	336	344	353	361	369	377	385	394	402	410	418	426	435	443

TABLE 78-2 Classification of Weight Status and Risk of Disease

	BMI (kg/m²)	Obesity Class	Risk of Disease
Underweight	<18.5		
Healthy weight	18.5–24.9		
Overweight	25.0–29.9		Increased
Obesity	30.0–34.9	I	High
Obesity	35.0–39.9	II	Very high
Extreme Obesity	≥40	III	Extremely high

Source: Adapted from National Institutes of Health, National Heart, Lung, and Blood Institute: *Clinical Guidelines on the Identification, Evaluation, and Treatment of Overweight and Obesity in Adults.* U.S. Department of Health and Human Services, Public Health Service, 1998.

adipose tissue and should be performed in the horizontal plane above the iliac crest (Table 78-3).

Physical fitness

Several prospective studies have demonstrated that physical fitness, reported by questionnaire or measured by a maximal treadmill exercise test, is an important predictor of all-cause mortality rate independent of BMI and body composition. These observations highlight the importance of taking an exercise history during examination as well as emphasizing physical activity as a treatment approach.

Obesity-associated comorbid conditions

The evaluation of comorbid conditions should be based on presentation of symptoms, risk factors, and index of suspicion. All patients

TABLE 78-3 Ethnic-Specific Values for Waist Circumference

Ethnic Group	Waist Circumference
Europeans	
Men	>94 cm (37 in)
Women	>80 cm (31.5 in)
South Asians and Chinese	
Men	>90 cm (35 in)
Women	>80 cm (31.5 in)
Japanese	
Men	>85 cm (33.5 in)
Women	>90 cm (35 in)
Ethnic South and Central Americans	Use south Asian recommendations until more specific data are available.
Sub-Saharan Africans	Use European data until more specific data are available.
Eastern Mediterranean and Middle East (Arab) populations	Use European data until more specific data are available.

Source: From KGMM Alberti et al for the IDF Epidemiology Task Force Consensus Group: Lancet 366:1059, 2005.

TABLE 78-4 Obesity-Related Organ Systems Review

Cardiovascular
- Hypertension
- Congestive heart failure
- Cor pulmonale
- Varicose veins
- Pulmonary embolism
- Coronary artery disease

Endocrine
- Metabolic syndrome
- Type 2 diabetes
- Dyslipidemia
- Polycystic ovarian syndrome

Musculoskeletal
- Hyperuricemia and gout
- Immobility
- Osteoarthritis (knees and hips)
- Low back pain
- Carpal tunnel syndrome

Psychological
- Depression/low self-esteem
- Body image disturbance
- Social stigmatization

Integument
- Striae distensae
- Stasis pigmentation of legs
- Lymphedema
- Cellulitis
- Intertrigo, carbuncles
- Acanthosis nigricans
- Acrochordon (skin tags)
- Hidradenitis suppurativa

Respiratory
- Dyspnea
- Obstructive sleep apnea
- Hypoventilation syndrome
- Pickwickian syndrome
- Asthma

Gastrointestinal
- Gastroesophageal reflux disease
- Nonalcoholic fatty liver disease
- Cholelithiasis
- Hernias
- Colon cancer

Genitourinary
- Urinary stress incontinence
- Obesity-related glomerulopathy
- Hypogonadism (male)
- Breast and uterine cancer
- Pregnancy complications

Neurologic
- Stroke
- Idiopathic intracranial hypertension
- Meralgia paresthetica
- Dementia

should have a fasting lipid panel [total, low-density lipoprotein (LDL), and high-density lipoprotein (HDL) cholesterol and triglyceride levels] and fasting blood glucose along with blood pressure determination. Symptoms and diseases that are directly or indirectly related to obesity are listed in Table 78-4. Although individuals vary, the number and severity of organ-specific comorbid conditions usually rise with increasing levels of obesity. Patients at very high absolute risk include those with the following: established coronary heart disease; presence of other atherosclerotic diseases, such as peripheral arterial disease, abdominal aortic aneurysm, and symptomatic carotid artery disease; Type 2 diabetes; and sleep apnea.

Assessing the patient's readiness to change

An attempt to initiate lifestyle changes when the patient is not ready usually leads to frustration and may hamper future weight-loss efforts. Assessment includes patient motivation and support, stressful life events, psychiatric status, time availability and constraints, and appropriateness of goals and expectations. Readiness can be viewed as the balance of two opposing forces: (1) motivation, or the patient's desire to change, and (2) resistance, or the patient's resistance to change.

A helpful method to begin a readiness assessment is to "anchor" the patient's interest and confidence to change on a numerical scale. With this technique, the patient is asked to rate his or her level of interest and confidence on a scale from 0 to 10, with 0 being not so important (or confident) and 10 being very important (or confident) to lose weight at this time. This exercise helps establish readiness to change and also serves as a basis for further dialogue.

TREATMENT Obesity

THE GOAL OF THERAPY The primary goal of treatment is to improve obesity-related comorbid conditions and reduce the risk of developing future comorbidities. Information obtained from the history, physical examination, and diagnostic tests is used to determine risk and develop a treatment plan (Fig. 78-1). The decision of how aggressively to treat the patient and which modalities to use is determined by the patient's risk status, expectations, and available resources. Therapy for obesity always begins with lifestyle management and may include pharmacotherapy or surgery, depending on

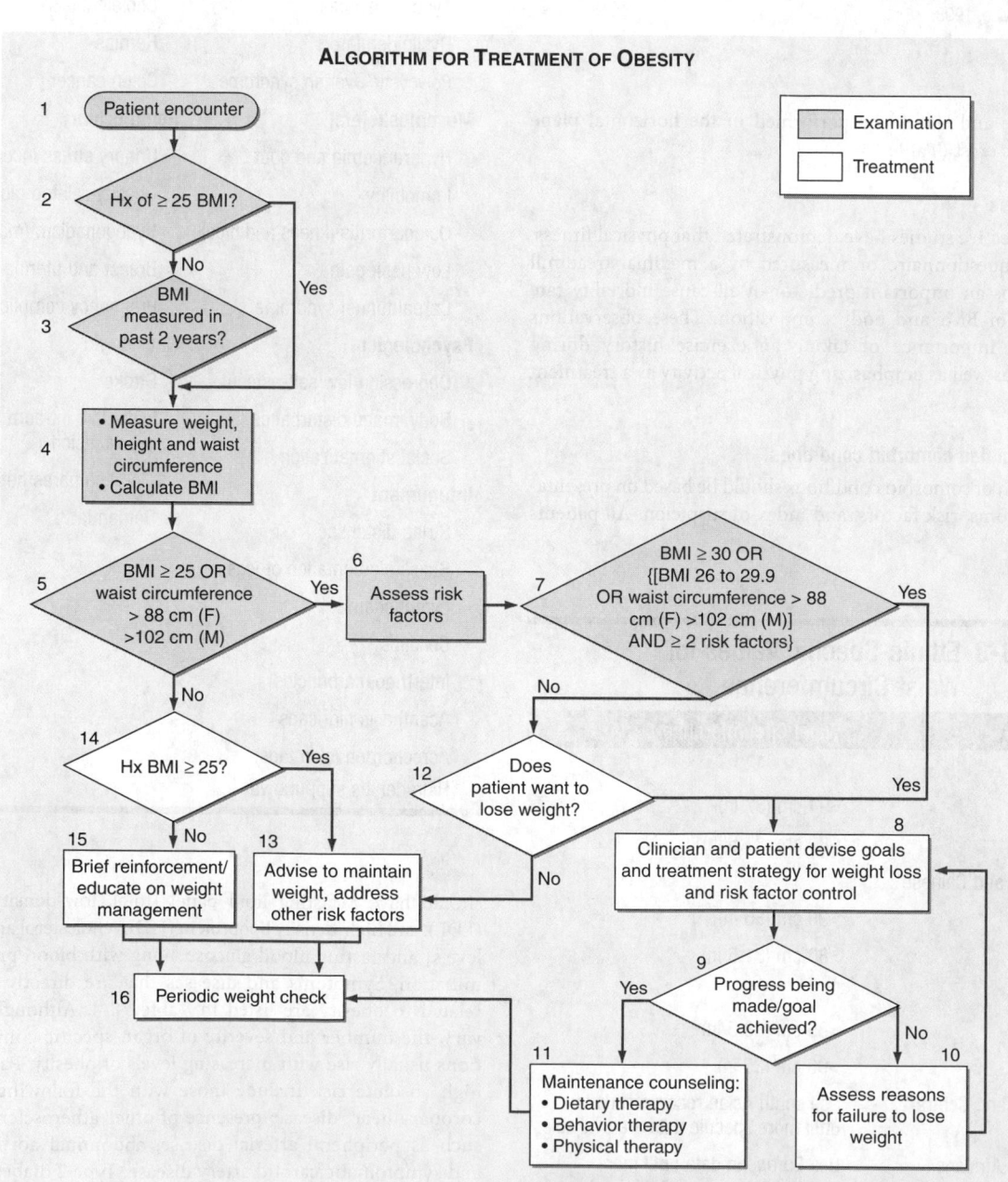

Figure 78-1 Treatment algorithm. This algorithm applies only to the assessment for overweight and obesity and subsequent decisions on that assessment. It does not reflect any initial overall assessment for other conditions that the physician may wish to perform. BMI, body mass index; Ht, height; Hx, history; Wt, weight. (*From National, Heart, Lung, and Blood Institute: Clinical guidelines on the identification, evaluation, and treatment of overweight and obesity in adults: The evidence report. Washington, DC, US Department of Health and Human Services, 1998.*)

TABLE 78-5 A Guide to Selecting Treatment

	BMI Category				
Treatment	25–26.9	27–29.9	30–35	35–39.9	≥40
Diet, exercise, behavior therapy	With comorbidities	With comorbidities	+	+	+
Pharmacotherapy		With comorbidities	+	+	+
Surgery				With comorbidities	+

Source: From National Heart, Lung, and Blood Institute, North American Association for the Study of Obesity (2000).

BMI risk category (Table 78-5). Setting an initial weight-loss goal of 10% over 6 months is a realistic target.

LIFESTYLE MANAGEMENT Obesity care involves attention to three essential elements of lifestyle: dietary habits, physical activity, and behavior modification. Because obesity is fundamentally a disease of energy imbalance, all patients must learn how and when energy is consumed (diet), how and when energy is expended (physical activity), and how to incorporate this information into their daily lives (behavior therapy). Lifestyle management has been shown to result in a modest (typically 3–5 kg) weight loss compared with no treatment or usual care.

Diet Therapy The primary focus of diet therapy is to reduce overall calorie consumption. The National Heart, Lung, and Blood Institute (NHLBI) guidelines recommend initiating treatment with a calorie deficit of 500–1000 kcal/d compared with the patient's habitual diet. This reduction is consistent with a goal of losing approximately 1–2 lb per week. This calorie deficit can be accomplished by suggesting substitutions or alternatives to the diet. Examples include choosing smaller portion sizes, eating more fruits and vegetables, consuming more whole-grain cereals, selecting leaner cuts of meat and skimmed dairy products, reducing fried foods and other added fats and oils, and drinking water instead of caloric beverages. It is important that the dietary counseling remain patient-centered and that the goals be practical, realistic, and achievable.

The macronutrient composition of the diet will vary with the patient's preference and medical condition. The 2005 U.S. Department of Agriculture Dietary Guidelines for Americans (Chap. 73), which focus on health promotion and risk reduction, can be applied to treatment of overweight or obese patients. The recommendations include maintaining a diet rich in whole grains, fruits, vegetables, and dietary fiber; consuming two servings (8 oz) of fish high in omega 3 fatty acids per week; decreasing sodium to <2300 mg/d; consuming 3 cups of milk (or equivalent low-fat or fat-free dairy products) per day; limiting cholesterol to <300 mg/d; and keeping total fat between 20 and 35% of daily calories and saturated fats to <10% of daily calories. Application of these guidelines to specific calorie goals can be found on the website *www.mypyramid.gov*. The revised Dietary Reference Intakes for Macronutrients released by the Institute of Medicine recommends 45–65% of calories from carbohydrates, 20–35% from fat, and 10–35% from protein. The guidelines also recommend daily fiber intake of 38 g (men) and 25 g (women) for persons over 50 years of age and 30 g (men) and 21 g (women) for those under age 50.

Since portion control is one of the most difficult strategies for patients to manage, the use of pre-prepared products such as meal replacements is a simple and convenient suggestion. Examples include frozen entrees, canned beverages, and bars. Use of meal replacements in the diet has been shown to result in a 7–8% weight loss.

An ongoing area of investigation is the use of low-carbohydrate, high-protein diets for weight loss. These diets are based on the concept that carbohydrates are the primary cause of obesity and lead to insulin resistance. Most low-carbohydrate diets (e.g., South Beach, Zone, and Sugar Busters!) recommend a carbohydrate level of approximately 40–46% of energy. The Atkins diet contains 5–15% carbohydrate, depending on the phase of the diet. Low-carbohydrate, high-protein diets appear to be more effective in lowering BMI; improving coronary heart disease risk factors, including an increase in HDL cholesterol and a decrease in triglyceride levels; and controlling satiety in the short term compared with low-fat diets. However, after 12 months, there is no significance difference among diets. Multiple studies have shown that sustained adherence to the diet rather than diet type is likely to be the best predictor of weight-loss outcome.

Another dietary approach to consider is the concept of energy density, which refers to the number of calories (energy) a food contains per unit of weight. People tend to ingest a constant volume of food regardless of caloric or macronutrient content. Adding water or fiber to a food decreases its energy density by increasing weight without affecting caloric content. Examples of foods with low-energy density include soups, fruits, vegetables, oatmeal, and lean meats. Dry foods and high-fat foods such as pretzels, cheese, egg yolks, potato chips, and red meat have a high-energy density. Diets containing low-energy dense foods have been shown to control hunger and result in decreased caloric intake and weight loss.

Occasionally, very low calorie diets (VLCDs) are prescribed as a form of aggressive dietary therapy. The primary purpose of a VLCD is to promote a rapid and significant (13–23 kg) short-term weight loss over a 3- to 6-month period. These propriety formulas typically supply ≤800 kcal, 50–80 g protein, and 100% of the recommended daily intake for vitamins and minerals. According to a review by the National Task Force on the Prevention and Treatment of Obesity, indications for initiating a VLCD include well-motivated individuals who are moderately to severely obese (BMI >30), have failed at more conservative approaches to weight loss, and have a medical condition that would be immediately improved with rapid weight loss. These conditions include poorly controlled Type 2 diabetes, hypertriglyceridemia, obstructive sleep apnea, and symptomatic peripheral edema. The risk for gallstone formation increases exponentially at rates of weight loss >1.5 kg/week (3.3 lb/week). Prophylaxis against gallstone formation with ursodeoxycholic acid, 600 mg/d, is effective in reducing this risk. Because of the need for close metabolic monitoring, these diets usually are prescribed by physicians specializing in obesity care.

Physical Activity Therapy Although exercise alone is only moderately effective for weight loss, the combination of dietary modification and exercise is the most effective behavioral approach for the treatment of obesity. The most important role of exercise appears to be in the maintenance of the weight loss. The 2008 Physical Activity Guidelines for Americans recommends that adults should engage in 150 min a week of moderate-intensity or 75 minutes a week of vigorous-intensity aerobic physical activity performed in episodes of at least 10 min, preferably spread throughout the week. The guidelines can be found at *www.health.gov/paguidelines*. Focusing on simple ways to add physical activity into the normal daily routine through leisure activities, travel, and domestic work should be suggested. Examples include walking, using the stairs, doing home and yard work, and engaging in sport activities. Asking the patient to wear a pedometer to monitor total accumulation of steps as part of the activities of daily living is a useful strategy. Step counts are highly correlated with activity level. Studies have demonstrated that lifestyle activities are as effective as structured exercise programs for improving cardiorespiratory fitness and weight loss. A high amount of physical activity (more than 300 min of moderate-intensity activity a week) is often needed to lose weight and sustain weight loss. These exercise recommendations are daunting to most patients and need to be implemented gradually. Consultation with an exercise physiologist or personal trainer may be helpful.

Behavioral Therapy Cognitive behavioral therapy is used to help change and reinforce new dietary and physical activity behaviors. Strategies include self-monitoring techniques (e.g., journaling, weighing, and measuring food and activity); stress management; stimulus control (e.g., using smaller plates, not eating in front of the television or in the car); social support; problem solving; and cognitive restructuring to help patients develop more positive and realistic thoughts about themselves. When recommending any behavioral lifestyle change, have the patient identify what, when, where, and how the behavioral change will be performed. The patient should keep a record of the anticipated behavioral change so that progress can be reviewed at the next office visit. Because these techniques are time-consuming to implement, they are often provided by ancillary office staff such as a nurse clinician or registered dietitian.

PHARMACOTHERAPY Adjuvant pharmacologic treatments should be considered for patients with a BMI >30 kg/m^2 or a BMI >27 kg/m^2 for those who also have concomitant obesity-related diseases and for whom dietary and physical activity therapy has not been successful. When an antiobesity medication is prescribed, patients should be actively engaged in a lifestyle program that provides the strategies and skills needed to use the drug effectively since this support increases total weight loss.

There are several potential targets of pharmacologic therapy for obesity. The most thoroughly explored treatment is suppression of appetite via centrally active medications that alter monoamine neurotransmitters. A second strategy is to reduce the absorption of selective macronutrients from the gastrointestinal (GI) tract, such as fat.

Centrally Acting Anorexiant Medications Appetite-suppressing drugs, or anorexiants, affect satiety—the absence of hunger after eating—and hunger—a biologic sensation that initiates eating. By increasing satiety and decreasing hunger, these agents help patients reduce caloric intake without a sense of deprivation. The target site for the actions of anorexiants is the ventromedial and lateral hypothalamic regions in the central nervous system (Chap. 77). Their biologic effect on appetite regulation is produced by augmenting the neurotransmission of three monoamines: norepinephrine; serotonin [5-hydroxytryptamine (5-HT)]; and, to a lesser degree, dopamine. The classic sympathomimetic adrenergic agents (benzphetamine, phendimetrazine, diethylpropion, mazindol, and phentermine) function by stimulating norepinephrine release or by blocking its reuptake. In contrast, sibutramine (Meridia) functions as a serotonin and norepinephrine reuptake inhibitor. Unlike other previously used anorexiants, sibutramine is not pharmacologically related to amphetamine and has no addictive potential.

Sibutramine was the only available anorexiant approved by the U.S. Food and Drug Administration (FDA) for long-term use until it was voluntarily withdrawn from the U.S. market by the manufacturer in October 2010, due to an increased risk of nonfatal myocardial infarction and nonfatal stroke among individuals with preexisting cardiovascular disease.

Peripherally Acting Medications Orlistat (Xenical) is a synthetic hydrogenated derivative of a naturally occurring lipase inhibitor, lipostatin, produced by the mold *Streptomyces toxytricini*. Orlistat is a potent, slowly reversible inhibitor of pancreatic, gastric, and carboxylester lipases and phospholipase A$_2$, which are required for the hydrolysis of dietary fat into fatty acids and monoacylglycerols. The drug acts in the lumen of the stomach and small intestine by forming a covalent bond with the active site of these lipases. Taken at a therapeutic dose of 120 mg tid, orlistat blocks the digestion and absorption of about 30% of dietary fat. After discontinuation of the drug, fecal fat usually returns to normal concentrations within 48–72 h.

Multiple randomized, double-blind, placebo-controlled studies have shown that after 1 year, orlistat produces a weight loss of about 9–10%, compared with a 4–6% weight loss in the placebo-treated groups. Because orlistat is minimally (<1%) absorbed from the GI tract, it has no systemic side effects. Tolerability to the drug is related to the malabsorption of dietary fat and subsequent passage of fat in the feces. GI tract adverse effects are reported in at least 10% of orlistat-treated patients. These effects include flatus with discharge, fecal urgency, fatty/oily stool, and increased defecation. These side effects generally are experienced early, diminish as patients control their dietary fat intake, and infrequently cause patients to withdraw from clinical trials. Psyllium mucilloid is helpful in controlling the orlistat-induced GI side effects when taken concomitantly with the medication. Serum concentrations of the fat-soluble vitamins D and E and β-carotene may be reduced, and vitamin supplements are recommended to prevent potential deficiencies. Orlistat was approved for over-the-counter use in 2007.

The Endocannabinoid System Cannabinoid receptors and their endogenous ligands have been implicated in a variety of physiologic functions, including feeding, modulation of pain, emotional behavior, and peripheral lipid metabolism. Cannabis and its main ingredient, Δ^9-tetrahydrocannabinol (THC), is an exogenous cannabinoid compound. Two endocannabinoids have been identified: anandamide and 2-arachidonyl glyceride. Two cannabinoid receptors have been identified: CB$_1$ (abundant in the brain) and CB$_2$ (present in immune cells). The brain endocannabinoid system is thought to control food intake by reinforcing motivation to find and consume foods with high incentive value and to regulate actions of other mediators of appetite. The first selective cannabinoid CB$_1$ receptor antagonist, rimonabant, was discovered in 1994. The medication antagonizes the orexigenic effect of THC and suppresses appetite. Several large prospective, randomized controlled trials have demonstrated the effectiveness of rimonabant as a weight-loss agent with concomitant improvements in waist circumference and cardiovascular risk factors. However, increased risk of neurologic and psychiatric side effects—seizures, depression, anxiety, insomnia, aggressiveness, and suicidal thoughts among patients randomized to rimonabant—resulted in a ruling against approval of the drug by the FDA in June 2007. Although the drug was available in 56 countries around the world in 2008, approval was officially withdrawn by the European Medicines Agency (EMEA) in January 2009, stating that the benefits of rimonabant no longer outweighed its risks. Development of CB_1 antagonists that do not enter the brain and selectively target the peripheral endocannabinoid system is needed.

Antiobesity Drugs in Development An emerging theme in pharmacotherapy for obesity is to target several points in the regulatory pathways that control body weight. Several combination drug therapies have completed phase III trials and have been submitted to the FDA for approval. Bupropion and naltrexone (Contrave), a dopamine and norepinephrine reuptake inhibitor and an opioid receptor antagonist, respectively, are combined to dampen the motivation/reinforcement that food brings (dopamine effect) and the pleasure/palatability of eating (opioid effect). Another formulation of bupropion with zonisamide (Empatic) combines bupropion with an anticonvulsant that has serotonergic and dopaminergic activity. Lastly, a formulation of phentermine and topiramate (Qnexa) combines a catecholamine releaser and an anticonvulsant, respectively, that have independently been shown to result in weight loss. The mechanism responsible for topiramate's weight loss is uncertain but is thought to be mediated through its modulation of γ-aminobutyric acid (GABA) receptors, inhibition of carbonic anhydrase, and antagonism of glutamate to reduce food intake. In October 2010, the FDA rejected Qnexa's initial application as a new drug, citing clinical concerns regarding the potential teratogenic risks of topiramate in women of childbearing age. An additional investigational drug, lorcaserin, a 5-HT_2C receptor agonist, has completed phase III trials as a single agent. The FDA rejected Lorcaserin's initial application as a new drug, citing clinical concerns that the weight loss efficacy in overweight and obese individuals without type 2 diabetes is marginal, and non-clinical concerns related to mammary adenocarcinomas in female rats.

SURGERY Bariatric surgery can be considered for patients with severe obesity (BMI ≥40 kg/m²) or those with moderate obesity (BMI ≥35 kg/m²) associated with a serious medical condition. Surgical weight loss functions by reducing caloric intake and, depending on the procedure, macronutrient absorption.

Weight-loss surgeries fall into one of two categories: restrictive and restrictive-malabsorptive (Fig. 78-2). Restrictive surgeries limit the amount of food the stomach can hold and slow the rate of gastric emptying. The vertical banded gastroplasty (VBG) is the prototype of this category but is currently performed on a very limited basis due to lack of effectiveness in long-term trials. Laparoscopic adjustable silicone gastric banding (LASGB) has replaced the VBG as the most commonly performed restrictive operation. The first banding device, the LAP-BAND, was approved for use in the United States in 2001, and the second, the REALIZE band, in 2007. In contrast to previous devices, the diameters of these bands are adjustable by way of their connection to a reservoir that is implanted under the skin. Injection or removal of saline into the reservoir tightens or loosens the

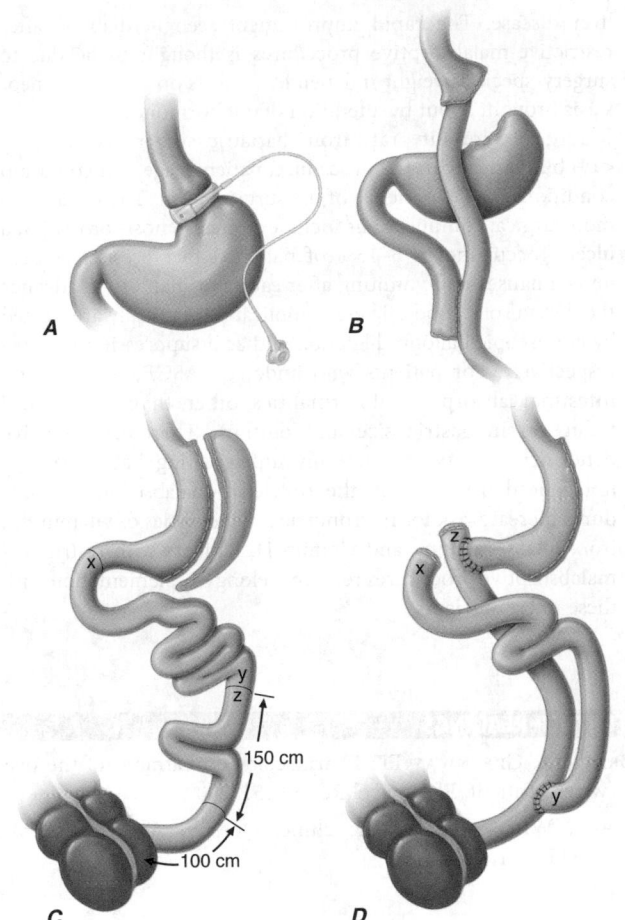

Figure 78-2 Bariatric surgical procedures. Examples of operative interventions used for surgical manipulation of the gastrointestinal tract. *A.* Laparoscopic gastric band (LAGB). *B.* The Roux-en-Y gastric bypass. *C.* Biliopancreatic diversion with duodenal switch. *D.* Biliopancreatic diversion. (*From ML Kendrick, GF Dakin: Mayo Clin Proc 815:518, 2006; with permission.*)

band's internal diameter, thus changing the size of the gastric opening.

The three restrictive-malabsorptive bypass procedures combine the elements of gastric restriction and selective malabsorption. These procedures include Roux-en-Y gastric bypass (RYGB), biliopancreatic diversion (BPD), and biliopancreatic diversion with duodenal switch (BPDDS) (Fig. 78-2). RYGB is the most commonly performed and accepted bypass procedure. It may be performed with an open incision or laparoscopically.

Although no recent randomized controlled trials compare weight loss after surgical and nonsurgical interventions, data from meta-analyses and large databases, primarily obtained from observational studies, suggest that bariatric surgery is the most effective weight-loss therapy for those with clinically severe obesity. These procedures generally produce a 30–35% average total body weight loss that is maintained in nearly 60% of patients at 5 years. In general, mean weight loss is greater after the combined restrictive-malabsorptive procedures than after the restrictive procedures. An abundance of data supports the positive impact of bariatric surgery on obesity-related morbid conditions, including diabetes mellitus, hypertension, obstructive sleep apnea, dyslipidemia, and nonalcoholic fatty liver disease. The rapid improvement seen in diabetes after restrictive-malabsorptive procedures is thought to be due to surgery-specific, weight-independent effects on glucose homeostasis brought about by alteration of gut hormones.

Surgical mortality rate from bariatric surgery is generally <1% but varies with the procedure, patient's age and comorbid conditions, and experience of the surgical team. The most common surgical complications include stomal stenosis or marginal ulcers (occurring in 5–15% of patients) that present as prolonged nausea and vomiting after eating or inability to advance the diet to solid foods. These complications typically are treated by endoscopic balloon dilatation and acid suppression therapy, respectively. For patients who undergo LASGB, there are no intestinal absorptive abnormalities other than mechanical reduction in gastric size and outflow. Therefore, selective deficiencies occur uncommonly unless eating habits become unbalanced. In contrast, the restrictive-malabsorptive procedures increase risk for micronutrient deficiencies of vitamin B_{12}, iron, folate, calcium, and vitamin D. Patients with restrictive-malabsorptive procedures require lifelong supplementation with these micronutrients.

FURTHER READINGS

BRAY GA, GREENWAY FL: Pharmacologic treatment of the overweight patient. Pharmacol Rev 59:151, 2007

———, WILSON JF: In the clinic: Obesity. Ann Intern Med 149:ITC4-1, 2008

DeMARIA EJ: Bariatric surgery for morbid obesity. N Engl J Med 356:2176, 2007

ECKEL RH: Nonsurgical management of obesity in adults. N Engl J Med 358:1941, 2008

KUSHNER RF: Roadmaps for clinical practice: Case studies in disease prevention and health promotion—assessment and management of adult obesity: A primer for physicians. Chicago, American Medical Association, 2003. Available online at www.ama-assn.org/ama/pub/category/10931.html

———: Anti-obesity drugs. Expert Opin Pharmacother 9:1339, 2008

McTIGUE KM et al: Screening and interventions for obesity in adults: Summary of the evidence for the U.S. Preventive Services Task Force. Ann Intern Med 139:933, 2003. (Appendix tables available at www.annals.org)

NATIONAL HEART, LUNG, AND BLOOD INSTITUTE, NORTH AMERICAN ASSOCIATION FOR THE STUDY OF OBESITY: Practical guide: Identification, evaluation, and treatment of overweight and obesity in adults. Bethesda, MD, National Institutes of Health pub number 00-4084, Oct. 2000. Available online at www.nhlbi.nih.gov/guidelines/obesity/practgde.htm

VETTER ML et al: Narrative review: Effect of bariatric surgery on type 2 diabetes mellitus. Ann Intern Med 150:94, 2009

WADDEN TA et al: Lifestyle modification for the management of obesity. Gastroenterology 132:2226, 2007

WEE CC: A 52-year-old woman with obesity: Review of bariatric surgery. JAMA 302:1097, 2009

CHAPTER **79**

Eating Disorders

B. Timothy Walsh
Evelyn Attia

Anorexia nervosa and bulimia nervosa are characterized by severe disturbances of eating behavior. The salient feature of *anorexia nervosa* (AN) is a voluntary restriction of food intake relative to caloric requirements leading to an inappropriately low body weight. *Bulimia nervosa* (BN) is characterized by recurrent episodes of binge eating followed by abnormal compensatory behaviors, such as self-induced vomiting. AN and BN are distinct clinical syndromes but share common features. Both disorders occur primarily among previously healthy young women who become overly concerned with body shape and weight. Many patients with BN have past histories of AN, and many patients with AN engage in binge eating and purging behavior. In the current diagnostic system, the critical distinction between AN and BN depends on body weight: patients with AN are, by definition, significantly underweight, whereas patients with BN have body weights in the normal range or above. *Binge eating disorder* (BED) is a more recently described syndrome characterized by repeated episodes of binge eating, similar to those of BN, in the absence of inappropriate compensatory behavior.

ANOREXIA NERVOSA

◼ EPIDEMIOLOGY

Among women, the lifetime prevalence of the full syndrome of AN is approximately 1%. AN is much less common in males. AN is more prevalent in cultures where food is plentiful and being thin is associated with attractiveness. Individuals who pursue interests that place a premium on thinness, such as ballet and modeling, are at greater risk. The incidence of AN has increased in recent decades.

◼ ETIOLOGY

The etiology of AN is unknown but appears to involve a combination of psychological, biologic, and cultural risk factors. Some factors, such as sexual or physical abuse and a family history of mood disturbance, are best viewed as nonspecific risk factors that increase vulnerability to a range of psychiatric disorders, including AN.

Patients who develop AN are inclined to be more obsessional and perfectionist than their peers. The disorder often begins as a diet not distinguishable at the outset from those undertaken by many adolescents and young women. As weight loss progresses, the fear of gaining weight grows; dieting becomes stricter; and psychological, behavioral, and medical aberrations increase. Eating disorders, including AN, may develop among individuals with type 1 diabetes mellitus and are associated with poorer glycemic control and an increased frequency of complications (Chap. 344).

Numerous physiologic disturbances, including abnormalities in a variety of neurotransmitter systems, have been described in AN (see below). It is difficult to distinguish neurochemical, metabolic, and hormonal changes that may have a role in the initiation or perpetuation of the syndrome from those that are secondary to the disorder. The resolution of most of these abnormalities with weight restoration argues against an etiologic role.

Genetic factors contribute to the risk of development of AN, as its incidence is greater in families with one affected member and the concordance in monozygotic twins is greater than in dizygotic twins. However, specific genes or risk factor loci have not been identified.

■ CLINICAL FEATURES

AN typically begins in mid to late adolescence, sometimes in association with a stressful life event such as leaving home for school (Table 79-1). The disorder occasionally develops in early puberty, before menarche, but seldom begins after age 40. Despite being underweight, patients with AN are irrationally afraid of gaining weight. They also exhibit a distortion of body image; despite being emaciated, patients with AN may believe that their body as a whole, or some part of their body, is too fat. Further weight loss is viewed by the patient as a fulfilling accomplishment, whereas weight gain is seen as a personal failure. Patients with AN rarely complain of hunger or fatigue and often exercise extensively. Despite the denial of hunger, one-quarter to one-half of patients with AN engage in eating binges. Patients tend to become socially withdrawn and increasingly committed to work or study, dieting, and exercise. As weight loss progresses, thoughts of food dominate mental life and

TABLE 79-1 Common Characteristics of Anorexia Nervosa, Bulimia Nervosa, and Binge Eating Disorder

	Anorexia Nervosa[a]	Bulimia Nervosa	Binge Eating Disorder[b]
Clinical Characteristics			
Onset	Mid-adolescence	Late adolescence/early adulthood	Late adolescence/early adulthood
Female:male	10:1	10:1	2:1
Lifetime prevalence	1% of women	1–3% of women	4% of men and women
Weight	Markedly decreased	Usually normal	Usually obese
Menstruation	Absent	Usually normal	Usually normal
Binge eating	25–50%	Required for diagnosis	Required for diagnosis
Mortality	~5% per decade	Low	Low
Physical and Laboratory Findings[a]			
Skin/extremities	Lanugo	Callus/abrasion on dorsum of hand	
	Acrocyanosis		
	Edema		
Cardiovascular	Bradycardia		
	Hypotension		
Gastrointestinal	Salivary gland enlargement	Salivary gland enlargement	
	Slow gastric emptying	Dental erosion	
	Constipation		
	Elevated liver enzymes		
Hematopoietic	Normochromic, normocytic anemia		
	Leukopenia		
Fluid/Electrolyte	Increased BUN, creatinine	Hypokalemia	
	Hypokalemia	Hypochloremia	
	Hypophosphatemia,	Alkalosis	
	Hypomagnesemia		
Endocrine	Hypoglycemia		
	Low estrogen or testosterone		
	Low LH and FSH		
	Low-normal thyroxine		
	Normal TSH		
	Increased cortisol		
Bone	Osteopenia		

[a]Patients with anorexia nervosa who frequently induce purging may also exhibit the physical and laboratory findings associated with bulimia nervosa.

[b]Obese patients with binge eating disorder are at risk for complications of obesity.

Abbreviations: BUN, blood urea nitrogen; FSH, follicle stimulating hormone; LH, luteinizing hormone; TSH, thyroid stimulating hormone.

idiosyncratic rules develop around eating. Patients with AN may obsessively collect cookbooks and recipes and be drawn to food-related occupations.

Physical features

Patients with AN typically have few physical complaints but may note cold intolerance. Gastrointestinal motility is diminished, leading to reduced gastric emptying and constipation. Some women who develop AN after menarche report that their menses ceased before significant weight loss occurred. Weight and height should be measured to allow calculation of body mass index (BMI; kg/m²). Vital signs may reveal bradycardia, hypotension, and mild hypothermia. Soft, downy hair growth (lanugo) sometimes occurs, as does alopecia. Salivary gland enlargement, which is associated with starvation as well as with binge eating and vomiting, may make the face appear surprisingly full in contrast to the marked general wasting. Acrocyanosis of the digits is common, and peripheral edema can be seen in the absence of hypoalbuminemia, particularly when the patient begins to regain weight. Consumption of large amounts of vegetables containing vitamin A can result in a yellow tint to the skin (*hypercarotenemia*), which is especially notable on the palms.

Laboratory abnormalities

Mild normochromic, normocytic anemia is frequent, as is mild to moderate leukopenia, with a disproportionate reduction of polymorphonuclear leukocytes. Dehydration may result in slightly increased levels of blood urea nitrogen and creatinine. Serum transaminase levels may increase, especially during the early phases of refeeding. The level of serum proteins is usually normal. Blood sugar is often low and serum cholesterol may be moderately elevated. Hypokalemia, often accompanied by alkalosis, suggests self-induced vomiting or use of diuretics. Hyponatremia is common and may result from excess fluid intake and disturbances in the secretion of antidiuretic hormone. Hypophosphatemia and hypomagnesemia may be present in severe AN, especially as part of a refeeding syndrome.

Endocrine abnormalities

The regulation of virtually every endocrine system is altered in AN, but the most striking changes occur in the reproductive system. Amenorrhea is hypothalamic in origin and reflects diminished production of gonadotropin-releasing hormone (GnRH). The resulting gonadotropin deficiency causes low plasma estrogen in women and reduced testosterone in men. The hypothalamic GnRH pulse generator is exquisitely sensitive, particularly in women, to body weight, stress, and exercise, each of which may contribute to *hypothalamic amenorrhea* in AN (Chap. 347).

Serum leptin levels are markedly reduced in AN as a result of undernutrition and decreased body-fat mass. The reduction in leptin is the primary factor responsible for the disturbances of the hypothalamic-pituitary-gonadal axis, and an important mediator of the other neuroendocrine abnormalities characteristic of AN (Chap. 77).

Serum cortisol and 24-h urine-free cortisol levels are generally elevated but without characteristic clinical signs of cortisol excess. Thyroid function tests resemble the pattern seen in euthyroid sick syndrome (Chap. 341). Thyroxine (T_4) and free T_4 levels are usually in the low-normal range, triiodothyronine (T_3) levels are reduced, and reverse T_3 (rT_3) is elevated. The level of thyroid-stimulating hormone (TSH) is normal or partially suppressed. Growth hormone is increased, but insulin-like growth factor 1 (IGF-1), which is produced mainly by the liver, is reduced, as in other conditions of starvation. Diminished bone density is routinely observed in AN and reflects the effects of multiple nutritional deficiencies,

TABLE 79-2 Diagnostic Features of Anorexia Nervosa

Refusal to maintain body weight at or above a minimally normal weight for age and height. (This includes a failure to achieve weight gain expected during a period of growth leading to an abnormally low body weight.)

Intense fear of weight gain or becoming fat.

Distortion of body image (e.g., feeling fat despite an objectively low weight or minimizing the seriousness of low weight).

Amenorrhea. (This criterion is met if menstrual periods occur only following hormone—e.g., estrogen—administration.)

reduced gonadal steroids, increased cortisol, and reduced IGF-1. The degree of bone-density reduction is proportional to the length of the illness, and patients are at risk for the development of symptomatic fractures. The occurrence of AN during adolescence may lead to the premature cessation of linear bone growth and a failure to achieve expected adult height.

Cardiac abnormalities

Cardiac output is reduced, and congestive heart failure occurs rarely during rapid refeeding. The electrocardiogram usually shows sinus bradycardia, reduced QRS voltage, and nonspecific ST-T-wave abnormalities. Some patients develop a prolonged QT_c interval, which may predispose to serious arrhythmias, particularly when electrolyte abnormalities are present.

◼ DIAGNOSIS

The diagnosis of AN is based on the presence of characteristic behavioral, psychological, and physical attributes (Table 79-2). Widely accepted diagnostic criteria are provided by the American Psychiatric Association's *Diagnostic and Statistical Manual of Mental Disorders* (DSM-IV). These criteria include maintenance of a less than minimally normal body weight for age and height. Weights less than 85% of that expected, roughly equivalent to a BMI of 18.5 kg/m², are commonly considered to meet this criterion, but a patient weighing somewhat more who meets all other diagnostic criteria would still merit the diagnosis of AN. The current diagnostic criteria require that women with AN not have spontaneous menses, patients who have other characteristics of AN but report menstrual activity probably merit the diagnosis.

The diagnosis of AN can usually be made confidently in a patient with a history of weight loss accomplished by restrictive dieting and excessive exercise accompanied by a marked reluctance to gain weight. Patients with AN often deny that they have a serious problem and may be brought to medical attention by concerned family or friends. Especially in atypical presentations, other causes of significant weight loss in previously healthy young people should be considered, including inflammatory bowel disease, gastric outlet obstruction, diabetes mellitus, CNS tumors, or neoplasm (Chap. 80).

◼ PROGNOSIS

The course and outcome of AN are highly variable. One-quarter to one-half of patients eventually recover fully, with few psychological or physical sequelae. However, many patients have persistent difficulties with weight maintenance, depression, and eating disturbances, including BN. The development of obesity following AN is rare. The long-term mortality of AN is among the highest associated with any psychiatric disorder. Approximately 5% of patients die per decade of follow-up, primarily due to the physical effects of chronic starvation or by suicide.

Virtually all of the physiologic abnormalities associated with AN are observed in other forms of starvation and markedly improve or disappear with weight gain. A worrisome exception is the reduction in bone mass, which may not recover fully, particularly if AN occurs during adolescence when peak bone mass is normally achieved.

TREATMENT Anorexia Nervosa

Because of the profound physiologic and psychological effects of starvation, there is a broad consensus that weight restoration to at least 90% of predicted weight is the primary goal in the treatment of AN. Unfortunately, because most patients resist this goal, the management of AN is often accompanied by frustration for the patient, the family, and the physician. Patients typically exaggerate their food intake and minimize their symptoms. Some patients resort to subterfuge to make their weights appear higher, for example, by water-loading before they are weighed. In attempting to engage the patient in treatment, it may be useful to elicit the patient's physical concerns (e.g., about osteoporosis, weakness, or fertility), and provide education about the importance of normalizing nutritional status in order to address those concerns. The physician should reassure the patient that weight gain will not be permitted to get out of control but simultaneously emphasize that weight restoration is medically and psychologically imperative.

The intensity of the initial treatment, including the need for hospitalization, is determined by the patient's current weight, the rapidity of recent weight loss, and the severity of medical and psychological complications (Fig. 79-1). Hospitalization

should be strongly considered for patients weighing <75% of that expected age and height, even if the results of routine blood studies are within normal limits. Acute medical problems, such as severe electrolyte imbalances, should be identified and addressed. Nutritional restoration can almost always be successfully accomplished by oral feeding, and parenteral methods are rarely required. For severely underweight patients, sufficient calories (approximately 1200–1800 kcal/d) should be provided initially in divided meals as food or liquid supplements to maintain weight and permit physiological stabilization. Calories can then be gradually increased to achieve a weight gain of 1–2 kg (2–4 lb) per week, typically requiring an intake of 3000–4000 kcal/d. Meals must be supervised, ideally by personnel who are firm regarding the necessity of food consumption, empathic regarding the challenges entailed, and reassuring about the patient's eventual recovery. Patients have great psychological difficulty complying with the need for increased caloric consumption, and the assistance of psychiatrists or psychologists experienced in the treatment of AN is usually necessary.

Less severely affected patients may be treated in a partial hospitalization program where medical and psychiatric supervision is available and several meals can be monitored each day. Outpatient treatment may suffice for mildly ill patients. Weight must be monitored at frequent intervals, and explicit goals agreed on for weight gain, with the understanding that more intensive treatment will be required if the level of care initially employed is not successful. For younger patients, the active involvement of the family in treatment is crucial regardless of treatment setting. Outpatient interventions that help parents refeed their child have been be quite successful at achieving weight restoration.

Psychiatric treatment focuses primarily on two issues. First, patients require much emotional support during the period of weight gain. They often intellectually agree with the need to gain weight, but strenuously resist increases in caloric intake, and often surreptitiously discard food that is provided. Second, patients must learn to base their self-esteem not on the achievement of an inappropriately low weight, but on the development of satisfying personal relationships and the attainment of reasonable academic and occupational goals. While this is often possible, some patients with AN develop other serious emotional and behavioral symptoms such as depression, self-mutilation, obsessive-compulsive behavior, and suicidal ideation. These symptoms may require additional therapeutic interventions, in the form of psychotherapy, medication, or hospitalization.

Medical complications occasionally occur during refeeding. Especially in the early stages of treatment, severely malnourished patients may develop a "refeeding syndrome" characterized by hypophosphatemia, hypomagnesemia, and cardiovascular instability. Acute gastric dilatation has been described when refeeding is rapid. As in other forms of malnutrition, fluid retention and peripheral edema may occur, but they generally do not require specific treatment in the absence of cardiac, renal, or hepatic dysfunction. Transient modest elevations in serum liver enzyme levels occasionally occur. Multivitamins should be given, and an adequate intake of vitamin D (400 IU/d) and calcium (1500 mg/d) should be provided.

No psychotropic medications are of established value in the treatment of AN, although there is recent preliminary evidence that the atypical antipsychotic medication olanzapine may assist some patients by increasing the rate of weight gain and decreasing obsessive thinking. Medications that may prolong the QT_c interval should be avoided. The alterations of cortisol and thyroid hormone metabolism do not require specific treatment and

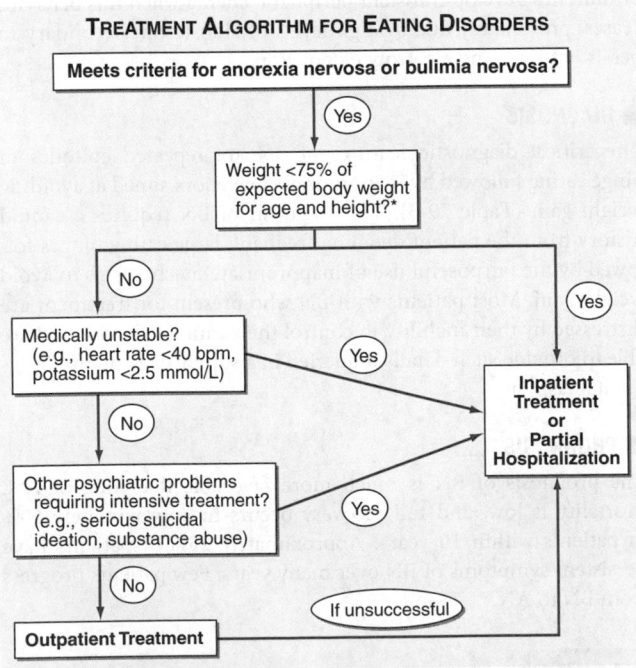

Figure 79-1 An algorithm for basic treatment decisions regarding patients with anorexia nervosa or bulimia nervosa. Based on the American Psychiatric Association practice guidelines for the treatment of patients with eating disorders. *Although outpatient management may be considered for patients with anorexia nervosa weighing more than 75% of expected, there should be a low threshold for using more intensive interventions if the weight loss has been rapid or if current weight is <80% of expected.

correct with weight gain. Estrogen treatment appears to offer no benefit to bone density in underweight patients, and the small benefit of bisphosphonate treatment appears to be outweighed by the potential risks of such agents in young women.

BULIMIA NERVOSA

■ EPIDEMIOLOGY

In women, the full syndrome of BN occurs with a lifetime prevalence of 1–3%. Variants of the disorder, such as occasional binge eating or purging, are much more common and occur in 5–10% of young women. The frequency of BN among men is less than one-tenth of that among women. The prevalence of BN increased dramatically in the early 1970s and 1980s but may have leveled off or declined somewhat in recent years.

■ ETIOLOGY

As with AN, the etiology of BN is likely to be multifactorial. Patients who develop BN describe a higher-than-expected prevalence of childhood and parental obesity, suggesting that a predisposition toward obesity may increase vulnerability to this eating disorder. The marked increase in the number of cases of BN during the past 30 years and the rarity of BN in underdeveloped countries imply that cultural factors are important.

■ CLINICAL FEATURES

The typical patient presenting for treatment of BN is a woman of normal weight in her mid-twenties who reports binge eating and purging 5–10 times a week for 5–10 years (Table 79-3). The disorder usually begins in late adolescence or early adulthood during or following a diet, often in association with depressed mood. The self-imposed caloric restriction leads to increased hunger and to overeating. In an attempt to avoid weight gain, the patient induces vomiting, takes laxatives or diuretics, or engages in some other form of compensatory behavior. During binges, patients with this disorder tend to consume large amounts of sweet foods with a high fat content, such as dessert items. The most frequent compensatory behaviors are self-induced vomiting and laxative abuse, but a wide variety of techniques have been described, including the omission of insulin injections by individuals with type 1 diabetes mellitus. Initially, patients may experience a sense of satisfaction that appealing food can be eaten without weight gain. However, as the disorder progresses, patients perceive diminished control over-eating. Binges increase in size and frequency and are provoked by a variety of stimuli, such as transient depression, anxiety, or a sense that too much food has been consumed in a normal meal. Between binges, patients restrict caloric intake, which increases hunger and sets the stage for the next binge. Typically, patients with BN are ashamed of their behavior and endeavor to keep their disorder hidden from family and friends. Like patients with AN, those with BN place an unusual emphasis on weight and shape as a basis for their self-esteem. Many patients with BN have mild symptoms of depression. Some patients exhibit serious mood and behavioral disturbances, such as suicide attempts, sexual promiscuity, and drug and alcohol abuse. Although vomiting may be triggered initially by manual stimulation of the gag reflex, most patients with BN develop the ability to induce vomiting at will. Rarely, patients resort to the regular use of syrup of ipecac. Laxatives and diuretics are frequently taken in impressive quantities, such as 30 or 60 laxative pills on a single occasion. The resulting fluid loss produces dehydration and a feeling of emptiness but has little impact on caloric balance.

The physical abnormalities associated with BN primarily result from the purging behavior. Painless bilateral salivary gland hypertrophy (sialadenosis) may be noted. A scar or callus on the dorsum of the hand may develop due to repeated trauma from the teeth among patients who manually stimulate the gag reflex. Recurrent vomiting and the exposure of the lingual surfaces of the teeth to stomach acid lead to loss of dental enamel and eventually to chipping and erosion of the front teeth. Laboratory abnormalities are surprisingly infrequent, but hypokalemia, hypochloremia, and hyponatremia are observed occasionally. Repeated vomiting may lead to alkalosis, whereas repeated laxative abuse may produce a mild metabolic acidosis. Serum amylase may be slightly elevated due to an increase in the salivary isoenzyme.

Serious physical complications resulting from BN are rare. Oligomenorrhea and amenorrhea are more frequent than among women without eating disorders. Arrhythmias occasionally occur secondary to electrolyte disturbances. Tearing of the esophagus and rupture of the stomach have been reported and constitute life-threatening events. Some patients who chronically abuse laxatives or diuretics develop transient peripheral edema when this behavior ceases, presumably due to high levels of aldosterone secondary to persistent fluid and electrolyte depletion.

■ DIAGNOSIS

The critical diagnostic features of BN are repeated episodes of binge eating followed by inappropriate behaviors aimed at avoiding weight gain (Table 79-3). The diagnosis of BN requires a candid history from the patient detailing frequent, large eating binges followed by the purposeful use of inappropriate mechanisms to avoid weight gain. Most patients with BN who present for treatment are distressed by their inability to control their eating behavior and are able to provide such details if queried in a supportive and nonjudgmental fashion.

■ PROGNOSIS

The prognosis of BN is much more favorable than that of AN. Mortality is low, and full recovery occurs in approximately 50% of patients within 10 years. Approximately 25% of patients have persistent symptoms of BN over many years. Few patients progress from BN to AN.

TABLE 79-3 Diagnostic Features of Bulimia Nervosa

Recurrent episodes of binge eating, which is characterized by the consumption of a large amount of food in a short period of time and a feeling that the eating is out of control.

Recurrent inappropriate behavior to compensate for the binge eating, such as self-induced vomiting.

The occurrence of both the binge eating and the inappropriate compensatory behavior at least twice weekly, on average, for 3 months.

Overconcern with body shape and weight.

Note: If the diagnostic criteria for anorexia nervosa are simultaneously met, only the diagnosis of anorexia nervosa is given.

TREATMENT   Bulimia Nervosa

BN can usually be treated on an outpatient basis (Fig. 79-1). Cognitive behavioral therapy (CBT) is a short-term (4–6 months) psychological treatment that focuses on the intense concern with shape and weight, the persistent dieting, and the binge eating and purging that characterize this disorder. Patients are directed to monitor the circumstances, thoughts, and emotions associated with binge/purge episodes, to eat regularly, and to challenge their assumptions linking weight to self-esteem. CBT produces symptomatic remission in 25–50% of patients.

Numerous double-blind, placebo-controlled trials have documented that antidepressant medications are useful in the treatment of BN but are probably somewhat less effective than CBT. Although efficacy has been established for virtually all chemical classes of antidepressants, only the selective serotonin reuptake inhibitor fluoxetine (Prozac) has been approved for use in BN by the U.S. Food and Drug Administration. Antidepressant medications are helpful even for patients with BN who are not depressed, and the dose of fluoxetine recommended for BN (60 mg/d) is higher than that typically used to treat depression. These observations suggest that different mechanisms may underlie the utility of these medications in BN and in depression.

A subset of patients does not respond to CBT, antidepressant medication, or their combination. More intensive forms of treatment, including hospitalization, may be required.

BINGE EATING DISORDER

Binge eating disorder (BED) is characterized by frequent episodes of eating unusually large amounts of food accompanied by feeling loss of control. In contrast to those with BN, patients with BED do not frequently engage in appropriate behavior to compensate for binge eating. In addition, BED is commonly associated with obesity (Table 79-1). BED occurs more frequently than AN and BN in both clinical and community population samples, and males constitute a greater fraction of affected individuals. Compared with obese individuals without BED, those with BED have higher rates of anxiety, depression, and health care use. A range of psychological treatments, such as CBT and interpersonal therapy (IPT) and medications, including antidepressants and weight-loss agents, appear helpful in reducing binge eating. Surprisingly, cessation of binge eating is not routinely followed by loss of weight.

GLOBAL CONSIDERATIONS

 Eating disorders are more common in cultures where food is available and thinness is idealized. Nevertheless, eating disorders have been reported across the world, including in many parts of Asia and Africa. Cultural variation may contribute to differing presentations of eating disorder symptoms. For example, in some cultural groups, the rationale for food refusal of low weight individuals who exhibit many symptoms of AN may not include the DSM IV criterion, "intense fear of gaining weight or becoming fat."

FURTHER READINGS

ATTIA E, WALSH BT: Behavioral management for anorexia nervosa. N Engl J Med 30:500, 2009

KATZMAN DK: Medical complications in adolescents with anorexia: A review of the literature. Int J Eat Disord 37(Suppl):S52, 2005

KESKI-RAHKONEN A et al: Epidemiology and course of anorexia nervosa in the community. Am J Psychiatry 164:1259, 2007

MEHLER PS: Clinical practice. Bulimia nervosa. N Engl J Med 349:875, 2003

MEHLER PS, MACKENZIE TD: Treatment of osteopenia and osteoporosis in anorexia nervosa: A systematic review of the literature. Int J Eat Disord 42:195, 2009

TREASURE J et al: Eating Disorders. Lancet 375:583, 2010

YAGER J et al: Practice guideline for the treatment of patients with eating disorders, 3rd ed, in *American Psychiatric Association Practice Guidelines for the Treatment of Psychiatric Disorders Compendium 2006*, American Psychiatric Association (ed). Arlington, Virginia, American Psychiatric Association, 2006

CHAPTER **80**
Involuntary Weight Loss

Russell G. Robertson
J. Larry Jameson

Involuntary weight loss (IWL) is frequently insidious and can have important implications, often serving as a harbinger of serious underlying disease. Clinically important weight loss is defined as the loss of 10 pounds (4.5 kg) or >5% of one's body weight over a period of 6–12 months. IWL is encountered in up to 8% of all adult outpatients and 27% of frail persons age 65 years and older. There is no identifiable cause in up to one-quarter of patients despite extensive investigation. Conversely, up to half of people who claim to have lost weight have no documented evidence of weight loss. People with no known cause of weight loss generally have a better prognosis than do those with known causes, particularly when the source is neoplastic. Weight loss in older persons is associated with a variety of deleterious effects, including hip fracture, pressure ulcers, impaired immune function, decreased functional status, and death. Not surprisingly, significant weight loss is associated with increased mortality, which can range from 9% to as high as 38% within 1 to 2.5 years in the absence of clinical awareness and attention.

■ PHYSIOLOGY OF WEIGHT REGULATION WITH AGING

(See also Chaps. 71 and 77) Among healthy aging people, total body weight peaks in the sixth decade of life and generally remains stable until the ninth decade, after which it gradually falls. In contrast, lean body mass (fat-free mass) begins to decline at a rate of 0.3 kg per year in the third decade, and the rate of decline increases further beginning at age 60 in men and age 65 in women. These changes in lean body mass largely reflect the age-dependent decline in growth hormone secretion and, consequently, circulating levels of insulin-like growth factor type I (IGF-I) that occur with normal aging. In the healthy elderly, an increase in fat tissue balances the loss in lean body mass until very old age, when loss of both fat and skeletal muscle occurs. Age-dependent changes also occur at the cellular level. Telomeres shorten, and body cell mass—the fat-free portion of cells—declines steadily with aging.

Between ages 20 and 80, mean energy intake is reduced by up to 1200 kcal/d in men and 800 kcal/d in women. Decreased hunger is a reflection of reduced physical activity and loss of lean body mass, producing lower demand for calories and food intake. Several important age-associated physiologic changes also predispose elderly persons to weight loss, such as declining chemosensory function (smell and taste), reduced efficiency of chewing, slowed gastric emptying, and alterations in the neuroendocrine axis, including changes in levels of leptin, cholecystokinin, neuropeptide Y, and other hormones and peptides. These changes are associated with early satiety and a decline in both appetite and the hedonistic appreciation of food. Collectively, they contribute to the "anorexia of aging."

■ CAUSES OF INVOLUNTARY WEIGHT LOSS

Most causes of IWL belong to one of four categories: (1) malignant neoplasms, (2) chronic inflammatory or infectious diseases, (3) metabolic disorders (e.g., hyperthyroidism and diabetes), or (4) psychiatric disorders (Table 80-1). Not infrequently, more than

TABLE 80-1 Causes of Involuntary Weight Loss

Cancer	Medications
Colon	Sedatives
Hepatobiliary	Antibiotics
Hematologic	Nonsteroidal anti-inflammatory drugs
Lung	
Breast	Serotonin reuptake inhibitors
Genitourinary	Metformin
Ovarian	Levodopa
Prostate	Angiotensin-converting enzyme inhibitors
Gastrointestinal disorders	
Malabsorption	Other drugs
Peptic ulcer	**Disorders of the mouth and teeth**
Inflammatory bowel disease	Caries
Pancreatitis	Dygeusia
Obstruction/constipation	**Age-related factors**
Pernicious anemia	Physiologic changes
Endocrine and metabolic	Visual impairment
Hyperthyroidism	Decreased taste and smell
Diabetes mellitus	Functional disabilities
Pheochromocytoma	**Neurologic**
Adrenal insufficiency	Stroke
Cardiac disorders	Parkinson's disease
Chronic ischemia	Neuromuscular disorders
Chronic congestive heart failure	Dementia
Respiratory disorders	**Social**
Emphysema	Isolation
Chronic obstructive pulmonary disease	Economic hardship
	Psychiatric and behavioral
Renal insufficiency	Depression
Rheumatologic disease	Anxiety
Infections	Paranoia
HIV	Bereavement
Tuberculosis	Alcoholism
Parasitic infection	Eating disorders
Subacute bacterial endocarditis	Increased activity or exercise
	Idiopathic

one of these causes can be responsible for IWL. In most series, IWL is caused by malignant disease in a quarter of patients and by organic disease in one-third, with the remainder due to psychiatric disease, medications, or uncertain causes.

The most common malignant causes of IWL are gastrointestinal, hepatobiliary, hematologic, lung, breast, genitourinary, ovarian, and prostate. Half of all patients with cancer lose some body weight; one-third lose more than 5% of their original body weight, and up to 20% of all cancer deaths are caused directly by cachexia (through immobility and/or cardiac/respiratory failure). The greatest incidence of weight loss is seen among patients with solid tumors. Malignancy that reveals itself through significant weight loss usually has a very poor prognosis.

In addition to malignancies, gastrointestinal causes are among the most prominent causes of IWL. Peptic ulcer disease, inflammatory bowel disease, dysmotility syndromes, chronic pancreatitis, celiac disease, constipation, and atrophic gastritis are some of the more common entities. Oral and dental problems are easily overlooked and may manifest with halitosis, poor oral hygiene, xerostomia, inability to chew, reduced masticatory force, nonocclusion, temporomandibular joint syndrome, edentulousness, and pain due to caries or abscesses.

Tuberculosis, fungal diseases, parasites, subacute bacterial endocarditis, and HIV are well-documented causes of IWL. Cardiovascular and pulmonary diseases cause unintentional weight loss through increased metabolic demand and decreased appetite and caloric intake. Uremia produces nausea, anorexia, and vomiting. Connective tissue diseases may increase metabolic demand and disrupt nutritional balance. As the incidence of diabetes mellitus increases with aging, the associated glucosuria can contribute to weight loss. Hyperthyroidism in the elderly may have less prominent sympathomimetic features and may present as "apathetic hyperthyroidism" or T_3 toxicosis (Chap. 341).

Neurologic injuries such as stroke, quadriplegia, and multiple sclerosis may lead to visceral and autonomic dysfunction that can impair caloric intake. Dysphagia from these neurologic insults is a common mechanism. Functional disability that compromises activities of daily living (ADLs) is a common cause of undernutrition in the elderly. Visual impairment from ophthalmic or central nervous system disorders such as a tremor can limit the ability of people to prepare and eat meals. IWL may be one of the earliest manifestations of Alzheimer's dementia.

Isolation and depression are significant causes of IWL that may manifest as an inability to care for oneself, including nutritional needs. A cytokine-mediated inflammatory metabolic cascade can be both a cause of and a manifestation of depression. Bereavement can be a cause of IWL and, when present, is more pronounced in men. More intense forms of mental illness such as paranoid disorders may lead to delusions about food and cause weight loss. Alcoholism can be a significant source of weight loss and malnutrition.

Elderly persons living in poverty may have to choose between purchasing food and purchasing medications. Institutionalization is an independent risk factor, as up to 30–50% of nursing home patients have inadequate food intake.

Medications can cause anorexia, nausea, vomiting, gastrointestinal distress, diarrhea, dry mouth, and changes in taste. This is particularly an issue in the elderly, many of whom take five or more medications.

■ ASSESSMENT

The four major manifestations of IWL are (1) anorexia (loss of appetite), (2) sarcopenia (loss of muscle mass), (3) cachexia (a syndrome that combines weight loss, loss of muscle and adipose tissue, anorexia, and weakness), and (4) dehydration. The current obesity epidemic adds complexity, as excess adipose tissue can mask the development of sarcopenia and delay awareness of the development of cachexia. If it is not possible to measure weight directly, a change in clothing size, corroboration of weight loss by a relative or friend, and a numeric estimate of weight loss provided by the patient are suggestive of true weight loss.

Initial assessment includes a comprehensive history and physical, a complete blood count, tests of liver enzyme levels, a C-reactive protein, erythrocyte sedimentation rate, renal function studies, thyroid function tests, chest radiography, and an abdominal ultrasound (Table 80-2). Age, sex, and risk factor–specific cancer screening tests, such as mammography and colonoscopy, should be performed (Chap. 82). Patients at risk should have HIV testing. All elderly patients with weight loss should undergo screening for dementia and depression by using instruments such as the Mini-Mental Status Examination and the Geriatric Depression Scale, respectively (Chap. 72). The Mini Nutritional Assessment (*www.mna-elderly.com*) and the Nutrition Screening Initiative (*www.aafp.org/afp/980301ap/edits.html*) are also available for the nutritional assessment of elderly patients. Almost all patients with a malignancy and >90% of those with other organic diseases have at least one laboratory abnormality. In patients presenting with substantial IWL, major organic and malignant diseases are unlikely when a baseline evaluation is completely normal. Careful follow-up rather than undirected testing is advised since the prognosis of weight loss of undetermined cause is generally favorable.

TABLE 80-2 Assessment and Testing for Involuntary Weight Loss

Indications	Laboratory
5% weight loss in 30 d	Complete blood count
10% weight loss in 180 d	Comprehensive electrolyte and metabolic panel, including liver and renal function tests
Body mass index <21	
25% of food left uneaten after 7 d	
Change in fit of clothing	Thyroid function tests
Change in appetite, smell, or taste	Erythrocyte sedimentation rate
	C-reactive protein
Abdominal pain, nausea, vomiting, diarrhea, constipation, dysphagia	Ferritin
	HIV testing, if indicated
Assessment	**Radiology**
Complete physical exam, including dental evaluation	Chest x-ray
Medication review	Abdominal ultrasound
Recommended cancer screening	
Mini-Mental State Examination*	
Mini-Nutritional Assessment*	
Nutrition Screening Initiative*	
Simplified Nutritional Assessment Questionnaire*	
Observation of eating*	
Activities of daily living*	
Instrumental activities of daily living*	

*May be more specific to assess weight loss in the elderly.

TREATMENT Unintentional Weight Loss

The first priority in managing weight loss is to identify and treat the underlying causes systematically. Treatment of underlying metabolic, psychiatric, infectious, or other systemic disorders may be sufficient to restore weight and functional status gradually. Medications that cause nausea or anorexia should be withdrawn or changed, if possible. For those with unexplained IWL, oral nutritional supplements such as high-energy drinks sometimes reverse weight loss. Advising patients to consume supplements between meals rather than with a meal may help minimize appetite suppression and facilitate increased overall intake. Orexigenic, anabolic, and anticytokine agents are under investigation. In selected patients, the antidepressant mirtazapine results in a significant increase in body weight, body fat mass, and leptin concentration. Patients with wasting conditions who can comply with an appropriate exercise program gain muscle protein mass, strength, and endurance and may be more capable of performing ADL.

FURTHER READINGS

ALIBHAI SM et al: An approach to the management of unintentional weight loss in elderly people. CMAJ 172:773, 2005

CHEN SP et al: Evaluating probability of cancer among older people with unexplained, unintentional weight loss. Arch Gerontol Geriatr 50 Suppl 1:S27, 2010

MILLER SL, WOLFE RR: The danger of weight loss in the elderly. J Nutr Health Aging 12:487, 2008

ROLLAND Y et al: Office management of weight loss in older persons. Am J Med 119:1019, 2006

VANDERSCHUEREN S et al: The diagnostic spectrum of unintentional weight loss. Eur J Intern Med 16:160, 2005

VISVANATHAN R, CHAPMAN IM: Undernutrition and anorexia in the older person. Gastroenterol Clin North Am 38:393, 2009

PART 7

Oncology and Hematology

PART 7

Oncology and Hematology

CHAPTER **81**

Approach to the Patient With Cancer

Dan L. Longo

The application of current treatment techniques (surgery, radiation therapy, chemotherapy, and biologic therapy) results in the cure of nearly two of three patients diagnosed with cancer. Nevertheless, patients experience the diagnosis of cancer as one of the most traumatic and revolutionary events that has ever happened to them. Independent of prognosis, the diagnosis brings with it a change in a person's self-image and in his or her role in the home and workplace. The prognosis of a person who has just been found to have pancreatic cancer is the same as the prognosis of the person with aortic stenosis who develops the first symptoms of congestive heart failure (median survival, ~8 months). However, the patient with heart disease may remain functional and maintain a self-image as a fully intact person with just a malfunctioning part, a diseased organ ("a bum ticker"). By contrast, the patient with pancreatic cancer has a completely altered self-image and is viewed differently by family and anyone who knows the diagnosis. He or she is being attacked and invaded by a disease that could be anywhere in the body. Every ache or pain takes on desperate significance. Cancer is an exception to the coordinated interaction among cells and organs. In general, the cells of a multicellular organism are programmed for collaboration. Many diseases occur because the specialized cells fail to perform their assigned task. Cancer takes this malfunction one step further. Not only is there a failure of the cancer cell to maintain its specialized function but it also strikes out on its own; the cancer cell competes to survive using natural mutability and natural selection to seek advantage over normal cells in a recapitulation of evolution. One consequence of the traitorous behavior of cancer cells is that the patient feels betrayed by his or her body. The cancer patient feels that he or she, and not just a body part, is diseased.

THE MAGNITUDE OF THE PROBLEM

No nationwide cancer registry exists; therefore, the incidence of cancer is estimated on the basis of the National Cancer Institute's Surveillance, Epidemiology, and End Results (SEER) database, which tabulates cancer incidence and death figures from nine sites, accounting for about 10% of the U.S. population, and from population data from the U.S. Census Bureau. In 2010, 1.530 million new cases of invasive cancer (789,620 men, 739,940 women) were diagnosed and 569,490 persons (299,200 men, 270,290 women) died from cancer. The percent distribution of new cancer cases and cancer deaths by site for men and women are shown in Table 81-1. Cancer incidence has been declining by about 2% each year since 1992.

The most significant risk factor for cancer overall is age; two-thirds of all cases were in those older than age 65 years. Cancer incidence increases as the third, fourth, or fifth power of age in different sites. For the interval between birth and age 39 years, 1 in 70 men and 1 in 48 women will develop cancer; for the interval

TABLE 81-1 Distribution of Cancer Incidence and Deaths for 2010

Sites	Male %	Male Number	Sites	Female %	Female Number
Cancer Incidence					
Prostate	28	217,730	Breast	28	207,090
Lung	15	116,750	Lung	14	105,770
Colorectal	9	72,090	Colorectal	10	70,480
Bladder	7	52,760	Endometrial	6	43,470
Melanoma	5	38,870	Thyroid	5	33,930
Lymphoma	4	35,380	Lymphoma	4	30,160
Kidney	4	35,370	Melanoma	4	29,260
Oral cavity	3	25,420	Kidney	3	22,870
Leukemia	3	24,690	Ovary	3	21,880
Pancreas	3	21,370	Pancreas	3	21,770
All others	19	149,190	All others	20	153,260
All sites	100	789,620	All sites	100	739,940
Cancer Deaths					
Lung	29	86,220	Lung	26	71,080
Prostate	11	32,050	Breast	15	39,840
Colorectal	9	26,580	Colorectal	9	24,790
Pancreas	6	18,770	Pancreas	7	18,030
Liver	4	12,720	Ovary	5	13,850
Leukemia	4	12,660	Lymphoma	4	9500
Esophagus	4	11,650	Leukemia	3	9180
Lymphoma	4	10,710	Endometrial	3	7950
Bladder	3	10,410	Liver	2	6190
Kidney	3	8210	CNS	2	5720
All others	23	69,220	All others	24	64,160
All sites	100	299,200	All sites	100	270,290

between ages 40 and 59 years, 1 in 12 men and 1 in 11 women will develop cancer; and for the interval between ages 60 and 79 years, 1 in 3 men and 1 in 5 women will develop cancer. Overall, men have a 44% risk of developing cancer at some time during their lives; women have a 38% lifetime risk.

Cancer is the second leading cause of death behind heart disease. Deaths from heart disease have declined 45% in the United States since 1950 and continue to decline. Cancer has overtaken heart disease as the number one cause of death in persons younger than age 85 years (Fig. 81-1). After a 70-year period of increase, cancer deaths began to decline in 1990-1991 (Fig. 81-2). Between 1990 and 2006, cancer deaths decreased by 21% among men and 12.3% among women. The five leading causes of cancer deaths are shown

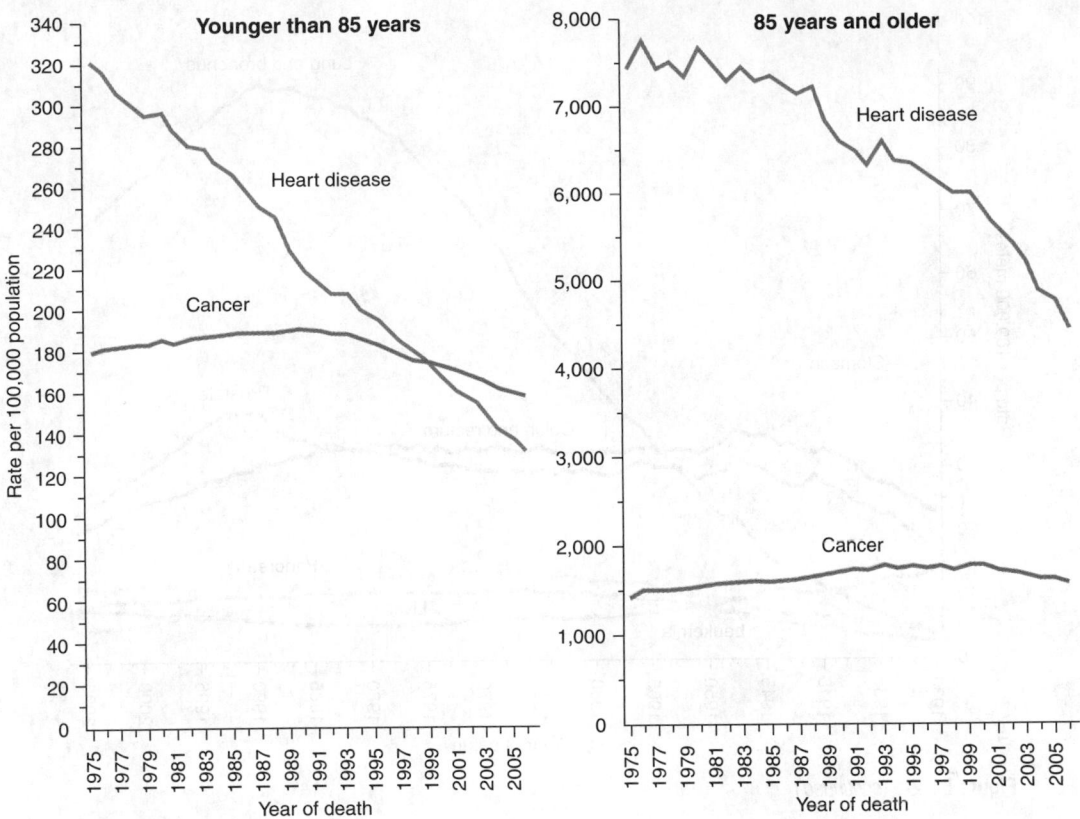

Figure 81-1 Death rates for heart disease and cancer among people younger and older than age 85 years. **A.** In people younger than age 85 years, cancer has overtaken heart disease as the largest cause of death. **B.** In people older than age 85 years, heart disease is by far the major cause of death. *(From Jemal et al.)*

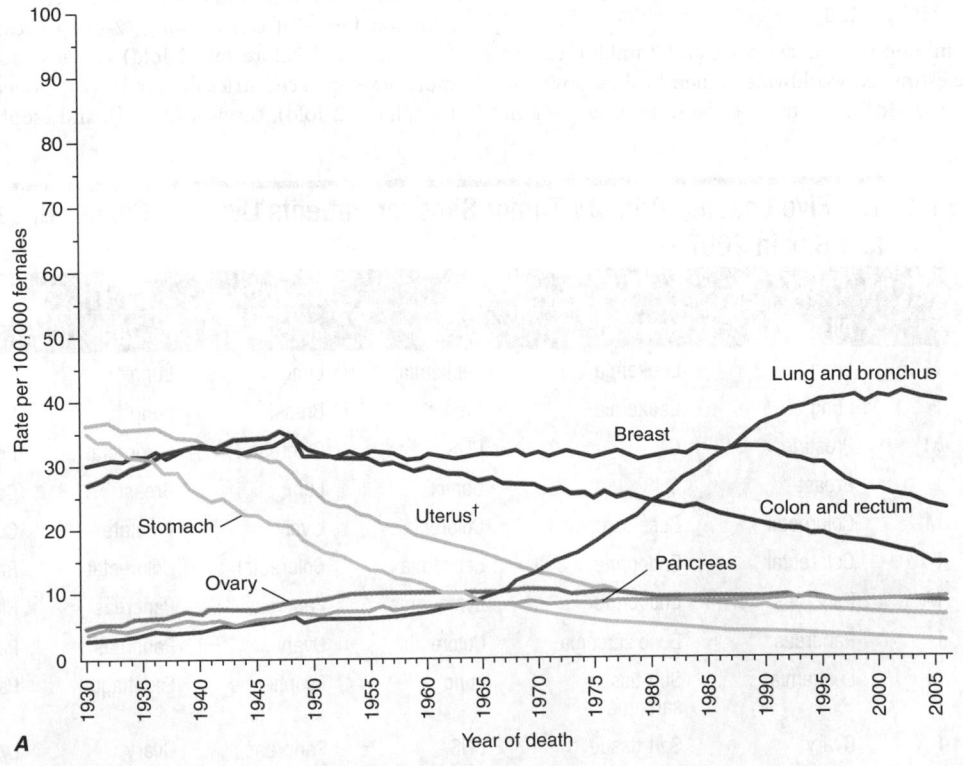

A

Figure 81-2 Sixty-five-year trend in cancer death rates for (*A*) women and (*B*) men by site in the United States, 1930–2006. Rates are per 100,000 age-adjusted to the 2000 U.S. standard population. *(From Jemal et al.)*

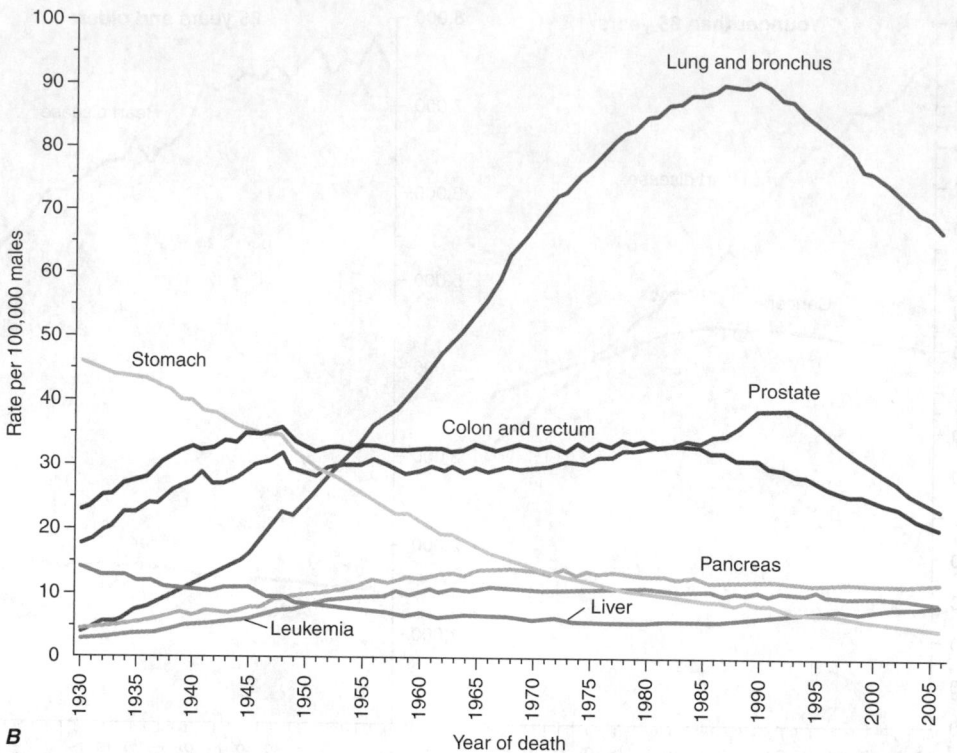

Figure 81-2 (*continued*)

for various populations in Table 81-2. The 5-year survival for white patients was 39% in 1960–1963 and 69% in 1999–2005. Cancers are more often deadly in blacks; the 5-year survival was 59% for the 1999–2005 interval. Incidence and mortality vary among racial and ethnic groups (Table 81-3). The basis for these differences is unclear.

■ CANCER AROUND THE WORLD

 In 2002, 11 million new cancer cases and 7 million cancer deaths were estimated worldwide. When broken down by region of the world, ~45% of cases were in Asia, 26% in

Europe, 14.5% in North America, 7.1% in Central/South America, 6% in Africa, and 1% in Australia/New Zealand (Fig. 81-3). Lung cancer is the most common cancer and the most common cause of cancer death in the world. Its incidence is highly variable, affecting only 2 per 100,000 African women but as many as 61 per 100,000 North American men. Breast cancer is the second most common cancer worldwide; however, it ranks fifth as a cause of death behind lung, stomach, liver, and colorectal cancer. Among the eight most common forms of cancer, lung (2-fold), breast (3-fold), prostate (2.5-fold), and colorectal (3-fold) cancers are more common in more developed countries than in less developed countries. By contrast, liver (2-fold), cervical (2-fold), and esophageal (2- to 3-fold)

TABLE 81-2 The Five Leading Primary Tumor Sites for Patients Dying of Cancer Based on Age and Sex in 2007

Rank		All Ages	Age, years				
			Under 20	20–39	40–59	60–79	>80
1	M	Lung	Leukemia	Leukemia	Lung	Lung	Lung
	F	Lung	Leukemia	Breast	Breast	Lung	Lung
2	M	Prostate	CNS	CNS	Colorectal	Colorectal	Prostate
	F	Breast	CNS	Cervix	Lung	Breast	Colorectal
3	M	Colorectal	Bone sarcoma	Colorectal	Liver	Prostate	Colorectal
	F	Colorectal	Endocrine	Leukemia	Colorectal	Colorectal	Breast
4	M	Pancreas	Endocrine	Lymphoma	Pancreas	Pancreas	Bladder
	F	Pancreas	Bone sarcoma	Colorectal	Ovary	Pancreas	Pancreas
5	M	Leukemia	Soft tissue sarcoma	Lung	Esophagus	Esophagus	Pancreas
	F	Ovary	Soft tissue sarcoma	CNS	Pancreas	Ovary	Lymphoma

Abbreviations: M, male; F, female.

TABLE 81-3 Cancer Incidence and Mortality in Racial and Ethnic Groups, U.S., 2002–2006

Site		White	Black	Asian/Pacific Islander	American Indian	Hispanic
Incidence per 100,000 Population						
All	M	550.1	626.8	334.5	318.4	430.3
	F	420.0	389.5	276.3	265.1	326.8
Breast		123.5	113.0	81.6	67.2	90.2
Colorectal	M	58.2	68.4	44.1	38.1	50.0
	F	42.6	51.7	33.1	30.7	35.1
Kidney	M	19.7	20.6	9.0	16.6	18.2
	F	10.3	10.6	4.5	10.6	10.3
Liver	M	8.0	12.5	21.4	8.9	15.9
	F	2.8	3.8	8.1	4.6	6.2
Lung	M	85.9	104.8	50.6	57.9	49.2
	F	57.1	50.7	27.6	41.3	26.5
Prostate		146.3	231.9	82.3	82.7	131.1
Deaths per 100,000 Population						
All	M	226.7	304.2	135.4	183.3	154.8
	F	157.3	183.7	95.1	140.1	103.9
Breast		23.9	33.0	12.5	17.6	15.5
Colorectal	M	21.4	31.4	13.8	20.0	16.2
	F	14.9	21.6	10.0	13.7	10.7
Kidney	M	6.1	6.0	2.4	9.0	5.2
	F	2.8	2.7	1.2	4.2	2.4
Liver	M	6.8	10.8	15.0	10.3	11.2
	F	2.9	3.9	6.6	6.5	5.1
Lung	M	69.9	90.1	36.9	48.0	33.9
	F	41.9	40.0	18.2	33.5	14.4
Prostate		23.6	56.3	10.6	20.0	19.6

Abbreviations: M, male; F, female.

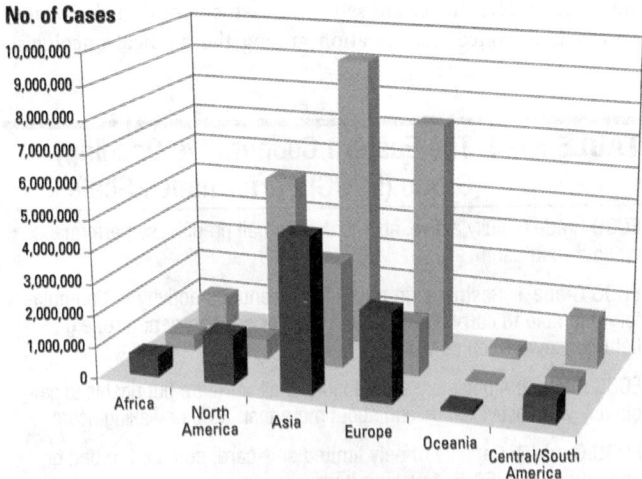

Figure 81-3 Worldwide overall annual cancer incidence, mortality and 5-year prevalence for the period of 1993–2001. *(From Kamangar et al.)*

cancers are more common in less developed countries. Stomach cancer incidence is similar in more and less developed countries but is much more common in Asia than North America or Africa. The most common cancers in Africa are cervical, breast, and liver cancers. It has been estimated that nine modifiable risk factors are responsible for more than one-third of cancers worldwide. These include smoking, alcohol consumption, obesity, physical inactivity, low fruit and vegetable consumption, unsafe sex, air pollution, indoor smoke from household fuels, and contaminated injections.

PATIENT MANAGEMENT

Important information is obtained from every portion of the routine history and physical examination. The duration of symptoms may reveal the chronicity of disease. The past medical history may alert the physician to the presence of underlying diseases that may affect the choice of therapy or the side effects of treatment. The social history may reveal occupational exposure to carcinogens or habits, such as smoking or alcohol consumption, that may influence the course of disease and its treatment. The family history may suggest an underlying familial cancer predisposition and point out the need to begin surveillance or other preventive therapy for unaffected siblings of the patient. The review of systems may suggest early symptoms of metastatic disease or a paraneoplastic syndrome.

■ DIAGNOSIS

The diagnosis of cancer relies most heavily on invasive tissue biopsy and should never be made without obtaining tissue; no noninvasive diagnostic test is sufficient to define a disease process as cancer. Although in rare clinical settings (e.g., thyroid nodules) fine-needle aspiration is an acceptable diagnostic procedure, the diagnosis generally depends on obtaining adequate tissue to permit careful evaluation of the histology of the tumor, its grade, and its invasiveness and to yield further molecular diagnostic information, such as the expression of cell-surface markers or intracellular proteins that typify a particular cancer, or the presence of a molecular marker, such as the t(8;14) translocation of Burkitt's lymphoma. Increasing evidence links the expression of certain genes with the prognosis and response to therapy (Chaps. 83 and 84).

Occasionally a patient will present with a metastatic disease process that is defined as cancer on biopsy but has no apparent primary site of disease. Efforts should be made to define the primary site based on age, sex, sites of involvement, histology and tumor markers, and personal and family history. Particular attention should be focused on ruling out the most treatable causes (Chap. 99).

Once the diagnosis of cancer is made, the management of the patient is best undertaken as a multidisciplinary collaboration among the primary care physician, medical oncologists, surgical oncologists, radiation oncologists, oncology nurse specialists, pharmacists, social workers, rehabilitation medicine specialists, and a number of other consulting professionals working closely with each other and with the patient and family.

■ DEFINING THE EXTENT OF DISEASE AND THE PROGNOSIS

The first priority in patient management after the diagnosis of cancer is established and shared with the patient is to determine the extent of disease. The curability of a tumor usually is inversely proportional to the tumor burden. Ideally, the tumor will be diagnosed before symptoms develop or as a consequence of screening efforts (Chap. 82). A very high proportion of such patients can be cured. However, most patients with cancer present with symptoms related to the cancer, caused either by mass effects of the tumor or by alterations associated with the production of cytokines or hormones by the tumor.

For most cancers, the extent of disease is evaluated by a variety of noninvasive and invasive diagnostic tests and procedures. This process is called *staging*. There are two types. *Clinical staging* is based on physical examination, radiographs, isotopic scans, CT scans, and other imaging procedures; *pathologic staging* takes into account information obtained during a surgical procedure, which might include intraoperative palpation, resection of regional lymph nodes and/or tissue adjacent to the tumor, and inspection and biopsy of organs commonly involved in disease spread. Pathologic staging includes histologic examination of all tissues removed during the surgical procedure. Surgical procedures performed may include a simple lymph node biopsy or more extensive procedures such as thoracotomy, mediastinoscopy, or laparotomy. Surgical staging may occur in a separate procedure or may be done at the time of definitive surgical resection of the primary tumor.

Knowledge of the predilection of particular tumors for spreading to adjacent or distant organs helps direct the staging evaluation.

Information obtained from staging is used to define the extent of disease either as localized, as exhibiting spread outside of the organ of origin to regional but not distant sites, or as metastatic to distant sites. The most widely used system of staging is the TNM (tumor, node, metastasis) system codified by the International Union Against Cancer and the American Joint Committee on Cancer. The TNM classification is an anatomically based system that categorizes the tumor on the basis of the size of the primary tumor lesion (T1–4, where a higher number indicates a tumor of larger size), the presence of nodal involvement (usually N0 and N1 for the absence and presence, respectively, of involved nodes, although some tumors have more elaborate systems of nodal grading), and the presence of metastatic disease (M0 and M1 for the absence and presence, respectively, of metastases). The various permutations of T, N, and M scores (sometimes including tumor histologic grade G) are then broken into stages, usually designated by the roman numerals I through IV. Tumor burden increases and curability decreases with increasing stage. Other anatomic staging systems are used for some tumors, e.g., the Dukes classification for colorectal cancers, the International Federation of Gynecologists and Obstetricians classification for gynecologic cancers, and the Ann Arbor classification for Hodgkin's disease.

Certain tumors cannot be grouped on the basis of anatomic considerations. For example, hematopoietic tumors such as leukemia, myeloma, and lymphoma are often disseminated at presentation and do not spread like solid tumors. For these tumors, other prognostic factors have been identified (Chaps. 109–111).

In addition to tumor burden, a second major determinant of treatment outcome is the physiologic reserve of the patient. Patients who are bedridden before developing cancer are likely to fare worse, stage for stage, than fully active patients. Physiologic reserve is a determinant of how a patient is likely to cope with the physiologic stresses imposed by the cancer and its treatment. This factor is difficult to assess directly. Instead, surrogate markers for physiologic reserve are used, such as the patient's age or Karnofsky performance status (Table 81-4) or Eastern Cooperative Oncology Group (ECOG) performance status (Table 81-5). Older patients and those with a Karnofsky performance status <70 or ECOG performance status ≥3 have a poor prognosis unless the poor performance is a reversible consequence of the tumor.

Increasingly, biologic features of the tumor are being related to prognosis. The expression of particular oncogenes, drug-resistance genes, apoptosis-related genes, and genes involved in metastasis are being found to influence response to therapy and prognosis. The presence of selected cytogenetic abnormalities may influence survival. Tumors with higher growth fractions, as assessed by expression of proliferation-related markers such as proliferating cell nuclear antigen, behave more aggressively than tumors with lower growth fractions. Information obtained from studying the tumor

TABLE 81-4 Karnofsky Performance Index

Performance Status	Functional Capability of the Patient
100	Normal; no complaints; no evidence of disease
90	Able to carry on normal activity; minor signs or symptoms of disease
80	Normal activity with effort; some signs or symptoms of disease
70	Cares for self; unable to carry on normal activity or do active work
60	Requires occasional assistance but is able to care for most needs
50	Requires considerable assistance and frequent medical care
40	Disabled; requires special care and assistance
30	Severely disabled; hospitalization is indicated although death is not imminent
20	Very sick; hospitalization necessary; active supportive treatment is necessary
10	Moribund, fatal processes progressing rapidly
0	Dead

itself will increasingly be used to influence treatment decisions. Host genes involved in drug metabolism can influence the safety and efficacy of particular treatments.

▪ MAKING A TREATMENT PLAN

From information on the extent of disease and the prognosis and in conjunction with the patient's wishes, it is determined whether the treatment approach should be curative or palliative in intent. Cooperation among the various professionals involved in cancer treatment is of the utmost importance in treatment planning. For some cancers, chemotherapy or chemotherapy plus radiation therapy delivered before the use of definitive surgical treatment (so-called neoadjuvant therapy) may improve the outcome, as seems to be the case for locally advanced breast cancer and head and neck cancers. In certain settings in which combined modality therapy is intended, coordination among the medical oncologist,

TABLE 81-5 The Eastern Cooperative Oncology Group (ECOG) Performance Scale

ECOG Grade 0: Fully active, able to carry on all predisease performance without restriction

ECOG Grade 1: Restricted in physically strenuous activity but ambulatory and able to carry out work of a light or sedentary nature, e.g., light housework, office work

ECOG Grade 2: Ambulatory and capable of all self-care but unable to carry out any work activities. Up and about more than 50% of waking hours

ECOG Grade 3: Capable of only limited self-care, confined to bed or chair more than 50% of waking hours

ECOG Grade 4: Completely disabled. Cannot carry on any self-care. Totally confined to bed or chair

ECOG Grade 5: Dead

Source: From MM Oken et al: Am J Clin Oncol 5:649, 1982.

radiation oncologist, and surgeon is crucial to achieving optimal results. Sometimes the chemotherapy and radiation therapy need to be delivered sequentially, and other times concurrently. Surgical procedures may precede or follow other treatment approaches. It is best for the treatment plan either to follow a standard protocol precisely or else to be part of an ongoing clinical research protocol evaluating new treatments. Ad hoc modifications of standard protocols are likely to compromise treatment results.

The choice of treatment approaches was formerly dominated by the local culture in both the university and the practice settings. However, it is now possible to gain access electronically to standard treatment protocols and to every approved clinical research study in North America through a personal computer interface with the Internet.[1]

The skilled physician also has much to offer the patient for whom curative therapy is no longer an option. Often a combination of guilt and frustration over the inability to cure the patient and the pressure of a busy schedule greatly limit the time a physician spends with a patient who is receiving only palliative care. Resist these forces. In addition to the medicines administered to alleviate symptoms (see below), it is important to remember the comfort that is provided by holding the patient's hand, continuing regular examinations, and taking time to talk.

■ MANAGEMENT OF DISEASE AND TREATMENT COMPLICATIONS

Because cancer therapies are toxic (Chap. 85), patient management involves addressing complications of both the disease and its treatment as well as the complex psychosocial problems associated with cancer. In the short term during a course of curative therapy, the patient's functional status may decline. Treatment-induced toxicity is less acceptable if the goal of therapy is palliation. The most common side effects of treatment are nausea and vomiting (see below), febrile neutropenia (Chap. 86), and myelosuppression (Chap. 85). Tools are now available to minimize the acute toxicity of cancer treatment.

New symptoms developing in the course of cancer treatment should always be assumed to be reversible until proven otherwise. The fatalistic attribution of anorexia, weight loss, and jaundice to recurrent or progressive tumor could result in a patient dying from a reversible intercurrent cholecystitis. Intestinal obstruction may be due to reversible adhesions rather than progressive tumor. Systemic infections, sometimes with unusual pathogens, may be a consequence of the immunosuppression associated with cancer therapy. Some drugs used to treat cancer or its complications (e.g., nausea) may produce central nervous system symptoms that look like metastatic disease or may mimic paraneoplastic syndromes such as the syndrome of inappropriate antidiuretic hormone. A definitive diagnosis should be pursued and may even require a repeat biopsy.

A critical component of cancer management is assessing the response to treatment. In addition to a careful physical examination in which all sites of disease are physically measured and recorded in a flow chart by date, response assessment usually requires periodic repeating of imaging tests that were abnormal at the time of staging. If imaging tests have become normal, repeat biopsy of previously involved tissue is performed to document complete response by pathologic criteria. Biopsies are not usually required if there is macroscopic residual disease. A *complete response* is defined as disappearance of all evidence of disease, and a *partial response* as >50% reduction in the sum of the products of the perpendicular diameters of all measurable lesions. The determination of partial response may also be based on a 30% decrease in the sums of the longest diameters of lesions (Response Evaluation Criteria in Solid Tumors, or RECIST, criteria). *Progressive disease* is defined as the appearance of any new lesion or an increase of >25% in the sum of the products of the perpendicular diameters of all measurable lesions (or an increase of 20% in the sums of the longest diameters by RECIST). Tumor shrinkage or growth that does not meet any of these criteria is considered *stable disease*. Some sites of involvement (e.g., bone) or patterns of involvement (e.g., lymphangitic lung or diffuse pulmonary infiltrates) are considered unmeasurable. No response is complete without biopsy documentation of their resolution, but partial responses may exclude their assessment unless clear objective progression has occurred.

Tumor markers may be useful in patient management in certain tumors. Response to therapy may be difficult to gauge with certainty. However, some tumors produce or elicit the production of markers that can be measured in the serum or urine, and in a particular patient, rising and falling levels of the marker are usually associated with increasing or decreasing tumor burden, respectively. Some clinically useful tumor markers are shown in Table 81-6. Tumor markers are not in themselves specific enough to permit a diagnosis of malignancy to be made, but once a malignancy has been diagnosed and shown to be associated with elevated levels of a tumor marker, the marker can be used to assess response to treatment.

The recognition and treatment of depression are important components of management. The incidence of depression in cancer patients is ~25% overall and may be greater in patients with greater debility. This diagnosis is likely in a patient with a depressed mood (dysphoria) and/or a loss of interest in pleasure (anhedonia) for at least 2 weeks. In addition, three or more of the following symptoms are usually present: appetite change, sleep problems, psychomotor retardation or agitation, fatigue, feelings of guilt or worthlessness, inability to concentrate, and suicidal ideation. Patients with these symptoms should receive therapy. Medical therapy with a serotonin reuptake inhibitor such as fluoxetine (10–20 mg/d), sertraline (50–150 mg/d), or paroxetine (10–20 mg/d) or a tricyclic antidepressant such as amitriptyline (50–100 mg/d) or desipramine (75–150 mg/d) should be tried, allowing 4–6 weeks for response. Effective therapy should be continued at least 6 months after resolution of symptoms. If therapy is unsuccessful, other classes of antidepressants may be used. In addition to medication, psychosocial interventions such as support groups, psychotherapy, and guided imagery may be of benefit.

Many patients opt for unproven or unsound approaches to treatment when it appears that conventional medicine is unlikely to be curative. Those seeking such alternatives are often well educated and may be early in the course of their disease. Unsound approaches are usually hawked on the basis of unsubstantiated anecdotes and not only cannot help the patient but may be harmful. Physicians should strive to keep communications open and nonjudgmental, so that patients are more likely to discuss with the physician what they are actually doing. The appearance of unexpected toxicity may be an indication that a supplemental therapy is being taken.[2]

---

[1]The National Cancer Institute maintains a database called PDQ (Physician Data Query) that is accessible on the Internet under the name CancerNet at *www.cancer.gov/cancertopics/pdq/cancerdatabase*. Information can be obtained through a facsimile machine using CancerFax by dialing 301-402-5874. Patient information is also provided by the National Cancer Institute in at least three formats: on the Internet via CancerNet at *www.cancer.gov*, through the CancerFax number listed above, or by calling 1-800-4-CANCER. The quality control for the information provided through these services is rigorous.

---

[2] Information about unsound methods may be obtained from the National Council Against Health Fraud, Box 1276, Loma Linda, CA 92354, or from the Center for Medical Consumers and Health Care Information, 237 Thompson Street, New York, NY 10012.

TABLE 81-6 Tumor Markers

Tumor Markers	Cancer	Nonneoplastic Conditions
Hormones		
Human chorionic gonadotropin	Gestational trophoblastic disease, gonadal germ cell tumor	Pregnancy
Calcitonin	Medullary cancer of the thyroid	
Catecholamines	Pheochromocytoma	
Oncofetal Antigens		
α Fetoprotein	Hepatocellular carcinoma, gonadal germ cell tumor	Cirrhosis, hepatitis
Carcinoembryonic antigen	Adenocarcinomas of the colon, pancreas, lung, breast, ovary	Pancreatitis, hepatitis, inflammatory bowel disease, smoking
Enzymes		
Prostatic acid phosphatase	Prostate cancer	Prostatitis, prostatic hypertrophy
Neuron-specific enolase	Small cell cancer of the lung, neuroblastoma	
Lactate dehydrogenase	Lymphoma, Ewing's sarcoma	Hepatitis, hemolytic anemia, many others
Tumor-Associated Proteins		
Prostate-specific antigen	Prostate cancer	Prostatitis, prostatic hypertrophy
Monoclonal immunoglobulin	Myeloma	Infection, MGUS
CA-125	Ovarian cancer, some lymphomas	Menstruation, peritonitis, pregnancy
CA 19-9	Colon, pancreatic, breast cancer	Pancreatitis, ulcerative colitis
CD30	Hodgkin's disease, anaplastic large cell lymphoma	—
CD25	Hairy cell leukemia, adult T cell leukemia/lymphoma	—

Abbreviation: MGUS, monoclonal gammopathy of uncertain significance.

■ LONG-TERM FOLLOW-UP/LATE COMPLICATIONS

At the completion of treatment, sites originally involved with tumor are reassessed, usually by radiography or imaging techniques, and any persistent abnormality is biopsied. If disease persists, the multidisciplinary team discusses a new salvage treatment plan. If the patient has been rendered disease-free by the original treatment, the patient is followed regularly for disease recurrence. The optimal guidelines for follow-up care are not known. For many years, a routine practice has been to follow the patient monthly for 6–12 months, then every other month for a year, every 3 months for a year, every 4 months for a year, every 6 months for a year, and then annually. At each visit, a battery of laboratory and radiographic and imaging tests were obtained on the assumption that it is best to detect recurrent disease before it becomes symptomatic. However, where follow-up procedures have been examined, this assumption has been found to be untrue. Studies of breast cancer, melanoma, lung cancer, colon cancer, and lymphoma have all failed to support the notion that asymptomatic relapses are more readily cured by salvage therapy than symptomatic relapses. In view of the enormous cost of a full battery of diagnostic tests and their manifest lack of impact on survival, new guidelines are emerging for less frequent

follow-up visits, during which the history and physical examination are the major investigations performed.

As time passes, the likelihood of recurrence of the primary cancer diminishes. For many types of cancer, survival for 5 years without recurrence is tantamount to cure. However, important medical problems can occur in patients treated for cancer and must be examined (Chap. 102). Some problems emerge as a consequence of the disease and some as a consequence of the treatment. An understanding of these disease- and treatment-related problems may help in their detection and management.

Despite these concerns, most patients who are cured of cancer return to normal lives.

■ SUPPORTIVE CARE

In many ways, the success of cancer therapy depends on the success of the supportive care. Failure to control the symptoms of cancer and its treatment may lead patients to abandon curative therapy. Of equal importance, supportive care is a major determinant of quality of life. Even when life cannot be prolonged, the physician must strive to preserve its quality. Quality-of-life measurements have become common endpoints of clinical research studies. Furthermore, palliative care has been shown to be cost-effective when approached in an organized fashion. A credo for oncology could be to cure sometimes, to extend life often, and to comfort always.

Pain

Pain occurs with variable frequency in the cancer patient: 25–50% of patients present with pain at diagnosis, 33% have pain associated with treatment, and 75% have pain with progressive disease. The pain may have several causes. In ~70% of cases, pain is caused by the tumor itself—by invasion of bone, nerves, blood vessels, or mucous membranes or obstruction of a hollow viscus or duct. In ~20% of cases, pain is related to a surgical or invasive medical procedure, to radiation injury (mucositis, enteritis, or plexus or spinal cord injury), or to chemotherapy injury (mucositis, peripheral neuropathy, phlebitis, steroid-induced aseptic necrosis of the femoral head). In 10% of cases, pain is unrelated to cancer or its treatment.

Assessment of pain requires the methodical investigation of the history of the pain, its location, character, temporal features, provocative and palliative factors, and intensity (Chap. 11); a review of the oncologic history and past medical history as well as personal and social history; and a thorough physical examination. The patient should be given a 10-division visual analogue scale on which to indicate the severity of the pain. The clinical condition is often dynamic, making it necessary to reassess the patient frequently. Pain therapy should not be withheld while the cause of pain is being sought.

A variety of tools are available with which to address cancer pain. About 85% of patients will have pain relief from pharmacologic intervention. However, other modalities, including antitumor therapy (such as surgical relief of obstruction, radiation therapy, and strontium-89 or samarium-153 treatment for bone pain), neurostimulatory techniques, regional analgesia, or neuroablative procedures are effective in an additional 12% or so. Thus, very few patients will have inadequate pain relief if appropriate measures are taken. A specific approach to pain relief is detailed in Chap. 9.

Nausea

Emesis in the cancer patient is usually caused by chemotherapy (Chap. 85). Its severity can be predicted from the drugs used to treat the cancer. Three forms of emesis are recognized on the basis of their timing with regard to the noxious insult. *Acute emesis*, the most common variety, occurs within 24 h of treatment. *Delayed emesis* occurs 1–7 days after treatment; it is rare, but, when present, usually follows cisplatin administration. *Anticipatory emesis* occurs before administration of chemotherapy and represents a conditioned response to visual and olfactory stimuli previously associated with chemotherapy delivery.

Acute emesis is the best understood form. Stimuli that activate signals in the chemoreceptor trigger zone in the medulla, the cerebral cortex, and peripherally in the intestinal tract lead to stimulation of the vomiting center in the medulla, the motor center responsible for coordinating the secretory and muscle contraction activity that leads to emesis. Diverse receptor types participate in the process, including dopamine, serotonin, histamine, opioid, and acetylcholine receptors. The serotonin receptor antagonists ondansetron and granisetron are the most effective drugs against highly emetogenic agents, but they are expensive.

As with the analgesia ladder, emesis therapy should be tailored to the situation. For mildly and moderately emetogenic agents, prochlorperazine, 5–10 mg PO or 25 mg PR, is effective. Its efficacy may be enhanced by administering the drug before the chemotherapy is delivered. Dexamethasone, 10–20 mg IV, is also effective and may enhance the efficacy of prochlorperazine. For highly emetogenic agents such as cisplatin, mechlorethamine, dacarbazine, and streptozocin, combinations of agents work best and administration should begin 6–24 h before treatment. Ondansetron, 8 mg PO every 6 h the day before therapy and IV on the day of therapy, plus dexamethasone, 20 mg IV before treatment, is an effective regimen. Addition of oral aprepitant (a substance P/neurokinin 1 receptor antagonist) to this regimen (125 mg on day 1, 80 mg on days 2 and 3) further decreases the risk of both acute and delayed vomiting. Like pain, emesis is easier to prevent than to alleviate.

Delayed emesis may be related to bowel inflammation from the therapy and can be controlled with oral dexamethasone and oral metoclopramide, a dopamine receptor antagonist that also blocks serotonin receptors at high dosages. The best strategy for preventing anticipatory emesis is to control emesis in the early cycles of therapy to prevent the conditioning from taking place. If this is unsuccessful, prophylactic antiemetics the day before treatment may help. Experimental studies are evaluating behavior modification.

Effusions

Fluid may accumulate abnormally in the pleural cavity, pericardium, or peritoneum. Asymptomatic malignant effusions may not require treatment. Symptomatic effusions occurring in tumors responsive to systemic therapy usually do not require local treatment but respond to the treatment for the underlying tumor. Symptomatic effusions occurring in tumors unresponsive to systemic therapy may require local treatment in patients with a life expectancy of at least 6 months.

Pleural effusions due to tumors may or may not contain malignant cells. Lung cancer, breast cancer, and lymphomas account for ~75% of malignant pleural effusions. Their exudative nature is usually gauged by an effusion/serum protein ratio of ≥0.5 or an effusion/serum lactate dehydrogenase ratio of ≥0.6. When the condition is symptomatic, thoracentesis is usually performed first. In most cases, symptomatic improvement occurs for <1 month. Chest tube drainage is required if symptoms recur within 2 weeks. Fluid is aspirated until the flow rate is <100 mL in 24 h. Then either 60 units of bleomycin or 1 g of doxycycline is infused into the chest tube in 50 mL of 5% dextrose in water; the tube is clamped; the patient is rotated on four sides, spending 15 min in each position; and, after 1–2 h, the tube is again attached to suction for another 24 h. The tube is then disconnected from suction and allowed to drain by gravity. If <100 mL drains over the next 24 h, the chest tube is pulled, and a radiograph taken 24 h later. If the chest tube continues to drain fluid at an unacceptably high rate, sclerosis can be repeated. Bleomycin may be somewhat more effective than doxycycline but is very expensive. Doxycycline is usually the drug of first choice. If neither doxycycline nor bleomycin is effective, talc can be used.

Symptomatic pericardial effusions are usually treated by creating a pericardial window or by stripping the pericardium. If the patient's condition does not permit a surgical procedure, sclerosis can be attempted with doxycycline and/or bleomycin.

Malignant ascites is usually treated with repeated paracentesis of small volumes of fluid. If the underlying malignancy is unresponsive to systemic therapy, peritoneovenous shunts may be inserted. Despite the fear of disseminating tumor cells into the circulation, widespread metastases are an unusual complication. The major complications are occlusion, leakage, and fluid overload. Patients with severe liver disease may develop disseminated intravascular coagulation.

Nutrition

Cancer and its treatment may lead to a decrease in nutrient intake of sufficient magnitude to cause weight loss and alteration of intermediary metabolism. The prevalence of this problem is difficult to estimate because of variations in the definition of cancer cachexia, but most patients with advanced cancer experience weight loss and decreased appetite. A variety of both tumor-derived factors (e.g., bombesin, adrenocorticotropic hormone) and host-derived factors (e.g., tumor necrosis factor, interleukins 1 and 6, growth hormone) contribute to the altered metabolism, and a vicious cycle is established in which protein catabolism, glucose intolerance, and lipolysis cannot be reversed by the provision of calories.

It remains controversial how to assess nutritional status and when and how to intervene. Efforts to make the assessment objective have included the use of a prognostic nutritional index based on albumin levels, triceps skinfold thickness, transferrin levels, and delayed-type hypersensitivity skin testing. However, a simpler approach has been to define the threshold for nutritional intervention as >10% unexplained body weight loss, serum transferrin level <1500 mg/L (150 mg/dL), and serum albumin <34 g/L (3.4 g/dL).

The decision is important, because it appears that cancer therapy is substantially more toxic and less effective in the face of malnutrition. Nevertheless, it remains unclear whether nutritional intervention can alter the natural history. Unless some pathology is affecting the absorptive function of the gastrointestinal tract, enteral nutrition provided orally or by tube feeding is preferred over parenteral supplementation. However, the risks associated with the tube may outweigh the benefits. Megestrol acetate, a progestational agent, has been advocated as a pharmacologic intervention to improve nutritional status. Research in this area may provide more tools in the future as cytokine-mediated mechanisms are further elucidated.

Psychosocial support

The psychosocial needs of patients vary with their situation. Patients undergoing treatment experience fear, anxiety, and depression.

Self-image is often seriously compromised by deforming surgery and loss of hair. Women who receive cosmetic advice that enables them to look better also feel better. Loss of control over how one spends time can contribute to the sense of vulnerability. Juggling the demands of work and family with the demands of treatment may create enormous stresses. Sexual dysfunction is highly prevalent and needs to be discussed openly with the patient. An empathetic health care team is sensitive to the individual patient's needs and permits negotiation where such flexibility will not adversely affect the course of treatment.

Cancer survivors have other sets of difficulties. Patients may have fears associated with the termination of a treatment they associate with their continued survival. Adjustments are required to physical losses and handicaps, real and perceived. Patients may be preoccupied with minor physical problems. They perceive a decline in their job mobility and view themselves as less desirable workers. They may be victims of job and/or insurance discrimination. Patients may experience difficulty reentering their normal past life. They may feel guilty for having survived and may carry a sense of vulnerability to colds and other illnesses. Perhaps the most pervasive and threatening concern is the ever-present fear of relapse (the Damocles syndrome).

Patients in whom therapy has been unsuccessful have other problems related to the end of life.

Death and dying

The most common causes of death in patients with cancer are infection (leading to circulatory failure), respiratory failure, hepatic failure, and renal failure. Intestinal blockage may lead to inanition and starvation. Central nervous system disease may lead to seizures, coma, and central hypoventilation. About 70% of patients develop dyspnea preterminally. However, many months usually pass between the diagnosis of cancer and the occurrence of these complications, and during this period the patient is severely affected by the possibility of death. The path of unsuccessful cancer treatment usually occurs in three phases. First, there is optimism at the hope of cure; when the tumor recurs, there is the acknowledgment of an incurable disease, and the goal of palliative therapy is embraced in the hope of being able to live with disease; finally, at the disclosure of imminent death, another adjustment in outlook takes place. The patient imagines the worst in preparation for the end of life and may go through stages of adjustment to the diagnosis. These stages include denial, isolation, anger, bargaining, depression, acceptance, and hope. Of course, patients do not all progress through all the stages or proceed through them in the same order or at the same rate. Nevertheless, developing an understanding of how the patient has been affected by the diagnosis and is coping with it is an important goal of patient management.

It is best to speak frankly with the patient and the family regarding the likely course of disease. These discussions can be difficult for the physician as well as for the patient and family. The critical features of the interaction are to reassure the patient and family that everything that can be done to provide comfort will be done. They will not be abandoned. Many patients prefer to be cared for in their homes or in a hospice setting rather than a hospital. The American College of Physicians has published a book called *Home Care Guide for Cancer: How to Care for Family and Friends at Home* that teaches an approach to successful problem-solving in home care. With appropriate planning, it should be possible to provide the patient with the necessary medical care as well as the psychological and spiritual support that will prevent the isolation and depersonalization that can attend in-hospital death.

The care of dying patients may take a toll on the physician. A "burnout" syndrome has been described that is characterized by fatigue, disengagement from patients and colleagues, and a loss of self-fulfillment. Efforts at stress reduction, maintenance of a balanced life, and setting realistic goals may combat this disorder.

End-of-life decisions

Unfortunately, a smooth transition in treatment goals from curative to palliative may not be possible in all cases because of the occurrence of serious treatment-related complications or rapid disease progression. Vigorous and invasive medical support for a reversible disease or treatment complication is assumed to be justified. However, if the reversibility of the condition is in doubt, the patient's wishes determine the level of medical care. These wishes should be elicited before the terminal phase of illness and reviewed periodically. Information about advance directives can be obtained from the American Association of Retired Persons, 601 E Street, NW, Washington, DC 20049, 202-434-2277 or Choice in Dying, 250 West 57th Street, New York, NY 10107, 212-366-5540. A full discussion of end-of-life management is in Chap. 9.

FURTHER READINGS

EDGE SB et al (eds): *American Joint Commission on Cancer Staging Manual*, 7th ed. New York, Springer, 2010

EISENHAUER EA et al: New response evaluation criteria in solid tumours: Revised RECIST guideline (version 1.1). Eur J Cancer 45:228, 2009

GREEN E et al: Cancer-related pain management: A report of evidence-based recommendations to guide practice. Clin J Pain 26:449, 2010

JEMAL A et al: Cancer statistics, 2010. CA Cancer J Clin 60:277, 2010

KAMANGAR F et al: Patterns of cancer incidence, mortality, and prevalence across five continents: Defining priorities to reduce cancer disparities in different geographic regions of the world. J Clin Oncol 24:2137, 2006

U.S. DEPARTMENT OF HEALTH AND HUMAN SERVICES: *Clinical Practice Guideline Number 9, Management of Cancer Pain*. U.S. Department of Health and Human Services, Agency for Health Care Policy and Research publication no. 94-0592, 1994

WALSH D et al: The symptoms of advanced cancer: Relationship to age, gender, and performance status in 1000 patients. Support Care Cancer 8:175, 2000

WICKHAM R: Best practice management of CINV in oncology patients: II. Antiemetic guidelines and rationale for use. J Support Oncol 8:10, 2010

CHAPTER 82

Prevention and Early Detection of Cancer

Jennifer M. Croswell
Otis W. Brawley
Barnett S. Kramer

Improved understanding of carcinogenesis has allowed cancer prevention and early detection (also known as cancer control) to expand beyond the identification and avoidance of carcinogens. Specific interventions to prevent cancer in those at risk, and effective screening for early detection of cancer, are the goals.

Carcinogenesis is not simply an event but a process, a continuum of discrete tissue and cellular changes over time resulting in more autonomous cellular processes. Prevention concerns the identification and manipulation of the biologic, environmental, and genetic factors in the causal pathway of cancer.

EDUCATION AND HEALTHFUL HABITS

Public education on the avoidance of identified risk factors for cancer and encouraging healthy habits contributes to cancer prevention and control. The clinician is a powerful messenger in this process. The patient-provider encounter provides an opportunity to teach patients about the hazards of smoking, the features of a healthy lifestyle, use of proven cancer screening methods, and sun avoidance.

■ SMOKING CESSATION

Tobacco smoking is a strong, modifiable risk factor for cardiovascular disease, pulmonary disease, and cancer. Smokers have an approximately 1 in 3 lifetime risk of dying prematurely from a tobacco-related cancer or cardiovascular or pulmonary disease. Tobacco use causes more deaths from cardiovascular disease than from cancer. Lung cancer and cancers of the larynx, oropharynx, esophagus, kidney, bladder, pancreas, and stomach are all tobacco-related.

The number of cigarettes smoked per day and the level of inhalation of cigarette smoke are correlated with risk of lung cancer mortality. Light- and low-tar cigarettes are not safer because smokers tend to inhale them more frequently and deeply.

Those who stop smoking have a 30–50% lower 10-year lung cancer mortality rate compared to those who continue smoking, despite the fact that some carcinogen-induced gene mutations persist for years after smoking cessation. Smoking cessation and avoidance have the potential to save more lives than any other public health activity.

The risk of tobacco smoke is not limited to the smoker. Environmental tobacco smoke, known as secondhand or passive smoke, causes lung cancer and other cardiopulmonary diseases in nonsmokers.

Tobacco prevention is a pediatric issue. More than 80% of adult American smokers began smoking before the age of 18 years. Approximately 20% of Americans in Grades 9 through 12 have smoked a cigarette in the past month. Counseling of adolescents and young adults is critical to prevent smoking. A clinician's simple advice to not start smoking or to quit smoking can be of benefit. Providers should query patients on tobacco use and offer smokers assistance in quitting.

Current approaches to smoking cessation recognize that smoking is an addiction (Chap. 395). The smoker who is quitting goes through a process with identifiable stages that include contemplation of quitting, an action phase in which the smoker quits, and a maintenance phase. Smokers who quit completely are more likely to be successful than those who gradually reduce the number of cigarettes smoked or change to lower-tar or lower-nicotine cigarettes. More than 90% of the Americans who have successfully quit smoking did so on their own, without participation in an organized cessation program, but cessation programs are helpful for some smokers. The Community Intervention Trial for Smoking Cessation (COMMIT) was a 4-year program showing that light smokers (<25 cigarettes per day) were more likely to benefit from simple cessation messages and cessation programs than those who did not receive an intervention. Quit rates were 30.6% in the intervention group and 27.5% in the control group. The COMMIT interventions were not successful in heavy smokers (>25 cigarettes per day). Heavy smokers may need an intensive broad-based cessation program that includes counseling, behavioral strategies, and pharmacologic adjuncts, such as nicotine replacement (gum, patches, sprays, lozenges, and inhalers), bupropion, and/or varenicline.

The health risks of cigars are similar to those of cigarettes. Smoking one or two cigars daily doubles the risk for oral and esophageal cancers; three or four cigars daily increases the risk of oral cancers more than eightfold and esophageal cancer fourfold. The risks of occasional use are unknown.

Smokeless tobacco also represents a substantial health risk. Chewing tobacco is a carcinogen linked to dental caries, gingivitis, oral leukoplakia, and oral cancer. The systemic effects of smokeless tobacco (including snuff) may increase risks for other cancers. Esophageal cancer is linked to carcinogens in tobacco dissolved in saliva and swallowed.

■ PHYSICAL ACTIVITY

Physical activity is associated with a decreased risk of colon and breast cancer. A variety of mechanisms have been proposed. However, such studies are prone to confounding factors such as recall bias, association of exercise with other health-related practices, and effects of preclinical cancers on exercise habits (reverse causality).

■ DIET MODIFICATION

International epidemiologic studies suggest that diets high in fat are associated with increased risk for cancers of the breast, colon, prostate, and endometrium. These cancers have their highest incidence and mortalities in western cultures, where fat comprises an average of one-third of the total calories consumed.

Despite correlations, dietary fat has not been proven to cause cancer. Case-control and cohort epidemiologic studies give conflicting results. In addition, diet is a highly complex exposure to many nutrients and chemicals. Low-fat diets are associated with many dietary changes beyond simple subtraction of fat. Other lifestyle changes are also associated with adherence to a low-fat diet.

In observational studies, dietary fiber is associated with a reduced risk of colonic polyps and invasive cancer of the colon. However, cancer-protective effects of increasing fiber and lowering dietary fat have not been proven in the context of a prospective clinical trial. The putative protective mechanisms are complex and speculative. Fiber binds oxidized bile acids and generates soluble fiber products, such as butyrate, that may have differentiating properties. Fiber does not increase bowel transit times. High-fiber diets could lower the risk of breast and prostate cancer by absorbing and inactivating dietary estrogenic and androgenic cancer promoters. However, two large prospective cohort studies of >100,000 health professionals showed no association between fruit and vegetable intake and risk of cancer.

The Polyp Prevention Trial randomly assigned 2000 elderly persons, who had polyps removed, to a low-fat, high-fiber diet versus routine diet for 4 years. No differences were noted in polyp formation.

The U.S. National Institutes of Health Women's Health Initiative, launched in 1994, was a long-term clinical trial enrolling >100,000 women aged 45–69 years. It placed women in 22 intervention groups. Participants received calcium/vitamin D supplementation; hormone-replacement therapy; and counseling to increase exercise, eat a low-fat diet with increased consumption of fruits, vegetables, and fiber, and cease smoking. The study showed that while dietary fat intake was lower in the diet intervention group, invasive breast cancers were not reduced over an 8-year follow-up period compared to the control group. No reduction was seen in the incidence of colorectal cancer in the dietary intervention arm. The difference in dietary fat averaged ~10% between the two groups. Evidence does not currently establish the anticarcinogenic value of vitamin, mineral, or nutritional supplements in amounts greater than those provided by a balanced diet.

■ ENERGY BALANCE

Risk of cancer appears to increase as body mass index increases to more than 25 kg/m². Obesity is associated with increased risk for cancers of the colon, breast (female postmenopausal), endometrium, kidney (renal cell), and esophagus, although causality has not been established.

In observational studies, relative risks of colon cancer are increased in obesity by 1.5–2 for men and 1.2–1.5 for women. Obese postmenopausal women have a 30–50% increased risk of breast cancer. A hypothesis for the association is that adipose tissue serves as a depot for aromatase that facilitates estrogen production.

■ SUN AVOIDANCE

Nonmelanoma skin cancers (basal cell and squamous cell) are induced by cumulative exposure to ultraviolet (UV) radiation. Intermittent acute sun exposure and sun damage have been linked to melanoma, but the evidence is inconsistent. Sunburns, especially in childhood and adolescence, may be associated with an increased risk of melanoma in adulthood. Reduction of sun exposure through use of protective clothing and changing patterns of outdoor activities can reduce skin cancer risk. Sunscreens decrease the risk of actinic keratoses, the precursor to squamous cell skin cancer, but melanoma risk may not be reduced. Sunscreens prevent burning, but they may encourage more prolonged exposure to the sun and may not filter out wavelengths of energy that cause melanoma.

Educational interventions to help individuals accurately assess their risk of developing skin cancer have some impact. Self-examination for skin pigment characteristics associated with skin cancer, such as freckling, may be useful in identifying people at high risk. Those who recognize themselves as being at risk tend to be more compliant with sun-avoidance recommendations. Risk factors for melanoma include a propensity to sunburn, a large number of benign melanocytic nevi, and atypical nevi.

CANCER CHEMOPREVENTION

Chemoprevention involves the use of specific natural or synthetic chemical agents to reverse, suppress, or prevent carcinogenesis before the development of invasive malignancy.

Cancer develops through an accumulation of tissue abnormalities associated with genetic and epigenetic changes that are potential points of intervention to prevent cancer. The initial changes are termed *initiation*. The alteration can be inherited or acquired through the action of physical, infectious, or chemical carcinogens. Like most human diseases, cancer arises from an interaction between genetics and environmental exposures (Table 82-1). Influences that cause the initiated cell to progress through the carcinogenic process and change phenotypically are termed *promoters*. Promoters include hormones such as androgens, linked to prostate

TABLE 82-1 Suspected Carcinogens

Carcinogens[a]	Associated Cancer or Neoplasm
Alkylating agents	Acute myeloid leukemia, bladder cancer
Androgens	Prostate cancer
Aromatic amines (dyes)	Bladder cancer
Arsenic	Cancer of the lung, skin
Asbestos	Cancer of the lung, pleura, peritoneum
Benzene	Acute myelocytic leukemia
Chromium	Lung cancer
Diethylstilbestrol (prenatal)	Vaginal cancer (clear cell)
Epstein-Barr virus	Burkitt's lymphoma, nasal T cell lymphoma
Estrogens	Cancer of the endometrium, liver, breast
Ethyl alcohol	Cancer of the liver, esophagus, head and neck
Helicobacter pylori	Gastric cancer, gastric MALT lymphoma
Hepatitis B or C virus	Liver cancer
Human immunodeficiency virus	Non-Hodgkin's lymphoma, Kaposi's sarcoma, squamous cell carcinomas (especially of the urogenital tract)
Human papilloma virus	Cervix cancer, head and neck cancer
Human T cell lymphotropic virus type I (HTLV-I)	Adult T cell leukemia/lymphoma
Immunosuppressive agents (azathioprine, cyclosporine, glucocorticoids)	Non-Hodgkin's lymphoma
Ionizing radiation (therapeutic or diagnostic)	Breast, bladder, thyroid, soft tissue, bone, hematopoietic, and many more
Nitrogen mustard gas	Cancer of the lung, head and neck, nasal sinuses
Nickel dust	Cancer of the lung, nasal sinuses
Phenacetin	Cancer of the renal pelvis and bladder
Polycyclic hydrocarbons	Cancer of the lung, skin (especially squamous cell carcinoma of scrotal skin)
Schistosomiasis	Bladder cancer (squamous cell)
Sunlight (ultraviolet)	Skin cancer (squamous cell and melanoma)
Tobacco (including smokeless)	Cancer of the upper aerodigestive tract, bladder
Vinyl chloride	Liver cancer (angiosarcoma)

[a]Agents that are thought to act as cancer initiators and/or promoters.

cancer, and estrogen, linked to breast and endometrial cancer. The distinction between an initiator and promoter is sometimes arbitrary; some components of cigarette smoke are "complete carcinogens," acting as both initiators and promoters. Cancer can be prevented or controlled through interference with the factors that cause cancer initiation, promotion, or progression. Compounds of interest in chemoprevention often have antimutagenic, hormone modulation, anti-inflammatory, antiproliferative, or pro-apoptotic activity (or a combination).

■ CHEMOPREVENTION OF CANCERS OF THE UPPER AERODIGESTIVE TRACT

Smoking causes diffuse epithelial injury in the oral cavity, neck, esophagus, and lung. Patients cured of squamous cell cancers of the lung, esophagus, oral cavity, and neck are at risk (as high as 5% per year) of developing second cancers of the upper aerodigestive tract. Cessation of cigarette smoking does not markedly decrease the cured cancer patient's risk of second malignancy, even though it does lower the cancer risk in those who have never developed a malignancy. Smoking cessation may halt the early stages of the carcinogenic process (such as metaplasia), but it may have no effect on late stages of carcinogenesis. This "field carcinogenesis" hypothesis for upper aerodigestive tract cancer has made "cured" patients an important population for chemoprevention of second malignancies.

Oral human papilloma virus (HPV) infection, particularly HPV-16, increases the risk for cancers of the oropharynx. This association exists even in the absence of other risk factors such as smoking or alcohol use (although the magnitude of increased risk appears greater than additive when HPV infection and smoking are both present). Oral HPV infection is believed to be largely sexually acquired. The introduction of the HPV vaccine might eventually reduce oropharyngeal cancer rates.

Oral leukoplakia, a premalignant lesion commonly found in smokers, has been used as an intermediate marker allowing demonstration of chemopreventive activity in smaller shorter-duration, randomized, placebo-controlled trials. Response was associated with upregulation of retinoic acid receptor-β (RAR-β). Therapy with high, relatively toxic doses of isotretinoin (13-*cis*-retinoic acid) causes regression of oral leukoplakia. However, the lesions recur when the therapy is withdrawn, suggesting the need for long-term administration. More tolerable doses of isotretinoin have not proven beneficial in the prevention of head and neck cancer. Isotretinoin also failed to prevent second malignancies in patients cured of early-stage non-small cell lung cancer; mortality rates were actually increased in current smokers.

Several large-scale trials have assessed agents in the chemoprevention of lung cancer in patients at high risk. In the α-tocopherol/β-carotene (ATBC) Lung Cancer Prevention Trial, participants were male smokers, ages 50–69 years at entry. Participants had smoked an average of one pack of cigarettes per day for 35.9 years. Participants received α-tocopherol, β-carotene, and/or placebo in a randomized, two-by-two factorial design. After median follow-up of 6.1 years, lung cancer incidence and mortality were statistically significantly increased in those receiving β-carotene. α-Tocopherol had no effect on lung cancer mortality, and no evidence suggested interaction between the two drugs. Patients receiving α-tocopherol had a higher incidence of hemorrhagic stroke.

The β-Carotene and Retinol Efficacy Trial (CARET) involved 17,000 American smokers and workers with asbestos exposure. Entrants were randomly assigned to one of four arms and received β-carotene, retinol, and/or placebo in a two-by-two factorial design. This trial also demonstrated harm from β-carotene: a lung cancer rate of 5 per 1000 subjects per year for those taking placebo and of 6 per 1000 subjects per year for those taking β-carotene.

The ATBC and CARET results demonstrate the importance of testing chemoprevention hypotheses thoroughly before their widespread implementation as the results contradict a number of observational studies. The Physicians' Health Trial showed no change in the risk of lung cancer for those taking β-carotene; however, fewer of its participants were smokers than those in the ATBC and CARET studies.

■ CHEMOPREVENTION OF COLON CANCER

Many colon cancer prevention trials are based on the premise that most colorectal cancers develop from adenomatous polyps. These trials use adenoma recurrence or disappearance as a surrogate endpoint (not yet validated) for colon cancer prevention. Early clinical trial results suggest that nonsteroidal anti-inflammatory drugs (NSAIDs), such as piroxicam, sulindac, and aspirin, may prevent adenoma formation or cause regression of adenomatous polyps. The mechanism of action of NSAIDs is unknown, but they are presumed to work through the cyclooxygenase pathway. Pooled findings from observational cohort studies demonstrate a relative reduction in colorectal cancer incidence of approximately 22%, and a relative reduction in colorectal adenoma incidence of about 28%, with regular aspirin use; however, in two randomized controlled trials (the Physicians' Health Study and the Women's Health Study), aspirin had no effect on colon cancer or adenoma incidence in persons with no previous history of colonic lesions, at up to 10 years of therapy. The randomized controlled trials did show an approximately 18% relative risk reduction for colonic adenoma incidence in persons with a previous history of adenomas after 1 year's therapy.

Cyclooxygenase-2 (COX-2) inhibitors have also been considered for colorectal cancer and polyp prevention. Trials with COX-2 inhibitors were initiated but an increased risk of cardiovascular events in those taking the COX-2 inhibitors was noted, suggesting that these agents are not suitable for chemoprevention in the general population.

Epidemiologic studies suggest that diets high in calcium lower colon cancer risk. Calcium binds bile and fatty acids, which cause proliferation of colonic epithelium. It is hypothesized that calcium reduces intraluminal exposure to these compounds. The randomized controlled Calcium Polyp Prevention Study found that calcium supplementation decreased the absolute risk of adenomatous polyp recurrence by 7% at 4 years; extended observational follow-up demonstrated a 12% absolute risk reduction 5 years after cessation of treatment. However, in the Women's Health Initiative, combined use of calcium carbonate and vitamin D twice daily did not reduce the incidence of invasive colorectal cancer compared with placebo after 7 years.

The Women's Health Initiative demonstrated that postmenopausal women taking estrogen plus progestin have a 44% lower risk of colorectal cancer compared to women taking placebo. Of >16,600 women randomized and followed for a median of 5.6 years, 43 invasive colorectal cancers occurred in the hormone group and 72 in the placebo group. The positive effect on colon cancer is mitigated by the modest increase in cardiovascular and breast cancer risks associated with combined estrogen plus progestin therapy.

A case-control study suggested that statins decrease the incidence of colorectal cancer; however, several subsequent case-control and cohort studies have not demonstrated an association between regular statin use and a reduced risk of colorectal cancer. No randomized controlled trials have addressed this hypothesis. A meta-analysis of statin use showed no protective effect of statins on overall cancer incidence or death.

■ CHEMOPREVENTION OF BREAST CANCER

Tamoxifen is an antiestrogen with partial estrogen agonistic activity in some tissues, such as endometrium and bone. One of its actions is to upregulate transforming growth factor β, which decreases breast cell proliferation. In randomized placebo-controlled trials to assess tamoxifen as adjuvant therapy for breast cancer, tamoxifen reduced the number of new breast cancers in the opposite breast by more than a third. In a randomized placebo-controlled prevention trial involving >13,000 women at high risk, tamoxifen decreased the risk of developing breast cancer by 49% (from 43.4 to 22 per 1000 women) after a median follow-up of nearly 6 years. Tamoxifen also reduced bone fractures; a small increase in risk of endometrial cancer, stroke, pulmonary emboli, and deep vein thrombosis was noted. The International Breast Cancer Intervention Study (IBIS-I) and the Italian Randomized Tamoxifen Prevention Trial also demonstrated a reduction in breast cancer incidence with tamoxifen use. Tamoxifen has been approved by the U.S. Food and Drug Administration for reduction of breast cancer in women at high risk for the disease (1.66% risk at 5 years based on the Gail risk model: *http://www.nci.nih.gov/cancertopics/pdq/genetics/breast-and-ovarian/ healthprofessional#Section_66*).

A trial comparing tamoxifen with another selective estrogen receptor modulator, raloxifene, showed that raloxifene is comparable to tamoxifen in cancer prevention. This trial only included postmenopausal women. Raloxifene was associated with more noninvasive breast cancer than tamoxifen; the drugs are similar in risks of other cancers, fractures, ischemic heart disease, and stroke. Because the aromatase inhibitors are even more effective than tamoxifen in adjuvant breast cancer therapy, it is hoped that they would be more effective in breast cancer prevention. However, no data are yet available on this point.

■ CHEMOPREVENTION OF PROSTATE CANCER

Finasteride is a 5-α-reductase inhibitor. It inhibits conversion of testosterone to dihydrotestosterone (DHT), a potent stimulator of prostate cell proliferation. The Prostate Cancer Prevention Trial (PCPT) randomly assigned men aged 55 years or older at average risk of prostate cancer to finasteride or placebo. All men in the trial were being regularly screened with PSA and digital rectal examination. After 7 years of therapy, the incidence of prostate cancer was 18.4% in the finasteride arm and 24.8% in the placebo arm, a statistically significant difference. However, the finasteride group had more patients with tumors of Gleason score 7 and higher compared to the placebo arm (6.4 vs 5.1%). The clinical significance of this finding, if any, is unknown. The observed increase in high-grade tumors was spurious and likely due to an increased sensitivity of PSA and digital rectal exam for high-grade tumors in men receiving finasteride.

Another 5-α-reductase inhibitor, dutasteride, has also been evaluated as a preventive agent for prostate cancer. The Reduction by Dutasteride of Prostate Cancer Events (REDUCE) trial was a randomized double-blind trial in which approximately 8200 men with an elevated PSA (2.5–10 ng/mL for men aged 50–60 years and 3–10 ng/mL for men aged 60 years or older) and negative prostate biopsy on enrollment received daily 0.5 mg dutasteride or placebo. A preliminary report from this trial noted a statistically significant 23% relative risk reduction in the incidence of biopsy-detected prostate cancer in the dutasteride arm at 4 years of treatment (659 cases vs 857 cases, respectively). Unlike the PCPT, no difference was observed in the rates of high-grade prostate cancer. Since all men in both the PCPT and REDUCE trials were being screened and since screening approximately doubles the rate of prostate cancer, it is not known if finasteride or dutasteride decrease the risk of prostate cancer in men who are not being screened.

Several favorable laboratory and observational studies led to the formal evaluation of selenium and α-tocopherol (vitamin E) as potential prostate cancer preventives. The Selenium and Vitamin E Cancer Prevention Trial (SELECT) assigned 35,533 men to receive 200 μg/d selenium, 400 IU/d α-tocopherol, selenium plus vitamin E, or placebo. After a median follow-up of 5.5 years, no significant difference in the prostate cancer incidence rate was observed for any group. In fact, compared to placebo, a trend toward an increased risk of developing prostate cancer was observed for those men taking vitamin E alone (hazard ratio 1.13, 95% confidence interval, 0.99–1.29)

■ VACCINES AND CANCER PREVENTION

A number of infectious agents cause cancer. Hepatitis B and C are linked to liver cancer; some human papilloma virus (HPV) strains are linked to cervical and head and neck cancer; and *Helicobacter pylori* is associated with gastric adenocarcinoma and gastric lymphoma. Vaccines to protect against these agents may reduce the risk of their associated cancers.

The hepatitis B vaccine is effective in preventing hepatitis and hepatomas due to chronic hepatitis B infection. Public health officials are encouraging widespread administration of the hepatitis B vaccine, especially in Asia, where the disease is epidemic.

A quadrivalent HPV vaccine (covering HPV strains 6, 11, 16, and 18) and a bivalent vaccine (covering HPV strains 16 and 18) are available for use in the United States. HPV types 16 and 18 cause cervical cancer, and types 6 and 11 cause genital papillomas. For females not previously infected with these HPV strains, the vaccines demonstrate high efficacy in preventing persistent strain-specific HPV infections. Trials that evaluated the vaccines' ability to prevent cervical cancer relied on surrogate outcome measures [cervical intraepithelial neoplasia (CIN) I, II, and III], and no cases of cervical cancer were observed in either the vaccine or control arms. The vaccines do not appear to impact preexisting infections; efficacy was markedly lower for populations that had previously been exposed to vaccine-specific HPV strains. The vaccine is recommended for girls and women ages 9–26 years. Reduction in these HPV types could prevent >70% of cervical cancers worldwide.

SURGICAL PREVENTION OF CANCER

Some organs in some individuals are at such high risk of developing cancer that surgical removal of the organ at risk may be considered. Women with severe cervical dysplasia are treated with conization and occasionally even hysterectomy. Colectomy is used to prevent colon cancer in patients with familial polyposis or ulcerative colitis.

Prophylactic bilateral mastectomy may be chosen for breast cancer prevention among women with genetic predisposition to breast cancer. In a prospective series of 139 women with *BRCA1* and *BRCA2* mutations, 76 chose to undergo prophylactic mastectomy and 63 chose close surveillance. At 3 years, no cases of breast cancer had been diagnosed in those opting for surgery, but 8 in the surveillance group had developed breast cancer. A larger (*n* = 639) retrospective cohort study reported that 3 patients developed breast cancer after prophylactic mastectomy compared with an expected incidence of 30–53 cases: a 90–94% reduction in breast cancer risk. The effect of the procedure on mortality is unknown.

Prophylactic oophorectomy may also be employed for the prevention of ovarian and breast cancers among high-risk women. A case-control study of women with *BRCA1* or *BRCA2* mutations found that 6 (2.8%) of 259 women who underwent bilateral prophylactic oophorectomy had stage I ovarian cancer at the time of surgery and 2 (0.8%) developed papillary serous peritoneal carcinoma over 9 years. By comparison, 58 (19.9%) of 292 women in the matched control group developed ovarian cancer: this corresponds to a 96% relative risk reduction for ovarian cancer with the use of prophylactic surgery. Studies of prophylactic oophorectomy for prevention of breast cancer in women with genetic mutations have shown relative risk reductions of approximately 50%.

At present, all of the evidence concerning the use of prophylactic mastectomy and oophorectomy for prevention of breast and ovarian cancer in high-risk women has been observational in nature; such studies are prone to a variety of biases, including case selection bias, family relationships between patients and controls, and inadequate information about hormone use. Thus, they may give an overestimate of the magnitude of benefit.

Orchiectomy is an effective method of androgen deprivation in prostate cancer.

■ CANCER SCREENING

Screening is a means of detecting disease early in asymptomatic individuals, with the goal of decreasing morbidity and mortality. While screening can potentially reduce disease-specific deaths and has been shown to do so in cervical, colon, and breast cancer, it is also subject to a number of biases that can suggest a benefit when actually there is none. Biases can even mask net harm. Early detection does not in itself confer benefit. To be of value, screening must detect disease earlier, and treatment of earlier disease must yield a better outcome than treatment at the onset of symptoms. Cause-specific mortality, rather than survival after diagnosis, is the preferred endpoint (see below).

Because screening is done on asymptomatic, healthy persons, it should offer substantial likelihood of benefit that outweighs harm. Screening tests and their appropriate use should be carefully evaluated before their use is widely encouraged in screening programs, as a matter of public policy.

A large and increasing number of genetic mutations and nucleotide polymorphisms have been associated with an increased risk of cancer. Testing for these genetic mutations could in theory define a high-risk population. However, most of the identified mutations have very low penetrance and individually provide minimal predictive accuracy. The ability to predict the development of a particular cancer may some day present therapeutic options as well as ethical dilemmas. It may eventually allow for early intervention to prevent a cancer or limit its severity. People at high risk may be ideal candidates for chemoprevention and screening; however, efficacy of these interventions in the high-risk population should be investigated. Currently, persons at high risk for a particular cancer can engage in intensive screening. While this course is clinically reasonable, it is not known if it saves lives in these populations.

The accuracy of screening

A screening test's accuracy or ability to discriminate disease is described by four indices: sensitivity, specificity, positive predictive value, and negative predictive value (Table 82-2). *Sensitivity*, also called the true positive rate, is the proportion of persons with the disease who test positive in the screen (i.e., the ability of the test to detect disease when it is present). *Specificity*, or 1 minus the false positive rate, is the proportion of persons who do not have the disease and test negative in the screening test (i.e., the ability of a test to correctly identify that the disease is not present). The *positive predictive value* is the proportion of persons who test positive and actually have the disease. Similarly, *negative predictive value* is the proportion testing negative who do not have the disease. The sensitivity and specificity of a test are independent of the underlying prevalence (or risk) of the disease in the population screened, but the predictive values depend strongly on the prevalence of the disease.

Screening is most beneficial, efficient, and economical when the target disease is common in the population being screened. To be valuable, the screening test should have a high specificity; sensitivity need not be very high.

TABLE 82-2 Assessment of the Value of a Diagnostic Test[a]

	Condition Present	Condition Absent
Positive test	a	b
Negative test	c	d

a = true positive
b = false positive
c = false negative
d = true negative

Sensitivity	The proportion of persons with the condition who test positive: $a/(a + c)$
Specificity	The proportion of persons without the condition who test negative: $d/(b + d)$
Positive predictive value (PPV)	The proportion of persons with a positive test who have the condition: $a/(a + b)$
Negative predictive value	The proportion of persons with a negative test who do not have the condition: $d/(c + d)$

Prevalence, sensitivity, and specificity determine PPV

$$PPV = \frac{prevalence \times sensitivity}{(prevalence \times sensitivity) + (1 - prevalence)(1 - specificity)}$$

[a]For diseases of low prevalence, such as cancer, poor specificity has a dramatic adverse effect on PPV such that only a small fraction of positive tests are true positives.

Potential biases of screening tests

Common biases of screening are lead time, length-biased sampling, and selection. These biases can make a screening test seem beneficial when actually it is not (or even causes net harm). Whether beneficial or not, screening can create the false impression of an epidemic by increasing the number of cancers diagnosed. It can also produce a shift in proportion of patients diagnosed at an early stage and inflated survival statistics without reducing mortality (i.e., the number of deaths from a given cancer relative to the number of those at risk for the cancer). In such a case, the *apparent* duration of survival (measured from date of diagnosis) increases without lives being saved or life expectancy changed.

Lead-time bias occurs when a test does not influence the natural history of the disease; the patient is merely diagnosed at an earlier date. When lead-time bias occurs, survival *appears* increased, but life is not really prolonged. The screening test only prolongs the time the subject is aware of the disease and spends as a patient.

Length-biased sampling occurs because screening tests generally can more easily detect slow-growing, less aggressive cancers than fast-growing cancers. Cancers diagnosed due to the onset of symptoms between scheduled screenings are on average more aggressive, and treatment outcomes are not as favorable. An extreme form of length bias sampling is termed *overdiagnosis*, the detection of "pseudo disease." The reservoir of some undetected slow-growing tumors is large. Many of these tumors fulfill the histologic criteria of cancer but will never become clinically significant or cause death. This problem is compounded by the fact that the most common cancers appear most frequently at ages when competing causes of death are more frequent.

Selection bias must be considered in assessing the results of any screening effort. The population most likely to seek screening may differ from the general population to which the screening test might be applied. In general, volunteers for studies are more health conscious and likely to have a better prognosis or lower mortality rate, irrespective of the screening result. This is termed the *healthy volunteer effect*.

Potential drawbacks of screening

Risks associated with screening include harm caused by the screening intervention itself, harm due to the further investigation of persons with positive tests (both true and false positives), and harm from the treatment of persons with a true-positive result, even if life is extended by treatment. The diagnosis and treatment of cancers that would never have caused medical problems can lead to the harm of unnecessary treatment and give patients the anxiety of a cancer diagnosis. The psychosocial impact of cancer screening can also be substantial when applied to the entire population.

Assessment of screening tests

Good clinical trial design can offset some biases of screening and demonstrate the relative risks and benefits of a screening test. A randomized controlled screening trial with cause-specific mortality as the endpoint provides the strongest support for a screening intervention. Overall mortality should also be reported to detect an adverse effect of screening and treatment on other disease outcomes (e.g., cardiovascular disease). In a randomized trial, two like populations are randomly established. One is given the usual standard of care (which may be no screening at all) and the other receives the screening intervention being assessed. The two populations are compared over time. Efficacy for the population studied is established when the group receiving the screening test has a better cause-specific mortality rate than the control group. Studies showing a reduction in the incidence of advanced-stage disease, an improved survival, or a stage shift are weaker (and possibly misleading) evidence of benefit. These latter criteria are necessary but not sufficient to establish the value of a screening test.

Although a randomized, controlled screening trial provides the strongest evidence to support a screening test, it is not perfect. Unless the trial is population-based, it does not remove the question of generalizability to the target population. Screening trials generally involve thousands of persons and last for years. Less definitive study designs are therefore often used to estimate the effectiveness of screening practices. However, every non-randomized study design is subject to strong confounders. In descending order of strength, evidence may also be derived from the findings of internally controlled trials using intervention allocation methods other than randomization (e.g., allocation by birth date, date of clinic visit); the findings of cohort or case-control analytic observational studies; or the results of multiple time series studies with or without the intervention.

Screening for specific cancers

Widespread screening for cervical, colon, and breast cancer is beneficial for certain age groups. A number of organizations have considered whether or not to endorse routine use of certain screening tests. Because these groups have not used the same criteria to judge whether a screening test should be endorsed, they have arrived at different recommendations. The American Cancer Society (ACS) and the U.S. Preventive Services Task Force (USPSTF) publish screening guidelines (Table 82-3); the American College of Physicians (ACP) and the American Academy of Family Practitioners (AAFP) generally follow/endorse the USPSTF recommendations. Special surveillance of those at high risk for a specific cancer because of a family history or a genetic risk factor may be prudent, but few studies have assessed the influence on mortality.

Breast cancer Breast self-examination, clinical breast examination by a caregiver, mammography, and MRI have all been variably advocated as useful screening tools.

A number of trials have suggested that annual or biennial screening with mammography or mammography plus clinical breast examination in normal-risk women older than age 50 years decreases breast cancer mortality. Each trial has been criticized for design flaws. In most trials, breast cancer mortality rate is decreased by 15–30%. Experts disagree on whether average-risk women aged 40–49 years should receive regular screening (Table 82-3). The U.K. Age Trial, the only randomized trial of breast cancer screening to specifically evaluate the impact of mammography in women aged 40–49 years, found no statistically significant difference in breast cancer mortality for screened women versus controls after about 11 years of follow-up (RR, 0.83; 95% CI, 0.66–1.04); however, less than 70% of women received screening in the intervention arm, potentially diluting the observed effect. A meta-analysis of eight large randomized trials showed a 15% relative reduction in mortality (RR, 0.85; 95% CI, 0.75–0.96) from mammography screening for women aged 39–49 years after 11–20 years of follow-up. This is equivalent to a number needed to invite to screening of 1904 over 10 years to prevent one breast cancer death. At the same time, nearly half of women aged 40–49 years screened annually will have false-positive mammograms necessitating further evaluation, often including biopsy. Estimates of overdiagnosis range from 10 to 40% of diagnosed invasive cancers.

No study of breast self-examination has shown it to decrease mortality. A randomized controlled trial of approximately 266,000 women in China demonstrated no difference in mortality between a group that received intensive breast self-exam instruction and reinforcement/reminders and controls at 10 years of follow-up. However, more benign breast lesions were discovered and more breast biopsies were performed in the self-examination arm.

Genetic screening for *BRCA1* and *BRCA2* mutations and other markers of breast cancer risk has identified a group of women at high risk for breast cancer. Unfortunately, when to begin and the optimal frequency of screening have not been defined. Mammography is less sensitive at detecting breast cancers in women carrying *BRCA1* and *-2* mutations, possibly because such cancers occur in younger women, in whom mammography is known to be less sensitive. MRI screening may be more sensitive than mammography in women at high risk due to genetic predisposition or in women with very dense breast tissue, but specificity may be lower. An increase in overdiagnosis may accompany the higher sensitivity. The impact of MRI on breast cancer mortality with or without concomitant use of mammography has not been evaluated in a randomized controlled trial.

Cervical cancer Screening with Papanicolaou smears decreases cervical cancer mortality. The cervical cancer mortality rate has fallen substantially since the widespread use of the Pap smear. Screening guidelines recommend regular Pap testing for all women who have reached the age of 21; some organizations advocate beginning earlier depending on sexual history. With the onset of sexual activity comes the risk of sexual transmission of HPV, the most common etiologic factor for cervical cancer. The recommended interval for Pap screening varies from 1 to 3 years. At age 30, women who have had three normal test results in a row may get screened every 2–3 years. An upper age limit at which screening ceases to be effective is not known, but women aged 65–70 years with no abnormal results in the previous 10 years may choose to stop screening. Screening should be discontinued in women who have undergone a hysterectomy for non-cancerous reasons.

Although the efficacy of the Papanicolaou smear in reducing cervical cancer mortality has never been directly confirmed in a randomized, controlled setting, a clustered randomized trial in India evaluated the impact of one-time cervical visual inspection and immediate colposcopy, biopsy, and/or cryotherapy (where indicated) versus counseling on cervical cancer deaths in women aged 30–59 years. After 7 years of follow-up, the age-standardized rate of death

TABLE 82-3 Screening Recommendations for Asymptomatic Normal-Risk Subjects[a]

Test or Procedure	USPSTF	ACS
Sigmoidoscopy	Adults 50–75 years: every 5 years ("A")[b] Adults 76–85 years: "C" Adults ≥85 years: "D"	Adults ≥50 years: Screen every 5 years
Fecal occult blood testing (FOBT)	Adults 50–75 years: Annually ("A") Adults 76–85 years: "C" Adults ≥85 years: "D"	Adults ≥50 years: Screen every year
Colonoscopy	Adults 50–75 years: every 10 years ("A") Adults 76–85 years: "C" Adults ≥85 years: "D"	Adults ≥50 years: Screen every 10 years
Fecal DNA testing	"I"	Adults ≥50 years: Screen, but interval uncertain
Fecal immunochemical testing (FIT)	"I"	Adults ≥50 years: Screen every year
CT colonography	"I"	Adults ≥50 years: Screen every 5 years
Digital rectal examination (DRE)	No recommendation	Men ≥50 years, with a 10-year life expectancy; men ≥45 years, if African-American, or men with a first-degree relative diagnosed with prostate cancer <65 years; ≥40, if has several relatives with prostate cancer <65 years: Discuss and offer (with PSA testing) annually
Prostate-specific antigen (PSA)	Men <75 years: "I" Men ≥75 years: "D"	As for DRE
Pap test	Women <65 years: Beginning 3 years after first intercourse or by age 21, screen at least every 3 years ("A") Women ≥65 years, with adequate, normal recent Pap screenings: "D" Women after total hysterectomy for noncancerous causes: "D"	Women <30 years: Beginning 3 years after first intercourse or by age 21. Yearly for standard Pap; every 2 years with liquid test. Women 30–70 years: Every 2–3 years if last 3 tests normal Women ≥70 years: May stop screening if no abnormal Pap in past 10 years Women after total hysterectomy for noncancerous causes: Do not screen
Breast self-examination	"D"	Women ≥20 years: Breast self-exam is an option
Breast clinical examination	Women ≥40 years: "I" (as a stand-alone without mammography)	Women 20–40 years: Perform every 3 years Women ≥40 years: Perform annually
Mammography	Women 40–49 years: The decision should be an individual one, and take patient context into account ("C") Women 50–74 years: every 2 years ("B") Women ≥75 years: ("I")	Women ≥40 years: Screen annually
Magnetic resonance imaging (MRI)	"I"	Women >20% lifetime risk of breast cancer: Screen with MRI plus mammography annually Women 15–20% lifetime risk of breast cancer: Discuss option of MRI plus mammography annually Women <15% lifetime risk of breast cancer: Do not screen annually with MRI
Complete skin examination	"I"	Self-examination monthly; clinical exam as part of routine cancer-related checkup

[a]Summary of the screening procedures recommended for the general population by the U.S. Preventive Services Task Force and the American Cancer Society. These recommendations refer to asymptomatic persons who have no risk factors, other than age or gender, for the targeted condition.
[b]USPSTF lettered recommendations are defined as follows: "A": The USPSTF strongly recommends that clinicians provide (the service) to eligible patients; "B": The USPSTF recommends that clinicians provide (this service) to eligible patients; "C": The USPSTF makes no recommendation for or against routine provision of (the service); "D": The USPSTF recommends against routinely providing [the service] to asymptomatic patients; "I": The USPSTF concludes that the evidence is insufficient to recommend for or against routinely providing (the service).
Abbreviations: ACS, American Cancer Society; USPSTF, U.S. Preventive Services Task Force.

due to cervical cancer was 39.6 per 100,000 person-years in the intervention group versus 56.7 per 100,000 person-years in controls.

Colorectal cancer Fecal occult blood testing (FOBT), digital rectal examination (DRE), rigid and flexible sigmoidoscopy, colonoscopy, and CT colonography have been considered for colorectal cancer screening. Annual FOBT could reduce colorectal cancer mortality by a third. The sensitivity for fecal occult blood is increased if specimens are re-hydrated before testing, but at the cost of lower specificity. The false-positive rate for rehydrated FOBT is high; 1–5% of persons tested have a positive test. Only 2–10% of those with occult blood in the stool have cancer and 20–30% have adenomas. The high false-positive rate of FOBT dramatically increases the number of colonoscopies performed.

Fecal immunochemical tests appear to have higher sensitivity for colorectal cancer than nonrehydrated FOBT tests. Fecal DNA testing is an emerging testing modality; it appears to have increased sensitivity and comparable specificity to FOBT and could potentially reduce harms associated with follow-up of false-positive tests. The body of evidence on the operating characteristics and effectiveness of fecal DNA tests in reducing colorectal cancer mortality is limited.

Two case-control studies suggest that regular screening of those older than age 50 years with sigmoidoscopy decreases mortality. This type of study is prone to selection biases. A quarter to a third of polyps can be discovered with the rigid sigmoidoscope; half are found with a 35-cm flexible scope and two-thirds to three-quarters are found with a 60-cm scope. Diagnosis of adenomatous polyps by sigmoidoscopy should lead to evaluation of the entire colon with colonoscopy. The most efficient interval for screening sigmoidoscopy is unknown, but 5 years is often recommended. Case-control studies suggest that intervals of up to 15 years may confer benefit.

One-time colonoscopy detects ~25% more advanced lesions (polyps >10 mm, villous adenomas, adenomatous polyps with high-grade dysplasia, invasive cancer) than one-time FOBT with sigmoidoscopy. Perforation rates are about 3/1000 for colonoscopy and 1/1000 for sigmoidoscopy. Debate continues on whether colonoscopy is too expensive and invasive for widespread use as a screening tool in standard-risk populations. Two observational studies suggest that efficacy of colonoscopy to decrease colorectal cancer mortality is restricted to the left side of the colon. CT colonography, if done at expert centers, appears to have a sensitivity for polyps ≥6 mm comparable to colonoscopy. However, the rate of extracolonic findings of abnormalities of uncertain significance that must nevertheless be worked up is high (~15–30%); the long-term cumulative radiation risk of repeated colonography screenings is also a concern.

Lung cancer Chest x-ray and sputum cytology have been evaluated in randomized lung cancer screening trials. No reduction in lung cancer mortality has been seen, although all controlled trials have had low statistical power. Preliminary (unpublished) findings from the National Lung Screening Trial, a randomized controlled trial of screening for lung cancer in approximately 53,000 persons aged 55-74 years with a 30+ pack-year smoking history, have shown a statistically significant 20% reduction in lung cancer mortality in the spiral CT arm (354 deaths) compared to the chest x-ray arm (442 deaths). However, the mortality benefits must be weighed against the disadvantages of spiral CT for a given population. These include the potential radiation risks associated with multiple scans, the discovery of incidental findings of unclear significance, and a high rate of false-positive test results. Both incidental findings and false-positive tests can lead to invasive diagnostic procedures associated with anxiety, expense, and complications (e.g., pneumo- or hemothorax after lung biopsy).

Ovarian cancer Adnexal palpation, transvaginal ultrasound, and serum CA-125 assay have been considered for ovarian cancer screening. These tests alone and in combination do not have sufficiently high sensitivity or specificity to be recommended for routine screening of ovarian cancer. The risks and costs associated with the high number of false-positive results is an impediment to routine use of these modalities for screening. A large randomized controlled trial has shown that of female participants receiving at least one false-positive serum CA-125 test, 14% underwent a major surgical procedure (e.g., laparotomy with oophorectomy) for benign disease. For transvaginal ultrasound, the rate was close to 40%.

Prostate cancer The most common prostate cancer screening modalities are DRE and serum prostate-specific antigen (PSA) assay. Newer serum tests, such as measurement of bound to free serum PSA, have yet to be fully evaluated. An emphasis on PSA screening has caused prostate cancer to become the most common non-skin cancer diagnosed in American males. This disease is prone to lead-time bias, length bias, and overdiagnosis, and substantial debate rages among experts as to whether it is effective. Prostate cancer screening clearly detects many asymptomatic cancers, but the ability to distinguish tumors that are lethal but still curable from those that pose little or no threat to health is limited. Men older than age 50 years have a high prevalence of indolent, clinically insignificant prostate cancers.

Two randomized controlled trials of the impact of PSA screening on prostate cancer mortality have been published. The Prostate, Lung, Colorectal, and Ovarian (PLCO) Cancer Screening Trial was a multicenter U.S. trial that randomized almost 77,000 men ages 55–74 years to receive annual PSA testing for 6 years or usual care. At 7 years of follow-up, no statistically significant difference in the number of prostate cancer deaths were noted between the arms (rate ratio, 1.13; 95% CI, 0.75–1.90). The data at 10 years (67% complete) showed similar results. Approximately 44% of men in the control arm received at least one PSA test during the trial, which may have potentially diluted an observed effect.

The European Randomized Study of Screening for Prostate Cancer (ERSPC) was a multinational study that randomized approximately 162,000 men between ages 50 and 74 years (with a predefined "core" screening group of men ages 55–69 years) to receive PSA testing every 4 years or no screening. Recruitment and randomization procedures and actual frequency of PSA testing varied by country. After a median follow-up of 9 years, a 20% relative reduction in the risk of prostate cancer death in the screened arm was noted in the "core" screening group (no difference in mortality was observed in the overall study population). The trial also found that 1140 men would need to be screened, and 48 additional cases treated to avert 1 death from prostate cancer.

The effectiveness of treatments for low-stage prostate cancer is under study. However, both surgery and radiation therapy may cause significant morbidity, such as impotence and urinary incontinence. Comparison of radical prostatectomy to "watchful waiting" in clinically diagnosed (not screen-detected) prostate cancers showed a small decrease in prostate cancer death rate in the surgery arm, but no statistically significant decrease in overall mortality was seen after 11 years of follow-up. Benefits were restricted to men younger than age 65 years. Urinary incontinence and sexual impotence were more common in the surgery arm. A man should have a life expectancy of at least 10 years to be eligible for screening. The USPSTF has found insufficient evidence to recommend prostate cancer screening for men younger than age 75 years; it recommends against screening for prostate cancer in men age 75 years or older ("D" recommendation) (Table 82-3).

Endometrial cancer Transvaginal ultrasound and endometrial sampling have been advocated as screening tests for endometrial cancer.

Benefit from routine screening has not been shown. Transvaginal ultrasound and endometrial sampling are indicated for workup of vaginal bleeding in postmenopausal women but are not considered as screening tests in symptomatic women.

Skin cancer   Visual examination of all skin surfaces by the patient or by a health care provider is used in screening for basal and squamous cell cancers and melanoma. No prospective randomized study has been performed to look for a mortality decrease. Unfortunately, screening is associated with a substantial rate of overdiagnosis.

FURTHER READINGS

ANDRIOLE GL et al: Mortality results from a randomized prostate-cancer screening trial. N Engl J Med 360:1310, 2009

ATKIN WS et al: Once-only flexible sigmoidoscopy screening in prevention of colorectal cancer: A multicentre randomised controlled trial. Lancet 375:1624, 2010

BACH PB et al: Computed tomography screening and lung cancer outcomes. JAMA 297:953, 2007

BARRETT-CONNOR E et al: Effects of raloxifene on cardiovascular events and breast cancer in postmenopausal women. N Engl J Med 355:125, 2006

KRAMER BS et al: Cancer screening: The clash of science and intuition. Annu Rev Med 60:125, 2009.

NELSON HD et al: Screening for breast cancer: An update for the U.S. Preventive Services Task Force. Ann Intern Med 151:727, 2009

PRENTICE RL et al: Low-fat dietary pattern and risk of invasive breast cancer. The Women's Health Initiative randomized controlled dietary modification trial. JAMA 295:629, 2006

SCHROEDER FH et al: Screening and prostate-cancer mortality in a randomized European study. N Engl J Med 360: 1320, 2009

■ WEB SITES

The U.S. Preventive Services Task Force: *http://www.ahrq.gov/clinic/uspstfix.htm*

The National Cancer Institute Cancernet: *http://www.cancer.gov/cancertopics*

CHAPTER **83**

Cancer Genetics

Pat J. Morin

Jeffrey M. Trent

Francis S. Collins

Bert Vogelstein

CANCER IS A GENETIC DISEASE

Cancer arises through a series of somatic alterations in DNA that result in unrestrained cellular proliferation. Most of these alterations involve actual sequence changes in DNA (i.e., mutations). They may originate as a consequence of random replication errors, exposure to carcinogens (e.g., radiation), or faulty DNA repair processes. While most cancers arise sporadically, familial clustering of cancers occurs in certain families that carry a germline mutation in a cancer gene.

HISTORICAL PERSPECTIVE

The idea that cancer progression is driven by sequential somatic mutations in specific genes has only gained general acceptance in the past 25 years. Before the advent of the microscope, cancer was believed to be composed of aggregates of mucus or other noncellular matter. By the middle of the nineteenth century, it became clear that tumors were masses of cells and that these cells arose from the normal cells of the tissue from which the cancer originated. However, the molecular basis for the uncontrolled proliferation of cancer cells was to remain a mystery for another century. During that time, a number of theories for the origin of cancer were postulated. The great biochemist Otto Warburg proposed the combustion theory of cancer, which stipulated that cancer was due to abnormal oxygen metabolism. In addition, some believed that all cancers were caused by viruses, and that cancer was in fact a contagious disease.

In the end, observations of cancer occurring in chimney sweeps, studies of x-rays, and the overwhelming data demonstrating cigarette smoke as a causative agent in lung cancer, together with Ames's work on chemical mutagenesis, provided convincing evidence that cancer originated through changes in DNA. Although the viral theory of cancer did not prove to be generally accurate (with the exception of human papillomaviruses, which can cause cervical cancer in human), the study of retroviruses led to the discovery of the first human *oncogenes* in the late 1970s. Soon after, the study of families with genetic predisposition to cancer was instrumental in the discovery of *tumor-suppressor genes*. The field that studies the type of mutations, as well as the consequence of these mutations in tumor cells, is now known as *cancer genetics*.

THE CLONAL ORIGIN AND MULTISTEP NATURE OF CANCER

Nearly all cancers originate from a single cell; this clonal origin is a critical discriminating feature between neoplasia and hyperplasia. Multiple cumulative mutational events are invariably required for the progression of a tumor from normal to fully malignant phenotype. The process can be seen as Darwinian microevolution in which, at each successive step, the mutated cells gain a growth advantage resulting in an increased representation relative to their neighbors (Fig. 83-1). Based on observations of cancer frequency increases during aging, as well as recent molecular genetics work, it is believed that 5 to 10 accumulated mutations are necessary for a cell to progress from the normal to the fully malignant phenotype.

We are beginning to understand the precise nature of the genetic alterations responsible for some malignancies and to get a sense of the order in which they occur. The best studied example is colon cancer, in which analyses of DNA from tissues extending from normal colon epithelium through adenoma to carcinoma have identified some of the genes mutated in the process (Fig. 83-2). Other malignancies are believed to progress in a similar step-wise fashion, although the order and identity of genes affected may be different.

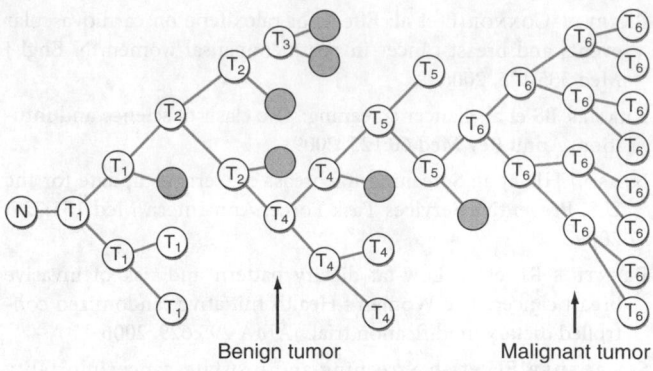

Benign tumor   Malignant tumor

Figure 83-1 Multistep clonal development of malignancy. In this diagram a series of five cumulative mutations (T1, T2, T4, T5, T6), each with a modest growth advantage acting alone, eventually results in a malignant tumor. Note that not all such alterations result in progression; for example, the T3 clone is a dead end. The actual number of cumulative mutations necessary to transform from the normal to the malignant state is unknown in most tumors. *(After P Nowell: Science 194:23, 1976, with permission.)*

TWO TYPES OF CANCER GENES: ONCOGENES AND TUMOR-SUPPRESSOR GENES

There are two major types of cancer genes. The first type comprises genes that positively influence tumor formation and are known as *oncogenes*. The second type of cancer genes negatively impact tumor growth and have been named *tumor-suppressor genes*. Both oncogenes and tumor-suppressor genes exert their effects on tumor growth through their ability to control cell division (cell birth) or cell death (apoptosis), although the mechanisms can be extremely complex. While tightly regulated in normal cells, oncogenes acquire mutations in cancer cells, and the mutations typically relieve this control and lead to increased activity of the gene products. This mutational event typically occurs in a single allele of the oncogene and acts in a dominant fashion. In contrast, the normal function of tumor-suppressor genes is usually to restrain cell growth, and this function is lost in cancer. Because of the diploid nature of mammalian cells, both alleles must be inactivated for a cell to completely lose the function of a tumor-suppressor gene, leading to a recessive mechanism at the cellular level. From these ideas and studies on the inherited form of retinoblastoma, Knudson and others formulated the *two-hit hypothesis*, which in its modern version states that both copies of a tumor-suppressor gene must be inactivated in cancer.

There is a subset of tumor-suppressor genes, the *caretaker genes*, which do not affect cell growth directly, but rather control the ability of the cell to maintain the integrity of its genome. Cells with a deficiency in these genes have an increased rate of mutations throughout their genomes, including in oncogenes and tumor-suppressor genes. This "mutator" phenotype was first hypothesized by Loeb to explain how the multiple mutational events required for tumorigenesis can occur in the lifetime of an individual. A mutator phenotype has now been observed in some forms of cancer, such as those associated with deficiencies in DNA mismatch repair. The great majority of cancers, however, do not harbor repair deficiencies, and their rate of mutation is similar to that observed in normal cells. Many of these cancers, however, appear to harbor a different kind of genetic instability, affecting the loss or gains of whole chromosomes or large parts thereof (as explained in more detail below).

ONCOGENES IN HUMAN CANCER

Work by Peyton Rous in the early 1900s revealed that a chicken sarcoma could be transmitted from animal to animal in cell-free extracts, suggesting that cancer could be induced by an agent acting positively to promote tumor formation. The agent responsible for the transmission of the cancer was a retrovirus (Rous sarcoma virus, RSV) and the oncogene responsible was identified 75 years later as *v-src*. Other oncogenes were also discovered through their presence in the genomes of retroviruses that are capable of causing cancers in chickens, mice, and rats. The cellular homologues of these viral genes are called protooncogenes and are often targets of mutation or aberrant regulation in human cancer. Whereas many oncogenes were discovered because of their presence in retroviruses, other oncogenes, particularly those involved in translocations characteristic of particular leukemias and lymphomas, were isolated through genomic approaches. Investigators cloned the sequences surrounding the chromosomal translocations observed cytogenetically and then deduced the nature of the genes that were the targets of these translocations (see below). Some of these were oncogenes known from retroviruses (like *ABL*, involved in chronic myeloid leukemia [CML]), while others were new (like *BCL2*, involved in B cell lymphoma). In the normal cellular environment, protooncogenes have crucial roles in cell proliferation and differentiation. Table 83-1 is a partial list of oncogenes known to be involved in human cancer.

The normal growth and differentiation of cells is controlled by growth factors that bind to receptors on the surface of the cell. The signals generated by the membrane receptors are transmitted inside the cells through signaling cascades involving kinases, G proteins, and other regulatory proteins. Ultimately, these signals affect the activity of transcription factors in the nucleus, which regulate the expression of genes crucial in cell proliferation, cell differentiation, and cell death. Oncogene products have been found to function at critical steps in these pathways (Chap. 84), and inappropriate activation of these pathways can lead to tumorigenesis.

MECHANISMS OF ONCOGENE ACTIVATION

■ POINT MUTATION

Point mutation is a common mechanism of oncogene activation. For example, mutations in one of the *RAS* genes (*HRAS*, *KRAS*, or *NRAS*) are present in up to 85% of pancreatic cancers and 45% of colon cancers but are less common in other cancer types, although they can occur at significant frequencies in

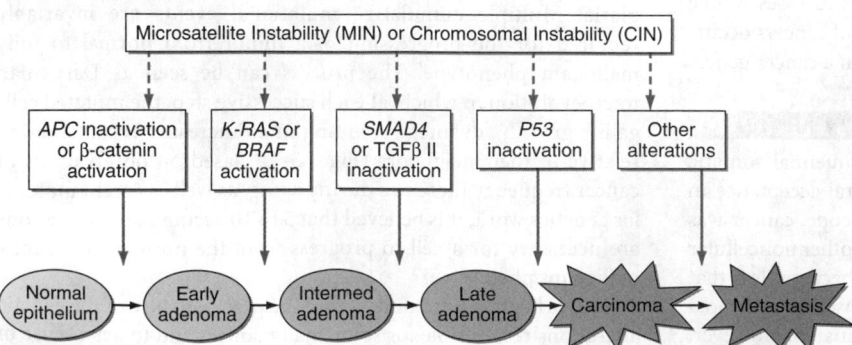

Figure 83-2 Progressive somatic mutational steps in the development of colon carcinoma. The accumulation of alterations in a number of different genes results in the progression from normal epithelium through adenoma to full-blown carcinoma. Genetic instability (microsatellite or chromosomal) accelerates the progression by increasing the likelihood of mutation at each step. Patients with familial polyposis are already one step into this pathway, since they inherit a germline alteration of the *APC* gene. TGF, transforming growth factor.

TABLE 83-1 Common Oncogenes Altered in Human Cancers

Oncogene	Function	Alteration in Cancer	Neoplasm
AKT1	Serine/threonine kinase	Amplification	Stomach
AKT2	Serine/threonine kinase	Amplification	Ovarian, breast, pancreatic
BRAF	Serine/threonine kinase	Point mutation	Melanoma, lung, colorectal
CTNNB1	Signal transduction	Point mutation	Colon, prostate, melanoma, skin, others
FOS	Transcription factor	Overexpression	Osteosarcomas
ERBB2	Receptor tyrosine kinase	Point mutation, amplification	Breast, ovary, stomach, neuroblastoma
JUN	Transcription factor	Overexpression	Lung
MET	Receptor tyrosine kinase	Point mutation, rearrangement	Osteocarcinoma, kidney, glioma
MYB	Transcription factor	Amplification	AML, CML, colorectal, melanoma
C-MYC	Transcription factor	Amplification	Breast, colon, gastric, lung
L-MYC	Transcription factor	Amplification	Lung, bladder
N-MYC	Transcription factor	Amplification	Neuroblastoma, lung
HRAS	GTPase	Point mutation	Colon, lung, pancreas
KRAS	GTPase	Point mutation	Melanoma, colorectal, AML
NRAS	GTPase	Point mutation	Various carcinomas, melanoma
REL	Transcription factor	Rearrangement, amplification	Lymphomas
WNT1	Growth factor	Amplification	Retinoblastoma

Abbreviations: AML, acute myeloid leukemia; CML, chronic myeloid leukemia.

CHAPTER 83

Cancer Genetics

leukemia, lung, and thyroid cancers. Remarkably—and in contrast to the diversity of mutations found in tumor-suppressor genes (see below)—most of the activated *RAS* genes contain point mutations in codons 12, 13, or 61 (these mutations reduce RAS GTPase activity, leading to constitutive activation of the mutant RAS protein). The restricted pattern of mutations observed in oncogenes compared to that of tumor-suppressor genes reflects the fact that gain-of-function mutations are less likely to occur than mutations that simply lead to loss of activity. Indeed, inactivation of a gene can in theory be accomplished through the introduction of a stop codon anywhere in the coding sequence, whereas activations require precise substitutions at residues that can somehow lead to an increase in the activity of the encoded protein. Importantly, the specificity of oncogene mutations provides diagnostic opportunities, as tests that identify mutations at defined positions are easier to design than tests aimed at detecting random changes in a gene.

■ DNA AMPLIFICATION

The second mechanism for activation of oncogenes is DNA sequence amplification, leading to overexpression of the gene product. This increase in DNA copy number may cause cytologically recognizable chromosome alterations referred to as *homogeneous staining regions* (HSRs) if integrated within chromosomes, or *double minutes* (dmins) if extrachromosomal. The recognition of DNA amplification is accomplished through various cytogenetic techniques such as comparative genomic hybridization (CGH) or fluorescence in situ hybridization (FISH), which allow the visualization of chromosomal aberrations using fluorescent dyes. In addition, noncytogenetic, microarray-based approaches are now available for identifying changes in copy number at high resolution. Newer short-tag–based sequencing approaches have been used to evaluate amplifications. When paired with next-generation sequencing instruments, this approach offers the highest degree of

resolution and quantification available. With both microarray and sequencing technologies, the entire genome can be surveyed for gains and losses of DNA sequences, thus pinpointing chromosomal regions likely to contain genes important in the development or progression of cancer.

Numerous genes have been reported to be amplified in cancer. Several of these genes, including *NMYC* and *LMYC*, were identified through their presence within the amplified DNA sequences of a tumor and had homology to known oncogenes. Because the region amplified often includes hundreds of thousands of base pairs, multiple oncogenes may be amplified in a single amplicon in some cancers (particularly in sarcomas). Indeed, *MDM2*, *GLI*, *CDK4*, and *SAS* at chromosomal location 12q13-15 have been shown to be simultaneously amplified in several types of sarcomas and other tumors. Amplification of a cellular gene is often a predictor of poor prognosis; for example, *ERBB2/HER2* and *NMYC* are often amplified in aggressive breast cancers and neuroblastoma, respectively.

■ CHROMOSOMAL REARRANGEMENT

Chromosomal alterations provide important clues to the genetic changes in cancer. The chromosomal alterations in human solid tumors such as carcinomas are heterogeneous and complex and occur as a result of the frequent chromosomal instability (CIN) observed in these tumors (see below). In contrast, the chromosome alterations in myeloid and lymphoid tumors are often simple translocations, i.e., reciprocal transfers of chromosome arms from one chromosome to another. Consequently, many detailed and informative chromosome analyses have been performed on hematopoietic cancers. The breakpoints of recurring chromosome abnormalities usually occur at the site of cellular oncogenes. Table 83-2 lists representative examples of recurring chromosome alterations in malignancy and the associated gene(s) rearranged or deregulated

665

TABLE 83-2 Representative Oncogenes at Chromosomal Translocations

Gene (Chromosome)	Translocation	Malignancy
ABL (9q34.1)–BCR (22q11)	(9;22)(q34;q11)	Chronic myeloid leukemia
ATF1 (12q13)–EWS (22q12)	(12;22)(q13;q12)	Malignant melanoma of soft parts
BCL1 (11q13.3)–IgH (14q32)	(11;14)(q13;q32)	Mantle cell lymphoma
BCL2 (18q21.3)–IgH (14q32)	(14;18)(q32;q21)	Follicular lymphoma
FLI1 (11q24)–EWS (22q12)	(11;22)(q24;q12)	Ewing's sarcoma
LCK (1p34)–TCRB (7q35)	(1;7)(p34;q35)	T cell acute lymphocytic leukemia
MYC (8q24)–IgH (14q32)	(8;14)(q24;q32)	Burkitt's lymphoma, B cell acute lympho-cytic leukemia
PAX3 (2q35)–FKHR/ALV (13q14)	(2;13)(q35;q14)	Alveolar rhab-domyosarcoma
PAX7 (1p36)–KHR/ALV(13q14)	(1;13)(p36;q14)	Alveolar rhab-domyosarcoma
REL (2p13)–NRG (2p11.2-14)	Inv(2(p13;p11.2-14)	Non-Hodgkin's lymphoma
RET (10q11.2)–PKAR1A (17q23)	(10;17)(q11.2;q23)	Thyroid carcinoma
TAL1(1p32)–TCTA (3p21)	(1;3)(p34;p21)	Acute T cell leukemia
TRK (1q23-1q24)–TPM3 (1q31)	Inv1(q23;q31)	Colon carcinoma
WT1 (11p13)–EWS (22q12)	(11;22)(p13;q12)	Desmoplastic small round cell tumor

Source: From Hesketh R: *The Oncogene and Tumour Suppressor Gene Facts Book*, 2nd ed. San Diego, Academic Press, 1997; with permission.

by the chromosomal rearrangement. Translocations are particularly common in lymphoid tumors, probably because these cell types have the capability to rearrange their DNA to generate antigen receptors. Indeed, antigen receptor genes are commonly involved in the translocations, implying that an imperfect regulation of receptor gene rearrangement may be involved in the pathogenesis. An interesting example is Burkitt's lymphoma, a B cell tumor characterized by a reciprocal translocation between chromosomes 8 and 14. Molecular analysis of Burkitt's lymphomas demonstrated that the breakpoints occurred within or near the *MYC* locus on chromosome 8 and within the immunoglobulin heavy chain locus on chromosome 14, resulting in the transcriptional activation of *MYC*. Enhancer activation by translocation, although not universal, appears to play an important role in malignant progression. In addition to transcription factors and signal transduction molecules, translocation may result in the overexpression of cell cycle regulatory proteins or proteins such as cyclins and of proteins that regulate cell death.

The first reproducible chromosome abnormality detected in human malignancy was the Philadelphia chromosome detected in CML. This cytogenetic abnormality is generated by reciprocal translocation involving the *ABL* oncogene on chromosome 9, encoding a tyrosine kinase, being placed in proximity to the *BCR* (breakpoint cluster region) gene on chromosome 22. Figure 83-3 illustrates the generation of the translocation and its protein product. The consequence of expression of the *BCR-ABL* gene product is the activation of signal transduction pathways leading to cell growth independent of normal external signals. Imatinib (marketed as Gleevec), a drug that specifically blocks the activity of *BCR-ABL*, has shown remarkable efficacy with little toxicity in patients with CML. It is hoped that knowledge of genetic alterations in other cancers will likewise lead to mechanism-based design and development of a new generation of chemotherapeutic agents.

CHROMOSOMAL INSTABILITY IN SOLID TUMORS

Solid tumors are generally highly aneuploid, containing an abnormal number of chromosomes; these chromosomes also exhibit structural alterations such as translocations, deletions, and amplifications. These abnormalities are collectively referred to as chromosomal instability (CIN). Normal cells possess several cell cycle checkpoints, essentially quality-control requirements that have to be met before subsequent events are allowed to take place. The

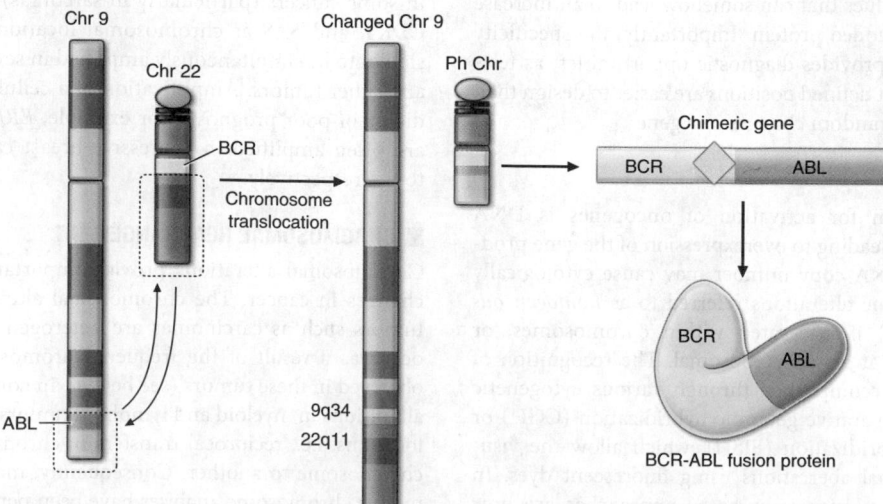

Figure 83-3 Specific translocation seen in chronic myelogenous leukemia (CML). The Philadelphia chromosome (Ph) is derived from a reciprocal translocation between chromosomes 9 and 22 with the breakpoint joining the sequences of the *ABL* oncogene with the *BCR* gene. The fusion of these DNA sequences allows the generation of an entirely novel fusion protein with modified function.

mitotic checkpoint, which ensures proper chromosome attachment to the mitotic spindle before allowing the sister chromatids to separate, is altered in certain cancers. The molecular basis of CIN remains unclear, although a number of mitotic checkpoint genes are found mutated or abnormally expressed in various tumors. The exact effects of these changes on the mitotic checkpoint are unknown, and both weakening and overactivation of the checkpoint have been proposed. The identification of the cause of CIN in tumors will likely be a formidable task, considering that several hundred genes are thought to control the mitotic checkpoint and other cellular processes ensuring proper chromosome segregation. Regardless of the mechanisms underlying CIN, the measurement of the number of chromosomal alterations present in tumors is now possible with both cytogenetic and molecular techniques, and several studies have shown that this information can be useful for prognostic purposes. In addition, since the mitotic checkpoint is essential for cellular viability, it may become a target for novel therapeutic approaches.

TUMOR-SUPPRESSOR GENE INACTIVATION IN CANCER

The first indication of the existence of tumor-suppressor genes came from experiments showing that fusion of mouse cancer cells with normal mouse fibroblasts led to a nonmalignant phenotype in the fused cells. The normal role of tumor-suppressor genes is to restrain cell growth, and the function of these genes is inactivated in cancer. The two major types of somatic lesions observed

in tumor-suppressor genes during tumor development are *point mutations* and *large deletions*. Point mutations in the coding region of tumor-suppressor genes will frequently lead to truncated protein products or otherwise nonfunctional proteins. Similarly, deletions lead to the loss of a functional product and sometimes encompass the entire gene or even the entire chromosome arm, leading to loss of heterozygosity (LOH) in the tumor DNA compared to the corresponding normal tissue DNA (Fig. 83-4). LOH in tumor DNA is considered a hallmark for the presence of a tumor-suppressor gene at a particular chromosomal location, and LOH studies have been useful in the positional cloning of many tumor-suppressor genes.

Gene silencing, an epigenetic change that leads to the loss of gene expression and occurs in conjunction with hypermethylation of the promoter and histone deacetylation, is another mechanism of tumor-suppressor gene inactivation. (An *epigenetic modification* refers to a change in the genome, heritable by cell progeny, that does not involve a change in the DNA sequence. The inactivation of the second X chromosome in female cells is an example of an epigenetic silencing that prevents gene expression from the inactivated chromosome). During embryologic development, regions of chromosomes from one parent are silenced and gene expression proceeds from the chromosome of the other parent. For most genes, expression occurs from both alleles or randomly from one allele or the other. The preferential expression of a particular

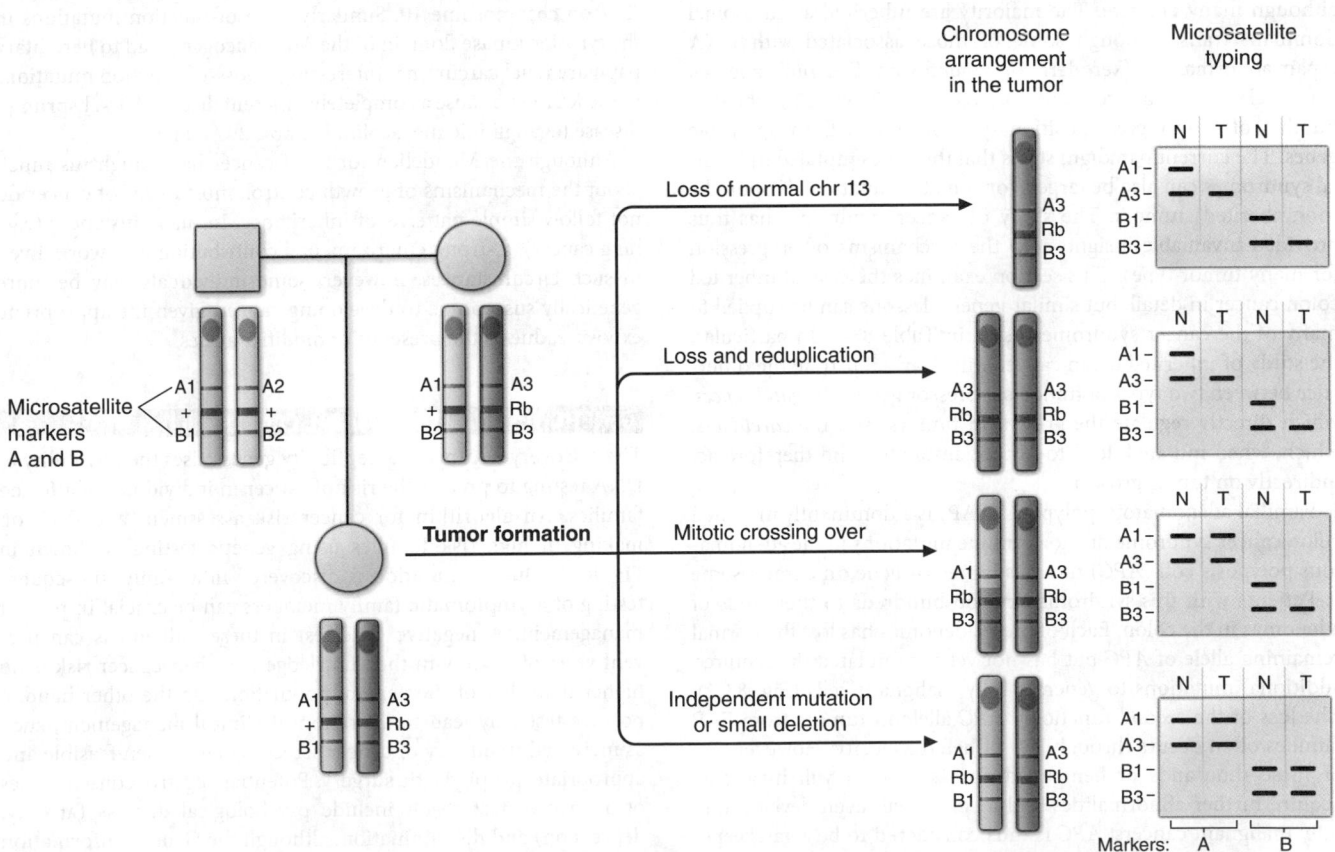

Figure 83-4 **Diagram of possible mechanisms for tumor formation in an individual with hereditary (familial) retinoblastoma.** On the left is shown the pedigree of an affected individual who has inherited the abnormal (Rb) allele from her affected mother. The normal allele is shown as a (+). The four chromosomes of her two parents are drawn to indicate their origin. Flanking the retinoblastoma locus are microsatellite markers (A and B) also analyzed in this family. Markers A3 and B3 are on the chromosome carrying the retinoblastoma disease gene. Tumor formation results when the normal allele, which this patient inherited from her father, is inactivated. On the right are shown four possible ways in which this could occur. In each case, the resulting chromosome 13 arrangement is shown, as well as the results of PCR typing using the microsatellite markers comparing normal tissue (N) with tumor tissue (T). Note that in the first three situations the normal allele (B1) has been lost in the tumor tissue, which is referred to as loss of heterozygosity (LOH) at this locus.

gene exclusively from the allele contributed by one parent is called *parental imprinting* and is thought to be regulated by covalent modifications of chromatin protein and DNA (often methylation) of the silenced allele.

The role of epigenetic control mechanisms in the development of human cancer is unclear. However, a general decrease in the level of DNA methylation has been noted as a common change in cancer. In addition, numerous genes, including some tumor-suppressor genes, appear to become hypermethylated and silenced during tumorigenesis. *VHL* and *p16INK4* are well-studied examples of such tumor-suppressor genes. Overall, epigenetic mechanisms may be responsible for reprogramming the expression of a large number of genes in cancer and, together with the mutation of specific genes, are likely to be crucial in the development of human malignancies.

FAMILIAL CANCER SYNDROMES

A small fraction of cancers occur in patients with a genetic predisposition. In these families, the affected individuals have a predisposing loss-of-function mutation in one allele of a tumor-suppressor gene. The tumors in these patients show a loss of the remaining normal allele as a result of somatic events (point mutations or deletions), in agreement with the two-hit hypothesis (Fig. 83-4). Thus, most cells of an individual with an inherited loss-of-function mutation in a tumor-suppressor gene are functionally normal, and only the rare cells that develop a mutation in the remaining normal allele will exhibit uncontrolled regulation.

Roughly 100 syndromes of familial cancer have been reported, although many are rare. The majority are inherited as autosomal dominant traits, although some of those associated with DNA repair abnormalities (xeroderma pigmentosum, Fanconi's anemia, ataxia telangiectasia) are autosomal recessive. Table 83-3 shows a number of cancer predisposition syndromes and the responsible genes. The current paradigm states that the genes mutated in familial syndromes can also be targets for somatic mutations in sporadic (noninherited) tumors. The study of cancer syndromes has thus provided invaluable insights into the mechanisms of progression for many tumor types. This section examines the case of inherited colon cancer in detail, but similar general lessons can be applied to many of the cancer syndromes listed in Table 83-3. In particular, the study of inherited colon cancer will clearly illustrate the difference between two types of tumor-suppressor genes: the *gatekeepers*, which directly regulate the growth of tumors, and the *caretakers*, which, when mutated, lead to genetic instability and therefore act indirectly on tumor growth.

Familial adenomatous polyposis (FAP) is a dominantly inherited colon cancer syndrome due to germline mutations in the adenomatous polyposis coli (*APC*) tumor-suppressor gene on chromosome 5. Patients with this syndrome develop hundreds to thousands of adenomas in the colon. Each of these adenomas has lost the normal remaining allele of *APC* but has not yet accumulated the required additional mutations to generate fully malignant cells (Fig. 83-2). The loss of the second functional *APC* allele in tumors from FAP families often occurs through loss of heterozygosity. However, out of these thousands of benign adenomas, several will invariably acquire further abnormalities and a subset will even develop into fully malignant cancers. *APC* is thus considered to be a gatekeeper for colon tumorigenesis: in the absence of mutation of this gatekeeper (or a gene acting within the same pathway), a colorectal tumor simply cannot form. Figure 83-5 shows germline and somatic mutations found in the *APC* gene. The function of the APC protein is still not completely understood, but it likely provides differentiation and apoptotic cues to colonic cells as they migrate up the crypts. Defects in this process may lead to abnormal accumulation of cells that should normally undergo apoptosis.

In contrast to patients with FAP, patients with hereditary nonpolyposis colon cancer (HNPCC, or Lynch syndrome) do not develop multiple polyposis but instead develop only one or a small number of adenomas that rapidly progress to cancer. Most HNPCC cases are due to mutations in one of four DNA mismatch repair genes (Table 83-3), which are components of a repair system that is normally responsible for correcting errors in freshly replicated DNA. Germline mutations in *MSH2* and *MLH1* account for more than 90% of HNPCC cases, while mutations in *MSH6* and *PMS2* are much less frequent. When a somatic mutation inactivates the remaining wild-type allele of a mismatch repair gene, the cell develops a hypermutable phenotype characterized by profound genomic instability, especially for the short repeated sequences called *microsatellites*. This microsatellite instability (MSI) favors the development of cancer by increasing the rate of mutations in many genes, including oncogenes and tumor-suppressor genes (Fig. 83-2). These genes can thus be considered caretakers. Interestingly, chromosomal instability (CIN) can also be found in colon cancer, but MSI and CIN appear to be mutually exclusive, suggesting that they represent alternative mechanisms for the generation of a mutator phenotype in this cancer (Fig. 83-2). Other cancer types rarely exhibit MSI but most exhibit CIN.

While most autosomal dominant inherited cancer syndromes are due to mutations in tumor-suppressor genes (Table 83-3), there are a few interesting exceptions. Multiple endocrine neoplasia type II, a dominant disorder characterized by pituitary adenomas, medullary carcinoma of the thyroid, and (in some pedigrees) pheochromocytoma, is due to gain-of-function mutations in the protooncogene *RET* on chromosome 10. Similarly, gain-of-function mutations in the tyrosine kinase domain of the *MET* oncogene lead to hereditary papillary renal carcinoma. Interestingly, loss-of-function mutations in the *RET* gene cause a completely different disease, Hirschsprung's disease (aganglionic megacolon [Chaps. 297 and 351]).

Although the Mendelian forms of cancer have taught us much about the mechanisms of growth control, most forms of cancer do not follow simple patterns of inheritance. In many instances (e.g., lung cancer), a strong environmental contribution is at work. Even in such circumstances, however, some individuals may be more genetically susceptible to developing cancer, given the appropriate exposure, due to the presence of modifier alleles.

GENETIC TESTING FOR FAMILIAL CANCER

The discovery of cancer susceptibility genes raises the possibility of DNA testing to predict the risk of cancer in individuals of affected families. An algorithm for cancer risk assessment and decision making in high-risk families using genetic testing is shown in Fig. 83-6. Once a mutation is discovered in a family, subsequent testing of asymptomatic family members can be crucial in patient management. A negative gene test in these individuals can prevent years of anxiety in the knowledge that their cancer risk is no higher than that of the general population. On the other hand, a positive test may lead to alteration of clinical management, such as increased frequency of cancer screening and, when feasible and appropriate, prophylactic surgery. Potential negative consequences of a positive test result include psychological distress (anxiety, depression) and discrimination, although the Genetic Information Nondiscrimination Act (GINA) makes it illegal for predictive genetic information to be used to discriminate in health insurance or employment. Testing should therefore not be conducted without counseling before and after disclosure of the test result. In addition, the decision to test should depend on whether effective interventions exist for the particular type of cancer to be tested. Despite these caveats, genetic cancer testing for some cancer syndromes already appears to have greater benefits than risks, and many

TABLE 83-3 Cancer Predisposition Syndromes and Associated Genes

Syndrome	Gene	Chromosome	Inheritance	Tumors
Ataxia telangiectasia	ATM	11q22-q23	AR	Breast
Autoimmune lymphoproliferative syndrome	FAS FASL	10q24 1q23	AD	Lymphomas
Bloom syndrome	BLM	15q26.1	AR	Several types
Cowden syndrome	PTEN	10q23	AD	Breast, thyroid
Familial adenomatous polyposis	APC	5q21	AD	Intestinal adenoma, colorectal
Familial melanoma	p16INK4	9p21	AD	Melanoma, pancreatic
Familial Wilms' tumor	WT1	11p13	AD	Kidney (pediatric)
Hereditary breast/ovarian cancer	BRCA1 BRCA2	17q21 13q12.3	AD	Breast, ovarian, colon, prostate
Hereditary diffuse gastric cancer	CDH1	16q22	AD	Stomach
Hereditary multiple exostoses	EXT1 EXT2	8q24 11p11-12	AD	Exostoses, chondrosarcoma
Hereditary prostate cancer	HPC1	1q24-25	AD	Prostate
Hereditary retinoblastoma	RB1	13q14.2	AD	Retinoblastoma, osteosarcoma
Hereditary nonpolyposis colon cancer (HNPCC)	MSH2 MLH1 MSH6 PMS2	2p16 3p21.3 2p16 7p22	AD	Colon, endometrial, ovarian, stomach, small bowel, ureter carcinoma
Hereditary papillary renal carcinoma	MET	7q31	AD	Papillary kidney
Juvenile polyposis	SMAD4	18q21	AD	Gastrointestinal, pancreatic
Li-Fraumeni	TP53	17p13.1	AD	Sarcoma, breast
Multiple endocrine neoplasia type 1	MEN1	11q13	AD	Parathyroid, endocrine, pancreas, and pituitary
Multiple endocrine neoplasia type 2a	RET	10q11.2	AD	Medullary thyroid carcinoma, pheochromocytoma
Neurofibromatosis type 1	NF1	17q11.2	AD	Neurofibroma, neurofibrosarcoma, brain
Neurofibromatosis type 2	NF2	22q12.2	AD	Vestibular schwannoma, meningioma, spine
Nevoid basal cell carcinoma syndrome (Gorlin's syndrome)	PTCH	9q22.3	AD	Basal cell carcinoma, medulloblastoma, jaw cysts
Tuberous sclerosis	TSC1 TSC2	9q34 16p13.3	AD	Angiofibroma, renal angiomyolipoma
von Hippel–Lindau	VHL	3p25-26	AD	Kidney, cerebellum, pheochromocytoma

Abbreviations: AD, autosomal dominant; AR, autosomal recessive.

companies now offer testing for various genes associated with the predisposition to breast cancer (*BRCA1* and *BRCA2*), melanoma (*p16INK4*), and colon cancer (*APC* and the HNPCC genes).

Because of the inherent problems of genetic testing such as cost, specificity, and sensitivity, it is not yet appropriate to offer these tests to the general population. However, testing may be appropriate in some subpopulations with a known increased risk, even without a defined family history. For example, two mutations in the breast cancer susceptibility gene *BRCA1*, 185delAG and 5382insC, exhibit a sufficiently high frequency in the Ashkenazi Jewish population that genetic testing of an individual of this ethnic group may be warranted.

As noted above, it is important that genetic test results be communicated to families by trained genetic counselors, especially for high-risk high-penetrance conditions such as the hereditary breast/ovarian cancer syndrome (*BRCA1/BRCA2*). To ensure that the families clearly understand its advantages and disadvantages and the impact it may have on disease management and psyche, genetic testing should never be done before counseling. Significant expertise is needed to communicate the results of genetic testing to families.

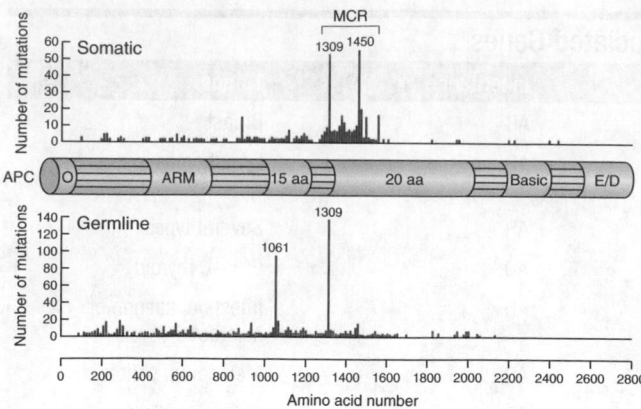

Figure 83-5 Germline and somatic mutations in the tumor-suppressor gene *APC*. *APC* encodes a 2843-amino-acid protein with 6 major domains: an oligomerization region (O), armadillo repeats (ARM), 15-amino-acid repeats (15 aa), 20-amino-acid repeats (20 aa), a basic region, and a domain involved in binding EB1 and the *Drosophila* discs large homologue (E/D). Shown are the positions within the *APC* gene of a total of 650 somatic and 826 germline mutations (from the *APC* database at *http://www.umd.be/APC*). The vast majority of these mutations result in the truncation of the APC protein. Germline mutations are found to be relatively evenly distributed up to codon 1600 except for two mutation hotspots at amino acids 1061 and 1309, which together account for one-third of the mutations found in familial adenomatous polyposis (FAP) families. Somatic *APC* mutations in colon tumors cluster in an area of the gene known as the *mutation cluster region* (MCR). The location of the MCR suggests that the 20-amino-acid domain plays a crucial role in tumor suppression.

For example, one common mistake is to misinterpret the result of negative genetic tests. For many cancer predisposition genes, the sensitivity of genetic testing is less than 70% (i.e., of 100 kindreds tested, disease-causing mutations can be identified in 70 at most). Therefore, such testing should in general begin with an affected member of the kindred (the youngest family member still alive who has had the cancer of interest). If a mutation is not identified in this individual, then the test should be reported as noninformative (Fig. 83-6) rather than negative (because it is possible that, for technical reasons, the mutation in this individual is not detectable by standard genetic assays). On the other hand, if a mutation can be identified in this individual, then testing of other family members can be performed, and the sensitivity of such subsequent tests will be 100% (because the mutation in the family is in this case known to be detectable by the method used).

MICRORNAs AND CANCER

MicroRNAs (miRNAs) are small noncoding RNAs 20–22 nucleotides in length that are involved in posttranscriptional gene regulation. Studies in chronic lymphocytic leukemia first suggested a link between miRNAs and cancer when *miR-15* and *miR-16* were found to be deleted or downregulated in the vast majority of tumors. Various miRNAs have since been found abnormally expressed in several human malignancies. Aberrant expression of miRNAs in cancer has been attributed to several mechanisms, such as chromosomal rearrangements, genomic copy number change, epigenetic modifications, defects in miRNA biogenesis pathway, and regulation by transcriptional factors.

Functionally, miRNAs have been suggested to contribute to tumorigenesis through their ability to regulate oncogenic signaling pathways. For example, *miR-15* and *miR-16* have been shown to target the *BCL2* oncogene, leading to its downregulation in leukemic cells and apoptosis. As another example of miRNAs' involvement in

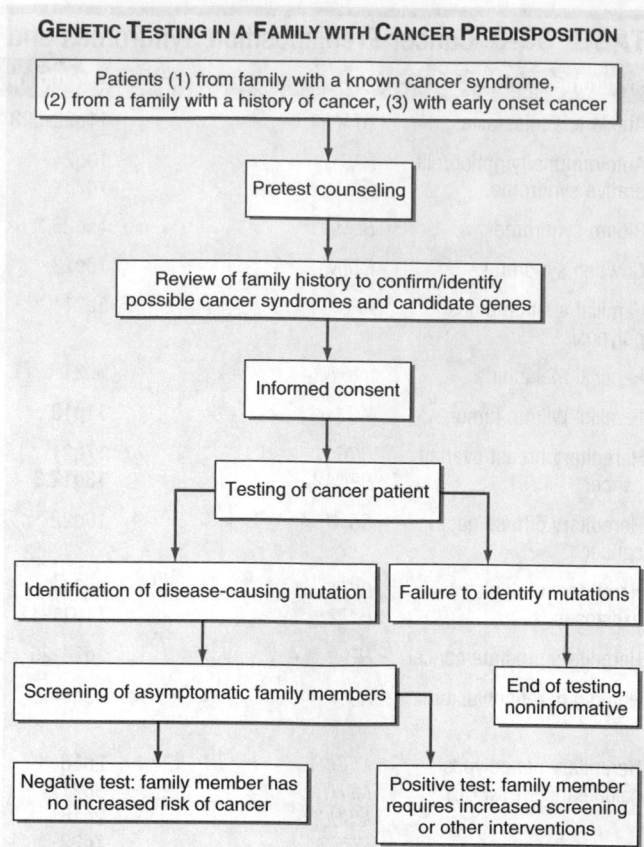

Figure 83-6 Algorithm for genetic testing in a family with cancer predisposition. The key step is the identification of a mutation in a cancer patient, which allows testing of asymptomatic family members. Asymptomatic family members who test positive may require increased screening or surgery, whereas others are at no greater risk for cancer than the general population.

oncogenic pathways, the p53 tumor suppressor can transcriptionally induce *miR-34* following genotoxic stress, and this induction is important in mediating p53 function. The expression of miRNAs is extremely specific and there is evidence that miRNA expression patterns may be useful in distinguishing lineage and differentiation state, as well as cancer diagnosis and outcome prediction. However, no miRNA gene has ever been observed to be mutated in a cancer, either in the germline or somatically. At present, the only absolutely reliable way to causally implicate a gene in the human neoplastic process is through evidence of its mutant status. Hundreds of other genes, besides miRNAs, are expressed at higher or lower levels in cancers compared to corresponding normal tissues, and the roles of any of these genes in human cancer remain conjectural.

VIRUSES IN HUMAN CANCER

Certain human malignancies are associated with viruses. Examples include Burkitt's lymphoma (Epstein-Barr virus), hepatocellular carcinoma (hepatitis viruses), cervical cancer [human papillomavirus (HPV)], and T cell leukemia (retroviruses). The mechanisms of action of these viruses are varied but always involve activation of growth-promoting pathways or inhibition of tumor-suppressor products in the infected cells. For example, HPV proteins E6 and E7 bind and inactivate cellular tumor suppressors p53 and pRB, respectively. Viruses are not sufficient for cancer development, but constitute one alteration in the multistep process of cancer progression.

GENE EXPRESSION IN CANCER

The tumorigenesis process, driven by alterations in tumor suppressors, oncogenes, and epigenetic regulation, is accompanied by changes in gene expression. The advent of powerful techniques for high-throughput gene expression profiling, based on sequencing or microarrays, has allowed the comprehensive study of gene expression in neoplastic cells. It is indeed possible to identify the expression levels of thousands of genes expressed in normal and cancer tissues. Figure 83-7 shows a typical microarray experiment examining gene expression in cancer. This global knowledge of gene expression allows the identification of differentially expressed genes and, in principle, the understanding of the complex molecular circuitry regulating normal and neoplastic behaviors. Such studies have led to molecular profiling of tumors, which has suggested general methods for distinguishing tumors of various biologic behaviors (molecular classification), elucidating pathways relevant to the development of tumors, and identifying molecular targets for the detection and therapy of cancer. The first practical applications of this technology have suggested that global gene expression profiling can provide prognostic information not evident from other clinical or laboratory tests. The Sanger Cancer Genome Project (http://www.sanger.ac.uk/genetics/CGP/) maintains a database dedicated to collect data on gene expression in normal and malignant tissues and make it available on the Internet. The Gene Expression Omnibus (GEO, http://www.ncbi.nlm.nih.gov/geo/) is another online data repository for expression profiling experiments.

GENOMEWIDE MUTATIONAL PROFILING IN CANCER

With the completion of the Human Genome Project and advances in sequencing technologies, systematic mutational analysis of the cancer genome has become possible. All protein-encoding genes known to be present in the human genome have been sequenced in breast, pancreatic, brain, and colorectal tumors. Interestingly it was found that there are generally 40 to 100 genetic alterations that affect protein sequence in a typical cancer, although statistical analyses suggested that only 8–15 are functionally involved in tumorigenesis. The picture that emerges from these studies is that most genes found mutated in tumors are actually mutated at relatively low frequencies (<5%), while a small number of genes (such as p53, KRAS) are mutated in a large proportion of tumors (Fig. 83-8). In the past, the focus of research has been on the frequently mutated genes, but it appears that the large number of genes that are infrequently mutated in cancer are major contributors to the cancer phenotype. Understanding the signaling pathways altered by mutations in these genes, as well as the functional relevance of these different mutations, represents the next challenge in the field. The Cancer Genome Atlas (http://cancergenome.nih.gov) is a coordinated effort from the National Cancer Institute and the National Human Genome Research Institute to systematically

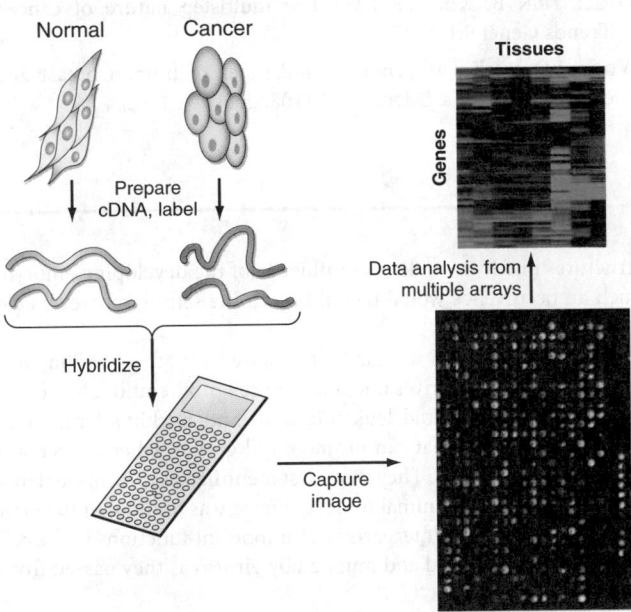

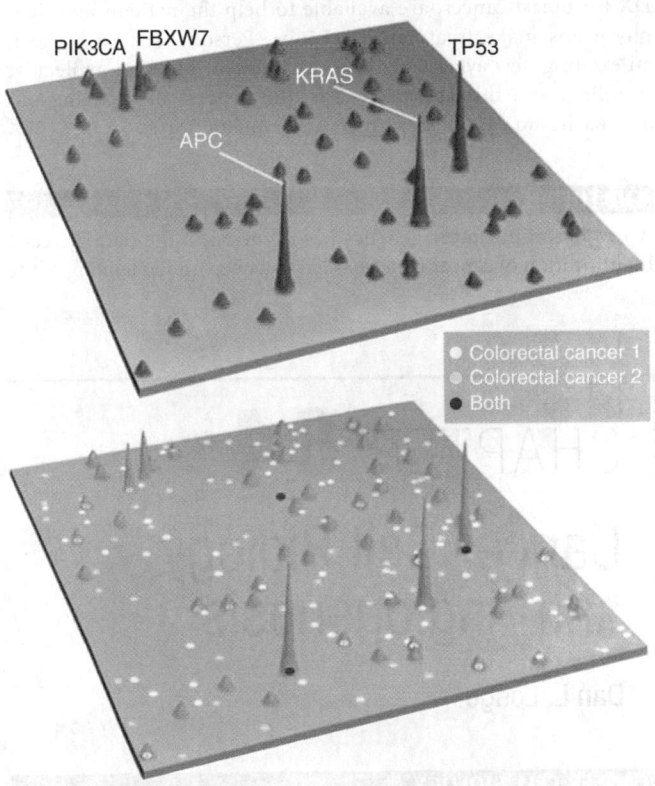

Figure 83-7   A microarray experiment. RNA is prepared from cells, reverse transcribed to cDNA, and labeled with fluorescent dyes (typically green for normal cells and red for cancer cells). The fluorescent probes are mixed and hybridized to a cDNA array. Each spot on the array is an oligonucleotide (or cDNA fragment) that represents a different gene. The image is then captured with a fluorescence camera; red spots indicate higher expression in tumor cells compared with reference, while green spots represent the lower expression in tumor cells. Yellow signals indicate equal expression levels in normal and tumor specimens. After clustering analysis of multiple arrays, the results are typically represented graphically using a visualization software, which shows, for each sample, a color-coded representation of gene expression for every gene on the array.

Figure 83-8   A two-dimensional maps of genes mutated in colorectal cancer. The two-dimensional landscape represent the positions of the RefSeq genes along the chromosomes and the height of the peaks represent the mutation frequency. On the top map, the taller peaks represent the genes that are commonly mutated in colon cancer while the large number of smaller hills indicates the genes that are mutated at lower frequency. On the lower map, the mutations of two individual tumors are indicated. Note that there is little overlap between the mutated genes of the two colorectal tumors shown. These differences may represent the basis for the heterogeneity in terms of behavior and responsiveness to therapy observed in human cancer. (From Wood et al: Science 318:1108, 2007, with permission.)

characterize the entire spectrum of genomic changes involved in human cancers.

PERSONALIZED CANCER TREATMENT BASED ON MOLECULAR PROFILES

Gene expression profiling and genomewide sequencing approaches have allowed for an unprecedented understanding of cancer at the molecular level. It has been suggested that individualized knowledge of pathways or genes deregulated in a given tumor (personalized genomics) may provide a guide for therapeutic options on this tumor, thus leading to personalized therapy. As tumor behavior is highly heterogeneous, even within a tumor type, personalized information-based medicine may provide a viable alternative to current one-size-fits-all therapy, especially in the case of tumors resistant to conventional therapeutic approaches. The success of this approach will be dependent on accumulated information on cancer behavior and phenotypes. For example, the identification of a particular mutation, such as that in *BRAF*, can indicate whether a certain tumor (such as melanoma) is likely to be susceptible to a specific drug that targets the mutant *BRAF* gene. Similarly, the identification of another mutation, in *KRAS*, can indicate that tumor is unlikely to be sensitive to an antibody targeting EGFR. Gene expression also offers the potential to predict drug sensitivities as well as provide prognostic information. Commercial diagnostic tests, such as Mammaprint and Oncotype DX for breast cancer, are available to help the patients and their physicians make treatment decisions. Personalized medicine is an exciting new avenue for cancer treatment based on molecular profiling, and this approach is in the process of changing our approaches to cancer therapy in fundamental ways.

THE FUTURE

A revolution in cancer genetics has occurred in the past 25 years. Identification of cancer genes has led to a deep understanding of the tumorigenesis process and has had important repercussions on all fields of cancer biology. In particular, the advancement of powerful techniques for genomewide expression profiling and mutation analyses has provided a detailed picture of the molecular defects present in individual tumors. In addition, individualized treatment based on the specific genetic alterations within some tumor types has already become possible. While these advances have not yet translated into overall changes in cancer prevention, prognosis, or treatment, it is expected that breakthroughs in these areas will continue to emerge and be applicable to an ever-increasing number of cancers.

FURTHER READINGS

FOULKES WD: Inherited susceptibility to common cancers. N Engl J Med 359:2148, 2008

LEY TJ et al: DNA sequencing of a cytogenetically normal acute myeloid leukaemia genome. Nature 456:66, 2008

MARKOWITZ SD, BERTAGNOLLI M: Molecular basis of colorectal cancer. N Engl J Med 361:2449, 2009

MOUSSES S et al: Using biointelligence to search the cancer genome: an epistemological perspective on knowledge recovery strategies to enable precision medical genomics. Oncogene 27:S58, 2009

SCHVARTZMAN JM et al: Mitotic chromosomal instability and cancer: mouse modelling of the human disease. Nat Rev Cancer 10:102, 2010

TIMP W et al: A new link between epigenetic progenitor lesions in cancer and the dynamics of signal transduction. Cell Cycle 8:383, 2009

VOGELSTEIN B, KINZLER KW: The multistep nature of cancer. Trends Genet 9:138, 1993

WOOD LD et al: The genomic landscapes of human breast and colorectal cancers. Science 318:1108, 2007

CHAPTER **84**

Cancer Cell Biology and Angiogenesis

Dan L. Longo

CANCER CELL BIOLOGY

Cancers are characterized by unregulated cell growth, tissue invasion, and metastasis. A neoplasm is *benign* when it grows in an unregulated fashion without tissue invasion. The presence of both features is characteristic of *malignant* neoplasms. Cancers are named based on their origin: those derived from epithelial tissue are called *carcinomas*, those derived from mesenchymal tissues are *sarcomas*, and those derived from hematopoietic tissue are *leukemias* or *lymphomas*.

Cancers nearly always arise as a consequence of genetic alterations. Choriocarcinoma may be an exception to this rule in that experimental insertion of a choriocarcinoma cell into an animal blastocyst can result in the neoplastic cell giving rise to normal body structures under the inductive influence of the developing embryo. Such an occurrence would be unlikely in the setting of irreversible genetic damage.

Occasional cancers appear to be caused by an alteration in a dominant gene that drives uncontrolled cell proliferation. Examples include chronic myeloid leukemia (*abl*) and Burkitt's lymphoma (*c-myc*). The genes that can promote cell growth when altered are often called *oncogenes*. They were first identified as critical elements of viruses that cause animal tumors; later it was found that the viral genes had normal counterparts with important functions in the cell and had been captured and mutated by viruses as they passed from host to host.

However, the vast majority of human cancers are characterized by multiple genetic abnormalities, each of which contributes to the loss of control of cell proliferation and differentiation and the acquisition of capabilities, such as tissue invasion and angiogenesis. Many cancers go through recognizable steps of progressively more abnormal phenotypes: hyperplasia, to adenoma, to dysplasia, to carcinoma in situ, to invasive cancer (Table 84-1). These properties are not found in the normal adult cell from which the tumor is derived. Indeed, normal cells have a large number of safeguards against uncontrolled proliferation and invasion.

In most organs, only primitive nonfunctional cells are capable of proliferating and the cells lose the capacity to proliferate as they differentiate and acquire functional capability. The expansion of

TABLE 84-1 Phenotypic Characteristics of Malignant Cells

Deregulated cell proliferation: Loss of function of negative growth regulators (suppressor oncogenes, i.e., Rb, p53), and increased action of positive growth regulators (oncogenes, i.e., *Ras, Myc*). Leads to aberrant cell cycle control and includes loss of normal checkpoint responses.

Failure to differentiate: Arrest at a stage before terminal differentiation. May retain stem cell properties. (Frequently observed in leukemias due to transcriptional repression of developmental programs by the gene products of chromosomal translocations.)

Loss of normal apoptosis pathways: Inactivation of p53, increases in Bcl-2 family members. This defect enhances the survival of cells with oncogenic mutations and genetic instability and allows clonal expansion and diversification within the tumor without activation of physiologic cell death pathways.

Genetic instability: Defects in DNA repair pathways leading to either single or oligo-nucleotide mutations (as in microsatellite instability, MIN) or more commonly chromosomal instability (CIN) leading to aneuploidy. Caused by loss of function of p53, BRCA1/2, mismatch repair genes, DNA repair enzymes, and the spindle checkpoint.

Loss of replicative senescence: Normal cells stop dividing in vitro after 25–50 population doublings. Arrest is mediated by the Rb, p16^{INK4a}, and p53 pathways. Further replication leads to telomere loss, with crisis. Surviving cells often harbor gross chromosomal abnormalities. Relevance to human in vivo cancer remains uncertain. Many human cancers express telomerase.

Increased angiogenesis: Due to increased gene expression of proangiogenic factors (VEGF, FGF, IL-8) by tumor or stromal cells, or loss of negative regulators (endostatin, tumstatin, thrombospondin).

Invasion: Loss of cell-cell contacts (gap junctions, cadherins) and increased production of matrix metalloproteinases (MMPs). Often takes the form of epithelial-to-mesenchymal transition (EMT), with anchored epithelial cells becoming more like motile fibroblasts.

Metastasis: Spread of tumor cells to lymph nodes or distant tissue sites. Limited by the ability of tumor cells to survive in a foreign environment.

Evasion of the immune system: Downregulation of MHC class I and II molecules; induction of T cell tolerance; inhibition of normal dendritic cell and/or T cell function; antigenic loss variants and clonal heterogeneity; increase in regulatory T cells.

Abbreviations: FGF, fibroblast growth factor; IL, interleukin; MHC, major histocompatibility complex; VEGF, vascular endothelial growth factor.

the primitive cells is linked to some functional need in the host through receptors that receive signals from the local environment or through hormonal influences delivered by the vascular supply. In the absence of such signals, the cells are at rest. We have a poor understanding of the signals that keep the primitive cells at rest. These signals, too, must be environmental, based on the observations that a regenerating liver stops growing when it has replaced the portion that has been surgically removed and regenerating bone marrow stops growing when the peripheral blood counts return to normal. Cancer cells clearly have lost responsiveness to such controls and do not recognize when they have overgrown the niche normally occupied by the organ from which they are derived. We know very little about this mechanism of growth regulation.

■ CELL CYCLE CHECKPOINTS

Normal cells have a number of control mechanisms that are targeted by specific genetic alterations in cancer. The progression of a cell through the cell division cycle is regulated at a number of checkpoints by a wide array of genes. In the first phase, G_1, preparations are made to replicate the genetic material. The cell stops before entering the DNA synthesis phase or S phase to take inventory. Are we ready to replicate our DNA? Is the DNA repair machinery in place to fix any mutations that are detected? Are the DNA replicating enzymes available? Is there an adequate supply of nucleotides? Is there sufficient energy? The main brake on the process is the retinoblastoma protein, Rb. When the cell determines that it is prepared to move ahead, sequential activation of cyclin-dependent kinases (CDKs) results in the inactivation of the brake, Rb, by phosphorylation. Phosphorylated Rb releases the S-phase-regulating transcription factor, E2F/DP1, and genes required for S phase progression are expressed. If the cell determines that it is unready to move ahead with DNA replication, a number of inhibitors are capable of blocking the action of the CDKs, including p21$^{Cip2/Waf1}$, p16^{Ink4a}, and p27^{Kip1}. *Nearly every cancer has one or more genetic lesions in the G_1 checkpoint that permits progression to S phase.*

At the end of S phase, when the cell has exactly duplicated its DNA content, a second inventory is taken at the S checkpoint. Have all of the chromosomes been fully duplicated? Were any segments of DNA copied more than once? Do we have the right number of chromosomes and the right amount of DNA? If so, the cell proceeds to G_2, in which the cell prepares for division by synthesizing mitotic spindle and other proteins needed to produce two daughter cells. When DNA damage is detected, the p53 pathway is normally activated. Called the guardian of the genome, p53 is a transcription factor that is normally present in the cell in very low levels. Its level is generally regulated through its rapid turnover. Normally p53 is bound to mdm2, which transports p53 out of the nucleus for degradation in the proteosome. When damage is sensed, the ATM (ataxia-telangiectasia mutated) pathway is activated; ATM phosphorylates mdm2, which no longer binds to p53, and p53 then stops cell cycle progression, directs the synthesis of repair enzymes, or if the damage is too great, initiates apoptosis of the cell to prevent the propagation of a damaged cell (Fig. 84-1).

A second method of activating p53 involves the induction by oncogenes of p14^{ARF} (p19 in the mouse). ARF competes with p53 for binding to mdm2, allowing p53 to escape the effects of mdm2 and accumulate in the cell. Then p53 stops cell cycle progression by activating CDK inhibitors such as p21 and/or initiating the apoptosis pathway. Mutations in the gene for p53 on chromosome 17p are found in more than 50% of human cancers. Most commonly these mutations are acquired in the malignant tissue in one allele and the second allele is deleted, leaving the cell unprotected from DNA-damaging agents. Some environmental exposures produce signature mutations in p53; for example, aflatoxin exposure leads to mutation of arginine to serine at codon 249 and leads to hepatocellular carcinoma. In rare instances, p53 mutations are in the germ line (Li-Fraumeni syndrome) and produce a familial cancer syndrome. The absence of p53 leads to chromosome instability and the accumulation of DNA damage including the acquisition of properties that give the abnormal cell a proliferative and survival advantage. *Like Rb dysfunction, most cancers have mutations that disable the p53 pathway.* Indeed, the importance of p53 and Rb in the development of cancer is underscored by the neoplastic transformation mechanism of human papillomavirus. This virus has two main oncogenes, E6 and E7. E6 acts to increase the rapid turnover of p53, and E7 acts to inhibit Rb function; inhibition of these two targets is sufficient to lead to neoplasia.

Another cell cycle checkpoint exists when the cell is undergoing division, the spindle checkpoint. The details of this checkpoint are still being discovered; however, it appears that if the spindle apparatus does not properly align the chromosomes for division, if the chromosome number is abnormal (i.e., greater or less than 4n), if the

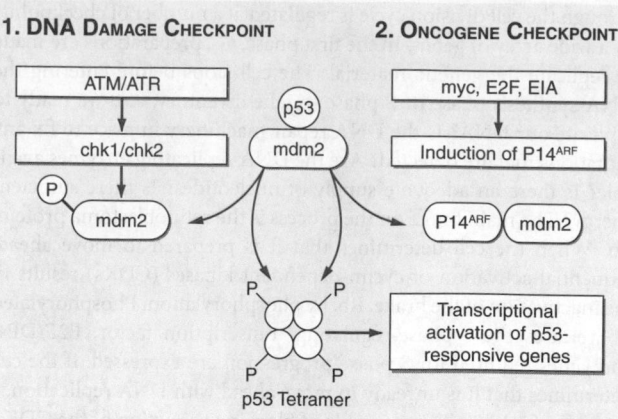

1. DNA DAMAGE CHECKPOINT

2. ONCOGENE CHECKPOINT

Figure 84-1 **Induction of p53 by the DNA damage and oncogene checkpoints.** In response to noxious stimuli, p53 and mdm2 are phosphorylated by the ataxia-telangiectasia mutated (ATM) and related ATR serine/threonine kinases, as well as the immediate downstream checkpoint kinases, Chk1 and Chk2. This causes dissociation of p53 from mdm2, leading to increased p53 protein levels and transcription of genes leading to cell cycle arrest (p21$^{Cip1/Waf1}$) or apoptosis (e.g., the proapoptotic Bcl-2 family members Noxa and Puma). Inducers of p53 include hypoxemia, DNA damage (caused by ultraviolet radiation, gamma irradiation, or chemotherapy), ribonucleotide depletion, and telomere shortening. A second mechanism of p53 induction is activated by oncogenes such as *Myc*, which promote aberrant G$_1$/S transition. This pathway is regulated by a second product of the Ink4a locus, p14^{ARF} (p19 in mice), which is encoded by an *alternative reading frame* of the same stretch of DNA that codes for p16^{Ink4a}. Levels of ARF are upregulated by *Myc* and E2F, and ARF binds to mdm2 and rescues p53 from its inhibitory effect. This *oncogene checkpoint* leads to the death or senescence (an irreversible arrest in G$_1$ of the cell cycle) of renegade cells that attempt to enter S phase without appropriate physiologic signals. Senescent cells have been identified in patients whose premalignant lesions harbor activated oncogenes, for instance, dysplastic nevi that encode an activated form of BRAF (see below), demonstrating that induction of senescence is a protective mechanism that operates in humans to prevent the outgrowth of neoplastic cells.

centromeres are not properly paired with their duplicated partners, the cell initiates a cell death pathway to prevent the production of aneuploid progeny. Abnormalities in the spindle checkpoint facilitate the development of aneuploidy. In some tumors, aneuploidy is a predominant genetic feature. In others, microsatellite instability is the primary genetic lesion. Microsatellite instability arises from defects in DNA mismatch repair genes. In general, tumors either have defects in chromosome number or microsatellite instability, but not both. Defects that lead to cancer include abnormal cell cycle checkpoints, inadequate DNA repair, and failure to preserve genome integrity.

Efforts are underway to therapeutically restore the defects in cell cycle regulation that characterize cancer.

■ CANCER AS AN ORGAN THAT IGNORES ITS NICHE

The fundamental cellular defects that create a malignant neoplasm act at the cellular level. However, that is not the entire story. Cancers behave as organs that have lost their specialized function and stopped responding to signals that normally limit their growth. Human cancers usually become clinically detectable when a primary mass is at least 1 cm in diameter—such a mass consists of about 10^9 cells. More commonly patients present with tumors that are 10^{10} cells or greater. A lethal tumor burden is about 10^{12} cells. If all tumor cells were dividing at the time of diagnosis, patients would reach a lethal tumor burden in a very short time. However,

human tumors grow by Gompertzian kinetics—this means that not every daughter cell produced by a cell division is itself capable of dividing. The growth fraction of a tumor declines exponentially with time. The growth fraction of the first malignant cell is 100%, and by the time a patient presents for medical care, the growth fraction is 2–3% or less. This fraction is similar to the growth fraction of normal bone marrow and normal intestinal epithelium, the most highly proliferative normal tissues in the human body, a fact that may explain the dose-limiting toxicities of agents that target dividing cells.

The implication of these data is that the tumor is slowing its own growth over time. How does it do this? The tumor cells have multiple genetic lesions that tend to promote proliferation, yet by the time the tumor is clinically detectable, its capacity for proliferation has declined. We need to better understand how a tumor stops its own growth. A number of factors can contribute to the failure of tumor cells to proliferate in vivo. Some cells are hypoxemic and have inadequate supply of nutrients and energy. Some have sustained too much genetic damage to complete the cell cycle and have lost the capacity to undergo apoptosis. However, an important subset is not actively dividing but retains the capacity to divide and starts dividing again when the tumor mass is reduced by treatments. Just as the bone marrow increases its rate of proliferation in response to bone marrow–damaging agents, so too does the tumor seem to sense when the tumor cell numbers have been reduced and responds by increasing growth rate. However, the marrow stops growing when it has reached its production goals. Tumors do not.

It is not in the long-term interest of a cancer to kill its host. It errs when it overshoots the limits imposed by the organ niche it occupies. Additional tumor cell vulnerabilities are likely to be detected when we learn more about how normal cells respond to "stop" signals from their environment and how tumor cells fail to heed such signals.

■ IS IN VITRO SENESCENCE RELEVANT TO CARCINOGENESIS?

When normal cells are placed in culture in vitro, most are not capable of sustained growth. Fibroblasts are an exception to this rule. When they are cultured, fibroblasts may divide 30–50 times and then they undergo what has been termed a "crisis" during which the majority of cells stop dividing (usually due to an increase in p21 expression, a CDK inhibitor), many die, and a small fraction emerge that have acquired genetic changes that permit their uncontrolled growth. The cessation of growth of normal cells in culture has been termed "senescence" and whether this phenomenon is relevant to any physiologic event in vivo is debated.

Among the cellular changes during in vitro propagation is telomere shortening. DNA polymerase is unable to replicate the tips of chromosomes, resulting in the loss of DNA at the specialized ends of chromosomes (called *telomeres*) with each replication cycle. At birth, human telomeres are 15- to 20-kb pairs long and are composed of tandem repeats of a six-nucleotide sequence (TTAGGG) that associates with specialized telomere-binding proteins to form a T-loop structure that protects the ends of chromosomes from being mistakenly recognized as damaged. The loss of telomeric repeats with each cell division cycle causes gradual telomere shortening, leading to growth arrest (called *senescence*) when one or more critically short telomeres trigger a p53-regulated DNA-damage checkpoint response. Cells can bypass this growth arrest if pRb and p53 are nonfunctional, but cell death ensues when the unprotected ends of chromosomes lead to chromosome fusions or other catastrophic DNA rearrangements. *The ability to bypass telomere-based growth limitations is thought to be a critical step in the evolution of most malignancies.* This occurs by the reactivation of telomerase expression in cancer cells. Telomerase is an enzyme that adds TTAGGG repeats onto the 3′ ends of chromosomes. It contains a catalytic subunit with reverse transcriptase activity (hTERT) and an RNA component that provides the template for telomere extension. Most normal somatic cells do not express sufficient telomerase to prevent telomere attrition with each cell division. Exceptions include stem cells (such as those found in hematopoietic tissues, gut and skin epithelium, and germ cells) that require extensive cell division to maintain tissue homeostasis. More than 90% of human cancers express high levels of telomerase that prevent telomere shortening to critical levels and allow indefinite cell proliferation. In vitro experiments indicate that inhibition of telomerase activity leads to tumor cell apoptosis. Major efforts are underway to develop methods to inhibit telomerase activity in cancer cells. The reverse transcriptase activity of telomerase is a prime target for small-molecule pharmaceuticals. In addition, the protein component of telomerase (hTERT) may act as a tumor-associated antigen and be targeted by vaccine approaches.

All of the known functions of telomerase relate to cell division. Thus, it is unclear how short telomeres interfere with the differentiated functions of normal cells. Nevertheless, a major growth industry in medical research has been discovering an association between short telomeres and human diseases ranging from diabetes and coronary artery disease to Alzheimer's disease. The picture is further complicated by the fact that rare genetic defects in the telomerase enzyme seem to cause pulmonary fibrosis, but not hematopoietic failure or defects in nutrient absorption in the gut, the sites that might be presumed to be most sensitive to defective cell proliferation. Much remains to be learned about how telomere shortening and telomere maintenance is related to human illness in general and cancer in particular.

SIGNAL TRANSDUCTION PATHWAYS IN CANCER CELLS

Signals that affect cell behavior come from adjacent cells, the stroma in which the cells are located, hormonal signals that originate remotely, and from the cells themselves (autocrine signaling). These signals generally exert their influence on the receiving cell through activation of signal transduction pathways that have as their end result the induction of activated transcription factors that mediate a change in cell behavior or function or the acquisition of effector machinery to accomplish a new task. Although signal transduction pathways can lead to a wide variety of outcomes, many such pathways rely on cascades of signals that sequentially activate different proteins or glycoproteins and lipids or glycolipids, and the activation steps often involve the addition or removal of one or more phosphate groups on a downstream target. Other chemical changes can result from signal transduction pathways, but phosphorylation and dephosphorylation play a major role. The protein kinases are generally of two distinct classes; one class acts on tyrosine residues and the other acts on serine/threonine residues. The tyrosine kinases often play critical roles in signal transduction pathways; they may be receptor tyrosine kinases or they may be linked to other cell-surface receptors through associated docking proteins (Fig. 84-2).

Normally, tyrosine kinase activity is short-lived and reversed by protein tyrosine phosphatases (PTPs). However, in many human cancers, tyrosine kinases or components of their downstream pathways are activated by mutation, gene amplification, or chromosomal translocations. Because these pathways regulate proliferation, survival, migration, and angiogenesis, they have been identified as important targets for cancer therapeutics.

Inhibition of kinase activity is effective in the treatment of a number of neoplasms. Lung cancers with mutations in the epidermal growth factor receptor are highly responsive to erlotinib and gefitinib (Table 84-2). Lung cancers with activation of the anaplastic lymphoma kinase (ALK) respond to crizotinib, an ALK inhibitor. A BRAF inhibitor is highly effective in melanomas and thyroid cancers in which BRAF is overexpressed. Janus kinase inhibitors are active in myeloproliferative syndromes in which JAK2 activation is a pathogenetic event. Imatinib is an effective agent in tumors that overexpress c-Abl (such as chronic myeloid leukemia), c-Kit (gastrointestinal stromal cell tumors), or platelet-derived growth factor receptor (PDGFR; chronic myelomonocytic leukemia); second-generation congeners, dasatinib, and nilotinib are even more effective. Sorafenib and sunitinib, agents that inhibit a large number of kinases, are being widely tested and have shown promising antitumor activity in renal cell cancer and hepatocellular carcinoma. Inhibitors of the mammalian target of rapamycin (mTOR) such as temsirolimus are also active in renal cell cancer. The list of active agents and treatment indications is growing rapidly. These new agents have ushered in a new era of personalized therapy. It is becoming more routine for resected tumors to be assessed for specific molecular changes that predict response and to have clinical decision-making guided by those results.

However, it must be acknowledged that none of these therapies is curative in any malignancy. The reasons for the failure to cure are not all defined. However, at least some causes of resistance are known. In some tumors, resistance to kinase inhibitors is related to an acquired mutation in the target kinase that inhibits drug binding. Many of these kinase inhibitors act as competitive inhibitors of the ATP-binding pocket. ATP is the phosphate donor in these phosphorylation reactions. Mutation in the BCR-ABL kinase in the ATP-binding pocket (such as the tyrosine to isoleucine change at codon 315) can prevent imatinib binding. Other resistance mechanisms include altering other signal transduction pathways to bypass the inhibited pathway. Some kinase inhibitors are less specific for an oncogenic target than was hoped, and toxicities related to off-target kinase inhibition limit the use of the agent at a dose that would inhibit the cancer-relevant kinase. As resistance mechanisms become better defined, rational strategies to overcome resistance will emerge.

Another strategy to enhance the antitumor effects of targeted agents is to use them in rational combinations with each other and in empiric combinations with chemotherapy agents that kill cells in ways distinct from targeted agents. For example, in the c-Kit overexpressing gastrointestinal stromal tumor (GIST), resistance to imatinib develops due to secondary mutations in c-Kit, and many of these tumors are susceptible to treatment with the multitargeted tyrosine kinase (TK) inhibitor sunitinib that has activity against c-Kit as well as the PDGF and vascular endothelial growth factor (VEGF) receptors. Sunitinib is approved by the U.S. Food and Drug Administration for treatment of patients with imatinib-resistant GIST or who are intolerant of imatinib (Table 84-2). Interestingly, tumors with mutations in exon 11 of c-Kit's juxtamembrane region are particularly sensitive to imatinib, whereas those with exon 9 mutations (extracellular domain) respond better to sunitinib than imatinib. In the future, primary therapy for GIST may be determined by the specific molecular defect in c-Kit.

While targeted therapies have not yet resulted in cures when used alone, their use in the adjuvant setting and when combined with other effective treatments has substantially increased the fraction of patients cured. For example, the addition of rituximab, an anti-CD20 antibody, to combination chemotherapy in patients with diffuse large B-cell lymphoma improves cure rates by 15–20%. The addition of trastuzumab, antibody to HER2, to combination chemotherapy in the adjuvant treatment of HER2-positive breast cancer reduces relapse rates by 50%.

Targeted therapies are being developed for the ras/mitogen-activated protein (MAP) kinase pathways, the hedgehog pathway, various angiogenesis pathways, and phospholipid signaling

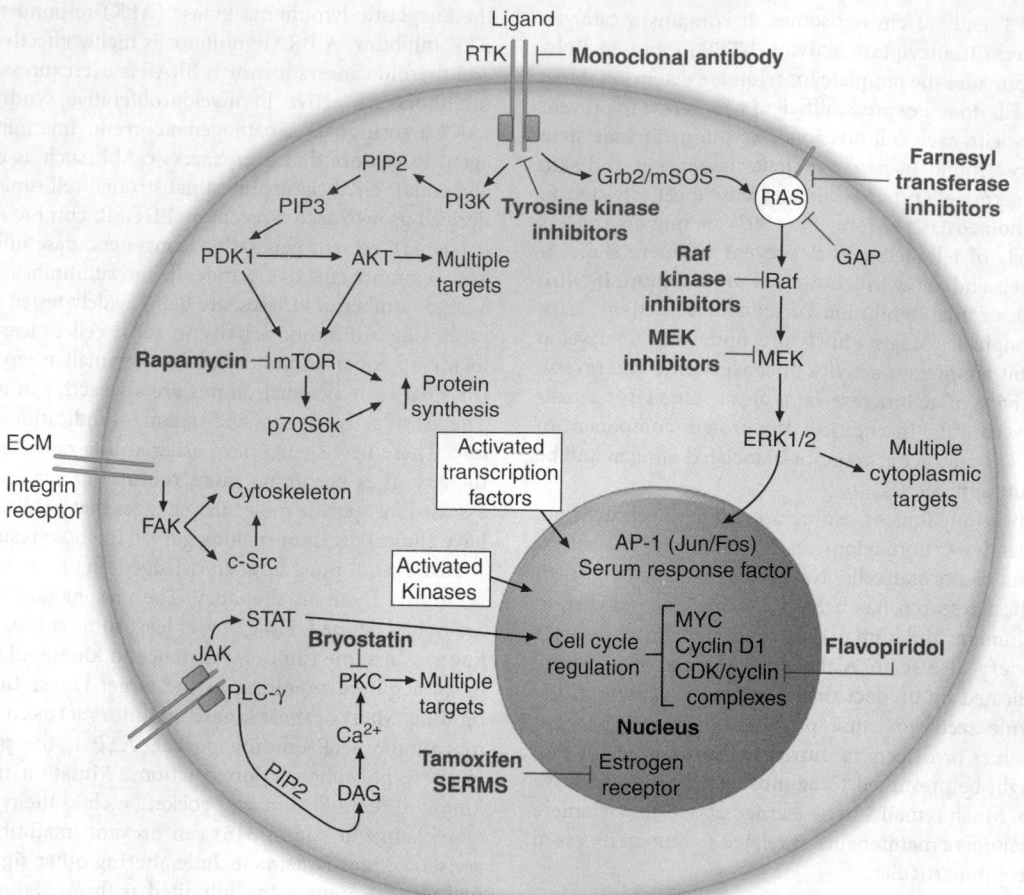

Figure 84-2 **Therapeutic targeting of signal transduction pathways in cancer cells.** Three major signal transduction pathways are activated by receptor tyrosine kinases (RTK). **1.** The protooncogene Ras is activated by the Grb2/mSOS guanine nucleotide exchange factor, which induces an association with Raf and activation of downstream kinases (MEK and ERK1/2). **2.** Activated PI3K phosphorylates the membrane lipid PIP$_2$ to generate PIP$_3$, which acts as a membrane-docking site for a number of cellular proteins including the serine/threonine kinases PDK1 and Akt. PDK1 has numerous cellular targets, including Akt and mTOR. Akt phosphorylates target proteins that promote resistance to apoptosis and enhance cell cycle progression, while mTOR and its target p70S6K upregulate protein synthesis to potentiate cell growth. **3.** Activation of PLC-γ leads the formation of diacylglycerol (DAG) and increased intracellular calcium, with activation of multiple isoforms of PKC and other enzymes regulated by the calcium/calmodulin system. Other important signaling pathways involve non-RTKs that are activated by cytokine or integrin receptors. Janus kinases (JAK) phosphorylate STAT (signal transducer and activator of transcription) transcription factors, which translocate to the nucleus and activate target genes. Integrin receptors mediate cellular interactions with the extracellular matrix (ECM), inducing activation of FAK (focal adhesion kinase) and c-Src, which activate multiple downstream pathways, including modulation of the cell cytoskeleton. Many activated kinases and transcription factors migrate into the nucleus, where they regulate gene transcription, thus completing the path from extracellular signals, such as growth factors, to a change in cell phenotype, such as induction of differentiation or cell proliferation. The nuclear targets of these processes include transcription factors (e.g., Myc, AP-1, and serum response factor) and the cell cycle machinery (CDKs and cyclins). Inhibitors of many of these pathways have been developed for the treatment of human cancers. Examples of inhibitors that are currently being evaluated in clinical trials are shown in purple type.

pathways such as the phosphatidylinositol-3-kinase (PI3K) and phospholipase C-gamma pathways, which are involved in a large number of cellular processes that are important in cancer development and progression.

One of the strategies for new drug development is to take advantage of so-called oncogene addiction. This situation (Fig. 84-3) is created when a tumor cell develops an activating mutation in an oncogene that becomes a dominant pathway with reduced contributions from auxiliary pathways. This dependency on a single pathway creates a cell that is vulnerable to inhibitors of the oncogene pathway. For example, cells harboring mutations in *BRAF* are very sensitive to MEK inhibitors.

Many transcription factors are activated by phosphorylation, which can be prevented by tyrosine- or serine/threonine kinase

inhibitors. The transcription factor NF-κB is a heterodimer composed of p65 and p50 subunits that associate with an inhibitor, IκB, in the cell cytoplasm. In response to growth factor or cytokine signaling, a multi-subunit kinase called IKK (IκB-kinase) phosphorylates IκB and directs its degradation by the ubiquitin/proteasome system. NF-κB, free of its inhibitor, translocates to the nucleus and activates target genes, many of which promote the survival of tumor cells. Novel drugs called *proteasome inhibitors* block the proteolysis of IκB, thereby preventing NF-κB activation. For unexplained reasons, this is selectively toxic to tumor cells. The antitumor effects of proteasome inhibitors are more complicated and involve the inhibition of the degradation of multiple cellular proteins. Proteasome inhibitors [bortezomib (Velcade)] have activity in patients with multiple myeloma, including partial and

TABLE 84-2 Some FDA-Approved Molecularly Targeted Agents for the Treatment of Cancer

Drug	Molecular Target	Disease	Mechanism of Action
All-*trans* retinoic acid (ATRA)	PML-RARα oncogene	Acute promyelocytic leukemia M3 AML; t(15;17)	Inhibits transcriptional repression by PML-RARα
Imatinib (Gleevec) Dasatinib (Sprycel) Nilotinib (Tasigna)	Bcr-Abl, c-Abl, c-Kit, PDGFR-α/β	Chronic myeloid leukemia; GIST	Blocks ATP binding to tyrosine kinase active site
Sunitinib (Sutent)	c-Kit, VEGFR-2, PDGFR-β, Flt-3	GIST; renal cell cancer	Inhibits activated c-Kit and PDGFR in GIST; inhibits VEGFR in RCC
Sorafenib (Nexavar)	RAF, VEGFR-2, PDGFR-α/β, Flt-3, c-Kit	RCC; hepatocellular carcinoma	Targets VEGFR pathways in RCC. Possible activity against BRAF in melanoma, colon cancer, and others
Erlotinib (Tarceva)	EGFR	Non-small cell lung cancer; pancreatic cancer	Competitive inhibitor of the ATP-binding site of the EGFR
Gefitinib (Iressa)	EGFR	Non-small cell lung cancer	Inhibitor of EGFR tyrosine kinase
Bortezomib (Velcade)	Proteasome	Multiple myeloma	Inhibits proteolytic degradation of multiple cellular proteins
Monoclonal Antibodies			
Trastuzumab (Herceptin)	HER2/neu (ERBB2)	Breast cancer	Binds HER2 on tumor cell surface and induces receptor internalization
Cetuximab (Erbitux)	EGFR	Colon cancer, squamous cell carcinoma of the head and neck	Binds extracellular domain of EGFR and blocks binding of EGF and TGF-α; induces receptor internalization. Potentiates the efficacy of chemotherapy and radiotherapy
Panitumumab (Vectibix)	EGFR	Colon cancer	Like cetuximab; likely to be very similar in clinical activity
Rituximab (Rituxan)	CD20	B cell lymphomas and leukemias that express CD20	Multiple potential mechanisms, including direct induction of tumor cell apoptosis and immune mechanisms
Alemtuzumab (Campath)	CD52	Chronic lymphocytic leukemia and CD52-expressing lymphoid tumors	Immune mechanisms
Bevacizumab (Avastin)	VEGF	Colon, lung, breast cancers; data pending in other tumors	Inhibits angiogenesis by high-affinity binding to VEGF

Abbreviations: AML, acute myeloid leukemia; EGFR, epidermal growth factor receptor; Flt-3, fms-like tyrosine kinase-3; GIST, gastrointestinal stromal tumor; PDGFR, platelet-derived growth factor receptor; PML-RARα, promyelocytic leukemia-retinoic acid receptor-alpha; RCC, renal cell cancer; t(15;17), translocation between chromosomes 15 and 17; TGF-α, transforming growth factor-alpha; VEGFR, vascular endothelial growth factor receptor.

complete remissions. Inhibitors of IKK are also in development, with the hope of more selectively blocking the degradation of IκB, thus "locking" NF-κB in an inhibitory complex and rendering the cancer cell more susceptible to apoptosis-inducing agents.

Estrogen receptors (ERs) and androgen receptors, members of the steroid hormone family of nuclear receptors, are targets of inhibition by drugs used to treat breast and prostate cancers, respectively. Tamoxifen, a partial agonist and antagonist of ER function, can mediate tumor regression in metastatic breast cancer and can prevent disease recurrence in the adjuvant setting. Tamoxifen binds to the ER and modulates its transcriptional activity, inhibiting activity in the breast but promoting activity in bone and uterine epithelium. Selective estrogen receptor modulators (SERMs) have been developed with the hope of a more beneficial modulation of ER activity, i.e., antiestrogenic activity in the breast, uterus, and ovary, but estrogenic for bone, brain, and cardiovascular tissues.

Aromatase inhibitors, which block the conversion of androgens to estrogens in breast and subcutaneous fat tissues, have demonstrated improved clinical efficacy compared with tamoxifen and are often used as first-line therapy in patients with ER-positive disease (Chap. 90).

EPIGENETIC INFLUENCES ON CANCER GENE TRANSCRIPTION

Chromatin structure regulates the hierarchical order of sequential gene transcription that governs differentiation and tissue homeostasis. Disruption of chromatin remodeling leads to aberrant gene expression and can induce proliferation of undifferentiated cells. *Epigenetics* is defined as changes that alter the pattern of gene expression that persist across at least one cell division but are not caused by changes in the DNA code. Epigenetic changes include alterations of chromatin structure mediated by methylation of

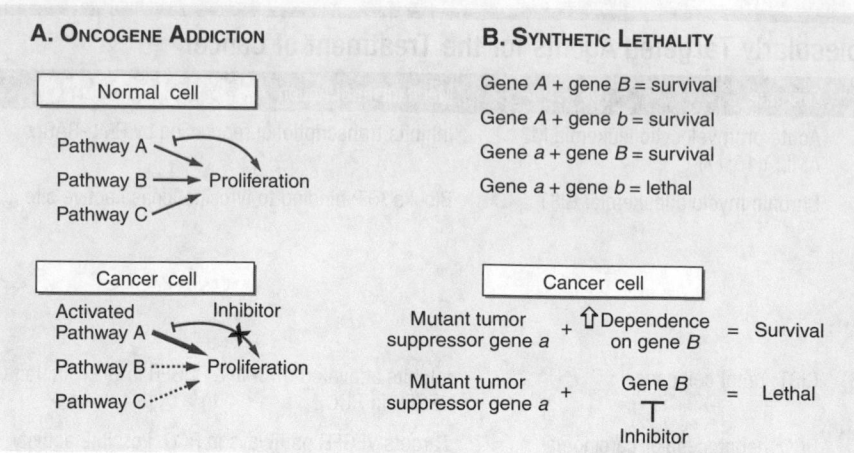

A. Oncogene Addiction

Normal cell

Pathway A
Pathway B → Proliferation
Pathway C

Cancer cell

Activated Pathway A — Inhibitor ✗
Pathway B ······→ Proliferation
Pathway C ·······

B. Synthetic Lethality

Gene *A* + gene *B* = survival
Gene *A* + gene *b* = survival
Gene *a* + gene *B* = survival
Gene *a* + gene *b* = lethal

Cancer cell

Mutant tumor suppressor gene *a* + ⇧Dependence on gene *B* = Survival

Mutant tumor suppressor gene *a* + Gene *B* ⊤ Inhibitor = Lethal

Figure 84-3 Oncogene addiction and synthetic lethality: keys to discovery of new anticancer drugs. Panel *A.* Normal cells receive environmental signals that activate signaling pathways (pathways A, B, and C) that together promote G_1 to S phase transition and passage through the cell cycle. Inhibition of one pathway (such as pathway A by a targeted inhibitor) has no significant effect due to redundancy provided by pathways B and C. In cancer cells, oncogenic mutations lead over time to dependency on the activated pathway, with loss of significant input from pathways B and C. The dependency or addiction of the cancer cell to pathway A makes it highly vulnerable to inhibitors that target components of this pathway. Clinically relevant examples include Bcr-Abl (CML), amplified HER2/*neu* (breast cancer), overexpressed or mutated EGF receptors (lung cancer), and mutated *BRAF* (melanoma). Panel *B.* Genes are said to have a synthetic lethal relationship when mutation of either gene alone is tolerated by the cell, but mutation of both genes leads to lethality. Thus, in the example, mutant *gene a* and *gene b* have a synthetic lethal relationship, implying that the loss of one gene makes the cell dependent on the function of the other gene. In cancer cells, loss of function of a tumor-suppressor gene (wild-type designated *gene A*; mutant designated *gene a*) may render the cancer cells dependent on an alternative pathway of which *gene B* is a component. As shown in the figure, if an inhibitor of *gene B* can be identified, this can cause death of the cancer cell, without harming normal cells (which maintain wild-type function for *gene A*). High-throughput screens can now be performed using isogenic cell line pairs in which one cell line has a defined defect in a tumor-suppressor pathway. Compounds can be identified that selectively kill the mutant cell line; targets of these compounds have a synthetic lethal relationship to the tumor-suppressor pathway, and are potentially important targets for future therapeutics. Note that this approach allows discovery of drugs that indirectly target deleted tumor-suppressor genes and hence greatly expands the list of physiologically relevant cancer targets.

cytosine residues in CpG dinucleotides, modification of histones by acetylation or methylation, or changes in higher-order chromosome structure (Fig. 84-4). The transcriptional regulatory regions of active genes often contain a high frequency of CpG dinucleotides (referred to as *CpG islands*), which are normally unmethylated. Expression of these genes is controlled by transient association with repressor or activator proteins that regulate transcriptional activation. However, hypermethylation of promoter regions is a common mechanism by which tumor-suppressor loci are epigenetically silenced in cancer cells. Thus one allele may be inactivated by mutation or deletion (as occurs in loss of heterozygosity), while expression of the other allele is epigenetically silenced. The mechanisms that target tumor-suppressor genes for this form of gene silencing are unknown.

Acetylation of the amino terminus of the core histones H3 and H4 induces an open chromatin conformation that promotes transcription initiation. Histone acetylases are components of coactivator complexes recruited to promoter/enhancer regions by sequence-specific transcription factors during the activation of genes (Fig. 84-4). Histone deacetylases (HDACs; at least 17 are encoded in the human genome) are recruited to genes by transcriptional repressors and prevent the initiation of gene transcription. Methylated cytosine residues in promoter regions become associated with methyl cytosine–binding proteins that recruit protein complexes

with HDAC activity. The balance between permissive and inhibitory chromatin structure is therefore largely determined by the activity of transcription factors in modulating the "histone code" and the methylation status of the genetic regulatory elements of genes.

The pattern of gene transcription is aberrant in all human cancers, and in many cases, epigenetic events are responsible. Unlike genetic events that alter DNA primary structure (e.g., deletions), epigenetic changes are potentially reversible and appear amenable to therapeutic intervention. In certain human cancers, including pancreatic cancer and multiple myeloma, the p16^{Ink4a} promoter is inactivated by methylation, thus permitting the unchecked activity of CDK4/cyclin D and rendering pRb nonfunctional. In sporadic forms of renal, breast, and colon cancer, the von Hippel–Lindau (*VHL*), breast cancer 1 (*BRCA1*), and serine/threonine kinase 11 (*STK11*) genes, respectively, are epigenetically silenced. Other targeted genes include the p15^{Ink4b} CDK inhibitor, glutathione-S-transferase (which detoxifies reactive oxygen species), and the E-cadherin molecule (important for junction formation between epithelial cells). Epigenetic silencing can occur in premalignant lesions and can affect genes involved in DNA repair, thus predisposing to further genetic damage. Examples include MLH1 (mut L homologue) in hereditary nonpolyposis colon cancer (HNPCC, also called Lynch's syndrome), which is critical for repair of mismatched bases that occur during DNA synthesis, and O^6-methylguanine-DNA methyltransferase, which removes alkylated guanine adducts from DNA and is often silenced in colon, lung, and lymphoid tumors.

Human leukemias often have chromosomal translocations that code for novel fusion proteins with enzymatic activities that alter chromatin structure. The promyelocytic leukemia–retinoic acid receptor (PML-RAR) fusion protein, generated by the t(15;17) observed in most cases of acute promyelocytic leukemia (APL), binds to promoters containing retinoic acid response elements and recruits HDAC to these promoters, effectively inhibiting gene expression. This arrests differentiation at the promyelocyte stage and promotes tumor cell proliferation and survival. Treatment with pharmacologic doses of all-*trans* retinoic acid (ATRA), the ligand for RARα, results in the release of HDAC activity and the recruitment of coactivators, which overcome the differentiation block. This induced differentiation of APL cells has improved treatment of these patients but also has led to a novel treatment toxicity when newly differentiated tumor cells infiltrate the lungs. However, ATRA represents a treatment paradigm for the reversal of epigenetic changes in cancer. For other leukemia-associated fusion proteins, such as acute myeloid leukemia (AML)-eight-twenty-one (ETO) and the MLL fusion proteins seen in AML and ALL, no ligand is known. Therefore, efforts are ongoing to determine the structural basis for interactions between translocation fusion proteins and chromatin-remodeling proteins and to use this information to rationally design

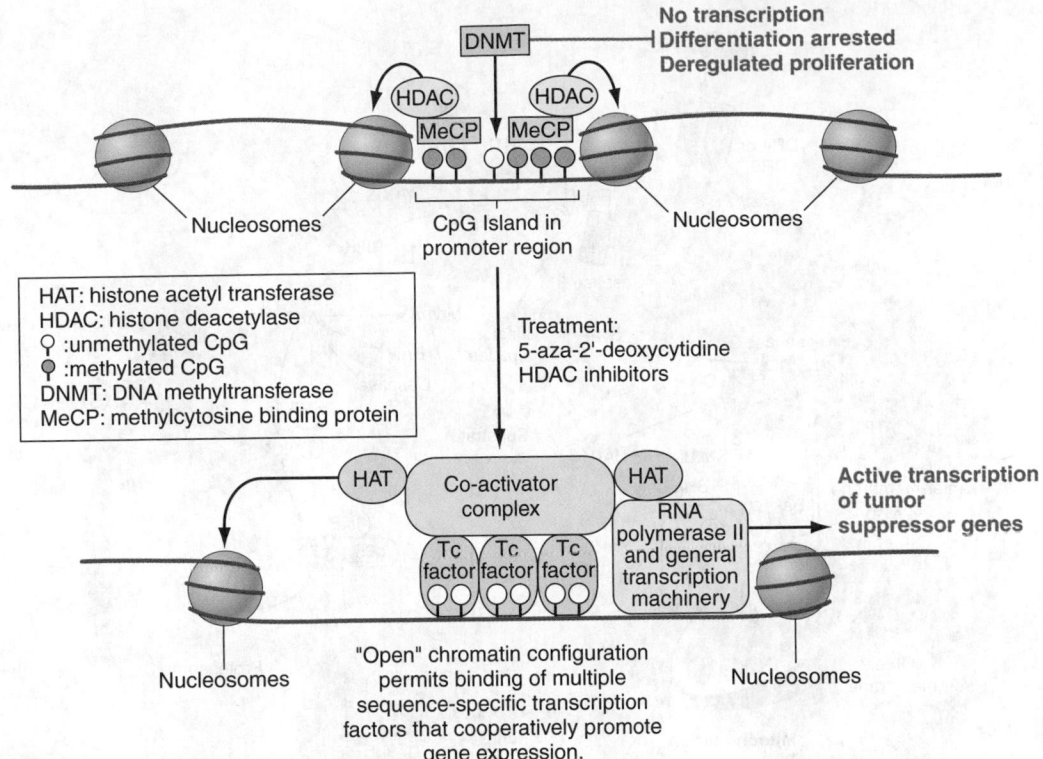

No transcription
Differentiation arrested
Deregulated proliferation

Nucleosomes

CpG Island in
promoter region

Nucleosomes

HAT: histone acetyl transferase
HDAC: histone deacetylase
♀ :unmethylated CpG
♀ :methylated CpG
DNMT: DNA methyltransferase
MeCP: methylcytosine binding protein

Treatment:
5-aza-2'-deoxycytidine
HDAC inhibitors

Active transcription
of tumor
suppressor genes

Co-activator
complex

Tc factor Tc factor Tc factor

RNA polymerase II
and general
transcription
machinery

Nucleosomes

"Open" chromatin configuration
permits binding of multiple
sequence-specific transcription
factors that cooperatively promote
gene expression.

Nucleosomes

Figure 84-4   Epigenetic regulation of gene expression in cancer cells. Tumor-suppressor genes are often epigenetically silenced in cancer cells. In the upper portion, a CpG island within the promoter and enhancer regions of the gene has been methylated, resulting in the recruitment of methyl-cytosine binding proteins (MeCP) and complexes with histone deacetylase (HDAC) activity. Chromatin is in a condensed, nonpermissive conformation that inhibits transcription. Clinical trials are under way utilizing the combination of demethylating agents such as 5-aza-2′-deoxycytidine plus HDAC inhibitors, which together confer an open, permissive chromatin structure (*lower portion*). Transcription factors bind to specific DNA sequences in promoter regions and, through protein-protein interactions, recruit co-activator complexes containing histone acetyl transferase (HAT) activity. This enhances transcription initiation by RNA polymerase II and associated general transcription factors. The expression of the tumor-suppressor gene commences, with phenotypic changes that may include growth arrest, differentiation, or apoptosis.

small molecules that will disrupt specific protein-protein associations. Drugs that block the enzymatic activity of HDAC are being tested. HDAC inhibitors have demonstrated antitumor activity in clinical studies against cutaneous T cell lymphoma (e.g., vorinostat) and some solid tumors. HDAC inhibitors may target cancer cells via a number of mechanisms, including upregulation of death receptors (DR4/5, FAS, and their ligands) and p21$^{Cip1/Waf1}$, as well as inhibition of cell cycle checkpoints.

Efforts are also under way to reverse the hypermethylation of CpG islands that characterizes many solid tumors. Drugs that induce DNA demethylation, such as 5-aza-2′-deoxycytidine, can lead to reexpression of silenced genes in cancer cells with restoration of function. However, 5-aza-2′-deoxycytidine has limited aqueous solubility and is myelosuppressive. Other inhibitors of DNA methyltransferases are in development. In ongoing clinical trials, inhibitors of DNA methylation are being combined with HDAC inhibitors. The hope is that by reversing coexisting epigenetic changes, the deregulated patterns of gene transcription in cancer cells will be at least partially reversed.

Another epigenetic form of gene regulation is microRNAs. These are short (average 22 nucleotides in length) RNA molecules that silence gene expression after transcription by binding and inhibiting the translation or promoting the degradation of mRNA transcripts. It is estimated that more than 1000 microRNAs are encoded in the human genome. Each tissue has a distinctive repertoire of microRNA expression and this pattern is altered in specific ways in cancers. However, specific correlations between microRNA expression and tumor biology and clinical behavior are just now emerging. Therapies targeting microRNAs are not currently at hand but represent a novel area of treatment development.

APOPTOSIS

Tissue homeostasis requires a balance between the death of aged, terminally differentiated cells and their renewal by proliferation of committed progenitors. Genetic damage to growth-regulating genes of stem cells could lead to catastrophic results for the host as a whole. However, genetic events causing activation of oncogenes or loss of tumor suppressors, which would be predicted to lead to unregulated cell proliferation, may instead activate signal transduction pathways that block aberrant cell proliferation. These pathways can lead to programmed cell death (*apoptosis*) or irreversible growth arrest (*senescence*). Much as a panoply of intra- and extracellular signals impinge upon the core cell cycle machinery to regulate cell division, so too these signals are transmitted to a core enzymatic machinery that regulates cell death and survival.

Apoptosis is induced by two main pathways (Fig. 84-5). The extrinsic pathway of apoptosis is activated by cross-linking members of the tumor necrosis factor (TNF) receptor superfamily, such as CD95 (Fas) and death receptors DR4 and DR5, by their ligands, Fas ligand or TRAIL (TNF-related apoptosis-inducing ligand), respectively. This induces the association of FADD (Fas-associated death domain) and procaspase-8 to death domain motifs of the receptors. Caspase-8 is activated and then cleaves and activates

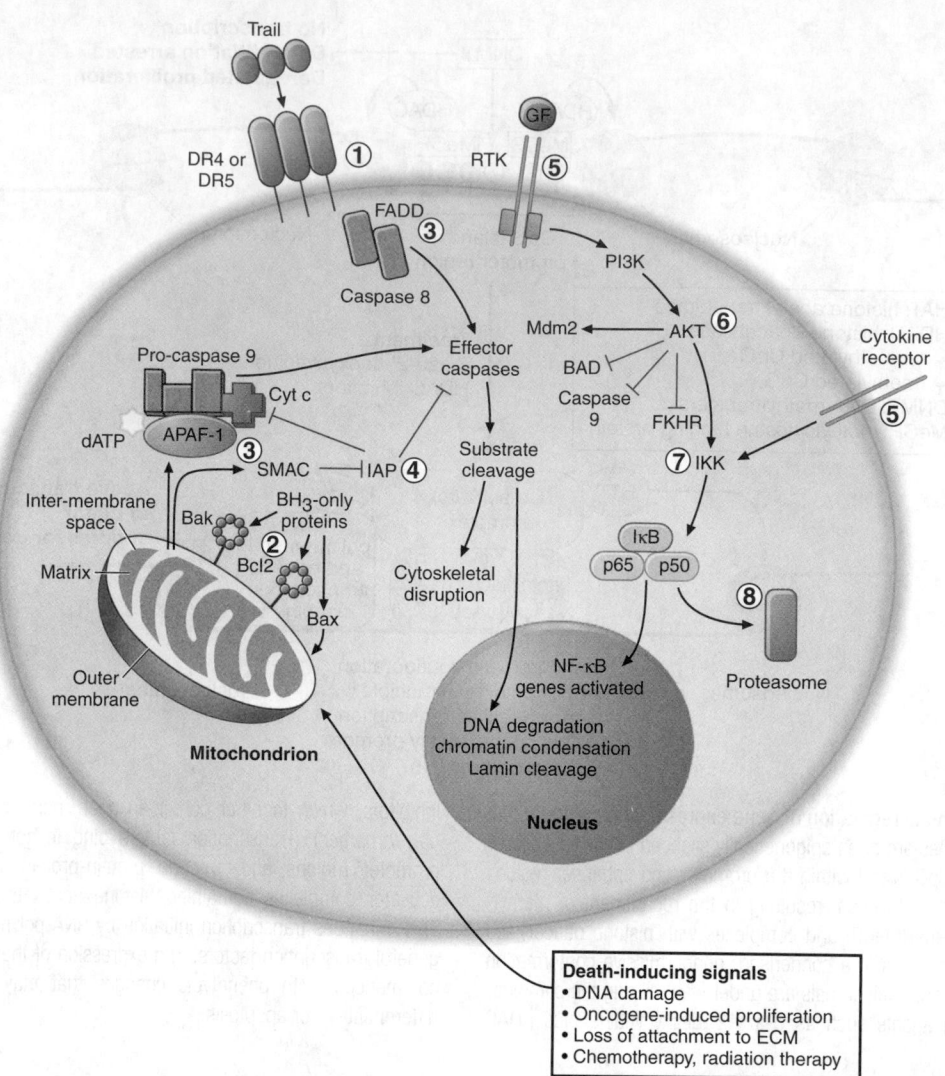

Death-inducing signals
- DNA damage
- Oncogene-induced proliferation
- Loss of attachment to ECM
- Chemotherapy, radiation therapy

Figure 84-5 Therapeutic strategies to overcome aberrant survival pathways in cancer cells. *1.* The extrinsic pathway of apoptosis can be selectively induced in cancer cells by TRAIL (the ligand for death receptors 4 and 5) or by agonistic monoclonal antibodies. *2.* Inhibition of antiapoptotic Bcl-2 family members with antisense oligonucleotides or inhibitors of the BH$_3$-binding pocket will promote formation of Bak- or Bax-induced pores in the mitochondrial outer membrane. *3.* Epigenetic silencing of APAF-1, caspase-8, and other proteins can be overcome using demethylating agents and inhibitors of histone deacetylases. *4.* Inhibitor of apoptosis proteins (IAP) blocks activation of caspases; small-molecule inhibitors of IAP function (mimicking SMAC action) should lower the threshold for apoptosis. *5.* Signal transduction pathways originating with activation of receptor tyrosine kinase receptors (RTKs) or cytokine receptors promote survival of cancer cells by a number of mechanisms. Inhibiting receptor function with monoclonal

antibodies, such as trastuzumab or cetuximab, or inhibiting kinase activity with small-molecule inhibitors can block the pathway. *6.* The Akt kinase phosphorylates many regulators of apoptosis to promote cell survival; inhibitors of Akt may render tumor cells more sensitive to apoptosis-inducing signals; however, the possibility of toxicity to normal cells may limit the therapeutic value of these agents. *7* and *8.* Activation of the transcription factor NF-κB (composed of p65 and p50 subunits) occurs when its inhibitor, IκB, is phosphorylated by IκB-kinase (IKK), with subsequent degradation of IκB by the proteasome. Inhibition of IKK activity should selectively block the activation of NF-κB target genes, many of which promote cell survival. Inhibitors of proteasome function are FDA approved and may work in part by preventing destruction of IκB, thus blocking NF-κB nuclear localization. NF-κB is unlikely to be the only target for proteasome inhibitors.

effector caspases-3 and -7, which then target cellular constituents (including caspase-activated DNAse, cytoskeletal proteins, and a number of regulatory proteins), inducing the morphologic appearance characteristic of apoptosis, which pathologists term "karyorrhexis." The intrinsic pathway of apoptosis is initiated by the release of cytochrome *c* and SMAC (second mitochondrial activator of caspases) from the mitochondrial intermembrane space in response to a variety of noxious stimuli, including DNA damage, loss of adherence to the extracellular matrix (ECM), oncogene-induced proliferation, and growth factor deprivation. Upon release into the cytoplasm, cytochrome *c* associates with dATP, procaspase-9, and the adaptor protein APAF-1, leading to

the sequential activation of caspase-9 and effector caspases. SMAC binds to and blocks the function of inhibitor of apoptosis proteins (IAP), negative regulators of caspase activation.

The release of apoptosis-inducing proteins from the mitochondria is regulated by pro- and antiapoptotic members of the Bcl-2 family. Antiapoptotic members (e.g., Bcl-2, Bcl-XL, and Mcl-1) associate with the mitochondrial outer membrane via their carboxyl termini, exposing to the cytoplasm a hydrophobic binding pocket composed of Bcl-2 homology (BH) domains 1, 2, and 3 that is crucial for their activity. Perturbations of normal physiologic processes in specific cellular compartments lead to the activation of BH3-only proapoptotic family members (such as

Bad, Bim, Bid, Puma, Noxa, and others) that can alter the conformation of the outer-membrane proteins Bax and Bak, which then oligomerize to form pores in the mitochondrial outer membrane resulting in cytochrome c release. If proteins comprised only by BH3 domains are sequestered by Bcl-2, Bcl-XL, or Mcl-1, pores do not form and apoptosis-inducing proteins are not released from the mitochondria. The ratio of levels of antiapoptotic Bcl-2 family members and the levels of proapoptotic BH3-only proteins at the mitochondrial membrane determines the activation state of the intrinsic pathway. The mitochondrion must therefore be recognized not only as an organelle with vital roles in intermediary metabolism and oxidative phosphorylation but also as a central regulatory structure of the apoptotic process.

The evolution of tumor cells to a more malignant phenotype requires the acquisition of genetic changes that subvert apoptosis pathways and promote cancer cell survival and resistance to anticancer therapies. However, cancer cells may be more vulnerable than normal cells to therapeutic interventions that target the apoptosis pathways that cancer cells depend upon. For instance, overexpression of Bcl-2 as a result of the t(14;18) translocation contributes to follicular lymphoma. Upregulation of Bcl-2 expression is also observed in prostate, breast, and lung cancers and melanoma. Targeting of antiapoptotic Bcl-2 family members has been accomplished by the identification of several low-molecular-weight compounds that bind to the hydrophobic pockets of either Bcl-2 or Bcl-XL and block their ability to associate with death-inducing BH3-only proteins. These compounds inhibit the antiapoptotic activities of Bcl-2 and Bcl-XL at nanomolar concentrations in the laboratory and are entering clinical trials.

Preclinical studies targeting death receptors DR4 and -5 have demonstrated that recombinant, soluble, human TRAIL or humanized monoclonal antibodies with agonist activity against DR4 or -5 can induce apoptosis of tumor cells while sparing normal cells. The mechanisms for this selectivity may include expression of decoy receptors or elevated levels of intracellular inhibitors (such as FLIP, which competes with caspase-8 for FADD) by normal cells but not tumor cells. Synergy has been shown between TRAIL-induced apoptosis and chemotherapeutic agents. For instance, some colon cancers encode mutated Bax protein as the result of mismatch repair (MMR) defects and are resistant to TRAIL. However, upregulation of Bak by chemotherapy restores the ability of TRAIL to activate the mitochondrial pathway of apoptosis. However, clinical studies have not yet shown that clinical activity correlates with activation of the extrinsic pathway of apoptosis.

Many of the signal transduction pathways perturbed in cancer promote tumor cell survival (Fig. 84-5). These include activation of the PI3K/Akt pathway, increased levels of the NF-κB transcription factor, and epigenetic silencing of genes such as APAF-1 and caspase-8. Each of these pathways is a target for therapeutic agents that, in addition to affecting cancer cell proliferation or gene expression, may render cancer cells more susceptible to apoptosis, thus promoting synergy when combined with other chemotherapeutic agents.

Some tumor cells resist drug-induced apoptosis by expression of one or more members of the ABC family of ATP-dependent efflux pumps that mediate the multidrug-resistance (MDR) phenotype. The prototype, P-glycoprotein (PGP), spans the plasma membrane 12 times and has two ATP-binding sites. Hydrophobic drugs (e.g., anthracyclines and vinca alkaloids) are recognized by PGP as they enter the cell and are pumped out. Numerous clinical studies have failed to demonstrate that drug resistance can be overcome using inhibitors of PGP. However, ABC transporters have different substrate specificities, and inhibition of a single family member may not be sufficient to overcome the MDR phenotype. Efforts to reverse PGP-mediated drug resistance continue.

■ METASTASIS

The three major features of tissue invasion are cell adhesion to the basement membrane, local proteolysis of the membrane, and movement of the cell through the rent in the membrane and the extracellular matrix (ECM). Malignant cells that gain access to the circulation must then repeat those steps at a remote site, find a hospitable niche in a foreign tissue, avoid detection by host defenses, and induce the growth of new blood vessels. Few drugs directly target the process of metastasis. Metalloproteinase inhibitors (see "Tumor Angiogenesis," below) represent an initial attempt to inhibit the migration of tumor cells into blood and lymphatic vessels. The rate-limiting step for metastasis is the ability for tumor cells to survive and expand in the novel microenvironment of the metastatic site, and multiple host-tumor interactions determine the ultimate outcome (Fig. 84-6).

The metastatic phenotype is likely restricted to a small fraction of tumor cells (Fig. 84-6). Some data suggest that cells with the appropriate capability express chemokine receptors. A number of candidate metastasis-suppressor genes have been identified. The loss of function of these genes enhances metastasis, and although the molecular mechanisms are in many cases uncertain, one common theme is enhancing the ability of the metastatic tumor cells to overcome apoptosis signals. Gene expression profiling is being used to study the metastatic process and other properties of tumor cells that may predict susceptibilities.

Bone metastases are extremely painful, cause fractures of weight-bearing bones, can lead to hypercalcemia, and are a major cause of morbidity for cancer patients. Osteoclasts and their monocyte-derived precursors express the surface receptor RANK (receptor activator of NF-κB), which is required for terminal differentiation and activation of osteoclasts. Osteoblasts and other stromal cells express RANK ligand, as both a membrane-bound and soluble cytokine. Osteoprotegerin (OPG), a soluble receptor for RANK ligand produced by stromal cells, acts as a decoy receptor to inhibit RANK activation. The relative balance of RANK ligand and OPG determines the activation state of RANK on osteoclasts. Many tumors increase osteoclast activity by secretion of substances such as parathyroid hormone (PTH), PTH-related peptide, interleukin (IL)-1, or Mip1 that perturb the homeostatic balance of bone remodeling by increasing RANK signaling. One example is multiple myeloma, where tumor cell–stromal cell interactions activate osteoclasts and inhibit osteoblasts, leading to the development of multiple lytic bone lesions. Inhibition of RANK ligand by an antibody (denosumab) can prevent further bone destruction. Bisphosphonates are also effective inhibitors of osteoclast function that are used in the treatment of cancer patients with bone metastases.

■ CANCER STEM CELLS

Only a small proportion of the cells within a tumor are capable of initiating colonies in vitro or forming tumors at high efficiency when injected into immunocompromised NOD/SCID mice. Acute and chronic myeloid leukemias (AML and CML) have a small population of cells (<1%) that have properties of stem cells, such as unlimited self-renewal and the capacity to cause leukemia when serially transplanted in mice. These cells have an undifferentiated phenotype (Thy1$^-$CD34$^+$CD38$^-$ and do not express other differentiation markers) and resemble normal stem cells in many ways, but are no longer under homeostatic control (Fig. 84-7). Solid tumors may also contain a population of stem cells. Cancer stem cells, like their normal counterparts, have unlimited proliferative capacity and paradoxically traverse the cell cycle at a very slow rate; cancer growth occurs largely due to expansion of the stem cell pool, the unregulated proliferation of an amplifying population, and failure

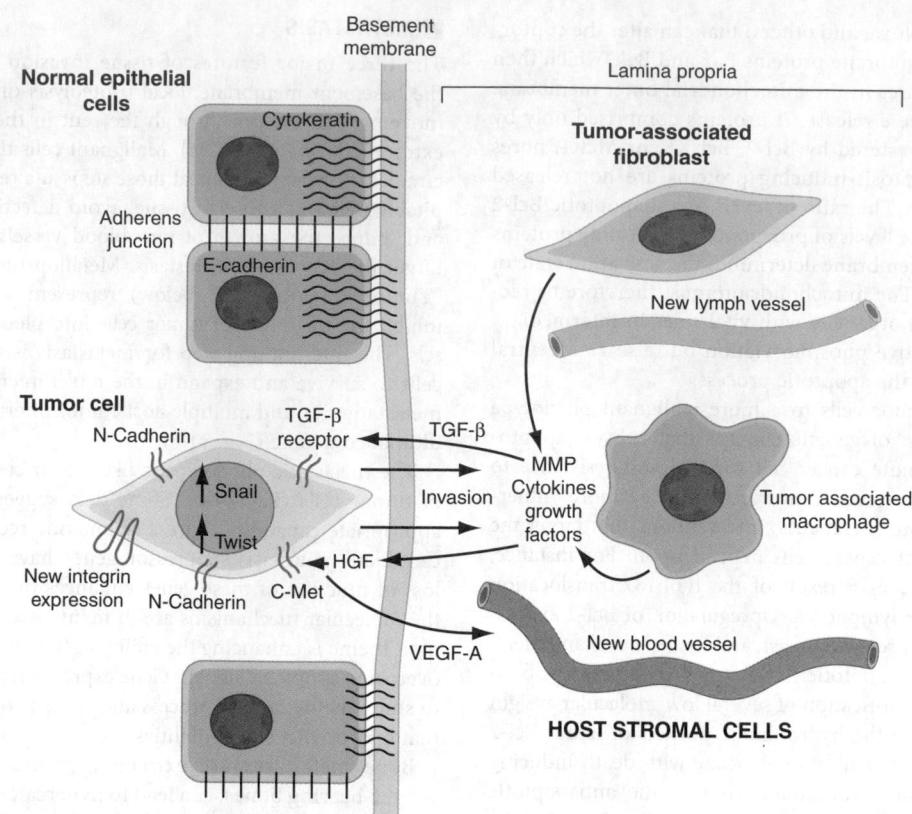

Figure 84-6 Oncogene signaling pathways are activated during tumor progression and promote metastatic potential. This figure shows a cancer cell that has undergone epithelial to mesenchymal transition (EMT) under the influence of several environmental signals. Critical components include activated transforming growth factor beta (TGF-β) and the hepatocyte growth factor (HGF)/c-Met pathways, as well as changes in the expression of adhesion molecules that mediate cell-cell and cell–extracellular matrix interactions. Important changes in gene expression are mediated by the Snail and Twist family of transcriptional repressors (whose expression is induced by the oncogenic pathways), leading to reduced expression of E-cadherin, a key component of adherens junctions between epithelial cells. This, in conjunction with upregulation of N-cadherin, a change in the pattern of expression of integrins (which mediate cell–extracellular matrix associations that are important for cell motility), and a switch in intermediate filament expression from cytokeratin to vimentin, results in the phenotypic change from adherent highly organized epithelial cells to motile and invasive cells with a fibroblast or mesenchymal morphology. EMT is thought to be an important step leading to metastasis in some human cancers. Host stromal cells, including tumor-associated fibroblasts and macrophages, play an important role in modulating tumor cell behavior through secretion of growth factors and proangiogenic cytokines, and matrix metalloproteinases that degrade the basement membrane. VEGF-A, -C, and -D are produced by tumor cells and stromal cells in response to hypoxemia or oncogenic signals, and induce production of new blood vessels and lymphatic channels through which tumor cells metastasize to lymph nodes or tissues.

of apoptosis pathways (Fig. 84-7). Slow cell cycle progression and high levels of expression of antiapoptotic Bcl-2 family members and drug efflux pumps of the MDR family render cancer stem cells less vulnerable to cancer chemotherapy or radiation therapy. Implicit in the cancer stem cell hypothesis is the idea that failure to cure most human cancers is due to the fact that current therapeutic agents do not kill the stem cells. If cancer stem cells can be identified and isolated, then aberrant signaling pathways that distinguish these cells from normal tissue stem cells can be identified and targeted.

ONCOGENE ADDICTION AND SYNTHETIC LETHALITY

The concepts of oncogene addiction and synthetic lethality have spurred new drug development targeting oncogene- and tumor-suppressor pathways. As discussed earlier in this chapter and outlined in Fig. 84-3, cancer cells become dependent upon signaling pathways containing activated oncogenes; this can effect proliferation (i.e., mutated Ras, BRAF, overexpressed Myc, or activated tyrosine kinases), survival (overexpression of Bcl-2 or NF-κB), cell metabolism (as occurs when hypoxemia-inducible factor (HIF)-1α and Akt increase dependence on glycolysis), and perhaps angiogenesis (production of VEGF,

e.g., renal cell cancer). In such cases, targeted inhibition of the pathway can lead to specific killing of the cancer cells. However, targeting defects in tumor-suppressor genes has been much more difficult, since the target of the mutation is often deleted. However, identifying genes that have a synthetic lethal relationship to tumor-suppressor pathways may allow targeting of proteins required uniquely by the tumor cells (Fig. 84-3, panel B). Several examples of this have been identified. For instance, the von Hippel–Lindau tumor-suppressor protein is inactivated in 60% of renal cell cancers, leading to overexpression of HIF-1α and the subsequent activation of downstream genes that promote angiogenesis, proliferation, survival, and altered glucose metabolism. HIF-1α mRNA has a complex 5′-terminus that indirectly requires the activity of mTOR (via activation of p70S6K and inhibition of 4E-BP) for efficient protein translation. Inhibitors of mTOR block HIF-1α translation and have significant clinical activity in renal cell cancer. In this case, mTOR is synthetic lethal to VHL loss (Fig. 84-3), and its inhibition results in selective killing of cancer cells. Conceptually, this provides a framework for genetic screens to identify other synthetic lethal combinations involving known tumor-suppressor genes, and development of novel therapeutic agents to target dependent pathways.

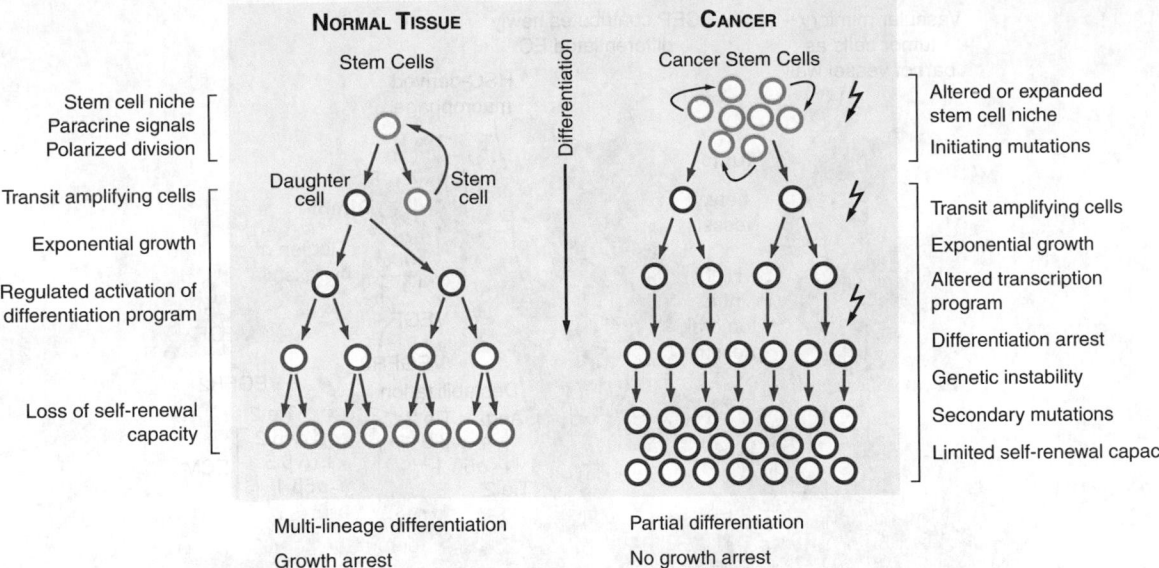

NORMAL TISSUE		CANCER

NORMAL TISSUE

Stem Cells

Stem cell niche
Paracrine signals
Polarized division

Daughter cell — Stem cell

Transit amplifying cells

Exponential growth

Regulated activation of differentiation program

Loss of self-renewal capacity

Differentiation

CANCER

Cancer Stem Cells

Altered or expanded stem cell niche

Initiating mutations

Transit amplifying cells

Exponential growth

Altered transcription program

Differentiation arrest

Genetic instability

Secondary mutations

Limited self-renewal capacity

Multi-lineage differentiation

Growth arrest

Maintenance of tissue architecture and homeostasis

Partial differentiation

No growth arrest

Loss of tissue architecture and homeostasis control

Figure 84-7   Cancer stem cells play a critical role in the initiation, progression, and resistance to therapy of malignant neoplasms. In normal tissues (left), homeostasis is maintained by asymmetric division of stem cells leading to one progeny cell that will differentiate and one cell that will maintain the stem cell pool. This occurs within highly specific niches unique to each tissue, such as in close apposition to osteoblasts in bone marrow, or at the base of crypts in the colon. Here, paracrine signals from stromal cells, such as sonic hedgehog or Notch-ligands, as well as upregulation of β-catenin and telomerase, help to maintain stem cell features of unlimited self-renewal while preventing differentiation or cell death. This occurs in part through upregulation of the transcriptional repressor Bmi-1 and inhibition of the p16^{Ink4a}/Arf and p53 pathways. Daughter cells leave the stem cells niche and enter a proliferative phase (referred to as *transit-amplifying*) for a specified number of cell divisions, during which time a developmental program is activated, eventually giving rise to fully differentiated cells that have lost proliferative potential. Cell renewal equals cell death, and homeostasis is maintained. In this hierarchical system, only stem cells are long-lived. The hypothesis is that cancers harbor stem cells that make up a small fraction

(i.e., 0.001–1%) of all cancer cells. These cells share several features with normal stem cells, including an undifferentiated phenotype, unlimited self-renewal potential, a capacity for some degree of differentiation; however, due to initiating mutations (mutations are indicated by lightning bolts), they are no longer regulated by environmental cues. The cancer stem cell pool is expanded, and rapidly proliferating progeny, through additional mutations, may attain stem cell properties, although most of this population is thought to have a limited proliferative capacity. Differentiation programs are dysfunctional due to reprogramming of the pattern of gene transcription by oncogenic signaling pathways. Within the cancer transit-amplifying population, genomic instability generates aneuploidy and clonal heterogeneity as cells attain a fully malignant phenotype with metastatic potential. The cancer stem cell hypothesis has led to the idea that current cancer therapies may be effective at killing the bulk of tumor cells but do not kill tumor stem cells, leading to a regrowth of tumors that is manifested as tumor recurrence or disease progression. Research is in progress to identify unique molecular features of cancer stem cells that can lead to their direct targeting by novel therapeutic agents.

TUMOR ANGIOGENESIS

The growth of primary and metastatic tumors to larger than a few millimeters requires the recruitment of blood vessels and vascular endothelial cells to support their metabolic requirements. The diffusion limit for oxygen in tissues is ~100 mm. A critical element in the growth of primary tumors and formation of metastatic sites is the *angiogenic switch*: the ability of the tumor to promote the formation of new capillaries from preexisting host vessels. The angiogenic switch is a phase in tumor development when the dynamic balance of pro- and antiangiogenic factors is tipped in favor of vessel formation by the effects of the tumor on its immediate environment. Stimuli for tumor angiogenesis include hypoxemia, inflammation, and genetic lesions in oncogenes or tumor suppressors that alter tumor cell gene expression. Angiogenesis consists of several steps, including the stimulation of endothelial cells (ECs) by growth factors, the degradation of the ECM by proteases, proliferation of ECs and migration into the tumor, and the eventual formation of new capillary tubes.

Tumor blood vessels are not normal; they have chaotic architecture and blood flow. Due to an imbalance of angiogenic regulators such as VEGF and angiopoietins (see below), tumor vessels are tortuous and dilated with an uneven diameter, excessive branching, and

shunting. Tumor blood flow is variable, with areas of hypoxemia and acidosis leading to the selection of variants that are resistant to hypoxemia-induced apoptosis (often due to the loss of p53 expression). Tumor vessel walls have numerous openings, widened interendothelial junctions, and discontinuous or absent basement membrane; this contributes to the high vascular permeability of these vessels and, together with lack of functional intratumoral lymphatics, causes increased interstitial pressure within the tumor (which also interferes with the delivery of therapeutics to the tumor; Figs. 84-8, 84-9, and 84-10). Tumor blood vessels lack perivascular cells such as pericytes and smooth-muscle cells that normally regulate flow in response to tissue metabolic needs.

Unlike normal blood vessels, the vascular lining of tumor vessels is not a homogeneous layer of ECs but often consists of a mosaic of ECs and tumor cells; the concept of cancer cell–derived vascular channels, which may be lined by ECM secreted by the tumor cells, is referred to as *vascular mimicry*. It is unclear whether tumor cells actually form structural elements of vascular channels or represent tumor cells in transit into or out of the vessel. However, the former is supported by evidence that in some human colon cancers, tumor cells can comprise up to 15% of vessel walls. The ECs of angiogenic blood vessels are unlike quiescent ECs found in adult vessels, where

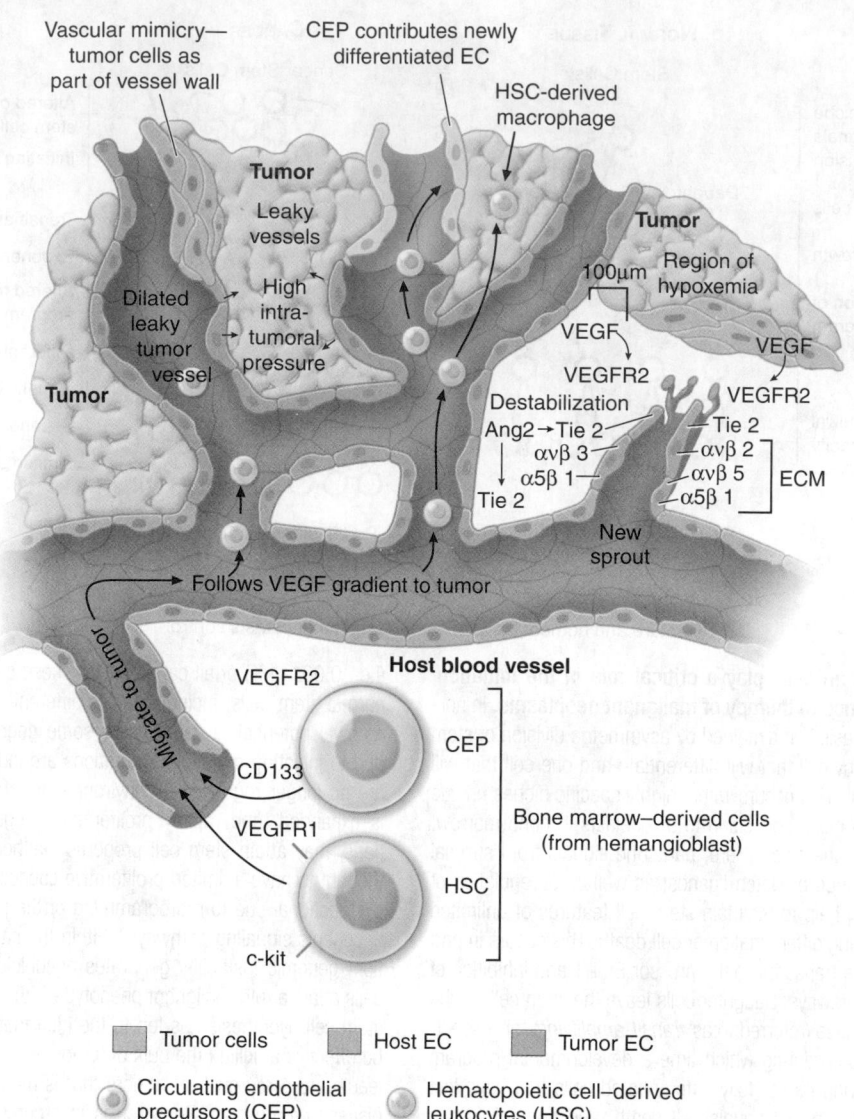

Figure 84-8 **Tumor angiogenesis** is a complex process involving many different cell types that must proliferate, migrate, invade, and differentiate in response to signals from the tumor microenvironment. Endothelial cells (ECs) sprout from host vessels in response to VEGF, bFGF, Ang2, and other proangiogenic stimuli. Sprouting is stimulated by VEGF/VEGFR2, Ang2/Tie-2, and integrin/extracellular matrix (ECM) interactions. Bone marrow–derived circulating endothelial precursors (CEPs) migrate to the tumor in response to VEGF and differentiate into ECs, while hematopoietic stem cells differentiate into leukocytes, including tumor-associated macrophages that secrete angiogenic growth factors and produce MMPs that remodel the ECM and release bound growth factors. Tumor cells themselves may directly form parts of vascular channels within tumors. The pattern of vessel formation is haphazard: vessels are tortuous, dilated, leaky, and branch in random ways. This leads to uneven blood flow within the tumor, with areas of acidosis and hypoxemia (which stimulate release of angiogenic factors) and high intratumoral pressures that inhibit delivery of therapeutic agents.

only 0.01% of ECs are dividing. During tumor angiogenesis, ECs are highly proliferative and express a number of plasma membrane proteins that are characteristic of activated endothelium, including growth factor receptors and adhesion molecules such as integrins.

■ MECHANISMS OF TUMOR VESSEL FORMATION

Tumors use a number of mechanisms to promote vascularization, subverting normal angiogenic processes for this purpose (Fig. 84-8). Primary or metastatic tumor cells sometimes arise in proximity to host blood vessels and grow around these vessels, parasitizing nutrients by co-opting the local blood supply. However, most tumor blood vessels arise by the process of *sprouting*, in which tumors secrete trophic angiogenic molecules, the most potent being VEGF, that induce the proliferation and migration of host ECs into

the tumor. Sprouting in normal and pathogenic angiogenesis is regulated by three families of transmembrane receptor tyrosine kinases (RTKs) expressed on ECs and their ligands (VEGFs, angiopoietins, ephrins; Fig. 84-9), which are produced by tumor cells, inflammatory cells, or stromal cells in the tumor microenvironment.

When tumor cells arise in or metastasize to an avascular area, they grow to a size limited by hypoxemia and nutrient deprivation. Hypoxemia, a key regulator of tumor angiogenesis, causes the transcriptional induction of the gene encoding VEGF by a process that involves stabilization of HIF-1α. Under normoxemic conditions, HIF-1α levels are maintained at a low level by proteasome-mediated destruction regulated by a ubiquitin E3-ligase encoded by the VHL tumor-suppressor locus. However, under hypoxemic conditions, HIF-1α is not hydroxylated and association with VHL

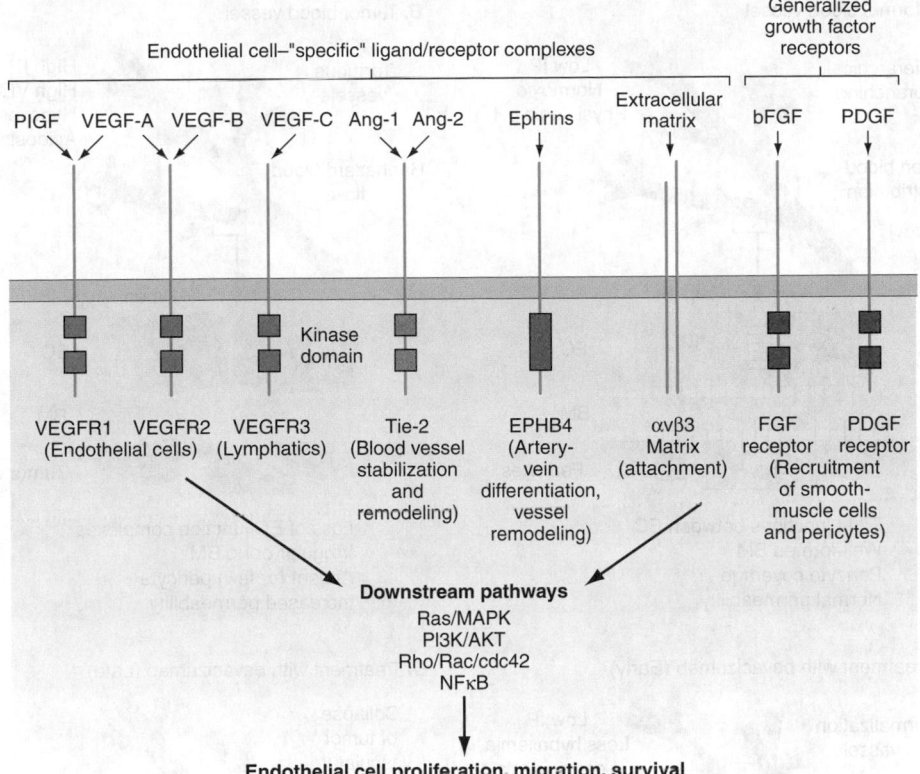

Figure 84-9 Critical molecular determinants of endothelial cell biology. Angiogenic endothelium expresses a number of receptors not found on resting endothelium. These include receptor tyrosine kinases (RTKs) and integrins that bind to the extracellular matrix and mediate endothelial cell (EC) adhesion, migration, and invasion. ECs also express RTK (i.e., the FGF and PDGF receptors) that are found on many other cell types. Critical functions mediated by activated RTK include proliferation, migration, and enhanced survival of endothelial cells, as well as regulation of the recruitment of perivascular cells and bloodborne circulating endothelial precursors and hematopoietic stem cells to the tumor. Intracellular signaling via EC-specific RTK utilizes molecular pathways that may be targets for future antiangiogenic therapies.

does not occur; therefore HIF-1 levels increase, and target genes including VEGF, nitric oxide synthetase (NOS), and Ang2 are induced. Loss of the *VHL* genes, as occurs in familial and sporadic renal cell carcinomas, results in HIF-1α stabilization and induction of VEGF. Most tumors have hypoxemic regions due to poor blood flow, and tumor cells in these areas stain positive for HIF-1α expression; in renal cancers with *VHL* deletion, all of the tumor cells express high levels of HIF-1α, and VEGF-induced angiogenesis leads to high microvascular density.

VEGF and its receptors are required for embryonic *vasculogenesis*, and normal (wound healing, corpus luteum formation) and pathologic angiogenesis (tumor angiogenesis, inflammatory conditions such as rheumatoid arthritis). VEGF-A is a heparin-binding glycoprotein with at least four isoforms (splice variants) that regulates blood vessel formation by binding to the RTKs VEGFR1 and VEGFR2, which are expressed on all ECs in addition to a subset of hematopoietic cells (Fig. 84-8). VEGFR2 regulates EC proliferation, migration, and survival, while VEGFR1 may act as an antagonist of R2 in ECs but is probably also important for angioblast differentiation during embryogenesis. Tumor vessels may be more dependent on VEGFR signaling for growth and survival than normal ECs. While VEGF signaling is a critical initiator of angiogenesis, this is a complex process regulated by additional signaling pathways (Fig. 84-9). The angiopoietin, Ang1, produced by stromal cells, binds to the EC RTK Tie-2 and promotes the interaction of ECs with the ECM and perivascular cells, such as pericytes and smooth-muscle cells, to form tight, nonleaky vessels. PDGF and basic fibroblast growth factor (bFGF) help to recruit these perivascular

cells. Ang1 is required for maintaining the quiescence and stability of mature blood vessels and prevents the vascular permeability normally induced by VEGF and inflammatory cytokines.

For tumor cell–derived VEGF to initiate sprouting from host vessels, the stability conferred by the Ang1/Tie2 pathway must be perturbed; this occurs by the secretion of Ang2 by ECs that are undergoing active remodeling. Ang2 binds to Tie2 and is a competitive inhibitor of Ang1 action: under the influence of Ang2, preexisting blood vessels become more responsive to remodeling signals, with less adherence of ECs to stroma and associated perivascular cells and more responsiveness to VEGF. Therefore, Ang2 is required at early stages of tumor angiogenesis for destabilizing the vasculature by making host ECs more sensitive to angiogenic signals. Since tumor ECs are blocked by Ang2, there is no stabilization by the Ang1/Tie2 interaction, and tumor blood vessels are leaky, hemorrhagic, and have poor association of ECs with underlying stroma. Sprouting tumor ECs express high levels of the transmembrane protein ephrin-B2 and its receptor, the RTK EPH, whose signaling appears to work with the angiopoietins during vessel remodeling. During embryogenesis, EPH receptors are expressed on the endothelium of primordial venous vessels while the transmembrane ligand ephrin-B2 is expressed by cells of primordial arteries; the reciprocal expression may regulate differentiation and patterning of the vasculature.

A number of ubiquitously expressed host molecules play critical roles in normal and pathologic angiogenesis. Proangiogenic cytokines, chemokines, and growth factors secreted by stromal cells or inflammatory cells make important contributions to

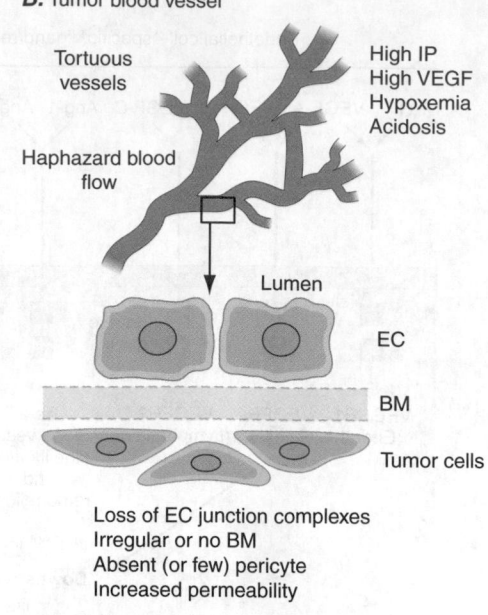

A. Normal blood vessel

Hierarchical branching

Low IP
Normoxic
Physiologic pH

Even blood distribution

Lumen

EC

BM

Pericytes

Tight junctions between EC
Well-formed BM
Pericyte coverage
Normal permeability

B. Tumor blood vessel

Tortuous vessels

High IP
High VEGF
Hypoxemia
Acidosis

Haphazard blood flow

Lumen

EC

BM

Tumor cells

Loss of EC junction complexes
Irregular or no BM
Absent (or few) pericyte
Increased permeability

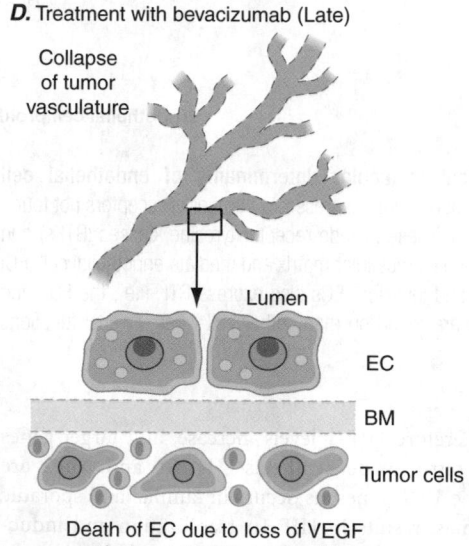

C. Treatment with bevacizumab (Early)

Normalization of vessels

Low IP
Less hypoxemia
Less acidosis

Improved blood flow

Lumen

EC

BM

Pericytes

More efficient delivery of chemotherapy and oxygen
Reduced permeability

D. Treatment with bevacizumab (Late)

Collapse of tumor vasculature

Lumen

EC

BM

Tumor cells

Death of EC due to loss of VEGF survival signals (plus chemotherapy or radiotherapy)
Apoptosis of tumor due to starvation and/or effects of chemotherapy.

Figure 84-10 Normalization of tumor blood vessels due to inhibition of VEGF signaling. *A.* Blood vessels in normal tissues exhibit a regular hierarchical branching pattern that delivers blood to tissues in a spatially and temporally efficient manner to meet the metabolic needs of the tissue (top). At the microscopic level, tight junctions are maintained between endothelial cells (ECs), which are adherent to a thick and evenly distributed basement membrane (BM). Pericytes form a surrounding layer that provides trophic signals to the EC and helps maintain proper vessel tone. Vascular permeability is regulated, interstitial fluid pressure is low, and oxygen tension and pH are physiologic. *B.* Tumors have abnormal vessels with tortuous branching and dilated, irregular interconnecting branches, causing uneven blood flow with areas of hypoxemia and acidosis. This harsh environment selects genetic events that result in resistant tumor variants, such as the loss of p53. High levels of VEGF (secreted by tumor cells) disrupt gap junction communication, tight junctions, and adherens junctions between EC via src-mediated phosphorylation of proteins such as connexin 43, zonula occludens-1, VE-cadherin, and α/β-catenins. Tumor vessels have thin, irregular BM, and pericytes are sparse or absent. Together, these molecular abnormalities result in a

vasculature that is permeable to serum macromolecules, leading to high tumor interstitial pressure, which can prevent the delivery of drugs to the tumor cells. This is made worse by the binding and activation of platelets at sites of exposed BM, with release of stored VEGF and microvessel clot formation, creating more abnormal blood flow and regions of hypoxemia. *C.* In experimental systems, treatment with bevacizumab or blocking antibodies to VEGFR2 leads to changes in the tumor vasculature that has been termed *vessel normalization*. During the first week of treatment, abnormal vessels are eliminated or pruned (dotted lines), leaving a more normal branching pattern. ECs partially regain features such as cell-cell junctions, adherence to a more normal BM, and pericyte coverage. These changes lead to a decrease in vascular permeability, reduced interstitial pressure, and a transient increase in blood flow within the tumor. Note that in murine models, this normalization period lasts only for ~5–6 days. *D.* After continued anti-VEGF/VEGFR therapy (which is often combined with chemo- or radiotherapy), ECs die, leading to tumor cell death (either due to direct effects of the chemotherapy or lack of blood flow).

neovascularization, including bFGF, transforming growth factor-α (TGF-α), TNF-α, and IL-8. In contrast to normal endothelium, angiogenic endothelium overexpresses specific members of the integrin family of ECM-binding proteins that mediate EC adhesion, migration, and survival. Specifically, expression of integrins $\alpha_v\beta_3$, $\alpha_v\beta_5$, and $\alpha_5\beta_1$ mediates spreading and migration of ECs and is required for angiogenesis induced by VEGF and bFGF, which in turn can upregulate EC integrin expression. The $\alpha_v\beta_3$ integrin physically associates with VEGFR2 in the plasma membrane and promotes signal transduction from each receptor to promote EC proliferation (via focal adhesion kinase, src, PI3K, and other pathways) and survival (by inhibition of p53 and increasing the Bcl-2/Bax expression ratio). In addition, $\alpha_v\beta_3$ forms cell-surface complexes with matrix metalloproteinases (MMPs), zinc-requiring proteases that cleave ECM proteins, leading to enhanced EC migration and the release of heparin-binding growth factors, including VEGF and bFGF. EC adhesion molecules can be upregulated (i.e., by VEGF, TNF-α) or downregulated (by TGF-β); this, together with chaotic blood flow, explains poor leukocyte-endothelial interactions in tumor blood vessels and may help tumor cells avoid immune surveillance.

Cells derived from hematopoietic progenitors in the host bone marrow contribute to tumor angiogenesis in a process linked to the secretion of VEGF and PlGF (placenta-derived growth factor) by tumor cells and their surrounding stroma. VEGF promotes the mobilization and recruitment of circulating endothelial cell precursors (CEPs) and hematopoietic stem cells (HSCs) to tumors where they co-localize and appear to cooperate in neovessel formation. CEPs express VEGFR2, while HSCs express VEGFR1, a receptor for VEGF and PlGF. Both CEPs and HSCs are derived from a common precursor, the hemangioblast. CEPs are thought to differentiate into ECs, whereas the role of HSC-derived cells (such as tumor-associated macrophages) may be to secrete angiogenic factors required for sprouting and stabilization of ECs (VEGF, bFGF, angiopoietins) and to activate MMPs, resulting in ECM remodeling and growth factor release. In mouse tumor models and in human cancers, increased numbers of CEPs and subsets of VEGFR-expressing HSCs can be detected in the circulation, which may correlate with increased levels of serum VEGF. It is not yet known whether levels of these cells have prognostic value or if changes during treatment correlate with inhibition of tumor angiogenesis. Whether CEPs and VEGFR1-expressing HSCs are required to maintain the long-term integrity of established tumor vessels is also unknown.

Lymphatic vessels also exist within tumors. Development of tumor lymphatics is associated with expression of VEGFR3 and its ligands VEGF-C and VEGF-D. The role of these vessels in tumor cell metastasis to regional lymph nodes remains to be determined, since, as discussed above, interstitial pressures within tumors are high and most lymphatic vessels may exit in a collapsed and non-functional state. However, VEGF-C levels correlate significantly with metastasis to regional lymph nodes in lung, prostate, and colorectal cancers.

■ ANTIANGIOGENIC THERAPY

ECs comprising the tumor vasculature are genetically stable and do not share genetic changes with tumor cells; the EC apoptosis pathways are therefore intact. Each EC of a tumor vessel helps provide nourishment to many tumor cells, and although tumor angiogenesis can be driven by a number of exogenous proangiogenic stimuli, experimental data indicate that at least in some tumor types, blockade of a single growth factor (e.g., VEGF) may inhibit tumor-induced vascular growth. Angiogenesis inhibitors function by targeting the critical molecular pathways involved in EC proliferation, migration, and/or survival, many of which are unique to the activated endothelium in tumors. Inhibition of growth factor and adhesion-dependent signaling pathways can induce EC apoptosis with concomitant inhibition of tumor growth. Different types of tumors use distinct molecular mechanisms to activate the angiogenic switch. Therefore, it is doubtful that a single antiangiogenic strategy will suffice for all human cancers; rather, a number of agents will be needed, each responding to distinct programs of angiogenesis used by different human cancers.

Bevacizumab, an antibody to VEGF, appears to potentiate the effects of many different types of active chemotherapeutic regimens used to treat a variety of different tumor types. It lacks single-agent antitumor activity and its strategy, the sopping up of locally produced VEGF after systemic administration, does not seem as likely to be effective as a therapy that interferes with the VEGF receptor on target cells. Bevacizumab appears to augment the antitumor effects of chemotherapy in colon cancer and additional testing in other tumor types is underway.

Bevacizumab is administered IV every 2–3 weeks (its half-life is nearly 20 days) and is generally well tolerated. Hypertension has been noted in most trials that utilize inhibitors of VEGF receptors, but only 10% of patients require treatment with antihypertensive agents and this rarely requires discontinuation of therapy. A mechanism for the hypertension may be a bevacizumab-induced decrease in vessel production of nitric oxide, resulting in vasoconstriction and increased blood pressure. Rare but serious side effects of bevacizumab include an increased risk of arterial thromboembolic events including stroke and myocardial infarction, usually in patients older than age 65 with a history of cardiovascular disease. An increased risk of hemorrhage was noted in lung cancer patients with a squamous histology and large central tumors near the major mediastinal blood vessels. Cavitation of the tumor with vessel rupture and massive hemoptysis lead to the exclusion of squamous cell cancers from treatment with bevacizumab. This potentially fatal side effect may actually reflect an increased activity of bevacizumab plus chemotherapy in squamous cell cancers. Other serious complications include bowel perforations that have been observed in 1–3% of patients (mainly those with colon and ovarian cancers).

The bevacizumab experience suggests that inhibition of the VEGF pathway will be most efficacious when combined with agents that directly target tumor cells. This also appears to be the case in the development of small-molecule inhibitors (SMI) that target VEGF receptor tyrosine kinase activity but are also inhibitory to other kinases that are expressed by tumor cells and important for their proliferation and survival. Sunitinib, FDA approved for the treatment of GIST (see above and Table 84-2), has activity directed against mutant c-Kit receptors, but also targets VEGFR and PDGFR, and has shown significant antitumor activity against metastatic renal cell carcinoma (RCC), presumably on the basis of its antiangiogenic activity. Similarly, sorafenib, originally developed as a Raf kinase inhibitor but with potent activity against VEGF and PDGF receptors, increases progression-free survival in RCC. Thus, agents that target both angiogenesis and tumor-specific signaling pathways may have greater efficacy against a broad range of cancers. A caveat is that RCC and GIST are highly dependent upon single signaling pathways (VEGF and c-Kit, respectively), whereas most solid tumors use a panoply of interconnected proliferation and survival pathways that are redundant and likely to be less amenable to single-agent targeting.

The success in targeting tumor angiogenesis has led to enhanced enthusiasm for the development of drugs that target other aspects of the angiogenic process; some of these therapeutic approaches are outlined in Fig. 84-11.

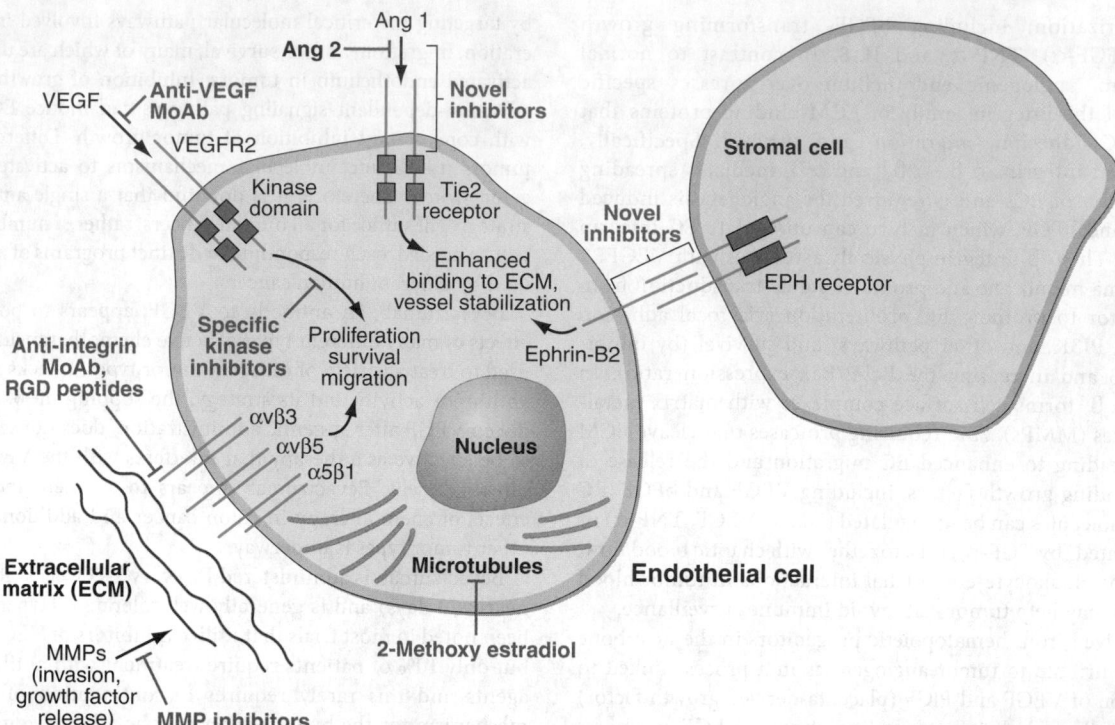

Figure 84-11 Knowledge of the molecular events governing tumor angiogenesis has led to a number of therapeutic strategies to block tumor blood vessel formation. The successful therapeutic targeting of VEGF is described in the text. Other endothelial cell–specific receptor tyrosine kinase pathways (e.g., angiopoietin/Tie2 and ephrin/EPH) are likely targets for the future. Ligation of the $\alpha_v\beta_3$ integrin is required for EC survival. Integrins are also required for EC migration and are important regulators of matrix metalloproteinase (MMP) activity, which modulates EC movement through the ECM as well as release of bound growth factors. Targeting of integrins includes development of blocking antibodies, small peptide inhibitors of integrin signaling, and arg-gly-asp–containing peptides that prevent integrin:ECM binding. Peptides derived from normal proteins by proteolytic cleavage, including endostatin and tumstatin, inhibit angiogenesis by mechanisms that include interfering with integrin function. Signal transduction pathways that are dysregulated in tumor cells indirectly regulate EC function. Inhibition of EGF-family receptors, whose signaling activity is upregulated in a number of human cancers (e.g., breast, colon, and lung cancers), results in downregulation of VEGF and IL-8, while increasing expression of the antiangiogenic protein thrombospondin-1. The Ras/MAPK, PI3K/Akt, and Src kinase pathways constitute important antitumor targets that also regulate the proliferation and survival of tumor-derived EC. The discovery that EC from normal tissues express tissue-specific "vascular addressins" on their cell surface suggests that targeting specific EC subsets may be possible.

SUMMARY

The explosion of information on tumor cell biology, metastasis, and angiogenesis has ushered in a new era of rational targeted therapy for cancer. Furthermore, it has become clear that specific molecular factors detected in individual tumors (specific gene mutations, gene-expression profiles, microRNA expression) can be used to tailor therapy and maximize antitumor effects.

ACKNOWLEDGEMENT
Robert G. Fenton contributed to this chapter in prior editions and important material from those prior chapters has been included here.

FURTHER READINGS

Bild AH et al: Oncogenic pathway signatures in human cancers as a guide to targeted therapies. Nature 439:353, 2006

Brough R et al: Searching for synthetic lethality in cancer. Curr Opin Genet Dev 21:34, 2011

Dai Y, Grant S: Targeting multiple arms of the apoptotic regulatory machinery. Cancer Res 67:2908, 2007

Finkel T et al: The common biology of cancer and ageing. Nature 448:767, 2007

Flaherty KT et al: Inhibition of mutated, activated BRAF in metastatic melanoma. N Engl J Med 363:809, 2010

Huber MA et al: Molecular requirements for epithelial-mesenchymal transition during tumor progression. Curr Opin Cell Biol 17:548, 2005

Nana-Sinkam SP, Croce CM: MicroRNA in chronic lymphocytic leukemia: Transitioning from laboratory-based investigation to clinical application. Cancer Genet Cytogenet 203:127, 2010

Panares RL, Garcia AA: Bevacizumab in the management of solid tumors. Expert Rev Anticancer Ther 7:434, 2007

Sharma SV et al: Epidermal growth factor receptor mutations in lung cancer. Nat Rev Cancer 7:169, 2007

Sherbenou DW, Drucker BJ: Applying the discovery of the Philadelphia chromosome. J Clin Invest 117:2068, 2007

Vousden KH, Lane DP: p53 in health and disease. Nat Rev Mol Cell Biol 8:275, 2007

CHAPTER 85

Principles of Cancer Treatment

Edward A. Sausville
Dan L. Longo

The goal of cancer treatment is first to eradicate the cancer. If this primary goal cannot be accomplished, the goal of cancer treatment shifts to palliation, the amelioration of symptoms, and preservation of quality of life while striving to extend life. The dictum *primum non nocere* may not always be the guiding principle of cancer therapy. When cure of cancer is possible, cancer treatments may be undertaken despite the certainty of severe and perhaps life-threatening toxicities. Every cancer treatment has the potential to cause harm, and treatment may be given that produces toxicity with no benefit. The therapeutic index of many interventions is quite narrow, and most treatments are given to the point of toxicity. Conversely, when the clinical goal is palliation, careful attention to minimizing the toxicity of potentially toxic treatments becomes a significant goal. Irrespective of the clinical scenario, the guiding principle of cancer treatment should be *primum succerrere*, "first hasten to help." Radical surgical procedures, large-field hyperfractionated radiation therapy, high-dose chemotherapy, and maximum tolerable doses of cytokines such as interleukin (IL) 2 are all used in certain settings where 100% of the patients will experience toxicity and side effects from the intervention and only a fraction of the patients will experience benefit. One of the challenges of cancer treatment is to use the various treatment modalities alone and together in a fashion that maximizes the chances for patient benefit.

Cancer treatments are divided into four main types: surgery, radiation therapy (including photodynamic therapy), chemotherapy (including hormonal therapy and molecularly targeted therapy), and biologic therapy (including immunotherapy and gene therapy). The modalities are often used in combination, and agents in one category can act by several mechanisms. For example, cancer chemotherapy agents can induce differentiation, and antibodies (a form of immunotherapy) can be used to deliver radiation therapy. Surgery and radiation therapy are considered local treatments, though their effects can influence the behavior of tumor at remote sites. Chemotherapy and biologic therapy are usually systemic treatments. *Oncology*, the study of tumors including treatment approaches, is a multidisciplinary effort with surgical-, radiotherapy-, and internal medicine–related areas of expertise. Treatments for patients with hematologic malignancies are often shared by hematologists and medical oncologists.

In many ways, cancer mimics an organ attempting to regulate its own growth. However, cancers have not set an appropriate limit on how much growth should be permitted. Normal organs and cancers share the property of having (1) a population of cells in cycle and actively renewing and (2) a population of cells not in cycle. In cancers, cells that are not dividing are heterogeneous; some have sustained too much genetic damage to replicate but have defects in their death pathways that permit their survival, some are starving for nutrients and oxygen, and some are out of cycle but poised to be recruited back into cycle and expand if needed (i.e., reversibly growth-arrested). Severely damaged and starving cells are unlikely to kill the patient. The problem is that the cells that are

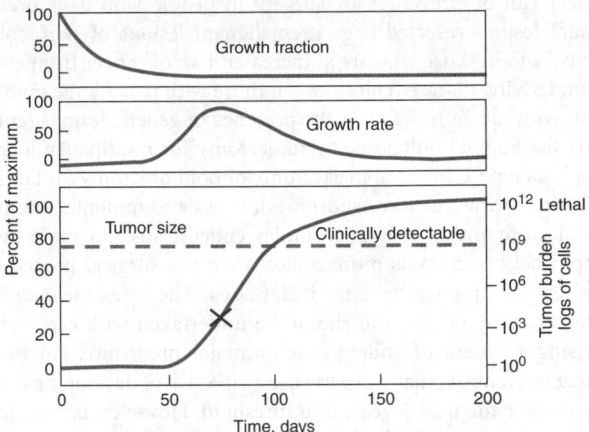

Figure 85-1 Gompertzian tumor growth. The growth fraction of a tumor declines exponentially over time *(top)*. The growth rate of a tumor peaks before it is clinically detectable *(middle)*. Tumor size increases slowly, goes through an exponential phase, and slows again as the tumor reaches the size at which limitation of nutrients or auto- or host regulatory influences can occur. The maximum growth rate occurs at 1/e, the point at which the tumor is about 37% of its maximum size *(marked with an X)*. Tumor becomes detectable at a burden of about 10^9 (1 cm³) cells and kills the patient at a tumor cell burden of about 10^{12} (1 kg). Efforts to treat the tumor and reduce its size can result in an increase in the growth fraction and an increase in growth rate.

reversibly not in cycle are capable of replenishing tumor cells physically removed or damaged by radiation and chemotherapy. These include *cancer stem cells*, whose properties are being elucidated. The stem cell fraction may define new targets for therapies that will retard their ability to reenter the cell cycle.

Tumors follow a Gompertzian growth curve (Fig. 85-1); the growth fraction of a neoplasm starts at 100% with the first transformed cell and declines exponentially over time until at the time of diagnosis, with a tumor burden of 1–5×10^9 tumor cells, the growth fraction is usually 1–4%. Thus, peak growth rate occurs before the tumor is detectable. A key feature of a successful tumor is the ability to stimulate the development of a new supporting stroma through angiogenesis and production of proteases to allow invasion through basement membranes and normal tissue barriers (Chap. 84). Specific cellular mechanisms promote entry or withdrawal of tumor cells from the cell cycle. For example, when a tumor recurs after surgery or chemotherapy, frequently its growth is accelerated and the growth fraction of the tumor is increased. This pattern is similar to that seen in regenerating organs. Partial resection of the liver results in the recruitment of cells into the cell cycle, and the resected liver volume is replaced. Similarly, chemotherapy-damaged bone marrow increases its growth to replace cells killed by chemotherapy. However, cancers do not recognize a limit on their expansion. Monoclonal gammopathy of uncertain significance may be an example of a clonal neoplasm with intrinsic features that stop its growth before a lethal tumor burden is reached. A fraction of patients with this disorder go on to develop fatal multiple myeloma, but probably this occurs because of the accumulation of additional genetic lesions. Elucidation of the mechanisms that regulate this "organ-like" behavior of tumors may provide additional clues to cancer control and treatment.

PRINCIPLES OF CANCER SURGERY

Surgery is used in cancer prevention, diagnosis, staging, treatment (for both localized and metastatic disease), palliation, and rehabilitation.

■ PROPHYLAXIS

Cancer can be prevented by surgery in people who have premalignant lesions resected (e.g., premalignant lesions of skin, colon, cervix) and in those who are at increased risk of cancer from either an underlying disease (colectomy in those with pancolonic involvement with ulcerative colitis), the presence of genetic lesions (colectomy for familial polyposis, thyroidectomy for multiple endocrine neoplasia type 2, bilateral mastectomy or oophorectomy for familial breast or ovarian cancer syndromes), or a developmental anomaly (orchiectomy in those with an undescended testis). In some cases, prophylactic surgery is more radical than the surgical procedures used to treat the cancer after it develops. The assessment of risk involves many factors and should be undertaken with care before advising a patient to undergo such a major procedure. For breast cancer prevention, many experts use a 20% risk of developing breast cancer over the next 5 years as a threshold. However, patient fears play a major role in defining candidates for cancer prevention surgery. Counseling and education may not be enough to allay the fears of someone who has lost close family members to a malignancy.

■ DIAGNOSIS

The underlying principle in cancer diagnosis is to obtain as much tissue as safely possible. Owing to tumor heterogeneity, pathologists are better able to make the diagnosis when they have more tissue to examine. In addition to light-microscopic inspection of a tumor for pattern of growth, degree of cellular atypia, invasiveness, and morphologic features that aid in the differential diagnosis, sufficient tissue is of value in searching for genetic abnormalities and protein expression patterns, such as hormone receptor expression in breast cancers, that may aid in differential diagnosis or provide information about prognosis or likely response to treatment. Efforts to define "personalized" information from the biology of each patient's tumor and pertinent to each patient's treatment plan are becoming increasingly important in selecting treatment options. Histologically similar tumors may have very different gene expression patterns when assessed by such techniques as microarray analysis using gene chips, with important differences in response to treatment. Such testing requires that the tissue be handled properly (e.g., immunologic detection of proteins is more effective in fresh-frozen tissue rather than in formalin-fixed tissue). Coordination among the surgeon, pathologist, and primary care physician is essential to ensure that the amount of information learned from the biopsy material is maximized.

These goals are best met by an *excisional biopsy* in which the entire tumor mass is removed with a small margin of normal tissue surrounding it. If an excisional biopsy cannot be performed, *incisional biopsy* is the procedure of second choice. A wedge of tissue is removed, and an effort is made to include the majority of the cross-sectional diameter of the tumor in the biopsy to minimize sampling error. The biopsy techniques that involve cutting into tumor carry with them a risk of facilitating the spread of the tumor. *Core-needle biopsy* usually obtains considerably less tissue, but this procedure often provides enough information to plan a definitive surgical procedure. *Fine-needle aspiration* generally obtains only a suspension of cells from within a mass. This procedure is minimally invasive, and if positive for cancer it may allow inception of systemic treatment when metastatic disease is evident, or it can provide a basis for planning a more meticulous and extensive surgical procedure.

■ STAGING

As noted in Chap. 81, an important component of patient management is defining the extent of disease. Radiographic and other imaging tests can be helpful in defining the clinical stage; however, pathologic staging requires defining the extent of involvement by documenting the histologic presence of tumor in tissue biopsies

obtained through a surgical procedure. Axillary lymph node sampling in breast cancer and lymph node sampling at laparotomy for testicular, colon, and other intraabdominal cancers may provide crucial information for treatment planning and may determine the extent and nature of primary cancer treatment.

■ TREATMENT

Surgery is the most effective means of treating cancer. Today about 40% of cancer patients are cured by surgery. Unfortunately, a large fraction of patients with solid tumors (perhaps 60%) have metastatic disease that is not accessible for removal. However, even when the disease is not curable by surgery alone, the removal of tumor can obtain important benefits, including local control of tumor, preservation of organ function, debulking that permits subsequent therapy to work better, and staging information on extent of involvement. Cancer surgery aiming for cure is usually planned to excise the tumor completely with an adequate margin of normal tissue (the margin varies with the tumor and the anatomy), touching the tumor as little as possible to prevent vascular and lymphatic spread, and minimizing operative risk. Extending the procedure to resect draining lymph nodes obtains prognostic information, but such resections alone generally do not improve survival.

Increasingly, laparoscopic approaches are being used to address primary abdominal and pelvic tumors. Lymph node spread may be assessed using the sentinel node approach, in which the first draining lymph node a spreading tumor would encounter is defined by injecting a dye into the tumor site at operation and then resecting the first node to turn blue. The sentinel node assessment is continuing to undergo clinical evaluation but appears to provide reliable information without the risks (lymphedema, lymphangiosarcoma) associated with resection of all the regional nodes. Advances in adjuvant chemotherapy and radiation therapy following surgery have permitted a substantial decrease in the extent of primary surgery necessary to obtain the best outcomes. Thus, lumpectomy with radiation therapy is as effective as modified radical mastectomy for breast cancer, and limb-sparing surgery followed by adjuvant radiation therapy and chemotherapy has replaced radical primary surgical procedures involving amputation and disarticulation for childhood rhabdomyosarcomas. More limited surgery is also being employed to spare organ function, as in larynx and bladder cancer. The magnitude of operations necessary to optimally control and cure cancer has also been diminished by technical advances; for example, the circular anastomotic stapler has allowed narrower (<2-cm) margins in colon cancer without compromise of local control rates, and many patients who would have had colostomies are able to maintain normal anatomy.

In some settings—e.g., bulky testicular cancer or stage III breast cancer—surgery is not the first treatment modality employed. After an initial diagnostic biopsy, chemotherapy and/or radiation therapy is delivered to reduce the size of the tumor and clinically control undetected metastatic disease. Such therapy is followed by a surgical procedure to remove residual masses; this is called *neoadjuvant therapy*. Because the sequence of treatment is critical to success and is different from the standard surgery-first approach, coordination among the surgical oncologist, radiation oncologist, and medical oncologist is crucial.

Surgery may be curative in a subset of patients with metastatic disease. Patients with lung metastases from osteosarcoma may be cured by resection of the lung lesions. In patients with colon cancer who have fewer than five liver metastases restricted to one lobe and no extrahepatic metastases, hepatic lobectomy may produce long-term disease-free survival in 25% of selected patients. Surgery can also be associated with systemic antitumor effects. In the setting of hormonally responsive tumors, oophorectomy and/or adrenalectomy may control estrogen production, and orchiectomy may reduce androgen production; both have effects on metastatic tumor growth. If resection of the primary lesion takes place in the presence of metastases, acceleration of metastatic growth may occur, perhaps based on the removal of a source of angiogenesis inhibitors and mass-related growth regulators in the tumor.

In selecting a surgeon or center for primary cancer treatment, consideration must be given to the volume of cancer surgeries undertaken by the site. Studies in a variety of cancers have shown that increased annual procedure volume appears to correlate with outcome. In addition, facilities with extensive support systems—e.g., for joint thoracic and abdominal surgical teams with cardiopulmonary bypass, if needed—may allow resection of certain tumors that would otherwise not be possible.

■ PALLIATION

Surgery is employed in a number of ways for supportive care: insertion of central venous catheters, control of pleural and pericardial effusions and ascites, caval interruption for recurrent pulmonary emboli, stabilization of cancer-weakened weight-bearing bones, and control of hemorrhage, among others. Surgical bypass of gastrointestinal, urinary tract, or biliary tree obstruction can alleviate symptoms and prolong survival. Surgical procedures may provide relief of otherwise intractable pain or reverse neurologic dysfunction (cord decompression). Splenectomy may relieve symptoms and reverse hypersplenism. Intrathecal or intrahepatic therapy relies on surgical placement of appropriate infusion portals. Surgery may correct other treatment-related toxicities such as adhesions or strictures.

■ REHABILITATION

Surgical procedures are also valuable in restoring a cancer patient to full health. Orthopedic procedures may be necessary to ensure proper ambulation. Breast reconstruction can make an enormous impact on the patient's perception of successful therapy. Plastic and reconstructive surgery can correct the effects of disfiguring primary treatment.

PRINCIPLES OF RADIATION THERAPY

■ PHYSICAL PROPERTIES AND BIOLOGIC EFFECTS

Radiation is a physical form of treatment that damages any tissue in its path; its selectivity for cancer cells may be due to defects in a cancer cell's ability to repair sublethal DNA and other damage. Radiation causes breaks in DNA and generates free radicals from cell water that may damage cell membranes, proteins, and organelles. Radiation damage is augmented dependent on only oxygen; hypoxemic cells are more resistant. Augmentation of oxygen is the basis for radiation sensitization. Sulfhydryl compounds interfere with free radical generation and may act as radiation protectors.

Most radiation-induced cell damage is due to the formation of hydroxyl radicals:

$$\text{Ionizing radiation} + H_2O \rightarrow H_2O^+ + e^-$$
$$H_2O^+ + H_2O \rightarrow H_3O^+ + OH^\bullet$$
$$OH^\bullet \rightarrow \text{cell damage}$$

The dose-response curve for cells has both linear and exponential components. The linear component is from double-strand DNA breaks produced by single hits. The exponential component represents breaks produced by multiple hits. Plotting the fraction of surviving cells against doses of x-rays or gamma radiation, the curve has a shoulder that reflects the cell's repair of sublethal damage, followed by a linear portion reflecting greater cell kill with larger doses. The features that make a particular cell more sensitive or more resistant to the biologic effects of radiation are not completely defined.

Therapeutic radiation is delivered in three ways: (1) *teletherapy*, with beams of radiation generated at a distance and aimed at the tumor within the patient; (2) *brachytherapy*, with encapsulated sources of radiation implanted directly into or adjacent to tumor tissues; and (3) *systemic therapy*, with radionuclides targeted in some fashion to a site of tumor. Teletherapy is the most commonly used form of radiation therapy.

X-rays and gamma rays are the forms of radiation most commonly used to treat cancer. They are both electromagnetic, nonparticulate waves that cause the ejection of an orbital electron when absorbed. This orbital electron ejection is called *ionization*. X-rays are generated by linear accelerators; gamma rays are generated from decay of atomic nuclei in radioisotopes such as cobalt and radium. These waves behave biologically as packets of energy, called *photons*. Particulate forms of radiation are also used in certain circumstances. Electron beams have a very low tissue penetrance and are used to treat skin conditions such as mycosis fungoides. Proton beams are becoming more widely available, and may be more able to delimit dose to tumor in certain anatomic locations. However, aside from these specialized uses, particulate forms of radiation such as neutrons, protons, and negative mesons, which should do more tissue damage because of their higher linear energy transfer and lesser dependence on oxygen, are in most applications not superior to X- or gamma rays in clinical studies reported thus far.

A number of parameters influence the damage done to tissue by radiation. Hypoxemic cells are relatively resistant. Nondividing cells are more resistant than dividing cells. In addition to these biologic parameters, physical parameters of the radiation are also crucial. The energy of the radiation determines its ability to penetrate tissue. Low-energy orthovoltage beams (150–400 kV) scatter when they strike the body, much like light diffuses when it strikes particles in the air. Such beams result in more damage to adjacent normal tissues and less radiation delivered to the tumor. Megavoltage radiation (>1 MeV) has very low lateral scatter; this produces a skin-sparing effect, more homogeneous distribution of the radiation energy, and greater deposit of the energy in the tumor, or *target volume*. The tissues that the beam passes through to get to the tumor are called the *transit volume*. The maximum dose in the target volume is often the cause of complications to tissues in the transit volume, and the minimum dose in the target volume influences the likelihood of tumor recurrence. Dose homogeneity in the target volume is the goal. Computational approaches and delivery of many beams to converge on a target lesion are the basis for "gamma knife" and related approaches to deliver high dose to small volumes of tumor, sparing normal tissue.

Radiation is quantitated on the basis of the amount of radiation absorbed in the patient; it is not based on the amount of radiation generated by the machine. The *rad* (radiation *a*bsorbed *d*ose) is defined as 100 ergs of energy per gram of tissue. The International System (SI) unit for rad is the Gray (Gy); 1 Gy = 100 rad. Radiation dose is measured by placing detectors at the body surface or calculating the dose based on radiating phantoms that resemble human form and substance. Radiation dose has three determinants: total absorbed dose, number of fractions, and time. A frequent error is to omit the number of fractions and the duration of treatment. This is analogous to saying that a runner completed a race in 20 s; without knowing how far he or she ran, the result is difficult to interpret. The time could be very good for a 200-m race or very poor for a 100-m race. Thus, a typical course of radiation therapy should be described as 4500 cGy delivered to a particular target (e.g., mediastinum) over 5 weeks in 180-cGy fractions. Most curative radiation treatment programs are delivered once a day, 5 days a week in 150- to 200-cGy fractions.

Certain drugs used in cancer treatment may also act as radiation sensitizers. For example, compounds that incorporate into DNA and alter its stereochemistry (e.g., halogenated pyrimidines, cisplatin) augment radiation effects, as does hydroxyurea, another DNA synthesis inhibitor.

■ APPLICATION TO PATIENTS

Teletherapy

Radiation therapy can be used alone or together with chemotherapy to produce cure of localized tumors and control of the primary site of disease in tumors that have disseminated. Therapy is planned based on the use of a simulator with the treatment field or fields designed to accommodate an individual patient's anatomic features. Individualized treatment planning employs lead shielding tailored to shape the field and limit the radiation exposure of normal tissue. Often the radiation is delivered from two or three different positions. Conformal three-dimensional treatment planning permits the delivery of higher doses of radiation to the target volume without increasing complications in the transit volume.

Radiation therapy is a component of curative therapy for a number of diseases, including breast cancer, Hodgkin's disease, head and neck cancer, prostate cancer, and gynecologic cancers. Radiation therapy can also palliate disease symptoms in a variety of settings: relief of bone pain from metastatic disease, control of brain metastases, reversal of spinal cord compression and superior vena caval obstruction, shrinkage of painful masses, and opening of threatened airways. In high-risk settings, radiation therapy can prevent the development of leptomeningeal disease and brain metastases in acute leukemia and lung cancer.

Brachytherapy

Brachytherapy involves placing a sealed source of radiation into or adjacent to the tumor and withdrawing the radiation source after a period of time precisely calculated to deliver a chosen dose of radiation to the tumor. This approach is often used to treat prostate tumors and cervical cancer. The difficulty with brachytherapy is the short range of radiation effects (the inverse square law) and the inability to shape the radiation to fit the target volume. Normal tissue may receive toxic exposure to the radiation, with attendant radiation enteritis or cystitis in cervix cancer or brain injury in brain tumors.

Radionuclides and radioimmunotherapy

Nuclear medicine physicians or radiation oncologists may administer radionuclides with therapeutic effects. Iodine 131 is used to treat thyroid cancer since iodine is naturally taken up preferentially by the thyroid; it emits gamma rays that destroy the normal thyroid as well as the tumor. Strontium 89 and samarium 153 are two radionuclides that are preferentially taken up in bone, particularly sites of new bone formation. Both are capable of controlling bone metastases and the pain associated with them, but the dose-limiting toxicity is myelosuppression.

Monoclonal antibodies and other ligands can be attached to radioisotopes by conjugation (for nonmetal isotopes) or by chelation (for metal isotopes), and the targeting moiety can result in the accumulation of the radionuclide preferentially in tumor. Iodine 131–labeled anti-CD20 and yttrium 90–labeled anti-CD20 are active in B cell lymphoma, and other labeled antibodies are being evaluated. Thyroid uptake of labeled iodine is blocked by cold iodine. Dose-limiting toxicity is myelosuppression.

Photodynamic therapy

Some chemical structures (porphyrins, phthalocyanines) are selectively taken up by cancer cells by mechanisms not fully defined. When light, usually delivered by a laser, is shone on cells containing these compounds, free radicals are generated and the cells die. Hematoporphyrins and light are being used with increasing frequency to treat skin cancer; ovarian cancer; and cancers of the lung, colon, rectum, and esophagus. Palliation of recurrent locally advanced disease can sometimes be dramatic and last many months.

■ TOXICITY

Though radiation therapy is most often administered to a local region, systemic effects, including fatigue, anorexia, nausea, and vomiting, may develop that are related in part to the volume of tissue irradiated, dose fractionation, radiation fields, and individual susceptibility. Bone is among the most radioresistant organs, radiation effects being manifested mainly in children through premature fusion of the epiphyseal growth plate. By contrast, the male testis, female ovary, and bone marrow are the most sensitive organs. Any bone marrow in a radiation field will be eradicated by therapeutic irradiation. Organs with less need for cell renewal, such as heart, skeletal muscle, and nerves, are more resistant to radiation effects. In radiation-resistant organs, the vascular endothelium is the most sensitive component. Organs with more self-renewal as a part of normal homeostasis, such as the hematopoietic system and mucosal lining of the intestinal tract, are more sensitive. Acute toxicities include mucositis, skin erythema (ulceration in severe cases), and bone marrow toxicity. Often these can be alleviated by interruption of treatment.

Chronic toxicities are more serious. Radiation of the head and neck region often produces thyroid failure. Cataracts and retinal damage can lead to blindness. Salivary glands stop making saliva, which leads to dental caries and poor dentition. Taste and smell can be affected. Mediastinal irradiation leads to a threefold increased risk of fatal myocardial infarction. Other late vascular effects include chronic constrictive pericarditis, lung fibrosis, viscus stricture, spinal cord transection, and radiation enteritis. A serious late toxicity is the development of second solid tumors in or adjacent to the radiation fields. Such tumors can develop in any organ or tissue and occur at a rate of about 1% per year beginning in the second decade after treatment. Some organs vary in susceptibility to radiation carcinogenesis. A woman who receives mantle field radiation therapy for Hodgkin's disease at age 25 years has a 30% risk of developing breast cancer by age 55 years. This is comparable in magnitude to genetic breast cancer syndromes. Women treated after age 30 years have little or no increased risk of breast cancer. No data suggest that a threshold dose of therapeutic radiation exists below which the incidence of second cancers is decreased. High rates of second tumors occur in people who receive as little as 1000 cGy.

PRINCIPLES OF CHEMOTHERAPY

Medical oncology is the subspecialty of internal medicine that cares for and designs treatment approaches to patients with cancer, in conjunction with surgical and radiation oncologists. The core skills of the medical oncologist include the use of drugs that may have a beneficial effect on the natural history of the patient's illness or favorably influence the patient's quality of life.

■ ENDPOINTS OF DRUG ACTION

The concept that systemically administered drugs may have a useful effect on cancers was historically derived from three sets of observations. Paul Ehrlich in the nineteenth century observed that different dyes reacted with different cell and tissue components. He hypothesized the existence of compounds that would be "magic bullets" that might bind to tumors, owing to the affinity of the agent for the tumor. A second observation was the toxic effects of certain mustard gas derivatives on the bone marrow during World War I, leading to the idea that smaller doses of these agents might be used to treat tumors of marrow-derived cells. Finally, the observation that certain tumors from hormone-responsive tissues, e.g. breast tumors, could shrink after oophorectomy led to the idea that endogenous substances promoting the growth of a tumor might be antagonized. Chemicals achieving each of the goals are actually or intellectually the forbearers of the currently used cancer chemotherapy agents.

Chemotherapy agents may be used for the treatment of active, clinically apparent cancer. Table 85-1, A lists those tumors considered curable by conventionally available chemotherapeutic agents when used to address disseminated or metastatic cancers. If a tumor is localized to a single site, serious consideration of surgery or primary radiation therapy should be given, as these treatment modalities may be curative as local treatments. Chemotherapy may be employed after the failure of these modalities to eradicate a local tumor or as part of multimodality approaches to offer primary treatment to a clinically localized tumor. In this event, it can allow organ preservation when given with radiation, as in the larynx or other upper airway sites; or sensitize tumors to radiation when given, e.g., to patients concurrently receiving radiation for lung or cervix cancer (Table 85-1, B). Chemotherapy can be administered as an adjuvant, i.e., in addition to surgery (Table 85-1, C) or radiation, after all clinically apparent disease has been removed. This use of chemotherapy may have curative potential in breast and colorectal neoplasms, as it attempts to eliminate clinically unapparent tumor that may have already disseminated. As noted above, small tumors frequently have high growth fractions and therefore may be intrinsically more susceptible to the action of antiproliferative agents. Chemotherapy is routinely used in "conventional" dose regimens. In general, these doses produce reversible acute side effects, primarily consisting of transient myelosuppression with or without gastrointestinal toxicity (usually nausea), which are readily managed. High-dose chemotherapy regimens are predicated on the observation that the dose-response curve for many anticancer agents is rather steep, and increased dose can produce markedly increased therapeutic effect, although at the cost of potentially life-threatening complications that require intensive support, usually in the form of hematopoietic stem cell support from the patient (*autologous*) or from donors matched for histocompatibility loci (*allogeneic*). High-dose regimens have definite curative potential in defined clinical settings (Table 85-1, D).

Karnofsky was among the first to champion the evaluation of a chemotherapeutic agent's benefit by carefully quantitating its effect on tumor size and using these measurements to objectively decide the basis for further treatment of a particular patient or further clinical evaluation of a drug's potential. A partial response (PR) is defined conventionally as a decrease by at least 50% in a tumor's bidimensional area; a complete response (CR) connotes disappearance of all tumor; progression of disease signifies an increase in size of existing lesions by >25% from baseline or best response or development of new lesions; and "stable" disease fits into none of the above categories. Newer evaluation systems such as RECIST (Response Evaluation Criteria In Solid Tumors) utilize unidimensional measurement, but the intent is similar in rigorously defining evidence for the activity of the agent in assessing its value to the patient.

If cure is not possible, chemotherapy may be undertaken with the goal of palliating some aspect of the tumor's effect on the host. Common tumors that may be meaningfully addressed with palliative intent are listed in Table 85-1, E. Usually, tumor-related symptoms may manifest as pain, weight loss, or some local symptom related to the tumor's effect on normal structures. Patients treated with palliative intent should be aware of their diagnosis and the limitations of the proposed treatments, have access to supportive care, and have suitable "performance status," according to assessment algorithms such as the one developed by Karnofsky or by the Eastern Cooperative Oncology Group (ECOG). ECOG performance status 0 (PS0) patients are without symptoms; PS1 patients are ambulatory but restricted in strenuous physical activity; PS2 patients are ambulatory but unable to work and are up and about 50% or more of the time; PS3 patients are capable of limited

TABLE 85-1 Curability of Cancers With Chemotherapy

A. Advanced Cancers With Possible Cure

Acute lymphoid and acute myeloid leukemia (pediatric/adult)

Hodgkin's disease (pediatric/adult)

Lymphomas—certain types (pediatric/adult)

Germ cell neoplasms

 Embryonal carcinoma

 Teratocarcinoma

 Seminoma or dysgerminoma

 Choriocarcinoma

Gestational trophoblastic neoplasia

Pediatric neoplasms

 Wilms' tumor

 Embryonal rhabdomyosarcoma

 Ewing's sarcoma

 Peripheral neuroepithelioma

 Neuroblastoma

Small cell lung carcinoma

Ovarian carcinoma

B. Advanced Cancers Possibly Cured by Chemotherapy and Radiation

Squamous carcinoma (head and neck)

Squamous carcinoma (anus)

Breast carcinoma

Carcinoma of the uterine cervix

Non-small cell lung carcinoma (stage III)

Small cell lung carcinoma

C. Cancers Possibly Cured With Chemotherapy as Adjuvant to Surgery

Breast carcinoma

Colorectal carcinoma[a]

Osteogenic sarcoma

Soft tissue sarcoma

D. Cancers Possibly Cured with "High-Dose" Chemotherapy With Stem Cell Support

Relapsed leukemias, lymphoid and myeloid

Relapsed lymphomas, Hodgkin's and non-Hodgkin's

Chronic myeloid leukemia

Multiple myeloma

E. Cancers Responsive With Useful Palliation, But Not Cure, by Chemotherapy

Bladder carcinoma

Chronic myeloid leukemia

Hairy cell leukemia

Chronic lymphocytic leukemia

Lymphoma—certain types

Multiple myeloma

Gastric carcinoma

Cervix carcinoma

Endometrial carcinoma

Soft tissue sarcoma

Head and neck cancer

Adrenocortical carcinoma

Islet-cell neoplasms

Breast carcinoma

Colorectal carcinoma

Renal carcinoma

F. Tumor Poorly Responsive in Advanced Stages to Chemotherapy

Pancreatic carcinoma

Biliary-tract neoplasms

Thyroid carcinoma

Carcinoma of the vulva

Non-small cell lung carcinoma

Prostate carcinoma

Melanoma

Hepatocellular carcinoma

Salivary gland cancer

[a]Rectum also receives radiation therapy.

self-care and are up <50% of the time; PS4 patients are totally confined to bed or chair and incapable of self-care. Only PS0, PS1, and PS2 patients are generally considered suitable for palliative (noncurative) treatment. If there is curative potential, even poor–performance status patients may be treated, but their prognosis is usually inferior to that of good–performance status patients treated with similar regimens.

An important perspective the primary care provider may bring to patients and their families facing incurable cancer is that, given the limited value of chemotherapeutic approaches at some point in the natural history, *palliative care* or *hospice-based* approaches, with meticulous and ongoing attention to symptom relief and with family, psychological, and spiritual support, should receive prominent attention as a valuable therapeutic plan (Chap. 9). Optimizing the quality of life rather than attempting to extend it becomes a valued intervention. Patients facing the impending progression of disease in a life-threatening way frequently choose to undertake toxic treatments of little to no potential value, and support provided by the primary caregiver in accessing palliative and hospice-based options in contrast to receiving toxic and ineffective regimen can be critical in providing a basis for patients to make sensible choices.

■ CANCER DRUGS: OVERVIEW AND PRINCIPLES FOR USE

Cancer drug treatments are of four broad types. *Conventional chemotherapy agents* were historically derived by the empirical observation that these "small molecules" (generally with molecular mass <1500 Da) could cause major regression of experimental tumors growing in animals. These agents mainly target DNA structure or segregation of DNA as chromosomes in mitosis. *Targeted agents* refer to small molecules or "biologicals" (generally macromolecules such as antibodies or cytokines) designed and developed to interact with a defined molecular target important in either maintaining the malignant state or selectively expressed by the tumor cells. As described in Chap. 84, successful tumors have activated biochemical pathways that lead to uncontrolled proliferation through the action of, e.g., oncogene products, loss of cell cycle inhibitors, or loss of cell death regulation, and have acquired the capacity to replicate chromosomes indefinitely, invade, metastasize, and evade the immune system. Targeted therapies seek to capitalize on the biology behind the aberrant cellular behavior as a basis for therapeutic effects. *Hormonal therapies* (the first form of targeted therapy) capitalize on the biochemical pathways underlying estrogen and androgen function and action as a therapeutic basis for approaching patients with tumors of breast, prostate, uterus, and ovarian origin. *Biologic therapies* are often macromolecules that have a particular target (e.g., antigrowth factor or cytokine antibodies) or may have the capacity to regulate growth of tumor cells or induce a host immune response to kill tumor cells. Thus, biologic therapies include not only antibodies but cytokines and gene therapies.

The usefulness of any drug is governed by the extent to which a given dose causes a useful result (therapeutic effect; in the case of anticancer agents, toxicity to tumor cells) as opposed to a toxic effect to the host. The *therapeutic index* is the degree of separation between toxic and therapeutic doses. Really useful drugs have large therapeutic indices, and this usually occurs when the drug target is expressed in the disease-causing compartment as opposed to the normal compartment. Classically, selective toxicity of an agent for an organ is governed by the expression of an agent's target or by differential accumulation into or elimination from compartments where toxicity is experienced or ameliorated, respectively. Currently used chemotherapeutic agents have the unfortunate property that their targets are present in both normal and tumor tissues. Therefore, they have relatively narrow therapeutic indices.

Figure 85-2 illustrates steps in cancer drug discovery and development. Following demonstration of antitumor activity in animal models, potentially useful anticancer agents are further evaluated to define an optimal schedule of administration and arrive at a drug formulation designed for a given route and schedule. Safety testing in two species on an analogous schedule of administration defines the starting dose for a phase I trial in humans. This is established as a fraction, usually one-sixth to one-tenth, of the dose just causing easily reversible toxicity in the more sensitive animal species. Escalating

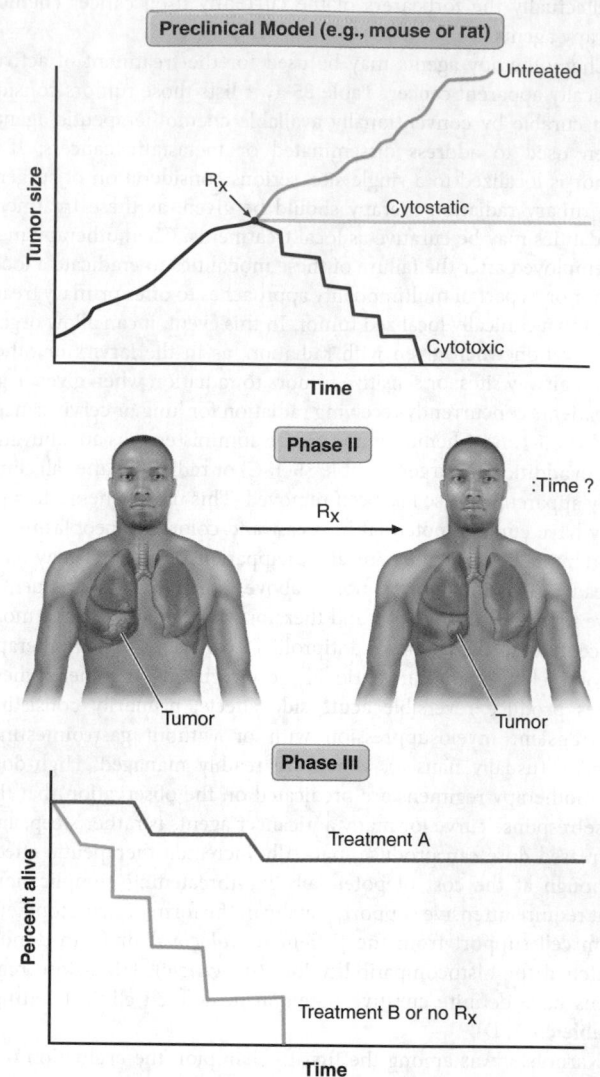

Figure 85-2 Steps in cancer drug discovery and development. Preclinical activity *(top)* in animal models of cancers may be used as evidence to support the entry of the drug candidate into phase I trials in humans to define a correct dose and observe any clinical antitumor effect that may occur. The drug may then be advanced to phase II trials directed against specific cancer types, with rigorous quantitation of antitumor effects *(middle)*. Phase III trials then may reveal activity superior to standard or no treatment *(lowest panel)*.

doses of the drug are then given during the human phase I trial until reversible toxicity is observed. Dose-limiting toxicity (DLT) defines a dose that conveys greater toxicity than would be acceptable in routine practice, allowing definition of a lower maximal tolerated dose (MTD). The occurrence of toxicity is, if possible, correlated with plasma drug concentrations. The MTD or a dose just lower than the MTD is usually the dose suitable for phase II trials, where a fixed dose is administered to a relatively homogeneous set of patients with a particular tumor type in an effort to define whether the drug causes regression of tumors. An "active" agent conventionally has PR rates of at least 20–25% with reversible non-life-threatening side effects, and it may then be suitable for study in phase III trials to assess efficacy in comparison to standard or no therapy.

Response, defined as tumor shrinkage, is but the most immediate indicator of drug effect. To be clinically valuable, responses must translate into clinical benefit. This is conventionally established by a beneficial effect on overall survival, or at least an increased time to further progression of disease. Active efforts are being made to quantitate effects of anticancer agents on quality of life. Cancer drug clinical trials conventionally use a toxicity grading scale where grade I toxicities do not require treatment, grade II often require symptomatic treatment but are not life-threatening, grade III toxicities are potentially life-threatening if untreated, grade IV toxicities are actually life-threatening, and grade V toxicities are those that result in the patient's death.

Development of "targeted agents" may proceed quite differently. While phase I–III trials are still conducted, molecular analysis of human tumors may allow the precise definition of target expression in a patient's tumor that is necessary for or relevant to the drug's action. This information might then allow selection of patients expressing the drug target for participation in all trial phases. These patients may then have a greater chance of developing a useful response to the drug by virtue of expressing the target in the tumor. Clinical trials may be designed to incorporate an assessment of the behavior of the target in relation to the drug (pharmacodynamic studies). Ideally, the plasma concentration that affects the drug target is known, so escalation to MTD may not be necessary. Rather, the correlation of host toxicity while achieving an "optimal biologic dose" becomes a more relevant endpoint for phase I and early phase II trials with targeted agents.

Useful cancer drug treatment strategies using conventional chemotherapy agents, targeted agents, hormonal treatments, or biologicals have one of two valuable outcomes. They can induce cancer cell death, resulting in tumor shrinkage with corresponding improvement in patient survival, or increase the time until the disease progresses. Another potential outcome is to induce cancer cell *differentiation* or dormancy with loss of tumor cell replicative potential and reacquisition of phenotypic properties resembling normal cells. Blocking tumor cell differentiation may be a key feature in the pathogenesis of certain leukemias.

Cell death is a closely regulated process. *Necrosis* refers to cell death induced, for example, by physical damage with the hallmarks of cell swelling and membrane disruption. *Apoptosis*, or programmed cell death, refers to a highly ordered process whereby cells respond to defined stimuli by dying, and it recapitulates the necessary cell death observed during the ontogeny of the organism. *Anoikis* refers to the death of epithelial cells after removal from the normal milieu of substrate, particularly from cell-to-cell contact. Cancer chemotherapeutic agents can cause both necrosis and apoptosis. Apoptosis is characterized by chromatin condensation (giving rise to "apoptotic

bodies"); cell shrinkage; and, in living animals, phagocytosis by surrounding stromal cells without evidence of inflammation. This process is regulated either by signal transduction systems that promote a cell's demise after a certain level of insult is achieved, or in response to specific cell-surface receptors that mediate cell death signals. Modulation of apoptosis by manipulation of signal transduction pathways has emerged as a basis for understanding the actions of drugs and designing new strategies to improve their use. *Autophagy* is a cellular response to injury where the cell does not initially die but catabolizes itself in a way that can lead to loss of replicative potential.

A general view of how cancer treatments work is that the interaction of a chemotherapeutic drug with its target induces a "cascade" of further signaling steps. These signals ultimately lead to cell death by triggering an "execution phase" where proteases, nucleases, and endogenous regulators of the cell death pathway are activated (Fig. 85-3).

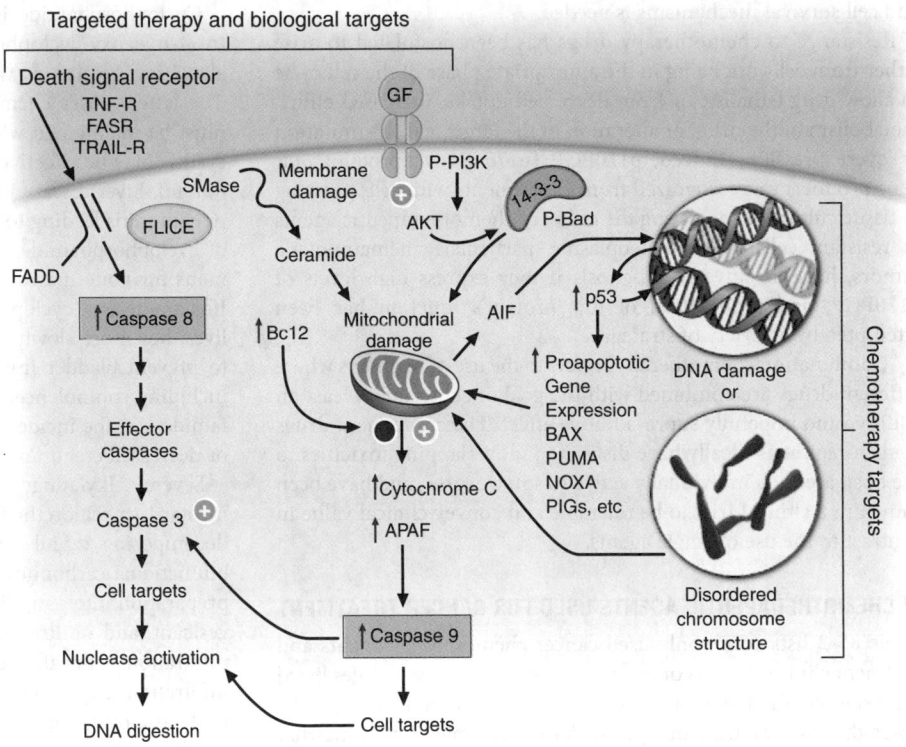

Figure 85-3 Integration of cell death responses. Cell death through an apoptotic mechanism requires active participation of the cell. In response to interruption of growth factor (GF) or propagation of certain cytokine death signals (e.g., tumor necrosis factor receptor, TNF-R), there is activation of "upstream" cysteine aspartyl proteases (caspases), which then directly digest cytoplasmic and nuclear proteins, resulting in activation of "downstream" caspases; these cause activation of nucleases, resulting in the characteristic DNA fragmentation that is a hallmark of apoptosis. Chemotherapy agents that create lesions in DNA or alter mitotic spindle function seem to activate aspects of this process by damage ultimately conveyed to the mitochondria, perhaps by activating the transcription of genes whose products can produce or modulate the toxicity of free radicals. In addition, membrane damage with activation of sphingomyelinases results in the production of ceramides that can have a direct action at mitochondria. The antiapoptotic protein bcl2 attenuates mitochondrial toxicity, while proapoptotic gene products such as bax antagonize the action of bcl2. Damaged mitochondria release cytochrome C and apoptosis-activating factor (APAF), which can directly activate caspase 9, resulting in propagation of a direct signal to other downstream caspases through protease activation. Apoptosis-inducing factor (AIF) is also released from the mitochondrion and then can translocate to the nucleus, bind to DNA, and generate free radicals to further damage DNA. An additional proapoptotic stimulus is the bad protein, which can heterodimerize with *bcl2* gene family members to antagonize apoptosis. Importantly, though, bad protein function can be retarded by its sequestration as phospho-bad through the 14-3-3 adapter proteins. The phosphorylation of bad is mediated by the action of the AKT kinase in a way that defines how growth factors that activate this kinase can retard apoptosis and promote cell survival.

Targeted agents differ from chemotherapy agents in that they do not indiscriminately cause macromolecular lesions but regulate the action of particular pathways. For example, the p210$^{bcr-abl}$ fusion protein tyrosine kinase drives chronic myeloid leukemia (CML), and HER-2/neu stimulates the proliferation of certain breast cancers. The tumor has been described as "addicted" to the function of these molecules in the sense that without the pathway's continued action, the tumor cell cannot survive. In this way, targeted agents may alter the "threshold" tumors have for undergoing apoptosis without actually creating any molecular lesions such as direct DNA strand breakage or altered membrane function.

While apoptotic mechanisms are important in regulating cellular proliferation and the behavior of tumor cells in vitro, in vivo it is unclear whether all of the actions of chemotherapeutic agents to cause cell death can be attributed to apoptotic mechanisms. However, changes in molecules that regulate apoptosis are correlated with clinical outcomes (e.g., *bcl2* overexpression in certain lymphomas conveys poor prognosis; proapoptotic *bax* expression is associated with a better outcome after chemotherapy for ovarian carcinoma). A better understanding of the relationship of cell death and cell survival mechanisms is needed.

Resistance to chemotherapy drugs has been postulated to arise either from cells not being in the appropriate phase of the cell cycle to allow drug lethality, or from decreased uptake, increased efflux, metabolism of the drug, or alteration of the target, e.g., by mutation or overexpression. Indeed, p170PGP (p170 P-glycoprotein; *mdr* gene product) was recognized from experiments with cells growing in tissue culture as mediating the efflux of chemotherapeutic agents in resistant cells. Certain neoplasms, particularly hematopoietic tumors, have an adverse prognosis if they express high levels of p170PGP, and modulation of this protein's function has been attempted by a variety of strategies.

"Combination chemotherapy" refers to the use of regimens where different drugs are combined with the goal of achieving at least an additive and hopefully supra-additive effect. The component drugs in such regimens ideally have distinct, nonoverlapping toxicities to the host, are each individually active to some degree, and have been shown in a clinical trial to be tolerable and convey clinical value in contrast to the use of single agents.

■ CHEMOTHERAPEUTIC AGENTS USED FOR CANCER TREATMENT

Table 85-2 lists commonly used cancer chemotherapy agents and pertinent clinical aspects of their use. The drugs and schedules listed are examples that have proved tolerable and useful; the specific doses that may be used in a particular patient may vary somewhat with the particular protocol, or plan, of treatment. Significant variation from these dose ranges should be carefully verified to avoid or anticipate toxicity. Not included in Table 85-2 are hormone receptor–directed agents, as the side effects are generally those expected from the interruption or augmentation of hormonal effect, and doses used in most cases are those that adequately saturate the intended hormone receptor. The drugs listed may be usefully grouped into three general categories: those affecting DNA, those affecting microtubules, and molecularly targeted agents.

Direct DNA-interactive agents

DNA replication occurs during the synthesis or S-phase of the cell cycle, with chromosome segregation of the replicated DNA occurring in the M, or mitosis, phase. The G_1 and G_2 "gap phases" precede S and M, respectively. Historically, chemotherapeutic agents have been divided into "phase-nonspecific" agents, which can act in any phase of the cell cycle, and "phase-specific" agents, which require the cell to be at a particular cell cycle phase to cause greatest effect. Once the agent has acted, cells may progress to "checkpoints"

in the cell cycle where the drug-related damage may be assessed and either repaired or allowed to initiate apoptosis. An important function of certain tumor-suppressor genes such as *p53* may be to modulate checkpoint function.

Formation of covalent DNA adducts Alkylating agents as a class are cell cycle phase–nonspecific agents. They break down, either spontaneously or after normal organ or tumor cell metabolism, to reactive intermediates that covalently modify bases in DNA. This leads to cross-linkage of DNA strands or the appearance of breaks in DNA as a result of repair efforts. "Broken" or cross-linked DNA is intrinsically unable to complete normal replication or cell division; in addition, it is a potent activator of cell cycle checkpoints and further activates cell-signaling pathways that can precipitate apoptosis. As a class, alkylating agents share similar toxicities: myelosuppression, alopecia, gonadal dysfunction, mucositis, and pulmonary fibrosis. They differ greatly in a spectrum of normal organ toxicities. As a class they share the capacity to cause "second" neoplasms, particularly leukemia, many years after use, particularly when used in low doses for protracted periods.

Cyclophosphamide is inactive unless metabolized by the liver to 4-hydroxy-cyclophosphamide, which decomposes into an alkylating species, as well as to chloroacetaldehyde and acrolein. The latter causes chemical cystitis; therefore, excellent hydration must be maintained while using cyclophosphamide. If severe, the cystitis may be effectively treated by mesna (2-*m*ercaptoethanesulfo*n*ate). Liver disease impairs drug activation. Sporadic interstitial pneumonitis leading to pulmonary fibrosis can accompany the use of cyclophosphamide, and high doses used in conditioning regimens for bone marrow transplant can cause cardiac dysfunction. Ifosfamide is a cyclophosphamide analogue also activated in the liver, but more slowly, and it requires coadministration of mesna to prevent bladder injury. Central nervous system (CNS) effects, including somnolence, confusion, and psychosis, can follow ifosfamide use; the incidence appears related to low body surface area or decreased creatinine clearance.

Several alkylating agents are less commonly used. Nitrogen mustard (mechlorethamine) is the prototypic agent of this class, decomposing rapidly in aqueous solution to potentially yield a bifunctional carbonium ion. It must be administered shortly after preparation into a rapidly flowing intravenous line. It is a powerful vesicant, and infiltration may be symptomatically ameliorated by infiltration of the affected site with 1/6 *M* thiosulfate. Even without infiltration, aseptic thrombophlebitis is frequent. It can be used topically as a dilute solution in cutaneous lymphomas, with a notable incidence of hypersensitivity reactions. It causes moderate nausea after intravenous administration. Bendamustine is a nitrogen mustard derivative with evidence of activity in chronic lymphocytic leukemia and certain lymphomas.

Chlorambucil causes predictable myelosuppression, azoospermia, nausea, and pulmonary side effects. Busulfan can cause profound myelosuppression, alopecia, and pulmonary toxicity but is relatively "lymphocyte sparing." Its routine use in treatment of CML has been curtailed in favor of imatinib (Gleevec) or dasatinib, but it is still employed in transplant preparation regimens. Melphalan shows variable oral bioavailability and undergoes extensive binding to albumin and α_1-acidic glycoprotein. Mucositis appears more prominently; however, it has prominent activity in multiple myeloma.

Nitrosoureas break down to carbamylating species that not only cause a distinct pattern of DNA base pair–directed toxicity but also can covalently modify proteins. They share the feature of causing relatively delayed bone marrow toxicity, which can be cumulative and long-lasting. Methyl CCNU (lomustine) causes direct glomerular as well as tubular damage, cumulatively related to dose and time of exposure.

TABLE 85-2 Commonly Used Cancer Chemotherapy Agents

Drug	Examples of Usual Doses	Toxicity	Interactions, Issues
Direct DNA-Interacting Agents			
Alkylators			
Cyclophosphamide	400–2000 mg/m² IV 100 mg/m² PO qd	Marrow (relative platelet sparing) Cystitis Common alkylator[a] Cardiac (high dose)	Liver metabolism required to activate to phos-phoramide mustard + acrolein Mesna protects against "high-dose" bladder damage
Mechlorethamine	6 mg/m² IV day 1 and day 8	Marrow Vesicant Nausea	Topical use in cutaneous lymphoma
Chlorambucil	1–3 mg/m² qd PO	Marrow Common alkylator[a]	
Melphalan	8 mg/m² qd × 5, PO	Marrow (delayed nadir) GI (high dose)	Decreased renal function delays clearance
Carmustine (BCNU)	200 mg/m² IV 150 mg/m² PO	Marrow (delayed nadir) GI, liver (high dose) Renal	
Lomustine (CCNU)	100–300 mg/m² PO	Marrow (delayed nadir)	
Ifosfamide	1.2 g/m² per day qd × 5 + mesna	Myelosuppressive Bladder Neurologic Metabolic acidosis Neuropathy	Isomeric analogue of cyclophosphamide More lipid soluble Greater activity vs testicular neoplasms and sarcomas Must use mesna
Procarbazine	100 mg/m² per day qd × 14	Marrow Nausea Neurologic Common alkylator[a]	Liver and tissue metabolism required Disulfiram-like effect with ethanol Acts as MAOI HBP after tyrosinase-rich foods
Dacarbazine (DTIC)	375 mg/m² IV day 1 and day 15	Marrow Nausea Flulike	Metabolic activation
Temozolomide	150–200 mg/m² qd × 5 q28d *or* 75 mg/m² qd × 6–7 weeks	Nausea/vomiting Headache/fatigue Constipation	Infrequent myelosuppression
Altretamine (formerly hexamethyl-melamine)	260 mg/m² per day qd × 14–21 as 4 divided oral doses	Nausea Neurologic (mood swing) Neuropathy Marrow (less)	Liver activation Barbiturates enhance/cimetidine diminishes
Cisplatin	20 mg/m² qd × 5 IV 1 q3–4 weeks or 100–200 mg/m² per dose IV q3–4 weeks	Nausea Neuropathy Auditory Marrow platelets > WBCs Renal Mg²⁺, Ca²⁺	Maintain high urine flow; osmotic diuresis, monitor intake/output K^+, Mg^{2+} Emetogenic—prophylaxis needed Full dose if CrCl > 60 mL/min and tolerate fluid push
Carboplatin	365 mg/m² IV q3–4 weeks as adjusted for CrCl	Marrow platelets > WBCs Nausea Renal (high dose)	Reduce dose according to CrCl: to AUC of 5–7 mg/mL per min [AUC = dose/(CrCl + 25)]
Oxaliplatin	130 mg/m² q3 weeks over 2 h *or* 85 mg/m² q2 weeks	Nausea Anemia	Acute reversible neurotoxicity; chronic sensory neurotoxicity cumulative with dose; reversible laryngopharyngeal spasm
Antitumor Antibiotics and Topoisomerase Poisons			
Bleomycin	15–25 mg/d qd × 5 IV bolus *or* continuous IV	Pulmonary Skin effects Raynaud's Hypersensitivity	Inactivate by bleomycin hydrolase (decreased in lung/skin) O_2 enhances pulmonary toxicity Cisplatin-induced decrease in CrCl may increase skin/lung toxicity Reduce dose if CrCl < 60 mL/min
Actinomycin D	10–15 µg/kg per day qd × 5 IV bolus	Marrow Nausea Mucositis Vesicant Alopecia	Radiation recall

(continued)

Principles of Cancer Treatment

TABLE 85-2 Commonly Used Cancer Chemotherapy Agents (*Continued*)

Drug	Examples of Usual Doses	Toxicity	Interactions, Issues
Etoposide (VP16-213)	100–150 mg/m² IV qd × 3–5d *or* 50 mg/m² PO qd × 21d *or* up to 1500 mg/m² per dose (high dose with stem cell support)	Marrow (WBCs > platelet) Alopecia Hypotension Hypersensitivity (rapid IV) Nausea Mucositis (high dose)	Hepatic metabolism—renal 30% Reduce doses with renal failure Schedule-dependent (5 day better than 1 day) Late leukemogenic Accentuate antimetabolite action
Topotecan	20 mg/m² IV q3–4 weeks over 30 min *or* 1.5–3 mg/m² q3–4 weeks over 24 h *or* 0.5 mg/m² per day over 21 days	Marrow Mucositis Nausea Mild alopecia	Reduce dose with renal failure No liver toxicity
Irinotecan (CPT II)	100–150 mg/m² IV over 90 min q3–4 weeks *or* 30 mg/m² per day over 120 h	Diarrhea: "early onset" with cramping, flushing, vomiting; "late onset" after several doses Marrow Alopecia Nausea Vomiting Pulmonary	Prodrug requires enzymatic clearance to active drug "SN 38" Early diarrhea likely due to biliary excretion Late diarrhea, use "high-dose" loperamide (2 mg q2–4 h)
Doxorubicin and daunorubicin	45–60 mg/m² dose q3–4 weeks *or* 10–30 mg/m² dose q week *or* continuous-infusion regimen	Marrow Mucositis Alopecia Cardiovascular acute/chronic Vesicant	Heparin aggregate; coadministration increases clearance Acetaminophen, BCNU increase liver toxicity Radiation recall
Idarubicin	10–15 mg/m² IV q 3 weeks *or* 10 mg/m² IV qd × 3	Marrow Cardiac (less than doxorubicin)	None established
Epirubicin	150 mg/m² IV q3 weeks	Marrow Cardiac	None established
Mitoxantrone	12 mg/m² qd × 3 *or* 12–14 mg/m² q3 weeks	Marrow Cardiac (less than doxorubicin) Vesicant (mild) Blue urine, sclerae, nails	Interacts with heparin Less alopecia, nausea than doxorubicin Radiation recall

Indirect DNA-Interacting Agents

Antimetabolites

Deoxycoformycin	4 mg/m² IV every other week	Nausea Immunosuppression Neurologic Renal	Excretes in urine Reduce dose for renal failure Inhibits adenosine deaminase
6-Mercaptopurine	75 mg/m² PO *or* up to 500 mg/m² PO (high dose)	Marrow Liver Nausea	Variable bioavailability Metabolize by xanthine oxidase Decrease dose with allopurinol Increased toxicity with thiopurine methyltransferase deficiency
6-Thioguanine	2–3 mg/kg per day for up to 3–4 weeks	Marrow Liver Nausea	Variable bioavailability Increased toxicity with thiopurine methyltransferase deficiency
Azathioprine	1–5 mg/kg per day	Marrow Nausea Liver	Metabolizes to 6MP, therefore reduce dose with allopurinol Increased toxicity with thiopurine methyltransferase deficiency
2-Chlorodeoxyaden-osine	0.09 mg/kg per day qd × 7 as continuous infusion	Marrow Renal Fever	Notable use in hairy cell leukemia
Hydroxyurea	20–50 mg/kg (lean body weight) PO qd *or* 1–3 g/d	Marrow Nausea Mucositis Skin changes Rare renal, liver, lung, CNS	Decrease dose with renal failure Augments antimetabolite effect

(continued)

TABLE 85-2 Commonly Used Cancer Chemotherapy Agents (*Continued*)

Drug	Examples of Usual Doses	Toxicity	Interactions, Issues
Methotrexate	15–30 mg PO or IM qd × 3–5 *or* 30 mg IV days 1 and 8 *or* 1.5–12g/m^2 per day (with leucovorin)	Marrow Liver/lung Renal tubular Mucositis	Rescue with leucovorin Excreted in urine Decrease dose in renal failure NSAIDs increase renal toxicity
5-Fluorouracil (5FU)	375 mg/m^2 IV qd × 5 *or* 600 mg/m^2 IV days 1 and 8	Marrow Mucositis Neurologic Skin changes	Toxicity enhanced by leucovorin Dihydropyrimidine dehydrogenase deficiency increases toxicity Metabolizes in tissues
Capecitabine	665 mg/m^2 bid continuous; 1250 mg/m^2 bid 2 weeks on / 1 off; 829 mg/m^2 bid 2 weeks on / 1 off + 60 mg/d leucovorin	Diarrhea Hand-foot syndrome	Prodrug of 5FU due to intratumoral metabolism
Cytosine arabinoside	100 mg/m^2 per day qd × 7 by continuous infusion *or* 1–3 g/m^2 dose IV bolus	Marrow Mucositis Neurologic (high dose) Conjunctivitis (high dose) Noncardiogenic pulmonary edema	Enhances activity of alkylating agents Metabolizes in tissues by deamination
Azacytidine	750 mg/m^2 per week or 75–200 mg/m^2 per day × 5–10 (bolus) or (continuous IV or subcutaneous)	Marrow Nausea Liver Neurologic Myalgia	Use limited to leukemia Altered methylation of DNA alters gene expression
Gemcitabine	1000 mg/m^2 IV weekly × 7	Marrow Nausea Hepatic Fever/"flu syndrome"	
Fludarabine phosphate	25 mg/m^2 IV qd × 5	Marrow Neurologic Lung	Dose reduction with renal failure Metabolized to F-ara converted to F-ara ATP in cells by deoxycytidine kinase
Asparaginase	25,000 IU/m^2 q3–4 weeks *or* 6000 IU/m^2 per day qod for 3–4 weeks *or* 1000–2000 IU/m^2 for 10–20 days	Protein synthesis Clotting factors Glucose Albumin Hypersensitivity CNS Pancreatitis Hepatic	Blocks methotrexate action
Pemetrexed	200 mg/m^2 q3 weeks	Anemia Neutropenia Thrombocytopenia	Supplement folate/B$_{12}$ Caution in renal failure
Antimitotic Agents			
Vincristine	1–1.4 mg/m^2 per week (frequently cap at 2 mg total dose)	Vesicant Marrow Neurologic GI: ileus/constipation; bladder hypotoxicity; SIADH Cardiovascular	Hepatic clearance Dose reduction for bilirubin >1.5 mg/dL Prophylactic bowel regimen
Vinblastine	6–8 mg/m^2 per week	Vesicant Marrow Neurologic (less common but similar spectrum to other vincas) Hypertension Raynaud's	Hepatic clearance Dose reduction as with vincristine
Vinorelbine	15–30 mg/m^2 per week	Vesicant Marrow Allergic/bronchospasm (immediate) Dyspnea/cough (subacute) Neurologic (less prominent but similar spectrum to other vincas)	Hepatic clearance

(*continued*)

TABLE 85-2 Commonly Used Cancer Chemotherapy Agents (*Continued*)

Drug	Examples of Usual Doses	Toxicity	Interactions, Issues
Paclitaxel	135–175 mg/m² per 24-h infusion *or* 175 mg/m² per 3-h infusion *or* 140 mg/m² per 96-h infusion *or* 250 mg/m² per 24-h infusion plus G-CSF	Hypersensitivity Marrow Mucositis Alopecia Sensory neuropathy CV conduction disturbance Nausea—infrequent	Premedicate with steroids, H₁ and H₂ blockers Hepatic clearance Dose reduction as with vincas
Docetaxel	100 mg/m² per 1-h infusion q3 weeks	Hypersensitivity Fluid retention syndrome Marrow Dermatologic Sensory neuropathy Nausea infrequent Some stomatitis	Premedicate with steroids, H₁ and H₂ blockers
Estramustine phosphate	14 mg/kg per day in 3–4 divided doses with water >2 h after meals Avoid Ca²⁺-rich foods	Nausea Vomiting Diarrhea CHF Thrombosis Gynecomastia	
Nab-paclitaxel (protein bound)	260 mg/m² q3 weeks	Neuropathy Anemia Neutropenia Thrombocytopenia	Caution in hepatic insufficiency
Ixabepilone	40 mg/m² q3 weeks	Myelosuppression Neuropathy	

Molecularly Targeted Agents

Retinoids

Tretinoin	45 mg/m² per day until complete response + anthracycline-based regimen in APL	Teratogenic Cutaneous	APL differentiation syndrome: pulmonary dysfunction/infiltrate, pleural/pericardial effusion, fever
Bexarotene	300–400 mg/m² per day, continuous	Hypercholesterolemia Hypertriglyceridemia Cutaneous Teratogenic	Central hypothyroidism

Targeted Toxins

Denileukin diftitox	9–18 μg/kg per day × 5 d q3 weeks	Nausea/vomiting Chills/fever Asthenia Hepatic	Acute hypersensitivity: hypotension, vasodilation, rash, chest tightness Vascular leak: hypotension, edema, hypoalbuminemia, thrombotic events (MI, DVT, CVA)

Tyrosine Kinase Inhibitors

Imatinib	400 mg/d, continuous	Nausea Periorbital edema	Myelosuppression not frequent in solid tumor indications
Gefitinib	250 mg PO per day	Rash Diarrhea	In U.S., only with prior documented benefit
Erlotinib	150 mg PO per day	Rash Diarrhea	1 h before, 2 h after meals
Dasatinib	70 mg PO bid; 100 mg PO per day	Liver changes Rash Neutropenia Thrombocytopenia	
Sorafenib	400 mg PO bid	Diarrhea Hand-foot syndrome Other rash	
Sunitinib	50 mg PO qd for 4 of 6 weeks	Fatigue Diarrhea Neutropenia	

(*continued*)

TABLE 85-2 Commonly Used Cancer Chemotherapy Agents (*Continued*)

Drug	Examples of Usual Doses	Toxicity	Interactions, Issues
Proteosome Inhibitors			
Bortezomib	1.3 mg/m² day 1,4	Neuropathy Thrombocytopenia	
Histone Deacetylase Inhibitors			
Vorinostat	400 mg/day	Fatigue Diarrhea Thrombocytopenia Embolism	
Romidepsin	14 mg/m² day 1, 8, 15	Nausea Vomiting Cytopenias Cardiac conduction	
mTOR Inhibitors			
Temsirolimus	25 mg weekly	Stomatitis Thrombocytopenia Nausea Anorexia, fatigue Metabolic (glucose, lipid)	
Everolimus	10 mg daily	Stomatitis Fatigue	
Miscellaneous			
Arsenic trioxide	0.16 mg/kg per day up to 50 days in APL	↑ QT$_c$ Peripheral neuropathy Musculoskeletal pain Hyperglycemia	APL differentiation syndrome (see under tretinoin)

[a]Common alkylator: alopecia, pulmonary, infertility, plus teratogenesis.

Abbreviations: APL, acute promyelocytic leukemia; AUC, area under the curve; CHF, congestive heart failure; CNS, central nervous system; CrCl, creatinine clearance; CV, cardiovascular; CVA, cerebrovascular accident; DVT, deep venous thrombosis; G-CSF, granulocyte colony-stimulating factor; GI, gastrointestinal; HBP, high blood pressure; MAOI, monoamine oxidase inhibitors; MI, myocardial infarction; 6MP, 6-mercaptopurine; mTOR, mammalian target of rapamycin; NSAIDs, nonsteroidal anti-inflammatory drugs; SIADH, syndrome of inappropriate antidiuretic hormone; WBCs, white blood cells.

Procarbazine is metabolized in the liver and possibly in tumor cells to yield a variety of free radical and alkylating species. In addition to myelosuppression, it causes hypnotic and other CNS effects, including vivid nightmares. It can cause a disulfiram-like syndrome on ingestion of ethanol. Altretamine (formerly hexamethylmelamine) and thiotepa can chemically give rise to alkylating species, although the nature of the DNA damage has not been well characterized in either case. Dacarbazine (DTIC) is activated in the liver to yield the highly reactive methyl diazonium cation. It causes only modest myelosuppression 21–25 days after a dose but causes prominent nausea on day 1. Temozolomide is structurally related to dacarbazine but was designed to be activated by nonenzymatic hydrolysis in tumors and is bioavailable orally.

Cisplatin was discovered fortuitously by observing that bacteria present in electrolysis solutions could not divide. Only the *cis* diamine configuration is active as an antitumor agent. It is hypothesized that in the intracellular environment, a chloride is lost from each position, being replaced by a water molecule. The resulting positively charged species is an efficient bifunctional interactor with DNA, forming Pt-based cross-links. Cisplatin requires administration with adequate hydration, including forced diuresis with mannitol to prevent kidney damage; even with the use of hydration, gradual decrease in kidney function is common, along with noteworthy anemia. Hypomagnesemia frequently attends cisplatin use and can lead to hypocalcemia and tetany. Other common toxicities include neurotoxocity with stocking-and-glove sensorimotor neuropathy. Hearing loss occurs in 50% of patients treated with conventional doses. Cisplatin is intensely emetogenic, requiring prophylactic antiemetics. Myelosuppression is less evident than with other alkylating agents. Chronic vascular toxicity (Raynaud's phenomenon, coronary artery disease) is a more unusual toxicity. Carboplatin displays less nephro-, oto-, and neurotoxicity. However, myelosuppression is more frequent, and as the drug is exclusively cleared through the kidney, adjustment of dose for creatinine clearance must be accomplished through use of various dosing nomograms. Oxaliplatin is a platinum analogue with noteworthy activity in colon cancers refractory to other treatments. It is prominently neurotoxic.

Antitumor antibiotics and topoisomerase poisons Antitumor antibiotics are substances produced by bacteria that in nature appear to provide a chemical defense against other hostile microorganisms. As a class they bind to DNA directly and can frequently undergo electron transfer reactions to generate free radicals in close proximity to DNA, leading to DNA damage in the form of single-strand breaks or cross-links. Topoisomerase poisons include natural products or semisynthetic species derived ultimately from plants, and they modify enzymes that regulate the capacity of DNA to unwind to allow normal replication or transcription. These include topoisomerase I, which creates single-strand breaks that then rejoin following the passage of the other DNA strand through the break. Topoisomerase II creates double-strand breaks through which another segment of DNA duplex passes before rejoining. DNA damage from these agents can occur in any cell cycle phase, but cells tend to arrest in S-phase or G_2 of the cell cycle in cells with p53 and Rb pathway lesions as the result of defective checkpoint mechanisms in cancer cells. Owing to the role of topoisomerase I in the procession of the replication fork, topoisomerase I poisons cause lethality if the topoisomerase I–induced lesions are made in S-phase.

Doxorubicin can intercalate into DNA, thereby altering DNA structure, replication, and topoisomerase II function. It can also undergo reduction reactions by accepting electrons into its quinone ring system, with the capacity to undergo reoxidation to form reactive oxygen radicals after reoxidation. It causes predictable myelosuppression, alopecia, nausea, and mucositis. In addition, it causes acute cardiotoxicity in the form of atrial and ventricular dysrhythmias, but these are rarely of clinical significance. In contrast, cumulative doses >550 mg/m² are associated with a 10% incidence of chronic cardiomyopathy. The incidence of cardiomyopathy appears to be related to schedule (peak serum concentration), with low-dose, frequent treatment or continuous infusions better tolerated than intermittent higher-dose exposures. Cardiotoxicity has been related to iron-catalyzed oxidation and reduction of doxorubicin, and not to topoisomerase action. Cardiotoxicity is related to peak plasma dose; thus, lower doses and continuous infusions are less likely to cause heart damage. Doxorubicin's cardiotoxicity is increased when given together with trastuzumab (Herceptin), the anti-HER2/neu antibody. Radiation recall or interaction with concomitantly administered radiation to cause local site complications is frequent. The drug is a powerful vesicant, with necrosis of tissue apparent 4–7 days after an extravasation; therefore, it should be administered into a rapidly flowing intravenous line. Dexrazoxane is an antidote to doxorubicin-induced extravasation. Doxorubicin is metabolized by the liver, so doses must be reduced by 50–75% in the presence of liver dysfunction. Daunorubicin is closely related to doxorubicin and was actually introduced first into leukemia treatment, where it remains part of curative regimens and has been shown preferable to doxorubicin owing to less mucositis and colonic damage. Idarubicin is also used in acute myeloid leukemia treatment and may be preferable to daunorubicin in activity. Encapsulation of daunorubicin into a liposomal formulation has attenuated cardiac toxicity and antitumor activity in Kaposi's sarcoma and ovarian cancer.

Bleomycin refers to a mixture of glycopeptides that have the unique feature of forming complexes with Fe^{2+} while also bound to DNA. It remains an important component of curative regimens for Hodgkin's disease and germ cell neoplasms. Oxidation of Fe^{2+} gives rise to superoxide and hydroxyl radicals. The drug causes little, if any, myelosuppression. The drug is cleared rapidly, but augmented skin and pulmonary toxicity in the presence of renal failure has led to the recommendation that doses be reduced by 50–75% in the face of a creatinine clearance <25 mL/min. Bleomycin is not a vesicant and can be administered intravenously, intramuscularly, or subcutaneously. Common side effects include fever and chills, facial flush, and Raynaud's phenomenon. Hypertension can follow rapid intravenous administration, and the incidence of anaphylaxis with early preparations of the drug has led to the practice of administering a test dose of 0.5–1 unit before the rest of the dose. The most feared complication of bleomycin treatment is pulmonary fibrosis, which increases in incidence at >300 cumulative units administered and is minimally responsive to treatment (e.g., glucocorticoids). The earliest indicator of an adverse effect is a decline in the DL_{CO}, although cessation of drug immediately upon documentation of a decrease in DL_{CO} may not prevent further decline in pulmonary

function. Bleomycin is inactivated by a bleomycin hydrolase, whose concentration is diminished in skin and lung. Because bleomycin-dependent electron transport is dependent on O_2, bleomycin toxicity may become apparent after exposure to transient very high P_{IO_2}. Thus, during surgical procedures, patients with prior exposure to bleomycin should be maintained on the lowest P_{IO_2} consistent with maintaining adequate tissue oxygenation.

Mitoxantrone is a synthetic compound that was designed to recapitulate features of doxorubicin but with less cardiotoxicity. It is quantitatively less cardiotoxic (comparing the ratio of cardiotoxic to therapeutically effective doses) but is still associated with a 10% incidence of cardiotoxicity at cumulative doses of >150 mg/m². It also causes alopecia. Cases of acute promyelocytic leukemia (APL) have arisen shortly after exposure of patients to mitoxantrone, particularly in the adjuvant treatment of breast cancer. While chemotherapy-associated leukemia is generally of the acute myeloid type, APL arising in the setting of prior mitoxantrone treatment had the typical t(15;17) chromosome translocation associated with APL, but the breakpoints of the translocation appeared to be at topoisomerase II sites that would be preferred sites of mitoxantrone action, clearly linking the action of the drug to the generation of the leukemia.

Etoposide was synthetically derived from the plant product podophyllotoxin; it binds directly to topoisomerase II and DNA in a reversible ternary complex. It stabilizes the covalent intermediate in the enzyme's action where the enzyme is covalently linked to DNA. This "alkali-labile" DNA bond was historically a first hint that an enzyme such as a topoisomerase might exist. The drug therefore causes a prominent G_2 arrest, reflecting the action of a DNA damage checkpoint. Prominent clinical effects include myelosuppression, nausea, and transient hypotension related to the speed of administration of the agent. Etoposide is a mild vesicant but is relatively free from other large-organ toxicities. When given at high doses or very frequently, topoisomerase II inhibitors may cause acute leukemia associated with chromosome 11q23 abnormalities in up to 1% of exposed patients.

Camptothecin was isolated from extracts of a Chinese tree and had notable antileukemia activity in preclinical mouse models. Early human clinical studies with the sodium salt of the hydrolyzed camptothecin lactone showed evidence of toxicity with little antitumor activity. Identification of topoisomerase I as the target of camptothecins and the need to preserve lactone structure allowed additional efforts to identify active members of this series. Topoisomerase I is responsible for unwinding the DNA strand by introducing single-strand breaks and allowing rotation of one strand about the other. In S-phase, topoisomerase I–induced breaks that are not promptly resealed lead to progress of the replication fork off the end of a DNA strand. The DNA damage is a potent signal for induction of apoptosis. Camptothecins promote the stabilization of the DNA linked to the enzyme in a so-called cleavable complex, analogous to the action of etoposide with topoisomerase II. Topotecan is a camptothecin derivative approved for use in gynecologic tumors and small cell lung cancer. Toxicity is limited to myelosuppression and mucositis. CPT-11, or irinotecan, is a camptothecin with evidence of activity in colon carcinoma. In addition to myelosuppression, it causes a secretory diarrhea related to the toxicity of a metabolite called SN-38. The diarrhea can be treated effectively with loperamide or octreotide.

Indirect effectors of DNA function: antimetabolites

A broad definition of antimetabolites would include compounds with structural similarity to precursors of purines or pyrimidines, or compounds that interfere with purine or pyrimidine synthesis. Antimetabolites can cause DNA damage indirectly, through misincorporation into DNA, abnormal timing or progression through

DNA synthesis, or altered function of pyrimidine and purine biosynthetic enzymes. They tend to convey greatest toxicity to cells in S-phase, and the degree of toxicity increases with duration of exposure. Common toxic manifestations include stomatitis, diarrhea, and myelosuppression. Second malignancies are not associated with their use.

Methotrexate inhibits dihydrofolate reductase, which regenerates reduced folates from the oxidized folates produced when thymidine monophosphate is formed from deoxyuridine monophosphate. Without reduced folates, cells die a "thymine-less" death. $N5$-tetrahydrofolate or $N5$-formyltetrahydrofolate (leucovorin) can bypass this block and rescue cells from methotrexate, which is maintained in cells by polyglutamylation. The drug and other reduced folates are transported into cells by the folate carrier, and high concentrations of drug can bypass this carrier and allow diffusion of drug directly into cells. These properties have suggested the design of "high-dose" methotrexate regimens with leucovorin rescue of normal marrow and mucosa as part of curative approaches to osteosarcoma in the adjuvant setting and hematopoietic neoplasms of children and adults. Methotrexate is cleared by the kidney via both glomerular filtration and tubular secretion, and toxicity is augmented by renal dysfunction and drugs such as salicylates, probenecid, and nonsteroidal anti-inflammatory agents that undergo tubular secretion. With normal renal function, 15 mg/m^2 leucovorin will rescue 10^{-8} to 10^{-6} M methotrexate in three to four doses. However, with decreased creatinine clearance, doses of 50–100 mg/m^2 are continued until methotrexate levels are $<5 \times 10^{-8}$ M. In addition to bone marrow suppression and mucosal irritation, methotrexate can cause renal failure itself at high doses owing to crystallization in renal tubules; therefore, high-dose regimens require alkalinization of urine with increased flow by hydration. Methotrexate can be sequestered in third-space collections and leach back into the general circulation, causing prolonged myelosuppression. Less-frequent adverse effects include reversible increases in transaminases and hypersensitivity-like pulmonary syndrome. Chronic low-dose methotrexate can cause hepatic fibrosis. When administered to the intrathecal space, methotrexate can cause chemical arachnoiditis and CNS dysfunction.

Pemetrexed is a novel folate-directed antimetabolite. It is "multitargeted" in that it inhibits the activity of several enzymes, including thymidylate synthetase, dihydrofolate reductase, and glycinamide ribonucleotide formyltransferase, thereby affecting the synthesis of both purine and pyrimidine nucleic acid precursors. To avoid significant toxicity to the normal tissues, patients receiving pemetrexed should also receive low-dose folate and vitamin B$_{12}$ supplementation. Pemetrexed has notable activity against certain lung cancers and, in combination with cisplatin, also against mesotheliomas. Palatrexate is an antifolate approved for use in T cell lymphoma that is very efficiently transported into cancer cells.

5-Fluorouracil (5FU) represents an early example of "rational" drug design in that it originated from the observation that tumor cells incorporate radiolabeled uracil more efficiently into DNA than normal cells, especially gut. 5FU is metabolized in cells to 5′FdUMP, which inhibits thymidylate synthetase (TS). In addition, misincorporation can lead to single-strand breaks, and RNA can aberrantly incorporate FUMP. 5FU is metabolized by dihydropyrimidine dehydrogenase, and deficiency of this enzyme can lead to excessive toxicity from 5FU. Oral bioavailability varies unreliably, but orally administered analogues of 5FU such as capecitabine have been developed that allow at least equivalent activity to many parenteral 5FU-based approaches. Intravenous administration of 5FU leads to bone marrow suppression after short infusions but to stomatitis after prolonged infusions. Leucovorin augments the activity of 5FU by promoting formation of the ternary covalent complex of 5FU, the reduced folate, and TS. Less-frequent toxicities include

CNS dysfunction, with prominent cerebellar signs, and endothelial toxicity manifested by thrombosis, including pulmonary embolus and myocardial infarction.

Cytosine arabinoside (ara-C) is incorporated into DNA after formation of ara-CTP, resulting in S-phase–related toxicity. Continuous infusion schedules allow maximal efficiency, with uptake maximal at 5–7 μM. Ara-C can be administered intrathecally. Adverse effects include nausea, diarrhea, stomatitis, chemical conjunctivitis, and cerebellar ataxia. Gemcitabine is a cytosine derivative that is similar to ara-C in that it is incorporated into DNA after anabolism to the triphosphate, rendering DNA susceptible to breakage and repair synthesis, which differs from that in ara-C in that gemcitabine-induced lesions are very inefficiently removed. In contrast to ara-C, gemcitabine appears to have useful activity in a variety of solid tumors, with limited nonmyelosuppressive toxicities. 6-Thioguanine and 6-mercaptopurine (6MP) are used in the treatment of acute lymphoid leukemia. Although administered orally, they display variable bioavailability. 6MP is metabolized by xanthine oxidase and therefore requires dose reduction when used with allopurinol.

Fludarabine phosphate is a prodrug of F-adenine arabinoside (F-ara-A), which in turn was designed to diminish the susceptibility of ara-A to adenosine deaminase. F-ara-A is incorporated into DNA and can cause delayed cytotoxicity even in cells with low growth fraction, including chronic lymphocytic leukemia and follicular B cell lymphoma. CNS and peripheral nerve dysfunction and T cell depletion leading to opportunistic infections can occur in addition to myelosuppression. 2-Chlorodeoxyadenosine is a similar compound with activity in hairy cell leukemia. 2-Deoxycoformycin inhibits adenosine deaminase, with resulting increase in dATP levels. This causes inhibition of ribonucleotide reductase as well as augmented susceptibility to apoptosis, particularly in T cells. Renal failure and CNS dysfunction are notable toxicities in addition to immunosuppression. Hydroxyurea inhibits ribonucleotide reductase, resulting in S-phase block. It is orally bioavailable and useful for the acute management of myeloproliferative states.

Asparaginase is a bacterial enzyme that causes breakdown of extracellular asparagine required for protein synthesis in certain leukemic cells. This effectively stops tumor cell DNA synthesis, as DNA synthesis requires concurrent protein synthesis. The outcome of asparaginase action is therefore very similar to the result of the small-molecule antimetabolites. As asparaginase is a foreign protein, hypersensitivity reactions are common, as are effects on organs such as pancreas and liver that normally require continuing protein synthesis. This may result in decreased insulin secretion with hyperglycemia, with or without hyperamylasemia and clotting function abnormalities. Close monitoring of clotting functions should accompany use of asparaginase. Paradoxically, owing to depletion of rapidly turning over anticoagulant factors, thromboses particularly affecting the CNS may also be seen with asparaginase.

Mitotic spindle inhibitors

Microtubules are cellular structures that form the mitotic spindle, and in interphase cells they are responsible for the cellular "scaffolding" along which various motile and secretory processes occur. Microtubules are composed of repeating noncovalent multimers of a heterodimer of α and β isoform of the protein tubulin. Vincristine binds to the tubulin dimer with the result that microtubules are disaggregated. This results in the block of growing cells in M-phase; however, toxic effects in G$_1$ and S-phase are also evident, reflecting effects on normal cellular activities of microtubules. Vincristine is metabolized by the liver, and dose adjustment in the presence of hepatic dysfunction is required. It is a powerful vesicant, and infiltration can be treated by local heat and infiltration of hyaluronidase. At clinically used intravenous doses, neurotoxicity in the form of glove-and-stocking neuropathy is frequent. Acute neuropathic effects include jaw pain, paralytic ileus, urinary retention, and the syndrome of inappropriate antidiuretic hormone secretion. Myelosuppression is not seen. Vinblastine is similar to vincristine, except that it tends to be more myelotoxic, with more frequent thrombocytopenia and also mucositis and stomatitis. Vinorelbine is a vinca alkaloid that appears to have differences in resistance patterns in comparison to vincristine and vinblastine; it may be administered orally.

The taxanes include paclitaxel and docetaxel. These agents differ from the vinca alkaloids in that the taxanes stabilize microtubules against depolymerization. The "stabilized" microtubules function abnormally and are not able to undergo the normal dynamic changes of microtubule structure and function necessary for cell cycle completion. Taxanes are among the most broadly active antineoplastic agents for use in solid tumors, with evidence of activity in ovarian cancer, breast cancer, Kaposi's sarcoma, and lung tumors. They are administered intravenously, and paclitaxel requires use of a Cremophor-containing vehicle that can cause hypersensitivity reactions. Premedication with dexamethasone (8–16 mg orally or intravenously 12 and 6 h before treatment) and diphenhydramine (50 mg) and cimetidine (300 mg), both 30 min before treatment, decreases but does not eliminate the risk of hypersensitivity reactions to the paclitaxel vehicle. Docetaxel uses a polysorbate 80 formulation, which can cause fluid retention in addition to hypersensitivity reactions, and dexamethasone premedication with or without antihistamines is frequently used. A protein-bound formulation of paclitaxel (called *nab-paclitaxel*) has at least equivalent antineoplastic activity and decreased risk of hypersensitivity reactions. Paclitaxel may also cause hypersensitivity reactions, myelosuppression, neurotoxicity in the form of glove-and-stocking numbness, and paresthesia. Cardiac rhythm disturbances were observed in phase I and II trials, most commonly asymptomatic bradycardia but also, much more rarely, varying degrees of heart block. These have not emerged as clinically significant in the majority of patients. Docetaxel causes comparable degrees of myelosuppression and neuropathy. Hypersensitivity reactions, including bronchospasm, dyspnea, and hypotension, are less frequent but occur to some degree in up to 25% of patients. Fluid retention appears to result from a vascular leak syndrome that can aggravate preexisting effusions. Rash can complicate docetaxel administration, appearing prominently as a pruritic maculopapular rash affecting the forearms, but it has also been associated with fingernail ridging, breakdown, and skin discoloration. Stomatitis appears to be somewhat more frequent than with paclitaxel.

Resistance to taxanes has been related to the emergence of efficient efflux of taxanes from tumor cells through the p170 P-glycoprotein (*mdr* gene product) or the presence of variant or mutant forms of tubulin. Epothilones represent a class of novel microtubule-stabilizing agents that have been conscientiously optimized for activity in taxane-resistant tumors. Ixabepilone has clear evidence of activity in breast cancers resistant to taxanes and anthracyclines such as doxorubicin. It retains acceptable expected side effects, including myelosuppression, and can also cause peripheral sensory neuropathy.

Estramustine was originally synthesized as a mustard derivative that might be useful in neoplasms that possessed estrogen receptors. However, no evidence of interaction with DNA was observed. Surprisingly, the drug caused metaphase arrest, and subsequent study revealed that it binds to microtubule-associated proteins, resulting in abnormal microtubule function. Estramustine binds to estramustine-binding proteins (EMBPs), which are notably present in prostate tumor tissue. The drug is used in patients with prostate cancer. Gastrointestinal and cardiovascular adverse effects related to the estrogen moiety occur in up to 10% of patients, including worsened heart failure and thromboembolic phenomena. Gynecomastia and nipple tenderness can also occur.

Hormonal agents

Steroid hormone receptor–related molecules have emerged as prominent targets for small molecules useful in cancer treatment. When bound to their cognate ligands, these receptors can alter gene transcription and, in certain tissues, induce apoptosis. The pharmacologic effect is a mirror or parody of the normal effects of the agents acting on nontransformed normal tissues, although the effects on tumors are mediated by indirect effects in some cases.

Glucocorticoids are generally given in "pulsed" high doses in leukemias and lymphomas, where they induce apoptosis in tumor cells. Cushing's syndrome or inadvertent adrenal suppression on withdrawal from high-dose glucocorticoids can be significant complications, along with infections common in immunosuppressed patients, in particular *Pneumocystis* pneumonia, which classically appears a few days after completing a course of high-dose glucocorticoids.

Tamoxifen is a partial estrogen receptor antagonist; it has a tenfold greater antitumor activity in breast cancer patients whose tumors express estrogen receptors than in those who have low or no levels of expression. It might be considered the prototypic "molecularly targeted" agent. Owing to its agonistic activities in vascular and uterine tissue, side effects include a somewhat increased risk of cardiovascular complications, such as thromboembolic phenomena, and a small increased incidence of endometrial carcinoma, which appears after chronic use (usually >5 years). Progestational agents—including medroxyprogesterone acetate, androgens including fluoxymesterone (Halotestin), and, paradoxically, estrogens—have approximately the same degree of activity in primary hormonal treatment of breast cancers that have elevated expression of estrogen receptor protein. Estrogen itself is not used often owing to prominent cardiovascular and uterotropic activity.

Aromatase refers to a family of enzymes that catalyze the formation of estrogen in various tissues, including the ovary and peripheral adipose tissue and some tumor cells. Aromatase inhibitors are of two types, the irreversible steroid analogues such as exemestane and the reversible inhibitors such as anastrozole or letrozole. Anastrozole is superior to tamoxifen in the adjuvant treatment of breast cancer in postmenopausal patients with estrogen receptor–positive tumors. Letrozole treatment affords benefit following tamoxifen treatment. Adverse effects of aromatase inhibitors may include an increased risk of osteoporosis.

Prostate cancer is classically treated by androgen deprivation. Diethylstilbestrol (DES) acting as an estrogen at the level of the hypothalamus to downregulate hypothalamic luteinizing hormone (LH) production results in decreased elaboration of testosterone by the testicle. For this reason, orchiectomy is equally as effective as moderate-dose DES, inducing responses in 80% of previously untreated patients with prostate cancer but without the prominent cardiovascular side effects of DES, including thrombosis and exacerbation of coronary artery disease. In the event that orchiectomy is not accepted by the patient, testicular androgen suppression can also be effected by luteinizing hormone–releasing hormone (LHRH) agonists such as leuprolide and goserelin. These agents cause tonic stimulation of the LHRH receptor, with the loss of its normal pulsatile activation resulting in decreased output of LH by the anterior pituitary. Therefore, as primary hormonal manipulation in prostate cancer, one can choose orchiectomy or leuprolide, but not both. The addition of androgen receptor blockers, including flutamide or bicalutamide, is of uncertain additional benefit in extending overall response duration; the combined use of orchiectomy or leuprolide plus flutamide is referred to as *total androgen blockade*.

Tumors that respond to a primary hormonal manipulation may frequently respond to second and third hormonal manipulations. Thus, breast tumors that had previously responded to tamoxifen have, on relapse, notable response rates to withdrawal of tamoxifen itself or to subsequent addition of an aromatase inhibitor or progestin. Likewise, initial treatment of prostate cancers with leuprolide plus flutamide may be followed after disease progression by response to withdrawal of flutamide. These responses may result from the removal of antagonists from mutant steroid hormone receptors that have come to depend on the presence of the antagonist as a growth-promoting influence.

Additional strategies to treat refractory breast and prostate cancers that possess steroid hormone receptors may also address adrenal capacity to produce androgens and estrogens, even after orchiectomy or oophorectomy, respectively. Thus, aminoglutethimide or ketoconazole can be used to block adrenal synthesis by interfering with the enzymes of steroid hormone metabolism. Administration of these agents requires concomitant hydrocortisone replacement and additional glucocorticoid doses administered in the event of physiologic stress.

Humoral mechanisms can also result in complications from an underlying malignancy producing the hormone. Adrenocortical carcinomas can cause Cushing's syndrome as well as syndromes of androgen or estrogen excess. Mitotane can counteract these by decreasing synthesis of steroid hormones. Islet cell neoplasms can cause debilitating diarrhea, treated with the somatostatin analogue octreotide. Prolactin-secreting tumors can be effectively managed by the dopaminergic agonist bromocriptine.

▪ TARGETED THERAPIES

A better understanding of cancer cell biology has suggested many new targets for cancer drug discovery and development. These include the products of oncogenes and tumor-suppressor genes, regulators of cell death pathways, mediators of cellular immortality such as telomerase, and molecules responsible for microenvironmental molding such as proteases or angiogenic factors. The essential difference in the development of agents that would target these processes is that the basis for discovery of the candidate drug is the a priori importance of the target in the biology of the tumor, rather than the initial detection of drug candidates based on the phenomenon of tumor cell regression in tissue culture or in animals. The following examples reflect the rapidly evolving clinical research activity in this area. Figure 85-4 summarizes how FDA-approved targeted agents act.

Hematopoietic neoplasms

Imatinib targets the ATP binding site of the p210$^{bcr-abl}$ protein tyrosine kinase that is formed as the result of the chromosome 9,22 translocation producing the Philadelphia chromosome in CML. Imatinib is superior to interferon plus chemotherapy in the initial treatment of the chronic phase of this disorder. It has lesser activity in the blast phase of CML, where the cells may have acquired additional mutations in p210$^{bcr-abl}$ itself or other genetic lesions. Its side effects are relatively tolerable in most patients and include hepatic dysfunction, diarrhea, and fluid retention. Rarely, patients receiving imatinib have decreased cardiac function, which may persist after discontinuation of the drug. The quality of response to imatinib

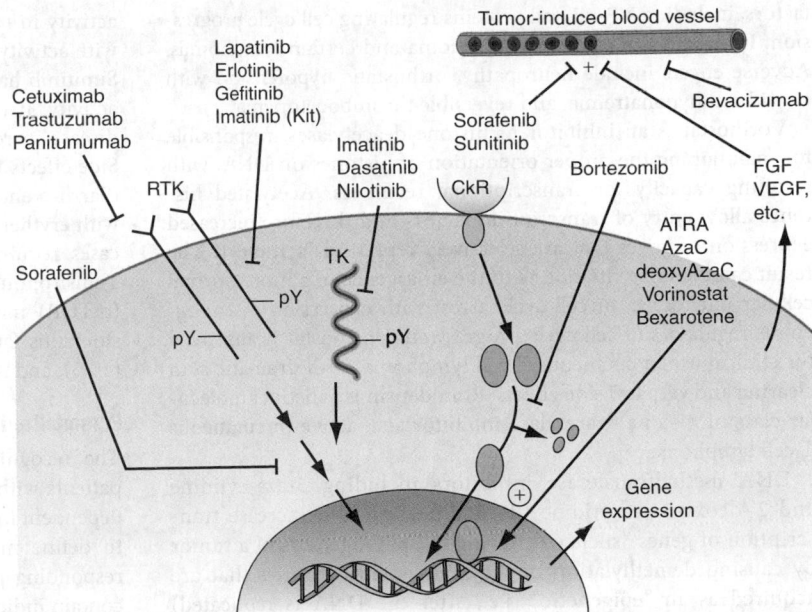

Figure 85-4   Site of action of targeted agents. Signals proceeding from growth factor–related receptor tyrosine kinases (RTKs) such as EGF-R, erbB2, or c-kit can be interrupted by lapatinib, erlotinib, gefitinib, and imatinib, acting at the ATP binding site; or by cetuximab, trastuzumab, or panitumumab acting at the receptor. Tyrosine kinases (TKs) that are not directly stimulated by growth factors such as p210 bcr-abl or src can be inhibited by imatinib, dasatinib, or nilotinib. Signals projected downstream from growth factor receptors can be affected by the multitargeted kinase inhibitor sorafenib, acting on c-raf, and, upon arrival at the nucleus, affect gene expression, which can be affected by the targeted transcriptional modulators vorinostat (targeting histone deacetylase), azacytidine derivatives (targeting DNA methyltransferase), or retinoid receptor modulators all-*trans*-retinoic acid (ATRA) or bexarotene. Cytokine receptors (CkRs) are one stimulus for degradation of the inhibitory subunit of the NFκB transcription factor by the proteosome. Bortezomib inhibits this process and can prevent activation of NFκB-dependent genes, among other growth-related effects. Sorafenib and sunitinib, acting as inhibitors of vascular endothelial growth factor (VEGF) receptors, can modulate tumor blood vessel function through their action on endothelial cells, while bevacizumab targets the same process by combining with VEGF itself.

enters into the decision about when to refer patients with CML for consideration of transplant approaches. Nilotinib is a tyrosine protein kinase inhibitor with a similar spectrum of activity to imatinib, but with increased potency and perhaps better tolerance by certain patients. Dasatinib, another inhibitor of the p210$^{bcr-abl}$ oncoproteins, is active in certain mutant variants of p210$^{bcr-abl}$ that are refractory to imatinib and arise during therapy with imatinib or are present de novo. Dasatinib also has inhibitory action against kinases belonging to the src tyrosine protein kinase family; this activity may contribute to its effects in hematopoietic tumors and suggest a role in solid tumors where src kinases are active. Only the T315I mutant is resistant to dasatinib; a new class of inhibitors called aurora kinase inhibitors is in development to address this problem.

All-*trans*-retinoic acid (ATRA) targets the PML-retinoic acid receptor (RAR) α fusion protein, which is the result of the chromosome 15,17 translocation pathogenic for most forms of APL. Administered orally, it causes differentiation of the neoplastic promyelocytes to mature granulocytes and attenuates the rate of hemorrhagic complications. Adverse effects include headache with or without pseudotumor cerebri and gastrointestinal and cutaneous toxicities. Another active retinoid is the synthetic retinoid X receptor ligand bexarotene, which has activity in cutaneous T cell lymphoma.

Bortezomib is an inhibitor of the proteasome, the multisubunit assembly of protease activities responsible for the selective degradation of proteins important in regulating activation of transcription factors, including NF-κB and proteins regulating cell cycle progression. It has activity in multiple myeloma and certain lymphomas. Adverse effects include neuropathy, orthostatic hypotension with or without hyponatremia, and reversible thrombocytopenia.

Vorinostat is an inhibitor of histone deacetylases, responsible for maintaining the proper orientation of histones on DNA, with resulting capacity for transcriptional readiness. Acetylated histones allow entry of transcription factors and therefore increased expression of genes that are selectively repressed in tumors. The result can be differentiation with the emergence of a more normal cellular phenotype, or cell cycle arrest with expression of endogenous regulators of cell cycle progression. Vorinostat is approved for clinical use in cutaneous T cell lymphoma, with dramatic skin clearing and very few side effects. Romidepsin is a distinct molecular class of histone deacetylase inhibitor also active in cutaneous T cell lymphoma.

DNA methyltransferase inhibitors including 5-aza-cytidine and 2′-deoxy-5-azacytidine (decitabine) can also increase transcription of genes "silenced" during the pathogenesis of a tumor by causing demethylation of the methylated cytosines that are acquired as an "epigenetic" (i.e., after the DNA is replicated) modification of DNA. These drugs were originally considered antimetabolites but have clinical value in myelodysplastic syndromes and certain leukemias when administered at low doses. Combinations of DNA methyltransferase inhibitors and histone deacetylase inhibitors may offer new approaches to regulate chromatin function.

Targeted toxins utilize macromolecules such as antibodies or cytokines with high affinity for defined tumor cell-surface molecules, such as a leukemia differentiation antigen, to which a therapeutic antibody can deliver a covalently linked potent cytotoxin, or a growth factor such as IL-2 to deliver a toxin (in the form of diphtheria toxin in denileukin diftitox) to cells bearing the IL-2 receptor. The value of such targeted approaches is that in addition to maximizing the therapeutic index by differential expression of the target in tumor (as opposed to nonrenewable normal cells), selection of patients for clinical use can capitalize on assessing the target in the tumor.

Solid tumors

Small-molecule epidermal growth factor (EGF) antagonists act at the ATP binding site of the EGF receptor tyrosine kinase. In early clinical trials, gefitinib showed evidence of responses in a small fraction of patients with non-small cell lung cancer (NSCLC). Side effects were generally acceptable, consisting mostly of rash and diarrhea. Subsequent analysis of responding patients revealed a high frequency of activating mutations in the EGF receptor. Often patients who developed resistance to gefitinib have acquired additional mutations in the enzyme, similar to what was seen in imatinib-resistant CML. Erlotinib is another EGF receptor tyrosine kinase antagonist with somewhat superior outcome in clinical trials in NSCLC. Even patients with wild-type EGF receptors may benefit from erlotinib treatment. Lapatinib is a combined EGF receptor and erbB2 tyrosine kinase antagonist with activity in breast cancers refractory to anti-erbB2 antibodies.

In addition to the p210$^{bcr-abl}$ kinase, imatinib also has activity against the c-kit tyrosine kinase, activated in gastrointestinal stromal sarcoma, and the platelet-derived growth factor receptor (PDGF-R), activated by translocation in certain sarcomas. Imatinib has found clinical utility in these neoplasms previously refractory to chemotherapeutic approaches.

"Multitargeted" kinase antagonists are small-molecule ATP site-directed antagonists that inhibit more than one protein kinase. Drugs of this type with prominent activity against the vascular endothelial growth factor receptor (VEGF-R) tyrosine kinase have

activity in renal cell carcinoma. Sorafenib is a VEGF-R antagonist with activity against the *raf* serine-threonine protein kinase as well. Sunitinib has anti-VEGF-R as well as anti-PDGF-R and anti-c-kit activity. It causes prominent responses as well as stabilization of disease in renal cell cancers and gastrointestinal stromal tumors. Side effects for both agents are mostly acceptable, with fatigue and diarrhea encountered with both agents. The "hand-foot syndrome" with erythema and desquamation of the distal extremities, in some cases requiring dose modification, may be seen with sorafenib. Temsirolimus and everolimus are mammalian target of rapamycin (mTOR) inhibitors with activity in renal cancers. They produce stomatitis, fatigue, and some hyperlipidemia (10%), myelosuppression (10%), and rare lung toxicity.

Personalized cancer treatment

The recognition that targeted therapies may benefit subsets of patients with an identical histologic diagnosis, but whose tumor is dependent for viability on the target's function, has spurred research to define molecular diagnostic approaches to define potentially responding patients. In addition, a patient's germ-line DNA may contain indicators of differential capacity to metabolize cancer chemotherapy agents and thus be susceptible to drug-induced toxicity. While efforts in this area are still a focus of both clinical and basic research, the following conclusions can be drawn, and are applicable to patients being initially managed in the primary care setting.

All patients undergoing initial diagnostic evaluation for breast cancer should have their tumor tested for the expression of the estrogen receptor (ER), progesterone receptor (PR), and the c-erbB2 (HER2; HER2/neu) oncoprotein by immunohistochemistry or fluorescence in situ hybridization (FISH). Patients expressing the ER and/or PR are candidates for adjuvant hormone receptor–directed therapies. Patients with evidence of abundant HER2 expression or HER2 gene amplification will likely derive benefit from trastuzumab. In addition, Oncotype Dx is a 21-gene expression test that has been approved by the FDA for defining patients without lymph node involvement but with ER+ tumors who may have the greatest chance of benefiting from adjuvant chemotherapy added to adjuvant estrogen therapy. The MammaPrint test is similar in intent for node-negative patients but without reference to ER expression status.

The value of characterizing the mutational status of the epidermal growth factor (EGF) receptor pathway in patients with lung cancer is also a matter of current clinical investigations. While the tyrosine kinase inhibitor erlotinib is approved for use in all patients with NSCLC who have had progression of disease despite treatment with platinum-based chemotherapy, subsets of patients, such as female Asian nonsmokers, have a high evidence of EGF-R mutations resulting in marked sensitivity to erlotinib. And it is possible that in the larger population of patients with NSCLC, such testing may allow selection of patients in whom initial use of erlotinib may also be considered. Conversely, a mutated K-ras oncogene in patients with lung adenocarcinoma is associated with no benefit from erlotinib treatment.

In patients with colon cancer, a mutated K-ras oncogene is clearly associated with no benefit to the use of the EGF-R–directed antibody cetuximab, and characterization of K-ras mutational status should be undertaken as part of the routine diagnostic evaluation of patients with newly diagnosed metastatic or newly recurrent colon cancer. Patients undergoing diagnostic evaluation for initial treatment of metastatic colon cancer might usefully undergo evaluation of their germ-line uridine diphosphate glucuronosyl transferase (UGT) 1A1 allele status, as the expression of variant alleles at that locus influences susceptibility to irinotecan-induced hematologic toxicity. Patients with known Gilbert's disease should receive irinotecan very cautiously or perhaps not at all.

ACUTE COMPLICATIONS OF CANCER CHEMOTHERAPY

Myelosuppression

The common cytotoxic chemotherapeutic agents almost invariably affect bone marrow function. Titration of this effect determines the MTD of the agent on a given schedule. The normal kinetics of blood cell turnover influences the sequence and sensitivity of each of the formed elements. Polymorphonuclear leukocytes (PMNs; $t_{1/2}$ = 6–8 h), platelets ($t_{1/2}$ = 5–7 days), and red blood cells (RBCs; $t_{1/2}$ = 120 days) respectively have most, less, and least susceptibility to usually administered cytotoxic agents. The nadir count of each cell type in response to classes of agents is characteristic. Maximal neutropenia occurs 6–14 days after conventional doses of anthracyclines, antifolates, and antimetabolites. Alkylating agents differ from each other in the timing of cytopenias. Nitrosoureas, DTIC, and procarbazine can display delayed marrow toxicity, first appearing 6 weeks after dosing.

Complications of myelosuppression result from the predictable sequelae of the missing cells' function. *Febrile neutropenia* refers to the clinical presentation of fever (one temperature ≥38.5°C or three readings ≥38°C but ≤38.5°C per 24 h) in a neutropenic patient with an uncontrolled neoplasm involving the bone marrow or, more usually, in a patient undergoing treatment with cytotoxic agents. Mortality from uncontrolled infection varies inversely with the neutrophil count. If the nadir neutrophil count is >1000/μL, there is little risk; if <500/μL, risk of death is markedly increased. Management of febrile neutropenia has conventionally included empirical coverage with antibiotics for the duration of neutropenia (Chap. 86). Selection of antibiotics is governed by the expected association of infections with certain underlying neoplasms; careful physical examination (with scrutiny of catheter sites, dentition, mucosal surfaces, and perirectal and genital orifices by gentle palpation); chest x-ray; and Gram stain and culture of blood, urine, and sputum (if any) to define a putative site of infection. In the absence of any originating site, a broadly acting β-lactam with anti-*Pseudomonas* activity, such as ceftazidime, is begun empirically. The addition of vancomycin to cover potential cutaneous sites of origin (until these are ruled out or shown to originate from methicillin-sensitive organisms) or metronidazole or imipenem for abdominal or other sites favoring anaerobes reflects modifications tailored to individual patient presentations. The coexistence of pulmonary compromise raises a distinct set of potential pathogens, including *Legionella*, *Pneumocystis*, and fungal agents that may require further diagnostic evaluations, such as bronchoscopy with bronchoalveolar lavage. Febrile neutropenic patients can be stratified broadly into two prognostic groups. The first, with expected short duration of neutropenia and no evidence of hypotension or abdominal or other localizing symptoms, may be expected to do well even with oral regimens, e.g., ciprofloxacin or moxifloxacin, or amoxicillin plus clavulanic acid. A less favorable prognostic group is patients with expected prolonged neutropenia, evidence of sepsis, and end organ compromise, particularly pneumonia. These patients require tailoring of their antibiotic regimen to their underlying presentation, with frequent empirical addition of antifungal agents if fever persists for 7 days without identification of an adequately treated organism or site.

Transfusion of granulocytes has no role in the management of febrile neutropenia, owing to their exceedingly short half-life, mechanical fragility, and clinical syndromes of pulmonary compromise with leukostasis after their use. Instead, colony-stimulating factors (CSFs) are used to augment bone marrow production of PMNs. Early-acting factors such as IL-1, IL-3, and stem cell factor have not been as useful clinically as late-acting, lineage-specific factors such as G-CSF (granulocyte colony-stimulating factor) or GM-CSF (granulocyte-macrophage colony-stimulating factor),

erythropoietin (EPO), thrombopoietin, IL-6, and IL-11. CSFs may easily become overused in oncology practice. The settings in which their use has been proved effective are limited. G-CSF, GM-CSF, EPO, and IL-11 are currently approved for use. The American Society of Clinical Oncology has developed practice guidelines for the use of G-CSF and GM-CSF (Table 85-3).

Primary prophylaxis (i.e., shortly after completing chemotherapy to reduce the nadir) administers G-CSF to patients receiving cytotoxic regimens associated with a 20% incidence of febrile neutropenia. "Dose-dense" regimens, where cycling of chemotherapy is intended to be completed without delay of administered doses, may also benefit, but such patients should be on a clinical trial. Administration of G-CSF in these circumstances has reduced the incidence of febrile neutropenia in several studies by about 50%. Most patients, however, receive regimens that do not have such a high risk of expected febrile neutropenia, and therefore most patients initially should not receive G-CSF or GM-CSF. Special circumstances—such as a documented history of febrile neutropenia with the regimen in a particular patient or categories of patients at increased risk, such as patients older than age 65 years with aggressive lymphoma treated with curative chemotherapy regimens; extensive compromise of marrow by prior radiation or chemotherapy; or active, open wounds or deep-seated infection—may support primary treatment with G-CSF or GM-CSF. Administration of G-CSF or GM-CSF to afebrile neutropenic patients or to patients with low-risk febrile neutropenia is not recommended, and patients receiving concomitant chemoradiation treatment, particularly those with thoracic neoplasms, likewise are not generally recommended for treatment. In contrast, administration of G-CSF to high-risk patients with febrile neutropenia and evidence of organ compromise including sepsis syndrome, invasive fungal infection, concurrent hospitalization at the time fever develops, pneumonia, profound neutropenia ($<0.1 \times 10^9$/L), or age >65 years is reasonable.

Secondary prophylaxis refers to the administration of CSFs in patients who have experienced a neutropenic complication from a prior cycle of chemotherapy; dose reduction or delay may be a reasonably considered alternative. G-CSF or GM-CSF is conventionally started 24–72 h after completion of chemotherapy and continued until a PMN count of 10,000/μL is achieved, unless a "depot" preparation of G-CSF such as pegfilgrastim is used, where one dose is administered at least 14 days before the next scheduled administration of chemotherapy. Also, patients with myeloid leukemias undergoing induction therapy may have a slight reduction in the duration of neutropenia if G-CSF is commenced after completion of therapy and may be of particular value in elderly patients, but the influence on long-term outcome has not been defined. GM-CSF probably has a more restricted utility than G-CSF, with its use currently limited to patients after autologous bone marrow transplants, although proper head-to-head comparisons with G-CSF have not been conducted in most instances. GM-CSF may be associated with more systemic side effects.

Dangerous degrees of thrombocytopenia do not frequently complicate the management of patients with solid tumors receiving cytotoxic chemotherapy (with the possible exception of certain carboplatin-containing regimens), but they are frequent in patients with certain hematologic neoplasms where marrow is infiltrated with tumor. Severe bleeding related to thrombocytopenia occurs with increased frequency at platelet counts <20,000/μL and is very prevalent at counts <5000/μL.

The precise "trigger" point at which to transfuse patients is being evaluated in a randomized study. This issue is important not only because of the costs of frequent transfusion, but unnecessary platelet transfusions expose the patient to the risks of allosensitization and loss of value from subsequent transfusion owing to rapid

TABLE 85-3 Indications for the Clinical Use of G-CSF or GM-CSF

Preventive Uses

With the first cycle of chemotherapy (so-called primary CSF administration)

Not needed on a routine basis

Use if the probability of febrile neutropenia is ≥20%

Use if patient has preexisting neutropenia or active infection

Age >65 years treated for lymphoma with curative intent or other tumor treated by similar regimens

Poor performance status

Extensive prior chemotherapy

Dose-dense regimens in a clinical trial or with strong evidence of benefit

With subsequent cycles if febrile neutropenia has previously occurred (so-called secondary CSF administration)

Not needed after short-duration neutropenia without fever

Use if patient had febrile neutropenia in previous cycle

Use if prolonged neutropenia (even without fever) delays therapy

Therapeutic Uses

Afebrile neutropenic patients

No evidence of benefit

Febrile neutropenic patients

No evidence of benefit

May feel compelled to use in the face of clinical deterioration from sepsis, pneumonia, or fungal infection, but benefit unclear

In bone marrow or peripheral blood stem cell transplantation

Use to mobilize stem cells from marrow

Use to hasten myeloid recovery

In acute myeloid leukemia

G-CSF of minor or no benefit

GM-CSF of no benefit and may be harmful

In myelodysplastic syndromes

Not routinely beneficial

Use intermittently in subset with neutropenia and recurrent infection

What Dose and Schedule Should Be Used?

G-CSF: 5 mg/kg per day subcutaneously

GM-CSF: 250 mg/m^2 per day subcutaneously

Peg-filgrastim: one dose of 6 mg 24 h after chemotherapy

When Should Therapy Begin and End?

When indicated, start 24–72 h after chemotherapy

Continue until absolute neutrophil count is 10,000/μL

Do not use concurrently with chemotherapy or radiation therapy

Abbreviations: G-CSF, granulocyte colony-stimulating factor; GM-CSF, granulocyte-macrophage colony-stimulating factor.
Source: From the American Society of Clinical Oncology.

platelet clearance, as well as the infectious and hypersensitivity risks inherent in any transfusion. Prophylactic transfusions to keep platelets >20,000/μL are reasonable in patients with leukemia who are stressed by fever or concomitant medical conditions (the threshold for transfusion is 10,000/μL in patients with solid tumors and no other bleeding diathesis or physiologic stressors such as fever or hypotension, a level that might also be reasonably considered for leukemia patients who are thrombocytopenic but not stressed or bleeding). In contrast, patients with myeloproliferative states may have functionally altered platelets despite normal platelet counts, and transfusion with normal donor platelets should be considered for evidence of bleeding in these patients. Careful review of medication lists to prevent exposure to nonsteroidal anti-inflammatory agents and maintenance of clotting factor levels adequate to support near-normal prothrombin and partial thromboplastin time tests are important in minimizing the risk of bleeding in the thrombocytopenic patient.

Certain cytokines in clinical investigation have shown an ability to increase platelets (e.g., IL-6, IL-1, thrombopoietin), but clinical benefit and safety are not yet proven. IL-11 (oprelvekin) is approved for use in the setting of expected thrombocytopenia, but its effects on platelet counts are small, and it is associated with side effects such as headache, fever, malaise, syncope, cardiac arrhythmias, and fluid retention.

Anemia associated with chemotherapy can be managed by transfusion of packed RBCs. Transfusion is not undertaken until the hemoglobin falls to <80 g/L (8 g/dL) or if compromise of end organ function occurs, or an underlying condition (e.g., coronary artery disease) calls for maintenance of hemoglobin >90 g/L (9 g/dL). Patients who are to receive therapy for >2 months on a "stable" regimen and who are likely to require continuing transfusions are also candidates for erythropoietin (EPO). Randomized trials in certain tumors have raised the possibility that EPO use may promote tumor-related adverse events. This information should be considered in the care of individual patients. In the event EPO treatment is undertaken, maintenance of hemoglobin of 90–100 g/L (9–10 g/dL) should be the target. In the setting of adequate iron stores and serum EPO levels <100 ng/mL, EPO, 150 U three times a week, can produce a slow increase in hemoglobin over about 2 months of administration. Depot formulations can be administered less frequently. It is unclear whether higher hemoglobin levels, up to 110–120 g/L (11–12 g/dL), are associated with improved quality of life to a degree that justifies the more intensive EPO use. Efforts to achieve levels at or above 120 g/L (12 g/dL) have been associated with increased thromboses and mortality rates. EPO may rescue hypoxemic cells from death and contribute to tumor radioresistance.

Nausea and vomiting

The most common side effect of chemotherapy administration is nausea, with or without vomiting. Nausea may be acute (within 24 h of chemotherapy), delayed (>24 h), or anticipatory of the receipt of chemotherapy. Patients may be likewise stratified for their risk of susceptibility to nausea and vomiting, with increased risk in young, female, heavily pretreated patients without a history of alcohol or drug use but with a history of motion or morning sickness. Antineoplastic agents vary in their capacity to cause nausea and vomiting. Highly emetogenic drugs (>90%) include mechlorethamine, streptozotocin, DTIC, cyclophosphamide at >1500 mg/m^2, and cisplatin; moderately emetogenic drugs (30–90% risk) include carboplatin, cytosine arabinoside (>1 mg/m^2), ifosfamide, conventional-dose cyclophosphamide, and anthracyclines; low-risk (10–30%) agents include fluorouracil, taxanes, etoposide, and bortezomib, with minimal risk (<10%) afforded by treatment with antibodies, bleomycin, busulfan, fludarabine, and vinca alkaloids. *Emesis* is a reflex caused by stimulation of the vomiting center in the medulla. Input to the vomiting center comes from the chemoreceptor trigger zone (CTZ) and afferents from the peripheral gastrointestinal tract, cerebral cortex, and heart. The different emesis "syndromes" require distinct management approaches. In addition, a conditioned reflex may contribute to anticipatory nausea arising after repeated cycles of chemotherapy. Accordingly, antiemetic agents differ in their locus and timing of action. Combining agents from different classes or the sequential use of different classes of agent is the cornerstone of successful management of chemotherapy-induced nausea and vomiting. Of great importance are the prophylactic administration of agents, and such psychological techniques as the maintenance of a supportive milieu, counseling, and relaxation to augment the action of antiemetic agents.

Serotonin antagonists (5-HT3) and neurokine (NK1) receptor antagonists are useful in "high-risk" chemotherapy regimens. The combination acts at both peripheral gastrointestinal as well as CNS sites that control nausea and vomiting. For example, the 5-HT3 blocker dolasetron (Anzamet), 100 mg intravenously or orally; dexamethasone, 12 mg; and the NK1 antagonist aprepitant, 125 mg orally, are combined on the day of administration of severely emetogenic regimens, with repetition of dexamethasone (8 mg) and aprepitant (80 mg) on days 2 and 3 for delayed nausea. Alternate 5-HT3 antagonists include ondansetron (Zofran), given as 0.15 mg/kg intravenously for three doses just before and at 4 and 8 h after chemotherapy; palonosetron (Aloxi) at 0.25 mg over 30 s, 30 min prechemotherapy; and granisetron (Kytril), given as a single dose of 0.01 mg/kg just before chemotherapy. Emesis from moderately emetic chemotherapy regimens may be prevented with a 5-HT3 antagonist and dexamethasone alone for patients not receiving doxorubicin and cyclophosphamide combinations; the latter combination requires the 5-HT3/dexamethasone/aprepitant on day 1 but aprepitant alone on days 2 and 3. Emesis from low-emetic-risk regimens may be prevented with 8 mg of dexamethasone alone, or with non-5-HT3, non-NK1 antagonist approaches including the following.

Antidopaminergic phenothiazines act directly at the CTZ and include prochlorperazine (Compazine), 10 mg intramuscularly or intravenously, 10–25 mg orally or 25 mg per rectum every 4–6 h for up to four doses; and thiethylperazine (Torecan), 10 mg by potentially all the above routes every 6 h. Haloperidol (Haldol) is a butyrophenone dopamine antagonist given at 1.0 to 1 mg intramuscularly or orally every 8 h. Antihistamines such as diphenhydramine (Benadryl) have little intrinsic antiemetic capacity but are frequently given to prevent or treat dystonic reactions that can complicate use of the antidopaminergic agents. Lorazepam (Ativan) is a short-acting benzodiazepine that provides an anxiolytic effect to augment the effectiveness of a variety of agents when used at 1–2 mg intramuscularly, intravenously, or orally every 4–6 h. Metoclopramide (Reglan) acts on peripheral dopamine receptors to augment gastric emptying and is used in high doses for highly emetogenic regimens (1–2 mg/kg intravenously 30 min before chemotherapy and every 2 h for up to three additional doses as needed); intravenous doses of 10–20 mg every 4–6 h as needed or 50 mg orally 4 h before and 8 and 12 h after chemotherapy are used for moderately emetogenic regimens. 5-9-Tetrahydrocannabinol (Marinol) is a rather weak antiemetic compared to other available agents, but it may be useful for persisting nausea and is used orally at 10 mg every 3–4 h as needed.

Diarrhea

Regimens that include fluorouracil infusions and/or irinotecan may produce severe diarrhea. Similar to the vomiting syndromes, chemotherapy-induced diarrhea may be immediate or can occur in a delayed fashion up to 48–72 h after the drugs. Careful attention to maintained hydration and electrolyte repletion, intravenously if necessary, along with antimotility treatments such as "high-dose" loperamide, commenced with 4 mg at the first occurrence of diarrhea, with 2 mg repeated every 2 h until 12 h without loose stools, not to exceed a total daily dose of 16 mg. Octreotide (100–150 μg), a somatostatin analogue, or opiate-based preparations may be considered for patients not responding to loperamide.

Mucositis

Irritation and inflammation of the mucous membranes particularly afflicting the oral and anal mucosa, but potentially involving the gastrointestinal tract, may accompany cytotoxic chemotherapy. Mucositis is due to damage to the proliferating cells at the base of the mucosal squamous epithelia or in the intestinal crypts. Topical therapies, including anesthetics and barrier-creating preparations, may provide symptomatic relief in mild cases. Palifermin or keratinocyte growth factor, a member of the fibroblast growth factor family, is effective in preventing severe mucositis in the setting of high-dose chemotherapy with stem cell transplantation for hematologic malignancies. It may also prevent or ameliorate mucositis from radiation.

Alopecia

Chemotherapeutic agents vary widely in causing alopecia, with anthracyclines, alkylating agents, and topoisomerase inhibitors reliably causing near-total alopecia when given at therapeutic doses. Antimetabolites are more variably associated with alopecia. Psychological support and the use of cosmetic resources are to be encouraged, and "chemo caps" that reduce scalp temperature to decrease the degree of alopecia should be discouraged, particularly during treatment with curative intent of neoplasms, such as leukemia or lymphoma, or in adjuvant breast cancer therapy. The richly vascularized scalp can certainly harbor micrometastatic or disseminated disease.

Gonadal dysfunction and pregnancy

Cessation of ovulation and azoospermia reliably result from alkylating agent– and topoisomerase poison–containing regimens. The duration of these effects varies with age and sex. Males treated for Hodgkin's disease with mechlorethamine- and procarbazine-containing regimens are effectively sterile, whereas fertility usually returns after regimens that include cisplatin, vinblastine, or etoposide and after bleomycin for testicular cancer. Sperm banking before treatment may be considered to support patients likely to be sterilized by treatment. Females experience amenorrhea with anovulation after alkylating agent therapy; they are likely to recover normal menses if treatment is completed before age 30 but unlikely to recover menses after age 35. Even those who regain menses usually experience premature menopause. As the magnitude and extent of decreased fertility can be difficult to predict, patients should be counseled to maintain effective contraception, preferably by barrier means, during and after therapy. Resumption of efforts to conceive should be considered in the context of the patient's likely prognosis. Hormone replacement therapy should be undertaken in women who do not have a hormonally responsive tumor. For those patients who have had a hormone-sensitive tumor primarily treated by a local modality, conventional practice would counsel against hormone replacement, but this issue is under investigation.

Chemotherapy agents have variable effects on the success of pregnancy. All agents tend to have increased risk of adverse outcomes when administered during the first trimester, and strategies to delay chemotherapy, if possible, until after this milestone should be considered if the pregnancy is to continue to term. Patients in their second or third trimester can be treated with most regimens for the common neoplasms afflicting women in their childbearing years, with the exception of antimetabolites, particularly antifolates, which have notable teratogenic or fetotoxic effects throughout pregnancy. The need for anticancer chemotherapy per se is infrequently a clear basis to recommend termination of a concurrent pregnancy, although each treatment strategy in this circumstance must be tailored to the individual needs of the patient. Chronic effects of cancer treatment are reviewed in Chap. 102.

BIOLOGIC THERAPY

The goal of biologic therapy is to manipulate the host–tumor interaction in favor of the host, potentially at an optimum biologic dose that might be different than an MTD. As a class, biologic therapies may be distinguished from molecularly targeted agents in that many biologic therapies require an active response (e.g., reexpression of silenced genes, or antigen expression) on the part of the tumor cell or on the part of the host (e.g., immunologic effects) to allow therapeutic effect. This may be contrasted with the more narrowly defined antiproliferative or apoptotic response that is the ultimate goal of molecularly targeted agents discussed above. However, there is much commonality in the strategies to evaluate and use molecularly targeted and biologic therapies.

■ IMMUNE MEDIATORS OF ANTITUMOR EFFECTS

Tumors have a variety of means of avoiding the immune system: (1) they are often only subtly different from their normal counterparts; (2) they are capable of downregulating their major histocompatibility complex antigens, effectively masking them from recognition by T cells; (3) they are inefficient at presenting antigens to the immune system; (4) they can cloak themselves in a protective shell of fibrin to minimize contact with surveillance mechanisms; and (5) they can produce a range of soluble molecules, including potential immune targets, that can distract the immune system from recognizing the tumor cell or can kill the immune effector cells. Some of the cell products initially polarize the immune response away from cellular immunity (shifting from T_H1 to T_H2 responses; Chap. 314) and ultimately lead to defects in T cells that prevent their activation and cytotoxic activity. Cancer treatment further suppresses host immunity. A variety of strategies are being tested to overcome these barriers.

Cell-mediated immunity

The strongest evidence that the immune system can exert clinically meaningful antitumor effects comes from allogeneic bone marrow transplantation. Adoptively transferred T cells from the donor expand in the tumor-bearing host, recognize the tumor as being foreign, and can mediate impressive antitumor effects (graft-versus-tumor effects). Three types of experimental interventions are being developed to take advantage of the ability of T cells to kill tumor cells.

1. Allogeneic T cells are transferred to cancer-bearing hosts in three major settings: in the form of allogeneic bone marrow transplantation, as pure lymphocyte transfusions following bone marrow recovery after allogeneic bone marrow transplantation, and as pure lymphocyte transfusions following immunosuppressive (but not myeloablative) therapy (so-called minitransplants). In each of these settings, the effector cells are donor T cells that recognize the tumor as being foreign, probably through minor histocompatibility differences. The main risk of such therapy is the development of graft-versus-host disease because of the minimal difference between the cancer and the normal host cells. This approach has been highly effective in certain hematologic cancers.

2. Autologous T cells are removed from the tumor-bearing host, manipulated in several ways in vitro, and given back to the patient. The two major classes of autologous T cell manipulation

are (a) to develop tumor antigen–specific T cells and expand them to large numbers over many weeks ex vivo before administration, and (b) to activate the cells with polyclonal stimulators such as anti-CD3 and anti-CD28 after a short period ex vivo and try to expand them in the host after adoptive transfer with stimulation by IL-2, for example. Short periods removed from the patient permit the cells to overcome the tumor-induced T cell defects, and such cells traffic and home to sites of disease better than cells that have been in culture for many weeks.

3. Tumor vaccines are aimed at boosting T cell immunity. The finding that mutant oncogenes that are expressed only intracellularly can be recognized as targets of T cell killing greatly expanded the possibilities for tumor vaccine development. No longer is it difficult to find something different about tumor cells. However, major difficulties remain in getting the tumor-specific peptides presented in a fashion to prime the T cells. Tumors themselves are very poor at presenting their own antigens to T cells at the first antigen exposure (*priming*). Priming is best accomplished by professional antigen-presenting cells (dendritic cells). Thus, a number of experimental strategies are aimed at priming host T cells against tumor-associated peptides. Vaccine adjuvants such as GM-CSF appear capable of attracting antigen-presenting cells to a skin site containing a tumor antigen. Such an approach has been documented to eradicate microscopic residual disease in follicular lymphoma and give rise to tumor-specific T cells. Purified antigen-presenting cells can be pulsed with tumor, its membranes, or particular tumor antigens and delivered as a vaccine. One such vaccine, Sipuleucel-T, is approved for use in patients with hormone-independent prostate cancer. In this approach, the patient undergoes leukapheresis, wherein mononuclear cells (that include antigen-presenting cells) are removed from the patient's blood. The cells are pulsed in a laboratory with an antigenic fusion protein comprising a protein frequently expressed by prostate cancer cells, prostate acid phosphatase, fused to GM-CSF, and matured to increase their capacity to present the antigen to immune effector cells. The cells are then returned to the patient, in a well-tolerated treatment. While no objective tumor response was documented, median survival was increased about 4 months. Tumor cells can also be transfected with genes that attract antigen-presenting cells. Vaccines against viruses that cause cancers are safe and effective. Hepatitis B vaccine prevents hepatocellular carcinoma, and a tetravalent human papilloma virus vaccine prevents infection by virus types currently accounting for 70% of cervical cancer. These vaccines are ineffective at treating patients who have developed a virus-induced cancer.

Antibodies

In general, antibodies are not very effective at killing cancer cells. Because the tumor seems to influence the host toward making antibodies rather than generating cellular immunity, it is inferred that antibodies are easier for the tumor to fend off. Many patients can be shown to have serum antibodies directed at their tumors, but these do not appear to influence disease progression. However, the ability to grow very large quantities of high-affinity antibody directed at a tumor by the hybridoma technique has led to the application of antibodies to the treatment of cancer.

Clinical antitumor efficacy has been obtained using antibodies where the antigen-combining regions are grafted onto human immunoglobulin gene products (chimerized or humanized) or derive de novo from mice bearing human immunoglobulin gene loci. Such humanized antibodies against the CD20 molecule expressed on B cell lymphomas (rituximab) and against the HER-2/neu receptor overexpressed on epithelial cancers, especially breast cancer (trastuzumab), have become reliable tools in the oncologist's armamentarium. Each used alone can cause tumor regression (rituximab more than trastuzumab), and both appear to potentiate the effects of combination chemotherapy given just after antibody administration. Antibodies to CD52 are active in chronic lymphoid leukemia and T cell malignancies. EGF-R–directed antibodies (such as cetuximab and panitumumab) have activity in colorectal cancer refractory to chemotherapy, particularly when utilized to augment the activity of an additional chemotherapy program, and in the primary treatment of head and neck cancers treated with radiation therapy. The mechanism of action is unclear. Direct effects on the tumor may mediate an antiproliferative effect as well as stimulate the participation of host mechanisms involving immune cell or complement-mediated response to tumor cell–bound antibody. Alternatively, the antibody may alter the release of paracrine factors promoting tumor cell survival.

The anti-VEGF antibody bevacizumab shows little evidence of antitumor effect when used alone, but when combined with chemotherapeutic agents it improves the magnitude of tumor shrinkage and time to disease progression in colorectal, lung, and breast cancer. The mechanism for the effect is unclear and may relate to the capacity of the antibody to alter delivery and tumor uptake of the active chemotherapeutic agent.

Side effects include infusion-related hypersensitivity reactions, usually limited to the first infusion, which can be managed with glucocorticoid and/or antihistamine prophylaxis. In addition, distinct syndromes have emerged with different antibodies. Anti-EGF-R antibodies produce an acneiform rash that poorly responds to steroid cream treatment. Trastuzumab (anti-HER2) can inhibit cardiac function, particularly in those patients with prior exposure to anthracyclines. Bevacizumab has a number of side effects of medical significance, including hypertension, thrombosis, proteinuria, hemorrhage, and gastrointestinal perforations with or without prior surgeries.

Conjugation of antibodies to drugs and toxins is discussed above; conjugates of antibodies with isotopes, photodynamic agents, and other killing moieties may also be effective. Radioconjugates targeting CD20 on lymphomas have been approved for use [ibritumomab tiuxetan (Zevalin), using yttrium-90 or ^{131}I-tositumomab]. Other conjugates are associated with problems that have not yet been solved (e.g., antigenicity, instability, poor tumor penetration).

Cytokines

There are >70 separate proteins and glycoproteins with biologic effects in humans: interferon (IFN) α, β, γ; IL-1 through -29 (so far); the tumor necrosis factor (TNF) family [including lymphotoxin, TNF-related apoptosis-inducing ligand (TRAIL), CD40 ligand, and others]; and the chemokine family. Only a fraction of these has been tested against cancer; only IFN-α and IL-2 are in routine clinical use.

About 20 different genes encode IFN-α, and their biologic effects are indistinguishable. Interferon induces the expression of many genes, inhibits protein synthesis, and exerts a number of different effects on diverse cellular processes. The two recombinant forms that are commercially available are IFN-α2a and -α2b. Interferon is not curative for any tumor but can induce partial responses in follicular lymphoma, hairy cell leukemia, CML, melanoma, and Kaposi's sarcoma. It has been used in the adjuvant setting in stage II

melanoma, multiple myeloma, and follicular lymphoma, with uncertain effects on survival. It produces fever, fatigue, a flulike syndrome, malaise, myelosuppression, and depression and can induce clinically significant autoimmune disease.

IL-2 must exert its antitumor effects indirectly through augmentation of immune function. Its biologic activity is to promote the growth and activity of T cells and natural killer (NK) cells. High doses of IL-2 can produce tumor regression in certain patients with metastatic melanoma and renal cell cancer. About 2–5% of patients may experience complete remissions that are durable, unlike any other treatment for these tumors. IL-2 is associated with myriad clinical side effects: intravascular volume depletion, capillary leak syndrome, adult respiratory distress syndrome, hypotension, fever, chills, skin rash, and impaired renal and liver function. Patients may require blood pressure support and intensive care to manage the toxicity. However, once the agent is stopped, most of the toxicities reverse completely within 3–6 days.

GENE THERAPIES

No gene therapy has been approved for routine clinical use. Several strategies are under evaluation, including the use of viruses that cannot replicate to express genes that can allow the action of drugs or directly inhibit cancer cell growth, viruses that can actually replicate but only in the context of the tumor cell, or viruses that can express antigens in the context of the tumor and therefore provoke a host-mediated immune response. Key issues in the success of these approaches will be in defining safe viral vector systems that escape host immune function and effectively target the tumor or tumor cell milieu. Other gene therapy strategies would utilize therapeutic oligonucleotides to target the expression of genes important in the maintenance of tumor cell viability.

ACKNOWLEDGMENTS

Stephen M. Hahn, MD, and Eli Glatstein, MD, contributed a chapter on radiation therapy in a prior edition, and some of their material has been incorporated into this chapter.

FURTHER READINGS

American Society of Clinical Oncology: 2006 Update of recommendations for the use of white blood cell growth factors: An evidence-based clinical practice guideline. J Clin Oncol 24:3187, 2006

Chabner BA, Longo DL (eds): *Cancer Chemotherapy and Biotherapy: Principles and Practice*, 5th ed. Philadelphia, Lippincott Williams & Wilkins, 2011

Ettinger DS et al: Antiemesis: Clinical practice guidelines in oncology. J Natl Compr Cancer Network 7:572, 2009

McDermott U, Settleman J: Personalized cancer therapy with selective kinase inhibitors: An emerging paradigm in medical oncology. J Clin Oncol 27: 5650, 2009

Olopade OI et al. Advances in breast cancer: Pathways to personalized medicine. Clin Cancer Res 14: 7988, 2008

Rizzo JD et al: ASCO special article: Use of epoetin and darbepoetin in patients with cancer: 2007 American Society of Clinical Oncology / American Society of Hematology Clinical Practice Guideline update. J Clin Oncol 26, 132, 2008

CHAPTER 86

Infections in Patients With Cancer

Robert Finberg

Infections are a common cause of death and an even more common cause of morbidity in patients with a wide variety of neoplasms. Autopsy studies show that most deaths from acute leukemia and half of deaths from lymphoma are caused directly by infection. With more intensive chemotherapy, patients with solid tumors have also become more likely to die of infection. Fortunately, an evolving approach to prevention and treatment of infectious complications of cancer has decreased infection-associated mortality rates and will probably continue to do so. This accomplishment has resulted from three major steps:

1. The concept of "early empirical" antibiotics reduced mortality rates among patients with leukemia and bacteremia from 84% in 1965 to 44% in 1972. This dramatic improvement is attributed to early intervention with appropriate antimicrobial therapy.
2. "Empirical" antifungal therapy has lowered the incidence of disseminated fungal infection; in trial settings, mortality rates now range from 7% to 21%. An antifungal agent is administered—on the basis of likely fungal infection—to neutropenic patients who, after 4–7 days of antibiotic therapy, remain febrile but have no positive cultures. In one study, the 7-day survival rate was ~85% among patients who had fever and neutropenia as a result of cancer chemotherapy and who required antifungal therapy.

3. Use of antibiotics for afebrile neutropenic patients as broad-spectrum prophylaxis against infections has decreased both mortality and morbidity even further. The current approach to treatment of severely neutropenic patients (e.g., those receiving high-dose chemotherapy for leukemia or high-grade lymphomas) is based on initial prophylactic therapy at the onset of neutropenia, with subsequent "empirical" antibacterial therapy targeting the organisms whose involvement is likely in light of physical findings (most often fever alone), and finally "empirical" antifungal therapy based on the known likelihood that fungal infection will become a serious issue after 4–7 days of broad-spectrum antibacterial therapy.

A physical predisposition to infection in patients with cancer (Table 86-1) can be a result of the neoplasm's production of a break in the skin. For example, a squamous cell carcinoma may cause local invasion of the epidermis, which allows bacteria to gain access to the subcutaneous tissue and permits the development of cellulitis. The artificial closing of a normally patent orifice can also predispose to infection; for example, obstruction of a ureter by a tumor can cause urinary tract infection, and obstruction of the bile duct can cause cholangitis. Part of the host's normal defense against infection depends on the continuous emptying of a viscus; without emptying, a few bacteria that are present as a result of bacteremia or local transit can multiply and cause disease.

A similar problem can affect patients whose lymph node integrity has been disrupted by radical surgery, particularly patients who have had radical node dissections. A common clinical problem following radical mastectomy is the development of cellulitis (usually caused by streptococci or staphylococci) because of lymphedema and/or inadequate lymph drainage. In most cases, this

TABLE 86-1 Disruption of Normal Barriers That May Predispose to Infections in Patients With Cancer

Type of Defense	Specific Lesion	Cells Involved	Organism	Cancer Association	Disease
Physical barrier	Breaks in skin	Skin epithelial cells	Staphylococci, streptococci	Head and neck, squamous cell carcinoma	Cellulitis, extensive skin infection
Emptying of fluid collections	Occlusion of orifices: ureters, bile duct, colon	Luminal epithelial cells	Gram-negative bacilli	Renal, ovarian, biliary tree, metastatic diseases of many cancers	Rapid, overwhelming bacteremia; urinary tract infection
Lymphatic function	Node dissection	Lymph nodes	Staphylococci, streptococci	Breast cancer surgery	Cellulitis
Splenic clearance of microorganisms	Splenectomy	Splenic reticuloendothelial cells	*Streptococcus pneumoniae, Haemophilus influenzae, Neisseria meningitidis, Babesia, Capnocytophaga canimorsus*	Hodgkin's disease, leukemia, idiopathic thrombocytopenic purpura	Rapid, overwhelming sepsis
Phagocytosis	Lack of granulocytes	Granulocytes (neutrophils)	Staphylococci, streptococci, enteric organisms, fungi	Hairy cell, acute myelocytic, and acute lymphocytic leukemias	Bacteremia
Humoral immunity	Lack of antibody	B cells	*S. pneumoniae, H. influenzae, N. meningitidis*	Chronic lymphocytic leukemia, multiple myeloma	Infections with encapsulated organisms, sinusitis, pneumonia
Cellular immunity	Lack of T cells	T cells and macrophages	*Mycobacterium tuberculosis, Listeria,* herpesviruses, fungi, intracellular parasites	Hodgkin's disease, leukemia, T cell lymphoma	Infections with intracellular bacteria, fungi, parasites

problem can be addressed by local measures designed to prevent fluid accumulation and breaks in the skin, but antibiotic prophylaxis has been necessary in refractory cases.

A life-threatening problem common to many cancer patients is the loss of the reticuloendothelial capacity to clear microorganisms after splenectomy, which may be performed as part of the management of hairy cell leukemia, chronic lymphocytic leukemia (CLL), and chronic myelocytic leukemia (CML) and in Hodgkin's disease. Even after curative therapy for the underlying disease, the lack of a spleen predisposes such patients to rapidly fatal infections. The loss of the spleen through trauma similarly predisposes the normal host to overwhelming infection throughout life. The splenectomized patient should be counseled about the risks of infection with certain organisms, such as the protozoan *Babesia* (Chap. 211) and *Capnocytophaga canimorsus*, a bacterium carried in the mouths of animals (Chaps. 146 and e24). Since encapsulated bacteria (*Streptococcus pneumoniae*, *Haemophilus influenzae*, and *Neisseria meningitidis*) are the organisms most commonly associated with postsplenectomy sepsis, splenectomized persons should be vaccinated (and revaccinated; Table 86-2 and Chap. 122) against the capsular polysaccharides of these organisms. Many clinicians recommend giving splenectomized patients a small supply of antibiotics effective against *S. pneumoniae*, *N. meningitidis*, and *H. influenzae* to avert rapid, overwhelming sepsis in the event that they cannot present for medical attention immediately after the onset of fever or other signs or symptoms of bacterial infection. A few amoxicillin/clavulanic acid tablets are a reasonable choice for this purpose.

The level of suspicion of infections with certain organisms should depend on the type of cancer diagnosed (Table 86-3). Diagnosis of multiple myeloma or CLL should alert the clinician to the possibility of hypogammaglobulinemia. While immunoglobulin replacement therapy can be effective, in most cases prophylactic antibiotics are a cheaper, more convenient method of eliminating bacterial infections in CLL patients with hypogammaglobulinemia. Patients with acute lymphocytic leukemia (ALL), patients with non-Hodgkin's lymphoma, and all cancer patients treated with high-dose glucocorticoids (or glucocorticoid-containing chemotherapy regimens) should receive antibiotic prophylaxis for *Pneumocystis* infection (Table 86-3) for the duration of their chemotherapy. In addition to exhibiting susceptibility to certain infectious organisms, patients with cancer are likely to manifest their infections in characteristic ways. For example, fever—generally a sign of infection in normal hosts—continues to be a reliable indicator in neutropenic patients. In contrast, patients receiving glucocorticoids and agents that impair T cell function and cytokine secretion may have serious infections in the absence of fever. Similarly, neutropenic patients commonly present with cellulitis without purulence and with pneumonia without sputum or even x-ray findings (see below).

TABLE 86-2 Vaccination of Cancer Patients Receiving Chemotherapy[a]

| Vaccine | Use in Indicated Patients | | |
	Intensive Chemotherapy	Hodgkin's Disease	Hematopoietic Stem Cell Transplantation
Diphtheria-tetanus[b]	Primary series and boosters as necessary	No special recommendation	3 doses given 6–12 months after transplantation
Poliomyelitis[c]	Complete primary series and boosters	No special recommendation	3 doses given 6–12 months after transplantation
Haemophilus influenzae type b conjugate	Primary series and booster for children	Immunization before treatment and booster 3 months afterward	3 doses given 6–12 months after transplantation
Human papillomavirus	3 doses for girls and women through 26 years of age	3 doses for girls and women through 26 years of age	3 doses for girls and women through 26 years of age
Hepatitis A	As indicated for normal hosts based on occupation and lifestyle	As indicated for normal hosts based on occupation and lifestyle	As indicated for normal hosts based on occupation and lifestyle
Hepatitis B	Same as for normal hosts	As indicated for normal hosts based on occupation and lifestyle	3 doses given 6–12 months after transplantation
23-Valent pneumococcal polysaccharide[d]	Every 5 years	Immunization before treatment and booster 3 months afterward	1 or 2 doses given 6–12 months after transplantation
4-Valent meningococcal vaccine[e]	Should be administered to splenectomized patients and patients living in endemic areas, including college students in dormitories	Should be administered to splenectomized patients and patients living in endemic areas, including college students in dormitories	Should be administered to splenectomized patients and patients living in endemic areas, including college students in dormitories
Influenza	Seasonal immunization	Seasonal immunization	Seasonal immunization
Measles/mumps/rubella	Contraindicated	Contraindicated during chemotherapy	After 24 months in patients without graft-versus-host disease
Varicella-zoster virus[f]	Contraindicated[g]	Contraindicated	Contraindicated

[a]The latest recommendations by the Advisory Committee on Immunization Practices and the CDC guidelines can be found at *http://www.cdc.gov/vaccines.*
[b]The Td (tetanus-diphtheria) combination was recommended for adults. Pertussis vaccine was not recommended for people >6 years of age in the past. However, recent data indicate that the Tdap (tetanus–diphtheria–acellular pertussis) product is both safe and efficacious in adults. A single Tdap booster is now recommended for adults.
[c]Live-virus vaccine is contraindicated; inactivated vaccine should be used.
[d]The 7- and 13-valent pneumococcal conjugate vaccines are currently recommended for children.
[e]Meningococcal conjugate vaccine (MCV4) is recommended for adults ≤55 years old and meningococcal polysaccharide vaccine (MPSV4) for those ≥56 years old.
[f]Includes both varicella vaccine for children and zoster vaccine for adults.
[g]Contact the manufacturer for more information on use in children with acute lymphocytic leukemia.

TABLE 86-3 Infections Associated With Specific Types of Cancer

Cancer	Underlying Immune Abnormality	Organisms Causing Infection
Multiple myeloma	Hypogammaglobulinemia	*Streptococcus pneumoniae, Haemophilus influenzae, Neisseria meningitidis*
Chronic lymphocytic leukemia	Hypogammaglobulinemia	*S. pneumoniae, H. influenzae, N. meningitidis*
Acute myelocytic or lymphocytic leukemia	Granulocytopenia, skin and mucous-membrane lesions	Extracellular gram-positive and gram-negative bacteria, fungi
Hodgkin's disease	Abnormal T cell function	Intracellular pathogens (*Mycobacterium tuberculosis, Listeria, Salmonella, Cryptococcus, Mycobacterium avium*)
Non-Hodgkin's lymphoma and acute lymphocytic leukemia	Glucocorticoid chemotherapy, T and B cell dysfunction	*Pneumocystis*
Colon and rectal tumors	Local abnormalities[a]	*Streptococcus bovis* (bacteremia)
Hairy cell leukemia	Abnormal T cell function	Intracellular pathogens (*M. tuberculosis, Listeria, Cryptococcus, M. avium*)

[a]The reason for this association is not well defined.

The use of monoclonal antibodies that target B and T cells as well as drugs that interfere with lymphocyte signal transduction events is associated with reactivation of latent infections. The use of rituximab, the antibody to CD20 (a B–cell surface protein), is associated with the development of reactivation tuberculosis as well as hepatitis B, cytomegalovirus (CMV) infection, and other latent infections. Like organ transplant recipients (Chap. 132), patients with positive purified protein derivative tests and underlying viral infection should be carefully monitored for reactivation disease.

SYSTEM-SPECIFIC SYNDROMES

■ SKIN-SPECIFIC SYNDROMES

Skin lesions are common in cancer patients, and the appearance of these lesions may permit the diagnosis of systemic bacterial or fungal infection. While cellulitis caused by skin organisms such as

Streptococcus or *Staphylococcus* is common, neutropenic patients—i.e., those with <500 functional polymorphonuclear leukocytes (PMNs)/μL—and patients with impaired blood or lymphatic drainage may develop infections with unusual organisms. Innocent-looking macules or papules may be the first sign of bacterial or fungal sepsis in immunocompromised patients (Fig. 86-1). In the neutropenic host, a macule progresses rapidly to ecthyma gangrenosum (Fig. e7-35), a usually painless, round, necrotic lesion consisting of a central black or gray-black eschar with surrounding erythema. Ecthyma gangrenosum, which is located in non-pressure areas (as distinguished from necrotic lesions associated with lack of circulation), is often associated with *Pseudomonas aeruginosa* bacteremia (Chap. 152) but may be caused by other bacteria.

Candidemia (Chap. 203) is also associated with a variety of skin conditions (Fig. e7-38) and commonly presents as a maculopapular rash. Punch biopsy of the skin may be the best method for diagnosis.

Cellulitis, an acute spreading inflammation of the skin, is most often caused by infection with group A *Streptococcus* or *Staphylococcus aureus*, virulent organisms normally found on the skin (Chap. 125). Although cellulitis tends to be circumscribed in normal hosts, it may spread rapidly in neutropenic patients. A tiny break in the skin may lead to spreading cellulitis, which is characterized by pain and erythema; in the affected patients, signs of infection (e.g., purulence) are often lacking. What might be a furuncle in a normal host may require amputation because of uncontrolled infection in a patient presenting with leukemia. A dramatic response to an infection that might be trivial in a normal host can mark the first sign of leukemia. Fortunately, granulocytopenic patients are likely to be infected with certain types of organisms (Table 86-4); thus the selection of an antibiotic regimen is somewhat easier than it might otherwise be (see "Antibacterial Therapy," below). It is essential

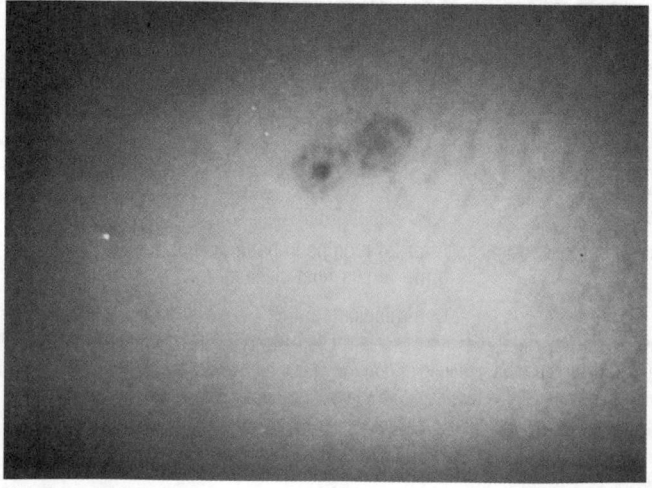
A

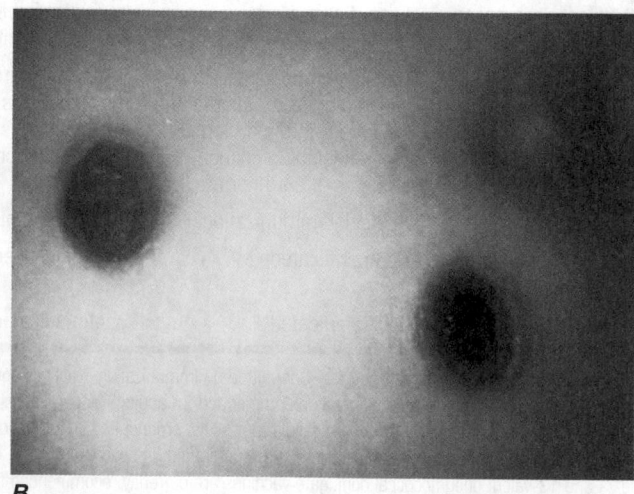
B

Figure 86-1 *A.* Papules related to *Escherichia coli* bacteremia in a neutropenic patient with acute lymphocytic leukemia. *B.* The same lesion the following day.

TABLE 86-4 Organisms Likely to Cause Infections in Granulocytopenic Patients

Gram-positive cocci	*Enterobacter* spp.
Staphylococcus epidermidis	*Serratia* spp.
Staphylococcus aureus	*Acinetobacter* spp.[a]
Viridans *Streptococcus*	*Citrobacter* spp.
Enterococcus faecalis	**Gram-positive bacilli**
Streptococcus pneumoniae	Diphtheroids
Gram-negative bacilli	JK bacillus[a]
Escherichia coli	**Fungi**
Klebsiella spp.	*Candida* spp.
Pseudomonas aeruginosa	*Aspergillus* spp.
Non-*aeruginosa Pseudomonas* spp.[a]	

[a]Often associated with intravenous catheters.

to recognize cellulitis early and to treat it aggressively. Patients who are neutropenic or have previously received antibiotics for other reasons may develop cellulitis with unusual organisms (e.g., *Escherichia coli, Pseudomonas,* or fungi). Early treatment, even of innocent-looking lesions, is essential to prevent necrosis and loss of tissue. Debridement to prevent spread may sometimes be necessary early in the course of disease, but it can often be performed after chemotherapy, when the PMN count increases.

Sweet's syndrome, or *febrile neutrophilic dermatosis,* was originally described in women with elevated white blood cell (WBC) counts. The disease is characterized by the presence of leukocytes in the lower dermis, with edema of the papillary body. Ironically, this disease now is usually seen in neutropenic patients with cancer, most often in association with acute leukemia but also in association with a variety of other malignancies. Sweet's syndrome usually presents as red or bluish-red papules or nodules that may coalesce and form sharply bordered plaques (Fig. e7-41). The edema may suggest vesicles, but on palpation the lesions are solid, and vesicles probably never arise in this disease. The lesions are most common on the face, neck, and arms. On the legs, they may be confused with erythema nodosum (Fig. e7-40). The development of lesions is often accompanied by high fevers and an elevated erythrocyte sedimentation rate. Both the lesions and the temperature elevation respond dramatically to glucocorticoid administration. Treatment begins with high doses of glucocorticoids (60 mg/d of prednisone) followed by tapered doses over the next 2–3 weeks.

Data indicate that *erythema multiforme* (Fig. e7-25) with mucous membrane involvement is often associated with herpes simplex virus (HSV) infection and is distinct from Stevens-Johnson syndrome, which is associated with drugs and tends to have a more widespread distribution. Since cancer patients are both immunosuppressed [and therefore susceptible to herpes infections) and heavily treated with drugs and therefore subject to Stevens-Johnson syndrome (Fig. e12-4)], both of these conditions are common in this population.

Cytokines, which are used as adjuvants or primary treatments for cancer, can themselves cause characteristic rashes, further complicating the differential diagnosis. This phenomenon is a particular problem in bone marrow transplant recipients (Chap. 132), who, in addition to having the usual chemotherapy-, antibiotic-, and cytokine-induced rashes, are plagued by graft-versus-host disease.

■ CATHETER-RELATED INFECTIONS

Because IV catheters are commonly used in cancer chemotherapy and are prone to infection (Chap. 131), they pose a major problem in the care of patients with cancer. Some catheter-associated infections can be treated with antibiotics, while in others the catheter must be removed (Table 86-5). If the patient has a "tunneled"

TABLE 86-5 Approach to Catheter Infections in Immunocompromised Patients

Clinical Presentation	Catheter Removal	Antibiotics	Comments
Evidence of Infection, Negative Blood Cultures			
Exit-site erythema	Not necessary if infection responds to treatment	Usually begin treatment for gram-positive cocci.	Coagulase-negative staphylococci are most common.
Tunnel-site erythema	Required	Treat for gram-positive cocci pending culture results.	Failure to remove the catheter may lead to complications.
Blood Culture–Positive Infections			
Coagulase-negative staphylococci	Line removal optimal but may be unnecessary if patient is clinically stable and responds to antibiotics	Usually start with vancomycin. (Linezolid, quinupristin/dalfopristin, and daptomycin are all appropriate.)	If there are no contraindications to line removal, this course of action is optimal. If the line is removed, antibiotics may not be necessary.
Other gram-positive cocci (e.g., *Staphylococcus aureus, Enterococcus*); gram-positive rods (*Bacillus, Corynebacterium* spp.)	Recommended	Treat with antibiotics to which the organism is sensitive, with duration based on the clinical setting.	The incidence of metastatic infections following *S. aureus* infection and the difficulty of treating enterococcal infection make line removal the recommended course of action. In addition, gram-positive rods do not respond readily to antibiotics alone.
Gram-negative bacteria	Recommended	Use an agent to which the organism is shown to be sensitive.	Organisms like *Stenotrophomonas, Pseudomonas,* and *Burkholderia* are notoriously hard to treat.
Fungi	Recommended	—	Fungal infections of catheters are extremely difficult to treat.

catheter (which consists of an entrance site, a subcutaneous tunnel, and an exit site), a red streak over the subcutaneous part of the line (the tunnel) is grounds for immediate device removal. Failure to remove catheters under these circumstances may result in extensive cellulitis and tissue necrosis.

More common than tunnel infections are exit-site infections, often with erythema around the area where the line penetrates the skin. Most authorities (Chap. 135) recommend treatment (usually with vancomycin) for an exit-site infection caused by coagulase-negative *Staphylococcus*. Treatment of coagulase-positive staphylococcal infection is associated with a poorer outcome, and it is advisable to remove the catheter if possible. Similarly, many clinicians remove catheters associated with infections due to *P. aeruginosa* and *Candida* species, since such infections are difficult to treat and bloodstream infections with these organisms are likely to be deadly. Catheter infections caused by *Burkholderia cepacia*, *Stenotrophomonas* spp., *Agrobacterium* spp., and *Acinetobacter baumannii* as well as *Pseudomonas* spp. other than *aeruginosa* are likely to be very difficult to eradicate with antibiotics alone. Similarly, isolation of *Bacillus*, *Corynebacterium*, and *Mycobacterium* spp. should prompt removal of the catheter.

■ GASTROINTESTINAL TRACT–SPECIFIC SYNDROMES

Upper gastrointestinal tract disease

Infections of the mouth The oral cavity is rich in aerobic and anaerobic bacteria (Chap. 164) that normally live in a commensal relationship with the host. The antimetabolic effects of chemotherapy cause a breakdown of host defenses, leading to ulceration of the mouth and the potential for invasion by resident bacteria. Mouth ulcerations afflict most patients receiving cytotoxic chemotherapy and have been associated with viridans streptococcal bacteremia. *Candida* infections of the mouth are very common. Fluconazole is clearly effective in the treatment of both local infections (thrush) and systemic infections (esophagitis) due to *Candida albicans*. Other azoles (e.g., voriconazole) as well as echinocandins offer similar efficacy as well as activity against the fluconazole-resistant organisms that are associated with extensive fluconazole treatment (Chap. 203).

Noma (*cancrum oris*), commonly seen in malnourished children, is a penetrating disease of the soft and hard tissues of the mouth and adjacent sites, with resulting necrosis and gangrene. It has a counterpart in immunocompromised patients and is thought to be due to invasion of the tissues by *Bacteroides*, *Fusobacterium*, and other normal inhabitants of the mouth. Noma is associated with debility, poor oral hygiene, and immunosuppression.

Viruses, particularly HSV, are a prominent cause of morbidity in immunocompromised patients, in whom they are associated with severe mucositis. The use of acyclovir, either prophylactically or therapeutically, is of value.

Esophageal infections The differential diagnosis of esophagitis (usually presenting as substernal chest pain upon swallowing) includes herpes simplex and candidiasis, both of which are readily treatable.

Lower gastrointestinal tract disease

Hepatic candidiasis (Chap. 203) results from seeding of the liver (usually from a gastrointestinal source) in neutropenic patients. It is most common among patients being treated for acute leukemia and usually presents symptomatically around the time the neutropenia resolves. The characteristic picture is that of persistent fever unresponsive to antibiotics, abdominal pain and tenderness or nausea, and elevated serum levels of alkaline phosphatase in a patient with hematologic malignancy who has recently recovered from neutropenia. The diagnosis of this disease (which may present in an indolent

manner and persist for several months) is based on the finding of yeasts or pseudohyphae in granulomatous lesions. Hepatic ultrasound or CT may reveal bull's-eye lesions. In some cases, MRI reveals small lesions not visible by other imaging modalities. The pathology (a granulomatous response) and the timing (with resolution of neutropenia and an elevation in granulocyte count) suggest that the host response to *Candida* is an important component of the manifestations of disease. In many cases, although organisms are visible, cultures of biopsied material may be negative. The designation *hepatosplenic candidiasis* or *hepatic candidiasis* is a misnomer because the disease often involves the kidneys and other tissues; the term *chronic disseminated candidiasis* may be more appropriate. Because of the risk of bleeding with liver biopsy, diagnosis is often based on imaging studies (MRI, CT). Treatment should be directed to the causative agent (usually *C. albicans* but sometimes *C. tropicalis* or other less common *Candida* spp).

Typhlitis

Typhlitis (also referred to as necrotizing colitis, neutropenic colitis, necrotizing enteropathy, ileocecal syndrome, and cecitis) is a clinical syndrome of fever and right-lower-quadrant tenderness in an immunosuppressed host. This syndrome is classically seen in neutropenic patients after chemotherapy with cytotoxic drugs. It may be more common among children than among adults and appears to be much more common among patients with acute myelocytic leukemia (AML) or ALL than among those with other types of cancer; a similar syndrome has been reported in patients infected with HIV type 1. Physical examination reveals right-lower-quadrant tenderness, with or without rebound tenderness. Associated diarrhea (often bloody) is common, and the diagnosis can be confirmed by the finding of a thickened cecal wall on CT, MRI, or ultrasonography. Plain films may reveal a right-lower-quadrant mass, but CT with contrast or MRI is a much more sensitive means of diagnosis. Although surgery is sometimes attempted to avoid perforation from ischemia, most cases resolve with medical therapy alone. The disease is sometimes associated with positive blood cultures (which usually yield aerobic gram-negative bacilli), and therapy is recommended for a broad spectrum of bacteria (particularly gram-negative bacilli, which are likely to be found in the bowel flora). Surgery is indicated in the case of perforation.

Clostridium difficile–induced diarrhea

Patients with cancer are predisposed to the development of *C. difficile* diarrhea (Chap. 129) as a consequence of chemotherapy alone. Thus, they may have positive toxin tests before receiving antibiotics. Obviously, such patients are also subject to *C. difficile*–induced diarrhea as a result of antibiotic pressure. *C. difficile* should always be considered as a possible cause of diarrhea in cancer patients who have received antibiotics.

■ CENTRAL NERVOUS SYSTEM–SPECIFIC SYNDROMES

Meningitis

The presentation of meningitis in patients with lymphoma or CLL, patients receiving chemotherapy (particularly with glucocorticoids) for solid tumors, and patients who have received bone marrow transplants suggests a diagnosis of cryptococcal or listerial infection. As noted previously, splenectomized patients are susceptible to rapid, overwhelming infection with encapsulated bacteria (including *S. pneumoniae*, *H. influenzae*, and *N. meningitidis*). Similarly, patients who are antibody-deficient (e.g., those with CLL, those who have received intensive chemotherapy, or those who have undergone bone marrow transplantation) are likely to have infections caused by these bacteria. Other cancer patients, however,

TABLE 86-6 Differential Diagnosis of Central Nervous System Infections in Patients With Cancer

Findings on CT or MRI	Underlying Predisposition	
	Prolonged Neutropenia	Defects in Cellular Immunity[a]
Mass lesions	*Aspergillus, Nocardia,* or *Cryptococcus* brain abscess	Toxoplasmosis EBV-LPD
Diffuse encephalitis	PML (JC virus)	Infection with VZV, CMV, HSV, HHV-6, JC virus (PML), *Listeria*

[a]High-dose glucocorticoid therapy, cytotoxic chemotherapy.
Abbreviations: CMV, cytomegalovirus; EBV-LPD, Epstein-Barr virus lymphoproliferative disease; HHV-6, human herpesvirus type 6; HSV, herpes simplex virus; PML, progressive multifocal leukoencephalopathy; VZV, varicella-zoster virus.

TABLE 86-7 Differential Diagnosis of Chest Infiltrates in Immunocompromised Patients

Infiltrate	Cause of Pneumonia	
	Infectious	Noninfectious
Localized	Bacteria (including *Legionella*, mycobacteria)	Local hemorrhage or embolism, tumor
Nodular	Fungi (e.g., *Aspergillus* or *Mucor*), *Nocardia*	Recurrent tumor
Diffuse	Viruses (especially CMV), *Chlamydia*, *Pneumocystis*, *Toxoplasma gondii*, mycobacteria	Congestive heart failure, radiation pneumonitis, drug-induced lung injury, diffuse alveolar hemorrhage (described after BMT)

Abbreviations: BMT, bone marrow transplantation; CMV, cytomegalovirus.

because of their defective cellular immunity, are likely to be infected with other pathogens (Table 86-3).

Encephalitis

The spectrum of disease resulting from viral encephalitis is expanded in immunocompromised patients. A predisposition to infections with intracellular organisms similar to those encountered in patients with AIDS (Chap. 189) is seen in cancer patients receiving (1) high-dose cytotoxic chemotherapy, (2) chemotherapy affecting T cell function (e.g., fludarabine), or (3) antibodies that eliminate T cells (e.g., anti-CD3, alemtuzumab, anti-CD52) or cytokine activity (anti-tumor necrosis factor agents or interleukin 1 receptor antagonists). Infection with varicella-zoster virus (VZV) has been associated with encephalitis that may be caused by VZV-related vasculitis. Chronic viral infections may also be associated with dementia and encephalitic presentations, and a diagnosis of progressive multifocal leukoencephalopathy (Chap. 381) should be considered when a patient who has received chemotherapy presents with dementia (Table 86-6). Other abnormalities of the central nervous system (CNS) that may be confused with infection include normal-pressure hydrocephalus and vasculitis resulting from CNS irradiation. It may be possible to differentiate these conditions by MRI.

Brain masses

Mass lesions of the brain most often present as headache with or without fever or neurologic abnormalities. Infections associated with mass lesions may be caused by bacteria (particularly *Nocardia*), fungi (particularly *Cryptococcus* or *Aspergillus*), or parasites (*Toxoplasma*). Epstein-Barr virus (EBV)–associated lymphoproliferative disease may also present as single or multiple mass lesions of the brain. A biopsy may be required for a definitive diagnosis.

■ PULMONARY INFECTIONS

Pneumonia (Chap. 257) in immunocompromised patients may be difficult to diagnose because conventional methods of diagnosis depend on the presence of neutrophils. Bacterial pneumonia in neutropenic patients may present without purulent sputum—or, in fact, without any sputum at all—and may not produce physical findings suggestive of chest consolidation (rales or egophony).

In granulocytopenic patients with persistent or recurrent fever, the chest x-ray pattern may help to localize an infection and thus to determine which investigative tests and procedures should be undertaken and which therapeutic options should be considered (Table 86-7). In this setting, a simple chest x-ray is a screening tool; because the impaired host response results in less evidence of consolidation or infiltration, high-resolution CT is recommended for the diagnosis of pulmonary infections. The difficulties encountered in the management of pulmonary infiltrates relate in part to the difficulties of performing diagnostic procedures on the patients involved. When platelet counts can be increased to adequate levels by transfusion, microscopic and microbiologic evaluation of the fluid obtained by endoscopic bronchial lavage is often diagnostic. Lavage fluid should be cultured for *Mycoplasma*, *Chlamydia*, *Legionella*, *Nocardia*, more common bacterial pathogens, and fungi. In addition, the possibility of *Pneumocystis* pneumonia should be considered, especially in patients with ALL or lymphoma who have not received prophylactic trimethoprim-sulfamethoxazole (TMP-SMX). The characteristics of the infiltrate may be helpful in decisions about further diagnostic and therapeutic maneuvers. Nodular infiltrates suggest fungal pneumonia (e.g., that caused by *Aspergillus* or *Mucor*). Such lesions may best be approached by visualized biopsy procedures.

Aspergillus species (Chap. 204) can colonize the skin and respiratory tract or cause fatal systemic illness. Although this fungus may cause aspergillomas in a previously existing cavity or may produce allergic bronchopulmonary disease, the major problem posed by this genus in neutropenic patients is invasive disease due to *A. fumigatus* or *A. flavus*. The organisms enter the host following colonization of the respiratory tract, with subsequent invasion of blood vessels. The disease is likely to present as a thrombotic or embolic event because of this ability of the fungi to invade blood vessels. The risk of infection with *Aspergillus* correlates directly with the duration of neutropenia. In prolonged neutropenia, positive surveillance cultures for nasopharyngeal colonization with *Aspergillus* may predict the development of disease.

Patients with *Aspergillus* infection often present with pleuritic chest pain and fever, which are sometimes accompanied by cough. Hemoptysis may be an ominous sign. Chest x-rays may reveal new focal infiltrates or nodules. Chest CT may reveal a characteristic halo consisting of a mass-like infiltrate surrounded by an area of low attenuation. The presence of a "crescent sign" on chest x-ray or chest CT, in which the mass progresses to central cavitation, is characteristic of invasive *Aspergillus* infection but may develop as the lesions are resolving.

In addition to causing pulmonary disease, *Aspergillus* may invade through the nose or palate, with deep sinus penetration. The appearance of a discolored area in the nasal passages or on the hard palate should prompt a search for invasive *Aspergillus*. This situation is likely to require surgical debridement. Catheter infections with *Aspergillus* usually require both removal of the catheter and antifungal therapy.

Diffuse interstitial infiltrates suggest viral, parasitic, or *Pneumocystis* pneumonia. If the patient has a diffuse interstitial pattern on chest x-ray, it may be reasonable, while considering invasive diagnostic procedures, to institute empirical treatment for *Pneumocystis* with TMP-SMX and for *Chlamydia*, *Mycoplasma*, and *Legionella* with a quinolone or an erythromycin derivative (e.g., azithromycin). Noninvasive procedures, such as staining of sputum smears for *Pneumocystis*, serum cryptococcal antigen tests, and urine testing for *Legionella* antigen, may be helpful. Serum galactomannan and β-D-glucan tests may be helpful in diagnosing *Aspergillus* infection, but their utility is limited by their lack of sensitivity. In transplant recipients who are seropositive for CMV, a determination of CMV load in the serum should be considered. Viral load studies (which allow physicians to quantitate viruses) have superseded simple measurement of serum IgG, which merely documents prior exposure to virus. Infections with viruses that cause only upper respiratory symptoms in immunocompetent hosts, such as respiratory syncytial virus (RSV), influenza viruses, and parainfluenza viruses, may be associated with fatal pneumonitis in immunocompromised hosts. Polymerase chain reaction testing now allows rapid diagnosis of viral pneumonia, which can lead to treatment in some cases (e.g., influenza).

Bleomycin is the most common cause of chemotherapy-induced lung disease. Other causes include alkylating agents (such as cyclophosphamide, chlorambucil, and melphalan), nitrosoureas [carmustine (BCNU), lomustine (CCNU), and methyl-CCNU], busulfan, procarbazine, methotrexate, and hydroxyurea. Both infectious and noninfectious (drug- and/or radiation-induced) pneumonitis can cause fever and abnormalities on chest x-ray; thus, the differential diagnosis of an infiltrate in a patient receiving chemotherapy encompasses a broad range of conditions (Table 86-7). The treatment of radiation pneumonitis (which may respond dramatically to glucocorticoids) or drug-induced pneumonitis is different from that of infectious pneumonia, and a biopsy may be important in the diagnosis. Unfortunately, no definitive diagnosis can be made in ~30% of cases, even after bronchoscopy.

Open-lung biopsy is the gold standard of diagnostic techniques. Biopsy via a visualized thoracostomy can replace an open procedure in many cases. When a biopsy cannot be performed, empirical treatment can be undertaken; a quinolone or an erythromycin derivative (azithromycin) and TMP-SMX are used in the case of diffuse infiltrates, and an antifungal agent is administered in the case of nodular infiltrates. The risks should be weighed carefully in these cases. If inappropriate drugs are administered, empirical treatment may prove toxic or ineffective; either of these outcomes may be riskier than biopsy.

■ CARDIOVASCULAR INFECTIONS

Patients with Hodgkin's disease are prone to persistent infections by *Salmonella*, sometimes (and particularly often in elderly patients) affecting a vascular site. The use of IV catheters deliberately lodged in the right atrium is associated with a high incidence of bacterial endocarditis, presumably related to valve damage followed by bacteremia. Nonbacterial thrombotic endocarditis has been described in association with a variety of malignancies (most often solid tumors) and may follow bone marrow transplantation as well.

The presentation of an embolic event with a new cardiac murmur suggests this diagnosis. Blood cultures are negative in this disease of unknown pathogenesis.

■ ENDOCRINE SYNDROMES

Infections of the endocrine system have been described in immunocompromised patients. *Candida* infection of the thyroid may be difficult to diagnose during the neutropenic period. It can be defined by indium-labeled WBC scans or gallium scans after neutrophil counts increase. CMV infection can cause adrenalitis with or without resulting adrenal insufficiency. The presentation of a sudden endocrine anomaly in an immunocompromised patient may be a sign of infection in the involved end organ.

■ MUSCULOSKELETAL INFECTIONS

Infection that is a consequence of vascular compromise, resulting in gangrene, can occur when a tumor restricts the blood supply to muscles, bones, or joints. The process of diagnosis and treatment of such infection is similar to that in normal hosts, with the following caveats:

1. *In terms of diagnosis*, a lack of physical findings resulting from a lack of granulocytes in the granulocytopenic patient should make the clinician more aggressive in obtaining tissue rather than relying on physical signs.
2. *In terms of therapy*, aggressive debridement of infected tissues may be required, but it is usually difficult to operate on patients who have recently received chemotherapy, both because of a lack of platelets (which results in bleeding complications) and because of a lack of WBCs (which may lead to secondary infection). A blood culture positive for *Clostridium perfringens*—an organism commonly associated with gas gangrene—can have a number of meanings (Chap. 142). Bloodstream infections with intestinal organisms such as *Streptococcus bovis* and *C. perfringens* may arise spontaneously from lower gastrointestinal lesions (tumor or polyps); alternatively, these lesions may be harbingers of invasive disease. The clinical setting must be considered in order to define the appropriate treatment for each case.

■ RENAL AND URETERAL INFECTIONS

Infections of the urinary tract are common among patients whose ureteral excretion is compromised (Table 86-1). *Candida*, which has a predilection for the kidney, can invade either from the bloodstream or in a retrograde manner (via the ureters or bladder) in immunocompromised patients. The presence of "fungus balls" or persistent candiduria suggests invasive disease. Persistent funguria (with *Aspergillus* as well as *Candida*) should prompt a search for a nidus of infection in the kidney.

Certain viruses are typically seen only in immunosuppressed patients. BK virus (polyomavirus hominis 1) has been documented in the urine of bone marrow transplant recipients and, like adenovirus, may be associated with hemorrhagic cystitis. BK-induced cystitis usually remits with decreasing immunosuppression. Anecdotal reports have described the treatment of infections due to adenovirus and BK virus with cidofovir.

ABNORMALITIES THAT PREDISPOSE TO INFECTION

(Table 86-1)

■ THE LYMPHOID SYSTEM

It is beyond the scope of this chapter to detail how all the immunologic abnormalities that result from cancer or from chemotherapy for cancer lead to infections. Disorders of the immune system are discussed in other sections of this book. As has been noted, patients with antibody deficiency are predisposed to overwhelming infection with encapsulated bacteria (including *S. pneumoniae, H. influenzae,* and *N. meningitidis*). Infections that result from the lack of a functional cellular immune system are described in Chap. 189. It is worth mentioning, however, that patients undergoing intensive chemotherapy for any form of cancer will have not only defects due to granulocytopenia but also lymphocyte dysfunction, which may be profound. Thus, these patients—especially those receiving glucocorticoid-containing regimens or drugs that inhibit either T cell activation (calcineurin inhibitors or drugs like fludarabine, which affect lymphocyte function) or cytokine induction—should be given prophylaxis for *Pneumocystis* pneumonia.

◼ THE HEMATOPOIETIC SYSTEM

Initial studies in the 1960s revealed a dramatic increase in the incidence of infections (fatal and nonfatal) among cancer patients with a granulocyte count of <500/μL. The use of prophylactic antibacterial agents has reduced the number of bacterial infections, but 35–78% of febrile neutropenic patients being treated for hematologic malignancies develop infections at some time during chemotherapy. Aerobic pathogens (both gram-positive and gram-negative) predominate in all series, but the exact organisms isolated vary from center to center. Infections with anaerobic organisms are uncommon. Geographic patterns affect the types of fungi isolated. Tuberculosis and malaria are common causes of fever in the developing world and may present in this setting as well.

Neutropenic patients are unusually susceptible to infection with a wide variety of bacteria; thus, antibiotic therapy should be initiated promptly to cover likely pathogens if infection is suspected. Indeed, early initiation of antibacterial agents is mandatory to prevent deaths. Like most immunocompromised patients, neutropenic patients are threatened by their own microbial flora, including gram-positive and gram-negative organisms found commonly on the skin and in the bowel (Table 86-4). Because treatment with narrow-spectrum agents leads to infection with organisms not covered by the antibiotics used, the initial regimen should target all pathogens likely to be initial causes of bacterial infection in neutropenic hosts. As noted in the algorithm shown in Fig. 86-2, administration of antimicrobial agents is routinely continued until neutropenia resolves—i.e., the granulocyte count is sustained above 500/μL for at least 2 days. In some cases, patients remain febrile after resolution of neutropenia. In these instances, the risk of sudden death from overwhelming bacteremia is greatly reduced, and the following diagnoses should be seriously considered: (1) fungal infection, (2) bacterial abscesses or undrained foci of infection, and (3) drug fever (including reactions to antimicrobial agents as well as to chemotherapy or cytokines). In the proper setting, viral infection or graft-versus-host disease should be considered. In clinical practice, antibacterial therapy is usually discontinued when the patient is no longer neutropenic and all evidence of bacterial disease has been eliminated. Antifungal agents are then discontinued if there is no evidence of fungal disease. If the patient remains febrile, a search for viral diseases or unusual pathogens is conducted while unnecessary cytokines and other drugs are systematically eliminated from the regimen.

TREATMENT   Infections in Cancer Patients

ANTIBACTERIAL THERAPY   Hundreds of antibacterial regimens have been tested for use in patients with cancer. The major risk of infection is related to the degree of neutropenia seen

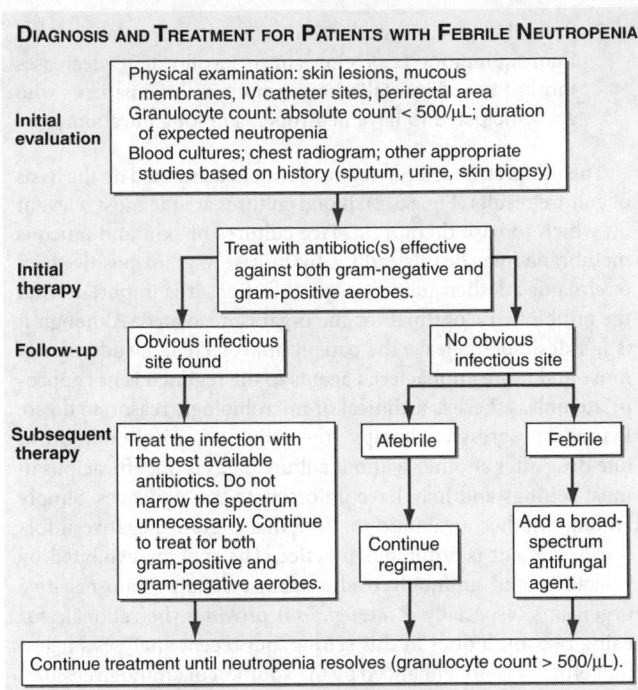

DIAGNOSIS AND TREATMENT FOR PATIENTS WITH FEBRILE NEUTROPENIA

Figure 86-2 Algorithm for the diagnosis and treatment of febrile neutropenic patients.

as a consequence of either the disease or the therapy. Many of the relevant studies have involved small populations in which the outcomes have generally been good, and most have lacked the statistical power to detect differences among the regimens studied. Each febrile neutropenic patient should be approached as a unique problem, with particular attention given to previous infections and recent antibiotic exposures. Several general guidelines are useful in the initial treatment of neutropenic patients with fever (Fig. 86-2):

1. In the initial regimen, it is necessary to use antibiotics active against both gram-negative and gram-positive bacteria (Table 86-4).
2. Monotherapy with an aminoglycoside or an antibiotic without good activity against gram-positive organisms (e.g., ciprofloxacin or aztreonam) is not adequate in this setting.
3. The agents used should reflect both the epidemiology and the antibiotic resistance pattern of the hospital.
4. If the pattern of resistance justifies its use, a single third-generation cephalosporin constitutes an appropriate initial regimen in many hospitals.
5. Most standard regimens are designed for patients who have not previously received prophylactic antibiotics. The development of fever in a patient who has received antibiotics affects the choice of subsequent therapy, which should target resistant organisms and organisms known to cause infections in patients being treated with the antibiotics already administered.
6. Randomized trials have indicated the safety of oral antibiotic regimens in the treatment of "low-risk" patients with fever and neutropenia. Outpatients who are expected to remain neutropenic for <10 days and who have no concurrent medical problems (such as hypotension, pulmonary compromise, or abdominal pain) can be classified as low risk and treated with a broad-spectrum oral regimen.

7. Several large-scale studies indicate that prophylaxis with a fluoroquinolone (ciprofloxacin or levofloxacin) decreases morbidity and mortality rates among afebrile patients who are anticipated to have neutropenia of long duration.

The initial antibacterial regimen should be refined on the basis of culture results (Fig. 86-2). Blood cultures are the most relevant on which to base therapy; surface cultures of skin and mucous membranes may be misleading. In the case of gram-positive bacteremia or another gram-positive infection, it is important that the antibiotic be optimal for the organism isolated. Although it is not desirable to leave the patient unprotected, the addition of more and more antibacterial agents to the regimen is not appropriate unless there is a clinical or microbiologic reason to do so. Planned progressive therapy (the serial, empirical addition of one drug after another without culture data) is not efficacious in most settings and may have unfortunate consequences. Simply adding another antibiotic for fear that a gram-negative infection is present is a dubious practice. The synergy exhibited by β-lactams and aminoglycosides against certain gram-negative organisms (especially *P. aeruginosa*) provides the rationale for using two antibiotics in this setting, but recent analyses suggest that efficacy is not enhanced by the addition of aminoglycosides, while toxicity may be increased. Mere "double coverage," with the addition of a quinolone or another antibiotic that is not likely to exhibit synergy, has not been shown to be of benefit and may cause additional toxicities and side effects. Cephalosporins can cause bone marrow suppression, and vancomycin is associated with neutropenia in some healthy individuals. Furthermore, the addition of multiple cephalosporins may induce β-lactamase production by some organisms; cephalosporins and double β-lactam combinations should probably be avoided altogether in *Enterobacter* infections.

ANTIFUNGAL THERAPY Fungal infections in cancer patients are most often associated with neutropenia. Neutropenic patients are predisposed to the development of invasive fungal infections, most commonly those due to *Candida* and *Aspergillus* species and occasionally those caused by *Fusarium*, *Trichosporon*, and *Bipolaris*. Cryptococcal infection, which is common among patients taking immunosuppressive agents, is uncommon among neutropenic patients receiving chemotherapy for AML. Invasive candidal disease is usually caused by *C. albicans* or *C. tropicalis* but can be caused by *C. krusei*, *C. parapsilosis*, and *C. glabrata*.

For decades it has been common clinical practice to add amphotericin B to antibacterial regimens if a neutropenic patient remains febrile despite 4–7 days of treatment with antibacterial agents. The rationale for this empirical addition is that it is difficult to culture fungi before they cause disseminated disease and that mortality rates from disseminated fungal infections in granulocytopenic patients are high. Before the introduction of newer azoles into clinical practice, amphotericin B was the mainstay of antifungal therapy. The insolubility of amphotericin B has resulted in the marketing of several lipid formulations that are less toxic than the amphotericin B deoxycholate complex. Echinocandins (e.g., caspofungin) are useful in the treatment of infections caused by azole-resistant *Candida* as well as in therapy for aspergillosis and have been shown to be equivalent to liposomal amphotericin B for the empirical treatment of patients with prolonged fever and neutropenia. Newer azoles have also been demonstrated to be effective in this setting. Although fluconazole is efficacious in the treatment of infections due to many *Candida* spp., its use against serious

fungal infections in immunocompromised patients is limited by its narrow spectrum: it has no activity against *Aspergillus* or against several non-*albicans Candida* spp. The broad-spectrum azoles (e.g., voriconazole and posaconazole) provide another option for the treatment of *Aspergillus* infection (Chap. 204), including CNS infection, in which amphotericin B has usually failed. Clinicians should be aware that the spectrum of each azole is somewhat different and that no drug can be assumed to be efficacious against all fungi. For example, while voriconazole is active against *Pseudallescheria boydii*, amphotericin B is not; however, voriconazole has no activity against *Mucor*. Posaconazole, which is administered orally, is useful as a prophylactic agent in patients with prolonged neutropenia. Studies in progress are assessing the use of these agents in combinations. For a full discussion of antifungal therapy, see Chap. 198.

ANTIVIRAL THERAPY The availability of a variety of agents active against herpes-group viruses, including some new agents with a broader spectrum of activity, has heightened focus on the treatment of viral infections, which pose a major problem in cancer patients. Viral diseases caused by the herpes group are prominent. Serious (and sometimes fatal) infections due to HSV and CMV are well documented, and VZV infections may be fatal to patients receiving chemotherapy. The roles of human herpesvirus (HHV)-6, HHV-7, and HHV-8 (Kaposi's sarcoma–associated herpesvirus) in cancer patients are still being defined (Chap. 182). While clinical experience is most extensive with acyclovir, which can be used therapeutically or prophylactically, a number of derivative drugs offer advantages over this agent (Table 86-8).

In addition to the herpes group, several respiratory viruses (especially RSV) may cause serious disease in cancer patients. While influenza vaccination is recommended (see below), it may be ineffective in this patient population. The availability of antiviral drugs with activity against influenza viruses gives the clinician additional options for the treatment of these patients (Table 86-9).

OTHER THERAPEUTIC MODALITIES Another way to address the problems of the febrile neutropenic patient is to replenish the neutrophil population. Although granulocyte transfusions are effective in the treatment of refractory gram-negative bacteremia, they do not have a documented role in prophylaxis. Because of the expense, the risk of leukoagglutinin reactions (which has probably been decreased by improved cell-separation procedures), and the risk of transmission of CMV from unscreened donors (which has been reduced by the use of filters), granulocyte transfusion is reserved for patients unresponsive to antibiotics. This modality is efficacious for documented gram-negative bacteremia refractory to antibiotics, particularly in situations where granulocyte numbers will be depressed for only a short period. The demonstrated usefulness of granulocyte colony-stimulating factor (G-CSF) in mobilizing neutrophils and advances in preservation techniques may make this option more useful than in the past.

A variety of cytokines, including G-CSF and granulocyte-macrophage colony-stimulating factor (GM-CSF), enhance granulocyte recovery after chemotherapy and consequently shorten the period of maximal vulnerability to fatal infections. Interferon γ has been demonstrated to be effective in some infections caused by intracellular organisms, presumably because of its ability to activate macrophages. The role of these cytokines in routine practice is still a matter of some debate. Most authorities recommend their use only when neutropenia is both severe and

TABLE 86-8 Antiviral Agents Active Against Herpesviruses

Agent	Description	Spectrum	Toxicity	Other Issues
Acyclovir	Inhibits HSV polymerase	HSV, VZV (± CMV, EBV)	Rarely has side effects; crystalluria can occur at high doses	Long history of safety; original antiviral agent
Famciclovir	Prodrug of penciclovir (a guanosine analogue)	HSV, VZV (± CMV)	Associated with cancer in rats	Longer effective half-life than acyclovir
Valacyclovir	Prodrug of acyclovir; better absorption	HSV, VZV (± CMV)	Associated with thrombotic microangiopathy in one study of immunocompromised patients	Better oral absorption and longer effective half-life than acyclovir; can be given as a single daily dose for prophylaxis
Ganciclovir	More potent polymerase inhibitor; more toxic than acyclovir	HSV, VZV, CMV, HHV-6	Bone marrow suppression	Neutropenia may respond to G-CSF or GM-CSF
Valganciclovir	Prodrug of ganciclovir; better absorption	HSV, VZV, CMV, HHV-6	Bone marrow suppression	—
Cidofovir	Nucleotide analogue of cytosine	HSV, VZV, CMV; good in vitro activity against adenovirus and others	Nephrotoxic marrow suppression	Given IV once a week
Foscarnet	Phosphonoformic acid; inhibits viral DNA polymerase	HSV, VZV, CMV, HHV-6	Nephrotoxic; electrolyte abnormalities common	IV only

Abbreviations: ±, agent has some activity but not enough for the treatment of infections; CMV, cytomegalovirus; EBV, Epstein-Barr virus; G-CSF, granulocyte colony-stimulating factor; GM-CSF, granulocyte-macrophage colony-stimulating factor; HHV, human herpesvirus; HSV, herpes simplex virus; VZV, varicella-zoster virus.

prolonged. The cytokines themselves may have adverse effects, including fever, hypoxemia, and pleural effusions or serositis in other areas (Chap. 314).

Once neutropenia has resolved, the risk of infection decreases dramatically. However, depending on what drugs they receive, patients who continue on chemotherapeutic protocols remain at high risk for certain diseases. Any patient receiving more than a maintenance dose of glucocorticoids (including many treatment regimens for diffuse lymphoma) should also receive prophylactic TMP-SMX because of the risk of *Pneumocystis* infection; those with ALL should receive such prophylaxis for the duration of chemotherapy.

TABLE 86-9 Other Antiviral Agents Useful in the Treatment of Infections in Cancer Patients

Agent	Description	Spectrum	Toxicity	Other Issues
Amantadine, rimantadine	Interfere with uncoating	Influenza A only	5–10% fewer CNS effects with rimantadine	May be given prophylactically
Zanamivir	Neuraminidase inhibitor	Influenza A and B	Usually well tolerated	Inhalation only
Oseltamivir	Neuraminidase inhibitor	Influenza A and B	Usually well tolerated	PO dosing
Pleconaril	Blocks enterovirus binding and uncoating	90% of enteroviruses, 80% of rhinoviruses	Generally well tolerated	Decreases duration of meningitis; available for compassionate use only
Interferons	Cytokines with broad spectrum of activity	Used locally for warts, systemically for hepatitis	Fever, myalgias, bone marrow suppression	Not shown to be helpful in CMV infection; use limited by toxicity
Ribavirin	Purine analogue (precise mechanism of action unknown)	Broad theoretical spectrum; documented use against RSV, Lassa fever virus, and hepatitis viruses (with interferon)	IV form causes anemia	Given by aerosol for RSV infection (efficacy in doubt); approved for use in children with heart/lung disease; given with interferon for hepatitis C

Abbreviations: CMV, cytomegalovirus; CNS, central nervous system; RSV, respiratory syncytial virus.

EFFECT OF THE ENVIRONMENT

Outbreaks of fatal *Aspergillus* infection have been associated with construction projects and materials in several hospitals. The association between spore counts and risk of infection suggests the need for a high-efficiency air-handling system in hospitals that care for large numbers of neutropenic patients. The use of laminar-flow rooms and prophylactic antibiotics has decreased the number of infectious episodes in severely neutropenic patients. However, because of the expense of such a program and the failure to show that it dramatically affects mortality rates, most centers do not routinely use laminar flow to care for neutropenic patients. Some centers use "reverse isolation," in which health care providers and visitors to a patient who is neutropenic wear gowns and gloves. Since most of the infections these patients develop are due to organisms that colonize the patients' own skin and bowel, the validity of such schemes is dubious, and limited clinical data do not support their use. Hand washing by all staff caring for neutropenic patients should be required to prevent the spread of resistant organisms.

The presence of large numbers of bacteria (particularly *P. aeruginosa*) in certain foods, especially fresh vegetables, has led some authorities to recommend a special "low-bacteria" diet. A diet consisting of cooked and canned food is satisfactory to most neutropenic patients and does not involve elaborate disinfection or sterilization protocols. However, there are no studies to support even this type of dietary restriction. Counseling of patients to avoid leftovers, deli foods, and unpasteurized dairy products is recommended.

PHYSICAL MEASURES

Although few studies address this issue, patients with cancer are predisposed to infections resulting from anatomic compromise (e.g., lymphedema resulting from node dissections after radical mastectomy). Surgeons who specialize in cancer surgery can provide specific guidelines for the care of such patients, and patients benefit from commonsense advice about how to prevent infections in vulnerable areas.

IMMUNOGLOBULIN REPLACEMENT

Many patients with multiple myeloma or CLL have immunoglobulin deficiencies as a result of their disease, and all allogeneic bone marrow transplant recipients are hypogammaglobulinemic for a period after transplantation. However, current recommendations reserve intravenous immunoglobulin replacement therapy for those patients with severe (<400 mg/dL), prolonged hypogammaglobulinemia. Antibiotic prophylaxis has been shown to be cheaper and is efficacious in preventing infections in most CLL patients with hypogammaglobulinemia. Routine use of immunoglobulin replacement is not recommended.

SEXUAL PRACTICES

The use of condoms is recommended for severely immunocompromised patients. Any sexual practice that results in oral exposure to feces is not recommended. Neutropenic patients should be advised to avoid any practice that results in trauma, as even microscopic cuts may result in bacterial invasion and fatal sepsis.

ANTIBIOTIC PROPHYLAXIS

Several studies indicate that the use of oral fluoroquinolones prevents infection and decreases mortality rates among severely neutropenic patients. Fluconazole prevents *Candida* infections when given prophylactically to patients receiving bone marrow transplants. The use of broader-spectrum antifungal agents (e.g., posaconazole) appears to be more efficacious. Prophylaxis for *Pneumocystis* is mandatory for patients with ALL and for all cancer patients receiving glucocorticoid-containing chemotherapy regimens.

VACCINATION OF CANCER PATIENTS

In general, patients undergoing chemotherapy respond less well to vaccines than do normal hosts. Their greater need for vaccines thus leads to a dilemma in their management. Purified proteins and inactivated vaccines are almost never contraindicated and should be given to patients even during chemotherapy. For example, all adults should receive diphtheria–tetanus toxoid boosters at the indicated times as well as seasonal influenza vaccine. However, if possible, vaccination should not be undertaken concurrent with cytotoxic chemotherapy. If patients are expected to be receiving chemotherapy for several months and vaccination is indicated (e.g., influenza vaccination in the fall), the vaccine should be given midcycle—as far apart in time as possible from the antimetabolic agents that will prevent an immune response. The meningococcal and pneumococcal polysaccharide vaccines should be given to patients before splenectomy, if possible. The *H. influenzae* type b conjugate vaccine should be administered to all splenectomized patients.

In general, live virus (or live bacterial) vaccines should not be given to patients during intensive chemotherapy because of the risk of disseminated infection. Recommendations on vaccination are summarized in Table 86-2.

FURTHER READINGS

GAFTER-GVILI A et al: Antibiotic prophylaxis for bacterial infections in afebrile neutropenic patients following chemotherapy. Cochrane Database Syst Rev 4:CD004386, 2009

GUPTA A et al: Infections in acute myeloid leukemia: An analysis of 382 febrile episodes. Med Oncol, published online October 15, 2009

MERMEL LA et al: Clinical practice guidelines for the diagnosis and management of intravenous catheter–related infection: 2009 update by the Infectious Diseases Society of America. Clin Infect Dis 49:1, 2009

PAUL M et al: Beta-lactam versus beta-lactam–aminoglycoside combination therapy in cancer patients with neutropenia. Cochrane Database Syst Rev 3:CD003038, 2010

PICKERING LK et al: Immunization programs for infants, children, adolescents, and adults: Clinical practice guidelines by the Infectious Diseases Society of America. Clin Infect Dis 49:817, 2009

TOMBLYN M et al: Guidelines for preventing infectious complications among hematopoietic cell transplantation recipients: A global perspective. Biol Blood Marrow Transplant 15:1143, 2009

ULLMANN AJ et al: Posaconazole or fluconazole for prophylaxis in severe graft-versus-host disease. N Engl J Med 356:335, 2007

VENTO S et al: Lung infections after cancer chemotherapy. Lancet Oncol 9:982, 2008

CHAPTER **87**

Cancer of the Skin

Walter J. Urba

Carl V. Washington

Hari Nadiminti

MELANOMA

Pigmented lesions are among the most common findings on skin examination. The challenge is to distinguish cutaneous melanomas, which account for the overwhelming majority of deaths resulting from skin cancer, from the remainder, which with rare exceptions are benign. Cutaneous melanoma can occur in adults of all ages, even young individuals, and people of all colors; it is located on the skin, where it is visible; and it has distinct clinical features that make it detectable at a time when complete surgical excision is possible. Examples of malignant and benign pigmented lesions are shown in Fig. 87-1.

■ EPIDEMIOLOGY

Melanoma is an aggressive malignancy of melanocytes: pigment-producing cells that originate from the neural crest and migrate to the skin, meninges, mucous membranes, upper esophagus, and eyes. Melanocytes in each of these locations have the potential for malignant transformation. In the United States, nearly 69,000 individuals were expected to develop melanoma and approximately 9,000 were expected to die in 2010. Although the overall incidence and mortality have increased over the last decades, the mortality rates for younger patients have flattened whereas those rates for individuals over age 65 have continued to increase. It is predominantly a malignancy of white-skinned people (98% of cases), and the incidence correlates with latitude of residence, providing strong evidence for the role of sun exposure. Men are affected slightly more than women (1.3:1), and the median age at diagnosis is the late fifties. Dark-skinned populations (such as those of India and Puerto Rico), blacks, and East Asians also develop melanoma, albeit at rates 10–20 times lower than those in whites. Cutaneous melanomas in these populations are diagnosed more often at a higher stage, and patients tend to have worse outcomes. Furthermore, in nonwhite populations, there is a much higher frequency of acral (subungual, plantar, palmar) and mucosal melanomas.

■ RISK FACTORS

The strongest risk factors for melanoma are the presence of multiple benign or atypical nevi and a family or personal history of melanoma (Table 87-1). The presence of melanocytic nevi, common or dysplastic, is a marker for increased risk of melanoma. Nevi have been referred to as precursor lesions because they can transform into melanomas; however, the actual risk for any specific nevus is exceedingly low. About one-quarter of melanomas are histologically associated with nevi, but the majority arise de novo. Table 87-2 lists the characteristic features of clinically atypical moles and the features that differentiate them from benign acquired nevi. The number of clinically atypical moles may vary from one to several hundred, and they usually differ from one another in appearance. The borders are often hazy and indistinct, and the pigment pattern is more highly varied than that in benign acquired nevi. Individuals with clinically atypical moles and a strong family history of melanoma have been

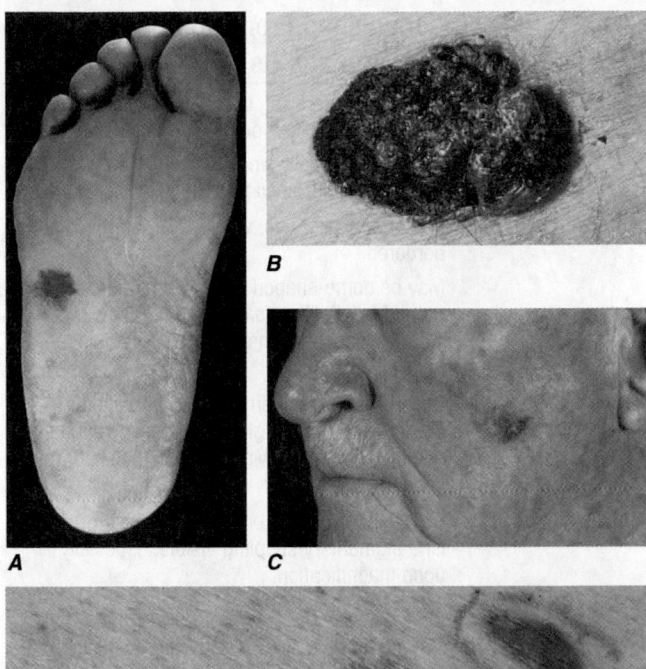
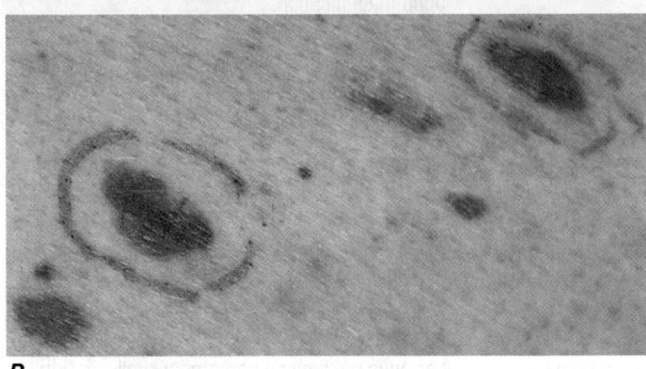

Figure 87-1 Atypical and malignant pigmented lesions. The most common melanoma is superficial spreading melanoma (not pictured). *A.* Acral lentiginous melanoma is the most common melanoma in blacks, Asians, and Hispanics and occurs as an enlarging hyperpigmented macule or plaque on the palms and soles. Lateral pigment diffusion is present. *B.* Nodular melanoma most commonly manifests as a rapidly growing, often ulcerated or crusted black nodule. *C.* Lentigo maligna melanoma occurs on sun-exposed skin as a large, hyperpigmented macule or plaque with irregular borders and variable pigmentation. *D.* Dysplastic nevi are irregularly pigmented and shaped nevomelanocytic lesions that may be associated with familial melanoma.

TABLE 87-1 Factors Associated With Increased Risk of Melanoma

Total body nevi (higher number = higher risk)

Family or personal history

Dysplastic nevi

Light skin/hair/eye color

Poor tanning ability

Freckling

UV exposure/sunburns/tanning booths

CDKN2A mutation

MC1R variants

TABLE 87-2 Pigmented Lesions That Must Be Distinguished From Cutaneous Melanoma and Its Precursors

Blue nevus	Gunmetal or cerulean blue, blue-gray. Stable over time. One-half occur on dorsa of hands and feet. Lesions are usually single, small, 3 mm–< 1 cm. Must be distinguished from nodular melanoma.
Compound nevus	Round or oval shape, well demarcated, smooth-bordered. May be dome-shaped or papillomatous; colors range from flesh-colored to very dark brown, with individual nevi being relatively homogeneous in color.
Hemangioma	Dome-shaped reddish, purple, blue nodule. Compression with a glass microscope slide may result in blanching. Must be distinguished from nodular melanoma.
Junctional nevus	Flat to barely raised brown lesion. Sharp border. Fine pigmentary stippling visible, especially upon magnification.
Lentigo	
Juvenile	Flat, uniformly medium or dark brown lesion with sharp border.
Solar	Solar lentigines are acquired lesions on sites of chronic solar exposure (face and backs of hands). Lesions are 2 mm–≥1 cm. Solar lentigines have reticulate pigmentation upon magnification.
Pigmented basal cell carcinoma	Papular border. May have central ulceration. Usually on a sun-exposed surface in an older patient. Patient usually has dark brown eyes and dark brown or black hair.
Pigmented dermatofibroma	Lesion is not well demarcated visually, is firm, and dimples downward when compressed laterally. Usually on extremities. Usually <6 mm.
Seborrheic keratosis	Rough, sharp-bordered lesions that feel waxy and "stuck on"; range in color from flesh to tan to dark brown. Presence of keratin plugs in surface is helpful for discriminating especially dark lesions from melanoma.
Subungual hematoma	Maroon (red-brown) coloration. As lesion grows out from nail fold, a curving clear area is seen.
Tattoo (medical or traumatic)	In medical tattoos, lesions are small pigmentary dots, often blue or green, which make a regular pattern (rectangle). Traumatic tattoos are irregular, and pigmentation may appear black.

reported to have a >50% lifetime risk for developing melanoma and warrant close follow-up with a dermatologist. Of the 90% of melanoma patients whose disease is regarded as sporadic (i.e., who lack a family history of melanoma), ~40% have clinically atypical moles, compared with an estimated 5–10% of the population at large.

Congenital melanocytic nevi, which are classified as small (≤1.5 cm), medium (1.5–20 cm), and giant (>20 cm), can be precursors for melanoma. The risk is highest for the giant melanocytic nevus, also called the bathing trunk nevus, which is a rare malformation that affects 1 in 30,000–100,000 individuals, with a lifetime risk of melanoma development estimated to be as high as 6%. At present there are no uniform management guidelines for giant congenital nevi, but because of the potential for malignancy, prophylactic excision early in life is prudent. This usually requires staged removal with coverage by split-thickness skin grafts. Surgery cannot remove all at-risk nevus cells, as some may penetrate into the

muscles or central nervous system (CNS) below the nevus. Small- to medium-size congenital melanocytic nevi affect approximately 1% of persons; the risk of melanoma developing in these lesions is not known but appears to be relatively low. The management of small- to medium-size congenital melanocytic nevi remains controversial.

Personal and family history

Perhaps the single greatest risk factor for melanoma is a personal history of melanoma. Once diagnosed, patients with melanoma require a lifetime of surveillance because their risk is 10 times that of the general population. First-degree relatives have a higher risk of developing melanoma than do individuals without a family history, but only 5–10% of all melanomas are truly familial. In familial melanoma, patients tend to be younger at first diagnosis, lesions are thinner, survival is improved, and multiple primary melanomas are common.

Genetic susceptibility

Approximately 20–40% of cases of hereditary melanoma (0.2–2% of all melanomas) are due to germ-line mutations in the cell cycle regulatory gene cyclin-dependent kinase inhibitor 2A (*CDKN2A*). In fact, 70% of all cutaneous melanomas have somatic mutations or deletions affecting the *CDKN2A* locus on chromosome 9p21. This locus encodes two distinct tumor suppressor proteins from alternate reading frames: p16 and ARF (p14^{ARF}). The p16 protein inhibits CDK4/6-mediated phosphorylation and inactivation of the retinoblastoma (RB) protein, whereas ARF inhibits MDM2 ubiquitin-mediated degradation of p53. The end result of the loss of *CDKN2A* is inactivation of two critical tumor suppressor pathways, RB and p53, which control entry of cells into the cell cycle. Several studies have shown an increased risk of pancreatic cancer among melanoma-prone families with *CDKN2A* mutations.

The melanocortin-1 receptor (*MC1R*) gene is also an inherited melanoma susceptibility factor. Solar radiation stimulates the production of melanocortin [α-melanocyte-stimulating hormone (α-MSH)], the ligand for *MC1R*, which is a G-protein-coupled receptor that signals via cyclic AMP and regulates the amount and type of pigment produced. *MC1R* is highly polymorphic, and among its 80 variants are those that result in partial loss of signaling and lead to the production of pheomelanin, which is not sun-protective and produces red hair. This red hair color (RHC) phenotype is associated with fair skin, red hair, freckles, increased sun sensitivity, and increased risk of melanoma.

■ CLINICAL CLASSIFICATION

Traditionally, four major types of cutaneous melanoma have been recognized (Table 87-3). In three of these types—*superficial spreading melanoma, lentigo maligna melanoma,* and *acral lentiginous melanoma*—the lesion has a period of superficial (so-called radial) growth during which it increases in size but does not penetrate deeply. It is during this period that the melanoma is most capable of being cured by surgical excision. The fourth type—*nodular melanoma*—does not have a recognizable radial growth phase and usually presents as a deeply invasive lesion that is capable of early metastasis. When tumors begin to penetrate deeply into the skin, they are in the so-called vertical growth phase. Melanomas with a radial growth phase are characterized by irregular and sometimes notched borders, variation in pigment pattern, and variation in color. An increase in size or in color is noted by the patient in 70% of early lesions. Bleeding, ulceration, and pain are late signs and are of little help in early recognition. Superficial spreading melanoma is the most common variant observed in the white population. The back is the most common site for melanoma in men. In women, the back and the lower leg (from knee to ankle) are common

TABLE 87-3 Classification of Malignant Melanoma

Type	Site	Average Age at Diagnosis, Years	Duration of Known Existence, Years	Color
Lentigo maligna melanoma	Sun-exposed surfaces, particularly malar region of cheek and temple	70	5–20 or longer*	In flat portions, shades of brown and tan predominate, but whitish gray occasionally present; in nodules, shades of reddish brown, bluish gray, bluish black
Superficial spreading melanoma	Any site (more common on upper back and, in women, lower legs)	40–50	1–7	Shades of brown mixed with bluish red (violaceous), bluish black, reddish brown, and often whitish pink, and the border of lesion is at least in part visibly and/or palpably elevated
Nodular melanoma	Any	40–50	Months–<5 years	Reddish blue (purple) or bluish black; either uniform in color or mixed with brown or black
Acral lentiginous melanoma	Palm, sole, nail bed, mucous membrane	60	1–10	In flat portions, dark brown predominantly; in raised lesions (plaques), brown-black or blue-black predominantly

*During much of this time, the precursor stage, lentigo maligna, is confined to the epidermis.

Source: Adapted from AJ Sober, in NA Soter, HP Baden (eds): *Pathophysiology of Dermatologic Diseases*. New York, McGraw-Hill, 1984.

CHAPTER 87

Cancer of the Skin

sites. Nodular melanomas are dark brown-black to blue-black nodules. Lentigo maligna melanoma usually is confined to chronically sun-damaged, sun-exposed sites (face, neck, back of hands) in older individuals. Acral lentiginous melanoma occurs on the palms, soles, nail beds, and mucous membranes. Although this type occurs in whites, it occurs most frequently (along with nodular melanoma) in blacks and East Asians. A fifth type of melanoma, *desmoplastic melanoma*, is associated with a fibrotic response, neural invasion, and a greater tendency for local recurrence. Occasionally, melanomas appear clinically to be amelanotic, in which case the diagnosis is established histologically after biopsy of a new or a changing skin nodule or because of suspicion of a basal cell carcinoma.

Although melanoma subtypes are clinically and histopathologically distinct, this classification does not have independent prognostic value and has fallen out of favor. Histologic subtype is not part of American Joint Committee on Cancer (AJCC) staging and often is not identified in current pathology reports. Future classification schemes will be based on molecular features of each melanoma (see below). The molecular analysis of individual melanomas will provide a basis for distinguishing benign nevi from melanomas, identify distinct subclasses of melanoma on the basis of the anatomic site, indicate the extent of ultraviolet (UV) exposure, and determine the mutational status of the tumor, which will help elucidate the molecular mechanisms of tumorigenesis and identify targets that will serve as a basis for selection of therapy.

◼ PATHOGENESIS AND MOLECULAR CLASSIFICATION

Considerable evidence from epidemiologic and molecular studies suggests that cutaneous melanomas arise via multiple pathways. There are both environmental and genetic components. UV solar radiation causes genetic changes in the skin, impairs cutaneous immune function, increases the production of growth factors, and induces the formation of DNA-damaging reactive oxygen species that affect keratinocytes and melanocytes. A comprehensive catalog of somatic mutations from a human melanoma revealed more than 33,000 base mutations with damage to almost 300 protein-coding segments compared with normal cells from the same patient. The dominant mutational signature reflected DNA damage due to UV light exposure. The melanoma also contained previously described driver mutations (i.e., mutations that confer selective clonal growth advantage and are implicated in oncogenesis). These driver mutations affect pathways that promote cell proliferation and inhibit normal pathways of apoptosis in response to DNA repair (see below). The altered melanocytes accumulate DNA damage, and selection occurs for all the attributes that constitute the malignant phenotype: invasion, metastasis, and angiogenesis.

An understanding of the molecular changes that occur during the transformation of normal melanocytes into malignant melanoma not only would help classify patients in similar prognostic groups but also would contribute to the understanding of etiology and help identify new therapeutic options. A genomewide assessment of melanomas classified into four groups based on their location and degree of exposure to the sun has confirmed that there are distinct genetic pathways in the development of melanoma. The four groups were melanomas on skin without chronic sun-induced damage, melanomas on skin with chronic sun-induced damage, mucosal melanomas, and acral melanomas. Remarkably, distinct patterns of DNA alterations were noted that varied with the site of origin and were independent of the histologic subtype of the tumor. What that work and research done by others have shown is that the overall pattern of mutation, amplification, and loss of cancer genes indicate that although the genetic changes are diverse,

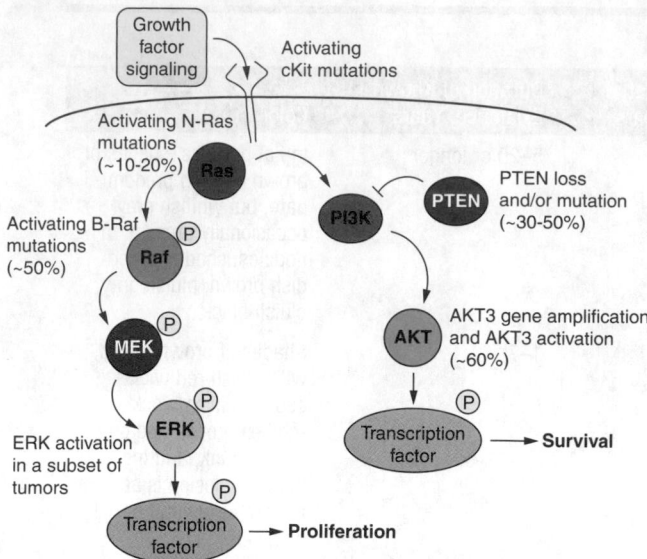

Figure 87-2 Major pathways involved in melanoma. The MAP kinase and AKT pathways, which promote proliferation and inhibit apoptosis, respectively, are subject to mutations in melanoma. ERK, extracellular signal-regulated kinase; MEK, methylethylketone; PTEN, pentaerythritol tetranitrate.

they have convergent effects on key biochemical pathways involved in proliferation, senescence, and apoptosis. The p16 mutation that leads to cell cycle arrest and the ARF mutation that results in defective apoptotic responses to genotoxic damage were described earlier. The proliferative pathways affected were the mitogen-activated protein (MAP) kinase and phosphatidylinositol 3′ kinase/AKT pathways (Fig. 87-2).

The RAS family and BRAF, members of the MAP kinase pathway, which classically mediates the transcription of genes involved in cell proliferation and survival, undergo somatic mutation in melanoma. N-RAS is mutated in approximately 20% of melanomas, and somatic activating BRAF mutations are found in most benign nevi and 40–60% of melanomas. Neither mutation by itself appears to be sufficient to cause melanoma; they often are accompanied by other mutations, (e.g., *CDKN2A*) or phosphatidylinositol 3′ kinase pathway (e.g., loss of PTEN). The BRAF mutation is almost always a point mutation (T→A nucleotide change) that results in a valine-to-glutamate amino acid substitution (V600E). V600E BRAF mutations do not have the standard UV signature mutation (pyrimidine dimer) but are present in most melanomas that arise on sites with intermittent sun exposure and are absent in melanomas from chronically sun-damaged skin.

Melanomas also contain mutations in AKT (primarily in AKT3) and PTEN (phosphatase and tensin homolog). AKT can be amplified, and PTEN may be deleted or undergo epigenetic silencing that leads to constitutive activation of the PI3K/AKT pathway and enhanced cell survival by antagonizing the intrinsic pathway of apoptosis. Loss of PTEN, which dysregulates AKT activity, and mutation of AKT3 prolong survival through inactivation of BAD, Bcl2-antagonist of cell death, and activation of the forkhead transcription factor FOXO1, which leads to synthesis of prosurvival genes. In melanoma, these two signaling pathways enhance tumorigenesis, chemoresistance, migration, and cell cycle dysregulation. Targeted agents are being employed that inhibit each pathway, but it is likely that effective antimelanoma therapy will require simultaneous inhibition of both MAPK and PI3K.

■ DIAGNOSIS

The main goal is to diagnose melanoma early in its natural history, before tumor invasion and life-threatening metastases have occurred. Early detection of melanoma may be facilitated by applying the ABCDEs: Asymmetry (benign lesions are usually symmetric); Border irregularity (most nevi have clear-cut borders); Color variegation (benign lesions usually have uniform light or dark pigment); Diameter >6 mm (the size of a pencil eraser); Evolving (any change in size, shape, color, or elevation or new symptoms such as bleeding, itching, and crusting). The aim of differential diagnosis is to distinguish benign pigmented lesions from melanoma and its precursor. If melanoma is a consideration, biopsy is appropriate. Some benign look-alikes may be removed in the process of trying to detect melanoma. Several factors may help distinguish benign nevi from atypical moles:

1. Size: Benign nevi usually are <6 mm in diameter; atypical moles usually are >6 mm in diameter.
2. Shape: Benign nevi usually are round with distinct borders and may be flat or elevated; atypical moles usually have irregular borders with pigment fading off at the edge.
3. Color: Benign nevi usually are uniformly brown or tan; atypical moles usually have variable mixtures of brown, tan, black, and reddish pigment and differ from one another.
4. Location: Benign nevi usually appear on sun-exposed skin above the waist, rarely involving scalp, breasts, or buttocks; atypical moles usually appear on sun-exposed skin, most often on the back, but can involve the scalp, breasts, or buttocks.
5. Number: Benign nevi are present in 85% of adults, with 10–40 moles scattered over the body; atypical nevi can be present in the hundreds.

The entire cutaneous surface, including the scalp and mucous membranes, as well as the nails should be examined in each patient. Bright room illumination is important, and a hand lens is helpful for evaluating variation in pigment pattern. Any suspicious lesions should be biopsied, evaluated by a specialist, or recorded by chart and/or photography for follow-up. A focused method for examining individual lesions, dermoscopy, employs low-level magnification of the epidermis and may allow a more precise visualization of patterns of pigmentation than is possible with the naked eye. Complete physical examination with attention to the regional lymph nodes is part of the initial evaluation in a patient with suspected melanoma. The patient should be advised to have other family members screened if either melanoma or clinically atypical moles (dysplastic nevi) are present. Patients who fit into high-risk groups should be instructed to perform monthly self-examinations.

Biopsy

Any pigmented cutaneous lesion that has changed in size or shape or has other features suggestive of malignant melanoma is a candidate for biopsy. The recommended technique is an excisional biopsy, which facilitates pathologic assessment of the lesion, permits accurate measurement of thickness if the lesion is melanoma, and constitutes treatment if the lesion is benign. For large lesions or lesions on anatomic sites where excisional biopsy may not be feasible (such as the face, hands, and feet), an incisional biopsy through the most nodular or darkest area of the lesion is acceptable; this should include the vertical growth phase of the primary tumor, if present. Incisional biopsy does not appear to facilitate the spread of melanoma. For suspicious lesions, every attempt should be made to preserve the ability to assess the deep and peripheral margins and to perform immunohistochemistry. Shave biopsies and cauterization should be avoided. The biopsy should be read by a pathologist experienced in pigmented lesions, and the minimal elements of the report should include Breslow thickness, mitoses per square millimeter for lesions ≤1mm, presence or absence of ulceration, and peripheral and deep margin status. Breslow thickness is the greatest thickness of a primary cutaneous melanoma measured on the slide from the top of the epidermal granular layer, or from the ulcer base, to the bottom of the tumor. To distinguish melanomas from benign nevi in cases with challenging histology, fluorescence in situ hybridization (FISH) with multiple probes can be helpful.

■ PROGNOSTIC FACTORS

The prognostic factors of greatest importance to a newly diagnosed patient are included in the staging classification (Table 87-4). The best predictor of metastatic risk is the lesion's Breslow thickness. The Clark level, which defines melanomas on the basis of the layer of skin to which a melanoma has invaded, does not add significant prognostic information and no longer is used. Other important factors recognized via the staging classification include presence of ulceration, evidence of nodal involvement, serum lactate dehydrogenase (LDH), and presence and site of distant metastases. The effects of these important prognostic factors on survival can be seen in Fig. 87-3, where survival is depicted according to stage (Table 87-4). Another determinant is anatomic site; favorable sites are the forearm and leg (excluding the feet), and unfavorable sites include the scalp, hands, feet, and mucous membranes. In general, women with stage I or II disease have better survival than men, perhaps in part because of earlier diagnosis; women frequently have melanomas on the lower leg, where self-recognition is more likely and the prognosis is better. The impact of age is not straightforward. Older individuals, especially men over 60, have worse prognoses, a finding that has been explained in part by a tendency toward later diagnosis (and thus thicker tumors) and in part by a higher proportion of acral melanomas in men. However, there is a greater risk of lymph node metastasis in young patients.

■ STAGING

Once the diagnosis of melanoma has been made, the tumor must be staged to determine the prognosis and treatment. The 2009 AJCC revised melanoma staging and classification are depicted in Table 87-4. The clinical stage of the patient is determined after the pathologic evaluation of the melanoma skin lesion and any clinical/radiologic assessment for metastatic disease. Pathologic staging also includes the pathologic evaluation of the regional lymph nodes obtained at sentinel lymph node biopsy or complete lymphadenectomy. All patients with melanoma should have a complete history and physical examination with attention to symptoms that may represent metastatic disease such as malaise, weight loss, headaches, visual difficulty, and pain. The physical examination should be directed to the site of the primary melanoma, looking for persistent disease or for dermal or subcutaneous nodules that could represent satellite or in-transit metastases. Physical examination also should include the regional draining lymph nodes, CNS, liver, and lungs. A complete blood count (CBC), complete metabolic panel, and LDH should be performed. Although these are low-yield tests for uncovering metastatic disease, a microcytic anemia would raise the possibility of bowel metastases, particularly in the small bowel, and an unexplained elevated LDH should prompt a more extensive evaluation, including CT scan or possibly a positron emission tomography (PET) (or CT/PET combined) scan. If signs or symptoms of metastatic disease are uncovered, appropriate diagnostic imaging should be performed. At initial presentation more than 80% of patients will have disease confined to the skin and a negative history and physical exam, in which case imaging generally is not indicated.

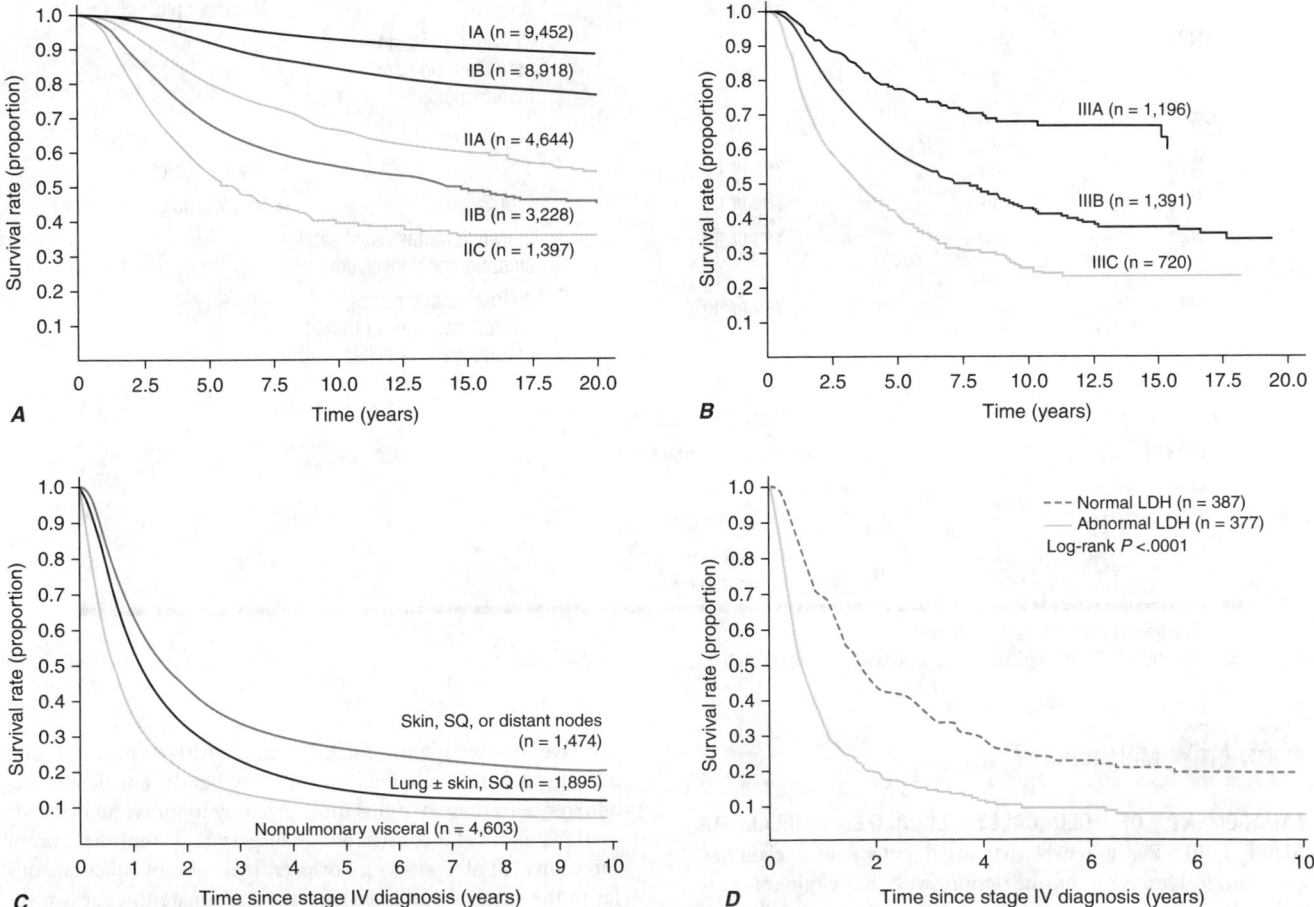

Figure 87-3 **Survival curves for patients with melanoma.** *A.* stage I and II disease; *B.* stage III disease; *C.* stage IV by site of metastatic disease; *D.* stage IV according to lactate dehydrogenase level. SQ, subcutaneous. *(From Balch et al, with permission.)*

TABLE 87-4 Staging Criteria for Melanoma

Pathologic and TNM Stage	Thickness, mm	Ulceration	No. Involved Lymph Nodes	Nodal Involvement
0				
Tis	In situ	No	0	None
IA				
T1a	<1	No, mitosis <1/mm	0	None
IB				
T1b	<1	Yes or mitosis >1/mm	0	None
T2a	1.01–2	No	0	None
IIA				
T2b	1.01–2	Yes	0	None
T3a	2.01–4	No	0	None
IIB				
T3b	2.01–4	Yes	0	None
T4a	>4	No	0	None
IIC				
T4b	>4	Yes	0	None
IIIA				
N1a	T1-4a	No	1	Microscopic
N2a	T1-4a	No	2 or 3	Microscopic
IIIB				
N1a	Any	Yes	1	Microscopic
N2a	Any	Yes	2 or 3	Microscopic
N1b	Any	Yes or no	1	Macroscopic
N2b	Any	Yes or no	2 or 3	Macroscopic
N2c	Any	Yes or no	In transit metastases/ satellites, no nodal involvement	
IIIC				
N1b	Any	Yes or no	1	Macroscopic
N2b	Any	Yes or no	2 or 3	Macroscopic
N2c	Any	Yes or no	In transit metastases/ satellites, no nodal involvement	
N3	Any	Yes or no	4+ metastatic nodes, matted nodes or in transit metastases/ satellites, with metastatic nodes	
IV		Distant metastasis		
M1a		Skin, subcutaneous		
M1b		Lung		
M1c		Other visceral site		
		Elevated lactate dehydrogenase		

Abbreviation: TNM, tumor-node metastasis.
Source: 2009 AJCC staging criteria and modified after Tsao et al: N Engl J Med 351:998, 2004

TREATMENT · Melanoma

MANAGEMENT OF CLINICALLY LOCALIZED MELANOMA (STAGE I, II) For a newly diagnosed cutaneous melanoma, wide surgical excision of the lesion with a margin of normal skin is necessary to remove all malignant cells and minimize possible local recurrence. The following margins are recommended for primary melanoma: in situ, 0.5 cm; invasive up to 1 mm thick, 1 cm; >1.01–2 mm,1–2 cm; >2 mm, 2 cm. For lesions on the face, hands, and feet, strict adherence to these margins must give way to individual considerations about the constraints of surgery and minimization of morbidity. In all instances, however, inclusion of subcutaneous fat in the surgical specimen facilitates adequate thickness measurement and assessment of surgical margins by the pathologist. Topical imiquimod also has been used, particularly for lentigo maligna, in cosmetically sensitive locations.

Sentinel lymph node biopsy (SLNB) is a valuable staging tool that has replaced elective regional nodal dissection for the evaluation of regional nodal status. SLNB provides prognostic information and helps identify patients at high risk for relapse who may be candidates for adjuvant therapy. The initial (sentinel) draining node(s) from the primary site is (are) identified by injecting a blue dye and a radioisotope around the primary site. The sentinel node(s) then is (are) identified by inspection of the nodal basin for the blue-stained node and/or the node with high uptake of the radioisotope. The identified nodes are removed and subjected to careful histopathologic processing with serial section with hematoxylin and eosin stains as well as immunohistochemical stains to identify melanocytes (e.g., S100, HMB45, and MelanA).

Not every patient is a candidate for a SLNB. Patients whose melanomas are ≤1 mm thick and have <1 mitotic figure/mm² have an excellent prognosis and generally do not need an SLNB unless they have high-risk features such as young age, an ulcerated primary, and positive deep margins. They usually can be referred for wide excision as definitive therapy. Most other patients with clinically negative lymph nodes should undergo an SLNB. Patients whose SLNB is negative are spared a complete node dissection and its attendant morbidities. They can simply be followed or considered for adjuvant therapy or a clinical trial as appropriate for the primary lesion. The current standard of care for all patients with a positive SLN is to perform a complete lymphadenectomy; however, ongoing clinical studies are attempting to determine whether patients with small-volume metastases in the sentinel node can be managed safely without additional surgery. Patients with microscopically positive lymph nodes should be considered for adjuvant therapy with interferon or enrolled in a clinical trial.

MANAGEMENT OF REGIONALLY METASTATIC MELANOMA (STAGE III)
Regional metastases may occur as a local recurrence at the edge of the scar or graft; as satellite metastases, which are separate from the scar but within 2–5 cm of the scar; as in-transit metastases, which are recurrences >5 cm from the scar; or, as in the most common case, as metastasis to a draining lymph node basin. Each of these recurrences is managed surgically, if possible, with the possibility of achieving long-term disease-free survival. An option for patients with extensive cutaneous regional recurrences in an extremity is isolated limb perfusion or infusion with melphalan and hyperthermia. High complete response rates have been reported, and responses are associated with significant palliation of symptoms.

After surgery, patients with regional metastases who are rendered free of disease may be at high risk for a local or distant recurrence. Therefore, some patients should be considered for adjuvant therapy. Adjuvant radiotherapy can reduce the risk of local recurrence after lymphadenectomy but does not affect overall survival. Patients with large (>3–4 cm) or multiple involved lymph nodes or extranodal spread on microscopic examination should be considered for radiation. Systemic adjuvant therapy is indicated primarily for patients with stage III disease, but high-risk, node-negative patients (>4 mm thick or ulcerated lesions) and patients with completely resected stage IV disease also may benefit. Interferon α2b (IFN-α2b), which is given for 1 year at 20 million units/m² intravenously 5 days a week for 4 weeks followed by 10 million units/m² subcutaneously three times a week for 11 months, is the only U.S. Food and Drug Administration (FDA)-approved agent for adjuvant therapy. High-dose IFN is associated with significant toxicity, including a flulike illness, decline in performance status, and the development of depression in a large fraction of patients. The toxicity can be managed in most patients

by appropriate therapy for symptoms, dose reduction, treatment interruption, and, for one-third of patients, early discontinuation of IFN. Adjuvant treatment with high-dose IFN has been associated with improved disease-free survival, but its impact on overall survival is unclear. Enrollment in a clinical trial is appropriate for these patients, many of whom will otherwise be observed without treatment either because they are poor candidates for IFN or because a patient (or his or her oncologist) does not believe the beneficial effects of IFN outweigh the toxicity.

TREATMENT | Metastatic Disease

When a patient with a history of melanoma develops signs or symptoms of recurrent disease, he or she should undergo restaging. This typically includes an MRI of the brain and total-body PET/CT or CT scans of the chest, abdomen, and pelvis. Distant metastases (stage IV), which may involve any organ, commonly include skin and lymph node metastases as well as visceral, bone, or brain metastases. Metastatic melanoma is generally incurable, and median survival ranges from 6 to15 months, depending on the organ involved (Fig. 87-3C, D). The prognosis is better for skin and subcutaneous metastases (Mla) than for lung (M1b) or other visceral metastases (Mlc). An elevated serum LDH in a patient with metastatic disease is a poor prognostic factor and puts the patient in stage Mlc regardless of the site of the metastases.

The only FDA-approved chemotherapy for melanoma is dacarbazine (DTIC). Other agents with modest activity include temozolomide (TMZ), cisplatin and carboplatin, the taxanes, paclitaxel and docetaxel alone or albumin-bound, and carmustine (BCNU), which have reported response rates of 12–20%. Although limited in efficacy, single-agent DTIC is still considered the standard treatment because drug combinations have never been shown to improve survival. Although not FDA-approved for melanoma, TMZ, which shares an active metabolite with DTIC, has been used widely because of its ease of oral administration, excellent tolerance, and penetration across the blood-brain barrier. Attempts to define superior combinations and identify new active agents are ongoing.

Interleukin 2 (IL-2)-based therapy has been associated with long-term disease-free survival (probable cures) in 5% of treated patients. Treatment usually consists of high-dose IL-2 alone, but some centers combine IL-2 with IFN-α and chemotherapy (biochemotherapy). IL-2 therapy generally is reserved for patients with a good performance status and administered at centers with experience managing IL-2-related toxicity. The mechanism by which IL-2 effects tumor regression has not been identified, but it is presumed that it induces melanoma-specific T cells that cause tumor regression. Based on this assumption, Rosenberg and his colleagues in the National Cancer Institute (NCI) Surgery Branch have used adoptive immunotherapy with in vitro-expanded tumor-infiltrating lymphocytes with high-dose IL-2. A series of studies of adoptive T cell therapy in patients who have been treated with nonmyeloablative chemotherapy (sometimes combined with total-body irradiation) have reported tumor regression in more than 50% of patients with IL-2-refractory melanoma. Multiple investigators have attempted to develop vaccination strategies against melanoma using purified tumor proteins, peptides, DNA vectors, dendritic cells, and unmodified or genetically altered tumor cells as immunogens to elicit melanoma-specific T cell responses, but none of these approaches has met with much clinical success.

A promising new approach is CTLA-4 blockade with a monoclonal antibody. CTLA-4 antibodies block the inhibitory signal produced when CTLA-4 is engaged on activated T cells, enhance T cell function, and cause tumor regression in animal models. Administration of anti-CTLA-4 (ipilimumab) to patients with previously treated metastatic melanoma in a randomized study was shown to improve overall survival compared to patients receiving a peptide vaccine. A novel spectrum of side effects that implies development of autoimmunity, so-called immune-related adverse events, has been noted. Patients who develop skin rashes, diarrhea and colitis, and hypophysitis, all of which can be managed, appear to have higher rates of tumor regression.

Targeted therapies are an exciting approach for patients with metastatic melanoma. The most promising available agents are those that target activating mutations in BRAF and c-kit, which result in constitutive activation of the MAP kinase pathway. V600E BRAF is the most common kinase mutation in melanoma. A highly selective oral BRAF inhibitor, PLX4032, has been developed, and tumor regression rates up to 70% have been reported in early clinical trials; to date, most remissions appear to be partial and of limited duration. Activating mutations in the c-kit receptor tyrosine kinase are also found in melanoma, but primarily in mucosal, acral lentiginous, and lentigo maligna melanoma. Since these tumors are found in only 5% of the patients with metastatic melanoma, the number of patients with c-kit mutations is exceedingly small. Nevertheless, if present, they are largely identical to mutations found in gastrointestinal stromal tumors (GISTs), and melanomas with activating c-kit mutations can have rather dramatic responses to imatinib. The availability of targeted therapies will require that selected patients have their tumors sent for molecular typing to determine their suitability for treatment with available agents or their eligibility for clinical trials of newly developed agents. Some patients with stage IV disease will experience long-term disease-free survival after surgical resection of their metastases (metastatectomy). Surgery often is performed in patients with metastatic disease involving a small number of sites, either before or after systemic therapy. These patients may have a solitary lung or brain metastasis, but surgery increasingly is being employed in patients with metastases at more than one site. After surgery, patients with no evidence of disease can be considered for INF therapy or a clinical trial because their risk of developing additional metastases is very high.

Current therapy for the overwhelming majority of patients is palliative, and so enrollment in a clinical trial is always an appropriate option, even for previously untreated patients. However, because most patients with stage IV disease are incurable, a major focus of care, particularly for patients with poor performance status, should be the timely integration of palliative care and hospice.

■ FOLLOW-UP

Skin examination and surveillance at least once a year is recommended for all patients with melanoma. The National Cancer Comprehensive Network (NCCN) guidelines for patients with stage IB–IV melanoma recommend a comprehensive history and physical examination every 3–6 months for 2 years, then every 3–12 months for 3 years, and annually thereafter, as clinically indicated. Particular attention should be paid to the draining lymph nodes in stage I–III patients as resection of lymph node recurrences may still be curative. A CBC, LDH, and chest x-ray are recommended at the physician's discretion. Routine imaging for metastatic disease is not recommended at this time because there is no discernible survival benefit to the early detection of metastatic disease.

■ PREVENTION

Primary melanoma prevention is based on protection from the sun, which includes wearing protective clothing, avoiding intense midday UV exposure and tanning booths, and routine application of a broad-spectrum ultraviolet-A/ultraviolet-B (UV-A/UV-B) sunblock with sun protection factor ≥15. This includes use of protective clothing and avoidance of intense midday UV exposure. Secondary prevention consists of education and screening. Patients should be educated in the clinical features of melanoma (ABCDEs) and advised to report any growth or other change in a pigmented lesion. Brochures are available from the American Cancer Society, the American Academy of Dermatology, the National Cancer Institute, and the Skin Cancer Foundation. Self-examination at 6- to 8-week intervals may enhance the likelihood of detecting change. Although the U.S. Preventive Services Task Force states that evidence is insufficient to recommend for or against skin cancer screening, a full-body skin cancer screening seems to be a simple, practical way to approach reducing the mortality rate for skin cancer. This is particularly true for patients with clinically atypical moles (dysplastic nevi) and those with a personal history of melanoma. Individuals with three or more primary melanomas and families with at least one invasive melanoma and two or more cases of melanoma and/or pancreatic cancer among first- or second-degree relatives on the same side of the family may benefit from genetic testing.

NONMELANOMA SKIN CANCER

Nonmelanoma skin cancer (NMSC) is the most common cancer in the United States, with an estimated annual incidence of 1.5–2 million cases. Basal cell carcinomas (BCCs) account for 70–80% of NMSCs. Squamous cell carcinomas (SCCs), though representing only ~20% of NMSCs, are more significant because of their ability to metastasize (Fig. 87-4). They account for most of the 2400 deaths annually. Incidence rates have risen dramatically over the last decade.

■ ETIOLOGY

The causes of BCC and SCC are multifactorial. Cumulative exposure to sunlight, principally the UV-B spectrum, is the most significant factor. Other factors associated with a higher incidence of skin cancer are male sex, older age, Celtic descent, a fair complexion, blond or red hair, blue or green eyes, a tendency to sunburn easily, and an outdoor occupation. The incidence of these tumors increases with decreasing latitude. Most tumors develop on sun-exposed areas of the head and neck. Tumors are more common on the left side of the body in the United States but on the right side in England, presumably owing to asymmetric exposure during driving. As the earth's protective ozone shield continues to thin, further increases in the incidence of skin cancer can be anticipated. In certain geographic areas, exposure to arsenic in well water or from industrial sources may increase the risk of BCC and SCC significantly. Skin cancer in affected individuals may be seen with or without other cutaneous markers of chronic arsenism (e.g., arsenical keratoses). Less common is exposure to the cyclic aromatic hydrocarbons in tar, soot, or shale. The risk of lip or oral SCC is increased with cigarette smoking. Human papillomaviruses and UV radiation may act as cocarcinogens.

Host factors associated with a higher risk of skin cancer include immunosuppression induced by disease or drugs. Solid-organ transplant recipients on chronic immunosuppressive therapy have a dramatically higher incidence of NMSCs. SCCs are most common, with a 65-fold increase in incidence, whereas BCCs have a tenfold increase in incidence. The frequency of skin cancer is proportional to the level and duration of immunosuppression as well as the extent of sun exposure both before and after transplantation. SCCs in this population also demonstrate more aggressive behavior with higher rates of local recurrence, metastasis, and mortality.

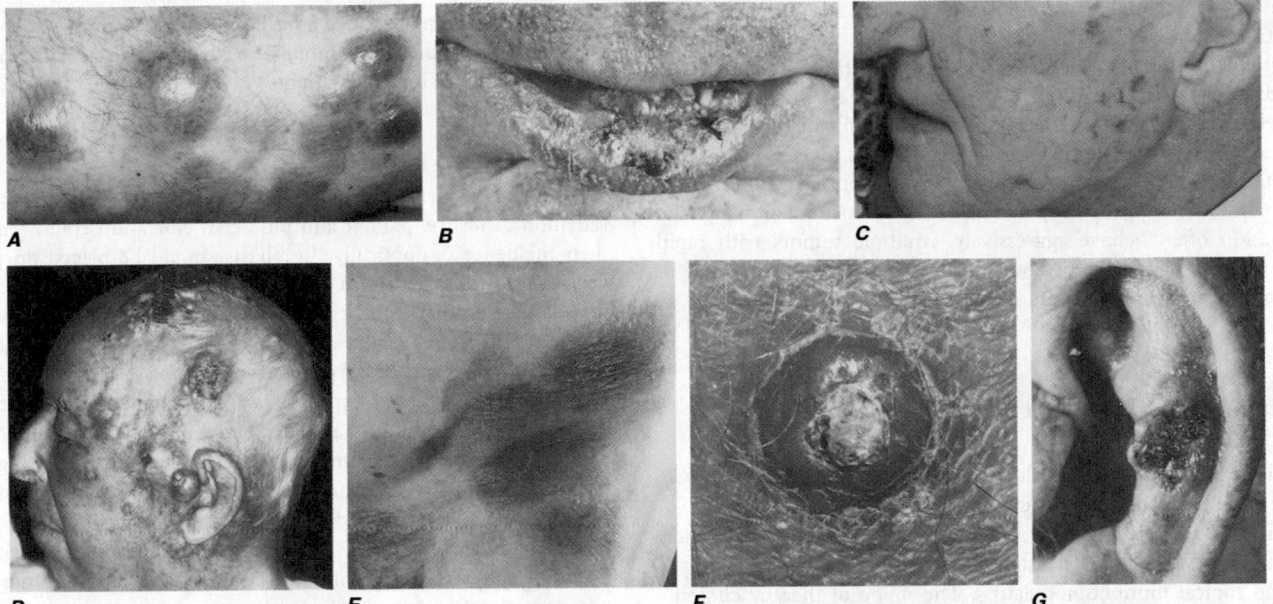

Figure 87-4 Cutaneous neoplasms. A. Non-Hodgkin's lymphoma involves the skin with typical violaceous, "plum-colored" nodules. **B.** Squamous cell carcinoma is seen here as a hyperkeratotic crusted and somewhat eroded plaque on the lower lip. Sun-exposed skin in areas such as the head, neck, hands, and arms represent other typical sites of involvement. **C.** Actinic keratoses consist of hyperkeratotic erythematous papules and patches on sun-exposed skin. They arise in middle-aged to older adults and have some potential for malignant transformation. **D.** Metastatic carcinoma to the skin is characterized by inflammatory, often ulcerated dermal nodules. **E.** Mycosis fungoides is a cutaneous T cell lymphoma, and plaque-stage lesions are seen in this patient. **F.** Keratoacanthoma is a low-grade squamous cell carcinoma that presents as an exophytic nodule with central keratinous debris. **G.** This basal cell carcinoma shows central ulceration and a pearly, rolled telangiectatic tumor border.

Skin cancer is not uncommon in patients infected with HIV, and tumors may be more aggressive in this setting. Other factors include ionizing radiation, thermal burn scars, and chronic ulcerations. Several heritable conditions are associated with skin cancer (e.g., albinism, xeroderma pigmentosum, Rombo's syndrome, Bazex-Dupré-Christol syndrome, and basal cell nevus syndrome). Background mutations in hedgehog pathway genes, primarily genes encoding patched homolog 1 (*PTCH1*) and smoothened homolog (*SMO*), occur in BCC. In fact, an oral hedgehog inhibitor has shown promise in clinical trials treating advanced inoperable or metastatic BCC.

■ CLINICAL PRESENTATION

NMSCs are often asymptomatic, but nonhealing ulceration, bleeding, or pain can occur in advanced lesions.

Basal cell carcinoma

BCC is a malignancy arising from epidermal basal cells. The least invasive of BCC subtypes, *superficial BCC*, classically consists of truncal erythematous scaling plaques that slowly enlarge. This BCC subtype may be confused with benign inflammatory dermatoses, especially nummular eczema and psoriasis. BCC also can present as a small, slowly growing pearly nodule, often with small telangiectatic vessels on its surface (*nodular BCC*). The occasional presence of melanin in this variant of nodular BCC (*pigmented BCC*) may lead to confusion clinically with melanoma. *Morpheaform (fibrosing) and micronodular BCC*, the most invasive subtypes, manifest as solitary, flat or slightly depressed, indurated whitish or yellowish plaques. Borders are typically indistinct, a feature associated with a greater potential for extensive subclinical spread.

Squamous cell carcinoma

Primary *cutaneous SCC* is a malignant neoplasm of keratinizing epidermal cells. SCC can grow rapidly and metastasize. The clinical features of SCC vary widely. Commonly, SCC appears as an ulcerated erythematous nodule or superficial erosion on the skin or lower lip, but it may present as a verrucous papule or plaque. Overlying telangiectasias are uncommon. The margins of this tumor may be ill defined, and fixation to underlying structures may occur. Cutaneous SCC may develop anywhere on the body but usually arises on sun-damaged skin. A related neoplasm, keratoacanthoma, typically appears as a dome-shaped papule with a central keratotic crater, expands rapidly, and commonly regresses without therapy. This lesion can be difficult to differentiate from SCC.

Actinic keratoses and *cheilitis*, both premalignant forms of SCC, present as hyperkeratotic papules on sun-exposed areas. The potential for malignant degeneration in untreated lesions ranges from 0.25 to 20%. *Bowen's disease*, the in situ form of SCC, presents as a scaling, erythematous plaque. Treatment of premalignant and in situ lesions reduces the subsequent risk of invasive disease.

■ NATURAL HISTORY

Basal cell carcinoma

The natural history of BCC is that of a slowly enlarging, locally invasive neoplasm. The degree of local destruction and risk of recurrence vary with the size, duration, location, and histologic subtype of the tumor; presence of recurrent disease; and various patient characteristics. Location on the central face, ears, or scalp may portend a higher risk. Small nodular, pigmented, cystic, or superficial BCCs respond well to most treatments. Large lesions and micronodular and morpheaform subtypes may be more aggressive. The metastatic potential of BCC has been estimated to be 0.0028–0.1%. Persons with either BCC or SCC have an increased risk of developing subsequent skin cancers that is estimated to be up to 40% in 5 years.

Squamous cell carcinoma

The natural history of SCC depends on both tumor and host characteristics. Tumors arising on sun-damaged skin have a lower metastatic potential than do those on protected surfaces. Cutaneous SCC metastasizes in 0.3–5.2% of individuals, most frequently to regional draining lymph nodes. Tumors occurring on the lower lip and ear have metastatic potentials approaching 13 and 11%, respectively. The metastatic potential of SCC arising in scars, chronic ulcerations, and genital or mucosal surfaces is higher. The overall metastatic rate for recurrent tumors may approach 30%. Large, poorly differentiated, deep tumors with perineural or lymphatic invasion often behave aggressively. Multiple tumors with rapid growth and aggressive behavior can be a therapeutic challenge in immunosuppressed patients.

TREATMENT   Basal Cell Carcinoma

The most frequently employed treatment modalities for BCC include electrodesiccation and curettage (ED&C), excision, cryosurgery, radiation therapy, laser therapy, Mohs micrographic surgery (MMS), topical 5-fluorouracil, photodynamic therapy, and topical immunomodulators. The mode of therapy chosen depends on tumor characteristics, patient age, medical status, preferences of the patient, and other factors. ED&C remains the method most commonly employed by dermatologists. This method is selected for low-risk tumors (e.g., a small primary tumor of a less aggressive subtype in a favorable location). Excision that offers the advantage of histologic control, usually is selected for more aggressive tumors or those in high-risk locations or, in many instances, for aesthetic reasons. Cryosurgery using liquid nitrogen may be used in certain low-risk tumors but requires specialized equipment (cryoprobes) to be employed effectively. Radiation therapy, although not used as often as a primary modality, offers an excellent chance for cure in many cases of BCC. It is useful in patients not considered surgical candidates and as a surgical adjunct in high-risk tumors. Younger patients may not be good candidates for radiation therapy because of the risks of long-term carcinogenesis and radiodermatitis. Despite rapidly advancing technology in laser development, its long-term efficacy in treating infiltrative or recurrent lesions is unknown. In contrast, MMS, a specialized type of surgical excision that permits the best histologic control and preservation of uninvolved tissue, is associated with cure rates >98%. It is the preferred modality for lesions that are recurrent, in a high-risk location, or are large and ill defined, and in which maximal tissue conservation is critical (e.g., the eyelids). Topical 5-fluorouracil therapy should be limited to superficial BCC. Topical immunomodulators (e.g., imiquimod) show promise in treating superficial and even smaller nodular BCCs. Intralesional chemotherapy (5-fluorouracil and interferon) and photodynamic therapy (which employs selective activation of a photoactive drug by visible light) have been used successfully in patients with numerous tumors. A topical endonuclease (T4N5 liposome lotion) has been shown to repair DNA and may decrease the rate of NMSC in xeroderma pigmentosum.

SQUAMOUS CELL CARCINOMA   Therapy for cutaneous SCC should be based on an analysis of risk factors influencing the biologic behavior of the tumor. These factors include the size, location, and degree of histologic differentiation of the tumor as well as the age and physical condition of the patient. Surgical excision, MMS, and radiation therapy are standard methods of treatment. Cryosurgery and ED&C have been used successfully for premalignant lesions and small primary tumors. Metastases are treated with lymph node dissection, irradiation, or both. 13-*cis*-retinoic acid (1 mg/kg PO qd) plus IFN-α (3 million U SC or IM qd) may produce a partial response in most patients. Systemic chemotherapy combinations that include cisplatin may also be palliative in some patients.

■ PREVENTION

As the vast majority of skin cancers are related to chronic UV radiation exposure, patient and physician education could reduce their incidence dramatically. Emphasis should be placed on preventive measures that begin early in life. Patients must understand that damage from UV-B begins early despite the fact that cancers develop years later. Regular use of sunscreens and protective clothing should be encouraged. Avoidance of tanning salons and midday (10 A.M. to 2 P.M.) sun exposure is recommended. Precancerous and in situ lesions should be treated early. Early detection of small tumors allows the use of simpler treatment modalities with higher cure rates and lower morbidity rates. In patients with a history of skin cancer, long-term follow-up for the detection of recurrence, metastasis, and new skin cancers should be emphasized. Chemoprophylaxis using synthetic retinoids as well as immunosuppression reduction in transplant patients may be useful in controlling new lesions in those with multiple tumors.

■ OTHER NONMELANOMA CUTANEOUS MALIGNANCIES

Neoplasms of cutaneous adnexa and sarcomas of fibrous, mesenchymal, fatty, and vascular tissues make up the remaining 1–2% of NMSCs (Table 87-1) *Merkel cell carcinoma* is a neural crest–derived (cytokeratin-20-positive), highly aggressive malignancy that exhibits mortality rates of about 33% at 3 years. Recent studies have implicated a novel oncogenic Merkel cell polyomavirus that is present in 80% of tumors. Prognosis largely depends on extent of disease: 90% survival with local disease, 52% with nodal involvement, and 10% with distant disease at 3 years. Incidence tripled from 1986 to 2001 with a current estimate of 1200 cases per year in the United States. It typically presents as an asymptomatic rapidly expanding red/pink tumor on sun-exposed skin of older white patients. Treatment is surgical excision with or without sentinel lymph node biopsy, often followed by adjuvant radiation.

Extramammary Paget's disease is an uncommon apocrine malignancy arising from stem cells of the epidermis that are characterized histologically by the presence of Paget cells. These tumors present as moist erythematous patches on anogenital or, less commonly, axillary skin of the elderly. Treatment may be challenging as these tumors characteristically extend far beyond clinical margins; surgical excision with MMS has the highest cure rates. Similarly, MMS is the treatment of choice in other rare cutaneous tumors with extensive subclinical extension such as *dermatofibromasarcoma protuberans*.

Kaposi's sarcoma (KS) is a soft tissue sarcoma of vascular origin that is induced by the human herpes virus 8. The incidence of KS was rare before the AIDS epidemic. AIDS-associated KS has decreased tenfold with the institution of highly active antiretroviral therapy.

ACKNOWLEDGMENT
Hensin Tsao, MD, and Arthur J. Sober, MD, contributed to this chapter in the 17th edition, and material from that chapter is included here.

FURTHER READINGS

ALAM M et al: Cutaneous squamous-cell carcinoma. N Engl J Med 344:975, 2001

BALCH CM et al: Final version of 2009 AJCC melanoma staging and classification. J Clin Oncol 27:6199, 2009

BERG D et al: Skin cancer in organ transplant recipients: Epidemiology, pathogenesis, and management. J Am Acad Dermatol 47:1, 2002

BERWICK M et al: Melanoma epidemiology and public health. Dermatol Clin 27:205, 2009

COIT DG et al: The NCCN melanoma clinical practice guidelines in oncology. J Natl Cancer Comp Netw 7:250, 2009

CURTIN JA et al: Distinct sets of genetic alterations in melanoma. N Engl J Med 353:2135, 2005

FENG H et al: Clonal integration of a polyomavirus in human Merkel cell carcinoma. Science 319:1096, 2008

FLAHERTY KT et al: Inhibition of mutated, activated BRAF in metastatic melanoma. N Engl J Med 363:809, 2010

HODI FS et al: Improved survival with ipilimumab in patients with metastatic melanoma. N Engl J Med 363:711, 2010

RUBIN AI et al: Basal-cell carcinoma. N Engl J Med 353:2262, 2005

SKULIC A et al: Malignant melanoma in the 21st century: The emerging molecular landscape. Mayo Clin Proc 83:825, 2008

CHAPTER **88**

Head and Neck Cancer

Everett E. Vokes

Epithelial carcinomas of the head and neck arise from the mucosal surfaces in the head and neck area and typically are squamous cell in origin. This category includes tumors of the paranasal sinuses, the oral cavity, and the nasopharynx, oropharynx, hypopharynx, and larynx. Tumors of the salivary glands differ from the more common carcinomas of the head and neck in etiology, histopathology, clinical presentation, and therapy. Thyroid malignancies are described in Chap. 341.

INCIDENCE AND EPIDEMIOLOGY

The number of new cases of head and neck cancers in the United States was 36,540 in 2010, accounting for about 3% of adult malignancies; 7880 people died from the disease. The worldwide incidence exceeds half a million cases annually. In North America and Europe, the tumors usually arise from the oral cavity, oropharynx, or larynx, whereas nasopharyngeal cancer is more commonly seen in the Mediterranean countries and in the Far East.

ETIOLOGY AND GENETICS

Alcohol and tobacco use are the most significant risk factors for head and neck cancer in the United States. Smokeless tobacco is an etiologic agent for oral cancers. Other potential carcinogens include marijuana and occupational exposures such as nickel refining, exposure to textile fibers, and woodworking.

Dietary factors may contribute. The incidence of head and neck cancer is higher in people with the lowest consumption of fruits and vegetables. Certain vitamins, including carotenoids, may be protective if included in a balanced diet. Supplements of retinoids such as *cis*-retinoic acid have not been shown to prevent head and neck cancers (or lung cancer) and may increase the risk in active smokers.

Some head and neck cancers have a viral etiology. Epstein-Barr virus (EBV) infection is frequently associated with nasopharyngeal cancer. Nasopharyngeal cancer occurs endemically in some countries of the Mediterranean and Far East, where EBV antibody titers can be measured to screen high-risk populations. Nasopharyngeal cancer has also been associated with consumption of salted fish.

In Western countries, the human papilloma virus (HPV) is associated with approximately 50% of tumors arising from the oropharynx, i.e., the tonsillar bed and base of tongue. Similar to cervical cancer, HPV 16 and 18 are the commonly associated viral subtypes. The incidence of oropharyngeal cancers is increasing in Western counties. Epidemiologically HPV-related oropharyngeal cancer occurs in a younger patient population and is associated with increased numbers of sexual partners and oral sexual practices.

No specific risk factors or environmental carcinogens have been identified for salivary gland tumors.

HISTOPATHOLOGY, CARCINOGENESIS, AND MOLECULAR BIOLOGY

Squamous cell head and neck cancers can be divided into well-differentiated, moderately well-differentiated, and poorly differentiated categories. Poorly differentiated tumors have a worse prognosis than well-differentiated tumors. For nasopharyngeal cancers, the less common differentiated squamous cell carcinoma is distinguished from nonkeratinizing and undifferentiated carcinoma (lymphoepithelioma) that contains infiltrating lymphocytes and is commonly associated with EBV.

Salivary gland tumors can arise from the major (parotid, submandibular, sublingual) or minor salivary glands (located in the submucosa of the upper aerodigestive tract). Most parotid tumors are benign, but half of submandibular and sublingual gland tumors and most minor salivary gland tumors are malignant. Malignant tumors include mucoepidermoid and adenoid cystic carcinomas and adenocarcinomas.

The mucosal surface of the entire pharynx is exposed to alcohol- and tobacco-related carcinogens and is at risk for the development of a premalignant or malignant lesion. Erythroplakia (a red patch) or leukoplakia (a white patch) can be histopathologically hyperplasia, dysplasia, carcinoma in situ, or carcinoma. However, most head and neck cancers do not present with a history of premalignant lesions. Multiple synchronous or metachronous cancers can also be observed. In fact, over time patients with early-stage head and neck cancer are at greater risk of dying from a second malignancy than from a recurrence of the primary disease.

Second head and neck malignancies are usually not therapy-induced; they reflect the exposure of the upper aerodigestive mucosa to the same carcinogens that caused the first cancer. These second primaries develop in the head and neck area, the lung, or the esophagus. Rarely, patients can develop a radiation therapy–induced sarcoma after having undergone prior radiotherapy for a head and neck cancer.

The molecular carcinogenesis of head and neck cancer is a developing story. Activation of oncogenes and inactivation of tumor suppressor genes (frequently of p53) have been described. Overexpression of the epidermal growth factor receptor (EGFR) is common and of prognostic importance.

Resected tumor specimens with histopathologically negative margins ("complete resection") can have residual tumor cells with persistent p53 mutations at the margins. Thus, a tumor-specific p53 mutation can be detected in some phenotypically "normal" surgical margins, indicating residual disease. Patients with such submicroscopic marginal involvement may have a worse prognosis than patients with truly negative margins.

Most head and neck cancers occur in patients older than age 50 years. HPV-related malignancies are frequently diagnosed in patients in their 40s while EBV-related nasopharyngeal cancer can occur in all ages, including teenagers. The manifestations vary according to the stage and primary site of the tumor. Patients with nonspecific signs and symptoms in the head and neck area should be evaluated with a thorough otolaryngologic exam, particularly if symptoms persist longer than 2–4 weeks.

Cancer of the nasopharynx typically does not cause early symptoms. However, on occasion it may cause unilateral serous otitis media due to obstruction of the eustachian tube, unilateral or bilateral nasal obstruction, or epistaxis. Advanced nasopharyngeal carcinoma causes neuropathies of the cranial nerves due to skull base involvement.

Carcinomas of the oral cavity present as nonhealing ulcers, changes in the fit of dentures, or painful lesions. Tumors of the tongue base or oropharynx can cause decreased tongue mobility and alterations in speech. Cancers of the oropharynx or hypopharynx rarely cause early symptoms, but they may cause sore throat and/or otalgia.

Hoarseness may be an early symptom of laryngeal cancer, and persistent hoarseness requires referral to a specialist for indirect laryngoscopy and/or radiographic studies. If a head and neck lesion treated initially with antibiotics does not resolve in a short period, further workup is indicated; to simply continue the antibiotic treatment may be to lose the chance of early diagnosis of a malignancy.

Advanced head and neck cancers in any location can cause severe pain, otalgia, airway obstruction, cranial neuropathies, trismus, odynophagia, dysphagia, decreased tongue mobility, fistulas, skin involvement, and massive cervical lymphadenopathy, which may be unilateral or bilateral. Some patients have enlarged lymph nodes even though no primary lesion can be detected by endoscopy or biopsy; these patients are considered to have carcinoma of unknown primary (Fig. 88-1). If the enlarged nodes are located in the upper neck and the tumor cells are of squamous cell histology, the malignancy probably arose from a mucosal surface in the head or neck. Tumor cells in supraclavicular lymph nodes may also arise from a primary site in the chest or abdomen.

The physical examination should include inspection of all visible mucosal surfaces and palpation of the floor of mouth and tongue and of the neck. In addition to tumors themselves, leukoplakia (a white mucosal patch) or erythroplakia (a red mucosal patch) may be observed; these "premalignant" lesions can represent hyperplasia, dysplasia, or carcinoma in situ and require biopsy. Further examination should be performed by a specialist. Additional staging procedures include CT of the head and neck to identify the extent of the disease. Patients with lymph node involvement should have chest radiography and a bone scan to screen for distant metastases. A positron emission tomographic scan may also be administered and can help to identify or exclude distant metastases. The definitive staging procedure is an endoscopic examination under anesthesia, which may include laryngoscopy, esophagoscopy, and bronchoscopy; during this procedure, multiple biopsy samples are obtained to establish a primary diagnosis, define the extent of primary disease, and identify any additional premalignant lesions or second primaries.

Head and neck tumors are classified according to the TNM system of the American Joint Committee on Cancer. This classification varies according to the specific anatomic subsite (Tables 88-1 and 88-2). Distant metastases are found in <10% of patients at initial diagnosis and are more common in patients with advanced lymph nodal stage; microscopic involvement of the lungs, bones, or liver is more common, particularly in patients with advanced neck lymph node disease. Modern imaging techniques may increase the number of patients with clinically detectable distant metastases in the future.

In patients with lymph node involvement and no visible primary, the diagnosis should be made by lymph node excision. If the results indicate squamous cell carcinoma, a panendoscopy should be performed, with biopsy of all suspicious-appearing areas and directed biopsies of common primary sites, such as the nasopharynx, tonsil, tongue base, and pyriform sinus.

TREATMENT Head and Neck Cancer

Patients with head and neck cancer can be grossly categorized into three clinical groups: those with localized disease, those with locally or regionally advanced disease, and those with recurrent and/or metastatic disease. Comorbidities associated with tobacco and alcohol abuse can affect treatment outcome and define long-term risks for patients who are cured of their disease.

LOCALIZED DISEASE Nearly one-third of patients have localized disease, that is, T1 or T2 (stage I or stage II) lesions without detectable lymph node involvement or distant metastases. These lesions are treated with curative intent by either surgery or radiation therapy. The choice of modality differs according to anatomic location and institutional expertise. Radiation therapy is often preferred for laryngeal cancer to preserve voice function, and surgery is preferred for small lesions in the oral cavity to avoid the long-term complications of radiation, such as xerostomia and dental decay. Overall 5-year survival is 60–90%. Most recurrences occur within the first 2 years following diagnosis and are usually local.

LOCALLY OR REGIONALLY ADVANCED DISEASE Locally or regionally advanced disease—disease with a large primary tumor and/or lymph node metastases—is the stage of presentation for >50% of patients. Such patients can also be treated with curative intent, but not with surgery or radiation therapy alone. Combined modality therapy including surgery, radiation therapy, and chemotherapy is most successful. It can be administered as induction chemotherapy (chemotherapy before surgery and/or radiotherapy) or as concomitant (simultaneous) chemotherapy and radiation therapy. The latter is currently most commonly used and best evidence–supported. In patients with intermediate stage (stage III and early stage IV) concomitant chemoradiotherapy is given postoperatively. It can be administered either as a primary

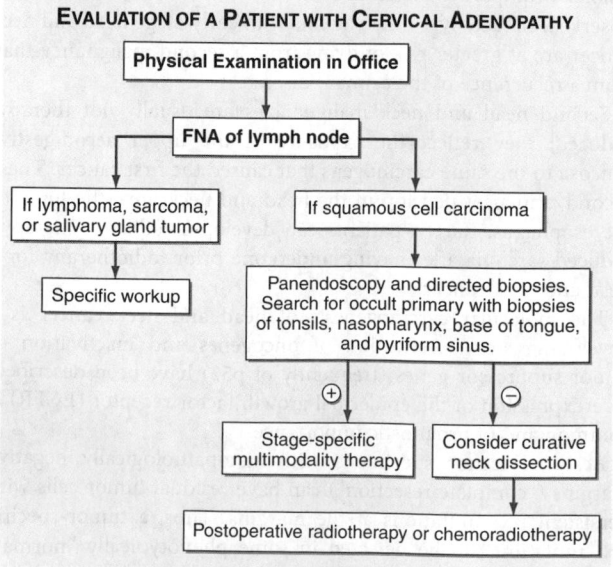

Figure 88-1 Evaluation of a patient with cervical adenopathy without a primary mucosal lesion; a diagnostic workup. FNA, fine-needle aspiration.

TABLE 88-1 TNM Classification for Head and Neck Cancer

Primary Tumor Site (Example)

T Grade	Oropharynx	Hypopharynx
T1	0–2 cm	0–2 cm
T2	2.1–4 cm	>1 site, 2.1–4 cm
T3	>4 cm	>4 cm or fixation of hemilarynx
T4a	Invasion of larynx, muscle of tongue, medial pterygoid, hard palate, mandible	Invasion of thyroid/cricoid cartilage, hyoid bone, thyroid gland, esophagus, or central compartment soft tissue invasion
T4b	Invasion of lateral pterygoid muscle, pterygoid plates, lateral nasopharynx, or skull base or encases carotid artery	Invasion of prevertebral fascia, encases carotid artery, or involvement of mediastinal structures

Regional Lymph Nodes (N)

NX	Regional lymph nodes cannot be assessed
N0	No regional lymph node metastasis
N1	Unilateral metastasis in lymph node(s), ≤3 cm in greatest dimension
N2	Single ipsilateral lymph node >3.1, ≤6 cm, or multiple ipsilateral, or contralateral lymph nodes ≤6 cm. Bilateral metastasis in lymph node(s), ≤6 cm in greatest dimension, above the supraclavicular fossa
N3	Lymph node >6 cm in greatest dimension

Stage Grouping

Stage			
Stage 0	Tis	N0	M0
Stage I	T1	N0	M0
Stage II	T2	N0	M0
Stage III	T3	N0	M0
	T1–T3	N1	M0
Stage IVA	T4a	N0	M0
	T4a	N1	M0
	T1–T4a	N2	M0
Stage IVB	T4b	Any N	M0
	Any T	N3	M0
Stage IVC	Any T	Any N	M1

TABLE 88-2 Definition of TNM-Nasopharynx

Primary Tumor (T)	Stage Grouping
Tis	Carcinoma in situ
T1	Tumor confined to the nasopharynx
T2	Tumor extends to parapharyngeal soft tissues
T3	Tumor involves bony structures of skull base and/or paranasal sinuses
T4	Tumor with intracranial extension and/or involvement of cranial nerves, infratemporal fossa, hypopharynx, orbit, or masticator space

Regional Lymph Nodes (N)

	The distribution and the prognostic impact of regional lymph node spread from nasopharynx cancer, particularly of the undifferentiated type, are different from those of other head and neck mucosal cancers and justify the use of a different N classification scheme.
N0	No regional lymph node metastasis
N1	Unilateral metastasis in lymph node(s), ≤6 cm in greatest dimension, above the supraclavicular fossa
N2	Bilateral metastasis in lymph node(s), ≤6 cm in greatest dimension, above the supraclavicular fossa
N3	Metastasis in lymph node(s), >6 cm and/or to supraclavicular fossa
N3a	Greater than 6 cm in dimension
N3b	Extension to the supraclavicular fossa

Anatomic Stage/Prognostic Groups

Nasopharynx

Stage			
Stage 0	Tis	N0	M0
Stage I	T1	N0	M0
Stage II	T1	N1	M0
	T2	N0–N1	M0
Stage III	T1	N2	M0
	T2	N2	M0
	T3	N0–N2	M0
Stage IVA	T4	N0–N2	M0
Stage IVB	Any T	N3	M0
Stage IVC	Any T	Any N	M1

treatment for patients with unresectable disease, to pursue an organ-preserving approach, or in the postoperative setting for intermediate-stage resectable tumors.

Induction chemotherapy In this strategy, patients receive chemotherapy [current standard is a three-drug regimen of docetaxel, cisplatin, and fluorouracil (5-FU)] before surgery and radiation therapy. Most patients who receive three cycles show tumor reduction, and the response is clinically "complete" in up to half. This "sequential" multimodality therapy allows for organ preservation (omission of surgery) in patients with laryngeal and hypopharyngeal cancer, and it has been shown to result in higher cure rates compared with radiotherapy alone.

Concomitant chemoradiotherapy With the concomitant strategy, chemotherapy and radiation therapy are given simultaneously rather than in sequence. Tumor recurrences from head and neck cancer develop most commonly locoregionally (in the head and neck area of the primary and draining lymph nodes). The concomitant approach is aimed at enhancing tumor cell killing by radiation therapy in the presence of chemotherapy (radiation enhancement). Toxicity (especially mucositis, grade 3 or 4 in 70–80%) is increased with concomitant chemoradiotherapy. However, meta-analyses of randomized trials document an improvement in 5-year survival of 8% with concomitant chemotherapy and radiation therapy. Results seem more favorable in recent trials as more active drugs or more intensive radiotherapy schedules are used. Five-year survival is 34–50%. In addition, concomitant chemoradiotherapy produces better laryngectomy-free survival (organ preservation) than radiation therapy alone in patients with advanced larynx cancer. The use of radiation therapy together with cisplatin has also produced improved survival in patients with advanced nasopharyngeal cancer. The outcome of HPV-related cancers seems to be especially favorable following cisplatin-based chemoradiotherapy.

The success of concomitant chemoradiotherapy in patients with unresectable disease has led to the testing of a similar approach in patients with resected intermediate-stage disease as a postoperative therapy. Concomitant chemoradiotherapy produces a significant improvement over postoperative radiation therapy alone for patients whose tumors demonstrate higher risk features, such as extracapsular spread beyond involved lymph nodes, involvement of multiple lymph nodes, or positive margins at the primary site following surgery.

A monoclonal antibody to the EGFR (cetuximab) increases survival rates when administered during radiotherapy. EGFR blockade results in radiation sensitization and has milder systemic side effects than traditional chemotherapy agents, although an acneiform skin rash is commonly observed. The integration of cetuximab into current standard chemoradiotherapy regimens is under investigation.

RECURRENT AND/OR METASTATIC DISEASE Ten percent of patients present with metastatic disease, and more than half of patients with locoregionally advanced disease have recurrence, frequently outside the head and neck region. Patients with recurrent and/or metastatic disease are, with few exceptions, treated with palliative intent. Some patients may require local or regional radiation therapy for pain control, but most are given chemotherapy. Response rates to chemotherapy average only 30–50%; the duration of response averages only 3 months, and the median survival time is 6–8 months. Therefore, chemotherapy provides transient symptomatic benefit. Drugs with single-agent activity in this setting include methotrexate, 5-FU, cisplatin, paclitaxel, and docetaxel. Combinations of cisplatin with 5-FU, carboplatin with 5-FU, and cisplatin or carboplatin with paclitaxel or docetaxel are frequently used.

EGFR-directed therapies, including monoclonal antibodies (e.g., cetuximab) and tyrosine kinase inhibitors (TKIs) of the EGFR signaling pathway (e.g., erlotinib or gefitinib) have single-agent activity of approximately 10%. Side effects are usually limited to an acneiform rash and diarrhea (for the TKIs). The addition of cetuximab to standard combination chemotherapy with cis- or carboplatin and 5-FU was shown to result in a significant increase in median survival.

COMPLICATIONS Complications from treatment of head and neck cancer are usually correlated to the extent of surgery and exposure of normal tissue structures to radiation. Currently, the extent of surgery has been limited or completely replaced by chemotherapy and radiation therapy as the primary approach. Acute complications of radiation include mucositis and dysphagia. Long-term complications include xerostomia, loss of taste, decreased tongue mobility, second malignancies, dysphagia, and neck fibrosis. The complications of chemotherapy vary with the regimen used but usually include myelosuppression, mucositis, nausea and vomiting, and nephrotoxicity (with cisplatin).

The mucosal side effects of therapy can lead to malnutrition and dehydration. Many centers address issues of dentition before starting treatment, and some place feeding tubes to ensure control of hydration and nutrition intake. About 50% of patients develop hypothyroidism from the treatment; thus, thyroid function should be monitored.

SALIVARY GLAND TUMORS

Most benign salivary gland tumors are treated with surgical excision, and patients with invasive salivary gland tumors are treated with surgery and radiation therapy. These tumors may recur regionally; adenoid cystic carcinoma has a tendency to recur along the nerve tracks. Distant metastases may occur as late as 10–20 years after the initial diagnosis. For metastatic disease, therapy is given with palliative intent, usually chemotherapy with doxorubicin and/or cisplatin. Identification of novel agents with activity in these tumors is a high priority.

FURTHER READINGS

ANG KK et al: Human papillomavirus and survival of patients with oropharyngeal cancer. N Engl J Med 363:24, 2010

BONNER JA et al: Radiotherapy plus cetuximab for locoregionally advanced head and neck cancer: 5-year survival data from a phase 3 randomised trial, and relation between cetuximab-induced rash and survival. Lancet 11:21, 2010

EDGE SB et al (eds): Pharynx, in *Cancer Staging Handbook: From the AJCC Cancer Staging Manual*, 7th ed, New York, Springer, 2009

HADDAD RI et al: Recent advances in head and neck cancer. N Engl J Med 359:1143, 2008

LONNEUX M et al: Positron emission tomography with [18F] fluorodeoxyglucose improves staging and patient management in patients with head and neck squamous cell carcinoma: a multicenter prospective study. J Clin Oncol 27:1190, 2010

PFISTER DG et al: American Society of Clinical Oncology clinical practice guideline for the use of larynx-preservation strategies in the treatment of laryngeal cancer. J Clin Oncol 24:3693, 2006

POINTREAU Y et al: Randomized trial of induction chemotherapy with cisplatin and 5-flourouracil with or without docetaxel for larynx preservation. J Natl Cancer Inst 101: 498, 2009

TOBIAS JS et al: Chemoradiotherapy for locally advanced head and neck cancer: 10-year follow-up of the UK Head and Neck (UKHAN1) trial. Lancet 11:66, 2010

VERMORKEN JB et al: Platinum-based chemotherapy plus cetuximab in head and neck cancer. N Engl J Med 359:1116, 2008

CHAPTER 89

Neoplasms of the Lung

Leora Horn
William Pao
David H. Johnson

Lung cancer is largely a disease of modern man and was considered quite rare before 1900, with fewer than 400 cases described in the medical literature. However, by the mid-twentieth century lung cancer had become epidemic and firmly established as the leading cause of cancer-related death in North America and Europe, killing more than three times as many men as prostate cancer and nearly twice as many women as breast cancer. This fact is particularly distressing since lung cancer is one of the most preventable of all of the common malignancies. Tobacco consumption is the primary cause of lung cancer, a fact firmly established in the mid-twentieth century and codified with the release of the U.S. Surgeon General's 1964 report on the health effects of tobacco smoking. Following the report, cigarette use started to decline in North America and parts of Europe, and with it so did the incidence of lung cancer. To date, the decline in lung cancer is seen most clearly in men; only recently has the decline become apparent among women in the United States. Unfortunately, in many parts of the world, especially in countries with developing economies, cigarette use continues to increase, and along with it, the incidence of lung cancers is also rising. While tobacco smoking remains the primary cause of lung cancer worldwide, more than 60% of new lung cancers occur in never smokers (smoked <100 cigarettes per lifetime) or former smokers (smoked ≥100 cigarettes per lifetime, quit ≥1 year), many of whom quit decades ago. Moreover, 1 in 5 women and 1 in 12 men diagnosed with lung cancer have never smoked. Given the magnitude of the problem, it is incumbent that every internist has a broad knowledge of lung cancer and its management.

EPIDEMIOLOGY

Lung cancer is the most common cause of cancer death among American men and women. More than 220,000 individuals will be diagnosed with lung cancer in the United States in 2010. The incidence of lung cancer peaked among men in the late 1980s and has plateaued in women. Lung cancer is rare below age 40, with rates increasing until age 80, after which the rate tapers off. The projected lifetime probability of developing lung cancer is estimated to be approximately 8% among males and approximately 6% among females. The incidence of lung cancer varies by racial and ethnic group, with the highest age-adjusted incidence rates among African Americans. The excess in age-adjusted rates among African Americans occurs only among men, but age-specific rates show that below age 50 mortality from lung cancer is more than 25% higher among African American than Caucasian women. Incidence and mortality rates among Hispanic and Native and Asian Americans are approximately 40–50% those of whites.

■ RISK FACTORS

While the large majority (80–90%) of lung cancers is caused by cigarette smoking, several other factors have been implicated, although none to the extent of tobacco. Cigarette smokers have a tenfold or greater increase in risk of this cancer compared to those who have never smoked. A deep sequencing study suggested that one genetic mutation is induced for every 15 cigarettes smoked. The risk of lung cancer is lower among persons who quit smoking than among those who continue smoking; former smokers have a ninefold increased risk of developing lung cancer compared to men who have never smoked versus the twentyfold excess in those who continue to smoke. The size of the risk reduction increases with the length of time the person has quit smoking, although generally even long-term former smokers have higher risks of lung cancer than those who never smoked. Cigarette smoking increases the risk of all the major lung cancer cell types. Environmental tobacco smoke (ETS) or secondhand smoke is also an established cause of lung cancer. The risk from ETS is less than from active smoking, with a 20–30% increase in lung cancer observed among never smokers married for many years to smokers, in comparison to the 2000% increase among continuing active smokers.

While cigarette smoking is the dominant cause of lung cancer, several other risk factors have been identified, including occupational exposures to asbestos, arsenic, bischloromethyl ether, hexavalent chromium, mustard gas, nickel (as in certain nickel-refining processes), and polycyclic aromatic hydrocarbons. Occupational studies also have provided insight into possible mechanisms of lung cancer induction. For example, the risk of lung cancer among asbestos-exposed workers is increased primarily among those with underlying asbestosis, raising the possibility that the scarring and inflammation produced by this fibrotic nonmalignant lung disease may in many cases (though likely not in all) be the trigger for asbestos-induced lung cancer. Several other occupational exposures have been associated with increased rates of lung cancer, but the causal nature of the association is not as clear.

The risk of lung cancer appears higher among individuals with low fruit and vegetable intake during adulthood. This observation led to hypotheses that specific nutrients, in particular retinoids and carotenoids, might have chemopreventive effects for lung cancer. However, randomized trials failed to validate this hypothesis. In fact, studies found the incidence of lung cancer was increased among smokers with supplementation. Ionizing radiation is also an established lung carcinogen, most convincingly demonstrated from studies showing increased rates of lung cancer among survivors of the atom bombs dropped on Hiroshima and Nagasaki and large excesses among workers exposed to alpha irradiation from radon in underground uranium mining. Prolonged exposure to low-level radon in homes might impart a risk of lung cancer equal or greater than that of ETS. Prior lung diseases such as chronic bronchitis, emphysema, and tuberculosis have been linked to increased risks of lung cancer as well.

Smoking cessation

Given the undeniable link between cigarette smoking and lung cancer (not even addressing other tobacco-related illnesses), physicians must promote tobacco abstinence. Physicians also must help their patients who smoke to stop smoking. Smoking cessation, even well into middle age, can minimize an individual's subsequent risk of lung cancer. Stopping tobacco use before middle age avoids more than 90% of the lung cancer risk attributable to tobacco. However, little health benefit is derived from just "cutting back." Importantly, smoking cessation can even be beneficial in individuals with an established diagnosis of lung cancer, as it is associated with improved survival, fewer side effects from therapy, and an overall improvement in quality of life. Moreover, smoking can alter the metabolism of many chemotherapy drugs, potentially adversely altering the toxicities and therapeutic benefits of the agents. Consequently, it is important to promote smoking cessation even *after* the diagnosis of lung cancer is established.

Physicians need to understand the essential elements of smoking cessation therapy. The individual must want to stop smoking and must be willing to work hard to achieve the goal of smoking abstinence. Self-help strategies alone only marginally affect quit rates, whereas individual and combined pharmacotherapies in combination with counseling can significantly increase rates of cessation. Therapy with an antidepressant (e.g., bupropion) or nicotine replacement therapy (varenicline, an $\alpha_4\beta_2$ nicotinic acetylcholine receptor partial agonist), are approved by the U.S. Food and Drug Administration (FDA) as first-line treatments for nicotine dependence. However, both drugs have been reported to increase suicidal ideation and must be used with caution. In a randomized trial, varenicline was more efficacious than bupropion or placebo. Prolonged use of varenicline beyond the initial induction phase proved useful in maintaining smoking abstinence. Clonidine and nortriptyline are recommended as second-line treatments (Chap. 395).

Inherited predisposition to lung cancer

Exposure to environmental carcinogens, such as those found in tobacco smoke, induce or facilitate the transformation from bronchoepithelial cells to the malignant phenotype. The contribution of carcinogens on transformation is modulated by polymorphic variations in genes that affect aspects of carcinogen metabolism. Certain genetic polymorphisms of the P450 enzyme system, specifically CYP1A1, or chromosome fragility are associated with the development of lung cancer. These genetic variations occur at relatively high frequency in the population but their contribution to an individual's lung cancer risk is generally low. However, because of their population frequency, the overall impact on lung cancer risk could be high. In addition, environmental factors, as modified by inherited modulators, likely affect specific genes by deregulating important pathways to enable the cancer phenotype.

First-degree relatives of lung cancer probands have a two- to threefold excess risk of lung cancer and other cancers, many of which are not smoking-related. These data suggest that specific genes and/or genetic variants may contribute to susceptibility to lung cancer. However, very few such genes have yet been identified. Individuals with inherited mutations in *RB* (patients with retinoblastoma living to adulthood) and *p53* (Li-Fraumeni syndrome) genes may develop lung cancer. Three genetic loci for lung cancer risk have been identified by genomewide association studies, including 5p15 (TERT-CLPTM1L), 15q25(CHRNA5-CHRNA-3 nicotinic acetylcholine receptor subunits), and 6p21 (BAT3-MSH5). A rare germline mutation (T790M) involving the epidermal growth factor receptor (EGFR) maybe be linked to lung cancer susceptibility in never smokers. Currently, however, no molecular criteria are used to select patients for more intense screening regimens or for specific chemopreventive strategies.

■ PATHOLOGY

The term *lung cancer* is used for tumors arising from the respiratory epithelium (bronchi, bronchioles, and alveoli). Mesotheliomas, lymphomas, and stromal tumors (sarcomas) are distinct from epithelial lung cancers. According to the World Health Organization classification, epithelial lung cancers consist of four major cell types: small cell lung cancer (SCLC) and the so-called non-small cell lung cancer (NSCLC) histologies including adenocarcinoma, squamous cell carcinoma, and large cell carcinoma (Fig. 89-1). These four histologies account for approximately 90% of all epithelial lung cancers. The remainder include undifferentiated carcinomas, carcinoids, bronchial gland tumors (including adenoid cystic carcinomas and mucoepidermoid tumors), and rarer tumor types. Tumors may occur as single or mixed-type histology.

All histologic types of lung cancer can be found in current and former smokers. Historically, the histologies associated with heavy

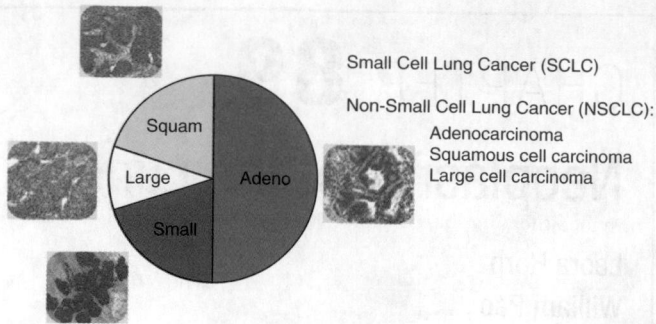

Figure 89-1 Traditional view of lung cancer.

tobacco use are squamous and small cell carcinomas. Squamous carcinoma was the most commonly diagnosed form of NSCLC; however, with the steady decline in cigarette consumption over the past four decades and changes in cigarette manufacturing (including use of different types of filters), adenocarcinoma has replaced squamous cell carcinoma as the most frequent histologic subtype in North America. The incidence of small cell carcinoma is also on the decline. In lifetime never smokers, all histologic forms of lung cancer can be found, although adenocarcinoma tends to predominate. Among women and young adults (<60 years), adenocarcinoma tends also to be the most common form of lung cancer.

Small cell carcinoma is a poorly differentiated neuroendocrine tumor that tends to occur as a central mass with endobronchial growth and is strongly associated with smoking. Small cell carcinoma cells have scant cytoplasm, small hyperchromatic nuclei with a fine ("salt and pepper") chromatin pattern and prominent nucleoli. Tumors might be arranged in diffuse sheets of cells or may show neuroendocrine patterns such as rosettes, trabeculae, or peripheral palisading of cells at the periphery of nests. There is often widespread cellular necrosis. Small cell carcinomas, more often than non-small cell carcinomas, may produce specific peptide hormones such as adrenocorticotrophic hormone (ACTH), arginine vasopressin (AVP), atrial natriuretic factor (ANF), and gastrin-releasing peptide (GRP). These hormones may be associated with distinctive paraneoplastic syndromes that prompt workup and eventual diagnosis (Chap. 100).

Squamous cell carcinomas of the lung are morphologically identical to extrapulmonary (i.e., head and neck) squamous cell carcinomas and require clinical correlation to differentiate. These tumors tend to occur centrally and are classically associated with a history of smoking. Histologically, the most common pattern is that of an infiltrating nest of tumor cells that lack intercellular bridges. Keratin can usually be seen when present.

Adenocarcinomas often occur in more peripheral lung locations and may be associated with a history of smoking. However, adenocarcinomas are the most common type of lung cancer occurring in never smokers. Histologically, the tissue may contain the presence of glands, papillary structure, bronchioloalveolar pattern, cellular mucin, or solid pattern if poorly differentiated. Variants of adenocarcinomas include signet-ring, clear cell, and mucinous and fetal adenocarcinomas. Bronchioloalveolar carcinoma (BAC) is a subtype of adenocarcinoma that grows along the alveoli without invasion and can present radiographically as a single mass, as a diffuse multinodular lesion, as a fluffy infiltrate, and on screening CT scans as a "ground-glass" opacity (GGO). Pure BAC is relatively rare. More common is adenocarcinoma with BAC features. BAC may present in a mucinous form, which tends to be multicentric, and a nonmucinous form, which tends to be solitary.

Large cell carcinomas tend to occur peripherally and are defined as poorly differentiated carcinomas of the lung composed of larger malignant cells without evidence of squamous, glandular differentiation, or features of small cell carcinoma by light microscopy. These tumors usually consist of sheets of large malignant cells, often with associated necrosis. Cytologically, the tumor is also arranged in syncytial groups and single cells. Variants of large cell, carcinoma include basaloid carcinoma, which may present as an endobronchial lesion and may resemble a high-grade neuroendocrine tumor, and lymphoepithelioma-like carcinoma, which is similar to the same-named tumor of other sites and is Epstein-Barr virus–related.

Historically, for treatment and prognostication purposes, the major distinction has been between SCLC and NSCLC, as these tumors have quite different natural histories and therapeutic approaches. SCLC is typically widely disseminated at diagnosis. Even if localized, it is rarely curable by surgery. By contrast, NSCLC can be potentially cured by resection in up to 30% of cases. Small cell cancers tend to respond more favorably to traditional cytotoxic chemotherapy agents. Intrinsic drug resistance is the norm for both SCLC and NSCLC. As knowledge of tumor biology improves, more sophisticated classification schemas are under development, including ones based in part on the presence of specific mutations and molecular alterations (Fig. 89-2). Recognition of these molecular distinctions may help guide therapy in the future.

IMMUNOHISTOCHEMISTRY

The diagnosis of lung cancer most often rests on the morphologic or cytologic features correlated with clinical and radiographic findings. Immunohistochemistry may be used to verify neuroendocrine differentiation within a tumor, with markers such as neuron-specific enolase (NSE), CD56 or neural cell adhesion molecule (NCAM), synaptophysin, chromogranin, and Leu7 (Table 89-1). Immunohistochemistry is also helpful in differentiating primary from metastatic adenocarcinomas. Thyroid transcription factor 1 (TTF-1), identified in tumors of thyroid and pulmonary origin, is positive in more than 70% of pulmonary adenocarcinomas and is a reliable indicator of primary lung cancer, provided a thyroid primary has been excluded. A negative TTF-1, however, does not exclude the possibility of a lung primary. TTF-1 is also positive in neuroendocrine tumors of pulmonary and extrapulmonary origin. Cytokeratins 7 and 20 used in combination can help narrow the differential diagnosis; nonsquamous NSCLC, SCLC, and mesothelioma may stain positive for CK7 and negative for CK20, while squamous cell lung cancer will be both CK7 and CK20 negative. Mesothelioma can be easily identified ultrastructurally, but it has historically been difficult to differentiate from adenocarcinoma through morphology and immunohistochemical staining. Several markers in the past few years have proven to be more helpful,

TABLE 89-1 Common Immunohistochemical Markers Used in the Diagnosis of Lung Tumors	
Histology	Positive Immunohistochemical Markers
Squamous cell carcinoma	Cytokeratin (CK) cocktail, e.g., AE1/AE3
	CK5/6
	CK7 rare
Adenocarcinoma	Cytokeratin cocktail, e.g., AE1/AE3
	CK7
	TTF-1
	Neuroendocrine markers rare, e.g., CD56, NSE
Large cell carcinoma	Cytokeratin
	TTF-1 rare
	Neuroendocrine markers rare (e.g., CD56, NSE)
Large cell neuroendocrine carcinoma	Cytokeratin cocktail, e.g., AE1/AE3
	TTF-1
	CD56
	Chromogranin
	Synaptophysin
Small cell carcinoma	Cytokeratin cocktail (tends to be patchy)
	TTF-1
	CD56
	Chromogranin
	Synaptophysin

Abbreviations: WT-1, Wilms' tumor gene 1; NSE, neuron-specific enolase; NCAM, neural cell adhesion molecule; TTF-1, thyroid transcription factor 1.

including CK5/6, calretinin, and Wilms' tumor gene 1 (WT-1), all of which show positivity in mesothelioma.

MOLECULAR PATHOGENESIS

Cancer is a disease involving dynamic changes in the genome. As proposed by Hanahan and Weinberg, virtually all cancer cells acquire six hallmark capabilities: self-sufficiency in growth signals, insensitivity to antigrowth signals, evading apoptosis, limitless replicative potential, sustained angiogenesis, and tissue invasion and metastasis. The order in which these hallmark capabilities are acquired appears quite variable and can differ from tumor to tumor. Events leading to acquisition of these hallmarks can vary widely; although broadly, cancers arise as a result of accumulations of gain-of-function mutations in oncogenes and loss-of-function mutations in tumor suppressor genes. Further complicating the study of lung cancer, the sequence of events that lead to disease is clearly different for the various histopathologic entities.

The exact cell of origin for lung cancers is not known. Whether one cell of origin leads to all histologic forms of lung cancer is unclear. However, at least for lung adenocarcinoma, type II epithelial cells (or alveolar epithelial

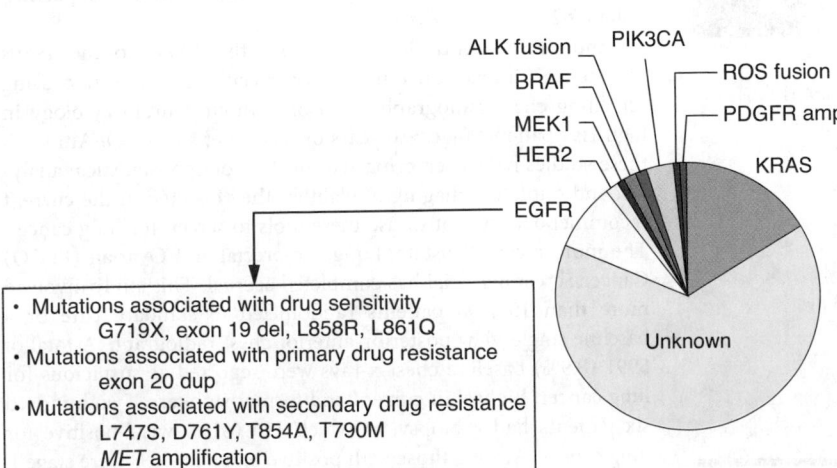

· Mutations associated with drug sensitivity
   G719X, exon 19 del, L858R, L861Q
· Mutations associated with primary drug resistance
   exon 20 dup
· Mutations associated with secondary drug resistance
   L747S, D761Y, T854A, T790M
   MET amplification

Figure 89-2 2010: Lung adenocarcinoma—multiple molecular subsets.

cells) have the capacity to give rise to tumors. For SCLC, cells of neuroendocrine origin have been implicated as precursors.

For cancers in general, one theory holds that a small subset of the cells within a tumor (i.e., "stem cells") are responsible for the full malignant behavior of the tumor. As part of this concept, the large bulk of the cells in a cancer are "offspring" of these cancer stem cells. While clonally related to the cancer stem cell subpopulation, most cells by themselves cannot regenerate the full malignant phenotype. The stem cell concept may explain the failure of standard medical therapies to eradicate lung cancers, even when there is a clinical complete response. Disease recurs because therapies do not eliminate the stem cell component, which may be more resistant to chemotherapy. Precise human lung cancer stem cells have yet to be identified.

Lung cancer cells harbor multiple chromosomal abnormalities, including mutations, amplifications, insertions, deletions, and translocations. One of the earliest set of oncogenes found to be aberrant was the MYC family of transcription factors (*MYC*, *MYCN*, and *MYCL*). *MYC* is most frequently activated via gene amplification or transcriptional dysregulation in both SCLC and NSCLC, whereas abnormalities of *MYCN* and *MYCL* generally occur in SCLC. Currently, there are no MYC-specific drugs.

To date, among lung cancer histologies, adenocarcinomas have been the most extensively catalogued for recurrent genomic gains and losses as well as for somatic mutations. While multiple different kinds of aberrations have been found, a major class involves "driver mutations"—mutations that occur in genes encoding signaling proteins that when aberrant, drive initiation and maintenance of tumor cells (Table 89-2). Importantly, driver mutations can serve as Achilles' heels for tumors if their gene products can be targeted appropriately. For example, one set of mutations involves the epidermal growth factor receptor (EGFR), which belongs to the ERBB (HER) family of protooncogenes, including *EGFR* (ERBB1), *Her2/neu* (ERBB2), *HER3* (ERBB3), and *HER4* (ERBB4). These genes encode cell-surface receptors consisting of an extracellular ligand-binding domain, a transmembrane structure, and an intracellular tyrosine kinase (TK) domain. The binding of ligand to receptor activates receptor dimerization and TK autophosphorylation, initiating a cascade of intracellular events, leading to increased

cell proliferation, angiogenesis, metastasis, and a decrease in apoptosis. Lung adenocarcinomas can arise when tumors express mutant *EGFR*. These same tumors display high sensitivity to small molecule EGFR tyrosine kinase inhibitors. Additional examples of driver mutations in lung adenocarcinoma include those involving the signaling molecules downstream of EGFR, e.g., the tyrosine kinase *HER2*; the GTPase, *KRAS*; the serine-threonine kinase, *BRAF*; and the lipid kinase, *PIK3CA*. In 2007, other subsets of lung adenocarcinoma were found to be defined by the presence of specific translocations fusing tyrosine kinases such as ALK and ROS to aberrant upstream partners. Notably, at least *EGFR*, *KRAS*, and *EML4-ALK* mutations are mutually exclusive, suggesting that acquisition of one of these driver mutations is sufficient to promote tumorigenesis. Thus far, potentially targetable driver mutations have mostly been identified in lung adenocarcinomas as opposed to lung cancers displaying other types of histologies.

A large number of tumor-suppressor genes (recessive oncogenes) have also been identified that are inactivated during the pathogenesis of lung cancer (Table 89-2). Such genes include *TP53*, *RB1*, *RASSF1A*, *CDKN2A/B*, *LKB1* (*STK11*), and *FHIT*. Nearly 90% of SCLCs harbor mutations in *TP53* and *RB1*. Several tumor-suppressor genes on chromosome 3p appear to be involved in nearly all lung cancers. Allelic loss for this region occurs very early in lung cancer pathogenesis, including in histologically normal smoking-damaged lung epithelium.

EARLY DETECTION AND SCREENING

The clinical outcome for lung cancer is related to the stage at diagnosis. Accordingly, it is presumed that early detection of occult tumors will lead to improved survival. Early detection is a process that involves screening tests, surveillance, diagnosis, and early treatment. By contrast, screening is defined as a systematic testing of asymptomatic individuals for preclinical disease. The majority of patients with lung cancer present with advanced disease, raising the question as to whether screening could detect lung tumors at earlier stages when they are theoretically more curable. In order for a screening program to be successful, the burden of disease within the population must be high, effective treatment must be available that can reduce mortality rate, and the test must be accessible, cost-effective, and both sensitive and specific. With any screening procedure, one must keep in mind the possible influence of lead-time bias (i.e., detecting the cancer earlier without an effect on survival), length time bias (i.e., indolent cancers are detected on screening and may actually not affect survival, while aggressive cancers are likely to cause symptoms earlier in patients and are less likely to be detected), and over diagnosis (i.e., diagnosing cancers so slow growing that they are unlikely to cause the death of the patient) (Chap. 82).

Randomized controlled trials from the 1960s to the 1980s reported no impact on lung cancer–specific mortality rate using screening chest radiographs with or without sputum cytology in high-risk patients (age >50 years or history of smoking). Although these studies have been criticized for their design, statistical analyses, and outdated imaging modalities, they resulted in the current recommendations not to use these tools to screen for lung cancer. The more recent Prostate, Lung, Colorectal and Ovarian (PLCO) Cancer Screening Trial has completed accrual. This study involved more than 150,000 patients randomized to standard care or a baseline single-view posterior-anterior chest radiograph. A total of 5991 (8.9%) baseline chest x-rays were reported as suspicious for lung cancer, highest in current and former smokers. Two hundred six patients had a biopsy, of which 126 (61%) were positive for lung cancer. Among those with positive biopsies, 52% were stage I, 12% were stage II, and 22% were stage III. Long-term follow-up is required to determine the effect on mortality rate, if any.

TABLE 89-2 List of Some Genes Somatically Altered in Different Histologic Subtypes of Lung Cancer

Histology	Oncogene	Tumor-Suppressor Genes
Adenocarcinoma	EGFR	TP53
	KRAS	CDKN2A/B (p16, p14)
	ALK	LKB1 (STK11)
Squamous cell carcinoma	EGFR	TP53
	PIK3CA	TP63
	IGF-1R	
Small cell carcinoma	MYC	TP53
	BCL-2	RB1
		FHIT
Large cell carcinoma (not well studied)		

Abbreviations: EGFR, epidermal growth factor receptor; ALK, anaplastic lymphoma kinase; IGF-1R, insulin-like growth factor 1 receptor; RB1, retinoblastoma protein 1.

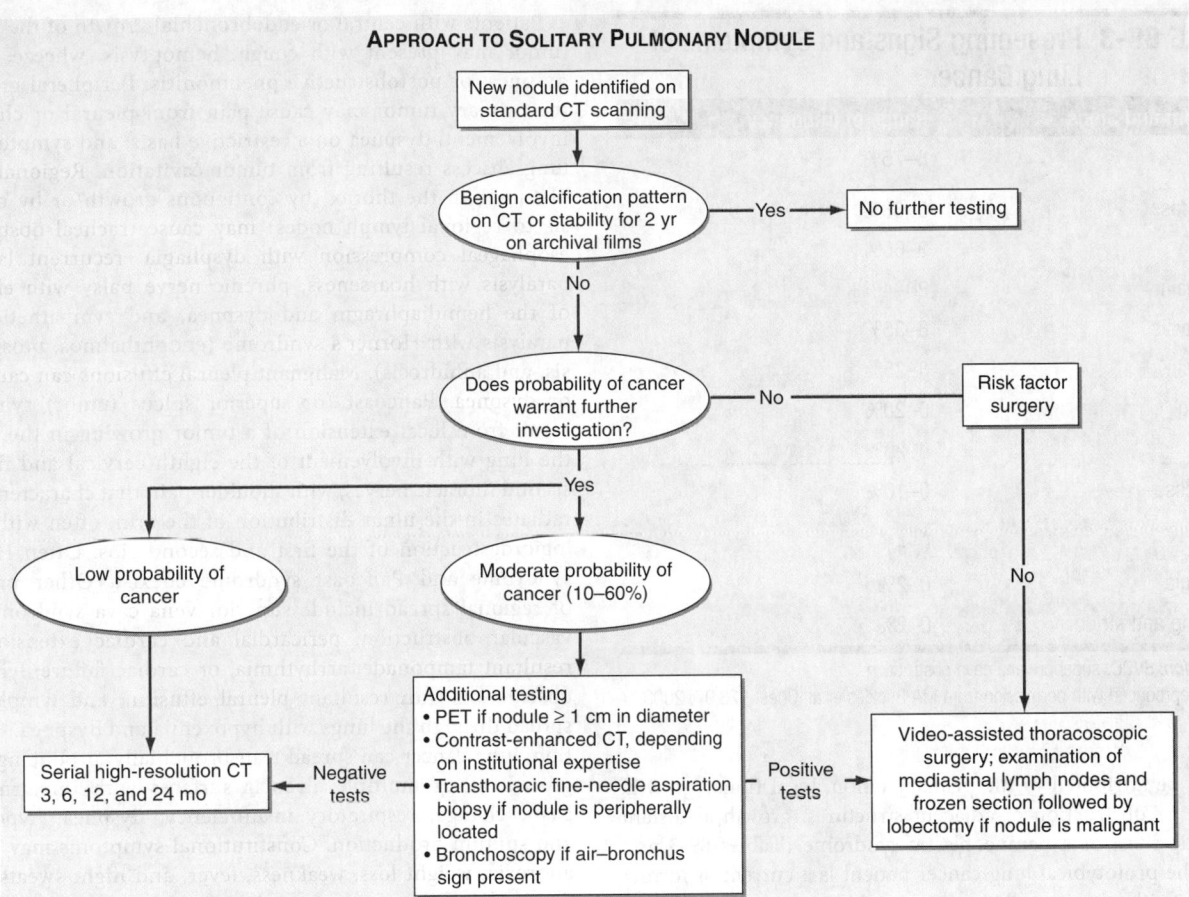

APPROACH TO SOLITARY PULMONARY NODULE

New nodule identified on standard CT scanning

Benign calcification pattern on CT or stability for 2 yr on archival films → Yes → No further testing

No

Does probability of cancer warrant further investigation? → No → Risk factor surgery

Yes

Low probability of cancer

Moderate probability of cancer (10–60%)

No

Additional testing
• PET if nodule ≥ 1 cm in diameter
• Contrast-enhanced CT, depending on institutional expertise
• Transthoracic fine-needle aspiration biopsy if nodule is peripherally located
• Bronchoscopy if air–bronchus sign present

Serial high-resolution CT 3, 6, 12, and 24 mo ← Negative tests

Positive tests → Video-assisted thoracoscopic surgery; examination of mediastinal lymph nodes and frozen section followed by lobectomy if nodule is malignant

Figure 89-3 Approach to solitary pulmonary nodule.

Low-dose, noncontrast, thin-slice helical or spiral chest CT has emerged as a possible new tool for lung cancer screening. In a spiral chest CT scan, only the pulmonary parenchyma is examined, thus negating the use of intravenous contrast and the necessity of a physician being present at the exam. The scan can usually be done quickly (within a breath) and involves low doses of radiation. However, the benefits of screening with such technology remain to be determined. The International Early Lung Cancer Action Project (I-ECLAP) screened 31,567 asymptomatic patients at high risk for lung cancer (age ≥60 years with history of at least a 10–pack-year smoking history) using low-dose baseline CT and annual screening in 27,456 study participants. Suspicious lesions requiring biopsies were indicated in 535 participants. Lung cancer was diagnosed in 484 participants; 405 at baseline, 74 on subsequent screening, and 5 participants due to symptoms between annual visits. Of the 484 participants who received a diagnosis of lung cancer, 412 (85%) were clinical stage I with an estimated 10-year survival rate of 88% regardless of treatment and 92% among the 302 participants who underwent resection within 1 month after diagnosis. A second trial randomized 1276 patients to low-dose CT screening and 1196 to baseline chest x-ray followed by yearly medical examination. At 3-year follow-up, this study found a trend toward more patients being diagnosed with stage I lung cancer in the low-dose CT arm, with no difference in the number of patients diagnosed with advanced lung cancer or lung cancer deaths. More mature data from all trials are required to determine whether screening reduces lung cancer mortality rates.

A major challenge confronting advocates of CT screening is the high false-positive rate; on initial screening of at-risk populations, false-positive rates range between 10 and 20% but can be as high as 50%, depending on the geographical region. Positive predictive values range from 2.8 to 11.6%. False positives can have a substantial impact on patients through the expense and risk of unneeded further evaluation and emotional stress. False-positive rates and positive predictive values are somewhat improved in annual follow-up CT scans, but there is still significant room for improvement. Based on extant data, it appears that nodules <0.5 mm are unlikely to be cancerous and those 5–10 mm in diameter (25–40% of noncalcified nodules detected) are of uncertain significance. The management of these patients usually consists of serial CT scans over time to see if the nodules grow, attempted fine-needle aspirates, or surgical resection (Fig. 89-3).

Two additional screening studies are ongoing, the National Lung Cancer Screening Trial (NLST), a prospective comparison of spiral CT and standard chest x-ray in 50,000 current or ex-smokers and a similar study in Europe comparing CT scanning with standard of care in subjects with a history of heavy smoking. Until these data and more mature data from the above-mentioned trials become available, routine CT screening for lung cancer cannot be recommended for any risk group. For those patients who want to be screened, physicians need to discuss the possible benefits and risks of screening. While lung cancers may be found, patients are at risk for more radiation exposure and false-positive results. The latter can result in multiple follow-up CTs and possible invasive procedures, with potential added costs, anxiety, and morbidity and mortality rates. There are no data on screening never smokers for lung cancer.

CLINICAL MANIFESTATIONS

More than half of all patients diagnosed with lung cancer present with advanced disease at the time of diagnosis. The majority of patients present with signs, symptoms, or laboratory abnormalities

TABLE 89-3 Presenting Signs and Symptoms of Lung Cancer

Symptom and Signs	Range of frequency
Cough	8–75%
Weight loss	0–68%
Dyspnea	3–60%
Chest pain	20–49%
Hemoptysis	6–35%
Bone pain	6–25%
Clubbing	0–20%
Fever	0–20%
Weakness	0–10%
SVCO	0–4%
Dysphagia	0–2%
Wheezing and stridor	0–2%

Abbreviation: SVCO, superior vena cava obstruction.
Source: Reproduced with permission from MA Beckles et al: Chest 123:97, 2003.

that can be attributed to the primary lesion, local tumor growth, invasion or obstruction of adjacent structures, growth at distant metastatic sites, or a paraneoplastic syndrome (Tables 89-3 and 89-4). The prototypical lung cancer patient is a current or former smoker of either sex, usually in the seventh decade of life. A history of chronic cough with or without hemoptysis in a current or former smoker with chronic obstructive pulmonary disease (COPD) aged 40 years or older should prompt a thorough investigation for lung cancer even in the face of a normal chest x-ray. A persistent pneumonia without constitutional symptoms and unresponsive to repeated courses of antibiotics also should prompt an evaluation for the underlying cause.

Lung cancer arising in a lifetime never smoker is more common in women and East Asians. Such patients also tend to be younger than their smoking counterparts at the time of diagnosis. The clinical presentation of lung cancer in never smokers tends to mirror that of current and former smokers.

TABLE 89-4 Clinical Findings Suggestive of Metastatic Disease

Symptoms elicited in history	• Constitutional: weight loss >10 lb
	• Musculoskeletal: focal skeletal pain
	• Neurologic: headaches, syncope, seizures, extremity weakness, recent change in mental status
Signs found on physical examination	• Lymphadenopathy (>1 cm)
	• Hoarseness, superior vena cava syndrome
	• Bone tenderness
	• Hepatomegaly (>13 cm span)
	• Focal neurologic signs, papilledema
	• Soft-tissue mass
Routine laboratory tests	• Hematocrit: <40% in men, <35% in women
	• Elevated alkaline phosphatase, GGT, SGOT, and calcium levels

Abbreviations: GGT, gamma-glutamyltransferase; SGOT, serum glutamic-oxaloacetic transaminase.
Source: Reproduced with permission from GA Silvestri et al: Chest 123(1 Suppl):147S, 2003.

Patients with central or endobronchial growth of the primary tumor may present with cough, hemoptysis, wheeze, stridor, dyspnea, or postobstructive pneumonitis. Peripheral growth of the primary tumor may cause pain from pleural or chest wall involvement, dyspnea on a restrictive basis, and symptoms of a lung abscess resulting from tumor cavitation. Regional spread of tumor in the thorax (by contiguous growth or by metastasis to regional lymph nodes) may cause tracheal obstruction, esophageal compression with dysphagia, recurrent laryngeal paralysis with hoarseness, phrenic nerve palsy with elevation of the hemidiaphragm and dyspnea, and sympathetic nerve paralysis with Horner's syndrome (enophthalmos, ptosis, miosis, and anhidrosis). Malignant pleural effusions can cause pain or dyspnea. Pancoast (or superior sulcus tumor) syndromes result from local extension of a tumor growing in the apex of the lung with involvement of the eighth cervical and first and second thoracic nerves, with shoulder pain that characteristically radiates in the ulnar distribution of the arm, often with radiologic destruction of the first and second ribs. Often Horner's syndrome and Pancoast syndrome coexist. Other problems of regional spread include superior vena cava syndrome from vascular obstruction; pericardial and cardiac extension with resultant tamponade, arrhythmia, or cardiac failure; lymphatic obstruction with resultant pleural effusion; and lymphangitic spread through the lungs with hypoxemia and dyspnea. In addition, lung cancer can spread transbronchially, producing tumor growth along multiple alveolar surfaces with impairment of gas exchange, respiratory insufficiency, dyspnea, hypoxemia, and sputum production. Constitutional symptoms may include anorexia, weight loss, weakness, fever, and night sweats. Apart from the brevity of symptom duration, these parameters fail to clearly distinguish SCLC from NSCLC or even from neoplasms metastatic to lungs.

Extrathoracic metastatic disease is found at autopsy in >50% of patients with squamous carcinoma, 80% of patients with adenocarcinoma and large cell carcinoma, and >95% of patients with SCLC. Approximately one-third of patients present with symptoms as a result of distant metastases. Lung cancer metastases may occur in virtually every organ system, and the site of metastatic involvement largely determines other symptoms. Patients with brain metastases may present with headache, nausea and vomiting, or neurologic deficits. Patients with bone metastases may present with pain, pathologic fractures, or cord compression. The latter may also occur with epidural metastases. Individuals with bone marrow invasion may present with cytopenias or leukoerythroblastosis. Those with liver metastases may present with hepatomegaly, right upper quadrant pain, anorexia, and weight loss. Liver dysfunction or biliary obstructions are rare. Adrenal metastases are common but rarely cause pain or adrenal insufficiency unless they are large.

Paraneoplastic syndromes are common in patients with lung cancer, especially those with SCLC, and may be the presenting finding or the first sign of recurrence. In addition, paraneoplastic syndromes may mimic metastatic disease and, unless detected, lead to inappropriate palliative rather than curative treatment. Often the paraneoplastic syndrome may be relieved with successful treatment of the tumor. In some cases, the pathophysiology of the paraneoplastic syndrome is known, particularly when a hormone with biologic activity is secreted by a tumor. However, in many cases the pathophysiology is not known. Systemic symptoms of anorexia, cachexia, weight loss (seen in 30% of patients), fever, and suppressed immunity are paraneoplastic syndromes of unknown etiology or at least not well defined. Weight loss greater than 10% of total body weight is considered a bad prognostic sign. Endocrine syndromes are seen in 12% of patients; hypercalcemia resulting from ectopic production of parathyroid hormone (PTH), or more commonly, PTH-related peptide, is the most common life-threatening metabolic complication of malignancy, primarily occurring with squamous cell carcinomas of the lung. Clinical symptoms include nausea, vomiting, abdominal pain, constipation, polyuria, thirst, and altered mental status.

Hyponatremia may be caused by the syndrome of inappropriate secretion of antidiuretic hormone (SIADH) or possibly atrial natriuretic peptide (ANP). SIADH resolves within 1–4 weeks of initiating chemotherapy in the vast majority of cases. During this period, serum sodium can usually be managed and maintained above 128 meq/L via fluid restriction. Demeclocycline can be a useful adjunctive measure when fluid restriction alone is insufficient. Of note, patients with ectopic ANP may have worsening hyponatremia if sodium intake is not concomitantly increased. Accordingly, if hyponatremia fails to improve or worsens after 3–4 days of adequate fluid restriction, plasma levels of ANP should be measured to determine the causative syndrome.

Ectopic secretion of ACTH by SCLC and pulmonary carcinoids usually results in additional electrolyte disturbances, especially hypokalemia, rather than the changes in body habitus that occur in Cushing's syndrome from a pituitary adenoma. Treatment with standard medications, such as metyrapone and ketoconazole, is largely ineffective due to extremely high cortisol levels. The most effective strategy for management of Cushing's syndrome is effective treatment of the underlying SCLC. Bilateral adrenalectomy may be considered in extreme cases.

Skeletal–connective tissue syndromes include clubbing in 30% of cases (usually NSCLCs) and hypertrophic primary osteoarthropathy in 1–10% of cases (usually adenocarcinomas). Patients may develop periostitis, causing pain, tenderness, and swelling over the affected bones and a positive bone scan. Neurologic–myopathic syndromes are seen in only 1% of patients but are dramatic and include the myasthenic Eaton-Lambert syndrome and retinal blindness with SCLC, while peripheral neuropathies, subacute cerebellar degeneration, cortical degeneration, and polymyositis are seen with all lung cancer types. Many of these are caused by autoimmune responses such as the development of anti–voltage-gated calcium channel antibodies in Eaton-Lambert syndrome. Patients with this disorder present with proximal muscle weakness, usually in the lower extremities, occasional autonomic dysfunction, and rarely with cranial nerve symptoms or involvement of the bulbar or respiratory muscles. Depressed deep tendon reflexes are frequently present. In contrast to patients with myasthenia gravis, strength improves with serial effort. Some patients who respond to chemotherapy will have resolution of the neurologic abnormalities. Thus, chemotherapy is the initial treatment of choice. Paraneoplastic encephalomyelitis and sensory neuropathies, cerebellar degeneration, limbic encephalitis, and brainstem encephalitis occur in SCLC in association with a variety of antineuronal antibodies such as anti-Hu, anti-CRMP5, and ANNA-3. Paraneoplastic cerebellar degeneration may be associated with anti-Hu, anti-Yo, or P/Q calcium channel autoantibodies. Coagulation, thrombotic, or other hematologic manifestations occur in 1–8% of patients and include migratory venous thrombophlebitis (Trousseau's syndrome), nonbacterial thrombotic (marantic) endocarditis with arterial emboli, and disseminated intravascular coagulation with hemorrhage, anemia, granulocytosis, and leukoerythroblastosis. Thrombotic

disease complicating cancer is usually a poor prognostic sign. Cutaneous manifestations such as dermatomyositis and acanthosis nigricans are uncommon (1%), as are the renal manifestations of nephrotic syndrome and glomerulonephritis (≤1%).

DIAGNOSING LUNG CANCER

Tissue sampling is required to confirm a diagnosis in all patients with suspected lung cancer. Tumor tissue may be obtained via minimally invasive techniques such as bronchial or transbronchial biopsy during fiberoptic bronchoscopy, by fine-needle aspiration (FNA) or percutaneous biopsy using image guidance, or via endobronchial ultrasound (EBUS)-guided biopsy. Depending on the location, lymph node sampling may occur via transesophageal endoscopic ultrasound guide biopsy (EUS), EBUS, or blind biopsy. In patients with clinically palpable lymph nodes, an FNA may be obtained. In patients with suspected metastatic disease, a diagnosis may be confirmed by percutaneous biopsy of a soft tissue mass, lytic bone lesion, bone marrow, pleural or liver lesion, or an adequate cell block obtained from a malignant pleural effusion. In patients with a suspected malignant pleural effusion, if the initial thoracentesis is negative, a repeat thoracentesis is recommended. While the majority of pleural effusions are due to malignant disease, particularly if they are exudative or bloody, some may be parapneumonic. In this case, patients should be considered for possible curative treatment.

The diagnostic yield of any biopsy depends on several factors, including location (accessibility) of the tumor, tumor size, tumor type, and technical aspects of the diagnostic procedure including the experience level of the bronchoscopist and pathologist. In general, central lesions, such as squamous cell carcinomas, small cell carcinomas, or endobronchial lesions, such as carcinoid tumors, are more readily diagnosed by bronchoscopic examination, while peripheral lesions such as adenocarcinomas and large cell carcinomas are more amenable to transthoracic FNA. Diagnostic accuracy for SCLC versus NSCLC for most specimens is excellent, with lesser accuracy for subtypes of NSCLC.

Bronchoscopic specimens include bronchial brush, bronchial wash, bronchioloalveolar lavage, and transbronchial FNA. Of these, transbronchial FNA consistently demonstrates the highest sensitivity, surpassed only by the use of a combination of bronchoscopic specimens. Overall sensitivity for combined use of bronchoscopic methods is approximately 80%, and together with tissue biopsy, the yield increases to 85–90%. Like transbronchial FNA specimens, transthoracic FNA specimens are also very good, yielding diagnostic material in 70–95% of cases. Sensitivity is highest for larger lesions and peripheral tumors. In general, FNA specimens, whether transbronchial, transthoracic, or endoscopic ultrasound-guided, are superior to other specimen types. This is primarily due to the higher percentage of tumor cells with fewer confounding factors, such as obscuring inflammation and reactive nonneoplastic cells. For more accurate histologic classification, mutation analysis, or for investigational purposes, reasonable efforts (e.g., a core-needle biopsy) should be made to obtain more tissue than what is contained in a routine cytology specimen obtained by FNA.

Sputum cytology is inexpensive and noninvasive but has a lower yield than other specimen types due to poor preservation of the cells and more variability in acquiring a good-quality specimen. The yield for sputum cytology is highest for larger and centrally located tumors such as squamous cell carcinoma and small cell carcinoma histology. The specificity for sputum cytology averages close to 100%, although sensitivity is generally less than 70%. The accuracy of sputum cytology improves with increased numbers of specimens analyzed. Consequently, analysis of at least three sputum specimens is recommended.

Lung cancer staging consists of two parts: first, a determination of the location of the tumor and possible metastatic sites (anatomic staging), and second, an assessment of a patient's ability to withstand various antitumor treatments (physiologic staging). All patients with lung cancer should have a complete history and physical examination, with evaluation of all other medical problems, determination of performance status, and history of weight loss. The most significant dividing line is between those patients who are candidates for surgical resection and those who are inoperable but will benefit from chemotherapy, radiation therapy, or both. Staging with regard to a patient's potential for surgical resection is principally applicable to NSCLC.

ANATOMIC STAGING OF PATIENTS WITH LUNG CANCER

The accurate staging of patients with NSCLC is essential for determining the appropriate treatment in patients with resectable disease and avoiding unnecessary surgical procedures in patients with advanced disease (Fig. 89-4). All patients with NSCLC should undergo initial radiographic imaging with CT scan, positron emission tomography (PET), or preferably CT-PET. PET scanning attempts to identify sites of malignancy based on glucose metabolism by measuring the uptake of fluorodeoxyglucose F18. Rapidly dividing cells, presumably in the lung tumors, will preferentially take up ^{18}F-FDG and appear as a "hot spot." To date, PET has been mostly used for staging and detection of metastases in lung cancer and in the detection of nodules >15 mm in diameter. Combined ^{18}F-FDG PET-CT imaging has been shown to improve the accuracy of staging in NSCLC compared to visual correlation of PET and CT or either study alone. CT-PET has been found to be superior in identifying pathologically enlarged mediastinal lymph nodes and

extrathoracic metastases. A standardized uptake value (SUV) of >2.5 on PET is highly suspicious for malignancy. False negatives can be seen in diabetes, in lesions <8 mm, in slow-growing tumors, and in concurrent infections such as tuberculosis. False positives can be seen in infections and granulomatous disease. Thus, PET should never be used alone to diagnose lung cancer, mediastinal involvement, or metastases. Confirmation with tissue biopsy is required. For brain metastases, MRI is the most effective method. MRI can also be useful in selected circumstances, such as for superior sulcus tumors, to rule out brachial plexus involvement, but in general does not play a major role in NSCLC staging.

In patients with NSCLC, the following are major contraindications to potential curative resection: extrathoracic metastases; superior vena cava syndrome; vocal cord and, in most cases, phrenic nerve paralysis; malignant pleural effusion; cardiac tamponade; tumor within 2 cm of the carina (potentially curable with combined chemoradiotherapy); metastasis to the contralateral lung; metastases to supraclavicular lymph nodes; contralateral mediastinal node metastases (potentially curable with combined chemoradiotherapy); and involvement of the main pulmonary artery. In situations where it will make a difference in treatment, abnormal scan findings require tissue confirmation of malignancy so that patients are not precluded from having potentially curative surgery.

The best predictor of metastatic disease remains a careful history and physical examination. If signs, symptoms, or findings from physical examination suggest the presence of malignancy, then sequential imaging starting with the most appropriate study should be performed. If the findings from the clinical evaluation are negative, then imaging studies beyond CT-PET are unnecessary and the search for metastatic disease is complete. More controversial is how one should assess patients with known stage III disease. Because these patients are more likely to have asymptomatic occult

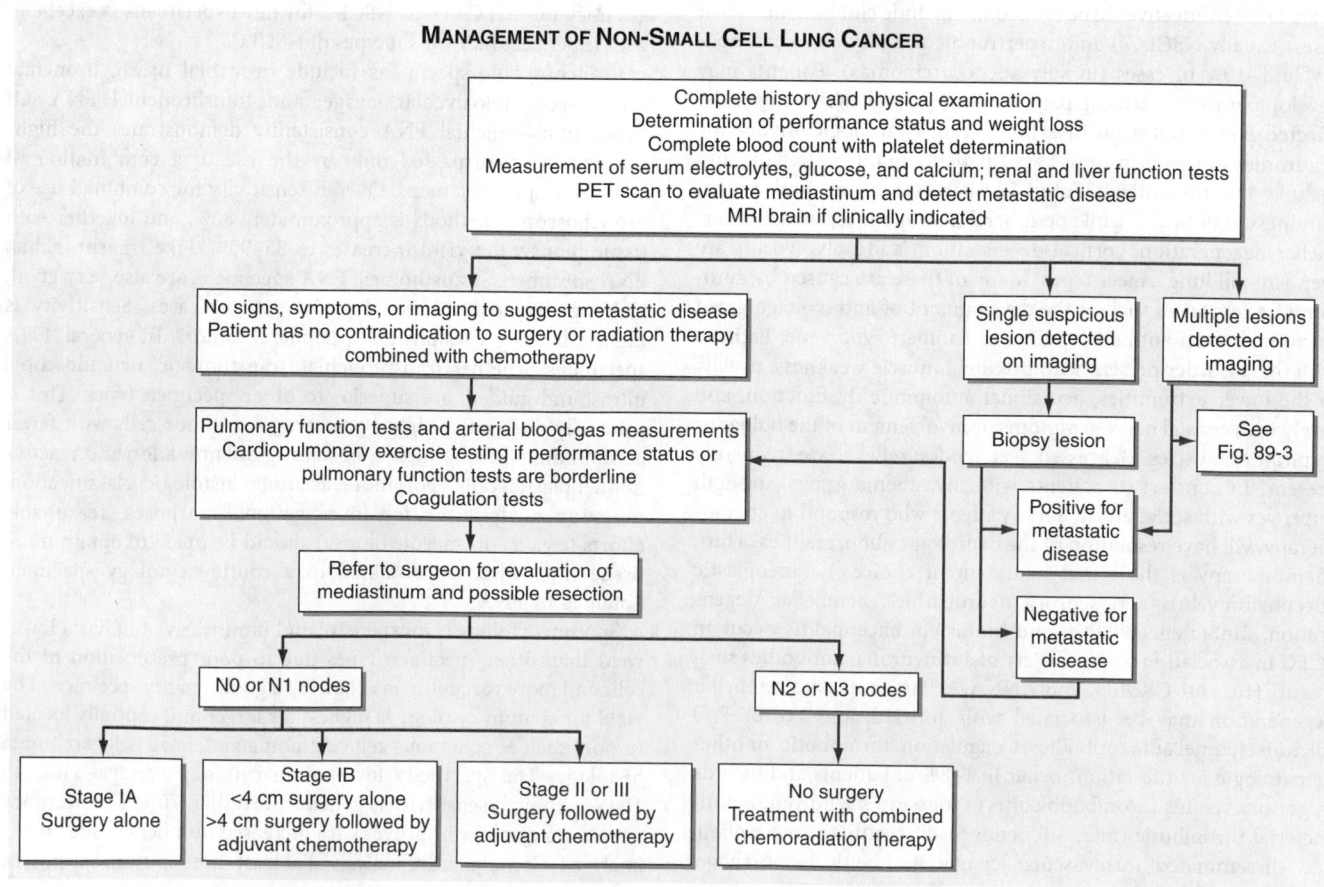

Figure 89-4 Algorithm for management of non-small cell lung cancer.

metastatic disease, current guidelines recommend a more extensive imaging evaluation, including imaging of the brain with either CT scan or MRI. In patients in whom distant metastatic disease has been ruled out, lymph node status needs to be assessed via a combination of radiographic imaging and/or minimally invasive techniques such as those mentioned above and/or invasive techniques such as mediastinoscopy, mediastinotomy, thoracoscopy, and thoracotomy. About a quarter to a half of patients diagnosed with NSCLC will have mediastinal lymph node metastases at the time of diagnosis. Lymph node sampling is recommended in all patients with enlarged nodes detected by CT or PET scan and in patients with large tumors or tumors occupying the inner third of the lung. The extent of mediastinal lymph node involvement is important in determining the appropriate treatment strategy: surgical resection followed by adjuvant chemotherapy versus combined chemoradiotherapy alone (see below). A standard nomenclature for referring to the location of lymph nodes involved with lung cancer has evolved (Fig. 89-5).

There are limited data on the use of CT-PET in the staging of patients with SCLC (Fig. 89-6). Current staging recommendations include a CT scan of the chest and abdomen (because of the high frequency of hepatic and adrenal involvement), MRI of the brain (positive in 10% of asymptomatic patients), and radionuclide (bone) scan if symptoms or signs suggest disease involvement in these areas. Bone marrow biopsies and aspirations are rarely performed given the low incidence of isolated bone marrow metastases. Confirmation of metastatic disease, ipsilateral or contralateral lung nodules, or metastases beyond the mediastinum may be achieved by the same modalities recommended above for patients with NSCLC.

If a patient has signs or symptoms of spinal cord compression (pain, weakness, paralysis, urinary retention), a spinal CT or MRI scan and examination of the cerebrospinal fluid cytology should be performed. If metastases are evident on imaging, a neurosurgeon should be consulted for possible palliative surgical resection and/or a radiation oncologist should be consulted for palliative radiotherapy to the site of compression. If signs of symptoms of leptomeningitis develop at any time in a patient with lung cancer, an MRI of the brain and spinal cord should be performed as well as a spinal tap for detection of malignant cells. If the spinal tap is negative, a repeat spinal tap should be considered. There is currently no approved therapy for the treatment of leptomeningeal disease.

■ THE STAGING SYSTEM FOR NON-SMALL CELL LUNG CANCER

The TNM International Staging System provides useful prognostic information and is used to stage all patients with NSCLC. The various T (tumor size), N (regional node involvement) and M (presence or absence of distant metastasis) are combined to form different stage groups (Table 89-5). The former tumor node metastasis (TNM) staging system for lung cancer (sixth edition) was developed based on a relatively small database of patients from a single institution. In 1999, the International Association for the Study of Lung Cancer established the lung cancer staging project and collected data on more than 68,000 cases from 46 sources in more than 19 countries to develop the new TNM (seventh edition) staging system, which has come into use as of 2010. As seen in Tables 89-5 and 89-6, the major distinction between the sixth and seventh edition staging system is within the T classification; T1 tumors are divided into tumors ≤2 cm in size, as these patients were found to have a better prognosis compared to tumors >2 cm but ≤3 cm. T2 tumors are divided into those that are >3 cm but ≤5 cm and those that are >5 cm but ≤7 cm. T3 tumors are >7 cm. T4 tumors include those that have additional nodules in the same lobe or tumors that have a malignant pleural effusion. No changes have been made to the current classification of lymph node involvement (N). Patients with metastasis may be classified as M1a, malignant pleural or pericardial effusion, pleural nodules or nodules in the contralateral lung, or M1b distant metastasis (e.g., bone, liver, adrenal, or brain metastasis). Based on these data, approximately one-third of patients have localized disease that can be treated with curative attempt (surgery or radiotherapy), one-third have local or regional disease that may or may not be amenable to a curative attempt, and one-third have metastatic disease at the time of diagnosis.

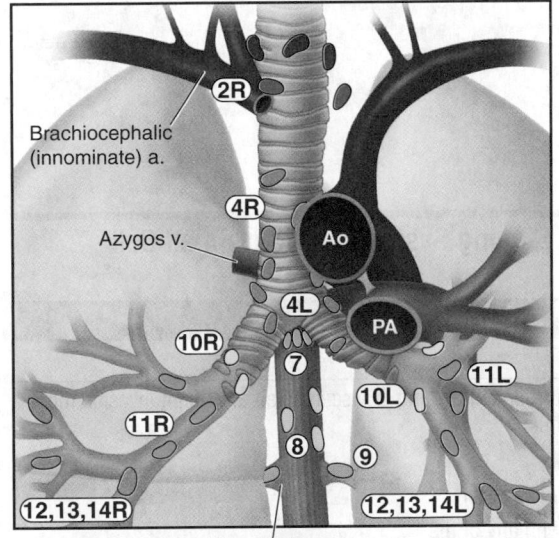

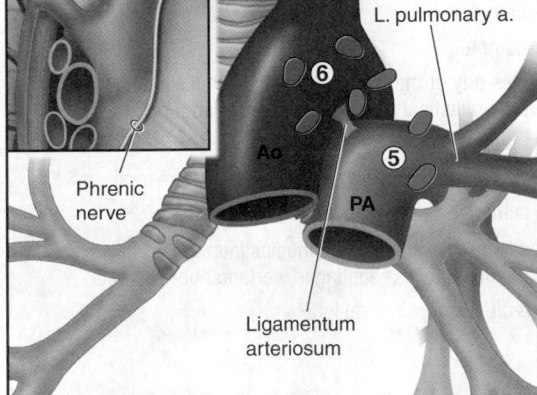

Superior Mediastinal Nodes

● 1. Highest Mediastinal

● 2. Upper Paratracheal

● 3. Prevascular and Retrotracheal

● 4. Lower Paratracheal
   (including Azygos Nodes)

   N2 = single digit, ipsilateral
   N3 = single digit, contralateral
        or supraclavicular

Aortic Nodes

● 5. Subaortic (A-P window)

● 6. Para-aortic (ascending
   aorta or phrenic)

Inferior Mediastinal Nodes

● 7. Subcarinal

● 8. Paraesophageal (below carina)

● 9. Pulmonary Ligament

N1 Nodes

○ 10. Hilar

● 11. Interlobar

● 12. Lobar

● 13. Segmental

● 14. Subsegmental

Figure 89-5 Lymph node stations in staging non-small cell lung cancer.

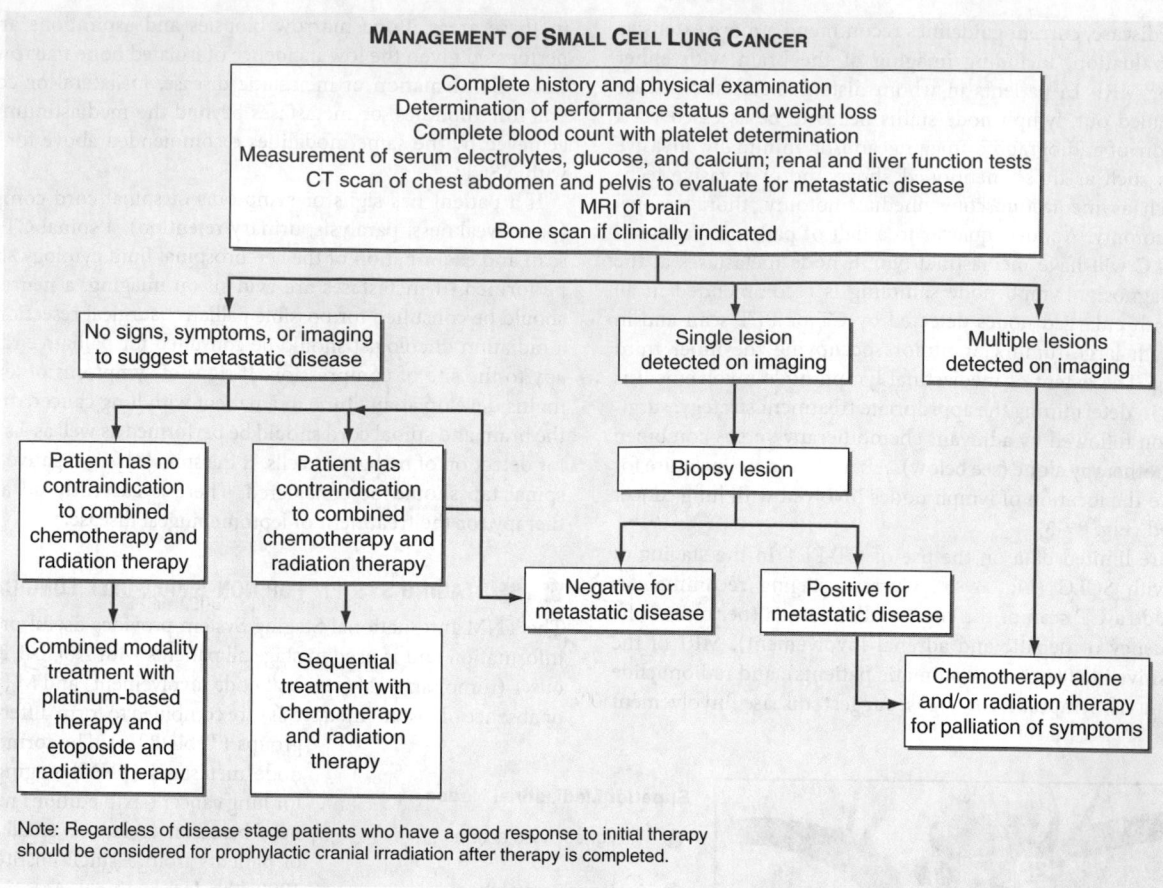

MANAGEMENT OF SMALL CELL LUNG CANCER

Note: Regardless of disease stage patients who have a good response to initial therapy should be considered for prophylactic cranial irradiation after therapy is completed.

Figure 89-6 Algorithm for management of small cell lung cancer.

TABLE 89-5 Comparison of the Sixth and Seventh Edition TNM Staging Systems for Non-Small Cell Lung Cancer

	Sixth Edition	Seventh Edition
Tumor (T)		
T1	Tumor ≤3 cm diameter without invasion more proximal than lobar bronchus	Tumor ≤3 cm diameter, surrounded by lung or visceral pleura, without invasion more proximal than lobar bronchus
T1a		Tumor ≤2 cm in diameter
T1b		Tumor >2 cm but ≤3 cm in diameter
T2	Tumor >3 cm diameter OR tumor of any size with any of the following: Visceral pleural invasion Atelectasis of less than entire lung Proximal extent at least 2 cm from carina	Tumor >3 cm but ≤7 cm with any of the following: Involves main bronchus, ≥2 cm distal to carina Invades visceral pleura Associated with atelectasis or obstructive pneumonitis extending to hilar region but not involving the entire lung
T2a		Tumor >3 cm but ≤5 cm in diameter
T2b		Tumor >5 cm but ≤7 cm in diameter
T3	Tumor of any size that invades any of the following: chest wall, diaphragm, mediastinal pleura, parietal pericardium Tumor <2 cm distal to carina	Tumor >7 cm or directly invades any of the following: chest wall (including superior sulcus tumors), phrenic nerve, mediastinal pleura, parietal pericardium Tumor <2 cm distal to carina but without involvement of carina Tumor with associated atelectasis or obstructive pneumonitis of entire lung Separate tumor nodule(s) in same lobe
T4	Tumor of any size that invades any of the following: mediastinum, heart or great vessels, trachea, esophagus, vertebral body, carina Tumor with malignant pleural or pericardial effusion Separate tumor nodules in same lobe	Tumor of any size that invades any of the following: mediastinum, heart or great vessels, trachea, recurrent laryngeal nerve, esophagus, vertebral body, carina Separate tumor nodule(s) in a different ipsilateral lobe

(continued)

TABLE 89-5 Comparison of the Sixth and Seventh Edition TNM Staging Systems for Non-Small Cell Lung Cancer (*Continued*)

Nodes (N)		
N0	No regional lymph node metastasis	No regional lymph node metastasis
N1	Metastasis in ipsilateral peribronchial and/or hilar lymph node(s)	Metastasis in ipsilateral peribronchial and/or hilar lymph node(s) and intrapulmonary node(s), including involvement by direct extensions
N2	Metastasis in ipsilateral mediastinal and/or subcarinal lymph node(s)	Metastasis in ipsilateral mediastinal and/or subcarinal lymph node(s)
N3	Metastasis in contralateral mediastinal, contralateral hilar, ipsilateral or contralateral scalene or supraclavicular lymph node(s)	Metastasis in contralateral mediastinal, hilar, ipsilateral or contralateral scalene or supraclavicular lymph node(s)
Metastasis (M)		
M0	No distant metastasis	No distant metastasis
M1	Distant metastasis (includes tumor nodules in different lobe from primary)	Distant metastasis
M1a		Separate tumor nodules in a contralateral lobe
		Tumor with pleural nodules or malignant pleural or pericardial effusion
M1b		Distant metastasis

Source: Reproduced with permission from P Goldstraw et al: J Thorac Oncol 2:706, 2007.

■ THE STAGING SYSTEM FOR SMALL CELL LUNG CANCER

Small cell lung cancer has a distinct two-stage system. Patients with limited-stage disease (LD) have cancer that is confined to the ipsilateral hemithorax and can be encompassed within a tolerable radiation port. Thus, contralateral supraclavicular nodes, recurrent laryngeal nerve involvement, and superior vena caval obstruction can all be part of limited-stage disease. Patients with extensive-stage disease (ED) have overt metastatic disease by imaging or physical examination. Cardiac tamponade, malignant pleural effusion, and bilateral pulmonary parenchymal involvement generally qualify disease as extensive-stage, because the involved organs cannot be encompassed safely or effectively within a single radiation therapy port. Sixty to 70% of patients are diagnosed with extensive disease at presentation.

■ PHYSIOLOGIC STAGING

Patients with lung cancer often have other comorbid conditions related to smoking, including cardiovascular disease and COPD. To improve their preoperative condition, correctable problems (e.g., anemia, electrolyte and fluid disorders, infections, cardiac disease, and arrhythmias) should be addressed, appropriate chest physical therapy instituted, and patients should be encouraged to stop smoking. Since it is not always possible to predict whether a lobectomy or pneumonectomy will be required until the time of operation, a conservative approach is to restrict surgical resection to patients who could potentially tolerate a pneumonectomy. Patients with an FEV_1 (forced expiratory volume in 1 s) of greater than 2 L or greater than 80% of predicted can tolerate a pneumonectomy, and those with an FEV_1 greater than 1.5 L have adequate reserve for a lobectomy. In patients with borderline lung function but a resectable tumor, cardiopulmonary exercise testing could be performed as part of the physiologic evaluation. This test allows an estimate of the maximal oxygen consumption (Vo_2max). A Vo_2max <15 mL/(kg·min) predicts for a higher risk of postoperative complications. Patients deemed unable to tolerate lobectomy or pneumonectomy from a pulmonary functional standpoint may be candidates for more limited resections, such as wedge or anatomic segmental resection, although such procedures are associated with significantly higher rates of local recurrence and a trend toward decreased overall survival. All patients should be assessed for cardiovascular risk using American College of Cardiology and American Heart Association guidelines. A myocardial infarction within the past 3 months is a contraindication to thoracic surgery because 20% of patients will die of reinfarction. An infarction in the past 6 months is a relative contraindication. Other major contraindications include uncontrolled arrhythmias, an FEV_1 of less than 1 L, CO_2 retention (resting PCO_2 >45 mmHg), DL_{CO} <40%, and severe pulmonary hypertension.

TABLE 89-6 Comparison of Survival by Stage in TNM Sixth and Seventh Editions

Stage	TNM Sixth Edition	TNM Seventh Edition	5-Year Survival (%)*
IA	T1N0M0	T1a-T1bN0M0	73
IB	T2N0M0	T2aN0M0	58
IIA	T1N1M0	T1a-T2aN1M0 or T2bN0M0	46
IIB	T2N1M0 or T3N0M0	T2bN1M0 or T3N0M0	36
IIIA	T3N1M0 or T1-3N2M0	T1a-T3N2M0 or T3N1M0 or T4N0-1M0	24
IIIB	Any T N3M0 T4 Any N M0	T4N2M0 or T1a-T4N3M0	9
IV	Any T Any N M1	Any T Any N M1a or M1b	13

*Survival according to the seventh edition.

The overall treatment approach to patients with NSCLC is shown in Fig. 89-4.

MANAGEMENT OF OCCULT AND STAGE 0 CARCINOMAS Patients with severe atypia on sputum cytology have an increased risk of developing lung cancer compared to those without atypia. In the uncommon circumstance where malignant cells are identified in a sputum or bronchial washing specimen but the chest imaging appears normal (TX tumor stage), the lesion must be localized. More than 90% of tumors can be localized by meticulous examination of the bronchial tree with a fiberoptic bronchoscope under general anesthesia and collection of a series of differential brushings and biopsies. Surgical resection following bronchoscopic localization improves survival compared to no treatment. Close follow-up of these patients is indicated because of the high incidence of second primary lung cancers (5% per patient per year).

SOLITARY PULMONARY NODULE AND "GROUND-GLASS" OPACITIES A solitary pulmonary nodule is defined as an x-ray density completely surrounded by normal aerated lung with circumscribed margins, of any shape, usually 1–6 cm at greatest diameter. The approach to a patient with a solitary pulmonary nodule is based on an estimate of the probability of cancer, determined according to the patient's smoking history, age, and characteristics on imaging (Table 89-7). Prior chest x-rays and CT scans should be obtained if available for comparison. A PET scan may be useful if the lesion is greater than 7–8 mm in diameter. If no diagnosis is apparent, Mayo Clinic investigators reported that clinical characteristics (age, cigarette smoking status, and prior cancer diagnosis) and three radiologic characteristics (nodule diameter, spiculation, and upper lobe location) were independent predictors of malignancy. At present, only two radiographic criteria are thought to predict the benign nature of a solitary pulmonary nodule: lack of growth over a period >2 years and certain characteristic patterns of calcification. Calcification alone, however, does not exclude malignancy; a dense central nidus, multiple punctate foci, and "bull's-eye" (granuloma) and "popcorn ball" (hamartoma) calcifications are highly suggestive of a benign lesion. In contrast, a relatively large lesion, lack of or asymmetric calcification, chest symptoms, associated atelectasis, pneumonitis, or growth of the lesion revealed by comparison with an old x-ray or CT scan or a positive PET scan are suggestive of a malignant process and warrant further attempts to establish a histologic diagnosis. An algorithm for assessing these lesions is shown in Fig. 89-3.

Since the advent of screening CTs, small GGOs have often been observed, particularly as the increased sensitivity of CTs enables detection of smaller lesions. Many of these GGOs, when biopsied, are found to be BAC. Some of the GGOs are semiopaque and referred to as "partial" GGOs. These are often more slow-growing and harbor atypical adenomatous hyperplasia histology, and are thought to be precursors to adenocarcinoma. By contrast, "solid" GGOs have faster growth rates and are usually typical adenocarcinoma histologically.

MANAGEMENT OF STAGES I AND II NSCLC

Surgical Resection for Stages I and II NSCLC Surgical resection by an experienced surgeon is the treatment of choice for patients with clinical stage I or II NSCLC who are able to tolerate the procedure. A retrospective review indicated that operative mortality rates for patients whose tumors were resected by noncardiothoracic or cardiothoracic surgeons were lower compared to general surgeons (5.8% vs 5.6% vs 7.6%, $p = .001$). The extent of resection is a matter of surgical judgment based on findings at exploration. A clinical trial in patients with stage IA NSCLC found that lobectomy was superior to wedge resection in reducing the rate of local recurrence, with a trend toward improvement in overall survival. A retrospective review of the Surveillance, Epidemiology, and End Results (SEER) database also reported a survival benefit for lobectomy compared to wedge resection. A limited resection, wedge resection, and segmentectomy [potentially by video-assisted thoracic surgery (VATS)] may be more appropriate in patients with comorbidities, including compromised pulmonary reserve and small peripheral lesions. Pneumonectomy is reserved for patients with very central tumors and should only be performed in patients with excellent pulmonary reserve. The 5-year survival rates are 60–80% for patients with stage I NSCLC and 40–50% for patients with stage II NSCLC.

Accurate pathologic staging requires adequate segmental, hilar, and mediastinal lymph node sampling. Mediastinal lymph node dissection provides for a significantly larger amount of material, which can refine pathologic (nodal) stage. On the right side, mediastinal stations 2R, 4R, 7, 8R, and 9R should be dissected; on the left side, stations 5, 6, 7, 8L, and 9L should be dissected (Fig. 89-5). Hilar lymph nodes are typically resected and sent with the specimen, although it is helpful to specifically dissect and label level 10 lymph nodes when possible. On the left side, level 2 and sometimes level 4 lymph nodes are generally obscured by the aorta. Although the therapeutic benefit of nodal dissection versus nodal sampling remains controversial, in a recent pooled analysis of three trials, 4-year survival was superior in patients undergoing resection with stages I–IIIA NSCLC who had complete mediastinal lymph node dissection compared with lymph node sampling. Moreover, a complete mediastinal lymphadenectomy adds little morbidity to a pulmonary resection for lung cancer. Thus, the recommendation at this time is that patients should have a complete mediastinal node dissection.

Radiation Therapy in Stages I and II NSCLC There is currently no role for adjuvant radiation therapy in patients following resection of stage I or II NSCLC. Patients with stage I or

---

TABLE 89-7 Assessment of Risk of Cancer in Patients With Solitary Pulmonary Nodules

| Variable | Risk | | |
	Low	Intermediate	High
Diameter (cm)	<1.5	1.5–2.2	≥2.3
Age (years)	<45	45–60	>60
Smoking status	Never smoker	Current smoker (<20 cigarettes/d)	Current smoker (>20 cigarettes/d)
Smoking cessation status	Quit ≥7 years ago or quit	Quit <7 years ago	Never quit
Characteristics of nodule margins	Smooth	Scalloped	Corona radiata or spiculated

Source: Reproduced with permission from D Ost et al: N Engl J Med 348:2535, 2003.

II disease who refuse or are not candidates for pulmonary resection should be considered for radiation therapy with curative intent. The decision to administer high-dose radiotherapy is based on the extent of disease and the volume of the chest that requires radiation. A systematic review reported 5-year survival rates of 13–39% in patients with stage I or II NSCLC treated with radical radiotherapy. Stereotactic radiation therapy and cryoablation are relatively new techniques that are being used in the treatment of patients with isolated pulmonary nodules who are not candidates for or refuse surgical resection, but their use may be limited by tumor size: ≤5 cm for stereotactic radiotherapy and ≤3 cm for cryoablation therapy.

Chemotherapy in Stages I and II NSCLC A multitude of trials have evaluated the role of adjuvant chemotherapy in patients with resected stage IA–IIIA NSCLC with conflicting results (Table 89-8). A meta-analysis, the Lung Adjuvant Cisplatin Evaluation Study (LACE), reported a 5.4% improvement in 5-year survival for adjuvant chemotherapy compared to surgery alone in patients with stage I–IIIA NSCLC. The effect of cisplatin plus vinorelbine appeared marginally better than other cisplatin-based doublet regimens. The analysis, however, reported a harmful effect for chemotherapy in patients with stage IA disease, with questionable benefit in patients with stage IB disease. Chemotherapy also appeared to be detrimental in patients with poor performance status (ECOG PS2). The results of these studies have led to the recommendation for adjuvant chemotherapy only in patients with stage II or III NSCLC. Chemotherapy should start 6 to 8 weeks after surgery, if the patient has recovered, and should be administered for four cycles. All patients should be treated with a cisplatin-based regimen. Carboplatin is a reasonable consideration in patients who are unlikely to tolerate cisplatin for reasons such as reduced renal function, presence of neuropathy, or hearing impairment.

The treatment of patients with stage IB NSCLC remains controversial. Retrospective subset analyses of randomized phase III trials have reported no benefit for adjuvant chemotherapy in patients with stage IB disease. The only trial to evaluate adjuvant chemotherapy in patients with stage IB NSCLC reported no improvement in overall survival; however, a retrospective analysis of the trial reported a benefit in patients with tumors that were ≥4 cm. At this time, the risks and benefits of chemotherapy should be considered on an individual patient basis.

Four trials have evaluated neoadjuvant chemotherapy (chemotherapy before surgery) in patients with stage I–III NSCLC, of which three reported a trend toward improvement in progression-free and overall survival. However, at this time, no data support the use of neoadjuvant chemotherapy in NSCLC patients.

All patients with resected NSCLC are at high risk of recurrence or developing a second primary lung cancer. Thus, it is reasonable to follow these patients with regular imaging. The most appropriate modality and frequency has not been defined. Given that the majority of patients recur within the first 2 years after therapy, one guideline suggests CT scans of the chest with contrast every 6 months for the first 2 years after surgery, followed by yearly CT scans of the chest without contrast thereafter.

MANAGEMENT OF STAGE III NSCLC The interpretation of the results of clinical trials involving patients with stage III NSCLC has been clouded by a number of issues, including changing diagnostic techniques, different staging systems, and heterogeneous patient populations. In prior studies, patients may have had tumors ranging from nonbulky stage IIIA (clinical N1 nodes with N2 nodes discovered only at the time of surgery, despite a negative mediastinoscopy) to bulky N2 nodes (lymph nodes >2 cm clearly visible on imaging, or multilevel ipsilateral mediastinal nodes) to clearly inoperable nodes.

Surgery followed by adjuvant chemotherapy is the treatment of choice for patients with stage IIIA disease due to hilar nodal involvement (T3N1). Surgery for N2 disease is more controversial. A randomized phase III trial demonstrated an improvement in progression-free survival but no improvement in overall survival when patients with pathologically staged N2 NSCLC were treated with concurrent chemoradiotherapy (cisplatin and etoposide) and 45 Gy of radiation followed by surgery compared to chemotherapy and 61 Gy of radiotherapy without surgery. Treatment-related mortality is greater in the surgery arm (8% vs 2%), with the majority of deaths occurring in patients undergoing pneumonectomy. In subset analysis, the investigators found survival was improved if a lobectomy was performed but not pneumonectomy compared to chemoradiotherapy alone.

TABLE 89-8 Adjuvant Chemotherapy Trials in Non-Small Cell Lung Cancer

Trial	Stage	Treatment	N	5-Year Survival	p
IALT	I–III	Cisplatin-based	932	44.5	<.03
		Control	835	40.4	
BR10	IB–II	Cisplatin + vinorelbine	242	69	.03
		Control	240	54	
ANITA	IB–IIIA	Cisplatin + vinorelbine	407	60	.017
		Control	433	58	
ALPI	I–III	MVP	548	50	.49
		Control	540	45	
BLT	I–III	Cisplatin-based	192	60	.90
		Control	189	58	
CALGB	IB	Carboplatin + paclitaxel	173	59	.10
			171	57	

Abbreviations: IALT, International Adjuvant Lung Cancer Trial; ANITA, Adjuvant Navelbine International Trialist Association; ALPI, Adjuvant Lung Cancer Project Italy; BLT, Big Lung Trial; CALGB, Cancer and Lung Cancer Group B; MVP, mitomycin, vindesine, and cisplatin.

In spite of a careful preoperative staging evaluation, as many as a quarter of patients will be found to have metastases to N2 nodes on frozen-section examination at the time of thoracotomy or on final pathologic examination of the surgical specimen. For patients with an occult, single-station mediastinal node metastasis recognized at thoracotomy in which a complete resection of the nodes and primary tumor is technically possible, most thoracic surgeons proceed with the planned lung resection and a mediastinal lymphadenectomy. If a complete resection is not possible or there is multistation or bulky nodal disease or extracapsular nodal disease, then the planned lung resection should be aborted. These patients can then be considered for combined chemoradiotherapy as described below. Although incomplete resection rarely results in long-term survival, collected results indicate that surgery alone in stage IIIA disease (N2 disease) is associated with a 14–30% 5-year survival. The best survival rate is seen in cases with minimal N2 disease and complete resection.

Chemotherapy plus radiation therapy is the treatment of choice for patients with N3 nodal involvement or bulky stage IIIA disease. In general, patients with histologically involved lymph nodes >2 cm in short-axis diameter measured by CT, who have extranodal involvement or multistation disease along with groups of multiple smaller lymph nodes involved, are considered to have bulky, unresectable disease. Randomized phase III trials initially demonstrated an improvement in median and long-term survival for chemotherapy followed by radiation therapy, compared with radiation therapy alone. Subsequent trials demonstrated administering concurrent chemotherapy and radiation therapy results in improved survival compared to sequential therapy, albeit with more side effects, such as fatigue, esophagitis, and neutropenia. Therefore, combined modality treatment with chemotherapy and radiation therapy is recommended in patients who are able to tolerate the treatment.

Superior Sulcus or Pancoast Tumors Superior sulcus tumors arise in the apex of the lung and invade adjacent structures producing Pancoast's syndrome: Horner's syndrome, shoulder and/or arm pain, and weakness and atrophy of the muscles of the hand. Patients with these tumors should undergo the same staging procedures as all patients with stage II or III NSCLC. Neoadjuvant chemotherapy or combined chemotherapy and radiation therapy is typically reserved for those patients with N0 or N1 involvement. This approach results in a 33-month median survival and 44% 5-year survival for all patients, and a 94-month median survival and 54% 5-year survival in patients with an R0 resection. For patients with Pancoast tumors that have metastatic disease at the time of presentation, radiation therapy with or without chemotherapy may be offered for palliation of symptoms.

TREATMENT OF METASTATIC NON-SMALL CELL LUNG CANCER

Approximately two-thirds of NSCLC patients present with advanced disease (stage IIIB with a pleural effusion or stage IV) at the time of diagnosis. These patients have a median survival of 4–5 months and a 1-year survival of 10% when managed with best supportive care alone. In addition, a significant number of patients who present with early-stage NSCLC eventually relapse with distant disease. Patients who have recurrent disease have a better prognosis than those presenting with metastatic disease at the time of diagnosis. Standard medical management, the judicious use of pain medications, and the appropriate use of radiotherapy and chemotherapy form the cornerstone of management.

Chemotherapy palliates symptoms, improves the quality of life, and improves survival in patients with stage IV NSCLC, particularly in patients with good performance status. In

addition, economic analysis has found chemotherapy to be cost-effective palliation for stage IV NSCLC. However, the use of chemotherapy for NSCLC requires clinical experience and careful judgment to balance potential benefits and toxicities.

First-Line Chemotherapy for Metastatic or Recurrent Non-Small Cell Lung Cancer The first indication of the benefit of chemotherapy in patients with advanced NSCLC came from a meta-analysis published in 1995 that reported a survival advantage in patients treated with cisplatin-based chemotherapy compared to those receiving supportive care alone (HR = 0.73, $p < .0001$). This led to a multitude of clinical trials comparing different cisplatin-based regimens in patients with advanced NSCLC all reporting a similar magnitude of benefit; 20–30% response rate and an 8- to 10-month median survival (Table 89-9). Chemotherapy was well tolerated in all studies in patients with a good performance status, ECOG PS 0–1.

TABLE 89-9 First-Line Chemotherapy Trials for Metastatic Non-Small Cell Lung Cancer

Trial	Regimen	N	RR (%)	Median Survival (months)
ECOG1594	Cisplatin + paclitaxel	288	21	7.8
	Cisplatin + gemcitabine	288	22	8.1
	Cisplatin + docetaxel	289	17	7.4
	Carboplatin + paclitaxel	290	17	8.1
TAX-326	Cisplatin + docetaxel	406	32	11.3
	Cisplatin + vinorelbine	394	25	10.1
	Carboplatin + docetaxel	404	24	9.4
EORTC	Cisplatin + paclitaxel	159	32	8.1
	Cisplatin + gemcitabine	160	37	8.9
	Paclitaxel + gemcitabine	161	28	6.7
ILCP	Cisplatin + gemcitabine	205	30	9.8
	Carboplatin + paclitaxel	204	32	9.9
	Cisplatin + vinorelbine	203	30	9.5
SWOG	Cisplatin + vinorelbine	202	28	8.0
	Carboplatin + paclitaxel	206	25	8.0
FACS	Cisplatin + irinotecan	145	31	13.9
	Carboplatin + paclitaxel	145	32	12.3
	Cisplatin + gemcitabine	146	30	14.0
	Cisplatin + vinorelbine	145	33	11.4
Scagliotti	Cisplatin + gemcitabine	863	28	10.3
	Cisplatin + pemetrexed	862	31	10.3
iPASS*	Carboplatin + paclitaxel	608	32	17.3
	Gefitinib	609	43	18.6

*Enrolled selected patients: 18 years of age or older, had histologic or cytologically confirmed stage IIIB or IV non-small cell lung cancer with histologic features of adenocarcinoma (including bronchioloalveolar carcinoma), were nonsmokers (defined as patients who had smoked <100 cigarettes in their lifetime) or former light smokers (those who had stopped smoking at least 15 years previously and had a total of ≤10 pack-years of smoking), and had had no previous chemotherapy or biologic or immunologic therapy.

Abbreviations: ECOG, Eastern Cooperative Oncology Group; EORTC, European Organization for Research and Treatment of Cancer; ILCP, Italian Lung Cancer Project; SWOG, South-Western Oncology Group; FACS, Follow-up After Colorectal Surgery; iPASS, Iressa Pan-Asian Study.

An ongoing debate in the treatment of patients with NSCLC is the appropriate duration of platinum-based chemotherapy. Several large phase III randomized trials have failed to show a benefit for increasing the duration of platinum-based doublet chemotherapy beyond four to six cycles. In fact, longer duration of chemotherapy has been associated with increased toxicities and impaired quality of life. Therefore, prolonged therapy (beyond four to six cycles) with platinum-based regimens is not recommended in patients with advanced NSCLC.

Tumor histology has emerged as an important consideration in the treatment of patients with NSCLC. A randomized phase III trial found that patients with nonsquamous NSCLC had an improved survival when treated with cisplatin and pemetrexed compared to cisplatin and gemcitabine, while patients with squamous carcinoma had an improved survival when treated with cisplatin and gemcitabine. This difference in survival is thought to be related to the differential expression of thymidylate synthase, one of the targets of pemetrexed, between tumor types. Bevacizumab, a monoclonal antibody against VEGF, when combined with chemotherapy improves response rate, progression-free survival, and overall survival in patients with advanced disease (see below). However, bevacizumab cannot be given to patients with squamous cell histology NSCLC because of the risk of serious hemorrhagic effects.

Second-Line Chemotherapy and Beyond
As first-line chemotherapy regimens improve, a substantial number of patients will maintain a good performance status and a desire for further therapy when they develop recurrent disease. At present only three drugs are FDA-approved for second-line therapy of NSCLC in the United States, i.e., docetaxel, pemetrexed, and erlotinib. In general, these agents have similar overall response rates of 5–10% (depending on the patient's prior exposure to taxanes and platinum) and yield median survivals of 6–8 months. However, the available drugs have distinct toxicity profiles that can influence their use in the second-line setting. Hematologic toxicity including febrile neutropenia is greater for docetaxel compared with pemetrexed and erlotinib, whereas nonhematologic toxicity, namely rash and diarrhea, is greater with erlotinib. Most of the survival benefit for any of these agents is realized in those patients who maintain a good performance status.

AGENTS THAT INHIBIT ANGIOGENESIS
Bevacizumab was the first antiangiogenic agent approved for the treatment of patients with advanced NSCLC in the United States. This drug primarily acts by sponging up VEGF and blocking the growth of new blood vessels, which are required for tumor viability. Two randomized phase III trials of chemotherapy with or without bevacizumab had conflicting results. The first trial, conducted in North America, compared carboplatin/paclitaxel with or without bevacizumab in patients with recurrent or advanced nonsquamous NSCLC and reported a significant improvement in response rate, progression-free survival, and overall survival for chemotherapy-plus-bevacizumab–treated patients compared to chemotherapy alone. Toxicities were more frequent in bevacizumab-treated patients. The second trial, conducted in Europe, compared cisplatin/gemcitabine with or without bevacizumab in patients with recurrent or advanced non-squamous NSCLC and reported a significant improvement in progression-free survival but no improvement in overall survival for bevacizumab-treated patients. Therefore, at this time carboplatin/paclitaxel and bevacizumab is an approved regimen for first-line treatment of nonsquamous NSCLC in the United States but not in Europe.

AGENTS THAT INHIBIT THE EPIDERMAL GROWTH FACTOR RECEPTOR
Erlotinib and gefitinib are oral small-molecule kinase inhibitors that inhibit signaling via EGFR. These were the first EGFR inhibitors to be approved for the treatment of patients with NSCLC. A randomized phase III trial compared erlotinib to placebo in previously treated patients with advanced NSCLC and reported an improvement in overall survival for erlotinib compared to placebo. Gefitinib received premarketing approval by the FDA after impressive results seen in phase II trials in patients with previously treated NSCLC; however, a randomized phase III trial found no difference in overall survival between patients treated with gefitinib compared to placebo. These results led to a U.S. FDA-mandated change in the gefitinib indication to include only patients who have previously benefited from this drug. However, gefitinib is still available for the treatment of NSCLC patients in Europe and Asia. Clinical features that have been shown to correlate with responsiveness to EGFR TKI treatment include female sex, never smoking status, adenocarcinoma histology, and Asian ethnicity. Somatic mutations in the kinase domain of EGFR and high EGFR copy number have also been shown to correlate with response and improved survival with oral EGFR inhibitors.

Two randomized phase III trials conducted in Asia have compared gefitinib to platinum-based chemotherapy in patients with NSCLC. The first trial compared first-line gefitinib to carboplatin/paclitaxel in never or light ex-smokers with newly diagnosed advanced NSCLC. Treatment with gefitinib was associated with a significant improvement in response rate and 12-month progression-free survival. In patients with tumors available for mutation analysis, treatment with gefitinib was favored over chemotherapy in patients with tumors that harbored an EGFR mutation and chemotherapy was favored in patients with tumors that were EGFR mutation negative. Quality of life favored treatment with gefitinib. The second trial enrolled only patients with tumors that were EGFR mutation positive and reported a significant improvement in progression-free survival and disease control for patients treated with gefitinib compared to cisplatin/docetaxel. These and related results suggest standard chemotherapy regimens or gefitinib and erlotinib could be considered for first-line therapy in a subset of advanced NSCLC patients with tumors that harbor the EGFR mutation.

Cetuximab is an intravenously administered chimeric antibody directed against EGFR. A randomized phase III trial evaluated treatment with cisplatin/vinorelbine with or without cetuximab in patients with advanced NSCLC and at least one EGFR-positive cell as determined by immunohistochemistry. The results showed no difference in progression-free survival but a significant improvement in response rate and overall survival in patients treated with cetuximab compared to placebo. A prespecified subgroup analysis showed no improvement in overall survival among patients of Asian ethnicity receiving cetuximab compared with placebo. However, a significant improvement in overall survival was noted among Caucasian patients receiving cetuximab; this appeared true regardless of histology. Contrary to patients with colon cancer, KRAS mutation status did not predict response to therapy with cetuximab, although the number of cases examined at the molecular level was suboptimal. Development of acneiform rash was associated with improved overall survival compared to patients with no rash. A second phase III trial in patients with advanced NSCLC with no required EGFR testing reported no difference in overall survival between patients randomized to carboplatin/paclitaxel or docetaxel with or without cetuximab.

MAINTENANCE THERAPY Maintenance chemotherapy in nonprogressing patients (patients with a complete response, partial response, or stable disease) is a controversial topic in the treatment of NSCLC patients. Two studies have investigated maintenance single-agent chemotherapy with docetaxel or pemetrexed in nonprogressing patients following treatment with first-line platinum-based chemotherapy. Both trials randomized patients to immediate single-agent therapy versus observation and reported improvements in progression-free and overall survival. In both trials, a significant portion of patients in the observation arm did not receive therapy with the agent under investigation upon disease progression; 37% of study patients never received docetaxel in the docetaxel study and 81% of patients never received pemetrexed in the pemetrexed study. In the trial of maintenance docetaxel versus observation, survival was identical to the treatment group in the subset of patients who received docetaxel on progression, indicating this is an active agent in NSCLC. These data are not available for the pemetrexed study. Currently maintenance pemetrexed is the only therapy approved by the U.S. FDA following platinum-based chemotherapy in patients with advanced NSCLC. However, maintenance chemotherapy is not without toxicity and at this time should be considered on an individual patient basis.

Two randomized controlled trials have reported improvements in progression-free survival from maintenance treatment with erlotinib compared to placebo in patients with advanced NSCLC following platinum-based chemotherapy.

TREATMENT Small Cell Lung Cancer

TREATMENT OF LIMITED DISEASE SMALL CELL LUNG CANCER

Surgery SCLC is a highly aggressive disease characterized by its rapid doubling time, high growth fraction, early development of disseminated disease, and dramatic response to first-line chemotherapy and radiation. Surgical resection is not routinely recommended for patients because even those patients with LD-SCLC still have occult micrometastases. If the histologic diagnosis of SCLC is made in patients on review of a resected surgical specimen, such patients should receive standard SCLC chemotherapy as described below. If one employs classic TNM staging categories, two retrospective series have reported high cure rates for adjuvant chemotherapy following resection in patients with stage I or II SCLC.

Chemotherapy Chemotherapy significantly prolongs survival in patients with SCLC. Combination chemotherapy with a platinum agent (cisplatin or carboplatin) and etoposide for four to six cycles is the mainstay of treatment and has not changed in almost three decades. Cyclophosphamide, doxorubicin (Adriamycin), and vincristine (CAV) may be an alternative for patients who are unable to tolerate a platinum-based regimen. Despite response rates to first-line therapy as high as 80%, the median survival ranges from 12 to 20 months for patients with LD and from 7 to 11 months for patients with ED. Regardless of disease extent, the majority of patients relapse and develop chemotherapy-resistant disease. Only 6–12% of patients with LD- and 2% of patients with ED-SCLC live beyond 5 years. The prognosis is especially poor for patients who relapse within the first 3 months of therapy; these patients are said to have platinum-*resistant disease*. Patients are said to have *sensitive disease* if they relapse more than 3 months after their initial therapy and are thought to have a somewhat better overall survival. Those patients with sensitive disease are thought to have the greatest potential benefit from second-line chemotherapy. Topotecan is the only FDA-approved agent with modest activity as second-line therapy in patients with SCLC.

Radiation Therapy Patients with LD-SCLC are treated with combined modality therapy with cisplatin and etoposide chemotherapy and radiation therapy. A retrospective analysis of patients with SCLC treated with once-daily fractionation found improved local control rates as the total dose delivered was increased from 30 to 50 Gy. Chemotherapy when given concurrently with radiation is more effective than sequential chemoradiation but is associated with significantly more esophagitis and hematologic toxicity. The addition of radiation therapy early on is preferred. Twice-daily (hyperfractionated) radiation has been shown to improve survival in patients with LD-SCLC but is associated with higher rates of grade 3 esophagitis and pulmonary toxicity. It is feasible to deliver once-daily radiation therapy doses up to at least 70 Gy when administered concurrently with cisplatin-based chemotherapy. This higher dose of once-daily radiotherapy may be equivalent or superior to the 45-Gy twice-daily radiotherapy dose. Patients should be carefully selected for concurrent chemoradiation therapy based on good performance status and pulmonary reserve.

Prophylactic Cranial Irradiation Prophylactic cranial irradiation (PCI) should be considered in all patients with LD- and ED-SCLC who have responded to initial therapy. A meta-analysis including 7 trials and 987 patients with LD-SCLC who had achieved a complete remission following primary chemotherapy reported a 5.4% improvement in overall survival for patients treated with PCI. In patients with ED-SCLC who had responded to first-line chemotherapy, PCI reduced the occurrence of symptomatic brain metastases and prolonged disease-free and overall survival compared to no radiation therapy. Long-term toxicities including deficits in cognition have been reported following PCI and are difficult to sort out from the effects of chemotherapy or normal aging.

Molecularly Tailored Lung Cancer Therapy In the past 40 years, clinical research in lung cancer has demonstrated that surgery, systemic chemotherapy, and radiation therapy can all be used to prolong patient survival and/or improve quality of life. However, conventional approaches, especially those that classify patients according to disease histology alone, appear to have reached a therapeutic plateau of effectiveness. One promising future approach to improve the outcome for patients with lung cancer is tailored therapy based on individualized phenotypic or genotypic tumor characteristics. Such a strategy is based upon an understanding of the molecular underpinnings of the disease, recognizing that although tumors may appear similar at the histologic level, they do differ from individual to individual. It is hoped that better outcomes can be achieved by matching the most appropriate therapy to a patient at the right time.

For example, one subset of lung cancer can be defined by somatic mutations in *EGFR*. *EGFR* mutations are almost exclusively found in lung adenocarcinoma and are more common in females, never smokers compared to former or current smokers, and in East Asians compared to Western populations (30–70% vs 8%). These mutations, primarily in-frame deletions in exon 19 and point mutations in exon 21 (L858R), result in constitutive activation of the receptor and are associated with very high response rates (60–90%) to the specific tyrosine kinase inhibitors gefitinib and erlotinib. Almost all patients with these dramatic responses, however, develop acquired resistance. In about half of patients, resistance can be attributed to the emergence of clones harboring a second-site mutation in exon 20 (T790M), which alters binding of drug to the receptor. About 20% of *EGFR* mutant tumors from patients with acquired resistance display amplification of a gene encoding a different tyrosine kinase, MET. As a result of these findings, many trials are being conducted in these patients using second-generation EGFR inhibitors that can overcome T790M-mediated resistance or MET inhibitors to target MET-dependent cells.

Another subset of lung adenocarcinoma can be defined by EML4-ALK fusion proteins. These translocations arise from a small inversion within chromosome 2p that leads to the formation of a fusion-gene comprising the N terminal of the echinoderm microtubule–associated protein-like 4 (EML4) gene and the intracellular tyrosine kinase domain of the anaplastic lymphoma kinase (ALK) gene. Patients with lung cancers harboring an ALK fusion protein have demonstrated dramatic responses to small-molecule ALK inhibitors in early clinical trials. The ALK fusion protein is relatively rare, occurring in 3–7% of NSCLCs. Clinical characteristics associated with EML4-ALK–positive lung cancer appears to be a younger age at diagnosis, minimal smoking history, male sex, and adenocarcinoma histology with signet-ring features.

Other biomarkers being explored include molecules that may predict outcomes with conventional chemotherapy. For example, low expression of the DNA repair gene excision repair cross-complementation group 1 (ERCC1) correlates with improved survival after treatment with platinum drugs, whereas tumors that have high expression of ERCC1 are less sensitive to therapy with a platinum agent. In the absence of treatment, lung cancer with low ERCC1 expression has a poorer prognosis.

Ribonucleotide reductase M1 (RRM1) encodes the regulatory subunit of ribonucleotide reductase, the rate-limiting enzyme in DNA synthesis. Ribonucleotide reductase converts ribonucleotide 5-diphosphate to deoxyribonucleotide 5-diphosphate. Notably, gemcitabine, an agent commonly used in the treatment of NSCLC, competes with ribonucleotide 5-diphosphate for incorporation into DNA. Levels of RRM1 expression are significantly and inversely correlated with disease response after two cycles of gemcitabine and carboplatin in patients with locally advanced NSCLC. In addition, low RRM1 mRNA expression levels are associated with a significantly longer median survival compared to high levels.

Thymidylate synthase (TS) catalyzes the methylation of dUMP to dTMP and is the rate-limiting irreversible step in de novo DNA synthesis. TS is one of the targets of the novel folate-based drug pemetrexed, an agent that is FDA-approved as second-line treatment in patients with NSCLC. TS expression is an independent prognostic and predictive factor in several cancers, including lung cancers, and overexpression of TS has been linked to resistance to pemetrexed, an agent commonly employed as second-line treatment in patients with non-squamous NSCLC. TS mRNA and protein levels are significantly higher in squamous cell carcinomas and small cell carcinomas of the lung as compared with adenocarcinomas. A randomized phase III trial reported that cisplatin plus gemcitabine was more effective in squamous cell carcinomas while, cisplatin plus pemetrexed was found to be more effective in adenocarcinomas and large cell carcinomas. Molecular markers are likely to play an increasing role in helping guide treatment decisions.

BENIGN LUNG NEOPLASMS

Benign tumors account for about 5% of all lung cancers. About half are hamartomas; the lungs are the site of about 90% of all hamartomas. The other half are bronchial adenomas.

■ HAMARTOMAS

Lung hamartomas are usually peripheral lung masses composed of normal pulmonary tissue components such as smooth muscle and collagen. They are more common in men than in women and have a peak incidence in the 60s. They are often incidental radiographic findings as solitary nodules. They have a pathognomonic "popcorn" pattern of calcification in some cases; however, without such a finding, resection is necessary to rule out malignancy, especially in smokers.

■ BRONCHIAL ADENOMAS

These are centrally located slow-growing endobronchial lesions that are generally carcinoid tumors (≥80%; Chap. 350), adenocystic tumors (so called cylindromas, 10–15%), or mucoepidermoid tumors (2–3%). Mean age at presentation is 45 years (range 15–60). Patients often give a history of chronic cough, intermittent hemoptysis, or repeated episodes of airway obstruction with atelectasis, or pneumonias with abscess formation due to endobronchial lesions obstructing the airway. They are usually visible at bronchoscopy but are highly vascular and may bleed profusely after a bronchoscopic biopsy. They are largely curable by surgical resection (local excision), but they may recur locally or become invasive and metastasize. Five-year survival after resection is 95% if the disease is localized. For bronchial adenomas that spread, the course of disease can become highly aggressive, such as SCLC, or somewhat slower, such as carcinoid tumors. Therapy is generally dictated by the pace of the disease.

FURTHER READINGS

Azzoli CG et al: American Society of Clinical Oncology clinical practice guideline update on chemotherapy for stage IV non-small cell lung cancer. J Clin Oncol 27:6251, 2009

Hanahan D, Weinberg RA: The hallmarks of cancer. Cell 100:57, 2000

Herbst RS et al: Lung cancer. N Engl J Med 359: 1367, 2008

Jackman DM, Johnson BE: Small-cell lung cancer. Lancet 366:1385, 2005

Kwak EL et al: Anaplastic lymphoma kinase inhibition in non-small-cell lung cancer. N Engl J Med 363:1693, 2010

Milroy R: New American College of Chest Physicians Lung Cancer Guidelines: An important addition to the lung cancer guidelines armamentarium. Chest 132:744, 2007

Ost D et al: The solitary pulmonary nodule. N Engl J Med 348:2535, 2003

CHAPTER 90

Breast Cancer

Marc E. Lippman

Breast cancer is a malignant proliferation of epithelial cells lining the ducts or lobules of the breast. In the year 2010, about 180,000 cases of invasive breast cancer and 40,000 deaths will occur in the United States. In addition, about 2000 men will be diagnosed with breast cancer. Epithelial malignancies of the breast are the most common cause of cancer in women (excluding skin cancer), accounting for about one-third of all cancer in women. As a result of improved treatment and earlier detection, mortality rate from breast cancer has begun to decrease very substantially in the United States. This chapter will not consider rare malignancies presenting in the breast, such as sarcomas and lymphomas, but will focus on the epithelial cancers. Human breast cancer is a clonal disease; a single transformed cell—the product of a series of somatic (acquired) or germ-line mutations—is eventually able to express full malignant potential. Thus, breast cancer may exist for a long period as either a noninvasive disease or an invasive but nonmetastatic disease. These facts have significant clinical ramifications.

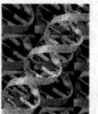

GENETIC CONSIDERATIONS

Not more than 10% of human breast cancers can be linked directly to germ-line mutations. Several genes have been implicated in familial cases. The Li-Fraumeni syndrome is characterized by inherited mutations in the p53 tumor-suppressor gene, which lead to an increased incidence of breast cancer, osteogenic sarcomas, and other malignancies. Inherited mutations in *PTEN* have also been reported in breast cancer.

Another tumor-suppressor gene, *BRCA-1*, has been identified at the chromosomal locus 17q21; this gene encodes a zinc finger protein, and the product therefore may function as a transcription factor. The gene appears to be involved in gene repair. Women who inherit a mutated allele of this gene from either parent have at least a 60–80% lifetime chance of developing breast cancer and about a 33% chance of developing ovarian cancer. The risk is higher among women born after 1940, presumably due to promotional effects of hormonal factors. Men who carry a mutant allele of the gene have an increased incidence of prostate cancer and breast cancer. A fourth gene, termed *BRCA-2*, which has been localized to chromosome 13q12, is also associated with an increased incidence of breast cancer in men and women.

Germ-line mutations in *BRCA-1* and *BRCA-2* can be readily detected; patients with these mutations can be counseled appropriately. All women with strong family histories for breast cancer should be referred to genetic screening programs, particularly women of Ashkenazi Jewish descent who have a high likelihood of a specific *BRCA-1* mutation (substitution of adenine for guanine at position 185).

Even more important than the role these genes play in inherited forms of breast cancer may be their role in sporadic breast cancer. A p53 mutation is present in nearly 40% of human breast cancers as an acquired defect. Acquired mutations in *PTEN* occur in about 10% of the cases. *BRCA-1* mutation in sporadic primary breast cancer has not been reported. However, decreased expression of *BRCA-1* mRNA (possibly via gene methylation) and abnormal cellular location of the *BRCA-1* protein have been found in some breast cancers. Loss of heterozygosity of *BRCA-1* and *BRCA-2* suggests that tumor-suppressor activity may be inactivated in sporadic cases of human breast cancer. Finally, increased expression of a dominant oncogene plays a role in about a quarter of human breast cancer cases. The product of this gene, a member of the epidermal growth factor receptor superfamily, is called *erbB2* (HER/2 neu) and is over-expressed in these breast cancers due to gene amplification; this overexpression can contribute to transformation of human breast epithelium and is the target of effective systemic therapy in adjuvant and metastatic disease settings.

EPIDEMIOLOGY

Breast cancer is a hormone-dependent disease. Women without functioning ovaries who never receive estrogen-replacement therapy do not develop breast cancer. The female-male ratio is about 150:1. For most epithelial malignancies, a log-log plot of incidence versus age shows a single-component straight-line increase with every year of life. A similar plot for breast cancer shows two components: a straight-line increase with age but with a decrease in slope beginning at the age of menopause. The three dates in a woman's life that have a major impact on breast cancer incidence are age at menarche, age at first full-term pregnancy, and age at menopause. Women who experience menarche at age 16 years have only 50–60% of the breast cancer risk of a woman having menarche at age 12 years; the lower risk persists throughout life. Similarly, menopause occurring 10 years before the median age of menopause (52 years), whether natural or surgically induced, reduces lifetime breast cancer risk by about 35%. Women who have a first full-term pregnancy by age 18 years have a 30–40% lower risk of breast cancer compared with nulliparous women. Thus, length of menstrual life—particularly the fraction occurring before first full-term pregnancy—is a substantial component of the total risk of breast cancer. These three factors (menarche, age of first full-term pregnancy, and menopause) can account for 70–80% of the variation in breast cancer frequency in different countries. A meta-analysis has shown that duration of maternal nursing correlates with substantial risk reduction independent of either parity or age at first full-term pregnancy.

International variation in incidence has provided some of the most important clues on hormonal carcinogenesis. A woman living to age 80 years in North America has one chance in nine of developing invasive breast cancer. Asian women have one-fifth to one-tenth the risk of breast cancer of women in North America or Western Europe. Asian women have substantially lower concentrations of estrogens and progesterone. These differences cannot be explained on a genetic basis because Asian women living in a Western environment have sex steroid hormone concentrations and risks identical to those of their Western counterparts. These migrant women, and more notably their daughters, also differ markedly in height and weight from Asian women in Asia; height and weight are critical regulators of age of menarche and have substantial effects on plasma concentrations of estrogens.

The role of diet in breast cancer etiology is controversial. While there are associative links between total caloric and fat intake and breast cancer risk, the exact role of fat in the diet is unproven. Increased caloric intake contributes to breast cancer risk in multiple ways: earlier menarche, later age at menopause, and increased post-menopausal estrogen concentrations reflecting enhanced aromatase activities in fatty tissues. Moderate alcohol intake also increases the risk by an unknown mechanism. Folic acid supplementation appears to modify risk in women who use alcohol but is not additionally protective in abstainers. Recommendations favoring abstinence from alcohol must be weighed against other social pressures and the possible cardioprotective effect of moderate alcohol intake.

Chronic low-dose aspirin use also appears associated with a decreased incidence of breast cancer.

Understanding the potential role of exogenous hormones in breast cancer is of extraordinary importance because millions of American women regularly use oral contraceptives and postmenopausal hormone replacement therapy. The most credible meta-analyses of oral contraceptive use suggest that these agents cause a small increased risk of breast cancer. By contrast, oral contraceptives offer a substantial protective effect against ovarian epithelial tumors and endometrial cancers. Hormone replacement therapy (HRT) has a powerful effect on breast cancer risk. Data from the Women's Health Initiative (WHI) trial showed that conjugated equine estrogens plus progestins increased the risk of breast cancer and adverse cardiovascular events but with decreases in bone fractures and colorectal cancer. On balance, there were more negative events with HRT; 6 to 7 years of HRT nearly doubled the risk of breast cancer. A parallel WHI trial with >12,000 women enrolled testing conjugated estrogens alone (ERT in women who have had hysterectomies) showed no significant increase in breast cancer incidence. A meta-analysis of nonrandomized HRT studies suggests that most of the previously attributed benefit of HRT can be accounted for by higher socioeconomic status among users, which is presumably associated with better access to health care and healthier behaviors. Certain potential benefits of HRT were not assessed in WHI. HRT is an area of rapid reevaluation, but it would appear (at least from breast cancer and cardiovascular disease vantage points) that there are serious concerns about long-term HRT use. HRT in women previously diagnosed with breast cancer increases recurrence rates. Rapid decrease in the number of women on HRT has already led to a coincident decrease in breast cancer incidence.

In addition to the other factors, radiation is a risk factor in younger women. Women who have been exposed before age 30 years to radiation in the form of multiple fluoroscopies (200–300 cGy) or treatment for Hodgkin's disease (>3600 cGy) have a substantial increase in risk of breast cancer, whereas radiation exposure after age 30 years appears to have a minimal carcinogenic effect on the breast.

EVALUATION OF BREAST MASSES IN MEN AND WOMEN

Because the breasts are a common site of potentially fatal malignancy in women, examination of the breast is an essential part of the physical examination. Unfortunately, internists frequently do not examine breasts in men, and, in women, they are apt to defer this evaluation to gynecologists. Because of the plausible association between early detection and improved outcome, it is the duty of every physician to identify breast abnormalities at the earliest possible stage and to institute a diagnostic workup. Women should be trained in breast self-examination (BSE). Although breast cancer in men is unusual, unilateral lesions should be evaluated in the same manner as in women, with the recognition that gynecomastia in men can sometimes begin unilaterally and is often asymmetric.

Virtually all breast cancer is diagnosed by biopsy of a nodule detected either on a mammogram or by palpation. Algorithms have been developed to enhance the likelihood of diagnosing breast cancer and reduce the frequency of unnecessary biopsy (Fig. 90-1).

■ THE PALPABLE BREAST MASS

Women should be strongly encouraged to examine their breasts monthly. A potentially flawed study from China has suggested that BSE does not alter survival, but given its safety, the procedure should still be encouraged. At worst, this practice increases the likelihood of detecting a mass at a smaller size when it can be treated with more limited surgery. Breast examination by the physician should be per-

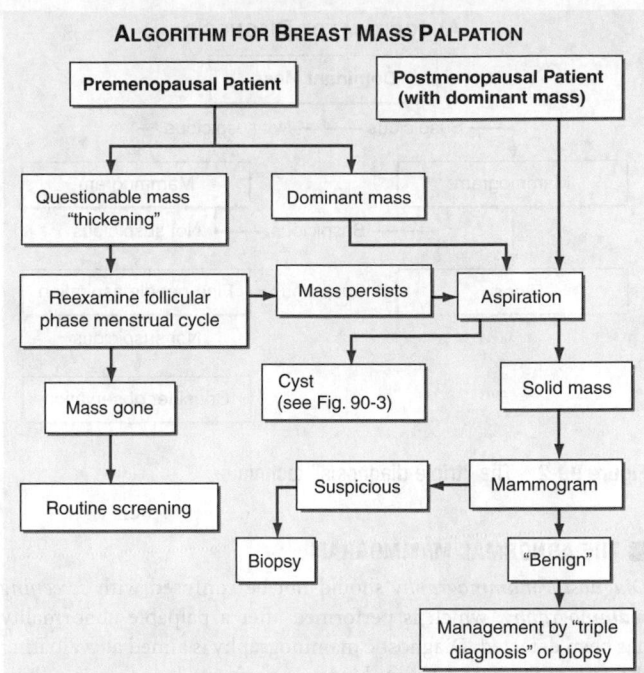

Figure 90-1   Approach to a palpable breast mass.

formed in good light so as to see retractions and other skin changes. The nipple and areolae should be inspected, and an attempt should be made to elicit nipple discharge. All regional lymph node groups should be examined, and any lesions should be measured. Physical examination alone cannot exclude malignancy. Lesions with certain features are more likely to be cancerous (hard, irregular, tethered or fixed, or painless lesions). A negative mammogram in the presence of a persistent lump in the breast does not exclude malignancy. Palpable lesions require additional diagnostic procedures, including biopsy.

In premenopausal women, lesions that are either equivocal or nonsuspicious on physical examination should be reexamined in 2–4 weeks, during the follicular phase of the menstrual cycle. Days 5–7 of the cycle are the best time for breast examination. A dominant mass in a postmenopausal woman or a dominant mass that persists through a menstrual cycle in a premenopausal woman should be aspirated by fine-needle biopsy or referred to a surgeon. If nonbloody fluid is aspirated, the diagnosis (cyst) and therapy have been accomplished together. Solid lesions that are persistent, recurrent, complex, or bloody cysts require mammography and biopsy, although in selected patients the so-called triple diagnostic techniques (palpation, mammography, aspiration) can be used to avoid biopsy (Figs. 90-1, 90-2, and 90-3). Ultrasound can be used in place of fine-needle aspiration to distinguish cysts from solid lesions. Not all solid masses are detected by ultrasound; thus, a palpable mass that is not visualized on ultrasound must be presumed to be solid.

Several points are essential in pursuing these management decision trees. First, risk-factor analysis is not part of the decision structure. No constellation of risk factors, by their presence or absence, can be used to exclude biopsy. Second, fine-needle aspiration should be used only in centers that have proven skill in obtaining such specimens and analyzing them. The likelihood of cancer is low in the setting of a "triple negative" (benign-feeling lump, negative mammogram, and negative fine-needle aspiration), but it is not zero. The patient and physician must be aware of a 1% risk of false negatives. Third, additional technologies such as MRI, ultrasound, and sestamibi imaging cannot be used to exclude the need for biopsy, although in unusual circumstances they may provoke a biopsy.

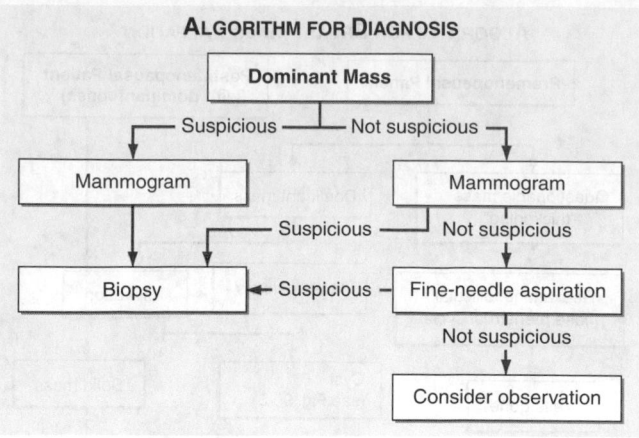

Figure 90-2 The "triple diagnosis" technique.

THE ABNORMAL MAMMOGRAM

Diagnostic mammography should not be confused with *screening mammography*, which is performed after a palpable abnormality has been detected. Diagnostic mammography is aimed at evaluating the rest of the breast before biopsy is performed or occasionally is part of the triple-test strategy to exclude immediate biopsy.

Subtle abnormalities that are first detected by screening mammography should be evaluated carefully by compression or magnified views. These abnormalities include clustered microcalcifications, densities (especially if spiculated), and new or enlarging architectural distortion. For some nonpalpable lesions, ultrasound may be helpful either to identify cysts or to guide biopsy. If there is no palpable lesion and detailed mammographic studies are unequivocally benign, the patient should have routine follow-up appropriate to the patient's age. It cannot be stressed too strongly that in the presence of a breast lump a negative mammogram does not rule out cancer.

If a nonpalpable mammographic lesion has a low index of suspicion, mammographic follow-up in 3–6 months is reasonable. Workup of indeterminate and suspicious lesions has been rendered more complex by the advent of stereotactic biopsies. Morrow and colleagues have suggested that these procedures are indicated for lesions that require biopsy but are likely to be benign—that is, for cases in which the procedure probably will eliminate additional surgery. When a lesion is more probably malignant, open biopsy should be performed with a needle localization technique. Others have proposed more widespread use of stereotactic core biopsies for nonpalpable lesions on economic grounds and because diagnosis

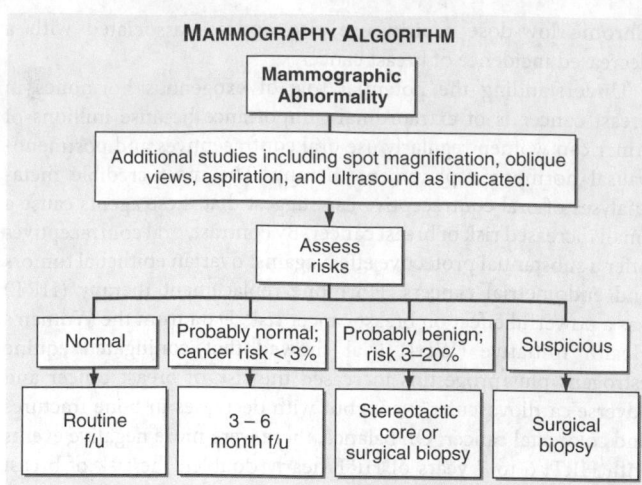

Figure 90-4 Approaches to abnormalities detected by mammogram.

leads to earlier treatment planning. However, stereotactic diagnosis of a malignant lesion does not eliminate the need for definitive surgical procedures, particularly if breast conservation is attempted. For example, after a breast biopsy with needle localization (i.e., local excision) of a stereotactically diagnosed malignancy, reexcision may still be necessary to achieve negative margins. To some extent, these issues are decided on the basis of referral pattern and the availability of the resources for stereotactic core biopsies. A reasonable approach is shown in Fig. 90-4.

BREAST MASSES IN THE PREGNANT OR LACTATING WOMAN

During pregnancy, the breast grows under the influence of estrogen, progesterone, prolactin, and human placental lactogen. Lactation is suppressed by progesterone, which blocks the effects of prolactin. After delivery, lactation is promoted by the fall in progesterone levels, which leaves the effects of prolactin unopposed. The development of a dominant mass during pregnancy or lactation should never be attributed to hormonal changes. A dominant mass must be treated with the same concern in a pregnant woman as any other. Breast cancer develops in 1 in every 3000–4000 pregnancies. Stage for stage, breast cancer in pregnant patients is no different from premenopausal breast cancer in nonpregnant patients. However, pregnant women often have more advanced disease because the significance of a breast mass was not fully considered and/or because of endogenous hormone stimulation. Persistent lumps in the breast of pregnant or lactating women *cannot* be attributed to benign changes based on physical findings; such patients should be promptly referred for diagnostic evaluation.

BENIGN BREAST MASSES

Only about 1 in every 5–10 breast biopsies leads to a diagnosis of cancer, although the rate of positive biopsies varies in different countries and clinical settings. (These differences may be related to interpretation, medicolegal considerations, and availability of mammograms.) The vast majority of benign breast masses are due to "fibrocystic" disease, a descriptive term for small fluid-filled cysts and modest epithelial cell and fibrous tissue hyperplasia. However, fibrocystic disease is a histologic, not a clinical, diagnosis, and women who have had a biopsy with benign findings are at greater risk of developing breast cancer than those who have not had a biopsy. The subset of women with ductal or lobular cell proliferation (about 30% of patients), particularly the small fraction (3%) with atypical hyperplasia, have a fourfold greater risk of developing breast cancer than those women who have not had a biopsy, and the increase in the risk is about ninefold for women in

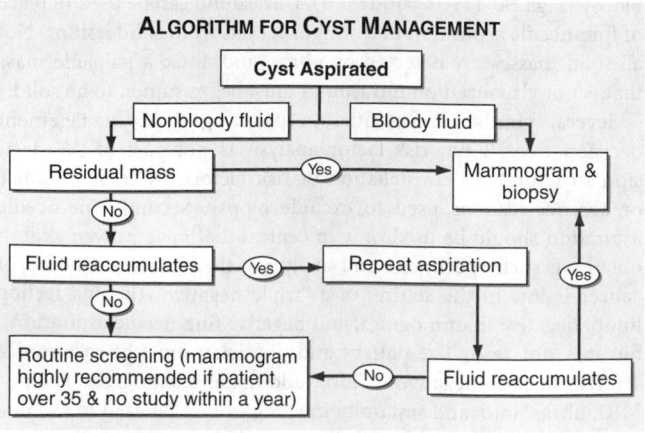

Figure 90-3 Management of a breast cyst.

this category who also have an affected first-degree relative. Thus, careful follow-up of these patients is required. By contrast, patients with a benign biopsy without atypical hyperplasia are at little risk and may be followed routinely.

SCREENING

Breast cancer is virtually unique among the epithelial tumors in adults in that screening (in the form of annual mammography) improves survival. Meta-analysis examining outcomes from every randomized trial of mammography conclusively shows a 25–30% reduction in the chance of dying from breast cancer with annual screening after age 50 years; the data for women between ages 40 and 50 years are almost as positive; however, since the incidence is much lower in younger women, there are more false positives. While controversy continues to surround the assessment of screening mammography, the preponderance of data strongly supports the benefits of screening mammography. New analyses of older randomized studies have occasionally suggested that screening may not work. While the design defects in some older studies cannot be retrospectively corrected, most experts, including panels of the American Society of Clinical Oncology and the American Cancer Society (ACS), continue to believe that screening conveys substantial benefit. Furthermore, the profound drop in breast cancer mortality rate seen over the past decade is unlikely to be solely attributable to improvements in therapy. It seems prudent to recommend annual or biannual mammography for women past the age of 40 years. Although no randomized study of BSE has ever shown any improvement in survival, its major benefit is identification of tumors appropriate for conservative local therapy. Better mammographic technology, including digitized mammography, routine use of magnified views, and greater skill in mammographic interpretation, combined with newer diagnostic techniques (MRI, magnetic resonance spectroscopy, positron emission tomography, etc.) may make it possible to identify breast cancers even more reliably and earlier. Screening by any technique other than mammography is not indicated; however, the ACS recommends younger women who are *BRCA-1* or *BRCA-2* carriers or their untested first-degree relative; history of radiation therapy to the chest between ages 10 and 30 years; a lifetime risk of breast cancer of at least 20%; or a history of Li-Fraumeni, Cowden, or Bannayan-Riley-Ruvalcaba syndromes benefit from MRI screening, where the higher sensitivity may outweigh the loss of specificity.

STAGING

Correct staging of breast cancer patients is of extraordinary importance. Not only does it permit an accurate prognosis, but in many cases therapeutic decision-making is based largely on the TNM (primary tumor, regional nodes, metastasis) classification (Table 90-1). Comparison with historic series should be undertaken with caution, as the staging has changed several times in the past 20 years. The current staging is complex and results in significant changes in outcome by stage as compared with prior staging systems.

TREATMENT   Breast Cancer

One of the most exciting aspects of breast cancer biology has been its recent subdivision into at least five subtypes based upon gene expression profiling.

1. **Luminal A**: The luminal tumors express cytokeratins 8 and 18, have the highest levels of estrogen receptor expression, tend to be low-grade, are most likely to respond to endocrine therapy, and have a favorable prognosis. They tend to be less responsive to chemotherapy.

2. **Luminal B**: Tumor cells are also of luminal epithelial origin, but with a gene expression pattern distinct from luminal A. Prognosis is somewhat worse that luminal A.

3. **Normal breast–like**: These tumors have a gene expression profile reminiscent of nonmalignant "normal" breast epithelium. Prognosis is similar to the luminal B group.

4. **HER2 amplified**: These tumors have amplification of the HER2 gene on chromosome 17q and frequently exhibit coamplification and overexpression of other genes adjacent to HER2. Historically the clinical prognosis of such tumors was poor. However, with the advent of trastuzumab, the clinical outcome of HER2-positive patients is markedly improving.

5. **Basal**: These estrogen-receptor/progesterone receptor-negative and HER2-negative tumors (so-called triple negative) are characterized by markers of basal/myoepithelial cells. They tend to be high-grade, and express cytokeratins 5/6 and 17 as well as vimentin, p63, CD10, α-smooth muscle actin, and epidermal growth factor receptor (EGFR). Patients with *BRCA* mutations also fall within this molecular subtype. They also have stem cell characteristics.

PRIMARY BREAST CANCER   Breast-conserving treatments, consisting of the removal of the primary tumor by some form of lumpectomy with or without irradiating the breast, result in a survival that is as good as (or slightly superior to) that after extensive surgical procedures, such as mastectomy or modified radical mastectomy, with or without further irradiation. Postlumpectomy breast irradiation greatly reduces the risk of recurrence in the breast. While breast conservation is associated with a possibility of recurrence in the breast, 10-year survival is at least as good as that after more extensive surgery. Postoperative radiation to regional nodes following mastectomy is also associated with an improvement in survival. Since radiation therapy can also reduce the rate of local or regional recurrence, it should be strongly considered following mastectomy for women with high-risk primary tumors (i.e., T2 in size, positive margins, positive nodes). At present, nearly one-third of women in the United States are managed by lumpectomy. Breast-conserving surgery is not suitable for all patients: it is not generally suitable for tumors >5 cm (or for smaller tumors if the breast is small), for tumors involving the nipple areola complex, for tumors with extensive intraductal disease involving multiple quadrants of the breast, for women with a history of collagen-vascular disease, and for women who either do not have the motivation for breast conservation or do not have convenient access to radiation therapy. However, these groups probably do not account for more than one-third of patients who are treated with mastectomy. Thus, a great many women still undergo mastectomy who could safely avoid this procedure and probably would if appropriately counseled.

An extensive intraductal component is a predictor of recurrence in the breast, and so are several clinical variables. Both axillary lymph node involvement and involvement of vascular or lymphatic channels by metastatic tumor in the breast are associated with a higher risk of relapse in the breast but are not contraindications to breast-conserving treatment. When these patients are excluded, and when lumpectomy with negative tumor margins is achieved, breast conservation is associated with a recurrence rate in the breast of substantially <10%. The survival of patients who have recurrence in the breast is somewhat worse than that of women who do not. Thus, recurrence in the breast is a negative prognostic variable for long-term survival. However, recurrence in the breast is not the *cause* of distant metastasis. If recurrence in the breast caused metastatic disease, then women treated

TABLE 90-1 Staging of Breast Cancer

Primary Tumor (T)

T0	No evidence of primary tumor
TIS	Carcinoma in situ
T1	Tumor ≤2 cm
T1a	Tumor >0.1 cm but ≤0.5 cm
T1b	Tumor >0.5 but ≤1 cm
T1c	Tumor >1 cm but ≤2 cm
T2	Tumor >2 cm but ≤5 cm
T3	Tumor >5 cm
T4	Extension to chest wall, inflammation, satellite lesions, ulcerations

Regional Lymph Nodes (N)

PN0(i−)	No regional lymph node metastasis histologically, negative IHC
PN0(i+)	No regional lymph node metastasis histologically, positive IHC, no IHC cluster greater than 0.2 mm
PN0(mol−)	No regional lymph node metastasis histologically, negative molecular findings (RT-PCR)
PN0(mol+)	No regional lymph node metastasis histologically, positive molecular findings (RT-PCR)
PN1	Metastasis in one to three axillary lymph nodes, or in internal mammary nodes with microscopic disease detected by sentinel lymph node dissection but not clinically apparent
PN1mi	Micrometastasis (>0.2 mm, none >2 mm)
PN1a	Metastasis in one to three axillary lymph nodes
PN1b	Metastasis in internal mammary nodes with microscopic disease detected by sentinel lymph node dissection but not *clinically apparent*[a]
PN1c	Metastasis in one to three axillary lymph nodes and in internal mammary lymph nodes with microscopic disease detected by sentinel lymph node dissection but not clinically apparent.[a] (If associated with greater than three positive axillary lymph nodes, the internal mammary nodes are classified as pN3b to reflect increased tumor burden.)
pN2	Metastasis in four to nine axillary lymph nodes, or in clinically apparent internal mammary lymph nodes in the *absence* of axillary lymph node metastasis
pN3	Metastasis in 10 or more axillary lymph nodes, or in infraclavicular lymph nodes, or in clinically apparent[a] ipsilateral internal mammary lymph nodes in the *presence* of 1 or more positive axillary lymph nodes; or in more than 3 axillary lymph nodes with clinically negative microscopic metastasis in internal mammary lymph nodes; or in ipsilateral subcarinal lymph nodes

Distant Metastasis (M)

M0	No distant metastasis
M1	Distant metastasis (includes spread to ipsilateral supraclavicular nodes)

Stage Grouping

Stage 0	TIS	N0	M0
Stage I	T1	N0	M0
Stage IIA	T0	N1	M0
	T1	N1	M0
	T2	N0	M0
Stage IIB	T2	N1	M0
	T3	N0	M0
Stage IIIA	T0	N2	M0
	T1	N2	M0
	T2	N2	M0
	T3	N1, N2	M0
Stage IIIB	T4	Any N	M0
	Any T	N3	M0
Stage IIIC	Any T	N3	M0
Stage IV	Any T	Any N	M1

[a]Clinically apparent is defined as detected by imaging studies (excluding lymphoscintigraphy) or by clinical examination.

Abbreviations: IHC, immunohistochemistry; RT-PCR, reverse transcriptase/polymerase chain reaction.

Source: Used with permission of the American Joint Committee on Cancer (AJCC), Chicago, Illinois. The original source for this material is the *AJCC Cancer Staging Manual*, 7th ed. New York, Springer, 2010; *www.springeronline.com.*

with lumpectomy, who have a higher rate of recurrence in the breast, should have poorer survival than women treated with mastectomy, and they do not. Most patients should consult with a radiation oncologist before making a final decision concerning local therapy. However, a multimodality clinic in which the surgeon, radiation oncologist, medical oncologist, and other caregivers cooperate to evaluate the patient and develop a treatment is usually considered a major advantage by patients.

Adjuvant Therapy The use of systemic therapy after local management of breast cancer substantially improves survival. More than half of the women who would otherwise die of metastatic breast cancer remain disease-free when treated with the appropriate systemic regimen. These data have grown more and more impressive with longer follow-up and more effective regimens.

Prognostic Variables The most important prognostic variables are provided by *tumor staging*. The size of the tumor and the status of the axillary lymph nodes provide reasonably accurate information on the likelihood of tumor relapse. The relation of pathologic stage to 5-year survival is shown in Table 90-2. For most women, the need for adjuvant therapy can be readily defined on this basis alone. In the absence of lymph node involvement, involvement of microvessels (either capillaries or lymphatic channels) in tumors is nearly equivalent to lymph node involvement. The greatest controversy concerns women with intermediate prognoses. *There is rarely justification for adjuvant chemotherapy in most women with tumors <1 cm in size whose axillary lymph nodes are negative. HER2-positive tumors are a potential exception.* Detection of breast cancer cells either in the circulation or bone marrow is associated with an increased relapse rate. The most exciting development in this area is the use of gene expression arrays to analyze patterns of tumor gene expression. Several groups have independently defined gene sets that reliably predict disease-free and overall survival far more accurately than any single prognostic variable including the Oncotype DX® analysis of 21 genes. Also the use of such standardized risk assessment tools such as Adjuvant! Online (*www.adjuvantonline.com*) are very helpful. These tools are highly recommended in otherwise ambiguous circumstances.

Estrogen and progesterone receptor status are of prognostic significance. Tumors that lack either or both of these receptors are more likely to recur than tumors that have them.

Several *measures of tumor growth rate* correlate with early relapse. S-phase analysis using flow cytometry is the most accurate measure. Indirect S-phase assessments using antigens associated with the cell cycle, such as PCNA (Ki67), are also valuable. Tumors with a high proportion (more than the median) of cells in S-phase pose a greater risk of relapse; chemotherapy offers the greatest survival benefit for these tumors. Assessment of DNA content in the form of ploidy is of modest value, with nondiploid tumors having a somewhat worse prognosis.

Histologic classification of the tumor has also been used as a prognostic factor. Tumors with a poor nuclear grade have a higher risk of recurrence than tumors with a good nuclear grade. Semiquantitative measures such as the Elston score improve the reproducibility of this measurement.

Molecular changes in the tumor are also useful. Tumors that overexpress *erbB2* (HER2/neu) or have a mutated p53 gene have a worse prognosis. Particular interest has centered on *erbB2* overexpression as measured by histochemistry or by fluorescence in situ hybridization. Tumors that overexpress *erbB2* are more likely to respond to higher doses of doxorubicin-containing regimens and predict those tumors that will respond to HER2/neu antibodies (trastuzumab) (herceptin) and HER2/neu kinase inhibitors.

To grow, tumors must generate a neovasculature (Chap. 84). The presence of more microvessels in a tumor, particularly when localized in so-called hot spots, is associated with a worse prognosis. This may assume even greater significance in light of blood vessel–targeting therapies such as bevacizumab (avastin). While the benefits of bevacizumab in metastatic disease have been modest, close attention should be paid to the soon-to-be reported studies evaluating its role in adjuvant therapy.

Other variables that have also been used to evaluate prognosis include proteins associated with invasiveness, such as type IV collagenase, cathepsin D, plasminogen activator, plasminogen activator receptor, and the metastasis-suppressor gene *nm23*. None of these has been widely accepted as a prognostic variable for therapeutic decision-making. One problem in interpreting these prognostic variables is that most of them have not been examined in a study using a large cohort of patients.

Adjuvant Regimens Adjuvant therapy is the use of systemic therapies in patients whose known disease has received local therapy but who are at risk of relapse. Selection of appropriate adjuvant chemotherapy or hormone therapy is highly controversial in some situations. Meta-analyses have helped to define broad limits for therapy but do not help in choosing optimal regimens or in choosing a regimen for certain subgroups of patients. A summary of recommendations is shown in Table 90-3. In general, premenopausal women for whom any form of adjuvant systemic therapy is indicated should receive multidrug chemotherapy. Antihormone therapy improves survival in premenopausal patients with positive estrogen receptors and should be added following completion of chemotherapy. Prophylactic castration may also be associated with a substantial survival benefit (primarily in estrogen receptor–positive patients) but is not widely used in this country.

Data on postmenopausal women are also controversial. The impact of adjuvant chemotherapy is quantitatively less clear-cut than in premenopausal patients, particularly in estrogen receptor–positive cases, although survival advantages have been shown. The first decision is whether chemotherapy or endocrine therapy should be used. While adjuvant endocrine therapy (aromatase inhibitors and tamoxifen) improves survival regardless of axillary lymph node status, the improvement in survival is modest for patients in whom multiple lymph nodes are involved. For this reason, it has been usual to give chemotherapy

TABLE 90-2 5-Year Survival Rate for Breast Cancer by Stage

Stage	5-Year Survival, %
0	99
I	92
IIA	82
IIB	65
IIIA	47
IIIB	44
IV	14

Source: Modified from data of the National Cancer Institute: Surveillance, Epidemiology, and End Results (SEER).

TABLE 90-3 Suggested Approaches to Adjuvant Therapy

Age Group	Lymph Node Status[a]	Estrogen Receptor (ER) Status	Tumor	Recommendation
Premenopausal	Positive	Any	Any	Multidrug chemotherapy + tamoxifen if ER-positive + trastuzumab in HER2/neu–positive tumors
Premenopausal	Negative	Any	>2 cm, or 1–2 cm with other poor prognostic variables	Multidrug chemotherapy + tamoxifen if ER-positive + trastuzumab in HER2/neu–positive tumors
Postmenopausal	Positive	Negative	Any	Multidrug chemotherapy + trastuzumab in HER2/neu–positive tumors
Postmenopausal	Positive	Positive	Any	Aromatase inhibitors and tamoxifen with or without chemotherapy + trastuzumab in HER2/neu–positive tumors
Postmenopausal	Negative	Positive	>2 cm, or 1–2 cm with other poor prognostic variables	Aromatase inhibitors and tamoxifen + trastuzumab in HER2/neu–positive tumors
Postmenopausal	Negative	Negative	>2 cm, or 1–2 cm with other poor prognostic variables	Consider multidrug chemotherapy + trastuzumab in HER2/neu–positive tumors

[a]As determined by pathologic examination.

to postmenopausal patients who have no medical contraindications and who have more than one positive lymph node; hormone therapy is commonly given subsequently. For postmenopausal women for whom systemic therapy is warranted but who have a more favorable prognosis (based more commonly on analysis such as the Oncotype DX methodology), hormone therapy may be used alone. Large clinical trials have shown superiority for aromatase inhibitors over tamoxifen alone in the adjuvant setting. Unfortunately the optimal plan is unclear. Tamoxifen for 5 years followed by an aromatase inhibitor, the reverse strategy, or even switching to an aromatase inhibitor after 2–3 years of tamoxifen has been shown to be better than tamoxifen alone. No valid information currently permits selection among the three clinically approved aromatase inhibitors. Large clinical trials currently underway will help address these questions. Concomitant use of bisphosphonates is almost always warranted; however, it is not finally settled as to whether their prophylactic use increases survival in addition to just decreasing recurrences in bone.

Most comparisons of adjuvant chemotherapy regimens show little difference among them, although small advantages for doxorubicin-containing regimens and "dose sense" regimens are usually seen.

One approach—so-called neoadjuvant chemotherapy—involves the administration of adjuvant therapy before definitive surgery and radiation therapy. Because the objective response rates of patients with breast cancer to systemic therapy in this setting exceed 75%, many patients will be "down-staged" and may become candidates for breast-conserving therapy. However, overall survival has not been improved using this approach. Patients who achieve a pathologic complete remission after neoadjuvant chemotherapy not unexpectedly have a substantially improved survival. The neoadjuvant setting also provides a wonderful opportunity for the evaluation of new agents.

Other adjuvant treatments under investigation include the use of taxanes, such as paclitaxel and docetaxel, and therapy based on alternative kinetic and biologic models. In such approaches, high doses of single agents are used separately in relatively dose-intensive cycling regimens. Node-positive patients treated with doxorubicin-cyclophosphamide for four cycles followed by four cycles of a taxane have a substantial improvement in survival as compared with women receiving doxorubicin-cyclophosphamide alone, particularly in women with estrogen receptor–negative tumors. In addition, administration of the same drug combinations at the same dose but at more frequent intervals (q2 weeks with cytokine support as compared with the standard q3 weeks) is even more effective. Among the 25% of women whose tumors overexpress HER2/neu, addition of trastuzumab given concurrently with a taxane and then for a year after chemotherapy produces significant improvement in survival. Though longer follow-up will be important, this is now the standard care for most women with HER2/neu–positive breast cancers. Cardiotoxicity, immediate and long-term, remains a concern, and further efforts to exploit non–anthracycline-containing regimens are being pursued. Very high dose therapy with stem cell transplantation in the adjuvant setting has not proved superior to standard-dose therapy and should not be routinely used.

A variety of exciting approaches are close to adoption and the literature needs to be followed attentively. These include the use of antiangiogenics such as bevacizumab. In addition, tyrosine kinase inhibitors such as lapatinib that target the HER2 kinase are very promising. Finally, as described in the next section, a novel class of agents targeting DNA repair—the so-called poly–ADP ribose polymerase [PARP] inhibitors—is likely to have a major impact on breast cancers either caused by *BRCA-1* or *-2* mutations or sharing similar defects in DNA repair in their etiology.

SYSTEMIC THERAPY OF METASTATIC DISEASE About one-third of patients treated for apparently localized breast cancer develop metastatic disease. Although a small number of these patients enjoy long remissions when treated with combinations of systemic and local therapy, most eventually succumb to metastatic disease. The median survival for all patients diagnosed with mestastatic breast cancer is less than 3 years. Soft tissue, bony, and visceral (lung and liver) metastases each account for approximately one-third of sites of initial relapses. However, by the time of death, most patients will have bony involvement. Recurrences can appear at any time after primary therapy. A very cruel fact about breast cancer recurrences is that at least half of all breast cancer recurrences occur >5 years after initial therapy.

Because the diagnosis of metastatic disease alters the outlook for the patient so drastically, it should rarely be made without a confirmatory biopsy. Every oncologist has seen patients with tuberculosis, gallstones, sarcoidosis, or other nonmalignant diseases misdiagnosed and treated as though they had metastatic breast cancer or even second malignancies such as multiple myeloma thought to be recurrent breast cancer. This is a catastrophic mistake and justifies biopsy for virtually every patient at the time of initial suspicion of metastatic disease.

The choice of therapy requires consideration of local therapy needs, the overall medical condition of the patient, and the hormone receptor status of the tumor, as well as clinical judgment. Because therapy of systemic disease is palliative, the potential toxicities of therapies should be balanced against the response rates. Several variables influence the response to systemic therapy. For example, the presence of estrogen and progesterone receptors is a strong indication for endocrine therapy. On the other hand, patients with short disease-free intervals, rapidly progressive visceral disease, lymphangitic pulmonary disease, or intracranial disease are unlikely to respond to endocrine therapy.

In many cases, systemic therapy can be withheld while the patient is managed with appropriate local therapy. Radiation therapy and occasionally surgery are effective at relieving the symptoms of metastatic disease, particularly when bony sites are involved. Many patients with bone-only or bone-dominant disease have a relatively indolent course. Under such circumstances, systemic chemotherapy has a modest effect, whereas radiation therapy may be effective for long periods. Other systemic treatments, such as strontium 89 and/or bisphosphonates, may provide a palliative benefit without inducing objective responses. Most patients with metastatic disease, and certainly all who have bone involvement, should receive concurrent bisphosphonates. Since the goal of therapy is to maintain well-being for as long as possible, emphasis should be placed on avoiding the most hazardous complications of metastatic disease, including pathologic fracture of the axial skeleton and spinal cord compression. New back pain in patients with cancer should be explored aggressively on an emergent basis; to wait for neurologic symptoms is a potentially catastrophic error. Metastatic involvement of endocrine organs can cause profound dysfunction, including adrenal insufficiency and hypopituitarism. Similarly, obstruction of the biliary tree or other impaired organ function may be better managed with a local therapy than with a systemic approach.

Endocrine Therapy Normal breast tissue is estrogen dependent. Both primary and metastatic breast cancer may retain this phenotype. The best means of ascertaining whether a breast cancer is hormone dependent is through analysis of estrogen and progesterone receptor levels on the tumor. Tumors that are positive for the estrogen receptor and negative for the progesterone receptor have a response rate of ~30%. Tumors that have both receptors have a response rate approaching 70%. If neither receptor is present, the objective response rates are <5%. Receptor analyses provide information as to the correct ordering of endocrine therapies as opposed to chemotherapy. Because of their lack of toxicity and because some patients whose receptor analyses are reported as negative respond to endocrine therapy, an endocrine treatment should be attempted in virtually every patient with metastatic breast cancer. Potential endocrine therapies are summarized in Table 90-4. The choice of endocrine therapy is usually determined by toxicity profile and availability. In most patients, the initial endocrine therapy should be an aromatase inhibitor rather than

TABLE 90-4 Endocrine Therapies for Breast Cancer

Therapy	Comments
Castration	For premenopausal women
Surgical	
LHRH agonists	
Antiestrogens	
Tamoxifen	Useful in pre- and postmenopausal women
"Pure" antiestrogens	Responses in tamoxifen-resistant and aromatase inhibitor–resistant patients
Surgical adrenalectomy	Rarely employed second-line choice
Aromatase inhibitors	Low toxicity; now first choice for metastatic disease
High-dose progestogens	Common fourth-line choice after AIs, tamoxifen and fulvestrant
Hypophysectomy	Rarely used
Additive androgens or estrogens	Plausible fourth-line therapies; potentially toxic

Abbreviations: AI, aromatase inhibitor; LHRH, luteinizing hormone–releasing hormone.

tamoxifen. For the subset of postmenopausal women who are estrogen receptor–positive but also HER2/neu positive, response rates to aromatase inhibitors are substantially higher than to tamoxifen. Newer "pure" antiestrogens that are free of agonistic effects are also effective. Cases in which tumors shrink in response to tamoxifen withdrawal (as well as withdrawal of pharmacologic doses of estrogens) have been reported. Endogenous estrogen formation may be blocked by analogues of luteinizing hormone–releasing hormone in premenopausal women. Additive endocrine therapies, including treatment with progestogens, estrogens, and androgens, may also be tried in patients who respond to initial endocrine therapy; the mechanism of action of these latter therapies is unknown. Patients who respond to one endocrine therapy have at least a 50% chance of responding to a second endocrine therapy. It is not uncommon for patients to respond to two or three sequential endocrine therapies; however, combination endocrine therapies do not appear to be superior to individual agents, and combinations of chemotherapy with endocrine therapy are not useful. The median survival of patients with metastatic disease is approximately 2 years, and many patients, particularly older persons and those with hormone-dependent disease, may respond to endocrine therapy for 3–5 years or longer.

Chemotherapy Unlike many other epithelial malignancies, breast cancer responds to multiple chemotherapeutic agents, including anthracyclines, alkylating agents, taxanes, and antimetabolites. Multiple combinations of these agents have been found to improve response rates somewhat, but they have had little effect on duration of response or survival. The choice among multidrug combinations frequently depends on whether adjuvant chemotherapy was administered and, if so, what type. While patients treated with adjuvant regimens such as cyclophosphamide, methotrexate, and fluorouracil (CMF regimens) may subsequently respond to the same combination in the metastatic disease setting, most oncologists use drugs to which the patients have not been previously exposed. Once patients have progressed after combination drug therapy, it is most common to treat them with single agents. Given the significant toxicity of most drugs, the use of a single effective agent will minimize toxicity by sparing the patient exposure to drugs that would be of little value. No method to select the drugs most efficacious for a given patient has been demonstrated to be useful.

Most oncologists use either an anthracycline or paclitaxel following failure with the initial regimen. However, the choice has to be balanced with individual needs. One randomized study has suggested docetaxel may be superior to paclitaxel. A nanoparticle formulation of paclitaxel (Abraxane) is also effective.

The use of a humanized antibody to *erbB2* [trastuzumab (Herceptin)] combined with paclitaxel can improve response rate and survival for women whose metastatic tumors overexpress *erbB2*. The magnitude of the survival extension is modest in patients with metastatic disease. Similarly, the use of bevacizumab (avastin) has improved the response rate and response duration to paclitaxel. Objective responses in previously treated patients may also be seen with gemcitabine, vinca alkaloids, capecitabine, Navelbine, and oral etoposide and a new class of agents, epothilones.

High-Dose Chemotherapy Including Autologous Bone Marrow Transplantation
Autologous bone marrow transplantation combined with high doses of single agents can produce objective responses even in heavily pretreated patients. However, such responses are rarely durable and do not alter the clinical course for most patients with advanced metastatic disease.

STAGE III BREAST CANCER Between 10 and 25% of patients present with so-called locally advanced, or stage III, breast cancer at diagnosis. Many of these cancers are technically operable, whereas others, particularly cancers with chest wall involvement, inflammatory breast cancers, or cancers with large matted axillary lymph nodes, cannot be managed with surgery initially. Although no randomized trials have proved the efficacy of neoadjuvant chemotherapy, this approach has gained widespread use. More than 90% of patients with locally advanced breast cancer show a partial or better response to multidrug chemotherapy regimens that include an anthracycline. Early administration of this treatment reduces the bulk of the disease and frequently makes the patient a suitable candidate for salvage surgery and/or radiation therapy. These patients should be managed in multimodality clinics to coordinate surgery, radiation therapy, and systemic chemotherapy. Such approaches produce long-term disease-free survival in about 30–50% of patients.

BREAST CANCER PREVENTION Women who have one breast cancer are at risk of developing a contralateral breast cancer at a rate of approximately 0.5% per year. When adjuvant tamoxifen is administered to these patients, the rate of development of contralateral breast cancers is reduced. In other tissues of the body, tamoxifen has estrogen-like effects that are beneficial: preservation of bone mineral density and long-term lowering of cholesterol. However, tamoxifen has estrogen-like effects on the uterus, leading to an increased risk of uterine cancer (0.75% incidence after 5 years on tamoxifen). Tamoxifen also increases the risk of cataract formation. The Breast Cancer Prevention Trial (BCPT) revealed a >49% reduction in breast cancer among women with a risk of at least 1.66% taking the drug for 5 years. Raloxifene has shown similar breast cancer prevention potency but may have different effects on bone and heart. The two agents have been compared in a prospective randomized prevention trial [the Study of Tamoxifen and Raloxifene (STAR) trial]. The agents are approximately equivalent in preventing breast cancer with fewer thromboembolic events and endometrial cancers with raloxifene; however, raloxifene did not reduce noninvasive

cancers as effectively as tamoxifen, so no clear winner has emerged. A newer selective estrogen receptor modulator (SERM), lasofoxifene has recently been shown to reduce cardiovascular events in addition to breast cancer and fractures, and further studies of this agent should be watched with interest. It should be recalled that prevention of contralateral breast cancers in women diagnosed with *onc* cancer is a reasonable surrogate for breast cancer prevention as these are second primaries not recurrences. In this regard, the aromatase inhibitors are all considerably more effective than tamoxifen; however, they are not approved for primary breast cancer prevention. It remains puzzling that agents with the safety profile of raloxifene, which can reduce breast cancer risk by 50% with additional benefits in preventing osteoporotic fracture, are still so infrequently prescribed.

NONINVASIVE BREAST CANCER Breast cancer develops as a series of molecular changes in the epithelial cells that lead to ever more malignant behavior. Increased use of mammography has led to more frequent diagnoses of noninvasive breast cancer. These lesions fall into two groups: ductal carcinoma in situ (DCIS) and lobular carcinoma in situ (lobular neoplasia). The management of both entities is controversial.

Ductal Carcinoma In Situ Proliferation of cytologically malignant breast epithelial cells within the ducts is termed *DCIS*. Atypical hyperplasia may be difficult to differentiate from DCIS. At least one-third of patients with untreated DCIS develop invasive breast cancer within 5 years. For many years, the standard treatment for this disease was mastectomy. However, treatment of this condition by lumpectomy and radiation therapy gives survival that is as good as the survival for invasive breast cancer treated by mastectomy. In one randomized trial, the combination of wide excision plus irradiation for DCIS caused a substantial reduction in the local recurrence rate as compared with wide excision alone with negative margins, though survival was identical in the two arms. No studies have compared either of these regimens to mastectomy. Addition of tamoxifen to any DCIS surgical/radiation therapy regimen further improves local control. Data for aromatase inhibitors in this setting are not available.

Several prognostic features may help to identify patients at high risk for local recurrence after either lumpectomy alone or lumpectomy with radiation therapy. These include extensive disease; age <40; and cytologic features such as necrosis, poor nuclear grade, and comedo subtype with overexpression of *erbB2*. Some data suggest that adequate excision with careful determination of pathologically clear margins is associated with a low recurrence rate. When surgery is combined with radiation therapy, recurrence (which is usually in the same quadrant) occurs with a frequency of ≤10%. Given the fact that half of these recurrences will be invasive, about 5% of the initial cohort will eventually develop invasive breast cancer. A reasonable expectation of mortality for these patients is about 1%, a figure that approximates the mortality rate for DCIS managed by mastectomy. Although this train of reasoning has not formally been proved valid, it is reasonable to recommend that patients who desire breast preservation, and in whom DCIS appears to be reasonably localized, be managed by adequate surgery with meticulous pathologic evaluation, followed by breast irradiation and tamoxifen. For patients with localized DCIS, axillary lymph node dissection is unnecessary. More controversial is the question of what management is optimal when there is any degree of invasion. Because of a significant likelihood (10–15%) of axillary lymph node involvement even when the primary lesion shows only microscopic invasion, it is prudent to do at least a level 1 and

2 axillary lymph node dissection for all patients with any degree of invasion, or sentinel node biopsy may be substituted. Further management is dictated by the presence of nodal spread.

Lobular Neoplasia Proliferation of cytologically malignant cells within the lobules is termed *lobular neoplasia*. Nearly 30% of patients who have had adequate local excision of the lesion develop breast cancer (usually infiltrating ductal carcinoma) over the next 15–20 years. Ipsilateral and contralateral cancers are equally common. Therefore, lobular neoplasia may be a premalignant lesion that suggests an elevated risk of subsequent breast cancer, rather than a form of malignancy itself, and aggressive local management seems unreasonable. Most patients should be treated with an SERM for 5 years and followed with careful annual mammography and semiannual physical examinations. Additional molecular analysis of these lesions may make it possible to discriminate between patients who are at risk of further progression and require additional therapy and those in whom simple follow-up is adequate.

MALE BREAST CANCER Breast cancer is about 1/150th as frequent in men as in women; 1720 men developed breast cancer in 2006. It usually presents as a unilateral lump in the breast and is frequently not diagnosed promptly. Given the small amount of soft tissue and the unexpected nature of the problem, locally advanced presentations are somewhat more common. When male breast cancer is matched to female breast cancer by age and stage, its overall prognosis is identical. Although gynecomastia may initially be unilateral or asymmetric, any unilateral mass in a man older than age 40 years should receive a careful workup including biopsy. On the other hand, bilateral symmetric breast development rarely represents breast cancer and is almost invariably due to endocrine disease or a drug effect. It should be kept in mind, nevertheless, that the risk of cancer is much greater in men with gynecomastia; in such men, gross asymmetry of the breasts should arouse suspicion of cancer. Male breast cancer is best managed by mastectomy and axillary lymph node dissection (modified radical mastectomy). Patients with locally advanced disease or positive nodes should also be treated with irradiation. Approximately 90% of male breast cancers contain estrogen receptors, and approximately 60% of cases with metastatic disease respond to endocrine therapy. No randomized studies have evaluated adjuvant therapy for male breast cancer. Two historic experiences suggest that the disease responds well to adjuvant systemic therapy, and, if not medically contraindicated, the same criteria for the use of adjuvant therapy in women should be applied to men.

The sites of relapse and spectrum of response to chemotherapeutic drugs are virtually identical for breast cancers in either sex.

FOLLOW-UP OF BREAST CANCER PATIENTS Despite the availability of sophisticated and expensive imaging techniques and a wide range of serum tumor marker tests, survival is not influenced by early diagnosis of relapse. Surveillance guidelines are given in Table 90-5. Despite pressure from patients and their families, routine CAT scans etc. are not recommended.

TABLE 90-5 Breast Cancer Surveillance Guidelines

Test	Frequency
Recommended	
History; eliciting symptoms; physical examination	q3–6 months × 3 years; q6–12 months × 2 years; then annually
Breast self-examination	Monthly
Mammography	Annually
Pelvic examination	Annually
Patient education about symptoms of recurrence	Ongoing
Coordination of care	Ongoing
Not Recommended	
Complete blood count	
Serum chemistry studies	
Chest radiographs	
Bone scans	
Ultrasound examination of the liver	
Computed tomography of chest, abdomen, or pelvis	
Tumor marker CA 15-3, CA 27-29	
Tumor marker CEA	

Source: Recommended Breast Cancer Surveillance Guidelines, ASCO Education Book, Fall, 1997.

FURTHER READINGS

CHLEBOWSKI RT et al: Breast cancer after use of estrogen plus progestin in postme nopausal women. N Engl J Med 360:6, 2009

CLARKE M et al: Adjuvant chemotherapy in oestrogen-receptor-poor breast cancer: Patient-level meta-analysis of randomised trials. Lancet 371:29, 2008

FOULKES WD et al: Triple-negative breast cancer. N Engl J Med 363:1938, 2010

GEYER CE et al: Lapatinib plus capecitabine for HER2-positive advanced breast cancer. N Engl J Med 355:2733, 2006

MANSEL RE et al: Randomized multicenter trial of sentinel node biopsy versus standard axillary treatment in operable breast cancer: The ALMANAC Trial. J Natl Cancer Inst98:599, 2006

MILLER K et al: Paclitaxel plus bevacizumab versus paclitaxel alone for metastatic breast cancer. N Engl J Med 357:26, 2007

OLIVOTTO IA et al: Population-based validation of the prognostic model ADJUVANT! for early breast cancer. J Clin Oncol 23:2716, 2005

PAIK S et al: Gene expression and benefit of chemotherapy in women with node-negative, estrogen receptor–positive breast cancer. J Clin Oncol 24:3726, 2006

SHIPITSIN M et al: Molecular definition of breast tumor heterogeneity. Cancer Cell 11:259, 2007

SORLIE T et al: Gene expression patterns of breast carcinomas distinguished tumor subclasses with clinical implications. Proc Natl Acad Sci USA 98:10869, 2001

SOTIRIOU C, PUSZTAI L: Gene-expression signatures in breast cancer. N Engl J Med360:8, 2009

CHAPTER 91

Gastrointestinal Tract Cancer

Robert J. Mayer

The gastrointestinal tract is the second most common noncutaneous site for cancer and the second major cause of cancer-related mortality in the United States.

ESOPHAGEAL CANCER

■ INCIDENCE AND ETIOLOGY

Cancer of the esophagus is a relatively uncommon but extremely lethal malignancy. The diagnosis was made in 16,640 Americans in 2010 and led to 14,500 deaths. Worldwide, the incidence, of esophageal cancer varies strikingly. It occurs frequently within a geographic region extending from the southern shore of the Caspian Sea on the west to northern China on the east and encompassing parts of Iran, Central Asia, Afghanistan, Siberia, and Mongolia. Familial increased risk has been seen in regions with high incidence, though gene associations are not yet defined. High-incidence "pockets" of the disease are also present in such disparate locations as Finland, Iceland, Curaçao, southeastern Africa, and northwestern France. In North America and western Europe, the disease is more common in blacks than whites and in males than females; it appears most often after age 50 and seems to be associated with a lower socioeconomic status.

A variety of causative factors have been implicated in the development of the disease (Table 91-1). In the United States, esophageal

TABLE 91-1 Some Etiologic Factors Believed to Be Associated With Esophageal Cancer

Excess alcohol consumption

Cigarette smoking

Other ingested carcinogens

Nitrates (converted to nitrites)

Smoked opiates

Fungal toxins in pickled vegetables

Mucosal damage from physical agents

Hot tea

Lye ingestion

Radiation-induced strictures

Chronic achalasia

Host susceptibility

Esophageal web with glossitis and iron deficiency (i.e., Plummer-Vinson or Paterson-Kelly syndrome)

Congenital hyperkeratosis and pitting of the palms and soles (i.e., tylosis palmaris et plantaris)

? Dietary deficiencies of selenium, molybdenum, zinc, and vitamin A

? Celiac sprue

Chronic gastric reflux (i.e., Barrett's esophagus) for adenocarcinoma

cancer cases are either squamous cell carcinomas or adenocarcinomas. The etiology of squamous cell esophageal cancer is related to excess alcohol consumption and/or cigarette smoking. The relative risk increases with the amount of tobacco smoked or alcohol consumed, with these factors acting synergistically. The consumption of whiskey is linked to a higher incidence than the consumption of wine or beer. Squamous cell esophageal carcinoma has also been associated with the ingestion of nitrites, smoked opiates, and fungal toxins in pickled vegetables, as well as mucosal damage caused by such physical insults as long-term exposure to extremely hot tea, the ingestion of lye, radiation-induced strictures, and chronic achalasia. The presence of an esophageal web in association with glossitis and iron deficiency (i.e., Plummer-Vinson or Paterson-Kelly syndrome) and congenital hyperkeratosis and pitting of the palms and soles (i.e., tylosis palmaris et plantaris) have each been linked with squamous cell esophageal cancer, as have dietary deficiencies of molybdenum, zinc, selenium, and vitamin A. Bisphosphonates may increase the risk in patients with Barrett's esophagus. Patients with head and neck cancer are at increased risk of squamous cell cancer of the esophagus.

For unclear reasons, the incidence of squamous cell esophageal cancer has decreased somewhat in both the black and white population in the United States over the past 30 years, while the rate of adenocarcinoma has risen dramatically, particularly in white males (M:F 6:1). Adenocarcinomas arise in the distal esophagus in the presence of chronic gastric reflux and gastric metaplasia of the epithelium (Barrett's esophagus), which is more common in obese persons. Adenocarcinomas arise within dysplastic columnar epithelium in the distal esophagus. Even before frank neoplasia is detectable, aneuploidy and p53 mutations are found in the dysplastic epithelium. These adenocarcinomas behave clinically like gastric adenocarcinoma and now account for >70% of esophageal cancers.

■ CLINICAL FEATURES

About 10% of esophageal cancers occur in the upper third of the esophagus (cervical esophagus), 35% in the middle third, and 55% in the lower third. Squamous cell carcinomas and adenocarcinomas cannot be distinguished radiographically or endoscopically.

Progressive dysphagia and weight loss of short duration are the initial symptoms in the vast majority of patients. Dysphagia initially occurs with solid foods and gradually progresses to include semisolids and liquids. By the time these symptoms develop, the disease is usually incurable, since difficulty in swallowing does not occur until >60% of the esophageal circumference is infiltrated with cancer. Dysphagia may be associated with pain on swallowing (odynophagia), pain radiating to the chest and/or back, regurgitation or vomiting, and aspiration pneumonia. The disease most commonly spreads to adjacent and supraclavicular lymph nodes, liver, lungs, pleura, and bone. Tracheoesophageal fistulas may develop as the disease advances, leading to severe suffering. As with other squamous cell carcinomas, hypercalcemia may occur in the absence of osseous metastases, probably from parathormone-related peptide secreted by tumor cells (Chap. 100).

■ DIAGNOSIS

Attempts at endoscopic and cytologic screening for carcinoma in patients with Barrett's esophagus, while effective as a means of detecting high-grade dysplasia, have not yet been shown to improve the prognosis in individuals found to have a carcinoma. Routine contrast radiographs effectively identify esophageal lesions large enough to cause symptoms. In contrast to benign esophageal leiomyomas, which result in esophageal narrowing with preservation of a normal mucosal pattern, esophageal carcinomas show ragged, ulcerating changes in the mucosa in association with deeper infiltration, producing a picture resembling achalasia. Smaller, potentially resectable tumors are often poorly visualized despite technically adequate esophagograms. Because of this, esophagoscopy should be performed in all patients suspected of having an esophageal abnormality, to visualize the tumor and to obtain histopathologic confirmation of the diagnosis. Because the population of persons at risk for squamous cell carcinoma of the esophagus (i.e., smokers and drinkers) also has a high rate of cancers of the lung and the head and neck region, endoscopic inspection of the larynx, trachea, and bronchi should also be done. A thorough examination of the fundus of the stomach (by retroflexing the endoscope) is imperative as well. Endoscopic biopsies of esophageal tumors fail to recover malignant tissue in one-third of cases because the biopsy forceps cannot penetrate deeply enough through normal mucosa pushed in front of the carcinoma. Taking multiple biopsies increases the yield. Cytologic examination of tumor brushings complements standard biopsies and should be performed routinely. The extent of tumor spread to the mediastinum and para-aortic lymph nodes should be assessed by CT scans of the chest and abdomen and by endoscopic ultrasound. Positron emission tomography scanning provides a useful assessment of resectability, offering accurate information regarding spread to mediastinal lymph nodes. Most patients have advanced disease at presentation.

TREATMENT   Esophageal Cancer

The prognosis for patients with esophageal carcinoma is poor. Fewer than 5% of patients survive 5 years after the diagnosis; thus, management focuses on symptom control. Surgical resection of all gross tumor (i.e., total resection) is feasible in only 45% of cases, with residual tumor cells frequently present at the resection margins. Such esophagectomies have been associated with a postoperative mortality rate of approximately 5% due to anastomotic fistulas, subphrenic abscesses, and respiratory complications. About 20% of patients who survive a total resection live 5 years. The efficacy of primary radiation therapy (5500–6000 cGy) for squamous cell carcinomas is similar to that of radical surgery, sparing patients perioperative morbidity but often resulting in less satisfactory palliation of obstructive symptoms. The evaluation of chemotherapeutic agents in patients with esophageal carcinoma has been hampered by ambiguity in the definition of "response" and the debilitated physical condition of many treated individuals. Nonetheless, significant reductions in the size of measurable tumor masses have been reported in 15–25% of patients given single-agent treatment and in 30–60% of patients treated with drug combinations that include cisplatin. Combination chemotherapy and radiation therapy as the initial therapeutic approach, either alone or followed by an attempt at operative resection, seems to be beneficial. When administered along with radiation therapy, chemotherapy produces a better survival outcome than radiation therapy alone. The use of preoperative chemotherapy and radiation therapy followed by esophageal resection appears to prolong survival as compared with controls in small, randomized trials, and some reports suggest that no additional benefit accrues when surgery is added if significant shrinkage of tumor has been achieved by the chemoradiation combination.

For the incurable, surgically unresectable patient with esophageal cancer, dysphagia, malnutrition, and the management of tracheoesophageal fistulas are major issues. Approaches to palliation include repeated endoscopic dilatation, the surgical placement of a gastrostomy or jejunostomy for hydration and feeding, and endoscopic placement of an expansive metal stent to bypass the tumor. Endoscopic fulguration of the obstructing tumor with lasers is the most promising of these techniques.

TUMORS OF THE STOMACH

■ GASTRIC ADENOCARCINOMA

Incidence and epidemiology

For unclear reasons, the incidence and mortality rates for gastric cancer have decreased markedly worldwide during the past 75 years. The mortality rate from gastric cancer in the United States has dropped in men from 28 to 5.8 per 100,000 persons, while in women the rate has decreased from 27 to 2.8 per 100,000. Nonetheless, 21,000 new cases of stomach cancer were diagnosed in the United States, and 10,570 Americans died of the disease in 2010. Gastric cancer incidence has decreased worldwide but remains high in Japan, China, Chile, and Ireland.

The risk of gastric cancer is greater among lower socioeconomic classes. Migrants from high- to low-incidence nations maintain their susceptibility to gastric cancer, while the risk for their offspring approximates that of the new homeland. These findings suggest that an environmental exposure, probably beginning early in life, is related to the development of gastric cancer, with dietary carcinogens considered the most likely factor(s).

Pathology

About 85% of stomach cancers are adenocarcinomas, with 15% due to lymphomas and gastrointestinal stromal tumors (GIST) and leiomyosarcomas. Gastric adenocarcinomas may be subdivided into two categories: a *diffuse type*, in which cell cohesion is absent, so that individual cells infiltrate and thicken the stomach wall without forming a discrete mass; and an *intestinal type*, characterized by cohesive neoplastic cells that form glandlike tubular structures. The diffuse carcinomas occur more often in younger patients, develop throughout the stomach (including the cardia), result in a loss of distensibility of the gastric wall (so-called linitis plastica, or "leather bottle" appearance), and carry a poorer prognosis. Diffuse cancers have defective intercellular adhesion, mainly as a consequence of loss of expression of E-cadherin. Intestinal-type lesions are frequently ulcerative, more commonly appear in the antrum and lesser curvature of the stomach, and are often preceded by a prolonged precancerous process, often initiated by *Helicobacter pylori* infection. While the incidence of diffuse carcinomas is similar in most populations, the intestinal type tends to predominate in the high-risk geographic regions and is less likely to be found in areas where the frequency of gastric cancer is declining. Thus, different etiologic factor(s) are likely involved in these two subtypes. In the United States, ~30% of gastric cancers originate in the distal stomach, ~20% arise in the midportion of the stomach, and ~37% originate in the proximal third of the stomach. The remaining 13% involve the entire stomach.

Etiology

The long-term ingestion of high concentrations of nitrates in dried, smoked, and salted foods appears to be associated with a higher risk. The nitrates are thought to be converted to carcinogenic nitrites by bacteria (Table 91-2). Such bacteria may be introduced exogenously through the ingestion of partially decayed foods, which are consumed in abundance worldwide by the lower socioeconomic classes. Bacteria such as *H. pylori* may also contribute to this effect by causing chronic gastritis, loss of gastric acidity, and bacterial growth in the stomach. The effect

TABLE 91-2 Nitrate-Converting Bacteria as a Factor in the Causation of Gastric Carcinoma[a]

Exogenous sources of nitrate-converting bacteria:

Bacterially contaminated food (common in lower socioeconomic classes, who have a higher incidence of the disease; diminished by improved food preservation and refrigeration)

? *Helicobacter pylori* infection

Endogenous factors favoring growth of nitrate-converting bacteria in the stomach:

Decreased gastric acidity

Prior gastric surgery (antrectomy) (15- to 20-year latency period)

Atrophic gastritis and/or pernicious anemia

? Prolonged exposure to histamine H_2-receptor antagonists

[a]Hypothesis: Dietary nitrates are converted to carcinogenic nitrites by bacteria.

of *H. pylori* eradication on the subsequent risk for gastric cancer in high-incidence areas is under investigation. Loss of acidity may occur when acid-producing cells of the gastric antrum have been removed surgically to control benign peptic ulcer disease or when achlorhydria, atrophic gastritis, and even pernicious anemia develop in the elderly. Serial endoscopic examinations of the stomach in patients with atrophic gastritis have documented replacement of the usual gastric mucosa by intestinal-type cells. This process of intestinal metaplasia may lead to cellular atypia and eventual neoplasia. Since the declining incidence of gastric cancer in the United States primarily reflects a decline in distal, ulcerating, intestinal-type lesions, it is conceivable that better food preservation and the availability of refrigeration to all socioeconomic classes have decreased the dietary ingestion of exogenous bacteria. *H. pylori* has not been associated with the diffuse, more proximal form of gastric carcinoma.

Several additional etiologic factors have been associated with gastric carcinoma. Gastric ulcers and adenomatous polyps have occasionally been linked, but data on a cause-and-effect relationship are unconvincing. The inadequate clinical distinction between benign gastric ulcers and small ulcerating carcinomas may, in part, account for this presumed association. The presence of extreme hypertrophy of gastric rugal folds (i.e., Ménétrier's disease), giving the impression of polypoid lesions, has been associated with a striking frequency of malignant transformation; such hypertrophy, however, does not represent the presence of true adenomatous polyps. Individuals with blood group A have a higher incidence of gastric cancer than persons with blood group O; this observation may be related to differences in the mucous secretion, leading to altered mucosal protection from carcinogens. A germ-line mutation in the E-cadherin gene (*CDH1*), inherited in an autosomal dominant pattern and coding for a cell adhesion protein, has been linked to a high incidence of occult diffuse-type gastric cancers in young asymptomatic carriers. Duodenal ulcers are not associated with gastric cancer.

In keeping with the stepwise model of carcinogenesis, K-*ras* mutations appear to be early events in intestinal-type gastric cancer. C-met expression is amplified in about 1 in 5 cases and correlates with advanced stage. About half of intestinal-type tumors have mutations in tumor suppressor genes such as *TP53, TP73, APC* (adenomatous polyposis coli), *TFF* (trefoid factor family), *DCC* (deleted in colon cancer), and *FHIT* (fragile histidine triad). Cyclin E overexpression is associated with progression from dysplasia.

Epigenetic changes (especially increased methylation) has been correlated with higher risk of invasive disease. Beta-catenin has been found in the nucleus of tumor cells at the leading edge of invasion.

Clinical features

Gastric cancers, when superficial and surgically curable, usually produce no symptoms. As the tumor becomes more extensive, patients may complain of an insidious upper abdominal discomfort varying in intensity from a vague, postprandial fullness to a severe, steady pain. Anorexia, often with slight nausea, is very common but is not the usual presenting complaint. Weight loss may eventually be observed, and nausea and vomiting are particularly prominent with tumors of the pylorus; dysphagia and early satiety may be the major symptoms caused by diffuse lesions originating in the cardia. There are no early physical signs. A palpable abdominal mass indicates long-standing growth and predicts regional extension.

Gastric carcinomas spread by direct extension through the gastric wall to the perigastric tissues, occasionally adhering to adjacent organs such as the pancreas, colon, or liver. The disease also spreads via lymphatics or by seeding of peritoneal surfaces. Metastases to intraabdominal and supraclavicular lymph nodes occur frequently, as do metastatic nodules to the ovary (Krukenberg's tumor), periumbilical region ("Sister Mary Joseph node"), or peritoneal cul-de-sac (Blumer's shelf palpable on rectal or vaginal examination); malignant ascites may also develop. The liver is the most common site for hematogenous spread of tumor.

The presence of iron-deficiency anemia in men and of occult blood in the stool in both sexes mandates a search for an occult gastrointestinal tract lesion. A careful assessment is of particular importance in patients with atrophic gastritis or pernicious anemia. Unusual clinical features associated with gastric adenocarcinomas include migratory thrombophlebitis, microangiopathic hemolytic anemia, diffuse seborrheic keratoses (so-called Leser-Trélat sign), and acanthosis nigricans.

Diagnosis

A double-contrast radiographic examination is the simplest diagnostic procedure for the evaluation of a patient with epigastric complaints. The use of double-contrast techniques helps to detect small lesions by improving mucosal detail. The stomach should be distended at some time during every radiographic examination, since decreased distensibility may be the only indication of a diffuse infiltrative carcinoma. Although gastric ulcers can be detected fairly early, distinguishing benign from malignant lesions radiographically is difficult. The anatomic location of an ulcer is not in itself an indication of the presence or absence of a cancer.

Gastric ulcers that appear benign by radiography present special problems. Some physicians believe that gastroscopy is not mandatory if the radiographic features are typically benign, if complete healing can be visualized by x-ray within 6 weeks, and if a follow-up contrast radiograph obtained several months later shows a normal appearance. However, we recommend gastroscopic biopsy and brush cytology for all patients with a gastric ulcer in order to exclude a malignancy. Malignant gastric ulcers must be recognized before they penetrate into surrounding tissues, because the rate of cure of early lesions limited to the mucosa or submucosa is >80%. Since gastric carcinomas are difficult to distinguish clinically or radiographically from gastric lymphomas, endoscopic biopsies should be made as deeply as possible, due to the submucosal location of lymphoid tumors.

The staging system for gastric carcinoma is shown in Table 91-3.

TABLE 91-3 Staging System for Gastric Carcinoma

Stage	TNM	Features	Data from ACS No. of Cases, %	Data from ACS 5-Year Survival, %
0	T_{is}N0M0	Node negative; limited to mucosa	1	90
IA	T1N0M0	Node negative; invasion of lamina propria or submucosa	7	59
IB	T2N0M0 T1N1M0	Node negative; invasion of muscularis propria	10	44
II	T1N2M0 T2N1M0	Node positive; invasion beyond mucosa but within wall *or*	17	29
	T3N0M0	Node negative; extension through wall		
IIIA	T2N2M0 T3N1-2M0	Node positive; invasion of muscularis propria or through wall	21	15
IIIB	T4N0-1M0	Node negative; adherence to surrounding tissue	14	9
IIIC	T4N2-3M0 T3N3M0	>3 nodes positive; invasion of serosa or adjacent structures 7 or more positive nodes; penetrates wall without invading serosa or adjacent structures		
IV	T4N2M0	Node positive; adherence to surrounding tissue *or*	30	3
	T1-4N0-2 M1	Distant metastases		

Abbreviation: ACS, American Cancer Society; TNM, tumor, node, metastasis.

TREATMENT ▶ **Gastric Adenocarcinoma**

Complete surgical removal of the tumor with resection of adjacent lymph nodes offers the only chance for cure. However, this is possible in less than a third of patients. A subtotal gastrectomy is the treatment of choice for patients with distal carcinomas, while total or near-total gastrectomies are required for more proximal tumors. The inclusion of extended lymph node dissection in these procedures appears to confer an added risk for complications without enhancing survival. The prognosis following complete surgical resection depends on the degree of tumor penetration into the stomach wall and is adversely influenced by regional lymph node involvement, vascular invasion, and abnormal DNA content (i.e., aneuploidy), characteristics found in the vast majority of American patients. As a result, the probability of survival after 5 years for the 25–30% of patients

able to undergo complete resection is ~20% for distal tumors and <10% for proximal tumors, with recurrences continuing for at least 8 years after surgery. In the absence of ascites or extensive hepatic or peritoneal metastases, even patients whose disease is believed to be incurable by surgery should be offered resection of the primary lesion. Reduction of tumor bulk is the best form of palliation and may enhance the probability of benefit from subsequent therapy.

Gastric adenocarcinoma is a relatively radioresistant tumor, and adequate control of the primary tumor requires doses of external beam irradiation that exceed the tolerance of surrounding structures, such as bowel mucosa and spinal cord. As a result, the major role of radiation therapy in patients has been palliation of pain. Radiation therapy alone after a complete resection does not prolong survival. In the setting of surgically unresectable disease limited to the epigastrium, patients treated with 3500–4000 cGy did not live longer than similar patients not receiving radiotherapy; however, survival was prolonged slightly when 5-fluorouracil (5-FU) plus leucovorin was given in combination with radiation therapy (3-year survival 50% vs 41% for radiation therapy alone). In this clinical setting, the 5-FU may be functioning as a radiosensitizer.

The administration of combinations of cytotoxic drugs to patients with advanced gastric carcinoma has been associated with partial responses in 30–50% of cases; responders appear to benefit from treatment. Such drug combinations have generally included cisplatin combined with epirubicin or docetaxel and infusional 5-FU, or with irinotecan. Despite this encouraging response rate, complete remissions are uncommon, the partial responses are transient, and the overall influence of multidrug therapy on survival has been unclear. The use of adjuvant chemotherapy alone following the complete resection of a gastric cancer has only minimally improved survival. However, combination chemotherapy administered before and after surgery (*perioperative treatment*) as well as postoperative chemotherapy combined with radiation therapy reduces the recurrence rate and prolongs survival.

■ PRIMARY GASTRIC LYMPHOMA

Primary lymphoma of the stomach is relatively uncommon, accounting for <15% of gastric malignancies and ~2% of all lymphomas. The stomach is, however, the most frequent extranodal site for lymphoma, and gastric lymphoma has increased in frequency during the past 30 years. The disease is difficult to distinguish clinically from gastric adenocarcinoma; both tumors are most often detected during the sixth decade of life; present with epigastric pain, early satiety, and generalized fatigue; and are usually characterized by ulcerations with a ragged, thickened mucosal pattern demonstrated by contrast radiographs. The diagnosis of lymphoma of the stomach may occasionally be made through cytologic brushings of the gastric mucosa but usually requires a biopsy at gastroscopy or laparotomy. Failure of gastroscopic biopsies to detect lymphoma in a given case should not be interpreted as being conclusive, since superficial biopsies may miss the deeper lymphoid infiltrate. The macroscopic pathology of gastric lymphoma may also mimic adenocarcinoma, consisting of either a bulky ulcerated lesion localized in the corpus or antrum or a diffuse process spreading throughout the entire gastric submucosa and even extending into the duodenum. Microscopically, the vast majority of gastric lymphoid tumors are non-Hodgkin's lymphomas of B cell origin; Hodgkin's disease involving the stomach is extremely uncommon. Histologically, these tumors may range from well-differentiated, superficial processes [mucosa-associated lymphoid tissue (MALT)] to high-grade, large-cell lymphomas. Like gastric adenocarcinoma, infection with *H. pylori* increases the risk for gastric lymphoma in general and MALT lymphomas in particular. Gastric lymphomas spread initially to regional lymph nodes (often to Waldeyer's ring) and may then disseminate. Gastric lymphomas are staged like other lymphomas (Chap. 110).

TREATMENT **Primary Gastric Lymphoma**

Primary gastric lymphoma is a far more treatable disease than adenocarcinoma of the stomach, a fact that underscores the need for making the correct diagnosis. Antibiotic treatment to eradicate *H. pylori* infection has led to regression of about 75% of gastric MALT lymphomas and should be considered before surgery, radiation therapy, or chemotherapy are undertaken in patients having such tumors. A lack of response to such antimicrobial treatment has been linked to a specific chromosomal abnormality, i.e., t(11;18). Responding patients should undergo periodic endoscopic surveillance because it remains unclear whether the neoplastic clone is eliminated or merely suppressed, although the response to antimicrobial treatment is quite durable. Subtotal gastrectomy, usually followed by combination chemotherapy, has led to 5-year survival rates of 40–60% in patients with localized high-grade lymphomas. The need for a major surgical procedure has been questioned, particularly in patients with preoperative radiographic evidence of nodal involvement, for whom chemotherapy [CHOP (cyclophosphamide, doxorubicin, vincristine, and prednisone)] plus rituximab is effective therapy. A role for radiation therapy is not defined because most recurrences develop at distant sites.

■ GASTRIC (NONLYMPHOID) SARCOMA

Leiomyosarcomas and GISTs make up 1–3% of gastric neoplasms. They most frequently involve the anterior and posterior walls of the gastric fundus and often ulcerate and bleed. Even those lesions that appear benign on histologic examination may behave in a malignant fashion. These tumors rarely invade adjacent viscera and characteristically do not metastasize to lymph nodes, but they may spread to the liver and lungs. The treatment of choice is surgical resection. Combination chemotherapy should be reserved for patients with metastatic disease. All such tumors should be analyzed for a mutation in the c-*kit* receptor. GISTs are unresponsive to conventional chemotherapy; yet ~50% of patients experience objective response and prolonged survival when treated with imatinib mesylate (Gleevec) (400–800 mg PO daily), a selective inhibitor of the c-*kit* tyrosine kinase. Many patients with GIST whose tumors have become refractory to imatinib subsequently benefit from sunitinib (Sutent), another inhibitor of the c-*kit* tyrosine kinase.

COLORECTAL CANCER

■ INCIDENCE

Cancer of the large bowel is second only to lung cancer as a cause of cancer death in the United States: 142,570 new cases occurred in 2010, and 51,370 deaths were due to colorectal cancer. The incidence rate has decreased significantly during the past 20 years, likely due to enhanced and more compliantly followed screening practices. Similarly, mortality rates in the United States have decreased by approximately 25%, resulting largely from improved treatment and earlier detection.

■ POLYPS AND MOLECULAR PATHOGENESIS

Most colorectal cancers, regardless of etiology, arise from adenomatous polyps. A polyp is a grossly visible protrusion from the mucosal surface and may be classified pathologically as a nonneoplastic hamartoma (*juvenile polyp*), a hyperplastic mucosal proliferation (*hyperplastic polyp*), or an adenomatous polyp. Only adenomas are clearly premalignant, and only a minority of such lesions becomes cancer. Adenomatous polyps may be found in the colons of ~30% of middle-aged and ~50% of elderly people; however, <1% of polyps ever become malignant. Most polyps produce no symptoms and remain clinically undetected. Occult blood in the stool is found in <5% of patients with polyps.

A number of molecular changes are noted in adenomatous polyps, dysplastic lesions, and polyps containing microscopic foci of tumor cells (carcinoma in situ), which are thought to reflect a multistep process in the evolution of normal colonic mucosa to life-threatening invasive carcinoma. These developmental steps toward carcinogenesis include, but are not restricted to, point mutations in the K-*ras* protooncogene; hypomethylation of DNA, leading to gene activation; loss of DNA (*allelic loss*) at the site of a tumor-suppressor gene [the adenomatous polyposis coli (*APC*) gene] on the long arm of chromosome 5 (5q21); allelic loss at the site of a tumor-suppressor gene located on chromosome 18q [the deleted in colorectal cancer (*DCC*) gene]; and allelic loss at chromosome 17p, associated with mutations in the p53 tumor-suppressor gene (see Fig. 83-2). Thus, the altered proliferative pattern of the colonic mucosa, which results in progression to a polyp and then to carcinoma, may involve the mutational activation of an oncogene followed by and coupled with the loss of genes that normally suppress tumorigenesis. It remains uncertain whether the genetic aberrations always occur in a defined order. Based on this model, however, cancer is believed to develop only in those polyps in which most (if not all) of these mutational events take place.

Clinically, the probability of an adenomatous polyp becoming a cancer depends on the gross appearance of the lesion, its histologic features, and its size. Adenomatous polyps may be pedunculated (stalked) or sessile (flat-based). Cancers develop more frequently in sessile polyps. Histologically, adenomatous polyps may be tubular, villous (i.e., papillary), or tubulovillous. Villous adenomas, most of which are sessile, become malignant more than three times as often as tubular adenomas. The likelihood that any polypoid lesion in the large bowel contains invasive cancer is related to the size of the polyp, being negligible (<2%) in lesions <1.5 cm, intermediate (2–10%) in lesions 1.5–2.5 cm, and substantial (10%) in lesions >2.5 cm in size.

Following the detection of an adenomatous polyp, the entire large bowel should be visualized endoscopically or radiographically, since synchronous lesions are noted in about one-third of cases. Colonoscopy should then be repeated periodically, even in the absence of a previously documented malignancy, since such patients have a 30–50% probability of developing another adenoma and are at a higher-than-average risk for developing a colorectal carcinoma. Adenomatous polyps are thought to require >5 years of growth before becoming clinically significant; colonoscopy need not be carried out more frequently than every 3 years.

■ ETIOLOGY AND RISK FACTORS

Risk factors for the development of colorectal cancer are listed in Table 91-4.

Diet

The etiology for most cases of large-bowel cancer appears to be related to environmental factors. The disease occurs more often in upper socioeconomic populations who live in urban areas. Mortality from colorectal cancer is directly correlated with per capita consumption of calories, meat protein, and dietary fat and oil as well as elevations in the serum cholesterol concentration and mortality from coronary artery disease. Geographic variations in incidence are

TABLE 91-4 Risk Factors for the Development of Colorectal Cancer

Diet: Animal fat

Hereditary syndromes (autosomal dominant inheritance)

  Polyposis coli

  Nonpolyposis syndrome (Lynch syndrome)

Inflammatory bowel disease

Streptococcus bovis bacteremia

Ureterosigmoidostomy

? Tobacco use

---

unrelated to genetic differences, since migrant groups tend to assume the large-bowel cancer incidence rates of their adopted countries. Furthermore, population groups such as Mormons and Seventh Day Adventists, whose lifestyle and dietary habits differ somewhat from those of their neighbors, have significantly lower-than-expected incidence and mortality rates for colorectal cancer. Colorectal cancer has increased in Japan since that nation has adopted a more "Western" diet. At least three hypotheses have been proposed to explain the relationship to diet, none of which is fully satisfactory.

Animal fats One hypothesis is that the ingestion of animal fats found in red meats and processed meat leads to an increased proportion of anaerobes in the gut microflora, resulting in the conversion of normal bile acids into carcinogens. This provocative hypothesis is supported by several reports of increased amounts of fecal anaerobes in the stools of patients with colorectal cancer. Diets high in animal (but not vegetable) fats are also associated with high serum cholesterol, which is also associated with enhanced risk for the development of colorectal adenomas and carcinomas.

Insulin resistance The large number of calories in Western diets coupled with physical inactivity has been associated with a higher prevalence of obesity. Obese persons develop insulin resistance with increased circulating levels of insulin, leading to higher circulating concentrations of insulin-like growth factor type I (IGF-I). This growth factor appears to stimulate proliferation of the intestinal mucosa.

Fiber Contrary to prior beliefs, the results of randomized trials and case-controlled studies have failed to show any value for dietary fiber or diets high in fruits and vegetables in preventing the recurrence of colorectal adenomas or the development of colorectal cancer. The weight of epidemiologic evidence, however, implicates diet as being the major etiologic factor for colorectal cancer, particularly diets high in animal fat and in calories.

■ HEREDITARY FACTORS AND SYNDROMES

Up to 25% of patients with colorectal cancer have a family history of the disease, suggesting a hereditary predisposition. Inherited large-bowel cancers can be divided into two main groups: the well-studied but uncommon polyposis syndromes and the more common nonpolyposis syndromes (Table 91-5).

Polyposis coli

Polyposis coli (familial polyposis of the colon) is a rare condition characterized by the appearance of thousands of adenomatous polyps throughout the large bowel. It is transmitted as an autosomal dominant trait; the occasional patient with no family history probably developed the condition due to a spontaneous mutation. Polyposis coli is associated with a deletion in the long arm of chromosome 5 [including the *APC* (adenomatous polyposis coli) gene] in both neoplastic (somatic mutation) and normal (germ-line mutation) cells. The loss of this genetic material (i.e., allelic loss) results in the absence of tumor-suppressor genes whose protein products would normally inhibit neoplastic growth. The presence of soft tissue and bony tumors, congenital hypertrophy of the retinal pigment epithelium, mesenteric desmoid tumors, and ampullary cancers in addition to the colonic polyps characterizes a subset of polyposis coli known as *Gardner's syndrome*. The appearance of malignant tumors of the central nervous system accompanying polyposis coli defines *Turcot's syndrome*. The colonic polyps in all these conditions are rarely present before puberty but are generally evident in affected individuals by age 25. If the polyposis is not treated surgically, colorectal cancer will develop in almost all patients before age 40. Polyposis coli results from a defect in the colonic mucosa, leading to an abnormal proliferative pattern and impaired DNA repair mechanisms. Once the multiple polyps are detected, patients should undergo a total colectomy. Medical therapy with nonsteroidal anti-inflammatory drugs

TABLE 91-5 Hereditable (Autosomal Dominant) Gastrointestinal Polyposis Syndromes

Syndrome	Distribution of Polyps	Histologic Type	Malignant Potential	Associated Lesions
Familial adenomatous polyposis	Large intestine	Adenoma	Common	None
Gardner's syndrome	Large and small intestines	Adenoma	Common	Osteomas, fibromas, lipomas, epidermoid cysts, ampullary cancers, congenital hypertrophy of retinal pigment epithelium
Turcot's syndrome	Large intestine	Adenoma	Common	Brain tumors
Nonpolyposis syndrome (Lynch syndrome)	Large intestine (often proximal)	Adenoma	Common	Endometrial and ovarian tumors
Peutz-Jeghers syndrome	Small and large intestines, stomach	Hamartoma	Rare	Mucocutaneous pigmentation; tumors of the ovary, breast, pancreas, endometrium
Juvenile polyposis	Large and small intestines, stomach	Hamartoma, rarely progressing to adenoma	Rare	Various congenital abnormalities

(NSAIDs) such as sulindac and cyclooxygenase-2 inhibitors such as celecoxib can decrease the number and size of polyps in patients with polyposis coli; however, this effect on polyps is only temporary, and NSAIDs are not proven to reduce the risk of cancer. Colectomy remains the primary therapy/prevention. The offspring of patients with polyposis coli, who often are prepubertal when the diagnosis is made in the parent, have a 50% risk for developing this premalignant disorder and should be carefully screened by annual flexible sigmoidoscopy until age 35. Proctosigmoidoscopy is a sufficient screening procedure because polyps tend to be evenly distributed from cecum to anus, making more-invasive and expensive techniques such as colonoscopy or barium enema unnecessary. Testing for occult blood in the stool is an inadequate screening maneuver. An alternative method for identifying carriers is testing DNA from peripheral blood mononuclear cells for the presence of a mutated *APC* gene. The detection of such a germ-line mutation can lead to a definitive diagnosis before the development of polyps.

Hereditary nonpolyposis colon cancer

Hereditary nonpolyposis colon cancer (HNPCC), also known as *Lynch syndrome*, is another autosomal dominant trait. It is characterized by the presence of three or more relatives with histologically documented colorectal cancer, one of whom is a first-degree relative of the other two; one or more cases of colorectal cancer diagnosed before age 50 in the family; and colorectal cancer involving at least two generations. In contrast to polyposis coli, HNPCC is associated with an unusually high frequency of cancer arising in the proximal large bowel. The median age for the appearance of an adenocarcinoma is <50 years, 10–15 years younger than the median age for the general population. Despite having a poorly differentiated histologic appearance, the proximal colon tumors in HNPCC have a better prognosis than sporadic tumors from patients of similar age. Families with HNPCC often include individuals with multiple primary cancers; the association of colorectal cancer with either ovarian or endometrial carcinomas is especially strong in women. It has been recommended that members of such families undergo biennial colonoscopy beginning at age 25 years, with intermittent pelvic ultrasonography and endometrial biopsy for afflicted women; such a screening strategy has not yet been validated. HNPCC is associated with germ-line mutations of several genes, particularly *hMSH2* on chromosome 2 and *hMLH1* on chromosome 3. These mutations lead to errors in DNA replication and are thought to result in DNA instability because of defective repair of DNA mismatches resulting in abnormal cell growth and tumor development. Testing tumor cells through molecular analysis of DNA or immunohistochemical staining of paraffin-fixed tissue for "microsatellite instability" (sequence changes reflecting defective mismatch repair) in patients younger than age 50 with colorectal cancer and a positive family history for colorectal or endometrial cancer may identify probands with HNPCC.

■ INFLAMMATORY BOWEL DISEASE

(Chap. 295) Large-bowel cancer is increased in incidence in patients with long-standing inflammatory bowel disease (IBD). Cancers develop more commonly in patients with ulcerative colitis than in those with granulomatous colitis, but this impression may result in part from the occasional difficulty of differentiating these two conditions. The risk of colorectal cancer in a patient with IBD is relatively small during the initial 10 years of the disease, but then it appears to increase at a rate of ~0.5–1% per year. Cancer may develop in 8–30% of patients after 25 years. The risk is higher in younger patients with pancolitis.

Cancer surveillance in patients with IBD is unsatisfactory. Symptoms such as bloody diarrhea, abdominal cramping, and obstruction, which may signal the appearance of a tumor, are similar to the complaints caused by a flare-up of the underlying disease. In patients with a history of IBD lasting ≥15 years who continue to experience exacerbations, the surgical removal of the colon can significantly reduce the risk for cancer and also eliminate the target organ for the underlying chronic gastrointestinal disorder. The value of such surveillance techniques as colonoscopy with mucosal biopsies and brushings for less-symptomatic individuals with chronic IBD is uncertain. The lack of uniformity regarding the pathologic criteria that characterize dysplasia and the absence of data that such surveillance reduces the development of lethal cancers have made this costly practice an area of controversy.

■ OTHER HIGH-RISK CONDITIONS

Streptococcus bovis bacteremia

For unknown reasons, individuals who develop endocarditis or septicemia from this fecal bacterium have a high incidence of occult colorectal tumors and, possibly, upper gastrointestinal cancers as well. Endoscopic or radiographic screening appears advisable.

Tobacco use

Cigarette smoking is linked to the development of colorectal adenomas, particularly after >35 years of tobacco use. No biologic explanation for this association has yet been proposed.

■ PRIMARY PREVENTION

Several orally administered compounds have been assessed as possible inhibitors of colon cancer. The most effective class of chemopreventive agents is aspirin and other NSAIDs, which are thought to suppress cell proliferation by inhibiting prostaglandin synthesis. Regular aspirin use reduces the risk of colon adenomas and carcinomas as well as death from large-bowel cancer; such use also appears to diminish the likelihood for developing additional premalignant adenomas following treatment for a prior colon carcinoma. This effect of aspirin on colon carcinogenesis increases with the duration and dosage of drug use. Oral folic acid supplements and oral calcium supplements reduce the risk of adenomatous polyps and colorectal cancers in case-controlled studies. The value of vitamin D as a form of chemo-prevention is under study. Antioxidant vitamins such as ascorbic acid, tocopherols, and β-carotene are ineffective at reducing the incidence of subsequent adenomas in patients who have undergone the removal of a colon adenoma. Estrogen-replacement therapy has been associated with a reduction in the risk of colorectal cancer in women, conceivably by an effect on bile acid synthesis and composition or by decreasing synthesis of IGF-I. The otherwise unexplained reduction in colorectal cancer mortality rate in women may be a result of the widespread use of estrogen replacement in postmenopausal individuals.

■ SCREENING

The rationale for colorectal cancer screening programs is that earlier detection of localized, superficial cancers in asymptomatic individuals will increase the surgical cure rate. Such screening programs are important for individuals having a family history of the disease in first-degree relatives. The relative risk for developing colorectal cancer increases to 1.75 in such individuals and may be even higher if the relative was afflicted before age 60. The prior use of proctosigmoidoscopy as a screening tool was based on the observation that 60% of early lesions are located in the rectosigmoid. For unexplained reasons, however, the proportion of large-bowel cancers arising in the rectum has been decreasing during the past several decades, with a corresponding increase in the proportion of cancers in the more proximal descending colon. As such, the potential for rigid proctosigmoidoscopy to detect a sufficient number of occult neoplasms to make the procedure cost-effective has been questioned. Flexible, fiberoptic sigmoidoscopes permit trained operators to visualize the colon for up to 60 cm, which enhances the capability for cancer detection. However, this technique still leaves the proximal half of the large bowel unscreened.

Most programs directed at the early detection of colorectal cancers have focused on digital rectal examinations and fecal occult blood testing. The digital examination should be part of any routine physical evaluation in adults older than age 40 years, serving as a screening test for prostate cancer in men, a component of the pelvic examination in women, and an inexpensive maneuver for the detection of masses in the rectum. The development of the Hemoccult test has greatly facilitated the detection of occult fecal blood. Unfortunately, even when performed optimally, the Hemoccult test has major limitations as a screening technique. About 50% of patients with documented colorectal cancers have a negative fecal Hemoccult test, consistent with the intermittent bleeding pattern of these tumors. When random cohorts of asymptomatic persons have been tested, 2–4% have Hemoccult-positive stools. Colorectal cancers have been found in <10% of these "test-positive" cases, with benign polyps being detected in an additional 20–30%. Thus, a colorectal neoplasm will not be found in most asymptomatic individuals with occult blood in their stool. Nonetheless, persons found to have Hemoccult-positive stool routinely undergo further medical evaluation, including sigmoidoscopy, barium enema, and/or colonoscopy—procedures that are not only uncomfortable and expensive but also associated with a small risk for significant complications. The added cost of these studies would appear justifiable if the small number of patients found to have occult neoplasms because of Hemoccult screening could be shown to have an improved prognosis and prolonged survival. Prospectively controlled trials showed a statistically significant reduction in mortality rate from colorectal cancer for individuals undergoing annual screening. However, this benefit only emerged after >13 years of follow-up and was extremely expensive to achieve, since all positive tests (most of which were false-positive) were followed by colonoscopy. Moreover, these colonoscopic examinations quite likely provided the opportunity for cancer prevention through the removal of potentially premalignant adenomatous polyps since the eventual development of cancer was reduced by 20% in the cohort undergoing annual screening.

Screening techniques for large-bowel cancer in asymptomatic persons remain unsatisfactory. Compliance with any screening strategy within the general population is poor. At present, the American Cancer Society suggests fecal Hemoccult screening annually and flexible sigmoidoscopy every 5 years beginning at age 50 for asymptomatic individuals having no colorectal cancer risk factors. The American Cancer Society has also endorsed a "total colon examination" (i.e., colonoscopy or double-contrast barium enema) every 10 years as an alternative to Hemoccult testing with periodic flexible sigmoidoscopy. Colonoscopy has been shown to be superior to double-contrast barium enema and also to have a higher sensitivity for detecting villous or dysplastic adenomas or cancers than the strategy employing occult fecal blood testing and flexible sigmoidoscopy. Whether colonoscopy performed every 10 years beginning after age 50 will prove to be cost-effective and whether it may be supplanted as a screening maneuver by sophisticated radiographic techniques ("virtual colonoscopy") remains unclear. More effective techniques for screening are needed, perhaps taking advantage of the molecular changes that have been described in these tumors. Analysis of fecal DNA for multiple mutations associated with colorectal cancer is being tested.

■ CLINICAL FEATURES

Presenting symptoms

Symptoms vary with the anatomic location of the tumor. Since stool is relatively liquid as it passes through the ileocecal valve into the right colon, cancers arising in the cecum and ascending colon may become quite large without resulting in any obstructive symptoms or noticeable alterations in bowel habits. Lesions of the right colon commonly ulcerate, leading to chronic, insidious blood loss without a change in the appearance of the stool. Consequently, patients with tumors of the ascending colon often present with symptoms such as fatigue, palpitations, and even angina pectoris and are found to have a hypochromic, microcytic anemia indicative of iron deficiency. Since the cancer may bleed intermittently, a random fecal occult blood test may be negative. As a result, the unexplained presence of iron-deficiency anemia in any adult (with the possible exception of a premenopausal, multiparous woman) mandates a thorough endoscopic and/or radiographic visualization of the entire large bowel (Fig. 91-1).

Since stool becomes more formed as it passes into the transverse and descending colon, tumors arising there tend to impede the passage of stool, resulting in the development of abdominal cramping, occasional obstruction, and even perforation. Radiographs of the abdomen often reveal characteristic annular, constricting lesions ("apple-core" or "napkin-ring") (Fig. 91-2).

Cancers arising in the rectosigmoid are often associated with hematochezia, tenesmus, and narrowing of the caliber of stool; anemia is an infrequent finding. While these symptoms may lead patients and their physicians to suspect the presence of hemorrhoids, the development of rectal bleeding and/or altered bowel habits demands a prompt digital rectal examination and proctosigmoidoscopy.

Staging, prognostic factors, and patterns of spread

The prognosis for individuals having colorectal cancer is related to the depth of tumor penetration into the bowel wall and the presence of both regional lymph node involvement and distant metastases. These variables are incorporated into the staging system introduced by Dukes and applied to a TNM classification method, in which

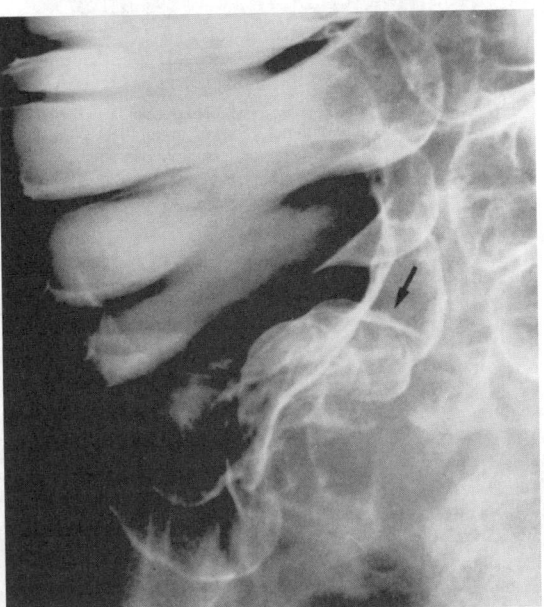

Figure 91-1 Double-contrast air-barium enema revealing a sessile tumor of the cecum in a patient with iron-deficiency anemia and guaiac-positive stool. The lesion at surgery was a stage II adenocarcinoma.

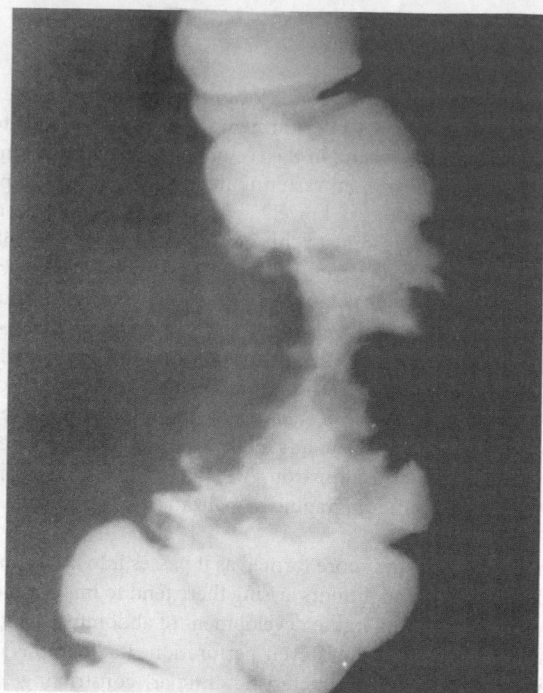

Figure 91-2   Annular, constricting adenocarcinoma of the descending colon. This radiographic appearance is referred to as an "apple-core" lesion and is always highly suggestive of malignancy.

T represents the depth of tumor penetration, N the presence of lymph node involvement, and M the presence or absence of distant metastases (Fig. 91-3). Superficial lesions that do not involve regional lymph nodes and do not penetrate through the submucosa (T1) or the muscularis (T2) are designated as *stage I* (T1–2N0M0) disease; tumors that penetrate through the muscularis but have not spread to lymph nodes are *stage II* disease (T3N0M0); regional lymph node involvement defines *stage III* (TXN_1M_0) disease; and metastatic spread to sites such as liver, lung, or bone indicates *stage IV* ($TXNXM_1$) disease. Unless gross evidence of metastatic disease is present, disease stage cannot be determined accurately before surgical resection and pathologic analysis of the operative specimens. It is not clear whether the detection of nodal metastases by special immunohistochemical molecular techniques has the same prognostic implications as disease detected by routine light microscopy.

Most recurrences after a surgical resection of a large-bowel cancer occur within the first 4 years, making 5-year survival a fairly reliable indicator of cure. The likelihood for 5-year survival in patients with colorectal cancer is stage-related (Fig. 91-3). That likelihood has improved during the past several decades when similar surgical stages have been compared. The most plausible explanation for this improvement is more thorough intraoperative and pathologic staging. In particular, more exacting attention to pathologic detail has revealed that the prognosis following the resection of a colorectal cancer is not related merely to the presence or absence of regional lymph node involvement. Prognosis may be more precisely gauged by the number of involved lymph nodes (one to three lymph nodes versus four or more lymph nodes) and the number of nodes examined. A minimum of 12 sampled lymph nodes is thought necessary to accurately define tumor stage, and the more nodes examined the better. Other predictors of a poor prognosis after a total surgical resection include tumor penetration through the bowel wall into pericolic fat, poorly differentiated histology, perforation and/or tumor adherence to adjacent organs (increasing the risk for an anatomically adjacent recurrence), and venous invasion by tumor (Table 91-6). Regardless of the clinicopathologic stage, a preoperative elevation of the plasma carcinoembryonic antigen (CEA) level predicts eventual tumor recurrence. The presence of aneuploidy and specific chromosomal deletions, such as allelic loss in chromosome 18q (involving the *DCC* gene) in tumor cells, appears to predict a higher risk for metastatic spread, particularly in patients with stage II (T3N0M0) disease. Conversely, the detection of microsatellite instability in tumor tissue indicates a more favorable outcome. In contrast to most other cancers, the prognosis in colorectal cancer

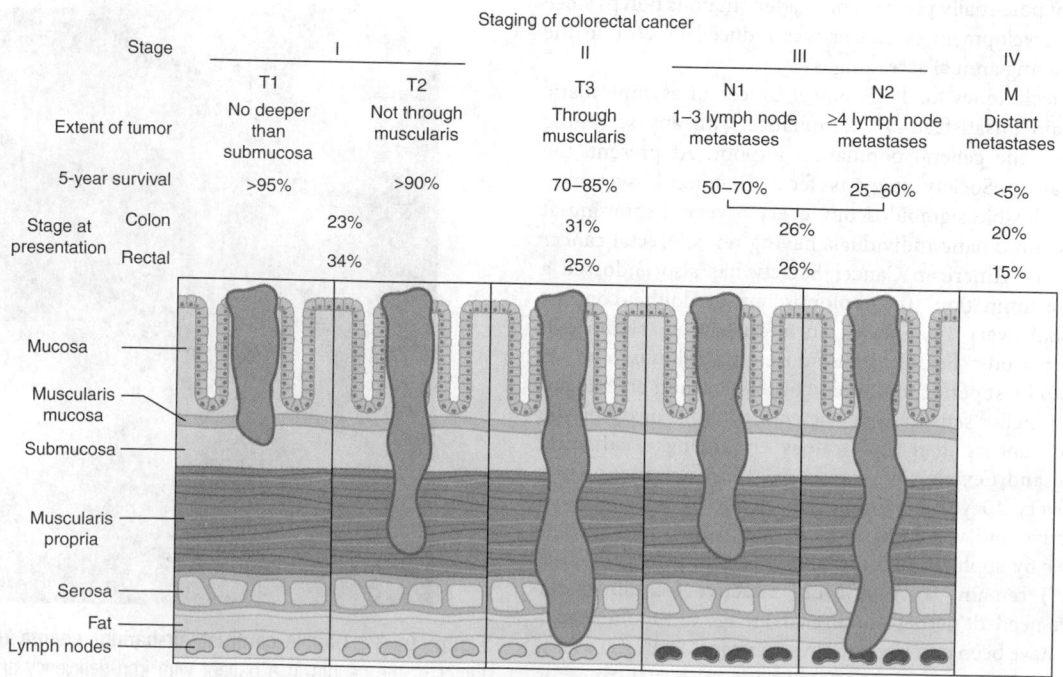

Figure 91-3   Staging and prognosis for patients with colorectal cancer.

TABLE 91-6 Predictors of Poor Outcome Following Total Surgical Resection of Colorectal Cancer

Tumor spread to regional lymph nodes

Number of regional lymph nodes involved

Tumor penetration through the bowel wall

Poorly differentiated histology

Perforation

Tumor adherence to adjacent organs

Venous invasion

Preoperative elevation of CEA titer (>5 ng/mL)

Aneuploidy

Specific chromosomal deletion (e.g., allelic loss on chromosome 18q)

Abbreviation: CEA, carcinoembryonic antigen.

is not influenced by the size of the primary lesion when adjusted for nodal involvement and histologic differentiation.

Cancers of the large bowel generally spread to regional lymph nodes or to the liver via the portal venous circulation. The liver represents the most frequent visceral site of metastasis; it is the initial site of distant spread in one-third of recurring colorectal cancers and is involved in more than two-thirds of such patients at the time of death. In general, colorectal cancer rarely spreads to the lungs, supraclavicular lymph nodes, bone, or brain without prior spread to the liver. A major exception to this rule occurs in patients having primary tumors in the distal rectum, from which tumor cells may spread through the paravertebral venous plexus, escaping the portal venous system and thereby reaching the lungs or supraclavicular lymph nodes without hepatic involvement. The median survival after the detection of distant metastases has ranged in the past from 6–9 months (hepatomegaly, abnormal liver chemistries) to 24–30 months (small liver nodule initially identified by elevated CEA level and subsequent CT scan), but effective systemic therapy is improving the prognosis.

Efforts to use gene expression profiles to identify patients at risk of recurrence or those particularly likely to benefit from adjuvant therapy have not yet yielded practice-changing results. Despite a burgeoning literature examining a host of prognostic factors, pathologic stage at diagnosis is the best predictor of long-term prognosis. Patients with lymphovascular invasion and high preoperative CEA levels are likely to have a more aggressive clinical course.

TREATMENT Colorectal Cancer

Total resection of tumor is the optimal treatment when a malignant lesion is detected in the large bowel. An evaluation for the presence of metastatic disease, including a thorough physical examination, chest radiograph, biochemical assessment of liver function, and measurement of the plasma CEA level, should be performed before surgery. When possible, a colonoscopy of the entire large bowel should be performed to identify synchronous neoplasms and/or polyps. The detection of metastases should not preclude surgery in patients with tumor-related symptoms such as gastrointestinal bleeding or obstruction, but it often prompts the use of a less radical operative procedure. At the time of laparotomy, the entire peritoneal cavity should be examined, with thorough inspection of the liver, pelvis, and hemidiaphragm and careful palpation of the full length of the large bowel. Following recovery from a complete resection, patients should be observed carefully for 5 years by semiannual physical examinations and yearly blood chemistry measurements. If a complete colonoscopy was not performed preoperatively, it should be carried out within the first several postoperative months. Some authorities favor measuring plasma CEA levels at 3-month intervals because of the sensitivity of this test as a marker for otherwise undetectable tumor recurrence. Subsequent endoscopic or radiographic surveillance of the large bowel, probably at triennial intervals, is indicated, since patients who have been cured of one colorectal cancer have a 3–5% probability of developing an additional bowel cancer during their lifetime and a >15% risk for the development of adenomatous polyps. Anastomotic ("suture-line") recurrences are infrequent in colorectal cancer patients, provided the surgical resection margins are adequate and free of tumor. The value of periodic CT scans of the abdomen, assessing for an early, asymptomatic indication of tumor recurrence, is an area of uncertainty, with some experts recommending the test be performed annually for the first 3 postoperative years.

Radiation therapy to the pelvis is recommended for patients with rectal cancer because it reduces the 20–25% probability of regional recurrences following complete surgical resection of stage II or III tumors, especially if they have penetrated through the serosa. This alarmingly high rate of local disease recurrence is believed to be due to the fact that the contained anatomic space within the pelvis limits the extent of the resection and because the rich lymphatic network of the pelvic side wall immediately adjacent to the rectum facilitates the early spread of malignant cells into surgically inaccessible tissue. The use of sharp rather than blunt dissection of rectal cancers (*total mesorectal excision*) appears to reduce the likelihood of local disease recurrence to ~10%. Radiation therapy, either pre- or postoperatively, reduces the likelihood of pelvic recurrences but does not appear to prolong survival. Combining postoperative radiation therapy with 5-fluorouracil-based chemotherapy lowers local recurrence rates and improves overall survival. Preoperative radiotherapy is indicated for patients with large, potentially unresectable rectal cancers; such lesions may shrink enough to permit subsequent surgical removal. Radiation therapy is not effective in the primary treatment of colon cancer.

Systemic therapy for patients with colorectal cancer has become more effective. 5-FU remains the backbone of treatment for this disease. Partial responses are obtained in 15–20% of patients. The probability of tumor response appears to be somewhat greater for patients with liver metastases when chemotherapy is infused directly into the hepatic artery, but intraarterial treatment is costly and toxic and does not appear to appreciably prolong survival. The concomitant administration of folinic acid (leucovorin) improves the efficacy of 5-FU in patients with advanced colorectal cancer, presumably by enhancing the binding of 5-FU to its target enzyme, thymidylate synthase. A threefold improvement in the partial response rate is noted when folinic acid is combined with 5-FU; however, the effect on survival is marginal, and the optimal dose schedule remains to be defined. 5-FU is generally administered intravenously but may also be given orally in the form of capecitabine (Xeloda) with seemingly similar efficacy.

Irinotecan (CPT-11), a topoisomerase 1 inhibitor, prolongs survival when compared to supportive care in patients whose disease has progressed on 5-FU. Furthermore, the addition of irinotecan to 5-FU and leucovorin (LV) improves response rates and survival of patients with metastatic disease. The *FOLFIRI regimen* is as follows: irinotecan, 180 mg/m² as a 90-min infusion on day 1; LV, 400 mg/m² as a 2-h infusion during irinotecan administration; immediately followed by 5-FU bolus, 400 mg/m², and 46-h continuous infusion of 2.4–3 g/m² every 2 weeks. Diarrhea is the major side effect from irinotecan. Oxaliplatin, a platinum analogue, also improves the response rate when added to 5-FU and LV as initial treatment of patients with metastatic disease. The *FOLFOX regimen* is the following: 2-h infusion of LV (400 mg/m² per day) followed by a 5-FU bolus (400 mg/m² per day) and 22-h infusion (1200 mg/m²) every 2 weeks, together with oxaliplatin, 85 mg/m² as a 2-h infusion on day 1. Oxaliplatin frequently causes a dose-dependent sensory neuropathy that often resolves following the cessation of therapy. FOLFIRI and FOLFOX are equal in efficacy. In metastatic disease, these regimens may produce median survivals of 2 years.

Monoclonal antibodies are also effective in patients with advanced colorectal cancer. Cetuximab (Erbitux) and panitumumab (Vectibix) are directed against the epidermal growth factor receptor (EGFR), a transmembrane glycoprotein involved in signaling pathways affecting growth and proliferation of tumor cells. Both cetuximab and panitumumab, when given alone, have been shown to benefit a small proportion of previously treated patients, and cetuximab appears to have therapeutic synergy with such chemotherapeutic agents as irinotecan, even in patients previously resistant to this drug; this suggests that cetuximab can reverse cellular resistance to cytotoxic chemotherapy. The antibodies are not effective in the subset of colon tumors that contain mutated K-*ras*. The use of both cetuximab and panitumumab can lead to an acne-like rash, with the development and severity of the rash being correlated with the likelihood of antitumor efficacy. Inhibitors of the EGFR tyrosine kinase such as erlotinib (Tarceva) do not appear to be effective in colorectal cancer.

Bevacizumab (Avastin) is a monoclonal antibody directed against the vascular endothelial growth factor (VEGF) and is thought to act as an anti-angiogenesis agent. The addition of bevacizumab to irinotecan-containing combinations and to FOLFOX initially appeared to improve the outcome observed with chemotherapy alone, but subsequent studies have been less convincing. The use of bevacizumab can lead to hypertension, proteinuria, and an increased likelihood of thromboembolic events.

Patients with solitary hepatic metastases without clinical or radiographic evidence of additional tumor involvement should be considered for partial liver resection, because such procedures are associated with 5-year survival rates of 25–30% when performed on selected individuals by experienced surgeons.

The administration of 5-FU and LV for 6 months after resection of tumor in patients with stage III disease leads to a 40% decrease in recurrence rates and 30% improvement in survival. The likelihood of recurrence has been further reduced when oxaliplatin has been combined with 5-FU and LV (e.g., FOLFOX); unexpectedly, the addition of irinotecan to 5-FU and LV as well as the addition of either bevacizumab or cetuximab to FOLFOX did not enhance outcome. Patients with stage II tumors do not appear to benefit applicably from adjuvant therapy with the use of such treatment generally restricted to those patients having biologic characteristics (e.g., perforated tumors, Ty lesions, lymphovascular invasion) that place them at higher than usual risk for recurrence. In rectal cancer, the delivery of preoperative or postoperative combined modality therapy (5-FU plus radiation therapy) reduces the risk of recurrence and increases the chance of cure for patients with stages II and III tumors, with the preoperative approach being better tolerated. The 5-FU acts as a radiosensitizer when delivered together with radiation therapy. Life-extending adjuvant therapy is used in only about half of patients older than age 65 years. This age bias is completely inappropriate as the benefits and likely the tolerance of adjuvant therapy in patients aged 65+ years appear similar to those seen in younger individuals.

TUMORS OF THE SMALL INTESTINE

Small-bowel tumors comprise <3% of gastrointestinal neoplasms. Because of their rarity, a correct diagnosis is often delayed. Abdominal symptoms are usually vague and poorly defined, and conventional radiographic studies of the upper and lower intestinal tract often appear normal. Small-bowel tumors should be considered in the differential diagnosis in the following situations: (1) recurrent, unexplained episodes of crampy abdominal pain; (2) intermittent bouts of intestinal obstruction, especially in the absence of IBD or prior abdominal surgery; (3) intussusception in the adult; and (4) evidence of chronic intestinal bleeding in the presence of negative conventional contrast radiographs. A careful small-bowel barium study is the diagnostic procedure of choice; the diagnostic accuracy may be improved by infusing barium through a nasogastric tube placed into the duodenum (enteroclysis).

■ BENIGN TUMORS

The histology of benign small-bowel tumors is difficult to predict on clinical and radiologic grounds alone. The symptomatology of benign tumors is not distinctive, with pain, obstruction, and hemorrhage being the most frequent symptoms. These tumors are usually discovered during the fifth and sixth decades of life, more often in the distal rather than the proximal small intestine. The most common benign tumors are adenomas, leiomyomas, lipomas, and angiomas.

Adenomas

These tumors include those of the islet cells and Brunner's glands as well as polypoid adenomas. *Islet cell adenomas* are occasionally located outside the pancreas; the associated syndromes are discussed in Chap. 350. *Brunner's gland adenomas* are not truly neoplastic but represent a hypertrophy or hyperplasia of submucosal duodenal glands. These appear as small nodules in the duodenal mucosa that secrete a highly viscous alkaline mucus. Most often, this is an incidental radiographic finding not associated with any specific clinical disorder.

Polypoid adenomas

About 25% of benign small-bowel tumors are polypoid adenomas (Table 91-5). They may present as single polypoid lesions or, less commonly, as papillary villous adenomas. As in the colon, the sessile or papillary form of the tumor is sometimes associated with a coexisting carcinoma. Occasionally, patients with Gardner's syndrome develop premalignant adenomas in the small bowel; such lesions are generally in the duodenum. Multiple polypoid tumors may occur throughout the small bowel (and occasionally the stomach and colorectum) in the Peutz-Jeghers syndrome. The polyps are usually hamartomas (juvenile polyps) having a low potential for malignant degeneration. Mucocutaneous melanin deposits as well as tumors of the ovary, breast, pancreas, and endometrium are also associated with this autosomal dominant condition.

Leiomyomas

These neoplasms arise from smooth-muscle components of the intestine and are usually intramural, affecting the overlying mucosa. Ulceration of the mucosa may cause gastrointestinal hemorrhage of varying severity. Cramping or intermittent abdominal pain is frequently encountered.

Lipomas

These tumors occur with greatest frequency in the distal ileum and at the ileocecal valve. They have a characteristic radiolucent appearance and are usually intramural and asymptomatic, but on occasion cause bleeding.

Angiomas

While not true neoplasms, these lesions are important because they frequently cause intestinal bleeding. They may take the form of telangiectasia or hemangiomas. Multiple intestinal telangiectasias occur in a nonhereditary form confined to the gastrointestinal tract or as part of the hereditary Osler-Rendu-Weber syndrome. Vascular tumors may also take the form of isolated hemangiomas, most commonly in the jejunum. Angiography, especially during bleeding, is the best procedure for evaluating these lesions.

■ MALIGNANT TUMORS

While rare, small-bowel malignancies occur in patients with long-standing regional enteritis and celiac sprue as well as in individuals with AIDS. Malignant tumors of the small bowel are frequently associated with fever, weight loss, anorexia, bleeding, and a palpable abdominal mass. After ampullary carcinomas (many of which arise from biliary or pancreatic ducts), the most frequently occurring small-bowel malignancies are adenocarcinomas, lymphomas, carcinoid tumors, and leiomyosarcomas.

Adenocarcinomas

The most common primary cancers of the small bowel are adenocarcinomas, accounting for ~50% of malignant tumors. These cancers occur most often in the distal duodenum and proximal jejunum, where they tend to ulcerate and cause hemorrhage or obstruction. Radiologically, they may be confused with chronic duodenal ulcer disease or with Crohn's disease if the patient has long-standing regional enteritis. The diagnosis is best made by endoscopy and biopsy under direct vision. Surgical resection is the treatment of choice.

Lymphomas

Lymphoma in the small bowel may be primary or secondary. A diagnosis of a primary intestinal lymphoma requires histologic confirmation in a clinical setting in which palpable adenopathy and hepatosplenomegaly are absent and no evidence of lymphoma is seen on chest radiograph, CT scan, or peripheral blood smear or on bone marrow aspiration and biopsy. Symptoms referable to the small bowel are present, usually accompanied by an anatomically discernible lesion. Secondary lymphoma of the small bowel consists of involvement of the intestine by a lymphoid malignancy extending from involved retroperitoneal or mesenteric lymph nodes (Chap. 110).

Primary intestinal lymphoma accounts for ~20% of malignancies of the small bowel. These neoplasms are non-Hodgkin's lymphomas; they usually have a diffuse, large-cell histology and are of T cell origin. Intestinal lymphoma involves the ileum, jejunum, and duodenum, in decreasing frequency—a pattern that mirrors the relative amount of normal lymphoid cells in these anatomic areas. The risk of small-bowel lymphoma is increased in patients with a prior history of malabsorptive conditions (e.g., celiac sprue), regional enteritis, and depressed immune function due to congenital immunodeficiency syndromes, prior organ transplantation, autoimmune disorders, or AIDS.

The development of localized or nodular masses that narrow the lumen results in periumbilical pain (made worse by eating) as well as weight loss, vomiting, and occasional intestinal obstruction. The diagnosis of small-bowel lymphoma may be suspected from the appearance on contrast radiographs of patterns such as infiltration and thickening of mucosal folds, mucosal nodules, areas of irregular ulceration, or stasis of contrast material. The diagnosis can be confirmed by surgical exploration and resection of involved segments. Intestinal lymphoma can occasionally be diagnosed by peroral intestinal mucosal biopsy, but since the disease mainly involves the lamina propria, full-thickness surgical biopsies are usually required.

Resection of the tumor constitutes the initial treatment modality. While postoperative radiation therapy has been given to some patients following a total resection, most authorities favor short-term (three cycles) systemic treatment with combination chemotherapy. The frequent presence of widespread intraabdominal disease at the time of diagnosis and the occasional multicentricity of the tumor often make a total resection impossible. The probability of sustained remission or cure is ~75% in patients with localized disease but is ~25% in individuals with unresectable lymphoma. In patients whose tumors are not resected, chemotherapy may lead to bowel perforation.

A unique form of small-bowel lymphoma, diffusely involving the entire intestine, was first described in oriental Jews and Arabs and is referred to as *immunoproliferative small intestinal disease* (IPSID), *Mediterranean lymphoma*, or α *heavy chain disease*. This is a B cell tumor. The typical presentation includes chronic diarrhea and steatorrhea associated with vomiting and abdominal cramps; clubbing of the digits may be observed. A curious feature in many patients with IPSID is the presence in the blood and intestinal secretions of an abnormal IgA that contains a shortened α heavy chain and is devoid of light chains. It is suspected that the abnormal α chains are produced by plasma cells infiltrating the small bowel. The clinical course of patients with IPSID is generally one of exacerbations and remissions, with death frequently resulting from either progressive malnutrition and wasting or the development of an aggressive lymphoma. The use of oral antibiotics such as tetracycline appears to be beneficial in the early phases of the disorder, suggesting a possible infectious etiology. Combination chemotherapy has been administered during later stages of the disease, with variable results. Results are better when antibiotics and chemotherapy are combined.

Carcinoid tumors

Carcinoid tumors arise from argentaffin cells of the crypts of Lieberkühn and are found from the distal duodenum to the ascending colon, areas embryologically derived from the midgut. More than 50% of intestinal carcinoids are found in the distal ileum, with most congregating close to the ileocecal valve. Most intestinal carcinoids are asymptomatic and of low malignant potential, but invasion and metastases may occur, leading to the carcinoid syndrome (Chap. 350).

Leiomyosarcomas

Leiomyosarcomas often are >5 cm in diameter and may be palpable on abdominal examination. Bleeding, obstruction, and perforation are common. Such tumors should be analyzed for the expression of mutant *c-kit* receptor (defining GIST), and in the presence of metastatic disease, justifying treatment with imatinib mesylate (Gleevec) or, in imatinib-refractory patients, sunitinib (Sutent).

CANCERS OF THE ANUS

Cancers of the anus account for 1–2% of the malignant tumors of the large bowel. Most such lesions arise in the anal canal, the anatomic area extending from the anorectal ring to a zone approximately halfway between the pectinate (or dentate) line and the anal verge. Carcinomas arising proximal to the pectinate line (i.e., in the transitional zone between the glandular mucosa of the rectum and the squamous epithelium of the distal anus) are known as *basaloid*, *cuboidal*, or *cloacogenic* tumors; about one-third of anal cancers have this histologic pattern. Malignancies arising distal to the pectinate line have squamous histology, ulcerate more frequently, and constitute ~55% of anal cancers. The prognosis for patients with basaloid and squamous cell cancers of the anus is identical when corrected for tumor size and the presence or absence of nodal spread.

The development of anal cancer is associated with infection by human papillomavirus, the same organism etiologically linked to cervical cancer. The virus is sexually transmitted. The infection may lead to anal warts (condyloma acuminata), which may progress to anal intraepithelial neoplasia and on to squamous cell carcinoma. The risk for anal cancer is increased among homosexual males, presumably related to anal intercourse. Anal cancer risk is increased in both men and women with AIDS, possibly because their immunosuppressed state permits more severe papillomavirus infection. Anal cancers occur most commonly in middle-aged persons and are more frequent in women than men. At diagnosis, patients may experience bleeding, pain, sensation of a perianal mass, and pruritus.

Radical surgery (abdominal-perineal resection with lymph node sampling and a permanent colostomy) was once the treatment of choice for this tumor type. The 5-year survival rate after such a procedure was 55–70% in the absence of spread to regional lymph nodes and <20% if nodal involvement was present. An alternative therapeutic approach combining external beam radiation therapy with concomitant chemotherapy has resulted in biopsy-proven disappearance of all tumor in

>80% of patients whose initial lesion was <3 cm in size. Tumor recurrences develop in <10% of these patients, meaning that ~70% of patients with anal cancers can be cured with nonoperative treatment. Surgery should be reserved for the minority of individuals who are found to have residual tumor after being managed initially with radiation therapy combined with chemotherapy.

FURTHER READINGS

ABBAS A et al: Management of anal cancer in 2010: Parts 1 and 2. Oncology 24:364 and 417, 2010

CUNNINGHAM D et al: Colorectal cancer. Lancet 375:1030, 2010

ENZINGER PC, MAYER RJ: Esophageal cancer. N Engl J Med 349:2241, 2003

HARTGRINK HH et al: Gastric cancer. Lancet 374:477, 2009

LIEBERMAN DA: Clinical practice. Screening for colorectal cancer. N Engl J Med 2009 361:1179, 2009

LYNCH HT, DE LA CHAPELLE A: Hereditary colorectal cancer. N Engl J Med 348:919, 2003

RADERER M, PAUL DE BOER J: Role of chemotherapy in gastric MALT lymphoma, diffuse large B-cell lymphoma and other lymphomas. Best Pract Clin Gastroenterol 24:19, 2010

ROSTRUM A et al: Nonsteroidal anti-inflammatory drugs and cyclooxygenase-2 inhibitors for primary prevention of colorectal cancer: A systematic review prepared for the US Preventive Services Task Force. Ann Intern Med 146:376, 2007

ROTHWELL PM et al: Long-term effect of aspirin on colorectal cancer incidence and mortality: 20-year follow-up of five randomised trials. Lancet 376:1741, 2010

SHAHEEN NJ et al: Radiofrequency ablation in Barrett's esophagus with dysplasia. N Engl J Med 360:2277, 2009

SHARMA P: Clinical practice. Barrett's esophagus. N Engl J Med 361:2548, 2009

SPECHLER SJ: Barrett's esophagus. N Engl J Med 346:836, 2002

UEMURA N et al: *Helicobacter pylori* infection and the development of gastric cancer. N Engl J Med 345:784, 2001

WOLPIN BM et al: Adjuvant treatment of colorectal cancer. CA Cancer Clin J 57:168, 2007

CHAPTER 92

Tumors of the Liver and Biliary Tree

Brian I. Carr

HEPATOCELLULAR CARCINOMA

■ INCIDENCE

Hepatocellular carcinoma (HCC) is one of the most common malignancies worldwide. The annual global incidence is approximately 1 million cases, with a male to female ratio of approximately 4:1 (1:1 without cirrhosis to 9:1 in many high-incidence countries). The incidence rate equals the death rate. In the United States, approximately 22,000 new cases are diagnosed annually, with 18,000 deaths. The death rates in males in low-incidence countries such as the United States are 1.9 per 100,000 per year; in intermediate areas such as Austria and South Africa, they range from 5.1–20; and in high-incidence areas such as in the Orient (China and Korea) as high as 23.1–150 per 100,000 per year (Table 92-1). The incidence of HCC in the United States is approximately 3 per 100,000 persons, with significant gender, ethnic, and geographic variations. These numbers are rapidly increasing and may be an underestimate. Approximately 4 million chronic hepatitis C virus (HCV) carriers are in the United States alone. Approximately 10% of them or 400,000 are likely to develop cirrhosis. Approximately 5% or 20,000 of these may develop HCC annually. Add to this the two other common predisposing factors—hepatitis B virus (HBV) and chronic alcohol consumption—and 60,000 new HCC cases annually seem possible. Future advances in HCC survival will likely depend in part on immunization strategies for HBV (and HCV) and earlier diagnosis by screening of patients at risk of HCC development.

Current directions

With the U.S. HCV epidemic, HCC is increasing in most states, and obesity-associated liver disease (nonalcoholic steatohepatitis [NASH]) is increasingly recognized as a cause.

■ EPIDEMIOLOGY

There are two general types of epidemiologic studies of HCC—those of country-based incidence rates (Table 92-1) and those of migrants. Endemic hot spots occur in areas of China and sub-Saharan Africa, which are associated both with high endemic hepatitis B carrier rates as well as mycotoxin contamination of foodstuffs (aflatoxin B_1), stored grains, drinking water, and soil. Environmental factors are important, for example, Japanese in Japan have a higher incidence than those living in Hawaii, who in turn have a higher incidence than those living in California.

■ ETIOLOGIC FACTORS

Chemical carcinogens

Causative agents for HCC have been studied along two general lines. First are agents identified as carcinogenic in experimental animals (particularly rodents) that are thought to be present in the human environment (Table 92-2). Second, is the association of HCC with various other clinical conditions. Probably the best-studied and most potent ubiquitous natural chemical carcinogen is a product of the *Aspergillus* fungus, called aflatoxin B_1. This mold and aflatoxin product can be found in a variety of stored grains in hot, humid places, where peanuts and rice are stored in unrefrigerated conditions. Aflatoxin contamination of foodstuffs correlates well with incidence rates in Africa and to some extent in China. In endemic areas of China, even farm animals such as ducks have HCC. The most potent carcinogens appear to be natural products of plants, fungi, and bacteria, such as bush trees containing pyrrolizidine alkaloids as well as tannic acid and safrole. Pollutants such as pesticides and insecticides are known rodent carcinogens.

TABLE 92-1 Age-Adjusted Incidence Rates for Hepatocellular Carcinoma

Country	Persons per 100,000 per Year	
	Male	Female
Argentina	6.0	2.5
Brazil, Recife	9.2	8.3
Brazil, Sao Paulo	3.8	2.6
Mozambique	112.9	30.8
South Africa, Cape: Black	26.3	8.4
South Africa, Cape: White	1.2	0.6
Senegal	25.6	9.0
Nigeria	15.4	3.2
Gambia	33.1	12.6
Burma	25.5	8.8
Japan	7.2	2.2
Korea	13.8	3.2
China, Shanghai	34.4	11.6
India, Bombay	4.9	2.5
India, Madras	2.1	0.7
Great Britain	1.6	0.8
France	6.9	1.2
Italy, Varese	7.1	2.7
Norway	1.8	1.1
Spain, Navarra	7.9	4.7

TABLE 92-2 Factors Associated With an Increased Risk of Developing HCC

Common	Unusual
Cirrhosis from any cause	Primary biliary cirrhosis
Hepatitis B or C chronic infection	Hemochromatosis
Ethanol chronic consumption	α_1 Antitrypsin deficiency
NASH/NAFL	Glycogen storage diseases
Aflatoxin B_1 or other mycotoxins	Citrullinemia
	Porphyria cutanea tarda
	Hereditary tyrosinemia
	Wilson's disease

Abbreviations: NAFL, nonalcoholic fatty liver; NASH, nonalcoholic steatohepatitis.

Hepatitis

Both case-control and cohort studies have shown a strong association between chronic hepatitis B carrier rates and increased incidence of HCC. In Taiwanese male postal carriers who were hepatitis B surface antigen (HBsAg)-positive, a 98-fold greater risk for HCC was found compared to HBsAg-negative individuals. The incidence of HCC in Alaskan natives is markedly increased related to a high prevalence of HBV infection. HBV-based HCC may involve rounds of hepatic destruction with subsequent proliferation and not necessarily frank cirrhosis. The increase in Japanese HCC incidence rates in the last three decades is thought to be from hepatitis C. A large-scale World Health Organization (WHO)-sponsored intervention study is currently underway in Asia involving HBV vaccination of the newborn. HCC in African blacks is not associated with severe cirrhosis but is poorly differentiated and very aggressive. Despite uniform HBV carrier rates among the South African Bantu, there is a ninefold difference in HCC incidence between Mozambicans living along the coast and inland. These differences are attributed to the additional exposure to dietary aflatoxin B_1 and other carcinogenic mycotoxins. A typical interval between HCV-associated transfusion and subsequent HCC is approximately 30 years. HCV-associated HCC patients tend to have more frequent and advanced cirrhosis, but in HBV-associated HCC, only half the patients have cirrhosis; the remainder having chronic active hepatitis (Chap. 306).

Other etiologic conditions

The 75–85% association of HCC with underlying cirrhosis has long been recognized, more typically with macronodular cirrhosis in Southeast Asia, but also with micronodular cirrhosis (alcohol) in Europe and the United States (Chap. 308). It is still not clear whether cirrhosis itself is a predisposing factor to the development of HCC or whether the underlying causes of the cirrhosis are actually the carcinogenic factors. However, ~20% of U.S. patients with HCC do not have underlying cirrhosis. Several underlying conditions are associated with an increased risk for cirrhosis-associated HCC (Table 92-2), including hepatitis, alcohol, autoimmune chronic active hepatitis, cryptogenic cirrhosis, and NASH. A less common association is with primary biliary cirrhosis and several metabolic diseases including hemochromatosis, Wilson disease, α_1-antitrypsin deficiency, tyrosinemia, porphyria cutanea tarda, glycogenesis types 1 and 3, citrullinemia. and orotic aciduria. The etiology of HCC in those 20% of patients who have no cirrhosis is currently unclear, and their HCC natural history is not well-defined.

Current directions

Many patients have multiple etiologies, and the interactions of either hepatitis or alcohol and smoking, or with aflatoxins, are just beginning to be explored.

◼ CLINICAL FEATURES

Symptoms

These include abdominal pain, weight loss, weakness, abdominal fullness and swelling, jaundice, and nausea (Table 92-3). Presenting signs and symptoms differ somewhat between high- and low-incidence areas. In high-risk areas, especially in South African blacks, the most common symptom is abdominal pain; by contrast, only 40–50% of Chinese and Japanese patients present with abdominal pain. Abdominal swelling may occur as a consequence of ascites due to the underlying chronic liver disease or may be due to a rapidly expanding tumor. Occasionally, central necrosis or acute hemorrhage into the peritoneal cavity leads to death. In countries with an active

TABLE 92-3 Hepatocellular Carcinoma Clinical Presentation (*n* = 547)

Symptom	Patient # (%)
No symptom	129(24)
Abdominal pain	219(40)
Other (workup of anemia and various diseases)	64(12)
Routine physical exam finding, elevated LFTs	129(24)
Weight loss	112(20)
Appetite loss	59 (11)
Weakness/malaise	83(15)
Jaundice	30(5)
Routine CT scan screening of known cirrhosis	92(17)
Cirrhosis symptoms (ankle swelling, abdominal bloating, increased girth, pruritus, GI bleed)	98(18)
Diarrhea	7 (1)
Tumor rupture	1
Patient Characteristics	
Mean age (yr)	56 ± 13
Male:Female	3:1
Ethnicity	
White	72 %
Middle Eastern	10 %
Asian	13 %
African American	5 %
Cirrhosis	81 %
No cirrhosis	19 %
Tumor Characteristics	
Hepatic tumor numbers	
1	20 %
2	25 %
3 or more	65 %
Portal vein invasion	75 %
Unilobar	25 %
Bilobar	75 %

Abbreviations: GI, gastrointestinal; LFT, liver function test.

surveillance program, HCC tends to be identified at an earlier stage, when symptoms may be due only to the underlying disease. Jaundice is usually due to obstruction of the intrahepatic ducts from underlying liver disease. Hematemesis may occur due to esophageal varices from the underlying portal hypertension. Bone pain is seen in 3–12% of patients, but necropsies show pathologic bone metastases in ~20% of patients. However, 25% of patients may be asymptomatic.

Physical signs

Hepatomegaly is the most common physical sign, occurring in 50–90% of the patients. Abdominal bruits are noted in 6–25%, and ascites occurs in 30–60% of patients. Ascites should be examined by cytology. Splenomegaly is mainly due to portal hypertension. Weight loss and muscle wasting are common, particularly with rapidly growing or large tumors. Fever is found in 10–50% of patients, from unclear cause. The signs of chronic liver disease may often be present, including jaundice, dilated abdominal veins, palmar erythema, gynecomastia, testicular atrophy, and peripheral edema. Budd-Chiari syndrome can occur due to HCC invasion of the hepatic veins, with tense ascites and a large tender liver (Chap. 308).

Paraneoplastic syndromes

Most paraneoplastic syndromes in HCC are biochemical abnormalities without associated clinical consequences. They include hypoglycemia (also caused by end-stage liver failure), erythrocytosis, hypercalcemia, hypercholesterolemia, dysfibrinogenemia, carcinoid syndrome, increased thyroxin-binding globulin, changes in secondary sex characteristics (gynecomastia, testicular atrophy, and precocious puberty), and porphyria cutanea tarda. Mild hypoglycemia occurs in rapidly growing HCC as part of terminal illness, and profound hypoglycemia may occur, although the cause is unclear. Erythrocytosis occurs in 3–12% of patients and hypercholesterolemia in 10–40%. A high percent of patients have thrombocytopenia or leukopenia, resulting from portal hypertension, and not from cancer infiltration of bone marrow, as in other tumor types.

▉ STAGING

Multiple clinical staging systems for HCC have been described. A widely used one has been the American Joint Commission for Cancer (AJCC)/tumor-node-metastasis (TNM) classification. However, the Cancer of the Liver Italian Program (CLIP) system is now popular as it takes the cirrhosis into account, based on the Okuda system (Table 92-4). Other staging systems have been proposed, and a consensus is needed. They are all based on combining the prognostic features of liver damage with those of tumor aggressiveness and include systems from Spain (Barcelona Clinic Liver Cancer [BCLC]), Japan, Hong Kong, and others (Chinese University Prognostic Index [CUPI], Japan Integrated Staging

[JIS], and SLiDe which stands for S, stage; Li, liver damage; De, des-γ-carboxy prothrombin). The best prognosis is for stage I, solitary tumors of less than 2-cm diameter without vascular invasion. Adverse prognostic features include ascites, jaundice, vascular invasion, and elevated α-fetoproteins (AFPs). Vascular invasion in particular has profound effects on prognosis and may be microscopic or macroscopic (visible on CT scans). Most large tumors have microscopic vascular invasion, so full staging can usually be made only after surgical resection. Stage III disease contains a mixture of lymph node–positive and -negative tumors. Stage III patients with positive lymph node disease have a poor prognosis, and few patients survive 1 year. The prognosis of stage IV is poor after either resection or transplantation and 1-year survival is rare. A working staging system based entirely on clinical grounds that incorporates the contribution of the underlying liver disease was originally developed by Okuda et al. (Table 92-4). Patients with Okuda stage III have a dire prognosis because they usually cannot be curatively resected, and the condition of their liver typically precludes chemotherapy.

New directions

Consensus is needed on staging. These systems will soon be upended by proteomics.

APPROACH TO THE PATIENT | Hepatocellular Carcinoma

HISTORY AND PHYSICAL The history is important in evaluating putative predisposing factors, including a history of hepatitis or jaundice, blood transfusion, or use of intravenous drugs. A family history of HCC or hepatitis should be sought and a detailed social history taken to include job descriptions for industrial exposure to possible carcinogenic drugs as well as contraceptive hormones. Physical examination should include assessing stigmata of underlying liver disease such as jaundice, ascites, peripheral edema, spider nevi, palmar erythema, and weight loss. Evaluation of the abdomen for hepatic size, masses or ascites, hepatic nodularity and tenderness, and splenomegaly is needed, as is assessment of overall performance status and psychosocial evaluation.

SEROLOGIC ASSAYS AFP is a serum tumor marker for HCC; however, it is only increased in approximately one-half of U.S. patients. The lens culinaris agglutinin-reactive fraction of AFP (AFP-L3) assay is thought to be more specific. The other widely used assay is that for des-γ-carboxy prothrombin (DCP), a protein induced by vitamin K absence (PIVKA-2). This protein is increased in as many as 80% of HCC patients but may also be elevated in patients with vitamin K deficiency; it is always elevated after Coumadin use. It may predict for portal vein invasion. Both AFP-L3 and DCP are FDA-approved. Many other assays have been developed, such as glypican-3, but none have greater aggregate sensitivity and specificity. In a patient presenting with either a new hepatic mass or other indications of recent hepatic decompensation, carcinoembryonic antigen (CEA), vitamin B_{12}, AFP, ferritin, PIVKA-2, and anti-mitochondrial Ab should be measured, and standard liver function tests should be performed, including prothrombin time (PT), partial thromboplastin time (PTT), albumin, transaminases, γ-glutamyl transpeptidase, and alkaline phosphatase. Decreases in platelet count and white blood cell count may reflect portal hypertension and associated hypersplenism. Hepatitis A, B, and C serology should be measured. If HBV or HCV serology is positive, quantitative measurements of HBV DNA or HCV RNA are needed.

TABLE 92-4 CLIP and Okuda Staging Systems for Hepatocellular Carcinoma

CLIP Classification

	Points		
Variables	0	1	2
i. Tumor number	Single	Multiple	–
Hepatic replacement by tumor (%)	<50	<50	>50
ii. Child-Pugh score	A	B	C
iii. α Fetoprotein level (ng/mL)	<400	≥400	–
iv. Portal vein thrombosis (CT)	No	Yes	–

CLIP stages (score = sum of points): CLIP 0, 0 points; CLIP 1, 1 point; CLIP 2, 2 points; CLIP 3, 3 points.

Okuda Classification

Tumor extent[a]		Ascites		Albumin (g/L)		Bilirubin (mg/dL)	
≥50%	<50	+	–	≤3	>3	≥ 3	<3
(+)	(–)	(+)	(–)	(+)	(–)	(+)	(–)

Okuda stages: stage 1, all (–); stage 2, 1 or 2 (+); stage 3, 3 or 4 (+)

Abbreviations: CLIP, Cancer of the Liver Italian Program.
[a]Extent of liver occupied by tumor

New Directions Newer biomarkers are being evaluated, especially tissue- and serum-based genomics profiling.

RADIOLOGY An ultrasound examination of the liver is an excellent screening tool. The two characteristic vascular abnormalities are hypervascularity of the tumor mass (neovascularization or abnormal tumor-feeding arterial vessels) and thrombosis by tumor invasion of otherwise normal portal veins. To determine tumor size and extent and the presence of portal vein invasion accurately, a helical/triphasic CT scan of the abdomen and pelvis, with fast-contrast bolus technique should be performed to detect the vascular lesions typical of HCC. Portal vein invasion is normally detected as an obstruction and expansion of the vessel. A chest CT is used to exclude metastases. MRI can also provide detailed information, especially with the newer contrast agents. Ethiodol (Lipiodol) is an ethiodized oil emulsion retained by liver tumors that can be delivered by hepatic artery injection (5–15 mL) for CT imaging 1 week later. For small tumors, Ethiodol injection is very helpful before biopsy because the histological presence of the dye constitutes proof that the needle biopsied the mass under suspicion. A prospective comparison of triphasic CT, gadolinium-enhanced MRI, ultrasound, and fluorodeoxyglucose positron emission tomography (FDG-PET) showed similar results for CT, MRI, and ultrasound; PET imaging was unsuccessful.

New Directions The altered tumor vascularity that is a consequence of molecularly targeted therapies is the basis for newer imaging techniques including contrast-enhanced ultrasound (CEUS) and dynamic MRI.

PATHOLOGIC DIAGNOSIS Histologic proof of the presence of HCC is obtained through a core liver biopsy of the liver mass under ultrasound guidance, as well as random biopsy of the underlying liver. Bleeding risk is increased compared to other cancers because (1) the tumors are hypervascular, and (2) patients often have thrombocytopenia and decreased liver-dependent clotting factors. Bleeding risk is further increased in the presence of ascites. Tracking of tumor has an uncommon problem. Fine-needle aspirates can provide sufficient material for diagnosis of cancer, but core biopsies are preferred. Tissue architecture allows the distinction between HCC and adenocarcinoma. Laparoscopic approaches can also be used. For patients suspected of having portal vein involvement, a core biopsy of the portal vein may be performed safely. If positive, this is regarded as an exclusion criterion for transplantation for HCC.

New Directions Immunohistochemistry has become mainstream. Prognostic subgroupings are being defined based on growth signaling pathway proteins and genotyping strategies. Furthermore, molecular profiling of the underlying liver has provided evidence for a "field-effect" of cirrhosis in generating recurrent or new HCCs after primary resection.

◼ SCREENING HIGH-RISK POPULATIONS

Screening has not been shown to save lives. Prospective studies in high-risk populations showed that ultrasound was more sensitive than AFP elevations. An Italian study in patients with cirrhosis identified a yearly HCC incidence of 3% but showed no increase in the rate of detection of potentially curable tumors with aggressive screening. Prevention strategies including universal vaccination against hepatitis are more likely to be effective than screening efforts. Despite absence of formal guidelines, most practitioners obtain 6-monthly AFP and CT (or ultrasound) when following high-risk patients (HBV carriers, HCV cirrhosis, family history of HCC).

Current directions

Cost-benefit analysis is not yet convincing, even though screening is intuitively sound. However, studies from areas of high HBV carrier rates have shown a survival benefit for screening as a result of earlier stage at diagnosis. Gamma-glutamyl transpeptidase appears useful for detecting small tumors.

TREATMENT ▶ **Hepatocellular Carcinoma**

Most HCC patients have two liver diseases, cirrhosis and HCC, each of which is an independent cause of death. The presence of cirrhosis usually places constraints on resection surgery, ablative therapies, and chemotherapy. Thus patient assessment and treatment planning has to take the severity of the nonmalignant liver disease into account. The clinical management choices for HCC can be complex (Fig. 92-1, Table 92-5, and Table 92-6). The natural history of HCC is highly variable. Patients presenting with advanced tumors (vascular invasion, symptoms, extrahepatic spread) have a median survival of ~4 months, with or without treatment. Treatment results from the literature are difficult to interpret. Survival is not always a measure of the efficacy of therapy because of the adverse effects on survival of the underlying liver disease. A multidisciplinary team, including a hepatologist, interventional radiologist, surgical oncologist, transplant surgeon, and medical oncologist, is important for the comprehensive management of HCC patients.

STAGES I AND II HCC Early-stage tumors are successfully treated using various techniques, including surgical resection, local ablation (thermal or radiofrequency [RFA]), and local injection therapies (Table 92-6). Because the majority of patients with HCC suffer from a field defect in the cirrhotic liver, they are at risk for subsequent multiple primary liver tumors. Many will also have significant underlying liver disease and may not tolerate major surgical loss of hepatic parenchyma, and they may be eligible for orthotopic liver transplant (OLTX). Living related donor transplants have increased in popularity resulting in absence of waiting for a transplant. An important principle in treating early-stage HCC is to use liver-sparing treatments and to focus on treatment of both the tumor and the cirrhosis.

Surgical Excision The risk of major hepatectomy is high (5–10% mortality rate) due to the underlying liver disease and the potential for liver failure, but acceptable in selected cases. Preoperative portal vein occlusion can sometimes be performed to cause atrophy of the HCC-involved lobe and compensatory hypertrophy of the noninvolved liver, permitting safer resection. Intraoperative ultrasound (US) is useful for planning the surgical approach. The US can image the proximity of major vascular structures that may be encountered during the dissection. In cirrhotic patients, any major liver surgery can result in liver failure. The Child-Pugh classification of liver failure is still a reliable prognosticator for tolerance of hepatic surgery and only Child A patients should be considered for surgical resection. Child B and C patients with stages I and II HCC should be referred for OLTX if appropriate, as well as patients with ascites or a recent history of variceal bleeding. Although open surgical excision is the most reliable, the patient may be better served with a laparoscopic approach to resection, using RFA or percutaneous ethanol injection (PEI). No adequate comparisons of these different techniques have been undertaken and the choice of treatment is usually based on physician skill.

Local Ablation Strategies Radiofrequency ablation (RFA) uses heat to ablate tumors. The maximum size of the probe arrays

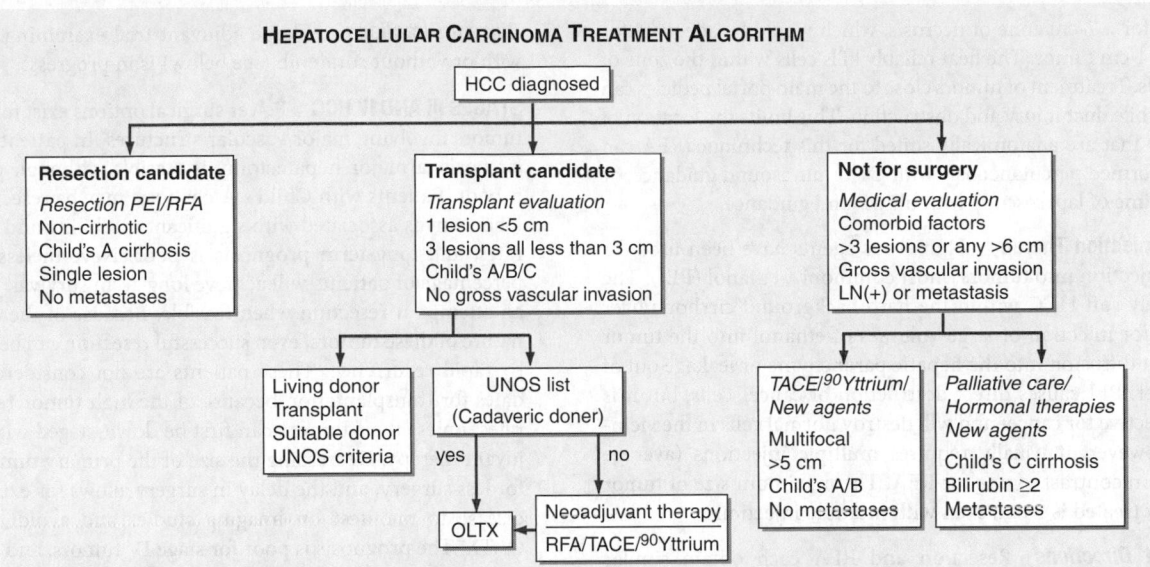

Figure 92-1   Hepatocellular carcinoma treatment algorithm. Treatment approach to patients with hepatocellular carcinoma. The initial clinical evaluation is aimed at assessing the extent of the tumor and the underlying functional compromise of the liver by cirrhosis. Patients are classified as having resectable disease, unresectable disease, or as transplantation candidates. LN, lymph node; OLTX, orthotopic liver transplantation; PEI, percutaneous ethanol injection; RFA, radiofrequency ablation; TACE, transarterial chemoembolization; UNOS, United Network for Organ Sharing. Child's A/B/C refers to the Child-Pugh classification of liver failure.

TABLE 92-5 Treatment Options for Hepatocellular Carcinoma

Surgery

Resection

Liver transplantation

Local Ablative Therapies

Cryosurgery

Radiofrequency ablation (RFA)

Percutaneous ethanol injection (PEI)

Regional Therapies: Hepatic Artery Transcatheter Treatments

Transarterial chemotherapy

Transarterial embolization

Transarterial chemoembolization

Transarterial drug-eluting beads

Transarterial radiotherapies:

^{90}Yttrium microspheres

^{131}Iodine - Ethiodol

Conformal External-Beam Radiation

Therapy systemic therapies

Molecularly targeted therapies (sorafenib, etc.)

Chemotherapy

Immunotherapy

Hormonal therapy + growth control

Supportive therapies

TABLE 92-6 Some Randomized Clinical Trials Involving Transhepatic Artery Chemoembolization (TACE) for Hepatocellular Carcinoma

Author	Year	Agents 1	Agents 2	Survival Effect
Kawaii	1992	Doxorubicin + Embo	Embo	No
Chang	1994	Cisplatin + Embo	Embo	No
Hatanaka	1995	Cisplatin, Doxorubicin + Embo	Same + Lipiodol	No
Uchino	1993	Cisplatin, Doxorubicin + oral FU	Same + Tamoxifen	No
Lin	1988	Embo	Embo + IV FU	No
Yoshikawa	1994	Epirubicin + Ethiodol	Epirubicin	No
Pelletier	1990	Doxorubicin + Gelfoam	None	No
Trinchet	1995	Cisplatin + Gelfoam	None	No
Bruix	1998	Coils and Gelfoam	None	No
Pelletier	1998	Cisplatin + Ethiodol	None	No
Trinchet	1995	Cisplatin + Gelfoam	None	No
Lo	2002	Cisplatin + Ethiodol	None	Yes
Llovet	2002	Doxorubicin + Ethiodol	None	Yes

Abbreviations: Embo, embolization; FU, 5-fluorouracil.

allows for a 7-cm zone of necrosis, which would be adequate for a 3- to 4-cm tumor. The heat reliably kills cells within the zone of necrosis. Treatment of tumors close to the main portal pedicles can lead to bile duct injury and obstruction. This limits the location of tumors that are anatomically suited for this technique. RFA can be performed percutaneously with CT or ultrasound guidance, or at the time of laparoscopy with ultrasound guidance.

Local Injection Therapy Numerous agents have been used for local injection into tumors, most commonly, ethanol (PEI). The relatively soft HCC within the hard background cirrhotic liver allows for injection of large volumes of ethanol into the tumor without diffusion into the hepatic parenchyma or leakage out of the liver. PEI causes direct destruction of cancer cells, but it is not selective for cancer and will destroy normal cells in the vicinity. However, it usually requires multiple injections (average three), in contrast to one for RFA. The maximum size of tumor reliably treated is 3 cm, even with multiple injections.

Current Directions Resection and RFA each obtain similar results.

Liver Transplantation (OLTX) A viable option for stages I and II tumors in the setting of cirrhosis is OLTX, with survival approaching that for noncancer cases. OLTX for patients with a single lesion ≤5 cm or three or fewer nodules, each ≤3 cm (Milan criteria), resulted in excellent tumor-free survival (≥70% at 5 years). For advanced HCC, OLTX has been abandoned due to high tumor recurrence rates. Priority scoring for OLTX previously led to HCC patients waiting too long for their OLTX, resulting in some tumors becoming too advanced during the patient's wait for a donated liver. A variety of therapies were used as a "bridge" to OLTX, including RFA, polyethylenimine, and transcatheter arterial chemoembolization (TACE). It seems clear that these pretransplant treatments allow patients to remain on the waiting list longer, giving them greater opportunities to be transplanted. What remains unclear, however, is whether this translates into prolonged survival after transplant. Further, it is not known whether patients who have had their tumor(s) treated preoperatively follow the recurrence pattern predicted by their tumor status at the time of transplant (i.e., post–local ablative therapy), or if they follow the course set by their tumor parameters present before such treatment. The United Network for Organ Sharing (UNOS) point system for priority scoring of OLTX recipients now includes additional points for patients with HCC. The success of living related donor liver transplantation programs has also led to patients receiving transplantation earlier for HCC and often with greater than minimal tumors.

Current Directions Expanded criteria for larger HCCs beyond the Milan criteria (one lesion <5 cm or three lesions, each less than 3 cm) are being increasingly accepted by various UNOS areas for OLTX with satisfactory longer-term survival. Furthermore, downstaging HCCs by medical therapy (TACE) is increasingly recognized as acceptable treatment before OLTX.

Adjuvant Therapy The role of adjuvant chemotherapy for patients after resection or OLTX remains unclear. Both adjuvant and neoadjuvant approaches have been studied, but no clear advantage in disease-free or overall survival has been found. However, a meta-analysis of several trials revealed a significant improvement in disease-free and overall survival. Although analysis of postoperative adjuvant systemic chemotherapy trials demonstrated no disease-free or overall survival advantage, single studies of TACE and neoadjuvant ^{131}I-Ethiodol showed enhanced survival post-resection.

Current Directions A large adjuvant trial examining resection with or without sorafenib (see below) is in progress.

STAGES III AND IV HCC Fewer surgical options exist for stage III tumors involving major vascular structures. In patients without cirrhosis, a major hepatectomy is feasible, although prognosis is poor. Patients with Child's A cirrhosis may be resected, but a lobectomy is associated with significant morbidity and mortality rates, and long-term prognosis is poor. Nevertheless, a small percentage of patients will achieve long-term survival, justifying an attempt at resection when feasible. Because of the advanced nature of these tumors, even successful resection can be followed by rapid recurrence. These patients are not considered candidates for transplantation because of the high tumor recurrence rates, unless their tumors can first be down-staged with neoadjuvant therapy. Decreasing the size of the primary tumor allows for less surgery, and the delay in surgery allows for extrahepatic disease to manifest on imaging studies and avoid unhelpful OLTX. The prognosis is poor for stage IV tumors, and no surgical treatment is recommended.

Systemic Chemotherapy A large number of controlled and uncontrolled clinical studies have been performed with most of the major classes of cancer chemotherapy. No single agent or combination of agents given systemically reproducibly leads to even a 25% response rate or has any effect on survival.

Regional Chemotherapy In contrast to the dismal results of systemic chemotherapy, a variety of agents given via the hepatic artery have activity for HCC confined to the liver (Table 92-6). Two randomized controlled trials have shown a survival advantage for TACE in a selected subset of patients. One used doxorubicin and the other used cisplatin. Despite the fact that increased hepatic extraction of chemotherapy has been shown for very few drugs, some drugs such as cisplatin, doxorubicin, mitomycin C, and possibly neocarzinostatin, produce substantial objective responses when administered regionally. Few data are available on continuous hepatic arterial infusion for HCC, although pilot studies with cisplatin have shown encouraging responses. Because the reports have not usually stratified responses or survival based on TNM staging, it is difficult to know long-term prognosis in relation to tumor extent. Most of the studies on regional hepatic arterial chemotherapy also use an embolizing agent such as Ethiodol, gelatin sponge particles (Gelfoam), starch (Spherex), or microspheres. Two products are composed of microspheres of defined size ranges—Embospheres (Biospheres) and Contour SE—using particles of 40–120, 100–300, 300–500, and 500–1000 μm in size. The optimal diameter of the particles for TACE has yet to be defined. Consistently higher objective response rates are reported for arterial administration of drugs together with some form of hepatic artery occlusion compared with any form of systemic chemotherapy to date. The widespread use of some form of embolization in addition to chemotherapy has added to its toxicities. These include a frequent, but transient fever, abdominal pain, and anorexia (all in >60% of patients). In addition, >20% of patients have increased ascites or transient elevation of transaminases. Cystic artery spasm and cholecystitis are also not uncommon. However, higher responses have also been obtained. The hepatic toxicities associated with embolization may be ameliorated by the use of degradable starch microspheres, with 50–60% response rates. Two randomized studies of TACE vs. placebo showed a survival advantage for treatment (Table 92-6). In addition, it is not clear that formal oncologic CT response criteria are adequate for HCC. A loss of vascularity on CT without size change may be an

TABLE 92-7 Targeted Therapies in HCC: Trials

Phase III	Target	Survival (mo)
Sorafenib vs placebo	Raf, VEGFR, PDGFR	10.7 vs. 7.9
Sorafenib vs placebo (Asians)	Raf, WGFR, PDGFR	6.5 vs. 4.2
Phase II		
Sorafenib		9
Sorafenib (Asians)		5
Sunitinib		9.8, 8 (2 trials)
Bevacizumab	VEGF	12.4
Bevacizumab plus erlotinib	VEGF plus EGFR	15.6
Bevacizumab plus capecitabine		8
Erlotinib	EGFR	13, 10.7 (2 trials)
Linifanib	VEGFR, PDGF	9.7
Brivanib	VEGFR, FGFR	10

Abbreviations: EGFR, epidermal growth factor receptor; FGFR, fibroblast growth factor receptor; PDGF, platelet-derived growth factor; PDGFR, platelet-derived growth factor receptor; Raf, rapidly accelerated fibrosarcoma; VEGF, vascular endothelial growth factor; VEGFR vascular endothelial growth factor receptor.

TABLE 92-8 Some Novel Medical Treatments for Hepatocellular Carcinoma

EGF receptor antagonists: Erlotinib, gefitinib, lapatinib, cetuximab, brivanib

Multi-kinase antagonists: sorafenib, sunitinib

VEGF antagonist: bevacizumab

VEGFR antagonist: ABT-869 (linifanib)

mTOR antagonists: sirolimus, temsirolimus, everolimus

Proteasome inhibitors: bortezomib

Vitamin K

^{131}I – Ethiodol (lipiodol)

^{131}I – Ferritin

^{90}Yttrium microspheres (TheraSphere, SIR-spheres)

^{166}Holmium, ^{188}Rhenium

Three-dimensional conformal radiation

Proton beam high-dose radiotherapy

Gamma knife, CyberKnife

New targets: inhibitors of cyclin dependent kinases (Cdk) and caspases

Abbreviations: EGF, epidermal growth factor; VEGF, vascular endothelial growth factor; VEGFR vascular endothelial growth factor receptor.

index of loss of viability and thus of response to TACE. A major problem that TACE trials have had in showing a survival advantage is that many HCC patients die of their underlying cirrhosis, not the tumor. However, improving quality of life is a legitimate goal of regional therapy.

New Therapies The major finding has been a survival advantage for oral sorafenib (Nexavar) vs. placebo controls in two randomized trials, leading to its approval by the FDA. However, tumor responses were negligible, and the survival in the treatment arm in Asians was below the placebo arm in the Western trial (Table 92-7). Furthermore, prolonged survival has been reported in phase II trials using newer agents, such as bevacizumab plus erlotinib. Several forms of *radiation therapy* have been used in the treatment of HCC, including external beam radiation and conformal radiation therapy. Radiation hepatitis remains a dose-limiting problem. The pure beta emitter ^{90}Yttrium attached to either glass or resin microspheres has been assessed in phase II trials of HCC and has encouraging survival effects with minimal toxicities. Randomized trials have yet to be performed. Vitamin K has been assessed in clinical trials at high dosage for its HCC-inhibitory actions. This idea is based on the characteristic biochemical defect in HCC of elevated plasma levels of immature prothrombin (DCP or PIVKA-2), due to a defect in the activity of prothrombin carboxylase, a vitamin K-dependent enzyme. Two vitamin K randomized controlled trials from Japan show decreased tumor occurrence.

Current Directions A number of new treatments are being evaluated for HCC (Table 92-8). These include the biologicals, such as Raf kinase and vascular endothelial growth factor (VEGF) inhibitors, ^{90}Yttrium looks promising without chemotherapy toxicities, and vitamin K_2 appears to prevent recurrences post-resection. The bottleneck of liver donors for OLTX is at last widening with increasing use of living donors, and criteria for OLTX for larger HCCs are slowly expanding. Patient participation in clinical trials assessing new therapies is encouraged (*www.clinicaltrials.gov*).

■ SUMMARY (TABLE 92-5)

The most common modes of patient presentation

1. A patient with known history of hepatitis, jaundice, or cirrhosis, with an abnormality on US or CT scan, or rising AFP or DCP (PIVKA-2)
2. A patient with an abnormal liver function test as part of a routine examination
3. Radiologic workup for liver transplant for cirrhosis
4. Symptoms of HCC including cachexia, abdominal pain, or fever

History and physical examination:

1. Clinical jaundice, asthenia, itching (scratches), tremors, or disorientation
2. Hepatomegaly, splenomegaly, ascites, peripheral edema, skin signs of liver failure

Clinical evaluation:

1. Blood tests: full blood count (splenomegaly), liver function tests, ammonia levels, electrolytes, AFP and DCP (PIVKA-2), Ca^{2+} and Mg^{2+}; hepatitis B, C, and D serology (and quantitative HBV DNA or HCV RNA, if either is positive); neurotensin (specific for fibrolamellar HCC)
2. Triphasic dynamic helical (spiral) CT scan of liver (if inadequate, then follow with an MRI); chest CT scan; upper and lower gastrointestinal endoscopy (for varices, bleeding, ulcers); and brain scan (only if symptoms suggest)
3. Core biopsy: of the tumor and separate biopsy of the underlying liver

Therapy (Tables 92-5 and 92-6):

1. HCC <2 cm: RFA, PEI, or resection
2. HCC >2 cm, no vascular invasion: liver resection, RFA, or OLTX
3. Multiple unilobar tumors or tumor with vascular invasion: TACE or sorafenib
4. Bilobar tumors, no vascular invasion: TACE with OLTX for patients with tumor response
5. Extrahepatic HCC or elevated bilirubin: sorafenib or bevacizumab plus erlotinib (combination agent trials are in progress)

OTHER PRIMARY LIVER TUMORS

■ FIBROLAMELLAR HCC (FL-HCC)

This rarer variant of HCC has a quite different biology than adult-type HCC. None of the known HCC causative factors seem important here. It is typically a disease of younger adults, often teenagers and predominantly females. It is AFP-negative, but patients typically have elevated blood neurotensin levels, normal liver function tests, and no cirrhosis. Radiology is similar for HCC, except that characteristic adult-type portal vein invasion is less common. Although it is often multifocal in the liver, and therefore not resectable, metastases are common, especially to lungs and locoregional lymph nodes, but survival is often much better than with adult-type HCC. Resectable tumors are associated with 5-year survival ≥50%. Patients often present with a huge liver or unexplained weight loss, fever, or elevated liver function tests on routine evaluations. These huge masses suggest quite slow growth for many tumors. Surgical resection is the best management option, even for metastases, as these tumors respond much less well to chemotherapy than adult-type HCC. Although several series of OLTX for FL-HCC have been reported, the patients seem to die from tumor recurrences, with a 2- to 5-year lag compared with OLTX for adult-type HCC. Anecdotal responses to gemcitabine plus cisplatin-TACE are reported.

Epithelioid hemangioendothelioma (EHE)

This rare vascular tumor of adults is also usually multifocal and can also be associated with prolonged survival, even in the presence of metastases, which are commonly in the lung. There is usually no underlying cirrhosis. Histologically, these tumors are usually of borderline malignancy and express factor VIII, confirming their endothelial origin. OLTX may produce prolonged survival.

Cholangiocarcinoma (CCC)

CCC typically refers to mucin-producing adenocarcinomas (different from HCC) that arise from the bile ducts. They are grouped by their anatomic site of origin, as intrahepatic, hilar (central, ~65% of CCCs), and peripheral (or distal, ~30% of CCCs). They arise on the basis of cirrhosis less frequently than HCC, excepting primary biliary cirrhosis. Nodular tumors arising at the bifurcation of the common bile duct are called *Klatskin* tumors and are often associated with a collapsed gallbladder, a finding that mandates visualization of the entire biliary tree. The approach to management of central and peripheral CCC is quite different. Incidence is increasing. Although most CCCs have no obvious cause, a number of predisposing factors have been identified. Predisposing diseases include primary sclerosing cholangitis (10–20% of primary sclerosing cholangitis [PSC] patients), an autoimmune disease, and liver fluke in Asians, especially *Opisthorchis viverrini* and *Clonorchis sinensis*. CCC seems also to be associated with any cause of chronic biliary inflammation and injury, with alcoholic liver disease,

choledocholithiasis, choledochal cysts (10%), and Caroli's disease (a rare inherited form of bile duct ectasia). CCC most typically presents as painless jaundice, often with pruritus or weight loss. Diagnosis is made by biopsy, percutaneously for peripheral liver lesions, or more commonly via endoscopic retrograde cholangiopancreatography (ERCP) under direct vision for central lesions. The tumors often stain positively for cytokeratins 7, 8, and 19 and negatively for cytokeratin 20. However, histology alone cannot usually distinguish CCC from metastases from colon or pancreas primary tumors. Serologic tumor markers appear to be nonspecific, but CEA, CA 19–9, and CA-125 are often elevated in CCC patients and are useful for following response to therapy. Radiologic evaluation typically starts with ultrasound, which is very useful in visualizing dilated bile ducts, and then proceeds with either MRI or magnetic resonance cholangiopancreatography (MRCP) or helical CT scans. Invasive cholangiopancreatography (ERCP) is then needed to define the biliary tree and obtain a biopsy or is needed therapeutically to decompress an obstructed biliary tree with internal stent placement. If that fails, then percutaneous biliary drainage will be needed, with the biliary drainage flowing into an external bag. Central tumors often invade the porta hepatis, and loco-regional lymph node involvement by tumor is frequent.

TREATMENT   Cholangiocarcinoma

Hilar CCC is resectable in ~30% of patients and usually involves bile duct resection and lymphadenectomy. Typical survival is approximately 24 months, with recurrences being mainly in the operative bed but with ~30% in the lungs and liver. Distal CCC, which involves the main ducts, is normally treated by resection of the extrahepatic bile ducts, often with pancreaticoduodenectomy. Survival is similar. Due to the high rates of locoregional recurrences or positive surgical margins, many patients receive postoperative adjuvant radiotherapy. Its effect on survival has not been assessed. Intraluminal brachyradiotherapy has also shown some promise. However, photodynamic therapy enhanced survival in one study. In this technique, sodium porfimer is injected intravenously and then subjected to intraluminal red light laser photoactivation. OLTX has been assessed for treatment of unresectable CCC. Five-year survival was ~20%, so enthusiasm waned. However, neoadjuvant radiotherapy with sensitizing chemotherapy has shown better survival rates for CCC treated by OLTX and is currently used by UNOS for perihilar CCC, size <3 cm with neither intrahepatic or extrahepatic metastases. Multiple chemotherapeutic agents have been assessed for activity and survival in unresectable CCC. Most have been inactive. However, both systemic and hepatic arterial gemcitabine have shown promising results. The combination of cisplatin plus gemcitabine has produced a survival advantage compared with gemcitabine alone and is considered standard therapy for unresectable CCC.

■ GALLBLADDER CANCER (GB CA)

GB Ca has an even worse prognosis than CCC, and with typical survival ~6 months or less. Women are affected much more commonly than men (4:1), unlike HCC or CCC, and GB Ca occurs more frequently than CCC. Most patients have a history of antecedent gallstones, but very few patients with gallstones develop GB Ca (~0.2%). It presents similarly to CCC and is often diagnosed unexpectedly during gallstone or cholecystitis surgery. Presentation is typically that of chronic cholecystitis, chronic right upper quadrant pain and weight loss. Useful but nonspecific serum markers include

CEA and CA 19-9. CT scans or MRCP typically reveal a gallbladder mass. The mainstay of treatment is surgical, either simple or radical cholecystectomy for stages I or II disease, respectively. Survival rates are near 100% at 5 years for stage I, and range from 60–90% at 5 years for stage II. More advanced GB Ca has worse survival, and many patients are unresectable. Adjuvant radiotherapy, used in the presence of local lymph node disease, has not been shown to enhance survival. Chemotherapy is not useful in advanced or metastatic GB Ca.

■ CARCINOMA OF THE AMPULLA OF VATER

This tumor arises within 2 cm of the distal end of the common bile duct and is mainly (90%) an adenocarcinoma. Locoregional lymph nodes are commonly involved (50%), and the liver is the most frequent site for metastases. The most common clinical presentation is jaundice, and many patients also have pruritus, weight loss, and epigastric pain. Initial evaluation is performed with an abdominal ultrasound to assess vascular involvement, biliary dilation, and liver lesions. This is followed by a CT scan, or MRI and especially MRCP. The most effective therapy is resection by pylorus-sparing pancreaticoduodenectomy, an aggressive procedure resulting in better survival rates than with local resection. Survival rates are ~25% at 5 years in operable patients with involved lymph nodes and ~50% in patients without involved nodes. Unlike CCC, approximately 80% of patients are thought to be resectable at diagnosis. Adjuvant chemotherapy or radiotherapy has not been shown to enhance survival. For metastatic tumors, chemotherapy is currently experimental.

■ TUMORS METASTATIC TO THE LIVER

These are predominantly from colon, pancreas, and breast primary tumors but can originate from any organ primary. Ocular melanomas are prone to liver metastasis. Tumor spread to the liver normally carries a poor prognosis for that tumor type. Colorectal and breast hepatic metastases were previously treated with continuous hepatic arterial infusion chemotherapy. However, more effective systemic drugs for each of these two cancers, especially the addition of oxaliplatin to colorectal cancer regimens, have reduced the use of hepatic artery infusion therapy. In a large randomized study of systemic versus infusional plus systemic chemotherapy for resected colorectal metastases to the liver, the patients receiving infusional therapy had no survival advantage, mainly due to extrahepatic tumor spread. ^{90}Yttrium resin beads are approved in the United States for treatment of colorectal hepatic metastases. The role of this modality, either alone or in combination with chemotherapy, is being evaluated in many centers. Palliation my be obtained from chemoembolization, PEI, or RFA.

■ BENIGN LIVER TUMORS

Three common benign tumors occur and all are found predominantly in women. They are *hemangiomas, adenomas,* and *focal nodular hyperplasia* (FNH). FNH is typically benign, and usually no treatment is needed. Hemangiomas are the most common and are entirely benign. Treatment is unnecessary unless their expansion causes symptoms. Adenomas are associated with contraceptive hormone use. They can cause pain and can bleed or rupture, causing acute problems. Their main interest for the physician is a low potential for malignant change and a 30% risk of bleeding. For this reason, considerable effort has gone into differentiating these three entities radiologically. On discovery of a liver mass, patients are usually advised to stop taking sex steroids, as adenoma regression may then occasionally occur. Adenomas can often be large masses ranging from 8–15 cm. Due to their size and definite, but low, malignant potential and potential for bleeding, adenomas are typically resected. The most useful diagnostic differentiating tool is a triphasic CT scan performed with HCC fast bolus protocol for arterial-phase imaging, together with subsequent delayed venous-phase imaging. Adenomas usually do not appear on the basis of cirrhosis, although both adenomas and HCCs are intensely vascular on the CT arterial phase and both can exhibit hemorrhage (40% of adenomas). However, adenomas have smooth, well-defined edges, and enhance homogeneously, especially in the portal venous phase on delayed images, when HCCs no longer enhance. FNHs exhibit a characteristic central scar that is hypovascular on the arterial-phase and hypervascular on the delayed-phase CT images. MRI is even more sensitive in depicting the characteristic central scar of FNH.

FURTHER READINGS

Carr BI et al: Therapeutic equivalence in survival for hepatic arterial chemoembolization and ^{90}Yttrium microspheres (Y90) treatments in unresectable HCC. Cancer 116:1305, 2010

Hoshida Y et al: Gene expression in fixed tissues and outcome in hepatocellular carcinoma. N Engl J Med 359:1995, 2008

Llovet JM et al: Sorafenib in advanced hepatocellular carcinoma. N Engl J Med 359:378, 2008

Mazzaferro V et al: Predicting survival after liver transplantation in patients with hepatocellular carcinoma beyond the Milan criteria: A retrospective, exploratory analysis. Lancet Oncol 10:35, 2009

Noda I et al: Regular surveillance by imaging for early detection and better prognosis of hepatocellular carcinoma in patients infected with hepatitis C virus. J Gastroenterol 45:105, 2010

Pancoska P et al: Network-based analysis of survival for unresectable hepatocellular carcinoma. Semin Oncol 37:170, 2010

Sherman M: Hepatocellular carcinoma: Epidemiology, surveillance and diagnosis. Semin Liver Dis 30:3, 2010

Valle J et al: Cisplatin plus gemcitabine versus gemcitabine for biliary tract cancer. N Engl J Med 362:1273, 2010

Villaneuva A et al: Hepatocellular carcinoma: Novel molecular approaches for diagnosis, prognosis and therapy. Annu Rev Med 61:317, 2010

CHAPTER 93
Pancreatic Cancer

Irene Chong
David Cunningham

Pancreatic cancer is the fourth leading cause of cancer death in the United States and is associated with a poor prognosis. Endocrine tumors affecting the pancreas are discussed in Chap. 350. Infiltrating ductal adenocarcinomas, the subject of this chapter, account for the vast majority of cases and arise most frequently in the head of pancreas. At the time of diagnosis 85–90% of patients have inoperable or metastatic disease, which is reflected in the 5-year survival rate of only 5% for all stages combined. An improved 5-year survival of up to 20% may be achieved when the tumor is detected at an early stage and when complete surgical resection is accomplished.

EPIDEMIOLOGY

Pancreatic cancer represents 3% of all newly diagnosed malignancies in the United States. The most common age group at diagnosis is 60–79 years for both sexes. Pancreatic cancer will be diagnosed in approximately 43,140 patients and account for 36,800 deaths in 2010. Over the past 30 years, 5-year survival rates have not improved substantially.

RISK FACTORS

Cigarette smoking may be the cause of up to 20–25% of all pancreatic cancers and is the most common environmental risk factor for this disease. Other risk factors are not well established due to inconsistent results from epidemiological studies, but include chronic pancreatitis and diabetes. It is difficult to evaluate whether these conditions are causally related, or develop as a consequence of cancer. Alcohol does not appear to be a risk factor unless excess consumption gives rise to chronic pancreatitis.

GENETIC CONSIDERATIONS

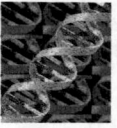 Pancreatic cancer is associated with a number of well-defined molecular hallmarks. The most frequent genetic aberrations comprise *KRAS* mutations, mostly affecting codon 12, which are observed in 60–75% of pancreatic cancers. The tumor-suppressor genes *p16*, *p53*, and *SMAD4* are frequently inactivated; the *p16* gene locus on chromosome 9p21 is deleted in up to 95% of tumors, the *p53* gene is inactivated by mutation or deleted in 50–70% of tumors, and the *SMAD4* gene is deleted in 55% of pancreatic tumors. Furthermore, *SMAD4* gene inactivation is associated with poorer survival in patients with surgically resected pancreatic adenocarcinoma. *IGF-1R* and focal adhesion kinase (*FAK*) interact to promote cell proliferation and survival, and their simultaneous inhibition synergistically inhibits pancreatic cell growth. Overexpression and/or aberrant activation of *c-Src* is frequently observed, which results in cell adhesion, enhanced migration, invasion, and cell proliferation. Survivin is overexpressed in more than 80% of pancreatic tumors, which results in resistance to apoptosis, and genomic sequencing has identified *PALB2* as a susceptibility gene for pancreatic cancer.

Up to 16% of pancreatic cancers are thought to be inherited. This occurs in three separate clinical settings: (1) familial multi-organ cancer syndromes, (2) genetically driven chronic diseases, and (3) familial pancreatic cancer with as yet unidentified genetic abnormalities, which comprise the largest proportion of inherited pancreatic cancer. The familial multi-organ cancer syndromes consist of Peutz-Jeghers syndrome, familial atypical multiple mole melanoma (FAMMM), familial breast-ovarian cancer associated with germline mutations in *BRCA1* and *BRCA2*, hereditary nonpolyposis colorectal cancer (HNPCC), familial adenomatous polyposis (FAP), and Li-Fraumeni syndrome. Peutz-Jeghers, associated with mutations in the *STK11* gene, carries the highest lifetime risk of pancreatic cancer with a relative risk of approximately 132-fold above that of the general population. Genetically driven chronic causes of pancreatic cancer include hereditary pancreatitis, cystic fibrosis, and ataxia telangiectasia. The absolute number of affected first-degree relatives is also correlated with increased cancer risk, and patients with at least two first-degree relatives with pancreatic cancer should be considered to have familial pancreatic cancer until proven otherwise.

SCREENING AND EARLY DETECTION

Screening is not routinely recommended as putative tumor markers such as Ca 19-9 and CEA have insufficient sensitivity, and computed tomography (CT) has inadequate resolution to detect pancreatic dysplasia. Endoscopic ultrasound (EUS) is a more promising screening tool, and preclinical efforts are focused on identifying biomarkers that may detect pancreatic cancer at an early stage. Consensus practice recommendations based largely on expert opinion have chosen a threshold of >tenfold increased risk for developing pancreatic cancer to select individuals who may benefit from screening. This includes family members with ≥3 first-degree relatives with pancreatic cancer, and patients with FAMMM, Peutz-Jeghers syndrome, or hereditary pancreatitis.

CLINICAL FEATURES
◼ CLINICAL PRESENTATION

Obstructive jaundice occurs frequently when the cancer is located in the head of pancreas. This may be accompanied by symptoms of abdominal discomfort, pruritus, lethargy, and weight loss. Less common presenting features include epigastric pain, backache, new onset diabetes mellitus, and acute pancreatitis caused by pressure effects on the pancreatic duct. Nausea and vomiting, resulting from gastroduodenal obstruction, may also be a symptom of this disease.

◼ PHYSICAL SIGNS

Patients can present with jaundice and cachexia, and scratch marks may be present. Of patients with operable tumors 25% have a palpable gall bladder (Courvoisier's sign). Physical signs related to the development of distant metastases include hepatomegaly, ascites, left supraclavicular lymphadenopathy (Virchow's node), and periumbilical lymphadenopathy (Sister Mary Joseph's nodes).

DIAGNOSIS
◼ DIAGNOSTIC IMAGING

Patients who present with clinical features suggestive of pancreatic cancer undergo imaging to confirm the presence of a tumor, and to establish whether the mass is likely to be inflammatory or malignant in nature. Other imaging objectives include the local and distant staging of the tumor, which will determine resectability and provide prognostic information. Dual phase, contrast-enhanced spiral CT is the imaging modality of choice (Fig. 93-1). It provides accurate

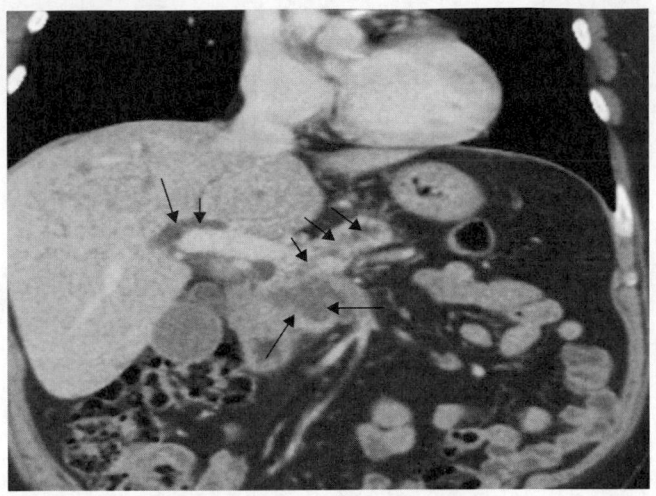

Figure 93-1 Coronal CT showing pancreatic cancer and dilated intrahepatic and pancreatic ducts (arrows).

visualization of surrounding viscera, vessels, and lymph nodes, thus determining tumor resectability. Intestinal infiltration, and liver and lung metastases are also reliably depicted on CT. There is no advantage of magnetic resonance imaging (MRI) over CT in predicting tumor resectability, but selected cases may benefit from MRI to characterize the nature of small indeterminate liver lesions and to evaluate the cause of biliary dilatation when no obvious mass is seen on CT. Endoscopic retrograde cholangiopancreatography (ERCP) is useful for revealing small pancreatic lesions, identifying stricture or obstruction in pancreatic or common bile ducts, and facilitates stent placement (Fig. 93-2). Magnetic resonance cholangiopancreatography (MRCP) is a noninvasive method for accurately depicting the level and degree of bile and pancreatic duct dilatation. EUS is highly sensitive in detecting lesions less than 3 cm in size, and is useful as a local staging tool for assessing vascular invasion and lymph node involvement. Positron-emission tomography with fluorodeoxyglucose positron emission tomography (FDG-PET) should be considered before surgery or radical chemoradiotherapy (CRT), as it is superior to conventional imaging in detecting distant metastases.

■ TISSUE DIAGNOSIS AND CYTOLOGY

Preoperative confirmation of malignancy is not always necessary in patients with radiological appearances consistent with operable pancreatic cancer. However, EUS-guided fine-needle aspiration is

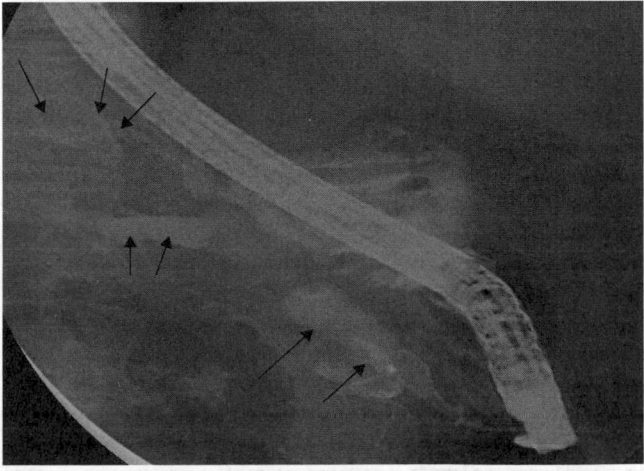

Figure 93-2 ERCP showing contrast in dilated pancreatic duct (arrows).

the technique of choice when there is any doubt, and also for use in patients who require neoadjuvant treatment. It has an accuracy of approximately 90% and has a smaller risk of intraperitoneal dissemination compared with the percutaneous route. Percutaneous biopsy of the pancreatic primary or liver metastases is only acceptable in patients with inoperable or metastatic disease. ERCP is a useful method for obtaining ductal brushings, but the diagnostic value of pancreatic juice sampling is only in the order of 25–30%.

■ SERUM MARKERS

Tumor-associated carbohydrate antigen 19-9 (CA 19-9) is elevated in approximately 70–80% of patients with pancreatic carcinoma, but is not recommended as a routine diagnostic or screening test as its sensitivity and specificity are inadequate for accurate diagnosis. Preoperative CA 19-9 levels correlate with tumor stage, and postresection CA 19-9 level has prognostic value. It is an indicator of asymptomatic recurrence in patients with completely resected tumors and is used as a biomarker of response in patients with advanced disease undergoing chemotherapy. A number of studies have established a high pretreatment CA 19-9 level as an independent prognostic factor.

STAGING

The American Joint Committee on Cancer (AJCC) tumor-node-metastasis (TNM) staging of pancreatic cancer takes into account the location and size of the tumor, the involvement of lymph nodes, and distant metastasis. This information is then combined to assign a stage (Fig. 93-3). From a practical standpoint, patients are grouped according to whether the cancer is resectable, locally advanced (unresectable, but without distant spread), or metastatic.

TREATMENT   Pancreatic Cancer

RESECTABLE DISEASE Approximately 10% of patients present with localized nonmetastatic disease that is potentially suitable for surgical resection. Approximately 30% of patients have R1 resection (microscopic residual disease) following surgery. Those who undergo R0 resection (no microscopic or macroscopic residual tumor), and who receive adjuvant treatment have the best chance of cure, with an estimated median survival of 20–23 months and a 5-year survival of approximately 20%. Outcomes are more favorable in patients with small (<3cm), well-differentiated tumors, and lymph node-negative disease.

Patients should have surgery in dedicated pancreatic centers that have lower postoperative morbidity and mortality rates. The standard surgical procedure for patients with tumors of the pancreatic head or uncinate process is a pylorus-preserving pancreaticoduodenectomy (modified Whipple's procedure). The procedure of choice for tumors of the pancreatic body and tail is a distal pancreatectomy, which routinely includes splenectomy.

Postoperative treatment, either chemotherapy or CRT, improves long-term outcomes in this group of patients. Adjuvant chemotherapy, comprising six cycles of fluorouracil (5FU) and folinic acid (FA) or gemcitabine, is common practice in Europe based on data from three randomized controlled trials (Table 93–1): Results from the European Study Group for Pancreatic Cancer 1 trial (ESPAC-1) revealed a median survival improvement from 14.7 months with surgery alone to 20.1 months with surgery plus adjuvant 5FU/FA, and patients did not benefit from CRT in this study. The Charité Onkologie trial (CONKO 001) found that the use of gemcitabine after complete resection significantly delayed the development of recurrent disease compared with surgery alone. The ESPAC-3 trial, which investigated the benefit of adjuvant 5FU/FA versus gemcitabine,

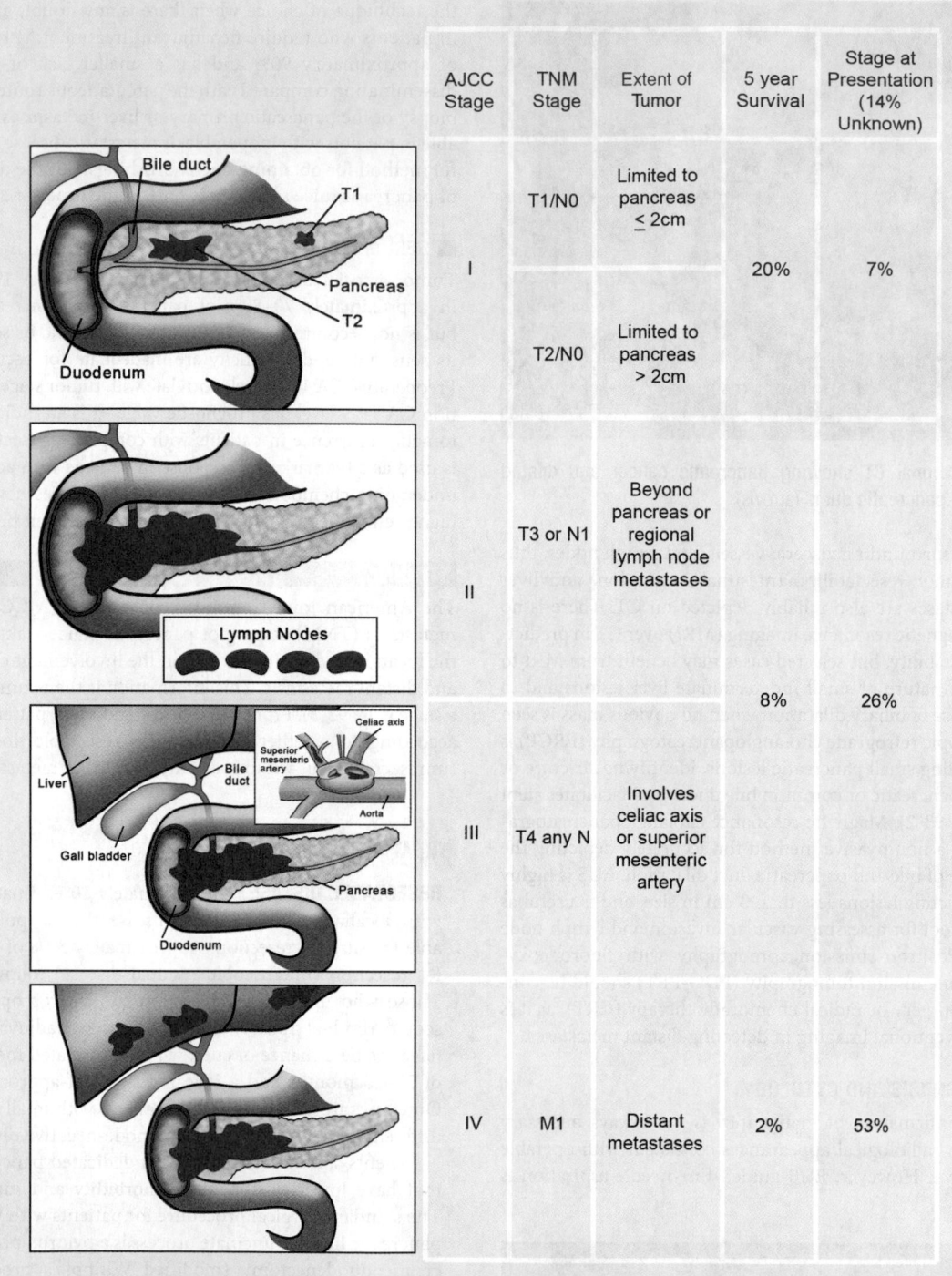

AJCC Stage	TNM Stage	Extent of Tumor	5 year Survival	Stage at Presentation (14% Unknown)
I	T1/N0	Limited to pancreas ≤ 2cm	20%	7%
	T2/N0	Limited to pancreas > 2cm		
II	T3 or N1	Beyond pancreas or regional lymph node metastases	8%	26%
III	T4 any N	Involves celiac axis or superior mesenteric artery		
IV	M1	Distant metastases	2%	53%

Figure 93-3   Staging of pancreatic cancer, and survival according to stage. *(Illustration by Stephen Millward.)*

TABLE 93-1 Phase III Studies of Adjuvant Chemotherapy in Resected Pancreatic Cancer

Study	Comparator Arm	Patient Number	Survival	
			PFS/DFS (months)	Median survival (months)
ESPAC 1 Neoptolemos et al. (2004)	Chemotherapy (Folinic acid + bolus 5FU) vs No chemotherapy	550	PFS 15.3 vs 9.4. (*p* = 0.02)	20.1 vs 14.7 (HR 0.71, 95% CI 0.55 to 0.92, *p* = 0.009)
CONKO 001 Oettle et al. (2007)	Gemcitabine vs Observation	368	Median DFS 13.4 vs 6.9 (*p* < 0.001)	22.1 vs 20.2 (*p* = 0.06)
ESPAC 3 Neoptolemos et al. (2010)	5FU/LV vs Gemcitabine	1088		23 vs 23.6 (HR 0.94, 95% CI 0.81 to 1.08, *p* = 0.39)

Abbreviations: CI, confidence interval; CONKO, charite ONKOlogie; DFS, disease free survival; ESPAC, European Study Group for Pancreatic Cancer; 5FU, fluorouracil; HR, hazard ratio; LV, leucovorin; PFS, progression-free survival.

TABLE 93-2 Selected Phase III Studies Evaluating Chemotherapy Treatment in Advanced Pancreatic Cancer

Study	Comparator Arm	Patient Number	Survival	
			PFS (months)	Median survival (months)
Moore M et al. (2007)	Gemcitabine vs Gemcitabine + erlotinib	569	3.55 vs 3.75 (HR 0.77, 95% CI 0.64 to 0.92, $p = 0.004$)	5.91 vs 6.24 (HR 0.82, 95% CI 0.69 to 0.99, $p = 0.038$)
GEM-CAP Cunningham et al. (2009)	Gemcitabine vs Gemcitabine + capecitabine (GEM-CAP)	533	3.8 vs 5.3 (HR 0.78, 95% CI 0.66 to 0.93, $p = 0.004$)	6.2 vs 7.1 (HR 0.86, 95% CI 0.72 to 1.02, $p = 0.08$)
GEM-CAP meta-analysis Cunningham et al. (2009)	Gemcitabine vs GEM-CAP	935		Overall survival in favor of GEM-CAP (HR 0.86, 95% CI 0.75 to 0.98, $p = 0.02$)

revealed no survival difference between the two drugs. However, the safety profile of adjuvant gemcitabine, with respect to the incidence of stomatitis and diarrhea, was superior to 5FU/FA.

A different treatment strategy using adjuvant 5FU based CRT following gemcitabine as advocated by the Radiation Therapy Oncology Group (RTOG) 97-04 trial is preferred in the United States. This approach may be most beneficial in patients with bulky tumors involving the pancreatic head, and in patients with R1 resection.

INOPERABLE LOCALLY ADVANCED DISEASE Approximately 30% of patients present with locally advanced unresectable but nonmetastatic pancreatic carcinoma. The median survival with gemcitabine is 9 months, and patients who respond to or achieve stable disease after 3–6 months of gemcitabine may derive benefit from consolidation radiotherapy.

METASTATIC DISEASE Approximately 60% of patients with pancreatic cancer present with metastatic disease. Patients with poor performance status do not benefit from chemotherapy. Gemcitabine is the standard treatment with a median survival of 6 months and a 1-year survival rate of only 20%. The toxicities associated with gemcitabine need to be weighed against the potential benefits of treatment.

Adding other drugs to gemcitabine to improve outcome has been generally unsuccessful with the exception of erlotinib, an oral HER1/EGFR tyrosine kinase inhibitor. The combination of erlotinib with gemcitabine resulted in an improved 1-year survival compared with gemcitabine alone (23% versus 17%, $p = 0.023$) (Table 93-2). Capecitabine, an oral fluoropyrimidine, has been combined with gemcitabine (GEM-CAP) in a phase III trial that showed an improvement in response rate and progression-free survival over single-agent gemcitabine, but no survival benefit. However, pooling of two other randomized controlled trials with this trial in a meta-analysis resulted in a survival advantage with GEM-CAP.

A trial in good performance status patients with metastatic pancreatic cancer showed improved survival with the combination of 5FU/FA, irinotecan and oxaliplatin (FOLFIRINOX) compared with gemcitabine, but with increased toxicity. Nab-paclitaxel (Abraxane), an albumin bound nano-particle formulation of paclitaxel, given with gemcitabine also shows promising activity.

FUTURE DIRECTIONS

The early detection and future treatment of pancreatic cancer relies on an improved understanding of molecular pathways involved in the development of this disease. This will ultimately lead to the discovery of novel agents, and the identification of patient groups who are likely to benefit most from targeted therapy.

FURTHER READINGS

CASCINU S, JELIC S: Pancreatic cancer: ESMO clinical recommendations for diagnosis, treatment and follow-up. Ann Oncol 20:37, 2009

CUNNINGHAM D et al: Phase III randomised comparison of gemcitabine versus gemcitabine plus capecitabine in patients with advanced pancreatic cancer. J Clin Oncol 27:5513, 2009

EDGE SB, BYRD DR (eds): *Exocrine and Endocrine Pancreas, AJCC Cancer Staging Manual*, 7th ed, New York, Springer, 2010, pp 241–249

MOORE MJ et al: Erlotinib plus gemcitabine compared with gemcitabine alone in patients with advanced pancreatic cancer: A phase III trial of the National Cancer Institute of Canada Clinical Trials Group. J Clin Oncol 26:1960, 2007

NEOPTOLEMOS JP et al: Adjuvant chemotherapy with fluorouracil plus folinic acid vs gemcitabine following pancreatic cancer resection: A randomised controlled trial. JAMA 304:1073, 2010

OETTLE H et al: Adjuvant chemotherapy with gemcitabine vs observation in patients undergoing curative-intent resection of pancreatic cancer: A randomized controlled trial. JAMA 297:267, 2007

CHAPTER 94

Bladder and Renal Cell Carcinomas

Howard I. Scher
Robert J. Motzer

BLADDER CANCER

A transitional cell epithelium lines the urinary tract from the renal pelvis to the ureter, urinary bladder, and the proximal two-thirds of the urethra. Cancers can occur at any point: 90% of malignancies develop in the bladder, 8% in the renal pelvis, and the remaining 2% in the ureter or urethra. Bladder cancer is the fourth most common cancer in men and the thirteenth in women, with an estimated 70,530 new cases and 14,680 deaths in the United States predicted for the year 2010. The almost 5:1 ratio of incidence to mortality reflects the higher frequency of the less lethal superficial variants compared to the more lethal invasive and metastatic variants. The incidence is three times higher in men than in women and twofold higher in whites than blacks, with a median age at diagnosis of 65 years.

Once diagnosed, urothelial tumors exhibit polychronotropism—the tendency to recur over time and in new locations in the urothelial tract. As long as urothelium is present, continuous monitoring of the tract is required.

EPIDEMIOLOGY

Cigarette smoking is believed to contribute to up to 50% of the diagnosed urothelial cancers in men and up to 40% in women. The risk of developing a urothelial malignancy in male smokers is increased two- to fourfold relative to nonsmokers and continues for 10 years or longer after cessation. Other implicated agents include the aniline dyes, the drugs phenacetin and chlornaphazine, and external beam radiation. Chronic cyclophosphamide exposure may also increase risk, whereas vitamin A supplements appear to be protective. Exposure to *Schistosoma haematobium*, a parasite found in many developing countries, is associated with an increase in both squamous and transitional cell carcinomas of the bladder.

PATHOLOGY

Clinical subtypes are grouped into three categories: 75% are superficial, 20% invade muscle, and 5% are metastatic at presentation. Staging of the tumor within the bladder is based on the pattern of growth and depth of invasion: Ta lesions grow as exophytic lesions; carcinoma in situ (CIS) lesions start on the surface and tend to invade. The revised tumor, node, metastasis (TNM) staging system is illustrated in Fig. 94-1. About half of invasive tumors presented originally as superficial lesions that later progressed. Tumors are also rated by grade. Grade I lesions (highly differentiated tumors) rarely progress to a higher stage, whereas grade III tumors do.

More than 95% of urothelial tumors in the United States are transitional cell in origin. Pure squamous cancers with keratinization constitute 3%, adenocarcinomas 2%, and small cell tumors (with paraneoplastic syndromes) <1%. Adenocarcinomas develop primarily in the urachal remnant in the dome of the bladder or in the periurethral tissues; some assume a signet cell histology. Lymphomas and melanomas are rare. Of the transitional cell tumors, low-grade papillary lesions that grow on a central stalk are most common. These tumors are very friable, have a tendency to bleed, are at high risk for recurrence, and yet rarely progress to the more lethal invasive variety. In contrast, CIS is a high-grade tumor that is considered a precursor of the more lethal muscle-invasive disease.

PATHOGENESIS

The multicentric nature of the disease and high rate of recurrence has led to the hypothesis of a field defect in the urothelium that results in a predisposition to cancer. Molecular genetic analyses suggest that the superficial and invasive lesions develop along distinct molecular pathways in which primary tumorigenic aberrations precede secondary changes associated with progression to a more advanced stage. Low-grade papillary tumors that do not tend to invade or metastasize harbor constitutive activation of the receptor-tyrosine kinase-Ras signal transduction pathway and

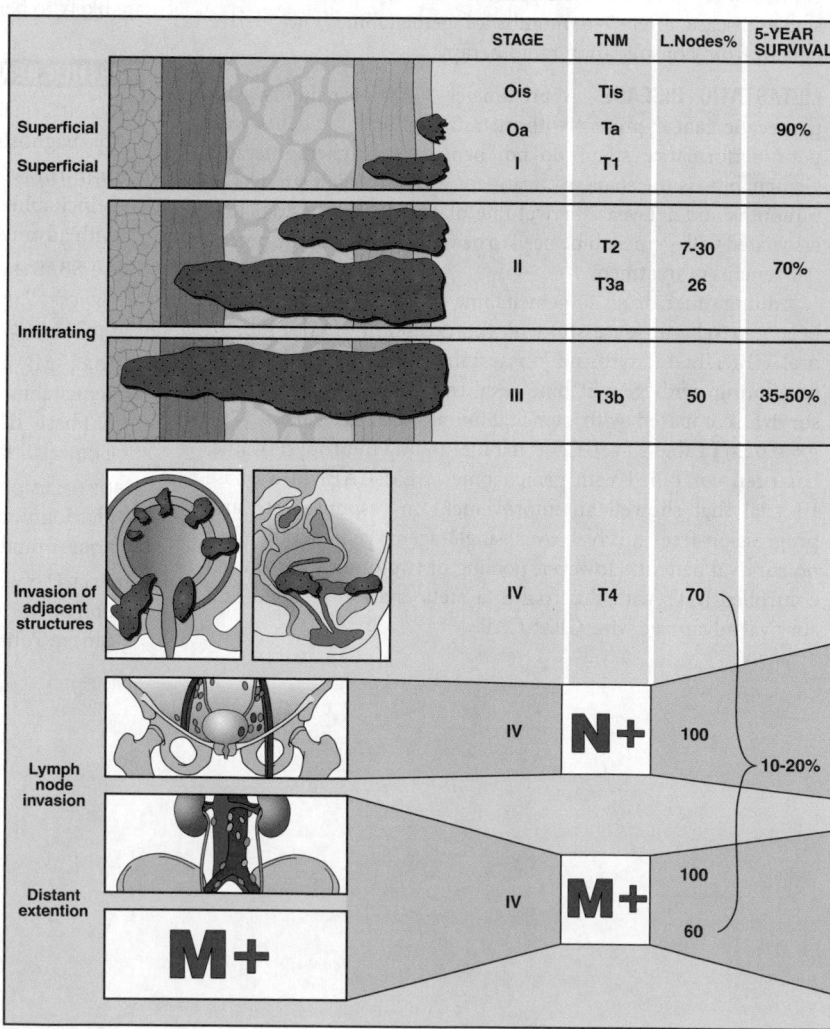

	STAGE	TNM	L.Nodes%	5-YEAR SURVIVAL
Superficial	Ois	Tis		
	Oa	Ta		90%
Superficial	I	T1		
Infiltrating	II	T2	7-30	70%
		T3a	26	
	III	T3b	50	35-50%
Invasion of adjacent structures	IV	T4	70	
Lymph node invasion	IV	N+	100	10-20%
Distant extention	IV	M+	100	
			60	

Figure 94-1 Bladder staging. TNM, tumor, node, metastasis.

a high frequency of fibroblast growth factor receptor 3 (FGFR3) mutations. In contrast, CIS and invasive tumors have a higher frequency of *TP53* and *RB* gene alternations. Within all clinical stages, including Tis, T1, and T2 or greater lesions, tumors with alterations in *p53*, *p21*, and/or *RB* have a higher probability of recurrence, metastasis, and death from disease.

CLINICAL PRESENTATION, DIAGNOSIS, AND STAGING

Hematuria occurs in 80–90% of patients and often reflects exophytic tumors. The bladder is the most common source of gross hematuria (40%), but benign cystitis (22%) is a more common cause than bladder cancer (15%) (Chap. 44). Microscopic hematuria is more commonly of prostate origin (25%); only 2% of bladder cancers produce microscopic hematuria. Once hematuria is documented, a urinary cytology, visualization of the urothelial tract by CT or intravenous pyelogram, and cystoscopy are recommended if no other etiology is found. Screening asymptomatic individuals for hematuria increases the diagnosis of tumors at an early stage but has not been shown to prolong life. After hematuria, irritative symptoms are the next most common presentation, which may reflect in situ disease. Obstruction of the ureters may cause flank pain. Symptoms of metastatic disease are rarely the first presenting sign.

The endoscopic evaluation includes an examination under anesthesia to determine whether a palpable mass is present. A flexible endoscope is inserted into the bladder, and bladder barbotage is performed. The visual inspection includes mapping the location, size, and number of lesions, as well as a description of the growth pattern (solid vs. papillary). An intraoperative video is often recorded. All visible tumors should be resected, and a sample of the muscle underlying the tumor should be obtained to assess the depth of invasion. Normal-appearing areas are biopsied at random to ensure no field defect. A notation is made as to whether a tumor was completely or incompletely resected. Selective catheterization and visualization of the upper tracts should be performed if the cytology is positive and no disease is visible in the bladder. Ultrasonography, CT, and/or MRI may help to determine whether a tumor extends to perivesical fat (T3) and to document nodal spread. Distant metastases are assessed by CT of the chest and abdomen, MRI, or radionuclide imaging of the skeleton.

TREATMENT   Bladder Cancer

Management depends on whether the tumor invades muscle and whether it has spread to the regional lymph nodes and beyond. The probability of spread increases with increasing T stage.

SUPERFICIAL DISEASE   At a minimum, the management of a superficial tumor is complete endoscopic resection with or without intravesical therapy. The decision to recommend intravesical therapy depends on the histologic subtype, number of lesions, depth of invasion, presence or absence of CIS, and antecedent history. Recurrences develop in upward of 50% of cases, of which 5–20% progress to a more advanced stage. In general, solitary papillary lesions are managed by transurethral surgery alone. CIS and recurrent disease are treated by transurethral surgery followed by intravesical therapy.

Intravesical therapies are used in two general contexts: as an adjuvant to a complete endoscopic resection to prevent recurrence or, less commonly, to eliminate disease that cannot be controlled by endoscopic resection alone. Intravesical treatments are advised for patients with recurrent disease, >40% involvement of the bladder surface by tumor, diffuse CIS, or T1 disease. The standard intravesical therapy, based on randomized

comparisons, is bacillus Calmette-Guerin (BCG) in six weekly instillations, followed by monthly maintenance administrations for ≥1 year. Other agents with activity include mitomycin-C, interferon (IFN), and gemcitabine. The side effects of intravesical therapies include dysuria, urinary frequency, and, depending on the drug, myelosuppression or contact dermatitis. Rarely, intravesical BCG may produce a systemic illness associated with granulomatous infections in multiple sites that requires antituberculin therapy.

Following the endoscopic resection, patients are monitored for recurrence at 3-month intervals during the first year. Recurrence may develop anywhere along the urothelial tract, including the renal pelvis, ureter, or urethra. A consequence of the "successful" treatment of tumors in the bladder is an increase in the frequency of extravesical recurrences (e.g., urethra or ureter). Those with persistent disease in the bladder or new tumors are generally considered for a second course of BCG or for intravesical chemotherapy with valrubicin or gemcitabine. In some cases, cystectomy is recommended, although the specific indications vary. Tumors in the ureter or renal pelvis are typically managed by resection during retrograde examination or, in some cases, by instillation through the renal pelvis. Tumors of the prostatic urethra may require cystectomy if the tumor cannot be resected completely.

INVASIVE DISEASE   The treatment of a tumor that has invaded muscle can be separated into control of the primary tumor and, depending on the pathologic findings at surgery, systemic chemotherapy to treat micrometastatic disease. Radical cystectomy is the standard, although in selected cases a bladder-sparing approach is used; this approach includes complete endoscopic resection; partial cystectomy; or a combination of resection, systemic chemotherapy, and external beam radiation therapy. In some countries, external beam radiation therapy is considered standard. In the United States, its role is limited to those patients deemed unfit for cystectomy, those with unresectable local disease, or as part of an experimental bladder-sparing approach.

Indications for cystectomy include muscle-invading tumors not suitable for segmental resection; low-stage tumors unsuitable for conservative management (e.g., due to multicentric and frequent recurrences resistant to intravesical instillations); high-grade tumors (T1G3) associated with CIS; and bladder symptoms, such as frequency or hemorrhage, that impair quality of life.

Radical cystectomy is major surgery that requires appropriate preoperative evaluation and management. The procedure involves removal of the bladder and pelvic lymph nodes and creation of a conduit or reservoir for urinary flow. Grossly abnormal lymph nodes are evaluated by frozen section. If metastases are confirmed, the procedure is often aborted. In males, radical cystectomy includes the removal of the prostate, seminal vesicles, and proximal urethra. Impotence is universal unless the nerves responsible for erectile function are preserved. In females, the procedure includes removal of the bladder, urethra, uterus, fallopian tubes, ovaries, anterior vaginal wall, and surrounding fascia.

Previously, urine flow was managed by directing the ureters to the abdominal wall, where it was collected in an external appliance. Currently, most patients receive either a continent cutaneous reservoir constructed from detubularized bowel or an orthotopic neobladder. Some 70% of men receive a neobladder. With a continent reservoir, 65–85% of men will be continent at night and 85–90% during the day. Cutaneous reservoirs are drained by intermittent catheterization; orthotopic neobladders are drained more naturally. Contraindications to a neobladder

TABLE 94-1 Survival Following Surgery for Bladder Cancer

Pathologic Stage	5-Year Survival, %	10-Year Survival, %
T2,N0	89	87
T3a,N0	78	76
T3b,N0	62	61
T4,N0	50	45
Any T,N1	35	34

TABLE 94-2 Management of Bladder Cancer

Nature of Lesion	Management Approach
Superficial	Endoscopic removal, usually with intravesical therapy
Invasive disease	Cystectomy ± systemic chemotherapy (before or after surgery)
Metastatic disease	Curative or palliative chemotherapy (based on prognostic factors) ± surgery

include renal insufficiency, an inability to self-catheterize, or an exophytic tumor or CIS in the urethra. Diffuse CIS in the bladder is a relative contraindication based on the risk of a urethral recurrence. Concurrent ulcerative colitis or Crohn's disease may hinder the use of resected bowel.

A partial cystectomy may be considered when the disease is limited to the dome of the bladder, a margin of at least 2 cm can be achieved, there is no CIS in other sites, and the bladder capacity is adequate after the tumor has been removed. This occurs in 5–10% of cases. Carcinomas in the ureter or in the renal pelvis are treated with nephroureterectomy with a bladder cuff to remove the tumor.

The probability of recurrence following surgery is predicted on the basis of pathologic stage, presence, or absence of lymphatic or vascular invasion, and nodal spread. Among those whose cancers recur, the recurrence develops in a median of 1 year (range 0.04–11.1 years). Long-term outcomes vary by pathologic stage and histology (Table 94-1). The number of lymph nodes removed is also prognostic, whether or not the nodes contained tumor.

Chemotherapy (described below) has been shown to prolong the survival of patients with invasive disease, but only when combined with definitive treatment of the bladder by radical cystectomy or radiation therapy. Thus, for the majority of patients, chemotherapy alone is inadequate to clear the bladder of disease. Experimental studies are evaluating bladder preservation strategies by combining chemotherapy and radiation therapy in patients whose tumors were endoscopically removed.

METASTATIC DISEASE The primary goal of treatment for metastatic disease is to achieve complete remission with chemotherapy alone or with a combined-modality approach of chemotherapy followed by surgical resection of residual disease, as is done routinely for the treatment of germ cell tumors. One can define a goal in terms of cure or palliation on the basis of the probability of achieving a complete response to chemotherapy using prognostic factors, such as Karnofsky Performance Status (KPS) (<80%), and whether the pattern of spread is nodal or visceral (liver, lung, or bone). For those with zero, one, or two risk factors, the probability of complete remission is 38, 25, and 5%, respectively, and median survival is 33, 13.4, and 9.3 months, respectively. Patients who are functionally compromised or who have visceral disease or bone metastases rarely achieve long-term survival. The toxicities also vary as a function of risk, and treatment-related mortality rates are as high as 3–4% using some combinations in these poor-risk patient groups.

CHEMOTHERAPY A number of chemotherapeutic drugs have shown activity as single agents; cisplatin, paclitaxel, and gemcitabine are considered most active. Standard therapy consists of two-, three-, or four-drug combinations. Overall response

rates of >50% have been reported using combinations such as methotrexate, vinblastine, doxorubicin, and cisplatin (M-VAC); cisplatin and paclitaxel (PT); gemcitabine and cisplatin (GC); or gemcitabine, paclitaxel, and cisplatin (GTC). M-VAC was considered standard, but the toxicities of neutropenia and fever, mucositis, diminished renal and auditory function, and peripheral neuropathy led to the development of alternative regimens. At present, GC is used more commonly than M-VAC, based on the results of a comparative trial of M-VAC versus GC that showed less neutropenia and fever, and less mucositis for the GC regimen. Anemia and thrombocytopenia were more common with GC. GTC is not more effective than GC.

Chemotherapy has also been evaluated in the neoadjuvant and adjuvant settings. In a randomized trial, patients receiving three cycles of neoadjuvant M-VAC followed by cystectomy had a significantly better median (6.2 years) and 5-year survival (57%) compared to cystectomy alone (median survival 3.8 years; 5-year survival 42%). Similar results were obtained in an international study of three cycles of cisplatin, methotrexate, and vinblastine (CMV) followed by either radical cystectomy or radiation therapy. The decision to administer adjuvant therapy is based on the risk of recurrence after cystectomy. Indications for adjuvant chemotherapy include the presence of nodal disease, extravesical tumor extension, or vascular invasion in the resected specimen. Another study of adjuvant therapy found that four cycles of CMV delayed recurrence, although an effect on survival was less clear. Additional trials are studying taxane- and gemcitabine-based combinations.

The management of bladder cancer is summarized in Table 94-2.

CARCINOMA OF THE RENAL PELVIS AND URETER

About 2500 cases of renal pelvis and ureter cancer occur each year; nearly all are transitional cell carcinomas similar to bladder cancer in biology and appearance. This tumor is also associated with chronic phenacetin abuse and with Balkan nephropathy, a chronic interstitial nephritis endemic in Bulgaria, Greece, Bosnia-Herzegovina, and Romania.

The most common symptom is painless gross hematuria, and the disease is usually detected on intravenous pyelogram during the workup for hematuria. Patterns of spread are like those in bladder cancer. For low-grade disease localized to the renal pelvis and ureter, nephroureterectomy (including excision of the distal ureter with a portion of the bladder) is associated with 5-year survival of 80–90%. More invasive or histologically poorly differentiated tumors are more likely to recur locally and to metastasize. Metastatic disease is treated with the chemotherapy used in bladder cancer, and the outcome is similar to that of metastatic transitional-cell cancer of bladder origin.

RENAL CELL CARCINOMA

Renal cell carcinomas account for 90–95% of malignant neoplasms arising from the kidney. Notable features include resistance to cytotoxic agents, infrequent responses to biologic response modifiers such as interleukin (IL) 2, robust activity to antiangiogenesis targeted agents, and a variable clinical course for patients with metastatic disease, including anecdotal reports of spontaneous regression.

■ EPIDEMIOLOGY

The incidence of renal cell carcinoma continues to rise and is now nearly 58,000 cases annually in the United States, resulting in 13,000 deaths. The male to female ratio is 2:1. Incidence peaks between the ages of 50 and 70 years, although this malignancy may be diagnosed at any age. Many environmental factors have been investigated as possible contributing causes; the strongest association is with cigarette smoking. Risk is also increased for patients who have acquired cystic disease of the kidney associated with end-stage renal disease, and for those with tuberous sclerosis. Most cases are sporadic, although familial forms have been reported. One is associated with von Hippel-Lindau (VHL) syndrome. VHL syndrome is an autosomal dominant disorder. Genetic studies identified the *VHL* gene on the short arm of chromosome 3. Approximately 35% of individuals with VHL disease develop clear cell renal cell carcinoma. Other associated neoplasms include retinal hemangioma, hemangioblastoma of the spinal cord and cerebellum, pheochromocytoma, neuroendocrine tumors and cysts, and cysts in the epididymis of the testis in men and the broad ligament in women. Subtypes vary according to low risk (type 1) or high risk (type 2) of developing pheochromocytoma.

■ PATHOLOGY AND GENETICS

Renal cell neoplasia represents a heterogeneous group of tumors with distinct histopathologic, genetic, and clinical features ranging from benign to high-grade malignant (Table 94-3). They are classified on the basis of morphology and histology. Categories include clear cell carcinoma (60% of cases), papillary tumors (5–15%), chromophobic tumors (5–10%), oncocytomas (5–10%), and collecting or Bellini duct tumors (<1%). Papillary tumors tend to be bilateral and multifocal. Chromophobic tumors have a more indolent clinical course, and oncocytomas are considered benign neoplasms. In contrast, Bellini duct carcinomas, which are thought to arise from

TABLE 94-3 Classification of Epithelial Neoplasms Arising From the Kidney

Carcinoma Type	Growth Pattern	Cell of Origin	Cytogenetics
Clear cell	Acinar or sarcomatoid	Proximal tubule	3p–
Papillary	Papillary or sarcomatoid	Proximal tubule	+7, +17, –Y
Chromophobic	Solid, tubular, or sarcomatoid	Cortical collecting duct	Hypodiploid
Oncocytic	Tumor nests	Cortical collecting duct	Undetermined
Collecting duct	Papillary or sarcomatoid	Medullary collecting duct	Undetermined

the collecting ducts within the renal medulla, are very rare but very aggressive. Clear cell tumors, the predominant histology, are found in >80% of patients who develop metastases. Clear cell tumors arise from the epithelial cells of the proximal tubules and usually show chromosome 3p deletions. Deletions of 3p21–26 (where the *VHL* gene maps) are identified in patients with familial as well as sporadic tumors. *VHL* encodes a tumor-suppressor protein that is involved in regulating the transcription of vascular endothelial growth factor (VEGF), platelet-derived growth factor (PDGF), and a number of other hypoxia-inducible proteins. Inactivation of *VHL* leads to overexpression of these agonists of the VEGF and PDGF receptors, which promote tumor angiogenesis and tumor growth. Agents that inhibit proangiogenic growth factor activity show antitumor effects.

■ CLINICAL PRESENTATION

The presenting signs and symptoms include hematuria, abdominal pain, and a flank or abdominal mass. This classic triad occurs in 10–20% of patients. Other symptoms are fever, weight loss, anemia, and a varicocele. The tumor is most commonly detected as an incidental finding on a radiograph. Widespread use of radiologic cross-sectional imaging procedures (CT, ultrasound, MRI) contributes to earlier detection, including incidental renal masses detected during evaluation for other medical conditions. The increasing number of incidentally discovered low-stage tumors has contributed to an improved 5-year survival for patients with renal cell carcinoma and increased use of nephron-sparing surgery (partial nephrectomy). A spectrum of paraneoplastic syndromes has been associated with these malignancies, including erythrocytosis, hypercalcemia, nonmetastatic hepatic dysfunction (Stauffer syndrome), and acquired dysfibrinogenemia. Erythrocytosis is noted at presentation in only about 3% of patients. Anemia, a sign of advanced disease, is more common.

The standard evaluation of patients with suspected renal cell tumors includes a CT scan of the abdomen and pelvis, chest radiograph, urine analysis, and urine cytology. If metastatic disease is suspected from the chest radiograph, a CT of the chest is warranted. MRI is useful in evaluating the inferior vena cava in cases of suspected tumor involvement or invasion by thrombus. In clinical practice, any solid renal masses should be considered malignant until proven otherwise; a definitive diagnosis is required. If no metastases are demonstrated, surgery is indicated, even if the renal vein is invaded. The differential diagnosis of a renal mass includes cysts, benign neoplasms (adenoma, angiomyolipoma, oncocytoma), inflammatory lesions (pyelonephritis or abscesses), and other primary or metastatic cancers. Other malignancies that may involve the kidney include transitional cell carcinoma of the renal pelvis, sarcoma, lymphoma, and Wilms' tumor. All of these are less common causes of renal masses than is renal cell cancer.

■ STAGING AND PROGNOSIS

Staging is based on the American Joint Committee on Cancer (AJCC) staging system (Fig. 94-2). Stage I tumors are <7 cm in greatest diameter and confined to the kidney, stage II tumors are ≥7 cm and confined to the kidney, stage III tumors extend through the renal capsule but are confined to Gerota's fascia (IIIa) or involve a single hilar lymph node (N1), and stage IV disease includes tumors that have invaded adjacent organs (excluding the adrenal gland) or involve multiple lymph nodes or distant metastases. The rate of 5-year survival varies by stage: >90% for stage I, 85% for stage II, 60% for stage III, and 10% for stage IV.

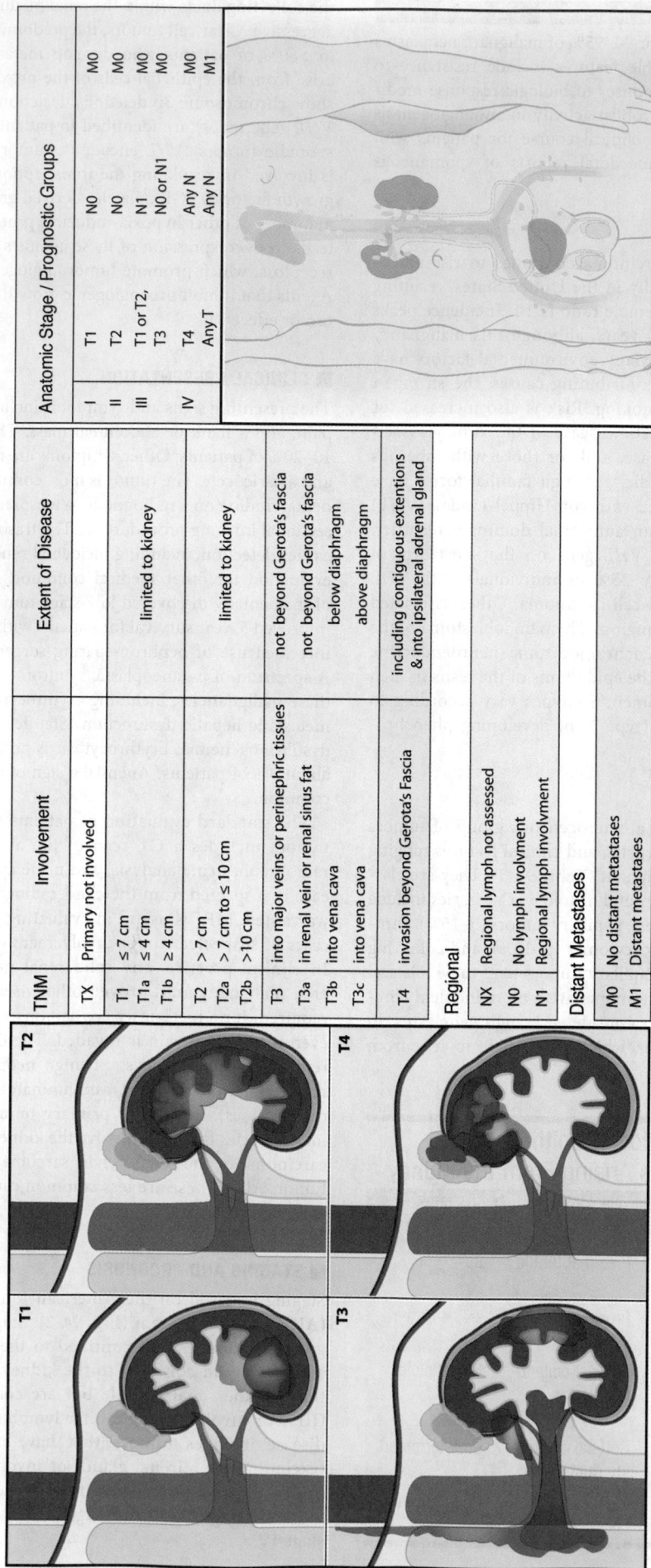

TNM	Involvement	Extent of Disease		Anatomic Stage / Prognostic Groups			
TX	Primary not involved			I	T1	N0	M0
T1	≤ 7 cm	limited to kidney		II	T2	N0	M0
T1a	≤ 4 cm			III	T1 or T2,	N1	M0
T1b	≥ 4 cm				T3	N0 or N1	M0
T2	> 7 cm	limited to kidney		IV	T4	Any N	M0
T2a	> 7 cm to ≤ 10 cm				Any T	Any N	M1
T2b	>10 cm						
T3	into major veins or perinephric tissues	not beyond Gerota's fascia					
T3a	in renal vein or renal sinus fat	not beyond Gerota's fascia					
T3b	into vena cava	below diaphragm					
T3c	into vena cava	above diaphragm					
T4	invasion beyond Gerota's Fascia	including contiguous extentions & into ipsilateral adrenal gland					

Regional

NX	Regional lymph not assessed
N0	No lymph involvment
N1	Regional lymph involvment

Distant Metastases

M0	No distant metastases
M1	Distant metastases

Figure 94-2 Renal cell carcinoma staging. TNM, tumor, node, metastasis

LOCALIZED TUMORS The standard management for stage I or II tumors and selected cases of stage III disease is radical nephrectomy. This procedure involves en bloc removal of Gerota's fascia and its contents, including the kidney, the ipsilateral adrenal gland, and adjacent hilar lymph nodes. The role of a regional lymphadenectomy is controversial. Extension into the renal vein or inferior vena cava (stage III disease) does not preclude resection even if cardiopulmonary bypass is required. If the tumor is resected, half of these patients have prolonged survival.

Nephron-sparing approaches via open or laparoscopic surgery may be appropriate for patients who have only one kidney, depending on the size and location of the lesion. A nephron-sparing approach can also be used for patients with bilateral tumors, accompanied by a radical nephrectomy on the opposite side. Partial nephrectomy techniques are applied electively to resect small masses for patients with a normal contralateral kidney. Adjuvant therapy following this surgery does not improve outcome, even in cases with a poor prognosis.

ADVANCED DISEASE Surgery has a limited role for patients with metastatic disease. However, long-term survival may occur in patients who relapse after nephrectomy in a solitary site that can be removed. One indication for nephrectomy with metastases at initial presentation is to alleviate pain or hemorrhage of a primary tumor. Also, a cytoreductive nephrectomy before systemic treatment improves survival for carefully selected patients with stage IV tumors.

Metastatic renal cell carcinoma is highly refractory to chemotherapy. Cytokine therapy with IL-2 or IFN-α produces regressions in 10–20% of patients. IL-2 produces durable complete remission in a small proportion of cases. In general, cytokine therapy is considered unsatisfactory for most patients.

The situation changed dramatically when two large-scale randomized trials established a role for antiangiogenic therapy in this disease, as predicted by the genetic studies. These trials separately evaluated two orally administered antiangiogenic agents, sorafenib and sunitinib, that inhibited receptor tyrosine kinase signaling through the VEGF and PDGF receptors. Both showed efficacy as second-line treatment following progression during cytokine treatment, resulting in approval by regulatory authorities for the treatment of advanced renal cell carcinoma. A randomized phase 3 trial comparing sunitinib to IFN-α showed superior efficacy for sunitinib with an acceptable safety profile. The trial resulted in a change in the standard first-line treatment from IFN to sunitinib. Sunitinib is usually given orally at a dose of 50 mg/d for 4 weeks out of 6. Diarrhea is the main toxicity. Sorafenib is usually given orally at a dose of 400 mg bid. In addition to diarrhea, toxicities include rash, fatigue, and hand-foot syndrome. Temsirolimus and everolimus, inhibitors of the mammalian target of rapamycin (mTOR), show activity in patients with untreated poor-prognosis tumors and in sunitinib/sorafenib refractory tumors.

The prognosis of metastatic renal cell carcinoma is variable. In one analysis, no prior nephrectomy, a KPS <80, low hemoglobin, high corrected calcium, and abnormal lactate dehydrogenase were poor prognostic factors. Patients with zero, one or two, and three or more factors had a median survival of 24, 12, and 5 months, respectively. These tumors may follow an unpredictable and protracted clinical course. It may be best to document progression before considering systemic treatment.

FURTHER READINGS

Bladder Cancer: NCCN Clinical Practice Guidelines in Oncology, version 1.2011 *www.nccn.org*

CHENG L et al: Bladder cancer: Translating molecular genetic insights into clinical practice. Hum Pathol 42:455, 2011

HUTSON TE et al: Targeted therapies for metastatic renal cell carcinoma: An overview of toxicity and dosing strategies. Oncologist 13:1084, 2008

IYER G et al: Novel strategies for treating relapsed/refractory urothelial carcinoma. Expert Rev Anticancer Ther 10:1917, 2010

LINEHAN WM et al: Molecular diagnosis and therapy of kidney cancer. Annu Rev Med 61:329, 2010

MOTZER RJ et al: Efficacy of everolimus in advanced renal cell carcinoma: A double-blind, randomised, placebo-controlled phase III trial. Lancet 372:449, 2008

MULDERS P: Vascular endothelial growth factor and mTOR pathways in renal cell carcinoma: Differences and synergies of two targeted mechanisms. BJU Int 104:158, 2009

PAL SK et al: Breaking through a plateau in renal cell carcinoma therapeutics: Development and incorporation of biomarkers. Mol Cancer Ther 9:3115, 2010

ROUPRÊT M et al: European guidelines for the diagnosis and management of upper urinary tract urothelial cell carcinomas: 2011 update. Eur Urol 59:584, 2011

SOLSONA E et al: Feasibility of radical transurethral resection as monotherapy for selected patients with muscle invasive bladder cancer. J Urol 184:475, 2010

ZLOTTA AR et al: BCAN Think Tank session 1: Overview of risks for and causes of bladder cancer. Urol Oncol 28:329, 2010

Benign and Malignant Diseases of the Prostate

Howard I. Scher

Benign and malignant changes in the prostate increase with age. Autopsies of men in the eighth decade of life show hyperplastic changes in >90% and malignant changes in >70% of individuals. The high prevalence of these diseases among the elderly, who often have competing causes of morbidity and mortality, mandates a risk-adapted approach to diagnosis and treatment. This can be achieved by considering these diseases as a series of states. Each state represents a distinct clinical milestone for which therapy(ies) may be recommended based on current symptoms, the risk of developing symptoms, or death from disease in relation to death from other causes within a given time frame (Fig. 95-1). For benign proliferative disorders, symptoms of urinary frequency, infection, and potential for obstruction are weighed against the side effects and complications of medical or surgical intervention. For prostate malignancies, the risks of developing the disease, symptoms, or death from cancer are balanced against the morbidities of the recommended treatments and preexisting comorbidities.

ANATOMY AND PATHOLOGY

The prostate is located in the pelvis and is surrounded by the rectum, the bladder, the periprostatic and dorsal vein complexes and neurovascular bundles that are responsible for erectile function, and the urinary sphincter that is responsible for passive urinary control. The prostate is composed of branching tubuloalveolar glands arranged in lobules surrounded by fibromuscular stroma. The acinar unit includes an epithelial compartment made up of epithelial, basal, and neuroendocrine cells and separated by a basement membrane, a stromal compartment that includes fibroblasts and smooth-muscle cells. Prostate-specific antigen (PSA) and prostatic acid phosphatase (PAP) are produced in the epithelial cells. Both prostate epithelial cells and stromal cells express androgen receptors (ARs) and depend on androgens for growth. Testosterone, the major circulating androgen, is converted by the enzyme 5α-reductase to dihydrotestosterone in the gland.

The periurethral portion of the gland increases in size during puberty and after the age of 55 years due to the growth of nonmalignant cells in the transition zone of the prostate that surrounds the urethra. Most cancers develop in the peripheral zone, and cancers in this location can often be palpated during a digital rectal examination (DRE).

PROSTATE CANCER

In 2010 approximately 217,730 prostate cancer cases were diagnosed, and 32,050 men died from prostate cancer in the United States. The absolute number of prostate cancer deaths has decreased in the past 5 years, which has been attributed by some to the widespread use of PSA-based detection strategies. However, the benefit of screening on survival is unclear. The paradox of management is that although 1 in 6 men will eventually be diagnosed with the disease, and the disease remains the second leading cause of cancer deaths in men, only 1 man in 30 with prostate cancer will die of his disease.

■ EPIDEMIOLOGY

Epidemiologic studies show that the risk of being diagnosed with prostate cancer increases by a factor of two if one first-degree relative is affected and by four if two or more are affected. Current estimates are that 40% of early-onset and 5–10% of all prostate cancers are hereditary. Prostate cancer affects ethnic groups differently. Matched for age, African-American males compared to white males have both a greater number of typically multifocal and highly unstable prostatic intraepithelial neoplasia (PIN) lesions, which are precursors to cancer, and larger tumors, possibly related to the higher levels of testosterone seen in African American males. Polymorphic variants of the AR, the cytochrome P450 C17, and the steroid 5α-reductase type II (SRD5A2) genes have also been implicated in the variations in incidence.

The prevalence of autopsy-detected cancers is similar around the world, while the incidence of clinical disease varies. Thus, environmental factors may play a role. High consumption of dietary fats,

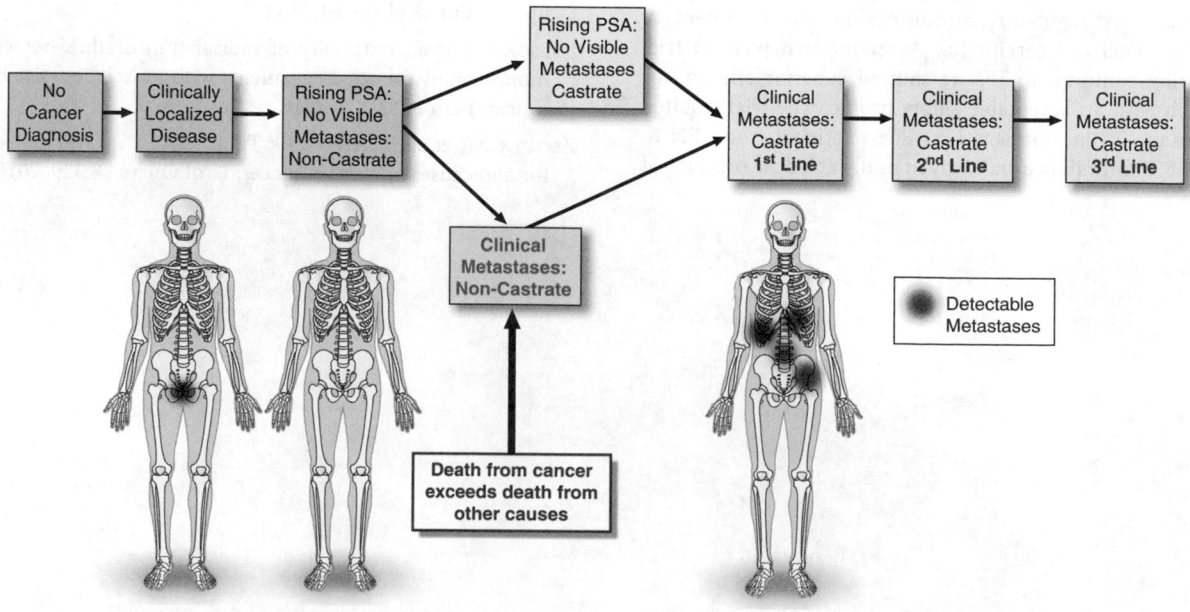

Figure 95-1 Clinical states of prostate cancer. PSA, prostate-specific antigen.

such as α-linoleic acid, or the polycyclic aromatic hydrocarbons that form when red meats are cooked is believed to increase risk. Similar to breast cancer in Asian women, the risk of prostate cancer in Asian men increases when they move to Western environments. Protective factors include consumption of the isoflavonoid genistein (which inhibits 5α-reductase) found in many legumes, cruciferous vegetables that contain the isothiocyanate sulforaphane, retinoids such as lycopene found in tomatoes, and inhibitors of cholesterol biosynthesis (e.g., statin drugs). The development of prostate cancer is a multistep process. One early change is hypermethylation of the GSTP1 gene promoter, which leads to loss of function of a gene that detoxifies carcinogens. The finding that many prostate cancers develop adjacent to a lesion termed PIA (proliferative inflammatory atrophy) suggests a role for inflammation.

■ DIAGNOSIS AND TREATMENT BY CLINICAL STATE

The prostate cancer continuum—from the appearance of a preneoplastic and invasive lesion localized to the prostate, to a metastatic lesion that results in symptoms and, ultimately, mortality—can span decades. To facilitate disease management, competing risks are considered in the context of a series of clinical states (Fig. 95-1). The states are defined operationally on the basis of whether or not a cancer diagnosis has been established and, for those with a diagnosis, whether or not metastases are detectable on imaging studies and the measured level of testosterone in the blood. With this approach, an individual resides in only one state and remains in that state until he has progressed. At each assessment, the decision to offer treatment and the specific form of treatment is based on the risk posed by the cancer relative to competing causes of mortality that may be present in that individual. It follows that the more advanced the disease, the greater the need for treatment.

For those without a cancer diagnosis, the decision to undergo testing to detect a cancer is based on the individual's estimated life expectancy and, separately, the probability that a clinically significant cancer may be present. For those with a prostate cancer diagnosis, the states model considers the probability of developing symptoms or dying from disease. Thus, a patient with localized prostate cancer who has had all cancer removed surgically remains in the state of localized disease as long as the PSA remains undetectable. The time within a state becomes a measure of the efficacy of an intervention, though the effect may not be assessable for years. As many men with active cancer are not at risk for developing metastases, symptoms, or death, the states model allows a distinction between *cure*—the elimination of all cancer cells, the primary therapeutic objective when treating most cancers—and *cancer control*, in which the tempo of the illness is altered and symptoms controlled until the patient dies of other causes. These can be equivalent therapeutically from a patient standpoint if the patient has not experienced symptoms of the disease or the treatment needed to control it. Even when a recurrence is documented, immediate therapy is not always necessary. Rather, as at the time of diagnosis, the need for intervention is based on the tempo of the illness as it unfolds in the individual, relative to the risk-to-benefit ratio of the therapy being considered.

■ NO CANCER DIAGNOSIS

Prevention

The results from several large double-blind, randomized chemoprevention trials have established 5α-reductase inhibitors (5ARI) as the predominant therapy to reduce the future risk of a prostate cancer diagnosis. The Prostate Cancer Prevention Trial (PCPT), in which men older than age 55 years received the 5α-reductase inhibitor finasteride, which inhibits the type 1 isoform, or a placebo, showed a 25% (95% confidence interval 19–31%) reduction in the period prevalence of prostate cancer across all age groups in favor of finasteride (18.4%) over placebo (24.4%). In REDUCE (Reduction by Dutasteride of Prostate Cancer Events Trial), a similar 23% reduction in the 4-year period prevalence was observed in favor of dutasteride ($p = 0.001$). Dutasteride inhibits both the type 1 and type 2 5ARI isoforms. These results contrast with those of the Selenium and Vitamin E Cancer Prevention Trial (SELECT) in which African American men aged ≥50 years and others aged ≥55 years were enrolled, which showed no difference in cancer incidence in patients receiving vitamin E (4.6%) or selenium (4.9%) alone or in combination (4.6%) relative to placebo (4.4%). A similar lack of benefit for vitamin E, vitamin C, and selenium was seen in the Physicians Health Study II.

Physical examination

The need to pursue a diagnosis of prostate cancer is based on symptoms, an abnormal DRE, or, more typically, a change in or an elevated serum PSA. The urologic history should focus on symptoms of outlet obstruction, continence, potency, or change in ejaculatory pattern.

The DRE focuses on prostate size and consistency and abnormalities within or beyond the gland. Many cancers occur in the peripheral zone and can be palpated on DRE. Carcinomas are characteristically hard, nodular, and irregular, while induration may also be due to benign prostatic hypertrophy (BPH) or calculi. Overall, 20–25% of men with an abnormal DRE have cancer.

Prostate-specific antigen

PSA (kallikrein-related peptidase 3; *KLK3*) is a kallikrein-related serine protease that causes liquefaction of seminal coagulum. It is produced by both nonmalignant and malignant epithelial cells and, as such, is prostate-specific, not prostate cancer–specific, and serum levels may also increase from prostatitis and BPH. Serum levels are not affected by DRE but the performance of a prostate biopsy can increase PSA levels up to tenfold for 8–10 weeks. PSA circulating in the blood is inactive and mainly occurs as a complex with the protease inhibitor α$_1$-antichymotrypsin *SERPIN A3* and as free unbound PSA forms. The formation of complexes between PSA, α$_2$-macroglobulin, or other protease inhibitors is less significant. Free PSA is rapidly eliminated from the blood by glomerular filtration with an estimated half-life of 12-18 hours. Elimination of PSA bound to α$_1$-antichymotrypsin is slow (estimated half-life of 1-2 weeks) as it is too large to be cleared by the kidneys. Levels should be undetectable after about six weeks if the prostate has been removed. Immunohistochemical staining for PSA can be used to establish a prostate cancer diagnosis.

PSA testing was approved by the U.S. FDA in 1994 for early detection of prostate cancer, and the widespread use of the test has played a significant role in the proportion of men diagnosed with early-stage cancers: more than 70–80% of newly diagnosed cancers are organ confined. The level of PSA in blood is strongly associated with the risk and outcome of prostate cancer. A single PSA measured at age 60 is associated (AUC of 0.90) with lifetime risk of death from prostate cancer. Most (90%) prostate cancer deaths occur among men with PSA levels in top quartile (>2 ng/mL), although only a minority of men with PSA >2 ng/mL will develop lethal prostate cancer. Despite this and mortality rate reductions reported from large randomized prostate cancer screening trials, routine use of the test remains controversial. The American Cancer Society (ACS) recommends that physicians offer PSA testing and a DRE on an annual basis for men older than age 50 years with an anticipated survival of >10 years; this includes men up to age 76 years. For African Americans and men with a family history of prostate cancer, testing is advised to begin at age 45 years. The American Urologic Association recommendations are similar, with the proviso that the risks and benefits of the performance of these tests are not defined. The American College of Physicians recommends that physicians "describe the potential benefits and known harms of screening" and to "individualize the decision to screen." The National Comprehensive Cancer Network (NCCN) guidelines mirror those of the ACS, with the proviso that "physicians and potential participants must thoroughly discuss the pros and cons of screening." The NCCN also advises that men who opt to participate obtain a baseline PSA and DRE in their values and use the value to stratify future risk. As PSA values may fluctuate for no apparent reason, it is advised that isolated abnormal values should be confirmed before proceeding with further testing.

The PSA criteria used to recommend a diagnostic prostate biopsy have evolved over time. However, based on the commonly used outpoint for prostate biopsy CPSA≥4 mg/mL, most men with a PSA elevation do not have histologic widence of prostate cancer at biopsy, and commonly, many men with PSA levels below this cut point harbor cancer cells in their prostate. The goal is to increase the sensitivity of the test for younger men more likely to die of the disease and to reduce the frequency of detecting cancers of low malignant potential in elderly men more likely to die of other causes. Previously, the threshold for performance of a biopsy was 4.0 ng/mL, which has been reduced to 3 mg/mL or 2.6 ng/mL for men aged <60 years by many groups based on the finding that nearly half of the men with PSAs who reached this level increased to 4 ng/mL within a relatively short (4-year) time frame and that, once diagnosed, in nearly one-third it had spread beyond the confines of the gland.

Most PSA is complexed to α_1-antichymotrypsin (ACT); only a small percentage is "free," and lower in men with cancer. Free and complexed PSA measurements are used when levels are between 4 and 10 ng/mL to decide whether a biopsy is needed. The risk of cancer is under 10% if the free PSA is >25% but as high as 56% for those with a free PSA <10%. PSA density (PSAD) measurements were developed to correct for the contribution of BPH to the total PSA level. PSAD is calculated by dividing the serum PSA by the prostate weight estimated from transrectal ultrasound (TRUS). Values <0.10 ng/mL per cm³ are consistent with BPH, while those >0.15 ng/mL per cm³ suggest cancer. *PSA dynamics* is the rate of change in PSA levels over time and is expressed most commonly as the *PSA velocity* or *PSA doubling time*. It is particularly useful for men with seemingly normal values that are rising. For men with a PSA level higher than 4 ng/mL, rates of rise >0.75 ng/mL per year suggest cancer, while for those with lower PSA levels, rates >0.5 ng/mL per year should be used to advise a biopsy. As an example, an increase from 2.5 to 3.2 ng/mL in a 1-year period would warrant further testing.

PSA-based detection strategies have changed the clinical spectrum of the disease. Now, 95–99% of newly diagnosed cancers are clinically localized, 40% are not palpable, and of these, 70% are pathologically organ-confined. However, the benefits of PSA screening remain controversial due to the overdetection of cancers with low malignant potential that may lead to overtreatment and unnecessary morbidity. To this end, the U.S. Prostate, Lung, Colorectal and Ovarian (PLCO) Cancer Screening trial found no mortality benefit from combined PSA screening and DRE in 76,693 randomized men (annual exam vs. standard care) with a median follow-up of 11 years. However, important caveats about the PLCO study include (1) many screening participants had already undergone PSA screening before the trial; (2) contamination from PSA testing among controls increased from 40% in year one to 52% in year six and; (3) and the biopsy compliance was low. These factors make interpretation difficult. A subgroup analysis of this trial showed a reduction in cancer mortality among screened men with little or no comorbidity. The European Randomized Study of Screening for Prostate Cancer (ERSPC) trial followed 182,000 men a median of 9 years randomized either to PSA screening every 4 years or to a group not receiving regular PSA screening. In this study, PSA screening without DRE corresponded to a 20% relative reduction of the rate of death from prostate cancer. A report from the Swedish subgroup of this study based on 14 years

follow-up suggested that PSA screening may reduce cancer-specific mortality by nearly half with less overdiagnosis and treatment than was noted in the European Study as a whole. Men remain advised to make an informed decision on an individual basis about whether to undergo testing.

A diagnostic algorithm based on the DRE and PSA findings is illustrated in Fig. 95-2. In general, a biopsy is recommended if the DRE or PSA is abnormal. Twenty-five percent of men with a PSA >4 ng/mL and an abnormal DRE have cancer, as do 17% of men with a PSA of 2.5–4 ng/mL and normal DRE.

Prostate biopsy

A diagnosis of cancer is established by a TRUS-guided needle biopsy. Direct visualization by ultrasound or MRI assures that all areas of the gland are sampled. A minimum of six separate cores, three from the right and three from the left, is advised, as is a separate biopsy of the transition zone if clinically indicated. Contemporary schemas advise an extended-pattern 12- to 14-core biopsy that includes the sextant sampling above plus 6 cores from the lateral peripheral zones as well as a lesion-directed palpable nodule or suspicious image-guided sampling. Patients with prostatitis should have a course of antibiotics before biopsy. Men with an abnormal PSA and negative biopsy are advised to undergo a repeat biopsy.

Each core of the biopsy is examined for the presence of cancer, and the amount of cancer is quantified based on the length of the tumor within the core and the percentage of the core involved.

Pathology

The noninvasive proliferation of epithelial cells within ducts is termed *prostatic intraepithelial neoplasia*. PIN is a precursor of cancer, but not all PIN lesions develop into invasive cancers. Of the cancers identified, >95% are adenocarcinomas; the rest are squamous or transitional cell tumors or, rarely, carcinosarcomas. Metastases to the prostate are rare, but in some cases colon cancers or transitional cell tumors of the bladder invade the gland by direct extension.

When prostate cancer is diagnosed, a measure of histologic aggressiveness is assigned using the *Gleason grading system*, in which the dominant and secondary glandular histologic patterns are scored from 1 (well-differentiated) to 5 (undifferentiated) and summed to give a total score of 2–10 for each tumor. The most poorly differentiated area of tumor (i.e., the area with the highest histologic grade) often determines biologic behavior. The presence or absence of perineural invasion and extracapsular spread are also recorded.

Prostate cancer staging

The TNM staging system includes categories for cancers that are palpable on DRE, those identified solely on the basis of an abnormal PSA (T1c), those that are palpable but clinically confined to the gland (T2), and those that have extended outside the gland (T3 and T4) (Table 95-1, Fig. 95-3). DRE alone is inaccurate in determining the extent of disease within the gland, the presence or absence of capsular invasion, involvement of seminal vesicles, and extension of disease to lymph nodes. Because of the inadequacy of DRE for staging, the TNM staging system was modified to include the results of imaging. Unfortunately, no single test has proven to accurately indicate the stage or the presence of organ-confined disease, seminal vesicle involvement, or lymph node spread.

TRUS is the imaging technique most frequently used to assess the primary tumor, but its chief use is directing prostate biopsies, not staging. No TRUS finding consistently indicates cancer with certainty. CT lacks sensitivity and specificity to detect extraprostatic extension and is inferior to MRI in visualization of lymph nodes. In general, MRI performed with an endorectal coil is superior to CT to detect cancer in the prostate and to assess local disease extent.

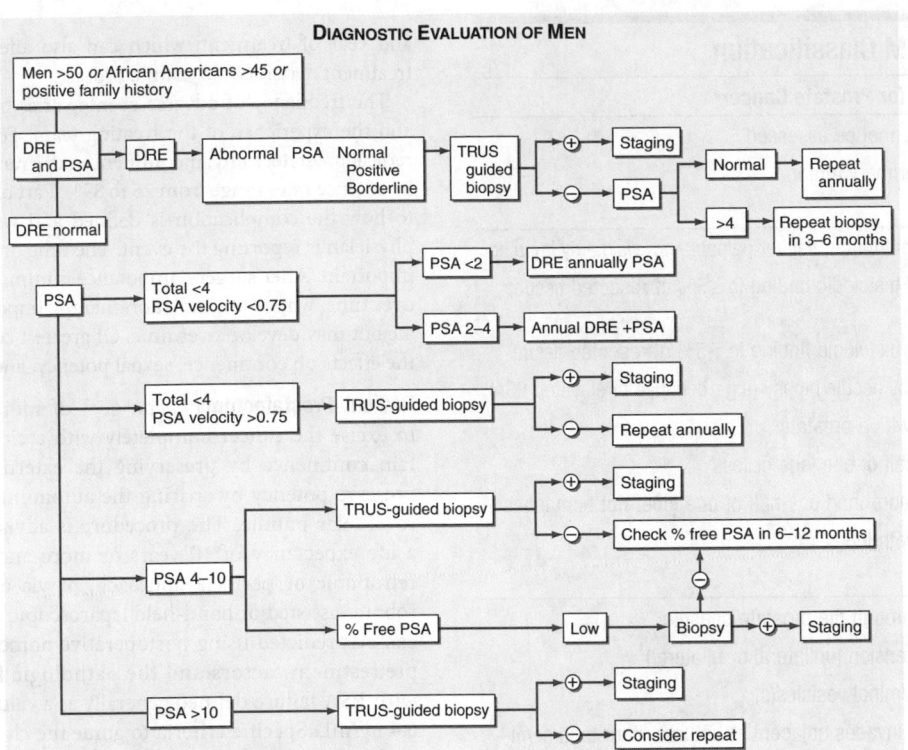

DIAGNOSTIC EVALUATION OF MEN

Figure 95-2 **Algorithm for diagnostic evaluation of men** based on digital rectal examination (DRE) and prostate-specific antigen (PSA) levels; TRUS, transrectal ultrasound.

T1-weighted images produce a high signal in the periprostatic fat, periprostatic venous plexus, perivesicular tissues, lymph nodes, and bone marrow. T2-weighted images demonstrate the internal architecture of the prostate and seminal vesicles. Most cancers have a low signal, while the normal peripheral zone has a high signal, although the technique lacks sensitivity and specificity. MRI is also useful for the planning of surgery and radiation therapy.

Radionuclide bone scans (bone scintigraphy) are used to evaluate spread to osseous sites. This test is sensitive but relatively nonspecific because areas of increased uptake are not always related to metastatic disease. Healing fractures, arthritis, Paget's disease, and other conditions will also cause abnormal uptake. True-positive bone scans are rare if the PSA is <8 ng/mL and uncommon when the PSA is <10 ng/mL unless the tumor is high-grade.

TREATMENT **Prostate Cancer**

CLINICALLY LOCALIZED DISEASE Localized prostate cancers are those that appear to be nonmetastatic after staging studies are performed. Patients with localized disease are managed by radical prostatectomy, radiation therapy, or active surveillance. Choice of therapy requires the consideration of several factors: the presence of symptoms, the probability that the untreated tumor will adversely affect the quality or duration of survival and thus require treatment, and the probability that the tumor can be cured by single-modality therapy directed at the prostate or requires both local and systemic therapy to achieve cure. As most of the tumors detected are deemed clinically significant, most men undergo treatment.

Data from the literature do not provide clear evidence for the superiority of any one treatment relative to another. Comparison of outcomes of various forms of therapy is limited by the lack of prospective trials, referral bias, the experience of the treating teams and differences in endpoints and cancer control definitions. Often, PSA relapse–free survival is used because an effect on metastatic progression or survival may not be apparent for years. After radical surgery to remove all prostate tissue, PSA should become undetectable in the blood within 4 weeks, based on the PSA half-life in the blood of 3 days. If PSA remains detectable, the patient is considered to have persistent disease. After radiation therapy, in contrast, PSA does not become undetectable because the remaining nonmalignant elements of the gland continue to produce PSA even if all cancer cells have been eliminated. Similarly, cancer control is not well defined for a patient managed by active surveillance because PSA levels will continue to rise in the absence of therapy. Other outcomes are time to objective progression (local or systemic) and cancer-specific and overall survival; however, these outcomes may take years to assess.

The more advanced the disease, the lower the probability of local control and the higher the probability of systemic relapse. More important is that within the categories of T1, T2, and T3 disease are tumors with a range of prognoses. Some T3 tumors are curable with therapy directed solely at the prostate, and some T1 lesions have a high probability of systemic relapse that requires the integration of local and systemic therapy to achieve cure. For T1c tumors in particular, stage alone is inadequate to predict outcome and select treatment; other factors must be considered.

To better assess risk and guide treatment selection, many groups have developed prognostic models or nomograms that use a combination of the initial T stage, Gleason score, and baseline PSA. Some use discrete cut points (PSA <10 or ≥10 ng/mL; Gleason score of ≤6, 7, or ≥8); others employ nomograms that use PSA and Gleason score as continuous variables. More than 100 nomograms have been reported to predict the probability that a clinically significant cancer is present, disease extent (organ-confined vs. non–organ-confined, node-negative or -positive), or the probability of success of treatment for specific local therapies using pretreatment variables. Considerable controversy exists over what constitutes "high risk" based on a predicted probability of success or

TABLE 95-1 TNM Classification

TNM Staging System for Prostate Cancer[a]

Tx	Primary tumor cannot be assessed
T0	No evidence of primary tumor

Localized Disease

T1	Clinically inapparent tumor, neither palpable nor visible by imaging
T1a	Tumor incidental histologic finding in ≤5% of resected tissue; not palpable
T1b	Tumor incidental histologic finding in >5% of resected tissue
T1c	Tumor identified by needle biopsy (e.g., because of elevated PSA)
T2	Tumor confined within prostate[b]
T2a	Tumor involves half of one lobe or less
T2b	Tumor involves more than one half of one lobe, not both lobes
T2c	Tumor involves both lobes

Local Extension

T3	Tumor extends through the prostate capsule[c]
T3a	Extracapsular extension (unilateral or bilateral)
T3b	Tumor invades seminal vesicles(s)
T4	Tumor is fixed or invades adjacent structures other than seminal vesicles such as external sphincter, rectum, bladder, levator muscles, and/or pelvic wall.

Metastatic Disease

N1	Positive regional lymph nodes
M1	Distant metastases

[a]Revised from SB Edge et al (eds): *AJCC Cancer Staging Manual*, 7th ed. New York, Springer, 2010.

[b]Tumor found in one or both lobes by needle biopsy, but not palpable or reliably visible by imaging, is classified as T1c.

[c]Invasion into the prostatic apex or into (but not beyond) the prostatic capsule is classified not as T3 but as T2.

Abbreviation: PSA, prostate-specific antigen.

failure. In these situations, nomograms and predictive models can only go so far. Exactly what probability of success or failure would lead a physician to recommend and a patient to seek alternative approaches is controversial. As an example, it may be appropriate to recommend radical surgery for a younger patient with a low probability of cure. Nomograms are being refined continually to incorporate additional clinical parameters, biologic determinants,

and year of treatment, which can also affect outcomes, making treatment decisions a dynamic process.

The frequency of adverse events varies by treatment modality and the experience of the treating team. For example, following radical prostatectomy, incontinence rates range from 2 to 47% and impotence rates range from 25 to 89%. Part of the variability relates to how the complication is defined and whether the patient or physician is reporting the event. The time of the assessment is also important. After surgery, impotence is immediate but may reverse over time, while with radiation therapy impotence is not immediate but may develop over time. Of greatest concern to patients are the effects on continence, sexual potency, and bowel function.

Radical Prostatectomy The goal of radical prostatectomy is to excise the cancer completely with a clear margin, to maintain continence by preserving the external sphincter, and to preserve potency by sparing the autonomic nerves in the neurovascular bundle. The procedure is advised for patients with a life expectancy of 10 years or more and is performed via a retropubic or perineal approach, or via a minimally invasive robotic-assisted or hand-held laparoscopic approach. Outcomes can be predicted using postoperative nomograms that consider pretreatment factors and the pathologic findings at surgery, with PSA failure defined generally as a value greater than 0.2 or 0.4 ng/mL. Specific criteria to guide the choice of one approach over another are lacking. Minimally invasive approaches offer the advantage of a shorter hospital stay and a more rapid recovery with the trade-off of higher rates of incontinence and erectile dysfunction. Cancer control rates are comparable.

Neoadjuvant hormonal therapy has also been explored in an attempt to improve the outcomes of surgery for high-risk patients using a variety of definitions. The results of several large trials testing 3 or 8 months of androgen depletion before surgery showed that serum PSA levels decreased by 96%, prostate volumes decreased by 34%, and margin positivity rates decreased from 41 to 17%. Unfortunately, hormones did not produce an improvement in PSA relapse–free survival. Thus, neoadjuvant hormonal therapy is not recommended.

Factors associated with incontinence include older age and urethral length, which impacts the ability to preserve the urethra beyond the apex and the distal sphincter. The specific surgical technique, open vs. laparoscopic vs. robotic, as well as the skill and experience of the surgeon are also factors. In a series treated at an academic center, 6% of patients had mild stress urinary incontinence (SUI) (requiring 1 pad/day), 2% moderate SUI (>1 pad/day), and 0.3% severe SUI (requiring an artificial

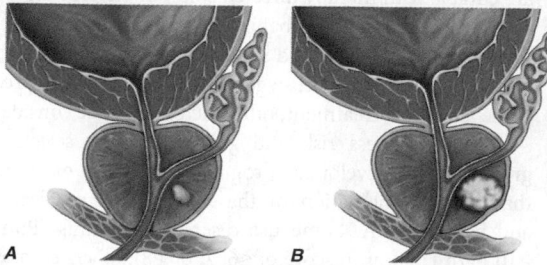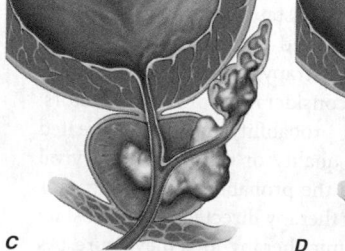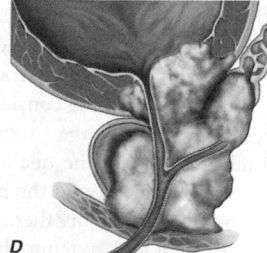

Figure 95-3 T stages of prostate cancer. *(A)* T1—Clinically inapparent tumor, neither palpable nor visible by imaging; *(B)* T2—Tumor confined within prostate; *(C)* T3—Tumor extends through prostate capsule and may invade the seminal vesicles; *(D)* T4—Tumor is fixed or invades adjacent structures. Eighty percent of patients present with local disease (T1 and T2), which is associated with a 5-year survival rate of 100%. An additional 12% of patients present with regional disease (T3 and T4 without metastases),

which is also associated with a 100% survival rate after 5 years. Four percent of patients present with distant disease (T4 with metastases), which is associated with a 30% 5-year survival rate. (Three percent of patients are ungraded.) *(Data from AJCC, http://seer.cancer.gov/statfacts/html/prost.html. Figure © Memorial Sloan-Kettering Cancer Center Medical Graphics; used with permission.)*

urinary sphincter). At 1 year, 92% were completely continent. In contrast, the results in a Medicare population treated at multiple centers showed that at 3, 12, and 24 months following surgery, 58, 35, and 42%, respectively, wore pads in their underwear, and 24, 11, and 15% reported "a lot" of urine leakage.

Recovery of erectile function is associated with younger age, quality of erections before surgery, and the absence of damage to the neurovascular bundles. In general, erectile function begins to return in a median of 4–6 months if both bundles are preserved. Potency is reduced by half if at least one nerve bundle is sacrificed. In cases where cancer control requires the removal of both bundles, sural nerve grafts have shown no utility. Overall, with the availability of drugs such as sildenafil, intraurethral inserts of alprostadil, and intracavernosal injections of vasodilators, many patients recover satisfactory sexual function.

Radiation Therapy Radiation therapy is given by external beam, by radioactive sources implanted into the gland, or by a combination of the two techniques.

External Beam Radiation Therapy Contemporary external beam radiation therapy requires three-dimensional conformal treatment plans intensity-modulated radiation therapy (IMRT) to maximize the dose to the prostate and to minimize the exposure of the surrounding normal tissue. IMRT permits shaping of the dose, and allows the delivery of higher doses to the prostate and a further reduction in normal tissue exposure than 3D-conformal treatment alone. These advances have enabled the safe administration of doses >80 Gy, higher local control rates, and fewer side effects.

Cancer control after radiation therapy has been defined by various criteria, including a decline in PSA to <0.5 or 1 ng/mL, "nonrising" PSA values, and a negative biopsy of the prostate 2 years after completion of treatment. The current standard definition of biochemical failure (the Phoenix definition) is a rise in PSA by ≥2 ng/mL higher than the lowest PSA achieved. The date of failure is "at call" and not backdated.

Radiation dose is important and a minimum of 75.6 to 79 or 80 Gy advised. In a representative study, a PSA nadir of <1.0 ng/mL in 90% of patients receiving 75.6 or 81.0 Gy vs. 76% and 56% of those receiving 70.2 and 64.8 Gy, and positive biopsy rates at 2.5 years were 4% for those treated with 81 Gy vs. 27 and 36% for those receiving 75.6 or 70.2 Gy.

Overall, radiation therapy is associated with a higher frequency of bowel complications (mainly diarrhea and proctitis) than surgery. The frequency relates directly to the volume of the anterior rectal wall receiving full-dose treatment. In one series, Grade 3 rectal or urinary toxicities were seen in 2.1% of patients who received a median dose of 75.6 Gy, while Grade 3 urethral strictures requiring dilatation developed in 1% of cases, all of whom had undergone a transurethral resection of the prostate (TURP). Pooled data show that the frequency of Grade 3 and 4 toxicities is 6.9 and 3.5%, respectively, for patients who received >70 Gy. The frequency of erectile dysfunction is related to the quality of erections pretreatment, the dose administered, and the time of assessment. Postradiation erectile dysfunction is related to a disruption of the vascular supply and not the nerve fibers.

Neoadjuvant hormone therapy before radiation therapy has been studied. The aim is to decrease the size of the prostate and, consequently, to reduce the exposure of normal tissues to full-dose radiation, to increase local control rates, and to decrease the rate of systemic failure. Short-term hormone therapy can reduce toxicities and improve local control rates, but long-term treatment (2–3 years) is needed to prolong the time to PSA failure and lower the risk of metastatic disease. The impact on survival

has been less clear. The decision to treat the pelvic lymph nodes is based on the nomogram-predicted risk of nodal spread.

Brachytherapy Brachytherapy is the direct implantation of radioactive sources (seeds) into the prostate. It is based on the principle that the deposition of radiation energy in tissues decreases as a function of the square of the distance from the source (Chap. 85). The goal is to deliver intensive irradiation to the prostate, minimizing the exposure of the surrounding tissues. The current standard technique achieves a more homogeneous dose distribution by placing seeds according to a customized template based on CT and ultrasonographic assessment of the tumor and computer-optimized dosimetry. The implantation is performed transperineally as a one-day procedure with real-time imaging.

Improvements in brachytherapy techniques have resulted in fewer complications and a marked reduction in local failure rates. In a series of 197 patients followed for a median of 3 years, 5-year actuarial PSA relapse–free survival for patients with pretherapy PSA levels of 0–4, 4–10, and >10 ng/mL were 98, 90, and 89%, respectively. In a separate report of 201 patients who underwent posttreatment biopsies, 80% were negative, 17% were indeterminate, and 3% were positive. The results did not change with longer follow-up. Nevertheless, many physicians feel that implantation is best reserved for patients with good or intermediate prognostic features.

Brachytherapy is well tolerated, although most patients experience urinary frequency and urgency that can persist for several months. Incontinence has been seen in 2–4% of cases. Higher complication rates are observed in patients who have undergone a prior TURP, while those with obstructive symptoms at baseline are at a higher risk for retention and persistent voiding symptoms. Proctitis has been reported in <2% of patients.

Active Surveillance While prostate cancer is the most common form of cancer affecting men in the United States, patients are being diagnosed earlier and more frequently present with early-stage disease. Active surveillance, described previously as *watchful waiting* or *deferred therapy*, is the policy of monitoring the illness at fixed intervals with DREs, PSA measurements, and repeat prostate biopsies as indicated until histopathologic or serologic changes correlative of progression warrant treatment with curative intent. It evolved from studies that evaluated predominantly elderly men with well-differentiated tumors who demonstrated no clinically significant progression for protracted periods, recognition of the contrast between incidence and disease-specific mortality, the high prevalence of autopsy cancers and an effort to reduce overtreatment. A recent screening study estimated that between 50 and 100 men with low-risk disease would need to be treated to prevent one prostate cancer–specific death.

Arguing against active surveillance are the results of a Swedish randomized trial of radical prostatectomy vs. active surveillance. With a median follow-up of 6.2 years, men treated by radical surgery had a lower risk of prostate cancer death relative to active surveillance patients (4.6 vs. 8.9%) and a lower risk of metastatic progression (hazard ratio 0.63). Case selection is critical, and determining clinical parameters predictive of cancer aggressiveness that can be used to reliably select men most likely to benefit from active surveillance is an area of intense study. In one prostatectomy series, it was estimated that 10–15% of those treated had "insignificant" disease. One set of criteria includes men with T1c tumors that are Gleason grade 6 or less involving 3 or fewer cores, each of them having less than 50% involvement by tumor and a PSAD of 0.15.

Concerns include the limited ability to predict pathologic findings by needle biopsy even when multiple cores are obtained, the recognized multifocality of the disease, and the possibility of a missed opportunity to cure the disease. Nomograms to help predict which patients can safely be managed by active surveillance continue to be refined, and as their predictive accuracy improves, it can be anticipated that more patients will be candidates.

RISING PSA This state consists of patients in whom the sole manifestation of disease is a rising PSA after surgery and/or radiation therapy. By definition, there is no evidence of disease on scan. For these patients, the central issue is whether the rise in PSA results from persistent disease in the primary site, systemic disease, or both. In theory, disease in the primary site may still be curable by additional local treatment: external beam radiation for patients who had undergone surgery and prostatectomy for patients who had undergone radiation therapy.

The decision to recommend radiation therapy after prostatectomy is guided by the pathologic findings at surgery, as imaging studies such as CT and bone scan are typically uninformative. Some recommend a Prostascint scan—imaging with a radiolabeled antibody to prostate-specific membrane antigen (PSMA), which is highly expressed on prostate epithelial cells—to help with this distinction. Antibody localization to the prostatic fossa suggests local recurrence; localization to extrapelvic sites predicts failure of radiation therapy. Others recommend that a biopsy of the urethrovesical anastomosis be obtained before considering radiation. Factors that predict for response to salvage radiation therapy are a positive surgical margin, lower Gleason grade, long interval from surgery to PSA failure, slow PSA doubling time, and low (<0.5–1 ng/mL) PSA value at the time of radiation treatment. Radiation therapy is generally not recommended if the PSA was persistently elevated after surgery, which usually indicates that the disease had spread outside of the area of the prostate bed and is unlikely to be controlled with radiation therapy. As is the case for other disease states, nomograms to predict the likelihood of success are also available.

For patients with a rising PSA after radiation therapy, salvage prostatectomy can be considered if the disease was "curable" at the outset, if persistent disease has been documented by a biopsy of the prostate, and if no metastatic disease is seen on imaging studies. Unfortunately, case selection is poorly defined in most series, and morbidities are significant. As currently performed, virtually all patients are impotent after salvage radical prostatectomy, and approximately 45% have either total urinary incontinence or stress incontinence. Major bleeding, bladder neck contractures, and rectal injury are not uncommon.

More frequently, the rise in PSA after surgery or radiation therapy indicates subclinical or micrometastatic disease. In these cases, the need for treatment depends, in part, on the estimated probability that the patient will show evidence of metastatic disease on a scan and in what time frame. That immediate therapy is not always required was shown in a series where patients received no systemic therapy until metastatic disease was documented. Overall, the median time to metastatic progression was 8 years, and 63% of the patients with rising PSA values remained free of metastases at 5 years. Factors associated with progression included the primary tumor's Gleason grade, time to recurrence, and PSA doubling time. For those with Gleason grade ≥8 tumors, the probability of metastatic progression was 37, 51, and 71% at 3, 5, and 7 years, respectively. If the time to recurrence was <2 years and PSA doubling time was long (>10 months), the proportion with metastatic disease at the same time intervals was 23, 32, and 53%, vs. 47, 69, and 79% if the doubling time was short (<10 months). PSA doubling times are also prognostic for survival. In one series, all patients who succumbed to disease had PSA doubling times of 3 months or less. Most physicians advise treatment when PSA doubling times are 12 months or less. A difficulty with predicting the risk of metastatic spread, symptoms, or death from disease in the rising PSA state is that most patients receive some form of therapy before the development of metastases. Nevertheless, predictive models continue to be refined.

METASTATIC DISEASE: NONCASTRATE The state of *noncastrate metastatic disease* includes men with metastases visible on an imaging study and noncastrate levels of testosterone (>150 ng/dL). The patient may be newly diagnosed or have a recurrence after treatment for localized disease. Symptoms of metastatic disease include pain from osseous spread, although many patients are asymptomatic despite extensive spread. Less common are symptoms related to marrow compromise (myelophthisis), coagulopathy, or spinal cord compression.

Standard treatment is to deplete/lower androgens by medical or surgical means and/or to block androgen binding to the AR with antiandrogens. More than 90% of male hormones originate in the testes; <10% are synthesized in the adrenal gland. Surgical orchiectomy is the "gold standard" but is least acceptable to patients (Fig. 95-4).

Testosterone-Lowering Agents Medical therapies that lower testosterone levels include the gonadotropin-releasing hormone (GnRH) agonists/antagonists, 17,20-lyase inhibitors, cyp-17 inhibitors, estrogens, and progestational agents. Estrogens such as diethylstilbestrol (DES) have fallen out of favor due to the risk of vascular complications such as fluid retention, phlebitis, emboli, and stroke. GnRH analogues (leuprolide acetate and goserelin acetate) initially produce a rise in luteinizing hormone and follicle-stimulating hormone followed by a downregulation of receptors in the pituitary gland, which effects a chemical castration. They were approved on the basis of randomized comparisons showing an improved safety profile (specifically, reduced cardiovascular toxicities) relative to DES, with equivalent potency. The initial rise in testosterone may result in a clinical flare of the disease. These agents are therefore contraindicated in men with significant obstructive symptoms, cancer-related pain, or spinal cord compromise. GnRH antagonists such as degarelix achieve castrate levels of testosterone within 48 hours without the initial rise in serum testosterone.

Agents that lower testosterone are associated with an androgen-depletion syndrome that includes hot flushes, weakness, fatigue, impotence, sarcopenia, anemia, change in personality, and depression. Changes in lipids, obesity, insulin resistance, along with an increased risk of diabetes and cardiovascular disease can also occur. A decrease in bone density can also occur that worsens over time and results in an increase risk of clinical fractures. This is a particular concern in men with preexisting osteopenia that results from hypogonadism, steroid or alcohol use, and which is significantly underappreciated. Baseline fracture risk can be assessed using the FRAX scale, and to minimize fracture risk patients are advised calcium and vitamin D supplementation, along with a bisphosphonate or the recently approved RANK-ligand inhibitor, denosumab.

Antiandrogens Nonsteroidal antiandrogens such as flutamide, bicalutamide, and nilutamide block the ligand binding to the AR and were initially approved to block the flare associated with the rise in serum testosterone associated with GnRH agonist/antagonist therapy. Given alone, testosterone levels remain the same or increase while relative to testosterone-lowering therapies, cause fewer hot flushes, less of an effect on libido, less muscle wasting, fewer personality changes, and less bone loss. Gynecomastia remains a significant problem but can be alleviated in part by tamoxifen.

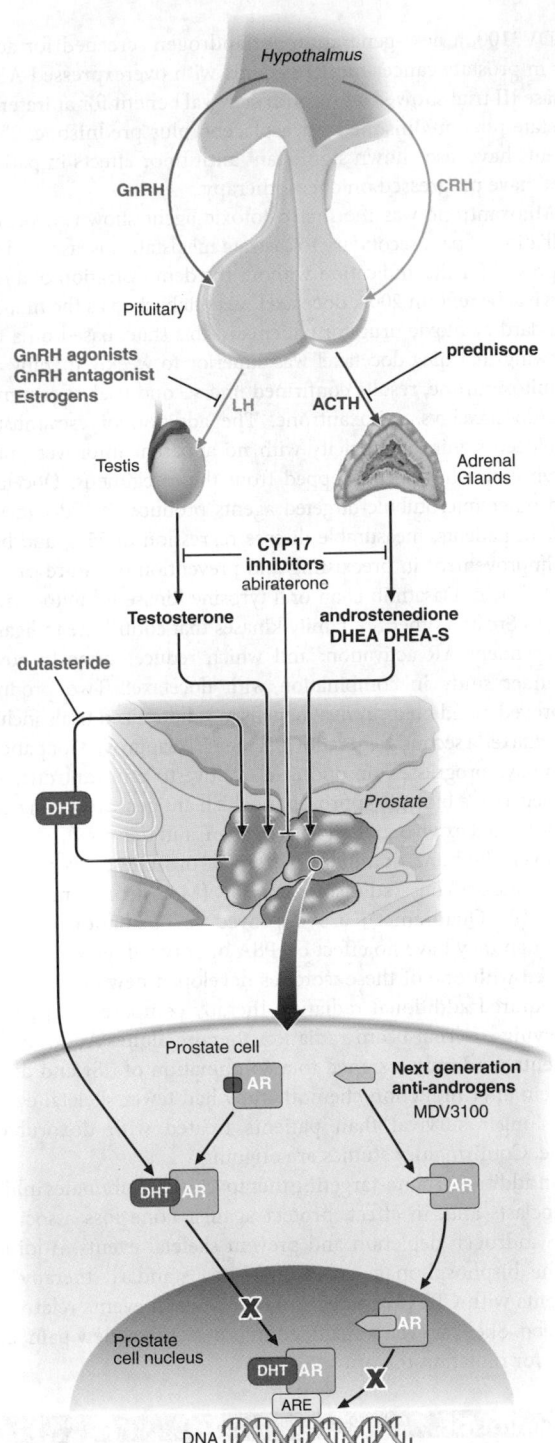

Figure 95-4 Sites of action of different hormone therapies.

monotherapies, and are no longer recommended. In practice, most patients who are treated with a GnRH analogue receive an antiandrogen for the first 2–4 weeks of treatment to protect against the flare.

Intermittent Androgen Deprivation Therapy (IADT) Another way to reduce the side effects of androgen depletion is to administer antiandrogens on an intermittent basis. This was proposed as a way to prevent the selection of cells that are resistant to androgen depletion. The hypothesis is that by allowing endogenous testosterone levels to rise, the cells that survive androgen depletion will induce a normal differentiation pathway. In this way, the surviving cells that are allowed to proliferate in the presence of androgen will retain sensitivity to subsequent androgen depletion. Applied in the clinic, androgen depletion is continued for 2–6 months beyond the point of maximal response. Once treatment is stopped, endogenous testosterone levels increase, and the symptoms associated with hormone treatment abate. PSA levels also begin to rise, and at some level treatment is restarted. With this approach, multiple cycles of regression and proliferation have been documented in individual patients. It is unknown whether the intermittent approach increases, decreases, or does not change the overall duration of sensitivity to androgen depletion. The approach is safe, but long-term data are needed to assess the course in men with low PSA levels. A trial to address this question is ongoing.

Outcomes of Androgen Depletion The antiprostate cancer effects of the various androgen depletion strategies are similar, and the clinical course is predictable: an initial response, then a period of stability in which tumor cells are dormant and nonproliferative, followed after a variable period of time by a rise in PSA and regrowth that is visible on a scan as a castration-resistant lesion. Androgen depletion is not curative because cells that survive castration are present when the disease is first diagnosed. Considered by disease manifestation, PSA levels return to normal in 60–70% of patients, and measurable disease regression occurs in 50%; improvements in bone scan occur in 25% of cases, but the majority remains stable. Duration of survival is inversely proportional to disease extent at the time androgen depletion is first started, while the degree of PSA decline at 6 months has been shown to be prognostic. In a large-scale trial, PSA nadir proved prognostic.

An active question is whether hormones should be given in the adjuvant setting after surgery or radiation treatment of the primary tumor, or at the time that a PSA recurrence is documented, or to wait until metastatic disease or symptoms of disease are manifest. Trials in support of early therapy have often been underpowered relative to the reported benefit or have been criticized for methodologic grounds. One trial, although it showed a survival benefit for patients treated with radiation therapy and 3 years of androgen depletion relative to radiation alone, was criticized for the poor outcomes of the control group. Another showing a survival benefit for patients with positive lymph nodes who were randomized to immediate medical or surgical castration compared to observation ($p = .02$) was criticized because the confidence intervals around the 5- and 8-year survival distributions for the two groups overlapped. A large randomized study comparing early to late hormone treatment (orchiectomy or GnRH analogue) in patients with locally advanced or asymptomatic metastatic disease showed that patients treated early were less likely to progress from M0 to M1 disease, to develop pain, and to die of prostate cancer. This trial was criticized because therapy was delayed "too long" in the late-treatment group. When patients treated by radical surgery, radiation therapy, or active surveillance were randomly assigned to receive bicalutamide 150 mg or placebo, hormone treatment produced a significant reduction in the proportion of patients

Most reported randomized trials suggest that the cancer-specific outcomes are inferior when antiandrogens are used alone. Bicalutamide, even at 150 mg (three times the recommended dose), was associated with a shorter time to progression and inferior survival compared to surgical castration for patients with established metastatic disease. Nevertheless, some men may accept the trade-off of a potentially inferior cancer outcome for an improved quality of life.

Combined androgen blockade, the administration of an antiandrogen plus a GnRH analogue or surgical orchiectomy, or triple androgen blockade, which includes the addition of a 5ARI, have not been shown to be superior to androgen depletion who developed osseous metastases at 2 years (9% for bicalutamide; 13.8% for placebo). This result has not gained acceptance in part because too many "good-risk" patients were treated and because no effect on survival was demonstrated. These criticisms are valid; however, the net influence on survival from early hormone intervention is similar to that observed in patients with breast cancer, for which adjuvant hormonal therapy is routinely given. It is of note that the American Society of Clinical Oncology Guidelines do not support immediate therapy.

METASTATIC DISEASE: CASTRATE Castration-resistant prostate cancer (CRPC), a disease that progresses despite androgen suppression by medical or surgical therapies where the measured levels of testosterone are 50 ng/mL or lower, continues to express the androgen receptor (AR) and is dependent on signaling through the receptor for growth. CRPC can manifest in many ways. For some it is a rise in PSA with no change in radiographs and no new symptoms. In others it is a rising PSA and progression in bone with or without symptoms of disease. Still others will show soft tissue disease with or without osseous metastases, and others have visceral spread. The prognosis, which is highly variable, can be predicted using nomograms designed for CRPC. The important point is that despite the failure of first-line hormone treatment, these tumors remain androgen driven and are not "hormone-refractory": the majority of these tumors remain sensitive to second- and third-line hormonal treatments. The rising PSA is an indication of continued signaling through the AR axis.

The manifestations of disease in this patient group limit the ability to reliably assess treatment effects because the traditional measures of outcome such as tumor regression do not apply. Bone scans can be inaccurate for assessing changes in osseous disease, and no PSA-based outcome is a true surrogate for survival benefit. It is essential to define therapeutic objectives before initiating treatment, as there are defined standards of care for different disease manifestations. Therapeutic objectives need not be defined by survival only as useful endpoints also include relief of symptoms and delay of metastases or new symptoms of disease.

Management of pain secondary to osseous metastatic disease is a critical part of therapy. Optimal palliation requires assessing whether the symptoms and metastases are focal or diffuse and whether disease threatens the spinal cord, the cauda equina, or the base of the skull. Neurologic symptoms require emergency evaluation because loss of function may be permanent if not addressed quickly. Single sites of pain and areas of neurologic involvement are best treated with external beam radiation. As the disease is often diffuse, palliation at one site often is followed by the emergence of symptoms in a separate site that had not received radiation.

It is also essential to ensure that a castrate status be documented. Patients receiving an antiandrogen alone, whose serum testosterone levels are elevated, should be treated first with a GnRH analogue or orchiectomy and observed for response. Patients on an antiandrogen in combination with a GnRH analogue should have the antiandrogen discontinued, as approximately 20% will respond to the selective discontinuation of the antiandrogen. Any withdrawal response occurs within weeks of stopping flutamide but may take 8–12 weeks with nilutamide and bicalutamide because of their long terminal half-lives. Ketoconazole, 600 to 1200 mg daily in combination with hydrocortisone, which inhibits adrenal androgen production, also has activity in this setting, but has not been formally evaluated in definitive phase III trials.

Hormonal agents in late phase III development that target specific pathogenetic mechanisms of AR function reactivation include abiraterone acetate, a novel CYP17 inhibitor that blocks androgen synthesis in the adrenal gland, testis, and tumor; and

MDV3100, a next-generation antiandrogen screened for activity in prostate cancer model systems with overexpressed AR. A phase III trial showed a 4-month survival benefit for abiraterone acetate plus prednisone over a placebo plus prednisone. These agents have also shown significant antitumor effects in patients who have progressed on chemotherapy.

Mitoxantrone was the first cytotoxic agent shown to provide palliation of pain secondary to castrate metastatic disease, and was approved for this indication without the demonstration of a clear survival benefit. In 2004, docetaxel was established as the first-line standard cytotoxic drug for patients in this state, based on a trial showing that q3w docetaxel was superior to weekly therapy and to mitoxantrone, results confirmed in a second trial of estramustine/docetaxel vs. mitoxantrone. The addition of estramustine produced significant toxicity with no apparent improvement in survival and has been dropped from these regimens. Docetaxel and other microtubule-targeted agents produce PSA declines in 50% of patients, measurable disease regression in 25%, and both an improvement in preexisting and prevention of future cancer-related pain. Dasatinib is an oral tyrosine kinase inhibitor which targets Src and other Src family kinases that contribute to ligand-independent AR activation, and which reduces bone turnover, is under study in combination with docetaxel. Two products approved based on a survival benefit in randomized trials include cabazitaxel, a second-generation taxane FDA-approved for patients who have progressed on docetaxel relative to mitoxantrone, and sipuleucel-t, a biologic approach in which antigen-presenting cells are activated ex vivo, pulsed with antigen, and reinfused.

Given the bone-dominant pattern of prostate cancer spread, two bone-seeking radioisotopes, ^{89}Sr (Metastron) and ^{153}Sm-EDTMP (Quadramet), are approved for palliation of pain, although they have no effect on PSA or survival. Fewer patients treated with one of these isotopes developed new areas of pain or required additional radiation therapy compared to patients receiving external beam radiation therapy alone. Additionally, patients randomly assigned to a combination of ^{89}Sr and doxorubicin after induction chemotherapy had fewer skeletal events and longer survival than patients treated with doxorubicin alone. Confirmatory studies are ongoing.

An additional bone-targeting therapy, bisphosphonates inhibit osteoclasts and, in effect, protect against bone loss associated with androgen depletion and prevent skeletal events. Addition of the bisphosphonate zoledronate to "standard therapy" in patients with CRPC resulted in fewer skeletal events relative to placebo. Skeletal events included microfractures, new pain, and need for radiation therapy.

BENIGN DISEASE

■ SYMPTOMS

Benign proliferative disease may produce hesitancy, intermittent voiding, a diminished stream, incomplete emptying, and postvoid leakage. The severity of these symptoms can be quantitated with the self-administered American Urological Association Symptom Index (Table 95-2), although the degree of symptoms does not always relate to gland size. Resistance to urine flow reduces bladder compliance, leading to nocturia, urgency, and, ultimately, urinary retention. Episodes of urinary retention may be precipitated by infection, tranquilizing drugs, antihistamines, and alcohol. Prostatitis often produces pain or induration. Typically, the symptoms remain stable over time and obstruction does not occur.

■ DIAGNOSTIC PROCEDURES AND TREATMENT

Asymptomatic patients do not require treatment regardless of the size of the gland, while those with an inability to urinate, gross hematuria,

TABLE 95-2 AUA Symptom Index

Questions to Be Answered	AUA Symptom Score (Circle 1 Number on Each Line)					
	Not at All	Less Than 1 Time in 5	Less Than Half the Time	About Half the Time	More Than Half the Time	Almost Always
Over the past month, how often have you had a sensation of not emptying your bladder completely after you finished urinating?	0+	1	2	3	4	5
Over the past month, how often have you had to urinate again less than 2 h after you finished urinating?	0	1	2	3	4	5
Over the past month, how often have you found you stopped and started again several times when you urinated?	0	1	2	3	4	5
Over the past month, how often have you found it difficult to postpone urination?	0	1	2	3	4	5
Over the past month, how often have you had a weak urinary stream?	0	1	2	3	4	5
Over the past month, how often have you had to push or strain to begin urination?	0	1	2	3	4	5
Over the past month, how many times did you most typically get up to urinate from the time you went to bed at night until the time you got up in the morning?	(None)	(1 time)	(2 times)	(3 times)	(4 times)	(5 times)
Sum of 7 circled numbers (AUA Symptom Score): ____						

Abbreviation: AUA, American Urological Association.
Source: MJ Barry et al: J Urol 148:1549, 1992. Used with permission.

recurrent infection, or bladder stones may require surgery. In patients with symptoms, uroflowmetry can identify those with normal flow rates who are unlikely to benefit from surgery and those with high postvoid residuals who may need other interventions. Pressure-flow studies detect primary bladder dysfunction. Cystoscopy is recommended if hematuria is documented and to assess the urinary outflow tract before surgery. Imaging of the upper tracts is advised for patients with hematuria, a history of calculi, or prior urinary tract problems.

Medical therapies for BPH include 5α-reductase inhibitors and α-adrenergic blockers. Finasteride (10 mg/d PO) and other 5α-reductase inhibitors that block the conversion of testosterone to dihydrotestosterone decrease prostate size, increase urine flow rates, and improve symptoms. Of note is that in the REDUCE trial, a reduction in BPH outcomes including acute urinary retention and BPH-related surgery was observed. Noteworthy is that these agents lower baseline PSA levels by 50%, an important consideration when using PSA to guide biopsy recommendations. α-Adrenergic blockers such as terazosin (1–10 mg PO at bedtime) act by relaxing the smooth muscle of the bladder neck and increasing peak urinary flow rates. No data show that these agents influence the progression of the disease.

Surgical approaches include TURP, transurethral incision, or removal of the gland via a retropubic, suprapubic, or perineal approach. Also utilized are TULIP (transurethral ultrasound-guided laser-induced prostatectomy), stents, and hyperthermia.

FURTHER READINGS

Andriole GL et al: Mortality results from a randomized prostate-cancer screening trial. N Engl J Med 360:1310, 2009

——: Reduce study group. Effect of dutasteride on the risk of prostate cancer. N Engl J Med 362:1192, 2010

Chen Y et al: Targeting the androgen receptor pathway in prostate cancer. Curr Opin Pharmacol 8:440, 2008

Hugosson J et al: Mortality results from the Göteborg randomised population-based prostate-cancer screening trial. Lancet Oncol 11:725, 2010

Klotz L et al: Clinical results of long-term follow-up of a large, active surveillance cohort with localized prostate cancer. J Clin Oncol 28:126, 2010

Lilja H et al: Prediction of significant prostate cancer diagnosed 20 to 30 years later with a single measure of prostate-specific antigen at or before age 50. Cancer 117:1210, 2011

Loblaw DA et al: Initial hormonal management of androgen-sensitive metastatic, recurrent or progressive prostate cancer: 2006 update of an American Society of Clinical Oncology practice guideline. J Clin Oncol 25:1596, 2007

Lowrance WT et al: Minimally invasive vs open radical prostatectomy. JAMA 303:619, 2010

Sausville J, Naslud M: Benign prostatic hyperplasia and prostate cancer: An overview for primary care physicians. Int J Clin Pract 64:1740, 2010

Scher HI, Heller G: Clinical states in prostate cancer: Toward a dynamic model of disease progression. Urology 55:323, 2000

Schröder FH et al: Screening and prostate-cancer mortality in a randomized European Study. N Engl J Med 360:1320, 2009

Tannock IM et al: Docetaxel plus prednisone or mitoxantrone plus prednisone for advanced prostate cancer. N Engl J Med 351:1502, 2004

Thompson IM et al: Chemoprevention of prostate cancer. J Urol 182:499, 2009

Vickers AJ et al: Finasteride to prevent prostate cancer: Should all men or only a high-risk subgroup be treated? J Clin Oncol 28:1112, 2010

Zelefsky MJ et al: Metastasis after radical prostatectomy or external beam radiotherapy for patients with clinically localized prostate cancer: A comparison of clinical cohorts adjusted for case mix. J Clin Oncol 2010; 28:1508, 2010

CHAPTER **96**

Testicular Cancer

Robert J. Motzer

George J. Bosl

Primary germ cell tumors (GCTs) of the testis arising by the malignant transformation of primordial germ cells constitute 95% of all testicular neoplasms. Infrequently, GCTs arise from an extragonadal site, including the mediastinum, retroperitoneum, and, very rarely, the pineal gland. This disease is notable for the young age of the afflicted patients, the totipotent capacity for differentiation of the tumor cells, and its curability; approximately 95% of newly diagnosed patients are cured. Experience in the management of GCTs leads to improved outcome.

INCIDENCE AND EPIDEMIOLOGY

In 2010, 8480 new cases of testicular GCT were diagnosed in the United States and 350 men died. The tumor occurs most frequently in men between the ages of 20 and 40 years. A testicular mass in a male ≥50 years should be regarded as a lymphoma until proved otherwise. GCT is at least four to five times more common in white than in African-American males, and a higher incidence has been observed in Scandinavia and New Zealand than in the United States.

ETIOLOGY AND GENETICS

Cryptorchidism is associated with a several-fold higher risk of GCT. Abdominal cryptorchid testes are at a higher risk than inguinal cryptorchid testes. Orchiopexy should be performed before puberty, if possible. Early orchiopexy reduces the risk of GCT and improves the ability to save the testis. An abdominal cryptorchid testis that cannot be brought into the scrotum should be removed. Approximately 2% of men with GCTs of one testis will develop a primary tumor in the other testis. Testicular feminization syndromes increase the risk of testicular GCT, and Klinefelter's syndrome is associated with mediastinal GCT.

An isochromosome of the short arm of chromosome 12 [i(12p)] is pathognomonic for GCT of all histologic types. Excess 12p copy number, either in the form of i(12p) or as increased 12p on aberrantly banded marker chromosomes, occurs in nearly all GCTs, but the gene(s) on 12p involved in the pathogenesis are not yet defined.

CLINICAL PRESENTATION

A painless testicular mass is pathognomonic for a testicular malignancy. More commonly, patients present with testicular discomfort or swelling suggestive of epididymitis and/or orchitis. In this circumstance, a trial of antibiotics is reasonable. However, if symptoms persist or a residual abnormality remains, then testicular ultrasound examination is indicated.

Ultrasound of the testis is indicated whenever a testicular malignancy is considered and for persistent or painful testicular swelling. If a testicular mass is detected, a radical inguinal orchiectomy should be performed. Because the testis develops from the gonadal ridge, its blood supply and lymphatic drainage originate in the abdomen and descend with the testis into the scrotum. An inguinal approach is taken to avoid breaching anatomic barriers and permitting additional pathways of spread.

Back pain from retroperitoneal metastases is common and must be distinguished from musculoskeletal pain. Dyspnea from pulmonary metastases occurs infrequently. Patients with increased serum levels of human chorionic gonadotropin (hCG) may present with gynecomastia. A delay in diagnosis is associated with a more advanced stage and possibly worse survival.

The staging evaluation for GCT includes a determination of serum levels of α fetoprotein (AFP), hCG, and lactate dehydrogenase (LDH). After orchiectomy, a chest radiograph and a CT scan of the abdomen and pelvis should be performed. A chest CT scan is required if pulmonary nodules or mediastinal or hilar disease is suspected. Stage I disease is limited to the testis, epididymis, or spermatic cord. Stage II disease is limited to retroperitoneal (regional) lymph nodes. Stage III disease is disease outside the retroperitoneum, involving supradiaphragmatic nodal sites or viscera. The staging may be "clinical"—defined solely by physical examination, blood marker evaluation, and radiographs—or "pathologic"—defined by an operative procedure.

The regional draining lymph nodes for the testis are in the retroperitoneum, and the vascular supply originates from the great vessels (for the right testis) or the renal vessels (for the left testis). As a result, the lymph nodes that are involved first by a right testicular tumor are the interaortocaval lymph nodes just below the renal vessels. For a left testicular tumor, the first involved lymph nodes are lateral to the aorta (para-aortic) and below the left renal vessels. In both cases, further nodal spread is inferior, contralateral, and, less commonly, above the renal hilum. Lymphatic involvement can extend cephalad to the retrocrural, posterior mediastinal, and supraclavicular lymph nodes. Treatment is determined by tumor histology (seminoma versus nonseminoma) and clinical stage (Fig. 96-1).

PATHOLOGY

GCTs are divided into nonseminoma and seminoma subtypes. Nonseminomatous GCTs are most frequent in the third decade of life and can display the full spectrum of embryonic and adult cellular differentiation. This entity comprises four histologies: embryonal carcinoma, teratoma, choriocarcinoma, and endodermal sinus (yolk sac) tumor. Choriocarcinoma, consisting of both cytotrophoblasts and syncytiotrophoblasts, represents malignant trophoblastic differentiation and is invariably associated with secretion of hCG. Endodermal sinus tumor is the malignant counterpart of the fetal yolk sac and is associated with secretion of AFP. Pure embryonal carcinoma may secrete AFP or hCG, or both; this pattern is biochemical evidence of differentiation. Teratoma is composed of somatic cell types derived from two or more germ layers (ectoderm, mesoderm, or endoderm). Each of these histologies may be present alone or in combination with others. Nonseminomatous GCTs tend to metastasize early to sites such as the retroperitoneal lymph nodes and lung parenchyma. One-third of patients present with disease limited to the testis (stage I), one-third with retroperitoneal metastases (stage II), and one-third with more extensive supradiaphragmatic nodal or visceral metastases (stage III).

Seminoma represents approximately 50% of all GCTs, has a median age in the fourth decade, and generally follows a more indolent clinical course. Most patients (70%) present with stage I disease, approximately 20% with stage II disease, and 10% with stage III disease; lung or other visceral metastases are rare. When a tumor contains both seminoma and nonseminoma components, patient management is directed by the more aggressive nonseminoma component.

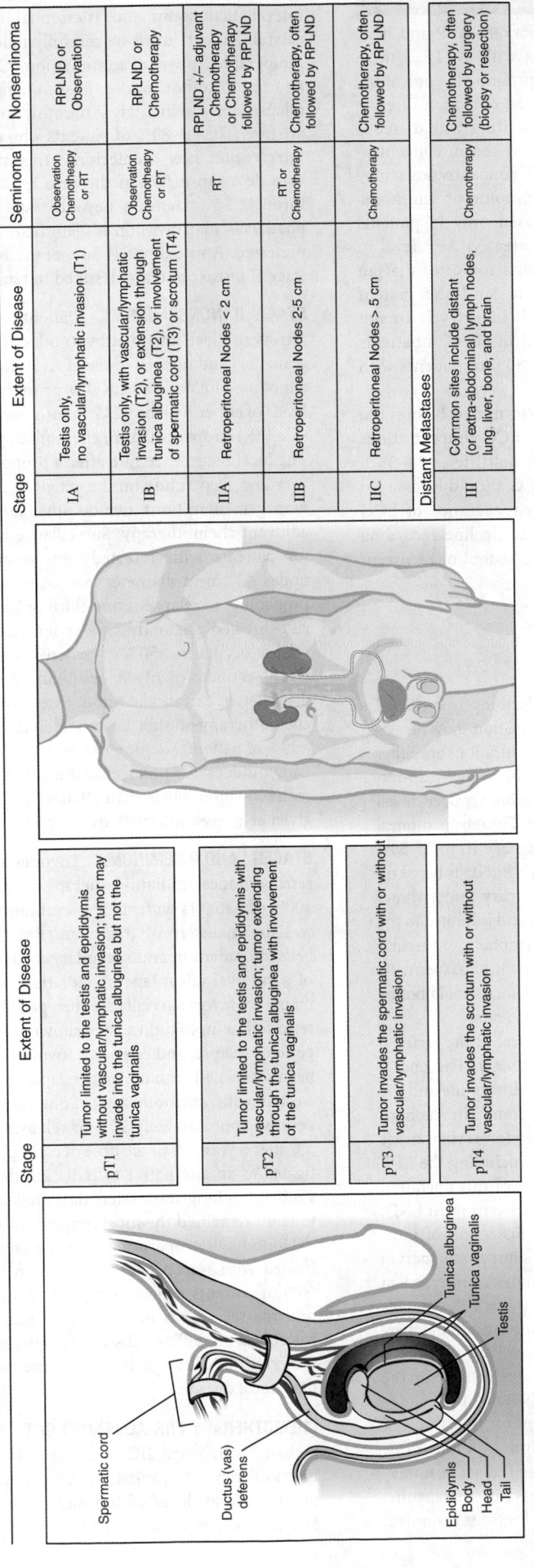

Stage	Extent of Disease
pT1	Tumor limited to the testis and epididymis without vascular/lymphatic invasion; tumor may invade into the tunica albuginea but not the tunica vaginalis
pT2	Tumor limited to the testis and epididymis with vascular/lymphatic invasion; tumor extending through the tunica albuginea with involvement of the tunica vaginalis
pT3	Tumor invades the spermatic cord with or without vascular/lymphatic invasion
pT4	Tumor invades the scrotum with or without vascular/lymphatic invasion

		Treatment Option	
Stage	Extent of Disease	Seminoma	Nonseminoma
IA	Testis only, no vascular/lymphatic invasion (T1)	Observation Chemotheapy or RT	RPLND or Observation
IB	Testis only, with vascular/lymphatic invasion (T2), or extension through tunica albuginea (T2), or involvement of spermatic cord (T3) or scrotum (T4)	Observation Chemotherapy or RT	RPLND or Chemotherapy
IIA	Retroperitoneal Nodes < 2 cm	RT	RPLND +/− adjuvant Chemotherapy or Chemotherapy followed by RPLND
IIB	Retroperitoneal Nodes 2–5 cm	RT or Chemotherapy	Chemotherapy, often followed by RPLND
IIC	Retroperitoneal Nodes > 5 cm	Chemotherapy	Chemotherapy, often followed by RPLND
Distant Metastases			
III	Common sites include distant (or extra-abdominal) lymph nodes, lung, liver, bone, and brain	Chemotherapy	Chemotherapy, often followed by surgery (biopsy or resection)

Figure 96–1 Germ cell tumor staging and treatment.

Careful monitoring of the serum tumor markers AFP and hCG is essential in the management of patients with GCT, as these markers are important for diagnosis, as prognostic indicators, in monitoring treatment response, and in the detection of early relapse. Approximately 70% of patients presenting with disseminated nonseminomatous GCT have increased serum concentrations of AFP and/or hCG. Although hCG concentrations may be increased in patients with either nonseminoma or seminoma histology, the AFP concentration is increased only in patients with nonseminoma. The presence of an increased AFP level in a patient whose tumor shows only seminoma indicates that an occult nonseminomatous component exists, and the patient should be treated for nonseminomatous GCT. LDH levels are not as specific as AFP or hCG but are increased in 50–60% patients with metastatic nonseminoma and in up to 80% of patients with advanced seminoma.

AFP, hCG, and LDH levels should be determined before and after orchiectomy. Increased serum AFP and hCG concentrations decay according to first-order kinetics; the half-life is 24–36 h for hCG and 5–7 days for AFP. AFP and hCG should be assayed serially during and after treatment. The reappearance of hCG and/or AFP or the failure of these markers to decline according to the predicted half-life is an indicator of persistent or recurrent tumor.

TREATMENT   Testicular Cancer

STAGE I NONSEMINOMA   If, after an orchiectomy (for clinical stage I disease), radiographs and physical examination show no evidence of disease and serum AFP and hCG concentrations are either normal or declining to normal according to the known half-life, patients may be managed by either a nerve-sparing retroperitoneal lymph node dissection (RPLND) or surveillance. The retroperitoneal lymph nodes are involved by GCT (pathologic stage II) in 20–50% of these patients. The choice of surveillance or RPLND is based on the pathology of the primary tumor. If the primary tumor shows no evidence for lymphatic or vascular invasion and is limited to the testis (T1), then either option is reasonable. If lymphatic or vascular invasion is present or the tumor extends into the tunica, spermatic cord, or scrotum (T2 through T4), then surveillance should not be offered. Either approach should cure >95% of patients.

RPLND is the standard operation for removal of the regional lymph nodes of the testis (retroperitoneal nodes). The operation removes the lymph nodes draining the primary site and the nodal groups adjacent to the primary landing zone. The standard (modified bilateral) RPLND removes all node-bearing tissue down to the bifurcation of the great vessels, including the ipsilateral iliac nodes. The major long-term effect of this operation is retrograde ejaculation and infertility. Nerve-sparing RPLND, usually accomplished by identification and dissection of individual nerve fibers, may avoid injury to the sympathetic nerves responsible for ejaculation. Normal ejaculation is preserved in ~90% of patients. Patients with pathologic stage I disease are observed, and only the <10% who relapse require additional therapy. If retroperitoneal nodes are found to be involved at RPLND, then a decision regarding adjuvant chemotherapy is made on the basis of the extent of retroperitoneal disease (see below).

Surveillance is an option in the management of clinical stage I disease when no vascular/lymphatic invasion is found (T1). Only 20–30% of patients have pathologic stage II disease, implying that most RPLNDs in this situation are not therapeutic. Surveillance and RPLND lead to equivalent long-term survival

rates. Patient compliance is essential if surveillance is to be successful. Patients must be carefully followed with periodic chest radiography, physical examination, CT scan of the abdomen, and serum tumor marker determinations. The median time to relapse is approximately 7 months, and late relapses (>2 years) are rare. The 70–80% of patients who do not relapse require no intervention after orchiectomy; treatment is reserved for those who do relapse. When the primary tumor is classified as T2 through T4 (extension beyond testis and epididymis or lymphatic/vascular invasion is identified), nerve-sparing RPLND is preferred. Approximately 50% of these patients have pathologic stage II disease and are destined to relapse without the RPLND.

STAGE II NONSEMINOMA   Patients with limited, ipsilateral retroperitoneal adenopathy (nodes usually ≤3 cm in largest diameter) and normal levels of AFP and hCG generally undergo a modified bilateral RPLND as primary management. Increased levels of either AFP or hCG or both imply metastatic disease outside the retroperitoneum; chemotherapy is used in this setting. The local recurrence rate after a properly performed RPLND is very low. Depending on the extent of disease, the postoperative management options include either surveillance or two cycles of adjuvant chemotherapy. Surveillance is the preferred approach for patients with resected "low-volume" metastases (tumor nodes ≤2 cm in diameter *and* <6 nodes involved) because the probability of relapse is one-third or less. For those who relapse, risk-directed chemotherapy is indicated (see below). Because relapse occurs in ≥50% of patients with "high-volume" metastases (>6 nodes involved, *or* any involved node >2 cm in largest diameter, *or* extranodal tumor extension), two cycles of adjuvant chemotherapy should be considered, as it results in a cure in ≥98% of patients. Regimens consisting of etoposide (100 mg/m^2 daily on days 1–5) plus cisplatin (20 mg/m^2 daily on days 1–5) with or without bleomycin (30 units per day on days 2, 9, and 16) given at 3-week intervals are effective and well tolerated.

STAGES I AND II SEMINOMA   Inguinal orchiectomy followed by retroperitoneal radiation therapy or surveillance cures nearly 100% of patients with stage I seminoma. Historically, radiation was the mainstay of treatment, But the reported association between radiation and secondary malignancies and the absence of a survival advantage of radiation over surveillance has led many to favor surveillance for patients committed to long-term follow-up. Studies have shown that approximately 15% of patients relapse, and rete testis involvement and size >4 cm have been associated with a higher relapse rate. The relapse is usually treated with chemotherapy. Long-term followup is essential, because approximately 30% of relapses occur after 2 years and 5% after 5 years. A single dose of carboplatin has also been investigated as an alternative to radiation therapy; the outcome was similar, but long-term safety data are lacking, and the retroperitoneum remained the most frequent site of relapse.

Nonbulky retroperitoneal disease (stage IIA and most IIB) is treated with retroperitoneal radiation therapy. Approximately 90% of patients achieve relapse-free survival with retroperitoneal masses <5 cm in diameter. Because at least one-third of patients with bulkier disease relapse, initial chemotherapy is preferred for all stage IIC and some stage IIB with bulkier or multifocal disease.

CHEMOTHERAPY FOR ADVANCED GCT   Regardless of histology, patients with stage IIC and stage III GCT are treated with chemotherapy. Combination chemotherapy programs based on cisplatin at doses of 100 mg/m^2 plus etoposide at doses of 500 mg/m^2 per cycle cure 70–80% of such patients, with or without bleomycin, depending on risk stratification (see below). A complete response (the complete disappearance of all clinical evidence of tumor on physical examination and radiography plus normal serum levels of AFP and hCG for ≥1 month) occurs after chemotherapy alone in ~60% of patients, and another 10–20% become disease-free with surgical resection of residual masses containing viable GCT. Lower doses of cisplatin result in inferior survival rates.

The toxicity of four cycles of the bleomycin, etoposide, and cisplatin (BEP) regimen is substantial. Nausea, vomiting, and hair loss occur in most patients, although nausea and vomiting have been markedly ameliorated by modern antiemetic regimens. Myelosuppression is frequent, and symptomatic bleomycin pulmonary toxicity occurs in ~5% of patients. Treatment-induced mortality due to neutropenia with septicemia or bleomycin-induced pulmonary failure occurs in 1–3% of patients. Dose reductions for myelosuppression are rarely indicated. Long-term permanent toxicities include nephrotoxicity (reduced glomerular filtration and persistent magnesium wasting), ototoxicity, and peripheral neuropathy. When bleomycin is administered by weekly bolus injection, Raynaud's phenomenon appears in 5–10% of patients. Other evidence of small blood vessel damage is seen less often, including transient ischemic attacks and myocardial infarction.

RISK-DIRECTED CHEMOTHERAPY Because not all patients are cured and treatment may cause significant toxicities, patients are stratified into "good-risk" and "poor-risk" groups according to pretreatment clinical features. For good-risk patients, the goal is to achieve maximum efficacy with minimal toxicity. For poor-risk patients, the goal is to identify more effective therapy with tolerable toxicity.

The International Germ Cell Cancer Consensus Group developed criteria to assign patients to three risk groups (good, intermediate, poor) (Table 96-1). The marker cut offs have been incorporated into the revised TNM (primary tumor, regional nodes, metastasis) staging of GCT. Hence, TNM stage groupings are now based on both anatomy (site and extent of disease) and biology (marker status and histology). Seminoma is either good or intermediate risk, based on the absence or presence of nonpulmonary visceral metastases. No poor-risk category exists for seminoma. Marker levels play no role in defining risk for seminoma. Nonseminomas have good-, intermediate-, and poor-risk categories based on the site of the primary tumor, the presence or absence of nonpulmonary visceral metastases, and marker levels.

For ~90% of patients with good-risk GCTs, four cycles of etoposide plus cisplatin (EP) or three cycles of BEP produce durable complete responses, with minimal acute and chronic toxicity. Pulmonary toxicity is absent when bleomycin is not used and is rare when therapy is limited to 9 weeks; myelosuppression with neutropenic fever is less frequent; and the treatment mortality rate is negligible. Approximately 75% of intermediate-risk patients and 45% of poor-risk patients achieve durable complete remission with four cycles of BEP, and no regimen has proved superior. More effective therapy is needed.

POSTCHEMOTHERAPY SURGERY Resection of residual metastases after the completion of chemotherapy is an integral part of therapy. If the initial histology is nonseminoma and the marker values have normalized, all sites of residual disease should be resected. In general, residual retroperitoneal disease requires a modified bilateral RPLND. Thoracotomy (unilateral or bilateral) and neck dissection are less frequently required to remove residual mediastinal, pulmonary parenchymal, or cervical nodal disease. Viable tumor (seminoma, embryonal carcinoma, yolk

TABLE 96-1 IGCCCG Risk Classification for Advanced Germ Cell Tumors

Risk	Nonseminoma	Seminoma
Good	Gonadal or retroperitoneal primary site	Any primary site
	Absent nonpulmonary visceral metastases	Absent nonpulmonary visceral metastases
	AFP <1000 ng/mL	
	Beta-hCG <5000 mIU/mL	Any LDH, hCG
	LDH <1.5 × upper limit or normal (ULN)	
Intermediate	Gonadal or retroperitoneal primary site	Any primary site
	Absent nonpulmonary visceral metastases	Presence of nonpulmonary visceral metastases
	AFP 1000–10,000 ng/mL	
	Beta-hCG 5000–50,000 mIU/mL	Any LDH, hCG
	LDH 1.5–10 × ULN	
Poor	Mediastinal primary site	No patients classified as poor prognosis
	Presence of nonpulmonary visceral metastases	
	AFP ≥10,000 ng/mL	
	Beta-hCG >50,000 mIU/mL	
	LDH > 10 × ULN	

Abbreviations: AFP, α fetoprotein; hCG, human chorionic gonadotropin; IGCCCG, International Germ Cell Consensus Classification Group; LDH, lactate dehydrogenase. ***Source:*** From International Germ Cell Cancer Consensus Group.

sac tumor, or choriocarcinoma) will be present in 15%, mature teratoma in 40%, and necrotic debris and fibrosis in 45% of resected specimens. The frequency of teratoma or viable disease is highest in residual mediastinal tumors. If necrotic debris or mature teratoma is present, no further chemotherapy is necessary. If viable tumor is present but is completely excised, two additional cycles of chemotherapy are given.

If the initial histology is pure seminoma, mature teratoma is rarely present, and the most frequent finding is necrotic debris. For residual retroperitoneal disease, a complete RPLND is technically difficult owing to extensive postchemotherapy fibrosis. Observation is recommended when no radiographic abnormality exists on CT scan. Positive findings on a positron emission tomography (PET) scan correlate with viable seminoma in residua, and mandate surgical excision or biopsy.

SALVAGE CHEMOTHERAPY Of patients with advanced GCT, 20–30% fail to achieve a durable complete response to first-line chemotherapy. A combination of vinblastine, ifosfamide, and cisplatin (VeIP) will cure approximately 25% of patients as a second-line therapy. Substitution of paclitaxel for vinblastine may be more effective in this setting. Patients are more likely to achieve a durable complete response if they had a testicular primary tumor and relapsed from a prior complete remission to first-line cisplatin-containing chemotherapy. In contrast, if the patient failed to achieve a complete response or has a primary mediastinal nonseminoma, then standard-dose salvage therapy is rarely beneficial. Treatment options for such patients include dose-intensive treatment, experimental therapies, and surgical resection.

Chemotherapy consisting of dose-intensive, high-dose carboplatin (≥1500 mg/m²) plus etoposide (≥1200 mg/m²), with or without cyclophosphamide, with peripheral blood stem cell support, induces a complete response in 25–40% of patients who have progressed after ifosfamide-containing salvage chemotherapy. Approximately one-half of the complete responses will be durable. High-dose therapy is standard of care for this patient population and has been suggested as treatment of choice for all patients with relapsed or refractory disease. Paclitaxel is also active in previously treated patients and shows promise in high-dose combination programs. Cure is still possible in some relapsed patients.

EXTRAGONADAL GCT AND MIDLINE CARCINOMA OF UNCERTAIN HISTOGENESIS

The prognosis and management of patients with extragonadal GCT depends on the tumor histology and site of origin. All patients with a diagnosis of extragonadal GCT should have a testicular ultrasound examination. Nearly all patients with retroperitoneal or mediastinal seminoma achieve a durable complete response to BEP or EP. The clinical features of patients with primary retroperitoneal nonseminoma GCT are similar to those of patients with a primary of testis origin, and careful evaluation will find evidence of a primary testicular GCT in about two-thirds of cases. In contrast, a primary mediastinal nonseminomatous GCT is associated with a poor prognosis; one-third of patients are cured with standard therapy (four cycles of BEP). Patients with newly diagnosed mediastinal nonseminoma are considered to have poor-risk disease and should be considered for clinical trials testing regimens of possibly greater efficacy. In addition, mediastinal nonseminoma is associated with hematologic disorders, including acute myelogenous leukemia, myelodysplastic syndrome, and essential thrombocytosis unrelated to previous chemotherapy. These hematologic disorders are very refractory to treatment. Nonseminoma of any primary site may change into other malignant histologies such as embryonal rhabdomyosarcoma or adenocarcinoma. This is called *malignant transformation.* i(12p) has been identified in the transformed cell type, indicating GCT clonal origin.

A group of patients with poorly differentiated tumors of unknown histogenesis, midline in distribution, and not associated with secretion of AFP or hCG has been described; a few (10–20%) are cured by standard cisplatin-containing chemotherapy. i(12p) is present in ~25% of such tumors (the fraction that are cisplatin-responsive), confirming their origin from primitive germ cells. This finding is also predictive of the response to cisplatin-based chemotherapy and resulting long-term survival. These tumors are heterogeneous; neuroepithelial tumors and lymphoma may also present in this fashion.

FERTILITY

Infertility is an important consequence of the treatment of GCTs. Preexisting infertility or impaired fertility is often present. Azoospermia and/or oligospermia are present at diagnosis in at least 50% of patients with testicular GCTs. Ejaculatory dysfunction is associated with RPLND, and germ cell damage may result from cisplatin-containing chemotherapy. Nerve-sparing techniques to preserve the retroperitoneal sympathetic nerves have made retrograde ejaculation less likely in the subgroups of patients who are candidates for this operation. Spermatogenesis does recur in some patients after chemotherapy. However, because of the significant risk of impaired reproductive capacity, semen analysis and cryopreservation of sperm in a sperm bank should be recommended to all patients before treatment.

FURTHER READINGS

Bosl GJ et al: Cancer of the testis, in *Cancer: Principles and Practice of Oncology*, 7th ed, VT DeVita et al (eds). Philadelphia, Lippincott Williams & Wilkins, 2008, pp 1463–1485

Ehrlich Y et al: Serum tumor markers in testicular cancer. Urol Oncol 3 Sep 2010 [Epub ahead of print]

Einhorn et al: High-dose chemotherapy and stem-cell rescue for metastatic germ-cell tumors. N Engl J Med 357:340, 2007

Feldman DR et al: Medical treatment of advanced testicular cancer. JAMA 299:672, 2008

International Germ Cell Cancer Consensus Group: International Germ Cell Consensus Classification: A prognostic factor-based staging system for metastatic germ cell cancers. J Clin Oncol 15:594, 1997

Sonpavde G et al: Management of recurrent testicular germ cell tumors. Oncologist 12:51, 2007

Travis LB et al: Testicular cancer survivorship: Research strategies and recommendations. J Natl Cancer Inst 102:1114, 2010

CHAPTER **97**
Gynecologic Malignancies

Michael V. Seiden

OVARIAN CANCER

◼ INCIDENCE AND PATHOLOGY

Ovarian cancer is the most lethal malignancy of gynecologic origin in the United States and other countries that have organized and effective cervical cancer screening programs. In 2010, 21,880 cases of ovarian cancer with 13,850 deaths are expected in the United States. The ovary is a complex and dynamic organ and, between the ages of approximately 11 and 50 years, is responsible for follicle maturation associated with egg maturation, ovulation, and cyclical sex steroid hormone production. These complex and linked biologic functions are coordinated through a variety of cells within the ovary, each of which possesses neoplastic potential. By far the most common and most lethal of the ovarian neoplasms arise from the ovarian epithelium found both on the surface of the ovary and in subsurface locations, known as cortical inclusion cysts, believed to be entrapped epithelium from the healing associated with prior follicle rupture during ovulation. The ovarian epithelium in good health appears as a simple epithelium, but with neoplastic transformation, it undergoes metaplastic changes into what is termed *müllerian epithelium.* The müllerian epithelium has a variety of subtypes each of which provide a specific phenotype of the tumor and in some cases different clinical presentations. Epithelial tumors are the most common ovarian neoplasm; they may be benign (50%), malignant (33%), or of borderline malignancy (16%). Age influences risk of malignancy; tumors in younger women are more likely benign. The most common of the ovarian epithelial malignancies are serous tumors (50%); tumors of mucinous (25%), endometrioid (15%), clear cell (5%), and transitional cell histology or Brenner tumor (1%) represent smaller proportions of epithelial ovarian tumors. In contrast, stromal tumors arise from the steroid hormone-producing cells and likewise have different phenotypes and clinical presentations largely dependent on the type and quantity of hormone production. Tumors arising in the germ cell are most similar in biology and behavior to testicular tumors in males (Chap. 96).

Tumors may also metastasize to the ovary from breast, colon, gastric, and pancreatic primaries. Bilateral ovarian masses from metastatic mucin-secreting gastrointestinal cancers are termed *Krukenberg tumors.*

■ OVARIAN CANCER OF EPITHELIAL ORIGIN

Epidemiology

A female has approximately a 1 in 72 lifetime risk (1.6%) of developing ovarian cancer, with the majority of affected women developing epithelial tumors. Epithelial tumors of the ovary have a peak incidence in women in their sixties, although age at presentation can range across the extremes of adult life, with cases being reported in women in their twenties to nineties. Known risk factors that increase the chance of subsequent ovarian cancer include epidemiologic, environmental, and genetic factors such as nulliparity, use of talc agents applied to the perineum, obesity, and probably hormone replacement therapy. Protective factors include the use of oral contraceptives, multiparity, and breast-feeding. These protective factors are thought to work through suppression of ovulation and perhaps reduction of ovarian inflammation and damage associated with the repair of the ovarian cortex associated with ovulation, and perhaps suppression of gonadotropins. Other protective factors, such as fallopian tube ligation are thought to protect the ovarian epithelium (or perhaps the distal fallopian tube fimbriae) from carcinogens that migrate from the vagina to the tubes and ovarian surface epithelium (see below).

Genetic risk factors

A variety of genetic syndromes substantially increases a woman's risk of developing ovarian cancer. Approximately 10% of women with ovarian cancer have a somatic mutation in one of two DNA repair genes: *BRCA1* (chromosome 17q12-21) or *BRCA2* (chromosome 13q12-13). Individuals inheriting a single copy of a mutant allele have a very high incidence of breast and ovarian cancer. Most of these women have a family history that is notable for multiple cases of breast and/or ovarian cancer, although inheritance through male members of the family can camouflage this genotype through several generations. The most common malignancy in these women is breast carcinoma, although women harboring germ-line *BRCA1* mutations have a marked increased risk of developing ovarian malignancies in their forties and fifties with a 30–50% lifetime risk of developing ovarian cancer. Women harboring a mutation in *BRCA2* have a lower penetrance of ovarian cancer with perhaps a 20–40% chance of developing this malignancy, with onset typically in their fifties or sixties. Women with a *BRCA2* mutation also are at slightly increased risk of pancreatic cancer. Screening studies in this select population suggest that current screening techniques, including serial evaluation of the CA-125 tumor marker and ultrasound, are insufficient at detecting early-stage and curable disease, so women with these germ-line mutations are advised to undergo prophylactic removal of ovaries and fallopian tubes typically after completing childbearing and ideally before ages 35–40. Early prophylactic oophorectomy also protects these women from subsequent breast cancer with a reduction of breast cancer risk of approximately 50%.

Ovarian cancer is also one form of cancer (along with colorectal and endometrial cancer) that may develop in women with Lynch syndrome, type II, caused by mutations in DNA mismatch repair genes (*MSH2, MLH1, MLH6, PMS1, PMS2*). Ovarian cancer may appear in women younger than 50 years of age in this syndrome.

Presentation

Neoplasms of the ovary tend to be painless unless they undergo torsion. Symptoms are therefore typically related to compression of local organs or due to symptoms from metastatic disease. Women with tumors localized to the ovary do have an increased incidence of symptoms including pelvic discomfort, bloating, and perhaps changes in a woman's typical urinary or bowel pattern. Unfortunately, these symptoms are frequently dismissed by either the woman or her health care team. It is believed that high-grade tumors metastasize early in the neoplastic process. Unlike other epithelial malignancies, these tumors tend to exfoliate throughout the peritoneal cavity and thus present with symptoms associated with disseminated intraperitoneal tumors. The most common symptoms at presentation include a multimonth period of progressive complaints that typically include some combination of heartburn, nausea, early satiety, indigestion, constipation, and abdominal pain. Signs include the rapid increase in abdominal girth due to the accumulation of ascites that typically alerts the patient and her physician that the concurrent gastrointestinal symptoms are likely associated with serious pathology. Radiologic evaluation typically demonstrates a complex adnexal mass and ascites. Laboratory evaluation demonstrates a markedly elevated CA-125, a shed mucin (Muc 16) associated with, but not specific for, ovarian cancer. Hematogenous and lymphatic spread are seen but are not the typical presentation. Ovarian cancers are divided into four stages, with stage I tumors confined to the ovary, stage II malignancies confined to the pelvis, and stage III confined to the peritoneal cavity (Table 97-1). These three stages are subdivided, with the most common presentation, stage IIIc, defined as tumors with bulky intraperitoneal disease. About 70% of women present with

TABLE 97-1 Staging and Survival in Gynecologic Malignancies

Stage	Ovarian	5-Year Survival, %	Endometrial	5-Year Survival, %	Cervix	5-Year Survival, %
0	—		—		Carcinoma in situ	100
I	Confined to ovary	90–95	Confined to corpus	89	Confined to uterus	85
II	Confined to pelvis	70–80	Involves corpus and cervix	73	Invades beyond uterus but not to pelvic wall	65
III	Intraabdominal spread	20–50	Extends outside the uterus but not outside the true pelvis	52	Extends to pelvic wall and/or lower third of vagina, or hydronephrosis	35
IV	Spread outside abdomen	1–5	Extends outside the true pelvis or involves the bladder or rectum	17	Invades mucosa of bladder or rectum or extends beyond the true pelvis	7

stage IIIc disease. Stage IV disease includes women with parenchymal metastases (liver, lung, spleen) or, alternatively, abdominal wall or pleural disease. The 30% not presenting with stage IIIc disease are roughly evenly distributed among the other stages.

Screening

Ovarian cancer is the fifth most lethal malignancy in women in the United States, curable in early stages, and seldom curable in advanced stages; hence, screening is of considerable interest. Furthermore the ovary is well visualized with a variety of imaging techniques, most notably transvaginal ultrasound. Early-stage tumors often produce proteins that can be measured in the blood such as CA-125 and HE-4. Nevertheless, the incidence of ovarian cancer in the middle-aged female population is low, with only approximately 1 in 2000 women between the ages of 50 and 60 carrying an asymptomatic and undetected tumor. Thus effective screening techniques must be sensitive but, more importantly, highly specific so to minimize the number of false positives. Even a screening test with 98% specificity and 50% sensitivity would have a positive predictive value of only about 1%. Despite these formidable barriers, ongoing studies are evaluating the utility of various screening strategies. However, screening for ovarian cancer is currently not recommended outside of a clinical trial.

TREATMENT   Ovarian Cancer

In women presenting with a localized ovarian mass, the principal diagnostic and therapeutic maneuver is to determine if the tumor is benign or malignant and, in the event that the tumor is malignant, whether the tumor arises in the ovary or is a site of metastatic disease. Metastatic disease to the ovary can be seen from primary tumors of the colon, appendix, stomach (Krukenberg tumors), and breast. Typically women undergo a unilateral salpingo-oophorectomy, and if pathology reveals a primary ovarian malignancy, then the procedure is followed by a hysterectomy, removal of the remaining tube and ovary, omentectomy, and pelvic node sampling along with some random biopsies of the peritoneal cavity. This extensive surgical procedure is performed because approximately 30% of tumors that by visual inspection appear to be confined to the ovary have already disseminated to the peritoneal cavity and/or surrounding lymph nodes.

If there is evidence of bulky intraabdominal disease, a comprehensive attempt at maximal tumor cytoreduction is attempted even if it involves partial bowel resection, splenectomy, and in certain cases more extensive upper abdominal surgery. The ability to debulk metastatic ovarian cancer to minimal visible disease is associated with an improved prognosis as compared to women left with visible disease. Patients without gross residual disease after resection have a median survival of 39 months, compared to 17 months for those left with macroscopic tumor. Once tumors have been surgically debulked, women receive therapy with a platinum agent typically with a taxane. Debate continues as to whether this therapy should be delivered intravenously or alternatively whether some of the therapy should be delivered directly into the peritoneal cavity via a catheter. Three randomized studies have demonstrated improved survival with intraperitoneal therapy, but this approach is still not widely accepted due to technical challenges associated with this delivery route and increased toxicity. In women who present with bulky disease, an alternative approach is to treat with platinum plus a taxane for several cycles (neoadjuvant therapy). Subsequent surgical procedures are more effective at leaving the patient without gross residual tumor, and survival is comparable to surgery followed by chemotherapy.

With optimal debulking surgery and platinum-based chemotherapy [usually carboplatin dosed to an area under the curve (AUC) of 7.5 plus paclitaxel 175 mg/m^2 by 3-h infusion in monthly cycles], 70% of women who present with advanced-stage tumors respond, and 40–50% experience a complete remission with normalization of their CA-125, CT scans, and physical examination. Unfortunately, only half the complete responders remain in remission. Disease recurs within 1 to 4 years from the completion of their primary therapy in half the complete responders. CA-125 levels often increase as a first sign of relapse; however, data are not clear that early intervention influences survival. Recurrent disease is effectively managed, but not cured, with a variety of chemotherapeutic agents. Eventually all of these women develop chemotherapy-refractory disease at which point refractory ascites, poor bowel motility, and obstruction or pseudoobstruction due to a tumor-infiltrated aperistaltic bowel are common. Limited surgery to relieve intestinal obstruction, localized radiation therapy to relieve pressure or pain from masses, or palliative chemotherapy may be helpful. Agents with >15% response rates include gemcitabine, topotecan, liposomal doxorubicin, and bevacizumab. Approximately 20% of ovarian cancers are HER2/neu positive, and trastuzumab may induce responses in this subset.

Five-year survival correlates with the stage of disease: stage I, 90–95%; stage II, 70–80%; stage III, 20–50%; stage IV, 1–5% (Table 97-1). Prognosis is also influenced by histologic grade: 5-year survival is 88% for well-differentiated tumors, 58% for moderately differentiated tumors, and 27% for poorly differentiated tumors. Histologic type has less influence on outcome. Patients with tumors of low malignant potential are managed by surgery; chemotherapy and radiation therapy do not improve survival.

■ OVARIAN SEX CORD AND STROMAL TUMORS

Epidemiology, presentation, and predisposing syndromes

Approximately 7% of ovarian neoplasms are stromal or sex cord tumors, with approximately 1800 cases expected each year in the United States. Ovarian stromal tumors or sex cord tumors are most common in women in their fifties or sixties, but tumors can present in the extremes of age, including the pediatric population. These tumors arise from the mesenchymal components of the ovary, including steroid-producing cells as well as fibroblasts. Essentially all of these tumors are of low malignant potential and present as unilateral solid masses. Three clinical presentations are common: the detection of an abdominal mass, abdominal pain due to ovarian torsion, intratumoral hemorrhage, or rupture or signs and symptoms due to hormonal production by these tumors.

The most common hormone-producing tumors include thecomas, granulosa cell tumor, or juvenile granulosa tumors in children. These estrogen-producing tumors often present with breast tenderness as well as isosexual precocious pseudopuberty in children, menometrorrhagia, oligomenorrhea, or amenorrhea in premenopausal women, or alternatively as postmenopausal bleeding in older women. In some women, estrogen-associated secondary malignancies, such as endometrial or breast cancer may present as synchronous malignancies. Alternatively, endometrial cancer may serve as the presenting malignancy with evaluation subsequently identifying a unilateral solid ovarian neoplasm that proves to be an occult granulosa cell tumor. Sertoli-Leydig tumors often present with hirsutism, virilization, and occasionally Cushing's syndrome due to increased production of testosterone, androstenedione, or other 17-ketosteroids. Hormonally inert tumors include fibroma that presents as a solitary mass often in association with ascites and occasionally hydrothorax also known as Meigs' syndrome. A subset of these tumors present in individuals with a variety of inherited disorders that predispose them to mesenchymal neoplasia. Associations include juvenile granulosa cell tumors and perhaps Sertoli-Leydig tumors with Ollier's disease (multiple enchondromatosis) or Maffucci's syndrome, ovarian sex cord tumors with annular tubules with Peutz-Jeghers syndrome, and fibromas with Gorlin disease.

TREATMENT Sex Cord Tumors

The mainstay of treatment for sex cord tumors is surgical resection. Most women present with tumors confined to the ovary. For the small subset of women who present with metastatic disease or develop evidence of tumor recurrence after primary resection, survival is still typically long, often in excess of a decade. Because these tumors are slow growing and relatively refractory to chemotherapy, women with metastatic disease are often debulked as disease is usually peritoneal based (as with epithelial ovarian cancer). Definitive data that surgical debulking of metastatic or recurrent disease prolongs survival are lacking, but ample data document women who have survived years or in some cases decades after resection of recurrent disease. In addition, large peritoneal-based metastases also have a proclivity for hemorrhage, sometimes with catastrophic complications. Chemotherapy is occasionally effective, and women tend to receive regimens designed to treat epithelial or germ cell tumors. These tumors often produce high levels of müllerian inhibiting substance (MIS), inhibin, and in the case of Sertoli-Leydig tumors α fetoprotein (AFP). These proteins are detectable in serum and can be used as tumor markers to monitor women for recurrent disease as the increase and decrease of these proteins in the serum tend to reflect the changing bulk of systemic tumor.

Germ cell tumors of the ovary

Germ cell tumors, like their counterparts in the testis, are cancers of germ cells. These totipotent cells contain the programming for differentiation to essentially all tissue types, and hence the germ cell tumors include a histologic menagerie of bizarre tumors, including benign teratomas and a variety of malignant tumors, such as immature teratomas, dysgerminomas, yolk sac malignancies, and choriocarcinomas. Benign teratoma (or dermoid cyst) is the most common germ cell neoplasm of the ovary and often presents in young woman. These tumors include a complex mixture of differentiated tissue including tissues from all three germ layers. In older women these differentiated tumors can develop malignant transformation, most commonly squamous cell carcinomas. Malignant germ cell tumors include dysgerminomas, yolk sac tumors, immature teratomas, as well as embryonal and choriocarcinomas. There are no known genetic abnormalities that unify these tumors. A subset of dysgerminomas harbor mutations in c-Kit oncogenes [as seen in gastrointestinal stromal tumors (GIST)], whereas a subset of germ cell tumors have isochromosome 12 abnormalities as seen in testicular malignancies. In addition, a subset of dysgerminomas is associated with dysgenetic ovaries. Identification of a dysgerminoma arising in genotypic XY gonads is important in that it highlights the need to identify and remove the contralateral gonad due to risk of gonadoblastoma.

Presentation

Germ cell tumors can present at all ages, but the peak age of presentation tends to be in females in their late teens or early twenties. Typically these tumors will become large ovarian masses, which eventually present as palpable low abdominal or pelvic masses. Like sex cord tumors, torsion or hemorrhage may present urgently or emergently as acute abdominal pain. Some of these tumors produce elevated levels of human chorionic gonadotropin (hCG) that can lead to isosexual precocious puberty when tumors present in younger girls. Unlike epithelial ovarian cancer, these tumors have a higher proclivity for nodal or hematogenous metastases. As with testicular tumors some of these tumors tend to produce AFP (yolk sac tumors) or hCG (embryonal and choriocarcinomas as well as some dysgerminomas) that are reliable tumor markers.

TREATMENT Germ Cell Tumors

Germ cell tumors typically present in women who are still of childbearing age, and because bilateral tumors are uncommon (except in dysgerminoma, 10–15%), the typical treatment is unilateral oophorectomy or salpingo-oophorectomy. Because nodal metastases to pelvic and para-aortic nodes are common and may affect treatment choices, these nodes should be carefully inspected, and if enlarged, should be resected if possible. Women with malignant germ cell tumors typically receive bleomycin, etoposide, and cisplatin (BEP) chemotherapy. In the majority of women, even those with advanced-stage disease, cure is expected. Close follow-up without adjuvant therapy of women with stage I tumors is reasonable if there is high confidence that the patient and health care team are committed to compulsive and careful follow-up, as chemotherapy at the time of tumor recurrence is likely to be curative.

Dysgerminoma is the ovarian counterpart of testicular seminoma. The 5-year disease-free survival is 100% in early-stage patients and 61% in stage III disease. Although the tumor is highly radiation-sensitive, radiation produces infertility in many patients. BEP chemotherapy is as effective or more so without causing infertility. The use of BEP following incomplete resection is associated with 95%, 2-year disease-free survival. This chemotherapy is now the treatment of choice for dysgerminoma.

FALLOPIAN TUBE CANCER

Transport of the egg to the uterus occurs via transit through the fallopian tube, with the distal ends of these tubes composed of fimbriae that drape about the ovarian surface and capture the egg as it erupts from the ovarian cortex. Fallopian tube malignancies typically have the same histologic pattern as ovarian malignancies, with the most common epithelial malignancy being of serous histology. Previous teaching was that these malignancies were rare, but more careful histologic examination suggests that many "ovarian malignancies" might actually arise in the distal fimbria of the fallopian tube. Data supporting this theory are strongest in the population of women who carry BRCA1 or BRCA2 somatic mutations. These women often present with adnexal masses, and like ovarian cancer, these tumors spread relatively early throughout the peritoneal cavity and respond to platinum and taxane therapy and have a natural history that is essentially identical to ovarian cancer (Table 97-1).

CERVICAL CANCER

■ GLOBAL CONSIDERATIONS

Cervical cancer is the second most common and most lethal malignancy in women worldwide likely due to the widespread infection with high-risk strains of human papillomavirus (HPV) and limited utilization or access to Pap smear screening in many nations throughout the world. Nearly 500,000 cases of cervical cancer are expected worldwide with approximately

240,000 deaths annually. Cancer incidence is particularly high in women residing in central and South America, the Caribbean, and southern and eastern Africa. Mortality rate is disproportionately high in Africa. In the United States, 12,200 women were diagnosed with cervical cancer and 4210 women died. Whereas efforts in developed countries have looked at high-technology screening techniques for HPV involving polymerase chain reaction and other molecular technologies, there is an urgent need for high-throughput low-technology strategies to identify and treat women bearing high-risk but treatable cervical dysplasia. The development of effective vaccines for high-risk HPV types makes it imperative to determine economical, socially acceptable, and logistically feasible strategies to deliver and distribute this vaccine to girls and perhaps boys before their engagement in sexual activity.

■ HPV INFECTION AND PREVENTIVE VACCINATION

HPV is the primary neoplastic-initiating event in the vast majority of women with invasive cervical cancer. This double-strand DNA virus infects epithelium near the transformation zone of the cervix. More than 60 types of HPV are known, with approximately 20 types having the ability to generate high-grade dysplasia and malignancy. HPV16 and 18 are the types most frequently associated with high-grade dysplasia and targeted by both FDA-approved vaccines. The large majority of sexually active adults are exposed to HPV, and most women clear the infection without specific intervention. The 8-kilobase HPV genome encodes seven early genes, most notably $E6$ and $E7$, which can bind to RB and $p53$, respectively. High-risk types of HPV encode $E6$ and $E7$ molecules that are particularly effective at inhibiting the normal cell cycle checkpoint functions of these regulatory proteins, leading to immortalization but not full transformation of cervical epithelium. A minority of woman will fail to clear the infection with subsequent HPV integration into the host genome. Over the course of as short as months but more typically years, some of these women develop high-grade dysplasia. The time from dysplasia to carcinoma is likely years to more than a decade and almost certainly requires the acquisition of other poorly defined genetic mutations within the infected and immortalized epithelium.

Risk factors include a high number of sexual partners, age of first intercourse, and history of venereal disease. Smoking is a cofactor; heavy smokers have a higher risk of dysplasia with HPV infection. HIV infection, especially when associated with low CD4+ T cell counts, is associated with a higher rate of high-grade dysplasia and likely a shorter latency period between infection and invasive disease.

Currently approved vaccines include the recombinant proteins to the late proteins, L1 and L2 of HPV-16 and -18. Vaccination of women before the initiation of sexual activity dramatically reduces the rate of HPV-16 and -18 infection and subsequent dysplasia. There is also partial protection against other HPV types, although vaccinated women are still at risk for HPV infection and still require standard Pap smear screening. Although no randomized trial data demonstrate the utility of Pap smears, the dramatic drop in cervical cancer incidence and death in developed countries employing wide-scale screening provides strong evidence for its effectiveness. The incorporation of HPV testing by polymerase chain reaction (PCR) or other molecular techniques increases the sensitivity of detecting cervical pathology but at the cost of lower sensitivity in that it identifies many women with transient infections who require no specific medical intervention.

■ CLINICAL PRESENTATIONS

The majority of cervical malignancies are squamous cell carcinomas associated with HPV. Adenocarcinomas are also HPV-related and arise deep in the endocervical canal; they are typically not seen by visual inspection of the cervix and thus often missed by Pap smear screening. A variety of rarer malignancies including atypical epithelial tumors, carcinoids, small cell carcinomas, sarcomas, and lymphomas have also been reported.

The principal role of Pap smear testing is the detection of asymptomatic preinvasive cervical dysplasia of squamous epithelial lining. Invasive carcinomas often have symptoms or signs including postcoital spotting or intermenstrual cycle bleeding or menometrorrhagia. Foul-smelling or persistent yellow discharge may also be seen. Presentations that include pelvic or sacral pain suggest lateral extension of the tumor into pelvic nerve plexus by either the primary tumor or a pelvic node and are signs of advanced-stage disease. Likewise, flank pain from hydronephrosis from ureteral compression or deep venous thrombosis from iliac vessel compression suggests either extensive nodal disease or direct extension of the primary tumor to the pelvic sidewall. The most common finding of physical exam is a visible tumor on the cervix.

TREATMENT   Cervical Cancer

Scans are not part of the formal clinical staging of cervical cancer yet are very useful in planning appropriate therapy. CT can detect hydronephrosis indicative of pelvic sidewall disease but is not accurate at evaluating other pelvic structures. MRI is more accurate at estimating uterine extension and paracervical extension of disease into soft tissues typically bordered by broad and cardinal ligaments that support the uterus in the central pelvis. Positron emission tomography (PET) scan may be the most accurate technique for evaluating the pelvis and more importantly nodal (pelvic, para-aortic, and scalene) sites for disease. This technique seems more prognostic (and probably accurate) than CT, MRI, or lymphangiogram, especially in the para-aortic region.

Stage I cervical tumors are confined to the cervix, whereas stage II tumors extend into the upper vagina or paracervical soft tissue (Fig. 97-1). Stage III tumors extend to the lower vagina or the pelvic sidewalls, whereas stage IV tumors invade the bladder or rectum or have spread to distant sites. Very small stage I cervical tumors can be treated with a variety of surgical procedures. In young women desiring to maintain fertility, radical trachelectomy removes the cervix with subsequent anastomosis of the upper vagina to the uterine corpus. Larger cervical tumors confined to the cervix can be treated with either surgical resection or radiation therapy in combination with cisplatin-based chemotherapy with a high chance of cure. Larger tumors that extend down the vagina or into the paracervical soft tissues or the pelvic sidewalls are treated with combination chemotherapy and radiation therapy. The treatment of recurrent or metastatic disease is unsatisfactory due to the relative resistance of these tumors to chemotherapy and currently available biological agents.

UTERINE CANCER

■ EPIDEMIOLOGY

Several different tumor types arise in uterine corpus. Most tumors arise in the glandular lining and are endometrial adeno-carcinomas. Tumors can also arise in the smooth muscle; most are benign (uterine leiomyoma), with a small minority of tumors being sarcomas. The endometrioid histologic subtype of endometrial cancer is the most common gynecologic malignancy in the United States. In 2010, it was diagnosed in 43,470 women and 7950 women died from the disease. Development of these tumors is a multistep process with estrogen playing an important early

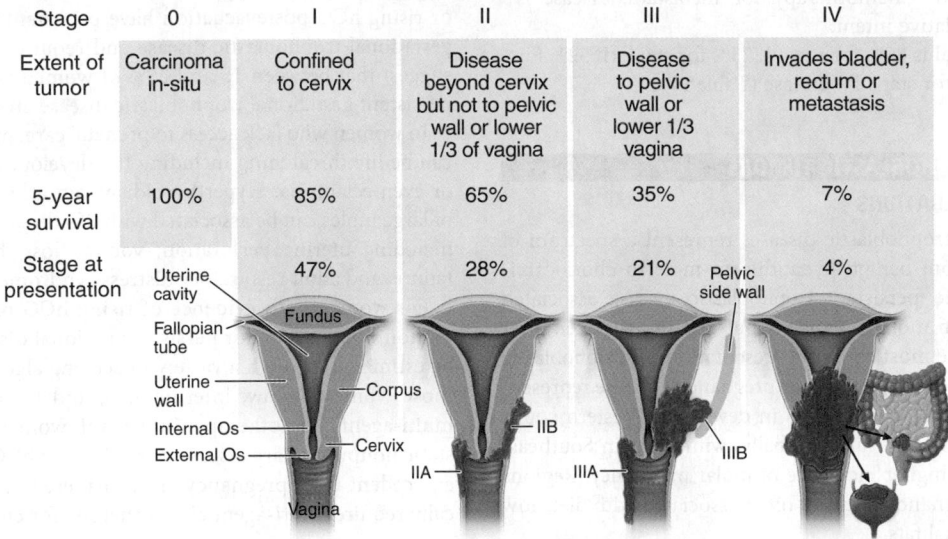

Staging of cervix cancer

Stage	0	I	II	III	IV
Extent of tumor	Carcinoma in-situ	Confined to cervix	Disease beyond cervix but not to pelvic wall or lower 1/3 of vagina	Disease to pelvic wall or lower 1/3 vagina	Invades bladder, rectum or metastasis
5-year survival	100%	85%	65%	35%	7%
Stage at presentation		47%	28%	21%	4%

Figure 97-1 Anatomic display of the stages of cervix cancer defined by location, extent of tumor, frequency of presentation, and 5-year survival.

role in driving endometrial gland proliferation. Relative overexposure to this class of hormones is a risk factor for the subsequent development of endometrioid tumors. In contrast progestins drive glandular maturation and are protective. Hence, women with high endogenous or pharmacologic exposure to estrogens, especially if unopposed by progesterone are at high risk for endometrial cancer. Obese women, women treated with unopposed estrogens, or women with estrogen-producing tumors (such as granulosa cell tumors of the ovary) are at higher risk for endometrial cancer. In addition, treatment with tamoxifen, which has antiestrogenic effects in breast tissue but estrogenic effects in uterine epithelium, is associated with an increased risk of endometrial cancer. Secondary events such as the loss of the PTEN or Cables tumor suppressor genes likely serve as secondary events in carcinogenesis. The molecular events that underlie less common endometrial cancers such as clear cell and papillary serous tumors of the uterine corpus are unknown.

Women with mutation in one of a series of DNA mismatch repair genes associated with the Lynch syndrome, also known as hereditary nonpolyposis colon cancer (HNPCC) syndrome, are at increased risk for endometrioid endometrial carcinoma. These individuals have germ-line mutations in *MSH2*, *MLH1*, and in rare cases *PMS1*, and *PMS2*. Individuals who carry these mutations typically have a family history of cancer and are at markedly increased risk for colon cancer and modestly increased risk for ovarian cancer and a variety of other tumors. Middle-aged women with HNPCC carry a 4% annual risk of endometrial cancer and a relative overall risk of approximately 200-fold as compared to age-matched women without HNPCC.

■ PATHOLOGY

Approximately 75–80% of endometrial cancers are adenocarcinomas. Prognosis depends on stage, histologic grade, and depth of myometrial invasion. Approximately 10% of patients have tumors with areas of squamous cell differentiation. When the tumor is well differentiated, it is called *adenoacanthoma*; when poorly differentiated, *adenosquamous* carcinoma. Less common histologies include mucinous carcinoma (5%) and a papillary serous tumor (<10%) that behaves like ovarian cancer.

■ PRESENTATIONS

The majority of women with tumors of the uterine corpus present with postmenopausal vaginal bleeding due to shedding of the malignant endometrial lining. Premenopausal women often will present with atypical bleeding between typical menstrual cycles. These signs typically bring a woman to the attention of a health care professional, and hence the majority of women present with early-stage disease in which the tumor is confined to the uterine corpus. Diagnosis is typically established by endometrial biopsy. Epithelial tumors may spread to pelvic or para-aortic lymph nodes. Pulmonary metastases can appear later in the natural history of this disease but are very uncommon at initial presentation. Serous tumors tend to have patterns of spread much more reminiscent of ovarian cancer with many patients presenting with omental disease and sometimes ascites. Some women presenting with uterine sarcomas will present with pelvic pain. Nodal metastases are uncommon with sarcomas, which are more likely to present with either intraabdominal disease or pulmonary metastases.

TREATMENT Uterine Cancer

Most women with endometrial cancer have disease that is localized to the uterus (75% are stage I, Table 97-1), and definitive treatment typically involves a hysterectomy with removal of the ovaries and fallopian tubes. The resection of lymph nodes does not improve outcome but does provide prognostic information. Node involvement defines stage III disease, present in 13% of patients. Tumor grade and depth of invasion are the two key prognostic variables in early-stage tumors, and women with low-grade and/or minimally invasive tumors are typically observed after definitive surgical therapy. Patients with high-grade tumors or tumors that are deeply invasive (stage IB, 13%) are at higher risk for pelvic recurrence or recurrence at the vaginal cuff, which is typically prevented by vaginal vault brachytherapy.

Women with regional metastases or metastatic disease (3% of patients) with low-grade tumors can be treated with progesterone. Poorly differentiated tumors are typically resistant to hormonal manipulation and thus are treated with chemotherapy.

The role of chemotherapy in the adjuvant setting is currently under investigation. Chemotherapy for metastatic disease is delivered with palliative intent.

Five-year survival is 89% for stage I, 73% for stage II, 52% for stage III, and 17% for stage IV disease (Table 97-1).

GESTATIONAL TROPHOBLASTIC TUMORS

■ GLOBAL CONSIDERATIONS

Gestational trophoblastic diseases represent a spectrum of neoplasia from benign hydatidiform mole to choriocarcinoma due to persistent trophoblastic disease associated most commonly with molar pregnancy but occasionally seen after normal gestation. The most common presentations of trophoblastic tumors are partial and complete molar pregnancies. These represent approximately 1 in 1500 conceptions in developed Western countries. The incidence widely varies globally, with areas in Southeast Asia having a much higher incidence of molar pregnancy. Regions with high molar pregnancy rates are often associated with diets low in carotene and animal fats.

■ RISK FACTORS

Trophoblastic tumors result from the outgrowth or persistence of placental tissue. They arise most commonly in the uterus but can also arise in other sites such as the fallopian tubes due to ectopic pregnancy. Risk factors include poorly defined dietary and environmental factors as well as conceptions at the extremes of reproductive age, with the incidence particularly high in females conceiving younger than age 16 or older than age 50. In older women, the incidence of molar pregnancy might be as high as one in three, likely due to increased risk of abnormal fertilization of the aged ova. Most trophoblastic neoplasms are associated with complete moles, diploid tumors with all genetic material from the paternal donor (known as parental disomy). This is thought to occur when a single sperm fertilizes an enucleate egg that subsequently duplicates the paternal DNA. Trophoblastic proliferation occurs with exuberant villous stroma. If pseudopregnancy extends out past the 12th week, fluid progressively accumulates within the stroma leading to "hydropic changes." There is no fetal development in complete moles.

Partial moles arise from the fertilization of an egg with two sperm, hence two-thirds of genetic material is paternal in these triploid tumors. Hydropic changes are less dramatic, and fetal development can often occur through late first trimester or early second trimester at which point spontaneous abortion is common. Laboratory findings will include excessively high hCG and high AFP. The risk of persistent gestational trophoblastic disease after partial mole is approximately 5%. Complete and partial moles can be noninvasive or invasive. Myometrial invasion occurs in no more than one in six complete moles and a lower portion of partial moles.

■ PRESENTATION OF INVASIVE TROPHOBLASTIC DISEASE

The clinical presentation of molar pregnancy is changing in developed countries due to the early detection of pregnancy with home pregnancy kits and the very early use of Doppler and ultrasound to evaluate the early fetus and uterine cavity for evidence of a viable fetus. Thus, in these countries, the majority of women presenting with trophoblastic disease have their moles detected early and have typical symptoms of early pregnancy including nausea, amenorrhea, and breast tenderness. With uterine evacuation of early complete and partial moles, most women experience spontaneous remission

of their disease as monitored by serial hCG levels. These women require no chemotherapy. Patients with persistent elevation of hCG or rising hCG postevacuation have persistent or actively growing gestational trophoblastic disease and require therapy. Most series suggest that between 15 and 25% of women will have evidence of persistent gestational trophoblastic disease after molar evacuation.

In women who lack access to prenatal care, presenting symptoms can be life threatening including the development of preeclampsia or even eclampsia. Hyperthyroidism can also be seen. Evacuation of large moles can be associated with life-threatening complications including uterine perforation, volume loss, high-output cardiac failure, and adult respiratory distress syndrome (ARDS).

For women with evidence of rising hCG or radiologic confirmation of metastatic or persistent regional disease, prognosis can be estimated through a variety of scoring algorithms that identify those women at low, intermediate, and high risk for requiring multi-agent chemotherapy. In general, women with widely metastatic nonpulmonary disease, very elevated hCG, and prior normal antecedent term pregnancy are considered at high risk and typically require multi-agent chemotherapy for cure.

TREATMENT	Invasive Trophoblastic Disease

The management for a persistent and rising hCG postevacuation of a molar conception is typically chemotherapy, although surgery can play an important role for disease that is persistently isolated in the uterus (especially if childbearing is complete) or to control hemorrhage. For women wishing to maintain fertility or with metastatic disease, the preferred treatment is chemotherapy. Chemotherapy is guided by the hCG level, which typically drops to undetectable levels with effective therapy. Single-agent treatment with methotrexate, or actinomycin D cures 90% of women with low-risk disease. Patients with high-risk disease (high hCG levels, presentation 4 or more months after pregnancy, brain or liver metastases, failure of methotrexate therapy) are typically treated with multi-agent chemotherapy [e.g., etoposide, methotrexate, and actinomycin D alternating with cyclophosphamide and vincristine (EMA-CO)], which is typically curative even in those women with extensive metastatic disease. Cisplatin, bleomycin, and either etoposide or vinblastine are also active combinations. Survival in high-risk disease exceeds 80%. Cured women may get pregnant again without evidence of increased fetal or maternal complications.

FURTHER READINGS

BERKOWITZ RS, GOLDSTEIN DP: Clinical practice. Molar pregnancy. N Engl J Med 360:1639, 2009

CLARKE-PEARSON DL: Clinical practice. Screening for ovarian cancer. N Engl J Med 361:170, 2009

JATOI I, ANDERSON WF: Management of women who have a genetic predisposition for breast cancer. Surg Clin North Am 88:845, 2008

KAHN JA: HPV vaccination for the prevention of cervical intraepithelial neoplasia. N Engl J Med 361:271, 2009

LEDERMANN JA, KRISTELEIT RS: Optimal treatment for relapsing ovarian cancer. Ann Oncol 21 Suppl 7:vii218, 2010

MOXLEY KM, MCMEEKIN DS: Endometrial carcinoma: A review of chemotherapy, drug resistance, and the search for new agents. Oncologist 15:1026, 2010

CHAPTER **98**

Soft Tissue and Bone Sarcomas and Bone Metastases

Shreyaskumar R. Patel
Robert S. Benjamin

Sarcomas are rare (<1% of all malignancies) mesenchymal neoplasms that arise in bone and soft tissues. These tumors are usually of mesodermal origin, although a few are derived from neuroectoderm, and they are biologically distinct from the more common epithelial malignancies. Sarcomas affect all age groups; 15% are found in children <15 years of age, and 40% occur after age 55 years. Sarcomas are one of the most common solid tumors of childhood and are the fifth most common cause of cancer deaths in children. Sarcomas may be divided into two groups, those derived from bone and those derived from soft tissues.

SOFT TISSUE SARCOMAS

Soft tissues include muscles, tendons, fat, fibrous tissue, synovial tissue, vessels, and nerves. Approximately 60% of soft tissue sarcomas arise in the extremities, with the lower extremities involved three times as often as the upper extremities. Thirty percent arise in the trunk, the retroperitoneum accounting for 40% of all trunk lesions. The remaining 10% arise in the head and neck.

■ INCIDENCE

Approximately 11,000 new cases of soft tissue sarcomas occurred in the United States in 2010. The annual age-adjusted incidence is 3 per 100,000 population, but the incidence varies with age. Soft tissue sarcomas constitute 0.7% of all cancers in the general population and 6.5% of all cancers in children.

■ EPIDEMIOLOGY

Malignant transformation of a benign soft tissue tumor is extremely rare, with the exception that malignant peripheral nerve sheath tumors (neurofibrosarcoma, malignant schwannoma) can arise from neurofibromas in patients with neurofibromatosis. Several etiologic factors have been implicated in soft tissue sarcomas.

Environmental factors

Trauma or previous injury is rarely involved, but sarcomas can arise in scar tissue resulting from a prior operation, burn, fracture, or foreign body implantation. Chemical carcinogens such as polycyclic hydrocarbons, asbestos, and dioxin may be involved in the pathogenesis.

Iatrogenic factors

Sarcomas in bone or soft tissues occur in patients who are treated with radiation therapy. The tumor nearly always arises in the irradiated field. The risk increases with time.

Viruses

Kaposi's sarcoma (KS) in patients with HIV type 1, classic KS, and KS in HIV-negative homosexual men is caused by human herpesvirus (HHV) 8 (Chap. 182). No other sarcomas are associated with viruses.

Immunologic factors

Congenital or acquired immunodeficiency, including therapeutic immunosuppression, increases the risk of sarcoma.

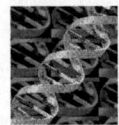 GENETIC CONSIDERATIONS

Li-Fraumeni syndrome is a familial cancer syndrome in which affected individuals have germ-line abnormalities of the tumor-suppressor gene p53 and an increased incidence of soft tissue sarcomas and other malignancies, including breast cancer, osteosarcoma, brain tumor, leukemia, and adrenal carcinoma (Chap. 83). Neurofibromatosis 1 (NF-1, peripheral form, von Recklinghausen's disease) is characterized by multiple neurofibromas and café au lait spots. Neurofibromas occasionally undergo malignant degeneration to become malignant peripheral nerve sheath tumors. The gene for NF-1 is located in the pericentromeric region of chromosome 17 and encodes neurofibromin, a tumor-suppressor protein with guanosine 5'-triphosphate (GTP)ase-activating activity that inhibits Ras function (Chap. 379). Germ-line mutation of the *Rb-1* locus (chromosome 13q14) in patients with inherited retinoblastoma is associated with the development of osteosarcoma in those who survive the retinoblastoma and of soft tissue sarcomas unrelated to radiation therapy. Other soft tissue tumors, including desmoid tumors, lipomas, leiomyomas, neuroblastomas, and paragangliomas, occasionally show a familial predisposition.

Ninety percent of synovial sarcomas contain a characteristic chromosomal translocation t(X;18)(p11;q11) involving a nuclear transcription factor on chromosome 18 called *SYT* and two breakpoints on X. Patients with translocations to the second X breakpoint (*SSX2*) may have longer survival than those with translocations involving *SSX1*.

Insulin-like growth factor (IGF) type II is produced by some sarcomas and may act as an autocrine growth factor and as a motility factor that promotes metastatic spread. IGF-II stimulates growth through IGF-I receptors, but its effects on motility are through different receptors. If secreted in large amounts, IGF-2 may produce hypoglycemia (Chaps. 100, 345).

■ CLASSIFICATION

Approximately 20 different groups of sarcomas are recognized on the basis of the pattern of differentiation toward normal tissue. For example, rhabdomyosarcoma shows evidence of skeletal muscle fibers with cross-striations; leiomyosarcomas contain interlacing fascicles of spindle cells resembling smooth muscle; and liposarcomas contain adipocytes. When precise characterization of the group is not possible, the tumors are called *unclassified sarcomas*. All of the primary bone sarcomas can also arise from soft tissues (e.g., extraskeletal osteosarcoma). The entity *malignant fibrous histiocytoma (MFH)* includes many tumors previously classified as fibrosarcomas or as pleomorphic variants of other sarcomas and is characterized by a mixture of spindle (fibrous) cells and round (histiocytic) cells arranged in a storiform pattern with frequent giant cells and areas of pleomorphism. As immunohistochemical suggestion of differentiation, particularly myogenic differentiation, may be found in a significant fraction of these patients, many are now characterized as poorly differentiated leiomyosarcomas, and the terms *undifferentiated pleomorphic sarcoma* and *myxofibrosarcoma* are replacing MFH and myxoid MFH.

For purposes of treatment, most soft tissue sarcomas can be considered together. However, some specific tumors have distinct features. For example, *liposarcoma* can have a spectrum of behaviors. Pleomorphic liposarcomas and dedifferentiated liposarcomas behave like other high-grade sarcomas; in contrast, well-differentiated liposarcomas (better termed *atypical lipomatous tumors*) lack metastatic potential, and myxoid liposarcomas metastasize infrequently, but, when they do, they have a predilection for unusual metastatic sites containing fat, such as the retroperitoneum, mediastinum, and subcutaneous tissue. Rhabdomyosarcomas, Ewing's sarcoma, and other small-cell sarcomas tend to be more aggressive and are more responsive to chemotherapy than other soft tissue sarcomas.

Gastrointestinal stromal cell tumors (GISTs), previously classified as gastrointestinal leiomyosarcomas, are now recognized as a distinct entity within soft tissue sarcomas. Its cell of origin resembles the interstitial cell of Cajal, which controls peristalsis. The majority of malignant GISTs have activating mutations of the c-*kit* gene that result in ligand-independent phosphorylation and activation of the KIT receptor tyrosine kinase, leading to tumorigenesis.

■ DIAGNOSIS

The most common presentation is an asymptomatic mass. Mechanical symptoms referable to pressure, traction, or entrapment of nerves or muscles may be present. All new and persistent or growing masses should be biopsied, either by a cutting needle (core-needle biopsy) or by a small incision, placed so that it can be encompassed in the subsequent excision without compromising a definitive resection. Lymph node metastases occur in 5%, except in synovial and epithelioid sarcomas, clear-cell sarcoma (melanoma of the soft parts), angiosarcoma, and rhabdomyosarcoma, where nodal spread may be seen in 17%. The pulmonary parenchyma is the most common site of metastases. Exceptions are GISTs, which metastasize to the liver; myxoid liposarcomas, which seek fatty tissue; and clear-cell sarcomas, which may metastasize to bones. Central nervous system metastases are rare, except in alveolar soft part sarcoma.

Radiographic evaluation

Imaging of the primary tumor is best with plain radiographs and MRI for tumors of the extremities or head and neck and by CT for tumors of the chest, abdomen, or retroperitoneal cavity. A radiograph and CT scan of the chest are important for the detection of lung metastases. Other imaging studies may be indicated, depending on the symptoms, signs, or histology.

■ STAGING AND PROGNOSIS

The histologic grade, relationship to fascial planes, and size of the primary tumor are the most important prognostic factors. The current American Joint Commission on Cancer (AJCC) staging system is shown in Table 98–1. Prognosis is related to the stage. Cure is common in the absence of metastatic disease, but a small number of patients with metastases can also be cured. Most patients with stage IV disease die within 12 months, but some patients may live with slowly progressive disease for many years.

TREATMENT   Soft Tissue Sarcomas

AJCC stage I patients are adequately treated with surgery alone. Stage II patients are considered for adjuvant radiation therapy. Stage III patients may benefit from adjuvant chemotherapy. Stage IV patients are managed primarily with chemotherapy, with or without other modalities.

SURGERY Soft tissue sarcomas tend to grow along fascial planes, with the surrounding soft tissues compressed to form a pseudocapsule that gives the sarcoma the appearance of a well-encapsulated lesion. This is invariably deceptive because "shelling out," or marginal excision, of such lesions results in a 50–90% probability of local recurrence. Wide excision with a negative margin, incorporating the biopsy site, is the standard surgical procedure for local disease. The adjuvant use of radiation therapy and/or chemotherapy improves the local control rate and permits the use of limb-sparing surgery with a local control rate (85–90%) comparable to that achieved by radical excisions and amputations. Limb-sparing approaches are indicated except when negative margins are not obtainable, when the risks of radiation are prohibitive, or when neurovascular structures are involved so that resection will result in serious functional consequences to the limb.

TABLE 98-1 AJCC Staging System for Sarcomas

Histologic Grade (G)	Tumor Size (T)	Node Status (N)	Metastases (M)
Well differentiated (G1)	≤5 cm (T1)	Not involved (N0)	Absent (M0)
Moderately differentiated (G2)	>5 cm (T2)	Involved (N1)	Present (M1)
Poorly differentiated (G3)	Superficial fascial involvement (Ta)		
Undifferentiated (G4)	Deep fascial involvement (Tb)		

Disease Stage	5-Year Survival, %
Stage I	98.8
A: G1,2; T1a,b; N0; M0	
B: G1,2; T2a; N0; M0	
Stage II	81.8
A: G1,2; T2b; N0; M0	
B: G3,4; T1; N0; M0	
C: G3,4; T2a; N0; M0	
Stage III G3,4; T2b; N0; M0	51.7
Stage IV	<20
A: any G; any T; N1; M0	
B: any G; any T; any N; M1	

RADIATION THERAPY External beam radiation therapy is an adjuvant to limb-sparing surgery for improved local control. Preoperative radiation therapy allows the use of smaller fields and smaller doses but results in a higher rate of wound complications. Postoperative radiation therapy must be given to larger fields, as the entire surgical bed must be encompassed, and in higher doses to compensate for hypoxia in the operated field. This results in a higher rate of late complications. Brachytherapy or interstitial therapy, in which the radiation source is inserted into the tumor bed, is comparable in efficacy (except in low-grade lesions), less time-consuming, and less expensive.

ADJUVANT CHEMOTHERAPY Chemotherapy is the mainstay of treatment for Ewing's primitive neuroectodermal tumors (PNET) and rhabdomyosarcomas. Meta-analysis of 14 randomized trials revealed a significant improvement in local control and disease-free survival in favor of doxorubicin-based chemotherapy. Overall survival improvement was 4% for all sites and 7% for the extremity site. An updated meta-analysis including four additional trials with doxorubicin and ifosfamide combination has reported a statistically significant 6% survival advantage in favor of chemotherapy. A chemotherapy regimen including an anthracycline and ifosfamide with growth factor support improved overall survival by 19% for high-risk (high-grade, ≥5 cm primary, or locally recurrent) extremity soft tissue sarcomas.

ADVANCED DISEASE Metastatic soft tissue sarcomas are largely incurable, but up to 20% of patients who achieve a complete response become long-term survivors. The therapeutic intent, therefore, is to produce a complete remission with chemotherapy (<10%) and/or surgery (30–40%). Surgical resection of metastases, whenever possible, is an integral part of the management. Some patients benefit from repeated surgical excision of metastases. The two most active chemotherapeutic agents are doxorubicin and ifosfamide. These drugs show a steep dose-response relationship in sarcomas. Gemcitabine with or without docetaxel has become an established second-line regimen and is particularly active in patients with leiomyosarcomas. Dacarbazine also has some modest activity. Taxanes have selective activity in angiosarcomas, and vincristine, etoposide, and irinotecan are effective in rhabdomyosarcomas and Ewing's sarcomas. Imatinib targets the KIT and platelet-derived growth factor (PDGF) tyrosine kinase activity and is standard therapy for advanced/metastatic GISTs and dermatofibrosarcoma protuberans. Imatinib is now also indicated as adjuvant therapy for completely resected primary GISTs.

BONE SARCOMAS

■ INCIDENCE AND EPIDEMIOLOGY

Bone sarcomas are rarer than soft tissue sarcomas; they accounted for only 0.2% of all new malignancies and 2600 new cases in the United States in 2010. Several benign bone lesions have the potential for malignant transformation. Enchondromas and osteochondromas can transform into chondrosarcoma; fibrous dysplasia, bone infarcts, and Paget's disease of bone can transform into either malignant fibrous histiocytoma or osteosarcoma.

■ CLASSIFICATION

Benign tumors

The common benign bone tumors include enchondroma, osteochondroma, chondroblastoma, and chondromyxoid fibroma, of cartilage origin; osteoid osteoma and osteoblastoma, of bone origin; fibroma and desmoplastic fibroma, of fibrous tissue origin; hemangioma, of vascular origin; and giant cell tumor, of unknown origin.

Malignant tumors

The most common malignant tumors of bone are plasma cell tumors (Chap. 111). The four most common malignant nonhematopoietic bone tumors are osteosarcoma, chondrosarcoma, Ewing's sarcoma, and malignant fibrous histiocytoma. Rare malignant tumors include chordoma (of notochordal origin), malignant giant cell tumor and adamantinoma (of unknown origin), and hemangioendothelioma (of vascular origin).

Musculoskeletal Tumor Society staging system

Sarcomas of bone are staged according to the Musculoskeletal Tumor Society staging system based on grade and compartmental localization. A Roman numeral reflects the tumor grade: stage I is low grade, stage II is high grade, and stage III includes tumors of any grade that have lymph node or distant metastases. In addition, the tumor is given a letter reflecting its compartmental localization. Tumors designated A are intracompartmental (i.e., confined to the same soft tissue compartment as the initial tumor), and tumors designated B are extracompartmental (i.e., extending into the adjacent soft tissue compartment or into bone). The tumor node metastasis (TNM) staging system is shown in Table 98-2.

TABLE 98-2 Staging System for Bone Sarcomas

Primary tumor (T)	TX	Primary tumor cannot be assessed
	T0	No evidence of primary tumor
	T1	Tumor ≤8 cm in greatest dimension
	T2	Tumor >8 cm in greatest dimension
	T3	Discontinuous tumors in the primary bone site
Regional lymph nodes (N)	NX	Regional lymph nodes cannot be assessed
	N0	No regional lymph node metastasis
	N1	Regional lymph node metastasis
Distant metastasis (M)	MX	Distant metastasis cannot be assessed
	M0	No distant metastasis
	M1	Distant metastasis
	M1a	Lung
	M1b	Other distant sites
Histologic grade (G)	GX	Grade cannot be assessed
	G1	Well differentiated—low grade
	G2	Moderately differentiated—low grade
	G3	Poorly differentiated—high grade
	G4	Undifferentiated—high grade (Ewing's is always classed G4)

Stage Grouping

Stage IA	T1	N0	M0	G1,2 low grade
Stage IB	T2	N0	M0	G1,2 low grade
Stage IIA	T1	N0	M0	G3,4 high grade
Stage IIB	T2	N0	M0	G3,4 high grade
Stage III	T3	N0	M0	Any G
Stage IVA	Any T	N0	M1a	Any G
Stage IVB	Any T	N1	Any M	Any G
	Any T	Any N	M1b	Any G

■ OSTEOSARCOMA

Osteosarcoma, accounting for almost 45% of all bone sarcomas, is a spindle cell neoplasm that produces osteoid (unmineralized bone) or bone. Approximately 60% of all osteosarcomas occur in children and adolescents in the second decade of life, and approximately 10% occur in the third decade of life. Osteosarcomas in the fifth and sixth decades of life are frequently secondary to either radiation therapy or transformation in a preexisting benign condition, such as Paget's disease. Males are affected 1.5–2 times as often as females. Osteosarcoma has a predilection for metaphyses of long bones; the most common sites of involvement are the distal femur, proximal tibia, and proximal humerus. The classification of osteosarcoma is complex, but 75% of osteosarcomas fall into the "classic" category, which include osteoblastic, chondroblastic, and fibroblastic osteosarcomas. The remaining 25% are classified as "variants" on the basis of (1) clinical characteristics, as in the case of osteosarcoma of the jaw, postradiation osteosarcoma, or Paget's osteosarcoma; (2) morphologic characteristics, as in the case of telangiectatic osteosarcoma, small cell osteosarcoma, or epithelioid osteosarcoma; or (3) location, as in parosteal or periosteal osteosarcoma. Diagnosis usually requires a synthesis of clinical, radiologic, and pathologic features. Patients typically present with pain and swelling of the affected area. A plain radiograph reveals a destructive lesion with a moth-eaten appearance, a spiculated periosteal reaction (sunburst appearance), and a cuff of periosteal new bone formation at the margin of the soft tissue mass (Codman's triangle). A CT scan of the primary tumor is best for defining bone destruction and the pattern of calcification, whereas MRI is better for defining intramedullary and soft tissue extension. A chest radiograph and CT scan are used to detect lung metastases. Metastases to the bony skeleton should be imaged by a bone scan, or by fluorodeoxyglucose positron emission tomography (FDG-PET). Almost all osteosarcomas are hypervascular. Angiography is not helpful for diagnosis, but it is the most sensitive test for assessing the response to preoperative chemotherapy. Pathologic diagnosis is established either with a core-needle biopsy, where feasible, or with an open biopsy with an appropriately placed incision that does not compromise future limb-sparing resection. Most osteosarcomas are high-grade. The most important prognostic factor for long-term survival is response to chemotherapy. Preoperative chemotherapy followed by limb-sparing surgery (which can be accomplished in >80% of patients) followed by postoperative chemotherapy is standard management. The effective drugs are doxorubicin, ifosfamide, cisplatin, and high-dose methotrexate with leucovorin rescue. The various combinations of these agents that have been used have all been about equally successful. Long-term survival rates in extremity osteosarcoma range from 60 to 80%. Osteosarcoma is radioresistant; radiation therapy has no role in the routine management. Malignant fibrous histiocytoma is considered a part of the spectrum of osteosarcoma and is managed similarly.

■ CHONDROSARCOMA

Chondrosarcoma, which constitutes ~20–25% of all bone sarcomas, is a tumor of adulthood and old age with a peak incidence in the fourth to sixth decades of life. It has a predilection for the flat bones, especially the shoulder and pelvic girdles, but can also affect the diaphyseal portions of long bones. Chondrosarcomas can arise de novo or as a malignant transformation of an enchondroma or, rarely, of the cartilaginous cap of an osteochondroma. Chondrosarcomas have an indolent natural history and typically present as pain and swelling. Radiographically, the lesion may have a lobular appearance with mottled or punctate or annular calcification of the cartilaginous matrix. It is difficult to distinguish low-grade chondrosarcoma from benign lesions by x-ray or histologic examination. The diagnosis is therefore influenced by clinical history and physical examination. A new onset of pain, signs of inflammation, and progressive increase in the size of the mass suggest malignancy. The histologic classification is complex, but most tumors fall within the classic category. Like other bone sarcomas, high-grade chondrosarcomas spread to the lungs. Most chondrosarcomas are resistant to chemotherapy, and surgical resection of primary or recurrent tumors, including pulmonary metastases, is the mainstay of therapy. This rule does not hold for two histologic variants. Dedifferentiated chondrosarcoma has a high-grade osteosarcoma or a malignant fibrous histiocytoma component that responds to chemotherapy. Mesenchymal chondrosarcoma, a rare variant composed of a small cell element, also is responsive to systemic chemotherapy and is treated like Ewing's sarcoma.

■ EWING'S SARCOMA

Ewing's sarcoma, which constitutes ~10–15% of all bone sarcomas, is common in adolescence and has a peak incidence in the second decade of life. It typically involves the diaphyseal region of long bones and also has an affinity for flat bones. The plain radiograph may show a characteristic "onion peel" periosteal reaction with a generous soft tissue mass, which is better demonstrated by CT or MRI. This mass is composed of sheets of monotonous, small, round, blue cells and can be confused with lymphoma, embryonal rhabdomyosarcoma, and small-cell carcinoma. The presence of p30/32, the product of the *mic-2* gene (which maps to the pseudoautosomal region of the X and Y chromosomes) is a cell-surface marker for Ewing's sarcoma (and other members of the Ewing's family of tumors, sometimes called PNETs). Most PNETs arise in soft tissues; they include peripheral neuroepithelioma, Askin's tumor (chest wall), and esthesioneuroblastoma. Glycogen-filled cytoplasm detected by staining with periodic acid–Schiff is also characteristic of Ewing's sarcoma cells. The classic cytogenetic abnormality associated with this disease (and other PNETs) is a reciprocal translocation of the long arms of chromosomes 11 and 22, t(11;22), which creates a chimeric gene product of unknown function with components from the *fli-1* gene on chromosome 11 and *ews* on 22. This disease is very aggressive, and it is therefore considered a systemic disease. Common sites of metastases are lung, bones, and bone marrow. Systemic chemotherapy is the mainstay of therapy, often being used before surgery. Doxorubicin, cyclophosphamide or ifosfamide, etoposide, vincristine, and dactinomycin are active drugs. Topotecan or irinotecan in combination with an alkylating agent are often used in relapsed patients. Targeted therapy with an anti-IGF1 receptor antibody appears to have promising activity in refractory cases. Local treatment for the primary tumor includes surgical resection, usually with limb salvage or radiation therapy. Patients with lesions below the elbow and below the mid-calf have a 5-year survival rate of 80% with effective treatment. Ewing's sarcoma at first presentation is a curable tumor, even in the presence of obvious metastatic disease, especially in children <11 years old.

TUMORS METASTATIC TO BONE

Bone is a common site of metastasis for carcinomas of the prostate, breast, lung, kidney, bladder, and thyroid and for lymphomas and sarcomas. Prostate, breast, and lung primaries account for 80% of all bone metastases. Metastatic tumors of bone are more common than primary bone tumors. Tumors usually spread to bone hematogenously, but local invasion from soft tissue masses also occurs. In descending order of frequency, the sites most often involved are the vertebrae, proximal femur, pelvis, ribs, sternum, proximal humerus, and skull. Bone metastases may be asymptomatic or may produce pain, swelling, nerve root or spinal cord compression, pathologic fracture, or myelophthisis (replacement of the marrow). Symptoms of hypercalcemia may be noted in cases of bony destruction.

Pain is the most frequent symptom. It usually develops gradually over weeks, is usually localized, and often is more severe at night. When patients with back pain develop neurologic signs or symptoms, emergency evaluation for spinal cord compression is indicated (Chap. 276). Bone metastases exert a major adverse effect on quality of life in cancer patients.

Cancer in the bone may produce osteolysis, osteogenesis, or both. Osteolytic lesions result when the tumor produces substances that can directly elicit bone resorption (vitamin D–like steroids, prostaglandins, or parathyroid hormone–related peptide) or cytokines that can induce the formation of osteoclasts (interleukin 1 and tumor necrosis factor). Osteoblastic lesions result when the tumor produces cytokines that activate osteoblasts. In general, purely osteolytic lesions are best detected by plain radiography, but they may not be apparent until they are >1 cm. These lesions are more commonly associated with hypercalcemia and with the excretion of hydroxyproline-containing peptides indicative of matrix destruction. When osteoblastic activity is prominent, the lesions may be readily detected using radionuclide bone scanning (which is sensitive to new bone formation), and the radiographic appearance may show increased bone density or sclerosis. Osteoblastic lesions are associated with higher serum levels of alkaline phosphatase and, if extensive, may produce hypocalcemia. Although some tumors may produce mainly osteolytic lesions (e.g., kidney cancer) and others mainly osteoblastic lesions (e.g., prostate cancer), most metastatic lesions produce both types of lesion and may go through stages where one or the other predominates.

In older patients, particularly women, it may be necessary to distinguish metastatic disease of the spine from osteoporosis. In osteoporosis, the cortical bone may be preserved, whereas cortical bone destruction is usually noted with metastatic cancer.

TREATMENT   Metastatic Bone Disease

Treatment of metastatic bone disease depends on the underlying malignancy and the symptoms. Some metastatic bone tumors are curable (lymphoma, Hodgkin's disease), and others are treated with palliative intent. Pain may be relieved by local radiation therapy. Hormonally responsive tumors are responsive to hormone inhibition (antiandrogens for prostate cancer, antiestrogens for breast cancer). Strontium 89 and samarium 153 are bone-seeking radionuclides that can exert antitumor effects and relieve symptoms. Bisphosphonates such as pamidronate may relieve pain and inhibit bone resorption, thereby maintaining bone mineral density and reducing risk of fractures in patients with osteolytic metastases from breast cancer and multiple myeloma. Careful monitoring of serum electrolytes and creatinine is recommended. Monthly administration prevents bone-related clinical events and may reduce the incidence of bone metastases in women with breast cancer. When the integrity of a weight-bearing bone is threatened by an expanding metastatic lesion that is refractory to radiation therapy, prophylactic internal fixation is indicated. Overall survival is related to the prognosis of the underlying tumor. Bone pain at the end of life is particularly common; an adequate pain relief regimen including sufficient amounts of narcotic analgesics is required. The management of hypercalcemia is discussed in Chap. 353.

FURTHER READINGS

BORDEN EC et al: Soft tissue sarcomas of adults: State of the translational science. Clin Cancer Res 9:1941, 2003

DEMATTEO R et al: Adjuvant imatinib mesylate after resection of localized primary GIST: A randomized double blind placebo controlled trial. Lancet 373:1097, 2009

HELMAN LJ, MELTZER P: Mechanisms of sarcoma development. Nat Rev Cancer 3:685, 2003

MOCELLIN S et al: Adult soft tissue sarcomas: Conventional therapies and molecularly targeted approaches. Cancer Treat Rev 32:9, 2006

PATEL SR, ZALCBERG J. Optimization of dose of Imatinib for the treatment of GIST—Lessons learned from the phase 3 trials. Eur J Cancer 44:501, 2008

PISTERS PW et al: Evidence-based recommendations for local therapy for soft tissue sarcomas. J Clin Oncol 25:1003, 2007

SCURR M, JUDSON I: How to treat the Ewing's family of sarcomas in adult patients. Oncologist 11:65, 2006

CHAPTER 99

Carcinoma of Unknown Primary

Gauri R. Varadhachary
James L. Abbruzzese

Carcinoma of unknown primary (CUP) is a biopsy-proven (mainly epithelial) malignancy for which the anatomic site of origin remains unidentified after an intensive search. CUP is one of the 10 most frequently diagnosed cancers worldwide, accounting for approximately 3–5% of all cancers. Most investigators do not include lymphomas, metastatic melanomas, and metastatic sarcomas that present without a known primary tumor as CUP because these cancers have specific stage- and histology-based treatments that guide management.

With the increasing availability of additional sophisticated imaging, invasive diagnostic techniques, and the emergence of effective targeted therapies in several cancers, an individualized management algorithm with an impact on quality of life and survival is critical. The reasons cancers present as CUP remain unclear. One hypothesis is that the primary tumor either regresses after seeding the metastasis or remains so small that it is not detected. It is possible that CUP falls on the continuum of cancer presentation where the primary has been contained or eliminated by the natural body defenses. Alternatively, CUP may represent a specific malignant event that results in an increase in metastatic spread or survival relative to the primary. Whether the CUP metastases truly define a clone that is genetically and phenotypically unique to this diagnosis remains to be determined.

CUP BIOLOGY

No characteristics that are unique to CUP relative to metastases from known primaries have been identified. Abnormalities in chromosomes 1 and 12 and other complex cytogenetic abnormalities have been reported. Aneuploidy has been described in 70% of CUP patients with metastatic adenocarcinoma or undifferentiated carcinoma. The overexpression of various genes, including *Ras*, *bcl-2* (40%), *her-2* (11%), and *p53* (26–53%), has been studied in CUP samples, but they have no effect on response to therapy or survival. The extent of angiogenesis in CUP relative to that in metastases from known primaries has also been evaluated, but no consistent findings have emerged.

■ CLINICAL EVALUATION

Obtaining a thorough medical history from CUP patients is essential, paying particular attention to previous surgeries, removed lesions, and family medical history to assess potential hereditary cancers. Physical examination, including a digital rectal examination in men and breast and pelvic examinations in women, should be performed. Determining the patient's performance status, nutritional status, comorbid illnesses, and cancer-induced complications is essential since these may affect treatment planning.

Role of serum tumor markers and cytogenetics

Most tumor markers, including CEA, CA-125, CA 19-9, and CA 15-3, when elevated, are nonspecific and not helpful in determining the primary tumor site. Men who present with adenocarcinoma and osteoblastic metastasis should undergo a prostate-specific antigen (PSA) test. In patients with undifferentiated or poorly differentiated carcinoma (especially with a midline tumor), elevated β-human chorionic gonadotropin (βhCG) and α fetoprotein (AFP) levels suggest the possibility of an extragonadal germ cell (testicular) tumor. Cytogenetic studies had a larger role in the past, although interpretation of these older studies can be challenging. In our opinion, with the availability of immunohistochemical stains, cytogenetic analyses are indicated only occasionally. We reserve them for undifferentiated neoplasms with inconclusive immunohistochemical stains and those for which a high suspicion of lymphoma exists.

Role of imaging studies

Chest x-rays are always obtained in CUP workups but are often negative, especially with low-volume disease. A CT scan of the chest, abdomen, and pelvis is indicated in the search for the primary, evaluate the extent of disease, and select the most favorable biopsy site. Older studies suggested that the primary tumor site is detected in 20–35% of patients who undergo a CT scan of the abdomen and pelvis, although by current definition these patients would not be considered as having CUP. Older studies also suggest a latent primary tumor prevalence of 20%; with more sophisticated imaging, this prevalence is ≤5% today.

Mammography should be performed in all women who present with metastatic adenocarcinoma, especially in those with adenocarcinoma and isolated axillary lymphadenopathy. MRI of the breast is a recognized follow-up modality in patients with suspected occult primary breast carcinoma following a negative mammography and sonography. The results of these imaging modalities can influence surgical management; a negative breast MRI result predicts a low tumor yield at mastectomy.

A conventional workup for a squamous cell carcinoma and cervical CUP (neck lymphadenopathy with no known primary tumor) includes a CT scan or MRI and invasive studies, including indirect and direct laryngoscopy, bronchoscopy, and upper endoscopy. Ipsilateral (or bilateral) tonsillectomy (with histopathology) has been recommended for these patients. Fluorodeoxyglucose positron emission tomography (FDG-PET) scans are useful in this patient population and may help guide the biopsy; determine the extent of disease; facilitate the appropriate treatment, including planning radiation fields; and help with disease surveillance. A smaller radiation field encompassing the primary (when found) and metastatic adenopathy decreases the risk of chronic xerostomia.

Several studies have evaluated the utility of PET in patients with cervical CUP. These trials have included a small number of patients; primary tumors were identified in ~21–30%.

The diagnostic contribution of PET to the evaluation of other CUP (outside of the neck adenopathy indication) is controversial. PET-CT can be helpful for patients who are candidates for surgical intervention for solitary metastatic disease because the presence of disease outside the primary site may affect surgical planning.

Invasive studies, including upper endoscopy, colonoscopy, and bronchoscopy, should be limited to symptomatic patients or those with laboratory, imaging or pathologic abnormalities that suggest that these techniques will result in a high yield in search for a primary cancer.

■ PATHOLOGIC DIAGNOSIS OF CUP

A detailed pathologic examination of the most accessible biopsied tissue specimen is mandatory in CUP patients. Pathologic evaluation typically consists of hematoxylin-and-eosin stains and immunohistochemical tests. Electron microscopy and cytogenetics are rarely useful.

Light microscopy evaluation

Adequate tissue obtained by fine-needle aspiration or core-needle biopsy should first be stained with hematoxylin and eosin and subjected to light microscopic examination. On light microscopy, 60–65% of CUP are adenocarcinoma, and 5% are squamous cell carcinoma. The remaining 30–35% are poorly differentiated adenocarcinoma, poorly differentiated carcinoma, poorly differentiated neoplasm. A small percentage of lesions are diagnosed as neuroendocrine cancers (2%), mixed tumors (adenosquamous, or sarcomatoid carcinomas), or undifferentiated neoplasms (Table 99-1).

Role of immunohistochemical analysis

Immunohistochemical stains are peroxidase-labeled antibodies against specific tumor antigens that are used to define tumor lineage. The number of available immunohistochemical stains is ever-increasing. However, in CUP cases, more is not necessarily better, and immunohistochemical stains should be used in conjunction with the patient's clinical presentation and imaging studies to select the best therapy. Communication between the clinician and pathologist is essential. No stain is 100% specific, and overinterpretation should be avoided. PSA and thyroglobulin tissue markers, which are positive in prostate and thyroid cancer, respectively, are the most specific of the current marker panel. However, these cancers rarely present as CUP, so the yield of these tests may be low. Fig. 99-1 delineates a simple algorithm for immunohistochemical staining in CUP cases. Table 99-2 lists additional tests that may be useful to further define the tumor lineage. A more comprehensive algorithm may improve the diagnostic accuracy but can make the process complex. With the use of immunohistochemical markers, electron microscopic analysis, which is time-consuming and expensive, is rarely needed.

TABLE 99-1 Major Histologies in CUP

Histology	Proportion, %
Well to moderately differentiated adenocarcinoma	60
Squamous cell cancer	5
Poorly differentiated adenocarcinoma, poorly differentiated carcinoma	30
Neuroendocrine	2
Undifferentiated malignancy	3

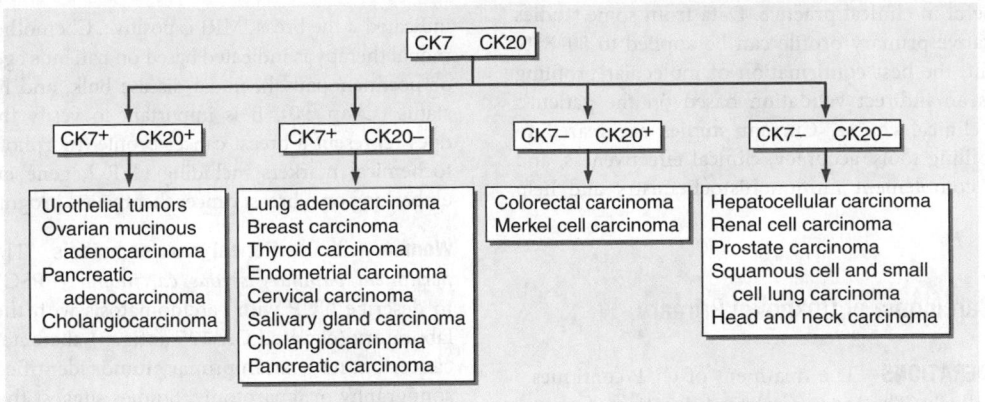

Figure 99-1 Approach to cytokeratin (CK7 and CK20) markers used in CUP.

There are >20 subtypes of cytokeratin (CK) intermediate filaments with different molecular weights and differential expression in various cell types and cancers. Monoclonal antibodies to specific CK subtypes have been used to help classify tumors according to their site of origin; commonly used CK stains in CUP are CK7 and CK20. CK7 is found in tumors of the lung, ovary, endometrium, and breast and not in those of the lower gastrointestinal tract, whereas CK20 is normally expressed in the gastrointestinal epithelium, urothelium, and Merkel cells. CK20+/CK7– strongly suggests a primary tumor of the colon; 75–95% of colon tumors show this pattern of staining. CK20–/CK7+ suggests cancer of the lung, breast, ovary, endometrium, and pancreaticobiliary tract; some of these can also be CK20+. The nuclear CDX-2 transcription factor, which is the product of a homeobox gene necessary for intestinal organogenesis, is often used to aid in the diagnosis of gastrointestinal adenocarcinomas.

TABLE 99-2 Additional Immunohistochemical Stains Useful in the Diagnosis of CUP

Tissue Marker	Diagnosis
Estrogen and progesterone receptors	Breast cancer
BRST-1	Breast cancer
Gross cystic disease fibrous protein-15	Breast cancer
Thyroid transcription factor 1	Lung and thyroid cancer
Thyroglobulin	Thyroid cancer
Chromogranin, synaptophysin, CD56	Neuroendocrine cancer
CDX-2	Gastrointestinal cancer
Calretinin, mesothelin	Mesothelioma
Leukocyte common antigen	Lymphoma
HMB-45, tyrosinase, Melan-A	Melanoma
URO-III, thrombomodulin	Bladder cancer
α Fetoprotein	Hepatocellular cancer, germ cell cancer
β-Human chronic gonadotropin	Germ cell cancer
Prostate specific antigen	Prostate cancer
WT-1, estrogen receptor (ER)	Müllerian/ovarian cancer
RCC, CD 10	Renal cell carcinoma

Thyroid transcription factor 1 (TTF-1) is a 38-kDa homeodomain-containing nuclear protein that plays a role in transcriptional activation during embryogenesis in the thyroid, diencephalon, and respiratory epithelium. TTF-1 nuclear staining is typically positive in lung and thyroid cancers. Approximately 68% of adenocarcinomas and 25% of squamous cell lung cancers stain positive for TTF-1, which helps differentiate a lung primary tumor from metastatic adenocarcinoma in a pleural effusion, the mediastinum, or the lung parenchyma.

Distinguishing pleural mesothelioma from lung adenocarcinoma can be challenging. Calretinin, Wilms' tumor gene-1 (WT-1), and mesothelin have been suggested as useful markers for mesothelioma.

Gross cystic disease fibrous protein-15, a 15-kDa monomer protein, is a marker of apocrine differentiation that is detected in 62–72% of breast carcinomas. UROIII, high-molecular-weight cytokeratin, thrombomodulin, and CK20 are the markers used to diagnose lesions of urothelial origin.

ROLE OF DNA MICROARRAY AND REVERSE TRANSCRIPTASE POLYMERASE CHAIN REACTION (RT-PCR) IN CUP

In the absence of a known primary, developing therapeutic strategies for CUP is challenging. The current diagnostic yield with imaging and immunochemistry is ~20–30% for CUP patients. The use of gene expression studies holds the promise of substantially increasing this yield. Gene expression profiles are most commonly generated using quantitative RT-PCR or DNA microarray.

Neural network programs have been used to develop predictive algorithms from the gene expression profiles. Typically, a training set of gene profiles from known cancers (preferably from metastatic sites) are used to train the software. The program can then be used to predict the putative origin of a test tumor, and presumably of true CUP. Comprehensive gene expression databases that have become available for common malignancies may also be useful in CUP. Investigators have used expression data from normal differentiated tissues to identify conserved expression profiles found in malignant tissue as a basis for predicting the tissue of origin (ToO). These approaches have been effective in blind testing against known primary cancers and their metastasis. However, because, by definition, the primary tumor site is not identifiable in CUP, validation of site prediction in this setting can be challenging, and any predictions currently must be supported by clinical and pathologic correlation. Prospective validation trials are currently evaluating the role of molecular studies identifying ToO in CUP and its impact on management. Early trials suggest that the profiling approach is feasible from archived formalin-fixed paraffin-embedded (FFPE) core-needle biopsies. Quantitative RT-PCR on fine-needle aspiration samples is very useful in clinical practice. Data from some studies suggest that a putative primary profile can be applied to 80–85% of cases. At present, the best confirmation of molecular profiling studies in CUP is an indirect validation based on the patient's presentation and clinical course. Current studies are geared to understanding profiling tools' accuracy, clinical effectiveness, and how these assays complement immunohistochemistry and help guide therapy.

| TREATMENT | Carcinoma of Unknown Primary |

GENERAL CONSIDERATIONS The treatment of CUP continues to evolve, albeit slowly. The median survival duration of most patients with disseminated CUP is ~6–10 months. Systemic chemotherapy is the primary treatment modality in most cases, but the careful integration of surgery, radiation therapy, and even periods of observation are important in the overall management of this condition (Figs. 99-2 and 99-3). Prognostic factors include performance status, site and number of metastases, response to chemotherapy, and serum lactate dehydrogenase (LDH) levels. Culine and colleagues developed a prognostic model using performance status and serum LDH levels, which allowed the assignment of patients into two subgroups with divergent outcomes. Future prospective trials using this prognostic model are warranted. Clinically, several CUP diagnoses fall into a favorable prognostic subset. Others, including those with disseminated CUP that do not fit a subset, have a more unfavorable prognosis.

TREATMENT OF FAVORABLE SUBSETS OF CUP

Women with isolated axillary adenopathy Women with isolated axillary adenopathy with adenocarcinoma or carcinoma are usually treated for stage II or III breast cancer based on pathologic findings. These patients should undergo a breast MRI if mammogram and ultrasound are negative. Radiation therapy to the ipsilateral breast is indicated if the breast MRI is positive. Chemotherapy and/or hormonal therapy is indicated based on patient's age (premenopausal or postmenopausal), nodal disease bulk, and hormone receptor status (Chap. 90). It is important to verify that the pathology does represent a breast cancer profile (morphology, immunohistochemical markers including HER-2, gene expression) before embarking on a breast cancer therapeutic program.

Women with peritoneal carcinomatosis The term *primary peritoneal papillary serous carcinoma* (PPSC) has been used to describe CUP with carcinomatosis with the pathologic and laboratory (elevated CA-125 antigen) characteristics of ovarian cancer but no ovarian primary tumor identified on transvaginal sonography or laparotomy. Studies suggest that ovarian cancer and PPSC, which are both of müllerian origin, have similar gene expression profiles. Similar to patients with ovarian cancer, patients with PPSC are candidates for cytoreductive surgery, followed by adjuvant taxane and platinum-based chemotherapy. In one retrospective study of 258 women with peritoneal carcinomatosis who had undergone cytoreductive surgery and chemotherapy, 22% of patients had a complete response to chemotherapy; the median survival duration was 18 months (range 11–24 months). However, not all peritoneal carcinomatosis in women is PPSC. Careful pathologic evaluation can help diagnose a colon cancer profile (CDX-2+, CK-20+, CK7–) or a pancreaticobiliary cancer.

Poorly differentiated carcinoma with midline adenopathy Men with poorly differentiated or undifferentiated carcinoma that presents as a midline adenopathy should be evaluated for extragonadal germ cell malignancy. If diagnosed and treated as such, they often experience a good response to treatment with platinum-based combination chemotherapy. Response rates of >50% have been noted, and 10–15% long-term survivors have been reported. Older patients (especially smokers) who present with mediastinal adenopathy are more likely to have a lung or head–and–neck cancer profile.

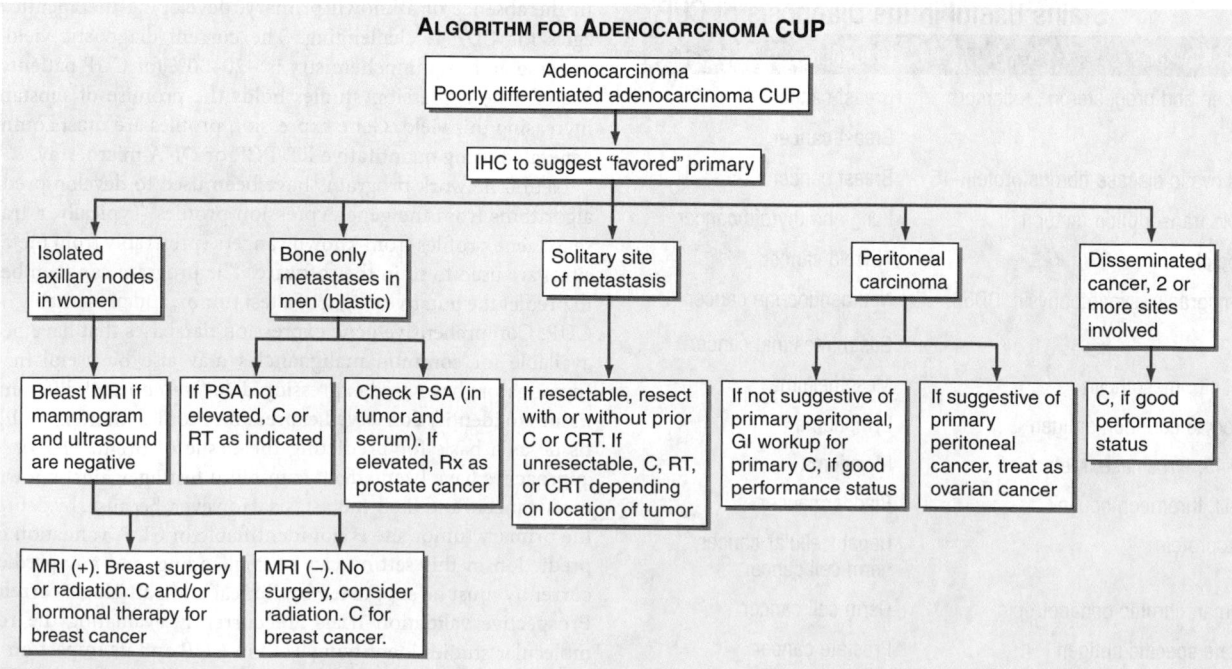

Figure 99-2 Treatment algorithm for adenocarcinoma and poorly differentiated adenocarcinoma CUP. C, chemotherapy; CRT, chemoradiation; GI, gastrointestinal; IHC, immunohistochemistry; MRI, magnetic resonance imaging; PSA, prostate-specific antigen; RT, radiation.

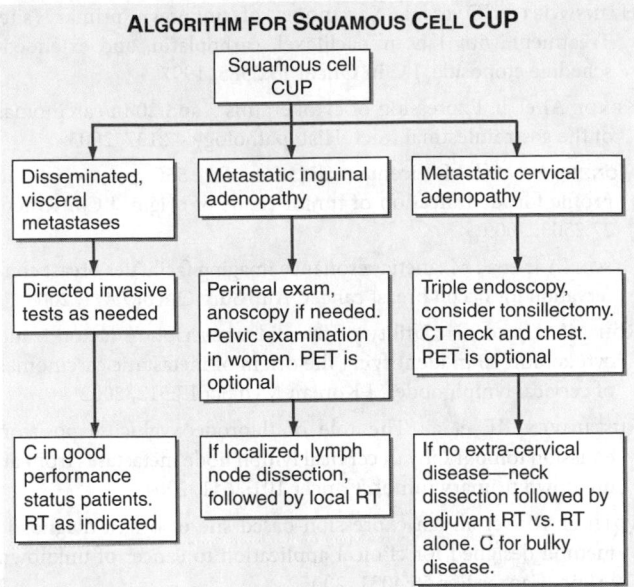

Figure 99-3 Treatment algorithm for squamous cell CUP. C, chemotherapy; CT, computed tomography; PET, positron emission tomography; RT, radiation.

Neuroendocrine carcinoma Low-grade neuroendocrine carcinoma often has an indolent course, and treatment decisions are based on symptoms and tumor bulk. Urine 5-HIAA and serum chromogranin may be elevated and can be followed as markers. Often the patient is treated with somatostatin analogues alone for hormone-related symptoms (diarrhea, flushing, nausea). Specific local therapies or systemic therapy would only be indicated if the patient is symptomatic with local pain secondary to significant growth of the metastasis or the hormone-related symptoms are not controlled with endocrine therapy. Patients with high-grade neuroendocrine carcinoma are treated as having small cell lung cancer and are responsive to chemotherapy; 20–25% show a complete response, and up to 10% patients survive more than 5 years.

Squamous cell carcinoma presenting as neck adenopathy Patients with early-stage squamous cell carcinoma involving the cervical lymph nodes are candidates for node dissection and radiation therapy, which can result in long-term survival. The role of chemotherapy in these patients is undefined, although chemoradiation therapy or induction chemotherapy is often used and is beneficial in bulky N2/N3 lymph node disease.

Solitary metastatic site Patients with solitary metastases can also experience good treatment outcomes. Some patients who present with locoregional disease are candidates for aggressive trimodality management; both prolonged disease-free interval and occasionally cure are possible.

Men with blastic skeletal metastases and elevated PSA Blastic bone-only metastasis is a rare presentation, and elevated serum PSA or tumor staining with PSA may provide confirmatory evidence of prostate cancer in these patients. Those with elevated levels are candidates for hormonal therapy for prostate cancer, although it is important to rule out other primary tumors (lung most common).

Management of Disseminated CUP Patients who present with liver, brain, and adrenal metastatic disease usually have a poor prognosis. Beside primary peritoneal carcinoma, carcinomatosis

presenting as CUP in other settings is not uncommon. Gastric, appendicular, colon, pancreas, and cholangiocarcinoma are all possible primaries, and imaging, endoscopy, and pathologic data help in the evaluation.

Traditionally, platinum-based combination chemotherapy regimens have been used to treat patients with CUP. In a phase II study by Hainsworth and colleagues, 55 mostly chemotherapy-naive patients were treated with paclitaxel, carboplatin, and oral etoposide every 3 weeks. The overall response rate was 47%, with median overall survival duration of 13.4 months. Briasoulis and colleagues reported similar response rates and survival durations in 77 patients with CUP, who had been treated with paclitaxel and carboplatin. In this study, patients with nodal or pleural disease and women with peritoneal carcinomatosis had higher response rates and overall survival durations of 13 and 15 months, respectively. Studies incorporating newer agents, including gemcitabine, irinotecan, and targeted agents, are showing higher response rates. In a phase II randomized trial by Culine and colleagues, 80 patients were randomly assigned to receive gemcitabine with cisplatin or irinotecan with cisplatin; 78 patients were assessable for efficacy and toxicity. Objective responses were observed in 21 patients (55%) in the gemcitabine and cisplatin arm and in 15 patients (38%) in the irinotecan and cisplatin arm. The median survival was 8 months for gemcitabine and cisplatin and 6 months for irinotecan and cisplatin.

The role of second-line chemotherapy in CUP is poorly defined. Gemcitabine as a single agent has shown a partial response rate of 8%, and 25% of patients had minor responses or stable disease, with improved symptoms. Combination chemotherapy as a second- and third-line treatment may result in a slightly improved response and therapy options should be guided by pathology and the patient's performance status.

Hainsworth and colleagues studied the combination of bevacizumab and erlotinib in 51 patients; 25% were chemotherapy-naive and had advanced bone or liver metastases, while the rest had been treated with 1 or 2 chemotherapy regimens. Responses were noted in 4 patients (8%), and 30 patients (59%) experienced stable disease or a minor response. The median overall survival was 8.9 months, with 42% of patients alive at 1 year.

Historically, patients with CUP have been treated with broad spectrum regimens that work for a variety of primary cancers; a "one treatment fits all" approach. With incremental improved responses over the past decade in known cancer types, we anticipate overall better response rates with newer regimens for selected CUP patients. With a more robust immunohistochemical panel (directed approach) and new molecular profiling tools, one may hope to create a more tailored treatment algorithm for CUP patients.

SUMMARY

Patients with CUP should undergo a directed diagnostic search for the primary tumor on the basis of clinical and pathologic data. Subsets of patients have prognostically favorable disease, as defined by clinical or histologic criteria, and may substantially benefit from aggressive treatment and expect prolonged survival. However, for most patients who present with advanced CUP, the prognosis remains poor, with early resistance to available cytotoxic therapy. The current focus has shifted away from empirical chemotherapeutic trials to understanding the metastatic phenotype, ToO profiling, and evaluating molecular targets in CUP patients. Our understanding of this challenging disease is growing steadily in the era of sophisticated diagnostics and therapeutics. A strategy that integrates information from a patient's clinical presentation including imaging and pathology with directed immunohistochemistry and molecular profiling in selected cases, will help us select the best treatment for our patients.

FURTHER READINGS

ABBRUZZESE JL et al: The biology of unknown primary tumors. Semin Oncol 20:238, 1993

BUGAT R et al: Summary of the standards, options and recommendations for the management of patients with carcinoma of unknown primary site. Br J Cancer 89:S59, 2003

CULINE S et al: Cisplatin in combination with either gemcitabine or irinotecan in carcinomas of unknown primary site: Results of a randomized phase II study—trial for the French Study Group on Carcinomas of Unknown Primary (GEFCAPI 01). J Clin Oncol 21:3479, 2003

DENNIS JL, OIEN KA: Hunting the primary: Novel strategies for defining the origin of tumours. J Pathol 205:236, 2005

GRECO FA. Therapy of adenocarcinoma of unknown primary: Are we making progress? J Natl Compr Cancer Netw 2008 10:1061, 2008.

HAINSWORTH JD et al: Carcinoma of unknown primary site: Treatment with 1-hour paclitaxel, carboplatin, and extended-schedule etoposide. J Clin Oncol 15:2385, 1997

KENDE AI et al: Expression of cytokeratins 7 and 20 in carcinomas of the gastrointestinal tract. Histopathology 42:137, 2003

MONZON FA et al: Multicenter validation of a 1,550-gene expression profile for identification of tumor tissue of origin. J Clin Oncol 27:2503, 2009

OLSON JA Jr et al: Magnetic resonance imaging facilitates breast conservation for occult breast cancer. Ann Surg Oncol 7:411, 2000

ROH MS, HONG SH: Utility of thyroid transcription factor-1 and cytokeratin 20 in identifying the origin of metastatic carcinomas of cervical lymph nodes. J Korean Med Sci 17:512, 2002

RUSTHOVEN KE et al: The role of fluorodeoxyglucose positron emission tomography in cervical lymph node metastases from an unknown primary tumor. Cancer 101:2641, 2004

TOTHILL RW et al: An expression-based site of origin diagnostic method designed for clinical application to cancer of unknown origin. Cancer Res 65:4031, 2005

VARADHACHARY GR et al: Molecular profiling of carcinoma of unknown primary and correlation with clinical evaluation. J Clin Oncol 26:4442, 2008

CHAPTER 100

Paraneoplastic Syndromes: Endocrinologic/ Hematologic

J. Larry Jameson
Dan L. Longo

In addition to local tissue invasion and metastasis, neoplastic cells can produce a variety of products that can stimulate hormonal, hematologic, dermatologic, and neurologic responses. *Paraneoplastic syndromes* is the term used to refer to the disorders that accompany benign or malignant tumors but are not directly related to mass effects or invasion. Tumors of neuroendocrine origin, such as small cell lung carcinoma (SCLC) and carcinoids, produce a wide array of peptide hormones and are common causes of paraneoplastic syndromes. However, almost every type of tumor has the potential to produce hormones or cytokines or to induce immunologic responses. Careful studies of the prevalence of paraneoplastic syndromes indicate that they are more common than is generally appreciated. The signs, symptoms, and metabolic alterations associated with paraneoplastic disorders may be overlooked in the context of a malignancy and its treatment. Consequently, atypical clinical manifestations in a patient with cancer should prompt consideration of a paraneoplastic syndrome. The most common endocrinologic and hematologic syndromes associated with underlying neoplasia will be discussed here.

ENDOCRINE PARANEOPLASTIC SYNDROMES

Etiology

Hormones can be produced from eutopic or ectopic sources. *Eutopic* refers to the expression of a hormone from its normal tissue of origin, whereas *ectopic* refers to hormone production from an atypical tissue source. For example, adrenocorticotropic hormone (ACTH) is expressed eutopically by the corticotrope cells of the anterior pituitary, but it can be expressed ectopically in SCLC. Many hormones are produced at low levels from a wide array of tissues in addition to the classic endocrine source. Thus, ectopic expression is often a quantitative change rather than an absolute change in tissue expression. Nevertheless, the term *ectopic expression* is firmly entrenched and conveys the abnormal physiology associated with hormone production by neoplastic cells. In addition to high levels of hormones, ectopic expression typically is characterized by abnormal regulation of hormone production (e.g., defective feedback control) and peptide processing (resulting in large, unprocessed precursors).

A diverse array of molecular mechanisms has been suggested to cause ectopic hormone production. In rare instances, genetic rearrangements explain aberrant hormone expression. For example, translocation of the *parathyroid hormone (PTH)* gene can result in high levels of PTH expression in tissues other than the parathyroid gland, apparently because the genetic rearrangement brings the *PTH* gene under the control of atypical regulatory elements. A related phenomenon is well documented in many forms of leukemia and lymphoma, in which somatic genetic rearrangements confer a growth advantage and alter cellular differentiation and function (Chap. 110). Although genetic rearrangements may cause selected cases of ectopic hormone production, this mechanism is probably rare, as many tumors are associated with excessive production of numerous peptides. Cellular dedifferentiation probably underlies most cases of ectopic hormone production. Many cancers are poorly differentiated, and certain tumor products, such as human chorionic gonadotropin (hCG), parathyroid hormone–related protein (PTHrP), and α fetoprotein, are characteristic of gene expression at earlier developmental stages. In contrast, the propensity of certain cancers to produce particular hormones (e.g., squamous cell carcinomas produce PTHrP) suggests that dedifferentiation is partial or that selective pathways are derepressed. These expression profiles probably reflect alterations in transcriptional repression, changes in DNA methylation, or other factors that govern cell differentiation.

In SCLC, the pathway of differentiation has been relatively well defined. The neuroendocrine phenotype is dictated in part by the basic-helix-loop-helix (bHLH) transcription factor human achaete-scute homologue 1 (hASH-1), which is expressed at abnormally high levels in SCLC associated with ectopic ACTH. The activity of hASH-1 is inhibited by hairy enhancer of split 1 (HES-1) and by Notch proteins, which also are capable of inducing growth arrest. Thus, abnormal expression of these developmental transcription factors appears to provide a link between cell proliferation and differentiation.

Ectopic hormone production would only be an epiphenomenon associated with cancer if it did not result in clinical manifestations. Excessive and unregulated production of hormones such as ACTH, PTHrP, and vasopressin can lead to substantial morbidity and complicate the cancer treatment plan. Moreover, the paraneoplastic endocrinopathies are sometimes the presenting feature of underlying malignancy and may prompt the search for an unrecognized tumor.

A large number of paraneoplastic endocrine syndromes have been described, linking overproduction of particular hormones with specific types of tumors. However, certain recurring syndromes emerge from this group (Table 100-1). The most common paraneoplastic endocrine syndromes include hypercalcemia from overproduction of PTHrP and other factors, hyponatremia from excess vasopressin, and Cushing's syndrome from ectopic ACTH.

TABLE 100-1 Paraneoplastic Syndromes Caused by Ectopic Hormone Production

Paraneoplastic Syndrome	Ectopic Hormone	Typical Tumor Types[a]
Common		
Hypercalcemia of malignancy	Parathyroid hormone-related protein (PTHrP)	Squamous cell (head and neck, lung, skin), breast, genitourinary, gastrointestinal
	1,25 dihydroxyvitamin D	Lymphomas
	Parathyroid hormone (PTH) (rare)	Lung, ovary
	Prostaglandin E2 (PGE2) (rare)	Renal, lung
Syndrome of inappropriate antidiuretic hormone secretion (SIADH)	Vasopressin	Lung (squamous, small cell), gastrointestinal, genitourinary, ovary
Cushing's syndrome	Adrenocorticotropic hormone (ACTH)	Lung (small cell, bronchial carcinoid, adenocarcinoma, squamous), thymus, pancreatic islet, medullary thyroid carcinoma
	Corticotropin-releasing hormone (CRH) (rare)	Pancreatic islet, carcinoid, lung, prostate
	Ectopic expression of gastric inhibitory peptide (GIP), luteinizing hormone (LH)/human chorionic gonadotropin (hCG), other G protein–coupled receptors (rare)	Macronodular adrenal hyperplasia
Less Common		
Non-islet cell hypoglycemia	Insulin-like growth factor (IGF-II)	Mesenchymal tumors, sarcomas, adrenal, hepatic, gastrointestinal, kidney, prostate
	Insulin (rare)	Cervix (small cell carcinoma)
Male feminization	hCG[b]	Testis (embryonal, seminomas), germinomas, choriocarcinoma, lung, hepatic, pancreatic islet
Diarrhea or intestinal hypermotility	Calcitonin[c]	Lung, colon, breast, medullary thyroid carcinoma
	Vasoactive intestinal peptide (VIP)	Pancreas, pheochromocytoma, esophagus
Rare		
Oncogenic osteomalacia	Phosphatonin [fibroblast growth factor 23 (FGF23)]	Hemangiopericytomas, osteoblastomas, fibromas, sarcomas, giant cell tumors, prostate, lung
Acromegaly	Growth hormone–releasing hormone (GHRH)	Pancreatic islet, bronchial and other carcinoids
	Growth hormone (GH)	Lung, pancreatic islet
Hyperthyroidism	Thyroid-stimulating hormone (TSH)	Hydatidiform mole, embryonal tumors, struma ovarii
Hypertension	Renin	Juxtaglomerular tumors, kidney, lung, pancreas, ovary

[a]Only the most common tumor types are listed. For most ectopic hormone syndromes, an extensive list of tumors has been reported to produce one or more hormones.
[b]hCG is produced eutopically by trophoblastic tumors. Certain tumors produce disproportionate amounts of the hCG α or hCG β subunit. High levels of hCG rarely cause hyperthyroidism because of weak binding to the TSH receptor. [c]Calcitonin is produced eutopically by medullary thyroid carcinoma and is used as a tumor marker.

■ HYPERCALCEMIA CAUSED BY ECTOPIC PRODUCTION OF PTHRP

(See also Chap. 353)

Etiology

Humoral hypercalcemia of malignancy (HHM) occurs in up to 20% of patients with cancer. HHM is most common in cancers of the lung, head and neck, skin, esophagus, breast, and genitourinary tract and in multiple myeloma and lymphomas. Although several distinct humoral causes of HHM occur, it is caused most commonly by overproduction of PTHrP. In addition to acting as a circulating humoral factor, bone metastases (e.g., breast, multiple myeloma) may produce PTHrP, leading to local osteolysis and hypercalcemia.

PTHrP is structurally related to PTH and binds to the PTH receptor, explaining the similar biochemical features of HHM and hyperparathyroidism. PTHrP plays a key role in skeletal development and regulates cellular proliferation and differentiation in other tissues, including skin, bone marrow, breast, and hair follicles. The mechanism of PTHrP induction in malignancy is incompletely understood; however, tumor-bearing tissues commonly associated with HHM normally produce PTHrP during development or cell renewal. PTHrP expression is stimulated by hedgehog pathways and Gli transcription factors that are active in many malignancies. Transforming growth factor β (TGF-β), which is produced by many tumors, also stimulates PTHrP, in part by activating the Gli pathway. Mutations in certain oncogenes, such as *Ras*, also can activate PTHrP expression. In adult T cell lymphoma, the transactivating Tax protein produced by human T cell lymphotropic virus I (HTLV-I) stimulates PTHrP promoter activity. Metastatic lesions to bone are more likely to produce PTHrP than are metastases in other tissues, suggesting that bone produces factors (e.g., TGF-β) that enhance PTHrP production or that PTHrP-producing metastases have a selective growth advantage in bone. Thus, PTHrP production can be stimulated by mutations in oncogenes, altered expression of viral or cellular transcription factors, and local growth factors.

Another relatively common cause of HHM is excess production of 1,25-dihydroxyvitamin D. Like granulomatous disorders associated with hypercalcemia, lymphomas can produce an enzyme that converts 25-hydroxyvitamin D to the more active 1,25-dihydroxyvitamin D, leading to enhanced gastrointestinal calcium absorption. Other causes of HHM include tumor-mediated production of osteolytic cytokines and inflammatory mediators.

Clinical Manifestations

The typical presentation of HHM is a patient with a known malignancy who is found to be hypercalcemic on routine laboratory tests. Less often, hypercalcemia is the initial presenting feature of malignancy. Particularly when calcium levels are markedly increased [>3.5 mmol/L (>14 mg/dL)], patients may experience fatigue, mental status changes, dehydration, or symptoms of nephrolithiasis.

Diagnosis

Features that favor HHM, as opposed to primary hyperparathyroidism, include known malignancy, recent onset of hypercalcemia, and very high serum calcium levels. Like hyperparathyroidism, hypercalcemia caused by PTHrP is accompanied by hypercalciuria and hypophosphatemia. Patients with HHM typically have metabolic alkalosis rather than hyperchloremic acidosis, as is seen in hyperparathyroidism. Measurement of PTH is useful to exclude primary hyperparathyroidism; the PTH level should be suppressed in HHM. An elevated PTHrP level confirms the diagnosis, and it is increased in ~80% of hypercalcemic patients with cancer. 1,25-Dihydroxyvitamin D levels may be increased in patients with lymphoma.

TREATMENT · Humoral Hypercalcemia of Malignancy

The management of HHM begins with removal of excess calcium in the diet, medications, or IV solutions. Oral phosphorus (e.g., 250 mg Neutra-Phos 3–4 times daily) should be given until serum phosphorus is >1 mmol/L (>3 mg/dL). Saline rehydration is used to dilute serum calcium and promote calciuresis. Forced diuresis with furosemide or other loop diuretics can enhance calcium excretion but provides relatively little value except in life-threatening hypercalcemia. When used, loop diuretics should be administered only after complete rehydration and with careful monitoring of fluid balance. Bisphosphonates such as pamidronate (60–90 mg IV), zoledronate (4–8 mg IV), and etidronate (7.5 mg/kg per day PO for 3–7 consecutive days) can reduce serum calcium within 1–2 days and suppress calcium release for several weeks. Bisphosphonate infusions can be repeated, or oral bisphosphonates can be used for chronic treatment. Dialysis should be considered in severe hypercalcemia when saline hydration and bisphosphonate treatments are not possible or are too slow in onset. Previously used agents such as calcitonin and mithramycin have little utility now that bisphosphonates are available. Calcitonin (2–8 U/kg SC every 6–12 h) should be considered when rapid correction of severe hypercalcemia is needed. Hypercalcemia associated with lymphomas, multiple myeloma, or leukemia may respond to glucocorticoid treatment (e.g., prednisone 40–100 mg PO in four divided doses).

■ ECTOPIC VASOPRESSIN: TUMOR-ASSOCIATED SIADH

(See also Chap. 45)

Etiology

Vasopressin is an antidiuretic hormone normally produced by the posterior pituitary gland. Ectopic vasopressin production by tumors is a common cause of the syndrome of inappropriate antidiuretic hormone (SIADH), occurring in at least half of patients with SCLC. SIADH also can be caused by a number of nonneoplastic conditions, including central nervous system (CNS) trauma, infections, and medications (Chap. 340). Compensatory responses to SIADH, such as decreased thirst, may mitigate the development of hyponatremia. However, with prolonged production of excessive vasopressin, the osmostat controlling thirst and hypothalamic vasopressin secretion may become reset. In addition, intake of free water, orally or intravenously, can quickly worsen hyponatremia because of reduced renal diuresis.

Tumors with neuroendocrine features, such as SCLC and carcinoids, are the most common sources of ectopic vasopressin production, but it also occurs in other forms of lung cancer and with CNS lesions, head and neck cancer, and genitourinary, gastrointestinal, and ovarian cancers. The mechanism of activation of the vasopressin gene in these tumors is unknown but often involves concomitant expression of the adjacent oxytocin gene, suggesting derepression of this locus.

Clinical Manifestations

Most patients with ectopic vasopressin secretion are asymptomatic and are identified because of the presence of hyponatremia on routine chemistry testing. Symptoms may include weakness, lethargy, nausea, confusion, depressed mental status, and seizures. The severity of symptoms reflects the rapidity of onset as well as the extent of hyponatremia. Hyponatremia usually develops slowly but may be exacerbated by the administration of IV fluids or the institution of new medications.

Diagnosis

The diagnostic features of ectopic vasopressin production are the same as those of other causes of SIADH (Chaps. 45 and 340). Hyponatremia and reduced serum osmolality occur in the setting of an inappropriately normal or increased urine osmolality. Urine sodium excretion is normal or increased unless volume depletion is present. Other causes of hyponatremia should be excluded, including renal, adrenal, or thyroid insufficiency. Physiologic sources of vasopressin stimulation (CNS lesions, pulmonary disease, nausea), adaptive circulatory mechanisms (hypotension, heart failure, hepatic cirrhosis), and medications, including many chemotherapeutic agents, also should be considered as possible causes of hyponatremia. Vasopressin measurements are not usually necessary to make the diagnosis.

TREATMENT Ectopic Vasopressin: Tumor-Associated SIADH

Most patients with ectopic vasopressin production develop hyponatremia over several weeks or months. The disorder should be corrected gradually unless mental status is altered or there is risk of seizures. Treatment of the underlying malignancy may reduce ectopic vasopressin production, but this response is slow if it occurs at all. Fluid restriction to less than urine output, plus insensible losses, is often sufficient to correct hyponatremia partially. However, strict monitoring of the amount and types of liquids consumed or administered intravenously is required for fluid restriction to be effective. Salt tablets and saline are not helpful unless volume depletion is also present. Demeclocycline (150–300 mg orally three to four times daily) can be used to inhibit vasopressin action on the renal distal tubule, but its onset of action is relatively slow (1–2 weeks). Conivaptan, a nonpeptide V_2-receptor antagonist, can be administered either PO (20–120 mg bid) or IV (10–40 mg) and is particularly effective when used in combination with fluid restriction in euvolemic hyponatremia. Severe hyponatremia (Na <115 meq/L) or mental status changes may require treatment with hypertonic (3%) or normal saline infusion together with furosemide to enhance free water clearance. The rate of sodium correction should be slow (0.5–1 meq/L per h) to prevent rapid fluid shifts and the possible development of central pontine myelinolysis.

◼ CUSHING'S SYNDROME CAUSED BY ECTOPIC ACTH PRODUCTION

(See also Chap. 342)

Etiology

Ectopic ACTH production accounts for 10–20% of cases of Cushing's syndrome. The syndrome is particularly common in neuroendocrine tumors. SCLC (>50%) is by far the most common cause of ectopic ACTH, followed by thymic carcinoid (15%), islet cell tumors (10%), bronchial carcinoid (10%), other carcinoids (5%), and pheochromocytomas (2%). Ectopic ACTH production is caused by increased expression of the proopiomelanocortin (POMC) gene, which encodes ACTH, along with melanocyte-stimulating hormone (MSH), β lipotropin, and several other peptides. In many tumors, there is abundant but aberrant expression of the POMC gene from an internal promoter, proximal to the third exon, which encodes ACTH. However, because this product lacks the signal sequence necessary for protein processing, it is not secreted. Increased production of ACTH arises instead from less abundant, but unregulated, POMC expression from the same promoter site used in the pituitary. However, because the tumors lack many of the enzymes needed to process the POMC polypeptide, it is typically released as multiple large, biologically inactive fragments along with relatively small amounts of fully processed, active ACTH.

Rarely, corticotropin-releasing hormone (CRH) is produced by pancreatic islet cell tumors, SCLC, medullary thyroid cancer, carcinoids, or prostate cancer. When levels are high enough, CRH can cause pituitary corticotrope hyperplasia and Cushing's syndrome. Tumors that produce CRH sometimes also produce ACTH, raising the possibility of a paracrine mechanism for ACTH production.

A distinct mechanism for ACTH-independent Cushing's syndrome involves ectopic expression of various G protein–coupled receptors in the adrenal nodules. Ectopic expression of the gastric inhibitory peptide (GIP) receptor is the best-characterized example of this mechanism. In this case, meals induce GIP secretion, which inappropriately stimulates adrenal growth and glucocorticoid production.

Clinical manifestations

The clinical features of hypercortisolemia are detected in only a small fraction of patients with documented ectopic ACTH production. Patients with ectopic ACTH syndrome generally exhibit less marked weight gain and centripetal fat redistribution, probably because the exposure to excess glucocorticoids is relatively short and because cachexia reduces the propensity for weight gain and fat deposition. The ectopic ACTH syndrome is associated with several clinical features that distinguish it from other causes of Cushing's syndrome (e.g., pituitary adenomas, adrenal adenomas, iatrogenic glucocorticoid excess). The metabolic manifestations of ectopic ACTH syndrome are dominated by fluid retention and hypertension, hypokalemia, metabolic alkalosis, glucose intolerance, and occasionally steroid psychosis. The very high ACTH levels often cause increased pigmentation, and melanotrope-stimulating hormone (MSH) activity derived from the POMC precursor peptide is also increased. The extraordinarily high glucocorticoid levels in patients with ectopic sources of ACTH can lead to marked skin fragility and easy bruising. In addition, the high cortisol levels often overwhelm the renal 11β-hydroxysteroid dehydrogenase type II enzyme, which normally inactivates cortisol and prevents it from binding to renal mineralocorticoid receptors. Consequently, in addition to the excess mineralocorticoids produced by ACTH stimulation of the adrenal gland, high levels of cortisol exert activity through the mineralocorticoid receptor, leading to severe hypokalemia.

Diagnosis

The diagnosis of ectopic ACTH syndrome is usually not difficult in the setting of a known malignancy. Urine free cortisol levels fluctuate but are typically greater than two to four times normal, and the plasma ACTH level is usually >22 pmol/L (>100 pg/mL). A suppressed ACTH level excludes this diagnosis and indicates an ACTH-independent cause of Cushing's syndrome (e.g., adrenal or exogenous glucocorticoid). In contrast to pituitary sources of ACTH, most ectopic sources of ACTH do not respond to glucocorticoid suppression. Therefore, high-dose dexamethasone (8 mg PO) suppresses 8:00 A.M. serum cortisol (50% decrease from baseline) in ~80% of pituitary ACTH-producing adenomas but fails to suppress ectopic ACTH in ~90% of cases. Bronchial and other carcinoids are well-documented exceptions to these general guidelines, as these ectopic sources of ACTH may exhibit feedback regulation indistinguishable from pituitary adenomas, including suppression by high-dose dexamethasone, and ACTH responsiveness to adrenal blockade with metyrapone. If necessary, petrosal sinus catheterization can be used to evaluate a patient with ACTH-dependent Cushing's syndrome when the source of ACTH is unclear. After

CRH stimulation, a 3:1 petrosal sinus:peripheral ACTH ratio strongly suggests a pituitary ACTH source. Imaging studies are also useful in the evaluation of suspected carcinoid lesions, allowing biopsy and characterization of hormone production using special stains.

TREATMENT	Cushing's Syndrome Caused by Ectopic ACTH Production

The morbidity associated with the ectopic ACTH syndrome can be substantial. Patients may experience depression or personality changes because of extreme cortisol excess. Metabolic derangements, including diabetes mellitus and hypokalemia, can worsen fatigue. Poor wound healing and predisposition to infections can complicate the surgical management of tumors, and opportunistic infections caused by organisms such as *Pneumocystis carinii* and mycoses are often the cause of death in patients with ectopic ACTH production. Depending on prognosis and treatment plans for the underlying malignancy, measures to reduce cortisol levels are often indicated. Treatment of the underlying malignancy may reduce ACTH levels but is rarely sufficient to reduce cortisol levels to normal. Adrenalectomy is not practical for most of these patients but should be considered if the underlying tumor is not resectable and the prognosis is otherwise favorable (e.g., carcinoid). Medical therapy with ketoconazole (300–600 mg PO bid), metyrapone (250–500 mg PO every 6 h), mitotane (3–6 g PO in four divided doses, tapered to maintain low cortisol production), or other agents that block steroid synthesis or action is often the most practical strategy for managing the hypercortisolism associated with ectopic ACTH production (Chap. 339). Glucocorticoid replacement should be provided to prevent adrenal insufficiency. Unfortunately, many patients eventually progress despite medical blockade.

■ TUMOR-INDUCED HYPOGLYCEMIA CAUSED BY EXCESS PRODUCTION OF IGF-II

(See also Chap. 345) Mesenchymal tumors, hemangiopericytomas, hepatocellular tumors, adrenal carcinomas, and a variety of other large tumors have been reported to produce excessive amounts of insulin-like growth factor type II (IGF-II) precursor, which binds weakly to insulin receptors and strongly to IGF-I receptors, leading to insulin-like actions. The gene encoding IGF-II resides on a chromosome 11p15 locus that is normally imprinted (that is, expression is exclusively from a single parental allele). Biallelic expression of the IGF-II gene occurs in a subset of tumors, suggesting loss of methylation and loss of imprinting as a mechanism for gene induction. In addition to increased IGF-II production, IGF-II bioavailability is increased due to complex alterations in circulating binding proteins. Increased IGF-II suppresses growth hormone (GH) and insulin, resulting in reduced IGF binding protein 3 (IGFBP-3), IGF-I, and acid-labile subunit (ALS). The reduction in ALS and IGFBP-3, which normally sequester IGF-II, causes it to be displaced to a small circulating complex that has greater access to insulin target tissues. For this reason, circulating IGF-II levels may not be markedly increased despite causing hypoglycemia. In addition to IGF-II–mediated hypoglycemia, tumors may occupy enough of the liver to impair gluconeogenesis.

In most cases, the tumor causing hypoglycemia is clinically apparent (usually >10 cm in size) and hypoglycemia develops in association with fasting. The diagnosis is made by documenting low serum glucose and suppressed insulin levels in association with symptoms of hypoglycemia. Serum IGF-II levels may not be increased (IGF-II

assays may not detect IGF-II precursors). Increased IGF-II mRNA expression is found in most of these tumors. Any medications associated with hypoglycemia should be eliminated. Treatment of the underlying malignancy, if possible, may reduce the predisposition to hypoglycemia. Frequent meals and IV glucose, especially during sleep or fasting, are often necessary to prevent hypoglycemia. Glucagon and glucocorticoids have also been used to enhance glucose production.

■ HUMAN CHORIONIC GONADOTROPIN

hCG is composed of α and β subunits and can be produced as intact hormone, which is biologically active, or as uncombined biologically inert subunits. Ectopic production of intact hCG occurs most often in association with testicular embryonal tumors, germ cell tumors, extragonadal germinomas, lung cancer, hepatoma, and pancreatic islet tumors. Eutopic production of hCG occurs with trophoblastic malignancies. hCG α subunit production is particularly common in lung cancer and pancreatic islet cancer. In men, high hCG levels stimulate steroidogenesis and aromatase activity in testicular Leydig cells, resulting in increased estrogen production and the development of gynecomastia. Precocious puberty in boys or gynecomastia in men should prompt measurement of hCG and consideration of a testicular tumor or another source of ectopic hCG production. Most women are asymptomatic. hCG is easily measured. Treatment should be directed at the underlying malignancy.

■ ONCOGENIC OSTEOMALACIA

Hypophosphatemic oncogenic osteomalacia, also called tumor-induced osteomalacia (TIO), is characterized by markedly reduced serum phosphorus and renal phosphate wasting, leading to muscle weakness, bone pain, and osteomalacia. Serum calcium and PTH levels are normal, and 1,25-dihydroxyvitamin D is low. Oncogenic osteomalacia is usually caused by benign mesenchymal tumors, such as hemangiopericytomas, fibromas, and giant cell tumors, often of the skeletal extremities or head. It has also been described in sarcomas and in patients with prostate and lung cancer. Resection of the tumor reverses the disorder, confirming its humoral basis. The circulating phosphaturic factor is called *phosphatonin*—a factor that inhibits renal tubular reabsorption of phosphate and renal conversion of 25-hydroxyvitamin D to 1,25-dihydroxyvitamin D. Phosphatonin has been identified as fibroblast growth factor 23 (FGF23). FGF23 levels are increased in some, but not all, patients with osteogenic osteomalacia. The disorder exhibits biochemical features similar to those seen with inactivating mutations in the *PHEX* gene, the cause of hereditary X-linked hypophosphatemia. The *PHEX* gene encodes a protease that inactivates FGF23. Treatment involves removal of the tumor, if possible, and supplementation with phosphate and vitamin D. Octreotide treatment reduces phosphate wasting in some patients with tumors that express somatostatin receptor subtype 2. Octreotide scans may also be useful in detecting these tumors.

HEMATOLOGIC SYNDROMES

The elevation of granulocyte, platelet, and eosinophil counts in most patients with myeloproliferative disorders is caused by the proliferation of the myeloid elements due to the underlying disease rather than to a paraneoplastic syndrome. The paraneoplastic hematologic syndromes in patients with solid tumors are less well characterized than are the endocrine syndromes because the ectopic hormone(s) or cytokines responsible have not been identified in most of these tumors (Table 100-2). The extent of the paraneoplastic syndromes parallels the course of the cancer.

TABLE 100-2 Paraneoplastic Hematologic Syndromes

Syndrome	Proteins	Cancers Typically Associated with Syndrome
Erythrocytosis	Erythropoietin	Renal cancers Hepatocarcinoma Cerebellar hemangioblastomas
Granulocytosis	G-CSF, GM-CSF, IL-6	Lung cancer Gastrointestinal cancer Ovarian cancer Genitourinary cancer Hodgkin's disease
Thrombocytosis	IL-6	Lung cancer Gastrointestinal cancer Breast cancer Ovarian cancer Lymphoma
Eosinophilia	IL-5	Lymphoma Leukemia Lung cancer
Thrombophlebitis	Unknown	Lung cancer Pancreatic cancer Gastrointestinal cancer Breast cancer Genitourinary cancer Ovarian cancer Prostate cancer Lymphoma

Abbreviations: G-CSF, granulocyte colony-stimulating factor; GM-CSF, granulocyte-macrophage CSF; IL, interleukin.

■ ERYTHROCYTOSIS

Ectopic production of erythropoietin by cancer cells causes most paraneoplastic erythrocytosis. The ectopically produced erythropoietin stimulates the production of red blood cells (RBCs) in the bone marrow and raises the hematocrit. Other lymphokines and hormones produced by cancer cells may stimulate erythropoietin release but have not been proved to cause erythrocytosis.

Most patients with erythrocytosis have an elevated hematocrit (>52% in men, >48% in women) that is detected on a routine blood count. Approximately 3% of patients with renal cell cancer, 10% of patients with hepatoma, and 15% of patients with cerebellar hemangioblastomas have erythrocytosis. In most cases the erythrocytosis is asymptomatic.

Patients with erythrocytosis due to a renal cell cancer, hepatoma, or CNS cancer should have measurement of red cell mass. If the red cell mass is elevated, the serum erythropoietin level should be measured. Patients with an appropriate cancer, elevated erythropoietin levels, and no other explanation for erythrocytosis (e.g., hemoglobinopathy that causes increased O_2 affinity; Chap. 57) have the paraneoplastic syndrome.

TREATMENT   Erythrocytosis

Successful resection of the cancer usually resolves the erythrocytosis. If the tumor cannot be resected or treated effectively with radiation therapy or chemotherapy, phlebotomy may control any symptoms related to erythrocytosis.

■ GRANULOCYTOSIS

Approximately 30% of patients with solid tumors have granulocytosis (granulocyte count >8000/μL). In about half of patients with granulocytosis and cancer, the granulocytosis has an identifiable nonparaneoplastic etiology (infection, tumor necrosis, glucocorticoid

administration, etc.). The other patients have proteins in urine and serum that stimulate the growth of bone marrow cells. Tumors and tumor cell lines from patients with lung, ovarian, and bladder cancers have been documented to produce granulocyte colony-stimulating factor (G-CSF), granulocyte-macrophage colony-stimulating factor (GM-CSF), and/or interleukin 6 (IL-6). However, the etiology of granulocytosis has not been characterized in most patients.

Patients with granulocytosis are nearly all asymptomatic, and the differential white blood cell count does not have a shift to immature forms of neutrophils. Granulocytosis occurs in 40% of patients with lung and gastrointestinal cancers, 20% of patients with breast cancer, 30% of patients with brain tumors and ovarian cancers, 20% of patients with Hodgkin's disease, and 10% of patients with renal cell carcinoma. Patients with advanced-stage disease are more likely to have granulocytosis than are those with early-stage disease.

Paraneoplastic granulocytosis does not require treatment. The granulocytosis resolves when the underlying cancer is treated.

■ THROMBOCYTOSIS

Some 35% of patients with thrombocytosis (platelet count >400,000/ μL) have an underlying diagnosis of cancer. IL-6, a candidate molecule for the etiology of paraneoplastic thrombocytosis, stimulates the production of platelets in vitro and in vivo. Some patients with cancer and thrombocytosis have elevated levels of IL-6 in plasma. Another candidate molecule is thrombopoietin, a peptide hormone that stimulates megakaryocyte proliferation and platelet production. The etiology of thrombocytosis has not been established in most cases.

Patients with thrombocytosis are nearly all asymptomatic. Thrombocytosis is not clearly linked to thrombosis in patients with cancer. Thrombocytosis is present in 40% of patients with lung and gastrointestinal cancers; 20% of patients with breast, endometrial, and ovarian cancers; and 10% of patients with lymphoma. Patients with thrombocytosis are more likely to have advanced-stage disease and have a poorer prognosis than do patients without thrombocytosis. Paraneoplastic thrombocytosis does not require treatment.

■ EOSINOPHILIA

Eosinophilia is present in ~1% of patients with cancer. Tumors and tumor cell lines from patients with lymphomas or leukemia may produce IL-5, which stimulates eosinophil growth. Activation of IL-5 transcription in lymphomas and leukemias may involve translocation of the long arm of chromosome 5, to which the genes for IL-5 and other cytokines map.

Patients with eosinophilia are typically asymptomatic. Eosinophilia is present in 10% of patients with lymphoma, 3% of patients with lung cancer, and occasional patients with cervical, gastrointestinal, renal, and breast cancer. Patients with markedly elevated eosinophil counts (>5000/μL) can develop shortness of breath and wheezing. A chest radiograph may reveal diffuse pulmonary infiltrates from eosinophil infiltration and activation in the lungs.

TREATMENT   Eosinophilia

Definitive treatment is directed at the underlying malignancy: Tumors should be resected or treated with radiation or chemotherapy. In most patients who develop shortness of breath related to eosinophilia, symptoms resolve with the use of oral or inhaled glucocorticoids.

■ THROMBOPHLEBITIS

Deep venous thrombosis and pulmonary embolism are the most common thrombotic conditions in patients with cancer. Migratory or recurrent thrombophlebitis may be the initial manifestation of cancer. Nearly 15% of patients who develop deep venous thrombosis or pulmonary embolism have a diagnosis of cancer (Chap. 117). The coexistence of peripheral venous thrombosis with visceral carcinoma, particularly pancreatic cancer, is called *Trousseau's syndrome*.

Pathogenesis

Patients with cancer are predisposed to thromboembolism because they are often at bed rest or immobilized, and tumors may obstruct or slow blood flow. Chronic IV catheters also predispose to clotting. In addition, clotting may be promoted by release of procoagulants or cytokines from tumor cells or associated inflammatory cells or by platelet adhesion or aggregation. The specific molecules that promote thromboembolism have not been identified.

In addition to cancer causing secondary thrombosis, primary thrombophilic diseases may be associated with cancer. For example, the antiphospholipid antibody syndrome is associated with a wide range of pathologic manifestations (Chap. 320). About 20% of patients with this syndrome have cancers. Among patients with cancer and antiphospholipid antibodies, 35–45% develop thrombosis.

Clinical Manifestations

Patients with cancer who develop deep venous thrombosis usually develop swelling or pain in the leg, and physical examination reveals tenderness, warmth, and redness. Patients who present with pulmonary embolism develop dyspnea, chest pain, and syncope, and physical examination shows tachycardia, cyanosis, and hypotension. Some 5% of patients with no history of cancer who have a diagnosis of deep venous thrombosis or pulmonary embolism will have a diagnosis of cancer within 1 year. The most common cancers associated with thromboembolic episodes include lung, pancreatic, gastrointestinal, breast, ovarian, and genitourinary cancers; lymphomas; and brain tumors. Patients with cancer who undergo surgical procedures requiring general anesthesia have a 20–30% risk of deep venous thrombosis.

Diagnosis

The diagnosis of deep venous thrombosis in patients with cancer is made by impedance plethysmography or bilateral compression ultrasonography of the leg veins. Patients with a noncompressible venous segment have deep venous thrombosis. If compression ultrasonography is normal and there is a high clinical suspicion for deep venous thrombosis, venography should be done to look for a luminal filling defect. Elevation of D-dimer is not as predictive of deep venous thrombosis in patients with cancer as it is in patients without cancer; elevations are seen in people over age 65 years without concomitant evidence of thrombosis, probably as a consequence of increased thrombin deposition and turnover in aging.

Patients with symptoms and signs suggesting a pulmonary embolism should be evaluated with a chest radiograph, electrocardiogram, arterial blood gas analysis, and ventilation-perfusion scan. Patients with mismatched segmental perfusion defects have a pulmonary embolus. Patients with equivocal ventilation-perfusion findings should be evaluated as described above for deep venous thrombosis in their legs. If deep venous thrombosis is detected, they should be anticoagulated. If deep venous thrombosis is not detected, they should be considered for a pulmonary angiogram.

Patients without a diagnosis of cancer who present with an initial episode of thrombophlebitis or pulmonary embolus need no additional tests for cancer other than a careful history and physical examination. In light of the many possible primary sites, diagnostic testing in asymptomatic patients is wasteful. However, if the clot is refractory to standard treatment or is in an unusual site or if the thrombophlebitis is migratory or recurrent, efforts to find an underlying cancer are indicated.

TREATMENT   Thrombophlebitis

Patients with cancer and a diagnosis of deep venous thrombosis or pulmonary embolism should be treated initially with IV unfractionated heparin or low-molecular-weight heparin for at least 5 days, and warfarin should be started within 1 or 2 days. The warfarin dose should be adjusted so that the international normalized ratio (INR) is 2–3. Patients with proximal deep venous thrombosis and a relative contraindication to heparin anticoagulation (hemorrhagic brain metastases or pericardial effusion) should be considered for placement of a filter in the inferior vena cava (Greenfield filter) to prevent pulmonary embolism. Warfarin should be administered for 3–6 months. An alternative approach is to use low-molecular-weight heparin for 6 months. Patients with cancer who undergo a major surgical procedure should be considered for heparin prophylaxis or pneumatic boots. Breast cancer patients undergoing chemotherapy and patients with implanted catheters should be considered for prophylaxis (1 mg/d warfarin).

Cutaneous paraneoplastic syndromes are discussed in Chap. 53. Neurologic paraneoplastic syndromes are discussed in Chap. 101.

ACKNOWLEDGMENT
The authors acknowledge the contributions of Bruce E. Johnson to prior versions of this chapter.

FURTHER READINGS

AL-TOURAH AJ et al: Paraneoplastic erythropoietin-induced polycythemia associated with small lymphocytic lymphoma. J Clin Oncol 24:2388, 2006

GOSDEN RG, FEINBERG AP: Genetics and epigenetics—nature's pen-and-pencil set. N Engl J Med 356:731, 2007

MUNDY GR, EDWARDS JR: PTH-related peptide (PTHrP) in hypercalcemia. J Am Soc Nephrol 19:672, 2008

PELOSOF LC, GERBER DE: Paraneoplastic syndromes: An approach to diagnosis and treatment. Mayo Clin Proc 85:838, 2010

RIKHOF B ET AL: The insulin-like growth factor system and sarcomas. J Pathol 217:469, 2009

SHAIKH A et al: Regulation of phosphate homeostasis by the phosphatonins and other novel mediators. Pediatr Nephrol 23:1203, 2008

STEWART AF: Clinical practice: Hypercalcemia associated with cancer. N Engl J Med 352:373, 2005

CHAPTER 101

Paraneoplastic Neurologic Syndromes

Josep Dalmau

Myrna R. Rosenfeld

Paraneoplastic neurologic disorders (PNDs) are cancer-related syndromes that can affect any part of the nervous system (Table 101-1). They are caused by mechanisms other than metastasis or by any of the complications of cancer such as coagulopathy, stroke, metabolic and nutritional conditions, infections, and side effects of cancer therapy. In 60% of patients the neurologic symptoms precede the cancer diagnosis. Clinically disabling PNDs occur in 0.5–1% of all cancer patients, but they affect 2–3% of patients with neuroblastoma or small cell lung cancer (SCLC) and 30–50% of patients with thymoma or sclerotic myeloma.

PATHOGENESIS

Most PNDs are mediated by immune responses triggered by neuronal proteins (onconeuronal antigens) expressed by tumors. In PNDs of the central nervous system (CNS), many antibody-associated immune responses have been identified (Table 101-2). These antibodies react with the patient's tumor, and their detection in serum or cerebrospinal fluid (CSF) usually predicts the presence of cancer. When the antigens are intracellular, most syndromes are

TABLE 101-2 Antibodies to Intracellular Antigens, Syndromes, and Associated Cancers

Antibody	Associated Neurologic Syndrome(s)	Tumors
Anti-Hu	Encephalomyelitis, subacute sensory neuronopathy	SCLC
Anti-Yo	Cerebellar degeneration	Ovary, breast
Anti-Ri	Cerebellar degeneration, opsoclonus	Breast, gynecologic, SCLC
Anti-Tr	Cerebellar degeneration	Hodgkin lymphoma
Anti-CV$_2$/CRMP5	Encephalomyelitis, chorea, optic neuritis, uveitis, peripheral neuropathy	SCLC, thymoma, other
Anti-Ma proteins	Limbic, hypothalamic, brainstem encephalitis	Testicular (Ma2), other (Ma)
Anti-amphiphysin	Stiff-person syndrome, encephalomyelitis	Breast, SCLC
Recoverin, bipolar cell antibodies, others[a]	Cancer-associated retinopathy (CAR)	SCLC (CAR), melanoma (MAR)
	Melanoma-associated retinopathy (MAR)	
Anti-GAD	Stiff-person, cerebellar syndromes	Infrequent tumor association (thymoma)

[a]A variety of target antigens have been identified.

Abbreviations: CRMP, collapsing response-mediator protein; SCLC, small cell lung cancer.

TABLE 101-1 Paraneoplastic Syndromes of the Nervous System

Classic Syndromes: Usually Occur With Cancer Association	Nonclassic Syndromes: May Occur With and Without Cancer Association
Encephalomyelitis	Brainstem encephalitis
Limbic encephalitis	Stiff-person syndrome
Cerebellar degeneration (adults)	Necrotizing myelopathy
Opsoclonus-myoclonus	Motor neuron disease
Subacute sensory neuronopathy	Guillain-Barré syndrome
Gastrointestinal paresis or pseudo-obstruction	Subacute and chronic mixed sensory-motor neuropathies
Dermatomyositis (adults)	Neuropathy associated with plasma cell dyscrasias and lymphoma
Lambert-Eaton myasthenic syndrome	Vasculitis of nerve
Cancer or melanoma associated retinopathy	Pure autonomic neuropathy
	Acute necrotizing myopathy
	Polymyositis
	Vasculitis of muscle
	Optic neuropathy
	BDUMP

Abbreviation: BDUMP, bilateral diffuse uveal melanocytic proliferation.

associated with extensive infiltrates of CD4+ and CD8+ T cells, microglial activation, gliosis, and variable neuronal loss. The infiltrating T cells are often in close contact with neurons undergoing degeneration, suggesting a primary pathogenic role. T cell–mediated cytotoxicity may contribute directly to cell death in these PNDs. Thus both humoral and cellular immune mechanisms participate in the pathogenesis of many PNDs. This complex immunopathogenesis may underlie the resistance of many of these conditions to therapy.

In contrast to the disorders associated with immune responses against intracellular antigens, those associated with antibodies to antigens expressed on the neuronal cell surface of the CNS or at neuromuscular synapses are more responsive to immunotherapy (Table 101-3, Fig. 101-1). These disorders occur with and without a cancer association, and there is increasing evidence that they are mediated by the antibodies.

Other PNDs are likely immune-mediated, although their antigens are unknown. These include several syndromes of inflammatory neuropathies and myopathies. In addition, many patients with typical PND syndromes are antibody-negative.

For still other PNDs, the cause remains quite obscure. These include, among others, several neuropathies that occur in the terminal stages of cancer and a number of neuropathies associated with plasma cell dyscrasias or lymphoma without evidence of inflammatory infiltrates or deposits of immunoglobulin, cryoglobulin, or amyloid.

TABLE 101-3 Antibodies to Cell Surface or Synaptic Antigens, Syndromes, and Associated Tumors

Antibody	Neurologic Syndrome	Tumor Type when Associated
Anti-AChR (muscle)[a]	Myasthenia gravis	Thymoma
Anti-AChR (neuronal)[a]	Autonomic neuropathy	SCLC
Anti-VGKC- related proteins[b] (LGI1, Caspr2)	Neuromyotonia, limbic encephalitis	Thymoma, SCLC
Anti-VGCC[c]	LEMS, cerebellar degeneration	SCLC
Anti-NMDAR[d]	Anti-NMDAR encephalitis	Teratoma
Anti-AMPAR[d]	Limbic encephalitis with relapses	SCLC, thymoma, breast
Anti-GABA$_B$R[d]	Limbic encephalitis, seizures	SCLC, neuroendocrine
Glycine receptor[d]	Encephalomyelitis with rigidity, stiff-person syndrome	Lung cancer

[a]A direct pathogenic role of these antibodies has been demonstrated.
[b]Anti-VGKC-related proteins are pathogenic for some types of neuromyotonia.
[c]Anti-VGCC antibodies are pathogenic for LEMS.
[d]These antibodies are strongly suspected to be pathogenic.

Abbreviations: AChR, acetylcholine receptor; AMPAR, α-amino-3-hydroxy-5-methylisoxazole-4-propionic acid receptor; GABA$_B$R, Gamma-amino-butyric acid B receptor; GAD, glutamic acid decarboxylase; LEMS, Lambert-Eaton myasthenic syndrome; NMDAR, N-methyl-D-aspartate receptor; SCLC, small cell lung cancer; VGCC, voltage-gated calcium channel; VGKC, voltage-gated potassium channel.

APPROACH TO THE PATIENT ▶ Paraneoplastic Neurologic Disorders

Three key concepts are important for the diagnosis and management of PNDs. First, it is common for symptoms to appear before the presence of a tumor is known; second, the neurologic syndrome usually develops rapidly, producing severe deficits in a short period of time; and third, there is evidence that prompt tumor control improves the neurologic outcome. Therefore, the major concern of the physician is to recognize a disorder promptly as paraneoplastic to identify and treat the tumor.

PND OF THE CENTRAL NERVOUS SYSTEM AND DORSAL ROOT GANGLIA When symptoms involve brain, spinal cord, or dorsal root ganglia, the suspicion of PND is usually based on a combination of clinical, radiologic, and CSF findings. In these cases, a biopsy of the affected tissue is often difficult to obtain, and although useful to rule out other disorders (e.g., metastasis, infection), neuropathologic findings are not specific for PND. Furthermore, there are no specific radiologic or electrophysiologic tests that are diagnostic of PND. The presence of antineuronal antibodies (Tables 101-2 and 101-3) may help in the diagnosis, but only 60–70% of PNDs of the CNS and less than 20% of those involving the peripheral nervous system have neuronal or neuromuscular antibodies that can be used as diagnostic tests.

MRI and CSF studies are important to rule out neurologic complications due to the direct spread of cancer, particularly metastatic and leptomeningeal disease. In most PNDs the MRI findings are nonspecific. Paraneoplastic limbic encephalitis is usually associated with characteristic MRI abnormalities in the mesial temporal lobes (see below), but similar findings can occur with other disorders [e.g., nonparaneoplastic autoimmune limbic encephalitis, and human herpesvirus type 6 (HHV-6) encephalitis] (Fig. 101-2). The CSF profile of patients with PND of the CNS or dorsal root ganglia typically consists of mild to moderate pleocytosis (<200 mononuclear cells, predominantly

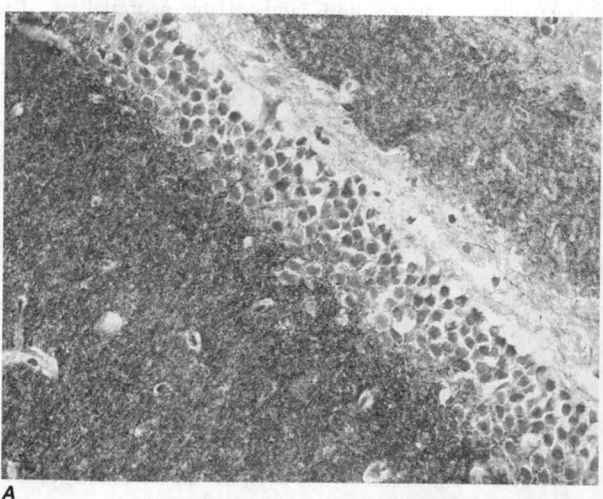
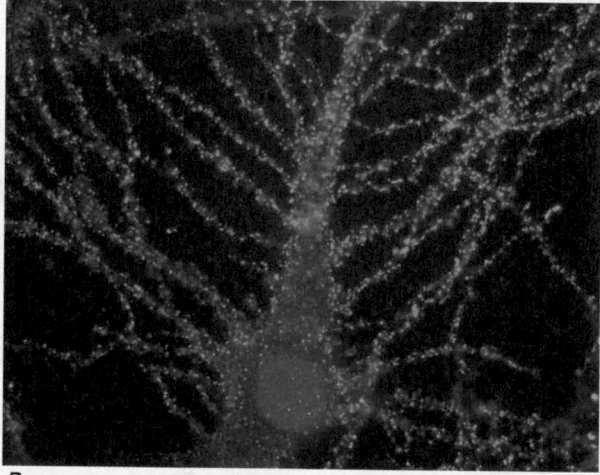
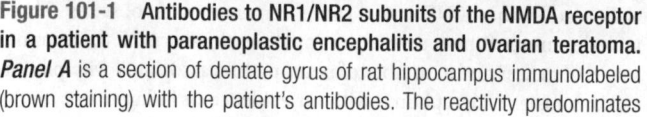

Figure 101-1 Antibodies to NR1/NR2 subunits of the NMDA receptor in a patient with paraneoplastic encephalitis and ovarian teratoma. *Panel A* is a section of dentate gyrus of rat hippocampus immunolabeled (brown staining) with the patient's antibodies. The reactivity predominates in the molecular layer, which is highly enriched in dendritic processes. Panel B shows the antibody reactivity with cultures of rat hippocampal neurons; the intense green immunolabeling is due to the antibodies against the NR1 subunits of NMDA receptors.

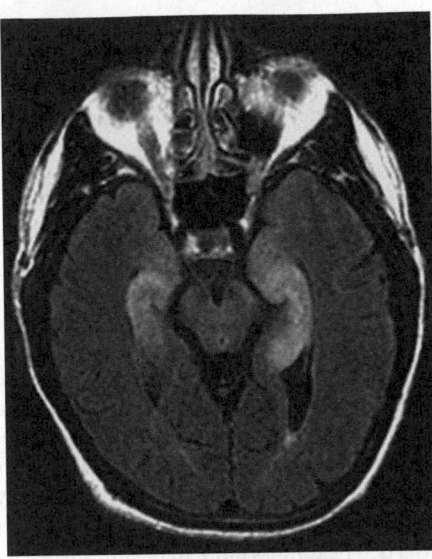

Figure 101-2 Fluid-attenuated inversion recovery sequence MRI of a patient with limbic encephalitis and LGI1 antibodies. Note the abnormal hyperintensity involving the medial aspect of the temporal lobes.

lymphocytes), an increase in the protein concentration, intrathecal synthesis of IgG, and a variable presence of oligoclonal bands.

PND OF NERVE AND MUSCLE If symptoms involve peripheral nerve, neuromuscular junction, or muscle, the diagnosis of a specific PND is usually established on clinical, electrophysiologic, and pathologic grounds. The clinical history, accompanying symptoms (e.g., anorexia, weight loss), and type of syndrome dictate the studies and degree of effort needed to demonstrate a neoplasm. For example, the frequent association of Lambert-Eaton myasthenic syndrome (LEMS) with SCLC should lead to a chest and abdomen CT or body positron emission tomography (PET) scan and, if negative, periodic tumor screening for at least 3 years after the neurologic diagnosis. In contrast, the weak association of polymyositis with cancer calls into question the need for repeated cancer screenings in this situation. Serum and urine immunofixation studies should be considered in patients with peripheral neuropathy of unknown cause; detection of a monoclonal gammopathy suggests the need for additional studies to uncover a B cell or plasma cell malignancy. In paraneoplastic neuropathies, diagnostically useful antineuronal antibodies are limited to anti-CV$_2$/CRMP5 and anti-Hu.

For any type of PND, if antineuronal antibodies are negative, the diagnosis relies on the demonstration of cancer and the exclusion of other cancer-related or independent neurologic disorders. Combined CT and PET scans often uncover tumors undetected by other tests. For germ-cell tumors of the testis and teratomas of the ovary ultrasound and MRI may reveal tumors undetectable by PET.

SPECIFIC PARANEOPLASTIC NEUROLOGIC SYNDROMES

■ PARANEOPLASTIC ENCEPHALOMYELITIS AND FOCAL ENCEPHALITIS

The term *encephalomyelitis* describes an inflammatory process with multifocal involvement of the nervous system, including brain, brainstem, cerebellum, and spinal cord. It is often associated with dorsal root ganglia and autonomic dysfunction. For any given patient, the clinical manifestations are determined by the areas predominantly involved, but pathologic studies almost always reveal abnormalities beyond the symptomatic regions. Several clinicopathologic syndromes may occur alone or in combination: (1) *cortical encephalitis*, which may present as "epilepsia partialis continua"; (2) *limbic encephalitis*, characterized by confusion, depression, agitation, anxiety, severe short-term memory deficits, partial complex seizures, and sometimes dementia (the MRI usually shows unilateral or bilateral medial temporal lobe abnormalities, best seen with T2 and fluid-attenuated inversion recovery sequences, and occasionally enhancing with gadolinium); (3) *brainstem encephalitis*, resulting in eye movement disorders (nystagmus, opsoclonus, supranuclear or nuclear paresis), cranial nerve paresis, dysarthria, dysphagia, and central autonomic dysfunction; (4) *cerebellar gait and limb ataxia*; (5) *myelitis*, which may cause lower or upper motor neuron symptoms, myoclonus, muscle rigidity, and spasms; and (6) *autonomic dysfunction* as a result of involvement of the neuraxis at multiple levels, including hypothalamus, brainstem, and autonomic nerves (see autonomic neuropathy). Cardiac arrhythmias, postural hypotension, or central hypoventilation are frequent causes of death in patients with encephalomyelitis.

Paraneoplastic encephalomyelitis and focal encephalitis are usually associated with SCLC, but many other cancers have also been reported. Patients with SCLC and these syndromes usually have anti-Hu antibodies in serum and CSF. Anti-CV$_2$/CRMP5 antibodies occur less frequently; some of these patients may develop chorea, uveitis, or optic neuritis. Antibodies to Ma proteins are associated with limbic, hypothalamic, and brainstem encephalitis and occasionally with cerebellar symptoms (Fig. 101-3); some patients develop

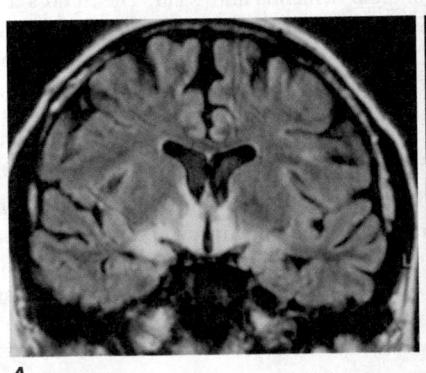
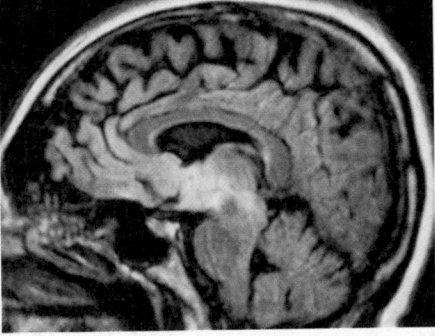
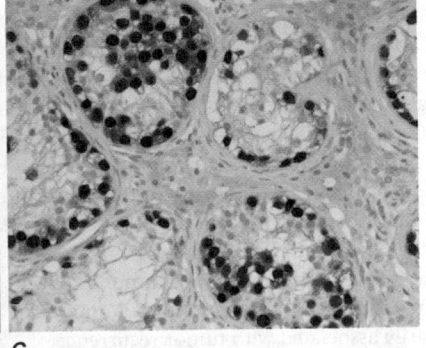

A *B* *C*

Figure 101-3 MRI and tumor of a patient with anti-Ma2-associated encephalitis. Panels *A* and *B* are fluid-attenuated inversion recovery MRI sequences showing abnormal hyperintensities in the medial temporal lobes, hypothalamus, and upper brainstem. *Panel C* corresponds to a section of the patient's orchiectomy incubated with a specific marker (Oct4) of germ-cell tumors. The positive (brown) cells correspond to an intratubular germ-cell neoplasm.

hypersomnia, cataplexy, and severe hypokinesia. MRI abnormalities are frequent, including those described with limbic encephalitis and variable involvement of the hypothalamus, basal ganglia, or upper brainstem. The oncologic associations of these antibodies are shown in Table 101-2.

TREATMENT   Encephalomyelitis and Focal Encephalitis

Most types of paraneoplastic encephalitis and encephalomyelitis respond poorly to treatment. Stabilization of symptoms or partial neurologic improvement may occasionally occur, particularly if there is a satisfactory response of the tumor to treatment. The roles of plasma exchange, intravenous immunoglobulin (IVIg), and immunosuppression have not been established. Approximately 30% of patients with anti-Ma2-associated encephalitis respond to treatment of the tumor (usually a germ-cell neoplasm of the testis) and immunotherapy.

■ ENCEPHALITIDES WITH ANTIBODIES TO CELL-SURFACE OR SYNAPTIC PROTEINS (TABLE 101-3)

These disorders are important for three reasons: (1) they can occur with and without tumor association, (2) some syndromes predominate in young individuals and children, and (3) despite the severity of the symptoms patients usually respond to treatment of the tumor, if found, and immunotherapy (glucocorticoids, plasma exchange, IVIg, rituximab, or cyclophosphamide).

Encephalitis with antibodies to voltage-gated potassium channels (VGKC)-related proteins (LGI1, Caspr2) predominates in men and frequently presents with memory loss and seizures (limbic encephalopathy), along with hyponatremia and sleep and autonomic dysfunction. Less commonly, patients develop neuromyotonia or a mixed clinical picture (Morvan's syndrome). Approximately 20% of patients with antibodies to VGKC-related proteins have an underlying tumor, usually SCLC or thymoma.

Encephalitis with N-methyl-D-aspartate (NMDA) receptor antibodies (Fig. 101-1) usually occurs in young women and children, but men and older patients of both sexes can be affected. The disorder has a characteristic pattern of symptom progression that includes a prodrome resembling a viral process, followed in a few days by the onset of severe psychiatric symptoms, memory loss, seizures, decreased level of consciousness, abnormal movements (orofacial, limb, and trunk dyskinesias, dystonic postures), autonomic instability, and frequent hypoventilation. The syndrome is often misdiagnosed as a viral or idiopathic encephalitis, neuroleptic malignant syndrome, or encephalitis lethargica, and many patients are initially evaluated by psychiatrists with the suspicion of drug abuse or an acute psychosis. The detection of an associated ovarian teratoma is age-dependant; 50% of female patients older than age 18 have uni- or bilateral ovarian teratomas, while less than 9% of girls younger than 14 years have a teratoma. In male patients the detection of a tumor is rare.

Encephalitis with α-amino-3-hydroxy-5-methylisoxazole-4-propionate (AMPA) receptor antibodies affects middle-aged women, who develop acute limbic dysfunction or less frequently prominent psychiatric symptoms; 70% of the patients have an underlying tumor in the lung, breast, or thymus. The neurologic disorder responds to treatment of the tumor and immunotherapy. Neurologic relapses may occur; these also respond to immunotherapy and are not necessarily associated with tumor recurrence.

Encephalitis with γ-aminobutyric acid type B (GABA$_B$) receptor antibodies usually presents with limbic encephalitis and seizures; 50% of the patients have SCLC or a neuroendocrine tumor of the lung. Neurologic symptoms often respond to immunotherapy and treatment of the tumor if found. Patients may have additional

antibodies to glutamic acid decarboxylase (GAD), of unclear significance. Other antibodies to nonneuronal proteins are often found in these patients as well as in patients with AMPA receptor antibodies, indicating a general tendency to autoimmunity.

■ PARANEOPLASTIC CEREBELLAR DEGENERATION

This disorder is often preceded by a prodrome that may include dizziness, oscillopsia, blurry or double vision, nausea, and vomiting. A few days or weeks later, patients develop dysarthria, gait and limb ataxia, and variable dysphagia. The examination usually shows downbeating nystagmus and, rarely, opsoclonus. Brainstem dysfunction, upgoing toes, or a mild neuropathy may occur, but more often the clinical features are restricted to the cerebellum. Early in the course, MRI studies are usually normal; later, the MRI typically reveals cerebellar atrophy. The disorder results from extensive degeneration of Purkinje cells, with variable involvement of other cerebellar cortical neurons, deep cerebellar nuclei, and spinocerebellar tracts. The tumors more frequently involved are SCLC, cancer of the breast and ovary, and Hodgkin lymphoma.

Anti-Yo antibodies in patients with breast and gynecologic cancers and anti-Tr antibodies in patients with Hodgkin lymphoma are the two immune responses typically associated with prominent or pure cerebellar degeneration. Antibodies to P/Q-type voltage-gated calcium channels (VGCC) occur in some patients with SCLC and cerebellar dysfunction; only some of these patients develop LEMS. A variable degree of cerebellar dysfunction can be associated with virtually any of the antibodies and PND of the CNS shown in Table 101-2.

A number of single case reports have described neurologic improvement after tumor removal, plasma exchange, IVIg, cyclophosphamide, rituximab, or glucocorticoids. However, large series of patients with antibody-positive paraneoplastic cerebellar degeneration show that this disorder rarely improves with any treatment.

■ PARANEOPLASTIC OPSOCLONUS-MYOCLONUS SYNDROME

Opsoclonus is a disorder of eye movement characterized by involuntary, chaotic saccades that occur in all directions of gaze; it is frequently associated with myoclonus and ataxia. Opsoclonus-myoclonus may be cancer-related or idiopathic. When the cause is paraneoplastic, the tumors involved are usually cancer of the lung and breast in adults and neuroblastoma in children. The pathologic substrate of opsoclonus-myoclonus is unclear, but studies suggest that disinhibition of the fastigial nucleus of the cerebellum is involved. Most patients do not have detectable antineuronal antibodies. A small subset of patients with ataxia, opsoclonus, and other eye-movement disorders develop anti-Ri antibodies; in rare instances muscle rigidity, autonomic dysfunction, and dementia also occur. The tumors most frequently involved in anti-Ri-associated syndromes are breast and ovarian cancer. If the tumor is not successfully treated, the neurologic syndrome in adults often progresses to encephalopathy, coma, and death. In addition to treating the tumor, symptoms may respond to immunotherapy (glucocorticoids, plasma exchange, and/or IVIg).

At least 50% of children with opsoclonus-myoclonus have an underlying neuroblastoma. Hypotonia, ataxia, behavioral changes, and irritability are frequent accompanying symptoms. Neurologic symptoms often improve with treatment of the tumor and glucocorticoids, adrenocorticotropic hormone (ACTH), plasma exchange, IVIg, and rituximab. Many patients are left with psychomotor retardation and behavioral and sleep problems.

■ PARANEOPLASTIC SYNDROMES OF THE SPINAL CORD

The number of reports of paraneoplastic spinal cord syndromes, such as *subacute motor neuronopathy* and *acute necrotizing myelopathy*, has decreased in recent years. This may represent a true decrease in incidence, due to improved and prompt oncologic interventions, or the identification of nonparaneoplastic etiologies.

Some patients with cancer develop *upper* or *lower motor neuron dysfunction* or both, resembling amyotrophic lateral sclerosis. It is unclear whether these disorders have a paraneoplastic etiology or simply coincide with the presence of cancer. There are isolated case reports of cancer patients with motor neuron dysfunction who had neurologic improvement after tumor treatment. A search for lymphoma should be undertaken in patients with a rapidly progressive motor neuron syndrome and a monoclonal protein in serum or CSF.

Paraneoplastic myelitis may present with upper or lower motor neuron symptoms, segmental myoclonus, and rigidity, and can be the first manifestation of encephalomyelitis.

Paraneoplastic myelopathy can also produce several syndromes characterized by prominent muscle stiffness and rigidity. The spectrum ranges from focal symptoms in one or several extremities (*stiff-limb syndrome* or *stiff-person syndrome*) to a disorder that also affects the brainstem (known as *encephalomyelitis with rigidity*) and likely has a different pathogenesis. Some patients with encephalomyelitis and rigidity have glycine receptor antibodies.

■ PARANEOPLASTIC STIFF-PERSON SYNDROME

This disorder is characterized by progressive muscle rigidity, stiffness, and painful spasms triggered by auditory, sensory, or emotional stimuli. Rigidity mainly involves the lower trunk and legs, but it can affect the upper extremities and neck. Symptoms improve with sleep and general anesthetics. Electrophysiologic studies demonstrate continuous motor unit activity. Antibodies associated with the stiff-person syndrome target proteins (GAD, amphiphysin) involved in the function of inhibitory synapses utilizing γ-aminobutyric acid (GABA) or glycine as neurotransmitters. Paraneoplastic stiff-person syndrome and amphiphysin antibodies are often related to SCLC and breast cancer. By contrast, antibodies to GAD may occur in some cancer patients but are much more frequently present in the nonparaneoplastic disorder.

| TREATMENT | Stiff-Person Syndrome |

Optimal treatment of stiff-person syndrome requires therapy of the underlying tumor, glucocorticoids, and symptomatic use of drugs that enhance GABA-ergic transmission (diazepam, baclofen, sodium valproate, tiagabine, vigabatrin). A benefit of IVIg has been demonstrated for the nonparaneoplastic disorder but remains to be established for the paraneoplastic syndrome.

■ PARANEOPLASTIC SENSORY NEURONOPATHY OR DORSAL ROOT GANGLIONOPATHY

This syndrome is characterized by sensory deficits that may be symmetric or asymmetric, painful dysesthesias, radicular pain, and decreased or absent reflexes. All modalities of sensation and any part of the body including face and trunk can be involved. Specialized sensations such as taste and hearing can also be affected. Electrophysiologic studies show decreased or absent sensory nerve potentials with normal or near-normal motor conduction velocities. Symptoms result from an inflammatory, likely immune-mediated, process that targets the dorsal root ganglia, causing neuronal loss, proliferation of satellite cells, and secondary degeneration of the posterior columns of the spinal cord. The dorsal and less frequently the anterior nerve roots and peripheral nerves may also be involved. This disorder often precedes or is associated with encephalomyelitis and autonomic dysfunction and has the same immunologic and oncologic associations, e.g., anti-Hu antibodies and SCLC.

| TREATMENT | Sensory Neuronopathy |

As with anti-Hu-associated encephalomyelitis, the therapeutic approach focuses on prompt treatment of the tumor. Glucocorticoids occasionally produce clinical stabilization or improvement. The benefit of IVIg and plasma exchange is not proved.

■ PARANEOPLASTIC PERIPHERAL NEUROPATHIES

These disorders may develop any time during the course of the neoplastic disease. Neuropathies occurring at late stages of cancer or lymphoma usually cause mild to moderate sensorimotor deficits due to axonal degeneration of unclear etiology. These neuropathies are often masked by concurrent neurotoxicity from chemotherapy and other cancer therapies. In contrast, the neuropathies that develop in the early stages of cancer frequently show a rapid progression, sometimes with a relapsing and remitting course, and evidence of inflammatory infiltrates and axonal loss or demyelination in biopsy studies. If demyelinating features predominate (Chap. 384), IVIg, plasma exchange, or glucocorticoids may improve symptoms. Occasionally anti-CV$_2$/CRMP5 antibodies are present; detection of anti-Hu suggests concurrent dorsal root ganglionitis.

Guillain-Barré syndrome and *brachial plexitis* have occasionally been reported in patients with lymphoma, but there is no clear evidence of a paraneoplastic association.

Malignant monoclonal gammopathies include: (1) multiple myeloma and sclerotic myeloma associated with IgG or IgA monoclonal proteins; and (2) Waldenström's macroglobulinemia, B cell lymphoma, and chronic B cell lymphocytic leukemia associated with IgM monoclonal proteins. These disorders may cause neuropathy by a variety of mechanisms, including compression of roots and plexuses by metastasis to vertebral bodies and pelvis, deposits of amyloid in peripheral nerves, and paraneoplastic mechanisms. The paraneoplastic variety has several distinctive features. Approximately half of patients with sclerotic myeloma develop a sensorimotor neuropathy with predominantly motor deficits, resembling a chronic inflammatory demyelinating neuropathy (Chap. 385); some patients develop elements of the POEMS syndrome (*p*olyneuropathy, *o*rganomegaly, *e*ndocrinopathy, *M* protein, *s*kin changes). Treatment of the plasmacytoma or sclerotic lesions usually improves the neuropathy. In contrast, the sensorimotor or sensory neuropathy associated with multiple myeloma rarely responds to treatment. Between 5 and 10% of patients with Waldenström's macroglobulinemia develop a distal symmetric sensorimotor neuropathy with predominant involvement of large sensory fibers. These patients may have IgM antibodies in their serum against myelin-associated glycoprotein and various gangliosides (Chap. 385). In addition to treating the Waldenström's macroglobulinemia, other therapies may improve the neuropathy, including plasma exchange, IVIg, chlorambucil, cyclophosphamide, fludarabine, or rituximab.

Vasculitis of the nerve and muscle causes a painful symmetric or asymmetric distal axonal sensorimotor neuropathy with variable proximal weakness. It predominantly affects elderly men and is associated with an elevated erythrocyte sedimentation rate and increased CSF protein concentration. SCLC and lymphoma are the primary tumors involved. Glucocorticoids and cyclophosphamide often result in neurologic improvement.

Peripheral nerve hyperexcitability (*neuromyotonia*, or *Isaacs' syndrome*) is characterized by spontaneous and continuous muscle fiber activity of peripheral nerve origin. Clinical features include cramps, muscle twitching (fasciculations or myokymia), stiffness, delayed muscle relaxation (pseudomyotonia), and spontaneous or evoked carpal or pedal spasms. The involved muscles may be hypertrophic, and some patients develop paresthesias and hyperhidrosis. CNS dysfunction, including mood changes, sleep disorder, or hallucinations, may occur. The electromyogram (EMG) shows fibrillations; fasciculations; and doublet, triplet, or multiplet single-unit (myokymic) discharges that have a high intraburst frequency. Approximately 20% of patients have serum antibodies to Caspr2-related proteins. The disorder often occurs without cancer; if paraneoplastic, benign, and malignant thymomas and SCLC are the usual tumors. Phenytoin, carbamazepine, and plasma exchange improve symptoms.

Paraneoplastic autonomic neuropathy usually develops as a component of other disorders, such as LEMS and encephalomyelitis. It may rarely occur as a pure or predominantly autonomic neuropathy with adrenergic or cholinergic dysfunction at the pre- or postganglionic levels. Patients can develop several life-threatening complications, such as gastrointestinal paresis with pseudoobstruction, cardiac dysrhythmias, and postural hypotension. Other clinical features include abnormal pupillary responses, dry mouth, anhidrosis, erectile dysfunction, and problems in sphincter control. The disorder occurs in association with several tumors, including SCLC, cancer of the pancreas or testis, carcinoid tumors, and lymphoma. Because autonomic symptoms can be the presenting feature of encephalomyelitis, serum anti-Hu and anti-CV_2/CRMP5 antibodies should be sought. Antibodies to ganglionic (alpha3-type) neuronal acetylcholine receptors are the cause of autoimmune autonomic ganglionopathy, a disorder that frequently occurs without cancer association (Chap. 375).

■ LAMBERT-EATON MYASTHENIC SYNDROME

LEMS is discussed in Chap. 386.

■ MYASTHENIA GRAVIS

Myasthenia gravis is discussed in Chap. 386.

■ POLYMYOSITIS-DERMATOMYOSITIS

Polymyositis and dermatomyositis are discussed in detail in Chap. 388.

■ ACUTE NECROTIZING MYOPATHY

Patients with this syndrome develop myalgias and rapid progression of weakness involving the extremities and the pharyngeal and respiratory muscles, often resulting in death. Serum muscle enzymes are elevated, and muscle biopsy shows extensive necrosis with minimal or absent inflammation and sometimes deposits of complement.

The disorder occurs as a paraneoplastic manifestation of a variety of cancers including SCLC and cancer of the gastrointestinal tract, breast, kidney, and prostate, among others. Glucocorticoids and treatment of the underlying tumor rarely control the disorder.

■ PARANEOPLASTIC VISUAL SYNDROMES

This group of disorders involves the retina and, less frequently, the uvea and optic nerves. The term *cancer-associated retinopathy* is used to describe paraneoplastic cone and rod dysfunction characterized by photosensitivity, progressive loss of vision and color perception, central or ring scotomas, night blindness, and attenuation of photopic and scotopic responses in the electroretinogram (ERG). The most commonly associated tumor is SCLC. Melanoma-associated retinopathy affects patients with metastatic cutaneous melanoma. Patients develop acute onset of night blindness and shimmering, flickering, or pulsating photopsias that often progress to visual loss. The ERG shows reduced b waves with normal dark adapted a waves. Paraneoplastic optic neuritis and uveitis are very uncommon and can develop in association with encephalomyelitis. Some patients with paraneoplastic uveitis harbor anti-CV_2/CRMP5 antibodies.

Some paraneoplastic retinopathies are associated with serum antibodies that specifically react with the subset of retinal cells undergoing degeneration, supporting an immune-mediated pathogenesis (Table 101-2). Paraneoplastic retinopathies usually fail to improve with treatment, although rare responses to glucocorticoids, plasma exchange, and IVIg have been reported.

FURTHER READINGS

ANTOINE JC, CAMDESSANCHÉ JP: Peripheral nervous system involvement in patients with cancer. Lancet Neurol 6:75, 2007

GRAUS F et al: Antibodies and neuronal autoimmune disorders of the CNS. J Neurol 257:509, 2010

LAI M et al: Investigation of LGI1 as the antigen in limbic encephalitis previously attributed to potassium channels: A case series. Lancet Neurol 9:776, 2010

ROSENFELD MR, DALMAU J: Update on paraneoplastic and autoimmune disorders of the central nervous system. Semin Neurol 30:320, 2010

TITULAER MJ et al: Screening for tumours in paraneoplastic syndromes: Report of an EFNS task force. Eur J Neurol 18:19, 2011

CHAPTER 102

Late Consequences of Cancer and Its Treatment

Carl E Freter
Dan L. Longo

Over 10 million Americans are cancer survivors. The vast majority of these people will bear some mark of their cancer and/or its treatment, and a large proportion will experience long-term consequences that include medical problems, psychosocial dysfunction, economic hardship, sexual dysfunction, and discrimination in employment and insurance. Many of these problems are directly related to cancer treatment.

As patients with more types of malignancies survive longer, the biologic toll that very imperfect therapies take in terms of morbidity and mortality rates is being recognized increasingly. These consequences of therapy confront the patients and the cancer specialists and general internists who manage them every day. Although long-term survivors of childhood leukemias, Hodgkin's lymphoma, and testicular cancer have increased knowledge about the consequences of cancer treatment, researchers and physicians keep learning more as patients survive longer with newer therapies. The pace of the development of therapies that mitigate treatment-related consequences has been slow, partly due to an understandable aversion to altering regimens that work and partly due to a lack of new, effective, less toxic therapeutic agents with less "collateral damage" to replace known agents with known toxicities. The types of damage from cancer treatment vary. Often, a final common pathway is irreparable damage to DNA. Surgery can create dysfunction, including blind gut loops that lead to absorption problems and loss of function of removed body parts. Radiation may damage end-organ function, for example, loss of potency in prostate cancer patients, pulmonary fibrosis, neurocognitive impairment, acceleration of atherosclerosis, and second cancers. Cancer chemotherapy may act as a carcinogen and has a kaleidoscope of other toxicities, as discussed in this chapter. Table 102-1 lists the long-term effects of treatment.

The first goal of therapy is to eradicate or control the malignancy. Late treatment consequences are, indeed, testimony to the increasing success of such treatment. Their occurrence sharply underlines the necessity to develop more effective therapies with less long-term morbidity and mortality. At the same time, a sense of perspective and relative risk is necessary; fear of long-term complications should not prevent the application of effective (particularly curative) cancer treatment.

CARDIOVASCULAR DYSFUNCTION

■ CHEMOTHERAPEUTIC AGENTS

The cardiovascular toxicity of cancer chemotherapeutic agents includes dysrhythmias, cardiomyopathic congestive heart failure (CHF), pericardial disease, and peripheral vascular disease. Because these cardiac toxicities are difficult to distinguish from disease that is not associated with cancer treatment, determining the clear etiologic implication of cancer chemotherapeutic agents may be difficult. Cardiovascular complications occurring in an unexpected clinical setting in patients who have undergone cancer therapy is often important in raising suspicion. Dose-dependent myocardial toxicity of anthracyclines with characteristic myofibrillar dropout is pathologically pathagnomonic on endomyocardial biopsy. Anthracycline cardiotoxity occurs through a root mechanism of chemical free-radical damage. Fe(III)-doxorubicin complexes damage DNA, nuclear and cytoplasmic membranes, and mitochondria. About 5% of patients receiving >450–550 mg/m² doxorubicin will develop CHF. Cardiotoxicity in relation to the dose of anthracycline is clearly not a step function but rather a continuous function, and occasional patients are seen with CHF at substantially lower doses. Advanced age, other concomitant cardiac disease, hypertension, diabetes, and thoracic radiation therapy are all important cofactors in promoting anthracycline-associated CHF. Anthracycline-related CHF is difficult to reverse; the mortality rate is as high as 50%, making prevention crucial. Some anthracyclines, such as mitoxantrone, are associated with less cardiotoxicity, and continuous infusion regimens or doxorubicin encapsulated in liposomes are associated with less cardiotoxicity. Dexrazoxane, an intracellular iron chelator, may limit anthracycline toxicity, but concern about limiting chemotherapeutic efficacy has limited its use. Monitoring patients for cardiac toxicity typically involves periodic gated nuclear cardiac blood pool ejection fraction testing [multi-gated acquisition scan (MUGA)] or cardiac ultrasonography. Cardiac MRI has been used but is not standard or widespread. Testing is performed more frequently at higher cumulative doses, with additional risk factors, certainly for any newly developing CHF or other symptoms of cardiac dysfunction.

Trastuzumab after anthracyclines is currently the next most commonly used cardiotoxic drug. Trastuzumab is commonly used in adjuvant therapy or for advanced HER2-positive breast cancer, sometimes in conjunction with anthracyclines, and is believed to result in additive or possibly synergistic toxicity. In contrast to anthracyclines, cardiotoxicity from trastuzumab is not dose-related, is usually reversible, is not associated with pathologic changes of anthracyclines on cardiac myofibrils, and has a different biochemical mechanism inhibiting intrinsic cardiac repair mechanisms. Toxicity is monitored routinely every three to

TABLE 102-1 Late Effects of Cancer Therapy

Surgical Procedure		Effect
Amputation		Functional loss
Lymph node dissection		Risk of lymphedema
Ostomy		Psychosocial impact
Splenectomy		Risk of sepsis
Adhesions		Risk of obstruction
Bowel anastomoses		Malabsorption syndromes
Radiation Therapy		Effect
Organ		
Bone		Premature termination of growth, osteonecrosis
Soft tissues		Atrophy, fibrosis
Brain		Neuropsychiatric deficits, cognitive dysfunction
Thyroid		Hypothyroidism, Graves' disease, cancer
Salivary glands		Dry mouth, caries, dysgeusia
Eyes		Cataracts
Heart		Pericarditis, myocarditis, coronary artery disease
Lung		Pulmonary fibrosis
Kidney		Decreased function, hypertension
Liver		Decreased function
Intestine		Malabsorption, stricture
Gonads		Infertility, premature menopause
Any		Secondary neoplasia
Chemotherapy		Effect
Organ	**Drug**	
Bone	Glucocorticoids	Osteoporosis, avascular necrosis
Brain	Methotrexate, cytarabine (Ara-C), others	Neuropsychiatric deficits, cognitive decline?
Peripheral nerves	Vincristine, platinum, taxanes	Neuropathy, hearing loss
Eyes	Glucocorticoids	Cataracts
Heart	Anthracyclines, trastuzumab	Cardiomyopathy
Lung	Bleomycin	Pulmonary fibrosis
	Methotrexate	Pulmonary hypersensitivity
Kidney	Platinum, others	Decreased function, hypomagnesemia
Liver	Various	Altered function
Gonads	Alkylating agents, others	Infertility, premature menopause
Bone marrow	Various	Aplasia, myelodysplasia, secondary leukemia

four doses with functional cardiac testing as described above for anthracyclines.

Other cardiotoxic drugs include lapatinib, phosphoramide mustards (cyclophosphamide), ifosfamide, interleukin 2, imatinib, and sunitinib.

■ RADIATION THERAPY

Radiation therapy that includes the heart can cause interstitial myocardial fibrosis, acute and chronic pericarditis, valvular disease, and accelerated premature atherosclerotic coronary artery disease. Repeated or high (>6000 cGy) radiation doses are associated with greater risk, as is concomitant or distant cardiotoxic cancer chemotherapy exposure. Symptoms of acute pericarditis, which peaks about 9 months after treatment, include dyspnea, chest pain, and fever. Chronic constrictive pericarditis may develop 5–10 years after radiation therapy. Cardiac valvular disease includes aortic insufficiency from fibrosis and papillary muscle dysfunction that results in mitral regurgitation. A three-fold increased risk of fatal myocardial infarction is associated with mantle field radiation, with accelerated coronary artery disease. Carotid radiation similarly increases the risk of embolic stroke.

TREATMENT | Chemotherapeutic/Radiation-Induced Cardiovascular Disease

Therapy for chemotherapeutic/radiation-induced cardiovascular disease is essentially the same as therapy for disease that is not associated with cancer treatment. Discontinuation of the offending agent is the first step. Diuretics, fluid and sodium restriction, and antiarylthmic agents are often useful for treating acute symptoms. Afterload reduction with angiotensin-converting enzyme (ACE) inhibitors or, in some cases, β-adrenergic blockers (carvedilol) often is of significant benefit, and digitalis may be helpful as well.

PULMONARY DYSFUNCTION

■ CHEMOTHERAPEUTIC AGENTS

Bleomycin generates activated free-radical oxygen species and causes pneumonitis associated with a radiographic or interstitial ground-glass appearance diffusely throughout both lungs, often worse in the lower lobes. This toxicity is dose-related and dose-limiting. The diffusion capacity of the lungs for carbon dioxide (DLCO) is a sensitive measure of toxicity and recovery, and a baseline value generally is obtained for future comparison before bleomycin therapy. Additive or synergistic risk factors include age, prior lung disease, and concomitant use of other chemotherapy, along with lung irradiation and high concentrations of inspired oxygen. Other chemotherapeutic agents notable for pulmonary toxicity include mitomycin, nitrosoureas, doxorubicin with radiation, gemcitabine combined with weekly docetaxel, methotrexate, and fludarabine. High-dose alkylating agents, cyclophosphamide, ifosfamide, and melphalan are used frequently in the hematopoietic stem cell transplant setting, often with whole-body radiation. This therapy may result in severe pulmonary fibrosis and/or pulmonary venoocclusive disease.

■ RADIATION THERAPY

Risk factors for radiation pneumonitis include advanced age, poor performance status, preexisting compromised pulmonary function, radiation volume, and dose. The dose "threshold" for lung damage is thought to be in the range of 5–20 Gy. Hypoxemia and dyspnea on exertion are characteristic. Fine, high-pitched "Velcro rales" may be an accompanying physical finding, and fever, cough,

and pleuritic chest pain are common symptoms. The DLCO is the most sensitive measure of pulmonary functional impairment, and ground-glass infiltrates often correspond with relatively sharp edges to the irradiated volume, although the pneumonitis may progress beyond the field and occasionally involve the contralateral unir-radiated lung.

TREATMENT | Pulmonary Dysfunction

Chemotherapy and radiation-induced pneumonitis are generally glucocorticoid-responsive, except in the case of nitrosoureas. Prednisone, 1 mg/kg, often is used to control acute symptoms and pulmonary dysfunction, with a generally slow taper. Prolonged glucocorticoid therapy requires gastrointestinal protection with proton pump inhibitors, management of hyperglycemia, heightened infection management, and prevention or treatment of steroid-induced osteoporosis. Antibiotics, bronchodilators, oxygen in only necessary doses, and diuretics may all play an important role in management of pneumonitis, and consultation with a pulmonologist should be undertaken routinely. Amifostine has been studied as a pulmonary radio-protectant, with inconclusive results, and is associated with skin rash, fatigue, and nausea; hence, it is not considered standard therapy at this time. Transforming growth factor β (TGF-β) is believed to be a major inducer of radiation fibrosis and represents a therapeutic target for development of anti-TGF-β therapies. As a general rule, patients who have received chest radiation therapy or bleomycin should receive supplemental O_2 when only absolutely necessary and at the lowest FiO_2 possible.

NEUROLOGIC DYSFUNCTION

■ CHEMOTHERAPEUTIC AGENTS

Chemotherapy and radiation-induced neurologic dysfunction are increasing in both incidence and severity as a result of improved supportive care leading to more aggressive regimens and longer cancer survival allowing the development of late toxicity. Direct effects on myelin, glial cells, and neurons have been implicated, with alterations in cellular cytoskeleton, axonal transport, and cellular metabolism as mechanisms.

Vinca alkaloids produce a characteristic "stocking-glove" neuropathy, with numbness and tingling advancing to loss of motor function, which is highly dose-related. Distal sensorimotor polyneuropathy prominently involves loss of deep tendon reflexes with initially loss of pain and temperature sensation, followed by proprioceptive and vibratory loss. This requires a careful patient history and physical examination by experienced oncologists to decide when the drug must be stopped due to toxicity. Milder toxicity often slowly resolves completely. Vinca alkaloids may be associated with jaw claudication, autonomic neuropathy, ileus, cranial nerve palsies, and, in severe cases, encephalopathy, seizures, and coma.

Cisplatin is associated with sensorimotor neuropathy as well as hearing loss, especially at doses >400 mg/m², requiring audiometry in patients with preexisting hearing compromise. Carboplatin often is substituted in such cases because of its lesser effect on hearing.

Neurocognitive dysfunction has been well described in child-hood survivors of acute lymphocytic leukemia (ALL) treatment, including intrathecal methotrexate or cytarabine in conjunction with prophylactic cranial irradiation. Methotrexate alone may cause acute leucoencephalopathy characterized by somnolence and confusion that is often reversible. Acute toxicity is dose-related, especially at doses > 3 g/m², with younger patients being at greater risk. Subacute methotrexate toxicity occurs weeks after therapy and often is ameliorated with glucocorticoid therapy. Chronic methotrexate toxicity (leucoencephalopathy) develops months or years after treatment and is characterized clinically as progressive loss of cognitive function and focal neurologic signs that are irreversible, are promoted by synchronous or metachronous radiation therapy, and are more pronounced at a younger age.

Neurocognitive decline after chemotherapy alone occurs notably in breast cancer patients receiving adjuvant chemotherapy; this has been referred to as "chemo brain." It is clinically associated with impaired memory, learning, attention, and speed of information processing. The magnitude of the problem has been difficult to assess in light of the fact that cognitive decline is a normal feature of aging. It is not entirely clear that women receiving adjuvant therapy for breast cancer have a more rapid cognitive decline than do age-matched controls. Furthermore, its causes are unexplained given the poor penetrance of chemotherapy agents into the central nervous system (CNS). No prevention or therapy has been developed. This entity is attracting the attention of investigators.

Many cancer patients experience intrusive or debilitating concerns about cancer recurrence after successful therapy. In addition, these patients may experience job, insurance, stress, relationship, financial, and sexual difficulties. Physicians need to ask about and address these issues explicitly with cancer survivors, with referral to the appropriate counseling or support systems. Suicidal ideation and suicide have an increased incidence in cancer patients and survivors.

■ RADIATION THERAPY

Acute radiation CNS toxicity occurs within weeks and is characterized by nausea, drowsiness, hypersomnia, and ataxia, symptoms that most often abate with time. Early-delayed toxicity occurring weeks to 3 months after therapy is associated with symptoms similar to those of acute toxicity and is pathologically associated with reversible demyelination. Chronic, late radiation injury occurs 9 months to up to 10 years after therapy. Focal necrosis is a common pathologic finding, and glucocorticoid therapy may be helpful. Diffuse radiation injury is associated with global CNS neurologic dysfunction and diffuse white matter changes on CT or MRI. Pathologically, small vessel changes are prominent. Glucocorticoids may be symptomatically useful but do not alter the course. Necrotizing encephalopathy is the most severe form of radiation injury and almost always is associated with chemotherapy, notably methotrexate.

Cranial radiation also may be associated with an array of endocrine abnormalities with disruption of normal pituitary-hypothalamic axis function. A high index of suspicion needs to be maintained to identify and treat this toxicity.

Radiation-associated spinal cord injury (myelopathy) is highly dose-dependent and rarely occurs with modern radiation therapy. An early, self-limited form involving electric sensations down the spine on neck flexion (Lhermitte's sign) is seen 6–12 weeks after treatment, and generally resolves over weeks. Peripheral nerve toxicity is quite rare owing to relative radiation resistance.

HEPATIC DYSFUNCTION
■ CHEMOTHERAPEUTIC AGENTS

Long-term hepatic damage from standard chemotherapy regimens is rare. Long-term methotrexate or high-dose chemotherapy alone or with radiation therapy—e.g., in preparative regimens for bone marrow transplantation—may result in venoocclusive disease of the liver. This potentially lethal complication classically presents with anicteric ascites, elevated alkaline phosphatase, and hepatosplenomegaly. Pathologically, venous congestion, epithelial cell proliferation, and hepatocyte atrophy progressing to frank fibrosis are noted. Frequent monitoring of liver function tests during any type of chemotherapy is necessary to avoid both idiosyncratic and expected toxicities. Ursodiol may prevent cholestasis in the setting of high-dose therapy before bone marrow transplant.

■ RADIATION THERAPY

Hepatic radiation damage depends on dose, volume, fractionation, preexisting liver disease, and synchronous or metachronous chemotherapy. In general, radiation doses to the liver >1500 cGy can produce hepatic dysfunction with a steep dose-injury curve. Radiation-induced liver disease (RILD) closely mimics hepatic venoocclusive disease.

RENAL/BLADDER DYSFUNCTION

Cisplatin produces reversible decrements in renal function but also may produce severe irreversible toxicity in the presence of renal disease and may predispose to accentuated damage with subsequent renal insults. Magnesium wasting with hypomagnesemia may be seen. Cyclophosphamide and ifosfamide, as prodrugs primarily activated in the liver, have cleavage products (acrolein) that can produce hemorrhagic cystitis. This can be prevented with the free-radical scavenger 2-mercaptoethane sulfonate (MESNA), which is required for ifosfamide administration. Hemorrhagic cystitis caused by these agents may predispose these patients to bladder cancer.

REPRODUCTIVE AND ENDOCRINE DYSFUNCTION
■ CHEMOTHERAPEUTIC AGENTS

Alkylating agents are associated with the highest rates of male and female infertility, which is directly dependent on age, dose, and duration of treatment. The age at treatment is an important determinant of fertility outcome, with prepubertal patients having the highest tolerance. Ovarian failure is age-related, and females who resume menses after treatment are still at increased risk for premature menopause. Males generally have reversible azospermia during lower-intensity alkylator chemotherapy, and long-term infertility is associated with total doses of cyclophosphamide >9 g/m^2 and with high-intensity therapy such as that used in hematopoietic stem cell transplantation. Males undergoing potentially sterilizing chemotherapy should be offered sperm banking. However, some cancers are associated with defective spermatogenesis. Gonadotropin-releasing hormone (GnRH) analogues to preserve ovarian function remain experimental. Assisted reproductive technologies may be helpful to couples with chemotherapy-induced infertility.

■ RADIATION THERAPY

The testicles and ovaries of prepubertal patients are less sensitive to radiation damage; spermatogenesis is affected by low doses of radiation, and complete azospermia occurs at 600–700 cGy. Leydig cell dysfunction, in contrast, occurs at <2000 cGy; hence, endocrine function is lost at much higher radiation doses than spermatogenesis. Erectile dysfunction occurs in up to 80% of men treated with external-beam radiation therapy for prostate cancer. Sildenafil (and congeners) may be useful in reversing erectile dysfunction. Ovarian function damage with radiation is age-related and occurs at doses of 150–500 cGY. Premature induction of menopause can have serious medical and psychological sequelae. Hormone replacement therapy often is contraindicated, as in estrogen receptor–positive breast cancer. Attention must be paid to maintenance of bone mass with calcium and vitamin D supplements and oral bisphosphonates; this is monitored by bone density determinations. Paroxetine, clonidine, pregabalin, and other drugs may be useful in symptomatically controlling hot flashes. In those without contraindications, estrogen may be used for periods <5 years at the lowest dose that relieves symptoms.

Long–term survivors of childhood cancer (e.g., ALL) who have received cranial radiation may have altered leptin biology and growth hormone deficiency, leading to obesity and reduced strength, exercise tolerance, and bone density.

Radiation therapy to the neck, for example, in Hodgkin's lymphoma, may lead to hypothyroidism, Graves' disease, thyroiditis, and thyroid malignancies. Thyroid-stimulating hormone (TSH) is followed routinely in these patients and suppressed with synthroid when elevated to prevent hypothyroidism and suppress the TSH drive, which may cause thyroid cancer.

OCULAR COMPLICATIONS

Cataracts may be caused by glucocorticoids, depending on the duration and dose; radiation therapy; and, uncommonly, tamoxifen. Orbital radiation therapy may cause blindness.

ORAL COMPLICATIONS

Radiation therapy can produce xerostomia (dry mouth) with an attendant increase in caries and poor dentition. Taste and appetite may be suppressed. Bisphosphonate use may result in osteonecrosis of the jaw.

RAYNAUD'S PHENOMENON

Up to 40% of patients treated with bleomycin may develop Raynaud's phenomenon. The mechanism is unknown.

SECOND MALIGNANCIES

Second malignancies in patients cured of cancer are a major cause of death, and treated cancer patients must be monitored for their occurrence. The induction of second malignancies is governed by the complex interplay of a number of factors, including age, sex, environmental exposures, genetic susceptibility, and cancer treatment itself. In a number of settings, the events leading to the primary cancer themselves increase the risk of second malignancies. Patients with lung cancer are at increased risk of esophageal and head and neck cancers, and vice versa, due to shared risk factors, including alcohol and tobacco abuse. Indeed, the risk of developing a second primary head and neck, esophageal, or lung cancer is also increased in these patients. Patients with breast cancer are at increased risk of cancer in the opposite breast. Patients with Hodgkin's lymphoma are at risk for non-Hodgkin's lymphomas. Genetic cancer syndromes, for example, multiple endocrine neoplasia and Li-Fraumeni, Lynch, Cowden, and Gardner's syndromes, are examples of genetically based second malignancies of specific types. Cancer treatment itself does not appear to be responsible for the risk of these secondary malignancies. Deficient DNA repair can greatly increase the risk of cancers from DNA-damaging agents, as in ataxia-telangectasia. Importantly, the risk of treatment-related second malignancies is at least additive and often is synergistic with combined chemotherapy and radiation therapy; hence, for such combined therapy treatment approaches, it is important to establish the necessity of each modality in the treatment program. All these patients require special surveillance or in some cases prophylactic surgery as part of appropriate treatment and follow-up.

■ CHEMOTHERAPEUTIC AGENTS

Chemotherapy is significantly associated with two fatal second malignancies: acute leukemia and myelodysplastic syndromes. Two types of leukemia have been described. In patients treated with alkylating agents, acute myeloid leukemia is associated with deletions in chromosomes 5 or 7. The lifetime risk is about 1–5%, is increased by radiation therapy, and increases with age. The incidence of these leukemias peaks at 4–6 years, with risk returning close to baseline at 10 years. The other type of acute myeloid leukemia is related to therapy with topoisomerase inhibitors, is associated with chromosome 10q23 translocations, has an incidence <1%, and generally occurs 1.5–3 years after treatment. Both of these acute leukemias are refractory to treatment and have a high mortality rate. The development of myelodysplastic syndromes is increased after chemotherapy, particularly chronic alkylating agent therapy, and these syndromes often are associated with leukemic progression with a dismal prognosis.

■ RADIATION THERAPY

Patients receiving radiation have an increasing and lifelong risk of second malignancies that is 1–2% per year in the second decade after treatment but increases to >25% after 25 years. These malignancies include cancers of the thyroid and breast, sarcomas, and CNS cancers, which often tend to be aggressive and have a poor prognosis. An example of organ-, age-, and sex-dependent radiation-induced secondary malignancy is breast cancer, in which the risk is small with radiation <age 30 but increases about twentyfold over baseline in women >30 years. A 25-year-old woman treated with mantle radiation for Hodgkin's lymphoma has a 29% actuarial risk of developing breast cancer by age 55.

■ HORMONAL THERAPY

Treatment of breast cancer with tamoxifen for 5 years or longer is associated with a 1–2% risk of endometrial cancer. Surveillance is generally effective at finding these cancers at an early stage. The risk of mortality from tamoxifen-induced endometrial cancer is low compared to the benefit of tamoxifen as adjuvant therapy for breast cancer.

■ IMMUNOSUPRESSIVE THERAPY

Immunosupressive therapy, as used in allogeneic bone marrow transplantation, particularly with T cell depletion and using antithymocyte globulin or other means, increases the risk of Epstein Barr virus–associated B cell lymphoproliferative disorder. The incidence at 10 years after T cell depletion is 9–12%. Discontinuation of immunosuppressive therapy, if possible, often is associated with complete disease regression.

RECOMMENDATIONS FOR FOLLOW-UP

All former cancer patients should be followed indefinitely. This is done most often by oncologists, but demographic changes suggest that more primary care physicians will need to be trained in the follow-up of treated cancer patients in remission. Cancer patients need to be educated about signs and symptoms of recurrence and potentially adverse effects related to therapy. Localized pain or palpable abnormality in a previously radiated field should prompt radiographic evaluation. Screening tests, when available and validated, should be used on a routine and regular basis, for example, mammography and Pap smear, particularly in patients receiving radiation to specific organs. Annual mammography should start no later than 10 years after breast radiation. Patients receiving radiation fields that encompass thyroid tissue should have regular thyroid exams and TSH testing. Patients treated with alkylating agents or topoisomerase inhibitors should have a complete blood count every 6–12 months, and cytopenias, abnormal

TABLE 102-2 Long-term Treatment Effects by Cancer Type

Cancer Type	Late Effects
Pediatric cancers	Majority have at least one late effect; 30% with moderate/severe problems Cardiovascular: radiation, anthracyclines Lungs: radiation Skeletal abnormalities: radiation Psychological, cognitive, and sexual problems Second neoplasms significant cause of death
Hodgkin's lymphoma	Thyroid dysfunction: radiation Premature coronary artery disease: radiation Gonadal dysfunction: chemotherapy Postsplenectomy sepsis Myelodysplasia Acute myeloid leukemia Non-Hodgkin's lymphomas Breast cancer, lung cancer, and melanoma Fatigue, psychological, and sexual problems Peripheral neuropathy
Non-Hodgkin's lymphoma	Myelodysplasia Acute leukemia Bladder cancer Peripheral neuropathy
Acute leukemia	Second malignancies: hematologic, solid tumors Neurophychiatric dysfunction Subnormal growth Thyroid abnormalities Infertility
Bone marrow stem cell transplantation	Infertility Graft-versus-host disease (allogeneic transplant) Psychosexual dysfunction
Head and neck cancer	Poor dentition, dry mouth, poor nutrition: radiation
Breast cancer	Tamoxifen: endometrial cancer, blood clots Aromatase inhibitors: osteoporosis, arthritis. Cardiomyopathy: anthracycline ± radiation, trastuzaumab Acute leukemia Hormone-deficiency symptoms: hot flashes, vaginal dryness, dyspareunia Psychosocial dysfunction "Chemo brain"
Testicular cancer	Raynaud's phenomenon Renal dysfunction Pulmonary dysfunction Retrograde ejaculation: surgery 15% sexual dysfunction
Colon cancer	Major risk is second colon cancer Quality of life high in survivors
Prostate cancer	Impotence Urinary incontinence (0–15%) Chronic prostatitis/cystitis: radiation

cells on peripheral smear, or macrocytosis should be evaluated with bone marrow biopsy and aspirate, along with cytogenetics, flow cytometry, or fluorescence in situ hybridization (FISH) studies as appropriate.

Cancer survival, as the population lives longer and expands, has become an increasingly recognized subject. The Institute of Medicine and the National Research Council of the National Academy of Sciences have published a monograph titled *From Cancer Patient to Cancer Survivor: Lost in Transition*. It proposes a plan to inform clinicians caring for cancer survivors in complete detail about their previous treatments, the complications of those treatments, signs and symptoms of late effects, and recommended screening and follow-up procedures. Table 102-2 describes long-term treatment effects by cancer type.

OUTLOOK

Clearly, the challenge for the future is to combine chemotherapy, targeted agents, biologic therapies, radiation, and surgery to produce better outcomes with less toxicity, including late effects of therapy. This is easily said and less easily accomplished. As treatment becomes more effective in new patient populations (ovarian, bladder, anal, and laryngeal cancers, for example), one can expect to discover new populations at risk for late effects. These populations will have to be followed carefully so that such effects are recognized and treated. Cancer survivors represent an underutilized resource for prevention studies. Childhood cancer survivors especially have multiple chronic health impairments. The incidence of these late treatment consequences appears to have no plateau with age, throwing in stark relief the necessity of close monitoring and therapies with fewer late consequences of treatment.

FURTHER READINGS

AHLES T et al: Neuropsychiatric impact of standard-dose chemotherapy in long-term survivors of breast cancer and lymphoma. J Clin Oncol 20:485, 2002

BOOKMAN MA et al: Late complications of curative treatment in Hodgkin's disease. JAMA 260:680, 1988

BROWN LM et al: Risk of second non-hematologic malignancies among 376,825 breast cancer survivors. Breast Cancer Res Treat 106:439, 2007

HEWITT M et al (eds): *From Cancer Patient to Cancer Survivor: Lost in Transition*. Committee on Cancer Survivorship: Improving Care and Quality of Life. Washington, DC, National Academies Press, 2006

LILES A et al: Monitoring pulmonary complications in long-term childhood cancer survivors for the primary care physician. Cleve Clin J Med 75:531, 2008

———: Factors affecting late mortality from heart disease after treatment of Hodgkin's disease. JAMA 270:1949, 1993

MURPHY BA: Advances in quality of life and symptom management for head and neck cancer patients. Curr Opin Oncol 21:242, 2009

NG AK et al: Secondary malignancies across the age spectrum. Semin Radiat Oncol 20:67, 2010

STUBBLEFIELD MD, O'DELL MW (eds): *Cancer Rehabilitation: Principles and Practice* . New York, Demos Medical, 2009

TRAVIS LB et al: Cumulative absolute breast cancer risk for young women treated for Hodgkin lymphoma. J Natl Cancer Inst 97:1428, 2005

CHAPTER **103**

Iron Deficiency and Other Hypoproliferative Anemias

John W. Adamson

Anemias associated with normocytic and normochromic red cells and an inappropriately low reticulocyte response (reticulocyte index <2–2.5) are *hypoproliferative anemias*. This category includes early iron deficiency (before hypochromic microcytic red cells develop), acute and chronic inflammation (including many malignancies), renal disease, hypometabolic states such as protein malnutrition and endocrine deficiencies, and anemias from marrow damage. Marrow damage states are discussed in Chap. 107.

Hypoproliferative anemias are the most common anemias, and anemia associated with chronic inflammation is the most common of these. The anemia of inflammation, similar to iron deficiency, is related in part to abnormal iron metabolism. The anemias associated with renal disease, inflammation, cancer, and hypometabolic states are characterized by an abnormal erythropoietin response to the anemia.

IRON METABOLISM

Iron is a critical element in the function of all cells, although the amount of iron required by individual tissues varies during development. At the same time, the body must protect itself from free iron, which is highly toxic in that it participates in chemical reactions that generate free radicals such as singlet O_2 or OH^-. Consequently, elaborate mechanisms have evolved that allow iron to be made available for physiologic functions while at the same time conserving this element and handling it in such a way that toxicity is avoided.

The major role of iron in mammals is to carry O_2 as part of hemoglobin. O_2 is also bound by myoglobin in muscle. Iron is a critical element in iron-containing enzymes, including the cytochrome system in mitochondria. Iron distribution in the body is shown in Table 103-1. Without iron, cells lose their capacity for electron transport and energy metabolism. In erythroid cells, hemoglobin synthesis is impaired, resulting in anemia and reduced O_2 delivery to tissue.

THE IRON CYCLE IN HUMANS

Figure 103-1 outlines the major pathways of internal iron exchange in humans. Iron absorbed from the diet or released from stores circulates in the plasma bound to *transferrin*, the iron transport protein. Transferrin is a bilobed glycoprotein with two iron binding sites. Transferrin that carries iron exists in two forms—*monoferric* (one iron atom) or *diferric* (two iron atoms). The turnover (half-clearance time) of transferrin-bound iron is very rapid—typically 60–90 min. Because almost all of the iron transported by transferrin is delivered to the erythroid marrow, the clearance time of transferrin-bound iron from the circulation is affected most by the plasma iron level and the erythroid marrow activity. When erythropoiesis is markedly stimulated, the pool of erythroid cells requiring iron increases and the clearance time of iron from the circulation decreases. The half-clearance time of iron in the presence of iron deficiency is as short as 10–15 min. With suppression of erythropoiesis, the plasma iron level typically increases and the half-clearance time may be prolonged to several hours. Normally, the iron bound to transferrin turns over 6–8 times per day. Assuming a normal plasma iron level of 80–100 μg/dL, the amount of iron passing through the transferrin pool is 20–24 mg/d.

The iron-transferrin complex circulates in the plasma until it interacts with specific *transferrin receptors* on the surface of marrow erythroid cells. Diferric transferrin has the highest affinity for transferrin receptors; apotransferrin (not carrying iron) has very little affinity. Although transferrin receptors are found on cells in many tissues within the body—and all cells at some time during development will display transferrin receptors—the cell having the

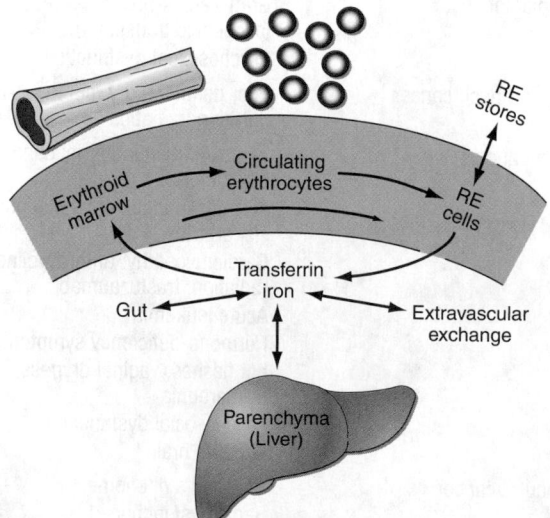

Figure 103-1 Internal iron exchange. Normally approximately 80% of iron passing through the plasma transferrin pool is recycled from broken-down red cells. Absorption of approximately 1 mg/d is required from the diet in men, and 1.4 mg/d in women to maintain homeostasis. As long as transferrin saturation is maintained between 20–60% and erythropoiesis is not increased, use of iron stores is not required. However, in the event of blood loss, dietary iron deficiency, or inadequate iron absorption, up to 40 mg/d of iron can be mobilized from stores. RE, reticuloendothelial.

TABLE 103-1 Body Iron Distribution

	Iron Content, mg	
	Adult Male, 80 kg	Adult Female, 60 kg
Hemoglobin	2500	1700
Myoglobin/enzymes	500	300
Transferrin iron	3	3
Iron stores	600–1000	0–300

greatest number of receptors (300,000 to 400,000/cell) is the developing erythroblast.

Once the iron-bearing transferrin interacts with its receptor, the complex is internalized via clathrin-coated pits and transported to an acidic endosome, where the iron is released at the low pH. The iron is then made available for heme synthesis while the transferrin-receptor complex is recycled to the surface of the cell, where the bulk of the transferrin is released back into circulation and the transferrin receptor reanchors into the cell membrane. At this point a certain amount of the transferrin receptor protein may be released into circulation and can be measured as soluble transferrin receptor protein. Within the erythroid cell, iron in excess of the amount needed for hemoglobin synthesis binds to a storage protein, *apoferritin*, forming *ferritin*. This mechanism of iron exchange also takes place in other cells of the body expressing transferrin receptors, especially liver parenchymal cells where the iron can be incorporated into heme-containing enzymes or stored. The iron incorporated into hemoglobin subsequently enters the circulation as new red cells are released from the bone marrow. The iron is then part of the red cell mass and will not become available for reutilization until the red cell dies.

In a normal individual, the average red cell life span is 120 days. Thus, 0.8–1% of red cells turn over each day. At the end of its life span, the red cell is recognized as senescent by the cells of the *reticuloendothelial (RE) system*, and the cell undergoes phagocytosis. Once within the RE cell, the hemoglobin from the ingested red cell is broken down, the globin and other proteins are returned to the amino acid pool, and the iron is shuttled back to the surface of the RE cell, where it is presented to circulating transferrin. It is the efficient and highly conserved recycling of iron from senescent red cells that supports steady state (and even mildly accelerated) erythropoiesis.

Because each milliliter of red cells contains 1 mg of elemental iron, the amount of iron needed to replace those red cells lost through senescence amounts to 20 mg/d (assuming an adult with a red cell mass of 2 L). Any additional iron required for daily red cell production comes from the diet. Normally, an adult male will need to absorb at least 1 mg of elemental iron daily to meet needs, while females in the childbearing years will need to absorb an average of 1.4 mg/d. However, to achieve a maximum proliferative erythroid marrow response to anemia, additional iron must be available. With markedly stimulated erythropoiesis, demands for iron are increased by as much as six- to eightfold. With extravascular hemolytic anemia, the rate of red cell destruction is increased, but the iron recovered from the red cells is efficiently reutilized for hemoglobin synthesis. In contrast, with intravascular hemolysis or blood loss anemia, the rate of red cell production is limited by the amount of iron that can be mobilized from stores. Typically, the rate of mobilization under these circumstances will not support red cell production more than 2.5 times normal. If the delivery of iron to the stimulated marrow is suboptimal, the marrow's proliferative response is blunted, and hemoglobin synthesis is impaired. The result is a hypoproliferative marrow accompanied by microcytic, hypochromic anemia.

Whereas blood loss or hemolysis places a demand on the iron supply, inflammatory conditions interfere with iron release from stores and can result in a rapid decrease in the serum iron (see below).

■ NUTRITIONAL IRON BALANCE

The balance of iron in humans is tightly controlled and designed to conserve iron for reutilization. There is no regulated excretory pathway for iron, and the only mechanisms by which iron is lost are blood loss (via gastrointestinal bleeding, menses, or other forms of bleeding) and the loss of epithelial cells from the skin, gut, and genitourinary tract. Normally, the only route by which iron comes into the body is via absorption from food or from medicinal iron taken orally. Iron may also enter the body through red-cell transfusions or injection of iron complexes. The margin between the amount of iron available for absorption and the requirement for iron in growing infants and the adult female is narrow; this accounts for the great prevalence of iron deficiency worldwide—currently estimated at one-half billion people.

The amount of iron required from the diet to replace losses averages approximately 10% of body iron content a year in men and 15% in women of childbearing age. Dietary iron content is closely related to total caloric intake (approximately 6 mg of elemental iron per 1000 calories). Iron bioavailability is affected by the nature of the foodstuff, with heme iron (e.g., red meat) being most readily absorbed. In the United States, the average iron intake in an adult male is 15 mg/d with 6% absorption; for the average female, the daily intake is 11 mg/d with 12% absorption. An individual with iron deficiency can increase iron absorption to approximately 20% of the iron present in a meat-containing diet but only 5–10% of the iron in a vegetarian diet. As a result, one-third of the female population in the United States has virtually no iron stores. Vegetarians are at an additional disadvantage because certain foodstuffs that include phytates and phosphates reduce iron absorption by approximately 50%. When ionizable iron salts are given together with food, the amount of iron absorbed is reduced. When the percentage of iron absorbed from individual food items is compared with the percentage for an equivalent amount of ferrous salt, iron in vegetables is only about one-twentieth as available, egg iron one-eighth, liver iron one-half, and heme iron one-half to two-thirds.

Infants, children, and adolescents may be unable to maintain normal iron balance because of the demands of body growth and lower dietary intake of iron. During the last two trimesters of pregnancy, daily iron requirements increase to 5–6 mg. That is the reason why iron supplements are strongly recommended for pregnant women in developed countries.

Iron absorption takes place largely in the proximal small intestine and is a carefully regulated process. For absorption, iron must be taken up by the luminal cell. That process is facilitated by the acidic contents of the stomach, which maintains the iron in solution. At the brush border of the absorptive cell, the ferric iron is converted to the ferrous form by a ferrireductase. Transport across the membrane is accomplished by divalent metal transporter type 1 [DMT-1, also known as natural resistance macrophage-associated protein type 2 (Nramp 2) or DCT-1]. DMT-1 is a general cation transporter. Once inside the gut cell, iron may be stored as ferritin or transported through the cell to be released at the basolateral surface to plasma transferrin through the membrane-embedded iron exporter, ferroportin. The function of ferroportin is negatively regulated by hepcidin, the principal iron regulatory hormone. In the process of release, iron interacts with another ferroxidase, hephaestin, which oxidizes the iron to the ferric form for transferrin binding. Hephaestin is similar to ceruloplasmin, the copper-carrying protein.

Iron absorption is influenced by a number of physiologic states. Erythroid hyperplasia stimulates iron absorption even in the face of normal or increased iron stores, and hepcidin levels are inappropriately low. The molecular mechanism underlying this relationship is not known. Thus, patients with anemias associated with high levels of ineffective erythropoiesis absorb excess amounts of dietary iron. Over time, this may lead to iron overload and tissue damage. In iron deficiency, hepcidin levels are low and iron is much more efficiently absorbed; the contrary is true in states of secondary iron overload. The normal individual can reduce iron absorption in situations of excessive intake or medicinal iron intake; however, while the percentage of iron absorbed goes down, the absolute amount goes up. This accounts for the acute iron toxicity occasionally seen when children ingest large numbers of iron tablets. Under these circumstances, the amount of iron absorbed exceeds the transferrin binding capacity of the plasma, resulting in free iron that affects critical organs such as cardiac muscle cells.

IRON-DEFICIENCY ANEMIA

Iron deficiency is one of the most prevalent forms of malnutrition. Globally, 50% of anemia is attributable to iron deficiency and accounts for approximately 841,000 deaths annually worldwide. Africa and parts of Asia bear 71% of the global mortality burden; North America represents only 1.4% of the total morbidity and mortality associated with iron deficiency.

■ STAGES OF IRON DEFICIENCY

The progression to iron deficiency can be divided into three stages (Fig. 103-2). The first stage is *negative iron balance*, in which the demands for (or losses of) iron exceed the body's ability to absorb iron from the diet. This stage results from a number of physiologic mechanisms, including blood loss, pregnancy (in which the demands for red cell production by the fetus outstrip the mother's ability to provide iron), rapid growth spurts in the adolescent, or inadequate dietary iron intake. Blood loss in excess of 10–20 mL of red cells per day is greater than the amount of iron that the gut can absorb from a normal diet. Under these circumstances the iron deficit must be made up by mobilization of iron from RE storage sites. During this period, iron stores—reflected by the serum ferritin level or the appearance of stainable iron on bone marrow aspirations—decrease. As long as iron stores are present and can be mobilized, the serum iron, total iron-binding capacity (TIBC), and red cell protoporphyrin levels remain within normal limits. At this stage, red cell morphology and indices are normal.

When iron stores become depleted, the serum iron begins to fall. Gradually, the TIBC increases, as do red cell protoporphyrin

levels. By definition, marrow iron stores are absent when the serum ferritin level is <15 μg/L. As long as the serum iron remains within the normal range, hemoglobin synthesis is unaffected despite the dwindling iron stores. Once the transferrin saturation falls to 15–20%, hemoglobin synthesis becomes impaired. This is a period of *iron-deficient erythropoiesis*. Careful evaluation of the peripheral blood smear reveals the first appearance of microcytic cells, and if the laboratory technology is available, one finds hypochromic reticulocytes in circulation. Gradually, the hemoglobin and hematocrit begin to fall, reflecting *iron-deficiency anemia*. The transferrin saturation at this point is 10–15%.

When moderate anemia is present (hemoglobin 10–13 g/dL), the bone marrow remains hypoproliferative. With more severe anemia (hemoglobin 7–8 g/dL), hypochromia and microcytosis become more prominent, target cells and misshapen red cells (poikilocytes) appear on the blood smear as cigar- or pencil-shaped forms, and the erythroid marrow becomes increasingly ineffective. Consequently, with severe prolonged iron-deficiency anemia, erythroid hyperplasia of the marrow develops, rather than hypoproliferation.

■ CAUSES OF IRON DEFICIENCY

Conditions that increase demand for iron, increase iron loss, or decrease iron intake or absorption can produce iron deficiency (Table 103-2).

■ CLINICAL PRESENTATION OF IRON DEFICIENCY

Certain clinical conditions carry an increased likelihood of iron deficiency. Pregnancy, adolescence, periods of rapid growth, and an intermittent history of blood loss of any kind should alert the clinician to possible iron deficiency. A cardinal rule is that the appearance of iron deficiency in an adult male means gastrointestinal blood loss until proven otherwise. Signs related to iron deficiency depend on the severity and chronicity of the anemia in addition to the usual signs of anemia—fatigue, pallor, and reduced exercise capacity. *Cheilosis* (fissures at the corners of the mouth) and *koilonychia* (spooning of the fingernails) are signs of advanced tissue iron deficiency. The diagnosis of iron deficiency is typically based on laboratory results.

	Normal	Negative iron balance	Iron-deficient erythropoiesis	Iron-deficiency anemia
Iron stores				
Erythron iron				
Marrow iron stores	1-3+	0-1+	0	0
Serum ferritin (μg/L)	50-200	<20	<15	<15
TIBC (μg/dL)	300-360	>360	>380	>400
SI (μg/dL)	50-150	NL	<50	<30
Saturation (%)	30-50	NL	<20	<10
Marrow sideroblasts (%)	40-60	NL	<10	<10
RBC protoporphyrin (μg/dL)	30-50	NL	>100	>200
RBC morphology	NL	NL	NL	Microcytic/ hypochromic

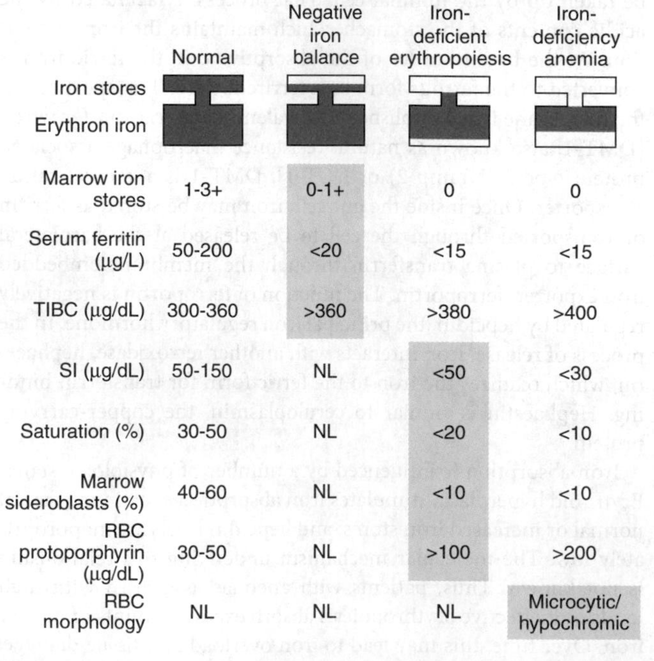

Figure 103-2 **Laboratory studies in the evolution of iron deficiency.** Measurements of marrow iron stores, serum ferritin, and total iron-binding capacity (TIBC) are sensitive to early iron-store depletion. Iron-deficient erythropoiesis is recognized from additional abnormalities in the serum iron (SI), percent transferrin saturation, the pattern of marrow sideroblasts, and the red cell protoporphyrin level. Patients with iron-deficiency anemia demonstrate all the same abnormalities plus hypochromic microcytic anemia. *(From Hillman and Finch, with permission.)*

TABLE 103-2 Causes of Iron Deficiency

Increased Demand for Iron

Rapid growth in infancy or adolescence

Pregnancy

Erythropoietin therapy

Increased Iron Loss

Chronic blood loss

Menses

Acute blood loss

Blood donation

Phlebotomy as treatment for polycythemia vera

Decreased Iron Intake or Absorption

Inadequate diet

Malabsorption from disease (sprue, Crohn's disease)

Malabsorption from surgery (postgastrectomy)

Acute or chronic inflammation

LABORATORY IRON STUDIES

Serum iron and total iron-binding capacity

The serum iron level represents the amount of circulating iron bound to transferrin. The TIBC is an indirect measure of the circulating transferrin. The normal range for the serum iron is 50–150 µg/dL; the normal range for TIBC is 300–360 µg/dL. Transferrin saturation, which is normally 25–50%, is obtained by the following formula: serum iron × 100 ÷ TIBC. Iron-deficiency states are associated with saturation levels below 20%. There is a diurnal variation in the serum iron. A transferrin saturation >50% indicates that a disproportionate amount of the iron bound to transferrin is being delivered to nonerythroid tissues. If this persists for an extended time, tissue iron overload may occur.

Serum ferritin

Free iron is toxic to cells, and the body has established an elaborate set of protective mechanisms to bind iron in various tissue compartments. Within cells, iron is stored complexed to protein as ferritin or hemosiderin. Apoferritin binds to free ferrous iron and stores it in the ferric state. As ferritin accumulates within cells of the RE system, protein aggregates are formed as hemosiderin. Iron in ferritin or hemosiderin can be extracted for release by the RE cells, although hemosiderin is less readily available. Under steady-state conditions, the serum ferritin level correlates with total body iron stores; thus, the serum ferritin level is the most convenient laboratory test to estimate iron stores. The normal value for ferritin varies according to the age and gender of the individual (Fig. 103-3). Adult males have serum ferritin values averaging 100 µg/L, while adult females have levels averaging 30 µg/L. As iron stores are depleted, the serum ferritin falls to <15 µg/L. Such levels are diagnostic of absent body iron stores.

Evaluation of bone marrow iron stores

Although RE cell iron stores can be estimated from the iron stain of a bone marrow aspirate or biopsy, the measurement of serum ferritin has largely supplanted bone marrow aspirates for determination of storage iron (Table 103-3). The serum ferritin level is a better indicator of iron overload than the marrow iron stain. However, in addition to storage iron, the marrow iron stain provides information about the effective delivery of iron to developing erythroblasts. Normally, when the marrow smear is stained for iron, 20–40% of developing erythroblasts—called *sideroblasts*—will have visible

TABLE 103-3 Iron Store Measurements

Iron Stores	Marrow Iron Stain, 0-4+	Serum Ferritin, µg/L
0	0	<15
1–300 mg	Trace to 1+	15–30
300–800 mg	2+	30–60
800–1000 mg	3+	60–150
1–2 g	4+	>150
Iron overload	—	>500–1000

ferritin granules in their cytoplasm. This represents iron in excess of that needed for hemoglobin synthesis. In states in which release of iron from storage sites is blocked, RE iron will be detectable, and there will be few or no sideroblasts. In the myelodysplastic syndromes, mitochondrial dysfunction can occur, and accumulation of iron in mitochondria appears in a necklace fashion around the nucleus of the erythroblast. Such cells are referred to as *ringed sideroblasts*.

Red cell protoporphyrin levels

Protoporphyrin is an intermediate in the pathway to heme synthesis. Under conditions in which heme synthesis is impaired, protoporphyrin accumulates within the red cell. This reflects an inadequate iron supply to erythroid precursors to support hemoglobin synthesis. Normal values are <30 µg/dL of red cells. In iron deficiency, values in excess of 100 µg/dL are seen. The most common causes of increased red cell protoporphyrin levels are absolute or relative iron deficiency and lead poisoning.

Serum levels of transferrin receptor protein

Because erythroid cells have the highest numbers of transferrin receptors of any cell in the body, and because transferrin receptor protein (TRP) is released by cells into the circulation, serum levels of TRP reflect the total erythroid marrow mass. Another condition in which TRP levels are elevated is absolute iron deficiency. Normal values are 4–9 µg/L determined by immunoassay. This laboratory test is becoming increasingly available and, along with the serum ferritin, has been proposed to distinguish between iron deficiency and the anemia of chronic inflammation (see below).

DIFFERENTIAL DIAGNOSIS

Other than iron deficiency, only three conditions need to be considered in the differential diagnosis of a hypochromic microcytic anemia (Table 103-4). The first is an inherited defect in globin chain synthesis: the thalassemias. These are differentiated from iron deficiency most readily by serum iron values; normal or increased serum iron levels and transferrin saturation are characteristic of the thalassemias. In addition, red blood cell distribution width (RDW) index is generally small in thalassemia and elevated in iron deficiency.

The second condition is the anemia of chronic inflammation with inadequate iron supply to the erythroid marrow. The distinction between true iron-deficiency anemia and the anemia associated with chronic inflammation is among the most common diagnostic problem encountered by clinicians (see below). Usually the anemia of chronic inflammation is normocytic and normochromic. The iron values usually make the differential diagnosis clear, as the ferritin level is normal or increased and the percent transferrin saturation and TIBC are typically below normal.

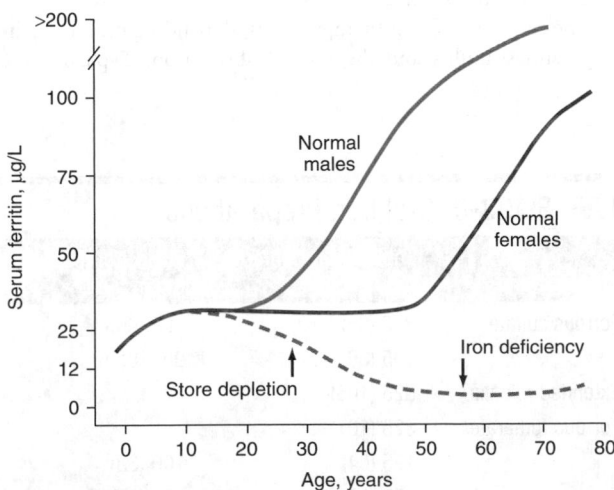

Figure 103-3 Serum ferritin levels as a function of sex and age. Iron store depletion and iron deficiency are accompanied by a decrease in serum ferritin level below 20 µg/L. *(From Hillman et al, with permission.)*

TABLE 103-4 Diagnosis of Microcytic Anemia

Tests	Iron Deficiency	Inflammation	Thalassemia	Sideroblastic Anemia
Smear	Micro/hypo	Normal micro/hypo	Micro/hypo with targeting	Variable
SI	<30	<50	Normal to high	Normal to high
TIBC	>360	<300	Normal	Normal
Percent saturation	<10	10–20	30–80	30–80
Ferritin (μg/L)	<15	30–200	50–300	50–300
Hemoglobin pattern on electrophoresis	Normal	Normal	Abnormal with β thalassemia; can be normal with α thalassemia	Normal

Abbreviations: SI, serum iron; TIBC, total iron-binding capacity.

Finally, the myelodysplastic syndromes represent the third and least common condition. Occasionally, patients with myelodysplasia have impaired hemoglobin synthesis with mitochondrial dysfunction, resulting in impaired iron incorporation into heme. The iron values again reveal normal stores and more than an adequate supply to the marrow, despite the microcytosis and hypochromia.

TREATMENT   Iron-Deficiency Anemia

The severity and cause of iron-deficiency anemia will determine the appropriate approach to treatment. As an example, symptomatic elderly patients with severe iron-deficiency anemia and cardiovascular instability may require red cell transfusions. Younger individuals who have compensated for their anemia can be treated more conservatively with iron replacement. The foremost issue for the latter patient is the precise identification of the cause of the iron deficiency.

For the majority of cases of iron deficiency (pregnant women, growing children and adolescents, patients with infrequent episodes of bleeding, and those with inadequate dietary intake of iron), oral iron therapy will suffice. For patients with unusual blood loss or malabsorption, specific diagnostic tests and appropriate therapy take priority. Once the diagnosis of iron-deficiency anemia and its cause is made, there are three major therapeutic approaches.

RED CELL TRANSFUSION Transfusion therapy is reserved for individuals who have symptoms of anemia, cardiovascular instability, continued and excessive blood loss from whatever source, and require immediate intervention. The management of these patients is less related to the iron deficiency than it is to the consequences of the severe anemia. Not only do transfusions correct the anemia acutely, but the transfused red cells provide a source of iron for reutilization, assuming they are not lost through continued bleeding. Transfusion therapy will stabilize the patient while other options are reviewed.

ORAL IRON THERAPY In the asymptomatic patient with established iron-deficiency anemia, treatment with oral iron is usually adequate. Multiple preparations are available, ranging from simple iron salts to complex iron compounds designed for sustained release throughout the small intestine (Table 103-5). Although the various preparations contain different amounts of iron, they are generally all absorbed well and are effective in treatment. Some come with other compounds designed to enhance iron absorption, such as ascorbic acid. It is not clear whether the benefits of such compounds justify their costs. Typically, for

iron replacement therapy, up to 300 mg of elemental iron per day is given, usually as three or four iron tablets (each containing 50–65 mg elemental iron) given over the course of the day. Ideally, oral iron preparations should be taken on an empty stomach, since food may inhibit iron absorption. Some patients with gastric disease or prior gastric surgery require special treatment with iron solutions, as the retention capacity of the stomach may be reduced. The retention capacity is necessary for dissolving the shell of the iron tablet before the release of iron. A dose of 200–300 mg of elemental iron per day should result in the absorption of iron up to 50 mg/d. This supports a red cell production level of two to three times normal in an individual with a normally functioning marrow and appropriate erythropoietin stimulus. However, as the hemoglobin level rises, erythropoietin stimulation decreases, and the amount of iron absorbed is reduced. The goal of therapy in individuals with iron-deficiency anemia is not only to repair the anemia, but also to provide stores of at least 0.5–1 g of iron. Sustained treatment for a period of 6–12 months after correction of the anemia will be necessary to achieve this.

Of the complications of oral iron therapy, gastrointestinal distress is the most prominent and is seen in 15–20% of patients. Abdominal pain, nausea, vomiting, or constipation may lead to noncompliance. Although small doses of iron or iron preparations with delayed release may help somewhat, the gastrointestinal side effects are a major impediment to the effective treatment of a number of patients.

The response to iron therapy varies, depending on the erythropoietin stimulus and the rate of absorption. Typically, the

TABLE 103-5 Oral Iron Preparations

Generic Name	Tablet (Iron Content), mg	Elixir (Iron Content), mg in 5 mL
Ferrous sulfate	325 (65)	300 (60)
	195 (39)	90 (18)
Extended release	525 (105)	
Ferrous fumarate	325 (107)	
	195 (64)	100 (33)
Ferrous gluconate	325 (39)	300 (35)
Polysaccharide iron	150 (150)	100 (100)
	50 (50)	

reticulocyte count should begin to increase within 4–7 days after initiation of therapy and peak at 1–1½ weeks. The absence of a response may be due to poor absorption, noncompliance (which is common), or a confounding diagnosis. A useful test in the clinic to determine the patient's ability to absorb iron is the *iron tolerance test*. Two iron tablets are given to the patient on an empty stomach, and the serum iron is measured serially over the subsequent 2 hours. Normal absorption will result in an increase in the serum iron of at least 100 μg/dL. If iron deficiency persists despite adequate treatment, it may be necessary to switch to parenteral iron therapy.

PARENTERAL IRON THERAPY Intravenous iron can be given to patients who are unable to tolerate oral iron; whose needs are relatively acute; or who need iron on an ongoing basis, usually due to persistent gastrointestinal blood loss. Parenteral iron use has been increasing rapidly in the last several years with the recognition that recombinant erythropoietin (EPO) therapy induces a large demand for iron—a demand that frequently cannot be met through the physiologic release of iron from RE sources or oral iron absorption. The safety of parenteral iron—particularly iron dextran—has been a concern. The serious adverse reaction rate to intravenous high-molecular weight iron dextran is 0.7%. Fortunately, newer iron complexes are available in the United States, such as sodium ferric gluconate (Ferrlecit) and iron sucrose (Venofer) that have much lower rates of adverse effects.

Parenteral iron is used in two ways: one is to administer the total dose of iron required to correct the hemoglobin deficit and provide the patient with at least 500 mg of iron stores; the second is to give repeated small doses of parenteral iron over a protracted period. The latter approach is common in dialysis centers, where it is not unusual for 100 mg of elemental iron to be given weekly for 10 weeks to augment the response to recombinant EPO therapy. The amount of iron needed by an individual patient is calculated by the following formula:

$$\text{Body weight (kg)} \times 2.3 \times (15 - \text{patient's hemoglobin, g/dL}) +$$
$$500 \text{ or } 1000 \text{ mg (for stores)}.$$

In administering intravenous iron dextran, anaphylaxis is a concern. Anaphylaxis is much rarer with the newer preparations. The factors that have correlated with an anaphylactic-like reaction include a history of multiple allergies or a prior allergic reaction to dextran (in the case of iron dextran). Generalized symptoms appearing several days after the infusion of a large dose of iron can include arthralgias, skin rash, and low-grade fever. These may be dose-related, but they do not preclude the further use of parenteral iron in the patient. To date, patients with sensitivity to iron dextran have been safely treated with iron gluconate. If a large dose of iron dextran is to be given (>100 mg), the iron preparation should be diluted in 5% dextrose in water or 0.9% NaCl solution. The iron solution can then be infused over a 60- to 90-minute period (for larger doses) or at a rate convenient for the attending nurse or physician. Although a test dose (25 mg) of parenteral iron dextran is recommended, in reality a slow infusion of a larger dose of parenteral iron solution will afford the same kind of early warning as a separately injected test dose. Early in the infusion of iron, if chest pain, wheezing, a fall in blood pressure, or other systemic symptoms occur, the infusion of iron should be stopped immediately.

OTHER HYPOPROLIFERATIVE ANEMIAS

In addition to mild to moderate iron-deficiency anemia, the hypoproliferative anemias can be divided into four categories: (1) chronic inflammation, (2) renal disease, (3) endocrine and

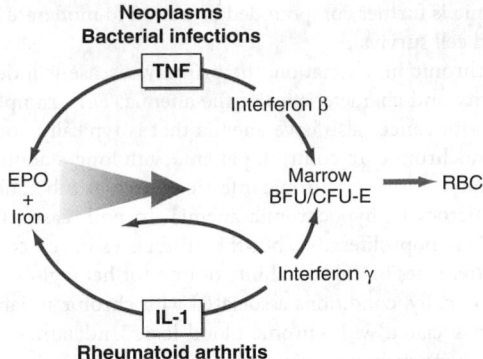

Figure 103-4 Suppression of erythropoiesis by inflammatory cytokines. Through the release of tumor necrosis factor (TNF) and interferon γ (IFN-γ), neoplasms and bacterial infections suppress erythropoietin (EPO) production and the proliferation of erythroid progenitors [erythroid burst-forming units and erythroid colony-forming units (BFU/CFU-E)]. The mediators in patients with vasculitis and rheumatoid arthritis include interleukin 1 (IL-1) and IFN-γ The red arrows indicate sites of inflammatory cytokine inhibitory effects.

nutritional deficiencies (hypometabolic states), and (4) marrow damage (Chap. 107). With chronic inflammation, renal disease, or hypometabolism, endogenous EPO production is inadequate for the degree of anemia observed. For the anemia of chronic inflammation, the erythroid marrow also responds inadequately to stimulation, due in part to defective *iron reutilization*. As a result of the lack of adequate EPO stimulation, an examination of the peripheral blood smear will disclose only an occasional polychromatophilic ("shift") reticulocyte. In cases of iron deficiency or marrow damage, appropriate elevations in endogenous EPO levels are typically found, and shift reticulocytes will be present on the blood smear.

◼ ANEMIA OF ACUTE AND CHRONIC INFLAMMATION/INFECTION (THE ANEMIA OF INFLAMMATION)

The anemia of inflammation—which encompasses inflammation, infection, tissue injury, and conditions (such as cancer) associated with the release of proinflammatory cytokines—is one of the most common forms of anemia seen clinically. It is the most important anemia in the differential diagnosis of iron deficiency, because many of the features of the anemia are brought about by inadequate iron delivery to the marrow, despite the presence of normal or increased iron stores. This is reflected by a low serum iron, increased red cell protoporphyrin, a hypoproliferative marrow, transferrin saturation in the range of 15–20%, and a normal or increased serum ferritin. The serum ferritin values are often the most distinguishing features between true iron-deficiency anemia and the iron-restricted erythropoiesis associated with inflammation. Typically, serum ferritin values increase threefold over basal levels in the face of inflammation. These changes are due to the effects of inflammatory cytokines and hepcidin, the key iron regulatory hormone, acting at several levels of erythropoiesis (Fig. 103-4).

Interleukin 1 (IL-1) directly decreases EPO production in response to anemia. IL-1, acting through accessory cell release of interferon γ (IFN-γ), suppresses the response of the erythroid marrow to EPO—an effect that can be overcome by EPO administration in vitro and in vivo. In addition, tumor necrosis factor (TNF), acting through the release of IFN-γ by marrow stromal cells, also suppresses the response to EPO. Hepcidin, made by the liver, is increased in inflammation and acts to suppress iron absorption and iron release from storage sites. The overall result is a chronic hypoproliferative anemia with classic changes in iron metabolism.

The anemia is further compounded by a mild to moderate shortening in red cell survival.

With chronic inflammation, the primary disease will determine the severity and characteristics of the anemia. For example, many patients with cancer also have anemia that is typically normocytic and normochromic. In contrast, patients with long-standing active rheumatoid arthritis or chronic infections such as tuberculosis will have a microcytic, hypochromic anemia. In both cases, the bone marrow is hypoproliferative, but the differences in red cell indices reflect differences in the availability of iron for hemoglobin synthesis. Occasionally, conditions associated with chronic inflammation are also associated with chronic blood loss. Under these circumstances, a bone marrow aspirate stained for iron may be necessary to rule out absolute iron deficiency. However, the administration of iron in this case will correct the iron deficiency component of the anemia and leave the inflammatory component unaffected.

The anemia associated with acute infection or inflammation is typically mild but becomes more pronounced over time. Acute infection can produce a decrease in hemoglobin levels of 2–3 g/dL within 1 or 2 days; this is largely related to the hemolysis of red cells near the end of their natural life span. The fever and cytokines released exert a selective pressure against cells with more limited capacity to maintain the red cell membrane. In most individuals the mild anemia is reasonably well tolerated, and symptoms, if present, are associated with the underlying disease. Occasionally, in patients with preexisting cardiac disease, moderate anemia (hemoglobin 10–11 g/dL) may be associated with angina, exercise intolerance, and shortness of breath. The erythropoietic profile that distinguishes the anemia of inflammation from the other causes of hypoproliferative anemias is shown in Table 103-6.

ANEMIA OF CHRONIC KIDNEY DISEASE (CKD)

Progressive CKD is usually associated with a moderate to severe hypoproliferative anemia; the level of the anemia correlates with the stage of CKD. Red cells are typically normocytic and normochromic, and reticulocytes are decreased. The anemia is primarily due to a failure of EPO production by the diseased kidney and a reduction in red cell survival. In certain forms of acute renal failure, the correlation between the anemia and renal function is weaker. Patients with the hemolytic-uremic syndrome increase erythropoiesis in response to the hemolysis, despite renal failure requiring dialysis. Polycystic kidney disease also shows a smaller degree of EPO deficiency for a given level of renal failure. By contrast, patients with diabetes or myeloma have more severe EPO deficiency for a given level of renal failure.

Assessment of iron status provides information to distinguish the anemia of CKD from the other forms of hypoproliferative anemia (Table 103-6) and to guide management. Patients with the anemia of CKD usually present with normal serum iron, TIBC, and ferritin levels. However, those maintained on chronic hemodialysis may develop iron deficiency from blood loss through the dialysis procedure. Iron must be replenished in these patients to ensure an adequate response to EPO therapy (see below).

ANEMIA IN HYPOMETABOLIC STATES

Patients who are starving, particularly for protein, and those with a variety of endocrine disorders that produce lower metabolic rates, may develop a mild to moderate hypoproliferative anemia. The release of EPO from the kidney is sensitive to the need for O_2, not just O_2 levels. Thus, EPO production is triggered at lower levels of blood O_2 content in disease states (such as hypothyroidism and starvation) where metabolic activity, and thus O_2 demand, is decreased.

Endocrine deficiency states

The difference in the levels of hemoglobin between men and women is related to the effects of androgen and estrogen on erythropoiesis. Testosterone and anabolic steroids augment erythropoiesis; castration and estrogen administration to males decrease erythropoiesis. Patients who are hypothyroid or have deficits in pituitary hormones also may develop a mild anemia. Pathogenesis may be complicated by other nutritional deficiencies because iron and folic acid absorption can be affected by these disorders. Usually, correction of the hormone deficiency reverses the anemia.

Anemia may be more severe in Addison's disease, depending on the level of thyroid and androgen hormone dysfunction; however, anemia may be masked by decreases in plasma volume. Once such patients are given cortisol and volume replacement, the hemoglobin level may fall rapidly. Mild anemia complicating hyperparathyroidism may be due to decreased EPO production as a consequence of the renal effects of hypercalcemia or to impaired proliferation of erythroid progenitors.

Protein starvation

Decreased dietary intake of protein may lead to mild to moderate hypoproliferative anemia; this form of anemia may be prevalent in the elderly. The anemia can be more severe in patients with a greater degree of starvation. In marasmus, where patients are both protein and calorie deficient, the release of EPO is impaired in proportion to the reduction in metabolic rate; however, the degree of

TABLE 103-6 Diagnosis of Hypoproliferative Anemias

Tests	Iron Deficiency	Inflammation	Renal Disease	Hypometabolic States
Anemia	Mild to severe	Mild	Mild to severe	Mild
MCV (fL)	60–90	80–90	90	90
Morphology	Normo-microcytic	Normocytic	Normocytic	Normocytic
SI	<30	<50	Normal	Normal
TIBC	>360	<300	Normal	Normal
Saturation (%)	<10	10–20	Normal	Normal
Serum ferritin (μg/L)	<15	30–200	115–150	Normal
Iron stores	0	2–4+	1–4+	Normal

Abbreviations: MCV, mean corpuscular volume; SI, serum iron; TIBC, total iron-binding capacity.

anemia may be masked by volume depletion and becomes apparent after refeeding. Deficiencies in other nutrients (iron, folate) may also complicate the clinical picture but may not be apparent at diagnosis. Changes in the erythrocyte indices on refeeding should prompt evaluation of iron, folate, and B$_{12}$ status.

Anemia in liver disease

A mild hypoproliferative anemia may develop in patients with chronic liver disease from nearly any cause. The peripheral blood smear may show spur cells and stomatocytes from the accumulation of excess cholesterol in the membrane from a deficiency of lecithin-cholesterol acyltransferase. Red cell survival is shortened, and the production of EPO is inadequate to compensate. In alcoholic liver disease, nutritional deficiencies are common and complicate the management. Folate deficiency from inadequate intake, as well as iron deficiency from blood loss and inadequate intake, can alter the red cell indices.

TREATMENT   Hypoproliferative Anemias

Many patients with hypoproliferative anemias experience recovery of normal hemoglobin levels when the underlying disease is appropriately treated. For those in whom such reversals are not possible—such as patients with end-stage kidney disease, cancer, and chronic inflammatory diseases—symptomatic anemia requires treatment. The two major forms of treatment are transfusions and EPO.

TRANSFUSIONS Thresholds for transfusion should be altered based on the patient's symptoms. In general, patients without serious underlying cardiovascular or pulmonary disease can tolerate hemoglobin levels above 8 g/dL and do not require intervention until the hemoglobin falls below that level. Patients with more physiologic compromise may need to have their hemoglobin levels kept above 11 g/dL. A typical unit of packed red cells increases the hemoglobin level by 1 g/dL. Transfusions are associated with certain infectious risks (Chap. 113), and chronic transfusions can produce iron overload. Importantly, the liberal use of blood has been associated with increased morbidity and mortality, particularly in the intensive care setting. Therefore, in the absence of documented tissue hypoxia, a conservative approach to the use of red cell transfusions is preferable.

ERYTHROPOIETIN (EPO) EPO is particularly useful in anemias in which endogenous EPO levels are inappropriately low, such as CKD or the anemia of chronic inflammation. Iron status must be evaluated and iron repleted to obtain optimal effects from EPO. In patients with CKD, the usual dose of EPO is 50–150 U/kg three times a week intravenously. Hemoglobin levels of 10–12 g/dL are usually reached within 4–6 weeks if iron levels are adequate; 90% of these patients respond. Once a target hemoglobin level is achieved, the EPO dose can be decreased. A decrease in hemoglobin level occurring in the face of EPO therapy usually signifies the development of an infection or iron depletion. Aluminum toxicity and hyperparathyroidism can also compromise the EPO response. When an infection intervenes, it is best to interrupt the EPO therapy and rely on transfusion to correct the anemia until the infection is adequately treated. The dose needed to correct the anemia in patients with cancer is higher, up to 300 U/kg three times a week, and only approximately 60% of patients respond. Because of evidence that tumor progression may result from EPO administration, the risks and benefits of using EPO in patients with chemotherapy-induced anemia must be weighed carefully, and the target hemoglobin should be that necessary to avoid transfusions.

Longer-acting preparations of EPO can reduce the frequency of injections. Darbepoetin alfa, a molecularly modified EPO with additional carbohydrate, has a half-life in the circulation that is three to four times longer than recombinant human EPO, permitting weekly or every other week dosing.

FURTHER READINGS

ANDREWS, NC. Forging a field: The golden age of iron biology. Blood 112:219, 2008

BAILIE GR et al: Parenteral iron use in the management of anemia in end-stage renal disease patients. Am J Kidney Dis 35:1, 2000

BRUGNARA C: Iron deficiency and erythropoiesis: New diagnostic approaches. Clin Chem 49:1573, 2003

FERRUCCI L et al: Proinflammatory state, hepcidin, and anemia in older persons. Blood 115:3810, 2010

GANZ T: Hepcidin, a key regulator of iron metabolism and mediator of inflammation. Blood 102:783, 2003

HILLMAN RS et al: *Hematology in Clinical Practice*, 5th ed, New York, McGraw-Hill, 2010

STOLTZFUS RF: Iron deficiency: Global prevalence and consequences. Food Nutr Bull 24:S99, 2003

THOMAS C et al: The diagnostic plot: A concept for identifying different states of iron deficiency and monitoring the response to epoetin therapy. Med Oncol 23:23, 2006

CHAPTER 104
Disorders of Hemoglobin

Edward J. Benz, Jr.

Hemoglobin is critical for normal oxygen delivery to tissues; it is also present in erythrocytes in such high concentrations that it can alter red cell shape, deformability, and viscosity. Hemoglobinopathies are disorders affecting the structure, function, or production of hemoglobin. These conditions are usually inherited and range in severity from asymptomatic laboratory abnormalities to death in utero. Different forms may present as hemolytic anemia, erythrocytosis, cyanosis, or vasoocclusive stigmata.

PROPERTIES OF THE HUMAN HEMOGLOBINS
■ HEMOGLOBIN STRUCTURE

Different hemoglobins are produced during embryonic, fetal, and adult life (Fig. 104-1). Each consists of a tetramer of globin polypeptide chains: a pair of α-like chains 141 amino acids long and a pair of β-like chains 146 amino acids long. The major adult hemoglobin, HbA, has the structure $\alpha_2\beta_2$. HbF ($\alpha_2\gamma_2$) predominates during most of gestation, and HbA_2 ($\alpha_2\delta_2$) is minor adult hemoglobin. Embryonic hemoglobins need not be considered here.

Each globin chain enfolds a single heme moiety, consisting of a protoporphyrin IX ring complexed with a single iron atom in the ferrous state (Fe^{2+}). Each heme moiety can bind a single oxygen molecule; a molecule of hemoglobin can transport up to four oxygen molecules.

The amino acid sequences of the various globins are highly homologous to one another. Each has a highly helical *secondary structure*. Their globular *tertiary structures* cause the exterior surfaces to be rich in polar (hydrophilic) amino acids that enhance solubility, and the interior to be lined with nonpolar groups, forming a hydrophobic pocket into which heme is inserted. The tetrameric *quaternary structure* of HbA contains two αβ dimers. Numerous tight interactions (i.e., $\alpha_1\beta_1$ contacts) hold the α and β chains together. The complete tetramer is held together by interfaces (i.e., $\alpha_1\beta_2$ contacts) between the α-like chain of one dimer and the non-α chain of the other dimer.

The hemoglobin tetramer is highly soluble but individual globin chains are insoluble. Unpaired globin precipitates, forming inclusions that damage the cell. Normal globin chain synthesis is balanced so that each newly synthesized α or non-α globin chain will have an available partner with which to pair.

Solubility and reversible oxygen binding are the key properties deranged in hemoglobinopathies. Both depend most on the hydrophilic surface amino acids, the hydrophobic amino acids lining the heme pocket, a key histidine in the F helix, and the amino acids forming the $\alpha_1\beta_1$ and $\alpha_1\beta_2$ contact points. Mutations in these strategic regions tend to be the ones that alter oxygen affinity or solubility.

■ FUNCTION OF HEMOGLOBIN

To support oxygen transport, hemoglobin must bind O_2 efficiently at the partial pressure of oxygen (PO_2) of the alveolus, retain it, and release it to tissues at the PO_2 of tissue capillary beds. Oxygen acquisition and delivery over a relatively narrow range of oxygen tensions depend on a property inherent in the tetrameric arrangement of heme and globin subunits within the hemoglobin molecule called *cooperativity* or *heme-heme interaction*.

At low oxygen tensions, the hemoglobin tetramer is fully deoxygenated (Fig. 104-2). Oxygen binding begins slowly as O_2 tension rises. However, as soon as some oxygen has been bound by the tetramer, an abrupt increase occurs in the slope of the curve. Thus, hemoglobin molecules that have bound some oxygen develop a higher oxygen affinity, greatly accelerating their ability to combine with more oxygen. This S-shaped oxygen equilibrium curve (Fig. 104-2), along which substantial amounts of oxygen loading and unloading can occur over a narrow range of oxygen tensions, is physiologically more useful than the high-affinity hyperbolic curve of individual monomers.

Oxygen affinity is modulated by several factors. The Bohr effect is the ability of hemoglobin to deliver more oxygen to tissues at low pH. It arises from the stabilizing action of protons on deoxyhemoglobin, which binds protons more readily than oxyhemoglobin because the latter is a weaker acid (Fig. 104-2). Thus, hemoglobin has a lower oxygen affinity at low pH. The major small molecule that alters oxygen affinity in humans is 2,3-bisphosphoglycerate (2,3-BPG, formerly 2,3-DPG), which lowers oxygen affinity when bound to hemoglobin. HbA has a reasonably high affinity for 2,3-BPG. HbF does not bind 2,3-BPG, so it tends to have a higher oxygen affinity in vivo. Hemoglobin also binds nitric oxide reversibly; this interaction influences vascular tone, but its clinical relevance remains controversial.

Proper oxygen transport depends on the tetrameric structure of the proteins, the proper arrangement of the charged amino acids, and interaction with protons or 2,3-BPG.

■ DEVELOPMENTAL BIOLOGY OF HUMAN HEMOGLOBINS

Red cells first appearing at about 6 weeks after conception contain the embryonic hemoglobins Hb Portland ($\zeta_2\gamma_2$), Hb Gower I ($\zeta_2\epsilon_2$), and Hb Gower II ($\alpha_2\epsilon_2$). At 10–11 weeks, fetal hemoglobin (HbF; $\alpha_2\gamma_2$) becomes predominant. The switch to nearly exclusive synthesis of adult hemoglobin (HbA; $\alpha_2\beta_2$) occurs at about 38 weeks (Fig. 104-1). Fetuses and newborns therefore require α-globin but not β-globin for normal gestation. A major advance in understanding the HbF to HbA transition has been the demonstration that the transcription factor Bcl11a plays a pivotal role in its regulation. Small amounts of HbF are produced during postnatal life. A few red cell clones called *F cells* are progeny of a small pool of immature committed erythroid precursors (BFU-e) that retain the ability to produce HbF. Profound erythroid stresses, such as severe hemolytic anemias, bone marrow transplantation, or cancer chemotherapy, cause more of the F-potent

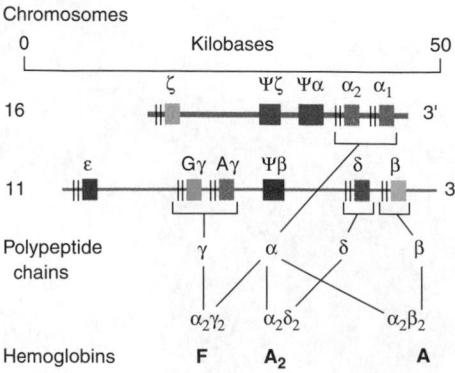

Figure 104-1 **The globin genes.** The α-like genes (α,ζ) are encoded on chromosome 16; the β-like genes (β,γ,δ,ε) are encoded on chromosome 11. The ζ and ε genes encode embryonic globins.

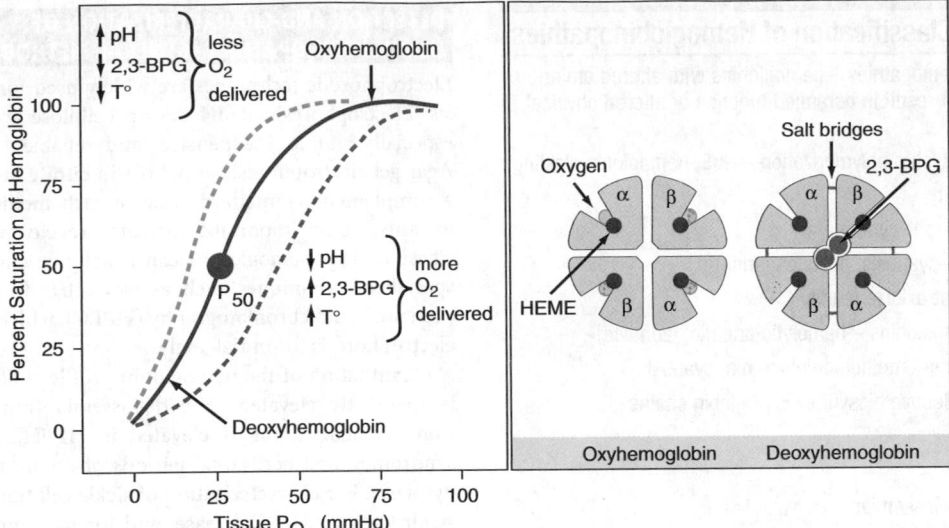

Figure 104-2 Hemoglobin-oxygen dissociation curve. The hemoglobin tetramer can bind up to four molecules of oxygen in the iron-containing sites of the heme molecules. As oxygen is bound, 2,3-BPG and CO_2 are expelled. Salt bridges are broken, and each of the globin molecules changes its conformation to facilitate oxygen binding. Oxygen release to the tissues is the reverse process, salt bridges being formed and 2,3-BPG and CO_2 bound. Deoxyhemoglobin does not bind oxygen efficiently until the cell returns to conditions of higher pH, the most important modulator of O_2 affinity (Bohr effect). When acid is produced in the tissues, the dissociation curve shifts to the right, facilitating oxygen release and CO_2 binding. Alkalosis has the opposite effect, reducing oxygen delivery.

BFU-e to be recruited. HbF levels thus tend to rise in some patients with sickle cell anemia or thalassemia. This phenomenon probably explains the ability of hydroxyurea to increase levels of HbF in adults. Agents such as butyrate and histone deacetylase inhibitors can also activate fetal globin genes partially after birth.

■ GENETICS AND BIOSYNTHESIS OF HUMAN HEMOGLOBIN

The human hemoglobins are encoded in two tightly linked gene clusters; the α-like globin genes are clustered on chromosome 16 and the β-like genes on chromosome 11 (Fig. 104-1). The α-like cluster consists of two α-globin genes and a single copy of the ζ gene. The non-α gene cluster consists of a single ε gene, the Gγ and Aγ fetal globin genes, and the adult δ and β genes.

Important regulatory sequences flank each gene. Immediately upstream are typical promoter elements needed for the assembly of the transcription initiation complex. Sequences in the 5′ flanking region of the γ and the β genes appear to be crucial for the correct developmental regulation of these genes, while elements that function like classic enhancers and silencers are in the 3′ flanking regions. The locus control region (LCR) elements located far upstream appear to control the overall level of expression of each cluster. These elements achieve their regulatory effects by interacting with trans-acting transcription factors. Some of these factors are ubiquitous (e.g., Sp1 and YY1), while others are more or less limited to erythroid cells or hematopoietic cells (e.g., GATA-1, NFE-2, and EKLF). The LCR controlling the α-globin gene cluster is modulated by a SWI/SNF-like protein called *ATRX*; this protein appears to influence chromatin remodeling and DNA methylation. The association of α thalassemia with mental retardation and myelodysplasia in some families appears to be related to mutations in the ATRX pathway. This pathway also modulates genes specifically expressed during erythropoiesis, such as those that encode the enzymes for heme biosynthesis. Normal red blood cell (RBC) differentiation requires the coordinated expression of the globin genes with the genes responsible for heme and iron metabolism. RBC precursors contain a protein, α-hemoglobin-stabilizing protein (AHSP), that enhances the folding and solubility of α globin, which is otherwise easily denatured, leading to insoluble precipitates. These precipitates play an important role in the thalassemia syndromes and certain unstable hemoglobin disorders. Polymorphic variation in the amounts and/or functional capacity of AHSP might explain some of the clinical variability seen in patients inheriting identical thalassemia mutations.

CLASSIFICATION OF HEMOGLOBINOPATHIES

There are five major classes of hemoglobinopathies (Table 104-1). *Structural hemoglobinopathies* occur when mutations alter the amino acid sequence of a globin chain, altering the physiologic properties of the variant hemoglobins and producing the characteristic clinical abnormalities. The most clinically relevant variant hemoglobins polymerize abnormally, as in sickle cell anemia, or exhibit altered solubility or oxygen-binding affinity. *Thalassemia syndromes* arise from mutations that impair production or translation of globin mRNA, leading to deficient globin chain biosynthesis. Clinical abnormalities are attributable to the inadequate supply of hemoglobin and the imbalances in the production of individual globin chains, leading to premature destruction of erythroblasts and RBC. *Thalassemic hemoglobin variants* combine features of thalassemia (e.g., abnormal globin biosynthesis) and of structural hemoglobinopathies (e.g., an abnormal amino acid sequence). *Hereditary persistence of fetal hemoglobin* (HPFH) is characterized by synthesis of high levels of fetal hemoglobin in adult life. *Acquired hemoglobinopathies* include modifications of the hemoglobin molecule by toxins (e.g., acquired methemoglobinemia) and clonal abnormalities of hemoglobin synthesis (e.g., high levels of HbF production in preleukemia and α thalassemia in myeloproliferative disorders).

■ EPIDEMIOLOGY

Hemoglobinopathies are especially common in areas in which malaria is endemic. This clustering of hemoglobinopathies is assumed to reflect a selective survival advantage for the abnormal RBC, which presumably provide a less hospitable environment during the obligate RBC stages of the parasitic life cycle. Very young children with α thalassemia are *more* susceptible to infection with the nonlethal *Plasmodium vivax*. Thalassemia might then favor a natural protection against infection with the more lethal *P. falciparum*.

TABLE 104-1 Classification of Hemoglobinopathies

I. Structural hemoglobinopathies—hemoglobins with altered amino acid sequences that result in deranged function or altered physical or chemical properties

  A. Abnormal hemoglobin polymerization—HbS, hemoglobin sickling

  B. Altered O2 affinity

    1. High affinity—polycythemia

    2. Low affinity—cyanosis, pseudoanemia

  C. Hemoglobins that oxidize readily

    1. Unstable hemoglobins—hemolytic anemia, jaundice

    2. M hemoglobins—methemoglobinemia, cyanosis

II. Thalassemias—defective biosynthesis of globin chains

  A. α Thalassemias

  B. β Thalassemias

  C. δβ, γδβ, αβ Thalassemias

III. Thalassemic hemoglobin variants—structurally abnormal Hb associated with co-inherited thalassemic phenotype

  A. HbE

  B. Hb Constant Spring

  C. Hb Lepore

IV. Hereditary persistence of fetal hemoglobin—persistence of high levels of HbF into adult life

V. Acquired hemoglobinopathies

  A. Methemoglobin due to toxic exposures

  B. Sulfhemoglobin due to toxic exposures

  C. Carboxyhemoglobin

  D. HbH in erythroleukemia

  E. Elevated HbF in states of erythroid stress and bone marrow dysplasia

---

Thalassemias are the most common genetic disorders in the world, affecting nearly 200 million people worldwide. About 15% of American blacks are silent carriers for α thalassemia; α-thalassemia trait (minor) occurs in 3% of American blacks and in 1–15% of persons of Mediterranean origin. β-Thalassemia has a 10–15% incidence in individuals from the Mediterranean and Southeast Asia and 0.8% in American blacks. The number of severe cases of thalassemia in the United States is about 1000. Sickle cell disease is the most common structural hemoglobinopathy, occurring in heterozygous form in ~8% of American blacks and in homozygous form in 1 in 400. Between 2 and 3% of American blacks carry a hemoglobin C allele.

■ INHERITANCE AND ONTOGENY

Hemoglobinopathies are autosomal codominant traits—compound heterozygotes who inherit a different abnormal mutant allele from each parent exhibit composite features of each. For example, patients inheriting sickle β thalassemia exhibit features of β thalassemia and sickle cell anemia. The α chain is present in HbA, HbA_2, and HbF; α-chain mutations thus cause abnormalities in all three. The α-globin hemoglobinopathies are symptomatic in utero and after birth because normal function of the α-globin gene is required throughout gestation and adult life. In contrast, infants with β-globin hemoglobinopathies tend to be asymptomatic until 3–9 months of age, when HbA has largely replaced HbF. Prevention or partial reversion of the switch should thus be an effective therapeutic strategy for β-chain hemoglobinopathies.

DETECTION AND CHARACTERIZATION OF HEMOGLOBINOPATHIES–GENERAL METHODS

Electrophoretic techniques are widely used for hemoglobin analysis. Electrophoresis at pH 8.6 on cellulose acetate membranes is especially simple, inexpensive, and reliable for initial screening. Agar gel electrophoresis at pH 6.1 in citrate buffer is often used as a complementary method because each method detects different variants. Some important variants are electrophoretically silent. These mutant hemoglobins can usually be characterized by more specialized techniques such as isoelectric focusing and/or high-pressure liquid chromatography (HPLC), which is rapidly replacing electrophoresis for initial analysis.

Quantitation of the hemoglobin profile is often desirable. HbA_2 is frequently elevated in β-thalassemia trait and depressed in iron deficiency. HbF is elevated in HPFH, some β-thalassemia syndromes, and occasional periods of erythroid stress or marrow dysplasia. For characterization of sickle cell trait, sickle thalassemia syndromes, or HbSC disease, and for monitoring the progress of exchange transfusion therapy to lower the percentage of circulating HbS, quantitation of individual hemoglobins is also required. In most laboratories, quantitation is performed only if the test is specifically ordered. Complete characterization, including amino acid sequencing or gene cloning and sequencing, is readily available from several reference laboratories.

Because some variants can comigrate with HbA or HbS (sickle hemoglobin), electrophoretic assessment should always be regarded as incomplete unless functional assays for hemoglobin sickling, solubility, or oxygen affinity are also performed, as dictated by the clinical presentation. The best sickling assays involve measurement of the degree to which the hemoglobin sample becomes insoluble, or gelated, as it is deoxygenated (i.e., sickle solubility test). Unstable hemoglobins are detected by their precipitation in isopropanol or after heating to 50°C. High-O_2 affinity and low-O_2 affinity variants are detected by quantitating the P_{50}, the partial pressure of oxygen at which the hemoglobin sample becomes 50% saturated with oxygen. Direct tests for the percentage carboxyhemoglobin and methemoglobin, employing spectrophotometric techniques, can readily be obtained from most clinical laboratories on an urgent basis.

Laboratory evaluation remains an adjunct, rather than the primary diagnostic aid. Diagnosis is best established by recognition of a characteristic history, physical findings, peripheral blood smear morphology, and abnormalities of the complete blood cell count (e.g., profound microcytosis with minimal anemia in thalassemia trait).

STRUCTURALLY ABNORMAL HEMOGLOBINS

■ SICKLE CELL SYNDROMES

The sickle cell syndromes are caused by a mutation in the β-globin gene that changes the sixth amino acid from glutamic acid to valine. HbS ($\alpha_2\beta_2^{6\ Glu\rightarrow Val}$) polymerizes reversibly when deoxygenated to form a gelatinous network of fibrous polymers that stiffen the RBC membrane, increase viscosity, and cause dehydration due to potassium leakage and calcium influx (Fig. 104-3). These changes also produce the sickle shape. Sickled cells lose the pliability needed to traverse small capillaries. They possess altered "sticky" membranes that are abnormally adherent to the endothelium of small venules. These abnormalities provoke unpredictable episodes of microvascular vasoocclusion and premature RBC destruction (hemolytic anemia). Hemolysis occurs because the spleen destroys the abnormal RBC. The rigid adherent cells clog small capillaries and venules, causing tissue ischemia, acute pain, and gradual end-organ damage. This venooclusive component usually dominates the clinical course. Prominent manifestations include episodes of ischemic pain (i.e., painful crises) and ischemic malfunction or frank infarction in the spleen, central nervous system, bones, liver, kidneys, and lungs (Fig. 104-3).

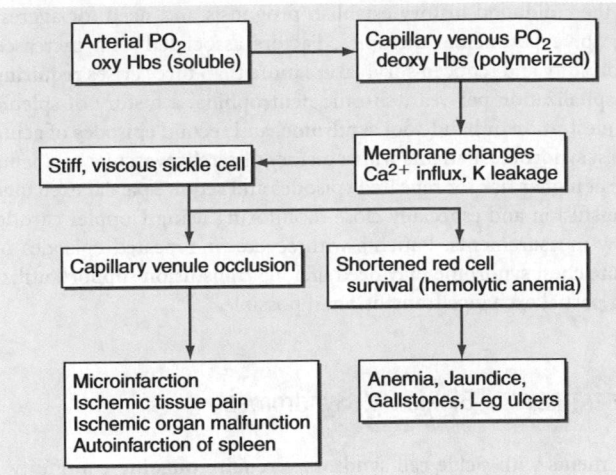

Figure 104-3 Pathophysiology of sickle cell crisis.

Several sickle syndromes occur as the result of inheritance of HbS from one parent and another hemoglobinopathy, such as β thalassemia or HbC ($\alpha_2\beta_2^{6\ Glu\rightarrow Lys}$), from the other parent. The prototype disease, sickle cell anemia, is the homozygous state for HbS (Table 104-2).

Clinical manifestations of sickle cell anemia

Most patients with sickling syndromes suffer from hemolytic anemia, with hematocrits from 15 to 30%, and significant reticulocytosis. Anemia was once thought to exert protective effects against vasoocclusion by reducing blood viscosity. However, natural history and drug therapy trials suggest that an *increase* in the hematocrit and feedback inhibition of reticulocytosis might be beneficial, even at the expense of increased blood viscosity. The role of adhesive reticulocytes in vasoocclusion might account for these paradoxical effects.

Granulocytosis is common. The white count can fluctuate substantially and unpredictably during and between painful crises, infectious episodes, and other intercurrent illnesses.

Vasoocclusion causes protean manifestations. Intermittent episodes of vasoocclusion in connective and musculoskeletal structures produce ischemia manifested by acute pain and tenderness, fever, tachycardia, and anxiety. These recurrent episodes, called *painful crises*, are the most common clinical manifestation. Their frequency

and severity vary greatly. Pain can develop almost anywhere in the body and may last from a few hours to 2 weeks. Repeated crises requiring hospitalization (>3 per year) correlate with reduced survival in adult life, suggesting that these episodes are associated with accumulation of chronic end organ damage. Provocative factors include infection, fever, excessive exercise, anxiety, abrupt changes in temperature, hypoxia, or hypertonic dyes.

Repeated micro-infarction can destroy tissues having microvascular beds prone to sickling. Thus, the spleen is frequently lost within the first 18–36 months of life, causing susceptibility to infection, particularly by pneumococci. Acute venous obstruction of the spleen (*splenic sequestration crisis*), a rare occurrence in early childhood, may require emergency transfusion and/or splenectomy to prevent trapping of the entire arterial output in the obstructed spleen. Occlusion of retinal vessels can produce hemorrhage, neovascularization, and eventual detachments. Renal papillary necrosis invariably produces isosthenuria. More widespread renal necrosis leads to renal failure in adults, a common late cause of death. Bone and joint ischemia can lead to aseptic necrosis, especially of the femoral or humeral heads; chronic arthropathy; and unusual susceptibility to osteomyelitis, which may be caused by organisms, such as *Salmonella*, rarely encountered in other settings. The *hand-foot syndrome* is caused by painful infarcts of the digits and dactylitis. Stroke is especially common in children; a small subset tend to suffer repeated episodes. Stroke is less common in adults and is often hemorrhagic. A particularly painful complication in males is priapism, due to infarction of the penile venous outflow tracts; permanent impotence is a frequent consequence. Chronic lower leg ulcers probably arise from ischemia and superinfection in the distal circulation.

Acute chest syndrome is a distinctive manifestation characterized by chest pain, tachypnea, fever, cough, and arterial oxygen desaturation. It can mimic pneumonia, pulmonary emboli, bone marrow infarction and embolism, myocardial ischemia, or in situ lung infarction. Acute chest syndrome is thought to reflect in situ sickling within the lung, producing pain and temporary pulmonary dysfunction. Often it is difficult or impossible to distinguish among other possibilities. Pulmonary infarction and pneumonia are the most frequent underlying or concomitant conditions in patients with this syndrome. Repeated episodes of acute chest pain correlate with reduced survival. Acutely, reduction in arterial oxygen saturation is especially ominous because it promotes sickling on a massive scale. Chronic acute or subacute pulmonary crises lead to pulmonary hypertension and cor pulmonale, an increasingly common cause of death as patients survive longer. Considerable controversy exists about the possible role played by free plasma HbS in scavenging NO_2, thus raising pulmonary vascular tone. Trials of sildenafil to restore NO_2 levels were terminated because of adverse effects.

Sickle cell syndromes are remarkable for their clinical heterogeneity. Some patients remain virtually asymptomatic into or even through adult life, while others suffer repeated crises requiring hospitalization from early childhood. Patients with sickle thalassemia and sickle-HbE tend to have similar, slightly milder, symptoms, perhaps because of the ameliorating effects of production of other hemoglobins within the RBC. Hemoglobin SC disease, one of the more common variants of sickle cell anemia, is

TABLE 104-2 Clinical Features of Sickle Hemoglobinopathies

Condition	Clinical Abnormalities	Hemoglobin Level g/L (g/dL)	MCV, fL	Hemoglobin Electrophoresis
Sickle cell trait	None; rare painless hematuria	Normal	Normal	Hb S/A:40/60
Sickle cell anemia	Vasoocclusive crises with infarction of spleen, brain, marrow, kidney, lung; aseptic necrosis of bone; gallstones; priapism; ankle ulcers	70–100 (7–10)	80–100	Hb S/A:100/0 Hb F:2–25%
S/β° thalassemia	Vasoocclusive crises; aseptic necrosis of bone	70–100 (7–10)	60–80	Hb S/A:100/0 Hb F:1–10%
S/β+ thalassemia	Rare crises and aseptic necrosis	100–140 (10–14)	70–80	Hb S/A:60/40
Hemoglobin SC	Rare crises and aseptic necrosis; painless hematuria	100–140 (10–14)	80–100	Hb S/A:50/0 Hb C:50%

frequently marked by lesser degrees of hemolytic anemia and a greater propensity for the development of retinopathy and aseptic necrosis of bones. In most respects, however, the clinical manifestations resemble sickle cell anemia. Some rare hemoglobin variants actually aggravate the sickling phenomenon.

The clinical variability in different patients inheriting the same disease-causing mutation (sickle hemoglobin) has made sickle cell disease the focus of efforts to identify modifying genetic polymorphisms in other genes that might account for the heterogeneity. The complexity of the data obtained thus far has dampened the expectation that genomewide analysis will yield individualized profiles that predict a patient's clinical course. Nevertheless, a number of interesting patterns have emerged from these modifying gene analyses. For example, genes affecting the inflammatory response or cytokine expression appear to be modifying candidates. Genes that affect transcriptional regulation of lymphocytes may be involved. Thus, it appears likely that key polymorphic changes in the patient's inflammatory response to the damages provoked by sickle red cells or in the response to chronic or recurrent infections may prove to be important for prognosticating the clinical severity of disease.

Clinical manifestations of sickle cell trait

Sickle cell trait is usually asymptomatic. Anemia and painful crises are rare. An uncommon but highly distinctive symptom is painless hematuria often occurring in adolescent males, probably due to papillary necrosis. Isosthenuria is a more common manifestation of the same process. Sloughing of papillae with urethral obstruction has been reported, as have isolated cases of massive sickling or sudden death due to exposure to high altitudes or extremes of exercise and dehydration. Avoidance of dehydration or extreme physical stress should be advised.

Diagnosis

Sickle cell syndromes are suspected on the basis of hemolytic anemia, RBC morphology (Fig. 104-4), and intermittent episodes of ischemic pain. Diagnosis is confirmed by hemoglobin electrophoresis and the sickling tests already discussed. Thorough characterization of the exact hemoglobin profile of the patient is important, because sickle thalassemia and hemoglobin SC disease have distinct prognoses or clinical features. Diagnosis is usually established in childhood, but occasional patients, often with compound heterozygous states, do not develop symptoms until the onset of puberty, pregnancy, or early adult life. Genotyping of family members and potential parental partners is critical for genetic counseling. Details

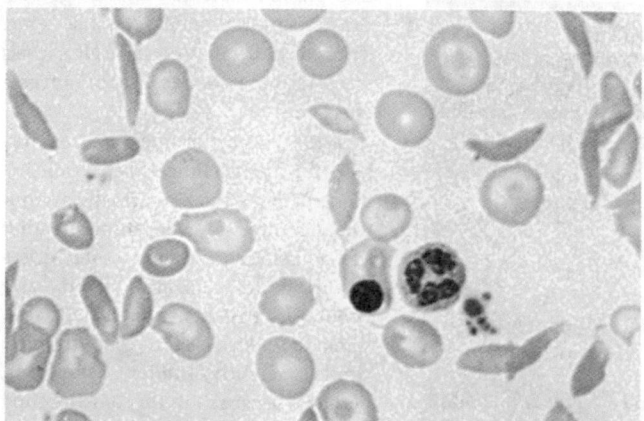

Figure 104-4 Sickle cell anemia. The elongated and crescent-shaped red blood cells seen on this smear represent circulating irreversibly sickled cells. Target cells and a nucleated red blood cell are also seen.

of the childhood history establish prognosis and need for aggressive or experimental therapies. Factors associated with increased morbidity and reduced survival are more than three crises requiring hospitalization per year, chronic neutrophilia, a history of splenic sequestration or hand-foot syndrome, and second episodes of acute chest syndrome. Patients with a history of cerebrovascular accidents are at higher risk for repeated episodes and require partial exchange transfusion and especially close monitoring using Doppler carotid flow measurements. Patients with severe or repeated episodes of acute chest syndrome may need lifelong transfusion support, utilizing partial exchange transfusion, if possible.

TREATMENT Sickle Cell Syndromes

Patients with sickle cell syndromes require ongoing continuity of care. Familiarity with the pattern of symptoms provides the best safeguard against excessive use of the emergency room, hospitalization, and habituation to addictive narcotics. Additional preventive measures include regular slit-lamp examinations to monitor development of retinopathy; antibiotic prophylaxis appropriate for splenectomized patients during dental or other invasive procedures; and vigorous oral hydration during or in anticipation of periods of extreme exercise, exposure to heat or cold, emotional stress, or infection. Pneumococcal and *Haemophilus influenzae* vaccines are less effective in splenectomized individuals. Thus, patients with sickle cell anemia should be vaccinated early in life.

The management of acute painful crisis includes vigorous hydration, thorough evaluation for underlying causes (such as infection), and aggressive analgesia administered by a standing order and/or patient-controlled analgesia (PCA) pump. Morphine (0.1–0.15 mg/kg every 3–4 h) should be used to control severe pain. Bone pain may respond as well to ketorolac (30–60 mg initial dose, then 15–30 mg every 6–8 h). Inhalation of nitrous oxide can provide short-term pain relief, but great care must be exercised to avoid hypoxia and respiratory depression. Nitrous oxide also elevates O_2 affinity, reducing O_2 delivery to tissues. Its use should be restricted to experts. Many crises can be managed at home with oral hydration and oral analgesia. Use of the emergency room should be reserved for especially severe symptoms or circumstances in which other processes, e.g., infection, are strongly suspected. Nasal oxygen should be employed as appropriate to protect arterial saturation. Most crises resolve in 1–7 days. Use of blood transfusion should be reserved for extreme cases: transfusions do not shorten the duration of the crisis.

No tests are definitive to diagnose acute painful crisis. Critical to good management is an approach that recognizes that most patients reporting crisis symptoms do indeed have crisis or another significant medical problem. Diligent diagnostic evaluation for underlying causes is imperative, even though these are found infrequently. In adults, the possibility of aseptic necrosis or sickle arthropathy must be considered, especially if pain and immobility become repeated or chronic at a single site. Nonsteroidal anti-inflammatory agents are often effective for sickle cell arthropathy.

Acute chest syndrome is a medical emergency that may require management in an intensive care unit. Hydration should be monitored carefully to avoid the development of pulmonary edema, and oxygen therapy should be especially vigorous for protection of arterial saturation. Diagnostic evaluation for pneumonia and pulmonary embolism should be especially thorough, since these may occur with atypical symptoms. Critical interventions are transfusion to maintain a hematocrit >30, and emergency exchange transfusion if arterial saturation drops to <90%. As patients with sickle cell syndrome increasingly survive into their fifth and sixth decades, end-stage renal failure and pulmonary hypertension are becoming increasingly prominent causes of end-stage morbidity. A sickle cell cardiomyopathy and/or premature coronary artery disease may compromise cardiac function in later years. Sickle cell patients have received kidney transplants, but they often experience an increase in the frequency and severity of crises, possibly due to increased infection as a consequence of immunosuppression.

The most significant advance in the therapy of sickle cell anemia has been the introduction of hydroxyurea as a mainstay of therapy for patients with severe symptoms. Hydroxyurea (10–30 mg/kg per day) increases fetal hemoglobin and may also exert beneficial affects on RBC hydration, vascular wall adherence, and suppression of the granulocyte and reticulocyte counts; dosage is titrated to maintain a white cell count between 5000 and 8000 per μL. White cells and reticulocytes may play a major role in the pathogenesis of sickle cell crisis, and their suppression may be an important benefit of hydroxyurea therapy.

Hydroxyurea should be considered in patients experiencing repeated episodes of acute chest syndrome or with more than three crises per year requiring hospitalization. The utility of this agent for reducing the incidence of other complications (priapism, retinopathy) is under evaluation, as are the long-term side effects. Hydroxyurea offers broad benefits to most patients whose disease is severe enough to impair their functional status, and it may improve survival. HbF levels increase in most patients within a few months.

The antitumor drug 5-azacytidine was the first agent found to elevate HbF. It never achieved widespread use because of concerns about acute toxicity and carcinogenesis. However, low doses of the related agent 5-deoxyazacytidine (decitabine) can elevate HbF with more acceptable toxicity.

Bone marrow transplantation can provide definitive cures but is known to be effective and safe only in children. Partially myeloablative conditioning regimens ("mini" transplants) may allow more widespread use of this modality. Prognostic features justifying bone marrow transplant are the presence of repeated crises early in life, a high neutrophil count, or the development of hand-foot syndrome. Children at risk for stroke can now be identified through the use of Doppler ultrasound techniques. Prophylactic exchange transfusion appears to substantially reduce the risk of stroke in this population. Children who do suffer a cerebrovascular accident should be maintained for at least 3–5 years on a program of vigorous exchange transfusion, as the risk of second strokes is extremely high.

Gene therapy for sickle cell anemia is being intensively pursued, but no safe measures are currently available. Agents blocking RBC dehydration or vascular adhesion, such as clotrimazole or magnesium, may have value as an adjunct to hydroxyurea therapy, pending the completion of ongoing trials. Combinations of clotrimazole and magnesium are being evaluated.

■ UNSTABLE HEMOGLOBINS

Amino acid substitutions that reduce solubility or increase susceptibility to oxidation produce unstable hemoglobins that precipitate, forming inclusion bodies injurious to the RBC membrane. Representative mutations are those that interfere with contact points between the α and β subunits [e.g., Hb Philly ($\beta^{35Tyr \to Phe}$)], alter the helical segments [e.g., Hb Genova ($\beta^{28Leu \to Pro}$)], or disrupt

TABLE 104-3 Representative Abnormal Hemoglobins With Altered Synthesis or Function

Designation	Mutation	Population	Main Clinical Effects[a]
Sickle or S	$\beta^{6Glu \to Val}$	African	Anemia, ischemic infarcts
C	$\beta^{6Glu \to Lys}$	African	Mild anemia; interacts with HbS
E	$\beta^{26Glu \to Lys}$	Southeast Asian	Microcytic anemia, splenomegaly, thalassemic phenotype
Köln	$\beta^{98Val \to Met}$	Sporadic	Hemolytic anemia, Heinz bodies when splenectomized
Yakima	$\beta^{99Asp \to His}$	Sporadic	Polycythemia
Kansas	$\beta^{102Asn \to Lys}$	Sporadic	Mild anemia
M. Iwata	$\alpha^{87His \to Tyr}$	Sporadic	Methemoglobinemia

[a]See text for details.

interactions of the hydrophobic pockets of the globin subunits with heme [e.g., Hb Koln ($\beta^{98Val \to Met}$)] (Table 104-3). The inclusions, called *Heinz bodies*, are clinically detectable by staining with supravital dyes such as crystal violet. Removal of these inclusions by the spleen generates pitted, rigid cells that have shortened life spans, producing hemolytic anemia of variable severity, sometimes requiring chronic transfusion support. Splenectomy may be needed to correct the anemia. Leg ulcers and premature gallbladder disease due to bilirubin loading are frequent stigmata.

Unstable hemoglobins occur sporadically, often by spontaneous new mutations. Heterozygotes are often symptomatic because a significant Heinz body burden can develop even when the unstable variant accounts for only a portion of the total hemoglobin. Symptomatic unstable hemoglobins tend to be β-globin variants, because sporadic mutations affecting only one of the four α globins would generate only 20–30% abnormal hemoglobin.

■ HEMOGLOBINS WITH ALTERED OXYGEN AFFINITY

High-affinity hemoglobins [e.g., Hb Yakima ($\beta^{99Asp \to His}$)] bind oxygen more readily but deliver less O_2 to tissues at normal capillary PO_2 levels (Fig. 104-2). Mild tissue hypoxia ensues, stimulating RBC production and erythrocytosis (Table 104-3). In extreme cases, the hematocrits can rise to 60–65%, increasing blood viscosity and producing typical symptoms (headache, somnolence, or dizziness). Phlebotomy may be required. Typical mutations alter interactions within the heme pocket or disrupt the Bohr effect or salt-bond site. Mutations that impair the interaction of HbA with 2,3-BPG can increase O_2 affinity because 2,3-BPG binding lowers O_2 affinity.

Low-affinity hemoglobins [e.g., Hb Kansas ($\beta^{102Asn \to Lys}$)] bind sufficient oxygen in the lungs, despite their lower oxygen affinity, to achieve nearly full saturation. At capillary oxygen tensions, they lose sufficient amounts of oxygen to maintain homeostasis at a low hematocrit (Fig. 104-2) (*pseudoanemia*). Capillary hemoglobin desaturation can also be sufficient to produce clinically apparent cyanosis. Despite these findings, patients usually require no specific treatment.

■ METHEMOGLOBINEMIAS

Methemoglobin is generated by oxidation of the heme iron moieties to the ferric state, causing a characteristic bluish-brown muddy color resembling cyanosis. Methemoglobin has such high oxygen affinity that virtually no oxygen is delivered. Levels >50–60% are often fatal.

Congenital methemoglobinemia arises from globin mutations that stabilize iron in the ferric state [e.g., HbM Iwata ($\alpha^{87His\rightarrow Tyr}$), Table 104-3] or from mutations that impair the enzymes that reduce methemoglobin to hemoglobin (e.g., methemoglobin reductase, NADP diaphorase). Acquired methemoglobinemia is caused by toxins that oxidize heme iron, notably nitrate and nitrite-containing compounds, including drugs commonly used in cardiology and anesthesiology.

■ DIAGNOSIS AND MANAGEMENT OF PATIENTS WITH UNSTABLE HEMOGLOBINS, HIGH-AFFINITY HEMOGLOBINS, AND METHEMOGLOBINEMIA

Unstable hemoglobin variants should be suspected in patients with nonimmune hemolytic anemia, jaundice, splenomegaly, or premature biliary tract disease. Severe hemolysis usually presents during infancy as neonatal jaundice or anemia. Milder cases may present in adult life with anemia or only as unexplained reticulocytosis, hepatosplenomegaly, premature biliary tract disease, or leg ulcers. Because spontaneous mutation is common, family history of anemia may be absent. The peripheral blood smear often shows anisocytosis, abundant cells with punctate inclusions, and irregular shapes (i.e., poikilocytosis).

The two best tests for diagnosing unstable hemoglobins are the Heinz body preparation and the isopropanol or heat stability test. Many unstable Hb variants are electrophoretically silent. A normal electrophoresis does not rule out the diagnosis.

Severely affected patients may require transfusion support for the first 3 years of life, because splenectomy before age 3 is associated with a significantly higher immune deficit. Splenectomy is usually effective thereafter, but occasional patients may require lifelong transfusion support. After splenectomy, patients can develop cholelithiasis and leg ulcers, hypercoagulable states, and susceptibility to overwhelming sepsis. Splenectomy should be avoided or delayed unless it is the only alternative. Precipitation of unstable hemoglobins is aggravated by oxidative stress, e.g., infection and antimalarial drugs, which should be avoided where possible.

High-O$_2$ affinity hemoglobin variants should be suspected in patients with erythrocytosis. The best test for confirmation is measurement of the P$_{50}$. A high-O$_2$ affinity Hb causes a significant left shift (i.e., lower numeric value of the P$_{50}$); confounding conditions, e.g., tobacco smoking or carbon monoxide exposure, can also lower the P$_{50}$.

High-affinity hemoglobins are often asymptomatic; rubor or plethora may be telltale signs. When the hematocrit reaches to 55–60%, symptoms of high blood viscosity and sluggish flow (headache, lethargy, dizziness, etc.) may be present. These persons may benefit from judicious phlebotomy. Erythrocytosis represents an appropriate attempt to compensate for the impaired oxygen delivery by the abnormal variant. Overzealous phlebotomy may stimulate increased erythropoiesis or aggravate symptoms by thwarting this compensatory mechanism. The guiding principle of phlebotomy should be to improve oxygen delivery by reducing blood viscosity and increasing blood flow rather than restoration of a normal hematocrit. Modest iron deficiency may aid in control.

Low-affinity hemoglobins should be considered in patients with cyanosis or a low hematocrit with no other reason apparent after thorough evaluation. The P$_{50}$ test confirms the diagnosis. Counseling and reassurance are the interventions of choice.

Methemoglobin should be suspected in patients with hypoxic symptoms who appear cyanotic but have a PaO$_2$ sufficiently high that hemoglobin should be fully saturated with oxygen. A history of nitrite or other oxidant ingestions may not always be available; some exposures may be inapparent to the patient, and others may

result from suicide attempts. The characteristic muddy appearance of freshly drawn blood can be a critical clue. The best diagnostic test is methemoglobin assay, which is usually available on an emergency basis.

Methemoglobinemia often causes symptoms of cerebral ischemia at levels >15%; levels >60% are usually lethal. Intravenous injection of 1 mg/kg of methylene blue is effective emergency therapy. Milder cases and follow-up of severe cases can be treated orally with methylene blue (60 mg three to four times each day) or ascorbic acid (300–600 mg/d).

THALASSEMIA SYNDROMES

The thalassemia syndromes are inherited disorders of α- or β-globin biosynthesis. The reduced supply of globin diminishes production of hemoglobin tetramers, causing hypochromia and microcytosis. Unbalanced accumulation of α and β subunits occurs because the synthesis of the unaffected globins proceeds at a normal rate. Unbalanced chain accumulation dominates the clinical phenotype. Clinical severity varies widely, depending on the degree to which the synthesis of the affected globin is impaired, altered synthesis of other globin chains, and coinheritance of other abnormal globin alleles.

■ CLINICAL MANIFESTATIONS OF β-THALASSEMIA SYNDROMES

Mutations causing thalassemia can affect any step in the pathway of globin gene expression: transcription, processing of the mRNA precursor, translation, and posttranslational metabolism of the β-globin polypeptide chain. The most common forms arise from mutations that derange splicing of the mRNA precursor or prematurely terminate translation of the mRNA.

Hypochromia and microcytosis characterize all forms of β thalassemia because of the reduced amounts of hemoglobin tetramers (Fig. 104-5). In heterozygotes (β-thalassemia trait), this is the only abnormality seen. Anemia is minimal. In more severe homozygous states, unbalanced α- and β-globin accumulation causes accumulation of highly insoluble unpaired α chains. They form toxic inclusion bodies that kill developing erythroblasts in the marrow. Few of the proerythroblasts beginning erythroid maturation survive. The surviving RBCs bear a burden of inclusion bodies that are detected in the spleen, shortening the RBC life span and producing severe hemolytic anemia. The resulting profound anemia stimulates erythropoietin release and compensatory erythroid hyperplasia, but the marrow response is sabotaged by the ineffective erythropoiesis. Anemia persists. Erythroid hyperplasia can become exuberant and

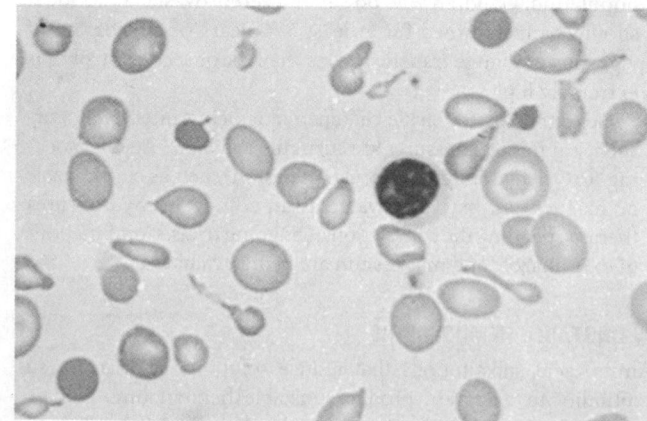

Figure 104-5 β-Thalassemia intermedia. Microcytic and hypochromic red blood cells are seen that resemble the red blood cells of severe iron deficiency anemia. Many elliptical and teardrop-shaped red blood cells are noted.

produce masses of extramedullary erythropoietic tissue in the liver and spleen.

Massive bone marrow expansion deranges growth and development. Children develop characteristic "chipmunk" facies due to maxillary marrow hyperplasia and frontal bossing. Thinning and pathologic fracture of long bones and vertebrae may occur due to cortical invasion by erythroid elements and profound growth retardation. Hemolytic anemia causes hepatosplenomegaly, leg ulcers, gallstones, and high-output congestive heart failure. The conscription of caloric resources to support erythropoiesis leads to inanition, susceptibility to infection, endocrine dysfunction, and in the most severe cases, death during the first decade of life. Chronic transfusions with RBCs improve oxygen delivery, suppress the excessive ineffective erythropoiesis, and prolong life, but the inevitable side effects, notably iron overload, usually prove fatal by age 30 years.

Severity is highly variable. Known modulating factors are those that ameliorate the burden of unpaired α-globin inclusions. Alleles associated with milder synthetic defects and coinheritance of α-thalassemia trait reduce clinical severity by reducing accumulation of excess α globin. HbF persists to various degrees in β thalassemias. γ-Globin gene chains can substitute for β chains, generating more hemoglobin and reducing the burden of α-globin inclusions. The terms β-*thalassemia major* and β-*thalassemia intermedia* are used to reflect the clinical heterogeneity. Patients with β-thalassemia major require intensive transfusion support to survive. Patients with β-thalassemia intermedia have a somewhat milder phenotype and can survive without transfusion. The terms β-*thalassemia minor* and β-*thalassemia trait* describe asymptomatic heterozygotes for β thalassemia.

■ THALASSEMIA SYNDROMES

The four classic α thalassemias, most common in Asians, are α-thalassemia-2 trait, in which one of the four α-globin loci is deleted; α-thalassemia-1 trait, with two deleted loci; HbH disease, with three loci deleted; and hydrops fetalis with Hb Barts, with all four loci deleted (Table 104-4). Nondeletion forms of α thalassemia also exist.

α-*Thalassemia-2 trait* is an asymptomatic, silent carrier state. α-*Thalassemia-1 trait* resembles β-thalassemia minor. Offspring doubly heterozygous for α-thalassemia-2 and α-thalassemia-1 exhibit a more severe phenotype called *HbH disease*. Heterozygosity for a deletion that removes both genes from the same chromosome (*cis* deletion) is common in Asians and in those from the Mediterranean region, as is homozygosity for α-thalassemia-2 (*trans* deletion). Both produce asymptomatic hypochromia and microcytosis.

In *HbH disease*, HbA production is only 25–30% normal. Fetuses accumulate some unpaired γ chains (Hb Barts; γ-chain tetramers). In adults, unpaired β chains accumulate and are soluble enough to form β_4 tetramers called HbH. HbH forms few inclusions in erythroblasts and precipitates in circulating RBC. Patients with HbH disease have thalassemia intermedia characterized by moderately severe hemolytic anemia but milder ineffective erythropoiesis. Survival into midadult life without transfusions is common.

The homozygous state for the α-thalassemia-1 *cis* deletion (hydrops fetalis) causes total absence of α-globin synthesis. No physiologically useful hemoglobin is produced beyond the embryonic stage. Excess γ globin forms tetramers called *Hb Barts* (γ_4), which has a very high oxygen affinity. It delivers almost no O_2 to fetal tissues, causing tissue asphyxia, edema (hydrops fetalis), congestive heart failure, and death in utero. α-Thalassemia-2 trait is common (15–20%) among people of African descent. The *cis* α-thalassemia-1 deletion is almost never seen, however. Thus, α-thalassemia-2 and the *trans* form of α-thalassemia-1 are very common, but HbH disease and hydrops fetalis are rare.

It has been known for some time that some patients with myelodysplasia or erythroleukemia produce RBC clones containing HbH. This phenomenon is due to mutations in the ATRX pathway that affect the LCR of the α-globin gene cluster.

■ DIAGNOSIS AND MANAGEMENT OF THALASSEMIAS

The diagnosis of β-thalassemia major is readily made during childhood on the basis of severe anemia accompanied by the characteristic signs of massive ineffective erythropoiesis: hepatosplenomegaly, profound microcytosis, a characteristic blood smear (Fig. 104-5), and elevated levels of HbF, HbA_2, or both. Many patients require chronic hypertransfusion therapy designed to maintain a hematocrit of at least 27–30% so that erythropoiesis is suppressed. Splenectomy is required if the annual transfusion requirement (volume of RBCs per kilogram of body weight per year) increases by >50%. Folic acid supplements may be useful. Vaccination with Pneumovax in anticipation of eventual splenectomy is advised, as is close monitoring for infection, leg ulcers, and biliary tract disease. Many patients develop endocrine deficiencies as a result of iron overload. Early endocrine evaluation is required for glucose intolerance, thyroid dysfunction, and delayed onset of puberty or secondary sexual characteristics.

Patients with β-thalassemia intermedia exhibit similar stigmata but can survive without chronic hypertransfusion. Management is particularly challenging because a number of factors can aggravate the anemia, including infection, onset of puberty, and development of splenomegaly and hypersplenism. Some patients may eventually benefit from splenectomy. The expanded erythron can cause absorption of excessive dietary iron and hemosiderosis, even without transfusion.

β-Thalassemia minor (i.e., thalassemia trait) usually presents as profound microcytosis and hypochromia with target cells, but only minimal or mild anemia. The mean corpuscular volume is rarely >75 fL; the hematocrit

TABLE 104-4 The α Thalassemias

Condition	Hemoglobin A, %	Hemoglobin H (β4), %	Hemoglobin Level, g/L (g/dL)	MCV, fL
Normal	97	0	150 (15)	90
Silent thalassemia: −α/αα	98–100	0	150 (15)	90
Thalassemia trait: −α/−α homozygous α-thal-2[a] or −−/αα heterozygous α-thal-1[a]	85–95	Rare red blood cell inclusions	120–130 (12–13)	70–80
Hemoglobin H disease: −−/−α heterozygous α-thal-1/α-thal-2	70–95	5–30	60–100 (6–10)	60–70
Hydrops fetalis: −−/−− homozygous α-thal-1	0	5–10b	Fatal in utero or at birth	

[a]When both α alleles on one chromosome are deleted, the locus is called α-thal-1; when only a single α allele on one chromosome is deleted, the locus is called α-thal-2.

[b]90–95% of the hemoglobin is hemoglobin Barts (tetramers of γ chains).

is rarely <30–33%. Hemoglobin analysis classically reveals an elevated HbA$_2$ (3.5–7.5%), but some forms are associated with normal HbA$_2$ and/or elevated HbF. Genetic counseling and patient education are essential. Patients with β-thalassemia trait should be warned that their blood picture resembles iron deficiency and can be misdiagnosed. They should eschew empirical use of iron, yet iron deficiency can develop during pregnancy or from chronic bleeding.

Persons with α-thalassemia trait may exhibit mild hypochromia and microcytosis usually without anemia. HbA$_2$ and HbF levels are normal. Affected individuals usually require only genetic counseling. HbH disease resembles β-thalassemia intermedia, with the added complication that the HbH molecule behaves like moderately unstable hemoglobin. Patients with HbH disease should undergo splenectomy if excessive anemia or a transfusion requirement develops. Oxidative drugs should be avoided. Iron overload leading to death can occur in more severely affected patients.

■ PREVENTION

Antenatal diagnosis of thalassemia syndromes is now widely available. DNA diagnosis is based on PCR amplification of fetal DNA, obtained by amniocentesis or chorionic villus biopsy followed by hybridization to allele-specific oligonucleotides probes or direct DNA sequencing.

THALASSEMIC STRUCTURAL VARIANTS

Thalassemic structural variants are characterized by both defective synthesis and abnormal structure.

■ HEMOGLOBIN LEPORE

Hb Lepore [α$_2$(δβ)$_2$] arises by an unequal crossover and recombination event that fuses the proximal end of the δ-gene with the distal end of the closely linked β-gene. It is common in the Mediterranean basin. The resulting chromosome contains only the fused δβ gene. The Lepore (δβ) globin is synthesized poorly because the fused gene is under the control of the weak δ-globin promoter. Hb Lepore alleles have a phenotype like β thalassemia, except for the added presence of 2–20% Hb Lepore. Compound heterozygotes for Hb Lepore and a classic β-thalassemia allele may also have severe thalassemia.

■ HEMOGLOBIN E

HbE (i.e., α$_2$β$_2^{26Glu→Lys}$) is extremely common in Cambodia, Thailand, and Vietnam. The gene has become far more prevalent in the United States as a result of immigration of Asian persons, especially in California, where HbE is the most common variant detected. HbE is mildly unstable but not enough to affect RBC life span significantly. Heterozygotes resemble individuals with a mild β-thalassemia trait. Homozygotes have somewhat more marked abnormalities but are asymptomatic. Compound heterozygotes for HbE and a β-thalassemia gene can have β-thalassemia intermedia or β-thalassemia major, depending on the severity of the coinherited thalassemic gene.

The β^E allele contains a single base change in codon 26 that causes the amino acid substitution. However, this mutation activates a cryptic RNA splice site, generating a structurally abnormal globin mRNA that cannot be translated from about 50% of the initial pre-mRNA molecules. The remaining 40–50% are normally spliced and generate functional mRNA that is translated into β^E-globin because the mature mRNA carries the base change that alters codon 26.

Genetic counseling of the persons at risk for HbE should focus on the interaction of HbE with β thalassemia rather than

HbE homozygosity, a condition associated with asymptomatic microcytosis, hypochromia, and hemoglobin levels rarely <100 g/L (<10 g/dL).

■ HEREDITARY PERSISTENCE OF FETAL HEMOGLOBIN

HPFH is characterized by continued synthesis of high levels of HbF in adult life. No deleterious effects are apparent, even when all of the hemoglobin produced is HbF. These rare patients demonstrate convincingly that prevention or reversal of the fetal to adult hemoglobin switch would provide effective therapy for sickle cell anemia and β thalassemia.

■ ACQUIRED HEMOGLOBINOPATHIES

The two most important acquired hemoglobinopathies are carbon monoxide poisoning and methemoglobinemia (see above). Carbon monoxide has a higher affinity for hemoglobin than does oxygen; it can replace oxygen and diminish O$_2$ delivery. Chronic elevation of carboxyhemoglobin levels to 10 or 15%, as occurs in smokers, can lead to secondary polycythemia. Carboxyhemoglobin is cherry red in color and masks the development of cyanosis usually associated with poor O$_2$ delivery to tissues.

Abnormalities of hemoglobin biosynthesis have also been described in blood dyscrasias. In some patients with myelodysplasia, erythroleukemia, or myeloproliferative disorders, elevated HbF or a mild form of HbH disease may also be seen. The abnormalities are not severe enough to alter the course of the underlying disease.

TREATMENT   Transfusional Hemosiderosis

Chronic blood transfusion can lead to bloodborne infection, alloimmunization, febrile reactions, and lethal iron overload (Chap. 113). A unit of packed RBCs contains 250–300 mg iron (1 mg/mL). The iron assimilated by a single transfusion of two units of packed RBCs is thus equal to a 1- to 2-year intake of iron. Iron accumulates in chronically transfused patients because no mechanisms exist for increasing iron excretion: an expanded erythron causes especially rapid development of iron overload because accelerated erythropoiesis promotes excessive absorption of dietary iron. Vitamin C should not be supplemented because it generates free radicals in iron excess states.

Patients who receive >100 units of packed RBCs usually develop hemosiderosis. The ferritin level rises, followed by early endocrine dysfunction (glucose intolerance and delayed puberty), cirrhosis, and cardiomyopathy. Liver biopsy shows both parenchymal and reticuloendothelial iron. The superconducting quantum-interference device (SQUID) is accurate at measuring hepatic iron but not widely available. Cardiac toxicity is often insidious. Early development of pericarditis is followed by dysrhythmia and pump failure. The onset of heart failure is ominous, often presaging death within a year (Chap. 357).

The decision to start long-term transfusion support should also prompt one to institute therapy with iron-chelating agents. Desferoxamine (Desferal) is for parenteral use. Its iron-binding kinetics require chronic slow infusion via a metering pump. The constant presence of the drug improves the efficiency of chelation and protects tissues from occasional releases of the most toxic fraction of iron—low-molecular-weight iron—which may not be sequestered by protective proteins.

Desferoxamine is relatively nontoxic. Occasional cataracts, deafness, and local skin reactions, including urticaria, occur.

Skin reactions can usually be managed with antihistamines. Negative iron balance can be achieved, even in the face of a high transfusion requirement, but this alone does not prevent long-term morbidity and mortality in chronically transfused patients. Irreversible end-organ deterioration develops at relatively modest levels of iron overload, even if symptoms do not appear for many years thereafter. To enjoy a significant survival advantage, chelation must begin before 5–8 years of age in β-thalassemia major.

Deferasirox is an oral iron-chelating agent. Single daily doses of 20 to 30 mg/kg deferasirox produced reductions in liver iron concentration comparable to desferoxamine in long-term transfused adult and pediatric patients. Deferasirox produces some elevations in liver enzymes and slight but persistent increases in serum creatinine, without apparent clinical consequence. Other toxicities are similar to those of desferoxamine. Its toxicity profile is acceptable, although long-term effects are still being evaluated.

EXPERIMENTAL THERAPIES

■ BONE MARROW TRANSPLANTATION, GENE THERAPY, AND MANIPULATION OF HBF

Bone marrow transplantation provides stem cells able to express normal hemoglobin; it has been used in a large number of patients with β thalassemia and a smaller number of patients with sickle cell anemia. Early in the course of disease, before end-organ damage occurs, transplantation is curative in 80–90% of patients. In highly experienced centers, the treatment-related mortality is <10%. Since survival into adult life is possible with conventional therapy, the decision to transplant is best made in consultation with specialized centers.

Gene therapy of thalassemia and sickle cell disease has proved to be an elusive goal. Uptake of gene vectors into the nondividing hematopoietic stem cells has been inefficient. Lentiviral-type vectors that can transduce nondividing cells may solve this problem.

Reestablishing high levels of fetal hemoglobin synthesis should ameliorate the symptoms of β chain hemoglobinopathies. Cytotoxic agents such as hydroxyurea and cytarabine promote high levels of HbF synthesis, probably by stimulating proliferation of the primitive HbF-producing progenitor cell population (i.e., F cell progenitors). Unfortunately, this regimen has not yet been effective in β thalassemia. Butyrates stimulate HbF production, but only transiently. Pulsed or intermittent administration has been found to sustain HbF induction in the majority of patients with sickle cell disease. It is unclear whether butyrates will have similar activity in patients with β thalassemia.

APLASTIC AND HYPOPLASTIC CRISIS IN PATIENTS WITH HEMOGLOBINOPATHIES

Patients with hemolytic anemias sometimes exhibit an alarming decline in hematocrit during and immediately after acute illnesses. Bone marrow suppression occurs in almost everyone during acute inflammatory illnesses. In patients with short RBC life spans, suppression can affect RBC counts more dramatically. These hypoplastic crises are usually transient and self-correcting before intervention is required.

Aplastic crisis refers to a profound cessation of erythroid activity in patients with chronic hemolytic anemias. It is associated with a rapidly falling hematocrit. Episodes are usually self-limited. Aplastic crises are caused by infection with a particular strain of parvovirus, B19A. Children infected with this virus usually develop permanent immunity. Aplastic crises do not often recur and are rarely seen in adults. Management requires close monitoring of the hematocrit and reticulocyte count. If anemia becomes symptomatic, transfusion support is indicated. Most crises resolve spontaneously within 1–2 weeks.

FURTHER READINGS

ATAGA KI, ORRINGA EP: Hypercoagulability in sickle cell disease: A curious paradox. Am J Med 115:721, 2003

DeSIMONE J et al: Maintenance of elevated fetal hemoglobin levels by decitabine during dose interval treatment of sickle cell anemia. Blood 99:3905, 2002

NEUFELD EJ: Oral chelators deferasirox and deferiprone for transfusional iron overload in thalassemia major: New data, new questions. Blood 107:3436, 2006

PRABHAKAR H et al: Sickle cell disease in the United States: Looking back and forward at 100 years of progress in management and survival. Am J Hematol 85:346, 2010

QUEK L, THEIN SL: Molecular therapies in beta-thalassaemia. Br J Haematol 136:353, 2007

SMIERS FJ et al: Hematopoietic stem cell transplantation for hemoglobinopathies: Current practice and emerging trends. Pediatr Clin North Am 57:181, 2010

STEINBERG MH: Pathophysiologically based drug treatment of sickle cell disease. Trends Pharmacol Sci 27:204, 2006

SWITZER JA et al: Pathophysiology and treatment of stroke in sickle-cell disease: Present and future. Lancet Neurol 5:501, 2006

WARE RE et al: Predictors of fetal hemoglobin response in children with sickle cell anemia receiving hydroxyurea therapy. Blood 99:10, 2002

WEATHERALL DJ: The inherited diseases of hemoglobin are an emerging global health burden. Blood 115:4331, 2010

CHAPTER 105

Megaloblastic Anemias

A. Victor Hoffbrand

The megaloblastic anemias are a group of disorders characterized by the presence of distinctive morphologic appearances of the developing red cells in the bone marrow. The marrow is usually cellular and the anemia is based on ineffective erythropoiesis. The cause is usually a deficiency of either cobalamin (vitamin B_{12}) or folate, but megaloblastic anemia may occur because of genetic or acquired abnormalities that affect the metabolism of these vitamins or because of defects in DNA synthesis not related to cobalamin or folate (Table 105-1). Cobalamin and folate absorption and metabolism are described next, followed by the biochemical basis, clinical and laboratory features, causes, and treatment of megaloblastic anemia.

COBALAMIN

Cobalamin (vitamin B_{12}) exists in a number of different chemical forms. All have a cobalt atom at the center of a corrin ring. In nature, the vitamin is mainly in the 2-deoxyadenosyl (ado) form, which is located in mitochondria. It is the cofactor for the enzyme methylmalonyl coenzyme A (CoA) mutase. The other major natural cobalamin is methylcobalamin, the form in human plasma and in cell cytoplasm. It is the cofactor for methionine synthase. There are also minor amounts of hydroxocobalamin to which methyl- and adocobalamin are converted rapidly by exposure to light.

Dietary sources and requirements

Cobalamin is synthesized solely by microorganisms. Ruminants obtain cobalamin from the foregut, but the only source for humans is food of animal origin, e.g., meat, fish, and dairy products. Vegetables, fruits, and other foods of nonanimal origin are free from cobalamin unless they are contaminated by bacteria. A normal Western diet contains 5–30 µg of cobalamin daily. Adult daily losses (mainly in the urine and feces) are 1–3 µg (~0.1% of body stores), and as the body does not have the ability to degrade cobalamin, daily requirements are also about 1–3 µg. Body stores are of the order of 2–3 mg, sufficient for 3–4 years if supplies are completely cut off.

TABLE 105-1 Causes of Megaloblastic Anemia

Cobalamin deficiency or abnormalities of cobalamin metabolism (see Tables 105-3, 105-4)

Folate deficiency or abnormalities of folate metabolism (see Table 105-5)

Therapy with antifolate drugs (e.g., methotrexate)

Independent of either cobalamin or folate deficiency and refractory to cobalamin and folate therapy:

  Some cases of acute myeloid leukemia, myelodysplasia

  Therapy with drugs interfering with synthesis of DNA [e.g., cytosine arabinoside, hydroxyurea, 6-mercaptopurine, azidothymidine (AZT)]

  Orotic aciduria (responds to uridine)

  Thiamine-responsive

Absorption

Two mechanisms exist for cobalamin absorption. One is passive, occurring equally through buccal, duodenal, and ileal mucosa; it is rapid but extremely inefficient, with <1% of an oral dose being absorbed by this process. The normal physiologic mechanism is active; it occurs through the ileum and is efficient for small (a few micrograms) oral doses of cobalamin, and it is mediated by gastric intrinsic factor (IF). Dietary cobalamin is released from protein complexes by enzymes in the stomach, duodenum, and jejunum; it combines rapidly with a salivary glycoprotein that belongs to the family of cobalamin-binding proteins known as haptocorrins (HCs). In the intestine, the haptocorrin is digested by pancreatic trypsin and the cobalamin is transferred to IF.

IF (gene at chromosome 11q13 coding for 9 exons) is produced in the gastric parietal cells of the fundus and body of the stomach, and its secretion parallels that of hydrochloric acid. Normally, there is a vast excess of IF. The IF-cobalamin complex passes to the ileum, where IF attaches to a specific receptor (cubilin) on the microvillus membrane of the enterocytes. Cubilin also is present in yolk sac and renal proximal tubular epithelium. Cubulin appears to traffic by means of amnionless (AMN), an endocytic receptor protein that directs sublocalization and endocytosis of cubulin with its ligand IF-cobalamin complex. The cobalamin-IF complex enters the ileal cell, where IF is destroyed. After a delay of about 6 h, the cobalamin appears in portal blood attached to transcobalamin (TC) II.

Between 0.5 and 5 µg of cobalamin enter the bile each day. This binds to IF, and a major portion of biliary cobalamin normally is reabsorbed together with cobalamin derived from sloughed intestinal cells. Because of the appreciable amount of cobalamin undergoing enterohepatic circulation, cobalamin deficiency develops more rapidly in individuals who malabsorb cobalamin than it does in vegans, in whom reabsorption of biliary cobalamin is intact.

Transport

Two main cobalamin transport proteins exist in human plasma; they both bind cobalamin—one molecule for one molecule. One HC, known as TC I, is closely related to other cobalamin-binding HCs in milk, gastric juice, bile, saliva, and other fluids. The gene TCNL is at chromosome 11q11-q12.3 and has 9 exons. These HCs differ from each other only in the carbohydrate moiety of the molecule. TC I is derived primarily from the specific granules in neutrophils. Normally, it is about two-thirds saturated with cobalamin, which it binds tightly. TC I does not enhance cobalamin entry into tissues. Glycoprotein receptors on liver cells are involved in the removal of TC I from plasma, and TC I may play a role in the transport of cobalamin analogues (which it binds more effectively than IF) to the liver for excretion in bile.

The other major cobalamin transport protein in plasma is TC II. The gene is on chromosome 22q11-q13.1. As for IF and HC, there are 9 exons. The three proteins are likely to have a common ancestral origin. TC II is synthesized by liver and by other tissues, including macrophages, ileum, and vascular endothelium. It normally carries only 20–60 ng of cobalamin per liter of plasma and readily gives up cobalamin to marrow, placenta, and other tissues, which it enters by receptor-mediated endocytosis involving the TC II receptor and megalin (encoded by the LRP-2 gene). The TC II cobalamin is internalized by endocytosis via clathrin-coated pits; the complex is degraded, but the receptor probably is recycled to the cell membrane as is the case for transferrin. Export of "free" cobalamin is via the ATP-binding cassette drug transporter alias multidrug resistance protein 1.

Dietary folate

Folic (pteroylglutamic) acid is a yellow, crystalline, water-soluble substance. It is the parent compound of a large family of natural folate compounds, which differ from it in three respects: (1) they are partly or completely reduced to di- or tetrahydrofolate (THF) derivatives, (2) they usually contain a single carbon unit (Table 105-2), and (3) 70–90% of natural folates are folate-polyglutamates.

Most foods contain some folate. The highest concentrations are found in liver, yeast, spinach, other greens, and nuts (>100 μg/100 g). The total folate content of an average Western diet is ~250 μg daily, but the amount varies widely according to the type of food eaten and the method of cooking. Folate is easily destroyed by heating, particularly in large volumes of water. Total-body folate in the adult is ~10 mg, with the liver containing the largest store. Daily adult requirements are ~100 μg, and so stores are sufficient for only 3–4 months in normal adults and severe folate deficiency may develop rapidly.

Absorption

Folates are absorbed rapidly from the upper small intestine. The absorption of folate polyglutamates is less efficient than that of monoglutamates; on average, ~50% of food folate is absorbed. Polyglutamate forms are hydrolyzed to the monoglutamate derivatives either in the lumen of the intestine or within the mucosa. All dietary folates are converted to 5-methylTHF (5-MTHF) within the small-intestinal mucosa before entering portal plasma. The monoglutamates are actively transported across the enterocyte by a carrier-mediated mechanism. Pteroylglutamic acid at doses >400 μg is absorbed largely unchanged and converted to natural folates in the liver. Lower doses are converted to 5-MTHF during absorption through the intestine.

About 60–90 μg of folate enters the bile each day and is excreted into the small intestine. Loss of this folate, together with the folate of sloughed intestinal cells, accelerates the speed with which folate deficiency develops in malabsorption conditions.

Transport

Folate is transported in plasma; about one-third is loosely bound to albumin, and two-thirds is unbound. In all body fluids (plasma, cerebrospinal fluid, milk, bile) folate is largely, if not entirely, 5-MTHF in the monoglutamate form. Two types of folate-binding protein are involved in the entry of MTHF into cells. A high-affinity proton-coupled folate receptor (PCFT/HCP1) takes folate into cells by endocytosis and is internalized by clathrin-coated pits or in a vesicle (caveola), which is then acidified, releasing folate. It accounts for the bulk of folate absorption. Folate then is carried by the membrane folate transporter into the cytoplasm. The high-affinity receptor is attached to the outer surface of the cell membrane by glycosyl phosphatidylinositol linkages. It may be involved in transport of oxidized folates and folate breakdown products to the liver for excretion in bile. An independent low-affinity reduced-folate carrier also mediates uptake of physiologic folates into cells but also regulates the uptake of methotrexate.

Biochemical functions

Folates (as the intracellular polyglutamate derivatives) act as coenzymes in the transfer of single-carbon units (Fig. 105-1 and Table 105-2). Two of these reactions are involved in purine synthesis and one in pyrimidine synthesis necessary for DNA and RNA replication. Folate is also a coenzyme for methionine synthesis, in which methylcobalamin is also involved and in which THF is regenerated. THF is the acceptor of single carbon units newly entering the active pool via conversion of serine to glycine. Methionine, the other product of the methionine synthase reaction, is the precursor for S-adenosylmethionine (SAM), the universal methyl donor involved in >100 methyltransferase reactions (Fig. 105-1).

During thymidylate synthesis, 5,10-methylene-THF is oxidized to DHF (dihydrofolate). The enzyme DHF reductase converts this to THF. The drugs methotrexate, pyrimethamine, and (mainly in bacteria) trimethoprim inhibit DHF reductase and so prevent formation of active THF coenzymes from DHF. A small fraction of the folate coenzyme is not recycled during thymidylate synthesis but is degraded.

TABLE 105-2 Biochemical Reactions of Folate Coenzymes

Reaction	Coenzyme Form of Folate Involved	Single Carbon Unit Transferred	Importance
Formate activation	THF	$-CHO$	Generation of 10-formyl-THF
Purine synthesis			
Formation of glycinamide ribonucleotide	5,10-MethyleneTHF	$-CHO$	Formation of purines needed for DNA, RNA synthesis, but reactions probably not rate-limiting
Formylation of aminoimidazole carboxamide ribonucleotide (AICAR)	10-Formyl (CHO)THF		
Pyrimidine synthesis			
Methylation of deoxyuridine monophosphate (dUMP) to thymidine monophosphate (dTMP)	5,10-MethyleneTHF	$-CH_3$	Rate limiting in DNA synthesis Oxidizes THF to DHF Some breakdown of folate at the C-9–N-10 bond
Amino acid interconversion			
Serine–glycine interconversion	THF	$=CH_2$	Entry of single carbon units into active pool
Homocysteine to methionine	5-Methyl(M)THF	$-CH_3$	Demethylation of 5-MTHF to THF; also requires cobalamin, flavine adenine dinucleotide, ATP, and adenosylmethionine
Forminoglutamic acid to glutamic acid in histidine catabolism	THF	$-HN-CH=$	

Abbreviations: DHF, dihydrofolate; THF, tetrahydrofolate.

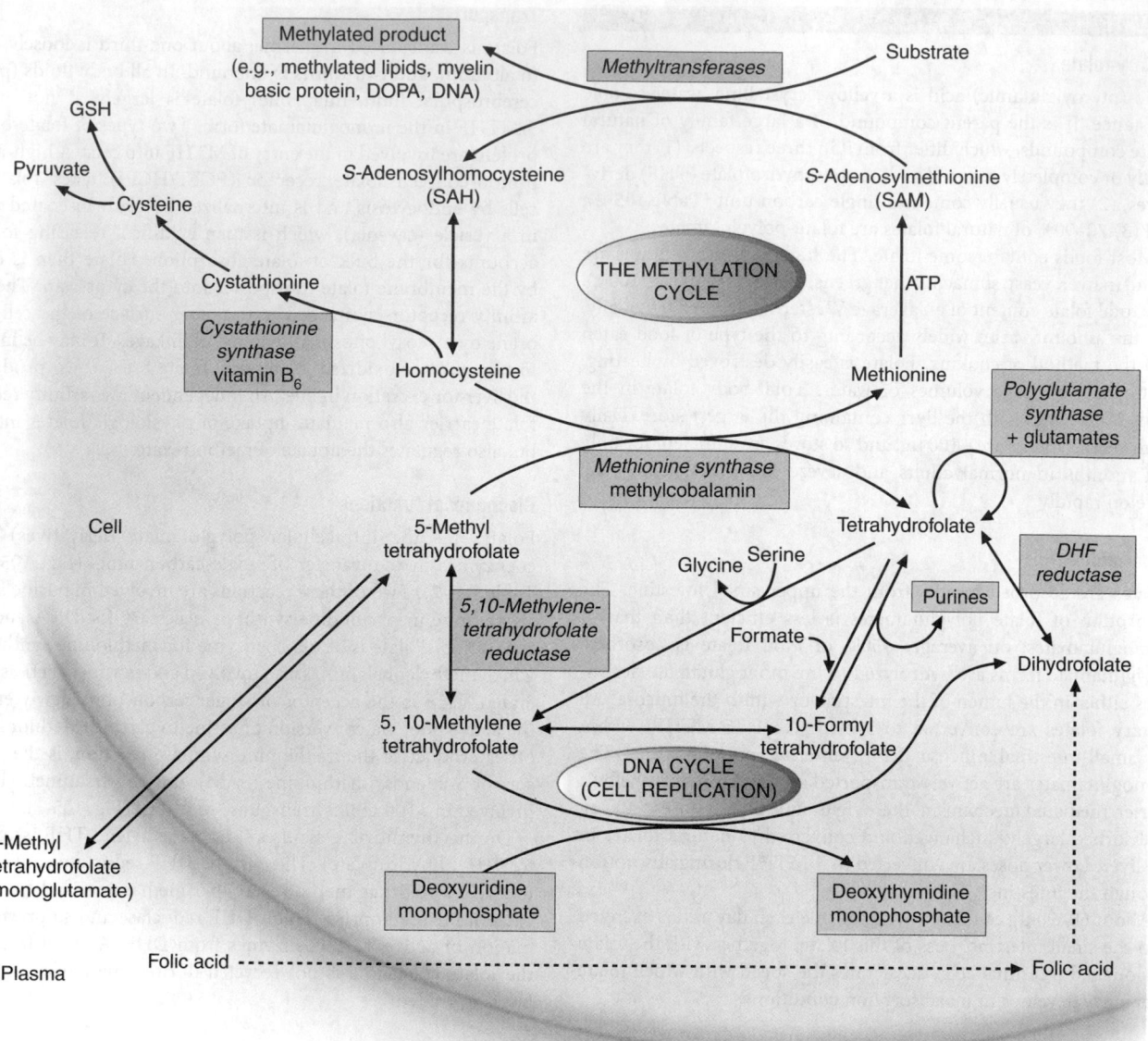

Figure 105-1 **The role of folates in DNA synthesis** and in formation of *S*-adenosylmethionine (SAM), which is involved in numerous methylation reactions. *[Reprinted from AV Hoffbrand et al (eds), Postgraduate Haematology, 5th ed, Oxford, UK, Blackwell Publishing, 2005; with permission.]*

BIOCHEMICAL BASIS OF MEGALOBLASTIC ANEMIA

The common feature of all megaloblastic anemias is a defect in DNA synthesis that affects rapidly dividing cells in the bone marrow. All conditions that give rise to megaloblastic changes have in common a disparity in the rate of synthesis or availability of the four immediate precursors of DNA: the deoxyribonucleoside triphosphates (dNTPs)—dA(adenine)TP and dG(guanine)TP (purines), dT(thymine)TP and dC(cytosine)TP (pyrimidines). In deficiencies of either folate or cobalamin, there is failure to convert deoxyuridine monophosphate (dUMP) to deoxythymidine monophosphate (dTMP), the precursor of dTTP (Fig. 105-1). This is the case because folate is needed as the coenzyme 5,10-methylene-THF polyglutamate for conversion of dUMP to dTMP; the availability of 5,10-methylene-THF is reduced in either cobalamin or folate deficiency. An alternative theory for megaloblastic anemia in cobalamin or folate deficiency is misincorporation of uracil into DNA because of a buildup of deoxyuridine triphosphate (dUTP) at the DNA replication fork as a consequence of the block in conversion of dUMP to dTMP.

Cobalamin-folate relations

Folate is required for many reactions in mammalian tissues. Only two reactions in the body are known to require cobalamin. Methylmalonyl CoA isomerization requires adocobalamin, and the methylation of homocysteine to methionine requires both methylcobalamin and 5-MTHF (Fig. 105-1). This reaction is the first step in the pathway by which 5-MTHF, which enters bone marrow and other cells from plasma, is converted into all the intracellular folate coenzymes. The coenzymes are all polyglutamated (the larger size aiding retention in the cell), but the enzyme folate polyglutamate synthase can use only THF, not MTHF, as substrate. In cobalamin deficiency, MTHF accumulates in plasma, and intracellular folate concentrations fall due to failure of formation of THF, the substrate on which folate polyglutamates are built. This has been termed *THF starvation*, or the *methylfolate trap*.

This theory explains the abnormalities of folate metabolism that occur in cobalamin deficiency [high serum folate, low cell folate, positive purine precursor aminoimidazole carboxamide ribonucleotide (AICAR) excretion; Table 105-2] and also why the anemia of cobalamin deficiency responds to folic acid in large doses.

CLINICAL FEATURES

Many symptomless patients are detected through the finding of a raised mean corpuscular volume (MCV) on a routine blood count. The main clinical features in more severe cases are those of anemia. Anorexia is usually marked, and there may be weight loss, diarrhea, or constipation. Glossitis, angular cheilosis, a mild fever in more severely anemic patients, jaundice (unconjugated), and reversible melanin skin hyperpigmentation also may occur with a deficiency of either folate or cobalamin. Thrombocytopenia sometimes leads to bruising, and this may be aggravated by vitamin C deficiency or alcohol in malnourished patients. The anemia and low leukocyte count may predispose to infections, particularly of the respiratory and urinary tracts. Cobalamin deficiency has also been associated with impaired bactericidal function of phagocytes.

General tissue effects of cobalamin and folate deficiencies

Epithelial surfaces After the marrow, the next most frequently affected tissues are the epithelial cell surfaces of the mouth, stomach, and small intestine and the respiratory, urinary, and female genital tracts. The cells show macrocytosis, with increased numbers of multinucleate and dying cells. The deficiencies may cause cervical smear abnormalities.

Complications of pregnancy The gonads are also affected, and infertility is common in both men and women with either deficiency. Maternal folate deficiency has been implicated as a cause of prematurity, and both folate deficiency and cobalamin deficiency have been implicated in recurrent fetal loss and neural tube defects, as discussed below.

Neural tube defects Folic acid supplements at the time of conception and in the first 12 weeks of pregnancy reduce by ~70% the incidence of neural tube defects (NTDs) (anencephaly, meningomyelocele, encephalocele, and spina bifida) in the fetus. Most of this protective effect can be achieved by taking folic acid, 0.4 mg daily at the time of conception.

The incidence of cleft palate and harelip also can be reduced by prophylactic folic acid. There is no clear simple relationship between maternal folate status and these fetal abnormalities, although overall the lower the maternal folate, the greater the risk to the fetus. NTDs also can be caused by antifolate and antiepileptic drugs.

An underlying maternal folate metabolic abnormality has also been postulated. One abnormality has been identified: reduced activity of the enzyme 5,10-methylene-THF reductase (MTHFR) (Fig. 105-1) caused by a common C677T polymorphism in the *MTHFR* gene. In one study, the prevalence of this polymorphism was found to be higher in the parents of NTD fetuses and in the fetuses themselves: Homozygosity for the TT mutation was found in 13% compared with 5% in control subjects. The polymorphism codes for a thermolabile form of MTHFR. The homozygous state results in a lower mean serum and red cell folate level compared with control subjects, as well as significantly higher serum homocysteine levels. Tests for mutations in other enzymes possibly associated with NTDs, e.g., methionine synthase and serine–glycine hydroxymethylase, have been negative. Autoantibodies to folate receptors were suggested to be more common in mothers of NTD babies, but this has been disproved.

Cardiovascular disease Children with severe homocystinuria (blood levels ≥100 μmol/L) due to deficiency of one of three enzymes, methionine synthase, MTHFR, or cystathionine synthase (Fig. 105-1), have vascular disease, e.g., ischemic heart disease, cerebrovascular disease, or pulmonary embolus as teenagers or in young adulthood. Lesser degrees of raised serum homocysteine and low levels of serum folate and homozygous inherited mutations of MTHFR have been found to be associated with cerebrovascular, peripheral vascular, and coronary heart disease and with deep vein thrombosis. Prospective randomized trials of lowering homocysteine levels with supplements of folic acid, vitamin B_{12}, and vitamin B_6 against placebo over a 5-year period in patients with vascular disease or diabetes have not, however, shown a reduction of major cardiovascular events, nor have these supplements reduced the risk of recurrent cardiovascular disease after an acute myocardial infarct. It is possible that these trials were not sufficiently powered to detect a small (e.g., 10%) benefit or that another underlying factor is responsible for both the vascular damage and the raised homocysteine. Alternatively, the beneficial effects of lowering homocysteine were offset in these trials by the vitamins stimulating endothelial cell proliferation. Meta-analysis has suggested that folic acid supplementation reduces the risk of stroke by 18%. The results of longer and larger trials are needed to resolve these uncertainties.

Malignancy Prophylactic folic acid in pregnancy has been found in some but not all studies to reduce the subsequent incidence of acute lymphoblastic leukemia (ALL) in childhood. A significant negative association has also been found with the *MTHFR* C677T polymorphism and leukemias with mixed lineage leukemia (MLL) translocations, but a positive association with hyperdiploidy in infants with ALL or acute myeloid leukemia or with childhood ALL. A second polymorphism in the *MTHFR* gene, A1298C, is also strongly associated with hyperdiploid leukemia. There are various positive and negative associations between polymorphisms in folate-dependent enzymes and the incidence of adult ALL. The C677T polymorphism is thought to lead to increased thymidine pools and "better quality" of DNA synthesis by shunting 1-carbon groups toward thymidine and purine synthesis. This may explain its reported association with a lower risk for colorectal cancer. Most but not all studies suggest that prophylactic folic acid also protects against colon adenomas. Other tumors that have been associated with folate polymorphisms or status include follicular lymphoma, breast cancer, and gastric cancer. Because folic acid may "feed" tumors, it probably should be avoided in those with established tumors unless there is severe megaloblastic anemia due to folate deficiency.

Neurologic manifestations Cobalamin deficiency may cause a bilateral peripheral neuropathy or degeneration (demyelination) of the posterior and pyramidal tracts of the spinal cord and, less frequently, optic atrophy or cerebral symptoms.

The patient, more frequently male, presents with paresthesias, muscle weakness, or difficulty in walking and sometimes dementia, psychotic disturbances, or visual impairment. Long-term nutritional cobalamin deficiency in infancy leads to poor brain development and impaired intellectual development. Folate deficiency has been suggested to cause organic nervous disease, but this is uncertain, although methotrexate injected into the cerebrospinal fluid may cause brain or spinal cord damage.

An important clinical problem is the nonanemic patient with neurologic or psychiatric abnormalities and a low or borderline serum cobalamin level. In such patients, it is necessary to try to establish whether there is significant cobalamin deficiency, e.g., by careful examination of the blood film, tests for serum gastrin level and for antibodies to IF or parietal cells, along with serum methylmalonic acid (MMA) measurement if available. A trial of cobalamin therapy for at least 3 months will usually also be needed to determine whether the symptoms improve.

The biochemical basis for cobalamin neuropathy remains obscure. Its occurrence in the absence of methylmalonic aciduria in TC II deficiency suggests that the neuropathy is related to the defect in homocysteine-methionine conversion. Accumulation of *S*-adenosylhomocysteine in the brain, resulting in inhibition of transmethylation reactions, has been suggested.

Psychiatric disturbance is common in both folate and cobalamin deficiencies. This, like the neuropathy, has been attributed to a failure of the synthesis of SAM, which is needed in methylation of biogenic amines (e.g., dopamine) as well as that of proteins, phospholipids, and neurotransmitters in the brain (Fig. 105-1). Associations between lower serum folate or cobalamin levels and higher homocysteine levels and the development of decreased cognitive function and dementia in Alzheimer's disease have been reported. A 2-year double-blind placebo-controlled randomized clinical trial involving healthy subjects >65 years old given folate, cobalamin, and vitamin B_6 supplements showed no benefit for cognitive performance, whereas a 3-year (FACIT) study did show benefit.

HEMATOLOGIC FINDINGS

Peripheral blood

Oval macrocytes, usually with considerable anisocytosis and poikilocytosis, are the main feature (Fig. 105-2A). The MCV is usually >100 fL unless a cause of microcytosis (e.g., iron deficiency or thalassemia trait) is present. Some of the neutrophils are hypersegmented (more than five nuclear lobes). There may be leukopenia due to a reduction in granulocytes and lymphocytes, but this is usually >1.5 × 10⁹/L; the platelet count may be moderately reduced, rarely to <40 × 10⁹/L. The severity of all these changes parallels the degree of anemia. In a nonanemic patient, the presence of a few macrocytes and hypersegmented neutrophils in the peripheral blood may be the only indication of the underlying disorder.

Bone marrow

In a severely anemic patient, the marrow is hypercellular with an accumulation of primitive cells due to selective death by apoptosis of more mature forms. The erythroblast nucleus maintains a primitive appearance despite maturation and hemoglobinization of the cytoplasm. The cells are larger than normoblasts, and an increased number of cells with eccentric lobulated nuclei or nuclear fragments may be present (Fig. 105-2B). Giant and abnormally shaped metamyelocytes and enlarged hyperpolyploid megakaryocytes are characteristic. In less anemic patients, the changes in the marrow may be difficult to recognize. The terms *intermediate,*

mild, and *early* have been used. The term *megaloblastoid* does not mean mildly megaloblastic. It is used to describe cells with both immature-appearing nuclei and defective hemoglobinization and is usually seen in myelodysplasia.

Chromosomes

Bone marrow cells, transformed lymphocytes, and other proliferating cells in the body show a variety of changes, including random breaks, reduced contraction, spreading of the centromere, and exaggeration of secondary chromosomal constrictions and overprominent satellites. Similar abnormalities may be produced by antimetabolite drugs (e.g., cytosine arabinoside, hydroxyurea, and methotrexate) that interfere with either DNA replication or folate metabolism and that also cause megaloblastic appearances.

Ineffective hematopoiesis

There is an accumulation of unconjugated bilirubin in plasma due to the death of nucleated red cells in the marrow (ineffective erythropoiesis). Other evidence for this includes raised urine urobilinogen, reduced haptoglobins and positive urine hemosiderin, and a raised serum lactate dehydrogenase. A weakly positive direct antiglobulin test due to complement can lead to a false diagnosis of autoimmune hemolytic anemia.

CAUSES OF COBALAMIN DEFICIENCY

Cobalamin deficiency is usually due to malabsorption. The only other cause is inadequate dietary intake.

Inadequate dietary intake

Adults Dietary cobalamin deficiency arises in vegans who omit meat, fish, eggs, cheese, and other animal products from their diet. The largest group in the world consists of Hindus, and it is likely that many millions of Indians are at risk of deficiency of cobalamin on a nutritional basis. Subnormal serum cobalamin levels are found in up to 50% of randomly selected, young, adult Indian vegans, but the deficiency usually does not progress to megaloblastic anemia since the diet of most vegans is not totally lacking in cobalamin and the enterohepatic circulation of cobalamin is intact. Dietary

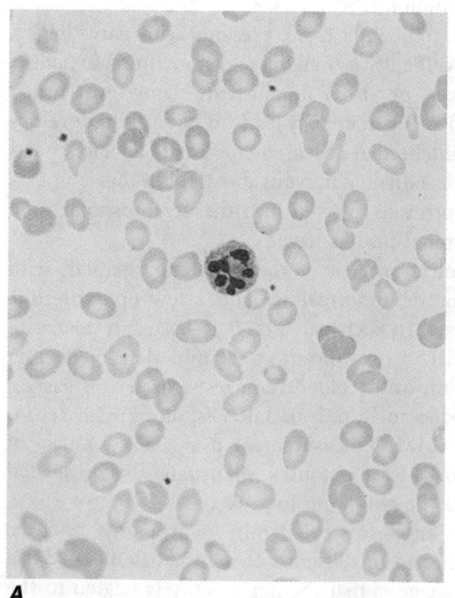
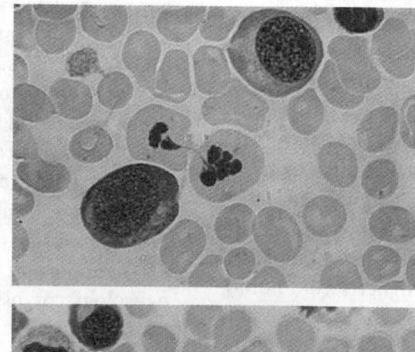
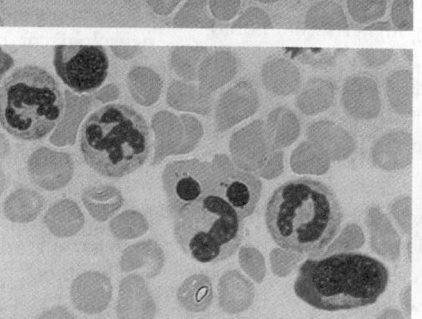
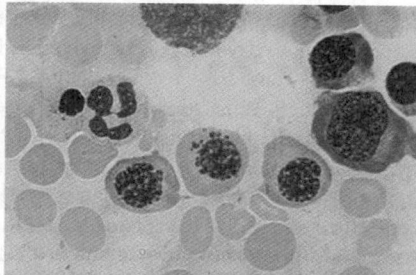
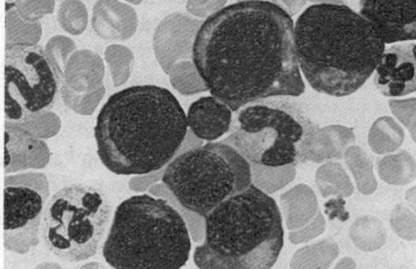

A

B

Figure 105-2 A. The peripheral blood in severe megaloblastic anemia. **B.** The bone marrow in severe megaloblastic anemia. *[Reprinted from AV Hoffbrand et al (eds), Postgraduate Haematology, 5th ed, Oxford, UK, Blackwell Publishing, 2005; with permission.]*

cobalamin deficiency may also arise rarely in nonvegetarian individuals who exist on grossly inadequate diets because of poverty or psychiatric disturbance.

Infants Cobalamin deficiency has been described in infants born to severely cobalamin-deficient mothers. These infants develop megaloblastic anemia at about 3–6 months of age, presumably because they are born with low stores of cobalamin and because they are fed breast milk with low cobalamin content. The babies have also shown growth retardation, impaired psychomotor development, and other neurologic sequelae.

Gastric causes of cobalamin malabsorption

See Tables 105-3 and 105-4.

Pernicious anemia Pernicious anemia (PA) may be defined as a severe lack of IF due to gastric atrophy. It is a common disease in north Europeans but occurs in all countries and ethnic groups. The overall incidence is about 120 per 100,000 population in the United Kingdom (UK). The ratio of incidence in men and women among whites is ~1:1.6, and the peak age of onset is 60 years, with only 10% of patients being <40 years of age. However, in some ethnic groups, notably black individuals and Latin Americans, the age at onset of PA is generally lower. The disease occurs more commonly than by chance in close relatives and in persons with other organ-specific autoimmune diseases, e.g., thyroid diseases, vitiligo, hypoparathyroidism, and Addison's disease. It is also associated with hypogammaglobulinemia, with premature graying or blue eyes, and persons of blood group A. An association with human leukocyte antigen (HLA) 3 has been reported in some but not all series and, in those with endocrine disease, with HLA-B8, -B12, and -BW15. Life expectancy is normal in women once regular treatment has begun. Men have a slightly subnormal life expectancy as a result of a higher incidence of carcinoma of the stomach than in control subjects. Gastric output of hydrochloric acid, pepsin, and IF is severely reduced. The serum gastrin level is raised, and serum pepsinogen I levels are low.

Gastric biopsy This usually shows atrophy of all layers of the body and fundus, with loss of glandular elements, an absence of parietal and chief cells and replacement by mucous cells, a mixed inflammatory cell infiltrate, and perhaps intestinal metaplasia. The infiltrate of plasma cells and lymphocytes contains an excess of CD4 cells.

TABLE 105-3 Causes of Cobalamin Deficiency Sufficiently Severe to Cause Megaloblastic Anemia

Nutritional	Vegans
Malabsorption	Pernicious anemia
Gastric causes	Congenital absence of intrinsic factor or functional abnormality
	Total or partial gastrectomy
Intestinal causes	Intestinal stagnant loop syndrome: jejunal diverticulosis, ileocolic fistula, anatomic blind loop, intestinal stricture, etc.
	Ileal resection and Crohn's disease
	Selective malabsorption with proteinuria
	Tropical sprue
	Transcobalamin II deficiency
	Fish tapeworm

TABLE 105-4 Malabsorption of Cobalamin May Occur in the Following Conditions But Is Not Usually Sufficiently Severe and Prolonged to Cause Megaloblastic Anemia

Gastric causes
  Simple atrophic gastritis (food cobalamin malabsorption)
  Zollinger–Ellison syndrome
  Gastric bypass surgery
  Use of proton pump inhibitors
Intestinal causes
  Gluten-induced enteropathy
  Severe pancreatitis
  HIV infection
  Radiotherapy
  Graft-versus-host disease
Deficiencies of cobalamin, folate, protein, ?riboflavin, ?nicotinic acid
Therapy with colchicine, para-aminosalicylate, neomycin, slow-release potassium chloride, anticonvulsant drugs, metformin, phenformin, cytotoxic drugs
Alcohol

The antral mucosa is usually well preserved. *Helicobacter pylori* infection occurs infrequently in PA, but it has been suggested that *H. pylori* gastritis occurs at an early phase of atrophic gastritis and presents in younger patients as iron-deficiency anemia but in older patients as PA. *H. pylori* is suggested to stimulate an autoimmune process directed against parietal cells, with the *H. pylori* infection then being gradually replaced, in some individuals, by an autoimmune process.

Serum antibodies Two types of IF immunoglobulin G antibody may be found in the sera of patients with PA. One, the "blocking," or type I, antibody, prevents the combination of IF and cobalamin, whereas the "binding," or type II, antibody prevents attachment of IF to ileal mucosa. Type I occurs in the sera of ~55% of patients, and type II in 35%. IF antibodies cross the placenta and may cause temporary IF deficiency in a newborn infant. Patients with PA also show cell-mediated immunity to IF. Type I antibody has been detected rarely in the sera of patients without PA but with thyrotoxicosis, myxedema, Hashimoto's disease, or diabetes mellitus and in relatives of PA patients. IF antibodies also have been detected in gastric juice in ~80% of PA patients. These gastric antibodies may reduce absorption of dietary cobalamin by combining with small amounts of remaining IF.

Parietal cell antibody is present in the sera of almost 90% of adult patients with PA but is frequently present in other subjects. Thus, it occurs in as many as 16% of randomly selected female subjects age >60 years. The parietal cell antibody is directed against the α and β subunits of the gastric proton pump (H^+,K^+-ATPase).

Juvenile pernicious anemia

This usually occurs in older children and resembles PA of adults. Gastric atrophy, achlorhydria, and serum IF antibodies are all present, although parietal cell antibodies are usually absent. About one-half of these patients show an associated endocrinopathy such as autoimmune thyroiditis, Addison's disease, or hypoparathyroidism; in some, mucocutaneous candidiasis occurs.

Congenital intrinsic factor deficiency or functional abnormality

An affected child usually presents with megaloblastic anemia in the first to third year of life; a few have presented as late as the second decade. The child usually has no demonstrable IF but has a normal gastric mucosa and normal secretion of acid. The inheritance is autosomal recessive. Parietal cell and IF antibodies are absent. Variants have been described in which the child is born with IF that can be detected immunologically but is unstable or functionally inactive, unable to bind cobalamin or to facilitate its uptake by ileal receptors.

Gastrectomy

After total gastrectomy, cobalamin deficiency is inevitable, and prophylactic cobalamin therapy should be commenced immediately after the operation. After partial gastrectomy, 10–15% of patients also develop this deficiency. The exact incidence and time of onset are most influenced by the size of the resection and the preexisting size of cobalamin body stores.

Food cobalamin malabsorption

Failure of release of cobalamin from binding proteins in food is believed to be responsible for this condition, which is more common in the elderly. It is associated with low serum cobalamin levels, with or without raised serum levels of MMA and homocysteine. Typically, these patients have normal cobalamin absorption, as measured with crystalline cobalamin, but show malabsorption when a modified test using food-bound cobalamin is used. The frequency of progression to severe cobalamin deficiency and the reasons for this progression are not clear.

Intestinal causes of cobalamin malabsorption

Intestinal stagnant loop syndrome Malabsorption of cobalamin occurs in a variety of intestinal lesions in which there is colonization of the upper small intestine by fecal organisms. This may occur in patients with jejunal diverticulosis, enteroanastomosis, or an intestinal stricture or fistula or with an anatomic blind loop due to Crohn's disease, tuberculosis, or an operative procedure.

Ileal resection Removal of ≥1.2 m of terminal ileum causes malabsorption of cobalamin. In some patients after ileal resection, particularly if the ileocecal valve is incompetent, colonic bacteria may contribute further to the onset of cobalamin deficiency.

Selective malabsorption of cobalamin with proteinuria (Imerslund syndrome: Imerslund-Gräsbeck syndrome; congenital cobalamin malabsorption; autosomal recessive megaloblastic anemia, MGA1) This autosomally recessive disease is the most common cause of megaloblastic anemia due to cobalamin deficiency in infancy in Western countries. More than 200 cases have been reported, with familial clusters in Finland, Norway, the Middle East, and North Africa. The patients secrete normal amounts of IF and gastric acid but are unable to absorb cobalamin. In Finland, impaired synthesis, processing, or ligand binding of cubilin due to inherited mutations is found. In Norway, mutation of the gene for AMN has been reported. Other tests of intestinal absorption are normal. Over 90% of these patients show nonspecific proteinuria, but renal function is otherwise normal and renal biopsy has not shown any consistent renal defect. A few have shown aminoaciduria and congenital renal abnormalities, such as duplication of the renal pelvis.

Tropical sprue Nearly all patients with acute and subacute tropical sprue show malabsorption of cobalamin; this may persist as the principal abnormality in the chronic form of the disease, when the patient may present with megaloblastic anemia or neuropathy due to cobalamin deficiency. Absorption of cobalamin usually improves after antibiotic therapy and, in the early stages, folic acid therapy.

Fish tapeworm infestation The fish tapeworm (*Diphyllobothrium latum*) lives in the small intestine of humans and accumulates cobalamin from food, rendering the cobalamin unavailable for absorption. Individuals acquire the worm by eating raw or partly cooked fish. Infestation is common around the lakes of Scandinavia, Germany, Japan, North America, and Russia. Megaloblastic anemia or cobalamin neuropathy occurs only in those with a heavy infestation.

Gluten-induced enteropathy Malabsorption of cobalamin occurs in ~30% of untreated patients (presumably those in whom the disease extends to the ileum). Cobalamin deficiency is not severe in these patients and is corrected with a gluten-free diet.

Severe chronic pancreatitis In this condition, lack of trypsin is thought to cause dietary cobalamin attached to gastric non-IF (R) binder to be unavailable for absorption. It also has been proposed that in pancreatitis, the concentration of calcium ions in the ileum falls below the level needed to maintain normal cobalamin absorption.

HIV infection Serum cobalamin levels tend to fall in patients with HIV infection and are subnormal in 10–35% of those with AIDS. Malabsorption of cobalamin not corrected by IF has been shown in some, but not all, patients with subnormal serum cobalamin levels. Cobalamin deficiency sufficiently severe to cause megaloblastic anemia or neuropathy is rare.

Zollinger–Ellison syndrome Malabsorption of cobalamin has been reported in the Zollinger–Ellison syndrome. It is thought that there is a failure to release cobalamin from R-binding protein due to inactivation of pancreatic trypsin by high acidity, as well as interference with IF binding of cobalamin.

Radiotherapy Both total-body irradiation and local radiotherapy to the ileum (e.g., as a complication of radiotherapy for carcinoma of the cervix) may cause malabsorption of cobalamin.

Graft-versus-host disease This commonly affects the small intestine. Malabsorption of cobalamin due to abnormal gut flora, as well as damage to ileal mucosa, is common.

Drugs The drugs that have been reported to cause malabsorption of cobalamin are listed in Table 105-4. Megaloblastic anemia due to these drugs is, however, rare.

Abnormalities of cobalamin metabolism

Congenital transcobalamin II deficiency or abnormality Infants with TC II deficiency usually present with megaloblastic anemia within a few weeks of birth. Serum cobalamin and folate levels are normal, but the anemia responds to massive (e.g., 1 mg three times weekly) injections of cobalamin. Some cases show neurologic complications. The protein may be present but functionally inert. Genetic abnormalities found include mutations of an intra-exonic cryptic splice site, extensive deletion, single nucleotide deletion, nonsense mutation, and an RNA editing defect. Malabsorption of cobalamin occurs in all cases, and serum immunoglobulins are usually reduced. Failure to institute adequate cobalamin therapy or treatment with folic acid may lead to neurologic damage.

Congenital methylmalonic acidemia and aciduria Infants with this abnormality are ill from birth with vomiting, failure to thrive, severe metabolic acidosis, ketosis, and mental retardation. Anemia, if present, is normocytic and normoblastic. The condition may be due to a functional defect in either mitochondrial methylmalonyl CoA mutase or its cofactor adocobalamin. Mutations in the methylmalonyl CoA mutase are not responsive, or only poorly responsive, to treatment with cobalamin. A proportion of infants with failure of adocobalamin synthesis respond to cobalamin in large doses. Some children have combined methylmalonic aciduria and homocystinuria due to defective formation of both cobalamin coenzymes. This usually presents in the first year of life with feeding difficulties, developmental delay, microcephaly, seizures, hypotonia, and megaloblastic anemia.

Acquired abnormality of cobalamin metabolism: nitrous oxide inhalation Nitrous oxide irreversibly oxidizes methylcobalamin to an inactive precursor; this inactivates methionine synthase. Megaloblastic anemia has occurred in patients undergoing prolonged N_2O anesthesia (e.g., in intensive care units). A neuropathy resembling cobalamin neuropathy has been described in dentists and anesthetists who are exposed repeatedly to N_2O. Methylmalonic aciduria does not occur as adocobalamin is not inactivated by N_2O.

CAUSES OF FOLATE DEFICIENCY

(Table 105-5)

Nutritional

Dietary folate deficiency is common. Indeed, in most patients with folate deficiency a nutritional element is present. Certain individuals are particularly prone to have diets containing inadequate amounts of folate (Table 105-5). In the United States and other countries where fortification of the diet with folic acid has been adopted, the prevalence of folate deficiency has dropped dramatically and is now almost restricted to high-risk groups with increased folate needs. Nutritional folate deficiency occurs in kwashiorkor and scurvy and in infants with repeated infections or those who are fed solely on goats' milk, which has a low folate content.

Malabsorption

Malabsorption of dietary folate occurs in tropical sprue and in gluten-induced enteropathy. In the rare congenital syndrome of selective malabsorption of folate due to mutation of the protein-coupled folate transporter (PCFT), there is an associated defect of folate transport into the cerebrospinal fluid, and these patients show megaloblastic anemia, which responds to physiologic doses of folic acid given parenterally but not orally. They also show mental retardation, convulsions, and other central nervous system abnormalities. Minor degrees of malabsorption may also occur after jejunal resection or partial gastrectomy, in Crohn's disease, and in systemic infections, but in these conditions, if severe deficiency occurs, it is usually largely due to poor nutrition. Malabsorption of folate has been described in patients receiving salazopyrine, cholestyramine, and triamterene.

Excess utilization or loss

Pregnancy Folate requirements are increased by 200–300 µg to ~400 µg daily in a normal pregnancy, partly because of transfer of the vitamin to the fetus but mainly because of increased folate catabolism due to cleavage of folate coenzymes in rapidly proliferating tissues. Megaloblastic anemia due to this deficiency is prevented by prophylactic folic acid therapy. It occurred in 0.5% of pregnancies in the UK and other Western countries before prophylaxis with folic acid, but the incidence is much higher in countries where the general nutritional status is poor.

Prematurity A newborn infant, whether full term or premature, has higher serum and red cell folate concentrations than does an adult. However, a newborn infant's demand for folate has been estimated to be up to 10 times that of adults on a weight basis, and the neonatal folate level falls rapidly to the lowest values at about 6 weeks of age. The falls are steepest and are liable to reach subnormal levels in premature babies, a number of whom develop megaloblastic anemia responsive to folic acid at about 4–6 weeks of age. This occurs particularly in the smallest babies (<1500 g birth weight) and those who have feeding difficulties or infections or have undergone multiple exchange transfusions. In these babies, prophylactic folic acid should be given.

Hematologic disorders Folate deficiency frequently occurs in chronic hemolytic anemia, particularly in sickle cell disease, autoimmune hemolytic anemia, and congenital spherocytosis. In these and other conditions of increased cell turnover (e.g., myelofibrosis, malignancies), folate deficiency arises because it is not completely reutilized after performing coenzyme functions.

Inflammatory conditions Chronic inflammatory diseases such as tuberculosis, rheumatoid arthritis, Crohn's disease, psoriasis, exfoliative dermatitis, bacterial endocarditis, and chronic bacterial infections cause deficiency by reducing the appetite and increasing the demand for folate. Systemic infections also may cause malabsorption of folate. Severe deficiency is virtually confined to the patients with the most active disease and the poorest diet.

Homocystinuria This is a rare metabolic defect in the conversion of homocysteine to cystathionine. Folate deficiency occurring in most

---

TABLE 105-5 Causes of Folate Deficiency

Dietary[a]

Particularly in: old age, infancy, poverty, alcoholism, chronic invalids, and the psychiatrically disturbed; may be associated with scurvy or kwashiorkor

Malabsorption

Major causes of deficiency

Tropical sprue, gluten-induced enteropathy in children and adults, and in association with dermatitis herpetiformis, specific malabsorption of folate, intestinal megaloblastosis caused by severe cobalamin or folate deficiency

Minor causes of deficiency

Extensive jejunal resection, Crohn's disease, partial gastrectomy, congestive heart failure, Whipple's disease, scleroderma, amyloid, diabetic enteropathy, systemic bacterial infection, lymphoma, salazopyrine

Excess utilization or loss

Physiologic

Pregnancy and lactation, prematurity

Pathologic

Hematologic diseases: chronic hemolytic anemias, sickle cell anemia, thalassemia major, myelofibrosis

Malignant diseases: carcinoma, lymphoma, leukemia, myeloma

Inflammatory diseases: tuberculosis, Crohn's disease, psoriasis, exfoliative dermatitis, malaria

Metabolic disease: homocystinuria

Excess urinary loss: congestive heart failure, active liver disease

Hemodialysis, peritoneal dialysis

Antifolate drugs[b]

Anticonvulsant drugs (phenytoin, primidone, barbiturates), sulphasalazine

Nitrofurantoin, tetracycline, antituberculosis (less well documented)

Mixed causes

Liver diseases, alcoholism, intensive care units

[a]In severely folate-deficient patients with causes other than those listed under Dietary, poor dietary intake is often present.
[b]Drugs inhibiting dihydrofolate reductase are discussed in the text.

of these patients may be due to excessive utilization because of compensatory increased conversion of homocysteine to methionine.

Long-term dialysis As folate is only loosely bound to plasma proteins, it is easily removed from plasma by dialysis. In patients with anorexia, vomiting, infections, and hemolysis, folate stores are particularly likely to become depleted. Routine folate prophylaxis is now given.

Congestive heart failure, liver disease Excess urinary folate losses of >100 μg per day may occur in some of these patients. The explanation appears to be release of folate from damaged liver cells.

Antifolate drugs

A large number of epileptics who are receiving long-term therapy with phenytoin or primidone, with or without barbiturates, develop low serum and red cell folate levels. The exact mechanism is unclear. Alcohol may also be a folate antagonist, as patients who are drinking spirits may develop megaloblastic anemia that will respond to normal quantities of dietary folate or to physiologic doses of folic acid only if alcohol is withdrawn. Macrocytosis of red cells is associated with chronic alcohol intake even when folate levels are normal. Inadequate folate intake is the major factor in the development of deficiency in spirit-drinking alcoholics. Beer is relatively folate-rich in some countries, depending on the technique used for brewing.

The drugs that inhibit DHF reductase include methotrexate, pyrimethamine, and trimethoprim. Methotrexate has the most powerful action against the human enzyme, whereas trimethoprim is most active against the bacterial enzyme and is likely to cause megaloblastic anemia only when used in conjunction with sulphamethoxazole in patients with preexisting folate or cobalamin deficiency. The activity of pyrimethamine is intermediate. The antidote to these drugs is folinic acid (5-formyl-THF).

Congenital abnormalities of folate metabolism

Some infants with congenital defects of folate enzymes (e.g., cyclohydrolase or methionine synthase) have had megaloblastic anemia.

DIAGNOSIS OF COBALAMIN AND FOLATE DEFICIENCIES

The diagnosis of cobalamin or folate deficiency has traditionally depended on the recognition of the relevant abnormalities in the peripheral blood and analysis of the blood levels of the vitamins.

Serum cobalamin

This is measured by an automated enzyme-linked immunosorbent assay (ELISA). Normal serum levels range from 118–148 pmol/L (160–200 ng/L) to ~738 pmol/L (1000 ng/L). In patients with megaloblastic anemia due to cobalamin deficiency, the level is usually <74 pmol/L (100 ng/L). In general, the more severe the deficiency, the lower the serum cobalamin level. In patients with spinal cord damage due to the deficiency, levels are very low even in the absence of anemia. Values between 74 and 148 pmol/L (100 and 200 ng/L) are regarded as borderline. They may occur, for instance, in pregnancy, in patients with megaloblastic anemia due to folate deficiency. They may also be due to heterozygous, homozygous, or compound heterozygous mutations of the gene *TCN1* that codes for haptocorrin (transcobalamin I). There is no clinical or rematologic abnormality. The serum cobalamin level is sufficiently robust, cost-effective, and most convenient to rule out cobalamin deficiency in the vast majority of patients suspected of having this problem.

Serum methylmalonate and homocysteine

In patients with cobalamin deficiency sufficient to cause anemia or neuropathy, the serum MMA level is raised. Sensitive methods for measuring MMA and homocysteine in serum have been introduced

and recommended for the early diagnosis of cobalamin deficiency, even in the absence of hematologic abnormalities or subnormal levels of serum cobalamin. Serum MMA levels fluctuate, however, in patients with renal failure. Mildly elevated serum MMA and/or homocysteine levels occur in up to 30% of apparently healthy volunteers, with serum cobalamin levels up to 258 pmol/L (350 ng/L) and normal serum folate levels; 15% of elderly subjects, even with cobalamin levels >258 pmol/L (>350 ng/L), have this pattern of raised metabolite levels. These findings bring into question the exact cutoff points for normal MMA and homocysteine levels. It is also unclear at present whether these mildly raised metabolite levels have clinical consequences.

Serum homocysteine is raised in both early cobalamin and folate deficiency but may be raised in other conditions, e.g., chronic renal disease, alcoholism, smoking, pyridoxine deficiency, hypothyroidism, and therapy with steroids, cyclosporine, and other drugs. Levels are also higher in serum than in plasma, in men than in premenopausal women, in women taking hormone replacement therapy or in oral contraceptive users, and in elderly persons and patients with several inborn errors of metabolism affecting enzymes in trans-sulfuration pathways of homocysteine metabolism. Thus, homocysteine levels are not used for diagnosis of cobalamin or folate deficiency.

Other tests

Studies of cobalamin absorption once were widely used, but difficulty in obtaining radioactive cobalamin and ensuring that IF preparations are free of viruses has made these tests obsolete. Tests to diagnose PA include serum gastrin, which is raised, and serum pepsinogen I, which is low in PA (90–92%) but also in other conditions. Tests for IF and parietal cell antibodies are also used as well as tests for individual intestinal diseases.

Serum folate

This is also measured by an ELISA technique. In most laboratories, the normal range is from 11 nmol/L (2 μg/L) to ~82 nmol/L (15 μg/L). The serum folate level is low in all folate-deficient patients. It also reflects recent diet. Because of this, serum folate may be low before there is hematologic or biochemical evidence of deficiency. Serum folate rises in severe cobalamin deficiency because of the block in conversion of MTHF to THF inside cells; raised levels have also been reported in the intestinal stagnant loop syndrome due to absorption of bacterially synthesized folate.

Red cell folate

The red cell folate assay is a valuable test of body folate stores. It is less affected than the serum assay by recent diet and traces of hemolysis. In normal adults, concentrations range from 880–3520 μmol/L (160–640 μg/L) of packed red cells. Subnormal levels occur in patients with megaloblastic anemia due to folate deficiency but also in nearly two-thirds of patients with severe cobalamin deficiency. False-normal results may occur if a folate-deficient patient has received a recent blood transfusion or if a patient has a raised reticulocyte count.

TREATMENT Megaloblastic Anemia

It is usually possible to establish which of the two deficiencies, folate or cobalamin, is the cause of the anemia and to treat only with the appropriate vitamin. In patients who enter the hospital severely ill, however, it may be necessary to treat with both vitamins in large doses once blood samples have been taken for cobalamin and folate assays and a bone marrow biopsy has been performed (if deemed necessary). Transfusion is usually unnecessary and inadvisable. If it is essential, packed red cells should be given slowly, one or two units only, with the usual treatment for heart failure if present. Potassium supplements have been recommended to obviate the danger of the hypokalemia but are not necessary. Occasionally, an excessive rise in platelets occurs after 1–2 weeks of therapy. Antiplatelet therapy, e.g., aspirin, should be considered if the platelet count rises to >800 × 10⁹/L.

COBALAMIN DEFICIENCY   It is usually necessary to treat patients who have developed cobalamin deficiency with lifelong regular cobalamin injections. In the UK, the form used is hydroxocobalamin; in the United States, cyanocobalamin. In a few instances, the underlying cause of cobalamin deficiency can be permanently corrected, e.g., fish tapeworm, tropical sprue, or an intestinal stagnant loop that is amenable to surgery. The indications for starting cobalamin therapy are a well-documented megaloblastic anemia or other hematologic abnormalities and neuropathy due to the deficiency. Patients with borderline serum cobalamin levels but no hematologic or other abnormality may be followed to make sure that the cobalamin deficiency does not progress (see below). If malabsorption of cobalamin or rises in serum MMA levels have been demonstrated, however, these patients also should be given regular maintenance cobalamin therapy. Cobalamin should be given routinely to all patients who have had a total gastrectomy or ileal resection. Patients who have undergone gastric reduction for control of obesity or who are receiving long-term treatment with proton pump inhibitors should be screened and, if necessary, given cobalamin replacement.

Replenishment of body stores should be complete with six 1000-μg IM injections of hydroxocobalamin given at 3- to 7-day intervals. More frequent doses are usually used in patients with cobalamin neuropathy, but there is no evidence that they produce a better response. Allergic reactions are rare and may require desensitization or antihistamine or glucocorticoid cover. For maintenance therapy, 1000 μg hydroxocobalamin IM once every 3 months is satisfactory. Because of the poorer retention of cyanocobalamin, protocols generally use higher and more frequent doses, e.g., 1000 μg IM, monthly, for maintenance treatment.

Because a small fraction of cobalamin can be absorbed passively through mucous membranes even when there is complete failure of physiologic IF-dependent absorption, large daily oral doses (1000–2000 μg) of cyanocobalamin have been used in PA for replacement and maintenance of normal cobalamin status in, e.g., food malabsorption of cobalamin. Sublingual therapy has also been proposed for those in whom injections are difficult because of a bleeding tendency and who may not tolerate oral therapy. If oral therapy is used, it is important to monitor compliance, particularly with elderly, forgetful patients.

For treatment of patients with subnormal serum B$_{12}$ levels with a normal MCV and no hypersegmentation of neutrophils, a negative IF antibody test in the absence of tests of B$_{12}$ absorption is problematic. Some (perhaps 15%) cases may be due to TC I (HC) deficiency. Homocysteine and/or MMA measurements may help, but in the absence of these tests and with otherwise normal gastrointestinal function, repeat serum B$_{12}$ assay after 6–12 months may help one decide whether to start cobalamin therapy.

FOLATE DEFICIENCY   Oral doses of 5–15 mg folic acid daily are satisfactory, as sufficient folate is absorbed from these extremely large doses even in patients with severe malabsorption. The length of time therapy must be continued depends on the underlying disease. It is customary to continue therapy for about 4 months, when all folate-deficient red cells will have been eliminated and replaced by new folate-replete populations.

Before large doses of folic acid are given, cobalamin deficiency must be excluded and, if present, corrected; otherwise cobalamin neuropathy may develop despite a response of the anemia of cobalamin deficiency to folate therapy. Studies in the United States, however, suggest that there is no increase in the proportion of individuals with low serum cobalamin levels and no anemia since food fortification with folic acid, but it is unknown if there has been a change in incidence of cobalamin neuropathy.

Long-term folic acid therapy is required when the underlying cause of the deficiency cannot be corrected and the deficiency is likely to recur, e.g., in chronic dialysis or hemolytic anemias. It may also be necessary in gluten-induced enteropathy that does not respond to a gluten-free diet. Where mild but chronic folate deficiency occurs, it is preferable to encourage improvement in the diet after correcting the deficiency with a short course of folic acid. In any patient receiving long-term folic acid therapy, it is important to measure the serum cobalamin level at regular (e.g., once-yearly) intervals to exclude the coincidental development of cobalamin deficiency.

Folinic Acid (5-Formyl-THF)   This is a stable form of fully reduced folate. It is given orally or parenterally to overcome the toxic effects of methotrexate or other DHF reductase inhibitors.

PROPHYLACTIC FOLIC ACID   In many countries, food is fortified with folic acid (in grain or flour) to prevent neural tube defects. It is also used in chronic dialysis patients and in parenteral feeds. Prophylactic folic acid has been used to reduce homocysteine levels to prevent cardiovascular disease, but further data are needed to assess the benefit for this and for cognitive function in the elderly.

Pregnancy   Folic acid, 400 μg daily, should be given as a supplement before and throughout pregnancy. In women who have had a previous fetus with a neural tube defect, 5 mg daily is recommended when pregnancy is contemplated and throughout the subsequent pregnancy.

Infancy and Childhood   The incidence of folate deficiency is so high in the smallest premature babies during the first 6 weeks of life that folic acid (e.g., 1 mg daily) should be given routinely to those weighing <1500 g at birth and to larger premature babies who require exchange transfusions or develop feeding difficulties, infections, or vomiting and diarrhea.

The World Health Organization currently recommends routine supplementation with iron and folic acid in children in countries where iron deficiency is common and child mortality, largely due to infectious diseases, is high. However, some studies suggest that in areas where malaria rates are high, this approach may increase the incidence of severe illness and death. Even where malaria is rare, there appears to be no survival benefit.

MEGALOBLASTIC ANEMIA NOT DUE TO COBALAMIN OR FOLATE DEFICIENCY OR ALTERED METABOLISM

This may occur with many antimetabolic drugs (e.g., hydroxyurea, cytosine arabinoside, 6-mercaptopurine) that inhibit DNA replication. Antiviral nucleoside analogues used in treatment of HIV infection may also cause macrocytosis and megaloblastic marrow changes. In the rare disease orotic aciduria, two consecutive enzymes in purine synthesis are defective. The condition responds to therapy with uridine, which bypasses the block. In thiamine-responsive megaloblastic anemia, there is a genetic defect in the high-affinity thiamine transport (*SLC19A2*) gene. This causes defective RNA ribose synthesis through impaired activity of transketolase, a thiamine-dependent enzyme in the pentose cycle. This leads to reduced nucleic acid production. It may be associated with diabetes mellitus and deafness and the presence of many ringed sideroblasts in the marrow. The explanation is unclear for megaloblastic changes in the marrow in some patients with acute myeloid leukemia and myelodysplasia.

FURTHER READINGS

ALBERT CM et al: Effect of folic acid and B vitamins on risk of cardiovascular events and total mortality among women at high risk for cardiovascular disease: A randomized trial. JAMA 299: 2027, 2008

CARMEL R: How I treat cobalamin (vitamin B12) deficiency. Blood 12:2214, 2008

DALI-YOUCEF N et al: An update on cobalamin deficiency in adults. Q J Med 102:17, 2009

DURGA J et al: Effect of 3-year folic acid supplementation on cognitive function in older adults in the FACIT trial: A randomized double-blind, controlled trial. Lancet 369:208, 2007

LONN E et al: Homocysteine lowering with folic acid and B vitamins in vascular disease. N Engl J Med 354:1567, 2006

MCMAHON JA et al: A controlled trial of homocysteine lowering and cognitive performance. N Engl J Med 354:2764, 2006

MORRIS MS et al: Folate and vitamin B-12 status in relation to anemia, macrocytosis, and cognitive impairment in older Americans in the age of folic acid fortification. Am J Clin Nutr 85:193, 2007

QUADROS EV: Advances in the understanding of cobalamin assimilation and metabolism. Br J Haematol 148:195, 2010

—— et al: The protein and the gene encoding the receptor for the cellular uptake of transcobalamin-bound cobalamin. Blood 113:186, 2008

ULRICH CM: Folate and cancer prevention—where to next? Cancer Epidemiol Biomarkers Prev 17:2226, 2008

CHAPTER **106**

Hemolytic Anemias and Anemia Due to Acute Blood Loss

Lucio Luzzatto

■ DEFINITIONS

A finite life span is a distinct characteristic of red cells. Hence, a logical, time-honored classification of anemias is in three groups: (1) decreased production of red cells, (2) increased destruction of red cells, (3) acute blood loss. Decreased production is covered in Chaps. 103, 105, and 107; increased destruction and acute blood loss are covered in this chapter.

All patients who are anemic as a result of either increased destruction or acute blood loss have two important elements in common: the anemia results from overconsumption of red cells from the peripheral blood, yet the supply of cells from the bone marrow (in the absence of coexisting marrow disease) is usually increased, as reflected by a reticulocytosis. On the other hand, physical loss of red cells from the bloodstream—which in most cases also means physical loss *from* the body—is fundamentally different from destruction of red cells *within* the body. Therefore the clinical aspects and the pathophysiology of anemia in these two groups of patients are quite different, and they will be considered separately.

HEMOLYTIC ANEMIAS

With respect to primary etiology, anemias due to increased destruction of red cells, which we know as hemolytic anemias (HAs), may be *inherited* or *acquired* (Table 106-1). From the clinical point of view they may be more *acute* or more *chronic*, they may vary from mild to very severe, and the site of hemolysis may be predominantly *intravascular* or *extravascular*. With respect to mechanisms, HAs may be due to *intracorpuscular* causes or to *extracorpuscular* causes. But before reviewing the individual types of HA it is appropriate to consider what they have in common.

■ GENERAL CLINICAL AND LABORATORY FEATURES

The clinical presentation of a patient with anemia is greatly influenced in the first place by whether the onset is abrupt or gradual, and HAs are no exception. A patient with autoimmune HA or with favism may be a medical emergency, whereas a patient with mild hereditary spherocytosis or with cold agglutinin disease may be diagnosed after years. This is due in large measure to the remarkable ability of the body to adapt to anemia when it is slowly progressing (Chap. 57).

What differentiates HAs from other anemias is that the patient has signs and symptoms arising directly from hemolysis

TABLE 106-1 Classification of Hemolytic Anemias*

	Intracorpuscular Defects	Extracorpuscular Factors
Hereditary	Hemoglobinopathies Enzymopathies Membrane-cytoskeletal defects	Familial (atypical) hemolytic uremic syndrome
Acquired	Paroxysmal nocturnal hemoglobinuria (PNH)	Mechanical destruction (microangiopathic) Toxic agents Drugs Infectious Autoimmune

*Hereditary causes correlate with intracorpuscular defects because these defects are due to inherited mutations. The one exception is PNH because the defect is due to an acquired somatic mutation. Similarly, acquired causes correlate with extracorpuscular factors because mostly these factors are exogenous. The one exception is familial hemolytic uremic syndrome (HUS; often referred to as atypical HUS) because here an inherited abnormality allows complement activation to be excessive, with bouts of production of membrane attack complex capable of destroying normal red cells.

TABLE 106-2 Some Common Features of Hemolytic Disorders

General examination	Jaundice, pallor
Other physical findings	Spleen may be enlarged; bossing of skull in severe congenital cases
Hemoglobin level	From normal to severely reduced
MCV, MCH	Usually increased
Reticulocytes	Increased
Bilirubin	Increased (mostly unconjugated)
LDH	Increased (up to 10× normal with intravascular hemolysis)
Haptoglobin	Reduced to absent (if hemolysis is part intravascular)

Abbreviations: LDH, lactate dehydrogenase; MCH, mean corpuscular hemoglobin; MCV, mean corpuscular volume.

(Table 106-2). At the clinical level, the main sign is *jaundice*; in addition, the patient may report discoloration of the urine. In many cases of HA, the spleen is enlarged because it is a preferential site of hemolysis, and in some cases the liver may be enlarged as well. In all severe congenital forms of HA, there also may be skeletal changes due to overactivity of the bone marrow (although they are never as severe as they are in thalassemia).

The laboratory features of HA are related to hemolysis per se and the erythropoietic response of the bone marrow. Hemolysis regularly produces in the serum an increase in unconjugated bilirubin and aspartate transaminase (AST); urobilinogen will be increased in both urine and stool. If hemolysis is mainly intravascular, the telltale sign is hemoglobinuria (often associated with hemosiderinuria); in the serum there is increased hemoglobin, lactate dehydrogenase (LDH) is increased, and haptoglobin is reduced. In contrast, the bilirubin level may be normal or only mildly elevated. The main sign of the erythropoietic response by the bone marrow is an increase in reticulocytes (Table 106-2); a test all too often neglected in the initial workup of a patient with anemia. Usually the increase will be reflected in both the percentage of reticulocytes (the more commonly quoted figure) and the absolute reticulocyte count (the more definitive parameter). The increased number of reticulocytes is associated with an increased mean corpuscular volume (MCV) in the blood count. On the blood smear, this is reflected in the presence of macrocytes; there is also polychromasia and sometimes one sees nucleated red cells. In most cases, a bone marrow aspirate is not necessary in the diagnostic workup; if it is done, it will show erythroid hyperplasia. In practice, once a HA is suspected, specific tests will usually be required for a definitive diagnosis of a specific type of HA.

GENERAL PATHOPHYSIOLOGY

The mature red cell is the product of a developmental pathway that brings the phenomenon of differentiation to an extreme. An orderly sequence of events produces synchronous changes whereby the gradual accumulation of a huge amount of hemoglobin in the cytoplasm (to a final level of 340 g/L, i.e. about 5 m*M*) goes hand in hand with the gradual loss of cellular organelles and of biosynthetic abilities. In the end, the erythroid cell undergoes a process that has features of apoptosis, including nuclear pyknosis and actual loss of the nucleus. However, the final result is more altruistic than suicidal; the cytoplasmic body, instead of disintegrating, is now able to provide oxygen to all cells in the human organism for some remaining 120 days of the red cell "life" span.

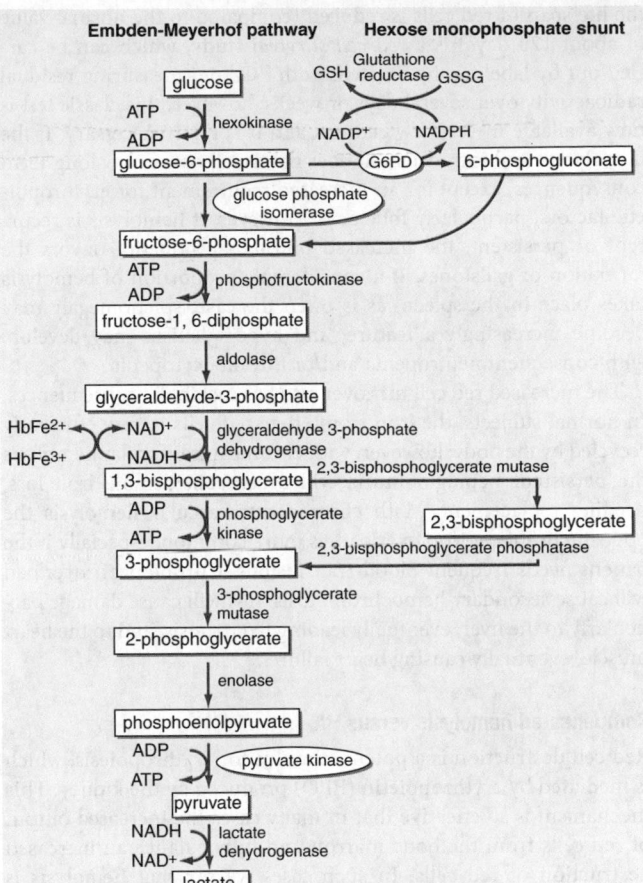

Figure 106-1 RBC metabolism. The Embden-Meyerhof pathway (glycolysis) generates ATP for energy and membrane maintenance. The generation of NADPH maintains hemoglobin in a reduced state. The hexose monophosphate shunt generates NADPH that is used to reduce glutathione, which protects the red cell against oxidant stress. Regulation of 2,3-bisphosphoglycerate levels is a critical determinant of oxygen affinity of hemoglobin. Enzyme deficiency states in order of prevalence: glucose-6-phosphate dehydrogenase (G6PD) > pyruvate kinase > glucose-6-phosphate isomerase > rare deficiencies of other enzymes in the pathway. The more common enzyme deficiencies are encircled.

As a result of this unique process of differentiation and maturation, intermediary metabolism is drastically curtailed in mature red cells (Fig. 106-1); for instance, cytochrome-mediated oxidative phosphorylation has been lost with the loss of mitochondria (through a process of physiologic autophagy); therefore, there is no backup to anaerobic glycolysis for the production of adenosine triphosphate (ATP). Also the capacity of making protein has been lost with the loss of ribosomes. This places the cell's limited metabolic apparatus at risk, because if any protein component deteriorates, it cannot be replaced, as it would be in most other cells, and in fact the activity of most enzymes gradually decreases as red cells age. Another consequence of the relative simplicity of red cells is that they have a very limited range of ways to manifest distress under hardship: in essence, any sort of metabolic failure will eventually lead either to structural damage to the membrane or to failure of the cation pump. In either case, the life span of the red cell is reduced, which is the definition of a *hemolytic disorder*. If the rate of red cell destruction exceeds the capacity of the bone marrow to produce more red cells, the hemolytic disorder will manifest as HA.

Thus, the essential pathophysiologic process common to all HAs is an increased red cell turnover. The gold standard for proving that the life span of red cells is reduced (compared to the normal value of about 120 days) is a *red cell survival* study, which can be carried out by labeling the red cells with ^{51}Cr and measuring residual radioactivity over several days or weeks; however, this classic test is now available in very few centers, and it is rarely necessary. If the hemolytic event is transient, it does not usually cause any long-term consequences, except for an increased requirement for erythropoietic factors, particularly folic acid. However, if hemolysis is recurrent or persistent, the increased bilirubin production favors the formation of gallstones. If a considerable proportion of hemolysis takes place in the spleen, as is often the case, splenomegaly may become increasingly a feature, and hypersplenism may develop, with consequent neutropenia and/or thrombocytopenia.

The increased red cell turnover also has metabolic consequences. In normal subjects, the iron from effete red cells is very efficiently recycled by the body; however, with chronic intravascular hemolysis the persistent hemoglobinuria will cause considerable iron loss, needing replacement. With chronic extravascular hemolysis the opposite problem, iron overload, is more common, especially if the patient needs frequent blood transfusions. Chronic iron overload will cause secondary hemochromatosis: this will cause damage particularly to the liver, eventually leading to cirrhosis, and to the heart muscle, eventually causing heart failure.

Compensated hemolysis versus HA

Red cell destruction is a potent stimulus for erythropoiesis, which is mediated by erythropoietin (EPO) produced by the kidney. This mechanism is so effective that in many cases the increased output of red cells from the bone marrow can fully balance an increased destruction of red cells. In such cases we say that hemolysis is *compensated*. The pathophysiology of compensated hemolysis is similar to what we have just described, except there is no anemia. This notion is important from the diagnostic point of view, because a patient with a hemolytic condition, even an inherited one, may present without anemia. It is also important from the point of view of management, because compensated hemolysis may become "decompensated"—i.e., anemia may suddenly appear—in certain circumstances, for instance pregnancy, folate deficiency, or renal failure, interfering with adequate EPO production. Another general feature of chronic HAs is seen when any intercurrent condition, for instance an acute infection, depresses erythropoiesis. When this happens, in view of the increased rate of red cell turnover, the effect

will be predictably much more marked than in a person who does not have hemolysis. The most dramatic example is infection by parvovirus B19, which may cause a rather precipitous fall in hemoglobin; an occurrence sometimes referred to as *aplastic crisis*.

■ INHERITED HEMOLYTIC ANEMIAS

There are three essential components in the red cell: (1) hemoglobin, (2) the membrane-cytoskeleton complex, and (3) the metabolic machinery necessary to keep (1) and (2) in working order. Diseases caused by abnormalities of hemoglobin, or hemoglobinopathies, are covered in Chap. 104. Here we will deal with diseases of the other two components.

Hemolytic anemias due to abnormalities of the membrane-cytoskeleton complex

The detailed architecture of the red cell membrane is complex, but its basic design is relatively simple (Fig. 106-2). The lipid bilayer incorporates phospholipids and cholesterol, and it is spanned by a number of proteins that have their hydrophobic transmembrane domains embedded in the membrane. Most of these proteins have hydrophilic domains extending toward both the outside and the inside of the cell. Other proteins are tethered to the membrane through a glycosylphosphatidylinositol (GPI) anchor, and they have only an extracellular domain. These proteins are arranged roughly perpendicular to or lying across the membrane: they include ion channels, receptors for complement components, receptors for other ligands, and some of unknown function. The most abundant of these proteins are glycophorins and the so-called band 3, an anion transporter. The extracellular domains of many of these proteins are heavily glycosylated, and they carry antigenic determinants that correspond to blood groups. Underneath the membrane, and tangential to it, is a network of other proteins that make up the cytoskeleton: the main cytoskeletal protein is spectrin, the basic unit of which is a dimer of α-spectrin and β-spectrin. The membrane is physically linked to the cytoskeleton by a third set of proteins (including ankyrin and the so-called band 4.1 and band 4.2), which thus make these two structures intimately connected to each other.

The membrane-cytoskeleton complex is indeed so integrated that, not surprisingly, an abnormality of almost any of its components will be disturbing or disruptive, causing structural failure, which results ultimately in hemolysis. These abnormalities are almost invariably inherited mutations; thus, diseases of the

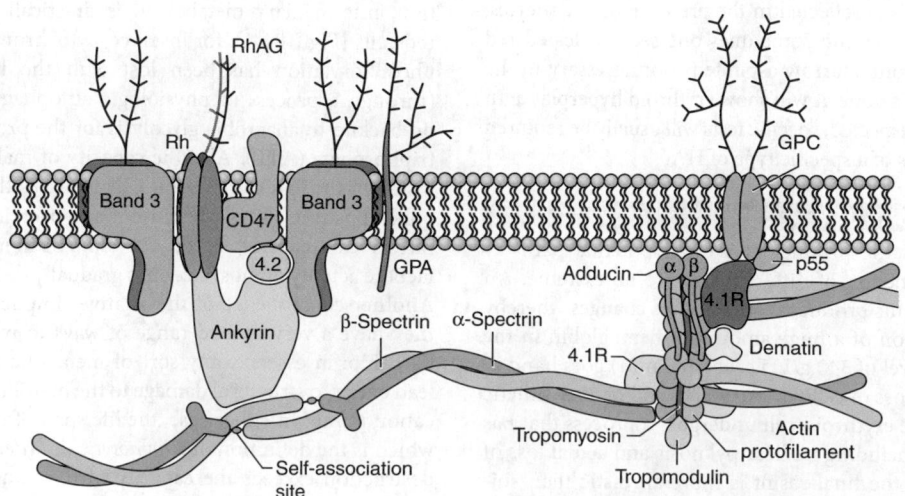

Figure 106-2 **Diagram of red cell membrane-cytoskeleton.** (For explanation see text.) *(From N Young et al: Clinical Hematology. Copyright Elsevier, 2006; with permission.)*

membrane-cytoskeleton complex belong to the category of inherited HAs. Before the red cells lyse, they often exhibit more or less specific morphologic changes that alter the normal biconcave disk shape. Thus, the majority of the diseases in this group have been known for over a century as *hereditary spherocytosis* and *hereditary elliptocytosis*.

Hereditary spherocytosis (HS)   This is a relatively common type of HA, with an estimated frequency of at least 1 in 5000. Its identification is credited to Minkowksy and Chauffard, who at the end of the nineteenth century reported families in which HS was inherited as an autosomal dominant condition (Fig 106-3*A*). From this seminal work, HS came to be defined as an inherited form of HA associated with the presence of spherocytes in the peripheral blood. In addition, in vitro studies revealed that the red cells were abnormally susceptible to lysis in hypotonic media: indeed, the presence of *osmotic fragility* became the main diagnostic test for HS. Today we know that HS, thus defined, is genetically heterogeneous; i.e., it can arise from a variety of mutations in one of several genes (Table 106-3). Whereas classically the inheritance of HS is autosomal dominant (with the patients being heterozygous), some severe forms are instead autosomal recessive (with the patient being homozygous).

Clinical presentation and diagnosis   The spectrum of clinical severity of HS is broad. Severe cases may present in infancy with severe anemia, whereas mild cases may present in young adults or even later in life. In women, HS is sometimes first diagnosed when anemia is investigated during pregnancy. The main clinical findings are jaundice, an enlarged spleen, and often gallstones; indeed, it is often the finding of gallstones in a young person that triggers diagnostic investigations.

The variability in clinical manifestations that is observed among patients with HS is largely due to the different underlying molecular lesions (Table 106-3). Not only are mutations of several genes involved, but individual mutations of the same gene can also give very different clinical manifestations. In milder cases hemolysis is often compensated (see above), and this may cause variation in time, even in the same patient, due to the fact that intercurrent conditions (e.g., infection) cause decompensation. The anemia is usually normocytic, with the characteristic morphology that gives the disease its name. A characteristic feature is an increase in mean corpuscular hemoglobin concentration (MCHC): this is almost the only condition in which an increased MCHC is seen.

When there is a family history (Fig. 106-3*A*) it is usually easy to suspect the diagnosis, but there may be no family history for at least two reasons. (1) The patient may have a de novo mutation, i.e., a mutation that has taken place in a germ cell of one of his or her parents or early after zygote formation. (2) The patient may have a recessive form of HS (Table 106-3). In most cases, the diagnosis can be made on the basis of red cell morphology and of a test for osmotic fragility, a modified version of which is called the "pink test." In some cases, a definitive diagnosis can be obtained only by molecular studies demonstrating a mutation in one of the genes underlying HS. This is usually carried out in laboratories with special expertise in this area.

| **TREATMENT** | Hereditary Spherocytosis |

We don't have a causal treatment for HS; i.e., no way has yet been found to correct the basic defect in the membrane-cytoskeleton structure. However, it has been apparent for a long time that the spleen plays a special role in HS through a dual mechanism. On one hand, like in many other HAs, the spleen itself is a major

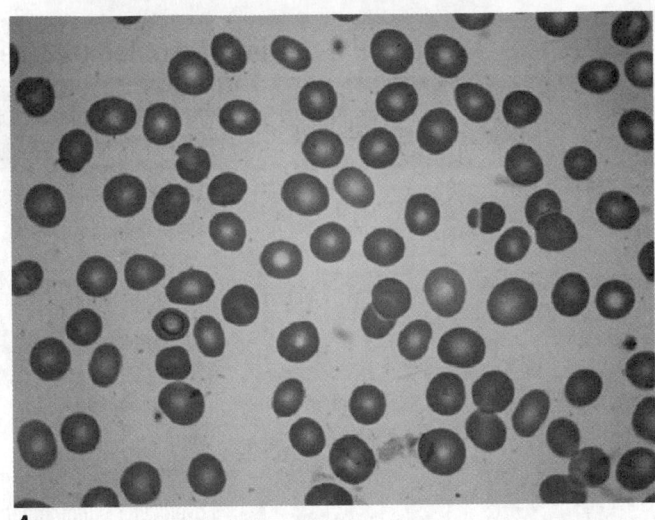

A

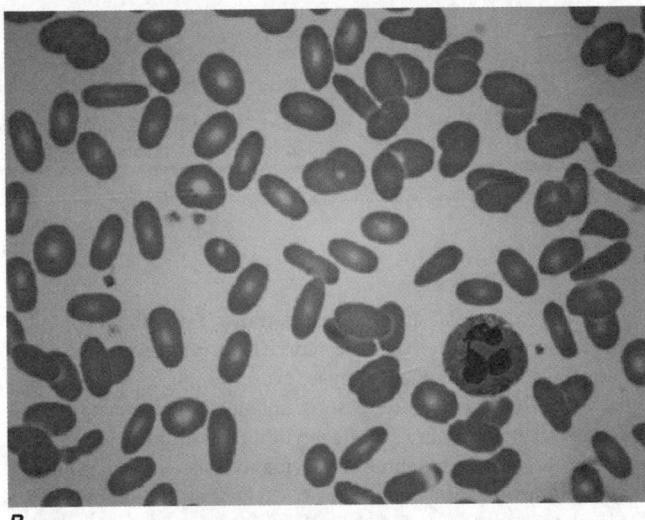

B

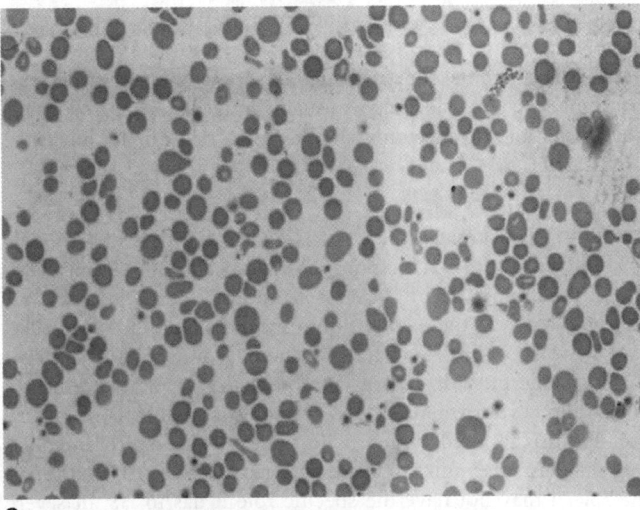

C

Figure 106-3   Peripheral blood smear from patients with membrane-cytoskeleton abnormalities. *A.* Hereditary spherocytosis. *B.* Hereditary elliptocytosis, heterozygote. *C.* Elliptocytosis, with both alleles of the α-spectrin gene mutated.

TABLE 106-3 Inherited Diseases of the Red Cell Membrane-Cytoskeleton

Gene	Chromosomal Location	Protein Produced	Disease(s) with Certain Mutations (Inheritance)	Comments
SPTA1	1q22-q23	α-Spectrin	HS (recessive)	Rare
			HE (dominant)	Mutations of this gene account for about 65% of HE. More severe forms may be due to coexistence of an otherwise silent mutant allele
SPTB	14q23-q24.1	β-Spectrin	HS (dominant)	Rare
			HE (dominant)	Mutations of this gene account for about 30% of HE, including some severe forms
ANK1	8p11.2	Ankyrin	HS (dominant)	May account for majority of HS
SLC4A1	17q21	Band 3 (anion channel)	HS (dominant)	Mutations of this gene may account for about 25% of HS
			Southeast Asia ovalocytosis (dominant)	Polymorphic mutation (deletion of 9 amino acids); clinically asymptomatic; protective against Plasmodium falciparum
			Stomatocytosis	Certain specific missense mutations shift protein function from anion exchanger to cation conductance
EPB41	1p33-p34.2	Band 4.1	HE (dominant)	Mutations of this gene account for about 5% of HE: mostly with prominent morphology but no hemolysis in heterozygotes; severe hemolysis in homozygotes
EPB42	15q15-q21	Band 4.2	HS (recessive)	Mutations of this gene account for about 3% of HS.
RHAG	6p21.1-p11	Rhesus antigen	Chronic nonspherocytic hemolytic anemia	Very rare; associated with total loss of all Rh antigens

Abbreviations: HE, hereditary elliptocytosis; HS, hereditary spherocytosis.

site of destruction; on the other hand, transit through the splenic circulation makes the defective red cells more spherocytic and therefore accelerates their demise, even though lysis may take place elsewhere. For these reasons, splenectomy has long been regarded as a prime, almost obligatory therapeutic measure in HS. Therefore, current guidelines (not evidence-based) are as follows. (1) Avoid splenectomy in mild cases. (2) Delay splenectomy until at least 4 years of age, after the risk of severe sepsis has peaked. (3) Antipneumococcal vaccination before splenectomy is imperative, whereas penicillin prophylaxis postsplenectomy is controversial. (4) There is no doubt that HS patients often may require cholecystectomy, in which case the practice has been to also carry out a splenectomy at the same time. Today the decision regarding this combined surgery should not be regarded as automatic: cholecystectomy is usually done via the laparoscopic approach and splenectomy should be carried out if clinically indicated.

Hereditary elliptocytosis (HE) HE is at least as heterogeneous as HS, both from the genetic point of view (Table 106-3) and from the clinical point of view. Again it is the shape of the red cells that gives the name to these conditions, but there is no direct correlation between the elliptocytic morphology and clinical severity. In fact, some mild or even asymptomatic cases may have nearly 100% elliptocytes, whereas in severe cases it is all sorts of bizarre poikilocytes that predominate. Clinical features and recommended management are similar to those outlined above for HS. Although the spleen may not have the specific role it has in HS, in severe cases splenectomy may be beneficial. The prevalence of HE causing clinical disease is similar to that of HS. However, an asymptomatic form, referred to as *Southeast Asia ovalocytosis,* has a frequency of up to 7% in certain populations, presumably as a result of malaria selection.

Disorders of cation transport

These rare conditions with autosomal dominant inheritance are characterized by increased intracellular sodium in red cells, with concomitant loss of potassium: indeed, they are sometimes discovered through the incidental finding, in a blood test, of high serum K^+ (*pseudohyperkalemia*). In patients from some families, the cation transport disturbance is associated with gain of water: as a result the red cells are overhydrated (low MCHC), and on a blood smear the normally round-shaped central pallor is replaced by a linear-shaped central pallor, which has earned this disorder the name *stomatocytosis.* In patients from other families, the red cells are instead dehydrated (high MCHC), and their consequent rigidity has earned this disorder the name *xerocytosis.* In these disorders, one would suspect that the primary defect may be in a cation transporter. In most cases this has not yet been demonstrated, but interestingly, certain missense mutations of the *SLC4A1* gene encoding band 3 (Table 106-3) give stomatocytosis. Hemolysis can vary from relatively mild to quite severe. From the practical point of view it is important to know that splenectomy is contraindicated, as it has been followed in a majority of cases by severe thromboembolic complications.

Enzyme abnormalities

When there is an important defect in the membrane or in the cytoskeleton, hemolysis is a direct consequence of the fact that the very structure of the red cell is abnormal. Instead, when one of the enzymes is defective, the consequences will depend on the precise role of that enzyme in the metabolic machinery of the red cell, which, in first approximation, has two important functions: (1) to provide energy in the form of ATP, and (2) to prevent oxidative damage to hemoglobin and to other proteins.

Abnormalities of the glycolytic pathway Since red cells, in the course of their differentiation, have sacrificed not only their nucleus and their ribosomes but also their mitochondria, they rely exclusively

TABLE 106-4 Red Cell Ezyme Abnormalities Causing Hemolysis

	Enzyme (Acronym)	Chromosomal Location	Prevalence of Enzyme Deficiency (Rank)	Clinical Manifestations Extra-Red Cell	Comments
GLYCOLYTIC PATHWAY	Hexokinase (HK)	10q22	Very rare		Other isoenzymes known
	Glucose 6-phosphate isomerase (G6PI)	19q31.1	Rare (4)*	NM, CNS	
	Phosphofructokinase (PFK)	12q13	Very rare	Myopathy	
	Aldolase	16q22-24	Very rare		
	Triose phosphate isomerase (TPI)	12p13	Very rare	CNS (severe), NM	
	Glyceraldehyde 3-phosphate dehydrogenase (GAPD)	12p13.31-p13.1	Very rare	Myopathy	
	Diphosphoglycerate mutase (DPGM)	7q31-q34	Very rare		Erythrocytosis rather than hemolysis
	Phosphoglycerate kinase (PGK)	Xq13	Very rare	CNS, NM	May benefit from splenectomy
	Pyruvate kinase (PK)	1q21	Rare (2)*		May benefit from splenectomy
REDOX	Glucose 6-phosphate dehydrogenase (G6PD)	Xq28	Common (1)*	Very rarely granulocytes	In almost all cases only AHA from exogenous trigger
	Glutathione synthase	20q11.2	Very rare	CNS	
	γ-Glutamylcysteine synthase	6p12	Very rare	CNS	
	Cytochrome b5 reductase	22q13.31-qter	Rare	CNS	Methemoglobinemia rather than hemolysis
NUCLEOTIDE METABOLISM	Adenylate kinase (AK)	9q34.1	Very rare	CNS	
	Pyrimidine 5′-nucleotidase (P5N)	3q11-q12	Rare (3)*		May benefit from splenectomy

*The numbers from (1) to (4) indicate the ranking order of these enzymopathies in terms of frequency.
Abbreviations: AHA, acquired hemolytic anemia; CNS, central nervous system.

on the anaerobic portion of the glycolytic pathway for producing energy in the form of ATP. Most of the ATP is required by the red cell for cation transport against a concentration gradient across the membrane. If this fails, due to a defect of any of the enzymes of the glycolytic pathway, the result will be hemolytic disease (Table 106-4).

Pyruvate kinase deficiency Abnormalities of the glycolytic pathway are all inherited and all rare. Among them, deficiency of pyruvate kinase (PK) is the less rare, with an estimated prevalence of the order of 1:10,000. The clinical picture is that of an HA that often presents in the newborn with neonatal jaundice; the jaundice persists, and it is usually associated with a very high reticulocytosis. The anemia is of variable severity; sometimes it is so severe as to require regular blood transfusion treatment; sometimes it is mild, bordering on a nearly compensated hemolytic disorder. As a result, the diagnosis may be delayed, and in some cases it is made in young adults; for instance, in a woman, during her first pregnancy, when the anemia may get worse. In part, the delay in diagnosis is due to the fact that the anemia is remarkably well tolerated, because the metabolic block at the last step in glycolysis causes an increase in bisphosphoglycerate (or DPG), a major effector of the hemoglobin-oxygen dissociation curve; thus, the oxygen delivery to the tissues is enhanced.

TREATMENT Pryuvate Kinase Deficiency

The management of PK deficiency is mainly supportive. In view of the marked increase in red cell turnover, oral folic acid supplements should be given constantly. Blood transfusion should be used as necessary, and iron chelation may have to be added if the blood transfusion requirement is high enough to cause iron overload. In these patients, who have more severe disease, splenectomy may be beneficial. There is a single case report of curative treatment of PK deficiency by bone marrow transplantation from an HLA-identical PK-normal sibling. This seems a viable option for severe cases when a sibling donor is available.

Other glycolytic enzyme abnormalities All of these defects are rare to very rare (Table 106-4), and all cause HA with varying degrees of severity. It is not unusual for the presentation to be in the guise of severe neonatal jaundice, which may require exchange transfusion. If the anemia is less severe, it may present later in life, or it may even remain asymptomatic and be detected incidentally when a blood count is done for unrelated reasons. The spleen is often enlarged. When other systemic manifestations occur, they involve the central nervous system, sometimes entailing severe mental retardation (particularly in the case of triose phosphate isomerase deficiency), or the neuromuscular system, or both. The *diagnosis* of HA is usually not difficult, thanks to the triad of normo-macrocytic anemia, reticulocytosis, and hyperbilirubinemia. Enzymopathies should be considered in the differential diagnosis of any chronic Coombs-negative hemolytic anemia. In most cases of glycolytic enzymopathies, the morphologic abnormalities of red cells characteristically seen in membrane disorders are conspicuous by their absence. A definitive diagnosis can be made only by demonstrating the deficiency of an individual enzyme by quantitative assays carried out in only a few specialized laboratories. If a particular molecular abnormality is already known in the family, then of course one could test directly for that at the DNA level, bypassing the need for enzyme assays.

Abnormalities of redox metabolism

G6PD deficiency Glucose 6-phosphate dehydrogenase (G6PD) is a housekeeping enzyme critical in the redox metabolism of all aerobic cells (Fig. 106-1). In red cells its role is even more critical, because it is the only source of NADPH that directly and via glutathione (GSH) defends these cells against oxidative stress. G6PD deficiency is a prime example of an HA due to interaction between an intracorpuscular cause and an extracorpuscular cause, because in the majority of cases, hemolysis is triggered by an exogenous agent. Although a decrease in G6PD activity is noted in most tissues of G6PD-deficient subjects, the decrease is less marked than in red cells, and it does not seem to have a clinical impact.

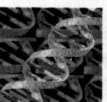

GENETIC CONSIDERATIONS

The G6PD gene is X-linked, and this has important implications. First, as males have only one G6PD gene (i.e., they are hemizygous for this gene), they must be either normal or G6PD-deficient. By contrast, females, having two G6PD genes, can be either normal or deficient (homozygous), or intermediate (heterozygous). As a result of the phenomenon of X-chromosome inactivation, heterozygous females are genetic mosaics, with a highly variable ratio of G6PD-normal to G6PD-deficient cells and an equally variable degree of clinical expression: some heterozygotes can be just as affected as hemizygous males. The enzymatically active form of G6PD is either a dimer or a tetramer of a single protein subunit of 514 amino acids. G6PD-deficient subjects have been found invariably to have mutations in the coding region of the G6PD gene (Fig. 106-4). Almost all of some 150 different mutations known are single missense point mutations, entailing single amino acid replacements in the G6PD protein. In most cases, these mutations cause G6PD deficiency by decreasing

the in vivo stability of the protein; thus, the physiologic decrease in G6PD activity that takes place with red cell aging is greatly accelerated. In some cases an amino acid replacement can also affect the catalytic function of the enzyme.

Among these mutations, those underlying *chronic nonspherocytic hemolytic anemia* (CNSHA; see "Clinical Manifestations," below) are a discrete subset. This much more severe clinical phenotype can be ascribed in some cases to adverse qualitative changes (for instance, a decreased affinity for the substrate, glucose 6-phosphate) or simply to the fact that the enzyme deficit is more extreme because of a more severe instability of the enzyme. For instance, a cluster of mutations map at or near the dimer interface, and clearly they compromise severely the formation of the dimer.

Epidemiology G6PD deficiency is widely distributed in tropical and subtropical parts of the world (Africa, Southern Europe, the Middle East, Southeast Asia, and Oceania) (Fig. 106-5) and wherever people from those areas have migrated. A conservative estimate is that at least 400 million people have a G6PD deficiency gene. In several of these areas the frequency of a G6PD deficiency gene may be as high as 20% or more. It would be quite extraordinary for a trait that causes significant pathology to spread widely and reach high frequencies in many populations without conferring some biologic advantage. Indeed, G6PD is one of the best characterized examples of genetic polymorphisms in the human species. Clinical field studies and in vitro experiments strongly support the view that G6PD deficiency has been selected by *Plasmodium falciparum* malaria, by virtue of the fact that it confers a relative resistance against this highly lethal infection. Whether this protective effect is exerted mainly in hemizygous males or in females heterozygous for G6PD deficiency is still not quite clear. Different G6PD variants underlie G6PD deficiency in different parts of the world. Some of the more widespread variants are G6PD Mediterranean on the shores of that sea, in the Middle East, and in India; G6PD A–in Africa and in Southern Europe; G6PD Vianchan and G6PD Mahidol in Southeast Asia; G6PD Canton in China; and G6PD Union worldwide. The heterogeneity of polymorphic G6PD variants is proof of their independent origin, and it supports the notion that they have been selected by a common environmental agent, in keeping with the concept of convergent evolution (Fig. 106-5).

Clinical manifestations The vast majority of people with G6PD deficiency remain clinically asymptomatic throughout their lifetime; however, all of them have an increased risk of developing neonatal jaundice (NNJ), and a risk of developing acute hemolytic anemia (AHA) when challenged by a number of oxidative agents. NNJ related to G6PD deficiency is very rarely present at birth. The peak incidence of clinical onset is between day 2 and day 3, and in most cases the anemia is not severe. However, NNJ can be very severe in some G6PD-deficient babies, especially in association with prematurity, infection, and/or environmental factors (such as naphthalene-camphor balls used in babies' bedding and clothing), and the risk of severe NNJ is also increased by the coexistence of a monoallelic or biallelic mutation in the uridyl transferase gene (*UGT1A1*; the same mutations are associated with the Gilbert syndrome). If inadequately managed, NNJ associated with G6PD deficiency can produce kernicterus and permanent neurologic damage.

AHA can develop as a result of three types of triggers: (1) fava beans, (2) infections, and (3) drugs (Table 106-5). Typically, a hemolytic attack starts with malaise, weakness, and abdominal or lumbar pain. After an interval of several hours to 2–3 days, the patient develops jaundice and often dark urine, due to hemoglobinuria. The onset can be extremely abrupt, especially with favism in children. The anemia is from moderate to extremely

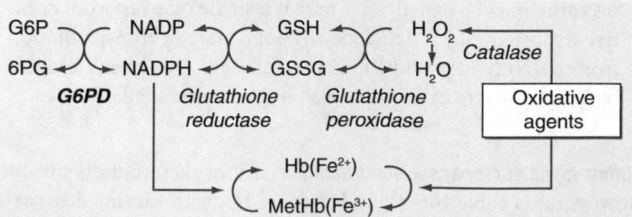

Figure 106-4 Diagram of redox metabolism in the red cell. G6P, glucose 6-phosphate; 6PG, 6-phosphogluconate; G6PD, glucose 6-phosphate dehydrogenase; GSH, reduced glutathione; GSSG, oxidized glutathione; Hb, hemoglobin; MetHb, methemoglobin; NADP, nicotinamide adenine dinucleotide phosphate; NADPH, reduced nicotinamide adenine dinucleotide phosphate.

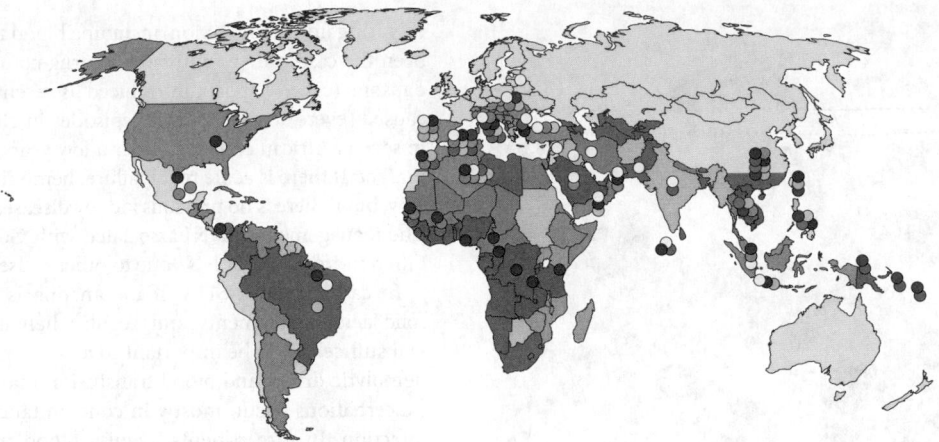

Figure 106-5 Epidemiology of G6PD deficiency throughout the world. The different shadings indicate increasingly high levels of prevalence, up to about 20%; the different colored symbols indicate individual genetic variants of G6PD, each one having a different mutation. *[From L Luzzatto et al, in C Scriver et al (eds): The Metabolic & Molecular Bases of Inherited Disease, 8th ed. New York, McGraw Hill, 2001.]*

severe. It is usually normocytic and normochromic, and it is due partly to intravascular hemolysis. Hence, it is associated with hemoglobinemia, hemoglobinuria, high LDH, and low or absent plasma haptoglobin. The blood film shows anisocytosis, polychromasia, and spherocytes (Fig. 106-6). The most typical feature is the presence of bizarre poikilocytes, with red cells that appear to have unevenly distributed hemoglobin ("hemighosts") and red cells that appear to have had parts of them bitten away ("bite cells" or "blister cells"). A classical test, now rarely carried out, is supravital staining with methyl violet that, if done promptly, reveals the presence of Heinz bodies, consisting of precipitates of denatured hemoglobin and regarded as a signature of oxidative damage to red cells (except for the rare occurrence of an unstable hemoglobin). LDH is high and so is the unconjugated bilirubin, indicating that there is also extravascular hemolysis. The most serious threat from AHA in adults is

the development of acute renal failure (this is exceedingly rare in children). Once the threat of acute anemia is over, and in the absence of comorbidity, full recovery from AHA associated with G6PD deficiency is the rule.

A very small minority of subjects with G6PD deficiency have *chronic nonspherocytic hemolytic anemia* (CNSHA) of variable severity. The patient is always a male, usually with a history of NNJ, who may present with anemia, unexplained jaundice, or because of gallstones later in life. The spleen may be enlarged. The severity of anemia ranges in different patients from borderline to transfusion-dependent. The anemia is usually normo-macrocytic, with reticulocytosis. Bilirubin and LDH are increased. Although hemolysis is, by definition, chronic in these patients, they are also vulnerable to acute oxidative damage, and therefore the same agents that can cause acute HA in people with the ordinary type of G6PD deficiency will cause severe exacerbations in people with the severe

TABLE 106-5 Drugs That Carry Risk of Clinical Hemolysis in Persons With G6PD Deficiency

	Definite Risk	Possible Risk	Doubtful Risk
Antimalarials	Primaquine	Chloroquine	Quinine
	Dapsone/chlorproguanil*		
Sulphonamides/sulphones	Sulfamethoxazole	Sulfasalazine	Sulfisoxazole
	Others	Sulfadimidine	Sulfadiazine
	Dapsone		
Antibacterial/antibiotics	Cotrimoxazole	Ciprofloxacin	Chloramphenicol
	Nalidixic acid	Norfloxacin	*p*-Aminosalicylic acid
	Nitrofurantoin		
	Niridazole		
Antipyretic/analgesics	Acetanilide	Acetylsalicylic acid high dose (>3 g/d)	Acetylsalicylic acid (<3 g/d)
	Phenazopyridine		Acetaminophen
			Phenacetin
Other	Naphthalene	Vitamin K analogues	Doxorubicin
	Methylene blue	Ascorbic acid >1 g	Probenecid
		Rasburicase	

*Marketed as Lapdap from 2003 to 2008.

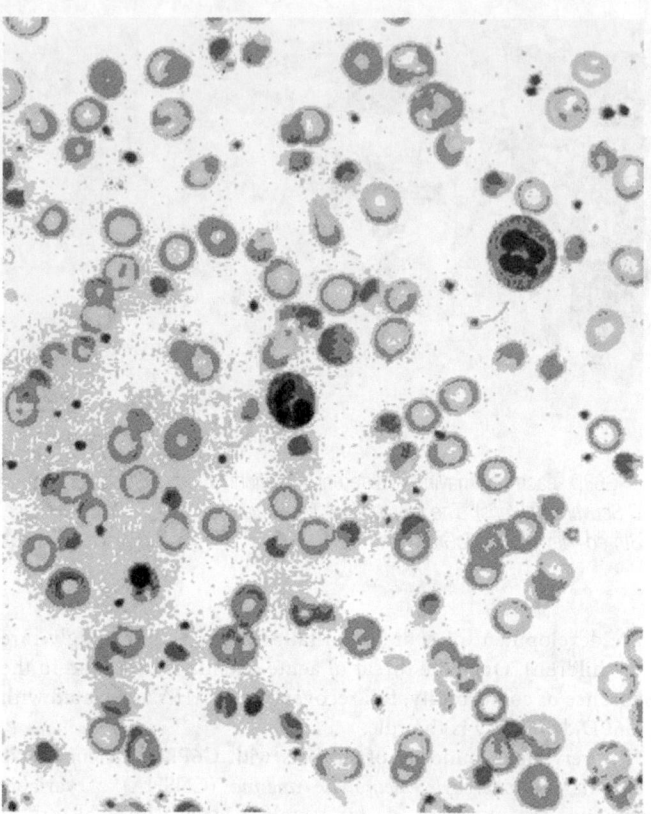

Figure 106-6 Peripheral blood smear from a 5-year-old G6PD-deficient boy with acute favism.

form of G6PD deficiency. In some cases of CNSHA, the deficiency of G6PD is so severe in granulocytes that it becomes rate-limiting for their oxidative burst, with consequent increased susceptibility to some bacterial infections.

Laboratory diagnosis The suspicion of G6PD deficiency can be confirmed by semiquantitative methods often referred to as screening tests, which are suitable for population studies and can correctly classify male subjects, in the steady state, as G6PD-normal or G6PD-deficient. However, in clinical practice, a diagnostic test is usually needed when the patient has had a hemolytic attack. This implies that the oldest, most G6PD-deficient red cells have been selectively destroyed, and young red cells, having higher G6PD activity, are being released into the circulation. Under these conditions, only a quantitative test can give a definitive result. In males, this test will identify normal hemizygotes and G6PD-deficient hemizygotes; among females, some heterozygotes will be missed, but those who are at most risk of hemolysis will be identified.

TREATMENT G6PD Deficiency

The acute hemolytic anemia of G6PD deficiency is largely preventable by avoiding exposure to triggering factors of previously screened subjects. Of course, the practicability and cost-effectiveness of screening depends on the prevalence of G6PD deficiency in each community. Favism is entirely preventable in G6PD-deficient subjects by not eating fava beans. Drug-induced hemolysis can be prevented by testing for G6PD deficiency before prescribing; in most cases, one can use alternative drugs. When AHA develops and once its cause is recognized, in most cases no specific treatment is needed. However, if the anemia is severe, it may be a medical emergency, especially in children,

requiring immediate action, including blood transfusion. This has been the case with an antimalarial drug combination containing dapsone (called Lapdap, introduced as recently as 2003) that has caused severe acute hemolytic episodes in children with malaria in several African countries; after a few years, it was taken off the market. If there is acute renal failure, hemodialysis may be necessary, but if there is no previous kidney disease, recovery is the rule. The management of NNJ associated with G6PD deficiency is no different from that of NNJ due to other causes.

In cases with CNSHA, if the anemia is not severe, regular folic acid supplements and regular hematologic surveillance will suffice. It will be important to avoid exposure to potentially hemolytic drugs, and blood transfusion may be indicated when exacerbations occur, mostly in concomitance with intercurrent infection. In rare patients, regular blood transfusions may be required, in which case appropriate iron chelation should be instituted. Unlike in hereditary spherocytosis, there is no evidence of selective red cell destruction in the spleen; however, in practice, splenectomy has proven beneficial in severe cases.

Other abnormalities of the redox system As mentioned above, GSH is a key player in the defense against oxidative stress. Inherited defects of GSH metabolism are exceedingly rare, but each one of them can give rise to chronic HA (Table 106-4). A rare, peculiar, usually self-limited severe HA of the first month of life, called *infantile poikilocytosis*, may be associated with deficiency of glutathione peroxidase (GSHPx) due not to an inherited abnormality but to transient nutritional deficiency of selenium, an element essential for the activity of GSHPx.

Pyrimidine 5′-nucleotidase (P5N) deficiency P5N is a key enzyme in the catabolism of nucleotides arising from the degradation of nucleic acids that takes place in the final stages of erythroid cell maturation. How exactly its deficiency causes HA is not well understood, but a highly distinctive feature of this condition is a morphologic abnormality of the red cells known as *basophilic stippling*. The condition is rare, but it probably ranks third in frequency among red cell enzyme defects (after G6PD deficiency and PK deficiency). The anemia is lifelong, of variable severity, and may benefit from splenectomy.

Familial (atypical) hemolytic uremic syndrome (aHUS)

This phrase is used to designate a group of rare disorders, mostly affecting children, characterized by microangiopathic HA with presence of fragmented erythrocytes in the peripheral blood smear, thrombocytopenia (usually mild), and acute renal failure. (The word *atypical* is part of the phrase because it is the HUS caused by infection with *Escherichia coli* producing the Shiga toxin that is regarded as typical). The genetic basis of aHUS has been elucidated only recently. Studies of more than 100 families have revealed that those family members who have developed HUS have mutations in any one of several genes encoding complement regulatory proteins: complement factor H (*CFH*), CD46 or membrane cofactor protein (*MCP*), complement factor I (*CFI*), complement component C3, complement factor B (*CFB*), and thrombomodulin. Thus, whereas all other inherited HAs are due to intrinsic red cell abnormalities, this group is unique in that hemolysis results from an inherited defect external to red cells (Table 106-1). Because the regulation of the complement cascade has considerable redundancy, in the steady state any of the above abnormalities can be tolerated. However, when an intercurrent infection or some other trigger activates complement through the alternative pathway, the deficiency of one of the complement regulators becomes critical. Endothelial cells get damaged, especially in the kidney, and at the same time and partly as a result of this, there will be brisk hemolysis [thus, the more common Shiga toxin–related HUS (Chap. 149) can be regarded as a phenocopy of aHUS]. Atypical HUS is a severe disease with up to 15% mortality in the acute phase and up to 50% of cases progressing to end-stage renal disease. Atypical HUS often undergoes spontaneous remission, and the best tested form of treatment is plasma exchange, which supplies the deficient complement regulator. Because the basis of aHUS is an inherited abnormality, it is not surprising that given exposure to an appropriate trigger, the syndrome will tend to recur: when it does, the prognosis is always serious. In some cases, kidney (and liver) transplantation has been carried out, but the role of these procedures is controversial.

ACQUIRED HEMOLYTIC ANEMIA

Mechanical destruction of red cells

Although red cells are characterized by the remarkable deformability that enables them to squeeze through capillaries narrower than themselves for thousands of times in their lifetime, there are at least two situations in which they succumb to shear, if not to wear and tear. The result is intravascular hemolysis, resulting in hemoglobinuria. One situation is acute and self-inflicted, *march hemoglobinuria*. Why sometimes a marathon runner may develop this complication, whereas on another occasion this does not happen, we don't know (perhaps her or his footwear needs attention). A similar syndrome may develop after prolonged barefoot ritual dancing. The other situation is chronic and iatrogenic (it has been called *microangiopathic hemolytic anemia*); it takes place in patients with prosthetic heart valves, especially when paraprosthetic regurgitation is present. If the hemolysis consequent to mechanical trauma to the red cells is mild, and provided the supply of iron is adequate, it may be largely compensated. If more than mild anemia develops, reintervention to correct regurgitation may be required.

Toxic agents and drugs

A number of chemicals with oxidative potential, whether medicinal or not, can cause hemolysis even in people who are not G6PD-deficient (see above). Examples are hyperbaric oxygen (or 100% oxygen), nitrates, chlorates, methylene blue, dapsone, cisplatin, and numerous aromatic (cyclic) compounds. Other chemicals may be hemolytic through a nonoxidative, largely unknown mechanism; examples are arsine, stibine, copper, and lead. The HA caused by lead poisoning is characterized by basophilic stippling. It is in fact a phenocopy of that seen in P5N deficiency (see above), suggesting it is mediated at least in part by lead inhibiting this enzyme.

In these cases, hemolysis appears to be mediated by a direct chemical action on red cells. But drugs can cause hemolysis through at least two other mechanisms. (1) A drug can behave as a hapten and induce antibody production. In rare subjects this happens, for instance, with penicillin. Upon a subsequent exposure, red cells are caught, as innocent bystanders, in the reaction between penicillin and antipenicillin antibodies. Hemolysis will subside as soon as penicillin administration is stopped. (2) A drug can trigger, perhaps through mimicry, the production of an antibody against a red cell antigen. The best known example is methyldopa, an antihypertensive agent no longer in use, which in a small fraction of patients stimulated the production of the Rhesus antibody anti-e. In patients who have this antigen the anti-e is a true autoantibody, which would then cause an autoimmune HA (see below). Usually this would gradually subside once methyldopa was discontinued.

Severe intravascular hemolysis can be caused by the venom of certain snakes (cobras and vipers); and HA can also follow spider bites.

Infection

By far, the most frequent infectious cause of HA, in endemic areas, is malaria (Chap. 210). In other parts of the world, the most frequent cause is probably Shiga toxin–producing *Escherichia coli* O157:H7, now recognized as the main etiologic agent of the hemolytic-uremic syndrome, more common in children than in adults (Chap. 149). Life-threatening intravascular hemolysis, due to a toxin with lecithinase activity, occurs with *Clostridium perfringens* sepsis, particularly following open wounds, septic abortion, or as a disastrous accident due to a contaminated blood unit. Occasionally, HA is seen, especially in children, with sepsis or endocarditis from a variety of organisms.

Autoimmune hemolytic anemia (AIHA)

Except for countries where malaria is endemic, AIHA is the most common form of *acquired hemolytic anemia*. In fact, not quite appropriately, the two phrases are sometimes used as synonymous.

Pathophysiology AIHA is caused by an autoantibody directed against a red cell antigen, i.e., a molecule present on the surface of red cells. The autoantibody binds to the red cells. Once a red cell is coated by antibody, it will be destroyed by one or more mechanisms. In most cases the Fc portion of the antibody will be recognized by the Fc receptor of macrophages, and this will trigger erythrophagocytosis (Fig. 106-7). Thus, destruction of red cells will take place wherever macrophages are abundant, i.e., in the spleen, liver, and bone marrow. Because of the special anatomy of the spleen, it is particularly efficient in trapping antibody-coated red cells, and often this is the predominant site of red cell destruction. Although in severe cases even circulating monocytes can take part in this process, most of the phagocytosis-mediated red cell destruction takes place in the organs just mentioned, and it is therefore called *extravascular hemolysis*. In some cases, the nature of the antibody (usually an IgM antibody) is such that the antigen-antibody complex on the surface of red cells is able to activate complement (C). As a result, a large amount of membrane attack complex will form, and the red cells may be destroyed directly; this is known as *intravascular hemolysis*.

Clinical features The onset of AIHA is very often abrupt and can be dramatic. The hemoglobin level can drop, within days, to as low as 4 g/dL; the massive red cell removal will produce jaundice; and sometimes the spleen is enlarged. When this triad is present, the suspicion of AIHA must be high. When hemolysis is (in part) intravascular, the telltale sign will be hemoglobinuria, which the patient may report or for which the physician must inquire/test. The diagnostic test for AIHA is the antiglobulin test worked out in 1945 by R. R. A. Coombs and known since by his name. The beauty of this test is that it directly detects the pathogenetic mediator of the disease, i.e., the presence of antibody on the red cells themselves. When the test is positive, it clinches the diagnosis, and when it is negative, the diagnosis is unlikely. However, the sensitivity of the Coombs test varies depending on the technology that is used, and in doubtful cases a repeat in a specialized lab is advisable; the term "Coombs-negative AIHA" is a last resort. In some cases, the autoantibody has a defined identity: it may be specific for an antigen belonging to the Rhesus system (it is often anti-e). In many cases it is regarded as "unspecific" because it reacts with virtually all types of red cells.

As in autoimmune diseases in general, the real cause of AIHA remains obscure. However, from the clinical point of view, an important feature is that AIHA can appear to be isolated, or it can develop as part of a more general autoimmune disease, particularly systemic lupus erythematosus, of which sometimes it may be the first manifestation. Therefore, when AIHA is diagnosed, a full screen for autoimmune disease is imperative. In some cases, AIHA can be associated, on first presentation or subsequently, with autoimmune thrombocytopenia (Evans's syndrome).

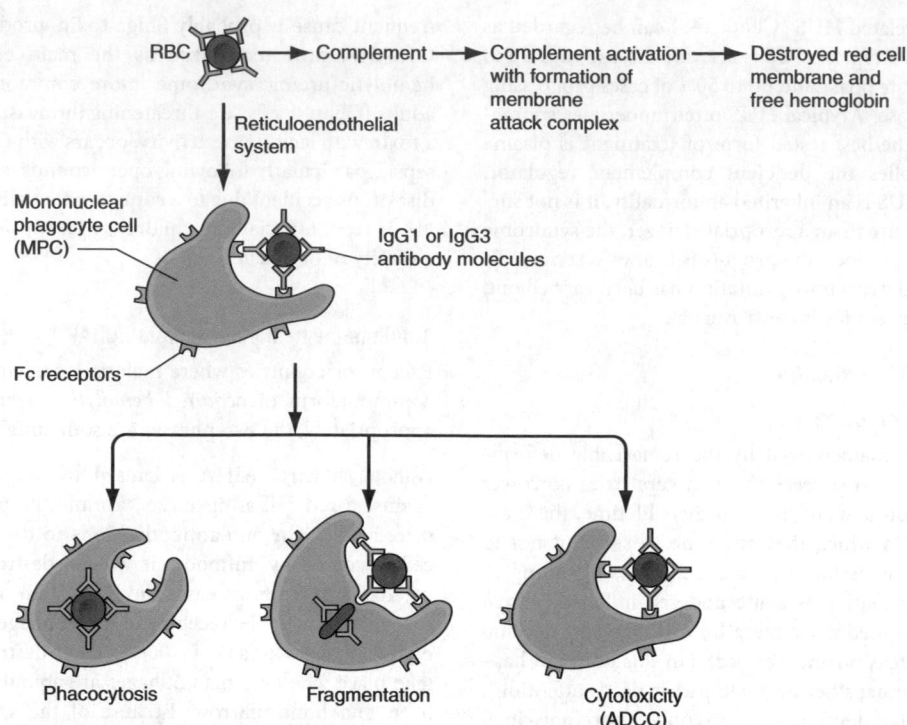

RBC → Complement → Complement activation with formation of membrane attack complex → Destroyed red cell membrane and free hemoglobin

Reticuloendothelial system

Mononuclear phagocyte cell (MPC)

IgG1 or IgG3 antibody molecules

Fc receptors

Phagocytosis   Fragmentation   Cytotoxicity (ADCC)

Figure 106-7   Mechanism of antibody-mediated immune destruction of red cells. *(From N Young et al: Clinical Hematology. Philadelphia, Elsevier, 2006; with permission.)*

TREATMENT   Autoimmune Hemolytic Anemia

Severe acute AIHA can be a medical emergency. The immediate treatment almost invariably includes transfusion of red cells. This may pose a special problem because if the antibody involved is unspecific, all the blood units cross-matched will be incompatible. In these cases it is often correct, paradoxically, to transfuse incompatible blood, the rationale being that the transfused red cells will be destroyed no less but no more than the patient's own red cells, but in the meantime the patient stays alive. Clearly, this rather unique situation requires good liaison and understanding between the clinical unit treating the patient and the blood transfusion/serology lab. Apart from emergency blood transfusion, the first-line treatment of AIHA is by using corticosteroids. In at least one-half of the cases, prednisone (1 mg/kg per day) will produce a remission promptly. Whereas some patients are then apparently cured, relapses are not uncommon. Although unfortunately most of the management of AIHA is not evidence-based, for patients who do not respond and for those who have relapsed (or who require more than 15 mg/d of prednisone to prevent relapse), it is highly recommended to consider a second-line treatment option, which might be either splenectomy or rituximab (anti-CD20). Splenectomy, although it does not cure the disease, can produce significant benefit by removing a major site of hemolysis, thus improving the anemia and/or reducing the need for other therapies (e.g., the dose of prednisone). Rituximab has emerged as a significant alternative to splenectomy because it can produce remissions in up to 80% of patients and it can be used repeatedly, even though progressive multifocal leukoencephalopathy is a dreaded if rare side effect. Azathioprine, cyclophosphamide, cyclosporine, and IV immunoglobulin have become third-line agents since the introduction of rituximab. In severe refractory cases, either auto- or allohematopoietic stem cell transplantation has been used, sometimes successfully.

Paroxysmal cold hemoglobinuria (PCH)   PCH is a rather rare form of AIHA occurring mostly in children, usually triggered by a viral infection, usually self-limited, and characterized by the involvement of the so-called Donath-Landsteiner antibody. In vitro this antibody has unique serologic features: it has anti-P specificity and it binds to red cells only at a low temperature (optimally at 4°C), but when the temperature is shifted to 37°C, lysis of red cells takes place in the presence of complement. Consequently, in vivo there is intravascular hemolysis, resulting in hemoglobinuria. Clinically, the differential diagnosis must include other causes of hemoglobinuria (Table 106-6), but the presence of the Donath-Landsteiner antibody will prove PCH. Active supportive treatment, including blood transfusion, is needed to control the anemia; subsequently, recovery is the rule.

Cold agglutinin disease (CAD)   This designation is used for a form of chronic AIHA that usually affects the elderly and has special clinical and pathologic features. First, the term *cold* refers to the fact that the autoantibody involved reacts with red cells poorly or not at all at 37°C, whereas it reacts strongly at lower temperatures.[1] As a result, hemolysis is more prominent the more the body is exposed to the cold. The antibody is usually IgM with an anti-I specificity (the I antigen is present on the red cells of almost everybody), and it may have a very high titer (1:100,000 or more has been observed). Second, the antibody is produced by an expanded clone of B lymphocytes, and sometimes its concentration in the plasma is high enough to show up as a spike in plasma protein electrophoresis; i.e., as a monoclonal gammopathy. Third, since the antibody is IgM, CAD is related to Waldenström macroglobulinemia (WM) (Chap. 111), although in most cases the other clinical features of this disease are not present. Thus, CAD must be regarded as a form of WM, i.e., as a low-grade mature B cell lymphoma that manifests at an earlier stage precisely because the unique biologic properties of the IgM that it produces give the clinical picture of chronic HA.

---

[1]In the past this type of antibody was called a cold antibody, whereas the antibodies causing the more common form of AIHA were called warm antibodies.

TABLE 106-6 Diseases/Clinical Situations With Predominantly Intravascular Hemolysis

	Onset/Time Course	Main Mechanism	Appropriate Diagnostic Procedure	Comments
Mismatched blood transfusion	Abrupt	Nearly always ABO incompatibility	Repeat cross-match	
Paroxysmal nocturnal hemoglobinuria (PNH)	Chronic with acute exacerbations	Complement (C)-mediated destruction of CD59(–) red cells	Flow cytometry to display a CD59(–) red cell population	Exacerbations due to C activation through any pathway
Paroxysmal cold hemoglobinuria (PCH)	Acute	Immune lysis of normal red cells	Test for Donath-Landsteiner antibody	Often triggered by viral infection
Septicemia	Very acute	Exotoxins produced by *Clostridium perfringens*	Blood cultures	Other organisms may be responsible
Microangiopathic	Acute or chronic	Red cell fragmentation	Red cell morphology on blood smear	Different causes ranging from endothelial damage to hemangioma to leaky prosthetic heart valve
March hemoglobinuria	Abrupt	Mechanical destruction	Targeted history taking	
Favism	Acute	Destruction of older fraction of G6PD-deficient red cells	G6PD assay	Triggered by ingestion of large dish of fava beans; but trigger can be infection or drug instead

In mild forms of CAD, avoidance of exposure to cold may be all that is needed to enable the patient to have a reasonably comfortable quality of life, but in more severe forms the management of CAD is not easy. Blood transfusion is not very effective because donor red cells are I-positive and will be rapidly removed. Immunosuppressive/cytotoxic treatment with azathioprine or cyclophosphamide can reduce the antibody titer, but clinical efficacy is limited and, in view of the chronic nature of the disease, the side effects may prove, in the long run, unacceptable. Unlike in AIHA, prednisone and splenectomy are ineffective. Plasma exchange is in theory a rational approach, but it is laborious and must be carried out at frequent intervals if it is to be beneficial. Since the advent of rituximab, the picture has changed significantly for those 60% of patients with CAD who respond to this agent. Given the long clinical course of CAD, it remains to be seen with what periodicity rituximab will need to be administered.

Paroxysmal nocturnal hemoglobinuria (PNH)

PNH is an acquired chronic HA characterized by persistent intravascular hemolysis (Table 106-6) subject to recurrent exacerbations. In addition to hemolysis, there is often pancytopenia and a distinct tendency to venous thrombosis. This triad makes PNH a truly unique clinical condition. However, when not all of these three features are manifest on presentation, the diagnosis is often delayed, although it can be always made by appropriate laboratory investigations (see below).

PNH has about the same frequency in men and in women, and it is encountered in all populations throughout the world, but it is a rare disease. Its prevalence is estimated to be between 1 and 5 per million (it may be somewhat less rare in Southeast Asia and in the Far East). There is no evidence of inherited susceptibility. PNH has never been reported as a congenital disease, but it can present in small children or as late as in the seventies, although most patients are young adults.

Clinical features The patient may seek medical attention because, one morning, she or he has "passed blood instead of urine" (Fig. 106-8). This distressing or frightening event may be regarded as the classical presentation; however, more frequently, this symptom is not noticed or is suppressed. Indeed, the patient often presents simply as a problem in the differential diagnosis of *anemia*,

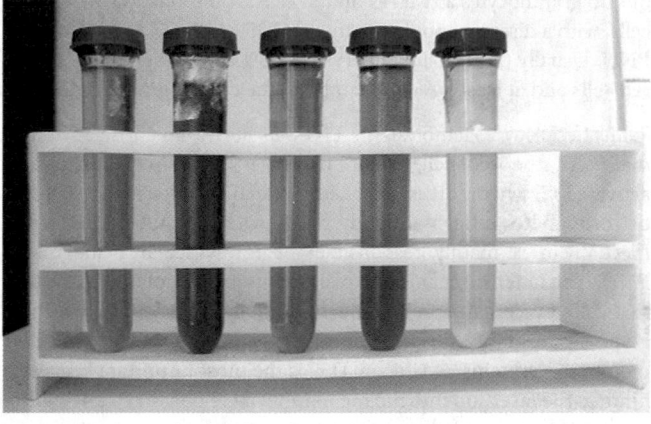

Figure 106-8 Consecutive urine samples from a patient with paroxysmal nocturnal hemoglobinuria (PNH). The variation in the severity of hemoglobinuria within hours is probably unique to this condition.

whether symptomatic or discovered incidentally. Sometimes, the anemia is associated from the outset with neutropenia, or thrombocytopenia, or both, thus signaling an element of bone marrow failure (see below). Some patients may present with recurrent attacks of severe abdominal pain, defying a specific diagnosis and eventually found to be related to thrombosis. When thrombosis affects the hepatic veins, it may produce acute hepatomegaly and ascites, i.e., a full-fledged Budd-Chiari syndrome, which in the absence of liver disease ought to raise the suspicion of PNH.

The *natural history* of PNH can extend over decades. Without treatment, the median survival is estimated to be about 8–10 years. In the past, the most common cause of death has been venous thrombosis, followed by infection secondary to severe neutropenia and hemorrhage secondary to severe thrombocytopenia. PNH may evolve into aplastic anemia (AA), and PNH may manifest itself in patients who previously had AA. Rarely (estimated 1–2% of all cases), PNH may terminate in acute myeloid leukemia. On the other hand, full spontaneous recovery from PNH has been well documented, albeit rarely.

Laboratory investigations and diagnosis The most consistent blood finding is anemia, which may range from mild to moderate to very severe. The anemia is usually normo-macrocytic, with unremarkable red cell morphology; if the MCV is high, it is usually largely accounted for by reticulocytosis, which may be quite marked (up to 20%, or up to 400,000/μL). The anemia may become microcytic if the patient is allowed to become iron-deficient as a result of chronic urinary blood loss through hemoglobinuria. Unconjugated bilirubin is mildly or moderately elevated, LDH is typically markedly elevated (values in the thousands are common), and haptoglobin is usually undetectable. All these findings make the diagnosis of HA compelling. Hemoglobinuria, the telltale sign of intravascular hemolysis (Table 106-6), may be overt in a random urine sample. If it is not, it may be helpful to obtain serial urine samples, since hemoglobinuria can vary dramatically from day to day, and even from hour to hour (Fig. 106-8). The bone marrow is usually cellular, with marked to massive erythroid hyperplasia, often with mild to moderate dyserythropoietic features (these do not justify confusing PNH with myelodysplastic syndrome). At some stage of the disease, the marrow may become hypocellular or even frankly aplastic (see below).

The definitive diagnosis of PNH must be based on the demonstration that a substantial proportion of the patient's red cells have an increased susceptibility to complement (C), due to the deficiency on their surface of proteins (particularly CD59 and CD55) that normally protect the red cells from activated C. The sucrose hemolysis test is unreliable, and the acidified serum (Ham) test is carried out in few labs. The gold standard today is flow cytometry, which can be carried out on granulocytes as well as on red cells. A bimodal distribution of cells, with a discrete population that is CD59-, CD55-, is diagnostic of PNH. Usually this population is at least 5% of the total in the case of red cells and at least 20% of the total in the case of granulocytes.

Pathophysiology Hemolysis in PNH is due to an intrinsic abnormality of the red cell, which makes it exquisitely sensitive to activated C, whether it is activated through the alternative pathway or through an antigen-antibody reaction (Fig. 106-9). The former mechanism is mainly responsible for intravascular hemolysis in PNH. The latter mechanism explains why the hemolysis can be dramatically exacerbated in the course of a viral or bacterial infection. Hypersusceptibility to C is due to deficiency of several protective membrane proteins, of which CD59 is the most important because it hinders the insertion into the membrane of C9 polymers. The molecular basis for the deficiency of these proteins has been pinpointed not to a defect in any of the respective genes, but rather to the shortage of a unique glycolipid molecule, glycosylphosphatidyl-inositol (GPI), which, through a peptide bond, anchors these proteins to the surface membrane of cells. The shortage of GPI is due in turn to a mutation in an X-linked gene, called *PIG-A*, required for an early step in GPI biosynthesis. In virtually each patient, the PIG-A mutation is different. This is not surprising, since these mutations are not inherited: rather, each one takes place de novo in a hematopoietic stem cell (i.e., they are somatic mutations). As a result, the patient's marrow is a mosaic of mutant and nonmutant cells, and the peripheral blood always contains both PNH cells and normal (non-PNH) cells. Thrombosis is one of the most immediately life-threatening complications of PNH and yet one of the least understood in its pathogenesis. It could be that deficiency of CD59 on the PNH platelet causes inappropriate platelet activation; however, other mechanisms are possible.

Bone marrow failure (BMF) and relationship between PNH and aplastic anemia (AA) It is not unusual that patients with firmly established PNH have a previous history of well-documented AA. On the other hand, sometimes a patient with PNH becomes less hemolytic and more pancytopenic and ultimately has the clinical picture of AA. Since AA is probably an organ-specific autoimmune disease, in which T cells cause damage to hematopoietic stem cells, the same may be true of PNH, with the specific proviso that the damage spares PNH stem cells. Skewing of the T cell repertoire in patients with PNH lends some support to this notion. In addition, there is evidence in mouse models that PNH stem cells do not expand when the rest of the bone marrow is normal, and by using high-sensitivity flow cytometry technology, very rare PNH cells harboring PIG-A mutations can be demonstrated in normal people. In view of these facts, it seems that an element of BMF in PNH is the rule rather than the exception. An extreme view is that PNH is a form of AA in which BMF is masked by the massive expansion of the PNH clone that populates the patient's bone marrow. The mechanism whereby PNH stem cells escape the damage suffered by non-PNH stem cells is not yet known.

> **TREATMENT** **Paroxysmal Nocturnal Hemoglobinuria**

Unlike other acquired HAs, PNH may be a lifelong condition; standard care was formerly supportive treatment only, including transfusion of filtered red cells[2] whenever necessary, which, for some patients, means quite frequently. Folic acid supplements (at least 3 mg/d) are mandatory, and the serum iron should be checked periodically and iron supplements administered as appropriate. Long-term glucocorticoids are not indicated because there is no evidence that they have any effect on chronic hemolysis: in fact they are contraindicated because of their many dangerous side effects. A major advance in the management of PNH has been the development of a humanized monoclonal antibody, eculizumab, directed against the complement component C5. In an international, multicenter, placebo-controlled randomized trial of 87 patients (so far the only controlled therapeutic trial in PNH) who had been selected on grounds of having severe hemolysis making them transfusion-dependent, eculizumab proved effective and was licensed in 2007 (Fig. 106-10). By blocking the complement cascade downstream of C5, eculizumab abrogates complement-dependent intravascular hemolysis in all PNH patients, which in itself significantly improves their quality of life. One would expect that, as a result, the need for blood transfusion would be also abrogated, and this indeed is the case in about one-half of the patients, in many of whom there is also a rise in hemoglobin levels. In the remaining patients, the anemia remains sufficiently severe to require blood transfusion, apparently because of ongoing extravascular hemolysis of red cells opsonized by complement (C3) fragments. Based on its half-life, eculizumab must be administered intravenously every 14 days. The only form of treatment that currently can provide a definitive cure for PNH is allogeneic bone marrow transplantation (BMT). When an HLA-identical sibling is available, BMT should be offered to any young patient with severe PNH; the availability of eculizumab has probably decreased significantly the proportion of those who take up this option.

For patients with the PNH-AA syndrome, immunosuppressive treatment with antilymphocyte globulin (ALG or ATG) and cyclosporine A may be indicated. Although no formal trial has ever been conducted, this approach has helped particularly to relieve severe thrombocytopenia and/or neutropenia in patients in whom these were the main problem(s). By contrast, there is often little immediate effect on hemolysis. Any patient who has had venous thrombosis or who has a genetically determined thrombophilic state in addition to PNH should be on regular anticoagulant prophylaxis.

---

[2]Now that filters with excellent retention of white cells are routinely used, the traditional washing of red cells, aiming to avoid white cell reactions triggering hemolysis, is no longer necessary and is wasteful

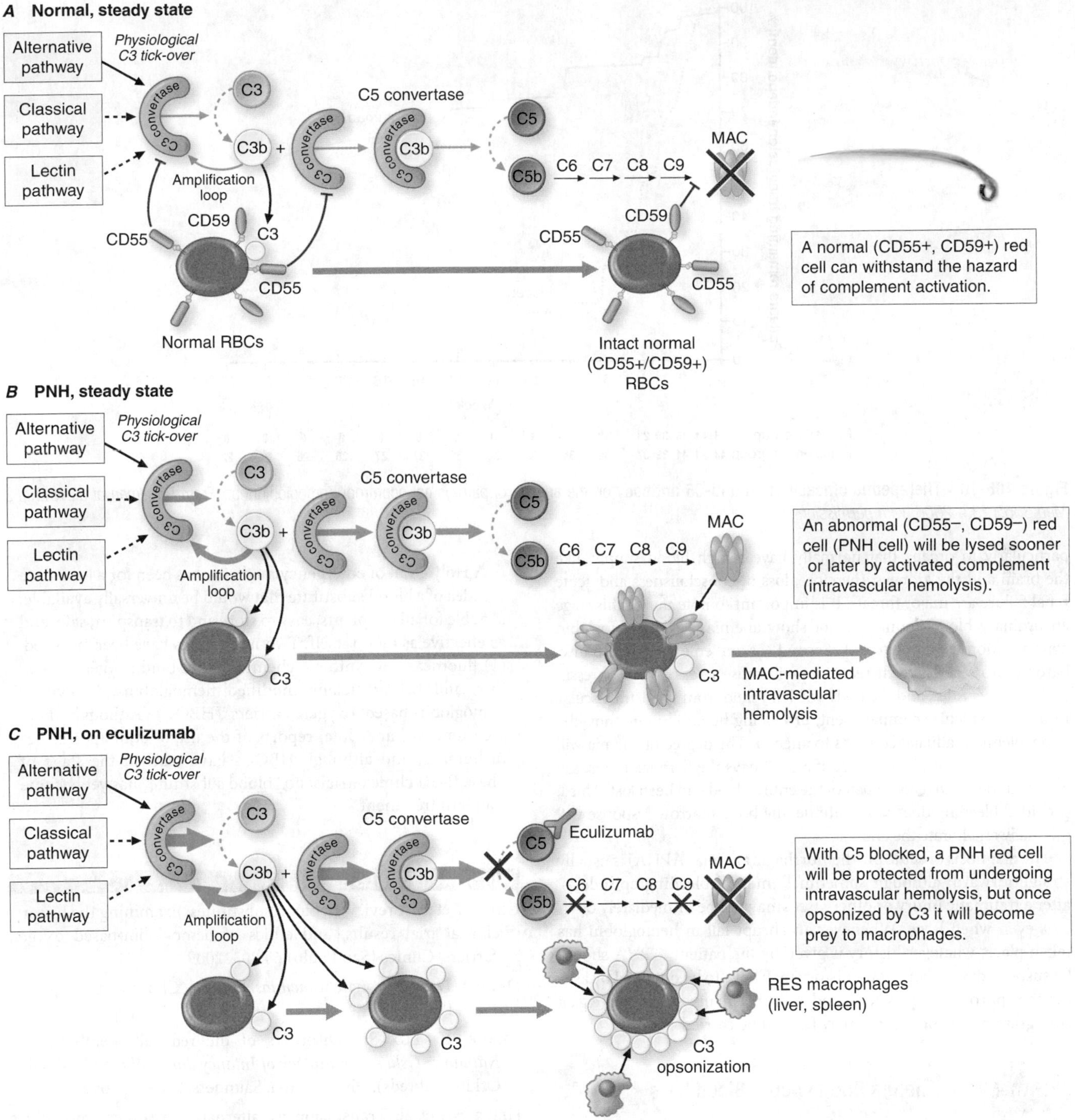

A   Normal, steady state

A normal (CD55+, CD59+) red cell can withstand the hazard of complement activation.

B   PNH, steady state

An abnormal (CD55−, CD59−) red cell (PNH cell) will be lysed sooner or later by activated complement (intravascular hemolysis).

C   PNH, on eculizumab

With C5 blocked, a PNH red cell will be protected from undergoing intravascular hemolysis, but once opsonized by C3 it will become prey to macrophages.

Figure 106-9   The complement cascade and the fate of red cells. *A.* Normal red cells are protected from complement activation and subsequent hemolysis by CD55 and CD59. These two proteins, being GPI-linked, are missing from the surface of PNH red cells as a result of a somatic mutation of the X-linked *PIG-A* gene that encodes a protein required for an early step of the GPI molecule biosynthesis. *B.* In the steady state, PNH erythrocytes suffer from spontaneous (tick-over) complement activation, with consequent intravascular hemolysis through formation of the membrane attack complex (MAC); when extra complement is activated through the classical pathway, an exacerbation of hemolysis will result. *C.* On eculizumab, PNH erythrocytes are protected from hemolysis from the inhibition of C5 cleavage; however, upstream complement activation may lead to C3 opsonization and possible extravascular hemolysis. GPI, glycosylphosphatidylinositol; PNH, paroxysmal nocturnal hemoglobinuria. *(From L Luzzatto, et al: Haematologica 95:523, 2010.)*

ANEMIA DUE TO ACUTE BLOOD LOSS

Blood loss causes anemia by two main mechanisms. First, by the direct loss of red cells, and second, because if the loss of blood is protracted, it will gradually deplete the iron stores, eventually resulting in iron deficiency. The latter type of anemia is covered in Chap. 103. Here we are concerned with the former type, i.e., the *posthemorrhagic anemia*, which follows *acute* blood loss. This can be *external* (as after trauma, or obstetric hemorrhage) or *internal* (e.g., from bleeding in the gastrointestinal tract, rupture of the spleen, rupture of an ectopic pregnancy, subarachnoid hemorrhage). In any of these cases, i.e., after the sudden loss of a large amount of blood, there are three clinical/pathophysiologic stages. First, the dominant feature is hypovolemia, which poses a threat

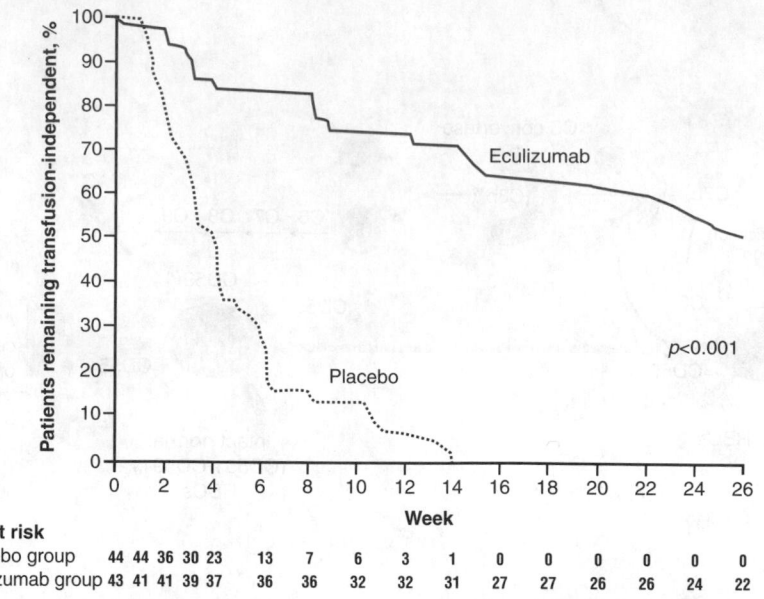

Figure 106-10 **Therapeutic efficacy of an anti-C5 antibody** on the anemia of paroxysmal nocturnal hemoglobinuria. *(From P Hillmen et al: N Engl J Med 355:1233, 2006; with permission.)*

particularly to organs that normally have a high blood supply, like the brain and the kidneys; therefore, loss of consciousness and acute renal failure are major threats. It is important to note that at this stage an ordinary blood count will not show anemia, as the hemoglobin concentration is not affected. Second, as an emergency response, baroreceptors and stretch receptors will cause release of vasopressin and other peptides, and the body will shift fluid from the extravascular to the intravascular compartment, producing hemodilution; thus, the hypovolemia gradually converts to anemia. The degree of anemia will reflect the amount of blood lost: if after 3 days the hemoglobin is, say 7 g/dL, it means that about half of the entire blood had been lost. Third, provided bleeding does not continue, the bone marrow response will gradually ameliorate the anemia.

The diagnosis of acute posthemorrhagic anemia (APHA) is usually straightforward; although sometimes internal bleeding episodes—after a traumatic injury or otherwise—may not be immediately obvious, even when large. Whenever an abrupt fall in hemoglobin has taken place, whatever history is given by the patient, APHA should be suspected: supplementary history may have to be obtained by asking the appropriate questions, and appropriate investigations (e.g., a sonogram or an endoscopy) may have to be carried out.

> **TREATMENT** Anemia Due to Acute Blood Loss

With respect to treatment, a two-pronged approach is imperative. (1) In many cases the blood lost needs to be replaced promptly. Unlike with many chronic anemias, when finding and correcting the cause of the anemia is the first priority and blood transfusion may not be even necessary because the body is adapted to the anemia, with acute blood loss the reverse is true; i.e., since the body is not adapted to the anemia, blood transfusion takes priority. (2) While the emergency is being confronted, it is imperative to stop the hemorrhage and to eliminate its source.

A special type of APHA is blood loss during and immediately after surgery, which can be substantial (for instance, up to 2 L in the case of a radical prostatectomy). Of course, with elective surgical procedures, the patient's own stored blood may be available (through preoperative autologous blood donation), and in any case blood loss is carefully monitored. Since this blood loss is iatrogenic, ever more effort should be invested in optimizing transfusion management.

A Holy Grail of emergency medicine has been for a long time the idea of a blood substitute that would be universally available, suitable for all recipients, easy to store and to transport, safe, and as effective as blood itself. Two main paths have been pursued: (1) fluorocarbon synthetic chemicals that bind oxygen reversibly, and (2) artificially modified hemoglobins, known as hemoglobin-based oxygen carriers (HBOC). Although there are numerous anecdotal reports of the use of both approaches in humans, and although HBOCs have reached the stage of phase II–III clinical trials, no "blood substitute" has yet become standard treatment.

FURTHER READINGS

CHEN JY et al: A review of blood substitutes: Examining the history, clinical trial results, and ethics of hemoglobin-based oxygen carriers. Clinics (Sao Paulo) 64:803, 2009

DACIE J: *The Haemolytic Anaemias*. London, Churchill Livingstone, 1985–1995

GRACE RF, LUX SE: Disorders of the red cell membrane, in *Nathan & Oski's Hematology of Infancy and Childhood*, 7th ed, S Orkin et al (eds). Philadelphia, Saunders, 2009, pp. 659–837

HEIER HE et al: Transfusion vs. alternative treatment modalities in acute bleeding: A systematic review. Acta Anaesthesiol Scand 509:20, 2006

HILLMEN P et al: The complement inhibitor eculizumab in paroxysmal nocturnal hemoglobinuria. N Engl J Med 355:1233, 2006

KAUSHANSKY K et al (eds): *Williams Hematology*, 8th ed. New York, McGraw Hill, 2010

LECHNER K, JAGER U: How I treat autoimmune hemolytic anemias in adults. Blood 116:1831, 2010

LUZZATTO L: The rise and fall of the antimalarial Lapdap: A lesson in pharmacogenetics. Lancet 376:739, 2010

LUZZATTO L, ARATEN D: Paroxysmal nocturnal hemoglobinuria, in *Clinical Hematology*, NS Young et al (eds). Philadelphia, Mosby, 2006, pp. 326–339

NORIS M, REMUZZI G: Atypical hemolytic-uremic syndrome. N Engl J Med 361:1676, 2009

CHAPTER 107

Aplastic Anemia, Myelodysplasia, and Related Bone Marrow Failure Syndromes

Neal S. Young

The hypoproliferative anemias are normochromic, normocytic, or macrocytic and are characterized by a low reticulocyte count. Deficient production of red blood cells (RBCs) occurs with marrow damage and dysfunction, which may be secondary to infection, inflammation, and cancer. Hypoproliferative anemia is also a prominent feature of hematologic diseases that are described as bone marrow failure states; these include aplastic anemia, myelodysplastic syndrome (MDS), pure red cell aplasia (PRCA), and myelophthisis. Anemia in these disorders is often not a solitary or even the major hematologic finding. More frequent in bone marrow failure is pancytopenia: anemia, leukopenia, and thrombocytopenia. Low blood counts in the marrow failure diseases result from deficient hematopoiesis, as distinguished from blood count depression due to peripheral destruction of red cells (hemolytic anemias), platelets [idiopathic thrombocytopenic purpura (ITP) or due to splenomegaly], and granulocytes (as in the immune leukopenias).

Hematopoietic failure syndromes are classified by dominant morphologic features of the bone marrow (Table 107-1). Although practical distinction among these syndromes usually is clear, they can occur secondary to other diseases, and some processes are so closely related that the diagnosis may be complex. Patients may seem to suffer from two or three related diseases simultaneously, or one diagnosis may appear to evolve into another. Many of these syndromes share an immune-mediated mechanism of marrow destruction and some element of genomic instability resulting in a higher rate of malignant transformation.

It is important that the internist and general practitioner recognize the marrow failure syndromes, as their prognosis may be poor if the patient is untreated; effective therapies are often available but sufficiently complex in their choice and delivery so as to warrant the care of a hematologist or oncologist.

APLASTIC ANEMIA

■ DEFINITION

Aplastic anemia is pancytopenia with bone marrow hypocellularity. Acquired aplastic anemia is distinguished from iatrogenic marrow aplasia, marrow hypocellularity after intensive cytotoxic chemotherapy for cancer. Aplastic anemia can also be constitutional: The genetic diseases Fanconi's anemia and dyskeratosis congenita, although frequently associated with typical physical anomalies and the development of pancytopenia early in life, can also present as marrow failure in normal-appearing adults. Acquired aplastic anemia is often stereotypical in its manifestations, with the abrupt onset of low blood counts in a previously well young adult; seronegative hepatitis or a course of an incriminated medical drug may precede the onset. The diagnosis in these instances is uncomplicated. Sometimes blood count depression is moderate or incomplete, resulting in anemia, leukopenia, and

TABLE 107-1 Differential Diagnosis of Pancytopenia

Pancytopenia with Hypocellular Bone Marrow

Acquired aplastic anemia

Constitutional aplastic anemia (Fanconi's anemia, dyskeratosis congenita)

Some myelodysplasia

Rare aleukemic leukemia

Some acute lymphoid leukemia

Some lymphomas of bone marrow

Pancytopenia with Cellular Bone Marrow

Primary bone marrow diseases	Secondary to systemic diseases
Myelodysplasia	Systemic lupus erythematosus
Paroxysmal nocturnal hemoglobinuria	Hypersplenism
Myelofibrosis	B_{12}, folate deficiency
Some aleukemic leukemia	Overwhelming infection
Myelophthisis	Alcohol
Bone marrow lymphoma	Brucellosis
Hairy cell leukemia	Sarcoidosis
	Tuberculosis
	Leishmaniasis

Hypocellular Bone Marrow ± Cytopenia

Q fever

Legionnaires' disease

Anorexia nervosa, starvation

Mycobacterium

thrombocytopenia in some combination. Aplastic anemia is related to both paroxysmal nocturnal hemoglobinuria (PNH; Chap. 106) and to MDS, and in some cases a clear distinction among these disorders may not be possible.

■ EPIDEMIOLOGY

The incidence of acquired aplastic anemia in Europe and Israel is two cases per million persons annually. In Thailand and China, rates of five to seven per million have been established. In general, men and women are affected with equal frequency, but the age distribution is biphasic, with the major peak in the teens and twenties and a second rise in older adults.

■ ETIOLOGY

The origins of aplastic anemia have been inferred from several recurring clinical associations (Table 107-2); unfortunately, these relationships are not reliable in an individual patient and may not be etiologic. In addition, although most cases of aplastic anemia are idiopathic, little other than history separates these cases from those with a presumed etiology such as a drug exposure.

Radiation

Marrow aplasia is a major acute sequela of radiation. Radiation damages DNA; tissues dependent on active mitosis are particularly susceptible. Nuclear accidents can involve not only power plant workers but also employees of hospitals, laboratories, and industry

TABLE 107-2 Classification of Aplastic Anemia and Single Cytopenias

Acquired	Inherited
Aplastic Anemia	
Secondary	Fanconi's anemia
Radiation	Dyskeratosis congenita
Drugs and chemicals	Shwachman-Diamond syndrome
Regular effects	Reticular dysgenesis
Idiosyncratic reactions	Amegakaryocytic thrombocytopenia
Viruses	Familial aplastic anemias
Epstein-Barr virus (infectious mononucleosis)	Preleukemia (monosomy 7, etc.)
Hepatitis (non-A, non-B, non-C hepatitis)	Nonhematologic syndrome (Down, Dubowitz, Seckel)
Parvovirus B19 (transient aplastic crisis, PRCA)	
HIV-1 (AIDS)	
Immune diseases	
Eosinophilic fasciitis	
Hyperimmunoglobulinemia	
Thymoma/thymic carcinoma	
Graft-versus-host disease in immunodeficiency	
Paroxysmal nocturnal hemoglobinuria	
Pregnancy	
Idiopathic	
Cytopenias	
PRCA (see Table 107-4)	Congenital PRCA (Diamond-Blackfan anemia)
Neutropenia/agranulocytosis	
Idiopathic	Kostmann's syndrome
Drugs, toxins	Shwachman-Diamond syndrome
Pure white cell aplasia	Reticular dysgenesis
Thrombocytopenia	
Drugs, toxins	Amegakaryocytic thrombocytopenia
Idiopathic amegakaryocytic	Thrombocytopenia with absent radii

Abbreviation: PRCA, pure red cell aplasia.

(food sterilization, metal radiography, etc.), as well as innocents exposed to stolen, misplaced, or misused sources. Whereas the radiation dose can be approximated from the rate and degree of decline in blood counts, dosimetry by reconstruction of the exposure can help to estimate the patient's prognosis and also to protect medical personnel from contact with radioactive tissue and excreta. MDS and leukemia, but probably not aplastic anemia, are late effects of radiation.

Chemicals

Benzene is a notorious cause of bone marrow failure: epidemiologic, clinical, and laboratory data link benzene to aplastic anemia, acute leukemia, and blood and marrow abnormalities. For leukemia, incidence is correlated with cumulative exposure, but susceptibility

must also be important, as only a minority of even heavily exposed workers develop myelotoxicity. The employment history is important, especially in industries where benzene is used for a secondary purpose, usually as a solvent. Benzene-related blood diseases have declined with regulation of industrial exposure. Although benzene is no longer generally available as a household solvent, exposure to its metabolites occurs in the normal diet and in the environment. The association between marrow failure and other chemicals is much less well substantiated.

Drugs

(Table 107-3) Many chemotherapeutic drugs have marrow suppression as a major toxicity; effects are dose dependent and will occur in all recipients. In contrast, idiosyncratic reactions to a large and diverse group of drugs may lead to aplastic anemia without a clear dose-response relationship. These associations rested largely on accumulated case reports until a large international study in Europe in the 1980s quantitated drug relationships, especially for

TABLE 107-3 Some Drugs and Chemicals Associated With Aplastic Anemia

Agents that regularly produce marrow depression as major toxicity in commonly employed doses or normal exposures:

  Cytotoxic drugs used in cancer chemotherapy: *alkylating agents*, *antimetabolites*, *antimitotics*, some antibiotics

Agents that frequently but not inevitably produce marrow aplasia:

  Benzene

Agents associated with aplastic anemia but with a relatively low probability:

  Chloramphenicol

  Insecticides

  Antiprotozoals: *quinacrine* and chloroquine, mepacrine

  Nonsteroidal anti-inflammatory drugs (including *phenylbutazone*, indomethacin, ibuprofen, sulindac, aspirin)

  Anticonvulsants (*hydantoins*, *carbamazepine*, phenacemide, felbamate)

  Heavy metals (*gold*, arsenic, bismuth, mercury)

  Sulfonamides: some antibiotics, antithyroid drugs (methimazole, methylthiouracil, propylthiouracil), antidiabetes drugs (tolbutamide, chlorpropamide), carbonic anhydrase inhibitors (acetazolamide and methazolamide)

  Antihistamines (*cimetidine*, chlorpheniramine)

  D-Penicillamine

  Estrogens (in pregnancy and in high doses in animals)

Agents whose association with aplastic anemia is more tenuous:

  Other antibiotics (streptomycin, tetracycline, methicillin, mebendazole, trimethoprim/sulfamethoxazole, flucytosine)

  Sedatives and tranquilizers (chlorpromazine, prochlorperazine, piperacetazine, chlordiazepoxide, meprobamate, methyprylon)

  Allopurinol

  Methyldopa

  Quinidine

  Lithium

  Guanidine

  Potassium perchlorate

  Thiocyanate

  Carbimazole

Note: Terms set in italics show the most consistent association with aplastic anemia.

nonsteroidal analgesics, sulfonamides, thyrostatic drugs, some psychotropics, penicillamine, allopurinol, and gold. Association does not equal causation: A drug may have been used to treat the first symptoms of bone marrow failure (antibiotics for fever or the preceding viral illness) or provoked the first symptom of a preexisting disease (petechiae by nonsteroidal anti-inflammatory agents administered to the thrombocytopenic patient). In the context of total drug use, idiosyncratic reactions, although individually devastating, are rare events. Risk estimates are usually lower when determined in population-based studies; furthermore, the low absolute risk is also made more obvious: even a ten- or twenty-fold increase in risk translates, in a rare disease, to but a handful of drug-induced aplastic anemia cases among hundreds of thousands of exposed persons.

Infections

Hepatitis is the most common preceding infection, and posthepatitis marrow failure accounts for approximately 5% of etiologies in most series. Patients are usually young men who have recovered from a bout of liver inflammation 1 to 2 months earlier; the subsequent pancytopenia is very severe. The hepatitis is seronegative (non-A, non-B, non-C) and possibly due to an as yet undiscovered infectious agent. Fulminant liver failure in childhood also follows seronegative hepatitis, and marrow failure occurs at a high rate in these patients. Aplastic anemia can rarely follow infectious mononucleosis. Parvovirus B19, the cause of transient aplastic crisis in hemolytic anemias and of some PRCAs (see below), does not usually cause generalized bone marrow failure. Mild blood count depression is frequent in the course of many viral and bacterial infections but resolves with the infection.

Immunologic diseases

Aplasia is a major consequence and the inevitable cause of death in *transfusion-associated graft-versus-host disease* (GVHD) that can occur after infusion of nonirradiated blood products to an immunodeficient recipient. Aplastic anemia is strongly associated with the rare collagen vascular syndrome *eosinophilic fasciitis* that is characterized by painful induration of subcutaneous tissues (Chap. 323). Pancytopenia with marrow hypoplasia can also occur in systemic lupus erythematosus (SLE).

Pregnancy

Aplastic anemia very rarely may occur and recur during pregnancy and resolve with delivery or with spontaneous or induced abortion.

Paroxysmal nocturnal hemoglobinuria

An acquired mutation in the *PIG-A* gene in a hematopoietic stem cell is required for the development of PNH, but *PIG-A* mutations probably occur commonly in normal individuals. If the PIG-A mutant stem cell proliferates, the result is a clone of progeny deficient in glycosylphosphatidylinositol-linked cell surface membrane proteins (Chap. 106). Small clones of deficient cells can be detected by sensitive flow cytometry tests in approximately one-half of patients with aplastic anemia at the time of presentation [and PNH cells are also seen in MDS (see below)]. Functional studies of bone marrow from PNH patients, even those with mainly hemolytic manifestations, show evidence of defective hematopoiesis. Patients with an initial clinical diagnosis of PNH, especially younger individuals, may later develop frank marrow aplasia and pancytopenia; patients with an initial diagnosis of aplastic anemia may suffer from hemolytic PNH years after recovery of blood counts.

Constitutional disorders

Fanconi's anemia, an autosomal recessive disorder, manifests as congenital developmental anomalies, progressive pancytopenia, and an increased risk of malignancy. Chromosomes in Fanconi's anemia are peculiarly susceptible to DNA cross-linking agents, the basis for a diagnostic assay. Patients with Fanconi's anemia typically have short stature, café au lait spots, and anomalies involving the thumb, radius, and genitourinary tract. At least 12 different genetic defects (all but one with an identified gene) have been defined; the most common, type A Fanconi's anemia, is due to a mutation in *FANCA*. Most of the Fanconi's anemia gene products form a protein complex that activates FANCD2 by monoubiquitination to play a role in the cellular response to DNA damage and especially interstrand cross-linking.

Dyskeratosis congenita is characterized by mucous membrane leukoplakia, dystrophic nails, reticular hyperpigmentation, and the development of aplastic anemia in childhood. Dyskeratosis is due to mutations in genes of the telomere repair complex, which acts to maintain telomere length in replicating cells: The X-linked variety is due to mutations in the *DKC1* (*dyskerin*) gene; the more unusual autosomal dominant type is due to mutation in *TERC*, which encodes an RNA template, and *TERT*, which encodes the catalytic reverse transcriptase, telomerase. Mutations in TNF2, a component of the shelterin, proteins that bind the telomere DNA, also occur in dyskeratosis.

In Shwachman-Diamond syndrome, marrow failure is seen with pancreatic insufficiency and malabsorption; most patients have compound heterozygous mutations in *SBDS* that may affect marrow stroma function.

Mutations in *TERT*, *TERC*, *TNF2*, and *SBDS* also can occur in patients with apparently acquired aplastic anemia (TERT and TERC mutations also are etiologic in familial pulmonary fibrosis and in some hepatic cirrhosis).

PATHOPHYSIOLOGY

Bone marrow failure results from severe damage to the hematopoietic cell compartment. In aplastic anemia, replacement of the bone marrow by fat is apparent in the morphology of the biopsy specimen (Fig. 107-1) and MRI of the spine. Cells bearing the CD34 antigen, a marker of early hematopoietic cells, are greatly diminished, and in functional studies, committed and primitive progenitor cells are virtually absent; in vitro assays have suggested that the stem cell pool is reduced to ≤1% of normal in severe disease at the time of presentation.

An intrinsic stem cell defect exists for the constitutional aplastic anemias: Cells from patients with Fanconi's anemia exhibit chromosome damage and death on exposure to certain chemical agents. Telomeres are short in some patients with aplastic anemia, due to heterozygous mutations in genes of the telomere repair complex. Variable penetrance means that *TERT* and *TERC* mutations represent risk factors for marrow failure, as family members with the same mutations may have normal or only slight hematologic abnormalities but more subtle evidence of (compensated) hematopoietic insufficiency.

Drug injury

Extrinsic damage to the marrow follows massive physical or chemical insults such as high doses of radiation and toxic chemicals. For the more common idiosyncratic reaction to modest doses of medical drugs, altered drug metabolism has been invoked as a likely mechanism. The metabolic pathways of many drugs and chemicals, especially if they are polar and have limited water solubility, involve enzymatic degradation to highly reactive electrophilic compounds; these intermediates are toxic because of their propensity to bind to cellular macromolecules. For example, derivative hydroquinones and quinolones are responsible for benzene-induced tissue injury. Excessive generation of toxic intermediates or failure to detoxify

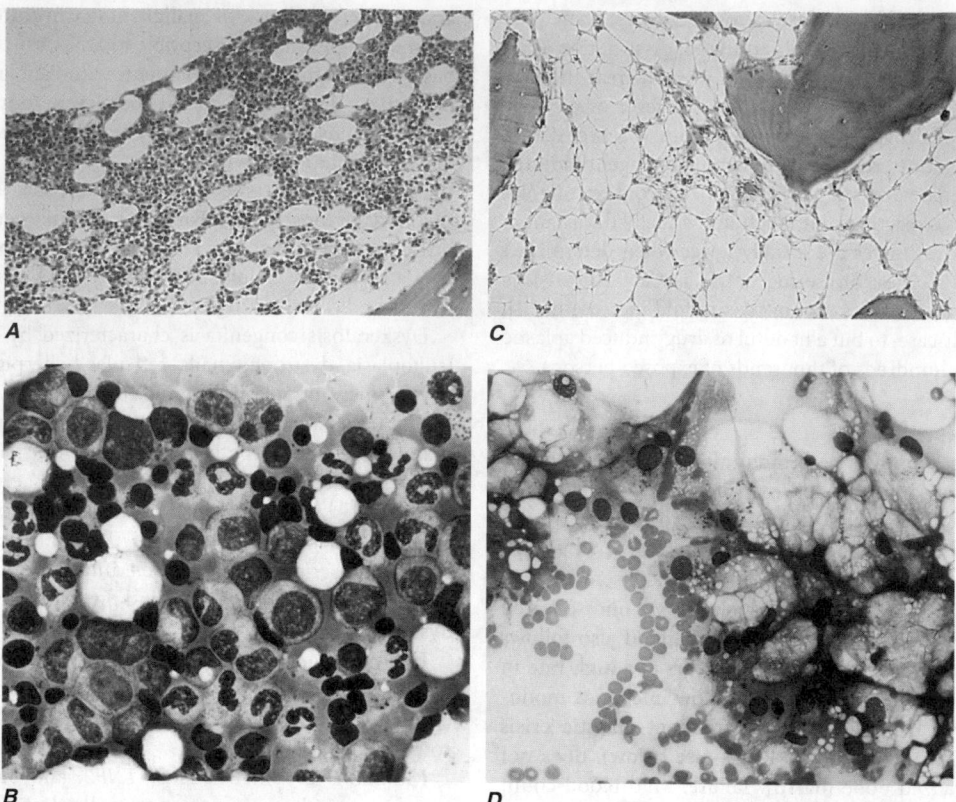

Figure 107-1 **A.** Normal bone marrow biopsy. **B.** Normal bone marrow aspirate smear. The marrow is normally 30–70% cellular, and there is a heterogeneous mix of myeloid, erythroid, and lymphoid cells. **C.** Aplastic anemia biopsy. **D.** Marrow smear in aplastic anemia. The marrow shows replacement of hematopoietic tissue by fat and only residual stromal and lymphoid cells.

the intermediates may be genetically determined and apparent only on specific drug challenge; the complexity and specificity of the pathways imply multiple susceptibility loci and would provide an explanation for the rarity of idiosyncratic drug reactions.

Immune-mediated injury

The recovery of marrow function in some patients prepared for bone marrow transplantation with antilymphocyte globulin (ALO) first suggested that aplastic anemia might be immune mediated. Consistent with this hypothesis was the frequent failure of simple bone marrow transplantation from a syngeneic twin, without conditioning cytotoxic chemotherapy, which also argued both *against* simple stem cell absence as the cause and *for* the presence of a host factor producing marrow failure. Laboratory data support an important role for the immune system in aplastic anemia. Blood and bone marrow cells of patients can suppress normal hematopoietic progenitor cell growth, and removal of T cells from aplastic anemia bone marrow improves colony formation in vitro. Increased numbers of activated cytotoxic T cell clones are observed in aplastic anemia patients and usually decline with successful immunosuppressive therapy; cytokine measurements show a T_H1 immune response [interferon γ (IFN γ) and tumor necrosis factor (TNF)]. Interferon and induce Fas expression on CD34 cells, leading to apoptotic cell death; localization of activated T cells to bone marrow and local production of their soluble factors are probably important in stem cell destruction.

Early immune system events in aplastic anemia are not well understood. An oligoclonal, T cell response implies an antigenic stimulus. Many different exogenous antigens appear capable of initiating a pathologic immune response, but at least some of the T cells may recognize true self-antigens. The rarity of aplastic anemia despite common exposures (medicines, seronegative hepatitis) suggests that genetically determined features of the immune response can convert a normal physiologic response into a sustained abnormal autoimmune process, including polymorphisms in histocompatibility antigens, cytokine genes, and genes that regulate T cell polarization and effector function.

■ CLINICAL FEATURES

History

Aplastic anemia can appear with seeming abruptness or have a more insidious onset. Bleeding is the most common early symptom; a complaint of days to weeks of easy bruising, oozing from the gums, nose bleeds, heavy menstrual flow, and sometimes petechiae will have been noticed. With thrombocytopenia, massive hemorrhage is unusual, but small amounts of bleeding in the central nervous system can result in catastrophic intracranial or retinal hemorrhage. Symptoms of anemia are also frequent, including lassitude, weakness, shortness of breath, and a pounding sensation in the ears. Infection is an unusual first symptom in aplastic anemia (unlike in agranulocytosis, where pharyngitis, anorectal infection, or frank sepsis occur early). A striking feature of aplastic anemia is the restriction of symptoms to the hematologic system, and patients often feel and look remarkably well despite drastically reduced blood counts. Systemic complaints and weight loss should point to other etiologies of pancytopenia. Prior drug use, chemical exposure, and preceding viral illnesses must often be elicited with repeated questioning. A family history of hematologic diseases or blood abnormalities, and of pulmonary or liver fibrosis, may indicate a constitutional etiology of marrow failure.

Physical examination

Petechiae and ecchymoses are typical, and retinal hemorrhages may be present. Pelvic and rectal examinations can often be deferred but, when performed, should be undertaken with great gentleness to avoid trauma; these will often show bleeding from the cervical os and blood in the stool. Pallor of the skin and mucous membranes is common except in the most acute cases or those already transfused. Infection on presentation is unusual but may occur if the patient has been symptomatic for a few weeks. Lymphadenopathy and splenomegaly are highly atypical of aplastic anemia. Café au lait spots and short stature suggest Fanconi's anemia; peculiar nails and leukoplakia suggest dyskeratosis congenita.

■ LABORATORY STUDIES

Blood

The smear shows large erythrocytes and a paucity of platelets and granulocytes. Mean corpuscular volume (MCV) is commonly increased. Reticulocytes are absent or few, and lymphocyte numbers may be normal or reduced. The presence of immature myeloid forms suggests leukemia or MDS; nucleated RBCs suggest marrow fibrosis or tumor invasion; abnormal platelets suggest either peripheral destruction or MDS.

Bone marrow

The bone marrow is usually readily aspirated but dilute on smear, and the fatty biopsy specimen may be grossly pale on withdrawal; a "dry tap" instead suggests fibrosis or myelophthisis. In severe aplasia the smear of the aspirated specimen shows only red cells, residual lymphocytes, and stromal cells; the biopsy (which should be >1 cm in length) is superior for determination of cellularity and shows mainly fat under the microscope, with hematopoietic cells occupying <25% of the marrow space; in the most serious cases the biopsy is virtually 100% fat. The correlation between marrow cellularity and disease severity is imperfect, in part because marrow cellularity declines physiologically with aging. Additionally, some patients with moderate disease by blood counts will have empty iliac crest biopsies, while "hot spots" of hematopoiesis may be seen in severe cases. If an iliac crest specimen is inadequate, cells may also be obtained by aspiration from the sternum. Residual hematopoietic cells should have normal morphology, except for mildly megaloblastic erythropoiesis; megakaryocytes are invariably greatly reduced and usually absent. Granulomas may indicate an infectious etiology of the marrow failure.

Ancillary studies

Chromosome breakage studies of peripheral blood using diepoxybutane or mitomycin C should be performed on children and younger adults to exclude Fanconi's anemia. Very short telomere length (available commercially) strongly suggests the presence of a telomerase or shelterin mutation, which can be pursued by family studies and nucleotide sequencing. Chromosome studies of bone marrow cells are often revealing in MDS and should be negative in typical aplastic anemia. Flow cytometry offers a sensitive diagnostic test for PNH. Serologic studies may show evidence of viral infection, such as Epstein-Barr virus and HIV. Posthepatitis aplastic anemia is seronegative. The spleen size should be determined by CT scanning or ultrasound if the physical examination of the abdomen is unsatisfactory. MRI may be helpful to assess the fat content of a few vertebrae in order to distinguish aplasia from MDS.

■ DIAGNOSIS

The diagnosis of aplastic anemia is usually straightforward, based on the combination of pancytopenia with a fatty bone marrow.

Aplastic anemia is a disease of the young and should be a leading diagnosis in the pancytopenic adolescent or young adult. When pancytopenia is secondary, the primary diagnosis is usually obvious from either history or physical examination: the massive spleen of alcoholic cirrhosis, the history of metastatic cancer or SLE, or miliary tuberculosis on chest radiograph (Table 107-1).

Diagnostic problems can occur with atypical presentations and among related hematologic diseases. Although pancytopenia is most common, some patients with bone marrow hypocellularity have depression of only one or two of three blood lines, with later progression to pancytopenia. The bone marrow in constitutional aplastic anemia is indistinguishable morphologically from the aspirate in acquired disease. The diagnosis can be suggested by family history, abnormal blood counts since childhood, or the presence of associated physical anomalies. Aplastic anemia may be difficult to distinguish from the hypocellular variety of MDS: MDS is favored by finding morphologic abnormalities, particularly of megakaryocytes and myeloid precursor cells, and typical cytogenetic abnormalities (see below).

■ PROGNOSIS

The natural history of severe aplastic anemia is rapid deterioration and death. Provision first of RBC and later of platelet transfusions and effective antibiotics are of some benefit, but few patients show spontaneous recovery. The major prognostic determinant is the blood count. Historically, severe disease was defined by the presence of two of three parameters: absolute neutrophil count <500/μL, platelet count <20,000/μL, and corrected reticulocyte count <1% (or absolute reticulocyte count <60,000/μL). In the era of effective immunosuppressive therapies, absolute numbers of reticulocytes (>25,000/uL) and lymphocytes (>1000/uL) may be a better predictor of response to treatment and long-term outcome.

TREATMENT   Aplastic Anemia

Severe acquired aplastic anemia can be cured by replacement of the absent hematopoietic cells (and the immune system) by stem cell transplant, or it can be ameliorated by suppression of the immune system to allow recovery of the patient's residual bone marrow function. Hematopoietic growth factors have limited usefulness, and glucocorticoids are of no value. Suspect exposures to drugs or chemicals should be discontinued; however, spontaneous recovery of severe blood count depression is rare, and a waiting period before beginning treatment may not be advisable unless the blood counts are only modestly depressed.

HEMATOPOIETIC STEM CELL TRANSPLANTATION   This is the best therapy for the younger patient with a fully histocompatible sibling donor (Chap. 114). Human leukocyte antigen (HLA) typing should be ordered as soon as the diagnosis of aplastic anemia is established in a child or younger adult. In transplant candidates, transfusion of blood from family members should be avoided so as to prevent sensitization to histocompatibility antigens, but limited numbers of blood products probably do not greatly affect outcome. For allogeneic transplant from fully matched siblings, long-term survival rates for children are approximately 90%. Transplant morbidity and mortality are increased among adults, due mainly to the higher risk of chronic GVHD and serious infections.

Most patients do not have a suitable sibling donor. Occasionally, a full phenotypic match can be found within the family and serve as well. Far more available are other alternative donors, either unrelated but histocompatible volunteers or closely but not perfectly matched family members. High resolution matching at HLA, as well as more effective conditioning regimens and GVHD prophylaxis, have led to improving survival rates in those patients who do proceed to alternative donor transplant, in some series approximating results with conventional sibling donors. Patients will be at risk for late complications, especially a higher rate of cancer, if radiation is used as a component of conditioning.

IMMUNOSUPPRESSION The standard regimen of ATG in combination with cyclosporine induces hematologic recovery (independence from transfusion and a leukocyte count adequate to prevent infection) in 60–70% of patients. Children do especially well, while older adult patients often suffer complications due to the presence of comorbidities. An early robust hematologic response correlates with long-term survival. Improvement in granulocyte number is generally apparent within 2 months of treatment. Most recovered patients continue to have some degree of blood count depression, the MCV remains elevated, and the bone marrow cellularity returns toward normal very slowly if at all. Relapse (recurrent pancytopenia) is frequent, often occurring as cyclosporine is discontinued; most, but not all, patients respond to reinstitution of immunosuppression, but some responders become dependent on continued cyclosporine administration. Development of MDS, with typical marrow morphologic or cytogenetic abnormalities, occurs in approximately 15% of treated patients, usually but not invariably associated with a return of pancytopenia, and some patients develop leukemia. A laboratory diagnosis of PNH can generally be made at the time of presentation of aplastic anemia by flow cytometry; recovered patients may have frank hemolysis if the PNH clone expands. Bone marrow examinations should be performed if there is an unfavorable change in blood counts.

Horse ATG and rabbit antilymphocyte globulin (ALG) are administered as intravenous infusions over 4 or 5 days, respectively. ATG binds to peripheral blood cells; therefore, platelet and granulocyte numbers may decrease further during active treatment. Serum sickness, a flulike illness with a characteristic cutaneous eruption and arthralgia, often develops approximately 10 days after initiating treatment. Methylprednisolone, 1 mg/kg per d for 2 weeks, can ameliorate the immune consequences of heterologous protein infusion. Excessive or extended glucocorticoid therapy is associated with avascular joint necrosis. Cyclosporine is administered orally at an initial high dose, with subsequent adjustment according to blood levels obtained every 2 weeks, rough levels should be between 150 and 200 ng/mL. The most important side effects are nephrotoxicity, hypertension, seizures, and opportunistic infections, especially *Pneumocystis carinii* (prophylactic treatment with monthly inhaled pentamidine is recommended).

Most patients with aplastic anemia lack a suitable marrow donor, and immunosuppression is the treatment of choice. Overall survival is equivalent with transplantation and immunosuppression. However, successful transplant cures marrow failure, whereas patients who recover adequate blood counts after immunosuppression remain at risk of relapse and malignant evolution. Because of excellent results in children and younger adults, allogeneic transplant should be performed if a suitable sibling donor is available. Increasing age and the severity of neutropenia are the most important factors weighing in the decision between transplant and immunosuppression in adults who have a matched family donor: Older patients do better with ATG and cyclosporine, whereas transplant is preferred if granulocytopenia is profound. Some patients may prefer immunosuppression; transplant is used for failure to recover blood counts or occurrence of late complications.

Outcomes following both transplant and immunosuppression have improved with time. High doses of cyclophosphamide, without stem cell rescue, have been reported to produce durable hematologic recovery, without relapse or evolution to MDS, but this treatment can produce sustained severe fatal neutropenia, and response is often delayed.

OTHER THERAPIES The effectiveness of androgens has not been verified in controlled trials, but occasional patients will respond or even demonstrate blood count dependence on continued therapy. Sex hormones upregulate telomerase gene activity in vitro, possibly also their mechanism of action in improving marrow function. For patients with moderate disease or those with severe pancytopenia in whom immunosuppression has failed, a 3–4-month trial is appropriate. Hematopoietic growth factors (HGFs) are not recommended as initial therapy for severe aplastic anemia, and even their roles as adjuncts to immunosuppression are not clear.

SUPPORTIVE CARE Meticulous medical attention is required so that the patient may survive to benefit from definitive therapy or, having failed treatment, to maintain a reasonable existence in the face of pancytopenia. First and most important, infection in the presence of severe neutropenia must be aggressively treated by prompt institution of parenteral, broad-spectrum antibiotics, usually ceftazidime or a combination of an aminoglycoside, cephalosporin, and semisynthetic penicillin. Therapy is empirical and must not await results of culture, although specific foci of infection such as oropharyngeal or anorectal abscesses, pneumonia, sinusitis, and typhlitis (necrotizing colitis) should be sought on physical examination and with radiographic studies. When indwelling plastic catheters become contaminated, vancomycin should be added. Persistent or recrudescent fever implies fungal disease: *Candida* and *Aspergillus* are common, especially after several courses of antibacterial antibiotics. A major reason for the improved prognosis in aplastic anemia has been the development of better antifungal drugs and the timely institution of such therapy when infection is suspected. Granulocyte transfusions using granulocyte colony-stimulating factor (G-CSF)–mobilized peripheral blood may be effective in the treatment of overwhelming or refractory infections. Hand washing, the single best method of preventing the spread of infection, remains a neglected practice. Nonabsorbed antibiotics for gut decontamination are poorly tolerated and not of proven value. Total reverse isolation does not reduce mortality from infections.

Both platelet and erythrocyte numbers can be maintained by transfusion. Alloimmunization historically limited the usefulness of platelet transfusions and is now minimized by several strategies, including use of single donors to reduce exposure and physical or chemical methods to diminish leukocytes in the product; HLA-matched platelets are often effective in patients refractory to random donor products. Inhibitors of fibrinolysis such as aminocaproic acid have not been shown to relieve mucosal oozing; the use of low-dose glucocorticoids to induce "vascular stability" is unproven and not recommended. Whether platelet transfusions are better used prophylactically or only as needed remains unclear. Any rational regimen of prophylaxis requires transfusions once or twice weekly to maintain the platelet count >10,000/µL (oozing from the gut, and presumably also from other vascular beds, increases precipitously at counts <5000/µL). Menstruation should be suppressed either by oral estrogens or nasal follicle-stimulating hormone/luteinizing hormone (FSH/LH) antagonists. Aspirin and other nonsteroidal anti-inflammatory agents inhibit platelet function and must be avoided.

Red blood cells should be transfused to maintain a normal level of activity, usually at a hemoglobin value of 70 g/L (90 g/L if there is underlying cardiac or pulmonary disease); a regimen of 2 units every 2 weeks will replace normal losses in a patient without a functioning bone marrow. In chronic anemia, the iron chelators, deferoxamine and deferasirox, should be added at approximately the fiftieth transfusion to avoid secondary hemochromatosis.

PURE RED CELL APLASIA

Other, more restricted forms of marrow failure occur, in which only a single circulating cell type is affected and the marrow shows corresponding absence or decreased numbers of specific precursor cells: aregenerative anemia as in PRCA (see below), thrombocytopenia with amegakaryocytosis (Chap. 115), and neutropenia without marrow myeloid cells in agranulocytosis (Chap. 60). In general, and in contrast to aplastic anemia and MDS, the unaffected lineages appear quantitatively and qualitatively normal. Agranulocytosis, the most frequent of these syndromes, is usually a complication of medical drug use (with agents similar to those related to aplastic anemia), either by a mechanism of direct chemical toxicity or by immune destruction. Agranulocytosis has an incidence similar to aplastic anemia but is especially frequent among older adults and in women. The syndrome should resolve with discontinuation of exposure, but significant mortality is attached to neutropenia in the older and often previously unwell patient. Both pure white cell aplasia (agranulocytosis without incriminating drug exposure) and amegakaryocytic thrombocytopenia are exceedingly rare and, like PRCA, appear to be due to destructive antibodies or lymphocytes and can respond to immunosuppressive therapies. In all the single lineage failure syndromes, progression to pancytopenia or leukemia is unusual.

DEFINITION AND DIFFERENTIAL DIAGNOSIS

PRCA is characterized by anemia, reticulocytopenia, and absent or rare erythroid precursor cells in the bone marrow. The classification of PRCA is shown in Table 107-4. In adults, PRCA is acquired. An identical syndrome can occur constitutionally: Diamond-Blackfan anemia, or congenital PRCA, is diagnosed at birth or in early childhood and often responds to glucocorticoid treatment; mutations in ribosomal RNA processing genes are etiologic. Temporary red cell failure occurs in transient aplastic crisis of hemolytic anemias due to acute parvovirus infection (Chap. 184) and in transient erythroblastopenia of childhood, which affects normal children.

CLINICAL ASSOCIATIONS AND ETIOLOGY

PRCA has important associations with immune system diseases. A small minority of cases occur with a thymoma. More frequently, red cell aplasia can be the major manifestation of large granular lymphocytosis or may occur in chronic lymphocytic leukemia. Some patients may be hypogammaglobulinemic. Infrequently (compared to agranulocytosis), PRCA can be due to an idiosyncratic drug reaction. Subcutaneous administration of erythropoietin (EPO) has provoked PRCA mediated by neutralizing antibodies.

Like aplastic anemia, PRCA results from diverse mechanisms. Antibodies to RBC precursors are frequently present in the blood, but T cell inhibition is probably the more common immune mechanism. Cytotoxic lymphocyte activity restricted by histocompatibility locus or specific for human T cell leukemia/lymphoma

TABLE 107-4 Classification of Pure Red Cell Aplasia

Self-limited
  Transient erythroblastopenia of childhood
  Transient aplastic crisis of hemolysis (acute B19 parvovirus infection)
Fetal red blood cell aplasia
  Nonimmune hydrops fetalis (in utero B19 parvovirus infection)
Hereditary pure red cell aplasia
  Congenital pure red cell aplasia (Diamond-Blackfan syndrome)
Acquired pure red cell aplasia
  Thymoma and malignancy
    Thymoma
    Lymphoid malignancies (and more rarely other hematologic diseases)
    Paraneoplastic to solid tumors
  Connective tissue disorders with immunologic abnormalities
    Systemic lupus erythematosus, juvenile rheumatoid arthritis, rheumatoid arthritis
    Multiple endocrine gland insufficiency
  Virus
    Persistent B19 parvovirus, hepatitis, adult T cell leukemia virus, Epstein-Barr virus
  Pregnancy
  Drugs
    Especially phenytoin, azathioprine, chloramphenicol, procainamide, isoniazid
    Erythropoietin
Idiopathic

virus I–infected cells, as well as natural killer cell activity inhibitory of erythropoiesis, have been demonstrated in particularly well-studied individual cases.

PERSISTENT PARVOVIRUS B19 INFECTION

Chronic parvovirus infection is an important, treatable cause of PRCA. This common virus causes a benign exanthem of childhood (fifth disease) and a polyarthralgia/arthritis syndrome in adults. In patients with underlying hemolysis (or any condition that increases demand for RBC production), parvovirus infection can cause a transient aplastic crisis and an abrupt but temporary worsening of the anemia due to failed erythropoiesis. In normal individuals, acute infection is resolved by production of neutralizing antibodies to the virus, but in the setting of congenital, acquired, or iatrogenic immunodeficiency, persistent viral infection may occur. The bone marrow shows red cell aplasia and the presence of giant pronormoblasts (Fig. 107-2), which is the cytopathic sign of B19 parvovirus infection. Viral tropism for human erythroid progenitor cells is due to its use of erythrocyte P antigen as a cellular receptor for entry. Direct cytotoxicity of virus causes anemia if demands on erythrocyte production are high; in normal individuals, the temporary cessation of red cell production is not clinically apparent, and skin and joint symptoms are mediated by immune complex deposition.

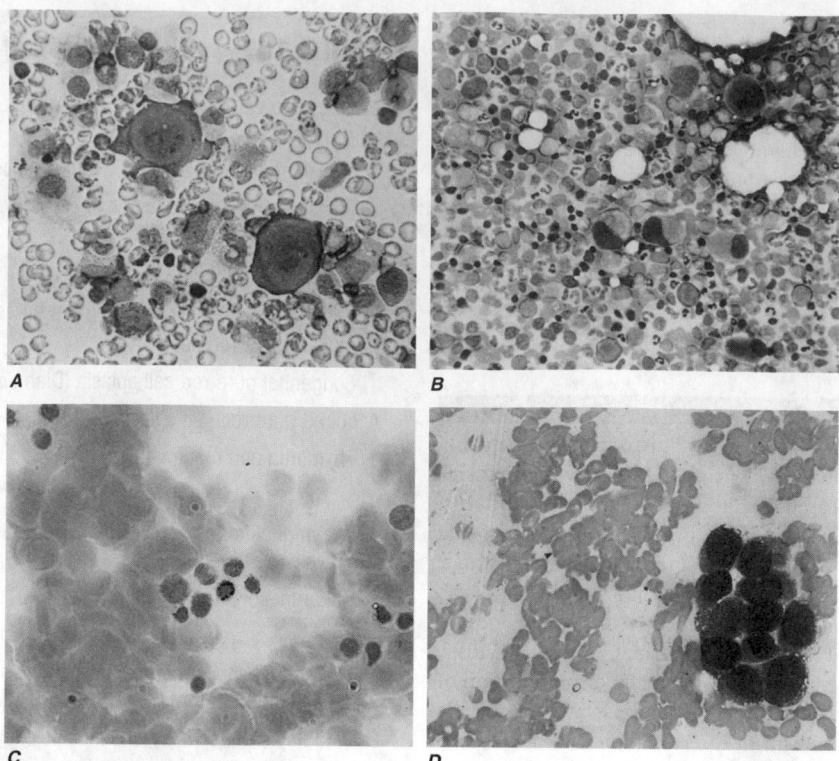

Figure 107-2 Pathognomonic cells in marrow failure syndromes.
A. Giant pronormoblast, the cytopathic effect of B19 parvovirus infection of the erythroid progenitor cell. **B.** Uninuclear megakaryocyte and microblastic erythroid precursors typical of the 5q–myelodysplasia syndrome. **C.** Ringed sideroblast showing perinuclear iron granules. **D.** Tumor cells present on a touch preparation made from the marrow biopsy of a patient with metastatic carcinoma.

TREATMENT **Pure Red Cell Aplasia**

History, physical examination, and routine laboratory studies may disclose an underlying disease or a drug exposure. Thymoma should be sought by radiographic procedures. Tumor excision is indicated, but anemia does not necessarily improve with surgery. The diagnosis of parvovirus infection requires detection of viral DNA sequences in the blood (IgG and IgM antibodies are commonly absent). The presence of erythroid colonies has been considered predictive of response to immunosuppressive therapy in idiopathic PRCA.

Red cell aplasia is compatible with long-term survival with supportive care alone: a combination of erythrocyte transfusions and iron chelation. For persistent B19 parvovirus infection, almost all patients respond to intravenous immunoglobulin therapy (e.g., 0.4 g/kg daily for 5 days), although relapse and retreatment may be expected, especially in patients with AIDS. The majority of patients with idiopathic PRCA respond favorably to immunosuppression. Most first receive a course of glucocorticoids. Also effective are cyclosporine, ATG, azathioprine, cyclophosphamide, and the monoclonal antibody daclizumab, an antibody to the high affinity IL-2 receptor. PRCA developing on EPO therapy should be treated with immunosuppression and withdrawal of EPO.

MYELODYSPLASIA

■ DEFINITION

Myelodysplasia or the MDSs are a heterogeneous group of hematologic disorders broadly characterized by cytopenias associated with a dysmorphic (or abnormal appearing) and usually cellular bone marrow, and by consequent ineffective blood cell production. A clinically useful nosology of these entities was first developed by the French-American-British Cooperative Group in 1983. Five entities were defined: refractory anemia (RA), refractory anemia with ringed sideroblasts (RARS), refractory anemia with excess blasts (RAEB), refractory anemia with excess blasts in transformation (RAEB-t), and chronic myelomonocytic leukemia (CMML). The World Health Organization (WHO) classification (2002) recognized that the distinction between RAEB-t and acute myeloid leukemia is arbitrary and groups them together as acute leukemia, that CMML behaves as a myeloproliferative disease, and separated refractory anemias with dysmorphic change restricted to erythroid lineage from those with multilineage changes. In a revision, specific categories for unilineage dysplasias were added (Table 107-5).

The diagnosis of MDS may be a challenge, as sometimes subtle clinical and pathologic features must be distinguished in a usually older adult patient >70 years of age with comorbidities; furthermore, precise diagnostic categorization requires a hematopathologist knowledgeable in the latest classification scheme. Nonetheless, it is important that the internist and primary care physician be sufficiently familiar with MDS to expedite referral to a hematologist, both because many new therapies are now available to improve hematopoietic function and the judicious use of supportive care can improve the patient's quality of life.

■ EPIDEMIOLOGY

Idiopathic MDS is a disease of the older adult; the mean age at onset is older than 70 years. There is a slight male preponderance. MDS is a relatively common form of bone marrow failure, with reported incidence rates of 35 to >100 per million persons in the general population and 120 to >500 per million in the older adult. MDS is rare in children, but monocytic leukemia can be seen. Secondary or therapy-related MDS is not age related. Rates of MDS have increased over time, due to the recognition of the syndrome by physicians and the aging of the population.

TABLE 107-5 World Health Organization (WHO) Classification of Myelodysplastic Syndromes/Neoplasms

Name	WHO Estimated Proportion of Patients with MDS	Peripheral Blood: Key Features	Bone Marrow: Key Features
Refractory cytopenias with unilineage dysplasia (RCUD):			
Refractory anemia (RA)	10-20%	Anemia <1% of blasts	Unilineage erythroid dysplasia (in ≥10% of cells) <5% blasts
Refractory neutropenia (RN)	<1%	Neutropenia <1% blasts	Unilineage granulocytic dysplasia <5% blasts
Refractory thrombocytopenia (RT)	<1%	Thrombocytopenia <1% blasts	Unilineage megakaryocytic dysplasia <5% blasts
Refractory anemia with ring sideroblasts (RARS)	3-11%	Anemia No blasts	Unilineage erythroid dysplasia ≥15% of erythroid precursors are ring sideroblasts <5% blasts
Refractory cytopenias with multilineage dysplasia (RCMD)	30%	Cytopenia(s) <1% blasts No Auer rods	Multilineage dysplasia ± ring sideroblasts <5% blasts No Auer rods
Refractory anemia with excess blasts, Type 1 (RAEB-1)	40%	Cytopenia(s) <5% blasts No Auer rods	Unilineage or multilineage dysplasia
Refractory anemia with excess blasts, type 2 (RAEB-2)		Cytopenia(s) 5-19% blasts ± Auer rods	Unilineage or multilineage dysplasia 10-19% blasts ± Auer rods
MDS associated with isolated Del(5q) (Del(5q)	Uncommon	Anemia Normal or high platelet count <1% blasts	Isolated 5q31 chromosome deletion Anemia; hypolobated megakaryocytes <5% blasts
Childhood MDS, including refractory cytopenia of childhood (*provisional*) (RCC)	<1 %	Pancytopenia	<5% marrow blasts for RCC Marrow usually hypocellular
MDS, unclassifiable (MDS-U)	?	Cytopenia ≤1% blasts	Does not fit other categories Dysplasia <5% blasts If no dysplasia, MDS-associated karyotype

Note: If peripheral blood blasts are 2–4%, the diagnosis is RAEB-1 even if marrow blasts are less than 5%. If Auer rods are present, the WHO considers the diagnosis RAEB-2 if the blast proportion is less than 20% (even if less than 10%), AML if at least 20% blasts. For all subtypes, peripheral blood monocytes are less than 1 × 10⁹/L. Bicytopenia may be observed in RCUD subtypes, but pancytopenia with unilineage marrow dysplasia should be classified as MDS-U. Therapy-related MDS (t-MDS), whether due to alkylating agents, topoisomerase II (t-MDS/t-AML) in the WHO classification of AML and precursor lesions. The listing in this table excludes MDS/myeloproliferative neoplasm overlap categories, such as chronic myelomonocytic leukemia, juvenile myelomonocytic leukemia, and the provisional entity RARS with thrombocytosis.

Abbreviation: MDS, myelodysplastic syndrome.

ETIOLOGY AND PATHOPHYSIOLOGY

MDS is associated with environmental exposures such as radiation and benzene; other risk factors have been reported inconsistently. Secondary MDS occurs as a late toxicity of cancer treatment, usually with a combination of radiation and the radiomimetic alkylating agents such as busulfan, nitrosourea, or procarbazine (with a latent period of 5–7 years) or the DNA topoisomerase inhibitors (2 years). Both acquired aplastic anemia following immunosuppressive treatment and Fanconi's anemia can evolve into MDS.

MDS is a clonal hematopoietic stem cell disorder leading to impaired cell proliferation and differentiation. Cytogenetic abnormalities are found in approximately one-half of patients, and some of the same specific lesions are also seen in frank leukemia; aneuploidy is more frequent than translocations. Both presenting and evolving hematologic manifestations result from the accumulation of multiple genetic lesions: loss of tumor suppressor genes, activating oncogene mutations, or other harmful alterations. Cytogenetic abnormalities are not random (loss of all or part of 5, 7, and 20, trisomy of 8) and may be related to etiology (11q23 following topoisomerase II inhibitors); CMML is often associated with t(5;12) that creates a chimeric *tel-PDGFβ* gene. The type and number of

cytogenetic abnormalities strongly correlate with the probability of leukemic transformation and survival. Mutations of N-*ras* (an oncogene), *p53* and *IRF-1* (tumor suppressor genes), *Bcl-2* (an antiapoptotic gene), and others have been reported in some patients but likely occur late in the sequence leading to leukemic transformation. Apoptosis of marrow cells is increased in early stage and low-risk categories of MDS, presumably due to these acquired genetic alterations or possibly to an overlaid immune response. An immune pathophysiology has been suggested for trisomy 8 MDS, which often responds clinically to immunosuppressive therapy. Such patients have T cell activity directed to the cytogenetically aberrant clone. Sideroblastic anemia may be related to mutations in mitochondrial genes; ineffective erythropoiesis and disordered iron metabolism are the functional consequences of the genetic alterations.

CLINICAL FEATURES

Anemia dominates the early course. Most symptomatic patients complain of the gradual onset of fatigue and weakness, dyspnea, and pallor, but at least one-half the patients are asymptomatic, and their MDS is discovered only incidentally on routine blood counts. Previous chemotherapy or radiation exposure is an important historic fact. Fever and weight loss should point to a myeloproliferative rather than myelodysplastic process. Children with Down syndrome are susceptible to MDS, and a family history may indicate a hereditary form of sideroblastic anemia or Fanconi's anemia.

The physical examination is remarkable for signs of anemia; approximately 20% of patients have splenomegaly. Some unusual skin lesions, including Sweet's syndrome (febrile neutrophilic dermatosis), occur with MDS. Autoimmune syndromes are not infrequent.

■ LABORATORY STUDIES

Blood

Anemia is present in the majority of cases, either alone or as part of bi- or pancytopenia; isolated neutropenia or thrombocytopenia is more unusual. Macrocytosis is common, and the smear may be dimorphic with a distinctive population of large red blood cells. Platelets are also large and lack granules. In functional studies, they may show marked abnormalities, and patients may have bleeding symptoms despite seemingly adequate numbers. Neutrophils are hypogranulated; have hyposegmented, ringed, or abnormally segmented nuclei; contain Döhle bodies; and may be functionally deficient. Circulating myeloblasts usually correlate with marrow blast numbers, and their quantitation is important for classification and prognosis. The total white blood cell count (WBC) is usually normal or low, except in chronic myelomonocytic leukemia. As in aplastic anemia, MDS can be associated with a clonal population of PNH cells.

Bone marrow

The bone marrow is usually normal or hypercellular, but in 20% of cases it is sufficiently hypocellular to be confused with aplasia. No single characteristic feature of marrow morphology distinguishes MDS, but the following are commonly observed: dyserythropoietic changes (especially nuclear abnormalities) and ringed sideroblasts in the erythroid lineage; hypogranulation and hyposegmentation in granulocytic precursors, with an increase in myeloblasts; and megakaryocytes showing reduced numbers or disorganized nuclei. Megaloblastic nuclei associated with defective hemoglobinization in the erythroid lineage are common. Prognosis strongly correlates with the proportion of marrow blasts. Cytogenetic analysis and fluorescent in situ hybridization can identify chromosomal abnormalities.

■ DIFFERENTIAL DIAGNOSIS

Deficiencies of vitamin B_{12} or folate should be excluded by appropriate blood tests; vitamin B_6 deficiency can be assessed by a therapeutic trial of pyridoxine if the bone marrow shows ringed sideroblasts. Marrow dysplasia can be observed in acute viral infections, drug reactions, or chemical toxicity but should be transient. More difficult are the distinctions between hypocellular MDS and aplasia or between refractory anemia with excess blasts and early acute leukemia. The WHO considers the presence of 20% blasts in the marrow as the criterion that separates acute myeloid leukemia (AML) from MDS.

■ PROGNOSIS

The median survival varies greatly from years for patients with 5q– or sideroblastic anemia to a few months in refractory anemia with excess blasts or severe pancytopenia associated with monosomy 7; an International Prognostic Scoring System (IPSS; Table 107-6) assists in making predictions. Most patients die as a result of complications of pancytopenia and not due to leukemic transformation; perhaps one-third will succumb to other diseases unrelated to their MDS. Precipitous worsening of pancytopenia, acquisition of new chromosomal abnormalities on serial cytogenetic determination, increase in the number of blasts, and marrow fibrosis are all poor prognostic indicators. The outlook in therapy-related MDS, regardless of type, is extremely poor, and most patients will progress within a few months to refractory AML.

TREATMENT Myelodysplasia

Historically, the therapy of MDS has been unsatisfactory. Only stem cell transplantation offers cure. Survival rates of 50% at 3 years have been reported, but older patients are particularly prone to develop treatment-related mortality and morbidity. Results of transplant using matched unrelated donors are comparable, although most series contain younger and more highly selected cases. However, multiple new drugs have been approved for use in MDS. Several regimens appear to not only improve blood counts but to delay onset of leukemia and to improve survival. The choice of therapy and implementation of treatment are complicated and require hematologic expertise.

MDS has been regarded as particularly refractory to cytotoxic chemotherapy regimens but is probably no more resistant to

TABLE 107-6 International Prognostic Scoring System (IPSS)

Prognostic Variable	Score Value				
	0	0.5	1	1.5	2
Bone marrow blasts (%)	<5%	5–10%		11–20%	21–30%
Karyotype[a]	Good	Intermediate	Poor		
Cytopenia[b] (lineages affected)	0 or 1	2 or 3			
Risk Group Scores	**Score**				
Low	0				
Intermediate-1	0.5–1				
Intermediate-2	1.5–2				
High	≥2.5				

[a]Good, normal, -Y, del(5q), del (20q); poor, complex (≥3 abnormalities) or chromosome 7 abnormalities; intermediate, all other abnormalities.
[b]Cytopenias defined as Hb <100 g/L, platelet count <100,000/μL, absolute neutrophil count <1500/μL.

effective treatment than AML in the older adult, in whom drug toxicity is often fatal and remissions, if achieved, are brief.

Low doses of cytotoxic drugs have been administered for their "differentiating" potential, and from this experience has emerged drug therapies based on pyrimidine analogues. Azacitidine is directly cytotoxic but also inhibits DNA methylation, thereby altering gene expression; however, demethylation status has not correlated well with clinical effects Azacitidine improves blood counts and also survival in a minority of MDS patients, compared to best supportive care. Azacitidine has been administered subcutaneously, daily for 7 days, at 4-week intervals, for at least four cycles before assessing for response. Decitabine is closely related to azacitidine and more potent. Similar to azacitidine, approximately 20% of patients show responses in blood counts, with a duration of response of almost a year. Activity may be higher in more advanced MDS subtypes. Decitabine is administered by continuous intravenous infusion, every 8 hours for 3 days, in repeating cycles. The optimal dose regimens for both azacitidine and decitabine are still being determined in clinical research protocols. The major toxicity of both azacitidine and decitabine is myelosuppression, leading to worsened blood counts. Other symptoms associated with cancer chemotherapy frequently occur.

Lenalidomide, a thalidomide derivative with a more favorable toxicity profile, is particularly effective in reversing anemia in MDS patients with 5q–syndrome; not only do a high proportion of these patients become transfusion independent with normal or near-normal hemoglobin levels, but their cytogenetics also become normal. The drug has many biologic activities, and it is unclear which is critical for clinical efficacy. Lenalidomide is administered orally. Most patients will improve within 3 months of initiating therapy. Toxicities include myelosuppression (worsening thrombocytopenia and neutropenia, necessitating blood count monitoring) and an increased risk of deep vein thrombosis and pulmonary embolism.

ATG and cyclosporine, as employed in aplastic anemia, also may produce sustained independence from transfusion and improve survival. Immunosuppression with ATG or, in more recent studies, the anti-CD52 monoclonal antibody Campath is especially effective in younger MDS patients (younger than age 60 years) with more favorable IPSS scores and who bear the histocompatability antigen HLA-DR15.

HGFs can improve blood counts but, as in most other marrow failure states, have been most beneficial to patients with the least severe pancytopenia. G-CSF treatment alone failed to improve survival in a controlled trial. EPO alone or in combination with G-CSF can improve hemoglobin levels, but mainly in those with low serum EPO levels who have no or only a modest need for transfusions, and retrospective analysis suggests improved survival with treatment

The same principles of supportive care described for aplastic anemia apply to MDS. Despite improvements in drug therapy, many patients will be anemic for years. RBC transfusion support should be accompanied by iron chelation to prevent secondary hemochromatosis.

MYELOPHTHISIC ANEMIAS

Fibrosis of the bone marrow (see Fig. 103-2), usually accompanied by a characteristic blood smear picture called *leukoerythroblastosis*, can occur as a primary hematologic disease, called *myelofibrosis* or *myeloid metaplasia* (Chap. 108), and as a secondary process, called *myelophthisis*. Myelophthisis, or secondary myelofibrosis, is reactive. Fibrosis can be a response to invading tumor cells, usually an epithelial cancer of breast, lung, a prostate origin or neuroblastoma. Marrow fibrosis may occur with infection of mycobacteria (both *Mycobacterium tuberculosis*

and *M. avium*), fungi, or HIV, and in sarcoidosis. Intracellular lipid deposition in Gaucher's disease and obliteration of the marrow space related to absence of osteoclast remodeling in congenital osteopetrosis also can produce fibrosis. Secondary myelofibrosis is a late consequence of radiation therapy or treatment with radiomimetic drugs. Usually the infectious or malignant underlying processes are obvious. Marrow fibrosis can also be a feature of a variety of hematologic syndromes, especially chronic myeloid leukemia, multiple myeloma, lymphomas, myeloma, and hairy cell leukemia.

The pathophysiology has three distinct features: proliferation of fibroblasts in the marrow space (myelofibrosis); the extension of hematopoiesis into the long bones and into extramedullary sites, usually the spleen, liver, and lymph nodes (myeloid metaplasia); and ineffective erythropoiesis. The etiology of the fibrosis is unknown but most likely involves dysregulated production of growth factors: Platelet-derived growth factor and transforming growth factor β have been implicated. Abnormal regulation of other hematopoietins would lead to localization of blood-producing cells in nonhematopoietic tissues and uncoupling of the usually balanced processes of stem cell proliferation and differentiation. Myelofibrosis is remarkable for pancytopenia despite very large numbers of circulating hematopoietic progenitor cells.

Anemia is dominant in secondary myelofibrosis, usually normocytic and normochromic. The diagnosis is suggested by the characteristic leukoerythroblastic smear (see Fig. 108-1). Erythrocyte morphology is highly abnormal, with circulating nucleated RBCs, teardrops, and shape distortions. WBC numbers are often elevated, sometimes mimicking a leukemoid reaction, with circulating myelocytes, promyelocytes, and myeloblasts. Platelets may be abundant and are often of giant size. Inability to aspirate the bone marrow, the characteristic "dry tap," can allow a presumptive diagnosis in the appropriate setting before the biopsy is decalcified.

The course of secondary myelofibrosis is determined by its etiology, usually a metastatic tumor or an advanced hematologic malignancy. Treatable causes must be excluded, especially tuberculosis and fungus. Transfusion support can relieve symptoms.

FURTHER READINGS

ADES L ET AL: Efficacy and safety of lenalidomide in intermediate-2 or high-risk myelodysplastic syndromes with 5q deletion: Results of a phase 2 study. Blood 113:3947, 2009

BAGBY GC, ALTER BP: Fanconi anemia. Semin Hematol 43:147, 2006

CALADO RT, YOUNG NS: Telomere diseases. N Engl J Med 361:2353, 2009

ESTEY E et al: Acute myeloid leukemia and myelodysplastic syndromes in older patients. J Clin Oncol 25:1908, 2007

FENAUX P et al: Efficacy of azacitidine compared with that of standard care regimens in the treatment of higher-risk myelodysplastic syndromes: A randomized, open-label, phase III trial. Lancet Oncol 10:223, 2009

FLYGARE J, KARLSSON S: Diamond-Blackfan anemia: Erythropoiesis lost in translation. Blood 109:3152, 2007

JADERSTEN M et al: Erythropoietin and granulocyte-colony stimulating factor treatment associated with improved survival in myelodysplastic syndromes. J Clin Oncol 26:3607, 2008

MA X et al: Myelodysplastic syndromes: Incidence and survival in the United States. Cancer 109:1536, 2007

YOUNG NS, BROWN KE: Parvovirus B19. N Engl J Med 350:586, 2004

—— et al: Current concepts in the pathophysiology and treatment of aplastic anemia. Blood 108:2509, 2006

CHAPTER 108

Polycythemia Vera and Other Myeloproliferative Diseases

Jerry L. Spivak

The World Health Organization (WHO) classification of the chronic myeloproliferative diseases (MPDs) includes eight disorders, some of which are rare or poorly characterized (Table 108-1) but all of which share an origin in a multipotent hematopoietic progenitor cell; overproduction of one or more of the formed elements of the blood without significant dysplasia; a predilection to extramedullary hematopoiesis, myelofibrosis; and transformation at varying rates to acute leukemia. Within this broad classification, however, significant phenotypic heterogeneity exists. Some diseases such as chronic myelogenous leukemia (CML), chronic neutrophilic leukemia (CNL), and chronic eosinophilic leukemia (CEL) express primarily a myeloid phenotype, while in others such as polycythemia vera (PV), primary myelofibrosis (PMF), and essential thrombocytosis (ET), erythroid or megakaryocytic hyperplasia predominates. The latter three disorders, in contrast to the former three, also appear capable of transforming into each other.

Such phenotypic heterogeneity has a genetic basis; CML is the consequence of the balanced translocation between chromosomes 9 and 22 [t(9;22)(q34;11)]; CNL has been associated with a t(15;19) translocation; and CEL occurs with a deletion or balanced translocations involving the *PDGFRα* gene. By contrast, to a greater or lesser extent, PV, PMF, and ET are characterized by expression of a *JAK2* mutation, V617F that causes constitutive activation of this tyrosine kinase that is essential for the function of the erythropoietin and thrombopoietin receptors but not the granulocyte colony-stimulating factor receptor. This essential distinction is also reflected in the natural history of CML, CNL, and CEL, which is usually measured in years, and their high rate of transformation into acute leukemia. By contrast, the natural history of PV, PMF, and ET is usually measured in decades, and transformation to acute leukemia is uncommon in the absence of exposure to mutagenic agents. This chapter, therefore, will focus only on PV, PMF, and ET,

because their clinical overlap is substantial but their clinical courses are distinctly different.

Other chronic myeloproliferative disorders will be discussed in Chap. 109.

POLYCYTHEMIA VERA

PV is a clonal disorder involving a multipotent hematopoietic progenitor cell in which phenotypically normal red cells, granulocytes, and platelets accumulate in the absence of a recognizable physiologic stimulus. The most common of the chronic myeloproliferative disorders, PV occurs in 2 per 100,000 persons, sparing no adult age group and increasing with age to rates as high as 18/100,000. Familial transmission occurs but is infrequent and women predominate among sporadic cases.

■ ETIOLOGY

The etiology of PV is unknown. Although nonrandom chromosome abnormalities such as 20q and trisomy 8 and 9 have been documented in up to 30% of untreated PV patients, unlike CML, no consistent cytogenetic abnormality has been associated with the disorder. However, a mutation in the autoinhibitory, pseudokinase domain of the tyrosine kinase JAK2—that replaces valine with phenylalanine (V617F), causing constitutive activation of the kinase—appears to have a central role in the pathogenesis of PV.

JAK2 is a member of an evolutionarily well-conserved, nonreceptor tyrosine kinase family and serves as the cognate tyrosine kinase for the erythropoietin and thrombopoietin receptors. It also functions as an obligate chaperone for these receptors in the Golgi apparatus and is responsible for their cell-surface expression. The conformational change induced in the erythropoietin and thrombopoietin receptors following binding to erythropoietin or thrombopoietin leads to JAK2 autophosphorylation, receptor phosphorylation, and phosphorylation of proteins involved in cell proliferation, differentiation, and resistance to apoptosis. Transgenic animals lacking *JAK2* die as embryos from severe anemia. Constitutive activation of JAK2 can explain the erythropoietin-independent erythroid colony formation, and the hypersensitivity of PV erythroid progenitor cells to erythropoietin and other hematopoietic growth factors, their resistance to apoptosis in vitro in the absence of erythropoietin, their rapid terminal differentiation, and their increase in Bcl-X_L expression, all of which are characteristic in PV.

Importantly, the *JAK2* gene is located on the short arm of chromosome 9, and loss of heterozygosity on chromosome 9p, due to mitotic recombination is the most common cytogenetic abnormality in PV. The segment of 9p involved contains the *JAK2* locus; loss of heterozygosity in this region leads to homozygosity for the mutant *JAK2* V617F. More than 90% of PV patients express this mutation, as do approximately 50% of PMF and ET patients. Homozygosity for the mutation occurs in approximately 30% of PV patients and 60% of PMF patients; homozygosity is rare in ET. Over time, a portion of PV *JAK2* V617F heterozygotes become homozygotes due to mitotic recombination, but usually not after 10 years of the disease. PV patients who do not express *JAK2* V617F are not clinically different from those who do, nor do *JAK2* V617F heterozygotes differ clinically from homozygotes. Interestingly, predisposition to acquire mutations in *JAK2* appears to be associated with a specific *JAK2* haplotype, GGCC. *JAK2* V617F is the basis for many of the phenotypic and biochemical characteristics of PV such as elevation of the leukocyte alkaline phosphatase (LAP) score; however, it cannot solely account for the entire PV phenotype and is probably not the initiating lesion in the three MPDs. First, some PV patients with the same phenotype and documented clonal disease lack this mutation. Second, ET and PMF patients have the

TABLE 108-1 WHO classification of Chronic Myeloproliferative Disorders

Chronic myelogenous leukemia, bcr-abl–positive

Chronic neutrophilic leukemia

Chronic eosinophilic leukemia, not otherwise specified

Polycythemia vera

Primary myelofibrosis

Essential thrombocytosis

Mastocytosis

Myeloproliferative neoplasms, unclassifiable

same mutation but different clinical phenotypes. Third, familial PV can occur without the mutation, even when other members of the same family express it. Fourth, not all the cells of the malignant clone express *JAK2* V617F. Fifth, *JAK2* V617F has been observed in patients with long-standing idiopathic erythrocytosis. Sixth, in some patients, *JAK2* V617F appears to be acquired after another mutation. Finally, in some *JAK2* V617F-positive PV or ET patients, acute leukemia can occur in a *JAK2* V617F-negative progenitor cell. However, while *JAK2* V617F alone may not be sufficient to cause PV, it is essential for the transformation of ET to PV, though not for its transformation to PMF.

■ CLINICAL FEATURES

Although splenomegaly may be the initial presenting sign in PV, most often the disorder is first recognized by the incidental discovery of a high hemoglobin or hematocrit. With the exception of aquagenic pruritus, no symptoms distinguish PV from other causes of erythrocytosis.

Uncontrolled erythrocytosis causes hyperviscosity, leading to neurologic symptoms such as vertigo, tinnitus, headache, visual disturbances, and transient ischemic attacks (TIAs). Systolic hypertension is also a feature of the red cell mass elevation. In some patients, venous or arterial thrombosis may be the presenting manifestation of PV. Any vessel can be affected; but cerebral, cardiac, or mesenteric vessels are most commonly involved. Intraabdominal venous thrombosis is particularly common in young women and may be catastrophic if a sudden and complete obstruction of the hepatic vein occurs. Indeed, PV should be suspected in any patient who develops hepatic vein thrombosis. Digital ischemia, easy bruising, epistaxis, acid-peptic disease, or gastrointestinal hemorrhage may occur due to vascular stasis or thrombocytosis. Erythema, burning, and pain in the extremities, a symptom complex known as erythromelalgia, is another complication of the thrombocytosis of PV due to increased platelet stickiness. Given the large turnover of hematopoietic cells, hyperuricemia with secondary gout, uric acid stones, and symptoms due to hypermetabolism can also complicate the disorder.

■ DIAGNOSIS

When PV presents with erythrocytosis in combination with leukocytosis, thrombocytosis, or both, the diagnosis is apparent. However, when patients present with an elevated hemoglobin or hematocrit alone, or with thrombocytosis alone, the diagnostic evaluation is more complex because of the many diagnostic possibilities (Table 108-2). Furthermore, unless the hemoglobin level is ≥20 g/DL (hematocrit ≥60%), it is not possible to distinguish true erythrocytosis from disorders causing plasma volume contraction. Uniquely in PV, in contrast to other causes for true erythrocytosis, an expanded plasma volume can mask the elevated red cell mass; thus, red cell mass and plasma volume determinations are mandatory to establish the presence of an absolute erythrocytosis and to distinguish this from relative erythrocytosis due to a reduction in plasma volume alone (also known as *stress* or *spurious erythrocytosis* or *Gaisböck's syndrome*). This is true even with the finding of *JAK2* V617F mutation, because not every patient with PV expresses this mutation, while patients without PV do. Figure 57-18 illustrates a diagnostic algorithm for the evaluation of suspected erythrocytosis.

Once absolute erythrocytosis has been established, its cause must be determined. An elevated plasma erythropoietin level suggests either a hypoxic cause for erythrocytosis or autonomous erythropoietin production, in which case assessment of pulmonary function and an abdominal CT scan to evaluate renal and hepatic anatomy are appropriate. A normal erythropoietin level, however,

TABLE 108-2 Causes of Erythrocytosis

Relative Erythrocytosis

Hemoconcentration secondary to dehydration, diuretics, ethanol abuse, androgens or tobacco abuse

Absolute Erythrocytosis

Hypoxia	**Tumors**
Carbon monoxide intoxication	Hypernephroma
High oxygen-affinity hemoglobin	Hepatoma
	Cerebellar hemangioblastoma
High altitude	Uterine myoma
Pulmonary disease	Adrenal tumors
Right to left cardiac or vascular shunts	Meningioma
	Pheochromocytoma
Sleep apnea syndrome	**Drugs**
Hepatopulmonary syndrome	Androgens
Renal Disease	Recombinant erythropoietin
Renal artery stenosis	**Familial (with normal hemoglobin function)**
Focal sclerosing or membranous glomerulonephritis	Erythropoietin receptor mutation
Postrenal transplantation	VHL mutations (Chuvash polycythemia)
Renal cysts	2,3-BPG mutation
Bartter's syndrome	**Polycythemia vera**

Abbreviations: 2,3-BPG, 2,3-bisphosphoglycerate; VHL, von Hippel-Lindau.

does not exclude a secondary cause for erythrocytosis or PV. In PV, in contrast to hypoxic erythrocytosis, the arterial oxygen saturation is normal. However, a normal oxygen saturation does not exclude a high-affinity hemoglobin as a cause for erythrocytosis; documentation of previous hemoglobin levels and a family study are important in this regard.

Other laboratory studies that may aid in diagnosis include the red cell count, mean corpuscular volume, and red cell distribution width (RDW). Only three situations cause microcytic erythrocytosis: β-thalassemia trait, hypoxic erythrocytosis, and PV. With β-thalassemia trait the RDW is normal, whereas with hypoxic erythrocytosis and PV, the RDW is usually elevated due to iron deficiency. Today, an assay for *JAK2* V617F has superseded other tests for establishing the diagnosis of PV. Of course, in patients with associated acid-peptic disease, occult gastrointestinal bleeding may lead to presentation with hypochromic, microcytic anemia, masking the presence of PV.

A bone marrow aspirate and biopsy provide no specific diagnostic information since these may be normal or indistinguishable from ET or PMF, and unless there is a need to exclude some other disorder, these procedures need not be done. Although the presence of a cytogenetic abnormality such as trisomy 8 or 9 or 20q− in the setting of an expanded red cell mass supports a clonal etiology, no specific cytogenetic abnormality is associated with PV, and the absence of a cytogenetic marker does not exclude the diagnosis.

■ COMPLICATIONS

Many of the clinical complications of PV relate directly to the increase in blood viscosity associated with red cell mass elevation and indirectly to the increased turnover of red cells, leukocytes, and platelets with the attendant increase in uric acid and cytokine production. The latter appears to be responsible for constitutional symptoms, while peptic ulcer disease may be due to *Helicobacter pylori* and the pruritus associated with this disorder may be a consequence of basophil activation by *JAK2* V617F. A sudden increase in spleen size can be associated with splenic infarction. Myelofibrosis appears to be part of the natural history of the disease but is a reactive, reversible process that does not itself impede hematopoiesis and by itself has no prognostic significance. In some patients, however, the myelofibrosis is accompanied by significant extramedullary hematopoiesis, hepatosplenomegaly, and transfusion-dependent anemia, which are manifestations of stem cell failure. The organomegaly can cause significant mechanical discomfort, portal hypertension, and progressive cachexia. Although the incidence of acute nonlymphocytic leukemia is increased in PV, the incidence of acute leukemia in patients not exposed to chemotherapy or radiation is low, and the development of leukemia is related to the development of extramedullary hematopoiesis, hepatosplenomegaly, and transfusion-dependent anemia or exposure to chemotherapy. Importantly, chemotherapy alone, including hydroxyurea, has been associated with acute leukemia that develops in *JAK2* V617F–negative stem cells. *Erythromelalgia* is a curious syndrome of unknown etiology associated with thrombocytosis, primarily involving the lower extremities and usually manifested by erythema, warmth, and pain of the affected appendage and occasionally digital infarction. It occurs with a variable frequency in MPD patients and is usually responsive to salicylates. Some of the central nervous system symptoms observed in patients with PV such as ocular migraine, appear to represent a variant of erythromelalgia.

If left uncontrolled, erythrocytosis can lead to thrombosis involving vital organs such as the liver, heart, brain, or lungs. Patients with massive splenomegaly are particularly prone to thrombotic events because the associated increase in plasma volume masks the true extent of the red cell mass elevation as measured by the hematocrit or hemoglobin level. A "normal" hematocrit or hemoglobin level in a PV patient with massive splenomegaly should be considered indicative of an elevated red cell mass until proven otherwise.

TREATMENT   Polycythemia Vera

PV is generally an indolent disorder, the clinical course of which is measured in decades, and its management should reflect its tempo. Thrombosis due to erythrocytosis is the most significant complication, and maintenance of the hemoglobin level at ≤140 g/L (14 g/dL; hematocrit <45%) in men and ≤120 g/L (12 g/dL; hematocrit <42%) in women is mandatory to avoid thrombotic complications. Phlebotomy serves initially to reduce hyperviscosity by bringing the red cell mass into the normal range. Periodic phlebotomies thereafter serve to maintain the red cell mass within the normal range and to induce a state of iron deficiency that prevents an accelerated reexpansion of the red cell mass. In most PV patients, once an iron-deficient state is achieved, phlebotomy is usually only required at 3-month intervals. Neither phlebotomy nor iron deficiency increases the platelet count relative to the effect of the disease itself, and thrombocytosis is not correlated with thrombosis in PV, in contrast to the strong correlation between erythrocytosis and thrombosis in this disease. The use of salicylates as a tonic against thrombosis in PV patients is not only potentially harmful if the red cell mass is not controlled by phlebotomy, but also an unproven remedy. Anticoagulants are only indicated when a thrombosis has occurred and can be difficult to monitor owing to the artifactual imbalance between the test tube anticoagulant and plasma that occurs when blood from these patients is assayed for prothrombin or partial thromboplastin activity if the red cell mass is substantially elevated. Asymptomatic hyperuricemia (<10 mg%) requires no therapy, but allopurinol

should be administered to avoid further elevation of the uric acid when chemotherapy is employed to reduce splenomegaly or leukocytosis or to treat pruritus. Generalized pruritus intractable to antihistamines or antidepressants such as doxepin can be a major problem in PV; interferon α (IFN-α), psoralens with ultraviolet light in the A range (PUVA) therapy, and hydroxyurea are other methods of palliation. Asymptomatic thrombocytosis requires no therapy unless the platelet count is sufficiently high to cause an acquired form of von Willebrand's disease due to adsorption and proteolysis of high-molecular-weight von Willebrand factor (vWF) multimers by the expanded platelet mass. Symptomatic splenomegaly can be treated with IFN-α, although the drug can be associated with significant side effects when used chronically. Pegylated IFN-α produces complete remissions in PV patients, and its role in this disorder may be expanding. Anagrelide, a phosphodiesterase inhibitor, can reduce the platelet count and, if tolerated, is preferable to hydroxyurea because it lacks marrow toxicity and actually is protective against venous thrombosis. A reduction in platelet number may be necessary for the treatment of erythromelalgia or ocular migraine if salicylates are not effective or if the platelet count is sufficiently high to cause a hemorrhagic diathesis but only to the degree that symptoms are alleviated. Alkylating agents and radioactive sodium phosphate (^{32}P) are leukemogenic in PV, and their use should be avoided. If a cytotoxic agent must be used, hydroxyurea is preferred, but this drug does not prevent either thrombosis or myelofibrosis in this disorder, is itself leukemogenic, and should only be used for as short a time as possible. In some patients, massive splenomegaly unresponsive to reduction by therapy and associated with intractable weight loss will require splenectomy. In some patients with end-stage disease, pulmonary hypertension may develop due to fibrosis and extramedullary hematopoiesis. Allogeneic bone marrow transplantation may be curative in young patients. Several *JAK2* inhibitors are undergoing clinical trial; to date, these agents have been demonstrated to alleviate constitutional symptoms and to rapidly reduce spleen size without significant effects on blood counts or the *JAK2* V617F neutrophil allele burden, suggesting that they may at least have an important palliative role.

Most patients with PV can live long lives without functional impairment when their red cell mass is effectively managed with phlebotomy alone. Chemotherapy is never indicated to control the red cell mass unless venous access is inadequate.

PRIMARY MYELOFIBROSIS

Chronic PMF (other designations include idiopathic myelofibrosis, *agnogenic myeloid metaplasia* or *myelofibrosis with myeloid metaplasia*) is a clonal disorder of a multipotent hematopoietic progenitor cell of unknown etiology characterized by marrow fibrosis, extramedullary hematopoiesis, and splenomegaly. PMF is the least common chronic MPD, and establishing this diagnosis in the absence of a specific clonal marker is difficult because myelofibrosis and splenomegaly are also features of both PV and CML. Furthermore, myelofibrosis and splenomegaly also occur in a variety of benign and malignant disorders (Table 108-3), many of which are amenable to specific therapies not effective in PMF. In contrast to the other chronic MPDs and so-called acute or malignant myelofibrosis, which can occur at any age, PMF primarily afflicts men in their sixth decade or later.

■ ETIOLOGY

The etiology of PMF is unknown. Nonrandom chromosome abnormalities such as 9p, 20q–, 13q–, trisomy 8 or 9, or partial trisomy 1q are common, but no cytogenetic abnormality specific to the disease

TABLE 108-3 Disorders Causing Myelofibrosis

Malignant	Nonmalignant
Acute leukemia (lymphocytic, myelogenous, megakaryocytic)	HIV infection
	Hyperparathyroidism
Chronic myelogenous leukemia	Renal osteodystrophy
Hairy cell leukemia	Systemic lupus erythematosus
Hodgkin's disease	Tuberculosis
Idiopathic myelofibrosis	Vitamin D deficiency
Lymphoma	Thorium dioxide exposure
Multiple myeloma	Gray platelet syndrome
Myelodysplasia	
Metastatic carcinoma	
Polycythemia vera	
Systemic mastocytosis	

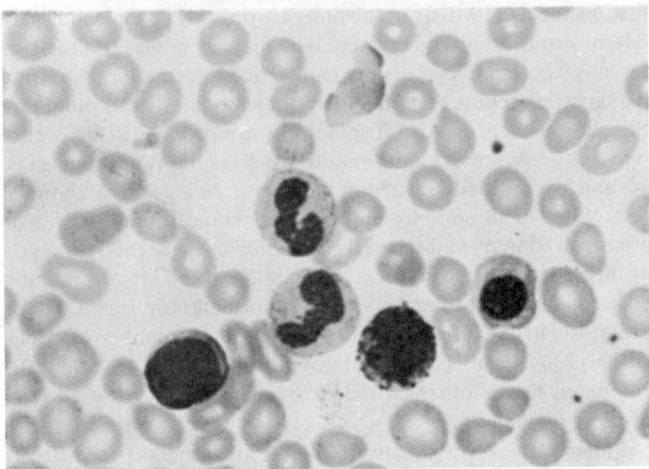

Figure 108-1 Teardrop-shaped red blood cells indicative of membrane damage from passage through the spleen, a nucleated red blood cell, and immature myeloid cells indicative of extramedullary hematopoiesis are noted. This peripheral blood smear is related to any cause of extramedullary hematopoiesis.

has been identified. *JAK2* V617F is present in approximately 50% of PMF patients and mutations in the thrombopoietin receptor *Mpl* occur in about 5%. The degree of myelofibrosis and the extent of extramedullary hematopoiesis are also not related. Fibrosis in this disorder is associated with overproduction of transforming growth factor β and tissue inhibitors of metalloproteinases, while osteosclerosis is associated with overproduction of osteoprotegerin, an osteoclast inhibitor. Marrow angiogenesis occurs due to increased production of vascular endothelial growth factor. Importantly, fibroblasts in PMF are polyclonal and not part of the neoplastic clone.

■ CLINICAL FEATURES

No signs or symptoms are specific for PMF. Many patients are asymptomatic at presentation, and the disease is usually detected by the discovery of splenic enlargement and/or abnormal blood counts during a routine examination. However, in contrast to its companion MPDs, night sweats, fatigue, and weight loss are common presenting complaints. A blood smear will show the characteristic features of extramedullary hematopoiesis: teardrop-shaped red cells, nucleated red cells, myelocytes, and promyelocytes; myeloblasts may also be present (Fig. 108-1). Anemia, usually mild initially, is the rule, while the leukocyte and platelet counts are either normal or increased, but either can be depressed. Mild hepatomegaly may accompany the splenomegaly but is unusual in the absence of splenic enlargement; isolated lymphadenopathy should suggest another diagnosis. Both serum lactate dehydrogenase and alkaline phosphatase levels can be elevated. The LAP score can be low, normal, or high. Marrow is usually inaspirable due to the myelofibrosis (Fig. 108-2), and bone x-rays may reveal osteosclerosis. Exuberant extramedullary hematopoiesis can cause ascites; portal, pulmonary, or intracranial hypertension; intestinal or ureteral obstruction; pericardial tamponade; spinal cord compression; or skin nodules. Splenic enlargement can be sufficiently rapid to cause splenic infarction with fever and pleuritic chest pain. Hyperuricemia and secondary gout may ensue.

■ DIAGNOSIS

While the clinical picture described above is characteristic of PMF, all of the clinical features described can also be observed in PV or CML. Massive splenomegaly commonly masks erythrocytosis in PV, and reports of intraabdominal thromboses in PMF most likely represent instances of unrecognized PV. In some patients with PMF, erythrocytosis has developed during the course of the

disease. Furthermore, since many other disorders have features that overlap with PMF but respond to distinctly different therapies, the diagnosis of PMF is one of exclusion, which requires that the disorders listed in Table 108-3 be ruled out. A diagnostic algorithm has been proposed but does not distinguish one disease causing myeloid metaplasia from another.

The presence of teardrop-shaped red cells, nucleated red cells, myelocytes, and promyelocytes establishes the presence of extramedullary hematopoiesis, while the presence of leukocytosis, thrombocytosis with large and bizarre platelets, and circulating myelocytes suggests the presence of an MPD as opposed to a secondary form of myelofibrosis (Table 108-3). Marrow is usually not aspirable due to increased marrow reticulin, but marrow biopsy will reveal a hypercellular marrow with trilineage hyperplasia and, in particular, increased numbers of megakaryocytes in clusters and with large, dysplastic nuclei. However, there are no characteristic morphologic abnormalities of the bone marrow

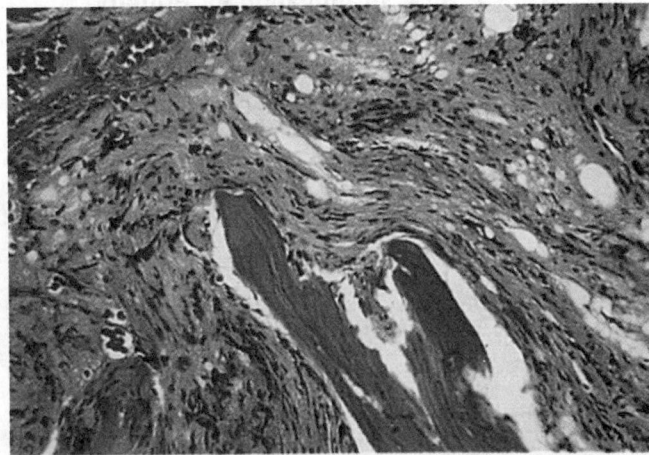

Figure 108-2 This marrow section shows the marrow cavity replaced by fibrous tissue composed of reticulin fibers and collagen. When this fibrosis is due to a primary hematologic process, it is called *myelofibrosis*. When the fibrosis is secondary to a tumor or a granulomatous process, it is called *myelophthisis*.

that distinguish PMF from the other chronic MPDs. Splenomegaly due to extramedullary hematopoiesis may be sufficiently massive to cause portal hypertension and variceal formation. In some patients, exuberant extramedullary hematopoiesis can dominate the clinical picture. An intriguing feature of PMF is the occurrence of autoimmune abnormalities such as immune complexes, antinuclear antibodies, rheumatoid factor, or a positive Coombs' test. Whether these represent a host reaction to the disorder or are involved in its pathogenesis is unknown. Cytogenetic analysis of blood is useful both to exclude CML and for prognostic purposes, because complex karyotype abnormalities portend a poor prognosis in PMF. For unknown reasons, the number of circulating CD34+ cells is markedly increased in PMF (>15,000/μL) compared to the other chronic MPDs, unless they too develop myeloid metaplasia.

Importantly, approximately 50% of PMF patients, like patients with its companion myeloproliferative disorders PV and ET, express the *JAK2* V617F mutation, often as homozygotes. Such patients had a poorer survival in one retrospective study but not in another, where they were found to be older and to have higher hematocrits than those patients who were *JAK2* V617F–negative. Those patients with an *MPL* mutation tend to be more anemic than those without this mutation.

■ COMPLICATIONS

Survival in PMF varies according to specific clinical features (Table 108-4) but is shorter than in patients with PV or ET. The natural history of PMF is one of increasing marrow failure with transfusion-dependent anemia and increasing organomegaly due to extramedullary hematopoiesis. As with CML, PMF can evolve from a chronic phase to an accelerated phase with constitutional symptoms and increasing marrow failure. About 10% of patients spontaneously transform to an aggressive form of acute leukemia for which therapy is usually ineffective. Important prognostic factors for disease acceleration include anemia, leukocytosis, thrombocytopenia, the presence of circulating myeloblasts, older age, the presence of complex cytogenetic abnormalities, and constitutional symptoms such as unexplained fever, night sweats, or weight loss.

TABLE 108-4 Risk Stratification for Primary Myelofibrosis

Risk Factors	Frequency of Occurrence (%)
Age >65 years	45
Constitutional symptoms	26
Hemoglobin <10 g/dL	35
WBC >25 × 109/L	10
Blood blasts >10%	36

Risk Groups	No. of Factors	Proportion of Patients (%)	Median Survival (years)
Low	0	22	11
Intermediate-1	1	29	8
Intermediate-2	2	28	4
High	≥3	21	2

Source: From F Cervantes et al: Blood 113:2895, 2009.

TREATMENT Primary Myelofibrosis

No specific therapy exists for PMF. Anemia may be due to gastrointestinal blood loss, may be exacerbated by folic acid deficiency, and in rare instances, pyridoxine therapy has been effective. However, anemia is more often due to ineffective erythropoiesis uncompensated by extramedullary hematopoiesis in the spleen and liver. Neither recombinant erythropoietin nor androgens such as Danazol have proved consistently effective as therapy for the anemia. Erythropoietin may worsen splenomegaly and will be ineffective if the serum erythropoietin level is >125 mU/L. A red cell splenic sequestration study can establish the presence of hypersplenism, for which splenectomy is indicated. Splenectomy may also be necessary if splenomegaly impairs alimentation and should be performed before cachexia sets in. In this situation, splenectomy should not be avoided because of concern over rebound thrombocytosis, loss of hematopoietic capacity, or compensatory hepatomegaly. However, for unexplained reasons, splenectomy increases the risk of blastic transformation. Splenic irradiation is, at best, temporarily palliative and associated with a significant risk of neutropenia, infection, and operative hemorrhage. Allopurinol can control significant hyperuricemia, and hydroxyurea has proved useful for controlling organomegaly in some patients. The role of IFN-α is still undefined; its side effects are more pronounced in the older individuals who are usually afflicted with this disorder and it should be used at lower doses. Glucocorticoids have been used to control constitutional symptoms and autoimmune complications and may ameliorate anemia alone, or in combination with low-dose thalidomide (50–100 mg/d); such therapy may also palliate splenomegaly. Allogeneic bone marrow transplantation is the only curative treatment and should be considered in younger patients; reduced-intensity conditioning regimens may permit hematopoietic cell transplantation to be extended to older individuals. *JAK2* inhibitors have been effective in alleviating constitutional symptoms and splenomegaly in PMF patients and are currently used in phase III clinical trials. While their effects are reversible, these agents may offer a less toxic and more effective means of palliation in this disorder.

ESSENTIAL THROMBOCYTOSIS

Essential thrombocytosis (other designations include *essential thrombocythemia, idiopathic thrombocytosis, primary thrombocytosis,* and *hemorrhagic thrombocythemia*) is a clonal disorder of unknown etiology involving a multipotent hematopoietic progenitor cell manifested clinically by overproduction of platelets without a definable cause. ET is an uncommon disorder, with an incidence of 1–2/100,000 and a distinct female predominance. No clonal marker is available to consistently distinguish ET from the more common nonclonal, reactive forms of thrombocytosis (Table 108-5), making its diagnosis difficult. Once considered a disease of the elderly and responsible for significant morbidity due to hemorrhage or thrombosis, with the widespread use of electronic cell counters, it is now clear that ET can occur at any age in adults and often without symptoms or disturbances of hemostasis. There is an unexplained female predominance in contrast to PMF or the reactive forms of thrombocytosis where no sex difference exists. Because no specific clonal marker is available, clinical criteria have been proposed to distinguish ET from the other chronic MPDs, which may also present with thrombocytosis but have differing prognoses and therapies (Table 108-5). These criteria do not establish clonality; therefore, they are truly useful only in identifying disorders such as CML,

TABLE 108-5 Causes of Thrombocytosis

Tissue inflammation: collagen vascular disease, inflammatory bowel disease	Hemorrhage
Malignancy	Iron deficiency anemia
Infection	Surgery
Myeloproliferative disorders: polycythemia vera, primary myelofibrosis, essential thrombocytosis, chronic myelogenous leukemia	Rebound: Correction of vitamin B_{12} or folate deficiency, post-ethanol abuse
Myelodysplastic disorders: 5q-syndrome, idiopathic refractory sideroblastic anemia	Hemolysis
Postsplenectomy or hyposplenism	Familial: Thrombopoietin overproduction, constitutive Mpl activation

PV, or myelodysplasia, which can masquerade as ET, as opposed to actually establishing the presence of ET. Furthermore, as with "idiopathic" erythrocytosis, nonclonal benign forms of thrombocytosis exist (such as hereditary overproduction of thrombopoietin) that are not widely recognized because we currently lack adequate diagnostic tools. Approximately 50% of ET patients carry the *JAK2* V617F mutation but its absence does not exclude the disorder.

■ ETIOLOGY

Megakaryocytopoiesis and platelet production depend upon thrombopoietin and its receptor *Mpl*. As in the case of early erythroid and myeloid progenitor cells, early megakaryocytic progenitors require the presence of interleukin 3 (IL-3) and stem cell factor for optimal proliferation in addition to thrombopoietin. Their subsequent development is also enhanced by the chemokine stromal cell-derived factor 1 (SDF-1). However, megakaryocyte maturation requires thrombopoietin.

Megakaryocytes are unique among hematopoietic progenitor cells because reduplication of their genome is endomitotic rather than mitotic. In the absence of thrombopoietin, endomitotic megakaryocytic reduplication and, by extension, the cytoplasmic development necessary for platelet production are impaired. Like erythropoietin, thrombopoietin is produced in both the liver and the kidneys, and an inverse correlation exists between the platelet count and plasma thrombopoietic activity. Like erythropoietin levels, plasma levels of thrombopoietin are controlled largely by the size of its progenitor cell pool. In contrast to erythropoietin, but like its myeloid counterparts, granulocyte- and granulocyte-macrophage colony-stimulating factors, thrombopoietin not only enhances the proliferation of its target cells but also enhances the reactivity of their end-stage product, the platelet. In addition to its role in thrombopoiesis, thrombopoietin also enhances the survival of multipotent hematopoietic stem cells.

The clonal nature of ET was established by analysis of glucose-6-phosphate dehydrogenase isoenzyme expression in patients hemizygous for this gene, by analysis of X-linked DNA polymorphisms in informative female patients, and by the expression in patients of nonrandom, though variable, cytogenetic abnormalities. Although thrombocytosis is its principal manifestation, like the other chronic MPDs, a multipotent hematopoietic progenitor cell is involved in ET. Furthermore, a number of families have been described in which ET was inherited, in one instance as an autosomal dominant

trait. In addition to ET, PMF and PV have also been observed in some kindreds.

■ CLINICAL FEATURES

Clinically, ET is most often identified incidentally when a platelet count is obtained during the course of a routine medical evaluation. Occasionally, review of previous blood counts will reveal that an elevated platelet count was present but overlooked for many years. No symptoms or signs are specific for ET, but these patients can have hemorrhagic and thrombotic tendencies expressed as easy bruising for the former and microvascular occlusions for the latter such as erythromelalgia, ocular migraine, or TIAs. Physical examination is generally unremarkable except occasionally for mild splenomegaly. Massive splenomegaly is indicative of another MPD, in particular PV, PMF, or CML.

Anemia is unusual, but a mild neutrophilic leukocytosis is not. The blood smear is most remarkable for the number of platelets present, some of which may be very large. The large mass of circulating platelets may prevent the accurate measurement of serum potassium due to release of platelet potassium upon blood clotting. This type of hyperkalemia is a laboratory artifact and not associated with electrocardiographic abnormalities. Similarly, arterial oxygen measurements can be inaccurate unless thrombocythemic blood is collected on ice. The prothrombin and partial thromboplastin times are normal, while abnormalities of platelet function such as a prolonged bleeding time and impaired platelet aggregation can be present. However, in spite of much study, no platelet function abnormality is characteristic of ET, and no platelet function test predicts the risk of clinically significant bleeding or thrombosis.

The elevated platelet count may hinder marrow aspiration, but marrow biopsy usually reveals megakaryocyte hyperplasia and hypertrophy, as well as an overall increase in marrow cellularity. If marrow reticulin is increased, another diagnosis should be considered. The absence of stainable iron demands an explanation because iron deficiency alone can cause thrombocytosis, and absent marrow iron in the presence of marrow hypercellularity is a feature of PV.

Nonrandom cytogenetic abnormalities occur in ET but are uncommon, and no specific or consistent abnormality is notable, even those involving chromosomes 3 and 1, where the genes for thrombopoietin and its receptor *Mpl*, respectively, are located.

■ DIAGNOSIS

Thrombocytosis is encountered in a broad variety of clinical disorders (Table 108-5) in many of which production of cytokines is increased. The absolute level of the platelet count is not a useful diagnostic aid for distinguishing between benign and clonal causes of thrombocytosis. About 50% of ET patients express the *JAK2* V617F mutation. When *JAK2* V617F is absent, cytogenetic evaluation is mandatory to determine if the thrombocytosis is due to CML or a myelodysplastic disorder such as the 5q– syndrome. Because the bcr-abl translocation can be present in the absence of the Ph chromosome, and because bcr-abl reverse transcriptase polymerase chain reaction is associated with false-positive results, fluorescence in situ hybridization (FISH) analysis for bcr-abl is the preferred assay in patients with thrombocytosis in whom a cytogenetic study for the Ph chromosome is negative. Anemia and ringed sideroblasts are not features of ET, but they are features of idiopathic refractory sideroblastic anemia, and in some of these patients the thrombocytosis occurs in association with *JAK2* V617F expression. Massive splenomegaly should suggest the presence of another MPD, and in this setting a red cell mass determination should be performed because splenomegaly can mask the presence of erythrocytosis. Importantly, what appears to be ET can evolve into PV or PMF after a period of many years, revealing the true nature of the underlying MPD.

There is sufficient overlap of the *JAK2* V617F neutrophil allele burden between ET and PV that this cannot be used as a distinguishing diagnostic feature; only a red cell mass and plasma volume determination can distinguish PV from ET and importantly in this regard, 64% of *JAK2* V617F–positive ET patients actually were found to have PV when red cell mass and plasma volume determinations were performed.

■ COMPLICATIONS

Perhaps no other condition in clinical medicine has caused otherwise astute physicians to intervene inappropriately more often than thrombocytosis, particularly if the platelet count is $>1 \times 10^6/\mu L$. It is commonly believed that a high platelet count causes intravascular stasis and thrombosis; however, no controlled clinical study has ever established this association, and in patients younger than age 60 years, the incidence of thrombosis was not greater in patients with thrombocytosis than in age-matched controls.

To the contrary, very high platelet counts are associated primarily with hemorrhage due to acquired von Willebrand disease. This is not meant to imply that an elevated platelet count cannot cause symptoms in an ET patient, but rather that the focus should be on the patient, not the platelet count. For example, some of the most dramatic neurologic problems in ET are migraine-related and respond only to lowering of the platelet count, while other symptoms such as erythromelalgia respond simply to platelet cyclooxygenase 1 inhibitors such as aspirin or ibuprofen, without a reduction in platelet number. Still others may represent an interaction between an atherosclerotic vascular system and a high platelet count, and others may have no relationship to the platelet count whatsoever. Recognition that PV can present with thrombocytosis alone as well as the discovery of previously unrecognized causes of hypercoagulability (Chap. 117) make the older literature on the complications of thrombocytosis unreliable.

TREATMENT	Essential Thrombocytosis

Survival of patients with ET is not different than for the general population. An elevated platelet count in an asymptomatic patient without cardiovascular risk factors requires no therapy. Indeed, before any therapy is initiated in a patient with thrombocytosis, the cause of symptoms must be clearly identified as due to the elevated platelet count. When the platelet count rises above $1 \times 10^6/\mu L$, a substantial quantity of high-molecular-weight von Willebrand multimers are removed from the circulation and destroyed by the enlarged platelet mass, resulting in an acquired form of von Willebrand's disease. This can be identified by a reduction in ristocetin cofactor activity. In this situation, aspirin could promote hemorrhage. Bleeding in this situation usually responds to ε-aminocaproic acid, which can be given prophylactically before and after elective surgery. Plateletpheresis is at best a temporary and inefficient remedy that is rarely required.

Importantly, ET patients treated with ^{32}P or alkylating agents are at risk of developing acute leukemia without any proof of benefit; combining either therapy with hydroxyurea increases this risk. If platelet reduction is deemed necessary on the basis of symptoms refractory to salicylates alone, IFN-α, the quinazoline derivative, anagrelide, or hydroxyurea can be used to reduce the platelet count, but none of these is uniformly effective nor without significant side effects. Hydroxyurea and aspirin are more effective than anagrelide and aspirin for prevention of TIAs but not more effective for the prevention of other types of arterial thrombosis and are actually less effective for venous thrombosis. The effectiveness of hydroxyurea in preventing TIAs is because it is an NO donor. Normalizing the platelet count also does not prevent either arterial or venous thrombosis. The risk of gastrointestinal bleeding is also higher when aspirin is combined with anagrelide.

As more clinical experience is acquired, ET appears more benign than previously thought. Evolution to acute leukemia is more likely to be a consequence of therapy than of the disease itself. In managing patients with thrombocytosis, the physician's first obligation is to do no harm.

FURTHER READINGS

ALCHALBY H et al: Impact of JAK2V617F mutation status, allele burden, and clearance after allogeneic stem cell transplantation for myelofibrosis. Blood 116:3572, 2010

BUSS DH et al: The incidence of thrombotic and hemorrhagic disorders in association with extreme thrombocytosis: An analysis of 129 cases. Am J Hematol 20:365, 1985

CASSINAT B et al: Classification of myeloproliferative disorders in the JAK2 era: Is there a role for red cell mass? Leukemia 22:452, 2002

CERVANTES F et al: New prognostic scoring system for primary myelofibrosis based on a study of the International Working Group for Myelofibrosis Research and Treatment. Blood 113:2895, 2009

JONES AV et al: JAK2 haplotype is a major risk factor for the development of myeloproliferative neoplasms. Nat Genet 41:446, 2009

KILADJIAN JJ et al: Pegylated interferon-alfa-2a induces complete hematologic and molecular responses with low toxicity in polycythemia vera. Blood 112:3065, 2008

REILLY JT: Idiopathic myelofibrosis: Pathogenesis to treatment. Hematol Oncol 24:56, 2006

SPIVAK JL: Polycythemia vera: Myths, mechanisms, and management. Blood 100:4272, 2002

———: Narrative review: Thrombocytosis, polycythemia vera, and JAK2 mutations: The phenotypic mimicry of chronic myeloproliferation. Ann Intern Med 152:300, 2010

VERSTOVSEK S et al: Safety and efficacy of INCB018424, a JAK1 and JAK2 inhibitor, in myelofibrosis. N Engl J Med 363:1117, 2010

CHAPTER **109**

Acute and Chronic Myeloid Leukemia

Meir Wetzler
Guido Marcucci
Clara D. Bloomfield

The myeloid leukemias are a heterogeneous group of diseases characterized by infiltration of the blood, bone marrow, and other tissues by neoplastic cells of the hematopoietic system. In 2010 the estimated number of new myeloid leukemia cases in the United States was 17,200. These leukemias comprise a spectrum of malignancies that, untreated, range from rapidly fatal to slowly growing. Based on their untreated course, the myeloid leukemias have traditionally been designated acute or chronic.

ACUTE MYELOID LEUKEMIA

■ INCIDENCE

The incidence of acute myeloid leukemia (AML) is ~3.5 per 100,000 people per year, and the age-adjusted incidence is higher in men than in women (4.3 vs 2.9). AML incidence increases with age; it is 1.7 in individuals aged <65 years and 15.9 in those aged >65 years. The median age at diagnosis is 67 years.

■ ETIOLOGY

Heredity, radiation, chemical and other occupational exposures, and drugs have been implicated in the development of AML. No direct evidence suggests a viral etiology.

Heredity

Certain syndromes with somatic cell chromosome aneuploidy, such as trisomy 21 noted in Down syndrome, are associated with an increased incidence of AML. Inherited diseases with defective DNA repair, e.g., Fanconi anemia, Bloom syndrome, and ataxia-telangiectasia, are also associated with AML. Congenital neutropenia (Kostmann syndrome) is a disease with mutations in the granulocyte colony-stimulating factor (G-CSF) receptor and, often, neutrophil elastase that may evolve into AML. Myeloproliferative syndromes may also evolve into AML (Chap. 108). Germ-line mutations of CCAAT/enhancer-binding protein α (*CEBPA*), runt-related transcription factor 1 (*RUNX1*), and tumor protein p53 (*TP53*) have also been associated with a higher predisposition to AML in some series.

Radiation

High-dose radiation, like that experienced by survivors of the atomic bombs in Japan or nuclear reactor accidents, increase the risk of myeloid leukemias that peak 5–7 years after exposure. Therapeutic radiation alone seems to add little risk of AML but can increase the risk in people also exposed to alkylating agents.

Chemical and other exposures

Exposure to benzene, a solvent used in the chemical, plastic, rubber, and pharmaceutical industries, is associated with an increased incidence of AML. Smoking and exposure to petroleum products, paint, embalming fluids, ethylene oxide, herbicides, and pesticides have also been associated with an increased risk of AML.

Drugs

Anticancer drugs are the leading cause of therapy-associated AML. Alkylating agent–associated leukemias occur on average 4–6 years after exposure, and affected individuals have aberrations in chromosomes 5 and 7. Topoisomerase II inhibitor–associated leukemias occur 1–3 years after exposure, and affected individuals often have aberrations involving chromosome 11q23. Chloramphenicol, phenylbutazone, and, less commonly, chloroquine and methoxypsoralen can result in bone marrow failure that may evolve into AML.

■ CLASSIFICATION

The current categorization of AML uses the World Health Organization (WHO) classification (Table 109-1), which includes different biologically distinct groups based on clinical features and cytogenetic and molecular abnormalities in addition to morphology. In contrast to the previously used French-American-British (FAB) schema, the WHO classification places limited reliance on cytochemistry. Since some of the recent literature and some ongoing studies use the FAB classification, a description of this system is also provided in Table 109-1. A major difference between the WHO and FAB systems is the blast cutoff for a diagnosis of AML as opposed to myelodysplastic syndrome (MDS); it is 20% in the WHO classification and 30% in the FAB. AML with 20–30% blasts as defined by the WHO classification can benefit from therapies for MDS (such as decitabine or 5-azacytidine) that were approved by the U.S. Food and Drug Administration (FDA) based on trials using the FAB criteria. Selected components of the WHO classification are outlined below.

Immunophenotype and relevance to the WHO classification

The immunophenotype of human leukemia cells can be studied by multiparameter flow cytometry after the cells are labeled with monoclonal antibodies to cell-surface antigens. This can be important for separating AML from acute lymphoblastic leukemia (ALL) and identifying some types of AML. For example, AML with minimal differentiation that is characterized by immature morphology and no lineage-specific cytochemical reactions may be diagnosed by flow-cytometric demonstration of the myeloid-specific antigens cluster designation (CD) 13 and/or 117. Similarly, acute megakaryoblastic leukemia can often be diagnosed only by expression of the platelet-specific antigens CD41 and/or CD61. While flow cytometry is useful, widely used, and in some cases essential for the diagnosis of AML, it is supportive only in establishing the different subtypes of AML through the WHO classification.

Clinical features and relevance to the WHO classification

The WHO classification considers clinical features in subdividing AML. For example, it identifies therapy-related AML as a separate entity that develops following prior therapy (e.g., alkylating agents, topoisomerase II inhibitors, ionizing radiation). It also identifies AML with myelodysplasia-related changes based in part upon medical history of an antecedent MDS or myelodysplastic/myeloproliferative neoplasm. The clinical features likely contribute to the prognosis of AML and have therefore been included in the classification.

Genetic findings and relevance to the WHO classification

The WHO classification is the first AML classification to incorporate genetic (chromosomal and molecular) information. Indeed, AML is first subclassified based on the presence or absence of specific recurrent genetic abnormalities. For example, AML FAB M3 is now designated *acute promyelocytic leukemia* (APL), based on the

TABLE 109-1 AML Classification Systems

World Health Organization Classification[a]

AML with recurrent genetic abnormalities

AML with t(8;21)(q22;q22);*RUNX1-RUNX1T1*[b]

AML with inv(16)(pl3.1q22) or t(16;16)(p13.1;q22);*CBFB-MYH11*[b]

Acute promyelocytic leukemia with t(15;17)(q22;q12); *PML-RARA*[b]

AML with t(9;11)(p22;q23); *MLLT3-MLL*

AML with t(6;9)(p23;q34); *DEK-NUP214*

AML with inv(3)(q21q26.2) or t(3;3)(q21;q26.2); *RPN1-EVI1*

AML (megakaryoblastic) with t(1;22)(p13;q13); *RBM15-MKL1*

Provisional entity: AML with mutated NPM1

Provisional entity: AML with mutated CEBPA

AML with myelodysplasia-related changes

Therapy-related myeloid neoplasms

AML not otherwise specified

AML with minimal differentiation

AML without maturation

AML with maturation

Acute myelomonocytic leukemia

Acute monoblastic and monocytic leukemia

Acute erythroid leukemia

Acute megakaryoblastic leukemia

Acute basophilic leukemia

Acute panmyelosis with myelofibrosis

Myeloid sarcoma

Myeloid proliferations related to Down syndrome

Transient abnormal myelopoiesis

Myeloid leukemia associated with Down syndrome

Blastic plasmacytoid dendritic cell neoplasm

Acute leukemia of ambiguous lineage

Acute undifferentiated leukemia

Mixed phenotype acute leukemia with t(9;22)(q34;q11,20); *BCR-ABL11*

Mixed phenotype acute leukemia with t(v;11q23); *MLL* rearranged

Mixed phenotype acute leukemia, B/myeloid, NOS

Mixed phenotype acute leukemia, T/myeloid, NOS

Provisional entity: Natural killer (NK)-cell lymphoblastic leukemia/ lymphoma

French-American-British (FAB) Classification[c]

M0: Minimally differentiated leukemia

Ml: Myeloblastic leukemia without maturation

M2: Myeloblastic leukemia with maturation

M3: Hypergranular promyelocytic leukemia

M4: Myelomonocytic leukemia

M4Eo: Variant: Increase in abnormal marrow eosinophils

M5: Monocytic leukemia

M6: Erythroleukemia (DiGuglielmo's disease)

M7: Megakaryoblastic leukemia

[a]From SH Swerdlow et al (eds): *World Health Organization Classification of Tumours of Haematopoietic and Lymphoid Tissues.* Lyon, IARC Press, 2008.
[b]Diagnosis is AML regardless of blast count.
[c]From JM Bennett et al: Ann Intern Med 103:620, 1985.
Abbreviation: AML, acute myeloid leukemia.

---

presence of either the t(15;17)(q22;q12) cytogenetic rearrangement or the *PML-RARA* fusion product of the translocation. A similar approach is taken with regard to core binding factor (CBF) AML that is now designated based on the presence of t(8;21)(q22;q22) or inv(16)(p13q22) or the respective fusion products *RUNX1-RUNX1T1* and *CBFB-MYH11*. Thus, the WHO classification separates recurrent cytogenetic and/or molecular types of AML and forces the clinician to take the appropriate steps to correctly identify the entity and thus tailor treatment(s) accordingly.

Chromosomal analyses Chromosomal analysis of the leukemic cell provides the most important pretreatment prognostic information in AML. The WHO classification incorporates cytogenetics in the AML classification by recognizing a category of AML with recurrent genetic abnormalities and a category of AML with myelodysplasia-related changes (Table 109-1). The latter category is diagnosed in part by AML with selected myelodysplasia-related cytogenetic abnormalities (e.g., complex karyotypes and unbalanced and balanced changes involving among others, chromosomes 5, 7, and 11). Only one cytogenetic abnormality has been invariably associated with specific morphologic features: t(15;17)(q22;q12) with APL. Other chromosomal abnormalities have been associated primarily with one morphologic/immunophenotypic group, including

inv(16)(p13q22) with AML with abnormal bone marrow eosinophils; t(8;21)(q22;q22) with slender Auer rods, expression of CD19 and increased normal eosinophils; and t(9;11)(p22;q23), and other translocations involving 11q23, with monocytic features. Recurring chromosomal abnormalities in AML may also be associated with specific clinical characteristics. More commonly associated with younger age are t(8;21) and t(l5;17), and with older age, del(5q) and del(7q). Myeloid sarcomas (see below) are associated with t(8;21), and disseminated intravascular coagulation (DIC) with t(15;17).

Molecular classification

Molecular study of many recurring cytogenetic abnormalities has revealed genes that may be involved in leukemogenesis; this information is increasingly being incorporated into the WHO classification. For instance, t(15;17) results in the fusion gene *PML-RARA* that encodes a chimeric protein, promyelocytic leukemia (Pml)–retinoic acid receptor α (Rarα), which is formed by the fusion of the retinoic acid receptor α (*RARA*) gene from chromosome 17, and the promyelocytic leukemia (*PML*) gene from chromosome 15. The *RARA* gene encodes a member of the nuclear hormone receptor family of transcription factors. After binding retinoic acid, *RARA* can promote expression of a variety of genes. The 15;17 translocation juxtaposes *PML* with *RARA* in a head-to-tail configuration that is under the transcriptional control of *PML*. Three different breakpoints in the *PML* gene lead to various fusion protein isoforms. The Pml-Rarα fusion protein tends to suppress gene transcription and blocks differentiation of the cells. Pharmacologic doses of the Rarα ligand, all-*trans*-retinoic acid (tretinoin), relieve the block and promote hematopoietic cell differentiation (see below). Similar examples of molecular subtypes of the disease included in the category of AML with recurrent genetic abnormalities are those characterized by the leukemogenic fusion genes *RUNX1-RUNX1T1*, *CBFB-MYH11*, *MLLT3-MLL*, and *DEK-NUP214* resulting, respectively, from t(8;21), inv(16), t(9;11), and t(6;9)(p23;q34).

Two new provisional entities defined by the presence of gene mutations, rather than macroscopic chromosomal abnormalities, have been recently added to the category of AML with recurrent genetic abnormalities: *AML with mutated nucleophosmin* (*NPM1*) and *AML with mutated CEBPA*. AML with fms-related tyrosine kinase 3 (*FLT3*) mutations is not considered a distinct entity, although determining the presence of such mutations is recommended by WHO in patients with cytogenetically normal AML (CN-AML) because the relatively frequent *FLT3*-internal tandem duplication (ITD) carries a negative prognostic significance and therefore is clinically relevant (Table 109-2). *FLT3* encodes a tyrosine kinase receptor important in the development of myeloid and lymphoid lineages. Activating mutations of *FLT3* are present in ~30% of adult AML patients due to ITD in the juxtamembrane domain or mutations of the activating loop of the kinase. Continuous activation of the *FLT3*-encoded protein provides increased proliferation and antiapoptotic signals to the myeloid progenitor cell. *FLT3*-ITD, the more common of the *FLT3* mutations, occurs preferentially in patients with CN-AML. The importance of identifying *FLT3*-ITD at diagnosis relates to the fact that it not only is useful in prognostication but also may predict response to specific treatment such as the tyrosine kinase inhibitors that are being tested in clinical trials.

Other molecular prognostic factors (Table 109-2) in AML include v-kit Hardy-Zuckerman 4 feline sarcoma viral oncogene homolog (*KIT*) mutations that are found in 25–30% of t(8;21) or inv(16) patients. Others include Wilms' tumor 1 (*WT1*) mutations found in 10–13% of CN-AML and overexpression of genes such as brain and acute leukemia, cytoplasmic (*BAALC*), ets erythroblastosis virus E26

oncogene homologue (avian) (*ERG*), meningioma (disrupted in balanced translocation) 1 (*MN1*), and MDS1 and EVI1 complex locus (*MECOM*, also known as *EVI1*), which predict for poor outcome in CN-AML. The applicability of screening for these molecular aberrations to AML classification and clinical practice is being tested.

With progress in genomics technology including genomewide investigation of gene mutations and expression levels, additional aberrations are being discovered, underscoring the molecular heterogeneity of AML. The applicability of gene expression profiling to diagnosis and outcome prediction of cytogenetic and molecular subsets of AML patients and to clinical management of AML is under active investigation. MicroRNAs, naturally occurring noncoding RNAs, have been shown to regulate the expression of proteins involved in hematopoietic differentiation and survival pathways by degradation or translation inhibition of target coding RNAs. Deregulated expression levels of microRNAs have been shown to associate with specific cytogenetic and molecular subsets of AML and predict outcome in CN-AML. Finally, massive parallel sequencing of the whole genome from AML patients' blasts is revealing previously unrecognized mutations of genes that are involved in metabolic pathways that have not been previously hypothesized to be disrupted in AML, such as mutations in the isocitrate dehydrogenase 1 (NADP+), soluble (*IDH1*) and isocitrate dehydrogenase 2 (NADP+), and mitochondrial (*IDH2*) genes.

It is likely that once the biologic and clinical significance of these emerging genetic aberrations is understood, AML will be primarily classified molecularly to define specific entities and stratify patients to a corresponding, optimal targeting therapy.

CLINICAL PRESENTATION

Symptoms

Patients with AML most often present with nonspecific symptoms that begin gradually or abruptly and are the consequence of anemia, leukocytosis, leukopenia or leukocyte dysfunction, or thrombocytopenia. Nearly half have had symptoms for ≤3 months before the leukemia was diagnosed.

Half mention fatigue as the first symptom, but most complain of fatigue or weakness at the time of diagnosis. Anorexia and weight loss are common. Fever with or without an identifiable infection is the initial symptom in ~10% of patients. Signs of abnormal hemostasis (bleeding, easy bruising) are noted first in 5% of patients. On occasion, bone pain, lymphadenopathy, nonspecific cough, headache, or diaphoresis is the presenting symptom.

Rarely patients may present with symptoms from a myeloid sarcoma that is a tumor mass consisting of myeloid blasts occurring at anatomic sites other than bone marrow. Sites involved are most commonly the skin, lymph node, gastrointestinal tract, soft tissue, and testis. This rare presentation, often characterized by chromosome aberrations [e.g., monosomy 7, trisomy 8, *MLL* rearrangement, inv(16), trisomy 4, t(8;21)] may precede or coincide with AML.

Physical findings

Fever, splenomegaly, hepatomegaly, lymphadenopathy, sternal tenderness, and evidence of infection and hemorrhage are often found at diagnosis. Significant gastrointestinal bleeding, intrapulmonary hemorrhage, or intracranial hemorrhage occur most often in APL. Bleeding associated with coagulopathy may also occur in monocytic AML and with extreme degrees of leukocytosis or thrombocytopenia in other morphologic subtypes. Retinal hemorrhages are detected in 15% of patients. Infiltration of the gingivae, skin, soft tissues, or the meninges with leukemic blasts at diagnosis is characteristic of the monocytic subtypes and those with 11q23 chromosomal abnormalities.

TABLE 109-2 Molecular Prognostic Markers in AML

Marker	Marker Location	Prognostic Impact
NPM1 mutation	5q35	Favorable
CEBPA mutation	19q13.1	Favorable
FLT3-ITD	13q12	Adverse
WT1 mutation	11p13	Adverse
KIT mutation	4q11-q12	Adverse
BAALC overexpression	8q22.3	Adverse
ERG overexpression	21q22.3	Adverse
MN1 overexpression	22q12.1	Adverse
EVI1 overexpression	3q26	Adverse

Abbreviations: AML, acute myeloid leukemia; ITD, internal tandem duplication.

Hematologic findings

Anemia is usually present at diagnosis and can be severe. The degree varies considerably, irrespective of other hematologic findings, splenomegaly, or duration of symptoms. The anemia is usually normocytic normochromic. Decreased erythropoiesis often results in a reduced reticulocyte count, and red blood cell (RBC) survival is decreased by accelerated destruction. Active blood loss also contributes to the anemia.

The median presenting leukocyte count is about 15,000/μL. Between 25 and 40% of patients have counts <5000/μL, and 20% have counts >100,000/μL. Fewer than 5% have no detectable leukemic cells in the blood. The morphology of the malignant cell varies in different subsets. In AML, the cytoplasm often contains primary (non-specific) granules, and the nucleus shows fine, lacy chromatin with one or more nucleoli characteristic of immature cells. Abnormal rod-shaped granules called Auer rods are not uniformly present, but when they are, myeloid lineage is virtually certain (Fig. 109-1). Poor neutrophil function may be noted functionally by impaired phagocytosis and migration and morphologically by abnormal lobulation and deficient granulation.

Platelet counts <100,000/μL are found at diagnosis in ~75% of patients, and about 25% have counts <25,000/μL. Both morphologic and functional platelet abnormalities can be observed, including large and bizarre shapes with abnormal granulation

and inability of platelets to aggregate or adhere normally to one another.

Pretreatment evaluation

Once the diagnosis of AML is suspected, a rapid evaluation and initiation of appropriate therapy should follow (Table 109-3). In addition to clarifying the subtype of leukemia, initial studies should evaluate the overall functional integrity of the major organ systems, including the cardiovascular, pulmonary, hepatic, and renal systems. Factors that have prognostic significance, either for achieving complete remission (CR) or for predicting the duration of CR, should also be assessed before initiating treatment, including cytogenetics and molecular markers (at least *NMP1* and *CEBPA* mutations and *FLT3*-ITD in CN-AML). Leukemic cells should be obtained from all patients and cryopreserved for future use as new tests and therapeutics become available. All patients should be evaluated for infection.

Most patients are anemic and thrombocytopenic at presentation. Replacement of the appropriate blood components, if necessary, should begin promptly. Because qualitative platelet dysfunction or the presence of an infection may increase the likelihood of bleeding, evidence of hemorrhage justifies the immediate use of platelet transfusion, even if the platelet count is only moderately decreased.

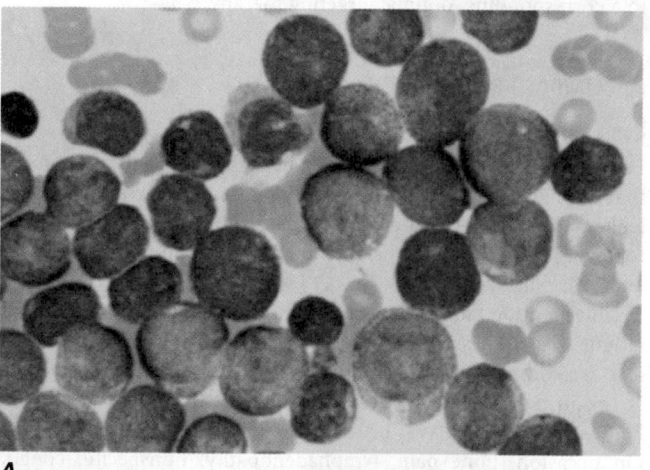

A

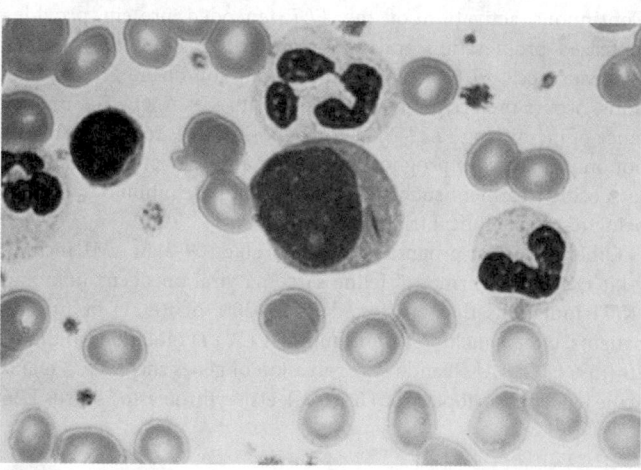

B

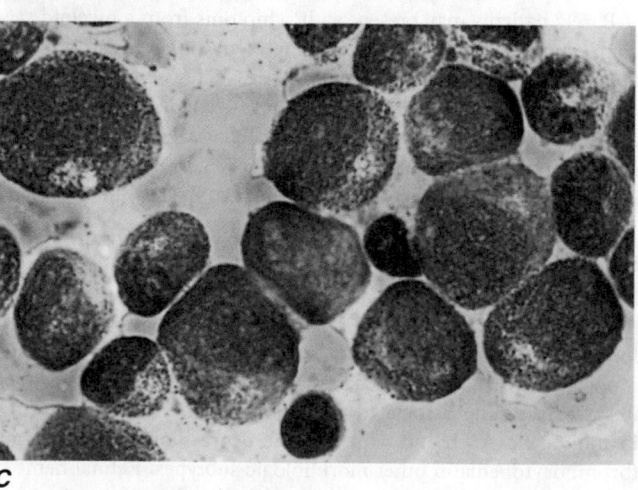

C

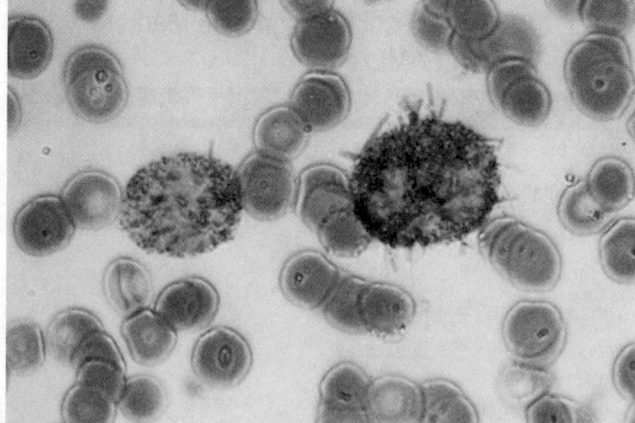

D

Figure 109-1 Morphology of AML cells. *A.* Uniform population of primitive myeloblasts with immature chromatin, nucleoli in some cells, and primary cytoplasmic granules. ***B.*** Leukemic myeloblast containing an Auer rod. ***C.*** Promyelocytic leukemia cells with prominent cytoplasmic primary granules. ***D.*** Peroxidase stain shows dark blue color characteristic of peroxidase in granules in AML.

TABLE 109-3 Initial Diagnostic Evaluation and Management of Adult Patients With AML

History

Increasing fatigue or decreased exercise tolerance (anemia)

Excess bleeding or bleeding from unusual sites (DIC, thrombocytopenia)

Fevers or recurrent infections (granulocytopenia)

Headache, vision changes, nonfocal neurologic abnormalities (CNS leukemia or bleed)

Early satiety (splenomegaly)

Family history of AML (Fanconi, Bloom, or Kostmann syndromes or ataxia-telangiectasia)

History of cancer (exposure to alkylating agents, radiation, topoisomerase II inhibitors)

Occupational exposures (radiation, benzene, petroleum products, paint, smoking, pesticides)

Physical Examination

Performance status (prognostic factor)

Ecchymosis and oozing from IV sites (DIC, possible acute promyelocytic leukemia)

Fever and tachycardia (signs of infection)

Papilledema, retinal infiltrates, cranial nerve abnormalities (CNS leukemia)

Poor dentition, dental abscesses

Gum hypertrophy (leukemic infiltration, most common in monocytic leukemia)

Skin infiltration or nodules (leukemia infiltration, most common in monocytic leukemia)

Lymphadenopathy, splenomegaly, hepatomegaly

Back pain, lower extremity weakness [spinal granulocytic sarcoma, most likely in t(8;21) patients]

Laboratory and Radiologic Studies

CBC with manual differential cell count

Chemistry tests (electrolytes, creatinine, BUN, calcium, phosphorus, uric acid, hepatic enzymes, bilirubin, LDH, amylase, lipase)

Clotting studies (prothrombin time, partial thromboplastin time, fibrinogen, D-dimer)

Viral serologies (CMV, HSV-1, varicella-zoster)

RBC type and screen

HLA typing for potential allogeneic HSCT

Bone marrow aspirate and biopsy (morphology, cytogenetics, flow cytometry, molecular studies for *NPM1* and *CEBPA* mutations and *FLT3*-ITD)

Cryopreservation of viable leukemia cells

Echocardiogram or heart scan

PA and lateral chest radiograph

Placement of central venous access device

Interventions for Specific Patients

Dental evaluation (for those with poor dentition)

Lumbar puncture (for those with symptoms of CNS involvement)

Screening spine MRI (for patients with back pain, lower extremity weakness, paresthesias)

Social work referral for patient and family psychosocial support

Counseling for All Patients

Provide patient with information regarding their disease, financial counseling, and support group contacts.

Abbreviations: AML, acute myeloid leukemia; BUN, blood urea nitrogen; CBC, complete blood count; CMV, cytomegalovirus; CNS, central nervous system; DIC, disseminated intravascular coagulation; HLA, human leukocyte antigen; HSCT, hematopoietic stem cell transplant; HSV, herpes simplex virus; LDH, lactate dehydrogenase; PA, posteroanterior; RBC, red blood (cell) count.

About 50% of patients have a mild to moderate elevation of serum uric acid at presentation. Only 10% have marked elevations, but renal precipitation of uric acid and the nephropathy that may result is a serious but uncommon complication. The initiation of chemotherapy may aggravate hyperuricemia, and patients are usually started immediately on allopurinol and hydration at diagnosis. Rasburicase (recombinant uric oxidase) is also useful for treating uric acid nephropathy and often can normalize the serum uric acid level within hours with a single dose of treatment. The presence of high concentrations of lysozyme, a marker for monocytic differentiation, may be etiologic in renal tubular dysfunction, which could worsen other renal problems that arise during the initial phases of therapy.

◼ PROGNOSTIC FACTORS

Many factors influence the likelihood of entering CR, the length of CR, and the curability of AML. CR is defined after examination of both blood and bone marrow. The blood neutrophil count must be ≥1000/μL and the platelet count ≥100,000/μL. Hemoglobin concentration is not considered in determining CR. Circulating blasts should be absent. While rare blasts may be detected in the blood during marrow regeneration, they should disappear on successive studies. The bone marrow should contain <5% blasts, and Auer rods should be absent. Extramedullary leukemia should not be present.

For patients in morphologic CR, immunophenotyping to detect minute populations of blasts, reverse transcriptase polymerase chain reaction (RT-PCR) to detect AML-associated molecular abnormalities, and either metaphase cytogenetics or interphase cytogenetics by fluorescence in situ hybridization (FISH) to detect AML-associated cytogenetic aberrations are currently being investigated to assess whether residual disease that has clinical significance is present following treatment. Detection of minimal residual disease may become a reliable discriminator between patients in CR who do or do not require additional and/or alternative therapies. In APL, detection of the *PML-RARA* fusion gene transcript by RT-PCR in bone marrow and/or blood during CR predicts relapse, and this assay is being routinely used in the clinic to anticipate clinical relapse and initiate timely salvage treatment. In other types of AML, the clinical relevance of minimal residual disease requires further investigation.

Age at diagnosis is among the most important risk factors. Advancing age is associated with a poorer prognosis, in part because of its influence on the patient's ability to survive induction therapy. Age also influences outcome because AML in older patients differs biologically. The leukemic cells in elderly patients more commonly express the multidrug resistance 1 (MDR1) efflux pump that conveys resistance to natural product–derived agents such as the anthracyclines (see below). With each successive decade of age, a greater proportion of patients have more resistant disease. Chronic and intercurrent diseases impair tolerance to rigorous therapy; acute medical problems at diagnosis reduce the likelihood of survival. Performance status, independent of age, also influences ability to survive induction therapy and thus respond to treatment.

A prolonged symptomatic interval with cytopenias preceding diagnosis or a history of an antecedent hematologic disorder is another pretreatment clinical feature associated with a lower CR rate and shorter survival time. The CR rate is lower in patients who have had anemia, leukopenia, and/or thrombocytopenia for >3 months before the diagnosis of AML when compared to those without such a history. Responsiveness to chemotherapy declines as the duration of the antecedent disorder(s) increases. AML developing after treatment with cytotoxic agents for other malignancies is usually difficult to treat successfully.

A high presenting leukocyte count in some series is an independent prognostic factor for attaining a CR. Among patients with hyperleukocytosis (>100,000/μL), early central nervous system bleeding and pulmonary leukostasis contribute to poor outcome with initial therapy.

Chromosome findings at diagnosis are currently the most important independent prognostic factor. Patients with t(15;17) have a very good prognosis (approximately 85% cured), and those with t(8;21) and inv(16) a good prognosis (approximately 55% cured), while those with no cytogenetic abnormality have a moderately favorable outcome (approximately 40% cured). Patients with a complex karyotype, t(6;9), inv(3), or -7 have a very poor prognosis.

For those patients lacking prognostic cytogenetic abnormalities, such as those with CN-AML, outcome prediction utilizes molecular genetic abnormalities. *NPM1* mutations without concurrent presence of *FLT3*-ITD, and *CEBPA* mutations, especially if concurrently present in two different alleles, have been shown to predict favorable outcome, whereas *FLT3*-ITD predicts poor outcome. Given the prognostic importance of *NPM1* and *CEBPA* mutations and *FLT3*-ITD, molecular assessment of these genes at diagnosis have been incorporated in AML management guidelines by the National Comprehensive Cancer Network (NCCN) and the European Leukemia Net (ELN). Other molecular aberrations (Table 109-2) may in the future be utilized for prognostication.

In addition to pretreatment variables such as age, leukocyte count, and cytogenetics and/or molecular genetic aberrations, several treatment factors correlate with prognosis in AML, including, most importantly, achievement of CR. In addition, patients who achieve CR after one induction cycle have longer CR durations than those requiring multiple cycles.

| TREATMENT | Acute Myeloid Leukemia |

Treatment of the newly diagnosed patient with AML is usually divided into two phases, induction and postremission management (Fig. 109-2). The initial goal is to quickly induce CR. Once CR is obtained, further therapy must be used to prolong survival and achieve cure. The initial induction treatment and subsequent postremission therapy are often chosen based on the patient's age. Intensifying therapy with traditional chemotherapy agents such as cytarabine and anthracyclines in younger patients (<60 years) appears to increase the cure rate of AML. In older patients the benefit of intensive therapy is controversial; novel therapies are being pursued.

INDUCTION CHEMOTHERAPY The most commonly used CR induction regimens (for patients other than those with APL) consist of combination chemotherapy with cytarabine and an anthracycline. Cytarabine is a cell cycle S-phase–specific antimetabolite that becomes phosphorylated intracellularly to an active triphosphate form that interferes with DNA synthesis. Anthracyclines are DNA intercalators. Their primary mode of action is thought to be inhibition of topoisomerase II, leading to DNA breaks. Cytarabine is usually administered as a continuous intravenous infusion for 7 days. Anthracycline therapy generally consists of daunorubicin intravenously on days 1, 2, and 3 (the 7 and 3 regimen). Treatment with idarubicin for 3 days in conjunction with cytarabine by 7-day continuous infusion is at least as effective as daunorubicin in younger patients. The addition of etoposide may improve the CR duration. When combined with cytarabine in a 7 and 3 regimen, a higher dose of anthracycline (i.e., daunorubicin 90 mg/m^2) improves outcome compared with a lower dose (i.e., daunorubicin 45 mg/m^2).

After induction chemotherapy, if persistence of leukemia is documented, the patient is usually re-treated with cytarabine and an anthracycline in doses similar to those given initially, but for 5 and 2 days, respectively. Our recommendation, however, is to consider changing therapy in this setting.

With the 7 and 3 cytarabine/daunorubicin regimen outlined above, 65–75% of adults with de novo AML younger than age 60 years achieve CR. Two-thirds achieve CR after a single course of therapy, and one-third require two courses. About 50% of patients who do not achieve CR have a drug-resistant leukemia, and 50% do not achieve CR because of fatal complications of bone marrow aplasia or impaired recovery of normal stem cells.

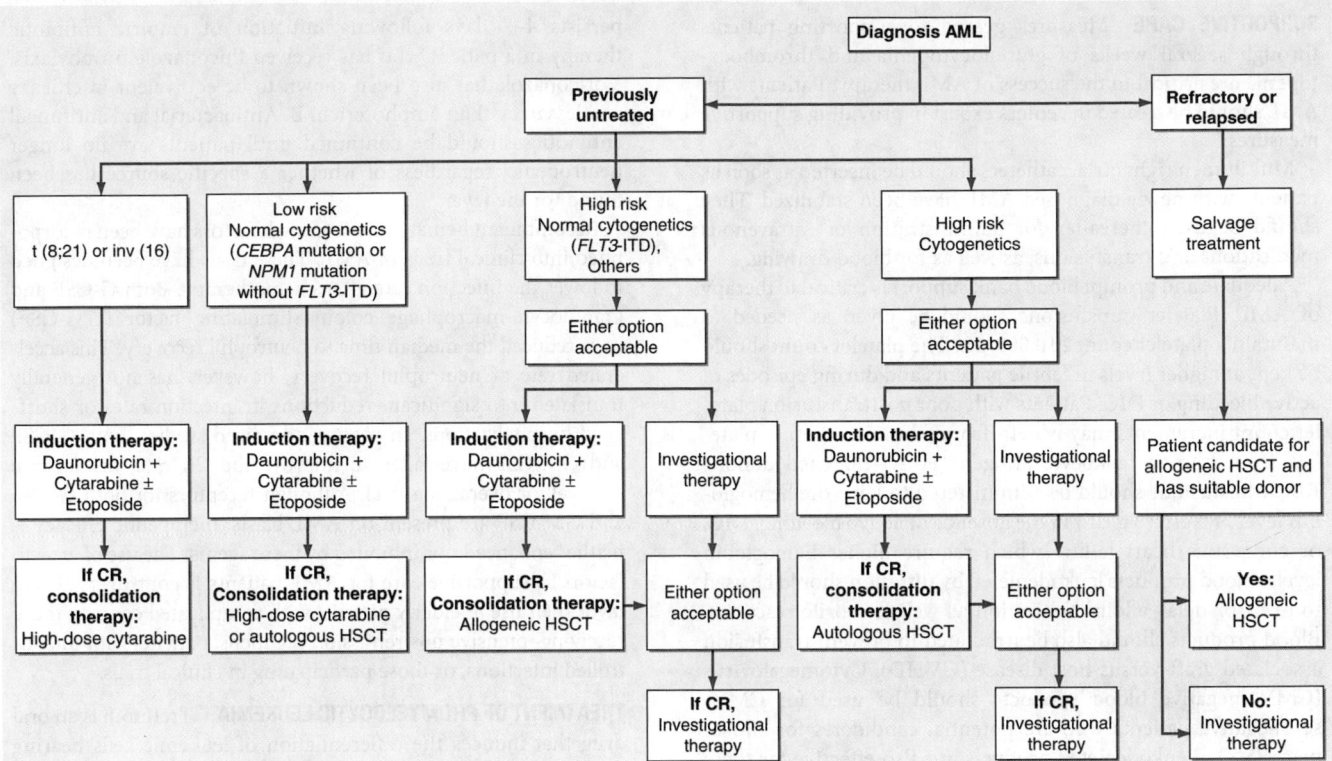

Figure 109-2 Flow chart for the therapy of newly diagnosed acute myeloid leukemia. For all forms of AML except acute promyelocytic leukemia (APL), standard therapy includes a 7-day continuous infusion of cytarabine (100–200 mg/m² per day) and a 3-day course of daunorubicin (60–90 mg/m² per day) with or without 3 days of etoposide (only with daunorubicin 60 mg/m² per day) or novel therapies based on their predicted risk of relapse (i.e., risk-stratified therapy). Idarubicin (12–13 mg/m² per day) could be used in place of daunorubicin (not shown). Patients who achieve complete remission undergo postremission consolidation therapy, including sequential courses of high-dose cytarabine, autologous hematopoietic stem cell transplant (HSCT), allogeneic HSCT, or novel therapies, based on their predicted risk of relapse (i.e., risk-stratified therapy). Patients with APL (see text for treatment) usually receive tretinoin together with anthracycline-based chemotherapy for remission induction and then arsenic trioxide followed by consolidation with anthracycline-based chemotherapy and possibly maintenance with tretinoin. The role of cytarabine in APL induction and consolidation is controversial.

Higher induction treatment–related mortality rate and frequency of resistant disease have been observed with increasing age and in patients with prior hematologic disorders (MDS or myeloproliferative syndromes) or chemotherapy treatment for another malignancy.

Patients who fail to attain CR after two induction courses should be treated with an allogeneic hematopoietic stem cell transplant (HSCT) if an appropriate donor exists. Whether achievement of cytoreduction of disease burden with a salvage treatment should be attempted before a patient with refractory disease after two induction courses can proceed to HSCT is controversial.

High-dose cytarabine-based regimens have high CR rates after a single cycle of therapy. When given in high doses, more cytarabine may enter the cells, saturate the cytarabine-inactivating enzymes, and increase the intracellular levels of 1-β-D-arabinofuranylcytosine-triphosphate, the active metabolite incorporated into DNA. Thus, higher doses of cytarabine may increase the inhibition of DNA synthesis and thereby overcome resistance to standard-dose cytarabine. In two randomized studies, high-dose cytarabine with an anthracycline produced CR rates similar to those achieved with standard 7 and 3 regimens. However, the CR duration was longer after high-dose cytarabine than after standard-dose cytarabine.

The hematologic toxicity of high-dose cytarabine-based induction regimens has typically been greater than that associated with 7 and 3 regimens. Toxicity with high-dose cytarabine includes myelosuppression, pulmonary toxicity, and significant and occasionally irreversible cerebellar toxicity. All patients treated with high-dose cytarabine must be closely monitored for cerebellar toxicity. Full cerebellar testing should be performed before each dose, and further high-dose cytarabine should be withheld if evidence of cerebellar toxicity develops. This toxicity occurs more commonly in patients with renal impairment and in those older than age 60 years. The increased toxicity observed with high-dose cytarabine has limited the use of this therapy in elderly AML patients.

Because of the negative impact of age on outcome when treatment with conventional chemotherapy is administered, clinical trials in elderly patients have focused upon new agents or alternative approaches such as reduced-intensity allogeneic HSCT. Among these, one promising therapy is decitabine, a nucleoside analogue that inhibits DNA methyltransferase, reverses aberrant DNA methylation, and subsequently induces transcription of otherwise silenced tumor suppressor genes in AML cells. Interestingly, this effect on inhibiting DNA methyltransferase occurs at a much lower dose than previously used with this agent to produce a cytotoxic effect in AML. Low-dose decitabine yields complete responses in older patients with AML, including those with unfavorable karyotypes. Other agents with relatively favorable toxicity profiles such as clofarabine have activity in older patients with AML.

SUPPORTIVE CARE Measures geared to supporting patients through several weeks of granulocytopenia and thrombocytopenia are critical to the success of AML therapy. Patients with AML should be treated in centers expert in providing supportive measures.

Multilumen right atrial catheters should be inserted as soon as patients with newly diagnosed AML have been stabilized. They should be used thereafter for administration of intravenous medications and transfusions, as well as for blood drawing.

Adequate and prompt blood bank support is critical to therapy of AML. Platelet transfusions should be given as needed to maintain a platelet count ≥10,000/μL. The platelet count should be kept at higher levels in febrile patients and during episodes of active bleeding or DIC. Patients with poor posttransfusion platelet count increments may benefit from administration of platelets from human leukocyte antigen (HLA)–matched donors. RBC transfusions should be administered to keep the hemoglobin level >80 g/L (8 g/dL) in the absence of active bleeding, DIC, or congestive heart failure which require higher hemoglobin levels. Blood products leukodepleted by filtration should be used to avert or delay alloimmunization as well as febrile reactions. Blood products should also be irradiated to prevent transfusion associated graft-versus-host disease (GVHD). Cytomegalovirus (CMV)-negative blood products should be used for CMV-seronegative patients who are potential candidates for allogeneic HSCT. Leukodepleted products are also effective for these patients if CMV-negative products are not available.

Infectious complications remain the major cause of morbidity and death during induction and postremission chemotherapy for AML. Antibacterial (i.e., quinolones) and antifungal (e.g, fluconazole, posaconazole) prophylaxis in the absence of fever is likely to be beneficial. For patients who are herpes simplex virus– or varicella zoster–seropositive, antiviral prophylaxis should be initiated.

Fever develops in most patients with AML, but infections are documented in only half of febrile patients. Early initiation of empirical broad-spectrum antibacterial and antifungal antibiotics has significantly reduced the number of patients dying of infectious complications (Chap. 86). An antibiotic regimen adequate to treat gram-negative organisms should be instituted at the onset of fever in a granulocytopenic patient after clinical evaluation, including a detailed physical examination with inspection of the indwelling catheter exit site and a perirectal examination, as well as procurement of cultures and radiographs aimed at documenting the source of fever. Specific antibiotic regimens should be based on antibiotic sensitivity data obtained from the institution at which the patient is being treated. Acceptable regimens for empiric antibiotic therapy include monotherapy with imipenem-cilastin, meropenem, piperacillin/tazobactam, or an extended-spectrum antipseudomonal cephalosporin (cefepime or ceftazidime); an aminoglycoside in combination with an antipseudomonal penicillin (e.g., piperacillin); an aminoglycoside in combination with an extended-spectrum antipseudomonal cephalosporin; and ciprofloxacin in combination with an antipseudomonal penicillin. Aminoglycosides should be avoided if possible in patients with renal insufficiency. Empirical vancomycin should be initiated in neutropenic patients with catheter-related infections, blood cultures positive for gram-positive bacteria before final identification and susceptibility testing, hypotension or shock, and increased risk for viridans group streptococcal bacteremia.

Caspofungin (or similar echinocandin) or liposomal amphotericin B should be considered for antifungal treatment if fever persists 4–7 days following initiation of empiric antibiotic therapy in a patient who has received fluconazole prophylaxis. Voriconazole has also been shown to be equivalent in efficacy and less toxic than amphotericin B. Antibacterial and antifungal antibiotics should be continued until patients are no longer neutropenic, regardless of whether a specific source has been found for the fever.

Recombinant hematopoietic growth factors have been incorporated into clinical trials in AML. These trials have been designed to lower the infection rate after chemotherapy. Both G-CSF and granulocyte-macrophage colony-stimulating factor (GM-CSF) have reduced the median time to neutrophil recovery. This accelerated rate of neutrophil recovery, however, has not generally translated into significant reductions in infection rates or shortened hospitalizations. In most randomized studies, both G-CSF and GM-CSF have failed to improve the CR rate, disease-free survival, or overall survival. Although receptors for both G-CSF and GM-CSF are present on AML blasts, therapeutic efficacy is neither enhanced nor inhibited by these agents. The use of growth factors as supportive care for AML patients is controversial. We favor their use in elderly patients with complicated courses, those receiving intensive postremission regimens, patients with uncontrolled infections, or those participating in clinical trials.

TREATMENT OF PROMYELOCYTIC LEUKEMIA Tretinoin is an oral drug that induces the differentiation of leukemic cells bearing the t(15;17). APL is responsive to cytarabine and daunorubicin, but about 10% of patients treated with these drugs die from DIC induced by the release of granule components by dying tumor cells. Tretinoin does not produce DIC but produces another complication called the APL differentiation syndrome. Occurring within the first 3 weeks of treatment, it is characterized by fever, fluid retention, dyspnea, chest pain, pulmonary infiltrates, pleural and pericardial effusions, and hypoxemia. The syndrome is related to adhesion of differentiated neoplastic cells to the pulmonary vasculature endothelium. Glucocorticoids, chemotherapy, and/or supportive measures can be effective for management of the APL differentiation syndrome. Temporary discontinuation of tretinoin is necessary in cases of severe APL differentiation syndrome (i.e., patients developing renal failure or requiring admission to the intensive care unit due to respiratory distress). The mortality rate of this syndrome is about 10%.

Tretinoin (45 mg/m² per day orally until remission is documented) plus concurrent anthracycline-based chemotherapy appears to be among the most effective treatments for APL leading to CR rates of 90–95%. The addition of cytarabine, although not demonstrated to increase the CR rate, seemingly decreases the risk for relapse. Following achievement of CR, patients should receive at least two cycles of anthracycline-based chemotherapy.

Given the progress made in APL resulting in high cure rates, the goals are to identify patients with very low risk of relapse where attempts are being made to decrease the amount of therapy administered and to identify patients at greatest risk of relapse in order to develop new approaches to increase cure.

Arsenic trioxide has significant antileukemic activity and is being explored as part of initial treatment in clinical trials of APL. In a randomized trial, arsenic trioxide improved outcome if utilized after achievement of CR and before consolidation therapy with anthracycline-based chemotherapy. Additionally, studies combining arsenic trioxide with tretinoin in the absence of chemotherapy are ongoing and preliminarily have shown promise in those patients "unfit" to receive chemotherapy. Furthermore, combinations of arsenic trioxide, tretinoin, and/or chemotherapy and/or gemtuzumab ozogamicin, a monoclonal CD33 antibody linked to the cytotoxic agent calicheamicin, have shown favorable response in high-risk APL patients (i.e., those presenting with a leukocyte count ≥10,000/μL) at diagnosis. Patients receiving arsenic trioxide are at risk of APL differentiation syndrome, especially when it is administered during induction or salvage treatment after disease relapse. In addition, arsenic trioxide may prolong the QT interval, increasing the risk of cardiac arrhythmias.

Assessment of residual disease by RT-PCR amplification of the t(15;17) chimeric gene product *PML-RARA* following the final cycle of chemotherapy is an important step in the management of APL patients. Disappearance of the signal is associated with long-term disease-free survival; its persistence documented by two consecutive tests performed 2 weeks apart invariably predicts relapse. Sequential monitoring of RT-PCR for t(15;17) is now considered standard for postremission monitoring of APL.

Patients who continue in molecular remission may benefit from maintenance therapy with tretinoin. Patients in molecular, cytogenetic, or clinical relapse should be salvaged with arsenic trioxide; it produces meaningful responses in up to 85% of patients and can be followed by HSCT.

POSTREMISSION THERAPY Induction of a durable first CR is critical to long-term disease-free survival in AML. However, without further therapy, virtually all patients experience relapse. Once relapse has occurred, AML is generally curable only by HSCT.

Postremission therapy is designed to eradicate residual leukemic cells to prevent relapse and prolong survival. Postremission therapy in AML is often based on age (younger than ages 55–65 years and older than ages 55–65 years). For younger patients, most studies include intensive chemotherapy and allogeneic or autologous HSCT. High-dose cytarabine is more effective than standard-dose cytarabine. The Cancer and Leukemia Group B (CALGB), for example, compared the duration of CR in patients randomly assigned postremission to four cycles of high (3 g/m², every 12 hours on days 1, 3, and 5), intermediate (400 mg/m² for 5 days by continuous infusion), or standard (100 mg/m² per day for 5 days by continuous infusion) doses of cytarabine. A dose-response effect for cytarabine in patients with AML who were aged ≤60 years was demonstrated. High-dose cytarabine significantly prolonged CR and increased the fraction cured in patients with favorable [t(8;21) and inv(16)] and normal cytogenetics, but it had no significant effect on patients with other abnormal karyotypes. For older patients, exploration of attenuated intensive therapy that includes either chemotherapy or reduced-intensity allogeneic HSCT has been pursued. Postremission therapy is a setting for introduction of new agents (Table 109-4).

Allogeneic HSCT is used in patients ages <70–75 years with an HLA-compatible donor who have high-risk cytogenetics. In patients with CN-AML and high-risk molecular features such as *FLT3*-ITD, allogeneic HSCT is best applied in the context of clinical trials, as the impact of aggressive therapy on outcome is unknown. Relapse following allogeneic HSCT occurs in only a small fraction of patients, but treatment-related toxicity is relatively high; complications include venoocclusive disease, GVHD, and infections. Autologous HSCT can be administered in young and older patients and uses the same preparative regimens. Patients subsequently receive their own stem cells collected while in remission. The toxicity is relatively low with autologous HSCT (5% mortality rate), but the relapse rate is higher than with allogeneic HSCT, due to the absence of the graft-versus-leukemia (GVL) effect seen with allogeneic HSCT and possible contamination of the autologous stem cells with

TABLE 109-4 Selected New Agents Under Study for the Treatment of Adults With AML

Class of Drugs	Examples of Agents in Class
Tyrosine kinase inhibitors	PKC412, MLN518, SU11248, CHIR-258, imatinib (STI571, Gleevec), dasatinib, AMN107
Demethylating agents	Decitabine, 5-azacytidine
Histone deacetylase inhibitors	Suberoylanilide hydroxamic acid (SAHA), MS275, LBH589, valproic acid
Heavy metals	Arsenic trioxide
Farnesyl transferase inhibitors	R115777, SCH66336
HSP-90 antagonists	17-allylaminogeldanamycin (17-AAG), DMAG, or derivatives
Cell cycle inhibitors	Flavopiridol, CYC202 (R-Roscovitine), SNS-032
Nucleoside analogues	Clofarabine, troxacitabine
Humanized antibodies	Anti-CD33 (SGN33), anti-KIR
Toxin-conjugated antibodies	Gemtuzumab ozogamicin
Proteasome inhibitors	Bortezomib
Aurora inhibitors	AZD1152, MLN-8237, AT9283
Immunomodulatory	Lenalidomide, IL-2, histamine dihydrochloride

Abbreviations: AML, acute myeloid leukemia; IL-2, interleukin.

residual tumor cells. Purging tumor from the autologous stem cells has not lowered the relapse rate with autologous HSCT.

Randomized trials comparing intensive chemotherapy and autologous and allogeneic HSCT have shown improved duration of remission with allogeneic HSCT compared to autologous HSCT or chemotherapy alone. However, overall survival is generally not different; the improved disease control with allogeneic HSCT is erased by the increase in fatal toxicity. While stem cells were previously harvested from the bone marrow, virtually all efforts currently collect these from the blood following mobilization regimens. Prognostic factors may help select patients in first CR for whom transplant is most effective.

Our approach includes allogeneic HSCT if feasible in first CR for patients with high-risk karyotypes (Fig. 109-2). Patients with CN-AML who have other poor risk factors (e.g., an antecedent hematologic disorder, or failure to attain remission with a single induction course) and patients lacking a favorable genotype (e.g., patients who do not have *CEBPA* mutations or *NPM1* mutations without *FLT3*-ITD) are also potential candidates. If a suitable HLA donor does not exist, investigational therapeutic approaches are considered. As *FLT3*-ITD can be targeted with emerging novel inhibitors, patients with this molecular abnormality should be considered for clinical trials with these agents whenever possible. New transplant strategies, including reduced-intensity HSCT, are being explored for consolidation of high-risk AML patients (Chap. 114). Patients with t(8;21) and inv(16) are treated with repetitive doses of high-dose cytarabine, which offers a high frequency of cure without the morbidity of transplant. In AML patients with t(8;21) and inv(16), those with

KIT mutations, who have a worse prognosis, may be considered for novel investigational studies.

Autologous HSCT is generally applied to AML patients only in the context of a clinical trial or when the risk of repetitive intensive chemotherapy represents a higher risk than the autologous HSCT (e.g., in patients with severe platelet alloimmunization).

RELAPSE Once relapse occurs, patients are rarely cured with further standard-dose chemotherapy. Patients eligible for allogeneic HSCT should receive transplants expeditiously at the first sign of relapse. Long-term disease-free survival is approximately the same (30–50%) with allogeneic HSCT in first relapse or in second remission. Autologous HSCT rescues about 20% of relapsed patients with AML who have chemosensitive disease. The most important factors predicting response at relapse are the length of the previous CR, whether initial CR was achieved with one or two courses of chemotherapy, and the type of postremission therapy.

Because of the poor outcome of patients in early first relapse (<12 months), it is justified (for patients without HLA-compatible donors) to explore innovative approaches, such as new drugs or immunotherapies (Table 109-4). Patients with longer first CR (>12 months) generally relapse with drug-sensitive disease and have a higher chance of attaining a CR. However, cure is uncommon, and treatment with novel approaches should be considered if allogeneic HSCT is not possible. New agents that may have clinical activity in AML are needed and many are being tested in clinical trials (Table 109-4).

For elderly patients (age >60 years) for whom clinical trials are not available, gemtuzumab ozogamicin is another alternative. The CR rate with this agent is ~30%. However, its effectiveness in early relapsing (<6 months) or refractory AML patients is limited, possibly due to calicheamicin being a potent MDR1 substrate. Toxicity, including myelosuppression, infusion toxicity, and venoocclusive disease, can be observed with gemtuzumab ozogamicin. Pretreatment with glucocorticoids can diminish many of the associated infusion reactions. Studies are examining this treatment in combination with chemotherapy for both young and older patients with previously untreated AML. This agent has been withdrawn from the U.S. market at the request of the U.S. Food and Drug Administration due to concerns about the product's safety and clinical benefit as shown in trials subsequent to those leading to its accelerated approval.

CHRONIC MYELOID LEUKEMIA

■ INCIDENCE

The incidence of chronic myeloid leukemia (CML) is 1.5 per 100,000 people per year, and the age-adjusted incidence is higher in men than in women (1.9 vs 1.1). The incidence of CML increases slowly with age until the middle forties, when it starts to rise rapidly. The incidence of CML for females decreased slightly (1.8%) between 1994 and 2006 as compared to 1975–1994.

■ DEFINITION

The diagnosis of CML is established by identifying a clonal expansion of a hematopoietic stem cell possessing a reciprocal translocation between chromosomes 9 and 22. This translocation results in the head-to-tail fusion of the breakpoint cluster region (*BCR*) gene on chromosome 22q11 with the *ABL1* (named after the abelson murine leukemia virus) gene located on chromosome 9q34. Untreated, the disease is characterized by the inevitable transition from a chronic phase to an accelerated phase and on to blast crisis in a median time of 4 years.

■ ETIOLOGY

No clear correlation with exposure to cytotoxic drugs has been found, and no evidence suggests a viral etiology. In the pre-imatinib era, cigarette smoking accelerated the progression to blast crisis and therefore adversely affected survival in CML. Atomic bomb survivors had an increased incidence; the development of a CML cell mass of 10,000/μL took 6.3 years. No increase in CML incidence was found in the survivors of the Chernobyl accident, suggesting that only large doses of radiation can induce CML.

■ PATHOPHYSIOLOGY

The product of the fusion gene resulting from the t(9;22) plays a central role in the development of CML. This chimeric gene is transcribed into a hybrid *BCR-ABL1* mRNA in which exon 1 of *ABL1* is replaced by variable numbers of 5′ *BCR* exons. Bcr-Abl fusion proteins, p210$^{BCR-ABL1}$, are produced that contain NH_2-terminal domains of Bcr and the COOH-terminal domains of Abl. A rare breakpoint, occurring within the 3′ region of the *BCR* gene, yields a fusion protein of 230 kDa, p230$^{BCR-ABL1}$. Bcr-Abl fusion proteins can transform hematopoietic progenitor cells in vitro. Furthermore, reconstituting lethally irradiated mice with bone marrow cells infected with retrovirus carrying the gene encoding the p210$^{BCR-ABL1}$ leads to the development of a myeloproliferative syndrome resembling CML in 50% of the mice. Specific antisense oligomers to the *BCR-ABL1* junction inhibit the growth of t(9;22)-positive leukemic cells without affecting normal colony formation.

The mechanism(s) by which p210$^{BCR-ABL1}$ promotes the transition from the benign state to the fully malignant one is still unclear. Messenger RNA for *BCR-ABL1* can occasionally be detected in normal individuals. However, attachment of the *BCR* sequences to *ABL1* results in three critical functional changes: (1) the Abl protein becomes constitutively active as a tyrosine kinase (TK) enzyme, activating downstream kinases that prevent apoptosis; (2) the DNA-protein-binding activity of Abl is attenuated; and (3) the binding of Abl to cytoskeletal actin microfilaments is enhanced.

Disease progression

The events associated with transition to the acute phase, a common occurrence in the pre-imatinib era, were extensively studied. Chromosomal instability of the malignant clone resulting, for example, in the acquisition of an additional t(9;22), trisomy 8, or 17p- (*TP53* loss) is a basic feature of CML. Acquisition of these additional genetic and/or molecular abnormalities is critical to the phenotypic transformation. Heterogeneous structural alterations of the *TP53* gene, as well as structural alterations and lack of protein production of the retinoblastoma 1 (*RB1*) gene and the catalytic component of telomerase, have been associated with disease progression in a subset of patients. Rare patients show alterations in the rat sarcoma viral oncogene homologue (*RAS*). Sporadic reports also document the presence of an altered v-myc myelocytomatosis viral oncogene homologue (avian) (*MYC*) gene. Progressive de novo DNA methylation at the *BCR-ABL1* locus and hypomethylation of the *LINE-1* retrotransposon promoter herald blastic transformation. Further, interleukin 1β may be involved in the progression of CML to the blastic phase. In addition, functional inactivation of the tumor suppressor protein phosphatase A2 may be required for blastic transformation. Finally, CML that develops resistance to imatinib is at an increased risk of progressing to accelerated/blast crisis. Multiple pathways to disease transformation exist, but the exact timing and relevance of each remain unclear.

■ CLINICAL PRESENTATION

Symptoms

The clinical onset of the chronic phase is generally insidious. Accordingly, some patients are diagnosed, while still asymptomatic, during health-screening tests; other patients present with fatigue, malaise, and weight loss or have symptoms resulting from splenic enlargement, such as early satiety and left upper quadrant pain or mass. Less common are features related to granulocyte or platelet dysfunction, such as infections, thrombosis, or bleeding. Occasionally, patients present with leukostatic manifestations due to severe leukocytosis or thrombosis such as vasoocclusive disease, cerebrovascular accidents, myocardial infarction, venous thrombosis, priapism, visual disturbances, and pulmonary insufficiency. Patients with p230*BCR-ABL1*-positive CML have a more indolent course.

Progression of CML is associated with worsening symptoms. Unexplained fever, significant weight loss, increasing dose requirement of the drugs controlling the disease, bone and joint pain, bleeding, thrombosis, and infections suggest transformation into accelerated or blastic phases. Less than 10–15% of newly diagnosed patients present with accelerated disease or with de novo blastic phase CML.

Physical findings

Minimal to moderate splenomegaly is the most common physical finding; mild hepatomegaly is found occasionally. Persistent splenomegaly despite continued therapy is a sign of disease acceleration. Lymphadenopathy and myeloid sarcomas are unusual except late in the course of the disease; when they are present, the prognosis is poor.

Hematologic findings

Elevated white blood (cell) counts (WBCs), with increases in both immature and mature granulocytes, are present at diagnosis. Usually <5% circulating blasts and <10% blasts and promyelocytes are noted, with the majority of cells being myelocytes, metamyelocytes, and band forms. Cycling of the counts may be observed in patients followed without treatment. Platelet counts are almost always elevated at diagnosis, and a mild degree of normocytic normochromic anemia is present. Leukocyte alkaline phosphatase is low in CML cells. Phagocytic functions are usually normal at diagnosis and remain normal during the chronic phase. Histamine production secondary to basophilia is increased in later stages, causing pruritus, diarrhea, and flushing.

At diagnosis, bone marrow cellularity is increased, with an increased myeloid-to-erythroid ratio. The marrow blast percentage is generally normal or slightly elevated. Marrow or blood basophilia, eosinophilia, and monocytosis may be present. While collagen fibrosis in the marrow is unusual at presentation, significant degrees of reticulin stain–measured fibrosis are noted in about half of the patients.

Disease acceleration is defined by the development of increasing degrees of anemia unaccounted for by bleeding or therapy; cytogenetic clonal evolution; or blood or marrow blasts between 10 and 20%, blood or marrow basophils ≥20%, or platelet count <100,000/μL. *Blast crisis* is defined as acute leukemia, with blood or marrow blasts ≥20%. Hyposegmented neutrophils may appear (Pelger-Huët anomaly). Blast cells can be classified as myeloid, lymphoid, erythroid, or undifferentiated, based on morphologic, cytochemical, and immunologic features. Occurrence of de novo blast crisis or following imatinib therapy is rare.

Chromosomal findings

The cytogenetic hallmark of CML, found in 90–95% of patients, is the t(9;22)(q34;q11.2). Originally, this was recognized by the presence of a shortened chromosome 22 (22q-), designated as the *Philadelphia chromosome*, that arises from the reciprocal t(9;22). Some patients may have complex translocations (designated as *variant translocations*) involving three, four, or five chromosomes

(usually including chromosomes 9 and 22). However, the molecular consequences of these changes are similar to those resulting from the typical t(9;22). All patients should have evidence of the translocation molecularly or by cytogenetics or FISH to make a diagnosis of CML.

■ PROGNOSTIC FACTORS

The clinical outcome of patients with CML is variable. Before imatinib mesylate, death was expected in 10% of patients within 2 years and in about 20% yearly thereafter, and the median survival time was ~4 years. Therefore, several prognostic models that identify different risk groups in CML were developed. The most commonly used staging systems have been derived from multivariate analyses of prognostic factors. The *Sokal index* identified percentage of circulating blasts, spleen size, platelet count, age, and cytogenetic clonal evolution as the most important prognostic indicators. This system was developed based on chemotherapy-treated patients. The *Hasford system* was developed based on interferon (IFN) α–treated patients. It identified percentage of circulating blasts, spleen size, platelet count, age, and percentage of eosinophils and basophils as the most important prognostic indicators. This system differs from the Sokal index by ignoring clonal evolution and incorporating percentage of eosinophils and basophils. When applied to a data set of 272 patients treated with IFN-α, the Hasford system was better than the Sokal score for predicting survival time; it identified more low-risk patients but left only a small number of cases in the high-risk group. Preliminary results suggest that both the Sokal and the Hasford systems are applicable to imatinib-treated patients.

TREATMENT   Chronic Myeloid Leukemia

The therapy of CML is changing rapidly because we have a proven curative treatment (allogeneic transplantation) that has significant toxicity and a new targeted treatment (imatinib) with outstanding outcome based on 8-year follow-up data. We recommend starting with TK inhibitors and reserving allogeneic transplantation for those who develop imatinib resistance.

At present, the goal of therapy in CML is to achieve prolonged, durable, nonneoplastic, nonclonal hematopoiesis, which entails the eradication of any residual cells containing the *BCR-ABL1* transcript. Hence, the goal is complete molecular remission and cure. A proposed imatinib treatment algorithm for the newly diagnosed CML patient is presented in Table 109-5.

IMATINIB MESYLATE   Imatinib mesylate (Gleevec) functions through competitive inhibition at the ATP-binding site of the Abl kinase in the inactive conformation, which leads to inhibition of tyrosine phosphorylation of proteins involved in Bcr-Abl signal transduction. It shows specificity for Bcr-Abl, the receptor for platelet-derived growth factor, and Kit TK. Imatinib induces apoptosis in cells expressing Bcr-Abl.

In newly diagnosed CML, imatinib (400 mg/d) is more effective than IFN-α and cytarabine. The complete hematologic remission rate of patients treated with imatinib was 95% compared to 56% in patients treated with IFN-α and cytarabine. Similarly, the complete cytogenetic remission rate at 18 months was 76% with imatinib compared to 15% with IFN-α and cytarabine. The rate of complete cytogenetic remission in imatinib-treated patients differed by Sokal score: the rate in those with low-risk disease was 89% compared with 82% for patients with intermediate-risk disease and 69% for those with high-risk disease.

TABLE 109-5 Imatinib Treatment Milestones for Newly Diagnosed CML Patients

| Time Months | NCCN[a] | | ELN[b] | |
	Expected[c]	Failure[d]	Suboptimal[e]	Failure[d]
3	Complete hematologic remission[f]	No complete hematologic remission	Minor cytogenetic remission	No cytogenetic remission; new mutations
6	Any cytogenetic remission	No cytogenetic remission	Partial cytogenetic remission	Minimal cytogenetic remission[g]; new mutations
12	Complete[h] or partial[i] cytogenetic remission	Minor[j] or no cytogenetic remission	Less than major molecular response	Less than partial cytogenetic remission; new mutations
18	Complete cytogenetic remission	Partial, minor, or no cytogenetic remission		
Anytime	Loss of previously achieved hematologic, cytogenetic, or molecular remission; new mutations[d]			

[a]National Comprehensive Cancer Network.
[b]European Leukemia Net.
[c]Denotes that at the indicated milestone, patients should stay on the same dose.
[d]Denotes that at the indicated milestones, for patients on 400 mg/d, one can either increase the dose to a maximum of 600–800 mg, as tolerated, or probably switch to another TK inhibitor.
[e]Denotes that the patients may still have substantial long-term benefit from continuing a specific treatment, but chances are reduced and therefore these patients may be eligible for alternative treatments.
[f]Complete hematologic remission, white blood cell count <10,000/μL, normal morphology, hemoglobin and platelet counts, and disappearance of splenomegaly.
[g]Minimal cytogenetic remission, 66–95% bone marrow metaphases with t(9;22).
[h]Complete cytogenetic remission, no bone marrow metaphases with t(9;22).
[i]Partial cytogenetic remission, 1–35% bone marrow metaphases with t(9;22).
[j]Minor cytogenetic remission, 36–85% bone marrow metaphases with t(9;22).
Abbreviation: CML, chronic myeloid leukemia.

All imatinib-treated patients who achieved major molecular remission (26%), defined as ≥3 log reduction in *BCR-ABL1* transcript level at 18 months compared to pretreatment level, were progression-free at 5 years. The progression-free survival (PFS) at 5 years for patients achieving complete cytogenetic remission but less pronounced molecular remission is 98%. The 5-year PFS for patients not achieving complete cytogenetic remission at 18 months was 87%. These results have led to a consensus that molecular responses can be used as a treatment goal in CML. Specific milestones have been developed for chronic-phase CML patients (Table 109-5). They differ between the Americans (NCCN) and the Europeans (ELN), with more strict milestones by the latter. For example, in the NCCN milestones, chronic-phase CML patients who do not achieve any cytogenetic remission following 6 months of imatinib should be offered other treatment approaches while in the ELN milestones, the same recommendation is offered following 3 months of imatinib treatment. We favor the ELN approach and expect the NCCN milestones to align with the ELN ones in the very near future.

Progression to accelerated/blastic phases of the disease was noted in 3% of patients treated with imatinib as compared to 8.5% of patients treated with IFN-α and cytarabine during the first year. Over time, the annual incidence of disease progression on imatinib decreased gradually to <1% during the fourth year and beyond, and no patient who achieved major molecular response by 12 months progressed to the accelerated/blastic phases of the disease.

Treatment is currently recommended for life unless patients are enrolled in a clinical trial with a specific question of treatment discontinuation. An early trial evaluating the effect of imatinib discontinuation after at least 2 years of complete molecular remission revealed molecular relapse in 6 of 12 patients. Interestingly, 6 of 10 patients who were treated with IFN-α before imatinib maintained molecular remission, while both patients who were not exposed to IFN-α relapsed. These results raised the hypothesis that IFN-α may have a protective effect against relapse, possibly by eradicating the leukemia-initiating cells. This hypothesis is supported by the randomized trial comparing imatinib to imatinib plus IFN-α; preliminary results from this trial revealed better major molecular response for the combination although a significant number of patients discontinued IFN-α treatment during the first year due to toxicity. Finally, a recent IFN-α maintenance study, following imatinib discontinuation, demonstrated maintained molecular remission in 15 (75%) of 20 patients. IFN's mechanism of action in this situation is unclear.

Imatinib is administered orally. The main side effects are fluid retention, nausea, muscle cramps, diarrhea, and skin rashes. The management of these side effects is usually supportive. Myelosuppression is the most common hematologic side effect. Myelosuppression, while rare, may require holding drug and/or growth factor support. Doses <300 mg/d seem ineffective and may lead to development of resistance.

Four mechanisms of resistance to imatinib have been described to date. These are (1) gene amplification, (2) mutations at the kinase site, (3) enhanced expression of multidrug exporter proteins, and (4) alternative signaling pathways functionally compensating for the imatinib-sensitive mechanisms. All four mechanisms are being targeted in clinical trials.

BCR-ABL1 gene amplification and decreased intracellular imatinib concentrations are addressed by intensifying the therapy with higher (up to 800 mg/d) imatinib doses. Three randomized trials have been published so far. The first randomized study compared 400 mg/d to 800 mg/d in newly diagnosed CML patients and revealed improved major molecular responses at 3, 6, and 9 months but similar results at 12 months. A similar study comparing 600 mg/d to 800 mg/d showed a borderline benefit for the higher dose based on both cytogenetic and major molecular responses at 12 months, while a third study, concentrating only on high-risk (Sokal) patients failed to show any significant difference between 400 mg/d and 800 mg/d at 12 months. All these studies have too short follow-up to evaluate dosing effect on survival.

Mutations at the kinase domain occur in approximately half of imatinib-resistant chronic-phase cases and even more frequently in the more advanced phases of the disease. These mutations are being targeted by novel TK inhibitors that have a different conformation than imatinib, demonstrating activity against most imatinib-resistant mutations. Nilotinib (Tasigma), like imatinib, binds to the kinase domain in the inactive conformation. Dasatinib (Sprycel) binds to the kinase domain in the open conformation and also inhibits the SRC (sarcoma) family of kinases, addressing the last mechanism of resistance. CML with the T315I mutation is resistant to imatinib, nilotinib, and dasatinib. In addition, nilotinib is also resistant to E255K/V and Y253F/H while dasatinib is also resistant to X299L and F317L.

Dasatinib is approved by the FDA at a dose of 100 mg/day for the treatment of all stages of CML with resistance or intolerance to prior therapy, including imatinib. Nilotinib is approved by the FDA at a dose of 400 mg twice daily for the treatment of chronic- and accelerated-phase CML with resistance or intolerance to prior therapy, including imatinib. Both are oral agents, dasatinib is given once daily while nilotinib is given twice daily with food restrictions before and after dosing. Their toxicity profiles are similar to imatinib with small but significant differences. Dasatinib causes pleural effusions in 22% of patients, with 7% developing grade 3–4 toxicity. Nilotinib was associated with sudden death in 6 of approximately 550 CML patients. A suspected relationship to nilotinib was reported in two of these cases and led to a requirement for additional cardiac monitoring while using this drug. A randomized trial in chronic-phase imatinib-resistant CML patients showed superiority of switching to dasatinib over increasing imatinib to 800 mg/day. Finally, randomized trials have demonstrated that either nilotinib or dasatinib are more effective than imatinib as first-line treatment in newly diagnosed chronic-phase CML patients in time to complete hematologic and cytogenetic remission and major molecular response at 1 year and led to their approval for the first line setting. Similar results are likely with bosutinib, another Src and Abl TK inhibitor. These studies are expanding the armamentarium for newly diagnosed CML patients.

These new agents have already changed the treatment algorithm of CML. For example, patients who do not achieve any cytogenetic remission at 6 months (or 3 months by ELN) on imatinib are now offered dasatinib, nilotinib, or HSCT. IFN-α is FDA approved for CML but is only offered if all other options have failed.

The encouraging results with imatinib have led clinicians to offer it as first-line therapy for newly diagnosed CML patients, including those who otherwise would have benefited from transplant (e.g., young patients with a matched sibling donor). Prior exposure to imatinib does not affect transplant outcome. Similar data, in smaller series, were also described for dasatinib and nilotinib treatment before HSCT. However, delaying HSCT for high-risk patients (Sokal/Hasford criteria) may result in disease progression. HSCT after disease progression is associated with poorer outcome. Therefore, we recommend close monitoring of TK inhibitors response in these patients.

TABLE 109-6 Novel Agents for BCR-ABL With T315I and Patients Who Failed All Currently Available Tyrosine Kinase Inhibitors

Agent	Mechanism of Action
Omacetaxine (formerly known as homoharringtonine)	Protein translation inhibitor
XL228	Dual Src/Abl inhibitor with potential effect against T315I mutation
FTY720 (also known as fingolimod)	Activation of protein phosphatase 2A that is essential for *ABL1*-mediated leukemogenesis
AP24534	Pan-Bcr-Abl inhibitor that inhibits T315I
DCC-2036	Non-ATP-competitive Abl inhibition, avoids the steric clash with T315I mutation
PH-739358	Aurora kinase inhibitor that is also active against T315I mutation
Sorafenib	Raf kinase inhibitor that down regulates down stream Bcr-Abl targets

NEW AGENTS Several new agents are now in development for CML with T315I and patients who fail all currently available TK inhibitors. These include omacetaxine, XL228, FTY720, AP24534, DCC-2036, PH-739358, and sorafenib (Table 109-6).

ALLOGENEIC HSCT Allogeneic HSCT is complicated by early mortality owing to the transplant procedure. Outcome of HSCT depends on multiple factors, including (1) the patient (e.g., age and phase of disease); (2) the type of donor [e.g., syngeneic (monozygotic twins) or HLA-compatible allogeneic, related or unrelated]; (3) the preparative regimen (myeloablative or reduced-intensity); (4) GVHD; and (5) posttransplantation treatment.

Posttransplantation Treatment Posttransplant *BCR-ABL1* transcript levels have served as early predictors for hematologic relapse following HSCT. These should facilitate risk-adapted approaches with immunosuppression or TK inhibitor(s), or a combination of the two. Donor leukocyte infusions (without any preparative chemotherapy or GVHD prophylaxis) can induce hematologic and cytogenetic remissions in patients with CML who have relapsed after allogeneic HSCT but carry the risk of significant GVHD.

Imatinib can control CML that has recurred after allogeneic HSCT but is sometimes associated with myelosuppression and recurrence of severe GVHD. Imatinib after allogeneic HSCT is being studied for prevention of relapse in patients with advanced disease at the time of transplantation (i.e., patients at high risk for relapse), patients undergoing reduced-intensity transplants, or patients with slow reduction of *BCR-ABL1* message following transplantation. Imatinib has also been combined with donor lymphocytes to induce rapid molecular remissions in CML patients with disease relapse after allogeneic HSCT. Of interest are studies with newer TK inhibitors following transplantation for imatinib-resistant CML.

INTERFERON Before imatinib, when allogeneic HSCT was not feasible, IFN-α therapy was the treatment of choice. Only longer follow-up of patients treated with imatinib will prove whether IFN-α will still have a role in the treatment of CML. Its mode(s) of action in CML is still unknown.

CHEMOTHERAPY Initial management of patients with chemotherapy is currently reserved for rapid lowering of WBCs, reduction of symptoms, and reversal of symptomatic splenomegaly. Hydroxyurea, a ribonucleotide reductase inhibitor, induces rapid disease control. The initial dose is 1–4 g/d; the dose should be halved with each 50% reduction of the leukocyte count. Unfortunately, cytogenetic remissions with hydroxyurea are uncommon. Busulphan, an alkylating agent that acts on early progenitor cells, has a more prolonged effect. However, we do not recommend its use because of its serious side effects, which include unexpected, and occasionally fatal, myelosuppression in 5–10% of patients; pulmonary, endocardial, and marrow fibrosis; and an Addison-like wasting syndrome.

AUTOLOGOUS HSCT Autologous HSCT could potentially cure CML if cells are collected at complete molecular remission. However, since patients who achieve this degree of response do not relapse, this treatment modality has been abandoned by most groups.

LEUKAPHERESIS AND SPLENECTOMY Intensive leukapheresis may control the blood counts in chronic-phase CML; however, it is expensive and cumbersome. It is useful in emergencies where leukostasis-related complications such as pulmonary failure or cerebrovascular accidents are likely. It may also have a role in the treatment of pregnant women, in whom it is important to avoid potentially teratogenic drugs.

Splenectomy was used in CML in the past because of the suggestion that evolution to the acute phase might occur in the spleen. However, this does not appear to be the case, and splenectomy is now reserved for symptomatic relief of painful splenomegaly unresponsive to imatinib or chemotherapy, or for significant anemia or thrombocytopenia associated with hypersplenism. Splenic radiation is used rarely to reduce the size of the spleen.

MINIMAL RESIDUAL DISEASE The kinetics of *BCR-ABL1* transcript elimination is currently replacing qualitative detection of the *BCR-ABL1* message as an index of tumor burden, in spite of a lack of standard acceptable methodology. A consensus panel has proposed ways to harmonize the different methods and to use a conversion factor so that individual laboratories will be able to express *BCR-ABL1* transcript levels on an agreed upon scale.

Slow reduction of *BCR-ABL1* transcripts following HSCT correlates with the possibility of hematologic relapse. However, the definition of "slow reduction" depends on the preparative regimen (reduced-intensity vs fully myeloablative) and the selection of time points to measure the transcript levels. While persistent RT-PCR positivity at 6 months was regarded as an indication for additional therapy in the past, current studies utilize periods between engraftment and day 100 for evaluating the clearance rate of *BCR-ABL1* transcripts and recommending additional therapies. Large trials with longer follow-up are needed to establish consensus guidelines.

The randomized trial of imatinib versus IFN-α and cytarabine (IRIS) was the first to establish the concept of $\log_{10}$ reduction of *BCR-ABL1* transcript from a standardized baseline for untreated patients. This measurement unit was developed instead of either the transcript numbers expressed per microgram of leukocyte RNA or the ratio of *BCR-ABL1* to a housekeeping gene on a log scale. In this randomized trial, patients who achieved ≥3 log reduction of *BCR-ABL1* message had an extremely low probability of relapse, with a median follow-up of 96 months.

These studies also established the value and convenience of using peripheral blood instead of bone marrow testing as a means to assess disease status in patients who achieve complete cytogenetic responses. However, one still needs to consider following CML patients in complete cytogenetic remission and at least major molecular remission with occasional cytogenetic bone marrow testing. This should be performed if they develop cytopenia late in the treatment course as such patients are at risk of developing cytogenetic aberrations, especially monosomy 7, in t(9;22)-negative cells and secondary MDS/AML. Other aberrations in the t(9;22)-negative cells are frequently transient, and their clinical significance is unclear. Development of secondary MDS/AML is rare.

TREATMENT OF BLAST CRISIS Treatments for primary blast crisis, including imatinib, are generally ineffective. Only 52% of patients treated with imatinib achieved hematologic remission (21% complete hematologic remission), and the median overall survival was 6.6 months. Patients who achieve complete hematologic remission or whose disease returns to a second chronic phase should be considered for allogeneic HSCT. Other approaches include induction chemotherapy tailored to the phenotype of the blast cell followed by TK inhibitors, with or without additional chemotherapy and HSCT. Blast crisis following initial therapy with imatinib carries a dismal prognosis even if treated with dasatinib or nilotinib.

FURTHER READINGS

AML

DÖHNER H et al: Diagnosis and management of acute myeloid leukemia in adults: Recommendations from an international expert panel, on behalf of the European Leukemia Net. Blood 115:453, 2010

NATIONAL COMPREHENSIVE CANCER NETWORK: Acute myeloid leukemia. Clinical Practice Guidelines in Oncology, Version 2. 2010. *http://www.nccn.org/professionals/physician_gls/PDF/cml.pdf*

SANZ MA et al: Management of acute promyelocytic leukemia: Recommendations from an expert panel on behalf of the European Leukemia Net. Blood 113:1875, 2009

VARDIMAN JW et al: The 2008 revision of the World Health Organization (WHO) classification of myeloid neoplasms and acute leukemia: Rationale and important changes. Blood 114:937, 2009

CML

BACCARANI M et al: Chronic myeloid leukemia: An update of concepts and management recommendations of European Leukemia Net. J Clin Oncol 27:6041, 2009

IRVINE DA et al: Optimising chronic myeloid leukaemia therapy in the face of resistance to tyrosine kinase inhibitors—a synthesis of clinical and laboratory data. Blood Rev 24:1, 2010

KANTARJIAN H et al: Dasatinib versus imatinib in newly diagnosed chronic-phase chronic myeloid leukemia. N Engl J Med 362:2260, 2010

NATIONAL COMPREHENSIVE CANCER NETWORK: Chronic myelogenous leukemia. Clinical Practice Guidelines in Oncology, Version 2. 2010. *http://www.nccn.org/professionals/physician_gls/PDF/cml.pdf*

SAGLIO G et al: Nilotinib versus imatinib for newly diagnosed chronic myeloid leukemia. N Engl J Med 362:2251, 2010

CHAPTER 110

Malignancies of Lymphoid Cells

Dan L. Longo

Malignancies of lymphoid cells range from the most indolent to the most aggressive human malignancies. These cancers arise from cells of the immune system at different stages of differentiation, resulting in a wide range of morphologic, immunologic, and clinical findings. Insights on the normal immune system have allowed a better understanding of these sometimes confusing disorders.

Some malignancies of lymphoid cells almost always present as leukemia (i.e., primary involvement of bone marrow and blood), while others almost always present as lymphomas (i.e., solid tumors of the immune system). However, other malignancies of lymphoid cells can present as either leukemia or lymphoma. In addition, the clinical pattern can change over the course of the illness. This change is more often seen in a patient who seems to have a lymphoma and then develops the manifestations of leukemia over the course of the illness.

BIOLOGY OF LYMPHOID MALIGNANCIES: CONCEPTS OF THE WHO CLASSIFICATION OF LYMPHOID MALIGNANCIES

The classification of lymphoid cancers evolved steadily throughout the twentieth century. The distinction between leukemia and lymphoma was made early, and separate classification systems were developed for each. Leukemias were first divided into acute and chronic subtypes based on average survival. Chronic leukemias were easily subdivided into those of lymphoid or myeloid origin based on morphologic characteristics. However, a spectrum of diseases that were formerly all called *chronic lymphoid leukemia* has become apparent (Table 110-1). The acute leukemias were usually malignancies of blast cells with few identifying characteristics. When cytochemical stains became available, it was possible to divide these objectively into myeloid malignancies and acute leukemias of lymphoid cells. Acute leukemias of lymphoid cells have been subdivided based on morphologic characteristics by the French-American-British (FAB) group (Table 110-2). Using this system, lymphoid malignancies of small uniform blasts (e.g., typical childhood acute lymphoblastic leukemia) were called L1, lymphoid malignancies with larger and more variable size cells were called

TABLE 110-1 Lymphoid Disorders That Can Present as "Chronic Leukemia" and Be Confused With Typical B Cell Chronic Lymphoid Leukemia

Follicular lymphoma	Prolymphocytic leukemia (B cell or T cell)
Splenic marginal zone lymphoma	
Nodal marginal zone lymphoma	Lymphoplasmacytic lymphoma
Mantle cell lymphoma	Sézary's syndrome
Hairy cell leukemia	Smoldering adult T cell leukemia/lymphoma

TABLE 110-2 Classification of Acute Lymphoid Leukemia (ALL)

Immunologic Subtype	% of Cases	FAB Subtype	Cytogenetic Abnormalities
Pre-B ALL	75	L1, L2	t(9;22), t(4;11), t(1;19)
T cell ALL	20	L1, L2	14q11 or 7q34
B cell ALL	5	L3	t(8;14), t(8;22), t(2;8)

Abbreviation: FAB, French-American-British classification.

L2, and lymphoid malignancies of uniform cells with basophilic and sometimes vacuolated cytoplasm were called L3 (e.g., typical Burkitt's lymphoma cells). Acute leukemias of lymphoid cells have also been subdivided based on immunologic (i.e., T cell vs. B cell) and cytogenetic abnormalities (Table 110-2). Major cytogenetic subgroups include the t(9;22) (e.g., Philadelphia chromosome–positive acute lymphoblastic leukemia) and the t(8;14) found in the L3 or Burkitt's leukemia.

Non-Hodgkin's lymphomas were separated from Hodgkin's disease by recognition of the Sternberg-Reed cells early in the twentieth century. The histologic classification for non-Hodgkin's lymphomas has been one of the most contentious issues in oncology. Imperfect morphologic systems were supplanted by imperfect immunologic systems, and poor reproducibility of diagnosis has hampered progress. In 1999, the World Health Organization (WHO) classification of lymphoid malignancies was devised through a process of consensus development among international leaders in hematopathology and clinical oncology. The WHO classification takes into account morphologic, clinical, immunologic, and genetic information and attempts to divide non-Hodgkin's lymphomas and other lymphoid malignancies into clinical/pathologic entities that have clinical and therapeutic relevance. This system is presented in Table 110-3. This system is clinically relevant and has a higher degree of diagnostic accuracy than those used previously. The possibilities for subdividing lymphoid malignancies are extensive. However, Table 110-3 presents in bold those malignancies that occur in at least 1% of patients. Specific lymphoma subtypes will be dealt with in more detail below. Lymphomas associated with HIV infection are discussed in Chap. 189.

GENERAL ASPECTS OF LYMPHOID MALIGNANCIES

■ ETIOLOGY AND EPIDEMIOLOGY

The relative frequency of the various lymphoid malignancies is shown in Fig. 110-1. Chronic lymphoid leukemia (CLL) is the most prevalent form of leukemia in Western countries. It occurs most frequently in older adults and is exceedingly rare in children. In 2010, 14,990 new cases were diagnosed in the United States, but because of the prolonged survival associated with this disorder, the total prevalence is many times higher. CLL is more common in men than in women and more common in whites than in blacks. This is an uncommon malignancy in Asia. The etiologic factors for typical CLL are unknown.

In contrast to CLL, acute lymphoid leukemias (ALLs) are predominantly cancers of children and young adults. The L3 or Burkitt's leukemia occurring in children in developing countries seems to be associated with infection by the Epstein-Barr virus (EBV) in infancy. However, the explanation for the etiology of more common subtypes of ALL is much less certain. Childhood ALL occurs more often in higher socioeconomic subgroups. Children

TABLE 110-3 WHO Classification of Lymphoid Malignancies

B Cell	T Cell	Hodgkin's Disease
Precursor B cell neoplasm **Precursor B lymphoblastic leukemia/lymphoma (precursor B cell acute lymphoblastic leukemia)**	Precursor T cell neoplasm **Precursor T lymphoblastic lymphoma/leukemia (precursor T cell acute lymphoblastic leukemia)**	Nodular lymphocyte-predominant Hodgkin's disease
Mature (peripheral) B cell neoplasms	Mature (peripheral) T cell neoplasms	Classical Hodgkin's disease
B cell chronic lymphocytic leukemia/small lymphocytic lymphoma	T cell prolymphocytic leukemia	Nodular sclerosis Hodgkin's disease
B cell prolymphocytic leukemia	T cell granular lymphocytic leukemia	Lymphocyte-rich classic Hodgkin's disease
Lymphoplasmacytic lymphoma	Aggressive NK cell leukemia	Mixed-cellularity Hodgkin's disease
Splenic marginal zone B cell lymphoma (± villous lymphocytes)	Adult T cell lymphoma/leukemia (HTLV-I+)	Lymphocyte-depletion Hodgkin's disease
Hairy cell leukemia	Extranodal NK/T cell lymphoma, nasal type	
Plasma cell myeloma/plasmacytoma	Enteropathy-type T cell lymphoma	
Extranodal marginal zone B cell lymphoma of MALT type	Hepatosplenic γδ T cell lymphoma	
Mantle cell lymphoma	Subcutaneous panniculitis-like T cell lymphoma	
Follicular lymphoma	**Mycosis fungoides/Sézary's syndrome**	
Nodal marginal zone B cell lymphoma (± monocytoid B cells)	Anaplastic large cell lymphoma, primary cutaneous type	
Diffuse large B cell lymphoma	**Peripheral T cell lymphoma, not otherwise specified (NOS)**	
Burkitt's lymphoma/Burkitt's cell leukemia	**Angioimmunoblastic T cell lymphoma**	
	Anaplastic large cell lymphoma, primary systemic type	

Note: Malignancies in bold occur in at least 1% of patients.
Abbreviations: HTLV, human T cell lymphotropic virus; MALT, mucosa-associated lymphoid tissue; NK, natural killer; WHO, World Health Organization.
Source: Adapted from Harris et al.

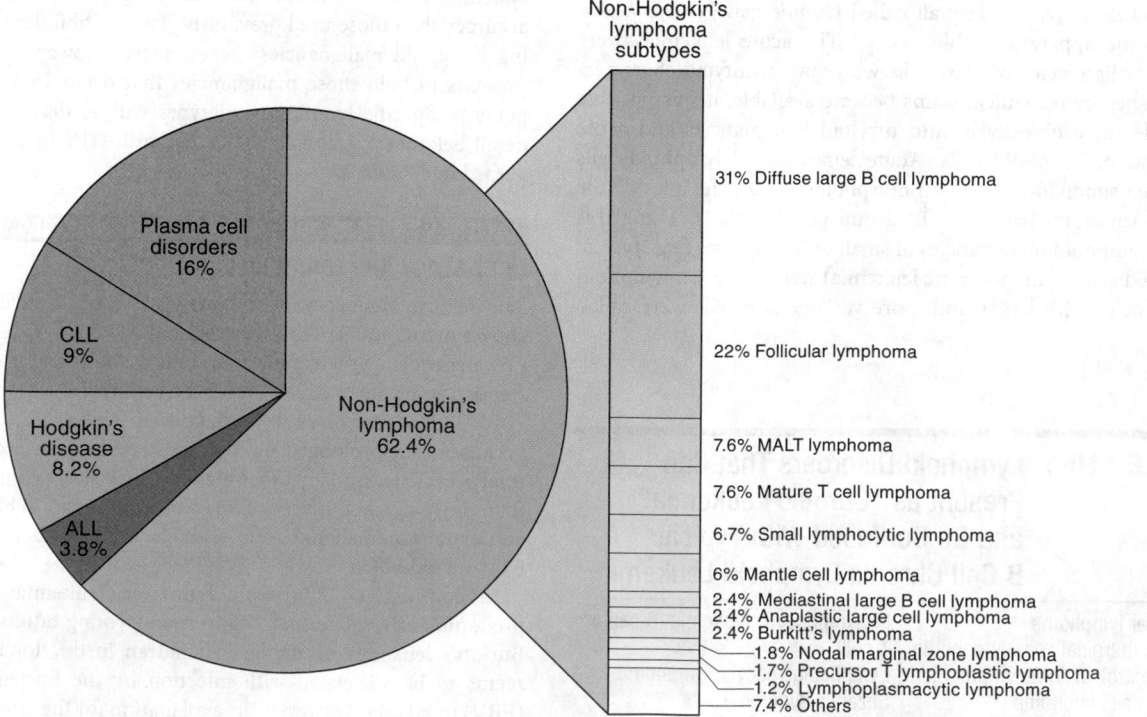

Figure 110-1 **Relative frequency of lymphoid malignancies.** ALL, acute lymphoid leukemia; CLL, chronic lymphoid leukemia; MALT, mucosa-associated lymphoid tissue.

with trisomy 21 (Down syndrome) have an increased risk for childhood ALL as well as acute myeloid leukemia (AML). Exposure to high-energy radiation in early childhood increases the risk of developing T cell ALL.

The etiology of ALL in adults is also uncertain. ALL is unusual in middle-aged adults but increases in incidence in the elderly. However, AML is still much more common in older patients. Environmental exposures, including certain industrial exposures, exposure to agricultural chemicals, and smoking, might increase the risk of developing ALL as an adult. ALL was diagnosed in 5330 persons and AML in 12,330 persons in the United States in 2010.

The preponderance of evidence suggests that Hodgkin's disease is of B cell origin. The incidence of Hodgkin's disease appears fairly stable, with 8490 new cases diagnosed in 2010 in the United States. Hodgkin's disease is more common in whites than in blacks and more common in males than in females. A bimodal distribution of age at diagnosis has been observed, with one peak incidence occurring in patients in their twenties and the other in those in their eighties. Some of the late age peak may be attributed to confusion among entities with similar appearance such as anaplastic large cell lymphoma and T cell–rich B cell lymphoma. Patients in the younger age groups diagnosed in the United States largely have the nodular sclerosing subtype of Hodgkin's disease. Elderly patients, patients infected with HIV, and patients in Third World countries more commonly have mixed-cellularity Hodgkin's disease or lymphocyte-depleted Hodgkin's disease. Infection by HIV is a risk factor for developing Hodgkin's disease. In addition, an association between infection by EBV and Hodgkin's disease has been suggested. A monoclonal or oligoclonal proliferation of EBV-infected cells in 20–40% of the patients with Hodgkin's disease has led to proposals for this virus having an etiologic role in Hodgkin's disease. However, the matter is not settled definitively.

For unknown reasons, non-Hodgkin's lymphomas increased in frequency in the United States at the rate of 4% per year and increased 2–8% per year globally between 1950 and the late 1990s. The rate of increase in the past few years seems to be decreasing. About 65,540 new cases of non-Hodgkin's lymphoma were diagnosed in the United States in 2010 and nearly 360,000 cases worldwide. Non-Hodgkin's lymphomas are more frequent in the elderly and more frequent in men. Patients with both primary and secondary immunodeficiency states are predisposed to developing non-Hodgkin's lymphomas. These include patients with HIV infection; patients who have undergone organ transplantation; and patients with inherited immune deficiencies, the sicca syndrome, and rheumatoid arthritis.

The incidence of non-Hodgkin's lymphomas and the patterns of expression of the various subtypes differ geographically. T cell lymphomas are more common in Asia than in Western countries, while certain subtypes of B cell lymphomas such as follicular lymphoma are more common in Western countries. A specific subtype of non-Hodgkin's lymphoma known as the angiocentric nasal T/natural killer (NK) cell lymphoma has a striking geographic occurrence, being most frequent in Southern Asia and parts of Latin America. Another subtype of non-Hodgkin's lymphoma associated with infection by human T cell lymphotropic virus (HTLV) I is seen particularly in southern Japan and the Caribbean (Chap. 188).

A number of environmental factors have been implicated in the occurrence of non-Hodgkin's lymphoma, including infectious agents, chemical exposures, and medical treatments. Several studies have demonstrated an association between exposure to agricultural chemicals and an increased incidence in non-Hodgkin's lymphoma. Patients treated for Hodgkin's disease can develop non-Hodgkin's lymphoma; it is unclear whether this is a consequence of the Hodgkin's disease or its treatment. However, a number of

TABLE 110-4 Infectious Agents Associated With the Development of Lymphoid Malignancies

Infectious Agent	Lymphoid Malignancy
Epstein-Barr virus	Burkitt's lymphoma Post–organ transplant lymphoma Primary CNS diffuse large B cell lymphoma Hodgkin's disease Extranodal NK/T cell lymphoma, nasal type
HTLV-I	Adult T cell leukemia/lymphoma
HIV	Diffuse large B cell lymphoma Burkitt's lymphoma
Hepatitis C virus	Lymphoplasmacytic lymphoma
Helicobacter pylori	Gastric MALT lymphoma
Human herpesvirus 8	Primary effusion lymphoma Multicentric Castleman's disease

Abbreviations: CNS, central nervous system; HIV, human immunodeficiency virus; HTLV, human T cell lymphotropic virus; MALT, mucosa-associated lymphoid tissue; NK, natural killer.

non-Hodgkin's lymphomas are associated with infectious agents (Table 110-4). HTLV-I infects T cells and leads directly to the development of adult T cell lymphoma (ATL) in a small percentage of infected patients. The cumulative lifetime risk of developing lymphoma in an infected patient is 2.5%. The virus is transmitted by infected lymphocytes ingested by nursing babies of infected mothers, bloodborne transmission, or sexually. The median age of patients with ATL is ~56 years, emphasizing the long latency. HTLV-I is also the cause of tropical spastic paraparesis—a neurologic disorder that occurs somewhat more frequently than lymphoma and with shorter latency and usually from transfusion-transmitted virus (Chap. 188).

EBV is associated with the development of Burkitt's lymphoma in Central Africa and the occurrence of aggressive non-Hodgkin's lymphomas in immunosuppressed patients in Western countries. The majority of primary central nervous system (CNS) lymphomas are associated with EBV. EBV infection is strongly associated with the occurrence of extranodal nasal T/NK cell lymphomas in Asia and South America. Infection with HIV predisposes to the development of aggressive, B cell non-Hodgkin's lymphoma. This may be through overexpression of interleukin 6 by infected macrophages. Infection of the stomach by the bacterium *Helicobacter pylori* induces the development of gastric MALT (mucosa-associated lymphoid tissue) lymphomas. This association is supported by evidence that patients treated with antibiotics to eradicate *H. pylori* have regression of their MALT lymphoma. The bacterium does not transform lymphocytes to produce the lymphoma; instead, a vigorous immune response is made to the bacterium, and the chronic antigenic stimulation leads to the neoplasia. MALT lymphomas of the skin may be related to *Borrelia* sp. infections, those of the eyes to *Chlamydophila psittaci*, and those of the small intestine to *Campylobacter jejuni*.

Chronic hepatitis C virus infection has been associated with the development of lymphoplasmacytic lymphoma. Human herpesvirus 8 is associated with primary effusion lymphoma in HIV-infected persons and multicentric Castleman's disease, a diffuse lymphadenopathy associated with systemic symptoms of fever, malaise, and weight loss.

In addition to infectious agents, a number of other diseases or exposures may predispose to developing lymphoma (Table 110-5).

TABLE 110-5 Diseases or Exposures Associated with Increased Risk of Development of Malignant Lymphoma

Inherited immunodeficiency disease	Autoimmune disease
Klinefelter's syndrome	Sjögren's syndrome
Chédiak-Higashi syndrome	Celiac sprue
Ataxia-telangiectasia syndrome	Rheumatoid arthritis and
Wiskott-Aldrich syndrome	systemic lupus erythematosus
Common variable	Chemical or drug exposures
immunodeficiency disease	Phenytoin
Acquired immunodeficiency diseases	Dioxin, Phenoxy herbicides
Iatrogenic immunosuppression	Radiation
HIV-1 infection	Prior chemotherapy and
Acquired hypogammaglobulinemia	radiation therapy

■ IMMUNOLOGY

All lymphoid cells are derived from a common hematopoietic progenitor that gives rise to lymphoid, myeloid, erythroid, monocyte, and megakaryocyte lineages. Through the ordered and sequential activation of a series of transcription factors, the cell first becomes committed to the lymphoid lineage and then gives rise to B and T cells. About 75% of all lymphoid leukemias and 90% of all lymphomas are of B cell origin. A cell becomes committed to B cell development when it begins to rearrange its immunoglobulin genes. The sequence of cellular changes, including changes in cell-surface phenotype, that characterizes normal B cell development is shown in Fig. 110-2. A cell becomes committed to T cell differentiation upon migration to the thymus and rearrangement of T cell antigen receptor genes. The sequence of the events that characterize T cell development is depicted in Fig. 110-3.

Although lymphoid malignancies often retain the cell-surface phenotype of lymphoid cells at particular stages of differentiation, this information is of little consequence. The so-called stage of differentiation of a malignant lymphoma does not predict its natural history. For example, the clinically most aggressive lymphoid leukemia is Burkitt's leukemia, which has the phenotype of a mature follicle center IgM-bearing B cell. Leukemias bearing the immunologic cell-surface phenotype of more primitive cells (e.g., pre-B ALL, CD10+) are less aggressive and more amenable to curative therapy than the

"more mature" appearing Burkitt's leukemia cells. Furthermore, the apparent stage of differentiation of the malignant cell does not reflect the stage at which the genetic lesions that gave rise to the malignancy developed. For example, follicular lymphoma has the cell-surface phenotype of a follicle center cell, but its characteristic chromosomal translocation, the t(14;18), which involves juxtaposition of the antiapoptotic bcl-2 gene next to the immunoglobulin heavy chain gene (see below), had to develop early in ontogeny as an error in the process of immunoglobulin gene rearrangement. Why the subsequent steps that led to transformation became manifest in a cell of follicle center differentiation is not clear.

The major value of cell-surface phenotyping is to aid in the differential diagnosis of lymphoid tumors that appear similar by light microscopy. For example, benign follicular hyperplasia may resemble follicular lymphoma; however, the demonstration that all the cells bear the same immunoglobulin light chain isotype strongly suggests the mass is a clonal proliferation rather than a polyclonal response to an exogenous stimulus.

Malignancies of lymphoid cells are associated with recurring genetic abnormalities. While specific genetic abnormalities have not been identified for all subtypes of lymphoid malignancies, it is presumed that they exist. Genetic abnormalities can be identified at a variety of levels including gross chromosomal changes (i.e., translocations, additions, or deletions); rearrangement of specific genes that may or may not be apparent from cytogenetic studies;

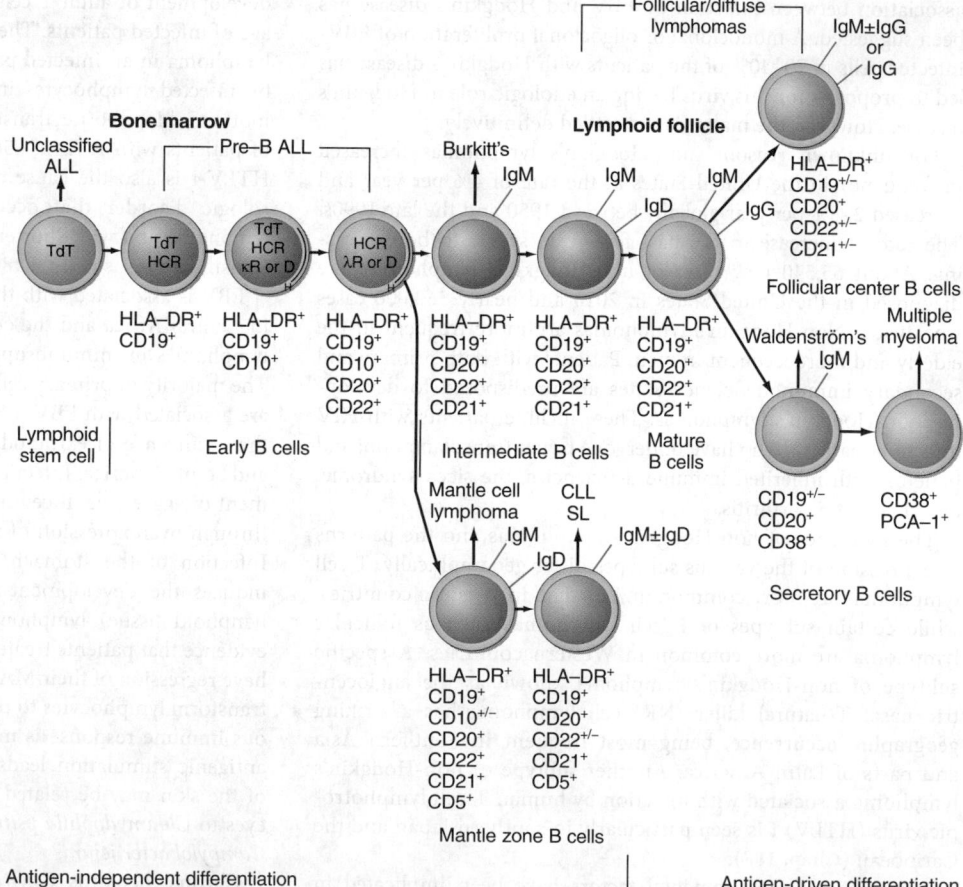

Figure 110-2 **Pathway of normal B cell differentiation and relationship to B cell lymphomas.** HLA-DR, CD10, CD19, CD20, CD21, CD22, CD5, and CD38 are cell markers used to distinguish stages of development. Terminal transferase (TdT) is a cellular enzyme. Immunoglobulin heavy chain gene rearrangement (HCR) and light chain gene rearrangement or deletion (κR or D, λR or D) occur early in B cell development. The approximate normal stage of differentiation associated with particular lymphomas is shown. ALL, acute lymphoid leukemia; CLL, chronic lymphoid leukemia; SL, small lymphocytic lymphoma.

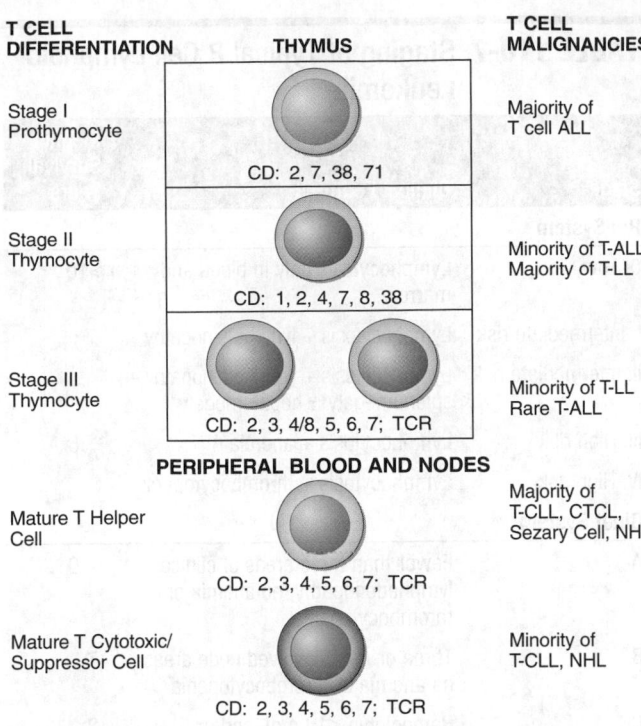

T CELL DIFFERENTIATION	THYMUS	T CELL MALIGNANCIES
Stage I Prothymocyte	CD: 2, 7, 38, 71	Majority of T cell ALL
Stage II Thymocyte	CD: 1, 2, 4, 7, 8, 38	Minority of T-ALL Majority of T-LL
Stage III Thymocyte	CD: 2, 3, 4/8, 5, 6, 7; TCR	Minority of T-LL Rare T-ALL

PERIPHERAL BLOOD AND NODES

| Mature T Helper Cell | CD: 2, 3, 4, 5, 6, 7; TCR | Majority of T-CLL, CTCL, Sezary Cell, NHL |
| Mature T Cytotoxic/ Suppressor Cell | CD: 2, 3, 4, 5, 6, 7; TCR | Minority of T-CLL, NHL |

Figure 110-3 Pathway of normal T cell differentiation and relationship to T cell lymphomas. CD1, CD2, CD3, CD4, CD5, CD6, CD7, CD8, CD38, and CD71 are cell markers used to distinguish stages of development. T cell antigen receptors (TCR) rearrange in the thymus, and mature T cells emigrate to nodes and peripheral blood. ALL, acute lymphoid leukemia; T-ALL, T cell ALL; T-LL, T cell lymphoblastic lymphoma; T-CLL, T cell chronic lymphoid leukemia; CTCL, cutaneous T cell lymphoma; NHL, non-Hodgkin's lymphoma.

TABLE 110-6 Cytogenetic Translocation and Associated Oncogenes Often Seen in Lymphoid Malignancies

Disease	Cytogenetic Abnormality	Oncogene
CLL/small lymphocytic lymphoma	t(14;15)(q32;q13)	—
MALT lymphoma	t(11;18)(q21;q21)	API2/MALT, BCL-10
Precursor B cell acute lymphoid leukemia	t(9;22)(q34;q11) or variant t(4;11)(q21;q23)	BCR/ABL AF4, ALLI
Precursor acute lymphoid leukemia	t(9;22) t(1;19) t(17;19) t(5;14)	BCR, ABL E2A, PBX HLF, E2A HOX11L2, CTIP2
Mantle cell lymphoma	t(11;14)(q13;q32)	BCL-1, IgH
Follicular lymphoma	t(14;18)(q32;q21)	BCL-2, IgH
Diffuse large cell lymphoma	t(3;-)(q27;-)[a] t(17;-)(p13;-)	BCL-6 p53
Burkitt's lymphoma, Burkitt's leukemia	t(8;-)(q24;-)[a]	C-MYC
CD30+ Anaplastic large cell lymphoma	t(2;5)(p23;q35)	ALK
Lymphoplasmacytoid lymphoma	t(9;14)(p13;q32)	PAX5, IgH

[a]Numerous sites of translocation may be involved with these genes.
Abbreviations: CLL, chronic lymphoid leukemia; IgH, immunoglobulin heavy chain; MALT, mucosa-associated lymphoid tissue.

and overexpression, underexpression, or mutation of specific oncogenes. Altered expression or mutation of specific proteins is particularly important. Many lymphomas contain balanced chromosomal translocations involving the antigen receptor genes; immunoglobulin genes on chromosomes 2, 14, and 22 in B cells; and T cell antigen receptor genes on chromosomes 7 and 14 in T cells. The rearrangement of chromosome segments to generate mature antigen receptors must create a site of vulnerability to aberrant recombination. B cells are even more susceptible to acquiring mutations during their maturation in germinal centers; the generation of antibody of higher affinity requires the introduction of mutations into the variable region genes in the germinal centers. Other nonimmunoglobulin genes, e.g., bcl-6, may acquire mutations as well.

In the case of diffuse large B cell lymphoma, the translocation t(14;18) occurs in ~30% of patients and leads to overexpression of the bcl-2 gene found on chromosome 18. Some other patients without the translocation also overexpress the BCL-2 protein. This protein is involved in suppressing apoptosis—i.e., the mechanism of cell death most often induced by cytotoxic chemotherapeutic agents. A higher relapse rate has been observed in patients whose tumors overexpress the BCL-2 protein, but not in those patients whose lymphoma cells show only the translocation. Thus, particular genetic mechanisms have clinical ramifications.

Table 110-6 presents the best documented translocations and associated oncogenes for various subtypes of lymphoid malignancies. In some cases, such as the association of the t(14;18) in follicular lymphoma, the t(2;5) in anaplastic large T/null cell lymphoma, the t(8;14) in Burkitt's lymphoma, and the t(11;14) in mantle cell lymphoma, the great majority of tumors in patients with these diagnoses display these abnormalities. In other types of lymphoma

where a minority of the patients have tumors expressing specific genetic abnormalities, the defects may have prognostic significance. No specific genetic abnormalities have been identified in Hodgkin's disease other than aneuploidy.

In typical B cell CLL, trisomy 12 conveys a poorer prognosis. In ALL in both adults and children, genetic abnormalities have important prognostic significance. Patients whose tumor cells display the t(9;22) and translocations involving the MLL gene on chromosome 11q23 have a much poorer outlook than patients who do not have these translocations. Other genetic abnormalities that occur frequently in adults with ALL include the t(4;11) and the t(8;14). The t(4;11) is associated with younger age, female predominance, high white cell counts, and L1 morphology. The t(8;14) is associated with older age, male predominance, frequent CNS involvement, and L3 morphology. Both are associated with a poor prognosis. In childhood ALL, hyperdiploidy has been shown to have a favorable prognosis.

Gene profiling using array technology allows the simultaneous assessment of the expression of thousands of genes. This technology provides the possibility to identify new genes with pathologic importance in lymphomas, the identification of patterns of gene expression with diagnostic and/or prognostic significance, and the identification of new therapeutic targets. Recognition of patterns of gene expression is complicated and requires sophisticated mathematical techniques. Early successes using this technology in lymphoma include the identification of previously unrecognized subtypes of diffuse large B cell lymphoma whose gene expression patterns resemble either those of follicular center B cells or activated peripheral blood B cells. Patients whose lymphomas have a germinal center B cell pattern of gene expression have a considerably better prognosis than those whose lymphomas have a pattern resembling activated peripheral blood B cells. This improved prognosis is independent of other known prognostic factors. Similar information is being generated in follicular lymphoma and mantle cell lymphoma. The challenge remains to provide information from such techniques in a clinically useful time frame.

APPROACH TO THE PATIENT: Lymphoid Cell Malignancies

Regardless of the type of lymphoid malignancy, the initial evaluation of the patient should include performance of a careful history and physical examination. These will help confirm the diagnosis, identify those manifestations of the disease that might require prompt attention, and aid in the selection of further studies to optimally characterize the patient's status to allow the best choice of therapy. It is difficult to overemphasize the importance of a carefully done history and physical examination. They might provide observations that lead to reconsidering the diagnosis, provide hints at etiology, clarify the stage, and allow the physician to establish rapport with the patient that will make it possible to develop and carry out a therapeutic plan.

For patients with ALL, evaluation is usually completed after a complete blood count, chemistry studies reflecting major organ function, a bone marrow biopsy with genetic and immunologic studies, and a lumbar puncture. The latter is necessary to rule out occult CNS involvement. At this point, most patients would be ready to begin therapy. In ALL, prognosis is dependent upon the genetic characteristics of the tumor, the patient's age, the white cell count, and the patient's overall clinical status and major organ function.

In CLL, the patient evaluation should include a complete blood count, chemistry tests to measure major organ function, serum protein electrophoresis, and a bone marrow biopsy. However, some physicians believe that the diagnosis would not always require a bone marrow biopsy. Patients often have imaging studies of the chest and abdomen looking for pathologic lymphadenopathy. Patients with typical B cell CLL can be subdivided into three major prognostic groups. Those patients with only blood and bone marrow involvement by leukemia but no lymphadenopathy, organomegaly, or signs of bone marrow failure have the best prognosis. Those with lymphadenopathy and organomegaly have an intermediate prognosis, and patients with bone marrow failure, defined as hemoglobin <100 g/L (10 g/dL) or platelet count <100,000/μL, have the worst prognosis. The pathogenesis of the anemia or thrombocytopenia is important to discern. The prognosis is adversely affected when either or both of these abnormalities are due to progressive marrow infiltration and loss of productive marrow. However, either or both may be due to autoimmune phenomena or to hypersplenism that can develop during the course of the disease. These destructive mechanisms are usually completely reversible (glucocorticoids for autoimmune disease; splenectomy for hypersplenism) and do not influence disease prognosis.

Two popular staging systems have been developed to reflect these prognostic groupings (Table 110-7). Patients with typical B cell CLL can have their course complicated by immunologic abnormalities, including autoimmune hemolytic anemia, autoimmune thrombocytopenia, and hypogammaglobulinemia. Patients with hypogammaglobulinemia benefit from regular (monthly) γ globulin administration. Because of expense, γ globulin is often withheld until the patient experiences a significant

TABLE 110-7 Staging of Typical B Cell Lymphoid Leukemia

Stage	Clinical Features	Median Survival, Years
Rai System		
0: Low risk	Lymphocytosis only in blood and marrow	>10
I: Intermediate risk	Lymphocytosis + lymphadenopathy	7
II: Intermediate risk	Lymphocytosis + lymphadenopathy + splenomegaly ± hepatomegaly	
III: High risk	Lymphocytosis + anemia	1.5
IV: High risk	Lymphocytosis + thrombocytopenia	
Binet System		
A	Fewer than three areas of clinical lymphadenopathy; no anemia or thrombocytopenia	>10
B	Three or more involved node areas; no anemia or thrombocytopenia	7
C	Hemoglobin ≤10 g/dL and/or platelets <100,000/μL	2

infection. These abnormalities do not have a clear prognostic significance and should not be used to assign a higher stage.

Two other features may be used to assess prognosis in B cell CLL, but neither has yet been incorporated into a staging classification. At least two subsets of CLL have been identified based on the cytoplasmic expression of ZAP-70; expression of this protein, which is usually expressed in T cells, identifies a subgroup with poorer prognosis. A less powerful subsetting tool is CD38 expression. CD38+ tumors tend to have a poorer prognosis than CD38– tumors.

The initial evaluation of a patient with Hodgkin's disease or non-Hodgkin's lymphoma is similar. In both situations, the determination of an accurate anatomic stage is an important part of the evaluation. Staging is done using the Ann Arbor staging system originally developed for Hodgkin's disease (Table 110-8).

Evaluation of patients with Hodgkin's disease will typically include a complete blood count; erythrocyte sedimentation rate; chemistry studies reflecting major organ function; CT scans of the chest, abdomen, and pelvis; and a bone marrow biopsy. Neither a positron emission tomography (PET) scan nor a gallium scan is absolutely necessary for primary staging, but one performed at the completion of therapy allows evaluation of persisting radiographic abnormalities, particularly the mediastinum. Knowing that the PET scan or gallium scan is abnormal before treatment can help in this assessment. In most cases, these studies will allow assignment of anatomic stage and the development of a therapeutic plan.

In patients with non-Hodgkin's lymphoma, the same evaluation described for patients with Hodgkin's disease is usually carried out. In addition, serum levels of lactate dehydrogenase (LDH) and β₂-microglobulin and serum protein electrophoresis are often included in the evaluation. Anatomic stage is assigned in the same manner as used for Hodgkin's disease. However, the prognosis of patients with non-Hodgkin's lymphoma is best assigned using the International Prognostic Index (IPI) (Table 110-9). This is a powerful predictor of

TABLE 110-8 The Ann Arbor Staging System for Hodgkin's Disease

Stage	Definition
I	Involvement of a single lymph node region or lymphoid structure (e.g., spleen, thymus, Waldeyer's ring)
II	Involvement of two or more lymph node regions on the same side of the diaphragm (the mediastinum is a single site; hilar lymph nodes should be considered "lateralized" and, when involved on both sides, constitute stage II disease)
III	Involvement of lymph node regions or lymphoid structures on both sides of the diaphragm
III$_1$	Subdiaphragmatic involvement limited to spleen, splenic hilar nodes, celiac nodes, or portal nodes
III$_2$	Subdiaphragmatic involvement includes paraaortic, iliac, or mesenteric nodes plus structures in III$_1$
IV	Involvement of extranodal site(s) beyond that designated as "E" More than one extranodal deposit at any location Any involvement of liver or bone marrow
A	No symptoms
B	Unexplained weight loss of >10% of the body weight during the 6 months before staging investigation Unexplained, persistent, or recurrent fever with temperatures >38°C during the previous month Recurrent drenching night sweats during the previous month
E	Localized, solitary involvement of extralymphatic tissue, excluding liver and bone marrow

TABLE 110-9 International Prognostic Index for NHL

Five clinical risk factors:

Age ≥ 60 years

Serum lactate dehydrogenase levels elevated

Performance status ≥2 (ECOG) or ≤ 70 (Karnofsky)

Ann Arbor stage III or IV

>1 site of extranodal involvement

Patients are assigned a number for each risk factor they have

Patients are grouped differently based upon the type of lymphoma

For diffuse large B cell lymphoma:

0, 1 factor = low risk:	35% of cases; 5-year survival, 73%
2 factors = low-intermediate risk:	27% of cases; 5-year survival, 51%
3 factors = high-intermediate risk:	22% of cases; 5-year survival, 43%
4, 5 factors = high risk:	16% of cases; 5-year survival, 26%

For diffuse large B cell lymphoma treated with R-CHOP:

0 factor = very good:	10% of cases; 5-year survival, 94%
1, 2 factors = good:	45% of cases; 5-year survival, 79%
3, 4, 5 factors = poor:	45% of cases; 5-year survival, 55%

Abbreviations: ECOG, Eastern Cooperative Oncology Group; R-CHOP, rituximab, cyclophosphamide, doxorubicin, vincristine, prednisone.

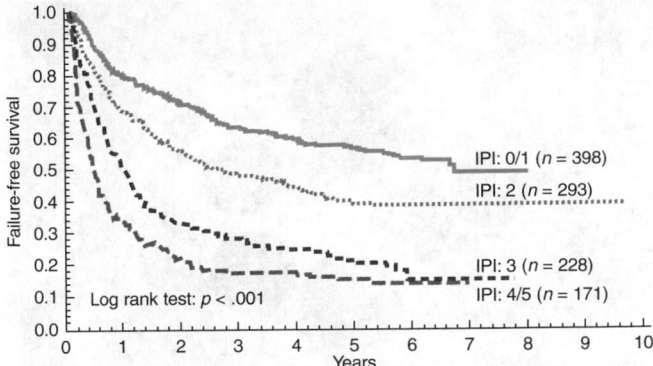

Figure 110-4 Relationship of International Prognostic Index (IPI) to survival. Kaplan-Meier survival curves for 1300 patients with various kinds of lymphoma stratified according to the IPI.

outcome in all subtypes of non-Hodgkin's lymphoma. Patients are assigned an IPI score based on the presence or absence of five adverse prognostic factors and may have none or all five of these adverse prognostic factors. Figure 110-4 shows the prognostic significance of this score in 1300 patients with all types of non-Hodgkin's lymphoma. With the addition of rituximab to CHOP (cyclophosphamide, doxorubicin, vincristine, and prednisone), treatment outcomes have improved and the original IPI has lost some of its discrimination power. A revised IPI has been proposed that better predicts outcome of rituximab plus chemotherapy-based programs (Table 110-9). CT scans are routinely used in the evaluation of patients with all subtypes of non-Hodgkin's lymphoma, but PET and gallium scans are much more useful in aggressive subtypes such as diffuse large B cell lymphoma than in more indolent subtypes such as follicular lymphoma or small lymphocytic lymphoma. While the IPI does divide patients with follicular lymphoma into subsets with distinct prognoses, the distribution of such patients is skewed toward lower-risk categories. A follicular lymphoma–specific IPI (FLIPI) has been proposed that replaces performance status with hemoglobin level [<120 g/L (<12 g/dL)] and number of extranodal sites with number of nodal sites (more than four). Low risk (zero or one factor) was assigned to 36% of patients, intermediate risk (two factors) to 37%, and poor risk (more than two factors) to 27% of patients.

CLINICAL FEATURES, TREATMENT, AND PROGNOSIS OF SPECIFIC LYMPHOID MALIGNANCIES

■ PRECURSOR CELL B CELL NEOPLASMS

Precursor B cell lymphoblastic leukemia/lymphoma

The most common cancer in childhood is B cell ALL. Although this disorder can also present as a lymphoma in either adults or children, presentation as lymphoma is rare.

The malignant cells in patients with precursor B cell lymphoblastic leukemia are most commonly of pre–B cell origin. Patients typically present with signs of bone marrow failure such as pallor, fatigue, bleeding, fever, and infection related to peripheral blood cytopenias. Peripheral blood counts regularly show anemia and thrombocytopenia but might show leukopenia, a normal leukocyte count, or leukocytosis based largely on the number of circulating malignant cells (Fig. 110-5). Extramedullary sites of disease are frequently involved in

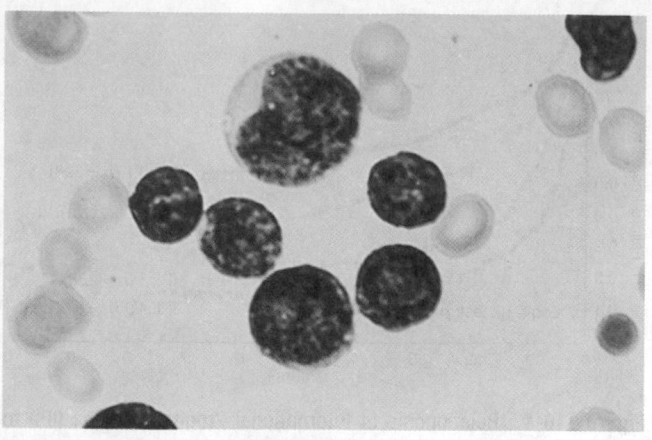

Figure 110-5 Acute lymphoblastic leukemia. The cells are heterogeneous in size, have round or convoluted nuclei, high nuclear/cytoplasmic ratio, and absence of cytoplasmic granules.

patients who present with leukemia, including lymphadenopathy, hepato- or splenomegaly, CNS disease, testicular enlargement, and/or cutaneous infiltration.

The diagnosis is usually made by bone marrow biopsy, which shows infiltration by malignant lymphoblasts. Demonstration of a pre–B cell immunophenotype (Fig. 110-2) and, often, characteristic cytogenetic abnormalities (Table 110-6) confirm the diagnosis. An adverse prognosis in patients with precursor B cell ALL is predicted by a very high white cell count, the presence of symptomatic CNS disease, and unfavorable cytogenetic abnormalities. For example, t(9;22), frequently found in adults with B cell ALL, has been associated with a very poor outlook. The bcr/abl kinase inhibitors have improved the prognosis.

TREATMENT ▶ Precursor B Cell Lymphoblastic Leukemia

The treatment of patients with precursor B cell ALL involves remission induction with combination chemotherapy, a consolidation phase that includes administration of high-dose systemic therapy and treatment to eliminate disease in the CNS, and a period of continuing therapy to prevent relapse and effect cure. The overall cure rate in children is 90%, while ~50% of adults are long-term disease-free survivors. This reflects the high proportion of adverse cytogenetic abnormalities seen in adults with precursor B cell ALL.

Precursor B cell lymphoblastic lymphoma is a rare presentation of precursor B cell lymphoblastic malignancy. These patients often have a rapid transformation to leukemia and should be treated as though they had presented with leukemia. The few patients who present with the disease confined to lymph nodes have a high cure rate.

■ MATURE (PERIPHERAL) B CELL NEOPLASMS

B cell chronic lymphoid leukemia/small lymphocytic lymphoma

B cell CLL/small lymphocytic lymphoma represents the most common lymphoid leukemia, and when presenting as a lymphoma, it accounts for ~7% of non-Hodgkin's lymphomas. Presentation can be as either leukemia or lymphoma. The major clinical characteristics of B cell CLL/small lymphocytic lymphoma are presented in Table 110-10.

The diagnosis of typical B cell CLL is made when an increased number of circulating lymphocytes (i.e., >4 × 10⁹/L and usually >10 × 10⁹/L) is found (Fig. 110-6) that are monoclonal B cells expressing the CD5 antigen. Finding bone marrow infiltration by the same cells confirms the diagnosis. The peripheral blood smear in such patients typically shows many "smudge" or "basket" cells, nuclear

TABLE 110-10 Clinical Characteristics of Patients With Common Types of Non-Hodgkin's Lymphomas (NHL)

Disease	Median Age, years	Frequency in Children	% Male	Stage I/II vs III/IV, %	B Symptoms, %	Bone Marrow Involvement, %	Gastrointestinal Tract Involvement, %	% Surviving 5 years
B cell chronic lymphocytic leukemia/small lymphocytic lymphoma	65	Rare	53	9 vs 91	33	72	3	51
Mantle cell lymphoma	63	Rare	74	20 vs 80	28	64	9	27
Extranodal marginal zone B cell lymphoma of MALT type	60	Rare	48	67 vs 33	19	14	50	74
Follicular lymphoma	59	Rare	42	33 vs 67	28	42	4	72
Diffuse large B cell lymphoma	64	~25% of childhood NHL	55	54 vs 46	33	16	18	46
Burkitt's lymphoma	31	~30% of childhood NHL	89	62 vs 38	22	33	11	45
Precursor T cell lymphoblastic lymphoma	28	~40% of childhood NHL	64	11 vs 89	21	50	4	26
Anaplastic large T/null cell lymphoma	34	Common	69	51 vs 49	53	13	9	77
Peripheral T cell non-Hodgkin's lymphoma	61	~5% of childhood NHL	55	20 vs 80	50	36	15	25

Abbreviation: MALT, mucosa-associated lymphoid tissue.

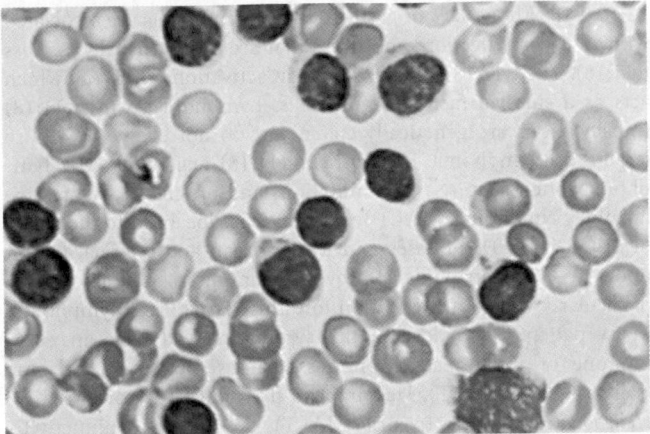

Figure 110-6   Chronic lymphocytic leukemia. The peripheral white blood cell count is high due to increased numbers of small, well-differentiated, normal-appearing lymphocytes. The leukemia lymphocytes are fragile, and substantial numbers of broken, smudged cells are usually also present on the blood smear.

remnants of cells damaged by the physical shear stress of making the blood smear. If cytogenetic studies are performed, trisomy 12 is found in 25–30% of patients. Abnormalities in chromosome 13 are also seen.

If the primary presentation is lymphadenopathy and a lymph node biopsy is performed, pathologists usually have little difficulty in making the diagnosis of small lymphocytic lymphoma based on morphologic findings and immunophenotype. However, even in these patients, 70–75% will be found to have bone marrow involvement and circulating monoclonal B lymphocytes are often present.

The differential diagnosis of typical B cell CLL is extensive (Table 110-1). Immunophenotyping will eliminate the T cell disorders and can often help sort out other B cell malignancies. For example, only mantle cell lymphoma and typical B cell CLL are usually CD5 positive. Typical B cell small lymphocytic lymphoma can be confused with other B cell disorders, including lymphoplasmacytic lymphoma (i.e., the tissue manifestation of Waldenström's macroglobulinemia), nodal marginal zone B cell lymphoma, and mantle cell lymphoma. In addition, some small lymphocytic lymphomas have areas of large cells that can lead to confusion with diffuse large B cell lymphoma. An expert hematopathologist is vital for making this distinction.

Typical B cell CLL is often found incidentally when a complete blood count is done for another reason. However, complaints that might lead to the diagnosis include fatigue, frequent infections, and new lymphadenopathy. The diagnosis of typical B cell CLL should be considered in a patient presenting with an autoimmune hemolytic anemia or autoimmune thrombocytopenia. B cell CLL has also been associated with red cell aplasia. When this disorder presents as lymphoma, the most common abnormality is asymptomatic lymphadenopathy, with or without splenomegaly. The staging systems predict prognosis in patients with typical B cell CLL (Table 110-7). The evaluation of a new patient with typical B cell CLL/small lymphocytic lymphoma will include many of the studies (Table 110-11) that are used in patients with other non-Hodgkin's lymphomas. In addition, particular attention needs to be given to detecting immune abnormalities such as autoimmune hemolytic anemia, autoimmune thrombocytopenia, hypogammaglobulinemia, and red cell aplasia. Molecular analysis of immunoglobulin gene sequences in CLL has demonstrated that about half the patients have tumors expressing mutated immunoglobulin genes and half have tumors expressing unmutated or germ-line immunoglobulin sequences. Patients with unmutated immunoglobulins tend to have

TABLE 110-11	Staging Evaluation for Non-Hodgkin's Lymphoma

Physical examination
Documentation of B symptoms
Laboratory evaluation
    Complete blood counts
    Liver function tests
    Uric acid
    Calcium
    Serum protein electrophoresis
    Serum β_2-microglobulin
Chest radiograph
CT scan of abdomen, pelvis, and usually chest
Bone marrow biopsy
Lumbar puncture in lymphoblastic, Burkitt's, and diffuse large B cell lymphoma with positive marrow biopsy
Gallium scan (SPECT) or PET scan in large cell lymphoma

Abbreviations: PET, positron emission tomography; SPECT, single photon emission CT.

a more aggressive clinical course and are less responsive to therapy. Unfortunately, immunoglobulin gene sequencing is not routinely available. CD38 expression is said to be low in the better-prognosis patients expressing mutated immunoglobulin and high in poorer-prognosis patients expressing unmutated immunoglobulin, but this test has not been confirmed as a reliable means of distinguishing the two groups. ZAP-70 expression correlates with the presence of unmutated immunoglobulin genes, but the assay is not yet standardized and widely available.

TREATMENT	B Cell Chronic Lymphoid Leukemia/Small Lymphocytic Lymphoma

Patients whose presentation is typical B cell CLL with no manifestations of the disease other than bone marrow involvement and lymphocytosis (i.e., Rai stage 0 and Binet stage A; Table 110-7) can be followed without specific therapy for their malignancy. These patients have a median survival >10 years, and some will never require therapy for this disorder. If the patient has an adequate number of circulating normal blood cells and is asymptomatic, many physicians would not initiate therapy for patients in the intermediate stage of the disease manifested by lymphadenopathy and/or hepatosplenomegaly. However, the median survival for these patients is ~7 years, and most will require treatment in the first few years of follow-up. Patients who present with bone marrow failure (i.e., Rai stage III or IV or Binet stage C) will require initial therapy in almost all cases. These patients have a serious disorder with a median survival of only 1.5 years. It must be remembered that immune manifestations of typical B cell CLL should be managed independently of specific antileukemia therapy. For example, glucocorticoid therapy for autoimmune cytopenias and γ globulin replacement for patients with hypogammaglobulinemia should be used whether or not antileukemia therapy is given.

Patients who present primarily with lymphoma and have a low IPI score have a 5-year survival of ~75%, but those with a high IPI score have a 5-year survival of <40% and are more likely to require early therapy.

The most common treatments for patients with typical B cell CLL/small lymphocytic lymphoma have been chlorambucil or fludarabine, alone or in combination. Chlorambucil can be administered orally with few immediate side effects, while fludarabine is administered IV and is associated with significant immune suppression. However, fludarabine is by far the more active agent and is the only drug associated with a significant incidence of complete remission. The combination of rituximab (375–500 mg/m² day 1), fludarabine (25 mg/m² days 2–4 on cycle 1 and 1–3 in subsequent cycles), and cyclophosphamide (250 mg/m² with fludarabine) achieves complete responses in 69% of patients, and those responses are associated with molecular remissions in half of the cases. Half the patients experience grade III or IV neutropenia. For young patients presenting with leukemia requiring therapy, regimens containing fludarabine are the treatment of choice. Because fludarabine is an effective second-line agent in patients with tumors unresponsive to chlorambucil, the latter agent is often chosen in elderly patients who require therapy. Bendamustine, an alkylating agent structurally related to nitrogen mustard, is highly effective and is vying with fludarabine as the primary treatment of choice. Patients who present with lymphoma (rather than leukemia) are also highly responsive to bendamustine and some patients will receive a combination chemotherapy regimen used in other lymphomas such as CVP (cyclophosphamide, vincristine, and prednisone) or CHOP (cyclophosphamide, doxorubicin, vincristine, and prednisone) plus rituximab. Alemtuzumab (anti-CD52) is an antibody with activity in the disease, but it kills both B and T cells and is associated with more immune compromise than rituximab. Young patients with this disease can be candidates for bone marrow transplantation. Allogeneic bone marrow transplantation can be curative but is associated with a significant treatment-related mortality rate. Mini-transplants using immunosuppressive rather than myeloablative doses of preparative drugs are being studied (Chap. 114). The use of autologous transplantation in patients with this disorder has been discouraging.

Extranodal marginal zone B cell lymphoma of malt type

Extranodal marginal zone B cell lymphoma of MALT type (MALT lymphoma) makes up ~8% of non-Hodgkin's lymphomas. This small cell lymphoma presents in extranodal sites. It was previously considered a small lymphocytic lymphoma or sometimes a pseudolymphoma. The recognition that the gastric presentation of this lymphoma was associated with *H. pylori* infection was an important step in recognizing it as a separate entity. The clinical characteristics of MALT lymphoma are presented in Table 110-10.

The diagnosis of MALT lymphoma can be made accurately by an expert hematopathologist based on a characteristic pattern of infiltration of small lymphocytes that are monoclonal B cells and CD5 negative. In some cases, transformation to diffuse large B cell lymphoma occurs, and both diagnoses may be made in the same biopsy. The differential diagnosis includes benign lymphocytic infiltration of extranodal organs and other small cell B cell lymphomas.

MALT lymphoma may occur in the stomach, orbit, intestine, lung, thyroid, salivary gland, skin, soft tissues, bladder, kidney, and CNS. It may present as a new mass, be found on routine imaging studies, or be associated with local symptoms such as upper abdominal discomfort in gastric lymphoma. Most MALT lymphomas are gastric in origin. At least two genetic forms of gastric MALT exist: one (accounting for ~50% of cases) characterized by t(11;18)(q21;q21) that juxtaposes the amino terminal of the *API2* gene with the carboxy terminal of the *MALT1* gene creating an API2/MALT1 fusion product, and the other characterized by multiple sites of genetic instability including trisomies of chromosomes 3, 7,

12, and 18. About 95% of gastric MALT lymphomas are associated with *H. pylori* infection, and those that are do not usually express t(11;18). The t(11;18) usually results in activation of NF-κB, which acts as a survival factor for the cells. Lymphomas with t(11;18) translocations are genetically stable and do not evolve to diffuse large B cell lymphoma. By contrast, t(11;18)-negative MALT lymphomas often acquire *BCL6* mutations and progress to aggressive histology lymphoma. MALT lymphomas are localized to the organ of origin in ~40% of cases and to the organ and regional lymph nodes in ~30% of patients. However, distant metastasis can occur—particularly with transformation to diffuse large B cell lymphoma. Many patients who develop this lymphoma will have an autoimmune or inflammatory process such as Sjögren's syndrome (salivary gland MALT), Hashimoto's thyroiditis (thyroid MALT), *Helicobacter* gastritis (gastric MALT), *C. psittaci* conjunctivitis (ocular MALT), or *Borrelia* skin infections (cutaneous MALT).

Evaluation of patients with MALT lymphoma follows the pattern (Table 110-11) for staging a patient with non-Hodgkin's lymphoma. In particular, patients with gastric lymphoma need to have studies performed to document the presence or absence of *H. pylori* infection. Endoscopic studies including ultrasound can help define the extent of gastric involvement. Most patients with MALT lymphoma have a good prognosis, with a 5-year survival of ~75%. In patients with a low IPI score, the 5-year survival is ~90%, while it drops to ~40% in patients with a high IPI score.

TREATMENT Mucosa-Associated Lymphoid Tissue Lymphoma

MALT lymphoma is often localized. Patients with gastric MALT lymphomas who are infected with *H. pylori* can achieve remission in the 80% of cases with eradication of the infection. These remissions can be durable, but molecular evidence of persisting neoplasia is not infrequent. After *H. pylori* eradication, symptoms generally improve quickly but molecular evidence of persistent disease may be present for 12–18 months. Additional therapy is not indicated unless progressive disease is documented. Patients with more extensive disease or progressive disease are most often treated with single-agent chemotherapy such as chlorambucil. Combination regimens that include rituximab are also highly effective. Coexistent diffuse large B cell lymphoma must be treated with combination chemotherapy (see below). The additional acquired mutations that mediate the histologic progression also convey *Helicobacter* independence to the growth.

Mantle cell lymphoma

Mantle cell lymphoma makes up ~6% of all non-Hodgkin's lymphomas. This lymphoma was previously placed in a number of other subtypes. Its existence was confirmed by the recognition that these lymphomas have a characteristic chromosomal translocation, t(11;14), between the immunoglobulin heavy chain gene on chromosome 14 and the *bcl-1* gene on chromosome 11, and regularly overexpress the BCL-1 protein, also known as cyclin D1. Table 110-10 shows the clinical characteristics of mantle cell lymphoma.

The diagnosis of mantle cell lymphoma can be made accurately by an expert hematopathologist. As with all subtypes of lymphoma, an adequate biopsy is important. The differential diagnosis of mantle cell lymphoma includes other small cell B cell lymphomas. In particular, mantle cell lymphoma and small lymphocytic lymphoma share a characteristic expression of CD5. Mantle cell lymphoma usually has a slightly indented nucleus.

The most common presentation of mantle cell lymphoma is with palpable lymphadenopathy, frequently accompanied by systemic symptoms. The median age is 63 years and men are affected four times as commonly as women. Approximately 70% of patients will be stage IV at the time of diagnosis, with frequent bone marrow and peripheral blood involvement. Of the extranodal organs that can be involved, gastrointestinal involvement is particularly important to recognize. Patients who present with lymphomatosis polyposis in the large intestine usually have mantle cell lymphoma. Table 110-11 outlines the evaluation of patients with mantle cell lymphoma. Patients who present with gastrointestinal tract involvement often have Waldeyer's ring involvement, and vice versa. The 5-year survival for all patients with mantle cell lymphoma is ~25%, with only occasional patients who present with a high IPI score surviving 5 years and ~50% of patients with a low IPI score surviving 5 years.

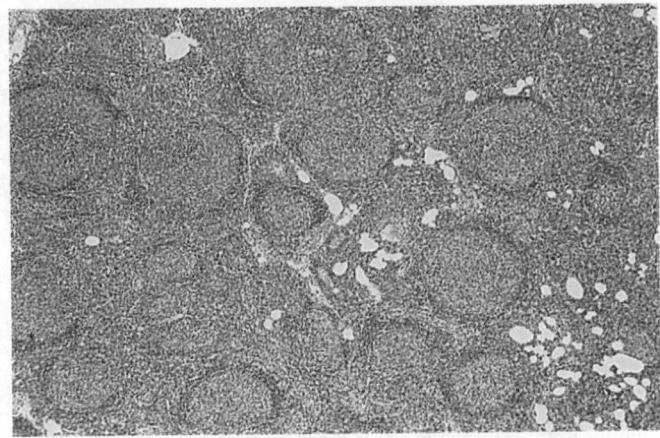

Figure 110-7 Follicular lymphoma. The normal nodal architecture is effaced by nodular expansions of tumor cells. Nodules vary in size and contain predominantly small lymphocytes with cleaved nuclei along with variable numbers of larger cells with vesicular chromatin and prominent nucleoli.

TREATMENT ▶ Mantle Cell Lymphoma

Current therapies for mantle cell lymphoma are evolving. Patients with localized disease might be treated with combination chemotherapy followed by radiotherapy; however, these patients are exceedingly rare. For the usual presentation with disseminated disease, standard lymphoma treatments have been unsatisfactory, with the minority of patients achieving complete remission. Aggressive combination chemotherapy regimens followed by autologous or allogeneic bone marrow transplantation are frequently offered to younger patients. For the occasional elderly, asymptomatic patient, observation followed by single-agent chemotherapy might be the most practical approach. An intensive combination chemotherapy regimen originally used in the treatment of acute leukemia, HyperC-VAD (cyclophosphamide, vincristine, doxorubicin, dexamethasone, cytarabine, and methotrexate), in combination with rituximab, seems to be associated with better response rates—particularly in younger patients. Alternating two regimens, HyperC-VAD with rituximab added (R-HyperC-VAD) and rituximab plus high-dose methotrexate and cytarabine can achieve complete responses in >80% of patients and 8-year survival of 56%, comparable to regimens employing high-dose therapy and autologous hematopoietic stem cell transplantation. Bortezomib, temsirolimus, and bendamustine are single agents that induce transient partial responses in a minority of patients and are being added to primary combinations.

Follicular lymphoma

Follicular lymphomas make up 22% of non-Hodgkin's lymphomas worldwide and at least 30% of non-Hodgkin's lymphomas diagnosed in the United States. This type of lymphoma can be diagnosed accurately on morphologic findings alone and has been the diagnosis in the majority of patients in therapeutic trials for "low-grade" lymphoma in the past. The clinical characteristics of follicular lymphoma are presented in Table 110-10.

Evaluation of an adequate biopsy by an expert hematopathologist is sufficient to make a diagnosis of follicular lymphoma. The tumor is composed of small cleaved and large cells in varying proportions organized in a follicular pattern of growth (Fig. 110-7). Confirmation of B cell immunophenotype and the existence of the t(14;18) and abnormal expression of BCL-2 protein are confirmatory. The major differential diagnosis is between lymphoma and reactive follicular hyperplasia. The coexistence of diffuse large B cell lymphoma must be considered. Patients with follicular lymphoma are often subclassified into those with predominantly small

cells, those with a mixture of small and large cells, and those with predominantly large cells. While this distinction cannot be made simply or very accurately, these subdivisions do have prognostic significance. Patients with follicular lymphoma with predominantly large cells have a higher proliferative fraction, progress more rapidly, and have a shorter overall survival with simple chemotherapy regimens.

The most common presentation for follicular lymphoma is with new, painless lymphadenopathy. Multiple sites of lymphoid involvement are typical, and unusual sites such as epitrochlear nodes are sometimes seen. However, essentially any organ can be involved, and extranodal presentations do occur. Most patients do not have fevers, sweats, or weight loss, and an IPI score of 0 or 1 is found in ~50% of patients. Fewer than 10% of patients have a high (i.e., 4 or 5) IPI score. The staging evaluation for patients with follicular lymphoma should include the studies included in Table 110-11.

TREATMENT ▶ Follicular Lymphoma

Follicular lymphoma is one of the malignancies most responsive to chemotherapy and radiotherapy. In addition, tumors in as many as 25% of the patients undergo spontaneous regression—usually transient—without therapy. In an asymptomatic patient, no initial treatment and watchful waiting can be an appropriate management strategy and is particularly likely to be adopted for older patients with advanced-stage disease. For patients who do require treatment, single-agent chlorambucil or cyclophosphamide or combination chemotherapy with CVP or CHOP are most frequently used. With adequate treatment, 50–75% of patients will achieve a complete remission. While most patients relapse (median response duration is ~2 years), at least 20% of complete responders will remain in remission for >10 years. For the rare patient (15%) with localized follicular lymphoma, involved field radiotherapy produces long-term disease-free survival in the majority.

A number of therapies have been shown to be active in the treatment of patients with follicular lymphoma. These include cytotoxic agents such as fludarabine, biologic agents such as interferon α, monoclonal antibodies with or without radionuclides, and lymphoma vaccines. In patients treated with a doxorubicin-containing combination chemotherapy regimen, interferon α given to patients in complete remission seems to prolong survival, but interferon toxicities can affect quality of life. The monoclonal antibody rituximab can cause objective responses in 35–50% of patients with relapsed follicular lymphoma, and radiolabeled antibodies appear to have response rates well in excess of 50%. The addition of rituximab to CHOP and other effective combination chemotherapy programs is beginning to show prolonged overall survival and a decreased risk of histologic progression. Complete remissions can be noted in 85% or more of patients treated with R-CHOP and median remission durations can exceed 6 or 7 years. Maintenance intermittent rituximab therapy can prolong remissions even further, though it is not completely clear that overall survival is prolonged. Some trials with tumor vaccines have been encouraging. Both autologous and allogeneic hematopoietic stem cell transplantation yield high complete response rates in patients with relapsed follicular lymphoma, and long-term remissions can occur in 40% or more of patients.

Patients with follicular lymphoma with a predominance of large cells have a shorter survival when treated with single-agent chemotherapy but seem to benefit from receiving an anthracycline-containing combination chemotherapy regimen plus rituximab. When their disease is treated aggressively, the overall survival for such patients is no lower than for patients with other follicular lymphomas, and the failure-free survival is superior.

Patients with follicular lymphoma have a high rate of histologic transformation to diffuse large B cell lymphoma (5–7% per year). This is recognized ~40% of the time during the course of the illness by repeat biopsy and is present in almost all patients at autopsy. This transformation is usually heralded by rapid growth of lymph nodes—often localized—and the development of systemic symptoms such as fevers, sweats, and weight loss. Although these patients have a poor prognosis, aggressive combination chemotherapy regimens can sometimes cause a complete remission in the diffuse large B cell lymphoma, at times leaving the patient with persisting follicular lymphoma. With more frequent use of R-CHOP to treat follicular lymphoma at diagnosis, it appears that the rate of histologic progression is decreasing.

Diffuse large B cell lymphoma

Diffuse large B cell lymphoma is the most common type of non-Hodgkin's lymphoma, representing approximately one-third of all cases. This lymphoma makes up the majority of cases in previous clinical trials of "aggressive" or "intermediate-grade" lymphoma. Table 110-10 shows the clinical characteristics of diffuse large B cell lymphoma.

The diagnosis of diffuse large B cell lymphoma can be made accurately by an expert hematopathologist (Fig. 110-8). Cytogenetic and molecular genetic studies are not necessary for diagnosis, but some evidence has accumulated that patients whose tumors overexpress the BCL-2 protein might be more likely to relapse than others. Patients with prominent mediastinal involvement are sometimes diagnosed as a separate subgroup having primary mediastinal diffuse large B cell lymphoma. This latter group of patients has a younger median age (i.e., 37 years) and a female predominance (66%). Subtypes of diffuse large B cell lymphoma, including those with an immunoblastic subtype and tumors with extensive fibrosis, are recognized by pathologists but do not appear to have important independent prognostic significance.

Diffuse large B cell lymphoma can present as either primary lymph node disease or at extranodal sites. More than 50% of patients will have some site of extranodal involvement at diagnosis, with the

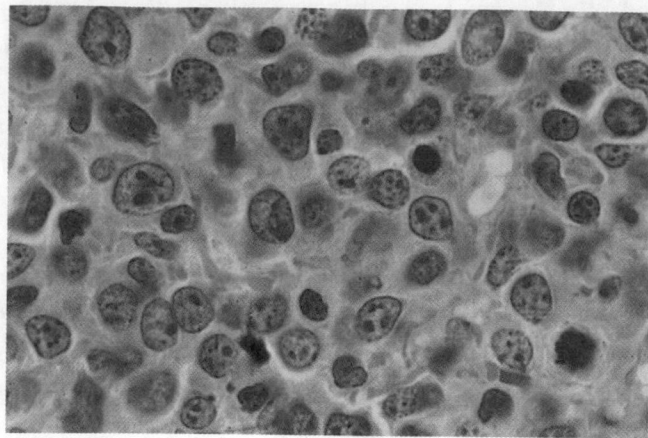

Figure 110-8 Diffuse large B cell lymphoma. The neoplastic cells are heterogeneous but predominantly large cells with vesicular chromatin and prominent nucleoli.

most common sites being the gastrointestinal tract and bone marrow, each being involved in 15–20% of patients. Essentially any organ can be involved, making a diagnostic biopsy imperative. For example, diffuse large B cell lymphoma of the pancreas has a much better prognosis than pancreatic carcinoma but would be missed without biopsy. Primary diffuse large B cell lymphoma of the brain is being diagnosed with increasing frequency. Other unusual subtypes of diffuse large B cell lymphoma such as pleural effusion lymphoma and intravascular lymphoma have been difficult to diagnose and associated with a very poor prognosis.

Table 110-11 shows the initial evaluation of patients with diffuse large B cell lymphoma. After a careful staging evaluation, ~50% of patients will be found to have stage I or II disease and ~50% will have widely disseminated lymphoma. Bone marrow biopsy shows involvement by lymphoma in ~15% of cases, with marrow involvement by small cells more frequent than by large cells.

TREATMENT **Diffuse Large B Cell Lymphoma**

The initial treatment of all patients with diffuse large B cell lymphoma should be with a combination chemotherapy regimen. The most popular regimen in the United States is CHOP plus rituximab, although a variety of other anthracycline-containing combination chemotherapy regimens appear to be equally efficacious. Patients with stage I or nonbulky stage II disease can be effectively treated with three to four cycles of combination chemotherapy with or without subsequent involved field radiotherapy. The need for radiation therapy is unclear. Cure rates of 70–80% in stage II disease and 85–90% in stage I disease can be expected.

For patients with bulky stage II, stage III, or stage IV disease, six to eight cycles of CHOP plus rituximab are usually administered. A large randomized trial showed the superiority of CHOP combined with rituximab over CHOP alone in elderly patients. A frequent approach would be to administer four cycles of therapy and then reevaluate. If the patient has achieved a complete remission after four cycles, two more cycles of treatment might be given and then therapy discontinued. Using this approach, 70–80% of patients can be expected to achieve a complete remission, and 50–70% of complete responders will be cured. The chances for a favorable response to treatment are predicted by the IPI. In fact, the IPI was developed based on the outcome of patients with diffuse large B cell lymphoma treated with CHOP-like regimens. For the 35% of patients with a low IPI score of 0–1, the 5-year survival is >70%, while for the 20% of patients with a high IPI score of 4–5, the 5-year survival is ~20%. The addition of rituximab to CHOP has improved each of those numbers by ~15%. A number of other factors, including molecular features of the tumor, levels of circulating cytokines and soluble receptors, and other surrogate markers, have been shown to influence prognosis. However, they have not been validated as rigorously as the IPI and have not been uniformly applied clinically.

Because a number of patients with diffuse large B cell lymphoma are either initially refractory to therapy or relapse after apparently effective chemotherapy, 30–40% of patients will be candidates for salvage treatment at some point. Alternative combination chemotherapy regimens can induce complete remission in as many as 50% of these patients, but long-term disease-free survival is seen in ≤10%. Autologous bone marrow transplantation is superior to salvage chemotherapy at usual doses and leads to long-term disease-free survival in ~40% of patients whose lymphomas remain chemotherapy-sensitive after relapse.

Burkitt's lymphoma/leukemia

Burkitt's lymphoma/leukemia is a rare disease in adults in the United States, making up <1% of non-Hodgkin's lymphomas, but it makes up ~30% of childhood non-Hodgkin's lymphoma. Burkitt's leukemia, or L3 ALL, makes up a small proportion of childhood and adult acute leukemias. Table 110-10 shows the clinical features of Burkitt's lymphoma.

Burkitt's lymphoma can be diagnosed morphologically by an expert hematopathologist with a high degree of accuracy. The cells are homogeneous in size and shape (Fig. 110-9). Demonstration of a very high proliferative fraction and the presence of the t(8;14) or one of its variants, t(2;8) (*c-myc* and the λ light chain gene) or t(8;22) (*c-myc* and the κ light chain gene), can be confirmatory. Burkitt's cell leukemia is recognized by the typical monotonous mass of medium-sized cells with round nuclei, multiple nucleoli, and basophilic cytoplasm with cytoplasmic vacuoles. Demonstration of surface expression of immunoglobulin and one of the above-noted cytogenetic abnormalities is confirmatory.

Three distinct clinical forms of Burkitt's lymphoma are recognized; endemic, sporadic, and immunodeficiency-associated.

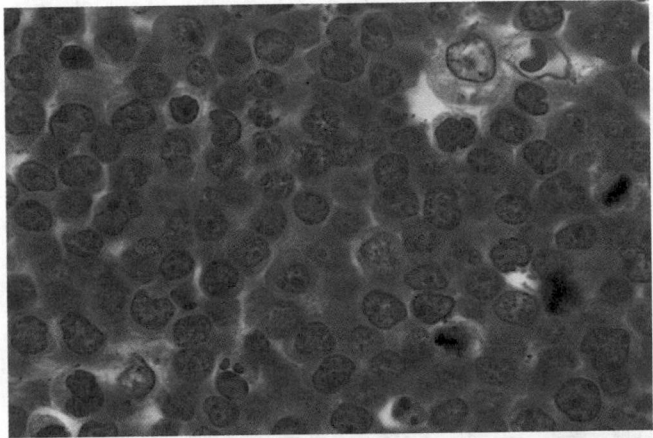

Figure 110-9 Burkitt's lymphoma. The neoplastic cells are homogeneous, medium-sized B cells with frequent mitotic figures, a morphologic correlate of high growth fraction. Reactive macrophages are scattered through the tumor and their pale cytoplasm in a background of blue-staining tumor cells give the tumor a so-called starry sky appearance.

Endemic and sporadic Burkitt's lymphomas occur frequently in children in Africa, and the sporadic form in Western countries. Immunodeficiency-associated Burkitt's lymphoma is seen in patients with HIV infection.

Pathologists sometimes have difficulty distinguishing between Burkitt's lymphoma and diffuse large B cell lymphoma. In the past, a separate subgroup of non-Hodgkin's lymphoma intermediate between the two was recognized. When tested, this subgroup could not be diagnosed accurately. Distinction between the two major types of B cell aggressive non-Hodgkin's lymphoma can sometimes be made based on the extremely high proliferative fraction seen in patients with Burkitt's lymphoma (i.e., essentially 100% of tumor cells are in cycle) caused by *c-myc* deregulation.

Most patients in the United States with Burkitt's lymphoma present with peripheral lymphadenopathy or an intraabdominal mass. The disease is rapidly progressive and has a propensity to metastasize to the CNS. Initial evaluation should always include an examination of cerebrospinal fluid to rule out metastasis in addition to the other staging evaluations noted in Table 110-11. Once the diagnosis of Burkitt's lymphoma is suspected, a diagnosis must be made promptly and staging evaluation must be accomplished expeditiously. This is the most rapidly progressive human tumor, and any delay in initiating therapy can adversely affect the patient's prognosis.

TREATMENT   Burkitt's Lymphoma

Treatment of Burkitt's lymphoma in both children and adults should begin within 48 h of diagnosis and involves the use of intensive combination chemotherapy regimens incorporating high doses of cyclophosphamide. Prophylactic therapy to the CNS is mandatory. Burkitt's lymphoma was one of the first cancers shown to be curable by chemotherapy. Today, cure can be expected in 70–80% of both children and young adults when effective therapy is administered precisely. Salvage therapy has been generally ineffective in patients failing the initial treatment, emphasizing the importance of the initial treatment approach.

Other B cell lymphoid malignancies

B cell prolymphocytic leukemia involves blood and marrow infiltration by large lymphocytes with prominent nucleoli. Patients typically have a high white cell count, splenomegaly, and minimal lymphadenopathy. The chances for a complete response to therapy are poor.

Hairy cell leukemia is a rare disease that presents predominantly in older males. Typical presentation involves pancytopenia, although occasional patients will have a leukemic presentation. Splenomegaly is usual. The malignant cells appear to have "hairy" projections on light and electron microscopy and show a characteristic staining pattern with tartrate-resistant acid phosphatase. Bone marrow is typically not able to be aspirated, and biopsy shows a pattern of fibrosis with diffuse infiltration by the malignant cells. Patients with this disorder are prone to unusual infections, including infection by *Mycobacterium avium intracellulare*, and to vasculitic syndromes. Hairy cell leukemia is responsive to chemotherapy with interferon α, pentostatin, or cladribine, with the latter being the usually preferred treatment. Clinical complete remissions with cladribine occur in the majority of patients, and long-term disease-free survival is frequent.

Splenic marginal zone lymphoma involves infiltration of the splenic white pulp by small, monoclonal B cells. This is a rare disorder that can present as leukemia as well as lymphoma. Definitive diagnosis is often made at splenectomy, which is also an effective therapy. This is an extremely indolent disorder, but when chemotherapy is required, the most usual treatment has been chlorambucil.

Lymphoplasmacytic lymphoma is the tissue manifestation of Waldenström's macroglobulinemia (Chap. 111). This type of lymphoma has been associated with chronic hepatitis C virus infection, and an etiologic association has been proposed. Patients typically present with lymphadenopathy, splenomegaly, bone marrow involvement, and occasionally peripheral blood involvement. The tumor cells do not express CD5. Patients often have a monoclonal IgM protein, high levels of which can dominate the clinical picture with the symptoms of hyperviscosity. Treatment of lymphoplasmacytic lymphoma can be aimed primarily at reducing the abnormal protein, if present, but will usually also involve chemotherapy. Chlorambucil, fludarabine, and cladribine have been utilized. The median 5-year survival for patients with this disorder is ~60%.

Nodal marginal zone lymphoma, also known as *monocytoid B cell lymphoma*, represents ~1% of non-Hodgkin's lymphomas. This lymphoma has a slight female predominance and presents with disseminated disease (i.e., stage III or IV) in 75% of patients. Approximately one-third of patients have bone marrow involvement, and a leukemic presentation occasionally occurs. The staging evaluation and therapy should use the same approach as used for patients with follicular lymphoma. Approximately 60% of the patients with nodal marginal zone lymphoma will survive 5 years after diagnosis.

■ PRECURSOR T CELL MALIGNANCIES

Precursor T cell lymphoblastic leukemia/lymphoma

Precursor T cell malignancies can present either as ALL or as an aggressive lymphoma. These malignancies are more common in children and young adults, with males more frequently affected than females.

Precursor T cell ALL can present with bone marrow failure, although the severity of anemia, neutropenia, and thrombocytopenia is often less than in precursor B cell ALL. These patients sometimes have very high white cell counts, a mediastinal mass, lymphadenopathy, and hepatosplenomegaly. Precursor T cell lymphoblastic lymphoma is most often found in young men presenting with a large mediastinal mass and pleural effusions. Both presentations have a propensity to metastasize to the CNS, and CNS involvement is often present at diagnosis.

| TREATMENT | Precursor T Cell Lymphoblastic Leukemia/Lymphoma |

Children with precursor T cell ALL seem to benefit from very intensive remission induction and consolidation regimens. The majority of patients treated in this manner can be cured. Older children and young adults with precursor T cell lymphoblastic lymphoma are also often treated with "leukemia-like" regimens. Patients who present with localized disease have an excellent prognosis. However, advanced age is an adverse prognostic factor. Adults with precursor T cell lymphoblastic lymphoma who present with high LDH levels or bone marrow or CNS involvement are often offered bone marrow transplantation as part of their primary therapy.

■ MATURE (PERIPHERAL) T CELL DISORDERS

Mycosis fungoides

Mycosis fungoides is also known as *cutaneous T cell lymphoma*. This lymphoma is more often seen by dermatologists than internists.

The median age of onset is in the midfifties, and the disease is more common in males and in blacks.

Mycosis fungoides is an indolent lymphoma with patients often having several years of eczematous or dermatitic skin lesions before the diagnosis is finally established. The skin lesions progress from patch stage to plaque stage to cutaneous tumors. Early in the disease, biopsies are often difficult to interpret, and the diagnosis may only become apparent by observing the patient over time. In advanced stages, the lymphoma can spread to lymph nodes and visceral organs. Patients with this lymphoma may develop generalized erythroderma and circulating tumor cells, called *Sézary's syndrome*.

Rare patients with localized early-stage mycosis fungoides can be cured with radiotherapy, often total-skin electron beam irradiation. More advanced disease has been treated with topical glucocorticoids, topical nitrogen mustard, phototherapy, psoralen with ultraviolet A (PUVA), extracorporeal photopheresis, retinoids (bexarotene), electron beam radiation, interferon, antibodies, fusion toxins, histone deacetylase inhibitors, and systemic cytotoxic therapy. Unfortunately, these treatments are palliative.

Adult T cell lymphoma/leukemia

Adult T cell lymphoma/leukemia is one manifestation of infection by the HTLV-I retrovirus. Patients can be infected through transplacental transmission, mother's milk, blood transfusion, and by sexual transmission of the virus. Patients who acquire the virus from their mother through breast milk are most likely to develop lymphoma, but the risk is still only 2.5% and the latency averages 55 years. Nationwide testing for HTLV-I antibodies and the aggressive implementation of public health measures could theoretically lead to the disappearance of adult T cell lymphoma/leukemia. Tropical spastic paraparesis, another manifestation of HTLV-I infection (Chap. 188), occurs after a shorter latency (1–3 years) and is most common in individuals who acquire the virus during adulthood from transfusion or sex.

The diagnosis of adult T cell lymphoma/leukemia is made when an expert hematopathologist recognizes the typical morphologic picture, a T cell immunophenotype (i.e., CD4 positive), and the presence in serum of antibodies to HTLV-I. Examination of the peripheral blood will usually reveal characteristic, pleomorphic abnormal CD4-positive cells with indented nuclei, which have been called "flower" cells (Fig. 110-10).

A subset of patients have a smoldering clinical course and long survival, but most patients present with an aggressive disease manifested by lymphadenopathy, hepatosplenomegaly, skin infiltration,

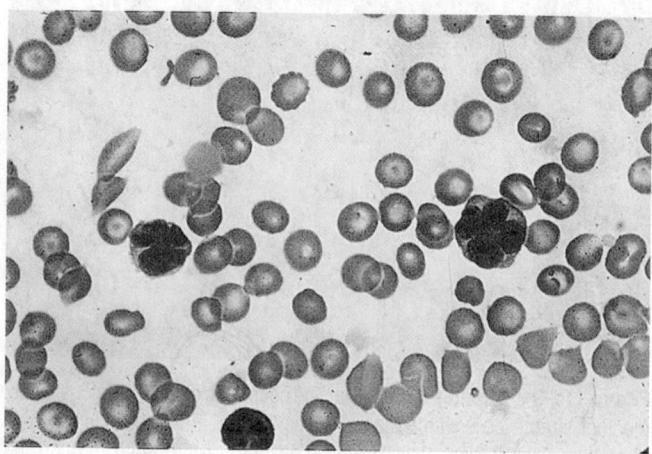

Figure 110-10 Adult T cell leukemia/lymphoma. Peripheral blood smear showing leukemia cells with typical "flower-shaped" nucleus.

pulmonary infiltrates, hypercalcemia, lytic bone lesions, and elevated LDH levels. The skin lesions can be papules, plaques, tumors, and ulcerations. Lung lesions can be either tumor or opportunistic infection in light of the underlying immunodeficiency in the disease. Bone marrow involvement is not usually extensive, and anemia and thrombocytopenia are not usually prominent. Although treatment with combination chemotherapy regimens can result in objective responses, true complete remissions are unusual, and the median survival of patients is ~7 months. A small phase II study reported a high response rate with interferon plus zidovudine and arsenic trioxide.

Anaplastic large T/null cell lymphoma

Anaplastic large T/null cell lymphoma was previously usually diagnosed as undifferentiated carcinoma or malignant histiocytosis. Discovery of the CD30 (Ki-1) antigen and the recognition that some patients with previously unclassified malignancies displayed this antigen led to the identification of a new type of lymphoma. Subsequently, discovery of the t(2;5) and the resultant frequent overexpression of the anaplastic lymphoma kinase (ALK) protein confirmed the existence of this entity. This lymphoma accounts for ~2% of all non-Hodgkin's lymphomas. Table 110-10 shows the clinical characteristics of patients with anaplastic large T/null cell lymphoma.

The diagnosis of anaplastic large T/null cell lymphoma is made when an expert hematopathologist recognizes the typical morphologic picture and a T cell or null cell immunophenotype with CD30 positivity. Documentation of the t(2;5) and/or overexpression of ALK protein confirm the diagnosis. Some diffuse large B cell lymphomas can also have an anaplastic appearance but have the same clinical course or response to therapy as other diffuse large B cell lymphomas.

Patients with anaplastic large T/null cell lymphoma are typically young (median age, 33 years) and male (~70%). Some 50% of patients present in stage I/II, and the remainder with more extensive disease. Systemic symptoms and elevated LDH levels are seen in about one-half of patients. Bone marrow and the gastrointestinal tract are rarely involved, but skin involvement is frequent. Some patients with disease confined to the skin have a different and more indolent disorder that has been termed *cutaneous anaplastic large T/null cell lymphoma* and might be related to lymphomatoid papulosis.

> **TREATMENT**   Anaplastic Large T/Null Cell Lymphoma

Treatment regimens appropriate for other aggressive lymphomas, such as diffuse large B cell lymphoma, should be utilized in patients with anaplastic large T/null cell lymphoma, with the exception that the B cell–specific antibody, rituximab, is omitted. Surprisingly, given the anaplastic appearance, this disorder has the best survival rate of any aggressive lymphoma. The 5-year survival is >75%. While traditional prognostic factors such as the IPI predict treatment outcome, overexpression of the ALK protein is an important prognostic factor, with patients overexpressing this protein having a superior treatment outcome. The ALK inhibitor crizotinib appears highly active as well.

Peripheral T cell lymphoma

The peripheral T cell lymphomas make up a heterogeneous morphologic group of aggressive neoplasms that share a mature T cell immunophenotype. They represent ~7% of all cases of non-Hodgkin's lymphoma. A number of distinct clinical syndromes are included in this group of disorders. Table 110-10 shows the clinical characteristics of patients with peripheral T cell lymphoma.

The diagnosis of peripheral T cell lymphoma, or any of its specific subtypes, requires an expert hematopathologist, an adequate biopsy, and immunophenotyping. Most peripheral T cell lymphomas are CD4+, but a few will be CD8+, both CD4+ and CD8+, or have an NK cell immunophenotype. No characteristic genetic abnormalities have yet been identified, but translocations involving the T cell antigen receptor genes on chromosomes 7 or 14 may be detected. The differential diagnosis of patients suspected of having peripheral T cell lymphoma includes reactive T cell infiltrative processes. In some cases, demonstration of a monoclonal T cell population using T cell receptor gene rearrangement studies will be required to make a diagnosis.

The initial evaluation of a patient with a peripheral T cell lymphoma should include the studies in Table 110-11 for staging patients with non-Hodgkin's lymphoma. Unfortunately, patients with peripheral T cell lymphoma usually present with adverse prognostic factors, with >80% of patients having an IPI score ≥2 and >30% having an IPI score ≥4. As this would predict, peripheral T cell lymphomas are associated with a poor outcome, and only 25% of the patients survive 5 years after diagnosis. Treatment regimens are the same as those used for diffuse large B cell lymphoma (omitting rituximab), but patients with peripheral T cell lymphoma have a poorer response to treatment. Because of this poor treatment outcome, hematopoietic stem cell transplantation is often considered early in the care of young patients.

A number of specific clinical syndromes are seen in the peripheral T cell lymphomas. *Angioimmunoblastic T cell lymphoma* is one of the more common subtypes, making up ~20% of T cell lymphomas. These patients typically present with generalized lymphadenopathy, fever, weight loss, skin rash, and polyclonal hypergammaglobulinemia. In some cases, it is difficult to separate patients with a reactive disorder from those with true lymphoma.

Extranodal T/NK cell lymphoma of nasal type has also been called *angiocentric lymphoma* and was previously termed *lethal midline granuloma*. This disorder is more frequent in Asia and South America than in the United States and Europe. EBV is thought to play an etiologic role. Although most frequent in the upper airway, it can involve other organs. The course is aggressive, and patients frequently have the hemophagocytic syndrome. When marrow and blood involvement occur, distinction between this disease and leukemia might be difficult. Some patients will respond to aggressive combination chemotherapy regimens, but the overall outlook is poor.

Enteropathy-type intestinal T cell lymphoma is a rare disorder that occurs in patients with untreated gluten-sensitive enteropathy. Patients are frequently wasted and sometimes present with intestinal perforation. The prognosis is poor. *Hepatosplenic γδ T cell lymphoma* is a systemic illness that presents with sinusoidal infiltration of the liver, spleen, and bone marrow by malignant T cells. Tumor masses generally do not occur. The disease is associated with systemic symptoms and is often difficult to diagnose. Treatment outcome is poor. *Subcutaneous panniculitis-like T cell lymphoma* is a rare disorder that is often confused with panniculitis. Patients present with multiple subcutaneous nodules, which progress and can ulcerate. Hemophagocytic syndrome is common. Response to therapy is poor. The development of the hemophagocytic syndrome (profound anemia, ingestion of erythrocytes by monocytes and macrophages) in the course of any peripheral T cell lymphoma is generally associated with a fatal outcome.

■ HODGKIN'S DISEASE

Classical Hodgkin's disease

Hodgkin's disease occurs in 8000 patients in the United States each year, and the disease does not appear to be increasing in frequency.

Most patients present with palpable lymphadenopathy that is nontender; in most patients, these lymph nodes are in the neck, supraclavicular area, and axilla. More than half the patients will have mediastinal adenopathy at diagnosis, and this is sometimes the initial manifestation. Subdiaphragmatic presentation of Hodgkin's disease is unusual and more common in older males. One-third of patients present with fevers, night sweats, and/or weight loss—B symptoms in the Ann Arbor staging classification (Table 110-8). Occasionally, Hodgkin's disease can present as a fever of unknown origin. This is more common in older patients who are found to have mixed-cellularity Hodgkin's disease in an abdominal site. Rarely, the fevers persist for days to weeks, followed by afebrile intervals and then recurrence of the fever. This pattern is known as *Pel-Ebstein fever*. Hodgkin's disease can occasionally present with unusual manifestations. These include severe and unexplained itching, cutaneous disorders such as erythema nodosum and ichthyosiform atrophy, paraneoplastic cerebellar degeneration and other distant effects on the CNS, nephrotic syndrome, immune hemolytic anemia and thrombocytopenia, hypercalcemia, and pain in lymph nodes on alcohol ingestion.

The diagnosis of Hodgkin's disease is established by review of an adequate biopsy specimen by an expert hematopathologist. In the United States, most patients have nodular sclerosing Hodgkin's disease, with a minority of patients having mixed-cellularity Hodgkin's disease. Lymphocyte-predominant and lymphocyte-depleted Hodgkin's disease are rare. Mixed-cellularity Hodgkin's disease or lymphocyte-depletion Hodgkin's disease are seen more frequently in patients infected by HIV (Fig. 110-11). Hodgkin's disease is a tumor characterized by rare neoplastic cells of B cell origin (immunoglobulin genes are rearranged but not expressed) in a tumor mass that is largely polyclonal inflammatory infiltrate, probably a reaction to cytokines produced by the tumor cells. The differential diagnosis of a lymph node biopsy suspicious for Hodgkin's disease includes inflammatory processes, mononucleosis, non-Hodgkin's lymphoma, phenytoin-induced adenopathy, and nonlymphomatous malignancies.

The staging evaluation for a patient with Hodgkin's disease would typically include a careful history and physical examination; complete blood count; erythrocyte sedimentation rate; serum chemistry studies including LDH; chest radiograph; CT scan of the chest, abdomen, and pelvis; and bone marrow biopsy. Many patients would also have a PET scan or a gallium scan. Although

rarely utilized, a bipedal lymphangiogram can be helpful. PET and gallium scans are most useful to document remission. Staging laparotomies were once popular for most patients with Hodgkin's disease but are now done rarely because of an increased reliance on systemic rather than local therapy.

TREATMENT **Classical Hodgkin's Disease**

Patients with localized Hodgkin's disease are cured >90% of the time. In patients with good prognostic factors, extended-field radiotherapy has a high cure rate. Increasingly, patients with all stages of Hodgkin's disease are treated initially with chemotherapy. Patients with localized or good-prognosis disease receive a brief course of chemotherapy followed by radiotherapy to sites of node involvement. Patients with more extensive disease or those with B symptoms receive a complete course of chemotherapy. The most popular chemotherapy regimens used in Hodgkin's disease include doxorubicin, bleomycin, vinblastine, and dacarbazine (ABVD) and mechlorethamine, vincristine, procarbazine, and prednisone (MOPP), or combinations of the drugs in these two regimens. Today, most patients in the United States receive ABVD, but a weekly chemotherapy regimen administered for 12 weeks called *Stanford V* is becoming increasingly popular, but includes radiation therapy, which has been associated with life-threatening late toxicities such as premature coronary artery disease and second solid tumors. In Europe, a high-dose regimen called *BEACOPP* incorporating alkylating agents has become popular and might have a better response rate in very high risk patients. Long-term disease-free survival in patients with advanced disease can be achieved in >75% of patients who lack systemic symptoms and in 60–70% of patients with systemic symptoms.

Patients who relapse after primary therapy of Hodgkin's disease can frequently still be cured. Patients who relapse after initial treatment with only radiotherapy have an excellent outcome when treated with chemotherapy. Patients who relapse after an effective chemotherapy regimen are usually not curable with subsequent chemotherapy administered at standard doses. However, patients with a long initial remission can be an exception to this rule. Autologous bone marrow transplantation can cure half of patients who fail effective chemotherapy regimens.

Because of the very high cure rate in patients with Hodgkin's disease, long-term complications have become a major focus for clinical research. In fact, in some series of patients with early-stage disease, more patients died from late complications of therapy than from Hodgkin's disease itself. This is particularly true in patients with localized disease. The most serious late side effects include second malignancies and cardiac injury. Patients are at risk for the development of acute leukemia in the first 10 years after treatment with combination chemotherapy regimens that contain alkylating agents plus radiation therapy. The risk for development of acute leukemia appears to be greater after MOPP-like regimens than with ABVD. The risk of development of acute leukemia after treatment for Hodgkin's disease is also related to the number of exposures to potentially leukemogenic agents (i.e., multiple treatments after relapse) and the age of the patient being treated, with those aged >60 years at particularly high risk. The development of carcinomas as a complication of treatment for Hodgkin's disease has become a major problem. These tumors usually occur ≥10 years after treatment and are associated with use of radiotherapy. For this reason, young women treated with thoracic radiotherapy for Hodgkin's disease should institute screening mammograms

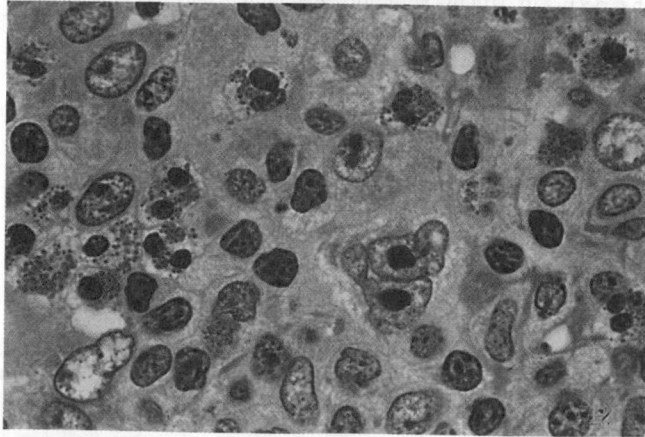

Figure 110-11   Mixed-cellularity Hodgkin's disease. A Reed-Sternberg cell is present near the center of the field; a large cell with a bilobed nucleus and prominent nucleoli giving an "owl's eyes" appearance. The majority of the cells are normal lymphocytes, neutrophils, and eosinophils that form a pleomorphic cellular infiltrate.

5–10 years after treatment, and all patients who receive thoracic radiotherapy for Hodgkin's disease should be discouraged from smoking. Thoracic radiation also accelerates coronary artery disease, and patients should be encouraged to minimize risk factors for coronary artery disease such as smoking and elevated cholesterol levels. Cervical radiation therapy increases the risk of carotid atherosclerosis and stroke.

A number of other late side effects from the treatment of Hodgkin's disease are well known. Patients who receive thoracic radiotherapy are at very high risk for the eventual development of hypothyroidism and should be observed for this complication; intermittent measurement of thyrotropin should be made to identify the condition before it becomes symptomatic. Lhermitte's syndrome occurs in ~15% of patients who receive thoracic radiotherapy. This syndrome is manifested by an "electric shock" sensation into the lower extremities on flexion of the neck. Infertility is a concern for all patients undergoing treatment for Hodgkin's disease. In both women and men, the risk of permanent infertility is age-related, with younger patients more likely to recover fertility. In addition, treatment with ABVD rather than MOPP increases the chances to retain fertility.

Nodular lymphocyte-predominant Hodgkin's disease

Nodular lymphocyte-predominant Hodgkin's disease is now recognized as an entity distinct from classical Hodgkin's disease. Previous classification systems recognized that biopsies from a subset of patients diagnosed as having Hodgkin's disease contained a predominance of small lymphocytes and rare Reed-Sternberg cells (Fig. 110-11). A subset of these patients have tumors with nodular growth pattern and a clinical course that varied from that of patients with classical Hodgkin's disease. This is an unusual clinical entity and represents <5% of cases of Hodgkin's disease.

Nodular lymphocyte-predominant Hodgkin's disease has a number of characteristics that suggest its relationship to non-Hodgkin's lymphoma. These include a clonal proliferation of B cells and a distinctive immunophenotype; tumor cells express J chain and display CD45 and epithelial membrane antigen (EMA) and do not express two markers normally found on Reed-Sternberg cells, CD30 and CD15. This lymphoma tends to have a chronic, relapsing course and sometimes transforms to diffuse large B cell lymphoma.

The treatment of patients with nodular lymphocyte-predominant Hodgkin's disease is controversial. Some clinicians favor no treatment and merely close follow-up. In the United States, most physicians will treat localized disease with radiotherapy and disseminated disease with regimens utilized for patients with classical Hodgkin's disease. Regardless of the therapy utilized, most series report a long-term survival of >80%.

LYMPHOMA-LIKE DISORDERS

The most common condition that pathologists and clinicians might confuse with lymphoma is reactive, atypical lymphoid hyperplasia. Patients might have localized or disseminated lymphadenopathy and might have the systemic symptoms characteristic of lymphoma. Underlying causes include a drug reaction to phenytoin or carbamazepine. Immune disorders such as rheumatoid arthritis and lupus erythematosus, viral infections such as cytomegalovirus

and EBV, and bacterial infections such as cat-scratch disease may cause adenopathy (Chap. 59). In the absence of a definitive diagnosis after initial biopsy, continued follow-up, further testing, and repeated biopsies, if necessary, are the appropriate approach rather than instituting therapy.

Specific conditions that can be confused with lymphoma include *Castleman's disease*, which can present with localized or disseminated lymphadenopathy; some patients have systemic symptoms. The disseminated form is often accompanied by anemia and polyclonal hypergammaglobulinemia, and the condition has been associated with overproduction of interleukin 6, possibly produced by human herpesvirus 8. Patients with localized disease can be treated effectively with local therapy, while the initial treatment for patients with disseminated disease is usually with systemic glucocorticoids. IL-6-directed therapy is being developed.

Sinus histiocytosis with massive lymphadenopathy (Rosai-Dorfman's disease) usually presents with bulky lymphadenopathy in children or young adults. The disease is usually nonprogressive and self-limited, but patients can manifest autoimmune hemolytic anemia.

Lymphomatoid papulosis is a cutaneous lymphoproliferative disorder that is often confused with anaplastic large cell lymphoma involving the skin. The cells of lymphomatoid papulosis are similar to those seen in lymphoma and stain for CD30, and T cell receptor gene rearrangements are sometimes seen. However, the condition is characterized by waxing and waning skin lesions that usually heal, leaving small scars. In the absence of effective communication between the clinician and the pathologist regarding the clinical course in the patient, this disease will be misdiagnosed. Since the clinical picture is usually benign, misdiagnosis is a serious mistake.

ACKNOWLEDGMENT

James Armitage was a coauthor of this chapter in prior editions, and substantial material from those editions has been included here.

FURTHER READINGS

ANSEL SM, ARMITAGE JO: Management of Hodgkin lymphoma. Mayo Clin Proc 81:419, 2006

ARMITAGE JO: Early-stage Hodgkin's lymphoma. N Engl J Med 363:653, 2010

BREPOELS L et al: PET and PET/CT for response evaluation in lymphoma: Current practice and developments. Leuk Lymphoma 48:270, 2007

CABANILLAS F: Front-line therapy of diffuse large B-cell lymphoma. Curr Opin Oncol 22:642, 2010

HARRIS NL et al: World Health Organization classification of neoplastic diseases of the hematopoietic and lymphoid tissues: Report of the Clinical Advisory Committee Meeting, Airlie House, Virginia, November, 1997. J Clin Oncol 17:3835, 1999

LONGO DL (ed): Hodgkin's lymphoma. Cancer J 15:114, 2009

SEHN LH et al: The revised International Prognostic Index (R-IPI) is a better predictor of outcome than the standard IPI for patients with diffuse large B-cell lymphoma treated with R-CHOP. Blood 109:1857, 2007

STATHIS A et al: Treatment of gastric marginal zone lymphoma of MALT type. Expert Opin Pharmacother 11:2141, 2010

CHAPTER 111

Plasma Cell Disorders

Nikhil C. Munshi

Dan L. Longo

Kenneth C. Anderson

The *plasma cell disorders* are monoclonal neoplasms related to each other by virtue of their development from common progenitors in the B lymphocyte lineage. Multiple myeloma, Waldenström's macroglobulinemia, primary amyloidosis (Chap. 112), and the heavy chain diseases comprise this group and may be designated by a variety of synonyms such as *monoclonal gammopathies, paraproteinemias, plasma cell dyscrasias,* and *dysproteinemias.* Mature B lymphocytes destined to produce IgG bear surface immunoglobulin molecules of both M and G heavy chain isotypes with both isotypes having identical idiotypes (variable regions). Under normal circumstances, maturation to antibody-secreting plasma cells and their proliferation is stimulated by exposure to the antigen for which the surface immunoglobulin is specific; however, in the plasma cell disorders the control over this process is lost. The clinical manifestations of all the plasma cell disorders relate to the expansion of the neoplastic cells, to the secretion of cell products (immunoglobulin molecules or subunits, lymphokines), and to some extent to the host's response to the tumor. Normal development of B lymphocytes is discussed in Chap. 314.

There are three categories of structural variation among immunoglobulin molecules that form antigenic determinants, and these are used to classify immunoglobulins (Chap. 314). *Isotypes* are those determinants that distinguish among the main classes of antibodies of a given species and are the same in all normal individuals of that species. Therefore, isotypic determinants are, by definition, recognized by antibodies from a distinct species (heterologous sera) but not by antibodies from the same species (homologous sera). There are five heavy chain isotypes (M, G, A, D, E) and two light chain isotypes (κ, λ). *Allotypes* are distinct determinants that reflect regular small differences between individuals of the same species in the amino acid sequences of otherwise similar immunoglobulins. These differences are determined by allelic genes; by definition, they are detected by antibodies made in the same species. *Idiotypes* are the third category of antigenic determinants. They are unique to the molecules produced by a given clone of antibody-producing cells. Idiotypes are formed by the unique structure of the antigen-binding portion of the molecule.

Antibody molecules (Fig. 314-8) are composed of two heavy chains (~50,000 mol wt) and two light chains (~25,000 mol wt). Each chain has a constant portion (limited amino acid sequence variability) and a variable region (extensive sequence variability). The light and heavy chains are linked by disulfide bonds and are aligned so that their variable regions are adjacent to one another. This variable region forms the antigen recognition site of the antibody molecule; its unique structural features form a particular set of determinants, or idiotypes, that are reliable markers for a particular clone of cells because each antibody is formed and secreted by a single clone. Each chain is specified by distinct genes, synthesized separately, and assembled into an intact antibody molecule after translation. Because of the mechanics of the gene rearrangements necessary to specify the immunoglobulin variable regions (VDJ

joining for the heavy chain, VJ joining for the light chain), a particular clone rearranges only one of the two chromosomes to produce an immunoglobulin molecule of only one light chain isotype and only one allotype (allelic exclusion). After exposure to antigen, the variable region may become associated with a new heavy chain isotype (class switch). Each clone of cells performs these sequential gene arrangements in a unique way. This results in each clone producing a unique immunoglobulin molecule. In most plasma cells, light chains are synthesized in slight excess, secreted as free light chains, and are cleared by the kidney, but <10 mg of such light chains is excreted per day.

Electrophoretic analysis permits separation of components of the serum proteins (Fig. 111-1). The immunoglobulins move heterogeneously in an electric field and form a broad peak in the gamma region. The γ globulin region of the electrophoretic pattern is usually increased in the sera of patients with plasma cell tumors. There is a sharp spike in this region called an *M component* (M for monoclonal). Less commonly, the M component may appear in the β_2 or α_2 globulin region. The monoclonal antibody must be present at a concentration of at least 5 g/L (0.5 g/dL) to be accurately quantitated by this method. This corresponds to ~10^9 cells producing the antibody. Confirmation that such an M component is truly monoclonal and the type of immunoglobulin is determined by immunoelectrophoresis that reveals a single heavy and/or light chain type. Hence immunoelectrophoresis and electrophoresis provide qualitative and quantitative assessment of the M component, respectively. Once the presence of an M component has been confirmed, electrophoresis provides the more practical information for managing patients with monoclonal gammopathies. In a given patient, the amount of M component in the serum is a reliable measure of the tumor burden. This makes the M component an excellent tumor marker, yet it is not specific enough to be used to screen asymptomatic patients. In addition to the plasma cell disorders, M components may be detected in other lymphoid neoplasms such as chronic lymphocytic leukemia and lymphomas of B or T cell origin; nonlymphoid neoplasms such as chronic myeloid leukemia, breast cancer, and colon cancer; a variety of nonneoplastic conditions such as cirrhosis, sarcoidosis, parasitic diseases, Gaucher disease, and pyoderma gangrenosum; and a number of autoimmune conditions, including rheumatoid arthritis, myasthenia gravis, and cold agglutinin disease. At least two very rare skin diseases—lichen myxedematosus, or papular mucinosis, and necrobiotic xanthogranuloma—are associated with a monoclonal gammopathy. In papular mucinosis, highly cationic IgG is deposited in the dermis of patients. This organ specificity may reflect the specificity of the antibody for some antigenic component of the dermis. Necrobiotic xanthogranuloma is a histiocytic infiltration of the skin, usually of the face, that produces red or yellow nodules that can enlarge to plaques. Some 10% progress to myeloma. Five percent of patients with sensory motor neuropathy are associated with monoclonal protein.

The nature of the M component is variable in plasma cell disorders. It may be an intact antibody molecule of any heavy chain subclass, or it may be an altered antibody or fragment. Isolated light or heavy chains may be produced. In some plasma cell tumors such as extramedullary or solitary bone plasmacytomas, less than one-third of patients will have an M component. In ~20% of myelomas, only light chains are produced and in most cases are secreted in the urine as Bence Jones proteins. The frequency of myelomas of a particular heavy chain class is roughly proportional to the serum concentration, and therefore IgG myelomas are more common than IgA and IgD myelomas. In approximately 1% of patients with myeloma, biclonal or triclonal gammopathy is observed.

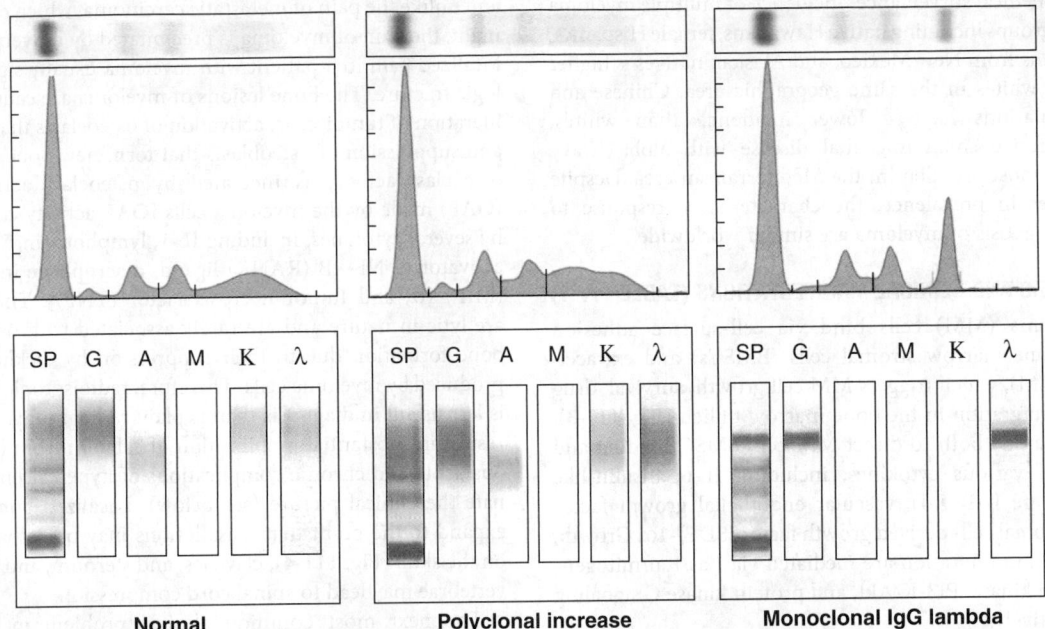

SP G A M K λ	SP G A M K λ	SP G A M K λ
Normal	**Polyclonal increase**	**Monoclonal IgG lambda**

Figure 111-1   Representative patterns of serum electrophoresis and immunofixation. The upper panels represent agarose gel, middle panels are the densitometric tracing of the gel, and lower panels are immunofixation patterns. Panel on the left illustrates the normal pattern of serum protein on electrophoresis. Since there are many different immunoglobulins in the serum, their differing mobilities in an electric field produce a broad peak. In conditions associated with increases in polyclonal immunoglobulin, the broad peak is more prominent (middle panel). In monoclonal gammopathies, the predominance of a product of a single cell produces a "church spire" sharp peak, usually in the γ globulin region (right panel). The immunofixation (lower panel) identifies the type of immunoglobulin. For example, normal and polyclonal increase in immunoglobulins produce no distinct bands; however, the right panel shows distinct bands in IgG and lambda protein lanes, confirming the presence of IgG lambda monoclonal protein. *(Courtesy of Dr. Neal I Lindeman; with permission.)*

MULTIPLE MYELOMA

■ DEFINITION

Multiple myeloma represents a malignant proliferation of plasma cells derived from a single clone. The tumor, its products, and the host response to it result in a number of organ dysfunctions and symptoms, including bone pain or fracture, renal failure, susceptibility to infection, anemia, hypercalcemia, and occasionally clotting abnormalities, neurologic symptoms, and manifestations of hyperviscosity.

■ ETIOLOGY

The cause of myeloma is not known. Myeloma occurred with increased frequency in those exposed to the radiation of nuclear warheads in World War II after a 20-year latency. Myeloma has been seen more commonly than expected among farmers, wood workers, leather workers, and those exposed to petroleum products. A variety of chromosomal alterations with prognostic significance has been found in patients with myeloma; 13q14 deletions, 17p13 deletions, and translocations t(11;14)(q13;q32) and t(4;14) (p16;q32) predominate, and evidence is strong that errors in switch recombination—the genetic mechanism to change antibody heavy chain isotype—participate in the transformation process. However, no common molecular pathogenetic pathway has yet emerged. The neoplastic event in myeloma may involve cells earlier in B cell differentiation than the plasma cell. Interleukin (IL)-6 may play a role in driving myeloma cell proliferation. It remains difficult to distinguish benign from malignant plasma cells on the basis of morphologic criteria in all but a few cases (Fig. 111-2).

■ INCIDENCE AND PREVALENCE

Estimated 20,180 new cases of myeloma were diagnosed in 2010, and 10,650 people died from the disease in the United States. Myeloma increases in incidence with age. The median age at diagnosis is 70 years; it is uncommon under age 40. Males are more commonly affected than females, and blacks have nearly twice the incidence of whites. Myeloma accounts for ~1% of all malignancies in whites and 2% in blacks, and 13% of all hematologic cancers in whites and 33% in blacks.

■ GLOBAL CONSIDERATIONS

The incidence of myeloma is highest in African Americans and Pacific islanders; intermediate in Europeans and North American whites; and lowest in developing countries including Asia. The higher incidence in more developed countries may result from the combination of a longer life expectancy and

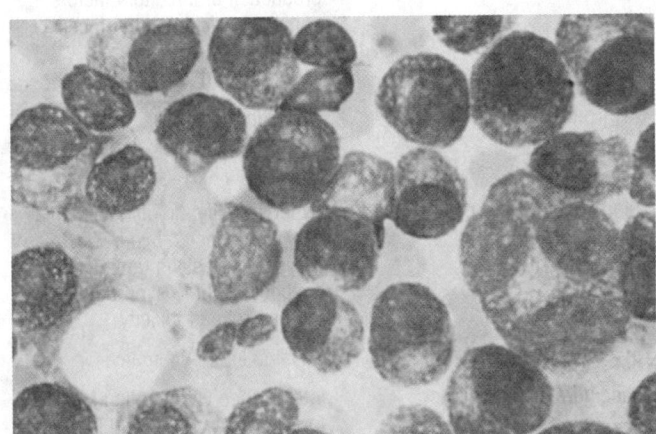

Figure 111-2   Multiple myeloma (marrow). The cells bear characteristic morphologic features of plasma cells, round or oval cells with an eccentric nucleus composed of coarsely clumped chromatin, a densely basophilic cytoplasm, and a perinuclear clear zone containing the Golgi apparatus. Binucleate and multinucleate malignant plasma cells can be seen.

more frequent medical surveillance. Incidence of multiple myeloma in other ethnic groups including native Hawaiians, female Hispanics, American Indians from New Mexico, and Alaskan natives is higher relative to U.S. whites in the same geographic area. Chinese and Japanese populations have a lower incidence than whites. Immunoproliferative small intestinal disease with alpha heavy chain disease is most prevalent in the Mediterranean area. Despite these differences in prevalence, the characteristics, response to therapy, and prognosis of myeloma are similar worldwide.

■ PATHOGENESIS AND CLINICAL MANIFESTATIONS (TABLE 111-1)

Multiple myeloma (MM) cells bind via cell-surface adhesion molecules to bone marrow stromal cells (BMSCs) and extracellular matrix (ECM), which triggers MM cell growth, survival, drug resistance, and migration in the bone marrow milieu (Fig. 111-3). These effects are due both to direct MM cell–BMSC binding and to induction of various cytokines, including IL-6, insulin-like growth factor type I (IGF-I), vascular endothelial growth factor (VEGF), and stromal cell–derived growth factor (SDF)-1α. Growth, drug resistance, and migration are mediated via Ras/Raf/mitogen-activated protein kinase, PI3-K/Akt, and protein kinase C signaling cascades, respectively.

Bone pain is the most common symptom in myeloma, affecting nearly 70% of patients. The pain usually involves the back and ribs,

TABLE 111-1 Clinical Features of Multiple Myeloma

Clinical Finding	Underlying Cause and Pathogenetic Mechanism
Hypercalcemia, osteoporosis, pathologic fractures, lytic bone lesions, bone pain	Tumor expansion, production of osteoclast activating factor by tumor cells, osteoblast inhibitory factors
Renal failure	Hypercalcemia, light chain deposition, amyloidosis, urate nephropathy, drug toxicity (nonsteroidal anti-inflammatory agents, bisphosphonates), contrast dye
Easy fatigue/anemia	Bone marrow infiltration, production of inhibitory factors, hemolysis, decreased red cell production, decreased erythropoietin levels
Recurrent infections	Hypogammaglobulinemia, low CD4 count, decreased neutrophil migration
Neurologic symptoms	Hyperviscosity, cryoglobulinemia, amyloid deposits, hypercalcemia, nerve compression, antineuronal antibody, POEMS syndrome, therapy-related toxicity
Nausea and vomiting	Renal failure, hypercalcemia
Bleeding/clotting disorder	Interference with clotting factors, antibody to clotting factors, amyloid damage of endothelium, platelet dysfunction, antibody coating of platelet, therapy-related hypercoagulable defects

Abbreviation: POEMS, polyneuropathy, organomegaly, endocrinopathy, multiple myeloma, and skin changes.

and unlike the pain of metastatic carcinoma, which often is worse at night, the pain of myeloma is precipitated by movement. Persistent localized pain in a patient with myeloma usually signifies a pathologic fracture. The bone lesions of myeloma are caused by the proliferation of tumor cells, activation of osteoclasts that destroy bone, and suppression of osteoblasts that form new bone. The increased osteoclast activity is mediated by osteoclast activating factors (OAF) made by the myeloma cells [OAF activity can be mediated by several cytokines, including IL-1, lymphotoxin, VEGF, receptor activator of NF-κB (RANK) ligand, macrophage inhibitory factor (MIP)-1α, and tumor necrosis factor (TNF)]. The bone lesions are lytic in nature and are rarely associated with osteoblastic new bone formation due to their suppression by dickhoff-1 (DKK-1) produced by myeloma cells. Therefore, radioisotopic bone scanning is less useful in diagnosis than is plain radiography. The bony lysis results in substantial mobilization of calcium from bone, and serious acute and chronic complications of hypercalcemia may dominate the clinical picture (see below). Localized bone lesions may expand to the point that mass lesions may be palpated, especially on the skull (Fig. 111-4), clavicles, and sternum, and the collapse of vertebrae may lead to spinal cord compression.

The next most common clinical problem in patients with myeloma is susceptibility to bacterial infections. The most common infections are pneumonias and pyelonephritis, and the most frequent pathogens are *Streptococcus pneumoniae*, *Staphylococcus aureus*, and *Klebsiella pneumoniae* in the lungs and *Escherichia coli* and other gram-negative organisms in the urinary tract. In ~25% of patients, recurrent infections are the presenting features, and >75% of patients will have a serious infection at some time in their course. The susceptibility to infection has several contributing causes. First, patients with myeloma have diffuse hypogammaglobulinemia if the M component is excluded. The hypogammaglobulinemia is related to both decreased production and increased destruction of normal antibodies. Moreover, some patients generate a population of circulating regulatory cells in response to their myeloma that can suppress normal antibody synthesis. In the case of IgG myeloma, normal IgG antibodies are broken down more rapidly than normal because the catabolic rate for IgG antibodies varies directly with the serum concentration. The large M component results in fractional catabolic rates of 8–16% of the normal 2%. These patients have very poor antibody responses, especially to polysaccharide antigens such as those on bacterial cell walls. Most measures of T cell function in myeloma are normal, but a subset of CD4+ cells may be decreased. Granulocyte lysozyme content is low, and granulocyte migration is not as rapid as normal in patients with myeloma, probably the result of a tumor product. There are also a variety of abnormalities in complement functions in myeloma patients. All these factors contribute to the immune deficiency of these patients. Some commonly used therapeutic agents, e.g., dexamethasone, suppress immune responses and increase susceptibility to infection.

Renal failure occurs in nearly 25% of myeloma patients, and some renal pathology is noted in more than 50%. Many factors contribute to this. Hypercalcemia is the most common cause of renal failure. Glomerular deposits of amyloid, hyperuricemia, recurrent infections, frequent use of nonsteroidal anti-inflammatory agents for pain control, use of iodinated contrast dye for imaging, bisphosphonate use, and occasional infiltration of the kidney by myeloma cells all may contribute to renal dysfunction. However, tubular damage associated with the excretion of light chains is almost always present. Normally, light chains are filtered, reabsorbed in the tubules, and catabolized. With the increase in the amount of light chains presented to the tubule, the tubular cells become overloaded with these proteins, and tubular damage results either directly from light chain toxic effects or indirectly from the release of intracellular lysosomal enzymes. The earliest manifestation of this tubular damage

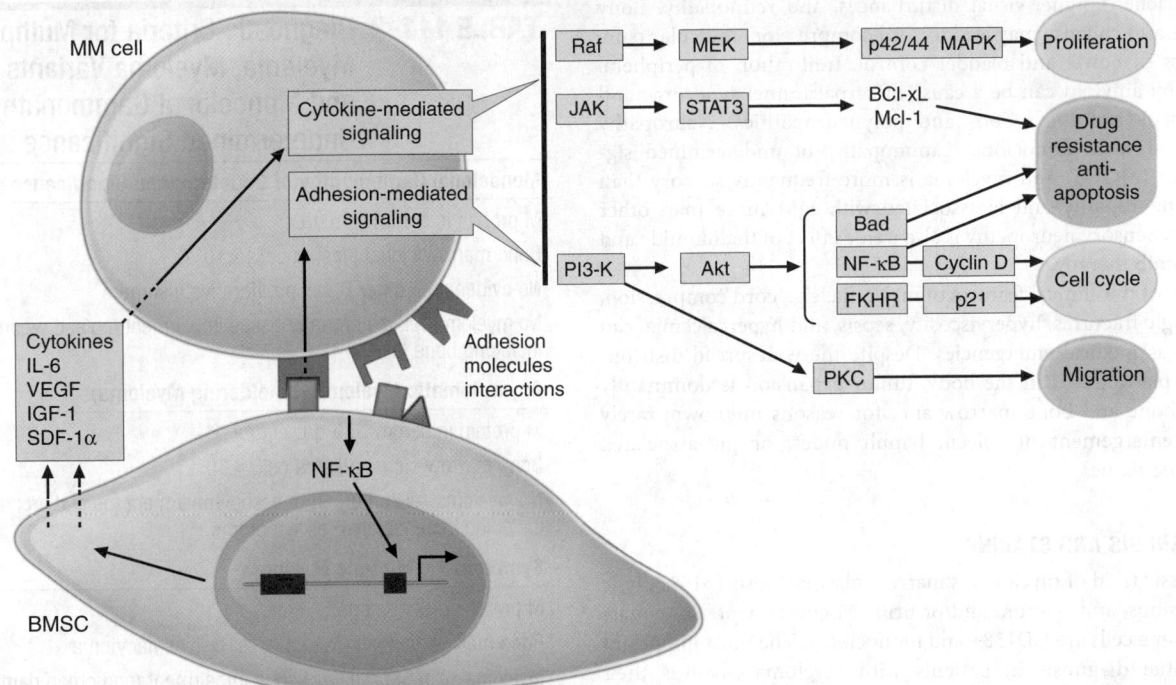

Figure 111-3 Pathogenesis of multiple myeloma. Multiple myeloma cells interact with bone marrow stromal cells and extracellular matrix proteins via adhesion molecules, triggering adhesion-mediated signaling as well as cytokine production. This triggers cytokine-mediated signaling that provides growth, survival, and antiapoptotic effects as well as development of drug resistance. HSP, heparin sulfate proteoglycan.

is the adult Fanconi syndrome (a type 2 proximal renal tubular acidosis), with loss of glucose and amino acids, as well as defects in the ability of the kidney to acidify and concentrate the urine. The proteinuria is not accompanied by hypertension, and the protein is nearly all light chains. Generally, very little albumin is in the urine because glomerular function is usually normal. When the glomeruli are involved, nonselective proteinuria is also observed. Patients with myeloma also have a decreased anion gap [i.e., $Na^+ - (Cl^- + HCO_3^-)$] because the M component is cationic, resulting in retention of chloride. This is often accompanied by hyponatremia that is felt to be artificial (pseudohyponatremia) because each volume of serum has less water as a result of the increased protein. Renal dysfunction due to light chain deposition disease, light chain cast nephropathy, and amyloidosis is partially reversible with effective therapy. Myeloma patients are susceptible to developing acute renal failure if they become dehydrated.

Normocytic and normochromic anemia occurs in ~80% of myeloma patients. It is usually related to the replacement of normal marrow by expanding tumor cells, to the inhibition of hematopoiesis by factors made by the tumor, and to reduced production of erythropoietin by the kidney. In addition, mild hemolysis may contribute to the anemia. A larger than expected fraction of patients may have megaloblastic anemia due to either folate or vitamin B_{12} deficiency. Granulocytopenia and thrombocytopenia are very rare except when therapy-induced. Clotting abnormalities may be seen due to the failure of antibody-coated platelets to function properly or to the interaction of the M component with clotting factors I, II, V, VII, or VIII. Deep venous thrombosis is also observed with use of thalidomide or lenalidomide in combination with dexamethasone. Raynaud's phenomenon and impaired circulation may result if the M component forms cryoglobulins, and hyperviscosity syndromes may develop depending on the physical properties of the M component (most common with IgM, IgG3, and IgA paraproteins). Hyperviscosity is defined on the basis of the relative viscosity of serum as compared with water. Normal relative serum viscosity is 1.8 (i.e., serum is normally almost twice as viscous as water). Symptoms of hyperviscosity occur at a level greater than 4 centipoise (cP), which is usually reached at paraprotein concentrations of ~40 g/L (4 g/dL) for IgM, 50 g/L (5 g/dL) for IgG3, and 70 g/L (7 g/dL) for IgA.

Although neurologic symptoms occur in a minority of patients, they may have many causes. Hypercalcemia may produce lethargy, weakness, depression, and confusion. Hyperviscosity may lead

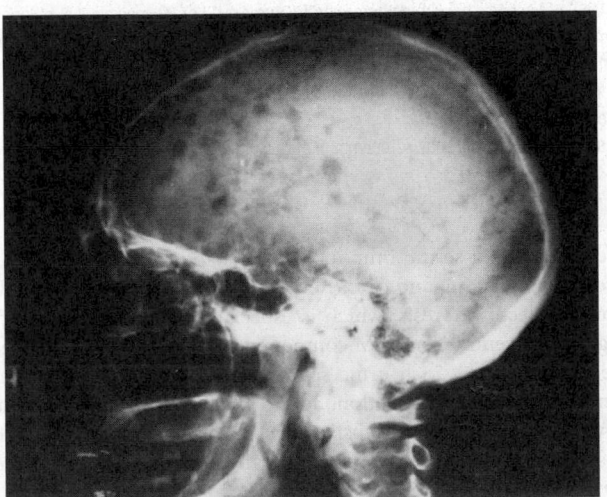

Figure 111-4 Bony lesions in multiple myeloma. The skull demonstrates the typical "punched out" lesions characteristic of multiple myeloma. The lesion represents a purely osteolytic lesion with little or no osteoblastic activity. *(Courtesy of Dr. Geraldine Schechter; with permission.)*

to headache, fatigue, visual disturbances, and retinopathy. Bony damage and collapse may lead to cord compression, radicular pain, and loss of bowel and bladder control. Infiltration of peripheral nerves by amyloid can be a cause of carpal tunnel syndrome and other sensorimotor mono- and polyneuropathies. Neuropathy associated with monoclonal gammopathy of undetermined significance (MGUS) and myeloma is more frequently sensory than motor neuropathy and is associated with IgM more than other isotypes. Sensory neuropathy is also a side effect of thalidomide and bortezomib therapy.

Many of the clinical features of myeloma, e.g., cord compression, pathologic fractures, hyperviscosity, sepsis, and hypercalcemia, can present as medical emergencies. Despite the widespread distribution of plasma cells in the body, tumor expansion is dominantly within bone and bone marrow and, for reasons unknown, rarely causes enlargement of spleen, lymph nodes, or gut-associated lymphatic tissue.

◼ DIAGNOSIS AND STAGING

The classic triad of myeloma is marrow plasmacytosis (>10%), lytic bone lesions, and a serum and/or urine M component. Bone marrow plasma cells are CD138+ and monoclonal. The most important differential diagnosis in patients with myeloma involves their separation from individuals with MGUS or smoldering multiple myeloma (SMM). MGUS are vastly more common than myeloma, occurring in 1% of the population older than age 50 years and in up to 10% of individuals older than age 75 years. The diagnostic criteria for MGUS, SMM, and myeloma are described in Table 111-2. When bone marrow cells are exposed to radioactive thymidine in order to quantitate dividing cells, patients with MGUS always have a labeling index <1%, whereas patients with myeloma always have a labeling index >1%. Although ~1% per year of patients with MGUS go on to develop myeloma, all myeloma is preceded by MGUS. Non-IgG subtype, abnormal kappa/lambda free light chain ratio, and serum M protein >15 g/L (1.5 g/dL) are associated with higher incidence of progression of MGUS to myeloma. The features responsible for higher risk of progression from smoldering myeloma to MM are bone marrow plasmacytosis >30%, abnormal kappa/lambda free light chain ratio, and serum M protein >30 g/L (3 g/dL). Typically, patients with MGUS and smoldering myeloma require no therapy. There are two important variants of myeloma, solitary bone plasmacytoma and extramedullary plasmacytoma. These lesions are associated with an M component in <30% of the cases, they may affect younger individuals, and both are associated with median survivals of ≥10 years. Solitary bone plasmacytoma is a single lytic bone lesion without marrow plasmacytosis. Extramedullary plasmacytomas usually involve the submucosal lymphoid tissue of the nasopharynx or paranasal sinuses without marrow plasmacytosis. Both tumors are highly responsive to local radiation therapy. If an M component is present, it should disappear after treatment. Solitary bone plasmacytomas may recur in other bony sites or evolve into myeloma. Extramedullary plasmacytomas rarely recur or progress.

The clinical evaluation of patients with myeloma includes a careful physical examination searching for tender bones and masses. Chest and bone radiographs may reveal lytic lesions or diffuse osteopenia. MRI offers a sensitive means to document extent of bone marrow infiltration and cord or root compression in patients with pain syndromes. A complete blood count with differential may reveal anemia. Erythrocyte sedimentation rate is elevated. Rare patients (~2%) may have plasma cell leukemia with >2000 plasma cells/μL. This may be seen in disproportionate frequency in IgD (12%) and IgE (25%) myelomas. Serum calcium, urea nitrogen, creatinine, and uric acid levels may be elevated. Protein electrophoresis and

TABLE 111-2 Diagnostic Criteria for Multiple Myeloma, Myeloma Variants, and Monoclonal Gammopathy of Undetermined Significance

Monoclonal Gammopathy of Undetermined Significance (MGUS)

M protein in serum <30 g/L

Bone marrow clonal plasma cells <10%

No evidence of other B cell proliferative disorders

No myeloma-related organ or tissue impairment (no end organ damage, including bone lesions)[a]

Asymptomatic Myeloma (Smoldering Myeloma)

M protein in serum ≥30 g/L *and/or*

Bone marrow clonal plasma cells ≥10%

No myeloma-related organ or tissue impairment (no end organ damage, including bone lesions)[a] or symptoms

Symptomatic Multiple Myeloma

M protein in serum and/or urine

Bone marrow (clonal) plasma cells[b] or plasmacytoma

Myeloma-related organ or tissue impairment (end organ damage, including bone lesions)

Nonsecretory Myeloma

No M protein in serum and/or urine with immunofixation

Bone marrow clonal plasmacytosis ≥10% or plasmacytoma

Myeloma-related organ or tissue impairment (end organ damage, including bone lesions)[a]

Solitary Plasmacytoma of Bone

No M protein in serum and/or urine[c]

Single area of bone destruction due to clonal plasma cells

Bone marrow not consistent with multiple myeloma

Normal skeletal survey (and MRI of spine and pelvis if done)

No related organ or tissue impairment (no end organ damage other than solitary bone lesion)[a]

[a]Myeloma-related organ or tissue impairment (end organ damage) (ROTI): Calcium levels increased: serum calcium >0.25 mmol/L above the upper limit of normal or >2.75 mmol/L; renal insufficiency: creatinine >173 mmol/L; anemia: hemoglobin 2 g/dL below the lower limit of normal or hemoglobin <10 g/dL; bone lesions: lytic lesions or osteoporosis with compression fractures (MRI or CT may clarify); other: symptomatic hyperviscosity, amyloidosis, recurrent bacterial infections (>2 episodes in 12 months).
[b]If flow cytometry is performed, most plasma cells (>90%) will show a "neoplastic" phenotype.
[c]A small M component may sometimes be present.

measurement of serum immunoglobulins and free light chains are useful for detecting and characterizing M spikes, supplemented by immunoelectrophoresis, which is especially sensitive for identifying low concentrations of M components not detectable by protein electrophoresis. A 24-h urine specimen is necessary to quantitate Bence Jones protein excretion. Serum alkaline phosphatase is usually normal even with extensive bone involvement because of the absence of osteoblastic activity. It is also important to quantitate serum β_2-microglobulin (see below).

The serum M component will be IgG in 53% of patients, IgA in 25%, and IgD in 1%; 20% of patients will have only light chains in serum and urine. Dipsticks for detecting proteinuria are not reliable at identifying light chains, and the heat test for detecting Bence

Jones protein is falsely negative in ~50% of patients with light chain myeloma. Fewer than 1% of patients have no identifiable M component; these patients usually have light chain myeloma in which renal catabolism has made the light chains undetectable in the urine. In most of these patients, light chains can now be detected by serum free light chain assay. IgD myeloma may also present as light chain myeloma. About two-thirds of patients with serum M components also have urinary light chains. The light chain isotype may have an impact on survival. Patients secreting lambda light chains have a significantly shorter overall survival than those secreting kappa light chains. Whether this is due to some genetically important determinant of cell proliferation or because lambda light chains are more likely to cause renal damage and form amyloid than are kappa light chains is unclear. The heavy chain isotype may have an impact on patient management as well. About half of patients with IgM paraproteins develop hyperviscosity compared with only 2–4% of patients with IgA and IgG M components. Among IgG myelomas, it is the IgG3 subclass that has the highest tendency to form both concentration- and temperature-dependent aggregates, leading to hyperviscosity and cold agglutination at lower serum concentrations.

The staging systems for patients with myeloma (Table 111-3) are functional systems for predicting survival and are based on a variety of clinical and laboratory tests, unlike the anatomic staging systems for solid tumors. The Durie-Salmon staging system used previously has been found not to predict prognosis after treatment with high-dose therapy or the novel targeted therapies that have emerged.

Serum β_2-microglobulin is the single most powerful predictor of survival and can substitute for staging. β_2-Microglobulin is a protein of 11,000 mol wt with homologies to the constant region of immunoglobulins that is the light chain of the class I major histocompatibility antigens (HLA-A, -B, -C) on the surface of every cell. Patients with β_2-microglobulin levels <0.004 g/L have a median survival of 43 months and those with levels >0.004 g/L only 12 months. Serum β_2-microglobulin and albumin levels are the basis for a three-stage International Staging System (ISS) (Table 111-3). It is also felt that once the diagnosis of myeloma is firm, histologic features of atypia may also exert an influence on prognosis. High labeling index and high levels of lactate dehydrogenase are also associated with poor prognosis.

Other factors that may influence prognosis are the presence and number of cytogenetic abnormalities, hypodiploidy, chromosome 13q and 17p deletion, translocations t(4;14) and t(14;16); circulating plasma cells; performance status; as well as serum levels of soluble IL-6 receptor, C-reactive protein, hepatocyte growth factor, C-terminal cross-linked telopeptide of collagen I, transforming growth factor (TGF)-β, and syndecan-1. Microarray profiling and comparative genomic hybridization have formed the basis for RNA- and DNA-based prognostic staging systems, respectively. The ISS system is the most widely used method of assessing prognosis (Table 111-3).

TABLE 111-3 International Staging System

	Stage	Median Survival, Months
β_2M < 3.5, alb ≥ 3.5	I (28%)	62
β_2M < 3.5, alb < 3.5 *or* β_2M = 3.5–5.5	II (39%)	44
β_2M > 5.5	III (33%)	29

Note: (#), % patients presenting at each stage.
Abbreviations: β_2M, serum β_2-microglobulin in mg/L; alb, serum albumin in g/Dl.

About 10% of patients with myeloma will have an indolent course (smoldering myeloma) demonstrating only very slow progression of disease over many years. Such patients only require antitumor therapy when the disease becomes symptomatic with development of anemia, hypercalcemia, progressive lytic bone lesions, renal dysfunction, progressive rise in serum myeloma protein levels and/or Bence Jones proteinuria, or recurrent infections. Patients with solitary bone plasmacytomas and extramedullary plasmacytomas may be expected to enjoy prolonged disease-free survival after local radiation therapy to a dose of around 40 Gy. There is a low incidence of occult marrow involvement in patients with solitary bone plasmacytoma. Such patients are usually detected because their serum M component falls slowly or disappears initially only to return after a few months. These patients respond well to systemic therapy.

Patients with symptomatic and/or progressive myeloma require therapeutic intervention. In general, such therapy is of two sorts: systemic therapy to control the progression of myeloma and symptomatic supportive care to prevent serious morbidity from the complications of the disease. Therapy can significantly prolong survival and improve the quality of life for myeloma patients.

The initial standard treatment for newly diagnosed myeloma is dependent on whether or not the patient is a candidate for high-dose chemotherapy with autologous stem cell transplant.

In patients who are transplant candidates, alkylating agents such as melphalan should be avoided since they damage stem cells, leading to decreased ability to collect stem cells for autologous transplant. Newer agents combined with pulsed glucocorticoids have now become standard of care as induction therapy in newly diagnosed patients. Two phase II studies have combined thalidomide with dexamethasone as initial therapy for newly diagnosed multiple myeloma in transplant candidates and reported rapid responses in two-thirds of patients, while allowing for successful harvesting of peripheral blood stem cells for transplantation. A randomized phase III trial showed significantly higher response rates for thalidomide (200 mg PO qhs) plus dexamethasone (40 mg for 4 days every 2 weeks) compared to dexamethasone alone, setting the stage for use of this combination as standard therapy in newly diagnosed patients. Importantly, novel agents bortezomib, a proteasome inhibitor, and lenalidomide, an immunomodulatory derivative of thalidomide, have similarly been combined with dexamethasone and obtained high response rates (>80%) without compromising stem cell collection for transplantation. Their superior toxicity profile with improved efficacy has made them the preferred agents for induction therapy. Efforts to improve the fraction of patients responding and the degree of response have involved adding agents to the treatment program. Combination of lenalidomide, bortezomib, and dexamethasone achieves close to 100% response rate, and other similar three-drug combinations (bortezomib, thalidomide, and dexamethasone or bortezomib, cyclophosphamide, and dexamethasone) achieve >90% response rate. Initial therapy is continued until maximal cytoreduction.

In patients who are not transplant candidates, besides the options available for transplant candidates, therapy consisting of intermittent pulses of an alkylating agent, melphalan with prednisone, has been utilized. The usual doses of melphalan/prednisone (MP) are melphalan, 0.25 mg/kg per day, and prednisone, 1 mg/kg per day for 4 days. Doses may need adjustment due to unpredictable absorption and based on marrow tolerance.

However, a number of studies have combined novel agents with MP combination and reported superior response and survival outcome. In patients >65 years old, combining thalidomide with MP (MPT) obtains higher response rates and overall survival compared to MP alone. Similarly, significantly improved response (71 vs 35%) and overall survival (3-year survival 72 vs 59%) were observed with combination of bortezomib with MP compared to MP alone. Lenalidomide added to MP followed by lenalidomide maintenance also prolonged progression-free survival compared to MP alone. These combinations of novel agents with MP also achieve high complete response rates (MPT ~ 15%; MPV ~ 30%, MPR ~ 20%, and MP ~ 2-4%). Patients responding to therapy generally have a prompt and gratifying reduction in bone pain, hypercalcemia, and anemia and often have fewer infections. Improvement in the serum M component may lag behind the symptomatic improvement. The fall in M component depends on the rate of tumor kill and the fractional catabolic rate of immunoglobulin, which in turn depends on the serum concentration (for IgG). Light chain excretion, with a functional half-life of ~6 h, may fall within the first week of treatment. Since urine light chain levels may relate to renal tubular function, they are not a reliable measure of tumor cell kill; however, improvements in serum free light chain measurement are often seen sooner. Although patients may not achieve complete remission, clinical responses may last long periods of time. The important feature of the level of the M protein is not how far or how fast it falls but the rate of its increase after therapy.

Randomized studies comparing standard-dose therapy to high-dose melphalan therapy (HDT) with hematopoietic stem cell support have shown that HDT can achieve high overall response rates and prolonged progression-free and overall survival; however, few, if any, patients are cured. Although complete responses are rare (<5%) with standard-dose chemotherapy, HDT achieves 25–40% complete responses. In randomized studies, HDT produced better median event-free survival in four of five studies, higher complete response rate in four of five trials, and better overall survival in three of five studies. A randomized study failed to show any significant difference in overall survival between early transplant after induction therapy versus delayed transplant at relapse. These data allow an option to delay transplant, especially with the availability of more agents and combinations. Two successive HDTs (tandem transplants) are more effective than single HDT in the subset of patients who do not achieve a complete or very good partial response to the first transplant. Allogeneic transplants may also produce high response rates, but treatment-related mortality may be as high as 40%. Nonmyeloablative allogeneic transplantation is now under evaluation to reduce toxicity, while permitting an immune graft-vs-myeloma effect.

Oral prednisone maintenance therapy was effective in a single trial after standard-dose chemotherapy. Maintenance therapy prolongs remissions following standard-dose regimens as well as HDT. Thalidomide administered post-HDT prolongs relapse-free survival. Phase III studies have demonstrated improved outcome in patients receiving lenalidomide compared to placebo as maintenance therapy after HDT, and another phase III study showed prolonged progression-free survival after MP lenalidomide and lenalidomide maintenance therapy in nontransplant candidates.

Relapsed myeloma can be treated with novel agents including lenalidomide and/or bortezomib. These agents target not only the tumor cell but also the tumor cell–bone marrow interaction and the bone marrow milieu. These agents in combination with dexamethasone can achieve up to 60% partial responses and 10–15% complete responses in patients with relapsed disease. The combination of bortezomib and liposomal doxorubicin is active in relapsed myeloma. Thalidomide, if not used as initial therapy, can achieve responses in refractory cases. High-dose melphalan and stem cell transplant, if not used earlier, also have activity in patients with refractory disease.

The median overall survival of patients with myeloma is 7–8 years, with subsets of younger patients surviving more than 10 years. The major causes of death are progressive myeloma, renal failure, sepsis, or therapy-related myelodysplasia. Nearly a quarter of patients die of myocardial infarction, chronic lung disease, diabetes, or stroke—all intercurrent illnesses related more to the age of the patient group than to the tumor.

Supportive care directed at the anticipated complications of the disease may be as important as primary antitumor therapy. The hypercalcemia generally responds well to bisphosphonates, glucocorticoid therapy, hydration, and natriuresis. Calcitonin may add to the inhibitory effects of glucocorticoids on bone resorption. Bisphosphonates (e.g., pamidronate 90 mg or zoledronate 4 mg once a month) reduce osteoclastic bone resorption and preserve performance status and quality of life, decrease bone-related complications, and may also have antitumor effects. Osteonecrosis of the jaw and renal dysfunction can occur in a minority of cases. Treatments aimed at strengthening the skeleton, such as fluorides, calcium, and vitamin D, with or without androgens, have been suggested but are not of proven efficacy. Iatrogenic worsening of renal function may be prevented by maintaining a high fluid intake to prevent dehydration and to help excrete light chains and calcium. In the event of acute renal failure, plasmapheresis is ~10 times more effective at clearing light chains than peritoneal dialysis; however, its role in reversing renal failure remains controversial. Importantly, reducing the protein load by effective antitumor therapy with agents such as bortezomib may result in functional improvement. Urinary tract infections should be watched for and treated early. Plasmapheresis may be the treatment of choice for hyperviscosity syndromes. Although the pneumococcus is a dreaded pathogen in myeloma patients, pneumococcal polysaccharide vaccines may not elicit an antibody response. Prophylactic administration of IV γ globulin preparations is used in the setting of recurrent serious infections. Chronic oral antibiotic prophylaxis is probably not warranted. Patients developing neurologic symptoms in the lower extremities, severe localized back pain, or problems with bowel and bladder control may need emergency MRI and radiation therapy for cord compression. Most bone lesions respond to analgesics and chemotherapy, but certain painful lesions may respond most promptly to localized radiation. The anemia associated with myeloma may respond to erythropoietin along with hematinics (iron, folate, cobalamin). The pathogenesis of the anemia should be established and specific therapy instituted, where possible.

WALDENSTRÖM'S MACROGLOBULINEMIA

In 1948, Waldenström described a malignancy of lymphoplasmacytoid cells that secreted IgM. In contrast to myeloma, the disease was associated with lymphadenopathy and hepatosplenomegaly, but the major clinical manifestation was the hyperviscosity syndrome. The disease resembles the related diseases chronic lymphocytic leukemia, myeloma, and lymphocytic lymphoma. It originates from a post–germinal center B cell that has undergone somatic mutations and antigenic selection in the lymphoid follicle and has the characteristics of an IgM-bearing memory B cell. Waldenström's macroglobulinemia and IgM myeloma follow a similar clinical course, but therapeutic options are different. The diagnosis of IgM myeloma is usually reserved for patients with lytic bone lesions and predominant infiltration with CD138+ plasma cells in the bone marrow. Such patients are at greater risk of pathologic fractures than patients with Waldenström's macroglobulinemia.

The cause of macroglobulinemia is unknown. The disease is similar to myeloma in being slightly more common in men and occurring with increased incidence with age (median 64 years). There have been reports that the IgM in some patients with macroglobulinemia may have specificity for myelin-associated glycoprotein (MAG), a protein that has been associated with demyelinating disease of the peripheral nervous system and may be lost earlier and to a greater extent than the better known myelin basic protein in patients with multiple sclerosis. Sometimes patients with macroglobulinemia develop a peripheral neuropathy, and half of these patients are positive for anti-MAG antibody. The neuropathy may precede the appearance of the neoplasm. There is speculation that the whole process begins with a viral infection that may elicit an antibody response that cross-reacts with a normal tissue component.

Like myeloma, the disease involves the bone marrow, but unlike myeloma, it does not cause bone lesions or hypercalcemia. Bone marrow shows >10% infiltration with lymphoplasmacytic cells (surface IgM+, CD19+, CD20+, and CD22+, rarely CD5+, but CD10– and CD23–) with increase in number of mast cells. Like myeloma, M component is present in the serum in excess of 30 g/L (3 g/dL), but unlike myeloma, the size of the IgM paraprotein results in little renal excretion, and only ~20% of patients excrete light chains. Therefore, renal disease is not common. The light chain isotype is kappa in 80% of the cases. Patients present with weakness, fatigue, and recurrent infections, similar to myeloma patients, but epistaxis, visual disturbances, and neurologic symptoms such as peripheral neuropathy, dizziness, headache, and transient paresis are much more common in macroglobulinemia. Physical examination reveals adenopathy and hepatosplenomegaly, and ophthalmoscopic examination may reveal vascular segmentation and dilation of the retinal veins characteristic of hyperviscosity states. Patients may have a normocytic, normochromic anemia, but rouleaux formation and a positive Coombs' test are much more common than in myeloma. Malignant lymphocytes are usually present in the peripheral blood. About 10% of macroglobulins are cryoglobulins. These are pure M components and are not the mixed cryoglobulins seen in rheumatoid arthritis and other autoimmune diseases. Mixed cryoglobulins are composed of IgM or IgA complexed with IgG, for which they are specific. In both cases, Raynaud's phenomenon and serious vascular symptoms precipitated by the cold may occur, but mixed cryoglobulins are not commonly associated with malignancy. Patients suspected of having a cryoglobulin based on history and physical examination should have their blood drawn into a warm syringe and delivered to the laboratory in a container of warm water to avoid errors in quantitating the cryoglobulin.

TREATMENT   Waldenström's Macroglobulinemia

Control of serious hyperviscosity symptoms such as an altered state of consciousness or paresis can be achieved acutely by plasmapheresis because 80% of the IgM paraprotein is intravascular. The median survival is ~50 months, similar to that of multiple myeloma. However, many individuals with Waldenström's macroglobulinemia have indolent disease that does not require therapy. Pretreatment parameters including older age, male sex, general symptoms, and cytopenias define a high-risk population. Fludarabine (25 mg/m² per day for 5 days every 4 weeks) or cladribine (0.1 mg/kg per day for 7 days every 4 weeks) are highly effective single agents. About 80% of patients respond to chemotherapy, and their median survival is >3 years. Rituximab (anti-CD20) can produce responses alone or combined with chemotherapy. As in multiple myeloma, the introduction of novel agents such as bortezomib, bendamustine, and lenalidomide have improved patient outcome.

POEMS SYNDROME

The features of this syndrome are *p*olyneuropathy, *o*rganomegaly, *e*ndocrinopathy, *m*ultiple myeloma, and *s*kin changes (POEMS). Patients usually have a severe, progressive sensorimotor polyneuropathy associated with sclerotic bone lesions from myeloma. Polyneuropathy occurs in ~1.4% of myelomas, but the POEMS syndrome is only a rare subset of that group. Unlike typical myeloma, hepatomegaly and lymphadenopathy occur in about two-thirds of patients, and splenomegaly is seen in one-third. The lymphadenopathy frequently resembles Castleman's disease histologically, a condition that has been linked to IL-6 overproduction. The endocrine manifestations include amenorrhea in women and impotence and gynecomastia in men. Hyperprolactinemia due to loss of normal inhibitory control by the hypothalamus may be associated with other central nervous system manifestations such as papilledema and elevated cerebrospinal fluid pressure and protein. Type 2 diabetes mellitus occurs in about one-third of patients. Hypothyroidism and adrenal insufficiency are occasionally noted. Skin changes are diverse: hyperpigmentation, hypertrichosis, skin thickening, and digital clubbing. Other manifestations include peripheral edema, ascites, pleural effusions, fever, and thrombocytosis. Not all the components of POEMS syndrome may be present initially.

The pathogenesis of the disease is unclear, but high circulating levels of the proinflammatory cytokines IL-1, IL-6, VEGF, and TNF have been documented, and levels of the inhibitory cytokine TGF-β are lower than expected. Treatment of the myeloma may result in an improvement in the other disease manifestations.

Patients are often treated similarly to those with myeloma. Plasmapheresis does not appear to be of benefit in POEMS syndrome. Patients presenting with isolated sclerotic lesions may have resolution of neuropathic symptoms after local therapy for plasmacytoma with radiotherapy. Similar to multiple myeloma, novel agents as well as high-dose therapy with autologous stem cell transplant have been pursued in selected patients and have been associated with prolonged progression-free survival.

HEAVY CHAIN DISEASES

The heavy chain diseases are rare lymphoplasmacytic malignancies. Their clinical manifestations vary with the heavy chain isotype. Patients have absence of light chain and secrete a defective heavy chain that usually has an intact Fc fragment and a deletion in the Fd region. Gamma, alpha, and mu heavy chain diseases have been described, but no reports of delta or epsilon heavy chain diseases have appeared. Molecular biologic analysis of these tumors has revealed structural genetic defects that may account for the aberrant chain secreted.

■ GAMMA HEAVY CHAIN DISEASE (FRANKLIN'S DISEASE)

This disease affects individuals of widely different age groups and countries of origin. It is characterized by lymphadenopathy, fever, anemia, malaise, hepatosplenomegaly, and weakness. It is frequently associated with autoimmune diseases, especially rheumatoid arthritis. Its most distinctive symptom is palatal edema, resulting from involvement of nodes in Waldeyer's ring, and this may progress to produce respiratory compromise. The diagnosis depends on the demonstration of an anomalous serum M component [often <20 g/L (<2 g/dL)] that reacts with anti-IgG but not anti–light chain reagents. *The M component is typically present in both serum and urine.* Most of the paraproteins have been of the γ_1 subclass, but other subclasses have been seen. The patients may have thrombocytopenia, eosinophilia, and nondiagnostic bone marrow that may show increased numbers of lymphocytes or plasma cells that do not stain for light chain. Patients usually have a rapid downhill course and die of infection; however, some patients have survived 5 years with chemotherapy. Therapy is indicated when symptomatic and involves chemotherapeutic combinations used in low-grade lymphoma. Rituximab has also been reported to show efficacy.

■ ALPHA HEAVY CHAIN DISEASE (SELIGMANN'S DISEASE)

This is the most common of the heavy chain diseases. It is closely related to a malignancy known as *Mediterranean lymphoma*, a disease that affects young persons in parts of the world where intestinal parasites are common, such as the Mediterranean, Asia, and South America. The disease is characterized by an infiltration of the lamina propria of the small intestine with lymphoplasmacytoid cells that secrete truncated alpha chains. Demonstrating alpha heavy chains is difficult because the alpha chains tend to polymerize and appear as a smear instead of a sharp peak on electrophoretic profiles. Despite the polymerization, hyperviscosity is not a common problem in alpha heavy chain disease. Without J chain–facilitated dimerization, viscosity does not increase dramatically. Light chains are absent from serum and urine. The patients present with chronic diarrhea, weight loss, and malabsorption and have extensive mesenteric and paraaortic adenopathy. Respiratory tract involvement occurs rarely. Patients may vary widely in their clinical course. Some may develop diffuse aggressive histologies of malignant lymphoma. Chemotherapy may produce long-term remissions. Rare patients appear to have responded to antibiotic therapy, raising the question of the etiologic role of antigenic stimulation, perhaps by some chronic intestinal infection. Chemotherapy plus antibiotics may be more effective than chemotherapy alone. Immunoproliferative small-intestinal disease (IPSID) is recognized as an infectious pathogen–associated human lymphoma that has association with *Campylobacter jejuni*. It involves mainly the proximal small intestine resulting in malabsorption, diarrhea, and abdominal pain. IPSID is associated with excessive plasma cell differentiation and produces truncated alpha heavy chain proteins lacking the light chains as well as the first constant domain. Early-stage IPSID responds to antibiotics (30–70% complete remission). Most untreated IPSID patients progress to lymphoplasmacytic and immunoblastic lymphoma. Patients not responding to antibiotic therapy are considered for treatment with combination chemotherapy used to treat low-grade lymphoma.

■ MU HEAVY CHAIN DISEASE

The secretion of isolated mu heavy chains into the serum appears to occur in a very rare subset of patients with chronic lymphocytic leukemia. The only features that may distinguish patients with mu heavy chain disease are the presence of vacuoles in the malignant lymphocytes and the excretion of kappa light chains in the urine. The diagnosis requires ultracentrifugation or gel filtration to confirm the nonreactivity of the paraprotein with the light chain reagents, because some intact macroglobulins fail to interact with these serums. The tumor cells seem to have a defect in the assembly of light and heavy chains, because they appear to contain both in their cytoplasm. There is no evidence that such patients should be treated differently from other patients with chronic lymphocytic leukemia (Chap. 110).

FURTHER READINGS

DIMOPOULOS M et al: Consensus recommendations for standard investigative workup: Report of the International Myeloma Workshop Consensus Panel 3. Blood 117:4701, 2011

FACON T et al: Frontline treatment in elderly patients with multiple myeloma. Semin Hematol 46:133, 2009

HAROUSSEAU JL, MOREAU P: Autologous hematopoietic stem-cell transplantation for multiple myeloma. N Engl J Med 360:2645, 2009

HIDESHIMA T et al: Understanding multiple myeloma pathogenesis in the bone marrow to identify new therapeutic targets. Nat Rev Cancer 7:585, 2007

THE INTERNATIONAL MYELOMA WORKING GROUP: Criteria for the classification of monoclonal gammopathies, multiple myeloma and related disorders: A report of the International Myeloma Working Group. Br J Haematol 121:749, 2003

JAGANNATH S et al: The current status and future of multiple myeloma in the clinic. Clin Lymphoma Myeloma Leuk 10:28, 2010

KYLE RA et al: Prevalence of monoclonal gammopathy of undetermined significance. N Engl J Med 354:1362, 2006

—— et al: Clinical course and prognosis of smoldering (asymptomatic) multiple myeloma. N Engl J Med 356:2582, 2007

MUNSHI NC et al: Consensus recommendations for risk stratification in multiple myeloma: Report of the International Myeloma Workshop Consensus Panel 2. Blood 117:4696, 2011

RAJKUMAR SV et al: Front-line treatment in younger patients with multiple myeloma. Semin Hematol 46:118, 2009

TREON SP: How I treat Waldenström macroglobulinemia. Blood 114:2375, 2009

—— et al: Advances in the biology and treatment of Waldenström's macroglobulinemia: A report from the 5th International Workshop on Waldenström's Macroglobulinemia, Stockholm, Sweden. Clin Lymphoma Myeloma 9:10, 2009

WAHNER-ROEDLER DL et al: Gamma-heavy chain disease: Review of 23 cases. Medicine 82:236, 2003

CHAPTER 112

Amyloidosis

David C. Seldin
Martha Skinner

GENERAL PRINCIPLES

Amyloidosis is the term for diseases caused by the extracellular deposition of insoluble polymeric protein fibrils in tissues and organs. These diseases are a subset of a growing group of disorders attributed to misfolding of proteins. Among these are Alzheimer's disease and other neurodegenerative diseases, transmissible prion diseases, and genetic diseases caused by mutations that lead to misfolding, aggregation, and protein loss of function, such as certain of the cystic fibrosis mutations. Amyloid fibrils share a common β-pleated sheet structural conformation that confers unique staining properties. The term *amyloid* was coined by the pathologist Rudolf Virchow around 1854, who thought such deposits were cellulose-like under the microscope.

Amyloid diseases are defined by the biochemical nature of the protein in the fibril deposits and are classified according to whether they are systemic or localized, acquired or inherited, and by their clinical patterns (Table 112-1). The accepted nomenclature is *AX*, where *A* indicates amyloidosis and *X* represents the protein in the fibril. *AL* is amyloid composed of immunoglobulin light chains (LCs), and has been called *primary systemic amyloidosis*; it arises from a clonal B cell disorder and may be associated with myeloma or lymphoma. *AF* groups the *familial amyloidoses*, most commonly due to mutations in transthyretin, the transport protein for thyroid hormone and retinol-binding protein. *AA* amyloid is composed of the acute-phase reactant serum amyloid A protein and occurs in the setting of chronic inflammatory or infectious diseases and has been termed *secondary amyloidosis*. $A\beta_2M$ is amyloid composed of β_2-microglobulin and occurs in individuals with end-stage renal disease (ESRD) of long duration. $A\beta$ is the most common form of localized amyloidosis. $A\beta$ is deposited in the brain in Alzheimer's disease and is derived from abnormal proteolytic processing of the amyloid precursor protein (APP).

Diagnosis and treatment of the amyloidoses rest upon the pathologic diagnosis of amyloid deposits and immunohistochemical or biochemical identification of amyloid type (Fig. 112-1). In the systemic amyloidoses, the involved organs can be biopsied, but amyloid deposits may be found in any tissue of the body. Historically, blood vessels of the gingiva or rectal mucosa were examined, but the most easily accessible tissue, positive in more than 80% of patients with systemic amyloidosis, is fat. After local anesthesia, needle aspiration of fat from the abdominal wall can be expelled onto a slide and stained, avoiding even a minor surgical procedure. If this material is negative, biopsy of kidney, heart, liver, or gastrointestinal tract can be considered. The regular β-sheet

TABLE 112-1 Amyloid Fibril Proteins and Their Clinical Syndromes

Term	Precursor	Clinical Syndrome	Clinical Involvement
Systemic Amyloidoses			
AL	Immunoglobulin light chain	Primary or myeloma associated[a]	Any
AH	Immunoglobulin heavy chain	Primary or myeloma associated (rare)	Any
AA	Serum amyloid A protein	Secondary; reactive[b]	Renal, any
$A\beta_2M$	β_2-Microglobulin	Hemodialysis-associated	Synovial membrane, bone
ATTR	Transthyretin	Familial (mutant) Senile systemic (wild type)	Cardiac, peripheral and autonomic nerves
AApoAI	Apolipoprotein AI	Familial	Hepatic, renal
AApoAII	Apolipoprotein AII	Familial	Renal
AGel	Gelsolin	Familial	Corneas, cranial nerves, renal
AFib	Fibrinogen Aα	Familial	Renal
ALys	Lysozyme	Familial	Renal
ALECT2	Leukocyte chemotactic factor 2	?	Renal
Localized Amyloidoses			
$A\beta$	Amyloid β protein	Alzheimer's disease; Down syndrome	CNS
ACys	Cystatin C	Cerebral amyloid angiopathy	CNS, vascular
APrP	Prion protein	Spongiform encephalopathies	CNS
AIAPP	Islet amyloid polypeptide (amylin)	Diabetes-associated	Pancreas
ACal	Calcitonin	Medullary carcinoma of the thyroid	Thyroid
AANF	Atrial natriuretic factor	Age-related	Cardiac atria
APro	Prolactin	Endocrinopathy	Pituitary

[a]Localized deposits can occur in skin, conjunctiva, urinary bladder, and tracheobronchial tree.
[b]Secondary to chronic inflammation or infection, or to a hereditary periodic fever syndrome, e.g., familial Mediterranean fever.

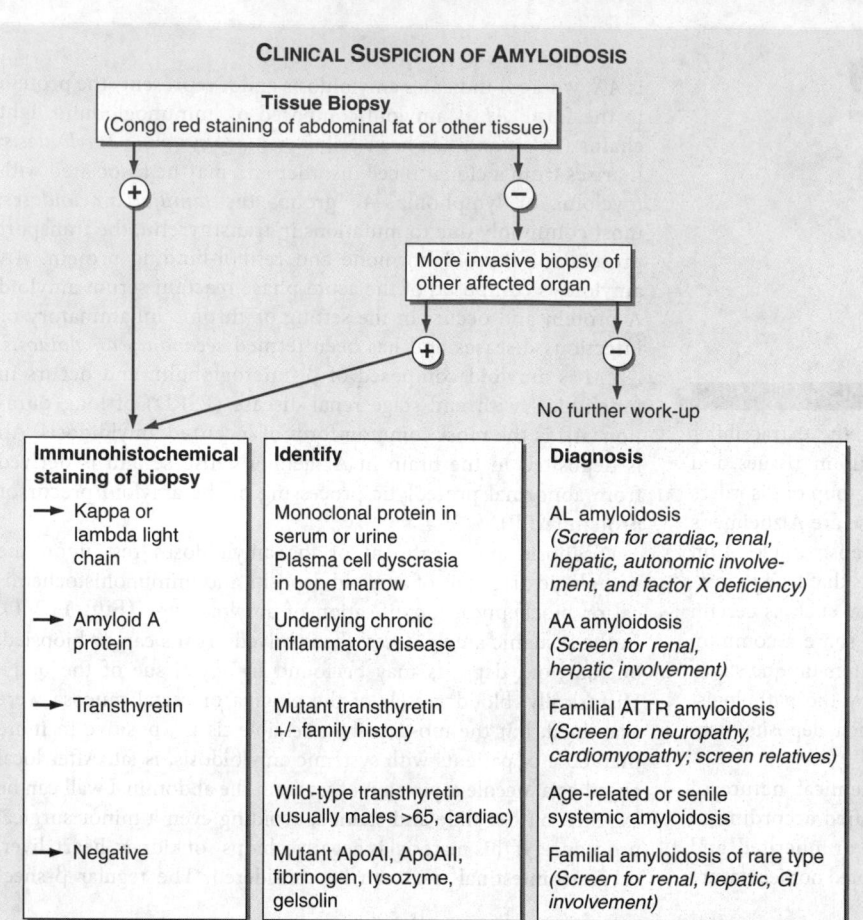

CLINICAL SUSPICION OF AMYLOIDOSIS

Tissue Biopsy
(Congo red staining of abdominal fat or other tissue)

+ / −

More invasive biopsy of
other affected organ

+ / −

No further work-up

Immunohistochemical staining of biopsy	Identify	Diagnosis
→ Kappa or lambda light chain	Monoclonal protein in serum or urine Plasma cell dyscrasia in bone marrow	AL amyloidosis (Screen for cardiac, renal, hepatic, autonomic involvement, and factor X deficiency)
→ Amyloid A protein	Underlying chronic inflammatory disease	AA amyloidosis (Screen for renal, hepatic involvement)
→ Transthyretin	Mutant transthyretin +/- family history	Familial ATTR amyloidosis (Screen for neuropathy, cardiomyopathy; screen relatives)
	Wild-type transthyretin (usually males >65, cardiac)	Age-related or senile systemic amyloidosis
→ Negative	Mutant ApoAI, ApoAII, fibrinogen, lysozyme, gelsolin	Familial amyloidosis of rare type (Screen for renal, hepatic, GI involvement)

Figure 112-1 Algorithm for the diagnosis of amyloidosis and determination of type: Clinical suspicion: unexplained nephropathy, cardiomyopathy, neuropathy, enteropathy, arthropathy, and macroglossia. ApoAI, apolipoprotein AI; ApoAII, apolipoprotein AII; GI, gastrointestinal.

structure of amyloid deposits exhibits a unique green birefringence by polarized light microscopy when stained with Congo red dye; the 10-nm-diameter fibrils can be seen directly by electron microscopy of paraformaldehyde-fixed tissue. Once amyloid is found, the protein type must be determined, usually by immunohistochemistry, immunoelectron microscopy, or by extraction and biochemical analysis by mass spectrometry or other technique. Careful evaluation of the patient's history, physical findings, and clinical presentation, including age and ethnic origin, organ system involvement, underlying diseases, and family history, can provide helpful clues to the type of amyloid.

The mechanisms of fibril formation and tissue toxicity remain controversial. Factors that contribute to fibrillogenesis include variant or unstable protein structure, extensive β-sheet conformation of the precursor protein, proteolytic processing of the precursor protein, association with components of the serum or extracellular matrix (e.g., amyloid P-component, apolipoprotein E, or glycosaminoglycans), and local physical properties, including pH of the tissue. Monomeric proteins appear to go through an oligomeric aggregation step and then form higher order polymers. Once the polymers reach a critical size, they become insoluble and deposit in extracellular tissue sites as fibrils. These large macromolecular deposits interfere with organ function and, due to cellular uptake of oligomeric amyloid precursors, may be toxic to target cells.

The clinical syndromes of the amyloidoses are associated with relatively nonspecific alterations in routine laboratory tests. Blood

counts are usually normal, although the erythrocyte sedimentation rate is frequently elevated. Patients with renal involvement will usually have proteinuria, which can be as much as 30 g/d, producing hypoalbuminemia that can be profound. Patients with cardiac involvement will often have elevation of brain natriuretic peptide (BNP), pro-BNP, and troponin. These can be useful for monitoring disease activity and have been proposed as prognostic factors; they can be falsely elevated in the presence of renal insufficiency. Patients with liver involvement, even when it is advanced, usually develop cholestasis with an elevated alkaline phosphatase but minimal elevation of the transaminases and preservation of synthetic function. In AL amyloidosis, endocrinopathies can occur, with laboratory testing demonstrating hypothyroidism, hypoadrenalism, or even hypopituitarism. None of these findings are specific for amyloidosis. Thus, a diagnosis of amyloidosis rests upon a tissue biopsy that, after Congo red staining, shows "apple-green" birefringence on polarization microscopy.

AL AMYLOIDOSIS

■ ETIOLOGY AND INCIDENCE

AL amyloidosis is most frequently caused by a clonal expansion of plasma cells in the bone marrow that secrete a monoclonal immunoglobulin LC that deposits as amyloid fibrils in tissues. It may be purely serendipitous whether the clonal plasma cells produce a LC that misfolds and leads to AL amyloidosis, or folds properly, allowing the cells to inexorably expand over time and develop into multiple myeloma (Chap. 111). It is also possible that the two processes have diverse molecular etiologies. AL amyloidosis can occur with multiple myeloma or other B lymphoproliferative diseases, including non-Hodgkin's lymphoma (Chap. 110) and Waldenström's macroglobulinemia (Chap. 111). AL amyloidosis is the most common type of systemic amyloidosis in North America. Its incidence has been estimated at 4.5 per 100,000; however, ascertainment continues to be inadequate, and the true incidence may be much higher. AL amyloidosis, like other plasma cell diseases, usually occurs after age 40 and is often rapidly progressive and fatal if untreated.

■ PATHOLOGY AND CLINICAL FEATURES OF AL AMYLOIDOSIS

Amyloid deposits are usually widespread in AL amyloidosis and can be present in the interstitium of any organ outside of the central nervous system. The amyloid fibril deposits are composed of intact 23-kDa monoclonal Ig LCs or smaller fragments, 11–18 kDa in size, representing the variable (V) region alone, or the V region and a portion of the constant (C) region. Although all kappa and lambda LC subtypes have been identified in AL amyloid fibrils, lambda subtypes predominate. The lambda 6 subtype appears to have unique structural properties that predispose it to fibril formation, often in the kidney.

AL amyloidosis is usually a rapidly progressive disease that presents with a pleiotropic set of clinical syndromes, recognition of which is key to initiating appropriate workup. Nonspecific symptoms of fatigue and weight loss are common; however, the diagnosis is rarely considered until symptoms referable to a specific organ develop. The kidneys are the most frequently affected organ, in 70–80% of patients. Renal amyloidosis is usually manifested as proteinuria, often in the nephrotic range and associated with significant hypoalbuminemia, secondary hypercholesterolemia, and edema or anasarca. In some patients, tubular rather than glomerular deposition of amyloid can produce azotemia without significant proteinuria. The heart is the second most commonly affected organ, in 50–60% of patients, and the leading cause of mortality. Early on, the electrocardiogram may show low voltage in the limb leads, with a pseudo-infarct pattern. Eventually, the echocardiogram will display concentrically thickened ventricles and diastolic dysfunction, leading to a restrictive cardiomyopathy; systolic function is preserved until late in the disease. A "sparkly" appearance is usually not seen using modern high-resolution echocardiography equipment. Cardiac MRI can show an increased wall thickness and also a characteristic subendocardial enhancement with gadolinium. Nervous system symptoms include a peripheral sensory neuropathy and/or autonomic dysfunction with gastrointestinal motility disturbances (early satiety, diarrhea, constipation) and orthostatic hypotension. Macroglossia, with an enlarged, indented, or immobile tongue, is pathognomonic of AL amyloidosis but is seen only in ~10% of patients. Liver involvement causes cholestasis and hepatomegaly. The spleen is frequently involved, and there may be functional hyposplenism in the absence of significant splenomegaly. Many patients have "easy bruising" due to amyloid deposits in capillaries or to deficiency of clotting factor X, which can bind to amyloid fibrils; cutaneous ecchymoses appear, particularly around the eyes, giving the "raccoon-eye" sign. Other findings include nail dystrophy, alopecia, and amyloid arthropathy with thickening of synovial membranes in wrists and shoulders (Fig. 112-2). The presence of a multisystem illness or general fatigue along with any of these clinical syndromes should prompt a workup for amyloidosis.

◼ DIAGNOSIS

Identification of the underlying B lymphoproliferative process and clonal LC is key to the diagnosis of AL amyloidosis. The serum protein electrophoresis (SPEP) and urine protein electrophoresis (UPEP) are NOT useful screening tests if AL amyloidosis is suspected because the clonal LC or whole immunoglobulin, unlike in multiple myeloma, is often not present in sufficient quantity in the serum to produce a monoclonal "M-spike" or in the urine to cause LC (Bence Jones) proteinuria. However, more than 90% of patients have a serum or urine monoclonal LC or whole immunoglobulin that can be detected by immunofixation electrophoresis of serum (SIFE) or urine (UIFE) (Fig. 112-3A). Assaying for free immunoglobulin LCs circulating in the serum unbound to heavy

chains using commercially available nephelometric (FreeLite©) assay demonstrates an elevation and abnormal free kappa:lambda ratio in more than 75% of patients. Examining the ratio as well as the absolute amount is essential, because in renal insufficiency LC clearance is reduced, and both types of LCs will be elevated. In addition, an increased percentage of plasma cells in the bone marrow, typically 5–30% of nucleated cells, is noted in about 90% of patients. Kappa or lambda clonality can be demonstrated by flow cytometry, immunohistochemical staining, or by in situ hybridization for LC mRNA (Fig. 112-3B).

A monoclonal serum protein by itself is not diagnostic of amyloidosis, since monoclonal gammopathy of uncertain significance (MGUS) is common in older patients (Chap. 111). However, when MGUS is present in patients with biopsy-proven amyloidosis, the AL type should be strongly suspected. Similarly, patients thought to have "smoldering myeloma" because of modest elevation of bone marrow plasma cells should be screened for AL amyloidosis if they have evidence of organ dysfunction. Accurate typing is essential for appropriate treatment. Immunohistochemical staining of the amyloid deposits is useful if they bind one light chain antibody in preference to the other; some AL deposits bind many antisera nonspecifically. Immunoelectron microscopy is more reliable and mass-spectrometry-based microsequencing of small amounts of protein extracted from fibril deposits can also be done. In ambiguous cases, other forms of amyloidosis should be thoroughly excluded with appropriate genetic and other testing.

TREATMENT   AL Amyloidosis

Extensive multisystem involvement typifies AL amyloidosis, and median survival with no treatment is usually only about 1–2 years from the time of diagnosis. Current therapies target the clonal bone marrow plasma cells using approaches employed for multiple myeloma. Treatment with cyclic oral melphalan and prednisone can decrease the plasma cell burden but produces complete hematologic remission in only a few percent of patients and minimal organ responses and improvement in survival (median 2 years), and it is no longer widely used. The substitution of dexamethasone for prednisone produces a higher response rate and more durable remissions, although dexamethasone is not always well tolerated by patients with significant edema or cardiac disease. High-dose intravenous melphalan followed by autologous stem cell transplantation (HDM/SCT) produces complete hematologic responses in about 40% of treated patients, as measured by complete loss (CR) of clonal plasma cells in the bone marrow and disappearance of the monoclonal

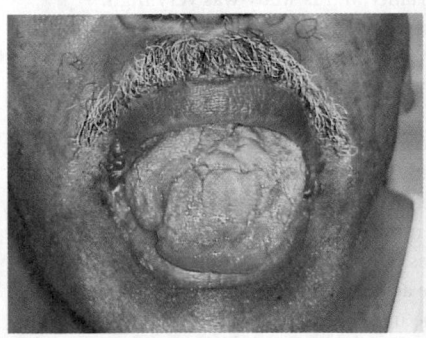
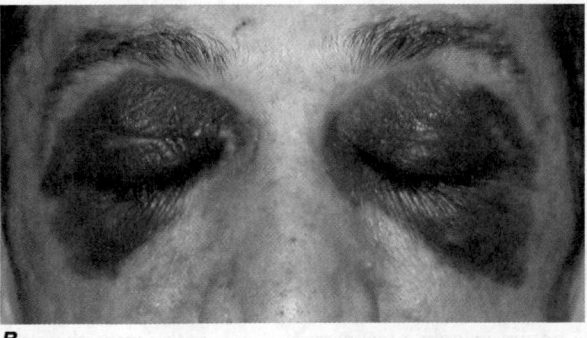
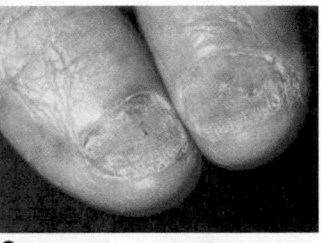

Figure 112-2 Clinical signs of AL amyloidosis. *A.* Macroglossia. *B.* Periorbital ecchymoses. *C.* Fingernail dystrophy.

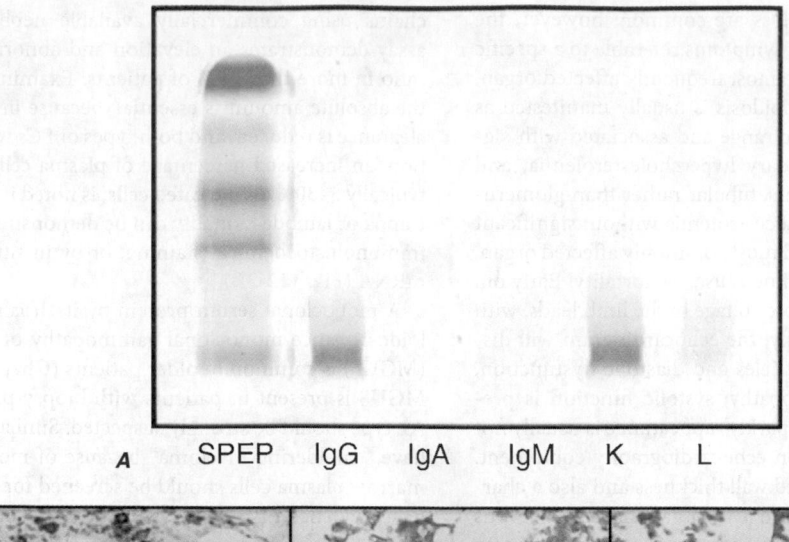

SPEP   IgG   IgA   IgM   K   L

A

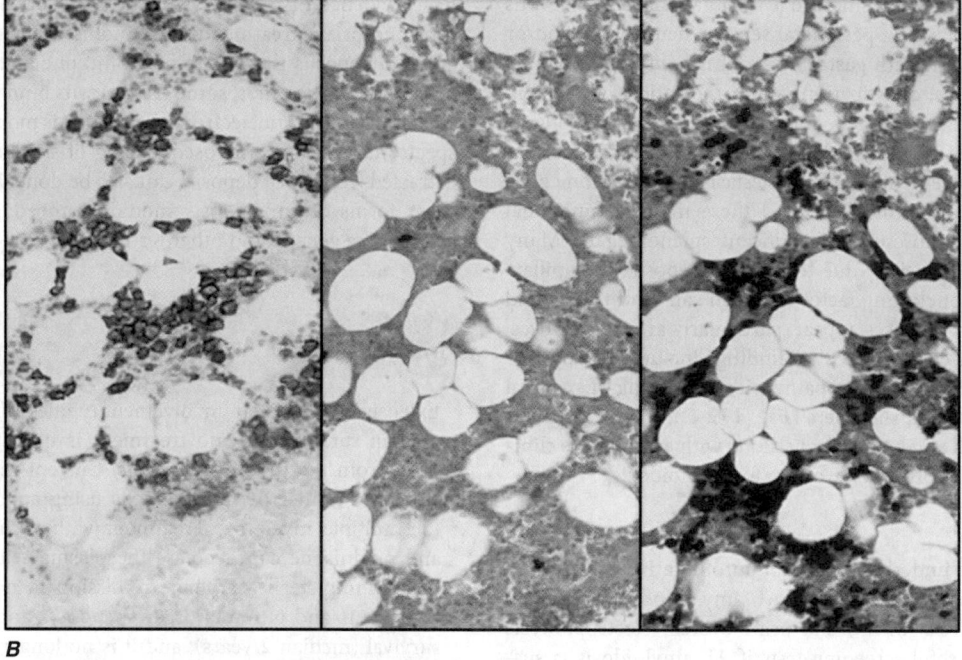

B

Figure 112-3 Laboratory features of AL amyloidosis. A. Serum immunofixation electrophoresis reveals an IgGκ monoclonal protein in this example; the serum protein electrophoresis is often normal. **B.** Bone marrow biopsy sections from another patient, stained with antibody to CD138 (syndecan, highly expressed on plasma cells) by immunohistochemistry (left panel). The middle and right panels are stained using in situ hybridization with fluorescein-tagged probes (Ventana Medical Systems) binding to κ and λ mRNA respectively in plasma cells. (*Photomicrograph courtesy of C. O'Hara; with permission.*)

LC by IFE and assay for free LCs. Hematologic responses can be followed in the subsequent 6–12 months by improvement in organ function and quality of life. The CRs after HDM/SCT appear to be more durable than those seen in multiple myeloma, with remissions continuing in some patients beyond 15 years without additional treatment. Unfortunately, only about half of AL amyloidosis patients are eligible for such aggressive treatment, and even at specialized treatment centers, peritransplant mortality is higher than for other hematologic diseases because of impaired organ function. Amyloid cardiomyopathy, poor nutritional status, impaired performance status, and multiple-organ disease contribute to excess morbidity and mortality. The bleeding diathesis due to adsorption of clotting factor X to amyloid fibrils also confers high mortality during myelosuppressive therapy; however, this syndrome occurs in only a few percent of patients. The single randomized multicenter trial comparing

oral melphalan and dexamethasone to HDM/SCT to date failed to show a benefit to dose-intensive treatment, although the transplant-related mortality in this study was very high.

For patients with impaired cardiac function or arrhythmias due to amyloid involvement of the myocardium, median survival is only about 6 months without treatment, and stem cell mobilization and high-dose chemotherapy are dangerous. In these patients, cardiac transplantation can be performed, followed by treatment with HDM/SCT to prevent amyloid deposition in the transplanted heart or other organs.

Recently, novel agents have been investigated for treatment of plasma cell diseases. The immunomodulators thalidomide and lenalidomide have activity; lenalidomide is well tolerated in doses lower than those used for myeloma and, in combination with dexamethasone, produces complete hematologic remissions and improvement in organ function. The proteasome inhibitor bortezomib has also been found to be effective in single- and multicenter trials. Combination therapy trials are now under development, and studies are examining the as yet unproven role of induction and maintenance treatment. Clinical trials are essential for improving therapy for this rare disease.

Supportive care is important for patients with any type of amyloidosis. For nephrotic syndrome, diuretics and supportive stockings can ameliorate edema; angiotensin-converting enzyme inhibitors should be used with caution and have not been shown to slow renal disease progression. Congestive heart failure due to amyloid cardiomyopathy is also best treated with diuretics; it is important to note that digitalis, calcium channel blockers, and beta blockers are relatively contraindicated as they can interact with amyloid fibrils and produce heart block and worsening heart failure. Amiodarone has been used for atrial and ventricular arrhythmias. Automatic implantable defibrillators have reduced effectiveness due to the thickened myocardium, but they can benefit some patients. Atrial ablation is an effective approach for atrial fibrillation. For conduction abnormalities, ventricular pacing may be indicated. Atrial contractile dysfunction is common in amyloid cardiomyopathy and is an indication for anticoagulation even in the absence of atrial fibrillation. Autonomic neuropathy can be treated with α agonists such as midodrine to support the blood pressure; gastrointestinal dysfunction may respond to motility or bulk agents. Nutritional supplementation, either orally or parenterally, is also important.

In localized AL, amyloid deposits can be produced by clonal plasma cells infiltrating local sites in the airways, bladder, skin, or lymph nodes (Table 112-1). Deposits may respond to surgical intervention or radiation therapy; systemic treatment is generally not appropriate. Patients should be referred to a center familiar with management of these rare manifestations of amyloidosis.

AA AMYLOIDOSIS

■ ETIOLOGY AND INCIDENCE

AA amyloidosis can occur in association with almost any chronic inflammatory state [e.g., rheumatoid arthritis, inflammatory bowel disease, familial Mediterranean fever (Chap. 330) or other periodic fever syndromes] or chronic infections such as tuberculosis or subacute bacterial endocarditis. In the United States and Europe, AA amyloidosis has become less common, occurring in <2% of patients with these diseases, presumably because of advances in anti-inflammatory and antimicrobial therapies. It has also been described in association with Castleman's disease, and patients with AA amyloidosis should have CT scanning to look for such tumors, as well as serologic and microbiologic studies. AA amyloidosis can also be seen without any identifiable underlying disease. AA is the only type of systemic amyloidosis that occurs in children.

■ PATHOLOGY AND CLINICAL FEATURES

Deposits are more limited in AA amyloidosis than in AL amyloidosis; they usually begin in the kidneys. Hepatomegaly, splenomegaly, and autonomic neuropathy can also occur as the disease progresses; cardiomyopathy occurs albeit rarely. However, the symptoms and signs cannot be reliably distinguished from those of AL amyloidosis. AA amyloid fibrils are usually composed of an 8-kDa, 76-amino-acid N-terminal portion of a 12-kDa precursor protein, serum amyloid A (SAA). SAA is an acute-phase apoprotein synthesized in the liver and transported by high-density lipoprotein, HDL3, in the plasma. Several years of an underlying inflammatory disease causing chronic elevation of SAA usually precedes fibril formation, although infections can lead to AA deposition more rapidly.

TREATMENT **AA Amyloidosis**

The primary therapy in AA amyloidosis is treatment of the underlying inflammatory or infectious disease. Treatment that suppresses or eliminates the inflammation or infection also decreases the SAA protein concentration. For familial Mediterranean fever, colchicine in a dose of 1.2–1.8 mg/d is the appropriate treatment. Colchicine has not been helpful for AA amyloidosis of other causes or for other amyloidoses. TNF and IL-1 antagonists can also be effective in syndromes related to cytokine elevation. For this disease, there is also a fibril-specific agent. Eprodisate was designed to interfere with the interaction of AA amyloid protein with glycosaminoglycans in tissues and prevent or disrupt fibril formation. This drug is well tolerated and delays progression of AA renal disease, regardless of the underlying inflammatory process. Eprodisate is awaiting FDA approval.

AF AMYLOIDOSIS

The familial amyloidoses are autosomal dominant diseases in which a variant plasma protein forms amyloid deposits, beginning in midlife. These diseases are rare, with an estimated incidence of <1 per 100,000 in the United States, although there are isolated areas of Portugal, Sweden, and Japan where founder effects have led to a much higher incidence of the disease. The most common form of AF is caused by mutation of the abundant plasma protein transthyretin (TTR, also known as *prealbumin*). More than 100 TTR mutations are known, and most are associated with ATTR amyloidosis. One variant, V122I, has a carrier frequency that may be as high as 4% in the African-American population and is associated with late-onset cardiac amyloidosis. The actual incidence and penetrance of disease in the African-American population is the subject of ongoing research, but it would be wise to consider this in the differential diagnosis of African-American patients who present with concentric cardiac hypertrophy and evidence of diastolic dysfunction, particularly in the absence of a history of hypertension. Even wild-type TTR can form fibrils, leading to so-called senile systemic amyloidosis (SSA) in older patients. It can be found in up to 25% of autopsies in patients older than age 80 years, and it can produce a clinical syndrome of amyloid cardiomyopathy that is similar to that occurring in younger patients carrying a mutant TTR. Other familial amyloidoses, caused by variant apolipoproteins AI or AII, gelsolin, fibrinogen Aα, or lysozyme, are reported in only a few families worldwide. New amyloidogenic serum proteins continue to be identified periodically, including recently the leukocyte chemotactic factor LECT2.

In ATTR and in other forms of familial amyloidosis, the variant structure of the precursor protein is the key factor in fibril formation. The role of aging is intriguing, since patients born with the variant proteins do not have clinically apparent disease until middle age, despite the lifelong presence of the abnormal protein. Further evidence of an age-related "trigger" is the occurrence of SSA in the elderly, caused by the deposition of fibrils derived from normal TTR.

■ CLINICAL FEATURES AND DIAGNOSIS

AF amyloidosis has a variable presentation but is usually consistent within affected kindreds with the same mutant protein. A family history makes AF more likely, but many patients present sporadically with new mutations. ATTR usually presents as a syndrome of familial amyloidotic polyneuropathy or familial amyloidotic cardiomyopathy. Peripheral neuropathy usually begins as a lower-extremity sensory and motor neuropathy and progresses to the upper extremities. Autonomic neuropathy is manifest by gastrointestinal symptoms of diarrhea with weight loss and orthostatic hypotension. Patients with TTR V30M, the most common mutation, have normal echocardiograms but may have conduction defects and require a pacemaker. Patients with TTR T60A and several other mutations have myocardial thickening similar to that caused by AL amyloidosis, although heart failure is less common and the prognosis is better. Vitreous opacities caused by amyloid deposits are pathognomonic of ATTR amyloidosis.

Typical syndromes associated with other forms of AF included renal amyloidosis with mutant fibrinogen, lysozyme, or apolipoproteins, or hepatic amyloidosis with apolipoprotein AI, and amyloidosis of cranial nerves and cornea with gelsolin.

Patients with AF amyloidosis can present with clinical syndromes that mimic those of patients with AL, and AF carriers can develop AL, or conversely, AF patients can develop a MGUS. Thus, it is important to screen for both plasma cell disorders and for mutations in some patients with amyloidosis. Variant TTR proteins can usually be detected by isoelectric focusing, but DNA sequencing is now standard for diagnosis of ATTR and the other AF mutations.

TREATMENT   ATTR Amyloidosis

Without intervention, survival after ATTR disease onset is 5–15 years. Orthotopic liver transplantation removes the major source of variant TTR production and replaces it with a source of normal TTR; it also arrests disease progression and leads to improvement in autonomic and peripheral neuropathy in some patients. Cardiomyopathy often does not improve, and in some patients it can worsen after liver transplantation, perhaps due to deposition of wild-type TTR as seen in SSA. Compounds have been identified that stabilize TTR in a nonpathogenic tetrameric conformation in vitro and are undergoing clinical testing in multicenter trials.

Aβ_2M AMYLOIDOSIS

Aβ_2M amyloidosis is composed of β_2-microglobulin, the invariant chain of class I human leukocyte antigens, and produces rheumatologic manifestations in patients on long-term hemodialysis. β_2-Microglobulin is excreted by the kidney, and levels become elevated in ESRD. The molecular mass of β_2M is 11.8 kDa, above the cutoff of some dialysis membranes. The incidence of this disease appears to be declining with newer high-flow dialysis techniques.

Aβ_2M amyloidosis usually presents with carpal tunnel syndrome, persistent joint effusions, spondyloarthropathy, or cystic bone lesions. Carpal tunnel syndrome is often the first symptom of disease. In the past, persistent joint effusions accompanied by mild discomfort were seen in up to 50% of patients on dialysis for more than 12 years. Involvement is bilateral, and large joints (shoulders, knees, wrists, and hips) are more frequently affected. The synovial fluid is noninflammatory, and β_2M amyloid can be found if the sediment is stained with Congo red. Although less common, visceral β_2M amyloid deposits do occasionally occur in the gastrointestinal tract, heart, tendons, and subcutaneous tissues of the buttocks. There is no specific therapy for Aβ_2M amyloidosis, but cessation of dialysis after renal allografting may lead to symptomatic improvement.

SUMMARY

A diagnosis of amyloidosis should be considered in patients with unexplained nephropathy, cardiomyopathy (particularly with diastolic dysfunction), neuropathy (either peripheral or autonomic), enteropathy, or the pathognomonic soft tissue findings of macroglossia or periorbital ecchymoses. Pathologic identification of amyloid fibrils can be made using Congo red staining of aspirated abdominal fat or of an involved organ biopsy specimen. Accurate typing using a combination of immunologic, biochemical, and genetic testing is essential to choosing the appropriate therapy (see algorithm for workup, Fig. 112-1). Tertiary referral centers can provide specialized diagnostic techniques and access to clinical trials for patients with these rare diseases.

FURTHER READINGS

Benson MD et al: Leukocyte chemotactic factor 2: A novel renal amyloid protein. Kidney Int 74:218, 2008

Connors L et al: Cardiac amyloidosis in African Americans: Comparison of clinical and laboratory features of transthyretin V122I amyloidosis and immunoglobulin light chain amyloidosis. Am Heart J 158:607, 2009

Dember L et al: Eprodisate for the treatment of renal disease in AA amyloidosis. N Engl J Med 356:2349, 2007

Dey BR et al: Cardiac transplantation followed by dose-intensive melphalan and autologous stem-cell transplantation for light chain amyloidosis and heart failure. Transplantation 90:905, 2010

Merlini G, Bellotti V: Molecular mechanisms of amyloidosis. N Engl J Med 349:583, 2003

Sanchorawala V et al: Long-term outcome of patients with AL amyloidosis treated with high-dose melphalan and stem-cell transplantation. Blood 110:3561, 2007

Skinner M et al: High-dose melphalan and autologous stem-cell transplantation in patients with AL amyloidosis: An 8-year study. Ann Intern Med 140:85, 2004

CHAPTER 113

Transfusion Biology and Therapy

Jeffery S. Dzieczkowski

Kenneth C. Anderson

BLOOD GROUP ANTIGENS AND ANTIBODIES

The study of red blood cell (RBC) antigens and antibodies forms the foundation of transfusion medicine. Serologic studies initially characterized these antigens, but now the molecular composition and structure of many are known. Antigens, either carbohydrate or protein, are assigned to a blood group system based on the structure and similarity of the determinant epitopes. Other cellular blood elements and plasma proteins are also antigenic and can result in *alloimmunization*, the production of antibodies directed against the blood group antigens of another individual. These antibodies are called *alloantibodies*.

Antibodies directed against RBC antigens may result from "natural" exposure, particularly to carbohydrates that mimic some blood group antigens. Those antibodies that occur via natural stimuli are usually produced by a T cell–independent response (thus, generating no memory) and are IgM isotype. *Autoantibodies* (antibodies against autologous blood group antigens) arise spontaneously or as the result of infectious sequelae (e.g., from *Mycoplasma pneumoniae*) and are also often IgM. These antibodies are often clinically insignificant due to their low affinity for antigen at body temperature. However, IgM antibodies can activate the complement cascade and result in hemolysis. Antibodies that result from allogeneic exposure, such as transfusion or pregnancy, are usually IgG. IgG antibodies commonly bind to antigen at warmer temperatures and may hemolyze RBCs. Unlike IgM antibodies, IgG antibodies can cross the placenta and bind fetal erythrocytes bearing the corresponding antigen, resulting in hemolytic disease of the newborn, or *hydrops fetalis*.

Alloimmunization to leukocytes, platelets, and plasma proteins may also result in transfusion complications such as fevers and urticaria but generally does not cause hemolysis. Assay for these other alloantibodies is not routinely performed; however, they may be detected using special assays.

◼ ABO ANTIGENS AND ANTIBODIES

The first blood group antigen system, recognized in 1900, was ABO, the most important in transfusion medicine. The major blood groups of this system are A, B, AB, and O. O type RBCs lack A or B antigens. These antigens are carbohydrates attached to a precursor backbone, may be found on the cellular membrane either as glycosphingolipids or glycoproteins, and are secreted into plasma and body fluids as glycoproteins. H substance is the immediate precursor on which the A and B antigens are added. This H substance is formed by the addition of fucose to the glycolipid or glycoprotein backbone. The subsequent addition of *N*-acetylgalactosamine creates the A antigen, while the addition of galactose produces the B antigen.

The genes that determine the A and B phenotypes are found on chromosome 9p and are expressed in a Mendelian codominant manner. The gene products are glycosyl transferases, which confer the enzymatic capability of attaching the specific antigenic carbohydrate. Individuals who lack the "A" and "B" transferases are phenotypically type "O," while those who inherit both transferases are type "AB." Rare individuals lack the H gene, which codes for fucose transferase, and cannot form H substance. These individuals are homozygous for the silent h allele (hh) and have Bombay phenotype (O_h).

The ABO blood group system is important because essentially all individuals produce antibodies to the ABH carbohydrate antigen that they lack. The naturally occurring anti-A and anti-B antibodies are termed *isoagglutinins*. Thus, type A individuals produce anti-B, while type B individuals make anti-A. Neither isoagglutinin is found in type AB individuals, while type O individuals produce both anti-A and anti-B. Thus, persons with type AB are "universal recipients" because they do not have antibodies against any ABO phenotype, while persons with type O blood can donate to essentially all recipients because their cells are not recognized by any ABO isoagglutinins. The rare individuals with Bombay phenotype produce antibodies to H substance (which is present on all red cells except those of hh phenotype) as well as to both A and B antigens and are therefore compatible only with other hh donors.

In most people, A and B antigens are secreted by the cells and are present in the circulation. Nonsecretors are susceptible to a variety of infections (e.g., *Candida albicans*, *Neisseria meningitidis*, *Streptococcus pneumoniae*, *Haemophilus influenzae*) as many organisms may bind to polysaccharides on cells. Soluble blood group antigens may block this binding.

◼ RH SYSTEM

The Rh system is the second most important blood group system in pretransfusion testing. The Rh antigens are found on a 30- to 32-kDa RBC membrane protein that has no defined function. Although >40 different antigens in the Rh system have been described, five determinants account for the vast majority of phenotypes. The presence of the D antigen confers Rh "positivity," while persons who lack the D antigen are Rh negative. Two allelic antigen pairs, E/e and C/c, are also found on the Rh protein. The three Rh genes, E/e, D, and C/c, are arranged in tandem on chromosome 1 and inherited as a haplotype, i.e., cDE or Cde. Two haplotypes can result in the phenotypic expression of two to five Rh antigens.

The D antigen is a potent alloantigen. About 15% of individuals lack this antigen. Exposure of these Rh-negative people to even small amounts of Rh-positive cells, by either transfusion or pregnancy, can result in the production of anti-D alloantibody.

◼ OTHER BLOOD GROUP SYSTEMS AND ALLOANTIBODIES

More than 100 blood group systems are recognized, composed of more than 500 antigens. The presence or absence of certain antigens has been associated with various diseases and anomalies; antigens also act as receptors for infectious agents. Alloantibodies of importance in routine clinical practice are listed in Table 113-1.

Antibodies to *Lewis system* carbohydrate antigens are the most common cause of incompatibility during pretransfusion screening. The Lewis gene product is a fucosyl transferase and maps to chromosome 19. The antigen is not an integral membrane structure but is adsorbed to the RBC membrane from the plasma. Antibodies to Lewis antigens are usually IgM and cannot cross the placenta. Lewis antigens may be adsorbed onto tumor cells and may be targets of therapy.

TABLE 113-1 RBC Blood Group Systems and Alloantigens

Blood Group System	Antigen	Alloantibody	Clinical Significance
Rh (D, C/c, E/e)	RBC protein	IgG	HTR, HDN
Lewis (Le^a, Le^b)	Oligosaccharide	IgM/IgG	Rare HTR
Kell (K/k)	RBC protein	IgG	HTR, HDN
Duffy (Fy^a/Fy^b)	RBC protein	IgG	HTR, HDN
Kidd (Jk^a/Jk^b)	RBC protein	IgG	HTR (often delayed), HDN (mild)
I/i	Carbohydrate	IgM	None
MNSsU	RBC protein	IgM/IgG	Anti-M rare HDN, anti-S, -s, and -U HDN, HTR

Abbreviations: RBC, red blood cell; HDN, hemolytic disease of the newborn; HTR, hemolytic transfusion reaction.

I system antigens are also oligosaccharides related to H, A, B, and Le. I and i are not allelic pairs but are carbohydrate antigens that differ only in the extent of branching. The i antigen is an unbranched chain that is converted by the I gene product, a glycosyltransferase, into a branched chain. The branching process affects all the ABH antigens, which become progressively more branched in the first 2 years of life. Some patients with cold agglutinin disease or lymphomas can produce anti-I autoantibodies that cause RBC destruction. Occasional patients with mononucleosis or *Mycoplasma* pneumonia may develop cold agglutinins of either anti-I or anti-i specificity. Most adults lack i expression; thus, finding a donor for patients with anti-i is not difficult. Even though most adults express I antigen, binding is generally low at body temperature. Thus, administration of warm blood prevents isoagglutination.

The *P system* is another group of carbohydrate antigens controlled by specific glycosyltransferases. Its clinical significance is in rare cases of syphilis and viral infection that lead to paroxysmal cold hemoglobinuria. In these cases, an unusual autoantibody to P is produced that binds to RBCs in the cold and fixes complement upon warming. Antibodies with these biphasic properties are called *Donath-Landsteiner antibodies*. The P antigen is the cellular receptor of parvovirus B19 and also may be a receptor for *Escherichia coli* binding to urothelial cells.

The *MNSsU system* is regulated by genes on chromosome 4. M and N are determinants on glycophorin A, an RBC membrane protein, and S and s are determinants on glycophorin B. Anti-S and anti-s IgG antibodies may develop after pregnancy or transfusion and lead to hemolysis. Anti-U antibodies are rare but problematic; virtually every donor is incompatible because nearly all persons express U.

The *Kell* protein is very large (720 amino acids), and its secondary structure contains many different antigenic epitopes. The immunogenicity of Kell is third behind the ABO and Rh systems. The absence of the Kell precursor protein (controlled by a gene on X) is associated with acanthocytosis, shortened RBC survival, and a progressive form of muscular dystrophy that includes cardiac defects. This rare condition is called the *McLeod phenotype*. The K_x gene

is linked to the 91-kDa component of the NADPH-oxidase on the X chromosome, deletion or mutation of which accounts for about 60% of cases of chronic granulomatous disease.

The *Duffy* antigens are codominant alleles, Fy^a and Fy^b, that also serve as receptors for *Plasmodium vivax*. More than 70% of persons in malaria-endemic areas lack these antigens, probably from selective influences of the infection on the population.

The *Kidd* antigens, Jk^a and Jk^b, may elicit antibodies transiently. A delayed hemolytic transfusion reaction that occurs with blood tested as compatible is often related to delayed appearance of anti-Jk^a.

PRETRANSFUSION TESTING

Pretransfusion testing of a potential recipient consists of the "type and screen." The "forward type" determines the ABO and Rh phenotype of the recipient's RBC by using antisera directed against the A, B, and D antigens. The "reverse type" detects isoagglutinins in the patient's serum and should correlate with the ABO phenotype, or forward type.

The alloantibody screen identifies antibodies directed against other RBC antigens. The alloantibody screen is performed by mixing patient serum with type O RBCs that contain the major antigens of most blood group systems and whose extended phenotype is known. The specificity of the alloantibody is identified by correlating the presence or absence of antigen with the results of the agglutination.

Cross-matching is ordered when there is a high probability that the patient will require a packed RBC (PRBC) transfusion. Blood selected for cross-matching must be ABO compatible and lack antigens for which the patient has alloantibodies. Nonreactive cross-matching confirms the absence of any major incompatibility and reserves that unit for the patient.

In the case of Rh-negative patients, every attempt must be made to provide Rh-negative blood components to prevent alloimmunization to the D antigen. In an emergency, Rh-positive blood can be safely transfused to an Rh-negative patient who lacks anti-D; however, the recipient is likely to become alloimmunized and produce anti-D. Rh-negative women of childbearing age who are transfused with products containing Rh-positive RBCs should receive passive immunization with anti-D (RhoGam or WinRho) to reduce or prevent sensitization.

BLOOD COMPONENTS

Blood products intended for transfusion are routinely collected as whole blood (450 mL) in various anticoagulants. Most donated blood is processed into components: PRBCs, platelets, and fresh-frozen plasma (FFP) or cryoprecipitate (Table 113-2). Whole blood is first separated into PRBCs and platelet-rich plasma by slow centrifugation. The platelet-rich plasma is then centrifuged at high speed to yield one unit of random donor (RD) platelets and one unit of FFP. Cryoprecipitate is produced by thawing FFP to precipitate the plasma proteins, then separated by centrifugation.

Apheresis technology is used for the collection of multiple units of platelets from a single donor. These single-donor apheresis platelets (SDAP) contain the equivalent of at least six units of RD platelets and have fewer contaminating leukocytes than pooled RD platelets.

Plasma may also be collected by apheresis. Plasma derivatives such as albumin, intravenous immunoglobulin, antithrombin, and coagulation factor concentrates are prepared from pooled plasma from many donors and are treated to eliminate infectious agents.

TABLE 113-2 Characteristics of Selected Blood Components

Component	Volume, mL	Content	Clinical Response
PRBC	180–200	RBCs with variable leukocyte content and small amount of plasma	Increase hemoglobin 10 g/L and hematocrit 3%
Platelets	50–70	5.5×10^{10}/RD unit	Increase platelet count 5000–10,000/µL
	200–400	$\geq 3 \times 10^{11}$/SDAP product	CCI $\geq 10 \times 10^9$/L within 1 h and $\geq 7.5 \times 10^9$/L within 24 h posttransfusion
FFP	200–250	Plasma proteins—coagulation factors, proteins C and S, antithrombin	Increases coagulation factors about 2%
Cryoprecipitate	10–15	Cold-insoluble plasma proteins, fibrinogen, factor VIII, vWF	Topical fibrin glue, also 80 IU factor VIII

Abbreviations: CCI, corrected count increment; FFP, fresh-frozen plasma; PRBC, packed red blood cells; RBC, red blood cell; RD, random donor; SDAP, single-donor apheresis platelets; vWF, von Willebrand factor.

■ WHOLE BLOOD

Whole blood provides both oxygen-carrying capacity and volume expansion. It is the ideal component for patients who have sustained acute hemorrhage of ≥25% total blood volume loss. Whole blood is stored at 4°C to maintain erythrocyte viability, but platelet dysfunction and degradation of some coagulation factors occurs. In addition, 2,3-bisphosphoglycerate levels fall over time, leading to an increase in the oxygen affinity of the hemoglobin and a decreased capacity to deliver oxygen to the tissues, a problem with all red cell storage. Fresh whole blood avoids these problems, but it is typically used only in emergency settings (i.e., military). Whole blood is not readily available, since it is routinely processed into components.

■ PACKED RED BLOOD CELLS

This product increases oxygen-carrying capacity in the anemic patient. Adequate oxygenation can be maintained with a hemoglobin content of 70 g/L in the normovolemic patient without cardiac disease; however, comorbid factors may necessitate transfusion at a higher threshold. The decision to transfuse should be guided by the clinical situation and not by an arbitrary laboratory value. In the critical care setting, liberal use of transfusions to maintain near-normal levels of hemoglobin has not proven advantageous. In most patients requiring transfusion, levels of hemoglobin of 100 g/L are sufficient to keep oxygen supply from being critically low.

PRBCs may be modified to prevent certain adverse reactions. The majority of cellular blood products are now leukocyte reduced and universal prestorage leukocyte reduction has been recommended. Prestorage filtration appears superior to bedside filtration as smaller amounts of cytokines are generated in the stored product. These PRBC units contain $<5 \times 10^6$ donor white blood cells (WBCs), and their use lowers the incidence of posttransfusion fever, cytomegalovirus (CMV) infections, and alloimmunization. Other theoretical benefits include less immunosuppression in the recipient and lower

risk of infections. Plasma, which may cause allergic reactions, can be removed from cellular blood components by washing.

■ PLATELETS

Thrombocytopenia is a risk factor for hemorrhage, and platelet transfusion reduces the incidence of bleeding. The threshold for prophylactic platelet transfusion is 10,000/µL. In patients without fever or infections, a threshold of 5000/µL may be sufficient to prevent spontaneous hemorrhage. For invasive procedures, 50,000/µL platelets is the usual target level.

Platelets are given either as pools prepared RDs or as SDAPs from a single donor. In an unsensitized patient without increased platelet consumption [splenomegaly, fever, disseminated intravascular coagulation (DIC)], two units of transfused RD per square-meter body surface area (BSA) is anticipated to increase the platelet count by approximately 10,000/uL. Patients who have received multiple transfusions may be alloimmunized to many HLA- and platelet-specific antigens and have little or no increase in their posttransfusion platelet counts. Patients who may require multiple transfusions are best served by receiving SDAP and leukocyte-reduced components to lower the risk of alloimmunization.

Refractoriness to platelet transfusion may be evaluated using the corrected count increment (CCI):

$$ \text{CCI} = \frac{\text{posttransfusion count (/µL)} - \text{pretransfusion count (/µL)}}{\text{number of platelets transfused} \times 10^{-11}} \times \text{BSA (m}^2) $$

where BSA is body surface area measured in square meters. The platelet count performed 1 h after the transfusion is acceptable if the CCI is 10×10^9/mL, and after 18–24 h an increment of 7.5×10^9/mL is expected. Patients who have suboptimal responses are likely to have received multiple transfusions and have antibodies directed against class I HLA antigens. Refractoriness can be investigated by detecting anti-HLA antibodies in the recipient's serum. Patients who are sensitized will often react with 100% of the lymphocytes used for the HLA-antibody screen, and HLA-matched SDAPs should be considered for those patients who require transfusion. Although ABO-identical HLA-matched SDAPs provide the best chance for increasing the platelet count, locating these products is difficult. Platelet cross-matching is available in some centers. Additional clinical causes for a low platelet CCI include fever, bleeding, splenomegaly, DIC, or medications in the recipient.

■ FRESH-FROZEN PLASMA

FFP contains stable coagulation factors and plasma proteins: fibrinogen, antithrombin, albumin, as well as proteins C and S. Indications for FFP include correction of coagulopathies, including the rapid reversal of warfarin; supplying deficient plasma proteins; and treatment of thrombotic thrombocytopenic purpura. FFP should not be routinely used to expand blood volume. FFP is an acellular component and does not transmit intracellular infections, e.g., CMV. Patients who are IgA-deficient and require plasma support should receive FFP from IgA-deficient donors to prevent anaphylaxis (see below).

■ CRYOPRECIPITATE

Cryoprecipitate is a source of fibrinogen, factor VIII, and von Willebrand factor (vWF). It is ideal for supplying fibrinogen to the volume-sensitive patient. When factor VIII concentrates are not available, cryoprecipitate may be used since each unit contains approximately 80 units of factor VIII. Cryoprecipitate may also supply vWF to patients with dysfunctional (type II) or absent (type III) von Willebrand disease.

■ PLASMA DERIVATIVES

Plasma from thousands of donors may be pooled to derive specific protein concentrates, including albumin, intravenous immunoglobulin, antithrombin, and coagulation factors. In addition, donors who have high-titer antibodies to specific agents or antigens provide hyperimmune globulins, such as anti-D (RhoGam, WinRho), and antisera to hepatitis B virus (HBV), varicella-zoster virus, CMV, and other infectious agents.

ADVERSE REACTIONS TO BLOOD TRANSFUSION

Adverse reactions to transfused blood components occur despite multiple tests, inspections, and checks. Fortunately, the most common reactions are not life threatening, although serious reactions can present with mild symptoms and signs. Some reactions can be reduced or prevented by modified (filtered, washed, or irradiated) blood components. When an adverse reaction is suspected, the transfusion should be stopped and reported to the blood bank for investigation.

Transfusion reactions may result from immune and nonimmune mechanisms. Immune-mediated reactions are often due to preformed donor or recipient antibody; however, cellular elements may also cause adverse effects. Nonimmune causes of reactions are due to the chemical and physical properties of the stored blood component and its additives.

Transfusion-transmitted viral infections are increasingly rare due to improved screening and testing. As the risk of viral infection is reduced, the relative risk of other reactions increases, such as hemolytic transfusion reactions and sepsis from bacterially contaminated components. Pretransfusion quality assurance improvements further increase the safety of transfusion therapy. Infections, like any adverse transfusion reaction, must be brought to the attention of the blood bank for appropriate studies (Table 113-3).

■ IMMUNE-MEDIATED REACTIONS

Acute hemolytic transfusion reactions

Immune-mediated hemolysis occurs when the recipient has preformed antibodies that lyse donor erythrocytes. The ABO isoagglutinins are responsible for the majority of these reactions, although alloantibodies directed against other RBC antigens, i.e., Rh, Kell, and Duffy, may result in hemolysis.

Acute hemolytic reactions may present with hypotension, tachypnea, tachycardia, fever, chills, hemoglobinemia, hemoglobinuria, chest and/or flank pain, and discomfort at the infusion site. Monitoring the patient's vital signs before and during the transfusion is important to identify reactions promptly. When acute hemolysis is suspected, the transfusion must be stopped immediately, intravenous access maintained, and the reaction reported to the blood bank. A correctly labeled posttransfusion blood sample and any untransfused blood should be sent to the blood bank for analysis. The laboratory evaluation for hemolysis includes the measurement of serum haptoglobin, lactate dehydrogenase (LDH), and indirect bilirubin levels.

The immune complexes that result in RBC lysis can cause renal dysfunction and failure. Diuresis should be induced with intravenous fluids and furosemide or mannitol. Tissue factor released from the lysed erythrocytes may initiate DIC. Coagulation studies including prothrombin time (PT), activated partial thromboplastin time (aPTT), fibrinogen, and platelet count should be monitored in patients with hemolytic reactions.

TABLE 113-3 Risks of Transfusion Complications

	Frequency, Episodes: Unit
Reactions	
Febrile (FNHTR)	• 1–4:100
Allergic	• 1–4:100
Delayed hemolytic	• 1:1000
TRALI	• 1:5000
Acute hemolytic	• 1:12,000
Fatal hemolytic	• 1:100,000
Anaphylactic	• 1:150,000
Infections[a]	
Hepatitis B	• 1:220,000
Hepatitis C	• 1:1,800,000
HIV-1, -2	• 1:2,300,000
HTLV-I and -II	• 1:2,993,000
Malaria	• 1:4,000,000
Other complications	
RBC allosensitization	• 1:100
HLA allosensitization	• 1:10
Graft-versus-host disease	Rare

[a]Infectious agents rarely associated with transfusion, theoretically possible or of unknown risk include West Nile virus, hepatitis A virus, parvovirus B-19, *Babesia microti* (babesiosis), *Borrelia burgdorferi* (Lyme disease), *Anaplasma phagocytophilum* (human granulocytic ehrlichiosis), *Trypanosoma cruzi* (Chagas disease), *Treponema pallidum*, and human herpesvirus-8.
Abbreviations: FNHTR, febrile nonhemolytic transfusion reaction; TRALI, transfusion-related acute lung injury; HTLV, human T lymphotropic virus; RBC, red blood cell.

Errors at the patient's bedside, such as mislabeling the sample or transfusing the wrong patient, are responsible for the majority of these reactions. The blood bank investigation of these reactions includes examination of the pre- and posttransfusion samples for hemolysis and repeat typing of the patient samples; direct antiglobulin test (DAT), sometimes called the *direct Coombs test*, of the posttransfusion sample; repeating the cross-matching of the blood component; and checking all clerical records for errors. DAT detects the presence of antibody or complement bound to RBCs in vivo.

Delayed hemolytic and serologic transfusion reactions

Delayed hemolytic transfusion reactions (DHTRs) are not completely preventable. These reactions occur in patients previously sensitized to RBC alloantigens who have a negative alloantibody screen due to low antibody levels. When the patient is transfused with antigen-positive blood, an anamnestic response results in the early production of alloantibody that binds donor RBCs. The alloantibody is detectable 1–2 weeks following the transfusion, and the posttransfusion DAT may become positive due to circulating donor RBCs coated with antibody or complement. The transfused, alloantibody-coated erythrocytes are cleared by the reticuloendothelial system. These reactions are detected most commonly in the blood bank when a subsequent patient sample reveals a positive alloantibody screen or a new alloantibody in a recently transfused recipient.

No specific therapy is usually required, although additional RBC transfusions may be necessary. Delayed serologic transfusion reactions are similar to DHTR, as the DAT is positive and alloantibody is detected; however, RBC clearance is not increased.

Febrile nonhemolytic transfusion reaction

The most frequent reaction associated with the transfusion of cellular blood components is a febrile nonhemolytic transfusion reaction (FNHTR). These reactions are characterized by chills and rigors and a ≥1°C rise in temperature. FNHTR is diagnosed when other causes of fever in the transfused patient are ruled out. Antibodies directed against donor leukocyte and HLA antigens may mediate these reactions; thus, multiply transfused patients and multiparous women are felt to be at increased risk. Although anti-HLA antibodies may be demonstrated in the recipient's serum, investigation is not routinely done because of the mild nature of most FNHTR. The use of leukocyte-reduced blood products may prevent or delay sensitization to leukocyte antigens and thereby reduce the incidence of these febrile episodes. Cytokines released from cells within stored blood components may mediate FNHTR; thus, leukoreduction before storage may prevent these reactions.

Allergic reactions

Urticarial reactions are related to plasma proteins found in transfused components. Mild reactions may be treated symptomatically by temporarily stopping the transfusion and administering antihistamines (diphenhydramine, 50 mg orally or intramuscularly). The transfusion may be completed after the signs and/or symptoms resolve. Patients with a history of allergic transfusion reaction should be premedicated with an antihistamine. Cellular components can be washed to remove residual plasma for the extremely sensitized patient.

Anaphylactic reaction

This severe reaction presents after transfusion of only a few milliliters of the blood component. Symptoms and signs include difficulty breathing, coughing, nausea and vomiting, hypotension, bronchospasm, loss of consciousness, respiratory arrest, and shock. Treatment includes stopping the transfusion, maintaining vascular access, and administering epinephrine (0.5–1 mL of 1:1000 dilution subcutaneously). Glucocorticoids may be required in severe cases.

Patients who are IgA-deficient, <1% of the population, may be sensitized to this Ig class and are at risk for anaphylactic reactions associated with plasma transfusion. Individuals with severe IgA deficiency should therefore receive only IgA-deficient plasma and washed cellular blood components. Patients who have anaphylactic or repeated allergic reactions to blood components should be tested for IgA deficiency.

Graft-versus-host disease

Graft-versus-host disease (GVHD) is a frequent complication of allogeneic stem cell transplantation, in which lymphocytes from the donor attack and cannot be eliminated by an immunodeficient host. Transfusion-related GVHD is mediated by donor T lymphocytes that recognize host HLA antigens as foreign and mount an immune response, which is manifested clinically by the development of fever, a characteristic cutaneous eruption, diarrhea, and liver function abnormalities. GVHD can also occur when blood components that contain viable T lymphocytes are transfused to immunodeficient recipients or to immunocompetent recipients who share HLA antigens with the donor (e.g., a family donor). In addition to the aforementioned clinical features of GVHD, transfusion-associated GVHD (TA-GVHD) is characterized by marrow aplasia and pancytopenia. TA-GVHD is highly resistant to treatment with immunosuppressive therapies, including glucocorticoids, cyclosporine, antithymocyte globulin, and ablative therapy followed by allogeneic bone marrow transplantation. Clinical manifestations appear at 8–10 days, and death occurs at 3–4 weeks posttransfusion.

TA-GVHD can be prevented by irradiation of cellular components (minimum of 2500 cGy) before transfusion to patients at risk. Patients at risk for TA-GVHD include fetuses receiving intrauterine transfusions, selected immunocompetent (e.g., lymphoma patients) or immunocompromised recipients, recipients of donor units known to be from a blood relative, and recipients who have undergone marrow transplantation. Directed donations by family members should be discouraged (they are not less likely to transmit infection); lacking other options, the blood products from family members should always be irradiated.

Transfusion-related acute lung injury

Transfusion-related acute lung injury (TRALI) presents as acute respiratory distress, either during or within 6 h of transfusing the patient. The recipient develops symptoms of respiratory compromise and signs of noncardiogenic pulmonary edema, including bilateral interstitial infiltrates on chest x-ray. Treatment is supportive, and patients usually recover without sequelae. TRALI usually results from the transfusion of donor plasma that contains high-titer anti-HLA antibodies that bind recipient leukocytes. The leukocytes aggregate in the pulmonary vasculature and release mediators that increase capillary permeability. Testing the donor's plasma for anti-HLA antibodies can support this diagnosis. The implicated donors are frequently multiparous women, and transfusion of their plasma component should be avoided.

Posttransfusion purpura

This reaction presents as thrombocytopenia 7–10 days after platelet transfusion and occurs predominantly in women. Platelet-specific antibodies are found in the recipient's serum, and the most frequently recognized antigen is HPA-1a found on the platelet glycoprotein IIIa receptor. The delayed thrombocytopenia is due to the production of antibodies that react to both donor and recipient platelets. Additional platelet transfusions can worsen the thrombocytopenia and should be avoided. Treatment with intravenous immunoglobulin may neutralize the effector antibodies, or plasmapheresis can be used to remove the antibodies.

Alloimmunization

A recipient may become alloimmunized to a number of antigens on cellular blood elements and plasma proteins. Alloantibodies to RBC antigens are detected during pretransfusion testing, and their presence may delay finding antigen-negative cross-match-compatible products for transfusion. Women of childbearing age who are sensitized to certain RBC antigens (i.e., D, c, E, Kell, or Duffy) are at risk for bearing a fetus with hemolytic disease of the newborn. Matching for D antigen is the only pretransfusion selection test to prevent RBC alloimmunization.

Alloimmunization to antigens on leukocytes and platelets can result in refractoriness to platelet transfusions. Once alloimmunization has developed, HLA-compatible platelets from donors who share similar antigens with the recipient may be difficult to find. Hence, prudent transfusion practice is directed at preventing sensitization through the use of leukocyte-reduced cellular components, as well as limiting antigenic exposure by the judicious use of transfusions and use of SDAPs.

■ NONIMMUNOLOGIC REACTIONS

Fluid overload

Blood components are excellent volume expanders, and transfusion may quickly lead to volume overload. Monitoring the rate and volume of the transfusion and using a diuretic can minimize this problem.

Hypothermia

Refrigerated (4°C) or frozen (–18°C or below) blood components can result in hypothermia when rapidly infused. Cardiac dysrhythmias can result from exposing the sinoatrial node to cold fluid. Use of an in-line warmer will prevent this complication.

Electrolyte toxicity

RBC leakage during storage increases the concentration of potassium in the unit. Neonates and patients in renal failure are at risk for hyperkalemia. Preventive measures, such as using fresh or washed RBCs, are warranted for neonatal transfusions because this complication can be fatal.

Citrate, commonly used to anticoagulate blood components, chelates calcium and thereby inhibits the coagulation cascade. Hypocalcemia, manifested by circumoral numbness and/or tingling sensation of the fingers and toes, may result from multiple rapid transfusions. Because citrate is quickly metabolized to bicarbonate, calcium infusion is seldom required in this setting. If calcium or any other intravenous infusion is necessary, it must be given through a separate line.

Iron overload

Each unit of RBCs contains 200–250 mg of iron. Symptoms and signs of iron overload affecting endocrine, hepatic, and cardiac function are common after 100 units of RBCs have been transfused (total-body iron load of 20 g). Preventing this complication by using alternative therapies (e.g., erythropoietin) and judicious transfusion is preferable and cost effective. Chelating agents, such as deferoxamine and deferasirox, are available, but the response though is often suboptimal.

Hypotensive reactions

Transient hypotension may be noted among transfused patients who take angiotensin-converting enzyme (ACE) inhibitors. Since blood products contain bradykinin that is normally degraded by ACE, patients on ACE inhibitors may have increased bradykinin levels that cause hypotension in the recipient. The blood pressure typically returns to normal without intervention.

Immunomodulation

Transfusion of allogeneic blood is immunosuppressive. Multiply transfused renal transplant recipients are less likely to reject the graft, and transfusion may result in poorer outcomes in cancer patients and increase the risk of infections. Transfusion-related immunomodulation is thought to be mediated by transfused leukocytes. Leukocyte-depleted cellular products may cause less immunosuppression, though controlled data have not been obtained and are unlikely to be obtained as the blood supply becomes universally leukocyte-depleted.

◼ INFECTIOUS COMPLICATIONS

The blood supply is initially screened by selecting healthy donors without high-risk lifestyles, medical conditions, or exposure to transmissible pathogens, such as intravenous drug use or visiting malaria endemic areas. Multiple tests performed on donated blood to detect the presence of infectious agents using nucleic acid amplification testing (NAT) or evidence of prior infections by testing for antibodies to pathogens further reduce the risk of transfusion-acquired infections.

Viral infections

Hepatitis C virus   Blood donations are tested for antibodies to HCV and HCV RNA. The risk of acquiring HCV through transfusion is now calculated to be approximately 1 in 2,000,000 units. Infection with HCV may be asymptomatic or lead to chronic active hepatitis, cirrhosis, and liver failure.

Human immunodeficiency virus type 1   Donated blood is tested for antibodies to HIV-1, HIV-1 p24 antigen, and HIV RNA using NAT. Approximately a dozen seronegative donors have been shown to harbor HIV RNA. The risk of HIV-1 infection per transfusion episode is 1 in 2 million. Antibodies to HIV-2 are also measured in donated blood. No cases of HIV-2 infection have been reported in the United States since 1992.

Hepatitis B virus   Donated blood is screened for HBV using assays for hepatitis B surface antigen (HbsAg). NAT testing is not practical because of slow viral replication and lower levels of viremia. The risk of transfusion-associated HBV infection is several times greater than for HCV. Vaccination of individuals who require long-term transfusion therapy can prevent this complication.

Other hepatitis viruses   Hepatitis A virus is rarely transmitted by transfusion; infection is typically asymptomatic and does not lead to chronic disease. Other transfusion-transmitted viruses—TTV, SEN-V, and GBV-C—do not cause chronic hepatitis or other disease states. Routine testing does not appear to be warranted.

West Nile virus   Transfusion-transmitted WNV infections were documented in 2002. This RNA virus can be detected using NAT; routine screening began in 2003. WNV infections range in severity from asymptomatic to fatal, with the older population at greater risk.

Cytomegalovirus   This ubiquitous virus infects ≥50% of the general population and is transmitted by the infected "passenger" WBCs found in transfused PRBCs or platelet components. Cellular components that are leukocyte-reduced have a decreased risk of transmitting CMV, regardless of the serologic status of the donor. Groups at risk for CMV infections include immunosuppressed patients, CMV-seronegative transplant recipients, and neonates; these patients should receive leukocyte-depleted components or CMV seronegative products.

Human T lymphotropic virus (HTLV) type I   Assays to detect HTLV-I and -II are used to screen all donated blood. HTLV-I is associated with adult T cell leukemia/lymphoma and tropical spastic paraparesis in a small percentage of infected persons (Chap. 188). The risk of HTLV-I infection via transfusion is 1 in 641,000 transfusion episodes. HTLV-II is not clearly associated with any disease.

Parvovirus B-19   Blood components and pooled plasma products can transmit this virus, the etiologic agent of erythema infectiosum, or fifth disease, in children. Parvovirus B-19 shows tropism for erythroid precursors and inhibits both erythrocyte production and maturation. Pure red cell aplasia, presenting either as acute aplastic crisis or chronic anemia with shortened RBC survival, may occur in individuals with an underlying hematologic disease, such as sickle cell disease or thalassemia (Chap. 107). The fetus of a seronegative woman is at risk for developing hydrops from this virus.

Bacterial contamination

The relative risk of transfusion-transmitted bacterial infection has increased as the absolute risk of viral infections has dramatically decreased.

Most bacteria do not grow well at cold temperatures; thus, PRBCs and FFP are not common sources of bacterial contamination. However, some gram-negative bacteria can grow at 1° to 6°C. *Yersinia*, *Pseudomonas*, *Serratia*, *Acinetobacter*, and *Escherichia* species have all been implicated in infections related to PRBC transfusion. Platelet concentrates, which are stored at room temperature, are more likely to contain skin contaminants such as gram-positive organisms, including coagulase-negative staphylococci. It is estimated that 1 in 1000–2000 platelet components is contaminated with bacteria. The risk of death due to transfusion-associated sepsis has been calculated at 1 in 17,000 for single-unit platelets derived from whole blood donation and 1 in 61,000 for apheresis product. Since 2004, blood banks have instituted methods to detect contaminated platelet components.

Recipients of transfusion contaminated with bacteria may develop fever and chills, which can progress to septic shock and DIC. These reactions may occur abruptly, within minutes of initiating the transfusion, or after several hours. The onset of symptoms and signs is often sudden and fulminant, which distinguishes bacterial contamination from an FNHTR. The reactions, particularly those related to gram-negative contaminants, are the result of infused endotoxins formed within the contaminated stored component.

When these reactions are suspected, the transfusion must be stopped immediately. Therapy is directed at reversing any signs of shock, and broad-spectrum antibiotics should be given. The blood bank should be notified to identify any clerical or serologic error. The blood component bag should be sent for culture and Gram stain.

Other infectious agents

Various parasites, including those causing malaria, babesiosis, and Chagas disease, can be transmitted by blood transfusion. Geographic migration and travel of donors shift the incidence of these rare infections. Other agents implicated in transfusion transmission include dengue, chikungunya virus, variant Creutzfeldt-Jakob disease, *Anaplasma phagocytophilum*, and yellow fever vaccine virus and the list will grow. Tests for some pathogens are available, such as *Trypanosoma cruzi*, but not universally required. These infections should be considered in the transfused patient in the appropriate clinical setting.

ALTERNATIVES TO TRANSFUSION

Alternatives to allogeneic blood transfusions that avoid homologous donor exposures with attendant immunologic and infectious risks remain attractive. Autologous blood is the best option when transfusion is anticipated. However, the cost-benefit ratio of autologous transfusion remains high. No transfusion is a zero-risk event; clerical errors and bacterial contamination remain potential complications even with autologous transfusions. Additional methods of autologous transfusion in the surgical patient include preoperative hemodilution, recovery of shed blood from sterile surgical sites, and postoperative drainage collection. Directed or designated donation from friends and family of the potential recipient has not been safer than volunteer donor component transfusions. Such directed donations may in fact place the recipient at higher risk for complications such as GVHD and alloimmunization.

Granulocyte and granulocyte-macrophage colony-stimulating factors are clinically useful to hasten leukocyte recovery in patients with leukopenia related to high-dose chemotherapy. Erythropoietin stimulates erythrocyte production in patients with anemia of chronic renal failure and other conditions, thus avoiding or reducing the need for transfusion. This hormone can also stimulate erythropoiesis in the autologous donor to enable additional donation.

FURTHER READINGS

BRECHER ME, HAY SN: Bacterial contamination of blood components. Clin Microbiol Rev 18:195, 2005

CHAIWAT O, LANG JD: Early packed red blood cell transfusion and acute respiratory distress syndrome after trauma. Anesthesiology 110;351, 2009

GERBER DR: Transfusion of packed red blood cells in patient with ischemic heart disease. Crit Care Med 36:1068, 2008

HENDRICKSON JE, HILLYER CD: Noninfectious serious hazards for transfusion. Anesth Analg 108:759, 2009

LANGE MM et al: Leucocyte depletion of perioperative blood transfusion does not affect long-term survival and recurrence in patients with gastrointestinal cancer. Br J Surg 96;734, 2009

PETERSEN LR, BUSCH MP: Transfusion-transmitted arboviruses. Vox Sang 98;495, 2010

SLICHTER SJ, KAUFMAN RM: Dose of prophylactic platelet transfusions and prevention of hemorrhage. N Engl J Med 362;600, 2010

TRIULZI DJ: Transfusion-related acute lung injury: current concepts for the clinician. Anesth Analg 108;770, 2009

VAMVAKAS EC, BLAJCHMAN MA: Transfusion-related mortality: The ongoing risks of allogeneic blood transfusion and the available strategies for their prevention. Blood 113;3406, 2009

——— et al: *The Technical Manual*, 16th ed. Arlington, VA, American Association of Blood Banks, 2008

CHAPTER **114**

Hematopoietic Cell Transplantation

Frederick R. Appelbaum

Bone marrow transplantation was the original term used to describe the collection and transplantation of hematopoietic stem cells, but with the demonstration that the peripheral blood and umbilical cord blood are also useful sources of stem cells, *hematopoietic cell transplantation* has become the preferred generic term for this process. The procedure is usually carried out for one of two purposes: (1) to replace an abnormal but nonmalignant lymphohematopoietic system with one from a normal donor or (2) to treat malignancy by allowing the administration of higher doses of myelosuppressive therapy than would otherwise be possible. The use of hematopoietic cell transplantation has been increasing, both because of its efficacy in selected diseases and because of increasing availability of donors. The Center for International Blood and Marrow Transplant Research (*http://www.cibmtr.org*) estimates that about 65,000 transplants are performed each year.

THE HEMATOPOIETIC STEM CELL

Several features of the hematopoietic stem cell make transplantation clinically feasible, including its remarkable regenerative capacity, its ability to home to the marrow space following intravenous injection, and the ability of the stem cell to be cryopreserved (Chap. 66). Transplantation of a single stem cell can replace the entire lymphohematopoietic system of an adult mouse. In humans, transplantation of a few percent of a donor's bone marrow volume regularly results in complete and sustained replacement of the recipient's entire lymphohematopoietic system, including all red cells, granulocytes, B and T lymphocytes, and platelets, as well as cells comprising the fixed macrophage population, including Kupffer cells of the liver, pulmonary alveolar macrophages, osteoclasts, Langerhans cells of the skin, and brain microglial cells. The ability of the hematopoietic stem cell to home to the marrow following intravenous injection is mediated, in part, by an interaction between stromal cell–derived factor 1 (SDF1) produced by marrow stromal cells and the alpha-chemokine receptor CXCR4 found on stem cells. Homing is also influenced by the interaction of cell-surface molecules, termed *selectins*, on bone marrow endothelial cells with ligands, termed *integrins*, on early hematopoietic cells. Human hematopoietic stem cells can survive freezing and thawing with little, if any, damage, making it possible to remove and store a portion of the patient's own bone marrow for later reinfusion following treatment of the patient with high-dose myelotoxic therapy.

CATEGORIES OF HEMATOPOIETIC CELL TRANSPLANTATION

Hematopoietic cell transplantation can be described according to the relationship between the patient and the donor and by the anatomic source of stem cells. In ~1% of cases, patients have identical twins who can serve as donors. With the use of syngeneic donors, there is no risk of graft-versus-host disease (GVHD) which often complicates allogeneic transplantation, and unlike the use of autologous marrow, there is no risk that the stem cells are contaminated with tumor cells.

Allogeneic transplantation involves a donor and a recipient who are not genetically identical. Following allogeneic transplantation, immune cells transplanted with the stem cells or developing from them can react against the patient, causing GVHD. Alternatively, if the immunosuppressive preparative regimen used to treat the patient before transplant is inadequate, immunocompetent cells of the patient can cause graft rejection. The risks of these complications are greatly influenced by the degree of matching between donor and recipient for antigens encoded by genes of the major histocompatibility complex.

The human leukocyte antigen (HLA) molecules are responsible for binding antigenic proteins and presenting them to T cells. The antigens presented by HLA molecules may derive from exogenous sources (e.g., during active infections) or may be endogenous proteins. If individuals are not HLA-matched, T cells from one individual will react strongly to the mismatched HLA, or "major antigens," of the second. Even if the individuals are HLA-matched, the T cells of the donor may react to differing endogenous or "minor antigens" presented by the HLA of the recipient. Reactions to minor antigens tend to be less vigorous. The genes of major relevance to transplantation include HLA-A, -B, -C, and -D; they are closely linked and therefore tend to be inherited as haplotypes, with only rare crossovers between them. Thus, the odds that any one full sibling will match a patient are one in four, and the probability that the patient has an HLA-identical sibling is $1 - (0.75)^n$, where n equals the number of siblings.

With current techniques, the risk of graft rejection is 1–3%, and the risk of severe, life-threatening acute GVHD is ~15% following transplantation between HLA-identical siblings. The incidence of graft rejection and GVHD increases progressively with the use of family member donors mismatched for one, two, or three antigens. While survival following a one-antigen mismatched transplant is not markedly altered, survival following two- or three-antigen mismatched transplants is significantly reduced, and such transplants should be performed only as part of clinical trials.

Since the formation of the National Marrow Donor Program and other registries, it has become possible to identify HLA-matched unrelated donors for many patients. The genes encoding HLA antigens are highly polymorphic, and thus the odds of any two unrelated individuals being HLA-identical are extremely low, somewhat less than 1 in 10,000. However, by identifying and typing >14 million volunteer donors, HLA-matched donors can now be found for ~50% of patients for whom a search is initiated. It takes, on average, 3–4 months to complete a search and schedule and initiate an unrelated donor transplant. With improvements in HLA-typing and supportive care measures, survival following matched unrelated donor transplantation is essentially the same as that seen with HLA-matched siblings.

Autologous transplantation involves the removal and storage of the patient's own stem cells with subsequent reinfusion after the patient receives high-dose myeloablative therapy. Unlike allogeneic transplantation, there is no risk of GVHD or graft rejection with autologous transplantation. On the other hand, autologous transplantation lacks a graft-versus-tumor (GVT) effect, and the autologous stem cell product can be contaminated with tumor cells, which could lead to relapse. A variety of techniques have been developed to "purge" autologous products of tumor cells. Some use antibodies directed at tumor-associated antigens plus complement, antibodies linked to toxins, or antibodies conjugated to immunomagnetic beads. In vitro incubation with certain chemotherapeutic agents such as 4-hydroperoxycyclophosphamide and long-term culture of bone marrow have also been shown to diminish tumor cell numbers in stem cell products. Another technique is positive selection of stem cells using antibodies to CD34, with subsequent column adherence or flow techniques to select normal stem cells while leaving tumor cells behind. All these approaches can reduce the number of tumor cells from 1000- to 10,000-fold and are clinically feasible; however, no prospective randomized trials have yet shown that any of these approaches results in a decrease in relapse rates or improvements in disease-free or overall survival.

Bone marrow aspirated from the posterior and anterior iliac crests has traditionally been the source of hematopoietic stem cells for transplantation. Typically, anywhere from 1.5 to 5×10^8 nucleated marrow cells per kilogram are collected for allogeneic transplantation. Several studies have found improved survival in the settings of both matched sibling and unrelated transplantation by transplanting higher numbers of bone marrow cells.

Hematopoietic stem cells circulate in the peripheral blood but in very low concentrations. Following the administration of certain hematopoietic growth factors, including granulocyte colony-stimulating factor (G-CSF) or granulocyte-macrophage colony-stimulating factor (GM-CSF), and during recovery from intensive chemotherapy, the concentration of hematopoietic progenitor cells in blood, as measured either by colony-forming units or expression of the CD34 antigen, increases markedly. This has made it possible to harvest adequate numbers of stem cells from the peripheral blood for transplantation. Donors are typically treated with 4 or 5 days of hematopoietic growth factor, following which stem cells are collected in one or two 4-h pheresis sessions. In the autologous setting, transplantation of $>2.5 \times 10^6$ CD34 cells per kilogram, a number that can be collected in most circumstances, leads to rapid and sustained engraftment in virtually all cases. In the 10–20% of patients who fail to mobilize sufficient CD34+ cells with growth factor alone, the addition of plerixafor, an antagonist of CXCR4, may be useful. Compared to the use of autologous marrow, use of peripheral blood stem cells results in more rapid hematopoietic recovery, with granulocytes recovering to 500/μL by day 12 and platelets recovering to 20,000/μL by day 14. While this more rapid recovery diminishes the morbidity rate of transplantation, no studies show improved survival.

Hesitation in studying the use of peripheral blood stem cells for allogeneic transplantation was because peripheral blood stem cell products contain as much as 1 log more T cells than are contained in the typical marrow harvest; in animal models, the incidence of GVHD is related to the number of T cells transplanted. Nonetheless, clinical trials have shown that the use of growth factor–mobilized peripheral blood stem cells from HLA-matched family members leads to faster engraftment without an increase in acute GVHD. Chronic GVHD may be increased with peripheral blood stem cells, but in trials conducted so far, this has been more than balanced by reductions in relapse rates and nonrelapse mortality rates, with the use of peripheral blood stem cells resulting in improved overall survival. Randomized trials are now evaluating the use of peripheral blood versus bone marrow for matched unrelated donor transplantation.

Umbilical cord blood contains a high concentration of hematopoietic progenitor cells, allowing for its use as a source of stem cells for transplantation. Cord blood transplantation from family members has been explored in the setting where the immediate need for transplantation precludes waiting the 9 or so months generally required for the baby to mature to the point of donating marrow. Use of cord blood results in slower engraftment and peripheral count recovery than seen with marrow but a low incidence of GVHD, perhaps reflecting the low number of T cells in cord blood. Several banks have been developed to harvest and store cord blood for possible transplantation to unrelated patients from material that would otherwise be discarded. A summary of the first 562 unrelated cord blood transplants, facilitated by the New York Blood Center, reported engraftment in ~85% of patients but at a slower pace than seen with marrow. Severe GVHD was seen in 23% of patients. The risk of graft failure and transplant-related mortality were related to the dose of cord blood cells per kilogram, thus limiting the application of single cord blood transplantation for the treatment of larger adolescent and adult patients. Subsequent trials suggest that the use of double cord transplants diminishes the risk of graft failure and early mortality even though only one of the donors ultimately engrafts.

THE TRANSPLANT PREPARATIVE REGIMEN

The treatment regimen administered to patients immediately preceding transplantation is designed to eradicate the patient's underlying disease and, in the setting of allogeneic transplantation, immunosuppress the patient adequately to prevent rejection of the transplanted marrow. The appropriate regimen therefore depends on the disease setting and source of marrow. For example, when transplantation is performed to treat severe combined immunodeficiency and the donor is a histocompatible sibling, no treatment is needed because no host cells require eradication and the patient is already too immunoincompetent to reject the transplanted marrow. For aplastic anemia, there is no large population of cells to eradicate, and high-dose cyclophosphamide plus antithymocyte globulin are sufficient to immunosuppress the patient adequately to accept the marrow graft. In the setting of thalassemia and sickle cell anemia, high-dose busulfan is frequently added to cyclophosphamide in order to eradicate hyperplastic host hematopoiesis. A variety of different regimens have been developed to treat malignant diseases. Most of these regimens include agents that have high activity against the tumor in question at conventional doses and have myelosuppression as their predominant dose-limiting toxicity. Therefore, these regimens commonly include busulfan, cyclophosphamide, melphalan, thiotepa, carmustine, etoposide, and total-body irradiation in various combinations.

Although high-dose treatment regimens have typically been used in transplantation, the understanding that much of the antitumor effect of transplantation derives from an immunologically mediated GVT response has led investigators to ask if reduced-intensity conditioning regimens might be effective and more tolerable. Evidence for a GVT effect comes from studies showing that posttransplant relapse rates are lowest in patients who develop acute and chronic GVHD, higher in those without GVHD, and higher still in recipients of T cell–depleted allogeneic or syngeneic marrow. The demonstration that complete remissions can be obtained in many patients who have relapsed posttransplant by simply administering viable lymphocytes from the original donor further strengthens the argument for a potent GVT effect. Accordingly, a variety of less-intensive nonmyeloablative regimens have been studied, ranging in intensity from the very minimum required to achieve engraftment (e.g., fludarabine plus 200 cGy total-body irradiation) to regimens of more immediate intensity (e.g., fludarabine plus melphalan). Studies to date document that engraftment can be readily achieved with less toxicity than seen with conventional transplantation. Furthermore, the severity of acute GVHD appears to be decreased because less tissue damage is done by the lower doses of drugs in the preparative regimen. Complete sustained responses have been documented in many patients, particularly those with more indolent hematologic malignancies. The role of reduced-intensity conditioning in any disease, however, has not been fully defined.

■ THE TRANSPLANT PROCEDURE

Marrow is usually collected from the donor's posterior and sometimes anterior iliac crests, with the donor under general or spinal anesthesia. Typically, 10–15 mL/kg of marrow is aspirated, placed in heparinized media, and filtered through 0.3- and 0.2-mm screens to remove fat and bony spicules. The collected marrow may undergo further processing depending on the clinical situation, such as the removal of red cells to prevent hemolysis in ABO-incompatible transplants, the removal of donor T cells to prevent GVHD, or attempts to remove possible contaminating tumor cells in autologous transplantation. Marrow donation is safe, with only very rare complications reported.

Peripheral blood stem cells are collected by leukapheresis after the donor has been treated with hematopoietic growth factors or, in the setting of autologous transplantation, sometimes after treatment with a combination of chemotherapy and growth factors. Stem cells for transplantation are generally infused through a large-bore central venous catheter. Such infusions are usually well tolerated, although occasionally patients develop fever, cough, or shortness of breath. These symptoms usually resolve with slowing of the infusion. When the stem cell product has been cryopreserved using dimethyl sulfoxide, patients more often experience short-lived nausea or vomiting due to the odor and taste of the cryoprotectant.

■ ENGRAFTMENT

Peripheral blood counts usually reach their nadir several days to a week posttransplant as a consequence of the preparative regimen; then cells produced by the transplanted stem cells begin to appear in the peripheral blood. The rate of recovery depends on the source of stem cells, the use of posttransplant growth factors, and the form of GVHD prophylaxis employed. If marrow is the source of stem cells, recovery to 100 granulocytes/μL occurs by day 16 and to 500/μL by day 22. Use of G-CSF–mobilized peripheral blood stem cells speeds the rate of recovery by ~1 week when compared to marrow, whereas engraftment following cord blood transplantation is typically delayed by ~1 week compared to marrow. Use of a myeloid growth factor (G-CSF or GM-CSF) posttransplant can accelerate recovery by 3–5 days, while use of methotrexate to prevent GVHD delays engraftment by a similar period. Following allogeneic transplantation, engraftment can be documented using fluorescence in situ hybridization of sex chromosomes if donor and recipient are sex-mismatched, HLA-typing if HLA-mismatched, or restriction fragment length polymorphism analysis if sex- and HLA-matched.

■ COMPLICATIONS FOLLOWING HEMATOPOIETIC CELL TRANSPLANT

Early direct chemoradiotoxicities

The transplant preparative regimen may cause a spectrum of acute toxicities that vary according to intensity of the regimen and the specific agents used, but frequently results in nausea, vomiting, and mild skin erythema (Fig. 114-1). Regimens that include high-dose cyclophosphamide can result in hemorrhagic cystitis, which can usually be prevented by bladder irrigation or with the sulfhydryl compound mercaptoethanesulfonate (MESNA); rarely, acute hemorrhagic carditis is seen. Most high-dose preparative regimens will result in oral mucositis, which typically develops 5–7 days posttransplant and often requires narcotic analgesia. Use of a patient-controlled analgesic pump provides the greatest patient satisfaction and results in a lower cumulative dose of narcotic. Keratinocyte growth factor (palifermin) can shorten the duration of mucositis by several days following autologous transplantation. Patients begin losing their hair 5–6 days posttransplant and by 1 week are usually profoundly pancytopenic.

Depending on the intensity of the conditioning regimen, 3–10% of patients will develop sinusoidal obstruction syndrome of the liver, a syndrome that results from direct cytotoxic injury to hepatic-venular and sinusoidal endothelium, with subsequent

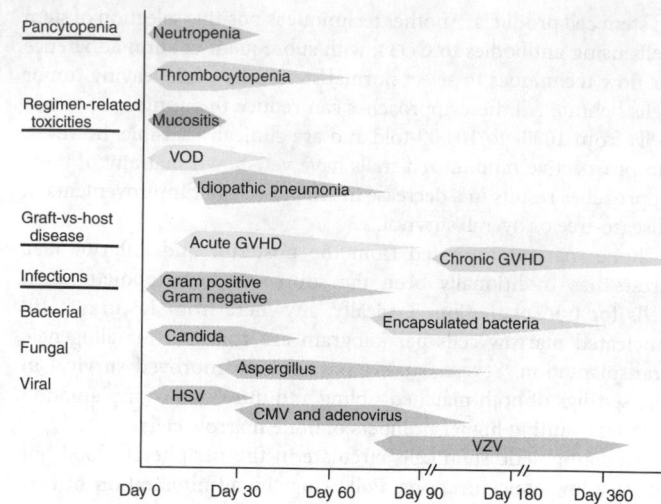

Figure 114-1   Major syndromes complicating marrow transplantation. VOD, venoocclusive disease; GVHD, graft-versus-host disease; HSV, herpes simplex virus; CMV, cytomegalovirus; VZV, varicella-zoster virus. The size of the shaded area roughly reflects the risk of the complication.

deposition of fibrin and the development of a local hypercoagulable state. This chain of events leads to the clinical symptoms of tender hepatomegaly, ascites, jaundice, and fluid retention. These symptoms can develop any time during the first month posttransplant, with the peak incidence at day 16. Predisposing factors include prior exposure to intensive chemotherapy, pretransplant hepatitis of any cause, and use of more intense conditioning regimens. The mortality rate of sinusoidal obstruction syndrome is ~30%, with progressive hepatic failure culminating in a terminal hepatorenal syndrome. Both thrombolytic and antithrombotic agents, such as tissue plasminogen activator, heparin, and prostaglandin E, have been studied as therapy, but none has proven of consistent major benefit in controlled trials, and all have significant toxicity. Early studies with defibrotide, a polydeoxyribonucleotide, seem encouraging.

Although most pneumonias developing posttransplant are caused by infectious agents, in ~5% of patients a diffuse interstitial pneumonia will develop that is thought to be the result of direct toxicity of high-dose preparative regimens. Bronchoalveolar lavage typically shows alveolar hemorrhage, and biopsies are typically characterized by diffuse alveolar damage, although some cases may have a more clearly interstitial pattern. High-dose glucocorticoids or antitumor necrosis factor therapies are sometimes used as treatment, although randomized trials testing their utility have not been reported.

Late direct chemoradiotoxicities

Late complications of the preparative regimen include decreased growth velocity in children and delayed development of secondary sex characteristics. These complications can be partly ameliorated with the use of appropriate growth and sex hormone replacement. Most men become azoospermic, and most postpubertal women will develop ovarian failure, which should be treated. Thyroid dysfunction, usually well compensated, is sometimes seen. Cataracts develop in 10–20% of patients and are most common in patients treated with total-body irradiation and those who receive glucocorticoid therapy posttransplant for treatment of GVHD. Aseptic necrosis of the femoral head is seen in 10% of patients and is particularly frequent in those receiving chronic glucocorticoid therapy. Both acute and late chemoradiotoxicities (except those due to glucocorticoids) are considerably less frequent in recipients of reduced- compared to high-dose preparative regimens.

Graft-versus-host disease

GVHD is the result of allogeneic T cells that are transferred with the donor's stem cell inoculum reacting with antigenic targets on host cells. GVHD developing within the first 3 months posttransplant is termed *acute GVHD*, while GVHD developing or persisting beyond 3 months posttransplant is termed *chronic GVHD*. Acute GVHD most often first becomes apparent 2–4 weeks posttransplant and is characterized by an erythematous maculopapular rash; persistent anorexia or diarrhea, or both; and by liver disease with increased serum levels of bilirubin, alanine and aspartate aminotransferase, and alkaline phosphatase. Since many conditions can mimic acute GVHD, diagnosis usually requires skin, liver, or endoscopic biopsy for confirmation. In all these organs, endothelial damage and lymphocytic infiltrates are seen. In skin, the epidermis and hair follicles are damaged; in liver, the small bile ducts show segmental disruption; and in intestines, destruction of the crypts and mucosal ulceration may be noted. A commonly used rating system for acute GVHD is shown in Table 114-1. Grade I acute GVHD is of little clinical significance, does not affect the likelihood of survival, and does not require treatment. In contrast, grades II to IV GVHD are associated with significant symptoms and a poorer probability of survival, and they require aggressive therapy. The incidence of acute GVHD is higher in recipients of stem cells from mismatched or unrelated donors, in older patients, and in patients unable to receive full doses of drugs used to prevent the disease.

One general approach to the prevention of GVHD is the administration of immunosuppressive drugs early after transplant. Combinations of methotrexate and either cyclosporine or tacrolimus are among the most effective and widely used regimens. Prednisone, anti–T cell antibodies, mycophenolate mofetil, and other immunosuppressive agents have also been or are being studied in various combinations. A second general approach to GVHD prevention is removal of T cells from the stem cell inoculum. While effective in preventing GVHD, T cell depletion is associated with an increased incidence of graft failure and of tumor recurrence posttransplant; as yet, little evidence suggests that T-cell depletion improves cure rates in any specific setting.

Despite prophylaxis, significant acute GVHD will develop in ~30% of recipients of stem cells from matched siblings and in as many as 60% of those receiving stem cells from unrelated donors. The disease is usually treated with glucocorticoids, additional immunosuppressants or monoclonal antibodies targeted against T cells or T cell subsets.

Between 20 and 50% of patients surviving >6 months after allogeneic transplantation will develop chronic GVHD. The disease is more common in older patients, in recipients of mismatched or unrelated stem cells, and in those with a preceding episode of acute GVHD. The disease resembles an autoimmune disorder with malar rash, sicca syndrome, arthritis, obliterative bronchiolitis, and bile duct degeneration and cholestasis. Single-agent prednisone or cyclosporine is standard treatment at present, although trials of other agents are under way. In most patients, chronic GVHD resolves, but it may require 1–3 years of immunosuppressive treatment before these agents can be withdrawn without the disease recurring. Because patients with chronic GVHD are susceptible to significant infection, they should receive prophylactic trimethoprim-sulfamethoxazole, and all suspected infections should be investigated and treated aggressively.

Graft failure

While complete and sustained engraftment is usually seen posttransplant, occasionally marrow function either does not return or, after a brief period of engraftment, is lost. Graft failure after autologous transplantation can be the result of inadequate numbers of stem cells being transplanted, damage during ex vivo treatment or storage, or exposure of the patient to myelotoxic agents posttransplant. Infections with cytomegalovirus (CMV) or human herpesvirus type 6 have also been associated with loss of marrow function. Graft failure after allogeneic transplantation can also be due to immunologic rejection of the graft by immunocompetent host cells. Immunologically based graft rejection is more common following use of less-immunosuppressive preparative regimens, in recipients of T cell–depleted stem cell products, and in patients receiving grafts from HLA-mismatched donors or cord blood.

Treatment of graft failure usually involves removing all potentially myelotoxic agents from the patient's regimen and attempting a short trial of a myeloid growth factor. Persistence of lymphocytes of host origin in allogeneic transplant recipients with graft failure indicates immunologic rejection. Reinfusion of donor stem cells in such patients is usually unsuccessful unless preceded by a second immunosuppressive preparative regimen. Standard high-dose preparative regimens are generally tolerated poorly if administered within 100 days of a first transplant because of cumulative toxicities. However, use of regimens combining, for example, anti-CD3 antibodies with high-dose glucocorticoids, fludarabine plus low-dose total-body irradiation, or cyclophosphamide plus antithymocyte globulin, has been effective in some cases.

TABLE 114-1 Clinical Staging and Grading of Acute Graft-Versus-Host Disease

Clinical Stage	Skin	Liver—Bilirubin, μmol/L (mg/dL)	Gut
1	Rash <25% body surface	34–51 (2–3)	Diarrhea 500–1000 mL/d
2	Rash 25–50% body surface	51–103 (3–6)	Diarrhea 1000–1500 mL/d
3	Generalized erythroderma	103–257 (6–15)	Diarrhea >1500 mL/d
4	Desquamation and bullae	>257 (>15)	Ileus

Overall Clinical Grade	Skin Stage	Liver Stage	Gut Stage
I	1–2	0	0
II	1–3	1	1
III	1–3	2–3	2–3
IV	2–4	2–4	2–4

Infection

Posttransplant patients, particularly recipients of allogeneic transplantation, require unique approaches to the problem of infection. Early after transplantation, patients are profoundly neutropenic, and because the risk of bacterial infection is so great, most centers initiate antibiotic treatment once the granulocyte count falls to <500/μL. Fluconazole prophylaxis at a dose of 200–400 mg/kg per day reduces the risk of candidal infections. Patients seropositive for herpes simplex should receive acyclovir prophylaxis. One approach to infection prophylaxis is shown in Table 114-2. Despite these prophylactic measures, most patients will develop fever and signs of infection posttransplant. The management of patients who become febrile despite bacterial and fungal prophylaxis is a difficult challenge and is guided by individual aspects of the patient and by the institution's experience.

The general problem of infection in the immunocompromised host is discussed in Chap. 132.

Once patients engraft, the incidence of bacterial infection diminishes; however, patients, particularly allogeneic transplant recipients, remain at significant risk of infection. During the period from engraftment until about 3 months posttransplant, the most common causes of infection are gram-positive bacteria, fungi (particularly *Aspergillus*), and viruses including CMV. CMV infection, which in the past was frequently seen and often fatal, can be prevented in seronegative patients transplanted from seronegative donors by the use of either seronegative blood products or products from which the white blood cells have been removed. In seropositive patients or patients transplanted from seropositive donors, the use of ganciclovir, either as prophylaxis beginning at the time of engraftment or initiated when CMV first reactivates as evidenced by development of antigenemia or viremia, can significantly reduce the risk of CMV disease. Foscarnet is effective for some patients who develop CMV antigenemia or infection despite the use of ganciclovir or who cannot tolerate the drug.

Pneumocystis jiroveci pneumonia, once seen in 5–10% of patients, can be prevented by treating patients with oral trimethoprim-sulfamethoxazole for 1 week pretransplant and resuming the treatment once patients have engrafted.

The risk of infection diminishes considerably beyond 3 months after transplant unless chronic GVHD develops, requiring continuous immunosuppression. Most transplant centers recommend continuing trimethoprim-sulfamethoxazole prophylaxis while patients are receiving any immunosuppressive drugs and also recommend careful monitoring for late CMV reactivation. In addition, many centers recommend prophylaxis against varicella zoster, using acyclovir for 1 year posttransplant. Patients should be revaccinated against tetanus, diphtheria, haemophilus influenza, polio, and pneumococcal pneumonia starting at 12 months posttransplant and against measles, mumps, and rubella at 24 months.

TREATMENT OF SPECIFIC DISEASES USING HEMATOPOIETIC CELL TRANSPLANTATION

TREATMENT Nonmalignant Diseases

IMMUNODEFICIENCY DISORDERS By replacing abnormal stem cells with cells from a normal donor, hematopoietic cell transplantation can cure patients of a variety of immunodeficiency disorders including severe combined immunodeficiency, Wiskott-Aldrich syndrome, and Chédiak-Higashi syndrome. The widest experience has been with severe combined immunodeficiency disease, where cure rates of 90% can be expected with HLA-identical donors and success rates of 50–70% have been reported using haplotype-mismatched parents as donors (Table 114-3).

APLASTIC ANEMIA Transplantation from matched siblings after a preparative regimen of high-dose cyclophosphamide and antithymocyte globulin can cure up to 90% of patients age <40 years with severe aplastic anemia. Results in older patients and in recipients of mismatched family member or unrelated marrow are less favorable; therefore, a trial of immunosuppressive therapy is generally recommended for such patients before considering transplantation. Transplantation is effective in all forms of aplastic anemia including, for example, the syndromes associated with paroxysmal nocturnal hemoglobinuria and Fanconi's anemia. Patients with Fanconi's anemia are abnormally sensitive to the toxic effects of alkylating agents and so less intensive preparative regimens must be used in their treatment (Chap. 107).

HEMOGLOBINOPATHIES Marrow transplantation from an HLA-identical sibling following a preparative regimen of busulfan and cyclophosphamide can cure 70–90% of patients with thalassemia major. The best outcomes can be expected if patients are transplanted before they develop hepatomegaly or portal fibrosis and if they have been given adequate iron chelation therapy. Among such patients, the probabilities of 5-year survival and disease-free survival are 95 and 90%, respectively. Although prolonged survival can be achieved with aggressive chelation therapy, transplantation is the only curative treatment for thalassemia. Transplantation is being studied as a curative approach to patients with sickle cell anemia. Two-year survival and disease-free survival rates of 90 and 80%, respectively, have been reported following matched sibling transplantation. Decisions about patient selection and the timing of transplantation remain difficult, but transplantation represents a reasonable option for younger patients who suffer repeated crises or other significant complications and who have not responded to other interventions (Chap. 104).

TABLE 114-2 Approach to Infection Prophylaxis in Allogeneic Transplant Recipients

Organism		Approach
Bacterial	Levofloxacin	750 mg PO or IV daily
Fungal	Fluconazole	400 mg PO qd to day 75 posttransplant
Pneumocystis carinii	Trimethoprim-sulfamethoxazole	1 double-strength tablet PO bid 2 days/week until day 180 or off immunosuppression
Viral		
Herpes simplex	Acyclovir	800 mg PO bid to day 30
Varicella-zoster	Acyclovir	800 mg PO bid to day 365
Cytomegalovirus	Ganciclovir	5 mg/kg IV bid for 7 days, then 5 (mg/kg)/d 5 days/week to day 100

TABLE 114-3 Estimated 5-Year Survival Rates Following Transplantation[*]

Disease	Allogeneic, %	Autologous, %
Severe combined immunodeficiency	90	N/A
Aplastic anemia	90	N/A
Thalassemia	90	N/A
Acute myeloid leukemia		
First remission	55–60	50
Second remission	40	30
Acute lymphocytic leukemia		
First remission	50	40
Second remission	40	30
Chronic myeloid leukemia		
Chronic phase	70	ID
Accelerated phase	40	ID
Blast crisis	15	ID
Chronic lymphocytic leukemia	50	ID
Myelodysplasia	45	ID
Multiple myeloma	30	35
Non-Hodgkin's lymphoma		
First relapse/second remission	40	40
Hodgkin's disease		
First relapse/ second remission	40	50
Breast cancer		
High-risk stage II	N/A	70
Stage IV	N/A	15

[*]These estimates are generally based on data reported by the International Bone Marrow Transplant Registry. The analysis has not been reviewed by their Advisory Committee.

Abbreviations: N/A, not applicable; ID, insufficient data.

OTHER NONMALIGNANT DISEASES Theoretically, hematopoietic cell transplantation should be able to cure any disease that results from an inborn error of the lymphohematopoietic system. Transplantation has been used successfully to treat congenital disorders of white blood cells such as Kostmann's syndrome, chronic granulomatous disease, and leukocyte adhesion deficiency. Congenital anemias such as Blackfan-Diamond anemia can also be cured with transplantation. Infantile malignant osteopetrosis is due to an inability of the osteoclast to resorb bone, and since osteoclasts derive from the marrow, transplantation can cure this rare inherited disorder.

Hematopoietic cell transplantation has been used as treatment for a number of storage diseases caused by enzymatic deficiencies, such as Gaucher's disease, Hurler's syndrome, Hunter's syndrome, and infantile metachromatic leukodystrophy. Transplantation for these diseases has not been uniformly successful, but treatment early in the course of these diseases, before irreversible damage to extramedullary organs has occurred, increases the chance for success.

Transplantation is being explored as a treatment for severe acquired autoimmune disorders. These trials are based on studies demonstrating that transplantation can reverse autoimmune disorders in animal models and on the observation that occasional patients with coexisting autoimmune disorders and hematologic malignancies have been cured of both with transplantation.

TREATMENT   Malignant Diseases

ACUTE LEUKEMIA Allogeneic hematopoietic cell transplantation cures 15–20% of patients who do not achieve complete response from induction chemotherapy for acute myeloid leukemia (AML) and is the only form of therapy that can cure such patients. Cure rates of 30–35% are seen when patients are transplanted in second remission or in first relapse. The best results with allogeneic transplantation are achieved when applied during first remission, with disease-free survival rates averaging 55–60%. Meta-analyses of studies comparing matched related donor transplantation to chemotherapy for adult AML patients age <60 years show a survival advantage with transplantation. This advantage is greatest for those with unfavorable-risk AML and lost in those with favorable-risk disease. The role of autologous transplantation in the treatment of AML is less well defined. The rates of disease recurrence with autologous transplantation are higher than those seen after allogeneic transplantation, and cure rates are somewhat less.

Similar to patients with AML, adults with acute lymphocytic leukemia who do not achieve a complete response to induction chemotherapy can be cured in 15–20% of cases with immediate transplantation. Cure rates improve to 30–50% in second remission, and therefore transplantation can be recommended for adults who have persistent disease after induction chemotherapy or who have subsequently relapsed. Transplantation in first remission results in cure rates about 55%. Transplantation appears to offer a clear advantage over chemotherapy for patients with high-risk disease, such as those with Philadelphia chromosome–positive disease. Debate continues about whether adults with standard-risk disease should be transplanted in first remission or whether transplantation should be reserved until relapse. Autologous transplantation is associated with a higher relapse rate but a somewhat lower risk of nonrelapse mortality when compared to allogeneic transplantation. There is no obvious role of autologous transplantation for ALL in first remission, and for second-remission patients, most experts recommend use of allogeneic stem cells if an appropriate donor is available.

CHRONIC LEUKEMIA Allogeneic hematopoietic cell transplantation is the only therapy shown to cure a substantial portion of patients with chronic myeloid leukemia (CML). Five-year disease-free survival rates are 15–20% for patients transplanted for blast crisis, 25–50% for accelerated-phase patients, and 60–70% for chronic-phase patients, with cure rates as high as 80% at selected centers. However, with the availability of imatinib mesylate, a remarkably effective, relatively nontoxic oral agent, most physicians favor reserving transplantation for those who fail to achieve a complete cytogenetic response with imatinib, relapse after an initial response, or are intolerant of the drug (Chap. 109).

Allogeneic transplantation using high-dose preparative regimen was rarely used for chronic lymphocytic leukemia (CLL), in large part because of the chronic nature of the disease and because of the age profile of patients. In those cases where it was studied, complete remissions were achieved in the majority of patients, with disease-free survival rates of ~50% at 3 years, despite the advanced stage of the disease at the time of transplant. The marked antitumor effects have resulted in the increased use and study of allogeneic transplantation using reduced-intensity conditioning for the treatment of CLL.

MYELODYSPLASIA Between 40 and 50% of patients with myelodysplasia appear to be cured with allogeneic transplantation. Results are better among younger patients and those with less advanced disease. However, some patients with myelodysplasia can live for extended periods without intervention, and so transplantation is generally recommended only for patients with disease categorized as intermediate risk I or greater according to the International Prognostic Scoring System (Chap. 107).

LYMPHOMA Patients with disseminated intermediate- or high-grade non-Hodgkin's lymphoma who have not been cured by first-line chemotherapy and are transplanted in first relapse or second remission can still be cured in 40–50% of cases. This represents a clear advantage over results obtained with conventional-dose salvage chemotherapy. It is unsettled whether patients with high-risk disease benefit from transplantation in first remission. Most experts favor the use of autologous rather than allogeneic transplantation for patients with intermediate- or high-grade non-Hodgkin's lymphoma, because fewer complications occur with this approach and survival appears equivalent. For patients with recurrent disseminated indolent non-Hodgkin's lymphoma, autologous transplantation results in high response rates and improved progression-free survival compared to salvage chemotherapy. However, late relapses are seen after transplantation. The role of autologous transplantation in the initial treatment of patients is under study. Reduced-intensity conditioning regimens followed by allogeneic transplantation result in high response rates in patients with indolent lymphomas, but the exact role of this approach remains to be defined.

The role of transplantation in Hodgkin's disease is similar to that in intermediate- and high-grade non-Hodgkin's lymphoma. With transplantation, 5-year disease-free survival is 20–30% in patients who never achieve a first remission with standard chemotherapy and up to 70% for those transplanted in second remission. Transplantation has no defined role in first remission in Hodgkin's disease.

MYELOMA Patients with myeloma who have progressed on first-line therapy can sometimes benefit from allogeneic or autologous transplantation. Autologous transplantation has been studied as part of the initial therapy of patients, and both disease-free survival and overall survival were improved with this approach in randomized trials. The use of autologous transplantation followed by nonmyeloablative allogeneic transplantation is the subject of ongoing research.

SOLID TUMORS Among women with metastatic breast cancer, 15–20% disease-free survival rates at 3 years have been reported, with better results seen in younger patients who have responded completely to standard-dose therapy before undergoing transplantation. Randomized trials have not shown superior survival for patients treated for metastatic disease with high-dose chemotherapy plus stem cell support. Randomized trials evaluating transplantation as treatment for primary breast cancer have yielded mixed results. No role for autologous transplantation has been established in the treatment of breast cancer.

Patients with testicular cancer who have failed first-line chemotherapy have been treated with autologous transplantation; ~10–20% of such patients apparently have been cured with this approach.

The use of high-dose chemotherapy with autologous stem cell support is being studied for several other solid tumors, including neuroblastoma and pediatric sarcomas. As in most other settings, the best results have been obtained in patients with limited amounts of disease and where the remaining tumor remains sensitive to conventional-dose chemotherapy. Few randomized trials of transplantation in these diseases have been completed.

Partial and complete responses have been reported following nonmyeloablative allogeneic transplantation for some solid tumors, most notably renal cell cancers. The GVT effect, well documented in the treatment of hematologic malignancies, may apply to selected solid tumors under certain circumstances.

POSTTRANSPLANT RELAPSE Patients who relapse following autologous transplantation sometimes respond to further chemotherapy and may be candidates for possible allogeneic transplantation, particularly if the remission following the initial autologous transplant was long. Several options are available for patients who relapse following allogeneic transplantation. Of particular interest are the response rates seen with infusion of unirradiated donor lymphocytes. Complete responses in as many as 75% of patients with chronic myeloid leukemia, 40% in myelodysplasia, 25% in AML, and 15% in myeloma have been reported. Major complications of donor lymphocyte infusions include transient myelosuppression and the development of GVHD. These complications depend on the number of donor lymphocytes given and the schedule of infusions, with less GVHD seen with lower dose, fractionated schedules.

FURTHER READINGS

APPELBAUM FR: Hematopoietic-cell transplantation at 50. N Engl J Med 357:1472, 2007

GYURKOCZA B et al: Allogeneic hematopoietic cell transplantation: The state of the art. Expert Rev Hematol 3:285, 2010

KORETH J et al: Allogeneic stem cell transplantation for acute myeloid leukemia in first complete remission: A systematic review and meta-analysis of prospective clinical trials. JAMA 301(22):2349, 2009

LEE SJ et al: High-resolution donor-recipient HLA matching contributes to the success of unrelated donor marrow transplantation. Blood 110:4576, 2007

TOMBLYN M et al: Guidelines for preventing infectious complications among hematopoietic cell transplantation recipients: A global perspective. Biol Blood Marrow Transplant 15:1143, 2009

CHAPTER 115

Disorders of Platelets and Vessel Wall

Barbara Konkle

Hemostasis is a dynamic process in which the platelet and the blood vessel wall play key roles. Platelets become activated upon adhesion to von Willebrand factor (VWF) and collagen in the exposed subendothelium after injury. Platelet activation is also mediated through shear forces imposed by blood flow itself, particularly in areas where the vessel wall is diseased, and is also affected by the inflammatory state of the endothelium. The activated platelet surface provides the major physiologic site for coagulation factor activation, which results in further platelet activation and fibrin formation. Genetic and acquired influences on the platelet and vessel wall, as well as on the coagulation and fibrinolytic systems, determine whether normal hemostasis, or bleeding or clotting symptoms, will result.

■ THE PLATELET

Platelets are released from the megakaryocyte, likely under the influence of flow in the capillary sinuses. The normal blood platelet count is 150,000–450,000/μL. The major regulator of platelet production is the hormone thrombopoietin (TPO), which is synthesized in the liver. Synthesis is increased with inflammation and specifically by interleukin 6. TPO binds to its receptor on platelets and megakaryocytes, by which it is removed from the circulation. Thus a reduction in platelet and megakaryocyte mass increases the level of TPO, which then stimulates platelet production. Platelets circulate with an average life span of 7 to 10 days. Approximately one-third of the platelets reside in the spleen, and this number increases in proportion to splenic size, although the platelet count rarely decreases to <40,000/μL as the spleen enlarges. Platelets are physiologically very active, but are anucleate, and thus have limited capacity to synthesize new proteins.

Normal vascular endothelium contributes to preventing thrombosis by inhibiting platelet function (Chap. 58). When vascular endothelium is injured, these inhibitory effects are overcome, and platelets adhere to the exposed intimal surface primarily through VWF, a large multimeric protein present in both plasma and in the extracellular matrix of the subendothelial vessel wall. Platelet adhesion results in the generation of intracellular signals that lead to activation of the platelet glycoprotein (Gp) IIb/IIIa ($\alpha_{IIb}\beta_3$) receptor and resultant platelet aggregation.

Activated platelets undergo release of their granule contents, which include nucleotides, adhesive proteins, growth factors, and procoagulants that serve to promote platelet aggregation and blood clot formation and influence the environment of the forming clot. During platelet aggregation, additional platelets are recruited to the site of injury, leading to the formation of an occlusive platelet thrombus. The platelet plug is stabilized by the fibrin mesh that develops simultaneously as the product of the coagulation cascade.

■ THE VESSEL WALL

Endothelial cells line the surface of the entire circulatory tree, totaling $1-6 \times 10^{13}$ cells, enough to cover a surface area equivalent to about six tennis courts. The endothelium is physiologically active, controlling vascular permeability, flow of biologically active molecules and nutrients, blood cell interactions with the vessel wall, the inflammatory response, and angiogenesis.

The endothelium normally presents an antithrombotic surface (Chap. 58) but rapidly becomes prothrombotic when stimulated, which promotes coagulation, inhibits fibrinolysis, and activates platelets. In many cases, endothelium-derived vasodilators are also platelet inhibitors (e.g., nitric oxide) and, conversely, endothelium-derived vasoconstrictors (e.g., endothelin) can also be platelet activators. The net effect of vasodilation and inhibition of platelet function is to promote blood fluidity, whereas the net effect of vasoconstriction and platelet activation is to promote thrombosis. Thus, blood fluidity and hemostasis is regulated by the balance of antithrombotic/prothrombotic and vasodilatory/vasoconstrictor properties of endothelial cells.

DISORDERS OF PLATELETS

■ THROMBOCYTOPENIA

Thrombocytopenia results from one or more of three processes: (1) decreased bone marrow production; (2) sequestration, usually in an enlarged spleen; and/or (3) increased platelet destruction. Disorders of production may be either inherited or acquired. In evaluating a patient with thrombocytopenia, a key step is to review the peripheral blood smear and to first rule out "pseudothrombocytopenia," particularly in a patient without an apparent cause for the thrombocytopenia. Pseudothrombocytopenia (Fig. 115-1B) is an in vitro artifact resulting from platelet agglutination via antibodies (usually IgG, but also IgM and IgA) when the calcium content is decreased by blood collection in ethylenediamine tetraacetic (EDTA) [the anticoagulant present in tubes (purple top) used to collect blood for complete blood counts (CBCs)]. If a low platelet count is obtained in EDTA-anticoagulated blood, a blood smear should be evaluated and a platelet count determined in blood collected into sodium citrate (blue top tube) or heparin (green top tube), or a smear of freshly obtained unanticoagulated blood, such as from a finger stick, can be examined.

> **APPROACH TO THE PATIENT** Thrombocytopenia
>
> The history and physical examination, results of the CBC, and review of the peripheral blood smear are all critical components in the initial evaluation of thrombocytopenic patients (Fig. 115-2). The overall health of the patient and whether he or she is receiving drug treatment will influence the differential diagnosis. A healthy young adult with thrombocytopenia will have a much more limited differential diagnosis than an ill hospitalized patient who is receiving multiple medications. Except in unusual inherited disorders, decreased platelet production usually results from bone marrow disorders that also affect red blood cell (RBC) and/or white blood cell (WBC)

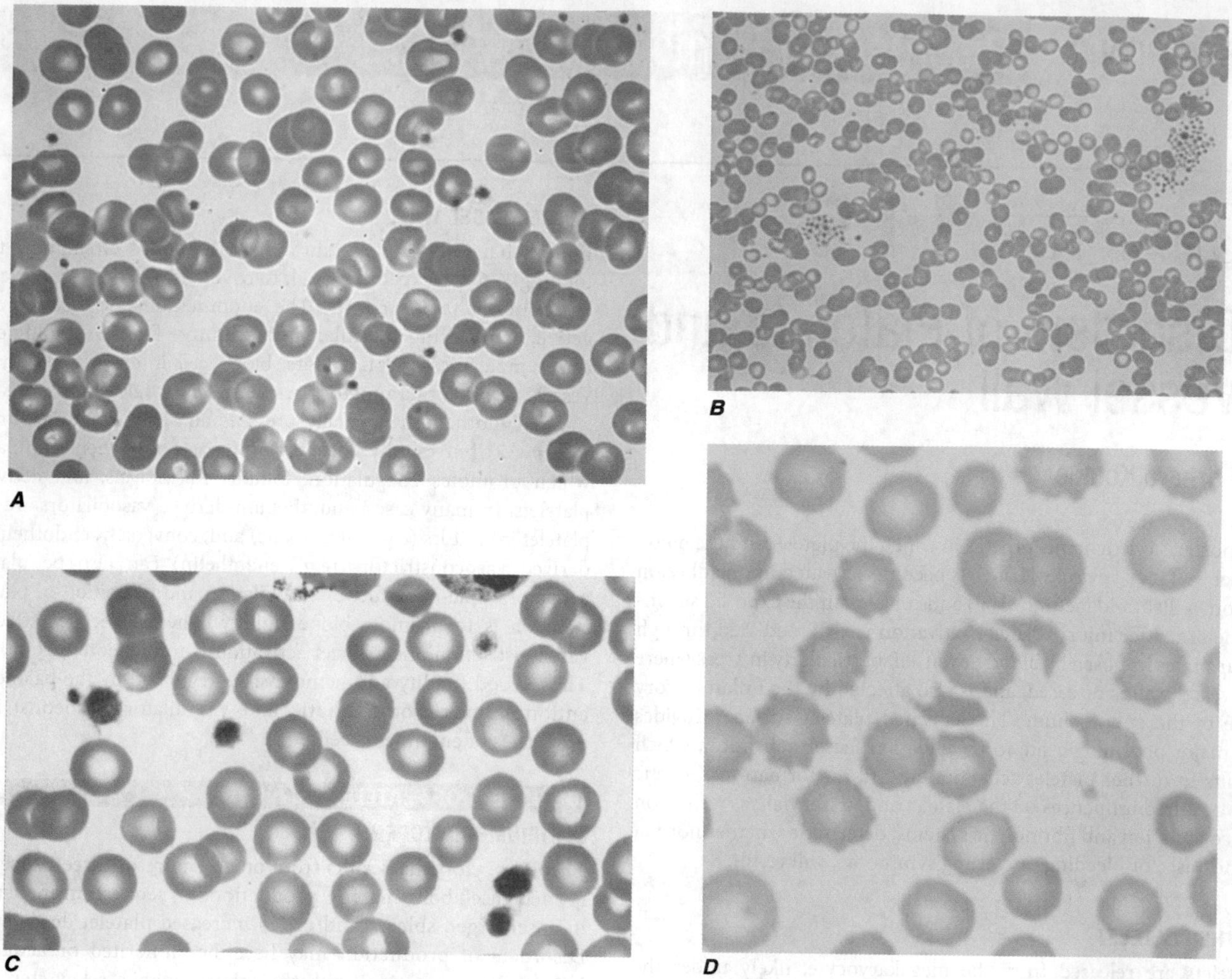

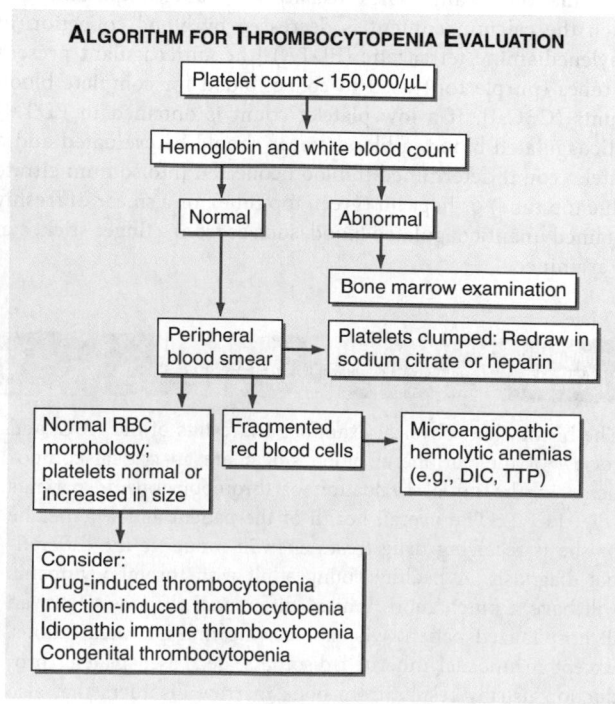

Figure 115-1 **Photomicrographs of peripheral blood smears: *A.*** Normal peripheral blood. ***B.*** Platelet clumping in pseudothrombocytopenia. ***C.*** Abnormal large platelet in autosomal dominant macrothrombocytopenia. ***D.*** Schistocytes and decreased platelets in microangiopathic hemolytic anemia.

ALGORITHM FOR THROMBOCYTOPENIA EVALUATION

Platelet count < 150,000/µL

↓

Hemoglobin and white blood count

↓

Normal — Abnormal

Abnormal → Bone marrow examination

Normal → Peripheral blood smear → Platelets clumped: Redraw in sodium citrate or heparin

Normal RBC morphology; platelets normal or increased in size

Fragmented red blood cells → Microangiopathic hemolytic anemias (e.g., DIC, TTP)

Consider:
Drug-induced thrombocytopenia
Infection-induced thrombocytopenia
Idiopathic immune thrombocytopenia
Congenital thrombocytopenia

Figure 115-2 Algorithm for evaluating the thrombocytopenic patient.

production. Because myelodysplasia can present with isolated thrombocytopenia, the bone marrow should be examined in patients presenting with isolated thrombocytopenia who are older than 60 years of age. While inherited thrombocytopenia is rare, any prior platelet counts should be retrieved and a family history regarding thrombocytopenia obtained. A careful history of drug ingestion should be obtained, including nonprescription and herbal remedies, as drugs are the most common cause of thrombocytopenia.

The physical examination can document an enlarged spleen, evidence of chronic liver disease, and other underlying disorders. Mild to moderate splenomegaly may be difficult to appreciate in many individuals due to body habitus and/or obesity but can be easily assessed by abdominal ultrasound. A platelet count of approximately 5000–10,000 is required to maintain vascular integrity in the microcirculation. When the count is markedly decreased, petechiae first appear in areas of increased venous pressure, the ankles and feet in an ambulatory patient. Petechiae are pin-point, nonblanching hemorrhages and are usually a sign of a decreased platelet number and not platelet dysfunction. Wet purpura, blood blisters that form on the oral mucosa, are thought to denote an increased risk of life-threatening hemorrhage in the thrombocytopenic patient. Excessive bruising is seen in disorders of both platelet number and function.

Infection-induced thrombocytopenia

Many viral and bacterial infections result in thrombocytopenia and are the most common noniatrogenic cause of thrombocytopenia. This may or may not be associated with laboratory evidence of disseminated intravascular coagulation (DIC), which is most commonly seen in patients with systemic infections with gram-negative bacteria. Infections can affect both platelet production and platelet survival. In addition, immune mechanisms can be at work, as in infectious mononucleosis and early HIV infection. Late in HIV infection, pancytopenia and decreased and dysplastic platelet production is more common. Immune-mediated thrombocytopenia in children usually follows a viral infection and almost always resolves spontaneously. This association of infection with ITP is less clear in adults.

Bone marrow examination is often requested for evaluation of occult infections. A study evaluating the role of bone marrow examination in fever of unknown origin in HIV-infected patients found that for 86% of patients, the same diagnosis was established by less-invasive techniques, notably blood culture. In some instances, however, the diagnosis can be made earlier; thus, a bone marrow examination and culture is recommended when the diagnosis is needed urgently or when other, less invasive methods have been unsuccessful.

Drug-induced thrombocytopenia

Many drugs have been associated with thrombocytopenia. A predictable decrease in platelet count occurs after treatment with many chemotherapeutic drugs due to bone marrow suppression (Chap. 85). Other, commonly used drugs that cause isolated thrombocytopenia are listed in Table 115-1, but all drugs should be suspect in a patient with thrombocytopenia without an apparent cause and should be stopped, or substituted, if possible. A helpful website, Platelets on the Internet (*http://www.ouhsc.edu/platelets/index.html*), lists drugs and supplements reported to have caused thrombocytopenia and the level of evidence supporting the association. Although not as well studied, herbal and over-the-counter preparations may also result in thrombocytopenia and should be discontinued in patients who are thrombocytopenic.

Classic drug-dependent antibodies are antibodies that react with specific platelet surface antigens, and result in thrombocytopenia only when the drug is present. Many drugs are capable of inducing these antibodies, but for some reason they are more common with quinine and sulfonamides. Drug-dependent antibody binding can be demonstrated by laboratory assays, showing antibody binding in the presence of, but not without, the drug present in the assay. The thrombocytopenia typically occurs after a period of initial exposure (median length 21 days), or upon reexposure, and usually resolves in 7–10 days after drug withdrawal. The thrombocytopenia caused by the platelet GpIIbIIIa inhibitory drugs, such as abciximab, differs in that it may occur within 24 h of initial exposure. This appears to be due to the presence of naturally occurring antibodies that cross-react with the drug bound to the platelet.

Heparin-induced thrombocytopenia

Drug-induced thrombocytopenia due to heparin differs from that seen with other drugs in two major ways. (1) The thrombocytopenia is not usually severe, with nadir counts rarely <20,000/μL. (2) Heparin-induced thrombocytopenia (HIT) is not associated with bleeding and, in fact, markedly increases the risk of thrombosis. HIT results from antibody formation to a complex of the platelet-specific protein platelet factor 4 (PF4) and heparin. The antiheparin/PF4 antibody can activate platelets through the FcγRIIa receptor and also activate monocytes and endothelial cells. Many patients exposed to heparin develop antibodies to heparin/PF4, but

TABLE 115-1 Drugs Reported as Definitely or Probably Causing Isolated Thrombocytopenia*

Abciximab	Ibuprofen
Acetaminophen	Iopanoic acid
Aminoglutethimide	Levamisole
Aminosalicylic acid	Linezolid
Amiodarone	Meclofenamate
Amphotericin B	Methicillin
Ampicillin	Methyldopa
Carbamazepine	Nalidixic acid
Chlorpropamide	Naproxen
Danazol	Oxyphenbutazone
Captopril	Phenytoin
Cimetidine	Piperacillin
Diatrizoate meglumine (Hypaque Meglumine®)	Procainamide
Diclofenac	Quinine
Digoxin	Quinidine
Dipyridamole	Rifampin
Eptifibatide	Simvastatin
Ethambutol	Sulfa-containing drugs
Famotidine	Tamoxifen
Fluconazole	Tirofiban
Furosemide	Trimethoprim/sulfamethoxazole
Glyburide	Valproic acid
Gold	Vancomycin
Hydrochlorothiazide	
Imipenem/Cilastatin	

*Reported in ≥ 2 patients

Source: Data from *http://www.ouhsc.edu/platelets/index.html*.

do not appear to have adverse consequences. A fraction of those who develop antibodies will develop HIT, and a portion of those (up to 50%) will develop thrombosis (HITT).

HIT can occur after exposure to low-molecular-weight heparin (LMWH) as well as unfractionated heparin (UFH), although it is about 10 times more common with the latter. Most patients develop HIT after exposure to heparin for 5–14 days (Fig. 115-3). It occurs before 5 days in those who were exposed to heparin in the prior few weeks or months (<~100 days) and have circulating antiheparin/PF4 antibodies. Rarely, thrombocytopenia and thrombosis begin several days after all heparin has been stopped (termed *delayed-onset HIT*). The 4 *T*'s have been recommended to be used in a diagnostic algorithm for HIT: *t*hrombocytopenia, *t*iming of platelet count drop, *t*hrombosis and other sequelae such as localized skin reactions, and o*t*her causes of thrombocytopenia not evident. A new scoring model based on broad expert opinion [the HIT Expert Probability (HEP) Score] has improved operating characteristics and should provide better utility as a scoring system.

Laboratory testing for HIT HIT (anti-heparin/PF4) antibodies can be detected using two types of assays. The most widely available

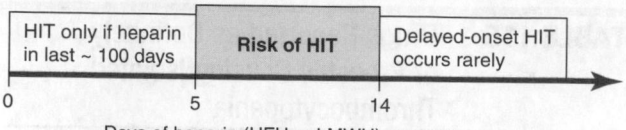

HIT only if heparin in last ~ 100 days	Risk of HIT	Delayed-onset HIT occurs rarely

0   5   14

Days of heparin (UFH or LMWH) exposure

Figure 115-3 Time course of heparin-induced thrombocytopenia (HIT) development after heparin exposure. The timing of development after heparin exposure is a critical factor in determining the likelihood of HIT in a patient. HIT occurs early after heparin exposure in the presence of preexisting heparin/platelet factor 4 (PF4) antibodies, which disappear from circulation by ~100 days following a prior exposure. Rarely, HIT may occur later after heparin exposure (termed delayed-onset HIT). In this setting, heparin/PF4 antibody testing is usually markedly positive. HIT can occur after exposure to either unfractionated (UFH) or low-molecular-weight heparin (LMWH).

is an enzyme-linked immunoassay (ELISA) with PF4/polyanion complex as the antigen. Since many patients develop antibodies but do not develop clinical HIT, the test has a low specificity for the diagnosis of HIT. This is especially true in patients who have undergone cardiopulmonary bypass surgery, where approximately 50% of patients develop these antibodies postoperatively. IgG-specific ELISAs increase specificity but may decrease sensitivity. The other assay is a platelet activation assay, which measures the ability of the patient's serum to activate platelets in the presence of heparin in a concentration-dependent manner. This test has lower sensitivity but higher specificity than the ELISA. However, HIT remains a clinical diagnosis.

TREATMENT **Heparin-Induced Thrombocytopenia**

Early recognition is key in treatment of HIT, with prompt discontinuation of heparin and use of alternative anticoagulants. Thrombosis is a common complication of HIT, even after heparin discontinuation, and can occur in both the venous and arterial systems. Patients with higher anti-heparin/PF4 antibody titers have a higher risk of thrombosis. In patients diagnosed with HIT, imaging studies to evaluate the patient for thrombosis (at least lower extremity duplex Dopplers) are recommended. Patients requiring anticoagulation should be switched from heparin to an alternative anticoagulant. The direct thrombin inhibitors (DTIs) argatroban and lepirudin are effective in HITT. The DTI bivalirudin and the antithrombin-binding pentasaccharide fondaparinux are also effective but not yet approved by the U.S. Food and Drug Administration (FDA) for this indication. Danaparoid, a mixture of glycosoaminoglycans with anti-Xa activity, has been used extensively for the treatment of HITT; it is no longer available in the United States but is in other countries. HIT antibodies cross-react with LMWH, and these preparations should not be used in the treatment of HIT.

Because of the high rate of thrombosis in patients with HIT, anticoagulation should be strongly considered, even in the absence of thrombosis. In patients with thrombosis, patients can be transitioned to warfarin, with treatment usually for 3–6 months. In patients without thrombosis, the duration of anticoagulation needed is undefined. An increased risk of thrombosis is present for at least 1 month after diagnosis; however, most thromboses occur early, and whether thrombosis occurs later if the patient is initially anticoagulated is unknown. Options

include continuing anticoagulation until a few days after platelet recovery or for one month. Introduction of warfarin alone in the setting of HIT or HITT may precipitate thrombosis, particularly venous gangrene, presumably due to clotting activation and severely reduced levels of proteins C and S. Warfarin therapy, if started, should be overlapped with a DTI or fondaparinux, and started after resolution of the thrombocytopenia and lessening of the prothrombotic state.

Immune thrombocytopenic purpura (ITP)

Immune thrombocytopenic purpura (ITP; also termed *idiopathic thrombocytopenic purpura*) is an acquired disorder in which there is immune-mediated destruction of platelets and possibly inhibition of platelet release from the megakaryocyte. In children, it is usually an acute disease, most commonly following an infection, and with a self-limited course. In adults, it usually runs a more chronic course. ITP is termed *secondary* if it is associated with an underlying disorder; autoimmune disorders, particularly systemic lupus erythematosus (SLE), and infections, such as HIV and hepatitis C, are common causes. The association of ITP with *Helicobacter pylori* infection is unclear.

ITP is characterized by mucocutaneous bleeding and a low, often very low, platelet count, with an otherwise normal peripheral blood cells and smear. Patients usually present either with ecchymoses and petechiae, or with thrombocytopenia incidentally found on a routine CBC. Mucocutaneous bleeding, such as oral mucosa, gastrointestinal, or heavy menstrual bleeding, may be present. Rarely, life-threatening, including central nervous system, bleeding can occur. Wet purpura (blood blisters in the mouth) and retinal hemorrhages may herald life-threatening bleeding.

Laboratory testing in ITP Laboratory testing for antibodies (serologic testing) is usually not helpful due to the low sensitivity and specificity of the current tests. Bone marrow examination can be reserved for older adults (usually >60 years) or those who have other signs or laboratory abnormalities not explained by ITP, or in patients who do not respond to initial therapy. The peripheral blood smear may show large platelets, with otherwise normal morphology. Depending on the bleeding history, iron deficiency anemia may be present.

Laboratory testing is performed to evaluate for secondary causes of ITP and should include testing for HIV infection and hepatitis C (and other infections if indicated); serologic testing for SLE, serum protein electrophoresis, and immunoglobulin levels to potentially detect hypogammaglobulinemia; selective testing for IgA deficiency or monoclonal gammopathies and, if anemia is present, direct antiglobulin testing (Coombs test) to rule out combined autoimmune hemolytic anemia with ITP (Evans syndrome).

TREATMENT **Immune Thrombocytopenic Purpura**

The treatment of ITP utilizes drugs that decrease reticuloendothelial uptake of the antibody-bound platelet, decrease antibody production, and/or increase platelet production. The diagnosis of ITP does not necessarily mean that treatment must be instituted. Patients with platelet counts greater than 30,000/μL appear not to have increased mortality related to the thrombocytopenia.

Initial treatment in patients without significant bleeding symptoms, severe thrombocytopenia (<5000/μL), or signs of impending bleeding (such as retinal hemorrhage or large oral mucosal hemorrhages) can be instituted as an outpatient using single agents. Traditionally, this has been prednisone at 1 mg/kg, although $Rh_0(D)$ immune globulin therapy (WinRho SDF), at 50–75 µg/kg, is also being used in this setting. $Rh_0(D)$ immune globulin must be used only in Rh-positive patients as the mechanism of action is production of limited hemolysis, with antibody-coated cells "saturating" the Fc receptors, inhibiting Fc receptor function. Monitoring patients for 8 h postinfusion is now advised by the FDA because of the rare complication of severe intravascular hemolysis. Intravenous gamma globulin (IVIgG), which is pooled, primarily IgG antibodies, also blocks the Fc receptor system, but appears to work primarily through different mechanism(s). IVIgG has more efficacy than anti-$Rh_0(D)$ in postsplenectomized patients. IVIgG is dosed at 2 g/kg total, given in divided doses over 2–5 days. Side effects are usually related to the volume of infusion and infrequently include aseptic meningitis and renal failure. All immunoglobulin preparations are derived from human plasma and undergo treatment for viral inactivation.

For patients with severe ITP and/or symptoms of bleeding, hospital admission and combined-modality therapy is given using high-dose glucocorticoids with IVIgG or anti-$Rh_0(D)$ therapy, and, as needed, additional immunosuppressive agents. Rituximab, an anti-CD20 (B cell) antibody, has shown efficacy in the treatment of refractory ITP.

Splenectomy has been used for treatment of patients who relapse after glucocorticoids are tapered. Splenectomy remains an important treatment option; however, more patients than previously thought will go into a remission over time. Observation, if the platelet count is high enough, or intermittent treatment with anti-$Rh_0(D)$ or IVIgG may be a reasonable approach to see if the ITP will resolve. Vaccination against encapsulated organisms (especially pneumococcus, but also meningococcus and *Haemophilus influenzae*, depending on patient age and potential exposure) is recommended before splenectomy. Accessory spleen(s) are a very rare cause of relapse.

Thrombopoietin receptor agonists are now available for the treatment of ITP. This approach stems from the finding that many patients with ITP do not have increased TPO levels, as was previously hypothesized. TPO levels reflect megakaryocyte mass, which is usually normal in ITP. TPO levels are not increased in the setting of platelet destruction. Two agents, one administered subcutaneously (romiplostim) and another orally (eltrombopag), have shown response in many patients with refractory ITP. Roles for these agents in ITP treatment are not fully defined but given the chronicity of treatment, they are generally reserved for patients with refractory disease

Inherited thrombocytopenia

Thrombocytopenia is rarely inherited, either as an isolated finding or as part of a syndrome, and may be inherited in an autosomal dominant, autosomal recessive, or X-linked pattern. Many forms of autosomal dominant thrombocytopenia are now known to be associated with mutations in the nonmuscle myosin heavy chain *MYH9* gene. Interestingly, these include the May-Hegglin anomaly, and Sebastian, Epstein's, and Fechtner syndromes, all of which have distinct distinguishing features. A common feature of these disorders is large platelets (Fig. 115-1C). Autosomal recessive disorders include congenital amegakaryocytic thrombocytopenia, thrombocytopenia with absent radii, and Bernard Soulier syndrome. The latter is primarily a functional platelet disorder due to absence of GPIb-IX-V, the VWF adhesion receptor. X-linked disorders include Wiskott-Aldrich syndrome and a dyshematopoietic syndrome resulting from a

mutation in GATA-1, an important transcriptional regulator of hematopoiesis.

◼ THROMBOTIC THROMBOCYTOPENIC PURPURA AND HEMOLYTIC UREMIC SYNDROME

Thrombotic thrombocytopenic microangiopathies are a group of disorders characterized by thrombocytopenia, a microangiopathic hemolytic anemia evident by fragmented RBCs (Fig. 115-1D) and laboratory evidence of hemolysis, and microvascular thrombosis. They include thrombotic thrombocytopenic purpura (TTP) and hemolytic uremic syndrome (HUS), as well as syndromes complicating bone marrow transplantation, certain medications and infections, pregnancy and vasculitis. In DIC, while thrombocytopenia and microangiopathy are seen, a coagulopathy predominates, with consumption of clotting factors and fibrinogen resulting in an elevated prothrombin time (PT), and often activated partial thromboplastin time (aPTT). The PT and aPTT are characteristically normal in TTP or HUS.

Thrombotic thrombocytopenic purpura (TTP)

TTP and HUS were previously considered overlap syndromes. However, in the past few years the pathophysiology of inherited and idiopathic TTP has become better understood and clearly differs from HUS. TTP was first described in 1924 by Eli Moschcowitz and characterized by a pentad of findings that include microangiopathic hemolytic anemia, thrombocytopenia, renal failure, neurologic findings, and fever. The full-blown syndrome is less commonly seen now, probably due to earlier diagnosis. The introduction of treatment with plasma exchange markedly improved the prognosis in patients, with a decrease in mortality from 85–100% to 10–30%.

The pathogenesis of inherited (Upshaw-Schulman syndrome) and idiopathic TTP is related to a deficiency of, or antibodies to, the metalloprotease ADAMTS13, that cleaves VWF. VWF is normally secreted as ultra-large multimers, which are then cleaved by ADAMTS13. The persistence of ultra-large VWF molecules is thought to contribute to pathogenic platelet adhesion and aggregation (Fig. 115-4). This defect alone, however, is not sufficient to result in TTP as individuals with a congenital absence of ADAMTS13 develop TTP only episodically. Additional provocative factors have not been defined. The level of ADAMTS13 activity, as well as antibodies, can now be detected by laboratory assays. However, assays with sufficient sensitivity and specificity to direct clinical management have yet to be clearly defined.

Idiopathic TTP appears to be more common in women than in men. No geographic or racial distribution has been defined. TTP is more common in patients with HIV infection and in pregnant women. TTP in pregnancy is not clearly related to ADAMTS13. Medication-related microangiopathic hemolytic anemia may be secondary to antibody formation (ticlopidine and possibly clopidogrel) or direct endothelial toxicity (cyclosporine, mitomycin C, tacrolimus, quinine), although this is not always so clear, and fear of withholding treatment, as well as lack of other treatment alternatives, results in broad application of plasma exchange. However, withdrawal, or reduction in dose, of endothelial toxic agents usually decreases the microangiopathy.

| TREATMENT | Thrombotic Thrombocytopenic Purpura |

TTP is a devastating disease if not diagnosed and treated promptly. In patients presenting with new thrombocytopenia, with or without evidence of renal insufficiency and other elements of classic TTP, laboratory data should be obtained

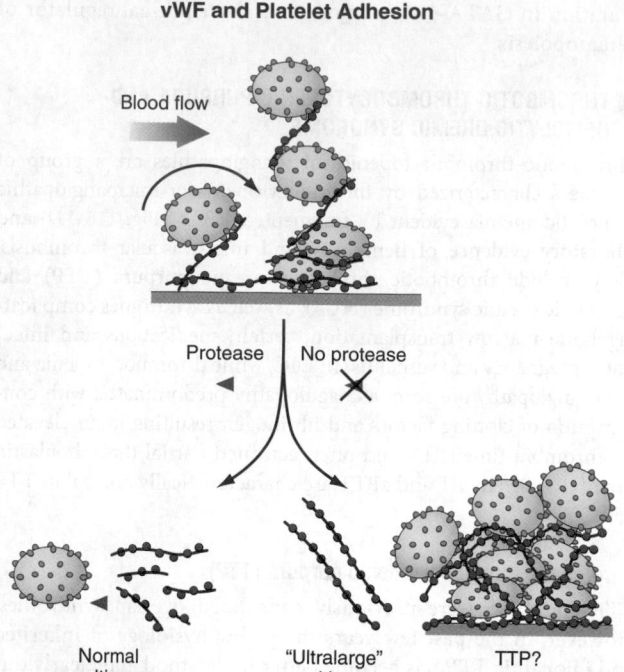

vWF and Platelet Adhesion

Blood flow

Protease   No protease

Normal   "Ultralarge"   TTP?
multimers   multimers

Figure 115-4   Pathogenesis of thrombotic thrombocytopenic purpura (TTP). Normally the ultra-high-molecular-weight multimers of von Willebrand factor (VWF) produced by the endothelial cells are processed into smaller multimers by a plasma metalloproteinase called ADAMTS13. In TTP the activity of the protease is inhibited, and the ultra-high-molecular-weight multimers of VWF initiate platelet aggregation and thrombosis.

to rule out DIC and to evaluate for evidence of microangiopathic hemolytic anemia. Findings to support the TTP diagnosis include an increased lactate dehydrogenase and indirect bilirubin, decreased haptoglobin, and increased reticulocyte count, with a negative direct antiglobulin test. The peripheral smear should be examined for evidence of schistocytes (Fig. 115-1D). Polychromasia is usually also present due to the increased number of young red blood cells, and nucleated RBCs are often present, which is thought to be due to infarction in the microcirculatory system of the bone marrow.

Plasma exchange remains the mainstay of treatment of TTP. ADAMTS 13 antibody-mediated TTP (idiopathic TTP) appears to respond best to plasma exchange. Plasma exchange is continued until the platelet count is normal and signs of hemolysis are resolved for at least 2 days. While never evaluated in clinical trial, the use of glucocorticoids seems a reasonable approach, but should only be used as an adjunct to plasma exchange. Additionally, other immunomodulatory therapies have been reported to be successful in refractory or relapsing TTP, including rituximab, vincristine, cyclophosphamide, and splenectomy. The role of rituximab in the treatment of this disorder needs to be defined. A significant relapse rate is noted, 25–45% within 30 days of initial "remission," and 12–40% with late relapses. Relapses may be more frequent in patients with severe ADAMTS 13 deficiency at presentation.

Hemolytic uremic syndrome

HUS is a syndrome characterized by acute renal failure, microangiopathic hemolytic anemia, and thrombocytopenia. It is seen predominantly in children and in most cases is preceded by an episode of diarrhea, often hemorrhagic in nature. *Escherichia coli* O157:H7 is the most frequent, although not only, etiologic serotype. HUS not associated with diarrhea (termed *DHUS*) is more heterogeneous in presentation and course. Some children who develop DHUS have been found to have mutations in genes encoding factor H, a soluble complement regulator, and membrane cofactor protein that is mainly expressed in the kidney.

TREATMENT   Hemolytic Uremic Syndrome

Treatment of HUS is primarily supportive. In D⁺HUS, many (~40%) children require at least some period of support with dialysis; however, the overall mortality is <5%. In D⁻HUS, the mortality is higher, approximately 26%. Plasma infusion or plasma exchange has not been shown to alter the overall course. ADAMTS13 levels are generally reported to be normal in HUS, although occasionally they have been reported to be decreased. As ADAMTS13 assays improve, they may help in defining a subset that better fit a TTP diagnosis, and may respond to plasma exchange.

■ THROMOBCYTOSIS

Thrombocytosis is almost always due either to (1) iron deficiency; (2) inflammation, cancer, or infection (reactive thrombocytosis); or (3) an underlying myeloproliferative process [essential thrombocythemia or polycythemia vera) (Chap. 108)] or, rarely, the 5q- myelodysplastic process (Chap. 107). Patients presenting with an elevated platelet count should be evaluated for underlying inflammation or malignancy, and iron deficiency should be ruled out. Thrombocytosis in response to acute or chronic inflammation has not been associated with an increased thrombotic risk. In fact, patients with markedly elevated platelet counts (>1.5 million), usually seen in the setting of a myeloproliferative disorder, have an increased risk of bleeding. This appears to be due, at least in part, to acquired von Willebrand disease (VWD) due to platelet-VWF adhesion and removal.

■ QUALITATIVE DISORDERS OF PLATELET FUNCTION

Inherited disorders of platelet function

Inherited platelet function disorders are thought to be relatively rare, although the prevalence of mild disorders of platelet function is unclear, in part because our testing for such disorders is suboptimal. Rare qualitative disorders include the autosomal recessive disorders Glanzmann's thrombasthenia (absence of the platelet GpIIbIIIa receptor) and Bernard Soulier syndrome (absence of the platelet GpIb-IX-V receptor). Both are inherited in an autosomal recessive fashion and present with bleeding symptoms in childhood.

Platelet storage pool disorder (SPD) is the classic autosomal dominant qualitative platelet disorder. This results from abnormalities of platelet granule formation. It is also seen as a part of inherited disorders of granule formation, such as Hermansky-Pudlak syndrome. Bleeding symptoms in SPD are variable, but often are mild. The most common inherited disorders of platelet function are disorders that prevent normal secretion of granule content. Few of the abnormalities have been dissected at the molecular level but these are likely due to multiple abnormalities. They are usually described as *secretion defects*. Bleeding symptoms are usually mild in nature.

Bleeding symptoms or prevention of bleeding in patients with severe platelet dysfunction frequently requires platelet transfusion. Care is taken to limit the risk of alloimmunization by limiting exposure, using apheresis leuko-depleted platelets for transfusion. Platelet disorders associated with milder bleeding symptoms frequently respond to desmopressin [1-deamino-8-D-arginine vasopressin (DDAVP)]. DDAVP increases plasma VWF and FVIII levels; it may also have a direct effect on platelet function. Particularly for mucosal bleeding symptoms, antifibrinolytic therapy (epsilon-aminocaproic acid or tranexamic acid) is used alone or in conjunction with DDAVP or platelet therapy.

Acquired disorders of platelet function

Acquired platelet dysfunction is common, usually due to medications, either intentionally as with antiplatelet therapy, or unintentionally as with high-dose penicillins. Acquired platelet dysfunction occurs in uremia. This is likely multifactorial but the resultant effect is defective adhesion and activation. The platelet defect is improved most by dialysis but may also be improved by increasing the hematocrit to 27–32%, giving DDAVP (0.3 μg/kg), or use of conjugated estrogens. Platelet dysfunction also occurs with cardiopulmonary bypass due to the effect of the artificial circuit on platelets, and bleeding symptoms respond to platelet transfusion. Platelet dysfunction seen with underlying hematologic disorders can result from nonspecific interference by circulating paraproteins or intrinsic platelet defects in myeloproliferative and myelodysplastic syndromes.

■ VON WILLEBRAND DISEASE

VWD vvVis the most common inherited bleeding disorder. Estimates from laboratory data suggest a prevalence of approximately 1%, but data based on symptomatic individuals suggest that it is closer to 0.1% of the population. VWF serves two roles: (1) as the major adhesion molecule that tethers the platelet to the exposed subendothelium; and (2) as the binding protein for FVIII, resulting in significant prolongation of the FVIII half-life in circulation. The platelet-adhesive function of VWF is critically dependent on the presence of large VWF multimers, while FVIII binding is not. Most of the symptoms of VWD are "platelet-like" except in more severe VWD when the FVIII is low enough to produce symptoms similar to those found in Factor VIII deficiency (hemophilia A).

VWD has been classified into three major types, with four subtypes of type 2 (Table 115-2; Fig. 115-5). By far the most common type of VWD is type 1 disease, with a parallel decrease in VWF protein, VWF function, and FVIII levels, accounting for at least 80% of cases. Patients have predominantly mucosal bleeding symptoms, although postoperative bleeding can also be seen. Bleeding symptoms are very uncommon in infancy and usually manifest later in childhood with excessive bruising and epistaxis. Since these symptoms occur commonly in childhood, the clinician should particularly note bruising at sites unlikely to be traumatized and/or prolonged epistaxis requiring medical attention. Menorrhagia is a common manifestation of VWD. Menstrual bleeding resulting in anemia should warrant an evaluation for VWD and, if negative, functional platelet disorders. Frequently, mild type 1 VWD first manifests with dental extractions, particularly wisdom tooth extraction, or tonsillectomy.

Not all patients with low VWF levels have bleeding symptoms. Whether patients bleed or not will depend on the overall hemostatic balance they have inherited, along with environmental influences

TABLE 115-2 Laboratory Diagnosis of von Willebrand Disease

Type	aPTT	VWF Antigen	VWF Activity	FVIII Activity	Multimer
1	NI or ↑	↓	↓	↓	Normal distribution, decreased in quantity
2A	NI or ↑	↓	↓↓	↓	Loss of high- and intermediate-MW multimers
2B[a]	NI or ↑	↓	↓↓	↓	Loss of high-MW multimers
2M	NI or ↑	↓	↓↓	↓	Normal distribution, decreased in quantity
2N	↑↑	NI or ↓[b]	NI or ↓[b]	↓↓	Normal distribution
3	↑↑	↓↓	↓↓	↓↓	Absent

[a]Usually also decreased platelet count.

[b]For type 2N, in the homozygous state, FVIII is very low; in the heterozygous state, only seen in conjunction with type 1 VWD.

Abbreviations: aPTT, activated partial thromboplastin time; F, Factor; MW, molecular weight; NI, normal; VWF, von Willebrand factor.

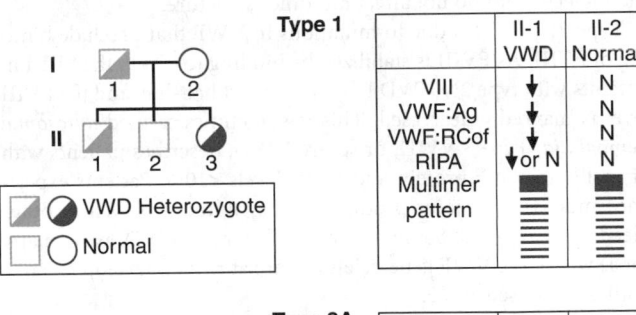

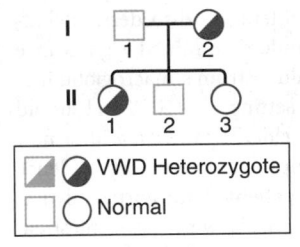

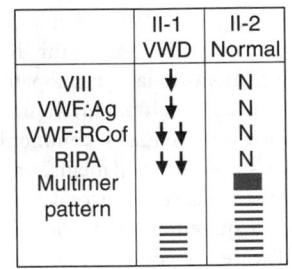

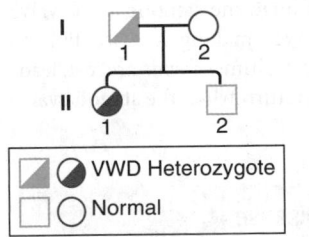

Figure 115-5 Pattern of inheritance and laboratory findings in von Willebrand disease. The assays of platelet function include a coagulation assay of Factor VIII bound and carried by von Willebrand factor (VWF), abbreviated as VIII; immunoassay of total VWF protein (VWF:Ag); bioassay of the ability of patient plasma to support ristocetin-induced agglutination of normal platelets (VWF:RCoF); and ristocetin-induced aggregation of patient platelets, abbreviated RIPA. The multimer pattern illustrates the protein bands present when plasma is electrophoresed in a polyacrylamide gel. The II-1 and II-2 columns refer to the phenotypes of the second-generation offspring.

and the type of hemostatic challenges they experience. Although the inheritance of VWD is autosomal, many factors modulate both VWF levels and bleeding symptoms. These have not all been defined, but include blood type, thyroid hormone status, race, stress, exercise, and hormonal (both endogenous and exogenous) influences. Patients with type O blood have VWF protein levels of approximately one-half that of patients with AB blood type; and, in fact, the normal range for patients with type O blood overlaps that which has been considered diagnostic for VWD. A mildly decreased VWF level should perhaps be viewed more as a risk factor for bleeding than as an actual disease.

Patients with Type 2 VWD have functional defects; thus, the VWF antigen measurement is significantly higher than the test of function. For types 2A, 2B and 2M, VWF activity is decreased, measured as ristocetin cofactor or collagen-binding activity. In type 2A VWD, the impaired function is due either to increased susceptibility to cleavage by ADAMTS13, resulting in loss of intermediate and high-molecular-weight multimers, or to decreased secretion of these multimers by the cell. Type 2B VWD results from gain of function mutations that result in increased spontaneous binding of VWF to platelets in circulation, with subsequent clearance of this complex by the reticuloendothelial system. The resulting VWF in the patients' plasma lacks the highest- molecular-weight multimers, and the platelet count is usually modestly reduced. Type 2M occurs as a consequence of a group of mutations that cause dysfunction of the molecule but do not affect multimer structure.

Type 2N VWD is due to mutations in VWF that preclude binding of FVIII. As FVIII is stabilized by binding to VWF, the FVIII in patients with type 2N VWD has a very short half-life, and the FVIII level is markedly decreased. This is sometimes termed *autosomal hemophilia*. Type 3 VWD, or severe VWD, describes patients with virtually no VWF protein and FVIII levels <10%. Patients experience mucosal and joint postoperative symptoms as well as other bleeding symptoms. Some patients with type 3 VWD, particularly those with large VWF gene deletions, are at risk of developing antibodies to infused VWF.

Acquired VWD is a rare disorder, most commonly seen in patients with underlying lymphoproliferative disorders, including monoclonal gammopathies of underdetermined significance (MGUS), multiple myeloma, and Waldenström's macroglobulinemia. It is seen most commonly in the setting of MGUS and should be suspected in patients, particularly elderly patients, with a new onset of severe mucosal bleeding symptoms. Laboratory evidence of acquired VWD is found in some patients with aortic valvular disease. Heyde's syndrome (aortic stenosis with gastrointestinal bleeding) is attributed to the presence of angiodysplasia of the gastrointestinal tract in patients with aortic stenosis. However, the shear stress on blood passing through the stenotic aortic valve appears to produce a change in VWF, making it susceptible to serum proteases. Consequently, large multimer forms are lost, leading to an acquired type 2 VWD, but return when the stenotic valve is replaced.

TREATMENT von Willebrand Disease

The mainstay of treatment for type 1 VWD is 1-deamino-8-D-arginine vasopressin (DDAVP, or desmopressin), which results in release of VWF and FVIII from endothelial stores. DDAVP can be given intravenously or by a high concentration intranasal spray (1.5 mg/mL). The peak activity when given intravenously is approximately 30 minutes, while it is 2 h when given intranasally. The usual dose is 0.3 μg/kg intravenously or 2 squirts (1 in each nostril) for patients >50 kg (1 squirt for those <50 kg). It is

recommended that patients with VWD be tested with DDAVP to assess their response before using it. In patients who respond well (increase in values of two- to fourfold), it can be used for procedures with minor to moderate risk of bleeding. Depending on the procedure, additional doses may be needed; it is usually given every 12–24 h. Less frequent dosing may result in less tachyphylaxis, which occurs when synthesis cannot compensate for the released stores. The major side effect of DDAVP is hyponatremia due to decreased free water clearance. This occurs most commonly in the very young and the very old, but fluid restriction should be advised for all patients for the 24 h following each dose.

Some patients with types 2A and 2M VWD respond to DDAVP such that it can be used for minor procedures. For the other subtypes, for type 3 disease, and for major procedures requiring longer periods of normal hemostasis, VWF replacement can be given. Virally inactivated VWF-containing factor concentrates are thought to be safer than cryoprecipitate as the replacement product.

Antifibrinolytic therapy using either ε-aminocaproic acid or tranexamic acid is an important therapy, either alone or in an adjunctive capacity, particularly for the prevention or treatment of mucosal bleeding. These agents are particularly useful in prophylaxis for dental procedures, with DDAVP for dental extractions and tonsillectomy, menorrhagia, and prostate procedures. It is contraindicated in the setting of upper urinary tract bleeding, due to the risk of ureteral obstruction.

DISORDERS OF THE VESSEL WALL

The vessel wall is an integral part of hemostasis, and separation of a fluid phase is artificial, particularly in disorders such as TTP or HIT that clearly involve the endothelium as well. Inflammation localized to the vessel wall, such as vasculitis, or inherited connective tissue disorders are abnormalities inherent to the vessel wall.

METABOLIC AND INFLAMMATORY DISORDERS

Acute febrile illnesses may result in vascular damage. This can result from immune complexes containing viral antigens or the viruses themselves. Certain pathogens, such as the rickettsiae causing Rocky Mountain spotted fever, replicate in endothelial cells and damage them. Vascular purpura may occur in patients with polyclonal gammopathies but more commonly in those with monoclonal gammopathies, including Waldenström's macroglobulinemia, multiple myeloma, and cryoglobulinemia. Patients with mixed cryoglobulinemia develop a more extensive maculopapular rash due to immune complex–mediated damage to the vessel wall.

Patients with scurvy (vitamin C deficiency) develop painful episodes of perifollicular skin bleeding as well as more systemic bleeding symptoms. Vitamin C is needed to synthesize hydroxyproline, an essential constituent of collagen. Patients with Cushing's syndrome or on chronic glucocorticoid therapy develop skin bleeding and easy bruising due to atrophy of supporting connective tissue. A similar phenomenon is seen with aging, where following minor trauma, blood spreads superficially under the epidermis. This has been termed *senile purpura*. It is most common on skin that has been previously damaged by sun exposure.

Henoch-Schönlein, or anaphylactoid, purpura is a distinct, self-limited type of vasculitis that occurs in children and young adults. Patients have an acute inflammatory reaction with IgA and complement components in capillaries, mesangial tissues, and small arterioles leading to increased vascular permeability and localized hemorrhage. The syndrome is often preceded by an upper respiratory infection, commonly with streptococcal pharyngitis, or is triggered by drug or food allergies. Patients develop a purpuric rash on the extensor surfaces of the arms and legs, usually accompanied by polyarthralgias or arthritis, abdominal pain, and hematuria from focal glomerulonephritis. All coagulation tests are normal but renal impairment may occur. Glucocorticoids can provide symptomatic relief but do not alter the course of the illness.

■ INHERITED DISORDERS OF THE VESSEL WALL

Patients with inherited disorders of the connective tissue matrix, such as Marfan's syndrome, Ehlers-Danlos syndrome, and pseudoxanthoma elasticum, frequently report easy bruising. Inherited vascular abnormalities can result in increased bleeding. This is notably seen in hereditary hemorrhagic telangiectasia (HHT, or Osler-Weber-Rendu disease), a disorder where abnormal telangiectatic capillaries result in frequent bleeding episodes, primarily from the nose and gastrointestinal tract. Arteriovenous malformation (AVM) in the lung, brain, and liver may also occur in HHT. The telangiectasia can often be visualized on the oral and nasal mucosa. Signs and symptoms develop over time. Expistaxis begins, on average, at the age of 12 and occurs in >95% of affected individuals by middle age. Two genes involved in the pathogenesis are *eng* (endoglin) on chromosome 9q33-34 (so-called HHT type 1), associated with pulmonary AVM in 40% of cases; and *alk1* (activin-receptor-like kinase *11*) on chromosome 12q13, associated with a much lower risk of pulmonary AVM.

ACKNOWLEDGMENT
Robert Handin, MD, contributed this chapter in the 16th edition and some materials from his chapter are included here.

FURTHER READINGS

ArEPALLY GM, ORTEL TL: Heparin-induced thrombocytopenia. Annu Rev Med 61:77, 2010

ASTER RH et al: Drug-induced immune thrombocytopenia: Pathogenesis, diagnosis and management. J Thromb Haemost 7:911, 2009

BUSSEL JB: Traditional and new approaches to the management of immune thrombocytopenia: Issues of when and who to treat. Hematol Oncol Clin North Am 23:1329, 2009

Diagnosis, Evaluation and Management of von Willebrand Disease. NIH Publication #08-5832. National Heart, Lung and Blood Institute, 2007, www.nhlbi.nih.gov

HAYWARD CPM: Diagnostic approach to platelet function disorders. Trans Apher Sci 38:65, 2008

ISRAELS SJ et al: Inherited disorders of platelet function and challenges to diagnosis of mucocutaneous bleeding. Haemophilia 16:152, 2010

KREMER HOVINGA JA et al: Survival and relapse in patients with thrombotic thrombocytopenic purpura. Blood 115:1500, 2010

RICE TW, WHEELER AP: Coagulopathy in critically ill patients. Chest 136:1622, 2009

CHAPTER 116

Coagulation Disorders

Valder R. Arruda

Katherine A. High

Deficiencies of coagulation factors have been recognized for centuries. Patients with genetic deficiencies of plasma coagulation factors exhibit life-long recurrent bleeding episodes into joints, muscles, and closed spaces, either spontaneously or following an injury. The most common inherited factor deficiencies are the hemophilias, X-linked diseases caused by deficiency of factor (F) VIII (hemophilia A) or factor IX (FIX, hemophilia B). Rare congenital bleeding disorders due to deficiencies of other factors, including FII (prothrombin), FV, FVII, FX, FXI, FXIII, and fibrinogen are commonly inherited in an autosomal recessive manner (Table 116-1). Advances in characterization of the molecular bases of clotting factor deficiencies have contributed to better understanding of the disease phenotypes and may eventually allow more targeted therapeutic approaches through the development of small molecules, recombinant proteins, or cell and gene-based therapies.

Commonly used tests of hemostasis provide the initial screening for clotting factor activity (Fig. 116-1), and disease phenotype often correlates with the level of clotting activity. An isolated abnormal prothrombin time (PT) suggests FVII deficiency, whereas a prolonged activated partial thromboplastin time (aPTT) indicates most commonly hemophilia or FXI

deficiency (Fig. 116-1). The prolongation of both PT and aPTT suggests deficiency of FV, FX, FII, or fibrinogen abnormalities. The addition of the missing factor at a range of doses to the subject's plasma will correct the abnormal clotting times; the result is expressed as a percentage of the activity observed in normal subjects.

Acquired deficiencies of plasma coagulation factors are more frequent than congenital disorders; the most common disorders include hemorrhagic diathesis of liver disease, disseminated intravascular coagulation (DIC), and vitamin K deficiency. In these disorders, blood coagulation is hampered by the deficiency of more than one clotting factor, and the bleeding episodes are the result of perturbation of both primary (coagulation) and secondary (e.g., platelet and vessel wall interactions) hemostasis.

The development of antibodies to coagulation plasma proteins, clinically termed *inhibitors*, is a relatively rare disease that often affects hemophilia A or B and FXI-deficient patients on repetitive exposure to the missing protein to control bleeding episodes. Inhibitors also occur among subjects without genetic deficiency of clotting factors (e.g., in the postpartum setting as a manifestation of underlying autoimmune or neoplastic disease or idiopathically). Rare cases of inhibitors to thrombin or FV have been reported in patients receiving topical bovine thrombin preparation as a local hemostatic agent in complex surgeries. The diagnosis of inhibitors is based on the same tests as those used to diagnose inherited plasma coagulation factor deficiencies. However, the addition of the missing protein to the plasma of a subject with an inhibitor does not correct the abnormal aPTT and/or PT tests. This is the major laboratory difference between deficiencies and inhibitors. Additional tests are required to measure the specificity of the inhibitor and its titer.

The treatment of these bleeding disorders often requires replacement of the deficient protein using recombinant or purified

TABLE 116-1 Genetic and Laboratory Characteristics of Inherited Coagulation Disorders

Clotting Factor Deficiency	Inheritance	Prevalence in General Population	Laboratory Abnormality[a]			Minimum Hemostatic Levels	Treatment	Plasma Half-Life
			aPTT	PT	TT			
Fibrinogen	AR	1 in 1,000,000	+	+	+	100 mg/dL	Cryoprecipitate	2–4 d
Prothrombin	AR	1 in 2,000,000	+	+	−	20–30%	FFP/PCC	3–4 d
Factor V	AR	1 in 1,000,000	+/−	+/−	−	15–20%	FFP	36 h
Factor VII	AR	1 in 500,000	−	+	−	15–20%	FFP/PCC	4–6 h
Factor VIII	X-linked	1 in 5,000	+	−	−	30%	FVIII concentrates	8–12 h
Factor IX	X-linked	1 in 30,000	+	−	−	30%	FIX concentrates	18–24 h
Factor X	AR	1 in 1,000,000	+/−	+/−	−	15–20%	FFP/PCC	40–60 h
Factor XI	AR	1 in 1,000,000	+	−	−	15–20%	FFP	40–70 h
Factor XII	AR	ND	+	−	−	[b]	[b]	60 h
HK	AR	ND	+	−	−	[b]	[b]	150 h
Prekallikrein	AR	ND	+	−	−	[b]	[b]	35 h
Factor XIII	AR	1 in 2,000,000	−	−	+/−	2–5%	Cryoprecipitate	11–14 d

[a]Values within normal range (−) or prolonged (+).

[b]No risk for bleeding; treatment is not indicated.

Abbreviations: aPTT, activated partial thromboplastin time; AR, autosomal recessive; FFP, fresh-frozen plasma; HK, high-molecular-weight kininogen; ND, not determined; PCC, prothrombin complex concentrates; PT, prothrombin time; TT, thrombin time.

plasma-derived products or fresh-frozen plasma (FFP). Therefore, it is imperative to arrive at a proper diagnosis to optimize patient care without unnecessary exposure to suboptimal treatment and the risks of bloodborne disease.

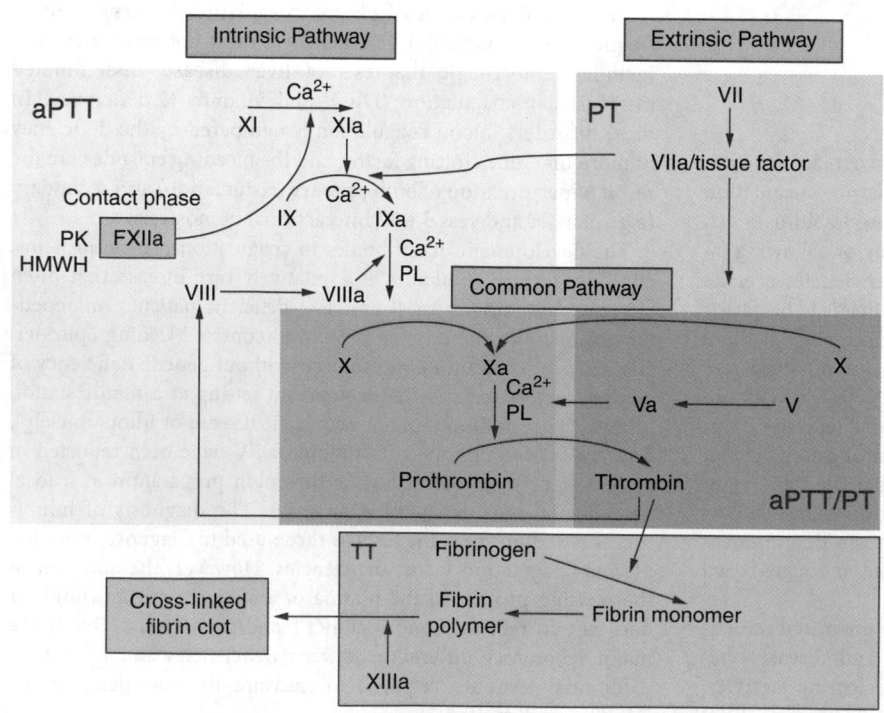

Figure 116-1   Coagulation cascade and laboratory assessment of clotting factor deficiency by activated partial prothrombin time (aPTT), prothrombin time (PT), and thrombin time (TT).

HEMOPHILIA

■ PATHOGENESIS AND CLINICAL MANIFESTATIONS

Hemophilia is an X-linked recessive hemorrhagic disease due to mutations in the *F8* gene (hemophilia A or classic hemophilia) or *F9* gene (hemophilia B). The disease affects 1 in 10,000 males worldwide, in all ethnic groups; hemophilia A represents 80% of all cases. Male subjects are clinically affected; women, who carry a single mutated gene, are generally asymptomatic. Family history of the disease is absent in ~30% of cases and in these cases, 80% of the mothers are carriers of the de novo mutated allele. More than 500 different mutations have been identified in the *F8* or *F9* genes of patients with hemophilia A or B, respectively. One of the most common hemophilia A mutations results from an inversion of the intron 22 sequence, and it is present in 40% of cases of severe hemophilia A. Advances in molecular diagnosis now permit precise identification of mutations, allowing accurate diagnosis of women carriers of the hemophilia gene in affected families.

Clinically, hemophilia A and hemophilia B are indistinguishable. The disease phenotype correlates with the residual activity of FVIII or FIX and can be classified as severe (<1%), moderate (1–5%), or mild (6–30%). In the severe and moderate forms, the disease is characterized by bleeding into the joints (hemarthrosis), soft tissues, and an upper respiratory infection, commonly with streptococcal pharyngitis, or is triggered by drug or food allergies. Patients develop a purpuric rash on the extensor surfaces of the arms and legs, usually accompanied by polyarthralgias or arthritis, abdominal pain, and hematuria from focal glomerulonephritis. All coagulation tests are normal but renal impairment may occur. Glucocorticoids can provide symptomatic relief but do not alter the course of the illness.

■ INHERITED DISORDERS OF THE VESSEL WALL

Patients with inherited disorders of the connective tissue matrix, such as Marfan's syndrome, Ehlers-Danlos syndrome, and pseudoxanthoma elasticum, frequently report easy bruising. Inherited vascular abnormalities can result in increased bleeding. This is notably seen in hereditary hemorrhagic telangiectasia (HHT, or Osler-Weber-Rendu disease), a disorder where abnormal telangiectatic capillaries result in frequent bleeding episodes, primarily from the nose and gastrointestinal tract. Arteriovenous malformation (AVM) in the lung, brain, and liver may also occur in HHT. The telangiectasia can often be visualized on the oral and nasal mucosa. Signs and symptoms develop over time. Expistaxis begins, on average, at the age of 12 and occurs in >95% of affected individuals by middle age. Two genes involved in the pathogenesis are *eng* (endoglin) on chromosome 9q33-34 (so-called HHT type 1), associated with pulmonary AVM in 40% of cases; and *alk1* (activin-receptor-like kinase *11*) on chromosome 12q13, associated with a much lower risk of pulmonary AVM.

ACKNOWLEDGMENT

Robert Handin, MD, contributed this chapter in the 16th edition and some materials from his chapter are included here.

FURTHER READINGS

AREPALLY GM, ORTEL TL: Heparin-induced thrombocytopenia. Annu Rev Med 61:77, 2010

ASTER RH et al: Drug-induced immune thrombocytopenia: Pathogenesis, diagnosis and management. J Thromb Haemost 7:911, 2009

BUSSEL JB: Traditional and new approaches to the management of immune thrombocytopenia: Issues of when and who to treat. Hematol Oncol Clin North Am 23:1329, 2009

Diagnosis, Evaluation and Management of von Willebrand Disease. NIH Publication #08-5832. National Heart, Lung and Blood Institute, 2007, www.nhlbi.nih.gov

HAYWARD CPM: Diagnostic approach to platelet function disorders. Trans Apher Sci 38:65, 2008

ISRAELS SJ et al: Inherited disorders of platelet function and challenges to diagnosis of mucocutaneous bleeding. Haemophilia 16:152, 2010

KREMER HOVINGA JA et al: Survival and relapse in patients with thrombotic thrombocytopenic purpura. Blood 115:1500, 2010

RICE TW, WHEELER AP: Coagulopathy in critically ill patients. Chest 136:1622, 2009

CHAPTER **116**

Coagulation Disorders

Valder R. Arruda

Katherine A. High

Deficiencies of coagulation factors have been recognized for centuries. Patients with genetic deficiencies of plasma coagulation factors exhibit life-long recurrent bleeding episodes into joints, muscles, and closed spaces, either spontaneously or following an injury. The most common inherited factor deficiencies are the hemophilias, X-linked diseases caused by deficiency of factor (F) VIII (hemophilia A) or factor IX (FIX, hemophilia B). Rare congenital bleeding disorders due to deficiencies of other factors, including FII (prothrombin), FV, FVII, FX, FXI, FXIII, and fibrinogen are commonly inherited in an autosomal recessive manner (Table 116-1). Advances in characterization of the molecular bases of clotting factor deficiencies have contributed to better understanding of the disease phenotypes and may eventually allow more targeted therapeutic approaches through the development of small molecules, recombinant proteins, or cell and gene-based therapies.

Commonly used tests of hemostasis provide the initial screening for clotting factor activity (Fig. 116-1), and disease phenotype often correlates with the level of clotting activity. An isolated abnormal prothrombin time (PT) suggests FVII deficiency, whereas a prolonged activated partial thromboplastin time (aPTT) indicates most commonly hemophilia or FXI

deficiency (Fig. 116-1). The prolongation of both PT and aPTT suggests deficiency of FV, FX, FII, or fibrinogen abnormalities. The addition of the missing factor at a range of doses to the subject's plasma will correct the abnormal clotting times; the result is expressed as a percentage of the activity observed in normal subjects.

Acquired deficiencies of plasma coagulation factors are more frequent than congenital disorders; the most common disorders include hemorrhagic diathesis of liver disease, disseminated intravascular coagulation (DIC), and vitamin K deficiency. In these disorders, blood coagulation is hampered by the deficiency of more than one clotting factor, and the bleeding episodes are the result of perturbation of both primary (coagulation) and secondary (e.g., platelet and vessel wall interactions) hemostasis.

The development of antibodies to coagulation plasma proteins, clinically termed *inhibitors*, is a relatively rare disease that often affects hemophilia A or B and FXI-deficient patients on repetitive exposure to the missing protein to control bleeding episodes. Inhibitors also occur among subjects without genetic deficiency of clotting factors (e.g., in the postpartum setting as a manifestation of underlying autoimmune or neoplastic disease or idiopathically). Rare cases of inhibitors to thrombin or FV have been reported in patients receiving topical bovine thrombin preparation as a local hemostatic agent in complex surgeries. The diagnosis of inhibitors is based on the same tests as those used to diagnose inherited plasma coagulation factor deficiencies. However, the addition of the missing protein to the plasma of a subject with an inhibitor does not correct the abnormal aPTT and/or PT tests. This is the major laboratory difference between deficiencies and inhibitors. Additional tests are required to measure the specificity of the inhibitor and its titer.

The treatment of these bleeding disorders often requires replacement of the deficient protein using recombinant or purified

TABLE 116-1 Genetic and Laboratory Characteristics of Inherited Coagulation Disorders

Clotting Factor Deficiency	Inheritance	Prevalence in General Population	Laboratory Abnormality[a]			Minimum Hemostatic Levels	Treatment	Plasma Half-Life
			aPTT	PT	TT			
Fibrinogen	AR	1 in 1,000,000	+	+	+	100 mg/dL	Cryoprecipitate	2–4 d
Prothrombin	AR	1 in 2,000,000	+	+	−	20–30%	FFP/PCC	3–4 d
Factor V	AR	1 in 1,000,000	+/−	+/−	−	15–20%	FFP	36 h
Factor VII	AR	1 in 500,000	−	+	−	15–20%	FFP/PCC	4–6 h
Factor VIII	X-linked	1 in 5,000	+	−	−	30%	FVIII concentrates	8–12 h
Factor IX	X-linked	1 in 30,000	+	−	−	30%	FIX concentrates	18–24 h
Factor X	AR	1 in 1,000,000	+/−	+/−	−	15–20%	FFP/PCC	40–60 h
Factor XI	AR	1 in 1,000,000	+	−	−	15–20%	FFP	40–70 h
Factor XII	AR	ND	+	−	−	[b]	[b]	60 h
HK	AR	ND	+	−	−	[b]	[b]	150 h
Prekallikrein	AR	ND	+	−	−	[b]	[b]	35 h
Factor XIII	AR	1 in 2,000,000	−	−	+/−	2–5%	Cryoprecipitate	11–14 d

[a]Values within normal range (−) or prolonged (+).

[b]No risk for bleeding; treatment is not indicated.

Abbreviations: aPTT, activated partial thromboplastin time; AR, autosomal recessive; FFP, fresh-frozen plasma; HK, high-molecular-weight kininogen; ND, not determined; PCC, prothrombin complex concentrates; PT, prothrombin time; TT, thrombin time.

plasma-derived products or fresh-frozen plasma (FFP). Therefore, it is imperative to arrive at a proper diagnosis to optimize patient care without unnecessary exposure to suboptimal treatment and the risks of bloodborne disease.

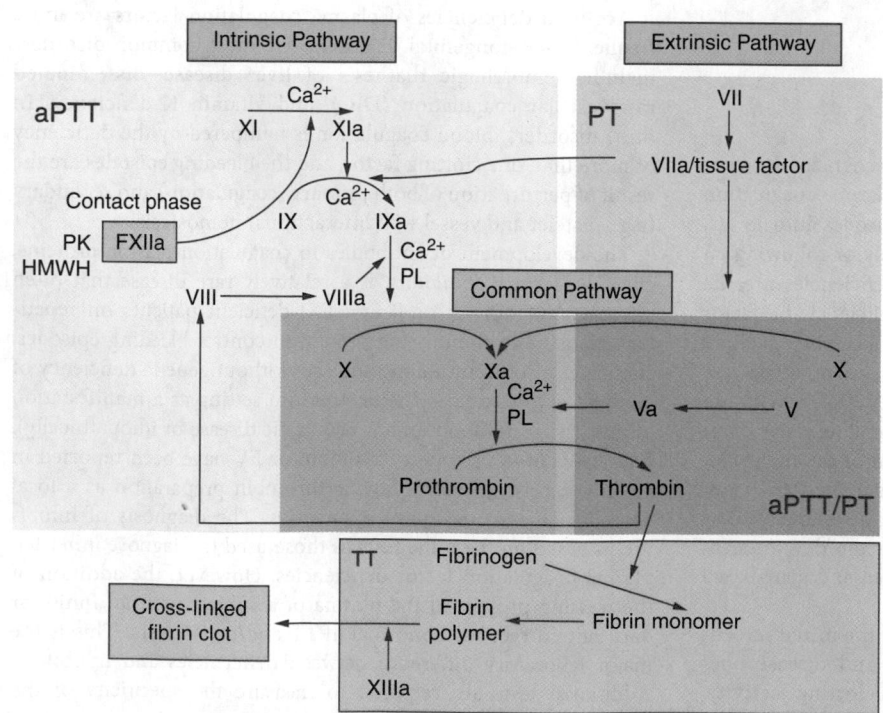

Figure 116-1 Coagulation cascade and laboratory assessment of clotting factor deficiency by activated partial prothrombin time (aPTT), prothrombin time (PT), and thrombin time (TT).

HEMOPHILIA

PATHOGENESIS AND CLINICAL MANIFESTATIONS

Hemophilia is an X-linked recessive hemorrhagic disease due to mutations in the *F8* gene (hemophilia A or classic hemophilia) or *F9* gene (hemophilia B). The disease affects 1 in 10,000 males worldwide, in all ethnic groups; hemophilia A represents 80% of all cases. Male subjects are clinically affected; women, who carry a single mutated gene, are generally asymptomatic. Family history of the disease is absent in ~30% of cases and in these cases, 80% of the mothers are carriers of the de novo mutated allele. More than 500 different mutations have been identified in the *F8* or *F9* genes of patients with hemophilia A or B, respectively. One of the most common hemophilia A mutations results from an inversion of the intron 22 sequence, and it is present in 40% of cases of severe hemophilia A. Advances in molecular diagnosis now permit precise identification of mutations, allowing accurate diagnosis of women carriers of the hemophilia gene in affected families.

Clinically, hemophilia A and hemophilia B are indistinguishable. The disease phenotype correlates with the residual activity of FVIII or FIX and can be classified as severe (<1%), moderate (1–5%), or mild (6–30%). In the severe and moderate forms, the disease is characterized by bleeding into the joints (hemarthrosis), soft tissues, and beyond middle age in the developing world. The life expectancy of a patient with severe hemophilia is only ~10 years shorter than the general male population. In patients with mild or moderate hemophilia, life expectancy is approaching that of the male population without coagulopathy. Elderly hemophilia patients have different problems compared to the younger generation; they have more severe arthropathy and chronic pain due to suboptimal treatment, and high rates of HCV and/or HIV infections.

Early data indicate that mortality from coronary artery disease is lower in hemophilia patients than the general male population. The underlying hypocoagulability probably provides a protective effect against thrombus formation, but it does not prevent the development of atherogenesis. Similar to the general population, these patients are exposed to cardiovascular risk factors such as age, obesity, and smoking. Moreover, physical inactivity, hypertension, and chronic renal disease are commonly observed in hemophilia patients. In HIV patients on combined antiretroviral therapy, there may be a further increase in the risk of cardiovascular disease. Therefore, these patients should be carefully considered for preventive and therapeutic approaches to minimize the risk of cardiovascular disease.

Excessive replacement therapy should be avoided, and it is prudent to slowly infuse factor concentrates. Continuous infusion of clotting factor is preferable to bolus dosing in patients with cardiovascular risk factors undergoing invasive procedures. The management of an acute ischemic event and coronary revascularization should include the collaboration of hematologists and internists. The early assumption that hemophilia would protect against occlusive vascular disease may change in this aging population.

Cancer is a common cause of mortality in aging hemophilia patients as they are at risk for HIV- and HCV-related malignancies. Hepatocellular carcinoma (HCC) is the most prevalent primary liver cancer and a common cause of death in HIV-negative patients. The recommendations for cancer screening for the general population should be the same for age-matched hemophilia patients. Among those with high-risk HCV, a semiannual or annual ultrasound and α fetoprotein is recommended for HCC. Screening for urogenital neoplasm in the presence of hematuria or hematochezia may be delayed due to the underlying bleeding disease, thus preventing early intervention. Multidisciplinary interaction should facilitate the attempts to ensure optimal cancer prevention and treatment recommendations for those with hemophilia.

Management of Carriers of Hemophilia Usually hemophilia carriers, with factor levels of ~50% of normal, have not been considered to be at risk for bleeding. However, a wide range of values (22–116%) have been reported due to random inactivation of the X chromosomes (*lyonization*). Therefore, it is important to measure the factor level of carriers to recognize those at risk of bleeding and to optimize preoperative and postoperative management. During pregnancy, both FVIII and FIX levels increase gradually until delivery. FVIII levels increase approximately two- to threefold compared to nonpregnant women, whereas a FIX increase is less pronounced. After delivery, there is a rapid fall in the pregnancy-induced rise of maternal clotting factor levels. This represents an imminent risk of bleeding that can be prevented by infusion of factor concentrate to levels of 50–70% for 3 days in the setting of vaginal delivery and up to 5 days for cesarean section. In mild cases, the use of DDAVP and/or antifibrinolytic drugs is recommended.

■ FACTOR XI DEFICIENCY

Factor XI is a zymogen of an active serine protease (FIXa) in the intrinsic pathway of blood coagulation that activates FIX (Fig. 116-1). There are two pathways for the formation of FXIa. In an aPTT-based assay, the protease is the result of activation by FXIIa in conjunction with high-molecular-weight kininogen and kallikrein. In vivo data suggest that thrombin is the physiologic activator of FXI. The generation of thrombin by the tissue-factor/factor VIIa pathway activates FXI on the platelet surface that contributes to additional thrombin generation after the clot has formed and thus augments resistance to fibrinolysis through a thrombin-activated fibrinolytic inhibitor (TAFI).

Factor XI deficiency is a rare bleeding disorder that occurs in the general population at a frequency of one in a million. However, the disease is highly prevalent among Ashkenazi and Iraqi Jewish populations, reaching a frequency of 6% as heterozygotes and 0.1 to 0.3% as homozygotes. More than 65 mutations in the FXI gene have been reported, whereas fewer mutations (two to three) are found among affected Jewish populations.

Normal FXI clotting activity levels range from 70 to 150 U/dL. In heterozygous patients with moderate deficiency, FXI ranges from 20 to 70 U/dL, whereas in homozygous or double heterozygote patients, FXI levels are <1–20 U/dL. Patients with FXI levels <10% of normal have a high risk of bleeding, but the disease phenotype does not always correlate with residual FXI clotting activity. A family history is indicative of the risk of bleeding in the propositus. Clinically, the presence of mucocutaneous hemorrhages such as bruises, gum bleeding, epistaxis, hematuria, and menorrhagia are common, especially following trauma. This hemorrhagic phenotype suggests that tissues rich in fibrinolytic activity are more susceptible to FXI deficiency. Postoperative bleeding is common but not always present, even among patients with very low FXI levels.

FXI replacement is indicated in patients with severe disease required to undergo a surgical procedure. A negative history of bleeding complications following invasive procedures does not exclude the possibility of an increased risk for hemorrhage.

TREATMENT   **Factor XI Deficiency**

The treatment of FXI deficiency is based on the infusion of FFP at doses of 15 to 20 mL/kg to maintain trough levels ranging from 10 to 20%. Because FXI has a half-life of 40–70 h, the replacement therapy can be given on alternate days. The use of antifibrinolytic drugs is beneficial to control bleeds, with the exception of hematuria or bleeds in the bladder. The development of an FXI inhibitor was observed in 10% of severely FXI-deficient patients who received replacement therapy. Patients with severe FXI deficiency who develop inhibitors usually do not bleed spontaneously. However, bleeding following a surgical procedure or trauma can be severe. In these patients, FFP and FXI concentrates should be avoided. The use of PCC/aPCC or recombinant activated FVII has been effective.

RARE BLEEDING DISORDERS

Collectively, the inherited disorders resulting from deficiencies of clotting factors other than FVIII, FIX, and FXI (Table 116-1) represent a group of rare bleeding diseases. The bleeding symptoms in these patients vary from asymptomatic (dysfibrinogenemia or FVII deficiency) to life-threatening (FX or FXIII deficiency). There is no pathognomonic clinical manifestation that suggests one specific disease, but overall, in contrast to hemophilia, hemarthrosis is a rare event and bleeding in the mucosal tract or after umbilical cord clamping is common. Individuals heterozygous for plasma coagulation deficiencies are often asymptomatic. The laboratory assessment for the specific deficient factor following screening with general coagulation tests (Table 116-1) will define the diagnosis.

Replacement therapy using FFP or prothrombin complex concentrates (containing prothrombin, FVII, FIX, and FX) provides adequate hemostasis in response to bleeds or as prophylactic treatment. The use of PCC should be carefully monitored and avoided in patients with underlying liver disease, or those at high risk for thrombosis because of the risk of disseminated intravascular coagulopathy.

■ FAMILIAL MULTIPLE COAGULATION DEFICIENCIES

There are several bleeding disorders characterized by the inherited deficiency of more than one plasma coagulation factor. To date, the genetic defects in two of these diseases have been characterized and they provide new insights into the regulation of hemostasis by gene-encoding proteins outside blood coagulation.

Combined deficiency of FV and FVIII

Patients with combined FV and FVIII deficiency exhibit ~5% of residual clotting activity of each factor. Interestingly, the disease phenotype is a mild bleeding tendency, often following trauma. An underlying mutation has been identified in the endoplasmic reticulum/Golgi intermediate compartment (*ERGIC-53*) gene, a mannose-binding protein localized in the Golgi apparatus that functions as a chaperone for both FV and FVIII. In other families, mutations in the multiple coagulation factor deficiency 2 (*MCFD2*) gene have been defined; this gene encodes a protein that forms a Ca^{2+}–dependent complex with *ERGIC-53* and provides cofactor activity in the intracellular mobilization of both FV and FVIII.

Multiple deficiencies of vitamin K–dependent coagulation factors

Two enzymes involved in vitamin K metabolism have been associated with combined deficiency of all vitamin K–dependent proteins, including the procoagulant proteins prothrombin, VII, IX, and X and the anticoagulant proteins C and S. Vitamin K is a fat-soluble vitamin that is a cofactor for carboxylation of the gamma carbon of the glutamic acid residues in the vitamin K–dependent factors, a critical step for calcium and phospholipid binding of these proteins (Fig. 116-2).

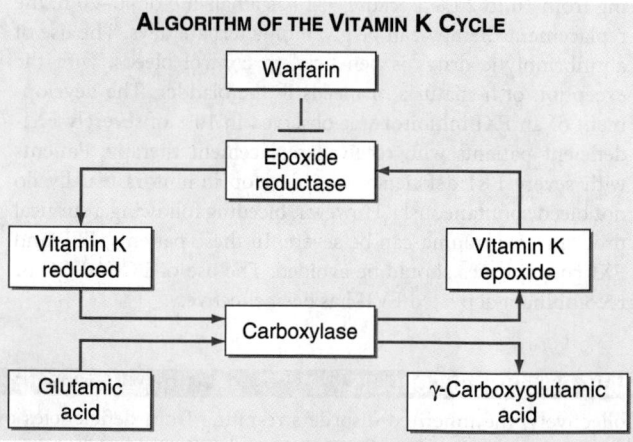

ALGORITHM OF THE VITAMIN K CYCLE

Figure 116-2   The vitamin K cycle. Vitamin K is a cofactor for the formation of γ-carboxyglutamic acid residues on coagulation proteins. Vitamin K–dependent γ-glutamylcarboxylase, the enzyme that catalyzes the vitamin K epoxide reductase, regenerates reduced vitamin K. Warfarin blocks the action of the reductase and competitively inhibits the effects of vitamin K.

The enzymes γ-glutamylcarboxylase and epoxide reductase are critical for the metabolism and regeneration of vitamin K. Mutations in the genes encoding the gamma-carboxylase (GGCX) or vitamin K epoxide reductase complex 1 (VKORC1) result in defective enzymes and thus in vitamin K–dependent factors with reduced activity, varying from 1 to 30% of normal. The disease phenotype is characterized by mild to severe bleeding episodes present from birth. Some patients respond to high doses of vitamin K. For severe bleeding, replacement therapy with FFP or PCC may be necessary for achieving full hemostatic control.

■ DISSEMINATED INTRAVASCULAR COAGULATION

Disseminated intravascular coagulation (DIC) is a clinicopathologic syndrome characterized by widespread intravascular fibrin formation in response to excessive blood protease activity that overcomes the natural anticoagulant mechanisms. There are several underlying pathologies associated with DIC (Table 116-2).

TABLE 116-2 Common Clinical Causes of Disseminated Intravascular Coagulation

Sepsis	**Immunologic disorders**
• Bacterial: Staphylococci, strep- tococci, pneumococci, meningococci, gram-negative bacilli	• Acute hemolytic transfusion reaction • Organ or tissue transplant rejection • Graft-versus-host disease
• Viral	
• Mycotic	
• Parasitic	
• Rickettsial	
Trauma and tissue injury	**Drugs**
• Brain injury (gunshot) • Extensive burns • Fat embolism • Rhabdomyolysis	• Fibrinolytic agents • Aprotinin • Warfarin (especially in neonates with protein C deficiency) • Prothrombin complex concentrates • Recreational drugs (amphetamines)
Vascular disorders	**Envenomation**
• Giant hemangiomas (Kasabach-Merritt syndrome) • Large vessel aneurysms (e.g., aorta)	• Snake • Insects
Obstetrical complications	**Liver disease**
• Abruptio placentae • Amniotic-fluid embolism • Dead fetus syndrome • Septic abortion	• Fulminant hepatic failure • Cirrhosis • Fatty liver of pregnancy
Cancer	**Miscellaneous**
• Adenocarcinoma (prostate, pancreas, etc.) • Hematologic malignancies (acute promyelocytic leukemia)	• Shock • Respiratory distress syndrome • Massive transfusion

The most common causes are bacterial sepsis, malignant disorders such as solid tumors or acute promyelocytic leukemia, and obstetric causes. DIC is diagnosed in almost one-half of pregnant women with abruptio placentae, or with amniotic fluid embolism. Trauma, particularly to the brain, can also result in DIC. The exposure of blood to phospholipids from damaged tissue, hemolysis, and endothelial damage are all contributing factors to the development of DIC in this setting. Purpura fulminans is a severe form of DIC resulting from thrombosis of extensive areas of the skin; it affects predominantly young children following viral or bacterial infection, particularly those with inherited or acquired hypercoagulability due to deficiencies of the components of the protein C pathway. Neonates homozygous for protein C deficiency also present high risk for purpura fulminans with or without thrombosis of large vessels.

The central mechanism of DIC is the uncontrolled generation of thrombin by exposure of the blood to pathologic levels of tissue factor (Fig. 116-3). Simultaneous suppression of physiologic anticoagulant mechanisms and abnormal fibrinolysis further accelerate the process. Together, these abnormalities contribute to systemic fibrin deposition in small and midsize vessels. The duration and intensity of the fibrin deposition can compromise the blood supply of many organs, especially the lung, kidney, liver, and brain, with consequent organ failure. The sustained activation of coagulation results in consumption of clotting factors and platelets, which in turn leads to systemic bleeding. This is further aggravated by secondary hyperfibrinolysis. Studies in animals demonstrate that the fibrinolytic system is indeed suppressed at the time of maximal activation of coagulation. Interestingly, in patients with acute promyelocytic leukemia, a severe hyperfibrinolytic state often occurs in addition to the coagulation activation. The release of several proinflammatory cytokines such as interleukin-6 and tumor necrosis factor α play central roles in mediating the coagulation defects in DIC and symptoms associated with systemic inflammatory response syndrome (SIRS).

Clinical manifestations of DIC are related to the magnitude of the imbalance of hemostasis, to the underlying disease, or to both. The most common findings are bleeding ranging from oozing from venipuncture sites, petechiae, and ecchymoses to severe hemorrhage from the gastrointestinal tract, lung, or into the CNS.

In chronic DIC, the bleeding symptoms are discrete and restricted to skin or mucosal surfaces. The hypercoagulability of DIC manifests as the occlusion of vessels in the microcirculation and resulting organ failure. Thrombosis of large vessels and cerebral embolism can also occur. Hemodynamic complications and shock are common among patients with acute DIC. The mortality ranges from 30 to >80% depending on the underlying disease, the severity of the DIC, and the age of the patient.

The diagnosis of clinically significant DIC is based on the presence of clinical and/or laboratory abnormalities of coagulation or thrombocytopenia. The laboratory diagnosis of DIC should prompt a search for the underlying disease if it is not already apparent. There is no single test that establishes the diagnosis of DIC. The laboratory investigation should include coagulation tests [aPTT, PT, thrombin time (TT)] and markers of fibrin degradation products (FDPs), in addition to platelet and red cell count and analysis of the blood smear. These tests should be repeated over a period of 6–8 hours because an initially mild abnormality can change dramatically in patients with severe DIC.

Common findings include the prolongation of PT and/or aPTT; platelet counts ≤100,000/μL³, or a rapid decline in platelet numbers; the presence of schistocytes (fragmented red cells) in the blood smear; and elevated levels of FDP. The most sensitive test for DIC is the FDP level. DIC is an unlikely diagnosis in the presence of normal levels of FDP. The D-dimer test is more specific for detection of fibrin—but not fibrinogen—degradation products and indicates that the cross-linked fibrin has been digested by plasmin. Because fibrinogen has a prolonged half-life, plasma levels diminish acutely only in severe cases of DIC. High-grade DIC is also associated with levels of antithrombin III or plasminogen activity <60% of normal.

Chronic DIC

Low-grade, compensated DIC can occur in clinical situations including giant hemangioma, metastatic carcinoma, or the dead fetus syndrome. Plasma levels of FDP or D-dimers are elevated. aPTT, PT, and fibrinogen values are within the normal range or high. Mild thrombocytopenia or normal platelet counts are also common findings. Red cell fragmentation is often detected but at a lower degree than in acute DIC.

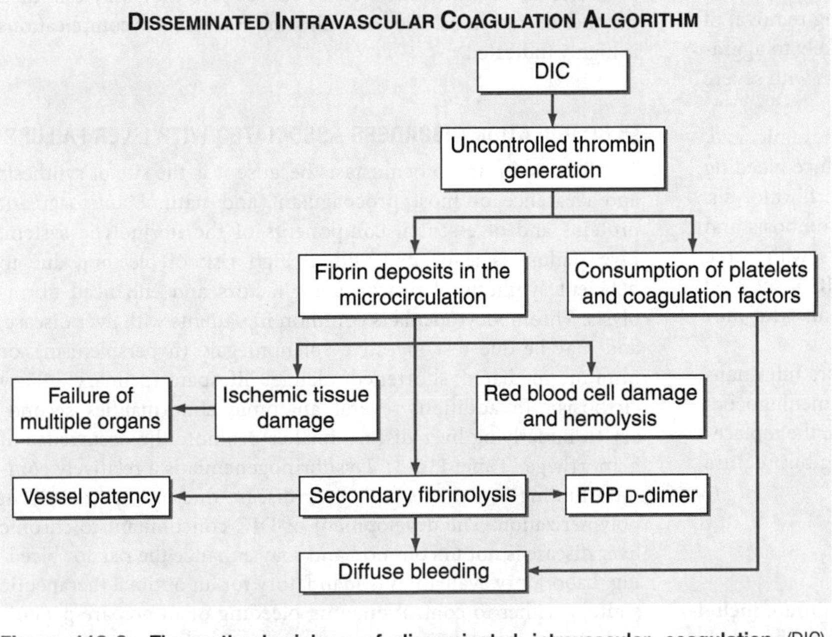

Differential diagnosis

The differential diagnosis between DIC and severe liver disease is challenging and requires serial measurements of the laboratory parameters of DIC. Patients with severe liver disease are at risk for bleeding and manifest laboratory features including thrombocytopenia (due to platelet sequestration, portal hypertension, or hypersplenism), decreased synthesis of coagulation factors and natural anticoagulants, and elevated levels of FDP due to reduced hepatic clearance. However, in contrast to DIC, these laboratory parameters in liver disease do not change rapidly. Other important differential findings include the presence of portal hypertension or other clinical or laboratory evidence of an underlying liver disease.

Microangiopathic disorders such as thrombotic thrombocytopenic purpura present an acute clinical onset of illness accompanied by thrombocytopenia, red cell fragmentation, and multiorgan failure. However, there is no consumption of clotting factors or hyperfibrinolysis.

DISSEMINATED INTRAVASCULAR COAGULATION ALGORITHM

Figure 116-3 The pathophysiology of disseminated intravascular coagulation (DIC). Interactions between coagulation and fibrinolytic pathways result in bleeding and thrombosis in the microcirculation in patients with DIC.

TREATMENT   Disseminated Intravascular Coagulation

The morbidity and mortality associated with DIC are primarily related to the underlying disease rather than the complications of the DIC. The control or elimination of the underlying cause should therefore be the primary concern. Patients with severe DIC require control of hemodynamic parameters, respiratory support, and sometimes invasive surgical procedures. Attempts to treat DIC without accompanying treatment of the causative disease are likely to fail.

MANAGEMENT OF HEMORRHAGIC SYMPTOMS The control of bleeding in DIC patients with marked thrombocytopenia (platelet counts <10,000–20,000/μL³) and low levels of coagulation factors will require replacement therapy. The PT (>1.5 times the normal) provides a good indicator of the severity of the clotting factor consumption. Replacement with FFP is indicated (1 unit of FFP increases most coagulation factors by 3% in an adult without DIC). Low levels of fibrinogen (<100 mg/dL) or brisk hyperfibrinolysis will require infusion of cryoprecipitate (plasma fraction enriched for fibrinogen, FVIII, and vWF). The replacement of 10 U of cryoprecipitate for every 2–3 U of FFP is sufficient to correct the hemostasis. The transfusion scheme must be adjusted according to the patient's clinical and laboratory evolution. Platelet concentrates at a dose of 1–2 U/10 kg body weight are sufficient for most DIC patients with severe thrombocytopenia.

Clotting factor concentrates are not recommended for control of bleeding in DIC because of the limited efficacy afforded by replacement of single factors (FVIII or FIX concentrates), and the high risk of products containing traces of aPCCs that further aggravate the disease.

REPLACEMENT OF COAGULATION OR FIBRINOLYSIS INHIBITORS Drugs to control coagulation such as heparin, ATIII concentrates, or antifibrinolytic drugs have all been tried in the treatment of DIC. Low doses of continuous infusion heparin (5–10 U/kg per h) may be effective in patients with low-grade DIC associated with solid tumor, acute promyelocytic leukemia, or in a setting with recognized thrombosis. Heparin is also indicated for the treatment of purpura fulminans during the surgical resection of giant hemangiomas and during removal of a dead fetus. In acute DIC, the use of heparin is likely to aggravate bleeding. To date, the use of heparin in patients with severe DIC has no proven survival benefit.

The use of antifibrinolytic drugs, EACA, or tranexamic acid, to prevent fibrin degradation by plasmin may reduce bleeding episodes in patients with DIC and confirmed hyperfibrinolysis. However, these drugs can increase the risk of thrombosis and concomitant use of heparin is indicated. Patients with acute promyelocytic leukemia or those with chronic DIC associated with giant hemangiomas are among the few patients who may benefit from this therapy.

The use of protein C concentrates to treat purpura fulminans associated with acquired protein C deficiency or meningococcemia has been proven efficacious. The results from the replacement of ATIII in early-phase studies are promising but require further study.

■ VITAMIN K DEFICIENCY

Vitamin K–dependent proteins are a heterogenous group, including clotting factor proteins and also proteins found in bone, lung, kidney, and placenta. Vitamin K mediates posttranslational modification of glutamate residues to γ-carboxylglutamate, a critical step for the activity of vitamin K–dependent proteins for calcium binding and proper assembly to phospholipid membranes (Fig. 116-2). Inherited deficiency of the functional activity of the enzymes involved in vitamin K metabolism, notably the GGCX or VKORC1 (see above), results in bleeding disorders. The amount of vitamin K in the diet is often limiting for the carboxylation reaction; thus recycling of the vitamin K is essential to maintain normal levels of vitamin K–dependent proteins. In adults, low dietary intake alone is seldom reason for severe vitamin K deficiency but may become common in association with the use of broad-spectrum antibiotics. Disease or surgical interventions that affect the ability of the intestinal tract to absorb vitamin K, either through anatomic alterations or by changing the fat content of bile salts and pancreatic juices in the proximal small bowel, can result in significant reduction of vitamin K levels. Chronic liver diseases such as primary biliary cirrhosis also deplete vitamin K stores. Neonatal vitamin K deficiency and the resulting hemorrhagic disease of the newborn have been almost entirely eliminated by routine administration of vitamin K to all neonates. Prolongation of PT values is the most common and earliest finding in vitamin K–deficient patients due to reduction in prothrombin, FVII, FIX, and FX levels. FVII has the shortest half-life among these factors that can prolong the PT before changes in the aPTT. Parenteral administration of vitamin K at a total dose of 10 mg is sufficient to restore normal levels of clotting factor within 8–10 h. In the presence of ongoing bleeding or a need for immediate correction before an invasive procedure, replacement with FFP or PCC is required. The latter should be avoided in patients with severe underlying liver disorders due to high risk of thrombosis. The reversal of excessive anticoagulant therapy with warfarin or warfarin-like drugs can be achieved by minimal doses of vitamin K (1 mg orally or by intravenous injection) for asymptomatic patients. This strategy can diminish the risk of bleeding while maintaining therapeutic anticoagulation for an underlying prothrombotic state.

In patients with life-threatening bleeds, the use of recombinant factor VIIa in nonhemophilia patients on anticoagulant therapy has been shown to be effective at restoring hemostasis rapidly, allowing emergency surgical intervention. However, patients with underlying vascular disease, vascular trauma and other comorbidities are at risk for thromboembolic complications that affect both arterial and venous systems. Thus, the use of factor VIIa in this setting is limited to administration of low doses given for only a limited number of injections. Close monitoring for vascular complications is highly indicated.

■ COAGULATION DISORDERS ASSOCIATED WITH LIVER FAILURE

The liver is central to hemostasis because it is the site of synthesis and clearance of most procoagulant and natural anticoagulant proteins and of essential components of the fibrinolytic system. Liver failure is associated with a high risk of bleeding due to deficient synthesis of procoagulant factors and enhanced fibrinolysis. Thrombocytopenia is common in patients with liver disease, and may be due to congestive splenomegaly (hypersplenism), or immune-mediated shortened platelet lifespan (primary biliary cirrhosis). In addition, several anatomic abnormalities secondary to underlying liver disease further promote the occurrence of hemorrhage (Table 116-3). Dysfibrinogenemia is a relatively common finding in patients with liver disease due to impaired fibrin polymerization. The development of DIC concomitant to chronic liver disease is not uncommon and may enhance the risk for bleeding. Laboratory evaluation is mandatory for an optimal therapeutic strategy, either to control ongoing bleeding or to prepare patients with liver disease for invasive procedures. Typically, these patients present with prolonged PT, aPTT, and TT depending on the degree of liver damage, thrombocytopenia, and normal or slight increase of

TABLE 116-3 Coagulation Disorders and Hemostasis in Liver Disease

Bleeding

Portal hypertension

    Esophageal varices

Thrombocytopenia

    Splenomegaly

    Chronic or acute DIC

Decreased synthesis of clotting factors

    Hepatocyte failure

    Vitamin K deficiency

Systemic fibrinolysis

DIC

Dysfibrinogenemia

Thrombosis

Decreased synthesis of coagulation inhibitors: protein C, protein S, antithrombin

    Hepatocyte failure

    Vitamin K deficiency (protein C, protein S)

Failure to clear activated coagulation proteins (DIC)

Dysfibrinogenemia

Iatrogenic: Transfusion of prothrombin complex concentrates

    Antifibrinolytic agents: EACA, tranexamic acid

Abbreviations: DIC, disseminated intravascular coagulation; EACA, ε-aminocaproic acid.

of FFP (5–10 mL/kg; each bag contains ~200 mL) is sufficient to ensure 10–20% of normal levels of clotting factors but not correction of PT or aPTT. Even high doses of FFP (20 mL/kg) do not correct the clotting times in all patients. Monitoring for clinical symptoms and clotting times will determine if repeated doses are required 8–12 h after the first infusion. Platelet concentrates are indicated when platelet counts are <10,000–20,000/μL³ to control an ongoing bleed or immediately before an invasive procedure if counts are <50,000/μL³. Cryoprecipitate is indicated only when fibrinogen levels are less than 100 mg/mL; dosing is six bags for a 70-kg patient daily. Prothrombin complex concentrate infusion in patients with liver failure should be avoided due to the high risk of thrombotic complications. The safety of the use of antifibrinolytic drugs to control bleeding in patients with liver failure is not yet well defined and should be avoided.

Liver disease and thromboembolism

The clinical bleeding phenotype of hemostasis in patients with stable liver disease is often mild or even asymptomatic. However, as the disease progresses, the hemostatic balance is less stable and more easily disturbed than in healthy individuals. Furthermore, the hemostatic balance is compromised by comorbid complications such as infections and renal failure (Fig. 116-4). Based on the clinical bleeding complications in patients with cirrhosis and laboratory evidence of hypocoagulation such as a prolonged PT/aPTT, it has long been assumed that these patients are protected against thrombotic disease. Cumulative clinical experience, however, has demonstrated that these patients are at risk for thrombosis, especially those with advanced liver disease. Although hypercoagulability could explain the occurrence of venous thrombosis, according to Virchow's triad, hemodynamic changes and damaged vasculature may also be a contributing factor, and both processes may potentially also occur in patients with liver disease. Liver-related

FDP. Fibrinogen levels are diminished only in fulminant hepatitis, decompensated cirrhosis or advanced liver disease, or in the presence of DIC. The presence of prolonged TT and normal fibrinogen and FDP levels suggest dysfibrinogenemia. FVIII levels are often normal or elevated in patients with liver failure, and decreased levels suggest superimposing DIC. Because FV is only synthesized in the hepatocyte and is not a vitamin K–dependent protein, reduced levels of FV may be an indicator of hepatocyte failure. Normal levels of FV and low levels of FVII suggest vitamin K deficiency. Vitamin K levels may be reduced in patients with liver failure due to compromised storage in hepatocellular disease, changes in bile acids or cholestasis that can diminish the absorption of vitamin K. Replacement of vitamin K may be desirable (10 mg given by slow intravenous injection) to improve hemostasis.

Treatment with FFP is the most effective to correct hemostasis in patients with liver failure. Infusion

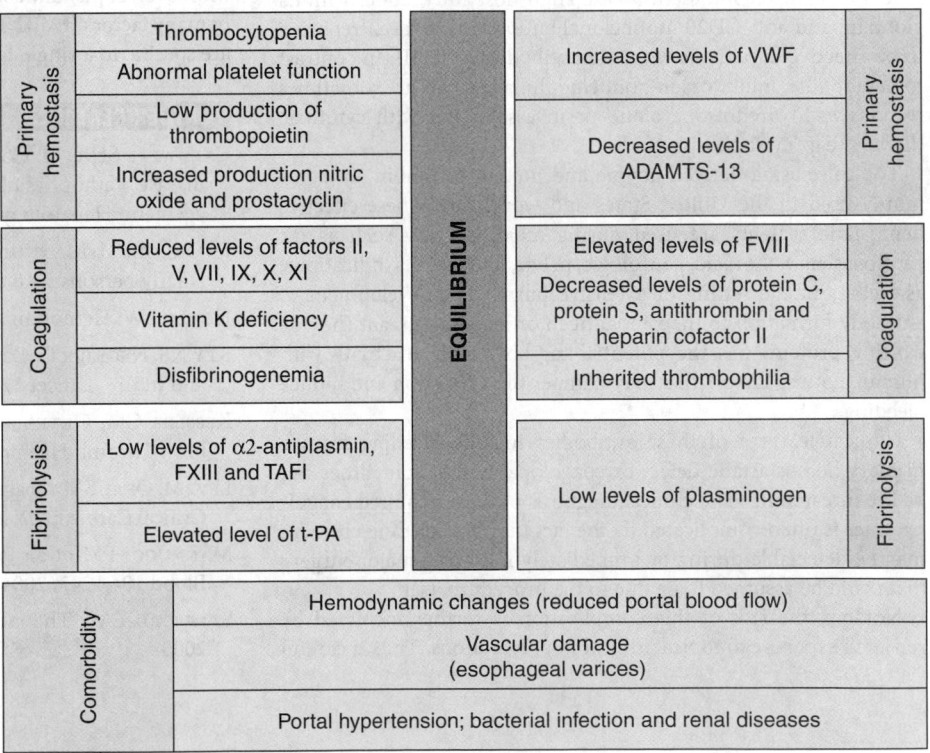

	BLEEDING		THROMBOSIS	
Primary hemostasis	Thrombocytopenia	**EQUILIBRIUM**	Increased levels of VWF	**Primary hemostasis**
	Abnormal platelet function			
	Low production of thrombopoietin		Decreased levels of ADAMTS-13	
	Increased production nitric oxide and prostacyclin			
Coagulation	Reduced levels of factors II, V, VII, IX, X, XI		Elevated levels of FVIII	**Coagulation**
	Vitamin K deficiency		Decreased levels of protein C, protein S, antithrombin and heparin cofactor II	
	Disfibrinogenemia		Inherited thrombophilia	
Fibrinolysis	Low levels of α2-antiplasmin, FXIII and TAFI		Low levels of plasminogen	**Fibrinolysis**
	Elevated level of t-PA			
Comorbidity	Hemodynamic changes (reduced portal blood flow)			
	Vascular damage (esophageal varices)			
	Portal hypertension; bacterial infection and renal diseases			

Figure 116-4 Balance of hemostasis in liver disease. TAFI, thrombin-activated fibriolytic inhibitor; t-PA, tissue plasminogen activator; VWF, von Willebrand factor.

thrombosis, in particular, thrombosis of the portal and mesenteric veins, is common in patients with advanced cirrhosis. Hemodynamic changes such as decreased portal flow, and evidence that inherited thrombophilia may enhance the risk for portal vein thrombosis in patients with cirrhosis suggest that hypercoagulability may play a role as well. Patients with liver disease develop deep vein thrombosis and pulmonary embolism at appreciable rates (ranging from 0.5 to 1.9%). The implication of these findings is relevant to the erroneous exclusion of thrombosis in patients with advanced liver disease, even in the presence of prolongation of routine clotting times, and caution should be advised on overcorrection of these laboratory abnormalities.

ACQUIRED INHIBITORS OF COAGULATION FACTORS

An acquired inhibitor is an immune-mediated disease characterized by the presence of an autoantibody against a specific clotting factor. FVIII is the most common target of antibody formation, but inhibitors to prothrombin, FV, FIX, FX, and FXI are also reported. The disease occurs predominantly in older adults (median age of 60 years), but occasionally in pregnant or postpartum women with no previous history of bleeding. In 50% of the patients with inhibitors, no underlying disease is identified at the time of diagnosis. In the remaining, the causes are autoimmune diseases, malignancies (lymphomas, prostate cancer), dermatologic diseases, and pregnancy. Bleeding episodes occur commonly in soft tissues, in the gastrointestinal or urinary tracts, and skin. In contrast to hemophilia, hemarthrosis is rare in these patients. Retroperitoneal hemorrhages and other life-threatening bleeding may appear suddenly. The overall mortality in untreated patients ranges from 8 to 22%, and most deaths occur within the first few weeks after presentation. The diagnosis is based on the prolonged aPTT with normal PT and TT. The aPTT remains prolonged after mixture of the test plasma with equal amounts of pooled normal plasma for 2 h at 37°C. The Bethesda assay using FVIII-deficient plasma as performed for inhibitor detection in hemophilia will confirm the diagnosis. Major bleeding is treated with high doses of human or porcine FVIII, PCC/PCCa, or recombinant FVIIa. High-dose intravenous gamma globulin, and anti-CD20 monoclonal antibody have been reported to be effective in patients with autoantibodies to FVIII. In contrast to hemophilia, inhibitors in nonhemophilia patients are sometimes responsive to prednisone alone or in association with cytotoxic therapy (e.g., cyclophosphamide).

Topical plasma-derived bovine and human thrombin are commonly used in the United States and worldwide. These effective hemostatic sealants are used during major surgery such as for cardiovascular, thoracic, neurologic, pelvic, and trauma indications, as well as in the setting of extensive burns. The development of antibody formation to the xenoantigen or its contaminant (bovine clotting protein) has the potential to show cross-reactivity with human clotting factors that may hamper their function and induce bleeding.

Clinical features of these antibodies include bleeding from a primary hemostastatic defect or coagulopathy that sometimes can be life threatening. The clinical diagnosis of these acquired coagulopathies is often complicated by the fact that the bleeding episodes may be detectable during or immediately following major surgery that could be assumed to be due to the procedure itself.

Notably, the risk of this complication is further increased by repeated exposure to topical thrombin preparations. Thus, a careful medical history of previous surgical interventions that may have occurred even decades earlier is critical to assessing risk.

The laboratory abnormalities are reflected by combined prolongation of the aPTT and PT that often fail to improve by transfusion of FFP and vitamin K. The abnormal laboratory tests cannot be corrected by mixing a test with equal parts of normal plasma that denotes the presence of inhibitory antibodies. The diagnosis of a specific antibody is obtained by the determination of the residual activity of human FV or other suspected human clotting factor. There are no commercially available assays specific for bovine thrombin coagulopathy.

There are no established treatment guidelines. Platelet transfusions have been utilized as a source of FV replacement for patients with FV inhibitors. Frequent injections of FFP and vitamin K supplementation may function as co-adjuvant rather than an effective treatment of the coagulopathy itself. Experience with recombinant FVIIa as a bypass agent is limited, and outcomes have been generally poor. Specific treatments to eradicate the antibodies based on immunosuppression with steroids, intravenous immunoglobulin, or serial plasmapheresis have been sporadically reported. Patients should be advised to avoid any topical thrombin sealant in the future.

Recently, novel plasma-derived and recombinant human thrombin preparations for topical hemostasis have been approved by the Food and Drug Administration. These preparations have demonstrated hemostatic efficacy with reduced immunogenicity compared to the first generation of bovine thrombin products.

The presence of lupus anticoagulant can be associated with venous or arterial thrombotic disease. However, bleeding has also been reported in lupus anticoagulant; it is due to the presence of antibodies to prothrombin, which results in hypoprothrombinemia. Both disorders show a prolonged PTT that do not correct on mixing. To distinguish acquired inhibitors from lupus anticoagulant, note that the dilute Russell's viper venom test and the hexagonal-phase phospholipids test will be negative in patients with an acquired inhibitor and positive in patients with lupus anticoagulants. Moreover, lupus anticoagulant interferes with the clotting activity of many factors (FVIII, FIX, FXII, FXI), whereas acquired inhibitors are specific to a single factor.

FURTHER READINGS

CALDWELL SH et al: Coagulation disorders and hemostasis in liver disease: Pathophysiology and critical assessment of current management. Hepatology 44:1039, 2006

FRANCHINI M, MANNUCCI PM: Co-morbidities and quality of life in elderly persons with haemophilia. Br J Haematol 148:522, 2010

HOYER LW: Hemophilia A. N Engl J Med 330:39, 1994

KEY NS, NEGRIER C: Coagulation factor concentrates: Past, present, and future. Lancet 370:439, 2007

KESSLER CM, ORTEL TL: Recent developments in topical thrombins. Thromb Haemost 101:15, 2009

LEVI M, OPAL SM: Coagulation abnormalities in critically ill patients. Critical Care 10:222, 2006

MANNUCCI PM et al: Recessively inherited coagulation disorders. Blood 104:1243, 2004

STAFFORD DW: The vitamin K cycle. J Thromb Haemost 3:1873, 2005

CHAPTER 117

Arterial and Venous Thrombosis

Jane E. Freedman

Joseph Loscalzo

OVERVIEW OF THROMBOSIS

GENERAL OVERVIEW

Thrombosis is defined as "hemostasis in the wrong place,"[1] and it is a major cause of morbidity and mortality in a wide range of arterial and venous diseases and patient populations. In 2009 in the United States, an estimated 785,000 people had a new coronary thrombotic event and about 470,000 had a recurrent ischemic episode. Each year, approximately 795,000 people have a new or recurrent stroke. Annually, more than 200,000 new cases of venous thromboembolism are found; 30% of these individuals die within 30 days, with one-fifth having sudden death due to pulmonary embolism.

In the nondiseased state, physiologic hemostasis reflects a delicate interplay between factors that promote and inhibit blood clotting, favoring the former. This response is crucial as it prevents uncontrolled hemorrhage and exsanguination following injury. In specific settings, the same processes that regulate normal hemostasis can cause pathological thrombosis leading to arterial or venous occlusion. Importantly, many commonly used therapeutic interventions may also alter the thrombotic–hemostatic balance adversely.

Hemostasis and thrombosis primarily involve the interplay among three factors: the vessel wall, coagulation proteins, and platelets. Many prevalent acute vascular diseases are due to thrombus formation within a vessel, including myocardial infarction, thrombotic cerebrovascular events, and venous thrombosis. Although the end result is vessel occlusion and tissue ischemia, the pathophysiologic processes governing these pathologies have similarities as well as distinct differences. While many of the pathways regulating thrombus formation are similar to those that regulate hemostasis, the processes triggering thrombosis and, often, perpetuating the thrombus are distinct. In venous thrombosis, primary hypercoagulable states reflecting defects in the proteins governing coagulation and/or fibrinolysis or secondary hypercoagulable states involving abnormalities of blood vessels and blood flow lead to thrombosis. By contrast, arterial thrombosis is highly dependent upon the state of the vessel wall, the platelet, and factors related to blood flow.

ARTERIAL THROMBOSIS

OVERVIEW OF ARTERIAL THROMBOSIS

In arterial thrombosis, the platelet and abnormalities of the vessel wall typically play a key role in vessel occlusion. Arterial thrombus forms via a series of sequential steps in which platelets adhere to the vessel wall, additional platelets are recruited, and thrombin is activated. The regulation of platelet adhesion, activation, aggregation, and recruitment will be described in detail below. In addition, while the primary function of platelets is regulation of hemostasis, our understanding of their role in other processes, such as immunity and inflammation, continues to grow.

[1] Macfarlane RG. Haemostasis: Introduction. Brit Med Bull 33:183, 1977.

ARTERIAL THROMBOSIS AND VASCULAR DISEASE

Arterial thrombosis is a major cause of morbidity and mortality both in the United States and, increasingly, worldwide. Coronary heart disease is estimated to cause about 1 of every 5 deaths in the United States. In addition to the 785,000 Americans who will have a new coronary event, an additional 195,000 silent first myocardial infarctions are projected to occur annually. Each year, about 795,000 people experience a new or recurrent stroke, although not all are caused by thrombotic occlusion of the vessel. Approximately 610,000 strokes are first events and 185,000 are recurrent events; it is estimated that 1 of every 18 deaths in the United States is due to stroke.

THE PLATELET

Many processes in platelets have parallels with other cell types, such as the presence of specific receptors and signaling pathways; however, unlike most cells, platelets lack a nucleus and are unable to adapt to changing biologic settings by altered gene transcription. Platelets sustain limited protein synthetic capacity from megakaryocyte-derived mRNA. Most of the molecules needed to respond to various stimuli, however, are maintained in storage granules and membrane compartments.

Platelets are disc-shaped, very small, anucleate cells (1–5 μm in diameter) that circulate in the blood at concentrations of 200–400,000/μL, with an average lifespan of 7–10 days. Platelets are derived from megakaryocytes, polyploidal hematopoietic cells found in the bone marrow. The primary regulator of platelet formation is thrombopoietin (TPO). The precise mechanism by which megakaryocytes produce and release fully formed platelets is unclear, but the process likely involves formation of proplatelets, pseudopod-like structures generated by the evagination of the cytoplasm from which platelets bud. Platelet granules are synthesized in megakaryocytes before thrombopoiesis and contain an array of prothrombotic, proinflammatory, and antimicrobial mediators. The two major types of platelet granules, alpha and dense, are distinguished by their size, abundance, and content. Alpha-granules contain soluble coagulation proteins, adhesion molecules, growth factors, integrins, cytokines, and inflammatory modulators. Platelet dense-granules are smaller than alpha-granules and less abundant. While alpha-granules contain proteins that may be more important in the inflammatory response, dense-granules contain high concentrations of small molecules, including ADP and serotonin, that influence platelet aggregation.

Platelet adhesion

(See Fig. 117-1) The formation of a thrombus is initiated by the adherence of platelets to the damaged vessel wall. Damage exposes subendothelial components responsible for triggering platelet reactivity, including collagen, von Willebrand factor, fibronectin, and other adhesive proteins, such as vitronectin and thrombospondin. The hemostatic response may vary, depending on the extent of damage, the specific proteins exposed, as well as flow conditions. Certain proteins are expressed on the platelet surface that subsequently regulate collagen-induced platelet adhesion, particularly under flow conditions, and include glycoprotein (GP) IV, GPVI, and the integrin $\alpha_2\beta_1$. The platelet GPIb-IX-V complex adhesive receptor is central both to platelet adhesion and to the initiation of platelet activation. Damage to the blood vessel wall exposes subendothelial von Willebrand factor and collagen to the circulating blood. The GPIb-IX-V complex binds to the exposed von Willebrand factor, causing platelets to adhere (Fig. 117-1). In addition, the engagement of the GPIb-IX-V complex with ligand induces signaling pathways that

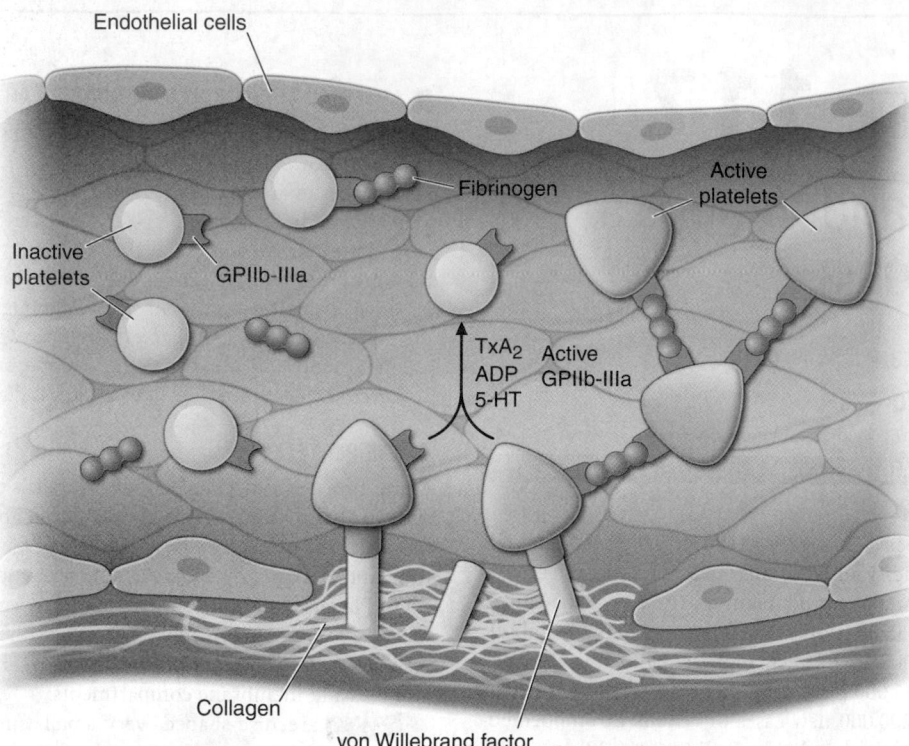

Figure 117-1 Platelet activation and thrombosis. Platelets circulate in an inactive form in the vasculature. Damage to the endothelium and/or external stimuli activates platelets that adhere to the exposed subendothelial von Willebrand factor and collagen. This adhesion leads to activation of the platelet, shape change, and the synthesis and release of TxA_2, 5-HT, and ADP. Platelet stimuli causes conformational change in the platelet integrin glycoprotein IIb/IIIa receptor leading to the high-affinity binding of fibrinogen and the formation of a stable platelet thrombus (TxA_2, thromboxane; 5-HT, serotonin).

lead to platelet activation. von Willebrand factor–bound GPIb-IX-V promotes a calcium-dependent conformational change in the GPIIb/IIIa receptor, transforming it from an inactive low-affinity state to an active high-affinity receptor for fibrinogen.

Platelet activation

The activation of platelets is controlled by a variety of surface receptors that regulate various functions in the activation process. Platelet receptors are stimulated by a wide variety of agonists and adhesive proteins that result in variable degrees of activation. In general terms, the stimulation of platelet receptors triggers two specific processes: (1) activation of internal signaling pathways that lead to further platelet activation and granule release and (2) the capacity of the platelet to bind to other adhesive proteins/platelets. Both of these processes contribute to the formation of a thrombus.

Many families and subfamilies of receptors are found on platelets that regulate a variety of platelet functions. These include the seven transmembrane receptor family, which is the main agonist-stimulated receptor family. Several seven transmembrane receptors are found on platelets, including the ADP receptors, prostaglandin receptors, lipid receptors, and chemokine receptors. Receptors for thrombin comprise the major seven transmembrane receptors found on platelets. Among this last group, the first identified was the protease activation receptor 1 (PAR1). The PAR class of receptors has a distinct mechanism of activation that involves specific cleavage of the N-terminus of thrombin, which, in turn, acts as a ligand for the receptor. Other PAR receptors are present on platelets, including PAR2 (not activated by thrombin) and PAR4. Adenosine receptors are responsible for transduction of ADP-induced signaling events, which are initiated by the binding of ADP to purinergic receptors on the platelet surface. There are several distinct ADP receptors, classified as $P2X_1$, $P2Y_1$, and $P2Y_{12}$ (Fig. 117-2). The activation of both the $P2Y_{12}$ and $P2Y_1$ receptors is essential for ADP-induced platelet aggregation. The thienopyridine derivatives, clopidogrel and prasugrel, are clinically utilized inhibitors of ADP-induced platelet aggregation.

Platelet aggregation

Activation of platelets results in a rapid series of signal transduction events, including tyrosine kinase, serine/threonine kinase, and lipid kinase activation. In unstimulated platelets, the major platelet integrin GPIIb/IIIa is maintained in an inactive conformation and functions as a low-affinity adhesion receptor for fibrinogen. This integrin is unique as it is only expressed on platelets. After stimulation, the interaction between fibrinogen and GPIIb/IIIa forms intercellular connections between platelets leading to the formation of a platelet aggregate (Fig. 117-1). A calcium-sensitive conformational change in the extracellular domain of GPIIb/IIIa enables the high-affinity binding of soluble plasma fibrinogen as a result of a complex network of inside-out signaling events. The GPIIb/IIIa receptor serves as a bidirectional conduit with GPIIb/IIIa–mediated signaling (outside-in) occurring immediately after the binding of fibrinogen. This leads to additional intracellular signaling that further stabilizes the platelet aggregate and transforms platelet aggregation from a reversible to an irreversible process (inside-out).

■ THE ROLE OF PLATELETS AND THROMBOSIS IN INFLAMMATION

Inflammation plays an important role during the acute thrombotic phase of acute coronary syndromes. Patients with acute coronary syndromes have not only increased interactions between platelets (homotypic aggregates), but also increased interactions between

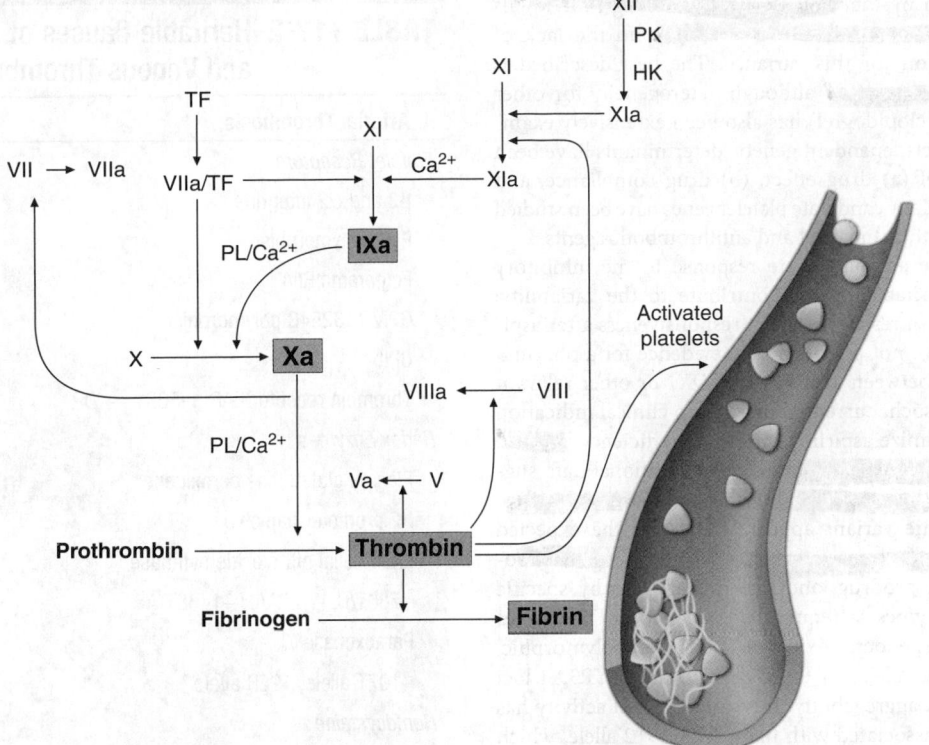

Figure 117-2 Summary of the coagulation pathways. Specific coagulation factors ("a" indicates activated form) are responsible for the conversion of soluble plasma fibrinogen into insoluble fibrin. This process occurs via a series of linked reactions in which the enzymatically active product subsequently converts the downstream inactive protein into an active serine protease. In addition, the activation of thrombin leads to stimulation of platelets HK, high-molecular-weight kininogen; PK, prekallikrein; TF, tissue factor.

platelets and leukocytes (heterotypic aggregates) detectable in circulating blood. These latter aggregates form when platelets are activated and adhere to circulating leukocytes. Platelets bind via P-selectin (CD62P) expressed on the surface of activated platelets to the leukocyte receptor, P-selectin glycoprotein ligand 1 (PSGL-1). This association leads to increased expression of CD11b/CD18 (Mac-1) on leukocytes, which itself supports interactions with platelets partially via bivalent fibrinogen linking this integrin with its platelet surface counterpart, GPIIb/IIIa. Platelet surface P-selectin also induces the expression of tissue factor on monocytes, which promotes fibrin formation.

In addition to platelet–monocyte aggregates, the immunomodulator, soluble CD40 ligand (CD40L or CD154), also reflects a link between thrombosis and inflammation. The CD40 ligand is a trimeric transmembrane protein of the tumor necrosis factor family and, with its receptor CD40, is an important contributor to the inflammatory process leading both to thrombosis and atherosclerosis. While many immunologic and vascular cells have been found to express CD40 and/or CD40 ligand, in platelets, CD40 ligand is rapidly translocated to the surface after stimulation and is upregulated in the newly formed thrombus. The surface-expressed CD40 ligand is cleaved from the platelet to generate a soluble fragment (soluble CD40 ligand).

Links have also been established among platelets, infection, immunity, and inflammation. Bacterial infections are associated with a transient increase in the risk of acute thrombotic events, such as acute myocardial infarction and stroke. In addition, platelets contribute significantly to the pathophysiology and high mortality rates of sepsis. The expression, functionality, and signaling pathways of toll-like receptors (TLRs) have been established in platelets. Stimulation of platelet TLR2 directly activates the platelet's thrombotic and inflammatory responses, and live bacteria induce a proinflammatory response in platelets in a TLR2-dependent manner, suggesting a mechanism by which specific bacteria and bacterial components can directly activate platelet-dependent thrombosis.

■ GENETICS OF ARTERIAL THROMBOSIS

Some studies have associated arterial thrombosis with genetic variants (Table 117-2A); however, in the area of genetic variability and platelet function, studies have primarily dealt with pharmacogenetics, the field of pharmacology dealing with the interindividual variability in drug response based on genetic determinants (Table 117-1). This

TABLE 117-1 Genetic Variation and Pharmacogenetic Responses to Platelet Inhibitors

Potential Gene Altered	Target Therapeutic Class	Specific Drug
P2Y1 and *P2Y12* *CYP2C19, CYP3A4, CYP3A5*	ADP receptor inhibitors	Clopidogrel, prasugrel
COX1, COX2	Cyclooxygenase inhibitors	Aspirin
PIA1/A2	Receptor inhibitors:	Abciximab, eptifibatide, tirofiban
INTB3, GPIbA	Glycoprotein IIb-IIIa receptor inhibitors	

focus has been driven by the wide variability among individuals in terms of response to antithrombotic drugs and the lack of a common explanation for this variance. The best described is the issue of "aspirin resistance," although heterogeneity for other antithrombotics (e.g., clopidogrel) has also been extensively examined. Primarily, platelet-dependent genetic determinants have been defined at the level of (a) drug effect, (b) drug compliance, and (c) drug metabolism. Many candidate platelet genes have been studied for their interaction with antiplatelet and antithrombotic agents.

Many patients have an inadequate response to the inhibitory effects of aspirin. Heritable factors contribute to the variability; however, ex vivo tests of residual platelet responsiveness after aspirin administration have not provided firm evidence for a pharmacogenetic interaction between aspirin and COX1 or other relevant platelet receptors. As such, currently, there is no clinical indication for genotyping to optimize aspirin's antiplatelet efficiency. For the platelet P2Y12 receptor inhibitor clopidogrel, additional data suggest that genetics may affect the drug's responsiveness and utility. The responsible genetic variant appears not to be the expected P2Y12 receptor but an enzyme responsible for drug metabolism. Clopidogrel is a prodrug, and liver metabolism by specific cytochrome P450 enzymes is required for activation. The genes encoding the CYP-dependent oxidative steps are polymorphic, and carriers of specific alleles of the CYP2C19 and CYP3A4 loci have increased platelet aggregability. Increased platelet activity has also been specifically associated with the CYP2C19*2 allele, which causes loss of platelet function in select patients. As these are common genetic variants, this observation has been shown to be clinically relevant in large studies.

VENOUS THROMBOSIS

■ OVERVIEW OF VENOUS THROMBOSIS

Coagulation is the process by which thrombin is activated and soluble plasma fibrinogen is converted into insoluble fibrin. These steps account for both normal hemostasis and the pathophysiologic processes influencing the development of venous thrombosis. The primary forms of venous thrombosis are deep-vein thrombosis (DVT) in the extremities and the subsequent embolization to the lungs (pulmonary embolism), referred to together as venous thromboembolic disease. Venous thrombosis occurs due to heritable causes (Table 117-2B) and acquired causes (Table 117-3).

■ DEEP VENOUS THROMBOSIS AND PULMONARY EMBOLISM

More than 200,000 new cases of venous thromboembolism occur each year. Of these cases, 30% die within 30 days and one-fifth suffer sudden death owing to pulmonary embolism; 30% go on to develop recurrent venous thromboembolism within 10 years. Data from the ARIC study reported a 9% 28-day fatality rate from deep venous thrombosis and a 15% fatality rate from pulmonary embolism. Pulmonary embolism in the setting of cancer has a 25% fatality rate. The mean incidence of first DVT in the general population is 5 per 10,000 person-years; the incidence is similar in males and females and increases dramatically with age from 2 to 3 per 10,000 person-years at 30–49 years of age to 20 at 70–79 years of age.

■ OVERVIEW OF THE COAGULATION CASCADE AND ITS ROLE IN VENOUS THROMBOSIS

Coagulation is defined as the formation of fibrin by a series of linked enzymatic reactions in which each reaction product converts the subsequent inactive zymogen into an active serine protease (Fig. 117-2). This coordinated sequence is called the coagulation cascade and is a key mechanism for regulating hemostasis. Central to the function of the coagulation cascade is the principle of amplification: owing

TABLE 117-2 Heritable Causes of Arterial and Venous Thrombosis

A. Arterial Thrombosis

Platelet Receptors

β3 and α2 integrins

P$_l$A2 polymorphism

Fc(gamma)RIIA

GPIV T13254C polymorphism

GPIb

Thrombin receptor PAR-1-5061 → D

Redox Enzymes

Plasma glutathione peroxidase

H2 promoter haplotype

Endothelial nitric oxide synthase

−786T/C, −922A/G, −1468T/A

Paraoxonase

−107T allele, 192R allele

Homocysteine

Cystathionine β-synthase 833T → C

5,10-methylene tetrahydrofolate reductase (MTHFR) 677C → T

B. Venous Thrombosis

Procoagulant Proteins

Fibrinogen

−455G/A, −854G/A

Prothrombin (20210G → A)

Protein C Anticoagulant Pathway

Factor V Leiden: 1691G → A (Arg506Gln)

Thrombomodulin 1481C → T (Ala455Val)

Fibrinolytic Proteins with Known Polymorphisms

Tissue plasminogen activator (tPA)

7351C/T, 20 099T/C in exon 6, 27 445T/A in intron 10

Plasminogen activator inhibitor (PAI-1)

4G/5G insertion/deletion polymorphism at position −675

Homocysteine

Cystathionine β-synthase 833T → C

5,10-methylene tetrahydrofolate reductase (MTHFR) 677C → T

to a series of linked enzymatic reactions, a small stimulus can lead to much greater quantities of fibrin, the end product that prevents hemorrhage at the site of vascular injury.

The coagulation cascade is primarily initiated by vascular injury exposing tissue factor to blood components (Fig. 117-2). Tissue factor may also be found in bloodborne cell-derived microparticles and, under pathophysiologic conditions, in leukocytes or platelets. Plasma factor VII (FVII) is the ligand for and is activated (FVIIa) by binding to tissue factor exposed at the site of vessel damage. The binding of FVII/VIIa to tissue factor activates the downstream conversion of factor X (FX) to active FX (FXa). In an alternative reaction, the FVII/FVIIa–tissue factor complex initially converts

TABLE 117-3 Acquired Causes of Venous Thrombosis

Surgery
  Neurosurgery
  Major abdominal surgery
Malignancy
  Antiphospholipid syndrome
Other
  Trauma
  Pregnancy
  Long-haul travel
  Obesity
  Oral contraceptives/hormone replacement
  Myeloproliferative disorders
  Polycythemia vera

FIX to FIXa, which then activates FX in conjunction with its cofactor factor VIII (FVIIIa). Factor Xa with its cofactor FVa converts prothrombin to thrombin, which then converts soluble plasma fibrinogen to insoluble fibrin, leading to clot or thrombus formation. Thrombin also activates FXIII to FXIIIa, a transglutaminase that covalently cross-links and stabilizes the fibrin clot.

Several antithrombotic factors also regulate coagulation; these include antithrombin, tissue factor pathway inhibitor (TFPI), heparin cofactor II, and protein C/protein S. Under normal conditions, these factors limit the production of thrombin to prevent the perpetuation of coagulation and thrombus formation. Typically, after the clot has caused occlusion at the damaged site and begins to expand toward adjacent uninjured vessel segments, the anticoagulant reactions governed by the normal endothelium become pivotal in limiting the extent of this hemostatically protective clot.

■ RISK FACTORS FOR VENOUS THROMBOSIS

The risk factors for venous thrombosis are primarily related to hypercoagulability, which can be genetic (Table 117-2) or acquired, or due to immobilization and venous stasis. Independent predictors for recurrence include increasing age, obesity, malignant neoplasm, and acute extremity paresis. Often, multiple risk factors are present in a single individual. Significant risk is incurred by major orthopedic, abdominal, or neurologic surgeries. Moderate risk is promoted by prolonged bedrest; certain types of cancer, pregnancy, hormone replacement therapy, or oral contraceptive use; and other sedentary conditions such as long-distance plane travel. It has been reported that the risk of developing a venous thromboembolic event doubles after air travel lasting 4 h, although the absolute risk remains low (1 in 6000). The relative risk of venous thromboembolism among pregnant or postpartum women is 4.3, and the overall incidence (absolute risk) is 199.7 per 100,000 woman-years.

■ GENETICS OF VENOUS THROMBOSIS

(See Table 117-2) Less common causes of venous thrombosis are those due to genetic variants. These abnormalities include loss-of-function mutations of endogenous anticoagulants as well as gain-of-function mutations of procoagulant proteins. Heterozygous antithrombin deficiency and homozygosity of the factor V Leiden mutation significantly increase the risk of venous thrombosis. While homozygous protein C or protein S deficiencies are rare

and may lead to fatal purpura fulminans, heterozygous deficiencies are associated with a moderate risk of thrombosis. Activated protein C impairs coagulation by proteolytic degradation of FVa. Patients resistant to the activity of activated protein C may have a point mutation in the FV gene located on chromosome 1, a mutant denoted factor V Leiden. Mildly increased risk has been attributed to elevated levels of procoagulant factors, as well as low levels of tissue factor pathway inhibitor. Polymorphisms of methylene tetrahydrofolate reductase as well as hyperhomocysteinemia have been shown to be independent risk factors for venous thrombosis, as well as arterial vascular disease; however, many of the initial descriptions of genetic variants and their associations with thromboembolism are being questioned in larger, more current studies.

■ FIBRINOLYSIS AND THROMBOSIS

Specific abnormalities in the fibrinolytic system have been associated with enhanced thrombosis. Factors such as elevated levels of tissue plasminogen activator (tPA) and plasminogen activator inhibitor type 1 (PAI-1) have been associated with decreased fibrinolytic activity and an increased risk of arterial thrombotic disease. Specific genetic variants have been associated with decreased fibrinolytic activity, including the 4G/5G insertion/deletion polymorphism in the (plasminogen activator type 1) PAI-1 gene. Additionally, the 311-bp Alu insertion/deletion in tPA's intron 8 has been associated with enhanced thrombosis; although genetic abnormalities have not been associated consistently with altered function or tPA levels, raising questions about the relevant pathophysiologic mechanism. Thrombin-activatable fibrinolysis inhibitor (TAFI) is a carboxypeptidase that regulates fibrinolysis; elevated plasma TAFI levels have been associated with an increased risk of both deep-vein thrombosis and cardiovascular disease.

The metabolic syndrome also is accompanied by altered fibrinolytic activity. This syndrome, which comprises abdominal fat (central obesity), altered glucose and insulin metabolism, dyslipidemia, and hypertension, has been associated with atherothrombosis. The mechanism for enhanced thrombosis appears to be due both to altered platelet function and to a procoagulant and hypofibrinolytic state. One of the most frequently documented prothrombotic abnormalities reported in this syndrome is an increase in plasma levels of PAI-1.

THE DISTINCTION BETWEEN ARTERIAL AND VENOUS THROMBOSIS

Although there is overlap, venous and arterial thrombosis are initiated differently and clot formation progresses by somewhat distinct pathways. In the setting of stasis or states of hypercoagulability, venous thrombosis is activated with the initiation of the coagulation cascade primarily due to exposure of tissue factor; this leads to the formation of thrombin and the subsequent conversion of fibrinogen to fibrin. In the artery, thrombin formation also occurs, but thrombosis is primarily promoted by the adhesion of platelets to an injured vessel and stimulated by exposed extracellular matrix (Figs. 117-1 and 117-2). There is wide variation in individual responses to vascular injury, an important determinant of which is the predisposition an individual has to arterial or venous thrombosis. This concept has been supported indirectly in prothrombotic animal models in which there is poor correlation between the propensity to develop venous versus arterial thrombosis.

Despite considerable progress in understanding the role of hypercoagulable states in venous thromboembolic disease, the contribution of hypercoagulability to arterial vascular disease is much less well understood. While specific thrombophilic conditions, such as factor V Leiden and the prothrombin G20210A mutation, are risk factors for DVT, pulmonary embolism, and other venous thromboembolic events, their contribution to arterial thrombosis is less well defined. In fact, to the contrary, many of these thrombophilic factors have not been found to be clinically important risk factors for arterial thrombotic events, such as acute coronary syndromes.

Clinically, although the pathophysiology is distinct, arterial and venous thrombosis do share common risk factors, including age, obesity, cigarette smoking, diabetes mellitus, arterial hypertension, hyperlipidemia, and metabolic syndrome. Select genetic variants, including those of the glutathione peroxidase gene, have also been associated with arterial and venous thrombo-occlusive disease. Importantly, arterial and venous thrombosis may both be triggered by pathophysiologic stimuli responsible for activating inflammatory and oxidative pathways.

The diagnosis and treatment of ischemic heart disease are discussed in Chap. 243. Stroke diagnosis and management are discussed in Chap. 275. The diagnosis and management of deep venous thrombosis and pulmonary embolus are discussed in Chap. 262.

ACKNOWLEDGMENT

The authors would like to thank Hannah Iafrati for her assistance with the figures.

FURTHER READINGS

ALEXANDER K, PETERSON ED: Managing the risks of antithrombotics and platelet inhibitors. Circulation 121:1960, 2010

DAVÍ G, PATRONO C: Platelet activation and atherothrombosis. N Engl J Med 13;357:2482, 2007

FREEDMAN JE: Translational therapeutics at the platelet vascular interface: oxidative stress and platelets. Arterioscler Thromb Vasc Biol 28:s11, 2008

FURIE B, FURIE BC: Mechanisms of thrombus formation. N Engl J Med 28;359:938, 2008

GURBEL PA, TANTRY US: Combination antithrombotic therapies. Circulation 121:569, 2010

LLOYD-JONES D et al. Heart disease and stroke statistics–2009 update. A report from the American Heart Association Statistics Committee and Stroke Statistics Subcommittee. Circulation 119:e21, 2009

TAPSON VF: Acute pulmonary embolism. N Engl J Med. 6;358:1037, 2008

CHAPTER **118**

Antiplatelet, Anticoagulant, and Fibrinolytic Drugs

Jeffrey I. Weitz

Arterial and venous thromboses are major causes of morbidity and mortality rates. Arterial thrombosis is the most common cause of acute myocardial infarction (MI), ischemic stroke, and limb gangrene, whereas deep-vein thrombosis (DVT) leads to pulmonary embolism (PE), which can be fatal, and to the postphlebitic syndrome. Most arterial thrombi are superimposed on disrupted atherosclerotic plaque because plaque rupture exposes thrombogenic material in the plaque core to the blood. This material then triggers platelet aggregation and fibrin formation, which results in the generation of a platelet-rich thrombus that can temporarily or permanently occlude blood flow. In contrast to arterial thrombi, venous thrombi rarely form at sites of obvious vascular disruption. Although they can develop after surgical trauma to veins or secondary to indwelling venous catheters, venous thrombi usually originate in the valve cusps of the deep veins of the calf or in the muscular sinuses, where they are triggered by stasis. Sluggish blood flow in these veins reduces the oxygen supply to the avascular valve cusps. Endothelial cells lining these valve cusps become activated and express adhesion molecules on their surface. Tissue factor–bearing leukocytes and microparticles adhere to these activated cells and induce coagulation. Local thrombus formation is exacerbated by reduced clearance of activated clotting factors as a result of impaired blood flow. If the thrombi extend into more proximal veins of the leg, thrombus fragments can dislodge, travel to the lungs, and produce a PE.

Arterial and venous thrombi are composed of platelets and fibrin, but the proportions differ. Arterial thrombi are rich in platelets because of the high shear in the injured arteries. In contrast,

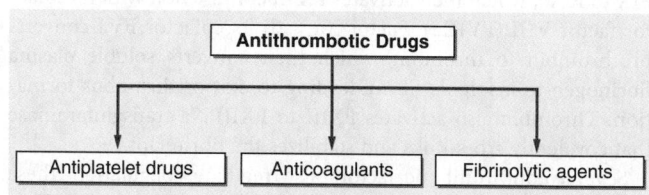

Figure 118-1 Classification of antithrombotic drugs.

venous thrombi, which form under low shear conditions, contain relatively few platelets and are predominantly composed of fibrin and trapped red cells. Because of the predominance of platelets, arterial thrombi appear white, whereas venous thrombi are red in color, reflecting the trapped red cells.

Antithrombotic drugs are used for prevention and treatment of thrombosis. Targeting the components of thrombi, these agents include (1) antiplatelet drugs, (2) anticoagulants, and (3) fibrinolytic agents (Fig. 118-1). With the predominance of platelets in arterial thrombi, strategies to inhibit or treat arterial thrombosis focus mainly on antiplatelet agents, although, in the acute setting, they often include anticoagulants and fibrinolytic agents. Anticoagulants are the mainstay of prevention and treatment of venous thromboembolism because fibrin is the predominant component of venous thrombi. Antiplatelet drugs are less effective than anticoagulants in this setting because of the limited platelet content of venous thrombi. Fibrinolytic therapy is used in selected patients with venous thromboembolism. For example, patients with massive or submassive PE can benefit from systemic or catheter-directed fibrinolytic therapy. The latter can also be used as an adjunct to anticoagulants for treatment of patients with extensive iliofemoral-vein thrombosis.

ANTIPLATELET DRUGS

■ ROLE OF PLATELETS IN ARTERIAL THROMBOSIS

In healthy vasculature, circulating platelets are maintained in an inactive state by nitric oxide (NO) and prostacyclin released by endothelial cells lining the blood vessels. In addition, endothelial cells also express CD39 on their surface, a membrane-associated ecto-adenosine diphosphatase (ADPase) that degrades ADP released from activated platelets. When

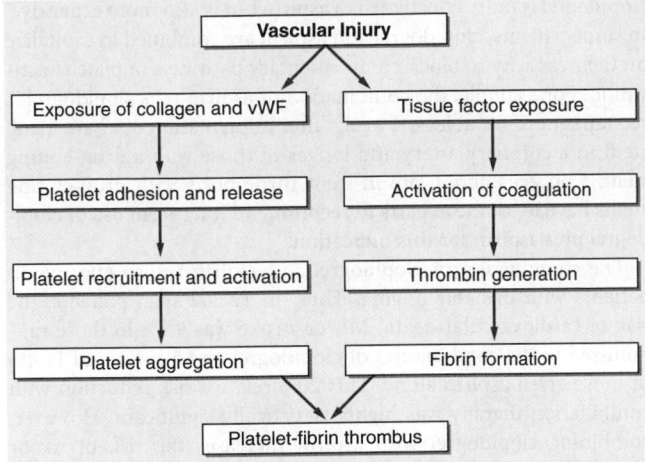

Figure 118-2 Coordinated role of platelets and the coagulation system in thrombogenesis. Vascular injury simultaneously triggers platelet activation and aggregation and activation of the coagulation system. Platelet activation is initiated by exposure of subendothelial collagen and von Willebrand factor (vWF), onto which platelets adhere. Adherent platelets become activated and release ADP and thromboxane A$_2$, platelet agonists that activate ambient platelets and recruit them to the site of injury. When platelets are activated, glycoprotein IIb/IIIa on their surface undergoes a conformational change that enables it to ligate fibrinogen and mediate platelet aggregation. Coagulation is triggered by tissue factor exposed at the site of injury. Tissue factor triggers thrombin generation. As a potent platelet agonist, thrombin amplifies platelet recruitment to the site of injury. Thrombin also converts fibrinogen to fibrin, and the fibrin strands then weave the platelet aggregates together to form a platelet/fibrin thrombus.

the vessel wall is damaged, release of these substances is impaired and subendothelial matrix is exposed. Platelets adhere to exposed collagen via $\alpha_2\beta_1$ and glycoprotein (GP)V1 and to von Willebrand factor (vWF) via GPIbα and GPIIb/IIIa ($\alpha_{IIb}\beta_3$)—receptors that are constitutively expressed on the platelet surface. Adherent platelets undergo a change in shape, secrete ADP from their dense granules, and synthesize and release thromboxane A$_2$. Released ADP and thromboxane A$_2$, which are platelet agonists, activate ambient platelets and recruit them to the site of vascular injury (Fig. 118-2).

Disruption of the vessel wall also exposes tissue factor–expressing cells to the blood. Tissue factor initiates coagulation. Activated platelets potentiate coagulation by binding clotting factors and supporting the assembly of activation complexes that enhance thrombin generation. In addition to converting fibrinogen to fibrin, thrombin also serves as a potent platelet agonist and recruits more platelets to the site of vascular injury.

When platelets are activated, GPIIb/IIIa, the most abundant receptor on the platelet surface, undergoes a conformational change that enables it to bind fibrinogen and, under high shear conditions, vWF. Divalent fibrinogen or multivalent vWF molecules bridge adjacent platelets together to form platelet aggregates. Fibrin strands, generated through the action of thrombin, then weave these aggregates together to form a platelet/fibrin mesh.

Antiplatelet drugs target various steps in this process. The commonly used drugs include aspirin, thienopyridines (clopidogrel, prasugrel, and ticlopidine), dipyridamole, and GPIIb/IIIa antagonists.

■ ASPIRIN

The most widely used antiplatelet agent worldwide is aspirin. As a cheap and effective antiplatelet drug, aspirin serves as the foundation of most antiplatelet strategies.

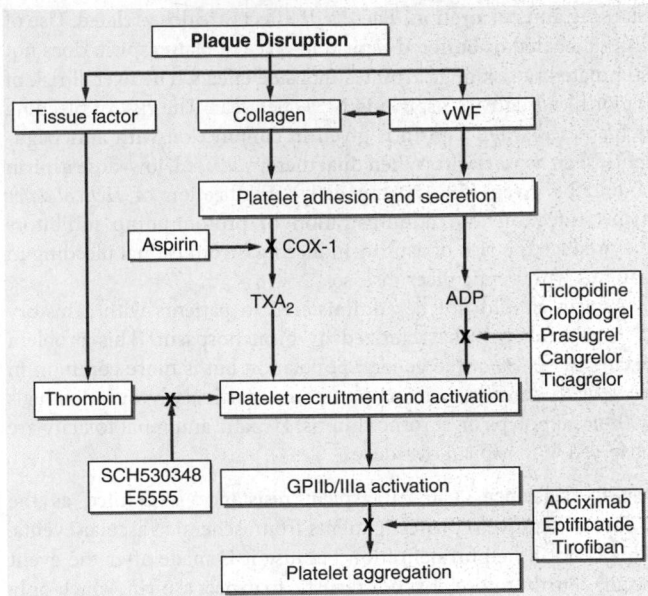

Figure 118-3 Site of action of antiplatelet drugs. Aspirin inhibits thromboxane A$_2$ (TXA$_2$) synthesis by irreversibly acetylating cyclooxygenase-1 (COX-1). Reduced TXA$_2$ release attenuates platelet activation and recruitment to the site of vascular injury. Ticlopidine, clopidogrel, and prasugrel irreversibly block P2Y$_{12}$, a key ADP receptor on the platelet surface; cangrelor and ticagrelor are reversible inhibitors of P2Y$_{12}$. Abciximab, eptifibatide, and tirofiban inhibit the final common pathway of platelet aggregation by blocking fibrinogen and von Willebrand factor binding to activated glycoprotein (GP) IIb/IIIa. SCH530348 and E5555 inhibit thrombin-mediated platelet activation by targeting protease-activated receptor-1 (PAR-1), the major thrombin receptor on human platelets.

Mechanism of action Aspirin produces its antithrombotic effect by irreversibly acetylating and inhibiting platelet cyclooxygenase (COX)-1 (Fig. 118-3), a critical enzyme in the biosynthesis of thromboxane A$_2$. At high doses (~1 g/d), aspirin also inhibits COX-2, an inducible COX isoform found in endothelial cells and inflammatory cells. In endothelial cells, COX-2 initiates the synthesis of prostacyclin, a potent vasodilator and inhibitor of platelet aggregation.

Indications Aspirin is widely used for secondary prevention of cardiovascular events in patients with coronary artery, cerebrovascular, or peripheral vascular disease. Compared with placebo, aspirin produces a 25% reduction in the risk of cardiovascular death, MI, or stroke. Aspirin is also used for primary prevention in patients whose estimated annual risk of MI is >1%, a point where its benefits are likely to outweigh harms. This includes patients older than age 40 years with two or more major risk factors for cardiovascular disease or those older than age 50 years with one or more such risk factors. Aspirin is equally effective in men and women. In men, aspirin mainly reduces the risk of MI, while in women aspirin lowers the risk of stroke.

Dosages Aspirin is usually administered at doses of 75–325 mg once daily. Higher doses of aspirin are not more effective than lower aspirin doses, and some analyses suggest reduced efficacy with higher doses. Because the side effects of aspirin are dose-related, daily aspirin doses of 75–100 mg are recommended for most indications. When rapid platelet inhibition is required, an initial aspirin dose of at least 160 mg should be given.

Side effects Most common side effects are gastrointestinal and range from dyspepsia to erosive gastritis or peptic ulcers with bleeding and perforation. These side effects are dose-related. Use of enteric-coated or buffered aspirin in place of plain aspirin does not eliminate the risk of gastrointestinal side effects. The overall risk of major bleeding with aspirin is 1–3% per year. The risk of bleeding is increased when aspirin is given in conjunction with anticoagulants, such as warfarin. When dual therapy is used, low-dose aspirin should be given (75–100 mg daily). Eradication of *Helicobacter pylori* infection and administration of proton pump inhibitors may reduce the risk of aspirin-induced gastrointestinal bleeding in patients with peptic ulcer disease.

Aspirin should not be administered to patients with a history of aspirin allergy characterized by bronchospasm. This problem occurs in ~0.3% of the general population but is more common in those with chronic urticaria or asthma, particularly in individuals with nasal polyps or chronic rhinitis. Hepatic and renal toxicity are observed with aspirin overdose.

Aspirin resistance Clinical aspirin resistance is defined as the failure of aspirin to protect patients from ischemic vascular events. This is not a helpful definition because it is made after the event occurs. Furthermore, it is not realistic to expect aspirin, which only blocks thromboxane A_2–induced platelet activation, to prevent all vascular events.

Aspirin resistance has also been described biochemically as failure of the drug to produce its expected inhibitory effects on tests of platelet function, such as thromboxane A_2 synthesis or arachidonic acid–induced platelet aggregation. However, the tests of platelet function used for diagnosis of biochemical aspirin resistance have not been well standardized. Furthermore, these tests are not proven to identify patients at risk of recurrent vascular events. In addition, resistance is not reversed by either giving higher doses of aspirin or adding other antiplatelet drugs. Thus, testing for aspirin resistance remains a research tool.

■ THIENOPYRIDINES

The thienopyridines include ticlopidine, clopidogrel, and prasugrel, drugs that target $P2Y_{12}$, a key ADP receptor on platelets.

Mechanism of action The thienopyridines are structurally related drugs that selectively inhibit ADP-induced platelet aggregation by irreversibly blocking $P2Y_{12}$ (Fig. 118-3). Ticlopidine and clopidogrel are prodrugs that require metabolism by the hepatic cytochrome P450 (CYP) enzyme system to acquire activity. Consequently, when given in usual doses, their onset of action is delayed for several days. Although prasugrel also is a prodrug that requires metabolic activation, its onset of action is more rapid than that of ticlopidine or clopidogrel, and prasugrel produces greater and more predictable inhibition of ADP-induced platelet aggregation. These characteristics reflect the rapid and complete absorption of prasugrel from the gut and its more efficient activation pathways. Whereas nearly all of the absorbed prasugrel undergoes metabolic activation in the liver, only 15% of absorbed clopidogrel is activated; the remainder is inactivated by esterases.

Indications Like aspirin, ticlopidine is more effective than placebo at reducing the risk of cardiovascular death, MI, and stroke in patients with atherosclerotic disease. Because of its delayed onset of action, ticlopidine is not recommended in patients with acute MI. Ticlopidine was used routinely as an adjunct to aspirin after coronary artery stenting and as an aspirin substitute in those intolerant to aspirin. Because clopidogrel is more potent than ticlopidine and has a better safety profile, clopidogrel has replaced ticlopidine.

When compared with aspirin in patients with recent ischemic stroke, MI, or peripheral arterial disease, clopidogrel reduced the risk of cardiovascular death, MI, and stroke by 8.7%. Therefore,

clopidogrel is more effective than aspirin but is also more expensive. In some patients, clopidogrel and aspirin are combined to capitalize on their capacity to block complementary pathways of platelet activation. For example, the combination of aspirin plus clopidogrel is recommended for at least 4 weeks after implantation of a bare metal stent in a coronary artery and longer in those with a drug-eluting stent. Concerns about late in-stent thrombosis with drug-eluting stents have led some experts to recommend long-term use of clopidogrel plus aspirin for this indication.

The combination of clopidogrel and aspirin is also effective in patients with unstable angina. Thus, in 12,562 such patients, the risk of cardiovascular death, MI, or stroke was 9.3% in those randomized to the combination of clopidogrel and aspirin and 11.4% in those given aspirin alone. This 20% relative risk reduction with combination therapy was highly statistically significant. However, combining clopidogrel with aspirin increases the risk of major bleeding to about 2% per year. This bleeding risk persists even if the daily dose of aspirin is ≤100 mg. Therefore, the combination of clopidogrel and aspirin should only be used when there is a clear benefit. For example, this combination has not proven to be superior to clopidogrel alone in patients with acute ischemic stroke or to aspirin alone for primary prevention in those at risk for cardiovascular events.

Prasugrel was compared with clopidogrel in 13,608 patients with acute coronary syndromes who were scheduled to undergo a percutaneous coronary intervention. The incidence of the primary efficacy endpoint, a composite of cardiovascular death, MI, and stroke, was significantly lower with prasugrel than with clopidogrel (9.9% and 12.1%, respectively), mainly reflecting a reduction in the incidence of nonfatal MI. The incidence of stent thrombosis also was significantly lower with prasugrel than with clopidogrel (1.1% and 2.4%, respectively). However, these advantages were at the expense of significantly higher rates of fatal bleeding (0.4% and 0.1%, respectively) and life-threatening bleeding (1.4% and 0.9%, respectively) with prasugrel. Because patients older than age 75 years and those with a history of prior stroke or transient ischemic attack have a particularly high risk of bleeding, prasugrel should generally be avoided in older patients, and the drug is contraindicated in those with a history of cerebrovascular disease. Caution is required if prasugrel is used in patients weighing less than 60 kg or in those with renal impairment.

Dosing Ticlopidine is given twice daily at a dose of 250 mg. The more potent clopidogrel is given once daily at a dose of 75 mg. Loading doses of clopidogrel are given when rapid ADP receptor blockade is desired. For example, patients undergoing coronary stenting are often given a loading dose of 300 mg, which affects inhibition of ADP-induced platelet aggregation in about 6 h. Loading doses of 600 or 900 mg produce an even more rapid effect. After a loading dose of 60 mg, prasugrel is given once daily at a dose of 10 mg. Patients older than age 75 years or weighing less than 60 kg should receive a lower daily prasugrel dose of 5 mg.

Side effects The most common side effects of ticlopidine are gastrointestinal. More serious are the hematologic side effects, which include neutropenia, thrombocytopenia, and thrombotic thrombocytopenic purpura. These side effects usually occur within the first few months of starting treatment. Therefore, blood counts must be carefully monitored when initiating therapy with ticlopidine. Gastrointestinal and hematologic side effects are rare with clopidogrel and prasugrel.

Thienopyridine resistance The capacity of clopidogrel to inhibit ADP-induced platelet aggregation varies among subjects. This variability reflects, at least in part, genetic polymorphisms in the CYP isoenzymes involved in the metabolic activation of clopidogrel.

Most important of these is *CYP2C19*. Clopidogrel-treated patients with the loss-of-function *CYP2C19*2* allele exhibit reduced platelet inhibition compared with those with the wild-type *CYP2C19*1* allele and experience a higher rate of cardiovascular events. This is important because estimates suggest that up to 25% of whites, 30% of African Americans, and 50% of Asians carry the loss-of-function allele, which would render them resistant to clopidogrel. Even patients with the reduced function *CYP2C19*3, *4*, or **5* alleles may derive less benefit from clopidogrel than those with the full-function *CYP2C19*1* allele. Concomitant administration of clopidogrel and proton pump inhibitors, which are inhibitors of *CYP2C19*, produces a small reduction in the inhibitory effects of clopidogrel on ADP-induced platelet aggregation. The extent to which this interaction increases the risk of cardiovascular events remains controversial.

In contrast to their effect on the metabolic activation of clopidogrel, *CYP2C19* polymorphisms appear to be less important determinants of the activation of prasugrel. Thus, no association was detected between the loss-of-function allele and decreased platelet inhibition or increased rate of cardiovascular events with prasugrel. The observation that genetic polymorphisms affecting clopidogrel absorption or metabolism influence clinical outcomes raises the possibilities that pharmacogenetic profiling may be useful to identify clopidogrel-resistant patients and that point-of-care assessment of the extent of clopidogrel-induced platelet inhibition may help detect patients at higher risk for subsequent cardiovascular events. It is unknown whether administration of higher doses of clopidogrel to such patients will overcome this resistance. Instead, prasugrel or newer $P2Y_{12}$ inhibitors may be better choices for these patients.

■ DIPYRIDAMOLE

Dipyridamole is a relatively weak antiplatelet agent on its own, but an extended-release formulation of dipyridamole combined with low-dose aspirin, a preparation known as *Aggrenox*, is used for prevention of stroke in patients with transient ischemic attacks.

Mechanism of action By inhibiting phosphodiesterase, dipyridamole blocks the breakdown of cyclic AMP. Increased levels of cyclic AMP reduce intracellular calcium and inhibit platelet activation. Dipyridamole also blocks the uptake of adenosine by platelets and other cells. This produces a further increase in local cyclic AMP levels because the platelet adenosine A_2 receptor is coupled to adenylate cyclase (Fig. 118-4).

Dosing Aggrenox is given twice daily. Each capsule contains 200 mg of extended-release dipyridamole and 25 mg of aspirin.

Side effects Because dipyridamole has vasodilatory effects, it must be used with caution in patients with coronary artery disease. Gastrointestinal complaints, headache, facial flushing, dizziness, and hypotension can also occur. These symptoms often subside with continued use of the drug.

Indications Dipyridamole plus aspirin was compared with aspirin or dipyridamole alone, or with placebo, in patients with an ischemic stroke or transient ischemic attack. The combination reduced the

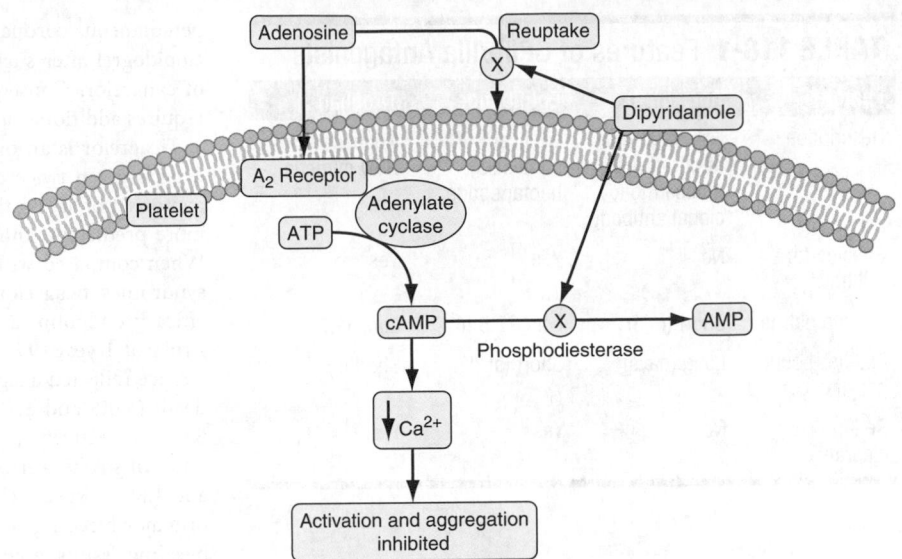

Figure 118-4   Mechanism of action of dipyridamole. Dipyridamole increases levels of cyclic AMP in platelets by (1) blocking the reuptake of adenosine and (2) inhibiting phosphodiesterase-mediated cyclic AMP degradation. By promoting calcium uptake, cyclic AMP reduces intracellular levels of calcium. This, in turn, inhibits platelet activation and aggregation.

risk of stroke by 22.1% compared with aspirin and by 24.4% compared with dipyridamole. A second trial compared dipyridamole plus aspirin with aspirin alone for secondary prevention in patients with ischemic stroke. Vascular death, stroke, or MI occurred in 13% of patients given combination therapy and in 16% of those treated with aspirin alone. Based on these data, Aggrenox was often used for stroke prevention. Another trial randomized 20,332 patients with noncardioembolic ischemic stroke to either Aggrenox or clopidogrel. The primary efficacy endpoint of recurrent stroke occurred in 9.0% of those given Aggrenox and in 8.8% of patients treated with clopidogrel. Although this difference was not statistically significant, the study failed to meet the prespecified margin to claim noninferiority of Aggrenox relative to clopidogrel. These results have dampened enthusiasm for the use of Aggrenox.

Because of its vasodilatory effects and the paucity of data supporting the use of dipyridamole in patients with symptomatic coronary artery disease, Aggrenox should not be used for stroke prevention in such patients. Clopidogrel is a better choice in this setting.

■ GPIIb/IIIa RECEPTOR ANTAGONISTS

As a class, parenteral GPIIb/IIIa receptor antagonists have an established niche in patients with acute coronary syndromes. The three agents in this class are abciximab, eptifibatide, and tirofiban.

Mechanism of action A member of the integrin family of adhesion receptors, GPIIb/IIIa is found on the surface of platelets and megakaryocytes. With about 80,000 copies per platelet, GPIIb/IIIa is the most abundant receptor. Consisting of a noncovalently linked heterodimer, GPIIb/IIIa is inactive on resting platelets. When platelets are activated, inside-outside signal transduction pathways trigger a conformational activation of the receptor. Once activated, GPIIb/IIIa binds adhesive molecules, such as fibrinogen and, under high shear conditions, vWF. Binding is mediated by the Arg-Gly-Asp (RGD) sequence found on the α chains of fibrinogen and on vWF, and by the Lys-Gly-Asp (KGD) sequence located within a unique dodecapeptide domain on the γ chains of fibrinogen. Once bound, fibrinogen and/or vWF bridge adjacent platelets together to induce platelet aggregation.

TABLE 118-1 Features of GPIIb/IIIa Antagonists

Feature	Abciximab	Eptifibatide	Tirofiban
Description	Fab fragment of humanized mouse monoclonal antibody	Cyclical KGD-containing heptapeptide	Nonpeptidic RGD mimetic
Specific for GPIIb/IIIa	No	Yes	Yes
Plasma half-life	Short (min)	Long (2.5 h)	Long (2.0 h)
Platelet-bound half-life	Long (days)	Short (s)	Short (s)
Renal clearance	No	Yes	Yes

Although abciximab, eptifibatide, and tirofiban all target the GPIIb/IIIa receptor, they are structurally and pharmacologically distinct (Table 118-1). Abciximab is a Fab fragment of a humanized murine monoclonal antibody directed against the activated form of GPIIb/IIIa. Abciximab binds to the activated receptor with high affinity and blocks the binding of adhesive molecules. In contrast to abciximab, eptifibatide and tirofiban are synthetic small molecules. Eptifibatide is a cyclic heptapeptide that binds GPIIb/IIIa because it incorporates the KGD motif, whereas tirofiban is a nonpeptidic tyrosine derivative that acts as an RGD mimetic. Abciximab has a long half-life and can be detected on the surface of platelets for up to 2 weeks. Eptifibatide and tirofiban have shorter half-lives.

In addition to targeting the GPIIb/IIIa receptor, abciximab also inhibits the closely related $\alpha_v\beta_3$ receptor, which binds vitronectin, and $\alpha_M\beta_2$, a leukocyte integrin. In contrast, eptifibatide and tirofiban are specific for GPIIb/IIIa. Inhibition of $\alpha_v\beta_3$ and $\alpha_M\beta_2$ may endow abciximab with anti-inflammatory and/or antiproliferative properties that extend beyond platelet inhibition.

Dosing All of the GPIIb/IIIa antagonists are given as an IV bolus followed by an infusion. Because they are cleared by the kidneys, the doses of eptifibatide and tirofiban must be reduced in patients with renal insufficiency.

Side effects In addition to bleeding, thrombocytopenia is the most serious complication. Thrombocytopenia is immune-mediated and is caused by antibodies directed against neoantigens on GPIIb/IIIa that are exposed upon antagonist binding. With abciximab, thrombocytopenia occurs in up to 5% of patients. Thrombocytopenia is severe in ~1% of these individuals. Thrombocytopenia is less common with the other two agents, occurring in ~1% of patients.

Indications Abciximab and eptifibatide are used in patients undergoing percutaneous coronary interventions, particularly those with acute MI. Tirofiban is used in high-risk patients with unstable angina. Eptifibatide also can be used for this indication.

■ NEW ANTIPLATELET AGENTS

New agents in advanced stages of development include cangrelor and ticagrelor, direct-acting reversible P2Y$_{12}$ antagonists, and SCH530348 (vorapaxar) and E5555 (atopaxar), orally active inhibitors of protease-activated receptor 1 (PAR-1), the major thrombin receptor on platelets (Fig. 118-3). Cangrelor is an adenosine analogue that binds reversibly to P2Y$_{12}$ and inhibits its activity. The drug has a half-life of 3–6 min and is given intravenously as a bolus followed by an infusion. When stopped, platelet function recovers within 60 min. Trials comparing cangrelor with placebo during

percutaneous coronary interventions or comparing cangrelor with clopidogrel after such procedures revealed little or no advantages of cangrelor. Consequently, identification of a role for cangrelor requires additional studies.

Ticagrelor is an orally active, reversible inhibitor of P2Y$_{12}$. The drug is given twice daily and it not only has a more rapid onset and offset of action than clopidogrel but also produces greater and more predictable inhibition of ADP-induced platelet aggregation. When compared with clopidogrel in patients with acute coronary syndromes, ticagrelor produced a greater reduction in the primary efficacy endpoint, a composite of cardiovascular death, MI, and stroke at 1 year (9.8% and 11.7%, respectively; $p = .001$). This difference reflected a significantly greater reduction in cardiovascular death (4.0% and 5.1%, respectively; $p = .001$) and MI (5.8% and 6.9%, respectively; $p = .005$) with ticagrelor than with clopidogrel. Rates of stroke were similar with ticagrelor and clopidogrel (1.5% and 1.3%, respectively) and there were no differences in the rates of major bleeding. When minor bleeding was added to the major bleeding results, however, ticagrelor showed an increase relative to clopidogrel (16.1% and 14.6%, respectively; $p = 0.008$). Ticagrelor also was superior to clopidogrel in the acute coronary syndrome patients who underwent percutaneous coronary interventions or aortocoronary bypass surgery. Although not yet licensed, ticagrelor is the first new antiplatelet drug to demonstrate a greater reduction in cardiovascular death than clopidogrel in patients with acute coronary syndromes.

SCH530348, an orally active inhibitor of PAR-1, is under investigation as an adjunct to aspirin or aspirin plus clopidogrel. Two large phase III trials are underway. E5555, a second oral PAR-1 antagonist, is earlier in development.

ANTICOAGULANTS

There are both parenteral and oral anticoagulants. Currently available parenteral anticoagulants include heparin, low-molecular-weight heparin (LMWH), and fondaparinux, a synthetic pentasaccharide. The only available oral anticoagulants are the vitamin K antagonists, of which warfarin is the agent most often used in North America.

Dabigatran etexilate, an oral thrombin inhibitor, and rivaroxaban, an oral Factor Xa inhibitor, are licensed in Europe and Canada for short-term thromboprophylaxis after elective hip or knee replacement surgery. Dabigatran etexilate was licensed in the United States and Canada as an alternative to warfarin for stroke prevention in patients with atrial fibrillation.

■ PARENTERAL ANTICOAGULANTS

Heparin

Heparin is a sulfated polysaccharide and is isolated from mammalian tissues rich in mast cells. Most commercial heparin is derived from porcine intestinal mucosa and is a polymer of alternating D-glucuronic acid and N-acetyl-D-glucosamine residues.

Mechanism of action Heparin acts as an anticoagulant by activating antithrombin (previously known as antithrombin III) and accelerating the rate at which antithrombin inhibits clotting enzymes, particularly thrombin and factor Xa. Antithrombin, the obligatory plasma cofactor for heparin, is a member of the serine protease inhibitor (serpin) superfamily. Synthesized in the liver and circulating in plasma at a concentration of $2.6 \pm 0.4\ \mu M$, antithrombin acts as a suicide substrate for its target enzymes.

To activate antithrombin, heparin binds to the serpin via a unique pentasaccharide sequence that is found on one-third of the chains of commercial heparin (Fig. 118-5). The remainder of the heparin chains that lack this pentasaccharide sequence have little or no anticoagulant activity. Once bound to antithrombin, heparin induces a conformational change in the reactive center loop of

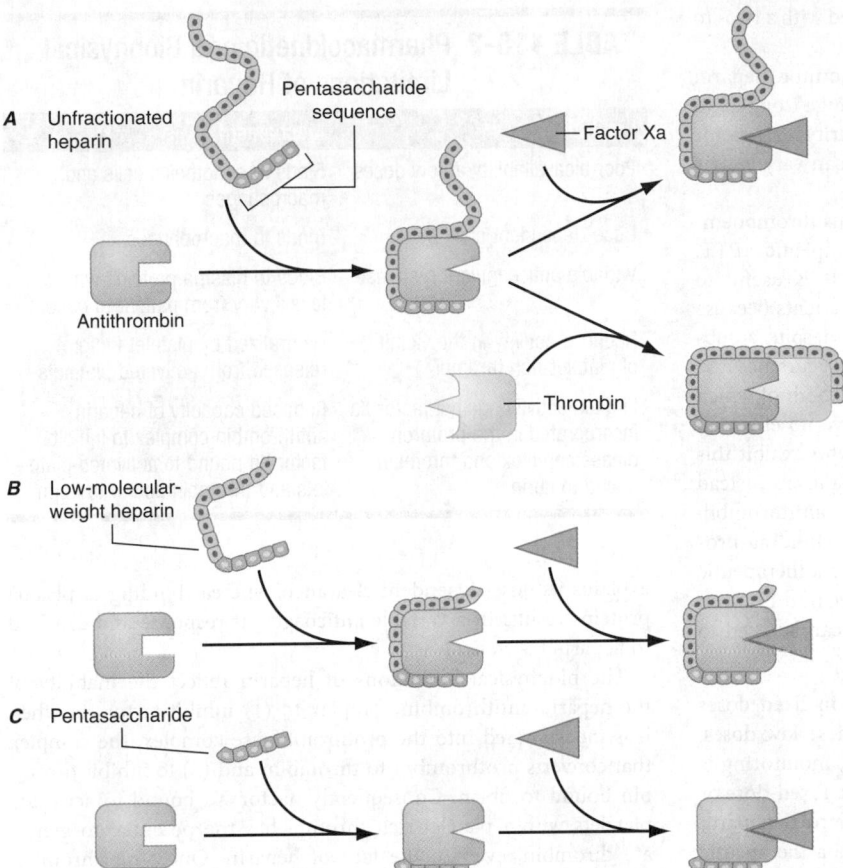

Figure 118-5 Mechanism of action of heparin, low-molecular-weight heparin (LMWH), and fondaparinux, a synthetic pentasaccharide. A. Heparin binds to antithrombin via its pentasaccharide sequence. This induces a conformational change in the reactive center loop of antithrombin that accelerates its interaction with factor Xa. To potentiate thrombin inhibition, heparin must simultaneously bind to antithrombin and thrombin. Only heparin chains composed of at least 18 saccharide units, which corresponds to a molecular weight of 5400, are of sufficient length to perform this bridging function. With a mean molecular weight of 15,000, all of the heparin chains are long enough to do this. **B.** LMWH has greater capacity to potentiate factor Xa inhibition by antithrombin than thrombin because, with a mean molecular weight of 4500–5000, at least half of the LMWH chains are too short to bridge antithrombin to thrombin. **C.** The pentasaccharide only accelerates factor Xa inhibition by antithrombin because the pentasaccharide is too short to bridge antithrombin to thrombin.

of tissue factor–bound factor VIIa, TFPI may contribute to the antithrombotic activity of heparin. Longer heparin chains induce the release of more TFPI than shorter chains.

Pharmacology Heparin must be given parenterally. It is usually administered SC or by continuous IV infusion. When used for therapeutic purposes, the IV route is most often employed. If heparin is given SC for treatment of thrombosis, the dose of heparin must be high enough to overcome the limited bioavailability associated with this method of delivery.

In the circulation, heparin binds to the endothelium and to plasma proteins other than antithrombin. Heparin binding to endothelial cells explains its dose-dependent clearance. At low doses, the half-life of heparin is short because it binds rapidly to the endothelium. With higher doses of heparin, the half-life is longer because heparin is cleared more slowly once the endothelium is saturated. Clearance is mainly extrarenal; heparin binds to macrophages, which internalize and depolymerize the long heparin chains and secrete shorter chains back into the circulation. Because of its dose-dependent clearance mechanism, the plasma half-life of heparin ranges from 30 to 60 min with bolus IV doses of 25 and 100 U/kg, respectively.

Once heparin enters the circulation, it binds to plasma proteins other than antithrombin, a phenomenon that reduces its anticoagulant activity. Some of the heparin-binding proteins found in plasma are acute-phase reactants whose levels are elevated in ill patients. Others, such as high-molecular-weight multimers of vWF, are released from activated platelets or endothelial cells. Activated platelets also release platelet factor 4 (PF4), a highly cationic protein that binds heparin with high affinity. The large amounts of PF4 found in the vicinity of platelet-rich arterial thrombi can neutralize the anticoagulant activity of heparin. This phenomenon may attenuate heparin's capacity to suppress thrombus growth.

antithrombin that renders it more readily accessible to its target proteases. This conformational change enhances the rate at which antithrombin inhibits Factor Xa by at least two orders of magnitude but has little effect on the rate of thrombin inhibition by antithrombin. To catalyze thrombin inhibition, heparin serves as a template that binds antithrombin and thrombin simultaneously. Formation of this ternary complex brings the enzyme in close apposition to the inhibitor, thereby promoting the formation of a stable covalent thrombin-antithrombin complex.

Only pentasaccharide-containing heparin chains composed of at least 18 saccharide units (which correspond to a molecular weight of 5400) are of sufficient length to bridge thrombin and antithrombin together. With a mean molecular weight of 15,000, and a range of 5000–30,000, almost all of the chains of unfractionated heparin are long enough to effect this bridging function. Consequently, by definition, heparin has equal capacity to promote the inhibition of thrombin and factor Xa by antithrombin and is assigned an anti-factor Xa to anti-factor IIa (thrombin) ratio of 1:1.

Heparin causes the release of tissue factor pathway inhibitor (TFPI) from the endothelium. A factor Xa–dependent inhibitor

Because the levels of heparin-binding proteins in plasma vary from person to person, the anticoagulant response to fixed or weight-adjusted doses of heparin is unpredictable. Consequently, coagulation monitoring is essential to ensure that a therapeutic response is obtained. This is particularly important when heparin is administered for treatment of established thrombosis because a subtherapeutic anticoagulant response may render patients at risk for recurrent thrombosis, whereas excessive anticoagulation increases the risk of bleeding.

Monitoring the anticoagulant effect Heparin therapy can be monitored using the activated partial thromboplastin time (aPTT) or anti-factor Xa level. Although the aPTT is the test most often employed for this purpose, there are problems with this assay. aPTT reagents vary in their sensitivity to heparin, and the type of coagulometer used for testing can influence the results. Consequently, laboratories must establish a therapeutic aPTT range with each reagent-coagulometer combination by measuring the aPTT and anti-factor Xa level in plasma samples collected from heparin-treated patients. For most of the aPTT reagents and coagulometers in current use, therapeutic heparin levels are achieved with a two- to threefold prolongation of the aPTT.

Anti-factor Xa levels also can be used to monitor heparin therapy. With this test, therapeutic heparin levels range from 0.3 to 0.7 units/mL. Although this test is gaining in popularity, anti-factor Xa assays have yet to be standardized, and results can vary widely between laboratories.

Up to 25% of heparin-treated patients with venous thromboembolism require >35,000 units/d to achieve a therapeutic aPTT. These patients are considered heparin resistant. It is useful to measure anti-factor Xa levels in heparin-resistant patients because many will have a therapeutic anti-factor Xa level despite a subtherapeutic aPTT. This dissociation in test results occurs because elevated plasma levels of fibrinogen and factor VIII, both of which are acute-phase proteins, shorten the aPTT but have no effect on anti-factor Xa levels. Heparin therapy in patients who exhibit this phenomenon is best monitored using anti-factor Xa levels instead of the aPTT. Patients with congenital or acquired antithrombin deficiency and those with elevated levels of heparin-binding proteins may also need high doses of heparin to achieve a therapeutic aPTT or anti-factor Xa level. If there is good correlation between the aPTT and the anti-factor Xa levels, either test can be used to monitor heparin therapy.

Dosing For prophylaxis, heparin is usually given in fixed doses of 5000 units SC two or three times daily. With these low doses, coagulation monitoring is unnecessary. In contrast, monitoring is essential when the drug is given in therapeutic doses. Fixed-dose or weight-based heparin nomograms are used to standardize heparin dosing and to shorten the time required to achieve a therapeutic anticoagulant response. At least two heparin nomograms have been validated in patients with venous thromboembolism and reduce the time required to achieve a therapeutic aPTT. Weight-adjusted heparin nomograms have also been evaluated in patients with acute coronary syndromes. After an IV heparin bolus of 5000 units or 70 units/kg, a heparin infusion rate of 12–15 units/kg per hour is usually administered. In contrast, weight-adjusted heparin nomograms for patients with venous thromboembolism use an initial bolus of 5000 units or 80 units/kg, followed by an infusion of 18 units/kg per hour. Thus, patients with venous thromboembolism appear to require higher doses of heparin to achieve a therapeutic aPTT than do patients with acute coronary syndromes. This may reflect differences in the thrombus burden. Heparin binds to fibrin, and the fibrin content of extensive deep-vein thrombi is greater than that of small coronary thrombi.

Heparin manufacturers in North America have traditionally measured heparin potency in USP units, with a unit defined as the concentration of heparin that prevents 1 mL of citrated sheep plasma from clotting for 1 h after calcium addition. In contrast, manufacturers in Europe measure heparin potency with anti-Xa assays using an international heparin standard for comparison. Because of problems with heparin contamination with oversulfated chondroitin sulfate, which the USP assay system does not detect, North American heparin manufacturers now use the anti-Xa assay to assess heparin potency. Although use of international units in place of USP units results in a 10% reduction in heparin doses, this change is unlikely to affect patient care because heparin has been dosed in international units in Europe for many years. Furthermore, heparin monitoring ensures a therapeutic anticoagulant response in high-risk situations, such as cardiopulmonary bypass surgery or percutaneous coronary intervention.

Limitations Heparin has pharmacokinetic and biophysical limitations (Table 118-2). The pharmacokinetic limitations reflect heparin's propensity to bind in a pentasaccharide-independent fashion to cells and plasma proteins. Heparin binding to endothelial cells

TABLE 118-2 Pharmacokinetic and Biophysical Limitations of Heparin

Limitations	Mechanism
Poor bioavailability at low doses	Binds to endothelial cells and macrophages
Dose-dependent clearance	Binds to macrophages
Variable anticoagulant response	Binds to plasma proteins whose levels vary from patient to patient
Reduced activity in the vicinity of platelet-rich thrombi	Neutralized by platelet factor 4 released from activated platelets
Limited activity against factor Xa incorporated in the prothrombinase complex and thrombin bound to fibrin	Reduced capacity of heparin-antithrombin complex to inhibit factor Xa bound to activated platelets and thrombin bound to fibrin

explains its dose-dependent clearance, whereas binding to plasma proteins results in a variable anticoagulant response and can lead to heparin resistance.

The biophysical limitations of heparin reflect the inability of the heparin-antithrombin complex to (1) inhibit factor Xa when it is incorporated into the prothrombinase complex, the complex that converts prothrombin to thrombin, and (2) to inhibit thrombin bound to fibrin. Consequently, factor Xa bound to activated platelets within platelet-rich thrombi has the potential to generate thrombin, even in the face of heparin. Once this thrombin binds to fibrin, it too is protected from inhibition by the heparin-antithrombin complex. Clot-associated thrombin can then trigger thrombus growth by locally activating platelets and amplifying its own generation through feedback activation of factors V, VIII, and XI. Further compounding the problem is the potential for heparin neutralization by the high concentrations of PF4 released from activated platelets within the platelet-rich thrombus.

Side effects The most common side effect of heparin is bleeding. Other complications include thrombocytopenia, osteoporosis, and elevated levels of transaminases.

Bleeding The risk of heparin-induced bleeding increases with higher heparin doses. Concomitant administration of drugs that affect hemostasis, such as antiplatelet or fibrinolytic agents, increases the risk of bleeding, as does recent surgery or trauma. Heparin-treated patients with serious bleeding can be given protamine sulfate to neutralize the heparin. Protamine sulfate, a mixture of basic polypeptides isolated from salmon sperm, binds heparin with high affinity, and the resultant protamine-heparin complexes are then cleared. Typically, 1 mg of protamine sulfate neutralizes 100 units of heparin. Protamine sulfate is given IV. Anaphylactoid reactions to protamine sulfate can occur, and drug administration by slow IV infusion is recommended to reduce the risk.

Thrombocytopenia Heparin can cause thrombocytopenia. Heparin-induced thrombocytopenia (HIT) is an antibody-mediated process that is triggered by antibodies directed against neoantigens on PF4 that are exposed when heparin binds to this protein. These antibodies, which are usually of the IgG isotype, bind simultaneously to the heparin-PF4 complex and to platelet Fc receptors. Such binding activates the platelets and generates platelet microparticles. Circulating microparticles are prothrombotic because they express anionic phospholipids on their surface and can bind clotting factors and promote thrombin generation.

The clinical features of HIT are illustrated in Table 118-3. Typically, HIT occurs 5–14 days after initiation of heparin

TABLE 118-3 Features of Heparin-Induced Thrombocytopenia

Features	Details
Thrombocytopenia	Platelet count of ≤100,000/μL or a decrease in platelet count of ≥50%
Timing	Platelet count falls 5–10 days after starting heparin
Type of heparin	More common with unfractionated heparin than low-molecular-weight heparin
Type of patient	More common in surgical patients and patients with cancer than general medical patients. More common in women than in men
Thrombosis	Venous thrombosis more common than arterial thrombosis

therapy, but it can manifest earlier if the patient has received heparin within the past 3 months. It is rare for the platelet count to fall below 100,000/μL in patients with HIT, and even a 50% decrease in the platelet count from the pretreatment value should raise the suspicion of HIT in those receiving heparin. HIT is more common in surgical patients than in medical patients and, like many autoimmune disorders, occurs more frequently in females than in males.

HIT can be associated with thrombosis, either arterial or venous. Venous thrombosis, which manifests as DVT and/or PE, is more common than arterial thrombosis. Arterial thrombosis can manifest as ischemic stroke or acute MI. Rarely, platelet-rich thrombi in the distal aorta or iliac arteries can cause critical limb ischemia.

The diagnosis of HIT is established using enzyme-linked assays to detect antibodies against heparin-PF4 complexes or with platelet activation assays. Enzyme-linked assays are sensitive but can be positive in the absence of any clinical evidence of HIT. The most specific diagnostic test is the serotonin release assay. This test is performed by quantifying serotonin release when washed platelets loaded with labeled serotonin are exposed to patient serum in the absence or presence of varying concentrations of heparin. If the patient serum contains the HIT antibody, heparin addition induces platelet activation and serotonin release.

Management of HIT is outlined in Table 118-4. Heparin should be stopped in patients with suspected or documented HIT, and an alternative anticoagulant should be administered to prevent or treat thrombosis. The agents most often used for this indication are

TABLE 118-4 Management of Heparin-Induced Thrombocytopenia

Stop all heparin

Give an alternative anticoagulant, such as lepirudin, argatroban, bivalirudin, or fondaparinux

Do not give platelet transfusions

Do not give warfarin until the platelet count returns to its baseline level. If warfarin is administered, give vitamin K to restore the INR to normal

Evaluate for thrombosis, particularly deep-vein thrombosis

Abbreviation: INR, International normalized ratio.

parenteral direct thrombin inhibitors, such as lepirudin, argatroban, or bivalirudin, or factor Xa inhibitors, such as fondaparinux.

Patients with HIT, particularly those with associated thrombosis, often have evidence of increased thrombin generation that can lead to consumption of protein C. If these patients are given warfarin without a concomitant parenteral anticoagulant to inhibit thrombin or thrombin generation, the further decrease in protein C levels induced by the vitamin K antagonist can trigger skin necrosis. To avoid this problem, patients with HIT should be treated with a direct thrombin inhibitor or fondaparinux until the platelet count returns to normal levels. At this point, low-dose warfarin therapy can be introduced, and the thrombin inhibitor can be discontinued when the anticoagulant response to warfarin has been therapeutic for at least 2 days.

Osteoporosis Treatment with therapeutic doses of heparin for >1 month can cause a reduction in bone density. This complication has been reported in up to 30% of patients given long-term heparin therapy, and symptomatic vertebral fractures occur in 2–3% of these individuals.

Heparin causes bone loss both by decreasing bone formation and by enhancing bone resorption. Thus, heparin affects the activity of both osteoblasts and osteoclasts.

Elevated levels of transaminases Therapeutic doses of heparin frequently cause modest elevation in the serum levels of hepatic transaminases, without a concomitant increase in the level of bilirubin. The levels of transaminases rapidly return to normal when the drug is stopped. The mechanism of this phenomenon is unknown.

Low-molecular-weight heparin

Consisting of smaller fragments of heparin, LMWH is prepared from unfractionated heparin by controlled enzymatic or chemical depolymerization. The mean molecular weight of LMWH is 5000, one-third the mean molecular weight of unfractionated heparin. LMWH has advantages over heparin (Table 118-5) and has replaced heparin for most indications.

Mechanism of action   Like heparin, LMWH exerts its anticoagulant activity by activating antithrombin. With a mean molecular weight of 5000, which corresponds to about 17 saccharide units, at least half of the pentasaccharide-containing chains of LMWH are too short to bridge thrombin to antithrombin (Fig. 118-5). However, these chains retain the capacity to accelerate factor Xa inhibition by antithrombin because this activity is largely the result of the conformational changes in antithrombin evoked by pentasaccharide binding. Consequently, LMWH catalyzes factor Xa inhibition by

TABLE 118-5 Advantages of LMWH Over Heparin

Advantage	Consequence
Better bioavailability and longer half-life after subcutaneous injection	Can be given subcutaneously once or twice daily for both prophylaxis and treatment
Dose-independent clearance	Simplified dosing
Predictable anticoagulant response	Coagulation monitoring is unnecessary in most patients
Lower risk of heparin-induced thrombocytopenia	Safer than heparin for short- or long-term administration
Lower risk of osteoporosis	Safer than heparin for extended administration

Abbreviation: LMWH, low-molecular-weight heparin.

antithrombin more than thrombin inhibition. Depending on their unique molecular weight distributions, LMWH preparations have anti-factor Xa to anti-factor IIa ratios ranging from 2:1 to 4:1.

Pharmacology Although usually given SC, LMWH also can be administered IV if a rapid anticoagulant response is needed. LMWH has pharmacokinetic advantages over heparin. These advantages reflect the fact that shorter heparin chains bind less avidly to endothelial cells, macrophages, and heparin-binding plasma proteins. Reduced binding to endothelial cells and macrophages eliminates the rapid, dose-dependent, and saturable mechanism of clearance that is a characteristic of unfractionated heparin. Instead, the clearance of LMWH is dose-independent and its plasma half-life is longer. Based on measurement of anti-factor Xa levels, LMWH has a plasma half-life of ~4 h. LMWH is cleared almost exclusively by the kidneys, and the drug can accumulate in patients with renal insufficiency.

LMWH exhibits about 90% bioavailability after SC injection. Because LMWH binds less avidly to heparin-binding proteins in plasma than heparin, LMWH produces a more predictable dose response, and resistance to LMWH is rare. With a longer half-life and more predictable anticoagulant response, LMWH can be given SC once or twice daily without coagulation monitoring, even when the drug is given in treatment doses. These properties render LMWH more convenient than unfractionated heparin. Capitalizing on this feature, studies in patients with venous thromboembolism have shown that home treatment with LMWH is as effective and safe as in-hospital treatment with continuous IV infusions of heparin. Outpatient treatment with LMWH streamlines care, reduces health care costs, and increases patient satisfaction.

Monitoring In the majority of patients, LMWH does not require coagulation monitoring. If monitoring is necessary, anti-factor Xa levels must be measured because most LMWH preparations have little effect on the aPTT. Therapeutic anti-factor Xa levels with LMWH range from 0.5 to 1.2 units/mL when measured 3–4 h after drug administration. When LMWH is given in prophylactic doses, peak anti-Factor Xa levels of 0.2–0.5 units/mL are desirable.

Indications for LMWH monitoring include renal insufficiency and obesity. LMWH monitoring in patients with a creatinine clearance of ≤50 mL/min is advisable to ensure that there is no drug accumulation. Although weight-adjusted LMWH dosing appears to produce therapeutic anti-factor Xa levels in patients who are overweight, this approach has not been extensively evaluated in those with morbid obesity. It may also be advisable to monitor the anticoagulant activity of LMWH during pregnancy because dose requirements can change, particularly in the third trimester. Monitoring should also be considered in high-risk settings, such as in patients with mechanical heart valves who are given LMWH for prevention of valve thrombosis, and when LMWH is used in treatment doses in infants or children.

Dosing The doses of LMWH recommended for prophylaxis or treatment vary depending on the LMWH preparation. For prophylaxis, once-daily SC doses of 4000–5000 units are often used, whereas doses of 2500–3000 units are given when the drug is administered twice daily. For treatment of venous thromboembolism, a dose of 150–200 units/kg is given if the drug is administered once daily. If a twice-daily regimen is employed, a dose of 100 units/kg is given. In patients with unstable angina, LMWH is given SC on a twice-daily basis at a dose of 100–120 units/kg.

Side effects The major complication of LMWH is bleeding. Meta-analyses suggest that the risk of major bleeding is lower with LMWH than with unfractionated heparin. HIT and osteoporosis are less common with LMWH than with unfractionated heparin.

Bleeding Like the situation with heparin, bleeding with LMWH is more common in patients receiving concomitant therapy with antiplatelet or fibrinolytic drugs. Recent surgery, trauma, or underlying hemostatic defects also increase the risk of bleeding with LMWH.

Although protamine sulfate can be used as an antidote for LMWH, protamine sulfate incompletely neutralizes the anticoagulant activity of LMWH because it only binds the longer chains of LMWH. Because longer chains are responsible for catalysis of thrombin inhibition by antithrombin, protamine sulfate completely reverses the anti-factor IIa activity of LMWH. In contrast, protamine sulfate only partially reverses the anti-factor Xa activity of LMWH because the shorter pentasaccharide-containing chains of LMWH do not bind to protamine sulfate. Consequently, patients at high risk for bleeding may be more safely treated with continuous IV unfractionated heparin than with SC LMWH.

Thrombocytopenia The risk of HIT is about fivefold lower with LMWH than with heparin. LMWH binds less avidly to platelets and causes less PF4 release. Furthermore, with lower affinity for PF4 than heparin, LMWH is less likely to induce the conformational changes in PF4 that trigger the formation of HIT antibodies.

LMWH should not be used to treat HIT patients because most HIT antibodies exhibit cross-reactivity with LMWH. This in vitro cross-reactivity is not simply a laboratory phenomenon because there are case reports of thrombosis when HIT patients are treated with LMWH.

Osteoporosis The risk of osteoporosis is lower with long-term LMWH than with heparin. For extended treatment, therefore, LMWH is a better choice than heparin because of the lower risk of osteoporosis and HIT.

Fondaparinux

A synthetic analogue of the antithrombin-binding pentasaccharide sequence, fondaparinux differs from LMWH in several ways (Table 118-6). Fondaparinux is licensed for thromboprophylaxis in general medical or surgical patients and in high-risk orthopedic patients and as an alternative to heparin or LMWH for initial treatment of patients with established venous thromboembolism. The drug is not yet licensed in the United States as an alternative for heparin or LMWH in patients with acute coronary syndromes.

Mechanism of action As a synthetic analogue of the antithrombin-binding pentasaccharide sequence found in heparin and LMWH,

TABLE 118-6 Comparison of LMWH and Fondaparinux

Features	LMWH	Fondaparinux
Number of saccharide units	15–17	5
Catalysis of factor Xa inhibition	Yes	Yes
Catalysis of thrombin inhibition	Yes	No
Bioavailability after subcutaneous administration (%)	90	100
Plasma half-life (h)	4	17
Renal excretion	Yes	Yes
Induces release of tissue factor pathway inhibitor	Yes	No
Neutralized by protamine sulfate	Partially	No

fondaparinux has a molecular weight of 1728. Fondaparinux binds only to antithrombin (Fig. 118-5) and is too short to bridge thrombin to antithrombin. Consequently, fondaparinux catalyzes factor Xa inhibition by antithrombin and does not enhance the rate of thrombin inhibition.

Pharmacology Fondaparinux exhibits complete bioavailability after SC injection. With no binding to endothelial cells or plasma proteins, the clearance of fondaparinux is dose independent and its plasma half-life is 17 h. The drug is given SC once daily. Because fondaparinux is cleared unchanged via the kidneys, it is contraindicated in patients with a creatinine clearance <30 mL/min and should be used with caution in those with a creatinine clearance <50 mL/min.

Fondaparinux produces a predictable anticoagulant response after administration in fixed doses because it does not bind to plasma proteins. The drug is given at a dose of 2.5 mg once daily for prevention of venous thromboembolism. For initial treatment of established venous thromboembolism, fondaparinux is given at a dose of 7.5 mg once daily. The dose can be reduced to 5 mg once daily for those weighing <50 kg and increased to 10 mg for those >100 kg. When given in these doses, fondaparinux is as effective as heparin or LMWH for initial treatment of patients with DVT or PE and produces similar rates of bleeding.

Fondaparinux is used at a dose of 2.5 mg once daily in patients with acute coronary syndromes. When this prophylactic dose of fondaparinux was compared with treatment doses of enoxaparin in patients with non-ST-segment elevation acute coronary syndromes, there was no difference in the rate of cardiovascular death, MI, or stroke at 9 days. However, the rate of major bleeding was 50% lower with fondaparinux than with enoxaparin, a difference that likely reflects the fact that the dose of fondaparinux was lower than that of enoxaparin. In acute coronary syndrome patients who require percutaneous coronary interventions, there is a risk of catheter thrombosis with fondaparinux, unless adjunctive heparin is given.

Side effects Fondaparinux does not cause HIT because it does not bind to PF4. In contrast to LMWH, there is no cross-reactivity of fondaparinux with HIT antibodies. Consequently, fondaparinux appears to be effective for treatment of HIT patients, although large clinical trials supporting its use are lacking.

The major side effect of fondaparinux is bleeding. There is no antidote for fondaparinux. Protamine sulfate has no effect on the anticoagulant activity of fondaparinux because it fails to bind to the drug. Recombinant activated factor VII reverses the anticoagulant effects of fondaparinux in volunteers, but it is unknown whether this agent will control fondaparinux-induced bleeding.

Parenteral direct thrombin inhibitors

Heparin and LMWH are indirect inhibitors of thrombin because their activity is mediated by antithrombin. In contrast, direct thrombin inhibitors do not require a plasma cofactor; instead, these agents bind directly to thrombin and block its interaction with its substrates. Approved parenteral direct thrombin inhibitors include lepirudin, argatroban, and bivalirudin (Table 118-7). Lepirudin and argatroban are licensed for treatment of patients with HIT, whereas bivalirudin is approved as an alternative to heparin in patients undergoing percutaneous coronary interventions, including those with HIT.

Lepirudin A recombinant form of hirudin, lepirudin is a bivalent direct thrombin inhibitor that interacts with both the active site and exosite 1, the substrate-binding site, on thrombin. For rapid anticoagulation, lepirudin is given by continuous IV infusion, but the drug can be given SC for thromboprophylaxis. Lepirudin has

TABLE 118-7 Comparison of the Properties of Lepirudin, Bivalirudin, and Argatroban

	Lepirudin	Bivalirudin	Argatroban
Molecular mass	7000	1980	527
Site(s) of interaction with thrombin	Active site and exosite 1	Active site and exosite 1	Active site
Renal clearance	Yes	No	No
Hepatic metabolism	No	No	Yes
Plasma half-life (min)	60	25	45

a plasma half-life of 60 min after IV infusion and is cleared by the kidneys. Consequently, lepirudin accumulates in patients with renal insufficiency. A high proportion of lepirudin-treated patients develop antibodies against the drug. Although these antibodies rarely cause problems, in a small subset of patients, they can delay lepirudin clearance and enhance its anticoagulant activity. Serious bleeding has been reported in some of these patients.

Lepirudin is usually monitored using the aPTT, and the dose is adjusted to maintain an aPTT that is 1.5–2.5 times the control. The aPTT is not an ideal test for monitoring lepirudin therapy because the clotting time plateaus with higher drug concentrations. Although the ecarin clotting time provides a better index of lepirudin dose than the aPTT, the ecarin clotting time has yet to be standardized.

Argatroban A univalent inhibitor that targets the active site of thrombin, argatroban is metabolized in the liver. Consequently, this drug must be used with caution in patients with hepatic insufficiency. Argatroban is not cleared via the kidneys, so this drug is safer than lepirudin for HIT patients with renal insufficiency.

Argatroban is administered by continuous IV infusion and has a plasma half-life of ~45 min. The aPTT is used to monitor its anticoagulant effect, and the dose is adjusted to achieve an aPTT 1.5–3 times the baseline value, but not to exceed 100 s. Argatroban also prolongs the international normalized ratio (INR), a feature that can complicate the transitioning of patients to warfarin. This problem can be circumvented by using the levels of factor X to monitor warfarin in place of the INR. Alternatively, argatroban can be stopped for 2–3 h before INR determination.

Bivalirudin A synthetic 20-amino-acid analogue of hirudin, bivalirudin is a divalent thrombin inhibitor. Thus, the N-terminal portion of bivalirudin interacts with the active site of thrombin, whereas its C-terminal tail binds to exosite 1, the substrate-binding domain on thrombin. Bivalirudin has a plasma half-life of 25 min, the shortest half-life of all the parenteral direct thrombin inhibitors. Bivalirudin is degraded by peptidases and is partially excreted via the kidneys. When given in high doses in the cardiac catheterization laboratory, the anticoagulant activity of bivalirudin is monitored using the activated clotting time. With lower doses, its activity can be assessed using the aPTT.

Studies comparing bivalirudin with heparin suggest that bivalirudin produces less bleeding. This feature plus its short half-life make bivalirudin an attractive alternative to heparin in patients undergoing percutaneous coronary interventions. Bivalirudin also has been used successfully in HIT patients who require percutaneous coronary interventions.

ORAL ANTICOAGULANTS

Current oral anticoagulant practice dates back almost 60 years to when the vitamin K antagonists were discovered as a result of investigations into the cause of hemorrhagic disease in cattle. Characterized by a decrease in prothrombin levels, this disorder is caused by ingestion of hay containing spoiled sweet clover. Hydroxycoumarin, which was isolated from bacterial contaminants in the hay, interferes with vitamin K metabolism, thereby causing a syndrome similar to vitamin K deficiency. Discovery of this compound provided the impetus for development of other vitamin K antagonists, including warfarin.

Warfarin

A water-soluble vitamin K antagonist initially developed as a rodenticide, warfarin is the coumarin derivative most often prescribed in North America. Like other vitamin K antagonists, warfarin interferes with the synthesis of the vitamin K–dependent clotting proteins, which include prothrombin (factor II) and factors VII, IX, and X. The synthesis of the vitamin K–dependent anticoagulant proteins, proteins C and S, is also reduced by vitamin K antagonists.

Mechanism of action All of the vitamin K–dependent clotting factors possess glutamic acid residues at their N termini. A posttranslational modification adds a carboxyl group to the γ-carbon of these residues to generate γ-carboxyglutamic acid. This modification is essential for expression of the activity of these clotting factors because it permits their calcium-dependent binding to negatively charged phospholipid surfaces. The γ-carboxylation process is catalyzed by a vitamin K–dependent carboxylase. Thus, vitamin K from the diet is reduced to vitamin K hydroquinone by vitamin K reductase (Fig. 118-6). Vitamin K hydroquinone serves as a cofactor for the carboxylase enzyme, which in the presence of carbon dioxide replaces the hydrogen on the γ-carbon of glutamic acid residues with a carboxyl group. During this process, vitamin K hydroquinone is oxidized to vitamin K epoxide, which is then reduced to vitamin K by vitamin K epoxide reductase.

Warfarin inhibits vitamin K epoxide reductase (VKOR), thereby blocking the γ-carboxylation process. This results in the synthesis of vitamin K–dependent clotting proteins that are only partially γ-carboxylated. Warfarin acts as an anticoagulant because these partially γ-carboxylated proteins have reduced or absent biologic activity. The onset of action of warfarin is delayed until the newly synthesized clotting factors with reduced activity gradually replace their fully active counterparts.

The antithrombotic effect of warfarin depends on a reduction in the functional levels of factor X and prothrombin, clotting factors that have half-lives of 24 and 72 h, respectively. Because of the delay in achieving an antithrombotic effect, initial treatment with warfarin is supported by concomitant administration of a rapidly acting parenteral anticoagulant, such as heparin, LMWH, or fondaparinux, in patients with established thrombosis or at high risk for thrombosis.

Pharmacology Warfarin is a racemic mixture of R and S isomers. Warfarin is rapidly and almost completely absorbed from the gastrointestinal tract. Levels of warfarin in the blood peak about 90 min after drug administration. Racemic warfarin has a plasma half-life of 36–42 h, and more than 97% of circulating warfarin is bound to albumin. Only the small fraction of unbound warfarin is biologically active.

Warfarin accumulates in the liver where the two isomers are metabolized via distinct pathways. CYP2C9 mediates oxidative metabolism of the more active S isomer (Fig. 118-6). Two relatively common variants, CYP2C9*2 and CYP2C9*3, encode an enzyme

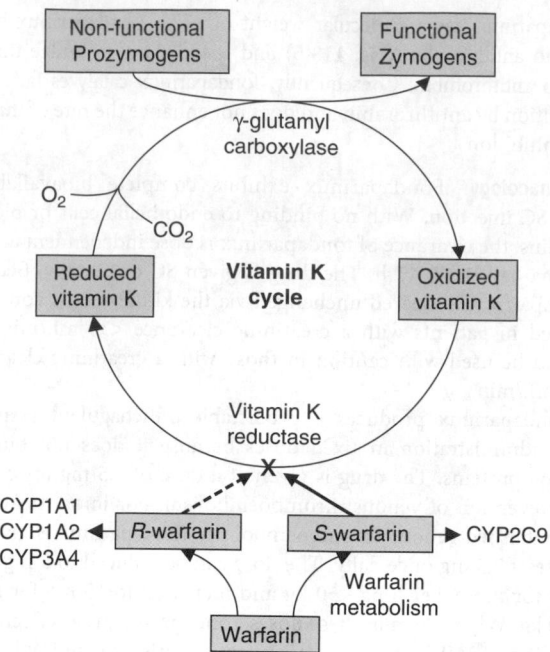

Figure 118-6 Mechanism of action of warfarin. A racemic mixture of S- and R-enantiomers, S-warfarin is most active. By blocking vitamin K epoxide reductase, warfarin inhibits the conversion of oxidized vitamin K into its reduced form. This inhibits vitamin K–dependent γ-carboxylation of factors II, VII, IX, and X because reduced vitamin K serves as a cofactor for a γ-glutamyl carboxylase that catalyzes the γ-carboxylation process, thereby converting prozymogens to zymogens capable of binding calcium and interacting with anionic phospholipid surfaces. S-warfarin is metabolized by CYP2C9. Common genetic polymorphisms in this enzyme can influence warfarin metabolism. Polymorphisms in the C1 subunit of vitamin K reductase (VKORC1) also can affect the susceptibility of the enzyme to warfarin-induced inhibition, thereby influencing warfarin dosage requirements.

with reduced activity. Patients with these variants require lower maintenance doses of warfarin. Approximately 25% of Caucasians have at least one variant allele of CYP2C9*2 or CYP2C9*3, whereas those variant alleles are less common in African Americans and Asians (Table 118-8). Heterozygosity for CYP2C9*2 or CYP2C9*3 decreases the warfarin dose requirement by 20–30% relative to that required in subjects with the wild-type CYP2C9*1/*1 alleles, whereas homozygosity for the CYP2C9*2 or CYP2C9*3 alleles reduces the warfarin dose requirement by 50–70%.

Consistent with their decreased warfarin dose requirement, subjects with at least one CYP2C9 variant allele are at increased risk for bleeding. Compared with individuals with no variant alleles, the relative risks for warfarin-associated bleeding in CYP2C9*2 or CYP2C9*3 carriers are 1.91 and 1.77, respectively.

Polymorphisms in VKORC1 also can influence the anticoagulant response to warfarin. Several genetic variations of VKORC1 are in strong linkage disequilibrium and have been designated as non-A haplotypes. VKORC1 variants are more prevalent than variants of CYP2C9. Asians have the highest prevalence of VKORC1 variants, followed by Caucasians and African Americans (Table 118-8). Polymorphisms in VKORC1 likely explain 30% of the variability in warfarin dose requirements. Compared with VKORC1 non-A/non-A homozygotes, the warfarin dose requirement decreases by 25 and 50% in A halotype heterozygotes and homozygotes, respectively. These findings prompted the Food and Drug Administration to amend the prescribing information for warfarin to indicate that lower initiation doses should be considered for patients with

TABLE 118-8 Frequencies of *CYP2C9* Genotypes and *VKORC1* Haplotypes in Different Populations and Their Effect on Warfarin Dose Requirements

Genotype/ haploptye	Frequency, %			Dose reduction compared with wild-type
	Caucasians	African Americans (A/A)	Asians (A)	
CYP2C9				
*1/*1	70	90	95	–
*1/*2	17	2	0	22
*1/*3	9	3	4	34
*2/*2	2	0	0	43
*2/*3	1	0	0	53
*3/*3	0	0	1	76
VKORC1				
Non-A/non-A	37	82	7	–
Non-A/A	45	12	30	26
A/A	18	6	63	50

CYP2C9 and *VKORC1* genetic variants. In addition to genotype data, other pertinent patient information has been incorporated into warfarin dosing algorithms. Although such algorithms help predict suitable warfarin doses, it remains unclear whether better dose identification improves patient outcome in terms of reducing hemorrhagic complications or recurrent thrombotic events.

In addition to genetic factors, the anticoagulant effect of warfarin is influenced by diet, drugs, and various disease states. Fluctuations in dietary vitamin K intake affect the activity of warfarin. A wide variety of drugs can alter absorption, clearance, or metabolism of warfarin. Because of the variability in the anticoagulant response to warfarin, coagulation monitoring is essential to ensure that a therapeutic response is obtained.

Monitoring Warfarin therapy is most often monitored using the prothrombin time, a test that is sensitive to reductions in the levels of prothrombin, factor VII, and factor X. The test is performed by adding thromboplastin, a reagent that contains tissue factor, phospholipid, and calcium, to citrated plasma and determining the time to clot formation. Thromboplastins vary in their sensitivity to reductions in the levels of the vitamin K–dependent clotting factors. Thus, less sensitive thromboplastins will trigger the administration of higher doses of warfarin to achieve a target prothrombin time. This is problematic because higher doses of warfarin increase the risk of bleeding.

The INR was developed to circumvent many of the problems associated with the prothrombin time. To calculate the INR, the patient's prothrombin time is divided by the mean normal prothrombin time, and this ratio is then multiplied by the international sensitivity index (ISI), an index of the sensitivity of the thromboplastin used for prothrombin time determination to reductions in the levels of the vitamin K–dependent clotting factors. Highly sensitive thromboplastins have an ISI of 1.0. Most current thromboplastins have ISI values that range from 1.0 to 1.4.

Although the INR has helped to standardize anticoagulant practice, problems persist. The precision of INR determination

varies depending on reagent-coagulometer combinations. This leads to variability in the INR results. Also complicating INR determination is unreliable reporting of the ISI by thromboplastin manufacturers. Furthermore, every laboratory must establish the mean normal prothrombin time with each new batch of thromboplastin reagent. To accomplish this, the prothrombin time must be measured in fresh plasma samples from at least 20 healthy volunteers using the same coagulometer that is used for patient samples.

For most indications, warfarin is administered in doses that produce a target INR of 2.0–3.0. An exception is patients with mechanical heart valves, where a target INR of 2.5–3.5 is recommended. Studies in atrial fibrillation demonstrate an increased risk of cardioembolic stroke when the INR falls to <1.7 and an increase in bleeding with INR values >4.5. These findings highlight the fact that vitamin K antagonists have a narrow therapeutic window. In support of this concept, a study in patients receiving long-term warfarin therapy for unprovoked venous thromboembolism demonstrated a higher rate of recurrent venous thromboembolism with a target INR of 1.5–1.9 compared with a target INR of 2.0–3.0.

Dosing Warfarin is usually started at a dose of 5–10 mg. Lower doses are used for patients with *CYP2C9* or *VKORC1* polymorphisms, which affect the pharmacodynamics or pharmacokinetics of warfarin and render patients more sensitive to the drug. The dose is then titrated to achieve the desired target INR. Because of its delayed onset of action, patients with established thrombosis or those at high risk for thrombosis are given concomitant treatment with a rapidly acting parenteral anticoagulant, such as heparin, LMWH, or fondaparinux. Initial prolongation of the INR reflects reduction in the functional levels of factor VII. Consequently, concomitant treatment with the parenteral anticoagulant should be continued until the INR has been therapeutic for at least 2 consecutive days. A minimum 5-day course of parenteral anticoagulation is recommended to ensure that the levels of prothrombin have been reduced into the therapeutic range with warfarin.

Because warfarin has a narrow therapeutic window, frequent coagulation monitoring is essential to ensure that a therapeutic anticoagulant response is obtained. Even patients with stable warfarin dose requirements should have their INR determined every 2–3 weeks. More frequent monitoring is necessary when new medications are introduced because so many drugs enhance or reduce the anticoagulant effects of warfarin.

Side effects Like all anticoagulants, the major side effect of warfarin is bleeding. A rare complication is skin necrosis. Warfarin crosses the placenta and can cause fetal abnormalities. Consequently, warfarin should not be used during pregnancy.

Bleeding At least half of the bleeding complications with warfarin occur when the INR exceeds the therapeutic range. Bleeding complications may be mild, such as epistaxis or hematuria, or more severe, such as retroperitoneal or gastrointestinal bleeding. Life-threatening intracranial bleeding can also occur.

To minimize the risk of bleeding, the INR should be maintained in the therapeutic range. In asymptomatic patients whose INR is between 3.5 and 4.5, warfarin should be withheld until the INR returns to the therapeutic range. If the INR is >4.5, a therapeutic INR can be achieved more rapidly by administration of low doses of sublingual vitamin K. A vitamin K dose of 1 mg is usually adequate for patients with an INR between 4.9 and 9, whereas 2–3 mg can be used for those with an INR >9. Higher doses of vitamin K can be administered if more rapid reversal of the INR is required or if the INR is excessively high. Although vitamin K administration results in a more rapid reduction in the INR compared with simply holding the warfarin, there is no evidence that vitamin K administration reduces the risk of hemorrhage.

Patients with serious bleeding need more aggressive treatment. These patients should be given 10 mg of vitamin K by slow IV infusion. Additional vitamin K should be given until the INR is in the normal range. Treatment with vitamin K should be supplemented with fresh-frozen plasma as a source of the vitamin K–dependent clotting proteins. For life-threatening bleeds, or if patients cannot tolerate the volume load, prothrombin complex concentrates can be used.

Warfarin-treated patients who experience bleeding when their INR is in the therapeutic range require investigation into the cause of the bleeding. Those with gastrointestinal bleeding often have underlying peptic ulcer disease or a tumor. Similarly, investigation of hematuria or uterine bleeding in patients with a therapeutic INR may unmask a tumor of the genitourinary tract.

Skin necrosis A rare complication of warfarin, skin necrosis usually is seen 2–5 days after initiation of therapy. Well-demarcated erythematous lesions form on the thighs, buttocks, breasts, or toes. Typically, the center of the lesion becomes progressively necrotic. Examination of skin biopsies taken from the border of these lesions reveals thrombi in the microvasculature.

Warfarin-induced skin necrosis is seen in patients with congenital or acquired deficiencies of protein C or protein S. Initiation of warfarin therapy in these patients produces a precipitous fall in plasma levels of proteins C or S, thereby eliminating this important anticoagulant pathway before warfarin exerts an antithrombotic effect through lowering of the functional levels of factor X and prothrombin. The resultant procoagulant state triggers thrombosis. Why the thrombosis is localized to the microvasculature of fatty tissues is unclear.

Treatment involves discontinuation of warfarin and reversal with vitamin K, if needed. An alternative anticoagulant, such as heparin or LMWH, should be given in patients with thrombosis. Protein C concentrates or recombinant activated protein C can be given to protein C–deficient patients to accelerate healing of the skin lesions; fresh-frozen plasma may be of value for those with protein S deficiency. Occasionally, skin grafting is necessary when there is extensive skin loss.

Because of the potential for skin necrosis, patients with known protein C or protein S deficiency require overlapping treatment with a parenteral anticoagulant when initiating warfarin therapy. Warfarin should be started in low doses in these patients, and the parenteral anticoagulant should be continued until the INR is therapeutic for at least 2–3 consecutive days.

Pregnancy Warfarin crosses the placenta and can cause fetal abnormalities or bleeding. The fetal abnormalities include a characteristic embryopathy, which consists of nasal hypoplasia and stippled epiphyses. The risk of embryopathy is highest if warfarin is given in the first trimester of pregnancy. Central nervous system abnormalities can also occur with exposure to warfarin at any time during pregnancy. Finally, maternal administration of warfarin produces an anticoagulant effect in the fetus that can cause bleeding. This is of particular concern at delivery when trauma to the head during passage through the birth canal can lead to intracranial bleeding. Because of these potential problems, warfarin is contraindicated in pregnancy, particularly in the first and third trimesters. Instead, heparin, LMWH, or fondaparinux can be given during pregnancy for prevention or treatment of thrombosis.

Warfarin does not pass into the breast milk. Consequently, warfarin can safely be given to nursing mothers.

Special problems Patients with a lupus anticoagulant or those who need urgent or elective surgery present special challenges. Although observational studies suggested that patients with thrombosis complicating the antiphospholipid antibody syndrome required higher intensity warfarin regimens to prevent recurrent thromboembolic events, two randomized trials showed that targeting an INR of 2.0–3.0 is as effective as higher intensity treatment and produces less bleeding. Monitoring warfarin therapy can be problematic in patients with antiphospholipid antibody syndrome if the lupus anticoagulant prolongs the baseline INR.

If patients receiving long-term warfarin treatment require an elective invasive procedure, warfarin can be stopped 5 days before the procedure to allow the INR to return to normal levels. Those at high risk for recurrent thrombosis can be bridged with once- or twice-daily SC injections of LMWH when the INR falls to <2.0. The last dose of LMWH should be given 12–24 h before the procedure, depending on whether LMWH is administered twice or once daily. After the procedure, treatment with warfarin can be restarted.

New oral anticoagulants

New oral anticoagulants that target thrombin or factor Xa are under development. These drugs have a rapid onset of action and have half-lives that permit once- or twice-daily administration. Designed to produce a predictable level of anticoagulation, these new oral agents are given in fixed doses without routine coagulation monitoring. Therefore, these drugs are more convenient to administer than warfarin.

Dabigatran etexilate, an oral thrombin inhibitor, and rivaroxaban, an oral factor Xa inhibitor, are licensed in Europe and Canada for short-term thromboprophylaxis after elective hip or knee replacement surgery. Phase III trials with apixaban, another oral factor Xa inhibitor, also have been completed in patients undergoing major orthopedic surgery (Table 118-9).

The RE-LY trial shows the promise of these new agents for long-term indications. This trial compared two different dose regimens of dabigatran etexilate (110 mg or 150 mg twice daily) with warfarin (dose-adjusted to achieve an INR between 2 and 3) for stroke prevention in 18,113 patients with nonvalvular atrial fibrillation. The annual rates of the primary efficacy outcome, stroke or systemic embolism, were 1.7% with warfarin, 1.5% with the lower dose dabigatran regimen, and 1.1% with the higher dose regimen. Thus, the lower dose dabigatran regimen was noninferior to warfarin,

TABLE 118-9 Comparison of the Features of New Oral Anticoagulants in Advanced Stages of Development

Features	Rivaroxaban	Apixaban	Dabigatran Etexilate
Target	Xa	Xa	IIa
Molecular weight	436	460	628
Prodrug	No	No	Yes
Bioavailability (%)	80	50	6
Time to peak (h)	3	3	2
Half-life (h)	9	9–14	12–17
Renal excretion (%)	65	25	80
Antidote	None	None	None

while the higher dose regimen was superior. Annual rates of major bleeding were 3.4% with warfarin compared with 2.7% and 3.1% with the lower and higher dose dabigatran regimens, respectively. Thus, the lower dose dabigatran regimen was associated with significantly less major bleeding than warfarin, while the rate of major bleeding with the higher dose regimen was not significantly different from that with warfarin. Rates of intracerebral bleeding were significantly lower with both doses of dabigatran than with warfarin, as were rates of life-threatening bleeding. There was no evidence of hepatotoxicity with dabigatran.

Based on the results of the RE-LY trial, dabigatran etexilate has been licensed in the United States and Canada for stroke prevention in patients with atrial fibrillation. The 150 mg twice daily dose of dabigatran is recommended for most patients. In the United States, a 75 mg twice daily dose is recommended for patients with a creatinine clearance of 30 to 50 mL/min, while in Canada, the 110 mg twice daily dose is recommended for those over the age of 80 years or for patients at high risk of bleeding. The drug is contraindicated in patients with a creatinine clearance less than 15 mL/min.

Dabigatran etexilate also was compared with warfarin in 2539 patients with acute venous thromboembolism. Patients were initially treated with heparin or LMWH and then randomized to a 6-month course of dabigatran (150 mg twice daily) or warfarin, which was dose-adjusted to achieve an INR of 2–3. The primary endpoint, a composite of recurrent venous thromboembolism or fatal pulmonary embolism, occurred in 2.4% of patients given dabigatran and in 2.1% of those treated with warfarin. Major bleeding occurred in 1.6 and 1.9% of patients given dabigatran and warfarin, respectively. Based on the results of this trial, unmonitored fixed-dose dabigatran appears to be noninferior to warfarin for treatment of patients with venous thromboembolism. Taken together with the results of the RE-LY trial, these findings suggest that the new oral anticoagulants will gradually replace warfarin.

FIBRINOLYTIC DRUGS

ROLE OF FIBRINOLYTIC THERAPY

Fibrinolytic drugs can be used to degrade thrombi and are administered systemically or can be delivered via catheters directly into the substance of the thrombus. Systemic delivery is used for treatment of acute MI, acute ischemic stroke, and most cases of massive PE. The goal of therapy is to produce rapid thrombus dissolution, thereby restoring antegrade blood flow. In the coronary circulation, restoration of blood flow reduces morbidity and mortality rates by limiting myocardial damage, whereas in the cerebral circulation, rapid thrombus dissolution decreases the neuronal death and brain infarction that produce irreversible brain injury. For patients with massive PE, the goal of thrombolytic therapy is to restore pulmonary artery perfusion.

Peripheral arterial thrombi and thrombi in the proximal deep veins of the leg are most often treated using catheter-directed thrombolytic therapy. Catheters with multiple side holes can be utilized to enhance drug delivery. In some cases, intravascular devices that fragment and extract the thrombus are used to hasten treatment. These devices can be used alone or in conjunction with fibrinolytic drugs.

MECHANISM OF ACTION

Currently approved fibrinolytic agents include streptokinase; acylated plasminogen streptokinase activator complex (anistreplase); urokinase; recombinant tissue-type plasminogen activator (rtPA), which is also known as alteplase or activase; and two recombinant derivatives of rtPA, tenecteplase and reteplase. All of these

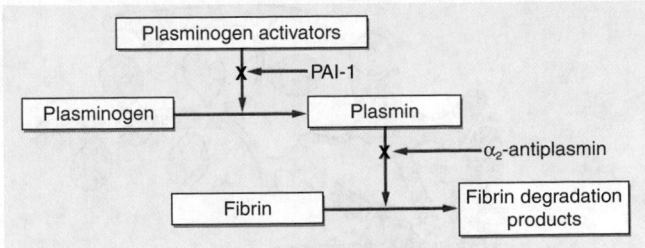

Figure 118-7 **The fibrinolytic system and its regulation.** Plasminogen activators convert plasminogen to plasmin. Plasmin then degrades fibrin into soluble fibrin degradation products. The system is regulated at two levels. Type 1 plasminogen activator inhibitor (PAI-1) regulates the plasminogen activators, whereas α_2-antiplasmin serves as the major inhibitor of plasmin.

agents act by converting the proenzyme, plasminogen, to plasmin, the active enzyme (Fig. 118-7). Plasmin then degrades the fibrin matrix of thrombi and produces soluble fibrin degradation products.

Endogenous fibrinolysis is regulated at two levels. Plasminogen activator inhibitors, particularly the type 1 form (PAI-1), prevent excessive plasminogen activation by regulating the activity of tPA and urokinase-type plasminogen activator (u-PA). Once plasmin is generated, it is regulated by plasmin inhibitors, the most important of which is α_2-antiplasmin. The plasma concentration of plasminogen is twofold higher than that of α_2-antiplasmin. Consequently, with pharmacologic doses of plasminogen activators, the concentration of plasmin that is generated can exceed that of α_2-antiplasmin. In addition to degrading fibrin, unregulated plasmin can also degrade fibrinogen and other clotting factors. This process, which is known as the *systemic lytic state*, reduces the hemostatic potential of the blood and increases the risk of bleeding.

The endogenous fibrinolytic system is geared to localize plasmin generation to the fibrin surface. Both plasminogen and tPA bind to fibrin to form a ternary complex that promotes efficient plasminogen activation. In contrast to free plasmin, plasmin generated on the fibrin surface is relatively protected from inactivation by α_2-antiplasmin, a feature that promotes fibrin dissolution. Furthermore, C-terminal lysine residues, exposed as plasmin degrades fibrin, serve as binding sites for additional plasminogen and tPA molecules. This creates a positive feedback that enhances plasmin generation. When used pharmacologically, the various plasminogen activators capitalize on these mechanisms to a lesser or greater extent.

Plasminogen activators that preferentially activate fibrin-bound plasminogen are considered fibrin-specific. In contrast, nonspecific plasminogen activators do not discriminate between fibrin-bound and circulating plasminogen. Activation of circulating plasminogen results in the generation of unopposed plasmin that can trigger the systemic lytic state. Alteplase and its derivatives are fibrin-specific plasminogen activators, whereas streptokinase, anistreplase, and urokinase are nonspecific agents.

STREPTOKINASE

Unlike other plasminogen activators, streptokinase is not an enzyme and does not directly convert plasminogen to plasmin. Instead, streptokinase forms a 1:1 stoichiometric complex with plasminogen. Formation of this complex induces a conformational change in plasminogen that exposes its active site (Fig. 118-8). This conformationally altered plasminogen then converts additional plasminogen molecules to plasmin.

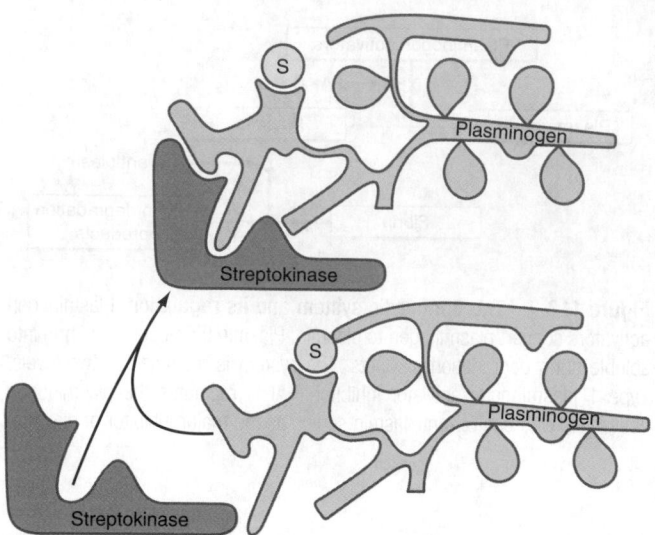

Figure 118-8 Mechanism of action of streptokinase. Streptokinase binds to plasminogen and induces a conformational change in plasminogen that exposes its active site. The streptokinase/plasmin(ogen) complex then serves as the activator of additional plasminogen molecules.

Streptokinase has no affinity for fibrin, and the streptokinase-plasminogen complex activates both free and fibrin-bound plasminogen. Activation of circulating plasminogen generates sufficient amounts of plasmin to overwhelm α_2-antiplasmin. Unopposed plasmin not only degrades fibrin in the occlusive thrombus but also induces a systemic lytic state.

When given systemically to patients with acute MI, streptokinase reduces mortality. For this indication, the drug is usually given as an IV infusion of 1.5 million units over 30–60 min. Patients who receive streptokinase can develop antibodies against the drug, as can patients with prior streptococcal infection. These antibodies can reduce the effectiveness of streptokinase.

Allergic reactions occur in ~5% of patients treated with streptokinase. These may manifest as a rash, fever, chills, and rigors. Although anaphylactic reactions can occur, these are rare. Transient hypotension is common with streptokinase and has been attributed to plasmin-mediated release of bradykinin from kininogen. The hypotension usually responds to leg elevation and administration of IV fluids and low doses of vasopressors, such as dopamine or norepinephrine.

ANISTREPLASE

To generate this drug, streptokinase is combined with equimolar amounts of Lys-plasminogen, a plasmin-cleaved form of plasminogen with a Lys residue at its N terminus. The active site of Lys-plasminogen that is exposed upon combination with streptokinase is then masked with an anisoyl group. After IV infusion, the anisoyl group is slowly removed by deacylation, giving the complex a half-life of ~100 min. This allows drug administration via a single bolus infusion.

Although it is more convenient to administer, anistreplase offers few mechanistic advantages over streptokinase. Like streptokinase, anistreplase does not distinguish between fibrin-bound and circulating plasminogen. Consequently, it too produces a systemic lytic state. Likewise, allergic reactions and hypotension are just as frequent with anistreplase as they are with streptokinase.

When anistreplase was compared with alteplase in patients with acute MI, reperfusion was obtained more rapidly with alteplase than with anistreplase. Improved reperfusion was associated with a trend toward better clinical outcomes and reduced mortality rate with alteplase. These results and the high cost of anistreplase have dampened the enthusiasm for its use.

UROKINASE

Urokinase is a two-chain serine protease derived from cultured fetal kidney cells with a molecular weight of 34,000. Urokinase converts plasminogen to plasmin directly by cleaving the Arg560-Val561 bond. Unlike streptokinase, urokinase is not immunogenic and allergic reactions are rare. Urokinase produces a systemic lytic state because it does not discriminate between fibrin-bound and circulating plasminogen.

Despite many years of use, urokinase has never been systemically evaluated for coronary thrombolysis. Instead, urokinase is often employed for catheter-directed lysis of thrombi in the deep veins or the peripheral arteries. Because of production problems, the availability of urokinase is limited.

ALTEPLASE

A recombinant form of single-chain tPA, alteplase has a molecular weight of 68,000. Alteplase is rapidly converted into its two-chain form by plasmin. Although single- and two-chain forms of tPA have equivalent activity in the presence of fibrin, in its absence, single-chain tPA has tenfold lower activity.

Alteplase consists of five discrete domains (Fig. 118-9); the N-terminal A chain of two-chain alteplase contains four of these domains. Residues 4 through 50 make up the finger domain, a region that resembles the finger domain of fibronectin; residues 50 through 87 are homologous with epidermal growth factor, whereas residues 92 through 173 and 180 through 261, which have homology to the kringle domains of plasminogen, are designated as the

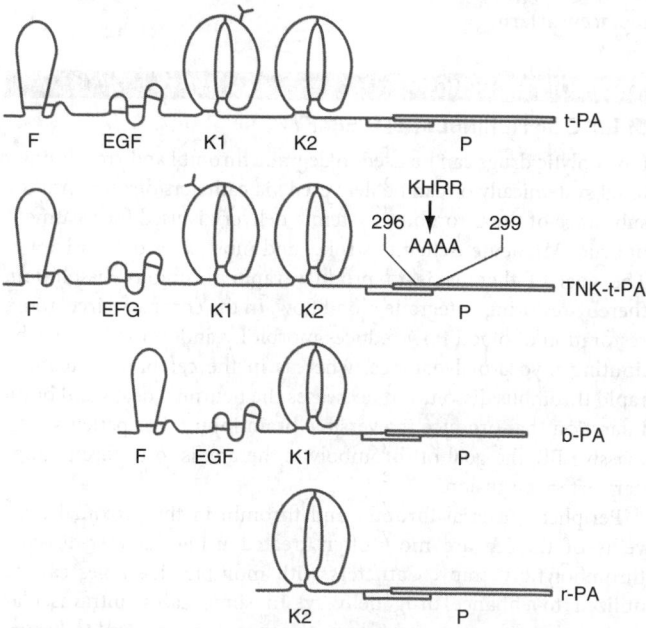

Figure 118-9 Domain structures of alteplase (tPA), tenecteplase (TNK-tPA), desmoteplase (b-PA), and reteplase (r-PA). The finger (F), epidermal growth factor (EGF), first and second kringles (K1 and K2, respectively), and protease (P) domains are illustrated. The glycosylation site (Y) on K1 has been repositioned in tenecteplase to endow it with a longer half-life. In addition, a tetra-alanine substitution in the protease domain renders tenecteplase resistant to PAI-1 inhibition. Desmoteplase differs from alteplase and tenecteplase in that it lacks a K2 domain. Reteplase is a truncated variant that lacks the F, EGF, and K1 domains.

first and second kringle, respectively. The fifth alteplase domain is the protease domain; it is located on the C-terminal B chain of two-chain alteplase.

The interaction of alteplase with fibrin is mediated by the finger domain and, to a lesser extent, by the second kringle domain. The affinity of alteplase for fibrin is considerably higher than that for fibrinogen. Consequently, the catalytic efficiency of plasminogen activation by alteplase is two to three orders of magnitude higher in the presence of fibrin than in the presence of fibrinogen. This phenomenon helps to localize plasmin generation to the fibrin surface.

Although alteplase preferentially activates plasminogen in the presence of fibrin, alteplase is not as fibrin-selective as was first predicted. Its fibrin specificity is limited because like fibrin, (DD)E, the major soluble degradation product of cross-linked fibrin, binds alteplase and plasminogen with high affinity. Consequently, (DD)E is as potent as fibrin as a stimulator of plasminogen activation by alteplase. Whereas plasmin generated on the fibrin surface results in thrombolysis, plasmin generated on the surface of circulating (DD)E degrades fibrinogen. Fibrinogenolysis results in the accumulation of fragment X, a high-molecular-weight clottable fibrinogen degradation product. Incorporation of fragment X into hemostatic plugs formed at sites of vascular injury renders them susceptible to lysis. This phenomenon may contribute to alteplase-induced bleeding.

A trial comparing alteplase with streptokinase for treatment of patients with acute MI demonstrated significantly lower mortality with alteplase than with streptokinase, although the absolute difference was small. The greatest benefit was seen in patients age <75 years with anterior MI who presented <6 h after symptom onset.

For treatment of acute MI or acute ischemic stroke, alteplase is given as an IV infusion over 60–90 min. The total dose of alteplase usually ranges from 90 to 100 mg. Allergic reactions and hypotension are rare, and alteplase is not immunogenic.

■ TENECTEPLASE

Tenecteplase is a genetically engineered variant of tPA and was designed to have a longer half-life than tPA and to be resistant to inactivation by PAI-1. To prolong its half-life, a new glycosylation site was added to the first kringle domain (Fig. 118-9). Because addition of this extra carbohydrate side chain reduced fibrin affinity, the existing glycosylation site on the first kringle domain was removed. To render the molecule resistant to inhibition by PAI-1, a tetra-alanine substitution was introduced at residues 296–299 in the protease domain, the region responsible for the interaction of tPA with PAI-1.

Tenecteplase is more fibrin-specific than tPA. Although both agents bind to fibrin with similar affinity, the affinity of tenecteplase for (DD)E is significantly lower than that of tPA. Consequently, (DD)E does not stimulate systemic plasminogen activation by tenecteplase to the same extent as tPA. As a result, tenecteplase produces less fibrinogenolysis than tPA.

For coronary thrombolysis, tenecteplase is given as a single IV bolus. In a large phase III trial that enrolled >16,000 patients, the 30-day mortality rate with single-bolus tenecteplase was similar to that with accelerated-dose tPA. Although rates of intracranial hemorrhage were also similar with both treatments, patients given tenecteplase had fewer noncerebral bleeds and a reduced need for blood transfusions than those treated with tPA. The improved safety profile of tenecteplase likely reflects its enhanced fibrin specificity.

■ RETEPLASE

Reteplase is a recombinant tPA derivative and is a single-chain variant that lacks the finger, epidermal growth factor, and first kringle domains (Fig. 118-9). This truncated derivative has a molecular weight of 39,000. Reteplase binds fibrin more weakly than tPA because it lacks the finger domain. Because it is produced in *Escherichia coli*, reteplase is not glycosylated. This endows it with a plasma half-life longer than that of tPA. Consequently, reteplase is given as two IV boluses, which are separated by 30 min. Clinical trials have demonstrated that reteplase is at least as effective as streptokinase for treatment of acute MI, but the agent is not superior to tPA.

■ NEW FIBRINOLYTIC AGENTS

Several new drugs are under investigation. These include desmoteplase (Fig. 118-9), a recombinant form of the full-length plasminogen activator isolated from the saliva of the vampire bat, and alfimeprase, a truncated form of fibrolase, an enzyme isolated from the venom of the southern copperhead snake. Clinical studies with these agents have been disappointing. Desmoteplase, which is more fibrin-specific than tPA, was investigated for treatment of acute ischemic stroke. Patients presenting 3–9 h after symptom onset were randomized to one of two doses of desmoteplase or to placebo. Overall response rates were low and no different with desmoteplase from with placebo. Mortality rate was higher in the desmoteplase arms.

Alfimeprase is a metalloproteinase that degrades fibrin and fibrinogen in a plasmin-independent fashion. In the circulation, alfimeprase is inhibited by α_2-macroglobulin. Consequently, the drug must be delivered via a catheter directly into the thrombus. Studies of alfimeprase for treatment of peripheral arterial occlusion or for restoration of flow in blocked central venous catheters were stopped due to lack of efficacy. The disappointing results with desmoteplase and alfimeprase highlight the challenges of introducing new fibrinolytic drugs.

CONCLUSIONS AND FUTURE DIRECTIONS

Arterial and venous thromboses reflect a complex interplay among the vessel wall, platelets, the coagulation system, and the fibrinolytic pathways. Activation of coagulation also triggers inflammatory pathways that may contribute to thrombogenesis. A better understanding of the biochemistry of blood coagulation and advances in structure-based drug design have identified new targets and resulted in the development of novel antithrombotic drugs. Well-designed clinical trials have provided detailed information on which drugs to use and when to use them. Despite these advances, however, thromboembolic disorders remain a major cause of morbidity and mortality rates. Therefore, the search for better targets and more potent antiplatelet, anticoagulant, and fibrinolytic drugs continues.

FURTHER READINGS

Connolly SJ et al: Dabigatran versus warfarin in patients with atrial fibrillation. N Engl J Med 361:1139, 2009

Eikelboom JW, Weitz JI: New anticoagulants. Circulation 121:1523, 2010

Greinacher A: Heparin-induced thrombocytopenia. J Thromb Haemost 7:9, 2009

International Warfarin Pharmacogenetics Consortium: Estimation of the warfarin dose with clinical and pharmacogenetic data. N Engl J Med 360:753, 2009

Mackman N: Triggers, targets and treatments of thrombosis. Nature 451:914, 2008

Mega JL et al: Cytochrome p-450 polymorphisms and response to clopidogrel. N Engl J Med 360:354, 2009

Rijken DC et al: New insights into the molecular mechanisms of the fibrinolytic system. J Thromb Haemost 7:4, 2009

VARENHORST C et al: Genetic variation of CYP2C19 affects both pharmacokinetic and pharmacodymamic responses to clopidogrel but not prasugrel in aspirin-treated patients with coronary artery disease. Eur Heart J 30:1744, 2009

WALLENTIN L et al: Ticagrelor versus clopidogrel in patients with acute coronary syndromes. N Engl J Med 361:1045, 2009

———: Effect of CYP2C19 and ABCB1 single nucleotide polymorphisms on outcomes of treatment with ticagrelor versus clopidogrel for acute coronary syndromes: A genetic substudy of the PLATO trial. Lancet 376:1320, 2010

WATSON SP: Platelet activation by extracellular matrix proteins in haemostasis and thrombosis. Curr Pharm Des 15:1358, 2009

WIVIOTT SD et al for the TRITON–TIMI 38 Investigators: Prasugrel versus clopidogrel in patients with acute coronary syndromes. N Engl J Med 357:2001, 2007

PART 8
Infectious Diseases

CHAPTER 119

Introduction to Infectious Diseases: Host–Pathogen Interactions

Lawrence C. Madoff
Dennis L. Kasper

Despite decades of dramatic progress in their treatment and prevention, infectious diseases remain a major cause of death and debility and are responsible for worsening the living conditions of many millions of people around the world. Infections frequently challenge the physician's diagnostic skill and must be considered in the differential diagnoses of syndromes affecting every organ system.

CHANGING EPIDEMIOLOGY OF INFECTIOUS DISEASES

With the advent of antimicrobial agents, some medical leaders believed that infectious diseases would soon be eliminated and become of historic interest only. Indeed, the hundreds of chemotherapeutic agents developed since World War II, most of which are potent and safe, include drugs effective not only against bacteria but also against viruses, fungi, and parasites. Nevertheless, we now realize that as we developed antimicrobial agents, microbes developed the ability to elude our best weapons and to counterattack with new survival strategies. Antibiotic resistance occurs at an alarming rate among all classes of mammalian pathogens. Pneumococci resistant to penicillin and enterococci resistant to vancomycin have become commonplace. Even *Staphylococcus aureus* strains resistant to vancomycin have appeared. Such pathogens present real clinical problems in managing infections that were easily treatable just a few years ago. Diseases once thought to have been nearly eradicated from the developed world—tuberculosis, cholera, and rheumatic fever, for example—have rebounded with renewed ferocity. Newly discovered and emerging infectious agents appear to have been brought into contact with humans by changes in the environment and by movements of human and animal populations. An example of the propensity for pathogens to escape from their usual niche is the alarming 1999 outbreak in New York of encephalitis due to West Nile virus, which had never previously been isolated in the Americas. In 2003, severe acute respiratory syndrome (SARS) was first recognized. This clinical entity was caused by a novel coronavirus that may have jumped from an animal host to become a significant human pathogen. For more than 10 years, the world's attention has been focused on H5N1 avian influenza, which spread rapidly through poultry farms in Asia, caused deaths in exposed humans, and reached Europe and Africa, heightening fears of a new influenza pandemic. When the pandemic came in 2009, however, it emerged unexpectedly in North America from an H1N1 strain whose origins were apparently in swine.

Many infectious agents have been discovered only in recent decades (Fig. 119-1). Ebola virus, human metapneumovirus, *Anaplasma phagocytophila* (the agent of human granulocytotropic anaplasmosis), and retroviruses such as HIV humble us despite our deepening understanding of pathogenesis at the most basic molecular level. Even in developed countries, infectious diseases have made a resurgence. Between 1980 and 1996, mortality rates from infectious diseases in the United States increased by 64% to levels not seen since the 1940s.

The role of infectious agents in the etiology of diseases once believed to be noninfectious is increasingly recognized. For example, it is accepted that *Helicobacter pylori* is the causative agent of peptic ulcer disease and perhaps of gastric malignancy. Human papillomavirus is likely to be the most important cause of invasive cervical cancer. Human herpesvirus type 8 is believed to be the cause of most cases of Kaposi's sarcoma. Epstein-Barr virus is a

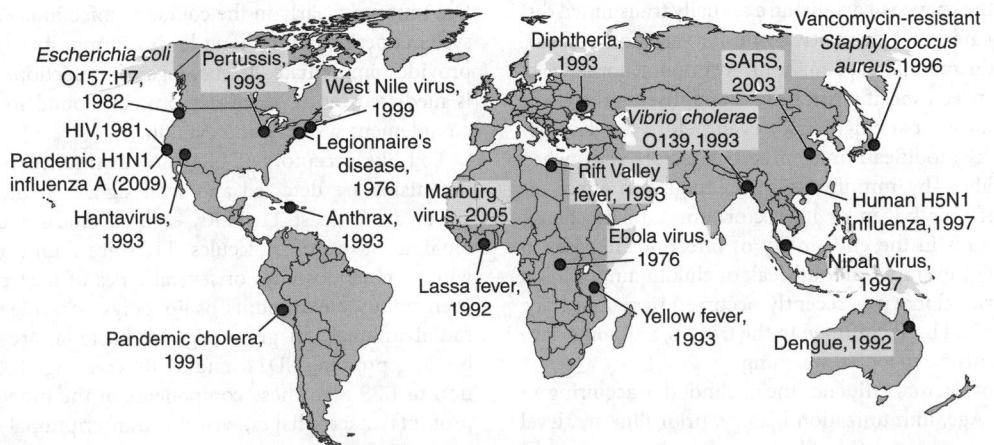

Figure 119-1 Map of the world showing examples of geographic locales where infectious diseases were noted to have emerged or resurged. (*Adapted from Addressing Emerging Infectious Disease Threats: A Prevention Strategy for the United States, Department of Health and Human Services, Centers for Disease Control and Prevention, 1994.*)

cause of certain lymphomas and may play a role in the genesis of Hodgkin's disease. The possibility certainly exists that other diseases of unknown cause, such as rheumatoid arthritis, sarcoidosis, or inflammatory bowel disease, have infectious etiologies. There is even evidence that atherosclerosis may have an infectious component. In contrast, there are data to suggest that decreased exposures to pathogens in childhood may be contributing to an increase in the observed rates of allergic diseases.

Medical advances against infectious diseases have been hindered by changes in patient populations. Immunocompromised hosts now constitute a significant proportion of the seriously infected population. Physicians immunosuppress their patients to prevent the rejection of transplants and to treat neoplastic and inflammatory diseases. Some infections, most notably that caused by HIV, immunocompromise the host in and of themselves. Lesser degrees of immunosuppression are associated with other infections, such as influenza and syphilis. Infectious agents that coexist peacefully with immunocompetent hosts wreak havoc in those who lack a complete immune system. AIDS has brought to prominence once-obscure organisms such as *Pneumocystis*, *Cryptosporidium parvum*, and *Mycobacterium avium*.

FACTORS INFLUENCING INFECTION

For any infectious process to occur, the pathogen and the host must first encounter each other. Factors such as geography, environment, climate, and behavior thus influence the likelihood of infection. Although the initial encounter between a susceptible host and a virulent organism frequently results in disease, some organisms can be harbored in the host for years before disease becomes clinically evident. For a complete view, individual patients must be considered in the context of the population to which they belong. Infectious diseases do not often occur in isolation; rather, they spread through a group exposed from a point source (e.g., a contaminated water supply) or from one individual to another (e.g., via respiratory droplets). Thus, the clinician must be alert to infections prevalent in the community as a whole. A detailed history, including information on travel, behavioral factors, exposures to animals or potentially contaminated environments, and living and occupational conditions, must be elicited. For example, the likelihood of infection by *Plasmodium falciparum* can be significantly affected by altitude, climate, terrain, season, and even time of day. Antibiotic-resistant strains of *P. falciparum* are localized to specific geographic regions, and a seemingly minor alteration in a travel itinerary can dramatically influence the likelihood of acquiring chloroquine-resistant malaria. If such important details in the history are overlooked, inappropriate treatment may result in the death of the patient. Likewise, the chance of acquiring a sexually transmitted disease can be greatly affected by a relatively minor variation in sexual practices, such as the method used for contraception. Knowledge of the relationship between specific risk factors and disease allows the physician to influence a patient's health even before the development of infection by modification of these risk factors and—when a vaccine is available—by immunization. Climate can affect the ecological niche of a pathogen or its vector, and climate change can lead to alterations in the endemicity of infectious diseases in different regions. For example, an outbreak of chikungunya caused by a mosquito-borne alphavirus recently occurred in central Italy; previous outbreaks had been confined to the tropics, and some have attributed this expansion to global warming.

Many specific host factors influence the likelihood of acquiring an infectious disease. Age, immunization history, prior illnesses, level of nutrition, pregnancy, coexisting illness, and perhaps emotional state all have some impact on the risk of infection after exposure to a potential pathogen. The importance of individual host defense mechanisms, either specific or nonspecific, becomes apparent in their absence, and our understanding of these immune mechanisms is enhanced by studies of clinical syndromes developing in immunodeficient patients (Table 119-1). For example, the higher attack rate of meningococcal disease among people with deficiencies in specific complement proteins of the so-called membrane attack complex (see "Adaptive Immunity," below) than in the general population underscores the importance of an intact complement system in the prevention of meningococcal infection. However, the genetic basis of susceptibility to infectious diseases is more complex than these examples of defects in any single gene would suggest. Human predisposition to infectious diseases involves a spectrum ranging from monogenic to polygenic traits that are the subject of ongoing study.

Medical care itself increases the patient's risk of acquiring an infection in several ways: (1) through contact with pathogens during hospitalization, (2) through breaching of the skin (with IV devices or surgical incisions) or mucosal surfaces (with endotracheal tubes or bladder catheters), (3) through introduction of foreign bodies, (4) through alteration of the natural flora with antibiotics, and (5) through treatment with immunosuppressive drugs.

Infection involves complicated interactions of microbe and host and inevitably affects both. In most cases, a pathogenic process consisting of several steps is required for the development of infections. Since the competent host has a complex series of barricades in place to prevent infection, the successful pathogen must use specific strategies at each of these steps. The specific strategies used by bacteria, viruses, and parasites (Chap. 120) have some remarkable conceptual similarities, but the strategic details are unique not only for each class of microorganism but also for individual species within a class.

THE IMMUNE RESPONSE

INNATE IMMUNITY

As they have co-evolved with microbes, higher organisms have developed mechanisms for recognizing and responding to microorganisms. Many of these mechanisms, referred to together as *innate immunity*, are evolutionarily ancient, having been conserved from insects to humans. In general, innate immune mechanisms exploit molecular patterns found specifically in pathogenic microorganisms. These "pathogen signatures" are recognized by host molecules that either directly interfere with the pathogen or initiate a response that does so. Innate immunity serves to protect the host without prior exposure to an infectious agent—i.e., before specific or adaptive immunity has had a chance to develop. Innate immunity also functions as a warning system that activates components of adaptive immunity early in the course of infection. The innate immune system does not confer long-lasting immunity to the host but rather provides immediate defense against infection. Innate immunity is mediated by cells, various proteins found in the host (i.e., the complement system), and cytokines.

Toll-like receptors (TLRs) are instructive in illustrating how organisms are detected and send signals to the immune system. There are at least 11 TLRs, each specific for detecting different biologic classes of molecules. TLRs are found on the surface and within the endosomes of several types of host cells. For example, even minuscule amounts of lipopolysaccharide (LPS), a molecule found uniquely in gram-negative bacteria, are detected by LPS-binding protein, CD14, and TLR4 (see Fig. 120-3). The interaction of LPS with these components of the innate immune system prompts macrophages, via the transcriptional activator nuclear factor κB (NF-κB), to produce cytokines that lead to inflammation and enzymes that enhance the clearance of microbes. These initial responses serve not only to limit infection but also to initiate specific or adaptive immune responses.

TABLE 119-1 Infections Associated With Selected Defects in Immunity

Host Defect	Disease or Therapy Associated With Defect	Common Etiologic Agent of Infection
Nonspecific Immunity		
Impaired cough	Rib fracture, neuromuscular dysfunction	Bacteria causing pneumonia, aerobic and anaerobic oral flora
Loss of gastric acidity	Achlorhydria, histamine blockade	*Salmonella* spp., enteric pathogens
Loss of cutaneous integrity	Penetrating trauma, athlete's foot	*Staphylococcus* spp., *Streptococcus* spp.
	Burn	*Pseudomonas aeruginosa*
	IV catheter	*Staphylococcus* spp., *Streptococcus* spp., gram-negative rods, coagulase-negative staphylococci
Implantable device	Heart valve	*Streptococcus* spp., coagulase-negative staphylococci, *Staphylococcus aureus*
	Artificial joint	*Staphylococcus* spp., *Streptococcus* spp., gram-negative rods
Loss of normal bacterial flora	Antibiotic use	*Clostridium difficile*, *Candida* spp.
Impaired clearance		
Poor drainage	Urinary tract infection	*Escherichia coli*
Abnormal secretions	Cystic fibrosis	Chronic pulmonary infection with *P. aeruginosa*
Inflammatory Response		
Neutropenia	Hematologic malignancy, cytotoxic chemotherapy, aplastic anemia, HIV infection	Gram-negative enteric bacilli, *Pseudomonas* spp., *Staphylococcus* spp., *Candida* spp.
Chemotaxis	Chédiak-Higashi syndrome, Job's syndrome, protein-calorie malnutrition	*S. aureus*, *Streptococcus pyogenes*, *Haemophilus influenzae*, gram-negative bacilli
	Leukocyte adhesion defects 1 and 2	Bacteria causing skin and systemic infections, gingivitis
Phagocytosis (cellular)	Systemic lupus erythematosus (SLE), chronic myelogenous leukemia, megaloblastic anemia	*Streptococcus pneumoniae*, *H. influenzae*
Splenectomy	—	*H. influenzae*, *S. pneumoniae*, other streptococci, *Capnocytophaga* spp., *Babesia microti*, *Salmonella* spp.
Microbicidal defect	Chronic granulomatous disease	Catalase-positive bacteria and fungi: staphylococci, *E. coli*, *Klebsiella* spp., *P. aeruginosa*, *Aspergillus* spp., *Nocardia* spp.
	Chédiak-Higashi syndrome	*S. aureus*, *S. pyogenes*
	Interferon γ receptor defect, interleukin 12 deficiency, interleukin 12 receptor defect	*Mycobacterium* spp., *Salmonella* spp.
Innate Immunity		
Complement system		
C3	Congenital liver disease, SLE, nephrotic syndrome	*S. aureus*, *S. pneumoniae*, *Pseudomonas* spp., *Proteus* spp.
C5	Congenital	*Neisseria* spp., gram-negative rods
C6, C7, C8	Congenital, SLE	*Neisseria meningitidis*, *N. gonorrhoeae*
Alternative pathway	Sickle cell disease	*S. pneumoniae*, *Salmonella* spp.
Toll-like receptor 4	Congenital	Gram-negative bacilli
Interleukin 1 receptor–associated kinase (IRAK) 4	Congenital	*S. pneumoniae*, *S. aureus*, other bacteria
Mannan-binding lectin	Congenital	*N. meningitidis*, other bacteria
Adaptive Immunity		
T lymphocyte deficiency/dysfunction	Thymic aplasia, thymic hypoplasia, Hodgkin's disease, sarcoidosis, lepromatous leprosy	*Listeria monocytogenes*, *Mycobacterium* spp., *Candida* spp., *Aspergillus* spp., *Cryptococcus neoformans*, herpes simplex virus, varicella-zoster virus
	AIDS	*Pneumocystis*, cytomegalovirus, herpes simplex virus, *Mycobacterium avium-intracellulare*, *C. neoformans*, *Candida* spp.
	Mucocutaneous candidiasis	*Candida* spp.
	Purine nucleoside phosphorylase deficiency	Fungi, viruses
B cell deficiency/dysfunction	Bruton's X-linked agammaglobulinemia	*S. pneumoniae*, other streptococci
	Agammaglobulinemia, chronic lymphocytic leukemia, multiple myeloma, dysglobulinemia	*H. influenzae*, *N. meningitidis*, *S. aureus*, *Klebsiella pneumoniae*, *E. coli*, *Giardia lamblia*, *Pneumocystis*, enteroviruses

(continued)

Host Defect	Disease or Therapy Associated With Defect	Common Etiologic Agent of Infection
Mixed T and B cell deficiency/dysfunction	Selective IgM deficiency	*S. pneumoniae, H. influenzae, E. coli*
	Selective IgA deficiency	*G. lamblia*, hepatitis virus, *S. pneumoniae, H. influenzae*
	Common variable hypogammaglobulinemia	*Pneumocystis*, cytomegalovirus, *S. pneumoniae, H. influenzae*, various other bacteria
	Ataxia-telangiectasia	*S. pneumoniae, H. influenzae, S. aureus*, rubella virus, *G. lamblia*
	Severe combined immunodeficiency	*S. aureus, S. pneumoniae, H. influenzae, Candida albicans, Pneumocystis*, varicella-zoster virus, rubella virus, cytomegalovirus
	Wiskott-Aldrich syndrome	Agents of infections associated with T and B cell abnormalities
	X-linked hyper-IgM syndrome	*Pneumocystis*, cytomegalovirus, *Cryptosporidium parvum*

Other receptor systems have been defined as important in regulating inflammation as well. The NOD-like receptors (i.e., the nucleotide-binding domain– and leucine-rich repeat–containing family of receptors, or NLRs) are cytoplasmic proteins that also recognize molecular patterns and activate inflammation through caspases, whose modification of proinflammatory cytokines such as interleukin (IL)-1 results in activation of NF-κB signaling to induce inflammatory molecules. The activated mediators of inflammation within the cytoplasm form multiprotein complexes called *inflammasomes*, which promote the inflammatory process.

■ **ADAPTIVE IMMUNITY**

Once in contact with the host immune system, the microorganism faces the host's tightly integrated cellular and humoral immune responses. Cellular immunity (Chap. 314), comprising T lymphocytes, macrophages, and natural killer cells, primarily recognizes and combats pathogens that proliferate intracellularly. Cellular immune mechanisms are important in immunity to all classes of infectious agents, including most viruses and many bacteria (e.g., *Mycoplasma, Chlamydophila, Listeria, Salmonella*, and *Mycobacterium*), parasites (e.g., *Trypanosoma, Toxoplasma*, and *Leishmania*), and fungi (e.g., *Histoplasma, Cryptococcus*, and *Coccidioides*). Usually, T lymphocytes are activated by dendritic cells, macrophages, and B lymphocytes, which present foreign antigens in the context of the host's own major histocompatibility complex antigen to the T cell receptor. Activated T cells may then act in several ways to fight infection. *Cytotoxic* CD8+ T cells may directly attack and lyse host cells that express foreign antigens. *Helper* CD4+ T cells stimulate the proliferation of B cells and the production of immunoglobulins. Antigen-presenting cells and T cells communicate with each other via a variety of signals, acting coordinately to instruct the immune system to respond in a specific fashion. T cells elaborate cytokines (e.g., interferon) that directly inhibit the growth of pathogens or stimulate killing by host macrophages and cytotoxic cells. Cytokines also augment the host's immunity by stimulating the inflammatory response (fever, the production of acute-phase serum components, and the proliferation of leukocytes). Cytokine stimulation does not always result in a favorable response in the host; septic shock (Chap. 271) and toxic shock syndrome (Chaps. 135 and 136) are among the conditions that are mediated by these inflammatory substances.

The immune system has also developed cells that specialize in controlling or downregulating immune responses. For example, T$_{reg}$ cells, a subgroup of CD4+ T cells, prevent autoimmune responses by other T cells and are thought to be important in downregulating immune responses to foreign antigens. There appear to be both naturally occurring and acquired T$_{reg}$ cells. One mechanism used by T$_{reg}$ cells to downregulate inflammation is the production of the anti-inflammatory cytokine IL-10.

The reticuloendothelial system, which clears circulating microorganisms, comprises monocyte-derived phagocytic cells (Kupffer cells) and Ito cells in the liver, alveolar macrophages in the lungs, macrophages and dendritic cells in the spleen, mesangial cells in the kidneys, microglia in the brain, and macrophages and dendritic cells in the lymph nodes. Although these tissue macrophages and polymorphonuclear leukocytes (PMNs) are capable of killing microorganisms without help, they function much more efficiently when pathogens are first *opsonized* (Greek, "prepared for eating") by components of the complement system such as C3b and/or by antibodies.

Extracellular pathogens, including most encapsulated bacteria (those surrounded by a complex polysaccharide coat), are attacked by the humoral immune system, which includes antibodies, the complement cascade, and phagocytic cells. *Antibodies* are complex glycoproteins (also called *immunoglobulins*) that are produced by mature B lymphocytes, circulate in body fluids, and are secreted on mucosal surfaces. Antibodies specifically recognize and bind to foreign antigens. One of the most impressive features of the immune system is the ability to generate an incredible diversity of antibodies capable of recognizing virtually every foreign antigen yet not reacting with self. In addition to being exquisitely specific for antigens, antibodies come in different structural and functional classes: IgG predominates in the circulation and persists for many years after exposure; IgM is the earliest specific antibody to appear in response to infection; secretory IgA is important in immunity at mucosal surfaces, while monomeric IgA appears in the serum; and IgE is important in allergic and parasitic diseases. Antibodies may directly impede the function of an invading organism, neutralize secreted toxins and enzymes, or facilitate the removal of the antigen (invading organism) by phagocytic cells. Immunoglobulins participate in cell-mediated immunity by promoting the antibody-dependent cellular cytotoxicity functions of certain T lymphocytes. Antibodies also promote the deposition of complement components on the surface of the invader.

The *complement* system (Chap. 314) consists of a group of serum proteins functioning as a cooperative, self-regulating cascade of enzymes that adhere to—and in some cases disrupt—the surface of invading organisms. Some of these surface-adherent proteins (e.g., C3b) can then act as opsonins for destruction of microbes by phagocytes. The later, "terminal" components (C7, C8, and C9) can directly kill some bacterial invaders (notably, many of the neisseriae) by forming a membrane attack complex and disrupting the integrity of the bacterial membrane, thus causing bacteriolysis. Other complement components, such as C5a, act as chemoattractants for PMNs (see below). Complement activation and deposition occur by either or both of two pathways: the *classic* pathway is activated primarily by immune complexes (i.e., antibody bound to antigen), and the *alternative* pathway is activated by microbial components, frequently in the absence of antibody. PMNs have receptors for both antibody and C3b, and antibody and complement function together to aid in the clearance of infectious agents.

PMNs, short-lived white blood cells that engulf and kill invading microbes, are first attracted to inflammatory sites by chemoattractants such as C5a, which is a product of complement activation at the site of infection. PMNs localize to the site of infection by adhering to cellular adhesion molecules expressed by endothelial cells. Endothelial cells express these receptors, called *selectins* (CD-62, ELAM-1), in response to inflammatory cytokines such as tumor necrosis factor α and IL-1. The binding of these selectin molecules to specific receptors on PMNs results in the adherence of the PMNs to the endothelium. Cytokine-mediated upregulation and expression of intercellular adhesion molecule 1 (ICAM-1) on endothelial cells then take place, and this latter receptor binds to β_2 integrins on PMNs, thereby facilitating diapedesis into the extravascular compartment. Once the PMNs are in the extravascular compartment, various molecules (e.g., arachidonic acids) further enhance the inflammatory process.

Infectious Diseases

The clinical manifestations of infectious diseases at presentation are myriad, varying from fulminant life-threatening processes to brief and self-limited conditions to indolent chronic maladies. A careful history is essential and must include details on underlying chronic diseases, medications, occupation, and travel. Risk factors for exposure to certain types of pathogens may give important clues to diagnosis. A sexual history may reveal risks for exposure to HIV and other sexually transmitted pathogens. A history of contact with animals may suggest numerous diagnoses, including rabies, Q fever, bartonellosis, *Escherichia coli* O157 infection, or cryptococcosis. Blood transfusions have been linked to diseases ranging from viral hepatitis to malaria to prion disease. A history of exposure to insect vectors (coupled with information about the season and geographic site of exposure) may lead to consideration of such diseases as Rocky Mountain spotted fever, other rickettsial diseases, tularemia, Lyme disease, babesiosis, malaria, trypanosomiasis, and numerous arboviral infections. Ingestion of contaminated liquids or foods may lead to enteric infection with *Salmonella, Listeria, Campylobacter,* amebas, cryptosporidia, or helminths. Since infectious diseases may involve many organ systems, a careful review of systems may elicit important clues as to the disease process.

The physical examination must be thorough, and attention must be paid to seemingly minor details, such as a soft heart murmur that might indicate bacterial endocarditis or a retinal lesion that suggests disseminated candidiasis or cytomegalovirus infection. Rashes are extremely important clues to infectious diagnoses and may be the only sign pointing to a specific etiology (Chaps. 17 and e7). Certain rashes are so specific as to be pathognomonic—e.g., the childhood exanthems (measles, rubella, varicella), the target lesion of erythema migrans (Lyme disease), ecthyma gangrenosum (*Pseudomonas aeruginosa*), and eschars (rickettsial diseases). Other rashes, although less specific, may be exceedingly important diagnostic indicators. The

prompt recognition of the early scarlatiniform and later petechial rashes of meningococcal infection or of the subtle embolic lesions of disseminated fungal infections in immunosuppressed patients can hasten life-saving therapy. Fever (Chaps. 16, 17, and 18) is a common manifestation of infection and may be its sole apparent indication. Sometimes the pattern of fever or its temporally associated findings may help refine the differential diagnosis. For example, fever occurring every 48–72 h is suggestive of malaria (Chap. 210). The elevation in body temperature in fever (through resetting of the hypothalamic setpoint mediated by cytokines) must be distinguished from elevations in body temperature from other causes such as drug toxicity (Chap. 18) or heat stroke (Chap. 16).

LABORATORY INVESTIGATIONS

Laboratory studies must be carefully considered and directed toward establishing an etiologic diagnosis in the shortest possible time, at the lowest possible cost, and with the least possible discomfort to the patient. Since mucosal surfaces and the skin are colonized with many harmless or beneficial microorganisms, cultures must be performed in a manner that minimizes the likelihood of contamination with this normal flora while maximizing the yield of pathogens. A sputum sample is far more likely to be valuable when elicited with careful coaching by the clinician than when collected in a container simply left at the bedside with cursory instructions. Gram's stains of specimens should be interpreted carefully and the quality of the specimen assessed. The findings on Gram's staining should correspond to the results of culture; a discrepancy may suggest diagnostic possibilities such as infection due to fastidious or anaerobic bacteria.

The microbiology laboratory must be an ally in the diagnostic endeavor. Astute laboratory personnel will suggest optimal culture and transport conditions or alternative tests to facilitate diagnosis. If informed about specific potential pathogens, an alert laboratory staff will allow sufficient time for these organisms to become evident in culture, even when the organisms are present in small numbers or are slow-growing. The parasitology technician who is attuned to the specific diagnostic considerations relevant to a particular case may be able to detect the rare, otherwise-elusive egg or cyst in a stool specimen. In cases where a diagnosis appears difficult, serum should be stored during the early acute phase of the illness so that a diagnostic rise in titer of antibody to a specific pathogen can be detected later. Bacterial and fungal antigens can sometimes be detected in body fluids, even when cultures are negative or are rendered sterile by antibiotic therapy. Nucleic acid amplification techniques allow the amplification of specific DNA and RNA sequences so that minute quantities of pathogens can be recognized in host specimens.

Infectious Diseases

Optimal therapy for infectious diseases requires a broad knowledge of medicine and careful clinical judgment. Life-threatening infections such as bacterial meningitis or sepsis, viral encephalitis, or falciparum malaria must be treated immediately, often before a specific causative organism is identified. Antimicrobial agents must be chosen empirically and must be active against the range of potential infectious agents consistent with the clinical scenario. In contrast, good clinical judgment sometimes dictates withholding of antimicrobial drugs in a self-limited process or until a specific diagnosis is made. The dictum *primum non nocere* should be adhered to, and it should be remembered that all antimicrobial agents carry a risk (and a cost). Direct toxicity may be encountered—e.g., ototoxicity due to aminoglycosides, lipodystrophy due to antiretroviral agents, and hepatotoxicity due to antituberculous agents such as isoniazid and rifampin. Allergic reactions are common and can be serious. Since superinfection sometimes follows eradication of the normal flora and colonization by a resistant organism, one invariant principle is that infectious disease therapy should be directed toward as narrow a spectrum of infectious agents as possible. Treatment specific for the pathogen should result in as little perturbation as possible of the host's microflora. Indeed, future therapeutic agents may act not by killing a microbe but by interfering with one or more of its virulence factors.

With few exceptions, abscesses require surgical or percutaneous drainage for cure. Foreign bodies, including medical devices, must generally be removed in order to eliminate an infection of the device or of the adjacent tissue. Other infections, such as necrotizing fasciitis, peritonitis due to a perforated organ, gas gangrene, and chronic osteomyelitis, require surgery as the primary means of cure; in these conditions, antibiotics play only an adjunctive role.

The role of immunomodulators in the management of infectious diseases has received increasing attention. Glucocorticoids have been shown to be of benefit in the adjunctive treatment of bacterial meningitis and in therapy for *Pneumocystis* pneumonia in patients with AIDS. The use of these agents in other infectious processes remains less clear and in some cases (in cerebral malaria, for example) is detrimental. Activated protein C (drotrecogin alfa, activated) is the first immunomodulatory agent widely available for the treatment of severe sepsis. Its usefulness demonstrates the interrelatedness of the clotting cascade and systemic immunity. Other agents that modulate the immune response include prostaglandin inhibitors, specific lymphokines, and tumor necrosis factor inhibitors. Specific antibody therapy plays a role in the treatment and prevention of many diseases. Specific immunoglobulins have long been known to prevent the development of symptomatic rabies and tetanus. Monoclonal antibodies targeting specific pathogens have been developed (e.g., for the treatment of respiratory syncytial virus infection). There is a pressing need for well-designed clinical trials to evaluate each new interventional modality.

PERSPECTIVE

The genetic simplicity of many infectious agents allows them to undergo rapid evolution and to develop selective advantages that result in constant variation in the clinical manifestations of infection. Moreover, changes in the environment and the host can predispose new populations to a particular infection. The dramatic march of West Nile virus from a single focus in New York City in 1999 to locations throughout the North American continent by the summer of 2002 caused widespread alarm, illustrating the fear that new plagues induce in the human psyche. The intentional release of deadly spores of *Bacillus anthracis* via the U.S. Postal Service awakened many from a sense of complacency regarding biologic weapons.

"The terror of the unknown is seldom better displayed than by the response of a population to the appearance of an epidemic, particularly when the epidemic strikes without apparent cause." Edward H. Kass made this statement in 1977 in reference to the newly discovered Legionnaire's disease, but it could apply equally to SARS, pandemic H1N1 influenza, or any other new and mysterious disease. The potential for infectious agents to emerge in novel and unexpected ways requires that physicians and public health officials be knowledgeable, vigilant, and open-minded in their approach to unexplained illness. The emergence of antimicrobial-resistant pathogens (e.g., enterococci that are resistant to all known antimicrobial agents and cause essentially untreatable infections) and the paucity of new classes of antimicrobial drugs have led some to conclude that we are entering the "postantibiotic era." Others have held to the perception that infectious diseases no longer represent as serious a concern to world health as they once did. The progress that science, medicine, and society as a whole have made in combating these maladies is impressive, and it is ironic that, as we stand on the threshold of an understanding of the most basic biology of the microbe, infectious diseases are posing renewed problems. We are threatened by the appearance of new diseases such as SARS, hepatitis C, and Ebola virus infection and by the reemergence of old foes such as tuberculosis, cholera, plague, and *Streptococcus pyogenes* infection. True students of infectious diseases were perhaps less surprised than anyone else by these developments. Those who know pathogens are aware of their incredible adaptability and diversity. As ingenious and successful as therapeutic approaches may be, our ability to develop methods to counter infectious agents so far has not matched the myriad strategies employed by the sea of microbes that surrounds us. Their sheer numbers and the rate at which they can evolve are daunting. Moreover, environmental changes, rapid global travel, population movements, and medicine itself—through its use of antibiotics and immunosuppressive agents—all increase the impact of infectious diseases. Although new vaccines, new antibiotics, improved global communication, and new modalities for treating and preventing infection will be developed, pathogenic microbes will continue to develop new strategies of their own, presenting us with an unending and dynamic challenge.

FURTHER READINGS

ALCAÏS A et al: Human genetics of infectious diseases: Between proof of principle and paradigm. J Clin Invest 119: 2506, 2009

ARMSTRONG G et al: Trends in infectious disease mortality in the United States during the 20th century. JAMA 281:61, 1999

BLASER MJ: Introduction to bacteria and bacterial diseases, in *Principles and Practice of Infectious Diseases*, 7th ed, GL Mandell et al (eds). Philadelphia, Elsevier, 2010, p 2539

HENDERSON DA: Countering the posteradication threat of smallpox and polio. Clin Infect Dis 34:79, 2002

HOFFMAN J et al: Phylogenetic perspectives in innate immunity. Science 284:1313, 1999

HUNG DT et al: Small-molecule inhibitor of *Vibrio cholerae* virulence and intestinal colonization. Science 310:670, 2005

NOVEL SWINE-ORIGIN INFLUENZA A (H1N1) VIRUS INVESTIGATION TEAM: Emergence of a novel swine-origin influenza A (H1N1) virus in humans. N Engl J Med 360:2605, 2009

PROMED-MAIL: The Program for Monitoring Emerging Diseases. *www.promedmail.org*

SHUMAN EK: Global climate change and infectious diseases. N Engl J Med 362:1061, 2010

VIRGIN HW: Pathogenesis of viral infections, in *Fields Virology*, DM Knipe, PM Howley (eds). Philadelphia, Lippincott Williams & Wilkins, 2007, pp 327–388

WEISS ST: Eat dirt—the hygiene hypothesis and allergic diseases. N Engl J Med 347:930, 2002

CHAPTER 120

Molecular Mechanisms of Microbial Pathogenesis

Gerald B. Pier

Over the past four decades, molecular studies of the pathogenesis of microorganisms have yielded an explosion of information about the various microbial and host molecules that contribute to the processes of infection and disease. These processes can be classified into several stages: microbial encounter with and entry into the host; microbial growth after entry; avoidance of innate host defenses; tissue invasion and tropism; tissue damage; and transmission to new hosts. *Virulence* is the measure of an organism's capacity to cause disease and is a function of the pathogenic factors elaborated by microbes. These factors promote *colonization* (the simple presence of potentially pathogenic microbes in or on a host), *infection* (attachment and growth of pathogens and avoidance of host defenses), and *disease* (often, but not always, the result of activities of secreted toxins or toxic metabolites). In addition, the host's inflammatory response to infection greatly contributes to disease and its attendant clinical signs and symptoms.

■ MICROBIAL ENTRY AND ADHERENCE

Entry sites

A microbial pathogen can potentially enter any part of a host organism. In general, the type of disease produced by a particular microbe is often a direct consequence of its route of entry into the body. The most common sites of entry are mucosal surfaces (the respiratory, alimentary, and urogenital tracts) and the skin. Ingestion, inhalation, and sexual contact are typical routes of microbial entry. Other portals of entry include sites of skin injury (cuts, bites, burns, trauma) along with injection via natural (i.e., vector-borne) or artificial (i.e., needle-stick injury) routes. A few pathogens, such as *Schistosoma* species, can penetrate unbroken skin. The conjunctiva can serve as an entry point for pathogens of the eye, which occasionally spread systemically from that site.

Microbial entry usually relies on the presence of specific factors needed for persistence and growth in a tissue. Fecal-oral spread via the alimentary tract requires a biologic profile consistent with survival in the varied environments of the gastrointestinal tract (including the low pH of the stomach and the high bile content of the intestine) as well as in contaminated food or water outside the host. Organisms that gain entry via the respiratory tract survive well in small moist droplets produced during sneezing and coughing. Pathogens that enter by venereal routes often survive best in the warm moist environment of the urogenital mucosa and have restricted host ranges (e.g., *Neisseria gonorrhoeae*, *Treponema pallidum*, and HIV).

The biology of microbes entering through the skin is highly varied. Some of these organisms can survive in a broad range of environments, such as the salivary glands or alimentary tracts of arthropod vectors, the mouths of larger animals, soil, and water. A complex biology allows protozoan parasites such as *Plasmodium*, *Leishmania*, and *Trypanosoma* spp. to undergo morphogenic changes that permit transmission of the organism to mammalian hosts during insect feeding for blood meals. Plasmodia are injected as infective sporozoites from the salivary glands during mosquito feeding. *Leishmania* parasites are regurgitated as promastigotes from the alimentary tract of sandflies and injected by bite into a susceptible host. Trypanosomes are first ingested from infected hosts by reduviid bugs; the pathogens then multiply in the gastrointestinal tract of the insects and are released in feces onto the host's skin during subsequent feedings. Most microbes that land directly on intact skin are destined to die, as survival on the skin or in hair follicles requires resistance to fatty acids, low pH, and other antimicrobial factors on the skin. Once it is damaged (and particularly if it becomes necrotic), the skin can be a major portal of entry and growth for pathogens and elaboration of their toxic products. Burn wound infections and tetanus are clear examples. After animal bites, pathogens resident in the animal's saliva gain access to the victim's tissues through the damaged skin. Rabies is the paradigm for this pathogenic process; rabies virus grows in striated muscle cells at the site of inoculation.

Microbial adherence

Once in or on a host, most microbes must anchor themselves to a tissue or tissue factor; the possible exceptions are organisms that directly enter the bloodstream and multiply there. Specific ligands or adhesins for host receptors constitute a major area of study in the field of microbial pathogenesis. Adhesins comprise a wide range of surface structures, not only anchoring the microbe to a tissue and promoting cellular entry where appropriate but also eliciting host responses critical to the pathogenic process (Table 120-1). Most microbes produce multiple adhesins specific for multiple host receptors. These adhesins are often redundant, are serologically variable, and act additively or synergistically with other microbial factors to promote microbial sticking to host tissues. In addition, some microbes adsorb host proteins onto their surface and utilize the natural host protein receptor for microbial binding and entry into target cells.

Viral adhesins All viral pathogens must bind to host cells, enter them, and replicate within them. Viral coat proteins serve as the ligands for cellular entry, and more than one ligand-receptor interaction may be needed; for example, HIV utilizes its envelope glycoprotein (gp) 120 to enter host cells by binding to both CD4 and one of two receptors for chemokines (designated CCR5 and CXCR4). Similarly, the measles virus H glycoprotein binds to both CD46 and the membrane-organizing protein moesin on host cells. The gB and gC proteins on herpes simplex virus bind to heparan sulfate, although this adherence is not essential for entry but rather serves to concentrate virions close to the cell surface; this step is followed by attachment to mammalian cells mediated by the viral gD protein, with subsequent formation of a homotrimer of viral gB protein or a heterodimer of viral gH and gL proteins that permits fusion of the viral envelope with the host cell membrane. Herpes simplex virus can use a number of eukaryotic cell surface receptors for entry, including the herpesvirus entry mediator (related to the tumor necrosis factor receptor), members of the immunoglobulin superfamily, the proteins nectin-1 and nectin-2, and modified heparan sulfate.

Bacterial adhesins Among the microbial adhesins studied in greatest detail are bacterial pili and flagella (Fig. 120-1). *Pili* or *fimbriae* are commonly used by gram-negative bacteria for attachment to host cells and tissues; recent studies have identified similar factors produced by gram-positive organisms such as group B streptococci. In electron micrographs, these hairlike projections (up to several hundred per cell) may be confined to one end of the organism (polar pili) or distributed more evenly over the surface. An individual cell may have pili with a variety of functions. Most pili are made up of a major

TABLE 120-1 Examples of Microbial Ligand-Receptor Interactions

Microorganism	Type of Microbial Ligand	Host Receptor
Viral Pathogens		
Influenza virus	Hemagglutinin	Sialic acid
Measles virus		
Vaccine strain	Hemagglutinin	CD46/moesin
Wild-type strains	Hemagglutinin	Signaling lymphocytic activation molecule (SLAM)
Human herpesvirus type 6	?	CD46
Herpes simplex virus	Glycoprotein C	Heparan sulfate
HIV	Surface glycoprotein	CD4 and chemokine receptors (CCR5 and CXCR4)
Epstein-Barr virus	Envelope protein	CD21 (CR2)
Adenovirus	Fiber protein	Coxsackie-adenovirus receptor (CAR)
Coxsackievirus	Viral coat proteins	CAR and major histocompatibility class I antigens
Bacterial Pathogens		
Neisseria spp.	Pili	Membrane co-factor protein (CD46)
Pseudomonas aeruginosa	Pili and flagella	Asialo-GM1
	Lipopolysaccharide	Cystic fibrosis transmembrane conductance regulator (CFTR)
Escherichia coli	Pili	Ceramides/mannose and digalactosyl residues
Streptococcus pyogenes	Hyaluronic acid capsule	CD44
Yersinia spp.	Invasin/accessory invasin locus	β_1 Integrins
Bordetella pertussis	Filamentous hemagglutinin	CR3
Legionella pneumophila	Adsorbed C3bi	CR3
Mycobacterium tuberculosis	Adsorbed C3bi	CR3; DC-SIGN[a]
Fungal Pathogens		
Blastomyces dermatitidis	WI-1	Possibly matrix proteins and integrins
Candida albicans	Int1p	Extracellular matrix proteins
Protozoal Pathogens		
Plasmodium vivax	Merozoite form	Duffy Fy antigen
Plasmodium falciparum	Erythrocyte-binding protein 175 (EBA-175)	Glycophorin A
Entamoeba histolytica	Surface lectin	*N*-Acetylglucosamine

[a]A novel dendritic cell–specific C-type lectin.

pilin protein subunit (molecular weight, 17,000–30,000) that polymerizes to form the pilus. Many strains of *Escherichia coli* isolated from urinary tract infections express mannose-binding type 1 pili, whose binding to integral membrane glycoproteins called *uroplakins* that coat the cells in the bladder epithelium is inhibited by D-mannose. Other strains produce the Pap (pyelonephritis-associated) or P pilus adhesin that mediates binding to digalactose (gal-gal) residues on globosides of the human P blood groups. Both of these types of pili have proteins located at the tips of the main pilus unit that are critical to the binding specificity of the whole pilus unit. Although immunization with the mannose-binding tip protein (FimH) of type 1 pili prevents experimental *E. coli* bladder infections in mice and monkeys, a human trial of this vaccine was not successful. *E. coli* cells causing diarrheal disease express pilus-like receptors for enterocytes on the small bowel, along with other receptors termed *colonization factors*.

The type IV pilus, a common type of pilus found in *Neisseria* species, *Moraxella* species, *Vibrio cholerae*, *Legionella pneumophila*, *Salmonella enterica* serovar Typhi, enteropathogenic *E. coli*, and *Pseudomonas aeruginosa*, mediates adherence of organisms to target surfaces. Type IV pili tend to have a relatively conserved amino-terminal region and a more variable carboxyl-terminal region. For some species (e.g., *N. gonorrhoeae*, *Neisseria meningitidis*, and enteropathogenic *E. coli*), the pili are critical for attachment to mucosal epithelial cells. For others, such as *P. aeruginosa*, the pili only partially mediate the cells' adherence to host tissues. *V. cholerae* cells appear to use two different types of pili for intestinal colonization. Whereas interference with this stage of colonization would appear to be an effective antibacterial strategy, attempts to develop pilus-based vaccines for human diseases have not been highly successful to date.

Flagella are long appendages attached at either one or both ends of the bacterial cell (polar flagella) or distributed over the entire cell surface (peritrichous flagella). Flagella, like pili, are composed of a polymerized or aggregated basic protein. In flagella, the protein

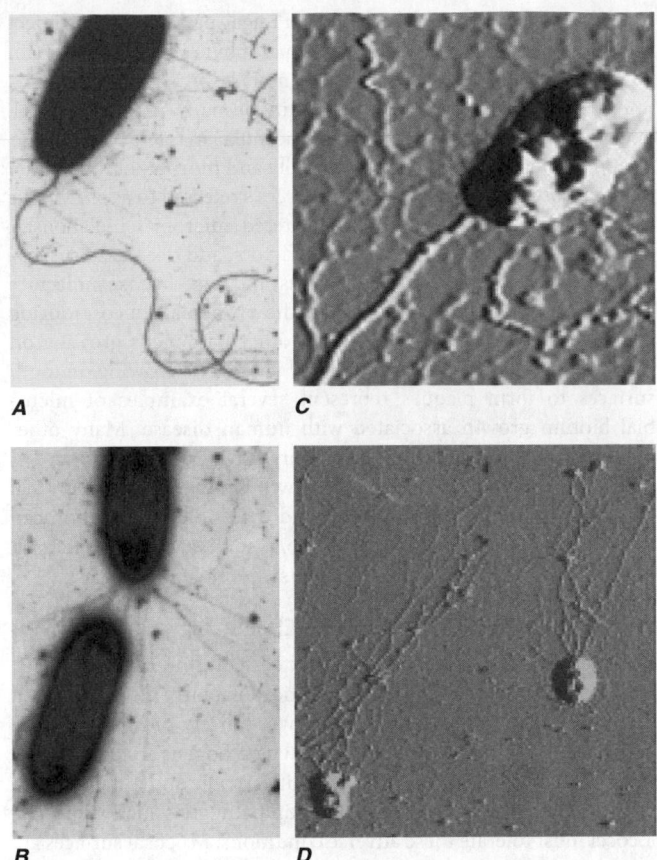

Figure 120-1 Bacterial surface structures. *A* and *B*. Traditional electron micrographic images of fixed cells of *Pseudomonas aeruginosa*. Flagella (*A*) and pili (*B*) project out from the bacterial poles. *C* and *D*. Atomic force microscopic image of live *P. aeruginosa* freshly planted onto a smooth mica surface. This technology reveals the fine, three-dimensional detail of the bacterial surface structures. *(Images courtesy of Drs. Martin Lee and Milan Bajmoczi, Harvard Medical School.)*

subunits form a tight helical structure and vary serologically with the species. Spirochetes such as *T. pallidum* and *Borrelia burgdorferi* have axial filaments similar to flagella running down the long axis of the center of the cell, and they "swim" by rotation around these filaments. Some bacteria can glide over a surface in the absence of obvious motility structures.

Other bacterial structures involved in adherence to host tissues include specific staphylococcal and streptococcal proteins that bind to human extracellular matrix proteins such as fibrin, fibronectin, fibrinogen, laminin, and collagen. Fibronectin appears to be a commonly used receptor for various pathogens; a particular amino acid sequence in fibronectin, Arg-Gly-Asp or RGD, is a critical target used by bacteria to bind to host tissues. Binding of a highly conserved *Staphylococcus aureus* surface protein, clumping factor A (ClfA), to fibrinogen has been implicated in many aspects of pathogenesis. However, attempts to interrupt this interaction and prevent *S. aureus* sepsis in low-birth-weight infants by administering an intravenous IgG preparation derived from the plasma of individuals with high titers of antibody to ClfA failed to show efficacy in a clinical trial completed in April 2006. The conserved outer-core portion of the lipopolysaccharide (LPS) of *P. aeruginosa* mediates binding to the cystic fibrosis transmembrane conductance regulator (CFTR) on airway epithelial cells—an event that appears to be critical for normal host resistance to infection. A number of bacterial pathogens, including coagulase-negative staphylococci, *S. aureus*, and

uropathogenic *E. coli* as well as *Yersinia pestis, Y. pseudotuberculosis, Y. enterocolitica, Bordetella* species, and *Acinetobacter baumannii*, express a surface polysaccharide composed of β-1-6-linked-poly-N-acetyl-D-glucosamine. One of its functions is to promote binding to materials used in catheters and other types of implanted devices. This polysaccharide may be a critical factor in the establishment of device-related infections by pathogens such as staphylococci and *E. coli*. High-powered imaging techniques (e.g., atomic force microscopy) have revealed that bacterial cells have a nonhomogeneous surface that is probably attributable to different concentrations of cell surface molecules, including microbial adhesins, at specific places on the cell surface (Fig. 120-1*D*).

Fungal adhesins Several fungal adhesins have been described that mediate colonization of epithelial surfaces, particularly adherence to structures like fibronectin, laminin, and collagen. The product of the *Candida albicans INT1* gene, Int1p, bears similarity to mammalian integrins that bind to extracellular matrix proteins. Transformation of normally nonadherent *Saccharomyces cerevisiae* with this gene allows these yeast cells to adhere to human epithelial cells. The agglutinin-like sequence (ALS) adhesins are large cell-surface glycoproteins mediating adherence of pathogenic *Candida* to host tissues. These adhesins possess a conserved three-domain structure composed of an N-terminal domain that mediates adherence to host tissue receptors, a central motif consisting of a number of repeats of a conserved sequence of 36 amino acids, and a C-terminal domain that varies in length and sequence and contains a glycosylphosphatidylinositol (GPI) anchor addition site that allows binding of the adhesin to the fungal cell wall. Variability in the number of central domains in different ALS proteins characterizes different adhesins with specificity for different host receptors. The ALS adhesins are expressed under certain environmental conditions—often associated with stress—and are crucial for pathogenesis of fungal infections.

For several fungal pathogens that initiate infections after inhalation of infectious material, the inoculum is ingested by alveolar macrophages, in which the fungal cells transform to pathogenic phenotypes. Like *C. albicans, Blastomyces dermatitidis* binds to CD11b/CD18 integrins as well as to CD14 on macrophages. *B. dermatitidis* produces a 120-kDa surface protein, designated WI-1, that mediates this adherence. The binding domain of WI-1 is homologous to the invasin protein of *Yersinia* that binds to the same type of host cell receptor. An unidentified factor on *Histoplasma capsulatum* also mediates binding of this fungal pathogen to the integrin surface proteins.

Eukaryotic pathogen adhesins Eukaryotic parasites use complicated surface glycoproteins as adhesins, some of which are lectins (proteins that bind to specific carbohydrates on host cells). For example, *Plasmodium vivax*, one of five *Plasmodium* species causing malaria, binds (via Duffy-binding protein) to the Duffy blood group carbohydrate antigen Fy on erythrocytes. *Entamoeba histolytica*, the third leading cause of death from parasitic diseases, expresses two proteins that bind to the disaccharide galactose/N-acetyl galactosamine. Reports indicate that children with mucosal IgA antibody to one of these lectins are resistant to reinfection with virulent *E. histolytica*. A major surface glycoprotein (gp63) of *Leishmania* promastigotes is needed for these parasites to enter human macrophages—the principal target cell of infection. This glycoprotein promotes complement binding but inhibits complement lytic activity, allowing the parasite to use complement receptors for entry into macrophages; gp63 also binds to fibronectin receptors on macrophages. In addition, the pathogen can express a carbohydrate that mediates binding to host cells. Evidence suggests that, as part of hepatic granuloma formation, *Schistosoma mansoni* expresses a carbohydrate epitope related to the Lewis X blood group antigen that promotes adherence of helminthic eggs to vascular endothelial cells under inflammatory conditions.

Host receptors

Host receptors are found both on target cells (such as epithelial cells lining mucosal surfaces) and within the mucus layer covering these cells. Microbial pathogens bind to a wide range of host receptors to establish infection (Table 120-1). Selective loss of host receptors for a pathogen may confer natural resistance to an otherwise susceptible population. For example, 70% of individuals in West Africa lack Fy antigens and are resistant to *P. vivax* infection. *S. enterica* serovar Typhi, the etiologic agent of typhoid fever, produces a pilus protein that binds to CFTR to enter the gastrointestinal submucosa after being ingested by enterocytes. As homozygous mutations in *CFTR* are the cause of the life-shortening disease cystic fibrosis, heterozygote carriers (e.g., 4–5% of individuals of European ancestry) may have had a selective advantage due to decreased susceptibility to typhoid fever. Genetic polymorphisms in CFTR besides those leading to cystic fibrosis have been associated with resistance to typhoid fever.

Numerous virus–target cell interactions have been described, and it is now clear that different viruses can use similar host cell receptors for entry. The list of certain and likely host receptors for viral pathogens is long. Among the host membrane components that can serve as receptors for viruses are sialic acids, gangliosides, glycosaminoglycans, integrins and other members of the immunoglobulin superfamily, histocompatibility antigens, and regulators and receptors for complement components. A notable example of the effect of host receptors on the pathogenesis of infection has emerged from studies comparing the binding of avian influenza A subtype H5N1 with that of influenza A strains expressing the H1 subtype of hemagglutinin. The H1 subtypes tend to be highly pathogenic and transmissible from human to human, and they bind to a receptor composed of two sugar molecules: sialic acid linked α-2-6 to galactose. This receptor is highly expressed in the airway epithelium; when virus is shed from this surface, its transmission via coughing and aerosol droplets is facilitated. In contrast, the H5N1 avian influenza virus binds to sialic acid linked α-2-3 to galactose, and this receptor is highly expressed in pneumocytes in the alveoli. Infection in the alveoli is thought to underlie the high mortality rate associated with avian influenza but also the low interhuman transmissibility of this strain, which is not readily transported to the airways from which it can be expelled by coughing.

■ MICROBIAL GROWTH AFTER ENTRY

Once established on a mucosal or skin site, pathogenic microbes must replicate before causing full-blown infection and disease. Within cells, viral particles release their nucleic acids, which may be directly translated into viral proteins (positive-strand RNA viruses), transcribed from a negative strand of RNA into a complementary mRNA (negative-strand RNA viruses), or transcribed into a complementary strand of DNA (retroviruses); for DNA viruses, mRNA may be transcribed directly from viral DNA, either in the cell nucleus or in the cytoplasm. To grow, bacteria must acquire specific nutrients or synthesize them from precursors in host tissues. Many infectious processes are usually confined to specific epithelial surfaces—e.g., H1 subtype influenza to the respiratory mucosa, gonorrhea to the urogenital epithelium, shigellosis to the gastrointestinal epithelium. While there are multiple reasons for this specificity, one important consideration is the ability of these pathogens to obtain from these specific environments the nutrients needed for growth and survival.

Temperature restrictions also play a role in limiting certain pathogens to specific tissues. Rhinoviruses, a cause of the common cold, grow best at 33°C and replicate in cooler nasal tissues but not in the lung. Leprosy lesions due to *Mycobacterium leprae* are found in and on relatively cool body sites. Fungal pathogens that infect the skin, hair follicles, and nails (dermatophyte infections) remain confined to the cooler, exterior, keratinous layer of the epithelium.

A topic of major interest is the ability of many bacterial, fungal, and protozoal species to grow in multicellular masses referred to as *biofilms*. These masses are biochemically and morphologically quite distinct from the free-living individual cells referred to as *planktonic cells*. Growth in biofilms leads to altered microbial metabolism, production of extracellular virulence factors, and decreased susceptibility to biocides, antimicrobial agents, and host defense molecules and cells. *P. aeruginosa* growing on the bronchial mucosa during chronic infection, staphylococci and other pathogens growing on implanted medical devices, and dental pathogens growing on tooth surfaces to form plaques represent several examples of microbial biofilm growth associated with human disease. Many other pathogens can form biofilms during in vitro growth. It is increasingly accepted that this mode of growth contributes to microbial virulence and induction of disease and that biofilm formation can also be an important factor in microbial survival outside the host, promoting transmission to additional susceptible individuals.

■ AVOIDANCE OF INNATE HOST DEFENSES

As microbes have probably interacted with mucosal/epithelial surfaces since the emergence of multicellular organisms, it is not surprising that multicellular hosts have a variety of innate surface defense mechanisms that can sense when pathogens are present and contribute to their elimination. The skin is acidic and is bathed with fatty acids toxic to many microbes. Skin pathogens such as staphylococci must tolerate these adverse conditions. Mucosal surfaces are covered by a barrier composed of a thick mucus layer that entraps microbes and facilitates their transport out of the body by such processes as mucociliary clearance, coughing, and urination. Mucous secretions, saliva, and tears contain antibacterial factors such as lysozyme and antimicrobial peptides as well as antiviral factors such as interferons (IFNs). Gastric acidity is inimical to the survival of many ingested pathogens, and most mucosal surfaces—particularly the nasopharynx, the vaginal tract, and the gastrointestinal tract—contain a resident flora of commensal microbes that interfere with the ability of pathogens to colonize and infect a host.

Pathogens that survive these factors must still contend with host endocytic, phagocytic, and inflammatory responses as well as with host genetic factors that determine the degree to which a pathogen can survive and grow. The list of genes whose variants, usually by single-nucleotide polymorphisms, can affect host susceptibility and resistance to infection is rapidly expanding. A classic example is a 32-bp deletion in the gene for the HIV-1 co-receptor known as chemokine receptor 5 (CCR5), which, when present in the homozygous state, confers high-level resistance to HIV-1 infection. The growth of viral pathogens entering skin or mucosal epithelial cells can be limited by a variety of host genetic factors, including production of IFNs, modulation of receptors for viral entry, and age- and hormone-related susceptibility factors; by nutritional status; and even by personal habits such as smoking and exercise.

Encounters with epithelial cells

Over the past decade, many bacterial pathogens have been shown to enter epithelial cells (Fig. 120-2); the bacteria often use specialized surface structures that bind to receptors, with consequent internalization. However, the exact role and the importance of this process in infection and disease are not well defined for most of these pathogens. Bacterial entry into host epithelial cells is seen as a means for dissemination to adjacent or deeper tissues or as a route to sanctuary to avoid ingestion and killing by professional phagocytes. Epithelial cell entry appears, for instance, to be a critical aspect of dysentery induction by *Shigella*.

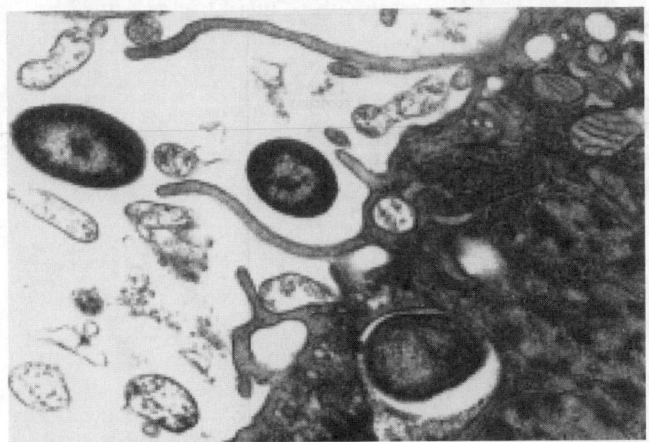

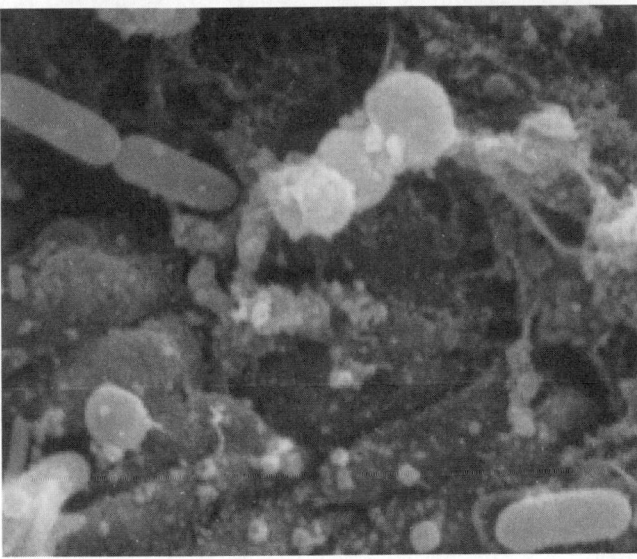

Figure 120-2   Entry of bacteria into epithelial cells. *A.* Internalization of *P. aeruginosa* by cultured airway epithelial cells expressing wild-type cystic fibrosis transmembrane conductance regulator, the cell receptor for bacterial ingestion. ***B.*** Entry of *P. aeruginosa* into murine tracheal epithelial cells after murine infection by the intranasal route.

Curiously, the less virulent strains of many bacterial pathogens are more adept at entering epithelial cells than are more virulent strains; examples include pathogens that lack the surface polysaccharide capsule needed to cause serious disease. Thus, for *Haemophilus influenzae*, *Streptococcus pneumoniae*, *Streptococcus agalactiae* (group B *Streptococcus*), and *Streptococcus pyogenes*, isogenic mutants or variants lacking capsules enter epithelial cells better than the wild-type, encapsulated parental forms that cause disseminated disease. These observations have led to the proposal that epithelial cell entry may be primarily a manifestation of host defense, resulting in bacterial clearance by both shedding of epithelial cells containing internalized bacteria and initiation of a protective and nonpathogenic inflammatory response. However, a possible consequence of this process could be the opening of a hole in the epithelium, potentially allowing uningested organisms to enter the submucosa. This scenario has been documented in murine *S. enterica* serovar Typhimurium infections and in experimental bladder infections with uropathogenic *E. coli*. In the latter system, bacterial pilus-mediated attachment to *uroplakins* induces exfoliation of the cells with attached bacteria. Subsequently, infection is produced by residual bacterial cells that invade the superficial bladder epithelium, where they can grow intracellularly into biofilm-like masses encased in an extracellular polysaccharide-rich matrix and surrounded by uroplakin. This mode of growth produces structures that have been referred to as *bacterial pods*. It is likely that at low bacterial inocula epithelial cell ingestion and subclinical inflammation are efficient means to eliminate pathogens, while at higher inocula a proportion of surviving bacterial cells enter the host tissue through the damaged mucosal surface and multiply, producing disease. Alternatively, failure of the appropriate epithelial cell response to a pathogen may allow the organism to survive on a mucosal surface where, if it avoids other host defenses, it can grow and cause a local infection. Along these lines, as noted above, *P. aeruginosa* is taken into epithelial cells by CFTR, a protein missing or nonfunctional in most severe cases of cystic fibrosis. The major clinical consequence of this disease is chronic airway-surface infection with *P. aeruginosa* in 80–90% of patients. The failure of airway epithelial cells to ingest and promote the removal of *P. aeruginosa* via a properly regulated inflammatory response has been proposed as a key component of the hypersusceptibility of these patients to chronic airway infection with this organism.

Encounters with phagocytes

Phagocytosis and inflammation   Phagocytosis of microbes is a major innate host defense that limits the growth and spread of pathogens. Phagocytes appear rapidly at sites of infection in conjunction with the initiation of inflammation. Ingestion of microbes by both tissue-fixed macrophages and migrating phagocytes probably accounts for the limited ability of most microbial agents to cause disease. A family of related molecules called *collectins*, *soluble defense collagens*, or *pattern-recognition molecules* are found in blood (mannose-binding lectins), in lung (surfactant proteins A and D), and most likely in other tissues as well and bind to carbohydrates on microbial surfaces to promote phagocyte clearance. Bacterial pathogens seem to be ingested principally by polymorphonuclear neutrophils, while eosinophils are frequently found at sites of infection by protozoan or multicellular parasites. Successful pathogens, by definition, must avoid being cleared by professional phagocytes. One of several antiphagocytic strategies employed by bacteria and by the fungal pathogen *Cryptococcus neoformans* is to elaborate large-molecular-weight surface polysaccharide antigens, often in the form of a capsule that coats the cell surface. Most pathogenic bacteria produce such antiphagocytic capsules. On occasion, proteins or polypeptides form capsule-like coatings for organisms such as group A streptococci and *Bacillus anthracis*.

As activation of local phagocytes in tissues is a key step in initiating inflammation and migration of additional phagocytes into infected sites, much attention has been paid to microbial factors that initiate inflammation. These are usually conserved factors critical to the microbes' survival and are referred to as *pathogen-associated molecular patterns* (PAMPs). Cellular responses to microbial encounters with phagocytes are governed largely by the structure of the microbial PAMPs that elicit inflammation, and detailed knowledge of these structures of bacterial pathogens has contributed greatly to our understanding of molecular mechanisms of microbial pathogenesis mediated by activation of host cell molecules such as Toll-like receptors (TLRs; Fig. 120-3). One of the best-studied systems involves the interaction of LPS from gram-negative bacteria and the GPI-anchored membrane protein CD14 found on the surface of professional phagocytes, including migrating and tissue-fixed macrophages and polymorphonuclear neutrophils. A soluble form of CD14 is also found in plasma and on mucosal surfaces. A plasma protein, LPS-binding protein, transfers

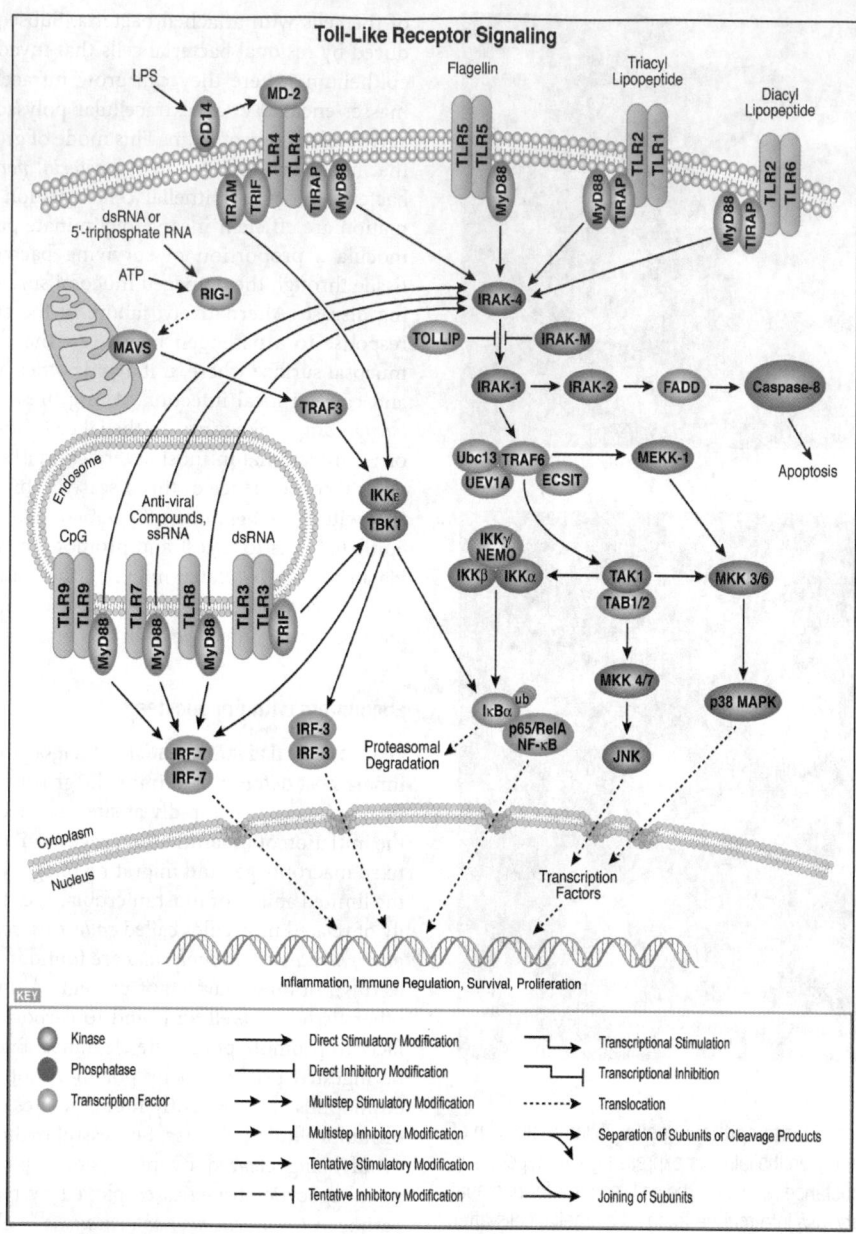

Toll-Like Receptor Signaling

Inflammation, Immune Regulation, Survival, Proliferation

KEY

⬤ Kinase	→ Direct Stimulatory Modification	Transcriptional Stimulation
⬤ Phosphatase	⊣ Direct Inhibitory Modification	Transcriptional Inhibition
⬤ Transcription Factor	⇢ Multistep Stimulatory Modification	···> Translocation
	⇥ Multistep Inhibitory Modification	Separation of Subunits or Cleavage Products
	--→ Tentative Stimulatory Modification	Joining of Subunits
	---┤ Tentative Inhibitory Modification	

Figure 120-3 Cellular signaling pathways for production of inflammatory cytokines in response to microbial products. Microbial cell-surface constituents interact with Toll-like receptors (TLRs), in some cases requiring additional factors such as MD-2, which facilitates the response to lipopolysaccharide (LPS) via TLR4. Although depicted as interacting with the TLRs on the cell surface, TLRs contain extracellular leucine-rich domains that become localized to the lumen of the phagosome upon uptake of bacterial cells. The internalized TLRs can bind to microbial products. The TLRs are oligomerized, usually forming homodimers, and then bind to the general adapter protein MyD88 via the C-terminal Toll/IL-1R (TIR) domains, which also bind to TIRAP (TIR domain-containing adapter protein), a molecule that participates in the transduction of signals from TLRs 1, 2, 4, and 6. The MyD88/TIRAP complex activates signal-transducing molecules such as IRAK-4 (IL-1Rc-associated kinase 4), which in turn activates IRAK-1. This activation can be blocked by IRAK-M and TOLLIP. IRAK-1 activates TRAF 6 (tumor necrosis factor receptor–associated factor 6), TAK-1 (transforming growth factor β–activating kinase 1), and TAB1/2 (TAK1-binding protein 1/2). This signaling complex associates with the ubiquitin-conjugating enzyme Ubc13 and the Ubc-like protein UEV1A to catalyze the formation of a polyubiquitin chain on TRAF6. Polyubiquitination of TRAF6 activates TAK1, which, along with TAB1/2 (a protein that binds to lysine residue 63 in polyubiquitin chains via a conserved zinc-finger domain), phosphorylates the inducible kinase complex: IKK-α, -β, and -γ. IKK-γ is also called NEMO [nuclear factor κB (NF-κB) essential modulator]. This large complex phosphorylates the inhibitory component of NF-κB, IκBα, resulting in release of IκBα from NF-κB. Phosphorylated (PP) IκB is then ubiquinated (ub) and degraded, and the two components of NF-κB, p50 or Rel and p65, translocate to the nucleus, where they bind to regulatory transcriptional sites on target genes, many of which encode inflammatory proteins. In addition to inducing NF-κB nuclear translocation, the TAK1/TAB1/2 complex activates MAP kinase transducers such as MKK 4/7 and MKK 3/6, which can lead to nuclear translocation of transcription factors such as AP1. TLR4 can also activate NF-κB nuclear translocation via the MyD88-independent TRIF (TIR-domain-containing adapter-inducing IFN-β) and TRAM (TRIF-related adapter molecule) cofactors. Intracellular TLRs 3, 7, 8, and 9 also use MyD88 and TRIF to activate IFN response factors 3 and 7 (IRF-3 and IRF-7), which also function as transcriptional factors in the nucleus. *[Pathway diagram reproduced courtesy of Cell Signaling Technology, Inc. (www.cellsignal.com).]*

LPS to membrane-bound CD14 on myeloid cells and promotes binding of LPS to soluble CD14. Soluble CD14/LPS/LPS-binding protein complexes bind to many cell types and may be internalized to initiate cellular responses to microbial pathogens. It has been shown that peptidoglycan and lipoteichoic acid from gram-positive bacteria and cell-surface products of mycobacteria and spirochetes can interact with CD14 (Fig. 120-3). Additional molecules, such as MD-2, also participate in the recognition of bacterial activators of inflammation.

GPI-anchored receptors do not have intracellular signaling domains; therefore, it is the TLRs that transduce signals for cellular activation due to LPS binding. Binding of microbial factors to TLRs to activate signal transduction occurs in the phagosome—and not on the surface—of dendritic cells that have internalized the microbe. This binding is probably due to the release of the microbial surface factor from the cell in the environment of the phagosome, where the liberated factor can bind to its cognate TLRs. TLRs initiate cellular activation through a series of signal-transducing molecules (Fig. 120-3) that lead to nuclear translocation of the transcription factor NF-κB, a master-switch for production of important inflammatory cytokines such as tumor necrosis factor α (TNF-α) and interleukin (IL) 1.

The initiation of inflammation can occur not only with LPS and peptidoglycan but also with viral particles and other microbial products such as polysaccharides, enzymes, and toxins. Bacterial flagella activate inflammation by binding of a conserved sequence to TLR5. Some pathogens (e.g., *Campylobacter jejuni, Helicobacter pylori,* and *Bartonella bacilliformis*) make flagella that lack this sequence and do not bind to TLR5; thus efficient host responses to infection are prevented. Bacteria also produce a high proportion of DNA molecules with unmethylated CpG residues that activate inflammation through TLR9. TLR3 recognizes double-stranded RNA, a pattern-recognition molecule produced by many viruses during their replicative cycle. TLR1 and TLR6 associate with TLR2 to promote recognition of acylated microbial proteins and peptides.

The myeloid differentiation factor 88 (MyD88) molecule and the Toll/IL-1R (TIR) domain-containing adapter protein (TIRAP) bind to the cytoplasmic domains of TLRs and also to receptors that are part of the IL-1 receptor families. Numerous studies have shown that MyD88/TIRAP-mediated transduction of signals from TLRs and other receptors is critical for innate resistance to infection, activating MAP-kinases and NF-κB and thereby leading to production of cytokines/chemokines. Mice lacking MyD88 are more susceptible than normal mice to infections with a broad range of pathogens. In one study, nine children homozygous for defective MyD88 genes had recurrent infections with *S. pneumoniae, S. aureus,* and *P. aeruginosa*—three bacterial species showing increased virulence in MyD88-deficient mice; however, unlike these mice, the MyD88-deficient children seemed to have no greater susceptibility to other bacteria, viruses, fungi, or parasites. Another component of the MyD88-dependent signaling pathway is a molecule known as IL-1 receptor–associated kinase 4 (IRAK-4). Individuals with a homozygous deficiency in genes encoding this protein are at increased risk for *S. pneumoniae* and *S. aureus* infections and, to some degree, for *P. aeruginosa* infections as well.

In addition to their role in MyD88-mediated signaling, some TLRs (e.g., TLR3 and TLR4) can activate signal transduction via a MyD88-independent pathway involving TIR domain-containing, adapter-inducing IFN-β (TRIF) and the TRIF-related adapter molecule (TRAM). Signaling through TRIF and TRAM activates the production of both NF-κB-dependent cytokines/chemokines and type 1 IFNs. The type 1 IFNs bind to the IFN-α receptor composed of two protein chains, IFNAR1 and IFNAR2. Humans produce three type 1 IFNs: IFN-α, IFN-β, and IFN-γ. These molecules activate another class of proteins known as the signal transducer and activator of transcription (STAT) complexes. The STAT factors are important in regulating immune system genes and thus play a critical role in responding to microbial infections.

Another intracellular complex of proteins found to be a major factor in the host cell response to infection is the inflammasome (Fig. 120-4), where inflammatory cytokines IL-1 and Il-18 are changed from their precursor to active forms prior to secretion by the cysteine protease caspase-1. Within the inflammasome are additional proteins that are members of the nucleotide binding and oligomerization domain (NOD)-like receptor (NLR) family. Like the TLRs, NOD proteins sense the presence of the conserved microbial factors released inside a cell. Recognition of these PAMPs by NLRs leads to caspase-1 activation and to secretion of active IL-1 and IL-18 by an unknown mechanism. Studies of mice indicate that as many as four inflammasomes with different components are formed: the IPAF inflammasome, the NALP1 inflammasome, the cryopyrin/NALP3 inflammasome, and an inflammasome triggered by *Francisella tularensis* infection (Fig. 120-4). The components depend on the type of stimulus driving inflammasome formation and activation.

Additional interactions of microbial pathogens and phagocytes Other ways that microbial pathogens avoid destruction by phagocytes include production of factors that are toxic to the phagocytes or that interfere with the chemotactic and ingestion function of phagocytes. Hemolysins, leukocidins, and the like are microbial proteins that can kill phagocytes that are attempting to ingest organisms elaborating these substances. For example, staphylococcal hemolysins inhibit macrophage chemotaxis and kill these phagocytes. Streptolysin O made by *S. pyogenes* binds to cholesterol in phagocyte membranes and initiates a process of internal degranulation, with the release of normally granule-sequestered toxic components into the phagocyte's cytoplasm. *E. histolytica*, an intestinal protozoan that causes amebic dysentery, can disrupt phagocyte membranes after direct contact via the release of protozoal phospholipase A and pore-forming peptides.

Microbial survival inside phagocytes Many important microbial pathogens use a variety of strategies to survive inside phagocytes (particularly macrophages) after ingestion. Inhibition of fusion of the phagocytic vacuole (the phagosome) containing the ingested microbe with the lysosomal granules containing antimicrobial substances (the lysosome) allows *Mycobacterium tuberculosis*, *S. enterica* serovar Typhi, and *Toxoplasma gondii* to survive inside macrophages. Some organisms, such as *Listeria monocytogenes*, escape into the phagocyte's cytoplasm to grow and eventually spread to other cells. Resistance to killing within the macrophage and subsequent growth are critical to successful infection by herpes-type viruses, measles virus, poxviruses, *Salmonella, Yersinia, Legionella, Mycobacterium, Trypanosoma, Nocardia, Histoplasma, Toxoplasma,* and *Rickettsia. Salmonella* species use a master regulatory system—in which the *PhoP/PhoQ* genes control other genes—to enter and survive within cells, with intracellular survival entailing structural changes in the cell envelope LPS.

■ TISSUE INVASION AND TISSUE TROPISM

Tissue invasion

Most viral pathogens cause disease by growth at skin or mucosal entry sites, but some pathogens spread from the initial site to deeper tissues. Virus can spread via the nerves (rabies virus) or plasma (picornaviruses) or within migratory blood cells (poliovirus, Epstein-Barr virus, and many others). Specific viral genes determine where and how individual viral strains can spread.

Bacteria may invade deeper layers of mucosal tissue via intracellular uptake by epithelial cells, traversal of epithelial cell junctions, or penetration through denuded epithelial surfaces. Among virulent

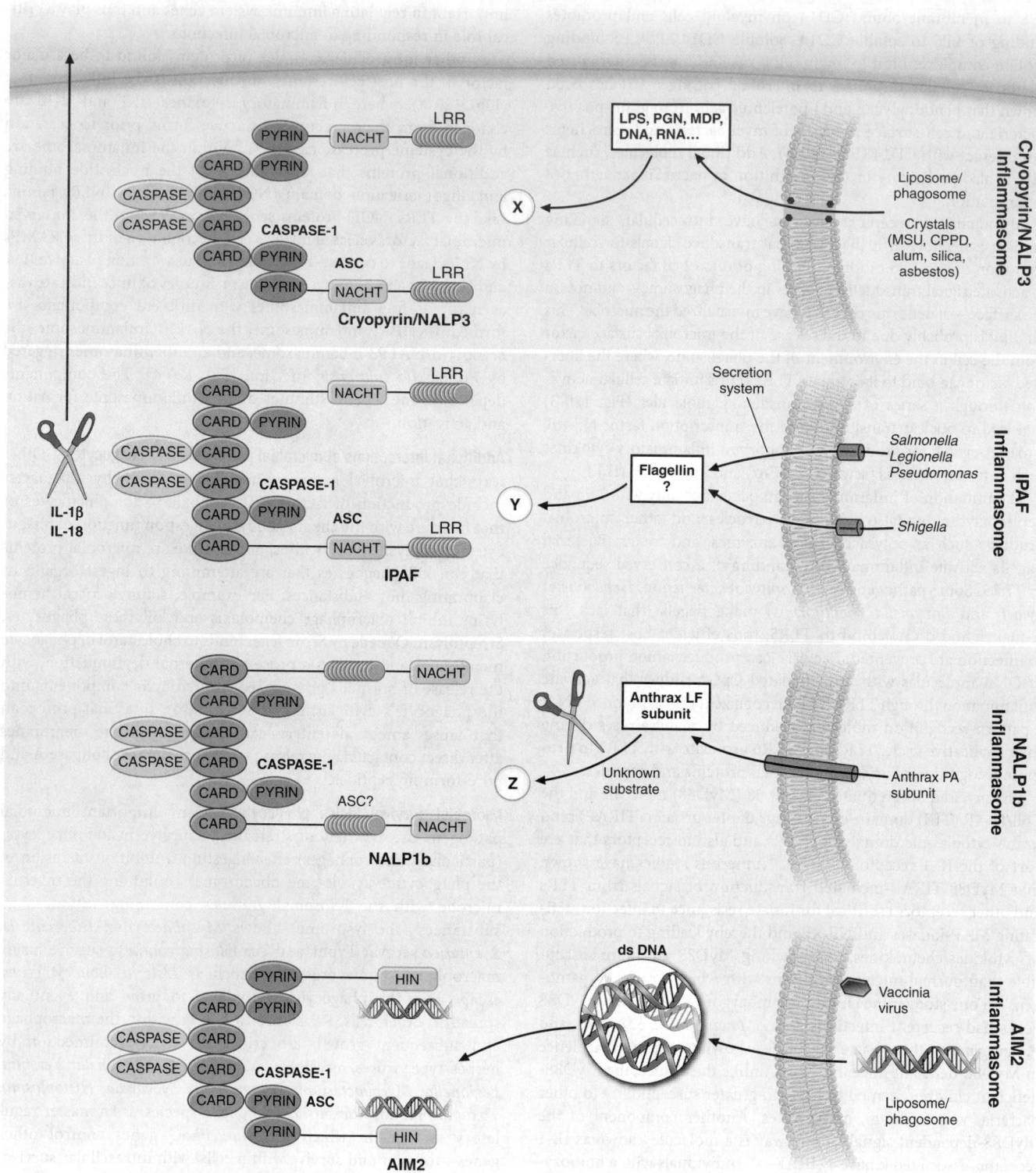

Figure 120-4 The NOD-like receptor (NLR) proteins NALP1b, cryopyrin/NALP3, and IPAF and the HIN-200 protein AIM2 assemble a caspase-1-activating inflammasome complex in response to specific microbial or bacterial factors. The murine NALP1b inflammasome recognizes the cytosolic presence of anthrax lethal toxin. The cryopyrin/NALP3 inflammasome recognizes multiple pathogen-associated molecular patterns (PAMPs) in combination with ATP or nigericin as well as crystalline substances including MSU, silica, and asbestos particles. The IPAF inflammasome senses *Salmonella* and *Legionella* flagellin and a yet-unidentified *Shigella flexneri* compound, all of which access the cytosol through a type III or IV secretion system. Cytosolic PAMPs may trigger assembly of a particular inflammasome complex by causing modifications in unknown host factors (X, Y, Z) that are monitored by specific NLR proteins. In contrast, AIM2 directly binds dsDNA in the cytosol to induce caspase-1 activation. The CARD/pyrin-containing adapter protein ASC is essential for all these inflammasome complexes, although its role in the NALP1b inflammasome remains to be formally established. Once activated, caspase-1 processes IL-1β and IL-18 precursors into the mature cytokines, which are secreted through an unknown mechanism. [*Figure and legend from Lamkanfi M, Dixit VM (2009) The Inflammasomes. PLoS Pathog 5(12): e1000510. doi:10.1371/journal.ppat.1000510.*]

Shigella strains and invasive *E. coli*, outer-membrane proteins are critical to epithelial cell invasion and bacterial multiplication. *Neisseria* and *Haemophilus* species penetrate mucosal cells by poorly understood mechanisms before dissemination into the bloodstream. Staphylococci and streptococci elaborate a variety of extracellular enzymes, such as hyaluronidase, lipases, nucleases, and hemolysins, that are probably important in breaking down cellular and matrix structures and allowing the bacteria access to deeper tissues and blood. Organisms that colonize the gastrointestinal tract can often translocate through the mucosa into the blood and, under circumstances in which host defenses are inadequate, cause bacteremia. *Y. enterocolitica* can invade the mucosa through the activity of the invasin protein. Some bacteria (e.g., *Brucella*) can be carried from a mucosal site to a distant site by phagocytic cells (e.g., polymorphonuclear neutrophils) that ingest but fail to kill the bacteria.

Fungal pathogens almost always take advantage of host immunocompromise to spread hematogenously to deeper tissues. The AIDS epidemic has resoundingly illustrated this principle: the immunodeficiency of many HIV-infected patients permits the development of life-threatening fungal infections of the lung, blood, and brain. Other than the capsule of *C. neoformans*, specific fungal antigens involved in tissue invasion are not well characterized. Both fungal pathogens and protozoal pathogens (e.g., *Plasmodium* species and *E. histolytica*) undergo morphologic changes to spread within a host. Malarial parasites grow in liver cells as merozoites and are released into the blood to invade erythrocytes and become trophozoites. *E. histolytica* is found as both a cyst and a trophozoite in the intestinal lumen, through which this pathogen enters the host, but only the trophozoite form can spread systemically to cause amebic liver abscesses. Other protozoal pathogens, such as *T. gondii*, *Giardia lamblia*, and *Cryptosporidium*, also undergo extensive morphologic changes after initial infection to spread to other tissues.

Tissue tropism

The propensity of certain microbes to cause disease by infecting specific tissues has been known since the early days of bacteriology, yet the molecular basis for this propensity is understood somewhat better for viral pathogens than for other agents of infectious disease. Specific receptor-ligand interactions clearly underlie the ability of certain viruses to enter cells within tissues and disrupt normal tissue function, but the mere presence of a receptor for a virus on a target tissue is not sufficient for tissue tropism. Factors in the cell, route of viral entry, viral capacity to penetrate into cells, viral genetic elements that regulate gene expression, and pathways of viral spread in a tissue all affect tissue tropism. Some viral genes are best transcribed in specific target cells, such as hepatitis B genes in liver cells and Epstein-Barr virus genes in B lymphocytes. The route of inoculation of poliovirus determines its neurotropism, although the molecular basis for this circumstance is not understood.

Compared with viral tissue tropism, the tissue tropism of bacterial and parasitic infections has not been as clearly elucidated, but studies of *Neisseria* species have provided insights. Both *N. gonorrhoeae*, which colonizes and infects the human genital tract, and *N. meningitidis*, which principally colonizes the human oropharynx but can spread to the brain, produce type IV pili (Tfp) that mediate adherence to host tissues. In the case of *N. gonorrhoeae*, the Tfp bind to a glucosamine-galactose-containing adhesin on the surface of cervical and urethral cells; in the case of *N. meningitidis*, the Tfp bind to cells in the human meninges in order to cross the blood-brain barrier. *N. meningitidis* expresses a capsular polysaccharide, while *N. gonorrhoeae* does not; however, there is no indication that this property plays a role in the different tissue tropisms displayed by these two bacterial species. *N. gonorrhoeae* can use cytidine monophosphate *N*-acetylneuraminic acid from host tissues to add *N*-acetylneuraminic acid (sialic acid) to its

lipooligosaccharide O side chain, and this alteration appears to make the organism resistant to host defenses. Lactate, present at high levels on genital mucosal surfaces, stimulates sialylation of gonococcal lipooligosaccharide. Bacteria with sialic acid sugars in their capsules, such as *N. meningitidis*, *E. coli* K1, and group B streptococci, have a propensity to cause meningitis, but this generalization has many exceptions. For example, all recognized serotypes of group B streptococci contain sialic acid in their capsules, but only one serotype (III) is responsible for most cases of group B streptococcal meningitis. Moreover, both *H. influenzae* and *S. pneumoniae* can readily cause meningitis, but these organisms do not have sialic acid in their capsules.

■ TISSUE DAMAGE AND DISEASE

Disease is a complex phenomenon resulting from tissue invasion and destruction, toxin elaboration, and host response. Viruses cause much of their damage by exerting a cytopathic effect on host cells and inhibiting host defenses. The growth of bacterial, fungal, and protozoal parasites in tissue, which may or may not be accompanied by toxin elaboration, can also compromise tissue function and lead to disease. For some bacterial and possibly some fungal pathogens, toxin production is one of the best-characterized molecular mechanisms of pathogenesis, while host factors such as IL-1, TNF-α, kinins, inflammatory proteins, products of complement activation, and mediators derived from arachidonic acid metabolites (leukotrienes) and cellular degranulation (histamines) readily contribute to the severity of disease.

Viral disease

Viral pathogens are well known to inhibit host immune responses by a variety of mechanisms. Immune responses can be affected by decreasing production of most major histocompatibility complex molecules (adenovirus E3 protein), by diminishing cytotoxic T cell recognition of virus-infected cells (Epstein-Barr virus EBNA1 antigen and cytomegalovirus IE protein), by producing virus-encoded complement receptor proteins that protect infected cells from complement-mediated lysis (herpesvirus and vaccinia virus), by making proteins that interfere with the action of IFN (influenza virus and poxvirus), and by elaborating superantigen-like proteins (mouse mammary tumor virus and related retroviruses and the rabies nucleocapsid). Superantigens activate large populations of T cells that express particular subsets of the T cell receptor β protein, causing massive cytokine release and subsequent host reactions. Another molecular mechanism of viral virulence involves the production of peptide growth factors for host cells, which disrupt normal cellular growth, proliferation, and differentiation. In addition, viral factors can bind to and interfere with the function of host receptors for signaling molecules. Modulation of cytokine production during viral infection can stimulate viral growth inside cells with receptors for the cytokine, and virus-encoded cytokine homologues (e.g., the Epstein-Barr virus BCRF1 protein, which is highly homologous to the immunoinhibitory IL-10 molecule) can potentially prevent immune-mediated clearance of viral particles. Viruses can cause disease in neural cells by interfering with levels of neurotransmitters without necessarily destroying the cells, or they may induce either programmed cell death (apoptosis) to destroy tissues or inhibitors of apoptosis to allow for prolonged viral infection of cells. For infection to spread, many viruses must be released from cells. In a newly identified function, viral protein U (Vpu) of HIV facilitates the release of virus, a process that is specific to certain cells. Mammalian cells produce a restriction factor involved in inhibiting the release of virus; for HIV, this factor is designated BST-2 (bone marrow stromal antigen 2)/HM1.24/CD317, or tetherin. Vpu of HIV interacts with tetherin, promoting release of infectious virus. Overall, disruption of normal cellular and tissue function due to viral infection, replication, and release promotes clinical disease.

Bacterial toxins

Among the first infectious diseases to be understood were those due to toxin-elaborating bacteria. Diphtheria, botulism, and tetanus toxins are responsible for the diseases associated with local infections due to *Corynebacterium diphtheriae*, *Clostridium botulinum*, and *Clostridium tetani*, respectively. Enterotoxins produced by *E. coli*, *Salmonella*, *Shigella*, *Staphylococcus*, and *V. cholerae* contribute to diarrheal disease caused by these organisms. Staphylococci, streptococci, *P. aeruginosa*, and *Bordetella* elaborate various toxins that cause or contribute to disease, including toxic shock syndrome toxin 1; erythrogenic toxin; exotoxins A, S, T and U; and pertussis toxin. A number of these toxins (e.g., cholera toxin, diphtheria toxin, pertussis toxin, *E. coli* heat-labile toxin, and *P. aeruginosa* exotoxin) have adenosine diphosphate ribosyl transferase activity; i.e., the toxins enzymatically catalyze the transfer of the adenosine diphosphate ribosyl portion of nicotinamide adenine diphosphate to target proteins and inactivate them. The staphylococcal enterotoxins, toxic shock syndrome toxin 1, and the streptococcal pyogenic exotoxins behave as superantigens, stimulating certain T cells to proliferate without processing of the protein toxin by antigen-presenting cells. Part of this process involves stimulation of the antigen-presenting cells to produce IL-1 and TNF-α, which have been implicated in many clinical features of diseases like toxic shock syndrome and scarlet fever. A number of gram-negative pathogens (*Salmonella*, *Yersinia*, and *P. aeruginosa*) can inject toxins directly into host target cells by means of a complex set of proteins referred to as the type III secretion system. Loss or inactivation of this virulence system usually greatly reduces the capacity of a bacterial pathogen to cause disease.

Endotoxin

The lipid A portion of gram-negative LPS has potent biologic activities that cause many of the clinical manifestations of gram-negative bacterial sepsis, including fever, muscle proteolysis, uncontrolled intravascular coagulation, and shock. The effects of lipid A appear to be mediated by the production of potent cytokines due to LPS binding to CD14 and signal transduction via TLRs, particularly TLR4. Cytokines exhibit potent hypothermic activity through effects on the hypothalamus; they also increase vascular permeability, alter the activity of endothelial cells, and induce endothelial-cell procoagulant activity. Numerous therapeutic strategies aimed at neutralizing the effects of endotoxin are under investigation, but so far the results have been disappointing. One drug, activated protein C, was found to reduce mortality rates by ~20% during severe sepsis, a condition that can be induced by endotoxin release during gram-negative bacterial sepsis.

Invasion

Many diseases are caused primarily by pathogens growing in tissue sites that are normally sterile. Pneumococcal pneumonia is mostly attributable to the growth of *S. pneumoniae* in the lung and the attendant host inflammatory response, although specific factors that enhance this process (e.g., pneumolysin) may be responsible for some of the pathogenic potential of the pneumococcus. Disease that follows bacteremia and invasion of the meninges by meningitis-producing bacteria such as *N. meningitidis*, *H. influenzae*, *E. coli* K1, and group B streptococci appears to be due solely to the ability of these organisms to gain access to these tissues, multiply in them, and provoke cytokine production leading to tissue-damaging host inflammation.

Specific molecular mechanisms accounting for tissue invasion by fungal and protozoal pathogens are less well described. Except for studies pointing to factors like capsule and melanin production by *C. neoformans* and possibly levels of cell wall glucans in some pathogenic fungi, the molecular basis for fungal invasiveness is not well defined. Melanism has been shown to protect the fungal cell against death caused by phagocyte factors such as nitric oxide, superoxide, and hypochlorite. Morphogenic variation and production of proteases (e.g., the *Candida* aspartyl proteinase) have been implicated in fungal invasion of host tissues.

If pathogens are effectively to invade host tissues (particularly the blood), they must avoid the major host defenses represented by complement and phagocytic cells. Bacteria most often avoid these defenses through their surface polysaccharides—either capsular polysaccharides or long O-side-chain antigens characteristic of the smooth LPS of gram-negative bacteria. These molecules can prevent the activation and/or deposition of complement opsonins or can limit the access of phagocytic cells with receptors for complement opsonins to these molecules when they are deposited on the bacterial surface below the capsular layer. Another potential mechanism of microbial virulence is the ability of some organisms to present the capsule as an apparent self antigen through molecular mimicry. For example, the polysialic acid capsule of group B *N. meningitidis* is chemically identical to an oligosaccharide found on human brain cells.

Immunochemical studies of capsular polysaccharides have led to an appreciation of the tremendous chemical diversity that can result from the linking of a few monosaccharides. For example, three hexoses can link up in more than 300 different, potentially serologically distinct ways, while three amino acids have only six possible peptide combinations. Capsular polysaccharides have been used as effective vaccines against meningococcal meningitis as well as against pneumococcal and *H. influenzae* infections and may prove to be of value as vaccines against any organisms that express a nontoxic, immunogenic capsular polysaccharide. In addition, most encapsulated pathogens become virtually avirulent when capsule production is interrupted by genetic manipulation; this observation emphasizes the importance of this structure in pathogenesis.

Host response

The inflammatory response of the host is critical for interruption and resolution of the infectious process but also is often responsible for the signs and symptoms of disease. Infection promotes a complex series of host responses involving the complement, kinin, and coagulation pathways. The production of cytokines such as IL-1, IL-18, TNF-α, and other factors regulated in part by the NF-κB transcription factor leads to fever, muscle proteolysis, and other effects. An inability to kill or contain the microbe usually results in further damage due to the progression of inflammation and infection. For example, in many chronic infections, degranulation of host inflammatory cells can lead to release of host proteases, elastases, histamines, and other toxic substances that can degrade host tissues. Chronic inflammation in any tissue can lead to the destruction of that tissue and to clinical disease associated with loss of organ function, such as sterility from pelvic inflammatory disease caused by chronic infection with *N. gonorrhoeae*.

The nature of the host response elicited by the pathogen often determines the pathology of a particular infection. Local inflammation produces local tissue damage, while systemic inflammation, such as that seen during sepsis, can result in the signs and symptoms of septic shock. The severity of septic shock is associated with the degree of production of host effectors. Disease due to intracellular parasitism results from the formation of granulomas, wherein the host attempts to wall off the parasite inside a fibrotic lesion surrounded by fused epithelial cells that make up so-called multinucleated giant cells. A number of pathogens, particularly anaerobic bacteria, staphylococci, and streptococci, provoke the formation of an abscess, probably because of the presence of zwitterionic surface polysaccharides such as the capsular polysaccharide of *Bacteroides fragilis*. The outcome of an infection depends on the balance between an effective host response that eliminates a pathogen and an excessive inflammatory response that is associated with an inability to eliminate a pathogen and with the resultant tissue damage that leads to disease.

■ TRANSMISSION TO NEW HOSTS

As part of the pathogenic process, most microbes are shed from the host, often in a form infectious for susceptible individuals. However, the rate of transmissibility may not necessarily be high, even if the disease is severe in the infected individual, as these traits are not linked. Most pathogens exit via the same route by which they entered: respiratory pathogens by aerosols from sneezing or coughing or through salivary spread, gastrointestinal pathogens by fecal-oral spread, sexually transmitted diseases by venereal spread, and vector-borne organisms by either direct contact with the vector through a blood meal or indirect contact with organisms shed into environmental sources such as water. Microbial factors that specifically promote transmission are not well characterized. Respiratory shedding is facilitated by overproduction of mucous secretions, with consequently enhanced sneezing and coughing. Diarrheal toxins such as cholera toxin, *E. coli* heat-labile toxins, and *Shigella* toxins probably facilitate fecal-oral spread of microbial cells in the high volumes of diarrheal fluid produced during infection. The ability to produce phenotypic variants that resist hostile environmental factors (e.g., the highly resistant cysts of *E. histolytica* shed in feces) represents another mechanism of pathogenesis relevant to transmission. Blood parasites such as *Plasmodium* species change phenotype after ingestion by a mosquito—a prerequisite for the continued transmission of this pathogen. Venereally transmitted pathogens may undergo phenotypic variation due to the production of specific factors to facilitate transmission, but shedding of these pathogens into the environment does not result in the formation of infectious foci.

In summary, the molecular mechanisms used by pathogens to colonize, invade, infect, and disrupt the host are numerous and diverse. Each phase of the infectious process involves a variety of microbial and host factors interacting in a manner that can result in disease. Recognition of the coordinated genetic regulation of virulence factor elaboration when organisms move from their natural environment into the mammalian host emphasizes the complex nature of the host-parasite interaction. Fortunately, the need for diverse factors in successful infection and disease implies that a variety of therapeutic strategies may be developed to interrupt this process and thereby prevent and treat microbial infections.

FURTHER READINGS

ARANA DM, PRIETO D: The role of the cell wall in fungal pathogenesis. Microb Biotechnol 2:308, 2009

CHAI LY et al: Fungal strategies for overcoming host innate immune response. Med Mycol 47:227, 2009

DIACOVICH L, GORVEL JP: Bacterial manipulation of innate immunity to promote infection. Nat Rev Microbiol 8:117, 2010

DUAN K et al: Chemical interactions between organisms in microbial communities. Contrib Microbiol 16:1, 2009

IMBERTY A, VARROT A: Microbial recognition of human cell surface glycoconjugates. Curr Opin Struct Biol 18:567, 2008

IWASAKI A, MEDZHITOV R: Regulation of adaptive immunity by the innate immune system. Science 327:291, 2010

KAWAI T, AKIRA S: The roles of TLRs, RLRs and NLRs in pathogen recognition. Int Immunol 21:317, 2009

KLINE KA et al: Bacterial adhesins in host-microbe interactions. Cell Host Microbe 5:580, 2009

STUTZ A et al: Inflammasomes: Too big to miss. J Clin Invest 119:3502, 2009

CHAPTER **121**

Approach to the Acutely Ill Infected Febrile Patient

Tamar F. Barlam
Dennis L. Kasper

The physician treating the acutely ill febrile patient must be able to recognize infections that require emergent attention. If such infections are not adequately evaluated and treated at initial presentation, the opportunity to alter an adverse outcome may be lost. In this chapter, the clinical presentations of and approach to patients with relatively common infectious disease emergencies are discussed. These infectious processes and their treatments are discussed in detail in other chapters.

APPROACH TO THE PATIENT | **Acute Febrile Illness**

Before the history is elicited and a physical examination performed, an immediate assessment of the patient's general appearance can yield valuable information. The perceptive physician's subjective sense that a patient is septic or toxic often proves accurate. Visible agitation or anxiety in a febrile patient can be a harbinger of critical illness.

HISTORY Presenting symptoms are frequently nonspecific. Detailed questions should be asked about the onset and duration of symptoms and about changes in severity or rate of progression over time. Host factors and comorbid conditions may enhance the risk of infection with certain organisms or of a more fulminant course than is usually seen. Lack of splenic function, alcoholism with significant liver disease, IV drug use, HIV infection, diabetes, malignancy, organ transplantation, and chemotherapy all predispose to specific infections and frequently to increased severity. The patient should be questioned about factors that might help identify a nidus for invasive infection, such as recent upper respiratory tract infections, influenza, or varicella; prior trauma; disruption of cutaneous barriers due to lacerations, burns, surgery, body piercing, or decubiti; and the presence of foreign bodies, such as nasal packing after rhinoplasty, tampons, or prosthetic joints. Travel, contact with pets or other animals, or activities that might result in tick or mosquito exposure can lead to diagnoses that would not otherwise be considered. Recent dietary intake, medication use, social or occupational contact with ill individuals, vaccination history, recent sexual contacts, and menstrual history may be relevant. A review of systems should focus on any neurologic signs or sensorium alterations, rashes or skin lesions, and focal pain or tenderness and should also include a general review of respiratory, gastrointestinal, or genitourinary symptoms.

PHYSICAL EXAMINATION A complete physical examination should be performed, with special attention to several areas that are sometimes given short shrift in routine examinations. Assessment of the patient's general appearance and vital signs, skin and soft tissue examination, and the neurologic evaluation are of particular importance.

The patient may appear either anxious and agitated or lethargic and apathetic. Fever is usually present, although elderly patients and compromised hosts [e.g., patients who are uremic or cirrhotic and those who are taking glucocorticoids or nonsteroidal anti-inflammatory drugs (NSAIDs)] may be afebrile despite serious underlying infection. Measurement of blood pressure, heart rate, and respiratory rate helps determine the degree of hemodynamic and metabolic compromise. The patient's airway must be evaluated to rule out the risk of obstruction from an invasive oropharyngeal infection.

The etiologic diagnosis may become evident in the context of a thorough skin examination (Chap. 17). Petechial rashes are typically seen with meningococcemia or Rocky Mountain spotted fever (RMSF; see Fig. e7-16); erythroderma is associated with toxic shock syndrome (TSS) and drug fever. The soft tissue and muscle examination is critical. Areas of erythema or duskiness, edema, and tenderness may indicate underlying necrotizing fasciitis, myositis, or myonecrosis. The neurologic examination must include a careful assessment of mental status for signs of early encephalopathy. Evidence of nuchal rigidity or focal neurologic findings should be sought.

DIAGNOSTIC WORKUP After a quick clinical assessment, diagnostic material should be obtained rapidly and antibiotic and supportive treatment begun. Blood (for cultures; baseline complete blood count with differential; measurement of serum electrolytes, blood urea nitrogen, serum creatinine, and serum glucose; and liver function tests) can be obtained at the time an IV line is placed and before antibiotics are administered. Three sets of blood cultures should be performed for patients with possible acute endocarditis. Asplenic patients should have a blood smear examined to confirm the presence of Howell-Jolly bodies (indicating the absence of splenic function) and a buffy coat examined for bacteria; these patients can have >10⁶ organisms per milliliter of blood (compared with 10^4/mL in patients with an intact spleen). Blood smears from patients at risk for severe parasitic disease, such as malaria or babesiosis (see Chap. e27), must be examined for the diagnosis and quantitation of parasitemia. Blood smears may also be diagnostic in ehrlichiosis and anaplasmosis.

Patients with possible meningitis should have cerebrospinal fluid (CSF) obtained before the initiation of antibiotic therapy. Focal findings, depressed mental status, or papilledema should be evaluated by brain imaging prior to lumbar puncture, which, in this setting, could initiate herniation. *Antibiotics should be administered before imaging but after blood for cultures has been drawn.* If CSF cultures are negative, blood cultures will provide the diagnosis in 50–70% of cases.

Focal abscesses necessitate immediate CT or MRI as part of an evaluation for surgical intervention. Other diagnostic procedures, such as wound cultures, should not delay the initiation of treatment for more than minutes. Once emergent evaluation, diagnostic procedures, and (if appropriate) surgical consultation (see below) have been completed, other laboratory tests can be conducted. Appropriate radiography, computed axial tomography, MRI, urinalysis, erythrocyte sedimentation rate (ESR) determination, and transthoracic or transesophageal echocardiography may all prove important.

TREATMENT   The Acutely Ill Patient

In the acutely ill patient, empirical antibiotic therapy is critical and should be administered without undue delay. Increased prevalence of antibiotic resistance in community-acquired bacteria must be considered when antibiotics are selected. Table 121-1 lists first-line treatments for infections considered in this chapter. In addition to the rapid initiation of antibiotic therapy, several of these infections require urgent surgical attention. Neurosurgical evaluation for subdural empyema, otolaryngologic surgery for possible mucormycosis, and cardiothoracic surgery for critically ill patients with acute endocarditis are as important as antibiotic therapy. For infections such as necrotizing fasciitis and clostridial myonecrosis, rapid surgical intervention supersedes other diagnostic or therapeutic maneuvers.

Adjunctive treatments may reduce morbidity and mortality rates and include dexamethasone for bacterial meningitis; IV immunoglobulin for TSS and necrotizing fasciitis caused by group A *Streptococcus*; low-dose hydrocortisone and fludrocortisone for septic shock; and drotrecogin alfa (activated), also known as recombinant human activated protein C, for meningococcemia and severe sepsis. Adjunctive therapies should usually be initiated within the first hours of treatment; however, dexamethasone for bacterial meningitis must be given before or at the time of the first dose of antibiotic.

SPECIFIC PRESENTATIONS

The infections considered below according to common clinical presentation can have rapidly catastrophic outcomes, and their immediate recognition and treatment can be life-saving. Recommended empirical therapeutic regimens are presented in Table 121-1.

■ SEPSIS WITHOUT AN OBVIOUS FOCUS OF PRIMARY INFECTION

These patients initially have a brief prodrome of nonspecific symptoms and signs that progresses quickly to hemodynamic instability with hypotension, tachycardia, tachypnea, respiratory distress, and altered mental status. Disseminated intravascular coagulation (DIC) with clinical evidence of a hemorrhagic diathesis is a poor prognostic sign.

Septic shock

(See also Chap. 271) Patients with bacteremia leading to septic shock may have a primary site of infection (e.g., pneumonia, pyelonephritis, or cholangitis) that is not evident initially. Elderly patients with comorbid conditions, hosts compromised by malignancy and neutropenia, and patients who have recently undergone a surgical procedure or hospitalization are at increased risk for an adverse outcome. Gram-negative bacteremia with organisms such

TABLE 121-1 Empirical Treatment for Common Infectious Disease Emergencies

Clinical Syndrome	Possible Etiologies	Treatment	Comments	See Chap.
Sepsis Without a Clear Focus				
Septic shock	*Pseudomonas* spp., gram-negative enteric bacilli, *Staphylococcus* spp., *Streptococcus* spp.	Vancomycin (1 g q12h) *plus* Gentamicin (5 mg/kg per day) *plus either* Piperacillin/tazobactam (3.375 g q4h) *or* Cefepime (2 g q12h)	Adjust treatment when culture data become available. Drotrecogin alfa (activated)[a] or low-dose hydrocortisone and fludrocortisone[b] may improve outcome in patients with septic shock.	135, 136, 149, 152, 271
Overwhelming post splenectomy sepsis	*Streptococcus pneumoniae, Haemophilus influenzae, Neisseria meningitidis*	Ceftriaxone (2 g q12h) *plus* Vancomycin (1 g q12h)	If a β-lactam-sensitive strain is identified, vancomycin can be discontinued.	271
Babesiosis	*Babesia microti* (U.S.), *B. divergens* (Europe)	**Either:** Clindamycin (600 mg tid) *plus* Quinine (650 mg tid) *or:* Atovaquone (750 mg q12h) *plus* Azithromycin (500-mg loading dose, then 250 mg/d)	Atovaquone and azithromycin are as effective as clindamycin and quinine and are associated with fewer side effects. Treatment with doxycycline (100 mg bid[c]) for potential co-infection with *Borrelia burgdorferi* or *Anaplasma* spp. may be prudent.	208, 211
Sepsis with Skin Findings				
Meningococcemia	*N. meningitidis*	Penicillin (4 mU q4h) *or* Ceftriaxone (2 g q12h)	Consider protein C replacement in fulminant meningococcemia.	143
Rocky Mountain spotted fever (RMSF)	*Rickettsia rickettsii*	Doxycycline (100 mg bid)	If both meningococcemia and RMSF are being considered, use ceftriaxone (2 g q12h) *plus* doxycycline (100 mg bid[c]) *or* chloramphenicol alone (50–75 mg/kg per day in four divided doses). If RMSF is diagnosed, doxycycline is the proven superior agent.	174
Purpura fulminans	*S. pneumoniae, H. influenzae, N. meningitidis*	Ceftriaxone (2 g q12h) *plus* Vancomycin (1 g q12h)	If a β-lactam–sensitive strain is identified, vancomycin can be discontinued.	134, 143, 145, 271
Erythroderma: toxic shock syndrome	Group A *Streptococcus, Staphylococcus aureus*	Vancomycin (1 g q12h) *plus* Clindamycin (600 mg q8h)	If a penicillin- or oxacillin-sensitive strain is isolated, these agents are superior to vancomycin (penicillin, 2 mU q4h; or oxacillin, 2 g q4h). The site of toxigenic bacteria should be debrided; IV immuno-globulin can be used in severe cases.[d]	135, 136
Sepsis with Soft Tissue Findings				
Necrotizing fasciitis	Group A *Streptococcus*, mixed aerobic/anaerobic flora, CA-MRSA[e]	Vancomycin (1 g q12h) *plus* Clindamycin (600 mg q8h) *plus* Gentamicin (5 mg/kg per day)	Urgent surgical evaluation is critical. If a penicillin- or oxacillin-sensitive strain is isolated, these agents are superior to vancomycin (penicillin, 2 mU q4h; or oxacillin, 2 g q4h).	125, 135, 136
Clostridial myonecrosis	*Clostridium perfringens*	Penicillin (2 mU q4h) *plus* Clindamycin (600 mg q8h)	Urgent surgical evaluation is critical.	142
Neurologic Infections				
Bacterial meningitis	*S. pneumoniae, N. meningitidis*	Ceftriaxone (2 g q12h) *plus* Vancomycin (1 g q12h)	If a β-lactam–sensitive strain is identified, vancomycin can be discontinued. If the patient is >50 years old or has comorbid disease, add ampicillin (2 g q4h) for *Listeria* coverage. Dexamethasone (10 mg q6h × 4 days) improves outcome in adult patients with meningitis (especially pneumococcal) and cloudy CSF, positive CSF Gram's stain, or a CSF leukocyte count >1000/mL.	381

(continued)

Clinical Syndrome	Possible Etiologies	Treatment	Comments	See Chap.
Brain abscess, suppurative intracranial infections	*Streptococcus* spp., *Staphylococcus* spp., anaerobes, gram-negative bacilli	Vancomycin (1 g q12h) *plus* Metronidazole (500 mg q8h) *plus* Ceftriaxone (2 g q12h)	Urgent surgical evaluation is critical. If a penicillin- or oxacillin-sensitive strain is isolated, these agents are superior to vancomycin (penicillin, 4 mU q4h; or oxacillin, 2 g q4h).	381
Cerebral malaria	*Plasmodium falciparum*	Artesunate (2.4 mg/kg IV at 0, 12, and 24 h; then once daily)[f] *or* Quinine (IV loading dose of 20 mg salt/kg; then 10 mg/kg q8h) *plus* Doxycycline (100 mg IV q12h)	Do not use glucocorticoids. Use IV quinidine if IV quinine is not available. During IV quinidine treatment, blood pressure and cardiac function should be monitored continuously and blood glucose monitored periodically.	208, 210
Spinal epidural abscess	*Staphylococcus* spp., gram-negative bacilli	Vancomycin (1 g q12h) *plus* Ceftriaxone (2 g q24h)	Surgical evaluation is essential. If a penicillin- or oxacillin-sensitive strain is isolated, these agents are superior to vancomycin (penicillin, 4 mU q4h; or oxacillin, 2 g q4h).	377

Focal Infections

Acute bacterial endocarditis	*S. aureus*, β-hemolytic streptococci, HACEK group,[g] *Neisseria* spp., *S. pneumoniae*	Ceftriaxone (2 g q12h) *plus* Vancomycin (1 g q12h)	Adjust treatment when culture data become available. Surgical evaluation is essential.	124

[a]Drotrecogin alfa (activated) is administered at a dose of 24 μg/kg per hour for 96 h. It has been approved for use in patients with severe sepsis and a high risk of death as defined by an Acute Physiology and Chronic Health Evaluation II (APACHE II) score of ≥25 and/or multiorgan failure.

[b]Hydrocortisone (50-mg IV bolus q6h) with fludrocortisone (50-μg tablet daily for 7 days) may improve outcomes of severe sepsis, particularly in the setting of relative adrenal insufficiency.

[c]Tetracyclines can be antagonistic in action to β-lactam agents. Adjust treatment as soon as the diagnosis is confirmed.

[d]The optimal dose of IV immunoglobulin has not been determined, but the median dose in observational studies is 2 g/kg (total dose administered over 1–5 days).

[e]Community-acquired methicillin-resistant *S. aureus*.

[f]In the United States, artesunate must be obtained by the Centers for Disease Control and Prevention. For patients diagnosed with severe malaria, full doses of parenteral antimalarial treatment should be started with whichever recommended antimalarial agent is first available.

[g]*Haemophilus aphrophilus, H. paraphrophilus, H. parainfluenzae, Aggregatibacter* (formerly *Actinobacillus*) *actinomycetemcomitans, Cardiobacterium hominis, Eikenella corrodens*, and *Kingella kingae*.

as *Pseudomonas aeruginosa* or *Escherichia coli* and gram-positive infection with organisms such as *Staphylococcus aureus*, including methicillin-resistant *S. aureus* (MRSA), or group A streptococci can present as intractable hypotension and multiorgan failure. Treatment can usually be initiated empirically on the basis of the presentation, host factors (Table 271-3), and local patterns of bacterial resistance. Worse outcomes are evident when antimicrobial treatment is delayed or the pathogenic etiology ultimately proves to be nonsusceptible to the initial regimen. Broad-spectrum antimicrobial agents are therefore recommended. Adjunctive therapy with either drotrecogin alfa (activated) or glucocorticoids should be considered for patients with severe sepsis.

Overwhelming infection in asplenic patients

(See also Chap. 271) Patients without splenic function are at risk for overwhelming bacterial sepsis. Asplenic adult patients succumb to sepsis at 58 times the rate of the general population. Most infections are thought to occur within the first 2 years after splenectomy, with a mortality rate of ~50%, but the increased risk persists throughout life. In asplenia, encapsulated bacteria cause the majority of infections. Adults, who are more likely to have antibody to these organisms, are at lower risk than children. *Streptococcus pneumoniae* is the most common isolate, causing 50–70% of cases, but the risk of

infection with *Haemophilus influenzae* or *Neisseria meningitidis* is also high. Severe clinical manifestations of infections due to *E. coli*, *S. aureus*, group B streptococci, *P. aeruginosa*, *Capnocytophaga*, *Bordetella holmesii*, *Babesia*, and *Plasmodium* have been described.

Babesiosis

(See also Chap. 211) A history of recent travel to endemic areas raises the possibility of infection with *Babesia*. Between 1 and 4 weeks after a tick bite, the patient experiences chills, fatigue, anorexia, myalgia, arthralgia, shortness of breath, nausea, and headache; ecchymosis and/or petechiae are occasionally seen. The tick that most commonly transmits *Babesia, Ixodes scapularis*, also transmits *Borrelia burgdorferi* (the agent of Lyme disease) and *Anaplasma*; co-infection can occur, resulting in more severe disease. Infection with the European species *Babesia divergens* is more frequently fulminant than that due to the U.S. species *Babesia microti. B. divergens* causes a febrile syndrome with hemolysis, jaundice, hemoglobinemia, and renal failure and is associated with a mortality rate of >50%. Severe babesiosis is especially common in asplenic hosts but does occur in hosts with normal splenic function, particularly those who are >60 years of age and those with underlying immunosuppressive conditions such as HIV infection or malignancy. Complications include renal failure, acute respiratory failure, and DIC.

Other sepsis syndromes

Tularemia (Chap. 158) is seen throughout the United States but occurs primarily in Arkansas, Missouri, South Dakota, and Oklahoma. This disease is associated with wild rabbit, tick, and tabanid fly contact. The typhoidal form can be associated with gram-negative septic shock and a mortality rate of >30%, especially in patients with underlying comorbid or immunosuppressive conditions. Plague occurs infrequently in the United States (Chap. 159), primarily after contact with ground squirrels, prairie dogs, or chipmunks, but is endemic in other parts of the world, with >90% of all cases occurring in Africa. The septic form is particularly rare and is associated with shock, multiorgan failure, and a 30% mortality rate. These infections should be considered in the appropriate epidemiologic setting. The Centers for Disease Control and Prevention lists *Francisella tularensis* and *Yersinia pestis* (the agents of tularemia and plague, respectively) along with *Bacillus anthracis* (the agent of anthrax) as important organisms that might be used for bioterrorism (Chap. 221).

■ SEPSIS WITH SKIN MANIFESTATIONS

(See also Chap. 17) Maculopapular rashes may reflect early meningococcal or rickettsial disease but are usually associated with nonemergent infections. Exanthems are usually viral. Primary HIV infection commonly presents with a rash that is typically maculopapular and involves the upper part of the body but can spread to the palms and soles. The patient is usually febrile and can have lymphadenopathy, severe headache, dysphagia, diarrhea, myalgias, and arthralgias. Recognition of this syndrome provides an opportunity to prevent transmission and to institute treatment and monitoring early on.

Petechial rashes caused by viruses are seldom associated with hypotension or a toxic appearance, although there can be exceptions (e.g., severe measles or arboviral infection). In other settings, petechial rashes require more urgent attention.

Meningococcemia

(See also Chap. 143) Almost three-quarters of patients with bacteremic *N. meningitidis* infection have a rash. Meningococcemia most often affects young children (i.e., those 6 months to 5 years old). In sub-Saharan Africa, the high prevalence of serogroup A meningococcal disease has been a threat to public health for more than a century. Thousands of deaths occur annually in this area, which is known as the "meningitis belt," and large epidemic waves occur approximately every 8–12 years. In the United States, sporadic cases and outbreaks occur in day-care centers, schools (grade school through college), and army barracks. Household contacts of index cases are at 400–800 times greater risk of disease than the general population. Patients may exhibit fever, headache, nausea, vomiting, myalgias, changes in mental status, and meningismus. However, the rapidly progressive form of disease is not usually associated with meningitis. The rash is initially pink, blanching, and maculopapular, appearing on the trunk and extremities, but then becomes hemorrhagic, forming petechiae. Petechiae are first seen at the ankles, wrists, axillae, mucosal surfaces, and palpebral and bulbar conjunctiva, with subsequent spread to the lower extremities and trunk. A cluster of petechiae may be seen at pressure points—e.g., where a blood pressure cuff has been inflated. In rapidly progressive meningococcemia (10–20% of cases), the petechial rash quickly becomes purpuric (see Fig. 51-5), and patients develop DIC, multiorgan failure, and shock. Of these patients, 50–60% die, and survivors often require extensive debridement or amputation of gangrenous extremities. Hypotension with petechiae for <12 h is associated with significant mortality. Cyanosis, coma, oliguria, metabolic acidosis, and elevated partial thromboplastin time are also associated with a fatal outcome. Correction of protein C deficiency may improve outcome. Antibiotics given in the office by the primary care provider before hospital evaluation and admission may improve prognosis; this observation suggests that early initiation of treatment may be life-saving.

Rocky Mountain spotted fever

(See also Chap. 174) RMSF is a tickborne disease caused by *Rickettsia rickettsii* that occurs throughout North and South America. Up to 40% of patients do not report a history of a tick bite, but a history of travel or outdoor activity (e.g., camping in tick-infested areas) can often be ascertained. For the first 3 days, headache, fever, malaise, myalgias, nausea, vomiting, and anorexia are documented. By day 3, half of patients have skin findings. Blanching macules develop initially on the wrists and ankles and then spread over the legs and trunk. The lesions become hemorrhagic and are frequently petechial. The rash spreads to palms and soles later in the course. The centripetal spread is a classic feature of RMSF but occurs in a minority of patients. Moreover, 10–15% of patients with RMSF never develop a rash. The patient can be hypotensive and develop noncardiogenic pulmonary edema, confusion, lethargy, and encephalitis progressing to coma. The CSF contains 10–100 cells/µL, usually with a predominance of mononuclear cells. The CSF glucose level is often normal; the protein concentration may be slightly elevated. Renal and hepatic injury and bleeding secondary to vascular damage are noted. Untreated infection has a mortality rate of 20–30%.

 Other rickettsial diseases cause significant morbidity and mortality worldwide. *Mediterranean spotted fever* caused by *Rickettsia conorii* is found in Africa, southwestern and south-central Asia, and southern Europe. Patients have fever, flu-like symptoms, and an inoculation eschar at the site of the tick bite. A maculopapular rash develops within 1–7 days, involving the palms and soles but sparing the face. Elderly patients or those with diabetes, alcoholism, uremia, or congestive heart failure are at risk for severe disease characterized by neurologic involvement, respiratory distress, and gangrene of the digits. Mortality rates associated with this severe form of disease approach 50%. *Epidemic typhus*, caused by *Rickettsia prowazekii*, is transmitted in louse-infested environments and emerges in conditions of extreme poverty, war, and natural disaster. Patients experience a sudden onset of high fevers, severe headache, cough, myalgias, and abdominal pain. A maculopapular rash develops (primarily on the trunk) in more than half of patients and can progress to petechiae and purpura. Serious signs include delirium, coma, seizures, noncardiogenic pulmonary edema, skin necrosis, and peripheral gangrene. Mortality rates approached 60% in the preantibiotic era and continue to exceed 10–15% in contemporary outbreaks. *Scrub typhus*, caused by *Orientia tsutsugamushi*—a separate genus in the family Rickettsiaceae—is transmitted by larval mites or chiggers and is one of the most common infections in southeastern Asia and the western Pacific. The organism is found in areas of heavy scrub vegetation (e.g., along riverbanks). Patients may have an inoculation eschar and may develop a maculopapular rash. Severe cases progress to pneumonia, meningoencephalitis, DIC, and renal failure. Mortality rates range from 1% to 35%.

If recognized in a timely fashion, rickettsial disease is very responsive to treatment. Doxycycline (100 mg twice daily for 3–14 days) is the treatment of choice for both adults and children. The newer macrolides and chloramphenicol may be suitable alternatives.

Purpura fulminans

(See also Chaps. 143 and 271) Purpura fulminans is the cutaneous manifestation of DIC and presents as large ecchymotic areas and hemorrhagic bullae. Progression of petechiae to purpura, ecchymoses, and gangrene is associated with congestive heart failure, septic shock, acute renal failure, acidosis, hypoxia, hypotension, and death. Purpura fulminans has been associated primarily with *N. meningitidis* but, in splenectomized patients, may be associated with *S. pneumoniae* and *H. influenzae*. Several small studies have suggested that correction of the protein C deficiency evident in meningococcal purpura fulminans with drotrecogin alfa (activated) may dramatically improve outcome.

Ecthyma gangrenosum

Septic shock caused by *P. aeruginosa* or *Aeromonas hydrophila* can be associated with ecthyma gangrenosum (see Figs. 152-1 and e7-35): hemorrhagic vesicles surrounded by a rim of erythema with central necrosis and ulceration. These gram-negative bacteremias are most common among patients with neutropenia, extensive burns, and hypogammaglobulinemia.

Other emergent infections associated with rash

Vibrio vulnificus and other noncholera *Vibrio* bacteremic infections (Chap. 156) can cause focal skin lesions and overwhelming sepsis in hosts with liver disease, diabetes, renal insufficiency, or other immunocompromising conditions. After ingestion of contaminated raw shellfish, there is a sudden onset of malaise, chills, fever, and hypotension. The patient develops bullous or hemorrhagic skin lesions, usually on the lower extremities, and 75% of patients have leg pain. The mortality rate can be as high as 50–60%, particularly when the patient presents with hypotension. Other infections, caused by agents such as *Aeromonas, Klebsiella*, and *E. coli*, can cause hemorrhagic bullae and death due to overwhelming sepsis in cirrhotic patients. *Capnocytophaga canimorsus* can cause septic shock in asplenic patients. Infection typically follows a dog bite. Patients present with fever, chills, myalgia, vomiting, diarrhea, dyspnea, confusion, and headache. Findings can include an exanthem or erythema multiforme (see Figs. 51-9 and e7-25), cyanotic mottling or peripheral cyanosis, petechiae, and ecchymosis. About 30% of patients with this fulminant form die of overwhelming sepsis and DIC, and survivors may require amputation because of gangrene.

Erythroderma

TSS (Chaps. 135 and 136) is usually associated with erythroderma. The patient presents with fever, malaise, myalgias, nausea, vomiting, diarrhea, and confusion. There is a sunburn-type rash that may be subtle and patchy but is usually diffuse and is found on the face, trunk, and extremities. Erythroderma, which desquamates after 1–2 weeks, is more common in *Staphylococcus*-associated than in *Streptococcus*-associated TSS. Hypotension develops rapidly—often within hours—after the onset of symptoms. Multiorgan failure is seen. Early renal failure may precede hypotension and distinguishes this syndrome from other septic shock syndromes. There may be no indication of a primary focal infection, although possible cutaneous or mucosal portals of entry for the organism can be ascertained when a careful history is taken. Colonization rather than overt infection of the vagina or a postoperative wound, for example, is typical with staphylococcal TSS, and the mucosal areas appear hyperemic but not infected. Streptococcal TSS is more often associated with skin or soft tissue infection (including necrotizing fasciitis), and patients are more likely to be bacteremic. The diagnosis of TSS is defined by the clinical criteria of fever, rash, hypotension, and multiorgan involvement. The mortality rate is 5% for menstruation-associated TSS, 10–15% for nonmenstrual TSS, and 30–70% for streptococcal TSS.

Viral hemorrhagic fevers

 Viral hemorrhagic fevers (Chaps. 196 and 197) are zoonotic illnesses caused by viruses that reside in either animal reservoirs or arthropod vectors. These diseases occur worldwide and are restricted to areas where the host species live. They are caused by four major groups of viruses: Arenaviridae (e.g., Lassa fever in Africa), Bunyaviridae (e.g., Rift Valley fever in Africa or hantavirus hemorrhagic fever with renal syndrome in Asia), Filoviridae (e.g., Ebola and Marburg virus infections in Africa), and Flaviviridae (e.g., yellow fever in Africa and South America and dengue in Asia, Africa, and the Americas). Lassa fever and Ebola and Marburg virus infections are also transmitted from person to person. The vectors for most viral fevers are found in rural areas; dengue and yellow fever are important exceptions. After a prodrome of fever, myalgias, and malaise, patients develop evidence of vascular damage, petechiae, and local hemorrhage. Shock, multifocal hemorrhaging, and neurologic signs (e.g., seizures or coma) predict a poor prognosis. Dengue (Chap. 196) is the most common arboviral disease worldwide. More than half a million cases of dengue hemorrhagic fever occur each year, with at least 12,000 deaths. Patients have a triad of symptoms: hemorrhagic manifestations, evidence of plasma leakage, and platelet counts <100,000/μL. Mortality rates are 10–20%. If dengue shock syndrome develops, mortality can reach 40%. Although supportive care to maintain blood pressure and intravascular volume with careful volume-replacement therapy is key, ribavirin also may be useful against Arenaviridae and Bunyaviridae.

■ SEPSIS WITH A SOFT TISSUE/MUSCLE PRIMARY FOCUS

See also Chap. 125.

Necrotizing fasciitis

This infection is characterized by extensive necrosis of the subcutaneous tissue and fascia. It may arise at a site of minimal trauma or postoperative incision and may also be associated with recent varicella, childbirth, or muscle strain. The most common causes of necrotizing fasciitis are group A streptococci alone (Chap. 136) and a mixed facultative and anaerobic flora (Chap. 125). Diabetes mellitus, peripheral vascular disease, and IV drug use are associated risk factors. Physical findings are minimal compared with the severity of pain and the degree of fever. The examination is often unremarkable except for soft tissue edema and erythema. The infected area is red, hot, shiny, swollen, and exquisitely tender. In untreated infection, the overlying skin develops blue-gray patches after 36 h, and cutaneous bullae and necrosis develop after 3–5 days. Necrotizing fasciitis due to a mixed flora, but not that due to group A streptococci, can be associated with gas production. Without treatment, pain decreases because of thrombosis of the small blood vessels and destruction of the peripheral nerves—an ominous sign. The mortality rate is 15–34% overall, >70% in association with TSS, and nearly 100% without surgical intervention. Necrotizing fasciitis may also be due to *Clostridium perfringens* (Chap. 142); in this condition, the patient is extremely toxic and the mortality rate is high. Within 48 h, rapid tissue invasion and systemic toxicity associated with hemolysis and death ensue. The distinction between this entity and clostridial myonecrosis is made by muscle biopsy. Necrotizing fasciitis caused by community-acquired MRSA has been reported. The MRSA-infected patients in one series required extensive surgical debridement, but there were no deaths.

Clostridial myonecrosis

(See also Chap. 142) Myonecrosis is often associated with trauma or surgery but can be spontaneous. The incubation period is usually 12–24 h long, and massive necrotizing gangrene develops within hours of onset. Systemic toxicity, shock, and death can occur within 12 h. The patient's pain and toxic appearance are out of proportion to physical findings. On examination, the patient is febrile, apathetic, tachycardic, and tachypneic and may express a feeling of impending doom. Hypotension and renal failure develop later, and hyperalertness is evident preterminally. The skin over the affected area is bronze-brown, mottled, and edematous. Bullous lesions with serosanguineous drainage and a mousy or sweet odor can develop. Crepitus can occur secondary to gas production in muscle tissue. The mortality rate is >65% with spontaneous myonecrosis, which is often associated with *Clostridium septicum* and underlying malignancy. The mortality rates associated with trunk and limb infection are 63% and 12%, respectively, and any delay in surgical treatment increases the risk of death.

◼ NEUROLOGIC INFECTIONS WITH OR WITHOUT SEPTIC SHOCK

Bacterial meningitis

(See also Chap. 381) Bacterial meningitis is one of the most common infectious disease emergencies involving the central nervous system. Although hosts with cell-mediated immune deficiency (including transplant recipients, diabetic patients, elderly patients, and cancer patients receiving certain chemotherapeutic agents) are at particular risk for *Listeria monocytogenes* meningitis, most cases in adults are due to *S. pneumoniae* (30–50%) and *N. meningitidis* (10–35%). The classic presentation of fever, meningismus, and altered mental status is seen in only one-half to two-thirds of patients. The elderly can present without fever or meningeal signs despite lethargy and confusion. Cerebral dysfunction is evidenced by confusion, delirium, and lethargy that can progress to coma. A fulminant presentation with sepsis and brain edema occurs in some cases; papilledema at presentation is unusual and suggests another diagnosis (e.g., an intracranial lesion). Focal signs, including cranial nerve palsies (IV, VI, VII), can be seen in 10–20% of cases; 50–70% of patients have bacteremia. A poor outcome is associated with coma, hypotension, meningitis due to *S. pneumoniae*, respiratory distress, a CSF glucose level of <0.6 mmol/L (<10 mg/dL), a CSF protein level of >2.5 g/L, a peripheral white blood cell count of <5000/μL, and a serum sodium level of <135 mmol/L. Rapid initiation of treatment is essential; the odds of an unfavorable outcome may increase by 30% for each hour that treatment is delayed.

Suppurative intracranial infections

(See also Chap. 381) In suppurative intracranial infections, rare intracranial lesions present along with sepsis and hemodynamic instability. Rapid recognition of the toxic patient with central neurologic signs is crucial to improvement of the dismal prognosis of these entities. *Subdural empyema* arises from the paranasal sinus in 60–70% of cases. Microaerophilic streptococci and staphylococci are the predominant etiologic organisms. The patient is toxic, with fever, headache, and nuchal rigidity. Of all patients, 75% have focal signs and 6–20% die. Despite improved survival rates, 15–44% of patients are left with permanent neurologic deficits. *Septic cavernous sinus thrombosis* follows a facial or sphenoid sinus infection; 70% of cases are due to staphylococci (including MRSA), and the remainder are due primarily to aerobic or anaerobic streptococci. A unilateral or retroorbital headache progresses to a toxic appearance and fever within days. Three-quarters of patients have unilateral periorbital edema that becomes bilateral and then progresses to ptosis, proptosis, ophthalmoplegia, and papilledema. The mortality rate is as high as 30%. *Septic thrombosis of the superior sagittal sinus* spreads from the ethmoid or maxillary sinuses and is caused by *S. pneumoniae*, other streptococci, and staphylococci. The fulminant course is characterized by headache, nausea, vomiting, rapid progression to confusion and coma, nuchal rigidity, and brainstem signs. If the sinus is totally thrombosed, the mortality rate exceeds 80%.

Brain abscess

(See also Chap. 381) Brain abscess often occurs without systemic signs. Almost half of patients are afebrile, and presentations are more consistent with a space-occupying lesion in the brain; 70% of patients have headache and/or altered mental status, 50% have focal neurologic signs, and 25% have papilledema. Abscesses can present as single or multiple lesions resulting from contiguous foci or hematogenous infection, such as endocarditis. The infection progresses over several days from cerebritis to an abscess with a mature capsule. More than half of infections are polymicrobial, with an etiology consisting of aerobic bacteria (primarily streptococcal species) and anaerobes. Abscesses arising hematogenously are especially apt to rupture into the ventricular space, causing a sudden and severe deterioration in clinical status and high mortality. Otherwise, mortality is low but morbidity is high (30–55%). Patients presenting with stroke and a parameningeal infectious focus, such as sinusitis or otitis, may have a brain abscess, and physicians must maintain a high level of suspicion. Prognosis worsens in patients with a fulminant course, delayed diagnosis, abscess rupture into the ventricles, multiple abscesses, or abnormal neurologic status at presentation.

Intracranial and spinal epidural abscesses

(See also Chap. 377) Spinal and intracranial epidural abscesses (SEAs and ICEAs) can result in permanent neurologic deficits, sepsis, and death. At-risk patients include those with diabetes mellitus; IV drug use; chronic alcohol abuse; recent spinal trauma, surgery, or epidural anesthesia; and other comorbid conditions, such as HIV infection. In the United States and Canada, where early treatment of otitis and sinusitis is typical, ICEA is rare but the number of cases of SEA is on the rise. In Africa and areas with limited access to health care, SEAs and ICEAs cause significant morbidity and mortality. ICEAs typically present as fever, mental status changes, and neck pain, while SEAs often present as fever, localized spinal tenderness, and back pain. ICEAs are typically polymicrobial, whereas SEAs are most often due to hematogenous seeding, with staphylococci the most common etiologic agent. Early diagnosis and treatment, which may include surgical drainage, minimize rates of mortality and permanent neurologic sequelae.

Cerebral malaria

(See also Chap. 210) This entity should be urgently considered if patients who have recently traveled to areas endemic for malaria present with a febrile illness and lethargy or other neurologic signs. Fulminant malaria is caused by *Plasmodium falciparum* and is associated with temperatures of >40°C (>104°F), hypotension, jaundice, adult respiratory distress syndrome, and bleeding. By definition, any patient with a change in mental status or repeated seizure in the setting of fulminant malaria has cerebral malaria. In adults, this nonspecific febrile illness progresses to coma over several days; occasionally, coma occurs within hours and death within 24 h. Nuchal rigidity and photophobia are rare. On physical examination, symmetric encephalopathy is typical, and upper motor neuron dysfunction with decorticate and decerebrate posturing can be seen in advanced disease. Unrecognized infection results in a 20–30% mortality rate.

Other focal syndromes with a fulminant course

Infection at virtually any primary focus (e.g., osteomyelitis, pneumonia, pyelonephritis, or cholangitis) can result in bacteremia and sepsis. TSS has been associated with focal infections such as septic arthritis, peritonitis, sinusitis, and wound infection. Rapid clinical deterioration and death can be associated with destruction of the primary site of infection, as is seen in endocarditis and in necrotizing infections of the oropharynx (in which edema suddenly compromises the airway).

Rhinocerebral mucormycosis

(See also Chap. 205) Patients with diabetes or immunocompromising conditions are at risk for invasive rhinocerebral mucormycosis. Patients present with low-grade fever, dull sinus pain, diplopia, decreased mental status, decreased ocular motion, chemosis, proptosis, dusky or necrotic nasal turbinates, and necrotic hard-palate lesions that respect the midline. Without rapid recognition and intervention, the process continues on an inexorable invasive course, with high mortality.

Acute bacterial endocarditis

(See also Chap. 124) This entity presents with a much more aggressive course than subacute endocarditis. Bacteria such as *S. aureus*, *S. pneumoniae*, *L. monocytogenes*, *Haemophilus* spp., and streptococci of groups A, B, and G attack native valves. Native-valve endocarditis caused by *S. aureus*, including MRSA, is increasing, particularly in health care settings. Mortality rates range from 10% to 40%. The host may have comorbid conditions such as underlying malignancy, diabetes mellitus, IV drug use, or alcoholism. The patient presents with fever, fatigue, and malaise <2 weeks after onset of infection. On physical examination, a changing murmur and congestive heart failure may be noted. Hemorrhagic macules on palms or soles (*Janeway lesions*) sometimes develop. Petechiae, Roth's spots, splinter hemorrhages, and splenomegaly are unusual. Rapid valvular destruction, particularly of the aortic valve, results in pulmonary edema and hypotension. Myocardial abscesses can form, eroding through the septum or into the conduction system and causing life-threatening arrhythmias or high-degree conduction block. Large friable vegetations can result in major arterial emboli, metastatic infection, or tissue infarction. Older patients with *S. aureus* endocarditis are especially likely to present with nonspecific symptoms—a circumstance that delays diagnosis and worsens prognosis. Rapid intervention is crucial for a successful outcome.

Inhalational anthrax

(See also Chap. 221) Inhalational anthrax, the most severe form of disease caused by *B. anthracis*, had not been reported in the United States for more than 25 years until the use of this organism as an agent of bioterrorism in 2001. Patients presented with malaise, fever, cough, nausea, drenching sweats, shortness of breath, and headache. Rhinorrhea was unusual. All patients had abnormal chest roentgenograms at presentation. Pulmonary infiltrates, mediastinal widening, and pleural effusions were the most common findings. Hemorrhagic meningitis was seen in 38% of these patients. Survival was more likely when antibiotics were given during the prodromal period and when multidrug regimens were used. In the absence of urgent intervention with antimicrobial agents and supportive care, inhalational anthrax progresses rapidly to hypotension, cyanosis, and death.

Avian influenza (H5N1) infection

 (See also Chap. 187) Human cases of avian influenza have occurred primarily in Southeast Asia, particularly Vietnam. Avian influenza should be considered in patients with severe respiratory tract illness, particularly if they have been exposed to poultry. Patients present with high fever, an influenza-like illness, and lower respiratory tract symptoms; this illness can progress rapidly to bilateral pneumonia, acute respiratory distress syndrome, multiorgan failure, and death. Early antiviral treatment with neuraminidase inhibitors should be initiated along with aggressive supportive measures. Unlike avian influenza, for which human-to-human transmission has been rare so far, a novel swine-associated influenza A/H1N1 virus has spread rapidly throughout the world. Early in the pandemic, there has been a sudden increase in severe pneumonia affecting a younger population. Patients most at risk of severe disease are children <5 years of age, elderly persons, patients with underlying chronic conditions, and pregnant women.

Hantavirus pulmonary syndrome

(See also Chap. 196) Hantavirus pulmonary syndrome has been documented in the United States (primarily the southwestern states), Canada, and South America. Most cases occur in rural areas and are associated with exposure to rodents. Patients present with a nonspecific viral prodrome of fever, malaise, myalgias, nausea, vomiting, and dizziness that may progress to pulmonary edema and respiratory failure. Hantavirus pulmonary syndrome causes myocardial depression and increased pulmonary vascular permeability; therefore, careful fluid resuscitation and use of pressor agents are crucial. Aggressive cardiopulmonary support during the first few hours of illness can be life-saving. The early onset of thrombocytopenia may help distinguish this syndrome from other febrile illnesses in an appropriate epidemiologic setting.

CONCLUSION

Acutely ill febrile patients with the syndromes discussed in this chapter require close observation, aggressive supportive measures, and—in most cases—admission to intensive care units. The most important task of the physician is to distinguish these patients from other infected febrile patients whose illness will not progress to fulminant disease. The alert physician must recognize the acute infectious disease emergency and then proceed with appropriate urgency.

FURTHER READINGS

DANTAS-TORRES F: Rocky Mountain spotted fever. Lancet Infect Dis 7:724, 2007

FITCH MT, VAN DE BEEK D: Emergency diagnosis and treatment of adult meningitis. Lancet Infect Dis 7:191, 2007

HASHAM S et al: Necrotising fasciitis. BMJ 330:830, 2005

HAYDEN FG et al: Clinical aspects of pandemic 2009 influenza A (H1N1) virus infection. N Engl J Med 362:1708, 2010

LAPPIN E, FERGUSON AJ: Gram-positive toxic shock syndromes. Lancet Infect Dis 9:281, 2009

NGUYEN HB et al: Severe sepsis and septic shock: Review of the literature and emergency department management guidelines. Ann Emerg Med 48:28, 2006

PRADILLA G et al: Epidural abscess of the CNS. Lancet Neurol 8:292, 2009

SPELMAN D et al: Guidelines for the prevention of sepsis in asplenic and hyposplenic patients. Intern Med J 38:349, 2008

STEPHENS DS et al: Epidemic meningitis, meningococcemia, and *Neisseria meningitidis*. Lancet 369:2196, 2007

TALAN DA et al (eds): *Infectious Disease Emergencies*. Infect Dis Clin North Am 22:1–187, 2008 [entire volume]

CHAPTER 122

Immunization Principles and Vaccine Use

Anne Schuchat
Lisa A. Jackson

Few medical interventions of the past century can rival the effect that immunization has had on longevity, economic savings, and quality of life. Seventeen diseases are now preventable through vaccines routinely administered to children and adults in the United States (Table 122-1), and most vaccine-preventable diseases of childhood are at historically low levels (Table 122-2). Health care providers deliver the vast majority of vaccines in the United States in the course of providing routine health services and therefore play an integral role in the nation's public health system.

■ VACCINE IMPACT

Direct and indirect effects

Immunizations against specific infectious diseases protect individuals against infection and thereby prevent symptomatic illnesses. Specific

TABLE 122-1 Diseases That Are Now Preventable With Vaccines Routinely Administered in the United States to Children and/or Adults

Condition	Target Population(s) for Routine Use
Pertussis	Children, adolescents, adults
Diphtheria	Children, adolescents, adults
Tetanus	Children, adolescents, adults
Poliomyelitis	Children
Measles	Children
Mumps	Children
Rubella, congenital rubella syndrome	Children
Hepatitis B	Children
Haemophilus influenzae type b infection	Children
Hepatitis A	Children
Influenza	Children, adolescents, adults
Varicella	Children
Invasive pneumococcal disease	Children, older adults
Meningococcal disease	Children, adolescents
Rotavirus infection	Infants
Human papillomavirus infection, cervical cancer	Adolescent girls and women
Zoster	Older adults

vaccines may blunt the severity of clinical illness (e.g., rotavirus vaccines and severe gastroenteritis) or reduce complications (e.g., zoster vaccines and postherpetic neuralgia). Some immunizations also reduce transmission of infectious disease agents from immunized people to others, thereby reducing the impact of infection spread. This indirect impact is known as *herd immunity*. The level of immunization in a population that is required to achieve indirect protection of unimmunized people varies substantially with the specific vaccine.

Since childhood vaccines have become widely available in the United States, major declines in rates of vaccine-preventable diseases among both children and adults have become evident (Table 122-2). For example, vaccination of children <5 years of age against seven types of *Streptococcus pneumoniae* led to a >90% overall reduction in invasive disease caused by those types. A series of vaccines targeting 10 vaccine-preventable childhood diseases in a single birth cohort leads to prevention of 33,000 premature deaths and 14 million illnesses and saves $42 billion (U.S.): $9 billion in direct medical savings and $33 billion in indirect societal savings.

Control, elimination, and eradication of vaccine-preventable diseases

Immunization programs are associated with the goals of controlling, eliminating, or eradicating a disease. *Control* of a vaccine-preventable disease reduces illness outcomes and often limits the disruptive impacts associated with outbreaks of disease in communities, schools, and institutions. Control programs can also reduce absences from work for ill persons and for parents caring for sick children, decrease absences from school, and limit health care utilization associated with treatment visits.

Elimination of a disease is a more demanding goal than control, usually requiring the reduction to zero of cases in a defined geographic area but sometimes defined as reduction in the indigenous sustained transmission of an infection in a geographic area. As of 2010, the United States had eliminated indigenous transmission of measles, rubella, poliomyelitis, and diphtheria. Importation of pathogens from other parts of the world continues to be important, and public health efforts are intended to react promptly to such cases and to limit forward spread of the infectious agent.

Eradication of a disease is achieved when its elimination can be sustained without ongoing interventions. The only vaccine-preventable disease that has been globally eradicated thus far is smallpox. Although smallpox vaccine is no longer given routinely, the disease has not naturally reemerged because all chains of human transmission were interrupted through earlier vaccination efforts and humans were the only natural reservoir of the virus. Currently, a major health initiative is targeting the global eradication of polio. Sustained transmission of polio has been eliminated from most nations but has never been interrupted in four countries: Afghanistan, India, Nigeria, and Pakistan. Detection of a case of disease that has been targeted for eradication or elimination is considered a sentinel event that could permit the infectious agent to become reestablished in the community or region. Hence, such episodes must be promptly reported to public health authorities.

Outbreak detection and control

Clusters of cases of a vaccine-preventable disease detected in an institution, a medical practice, or a community may signal important changes in the pathogen, vaccine, or environment. Several factors can give rise to increases in vaccine-preventable disease, including (1) low rates of immunization that result in an accumulation of susceptible people (e.g., measles resurgence among vaccination abstainers); (2) changes in the infectious agent that permit it to escape vaccine-induced protection (e.g., nonvaccine-type

TABLE 122-2 Decline in Vaccine-Preventable Diseases in the United States Following Widespread Implementation of National Vaccine Recommendations

Condition	Annual No. of Prevaccine Cases (Average)	No. of Cases Reported in 2010[a]	Reduction (%) in Cases After Widespread Vaccination
Smallpox	29,005	0	100
Diphtheria	21,053	0	100
Measles	530,217	61	≥99
Mumps	162,344	2,528	98
Pertussis	200,752	21,291	89
Polio (paralytic)	16,316	0	100
Rubella	47,745	6	>99
Congenital rubella syndrome	152	0	100
Tetanus	580	8	99
Haemophilus influenzae type b infection	20,000	270[b]	99
Hepatitis A	117,333	11,049	91
Hepatitis B (acute)	66,232	11,269	83
Invasive pneumococcal infection: all ages	63,067	44,000[c]	30
Invasive pneumococcal infection: <5 years of age	16,069	4,167[c]	74
Varicella	4,085,120	449,363	89.0

[a]Except for cases of hepatitis A, hepatitis B, and pneumococcal infection, for which 2008 figures are shown.
[b]Includes 16 type b infections and 254 infections caused by unknown types (<5 years of age).
[c]Data are from the CDC's Active Bacterial Core Surveillance Report; *www.cdc.gov/abcs/survreports/spneu08.pdf.*
Source: Adapted from Roush et al., with permission.

pneumococci); (3) waning of vaccine-induced immunity (e.g., pertussis among adolescents and adults vaccinated in early childhood); and (4) point-source introductions of large inocula (e.g., food-borne exposure to hepatitis A virus). Reporting episodes of outbreak-prone diseases to public health authorities can facilitate recognition of clusters that require further interventions.

Public health reporting Recognition of suspected cases of diseases targeted for elimination or eradication—along with other diseases that require urgent public health interventions, such as contact tracing, administration of chemo- or immunoprophylaxis, or epidemiologic investigation for common-source exposure)—is typically associated with special reporting requirements. Many diseases against which vaccines are routinely used, including measles, pertussis, *Haemophilus influenzae* invasive disease, and varicella, are nationally notifiable. Clinicians and laboratory staff have a responsibility to report some vaccine-preventable disease occurrences to local or state public health authorities according to specific case-definition criteria. All providers should be aware of state or city disease-reporting requirements and the best ways to contact public health authorities. A prompt response to vaccine-preventable disease outbreaks can greatly enhance the effectiveness of control measures.

Global considerations Several international health initiatives currently focus on reducing vaccine-preventable diseases in regions throughout the world. These efforts include improving access to new and underutilized vaccines, such as pneumococcal conjugate, rotavirus, human papillomavirus (HPV), and

meningococcal A conjugate vaccines. The American Red Cross, the World Health Organization (WHO), the United Nations Foundation, the United Nations Children's Fund (UNICEF), and the Centers for Disease Control and Prevention (CDC) are partners in the Measles Initiative, which targeted reduction of worldwide measles deaths by 90% from 2000 to 2010. During 2000–2008, global measles mortality rates declined by 78%—i.e., from an estimated 733,000 deaths in 2000 to 164,000 deaths in 2008. Rotary International, UNICEF, the CDC, and the WHO are leading partners in the global eradication of polio, an endeavor that reduced the annual number of paralytic polio cases from 350,000 in 1988 to <2000 in 2009. The GAVI Alliance and the Bill and Melinda Gates Foundation have brought substantial momentum to global efforts to reduce vaccine-preventable diseases, expanding on earlier efforts by the WHO, UNICEF, and governments in developed and developing countries.

Enhancing immunization in adults Although immunization has become a centerpiece of routine pediatric medical visits, it has not been as well integrated into routine health care visits for adults. This chapter focuses on immunization principles and vaccine use in adults. Accumulating evidence suggests that immunization coverage can be increased through efforts directed at consumer-, provider-, institution-, and system-level factors. The literature suggests that the application of multiple strategies is more effective at raising coverage rates than is the use of any single strategy.

Recommendations for adult immunizations The CDC's Advisory Committee on Immunization Practices (ACIP) is the main source of recommendations for use of vaccines licensed by the U.S. Food and Drug Administration (FDA) for children and adults in the U.S. civilian population. The ACIP is a federal advisory committee that consists of 15 voting members (experts in fields associated with immunization) appointed by the Secretary of the U.S. Department of Health and Human Services; 8 ex officio members representing federal agencies; and 26 nonvoting representatives of various liaison organizations, including major medical societies and managed-care organizations. The ACIP recommendations are available at *www.cdc.gov/vaccines/pubs/ACIP-list.htm.* These recommendations are harmonized to the greatest extent possible with vaccine recommendations made by other organizations, including the American College of Obstetricians and Gynecologists, the American Academy of Family Physicians, and the American College of Physicians.

Adult immunization schedules Immunization schedules for adults in the United States are updated annually and can be found online (*www.cdc.gov/vaccines/recs/schedules/adult-schedule.htm*). In January, the schedules are published in *American Family Physician*, the *Annals of Internal Medicine*, and *Morbidity and Mortality Weekly Report* (*www.cdc.gov/mmwr*). The adult immunization schedules for 2011 are summarized in Fig. 122-1. Additional information and specifications are contained in the footnotes to

Recommended Adult Immunization Schedule
UNITED STATES · 2011
Note: These recommendations *must* be read with the footnotes that follow
containing number of doses, intervals between doses, and other important information.

Recommended adult immunization schedule, by vaccine and age group

VACCINE ▼ AGE GROUP ▶	19–26 years	27–49 years	50–59 years	60–64 years	≥65 years
Influenza[1,*]	1 dose annually				
Tetanus, diphtheria, pertussis (Td/Tdap)[2,*]	Substitute 1-time dose of Tdap for Td booster; then boost with Td every 10 yrs				Td booster every 10 yrs
Varicella[3,*]	2 doses				
Human papillomavirus (PHV)[4,*]	3 doses (females)				
Zoster[5]				1 dose	
Measles, mumps, rubella (MMR)[6,*]	1 or 2 doses		1 dose		
Pneumococcal (polysaccharide)[7,8]	1 or 2 doses				1 dose
Meningococcal[9,*]	1 or more doses				
Hepatitis A[10,*]	2 doses				
Hepatitis B[11,*]	3 doses				

*Covered by the Vaccine Injury Compensation Program.

For all persons in this category who meet the age requirements and who lack evidence of immunity (e.g., lack documentation of vaccination or have no evidence of previous infection)

Recommended if some other risk factor is present (e.g., based on medical, occupational, lifestyle, or other indications)

No recommendation

Report all clinically significant postvaccination reactions to the Vaccine Adverse Event Reporting System (VAERS). Reporting forms and instructions on filing a VAERS report are available at http://www.vaers.hhs.gov or by telephone, 800-822-7967.

Information on how to file a Vaccine Injury Compensation Program claim is available at http://www.hrsa.gov/vaccinecompensation or by telephone, 800-338-2382. Information about filing a claim for vaccine injury is available through the U.S. Court of Federal Claims, 717 Madison Place, N.W., Washington, D.C. 20005; telephone, 202-357-6400.

Additional information about the vaccines in this schedule, extent of available data, and contraindications for vaccination also is available at http://www.cdc.gov/vaccines or from the CDC-INFO Contact Center at 800-CDC- INFO (800-232-4636) in English and Spanish, 24 hours a day, 7 days a week.

Vaccines that might be indicated for adults based on medical and other indications

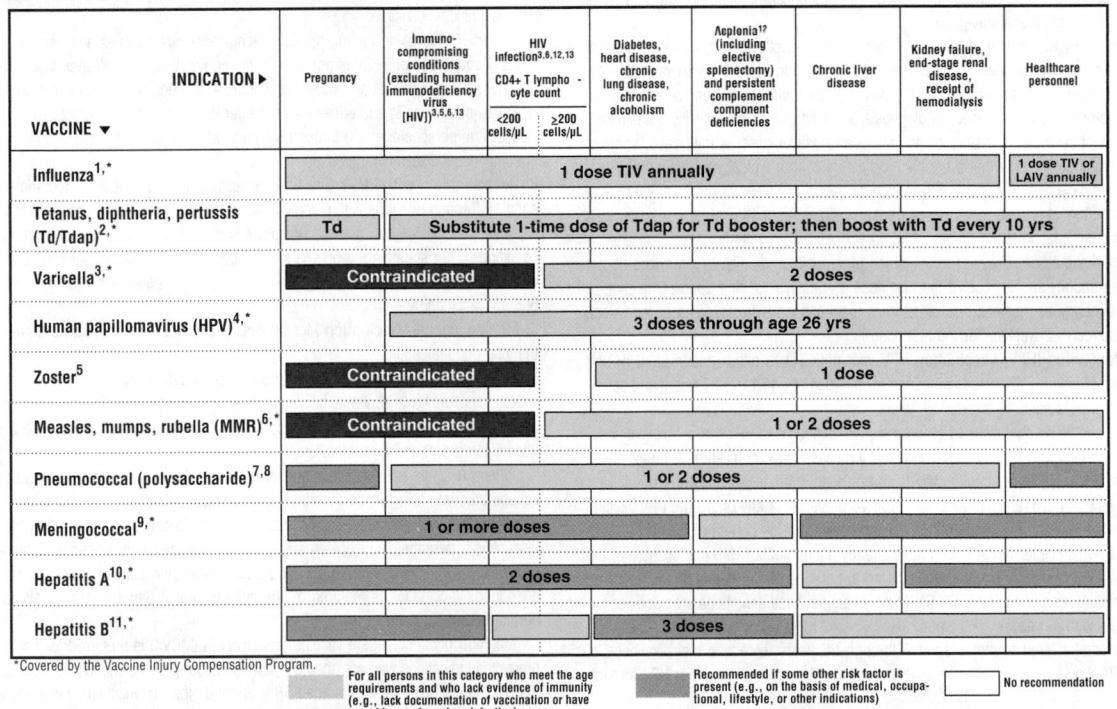

VACCINE ▼ INDICATION ▶	Pregnancy	Immuno-compromising conditions (excluding human immunodeficiency virus [HIV])[3,5,6,13]	HIV infection[3,6,12,13] CD4+ T lymphocyte count <200 cells/µL	HIV infection ≥200 cells/µL	Diabetes, heart disease, chronic lung disease, chronic alcoholism	Asplenia[17] (including elective splenectomy) and persistent complement component deficiencies	Chronic liver disease	Kidney failure, end-stage renal disease, receipt of hemodialysis	Healthcare personnel
Influenza[1,*]	1 dose TIV annually								1 dose TIV or LAIV annually
Tetanus, diphtheria, pertussis (Td/Tdap)[2,*]	Td	Substitute 1-time dose of Tdap for Td booster; then boost with Td every 10 yrs							
Varicella[3,*]	Contraindicated		2 doses						
Human papillomavirus (HPV)[4,*]		3 doses through age 26 yrs							
Zoster[5]	Contraindicated		1 dose						
Measles, mumps, rubella (MMR)[6,*]	Contraindicated		1 or 2 doses						
Pneumococcal (polysaccharide)[7,8]		1 or 2 doses							
Meningococcal[9,*]	1 or more doses								
Hepatitis A[10,*]	2 doses								
Hepatitis B[11,*]	3 doses								

*Covered by the Vaccine Injury Compensation Program.

For all persons in this category who meet the age requirements and who lack evidence of immunity (e.g., lack documentation of vaccination or have no evidence of previous infection)

Recommended if some other risk factor is present (e.g., on the basis of medical, occupational, lifestyle, or other indications)

No recommendation

These schedules indicate the recommended age groups and medical indications for which administration of currently licensed vaccines is commonly indicated for adults ages 19 years and older, as of February 4, 2011. For all vaccines being recommended on the adult immunization schedule, a vaccine series does not need to be restarted, regardless of the time that has elapsed between doses. Licensed combination vaccines may be used whenever any components of the combination are indicated and when the vaccine's other components are not contraindicated. For detailed recommendations on all vaccines, including those used primarily for travelers or that are issued during the year, consult the manufacturers' package inserts and the complete statements from the Advisory Committee on Immunization Practices (http:// www.cdc.gov/vaccines/pubs/acip-list.htm).

The recommendations in this schedule were approved by the Centers for Disease Control and Prevention's (CDC) Advisory Committee on Immunization Practices (ACIP), the American Academy of Family Physicians (AAFP), the American College of Obstetricians and Gynecologists (ACOG), and the American College of Physicians (ACP).

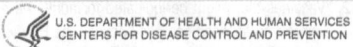

U.S. DEPARTMENT OF HEALTH AND HUMAN SERVICES
CENTERS FOR DISEASE CONTROL AND PREVENTION   CDC

Figure 122-1   Recommended adult immunization schedules, United States, 2011. For complete statements by the Advisory Committee on Immunization Practices (ACIP), visit *www.cdc.gov/vaccines/pubs/ACIP-list.htm.*

(continued)

Figure 122-1 (Continued)

1. Influenza vaccination Annual vaccination against influenza is recommended for all persons aged 6 months and older, including all adults. Healthy, nonpregnant adults aged less than 50 years without high-risk medical conditions can receive either intranasally administered live, attenuated influenza vaccine (FluMist), or inactivated vaccine. Other persons should receive the inactivated vaccine. Adults aged 65 years and older can receive the standard influenza vaccine or the high-dose (Fluzone) influenza vaccine. Additional information about influenza vaccination is available at *http://www.cdc.gov/vaccines/vpd-vac/flu/default.htm.*

2. Tetanus, diphtheria, and acellular pertussis (Td/Tdap) vaccination Administer a one-time dose of Tdap to adults aged less than 65 years who have not received Tdap previously or for whom vaccine status is unknown to replace one of the 10-year Td boosters, and as soon as feasible to all 1) postpartum women, 2) close contacts of infants younger than age 12 months (e.g., grandparents and child-care providers), and 3) healthcare personnel with direct patient contact. Adults aged 65 years and older who have not previously received Tdap and who have close contact with an infant aged less than 12 months also should be vaccinated. Other adults aged 65 years and older may receive Tdap. Tdap can be administered regardless of interval since the most recent tetanus or diphtheria-containing vaccine.

Adults with uncertain or incomplete history of completing a 3-dose primary vaccination series with Td-containing vaccines should begin or complete a primary vaccination series. For unvaccinated adults, administer the first 2 doses at least 4 weeks apart and the third dose 6–12 months after the second. If incompletely vaccinated (i.e., less than 3 doses), administer remaining doses. Substitute a one-time dose of Tdap for one of the doses of Td, either in the primary series or for the routine booster, whichever comes first.

If a woman is pregnant and received the most recent Td vaccination 10 or more years previously, administer Td during the second or third trimester. If the woman received the most recent Td vaccination less than 10 years previously, administer Tdap during the immediate postpartum period. At the clinician's discretion, Td may be deferred during pregnancy and Tdap substituted in the immediate postpartum period, or Tdap may be administered instead of Td to a pregnant woman after an informed discussion with the woman.

The ACIP statement for recommendations for administering Td as prophylaxis in wound management is available at *http://www.cdc.gov/vaccines/pubs/acip-list.htm.*

3. Varicella vaccination All adults without evidence of immunity to varicella should receive 2 doses of single-antigen varicella vaccine if not previously vaccinated or a second dose if they have received only 1 dose, unless they have a medical contraindication. Special consideration should be given to those who 1) have close contact with persons at high risk for severe disease (e.g., healthcare personnel and family contacts of persons with immunocompromising conditions) or 2) are at high risk for exposure or transmission (e.g., teachers; child-care employees; residents and staff members of institutional settings, including correctional institutions; college students; military personnel; adolescents and adults living in households with children; nonpregnant women of childbearing age; and international travelers).

Evidence of immunity to varicella in adults includes any of the following: 1) documentation of 2 doses of varicella vaccine at least 4 weeks apart; 2) U.S.-born before 1980 (although for healthcare personnel and pregnant women, birth before 1980 should not be considered evidence of immunity); 3) history of varicella based on diagnosis or verification of varicella by a healthcare provider (for a patient reporting a history of or having an atypical case, a mild case, or both, healthcare providers should seek either an epidemiologic link with a typical varicella case or to a laboratory-confirmed case or evidence of laboratory confirmation, if it was performed at the time of acute disease); 4) history of herpes zoster based on diagnosis or verification of herpes zoster by a healthcare provider; or 5) laboratory evidence of immunity or laboratory confirmation of disease.

Pregnant women should be assessed for evidence of varicella immunity. Women who do not have evidence of immunity should receive the first dose of varicella vaccine upon completion or termination of pregnancy and before discharge from the healthcare facility. The second dose should be administered 4–8 weeks after the first dose.

4. Human papillomavirus (HPV) vaccination HPV vaccination with either quadrivalent (HPV4) vaccine or bivalent vaccine (HPV2) is recommended for females at age 11 or 12 years and catch-up vaccination for females aged 13 through 26 years.

Ideally, vaccine should be administered before potential exposure to HPV through sexual activity; however, females who are sexually active should still be vaccinated consistent with age-based recommendations. Sexually active females who have not been infected with any of the four HPV vaccine types (types 6, 11, 16, and 18, all of which HPV4 prevents) or any of the two HPV vaccine types (types 16 and 18, both of which HPV2 prevents) receive the full benefit of the vaccination. Vaccination is less beneficial for females who have already been infected with one or more of the HPV vaccine types. HPV4 or HPV2 can be administered to persons with a history of genital warts, abnormal Papanicolaou test, or positive HPV DNA test, because these conditions are not evidence of previous infection with all vaccine HPV types.

HPV4 may be administered to males aged 9 through 26 years to reduce their likelihood of genital warts. HPV4 would be most effective when administered before exposure to HPV through sexual contact.

A complete series for either HPV4 or HPV2 consists of 3 doses. The second dose should be administered 1–2 months after the first dose; the third dose should be administered 6 months after the first dose.

Although HPV vaccination is not specifically recommended for persons with the medical indications described in Figure 2, "Vaccines that might be indicated for adults based on medical and other indications," it may be administered to these persons because the HPV vaccine is not a live-virus vaccine. However, the immune response and vaccine efficacy might be less for persons with the medical indications described in Figure 2 than in persons who do not have the medical indications described or who are immunocompetent.

5. Herpes zoster vaccination A single dose of zoster vaccine is recommended for adults aged 60 years and older regardless of whether they report a previous episode of herpes zoster.

Persons with chronic medical conditions may be vaccinated unless their condition constitutes a contraindication.

6. Measles, mumps, rubella (MMR) vaccination Adults born before 1957 generally are considered immune to measles and mumps. All adults born in 1957 or later should have documentation of 1 or more doses of MMR vaccine unless they have a medical contraindication to the vaccine, laboratory evidence of immunity to each of the three diseases, or documentation of provider-diagnosed measles or mumps disease. For rubella, documentation of provider-diagnosed disease is not considered acceptable evidence of immunity.

Measles component: A second dose of MMR vaccine, administered a minimum of 28 days after the first dose, is recommended for adults who 1) have been recently exposed to measles or are in an outbreak setting; 2) are students in postsecondary educational institutions; 3) work in a healthcare facility; or 4) plan to travel internationally. Persons who received inactivated (killed) measles vaccine or measles vaccine of unknown type during 1963–1967 should be revaccinated with 2 doses of MMR vaccine.

Mumps component: A second dose of MMR vaccine, administered a minimum of 28 days after the first dose, is recommended for adults who 1) live in a community experiencing a mumps outbreak and are in an affected age group; 2) are students in postsecondary educational institutions; 3) work in a healthcare facility; or 4) plan to travel internationally. Persons vaccinated before 1979 with either killed mumps vaccine or mumps vaccine of unknown type who are at high risk for mumps infection (e.g. persons who are working in a healthcare facility) should be revaccinated with 2 doses of MMR vaccine.

Rubella component: For women of childbearing age, regardless of birth year, rubella immunity should be determined. If there is no evidence of immunity, women who are not pregnant should be vaccinated. Pregnant women who do not have evidence of immunity should receive MMR vaccine upon completion or termination of pregnancy and before discharge from the healthcare facility.

Healthcare personnel born before 1957: For unvaccinated healthcare personnel born before 1957 who lack laboratory evidence of measles, mumps, and/or rubella immunity or laboratory confirmation of disease, healthcare facilities should 1) consider routinely vaccinating personnel with 2 doses of MMR vaccine at the appropriate interval (for measles and mumps) and 1 dose of MMR vaccine (for rubella), and 2) recommend 2 doses of MMR vaccine at the appropriate interval during an outbreak of measles or mumps, and 1 dose during an outbreak of rubella. Complete information about evidence of immunity is available at *http://www.cdc.gov/vaccines/recs/provisional/default.htm.*

7. Pneumococcal polysaccharide (PPSV) vaccination Vaccinate all persons with the following indications:

Medical: Chronic lung disease (including asthma); chronic cardiovascular diseases; diabetes mellitus; chronic liver diseases; cirrhosis; chronic alcoholism; functional or anatomic asplenia (e.g., sickle cell disease or splenectomy [if elective splenectomy is planned, vaccinate at least 2 weeks before surgery]); immunocompromising conditions (including chronic renal failure or nephrotic syndrome); and cochlear implants and cerebrospinal fluid leaks. Vaccinate as close to HIV diagnosis as possible.

Other: Residents of nursing homes or long-term care facilities and persons who smoke cigarettes. Routine use of PPSV is not recommended for American Indians/Alaska Natives or persons aged less than 65 years unless they have underlying medical conditions that are PPSV indications. However, public health authorities may consider recommending PPSV for American Indians/Alaska Natives and persons aged 50 through 64 years who are living in areas where the risk for invasive pneumococcal disease is increased

8. Revaccination with PPSV One-time revaccination after 5 years is recommended for persons aged 19 through 64 years with chronic renal failure or nephrotic syndrome; functional or anatomic asplenia (e.g., sickle cell disease or splenectomy); and for persons with immunocompromising conditions. For persons aged 65 years and older, one-time revaccination is recommended if they were vaccinated 5 or more years previously and were aged less than 65 years at the time of primary vaccination.

9. Meningococcal vaccination Meningococcal vaccine should be administered to persons with the following indications:

Medical: A 2-dose series of meningococcal conjugate vaccine is recommended for adults with anatomic or functional asplenia, or persistent complement component deficiencies. Adults with HIV infection who are vaccinated should also receive a routine 2-dose series. The 2 doses should be administered at 0 and 2 months.

Other: A single dose of meningococcal vaccine is recommended for unvaccinated first-year college students living in dormitories; microbiologists routinely exposed to isolates of *Neisseria meningitidis*; military recruits; and persons who travel to or live in countries in which meningococcal disease is hyperendemic or epidemic (e.g., the "meningitis belt" of sub-Saharan Africa during the dry season [December through June]), particularly if their contact with local populations will be prolonged. Vaccination is required by the government of Saudi Arabia for all travelers to Mecca during the annual Hajj.

Meningococcal conjugate vaccine, quadrivalent (MCV4) is preferred for adults with any of the preceding indications who are aged 55 years and younger; meningococcal polysaccharide vaccine (MPSV4) is preferred for adults aged 56 years and older. Revaccination with MCV4 every 5 years is recommended for adults previously vaccinated with MCV4 or MPSV4 who remain at increased risk for infection (e.g., adults with anatomic or functional asplenia, or persistent complement component deficiencies).

10. Hepatitis A vaccination Vaccinate persons with any of the following indications and any person seeking protection from hepatitis A virus (HAV) infection:

Behavioral: Men who have sex with men and persons who use injection drugs.

Occupational: Persons working with HAV-infected primates or with HAV in a research laboratory setting.

Medical: Persons with chronic liver disease and persons who receive clotting factor concentrates.

Other: Persons traveling to or working in countries that have high or intermediate endemicity of hepatitis A (a list of countries is available at *http://wwwn.cdc.gov/travel/contentdiseases.aspx*).

Figure 122-1 (*Continued*)

Unvaccinated persons who anticipate close personal contact (e.g., household or regular babysitting) with an international adoptee during the first 60 days after arrival in the United States from a country with high or intermediate endemicity should be vaccinated. The first dose of the 2-dose hepatitis A vaccine series should be administered as soon as adoption is planned, ideally 2 or more weeks before the arrival of the adoptee.

Single-antigen vaccine formulations should be administered in a 2-dose schedule at either 0 and 6–12 months (Havrix), or 0 and 6–18 months (Vaqta). If the combined hepatitis A and hepatitis B vaccine (Twinrix) is used, administer 3 doses at 0, 1, and 6 months; alternatively, a 4-dose schedule may be used, administered on days 0, 7, and 21–30, followed by a booster dose at month 12.

11. Hepatitis B vaccination Vaccinate persons with any of the following indications and any person seeking protection from hepatitis B virus (HBV) infection:

Behavioral: Sexually active persons who are not in a long-term, mutually monogamous relationship (e.g., persons with more than one sex partner during the previous 6 months); persons seeking evaluation or treatment for a sexually transmitted disease (STD); current or recent injection-drug users; and men who have sex with men.

Occupational: Healthcare personnel and public-safety workers who are exposed to blood or other potentially infectious body fluids.

Medical: Persons with end-stage renal disease, including patients receiving hemodialysis; persons with HIV infection; and persons with chronic liver disease.

Other: Household contacts and sex partners of persons with chronic HBV infection; clients and staff members of institutions for persons with developmental disabilities; and international travelers to countries with high or intermediate prevalence of chronic HBV infection (a list of countries is available at *http://wwwn.cdc.gov/travel/contentdiseases.aspx*).

Hepatitis B vaccination is recommended for all adults in the following settings: STD treatment facilities; HIV testing and treatment facilities; facilities providing drug-abuse treatment and prevention services; healthcare settings targeting services to injection-drug users or men who have sex with men; correctional facilities; end-stage renal disease programs and facilities for chronic hemodialysis patients; and institutions and nonresidential day-care facilities for persons with developmental disabilities.

Administer missing doses to complete a 3-dose series of hepatitis B vaccine to those persons not vaccinated or not completely vaccinated. The second dose should be administered 1 month after the first dose; the third dose should be given at least 2 months after the second dose (and at least 4 months after the first dose). If the combined hepatitis A and hepatitis B vaccine (Twinrix) is used, administer 3 doses at 0, 1, and 6 months; alternatively, a 4-dose Twinrix schedule, administered on days 0, 7, and 21 to 30, followed by a booster dose at month 12 may be used.

Adult patients receiving hemodialysis or with other immunocompromising conditions should receive 1 dose of 40 μg/mL (Recombivax HB) administered on a 3-dose schedule or 2 doses of 20 μg/mL (Engerix-B) administered simultaneously on a 4-dose schedule at 0, 1, 2, and 6 months.

12. Selected conditions for which Haemophilus influenzae type b (Hib) vaccine may be used 1 dose of Hib vaccine should be considered for persons who have sickle cell disease, leukemia, or HIV infection, or who have had a splenectomy, if they have not previously received Hib vaccine.

13. Immunocompromising conditions Inactivated vaccines generally are acceptable (e.g., pneumococcal, meningococcal, influenza [inactivated influenza vaccine]) and live vaccines generally are avoided in persons with immune deficiencies or immunocompromising conditions. Information on specific conditions is available at *http://www.cdc.gov/vaccines/pubs/acip-list.htm*.

---

these schedules. In the time between annual publications, additions and changes to schedules are published as Notices to Readers in *Morbidity and Mortality Weekly Report*.

■ IMMUNIZATION PRACTICE STANDARDS

Administering immunizations to adults involves a number of processes, such as deciding whom to vaccinate, assessing vaccine contraindications and precautions, providing vaccine information statements (VISs), ensuring appropriate storage and handling of vaccines, administering vaccines, and maintaining vaccine records. In addition, provider reporting of adverse events that follow vaccination is an essential component of the vaccine safety monitoring system.

Deciding whom to vaccinate

Every effort should be made to ensure that adults receive all indicated vaccines as expeditiously as possible. When adults present for care, their immunization history should be assessed and recorded, and this information should be used to identify needed vaccinations according to the most current version of the adult immunization schedule. Decision-support tools incorporated into electronic health records can provide prompts for needed vaccinations. Standing orders, which are often used for routinely indicated vaccines (e.g., influenza and pneumococcal vaccines), permit a nurse or another approved licensed practitioner to administer vaccines without a specific physician order, thus lowering barriers to adult immunization.

Assessing contraindications and regulations

Before vaccination, all patients should be screened for contraindications and precautions. A *contraindication* is a condition that is believed to substantially increase the risk of a serious adverse reaction to vaccination. A vaccine should not be administered when a contraindication is documented. For example, a history of an anaphylactic reaction to a dose of vaccine or to a vaccine component is a contraindication for further doses. A *precaution* is a condition that may increase the risk of an adverse event or that may compromise the ability of the vaccine to evoke immunity (e.g., administering measles vaccine to a person who has recently received a blood transfusion and may consequently have transient passive immunity to measles). Normally, a vaccine is not administered when a precaution is noted. However, situations may arise

when the benefits of vaccination outweigh the estimated risk of an adverse event, and the provider may decide to vaccinate the patient despite the precaution.

In some cases, contraindications and precautions are temporary and may lead to mere deferral of vaccination until a later time. For example, moderate or severe febrile illnesses are generally considered transient precautions to vaccination and result in postponement of vaccine administration until the acute phase has resolved; thus the superimposition of adverse effects of vaccination on the underlying illness and the mistaken attribution of a manifestation of the underlying illness to the vaccine are avoided. Contraindications and precautions to vaccines licensed in the United States for use in civilian adults are summarized in Table 122-3. It is important to recognize conditions that are *not* contraindications in order not to miss opportunities for vaccination. For example, in most cases, mild acute illness (with or without low-grade fever), a history of a mild to moderate local reaction to a previous dose of the vaccine, and breast-feeding are not contraindications to vaccination.

History of immediate hypersensitivity to a vaccine component A severe allergic reaction (e.g., anaphylaxis) to a previous dose of a vaccine or to one of its components is a contraindication to vaccination. While most vaccines have many components, substances to which individuals are most likely to have had a severe allergic reaction include egg protein, gelatin, and yeast. In addition, although natural rubber (latex) is not a vaccine component, some vaccines are supplied in vials or syringes that contain natural rubber. These vaccines can be identified by the product insert and should not be administered to persons who report a severe (anaphylactic) allergy to latex. The much more common local or contact hypersensitivity to latex is *not* a contraindication to administration of a vaccine supplied in a vial or syringe that contains latex. Vaccines that, as of April 2009, were sometimes supplied in a vial or syringe containing natural rubber included Havrix hepatitis A vaccine (syringe), Vaqta hepatitis A vaccine (vial and syringe), Engerix-B hepatitis B vaccine (syringe), Recombivax HB hepatitis B vaccine (vial), Boostrix Tdap vaccine (syringe), and Menomune meningococcal polysaccharide vaccine (vial).

Pregnancy Live-virus vaccines are contraindicated during pregnancy because of the possibility that vaccine virus replication will cause congenital infection or have other adverse effects on the fetus. Most live-virus vaccines, including varicella vaccine, are not secreted in breast milk; therefore, breast-feeding is not a contraindication for

TABLE 122-3 Contraindications and Precautions for Commonly Used Vaccines in Adults

Vaccine Formulation	Contraindications and Precautions
All vaccines	**Contraindication** Severe allergic reaction (e.g., anaphylaxis) after a previous vaccine dose or to a vaccine component **Precaution** Moderate or severe acute illness with or without fever; defer vaccination until illness resolves
Td	**Precautions** GBS within 6 weeks after a previous dose of TT-containing vaccine History of Arthus-type hypersensitivity reactions after a previous dose of TT-containing vaccine; defer vaccination until at least 10 years have elapsed since the last dose
Tdap	**Contraindication** History of encephalopathy (e.g., coma or prolonged seizures) not attributable to another identifiable cause within 7 days of administration of a vaccine with pertussis components, such as DTaP or Tdap **Precautions** GBS within 6 weeks after a previous dose of TT-containing vaccine Unstable neurologic condition (e.g., cerebrovascular events and acute encephalopathic conditions) History of Arthus-type hypersensitivity reactions after a previous dose of TT-containing and/or DT-containing vaccine, including MCV4; defer vaccination until at least 10 years have elapsed since the last dose Pregnancy
HPV	**Contraindication** History of immediate hypersensitivity to yeast (for Gardasil) **Precaution** Pregnancy. If a woman is found to be pregnant after initiation of the vaccination series, the remainder of the 3-dose regimen should be delayed until after completion of the pregnancy. If a vaccine dose has been administered during pregnancy, no intervention is needed. A vaccine-in-pregnancy registry has been established for Gardasil; patients and health care providers should report any exposure to quadrivalent HPV vaccine during pregnancy (telephone: 800-986-8999).
MMR	**Contraindications** History of immediate hypersensitivity reaction to gelatin[a] or neomycin Pregnancy Known severe immunodeficiency (e.g., hematologic and solid tumors; chemotherapy; congenital immunodeficiency; long-term immunosuppressive therapy; severe immunocompromise due to HIV infection) **Precaution** Recent (within 11 months) receipt of antibody-containing blood product
Varicella	**Contraindications** Pregnancy Known severe immunodeficiency History of immediate hypersensitivity reaction to gelatin[a] or neomycin **Precaution** Recent (within 11 months) receipt of antibody-containing blood product
Influenza, injectable, trivalent	**Contraindication** History of immediate hypersensitivity reaction to eggs[b] **Precautions** History of GBS within 6 weeks after a previous influenza vaccine dose Pregnancy is *not* a contraindication or precaution. This vaccine is recommended for women who will be pregnant during influenza season.
Influenza, live attenuated	**Contraindications** History of immediate hypersensitivity reaction to eggs[b] Age ≥50 years Pregnancy Immunosuppression, including that caused by medications or by HIV infection; known severe immunodeficiency (e.g., hematologic and solid tumors; chemotherapy; congenital immunodeficiency; long-term immunosuppressive therapy; severe immunocompromise due to HIV infection) Certain chronic medical conditions, such as diabetes mellitus; chronic pulmonary disease (including asthma); chronic cardiovascular disease (except hypertension); renal, hepatic, neurologic/neuromuscular, hematologic, or metabolic disorders Close contact with severely immunosuppressed persons who require a protected environment, such as isolation in a bone marrow transplantation unit Close contact with persons with lesser degrees of immunosuppression (e.g., persons receiving chemotherapy or radiation therapy who are not being cared for in a protective environment; persons with HIV infection) is *not* a contraindication or precaution. **Precaution** History of GBS within 6 weeks of a previous influenza vaccine dose

(continued)

TABLE 122-3 Contraindications and Precautions for Commonly Used Vaccines in Adults (*Continued*)

Vaccine Formulation	Contraindications and Precautions
Pneumococcal polysaccharide	None
Hepatitis A	**Precaution** Pregnancy
Hepatitis B	**Contraindication** History of immediate hypersensitivity to yeast
Meningococcal conjugate	**Contraindications** Age >55 years (licensed for use only among persons 2–55 years of age) History of severe allergic reaction to dry natural rubber (latex) or to DT-containing vaccines **Precautions** History of GBS
Meningococcal polysaccharide	**Contraindication** History of severe allergic reaction to dry natural rubber (latex)
Zoster	**Contraindications** Age <60 years Pregnancy Known severe immunodeficiency History of immediate hypersensitivity reaction to gelatin[a] or neomycin

[a]Extreme caution must be exercised in administering MMR, varicella, or zoster vaccine to persons with a history of an anaphylactic reaction to gelatin or gelatin-containing products. Before administration, skin testing for sensitivity to gelatin can be considered. However, no specific protocols for this purpose have been published.

[b]Protocols have been published for safely administering influenza vaccine to persons with egg allergies. See references 222–224 in Fiore AE et al: MMWR 57:1, 2008.

Abbreviations: DT, diphtheria toxoid; GBS, Guillain-Barré syndrome; HPV, human papillomavirus; MMR, measles, mumps, and rubella; Td, tetanus and diphtheria toxoids; Tdap, tetanus and diphtheria toxoids and acellular pertussis; TT, tetanus toxoid.

live-virus or other vaccines. Pregnancy is not a contraindication to administration of inactivated vaccines, but most are avoided during pregnancy because relevant safety data are limited. The only vaccine routinely recommended for women in the United States who are or will be pregnant during influenza season is trivalent inactivated influenza vaccine. Some other vaccines, such as tetanus and diphtheria toxoid (Td) vaccine and tetanus and diphtheria toxoid and acellular pertussis (Tdap) vaccine, may be given to pregnant women in certain circumstances. Resurgence of pertussis in some areas has prompted greater use of Tdap in pregnancy.

Immunosuppression Live-virus vaccines elicit an immune response due to replication of the attenuated (weakened) vaccine virus that is contained by the recipient's immune system. In persons with compromised immune function, enhanced replication of vaccine viruses is possible and could lead to disseminated infection with the vaccine virus. For this reason, live-virus vaccines are contraindicated for persons with severe immunosuppression, defined according to the specific vaccine on the basis—at least in part—of differences in the prevalence of conditions causing immunosuppression at the time of vaccine recommendation issuance. Severe immunosuppression may be caused by many disease conditions, including HIV infection and hematologic or generalized malignancy. In some of these conditions, all affected persons are severely immunocompromised. In others (e.g., HIV infection), the degree to which the immune system is compromised depends on the severity of the condition, which in turn depends on the stage of disease or treatment. Severe immunosuppression may also be due to therapy with immunosuppressive agents, including high-dose glucocorticoids. In this situation, the dose, duration, and route of administration may influence the degree of immunosuppression.

The definition of severe immunosuppression that is a contraindication to zoster vaccine—the most recently licensed live-virus vaccine for adults—may be used as a guide to conditions that are also contraindications to other live-virus vaccines. Recommendations

state that zoster vaccine should not be administered to persons with primary or acquired immunodeficiency, including the following:

1. Persons with leukemia, lymphomas, or other malignant neoplasms affecting the bone marrow or lymphatic system. However, patients whose leukemia is in remission and who have not received chemotherapy (e.g., alkylating drugs or antimetabolites) or radiation therapy for at least 3 months can receive zoster vaccine.
2. Persons with AIDS or other clinical manifestations of HIV infection, including persons with CD4+ T lymphocyte counts of ≤200/μL or ≤15% of total lymphocytes.
3. Persons receiving immunosuppressive therapy, including high-dose glucocorticoids (≥20 mg of prednisone per day or the equivalent) for ≥2 weeks. Zoster vaccination should be deferred for at least 1 month after discontinuation of such therapy. Short-term glucocorticoid therapy (<14 days); low to moderate glucocorticoid dosage (<20 mg of prednisone per day or the equivalent); topically applied glucocorticoids (e.g., those applied directly to the nose or skin or inhaled); intraarticular, bursal, or tendon glucocorticoid injections; and long-term alternate-day treatment with low to moderate doses of short-acting systemic glucocorticoids are not considered sufficiently immunosuppressive to cause concerns about vaccine safety and should not preclude the administration of zoster vaccine. Low doses of methotrexate (≤0.4 mg/kg per week), azathioprine (≤3.0 mg/kg per day), or 6-mercaptopurine (≤1.5 mg/kg per day) for treatment of rheumatoid arthritis, psoriasis, polymyositis, sarcoidosis, inflammatory bowel disease, and other conditions likewise do not constitute a contraindication.
4. Persons with clinical or laboratory evidence of other unspecified cellular immunodeficiency. However, persons with impaired humoral immunity (e.g., hypogammaglobulinemia or dysgammaglobulinemia) can receive zoster vaccine.
5. Persons undergoing hematopoietic stem cell transplantation. The experience of these patients with varicella-zoster virus–containing vaccines (e.g., zoster vaccine) is limited. Physicians

should assess the immune status of the recipient on a case-by-case basis to determine the relevant risks. If a decision is made to administer zoster vaccine, vaccination should take place no sooner than 24 months after transplantation.

6. Persons receiving recombinant human immune mediators and immune modulators, especially the anti–tumor necrosis factor agents adalimumab, infliximab, and etanercept. The safety and efficacy of zoster vaccine administered concurrently with these agents is unknown. If it is not possible to administer zoster vaccine to patients before initiation of therapy, physicians should assess immune status on a case-by-case basis to determine the relevant risks and benefits. Otherwise, vaccination should be deferred for at least 1 month after discontinuation of such therapy.

■ VACCINE INFORMATION STATEMENTS

A VIS is a one-page (two-sided) information sheet produced by the CDC that informs vaccine recipients (or their parents or legal representatives) about the benefits and risks of a vaccine. VISs are mandated by the National Childhood Vaccine Injury Act (NCVIA) of 1986 and—whether the vaccine recipient is a child or an adult—must be provided for any vaccine covered by the Vaccine Injury Compensation Program. As of June 2009, vaccines that are covered by the NCVIA and that are licensed for use in adults include Td, Tdap, hepatitis A, hepatitis B, HPV, inactivated influenza, live intranasal influenza, measles/mumps/rubella (MMR), meningococcal, polio, and varicella vaccines. When combination vaccines for which no separate VIS exists are given (e.g., hepatitis A and B combination vaccine), all relevant VISs should be provided. VISs also exist for some vaccines not covered by the NCVIA, such as pneumococcal polysaccharide, Japanese encephalitis, rabies, zoster, typhoid, and yellow fever vaccines. The use of these VISs is encouraged but is not mandated.

All current VISs are available on the internet at two websites: the CDC's Vaccines & Immunizations site (www.cdc.gov/vaccines) and the Immunization Action Coalition's site (www.immunize.org/vis/). (The latter site also includes translations of the VISs.) VISs from these sites can be downloaded and printed.

■ STORAGE AND HANDLING

Injectable vaccines are packaged in multidose vials, single-dose vials, or manufacturer-filled single-dose syringes. The live attenuated nasal-spray influenza vaccine is packaged in single-dose sprayers. Oral typhoid vaccine is packaged in capsules. Some vaccines, such as MMR, varicella, zoster, and meningococcal polysaccharide vaccines, come as lyophilized (freeze-dried) powders that must be reconstituted (i.e., mixed with a liquid diluent) before use. The lyophilized powder and the diluent come in separate vials. Diluents are not interchangeable but rather are specifically formulated for each type of vaccine; only the specific diluent provided by the manufacturer for each type of vaccine should be used. Once lyophilized vaccines have been reconstituted, their shelf-life is limited and they must be stored under appropriate temperature and light conditions. For example, varicella and zoster vaccines must be protected from light and administered within 30 minutes of reconstitution; MMR vaccine likewise must be protected from light but can be used up to 8 h after reconstitution. Single-dose vials of meningococcal polysaccharide vaccine must be used within 30 minutes of reconstitution, while multidose vials must be used within 35 days.

Vaccines are stored either at refrigerator temperature (2–8°C) or at freezer temperature (–15°C or colder). In general, inactivated vaccines (e.g., inactivated influenza, pneumococcal polysaccharide, and meningococcal conjugate vaccines) are stored at refrigerator temperature, while vials of lyophilized-powder live-virus vaccines (e.g., varicella, zoster, and MMR vaccines) are stored at freezer temperature. Diluents for lyophilized vaccines may be stored at refrigerator or room temperature. Live attenuated influenza vaccine—a live-virus liquid formulation administered by nasal spray—is stored at refrigerator temperature.

To avoid temperature fluctuations, vaccines should be placed in the body of a refrigerator and not in the door, in vegetable bins, on the floor, next to the wall, or next to the freezer—locations where temperatures may differ significantly. Frequent opening of a refrigerator door to retrieve food items can adversely affect the internal temperature of the unit and damage vaccines; thus food and drink should not be stored in the same refrigerator as vaccines. Frozen vaccines must be stored in the body (not the door) of a freezer that has its own external door separate from the refrigerator. They should not be stored in small "dormitory-style" refrigerators. The temperature of refrigerators and freezers used for vaccine storage must be monitored and the temperature recorded at least twice a day. Ideally, continuous thermometers are used that measure and record temperature all day and all night.

■ ADMINISTRATION OF VACCINES

Parenteral vaccines recommended for routine administration to adults in the United States are given by either the IM or the SC route. Most parenteral vaccines are given to adults by the IM route. Vaccines given by the SC route include live-virus vaccines such as varicella, zoster, and MMR vaccines as well as the inactivated meningococcal polysaccharide vaccine. The 23-valent pneumococcal polysaccharide vaccine may be given by either of these routes, but IM administration is preferred because it is associated with a lower risk of injection-site reactions.

Vaccines given to adults by the SC route are administered with a 5/8-inch needle into the upper outer-triceps area (Fig. 122-2). Vaccines administered to adults by the IM route are injected into the deltoid muscle (Fig. 122-2) with a needle whose length should be selected on the basis of the recipient's sex and weight to ensure adequate penetration into the muscle. Current guidelines indicate that, for men and women weighing <130 lbs (<60 kg), a 5/8-inch needle is sufficient; for women weighing 130–200 lbs (60–90 kg) and men weighing 130–260 lbs (60–118 kg), a 1- to 1.5-inch needle is needed; and for women weighing >200 lbs (>90 kg) and men weighing >260 lbs (>118 kg), a 1.5-inch needle is required.

Aspiration is the process of pulling back on the plunger of the syringe after skin penetration but prior to injection to ensure that the contents of the syringe are not injected into a blood vessel. Although this practice is advocated by some experts, aspiration is not required because of the lack of large blood vessels at the recommended vaccine injection sites.

Multiple vaccines can be administered at the same visit; indeed, administration of all needed vaccines at one visit is encouraged. Studies have shown that vaccines are as effective when administered simultaneously as they are individually, and simultaneous administration of multiple vaccines is not associated with an increased risk of adverse effects. If more than one vaccine must be administered in the same limb, the injection sites should be separated by 1–2 inches so that any local reactions can be differentiated. If a vaccine and an immune globulin preparation are administered simultaneously (e.g., Td vaccine and tetanus immune globulin), a separate anatomic site should be used for each injection.

For certain vaccines (e.g., HPV vaccine and hepatitis B vaccine), multiple doses are required for an adequate and persistent antibody response. The recommended vaccination schedule specifies the interval between doses. Many adults who receive the first dose in a multiple-dose vaccine series do not complete the series or do

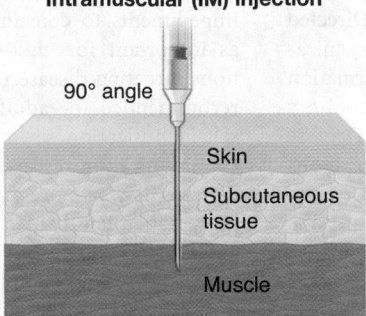

Subcutaneous (SC) injection   **Intramuscular (IM) injection**

45° angle   90° angle

Skin   Skin
Subcutaneous   Subcutaneous
tissue   tissue
Muscle   Muscle

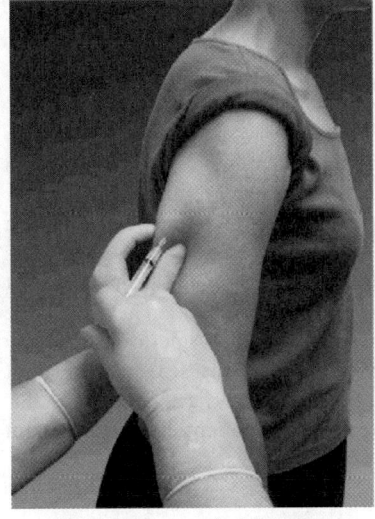
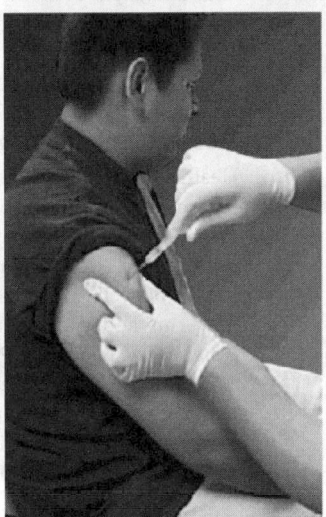

Subcutaneous administration   Intramuscular administration

Figure 122-2 Techniques for SC and IM administration of vaccines to adults. *(Adapted from materials provided by the Immunization Action Coalition; www.immunize.org.)*

not receive subsequent doses within the recommended interval; in these circumstances, vaccine efficacy and/or the duration of protection may be compromised. Providers should implement recall systems that will prompt patients to return for subsequent doses in a vaccination series at the appropriate intervals. With the exception of oral typhoid vaccination, an interruption in the schedule does not require restarting of the entire series or the addition of extra doses.

Syncope may follow vaccination, especially with adolescents and young adults. Serious injuries, including head trauma and motor vehicle accidents, have occurred. Vaccine administration procedures that minimize the impact of postvaccination syncope should be used. To avoid trauma when syncope does occur, patients should be seated during vaccination. The ACIP recommends that vaccine providers strongly consider observing patients for 15 minutes after they are vaccinated. If syncope develops, patients should be observed until the symptoms resolve.

Anaphylaxis is a rare complication of vaccination. All facilities providing immunizations should have an emergency kit containing aqueous epinephrine for administration in the event of a systemic anaphylactic reaction.

■ VACCINE SAFETY MONITORING AND ADVERSE EVENT REPORTING

Prelicensure evaluations of vaccine safety

Before vaccines are licensed by the FDA, they are evaluated in clinical trials with volunteers. These trials are conducted in three progressive phases. Phase 1 trials are small, usually involving fewer than 100 volunteers. Their purposes are to provide a basic evaluation of safety and to identify common adverse events. Phase 2 trials, which are larger and may involve several hundred participants, collect additional information on safety and are usually designed to evaluate immunogenicity as well. Data gained from phase 2 trials can be used to determine the composition of the vaccine, the number of doses required, and a profile of common adverse events. Vaccines that appear promising are evaluated in phase 3 trials, which typically involve several hundred to several thousand volunteers and are generally designed to demonstrate vaccine efficacy and provide additional information on vaccine safety.

Postlicensure monitoring of vaccine safety

After licensure, a vaccine's safety is assessed by several mechanisms. The NCVIA of 1986 requires health care providers to report certain adverse events that follow vaccination of children. As a mechanism for that reporting, the Vaccine Adverse Event Reporting System (VAERS) was established in 1990 and is jointly managed by the CDC and the FDA. This safety surveillance system collects reports of adverse events associated with vaccines currently licensed in the United States. *Adverse events* are defined as health effects that occur after immunization and that may or may not be related to the vaccine. While VAERS was established in response to the NCVIA, any adverse event following vaccination—whether in a child or an adult, and whether or not it is believed to have been caused by vaccination—may be reported through VAERS. In 2008, VAERS received >25,000 reports of adverse events following vaccination. Of those, 9.5% were reportedly serious, causing disability, hospitalization, life-threatening illness, or death.

Anyone can file a VAERS report, including health care providers, manufacturers, and vaccine recipients or their parents or guardians. VAERS reports may be submitted online (*http://vaers.hhs.gov/esub/index*) or by completing a paper form requested online, by phone (800-822-7967), or by fax (877-721-0366). The VAERS form asks for the following information: the type of vaccine received; the timing of vaccination; the time of onset of the adverse event; and the recipient's current illnesses or medications, history of adverse events following vaccination, and demographic characteristics (e.g., age and gender). This information is entered into a database. The individual who reported the adverse event then receives a confirmation letter by mail with a VAERS identification number that can be used if additional information is submitted later. In selected cases of serious adverse reaction, the patient's recovery status may be followed up at 60 days and 1 year after vaccination. The FDA and the CDC have access to VAERS data and use this information to monitor vaccine safety and conduct research studies. VAERS data (minus personal information) are also available to the public.

While the VAERS provides useful information on vaccine safety, this passive reporting system has important limitations. One is that it only collects information about events following vaccination; it does not assess whether a given type of event occurs more often than expected after vaccination. A second is that event reporting is incomplete and is biased toward events that are believed to be more likely to be due to vaccination and that occur relatively soon after vaccination. To obtain more systematic information on adverse events occurring in both vaccinated and unvaccinated persons, the Vaccine Safety Datalink project was initiated in 1991. Directed by the CDC, this project includes eight managed-care organizations in the United States; member databases include information on immunizations, medical conditions, demographics, laboratory results, and medication prescriptions. The Department of Defense oversees a similar system monitoring the safety of immunizations among active-duty military personnel. In addition, postlicensure evaluations of vaccine safety may be conducted by the vaccine manufacturer. In fact, such evaluations are often required by the FDA as a condition of vaccine licensure.

Maintenance of vaccine records

All vaccines administered should be fully documented in the patient's permanent medical record. Documentation should include the date of administration, the name or common abbreviation of the vaccine, the vaccine lot number and manufacturer, the administration site, the VIS edition, the date the VIS was provided, and the name of the person who administered the vaccine.

■ CONSUMER ACCESS TO AND DEMAND FOR IMMUNIZATION

By removing barriers to the consumer or patient, providers and health care institutions can improve vaccine use. Financial barriers have traditionally been important constraints, particularly among uninsured adults. Even for insured adults, out-of-pocket costs associated with newer, more expensive adult vaccines (e.g., zoster vaccine) are an obstacle to be overcome. After influenza vaccine was included by Medicare for all beneficiaries in 1993, coverage among persons ≥65 years of age doubled (from ~30% in 1989 to >60% in 1997; Fig. 122-3). Other strategies that enhance patients' access to vaccination include extended office hours (e.g., evening and weekend hours) and scheduled vaccination-only clinics where waiting times are reduced. Provision of vaccines outside the "medical home" (e.g., through occupational clinics, universities, and retail settings) can expand access for adults who do not make medical visits frequently. Increasing proportions of nonelderly adults are being vaccinated in these settings.

Health promotion efforts aimed at increasing the demand for immunization are common. Direct-to-consumer advertising by pharmaceutical companies has been used for some newer adolescent and adult vaccines. Efforts to raise consumer demand for vaccines have not increased immunization rates unless implemented in conjunction with other strategies that target strengthening of provider practices or reduction of consumer barriers.

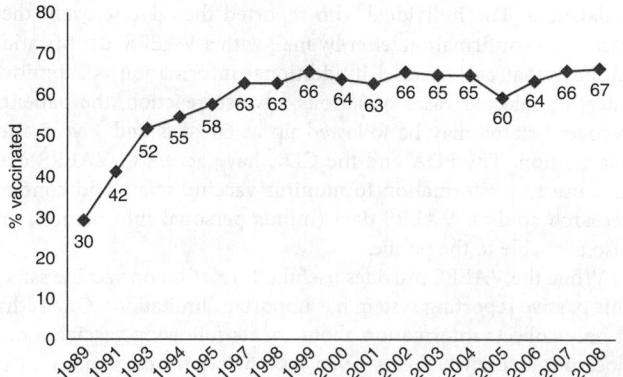

Figure 122-3 Influenza vaccination coverage among adults ≥65 years of age, United States, 1989–2008. *(From http://www.cdc.gov/FLU/PROFESSIONALS/VACCINATION/pdf/NHIS89_08fluvaxtrendtab.pdf.)*

Attitudes and beliefs related to vaccination can be considerable impediments to consumer demand. Many adults view vaccines as important for children but are less familiar with vaccinations targeting disease prevention in adults. Several vaccines are recommended for adults with certain medical risk factors, but self-identification as a high-risk individual is relatively rare. Communication research suggests that many adults with chronic diseases may be more motivated to receive a vaccine by a desire to protect their family members rather than to reduce their own risk. Some vaccines are explicitly recommended for persons at relatively low risk of serious complications, with the goal of reducing the risk of transmission to higher-risk contacts. For example, for parents and caretakers of newborns, vaccinations against influenza and pertussis are recommended.

■ STRATEGIES FOR PROVIDERS AND HEALTH CARE FACILITIES

Recommendation from the provider

Health care providers can have great influence on patients with regard to immunization. A recommendation from a doctor or nurse carries more weight than do recommendations from professional societies or endorsements by celebrities. Providers should be well informed about vaccine risks and benefits so that they can address patients' common concerns. The CDC, the American College of Physicians, and the American Academy of Family Physicians review and update the schedule for adult immunization on an annual basis and also have developed educational materials to facilitate provider–patient discussions about vaccination (*www.cdc.gov/vaccines*).

System supports

Medical offices can incorporate a variety of methods to ensure that providers consistently offer specific immunizations to patients with indications for specific vaccines. Decision-support tools have been incorporated into some electronic health records to alert the provider when specific vaccines are indicated. Manual or automated reminders and standing orders have been discussed (see "Deciding Whom to Vaccinate," above) and have consistently improved vaccination coverage in both office and hospital settings. Most clinicians' estimates of their own performance diverge from objective measurements of their patients' immunization coverage; quantitative assessment and feedback have been shown in pediatric practice to increase immunization performance significantly. Some health plans have instituted incentives for providers with high rates of immunization coverage. Specialty providers, including obstetrician–gynecologists, may be the only providers serving high-risk patients with indications for selected vaccines (e.g., HPV, influenza, or pneumococcal polysaccharide vaccine).

Immunization requirements

Vaccination against selected communicable diseases is required for attendance at many universities and colleges as well as for service in the U.S. military or in some occupational settings (e.g., child care, laboratory, veterinary, and health care). Immunizations are recommended and sometimes required for travel to certain countries (see Chap. 123).

Vaccination of health care staff

A particular area of focus for medical settings is vaccination of health care workers, including those with and without direct patient-care responsibilities. The Joint Commission (which accredits health care organizations), the CDC's Healthcare Infection Control Practices Advisory Committee, and the ACIP all recommend influenza vaccination of all health care personnel; new recommendations focus on requiring documentation of declination for providers that do not accept annual influenza vaccination. Some institutions and jurisdictions have added mandates on influenza vaccination of health care workers and have expanded on earlier requirements related to vaccination or proof of immunity for hepatitis B, measles, mumps, rubella, and varicella.

◼ VACCINATION IN NONMEDICAL SETTINGS

Rates of vaccination in medical offices are highest among young children and adults ≥65 years of age. People in these age groups make more office visits and are more likely to receive care in a consistent "medical home" than older children, adolescents, and nonelderly adults. Vaccination outside the medical home can expand access to those whose health care visits are limited and reduce the burden on busy clinical practices. In some locations, financial constraints related to inventory and storage requirements have led providers to stock few or no vaccines. Outside private office and hospital settings, vaccination may also occur at health department venues, workplaces, retail sites (including pharmacies and supermarkets), and schools or colleges.

When vaccines are given in nonmedical settings, it remains important for standards of immunization practice to be followed. Consumers should be provided with information on how to report adverse events (e.g., via provision of a VIS), and procedures should ensure that documentation of vaccine administration is forwarded to the primary care provider and the state or city public health immunization registry. Detailed documentation may be required for employment, school attendance, and travel. Personalized health records can help consumers keep track of their immunizations, and some occupational health clinics have incorporated automated immunization reports that help employees stay up-to-date with recommended vaccinations.

◼ PERFORMANCE MONITORING

Tracking of immunization coverage at national, state, institution, and practice levels can yield feedback to practitioners and programs and facilitate quality improvement. Healthcare Effectiveness Data and Information Set (HEDIS) measures related to adult immunization facilitate comparison of health plans. The CDC's National Immunization Survey and National Health Interview Survey provide selected information on immunization coverage among adults and track progress toward achievement of Healthy People 2020 targets for coverage among persons ≥65 years of age as well as among younger adults with conditions that increase risk. Influenza and pneumococcal vaccine coverage rates have been higher among persons ≥65 years of age (60–70%) than among high-risk 18- to 64-year-olds. Figures on state-specific immunization coverage with pneumococcal polysaccharide and influenza vaccines (as measured through the CDC's Behavioral Risk Factor Surveillance System) reveal substantial geographic variation in coverage. There are persistent disparities in adult immunization coverage rates between whites and racial and ethnic minorities. In contrast, racial and economic disparities in immunization of young children have been dramatically reduced during the past decade. Much of this progress is attributed to the Vaccines for Children

Program, which since 1994 has entitled uninsured children to receive free vaccines. Approximately 70% of African-American and Hispanic children are eligible for this program.

◼ FUTURE TRENDS

Although most vaccines developed in the twentieth century targeted common acute infectious diseases of childhood, more recently developed vaccines prevent chronic conditions prevalent among adults. Hepatitis B vaccine prevents hepatitis B–related cirrhosis and hepatocellular carcinoma, zoster vaccine prevents shingles and postherpetic neuralgia, and HPV vaccine prevents some types of cervical cancer as well as genital warts and anogenital cancers. New targets of vaccine development and research may further broaden the definition of vaccine-preventable disease. Research is ongoing on vaccines to prevent insulin-dependent diabetes mellitus, nicotine addiction, and Alzheimer's disease. Expanding strategies for vaccine development are incorporating molecular approaches such as DNA, vector, and peptide vaccines. New technologies, such as the use of transdermal and other needle-less routes of administration, are being applied to vaccine delivery.

FURTHER READINGS

BONHOEFFER J et al: Guidelines for collection, analysis, and presentation of vaccine safety data in surveillance systems. Vaccine 27:2289, 2009

CENTERS FOR DISEASE CONTROL AND PREVENTION: Progress toward interruption of wild poliovirus transmission worldwide, 2009. MMWR 59:545, 2010

PICKERING LK et al: Immunization programs for infants, children, adolescents, and adults: Clinical practice guidelines by the Infectious Diseases Society of America. Clin Infect Dis 49:817, 2009

PLOTKIN S et al (eds): Vaccines, 5th ed. Philadelphia, Saunders Elsevier, 2008

POLAND GA et al: Standards for adult immunization practices. Am J Prev Med 25:144, 2003

ROUSH SW et al: Historical comparisons of morbidity and mortality for vaccine-preventable diseases in the United States. JAMA 298:2155, 2007

SCHUCHAT A, BELL B: Monitoring the impact of vaccines postlicensure: New challenges, new opportunities. Expert Rev Vaccines 7:437, 2008

SMITH JC et al: Immunization policy development in the United States: The role of the Advisory Committee on Immunization Practices. Ann Intern Med 150:45, 2009

WHARTON M: Vaccine safety: Current systems and recent findings. Curr Opin Pediatr 22:88, 2010

WILLIS BC et al: Improving influenza, pneumococcal polysaccharide, and hepatitis B vaccination coverage among adults aged <65 years at high risk: A report on recommendations of the Task Force on Community Preventive Services. MMWR 54:1, 2005

CHAPTER 123

Health Recommendations for International Travel

Jay S. Keystone
Phyllis E. Kozarsky

According to the World Tourism Organization, international tourist arrivals grew exponentially from 25 million in 1950 to >900 million in 2008. Not only are more people traveling; travelers are seeking more exotic and remote destinations. Travel from industrialized to developing regions has been increasing, with Asia and the Pacific, Africa, and the Middle East now emerging destinations. Figure 123-1 summarizes the monthly incidence of health problems during travel in developing countries. Studies show that 50–75% of short-term travelers to the tropics or subtropics report some health impairment. Most of these health problems are minor: only 5% require medical attention, and <1% require hospitalization. Although infectious agents contribute substantially to morbidity among travelers, these pathogens account for only ~1% of deaths in this population. Cardiovascular disease and injuries are the most frequent causes of death among travelers from the United States, accounting for 49% and 22% of deaths, respectively. Age-specific rates of death due to cardiovascular disease are similar among travelers and nontravelers. In contrast, rates of death due to injury (the majority from motor vehicle, drowning, or aircraft accidents) are several times higher among travelers. If one excludes mortality due to cardiovascular disease and preexisting illness, motor vehicle accidents account for >40% of the remaining deaths.

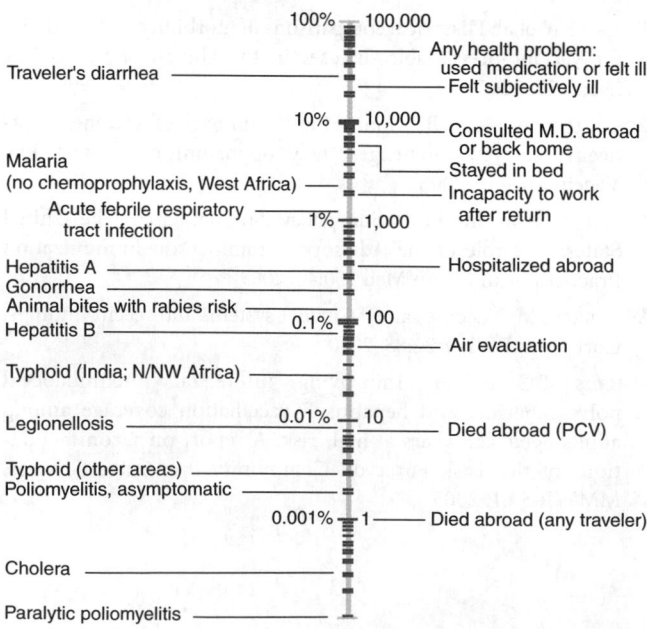

Figure 123-1 Incidence rate, per month, of health problems during a stay in developing countries. PCV, Peace Corps volunteer. *(From Steffen R, Lobel HO: Epidemiologic basis for the practice of travel medicine. J Wilderness Med 5:56, 1994. Reprinted with permission from Chapman and Hall, New York.)*

GENERAL ADVICE

Health maintenance recommendations are based not only on the traveler's destination but also on assessment of risk, which is determined by such variables as health status, specific itinerary, purpose of travel, season, and lifestyle during travel. Detailed information regarding country-specific risks and recommendations may be obtained from the Centers for Disease Control and Prevention (CDC) publication *Health Information for International Travel* (available at *wwwnc.cdc.gov/travel/*).

Fitness for travel is an issue of growing concern in view of the increased numbers of elderly and chronically ill individuals journeying to exotic destinations (see "Travel and Special Hosts," below). Since most commercial aircraft are pressurized to 2500 m (8000 ft) above sea level (corresponding to a Pa_{O_2} of ~55 mmHg), individuals with serious cardiopulmonary problems or anemia should be evaluated before travel. In addition, those who have recently had surgery, a myocardial infarction, a cerebrovascular accident, or a deep vein thrombosis may be at high risk for adverse events during flight. A summary of current recommendations regarding fitness to fly has been published by the Aerospace Medical Association Air Transport Medicine Committee (*www.asma.org/publications/*). A pretravel health assessment may be advisable for individuals considering particularly adventurous recreational activities, such as mountain climbing and scuba diving.

■ IMMUNIZATIONS FOR TRAVEL

Immunizations for travel fall into three broad categories: *routine* (childhood/adult boosters that are necessary regardless of travel), *required* (immunizations that are mandated by international regulations for entry into certain areas or for border crossings), and *recommended* (immunizations that are desirable because of travel-related risks). Required and recommended vaccines commonly given to travelers are listed in Table 123-1.

Routine immunizations

Diphtheria, tetanus, and polio Diphtheria (Chap. 138) continues to be a problem worldwide. Large outbreaks have occurred in countries that have reduced their public vaccination programs. Serologic surveys show that tetanus (Chap. 140) antitoxin is lacking in many North Americans, especially in women over the age of 50. The risk of polio (Chap. 191) to the international traveler is extremely low, and wild-type poliovirus has been eradicated from the Western Hemisphere and Europe. However, studies in the United States suggest that 12% of adult travelers are unprotected against at least one poliovirus serogroup. Foreign travel offers an ideal opportunity to have these immunizations updated. With the recent increase in pertussis among adults, the diphtheria–tetanus–acellular pertussis (Tdap) combination is now recommended for adults as a once-only replacement for the 10-year Td booster.

Measles Measles (rubeola) continues to be a major cause of morbidity and death in the developing world (Chap. 192). Several outbreaks of measles in the United States have been linked to imported cases. The group at highest risk consists of persons born after 1956 and vaccinated before 1980, in many of whom primary vaccination failed.

Influenza Influenza—possibly the most common vaccine-preventable infection in travelers—occurs year-round in the tropics and during the summer months in the Southern Hemisphere (coinciding with the winter months in the Northern Hemisphere). One prospective study showed that influenza developed in 1% of travelers to Southeast Asia per month of stay. Vaccination should

TABLE 123-1 Vaccines Commonly Used for Travel

Vaccine	Primary Series	Booster Interval
Cholera, live oral (CVD 103 - HgR)	1 dose	6 months
Hepatitis A (Havrix), 1440 enzyme immunoassay U/mL	2 doses, 6–12 months apart, IM	None required
Hepatitis A (VAQTA, AVAXIM, EPAXAL)	2 doses, 6–12 months apart, IM	None required
Hepatitis A/B combined (Twinrix)	3 doses at 0, 1, and 6–12 months *or* 0, 7, and 21 days plus booster at 1 year, IM	None required *except* 12 months (once only, for accelerated schedule)
Hepatitis B (Engerix B): accelerated schedule	3 doses at 0, 1, and 2 months *or* 0, 7, and 21 days plus booster at 1 year, IM	12 months, once only
Hepatitis B (Engerix B or Recombivax): standard schedule	3 doses at 0, 1, and 6 months, IM	None required
Immune globulin (hepatitis A prevention)	1 dose IM	Intervals of 3–5 months, depending on initial dose
Japanese encephalitis (JE-VAX)	3 doses, 1 week apart, SC	12–18 months (first booster), then 4 years
Japanese encephalitis (Ixiaro)	2 doses, 1 month apart, SC	Optimal booster schedule not yet determined
Meningococcus, quadrivalent [Menimmune (polysaccharide), Menactra, Menveo (conjugate)]	1 dose SC	>3 years (optimal booster schedule not yet determined)
Rabies (HDCV), rabies vaccine absorbed (RVA), or purified chick embryo cell vaccine (PCEC)	3 doses at 0, 7, and 21 or 28 days, IM	None required except with exposure
Typhoid Ty21a, oral live attenuated (Vivotif)	1 capsule every other day × 4 doses	5 years
Typhoid Vi capsular polysaccharide, injectable (Typhim Vi)	1 dose IM	2 years
Yellow fever	1 dose SC	10 years

be considered for all travelers to these regions, particularly those who are elderly or chronically ill. Travel-related influenza continues to occur during summer months in Alaska and the Northwest Territories of Canada among cruise-ship passengers and staff (Chap. 187). The speed of global spread of the pandemic H1N1 virus once again illustrates why influenza immunization is so important for travelers.

Pneumococcal infection Regardless of travel, pneumococcal vaccine should be administered routinely to the elderly and to persons at high risk of serious infection, including those with chronic heart, lung, or kidney disease and those who have been splenectomized or have sickle cell disease (Chap. 134).

Required immunizations

Yellow fever Documentation of vaccination against yellow fever (Chap. 196) may be required as a condition of entry into or passage through countries of sub-Saharan Africa and equatorial South America, where the disease is endemic or epidemic, or for entry into countries at risk of having the infection introduced. This vaccine is given only by state-authorized yellow fever centers, and its administration must be documented on an official International Certificate of Vaccination. A registry of U.S. clinics that provide the vaccine is available from the CDC (*wwwnc.cdc.gov/travel/*). Recent data suggest that fewer than 50% of travelers entering areas endemic for yellow fever are immunized. Severe adverse events associated with this vaccine have recently increased in incidence. First-time vaccine recipients may present with a syndrome characterized as either neurotropic (1 case per 125,000 doses) or viscerotropic (1 case per 250,000 doses; among persons 60–69 years of age, 1 case per 100,000 doses; and among persons ≥70 years of age, 1 case per 40,000 doses). Immunosuppression and thymic disease increase the risk of these adverse events (*www.cdc.gov/vaccines/pubs/vis/downloads/vis-yf.pdf*).

Meningococcal meningitis Protection against meningitis (using one of the quadrivalent vaccines) is required for entry into Saudi Arabia during the Hajj (Chap. 143).

Influenza Both seasonal and pandemic H1N1 vaccines (the latter, where available) were required for entry into Saudi Arabia during the Hajj in 2009.

Recommended immunizations

Hepatitis A and B Hepatitis A (Chap. 304) is one of the most common vaccine-preventable infections of travelers. The risk is six times greater for travelers who stray from the usual tourist routes. The mortality rate for hepatitis A increases with age, reaching almost 3% among individuals over age 50. Of the four hepatitis A vaccines currently available in North America (two in the United States), all are interchangeable and have an efficacy rate of >95%.

Long-stay overseas workers appear to be at considerable risk for hepatitis B infection (Chap. 304). The recommendation that all travelers be immunized against hepatitis B before departure is supported by two studies showing that 17% of the assessed travelers who received health care abroad had some type of injection; according to the World Health Organization, nonsterile equipment is used for up to 75% of all injections given in the developing world. A 3-week accelerated schedule of the combined hepatitis A and B vaccine has been approved in the United States. Virtually all travelers to less developed countries should be immunized against hepatitis A and B.

Typhoid fever The attack rate for typhoid fever (Chap. 153) is 1 case per 30,000 travelers per month of travel to the developing world. However, the attack rates in India, Senegal, and North Africa are tenfold higher and are especially high among travelers to relatively remote destinations and among VFRs (immigrants and their families returning to their homelands to visit friends or relatives). Between 1999 and 2006 in the United States, 66% of imported cases involved the latter group. Both of the available vaccines—one oral (live) and the other injectable (polysaccharide)—have efficacy rates of ~70%. In some countries, a combined hepatitis A/typhoid vaccine is available.

Meningococcal meningitis Although the risk of meningococcal disease among travelers has not been quantified, it is likely to be higher among travelers who live with poor indigenous populations in overcrowded conditions (Chap. 143). Because of its enhanced ability to prevent nasal carriage (compared with the older polysaccharide vaccine), a quadrivalent conjugate vaccine is the product of choice for immunization of persons traveling to sub-Saharan Africa during the dry season or to areas of the world where there are epidemics. The vaccine, which protects against serogroups A, C, Y, and W-135, has an efficacy rate of >90%.

Japanese encephalitis The risk of Japanese encephalitis (Chap. 196), an infection transmitted by mosquitoes in rural Asia and Southeast Asia, is ~1 case per 5000 travelers per month of stay in an endemic area. Most symptomatic infections among U.S. residents have involved military personnel or their families. The vaccine efficacy rate is >90%. The vaccine is recommended for persons staying >1 month in rural endemic areas or for shorter periods if their activities (e.g., camping, bicycling, hiking) in these areas will increase exposure risk. A new Vero cell vaccine is now available in the United States.

Cholera The risk of cholera (Chap. 156) is extremely low, with ~1 case per 500,000 journeys to endemic areas. Cholera vaccine, no longer available in the United States, was rarely recommended but was considered for aid and health care workers in refugee camps or in disaster-stricken/war-torn areas. A more effective oral cholera vaccine is available in other countries.

Rabies Domestic animals, primarily dogs, are the major transmitters of rabies in developing countries (Chap. 195). Several studies have shown that the risk of rabies posed by a dog bite in an endemic area translates into 1–3.6 cases per 1000 travelers per month of stay. Countries where canine rabies is highly endemic include Mexico, the Philippines, Sri Lanka, India, Thailand, and Vietnam. The three vaccines available in the United States provide >90% protection. Rabies vaccine is recommended for long-stay travelers, particularly children, and persons who may be occupationally exposed to rabies in endemic areas; however, in a large-scale study, almost 50% of potential exposures occurred within the first month of travel. Even after receipt of a preexposure rabies vaccine series, two postexposure doses are required. Travelers who have had the preexposure series do not require rabies immune globulin (which is often unavailable in developing countries) if they are exposed to the disease.

PREVENTION OF MALARIA AND OTHER INSECT-BORNE DISEASES

It is estimated that more than 30,000 American and European travelers develop malaria each year (Chap. 210). The risk to travelers is highest in Oceania and sub-Saharan Africa (estimated at 1:5 and 1:50 per month of stay, respectively, among persons not using chemoprophylaxis); intermediate in malarious areas on the Indian subcontinent and in Southeast Asia (1:250–1:1000 per month); and low in South and Central America (1:2500–1:10,000 per month). Of the more than 1000 cases of malaria reported annually in the United States, 90% of those due to *Plasmodium falciparum* occur in travelers returning or immigrating from Africa and Oceania. VFRs are at the highest risk of acquiring malaria. With the worldwide increase in chloroquine- and multidrug-resistant falciparum malaria, decisions about chemoprophylaxis have become more difficult. In addition, the spread of malaria due to primaquine- and chloroquine-resistant strains of *Plasmodium vivax* has added to the complexity of treatment, as has the recently described "monkey

malaria" of humans, which is caused by *P. knowlesi*. The case-fatality rate of falciparum malaria in the United States is 4%; however, *in only one-third of patients who die is the diagnosis of malaria considered before death.*

Several studies indicate that fewer than 50% of travelers adhere to basic recommendations for malaria prevention. Keys to the prevention of malaria include both personal protection measures against mosquito bites (especially between dusk and dawn) and malaria chemoprophylaxis. The former measures include the use of DEET-containing insect repellents, permethrin-impregnated bednets and clothing, screened sleeping accommodations, and protective clothing. Thus, in regions where infections such as malaria are transmitted, DEET products (25–50%) are recommended, even for children and infants at birth. Studies suggest that concentrations of DEET above ~50% do not offer a marked increase in protection time against mosquitoes. The CDC also recommends picaridin (icaridin), oil of lemon eucalyptus (PMD, para-menthane-3,8-diol), and IR3535 (ethyl butylacetylaminopropionate). In general, higher concentrations of active ingredient provide longer duration of protection, regardless of the active ingredient. Personal protection measures also help prevent other insect-transmitted illnesses, such as dengue fever (Chap. 196). Over the past decade, the incidence of dengue has increased, particularly in the Caribbean region, Latin America, and Southeast Asia. Both dengue and chikungunya viruses are transmitted by an urban-dwelling mosquito that bites primarily at dawn and dusk.

Table 123-2 lists the currently recommended drugs of choice for prophylaxis of malaria, by destination.

PREVENTION OF GASTROINTESTINAL ILLNESS

Diarrhea, the leading cause of illness in travelers (Chap. 128), is usually a short-lived, self-limited condition; however, 40% of affected individuals need to alter their scheduled activities, and another 20% are confined to bed. The most important determinant of risk is the destination. Incidence rates per 2-week stay have been reported to be as low as 8% in industrialized countries and as high as 55% in parts of

TABLE 123-2 Malaria Chemosuppressive Regimens, According to Geographic Area[a]

Geographic Area	Drug of Choice	Alternatives
Central America (north of Panama), Iraq, Turkey, northern Argentina, and Paraguay	Chloroquine	Atovaquone-proguanil[b] Doxycycline Mefloquine Primaquine (except Honduras)
South America, including Haiti, Dominican Republic, and Panama but not northern Argentina or Paraguay; Asia, including Southeast Asia; Africa; and Oceania	Doxycycline Atovaquone-proguanil Mefloquine	
Thai-Myanmar and Thai-Cambodian borders and central Vietnam	Atovaquone-proguanil Doxycycline	

[a]See CDC's *Health Information for International Travel 2010.*

[b]Malarone.

Note: See also Chap. 210.

Africa, Central and South America, and Southeast Asia. Infants and young adults are at particularly high risk. Recent reviews suggested that there is little correlation between dietary indiscretions and the occurrence of travelers' diarrhea. Earlier studies of U.S. students in Mexico showed that eating meals in restaurants and cafeterias or consuming food from street vendors was associated with increased risk.

Etiology

(See also Table 128-3) The most frequently identified pathogens causing travelers' diarrhea are toxigenic *Escherichia coli* and enteroaggregative *E. coli* (Chap. 149), although in some parts of the world (notably northern Africa and Southeast Asia) *Campylobacter* infections (Chap. 155) appear to predominate. Other common causative organisms include *Salmonella* (Chap. 153), *Shigella* (Chap. 154), rotavirus (Chap. 190), and norovirus (Chap. 190). The latter virus has caused numerous outbreaks on cruise ships. Except for giardiasis (Chap. 215), parasitic infections are uncommon causes of travelers' diarrhea. A growing problem for travelers is the development of antibiotic resistance among many bacterial pathogens. Examples include strains of *Campylobacter* resistant to quinolones and strains of *E. coli*, *Shigella*, and *Salmonella* resistant to trimethoprim-sulfamethoxazole.

Precautions

General food and water precautions include eating foods piping hot; avoiding foods that are raw, poorly cooked, or sold by street vendors; and drinking only boiled or commercially bottled beverages, particularly those that are carbonated. Heating kills diarrhea-causing organisms, whereas freezing does not; therefore, ice cubes made from unpurified water should be avoided. In spite of these recommendations, the literature has repeatedly documented dietary indiscretions by 98% of travelers within the first 72 h after arrival at their destination. The maxim "Boil it, cook it, peel it, or forget it!" is easy to remember but apparently difficult to follow.

Self-treatment

(See also Table 128-5) As travelers' diarrhea often occurs despite rigorous food and water precautions, travelers should carry medications for self-treatment. An antibiotic is useful in reducing the frequency of bowel movements and duration of illness in moderate to severe diarrhea. The standard regimen is a 3-day course of a quinolone taken twice daily (or, in the case of some newer formulations, once daily). However, studies have shown that a single double dose of a quinolone may be equally effective. For diarrhea acquired in areas such as Thailand, where >90% of *Campylobacter* infections are quinolone resistant, azithromycin may be a better alternative. Rifaximin, a poorly absorbed rifampin derivative, is highly effective against noninvasive bacterial pathogens such as toxigenic and enteroaggregative *E. coli*. The current approach to self-treatment of travelers' diarrhea is for the traveler to carry three once-daily doses of an antibiotic and to use as many doses as necessary to resolve the illness. If neither high fever nor blood in the stool accompanies the diarrhea, loperamide should be taken in combination with the antibiotic; studies have shown that this combination is more effective than an antibiotic alone.

Prophylaxis

Prophylaxis of travelers' diarrhea with bismuth subsalicylate is widely used but only ~60% effective. For certain individuals (e.g., athletes, persons with a repeated history of travelers' diarrhea, and persons with chronic diseases), a single daily dose of a quinolone, azithromycin, or rifaximin during travel of <1 month's duration is 75–90% efficacious in preventing travelers' diarrhea. Probiotics have been only ~20% effective as prophylaxis. In Europe and

Canada, an oral subunit cholera vaccine that cross-protects against enterotoxigenic *E. coli* has been shown to provide 30–50% protection against travelers' diarrhea.

Illness after return

Although extremely common, acute travelers' diarrhea is usually self-limited or amenable to antibiotic therapy. Persistent bowel problems after the traveler returns home have a less well-defined etiology and may require medical attention from a specialist. Infectious agents (e.g., *Giardia lamblia*, *Cyclospora cayetanensis*, *Entamoeba histolytica*) appear to be responsible for only a small proportion of cases with persistent bowel symptoms. By far the most common causes of persistent diarrhea after travel are postinfectious sequelae such as lactose intolerance or irritable bowel syndrome. A meta-analysis showed that postinfectious irritable bowel syndrome lasting months to years may occur in as many as 4–13% of cases. When no infectious etiology can be identified, a trial of metronidazole therapy for presumed giardiasis, a strict lactose-free diet for 1 week, or a several-week trial of high-dose hydrophilic mucilloid (plus an osmotic laxative such as lactulose or PEG 3350 for persons with alternating diarrhea and constipation) relieves the symptoms of many patients.

■ PREVENTION OF OTHER TRAVEL-RELATED PROBLEMS

Travelers are at high risk for *sexually transmitted diseases* (Chap. 130). Surveys have shown that large numbers engage in casual sex, and there is a reluctance to use condoms consistently. An increasing number of travelers are being diagnosed with *schistosomiasis* (Chap. 219). Travelers should be cautioned to avoid bathing, swimming, or wading in freshwater lakes, streams, or rivers in parts of northeastern South America, the Caribbean, Africa, and Southeast Asia. Prevention of *travel-associated injury* depends mostly on common-sense precautions. Riding on motorcycles (especially without helmets) and in overcrowded public vehicles is not recommended; in developing countries, individuals should not travel by road in rural areas after dark. In addition to its association with motor vehicle accidents, excessive alcohol use has been a significant factor in drownings, assaults, and injuries. Travelers are cautioned to avoid walking barefoot because of the risk of hookworm and *Strongyloides* infections (Chap. 217) and snakebites (Chap. 396).

■ THE TRAVELER'S MEDICAL KIT

A traveler's medical kit is strongly advisable. The contents may vary widely, depending on the itinerary, duration of stay, style of travel, and local medical facilities. While many medications are available abroad (often over the counter), directions for their use may be nonexistent or in a foreign language, or a product may be outdated or counterfeit. For example, a multicountry study in Southeast Asia showed that a mean of 53% (range, 21–92%) of antimalarial products were counterfeit or contained inadequate amounts of active drug. In the medical kit, the short-term traveler should consider carrying an analgesic; an antidiarrheal agent and an antibiotic for self-treatment of travelers' diarrhea; antihistamines; a laxative; oral rehydration salts; a sunscreen with a skin-protection factor of at least 30; a DEET-containing or equivalent insect repellent for the skin; an insecticide for clothing (permethrin); and, if necessary, an antimalarial drug. To these medications, the long-stay traveler might add a broad-spectrum general-purpose antibiotic (levofloxacin or azithromycin), an antibacterial eye and skin ointment, and a topical antifungal cream. Regardless of the duration of travel, a first-aid kit containing such items as scissors, tweezers, and bandages should be considered. A practical approach to self-treatment of infections in the long-stay traveler who carries a once-daily dose of antibiotics (e.g., levofloxacin) is to use 3 tablets "below the waist" (bowel and bladder infections) and 6 tablets "above the waist" (skin and respiratory infections).

TRAVEL AND SPECIAL HOSTS

■ PREGNANCY AND TRAVEL

(See also Chap. 7) A woman's medical history and itinerary, the quality of medical care at her destinations, and her degree of flexibility determine whether travel is wise during pregnancy. According to the American College of Obstetrics and Gynecology, the safest part of pregnancy in which to travel is between 18 and 24 weeks, when there is the least danger of spontaneous abortion or premature labor. Some obstetricians prefer that women stay within a few hundred miles of home after the 28th week of pregnancy in case problems arise. In general, however, healthy women may be advised that it is acceptable to travel.

Relative contraindications to international travel during pregnancy include a history of miscarriage, premature labor, incompetent cervix, or toxemia. General medical problems such as diabetes, heart failure, severe anemia, or a history of thromboembolic disease should also prompt the pregnant woman to postpone her travels. Finally, regions in which the pregnant woman and her fetus may be at excessive risk (e.g., those at high altitudes, those where live-virus vaccines are required, and those where multidrug-resistant malaria is endemic) are not ideal destinations during any trimester.

Malaria

Malaria during pregnancy carries a significant risk of morbidity and death. Levels of parasitemia are highest and failure to clear the parasites after treatment is most frequent among primigravidae. Severe disease, with complications such as cerebral malaria, massive hemolysis, and renal failure, is especially likely in pregnancy. Fetal sequelae include spontaneous abortion, stillbirth, preterm delivery, and congenital infection.

Enteric infections

Pregnant travelers must be extremely cautious regarding their food and beverage intake. Dehydration due to travelers' diarrhea can lead to inadequate placental blood flow. Infections such as toxoplasmosis, hepatitis E, and listeriosis can also cause serious sequelae in pregnancy.

The mainstay of therapy for travelers' diarrhea is rehydration. Loperamide may be used if necessary. For self-treatment, azithromycin may be the best option. Although quinolones are increasingly being used safely during pregnancy and rifaximin is poorly absorbed from the gastrointestinal tract, these drugs are not approved for this indication.

Because of the serious problems encountered when infants are given local foods and beverages, women are strongly encouraged to breast-feed when traveling with a neonate. A nursing mother with travelers' diarrhea should not stop breast-feeding but should increase her fluid intake.

Air travel and high-altitude destinations

Commercial air travel is not a risk to the healthy pregnant woman or to the fetus. The higher radiation levels reported at altitudes of >10,500 m (>35,000 ft) should pose no problem for the healthy pregnant traveler. Since each airline has a policy regarding pregnancy and flying, it is best to check with the specific carrier when booking reservations. Domestic air travel is usually permitted until the 36th week, whereas international air travel is generally curtailed after the 32nd week.

There are no known risks for pregnant women who travel to high-altitude destinations and stay for short periods. However, there are likewise no data on the safety of pregnant women at altitudes of >4500 m (15,000 ft).

■ THE HIV-INFECTED TRAVELER

(See also Chap. 189) The HIV-infected traveler is at special risk of serious infections due to a number of pathogens that may be more prevalent at travel destinations than at home. However, the degree of risk depends primarily on the state of the immune system at the time of travel. For persons whose CD4+ T cell counts are normal or >500/μL, data suggest no greater risk during travel than for persons without HIV infection. Individuals with AIDS (CD4+ T cell counts of <200/μL) and others who are symptomatic need special counseling and should visit a travel medicine practitioner before departure, especially when traveling to the developing world.

Several countries now routinely deny entry to HIV-positive individuals for prolonged stay, even though these restrictions do not appear to decrease rates of transmission of the virus. In general, HIV testing is required for individuals who wish to stay abroad >3 months or who intend to work or study abroad. Some countries will accept an HIV serologic test done within 6 months of departure, whereas others will not accept a blood test done at any time in the traveler's home country. Border officials often have the authority to make inquiries of individuals entering a country and to check the medications they are carrying. If antiretroviral drugs are identified, the person may be barred from entering the country. Information on testing requirements for specific countries is available from consular offices but is subject to frequent change.

Immunizations

All of the HIV-infected traveler's routine immunizations should be up to date (Chap. 122). The response to immunization may be impaired at CD4+ T cell counts of <200/μL and in some cases at even higher counts. Thus HIV-infected persons should be vaccinated as early as possible to ensure adequate immune responses to all vaccines. For patients receiving antiretroviral therapy, at least 3 months must elapse before regenerated CD4+ T cells can be considered fully functional; therefore, vaccination of these patients should be delayed. However, when the risk of illness is high or the sequelae of illness are serious, immunization is recommended. In certain circumstances, it may be prudent to check the adequacy of the serum antibody response before departure.

Because of the increased risk of infections due to *Streptococcus pneumoniae* and other bacterial pathogens that cause pneumonia following influenza, pneumococcal polysaccharide and influenza vaccines should be administered. The estimated rates of response to influenza vaccine are >80% among persons with asymptomatic HIV infection and <50% among those with AIDS.

In general, live attenuated vaccines are contraindicated for persons with immune dysfunction. Because measles (rubeola) can be a severe or lethal infection in HIV-positive patients, these patients should receive the measles vaccine (or the combination measles-mumps-rubella vaccine) unless the CD4+ T cell count is <200/μL. Between 18% and 58% of symptomatic HIV-infected vaccinees develop adequate antibody titers, and 50–100% of asymptomatic HIV-infected persons seroconvert.

It is recommended that the live yellow fever vaccine not be given to HIV-infected travelers. Although the potential adverse effects of a live vaccine in an HIV-infected individual are always a consideration, there appear to have been no reported cases of illness in those who have inadvertently received this vaccine. Nonetheless, if the CD4+ T cell count is <200/μL, an alternative itinerary that poses no risk of exposure to yellow fever is recommended. If the traveler is passing through or traveling to an area where the vaccine is required but the disease risk is low, a physician's waiver should be issued.

A transient increase in HIV viremia (lasting days to weeks) has been demonstrated in HIV-infected individuals following immunization against influenza, pneumococcal infection, and tetanus (Chap. 189). However, there is no evidence at this point that this transient increase is detrimental.

Gastrointestinal illness

Decreased levels of gastric acid, abnormal gastrointestinal mucosal immunity, other complications of HIV infection, and medications taken by HIV-infected patients make travelers' diarrhea especially problematic in these individuals. Travelers' diarrhea is likely to occur more frequently, be more severe, be accompanied by bacteremia, and be more difficult to treat. *Cryptosporidium*, *Isospora belli*, and *Microsporidium* infections, although uncommon, are associated with increased morbidity and mortality rates in AIDS patients.

The HIV-infected traveler must be careful to consume only appropriately prepared foods and beverages and may benefit from antibiotic prophylaxis for travelers' diarrhea. Sulfonamides (as used to prevent pneumocystosis) are ineffective because of widespread resistance.

Other travel-related infections

Data are lacking on the severity of many vector-borne diseases in HIV-infected individuals. Malaria is especially severe in asplenic persons and in those with AIDS. The HIV load doubles during malaria, with subsidence in ~8–9 weeks; the significance of this increase in viral load is unknown.

Visceral leishmaniasis (Chap. 212) has been reported in numerous HIV-infected travelers. Diagnosis may be difficult, given that splenomegaly and hyperglobulinemia are often lacking and serologic results are frequently negative. Sandfly bites may be prevented by evening use of insect repellents.

Certain respiratory illnesses, such as histoplasmosis and coccidioidomycosis, cause greater morbidity and mortality among patients with AIDS. Although tuberculosis is common among HIV-infected persons (especially in developing countries), its acquisition by the short-term HIV-infected traveler has not been reported as a major problem. From a prospective study, it is estimated that for nonmedical travelers the risk of tuberculosis infection is ~3% per year of travel.

Medications

Adverse events due to medications and drug interactions are common and raise complex issues for HIV-infected persons. Rates of cutaneous reaction (e.g., increased cutaneous sensitivity to sulfonamides) are unusually high among patients with AIDS. Since zidovudine is metabolized by hepatic glucuronidation, inhibitors of this process may elevate serum levels of the drug. Concomitant administration of the antimalarial drug mefloquine and the antiretroviral agent ritonavir may result in decreased plasma levels of ritonavir. In contrast, no significant influence of concomitant mefloquine administration on plasma levels of indinavir or nelfinavir was detected in two HIV-infected travelers. There is a strong theoretical concern that the antimalarial drugs lumefantrine (combined with artemisinin in Coartem) and halofantrine may interact with HIV protease inhibitors and nonnucleoside reverse transcriptase inhibitors since the latter are known to be potent inhibitors of cytochrome P450.

■ CHRONIC ILLNESS, DISABILITY, AND TRAVEL

Chronic health problems need not prevent travel, but special measures can make the journey safer and more comfortable.

Heart disease

Cardiovascular events are the main cause of deaths among travelers and of in-flight emergencies on commercial aircraft. Extra supplies of all medications should be kept in carry-on luggage, along with a copy of a recent electrocardiogram and the name and telephone number of the traveler's physician at home. Pacemakers are not affected by airport security devices, although electronic telephone checks of pacemaker function cannot be transmitted by international satellites. Travelers with electronic defibrillators should carry a note to that effect and ask for hand screening. A traveler may benefit from supplemental oxygen; since oxygen delivery systems are not standard, supplementary oxygen should be ordered by the traveler's physician well before flight time. Travelers may benefit from aisle seating and should walk, perform stretching and flexing exercises, consider wearing support hose, and remain hydrated during the flight to prevent venous thrombosis and pulmonary embolism.

Chronic lung disease

Chronic obstructive pulmonary disease is one of the most common diagnoses in patients who require emergency-department evaluation for symptoms occurring during airline flights. The best predictor of the development of in-flight problems is the sea-level Pa_{O_2}. A Pa_{O_2} of at least 72 mmHg corresponds to an in-flight arterial Pa_{O_2} of ~55 mmHg when the cabin is pressurized to 2500 m (8000 ft). If the traveler's baseline Pa_{O_2} is <72 mmHg, the provision of supplemental oxygen should be considered. Contraindications to flight include active bronchospasm, lower respiratory infection, lower-limb deep vein phlebitis, pulmonary hypertension, and recent thoracic surgery (within the preceding 3 weeks) or pneumothorax. Decreased outdoor activity at the destination should be considered if air pollution is excessive.

Diabetes mellitus

Alterations in glucose control and changes in insulin requirements are common problems among patients with diabetes who travel. Changes in time zone, in the amount and timing of food intake, and in physical activity demand vigilant assessment of metabolic control. The traveler with diabetes should pack medication (including a bottle of regular insulin for emergencies), insulin syringes and needles, equipment and supplies for glucose monitoring, and snacks in carry-on luggage. Insulin is stable for ~3 months at room temperature but should be kept as cool as possible. The name and telephone number of the home physician and a card and bracelet listing the patient's medical problems and the type and dose of insulin used should accompany the traveler. In traveling eastward (e.g., from the United States to Europe), the morning insulin dose on arrival may need to be decreased. The blood glucose can then be checked during the day to determine whether additional insulin is required. For flights westward, with lengthening of the day, an additional dose of regular insulin may be required.

Other special groups

Other groups for whom special travel measures are encouraged include patients undergoing dialysis, those with transplants, and those with other disabilities. Up to 13% of travelers have some disability, but few advocacy groups and tour companies dedicate themselves to this growing population. Medication interactions are a source of serious concern for these travelers, and appropriate medical information should be carried, along with the home physician's name and telephone number. Some travelers taking glucocorticoids carry stress doses in case they become ill. Immunization of these immunocompromised travelers may result in less than adequate protection. Thus the traveler and the physician must carefully consider which destinations are appropriate.

MEDICAL TOURISM

Travel for the purpose of obtaining health care abroad has recently received a great deal of attention in the medical literature and the media. According to the annual U.S. Department of Commerce in-flight survey, there were ~500,000 overseas trips during 2006 in which health treatment was at least one purpose of travel. Lower cost is usually cited as the motivation for this type of tourism, and an entire industry has flourished as a result of this phenomenon. However, the quality of facilities, assistance services, and care is neither uniform nor regulated; thus, in most instances, responsibility for assessing the suitability of an individual program or facility lies solely with the traveler. Persons considering this option must recognize that they are almost always at a disadvantage when being treated in a foreign country, particularly if there are complications. Concerns to be addressed include the quality of the health care facility and its staff; language and cultural differences that may impede accurate interpretation of both verbal and nonverbal communication; religious and ethical differences that may be encountered over issues such as efforts to preserve life and limb or care of the terminally ill; lack of familiarity with the local medical system; limited access of the care provider to the patient's medical history; the use of unfamiliar drugs and medicines; the relative difficulty of arranging follow-up care back in the United States; and the possibility that such follow-up care may be fraught with problems should there be complications. If serious issues arise, legal recourse may be difficult or impossible.

Patients planning to travel abroad to obtain health care, particularly when surgery is involved, should be immunized for hepatitis B and should consider having baseline hepatitis C and HIV tests preoperatively. Prevalence rates of hepatitis B and C and HIV infection vary considerably around the world and are generally higher in developing regions than in the United States and Western Europe. The latest information available on the safety of the blood supply outside the United States is the World Health Organization's Global Database on Blood Safety based on data from 2004–2005 (*www.who.int/bloodsafety/global_database/en*). Persons researching accreditation status of overseas facilities should note that, although these facilities may be part of a chain, they are surveyed and accredited individually. Accreditation resources include (1) the Joint Commission International (*www.jointcommissioninternational.org*), (2) the Australian Council for Healthcare Standards International (*www.achs.org.au/ACHSI*), and (3) the Canadian Council on Health Services (*www.cchsa.ca*).

PROBLEMS AFTER RETURN

The most common medical problems encountered by travelers after their return home are diarrhea, fever, respiratory illnesses, and skin diseases (Fig. 123-2). Frequently ignored problems are fatigue and emotional stress, especially in long-stay travelers. The approach to diagnosis requires some knowledge of geographic medicine, in particular the epidemiology and clinical presentation of infectious disorders. A geographic history should focus on the traveler's exact itinerary, including dates of arrival and departure; exposure history (food indiscretions, drinking-water sources, freshwater contact, sexual activity, animal contact, insect bites); location and style of travel (urban vs. rural, first-class hotel accommodation vs. camping); immunization history; and use of antimalarial chemosuppression.

■ DIARRHEA

See "Prevention of Gastrointestinal Illness," above.

■ FEVER

Fever in a traveler who has returned from a malarious area should be considered a medical emergency because death from *P. falciparum* malaria can follow an illness of only several days' duration. Although "fever from the tropics" does not always have a tropical cause, malaria should be the first diagnosis considered. The risk of *P. falciparum* malaria is highest among travelers returning from Africa or Oceania and among those who become symptomatic within the first 2 months after return. Other important causes of fever after travel include viral hepatitis (hepatitis A and E), typhoid fever, bacterial enteritis, arboviral infections (e.g., dengue fever), rickettsial infections (including tick and scrub typhus and Q fever), and—in rare instances—leptospirosis, acute HIV infection, and amebic liver abscess. A cooperative study by GeoSentinel (an emerging infectious disease surveillance group established by the CDC and the International Society of Travel Medicine) showed that, among 3907 febrile returned travelers, malaria was acquired most often from Africa, dengue from Southeast Asia and the Caribbean, typhoid fever from southern Asia, and rickettsial infections (tick typhus) from southern Africa (Table 123-3). In at least 25% of cases, no etiology can be found, and the fever resolves spontaneously. Clinicians should keep in mind that no present-day antimalarial agent guarantees protection from malaria and that some immunizations (notably, that against typhoid fever) are only partially protective.

When no specific diagnosis is forthcoming, the following investigations, where applicable, are suggested: complete blood count, liver function tests, thick/thin blood films or rapid diagnostic testing for malaria (repeated twice if necessary), urinalysis, urine and blood cultures (repeated once), chest x-ray, and collection of an acute-phase serum sample to be held for subsequent examination along with a paired convalescent-phase serum sample.

■ SKIN DISEASES

Pyodermas, sunburn, insect bites, skin ulcers, and cutaneous larva migrans are the most common skin conditions affecting travelers after their return home. In those with persistent skin ulcers, a diagnosis of cutaneous leishmaniasis, mycobacterial infection, or fungal infection should be considered. Careful, complete inspection of the skin is important in detecting the rickettsial eschar in a febrile patient or the central breathing hole in a "boil" due to myiasis.

■ EMERGING INFECTIOUS DISEASES

In recent years, travel and commerce have fostered the worldwide spread of HIV infection, led to the reemergence of cholera as a global health threat, and created considerable fear about the possible spread of severe acute respiratory syndrome (SARS) and avian influenza (H5N1). For travelers, there are more realistic concerns. One of the largest outbreaks of dengue fever ever documented is now raging in Latin America; chikungunya virus has spread rapidly from Africa to southern Asia and recently to southern Europe; schistosomiasis is being described in previously unaffected lakes in Africa; and antibiotic-resistant strains of sexually transmitted and enteric pathogens are emerging at an alarming rate in the developing world. In addition, concerns have been raised about the potential for bioterrorism involving not only standard strains of unusual agents but mutant strains as well. Time will tell whether travelers (as well as persons at home) will routinely be vaccinated against diseases such as anthrax and smallpox. As Nobel laureate Dr. Joshua Lederberg pointed out, "The microbe that felled one child in a distant continent yesterday can reach yours today and seed a global pandemic tomorrow." The vigilant clinician understands that the importance of a thorough travel history cannot be overemphasized.

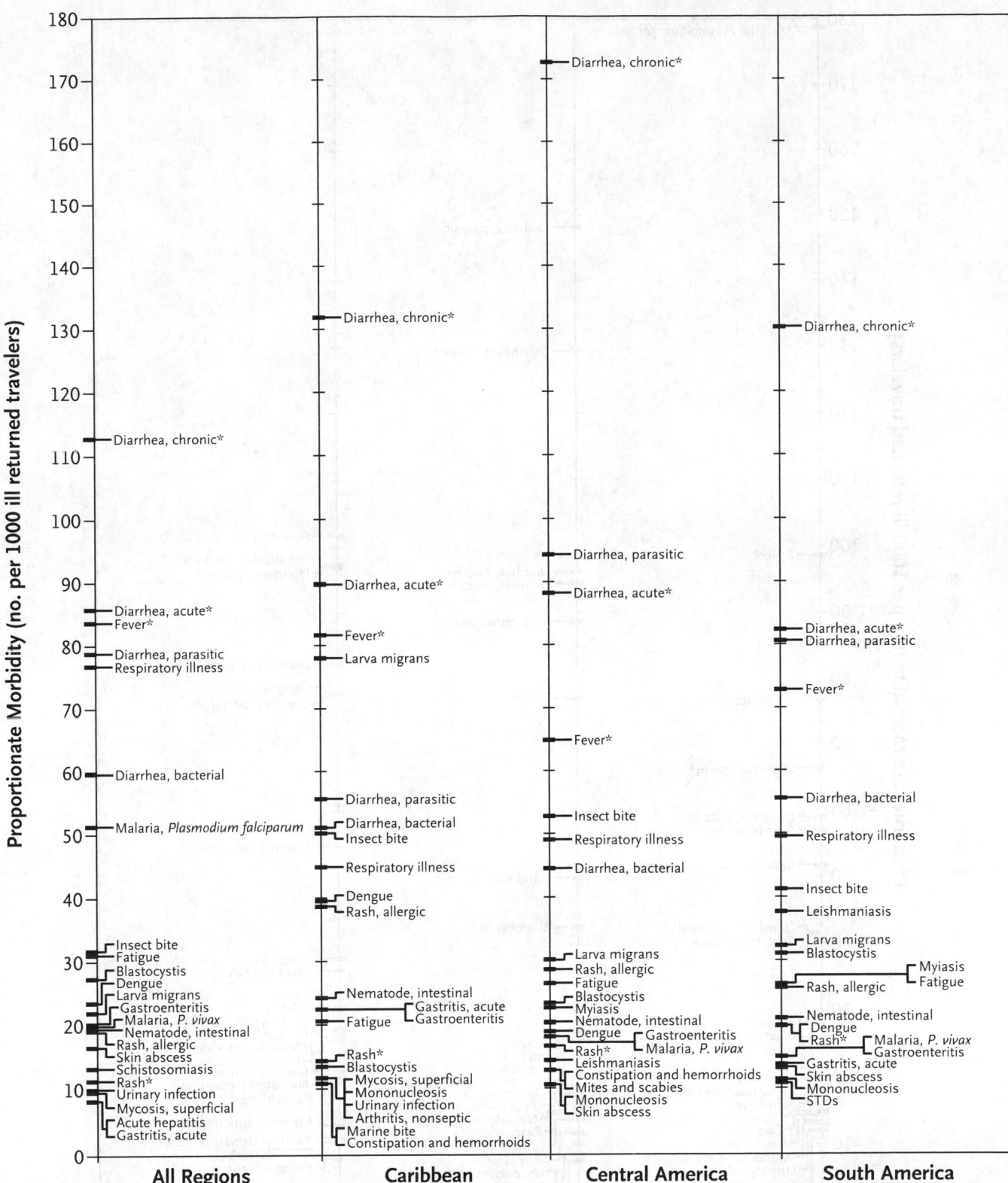

Figure 123-2 **Proportionate morbidity among ill travelers returning from the developing world, according to region of travel.** The proportions (not incidence rates) are shown for each of the top 22 specific diagnoses among all ill returned travelers within each region. STDs, sexually transmitted diseases. Asterisks indicate syndromic diagnoses for which specific etiologies could not be assigned. (*Reprinted with permission from Freedman et al. © 2006 Massachusetts Medical Society.*)

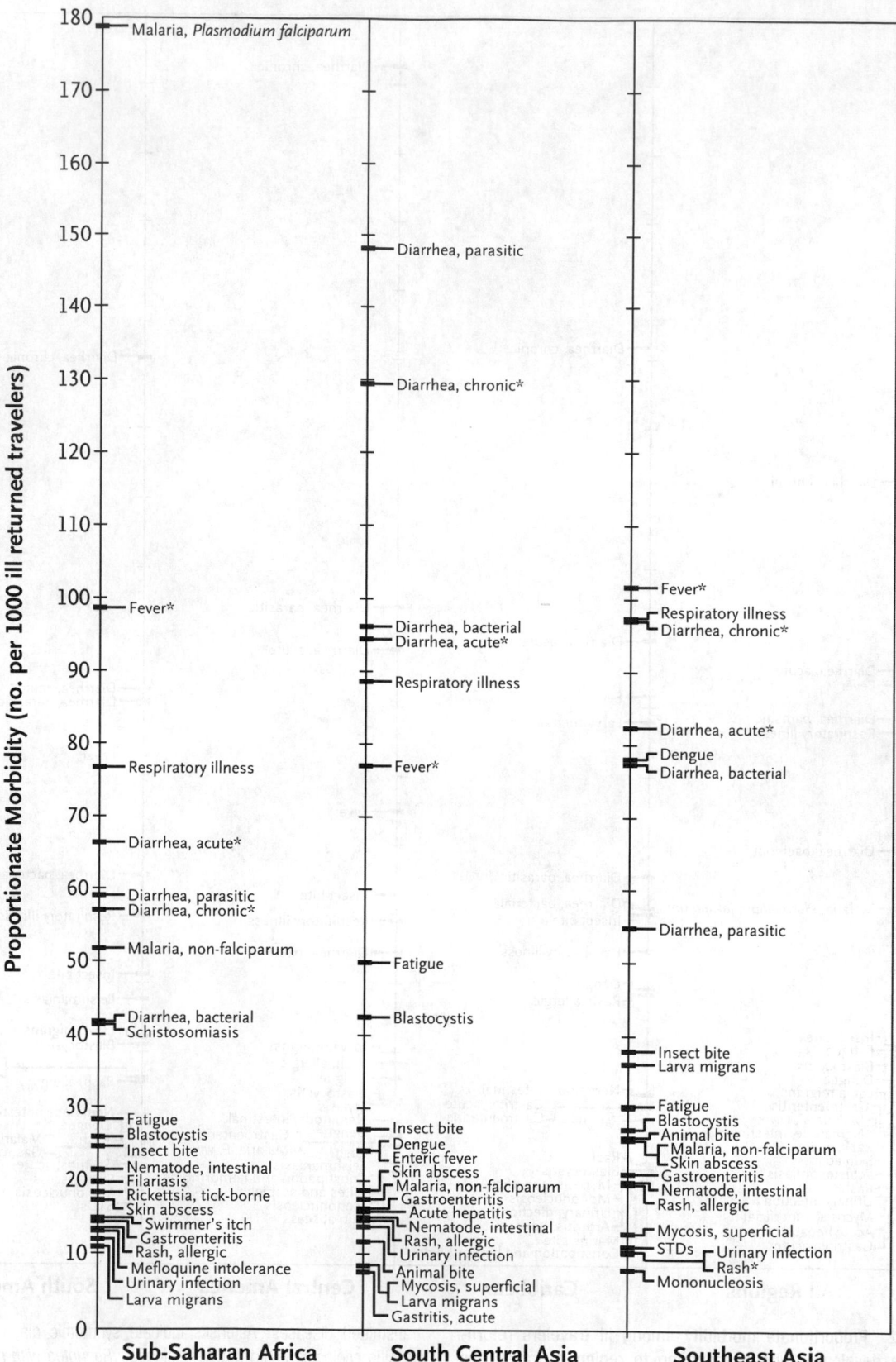

Figure 123-2 (*Continued*)

TABLE 123-3 Etiology and Geographic Distribution of Systemic Febrile Illness in Returned Travelers (n = 3907)

Etiology	Percentage of Cases					
	Carib	CAm	SAm	SSA	SCA	SEA
Malaria	<1	13	13	62	14	13
Dengue	23	12	14	<1	14	32
Mononucleosis	7	7	8	1	2	3
Rickettsia	0	0	0	6	1	2
Salmonella	2	3	2	<1	14	3

Note: Carib, Caribbean; CAm, Central America; SAm, South America; SSA, sub-Saharan Africa; SCA, south-central Asia; SEA, Southeast Asia. Bold type is for emphasis only.

Source: Revised from Table 2 in Freedman et al, 2006. Used with permission from the Massachusetts Medical Society.

FURTHER READINGS

Centers for Disease Control and Prevention: Health Information for International Travel 2010. Mosby, Philadelphia, 2009 (www.cdc.gov/travel)

CHEN LH et al: Controversies and misconceptions in malaria chemoprophylaxis for travelers. JAMA 297:2251, 2007

DUPONT HL et al: Expert review of the evidence base for self-therapy of travelers' diarrhea. J Travel Med 16:161, 2009

——— et al: Expert review of the evidence base for prevention of travelers' diarrhea. J Travel Med 16:149, 2009

FREEDMAN DO: Malaria prevention in short-term travelers. N Engl J Med 359:603, 2008

———et al (GeoSentinel Surveillance Network): Spectrum of disease and relation to place of exposure among ill returned travelers. N Engl J Med 354:119, 2006

JOHNSTON V et al: Fever in returned travellers presenting in the United Kingdom: Recommendations for investigation and initial management. J Infect 59:1, 2009

KEYSTONE JS et al: *Travel Medicine.* Mosby, Philadelphia, 2008

RYAN ET et al: Illness after international travel. N Engl J Med 347:505, 2002

SHERRARD AW, MCCARTHY AE: Travel patterns and health risks for patients infected with HIV. Travel Med Infect Dis 7:291, 2009

SOHAIL MR, FISCHER PR: Health risks to air travelers. Infect Dis Clin North Am 19:67, 2005

WILSON ME, CHEN LH: Dermatologic infectious diseases in international travelers. Curr Infect Dis Rep 6:54, 2004

WEBSITES

Chronic renal failure: *www.kidney.org*

Diabetes: *www.diabetesmonitor.com/other-14.htm*

Dialysis: *www.dialysisfinder.com*

Disability: *www.access-able.com*

HIV: *www.aegis.com*

CHAPTER 124

Infective Endocarditis

Adolf W. Karchmer

The prototypic lesion of infective endocarditis, the *vegetation* (Fig. 124-1), is a mass of platelets, fibrin, microcolonies of microorganisms, and scant inflammatory cells. Infection most commonly involves heart valves (either native or prosthetic) but may also occur on the low-pressure side of a ventricular septal defect, on the mural endocardium where it is damaged by aberrant jets of blood or foreign bodies, or on intracardiac devices themselves. The analogous process involving arteriovenous shunts, arterioarterial shunts (patent ductus arteriosus), or a coarctation of the aorta is called *infective endarteritis*.

Endocarditis may be classified according to the temporal evolution of disease, the site of infection, the cause of infection, or a predisposing risk factor such as injection drug use. While each classification criterion provides therapeutic and prognostic insight, none is sufficient alone. *Acute endocarditis* is a hectically febrile illness that rapidly damages cardiac structures, hematogenously seeds extracardiac sites, and, if untreated, progresses to death within weeks. *Subacute endocarditis* follows an indolent course; causes structural cardiac damage only slowly, if at all; rarely metastasizes; and is gradually progressive unless complicated by a major embolic event or ruptured mycotic aneurysm.

In developed countries, the incidence of endocarditis ranges from 2.6 to 7 cases per 100,000 population per year and has remained relatively stable during recent decades. While congenital heart diseases remain a constant predisposition, predisposing conditions in developed countries have shifted from chronic rheumatic heart disease (which remains a common predisposition in developing countries) to illicit IV drug use, degenerative valve disease, and intracardiac devices. The incidence of endocarditis is notably increased among the elderly. In developed countries, 30–35% of cases of native valve endocarditis (NVE) are associated with health care, and 16–30% of all cases of endocarditis involve prosthetic valves. The risk of prosthesis infection is greatest during the first 6–12 months after valve replacement; gradually declines to a low, stable rate thereafter; and is similar for mechanical and bioprosthetic devices.

■ ETIOLOGY

Although many species of bacteria and fungi cause sporadic episodes of endocarditis, a few bacterial species cause the majority of cases (Table 124-1). Because of their different portals of entry, the pathogens involved vary somewhat with the clinical types of endocarditis. The oral cavity, skin, and upper respiratory tract are the respective primary portals for the viridans streptococci, staphylococci, and HACEK organisms (*Haemophilus, Actinobacillus, Cardiobacterium, Eikenella,* and *Kingella; Haemophilus aphrophilus* and *Actinobacillus actinomycetemcomitans* have been reclassified into the genus *Aggregatibacter*). *Streptococcus gallolyticus*

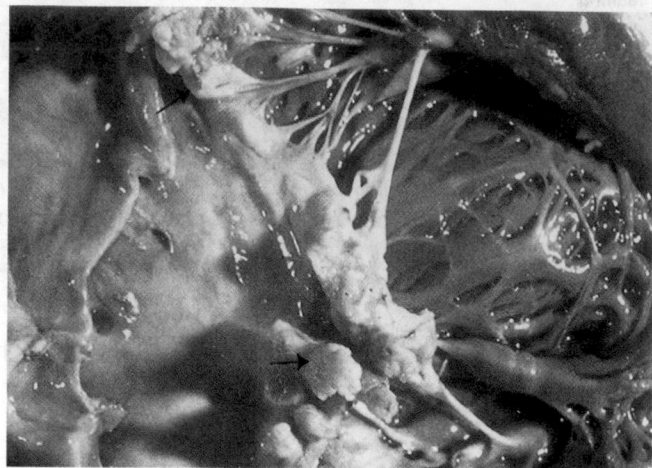

Figure 124-1 Vegetations (*arrows*) due to viridans streptococcal endocarditis involving the mitral valve.

(formerly *S. bovis*) originates from the gastrointestinal tract, where it is associated with polyps and colonic tumors, and enterococci enter the bloodstream from the genitourinary tract. Health care–associated NVE, commonly caused by *Staphylococcus aureus*, coagulase-negative staphylococci (CoNS), and enterococci, has a nosocomial onset (55%) or a community onset (45%) in patients who have had extensive contact with the health care system over the preceding 90 days. Endocarditis complicates 6–25% of episodes of catheter-associated *S. aureus* bacteremia; the higher rates are detected by careful transesophageal echocardiography (TEE) screening (see "Echocardiography," below).

Prosthetic valve endocarditis (PVE) arising within 2 months of valve surgery is generally nosocomial, the result of intraoperative contamination of the prosthesis or a bacteremic postoperative complication. This nosocomial origin is reflected in the primary microbial causes: *S. aureus*, CoNS, facultative gram-negative bacilli, diphtheroids, and fungi. The portals of entry and organisms causing cases beginning >12 months after surgery are similar to those in community-acquired NVE. PVE due to CoNS that presents 2–12 months after surgery often represents delayed-onset nosocomial infection. Regardless of the time of onset after surgery, at least 68–85% of CoNS strains that cause PVE are resistant to methicillin.

Transvenous pacemaker– or implanted defibrillator–associated endocarditis is usually nosocomial. The majority of episodes occur within weeks of implantation or generator change and are caused by *S. aureus* or CoNS, both of which are commonly resistant to methicillin.

Endocarditis occurring among injection drug users, especially that involving the tricuspid valve, is commonly caused by *S. aureus*, many strains of which are resistant to methicillin. Left-sided valve infections in addicts have a more varied etiology. In addition to the usual causes of endocarditis, these cases are caused by *Pseudomonas aeruginosa* and *Candida* species and sporadically by unusual organisms such as *Bacillus, Lactobacillus,* and *Corynebacterium* species. Polymicrobial endocarditis occurs among injection drug users. HIV infection in drug users does not significantly influence the causes of endocarditis.

PART 8

Infectious Diseases

TABLE 124-1 Organisms Causing Major Clinical Forms of Endocarditis

	Percentage of Cases							
	Native Valve Endocarditis		Prosthetic Valve Endocarditis at Indicated Time of Onset (Months) after Valve Surgery			Endocarditis in Injection Drug Users		
Organism	Community-Acquired (n =1718)	Health Care–Associated (n =788)	<2 (n = 144)	2–12 (n = 31)	>12 (n = 194)	Right-Sided (n = 346)	Left-Sided (n = 204)	Total (n = 675)[a]
Streptococci[b]	40	9	1	9	31	5	15	12
Pneumococci	2	—	—	—	—	—	—	—
Enterococci	9	13	8	12	11	2	24	9
Staphylococcus aureus	28	53[c]	22	12	18	77	23	57
Coagulase-negative staphylococci	5	12	33	32	11	—	—	—
Fastidious gram-negative coccobacilli (HACEK group)[d]	3	—	—	—	6	—	—	—
Gram-negative bacilli	1	2	13	3	6	5	13	7
Candida spp.	<1	2	8	12	1	—	12	4
Polymicrobial/miscellaneous	3	4	3	6	5	8	10	7
Diphtheroids	—	<1	6	—	3	—	—	0.1
Culture-negative	9	5	5	6	8	3	3	3

[a] The total number of cases is larger than the sum of right- and left-sided cases because the location of infection was not specified in some cases.

[b] Includes viridans streptococci; *Streptococcus gallolyticus*; other non–group A, groupable streptococci; and *Abiotrophia* spp. (nutritionally variant, pyridoxal-requiring streptococci).

[c] Methicillin resistance is common among these *S. aureus* strains.

[d] Includes *Haemophilus* spp., *Aggregatibacter actinomycetemcomitans*, *Cardiobacterium hominis*, *Eikenella* spp., and *Kingella* spp.

Note: Data are compiled from multiple studies.

From 5% to 15% of patients with endocarditis have negative blood cultures; in one-third to one-half of these cases, cultures are negative because of prior antibiotic exposure. The remainder of these patients are infected by fastidious organisms, such as nutritionally variant organisms (now designated *Granulicatella* and *Abiotrophia* species), HACEK organisms, *Coxiella burnetii*, and *Bartonella* species. Some fastidious organisms occur in characteristic geographic settings (e.g., *C. burnetii* and *Bartonella* species in Europe, *Brucella* species in the Middle East). *Tropheryma whipplei* causes an indolent, culture-negative, afebrile form of endocarditis.

■ PATHOGENESIS

The endothelium, unless damaged, is resistant to infection by most bacteria and to thrombus formation. Endothelial injury (e.g., at the site of impact of high-velocity blood jets or on the low-pressure side of a cardiac structural lesion) allows either direct infection by virulent organisms or the development of an uninfected platelet-fibrin thrombus—a condition called *nonbacterial thrombotic endocarditis* (NBTE). The thrombus subsequently serves as a site of bacterial attachment during transient bacteremia. The cardiac conditions most commonly resulting in NBTE are mitral regurgitation, aortic stenosis, aortic regurgitation, ventricular septal defects, and complex congenital heart disease. NBTE also arises as a result of a hypercoagulable state; this phenomenon gives rise to the clinical entity of *marantic endocarditis* (uninfected vegetations seen in patients with malignancy and chronic diseases) and to bland vegetations complicating systemic lupus erythematosus and the antiphospholipid antibody syndrome.

Organisms that cause endocarditis generally enter the bloodstream from mucosal surfaces, the skin, or sites of focal infection. Except for more virulent bacteria (e.g., *S. aureus*) that can adhere directly to intact endothelium or exposed subendothelial tissue, microorganisms in the blood adhere at sites of NBTE. If resistant to the bactericidal activity of serum and the microbicidal peptides released locally by platelets, the organisms proliferate and induce platelet deposition and a procoagulant state at the site by eliciting tissue factor from the endothelium or, in the case of *S. aureus*, from monocytes as well. Fibrin deposition combines with platelet aggregation and microorganism proliferation to generate an infected vegetation. The organisms that commonly cause endocarditis have surface adhesin molecules, collectively called microbial surface components recognizing adhesin matrix molecules (MSCRAMMs), that mediate adherence to NBTE sites or injured endothelium. Fibronectin-binding proteins present on many gram-positive bacteria, clumping factor (a fibrinogen- and fibrin-binding surface protein) on *S. aureus*, and glucans or FimA (a member of the family of oral mucosal adhesins) on streptococci facilitate adherence. Fibronectin-binding proteins are required for *S. aureus* invasion of intact endothelium; thus these surface proteins may facilitate infection of previously normal valves. In the absence of host defenses, organisms enmeshed in the growing platelet-fibrin vegetation proliferate to form dense microcolonies. Organisms deep in vegetations are metabolically inactive (nongrowing) and relatively resistant to killing by antimicrobial agents. Proliferating surface organisms are shed into the bloodstream continuously.

The pathophysiologic consequences and clinical manifestations of endocarditis—other than constitutional symptoms, which probably result from cytokine production—arise from damage to intracardiac structures; embolization of vegetation fragments, leading to infection or infarction of remote tissues; hematogenous infection of sites during bacteremia; and tissue injury due to the deposition of circulating immune complexes or immune responses to deposited bacterial antigens.

■ CLINICAL MANIFESTATIONS

The clinical syndrome of infective endocarditis is highly variable and spans a continuum between acute and subacute presentations. NVE (whether acquired in the community or in association with health care), PVE, and endocarditis due to injection drug use share clinical and laboratory manifestations (Table 124-2). The causative microorganism is primarily responsible for the temporal course of endocarditis. β-Hemolytic streptococci, *S. aureus*, and pneumococci typically result in an acute course, although *S. aureus* occasionally causes subacute disease. Endocarditis caused by *Staphylococcus lugdunensis* (a coagulase-negative species) or by enterococci may present acutely. Subacute endocarditis is typically caused by viridans streptococci, enterococci, CoNS, and the HACEK group. Endocarditis caused by *Bartonella* species, *T. whipplei*, or *C. burnetii* is exceptionally indolent.

The clinical features of endocarditis are nonspecific. However, these symptoms in a febrile patient with valvular abnormalities or a behavior pattern that predisposes to endocarditis (e.g.,

injection drug use) suggest the diagnosis, as do bacteremia with organisms that frequently cause endocarditis, otherwise-unexplained arterial emboli, and progressive cardiac valvular incompetence. In patients with subacute presentations, fever is typically low-grade and rarely exceeds 39.4°C (103°F); in contrast, temperatures of 39.4°–40°C (103°–104°F) are often noted in acute endocarditis. Fever may be blunted or absent in patients who are elderly or severely debilitated or who have marked cardiac or renal failure.

Cardiac manifestations

Although heart murmurs are usually indicative of the predisposing cardiac pathology rather than of endocarditis, valvular damage and ruptured chordae may result in new regurgitant murmurs. In acute endocarditis involving a normal valve, murmurs may be absent initially but ultimately are detected in 85% of cases. Congestive heart failure (CHF) develops in 30–40% of patients; it is usually a consequence of valvular dysfunction but occasionally is due to endocarditis-associated myocarditis or an intracardiac fistula. Heart failure due to aortic valve dysfunction progresses more rapidly than does that due to mitral valve dysfunction. Extension of infection beyond valve leaflets into adjacent annular or myocardial tissue results in perivalvular abscesses, which in turn may cause intracardiac fistulae with new murmurs. Abscesses may burrow from the aortic valve annulus through the epicardium, causing pericarditis, or into the upper ventricular septum, where they may interrupt the conduction system, leading to varying degrees of heart block. Perivalvular abscesses arising from the mitral valve rarely interrupt conduction pathways near the atrioventricular node or in the proximal bundle of His. Emboli to a coronary artery occur in 2% of patients and may result in myocardial infarction.

Noncardiac manifestations

The classic nonsuppurative peripheral manifestations of subacute endocarditis are related to the duration of infection and, with early diagnosis and treatment, have become infrequent. In contrast, septic embolization mimicking some of these lesions (subungual hemorrhage, Osler's nodes) is common in patients with acute *S. aureus* endocarditis (Fig. 124-2). Musculoskeletal pain usually remits promptly with treatment but must be distinguished from focal metastatic infections (e.g., spondylodiscitis), which may complicate 10–15% of cases. Hematogenously seeded focal infection is most often clinically evident in the skin, spleen, kidneys, skeletal

TABLE 124-2 Clinical and Laboratory Features of Infective Endocarditis

Feature	Frequency, %
Fever	80–90
Chills and sweats	40–75
Anorexia, weight loss, malaise	25–50
Myalgias, arthralgias	15–30
Back pain	7–15
Heart murmur	80–85
New/worsened regurgitant murmur	20–50
Arterial emboli	20–50
Splenomegaly	15–50
Clubbing	10–20
Neurologic manifestations	20–40
Peripheral manifestations (Osler's nodes, subungual hemorrhages, Janeway lesions, Roth's spots)	2–15
Petechiae	10–40
Laboratory manifestations	
Anemia	70–90
Leukocytosis	20–30
Microscopic hematuria	30–50
Elevated erythrocyte sedimentation rate	60–90
Elevated C-reactive protein level	>90
Rheumatoid factor	50
Circulating immune complexes	65–100
Decreased serum complement	5–40

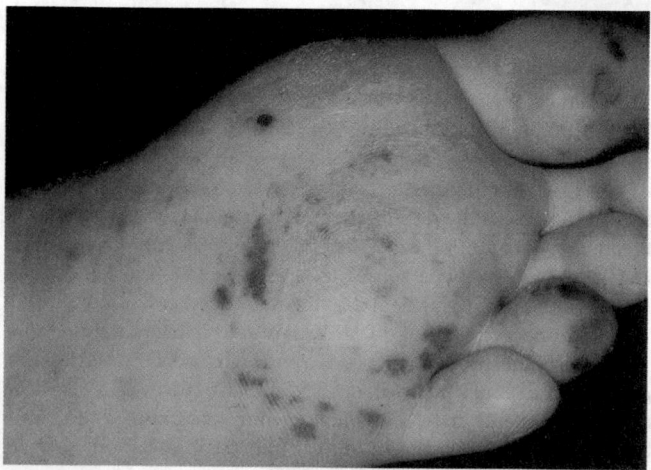

Figure 124-2 *Septic emboli* with hemorrhage and infarction due to acute *Staphylococcus aureus* endocarditis. *(Used with permission of L. Baden.)*

system, and meninges. Arterial emboli are clinically apparent in up to 50% of patients. Endocarditis caused by *S. aureus,* vegetations >10 mm in diameter (as measured by echocardiography), and infection involving the mitral valve are independently associated with an increased risk of embolization. Emboli occurring late during or after effective therapy do not in themselves constitute evidence of failed antimicrobial treatment. Cerebrovascular emboli presenting as strokes or occasionally as encephalopathy complicate 15–35% of cases of endocarditis. One-half of these events precede the diagnosis of endocarditis. The frequency of stroke is 8 per 1000 patient-days during the week prior to diagnosis; the figure falls to 4.8 and 1.7 per 1000 patient-days during the first and second weeks of effective antimicrobial therapy, respectively. This decline exceeds that which can be attributed to change in vegetation size. Only 3% of strokes occur after 1 week of effective therapy. Other neurologic complications include aseptic or purulent meningitis, intracranial hemorrhage due to hemorrhagic infarcts or ruptured mycotic aneurysms, and seizures. (*Mycotic aneurysms* are focal dilations of arteries occurring at points in the artery wall that have been weakened by infection in the vasa vasorum or where septic emboli have lodged.) Microabscesses in brain and meninges occur commonly in *S. aureus* endocarditis; surgically drainable intracerebral abscesses are infrequent.

Immune complex deposition on the glomerular basement membrane causes diffuse hypocomplementemic glomerulonephritis and renal dysfunction, which typically improve with effective antimicrobial therapy. Embolic renal infarcts cause flank pain and hematuria but rarely cause renal dysfunction.

Manifestations of specific predisposing conditions

Almost 50% of endocarditis cases associated with injection drug use are limited to the tricuspid valve and present with fever but with faint or no murmur. In 75% of cases, septic emboli cause cough, pleuritic chest pain, nodular pulmonary infiltrates, or occasionally pyopneumothorax. Infection of the aortic or mitral valves on the left side of the heart presents with the typical clinical features of endocarditis.

Health care–associated endocarditis has typical manifestations if it is not associated with a retained intracardiac device or masked by the symptoms of concurrent comorbid illness. Transvenous pacemaker– or implanted defibrillator–associated endocarditis may be associated with obvious or cryptic generator pocket infection and results in fever, minimal murmur, and pulmonary symptoms due to septic emboli.

Late-onset PVE presents with typical clinical features. In cases arising within 60 days of valve surgery (early onset), typical symptoms may be obscured by comorbidity associated with recent surgery. In both early-onset and more delayed presentations, paravalvular infection is common and often results in partial valve dehiscence, regurgitant murmurs, CHF, or disruption of the conduction system.

■ DIAGNOSIS

The Duke criteria

The diagnosis of infective endocarditis is established with certainty only when vegetations are examined histologically and microbiologically. Nevertheless, a highly sensitive and specific diagnostic schema—known as the *Duke criteria*—has been developed on the basis of clinical, laboratory, and echocardiographic findings (Table 124-3). Documentation of two major criteria, of one major criterion and three minor criteria, or of five minor criteria allows a clinical diagnosis of definite endocarditis. The diagnosis of endocarditis is rejected if an alternative diagnosis is

TABLE 124-3 The Duke Criteria for the Clinical Diagnosis of Infective Endocarditis[a]

Major Criteria

1. Positive blood culture

   Typical microorganism for infective endocarditis from two separate blood cultures
      Viridans streptococci, *Streptococcus gallolyticus,* HACEK group, *Staphylococcus aureus,* or
      Community-acquired enterococci in the absence of a primary focus, *or*

   Persistently positive blood culture, defined as recovery of a microorganism consistent with infective endocarditis from:
      Blood cultures drawn >12 h apart; *or*
      All of 3 or a majority of ≥4 separate blood cultures, with first and last drawn at least 1 h apart

   Single positive blood culture for *Coxiella burnetii* or phase I IgG antibody titer of >1:800

2. Evidence of endocardial involvement

   Positive echocardiogram[b]
      Oscillating intracardiac mass on valve or supporting structures or in the path of regurgitant jets or in implanted material, in the absence of an alternative anatomic explanation, *or*
      Abscess, *or*
      New partial dehiscence of prosthetic valve, *or*

   New valvular regurgitation (increase or change in preexisting murmur not sufficient)

Minor Criteria

1. Predisposition: predisposing heart condition or injection drug use
2. Fever ≥38.0°C (≥100.4°F)
3. Vascular phenomena: major arterial emboli, septic pulmonary infarcts, mycotic aneurysm, intracranial hemorrhage, conjunctival hemorrhages, Janeway lesions
4. Immunologic phenomena: glomerulonephritis, Osler's nodes, Roth's spots, rheumatoid factor
5. Microbiologic evidence: positive blood culture but not meeting major criterion as noted previously[c] or serologic evidence of active infection with organism consistent with infective endocarditis

[a]Definite endocarditis is defined by documentation of two major criteria, of one major criterion and three minor criteria, or of five minor criteria. See text for further details.

[b]Transesophageal echocardiography is recommended for assessing possible prosthetic valve endocarditis or complicated endocarditis.

[c]Excluding single positive cultures for coagulase-negative staphylococci and diphtheroids, which are common culture contaminants, and organisms that do not cause endocarditis frequently, such as gram-negative bacilli.

Note: HACEK, *Haemophilus* spp., *Aggregatibacter actinomycetemcomitans, Cardiobacterium hominis, Eikenella corrodens, Kingella* spp.

Source: Adapted from Li et al, with permission from the University of Chicago Press.

established, if symptoms resolve and do not recur with ≤4 days of antibiotic therapy, or if surgery or autopsy after ≤4 days of antimicrobial therapy yields no histologic evidence of endocarditis. Illnesses not classified as definite endocarditis or rejected as such are considered cases of possible infective endocarditis when either one major criterion and one minor criterion or three minor criteria are fulfilled. Requiring the identification of clinical features of endocarditis for classification as possible infective endocarditis increases the specificity of the schema without significantly reducing its sensitivity.

The roles of bacteremia and echocardiographic findings in the diagnosis of endocarditis are emphasized in the Duke criteria. The requirement for multiple positive blood cultures over time is consistent with the continuous low-density bacteremia characteristic of endocarditis. Among patients with untreated endocarditis who ultimately have a positive blood culture, 95% of all blood cultures are positive. The diagnostic criteria attach significance to the species of organism isolated from blood cultures. To fulfill a major criterion, the isolation of an organism that causes both endocarditis and bacteremia in the absence of endocarditis (e.g., *S. aureus*, enterococci) must take place repeatedly (i.e., persistent bacteremia) and in the absence of a primary focus of infection. Organisms that rarely cause endocarditis but commonly contaminate blood cultures (e.g., diphtheroids, CoNS) must be isolated repeatedly if their isolation is to serve as a major criterion.

Blood cultures

Isolation of the causative microorganism from blood cultures is critical for diagnosis, determination of antimicrobial susceptibility, and planning of treatment. In the absence of prior antibiotic therapy, three 2-bottle blood culture sets, separated from one another by at least 1 h, should be obtained from different venipuncture sites over 24 h. If the cultures remain negative after 48–72 h, two or three additional blood culture sets should be obtained, and the laboratory should be consulted for advice regarding optimal culture techniques. Pending culture results, empirical antimicrobial therapy should be withheld initially from hemodynamically stable patients with suspected subacute endocarditis, especially those who have received antibiotics within the preceding 2 weeks; thus, if necessary, additional blood culture sets can be obtained without the confounding effect of empirical treatment. Patients with acute endocarditis or with deteriorating hemodynamics who may require urgent surgery should be treated empirically immediately after three sets of blood cultures are obtained over several hours.

Non-blood-culture tests

Serologic tests can be used to implicate causally some organisms that are difficult to recover by blood culture: *Brucella, Bartonella, Legionella, Chlamydophila psittaci*, and *C. burnetii*. Pathogens can also be identified in vegetations by culture, microscopic examination with special stains (i.e., the periodic acid–Schiff stain for *T. whipplei*), or direct fluorescence antibody techniques and by the use of polymerase chain reaction (PCR) to recover unique microbial DNA or 16S rRNA that, when sequenced, allows identification of organisms.

Echocardiography

Echocardiography allows anatomic confirmation of infective endocarditis, sizing of vegetations, detection of intracardiac complications, and assessment of cardiac function (Fig. 124-3). Transthoracic echocardiography (TTE) is noninvasive and exceptionally specific; however, it cannot image vegetations <2 mm in diameter, and in 20% of patients it is technically inadequate because of emphysema or body habitus. TTE detects vegetations in only 65% of patients with definite clinical endocarditis. Moreover, TTE is not adequate for evaluating prosthetic valves or detecting intracardiac complications. TEE is safe and detects vegetations in >90% of patients with definite endocarditis; nevertheless, initial studies may be false-negative in 6–18% of endocarditis patients. When endocarditis is likely, a negative TEE result does not exclude the diagnosis but rather warrants repetition of the study in 7–10 days. TEE is the optimal method for the diagnosis of PVE or the detection of myocardial abscess, valve perforation, or intracardiac fistulae.

Experts favor echocardiographic evaluation of all patients with a clinical diagnosis of endocarditis; however, the test should not be used to screen patients with a low probability of endocarditis (e.g., patients with unexplained fever). An American Heart Association approach to the use of echocardiography for evaluation of patients with suspected endocarditis is illustrated in Fig. 124-4.

Other studies

Many laboratory studies that are not diagnostic—i.e., complete blood count, creatinine determination, liver function tests, chest radiography, and electrocardiography—are nevertheless important in the management of patients with endocarditis. The erythrocyte sedimentation rate, C-reactive protein level, and circulating immune complex titer are commonly increased in endocarditis (Table 124-2). Cardiac catheterization is useful primarily to assess coronary artery patency in older individuals who are to undergo surgery for endocarditis.

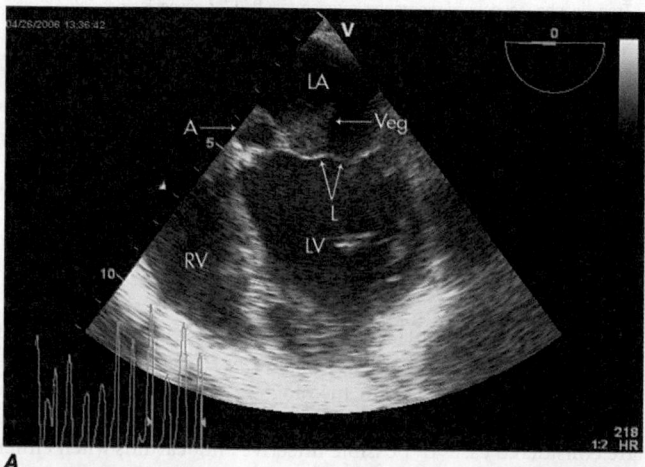

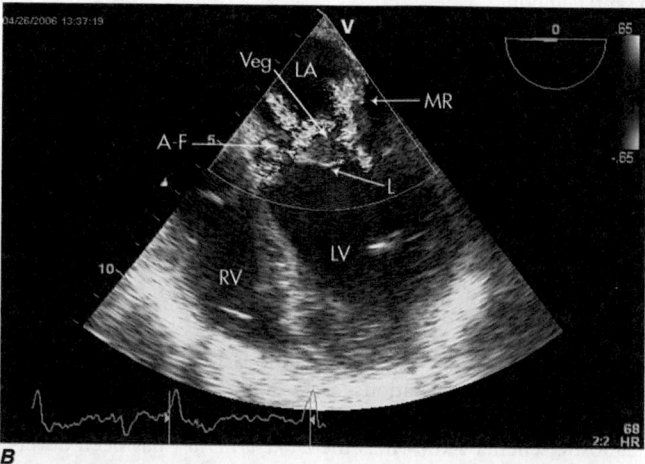

Figure 124-3 Imaging of a mitral valve infected with *Staphylococcus aureus* by low-esophageal four-chamber-view transesophageal echocardiography (TEE). *A.* Two-dimensional echocardiogram showing a large vegetation with an adjacent echolucent abscess cavity. *B.* Color-flow Doppler image showing severe mitral regurgitation through both the abscess-fistula and the central valve orifice. A, abscess; A-F, abscess-fistula; L, valve leaflets; LA, left atrium; LV, left ventricle; MR, mitral central valve regurgitation; RV, right ventricle; veg, vegetation. *(With permission of Andrew Burger, MD)*

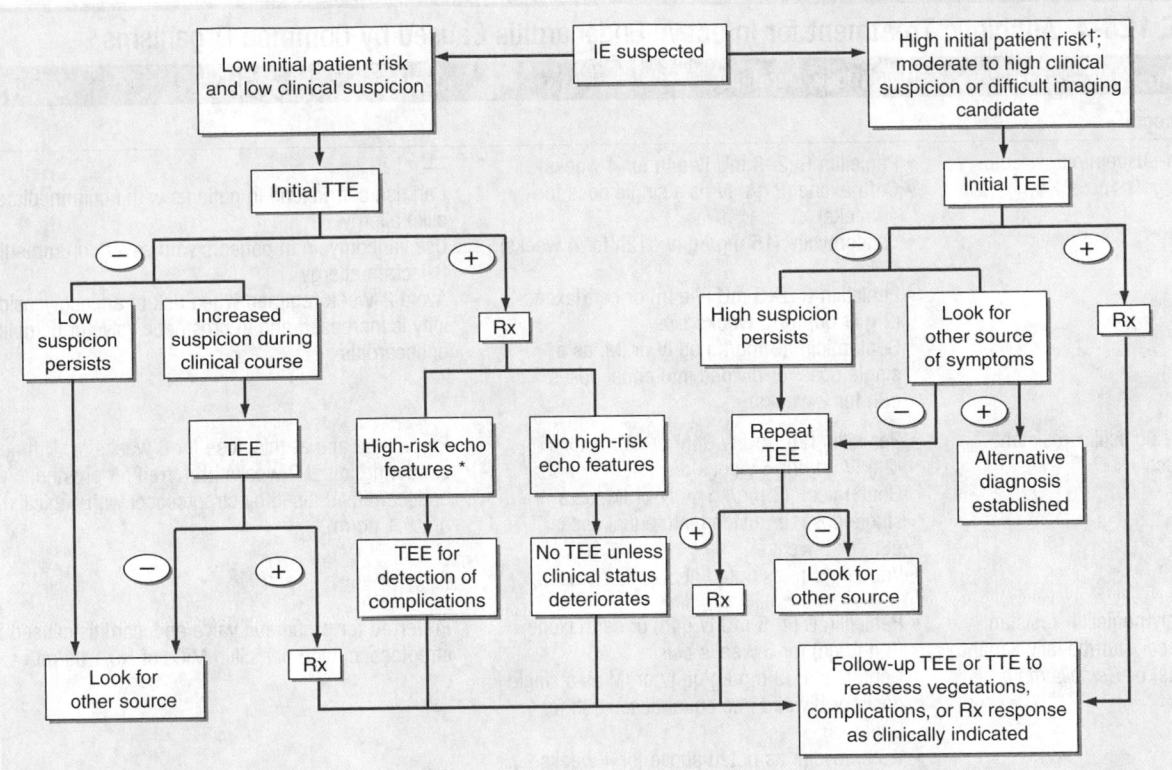

Figure 124-4 **The diagnostic use of transesophageal and transtra-cheal echocardiography (TEE and TTE, respectively).** †High initial patient risk for endocarditis as listed in Table 124-8 or evidence of intracardiac complications (new regurgitant murmur, new electrocardiographic conduction changes, or congestive heart failure). * High-risk echocardiographic features include large vegetations, valve insufficiency, paravalvular infection, or ventricular dysfunction. Rx indicates initiation of antibiotic therapy. *[Reproduced with permission from Diagnosis and Management of Infective Endocarditis and Its Complications (Circulation 1998; 98:2936-2948. © 1998 American Heart Association.)]*

TREATMENT Infective Endocarditis

ANTIMICROBIAL THERAPY It is difficult to eradicate bacteria from the vegetation because local host defenses are deficient and because the largely nongrowing, metabolically inactive bacteria are less easily killed by antibiotics. To cure endocarditis, all bacteria in the vegetation must be killed; therefore, therapy must be bactericidal and prolonged. Antibiotics are generally given parenterally to achieve serum concentrations that, through passive diffusion, lead to effective concentrations in the depths of the vegetation. To select effective therapy requires knowledge of the susceptibility of the causative microorganisms. The decision to initiate treatment empirically must balance the need to establish a microbiologic diagnosis against the potential progression of disease or the need for urgent surgery (see "Blood Cultures," above). Simultaneous infection at other sites (such as meningitis), allergies, end-organ dysfunction, interactions with concomitant medications, and risks of adverse events must be considered in the selection of therapy.

Although given for several weeks longer, the regimens recommended for the treatment of endocarditis involving prosthetic valves (except for staphylococcal infections) are similar to those used to treat NVE (Table 124-4). Recommended doses and durations of therapy should be adhered to unless alterations are required by end-organ dysfunction or adverse events.

Organism-specific therapies

Streptococci Optimal therapy for streptococcal endocarditis is based on the minimal inhibitory concentration (MIC) of penicillin for the causative isolate (Table 124-4). The 2-week penicillin/gentamicin or ceftriaxone/gentamicin regimens should not be used to treat complicated NVE or PVE. The regimen recommended for relatively penicillin-resistant streptococci is advocated for treatment of group B, C, or G streptococcal endocarditis. Nutritionally variant organisms (*Granulicatella* or *Abiotrophia* species) and *Gemella morbillorum* are treated with the regimen for moderately penicillin-resistant streptococci, as is PVE caused by these organisms or by streptococci with a penicillin MIC of >0.1 μg/mL (Table 124-4).

Enterococci Enterococci are resistant to oxacillin, nafcillin, and the cephalosporins and are only inhibited—not killed—by penicillin, ampicillin, teicoplanin (not available in the United States), and vancomycin. To kill enterococci requires the synergistic interaction of a cell wall–active antibiotic (penicillin, ampicillin, vancomycin, or teicoplanin) that is effective at achievable serum concentrations and an aminoglycoside (gentamicin or streptomycin) to which the isolate does not exhibit high-level resistance. An isolate's resistance to cell wall–active agents or its ability to replicate in the presence of gentamicin at ≥500 μg/mL or streptomycin at 1000–2000 μg/mL—a phenomenon called *high-level aminoglycoside resistance*—indicates that the ineffective antimicrobial agent cannot participate in the interaction to produce killing. High-level resistance to gentamicin predicts that tobramycin, netilmicin, amikacin, and kanamycin also will be ineffective. In fact, even when enterococci are not highly resistant to gentamicin, it is difficult to predict the ability of these other aminoglycosides to participate in synergistic killing; consequently, they should not in general

TABLE 124-4 Antibiotic Treatment for Infective Endocarditis Caused by Common Organisms[a]

Organism	Drug (Dose, Duration)	Comments
Streptococci		
Penicillin-susceptible[b] strepto-cocci, *S. gallolyticus*	• Penicillin G (2–3 mU IV q4h for 4 weeks) • Ceftriaxone (2 g/d IV as a single dose for 4 weeks) • Vancomycin[c] (15 mg/kg IV q12h for 4 weeks) • Penicillin G (2–3 mU IV q4h) or ceftriaxone (2 g IV qd) for 2 weeks *plus* Gentamicin[d] (3 mg/kg qd IV or IM, as a single dose[e] or divided into equal doses q8h for 2 weeks)	— Can use ceftriaxone in patients with nonimmediate peni-cillin allergy Use vancomycin in patients with severe or immediate β-lactam allergy Avoid 2-week regimen when risk of aminoglycoside tox-icity is increased and in prosthetic valve or complicated endocarditis
Relatively penicillin-resistant[f] streptococci	• Penicillin G (4 mU IV q4h) or ceftriaxone (2 g IV qd) for 4 weeks *plus* Gentamicin[d] (3 mg/kg qd IV or IM, as a single dose[e] or divided into equal doses q8h for 2 weeks) • Vancomycin[c] as noted above for 4 weeks	Penicillin alone at this dose for 6 weeks or with gentami-cin during initial 2 weeks preferred for prosthetic valve endocarditis caused by streptococci with penicillin MICs of ≤0.1 μg/mL —
Moderately penicillin-resistant[g] streptococci, nutritionally variant organisms, or *Gemella morbil-lorum*	• Penicillin G (4–5 mU IV q4h) or ceftriaxone (2 g IV qd) for 6 weeks *plus* Gentamicin[d] (3 mg/kg qd IV or IM as a single dose[e] or divided into equal doses q8h for 6 weeks) • Vancomycin[c] as noted above for 4 weeks	Preferred for prosthetic valve endocarditis caused by streptococci with penicillin MICs of >0.1 μg/mL —
Enterococci[h]		
	• Penicillin G (4–5 mU IV q4h) *plus* Gentamicin[d] (1 mg/kg IV q8h), both for 4–6 weeks • Ampicillin (2 g IV q4h) *plus* Gentamicin[d] (1 mg/kg IV q8h), both for 4–6 weeks • Vancomycin[c] (15 mg/kg IV q12h) *plus* Gentamicin[d] (1 mg/kg IV q8h), both for 4–6 weeks	Can use streptomycin (7.5 mg/kg q12h) in lieu of gentamicin if there is not high-level resistance to streptomycin — Use vancomycin plus gentamicin for penicillin-allergic patients, or desensitize to penicillin
Staphylococci		
Methicillin-susceptible, infecting native valves (no foreign devices)	• Nafcillin or oxacillin (2 g IV q4h for 4–6 weeks) • Cefazolin (2 g IV q8h for 4–6 weeks) • Vancomycin[c] (15 mg/kg IV q12h for 4–6 weeks)	Can use penicillin (4 mU q4h) if isolate is penicillin-susceptible (does not produce β-lactamase) Can use cefazolin regimen for patients with nonimmedi-ate penicillin allergy Use vancomycin for patients with immediate (urticarial) or severe penicillin allergy
Methicillin-resistant, infecting native valves (no foreign devices)	• Vancomycin[c] (15 mg/kg IV q8–12h for 4–6 weeks)	No role for routine use of rifampin
Methicillin-susceptible, infecting prosthetic valves	• Nafcillin or oxacillin (2 g IV q4h for 6–8 weeks) *plus* Gentamicin[d] (1 mg/kg IM or IV q8h for 2 weeks) *plus* Rifampin[i] (300 mg PO q8h for 6–8 weeks)	Use gentamicin during initial 2 weeks; determine susceptibility to gentamicin before initiating rifampin (see text); if patient is highly allergic to penicillin, use regimen for methicillin-resistant staphylococci; if β-lactam allergy is of the minor, nonimmediate type, can substitute cefa-zolin for oxacillin/nafcillin
Methicillin-resistant, infecting prosthetic valves	• Vancomycin[c] (15 mg/kg IV q12h for 6–8 weeks) *plus* Gentamicin[d] (1 mg/kg IM or IV q8h for 2 weeks) *plus* Rifampin[i] (300 mg PO q8h for 6–8 weeks)	Use gentamicin during initial 2 weeks; determine gentamicin susceptibility before initiating rifampin (see text)

(continued)

TABLE 124-4 Antibiotic Treatment for Infective Endocarditis Caused by Common Organisms[a] (*Continued*)

Organism	Drug (Dose, Duration)	Comments
HACEK Organisms		
	• Ceftriaxone (2 g/d IV as a single dose for 4 weeks)	Can use another third-generation cephalosporin at comparable dosage
	• Ampicillin/sulbactam (3 g IV q6h for 4 weeks)	—

[a]Doses are for adults with normal renal function. Doses of gentamicin, streptomycin, and vancomycin must be adjusted for reduced renal function. Ideal body weight is used to calculate doses of gentamicin and streptomycin per kilogram (men = 50 kg + 2.3 kg per inch over 5 feet; women = 45.5 kg + 2.3 kg per inch over 5 feet).

[b]MIC, ≤0.1 μg/mL.

[c]Vancomycin dose is based on actual body weight. Adjust for trough level of 10–15 μg/mL for streptococcal and enterococcal infections and 15–20 μg/mL for staphylococcal infections.

[d]Aminoglycosides should not be administered as single daily doses for enterococcal endocarditis and should be introduced as part of the initial treatment. Target peak and trough serum concentrations of divided-dose gentamicin 1 h after a 20- to 30-min infusion or IM injection are ~3.5 μg/mL and ≤1 μg/mL, respectively; target peak and trough serum concentrations of streptomycin (timing as with gentamicin) are 20–35 μg/mL and <10 μg/mL, respectively.

[e]Netilmicin (4 mg/kg qd, as a single dose) can be used in lieu of gentamicin.

[f]MIC, >0.1 μg/mL and <0.5 μg/mL.

[g]MIC, ≥0.5 μg/mL and <8 μg/mL.

[h]Antimicrobial susceptibility must be evaluated; see text.

[i]Rifampin increases warfarin and dicumarol requirements for anticoagulation.

be used to treat enterococcal endocarditis. High concentrations of ampicillin plus ceftriaxone or cefotaxime, by expanded binding of penicillin-binding proteins, kill *E. faecalis* in vitro and in animal models of endocarditis.

Enterococci causing endocarditis must be tested for high-level resistance to streptomycin and gentamicin, β-lactamase production, and susceptibility to penicillin and ampicillin (MIC, <8 μg/mL) and to vancomycin (MIC, ≤4 μg/mL). If the isolate produces β-lactamase, ampicillin/sulbactam or vancomycin can be used as the cell wall–active component; if the penicillin/ampicillin MIC is ≥8 μg/mL, vancomycin can be considered; and if the vancomycin MIC is ≥8 μg/mL, penicillin or ampicillin can be considered. In the absence of high-level resistance, gentamicin or streptomycin should be used as the aminoglycoside (Table 124-4). If there is high-level resistance to both these drugs, no aminoglycoside should be given; instead, an 8- to 12-week course of a single cell wall–active agent—or, for *E. faecalis*, high doses of ampicillin combined with ceftriaxone or cefotaxime—is suggested. If this alternative therapy fails or the isolate is resistant to all of the commonly used agents, surgical treatment is advised. The role of newer agents potentially active against multidrug-resistant enterococci [quinupristin/dalfopristin (*E. faecium* only), linezolid, and daptomycin] in the treatment of endocarditis has not been established. Although the dose of gentamicin used to achieve bactericidal synergy in treating enterococcal endocarditis is smaller than that used in standard therapy, nephrotoxicity is not uncommon during treatment for 4–6 weeks. Regimens in which the aminoglycoside component is discontinued at 2–3 weeks because of toxicity have been curative. Thus, discontinuation of the aminoglycoside is recommended when nephrotoxicity develops in patients who have responded satisfactorily to therapy. Alternatively, the ampicillin-ceftriaxone regimen can be used to treat *E. faecalis* endocarditis if nephrotoxicity develops or is exceptionally threatening.

Staphylococci The regimens used to treat staphylococcal endocarditis (Table 124-4) are based not on coagulase production but rather on the presence or absence of a prosthetic valve or foreign device, the native valve(s) involved, and the susceptibility of the isolate to penicillin, methicillin, and vancomycin.

All staphylococci are considered penicillin-resistant until shown not to produce penicillinase. Similarly, methicillin resistance has become so prevalent among staphylococci that therapy should be initiated with a regimen for methicillin-resistant organisms and subsequently revised if the strain proves to be susceptible to methicillin. The addition of 3–5 days of gentamicin (if the isolate is susceptible) to a β-lactam antibiotic to enhance therapy for native mitral or aortic valve endocarditis has been optional. While the addition of gentamicin minimally hastens eradication of bacteremia, it does not improve survival rates, and even abbreviated gentamicin therapy may be associated with nephrotoxicity and thus is not recommended. Gentamicin generally is not added to the vancomycin regimen in this setting.

For treatment of endocarditis caused by methicillin-resistant *S. aureus* (MRSA), vancomycin dosing to achieve trough concentrations of 15–20 μg/mL is recommended, with the recognition that this regimen may be associated with nephrotoxicity. Although resistance to vancomycin among staphylococci is rare, reduced vancomycin susceptibility among MRSA strains is increasingly encountered. Isolates with a vancomycin MIC of 4–16 μg/mL have intermediate susceptibility and are referred to as vancomycin-intermediate *S. aureus* (VISA). Isolates with an MIC of 2 μg/mL may harbor subpopulations with higher MICs. These isolates, called hetero-resistant VISA (hVISA), are not detectable by routine susceptibility testing. Because of the pharmacokinetics/pharmacodynamics of vancomycin, killing of MRSA with a vancomycin MIC of 2 μg/mL is unpredictable even with aggressive vancomycin dosing. Although not approved by the U.S. Food and Drug Administration, daptomycin [6 mg/kg (or, as some experts prefer, 8–10 mg/kg) IV once daily] has been recommended as an alternative to vancomycin, particularly for endocarditis caused by VISA, hVISA, and isolates with a vancomycin MIC of 2 μg/mL. These isolates should be tested to document daptomycin susceptibility. Treatment of endocarditis in which bacteremia persists despite this therapy is beyond the scope of this chapter and requires consultation with an infectious disease specialist. The efficacy of linezolid for left-sided MRSA endocarditis has not been established.

Methicillin-susceptible *S. aureus* endocarditis that is uncomplicated and limited to the tricuspid or pulmonic valve—a condition occurring almost exclusively in injection drug users—can often be treated with a 2-week course that combines oxacillin or nafcillin (but not vancomycin) with gentamicin. Patients with prolonged fever (≥5 days) during therapy or multiple septic pulmonary emboli should receive standard therapy. Right-sided endocarditis caused by MRSA is treated for 4 weeks with a standard vancomycin regimen or with daptomycin (6 mg/kg as a single daily dose).

Staphylococcal PVE is treated for 6–8 weeks with a multidrug regimen. Rifampin is an essential component because it kills staphylococci that are adherent to foreign material in a biofilm. Two other agents (selected on the basis of susceptibility testing) are combined with rifampin to prevent in vivo emergence of resistance. Because many staphylococci (particularly MRSA and *S. epidermidis*) are resistant to gentamicin, susceptibility to gentamicin or an alternative agent should be established before rifampin treatment is begun. If the isolate is resistant to gentamicin, then another aminoglycoside, a fluoroquinolone (chosen on the basis of susceptibility), or another active agent should be substituted for gentamicin.

Other organisms In the absence of meningitis, endocarditis caused by *S. pneumoniae* with a penicillin MIC of ≤1 μg/mL can be treated with IV penicillin (4 million units every 4 h), ceftriaxone (2 g/d as a single dose), or cefotaxime (at a comparable dosage). Infection caused by pneumococcal strains with a penicillin MIC of ≥2 μg/mL should be treated with vancomycin. Until the strain's susceptibility to penicillin is established, therapy should consist of vancomycin plus ceftriaxone, especially if concurrent meningitis is suspected. *P. aeruginosa* endocarditis is treated with an antipseudomonal penicillin (ticarcillin or piperacillin) and high doses of tobramycin (8 mg/kg per day in three divided doses). Endocarditis caused by Enterobacteriaceae is treated with a potent β-lactam antibiotic plus an aminoglycoside. Corynebacterial endocarditis is treated with penicillin plus an aminoglycoside (if the organism is susceptible to the aminoglycoside) or with vancomycin, which is highly bactericidal for most strains. Therapy for *Candida* endocarditis consists of amphotericin B plus flucytosine and early surgery; long-term (if not indefinite) suppression with an oral azole is advised. Caspofungin treatment of *Candida* endocarditis has been effective in sporadic cases; nevertheless, the role of echinocandins in this setting has not been established.

Empirical therapy In the design and execution of therapy without culture data (i.e., before culture results are known or when cultures are negative), clinical clues (e.g., site of infection, patient's predispositions) as well as epidemiologic clues to etiology must be considered. Thus, empirical therapy for acute endocarditis in an injection drug user should cover MRSA and gram-negative bacilli. Treatment with vancomycin plus gentamicin, initiated immediately after blood is obtained for cultures, covers these as well as many other potential causes. Similarly, treatment of health care–associated endocarditis must cover MRSA. In the treatment of culture-negative episodes, marantic endocarditis must be excluded and fastidious organisms sought by serologic testing. In the absence of prior antibiotic therapy, it is unlikely that *S. aureus*, CoNS, or enterococcal infection will present with negative blood cultures; thus, in this situation, recommended empirical therapy targets not these organisms but rather nutritionally variant organisms, the HACEK group, and *Bartonella* species. Pending the availability of diagnostic data, blood culture–negative subacute NVE is treated either with ampicillin-sulbactam (12 g every 24 h) or with ceftriaxone plus gentamicin; doxycycline (100 mg twice daily) is added for *Bartonella* coverage. Vancomycin, gentamicin, cefepime, and rifampin should be used if prosthetic valves in place for ≤1 year are involved. Empirical therapy for infected prosthetic valves in place for >1 year is similar to that for culture-negative PVE. If negative cultures have been confounded by prior antibiotic administration, broader empirical therapy may be indicated, with particular attention to pathogens likely to be inhibited by the specific prior therapy.

Outpatient antimicrobial therapy Fully compliant patients who have sterile blood cultures, no fever, and no clinical or echocardiographic findings that suggest an impending complication may complete therapy as outpatients. Careful follow-up and a stable home setting are necessary, as are predictable IV access and use of antimicrobial agents that are stable in solution.

Monitoring antimicrobial therapy The serum bactericidal titer—the highest dilution of the patient's serum during therapy that kills 99.9% of the standard inoculum of the infecting organism—is no longer recommended for assessment of standard regimens. However, in the treatment of endocarditis caused by unusual organisms, this measurement may provide a patient-specific assessment of in vivo antibiotic effect. Serum concentrations of aminoglycosides and vancomycin should be monitored.

Antibiotic toxicities, including allergic reactions, occur in 25–40% of patients and commonly arise during the third week of therapy. Blood tests to detect renal, hepatic, and hematologic toxicity should be performed periodically.

Blood cultures should be repeated daily until sterile, rechecked if there is recrudescent fever, and performed again 4–6 weeks after therapy to document cure. Blood cultures become sterile within 2 days after the start of appropriate therapy when infection is caused by viridans streptococci, enterococci, or HACEK organisms. In *S. aureus* endocarditis, β-lactam therapy results in sterile cultures in 3–5 days, whereas with MRSA endocarditis positive cultures may persist for 7–9 days with vancomycin treatment. MRSA bacteremia persisting despite an adequate dosage of vancomycin may indicate infection due to a strain with reduced vancomycin susceptibility and therefore may point to a need for alternative therapy. When fever persists for 7 days despite appropriate antibiotic therapy, patients should be evaluated for paravalvular abscess, extracardiac abscesses (spleen, kidney), or complications (embolic events). Recrudescent fever raises the question of these complications but also of drug reactions or complications of hospitalization. Vegetations become smaller with effective therapy; however, 3 months after cure, 50% are unchanged and 25% are slightly larger.

SURGICAL TREATMENT Intracardiac and central nervous system complications of endocarditis are important causes of morbidity and death. In some cases, effective treatment for these complications requires surgery. The indications for cardiac surgical treatment of endocarditis (Table 124-5) have been derived from observational studies and expert opinion. The strength of individual indications vary; thus, the risks and benefits as well as the timing of surgery must be individualized (Table 124-6). From 25% to 40% of patients with left-sided endocarditis undergo cardiac surgery during active infection, with slightly higher surgery rates with PVE than with NVE. Clinical events resulting from intracardiac complications, which are most reliably detected by TEE, justify most surgery. In the absence of randomized trials to evaluate a survival benefit for surgical intervention, the effect of surgery has been assessed in studies comparing populations of medically and surgically treated

TABLE 124-5 Indications for Cardiac Surgical Intervention in Patients With Endocarditis

Surgery required for optimal outcome

Moderate to severe congestive heart failure due to valve dysfunction

Partially dehisced unstable prosthetic valve

Persistent bacteremia despite optimal antimicrobial therapy

Lack of effective microbicidal therapy (e.g., fungal or *Brucella* endocarditis)

S. aureus prosthetic valve endocarditis with an intracardiac complication

Relapse of prosthetic valve endocarditis after optimal antimicrobial therapy

Surgery to be strongly considered for improved outcome[a]

Perivalvular extension of infection

Poorly responsive *S. aureus* endocarditis involving the aortic or mitral valve

Large (>10-mm diameter) hypermobile vegetations with increased risk of embolism

Persistent unexplained fever (≥10 days) in culture-negative native valve endocarditis

Poorly responsive or relapsed endocarditis due to highly antibiotic-resistant enterococci or gram-negative bacilli

[a]Surgery must be carefully considered; findings are often combined with other indications to prompt surgery.

patients matched for the necessity of surgery (indication), with adjustments for predictors of death (comorbidity) and time of the surgical intervention. Although study results vary, surgery for currently advised indications appears to convey a significant

survival benefit (27–55%) that becomes apparent only with follow-up for ≥6 months after the intervention. During the initial weeks after surgery, mortality risk is actually increased (disease-plus surgery-related mortality). With less demanding surgical indications, this combined mortality risk may erode potential long-term benefits. Benefit is greatest for NVE complicated by heart failure or myocardial abscess and is less clear for PVE; this difference may reflect sample size in the relevant studies.

Congestive heart failure Moderate to severe refractory CHF caused by new or worsening valve dysfunction is the major indication for cardiac surgical treatment of endocarditis. At 6 months of follow-up, patients with left-sided endocarditis and moderate to severe heart failure due to valve dysfunction who are treated only medically have a 50% mortality rate; the figure is 15% among matched patients who undergo surgery. The survival benefit with surgery is seen in both NVE and PVE. Surgery can relieve functional stenosis due to large vegetations or restore competence to damaged regurgitant valves by repair or replacement.

Perivalvular infection This complication, which is most common with aortic valve infection, occurs in 10–15% of native valve and 45–60% of prosthetic valve infections. It is suggested by persistent unexplained fever during appropriate therapy, new electrocardiographic conduction disturbances, and pericarditis. TEE with color Doppler is the test of choice to detect perivalvular abscesses (sensitivity, ≥85%). For optimal outcome, surgery is required, especially when fever persists, fistulae develop, prostheses are dehisced and unstable, and invasive infection relapses after appropriate treatment. Cardiac rhythm must be monitored since high-grade heart block may require insertion of a pacemaker.

Uncontrolled infection Continued positive blood cultures or otherwise-unexplained persistent fevers (in patients with either

TABLE 124-6 Timing of Cardiac Surgical Intervention in Patients With Endocarditis

Timing	Indication for Surgical Intervention	
	Strong Supporting Evidence	Conflicting Evidence, but Majority of Opinions Favor Surgery
Emergent (same day)	Acute aortic regurgitation plus preclosure of mitral valve	
	Sinus of Valsalva abscess ruptured into right heart	
	Rupture into pericardial sac	
Urgent (within 1–2 days)	Valve obstruction by vegetation	Major embolus plus persisting large vegetation (>10 mm in diameter)
	Unstable (dehisced) prosthesis	
	Acute aortic or mitral regurgitation with heart failure (New York Heart Association class III or IV)	
	Septal perforation	
	Perivalvular extension of infection with/without new electrocardiographic conduction system changes	
	Lack of effective antibiotic therapy	
Elective (earlier usually preferred)	Progressive paravalvular prosthetic regurgitation	Staphylococcal PVE
	Valve dysfunction plus persisting infection after ≥7–10 days of antimicrobial therapy	Early PVE (≤2 months after valve surgery)
	Fungal (mold) endocarditis	Fungal endocarditis (*Candida* spp.)
		Antibiotic-resistant organisms

Note: PVE, prosthetic valve endocarditis.

Source: Adapted from L Olaison, G Pettersson: Infect Dis Clin North Am 16:453, 2002.

blood culture–positive or –negative endocarditis) despite optimal antibiotic therapy may reflect uncontrolled infection and may warrant surgery. Surgical treatment is also advised for endocarditis caused by organisms for which experience indicates that effective antimicrobial therapy is lacking (e.g., yeasts, fungi, *P. aeruginosa*, other highly resistant gram-negative bacilli, *Brucella* species, and probably *C. burnetii*).

***S. aureus* endocarditis** The mortality rate for *S. aureus* PVE exceeds 50% with medical treatment but is reduced to 25% with surgical treatment. In patients with intracardiac complications associated with *S. aureus* PVE, surgical treatment reduces the mortality rate twentyfold. Surgical treatment should be considered for patients with *S. aureus* native aortic or mitral valve infection who have TTE-demonstrable vegetations and remain septic during the initial week of therapy. Isolated tricuspid valve endocarditis, even with persistent fever, rarely requires surgery.

Prevention of systemic emboli Death and persisting morbidity due to emboli are largely limited to patients suffering occlusion of cerebral or coronary arteries. Echocardiographic determination of vegetation size and anatomy, although predictive of patients at high risk of systemic emboli, does not identify those patients in whom the benefits of surgery to prevent emboli clearly exceed the risks of the surgical procedure. Net benefits from surgery to prevent emboli are most likely when other surgical benefits can be achieved simultaneously—e.g., repair of a moderately dysfunctional valve or debridement of a paravalvular abscess. Only 3.5% of patients undergo surgery solely to prevent systemic emboli. Valve repair avoiding insertion of a prosthesis makes the benefit-to-risk ratio of surgery to address vegetations more favorable.

Timing of cardiac surgery In general, when indications for surgical treatment of infective endocarditis are identified, surgery should not be delayed simply to permit additional antibiotic therapy, since this course of action increases the risk of death (Table 124-6). After 14 days of recommended antibiotic therapy, excised valves are culture-negative in 99% and 50% of patients with streptococcal and *S. aureus* endocarditis, respectively. Recrudescent endocarditis on a new implanted prosthetic valve follows surgery for active NVE and PVE in 2% and 6–15% of patients, respectively. These frequencies do not justify the risk of adverse outcome with delayed surgery, particularly in patients with severe heart failure, valve dysfunction, and staphylococcal infections. Delay is justified only when infection is controlled and CHF is resolved with medical therapy.

Among patients who have experienced a neurologic complication of endocarditis, further neurologic deterioration can occur as a consequence of cardiac surgery. The risk of neurologic deterioration is related to the type of neurologic complication and the interval between the complication and surgery. Whenever feasible, cardiac surgery should be delayed for 2–3 weeks after a nonhemorrhagic embolic infarction and for 4 weeks after a cerebral hemorrhage. A ruptured mycotic aneurysm should be treated before cardiac surgery.

Antibiotic therapy after cardiac surgery Bacteria visible in Gram-stained preparations of excised valves do not necessarily indicate a failure of antibiotic therapy. Organisms have been detected on Gram's stain—or their DNA has been detected by PCR—in excised valves from 45% of patients who have successfully completed the recommended therapy for endocarditis. In only 7% of these patients are the organisms, most of which are unusual and antibiotic resistant, cultured from the valve. Despite the detection of organisms or their DNA, relapse of

endocarditis after surgery is uncommon. Thus, when valve cultures are negative in uncomplicated NVE caused by susceptible organisms, the duration of preoperative plus postoperative treatment should equal the total duration of recommended therapy, with ~2 weeks of treatment administered after surgery. For endocarditis complicated by paravalvular abscess, partially treated PVE, or cases with culture-positive valves, a full course of therapy should be given postoperatively.

Extracardiac complications Splenic abscess develops in 3–5% of patients with endocarditis. Effective therapy requires either image-guided percutaneous drainage or splenectomy. Mycotic aneurysms occur in 2–15% of endocarditis patients; one-half of these cases involve the cerebral arteries and present as headaches, focal neurologic symptoms, or hemorrhage. Cerebral aneurysms should be monitored by angiography. Some will resolve with effective antimicrobial therapy, but those that persist, enlarge, or leak should be treated surgically if possible. Extracerebral aneurysms present as local pain, a mass, local ischemia, or bleeding; these aneurysms are treated by resection.

■ OUTCOME

Older age, severe comorbid conditions and diabetes, delayed diagnosis, involvement of prosthetic valves or the aortic valve, an invasive (*S. aureus*) or antibiotic-resistant (*P. aeruginosa*, yeast) pathogen, intracardiac and major neurologic complications, and an association with health care adversely affect outcome. Death and poor outcome often are related not to failure of antibiotic therapy but rather to the interactions of comorbidities and endocarditis-related end-organ complications. Overall survival rates for patients with NVE caused by viridans streptococci, HACEK organisms, or enterococci (susceptible to synergistic therapy) are 85–90%. For *S. aureus* NVE in patients who do not inject drugs, survival rates are 55–70%, whereas 85–90% of injection drug users survive this infection. PVE beginning within 2 months of valve replacement results in mortality rates of 40–50%, whereas rates are only 10–20% in later-onset cases.

■ PREVENTION

In the past, in an effort to prevent endocarditis (long a goal in clinical practice), expert committees have supported systemic antibiotic administration prior to many bacteremia-inducing procedures. In the absence of human trials, a reappraisal of the indirect evidence for antibiotic prophylaxis for endocarditis by the American Heart Association has culminated in guidelines that reverse prior recommendations and restrict prophylactic antibiotic use. At best, the benefit of antibiotic prophylaxis is minimal. Most endocarditis cases do not follow a procedure. In case-control studies, dental treatments—widely considered as predisposing to endocarditis—occur no more frequently before endocarditis than in matched controls. Furthermore, the frequency and magnitude of bacteremia associated with dental procedures and routine daily activities (e.g., tooth brushing and flossing) are similar. Because dental procedures are infrequent, exposure of cardiac structures to bacteremic oral-cavity organisms is notably greater from routine daily activities than from dental care. The relation of gastrointestinal and genitourinary procedures to subsequent endocarditis is more tenuous than that of dental procedures. In addition, cost-effectiveness and cost-benefit estimates suggest that antibiotic prophylaxis represents a poor use of resources.

Studies in animal models suggest that antibiotic prophylaxis may be effective. Thus it is possible that rare cases of endocarditis are prevented. Weighing the potential benefits, potential adverse events, and costs associated with antibiotic prophylaxis, the American

TABLE 124-7 Antibiotic Regimens for Prophylaxis of Endocarditis in Adults With High-Risk Cardiac Lesions[a,b]

A. Standard oral regimen
    1. Amoxicillin: 2 g PO 1 h before procedure
B. Inability to take oral medication
    1. Ampicillin: 2 g IV or IM within 1 h before procedure
C. Penicillin allergy
    1. Clarithromycin or azithromycin: 500 mg PO 1 h before procedure
    2. Cephalexin[c]: 2 g PO 1 h before procedure
    3. Clindamycin: 600 mg PO 1 h before procedure
D. Penicillin allergy, inability to take oral medication
    1. Cefazolin[c] or ceftriaxone[c]: 1 g IV or IM 30 min before procedure
    2. Clindamycin: 600 mg IV or IM 1 h before procedure

[a]Dosing for children: for amoxicillin, ampicillin, cephalexin, or cefadroxil, use 50 mg/kg PO; cefazolin, 25 mg/kg IV; clindamycin, 20 mg/kg PO, 25 mg/kg IV; clarithromycin, 15 mg/kg PO; and vancomycin, 20 mg/kg IV.

[b]For high-risk lesions, see Table 124-8. Prophylaxis is not advised for other lesions.

[c]Do not use cephalosporins in patients with immediate hypersensitivity (urticaria, angioedema, anaphylaxis) to penicillin.

Source: W Wilson et al: Circulation, published online 4/19/2007.

Heart Association and the European Society of Cardiology now recommend prophylactic antibiotics (Table 124-7) only for those patients at highest risk for severe morbidity or death from endocarditis (Table 124-8). Maintaining good dental hygiene is essential. Prophylaxis is recommended only when there is manipulation of gingival tissue or the periapical region of the teeth or perforation of the oral mucosa (including surgery on the respiratory tract). Prophylaxis is not advised for patients undergoing gastrointestinal or genitourinary tract procedures. High-risk patients should be treated before or when they undergo procedures on an infected genitourinary tract or on infected skin and soft tissue. The British Society for Antimicrobial Chemotherapy continues to recommend prophylaxis for at-risk patients undergoing selected gastrointestinal and genitourinary procedures. In contrast, the National Institute for Health and Clinical Excellence in the United Kingdom found no convincing evidence that antibiotic prophylaxis was cost effective and advised discontinuation of the practice (see *www.nice.org.uk/guidance/CG64*).

TABLE 124-8 High-Risk Cardiac Lesions for Which Endocarditis Prophylaxis Is Advised Before Dental Procedures

Prosthetic heart valves

Prior endocarditis

Unrepaired cyanotic congenital heart disease, including palliative shunts or conduits

Completely repaired congenital heart defects during the 6 months after repair

Incompletely repaired congenital heart disease with residual defects adjacent to prosthetic material

Valvulopathy developing after cardiac transplantation

Source: W Wilson et al: Circulation, published online 4/19/2007.

FURTHER READINGS

Aksoy O et al: Early surgery in patients with infective endocarditis: A propensity score analysis. Clin Infect Dis 44:364, 2007

Baddour LM et al: Diagnosis, antimicrobial therapy, and management of complications. A statement for healthcare professionals from the Committee on Rheumatic Fever, Endocarditis, and Kawasaki Disease, Council on Cardiovascular Disease in the Young, and the Councils on Clinical Cardiology, Stroke, and Cardiovascular Surgery and Anesthesia, American Heart Association. Circulation 111:e394, 2005

Bannay A et al: The impact of valve surgery on short- and long-term mortality in left-sided infective endocarditis: Do differences in methodological approaches explain previous conflicting results? Eur Heart J epub ahead of print, Feb 9, 2009 (*http://eurheartj.oxfordjournal.org/content/early/2009/02/09/eurheartj.ehp008*)

Benito N et al: Health care–associated native valve endocarditis: Importance of non-nosocomial acquisition. Ann Intern Med 150:586, 2009

Cosgrove SE et al: Initial low-dose gentamicin for *Staphylococcus aureus* bacteremia and endocarditis is nephrotoxic. Clin Infect Dis 48:713, 2009

Durack DT: Prevention of infective endocarditis, in *Principles and Practice of Infectious Diseases,* 7th ed, GL Mandell et al (eds). Philadelphia, Elsevier Churchill Livingstone, 2010, pp 1143–1151

Fowler VG Jr et al: Endocarditis and intravascular infections, in *Principles and Practice of Infectious Diseases,* 7th ed, GL Mandell et al (eds). Philadelphia, Elsevier Churchill Livingstone, 2010, pp 1067–1112

Habib G et al: Guidelines on the prevention, diagnosis, and treatment of infective endocarditis (new version 2009). Eur Heart J 30:2369, 2009

Murdoch DR et al: Clinical presentation, etiology, and outcome of infective endocarditis in the 21st century. Arch Intern Med 169:463, 2009

Rybak MJ et al: Vancomycin therapeutic guidelines: A summary of consensus recommendations from the Infectious Diseases Society of America, the American Society of Health-System Pharmacists, and the Society of Infectious Diseases Pharmacists. Clin Infect Dis 49:325, 2009

Thuny F et al: The timing of surgery influences mortality and morbidity in adults with severe complicated infective endocarditis: A propensity analysis. Eur Heart J epub ahead of print, March 26, 2009 (*http://eurheartj.oxfordjournal.org/content/early/2009/03/26/eurheartj.ehp089*)

Wilson W et al: Prevention of infective endocarditis. Guidelines from the American Heart Association. A guideline from the American Heart Association Rheumatic Fever, Endocarditis, and Kawasaki Disease Committee, Council on Cardiovascular Disease in the Young, and the Council on Clinical Cardiology, Council on Cardiovascular Surgery and Anesthesia, and the Quality of Care and Outcomes Research Interdisciplinary Working Group. Circulation 116:1736, 2007

CHAPTER 125

Infections of the Skin, Muscles, and Soft Tissues

Dennis L. Stevens

■ ANATOMIC RELATIONSHIPS: CLUES TO THE DIAGNOSIS OF SOFT TISSUE INFECTIONS

Skin and soft tissue infections have been common human afflictions for centuries. However, between 2000 and 2004, hospital admissions for skin and soft tissue infections rose by 27%, a remarkable increase that was attributable largely to the emergence of the USA300 clone of methicillin-resistant *Staphylococcus aureus* (MRSA). This chapter provides an anatomic approach to understanding the types of soft tissue infections and the diverse microbes responsible.

Protection against infection of the epidermis depends on the mechanical barrier afforded by the stratum corneum, since the epidermis itself is devoid of blood vessels (Fig. 125-1). Disruption of this layer by burns or bites, abrasions, foreign bodies, primary dermatologic disorders (e.g., herpes simplex, varicella, ecthyma gangrenosum), surgery, or vascular or pressure ulcer allows penetration of bacteria to the deeper structures. Similarly, the hair follicle can serve as a portal either for components of the normal flora (e.g., *Staphylococcus*) or for extrinsic bacteria (e.g., *Pseudomonas* in hottub folliculitis). Intracellular infection of the squamous epithelium with vesicle formation may arise from cutaneous inoculation, as in infection with herpes simplex virus (HSV) type 1; from the dermal capillary plexus, as in varicella and infections due to other viruses associated with viremia; or from cutaneous nerve roots, as in herpes zoster. Bacteria infecting the epidermis, such as *Streptococcus pyogenes*, may be translocated laterally to deeper structures via lymphatics, an event that results in the rapid superficial spread of erysipelas. Later, engorgement or obstruction of lymphatics causes

flaccid edema of the epidermis, another characteristic of erysipelas.

The rich plexus of capillaries beneath the dermal papillae provides nutrition to the stratum germinativum, and physiologic responses of this plexus produce important clinical signs and symptoms. For example, infective vasculitis of the plexus results in petechiae, Osler's nodes, Janeway lesions, and palpable purpura, which, if present, are important clues to the existence of endocarditis (Chap. 124). In addition, metastatic infection within this plexus can result in cutaneous manifestations of disseminated fungal infection (Chap. 203), gonococcal infection (Chap. 144), *Salmonella* infection (Chap. 153), *Pseudomonas* infection (i.e., ecthyma gangrenosum; Chap. 152), meningococcemia (Chap. 143), and staphylococcal infection (Chap. 135). The plexus also provides bacteria with access to the circulation, thereby facilitating local spread or bacteremia. The postcapillary venules of this plexus are a major site of polymorphonuclear leukocyte sequestration, diapedesis, and chemotaxis to the site of cutaneous infection.

Exaggeration of these physiologic mechanisms by excessive levels of cytokines or bacterial toxins causes leukostasis, venous occlusion, and pitting edema. Edema with purple bullae, ecchymosis, and cutaneous anesthesia suggests loss of vascular integrity and necessitates exploration of the deeper structures for evidence of necrotizing fasciitis or myonecrosis. An early diagnosis requires a high level of suspicion in instances of unexplained fever and of pain and tenderness in the soft tissue, even in the absence of acute cutaneous inflammation.

Table 125-1 indicates the chapters in which the infections described below are discussed in greater detail. Many of these infections are illustrated in the chapters cited or in Chap. e7 (Atlas of Rashes Associated With Fever).

■ INFECTIONS ASSOCIATED WITH VESICLES

(Table 125-1) Vesicle formation due to infection is caused by viral proliferation within the epidermis. In varicella and variola, viremia precedes the onset of a diffuse centripetal rash that progresses from macules to vesicles, then to pustules, and finally to scabs over the course of 1–2 weeks. Vesicles of varicella have a "dewdrop" appearance and develop in crops randomly about the trunk, extremities, and face over 3–4 days. Herpes zoster occurs in a single dermatome; the appearance of vesicles is preceded by pain for several days. Zoster may occur in persons of any age but is most common among immunosuppressed individuals and elderly patients, whereas most cases of varicella occur in young children. Vesicles due to HSV are found on or around the lips (HSV-1) or genitals (HSV-2) but may appear on the head and neck of young wrestlers (herpes gladiatorum) or on the digits of health care workers (herpetic whitlow). Recurrent herpes labialis (HSV-1) and herpes genitalis commonly follow primary infection. Coxsackievirus A16 characteristically causes vesicles on the hands, feet, and mouth of children. Orf is caused by a DNA virus related to smallpox virus and infects the fingers of individuals who work around goats and sheep. Molluscum contagiosum virus induces flaccid vesicles on the skin of healthy and immunocompromised individuals. Although variola (smallpox) in nature was eradicated as of 1977, recent terrorist events have renewed interest in this devastating infection (Chap. 221). Viremia beginning after an incubation period of 12 days is followed by a diffuse maculopapular rash, with rapid evolution to vesicles, pustules, and then scabs. Secondary cases can occur among close contacts.

Rickettsialpox begins after mite-bite inoculation of *Rickettsia akari* into the skin. A papule with a central vesicle evolves to form a 1- to 2.5-cm painless crusted black eschar with an erythematous halo and proximal adenopathy. While more common in the northeastern United States and the Ukraine in 1940–1950,

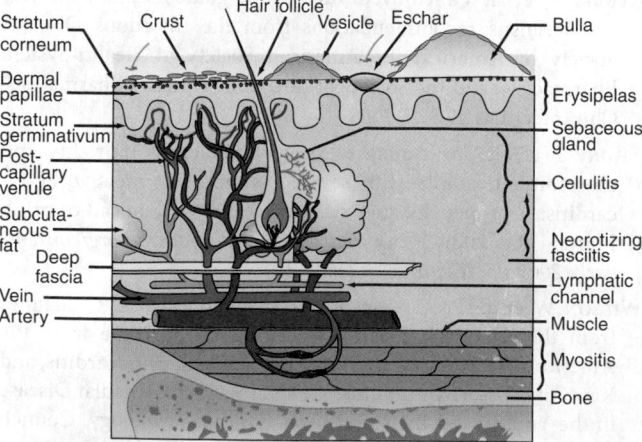

Figure 125-1 Structural components of the skin and soft tissue, superficial infections, and infections of the deeper structures. The rich capillary network beneath the dermal papillae plays a key role in the localization of infection and in the development of the acute inflammatory reaction.

TABLE 125-1 Skin and Soft Tissue Infections

Lesion, Clinical Syndrome	Infectious Agent	Chapter(s)
Vesicles		
Smallpox	Variola virus	221
Chickenpox	Varicella-zoster virus	180
Shingles (herpes zoster)	Varicella-zoster virus	180
Cold sores, herpetic whitlow, herpes gladiatorum	Herpes simplex virus	179
Hand-foot-and-mouth disease	Coxsackievirus A16	191
Orf	Parapoxvirus	183
Molluscum contagiosum	Pox-like virus	183
Rickettsialpox	*Rickettsia akari*	174
Blistering distal dactylitis	*Staphylococcus aureus* or *Streptococcus pyogenes*	135, 136
Bullae		
Staphylococcal scalded-skin syndrome	*S. aureus*	135
Necrotizing fasciitis	*S. pyogenes, Clostridium* spp., mixed aerobes and anaerobes	136, 142, 164
Gas gangrene	*Clostridium* spp.	142
Halophilic vibrio	*Vibrio vulnificus*	156
Crusted lesions		
Bullous impetigo/ecthyma	*S. aureus*	135
Impetigo contagiosa	*S. pyogenes*	136
Ringworm	Superficial dermatophyte fungi	206
Sporotrichosis	*Sporothrix schenckii*	206
Histoplasmosis	*Histoplasma capsulatum*	199
Coccidioidomycosis	*Coccidioides immitis*	200
Blastomycosis	*Blastomyces dermatitidis*	201
Cutaneous leishmaniasis	*Leishmania* spp.	212
Cutaneous tuberculosis	*Mycobacterium tuberculosis*	165
Nocardiosis	*Nocardia asteroides*	162
Folliculitis		
Furunculosis	*S. aureus*	135
Hot-tub folliculitis	*Pseudomonas aeruginosa*	152
Swimmer's itch	*Schistosoma* spp.	219
Acne vulgaris	*Propionibacterium acnes*	52
Papular and nodular lesions		
Fish-tank or swimming-pool granuloma	*Mycobacterium marinum*	167
Creeping eruption (cutaneous larva migrans)	*Ancylostoma braziliense*	216
Dracunculiasis	*Dracunculus medinensis*	218
Cercarial dermatitis	*Schistosoma mansoni*	219
Verruca vulgaris	Human papillomaviruses 1, 2, 4	185
Condylomata acuminata (anogenital warts)	Human papillomaviruses 6, 11, 16, 18	185
Onchocerciasis nodule	*Onchocerca volvulus*	218
Cutaneous myiasis	*Dermatobia hominis*	397
Verruca peruana	*Bartonella bacilliformis*	160
Cat-scratch disease	*Bartonella henselae*	160
Lepromatous leprosy	*Mycobacterium leprae*	166

(continued)

TABLE 125-1 Skin and Soft Tissue Infections (*Continued*)

Lesion, Clinical Syndrome	Infectious Agent	Chapter(s)
Secondary syphilis (papulosquamous and nodular lesions, condylomata lata)	*Treponema pallidum*	169
Tertiary syphilis (nodular gummatous lesions)	*T. pallidum*	169
Ulcers with or without eschars		
Anthrax	*Bacillus anthracis*	221
Ulceroglandular tularemia	*Francisella tularensis*	158, 221
Bubonic plague	*Yersinia pestis*	159, 221
Buruli ulcer	*Mycobacterium ulcerans*	167
Leprosy	*M. leprae*	166
Cutaneous tuberculosis	*M. tuberculosis*	165
Chancroid	*Haemophilus ducreyi*	145
Primary syphilis	*T. pallidum*	169
Erysipelas	*S. pyogenes*	136
Cellulitis	*Staphylococcus* spp., *Streptococcus* spp., various other bacteria	Various
Necrotizing fasciitis		
Streptococcal gangrene	*S. pyogenes*	136
Fournier's gangrene	Mixed aerobic and anaerobic bacteria	164
Staphylococcal necrotizing fasciitis	Methicillin-resistant *S. aureus*	135
Myositis and myonecrosis		
Pyomyositis	*S. aureus*	135
Streptococcal necrotizing myositis	*S. pyogenes*	136
Gas gangrene	*Clostridium* spp.	142
Nonclostridial (crepitant) myositis	Mixed aerobic and anaerobic bacteria	164
Synergistic nonclostridial anaerobic myonecrosis	Mixed aerobic and anaerobic bacteria	164

rickettsialpox has recently been described in Ohio, Arizona, and Utah. Blistering dactylitis is a painful, vesicular, localized *S. aureus* or group A streptococcal infection of the pulps of the distal digits of the hands.

■ INFECTIONS ASSOCIATED WITH BULLAE

(Table 125-1) Staphylococcal scalded-skin syndrome (SSSS) in neonates is caused by a toxin (exfoliatin) from phage group II *S. aureus*. SSSS must be distinguished from toxic epidermal necrolysis (TEN), which occurs primarily in adults, is drug-induced, and is associated with a higher mortality rate. Punch biopsy with frozen section is useful in making this distinction since the cleavage plane is the stratum corneum in SSSS and the stratum germinativum in TEN (Fig. 125-1). Intravenous γ-globulin is a promising treatment for TEN. Necrotizing fasciitis and gas gangrene also induce bulla formation (see "Necrotizing Fasciitis," below). Halophilic vibrio infection can be as aggressive and fulminant as necrotizing fasciitis; a helpful clue in its diagnosis is a history of exposure to waters of the Gulf of Mexico or the Atlantic seaboard or (in a patient with cirrhosis) the ingestion of raw seafood. The etiologic organism (*Vibrio vulnificus*) is highly susceptible to tetracycline.

■ INFECTIONS ASSOCIATED WITH CRUSTED LESIONS

(Table 125-1) Impetigo contagiosa is caused by *S. pyogenes*, and bullous impetigo is due to *S. aureus*. Both skin lesions may have an early bullous stage but then appear as thick crusts with a golden-brown color. Epidemics of impetigo caused by MRSA have been reported. Streptococcal lesions are most common among children 2–5 years of age, and epidemics may occur in settings of poor hygiene, particularly among children in lower socioeconomic settings in tropical climates. It is important to recognize impetigo contagiosa because of its relationship to poststreptococcal glomerulonephritis. Rheumatic fever is not a complication of skin infection caused by *S. pyogenes*. Superficial dermatophyte infection (ringworm) can occur on any skin surface, and skin scrapings with KOH staining are diagnostic. Primary infections with dimorphic fungi such as *Blastomyces dermatitidis* and *Sporothrix schenckii* can initially present as crusted skin lesions resembling ringworm. Disseminated infection with *Coccidioides immitis* can also involve the skin, and biopsy and culture should be performed on crusted lesions in patients from endemic areas. Crusted nodular lesions caused by *Mycobacterium chelonei* have been described in HIV-seropositive patients. Treatment with clarithromycin looks promising.

■ FOLLICULITIS

(Table 125-1) Hair follicles serve as portals for a number of bacteria, although *S. aureus* is the most common cause of localized folliculitis. Sebaceous glands empty into hair follicles and ducts and, if these portals are blocked, form sebaceous cysts that may resemble staphylococcal abscesses or may become secondarily infected.

Infection of sweat glands (hidradenitis suppurativa) can also mimic infection of hair follicles, particularly in the axillae. Chronic folliculitis is uncommon except in acne vulgaris, where constituents of the normal flora (e.g., *Propionibacterium acnes*) may play a role.

Diffuse folliculitis occurs in two settings. Hot-tub folliculitis is caused by *Pseudomonas aeruginosa* in waters that are insufficiently chlorinated and maintained at temperatures of 37–40°C. Infection is usually self-limited, although bacteremia and shock have been reported. Swimmer's itch occurs when a skin surface is exposed to water infested with freshwater avian schistosomes. Warm water temperatures and alkaline pH are suitable for mollusks that serve as intermediate hosts between birds and humans. Free-swimming schistosomal cercariae readily penetrate human hair follicles or pores but quickly die and elicit a brisk allergic reaction, causing intense itching and erythema.

■ PAPULAR AND NODULAR LESIONS

(Table 125-1) Raised lesions of the skin occur in many different forms. *Mycobacterium marinum* infections of the skin may present as cellulitis or as raised erythematous nodules. Erythematous papules are early manifestations of cat-scratch disease (with lesions developing at the primary site of inoculation of *Bartonella henselae*) and bacillary angiomatosis (also caused by *B. henselae*). Raised serpiginous or linear eruptions are characteristic of cutaneous larva migrans, which is caused by burrowing larvae of dog or cat hookworms (*Ancylostoma braziliense*) and which humans acquire through contact with soil that has been contaminated with dog or cat feces. Similar burrowing raised lesions are present in dracunculiasis caused by migration of the adult female nematode *Dracunculus medinensis*. Nodules caused by *Onchocerca volvulus* measure 1–10 cm in diameter and occur mostly in persons bitten by *Simulium* flies in Africa. The nodules contain the adult worm encased in fibrous tissue. Migration of microfilariae into the eyes may result in blindness. Verruga peruana is caused by *Bartonella bacilliformis*, which is transmitted to humans by the sandfly *Phlebotomus*. This condition can take the form of single gigantic lesions (several centimeters in diameter) or multiple small lesions (several millimeters in diameter). Numerous subcutaneous nodules may also be present in cysticercosis caused by larvae of *Taenia solium*. Multiple erythematous papules develop in schistosomiasis; each represents a cercarial invasion site. Skin nodules as well as thickened subcutaneous tissue are prominent features of lepromatous leprosy. Large nodules or gummas are features of tertiary syphilis, whereas flat papulosquamous lesions are characteristic of secondary syphilis. Human papillomavirus may cause singular warts (verruca vulgaris) or multiple warts in the anogenital area (condylomata acuminata). The latter are major problems in HIV-infected individuals.

■ ULCERS WITH OR WITHOUT ESCHARS

(Table 125-1) Cutaneous anthrax begins as a pruritic papule, which develops within days into an ulcer with surrounding vesicles and edema and then into an enlarging ulcer with a black eschar. Cutaneous anthrax may cause chronic nonhealing ulcers with an overlying dirty-gray membrane, although lesions may also mimic psoriasis, eczema, or impetigo. Ulceroglandular tularemia may have associated ulcerated skin lesions with painful regional adenopathy. Although buboes are the major cutaneous manifestation of plague, ulcers with eschars, papules, or pustules are also present in 25% of cases.

Mycobacterium ulcerans typically causes chronic skin ulcers on the extremities of individuals living in the tropics. *Mycobacterium leprae* may be associated with cutaneous ulcerations in patients with lepromatous leprosy related to Lucio's phenomenon, in which immune-mediated destruction of tissue bearing high concentrations

of *M. leprae* bacilli occurs, usually several months after initiation of effective therapy. *Mycobacterium tuberculosis* may also cause ulcerations, papules, or erythematous macular lesions of the skin in both normal and immunocompromised patients.

Decubitus ulcers are due to tissue hypoxemia secondary to pressure-induced vascular insufficiency and may become secondarily infected with components of the skin and gastrointestinal flora, including anaerobes. Ulcerative lesions on the anterior shins may be due to pyoderma gangrenosum, which must be distinguished from similar lesions of infectious etiology by histologic evaluation of biopsy sites. Ulcerated lesions on the genitals may be either painful (chancroid) or painless (primary syphilis).

■ ERYSIPELAS

(Table 125-1) Erysipelas is due to *S. pyogenes* and is characterized by an abrupt onset of fiery-red swelling of the face or extremities. The distinctive features of erysipelas are well-defined indurated margins, particularly along the nasolabial fold; rapid progression; and intense pain. Flaccid bullae may develop during the second or third day of illness, but extension to deeper soft tissues is rare. Treatment with penicillin is effective; swelling may progress despite appropriate treatment, although fever, pain, and the intense red color diminish. Desquamation of the involved skin occurs 5–10 days into the illness. Infants and elderly adults are most commonly afflicted, and the severity of systemic toxicity varies.

■ CELLULITIS

(Table 125-1) Cellulitis is an acute inflammatory condition of the skin that is characterized by localized pain, erythema, swelling, and heat. It may be caused by indigenous flora colonizing the skin and appendages (e.g., *S. aureus* and *S. pyogenes*) or by a wide variety of exogenous bacteria. Because the exogenous bacteria involved in cellulitis occupy unique niches in nature, a thorough history (including epidemiologic data) provides important clues to etiology. When there is drainage, an open wound, or an obvious portal of entry, Gram's stain and culture provide a definitive diagnosis. In the absence of these findings, the bacterial etiology of cellulitis is difficult to establish, and in some cases staphylococcal and streptococcal cellulitis may have similar features. Even with needle aspiration of the leading edge or a punch biopsy of the cellulitis tissue itself, cultures are positive in only 20% of cases. This observation suggests that relatively low numbers of bacteria may cause cellulitis and that the expanding area of erythema within the skin may be a direct effect of extracellular toxins or of the soluble mediators of inflammation elicited by the host.

Bacteria may gain access to the epidermis through cracks in the skin, abrasions, cuts, burns, insect bites, surgical incisions, and IV catheters. Cellulitis caused by *S. aureus* spreads from a central localized infection, such as an abscess, folliculitis, or an infected foreign body (e.g., a splinter, a prosthetic device, or an IV catheter). MRSA is rapidly replacing methicillin-sensitive *S. aureus* (MSSA) as a cause of cellulitis in both inpatient and outpatient settings. Cellulitis caused by MSSA or MRSA is usually associated with a focal infection, such as a furuncle, a carbuncle, a surgical wound, or an abscess. In contrast, cellulitis due to *S. pyogenes* is a more rapidly spreading, diffuse process that is frequently associated with lymphangitis and fever. Recurrent streptococcal cellulitis of the lower extremities may be caused by organisms of group A, C, or G in association with chronic venous stasis or with saphenous venectomy for coronary artery bypass surgery. Streptococci also cause recurrent cellulitis among patients with chronic lymphedema resulting from elephantiasis, lymph node dissection, or Milroy's disease. Recurrent staphylococcal cutaneous infections are more common among individuals who have eosinophilia and elevated serum levels of IgE (Job's syndrome) and among nasal carriers of staphylococci. Cellulitis caused by *Streptococcus agalactiae* (group B *Streptococcus*) occurs primarily in elderly patients and those with diabetes mellitus or peripheral vascular disease. *Haemophilus influenzae* typically causes periorbital cellulitis in children in association with sinusitis, otitis media, or epiglottitis. It is unclear whether this form of cellulitis will (like meningitis) become less common as a result of the impressive efficacy of the *H. influenzae* type b vaccine.

Many other bacteria also cause cellulitis. It is fortunate that these organisms occur in such characteristic settings that a good history provides useful clues to the diagnosis. Cellulitis associated with cat bites and, to a lesser degree, with dog bites is commonly caused by *Pasteurella multocida*, although in the latter case *Staphylococcus intermedius* and *Capnocytophaga canimorsus* (formerly DF-2) must also be considered. Sites of cellulitis and abscesses associated with dog bites and human bites also contain a variety of anaerobic organisms, including *Fusobacterium*, *Bacteroides*, aerobic and anaerobic streptococci, and *Eikenella corrodens*. *Pasteurella* is notoriously resistant to dicloxacillin and nafcillin but is sensitive to all other β-lactam antimicrobial agents as well as to quinolones, tetracycline, and erythromycin. Ampicillin/clavulanate, ampicillin/sulbactam, and cefoxitin are good choices for the treatment of animal or human bite infections. *Aeromonas hydrophila* causes aggressive cellulitis in tissues surrounding lacerations sustained in freshwater (lakes, rivers, and streams). This organism remains sensitive to aminoglycosides, fluoroquinolones, chloramphenicol, trimethoprim- sulfamethoxazole, and third-generation cephalosporins; it is resistant to ampicillin, however.

P. aeruginosa causes three types of soft tissue infection: ecthyma gangrenosum in neutropenic patients, hot-tub folliculitis, and cellulitis following penetrating injury. Most commonly, *P. aeruginosa* is introduced into the deep tissues when a person steps on a nail. Treatment includes surgical inspection and drainage, particularly if the injury also involves bone or joint capsule. Choices for empirical treatment while antimicrobial susceptibility data are awaited include an aminoglycoside, a third-generation cephalosporin (ceftazidime, cefoperazone, or cefotaxime), a semisynthetic penicillin (ticarcillin, mezlocillin, or piperacillin), or a fluoroquinolone (although drugs of the last class are not indicated for the treatment of children <13 years old).

Gram-negative bacillary cellulitis, including that due to *P. aeruginosa*, is most common among hospitalized, immunocompromised hosts. Cultures and sensitivity tests are critically important in this setting because of multidrug resistance (Chap. 152).

The gram-positive aerobic rod *Erysipelothrix rhusiopathiae* is most often associated with fish and domestic swine and causes cellulitis primarily in bone renderers and fishmongers. *E. rhusiopathiae* remains susceptible to most β-lactam antibiotics (including penicillin), erythromycin, clindamycin, tetracycline, and cephalosporins but is resistant to sulfonamides, chloramphenicol, and vancomycin. Its resistance to vancomycin, which is unusual among gram-positive bacteria, is of potential clinical significance since this agent is sometimes used in empirical therapy for skin infection. Fish food containing the water flea *Daphnia* is sometimes contaminated with *M. marinum*, which can cause cellulitis or granulomas on skin surfaces exposed to the water in aquariums or injured in swimming pools. Rifampin plus ethambutol has been an effective therapeutic combination in some cases, although no comprehensive studies have been undertaken. In addition, some strains of *M. marinum* are susceptible to tetracycline or to trimethoprim-sulfamethoxazole.

■ NECROTIZING FASCIITIS

(Table 125-1) Necrotizing fasciitis, formerly called streptococcal gangrene, may be associated with group A *Streptococcus* or mixed aerobic-anaerobic bacteria or may occur as part of gas gangrene

caused by *Clostridium perfringens*. Strains of MRSA that produce the Panton-Valentine leukocidin (PVL) toxin have been reported to cause necrotizing fasciitis. Early diagnosis may be difficult when pain or unexplained fever is the only presenting manifestation. Swelling then develops and is followed by brawny edema and tenderness. With progression, dark-red induration of the epidermis appears, along with bullae filled with blue or purple fluid. Later the skin becomes friable and takes on a bluish, maroon, or black color. By this stage, thrombosis of blood vessels in the dermal papillae (Fig. 125-1) is extensive. Extension of infection to the level of the deep fascia causes this tissue to take on a brownish-gray appearance. Rapid spread occurs along fascial planes, through venous channels and lymphatics. Patients in the later stages are toxic and frequently manifest shock and multiorgan failure.

Necrotizing fasciitis caused by mixed aerobic-anaerobic bacteria begins with a breach in the integrity of a mucous membrane barrier, such as the mucosa of the gastrointestinal or genitourinary tract. The portal can be a malignancy, a diverticulum, a hemorrhoid, an anal fissure, or a urethral tear. Other predisposing factors include peripheral vascular disease, diabetes mellitus, surgery, and penetrating injury to the abdomen. Leakage into the perineal area results in a syndrome called *Fournier's gangrene*, characterized by massive swelling of the scrotum and penis with extension into the perineum or the abdominal wall and legs.

Necrotizing fasciitis caused by *S. pyogenes* has increased in frequency and severity since 1985. There are two distinct clinical presentations: those with no portal of entry and those with a defined portal of entry. Infections in the first category often begin deep at the site of a nonpenetrating minor trauma, such as a bruise or a muscle strain. Seeding of the site via transient bacteremia is likely, although most patients deny antecedent streptococcal infection. The affected patients present with only severe pain and fever. Late in the course, the classic signs of necrotizing fasciitis, such as purple (violaceous) bullae, skin sloughing, and progressive toxicity, develop. In infections of the second type, *S. pyogenes* may reach the deep fascia from a site of cutaneous infection or penetrating trauma. These patients have early signs of superficial skin infection with progression to necrotizing fasciitis. In either case, toxicity is severe, and renal impairment may precede the development of shock. In 20–40% of cases, myositis occurs concomitantly, and, as in gas gangrene (see below), serum creatine phosphokinase levels may be markedly elevated. Necrotizing fasciitis due to mixed aerobic-anaerobic bacteria may be associated with gas in deep tissue, but gas usually is not present when the cause is *S. pyogenes* or MRSA. Prompt surgical exploration down to the deep fascia and muscle is essential. Necrotic tissue must be surgically removed, and Gram's staining and culture of excised tissue are useful in establishing whether group A streptococci, mixed aerobic-anaerobic bacteria, MRSA, or *Clostridium* species are present (see "Treatment," below).

■ MYOSITIS AND MYONECROSIS

(Table 125-1) Muscle involvement can occur with viral infection (e.g., influenza, dengue, or coxsackievirus B infection) or parasitic invasion (e.g., trichinellosis, cysticercosis, or toxoplasmosis). Although myalgia can occur in most of these infections, severe muscle pain is the hallmark of pleurodynia (coxsackievirus B), trichinellosis, and bacterial infection. Acute rhabdomyolysis predictably occurs with clostridial and streptococcal myositis but may also be associated with influenza virus, echovirus, coxsackievirus, Epstein-Barr virus, and *Legionella* infections.

Pyomyositis is usually due to *S. aureus*, is common in tropical areas, and generally has no known portal of entry. Cases of pyomyositis caused by MRSA producing the PVL toxin have been described among children in the United States. Muscle infection begins at the exact site of blunt trauma or muscle strain. Infection remains localized, and shock does not develop unless organisms produce toxic shock syndrome toxin 1 or certain enterotoxins and the patient lacks antibodies to the toxin produced by the infecting organisms. In contrast, *S. pyogenes* may induce primary myositis (referred to as *streptococcal necrotizing myositis*) in association with severe systemic toxicity. Myonecrosis occurs concomitantly with necrotizing fasciitis in ~50% of cases. Both are part of the streptococcal toxic shock syndrome.

Gas gangrene usually follows severe penetrating injuries that result in interruption of the blood supply and introduction of soil into wounds. Such cases of traumatic gangrene are usually caused by the clostridial species *C. perfringens*, *C. septicum*, and *C. histolyticum*. Rarely, latent or recurrent gangrene can occur years after penetrating trauma; dormant spores that reside at the site of previous injury are most likely responsible. Spontaneous nontraumatic gangrene among patients with neutropenia, gastrointestinal malignancy, diverticulosis, or recent radiation therapy to the abdomen is caused by several clostridial species, of which *C. septicum* is the most commonly involved. The tolerance of this anaerobe to oxygen probably explains why it can initiate infection spontaneously in normal tissue anywhere in the body.

Gas gangrene of the uterus, especially that due to *C. sordellii*, historically occurred as a consequence of illegal or self-induced abortion and nowadays also follows spontaneous abortion, vaginal delivery, and cesarean section. *C. sordellii* has also been implicated in medically induced abortion. Postpartum *C. sordellii* infections in young, previously healthy women present as a unique clinical picture: little or no fever, lack of a purulent discharge, refractory hypotension, extensive peripheral edema and effusions, hemoconcentration, and a markedly elevated white blood cell count. The infection is almost uniformly fatal, with death ensuing rapidly.

Synergistic nonclostridial anaerobic myonecrosis, also known as necrotizing cutaneous myositis and synergistic necrotizing cellulitis, is a variant of necrotizing fasciitis caused by mixed aerobic and anaerobic bacteria with the exclusion of clostridial organisms (see "Necrotizing Fasciitis," above).

■ DIAGNOSIS

This chapter has emphasized the physical appearance and location of lesions within the soft tissues as important diagnostic clues. The temporal progression of the lesions as well as the patient's travel history, animal exposure or bite history, age, underlying disease status, and lifestyle are also crucial considerations in narrowing the differential diagnosis. However, even the astute clinician may find it challenging to diagnose all infections of the soft tissues by history and inspection alone. Soft tissue radiography, computed tomography (Fig. 125-2), and magnetic resonance imaging may be useful in determining the depth of infection and should be performed when the patient has rapidly progressing lesions or evidence of a systemic inflammatory response syndrome. These tests are particularly valuable for defining a localized abscess or detecting gas in tissue. Unfortunately, they may reveal only soft tissue swelling and thus are not specific for fulminant infections such as necrotizing fasciitis or myonecrosis caused by group A *Streptococcus* (Fig. 125-2), where gas is not found in lesions.

Aspiration of the leading edge or punch biopsy with frozen section may be helpful if the results of imaging tests are positive, but false-negative results occur in ~80% of cases. There is some evidence that aspiration alone may be superior to injection and aspiration with normal saline. Frozen sections are especially useful in distinguishing SSSS from TEN and are quite valuable in cases of necrotizing fasciitis. Open surgical inspection, with debridement as indicated, is clearly the best way to determine the extent and severity of infection and to obtain material for Gram's staining and culture. Such an aggressive approach is important and may be

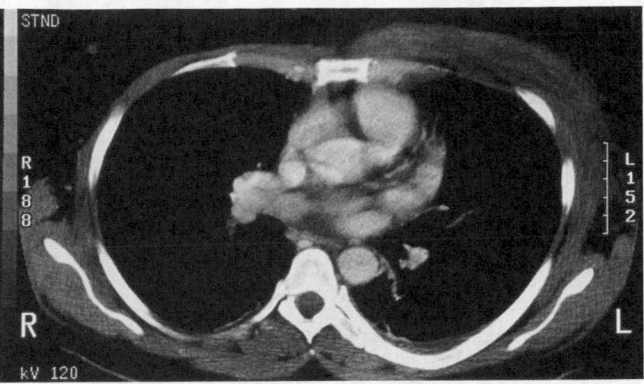

Figure 125-2 Computed tomography showing edema and inflammation of the left chest wall in a patient with necrotizing fasciitis and myonecrosis caused by group A *Streptococcus*.

lifesaving if undertaken early in the course of fulminant infections where there is evidence of systemic toxicity.

| TREATMENT | Infections of the Skin, Muscles, and Soft Tissues |

A full description of the treatment of all the clinical entities described herein is beyond the scope of this chapter. As a guide to the clinician in selecting appropriate treatment, the antimicrobial agents useful in the most common and the most fulminant cutaneous infections are listed in Table 125-2.

Furuncles, carbuncles, and abscesses caused by MRSA and MSSA are common, and their treatment depends upon the size of the lesion. Furuncles <2.5 cm in diameter are usually treated with moist heat. Those that are larger (4.5 cm of erythema and induration) require surgical drainage, and the occurrence of these larger lesions in association with fever, chills, or leukocytosis requires both drainage and antibiotic treatment. A study in children demonstrated that surgical drainage of abscesses (mean diameter, 3.8 cm) was as effective when used alone as when combined with trimethoprim-sulfamethoxazole treatment. However, the rate of recurrence of new lesions was lower in the group undergoing both drainage and antibiotic treatment.

Early and aggressive surgical exploration is essential in cases of suspected necrotizing fasciitis, myositis, or gangrene in order to (1) visualize the deep structures, (2) remove necrotic tissue, (3) reduce compartment pressure, and (4) obtain suitable material for Gram's staining and for aerobic and anaerobic cultures. Appropriate empirical antibiotic treatment for mixed aerobic-anaerobic infections could consist of ampicillin/sulbactam, cefoxitin, or the following combination: (1) clindamycin (600–900 mg intravenously every 8 h) or metronidazole (500 mg every 6 h) plus (2) ampicillin or ampicillin/sulbactam (1.5–3 g intravenously every 6 h) plus (3) gentamicin (1–1.5 mg/kg every 8 h). Group A streptococcal and clostridial infection of the fascia and/or muscle carries a mortality rate of 20–50% with penicillin treatment. In experimental models of streptococcal and clostridial necrotizing fasciitis/myositis, clindamycin has exhibited markedly superior efficacy, but no comparative clinical trials have been performed. A retrospective study of children with invasive group A streptococcal infection demonstrated higher survival rates with clindamycin treatment than with ß-lactam antibiotic therapy. Hyperbaric oxygen treatment may also be useful in gas

TABLE 125-2 Treatment of Common Infections of the Skin

Diagnosis/Condition	Primary Treatment	Alternative Treatment	See Also Chap(s).
Animal bite (prophylaxis or early infection)[a]	Amoxicillin/clavulanate, 875/125 mg PO bid	Doxycycline, 100 mg PO bid	**e24**
Animal bite[a] (established infection)	Ampicillin/sulbactam, 1.5–3 g IV q6h	Clindamycin, 600–900 mg IV q8h, *plus* Ciprofloxacin, 400 mg IV q12h, *or* Cefoxitin, 2 g IV q6h	**e24**
Bacillary angiomatosis	Erythromycin, 500 mg PO qid	Doxycycline, 100 mg PO bid	160
Herpes simplex (primary genital)	Acyclovir, 400 mg PO tid for 10 days	Famciclovir, 250 mg PO tid for 5–10 days, *or* Valacyclovir, 1000 mg PO bid for 10 days	179
Herpes zoster (immunocompetent host >50 years of age)	Acyclovir, 800 mg PO 5 times daily for 7–10 days	Famciclovir, 500 mg PO tid for 7–10 days, *or* Valacyclovir, 1000 mg PO tid for 7 days	180
Cellulitis (staphylococcal or streptococcal[b,c])	Nafcillin or oxacillin, 2 g IV q4–6h	Cefazolin, 1–2 g q8h, *or* Ampicillin/sulbactam, 1.5–3 g IV q6h, *or* Erythromycin, 0.5–1 g IV q6h, *or* Clindamycin, 600–900 mg IV q8h	135, 136
MRSA skin infection[d]	Vancomycin, 1 g IV q12h	Linezolid, 600 mg IV q12h	135
Necrotizing fasciitis (group A streptococcal[b])	Clindamycin, 600–900 mg IV q6–8h, *plus* Penicillin G, 4 million units IV q4h	Clindamycin, 600–900 mg IV q6–8h, *plus* Cephalosporin (first- or second-generation)	136
Necrotizing fasciitis (mixed aerobes and anaerobes)	Ampicillin, 2 g IV q4h, *plus* Clindamycin, 600–900 mg IV q6–8h, *plus* Ciprofloxacin, 400 mg IV q6–8h	Vancomycin, 1 g IV q6h, *plus* Metronidazole, 500 mg IV q6h, *plus* Ciprofloxacin, 400 mg IV q6–8h	164
Gas gangrene	Clindamycin, 600–900 mg IV q6–8h, *plus* Penicillin G, 4 million units IV q4–6h	Clindamycin, 600–900 mg IV q6–8h, *plus* Cefoxitin, 2 g IV q6h	142

[a]*Pasteurella multocida*, a species commonly associated with both dog and cat bites, is resistant to cephalexin, dicloxacillin, clindamycin, and erythromycin. *Eikenella corrodens*, a bacterium commonly associated with human bites, is resistant to clindamycin, penicillinase-resistant penicillins, and metronidazole but is sensitive to trimethoprim-sulfamethoxazole and fluoroquinolones.

[b]The frequency of erythromycin resistance in group A *Streptococcus* is currently ~5% in the United States but has reached 70–100% in some other countries. Most, but not all, erythromycin-resistant group A streptococci are susceptible to clindamycin. Approximately 90–95% of *Staphylococcus aureus* strains are sensitive to clindamycin.

[c]Severe hospital-acquired *S. aureus* infections or community-acquired *S. aureus* infections that are not responding to the ß-lactam antibiotics recommended in this table may be caused by methicillin-resistant strains, requiring a switch to vancomycin or linezolid.

[d]Some strains of methicillin-resistant *S. aureus* (MRSA) remain sensitive to tetracycline and trimethoprim-sulfamethoxazole. Daptomycin (4 mg/kg IV q24h) or tigecycline (100-mg loading dose followed by 50 mg IV q12h) are alternative treatments for MRSA.

gangrene due to clostridial species. Antibiotic treatment should be continued until all signs of systemic toxicity have resolved, all devitalized tissue has been removed, and granulation tissue has developed (Chaps. 136, 142, and 164).

In summary, infections of the skin and soft tissues are diverse in presentation and severity and offer a great challenge to the clinician. This chapter provides an approach to diagnosis and understanding of the pathophysiologic mechanisms involved in these infections. More in-depth information is found in chapters on specific infections.

FURTHER READINGS

Bisno AI, Stevens DL: Streptococcal infections in skin and soft tissues. N Engl J Med 334:240, 1996

Breman JG, Henderson DA: Diagnosis and management of smallpox. N Engl J Med 346:1300, 2002

Duong M et al: Randomized, controlled trial of antibiotics in the management of community-acquired skin abscesses in the pediatric patient. Ann Emerg Med 55:401, 2010

Fridkin SK et al: Methicillin-resistant *Staphylococcus aureus* disease in three communities. N Engl J Med 352:1436, 2005

PART 8

Infectious Diseases

MILLER LG et al: Necrotizing fasciitis caused by community-associated methicillin-resistant *Staphylococcus aureus* in Los Angeles. N Engl J Med 352:1445, 2005

NORRBY-TEGLUND A, STEVENS DL: Novel therapies in streptococcal toxic shock syndrome: Attenuation of virulence factor expression and modulation of host response. Curr Opin Infect Dis 11:285, 1998

STEVENS DL: Streptococcal toxic shock syndrome associated with necrotizing fasciitis. Annu Rev Med 51:271, 2000

———: Necrotizing soft tissue infections. Curr Treat Opt Infect Dis 2:359, 2000

——— et al: Practice guidelines for the diagnosis and management of skin and soft-tissue infections. Clin Infect Dis 41:1373, 2005

TALAN DA et al: Bacteriologic analysis of infected dog and cat bites. Emergency Medicine Animal Bite Infection Study Group. N Engl J Med 340:85, 1999

ZIMBELMAN J et al: Improved outcome of clindamycin compared with beta-lactam antibiotic treatment for invasive *Streptococcus pyogenes* infection. Pediatr Infect Dis J 18:1096, 1999

CHAPTER 126

Osteomyelitis

Alan D. Tice

Osteomyelitis, an infection of bone that leads to tissue destruction and often to debility, can be caused by a wide variety of bacteria (including mycobacteria) and fungi and may be associated with viral infections. Its management must be individualized and depends on numerous factors, including the causative organism, the specific bone involved, vascular supply, nerve function, foreign bodies, recent injury, the physiologic status of the host, and associated comorbidities. The spectrum of the disease can range from extensive (e.g., tibial and vertebral osteomyelitis) to localized (e.g., bone invasion associated with a tooth abscess). Two major classification systems for osteomyelitis are used in making decisions about medical therapy and surgery. Lee and Waldvogel categorized cases as acute or chronic, hematogenous or contiguous, and with or without vascular compromise. The Cierny and Mader classification system for long-bone osteomyelitis encompasses the location and extent of the infection as well as a number of other factors.

ETIOLOGY (TABLE 126-1)

The foremost bacterial cause of osteomyelitis is *Staphylococcus aureus*. Gram-negative organisms such as *Pseudomonas aeruginosa* and *Escherichia coli*, coagulase-negative staphylococci, enterococci, and propionibacteria may also be involved. *Mycobacterium tuberculosis* is a common cause of osteomyelitis in countries with limited medical resources; other mycobacterial species that infect bone include *M. marinum*, *M. chelonei*, and *M. fortuitum*. Fungal etiologies include *Candida*, *Coccidioides*, *Histoplasma*, and *Aspergillus* species. Noninfectious pathogenic mechanisms that may cause disease mimicking osteomyelitis include avascular necrosis, rheumatoid diseases, neuropathy with chronic trauma, gout, and malignancies.

The precipitating event(s) for osteomyelitis vary greatly. The prosthetic joint implants and stabilization devices that are increasingly being used in orthopedic surgery are associated with complex infections. Trauma is also a common cause of infection, especially when a wound is involved and there is contamination of bone or surrounding tissue along with significant tissue damage or destruction. Even in the absence of an open wound or a compound fracture, damaged tissue and extravasated blood may slow the circulation, establishing a favorable medium for the growth of bacteria that may reach the area through low-level bacteremia from the peripheral

TABLE 126-1 Microorganisms That Cause Osteomyelitis

Organism	Comment
Frequently Encountered Bacteria	
Staphylococcus aureus	Most likely bacterial pathogen
	Aggressive, invasive
	Often metastatic foci with bacteremia
	Consider surgery early
Staphylococci other than *S. aureus* (coagulase-negative)	Usually associated with foreign material or implants
	Biofllm production
Streptococci	May spread rapidly through soft tissues
Enterobacteriaceae (*Escherichia coli*, *Klebsiella*, others)	Considerable variation in antibiotic susceptibility
	Increasing antibiotic resistance with overuse
	May become resistant to antibiotics during therapy
Pseudomonas aeruginosa	Increasingly resistant to antibiotics
	Frequent successor to other bacteria when initial therapy fails
	May be related to contamination
Unusual Organisms	
Anaerobic bacteria	Usually mixed with aerobic bacteria
	May be synergistic
	Survival dependent on devitalized tissue
Bartonella henselae	Associated with cat scratches and probably with fleas
Brucella species	Prominent in developing countries, especially with unpasteurized milk
Fungi	*Candida* the most likely genus
	Considerable variation in susceptibility, depending on species
	Surgery may be helpful if infection is invasive
Mycobacterium tuberculosis	May involve any bone
	Vertebral osteomyelitis common in some countries
Mycobacteria other than *M. tuberculosis*	Need special culture media to recover
Viruses	Associated with some viral infections, including varicella and variola

venous circulation or from distal lymphatic channels. Bacteremia—whether due to endocarditis or due to seeding from other sites of infection (e.g., abscesses, boils, or vascular devices)—is also a frequent etiologic factor in osteomyelitis. Studies of *S. aureus* bacteremia indicate a rate of metastatic osteomyelitis approaching 28% if there is a prosthetic joint in place; *S. aureus* bacteremia can be complicated by the involvement of methicillin-resistant strains (MRSA), which are progressively replacing strains that are more susceptible to antibiotics. The overlapping circulations of the urinary tract and the spine may be a source of vertebral osteomyelitis due to urinary tract pathogens such as *E. coli* and *Klebsiella*. Additional predisposing factors include a poor arterial and venous supply, which may limit perfusion to bone to the point of an inadequate response and poor healing, even in patients with normal function. Host factors such as diabetes and its consequences contribute significantly to the development of osteomyelitis through impaired immunity with hyperglycemia, loss of sensation, vascular disease, and renal failure.

EPIDEMIOLOGY

In the United States, acute osteomyelitis affects ~0.1–1.8% of the otherwise healthy adult population. After a foot puncture, 30–40% of adults with diabetes develop osteomyelitis. In this country, there has been a major change in the profile of certain bacterial pathogens, with the emergence of MRSA strains over the last decade. MRSA has become a source of great concern in hospitals, especially after surgery. The morbidity and economic consequences appear to be greater for MRSA osteomyelitis than for osteomyelitis caused by methicillin-sensitive *S. aureus* strains. However, it is not clear that these poorer outcomes for MRSA are due to new or more destructive virulence factors. Rather, they may simply be the result of a delay in effective antimicrobial treatment.

The types and etiologies of osteomyelitis vary by region and with time. The United States has seen a rise in infections related to the increasing use of orthopedic surgery for correction of deformities and implantation of screws, pins, rods, plates, and prosthetic joints. With the aging of populations and the epidemics of obesity and diabetes in some countries, the frequency of these predisposing factors continues to increase, requiring adaptations in treatment approaches. Any type of instrumentation may lead to infection in a small proportion of cases. Osteomyelitis attributable to orthopedic devices and surgical interventions is considerably less common in countries with limited medical resources, where tuberculosis may be the dominant infection and brucellosis is not unusual. In many of these areas, agricultural injuries, industrial accidents, and war wounds are much more common than in wealthy countries, and the pathogens causing infection reflect those injuries. Osteomyelitis is more common in situations where wounds cannot promptly be debrided and repaired, microbiology laboratories are not readily available, and effective antimicrobial agents are in short supply.

PATHOGENESIS

The most common predisposing factor for osteomyelitis is an area of bone or contiguous surrounding tissue that is abnormal in terms of viability, blood supply, sensation, or edema. The damaged tissue not only compromises healthy circulation to the area but may slow the flow of venous blood and lymph, thereby providing nutrients to bacteria and fueling ongoing damage. Host factors such as poor nutrition and immunosuppression may also be relevant. Diabetes in adults poses the most significant risk. Diabetic neuropathy adds to the progression of osteomyelitis as the patient may be unaware of infection as it spreads into the bone; the consequences include thousands of amputations each year. Additional sources of immunosuppression, such as chemotherapy and treatment with glucocorticoids or tumor necrosis factor (TNF) inhibitors, also inhibit normal defense

mechanisms and thus predispose to more frequent and serious infections whose symptoms are diminished because of reduced inflammatory responses.

The bacteria involved in osteomyelitis perpetuate themselves by elaborating toxins that further damage tissues, including bone. *S. aureus* is particularly adept in this respect; it colonizes the nasal area in about one-third of healthy individuals and can produce a wide variety of cytokines, enzymes, and toxins that destroy tissue and affect neutrophil response. Some *S. aureus* bacteria survive uptake into the phagocytic vacuoles of macrophages and continue to cause disease and recrudescence by persistently eluding the usual defense mechanisms. This capacity for "hibernation" and persistence may allow *S. aureus* to remain dormant for decades before infection erupts at the sites of old injuries (e.g., shrapnel or other penetrating wounds).

Coagulase-negative staphylococci are generally not as virulent as *S. aureus* but have been found to persist by producing a biofilm that protects them from the host and apparently allows them to exist for many years on prosthetic joints, with minimal symptoms. The extent to which other organisms use biofilm to their advantage is unclear, but biofilm production probably plays a significant role in osteomyelitis, especially the chronic forms.

Multiple bacteria may be recovered from cultures, especially when there is an entry wound. Decisions about which ones to target in antibiotic therapy are often difficult. Common skin-dwelling and colonizing microbes usually do not need to be treated, and overtreatment in fact results in unnecessary toxicity and increases antimicrobial resistance among the organisms that survive. Anaerobic bacteria can often be recovered and may play a synergistic role with usual or unusual pathogens; specific therapy is sometimes beneficial in these situations.

The intrinsic factors of organisms that are responsible for persistence and bone destruction have not yet been identified. However, there is probably strain-to-strain variation in virulence factors produced by particular clones, with some strains consequently much more virulent than others. The prevention of biofilm production merits investigation in this regard.

APPROACH TO THE PATIENT: Osteomyelitis

The best approach to the care of a patient with significant osteomyelitis is to assemble a team of providers who can work together in considering the microbiology of the infection and make sound decisions about antibiotic therapy and surgery. The most effective program will include evaluation and management of antibiotics, microbiology, pharmacology, glucose levels, vascular disease, neuropathy, and renal function, with close follow-up by a knowledgeable physician who is interested in leading the team in coordinating care.

When osteomyelitis is suspected, a careful, methodical approach is needed (see "Clinical Manifestations and Diagnosis," below). Patients should be educated about the significance of an infection that involves bone, especially if risk factors cannot be eliminated. Blood tests, cultures, standard radiography, scans, biopsies, and surgery may all be necessary for a clear diagnosis and full delineation of the pathogen. Collection of this baseline information can be very important in both early and late decision-making.

Initial evaluations for osteomyelitis must be aggressive, as the infection can progress rapidly in the absence of antibiotic therapy effective against the wide variety of potential pathogens. Inadequacies in cultures, surgery, or temporizing measures may greatly exacerbate the damage caused by the infection.

Hospitalization may be indicated for rapid multispecialty evaluation, imaging, and stabilization of complex infections such as with a diabetic foot. Outpatient therapy may not be adequate for the teamwork and interventions needed. Early admission and procedures may actually shorten the length of hospital stay.

The physician should inform the patient about the value of all the necessary evaluations, the implications of surgery, and the possibility of a prolonged course of IV antibiotic therapy, whether in the hospital or at home. A patient's fear of amputation can lead to inordinate delays in seeking treatment that allow the infection to progress. Moreover, it is not unusual for a patient to refuse surgery and amputation even though such treatments will clearly increase the likelihood of a functional lifestyle. Therefore, it is best to prepare patients early on if there may be negative outcomes such as amputation and perhaps to set criteria and timelines for success or failure of therapy and interventions.

■ CLINICAL MANIFESTATIONS AND DIAGNOSIS

Diagnosis of acute osteomyelitis within the first few weeks of onset is important and is usually relatively easy. If the diagnosis is missed, however, the symptoms may become chronic, with slow progression or a dormant phase of several years.

A thorough history and physical examination are the mainstays of evaluation for osteomyelitis. A clear pattern of pain, swelling, and possibly drainage after surgery or injury should raise suspicion, but such indicators may not all be present, even in a patient with neuropathy, compromised circulation, chronic edema, organ failure, diabetes, or other predisposing factors. Direct questions about previous injuries, infections, surgeries, or hardware implantation—even decades earlier—can yield information critical in guiding empirical antibiotic therapy and surgery. A history of injury is particularly important, even if the skin was not broken and there were no clinical signs of bacteremia. It is not unusual for a soft tissue injury to serve as a nidus of secondary bone infection, presumably seeded by low-level bacteremia and often occurring without symptoms. Other sources of seeding may include boils, abscesses, cellulitis, or injection sites. A careful examination is essential in identifying additional predisposing factors and assessing the role of comorbidities such as neuropathy, arterial disease, venous insufficiency, and chronic trauma that can lead to severe accumulation of callus in insensate feet.

Careful consideration and assessment of disorders that may mimic or accompany osteomyelitis are essential. Arthritis, gout, ischemia, neuropathies, and recent surgery may be diagnosed when osteomyelitis is the real cause of symptoms on a cofactor. For example, chronic back pain may be attributed to degenerative arthritis, but there can be a substantial loss of neurologic function if the pain is actually due to diskitis with vertebral osteomyelitis.

Correctly diagnosing osteomyelitis early has crucial implications for later function, disability, treatment cost, and risk of a fatal outcome. A variety of tools must be used to definitively diagnose or conclusively rule out an infection. A standard x-ray is a good starting point that can reveal a variety of abnormalities (Fig. 126-1A) and may eliminate the need for further imaging studies. Bone loss, sequestra, periosteal elevation or swelling (which can develop early on), and shadows around foreign bodies are hallmarks of bone infection. However, these findings may also be found with other disorders, such as tumors, trauma, avascular necrosis, and gout. Standard two-dimensional images can be of limited value in assessing complex bones. The value of radiology may be limited by the time required for an infection to become apparent; actual dissolution or resorption of bone due to infection may not be apparent for several weeks or more.

Depending on the results of the initial x-ray, further investigations with invasive techniques may be appropriate. Collection of pus by needle aspiration through a clean area from a closed pocket not only documents bone infection but also permits recovery and evaluation of the pathogen(s). A culture of a wound swab may be of some value but is clearly less reliable in identifying the real culprit(s), which may be present in the bone but absent from its surface. Biopsy provides more accurate microbiologic information than needle aspiration and supplies tissue for pathology studies, which may be helpful. Some organisms that usually are not recovered (in a timely fashion or at all) by standard cultures may be rendered visible with special staining of tissue samples. Unfortunately, the size of the needle used for needle biopsy may not be appropriate for small bones of the hands or feet. Open surgical exploration, biopsy, and drainage, which can provide high-quality tissue samples for culture and pathology and offer a view of the infected bone and surrounding area, should also be considered. Necrotic tissue can be removed and circulation assessed with one procedure. Polymerase chain reaction and other sequencing technologies are increasingly being used to detect and identify specific organisms—and even to determine their susceptibilities—within hours instead of days or weeks. Information on specific strains of unusual organisms may be of value, especially in difficult cases.

Laboratory tests are useful in assessing osteomyelitis but usually do not yield specific information relevant to etiology or severity. Leukocytosis may be noted in acute infection but is less likely in chronic infection, which may also be associated with anemia. Determination of the erythrocyte sedimentation rate (ESR) is a simple, inexpensive aid to diagnosis; it serves as an indicator of response with *S. aureus* infections but is not as useful for gram-negative infections because the cytokines and inflammatory elements that result in elevations are different for gram-positive (*S. aureus*) than for gram-negative infections. C-reactive protein (CRP) measurement may be helpful, especially in the evaluation of children, but may not be as useful as an ESR determination in some cases. CRP changes occur earlier in response to bacterial infection. Both ESR and CRP determinations have significant limitations in multifactorial diseases, with elevated values reflecting conditions other than osteomyelitis. Additional laboratory tests for diseases associated with bone loss that may mimic or complicate osteomyelitis should include measurement of glucose levels and tests for renal failure, gout, vasculitis, and rheumatoid diseases.

Additional imaging studies may be of value if the diagnosis remains unclear. CT can delineate bone more clearly than standard radiography and offers three-dimensional displays that can be extremely useful in detecting abnormalities and devising a surgical approach. MRI (Fig. 126-1B–D) provides high-quality images of the soft tissue around the bone abnormality and may be essential in diagnosing an epidural abscess related to vertebral osteomyelitis. Technetium and leukocyte isotope scans offer insight into the activity of the disease process and the affected site(s). Although these additional screening tools may be helpful in evaluation and decision-making, they may not be cost-effective.

TREATMENT ▶ Osteomyelitis

Therapy for osteomyelitis is challenging because of the variety of causative organisms, the usual comorbidities, the need for a prolonged course and IV administration, the common physical limitations of the patient, and high costs. An aggressive therapeutic approach is warranted given the dire consequences of failure of medical therapy, which can include loss of limbs. The sooner the infection is diagnosed and treated, the better the outcome and the less damage done during delays in intervention. Antibiotic therapy should be used aggressively to stop disease progression and should be designed to avoid the development of

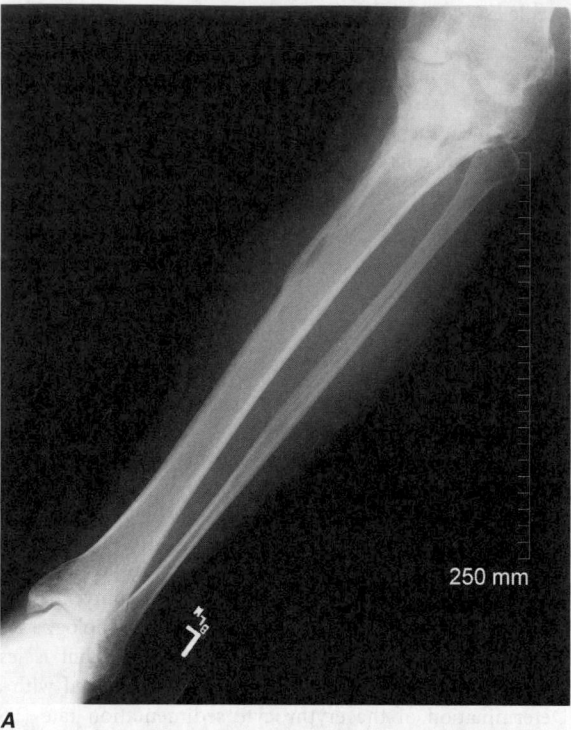

A

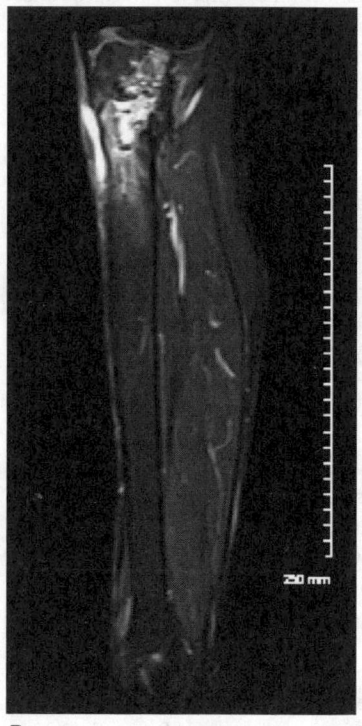

B

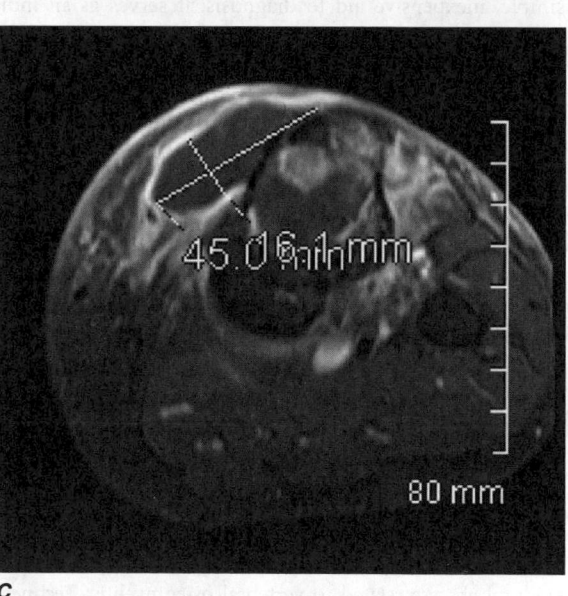

45.06 mm mm

80 mm

C

D

Figure 126-1 (**A**) Standard radiology image indicates infection with sclerosis of the proximal tibia and periosteal elevation and obvious bone destruction with an apparent cavity and the suggestion of a sequestrum in the proximal medial tibia. (**B, C**) Magnetic resonance images more clearly visualize the bone and soft tissue anatomy, confirming an extensive infection with destruction within the proximal tibia that has extended into the surrounding soft tissues and the joint as well as a ring of calcification most consistent with an abscess. (**D**) A longitudinal MRI shows the extent of longitudinal bone destruction and soft tissue involvement with contrast enhancement that suggests viable marrow from the middle to the distal tibial shaft.

resistant organisms. Early surgical intervention (e.g., debridement) can confirm the infection, identify and characterize the etiologic agent(s), and remove dead or devitalized tissue that may be providing bacteria with nutrients and allowing them to spread. A variety of antibiotics are available for most of the likely pathogens (Table 126-2), although the most common pathogen—*S. aureus*—continues to evolve mechanisms to elude these drugs. MRSA strains represent an increasing problem in both the hospital and the community. Staphylococci and Enterobacteriaceae resistant to even more antibiotics than MRSA appear to be evolving.

The most common targets for empirical antibiotic therapy are staphylococci, which are carried asymptomatically in and around the nares by nearly one-third of healthy people. The common β-lactam antibiotics provide excellent results against methicillin-sensitive *S. aureus* strains. Oxacillin and nafcillin are first-line agents but may elicit more adverse reactions than cephalosporins. Cefazolin is a reasonable alternative in the hospital, but ceftriaxone is preferred as an outpatient drug because it can be given (by the IV or IM route) only once a day.

TABLE 126-2 Antibiotics for the Treatment of Osteomyelitis

Organism	Antimicrobial Agent	Dosing	Comments
Methicillin-susceptible *Staphylococcus aureus*	Oxacillin or nafcillin	2 g IV q6h	May be more active than cephalosporins More difficult than cephalosporins to administer for long periods
	Cephalosporins	Cefazolin: 2 g IV q8h Ceftriaxone: 1–2 g IV q24h	Ceftriaxone advantageous with OPAT
	Clindamycin[a]	600–900 mg IV q8h	Not well studied for osteomyelitis Oral form possible (300–600 mg oral q8h) Resistance significant and increasing Toxicity different from that of β-lactam antibiotics
Methicillin-resistant *S. aureus*	Vancomycin	15 mg/kg IV q12h	Strains with an MIC of ≥2 μg/mL may not respond well.
	Daptomycin[a]	4–6 mg/kg IV q24h	Promising, but concern about adverse effects with prolonged therapy
	Linezolid[a]	600 mg IV or PO q12h	Effectiveness and adverse effects with prolonged therapy unclear Bacteriostatic
Streptococci	Penicillin	5 mU IV q6h or 20 mU/d by continuous infusion	Not all streptococci are susceptible Ceftriaxone (1 g/d IV or IM) and ampicillin (12 g/d IV) are alternatives
Enterococci	Penicillin plus gentamicin	As above 5 mg/kg daily IV	If strain is susceptible
	Vancomycin	As above	If strain is susceptible
Enterobacteriaceae (*E. coli*, *Klebsiella*, other)	Ceftriaxone or another cephalosporin Ciprofloxacin	As above 400 mg IV q8–12h	If strain is susceptible 500–750 mg q8–12h if strain is susceptible
Pseudomonas aeruginosa	Ciprofloxacin	As above	Resistance may develop during therapy; if strain is resistant, drugs to consider include cefepime and ceftazidime

[a]Not approved for use in osteomyelitis by the U.S. Food and Drug Administration.
Abbreviations: MIC, minimal inhibitory concentration; OPAT, outpatient parenteral antimicrobial therapy.

MRSA strains have been controlled with vancomycin for many years, but this drug appears to be losing its effectiveness against these microbes. New antibiotics have been designed to fill this need, although their efficacy has not been documented. In an outpatient setting, vancomycin does not appear to be as effective against methicillin-susceptible staphylococcal osteomyelitis as oxacillin or ceftriaxone. Publications about the value of daptomycin for osteomyelitis are encouraging. Tigecycline is active against MRSA but is only bacteriostatic and does not yet have a well-established outcomes record. Telavancin may also be of value against vancomycin-resistant staphylococci but has not yet been adequately tested for bone infections.

Additional antimicrobial agents for use against staphylococcal infections include linezolid, which offers the advantage of both oral and IV formulations but is bacteriostatic and has not yet been well studied. Moreover, its use—although apparently less expensive than that of other parenteral drugs—is limited by its cost. Clindamycin can also be used as both an IV and an oral agent, although antimicrobial resistance is a growing problem. Rifampin, a potential adjunct to other antistaphylococcal agents, is highly active in vitro and can penetrate phagocytic vacuoles to reach staphylococci therein. Unfortunately, resistance develops rapidly if rifampin is used alone, and clinical outcomes are not

always as good as anticipated. Other agents, such as aminoglycosides, folic acid inhibitors, and macrolides, may play a limited role; they generally are neither as effective nor as toxic as other available agents.

Fluoroquinolone antibiotics offer both IV and oral therapy options and are often included in the standard recommendation for treatment of many susceptible strains of Enterobacteriaceae and *Pseudomonas* species. Drugs of this class do, however, have some limitations in terms of emerging resistance (even during therapy) and may exert some adverse neuromuscular effects (e.g., tendon rupture and impaired healing) that may be particularly relevant to the prolonged courses of antibiotics usually needed to cure the infection. In general, fluoroquinolones should not be used to treat *S. aureus* infections because of these limitations and the availability of better-studied antibiotics.

The optimal route and duration of therapy for osteomyelitis remain controversial. The usual recommendations stem from a 1970 study in which cases of osteomyelitis were characterized and outcomes were evaluated in relation to the duration of IV therapy. Better outcomes appeared to be related to a course of ≥4 weeks in some types of infection. Even though the characteristics of the bacteria and the available antibiotics were quite different at that time, a 4- to 6-week course of IV therapy remains the standard and is the usual recommended minimum. This recommendation has been challenged in pediatric studies in light of increasing evidence that oral agents and shorter courses may be adequate. Because some of the active agents reach comparable levels when given by mouth, a switch from the recommended IV administration to oral therapy may be appropriate in some situations. The proper duration of antimicrobial therapy depends on a variety of factors, including the infecting organism, the bone involved, surgical procedures, and drug tolerance and safety. Prolonged courses may be justified by extensive disease, immunocompromise, poor clinical response, and vertebral osteomyelitis. Whether a bone infection has truly been cured becomes clear only over time; relapse is not uncommon and may occur years later, especially in patients with ongoing risk factors and comorbidities. The literature suggests that a 6-month follow-up period is adequate to determine the success of treatment. Patients should be followed for at least that long, even though antibiotics have been discontinued. The possibility of relapses and the potential for their prevention should not be overlooked.

Surgery is an important tool in the treatment of osteomyelitis, offering the benefits of direct observation, prompt removal of all devitalized tissue and bone, and drainage of the infection site. Nevertheless, it is not without risk, and loss of bone or other tissue may adversely affect function. In addition, because bone may regenerate to some degree when infection is eradicated, surgery is not always needed. Surgical approaches vary with the bone involved and the extent of disease. The Cierny-Mader classification system is helpful when three-dimensional imaging is done, and MRI may help determine the viability of bone or marrow. Residual dead spaces are a source of concern and may require tissue flaps and closure. Local antibiotics and impregnated cement or beads may be of value but not should not replace IV antibiotic therapy without further study. If surgery is performed and most or all of the infected bone is removed, a full 4- to 6-week course of IV therapy probably is not necessary. However, the precise duration that is required is not clear and most likely depends primarily on the other factors involved in individual cases. One week of IV therapy after surgery may be justified to ensure pathogen eradication and healing.

Outpatient parenteral antibiotic therapy (OPAT) is a valuable means of providing the long course of IV antibiotics that is considered the standard of care and has been proven efficacious over decades. Despite potential risks outside the hospital that patients and their providers must consider, OPAT is safe and effective when properly managed and administered. This approach is conducive to a better quality of life in a familiar setting, is considered safer because of the lack of exposure to hospital-related infections (which affect ~1 patient in every 20 admitted), is much less expensive than treatment administered in the hospital, and generally facilitates recovery, often allowing the patient to return to work or resume other day-to-day activities during the treatment course.

COMPLICATIONS

The complications of osteomyelitis are numerous and are most commonly related to loss of full function of the bone or supporting tissues. Fractures are more likely with progressive disease. Local spread and dissemination of infection are also possible. Misdiagnosis is particularly likely when another disease is complicating the infection. In rare instances, chronic inflammation and infection may lead to malignant transformation into squamous cell carcinoma or sarcoma.

PROGNOSIS

The outcomes of osteomyelitis vary tremendously depending on the bone involved, the predisposing factors, the underlying diseases, and

the treatment provided. Standard guidelines cannot be applied uniformly; e.g., a case of mandible infection arising from a tooth abscess may be cured with an extraction alone, whereas a case of vertebral osteomyelitis may require a prolonged course of IV therapy as it cannot be approached surgically without neurologic sequelae. For large bones, the 4- to 6-week course of IV therapy still seems reasonable, although recent studies suggest that with some new antimicrobial agents a shorter course of IV therapy, possibly with an early switch to oral therapy, may be sufficient. Determining the outcome even of long-bone osteomyelitis is complicated by uncertainty as to the duration of follow-up needed. The actual outcome in terms of debility and limb salvage may be as dependent on underlying and complicating factors and care as it is on antibiotic therapy.

PREVENTION

Osteomyelitis can be prevented in some instances by better infection-control measures, especially before surgery. Both mupirocin and chlorhexidine are of proven value in preventing operative infections, which are an increasing cause of bone infections associated with implanted material. Prompt treatment of bacteremia and elimination of sources of infection (e.g., boils or folliculitis) before surgery and in other situations may prevent infections. Aggressive surgical management of injuries may also help avoid the constellation of factors that lead to bone infections.

Awareness of persistent sites of infection and reasonable attempts at eradication may promote prevention. Many persistent infections that do not initially impair function or cause pain are ignored by patients; an example is provided by the classic problem of diabetic foot infections, with ulcers that burrow into the soles of insensate feet and often reach bones. Likewise, sacral ulcers are often overlooked or ignored both by physicians and by patients with neurologic impairment. Attempts to eradicate or close entry wounds are critical and should be undertaken early on.

FURTHER READINGS

BYREN I et al: Pharmacotherapy of diabetic foot osteomyelitis. Expert Opin Pharmacother 10:3033, 2009

FOWLER VG JR et al: *S. aureus* Endocarditis and Bacteremia Study Group. Daptomycin versus standard therapy for bacteremia and endocarditis caused by *Staphylococcus aureus*. N Engl J Med 355:653, 2006

LESENS O et al: Culture of per-wound bone specimen: A simplified approach for the medical management of diabetic foot osteomyelitis. Clin Microbiol Infect 17:285, 2011

LEW DP, WALDVOGEL FA: Osteomyelitis. Lancet 364:369, 2004

LIU C et al: Clinical practice guidelines by the Infectious Diseases Society of America for the treatment of methicillin-resistant *Staphylococcus aureus* infections in adults and children. Clin Infect Dis 52:1, 2011

NICOLAU DP, STEIN GE: Therapeutic options for diabetic foot infections: A review with an emphasis on tissue penetration characteristics. J Am Podiatr Med Assoc 100:52, 2010

PÄÄKKÖNEN M et al: Sensitivity of erythrocyte sedimentation rate and C-reactive protein in childhood bone and joint infections. Clin Orthop Relat Res 468:861, 2010

TICE AD et al: Practice guidelines for outpatient parenteral antimicrobial therapy. IDSA guidelines. Clin Infect Dis 38:1651, 2004

———et al: Outcomes of osteomyelitis among patients treated with outpatient parenteral antimicrobial therapy. Am J Med 114:723, 2003

ZIMMERLI W: Clinical practice. Vertebral osteomyelitis. N Engl J Med 362:1022, 2010

PART 8

Infectious Diseases

CHAPTER 127

Intraabdominal Infections and Abscesses

Miriam J. Baron
Dennis L. Kasper

Intraperitoneal infections generally arise because a normal anatomic barrier is disrupted. This disruption may occur when the appendix, a diverticulum, or an ulcer ruptures; when the bowel wall is weakened by ischemia, tumor, or inflammation (e.g., in inflammatory bowel disease); or with adjacent inflammatory processes, such as pancreatitis or pelvic inflammatory disease, in which enzymes (in the former case) or organisms (in the latter) may leak into the peritoneal cavity. Whatever the inciting event, once inflammation develops and organisms usually contained within the bowel or another organ enter the normally sterile peritoneal space, a predictable series of events takes place. Intraabdominal infections occur in two stages: peritonitis and—if the patient survives this stage and goes untreated—abscess formation. The types of microorganisms predominating in each stage of infection are responsible for the pathogenesis of disease.

PERITONITIS

Peritonitis is a life-threatening event that is often accompanied by bacteremia and sepsis syndrome (Chap. 271). The peritoneal cavity is large but is divided into compartments. The upper and lower peritoneal cavities are divided by the transverse mesocolon; the greater omentum extends from the transverse mesocolon and from the lower pole of the stomach to line the lower peritoneal cavity. The pancreas, duodenum, and ascending and descending colon are located in the anterior retroperitoneal space; the kidneys, ureters, and adrenals are found in the posterior retroperitoneal space. The other organs, including liver, stomach, gallbladder, spleen, jejunum, ileum, transverse and sigmoid colon, cecum, and appendix, are within the peritoneal cavity. The cavity is lined with a serous membrane that can serve as a conduit for fluids—a property exploited in peritoneal dialysis (Fig. 127-1). A small amount of serous fluid is normally present in the peritoneal space, with a protein content (consisting mainly of albumin) of <30 g/L and <300 white blood cells (WBCs, generally mononuclear cells) per microliter. In bacterial infections, leukocyte recruitment into the infected peritoneal cavity consists of an early influx of polymorphonuclear leukocytes (PMNs) and a prolonged subsequent phase of mononuclear cell migration. The phenotype of the infiltrating leukocytes during the course of inflammation is regulated primarily by resident-cell chemokine synthesis.

■ PRIMARY (SPONTANEOUS) BACTERIAL PERITONITIS

Peritonitis is either primary (without an apparent source of contamination) or secondary. The types of organisms found and the clinical presentations of these two processes are different. In adults, primary bacterial peritonitis (PBP) occurs most commonly in conjunction with cirrhosis of the liver (frequently the result of alcoholism). However, the disease has been reported in adults with metastatic malignant disease, postnecrotic cirrhosis, chronic active hepatitis, acute viral hepatitis, congestive heart failure, systemic lupus erythematosus, and lymphedema as well as in patients with no underlying disease. Although PBP virtually always develops in patients with

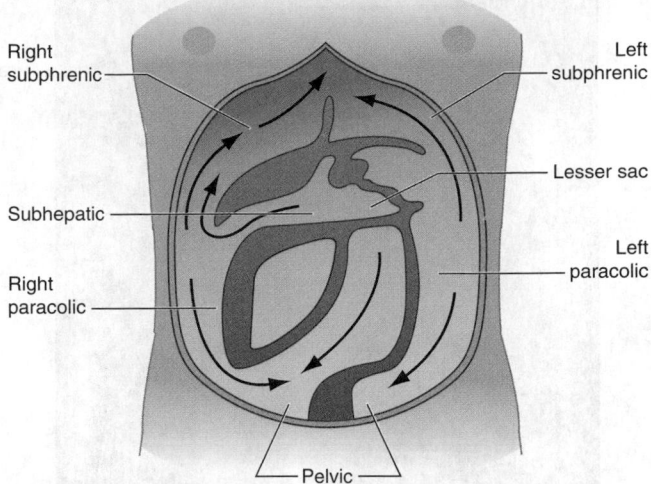

Figure 127-1 Diagram of the intraperitoneal spaces, showing the circulation of fluid and potential areas for abscess formation. Some compartments collect fluid or pus more often than others. These compartments include the pelvis (the lowest portion), the subphrenic spaces on the right and left sides, and Morrison's pouch, which is a posterosuperior extension of the subhepatic spaces and is the lowest part of the paravertebral groove when a patient is recumbent. The falciform ligament separating the right and left subphrenic spaces appears to act as a barrier to the spread of infection; consequently, it is unusual to find bilateral subphrenic collections. [Reprinted with permission from B Lorber (ed): Atlas of Infectious Diseases, vol VII: Intraabdominal Infections, Hepatitis, and Gastroenteritis. Philadelphia, Current Medicine, 1996, p 1.13.]

preexisting ascites, it is, in general, an uncommon event, occurring in ≤10% of cirrhotic patients. The cause of PBP has not been established definitively but is believed to involve hematogenous spread of organisms in a patient in whom a diseased liver and altered portal circulation result in a defect in the usual filtration function. Organisms multiply in ascites, a good medium for growth. The proteins of the complement cascade have been found in peritoneal fluid, with lower levels in cirrhotic patients than in patients with ascites of other etiologies. The opsonic and phagocytic properties of PMNs are diminished in patients with advanced liver disease.

The presentation of PBP differs from that of secondary peritonitis. The most common manifestation is fever, which is reported in up to 80% of patients. Ascites is found but virtually always predates infection. Abdominal pain, an acute onset of symptoms, and peritoneal irritation during physical examination can be helpful diagnostically, but the absence of any of these findings does not exclude this often-subtle diagnosis. Nonlocalizing symptoms (such as malaise, fatigue, or encephalopathy) without another clear etiology should also prompt consideration of PBP in a susceptible patient. It is vital to sample the peritoneal fluid of any cirrhotic patient with ascites and fever. The finding of >250 PMNs/μL is diagnostic for PBP, according to Conn (http://jac.oxfordjournals.org/cgi/content/full/47/3/369). This criterion does not apply to secondary peritonitis (see below). The microbiology of PBP is also distinctive. While enteric gram-negative bacilli such as *Escherichia coli* are most commonly encountered, gram-positive organisms such as streptococci, enterococci, or even pneumococci are sometimes found. In PBP, a single organism is typically isolated; anaerobes are found less frequently in PBP than in secondary peritonitis, in which a mixed flora including anaerobes is the rule. In fact, if PBP is suspected and

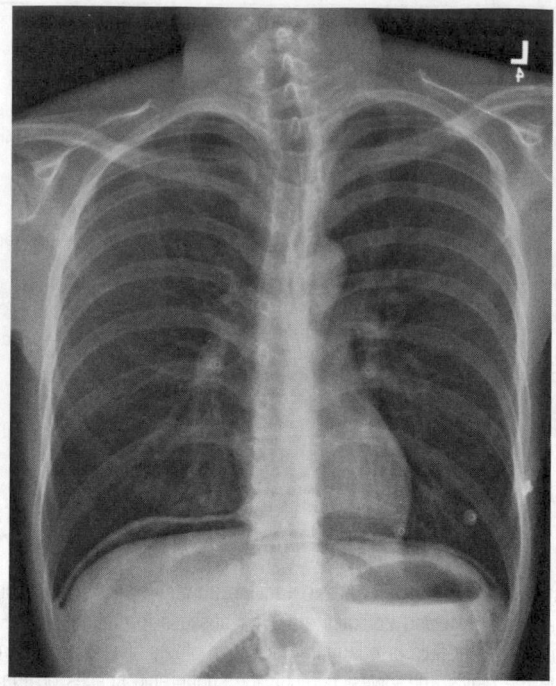

Figure 127-2 Pneumoperitoneum. Free air under the diaphragm on an upright chest film suggests the presence of a bowel perforation and associated peritonitis. *(Image courtesy of Dr. John Braver; with permission.)*

multiple organisms including anaerobes are recovered from the peritoneal fluid, the diagnosis must be reconsidered and a source of secondary peritonitis sought.

The diagnosis of PBP is not easy. It depends on the exclusion of a primary intraabdominal source of infection. Contrast-enhanced CT is useful in identifying an intraabdominal source for infection. It may be difficult to recover organisms from cultures of peritoneal fluid, presumably because the burden of organisms is low. However, the yield can be improved if 10 mL of peritoneal fluid is placed directly into a blood culture bottle. Since bacteremia frequently accompanies PBP, blood should be cultured simultaneously. No specific radiographic studies are helpful in the diagnosis of PBP. A plain film of the abdomen would be expected to show ascites. Chest and abdominal radiography should be performed in patients with abdominal pain to exclude free air, which signals a perforation (Fig. 127-2).

| TREATMENT | Primary Bacterial Peritonitis |

Treatment for PBP is directed at the isolate from blood or peritoneal fluid. Gram's staining of peritoneal fluid often gives negative results in PBP. Therefore, until culture results become available, therapy should cover gram-negative aerobic bacilli and gram-positive cocci. Third-generation cephalosporins such as cefotaxime (2 g q8h, administered IV) provide reasonable initial coverage in moderately ill patients. Broad-spectrum antibiotics, such as penicillin/β-lactamase inhibitor combinations (e.g., piperacillin/tazobactam, 3.375 g q6h IV for adults with normal renal function) or ceftriaxone (2 g q24h IV), are also options. Empirical coverage for anaerobes is not necessary. After the infecting organism is identified, therapy should be narrowed to target the specific pathogen. Patients with PBP usually respond within 72 h to appropriate antibiotic therapy. Antimicrobial treatment can be administered for as little as

5 days if rapid improvement occurs and blood cultures are negative, but a course of up to 2 weeks may be required for patients with bacteremia and for those whose improvement is slow. Persistence of WBCs in the ascitic fluid after therapy should prompt a search for additional diagnoses.

Prevention

Primary prevention One observational study raises the concern that proton pump inhibitor (PPI) therapy may increase the risk of PBP. No prospective studies have yet addressed whether avoidance of PPI therapy may prevent PBP.

Secondary prevention PBP has a high rate of recurrence. Up to 70% of patients experience a recurrence within 1 year. Antibiotic prophylaxis reduces this rate to <20% and improves short-term survival rates. Prophylactic regimens for adults with normal renal function include fluoroquinolones (ciprofloxacin, 750 mg weekly; norfloxacin, 400 mg/d) or trimethoprim-sulfamethoxazole (one double-strength tablet daily). However, long-term administration of broad-spectrum antibiotics in this setting has been shown to increase the risk of severe staphylococcal infections.

■ SECONDARY PERITONITIS

Secondary peritonitis develops when bacteria contaminate the peritoneum as a result of spillage from an intraabdominal viscus. The organisms found almost always constitute a mixed flora in which facultative gram-negative bacilli and anaerobes predominate, especially when the contaminating source is colonic. Early in the course of infection, when the host response is directed toward containment of the infection, exudate containing fibrin and PMNs is found. Early death in this setting is attributable to gram-negative bacillary sepsis and to potent endotoxins circulating in the bloodstream (Chap. 271). Gram-negative bacilli, particularly *E. coli*, are common bloodstream isolates, but *Bacteroides fragilis* bacteremia also occurs. The severity of abdominal pain and the clinical course depend on the inciting process. The organisms isolated from the peritoneum also vary with the source of the initial process and the normal flora at that site. Secondary peritonitis can result primarily from chemical irritation and/or bacterial contamination. For example, as long as the patient is not achlorhydric, a ruptured gastric ulcer will release low-pH gastric contents that will serve as a chemical irritant. The normal flora of the stomach comprises the same organisms found in the oropharynx (Chap. 164) but in lower numbers. Thus, the bacterial burden in a ruptured ulcer is negligible compared with that in a ruptured appendix. The normal flora of the colon below the ligament of Treitz contains ~10^{11} anaerobic organisms/g of feces but only 10^8 aerobes/g; therefore, anaerobic species account for 99.9% of the bacteria. Leakage of colonic contents (pH 7–8) does not cause significant chemical peritonitis, but infection is intense because of the heavy bacterial load.

Depending on the inciting event, local symptoms may occur in secondary peritonitis—for example, epigastric pain from a ruptured gastric ulcer. In appendicitis (Chap. 300), the initial presenting symptoms are often vague, with periumbilical discomfort and nausea followed in a number of hours by pain more localized to the right lower quadrant. Unusual locations of the appendix (including a retrocecal position) can complicate this presentation further. Once infection has spread to the peritoneal cavity, pain increases, particularly with infection involving the parietal peritoneum, which is innervated extensively. Patients usually lie motionless, often with knees drawn up to avoid stretching the nerve fibers of the peritoneal cavity. Coughing and sneezing, which increase pressure within the peritoneal cavity, are associated with sharp pain. There may or may not be pain localized to the infected or diseased organ from which secondary peritonitis has arisen. Patients with secondary peritonitis generally have abnormal findings on abdominal examination, with marked voluntary and involuntary guarding of the anterior abdominal musculature. Later findings include tenderness, especially rebound tenderness. In addition, there may be localized findings in the area of the inciting event. In general, patients are febrile, with marked leukocytosis and a left shift of the WBCs to band forms.

While recovery of organisms from peritoneal fluid is easier in secondary than in primary peritonitis, a tap of the abdomen is rarely the procedure of choice in secondary peritonitis. An exception is in cases involving trauma, where the possibility of a hemoperitoneum may need to be excluded early. Emergent studies (such as abdominal CT) to find the source of peritoneal contamination should be undertaken if the patient is hemodynamically stable; unstable patients may require surgical intervention without prior imaging.

TREATMENT Secondary Peritonitis

Treatment for secondary peritonitis includes early administration of antibiotics aimed particularly at aerobic gram-negative bacilli and anaerobes (see below). Mild to moderate disease can be treated with many drugs covering these organisms, including broad-spectrum penicillin/β-lactamase inhibitor combinations (e.g., ticarcillin/clavulanate, 3.1 g q4–6h IV), cefoxitin (2 g q4–6h IV), or a combination of a fluoroquinolone (e.g., levofloxacin, 750 mg q24h IV) or a third-generation cephalosporin (e.g., ceftriaxone, 2 g q24h IV) plus metronidazole (500 mg q8h IV). Patients in intensive care units should receive imipenem (500 mg q6h IV), meropenem (1 g q8h IV), or combinations of drugs, such as ampicillin plus metronidazole plus ciprofloxacin. The role of enterococci and *Candida* spp. in mixed infections is controversial. Secondary peritonitis usually requires both surgical intervention to address the inciting process and antibiotics to treat early bacteremia, to decrease the incidence of abscess formation and wound infection, and to prevent distant spread of infection. While surgery is rarely indicated in PBP in adults, it may be life-saving in secondary peritonitis. Recombinant human activated protein C has been shown to reduce mortality rates among patients with severe sepsis and may benefit some patients with secondary peritonitis.

Peritonitis may develop as a complication of abdominal surgeries. These infections may be accompanied by localizing pain and/or nonlocalizing symptoms such as fever, malaise, anorexia, and toxicity. As a nosocomial infection, postoperative peritonitis may be associated with organisms such as staphylococci, components of the gram-negative hospital microflora, and the microbes that cause PBP and secondary peritonitis, as described above.

■ PERITONITIS IN PATIENTS UNDERGOING CAPD

A third type of peritonitis arises in patients who are undergoing continuous ambulatory peritoneal dialysis (CAPD). Unlike PBP and secondary peritonitis, which are caused by endogenous bacteria, CAPD-associated peritonitis usually involves skin organisms. The pathogenesis of infection is similar to that of intravascular device–related infection, in which skin organisms migrate along the catheter, which both serves as an entry point and exerts the effects of a foreign body. Exit-site or tunnel infection may or may not accompany CAPD-associated peritonitis. Like PBP, CAPD-associated peritonitis is usually caused by a single organism. Peritonitis is, in fact, the most common reason for discontinuation of CAPD. Improvements in equipment design, especially the Y-set

connector, have resulted in a decrease from one case of peritonitis per 9 months of CAPD to one case per 24 months.

The clinical presentation of CAPD peritonitis resembles that of secondary peritonitis in that diffuse pain and peritoneal signs are common. The dialysate is usually cloudy and contains >100 WBCs/μL, >50% of which are neutrophils. The most common organisms are *Staphylococcus* spp., which accounted for ~45% of cases in one series. Historically, coagulase-negative staphylococcal species were identified most commonly in these infections, but more recently these isolates have been decreasing in frequency. *Staphylococcus aureus* is more often involved among patients who are nasal carriers of the organism than among those who are not, and this organism is the most common pathogen in overt exit-site infections. Gram-negative bacilli and fungi such as *Candida* spp. are also found. Vancomycin-resistant enterococci and vancomycin-intermediate *S. aureus* have been reported to produce peritonitis in CAPD patients. The finding of more than one organism in dialysate culture should prompt evaluation for secondary peritonitis. As with PBP, culture of dialysate fluid in blood culture bottles improves the yield. To facilitate diagnosis, several hundred milliliters of removed dialysis fluid should be concentrated by centrifugation before culture.

TREATMENT CAPD Peritonitis

Empirical therapy for CAPD peritonitis should be directed at *S. aureus*, coagulase-negative *Staphylococcus*, and gram-negative bacilli until the results of cultures are available. Guidelines issued in 2005 suggest that agents should be chosen on the basis of local experience with resistant organisms. In some centers, a first-generation cephalosporin such as cefazolin (for gram-positive bacteria) and a fluoroquinolone or a third-generation cephalosporin such as ceftazidime (for gram-negative bacteria) may be reasonable; in areas with high rates of infection with methicillin-resistant *S. aureus*, vancomycin should be used instead of cefazolin, and gram-negative coverage may need to be broadened. Broad coverage including vancomycin should be particularly considered for toxic patients and for those with exit-site infections. Loading doses are administered intraperitoneally; doses depend on the dialysis method and the patient's renal function. Antibiotics are given either continuously (i.e., with each exchange) or intermittently (i.e., once daily, with the dose allowed to remain in the peritoneal cavity for at least 6 h). If the patient is severely ill, IV antibiotics should be added at doses appropriate for the patient's degree of renal failure. The clinical response to an empirical treatment regimen should be rapid; if the patient has not responded after 48–96 h of treatment, catheter removal should be considered.

■ TUBERCULOUS PERITONITIS

See Chap. 165.

INTRAABDOMINAL ABSCESSES

■ INTRAPERITONEAL ABSCESSES

Abscess formation is common in untreated peritonitis if overt gram-negative sepsis either does not develop or develops but is not fatal. In experimental models of abscess formation, mixed aerobic and anaerobic organisms have been implanted intraperitoneally. Without therapy directed at anaerobes, animals develop intraabdominal abscesses. As in humans, these experimental abscesses may stud the peritoneal cavity, lie within the omentum or mesentery, or even develop on the surface of or within viscera such as the liver.

Pathogenesis and immunity

There is often disagreement about whether an abscess represents a disease state or a host response. In a sense, it represents both: while an abscess is an infection in which viable infecting organisms and PMNs are contained in a fibrous capsule, it is also a process by which the host confines microbes to a limited space, thereby preventing further spread of infection. In any event, abscesses do cause significant symptoms, and patients with abscesses can be quite ill. Experimental work has helped to define both the host cells and the bacterial virulence factors responsible—most notably in the case of *B. fragilis*. This organism, although accounting for only 0.5% of the normal colonic flora, is the anaerobe most frequently isolated from intraabdominal infections, is especially prominent in abscesses, and is the most common anaerobic bloodstream isolate. On clinical grounds, therefore, *B. fragilis* appears to be uniquely virulent. Moreover, *B. fragilis* acts alone to cause abscesses in animal models of intraabdominal infection, whereas most other *Bacteroides* species must act synergistically with a facultative organism to induce abscess formation.

Of the several virulence factors identified in *B. fragilis*, one is critical: the capsular polysaccharide complex (CPC) found on the bacterial surface. The CPC comprises at least eight distinct surface polysaccharides. Structural analysis of these polysaccharides has shown an unusual motif of oppositely charged sugars. Polysaccharides having these *zwitterionic* characteristics, such as polysaccharide A (PSA), evoke a host response in the peritoneal cavity that localizes bacteria into abscesses. *B. fragilis* and PSA have been found to adhere to primary mesothelial cells in vitro; this adherence, in turn, stimulates the production of tumor necrosis factor α (TNF-α) and intercellular adhesion molecule 1 (ICAM-1) by peritoneal macrophages. Although abscesses characteristically contain PMNs, the process of abscess induction depends on the stimulation of T lymphocytes by these unique zwitterionic polysaccharides. The stimulated CD4+ T lymphocytes secrete leukoattractant cytokines and chemokines. The alternative pathway of complement and fibrinogen also participate in abscess formation.

While antibodies to the CPC enhance bloodstream clearance of *B. fragilis*, CD4+ T cells are critical in immunity to abscesses. When administered subcutaneously, *B. fragilis* PSA has immunomodulatory characteristics and stimulates CD4+ T regulatory cells via an interleukin (IL) 2–dependent mechanism to produce IL-10. IL-10 downregulates the inflammatory response, thereby preventing abscess formation.

Clinical presentation

Of all intraabdominal abscesses, 74% are intraperitoneal or retroperitoneal and are not visceral. Most intraperitoneal abscesses result from fecal spillage from a colonic source, such as an inflamed appendix. Abscesses can also arise from other processes. They usually form within weeks of the development of peritonitis and may be found in a variety of locations—from omentum to mesentery, pelvis to psoas muscles, and subphrenic space to a visceral organ such as the liver, where they may develop either on the surface of the organ or within it. Periappendiceal and diverticular abscesses occur commonly. Diverticular abscesses are least likely to rupture. Infections of the female genital tract and pancreatitis are also among the more common causative events. When abscesses occur in the female genital tract—either as a primary infection (e.g., tuboovarian abscess) or as an infection extending into the pelvic cavity or peritoneum—*B. fragilis* figures

prominently among the organisms isolated. *B. fragilis* is not found in large numbers in the normal vaginal flora. For example, it is encountered less commonly in pelvic inflammatory disease and endometritis without an associated abscess. In pancreatitis with leakage of damaging pancreatic enzymes, inflammation is prominent. Therefore, clinical findings such as fever, leukocytosis, and even abdominal pain do not distinguish pancreatitis itself from complications such as pancreatic pseudocyst, pancreatic abscess (Chap. 313), or intraabdominal collections of pus. Especially in cases of necrotizing pancreatitis, in which the incidence of local pancreatic infection may be as high as 30%, needle aspiration under CT guidance is performed to sample fluid for culture. Many centers prescribe preemptive antibiotics for patients with necrotizing pancreatitis. Imipenem is frequently used for this purpose since it reaches high tissue levels in the pancreas (although it is not unique in this regard). If needle aspiration yields infected fluid in the setting of acute necrotizing pancreatitis, most experts agree that surgery is superior to percutaneous drainage. Infected pseudocysts that occur remotely from acute pancreatitis are unlikely to be associated with significant amounts of necrotic tissue and may be treated with either surgical or percutaneous catheter drainage in conjunction with appropriate antibiotic therapy.

Diagnosis

Scanning procedures have considerably facilitated the diagnosis of intraabdominal abscesses. Abdominal CT probably has the highest yield, although ultrasonography is particularly useful for the right upper quadrant, kidneys, and pelvis. Both indium-labeled WBCs and gallium tend to localize in abscesses and may be useful in finding a collection. Since gallium is taken up in the bowel, indium-labeled WBCs may have a slightly greater yield for abscesses near the bowel. Neither indium-labeled WBC nor gallium scans serve as a basis for a definitive diagnosis, however; both need to be followed by other, more specific studies, such as CT, if an area of possible abnormality is identified. Abscesses contiguous with or contained within diverticula are particularly difficult to diagnose with scanning procedures. Occasionally, a barium enema may detect a diverticular abscess not diagnosed by other procedures, although barium should not be injected if a perforation is suspected. If one study is negative, a second study sometimes reveals a collection. Although exploratory laparotomy has been less commonly used since the advent of CT, this procedure still must be undertaken on occasion if an abscess is strongly suspected on clinical grounds.

TREATMENT   Intraperitoneal Abscesses

An algorithm for the management of patients with intraabdominal (including intraperitoneal) abscesses is presented in Fig. 127-3. The treatment of intraabdominal infections involves the determination of the initial focus of infection, the administration of broad-spectrum antibiotics targeting the organisms involved, and the performance of a drainage procedure if one or more definitive abscesses have formed. Antimicrobial therapy, in general, is adjunctive to drainage and/or surgical correction of an underlying lesion or process in intraabdominal abscesses. Unlike the intraabdominal abscesses resulting from most causes, for which drainage of some kind is generally required, abscesses associated with diverticulitis usually wall off locally after rupture of a diverticulum, so that surgical intervention is not routinely required.

A number of agents exhibit excellent activity against aerobic gram-negative bacilli. Since death in intraabdominal sepsis is linked to gram-negative bacteremia, empirical therapy for

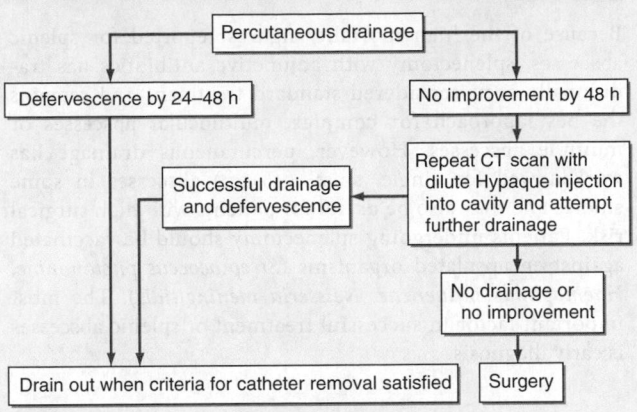

Figure 127-3 Algorithm for the management of patients with intraabdominal abscesses using percutaneous drainage. Antimicrobial therapy should be administered concomitantly. *[Reprinted with permission from B Lorber (ed): Atlas of Infectious Diseases, vol VII: Intra-abdominal Infections, Hepatitis, and Gastroenteritis. Philadelphia, Current Medicine, 1996, p 1.30, as adapted from OD Rotstein, RL Simmons, in SL Gorbach et al (eds): Infectious Diseases. Philadelphia, Saunders, 1992, p 668.]*

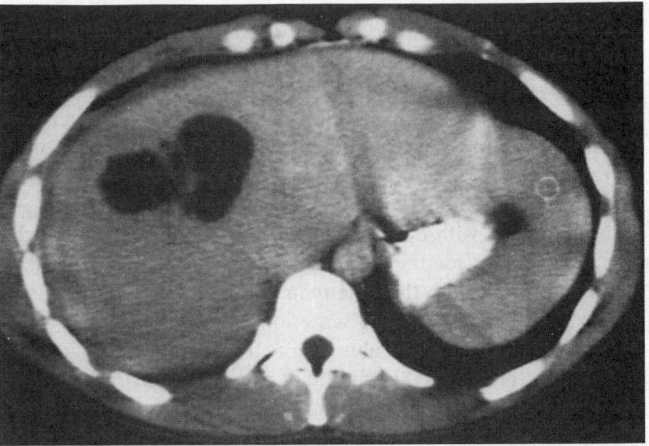

Figure 127-4 Multilocular liver abscess on CT scan. Multiple or multilocular abscesses are more common than solitary abscesses. *[Reprinted with permission from B Lorber (ed): Atlas of Infectious Diseases, Vol VII: Intra-abdominal Infections, Hepatitis, and Gastroenteritis. Philadelphia, Current Medicine, 1996, Fig. 1.22.]*

intraabdominal infection always needs to include adequate coverage of gram-negative aerobic, facultative, and anaerobic organisms. Even if anaerobes are not cultured from clinical specimens, they still must be covered by the therapeutic regimen. Empirical antibiotic therapy should be the same as that discussed above for secondary peritonitis.

■ VISCERAL ABSCESSES

Liver abscesses

The liver is the organ most subject to the development of abscesses. In one study of 540 intraabdominal abscesses, 26% were visceral. Liver abscesses made up 13% of the total number, or 48% of all visceral abscesses. Liver abscesses may be solitary or multiple; they may arise from hematogenous spread of bacteria or from local spread from contiguous sites of infection within the peritoneal cavity. In the past, appendicitis with rupture and subsequent spread of infection was the most common source for a liver abscess. Currently, associated disease of the biliary tract is most common. Pylephlebitis (suppurative thrombosis of the portal vein), usually arising from infection in the pelvis but sometimes from infection elsewhere in the peritoneal cavity, is another common source for bacterial seeding of the liver.

Fever is the most common presenting sign of liver abscess. Some patients, particularly those with associated disease of the biliary tract, have symptoms and signs localized to the right upper quadrant, including pain, guarding, punch tenderness, and even rebound tenderness. Nonspecific symptoms, such as chills, anorexia, weight loss, nausea, and vomiting, may also develop. Only 50% of patients with liver abscesses, however, have hepatomegaly, right-upper-quadrant tenderness, or jaundice; thus, one-half of patients have no symptoms or signs to direct attention to the liver. Fever of unknown origin (FUO) may be the only manifestation of liver abscess, especially in the elderly. Diagnostic studies of the abdomen, especially the right upper quadrant, should be a part of any FUO workup. The single most reliable laboratory finding is an elevated serum concentration of alkaline phosphatase, which is documented in 70% of patients with liver

abscesses. Other tests of liver function may yield normal results, but 50% of patients have elevated serum levels of bilirubin, and 48% have elevated concentrations of aspartate aminotransferase. Other laboratory findings include leukocytosis in 77% of patients, anemia (usually normochromic, normocytic) in 50%, and hypoalbuminemia in 33%. Concomitant bacteremia is found in one-third to one-half of patients. A liver abscess is sometimes suggested by chest radiography, especially if a new elevation of the right hemidiaphragm is seen; other suggestive findings include a right basilar infiltrate and a right pleural effusion.

Imaging studies are the most reliable methods for diagnosing liver abscesses. These studies include ultrasonography, CT (Fig. 127-4), indium-labeled WBC or gallium scan, and MRI. More than one such study may be required. Organisms recovered from liver abscesses vary with the source. In liver infection arising from the biliary tree, enteric gram-negative aerobic bacilli and enterococci are common isolates. Unless previous surgery has been performed, anaerobes are not generally involved in liver abscesses arising from biliary infections. In contrast, in liver abscesses arising from pelvic and other intraperitoneal sources, a mixed flora including both aerobic and anaerobic species is common; *B. fragilis* is the species most frequently isolated. With hematogenous spread of infection, usually only a single organism is encountered; this species may be *S. aureus* or a streptococcal species such as *S. milleri*. Results of cultures obtained from drain sites are not reliable for defining the etiology of infections. Liver abscesses may also be caused by *Candida* spp.; such abscesses usually follow fungemia in patients receiving chemotherapy for cancer and often present when PMNs return after a period of neutropenia. Amebic liver abscesses are not an uncommon problem (Chap. 209). Amebic serologic testing gives positive results in >95% of cases; thus, a negative result helps to exclude this diagnosis.

| TREATMENT | Liver Abscesses |

(Fig. 127-3) While drainage—either percutaneous (with a pigtail catheter kept in place) or surgical—is the mainstay of therapy for intraabdominal abscesses (including liver abscesses), there is growing interest in medical management alone for pyogenic liver abscesses. The drugs used for empirical therapy include the same ones used in intraabdominal sepsis and secondary bacterial peritonitis. Usually, blood cultures and a diagnostic aspirate of abscess contents should be obtained before the initiation of empirical therapy, with antibiotic choices adjusted when the results of Gram's staining and culture become available. Cases treated without definitive drainage generally require longer courses of antibiotic therapy. When percutaneous drainage was compared with open surgical drainage, the average length of hospital stay for the former was almost twice that for the latter, although both the time required for fever to resolve and the mortality rate were the same for the two procedures. The mortality rate was appreciable despite treatment, averaging 15%. Several factors predict the failure of percutaneous drainage and therefore may favor primary surgical intervention. These factors include the presence of multiple, sizable abscesses; viscous abscess contents that tend to plug the catheter; associated disease (e.g., disease of the biliary tract) requiring surgery; or the lack of a clinical response to percutaneous drainage in 4–7 days.

Treatment of candidal liver abscesses often entails initial administration of amphotericin B or liposomal amphotericin, with subsequent fluconazole therapy (Chap. 203). In some cases, therapy with fluconazole alone (6 mg/kg daily) may be used—e.g., in clinically stable patients whose infecting isolate is susceptible to this drug.

Splenic abscesses

Splenic abscesses are much less common than liver abscesses. The incidence of splenic abscesses has ranged from 0.14% to 0.7% in various autopsy series. The clinical setting and the organisms isolated usually differ from those for liver abscesses. The degree of clinical suspicion for splenic abscess needs to be high, as this condition is frequently fatal if left untreated. Even in the most recently published series, diagnosis was made only at autopsy in 37% of cases. While splenic abscesses may arise occasionally from contiguous spread of infection or from direct trauma to the spleen, hematogenous spread of infection is more common. Bacterial endocarditis is the most common associated infection (Chap. 124). Splenic abscesses can develop in patients who have received extensive immunosuppressive therapy (particularly those with malignancy involving the spleen) and in patients with hemoglobinopathies or other hematologic disorders (especially sickle cell anemia).

While ~50% of patients with splenic abscesses have abdominal pain, the pain is localized to the left upper quadrant in only one-half of these cases. Splenomegaly is found in ~50% of cases. Fever and leukocytosis are generally present; the development of fever preceded diagnosis by an average of 20 days in one series. Left-sided chest findings may include abnormalities to auscultation, and chest radiographic findings may include an infiltrate or a left-sided pleural effusion. CT scan of the abdomen has been the most sensitive diagnostic tool. Ultrasonography can yield the diagnosis but is less sensitive. Liver-spleen scan or gallium scan may also be useful. Streptococcal species are the most common bacterial isolates from splenic abscesses, followed by S. aureus—presumably reflecting the associated endocarditis. An increase in the prevalence of gram-negative aerobic isolates from splenic abscesses has been reported; these organisms often derive from a urinary tract focus, with associated bacteremia, or from another intraabdominal source. Salmonella species are seen fairly commonly, especially in patients with sickle cell hemoglobinopathy. Anaerobic species accounted for only 5% of isolates in the largest collected series, but the reporting of a number of "sterile abscesses" may indicate that optimal techniques for the isolation of anaerobes were not employed.

Because of the high mortality figures reported for splenic abscesses, splenectomy with adjunctive antibiotics has traditionally been considered standard treatment and remains the best approach for complex, multilocular abscesses or multiple abscesses. However, percutaneous drainage has worked well for single, small (<3-cm) abscesses in some studies and may also be useful for patients with high surgical risk. Patients undergoing splenectomy should be vaccinated against encapsulated organisms (*Streptococcus pneumoniae, Haemophilus influenzae, Neisseria meningitidis*). The most important factor in successful treatment of splenic abscesses is early diagnosis.

Perinephric and renal abscesses

Perinephric and renal abscesses are not common: The former accounted for only ~0.02% of hospital admissions and the latter for ~0.2% in Altemeier's series of 540 intraabdominal abscesses. Before antibiotics became available, most renal and perinephric abscesses were hematogenous in origin, usually complicating prolonged bacteremia, with S. aureus most commonly recovered. Now, in contrast, >75% of perinephric and renal abscesses arise from a urinary tract infection. Infection ascends from the bladder to the kidney, with pyelonephritis occurring prior to abscess development. Bacteria may directly invade the renal parenchyma from medulla to cortex. Local vascular channels within the kidney may also facilitate the transport of organisms. Areas of abscess developing within the parenchyma may rupture into the perinephric space. The kidneys and adrenal glands are surrounded by a layer of perirenal fat that, in turn, is surrounded by Gerota's fascia, which extends superiorly to the diaphragm and inferiorly to the pelvic fat. Abscesses extending into the perinephric space may track through Gerota's fascia into the psoas or transversalis muscles, into the anterior peritoneal cavity, superiorly to the subdiaphragmatic space, or inferiorly to the pelvis. Of the risk factors that have been associated with the development of perinephric abscesses, the most important is concomitant nephrolithiasis obstructing urinary flow. Of patients with perinephric abscess, 20–60% have renal stones. Other structural abnormalities of the urinary tract, prior urologic surgery, trauma, and diabetes mellitus have also been identified as risk factors.

The organisms most frequently encountered in perinephric and renal abscesses are E. coli, Proteus spp., and Klebsiella spp. E. coli, the aerobic species most commonly found in the colonic flora, seems to have unique virulence properties in the urinary tract, including factors promoting adherence to uroepithelial cells. The urease of Proteus spp. splits urea, thereby creating a more alkaline and more hospitable environment for bacterial proliferation. Proteus spp. are frequently found in association with large struvite stones caused by the precipitation of magnesium ammonium sulfate in an alkaline environment. These stones serve as a nidus for recurrent urinary tract infection. While a single bacterial species is usually recovered from a perinephric or renal abscess, multiple species may also be found. If a urine culture is not contaminated with periurethral flora and is found to contain more than one organism, a perinephric abscess or renal abscess should be considered in the differential diagnosis. Urine cultures may also be polymicrobial in cases of bladder diverticulum.

Candida spp. can cause renal abscesses. This fungus may spread to the kidney hematogenously or by ascension from the bladder. The hallmark of the latter route of infection is ureteral obstruction with large fungal balls.

The presentation of perinephric and renal abscesses is quite nonspecific. Flank pain and abdominal pain are common. At least 50% of patients are febrile. Pain may be referred to the groin or leg, particularly with extension of infection. The diagnosis of perinephric abscess, like that of splenic abscess, is frequently delayed, and the mortality rate in some series is appreciable, although lower than in the past. Perinephric or renal abscess should be most seriously considered when a patient presents with symptoms and signs of pyelonephritis and remains febrile after 4 or 5 days of treatment. Moreover, when a urine culture yields a polymicrobial flora, when a patient is known to have renal stones, or when fever and pyuria coexist with a sterile urine culture, these diagnoses should be entertained.

Renal ultrasonography and abdominal CT are the most useful diagnostic modalities. If a renal or perinephric abscess is diagnosed, nephrolithiasis should be excluded, especially when a high urinary pH suggests the presence of a urea-splitting organism.

TREATMENT   Perinephric and Renal Abscesses

Treatment for perinephric and renal abscesses, like that for other intraabdominal abscesses, includes drainage of pus and antibiotic therapy directed at the organism(s) recovered. For perinephric abscesses, percutaneous drainage is usually successful.

Psoas abscesses

The psoas muscle is another location in which abscesses are encountered. Psoas abscesses may arise from a hematogenous source, by contiguous spread from an intraabdominal or pelvic process, or by contiguous spread from nearby bony structures (e.g., vertebral bodies). Associated osteomyelitis due to spread from bone to muscle or from muscle to bone is common in psoas abscesses. When Pott's disease was common, *Mycobacterium tuberculosis* was a frequent cause of psoas abscess. Currently, either *S. aureus* or a mixture of enteric organisms including aerobic and anaerobic gram-negative bacilli is usually isolated from psoas abscesses in the United States. *S. aureus* is most likely to be isolated when a psoas abscess arises from hematogenous spread or a contiguous focus of osteomyelitis; a mixed enteric flora is the most likely etiology when the abscess has an intraabdominal or pelvic source. Patients with psoas abscesses frequently present with fever, lower abdominal or back pain, or pain referred to the hip or knee. CT is the most useful diagnostic technique.

TREATMENT   Psoas Abscesses

Treatment includes surgical drainage and the administration of an antibiotic regimen directed at the inciting organism(s).

Pancreatic abscesses

See Chap. 313.

ACKNOWLEDGMENT

The substantial contributions of Dori F. Zaleznik, MD, to this chapter in previous editions are gratefully acknowledged.

FURTHER READINGS

BAJAJ JS et al: Association of proton pump inhibitor therapy with spontaneous bacterial peritonitis in cirrhotic patients with ascites. Am J Gastroenterol 104:1130, 2009

BARIE PS et al: Benefit/risk of drotrecogin alpha [activated] in surgical patients with severe sepsis. Am J Surg 188:212, 2004

MEDDINGS L et al: A population-based study of pyogenic liver abscesses in the United States: mortality, and temporal trends. Am J Gastroenterol 105:117, 2010

NAVARRO LÓPEZ V et al: GTI-SEMI Group: Microbiology and outcome of iliopsoas abscess in 124 patients. Medicine (Baltimore) 88:120, 2009

PIRAINO B et al: Peritoneal dialysis–related infections recommendations: 2005 update. Perit Dial Int 25:107, 2005

SAAB S et al: Oral antibiotic prophylaxis reduces spontaneous bacterial peritonitis occurrence and improves short-term survival in cirrhosis: A meta-analysis. Am J Gastroenterol 104:993, 2009

SIFRI CD, MADOFF LC: Infections of the liver and biliary system, in *Principles and Practice of Infectious Diseases*, 7th ed, GL Mandell et al (eds). Philadelphia, Elsevier Churchill Livingstone, 2010, pp 1035–1044

SOLOMKIN JS, MAZUSKI J: Intra-abdominal sepsis: Newer interventional and antimicrobial therapies. Infect Dis Clin North Am 23:593, 2009

TZIANABOS AO et al: T cells activated by zwitterionic molecules prevent abscesses induced by pathogenic bacteria. J Biol Chem 275:6733, 2000

VAN RULER O et al: Comparison of on-demand vs planned relaparotomy strategy in patients with severe peritonitis: A randomized trial. JAMA 298:865, 2007

CHAPTER 127

Intraabdominal Infections and Abscesses

CHAPTER 128

Acute Infectious Diarrheal Diseases and Bacterial Food Poisoning

Regina C. LaRocque

Edward T. Ryan

Stephen B. Calderwood

Ranging from a mild annoyance to a devastating dehydrating illness, acute diarrheal disease is a leading cause of illness globally, with an estimated 4.6 billion episodes worldwide per year. Diarrheal disease ranks second only to lower respiratory infection as the most common infectious cause of death worldwide. Among children <5 years old, diarrheal disease is a particularly important cause of death. Every year nearly 2 million children in this age group die of diarrheal disease; the majority of these young children are impoverished and live in resource-poor areas. By contributing to malnutrition and thereby reducing resistance to other infectious agents, diarrheal disease is also an indirect factor in a far greater burden of disease.

The wide range of clinical manifestations of acute gastrointestinal illnesses is matched by the wide variety of infectious agents involved, including viruses, bacteria, and parasitic pathogens (Table 128-1). This chapter discusses factors that enable gastrointestinal pathogens to cause disease, reviews host defense mechanisms, and delineates an approach to the evaluation and treatment of patients presenting with acute diarrhea. Individual organisms causing acute gastrointestinal illnesses are discussed in detail in subsequent chapters.

PATHOGENIC MECHANISMS

Enteric pathogens have developed a variety of tactics to overcome host defenses. Understanding the virulence factors employed by these organisms is important in the diagnosis and treatment of clinical disease.

Inoculum size

The number of microorganisms that must be ingested to cause disease varies considerably from species to species. For *Shigella*, enterohemorrhagic *Escherichia coli*, *Giardia lamblia*, or *Entamoeba*, as few as 10–100 bacteria or cysts can produce infection, while 10^5–10^8 *Vibrio cholerae* organisms must be ingested orally to cause disease. The infective dose of *Salmonella* varies widely, depending on the species, host, and food vehicle. The ability of organisms to overcome host defenses has important implications for transmission; *Shigella*, enterohemorrhagic *E. coli*, *Entamoeba*, and *Giardia* can spread by person-to-person contact, whereas under some circumstances *Salmonella* may have to grow in food for several hours before reaching an effective infectious dose.

Adherence

Many organisms must adhere to the gastrointestinal mucosa as an initial step in the pathogenic process; thus, organisms that can compete with the normal bowel flora and colonize the mucosa have an important advantage in causing disease. Specific cell-surface proteins involved in attachment of bacteria to intestinal cells are important virulence determinants. *V. cholerae*, for example, adheres to the brush border of small-intestinal enterocytes via specific surface adhesins, including the toxin-coregulated pilus and other accessory colonization factors. Enterotoxigenic *E. coli*, which causes watery diarrhea, produces an adherence protein called *colonization factor antigen* that is necessary for colonization of the upper small intestine by the organism prior to the production of enterotoxin. Enteropathogenic *E. coli*, an agent of diarrhea in young children, and enterohemorrhagic *E. coli*, which causes hemorrhagic colitis and the hemolytic-uremic syndrome, produce virulence determinants that allow these organisms to attach to and efface the brush border of the intestinal epithelium.

Toxin production

The production of one or more exotoxins is important in the pathogenesis of numerous enteric organisms. Such toxins include *enterotoxins*, which cause watery diarrhea by acting directly on secretory mechanisms

TABLE 128-1 Gastrointestinal Pathogens Causing Acute Diarrhea

Mechanism	Location	Illness	Stool Findings	Examples of Pathogens Involved
Noninflammatory (enterotoxin)	Proximal small bowel	Watery diarrhea	No fecal leukocytes; mild or no increase in fecal lactoferrin	*Vibrio cholerae*, enterotoxigenic *Escherichia coli* (LT and/or ST), enteroaggregative *E. coli*, *Clostridium perfringens*, *Bacillus cereus*, *Staphylococcus aureus*, *Aeromonas hydrophila*, *Plesiomonas shigelloides*, rotavirus, norovirus, enteric adenoviruses, *Giardia lamblia*, *Cryptosporidium* spp., *Cyclospora* spp., microsporidia
Inflammatory (invasion or cytotoxin)	Colon or distal small bowel	Dysentery or inflammatory diarrhea	Fecal polymorphonuclear leukocytes; substantial increase in fecal lactoferrin	*Shigella* spp., *Salmonella* spp., *Campylobacter jejuni*, enterohemorrhagic *E. coli*, enteroinvasive *E. coli*, *Yersinia enterocolitica*, *Listeria monocytogenes*, *Vibrio parahaemolyticus*, *Clostridium difficile*, *A. hydrophila*, *P. shigelloides*, *Entamoeba histolytica*, *Klebsiella oxytoca*
Penetrating	Distal small bowel	Enteric fever	Fecal mononuclear leukocytes	*Salmonella typhi*, *Y. enterocolitica*

Abbreviations: LT, heat-labile enterotoxin; ST, heat-stable enterotoxin.
Source: After Steiner and Guerrant.

in the intestinal mucosa; *cytotoxins*, which cause destruction of mucosal cells and associated inflammatory diarrhea; and *neurotoxins*, which act directly on the central or peripheral nervous system.

The prototypical enterotoxin is cholera toxin, a heterodimeric protein composed of one A and five B subunits. The A subunit contains the enzymatic activity of the toxin, while the B subunit pentamer binds holotoxin to the enterocyte surface receptor, the ganglioside G_{M1}. After the binding of holotoxin, a fragment of the A subunit is translocated across the eukaryotic cell membrane into the cytoplasm, where it catalyzes the ADP-ribosylation of a GTP-binding protein and causes persistent activation of adenylate cyclase. The end result is an increase of cyclic AMP in the intestinal mucosa, which increases Cl^- secretion and decreases Na^+ absorption, leading to a loss of fluid and the production of diarrhea.

Enterotoxigenic strains of *E. coli* may produce a protein called *heat-labile enterotoxin* (LT) that is similar to cholera toxin and causes secretory diarrhea by the same mechanism. Alternatively, enterotoxigenic strains of *E. coli* may produce *heat-stable enterotoxin* (ST), one form of which causes diarrhea by activation of guanylate cyclase and elevation of intracellular cyclic GMP. Some enterotoxigenic strains of *E. coli* produce both LT and ST.

Bacterial cytotoxins, in contrast, destroy intestinal mucosal cells and produce the syndrome of dysentery, with bloody stools containing inflammatory cells. Enteric pathogens that produce such cytotoxins include *Shigella dysenteriae* type 1, *Vibrio parahaemolyticus*, and *Clostridium difficile*. *S. dysenteriae* type 1 and Shiga toxin–producing strains of *E. coli* produce potent cytotoxins and have been associated with outbreaks of hemorrhagic colitis and hemolytic-uremic syndrome.

Neurotoxins are usually produced by bacteria outside the host and therefore cause symptoms soon after ingestion. Included are the staphylococcal and *Bacillus cereus* toxins, which act on the central nervous system to produce vomiting.

Invasion

Dysentery may result not only from the production of cytotoxins but also from bacterial invasion and destruction of intestinal mucosal cells. Infections due to *Shigella* and enteroinvasive *E. coli* are characterized by the organisms' invasion of mucosal epithelial cells, intraepithelial multiplication, and subsequent spread to adjacent cells. *Salmonella* causes inflammatory diarrhea by invasion of the bowel mucosa but generally is not associated with the destruction of enterocytes or the full clinical syndrome of dysentery. *Salmonella typhi* and *Yersinia enterocolitica* can penetrate intact intestinal mucosa, multiply intracellularly in Peyer's patches and intestinal lymph nodes, and then disseminate through the bloodstream to cause enteric fever, a syndrome characterized by fever, headache, relative bradycardia, abdominal pain, splenomegaly, and leukopenia.

HOST DEFENSES

Given the enormous number of microorganisms ingested with every meal, the normal host must combat a constant influx of potential enteric pathogens. Studies of infections in patients with alterations in defense mechanisms have led to a greater understanding of the variety of ways in which the normal host can protect itself against disease.

Normal flora

The large numbers of bacteria that normally inhabit the intestine act as an important host defense by preventing colonization by potential enteric pathogens. Persons with fewer intestinal bacteria, such as infants who have not yet developed normal enteric colonization or patients receiving antibiotics, are at significantly greater risk of developing infections with enteric pathogens. The composition of the intestinal flora is as important as the number of organisms present. More than 99% of the normal colonic flora is made up of anaerobic bacteria, and the acidic pH and volatile fatty acids produced by these organisms appear to be critical elements in resistance to colonization.

Gastric acid

The acidic pH of the stomach is an important barrier to enteric pathogens, and an increased frequency of infections due to *Salmonella*, *G. lamblia*, and a variety of helminths has been reported among patients who have undergone gastric surgery or are achlorhydric for some other reason. Neutralization of gastric acid with antacids, proton pump inhibitors, or H_2 blockers—a common practice in the management of hospitalized patients—similarly increases the risk of enteric colonization. In addition, some microorganisms can survive the extreme acidity of the gastric environment; rotavirus, for example, is highly stable to acidity.

Intestinal motility

Normal peristalsis is the major mechanism for clearance of bacteria from the proximal small intestine. When intestinal motility is impaired (e.g., by treatment with opiates or other antimotility drugs, anatomic abnormalities, or hypomotility states), the frequency of bacterial overgrowth and infection of the small bowel with enteric pathogens is increased. Some patients whose treatment for *Shigella* infection consists of diphenoxylate hydrochloride with atropine (Lomotil) experience prolonged fever and shedding of organisms, while patients treated with opiates for mild *Salmonella* gastroenteritis have a higher frequency of bacteremia than those not treated with opiates.

Immunity

Both cellular immune responses and antibody production play important roles in protection from enteric infections. Humoral immunity to enteric pathogens consists of systemic IgG and IgM as well as secretory IgA. The mucosal immune system may be the first line of defense against many gastrointestinal pathogens. The binding of bacterial antigens to the luminal surface of M cells in the distal small bowel and the subsequent presentation of antigens to subepithelial lymphoid tissue lead to the proliferation of sensitized lymphocytes. These lymphocytes circulate and populate all of the mucosal tissues of the body as IgA-secreting plasma cells.

Genetic determinants

Host genetic variation influences susceptibility to diarrheal diseases. People with blood group O show increased susceptibility to disease due to *V. cholerae*, *Shigella*, *E. coli* O157, and norovirus. Polymorphisms in genes encoding inflammatory mediators have been associated with the outcome of infection with enteroaggregative *E. coli*, enterotoxin-producing *E. coli*, *Salmonella*, *C. difficile*, and *V. cholerae*.

> **APPROACH TO THE PATIENT**
>
> ### Infectious Diarrhea or Bacterial Food Poisoning
>
> The approach to the patient with possible infectious diarrhea or bacterial food poisoning is shown in Fig. 128-1.
>
> **HISTORY** The answers to questions with high discriminating value can quickly narrow the range of potential causes of diarrhea and help determine whether treatment is needed. Important elements of the narrative history are detailed in Fig. 128-1.

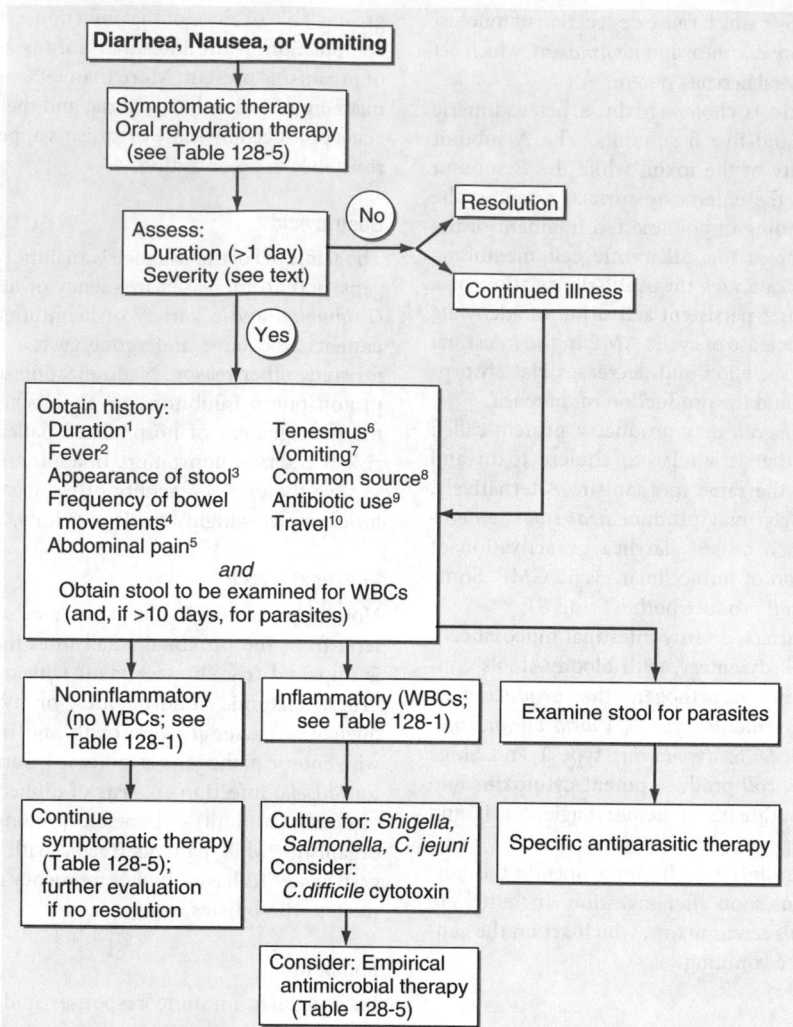

Figure 128-1 **Clinical algorithm for the approach to patients with community-acquired infectious diarrhea or bacterial food poisoning.** Key to superscripts: **1.** Diarrhea lasting >2 weeks is generally defined as chronic; in such cases, many of the causes of acute diarrhea are much less likely, and a new spectrum of causes needs to be considered. **2.** Fever often implies invasive disease, although fever and diarrhea may also result from infection outside the gastrointestinal tract, as in malaria. **3.** Stools that contain blood or mucus indicate ulceration of the large bowel. Bloody stools without fecal leukocytes should alert the laboratory to the possibility of infection with Shiga toxin–producing enterohemorrhagic *Escherichia coli.* Bulky white stools suggest a small-intestinal process that is causing malabsorption. Profuse "rice-water" stools suggest cholera or a similar toxigenic process. **4.** Frequent stools over a given period can provide the first warning of impending dehydration. **5.** Abdominal pain may be most severe in inflammatory processes like those due to *Shigella, Campylobacter,* and necrotizing toxins. Painful abdominal muscle cramps, caused by electrolyte loss, can develop in severe cases of cholera. Bloating is common in giardiasis. An appendicitis-like syndrome should prompt a culture for *Yersinia enterocolitica* with cold enrichment. **6.** Tenesmus (painful rectal spasms with a strong urge to defecate but little passage of stool) may be a feature of cases with proctitis, as in shigellosis or amebiasis. **7.** Vomiting implies an acute infection (e.g., a toxin-mediated illness or food poisoning) but can also be prominent in a variety of systemic illnesses (e.g., malaria) and in intestinal obstruction. **8.** Asking patients whether anyone else they know is sick is a more efficient means of identifying a common source than is constructing a list of recently eaten foods. If a common source seems likely, specific foods can be investigated. See text for a discussion of bacterial food poisoning. **9.** Current antibiotic therapy or a recent history of treatment suggests *Clostridium difficile* diarrhea (Chap. 129). Stop antibiotic treatment if possible and consider tests for *C. difficile* toxins. Antibiotic use may increase the risk of other infections, such as salmonellosis. **10.** See text (and Chap. 123) for a discussion of traveler's diarrhea. *(After Steiner and Guerrant; RL Guerrant, DA Bobak: N Engl J Med 325:327, 1991; with permission.)*

PHYSICAL EXAMINATION The examination of patients for signs of dehydration provides essential information about the severity of the diarrheal illness and the need for rapid therapy. Mild dehydration is indicated by thirst, dry mouth, decreased axillary sweat, decreased urine output, and slight weight loss. Signs of moderate dehydration include an orthostatic fall in blood pressure, skin tenting, and sunken eyes (or, in infants, a sunken fontanelle). Signs of severe dehydration include lethargy, obtundation, feeble pulse, hypotension, and frank shock.

DIAGNOSTIC APPROACH After the severity of illness is assessed, the clinician must distinguish between *inflammatory* and *non-inflammatory* disease. Using the history and epidemiologic features of the case as guides, the clinician can then rapidly evaluate the need for further efforts to define a specific etiology and for therapeutic intervention. Examination of a stool sample may supplement the narrative history. Grossly bloody or mucoid stool suggests an inflammatory process. A test for fecal leukocytes (preparation of a thin smear of stool on a glass

TABLE 128-2 Post-Diarrhea Complications of Acute Infectious Diarrheal Illness

Complication	Comments
Chronic diarrhea • Lactase deficiency • Small-bowel bacterial overgrowth • Malabsorption syndromes (tropical and celiac sprue)	Occurs in ~1% of travelers with acute diarrhea • Protozoa account for ~1/3 of cases
Initial presentation or exacerbation of inflammatory bowel disease	May be precipitated by traveler's diarrhea
Irritable bowel syndrome	Occurs in ~10% of travelers with traveler's diarrhea
Reactive arthritis (formerly known as Reiter's syndrome)	Particularly likely after infection with invasive organisms (*Shigella, Salmonella, Campylobacter, Yersinia*)
Hemolytic-uremic syndrome (hemolytic anemia, thrombocytopenia, and renal failure)	Follows infection with Shiga toxin–producing bacteria (*Shigella dysenteriae* type 1 and enterohemorrhagic *Escherichia coli*)
Guillain-Barré syndrome	Particularly likely after *Campylobacter* infection

slide, addition of a drop of methylene blue, and examination of the wet mount) can suggest inflammatory disease in patients with diarrhea, although the predictive value of this test is still debated. A test for fecal lactoferrin, which is a marker of fecal leukocytes, is more sensitive and is available in latex agglutination and enzyme-linked immunosorbent assay formats. Causes of acute infectious diarrhea, categorized as inflammatory and noninflammatory, are listed in Table 128-1.

POST-DIARRHEA COMPLICATIONS Chronic complications may follow the resolution of an acute diarrheal episode. The clinician should inquire about prior diarrheal illness if the conditions listed in Table 128-2 are observed.

EPIDEMIOLOGY

Travel history

Of the several million people who travel from temperate industrialized countries to tropical regions of Asia, Africa, and Central and South America each year, 20–50% experience a sudden onset of abdominal cramps, anorexia, and watery diarrhea; thus *traveler's diarrhea* is the most common travel-related infectious illness (Chap. 123). The time of onset is usually 3 days to 2 weeks after the traveler's arrival in a resource-poor area; most cases begin within the first 3–5 days. The illness is generally self-limited, lasting 1–5 days. The high rate of diarrhea among travelers to underdeveloped areas is related to the ingestion of contaminated food or water.

The organisms that cause traveler's diarrhea vary considerably with location (Table 128-3), as does the pattern of antimicrobial resistance. In all areas, enterotoxigenic and enteroaggregative strains of *E. coli* are the most common isolates from persons with the classic secretory traveler's diarrhea syndrome. Infection with *Campylobacter jejuni* is especially common in areas of Asia.

Location

Day-care centers have particularly high attack rates of enteric infections. Rotavirus is most common among children <2 years old, with attack rates of 75–100% among those exposed. *G. lamblia* is more common among older children, with somewhat lower attack rates. Other common organisms, often spread by fecal-oral contact, are *Shigella, C. jejuni,* and *Cryptosporidium.* A characteristic feature of infection among children attending day-care centers is the high rate of secondary cases among family members.

Similarly, hospitals are sites in which enteric infections are concentrated. Diarrhea is one of the most common manifestations of nosocomial infections. *C. difficile* is the predominant cause of nosocomial diarrhea among adults in the United States. *Klebsiella oxytoca* has been identified as a cause of antibiotic-associated hemorrhagic colitis. Viral pathogens, especially rotavirus, can spread rapidly in pediatric wards. Enteropathogenic *E. coli* has been associated with outbreaks of diarrhea in nurseries for newborns. One-third of elderly patients in chronic-care institutions

TABLE 128-3 Causes of Traveler's Diarrhea

Etiologic Agent	Approximate Percentage of Cases	Comments
BACTERIA	**50–75**	
Enterotoxigenic *Escherichia coli*	10–45	Single most important agent
Enteroaggregative *E. coli*	5–35	Emerging enteric pathogen with worldwide distribution
Campylobacter jejuni	5–25	More common in Asia
Shigella	0–15	Major cause of dysentery
Salmonella	0–15	
Others	0–5	Including *Aeromonas, Plesiomonas,* and *Vibrio cholerae*
VIRUSES	**0–20**	
Norovirus	0–10	Associated with cruise ships
Rotavirus	0–5	Particularly common among children
PARASITES	**0–10**	
Giardia lamblia	0–5	Affects hikers and campers who drink from freshwater streams; contaminates water supplies in Russia
Cryptosporidium	0–5	Resistant to chlorine treatment
Entamoeba histolytica	<1	
Cyclospora	<1	
OTHER	**0–10**	
Acute food poisoning[a]	0–5	
No pathogen identified	10–50	

[a]For etiologic agents, see Table 128-4.
Source: After Hill et al.

develop a significant diarrheal illness each year; more than one-half of these cases are caused by cytotoxin-producing *C. difficile*. Antimicrobial therapy can predispose to pseudomembranous colitis by altering the normal colonic flora and allowing the multiplication of *C. difficile* (Chap. 129).

Age

Globally, most morbidity and mortality from enteric pathogens involves children <5 years of age. Breast-fed infants are protected from contaminated food and water and derive some protection from maternal antibodies, but their risk of infection rises dramatically when they begin to eat solid foods. Exposure to rotavirus is universal, with most children experiencing their first infection in the first or second year of life. Older children and adults are more commonly infected with norovirus. Other organisms with higher attack rates among children than among adults include enterotoxigenic, enteropathogenic, and enterohemorrhagic *E. coli*; *Shigella*; *C. jejuni*; and *G. lamblia*.

Host immune status

Immunocompromised hosts are at elevated risk of acute and chronic infectious diarrhea. Individuals with defects in cell-mediated immunity (including those with AIDS) are at particularly high risk of invasive enteropathies, including salmonellosis, listeriosis, and cryptosporidiosis. Individuals with hypogammaglobulinemia are at particular risk of *C. difficile* colitis and giardiasis. Patients with cancer are more likely to develop *C. difficile* infection as a result of chemotherapy and frequent hospitalizations. Infectious diarrhea can be life-threatening in immunocompromised hosts, with complications including bacteremia and metastatic seeding of infection. Furthermore, dehydration may compromise renal function and increase the toxicity of immunosuppressive drugs.

Bacterial food poisoning

If the history and the stool examination indicate a noninflammatory etiology of diarrhea and there is evidence of a common-source outbreak, questions concerning the ingestion of specific foods and the time of onset of the diarrhea after a meal can provide clues to the bacterial cause of the illness. Potential causes of bacterial food poisoning are shown in Table 128-4.

Bacterial disease caused by an enterotoxin elaborated outside the host, such as that due to *Staphylococcus aureus* or *B. cereus*, has the shortest incubation period (1–6 h) and generally lasts <12 h. Most cases of staphylococcal food poisoning are caused by contamination from infected human carriers. Staphylococci can multiply at a wide range of temperatures; thus, if food is left to cool slowly and remains at room temperature after cooking, the organisms will have the opportunity to form enterotoxin. Outbreaks following picnics where potato salad, mayonnaise, and cream pastries have been served offer classic examples of staphylococcal food poisoning. Diarrhea, nausea, vomiting, and abdominal cramping are common, while fever is less so.

B. cereus can produce either a syndrome with a short incubation period—the *emetic* form, mediated by a staphylococcal type of enterotoxin—or one with a longer incubation period (8–16 h)—the *diarrheal* form, caused by an enterotoxin resembling *E. coli* LT, in which diarrhea and abdominal cramps are characteristic but vomiting is uncommon. The emetic form of *B. cereus* food poisoning is associated with contaminated fried rice; the organism is common in uncooked rice, and its heat-resistant spores survive boiling. If cooked rice is not refrigerated, the spores can germinate and produce toxin. Frying before serving may not destroy the preformed, heat-stable toxin.

Food poisoning due to *Clostridium perfringens* also has a slightly longer incubation period (8–14 h) and results from the survival of heat-resistant spores in inadequately cooked meat, poultry, or legumes. After ingestion, toxin is produced in the intestinal tract,

TABLE 128-4 Bacterial Food Poisoning

Incubation Period, Organism	Symptoms	Common Food Sources
1–6 h		
Staphylococcus aureus	Nausea, vomiting, diarrhea	Ham, poultry, potato or egg salad, mayonnaise, cream pastries
Bacillus cereus	Nausea, vomiting, diarrhea	Fried rice
8–16 h		
Clostridium perfringens	Abdominal cramps, diarrhea (vomiting rare)	Beef, poultry, legumes, gravies
B. cereus	Abdominal cramps, diarrhea (vomiting rare)	Meats, vegetables, dried beans, cereals
>16 h		
Vibrio cholerae	Watery diarrhea	Shellfish, water
Enterotoxigenic *Escherichia coli*	Watery diarrhea	Salads, cheese, meats, water
Enterohemorrhagic *E. coli*	Bloody diarrhea	Ground beef, roast beef, salami, raw milk, raw vegetables, apple juice
Salmonella spp.	Inflammatory diarrhea	Beef, poultry, eggs, dairy products
Campylobacter jejuni	Inflammatory diarrhea	Poultry, raw milk
Shigella spp.	Dysentery	Potato or egg salad, lettuce, raw vegetables
Vibrio parahaemolyticus	Dysentery	Mollusks, crustaceans

causing moderately severe abdominal cramps and diarrhea; vomiting is rare, as is fever. The illness is self-limited, rarely lasting >24 h.

Not all food poisoning has a bacterial cause. Nonbacterial agents of short-incubation food poisoning include capsaicin, which is found in hot peppers, and a variety of toxins found in fish and shellfish (Chap. 396).

LABORATORY EVALUATION

Many cases of noninflammatory diarrhea are self-limited or can be treated empirically, and in these instances the clinician may not need to determine a specific etiology. Potentially pathogenic *E. coli* cannot be distinguished from normal fecal flora by routine culture, and tests to detect enterotoxins are not available in most clinical laboratories. In situations in which cholera is a concern, stool should be cultured on selective media such as thiosulfate–citrate–bile salts–sucrose (TCBS) or tellurite-taurocholate-gelatin (TTG) agar. A latex agglutination test has made the rapid detection of rotavirus in stool practical for many laboratories, while reverse-transcriptase polymerase chain reaction and specific antigen enzyme immunoassays have been developed for the identification of norovirus. Stool specimens should be examined by immunofluorescence-based rapid assays or (less sensitive) standard microscopy for *Giardia* cysts or *Cryptosporidium* if the level of clinical suspicion regarding the involvement of these organisms is high.

TABLE 128-5 Treatment of Traveler's Diarrhea on the Basis of Clinical Features[a]

Clinical Syndrome	Suggested Therapy
Watery diarrhea (no blood in stool, no fever), 1 or 2 unformed stools per day without distressing enteric symptoms	Oral fluids (oral rehydration solution, Pedialyte, Lytren, or flavored mineral water) and saltine crackers
Watery diarrhea (no blood in stool, no fever), 1 or 2 unformed stools per day with distressing enteric symptoms	Bismuth subsalicylate (for adults): 30 mL or 2 tablets (262 mg/tablet) every 30 min for 8 doses; or loperamide[b]: 4 mg initially followed by 2 mg after passage of each unformed stool, not to exceed 8 tablets (16 mg) per day (prescription dose) or 4 caplets (8 mg) per day (over-the-counter dose); drugs can be taken for 2 days
Watery diarrhea (no blood in stool, no distressing abdominal pain, no fever), >2 unformed stools per day	Antibacterial drug[c] plus (for adults) loperamide[b] (see dose above)
Dysentery (passage of bloody stools) or fever (>37.8°C)	Antibacterial drug[c]
Vomiting, minimal diarrhea	Bismuth subsalicylate (for adults; see dose above)
Diarrhea in infants (<2 years old)	Fluids and electrolytes (oral rehydration solution, Pedialyte, Lytren); continue feeding, especially with breast milk; seek medical attention for moderate dehydration, fever lasting >24 h, bloody stools, or diarrhea lasting more than several days

[a]All patients should take oral fluids (Pedialyte, Lytren, or flavored mineral water) plus saltine crackers. If diarrhea becomes moderate or severe, if fever persists, or if bloody stools or dehydration develops, the patient should seek medical attention.

[b]Loperamide should not be used by patients with fever or dysentery; its use may prolong diarrhea in patients with infection due to *Shigella* or other invasive organisms.

[c]The recommended antibacterial drugs are as follows:

Travel to high-risk country other than Thailand:

Adults: (1) A fluoroquinolone such as ciprofloxacin, 750 mg as a single dose or 500 mg bid for 3 days; levofloxacin, 500 mg as a single dose or 500 mg qd for 3 days; or norfloxacin, 800 mg as a single dose or 400 mg bid for 3 days. (2) Azithromycin, 1000 mg as a single dose or 500 mg qd for 3 days. (3) Rifaximin, 200 mg tid or 400 mg bid for 3 days (not recommended for use in dysentery).

Children: Azithromycin, 10 mg/kg on day 1, 5 mg/kg on days 2 and 3 if diarrhea persists. Alternative agent: furazolidone, 7.5 mg/kg per day in four divided doses for 5 days.

Travel to Thailand (with risk of fluoroquinolone-resistant *Campylobacter*):

Adults: Azithromycin (at above dose for adults). Alternative agent: a fluoroquinolone (at above doses for adults).

Children: Same as for children traveling to other areas (see above).

Source: After Hill et al.

All patients with fever and evidence of inflammatory disease acquired outside the hospital should have stool cultured for *Salmonella*, *Shigella*, and *Campylobacter*. *Salmonella* and *Shigella* can be selected on MacConkey agar as non-lactose-fermenting (colorless) colonies or can be grown on *Salmonella-Shigella* agar or in selenite enrichment broth, both of which inhibit most organisms except these pathogens. Evaluation of nosocomial diarrhea should initially focus on *C. difficile*; stool culture for other pathogens in this setting has an extremely low yield and is not cost-effective. Toxins A and B produced by pathogenic strains of *C. difficile* can be detected by rapid enzyme immunoassays and latex agglutination tests (Chap. 129). Isolation of *C. jejuni* requires inoculation of fresh stool onto selective growth medium and incubation at 42°C in a microaerophilic atmosphere. In many laboratories in the United States, *E. coli* O157:H7 is among the most common pathogens isolated from visibly bloody stools. Strains of this enterohemorrhagic serotype can be identified in specialized laboratories by serotyping but also can be identified presumptively in hospital laboratories as lactose-fermenting, indole-positive colonies of sorbitol non-fermenters (white colonies) on sorbitol MacConkey plates. If the clinical presentation suggests the possibility of intestinal amebiasis, stool should be examined by a rapid antigen detection assay or by (less sensitive) microscopy.

TREATMENT Infectious Diarrhea or Bacterial Food Poisoning

In many cases, a specific diagnosis is not necessary or not available to guide treatment. The clinician can proceed with the information obtained from the history, stool examination, and evaluation of dehydration severity. Empirical regimens for the treatment of traveler's diarrhea are listed in Table 128-5.

The mainstay of treatment is adequate rehydration. The treatment of cholera and other dehydrating diarrheal diseases was revolutionized by the promotion of oral rehydration solution (ORS), the efficacy of which depends on the fact that glucose-facilitated absorption of sodium and water in the small intestine remains intact in the presence of cholera toxin. The use of ORS has reduced mortality rates for cholera from >50% (in untreated cases) to <1%. A number of ORS formulas have been used. Initial preparations were based on the treatment of patients with cholera and included a solution containing 3.5 g of sodium chloride, 2.5 g of sodium bicarbonate, 1.5 g of potassium chloride, and 20 g of glucose (or 40 g of sucrose) per liter of water. Such a preparation can still be used for the treatment of severe cholera. Many causes of secretory diarrhea, however, are associated with less electrolyte loss than occurs in cholera; beginning in 2002, the World Health Organization recommended a "reduced-osmolarity/reduced-salt" ORS that is better tolerated and more effective than classic ORS. This preparation contains 2.6 g of sodium chloride, 2.9 g of trisodium citrate, 1.5 g of potassium chloride, and 13.5 g of glucose (or 27 g of sucrose) per liter of water. ORS formulations containing rice or cereal as the carbohydrate source may be even more effective than glucose-based solutions. Patients who are severely dehydrated or in whom vomiting precludes the use of oral therapy should receive IV solutions such as Ringer's lactate.

Although most secretory forms of traveler's diarrhea (usually due to enterotoxigenic or enteroaggregative *E. coli* or to

Campylobacter) can be treated effectively with rehydration, bismuth subsalicylate, or antiperistaltic agents, antimicrobial agents can shorten the duration of illness from 3–4 days to 24–36 h. Changes in diet have not been shown to have an impact on the duration of illness, while the efficacy of probiotics continues to be debated. Most individuals who present with dysentery (bloody diarrhea and fever) should be treated empirically with an antimicrobial agent (e.g., a fluoroquinolone or a macrolide) pending microbiologic analysis of stool. Individuals with shigellosis should be treated with a 3- to 7-day course. Individuals with *Campylobacter* infection often benefit from antimicrobial treatment as well. Because of increasing resistance of *Campylobacter* to fluoroquinolones, especially in parts of Asia, a macrolide antibiotic such as erythromycin or azithromycin may be preferred for this infection.

Treatment of salmonellosis must be tailored to the individual patient. Since administration of antimicrobial agents often prolongs intestinal colonization with *Salmonella*, these drugs are usually reserved for individuals at high risk of complications from disseminated salmonellosis, such as young children, patients with prosthetic devices, elderly patients, and immunocompromised persons. Antimicrobial agents should not be administered to individuals (especially children) in whom enterohemorrhagic *E. coli* infection is suspected. Laboratory studies of enterohemorrhagic *E. coli* strains have demonstrated that a number of antibiotics induce replication of Shiga toxin–producing lambdoid bacteriophages, thereby significantly increasing toxin production by these strains. Clinical studies have supported these laboratory results, and antibiotics may increase by twentyfold the risk of hemolytic-uremic syndrome and renal failure during enterohemorrhagic *E. coli* infection. A clinical clue in the diagnosis of the latter infection is bloody diarrhea with low fever or none at all.

PROPHYLAXIS

Improvements in hygiene to limit fecal-oral spread of enteric pathogens will be necessary if the prevalence of diarrheal diseases is to be significantly reduced in developing countries. Travelers can reduce their risk of diarrhea by eating only hot, freshly cooked food; by avoiding raw vegetables, salads, and unpeeled fruit; and by drinking only boiled or treated water and avoiding ice. Historically, few travelers to tourist destinations adhere to these dietary restrictions. Bismuth subsalicylate is an inexpensive agent for the prophylaxis of traveler's diarrhea; it is taken at a dosage of 2 tablets (525 mg) four times a day. Treatment appears to be effective and safe for up to 3 weeks, but adverse events such as temporary darkening of the tongue and tinnitus can occur. A meta-analysis suggests that probiotics may lessen the likelihood of traveler's diarrhea by ~15%. Prophylactic antimicrobial agents, although effective, are not generally recommended for the prevention of traveler's diarrhea except when travelers are immunosuppressed or have other underlying illnesses that place them at high risk for morbidity from gastrointestinal infection. The risk of side effects and the possibility of

developing an infection with a drug-resistant organism or with more harmful, invasive bacteria make it more reasonable to institute an empirical short course of treatment if symptoms develop. If prophylaxis is indicated, the nonabsorbed antibiotic rifaximin can be considered for use in regions such as Latin America and Africa, where noninvasive *E. coli* predominates as the cause of traveler's diarrhea. Rifaximin is not effective against invasive enteropathogens.

The possibility of exerting a major impact on the worldwide morbidity and mortality associated with diarrheal diseases has led to intense efforts to develop effective vaccines against the common bacterial and viral enteric pathogens. An effective rotavirus vaccine is currently available. Vaccines against *S. typhi* and *V. cholerae* are also available, although the protection they offer is incomplete and/or short lived. At present, there is no effective commercially available vaccine against *Shigella*, enterotoxigenic *E. coli*, *Campylobacter*, nontyphoidal *Salmonella*, norovirus, or intestinal parasites.

ACKNOWLEDGMENTS
The substantial contributions of Joan R. Butterton, MD, an author of this chapter in previous editions, are gratefully acknowledged.

FURTHER READINGS

BOSCHI-PINTO C et al: Estimating child mortality due to diarrhea in developing countries. Bull WHO 86:710, 2008

CHRISTOPHER PR et al: Antibiotic therapy for *Shigella* dysentry. Cochrane Databse Syst Rev August 4;(8):CD006784, 2010

COHEN SH et al: Clinical pratice guidelines for *Clostridium Difficile* infection in adults: 2010 update by the Society for Healthcare Epidemiology of America (SHEA) and the infectious Diseases Society of America (IDSA). Infect Control Hosp Epidemiol 31:431, 2010

DUPONT HL: Clinical pratice. Bacterial diarrhea. N Engl J Med 361:1560, 2009

HILL DR et al: The practice of travel medicine: Guidelines by the Infectious Diseases Society of America. Clin Infect Dis 43:1499, 2006

——— et al: Management of travellers' diarrhea. BMJ 337:863, 2008

HOGENAUER C et al: *Klebsiella oxytoca* as a causative organism of antibiotic-associated hemorrhagic colitis. N Engl J Med 355:2418, 2006

SAZAWAL S et al: Efficacy of probiotics in prevention of acute diarrhoea: A meta-analysis of masked, randomised, placebo-controlled trials. Lancet Infect Dis 6:374, 2006

SHAH N et al: Global etiology of traveler's diarrhea: Systematic review from 1973 to the present. Am J Trop Med Hyg 80:609, 2009

SODHA SV et al: Foodborne disease, in *Mandell, Douglas, and Bennett's Principles and Practice of Infectious Diseases*, 7th ed, GL Mandell et al (eds). Philadelphia, Churchill Livingstone, 2010, pp 1413–1427

STEINER TS, GUERRANT RL: Principles and syndromes of enteric infection, in *Mandell, Douglas, and Bennett's Principles and Practice of Infectious Diseases*, 7th ed, GL Mandell et al (eds). Philadelphia, Churchill Livingstone, 2010, pp 1335–1351

CHAPTER 129

Clostridium difficile Infection, Including Pseudomembranous Colitis

Dale N. Gerding

Stuart Johnson

■ DEFINITION

Clostridium difficile infection (CDI) is a unique colonic disease that is acquired almost exclusively in association with antimicrobial use and the consequent disruption of the normal colonic flora. The most commonly diagnosed diarrheal illness acquired in the hospital, CDI results from the ingestion of spores of *C. difficile* that vegetate, multiply, and secrete toxins, causing diarrhea and pseudomembranous colitis (PMC).

■ ETIOLOGY AND EPIDEMIOLOGY

C. difficile is an obligately anaerobic, gram-positive, spore-forming bacillus whose spores are found widely in nature, particularly in the environment of hospitals and chronic-care facilities. CDI occurs most frequently in hospitals and nursing homes where the level of antimicrobial use is high and the environment is contaminated by *C. difficile* spores.

Clindamycin, ampicillin, and cephalosporins were the first antibiotics associated with CDI. The second- and third-generation cephalosporins, particularly cefotaxime, ceftriaxone, cefuroxime, and ceftazidime, are agents frequently responsible for this condition, and the fluoroquinolones (ciprofloxacin, levofloxacin, and moxifloxacin) are the most recent drug class to be implicated in hospital outbreaks. Penicillin/β-lactamase-inhibitor combinations such as ticarcillin/clavulanate and piperacillin/tazobactam pose significantly less risk. However, all antibiotics, including vancomycin and metronidazole (the agents most commonly used to treat CDI), have been found to carry a risk of subsequent CDI. Rare cases are reported in patients without prior antibiotic exposure.

C. difficile is acquired exogenously, most frequently in the hospital or nursing home, and is carried in the stool of symptomatic and asymptomatic patients. The rate of fecal colonization is often ≥20% among adult patients hospitalized for >1 week; in contrast, the rate is 1–3% among community residents. Community-onset CDI without recent hospitalization probably accounts for ≤10% of all cases. The risk of *C. difficile* acquisition increases in proportion to length of hospital stay. Asymptomatic fecal carriage of *C. difficile* in healthy neonates is very common, with rates often exceeding 50% during the first 6 months of life, but associated disease in this population is rare. Spores of *C. difficile* are found on environmental surfaces (where the organism can persist for months) and on the hands of hospital personnel who fail to practice good hand hygiene. Hospital epidemics of CDI have been attributed to a single *C. difficile* strain and to multiple strains present simultaneously. Other identified risk factors for CDI include older age, greater severity of underlying illness, gastrointestinal surgery, use of electronic rectal thermometers, enteral tube feeding, and antacid treatment.

Use of proton pump inhibitors may be a risk factor, but this risk is probably modest, and no firm data have implicated these agents in patients who are not already receiving antibiotics.

■ PATHOLOGY AND PATHOGENESIS

Spores of toxigenic *C. difficile* are ingested, survive gastric acidity, germinate in the small bowel, and colonize the lower intestinal tract, where they elaborate two large toxins: toxin A (an enterotoxin) and toxin B (a cytotoxin). These toxins initiate processes resulting in the disruption of epithelial-cell barrier function, diarrhea, and pseudomembrane formation. Toxin A is a potent neutrophil chemoattractant, and both toxins glucosylate the GTP-binding proteins of the Rho subfamily that regulate the actin cell cytoskeleton. Data from studies using molecular disruption of toxin genes in isogenic mutants suggest that toxin B is the essential virulence factor; this possibility, if confirmed, might account for the occurrence of clinical disease caused by toxin A–negative strains. Disruption of the cytoskeleton results in loss of cell shape, adherence, and tight junctions, with consequent fluid leakage. A third toxin, binary toxin CDT, was previously found in only ~6% of strains but is present in all isolates of the newly recognized epidemic strain (see "Global Considerations," below); this toxin is related to *C. perfringens* iota toxin. Its role in the pathogenesis of CDI has not yet been defined.

The pseudomembranes of PMC are confined to the colonic mucosa and initially appear as 1- to 2-mm whitish-yellow plaques. The intervening mucosa appears unremarkable, but, as the disease progresses, the pseudomembranes coalesce to form larger plaques and become confluent over the entire colon wall (Fig. 129-1). The whole colon is usually involved, but 10% of patients have rectal sparing. Viewed microscopically, the pseudomembranes have a mucosal attachment point and contain necrotic leukocytes, fibrin, mucus, and cellular debris. The epithelium is eroded and necrotic in focal areas, with neutrophil infiltration of the mucosa.

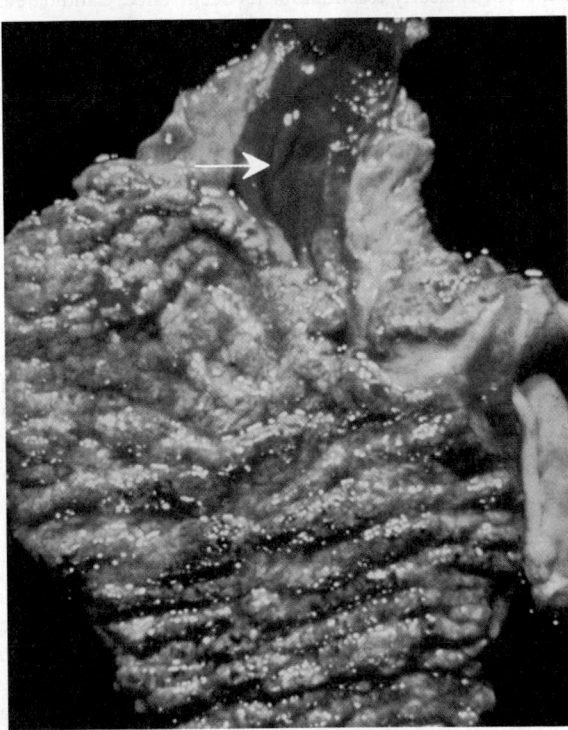

Figure 129-1 Autopsy specimen showing confluent pseudomembranes covering the cecum of a patient with pseudomembranous colitis. Note the sparing of the terminal ileum (*arrow*).

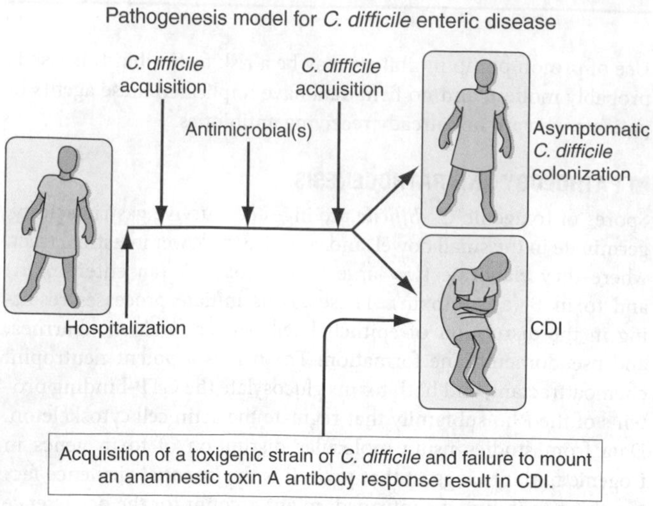

Pathogenesis model for *C. difficile* enteric disease

Acquisition of a toxigenic strain of *C. difficile* and failure to mount an anamnestic toxin A antibody response result in CDI.

Figure 129-2 **Pathogenesis model for hospital-acquired *Clostridium difficile* infection (CDI).** At least three events are integral to *C. difficile* pathogenesis. Exposure to antibiotics establishes susceptibility to infection. Once susceptible, the patient may acquire nontoxigenic (nonpathogenic) or toxigenic strains of *C. difficile* as a second event. Acquisition of toxigenic *C. difficile* may be followed by asymptomatic colonization or CDI, depending on one or more additional events, including an inadequate host anamnestic IgG response to *C. difficile* toxin A.

Patients colonized with *C. difficile* were initially thought to be at high risk for CDI. However, four prospective studies have shown that colonized patients actually have a decreased risk of subsequent CDI. At least three events are proposed as essential for the development of CDI (Fig. 129-2). Exposure to antimicrobial agents is the first event and establishes susceptibility to *C. difficile* infection. The second event is exposure to toxigenic *C. difficile*. Given that the majority of patients do not develop CDI after the first two events, a third event is clearly essential for its occurrence. Candidate third events include exposure to a *C. difficile* strain of particular virulence, exposure to antimicrobial agents especially likely to cause CDI, and an inadequate host immune response. The host anamnestic serum IgG antibody response to toxin A of *C. difficile* is the most likely third event that determines which patients develop diarrhea and which patients remain asymptomatic. The majority of humans first develop antibody to *C. difficile* toxins when colonized asymptomatically during the first year of life. Infants are thought not to develop symptomatic CDI because they lack suitable mucosal toxin receptors that develop later in life. In adulthood, serum levels of IgG antibody to toxin A increase more in response to infection in individuals who become asymptomatic carriers than in those who develop CDI. For persons who develop CDI, increasing levels of antitoxin A during treatment correlate with a lower risk of recurrence of CDI. A clinical trial using monoclonal antibodies to both toxin A and toxin B in addition to standard therapy showed rates of recurrence lower than those obtained with placebo plus standard therapy.

■ GLOBAL CONSIDERATIONS

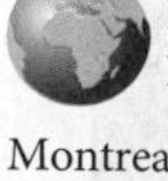

Rates and severity of CDI in the United States, Canada, and Europe have increased markedly since the year 2000. Rates in U.S. hospitals tripled between 2000 and 2005. Hospitals in Montreal, Quebec, have reported rates four times higher than the 1997 baseline, with directly attributable mortality of 6.9% (increased from 1.5%). An epidemic strain, variously known as toxinotype III, REA type BI, PCR ribotype 027, and pulsed-field type NAP1, is thought to account for much of the increase in incidence and has been found in North America, Europe, and Asia. The epidemic

organism is characterized by (1) an ability to produce 16–23 times as much toxin A and toxin B as control strains in vitro; (2) the presence of a third toxin (binary toxin CDT); and (3) high-level resistance to all fluoroquinolones. New strains have been and will probably continue to be implicated in outbreaks; their emergence may be explained in part by patterns of antibiotic use, particularly in hospitals.

■ CLINICAL MANIFESTATIONS

Diarrhea is the most common manifestation caused by *C. difficile*. Stools are almost never grossly bloody and range from soft and unformed to watery or mucoid in consistency, with a characteristic odor. Patients may have as many as 20 bowel movements per day. Clinical and laboratory findings include fever in 28% of cases, abdominal pain in 22%, and leukocytosis in 50%. When adynamic ileus (which is seen on x-ray in ~20% of cases) results in cessation of stool passage, the diagnosis of CDI is frequently overlooked. A clue to the presence of unsuspected CDI in these patients is unexplained leukocytosis, with ≥15,000 white blood cells (WBCs)/μL. Such patients are at high risk for complications of *C. difficile* infection, particularly toxic megacolon and sepsis.

C. difficile diarrhea recurs after treatment in ~15–30% of cases, and this figure may be increasing. Recurrences may represent either relapses due to the same strain or reinfections with a new strain. Susceptibility to recurrence of clinical CDI is likely a result of continued disruption of the normal fecal flora caused by the antibiotic used to treat CDI.

■ DIAGNOSIS

The diagnosis of CDI is based on a combination of clinical criteria: (1) diarrhea (≥3 unformed stools per 24 h for ≥2 days) with no other recognized cause plus (2) toxin A or B detected in the stool, toxin-producing *C. difficile* detected in the stool by polymerase chain reaction (PCR) or culture, or pseudomembranes seen in the colon. PMC is a more advanced form of CDI and is visualized at endoscopy in only ~50% of patients with diarrhea who have a positive stool culture and toxin assay for *C. difficile* (Table 129-1). Endoscopy is a rapid diagnostic tool in seriously ill patients with suspected PMC and an acute abdomen, but a negative result in this examination does not rule out CDI.

Despite the array of tests available for *C. difficile* and its toxins (Table 129-1), no single test has high sensitivity, high specificity, and rapid turnaround. Most laboratory tests for toxins, including enzyme immunoassays (EIAs), lack sensitivity. However, testing of multiple additional stool specimens is not recommended. PCR assays have now been approved for diagnostic testing and appear to be both rapid and sensitive while retaining high specificity. Empirical treatment is appropriate if CDI is strongly suspected on clinical grounds. Testing of asymptomatic patients is not recommended except for epidemiologic study purposes. In particular, so-called tests of cure following treatment are not recommended because many patients continue to harbor the organism and toxin after diarrhea has ceased and test results do not always predict recurrence of CDI. Thus these results should not be used to restrict placement of patients in long-term-care or nursing home facilities.

TREATMENT ▸ *Clostridium difficile* Infection

PRIMARY CDI When possible, discontinuation of any ongoing antimicrobial administration is recommended as the first step in treatment of CDI. Earlier studies indicated that 15–23% of patients respond to this simple measure. However, with the advent of the current epidemic strain and the associated rapid clinical deterioration of some patients, prompt initiation of specific CDI

PART 8 Infectious Diseases

1092

TABLE 129-1 Relative Sensitivity and Specificity of Diagnostic Tests for *Clostridium difficile* Infection (CDI)

Type of Test	Relative Sensitivity[a]	Relative Specificity[a]	Comment
Stool culture for *C. difficile*	++++	+++	Most sensitive test; specificity of ++++ if the *C. difficile* isolate tests positive for toxin; with clinical data, is diagnostic of CDI; turnaround time too slow for practical use
Cell culture cytotoxin test on stool	+++	++++	With clinical data, is diagnostic of CDI; highly specific but not as sensitive as stool culture; slow turnaround time
Enzyme immunoassay for toxin A or toxins A and B in stool	++ to +++	+++	With clinical data, is diagnostic of CDI; rapid results, but not as sensitive as stool culture or cell culture cytotoxin test
Enzyme immunoassay for *C. difficile* common antigen in stool	+++ to ++++	+++	Detects glutamate dehydrogenase found in toxigenic and nontoxigenic strains of *C. difficile* and other stool organisms; more sensitive and less specific than enzyme immunoassay for toxins; rapid results
PCR for *C. difficile* toxin B gene in stool	++++	++++	Detects toxigenic *C. difficile* in stool; newly approved for clinical testing, but appears to be more sensitive than enzyme immunoassay toxin testing and at least as specific
Colonoscopy or sigmoidoscopy	+	++++	Highly specific if pseudomembranes are seen; insensitive compared with other tests

[a] According to both clinical and test-based criteria.

Note: ++++, >90%; +++, 71–90%; ++, 51–70%; +, ~50%.

treatment has become the standard. General treatment guidelines include hydration and the avoidance of antiperistaltic agents and opiates, which may mask symptoms and possibly worsen disease. Nevertheless, antiperistaltic agents have been used safely with vancomycin or metronidazole for mild to moderate CDI.

All drugs, particularly vancomycin, should be given orally if possible. When IV metronidazole is administered, fecal bactericidal drug concentrations are achieved during acute diarrhea, and CDI treatment has been successful; however, in the presence of adynamic ileus, IV metronidazole treatment of PMC has failed. In previous randomized trials, diarrhea response rates to oral therapy with vancomycin or metronidazole were ≥94%, but four recent observational studies found that response rates for metronidazole had declined to 62–78%. Although the mean time to resolution of diarrhea is 2–4 days, the response to metronidazole may be much slower. Treatment should not be deemed a failure until a drug has been given for at least 6 days. On the basis of data for shorter courses of vancomycin, it is recommended that metronidazole and vancomycin be given for at least 10 days, although no controlled comparisons are available. Metronidazole is not approved for this indication by the U.S. Food and Drug Administration (FDA), but most patients with mild to moderate illness respond to 500 mg given by mouth three times a day for 10 days; extension of the treatment period may be needed for slow responders. In addition to the reports of increases in metronidazole failures, a prospective, randomized, double-blind, placebo-controlled study has demonstrated the superiority of vancomycin over metronidazole for treatment of severe CDI. The severity assessment score in that study included age as well as laboratory parameters (elevated temperature, low albumin level, or elevated WBC count), documentation of PMC by endoscopy, or treatment of CDI in the intensive care unit. Although a validated severity score is not yet available, it is important to initiate treatment with oral vancomycin for patients who appear seriously ill, particularly if they have a high WBC count (>15,000/μL) or a creatinine level that is ≥1.5 times

higher than the premorbid value (Table 129-2). Small randomized trials of nitazoxanide, bacitracin, rifaximin, and fusidic acid for treatment of CDI have been conducted. While these drugs have not yet been extensively studied, shown to be superior, or approved by the FDA for this indication, they provide potential alternatives to vancomycin and metronidazole.

RECURRENT CDI Overall, ~15–30% of patients experience recurrences of CDI, either as relapses caused by the original organism or as reinfections following treatment. Recurrence rates are higher among patients ≥65 years old, those who continue to take antibiotics while being treated for CDI, and those who remain in the hospital after the initial episode of CDI. Patients who have a first recurrence of CDI have a high rate of second recurrence (33–65%). In the first recurrence, re-treatment with metronidazole is comparable to treatment with vancomycin (Table 129-2). Recurrent disease, once thought to be relatively mild, has now been documented to pose a significant (11%) risk of serious complications (shock, megacolon, perforation, colectomy, or death within 30 days). There is no standard treatment for multiple recurrences, but long or repeated metronidazole courses should be avoided because of potential neurotoxicity. Approaches include the administration of vancomycin followed by the yeast *Saccharomyces boulardii*; the administration of vancomycin followed by a synthetic fecal bacterial enema; and the intentional colonization of the patient with a nontoxigenic strain of *C. difficile*. None of these biotherapeutic approaches has been approved by the FDA for use in the United States. Other strategies include (1) the use of vancomycin in tapering doses or with pulse dosing every other day for 2–8 weeks and (2) sequential treatment with vancomycin (125 mg four times daily for 10–14 days) followed by rifaximin (400 mg twice daily for 14 days). IV immunoglobulin, which has also been used with some success, presumably provides antibodies to *C. difficile* toxins.

SEVERE COMPLICATED OR FULMINANT CDI Fulminant (rapidly progressive and severe) CDI presents the most difficult

TABLE 129-2 Recommendations for the Treatment of *Clostridium difficile* Infection (CDI)

Clinical Setting	Treatment(s)	Comments
Initial episode, mild to moderate	Oral metronidazole (500 mg tid × 10–14 d)	
Initial episode, severe	Oral vancomycin (125 mg qid × 10–14 d)	Indicators of severe disease may include leukocytosis (≥15,000 white blood cells/μL) and a creatinine level ≥ 1.5 times the premorbid value.
Initial episode, severe complicated or fulminant	Vancomycin (500 mg PO or via nasogastric tube) plus metronidazole (500 mg IV q8h) *plus consider* Rectal instillation of vancomycin (500 mg in 100 mL of normal saline as a retention enema q6–8h)	Severe complicated or fulminant CDI is defined as severe CDI with the addition of hypotension, shock, ileus, or toxic megacolon. The duration of treatment may need to be >2 weeks and is dictated by response. Consider using IV tigecycline (50 mg q12h after a 100-mg loading dose) in place of metronidazole.
First recurrence	Same as for initial episode	
Second recurrence	Vancomycin in tapered/pulsed regimen	Typical taper/pulse regimen: 125 mg qid × 10–14 d, then bid × 1 week, then daily × 1 week, then q2–3d for 2–8 weeks
Multiple recurrences	Consider the following options: • Repeat vancomycin taper/pulse • Vancomycin (500 mg qid × 10 d) plus *Saccharomyces boulardii* (500 mg bid × 28 d) • Vancomycin (125 mg qid × 10–14 d); then stop vancomycin and start rifaximin (400 mg bid × 2 weeks) • Nitazoxanide (500 mg bid × 10 d) • Fecal transplantation • IV immunoglobulin (400 mg/kg)	The only controlled study of treatment for recurrent CDI used *S. boulardii* and showed borderline significance compared with placebo.

treatment challenge. Patients with fulminant disease often do not have diarrhea, and their illness mimics an acute surgical abdomen. Sepsis (hypotension, fever, tachycardia, leukocytosis) may result from severe CDI. An acute abdomen (with or without toxic megacolon) may include signs of obstruction, ileus, colon-wall thickening, and ascites on abdominal CT, often with peripheral-blood leukocytosis (≥20,000 WBCs/μL). With or without diarrhea, the differential diagnosis of an acute abdomen, sepsis, or toxic megacolon should include CDI if the patient has received antibiotics in the past 2 months. Cautious sigmoidoscopy or colonoscopy to visualize PMC and an abdominal CT examination are the best diagnostic tests in patients without diarrhea.

Medical management of fulminant CDI is suboptimal because of the difficulty of delivering metronidazole or vancomycin to the colon by the oral route in the presence of ileus (Table 129-2). The combination of vancomycin (given via nasogastric tube and by retention enema) plus IV metronidazole has been used with some success in uncontrolled studies, as has IV tigecycline in small-scale uncontrolled studies. Surgical colectomy may be life-saving if there is no response to medical management. If possible, colectomy should be performed before the serum lactate level reaches 5 mmol/L. The incidence of fulminant CDI requiring colectomy appears to be increasing in the evolving epidemic.

■ PROGNOSIS

The mortality rate attributed to CDI, previously found to be 0.6–3.5%, has reached 6.9% in recent outbreaks and is progressively higher with increasing age. Most patients recover, but recurrences are common.

■ PREVENTION AND CONTROL

Strategies for the prevention of CDI are of two types: those aimed at preventing transmission of the organism to the patient and those aimed at reducing the risk of CDI if the organism is transmitted. Transmission of *C. difficile* in clinical practice has been prevented by gloving of personnel, elimination of the use of contaminated electronic thermometers, and use of hypochlorite (bleach) solution for environmental decontamination of patients' rooms. Hand hygiene is critical; hand washing is recommended in CDI outbreaks because alcohol hand gels are not sporicidal. CDI outbreaks have been best controlled by restricting the use of specific antibiotics, such as clindamycin and second- and third-generation cephalosporins. Outbreaks of CDI due to clindamycin-resistant strains have resolved promptly when clindamycin use is restricted.

FURTHER READINGS

Cohen SH et al: Clinical practice guidelines for *Clostridium difficile* infection in adults: 2010 update by the Society of Healthcare Epidemiology of America (SHEA) and the Infectious Diseases Society of America (IDSA). Infect Control Hosp Epidemiol 31:431, 2010

Herpers BL et al: Intravenous tigecycline as adjunctive or alternative therapy for severe refractory *Clostridium difficile* infection. Clin Infect Dis 48:1732, 2009

Johnson S et al: Interruption of recurrent *Clostridium difficile*-associated diarrhea episodes by serial therapy with vancomycin and rifaximin. Clin Infect Dis 44:846, 2007

Kyne L et al: Asymptomatic carriage of *Clostridium difficile* and serum levels of IgG antibody against toxin A. N Engl J Med 342:390, 2000

Loo VG et al: A predominantly clonal multi-institutional outbreak of *Clostridium difficile*–associated diarrhea with high morbidity and mortality. N Engl J Med 353:2442, 2005

Lowy I et al: Treatment with monoclonal antibodies against *Clostridium difficile* toxins. N Engl J Med 362:197, 2010

Lyras D et al: Toxin B is essential for virulence of *Clostridium difficile*. Nature 458:1176, 2009

McDonald LC et al: *Clostridium difficile* infection in patients discharged from US short-stay hospitals, 1996-2003. Emerg Infect Dis 12:409, 2006

——— et al: An epidemic, toxin gene–variant strain of *Clostridium difficile*. N Engl J Med 353:2433, 2005

Pepin J et al: The management and outcomes of a first recurrence of *Clostridium difficile* associated disease in Quebec. Clin Infect Dis 42:758, 2006

Zar FA et al: A comparison of vancomycin and metronidazole for the treatment of *Clostridium difficile*–associated diarrhea, stratified by disease severity. Clin Infect Dis 45:302, 2007

CHAPTER **130**

Sexually Transmitted Infections: Overview and Clinical Approach

Jeanne M. Marrazzo
King K. Holmes

CLASSIFICATION AND EPIDEMIOLOGY

Worldwide, most adults acquire at least one sexually transmitted infection (STI), and many remain at risk for complications. Each year, for example, an estimated 6.2 million persons in the United States acquire a new genital human papillomavirus (HPV) infection, and many of these individuals are at risk for genital neoplasias. Certain STIs, such as syphilis, gonorrhea, HIV infection, hepatitis B, and chancroid, are most concentrated within "core populations" characterized by high rates of partner change, multiple concurrent partners, or "dense," highly connected sexual networks—e.g., involving sex workers and their clients, some men who have sex with men (MSM), and persons involved in the use of illicit drugs, particularly crack cocaine and methamphetamine. Other STIs are distributed more evenly throughout societies. For example, chlamydial infections, genital infections with HPV, and genital herpes can spread widely, even in relatively low-risk populations.

In general, the product of three factors determines the initial rate of spread of any STI within a population: rate of sexual exposure of susceptible to infectious people, efficiency of transmission per exposure, and duration of infectivity of those infected. Accordingly, efforts to prevent and control STIs aim to decrease the rate of sexual exposure of susceptibles to infected persons (e.g., through individual counseling and efforts to change the norms of sexual behavior and through a variety of STI control efforts aimed at reducing the proportion of the population infected), to decrease the duration of infectivity (through early diagnosis and curative or suppressive treatment), and to decrease the efficiency of transmission (e.g., through promotion of condom use and safer sexual practices, through use of effective vaccines, and recently through male circumcision).

 In all societies, STIs rank among the most common of all infectious diseases, with >30 infections now classified as predominantly sexually transmitted or as frequently sexually transmissible (Table 130-1). In developing countries, with three-quarters of the world's population and 90% of the world's STIs, factors such as population growth (especially in adolescent and young-adult age groups), rural-to-urban migration, wars, limited or no provision of reproductive health services for women, and poverty create exceptional vulnerability to disease resulting from unprotected sex. During the 1990s in China, Russia, the other states

TABLE 130-1 Sexually Transmitted and Sexually Transmissible Microorganisms

Bacteria	Viruses	Other[a]
Transmitted in Adults Predominantly by Sexual Intercourse		
Neisseria gonorrhoeae	HIV (types 1 and 2)	*Trichomonas vaginalis*
Chlamydia trachomatis	Human T-cell lymphotropic virus type I	*Phthirus pubis*
Treponema pallidum	Herpes simplex virus type 2	
Haemophilus ducreyi	Human papillomavirus (multiple genital	
Klebsiella (Calymmatobacterium)	genotypes)	
granulomatis	Hepatitis B virus[b]	
Ureaplasma urealyticum	Molluscum contagiosum virus	
Mycoplasma genitalium		
Sexual Transmission Repeatedly Described but Not Well Defined or Not the Predominant Mode		
Mycoplasma hominis	Cytomegalovirus	*Candida albicans*
Gardnerella vaginalis and other	Human T-cell lymphotropic virus type II	*Sarcoptes scabiei*
vaginal bacteria	Hepatitis C virus	
Group B *Streptococcus*	(?) Hepatitis D virus	
Mobiluncus spp.	Herpes simplex virus type 1	
Helicobacter cinaedi	(?) Epstein-Barr virus	
Helicobacter fennelliae	Human herpesvirus type 8	
Transmitted by Sexual Contact Involving Oral-Fecal Exposure; of Declining Importance in Men Who Have Sex with Men		
Shigella spp.	Hepatitis A virus	*Giardia lamblia*
Campylobacter spp.		*Entamoeba histolytica*

[a]Includes protozoa, ectoparasites, and fungi.
[b]Among U.S. patients for whom a risk factor can be ascertained, most hepatitis B virus infections are transmitted sexually.

of the former Soviet Union, and South Africa, internal social structures changed rapidly as borders opened to the West, unleashing enormous new epidemics of HIV infection and other STIs. Despite advances in the provision of highly effective antiretroviral therapy worldwide, HIV remains the leading cause of death in some developing countries, and HPV and hepatitis B virus (HBV) remain important causes of cervical and hepatocellular carcinoma, respectively—two of the most common malignancies in the developing world. Sexually transmitted herpes simplex virus (HSV) infections now cause most genital ulcer disease throughout the world and an increasing proportion of cases of genital herpes in developing countries with generalized HIV epidemics, where the positive-feedback loop between HSV and HIV transmission is a growing, intractable problem. Despite this consistent link, randomized trials evaluating the efficacy of antiviral therapy in suppressing HSV in both HIV-uninfected and HIV-infected persons have not demonstrated a protective effect against acquisition or transmission of HIV. Globally, ~350 million new cases of five curable STIs—gonorrhea, chlamydial infection, syphilis, chancroid, and trichomoniasis—were reported annually in the mid-1990s. Up to 50% of women of reproductive age in developing countries have bacterial vaginosis (arguably acquired sexually). All five of these curable infections have been associated with increased risk of HIV transmission or acquisition.

In the United States, the prevalence of antibody to HSV-2 began to fall in the late 1990s, especially among adolescents and young adults; the decline is presumably due to delayed sexual debut, increased condom use, and lower rates of multiple (≥4) sex partners, as is well documented by the U.S. Youth Risk Behavior Surveillance System. The estimated annual incidence of HBV infection has also declined dramatically since the mid-1980s; this decrease is probably attributable more to adoption of safer sexual practices and reduced needle sharing among injection drug users than to use of hepatitis B vaccine, for which coverage among young adults (including those at high risk for this infection) initially was very limited. Genital HPV remains the most common sexually transmitted pathogen in this country, infecting 60% of a cohort of initially HPV-negative, sexually active Washington state college women within 5 years in a study conducted from 1990 to 2000. The scale-up of HPV vaccine coverage among young women promises to lower the incidence of infection with the HPV types included in the vaccines.

In industrialized countries, fear of HIV infection since the mid-1980s, coupled with widespread behavioral interventions and better-organized systems of care for the curable STIs, initially helped curb the transmission of the latter diseases. However, foci of hyperendemic transmission persist in the southeastern United States and in most large U.S. cities. Rates of gonorrhea and syphilis remain higher in the United States than in any other Western industrialized country.

In the United States, the Centers for Disease Control and Prevention (CDC) has compiled reported rates of STIs since 1941. The incidence of reported gonorrhea peaked at 468 cases per 100,000 population in the mid-1970s, fell to a low of 112 cases per 100,000 in 2004, and remained relatively unchanged through 2008. Because of increased testing and more sensitive tests, the incidence of reported *Chlamydia trachomatis* infection has been increasing steadily since reporting began in 1984, reaching an all-time peak of 401 cases per 100,000 in 2008. The incidence of primary and secondary syphilis per 100,000 peaked at 71 cases in 1946, fell rapidly to 3.9 cases in 1956, ranged from ~10 to 15 cases through 1987 (with markedly increased rates among MSM men and African Americans), and then fell to a nadir of 2.1 cases in 2000–2001 (with rates falling most rapidly among heterosexual African Americans). Unfortunately, since 1996, with the introduction of highly active antiretroviral therapy, the increased use of "serosorting" (i.e., the avoidance of unprotected sex with HIV-serodiscordant partners but not with HIV-seroconcordant partners, a strategy that provides no

protection against STIs other than HIV infection), and an ongoing epidemic of methamphetamine use, gonorrhea, syphilis, and chlamydial infection have had a remarkable resurgence among MSM in North America and Europe, where outbreaks of a rare type of chlamydial infection (lymphogranuloma venereum; LGV) that had virtually disappeared during the AIDS era have occurred. These developments have resulted in a high degree of co-infection with HIV and other sexually transmitted pathogens (particularly syphilis and LGV), primarily among MSM.

MANAGEMENT OF COMMON SEXUALLY TRANSMITTED DISEASE (STD) SYNDROMES

Although other chapters discuss management of specific STIs, delineating treatment based on diagnosis of a specific infection, most patients are actually managed (at least initially) on the basis of presenting symptoms and signs and associated risk factors, even in industrialized countries. Table 130-2 lists some of the most common clinical STD syndromes and their microbial etiologies. Strategies for their management are outlined below. Chapters 188 and 189 address the management of infections with human retroviruses.

STD care and management begin with risk assessment and proceed to clinical assessment, diagnostic testing or screening, treatment, and prevention. Indeed, the routine care of any patient begins with risk assessment (e.g., for risk of heart disease, cancer). STD/HIV risk assessment is important in primary care, urgent care, and emergency care settings as well as in specialty clinics providing adolescent, HIV/AIDS, prenatal, and family planning services. STD/HIV risk assessment guides detection and interpretation of symptoms that could reflect an STD; decisions on screening or prophylactic/preventive treatment; risk reduction counseling and intervention (e.g., hepatitis B vaccination); and treatment of partners of patients with known infections. Consideration of routine demographic data (e.g., gender, age, area of residence) is a simple first step in STD/HIV risk assessment. For example, national guidelines strongly recommend routine screening of sexually active females ≤25 years of age for *C. trachomatis* infection. Table 130-3 provides a set of 10 STD/HIV risk-assessment questions that clinicians can pose verbally or that health care systems can adapt (with yes/no responses) into a routine self-administered questionnaire for use in clinics. The initial framing statement gives permission to discuss topics that may be perceived as sensitive or socially unacceptable by providers and patients alike.

Risk assessment is followed by clinical assessment (elicitation of information on specific current symptoms and signs of STDs). Confirmatory diagnostic tests (for persons with symptoms or signs) or screening tests (for those without symptoms or signs) may involve microscopic examination, culture, antigen detection tests, nucleic acid amplification tests (NAATs), or serology. Initial syndrome-based treatment should cover the most likely causes. For certain syndromes, results of rapid tests can narrow the spectrum of this initial therapy (e.g., saline microscopy of vaginal fluid for women with vaginal discharge, Gram's stain of urethral discharge for men with urethral discharge, rapid plasma reagin test for genital ulcer). After the institution of treatment, STD management proceeds to the "4 Cs" of prevention and control: contact tracing (see "Prevention and Control of STIs," below), ensuring compliance with therapy, and counseling on risk reduction, including condom promotion and provision.

Consistent with current guidelines, all adults should be screened for infection with HIV-1 at least once and more frequently if they are at risk for acquisition of this infection.

■ URETHRITIS IN MEN

Urethritis in men produces urethral discharge, dysuria, or both, usually without frequency of urination. Causes include *Neisseria gonorrhoeae*, *C. trachomatis*, *Mycoplasma genitalium*, *Ureaplasma urealyticum*, *Trichomonas vaginalis*, HSV, and adenovirus.

TABLE 130-2 Major STD Syndromes and Sexually Transmitted Microbial Etiologies

Syndrome	ST Microbial Etiologies
AIDS	HIV types 1 and 2
Urethritis: males	*Neisseria gonorrhoeae, Chlamydia trachomatis, Mycoplasma genitalium, Ureaplasma urealyticum* (?subspecies *urealyticum*), *Trichomonas vaginalis,* HSV
Epididymitis	*C. trachomatis, N. gonorrhoeae*
Lower genital tract infections: females	
Cystitis/urethritis	*C. trachomatis, N. gonorrhoeae,* HSV
Mucopurulent cervicitis	*C. trachomatis, N. gonorrhoeae, M. genitalium*
Vulvitis	*Candida albicans,* HSV
Vulvovaginitis	*C. albicans, T. vaginalis*
Bacterial vaginosis (BV)	BV-associated bacteria (see text)
Acute pelvic inflammatory disease	*N. gonorrhoeae, C. trachomatis,* BV-associated bacteria, *M. genitalium,* group B streptococci
Infertility	*N. gonorrhoeae, C. trachomatis,* BV-associated bacteria
Ulcerative lesions of the genitalia	HSV-1, HSV-2, *Treponema pallidum, Haemophilus ducreyi, C. trachomatis* (LGV strains), *Klebsiella (Calymmatobacterium) granulomatis*
Complications of pregnancy/ puerperium	Several agents implicated
Intestinal infections	
Proctitis	*C. trachomatis, N. gonorrhoeae,* HSV, *T. pallidum*
Proctocolitis or enterocolitis	*Campylobacter* spp., *Shigella* spp., *Entamoeba histolytica,* other enteric pathogens
Enteritis	*Giardia lamblia*
Acute arthritis with urogenital infection or viremia	*N. gonorrhoeae* (e.g., DGI), *C. trachomatis* (e.g., reactive arthritis), HBV
Genital and anal warts	HPV (30 genital types)
Mononucleosis syndrome	CMV, HIV, EBV
Hepatitis	Hepatitis viruses, *T. pallidum,* CMV, EBV
Neoplasias	
Squamous cell dysplasias and cancers of the cervix, anus, vulva, vagina, or penis	HPV (especially types 16, 18, 31, 45)
Kaposi's sarcoma, body-cavity lymphomas	HHV-8
T cell leukemia	HTLV-I
Hepatocellular carcinoma	HBV
Tropical spastic paraparesis	HTLV-I
Scabies	*Sarcoptes scabiei*
Pubic lice	*Pthirus pubis*

Abbreviations: CMV, cytomegalovirus; DGI, disseminated gonococcal infection; EBV, Epstein-Barr virus; HBV, hepatitis B virus; HHV-8, human herpesvirus type 8; HPV, human papillomavirus; HSV, herpes simplex virus; HTLV, human T cell lymphotropic virus; LGV, lymphogranuloma venereum.

TABLE 130-3 Ten-Question STD/HIV Risk Assessment

Framing Statement:

In order to provide the best care for you today and to understand your risk for certain infections, it is necessary for us to talk about your sexual behavior.

Screening Questions:

(1) Do you have any reason to think you might have a sexually transmitted infection? If so, what reason?

(2) For all adolescents <18 years old: Have you begun having any kind of sex yet?

STD History:

(3) Have you ever had any sexually transmitted infections or any genital infections? If so, which ones?

Sexual Preference:

(4) Have you had sex with men, women, or both?

Injection Drug Use:

(5) Have you ever injected yourself ("shot up") with drugs? (If yes, have you ever shared needles or injection equipment?)

(6) Have you ever had sex with a gay or bisexual man or with anyone who had ever injected drugs?

Characteristics of Partner(s):

(7) Has your sex partner(s) had any sexually transmitted infections? If so, which ones?

(8) Has your sex partner had other sex partners during the time you've been together?

STD Symptoms Checklist:

(9) Have you recently developed any of these symptoms?

For Men	For Women
(a) Discharge of pus (drip) from the penis	(a) Abnormal vaginal discharge (increased amount, abnormal odor, abnormal yellow color)
(b) Genital sores (ulcers) or rash	(b) Genital sores (ulcers), rash, or itching

Sexual Practices, Past 2 Months (for patients answering yes to any of the above questions, to guide examination and testing):

(10) Now I'd like to ask what parts of your body may have been sexually exposed to an STD (e.g., your penis, mouth, vagina, anus).

Query about Interest in STD Screening Tests (for patients answering no to all of the above questions):

(11) Would you like to be tested for HIV or any other STDs today? (If yes, clinician can explore which STD and why.)

Source: Adapted from JR Curtis, KK Holmes, in KK Holmes et al (eds): *Sexually Transmitted Diseases,* 4th ed. New York, McGraw-Hill, 2008.

Until recently, *C. trachomatis* caused ~30–40% of cases of nongonococcal urethritis (NGU), particularly in heterosexual men; however, the proportion of cases due to this organism has probably declined in some populations served by effective chlamydial-control programs, and older men with urethritis appear less likely to have chlamydial infection. HSV and *T. vaginalis* each cause a small proportion of NGU cases in the United States. Recently, multiple studies have consistently implicated *M. genitalium* as a probable cause of many *Chlamydia*-negative cases. Fewer studies than in the past have implicated *Ureaplasma*; the ureaplasmas have been differentiated into *U. urealyticum* and *U. parvum*, and a few studies suggest that *U. urealyticum*—but not *U. parvum*—is associated with NGU. Coliform bacteria can cause urethritis in men who practice insertive anal intercourse. The initial diagnosis of urethritis in men currently includes specific tests only for *N. gonorrhoeae* and *C. trachomatis*; it does not yet include testing for *Mycoplasma* or *Urealyticum* species. The following summarizes the approach to the patient with suspected urethritis:

1. *Establish the presence of urethritis.* If proximal-to-distal "milking" of the urethra does not express a purulent or mucopurulent discharge, even after the patient has not voided for several hours (or preferably overnight), a Gram's-stained smear of overt discharge or of an anterior urethral specimen obtained by passage of a small urethrogenital swab 2–3 cm into the urethra usually reveals ≥5 neutrophils per 1000× field in areas containing cells; in gonococcal infection, such a smear usually reveals gram-negative intracellular diplococci as well. Alternatively, the centrifuged sediment of the first 20–30 mL of voided urine—ideally collected as the first morning specimen—can be examined for inflammatory cells, either by microscopy showing ≥10 leukocytes per high-power field or by the leukocyte esterase test. Patients with symptoms who lack objective evidence of urethritis may have functional rather than organic problems and generally do not benefit from repeated courses of antibiotics.

2. *Evaluate for complications or alternative diagnoses.* A brief history and examination will exclude epididymitis and systemic complications, such as disseminated gonococcal infection (DGI) and reactive arthritis. Although digital examination of the prostate gland seldom contributes to the evaluation of sexually active young men with urethritis, men with dysuria who lack evidence of urethritis as well as sexually inactive men with urethritis should undergo prostate palpation, urinalysis, and urine culture to exclude bacterial prostatitis and cystitis.

3. *Evaluate for gonococcal and chlamydial infection.* An absence of typical gram-negative diplococci on Gram's-stained smear of urethral exudate containing inflammatory cells warrants a preliminary diagnosis of NGU, as this test is 98% sensitive for the diagnosis of gonococcal urethral infection. However, an increasing proportion of men with symptoms and/or signs of urethritis are simultaneously assessed for infection with *N. gonorrhoeae* and *C. trachomatis* by "multiplex" NAATs of first-voided urine. The urine specimen tested should comprise the first 10–15 mL of the stream, and patients should not have voided for the prior 2 h, if possible. Culture or NAAT for *N. gonorrhoeae* may be positive when Gram's staining is negative; certain strains of *N. gonorrhoeae* can result in negative urethral Gram's stains in up to 30% of cases of urethritis. Results of tests for gonococcal and chlamydial infection predict the patient's prognosis (with greater risk for recurrent NGU if neither chlamydiae nor gonococci are found than if either is detected) and can guide both the counseling given to the patient and the management of the patient's sexual partner(s).

4. *Treat urethritis promptly while test results are pending.*

TREATMENT   Urethritis in Men

Table 130-4 summarizes the steps in management of sexually active men with urethral discharge and/or dysuria.

In practice, if Gram's stain does not reveal gonococci, urethritis is treated with a regimen effective for NGU, such as azithromycin or doxycycline. Both are effective, although azithromycin may give better results in *M. genitalium* infection. If gonococci are demonstrated by Gram's stain or if no diagnostic tests are performed to exclude gonorrhea definitively, treatment should include a single-dose regimen for gonorrhea (Chap. 144) plus

TABLE 130-4 Management of Urethral Discharge in Men

Usual Causes	Usual Initial Evaluation
Chlamydia trachomatis *Neisseria gonorrhoeae* *Mycoplasma genitalium* *Ureaplasma urealyticum* *Trichomonas vaginalis* Herpes simplex virus	Demonstration of urethral discharge or pyuria Exclusion of local or systemic complications Urethral Gram's stain to confirm urethritis, detect gram-negative diplococci Test for *N. gonorrhoeae*, *C. trachomatis*

Initial Treatment for Patient and Partners

Treat gonorrhea (unless excluded):	plus	Treat chlamydial infection:
Ceftriaxone, 250 mg IM; *or* Cefpodoxime, 400 mg PO; *or* Cefixime, 400 mg PO[a]		Azithromycin, 1 g PO; *or* Doxycycline, 100 mg bid PO for 7 days

Management of Recurrence

Confirm objective evidence of urethritis. If patient was reexposed to untreated or new partner, repeat treatment of patient and partner.

If patient was not reexposed, consider infection with *T. vaginalis*[b] or doxycycline-resistant *M. genitalium* or *Ureaplasma*, and consider treatment with metronidazole, azithromycin, or both.

[a]Updates on the emergence of antimicrobial resistance in *N. gonorrhoeae* can be obtained from the Centers for Disease Control and Prevention at *http://www.cdc.gov/std.*
[b]In men, the diagnosis of *T. vaginalis* infection requires culture (or nucleic acid amplification test, where available) of early-morning first-voided urine sediment or of a urethral swab specimen obtained before voiding.

azithromycin or doxycycline treatment for *C. trachomatis*, which frequently causes urethral co-infection in men with gonococcal urethritis. Sexual partners should ideally be tested for gonorrhea and chlamydial infection; regardless of whether they are tested for these infections, however, they should receive the same regimen given to the male index case. Patients with confirmed persistence or recurrence of urethritis after treatment should be re-treated with the initial regimen if they did not comply with the original treatment or were reexposed to an untreated partner. Otherwise, an intraurethral swab specimen and a first-voided urine sample should be tested for *T. vaginalis* (currently best done by culture, although NAATs appear to be more sensitive and are likely to become commercially available in the future). If compliance with initial treatment is confirmed and reexposure to an untreated sex partner is deemed unlikely, the recommended treatment is with metronidazole or tinidazole (2 g by mouth in a single dose) plus azithromycin (1 g by mouth in a single dose); the azithromycin component is especially important if this drug has not been given during initial therapy.

■ EPIDIDYMITIS

Acute epididymitis, almost always unilateral, produces pain, swelling, and tenderness of the epididymis, with or without symptoms or signs of urethritis. This condition must be differentiated from testicular torsion, tumor, and trauma. Torsion, a surgical emergency, usually occurs in the second or third decade of life and produces a sudden onset of pain, elevation of the testicle within the scrotal sac, rotation of the epididymis from a posterior to an anterior position, and absence of blood flow on Doppler examination or ^{99m}Tc scan. Persistence of symptoms after a course of therapy for epididymitis suggests the possibility of testicular tumor or of a chronic granulomatous disease, such as tuberculosis. In sexually active men under age 35, acute epididymitis is caused most frequently by *C. trachomatis* and less commonly by *N. gonorrhoeae* and is usually associated with overt or subclinical urethritis. Acute epididymitis occurring in older men or following urinary tract instrumentation is usually caused by urinary pathogens. Similarly, epididymitis in men who have practiced insertive rectal intercourse is often caused by Enterobacteriaceae. These men usually have no urethritis but do have bacteriuria.

TREATMENT Epididymitis

Ceftriaxone (250 mg as a single dose IM) followed by doxycycline (100 mg by mouth twice daily for 10 days) constitutes effective treatment for epididymitis caused by *N. gonorrhoeae* or *C. trachomatis*. Fluoroquinolones are no longer recommended for treatment of gonorrhea in the United States because of the emergence of resistant strains of *N. gonorrhoeae*, especially (but not only) among MSM (Fig. 130-1). Oral levofloxacin (500 mg once daily for 10 days) is also effective for syndrome-based initial treatment of epididymitis when infection with Enterobacteriaceae is suspected; however, this regimen should be combined with effective therapy for possible gonococcal or chlamydial infection unless bacteriuria with Enterobacteriaceae is confirmed.

■ URETHRITIS AND THE URETHRAL SYNDROME IN WOMEN

C. trachomatis, *N. gonorrhoeae*, and occasionally HSV cause symptomatic urethritis—known as the urethral syndrome in women—that is characterized by "internal" dysuria (usually without urinary urgency or frequency), pyuria, and an absence of *Escherichia coli* and other uropathogens at counts of ≥10²/mL in urine. In contrast, the dysuria associated with vulvar herpes or vulvovaginal candidiasis (and perhaps with trichomoniasis) is often described as "external," being caused by painful contact of urine with the inflamed or ulcerated labia or introitus. Acute onset, association with urinary urgency or frequency, hematuria, or suprapubic bladder tenderness suggests bacterial cystitis. Among women with symptoms of acute bacterial cystitis, costovertebral pain and tenderness or fever suggests

acute pyelonephritis. The management of bacterial urinary tract infection (UTI) is discussed in Chap. 288.

Signs of vulvovaginitis, coupled with symptoms of external dysuria, suggest vulvar infection (e.g., with HSV or *Candida albicans*). Among dysuric women without signs of vulvovaginitis, bacterial UTI must be differentiated from the urethral syndrome by assessment of risk, evaluation of the pattern of symptoms and signs, and specific microbiologic testing. An STI etiology of the urethral syndrome is suggested by young age, more than one current sexual partner, a new partner within the past month, a partner with urethritis, or coexisting mucopurulent cervicitis (see below). The finding of a single urinary pathogen, such as *E. coli* or *Staphylococcus saprophyticus*, at a concentration of ≥10²/mL in a properly collected specimen of midstream urine from a dysuric woman with pyuria indicates probable bacterial UTI, whereas pyuria with <10² conventional uropathogens per milliliter of urine ("sterile" pyuria) suggests acute urethral syndrome due to *C. trachomatis* or *N. gonorrhoeae*. Gonorrhea and chlamydial infection should be sought by specific tests (e.g., NAATs on the first 10 mL of voided urine). Among dysuric women with sterile pyuria caused by infection with *N. gonorrhoeae* or *C. trachomatis*, appropriate treatment alleviates dysuria.

■ VULVOVAGINAL INFECTIONS

Abnormal vaginal discharge

If directly questioned about vaginal discharge during routine health checkups, many women acknowledge having nonspecific symptoms of vaginal discharge that do not correlate with objective signs of inflammation or with actual infection. However, unsolicited reporting of abnormal vaginal discharge does suggest bacterial vaginosis or trichomoniasis. Specifically, an abnormally increased amount or an abnormal odor of the discharge is associated with one or both of these conditions. Cervical infection with *N. gonorrhoeae* or *C. trachomatis* does not often cause an increased amount or abnormal odor of discharge; however, when these pathogens cause cervicitis, they—like *T. vaginalis*—often result in an increased number of neutrophils in vaginal fluid that thus takes on a yellow color. Vulvar conditions such as genital herpes or vulvovaginal candidiasis can cause vulvar pruritus, burning, irritation, or lesions as well as external dysuria (as urine passes over the inflamed vulva or areas of epithelial disruption) or vulvar dyspareunia.

Certain vulvovaginal infections may have serious sequelae. Trichomoniasis, bacterial vaginosis, and vulvovaginal candidiasis have all been associated with increased risk of acquisition of HIV infection. Vaginal trichomoniasis and bacterial vaginosis early in pregnancy independently predict premature onset of labor. Bacterial vaginosis can also lead to anaerobic bacterial infection of the endometrium and salpinges. Vaginitis may be an early and prominent feature of toxic shock syndrome, and recurrent or chronic vulvovaginal candidiasis develops with increased frequency among women with systemic illnesses, such as diabetes mellitus or HIV-related immunosuppression (although only a very small proportion of women with recurrent vulvovaginal candidiasis in industrialized countries actually have a serious predisposing illness).

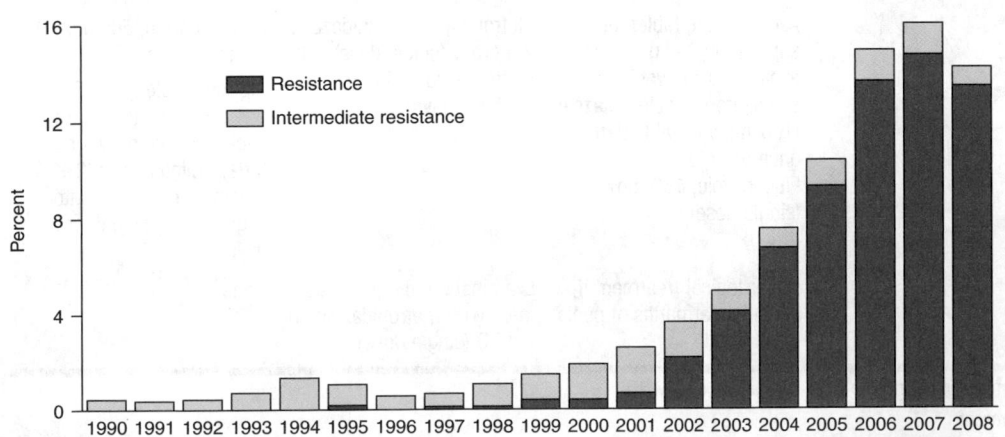

Figure 130-1 Percentage of *N. gonorrhoeae* isolates with intermediate resistance or resistance to ciprofloxacin, by year: Gonococcal Isolate Surveillance Project, United States, 1990–2008. Intermediate resistance is defined by ciprofloxacin minimal inhibitory concentrations (MICs) of 0.125–0.5 μg/mL and resistance by MICs of ≥1 μg/mL. *(From the Centers for Disease Control and Prevention: Sexually Transmitted Disease Surveillance, 2008. Atlanta, U.S. Department of Health and Human Services; November 2009.)*

Thus vulvovaginal symptoms or signs warrant careful evaluation, including pelvic examination, simple rapid diagnostic tests, and appropriate therapy specific for the anatomic site and type of infection. Unfortunately, a survey in the United States indicated that clinicians seldom perform the tests required to establish the cause of such symptoms. Further, comparison of telephone and office management of vulvovaginal symptoms has documented the inaccuracy of the former, and comparison of evaluations by nurse-midwives with those by physician-practitioners showed that the practitioners' clinical evaluations correlated poorly both with the nurses' evaluations and with diagnostic tests. The diagnosis and treatment of the three most common types of vaginal infection are summarized in Table 130-5.

Inspection of the vulva and perineum may reveal tender genital ulcerations or fissures (typically due to HSV infection or vulvovagi-

TABLE 130-5 Diagnostic Features and Management of Vaginal Infection

Feature	Normal Vaginal Examination	Vulvovaginal Candidiasis	Trichomonal Vaginitis	Bacterial Vaginosis
Etiology	Uninfected; lactobacilli predominant	*Candida albicans*	*Trichomonas vaginalis*	Associated with *Gardnerella vaginalis*, various anaerobic and/or noncultured bacteria, and mycoplasmas
Typical symptoms	None	Vulvar itching and/or irritation	Profuse purulent discharge; vulvar itching	Malodorous, slightly increased discharge
Discharge				
Amount	Variable; usually scant	Scant	Often profuse	Moderate
Color[a]	Clear or translucent	White	White or yellow	White or gray
Consistency	Nonhomogeneous, floccular	Clumped; adherent plaques	Homogeneous	Homogeneous, low viscosity; uniformly coats vaginal walls
Inflammation of vulvar or vaginal epithelium	None	Erythema of vaginal epithelium, introitus; vulvar dermatitis, fissures common	Erythema of vaginal and vulvar epithelium; colpitis macularis	None
pH of vaginal fluid[b]	Usually ≤4.5	Usually ≤4.5	Usually ≥5	Usually >4.5
Amine ("fishy") odor with 10% KOH	None	None	May be present	Present
Microscopy[c]	Normal epithelial cells; lactobacilli predominant	Leukocytes, epithelial cells; mycelia or pseudomycelia in up to 80% of *C. albicans* culture-positive persons with typical symptoms	Leukocytes; motile trichomonads seen in 80–90% of symptomatic patients, less often in the absence of symptoms	Clue cells; few leukocytes; no lactobacilli or only a few outnumbered by profuse mixed microbiota, nearly always including *G. vaginalis* plus anaerobic species on Gram's stain (Nugent's score ≥7)
Other laboratory findings		Isolation of *Candida* spp.	Isolation of T. *vaginalis* or positive NAAT[d]	
Usual treatment	None	Azole cream, tablet, or suppository—e.g., miconazole (100-mg vaginal suppository) or clotrimazole (100-mg vaginal tablet) once daily for 7 days Fluconazole, 150 mg orally (single dose)	Metronidazole or tinidazole, 2 g orally (single dose) Metronidazole, 500 mg PO bid for 7 days	Metronidazole, 500 mg PO bid for 7 days Metronidazole gel, 0.75%, one applicator (5 g) intravaginally once daily for 5 days Clindamycin, 2% cream, one full applicator vaginally each night for 7 days
Usual management of sexual partner	None	None; topical treatment if candidal dermatitis of penis is detected	Examination for STD; treatment with metronidazole, 2 g PO (single dose)	None

[a]Color of discharge is best determined by examination against the white background of a swab.

[b]A pH determination is not useful if blood is present.

[c]To detect fungal elements, vaginal fluid is digested with 10% KOH prior to microscopic examination; to examine for other features, fluid is mixed (1:1) with physiologic saline. Gram's stain is also excellent for detecting yeasts (less predictive of vulvovaginitis) and pseudomycelia or mycelin (strongly predictive of vulvovaginitis) and for distinguishing normal flora from the mixed flora seen in bacterial vaginosis, but it is less sensitive than the saline preparation for detection of *T. vaginalis*.

[d]NAAT, nucleic acid amplification test (where available).

Source: *The Practitioner's Handbook for the Management of Sexually Transmitted Diseases* accessed from *http://depts.washington.edu/nnptc/online_training/std_handbook/pdfs/ch6_vaginitis.pdf.*

nal candidiasis) or discharge visible at the introitus before insertion of a speculum (suggestive of bacterial vaginosis or trichomoniasis). Speculum examination permits the clinician to discern whether the discharge in fact looks abnormal and whether any abnormal discharge in the vagina emanates from the cervical os (mucoid and, if abnormal, yellow) or from the vagina (not mucoid, since the vaginal epithelium does not produce mucus). Symptoms or signs of abnormal vaginal discharge should prompt testing of vaginal fluid for pH, for a fishy odor when mixed with 10% KOH, and for certain microscopic features when mixed with saline (motile trichomonads and/or "clue cells") and with 10% KOH (pseudohyphae or hyphae indicative of vulvovaginal candidiasis). Additional objective laboratory tests useful for establishing the cause of abnormal vaginal discharge include rapid point-of-care tests for bacterial vaginosis, as described below, and a DNA probe test (the Affirm test) to detect *T. vaginalis* and *C. albicans* as well as the increased concentrations of *Gardnerella vaginalis* associated with bacterial vaginosis. Gram's staining of vaginal fluid can be used to score alterations in the vaginal microbiota but is employed primarily for research purposes and requires some familiarity with the morphotypes and scale involved.

TREATMENT Vaginal Discharge

Patterns of treatment for vaginal discharge vary widely. In developing countries, where clinics or pharmacies often dispense treatment based on symptoms alone without examination or testing, oral treatment with metronidazole—particularly with a 7-day regimen—provides reasonable coverage against both trichomoniasis and bacterial vaginosis, the usual causes of symptoms of vaginal discharge; metronidazole treatment of sex partners prevents reinfection of women with trichomoniasis, even though it does not help prevent the recurrence of bacterial vaginosis. Guidelines for syndromic management promulgated by the World Health Organization suggest consideration of treatment for cervical infection and for trichomoniasis, bacterial vaginosis, and vulvovaginal candidiasis in women with symptoms of abnormal vaginal discharge. However, it is important to note that the majority of chlamydial and gonococcal cervical infections produce no symptoms.

In industrialized countries, clinicians treating symptoms and signs of abnormal vaginal discharge should, at a minimum, differentiate between bacterial vaginosis and trichomoniasis, because optimal management of patients and partners differs for these two conditions (as discussed briefly below).

Vaginal trichomoniasis

(See also Chap. 215) Symptomatic trichomoniasis characteristically produces a profuse, yellow, purulent, homogeneous vaginal discharge and vulvar irritation, sometimes with visible inflammation of the vaginal and vulvar epithelium and petechial lesions on the cervix (the so-called strawberry cervix, usually evident only by colposcopy). The pH of vaginal fluid—normally <4.7—usually rises to ≥5. In women with typical symptoms and signs of trichomoniasis, microscopic examination of vaginal discharge mixed with saline reveals motile trichomonads in most culture-positive cases. However, saline microscopy probably detects only one-half of all cases, and, especially in the absence of symptoms or signs, culture is usually required for detection of the organism. NAAT for *T. vaginalis* is as sensitive as or more sensitive than culture, and NAAT of urine has disclosed surprisingly high prevalences of this pathogen among men at several STD clinics in the United States. Treatment of asymptomatic as well as symptomatic cases reduces rates of transmission and prevents later development of symptoms.

TREATMENT Vaginal Trichomoniasis

Only nitroimidazoles (e.g., metronidazole and tinidazole) consistently cure trichomoniasis. A single 2-g oral dose of metronidazole is effective and much less expensive than the alternatives. Tinidazole has a longer half-life than metronidazole, causes fewer gastrointestinal symptoms, and is especially useful in treating trichomoniasis that fails to respond to metronidazole. Treatment of sexual partners—facilitated by dispensing metronidazole to the female patient to give to her partner(s), with a warning about avoiding the concurrent use of alcohol—significantly reduces both the risk of reinfection and the reservoir of infection; treating the partner is the standard of care. Intravaginal treatment with 0.75% metronidazole gel is not reliable for vaginal trichomoniasis. Systemic use of metronidazole is recommended throughout pregnancy. In a large randomized trial, metronidazole treatment of trichomoniasis during pregnancy did not reduce—and in fact actually increased—the frequency of perinatal morbidity; thus routine screening of asymptomatic pregnant women for trichomoniasis is not recommended.

Bacterial vaginosis

Bacterial vaginosis (formerly termed *nonspecific vaginitis, Haemophilus vaginitis, anaerobic vaginitis,* or *Gardnerella-associated vaginal discharge*) is a syndrome of uncertain etiology that is characterized by symptoms of vaginal malodor and a slightly to moderately increased white discharge, which appears homogeneous, is low in viscosity, and evenly coats the vaginal mucosa. Bacterial vaginosis has been associated with increased risk of acquiring several other genital infections, including those caused by HIV, *C. trachomatis,* and *N. gonorrhoeae.* Other risk factors include recent unprotected vaginal intercourse, having a female sex partner, and vaginal douching. Although bacteria associated with bacterial vaginosis have been detected under the foreskin of uncircumcised men, metronidazole treatment of male partners has not reduced the rate of recurrence among affected women.

Among women with bacterial vaginosis, culture of vaginal fluid has shown markedly increased prevalences and concentrations of *G. vaginalis, Mycoplasma hominis,* and several anaerobic bacteria [e.g., *Mobiluncus, Prevotella* (formerly *Bacteroides*), and some *Peptostreptococcus* species] as well as an absence of hydrogen peroxide–producing *Lactobacillus* spp., that constitute most of the normal vaginal microbiota and help protect against certain cervical and vaginal infections. Broad-range polymerase chain reaction (PCR) amplification of 16S rDNA in vaginal fluid, with subsequent identification of specific bacterial species by various methods, has documented an even greater and unexpected bacterial diversity, including several unique species not previously cultivated [e.g., three species in the order Clostridiales that appear to be specific for bacterial vaginosis and are associated with metronidazole treatment failure (Fig. 130-2)]. Also detected are DNA sequences related to *Atopobium vaginae,* an organism that is strongly associated with bacterial vaginosis, is resistant to metronidazole, and is also associated with recurrent bacterial vaginosis after metronidazole treatment. Other genera newly implicated in bacterial vaginosis include *Megasphaera, Leptotrichia, Eggerthella,* and *Dialister.*

Bacterial vaginosis is conventionally diagnosed clinically with the Amsel criteria that include any three of the following four clinical abnormalities: (1) objective signs of increased white homogeneous vaginal discharge; (2) a vaginal discharge pH of >4.5; (3) liberation of a distinct fishy odor (attributable to volatile amines such as trimethylamine) immediately after vaginal secretions are mixed with

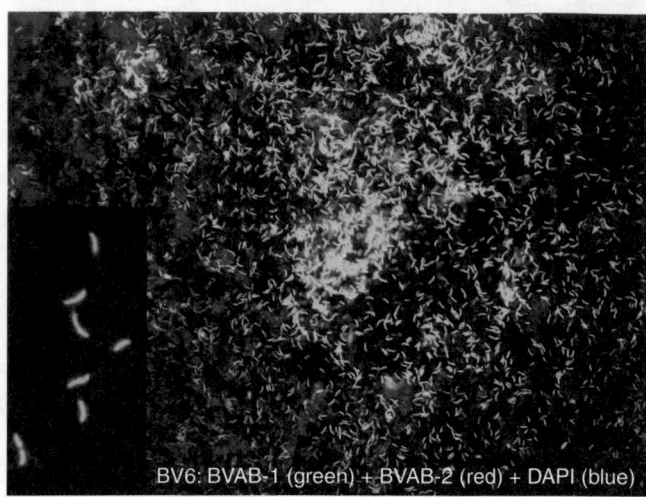

BV6: BVAB-1 (green) + BVAB-2 (red) + DAPI (blue)

Figure 130-2 Broad-range PCR amplification of 16S rDNA in vaginal fluid from a woman with bacterial vaginosis shows a field of bacteria hybridizing with probes for bacterial vaginosis–associated bacterium 1 (BVAB-1, visible as a thin, curved green rod) and for BVAB-2 (red). The inset shows that BVAB-1 has a morphology similar to that of *Mobiluncus* (curved rod). *(Reprinted with permission from DN Fredricks et al.)*

a 10% solution of KOH; and (4) microscopic demonstration of "clue cells" (vaginal epithelial cells coated with coccobacillary organisms, which have a granular appearance and indistinct borders; Fig. 130-3) on a wet mount prepared by mixing vaginal secretions with normal saline in a ratio of ~1:1.

TREATMENT   Bacterial Vaginosis

The standard dosage of oral metronidazole for the treatment of bacterial vaginosis is 500 mg twice daily for 7 days. The single 2-g oral dose of metronidazole recommended for trichomoniasis produces significantly lower short-term cure rates and should

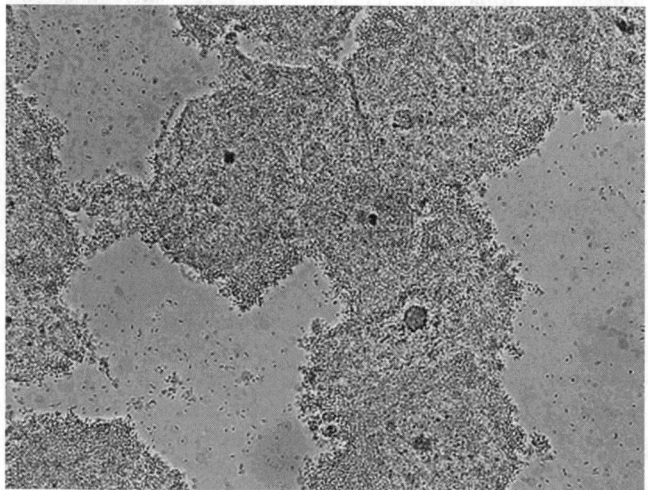

Figure 130-3 Wet mount of vaginal fluid showing typical clue cells from a woman with bacterial vaginosis. Note the obscured epithelial cell margins and the granular appearance attributable to many adherent bacteria (×400). *(Photograph provided by Lorna K. Rabe, reprinted with permission from S Hillier et al, in KK Holmes et al (eds). Sexually Transmitted Diseases, 4th ed. New York, McGraw-Hill, 2008.)*

not be used. Intravaginal treatment with 2% clindamycin cream [one full applicator (5 g containing 100 mg of clindamycin phosphate) each night for 7 nights] or with 0.75% metronidazole gel [one full applicator (5 g containing 37.5 mg of metronidazole) twice daily for 5 days] is also approved for use in the United States and does not elicit systemic adverse reactions; the response to both of these treatments is similar to the response to oral metronidazole. Other alternatives include oral clindamycin (300 mg twice daily for 7 days), clindamycin ovules (100 g intravaginally once at bedtime for 3 days), and oral tinidazole (1 g daily for 5 days or 2 g daily for 3 days). Unfortunately, recurrence over the long term (i.e., several months later) is distressingly common after either oral or intravaginal treatment. A randomized trial comparing intravaginal gel containing 37.5 mg of metronidazole with a suppository containing 500 mg of metronidazole plus nystatin (the latter not marketed in the United States) showed significantly higher rates of recurrence with the 37.5-mg regimen; this result suggests that higher metronidazole dosages may be important in topical intravaginal therapy. Recurrences can be significantly lessened with the twice-weekly use of suppressive intravaginal metronidazole gel. As stated above, treatment of male partners with metronidazole does not prevent recurrence of bacterial vaginosis.

Efforts to replenish numbers of vaginal lactobacilli that produce hydrogen peroxide and probably sustain vaginal health have been largely unsuccessful. While one randomized trial of orally ingested lactobacilli found reduced rates of recurrent bacterial vaginosis, this result has not yet been either confirmed or refuted, and a randomized multicenter trial in the United States found no benefit of repeated intravaginal inoculation of a vaginal peroxide-producing *Lactobacillus* species following treatment of bacterial vaginosis with metronidazole. A meta-analysis of 18 studies concluded that bacterial vaginosis during pregnancy substantially increased the risk of preterm delivery and of spontaneous abortion. However, most studies of topical intravaginal treatment of bacterial vaginosis with clindamycin during pregnancy have not reduced adverse pregnancy outcomes. Numerous trials of oral metronidazole treatment during pregnancy have given inconsistent results, and a 2007 Cochrane review concluded that antenatal treatment of women with bacterial vaginosis—even those with previous preterm delivery—did not reduce the risk of preterm delivery. The U.S. Preventive Services Task Force thus recommends against routine screening of pregnant women for bacterial vaginosis.

Vulvovaginal pruritus, burning, or irritation

Vulvovaginal candidiasis produces vulvar pruritus, burning, or irritation, generally without symptoms of increased vaginal discharge or malodor. Genital herpes can produce similar symptoms, with lesions sometimes difficult to distinguish from the fissures and inflammation caused by candidiasis. Signs of vulvovaginal candidiasis include vulvar erythema, edema, fissures, and tenderness. With candidiasis, a white scanty vaginal discharge sometimes takes the form of white thrush-like plaques or cottage cheese–like curds adhering loosely to the vaginal mucosa. *C. albicans* accounts for nearly all cases of symptomatic vulvovaginal candidiasis, which probably arise from endogenous strains of *C. albicans* that have colonized the vagina or the intestinal tract. Complicated vulvovaginal candidiasis includes cases that recur four or more times per year; are unusually severe; are caused by non-*albicans Candida* spp.; or occur in women with uncontrolled diabetes, debilitation, immunosuppression, or pregnancy.

In addition to compatible clinical symptoms, the diagnosis of vulvovaginal candidiasis usually involves the demonstration of pseudohyphae or hyphae by microscopic examination of vaginal fluid mixed with saline or 10% KOH or subjected to Gram's staining. Microscopic examination is less sensitive than culture but correlates better with symptoms. Culture is typically reserved for cases that do not respond to standard first-line antimycotic agents and is undertaken to rule out imidazole or azole resistance (often associated with *Candida glabrata*) or before the initiation of suppressive antifungal therapy for recurrent disease.

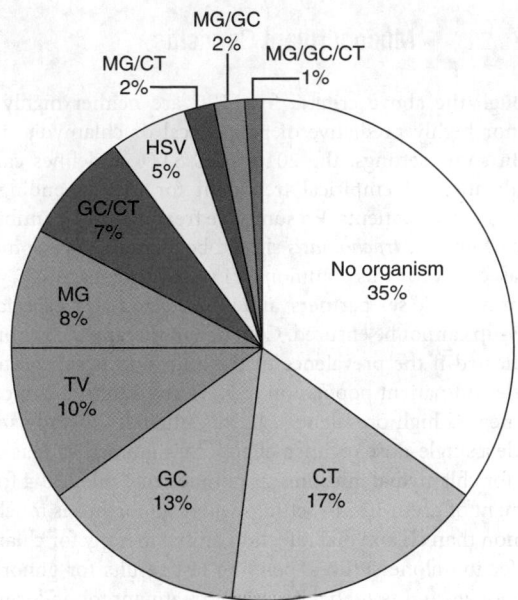

Figure 130-4 **Organisms detected among female STD clinic** patients with mucopurulent cervicitis (*n* = 167). GC, gonococcus; CT, *Chlamydia trachomatis*; MG, *Mycoplasma genitalium*; TV, *Trichomonas vaginalis*; HSV, herpes simplex virus. (*Courtesy of Dr. Lisa Manhart; with permission.*)

TREATMENT	Vulvovaginal Pruritus, Burning, or Irritation

Symptoms and signs of vulvovaginal candidiasis warrant treatment, usually intravaginal administration of any of several imidazole antibiotics (e.g., miconazole or clotrimazole) for 3–7 days or of a single dose of oral fluconazole (Table 130-5). Over-the-counter marketing of such preparations has reduced the cost of care and made treatment more convenient for many women with recurrent yeast vulvovaginitis. However, most women who purchase these preparations do not have vulvovaginal candidiasis, while many do have other vaginal infections that require different treatment. Therefore, only women with classic symptoms of vulvar pruritus and a history of previous episodes of yeast vulvovaginitis documented by an experienced clinician should self-treat. Short-course topical intravaginal azole drugs are effective for the treatment of uncomplicated vulvovaginal candidiasis (e.g., clotrimazole, two 100-mg vaginal tablets daily for 3 days; or miconazole, a 1200-mg vaginal suppository as a single dose). Single-dose oral treatment with fluconazole (150 mg) is also effective and is preferred by many patients. Management of complicated cases (see above) and those that do not respond to the usual intravaginal or single-dose oral therapy often involves prolonged or periodic oral therapy; this situation is discussed extensively in the 2010 CDC STD treatment guidelines (*http://www.cdc.gov/std/treatment*). Treatment of sexual partners is not routinely indicated.

Other causes of vaginal discharge or vaginitis

In the ulcerative vaginitis associated with staphylococcal toxic shock syndrome, *Staphylococcus aureus* should be promptly identified in vaginal fluid by Gram's stain and by culture. In desquamative inflammatory vaginitis, smears of vaginal fluid reveal neutrophils, massive vaginal epithelial-cell exfoliation with increased numbers of parabasal cells, and gram-positive cocci; this syndrome may respond to treatment with 2% clindamycin cream, often given in combination with topical steroid preparations for several weeks. Additional causes of vaginitis and vulvovaginal symptoms include retained foreign bodies (e.g., tampons), cervical caps, vaginal spermicides, vaginal antiseptic preparations or douches, vaginal epithelial atrophy (in postmenopausal women or during prolonged breast-feeding in the postpartum period), allergic reactions to latex condoms, vaginal aphthae associated with HIV infection or Behçet's syndrome, and vestibulitis (a poorly understood syndrome).

■ MUCOPURULENT CERVICITIS

Mucopurulent cervicitis (MPC) refers to inflammation of the columnar epithelium and subepithelium of the endocervix and of any contiguous columnar epithelium that lies exposed in an ectopic position on the ectocervix. MPC in women represents the "silent partner" of urethritis in men, being equally common and often caused by the same agents (*N. gonorrhoeae, C. trachomatis*, or—as shown by case-control studies—*M. genitalium*); however, MPC is more difficult than urethritis to recognize. As the most

common manifestation of these serious bacterial infections in women, MPC can be a harbinger or sign of upper genital tract infection, also known as *pelvic inflammatory disease* (PID; see below). In pregnant women, MPC can lead to obstetric complications. In a prospective study in Seattle of 167 consecutive patients with MPC [defined on the basis of yellow endocervical mucopus or ≥30 polymorphonuclear leukocytes (PMNs)/1000× microscopic field] who were seen at STD clinics during the 1980s, slightly more than one-third of cervicovaginal specimens tested for *C. trachomatis, N. gonorrhoeae, M. genitalium*, HSV, and *T. vaginalis* revealed no identifiable etiology (Fig. 130-4). More recently, a study in Baltimore using NAATs for these pathogens still failed to identify a microbiologic etiology in nearly one-half of the 133 women with MPC.

The diagnosis of MPC rests on the detection of cardinal signs at the cervix, including yellow mucopurulent discharge from the cervical os, endocervical bleeding upon gentle swabbing, and edematous cervical ectopy (see below); the latter two findings are somewhat more common with MPC due to chlamydial infection, but signs alone do not allow a distinction between the causative pathogens. Unlike the endocervicitis produced by gonococcal or chlamydial infection, cervicitis caused by HSV produces ulcerative lesions on the stratified squamous epithelium of the ectocervix as well as on the columnar epithelium. Yellow cervical mucus on a white swab removed from the endocervix indicates the presence of PMNs. Gram's staining may confirm their presence, although it adds relatively little to the diagnostic value of assessment for cervical signs. The presence of ≥20 PMNs/1000× microscopic field within strands of cervical mucus not contaminated by vaginal squamous epithelial cells or vaginal bacteria indicates endocervicitis. Detection of intracellular gram-negative diplococci in carefully collected endocervical mucus is quite specific but ≤50% sensitive for gonorrhea. Therefore, specific and sensitive tests for *N. gonorrhoeae* as well as for *C. trachomatis* (e.g., NAATs) are always indicated in the evaluation of MPC.

Although the above criteria for MPC are neither highly specific nor highly predictive of gonococcal or chlamydial infection in some settings, the 2010 CDC STD guidelines call for consideration of empirical treatment for MPC, pending test results, in most patients. Presumptive treatment with antibiotics active against *C. trachomatis* should be provided for women at increased risk for this common STI (risk factors: age <25 years, new or multiple sex partners, and unprotected sex), especially if follow-up cannot be ensured. Concurrent therapy for gonorrhea is indicated if the prevalence of this infection is substantial in the relevant patient population (e.g., young adults, a clinic with documented high prevalence). In this situation, therapy should include a single-dose regimen effective for gonorrhea plus treatment for chlamydial infection, as outlined in Table 130-4 for the treatment of urethritis. In settings where gonorrhea is much less common than chlamydial infection, initial therapy for chlamydial infection alone suffices, pending test results for gonorrhea. The etiology and potential benefit of treatment for endocervicitis not associated with gonorrhea or chlamydial infection have not been established. Although the antimicrobial susceptibility of *M. genitalium* is not yet well defined, the organism frequently persists after doxycycline therapy, and it currently seems reasonable to use azithromycin to treat possible *M. genitalium* infection in such cases. The sexual partner(s) of a woman with MPC should be examined and given a regimen similar to that chosen for the woman unless results of tests for gonorrhea or chlamydial infection in either partner warrant different therapy or no therapy.

■ CERVICAL ECTOPY

Cervical ectopy, often mislabeled "cervical erosion," is easily confused with infectious endocervicitis. Ectopy represents the presence of the one-cell-thick columnar epithelium extending from the endocervix out onto the visible ectocervix. In ectopy, the cervical os may contain clear or slightly cloudy mucus but usually not yellow mucopus. Colposcopy shows intact epithelium. Normally found during adolescence and early adulthood, ectopy gradually recedes through the second and third decades of life, as squamous metaplasia replaces the ectopic columnar epithelium. Oral contraceptive use favors the persistence or reappearance of ectopy, while smoking apparently accelerates squamous metaplasia. Cauterization of ectopy is not warranted. Ectopy may render the cervix more susceptible to infection with *N. gonorrhoeae*, *C. trachomatis*, or HIV.

■ PELVIC INFLAMMATORY DISEASE

The term *pelvic inflammatory disease* usually refers to infection that ascends from the cervix or vagina to involve the endometrium and/or fallopian tubes. Infection can extend beyond the reproductive tract to cause pelvic peritonitis, generalized peritonitis, perihepatitis, perisplenitis, or pelvic abscess. Rarely, infection not related to specific sexually transmitted pathogens extends secondarily to the pelvic organs (1) from adjacent foci of inflammation (e.g., appendicitis, regional ileitis, or diverticulitis) or bacterial vaginosis, (2) as a result of hematogenous dissemination (e.g., of tuberculosis or staphylococcal bacteremia), or (3) as a complication of certain tropical diseases (e.g., schistosomiasis). Intrauterine infection can be primary (spontaneously occurring and usually sexually transmitted) or secondary to invasive intrauterine surgical procedures [e.g., dilatation and curettage, termination of pregnancy, insertion of an intrauterine device (IUD), or hysterosalpingography] or to parturition.

Etiology

The agents most often implicated in acute PID include the primary causes of endocervicitis (e.g., *N. gonorrhoeae* and *C. trachomatis*) and organisms that can be regarded as components of an altered vaginal microbiota. In general, PID is most often caused by *N. gonorrhoeae* where there is a high incidence of gonorrhea—e.g., in inner-city populations in the United States. In case-control studies, *M. genitalium* has also been significantly associated with histopathologic diagnoses of endometritis and with salpingitis.

Anaerobic and facultative organisms (especially *Prevotella* species, peptostreptococci, *E. coli*, *Haemophilus influenzae*, and group B streptococci) as well as genital mycoplasmas have been isolated from the peritoneal fluid or fallopian tubes in a varying proportion (typically one-fourth to one-third) of women with PID studied in the United States. The difficulty of determining the exact microbial etiology of an individual case of PID—short of using invasive procedures for specimen collection—has implications for the approach to empirical antimicrobial treatment of this infection.

Epidemiology

In the United States, the estimated annual number of initial visits to physicians' offices for PID by women 15–44 years of age fell from an average of 400,000 during the 1980s to 250,000 in 1999 and then to 104,000 in 2008. Hospitalizations for acute PID in the United States also declined steadily throughout the 1980s and early 1990s but have remained fairly constant at 70,000–100,000 per year since 1995. Important risk factors for acute PID include the presence of endocervical infection or bacterial vaginosis, a history of salpingitis or of recent vaginal douching, and recent insertion of an IUD. Certain other iatrogenic factors, such as dilatation and curettage or cesarean section, can increase the risk of PID, especially among women with endocervical gonococcal or chlamydial infection or bacterial vaginosis. Symptoms of *N. gonorrhoeae*–associated and *C. trachomatis*–associated PID often begin during or soon after the menstrual period; this timing suggests that menstruation is a risk factor for ascending infection from the cervix and vagina. Experimental inoculation of the fallopian tubes of nonhuman primates has shown that repeated exposure to *C. trachomatis* leads to the greatest degree of tissue inflammation and damage; thus, immunopathology probably contributes to the pathogenesis of chlamydial salpingitis. Women using oral contraceptives appear to be at decreased risk of symptomatic PID, and tubal sterilization reduces the risk of salpingitis by preventing intraluminal spread of infection into the tubes.

Clinical manifestations

Endometritis: a clinical pathologic syndrome A study of women with clinically suspected PID who were undergoing both endometrial biopsy and laparoscopy showed that those with endometritis alone differed from those who also had salpingitis in significantly less often having lower quadrant, adnexal, or cervical motion or abdominal rebound tenderness; fever; or elevated C-reactive protein levels. In addition, women with endometritis alone differed from those with neither endometritis nor salpingitis in more often having gonorrhea, chlamydial infection, and risk factors such as douching or IUD use. Thus, women with endometritis alone were intermediate between those with neither endometritis nor salpingitis and those with salpingitis with respect to risk factors, clinical manifestations, cervical infection prevalence, and elevated C-reactive protein level. Women with endometritis alone are at lower risk of subsequent tubal occlusion and resulting infertility than are those with salpingitis.

Salpingitis Symptoms of nontuberculous salpingitis classically evolve from a yellow or malodorous vaginal discharge caused by MPC and/or bacterial vaginosis to midline abdominal pain and abnormal vaginal bleeding caused by endometritis and then to bilateral lower abdominal and pelvic pain caused by salpingitis, with nausea, vomiting, and increased abdominal tenderness if peritonitis develops.

The abdominal pain in nontuberculous salpingitis is usually described as dull or aching. In some cases, pain is lacking or atypical, but active inflammatory changes are found in the course of an unrelated evaluation or procedure, such as a laparoscopic evaluation for infertility. Abnormal uterine bleeding precedes or coincides with the onset of pain in ~40% of women with PID, symptoms of urethritis (dysuria) occur in 20%, and symptoms of proctitis (anorectal pain, tenesmus, and rectal discharge or bleeding) are occasionally seen in women with gonococcal or chlamydial infection.

Speculum examination shows evidence of MPC (yellow endocervical discharge, easily induced endocervical bleeding) in the majority of women with gonococcal or chlamydial PID. Cervical motion tenderness is produced by stretching of the adnexal attachments on the side toward which the cervix is pushed. Bimanual examination reveals uterine fundal tenderness due to endometritis and abnormal adnexal tenderness due to salpingitis that is usually, but not necessarily, bilateral. Adnexal swelling is palpable in about one-half of women with acute salpingitis, but evaluation of the adnexae in a patient with marked tenderness is not reliable. The initial temperature is >38°C in only about one-third of patients with acute salpingitis. Laboratory findings include elevation of the erythrocyte sedimentation rate (ESR) in 75% of patients with acute salpingitis and elevation of the peripheral white blood cell count in up to 60%.

Unlike nontuberculous salpingitis, genital tuberculosis often occurs in older women, many of whom are postmenopausal. Presenting symptoms include abnormal vaginal bleeding, pain (including dysmenorrhea), and infertility. About one-quarter of these women have had adnexal masses. Endometrial biopsy shows tuberculous granulomas and provides optimal specimens for culture.

Perihepatitis and periappendicitis Pleuritic upper abdominal pain and tenderness, usually localized to the right upper quadrant (RUQ), develop in 3–10% of women with acute PID. Symptoms of perihepatitis arise during or after the onset of symptoms of PID and may overshadow lower abdominal symptoms, thereby leading to a mistaken diagnosis of cholecystitis. In perhaps 5% of cases of acute salpingitis, early laparoscopy reveals perihepatic inflammation ranging from edema and erythema of the liver capsule to exudate with fibrinous adhesions between the visceral and parietal peritoneum. When treatment is delayed and laparoscopy is performed late, dense "violin-string" adhesions can be seen over the liver; chronic exertional or positional RUQ pain ensues when traction is placed on the adhesions. Although perihepatitis, also known as the *Fitz-Hugh–Curtis syndrome*, was for many years specifically attributed to gonococcal salpingitis, most cases are now attributed to chlamydial salpingitis. In patients with chlamydial salpingitis, serum titers of microimmunofluorescent antibody to *C. trachomatis* are typically much higher when perihepatitis is present than when it is absent.

Physical findings include RUQ tenderness and usually include adnexal tenderness and cervicitis, even in patients whose symptoms do not suggest salpingitis. Results of liver function tests and RUQ ultrasonography are nearly always normal. The presence of MPC and pelvic tenderness in a young woman with subacute pleuritic RUQ pain and normal ultrasonography of the gallbladder points to a diagnosis of perihepatitis.

Periappendicitis (appendiceal serositis without involvement of the intestinal mucosa) has been found in ~5% of patients undergoing appendectomy for suspected appendicitis and can occur as a complication of gonococcal or chlamydial salpingitis.

Among women with salpingitis, HIV infection is associated with increased severity of salpingitis and with tuboovarian abscess requiring hospitalization and surgical drainage. Nonetheless, among women with HIV infection and salpingitis, the clinical response to conventional antimicrobial therapy (coupled with drainage of tuboovarian abscess, when found) has usually been satisfactory.

Diagnosis

Treatment appropriate for PID must not be withheld from patients who have an equivocal diagnosis; it is better to err on the side of overdiagnosis and overtreatment. On the other hand, it is essential to differentiate between salpingitis and other pelvic pathology, particularly surgical emergencies such as appendicitis and ectopic pregnancy.

Nothing short of laparoscopy definitively identifies salpingitis, but routine laparoscopy to confirm suspected salpingitis is generally impractical. Most patients with acute PID have lower abdominal pain of <3 weeks' duration, pelvic tenderness on bimanual pelvic examination, and evidence of lower genital tract infection (e.g., MPC). Approximately 60% of such patients have salpingitis at laparoscopy, and perhaps 10–20% have endometritis alone. Among the patients with these findings, a rectal temperature >38°C, a palpable adnexal mass, and elevation of the ESR to >15 mm/h also raise the probability of salpingitis, which has been found at laparoscopy in 68% of patients with one of these additional findings, 90% of patients with two, and 96% of patients with three. However, only 17% of all patients with laparoscopy-confirmed salpingitis have had all three additional findings.

In a woman with pelvic pain and tenderness, increased numbers of PMNs (30 per 1000× microscopic field in strands of cervical mucus) or leukocytes outnumbering epithelial cells in vaginal fluid (in the absence of trichomonal vaginitis, that also produces PMNs in vaginal discharge) increase the predictive value of a clinical diagnosis of acute PID, as do onset with menses, history of recent abnormal menstrual bleeding, presence of an IUD, history of salpingitis, and sexual exposure to a male with urethritis. Appendicitis or another disorder of the gut is favored by the early onset of anorexia, nausea, or vomiting; the onset of pain later than day 14 of the menstrual cycle; or unilateral pain limited to the right or left lower quadrant. Whenever the diagnosis of PID is being considered, serum assays for human β-chorionic gonadotropin should be performed; these tests are usually positive with ectopic pregnancy. Ultrasonography and MRI can be useful for the identification of tuboovarian or pelvic abscess. MRI of the tubes can also show increased tubal diameter, intratubal fluid, or tubal wall thickening in cases of salpingitis.

The primary and uncontested value of laparoscopy in women with lower abdominal pain is for the exclusion of other surgical problems. Some of the most common or serious problems that may be confused with salpingitis (e.g., acute appendicitis, ectopic pregnancy, corpus luteum bleeding, ovarian tumor) are unilateral. Unilateral pain or pelvic mass, although not incompatible with PID, is a strong indication for laparoscopy unless the clinical picture warrants laparotomy instead. Atypical clinical findings such as the absence of lower genital tract infection, a missed menstrual period, a positive pregnancy test, or failure to respond to appropriate therapy, are other common indications for laparoscopy. Endometrial biopsy is relatively sensitive and specific for the diagnosis of endometritis, which correlates well with the presence of salpingitis.

Endocervical swab specimens should be examined by NAATs for *N. gonorrhoeae* and *C. trachomatis*. At a minimum, vaginal fluid should be evaluated for the presence of PMNs, and endocervical secretions ideally should be assessed by Gram's staining for PMNs and gram-negative diplococci that indicate gonococcal infection. The clinical diagnosis of PID made by expert gynecologists is confirmed by laparoscopy or endometrial biopsy in ~90% of women who also have cultures positive for *N. gonorrhoeae* or *C. trachomatis*. Even among women with no symptoms suggestive of acute PID who were attending an STD clinic or a gynecology clinic in Pittsburgh, endometritis was significantly associated with endocervical gonorrhea or chlamydial infection or with bacterial vaginosis, being detected in 26%, 27%, and 15% of women with these conditions, respectively.

The 2010 CDC guidelines recommend initiation of empirical treatment for PID in sexually active young women and other women at risk for PID if they are experiencing pelvic or lower abdominal pain, if no other cause for the pain can be identified, and if pelvic examination reveals one or more of the following criteria for PID: cervical motion tenderness, uterine tenderness, or adnexal tenderness. Women with suspected PID can be treated as either outpatients or inpatients. In the multicenter Pelvic Inflammatory Disease Evaluation and Clinical Health (PEACH) trial, 831 women with mild to moderately severe symptoms and signs of PID were randomized to receive either inpatient treatment with IV cefoxitin and doxycycline or outpatient treatment with a single IM dose of cefoxitin plus oral doxycycline. Short-term clinical and microbiologic outcomes and long-term outcomes were equivalent in the two groups. Nonetheless, hospitalization should be considered when (1) the diagnosis is uncertain and surgical emergencies such as appendicitis and ectopic pregnancy cannot be excluded, (2) the patient is pregnant, (3) pelvic abscess is suspected, (4) severe illness or nausea and vomiting preclude outpatient management, (5) the patient has HIV infection, (6) the patient is assessed as unable to follow or tolerate an outpatient regimen, or (7) the patient has failed to respond to outpatient therapy. Some experts also prefer to hospitalize adolescents with PID for initial therapy, although younger women do as well as older women on outpatient therapy.

Recommended combination regimens for ambulatory or parenteral management of PID are presented in Table 130-6. Women

TABLE 130-6   Combination Antimicrobial Regimens Recommended for Outpatient Treatment or for Parenteral Treatment of PID

Outpatient Regimens[a]	Parenteral Regimens
Ceftriaxone (250 mg IM once) *plus*	Initiate parenteral therapy with either of the following regimens; continue parenteral therapy until 48 h after clinical improvement; then change to outpatient therapy, as described in the text.
Doxycycline (100 mg PO bid for 14 days) *plus*[b]	
	Regimen A
Metronidazole (500 mg PO bid for 14 days)	Cefotetan (2 g IV q12h) *or* Cefoxitin (2 g IV q6h) *plus* Doxycycline (100 mg IV or PO q12h)
	Regimen B
	Clindamycin (900 mg IV q8h) *plus* Gentamicin (loading dose of 2 mg/kg IV or IM, then maintenance dose of 1.5 mg/kg q8h)

[a] See text for discussion of options in the patient who is intolerant of cephalosporins.
[b] The addition of metronidazole is recommended by some experts, particularly if bacterial vaginosis is present.
Source: Adapted from Centers for Disease Control and Prevention: MMWR Recomm Rep 59 (RR-12):1, 2010.

managed as outpatients should receive a combined regimen with broad activity, such as ceftriaxone (to cover possible gonococcal infection) followed by doxycycline (to cover possible chlamydial infection). Metronidazole can be added, if tolerated, to enhance activity against anaerobes; this addition should be strongly considered if bacterial vaginosis is documented. Although few methodologically sound clinical trials (especially with prolonged follow-up) have been conducted, one meta-analysis suggested a benefit of providing good coverage against anaerobes.

Neither doxycycline nor the fluoroquinolones provide reliable coverage for gonococcal infection today. Thus, adequate oral treatment of women with serious intolerance to cephalosporins is a challenge. If penicillins are an option, amoxicillin/clavulanic acid combined with doxycycline has effected short-term clinical response in one clinical trial. If fluoroquinolones are the only option and if the community prevalence and individual risk for gonorrhea are known to be low, oral levofloxacin (500 mg once daily) or ofloxacin (400 mg twice daily) for 14 days, with or without metronidazole, may be considered. In this case, it is imperative to perform a sensitive diagnostic test for gonorrhea (ideally, culture to test for antimicrobial susceptibility) before initiating therapy. For those women whose PID involves quinolone-resistant gonorrhea, treatment is uncertain but could include parenteral gentamicin or oral azithromycin, although the latter agent has not been studied for this purpose.

For hospitalized patients, the following two parenteral regimens have given nearly identical results in a multicenter randomized trial:

1. Doxycycline (100 mg twice daily, given IV or PO) plus cefotetan (2 g IV every 12 h) or cefoxitin (2 g IV every 6 h): Administration of these drugs should be continued by the IV route for at least 48 h after the patient's condition improves and then followed with oral doxycycline (100 mg twice daily) to complete 14 days of therapy.
2. Clindamycin (900 mg IV every 8 h) plus gentamicin (2 mg/kg IV or IM, followed by 1.5 mg/kg every 8 h) in patients with normal renal function: Once-daily dosing of gentamicin (with combination of the total daily dose into a single daily dose) has not been evaluated in PID but has been efficacious in other serious infections and could be substituted. Treatment with these drugs should be continued for at least 48 h after the patient's condition improves and then followed with oral doxycycline (100 mg twice daily) or clindamycin (450 mg four times daily) to complete 14 days of therapy. In cases with tuboovarian abscess, clindamycin rather than doxycycline for continued therapy provides better coverage for anaerobic infection.

FOLLOW-UP Hospitalized patients should show substantial clinical improvement within 3–5 days. Women treated as outpatients should be clinically reevaluated within 72 h. A follow-up telephone survey of women seen in an emergency department and given a prescription for 10 days of oral doxycycline for PID found that 28% never filled the prescription and 41% stopped taking the medication early (after an average of 4.1 days), often because of persistent symptoms, lack of symptoms, or side effects. Women not responding favorably to ambulatory therapy should be hospitalized for parenteral therapy and further diagnostic evaluations, including a consideration of laparoscopy. Male sex partners should be evaluated and treated empirically for gonorrhea and chlamydial infection. After completion of treatment, tests for persistent or recurrent infection with *N. gonorrhoeae* or *C. trachomatis* should be performed if symptoms persist or recur or if the patient has not complied with therapy or has been reexposed to an untreated sex partner.

SURGERY Surgery is necessary for the treatment of salpingitis only in the face of life-threatening infection (such as rupture or threatened rupture of a tuboovarian abscess) or for drainage of an abscess. Conservative surgical procedures are usually sufficient. Pelvic abscesses can often be drained by posterior colpotomy, and peritoneal lavage can be used for generalized peritonitis.

Prognosis

Late sequelae include infertility due to bilateral tubal occlusion, ectopic pregnancy due to tubal scarring without occlusion, chronic pelvic pain, and recurrent salpingitis. The overall postsalpingitis risk of infertility due to tubal occlusion in a large study in Sweden was 11% after one episode of salpingitis, 23% after two episodes, and 54% after three or more episodes. A University of Washington study found a sevenfold increase in the risk of ectopic pregnancy and an eightfold increase in the rate of hysterectomy after PID.

Prevention

A randomized controlled trial designed to determine whether selective screening for chlamydial infection reduces the risk of subsequent PID showed that women randomized to undergo screening had a 56% lower rate of PID over the following year than did women receiving the usual care without screening. This report helped prompt U.S. national guidelines for risk-based chlamydial screening of young women to reduce the incidence of PID and the prevalence of post-PID sequelae, while also reducing sexual transmission of *C. trachomatis*. The CDC and the U.S. Preventive Services Task Force recommend that sexually active women ≤25 years of age be screened for genital chlamydial infection annually. Despite this recommendation, screening coverage in many primary care settings remains low.

■ ULCERATIVE GENITAL OR PERIANAL LESIONS

Genital ulceration reflects a set of important STIs, most of which sharply increase the risk of sexual acquisition and shedding of HIV. In a 1996 study of genital ulcers in 10 of the U.S. cities with the highest rates of primary syphilis, PCR testing of ulcer specimens demonstrated HSV in 62% of patients, *Treponema pallidum* (the agent of chancroid) in 13%, and *Haemophilus ducreyi* (the agent of chancroid) in 12–20%. Today, genital herpes represents an even higher proportion of genital ulcers in the United States and other industrialized countries.

In Asia and Africa, chancroid (Fig. 130-5) was once considered the most common type of genital ulcer, followed in frequency by primary syphilis and then genital herpes (Fig. 130-6). With increased efforts to control chancroid and syphilis and widespread use of broad-spectrum antibiotics to treat STI-related syndromes, together with more frequent recurrences or persistence of genital herpes attributable to HIV infection, PCR testing of genital ulcers now clearly implicates genital herpes as the most common cause of genital ulceration in some developing countries. LGV caused by *C. trachomatis*; (Fig. 130-7) and donovanosis (granuloma inguinale, caused by *Klebsiella granulomatis*; see Fig. 161-1) continue to cause genital ulceration in developing countries. LGV virtually disappeared in industrialized countries during the first 20 years of the HIV pandemic, but outbreaks are again occurring in Europe (including the United Kingdom), in North America, and in Australia. In these outbreaks, LGV typically presents as proctitis in men who report unprotected receptive anal intercourse, very often in association with HIV and/or hepatitis C virus infection; the latter may be an acute infection acquired through the same exposure. Other causes of genital ulcers include (1) candidiasis and traumatized genital warts—both readily

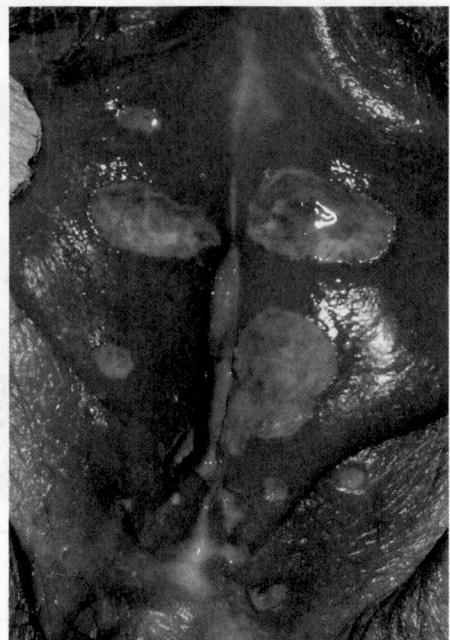

Figure 130-5 Chancroid: multiple, painful, punched-out ulcers with undermined borders on the labia occurring after autoinoculation.

recognized; (2) lesions due to genital involvement by more widespread dermatoses; (3) cutaneous manifestations of systemic diseases such as genital mucosal ulceration in Stevens-Johnson syndrome or Behçet's disease; (4) superinfections of lesions that may originally have been sexually acquired such as methicillin-resistant *S. aureus* complicating a genital ulcer due to HSV-2; and (5) localized drug reactions, such as the ulcers occasionally seen with topical paromomycin cream or boric acid preparations.

Diagnosis

Although most genital ulcerations cannot be diagnosed confidently on clinical grounds alone, clinical findings and epidemiologic considerations (Table 130-7) can usually guide initial management (Table 130-8) pending results of further tests. Clinicians should order a rapid serologic test for syphilis in all cases of genital ulcer. To evaluate lesions except those highly characteristic of infection with

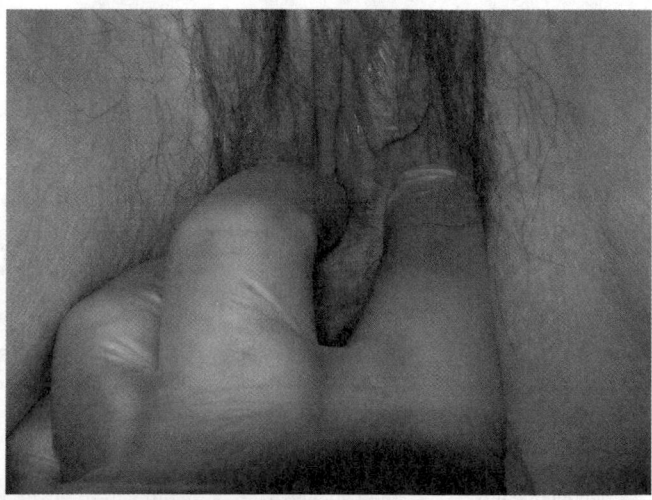

Figure 130-6 Genital herpes. A relatively mild, superficial ulcer is typically seen in episodic outbreaks. *(Courtesy of Michael Remington, University of Washington Virology Research Clinic.)*

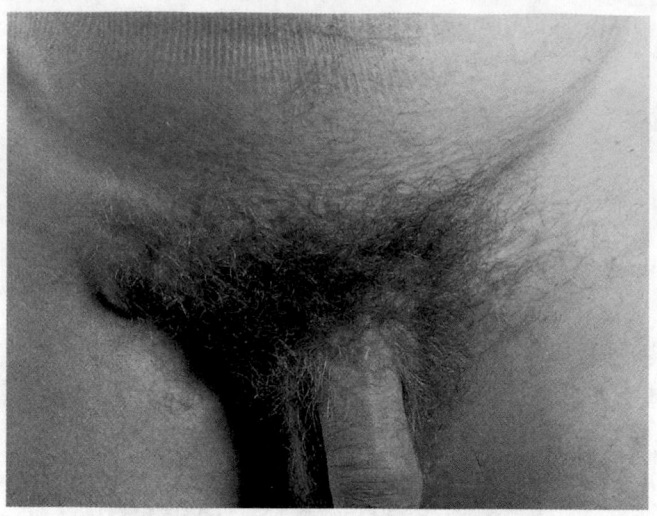

Figure 130-7 Lymphogranuloma venereum: striking tender lymphadenopathy occurring at the femoral and inguinal lymph nodes, separated by a groove made by Poupart's ligament. This "sign-of-the-groove" is not considered specific for LGV; for example, lymphomas may present with this sign.

HSV (i.e., those with herpetic vesicles), dark-field microscopy, direct immunofluorescence, and PCR for *T. pallidum* can be useful but are rarely available today in the United States. It is important to note that 30% of syphilitic chancres—the primary ulcer of syphilis—are associated with a nonreactive syphilis serology. All patients presenting with genital ulceration should be counseled and tested for HIV infection.

Typical vesicles or pustules or a cluster of painful ulcers preceded by vesiculopustular lesions suggests genital herpes. These typical clinical manifestations make detection of the virus optional; however, many patients want confirmation of the diagnosis, and differentiation of HSV-1 from HSV-2 has prognostic implications, since the latter causes more frequent genital recurrences.

Painless, nontender, indurated ulcers with firm, nontender inguinal adenopathy suggest primary syphilis. If results of dark-field examination and a rapid serologic test for syphilis are initially negative, presumptive therapy should be provided on the basis of the individual's risk. For example, with increasing rates of syphilis among MSM in the United States, most experts would not withhold therapy for this infection pending watchful waiting and/or subsequent detection of seroconversion. Repeated serologic testing for syphilis 1 or 2 weeks after treatment of seronegative primary syphilis usually demonstrates seroconversion.

"Atypical" or clinically trivial ulcers may be more common manifestations of genital herpes than classic vesiculopustular lesions. Specific tests for HSV in such lesions are therefore indicated (Chap. 179). Commercially available type-specific serologic tests for serum antibody to HSV-2 may give negative results, especially when patients present early with the initial episode of genital herpes or when HSV-1 is the cause of genital herpes (as is often the case today). Furthermore, a positive test for antibody to HSV-2 does not prove that the current lesions are herpetic, since nearly one-fifth of the general population of the United States (and no doubt a higher proportion of those at risk for other STIs) becomes seropositive for HSV-2 during early adulthood. Although even "type-specific" tests for HSV-2 that are commercially available in the United States are not 100% specific, a positive HSV-2 serology does enable the clinician to tell the patient that he or she has probably had genital herpes, should learn to recognize symptoms, should avoid sex during recurrences, and should consider use of condoms or suppressive antiviral therapy, both of which can reduce the risk of transmission to a sexual partner.

Demonstration of *H. ducreyi* by culture (or by PCR, when available) is most useful when ulcers are painful and purulent, especially if inguinal lymphadenopathy with fluctuance or overlying erythema is noted; if chancroid is prevalent in the community; or if the patient has recently had a sexual exposure elsewhere in a chancroid-endemic area (e.g., a developing country). Enlarged, fluctuant lymph nodes should be aspirated for culture or PCR to detect *H. ducreyi* as well as for Gram's staining and culture to rule out the presence of other pyogenic bacteria.

When genital ulcers persist beyond the natural history of initial episodes of herpes (2–3 weeks) or of chancroid or syphilis (up to

TABLE 130-7 Clinical Features of Genital Ulcers

Feature	Syphilis	Herpes	Chancroid	Lymphogranuloma Venereum	Donovanosis
Incubation period	9–90 days	2–7 days	1–14 days	3 days–6 weeks	1–4 weeks (up to 6 months)
Early primary lesions	Papule	Vesicle	Pustule	Papule, pustule, or vesicle	Papule
No. of lesions	Usually one	Multiple	Usually multiple, may coalesce	Usually one; often not detected, despite lymphadenopathy	Variable
Diameter	5–15 mm	1–2 mm	Variable	2–10 mm	Variable
Edges	Sharply demarcated, elevated, round, or oval	Erythematous	Undermined, ragged, irregular	Elevated, round, or oval	Elevated, irregular
Depth	Superficial or deep	Superficial	Excavated	Superficial or deep	Elevated
Base	Smooth, nonpurulent, relatively nonvascular	Serous, erythematous, nonvascular	Purulent, bleeds easily	Variable, nonvascular	Red and velvety, bleeds readily
Induration	Firm	None	Soft	Occasionally firm	Firm
Pain	Uncommon	Frequently tender	Usually very tender	Variable	Uncommon
Lymphadenopathy	Firm, nontender, bilateral	Firm, tender, often bilateral with initial episode	Tender, may suppurate, loculated, usually unilateral	Tender, may suppurate, loculated, usually unilateral	None; pseudobuboes

Source: From RM Ballard, in KK Holmes et al (eds): *Sexually Transmitted Diseases*, 4th ed. New York, McGraw-Hill, 2008.

TABLE 130-8 Initial Management of Genital or Perianal Ulcer

Usual causes

Herpes simplex virus (HSV)

Treponema pallidum (primary syphilis)

Haemophilus ducreyi (chancroid)

Usual initial laboratory evaluation

Dark-field exam (if available), direct FA, or PCR for *T. pallidum*; RPR, VDRL, or EIA test for syphilis (if negative but primary syphilis suspected, treat presumptively when indicated by epidemiologic and sexual risk assessment; repeat in 1 week); culture, direct FA, ELISA, or PCR for HSV; consider HSV-2-specific serology. In chancroid-endemic area: PCR or culture for *H. ducreyi*

Initial Treatment

Herpes confirmed or suspected (history or sign of vesicles):

Treat for genital herpes with acyclovir, valacyclovir, or famciclovir

Syphilis confirmed (dark-field, FA, or PCR showing *T. pallidum*, or RPR reactive):

Benzathine penicillin [2.4 million units IM once to patient, recent (e.g., within 3 months) seronegative partner(s), and all seropositive partners]

Chancroid confirmed or suspected (diagnostic test positive, or HSV and syphilis excluded, and persistent lesion):

Ciprofloxacin (500 mg PO as single dose) *or*

Ceftriaxone (250 mg IM as single dose) *or*

Azithromycin (1 g PO as single dose)

Abbreviations: FA, fluorescent antibody; PCR, polymerase chain reaction; RPR, rapid plasma reagin; EIA, enzyme immunoassay; ELISA, enzyme-linked immunosorbent assay; HSV, herpes simplex virus; VDRL, Venereal Disease Research Laboratory.

6 weeks) and do not resolve with syndrome-based antimicrobial therapy, then—in addition to the usual tests for herpes, syphilis, and chancroid—biopsy is indicated to exclude donovanosis, carcinoma, and other nonvenereal dermatoses. If not performed previously, HIV serology should be standard, since chronic, persistent genital herpes is common in AIDS.

TREATMENT   Ulcerative Genital or Perianal Lesions

Immediate syndrome-based treatment for acute genital ulcerations (after collection of all necessary diagnostic specimens at the first visit) is often appropriate before all test results become available, because patients with typical initial or recurrent episodes of genital or anorectal herpes can benefit from prompt oral antiviral therapy (Chap. 179); because early treatment of sexually transmitted causes of genital ulcers decreases further transmission; and because many patients do not return for test results and treatment. A thorough assessment of the patient's sexual-risk profile and medical history is critical in determining the course of initial management. The patient who has risk factors consistent with exposure to syphilis (e.g., a male patient who reports sex with other men or who has HIV infection) should generally receive initial treatment for syphilis. Empirical therapy for chancroid should be considered if there has been an exposure in an area of the world where chancroid occurs or if regional lymph node suppuration is evident. In resource-poor settings lacking ready access to diagnostic tests, this approach to syndromic treatment for syphilis and chancroid has

helped bring these two diseases under control. Finally, empirical antimicrobial therapy may be indicated if ulcers persist and the diagnosis remains unclear after a week of observation despite attempts to diagnose herpes, syphilis, and chancroid.

■ PROCTITIS, PROCTOCOLITIS, ENTEROCOLITIS, AND ENTERITIS

Sexually acquired *proctitis*, with inflammation limited to the rectal mucosa (the distal 10–12 cm), results from direct rectal inoculation of typical STD pathogens. In contrast, inflammation extending from the rectum to the colon (*proctocolitis*), involving both the small and the large bowel (*enterocolitis*), or involving the small bowel alone (*enteritis*) can result from ingestion of typical intestinal pathogens through oral-anal exposure during sexual contact. Anorectal pain and mucopurulent, bloody rectal discharge suggest proctitis or proctocolitis. Proctitis commonly produces tenesmus (causing frequent attempts to defecate, but not true diarrhea) and constipation, whereas proctocolitis and enterocolitis more often cause true diarrhea. In all three conditions, anoscopy usually shows mucosal exudate and easily induced mucosal bleeding (i.e., a positive "wipe test"), sometimes with petechiae or mucosal ulcers. Exudate should be sampled for Gram's staining and other microbiologic studies. Sigmoidoscopy or colonoscopy shows inflammation limited to the rectum in proctitis or disease extending at least up into the sigmoid colon in proctocolitis.

The AIDS era brought an extraordinary shift in the clinical and etiologic spectrum of intestinal infections among MSM. The number of cases of the acute intestinal STIs described above fell as high-risk sexual behaviors became less common in this group. At the same time, the number of AIDS-related opportunistic intestinal infections increased rapidly, many associated with chronic or recurrent symptoms. The incidence of these infections has since fallen with increasingly effective antiretroviral therapy. Two species initially isolated in association with intestinal symptoms in MSM are now known as *Helicobacter cinaedi* and *Helicobacter fennelliae*, and both have subsequently been isolated from the blood of HIV-infected men and other immunosuppressed persons, often in association with a syndrome of multifocal dermatitis and arthritis.

Acquisition of HSV, *N. gonorrhoeae*, or *C. trachomatis* (including LGV strains of *C. trachomatis*) during receptive anorectal intercourse causes most cases of infectious proctitis in women and MSM. Primary and secondary syphilis can also produce anal or anorectal lesions, with or without symptoms. Gonococcal or chlamydial proctitis typically involves the most distal rectal mucosa and the anal crypts and is clinically mild, without systemic manifestations. In contrast, primary proctitis due to HSV and proctocolitis due to the strains of *C. trachomatis* that cause LGV usually produce severe anorectal pain and often cause fever. Perianal ulcers and inguinal lymphadenopathy, most commonly due to HSV, can also occur in LGV or syphilis. Sacral nerve root radiculopathies, usually presenting as urinary retention, laxity of the anal sphincter, or constipation, may complicate primary herpetic proctitis. In LGV, rectal biopsy typically shows crypt abscesses, granulomas, and giant cells—findings resembling those in Crohn's disease; such findings should always prompt rectal culture and serology for LGV, which is a curable infection. Syphilis can also produce rectal granulomas, usually in association with infiltration by plasma cells or other mononuclear cells. Syphilis, LGV, and HSV infection involving the rectum can produce perirectal adenopathy that is sometimes mistaken for malignancy; syphilis, LGV, HSV infection, and chancroid involving the anus can produce inguinal adenopathy, because anal lymphatics drain to inguinal lymph nodes.

Diarrhea and abdominal bloating or cramping pain without anorectal symptoms and with normal findings on anoscopy and sigmoidoscopy occur with inflammation of the small intestine (enteritis) or with proximal colitis. In MSM without HIV infection, enteritis is often attributable to *Giardia lamblia*. Sexually acquired proctocolitis is most often due to *Campylobacter* or *Shigella* species.

| TREATMENT | Proctitis, Proctocolitis, Enterocolitis, and Enteritis |

Acute proctitis in persons who have practiced receptive anorectal intercourse is usually sexually acquired. Such patients should undergo anoscopy to detect rectal ulcers or vesicles and petechiae after swabbing of the rectal mucosa; to examine rectal exudates for PMNs and gram-negative diplococci; and to obtain rectal swab specimens for testing for rectal gonorrhea, chlamydial infection, herpes, and syphilis. Pending test results, patients with proctitis should receive empirical syndromic treatment—e.g., with ceftriaxone (a single IM dose of 125 mg for gonorrhea) plus doxycycline (100 mg by mouth twice daily for 7 days for possible chlamydial infection) plus treatment for herpes or syphilis if indicated.

PREVENTION AND CONTROL OF STIs

Prevention and control of STIs require the following:

1. Reduction of the average rate of sexual exposure to STIs through alteration of sexual risk behaviors and behavioral norms among both susceptible and infected persons in all population groups. The necessary changes include reduction in the total number of sexual partners and the number of concurrent sexual partners.
2. Reduction of the efficiency of transmission through the promotion of safer sexual practices, the use of condoms during casual or commercial sex, vaccination against HBV and HPV infection, male circumcision (which reduces risk of acquisition of HIV, chancroid, and perhaps other STIs), and a growing number of other approaches (e.g., early detection and treatment of other STIs to reduce the efficiency of sexual transmission of HIV). Longitudinal studies have shown that consistent condom use is associated with significant protection of both males and females against all STIs that have been examined, including HIV, HPV, and HSV infections as well as gonorrhea and chlamydial infection. The only exceptions are probably sexually transmitted *Pthirus pubis* and *Sarcoptes scabiei* infestations.
3. Shortening of the duration of infectivity of STIs through early detection and curative or suppressive treatment of patients and their sexual partners.

Financial and time constraints imposed by many clinical practices, along with the reluctance of some clinicians to ask questions about stigmatized sexual behaviors, often curtail screening and prevention services. As outlined in Fig. 130-8, the success of clinicians' efforts to detect and treat STIs depends in part on societal efforts to teach young people how to recognize symptoms of STIs; to motivate individuals with symptoms to seek care promptly; to educate persons who are at risk but have no symptoms about what tests they should undergo routinely; and to make high-quality, appropriate care accessible, affordable, and acceptable, especially to the young indigent patients most likely to acquire an STI.

Since many infected individuals develop no symptoms or fail to recognize and report symptoms, clinicians should routinely perform an STI risk assessment for teenagers and young adults as a guide to selective screening. As stated earlier, U.S. Preventive Services Task Force Guidelines recommend screening sexually active female patients ≤25 years of age for *C. trachomatis* whenever they present for health care (at least once a year); older women should be tested if they have more than one sexual partner, have begun a new sexual relationship since the previous test, or have another STI diagnosed. In women 25–29 years of age, chlamydial infection is uncommon but still may reach a

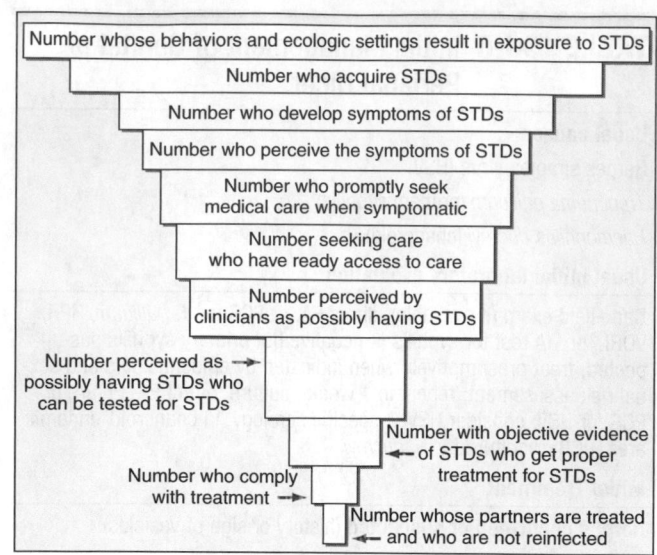

Figure 130-8 Critical control points for preventive and clinical interventions against sexually transmitted diseases (STDs). [*Adapted from HT Waller and MA Piot: Bull World Health Organ 41:75, 1969 and 43:1, 1970; and from "Resource allocation model for public health planning—a case study of tuberculosis control," Bull World Health Organ 48 (Suppl), 1973.*]

prevalence of 3–5% in some settings; information on a sex partner's concurrency provided by women in this age group (i.e., whether a male partner has had another sex partner during the time they have been together) is helpful in identifying women at increased risk. In the United States, widespread selective screening of young women for cervical *C. trachomatis* infection in some regions has been associated with a 50–60% drop in prevalence, and such screening also protects the individual woman from PID. Sensitive urine-based genetic amplification tests permit expansion of screening to men, teenage boys, and girls in settings where examination is not planned or is impractical (e.g., during pre-participation sports examinations or during initial medical evaluation of adolescent girls). Vaginal swabs—collected either by the health care provider at a pelvic examination or by the woman herself—are highly sensitive and specific for the diagnosis of chlamydial and gonococcal infection; they are now the preferred type of specimen for screening and diagnosis of these infections.

Although gonorrhea is now substantially less common than chlamydial infection in industrialized countries, screening tests for *N. gonorrhoeae* are still appropriate for women and teenage girls attending STD clinics and for sexually active teens and young women from areas of high gonorrhea prevalence. Multiplex NAATs that combine screening for *N. gonorrhoeae* and *C. trachomatis* in a single low-cost assay now facilitate the prevention and control of both infections in populations at high risk.

All patients with newly detected STIs or at high risk for STIs according to routine risk assessment as well as all pregnant women should be encouraged to undergo serologic testing for syphilis and HIV infection, with appropriate HIV counseling before and after testing. Randomized trials have shown that risk-reduction counseling of patients with STIs significantly lowers subsequent risk of acquiring an STI; such counseling should now be considered a standard component of STI management. Preimmunization serologic testing for antibody to HBV is indicated for unvaccinated persons who are known to be at high risk, such as homosexually active men and injection drug users. In most young persons, however, it is more cost-effective to vaccinate against HBV without serologic screening. It is important to recognize that, while immunization against HBV has contributed to marked reductions in the incidence of infection with this virus, the majority of new cases that do occur are acquired through sex. In 2006, the Advisory Committee on Immunization Practices (ACIP) of the CDC recommended the following: (1) Universal hepatitis B vaccination should be implemented for all unvaccinated adults in settings in which a high proportion of adults have risk factors for HBV infection (e.g., STD clinics, HIV testing and treatment facilities, drug-abuse treatment and prevention settings, health care settings targeting services to injection drug users or MSM, and correctional facilities). (2) In other primary care and specialty medical settings in which adults at risk for HBV infection receive care, health care providers should inform all patients about the health benefits of vaccination, the risk factors for HBV infection, and the persons for whom vaccination is recommended and should vaccinate adults who report risk factors for HBV infection as well as any adult who requests protection from HBV infection. To promote vaccination in all settings, health care providers should implement standing orders to identify adults recommended for hepatitis B vaccination, should administer hepatitis B vaccine as part of routine clinical services, should not require acknowledgment of an HBV infection risk factor for adult vaccination, and should use available reimbursement mechanisms to remove financial barriers to hepatitis B vaccination.

In 2007, the ACIP recommended routine immunization of 9- to 26-year-old girls and women with the quadrivalent HPV vaccine (against HPV types 6, 11, 16, and 18) approved by the U.S. Food and Drug Administration; the optimal age for recommended vaccination is 11–12 years because of the very high risk of HPV infection after sexual debut. In 2009, the ACIP added bivalent HPV vaccine (against types 6 and 11) as an option and expanded the groups in which immunization (with either quadrivalent or bivalent vaccine) is safe and effective to include boys and men 9–26 years old. HPV vaccines offering broader protection against additional oncogenic HPV types are anticipated.

Partner notification is the process of identifying and informing partners of infected patients about possible exposure to an STI and of examining, testing, and treating partners as appropriate. In a series of 22 reports concerning partner notification during the 1990s, index patients with gonorrhea or chlamydial infection named a mean of 0.75–1.6 partners, of whom one-fourth to one-third were infected; those with syphilis named 1.8–6.3 partners, with one-third to one-half infected; and those with HIV infection named 0.76–5.31 partners, with up to one-fourth infected. Persons who transmit infection or who have recently been infected and are still in the incubation period usually have no symptoms or only mild symptoms and seek medical attention only when notified of their exposure. Therefore, the clinician must encourage patients to participate in partner notification, must ensure that exposed persons are notified and treated, and must guarantee confidentiality to all involved. In the United States, local health departments often offer assistance in partner notification, treatment, and/or counseling. It seems both feasible and most useful to notify those partners exposed within the patient's likely period of infectiousness that is often considered the preceding 1 month for gonorrhea, 1–2 months for chlamydial infection, and up to 3 months for early syphilis.

Persons with a new-onset STI always have a *source* contact who gave them the infection; in addition, they may have a *secondary* (*spread* or *exposed*) contact with whom they had sex after becoming infected. The identification and treatment of these two types of contacts have different objectives. Treatment of the source contact (often a casual contact) benefits the community by preventing further transmission; treatment of the recently exposed secondary contact (typically a spouse or another steady sexual partner) prevents both the development of serious complications (such as PID) in the partner and reinfection of the index patient. A survey of a random sample of U.S. physicians found that most instructed patients to abstain from sex during treatment, to use condoms, and to inform their sex partners after being diagnosed with gonorrhea, chlamydial infection, or syphilis; physicians sometimes gave the patients drugs for their partners. However, follow-up of the partners by physicians was infrequent. A randomized trial compared patients' delivery of therapy to partners exposed to gonorrhea or chlamydial infection with conventional notification and advice to partners to seek evaluation for STD; patients' delivery of partners' therapy (PDPT), also known as *expedited partner therapy* (EPT), significantly reduced combined rates of reinfection of the index patient with *N. gonorrhoeae* or *C. trachomatis*. State-by-state variations in regulations governing this approach have not been well defined, but the 2010 CDC STD treatment guidelines and the EPT final report of 2006 (*http://www.cdc.gov/std/treatment/EPTFinalReport2006.pdf*) describe its potential use. Currently, EPT is commonly used by many practicing physicians. Its legal status varies by state, but EPT is now permissible in 22 states and potentially allowable in another 20. (Updated information on the legal status of EPT is available at *http://www.cdc.gov/std/ept*.)

In summary, clinicians and public health agencies share responsibility for the prevention and control of STIs. In the current health care environment, the role of primary care clinicians has become increasingly important in STI prevention as well as in diagnosis and treatment, and the resurgence of bacterial STIs like syphilis and LGV among MSM—particularly those co-infected with HIV—emphasizes the need for risk assessment and routine screening.

FURTHER READINGS

CELUM CL et al: Acyclovir and transmission of HIV-1 from persons infected with HIV-1 and HSV-2. N Engl J Med 362:427, 2010

CENTERS FOR DISEASE CONTROL AND PREVENTION: Sexually transmitted diseases treatment guidelines, 2010. MMWR Recomm Rep 59 (RR-12):1, 2010. Available at *http://www.cdc.gov/std/treatment*

FREDRICKS DN et al: Molecular identification of bacteria associated with bacterial vaginosis. N Engl J Med 353:1899, 2005

HOLMES KK et al (eds): *Sexually Transmitted Diseases*, 4th ed. New York, McGraw-Hill, 2008

MANHART LE, HOLMES KK: Randomized controlled trials of individual-level, population-level, and multilevel interventions for preventing sexually transmitted infections: What has worked? J Infect Dis 191(Suppl 1):S7, 2005

MARKOWITZ LE et al: Quadrivalent human papillomavirus vaccine: Recommendations of the Advisory Committee on Immunization Practices (ACIP). MMWR Recomm Rep 56(RR-2):1, 2007. Updated information available at *http://www.cdc.gov/vaccines/recs/acip/*

_____ et al: Seroprevalence of human papillomavirus vaccine types 6, 11, 16, and 18 in the United States: National Health and Nutrition Examination Survey 2003–2004. J Infect Dis 200:1059, 2009

MAST EE et al: A comprehensive immunization strategy to eliminate transmission of hepatitis B virus infection in the United States: Recommendations of the Advisory Committee on Immunization Practices (ACIP). Part II: Immunization of adults. MMWR Recomm Rep 55(RR-16):1, 2006

MORSE SA et al: *Atlas of Sexually Transmitted Diseases*, 4th ed. Elsevier, London, 2010

U.S. PREVENTIVE SERVICES TASK FORCE: Behavioral counseling to prevent sexually transmitted infections: U.S. Preventive Services Task Force recommendation statement. Ann Intern Med 149:491–6, W95, 2008

WORLD HEALTH ORGANIZATION: Sexually transmitted diseases diagnostics initiative. Geneva, WHO, 2001 (*http://www.who.int/std_diagnostics/*)

CHAPTER **131**

Health Care–Associated Infections

Robert A. Weinstein

The costs of hospital-acquired (nosocomial) and other health care–associated infections are great. It is estimated that these infections affect 1.7 million patients, cost ~$28–33 billion, and contribute to 99,000 deaths in U.S. hospitals annually. Although efforts to lower infection risks have been challenged by the growing numbers of immunocompromised patients, antibiotic-resistant bacteria, fungal and viral superinfections, and invasive devices and procedures, the viewpoint of consumer advocates—often termed "zero tolerance"—is that almost all health care–associated infections should be avoidable with strict application of evidence-based guidelines for prevention and control (Table 131-1). This chapter reviews health care–acquired and device-related infections as well as basic surveillance, prevention, control, and treatment activities.

ORGANIZATION, RESPONSIBILITIES, AND INCREASING SCRUTINY OF HEALTH CARE–ASSOCIATED INFECTIONS

The standards of the Joint Commission require all accredited hospitals to have an active program for surveillance, prevention, and control of nosocomial infections. Education of physicians in

TABLE 131-1 Sources of Infection Control Guidelines and Oversight

Organization	Role	Major Constituents	Website
Joint Commission	Regulatory	Hospitals, long-term-care facilities, laboratories	*www.jointcommission.org*
CAP	Regulatory	Laboratories	*www.cap.org*
OSHA	Regulatory	Workers	*www.osha.gov*
CMS	Regulatory	Medicare/Medicaid providers	*www.cms.hhs.gov*
PQRI	Regulatory and advisory	Eligible professionals	*www.cms.hhs.gov/pqri/*
HHS Action Plan	Regulatory and advisory	Health care and infection prevention personnel	*www.hhs.gov/ophs/initiatives/hai/*
CDC			
DHQP	Advisory	Health care facilities and personnel	*www.cdc.gov/ncidod/dhqp*
HICPAC	Advisory	Health care facilities and personnel	*www.cdc.gov/ncidod/dhqp/hicpac.html*
NIOSH	Advisory	Workers	*www.cdc.gov/niosh*
AHRQ	Advisory	Broad (e.g., health care personnel)	*www.ahrq.gov*
NQF	Advisory	Broad (e.g., health care personnel)	*www.qualityforum.org*
IOM	Advisory	Broad (e.g., health care personnel)	*www.iom.edu*
Federal Influenza Planning	Advisory	Health care and public health personnel	*pandemicflu.gov/professional/hospital/*
Trust for America's Health	Advisory	Broad (e.g., the public)	*healthyamericans.org*
CSTE	Advisory and professional society	Public health personnel	*www.cste.org*
IDSA	Professional society	Infectious disease physicians/researchers	*www.idsociety.org*
SHEA	Professional society	Health care epidemiologists	*www.shea-online.org*
HIS	Professional society	Health care epidemiologists	*www.his.org.uk/resource_library.cfm*
APIC	Professional society	Infection preventionists	*www.apic.org*
MedQIC	Quality improvement	Broad (e.g., health care personnel)	*www.qualitynet.org*
IHI	Quality improvement	Broad (e.g., health care personnel)	*www.ihi.org*
Leapfrog Group	Quality improvement	Broad (payers, consumers, employers, and health care personnel)	*www.leapfroggroup.org/for_hospitals*
NSQIP	Quality improvement	Surgery services	*www.acsnsqip.org*

Note: CAP, College of American Pathologists; OSHA, Occupational Safety & Health Administration; CMS, Centers for Medicare & Medicaid Services; PQRI, Physician Quality Reporting Initiative; HHS, Health and Human Services; CDC, Centers for Disease Control and Prevention; DHQP, Division of Healthcare Quality Promotion; HICPAC, Healthcare Infection Control Practices Advisory Committee; NIOSH, National Institute for Occupational Safety and Health; AHRQ, Agency for Healthcare Research and Quality; NQF, National Quality Forum; IOM, Institute of Medicine; CSTE, Council of State and Territorial Epidemiologists; IDSA, Infectious Diseases Society of America; SHEA, Society for Healthcare Epidemiology of America; HIS, Hospital Infection Society; APIC, Association for Professionals in Infection Control and Epidemiology; MedQIC, Medicare Quality Improvement Community; IHI, Institute for Healthcare Improvement; NSQIP, National Surgical Quality Improvement Program.

TABLE 131-2 Health Care–Acquired Conditions Not Eligible for Additional Federal Payment[a]

Vascular catheter–associated infections

Specific surgical-site infections (i.e., after coronary artery bypass graft surgery, certain orthopedic procedures, and certain bariatric surgeries)

Catheter-associated urinary tract infections

Decubitus ulcers (stages III and IV)

Fractures/other injuries from falls or trauma

Foreign objects retained after surgery

Air embolism

Blood incompatibilities

Venous thromboembolism (after hip or knee replacement)

Manifestations of poor glycemic control

[a]Based on the U.S. Federal Deficit Reduction Act of 2005. As of October 1, 2008, Medicare stopped paying additional money to hospitals for these 10 health care–acquired conditions. See *www.cms.hhs.gov/HospitalAcqCond/06_Hospital-Acquired_Conditions.asp* (last accessed November 16, 2009).

infection control and health care epidemiology is required in infectious disease fellowship programs and is available by online courses. Concerns over "patient safety" have led to federal legislation that prevents U.S. hospitals from upgrading Medicare charges to pay for hospital costs resulting from at least 10 specific nosocomial events (Table 131-2) and have prompted national efforts to improve, measure, and publicly report on processes of patient care (e.g., timely administration and appropriateness of perioperative antibiotic prophylaxis) and patient outcomes (e.g., surgical wound infection rates). In 2009, the U.S. Department of Health and Human Services released a major interagency Action Plan to Prevent Healthcare-Associated Infections that includes a list of 5-year national prevention targets, such as a 50% reduction in central-line bloodstream infections (see *www.hhs.gov/ophs/initiatives/hai/*).

SURVEILLANCE

Traditionally, infection preventionists have surveyed inpatients for infections acquired in hospitals (defined as those neither present nor incubating at the time of admission). Surveillance most often requires review of microbiology laboratory results, "shoe-leather" epidemiology on nursing wards, and application of standardized definitions of infection. More "high-tech" infection-control programs may use computerized hospital databases for algorithm-driven electronic surveillance (e.g., of vascular catheter and surgical wound infections). Commercial health care information systems that facilitate these functions are considered "value-added" products. Although infection surveillance in nursing homes and long-term acute-care hospitals (LTACHs) is still in its formative stage, the role of some facilities in the transmission of

antimicrobial-resistant pathogens will require their increased attention to infection surveillance and control.

Most hospitals aim surveillance at infections associated with high-level morbidity or expense. Quality-improvement activities in infection control have led to increased surveillance of personnel compliance with infection control policies (e.g., adherence to influenza vaccination recommendations). In the spirit of "what is measured improves," the majority of states now require public reporting of processes for prevention of health care–associated infection and/or patient outcomes (Fig. 131-1). These state laws have added new complexity to what hospitals measure and how they measure it. For example, in some locales, the surveillance pendulum is swinging back to use of "house-wide" surveillance, and many states now require that hospitals use the Centers for Disease Control and Prevention (CDC) National Healthcare Safety Network (NHSN) reporting system to provide uniform definitions and to facilitate transmission of data. (The NHSN is the successor to the National Nosocomial Infections Surveillance System, a program of the CDC that collected data from ~350 hospitals using standardized definitions of nosocomial infections. Increasing reliance on the NHSN by states to facilitate public reporting has led to participation by almost half of the ~5200 acute-care hospitals in the United States. This increased participation may represent a watershed in providing a more robust nationwide view of health care–associated infections.)

Results of surveillance are expressed as rates. In general, 5–10% of patients develop nosocomial infections. However, such broad statistics have little value unless qualified by duration of risk, by site of infection, by patient population, and by exposure to risk factors. Meaningful denominators for infection rates include the number of patients exposed to a specific risk (e.g., patients using mechanical ventilators) or the number of intervention days (e.g., 1000 patient-days on a ventilator). Temporal trends in rates should be reviewed, and rates should be compared with regional and national benchmarks. However, interhospital comparisons may be

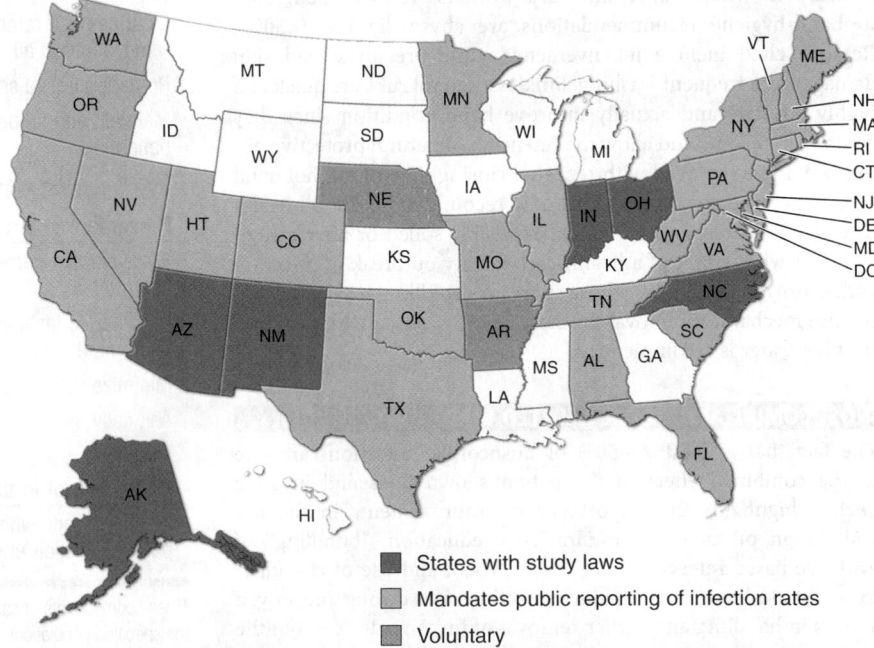

HAI reporting laws and regulations

■ States with study laws
■ Mandates public reporting of infection rates
■ Voluntary

Figure 131-1 Map indicating states with mandatory public reporting of health care–associated infections (HAIs), states with public-reporting study laws, and states with voluntary reporting laws. See *www.apic.org/am/images/maps/mandrpt_map.gif* (last accessed November 16, 2009).

misleading because of the wide range in risk factors and severity of underlying illnesses. Although systems for making adjustments for these factors either are rudimentary or have not been well validated, process measures (e.g., adherence to hand hygiene) do not usually require risk adjustment, and outcome measures (e.g., cardiac surgery wound infection rates) can identify hospitals with outlier infection rates (e.g., in the top deciles) for further evaluation. Moreover, temporal analysis of a hospital's infection rates can help to determine whether control measures are succeeding and where increased efforts should be focused.

EPIDEMIOLOGIC BASIS AND GENERAL MEASURES FOR PREVENTION AND CONTROL

Nosocomial infections follow basic epidemiologic patterns that can help to direct prevention and control measures. Nosocomial pathogens have reservoirs, are transmitted by largely predictable routes, and require susceptible hosts. Reservoirs and sources exist in the inanimate environment (e.g., tap water contaminated with *Legionella*) and in the animate environment (e.g., infected or colonized health care workers, patients, and hospital visitors). The mode of transmission usually is either cross-infection (e.g., indirect spread of pathogens from one patient to another on the inadequately cleaned hands of hospital personnel) or autoinoculation (e.g., aspiration of oropharyngeal flora into the lungs along an endotracheal tube). Occasionally, pathogens (e.g., group A streptococci and many respiratory viruses) are spread from person to person via large infectious droplets released by coughing or sneezing. Much less common—but often devastating in terms of epidemic risk—is true airborne spread of small or droplet nuclei (as in nosocomial chickenpox) or common-source spread by contaminated materials (e.g., contaminated intravenous fluids). Factors that increase host susceptibility include underlying conditions, abnormalities of innate defense (e.g., due to genetic polymorphisms; see Chap. 61), and the many medical-surgical interventions and procedures that bypass or compromise normal host defenses.

Hospitals' infection-control programs must determine general and specific control measures. Given the prominence of cross-infection, hand hygiene is the single most important preventive measure in hospitals. Health care workers' rates of adherence to hand-hygiene recommendations are abysmally low (<50%). Reasons cited include inconvenience, time pressures, and skin damage from frequent washing. Sinkless alcohol rubs are quick and highly effective and actually improve hand condition since they contain emollients and allow the retention of natural protective oils that would be removed with repeated rinsing. Use of alcohol hand rubs between patient contacts is now recommended for all health care workers except when hands are visibly soiled or after care of a patient who is part of a health-care facility outbreak of infection with *Clostridium difficile*, whose spores resist killing by alcohol and require mechanical removal. In these cases, washing with soap and running water is recommended.

NOSOCOMIAL AND DEVICE-RELATED INFECTIONS

The fact that at least 25–50% of nosocomial infections are due to the combined effect of the patient's own flora and invasive devices highlights the importance of improvements in the use and design of such devices. Intensive education, "bundling" of evidence-based interventions (Table 131-3), and use of checklists to facilitate adherence can reduce infection rates through improved asepsis in handling and earlier removal of invasive devices, but the maintenance of such gains requires ongoing efforts. It is especially noteworthy that turnover or shortages of trained personnel jeopardize safe and effective patient care and have been associated with increased infection rates.

Urinary tract infections

Urinary tract infections (UTIs) account for ~34% of nosocomial infections; up to 3% of bacteriuric patients develop bacteremia. Although UTIs contribute at most 15% to prolongation of hospital stay and may have an attributable cost in the range of only $1300, these infections are important reservoirs and sources for spread of antibiotic-resistant bacteria in hospitals. Almost all nosocomial UTIs are associated with preceding instrumentation or indwelling

---

TABLE 131-3 Examples of "Bundled Interventions" to Prevent Common Health Care–Associated Infections and Other Adverse Events

Prevention of Central Venous Catheter Infections

Educate personnel about catheter insertion and care.

Use chlorhexidine to prepare the insertion site.

Use maximal barrier precautions during catheter insertion.

Consolidate insertion supplies (e.g., in an insertion kit or cart).

Use a checklist to enhance adherence to the bundle.

Empower nurses to halt insertion if asepsis is breached.

Cleanse patients daily with chlorhexidine.

Ask daily: Is the catheter needed? Remove catheter if not needed or used.

Prevention of Ventilator-Associated Pneumonia and Complications

Elevate head of bed to 30–45 degrees.

Decontaminate oropharynx regularly with chlorhexidine.

Give "sedation vacation" and assess readiness to extubate daily.

Use peptic ulcer disease prophylaxis.

use deep-vein thrombosis prophylaxis (unless contraindicated).

Prevention of Surgical-Site Infections

Choose a surgeon wisely.

Administer prophylactic antibiotics within 1 h before surgery; discontinue within 24 h.

Limit any hair removal to the time of surgery; use clippers or do not remove hair at all.

Prepare surgical site with chlorhexidine-alcohol.

Maintain normal perioperative glucose levels (cardiac surgery patients).[a]

Maintain perioperative normothermia (colorectal surgery patients).[a]

Prevention of Urinary Tract Infections

Place bladder catheters only when absolutely needed (e.g., to relieve obstruction), not solely for the provider's convenience.

Use aseptic technique for catheter insertion and urinary tract instrumentation.

Minimize manipulation or opening of drainage systems.

Ask daily: Is the bladder catheter needed? Remove catheter if not needed.

Prevention of Pathogen Cross-Transmission

Cleanse hands with alcohol hand rub before and after all contacts with patients or their environments.

[a]These components of care are supported by clinical trials and experimental evidence in the specified populations; they may prove valuable for other surgical patients as well.

Source: Adapted from information presented at the following websites: *www.cdc.gov/ncidod/dhqp/gl_intravascular.html; www.cdc.gov/ncidod/dhqp/gl_hcpneumonia.html; www.cdc.gov/ncidod/dhqp/gl_surgicalsite.html; www.cdc.gov/ncidod/dhqp/dpac_uti_pc.html; www.ihi.org; www.qualitynet.org/medqic.*

bladder catheters, which create a 3–10% risk of infection each day. UTIs generally are caused by pathogens that spread up the periurethral space from the patient's perineum or gastrointestinal tract—the most common pathogenesis in women—or via intraluminal contamination of urinary catheters, usually due to cross-infection by caregivers who are irrigating catheters or emptying drainage bags. Pathogens come occasionally from inadequately disinfected urologic equipment and rarely from contaminated supplies.

Hospitals should closely monitor essential performance measures for preventing nosocomial UTIs (Table 131-3). Sealed catheter–drainage tube junctions can help to prevent breaks in the system. Prompts to clinicians to assess a patient's need for continued use of an indwelling bladder catheter can improve removal rates and may lessen the risk of UTI but also may be met with resistance by direct caregivers. Guidelines for managing postoperative urinary retention (e.g., with bladder scanners) also may limit the use or duration of catheterization. Other approaches to the prevention of UTIs have included use of topical meatal antimicrobial agents, drainage bag disinfectants, and anti-infective catheters. None of the latter three measures is considered routine.

Administration of systemic antimicrobial agents for other purposes decreases the risk of UTI during the first 4 days of catheterization, after which resistant bacteria or yeasts emerge as pathogens. Selective decontamination of the gut is also associated with a reduced risk. Again, however, neither approach is routine.

Irrigation of catheters, with or without antimicrobial agents, may actually increase the risk of infection. A condom catheter for men without bladder obstruction may be more acceptable than an indwelling catheter and may lessen the risk of UTI if maintained carefully. The role of suprapubic catheters in preventing infection is not well defined.

Treatment of UTIs is based on the results of quantitative urine cultures (Chap. 288). The most common pathogens are *Escherichia coli*, nosocomial gram-negative bacilli, enterococci, and *Candida*. Several caveats apply in the treatment of institutionally acquired infection. First, in patients with chronic indwelling bladder catheters, especially those in long-term-care facilities, "catheter flora"—microorganisms living on encrustations within the catheter lumen—may differ from actual urinary tract pathogens. Therefore, for suspected infection in the setting of chronic catheterization (especially in women), it is useful to replace the bladder catheter and to obtain a freshly voided urine specimen. Second, as in all nosocomial infections, at the time treatment is initiated on the basis of a positive culture, it is useful to repeat the culture to verify the persistence of infection. Third, the frequency with which UTIs occur may lead to the erroneous assumption that this site alone is the source of infection in a febrile hospitalized patient. Fourth, recovery of *Staphylococcus aureus* from urine cultures may result from hematogenous seeding and may indicate an occult systemic infection. Finally, although *Candida* is now the most common pathogen in nosocomial UTIs in patients on intensive care units (ICUs), treatment of candiduria is often unsuccessful and is recommended only when there is upper-pole or bladder-wall invasion, obstruction, neutropenia, or immunosuppression.

Pneumonia

Pneumonia accounts for ~13% of nosocomial infections. Ventilator-associated pneumonia, which occurs in 1 to >4 patients per 1000 ventilator-days, is responsible for a mean of 10 extra hospital days and $23,000 in extra costs per episode. Almost all cases of bacterial nosocomial pneumonia are caused by aspiration of endogenous or hospital-acquired oropharyngeal (and occasionally gastric) flora. Nosocomial pneumonias are associated with more deaths than are infections at any other body site. However, attributable mortality for ventilator-associated pneumonia—the most common and

lethal form of nosocomial pneumonia—is in the 6–14% range; this figure suggests that the risk of dying from nosocomial pneumonia is affected greatly by other factors, including comorbidities, inadequate antibiotic treatment, and the involvement of specific pathogens (particularly *Pseudomonas aeruginosa* or *Acinetobacter*). Surveillance and accurate diagnosis of pneumonia are often problematic in hospitals because many patients, especially those in the ICU, have abnormal chest roentgenographs, fever, and leukocytosis potentially attributable to multiple causes. Viral pneumonias, which are particularly important in pediatric and immunocompromised patients, are discussed in the virology section and in Chap. 257.

Risk factors for nosocomial pneumonia, particularly ventilator-associated pneumonia, include those events that increase colonization by potential pathogens (e.g., prior antimicrobial therapy, contaminated ventilator circuits or equipment, or decreased gastric acidity); those that facilitate aspiration of oropharyngeal contents into the lower respiratory tract (e.g., intubation, decreased levels of consciousness, or presence of a nasogastric tube); and those that reduce host defense mechanisms in the lung and permit overgrowth of aspirated pathogens (e.g., chronic obstructive pulmonary disease, extremes of age, or upper abdominal surgery).

Control measures for pneumonia (Table 131-3) are aimed at the remediation of risk factors in general patient care (e.g., minimizing aspiration-prone supine positioning) and at meticulous aseptic care of respirator equipment (e.g., disinfecting or sterilizing all inline reusable components such as nebulizers, replacing tubing/breathing circuits only if required because of malfunction or visible soiling—rather than on the basis of duration of use—to lessen the number of breaks in the system, and teaching aseptic technique for suctioning). Although the benefits of selective decontamination of the oropharynx and gut with nonabsorbable antimicrobial agents and/or use of short-course postintubation systemic antibiotics have been controversial, a randomized multicenter trial demonstrated lowered ICU mortality rates among patients on mechanical ventilation who underwent oropharyngeal decontamination.

Among the logical preventive measures that require further investigation are endotracheal intubation providing channels for subglottic drainage of secretions, which has been associated with reduced infection risks during short-term postoperative use, and noninvasive mechanical ventilation whenever feasible. Use of silver-coated endotracheal tubes may lessen risk of ventilator-associated pneumonia but is not considered routine. It is noteworthy that reducing the rate of ventilator-associated pneumonia often has not reduced overall ICU mortality; this fact suggests that this infection is a marker for patients with an otherwise-heightened risk of death.

The most likely pathogens for nosocomial pneumonia and treatment options are discussed in Chap. 257. Several considerations regarding diagnosis and treatment are worth emphasizing. First, clinical criteria for diagnosis (e.g., fever, leukocytosis, development of purulent secretions, new or changing radiographic infiltrates, changes in oxygen requirement or ventilator settings) have high sensitivity but relatively low specificity. These criteria are most useful for selecting patients for bronchoscopic or nonbronchoscopic procedures that yield lower respiratory tract samples protected from upper-tract contamination; quantitative cultures of such specimens have diagnostic sensitivities in the range of 80%. Second, early-onset nosocomial pneumonia, which manifests within the first 4 days of hospitalization, is most often caused by community-acquired pathogens such as *Streptococcus pneumoniae* and *Haemophilus* species, although some recent studies have challenged this view. Late-onset pneumonias most commonly are due to *S. aureus*, *P. aeruginosa*, *Enterobacter* species, *Klebsiella pneumoniae*, or *Acinetobacter*—a pathogen that is common in tropical countries and of increasing concern in ICUs in the United States. When invasive techniques are used to diagnose ventilator-associated pneumonia, the proportion of isolates accounted for by gram-negative bacilli decreases from 50–70% to 35–45%. Infection is polymicrobial in as many as 20–40% of cases. The role of anaerobic bacteria in ventilator-associated pneumonia is not well defined. Third, one multicenter study suggested that 8 days is an appropriate duration of therapy for nosocomial pneumonia, with a longer duration (15 days in that study) when the pathogen is *Acinetobacter* or *P. aeruginosa*. Finally, in febrile patients (particularly those who have endotracheal or gastric tubes inserted through the nares), more occult sources of respiratory tract infection, especially bacterial sinusitis and otitis media, should be considered.

Surgical wound infections

Wound infections account for ~17% of nosocomial infections but contribute up to 7–10 extra postoperative hospital days and from $3000 to $29,000 in extra costs, depending on the operative procedure and pathogen(s). The average wound infection has an incubation period of 5–7 days—longer than many postoperative stays. For this reason and because many procedures are now performed on an outpatient basis, the incidence of wound infections has become more difficult to assess. These infections usually are caused by the patient's endogenous or hospital-acquired skin and mucosal flora and occasionally are due to airborne spread of skin squames that may be shed into the wound from members of the operating-room team. True airborne spread of infection through droplet nuclei is rare in operating rooms unless there is a "disseminator" (e.g., of group A streptococci or staphylococci) among the staff. In general, the most common risks for postoperative wound infection are related to the surgeon's technical skill, the patient's underlying diseases (e.g., diabetes mellitus, obesity) or advanced age, and inappropriate timing of antibiotic prophylaxis. Additional risk factors include the presence of drains, prolonged preoperative hospital stays, shaving of the operative site by razor the day before surgery, a long duration of surgery, and infection at remote sites (e.g., untreated UTI).

The substantial literature related to risk factors for surgical-site infections and the recognized morbidity and cost of these infections have led to national prevention efforts—e.g., the Surgical Care Improvement Project (SCIP)—and to recommendations for "bundling" of evidence-based preventive measures (Table 131-3). Additional measures include attention to technical surgical issues and operating-room asepsis (e.g., avoiding open or prophylactic drains) as well as preoperative therapy for active infection. Reporting of surveillance results to surgeons has been associated with reductions in infection rates. Preoperative administration of intranasal mupirocin to patients colonized with *S. aureus*, preoperative antiseptic bathing, and supplemental intra- and postoperative oxygen remain controversial because of conflicting study results, but evidence seems to be mounting in favor of these interventions.

The process of diagnosing and treating wound infections begins with a careful assessment of the surgical site in the febrile postoperative patient. Clinical findings range from obvious cellulitis or abscess formation to subtler clues such as a sternal "click" following open-heart surgery. Diagnosis of deeper organ-space infections or subphrenic abscesses requires a high index of suspicion and the use of CT or MRI. Diagnosis of infections of prosthetic devices, such as orthopedic implants, may be particularly difficult and often requires the use of interventional radiographic techniques to obtain periprosthetic specimens for culture. Because cultures of periprosthetic joint tissue obtained at surgery may miss pathogens that are cloistered in prosthesis-adherent biofilms, cultures of sonicates from explanted prosthetic joints have been more sensitive, particularly for patients who have received antimicrobial agents within 2 weeks of surgery.

The most common pathogens in postoperative wound infections are *S. aureus*, coagulase-negative staphylococci, and enteric and anaerobic bacteria. In rapidly progressing postoperative infections, which manifest within 24–48 h of a surgical procedure, the level of suspicion regarding group A streptococcal or clostridial infection (Chaps. 136 and 142) should be high. Treatment of postoperative wound infections requires source control—drainage or surgical excision of infected or necrotic material—and antibiotic therapy aimed at the most likely or laboratory-confirmed pathogens.

Infections related to vascular access and monitoring

Intravascular device–related bacteremias cause ~14% of nosocomial infections; central vascular catheters (CVCs) account for most of these bloodstream infections. National estimates indicate that as many as 200,000 bloodstream infections associated with CVCs occur each year in the United States, with an attributable mortality of 12–25%, an excess mean length of hospital stay of 12 days, and an estimated cost of $3700 to $29,000 per episode; one-third to one-half of these episodes occur in ICUs. With increasing care of seriously ill patients in the community, vascular catheter–associated bloodstream infections acquired in outpatient settings are becoming more frequent. Broader surveillance for infections—outside ICUs and even outside hospitals—will be needed.

Catheter-related bloodstream infections derive largely from the cutaneous microflora of the insertion site, with pathogens migrating extraluminally to the catheter tip, usually during the first week after insertion. In addition, contamination of hubs of CVCs or of the ports of "needle-less" systems may lead to intraluminal infection over longer periods, particularly with surgically implanted or cuffed catheters. Intrinsic (during the manufacturing process) or extrinsic (on-site in a health care facility) contamination of infusate, although rare, is the most common cause of epidemic device-related bloodstream infection; extrinsic contamination may cause up to half of endemic bacteremias related to arterial infusions used for hemodynamic monitoring. The most common pathogens isolated from vascular device–associated bacteremias include coagulase-negative staphylococci, *S. aureus* (with ≥50% of isolates in the United States resistant to methicillin), enterococci, nosocomial gram-negative bacilli, and *Candida*. Many pathogens, especially staphylococci, produce extracellular polysaccharide biofilms that facilitate attachment to catheters and provide sanctuary from antimicrobial agents. "Quorum-sensing" proteins help bacterial cells communicate during biofilm development.

Infections related to vascular catheters and monitoring devices may be the most preventable of nosocomial infections. Evidence-based bundles of control measures (Table 131-3) have been strikingly effective, eliminating almost all infections in one ICU study. Hospitals should periodically monitor adherence to these performance indicators. Use of antimicrobial- or antiseptic-impregnated CVCs does not appear necessary if the prevention bundle is fully implemented.

Additional control measures for infections associated with vascular access include using a chlorhexidine-impregnated patch at the skin-catheter junction; bathing medical ICU patients daily with chlorhexidine; applying semitransparent access-site dressings (for ease of bathing and site inspection and protection of the site from secretions); avoiding the femoral site for catheterization because of an especially high risk of infection (most likely related to the density of the skin flora); moving peripheral catheters to a new site at specified intervals (e.g., every 72–96 h), which may be facilitated by use of an IV therapy team; and applying disposable transducers for pressure monitoring and aseptic technique for accessing transducers or other vascular ports.

Unresolved issues include the best frequency for rotation of CVC sites (given that guidewire-assisted catheter changes at the same site do not lessen and can even increase infection risk); the appropriate role of mupirocin ointment, a topical antibiotic with excellent antistaphylococcal activity, in site care; the relative degrees of risk posed by peripherally inserted central catheters (PICC lines); and the risk-benefit of prophylactic use of heparin (to avoid catheter thrombi, which may be associated with increased risk of infection) or of vancomycin or alcohol (as catheter flushes or "locks"—i.e., concentrated anti-infective solutions instilled into the catheter lumen) for high-risk patients.

Vascular device–related infection is suspected on the basis of the appearance of the catheter site or the presence of fever or bacteremia without another source in patients with vascular catheters. The diagnosis is confirmed by the recovery of the same species of microorganism from peripheral-blood cultures (preferably two cultures drawn from peripheral veins by separate venipunctures) and from semiquantitative or quantitative cultures of the vascular catheter tip. Less commonly used diagnostic measures include (1) differential faster time to positivity (>2 h) for blood drawn through the vascular access device compared with a sample from a peripheral vein and (2) differences in quantitative cultures (a threefold or greater "step-up") for blood samples drawn simultaneously from a peripheral vein and from a CVC. When infusion-related sepsis is considered (e.g., because of the abrupt onset of fever or shock temporally related to infusion therapy), a sample of the infusate or blood product should be retained for culture.

Therapy for vascular access–related infection is directed at the pathogen recovered from the blood and/or infected site. Important considerations in treatment are the need for an echocardiogram (to evaluate the patient for endocarditis), the duration of therapy, and the need to remove potentially infected catheters. In one report, approximately one-fourth of patients with intravascular catheter–associated *S. aureus* bacteremia who were studied by transesophageal echocardiography had evidence of endocarditis; this test may be useful in determining the appropriate duration of treatment.

Detailed consensus guidelines for the management of intravascular catheter–related infections have been published and recommend catheter removal in most cases of bacteremia or fungemia due to nontunneled CVCs. When attempting to salvage a potentially infected catheter, some clinicians use the "antibiotic lock" technique, which may facilitate penetration of infected biofilms, in addition to systemic antimicrobial therapy. In a single-center study of hemodialysis catheters, only about one-third of salvage attempts were successful, although delayed removal did not appear to increase the risk of complications.

Often, a potentially infected CVC may be exchanged over a guidewire. If cultures of the removed catheter tip are positive, the replacement catheter will be moved to a new site; if the tip cultures are negative, the replacement catheter may remain in the original site but may be at increased risk of subsequent infection due to this manipulation.

The authors of the consensus treatment guidelines advise that the decision to remove a tunneled catheter or implanted device suspected of being the source of bacteremia or fungemia should be based on the severity of the patient's illness, the strength of the evidence that the device is infected, the presence of local or systemic complications, an assessment of the specific pathogens, and the patient's response to antimicrobial therapy if the catheter or device is initially retained. For patients with track-site infection, successful therapy without catheter removal is unusual. For patients with suppurative venous thrombophlebitis, excision of the affected vein is usually required.

ISOLATION TECHNIQUES

Written policies for the isolation of infectious patients are a standard component of infection control programs. To replace its prior pathogen-specific guidelines, the CDC published recommendations in 2006 for the control of multidrug-resistant organisms in health care settings; in 2007, the CDC published a revised edition of its basic isolation guidelines to provide updated recommendations for all components of health care, including acute-care hospitals and long-term, ambulatory, and home-care settings (see "Further Readings," below).

Standard precautions are designed for the care of all patients in hospitals and aim to reduce the risk of transmission of microorganisms from both recognized and unrecognized sources. These precautions include gloving as well as hand cleansing for potential contact with (1) blood; (2) all other body fluids, secretions, and excretions, whether or not they contain visible blood; (3) nonintact skin; and (4) mucous membranes. Depending on exposure risks, standard precautions also include use of masks, eye protection, and gowns.

Precautions for the care of patients with potentially contagious clinical syndromes (e.g., acute diarrhea) or with suspected or diagnosed colonization or infection with transmissible pathogens are based on probable routes of transmission: *airborne*, *droplet*, or *contact*, for which personnel don at a minimum N95 respirators, surgical face masks, or glove and gown, respectively. Sets of precautions may be combined for diseases that have more than one route of transmission (e.g., contact and airborne isolation for varicella).

Because some prevalent antibiotic-resistant pathogens, particularly vancomycin-resistant enterococci (VRE), may be present on *intact* skin of patients in hospitals, some experts recommend gloving for all contact with patients who are acutely ill and/or from high-risk units, such as ICUs. Wearing gloves does not replace the need for hand hygiene because hands sometimes (in up to 20% of interactions) become contaminated during wearing or removal of gloves.

EPIDEMIC AND EMERGING PROBLEMS

Outbreaks and emerging pathogens are always big news but probably account for <5% of nosocomial infections. The investigation and control of nosocomial epidemics require that infection control personnel develop a case definition, confirm that an outbreak really exists (since apparent epidemics may be pseudo-outbreaks due to surveillance or laboratory artifacts), review aseptic practices and disinfectant use, determine the extent of the outbreak, perform an epidemiologic investigation to determine modes of transmission, work closely with microbiology personnel to culture for common sources or personnel carriers as appropriate and to type epidemiologically important isolates, and heighten surveillance to judge the effect of control measures. Control measures generally include reinforcing routine aseptic practices and hand hygiene during a search for compliance problems that may have fostered the outbreak, ensuring appropriate isolation of cases (and instituting cohort isolation and nursing if needed), and implementing further controls on the basis of the investigation's findings. Examples of some emerging and potential epidemic problems follow.

Viral respiratory infections: Pandemic influenza

Infections caused by the severe acute respiratory syndrome (SARS)–associated coronavirus challenged health care systems globally in 2003 (Chap. 186). Basic infection-control measures helped to keep the worldwide case and death counts at ~8000 and ~800, respectively, although SARS was unforgiving of lapses in protocol adherence or laboratory biosafety. The epidemiology of SARS—spread largely in households once patients were ill or in hospitals—contrasts markedly with that of influenza (Chap. 187), which is often contagious a day before symptom onset; can spread rapidly in the community among nonimmune persons; and even in its seasonal variety kills as many as 35,000 persons each year in the United States. Control of seasonal influenza has depended on (1) the use of effective vaccines, with increasingly broad evidence-based recommendations for vaccination of children, the general public, and health care workers; (2) the use of antiviral medications for early treatment and for prophylaxis as part of outbreak control, especially for high-risk patients and in high-risk settings like nursing homes or hospitals; and (3) infection control (surveillance and droplet precautions) for symptomatic patients.

With occurrence of localized outbreaks of avian (H5N1) influenza in Asia over the past few years, concerns about potential pandemic influenza led to recommendations for universal "respiratory hygiene and cough etiquette" (basically, "cover your cough"), as described and promoted in the CDC's 2007 *Guideline for Isolation Precautions*, and for "source containment" (e.g., use of face masks and spatial separation) for outpatients with potentially infectious respiratory illnesses; to re-examinations of the value in the 1918–1919 influenza pandemic of nonpharmacologic interventions, such as "social distancing" (e.g., closing schools and community venues); and to debate about the level of respiratory protection required for health care workers (i.e., whether to use the higher-efficiency N95 respirators recommended for airborne isolation rather than the surgical masks used for droplet precautions).

In the spring of 2009, a novel strain of influenza virus—H1N1 or "swine flu" virus—caused the first influenza pandemic in four decades. Interventions based on experience with seasonal influenza and prior pandemics included (1) aggressive use of infection control measures (e.g., droplet and contact precautions for suspected influenza cases); (2) hierarchical use of limited supplies of H1N1 monovalent influenza vaccine for pregnant woman, children, and adults with comorbidities (because of greater risk or worse H1N1 outcomes) and for health care and public safety workers (because of the perceived need to maintain a cohort of well essential-infrastructure workers); (3) prompt therapeutic use of neuraminidase inhibitors and emergency authorization for clinical use of experimental parenteral preparations from this class; and (4) prophylactic use of neuraminidase inhibitors in select settings (e.g., for exposed health care workers). Prominent among controversial infection-control issues were optimal respiratory protection (N95 respirators versus surgical masks) for health care workers entering influenza isolation rooms and the need to mandate influenza vaccination of health care workers because of the embarrassingly low rates of vaccination in this high-risk group.

Nosocomial diarrhea

A new, more virulent strain of *C. difficile*—BI/NAP1/027—has emerged in North America, and overall rates of *C. difficile*–associated diarrhea (Chap. 129) have increased, especially among older patients, in U.S. hospitals during the past few years. The potential role of exposure to newer fluoroquinolone antibiotics in driving these changes is being investigated. *C. difficile* control measures include judicious use of all antibiotics; heightened suspicion for "atypical" presentations (e.g., toxic megacolon or leukemoid reaction without diarrhea); and early diagnosis, treatment, and contact precautions.

Outbreaks of norovirus infection (Chap. 190) in U.S. and European health care facilities appear to be increasing in frequency, with the virus often introduced by ill visitors or staff. This pathogen should be suspected when nausea and vomiting are prominent aspects of bacterial culture–negative diarrheal syndromes. Contact precautions may need to be augmented by aggressive environmental cleaning (given the persistence of norovirus on inanimate objects), prevention of secondary cases in cleaning staff by an emphasis on the use of personal protective equipment and hand hygiene, and active exclusion of ill staff and visitors.

Chickenpox

Infection control practitioners institute a varicella exposure investigation and control plan whenever health care workers have been exposed to chickenpox (Chap. 180) or have worked while having or during the 24 h before developing chickenpox. The names of exposed workers and patients are obtained; medical histories are reviewed, and (if necessary) serologic tests for immunity are conducted; physicians are notified of susceptible exposed patients; postexposure prophylaxis with varicella-zoster immune globulin (VZIG) is considered for immunocompromised or pregnant contacts (see Table 180-1); varicella vaccine is recommended or preemptive use of acyclovir is considered as an alternative strategy in other susceptible persons; and susceptible exposed employees are furloughed during the at-risk period for disease (8–21 days or, if VZIG has been administered, 28 days). Routine varicella vaccination of children and susceptible employees has made nosocomial spread less common and problematic.

Tuberculosis

Important measures for the control of tuberculosis (Chap. 165) include prompt recognition, isolation, and treatment of cases; recognition of atypical presentations (e.g., lower-lobe infiltrates without cavitation); use of negative-pressure, 100% exhaust, private isolation rooms with closed doors and at least 6–12 air changes per hour; use of N95 respirators by caregivers entering isolation rooms; possible use of high-efficiency particulate air filter units and/or ultraviolet lights for disinfecting air when other engineering controls are not feasible or reliable; and follow-up skin-testing of susceptible personnel who have been exposed to infectious patients before isolation. The use of serologic tests, rather than skin tests, in the diagnosis of latent tuberculosis for infection control purposes remains controversial.

Group A streptococcal infections

The potential for an outbreak of group A streptococcal infection (Chap. 136) should be considered when even a single nosocomial case occurs. Most outbreaks involve surgical wounds and are due to the presence of an asymptomatic carrier in the operating room. Investigation can be confounded by carriage at extrapharyngeal sites such as the rectum and vagina. Health care workers in whom carriage has been linked to nosocomial transmission of group A streptococci are removed from the patient-care setting and are not permitted to return until carriage has been eliminated by antimicrobial therapy.

Fungal infections

Fungal spores are common in the environment, particularly on dusty surfaces. When dusty areas are disturbed during hospital repairs or renovation, the spores become airborne. Inhalation of spores by immunosuppressed (especially neutropenic) patients creates a risk of pulmonary and/or paranasal sinus infection and disseminated aspergillosis (Chap. 204). Routine surveillance among neutropenic patients for infections with filamentous fungi, such as *Aspergillus* and *Fusarium*, helps hospitals to determine whether they are facing unduly extensive environmental risks. As a matter of routine, hospitals should inspect and clean air-handling equipment, review all planned renovations with infection control personnel and subsequently construct appropriate barriers, remove immunosuppressed patients from renovation sites, and consider the use of high-efficiency particulate air intake filters for rooms housing immunosuppressed patients.

Legionellosis

Nosocomial *Legionella* pneumonia (Chap. 147) is most often due to contamination of potable water and predominantly affects immunosuppressed patients, particularly those receiving glucocorticoid medications. The risk varies greatly within and among geographic regions, depending on the extent of hospital hot-water contamination and on specific hospital practices (e.g., inappropriate use of nonsterile water in respiratory therapy equipment). Laboratory-based surveillance for nosocomial *Legionella* should be performed, and a diagnosis of legionellosis should probably be considered more often than it is. If nosocomial cases are detected, environmental samples (e.g., tap water) should be cultured. If cultures yield *Legionella* and if typing of clinical and environmental isolates reveals a correlation, eradication measures should be pursued. An alternative approach is to periodically culture tap water in wards housing high-risk patients. If *Legionella* is found, a concerted effort should be made to culture samples from all patients with nosocomial pneumonia for *Legionella*.

Antibiotic-resistant bacteria

Control of antibiotic resistance depends on close laboratory surveillance, with early detection of problems; on aggressive reinforcement of routine asepsis; on implementation of barrier precautions for all colonized and/or infected patients; on use of patient-surveillance cultures to more fully ascertain the extent of patient colonization; and on timely initiation of an epidemiologic investigation when rates increase. Molecular typing (e.g., pulsed-field gel electrophoresis) can help differentiate an outbreak due to a single strain (which necessitates an emphasis on hand hygiene and an evaluation of potential common-source exposures) from one that is polyclonal (which requires an emphasis on antibiotic prudence and device bundles; Table 131-3).

Currently, several antibiotic resistance problems are of particular concern. First, the emergence of community-associated methicillin-resistant *S. aureus* (CA-MRSA) has been dramatic in many countries, with as many as 50% of community-acquired "staph infections" in some U.S. cities now caused by strains resistant to β-lactam antibiotics (Chap. 135). The potential incursion of CA-MRSA into hospitals and the resulting impact on surveillance and control of nosocomial MRSA infections are of enormous concern. Second, in the ongoing global reemergence of nosocomial multidrug-resistant gram-negative bacilli, new problems include plasmid-mediated resistance to fluoroquinolones, metallo-β-lactamase–mediated resistance to carbapenems, strains of *K. pneumoniae* that contain carbapenemases (KPCs), and pan-resistant strains of *Acinetobacter*. Many multidrug-resistant gram-negative bacilli are susceptible only to colistin, a drug that is consequently being "rediscovered."

Third, there has been renewed recognition of the role of nursing homes, and now LTACHs, in the spread of resistant gram-negative bacilli such as KPCs. Fourth, there has been increasing community-based spread of *E. coli* strains harboring an enzyme, CTX-M, that renders them broadly resistant to β-lactam antibiotics; given the community focus of spread, these strains may be seen as a gram-negative version of CA-MRSA. Finally, clinical infections with MRSA strains exhibiting high-level vancomycin resistance due to VRE-derived plasmids have been reported in a few patients—almost all in the United States and most in Michigan—in the setting of prolonged or repeated treatment with vancomycin and/or VRE colonization. Much more common is vancomycin "MIC creep": increasing prevalence of MRSA strains that exhibit upper-limit susceptibility to vancomycin.

Colonized personnel who are implicated in nosocomial transmission of multidrug-resistant pathogens and patients who pose a threat can be decontaminated, depending on the pathogen. In a few ICUs, gastrointestinal decontamination of patients has been used successfully as a temporary emergency control measure for outbreaks of infection due to gram-negative bacilli. Other promising ICU control measures include daily bathing of patients with chlorhexidine and enforcement of environmental cleaning; in recent trials, the bathing intervention led to reduced risk of bacteremia in medical ICU

patients, and both of these measures reduced cross-transmission of VRE. "Search-and-destroy" methods—i.e., active surveillance cultures to detect and isolate the "resistance iceberg" of patients colonized with MRSA—in non-outbreak settings are credited with elimination of nosocomial MRSA in the Netherlands and Denmark.

Because the excessive use of broad-spectrum antibiotics underlies many resistance problems, "antibiotic stewardship" has been promulgated actively. The main tenets are to restrict the use of particular agents to narrowly defined indications in order to limit selective pressure on the nosocomial flora and, when broad-spectrum therapy is begun empirically in critically ill patients, to "de-escalate" treatment as soon as possible on the basis of the results of culture and susceptibility tests.

Bioterrorism and other "surge-event" preparedness

The horrific attack on the World Trade Center in New York City on September 11, 2001; the subsequent mailings of anthrax spores in the United States; and ongoing revelations of terrorist plans and activities in many countries, including the United States, have made bioterrorism a prominent source of concern to hospital infection-control programs. The essentials for hospital preparedness entail education, internal and external communication, and risk assessment. Up-to-date information is available from the CDC (see *www.bt.cdc.gov*).

EMPLOYEE HEALTH SERVICE ISSUES

An institution's employee health service is a critical component of its infection control efforts. New employees should be processed through the service, where a contagious-disease history can be taken; evidence of immunity to a variety of diseases, such as hepatitis B, chickenpox, measles, mumps, and rubella, can be sought; immunizations for hepatitis B, measles, mumps, rubella, and varicella can be given as needed and a reminder about the essential need for yearly influenza immunization can be imparted; baseline and "booster" PPD (purified protein derivative of tuberculin) skin-testing for tuberculosis can be performed; and education about personal responsibility for infection control can be initiated. Evaluations of employees should be codified to meet the requirements of accrediting and regulatory agencies.

The employee health service must have protocols for dealing with workers exposed to contagious diseases (e.g., influenza) and those percutaneously or mucosally exposed to the blood of patients infected with HIV or hepatitis B or C virus. For example, postexposure HIV prophylaxis with a combination of two or three antiretroviral agents is recommended; free consultation is available from the CDC PEPLine (1-888-HIV-4911). Protocols are also needed for dealing with caregivers who have common contagious diseases (such as chickenpox, group A streptococcal infection, influenza or another respiratory infection, or infectious diarrhea) and for those who have less common but high-visibility public health problems (such as chronic hepatitis B or C or HIV infection) for which exposure control guidelines have been published by the CDC and by the Society for Healthcare Epidemiology of America.

FURTHER READINGS

DAROUICHE R et al: Chlorhexidine-alcohol versus povidone-iodine for surgical-site antisepsis. N Engl J Med 362:18, 2010

JOHNSON LE et al: Resources for infection prevention and control on the World Wide Web. Clin Infect Dis 48:1585, 2009

MERMEL LA et al: Clinical practice guidelines for the diagnosis and management of intravascular catheter–related infection: 2009 update by the Infectious Diseases Society of America. Clin Infect Dis 49:1, 2009

Munoz-Price LS, Weinstein RA: *Acinetobacter* infection. N Engl J Med 358:1271, 2008

Peleg AY, Hooper DC: Hospital-acquired infections due to gram-negative bacteria. N Engl J Med 362:1804, 2010

Roberts RR et al: Hospital and societal costs of antimicrobial-resistant infections in a Chicago teaching hospital: Implications for antibiotic stewardship. Clin Infect Dis 49:1175, 2009

Rosenthal VD: Central line–associated bloodstream infections in limited-resource countries: A review of the literature. Clin Infect Dis 49:1899, 2009

Siegel JD et al: Management of Multidrug-Resistant Organisms in Healthcare Settings, 2006 (*www.cdc.gov/ncidod/dhqp/pdf/ar/mdroGuideline2006.pdf*)

——— et al: 2007 Guideline for Isolation Precautions: Preventing Transmission of Infectious Agents in Healthcare Settings (*www.cdc.gov/ncidod/dhqp/pdf/isolation2007.pdf*)

Yokoe DS et al: A compendium of strategies to prevent healthcare-associated infections in acute care hospitals. Infect Control Hosp Epidemiol 29:S12, 2008

CHAPTER **132**

Infections in Transplant Recipients

Robert Finberg
Joyce Fingeroth

This chapter considers aspects of infection unique to patients receiving transplanted organs. The evaluation of infections in transplant recipients involves consideration of both the donor and the recipient of the transplanted organ. Two central issues are of paramount importance: (1) Infectious agents (particularly viruses, but also bacteria, fungi, and parasites) can be introduced into the recipient by the donor organ. (2) Treatment of the recipient with medicine to prevent rejection can suppress normal immune responses, greatly increasing susceptibility to infection. Thus, what might have been a latent or asymptomatic infection in an immunocompetent donor or in the recipient prior to therapy can become a life-threatening problem when the recipient becomes immunosuppressed. The pretransplantation evaluation of each patient should be guided by an analysis of both (1) what infections the recipient is currently harboring, since organisms that exist in a state of latency or dormancy before the procedure may cause fatal disease when the patient receives immunosuppressive treatment; and (2) what organisms are likely to be transmitted by the donor organ, particularly those to which the recipient may be naïve.

■ PRETRANSPLANTATION EVALUATION

The donor

A variety of organisms have been transmitted by organ transplantation (Table 132-1). Transmission of infections that may have been latent or not clinically apparent in the donor has resulted in the development of specific donor-screening protocols. Serologic studies should be ordered to detect viruses such as herpes simplex virus types 1 and 2 (HSV-1, HSV-2), varicella-zoster virus (VZV), cytomegalovirus (CMV), Epstein-Barr virus (EBV), and Kaposi's sarcoma–associated herpesvirus (KSHV) as well as hepatitis A, B, and C viruses and HIV. In addition, when relevant, donors should be screened for viruses such as West Nile virus, rabies virus, human T lymphotropic virus type I, and lymphocytic choriomeningitis virus as well as for parasites such as *Toxoplasma gondii*, *Strongyloides stercoralis*, *Schistosoma* species, and *Trypanosoma cruzi* (the latter particularly in Latin America). Clinicians caring for prospective organ donors should examine chest radiographs for evidence of granulomatous disease (e.g., caused by mycobacteria or fungi) and should perform skin testing or obtain blood for immune cell–based assays that detect active or latent *Mycobacterium tuberculosis* infection. Evaluation for syphilis should also be performed. An investigation of the donor's dietary habits (e.g., consumption of raw meat or fish or of unpasteurized dairy products), occupations or avocations (e.g., gardening or spelunking), and travel history (e.g., travel to areas with endemic fungi) is also indicated and may mandate additional testing (Table 132-1).

The recipient

It is expected that the recipient will have been even more comprehensively assessed than the donor. Additional studies recommended for the recipient include evaluation for acute respiratory virus and gastrointestinal pathogens in the immediate pretransplantation period. An important caveat is that, because of immune dysfunction resulting from chemotherapy or underlying chronic disease, serologic testing of the recipient may prove less reliable than usual.

The donor cells/organ

Careful attention to the sterility of the medium used to process the donor organ, combined with meticulous microbiologic evaluation, reduces rates of transmission of bacteria (or, rarely, yeasts) that may be present or grow in the organ culture medium. From 2% to >20% of donor kidneys are estimated to be contaminated with bacteria—in most cases, with the organisms that colonize the skin or grow in the tissue culture medium used to bathe the donor organ while it awaits implantation. The reported rate of bacterial contamination of transplanted stem cells (bone marrow, peripheral blood, cord blood) is as high as 17% but most commonly is ~1%. The use of enrichment columns and monoclonal antibody depletion procedures results in a higher incidence of contamination. In one series of patients receiving contaminated stem cells, 14% had fever or bacteremia, but none died. Results of cultures performed at the time of cryopreservation and at the time of thawing were helpful in guiding therapy for the recipient.

INFECTIONS IN HEMATOPOIETIC STEM CELL TRANSPLANT RECIPIENTS

Transplantation of hematopoietic stem cells (HSCs) from bone marrow or from peripheral or cord blood for cancer, immunodeficiency, or autoimmune disease results in a transient state of complete immunologic incompetence. Immediately after myeloablative chemotherapy and transplantation, both innate immune cells (phagocytes, natural killer cells) and adaptive immune cells (T and B cells) are absent, and the host is extremely susceptible to infection. The reconstitution that follows transplantation has been likened to maturation of the immune system in neonates. The analogy does

TABLE 132-1 Common Pathogens Transmitted by Organ Transplantation: Frequent Sites of Reactivation and Disease[a]

	Blood	Lungs	Heart	Brain	Liver/Spleen	Skin
Bacteria/Mycobacteria						
Mycobacterium tuberculosis	±	+			±	
Atypical mycobacteria	+	+				
Brucella spp.	+					
Viruses						
Cytomegalovirus[b]	+	+	±	±	+	
Epstein-Barr virus[c]	+	+	±	±	+	
Herpes simplex virus		±		±	±	+
Human herpesvirus type 6	+	±		±		+
Kaposi's sarcoma–associated herpesvirus	+	±			±	+
Hepatitis B and C viruses					+	
Rabies virus[d]				+		
West Nile virus	+			+		
Lymphocytic choriomeningitis virus	+			+	±	
Fungi						
Candida albicans	+	+			+	+
Histoplasma capsulatum	+	+			+	+
Cryptococcus neoformans	+	+		+	±	±
Parasites						
Toxoplasma gondii[e]		+	+	+		
Strongyloides stercoralis[f,g]		+				
Trypanosoma cruzi[g]			+			
Plasmodium falciparum[g]	+					
Schistosoma spp.					+	
Prion Diseases						
Creutzfeldt-Jakob disease (CJD)[h]				+		
Variant CJD/bovine spongiform encephalopathy[i]				+		

[a]+, well documented; ±, less common.

[b]Cytomegalovirus reactivation is prone to occur in the transplanted organ. The same may be true for Kaposi's sarcoma–associated herpesvirus.

[c]Epstein-Barr virus reactivation usually presents as an extranodal proliferation of transformed B cells and can be present either as a diffuse disease or as a mass lesion in a single organ. It can occur in the allograft.

[d]Rabies virus has been transmitted through corneal transplants.

[e]T. gondii usually causes disease in the brain. In hematopoietic stem cell transplant recipients, acute pulmonary disease may also occur. Heart transplant recipients develop disease in the allograft.

[f]Strongyloides "hyperinfection" may present with pulmonary disease—often associated with gram-negative bacterial pneumonia.

[g]While transmission with organs has been described, it is unusual.

[h]CJD (sporadic and familial) has been transmitted with corneal transplants. Whether it can be transmitted with blood is not known.

[i]Variant CJD can be transmitted with transfused non-leukodepleted blood, posing a theoretical risk to transplant recipients.

not entirely predict infections seen in HSC transplant recipients, however, because the stem cells mature in an old host who has several latent infections already. The choice among the current variety of methods for obtaining stem cells is determined by availability and by the need to optimize the chances of cure for an individual recipient. One strategy is autologous HSC transplantation, in which the donor and the recipient are the same. After chemotherapy, stem cells are collected and are purged (ex vivo) of residual neoplastic populations. Allogeneic HSC transplantation has the advantage of providing a graft-versus-tumor effect. In this case, the recipient is matched to varying degrees for human leukocyte antigen (HLA) with a donor who may be related or unrelated. In some individuals, nonmyeloablative therapy (mini-allo transplantation) is used and permits recipient cells to persist for some time after transplantation while preserving the graft-versus-tumor effect and sparing the recipient myeloablative therapy. Cord-blood transplantation is increasingly utilized in adults; two independent cord-blood units are typically required for suitable neutrophil engraftment early after transplantation, even though only one of the units is likely to provide long-term engraftment. In each circumstance, a different balance is struck between the toxicity of conditioning therapy, the need for a maximal graft-versus-target effect, short-term and long-term infectious complications, and the risk of graft-versus-host disease (GVHD; acute versus chronic). The various approaches differ in terms of reconstitution speed, cell lineage, and likelihood of GVHD—all factors that can produce distinct effects on the risk of infection after transplantation (Table 132-2). Despite these caveats, most infections occur in a predictable time frame after transplantation (Table 132-3).

BACTERIAL INFECTIONS

In the first month after HSC transplantation, infectious complications are similar to those in granulocytopenic patients receiving chemotherapy for acute leukemia (Chap. 86). Because of the anticipated 1- to 4-week duration of neutropenia and the high rate of bacterial infection in this population, many centers give prophylactic antibiotics to patients upon initiation of myeloablative therapy. Quinolones decrease the incidence of gram-negative bacteremia among these patients. Bacterial infections are common in the first few days after HSC transplantation. The organisms involved are predominantly those found on the skin, mucosa, or IV catheters (Staphylococcus aureus, coagulase-negative staphylococci, streptococci) or aerobic bacteria that colonize the bowel (Escherichia coli, Klebsiella, Pseudomonas). Bacillus cereus, although rare, has emerged as a pathogen early after transplantation and can cause meningitis, which is unusual in these patients. Chemotherapy, use of broad-spectrum antibiotics, and delayed reconstitution of humoral immunity place HSC transplant patients at risk for diarrhea and colitis caused by Clostridium difficile overgrowth and toxin production.

Beyond the first few days of neutropenia, infections with nosocomial pathogens (e.g., vancomycin-resistant enterococci, Stenotrophomonas maltophilia,

TABLE 132-2 Risk of Infection, by Type of Hematopoietic Stem Cell Transplant

Type of Hematopoietic Stem Cell Transplant	Source of Stem Cells	Risk of Early Infection: Neutrophil Depletion	Risk of Late Infection: Impaired T and B Cell Function	Risk of Ongoing Infection: GVHD[a] and Iatrogenic Immunosuppression	Graft versus Tumor Effect
Autologous	Recipient (self)	High risk; neutrophil recovery sometimes prolonged	~ 1 year	Minimal to no risk of GVHD and late-onset severe infection	None (−)
Syngeneic (genetic twin)	Identical twin	Low risk; 1–2 weeks for recovery	~ 1 year	Minimal risk of GVHD and late-onset severe infection	+/−
Allogeneic related	Sibling	Low risk; 1–2 weeks for recovery	~ 1 year	Minimal to moderate risk of GVHD and late-onset severe infection	++
Allogeneic related	Child/parent (haploidentical)	Intermediate risk; 2–3 weeks for neutrophil recovery	1–2 years	Moderate risk of GVHD and late-onset severe infection	++++
Allogeneic unrelated adult	Unrelated donor	Intermediate risk; 2–3 weeks for neutrophil recovery	1–2 years	High risk of GVHD and late-onset severe infection	++++
Allogeneic unrelated cord blood	Unrelated cord blood units (×2)	Intermediate to high risk; neutrophil recovery sometimes prolonged	Prolonged	Minimal to moderate risk of GVHD and late-onset severe infection	++++
Allogeneic mini (nonmyeloablative)	Donor (transiently coexisting with recipient cells)	Low risk; neutrophil counts close to normal	1–2+ years	Variable risk of GVHD and late-onset severe infection[b]	++++ (but develops slowly)

[a]GVHD, graft-versus-host disease.

[b]Depending on the disparity of the match (major and minor histocompatibility antigens), GVHD may be severe or mild, the requirement for immunosuppression intense or minimal, and the risk of severe late infections coordinate with the degree of immunosuppression.

Acinetobacter species, and extended-spectrum β-lactamase-producing gram-negative organisms) as well as with filamentous bacteria (e.g., *Nocardia* species) become more common. Vigilance is indicated, particularly for patients with a history of active or known latent tuberc ulosis, even when they have been appropriately pretreated. Episodes of bacteremia due to encapsulated organisms mark the late posttransplantation period (>6 months after HSC reconstitution); patients who have undergone splenectomy and those with persistent hypogammaglobulinemia are at particular risk.

■ FUNGAL INFECTIONS

Beyond the first week after transplantation, fungal infections become increasingly common, particularly among patients who have received broad-spectrum antibiotics. As in most granulocytopenic patients, *Candida* infections are most commonly seen in this setting. However, with increased use of prophylactic fluconazole, infections with resistant fungi—in particular, *Aspergillus* and other molds (*Fusarium*, *Scedosporium*, *Penicillium*)—have become more common, prompting some centers to replace fluconazole with agents such as micafungin, voriconazole, and even posaconazole.

TABLE 132-3 Common Sources of Infections After Hematopoietic Stem Cell Transplantation

Infection Site	Period after Transplantation		
	Early (<1 Month)	Middle (1–4 Months)	Late (>6 Months)
Disseminated	Aerobic bacteria (gram-negative, gram-positive)	*Nocardia*, *Candida*, *Aspergillus*, EBV	Encapsulated bacteria (*Streptococcus pneumoniae*, *Haemophilus influenzae*, *Neisseria meningitidis*)
Skin and mucous membranes	HSV	HHV-6	VZV
Lungs	Aerobic bacteria (gram-negative, gram-positive), *Candida*, *Aspergillus*, other molds, HSV	CMV, seasonal respiratory viruses, *Pneumocystis*, *Toxoplasma*	*Pneumocystis*, *S. pneumoniae*
Gastrointestinal tract	*Clostridium difficile*	CMV, adenovirus	EBV, CMV
Kidney		BK virus, adenovirus	
Brain	HHV-6	HHV-6, *Toxoplasma*	*Toxoplasma*, JC virus (rare)
Bone marrow	HHV-6		

Abbreviations: CMV, cytomegalovirus; EBV, Epstein-Barr virus; HHV-6, human herpesvirus type 6; HSV, herpes simplex virus; VZV, varicella-zoster virus.

The role of antifungal prophylaxis with these different agents, in contrast to empirical treatment for suspected (based on positive β-D-glucan assay or galactomannan antigen test) or documented infection, remains controversial (Chap. 86). In patients with GVHD who require prolonged or indefinite courses of glucocorticoids and other immunosuppressive agents [e.g., cyclosporine, tacrolimus (FK 506, Prograf), mycophenolate mofetil (Cellcept), rapamycin (sirolimus, Rapamune), antithymocyte globulin, or anti-CD52 antibody (alemtuzumab, Campath, an antilymphocyte and antimonocyte monoclonal antibody)], there is a high risk of fungal infection (usually with *Candida* or *Aspergillus*), even after engraftment and resolution of neutropenia. These patients are also at high risk for reactivation of latent fungal infection (histoplasmosis, coccidioidomycosis, or blastomycosis) in areas where endemic fungi reside and after involvement in activities such as gardening or caving. Prolonged use of central venous catheters for parenteral nutrition (lipids) increases the risk of fungemia with *Malassezia*. Some centers administer prophylactic antifungal agents to these patients. Because of the high and prolonged risk of *Pneumocystis jiroveci* pneumonia (especially among patients being treated for hematologic malignancies), most patients receive maintenance prophylaxis with trimethoprim-sulfamethoxazole (TMP-SMX) starting 1 month after engraftment and continuing for at least 1 year.

■ PARASITIC INFECTIONS

The regimen just described for the fungal pathogen *Pneumocystis* may also protect patients seropositive for the parasite *T. gondii*, which can cause pneumonia, visceral disease (occasionally), and central nervous system (CNS) lesions (more commonly). The advantages of maintaining HSC transplant recipients on daily TMP-SMX for 1 year after transplantation include some protection against *Listeria monocytogenes* and nocardial disease as well as late infections with *Streptococcus pneumoniae* and *Haemophilus influenzae*, which stem from the inability of the immature immune system to respond to polysaccharide antigens.

With increasing international travel, parasitic diseases typically restricted to particular environmental niches may pose a risk of reactivation in certain patients after HSC transplantation. Thus, in recipients with an appropriate history who were not screened and/or treated before transplantation or in patients with recent exposures, evaluation for infection with *Strongyloides*, *Leishmania*, or various parasitic causes of diarrheal illness (*Giardia*, *Cryptosporidium*, microsporidia) may be warranted.

■ VIRAL INFECTIONS

HSC transplant recipients are susceptible to infection with a variety of viruses, including primary and reactivation syndromes caused by most human herpesviruses (Table 132-4) and acute infections caused by viruses that circulate in the community.

Herpes simplex virus

Within the first 2 weeks after transplantation, most patients who are seropositive for HSV-1 excrete the virus from the oropharynx. The ability to isolate HSV declines with time. Administration of prophylactic acyclovir (or valacyclovir) to seropositive HSC transplant recipients has been shown to reduce mucositis and prevent HSV pneumonia (a rare condition reported almost exclusively in allogeneic HSC transplant recipients). Both esophagitis (usually due to HSV-1) and anogenital disease (commonly caused by HSV-2) may be prevented with acyclovir prophylaxis. For further discussion, see Chap. 179.

TABLE 132-4 Herpesvirus Syndromes of Transplant Recipients

Virus	Reactivation Disease
Herpes simplex virus type 1	Oral lesions
	Esophageal lesions
	Pneumonia (only in HSC transplant recipients)
	Hepatitis (rare)
Herpes simplex virus type 2	Anogenital lesions
	Hepatitis (rare)
Varicella-zoster virus	Zoster (can disseminate)
Cytomegalovirus	Associated with graft rejection
	Fever and malaise
	Bone marrow failure
	Pneumonitis
	Gastrointestinal disease
Epstein-Barr virus	B cell lymphoproliferative disease/lymphoma
	Oral hairy leukoplakia (rare)
Human herpesvirus type 6	Fever
	Delayed monocyte/platelet engraftment
	Encephalitis (controversial)
Human herpesvirus type 7	Undefined
Kaposi's sarcoma–associated virus	Kaposi's sarcoma
	Primary effusion lymphoma (rare)
	Multicentric Castleman's disease (rare)
	Marrow aplasia (rare)

Abbreviation: HSC, hematopoietic stem cell.

Varicella-zoster virus

Reactivation of VZV manifests as herpes zoster and may occur within the first month but more commonly occurs several months after transplantation. Reactivation rates are ~40% for allogeneic HSC transplant recipients and 25% for autologous recipients. Localized zoster can spread rapidly in an immunosuppressed patient. Fortunately, disseminated disease can usually be controlled with high doses of acyclovir. Because of frequent dissemination among patients with skin lesions, acyclovir is given prophylactically in some centers to prevent severe disease. Low doses of acyclovir (400 mg orally, three times daily) appear to be effective in preventing reactivation of VZV. However, acyclovir can also suppress the development of VZV-specific immunity. Thus, its administration for only 6 months after transplantation does not prevent zoster from occurring when treatment is stopped. Administration of low doses of acyclovir for an entire year after transplantation is effective and may eliminate most cases of posttransplantation zoster. For further discussion, see Chap. 180.

Cytomegalovirus

The onset of CMV disease (interstitial pneumonia, bone marrow suppression, graft failure, hepatitis/colitis) usually begins 30–90 days after HSC transplantation, when the granulocyte count is adequate but immunologic reconstitution has not occurred. CMV disease rarely develops earlier than 14 days after transplantation and may become evident as late as 4 months after the procedure. It is of greatest concern in the second month after transplantation, particularly in allogeneic HSC transplant recipients. In cases in which the donor marrow is depleted of T cells (to prevent GVHD or eliminate a T cell tumor), the disease may be manifested earlier. The use of alemtuzumab to prevent GVHD in nonmyeloablative transplantation has been associated with an increase in CMV disease. Patients who receive ganciclovir for prophylaxis, preemptive treatment, or treatment (see below) may develop recurrent CMV infection even later than 4 months after transplantation, as treatment appears to delay the development of the normal immune response to CMV infection. Although CMV disease may present as isolated fever, granulocytopenia, thrombocytopenia, or gastrointestinal disease, the foremost cause of death from CMV infection in the setting of HSC transplantation is pneumonia.

With the standard use of CMV-negative or filtered blood products, primary CMV infection should be a major risk in allogeneic transplantation only when the donor is CMV-seropositive and the recipient is CMV-seronegative. Reactivation disease or superinfection with another strain from the donor is also common in CMV-positive recipients, and most seropositive patients who undergo HSC transplantation excrete CMV, with or without clinical findings. Serious CMV disease is much more common among allogeneic than autologous recipients and is often associated with GVHD. In addition to pneumonia and marrow suppression (and, less often, graft failure), manifestations of CMV disease in HSC transplant recipients include fever with or without arthralgias, myalgias, hepatitis, and esophagitis. CMV ulcerations occur in both the lower and the upper gastrointestinal tract, and it may be difficult to distinguish diarrhea due to GVHD from that due to CMV infection. The finding of CMV in the liver of a patient with GVHD does not necessarily mean that CMV is responsible for hepatic enzyme abnormalities. It is interesting that the ocular and neurologic manifestations of CMV infections, which are common in patients with AIDS, are uncommon in patients who develop disease after transplantation.

Management of CMV disease in HSC transplant recipients includes strategies directed at prophylaxis, preemptive therapy (suppression of silent replication), and treatment of disease. Prophylaxis results in a lower incidence of disease at the cost of treating many patients who otherwise would not require therapy. Because of the high fatality rate associated with CMV pneumonia in these patients and the difficulty of early diagnosis of CMV infection, prophylactic IV ganciclovir (or oral valganciclovir) has been used in some centers and has been shown to abort CMV disease during the period of maximal vulnerability (from engraftment to day 120 after transplantation). Ganciclovir also prevents HSV reactivation and reduces the risk of VZV reactivation; thus acyclovir prophylaxis should be discontinued when ganciclovir is administered. The foremost problem with the administration of ganciclovir relates to adverse effects, which include dose-related bone marrow suppression (thrombocytopenia, leukopenia, anemia, and pancytopenia). Because the frequency of CMV pneumonia is lower among autologous HSC transplant recipients (2–7%) than among allogeneic HSC transplant recipients (10–40%), prophylaxis in the former group will not become the rule until a less toxic oral antiviral agent becomes available.

Preemptive treatment of CMV—that is, initiation of therapy with drugs only after CMV is detected in blood, typically by a nucleic acid amplification test—is used at most centers. The preemptive approach has supplanted prophylactic therapy, or treatment of all seropositive (recipient and/or donor) HSC transplants with an antiviral agent (typically ganciclovir), because of toxic drug side effects (e.g., neutropenia and bone marrow suppression). Quantitative viral load assays, which are not dependent on circulating leukocytes, have supplanted older antigen-based assays for CMV. A positive test (or increasing viral load) prompts the initiation of preemptive therapy with ganciclovir. Preemptive approaches that target patients who

have polymerase chain reaction (PCR) evidence of CMV can still lead to unnecessary treatment of many individuals with drugs that have adverse effects on the basis of a laboratory test that is not highly predictive of disease; however, invasive disease, particularly in the form of pulmonary infection, is difficult to treat and is associated with high mortality rates. When prophylaxis or preemptive therapy is stopped, late manifestations of CMV replication may occur, although by then the HSC transplant patient is often equipped with improved graft function and is better able to combat disease.

CMV pneumonia in HSC transplant recipients (unlike that in other clinical settings) is often treated with both IV immunoglobulin (IVIg) and ganciclovir. In patients who cannot tolerate ganciclovir, foscarnet is a useful alternative, although it may produce nephrotoxicity and electrolyte imbalance. When neither ganciclovir nor foscarnet is clinically tolerated, cidofovir can be used; however, its efficacy is less well established, and its side effects include nephrotoxicity. Case reports have suggested that the immunosuppressive agent leflunomide may be active in this setting, but controlled studies are lacking. Transfusion of CMV-specific T cells from the donor has decreased viral load in a small series of patients; this result suggests that immunotherapy may play a role in the treatment of this disease in the future. For further discussion, see Chap. 182.

Human herpesviruses 6 and 7

Human herpesvirus type 6 (HHV-6), the cause of roseola in children, is a ubiquitous herpesvirus that reactivates (as determined by quantitative plasma PCR) in ~50% of HSC transplant recipients 2–4 weeks after transplantation. Reactivation is more common among patients requiring glucocorticoids for GVHD and among those receiving second transplants. Reactivation of HHV-6, primarily type B, may be associated with delayed monocyte and platelet engraftment. Limbic encephalitis developing after transplantation has been associated with HHV-6 in cerebrospinal fluid (CSF). The causality of the association is not well defined: in several cases, plasma viremia was detected long before the onset of encephalitis. Nevertheless, most patients with encephalitis had very high viral loads in plasma at the time of CNS illness, and viral antigen has been detected in hippocampal astrocytes. HHV-6 DNA is sometimes found in lung samples after transplantation. However, its role in pneumonitis is unclear, as co-pathogens are frequently present. While HHV-6 is susceptible to foscarnet or cidofovir (and possibly to ganciclovir) in vitro, the efficacy of antiviral treatment has not been well studied. Little is known about the related herpesvirus HHV-7 or its role in posttransplantation infection. For further discussion, see Chap. 182.

Epstein-Barr virus

Primary EBV infection can be fatal to HSC transplant recipients; EBV reactivation can cause EBV–B cell lymphoproliferative disease (EBV-LPD), which may also be fatal to patients taking immunosuppressive drugs. Latent EBV infection of B cells leads to several interesting phenomena in HSC transplant recipients. The marrow ablation that occurs as part of the HSC transplantation procedure may sometimes eliminate latent EBV from the host. Infection can then be reacquired immediately after transplantation by transfer of infected donor B cells. Rarely, transplantation from a seronegative donor may result in cure. The recipient is then at risk for a second primary infection.

EBV-LPD can develop in the recipient's B cells (if any survive marrow ablation) but is more likely to be a consequence of outgrowth of infected donor cells. Both lytic replication and latent replication of EBV are more likely during immunosuppression (e.g., they are associated with GVHD and the use of antibodies to T cells). Although less likely in autologous transplantation, reactivation can occur in T cell–depleted autologous recipients (e.g., patients being given antibodies to T cells for the treatment of a T cell lymphoma with marrow depletion). EBV-LPD, which can become apparent as early as 1–3 months after engraftment, can cause high fevers and cervical adenopathy resembling the symptoms of infectious mononucleosis but more commonly presents as an extranodal mass. The incidence of EBV-LPD among allogeneic HSC transplant recipients is 0.6–1%, which contrasts with figures of ~5% for renal transplant recipients and up to 20% for cardiac transplant patients. In all cases, EBV-LPD is more likely to occur with high-dose, prolonged immunosuppression, especially that caused by the use of antibodies to T cells, glucocorticoids, and calcineurin inhibitors (e.g., cyclosporine, tacrolimus). Ganciclovir, administered to preempt CMV disease, may reduce EBV lytic replication and thereby diminish the pool of B cells that can become newly infected and give rise to LPD. Increasing evidence indicates that replacement of calcineurin inhibitors with m-Tor inhibitors (e.g., rapamycin) exerts an antiproliferative effect on EBV-infected B cells that decreases the likelihood of developing LPD or unrelated proliferative disorders associated with transplant-related immunosuppression.

PCR can be used to monitor EBV production after HSC transplantation. High or increasing viral loads predict an enhanced likelihood of developing EBV-LPD and should prompt rapid reduction of immunosuppression and search for nodal or extra nodal disease. If reduction of immunosuppression does not have the desired effect, administration of a monoclonal antibody to CD20 (rituximab or others) for the treatment of B cell lymphomas that express this surface protein has elicited dramatic responses and currently constitutes first-line therapy for CD20-positive EBV-LPD. However, long-term suppression of new antibody responses accompanies therapy, and recurrences are not infrequent. Additional B cell–directed antibodies, including anti-CD22, are under study. The role of antiviral drugs is uncertain because no available agents have been documented to have activity against the different forms of latent EBV infection. Diminishing lytic replication and virion production in these patients would theoretically produce a statistical decrease in the frequency of latent disease by decreasing the number of virions available to cause additional infection. In case reports and small animal studies, ganciclovir and/or high-dose zidovudine (AZT), together with other agents, has been used to eradicate EBV-LPD and CNS lymphomas, another EBV-associated complication of transplantation. Both interferon and retinoic acid have been employed in the treatment of EBV-LPD, as has IVIg, but no large prospective studies have assessed the efficacy of any of these agents. Several additional drugs are undergoing preclinical evaluation. Standard chemotherapeutic regimens are used if disease persists after reduction of immunosuppressive agents and administration of antibodies. EBV-specific T cells generated from the donor have been used experimentally to prevent and to treat EBV-LPD in allogeneic recipients, and efforts are under way to increase the activity and specificity of ex vivo–generated T cells. For further discussion, see Chap. 181.

Human herpesvirus 8 (KSHV)

The EBV-related gammaherpesvirus KSHV, which is causally associated with Kaposi's sarcoma, primary effusion lymphoma, and multicentric Castleman's disease, has rarely resulted in disease in HSC transplant recipients, although some cases of virus-associated marrow aplasia have been reported in the peritransplantation period. The relatively low seroprevalence of KSHV in the population and the limited duration of profound T cell suppression after HSC transplantation provide a plausible explanation for the currently low incidence of KSHV disease compared with that in recipients of solid organ transplants and patients with HIV infection. For further discussion, see Chap. 182.

Other (nonherpes) viruses

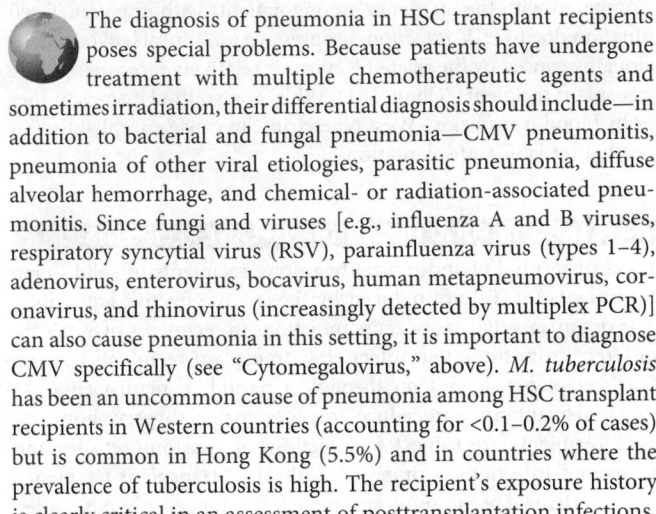 The diagnosis of pneumonia in HSC transplant recipients poses special problems. Because patients have undergone treatment with multiple chemotherapeutic agents and sometimes irradiation, their differential diagnosis should include—in addition to bacterial and fungal pneumonia—CMV pneumonitis, pneumonia of other viral etiologies, parasitic pneumonia, diffuse alveolar hemorrhage, and chemical- or radiation-associated pneumonitis. Since fungi and viruses [e.g., influenza A and B viruses, respiratory syncytial virus (RSV), parainfluenza virus (types 1–4), adenovirus, enterovirus, bocavirus, human metapneumovirus, coronavirus, and rhinovirus (increasingly detected by multiplex PCR)] can also cause pneumonia in this setting, it is important to diagnose CMV specifically (see "Cytomegalovirus," above). *M. tuberculosis* has been an uncommon cause of pneumonia among HSC transplant recipients in Western countries (accounting for <0.1–0.2% of cases) but is common in Hong Kong (5.5%) and in countries where the prevalence of tuberculosis is high. The recipient's exposure history is clearly critical in an assessment of posttransplantation infections.

Both RSV and parainfluenza viruses, particularly type 3, can cause severe or even fatal pneumonia in HSC transplant recipients. Infections with both of these agents sometimes occur as disastrous nosocomial epidemics. Therapy with palivizumab or ribavirin for RSV infection remains controversial. Influenza also occurs in HSC transplant recipients and generally mirrors the presence of infection in the community. Progression to pneumonia is more common when infection occurs early after transplantation and when the recipient is lymphopenic. Several drugs are available for the treatment of influenza. Amantadine and rimantadine have limited effects, primarily reducing symptoms and shortening the duration of illness caused by sensitive strains of influenza A virus. The neuraminidase inhibitors oseltamivir (oral) and zanamivir (aerosolized) are active against both influenza A virus and influenza B virus and are a reasonable treatment option. Parenteral forms of neuraminidase inhibitors such as peramivir (intravenous) are undergoing clinical trials. Peramivir is currently available through the Centers for Disease Control and Prevention (CDC) for the treatment of severe H1N1 influenza. An important preventive measure is immunization of household members, hospital staff members, and other frequent contacts. Adenoviruses can be isolated from HSC transplant recipients at rates varying from 5% to ≥18%. Like CMV infection, adenovirus infection usually occurs in the first to third month after transplantation and is often asymptomatic, although pneumonia, hemorrhagic cystitis/nephritis, severe gastroenteritis with hemorrhage, and fatal disseminated infection have been reported. A role for cidofovir therapy has been suggested, but the efficacy of this agent is unproven in adenovirus infection.

Although diverse respiratory viruses can sometimes cause severe pneumonia and respiratory failure in HSC transplant recipients, mild or even asymptomatic infection may be more common. For example, rhinoviruses and coronaviruses are frequent co-pathogens in HSC transplant recipients; however, whether they independently contribute to significant pulmonary infection is not known. At present, the overall contribution to the burden of lower respiratory tract disease in HSC transplant recipients for the secondary group of viral respiratory pathogens listed above is unknown.

Infections with parvovirus B19 (presenting as anemia or occasionally as pancytopenia) and disseminated enteroviruses (sometimes fatal) can occur. Parvovirus B19 infection can be treated with IVIg (Chap. 184). Intranasal pleconaril, a capsid-binding agent, is being studied for the treatment of enterovirus (and rhinovirus) infection.

Rotaviruses are a common cause of gastroenteritis in HSC transplant recipients. The polyomavirus BK virus is found at high titers in the urine of patients who are profoundly immunosuppressed. BK viruria may be associated with hemorrhagic cystitis in these patients. Compared with the incidence among patients with impaired T cell function due to HIV infection, progressive multifocal leukoencephalopathy caused by the related JC virus is relatively rare among HSC transplant recipients (Chap. 381). When transmitted by mosquitoes or by blood transfusion, West Nile virus can cause encephalitis and death after HSC transplantation.

INFECTIONS IN SOLID ORGAN TRANSPLANT RECIPIENTS

Rates of morbidity and mortality among recipients of solid organ transplants (SOTs) are reduced by the use of effective antibiotics. The organisms that cause acute infections in recipients of SOTs are different from those that infect HSC transplant recipients because SOT recipients do not go through a period of neutropenia. As the transplantation procedure involves major surgery, however, SOT recipients are subject to infections at anastomotic sites and to wound infections. Compared with HSC transplant recipients, SOT patients are immunosuppressed for longer periods (often permanently). Thus they are susceptible to many of the same organisms as patients with chronically impaired T cell immunity (Chap. 86, especially Table 86-1). Moreover, the persistent HLA mismatch between recipient immune cells (e.g., effector T cells) and the donor organ (allograft) places the organ at permanently increased risk of infection.

During the early period (<1 month after transplantation; Table 132-5), infections are most commonly caused by extracellular bacteria (staphylococci, streptococci, enterococci, E. coli, other gram-negative organisms), which often originate in surgical wound or anastomotic sites. The type of transplant largely determines the spectrum of infection. In subsequent weeks, the consequences of the administration of agents that suppress cell-mediated immunity become apparent, and acquisition—or, more commonly, reactivation—of viruses, mycobacteria, endemic fungi, and parasites (from the recipient or from the transplanted organ) can occur. CMV infection is often a problem, particularly in the first 6 months after transplantation, and may present as severe systemic disease or as infection of the transplanted organ. HHV-6 reactivation (assessed by plasma PCR) occurs within the first 2–4 weeks after transplantation and may be associated with fever, leukopenia, and very rare cases of encephalitis. Data suggest that replication of HHV-6 and HHV-7 may exacerbate CMV-induced disease. CMV is associated not only with generalized immunosuppression but also with organ-specific, rejection-related syndromes: glomerulopathy in kidney transplant recipients, bronchiolitis obliterans in lung transplant recipients, vasculopathy in heart transplant recipients, and the vanishing bile duct syndrome in liver transplant recipients. A complex interplay between increased CMV replication and enhanced graft rejection is well established: elevated immunosuppression leads to increased CMV replication, which is associated with graft rejection. For this reason, considerable attention has been focused on the diagnosis, prophylaxis, and treatment of CMV infection in SOT recipients. Early transmission of West Nile virus to transplant recipients from a donated organ or transfused blood has been reported; however, the risk of West Nile acquisition (at least in transfused blood) has been reduced by implementation of screening procedures. In rare instances, rabies virus and lymphocytic choriomeningitis virus have also been transmitted in this setting; although accompanied by distinct clinical syndromes, both viral infections have resulted in fatal encephalitis. As screening for unusual viruses is not routine, only vigilant assessment of the prospective donor is likely to prevent the use of an infected organ.

TABLE 132-5 Common Infections After Solid Organ Transplantation, by Site of Infection

Infected Site	Period after Transplantation		
	Early (<1 Month)	Middle (1–4 Months)	Late (>6 Months)
Donor organ	Bacterial and fungal infections of the graft, anastomotic site, and surgical wound	CMV infection	EBV infection (may present in allograft organ)
Systemic	Bacteremia and candidemia (often resulting from central venous catheter colonization)	CMV infection (fever, bone marrow suppression)	CMV infection, especially in patients given early posttransplantation prophylaxis; EBV proliferative syndromes (may occur in donor organs)
Lung	Bacterial aspiration pneumonia with prevalent nosocomial organisms associated with intubation and sedation (highest risk in lung transplantation)	*Pneumocystis* infection; CMV pneumonia (highest risk in lung transplantation); *Aspergillus* infection (highest risk in lung transplantation)	*Pneumocystis* infection; granulomatous lung diseases (nocardiae, reactivated fungal and mycobacterial diseases)
Kidney	Bacterial and fungal (*Candida*) infections (cystitis, pyelonephritis) associated with urinary tract catheters (highest risk in kidney transplantation)	Renal transplantation: BK virus infection (associated with nephropathy); JC virus infection	Renal transplantation: bacteria (late urinary tract infections, usually not associated with bacteremia); BK virus (nephropathy, graft failure, generalized vasculopathy)
Liver and biliary tract	Cholangitis	CMV hepatitis	CMV hepatitis
Heart		*Toxoplasma gondii* infection (highest risk in heart transplantation)	*T. gondii* (highest risk in heart transplantation)
Gastrointestinal tract	Peritonitis, especially after liver transplantation	Colitis secondary to *Clostridium difficile* infection (risk can persist)	Colitis secondary to *C. difficile* infection (risk can persist)
Central nervous system		*Listeria* (meningitis); *T. gondii* infection	*Listeria* meningitis; *Cryptococcus* meningitis; *Nocardia* abscess; JC virus–associated PML

Abbreviations: CMV, cytomegalovirus, EBV, Epstein-Barr virus, PML, progressive multifocal leukoencephalopathy.

Beyond 6 months after transplantation, infections characteristic of patients with defects in cell-mediated immunity—e.g., infections with *Listeria*, *Nocardia*, *Rhodococcus*, mycobacteria, various fungi, and other intracellular pathogens—may be a problem. International patients and global travelers may experience reactivation of dormant infections with trypanosomes, *Leishmania*, *Plasmodium*, *Strongyloides*, and other parasites. Reactivation of latent *M. tuberculosis* infection, while rare in Western nations, is far more common among persons from developing countries. The recipient is typically the source, although reactivation and spread from the donor organ can occur. While pulmonary disease remains most common, atypical sites may be involved and mortality rates can be high (up to 30%). Elimination of these late infections will not be possible until the patient develops specific tolerance to the transplanted organ in the absence of drugs that lead to generalized immunosuppression. Meanwhile, vigilance, prophylaxis/preemptive therapy (when indicated), and rapid diagnosis and treatment of infections can be lifesaving in SOT recipients, who, unlike most HSC transplant recipients, continue to be immunosuppressed.

SOT recipients are susceptible to EBV-LPD from as early as 2 months to many years after transplantation. The prevalence of this complication is increased by potent and prolonged use of T cell–suppressive drugs. Decreasing the degree of immunosuppression may in some cases reverse the condition. Among SOT patients, those with heart and lung transplants—who receive the most intensive immunosuppressive regimens—are most likely to develop EBV-LPD, particularly in the lungs. Although the disease usually originates in recipient B cells, several cases of donor origin, particularly in the transplanted organ, have been noted. High organ-specific content of B lymphoid tissues (e.g., bronchial-associated lymphoid tissue in the lung), anatomic factors (e.g., lack of access of host T cells to the transplanted organ because of disturbed lymphatics), and differences in major histocompatibility loci between the host T cells and the organ (e.g., lack of cell migration or lack of effective T cell/macrophage cooperation) may result in defective elimination of EBV-infected B cells. SOT recipients are also highly susceptible to the development of Kaposi's sarcoma and, less frequently, to the B cell–proliferative disorders associated with KSHV, such as primary effusion lymphoma and multicentric Castleman's disease. Kaposi's sarcoma is 550–1000 times more common in SOT recipients than in the general population, can develop very rapidly after transplantation, and can also occur in the allograft. However, because the seroprevalence of KSHV is very low in Western countries, Kaposi's sarcoma is not often observed.

Data suggest that a switch of immunosuppressive agents—from calcineurin inhibitors (cyclosporine, tacrolimus) to mTor pathway active agents (sirolimus, everolimus)—after adequate wound healing may significantly reduce the likelihood of developing Kaposi's sarcoma and perhaps of EBV-LPD and certain other posttransplantation malignancies.

◼ KIDNEY TRANSPLANTATION

(See Table 132-5)

Early infections

Bacteria often cause infections that develop in the period immediately after kidney transplantation. There is a role for perioperative antibiotic prophylaxis, and many centers give cephalosporins to decrease the risk of postoperative complications. Urinary tract infections developing soon after transplantation are usually related to anatomic alterations resulting from surgery. Such early infections may require prolonged treatment (e.g., 6 weeks of antibiotic administration for pyelonephritis). Urinary tract infections that occur >6 months after transplantation may be treated for shorter periods because they do not seem to be associated with the high rate of pyelonephritis or relapse seen with infections that occur in the first 3 months.

Daily prophylaxis with one double-strength tablet of TMP-SMX (800 mg of sulfamethoxazole; 160 mg of trimethoprim) for the first 4–6 months after transplantation decreases the incidence of early and middle-period infections (see below, Table 132-5, and Table 132-6).

Middle-period infections

Because of continuing immunosuppression, kidney transplant recipients are predisposed to lung infections characteristic of those in patients with T cell deficiency (i.e., infections with intracellular bacteria, mycobacteria, nocardiae, fungi, viruses, and parasites). A high mortality rate associated with *Legionella pneumophila* infection (Chap. 147) led to the closing of renal transplant units in hospitals with endemic legionellosis.

About 50% of all renal transplant recipients presenting with fever 1–4 months after transplantation have evidence of CMV disease; CMV itself accounts for the fever in more than two-thirds of cases and thus is the predominant pathogen during this period. CMV infection (Chap. 182) may also present as arthralgias, myalgias, or organ-specific symptoms. During this period, this infection may represent primary disease (in the case of a seronegative recipient of

TABLE 132-6 Prophylactic Regimens Commonly Used to Decrease Risk of Infection in Transplant Recipients

Risk Factor	Organism	Prophylactic Drug	Examination(s)*
Travel to or residence in area with known risk of endemic fungal infection	*Histoplasma, Blastomyces, Coccidioides*	Consider imidazoles based on clinical and laboratory assessment	Chest radiography, antigen testing, serology
Latent herpesviruses	HSV, VZV, CMV, EBV	Acyclovir after HSC transplantation to prevent HSV and VZV infection; ganciclovir for CMV (?EBV/?KSHV) in some settings	Serologic tests for HSV, VZV, CMV, HHV-6, EBV, KSHV; PCR
Latent fungi and parasites	*Pneumocystis jiroveci, Toxoplasma gondii*	Trimethoprim-sulfamethoxazole (dapsone or atovaquone)	Serologic test for *Toxoplasma*
History of exposure to active or latent tuberculosis	*Mycobacterium tuberculosis*	Isoniazid if recent conversion or positive chest imaging and/or no previous treatment	Chest imaging; TST and/or cell-based assay

*Serologic examination, TST (tuberculin skin test), and interferon assays may be less reliable after transplantation.

Abbreviations: CMV, cytomegalovirus; EBV, Epstein-Barr virus; HHV-6, human herpesvirus type 6; HSC, hematopoietic stem cell; HSV, herpes simplex virus; KSHV, Kaposi's sarcoma–associated herpesvirus; PCR, polymerase chain reaction; VZV, varicella-zoster virus.

a kidney from a seropositive donor) or may represent reactivation disease or superinfection. Patients may have atypical lymphocytosis. Unlike immunocompetent patients, however, they rarely have lymphadenopathy or splenomegaly. Therefore, clinical suspicion and laboratory confirmation are necessary for diagnosis. The clinical syndrome may be accompanied by bone marrow suppression (particularly leukopenia). CMV also causes glomerulopathy and is associated with an increased incidence of other opportunistic infections. Because of the frequency and severity of disease, a considerable effort has been made to prevent and treat CMV infection in renal transplant recipients. An immune globulin preparation enriched with antibodies to CMV was used by many centers in the past in an effort to protect the group at highest risk for severe infection (seronegative recipients of seropositive kidneys). However, with the development of effective oral antiviral agents, CMV immune globulin is no longer used. Ganciclovir (valganciclovir) is beneficial when prophylaxis is indicated and for the treatment of serious CMV disease. The availability of valganciclovir has allowed most centers to move to oral prophylaxis for transplant recipients. Infection with the other herpesviruses may become evident within 6 months after transplantation or later. Early after transplantation, HSV may cause either oral or anogenital lesions that are usually responsive to acyclovir. Large ulcerating lesions in the anogenital area may lead to bladder and rectal dysfunction as well as predisposing to bacterial infection. VZV may cause fatal disseminated infection in nonimmune kidney transplant recipients, but in immune patients reactivation zoster usually does not disseminate outside the dermatome; thus disseminated VZV infection is a less fearsome complication in kidney transplantation than in HSC transplantation. HHV-6 reactivation may take place and (although usually asymptomatic) may be associated with fever, rash, marrow suppression, or rarely encephalitis.

EBV disease is more serious; it may present as an extranodal proliferation of B cells that invade the CNS, nasopharynx, liver, small bowel, heart, and other organs, including the transplanted kidney. The disease is diagnosed by the finding of a mass of proliferating EBV-positive B cells. The incidence of EBV-LPD is higher among patients who acquire EBV infection from the donor and among patients given high doses of cyclosporine, tacrolimus, glucocorticoids, and anti–T cell antibodies. Disease may regress once immunocompetence is restored. KSHV infection can be transmitted with the donor kidney and result in development of Kaposi's sarcoma, although it more often represents reactivation of latent infection of the recipient. Kaposi's sarcoma often appears within 1 year after transplantation, although the range of onset is wide (1 month to ~20 years). Avoidance of immunosuppressive agents that inhibit calcineurin has been associated with less Kaposi's sarcoma, less EBV disease, and even less CMV replication. The use of rapamycin (sirolimus) has independently led to regression of Kaposi's sarcoma.

The papovaviruses BK virus and JC virus (polyomavirus hominis types 1 and 2) have been cultured from the urine of kidney transplant recipients (as they have from that of HSC transplant recipients) in the setting of profound immunosuppression. High levels of BK virus replication detected by PCR in urine and blood are predictive of pathology, especially in the setting of renal transplantation. JC virus may rarely cause similar disease in kidney transplantation. Urinary excretion of BK virus and BK viremia are associated with the development of ureteral strictures, polyomavirus-associated nephropathy (1–10% of renal transplant recipients), and (less commonly) generalized vasculopathy. Timely detection and early reduction of immunosuppression are critical and can reduce rates of graft loss related to polyomavirus-associated nephropathy from 90% to 10–30%. Therapeutic responses to IVIg, quinolones, leflunomide, and cidofovir have been reported, but the efficacy of these agents

has not been substantiated through adequate clinical study. Most centers approach the problem by reducing immunosuppression in an effort to enhance host immunity and decrease viral titers. JC virus is associated with rare cases of progressive multifocal leukoencephalopathy. Adenoviruses may persist and cause hemorrhagic nephritis/cystitis with continued immunosuppression in these patients, but disseminated disease as seen in HSC transplant recipients is much less common.

Kidney transplant recipients are also subject to infections with other intracellular organisms. These patients may develop pulmonary infections with *Mycobacterium*, *Aspergillus*, and *Mucor* species as well as infections with other pathogens in which the T cell/macrophage axis plays an important role. *Listeria monocytogenes* is a common cause of bacteremia ≥1 month after renal transplantation and should be seriously considered in renal transplant recipients presenting with fever and headache. Kidney transplant recipients may develop *Salmonella* bacteremia, which can lead to endovascular infections and require prolonged therapy. Pulmonary infections with *Pneumocystis* are common unless the patient is maintained on TMP-SMX prophylaxis. *Nocardia* infection (Chap. 162) may present in the skin, bones, and lungs or in the CNS, where it usually takes the form of single or multiple brain abscesses. Nocardiosis generally occurs ≥1 month after transplantation and may follow immunosuppressive treatment for an episode of rejection. Pulmonary manifestations most commonly consist of localized disease with or without cavities, but the disease may be disseminated. The diagnosis is made by culture of the organism from sputum or from the involved nodule. As with *Pneumocystis*, prophylaxis with TMP-SMX is often efficacious in the prevention of disease.

Toxoplasmosis can occur in seropositive patients but is less common than in other transplant settings, usually developing in the first few months after kidney transplantation. Again, TMP-SMX is helpful in prevention. In endemic areas, histoplasmosis, coccidioidomycosis, and blastomycosis may cause pulmonary infiltrates or disseminated disease.

Late infections

Late infections (>6 months after kidney transplantation) may involve the CNS and include CMV retinitis as well as other CNS manifestations of CMV disease. Patients (particularly those whose immunosuppression has been increased) are at risk for subacute meningitis due to *Cryptococcus neoformans*. Cryptococcal disease may present in an insidious manner (sometimes as a skin infection before the development of clear CNS findings). *Listeria* meningitis may have an acute presentation and requires prompt therapy to avoid a fatal outcome. TMP-SMX prophylaxis may reduce the frequency of *Listeria* infections.

Patients who continue to take glucocorticoids are predisposed to ongoing infection. "Transplant elbow," a recurrent bacterial infection in and around the elbow that is thought to result from a combination of poor tensile strength of the skin of steroid-treated patients and steroid-induced proximal myopathy, requires patients to push themselves up with their elbows to get out of chairs. Bouts of cellulitis (usually caused by *S. aureus*) recur until patients are provided with elbow protection.

Kidney transplant recipients are susceptible to invasive fungal infections, including those due to *Aspergillus* and *Rhizopus*, which may present as superficial lesions before dissemination. Mycobacterial infection (particularly that with *Mycobacterium marinum*) can be diagnosed by skin examination. Infection with *Prototheca wickerhamii* (an achlorophyllic alga) has been diagnosed by skin biopsy. Warts caused by human papillomaviruses (HPVs) are a late consequence of persistent immunosuppression; imiquimod or other forms of local therapy are usually satisfactory. Merkel cell carcinoma, a rare and aggressive neuroendocrine skin tumor the frequency of which is increased fivefold in elderly SOT (especially kidney) recipients, has been linked to a novel polyoma virus (Merkel cell polyomavirus).

Notably, although BK virus replication and virus-associated disease can be detected far earlier, the median time to clinical diagnosis of polyomavirus-associated nephropathy is ~300 days, qualifying it as a late-onset disease. With establishment of better screening procedures (e.g., blood PCR), it is likely that this disease will be detected earlier (see "Middle-Period Infections," above).

■ HEART TRANSPLANTATION

Early infections

Sternal wound infection and mediastinitis are early complications of heart transplantation. An indolent course is common, with fever or a mildly elevated white blood cell count preceding the development of site tenderness or drainage. Clinical suspicion based on evidence of sternal instability and failure to heal may lead to the diagnosis. Common microbial residents of the skin (e.g., *S. aureus*, including methicillin-resistant strains, and *Staphylococcus epidermidis*) as well as gram-negative organisms (e.g., *Pseudomonas aeruginosa*) and fungi (e.g., *Candida*) are often involved. In rare cases, mediastinitis in heart transplant recipients can also be due to *Mycoplasma hominis* (Chap. 175). Since this organism requires an anaerobic environment for growth and may be difficult to see on conventional medium, the laboratory should be alerted that *M. hominis* infection is suspected. *M. hominis* mediastinitis has been cured with a combination of surgical debridement (sometimes requiring muscle-flap placement) and the administration of clindamycin and tetracycline. Organisms associated with mediastinitis may sometimes be cultured from pericardial fluid.

Middle-period infections

T. gondii (Chap. 214) residing in the heart of a seropositive donor may be transmitted to a seronegative recipient. Thus serologic screening for *T. gondii* infection is important before and in the months after cardiac transplantation. Rarely, active disease can be introduced at the time of transplantation. The overall incidence of toxoplasmosis is so high in the setting of heart transplantation that some prophylaxis is always warranted. Although alternatives are available, the most frequently used agent is TMP-SMX, which prevents infection with *Pneumocystis* as well as with *Nocardia* and several other bacterial pathogens. CMV also has been transmitted by heart transplantation. *Toxoplasma*, *Nocardia*, and *Aspergillus* can cause CNS infections. *L. monocytogenes* meningitis should be considered in heart transplant recipients with fever and headache.

CMV infection is associated with poor outcomes after heart transplantation. The virus is usually detected 1–2 months after transplantation, causes early signs and laboratory abnormalities (usually fever and atypical lymphocytosis or leukopenia and thrombocytopenia) at 2–3 months, and can produce severe disease (e.g., pneumonia) at 3–4 months. An interesting observation is that seropositive recipients usually develop viremia faster than patients whose primary CMV infection is a consequence of transplantation. Between 40% and 70% of patients develop symptomatic CMV disease in the form of (1) CMV pneumonia, the most likely form to be fatal; (2) CMV esophagitis and gastritis, sometimes accompanied by abdominal pain with or without ulcerations and bleeding; and (3) the CMV syndrome, consisting of CMV in the blood along with fever, leukopenia, thrombocytopenia, and hepatic enzyme abnormalities. Ganciclovir is efficacious in the treatment of CMV infection; prophylaxis with ganciclovir or possibly with other antiviral agents, as described for renal transplantation, may reduce the overall incidence of CMV-related disease.

Late infections

EBV infection usually presents as a lymphoma-like proliferation of B cells late after heart transplantation, particularly in patients maintained on intense immunosuppressive therapy. A subset of heart and heart-lung transplant recipients may develop early fulminant EBV-LPD (within 2 months). Treatment includes the reduction of immunosuppression (if possible), the use of glucocorticoid and calcineurin inhibitor–sparing regimens, and the consideration of therapy with anti–B cell antibodies (rituximab and possibly others). Immunomodulatory and antiviral agents continue to be studied. Ganciclovir prophylaxis for CMV disease may indirectly reduce the risk of EBV-LPD through reduced spread of replicating EBV to naïve B cells. Aggressive chemotherapy is a last resort, as discussed earlier for HSC transplant recipients. KSHV-associated disease, including Kaposi's sarcoma and primary effusion lymphoma, has been reported in heart transplant recipients. GVHD prophylaxis with sirolimus may decrease the risk of both rejection and outgrowth of KSHV-infected cells. Antitumor therapy is discussed in Chap. 85. Prophylaxis for *Pneumocystis* infection is required for these patients (see "Lung Transplantation, Late Infections," below).

■ LUNG TRANSPLANTATION

Early Infections

It is not surprising that lung transplant recipients are predisposed to the development of pneumonia. The combination of ischemia and the resulting mucosal damage, together with accompanying denervation and lack of lymphatic drainage, probably contributes to the high rate of pneumonia (66% in one series). The prophylactic use of high doses of broad-spectrum antibiotics for the first 3–4 days after surgery may decrease the incidence of pneumonia. Gram-negative pathogens (Enterobacteriaceae and *Pseudomonas* species) are troublesome in the first 2 weeks after surgery (the period of maximal vulnerability). Pneumonia can also be caused by *Candida* (possibly as a result of colonization of the donor lung), *Aspergillus*, and *Cryptococcus*.

Mediastinitis may occur at an even higher rate among lung transplant recipients than among heart transplant recipients and most commonly develops within 2 weeks of surgery. In the absence of prophylaxis, pneumonitis due to CMV (which may be transmitted as a consequence of transplantation) usually presents between 2 weeks and 3 months after surgery, with primary disease occurring later than reactivation disease.

Middle-period infections

The incidence of CMV infection, either reactivated or primary, is 75–100% if either the donor or the recipient is seropositive for CMV. CMV-induced disease after solid organ transplantation appears to be most severe in recipients of lung and heart-lung transplants. Whether this severity relates to the mismatch in lung antigen presentation and host immune cells or is attributable to nonimmunologic factors is not known. More than half of lung transplant recipients with symptomatic CMV disease have pneumonia. Difficulty in distinguishing the radiographic picture of CMV infection from that of other infections or from organ rejection further complicates therapy. CMV can also cause bronchiolitis obliterans in lung transplants. The development of pneumonitis related to HSV has led to the prophylactic use of acyclovir. Such prophylaxis may also decrease rates of CMV disease, but ganciclovir is more active against CMV and is also active against HSV. The prophylaxis of CMV infection with IV ganciclovir—or increasingly with valganciclovir, the oral alternative—is recommended for lung transplant recipients. Antiviral alternatives are discussed in the earlier section on HSC transplantation. Although the overall incidence of serious disease is decreased during prophylaxis, late disease may occur when prophylaxis is stopped—a pattern observed increasingly in recent years. With recovery from peritransplantation complications and, in many cases, a decrease in immunosuppression, the recipient is often better equipped to combat late infection.

Late infections

The incidence of *Pneumocystis* infection (which may present with a paucity of findings) is high among lung and heart-lung transplant recipients. Some form of prophylaxis for *Pneumocystis* pneumonia is indicated in all organ transplant situations (Table 132-6). Prophylaxis with TMP-SMX for 12 months after transplantation may be sufficient to prevent *Pneumocystis* disease in patients whose immunosuppression is not increased.

As in other transplant recipients, infection with EBV may cause either a mononucleosis-like syndrome or EBV-LPD. The tendency of the B cell blasts to present in the lung appears to be greater after lung transplantation than after the transplantation of other organs, possibly because of a rich source of B cells in bronchial-associated lymphoid tissue. Reduction of immunosuppression and switching of regimens, as discussed in earlier sections, cause remission in some cases, but airway compression can be fatal and more rapid intervention may therefore become necessary. The approach to EBV-LPD is similar to that described in other sections.

■ LIVER TRANSPLANTATION

Early infections

As in other transplantation settings, early bacterial infections are a major problem after liver transplantation. Many centers administer systemic broad-spectrum antibiotics for the first 24 h or sometimes longer after surgery, even in the absence of documented infection. However, despite prophylaxis, infectious complications are common and correlate with the duration of the surgical procedure and the type of biliary drainage. An operation lasting >12 h is associated with an increased likelihood of infection. Patients who have a choledochojejunostomy with drainage of the biliary duct to a Roux-en-Y jejunal bowel loop have more fungal infections than those whose bile is drained via a choledochocholedochostomy with anastomosis of the donor common bile duct to the recipient common bile duct.

Peritonitis and intraabdominal abscesses are common complications of liver transplantation. Bacterial peritonitis or localized abscesses may result from biliary leaks. Early leaks are even more common with live-donor liver transplants. Peritonitis in liver transplant recipients is often polymicrobial, commonly involving enterococci, aerobic gram-negative bacteria, staphylococci, anaerobes, *Candida*, or sometimes other invasive fungi. Only one-third of patients with intraabdominal abscesses have bacteremia. Abscesses within the first month after surgery may occur not only in and around the liver but also in the spleen, pericolic area, and pelvis. Treatment includes antibiotic administration and drainage as necessary.

Liver transplant patients have a high incidence of fungal infections, and the occurrence of fungal (often candidal) infection correlates with preoperative use of glucocorticoids, long duration of treatment with antibacterial agents, and posttransplantation use of immunosuppressive agents. Many centers give fluconazole prophylactically in this setting.

Middle-period infections

The development of postsurgical biliary stricture predisposes patients to cholangitis. The incidence of strictures is increased in live-donor liver transplantation. Transplant recipients who develop cholangitis may have high spiking fevers and rigors but often lack the characteristic signs and symptoms of classic cholangitis, including abdominal pain and jaundice. Although these findings

may suggest graft rejection, rejection is typically accompanied by marked elevation of liver function enzymes. In contrast, in cholangitis in transplant recipients, results of liver function tests (with the possible exception of alkaline phosphatase levels) are often within the normal range. Definitive diagnosis of cholangitis in liver transplant recipients requires demonstration of aggregated neutrophils in bile duct biopsy specimens. Unfortunately, invasive studies of the biliary tract (either T-tube cholangiography or endoscopic retrograde cholangiopancreatography) may themselves lead to cholangitis. For this reason, many clinicians recommend an empirical trial of therapy with antibiotics covering gram-negative organisms and anaerobes before these procedures are undertaken as well as antibiotic coverage if procedures are eventually performed.

Reactivation of viral hepatitis is a common complication of liver transplantation (Chap. 304). Recurrent hepatitis B and C infections, for which transplantation may be performed, are problematic. To prevent hepatitis B virus reinfection, prophylaxis with an optimal antiviral agent or combination of agents (lamivudine, adefovir, entecavir) and hepatitis B immune globulin is currently recommended, although the optimal dose, route, and duration of therapy remain controversial. Success in preventing reinfection with hepatitis B virus has increased in recent years; in contrast, reinfection of the graft with hepatitis C virus occurs in all patients, with a variable time frame. Studies of aggressive pretransplantation treatment of selected recipients with antiviral agents and prophylactic/preemptive regimens are ongoing. However, early initiation of treatment for histologically documented disease with a combination of ribavirin and pegylated interferon has produced sustained responses at rates in the range of 25–40%. Several protease and polymerase inhibitors that block production of hepatitis C virus as well as a monoclonal antibody to the virus are undergoing preclinical and clinical trials.

As in other transplantation settings, reactivation disease with herpesviruses is common (Table 132-4). Herpesviruses can be transmitted in donor organs. Although CMV hepatitis occurs in ~4% of liver transplant recipients, it is usually not so severe as to require retransplantation. Without prophylaxis, CMV disease develops in the majority of seronegative recipients of organs from CMV-positive donors, but fatality rates are lower among liver transplant recipients than among lung or heart-lung transplant recipients. Disease due to CMV can also be associated with the vanishing bile duct syndrome after liver transplantation. Patients respond to treatment with ganciclovir; prophylaxis with oral forms of ganciclovir or high-dose acyclovir may decrease the frequency of disease. A role for HHV-6 reactivation in early posttransplantation fever and leukopenia has been proposed, although the more severe sequelae described in HSC transplantation are unusual. HHV-6 and HHV-7 appear to exacerbate CMV disease in this setting. EBV-LPD after liver transplantation shows a propensity for involvement of the liver, and such disease may be of donor origin. See previous sections for discussion of EBV infections in solid organ transplantation.

■ PANCREAS TRANSPLANTATION

Pancreas transplantation is most frequently performed together with or after kidney transplantation, although it may be performed alone. Transplantation of the pancreas can be complicated by early bacterial and yeast infections. Most pancreatic transplants are drained into the bowel, with the remaining transplants drained into the bladder. A cuff of duodenum is used in the anastomosis between the pancreatic graft and either the gut or the bladder. Bowel drainage poses a risk of early intraabdominal and allograft infections with enteric bacteria and yeasts. These infections can result in loss of the graft. Bladder drainage causes a high rate of urinary tract infection and sterile cystitis; however, infection can usually be cured with appropriate antimicrobial agents. In both procedures, prophylactic antimicrobial agents are commonly used at the time of surgery.

Aggressive immunosuppression is associated with late-onset systemic viral and fungal infections; thus many centers administer an antifungal drug and an antiviral agent (ganciclovir or a congener) for prophylaxis.

Issues related to the development of CMV infection, EBV-LPD, and infections with opportunistic pathogens in patients receiving a pancreatic transplant are similar to those in other SOT recipients.

■ MISCELLANEOUS INFECTIONS IN SOLID ORGAN TRANSPLANTATION

Indwelling IV catheter infections

The prolonged use of indwelling IV catheters for administration of medications, blood products, and nutrition is common in diverse transplantation settings and poses a risk of local and bloodstream infections. Significant insertion-site infection is most commonly caused by *S. aureus*. Bloodstream infection most frequently develops within a week of catheter placement or in patients who become neutropenic. Coagulase-negative staphylococci are the most common isolates from the blood.

For further discussion of differential diagnosis and therapeutic options, see Chap. 86.

Tuberculosis

The incidence of tuberculosis within the first 12 months after solid organ transplantation is greater than that observed after HSC transplantation (0.23–0.79%) and ranges broadly worldwide (1.2–15%), reflecting the prevalence of tuberculosis in local populations. Lesions suggesting prior tuberculosis on chest radiograph, older age, diabetes, chronic liver disease, GVHD, and intense immunosuppression are predictive of tuberculosis reactivation and development of disseminated disease in a host with latent disease. Tuberculosis has rarely been transmitted from the donor organ. In contrast to the low mortality rate among HSC transplant recipients, mortality rates among SOT patients are reported to be as high as 30%. Vigilance is indicated, as the presentation of disease is often extrapulmonary (gastrointestinal, genitourinary, central nervous, endocrine, musculoskeletal, laryngeal) and atypical, sometimes manifesting as a fever of unknown origin. A careful history and a direct evaluation of both the recipient and the donor prior to transplantation are optimal. Skin testing of the recipient with purified protein derivative may be unreliable because of chronic disease and/or immunosuppression, but newer cell-based assays that measure interferon and/or cytokine production may prove more sensitive in the future. Isoniazid toxicity has not been a significant problem except in the setting of liver transplantation. Therefore, appropriate prophylaxis should proceed. An assessment of the need to treat latent disease should include careful consideration of the possibility of a false-negative test result. Pending final confirmation of suspected tuberculosis, aggressive multidrug treatment in accordance with the guidelines of the CDC, the Infectious Diseases Society of America, and the American Thoracic Society is indicated because of the high mortality rates among these patients. Altered drug metabolism (e.g., upon co-administration of rifampin and certain immunosuppressive agents) can be managed with careful monitoring of drug levels and appropriate dose adjustment. Close follow-up of hepatic enzymes is warranted, particularly during treatment with isoniazid, pyrazinamide, and/or rifampin. Drug-resistant tuberculosis is especially problematic in these individuals (Chap. 165).

Virus-associated malignancies

In addition to malignancy associated with gammaherpesvirus infection (EBV, KSHV) and simple warts (HPV), other tumors that are virus-associated or suspected of being virus-associated are more likely to develop in transplant recipients, particularly those who require long-term immunosuppression, than in the general population. The interval to tumor development is usually >1 year. Transplant recipients develop nonmelanoma skin or lip cancers that, in contrast to de novo skin cancers, have a high ratio of squamous cells to basal cells. HPV may play a major role in these lesions. Cervical and vulvar carcinomas, quite clearly associated with HPV, develop with increased frequency in female transplant recipients. Among renal transplant recipients, rates of melanoma are modestly increased and rates of cancers of the kidney and bladder are increased.

VACCINATION OF TRANSPLANT RECIPIENTS

In addition to receiving antibiotic prophylaxis, transplant recipients should be vaccinated against likely pathogens (Table 132-7). In the case of HSC transplant recipients, optimal responses cannot be achieved until after immune reconstitution, despite previous immunization of both donor and recipient. Recipients of an allogeneic HSC transplant must be reimmunized if they are to be protected against pathogens. The situation is less clear-cut in the case of autologous transplantation. T and B cells in the peripheral blood may reconstitute the immune response if they are transferred in adequate numbers. However, cancer patients (particularly those with Hodgkin's disease, in whom vaccination has been extensively studied) who are undergoing chemotherapy do not respond normally to immunization, and titers of antibodies to infectious agents fall more rapidly than in healthy individuals. Therefore, even immunosuppressed patients who have not undergone HSC transplantation may need booster vaccine injections. If memory cells are specifically eliminated as part of a stem cell "cleanup" procedure, it will be necessary to reimmunize the recipient with a new primary series. Optimal times for immunizations of different transplant populations are being evaluated. Yearly immunization of household and other contacts (including health care personnel) against influenza benefits the patient by preventing local spread.

In the absence of compelling data as to optimal timing, it is reasonable to administer the pneumococcal and *H. influenzae* type b conjugate vaccines to both autologous and allogeneic HSC transplant recipients beginning 12 months after transplantation. A series that includes both the 13-valent pneumococcal conjugate vaccine and the 23-valent Pneumovax is now recommended (following CDC guidelines). The pneumococcal and *H. influenzae* type b vaccines are particularly important for patients who have undergone splenectomy. The *Neisseria meningitidis* polysaccharide conjugate vaccine (Menactra or Menveo) is also recommended. In addition, diphtheria, tetanus, acellular pertussis, and inactivated polio vaccines can all be given at these same intervals (12 months and, as required, 24 months after transplantation). Some authorities recommend a new primary series for tetanus/diphtheria/pertussis and inactivated polio vaccine beginning 12 months after transplantation. Vaccination to prevent hepatitis B and hepatitis A (both killed vaccines) also seems advisable. Live-virus measles/mumps/rubella (MMR) vaccine can be given to autologous HSC transplant recipients 24 months after transplantation and to most allogeneic HSC transplant recipients at the same point if they are not receiving maintenance therapy with immunosuppressive drugs and do not have ongoing GVHD. The risk of spread from a household contact is lower for MMR vaccine than for polio vaccine. Neither patients nor their household contacts should be vaccinated with vaccinia unless they have been exposed to the smallpox virus. Among patients who have active GVHD and/or are taking high maintenance doses of glucocorticoids, it may be prudent to avoid all live-virus vaccines.

TABLE 132-7 Vaccination of Hematopoietic Stem Cell (HSC) Transplant or Solid Organ Transplant (SOT) Recipients

| Vaccine | Type of Transplantation | |
	HSC Transplant	SOT*
Streptococcus pneumoniae, Haemophilus influenzae, Neisseria meningitidis	Immunize after transplantation. See CDC recommendations. (For pneumococcus, a new primary series may be indicated.)	Immunize before transplantation. See CDC recommendations. (For pneumococcus, a booster with polysaccharide vaccine every 5 years may be recommended.)
Influenza	Vaccinate in the fall. Vaccinate close contacts.	Vaccinate in the fall. Vaccinate close contacts.
Polio	Administer inactivated vaccine.	Administer inactivated vaccine.
Measles/mumps/rubella	Immunize 24 months after transplantation if GVHD is absent.	Immunize before transplantation with attenuated vaccine.
Diphtheria, pertussis, tetanus	Reimmunize after transplantation with primary series, DTaP. See CDC recommendations.	Immunize or boost before transplantation with Tdap; give boosters at 10 years or as required.
Hepatitis B and A	Reimmunize after transplantation. See CDC recommendations.	Immunize before transplantation.
Human papillomavirus	Recommendations are pending.	Recommendations are pending.

*Immunizations should be given before solid organ transplantation whenever possible.

Abbreviations: CDC, Centers for Disease Control and Prevention; DTaP, full-level diphtheria and tetanus toxoids and acellular pertussis, adsorbed; GVHD, graft-versus-host disease; Tdap, tetanus toxoid, reduced diphtheria toxoid, and acellular pertussis.

Note: Recommendations from the CDC should be checked regularly as they frequently change upon receipt of new clinical information and new formulations of specific vaccines.

In the case of SOT recipients, administration of all the usual vaccines and of the indicated booster doses should be completed before immunosuppression, if possible, to maximize responses. For patients taking immunosuppressive agents, the administration of pneumococcal vaccine should be repeated every 5 years. No data are available for the meningococcal vaccine, but it is probably reasonable to administer it along with the pneumococcal vaccine. *H. influenzae* conjugate vaccine is safe and should be efficacious in this population; therefore, its administration before transplantation is recommended. Booster doses of this vaccine are not recommended for adults. SOT recipients who continue to receive immunosuppressive drugs should not receive live-virus vaccines. A person in this group who is exposed to measles should be given measles immune globulin. Similarly, an immunocompromised patient who is seronegative for varicella and who comes into contact with a person who has chickenpox should be given varicella-zoster immune globulin as soon as possible, certainly within 96 h; if this is not possible, the patient should be started immediately on a 10- to 14-day course of acyclovir therapy. Upon the discontinuation of treatment, clinical disease may still occur in a small number of patients; thus vigilance is indicated. Rapid re-treatment with acyclovir should limit the symptoms of disease. Household contacts of transplant recipients can receive live attenuated VZV vaccine, but vaccinees should avoid direct contact with the patient if a rash develops. Virus-like particle (VLP) vaccines have been licensed for the prevention of infection with several HPV serotypes most commonly implicated in cervical and anal carcinomas and in anogenital and laryngeal warts. VLP vaccines are not live; however, no information is yet available about their immunogenicity or efficacy in transplant recipients.

Immunocompromised patients who travel may benefit from some but not all vaccines (Chaps. 122 and 123). In general, these patients should receive any killed or inactivated vaccine preparation appropriate to the area they are visiting; this recommendation includes the vaccines for Japanese encephalitis, hepatitis A and B, poliomyelitis, meningococcal infection, and typhoid. The live typhoid vaccines are not recommended for use in most immunocompromised patients, but inactivated or purified polysaccharide typhoid vaccine can be used. Live yellow fever vaccine should not be administered. On the other hand, primary immunization or boosting with the purified-protein hepatitis B vaccine is indicated if patients are likely to be exposed. Patients who will reside for >6 months in areas where hepatitis B is common (Africa, Southeast Asia, the Middle East, Eastern Europe, parts of South America, and the Caribbean) should receive hepatitis B vaccine. Inactivated hepatitis A vaccine should also be used in the appropriate setting (Chap. 122). A combined vaccine is now available that provides dual protection against hepatitis A and hepatitis B. If hepatitis A vaccine is not administered, travelers should consider receiving passive protection with immune globulin (the dose depending on the duration of travel in the high-risk area).

FURTHER READINGS

Aguado JM et al: Tuberculosis in solid-organ transplant recipients: Consensus statement of the Group for the Study of Infection in Transplant Recipients (GESTRA) of the Spanish Society of Infectious Diseases and Clinical Microbiology. Clin Infect Dis 48:1276, 2009

Allain J-P et al: Transfusion-transmitted infectious diseases. Biologicals 37:71, 2009

Jiang M et al: The role of polyomaviruses in human disease. Virology 384:266, 2009

Kotton CN: Zoonoses in solid-organ and hematopoietic stem cell transplant recipients. Clin Infect Dis 44:857, 2007

Neofytos D et al: Epidemiology and outcome of invasive fungal infection in adult hematopoietic stem cell transplant recipients: Analysis of Multicenter Prospective Antifungal Therapy (PATH) Alliance registry. Clin Infect Dis 48:265, 2009

Pappas PG et al: Invasive fungal infections among organ transplant recipients: Results of the Transplant-Associated Infection Surveillance Network (TRANSNET). Clin Infect Dis 50:1101, 2010

CHAPTER 133

Treatment and Prophylaxis of Bacterial Infections

Gordon L. Archer
Ronald E. Polk

The development of vaccines and drugs that prevent and cure bacterial infections was one of the twentieth century's major contributions to human longevity and quality of life. Antibacterial agents are among the most commonly prescribed drugs of any kind worldwide. Used appropriately, these drugs are lifesaving. However, their indiscriminate use drives up the cost of health care, leads to a plethora of side effects and drug interactions, and fosters the emergence of bacterial resistance, rendering previously valuable drugs useless. The rational use of antibacterial agents depends on an understanding of (1) the drugs' mechanisms of action, spectra of activity, pharmacokinetics, pharmacodynamics, toxicities, and interactions; (2) mechanisms underlying bacterial resistance; and (3) strategies that can be used by clinicians to limit resistance. In addition, patient-associated parameters, such as infection site, other drugs being taken, allergies, and immune and excretory status, are critically important to appropriate therapeutic decisions. This chapter provides specific data required for making an informed choice of antibacterial agent.

MECHANISMS OF ACTION

Antibacterial agents, like all antimicrobial drugs, are directed against unique targets not present in mammalian cells. The goal is to limit toxicity to the host and maximize chemotherapeutic activity affecting invading microbes only. *Bactericidal drugs* kill the bacteria that are within their spectrum of activity; *bacteriostatic drugs* only inhibit bacterial growth. While bacteriostatic activity is adequate for the treatment of most infections, bactericidal activity may be necessary for cure in patients with altered immune systems (e.g., neutropenia), protected infectious foci (e.g., endocarditis or meningitis), or specific infections (e.g., complicated *Staphylococcus aureus* bacteremia). The mechanisms of action of the antibacterial agents to be discussed in this section are summarized in Table 133-1 and are depicted in Fig. 133-1.

■ INHIBITION OF CELL-WALL SYNTHESIS

One major difference between bacterial and mammalian cells is the presence in bacteria of a rigid wall external to the cell membrane. The wall protects bacterial cells from osmotic rupture, which would result from the cell's usual marked hyperosmolarity (by up to 20 atm) relative to the host environment. The structure conferring cell-wall rigidity and resistance to osmotic lysis in both gram-positive and gram-negative bacteria is peptidoglycan, a large, covalently linked sacculus that surrounds the bacterium. In gram-positive bacteria, peptidoglycan is the only layered structure external to the cell membrane and is thick (20–80 nm); in gram-negative bacteria,

there is an outer membrane external to a very thin (1-nm) peptidoglycan layer.

Chemotherapeutic agents directed at any stage of the synthesis, export, assembly, or cross-linking of peptidoglycan lead to inhibition of bacterial cell growth and, in most cases, to cell death. Peptidoglycan is composed of (1) a backbone of two alternating sugars, N-acetylglucosamine and N-acetylmuramic acid; (2) a chain of four amino acids that extends down from the backbone (stem peptides); and (3) a peptide bridge that cross-links the peptide chains. Peptidoglycan is formed by the addition of subunits (a sugar with its five attached amino acids) that are assembled in the cytoplasm and transported through the cytoplasmic membrane to the cell surface. Subsequent cross-linking is driven by cleavage of the terminal stem-peptide amino acid.

Virtually all the antibiotics that inhibit bacterial cell-wall synthesis are bactericidal. That is, they eventually result in the cell's death due to osmotic lysis. However, much of the loss of cell-wall integrity following treatment with cell wall–active agents is due to the bacteria's own cell-wall remodeling enzymes (autolysins) that cleave peptidoglycan bonds in the normal course of cell growth. In the presence of antibacterial agents that inhibit cell-wall growth, autolysis proceeds without normal cell-wall repair; weakness and eventual cellular lysis occur. Antibacterial agents act to inhibit cell-wall synthesis in several ways, as described below.

Bacitracin Bacitracin, a cyclic peptide antibiotic, inhibits the conversion to its active form of the lipid carrier that moves the water-soluble cytoplasmic peptidoglycan subunits through the cell membrane to the cell exterior.

Glycopeptides Glycopeptides [vancomycin, teicoplanin, and telavancin (lipoglycopeptide)] are high-molecular-weight antibiotics that bind to the terminal D-alanine–D-alanine component of the stem peptide while the subunits are external to the cell membrane but still linked to the lipid carrier. This binding sterically inhibits the addition of subunits to the peptidoglycan backbone.

β-Lactam antibiotics β-Lactam antibiotics (penicillins, cephalosporins, carbapenems, and monobactams; Table 133-2) are characterized by a four-membered β-lactam ring and prevent the cross-linking reaction called *transpeptidation*. The energy for attaching a peptide cross-bridge from the stem peptide of one peptidoglycan subunit to another is derived from the cleavage of a terminal D-alanine residue from the subunit stem peptide. The cross-bridge amino acid is then attached to the penultimate D-alanine by transpeptidase enzymes. The β-lactam ring of the antibiotic forms an irreversible covalent acyl bond with the transpeptidase enzyme (probably because of the antibiotic's steric similarity to the enzyme's D-alanine–D-alanine target), preventing the cross-linking reaction. Transpeptidases and similar enzymes involved in cross-linking are called *penicillin-binding proteins* (PBPs) because they all have active sites that bind β-lactam antibiotics.

■ INHIBITION OF PROTEIN SYNTHESIS

Most of the antibacterial agents that inhibit protein synthesis interact with the bacterial ribosome. The difference between the composition of bacterial and mammalian ribosomes gives these compounds their selectivity.

Aminoglycosides Aminoglycosides (gentamicin, kanamycin, tobramycin, streptomycin, neomycin, and amikacin) are a group

TABLE 133-1 Mechanisms of Action of and Resistance to Major Classes of Antibacterial Agents

Letter for Fig. 133-1	Antibacterial Agent[a]	Major Cellular Target	Mechanism of Action	Major Mechanisms of Resistance
A	β-Lactams (penicillins, cephalosporins)	Cell wall	Inhibit cell-wall cross-linking	1. Drug inactivation (β-lactamase) 2. Insensitivity of target (altered penicillin-binding proteins) 3. Decreased permeability (altered gram-negative outer-membrane porins) 4. Active efflux
B	Vancomycin	Cell wall	Interferes with addition of new cell-wall subunits (muramyl pentapeptides)	Alteration of target (substitution of terminal amino acid of peptidoglycan subunit)
	Bacitracin	Cell wall	Prevents addition of cell-wall subunits by inhibiting recycling of membrane lipid carrier	Not defined
C	Macrolides (erythromycin)	Protein synthesis	Bind to 50S ribosomal subunit	1. Alteration of target (ribosomal methylation and mutation of 23S rRNA) 2. Active efflux
	Lincosamides (clindamycin)	Protein synthesis	Bind to 50S ribosomal subunit Block peptide chain elongation	1. Alteration of target (ribosomal methylation) 2. Active efflux
D	Chloramphenicol	Protein synthesis	Binds to 50S ribosomal subunit Blocks aminoacyl tRNA attachment	1. Drug inactivation (chloramphenicol acetyltransferase) 2. Active efflux
E	Tetracycline	Protein synthesis	Binds to 30S ribosomal subunit Blocks binding of aminoacyl tRNA	1. Decreased intracellular drug accumulation (active efflux) 2. Insensitivity of target
F	Aminoglycosides (gentamicin)	Protein synthesis	Bind to 30S ribosomal subunit Inhibit translocation of peptidyl-tRNA	1. Drug inactivation (aminoglycoside-modifying enzyme) 2. Decreased permeability through gram-negative outer membrane 3. Active efflux 4. Ribosomal methylation
G	Mupirocin	Protein synthesis	Inhibits isoleucine tRNA synthetase	Mutation of gene for target protein or acquisition of new gene for drug-insensitive target
H	Streptogramins [quinupristin/ dalfopristin (Synercid)]	Protein synthesis	Bind to 50S ribosomal subunit Block peptide chain elongation	1. Alteration of target (ribosomal methylation: dalfopristin) 2. Active efflux (quinupristin) 3. Drug inactivation (quinupristin and dalfopristin)
I	Linezolid	Protein synthesis	Binds to 50S ribosomal subunit Inhibits initiation of protein synthesis	Alteration of target (mutation of 23S rRNA)
J	Sulfonamides and trimethoprim	Cell metabolism	Competitively inhibit enzymes involved in two steps of folic acid biosynthesis	Production of insensitive targets [dihydropteroate synthetase (sulfonamides) and dihydrofolate reductase (trimethoprim)] that bypass metabolic block
K	Rifampin	Nucleic acid synthesis	Inhibits DNA-dependent RNA polymerase	Insensitivity of target (mutation of polymerase gene)
L	Metronidazole	Nucleic acid synthesis	Intracellularly generates short-lived reactive intermediates that damage DNA by electron transfer system	Not defined
M	Quinolones (ciprofloxacin)	DNA synthesis	Inhibit activity of DNA gyrase (A subunit) and topoisomerase IV	1. Insensitivity of target (mutation of gyrase genes) 2. Decreased intracellular drug accumulation (active efflux)
	Novobiocin	DNA synthesis	Inhibits activity of DNA gyrase (B subunit)	Not defined
N	Polymyxins (polymyxin B)	Cell membrane	Disrupt membrane permeability by charge alteration	Not defined
	Gramicidin	Cell membrane	Forms pores	Not defined
O	Daptomycin	Cell membrane	Forms channels that disrupt membrane potential	Alteration of membrane charge

[a] Compounds in parentheses are major representatives for the class.

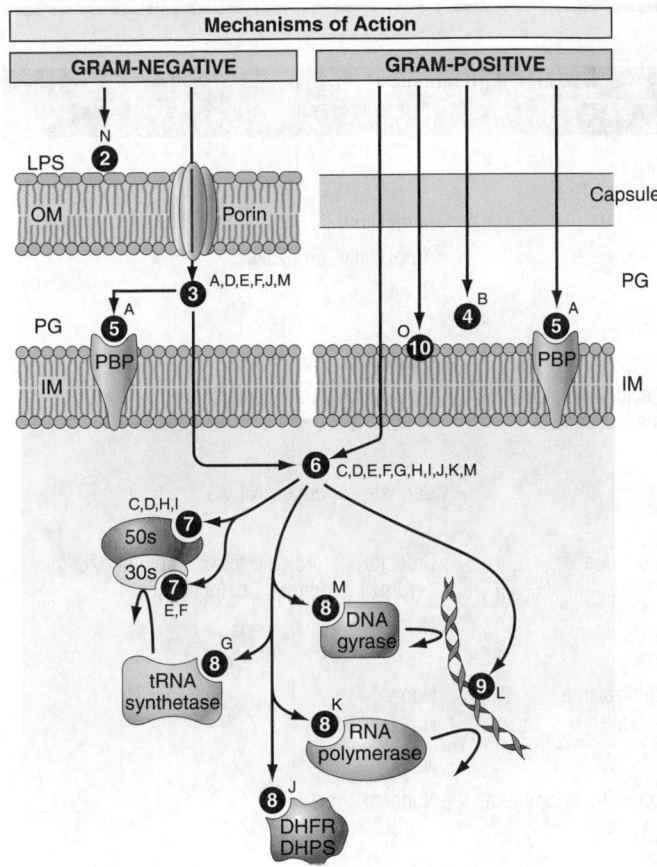

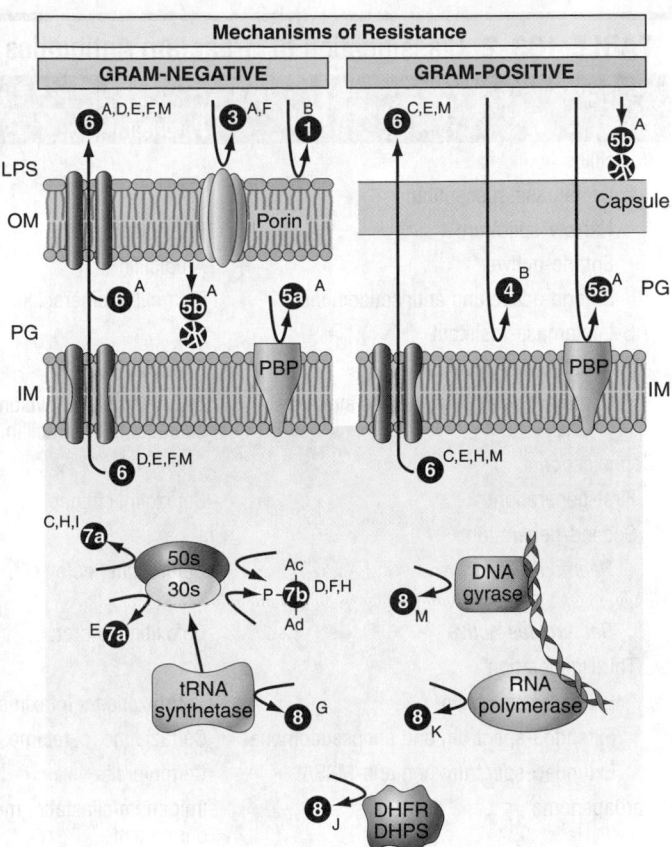

② Detergent action on lipid gram ⊖ outer membrane.

③ Penetration of hydrophilic drugs through porin channels in gram ⊖ outer membrane.

④ Free diffusion through gram ⊕ cell envelope with binding to cell wall PG **or**

⑤ Binding to cell membrane PBP. Drug confined to space external to IM.

⑥ Diffusion or transport of drugs with intracellular target through IM.

⑦ Binding to ribosomal target for protein synthesis inhibition.

⑧ Antibiotic interaction with target protein leading to metabolic (DHFR, DHPS), protein synthetic (tRNA synthetase), or nucleic acid (DNA gyrase, RNA polymerase) abnormalities.

⑨ Direct interaction of reactive intermediates with nucleic acid.

⑩ Insertion into cell membrane, disrupting membrane potential.

① **Intrinsic resistance:** Inability of antibiotic to penetrate gram ⊖ envelope (e.g., vancomycin).

③ Mutant porin channels **decrease** antimicrobial **penetration**.

④ **Production of insensitive target** by acquired gene mediating production of altered peptidoglycan.

⑤a **Production of β-lactam-insensitive PBP target** by mutation of gene or acquisition of new gene.

⑤b **Inactivation** of β-lactam antibiotic by β-lactamases in periplasm (gram ⊖) or surrounding medium (gram ⊕).

⑥ **Active efflux** of drugs from cytoplasm or from gram ⊖ periplasm.

⑦a Decreased ribosomal binding due to **target site alteration**.

⑦b **Inactivation** of drug by chemical modification leading to decreased ribosomal interaction.

⑧ Mutation of target gene or acquisition of new gene producing a **drug-insensitive target** protein.

Figure 133-1 **Mechanisms of action of and resistance to antibacterial agents.** Black lines trace the routes of drug interaction with bacterial cells, from entry to target site. The letters in each figure indicate specific antibacterial agents or classes of agents, as shown in Table 133-1. The numbers correspond to mechanisms listed beneath each panel. 50s and 30s, large and small ribosome subunits; Ac, acetylation; Ad, adenylation; DHFR, dihydrofolate reductase; DHPS, dihydropteroate synthetase; IM, inner (cytoplasmic) membrane; LPS, lipopolysaccharide; OM, outer membrane; P, phosphorylation; PBP, penicillin-binding protein; PG, peptidoglycan.

of structurally related compounds containing three linked hexose sugars. They exert a bactericidal effect by binding irreversibly to the 30S subunit of the bacterial ribosome and inhibiting translocation of peptidyl-tRNA from the A to the P site. Uptake of aminoglycosides and their penetration through the cell membrane constitute an aerobic, energy-dependent process. Thus, aminoglycoside activity is markedly reduced in an anaerobic environment. *Spectinomycin*, an aminocyclitol antibiotic, also acts on the 30S ribosomal subunit but has a different mechanism of action from the aminoglycosides and is bacteriostatic rather than bactericidal.

Macrolides, ketolides, and lincosamides *Macrolide antibiotics* (erythromycin, clarithromycin, and azithromycin) consist of a

large lactone ring to which sugars are attached. *Ketolide antibiotics*, including telithromycin, replace the cladinose sugar on the macrolactone ring with a ketone group. These drugs bind specifically to the 50S portion of the bacterial ribosome and inhibit protein chain elongation. Although structurally unrelated to the macrolides, *lincosamides* (clindamycin and lincomycin) bind to a site on the 50S ribosome nearly identical to the binding site for macrolides.

Streptogramins Streptogramins [quinupristin (streptogramin B) and dalfopristin (streptogramin A)], which are supplied as a combination in Synercid, are peptide macrolactones that also bind to the 50S ribosomal subunit and block protein synthesis. Streptogramin B binds to a ribosomal site similar to the binding site for macrolides

TABLE 133-2 Classification of β-Lactam Antibiotics

Class	Route of Administration	
	Parenteral	Oral
Penicillins		
β-Lactamase-susceptible		
Narrow-spectrum	Penicillin G	Penicillin V
Enteric-active	Ampicillin	Amoxicillin, ampicillin
Enteric-active and antipseudomonal	Ticarcillin, piperacillin	None
β-Lactamase-resistant		
Antistaphylococcal	Oxacillin, nafcillin	Cloxacillin, dicloxacillin
Combined with β-lactamase inhibitors	Ticarcillin plus clavulanic acid, ampicillin plus sulbactam, piperacillin plus tazobactam	Amoxicillin plus clavulanic acid
Cephalosporins		
First-generation	Cefazolin, cephapirin	Cephalexin, cefadroxil
Second-generation		
Haemophilus-active	Cefuroxime, cefonicid, ceforanide	Cefaclor, cefuroxime axetil, ceftibuten, cefdinir, cefprozil, cefditoren, cefpodoxime[a]
Bacteroides-active	Cefoxitin, cefotetan	None
Third-generation		
Extended-spectrum	Ceftriaxone, cefotaxime, ceftizoxime	None
Extended-spectrum and antipseudomonal	Ceftazidime, cefepime	None
Extended-spectrum and anti-MRSA[b]	Ceftobiprole	None
Carbapenems	Imipenem/cilastatin, meropenem, ertapenem, doripenem	None
Monobactams	Aztreonam	None

[a]Some sources classify cefpodoxime as a third-generation oral agent because of a marginally broader spectrum.
[b]Methicillin-resistant *Staphylococcus aureus*.

and lincosamides, whereas streptogramin A binds to a different ribosomal site, blocking the late phase of protein synthesis. The two streptogramins act synergistically to kill bacteria if the strain is susceptible to both components.

Chloramphenicol Chloramphenicol consists of a single aromatic ring and a short side chain. This antibiotic binds reversibly to the 50S portion of the bacterial ribosome at a site close to but not identical with the binding sites for the macrolides and lincosamides, inhibiting peptide bond formation by blocking attachment of the amino acid end of aminoacyl-tRNA to the ribosome.

Linezolid Linezolid is the only commercially available drug in the oxazolidinone class. Linezolid binds to the 50S ribosomal subunit and blocks the initiation of protein synthesis.

Tetracyclines and glycylcyclines Tetracyclines (tetracycline, doxycycline, and minocycline) and glycylcyclines (tigecycline) consist of four aromatic rings with various substituent groups. They interact reversibly with the bacterial 30S ribosomal subunit, blocking the binding of aminoacyl tRNA to the mRNA-ribosome complex. This mechanism is markedly different from that of the aminoglycosides, which also bind to the 30S subunit.

Mupirocin Mupirocin (pseudomonic acid) inhibits isoleucine tRNA synthetase by competing with bacterial isoleucine for its binding site on the enzyme and depleting cellular stores of isoleucine-charged tRNA.

■ INHIBITION OF BACTERIAL METABOLISM

The *antimetabolites* are all synthetic compounds that interfere with bacterial synthesis of folic acid. Products of the folic acid synthesis pathway function as coenzymes for the one-carbon transfer reactions that are essential for the synthesis of thymidine, all purines, and several amino acids. Inhibition of folate synthesis leads to cessation of bacterial cell growth and, in some cases, to bacterial cell death. The principal antibacterial antimetabolites are sulfonamides (sulfisoxazole, sulfadiazine, and sulfamethoxazole) and trimethoprim.

Sulfonamides Sulfonamides are structural analogues of *p*-aminobenzoic acid (PABA), one of the three structural components of folic acid (the other two being pteridine and glutamate). The first step in the synthesis of folic acid is the addition of PABA to pteridine by the enzyme dihydropteroic acid synthetase. Sulfonamides compete with PABA as substrates for the enzyme. The selective effect of sulfonamides is due to the fact that bacteria synthesize folic acid, while mammalian cells cannot synthesize the cofactor and must use exogenous supplies. However, the activity of sulfonamides can be greatly reduced by the presence of excess PABA or by the exogenous addition of end products of one-carbon transfer reactions (e.g., thymidine and purines). High concentrations of the latter substances may be present in some infections as a result of tissue and white cell breakdown, compromising sulfonamide activity.

Trimethoprim Trimethoprim is a diaminopyrimidine, a structural analogue of the pteridine moiety of folic acid. Trimethoprim is a competitive inhibitor of dihydrofolate reductase; this enzyme is responsible for reduction of dihydrofolic acid to tetrahydrofolic acid—the essential final component in the folic acid synthesis pathway. Like that of the sulfonamides, the activity of trimethoprim is compromised in the presence of exogenous thymine or thymidine.

INHIBITION OF NUCLEIC ACID SYNTHESIS OR ACTIVITY

Numerous antibacterial compounds have disparate effects on nucleic acids.

Quinolones The quinolones, including nalidixic acid and its fluorinated derivatives (ciprofloxacin, levofloxacin, and moxifloxacin), are synthetic compounds that inhibit the activity of the A subunit of the bacterial enzyme DNA gyrase as well as topoisomerase IV. DNA gyrase and topoisomerases are responsible for negative supercoiling of DNA—an essential conformation for DNA replication in the intact cell. Inhibition of the activity of DNA gyrase and topoisomerase IV is lethal to bacterial cells. The antibiotic *novobiocin* also interferes with the activity of DNA gyrase, but it interferes with the B subunit.

Rifampin Rifampin, used primarily against *Mycobacterium tuberculosis*, is also active against a variety of other bacteria. Rifampin binds tightly to the B subunit of bacterial DNA-dependent RNA polymerase, thus inhibiting transcription of DNA into RNA. Mammalian-cell RNA polymerase is not sensitive to this compound.

Nitrofurantoin Nitrofurantoin, a synthetic compound, causes DNA damage. The nitrofurans, compounds containing a single five-membered ring, are reduced by a bacterial enzyme to highly reactive, short-lived intermediates that are thought to cause DNA strand breakage, either directly or indirectly.

Metronidazole Metronidazole, a synthetic imidazole, is active only against anaerobic bacteria and protozoa. The reduction of metronidazole's nitro group by the bacterial anaerobic electron-transport system produces a transient series of reactive intermediates that are thought to cause DNA damage.

ALTERATION OF CELL-MEMBRANE PERMEABILITY

Polymyxins The polymyxins [polymyxin B and colistin (polymyxin E)] are cyclic, basic polypeptides. They behave as cationic, surface-active compounds that disrupt the permeability of both the outer and the cytoplasmic membranes of gram-negative bacteria.

Gramicidin A Gramicidin A is a polypeptide of 15 amino acids that acts as an ionophore, forming pores or channels in lipid bilayers.

Daptomycin Insertion of daptomycin, a bactericidal lipopeptide antibiotic, into the cell membrane of gram-positive bacteria forms a channel that causes depolarization of the membrane by efflux of intracellular ions, resulting in cell death.

MECHANISMS OF RESISTANCE

Some bacteria exhibit *intrinsic resistance* to certain classes of antibacterial agents (e.g., obligate anaerobic bacteria to aminoglycosides and gram-negative bacteria to vancomycin). In addition, bacteria that are ordinarily susceptible to antibacterial agents can acquire resistance. *Acquired resistance* is a major limitation to effective antibacterial chemotherapy. Resistance can develop by mutation of resident genes or by acquisition of new genes. New genes mediating resistance are usually spread from cell to cell by way of mobile genetic elements such as plasmids, transposons, and bacteriophages. The resistant bacterial populations flourish in areas of high antimicrobial use, where they enjoy a selective advantage over susceptible populations.

The major mechanisms used by bacteria to resist the action of antimicrobial agents are inactivation of the compound, alteration or overproduction of the antibacterial target through mutation of the target protein's gene, acquisition of a new gene that encodes a drug-insensitive target, decreased permeability of the cell envelope to the agent, failure to convert an inactive prodrug to its active derivative, and active efflux of the compound from the periplasm or interior

of the cell. Specific mechanisms of bacterial resistance to the major antibacterial agents are outlined below, summarized in Table 133-1, and depicted in Fig. 133-1.

β-LACTAM ANTIBIOTICS

Bacteria develop resistance to β-lactam antibiotics by a variety of mechanisms. Most common is the destruction of the drug by β-lactamases. The β-lactamases of gram-negative bacteria are confined to the periplasm, between the inner and outer membranes, while gram-positive bacteria secrete their β-lactamases into the surrounding medium. These enzymes have a higher affinity for the antibiotic than the antibiotic has for its target. Binding results in hydrolysis of the β-lactam ring. Genes encoding β-lactamases have been found in both chromosomal and extrachromosomal locations and in both gram-positive and gram-negative bacteria; these genes are often on mobile genetic elements. Many "advanced-generation" β-lactam antibiotics, such as ceftriaxone and cefepime, are stable in the presence of plasmid-mediated β-lactamases and are active against bacteria resistant to earlier-generation β-lactam antibiotics. However, extended-spectrum β-lactamases (ESBLs), either acquired on mobile genetic elements by gram-negative bacteria (e.g., *Klebsiella pneumoniae* and *Escherichia coli*) or present as stable chromosomal genes in other gram-negative species (e.g., *Enterobacter* spp.), have broad substrate specificity, hydrolyzing virtually all penicillins and cephalosporins. Carbapenems are generally resistant to ESBL hydrolysis and are the drugs of choice for the treatment of infections caused by ESBL-producing Enterobacteriaceae. However, Enterobacteriaceae (particularly *K. pneumoniae*) that produce carbapenemases and are resistant to virtually all β-lactam antibiotics have now emerged. One strategy that has been devised for circumventing resistance mediated by β-lactamases is to combine the β-lactam agent with an inhibitor that avidly binds the inactivating enzyme, preventing its attack on the antibiotic. Unfortunately, the inhibitors (e.g., clavulanic acid, sulbactam, and tazobactam) do not bind all chromosomal β-lactamases (e.g., that of *Enterobacter*) or carbapenemases and thus cannot be depended on to prevent the inactivation of β-lactam antibiotics by such enzymes. No β-lactam antibiotic or inhibitor has been produced that can resist all of the many β-lactamases that have been identified.

A second mechanism of bacterial resistance to β-lactam antibiotics is an alteration in PBP targets so that the PBPs have a markedly reduced affinity for the drug. While this alteration may occur by mutation of existing genes, the acquisition of new PBP genes (as in staphylococcal resistance to methicillin) or of new pieces of PBP genes (as in streptococcal, gonococcal, and meningococcal resistance to penicillin) is more important.

A final resistance mechanism is the coupling, in gram-negative bacteria, of a decrease in outer-membrane permeability with rapid efflux of the antibiotic from the periplasm to the cell exterior. Mutations of genes encoding outer-membrane protein channels called *porins* decrease the entry of β-lactam antibiotics into the cell, while additional proteins form channels that actively pump β-lactams out of the cell. Resistance of Enterobacteriaceae to some cephalosporins and resistance of *Pseudomonas* spp. to cephalosporins and piperacillin are the best examples of this mechanism.

VANCOMYCIN

Clinically important resistance to vancomycin was first described among enterococci in France in 1988. Vancomycin-resistant enterococci (VRE) have subsequently become disseminated worldwide. The genes encoding resistance are carried on plasmids that can transfer themselves from cell to cell and on transposons that can jump from plasmids to chromosomes. Resistance is mediated by enzymes that substitute D-lactate for D-alanine on the peptidoglycan stem peptide so that there is no longer an appropriate target for vancomycin binding. This alteration does not appear to affect cell-wall integrity, however. This type of acquired vancomycin resistance was confined for 14 years to enterococci—more specifically, to *Enterococcus faecium* rather than the more common pathogen *E. faecalis*. However, since 2002, *S. aureus* isolates that are highly resistant to vancomycin have been recovered from 11 patients in the United States. All of the isolates contain *vanA*, the gene that mediates vancomycin resistance in enterococci. In addition, since 1996, a few isolates of both *S. aureus* and *Staphylococcus epidermidis* that display a four- to eightfold reduction in susceptibility to vancomycin have been found worldwide; such *S. aureus* strains are termed vancomycin-intermediate-susceptibility *S. aureus*, or VISA. Many more isolates may contain subpopulations with reduced vancomycin susceptibility (heteroVISA, or hVISA). These isolates have not acquired the genes that mediate vancomycin resistance in enterococci but are mutant bacteria with markedly thickened cell walls. These mutants were apparently selected in patients who were undergoing prolonged vancomycin therapy. The failure of vancomycin therapy in some patients infected with *S. aureus* or *S. epidermidis* strains exhibiting only intermediate susceptibility to this drug is thought to have resulted from this resistance.

■ DAPTOMYCIN

In some *S. aureus* isolates with reduced susceptibility to daptomycin, a mutation in the *mprF* gene leads to an increase in the net positive charge of the bacterial membrane, repelling the antibiotic.

■ AMINOGLYCOSIDES

The most common aminoglycoside resistance mechanism is inactivation of the antibiotic. Aminoglycoside-modifying enzymes, usually encoded on plasmids, transfer phosphate, adenyl, or acetyl residues from intracellular molecules to hydroxyl or amino side groups on the antibiotic. The modified antibiotic is less active because of diminished binding to its ribosomal target. Modifying enzymes that can inactivate any of the available aminoglycosides have been found in both gram-positive and gram-negative bacteria. A second aminoglycoside resistance mechanism, which has been identified predominantly in clinical isolates of *Pseudomonas aeruginosa*, is decreased antibiotic uptake, presumably due to alterations in the bacterial outer membrane. A third, emerging form of resistance in gram-negative bacteria is methylation of the target 16S ribosomal RNA, which is mediated by plasmid-encoded methylases.

■ MACROLIDES, KETOLIDES, LINCOSAMIDES, AND STREPTOGRAMINS

Resistance in gram-positive bacteria, which are the usual target organisms for macrolides, ketolides, lincosamides, and streptogramins, can be due to the production of an enzyme—most commonly plasmid-encoded—that methylates ribosomal RNA, interfering with binding of the antibiotics to their target. Methylation mediates resistance to erythromycin, clarithromycin, azithromycin, clindamycin, and streptogramin B. Resistance to streptogramin B converts quinupristin/dalfopristin from a bactericidal to a bacteriostatic antibiotic. Streptococci can also actively cause the efflux of macrolides, and staphylococci can cause the efflux of macrolides, clindamycin, and streptogramin A. Ketolides such as telithromycin retain activity against most isolates of *Streptococcus pneumoniae* that are resistant to macrolides. In addition, staphylococci can inactivate streptogramin A by acetylation and streptogramin B by either acetylation or hydrolysis. Finally, mutations in 23S ribosomal RNA that alter the binding of macrolides to their targets have been found in both staphylococci and streptococci.

■ CHLORAMPHENICOL

Most bacteria resistant to chloramphenicol produce a plasmid-encoded enzyme, chloramphenicol acetyltransferase, that inactivates the compound by acetylation.

■ TETRACYCLINES AND TIGECYCLINE

The most common mechanism of tetracycline resistance in gram-negative bacteria is a plasmid-encoded active-efflux pump that is inserted into the cytoplasmic membrane and extrudes antibiotic from the cell. Resistance in gram-positive bacteria is due either to active efflux or to ribosomal alterations that diminish binding of the antibiotic to its target. Genes involved in ribosomal protection are found on mobile genetic elements. The parenteral tetracycline derivative tigecycline (a glycylcycline) is active against tetracycline-resistant bacteria because it is not removed by efflux and can bind to altered ribosomes.

■ MUPIROCIN

Although the topical compound mupirocin was introduced into clinical use relatively recently, resistance is already becoming widespread in some areas. The mechanism appears to be either mutation of the target isoleucine tRNA synthetase so that it is no longer inhibited by the antibiotic or plasmid-encoded production of a form of the target enzyme that binds mupirocin poorly.

■ TRIMETHOPRIM AND SULFONAMIDES

The most prevalent mechanism of resistance to trimethoprim and the sulfonamides in both gram-positive and gram-negative bacteria is the acquisition of plasmid-encoded genes that produce a new, drug-insensitive target—specifically, an insensitive dihydrofolate reductase for trimethoprim and an altered dihydropteroate synthetase for sulfonamides.

■ QUINOLONES

The most common mechanism of resistance to quinolones is the development of one or more mutations in target DNA gyrases and topoisomerase IV that prevent the antibacterial agent from interfering with the enzymes' activity. Some gram-negative bacteria develop mutations that both decrease outer-membrane porin permeability and cause active drug efflux from the cytoplasm. Mutations that result in active quinolone efflux are also found in gram-positive bacteria.

■ RIFAMPIN

Bacteria rapidly become resistant to rifampin by developing mutations in the B subunit of RNA polymerase that render the enzyme unable to bind the antibiotic. The rapid selection of resistant mutants is the major limitation to the use of this antibiotic against otherwise-susceptible staphylococci and requires that the drug be used in combination with another antistaphylococcal agent.

■ LINEZOLID

Enterococci, streptococci, and staphylococci can become resistant to linezolid in vitro by mutation of the 23S rRNA binding site. Clinical isolates of *E. faecium* and *E. faecalis* acquire resistance to linezolid readily by this mechanism, often during therapy. A new plasmid-encoded resistance gene has been found in staphylococci that methylates the linezolid ribosomal binding site. At least one outbreak of linezolid-resistant *S. aureus* infections caused by isolates carrying this gene has been described.

■ MULTIPLE ANTIBIOTIC RESISTANCE

The acquisition by one bacterium of resistance to multiple antibacterial agents is becoming increasingly common. The two major mechanisms are the acquisition of multiple unrelated resistance genes and the development of mutations in a single gene or gene complex that mediate resistance to a series of unrelated compounds. The construction of multiresistant strains by acquisition of multiple genes occurs by sequential steps of gene transfer and environmental selection in areas of high-level antimicrobial use. In contrast, mutations in a single gene can conceivably be selected in a single step. Bacteria that are multiresistant by virtue of the acquisition of new genes include hospital-associated strains of gram-negative bacteria, enterococci, and staphylococci and community-acquired strains of salmonellae, gonococci, and pneumococci. Mutations that confer resistance to multiple unrelated antimicrobial agents occur in the genes encoding outer-membrane porins and efflux proteins of gram-negative bacteria. These mutations decrease bacterial intracellular and periplasmic accumulation of β-lactams, quinolones, tetracyclines, chloramphenicol, and aminoglycosides. Multiresistant bacterial isolates pose increasing problems in U.S. hospitals; strains resistant to all available antibacterial chemotherapy have already been identified.

PHARMACOKINETICS OF ANTIBIOTICS

The *pharmacokinetic profile* of an antibacterial agent refers to its concentrations in serum and tissue versus time and reflects the processes of absorption, distribution, metabolism, and excretion. Important characteristics include peak and trough serum concentrations and mathematically derived parameters such as half-life, clearance, and distribution volume. Pharmacokinetic information is useful for estimating the appropriate antibacterial dose and frequency of administration, for adjusting dosages in patients with impaired excretory capacity, and for comparing one drug with another. In contrast, the *pharmacodynamic profile* of an antibiotic refers to the relationship between the pharmacokinetics of the antibiotic and its minimal inhibitory concentrations (MICs) for bacteria (see "Principles of Antibacterial Chemotherapy," below). For further discussion of basic pharmacokinetic principles, see Chap. 5.

■ ABSORPTION

Antibiotic *absorption* refers to the rate and extent of a drug's systemic bioavailability after oral, IM, or IV administration.

Oral administration

Most patients with infection are treated with oral antibacterial agents in the outpatient setting. Advantages of oral therapy over parenteral therapy include lower cost, generally fewer adverse effects (including complications of indwelling lines), and greater acceptance by patients. The percentage of an orally administered antibacterial agent that is absorbed (i.e., its *bioavailability*) ranges from as little as 10–20% (erythromycin and penicillin G) to nearly 100% [amoxicillin, clindamycin, metronidazole, doxycycline, trimethoprim-sulfamethoxazole (TMP-SMX), linezolid, and most fluoroquinolones]. These differences in bioavailability are not clinically important as long as drug concentrations at the site of infection are sufficient to inhibit or kill the pathogen. However, therapeutic efficacy may be compromised when absorption is reduced as a result of physiologic or pathologic conditions (such as the presence of food for some drugs or the shunting of blood away from the gastrointestinal tract in patients with hypotension), drug interactions (e.g., of quinolones and metal cations), or noncompliance. The oral route is usually used for patients with relatively mild infections in whom absorption is not thought to be compromised by the preceding conditions. In addition, the oral route can often be used in more severely ill patients after they have responded to parenteral therapy and can take oral medications.

Intramuscular administration

Although the IM route of administration usually results in 100% bioavailability, it is not as widely used in the United States as the oral and IV routes, in part because of the pain often associated with IM injections and the relative ease of IV access in the hospitalized patient. IM injection may be suitable for specific indications requiring an "immediate" and reliable effect (e.g., with long-acting forms of penicillin, including benzathine and procaine, and with single doses of ceftriaxone for acute otitis media or uncomplicated gonococcal infection).

Intravenous administration

The IV route is appropriate when oral antibacterial agents are not effective against a particular pathogen, when bioavailability is uncertain, or when larger doses are required than are feasible with the oral route. After IV administration, bioavailability is 100%; serum concentrations are maximal at the end of the infusion. For many patients in whom long-term antimicrobial therapy is required and oral therapy is not feasible, outpatient parenteral antibiotic therapy (OPAT), including the use of convenient portable pumps, may be cost-effective and safe. Alternatively, some oral antibacterial drugs (e.g., fluoroquinolones) are sufficiently active against many Enterobacteriaceae to provide potency equal to that of parenteral therapy; oral use of such drugs may allow the patient to return home from the hospital earlier or to avoid hospitalization entirely.

■ DISTRIBUTION

To be effective, concentrations of an antibacterial agent must exceed the pathogen's MIC. Serum antibiotic concentrations usually exceed the MIC for susceptible bacteria, but since most infections are extravascular, the antibiotic must also distribute to the site of the infection. Concentrations of most antibacterial agents in interstitial fluid are similar to free-drug concentrations in serum. However, when the infection is located in a "protected" site where penetration is poor, such as cerebrospinal fluid (CSF), the eye, the prostate, or infected cardiac vegetations, high parenteral doses or local administration for prolonged periods may be required for cure. In addition, even though an antibacterial agent may penetrate to the site of infection, its activity may be antagonized by factors in the local environment, such as an unfavorable pH or inactivation by cellular degradation products. For example, daptomycin's binding to pulmonary surfactant is believed to account for its poor efficacy in the treatment of pneumonia. In addition, the abscess milieu reduces the penetration and local activity of many antibacterial compounds, so that surgical drainage may be required for cure.

Most bacteria that cause human infections are located extracellularly. Intracellular pathogens such as *Legionella*, *Chlamydia*, *Brucella*, and *Salmonella* may persist or cause relapse if the antibacterial agent does not enter the cell. In general, β-lactams, vancomycin, and aminoglycosides penetrate cells poorly, whereas macrolides, ketolides, tetracyclines, metronidazole, chloramphenicol, rifampin, TMP-SMX, and quinolones penetrate cells well.

■ METABOLISM AND ELIMINATION

Like other drugs, antibacterial agents are disposed of by hepatic elimination (metabolism or biliary elimination), by renal excretion of the unchanged or metabolized form, or by a combination of the two processes. For most of the antibacterial drugs, metabolism leads to loss of in vitro activity, although some agents, such as cefotaxime, rifampin, and clarithromycin, have bioactive metabolites that may contribute to their overall efficacy.

The most practical application of information on the mode of excretion of an antibacterial agent is in adjusting dosage when elimination capability is impaired (Table 133-3). Direct, nonidiosyncratic toxicity from antibacterial drugs may result from failure to reduce the dosage given to patients with impaired elimination. For agents that are primarily cleared intact by glomerular filtration,

TABLE 133-3 Antibacterial Drug Dose Adjustments in Patients With Renal Impairment

Antibiotic	Major Route of Excretion	Dosage Adjustment with Renal Impairment
Aminoglycosides	Renal	Yes
Azithromycin	Biliary	No
Cefazolin	Renal	Yes
Cefepime	Renal	Yes
Ceftazidime	Renal	Yes
Ceftriaxone	Renal/biliary	Modest reduction in severe renal impairment
Ciprofloxacin	Renal/biliary	Only in severe renal insufficiency
Clarithromycin	Renal/biliary	Only in severe renal insufficiency
Daptomycin	Renal	Yes
Erythromycin	Biliary	Only when given in high IV doses
Levofloxacin	Renal	Yes
Linezolid	Metabolism	No
Metronidazole	Biliary	No
Nafcillin	Biliary	No
Penicillin G	Renal	Yes (when given in high IV doses)
Piperacillin	Renal	Only with Cl_{cr} of <40 mL/min
Quinupristin/ dalfopristin	Metabolism	No
Tigecycline	Biliary	No
TMP-SMX	Renal/biliary	Only in severe renal insufficiency
Vancomycin	Renal	Yes

Note: Cl_{cr}, creatinine clearance rate; TMP-SMX, trimethoprim-sulfamethoxazole.

drug clearance is correlated with creatinine clearance, and estimates of the latter can be used to guide dosage. For drugs, the elimination of which is primarily hepatic, no simple marker is useful for dosage adjustment in patients with liver disease. However, in patients with severe hepatic disease, residual metabolic capability is usually sufficient to preclude accumulation and toxic effects.

PRINCIPLES OF ANTIBACTERIAL CHEMOTHERAPY

The choice of an antibacterial compound for a particular patient and a specific infection involves more than just a knowledge of the agent's pharmacokinetic profile and in vitro activity. The basic tenets of chemotherapy, to be elaborated below, include the following: When appropriate, material containing the infecting organism(s) should be obtained before the start of treatment so that presumptive identification can be made by microscopic examination of stained specimens and the organism can be grown for definitive identification and susceptibility testing. Awareness of local susceptibility patterns is useful when the patient is treated empirically. Once the organism is identified and its susceptibility to antibacterial agents is determined, the regimen with the narrowest effective spectrum should be chosen. The choice of antibacterial agent is guided by the pharmacokinetic and adverse-reaction profile of active compounds, the site of infection, the immune status of the

host, and evidence of efficacy from well-performed clinical trials. If all other factors are equal, the least expensive antibacterial regimen should be chosen.

■ SUSCEPTIBILITY OF BACTERIA TO ANTIBACTERIAL DRUGS IN VITRO

Determination of the susceptibility of the patient's infecting organism to a panel of appropriate antibacterial agents is an essential first step in devising a chemotherapeutic regimen. Susceptibility testing is designed to estimate the susceptibility of a bacterial isolate to an antibacterial drug under standardized conditions. These conditions favor rapidly growing aerobic or facultative organisms and assess bacteriostasis only. Specialized testing is required for the assessment of bactericidal antimicrobial activity; for the detection of resistance among such fastidious organisms as obligate anaerobes, *Haemophilus* spp., and pneumococci; and for the determination of resistance phenotypes with variable expression, such as resistance to methicillin or oxacillin among staphylococci. Antimicrobial susceptibility testing is important when susceptibility is unpredictable, most often as a result of increasing acquired resistance among bacteria infecting hospitalized patients.

■ PHARMACODYNAMICS: RELATIONSHIP OF PHARMACOKINETICS AND IN VITRO SUSCEPTIBILITY TO CLINICAL RESPONSE

Bacteria have historically been considered *susceptible* to an antibacterial drug if the achievable peak serum concentration exceeds the MIC by approximately fourfold. Each antibiotic has a *breakpoint* concentration that separates susceptible from resistant bacteria (Fig. 133-2). When a majority of isolates of a given bacterial species are inhibited at concentrations below the breakpoint, the species is considered to be within the spectrum of the antibiotic.

The *pharmacokinetic-pharmacodynamic (PK-PD) profile* of an antibiotic refers to the quantitative relationships between the time course of antibiotic concentrations in serum and tissue, in vitro susceptibility (MIC), and microbial response (inhibition of growth or rate of killing). Three PK-PD parameters quantify these relationships: the ratio of the area under the plasma concentration vs. time curve to the MIC (AUC/MIC), the ratio of the maximal serum concentration to the MIC (C_{max}/MIC), and the time during a dosing

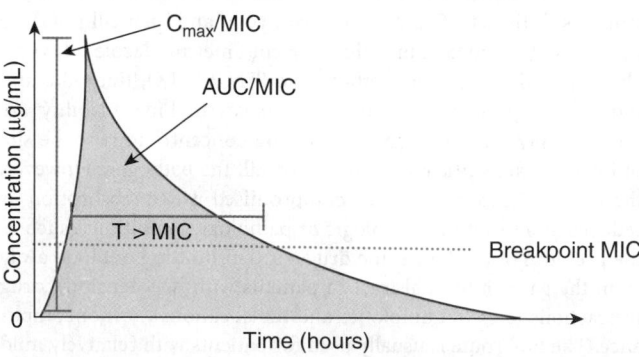

Figure 133-2 Relationship between the pharmacokinetic-pharmacodynamic (PK-PD) properties of an antibiotic and susceptibility. An organism is considered "susceptible" to an antibiotic if the drug's minimal inhibitory concentration (MIC) is below its "breakpoint" concentration (see text). PK-PD investigations explore various pharmacodynamic indices and clinical responses, including the ratio of the maximal serum concentration to the MIC (C_{max}/MIC), the ratio of the area under the serum concentration vs. time curve to the MIC (AUC/MIC), and the time during which serum concentrations exceed the MIC (*T* > MIC). See Table 133-4.

TABLE 133-4 Pharmacodynamic Indices of Major Antimicrobial Classes

Parameter Predicting Response	Drug or Drug Class
Time above the MIC	Penicillins, cephalosporins, carbapenems, aztreonam
24-h AUC/MIC	Aminoglycosides, fluoroquinolones, tetracyclines, vancomycin, macrolides, clindamycin, quinupristin/dalfopristin, tigecycline, daptomycin
Peak to MIC	Aminoglycosides, fluoroquinolones

Note: MIC, minimal inhibitory concentration; AUC, area under the concentration curve.

interval that plasma concentrations exceed the MIC ($T >$ MIC). The PK-PD profile of an antibiotic class is characterized as either *concentration dependent* (fluoroquinolones, aminoglycosides), such that an increase in antibiotic concentration leads to a more rapid rate of bacterial death, or *time dependent* (β-lactams), such that the reduction in bacterial density is proportional to the time that concentrations exceed the MIC. For concentration-dependent antibiotics, the C_{max}/MIC or AUC/MIC ratio correlates best with the reduction in microbial density in vitro and in animal investigations. Dosing strategies attempt to maximize these ratios by the administration of a large dose relative to the MIC for anticipated pathogens, often at long intervals (relative to the serum half-life). Once-daily dosing of aminoglycoside antibiotics is one practical consequence of these relationships. Another is the administration of larger doses of vancomycin than have been used in the past (e.g., >2 g/d for an adult with normal renal function) to increase the AUC/MIC ratio in an effort to improve the response rates of patients infected with methicillin-resistant *S. aureus* (MRSA). In contrast, dosage strategies for time-dependent antibiotics emphasize the maintenance of serum concentrations above the MIC for 30–50% of the dose interval. For example, some clinicians advocate prolonged—or even constant—infusions of some β-lactam antibiotics, such as the carbapenems and the β-lactam/β-lactamase inhibitors, to increase the $T >$ MIC between doses. The clinical implications of these pharmacodynamic relationships continue to be elucidated; their consideration has led to more rational antibacterial dosage regimens. Table 133-4 summarizes the pharmacodynamic properties of the major antibiotic classes.

■ STATUS OF THE HOST

Various host factors must be considered in the devising of antibacterial chemotherapy. The host's antibacterial *immune function* is of importance, particularly as it relates to opsonophagocytic function. Since the major host defense against acute, overwhelming bacterial infection is the polymorphonuclear leukocyte, patients with neutropenia must be treated aggressively and empirically with bactericidal drugs for suspected infection (Chap. 86). Likewise, patients who have deficient humoral immunity (e.g., those with chronic lymphocytic leukemia and multiple myeloma) and individuals with surgical or functional asplenia (e.g., those with sickle cell disease) should be treated empirically for infections with encapsulated organisms, especially the pneumococcus.

Pregnancy increases the risk of toxicity of certain antibacterial drugs for the mother (e.g., hepatic toxicity of tetracycline), affects drug disposition and pharmacokinetics, and—because of the risk of fetal toxicity—severely limits the choice of agents for treating infections. Certain antibacterial agents are contraindicated in pregnancy either because their safety has not been established (categories B and C) or because they are known to be toxic (categories D and X). Table 133-5 summarizes antibacterial drug safety in pregnancy.

In patients with *concomitant viral infections*, the incidence of adverse reactions to antibacterial drugs may be unusually high. For example, persons with infectious mononucleosis and those infected with HIV experience skin reactions more often to penicillins and folic acid synthesis inhibitors such as TMP-SMX, respectively.

In addition, the patient's age, sex, racial heritage, genetic background, concomitant drugs, and excretory status all determine the incidence and type of side effects that can be expected with certain antibacterial agents.

■ SITE OF INFECTION

The location of the infected site may play a major role in the choice and dose of antimicrobial drug. Patients with suspected *meningitis* should receive drugs that can cross the blood-CSF barrier; in addition, because of the relative paucity of phagocytes and opsonins at the site of infection, the agents should be bactericidal. β-Lactam drugs are the mainstay of therapy for most of these infections, even though they do not normally reach high concentrations in CSF. Their efficacy is based on the increased permeability of the blood-brain and blood-CSF barriers to hydrophilic molecules during inflammation and the low minimal bactericidal concentrations (MBCs) for most infectious organisms.

The vegetation, which is the major site of infection in *bacterial endocarditis*, is also a focus that is protected from normal host-defense mechanisms. Antibacterial therapy needs to be bactericidal, with the selected agent administered parenterally over a long period and at a dose that can eradicate the infecting organism. Likewise, *osteomyelitis* involves a site that is resistant to opsonophagocytic removal of infecting bacteria; furthermore, avascular bone (sequestrum) represents a foreign body that thwarts normal host-defense mechanisms. *Chronic prostatitis* is exceedingly difficult to cure because most antibiotics do not penetrate through the capillaries serving the prostate, especially when acute inflammation is absent. *Intraocular infections*, especially endophthalmitis, are difficult to treat because retinal capillaries lacking fenestration hinder drug penetration into the vitreous from blood. Inflammation does little to disrupt this barrier. Thus, direct injection into the vitreous is necessary in many cases. Antibiotic penetration into *abscesses* is usually poor, and local conditions (e.g., low pH or the presence of enzymes that hydrolyze the drug) may further antagonize antibacterial activity.

In contrast, *urinary tract infections* (UTIs), when confined to the bladder, are relatively easy to cure, in part because of the higher concentration of most antibiotics in urine than in blood. Since blood is the usual reference fluid in defining susceptibility (Fig. 133-2), even organisms found to be resistant to achievable serum concentrations may be susceptible to achievable urine concentrations. For drugs that are used only for the treatment of UTIs, such as the urinary tract antiseptics nitrofurantoin and methenamine salts, achievable urine concentrations are used to determine susceptibility.

■ COMBINATION CHEMOTHERAPY

One of the tenets of antibacterial chemotherapy is that if the infecting bacterium has been identified, the most specific chemotherapy possible should be used. The use of a single agent with a narrow spectrum of activity against the pathogen diminishes the alteration of normal flora and thus limits the overgrowth of resistant nosocomial organisms (e.g., *Candida albicans*, enterococci, *Clostridium difficile*, or MRSA), avoids the potential toxicity of multiple-drug regimens, and reduces cost. However, certain circumstances call for the use of more than one antibacterial agent. These are summarized below.

TABLE 133-5 Antibacterial Drugs in Pregnancy

Antibacterial Drug (Pregnancy Class[a])	Toxicity in Pregnancy	Recommendation
Aminoglycosides (C/D)	Possible 8th-nerve toxicity	Caution[b]
Chloramphenicol (C)	Gray syndrome in newborn	Caution at term
Fluoroquinolones (C)	Arthropathy in immature animals	Caution
Clarithromycin (C)	Teratogenicity in animals	Contraindicated
Ertapenem (B)	Decreased weight in animals	Caution
Erythromycin estolate (B)	Cholestatic hepatitis	Contraindicated
Imipenem/cilastatin (C)	Toxicity in some pregnant animals	Caution
Linezolid (C)	Embryonic and fetal toxicity in rats	Caution
Meropenem (B)	Unknown	Caution
Metronidazole (B)	None known, but carcinogenic in rats	Caution
Nitrofurantoin (B)	Hemolytic anemia in newborns	Caution; contraindicated at term[c]
Quinupristin/dalfopristin (B)	Unknown	Caution
Sulfonamides (C/D)	Hemolysis in newborn with G6PD[d] deficiency; kernicterus in newborn	Caution; contraindicated at term[c]
Telavancin (C)	Unknown (adverse development in animals)	Pregnancy test before use
Tetracyclines/tigecycline (D)	Tooth discoloration, inhibition of bone growth in fetus; hepatotoxicity	Contraindicated
Vancomycin (C)	Unknown	Caution

[a]**Category A:** Controlled studies in women fail to demonstrate a risk to the fetus; the possibility of fetal harm appears remote.

Category B: Either (1) animal reproduction studies have not demonstrated a fetal risk but there are no controlled studies in pregnant women or (2) animal reproduction studies have shown an adverse effect (other than a decrease in fertility) that was not confirmed in controlled studies of women in the first trimester (and there is no evidence of risk in later trimesters).

Category C: Studies in animals have revealed adverse effects on the fetus (teratogenic, embryocidal, or other), but no controlled studies of women have been conducted. Drug should be given only if the potential benefit justifies the potential risk to the fetus.

Category D: There is positive evidence of human fetal risk, but the benefits from use in pregnant women may nevertheless be acceptable (e.g., if the drug is needed in a life-threatening situation or for a serious disease against which safer drugs cannot be used or are ineffective).

[b]Use only for strong clinical indication in the absence of a suitable alternative.

[c]See Crider et al, 2009.

[d]G6PD, glucose-6-phosphate dehydrogenase.

1. *Prevention of the emergence of resistant mutants.* Spontaneous mutations occur at a detectable frequency in certain genes encoding the target proteins for some antibacterial agents. The use of these agents can eliminate the susceptible population, select out resistant mutants at the site of infection, and result in the failure of chemotherapy. Resistant mutants are usually selected when the MIC of the antibacterial agent for the infecting bacterium is close to achievable levels in serum or tissues and/or when the site of infection limits the access or activity of the agent. Among the most common examples are rifampin for staphylococci, imipenem for *Pseudomonas*, and fluoroquinolones for staphylococci and *Pseudomonas*. Small-colony variants of staphylococci resistant to aminoglycosides also emerge during monotherapy with these antibiotics. A second antibacterial agent with a mechanism of action different from that of the first is added in an attempt to prevent the emergence of resistant mutants (e.g., imipenem plus an aminoglycoside or a fluoroquinolone for systemic *Pseudomonas* infections). However, since resistant mutants have emerged following combination chemotherapy, this approach clearly is not uniformly successful.

2. *Synergistic or additive activity.* Synergistic or additive activity involves a lowering of the MIC or MBC of each or all of the drugs tested in combination against a specific bacterium. In *synergy*, each agent is more active when combined with a second drug than it would be alone, and the drugs' combined activity is therefore greater than the sum of the individual activities of each drug. In an *additive relationship*, the combined activity of the drugs is equal to the sum of their individual activities. Among the best examples of a synergistic or additive effect, confirmed both in vitro and by animal studies, are the enhanced bactericidal activities of certain β-lactam/aminoglycoside combinations against enterococci, viridans streptococci, and *P. aeruginosa*. The synergistic or additive activity of these combinations has also been demonstrated against selected isolates of enteric gram-negative bacteria and staphylococci. The combination of trimethoprim and sulfamethoxazole has synergistic or additive activity against many enteric gram-negative bacteria. Most other antimicrobial combinations display indifferent activity (i.e., the combination is *no better* than the more active of the two agents alone), and some combinations (e.g., penicillin plus tetracycline against pneumococci) may be antagonistic (i.e., the combination is *worse* than either drug alone).

3. *Therapy directed against multiple potential pathogens.* For certain infections, either a mixture of pathogens is suspected or the patient is desperately ill with an as-yet-unidentified infection (see "Empirical Therapy," below). In these situations, the most important of the likely infecting bacteria must be covered by therapy until culture and susceptibility results become available. Examples of the former infections are intraabdominal or brain abscesses and infections of limbs in diabetic patients with microvascular disease. The latter situations include fevers in neutropenic patients, acute pneumonia from aspiration of oral flora by hospitalized patients, and septic shock or sepsis syndrome.

EMPIRICAL THERAPY

In most situations, antibacterial therapy is begun before a specific bacterial pathogen has been identified. The choice of agent is guided by the results of studies identifying the usual pathogens at that site or in that clinical setting, by pharmacodynamic considerations, and by the resistance profile of the expected pathogens in a particular hospital or geographic area. Situations in which empirical therapy is appropriate include the following:

1. *Life-threatening infection.* Any suspected bacterial infection in a patient with a life-threatening illness should be treated presumptively. Therapy is usually begun with more than one agent and is later tailored to a specific pathogen if one is eventually identified. Early therapy with an effective antimicrobial regimen has consistently been demonstrated to improve survival rates.
2. *Treatment of community-acquired infections.* In most situations, it is appropriate to treat non-life-threatening infections without obtaining cultures. These situations include outpatient infections such as community-acquired upper and lower respiratory tract infections, cystitis, cellulitis or local wound infection, urethritis, and prostatitis. However, if any of these infections recurs or fails to respond to initial therapy, every effort should be made to obtain cultures to guide re-treatment.

CHOICE OF ANTIBACTERIAL THERAPY

Infections for which specific antibacterial agents are among the drugs of choice are detailed in Table 133-6. No attempt has been made to include all of the potential situations in which antibacterial agents may be used. A more detailed discussion of specific bacteria and infections that they cause can be found elsewhere in this volume.

The choice of antibacterial therapy increasingly involves an assessment of the acquired resistance of major microbial pathogens to the antimicrobial agents available to treat them. Resistance rates are dynamic (Table 133-6), both increasing and decreasing in response to the environmental pressure applied by antimicrobial use. For example, increased fluoroquinolone use in the community is associated with increasing rates of quinolone resistance in community-acquired strains of *S. pneumoniae, E. coli, Neisseria gonorrhoeae,* and *K. pneumoniae.* Fluoroquinolone resistance has also emerged rapidly among nosocomial isolates of *S. aureus* and *Pseudomonas* spp. as hospital use of this drug class has increased. It is important to note that, in many cases, wide variations in worldwide antimicrobial-resistance trends may not be reflected in the values recorded at U.S. hospitals. Therefore, the most important factor in choosing initial therapy for an infection in which the susceptibility of the specific pathogen(s) is not known is information on local resistance rates. This information can be obtained from local clinical microbiology laboratories in the annual hospital "antibiogram," from state health departments, or from publications of the Centers for Disease Control and Prevention (e.g., *Antimicrobial Resistance in Healthcare Settings; www.cdc.gov/ncidod/dhqp/ar.html*).

ADVERSE REACTIONS

Adverse drug reactions are frequently classified by mechanism as either *dose-related* ("toxic") or *unpredictable.* Unpredictable reactions are either idiosyncratic or allergic. Dose-related reactions include aminoglycoside-induced nephrotoxicity, linezolid-induced thrombocytopenia, penicillin-induced seizures, and vancomycin-induced anaphylactoid reactions. Many of these reactions can be avoided by reducing dosage in patients with impaired renal function, limiting the duration of therapy, or reducing the rate of administration. Adverse reactions to antibacterial agents are a common cause of morbidity, requiring alteration in therapy

and additional expense, and they occasionally result in death. The elderly, often those with the more severe infections, may be especially prone to certain adverse reactions. The most clinically relevant adverse reactions to common antibacterial drugs are listed in Table 133-7. For further discussion of adverse drug reactions, see Chap. 5.

DRUG INTERACTIONS

Antimicrobial drugs are a common cause of drug-drug interactions. Table 133-8 lists the most common and best-documented interactions of antibacterial agents with other drugs and characterizes the clinical relevance of these interactions. Coadministration of drugs paired in the table does not necessarily result in clinically important adverse consequences in all cases. The information in Table 133-8 is intended only to heighten awareness of the potential for an interaction. Additional sources should be consulted to identify appropriate options. For further discussion of drug interactions, see Chap. 5.

MACROLIDES AND KETOLIDES

Erythromycin, clarithromycin, and telithromycin inhibit CYP3A4, the hepatic P450 enzyme that metabolizes many drugs. In ~10% of patients receiving digoxin, concentrations increase significantly when erythromycin or telithromycin is coadministered, and this increase may lead to digoxin toxicity. Azithromycin has little effect on the metabolism of other drugs.

Many drugs, such as the azole antifungals, can also increase erythromycin serum concentrations, leading to prolongation of the QT interval and a fivefold increase in mortality rate. This example serves as a reminder that the true significance of drug-drug interactions may be subtle yet profound and that close attention to the evolving safety literature is important.

QUINUPRISTIN/DALFOPRISTIN

Quinupristin/dalfopristin is an inhibitor of CYP3A4. Its interactions with other drugs are similar to those of erythromycin.

LINEZOLID

Linezolid is a monoamine oxidase inhibitor. Its concomitant administration with sympathomimetics (e.g., phenylpropanolamine) and with foods with high concentrations of tyramine should be avoided. Many case reports describe serotonin syndrome following coadministration of linezolid with selective serotonin reuptake inhibitors.

TETRACYCLINES

The most important interaction involving tetracyclines is reduced absorption when these drugs are coadministered with divalent and trivalent cations, such as antacids, iron compounds, or dairy products.

SULFONAMIDES

Sulfonamides, including TMP-SMX, increase the hypoprothrombinemic effect of warfarin by inhibition of its metabolism or by protein-binding displacement. This interaction is a relatively common cause of bleeding in patients also taking warfarin, and the incidence may be increasing as more TMP-SMX is used to treat community-acquired infections caused by MRSA.

FLUOROQUINOLONES

Chelation of all fluoroquinolones with divalent and trivalent cations leads to a significant reduction in absorption. Scattered case reports suggest that quinolones can also potentiate the effects of warfarin, but

TABLE 133-6 Infections for Which Specific Antibacterial Agents Are Among the Drugs of Choice

Agent	Infections	Common Pathogen(s) (Resistance Rate, %)[a]
Penicillin G	Syphilis, yaws, leptospirosis, groups A and B streptococcal infections, pneumococcal infections, actinomycosis, oral and periodontal infections, meningococcal meningitis and meningococcemia, viridans streptococcal endocarditis, clostridial myonecrosis, tetanus, anthrax, rat-bite fever, *Pasteurella multocida* infections, and erysipeloid (*Erysipelothrix rhusiopathiae*)	*Neisseria meningitidis*[b] (intermediate,[c] 15–30; resistant, 0; geographic variation) Viridans streptococci (intermediate, 15–30; resistant, 5–10) *Streptococcus pneumoniae* (intermediate, 23; resistant, 17)
Ampicillin, amoxicillin	Salmonellosis, acute otitis media, *Haemophilus influenzae* meningitis and epiglottitis, *Listeria monocytogenes* meningitis, *Enterococcus faecalis* UTI	*Escherichia coli* (37) *H. influenzae* (35) *Salmonella* spp.[b] (30–50; geographic variation) *Enterococcus* spp. (24)
Nafcillin, oxacillin	*Staphylococcus aureus* (non-MRSA) bacteremia and endocarditis	*S. aureus* (46; MRSA) *Staphylococcus epidermidis* (78; MRSE)
Piperacillin plus tazobactam	Intraabdominal infections (facultative enteric gram-negative bacilli plus obligate anaerobes); infections caused by mixed flora (aspiration pneumonia, diabetic foot ulcers); infections caused by *Pseudomonas aeruginosa*	*P. aeruginosa* (6)
Cefazolin	*E. coli* UTI, surgical prophylaxis, *S. aureus* (non-MRSA) bacteremia and endocarditis	*E. coli* (7) *S. aureus* (46; MRSA)
Cefoxitin, cefotetan	Intraabdominal infections and pelvic inflammatory disease	*Bacteroides fragilis* (12)
Ceftriaxone	Gonococcal infections, pneumococcal meningitis, viridans streptococcal endocarditis, salmonellosis and typhoid fever, hospital-acquired infections caused by nonpseudomonal facultative gram-negative enteric bacilli	*S. pneumoniae* (intermediate, 16; resistant, 0) *E. coli* and *Klebsiella pneumoniae* (1; ESBL producers)
Ceftazidime, cefepime	Hospital-acquired infections caused by facultative gram-negative enteric bacilli and *Pseudomonas*	*P. aeruginosa* (16) (See ceftriaxone for ESBL producers)
Imipenem, meropenem	Intraabdominal infections, hospital-acquired infections (non-MRSA), infections caused by *Enterobacter* spp. and ESBL-producing gram-negative bacilli	*P. aeruginosa* (6) *Acinetobacter* spp. (35)
Aztreonam	Hospital-acquired infections caused by facultative gram-negative bacilli and *Pseudomonas* in penicillin-allergic patients	*P. aeruginosa* (16)
Vancomycin	Bacteremia, endocarditis, and other serious infections due to MRSA; pneumococcal meningitis; antibiotic-associated pseudomembranous colitis[d]	*Enterococcus* spp. (24)
Daptomycin	VRE infections; MRSA bacteremia	Rare
Gentamicin, amikacin, tobramycin	Combined with a penicillin for staphylococcal, enterococcal, or viridans streptococcal endocarditis; combined with a β-lactam antibiotic for gram-negative bacteremia; pyelonephritis	Gentamicin: *E. coli* (6) *P. aeruginosa* (17) *Acinetobacter* spp. (32)
Erythromycin, clarithromycin, azithromycin	*Legionella, Campylobacter*, and *Mycoplasma* infections; CAP; group A streptococcal pharyngitis in penicillin-allergic patients; bacillary angiomatosis (*Bartonella henselae*); gastric infections due to *Helicobacter pylori; Mycobacterium avium-intracellulare* infections	*S. pneumoniae* (28) *Streptococcus pyogenes*[b] (0–10; geographic variation) *H. pylori*[b] (2–20; geographic variation)
Clindamycin	Severe, invasive group A streptococcal infections; infections caused by obligate anaerobes; infections caused by susceptible staphylococci	*S. aureus* (nosocomial = 58; CA-MRSA = 10[b])
Doxycycline, minocycline	Acute bacterial exacerbations of chronic bronchitis, granuloma inguinale, brucellosis (with streptomycin), tularemia, glanders, melioidosis, spirochetal infections caused by *Borrelia* (Lyme disease and relapsing fever; doxycycline), infections caused by *Vibrio vulnificus*, some *Aeromonas* infections, infections due to *Stenotrophomonas* (minocycline), plague, ehrlichiosis, chlamydial infections (doxycycline), granulomatous skin infections due to *Mycobacterium marinum* (minocycline), rickettsial infections, mild CAP, skin and soft tissue infections caused by gram-positive cocci (CA-MRSA infections, leptospirosis, syphilis, actinomycosis in the penicillin-allergic patient)	*S. pneumoniae* (17) MRSA (5)

(continued)

Agent	Infections	Common Pathogen(s) (Resistance Rate, %)[a]
Trimethoprim-sulfamethoxazole	Community-acquired UTI; *S. aureus* skin and soft tissue infections (CA-MRSA)	*E. coli* (19) MRSA (3)
Sulfonamides	Nocardial infections, leprosy (dapsone, a sulfone), and toxoplasmosis (sulfadiazine)	UNK
Ciprofloxacin, levofloxacin, moxifloxacin	CAP (levofloxacin and moxifloxacin); UTI; bacterial gastroenteritis; hospital-acquired gram-negative enteric infections; *Pseudomonas* infections (ciprofloxacin and levofloxacin)	*S. pneumoniae* (1) *E. coli* (13) *P. aeruginosa* (23) *Salmonella* spp. (10–50; geographic variation) *Neisseria gonorrhoeae*[b] (0–5, non–West Coast U.S.; 10–15, California and Hawaii; 20–70, Asia, England, Wales)
Rifampin	Staphylococcal foreign body infections, in combination with other antistaphylococcal agents; *Legionella* pneumonia	Staphylococci rapidly develop resistance during rifampin monotherapy.
Metronidazole	Obligate anaerobic gram-negative bacteria (*Bacteroides* spp.): abscess in lung, brain, or abdomen; bacterial vaginosis; antibiotic-associated *Clostridium difficile* disease	UNK
Linezolid	VRE; staphylococcal skin and soft tissue infection (CA-MRSA)	Rare
Polymyxin E (colistin)	Hospital-acquired infection due to gram-negative bacilli resistant to all other chemotherapy: *P. aeruginosa*, *Acinetobacter* spp., *Stenotrophomonas maltophilia*	UNK
Quinupristin/dalfopristin	VRE	Vancomycin-resistant *E. faecalis*[b] (100) Vancomycin-resistant *E. faecium* (10)
Mupirocin	Topical application to nares to eradicate *S. aureus* carriage	UNK

[a]Unless otherwise noted, resistance rates are based on all isolates tested in 2008 in the clinical microbiology laboratory at Virginia Commonwealth University Medical Center. The rates are consistent with those reported by the National Nosocomial Infections Surveillance System (Am J Infect Control 32:470, 2004).

[b]Data from recent literature sources.

[c]Intermediate resistance.

[d]Drug is given orally for this indication.

Abbreviations: CA-MRSA, community-acquired methicillin-resistant *S. aureus*; CAP, community-acquired pneumonia; ESBL, extended-spectrum β-lactamase; MRSA, methicillin-resistant *S. aureus*; MRSE, methicillin-resistant *S. epidermidis*; UNK, resistance rates unknown: UTI, urinary tract infection; VRE, vancomycin-resistant enterococci.

this effect has not been observed in most controlled trials. Patients receiving glucocorticoids are at increased risk of tendon rupture.

■ RIFAMPIN

Rifampin is an excellent inducer of many cytochrome P450 enzymes and increases the hepatic clearance of a large number of drugs. Before rifampin is prescribed for any patient, a review of concomitant drug therapy is essential.

■ METRONIDAZOLE

Metronidazole has been reported to cause a disulfiram-like syndrome when alcohol is ingested. The true frequency and significance of this reaction are unknown, and it is not well documented; however, patients for whom metronidazole is prescribed are usually instructed to avoid alcohol. Inhibition of the metabolism of warfarin by metronidazole leads to significant rises in prothrombin times.

PROPHYLAXIS OF BACTERIAL INFECTIONS

Antibacterial agents are occasionally indicated for use in patients who have no evidence of infection but who have been or are expected to be exposed to bacterial pathogens under circumstances that constitute a major risk of infection. The basic tenets of antimicrobial prophylaxis are as follows: (1) The risk or potential severity of infection should outweigh the risk of side effects from the antibacterial agent. (2) The antibacterial agent should be given for the shortest period necessary to prevent target infections. (3) The antibacterial agent should be given before the expected period of risk (e.g., within 1 h of incision before elective surgery) or as soon as possible after contact with an infected individual (e.g., prophylaxis for meningococcal meningitis).

Table 133-9 lists the major indications for antibacterial prophylaxis in adults. The table includes only those indications that are widely accepted, supported by well-designed studies, or recommended by expert panels. Prophylaxis is also used but is less widely accepted for recurrent cellulitis in conjunction with lymphedema, recurrent pneumococcal meningitis in conjunction with deficiencies in humoral immunity or CSF leaks, traveler's diarrhea, gram-negative sepsis in conjunction with neutropenia, and spontaneous bacterial peritonitis in conjunction with ascites. The use of antibacterial agents in children to prevent rheumatic fever is also common practice.

The major use of antibacterial prophylaxis is to prevent infections following surgical procedures. Antibacterial agents are administered just before the surgical procedure—and, for long operations, during the procedure as well—to ensure high drug concentrations in serum and tissues during surgery. The objective is to eradicate bacteria originating from the air of the operating suite, the skin of the surgical team, or the patient's own flora that may contaminate the wound. In all but colorectal surgical procedures, prophylaxis is predominantly directed against staphylococci and cefazolin is

TABLE 133-7 Most Clinically Relevant Adverse Reactions to Common Antibacterial Drugs

Drug	Adverse Event	Comments
β-Lactams	Allergies in ~1–4% of treatment courses	Cephalosporins cause allergy in 2–4% of penicillin-allergic patients. Aztreonam is safe in β-lactam-allergic patients.
	Nonallergic skin reactions	Ampicillin "rash" is common among patients with Epstein-Barr virus infection.
	Diarrhea, including *Clostridium difficile* colitis (Chap. 129)	—
Vancomycin	Anaphylactoid reaction ("red man syndrome")	Give as a 1- to 2-h infusion.
	Nephrotoxicity, ototoxicity, allergy, neutropenia	Thought to be rare, but appear to be increasing as larger dosages are used
Telavancin	Taste disturbance, foamy urine, gastrointestinal distress	New drug; full spectrum of adverse reactions unclear
Aminoglycosides	Nephrotoxicity (generally reversible)	Greatest with prolonged therapy in the elderly or with preexisting renal insufficiency. Monitor serum creatinine every 2–3 days.
	Ototoxicity (often irreversible)	Risk factors similar to those for nephrotoxicity; both vestibular and hearing toxicities
Macrolides/ketolides	Gastrointestinal distress	Most common with erythromycin
	Ototoxicity	High-dose IV erythromycin
	Cardiac toxicity	QTc prolongation and torsades de pointes, especially when inhibitors of erythromycin metabolism are given simultaneously
	Hepatic toxicity (telithromycin)	Warning added to prescribing information (July 2006)
	Respiratory failure in patients with myasthenia gravis (telithromycin)	Warning added to prescribing information (July 2006)
Clindamycin	Diarrhea, including *C. difficile* colitis	—
Sulfonamides	Allergic reactions	Rashes (more common in HIV-infected patients); serious dermal reactions, including erythema multiforme, Stevens-Johnson syndrome, toxic epidermal necrolysis
	Hematologic reactions	Uncommon; include agranulocytosis and granulocytopenia (more common in HIV-infected patients), hemolytic and megaloblastic anemia, thrombocytopenia
	Renal insufficiency	Crystalluria with sulfadiazine therapy
Fluoroquinolones	Diarrhea, including *C. difficile* colitis	—
	Contraindicated for general use in patients <18 years old and pregnant women	Appear safe in treatment of pulmonary infections in children with cystic fibrosis
	Central nervous system adverse effects (e.g., insomnia)	—
	Miscellaneous: allergies, tendon rupture, dysglycemias, QTc prolongation	Rare, although warnings for tendon rupture have been added to prescribing information
Rifampin	Hepatotoxicity	Rare
	Orange discoloration of urine and body fluids	Common
	Miscellaneous: flu-like symptoms, hemolysis, renal insufficiency	Uncommon; usually related to intermittent administration
Metronidazole	Metallic taste	Common
Tetracyclines/glycylcyclines	Gastrointestinal distress	Up to 20% with tigecycline
	Esophageal ulceration	Doxycycline (take in A.M. with fluids)
Linezolid	Myelosuppression	Follows long-term treatment
	Ocular and peripheral neuritis	Follows long-term treatment
Daptomycin	Distal muscle pain or weakness	Weekly creatine phosphokinase measurements, especially in patients also receiving statins

TABLE 133-8 Interactions of Antibacterial Agents With Other Drugs

Antibiotic	Interacts with	Potential Consequence (Clinical Significance[a])
Erythromycin/clarithromycin/telithromycin	Theophylline	Theophylline toxicity (1)
	Carbamazepine	CNS depression (1)
	Digoxin	Digoxin toxicity (2)
	Triazolam/midazolam	CNS depression (2)
	Ergotamine	Ergotism (1)
	Warfarin	Bleeding (2)
	Cyclosporine/tacrolimus	Nephrotoxicity (1)
	Cisapride	Cardiac arrhythmias (1)
	Statins[b]	Rhabdomyolysis (2)
	Valproate	Valproate toxicity (2)
	Vincristine/vinblastine	Excess neurotoxicity (2)
Quinupristin/dalfopristin	Similar to erythromycin[c]	
Fluoroquinolones	Theophylline	Theophylline toxicity (2)[d]
	Antacids/sucralfate/iron	Subtherapeutic antibiotic levels (1)
Tetracycline	Antacids/sucralfate/iron	Subtherapeutic antibiotic levels (1)
Trimethoprim-sulfamethoxazole	Phenytoin	Phenytoin toxicity (2)
	Oral hypoglycemics	Hypoglycemia (2)
	Warfarin	Bleeding (1)
	Digoxin	Digoxin toxicity (2)
Metronidazole	Ethanol	Disulfiram-like reactions (2)
	Fluorouracil	Bone marrow suppression (1)
	Warfarin	Bleeding (2)
Rifampin	Warfarin	Clot formation (1)
	Oral contraceptives	Pregnancy (1)
	Cyclosporine/tacrolimus	Rejection (1)
	HIV-1 protease inhibitors	Increased viral load, resistance (1)
	Nonnucleoside reverse-transcriptase inhibitors	Increased viral load, resistance (1)
	Glucocorticoids	Loss of steroid effect (1)
	Methadone	Narcotic withdrawal symptoms (1)
	Digoxin	Subtherapeutic digoxin levels (1)
	Itraconazole	Subtherapeutic itraconazole levels (1)
	Phenytoin	Loss of seizure control (1)
	Statins	Hypercholesterolemia (1)
	Diltiazem	Subtherapeutic diltiazem levels (1)
	Verapamil	Subtherapeutic verapamil levels (1)

[a] 1 = a well-documented interaction with clinically important consequences; 2 = an interaction of uncertain frequency but of potential clinical importance.

[b] Lovastatin and simvastatin are most affected; pravastatin and atorvastatin are less prone to clinically important effects.

[c] The macrolide antibiotics and quinupristin/dalfopristin inhibit the same human metabolic enzyme, CYP3A4, and similar interactions are anticipated.

[d] Ciprofloxacin only. Levofloxacin and moxifloxacin do not inhibit theophylline metabolism.

Note: New interactions are commonly reported after marketing. Consult the most recent prescribing information for updates. CNS, central nervous system.

the drug most commonly recommended. Prophylaxis is intended to prevent wound infection or infection of implanted devices, not all infections that may occur during the postoperative period (e.g., UTIs or pneumonia). Prolonged prophylaxis (beyond 24 h) merely alters the normal flora and favors infections with organisms resistant to the antibacterial agents used. National efforts to reduce surgical-site infections were begun in 2002 by the Surgical Infection Prevention Project (SIPP) sponsored by the Centers for Medicare and Medicaid Services. Additional initiatives by the American

College of Surgeons–National Surgical Quality Improvement Program have been undertaken to further characterize best practices and to reduce surgical-site infections.

DURATION OF THERAPY AND TREATMENT FAILURE

Until recently, there was little incentive to establish the most appropriate duration of treatment; patients were instructed to take a 7- or 10-day course of treatment for most common infections. A number of recent investigations have evaluated shorter durations of therapy

TABLE 133-9 Prophylaxis of Bacterial Infections in Adults

Condition	Antibacterial Agent	Timing or Duration of Prophylaxis
Nonsurgical		
Cardiac lesions highly susceptible to bacterial endocarditis (prosthetic valves, previous endocarditis, congenital heart defects)	Amoxicillin	Before and after dental procedures that manipulate gingival tissue
Recurrent *S. aureus* infections	Mupirocin	5 days (intranasal)
Contact with patient with meningococcal meningitis	Rifampin	2 days
	Fluoroquinolone	Single dose
Bite wounds[a]	Amoxicillin/clavulanic acid (alternatives: amoxicillin, doxycycline, or moxifloxacin)	3–5 days
Recurrent cystitis	Trimethoprim-sulfamethoxazole or a fluoroquinolone or nitrofurantoin	3 times per week for up to 1 year or after sexual intercourse
Surgical		
Clean (cardiac, vascular, neurologic, or orthopedic surgery)	Cefazolin (vancomycin)[b]	Before and during procedure
Ocular	Topical combinations and subconjunctival cefazolin	During and at end of procedure
Clean-contaminated (head and neck, high-risk gastroduodenal or biliary tract surgery; high-risk cesarean section; hysterectomy)	Cefazolin (or clindamycin for head and neck)	Before and during procedure
Clean-contaminated (vaginal or abdominal hysterectomy)	Cefazolin or cefoxitin or cefotetan or ampicillin-sulbactam	Before and during procedure
Clean-contaminated (high-risk genitourinary surgery)	Fluoroquinolone	Before and during procedure
Clean-contaminated (colorectal surgery or appendectomy)	Oral: neomycin plus erythromycin or metronidazole	Before and during procedure
	Parenteral: cefoxitin *or* cefotetan *or* cefazolin plus metronidazole *or* ampicillin-sulbactam	
Dirty[a] (ruptured viscus)	Cefoxitin or cefotetan ± gentamicin, clindamycin + gentamicin, or another appropriate regimen directed at anaerobes and gram-negative aerobes	Before and for 3–5 days after procedure
Dirty[a] (traumatic wound)	Cefazolin	Before and for 3–5 days after trauma

[a] In these cases, use of antibacterial agents actually constitutes treatment of infection rather than prophylaxis.
[b] Vancomycin is recommended only in institutions that have a high incidence of infection with methicillin-resistant staphylococci.

than have been used in the past, including treatment of patients with community-acquired pneumonia (5 days) and those with ventilator-associated pneumonia (7 or 8 days). Table 133-10 lists common bacterial infections for which treatment duration guidelines have been established or for which there is sufficient clinical experience to establish treatment durations. The ultimate test of cure for a bacterial infection is the absence of relapse when therapy is discontinued. *Relapse* is defined as a recurrence of infection with the identical organism that caused the first infection. In general, therefore, the duration of therapy should be long enough to prevent relapse yet not excessive. Extension of therapy beyond the limit of effectiveness will increase the medication's side effects and encourage the selection of resistant bacteria. The art of treating bacterial infections lies in the ability to determine the appropriate duration of therapy for infections that are not covered by established guidelines. Re-treatment of serious infections for which therapy has failed usually requires a prolonged course (>4 weeks) with combinations of antibacterial agents.

STRATEGIES TO OPTIMIZE ANTIMICROBIAL USE

Antibiotic use is often not "rational," and it is easy to understand why. The diagnosis of bacterial infection is often uncertain, patients may expect or demand antimicrobial agents in this tenuous situation, and clinicians wish to provide effective therapy even when the cause remains uncertain. Furthermore, the rates of resistance for many bacterial pathogens are ever-changing, and even experts may not agree on the appropriate therapy or the clinical significance of resistance in some pathogens. Consequently, investigators report that ~50% of antibiotic use is in some way "inappropriate." Aside from the monetary cost of using unnecessary or expensive antibiotics, there are the more serious costs associated with excess morbidity from superinfections such as *C. difficile* disease, adverse drug reactions, drug interactions, and selection of resistant organisms. It is increasingly recognized that these costs add substantially to the overall costs of medical care.

At a time when fewer new antimicrobial drugs are entering the worldwide market than in the past, much has been written about the continued rise in rates of resistant microorganisms, its causes, and the solutions. The message seems clear: the use of existing and new antimicrobial agents must be more judicious and infection control efforts more effective if we are to slow or reverse trends in resistance. The phrase *antimicrobial stewardship* is used to describe the new attitude toward antibacterial agents that must be adopted to preserve their usefulness, and hospitals have been encouraged

TABLE 133-10 Duration of Therapy for Bacterial Infections

Duration of Therapy	Infections
Single dose	Gonococcal urethritis, streptococcal pharyngitis (penicillin G benzathine), primary and secondary syphilis (penicillin G benzathine)
3 days	Cystitis in young women, community- or travel-acquired diarrhea
3–10 days	Community-acquired pneumonia (3–5 days), community-acquired meningitis (pneumococcal or meningococcal), antibiotic-associated diarrhea (10 days), *Giardia* enteritis, cellulitis, epididymitis
2 weeks	*Helicobacter pylori*–associated peptic ulcer, neurosyphilis (penicillin IV), penicillin-susceptible viridans streptococcal endocarditis (penicillin plus aminoglycoside), disseminated gonococcal infection with arthritis, acute pyelonephritis, uncomplicated *S. aureus* catheter-associated bacteremia
3 weeks	Lyme disease, septic arthritis (nongonococcal)
4 weeks	Acute and chronic prostatitis, infective endocarditis (penicillin-resistant streptococcal)
>4 weeks	Acute and chronic osteomyelitis, *S. aureus* endocarditis, foreign-body infections (prosthetic-valve and joint infections), relapsing pseudomembranous colitis

by professional organizations to implement multidisciplinary antimicrobial stewardship programs. These programs are designed to improve the quality of patient care by adopting best practices at the local level to ensure that antimicrobial drugs are used only when necessary, at the most appropriate dosage, and for the most appropriate duration. While some newer antibacterial drugs undeniably represent important advances in therapy, many offer no advantage over older, less expensive agents. With rare exceptions, newer drugs are usually found to be no more effective than the comparison antibiotic in controlled trials, despite the "high prevalence of resistance" often touted to market the advantage of the new antibiotic over older therapies.

The following suggestions are intended to provide guidance through the antibiotic maze. First, objective evaluation of the merits of newer and older drugs is available. Online references such as the Johns Hopkins website (*www.hopkins-abxguide.org*) offer current and practical information regarding antimicrobial drugs and treatment regimens. Evidence-based practice guidelines for the treatment of most infections are available from the Infectious Diseases Society of America (*www.idsociety.org*). Furthermore, specialty texts such as *Principles and Practice of Infectious Diseases* are available online. Second, clinicians should become comfortable using a few drugs recommended by independent experts and professional organizations and should resist the temptation to use a new drug unless the merits are clear. A new antibacterial agent with a "broader spectrum and greater potency" or a "higher serum concentration-to-MIC ratio" will not necessarily be more clinically efficacious. Third, clinicians should become familiar with local bacterial susceptibility profiles available via annual "antibiograms" published by hospital clinical microbiology laboratories. It may not be necessary to use a new drug with "improved activity against *P. aeruginosa*" if that pathogen is rarely encountered or if it retains full susceptibility to older drugs. Fourth, a skeptical attitude toward manufacturers' claims is still appropriate. For example, rising rates of penicillin resistance in *S. pneumoniae* have been used to promote the use of broader-spectrum drugs, notably the fluoroquinolones. However, except in patients with meningitis, amoxicillin is still effective for infections caused by these "penicillin-resistant" strains. Finally, with regard to inpatient treatment with antibacterial drugs, a number of efforts to improve use are under study. The strategy of antibiotic "cycling" or rotation has not proved effective, but other strategies, such as reductions in the duration of therapy, hold promise. Adoption of other evidence-based strategies to improve antimicrobial use may be the best way to retain the utility of existing compounds. For example, appropriate empirical treatment of

the seriously ill patient with one or more broad-spectrum agents is important for improving survival rates, but therapy may often be simplified by switching to a narrower-spectrum agent or even an oral drug once the results of cultures and susceptibility tests become available. While there is an understandable temptation not to alter effective empirical broad-spectrum therapy, switching to a more specific agent once the patient's clinical condition has improved does not compromise outcome. A promising and active area of research includes the use of shorter courses of antimicrobial therapy, perhaps guided by markers of infection such as serum concentrations of procalcitonin. Many antibiotics that once were given for 7–14 days can be given for 3–5 days with no apparent loss of efficacy and no increase in relapse rates (Table 133-10). Shorter durations of therapy, once proven as effective as longer durations, offer an opportunity to decrease overall drug use and may result in decreased resistance. Adoption of new guidelines for shorter-course therapy will not undermine the care of patients, many unnecessary complications and expenses will be avoided, and the useful life of these valuable drugs will perhaps be extended.

FURTHER READINGS

Arias CA, Murray BE: Antibiotic-resistant bugs in the 21st century—a clinical super-challenge. N Engl J Med 360:439, 2009

Campbell DA et al: Surgical site infection prevention: The importance of operative duration and blood transfusion—results of the first American College of Surgeons–National Surgical Quality Improvement Program Best Practices Initiative. J Am Coll Surg 207:810, 2008

Centers for Disease Control and Prevention: Guidance for control of infections with carbapenem-resistant or carbapenemase-producing Enterobacteriaceae in acute care facilities. MMWR Morb Mortal Wkly Rep 58:256, 2009

Crider KS et al: Antibacterial medication use during pregnancy and risk of birth defects. National Birth Defects Prevention Study. Arch Pediatr Adolesc Med 163:978, 2009

Dellit TH et al: Infectious Diseases Society of America and the Society for Healthcare Epidemiology of America guidelines for developing an institutional program to enhance antimicrobial stewardship. Clin Infect Dis 44:159, 2007

Nishimura RA et al: ACC/AHA 2008 guideline update on valvular heart disease: Focused update on infective endocarditis. J Am Coll Cardiol 10:1016, 2008

ROBERTS RR et al: Hospital and societal costs of antimicrobial-resistant infections in a Chicago teaching hospital: Implications for antibiotic stewardship. Clin Infect Dis 49:1175, 2009

RUPNIK M et al: *Clostridium difficile* infection: New developments in epidemiology and pathogenesis. Nat Rev Microbiol 7:526, 2009

SÁNCHEZ GARCÍA M et al: Clinical outbreak of linezolid-resistant *Staphylococcus aureus* in an intensive care unit. JAMA 303:2260, 2010

SPELLBERG B et al: The epidemic of antibiotic-resistant infections: A call to action for the medical community from the Infectious Diseases Society of America. Clin Infect Dis 46:155, 2008

PART 8

Infectious Diseases

CHAPTER 134

Pneumococcal Infections

David Goldblatt
Katherine L. O'Brien

In the late nineteenth century, pairs of micrococci were first recognized in the blood of rabbits injected with human saliva by both Louis Pasteur working in France and George Sternberg, an American army physician. The important role of these micrococci in human disease was not appreciated at that time. By 1886, when the organism was designated "pneumokokkus" and *Diplococcus pneumoniae*, the pneumococcus had been isolated by many independent investigators, and its role in the etiology of pneumonia was well known. In the 1930s, pneumonia was the third leading cause of death in the United States (after heart disease and cancer) and was responsible for ~7% of all deaths both in the United States and in Europe. While pneumonia was caused by a host of pathogens, lobar pneumonia—a pattern more likely to be caused by the pneumococcus—accounted for approximately one-half of all pneumonia deaths in the United States in 1929. In 1974, the organism was reclassified as *Streptococcus pneumoniae*.

■ MICROBIOLOGY

Etiologic agent

Pneumococci are spherical gram-positive bacteria of the genus *Streptococcus*. Within this genus, cell division occurs along a single axis, and bacteria grow in chains or pairs—hence the name *Streptococcus*, from the Greek *streptos*, meaning "twisted," and *kokkos*, meaning "berry." At least 22 streptococcal species are recognized and are divided further into groups based on their hemolytic properties. *S. pneumoniae* belongs to the α-hemolytic group that characteristically produces a greenish color on blood agar because of the reduction of iron in hemoglobin (Fig. 134-1). The bacteria are fastidious and grow best in 5% CO_2 but require a source of catalase (e.g., blood) for growth on agar plates, where they develop mucoid (smooth/shiny) colonies. Pneumococci without a capsule produce colonies with a rough surface. Unlike that of other α-hemolytic streptococci, their growth is inhibited in the presence of optochin (ethyl hydrocuprein hydrochloride), and they are bile soluble.

In common with other gram-positive bacteria, pneumococci have a cell membrane beneath a cell wall, which in turn is covered by a polysaccharide capsule. Pneumococci are divided into serogroups or serotypes based on capsular polysaccharide structure, as distinguished with rabbit polyclonal antisera; capsules swell in the presence of specific antiserum (the Quellung reaction). The 91st and 92nd serotypes, 6C and 6D, have most recently been identified with monoclonal antibodies and by serologic, genetic, and biochemical means, respectively. Within the 92 serotypes there are 21 serogroups, each containing two to five serotypes with closely related capsules. The capsule protects the bacteria from phagocytosis by host cells in the absence of type-specific antibody and is arguably the most important determinant of pneumococcal virulence. Unencapsulated variants tend not to cause invasive disease.

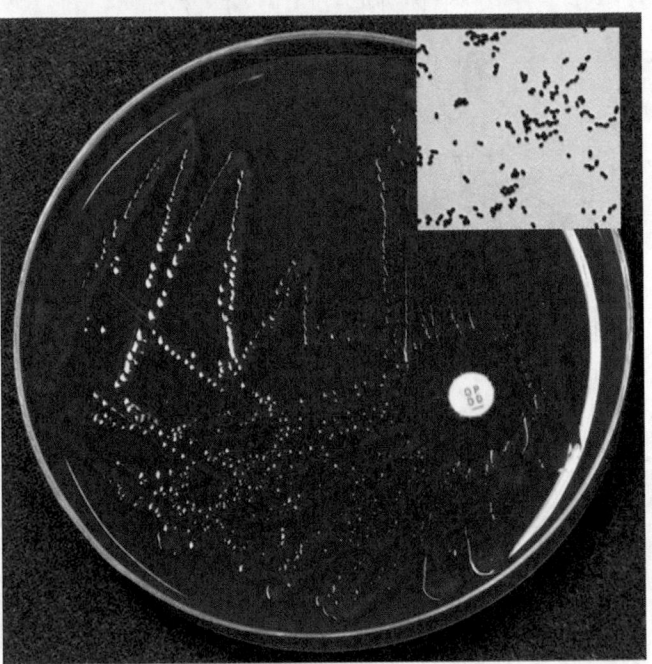

Figure 134-1   Pneumococci growing on blood agar, illustrating α hemolysis and optochin sensitivity (zone around optochin disk). *Inset:* Gram's stain, illustrating gram-positive diplococci. *(Photographs courtesy of Paul Turner, Shoklo Malaria Research Unit, Thailand.)*

Virulence factors   Within the cytoplasm, cell membrane, and cell wall, many molecules that may play a role in pneumococcal pathogenesis and virulence have been identified (Fig. 134-2). These proteins are often involved in direct interactions with host tissues or in concealment of the bacterial surface from host defense mechanisms. Pneumolysin is a secreted cytotoxin thought to result in cytolysis of cells and tissues, and LytA enhances pathogenesis. A number of cell wall proteins interfere with the complement pathway, thus inhibiting complement deposition and preventing lysis and/or opsonophagocytosis. The pneumococcal H inhibitor (Hic) impedes the formation of C3 convertase, while pneumococcal surface protein C (PspC), also known as choline-binding protein A (CbpA), binds factor H and is thought to accelerate the breakdown of C3. PspA and CbpA inhibit the deposition of or degrade C3b. The numerous pneumococcal proteins thought to be involved in adhesion include the ubiquitous surface-anchored sialidase (neuraminidase) NanA, which cleaves sialic acid on host cells and proteins, and pneumococcal surface adhesin A (PsaA). Pili recently recognized by electron microscopy may also play an important role in binding to cells. Some of the antigens mentioned above are potential vaccine candidates (see "Prevention," below).

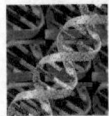 Although the capsule surrounding the cell wall of *S. pneumoniae* is the basis for categorization by serotype, the behavior and pathogenic potential of a serotype may also be related to the genetic origin of the strain. Molecular typing is therefore of considerable interest. Initially, techniques such as pulsed-field gel electrophoresis were used to determine genetic relatedness; such techniques have been superseded by sequencing of housekeeping genes to define a clone (multilocus

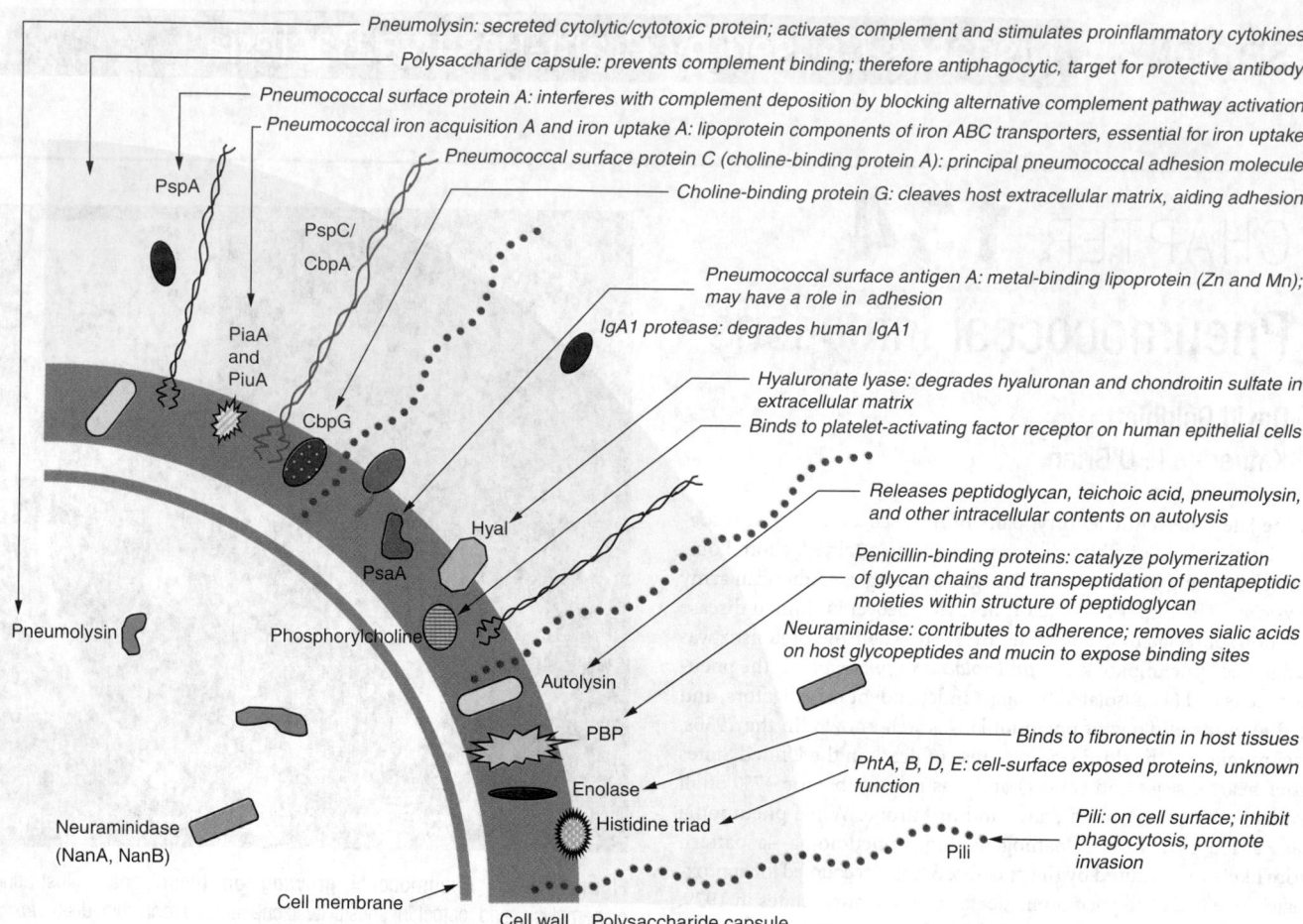

Pneumolysin: secreted cytolytic/cytotoxic protein; activates complement and stimulates proinflammatory cytokines

Polysaccharide capsule: prevents complement binding; therefore antiphagocytic, target for protective antibody

Pneumococcal surface protein A: interferes with complement deposition by blocking alternative complement pathway activation

Pneumococcal iron acquisition A and iron uptake A: lipoprotein components of iron ABC transporters, essential for iron uptake

Pneumococcal surface protein C (choline-binding protein A): principal pneumococcal adhesion molecule

Choline-binding protein G: cleaves host extracellular matrix, aiding adhesion

Pneumococcal surface antigen A: metal-binding lipoprotein (Zn and Mn); may have a role in adhesion

IgA1 protease: degrades human IgA1

Hyaluronate lyase: degrades hyaluronan and chondroitin sulfate in extracellular matrix

Binds to platelet-activating factor receptor on human epithelial cells

Releases peptidoglycan, teichoic acid, pneumolysin, and other intracellular contents on autolysis

Penicillin-binding proteins: catalyze polymerization of glycan chains and transpeptidation of pentapeptidic moieties within structure of peptidoglycan

Neuraminidase: contributes to adherence; removes sialic acids on host glycopeptides and mucin to expose binding sites

Binds to fibronectin in host tissues

PhtA, B, D, E: cell-surface exposed proteins, unknown function

Pili: on cell surface; inhibit phagocytosis, promote invasion

PspA
PspC/CbpA
PiaA and PiuA
CbpG
Hyal
PsaA
Pneumolysin
Phosphorylcholine
Autolysin
PBP
Enolase
Histidine triad
Pili
Neuraminidase (NanA, NanB)
Cell membrane
Cell wall   Polysaccharide capsule

Figure 134-2   Schematic diagram of the pneumococcal cell surface, with key antigens and their roles highlighted.

sequence typing, MLST). For *S. pneumoniae*, alleles at each of the loci *aroE*, *gdh*, *gki*, *recP*, *spi*, *xpt*, and *ddl* are sequenced and compared with all of the known alleles at that locus. Sequences identical to a known allele are assigned the same allele number, whereas those differing from any known allele—even at a single nucleotide site—are assigned new numbers. Software for assignment of alleles at each locus is available on the pneumococcal MLST Web site (*http://spneu-moniae.mlst.net/*), and the allelic profile of each isolate and its consequent sequence type are generated. With the advent of high-throughput and relatively inexpensive sequencing techniques, whole-genome sequencing will soon supersede MLST.

■ EPIDEMIOLOGY

Pneumococcal infections remain a significant global cause of morbidity and death, particularly among children and the elderly. Rapid and dramatic changes in the epidemiology of this disease during the past decade in several developed countries followed the licensure and routine childhood administration of pneumococcal polysaccharide–protein conjugate vaccine (PCV). With PCV introduction in developing and middle-income countries, additional profound changes in pneumococcal ecology and disease epidemiology are likely. The disease burden and serotype distribution in the PCV era may be different than expected because of concomitant secular trends in pneumococcal disease, the impact of antibiotic use on pneumococcal strain ecology, and surveillance system attributes that can themselves affect analysis of epidemiologic features.

Not all pneumococcal serotypes are equally likely to cause disease; serotype distribution varies by age, disease syndrome, and geography. Geographic differences may be driven by variation in

the burden of disease rather than by true serotype distribution differences. Most data on serotype distribution are related to pediatric invasive pneumococcal disease (IPD, defined as infection of a normally sterile site); much less information on global distribution is available on disease in adults. Among children <5 years of age, five to seven serotypes cause >60% of IPD cases in most parts of the world, seven serotypes (1, 5, 6A, 6B, 14, 19F, and 23F) account for ~60% of cases in all areas of the world, but in any given region these seven serotypes may not all rank as the most common disease strains (Fig. 134-3). Some serotypes (e.g., types 1 and 5) not only tend to cause disease in areas with a high disease burden but also cause waves of disease in lower-burden areas (e.g., Europe) or outbreaks (e.g., in military barracks; meningitis in sub-Saharan Africa). The broader range of serotypes causing disease among adults than among children is apparent from a comparison of the coverage of existing multiserotype vaccines in different age groups. For example, data from the United States for 2006–2007 on the serotypes causing IPD indicated that a polysaccharide vaccine containing 23 serotypes (PPV23) would cover 84% of cases among children <5 years of age and 76% of those among persons 18–64 years of age but only 65% of those among persons ≥65 years of age.

Pneumococci are intermittent inhabitants of the healthy human nasopharynx and are transmitted by respiratory droplets. In children, pneumococcal nasopharyngeal ecology varies by geographic region, socioeconomic status, climate, degree of crowding, and particularly intensity of exposure to other children, with children in day-care settings having higher rates of colonization. In developed-world settings, children serve as the major vectors of pneumococcal transmission. By 1 year of age, ~50% of children have had at least one

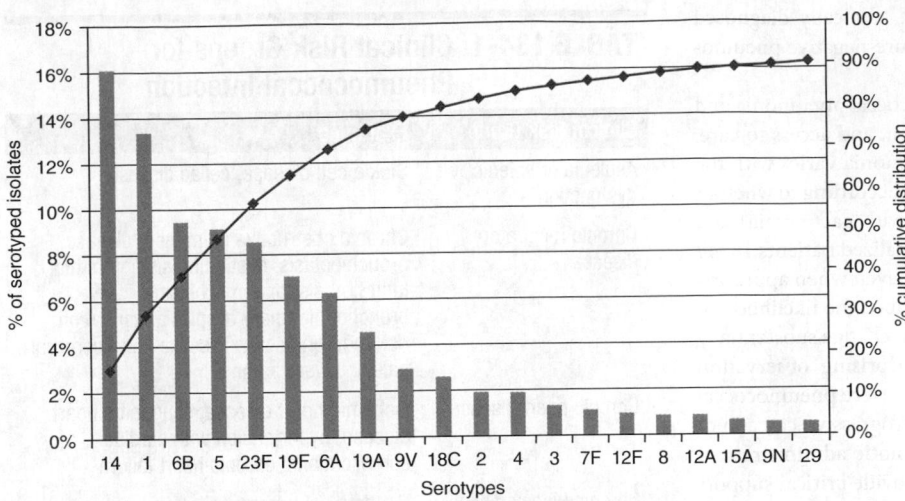

Figure 134-3 Meta-analysis of available global serotype data, adjusted for regional disease incidence. The red line shows cumulative incidence, as indicated on the right-hand Y axis. *(Source: Global Serotype Project Report for the Pneumococcal Advance Market Commitment Target Product Profile; available at http://www.vaccineamc.org/files/TPP_Codebook.pdf.)*

episode of pneumococcal colonization. Cross-sectional prevalence data show rates of pneumococcal carriage ranging from 20% to 50% for children <5 years of age and from 5% to 15% for young and middle-aged adults; Fig. 134-4 shows relevant data from the United Kingdom. Data on colonization rates among healthy elderly individuals are limited. In developing-world settings, pneumococcal acquisition occurs much earlier, sometimes within the first few days after birth, and nearly all infants have had at least one episode of colonization by 2 months of age. Cross-sectional studies show that up to the age of 5 years, 70–90% of children carry *S. pneumoniae* in the nasopharynx, and a significant proportion of adults (sometimes >40%) are also colonized. Their high rates of colonization make adults an important source of transmission and may affect community transmission dynamics.

IPD develops when *S. pneumoniae* invades the bloodstream and seeds other organs or directly reaches the cerebrospinal fluid (CSF) by local extension. Pneumonia may follow aspiration of pneumococci, although only 10–30% of such cases are associated with a positive blood culture (and thus contribute to the measured burden of IPD). The dramatic variation of IPD rates with age

is illustrated by data from the United States for 1998–1999, a period prior to PCV introduction. Rates of IPD were highest among children <2 years of age and among adults ≥65 years of age (188 and 60 cases per 100,000, respectively; Fig. 134-5). Since the introduction of PCV, IPD rates among infants and children in the United States have fallen by >75%, a decrease driven by the near elimination of vaccine-serotype IPD. A similar impact of PCV on vaccine-serotype IPD rates has been consistently observed in countries where PCV has been introduced into the routine pediatric vaccination schedule. However, changes in the non-vaccine-serotype IPD rate in various countries have been heterogeneous; the interpretation of this heterogeneity is a complex issue. In the United States, Canada, and Australia, rates of non-vaccine-serotype IPD have increased but the magnitude of the increase is generally small relative to

the substantial reductions in vaccine-serotype IPD. In contrast, in other settings (e.g., Alaska Native communities and the United Kingdom), the reduction in vaccine-serotype IPD has been offset by notable increases in rates of disease caused by non-vaccine serotypes. Explanations for the heterogeneity of findings include replacement disease resulting from vaccine pressure, changes in clinical case investigation, secular trends unrelated to PCV use, antibiotic pressure selecting for resistant organisms, changes in surveillance or reporting systems, rapidity of introduction, and inclusion of a catch-up campaign. The roles and relative importance of these hypothesized mechanisms in driving the observed non-vaccine-serotype IPD trends and in explaining the observed heterogeneity among populations are not yet fully understood.

Pneumonia is the most common of the serious pneumococcal disease syndromes and poses special challenges from a clinical and public health perspective. Most cases of pneumococcal pneumonia are not associated with bacteremia, and in these cases a definitive etiologic diagnosis is difficult. As a result, estimates of disease burden focus primarily on IPD rates and fail to include the major portion of the burden of serious pneumococcal disease. Among children, PCV trials designed to collect efficacy data on syndrome-based outcomes

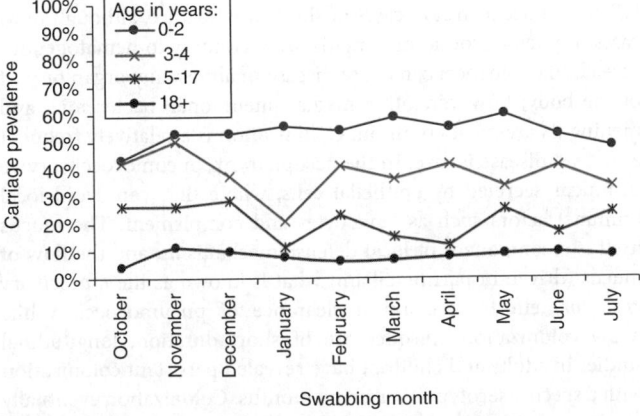

Figure 134-4 Prevalence of pneumococcal carriage in adults and children resident in the United Kingdom who had nasopharyngeal swabs collected monthly for 10 months (no seasonal trend; *t* test trend, >.05). *(Data adapted from D Goldblatt et al, 2005.)*

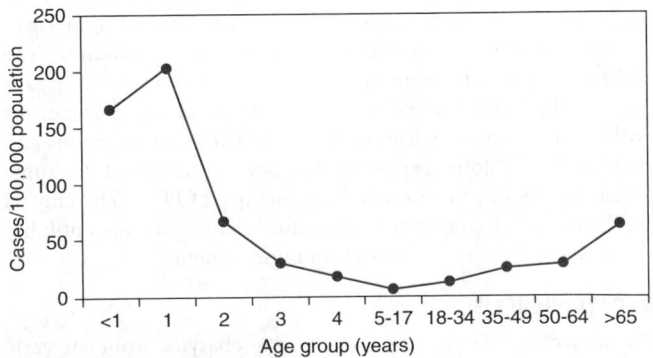

Figure 134-5 Rates of invasive pneumococcal disease before the introduction of pneumococcal conjugate vaccine, by age group: United States, 1998. *[Source: CDC, Active Bacterial Core Surveillance/Emerging Infectious Program Network, 2000. Data adapted from MMWR 49(RR-9), 2000.]*

(e.g., radiographically confirmed pneumonia, clinically diagnosed pneumonia) have revealed the burden of culture-negative pneumococcal pneumonia.

The case-fatality ratios (CFRs) for pneumococcal pneumonia and IPD vary by age, underlying medical condition, and access to care. In addition, the CFR for pneumococcal pneumonia varies with the severity of disease at presentation (rather than according to whether or not the pneumonia episode is associated with bacteremia) and with the patient's age (from <5% among hospitalized patients 18–44 years old to >12% among those >65 years old, even when appropriate and timely management is available). Notably, the likelihood of death in the first 24 h of hospitalization did not change substantially with the introduction of antibiotics; this surprising observation highlights the fact that the pathophysiology of severe pneumococcal pneumonia among adults reflects a rapidly progressive cascade of events that often unfolds irrespective of antibiotic administration. Management in an intensive care unit can provide critical support for the patient through the acute period, with lower CFRs.

Rates of pneumococcal disease vary by season, with higher rates in colder than in warmer months in temperate climates; by gender, with males more often affected than females; and by risk group, with risk factors including underlying medical conditions, behavioral issues, and ethnic group. In the United States, some Native American populations (including Alaska natives) and African Americans have higher rates of disease than the general population; the increased risk is probably attributable to socioeconomic conditions and the prevalence of underlying risk factors for pneumococcal disease. Medical conditions that increase the risk of pneumococcal infection are listed in Table 134-1. Outbreaks of disease are well recognized in crowded settings with susceptible individuals, such as infant day-care facilities, military barracks, and nursing homes. Furthermore, there is a clear association between preceding viral respiratory disease (especially but not exclusively influenza) and risk of secondary pneumococcal infections. The significant role of pneumococcal pneumonia in the morbidity and mortality associated with seasonal and pandemic influenza is increasingly recognized.

Reduced pneumococcal susceptibility to penicillin was first noted in 1967, but not until the 1990s did reduced antibiotic susceptibility emerge as a significant clinical and public health issue, with an increasing prevalence of pneumococcal isolates resistant to single or multiple classes of antibiotics and a rising absolute magnitude of minimal inhibitory concentrations (MICs). Strains with reduced susceptibility to penicillin G, cefotaxime, ceftriaxone, macrolides, and other antibiotics are now found worldwide and account for a significant proportion of disease-causing strains in many locations, especially among children. Vancomycin resistance has not yet been observed in clinical pneumococcal strains. Lack of antimicrobial susceptibility is clearly related to a subset of serotypes, many of which disproportionately cause disease among children. The vicious cycle of antibiotic exposure, selection of resistant organisms in the nasopharynx, and transmission of these organisms within the community leading to difficult-to-treat infections and increased antibiotic exposure has been interrupted to some extent by the introduction and routine use of PCV. The clinical implications of pneumococcal antimicrobial nonsusceptibility are addressed below in the section on treatment.

■ PATHOGENESIS

Pneumococci colonize the human nasopharynx from an early age; colonization acquisition events are generally described as asymptomatic, but evidence exists to associate acquisition with mild respiratory symptoms, especially in the very young. From the nasopharynx, the bacteria spread either via the bloodstream to distant sites (e.g., brain, joint, bones, peritoneal cavity) or locally to

TABLE 134-1 Clinical Risk Groups for Pneumococcal Infection

Clinical Risk Group	Examples
Asplenia or splenic dysfunction	Sickle cell disease, celiac disease
Chronic respiratory disease	Chronic obstructive pulmonary disease, bronchiectasis, cystic fibrosis, interstitial lung fibrosis, pneumoconiosis, bronchopulmonary dysplasia, aspiration risk, neuromuscular disease (e.g., cerebral palsy), severe asthma
Chronic heart disease	Ischemic heart disease, congenital heart disease, hypertension with cardiac complications, chronic heart failure
Chronic kidney disease	Nephrotic syndrome, chronic renal failure, renal transplantation
Chronic liver disease	Cirrhosis, biliary atresia, chronic hepatitis
Diabetes mellitus	Diabetes mellitus requiring insulin or oral hypoglycemic drugs
Immunocompromise/ immunosuppression	HIV infection, common variable immunodeficiency, leukemia, lymphoma, Hodgkin's disease, multiple myeloma, generalized malignancy, chemotherapy, organ or bone marrow transplantation, systemic glucocorticoid treatment for >1 month at a dose equivalent to ≥20 mg/day (children, ≥1 mg/kg per day)
Cochlear implants	. . .
Cerebrospinal fluid leaks	. . .
Miscellaneous	Infancy and old age; prior hospitalization; alcoholism; malnutrition; cigarette smoking; day-care center attendance; residence in military training camps, prisons, homeless shelters

Note: Groups for whom pneumococcal vaccines are recommended by the Advisory Committee on Immunization Practices can be found at *http://www.cdc.gov/vaccines/recs/schedules/default.htm.*

mucosal surfaces where they can cause otitis media or pneumonia. Direct spread from the nasopharynx to the central nervous system (CNS) can occur in rare cases of skull base fracture, although most cases of pneumococcal meningitis are secondary to hematogenous spread. Pneumococci can cause disease in almost any organ or part of the body; however, otitis media, pneumonia, bacteremia, and meningitis are most common. Colonization is a relatively frequent event, yet disease is rare. In the nasopharynx, pneumococci survive in mucus secreted by epithelial cells, where they can avoid local immune factors such as leukocytes and complement. The mucus itself is a component of local defense mechanisms, and the flow of mucus (driven in part by cilia in what is known as the *mucociliary escalator*) effects mechanical clearance of pneumococci. While many colonization episodes are of short duration, longitudinal studies in adults and children have revealed persistent colonization with a specific serotype over many months. Colonization eventually results in the development of capsule-specific serum IgG, which is thought to play a role in mediating clearance of bacteria from the nasopharynx. IgG antibodies to surface exposed cell wall or secreted proteins also appear in the circulation in an age-dependent fashion or after colonization; the biological role of these antibodies is less clear. Recent acquisition of a new colonizing serotype is more likely to be associated with subsequent invasion, presumably as a result of the absence of type-specific immunity. Intercurrent viral infections make the host more susceptible to pneumococcal colonization, and pneumococcal disease in a colonized individual often follows perturbation of the nasopharyngeal mucosa by such infections. Local cytokine production after a viral infection is thought to upregulate adhesion factors in the respiratory epithelium, allowing pneumococci to adhere via a variety of surface adhesin molecules, including PsaA, PspA, CbpA, PspC, Hyl, pneumolysin, and the neuraminidases (Fig. 134-2). Adhesion coupled with inflammation induced by pneumococcal factors such as peptidoglycans and teichoic acids results in invasion. It is the inflammation induced by various bacterium-derived factors that is responsible for the pathology associated with pneumococcal infection. Cell wall–derived teichoic acids and peptidoglycans induce a variety of cytokines, including the proinflammatory cytokines interleukin (IL) 1, IL-6, and tumor necrosis factor (TNF), and activate complement via the alternative pathway. Polymorphonuclear leukocytes are thus attracted, and an intense inflammatory response is initiated. Pneumolysin is also important in local pathology, inducing proinflammatory cytokine production by local monocytes.

The pneumococcal capsule, consisting of polysaccharides with antiphagocytic properties due to resistance to the deposition of complement, plays an important role in pathogenesis. While most capsular types can cause human disease, certain capsular types are more commonly isolated from sites of infection. The reason for the dominance of some serotypes over others in IPD, as depicted in Fig. 134-3, is unclear.

■ HOST DEFENSE MECHANISMS

Innate immunity

As described above, intact respiratory epithelium and a host of nonspecific or innate immune factors (e.g., mucus, splenic function, complement, neutrophils, and macrophages) constitute the first line of defense against pneumococci. Physical factors such as the cough reflex and the mucociliary escalator are important in clearing bacteria from the lungs. Immunologic factors are critical as well: C-reactive protein (CRP) binds phosphorylcholine in the pneumococcal cell wall, inducing complement activation and leading to bacterial clearance; Toll-like receptor 2 (TLR2) recognizes both pneumococcal lipoteichoic acid and cell wall peptidoglycan; and in animal models, the absence of host TLR2 leads to more severe infection and impaired clearance of nasopharyngeal colonization. TLR4 appears to be necessary for the proinflammatory effect of pneumolysin on macrophages. The importance of TLR recognition is underlined by descriptions of an inherited deficiency of human IL-1 receptor–associated kinase 4 (IRAK-4) that manifests as an unusual susceptibility to infection with bacteria, including *S. pneumoniae*. IRAK-4 is essential for the normal functioning of several TLRs. Other factors that interfere with these nonspecific mechanisms (e.g., viral infections, cystic fibrosis, bronchiectasis, complement deficiency, and chronic obstructive pulmonary disease) all predispose to the development of pneumococcal pneumonia. Patients who lack a spleen or have abnormal splenic function (e.g., persons with sickle cell disease) are at high risk of developing overwhelming pneumococcal disease.

Acquired immunity

Acquired immunity induced via contact following colonization or through cross-reactive antigens rests largely on the development of serum IgG antibody specific for the pneumococcal capsular polysaccharide. Nearly all polysaccharides are T cell–independent antigens; B cells can make antibodies to such antigens without T cell help. However, in children <1–2 years old, such B cell responses are poorly developed. This delayed ontogeny of capsule-specific IgG

in young children is associated with susceptibility to pneumococcal infection (Fig. 134-5). The extremely high risk of pneumococcal infection in the absence of serum immunoglobulin (i.e., in conditions such as agammaglobulinemia) highlights the important role of capsular antibody in protection against disease. Each serotype's capsule is chemically distinct; thus immunity tends to be serotype specific, although some cross-immunity exists. For example, conjugate vaccine–induced antibodies to serotype 6B prevent infection due to serotype 6A. However, cross-protection against serotypes within serogroups is not universal; for instance, antibodies to serotype 19F do not appear to confer protection against disease caused by serotype 19A. Antibodies to surface exposed or secreted pneumococcal proteins (such as pneumolysin, PsaA, and PspA) also appear in the circulation with increasing age of the host, but their functional significance remains unclear. Although data from murine models suggest that CD4+ T cells may play a role in preventing pneumococcal colonization and disease, these data have not yet been replicated in humans.

APPROACH TO THE PATIENT **Pneumococcal Infections**

There is no pathognomonic presentation of pneumococcal disease; patients may present with a range of syndromes and with more than one clinical syndrome (e.g., pneumonia and meningitis). *S. pneumoniae* can infect nearly any body tissue, manifesting as disease ranging in severity from mild and self-limited to life-threatening. The differential diagnosis of common clinical syndromes such as pneumonia, otitis media, fever of unknown origin, and meningitis should always include pneumococcal infection. A microbiologically confirmed diagnosis is made in only a minority of pneumococcal cases since, in most circumstances (and especially in pneumonia and otitis media), fluid from the site of infection is not available for etiologic determination. Empirical therapy that includes appropriate treatment for *S. pneumoniae* is often indicated.

Algorithms for assessment and management of ill children have been developed for use in the developing world or in other settings where evaluation by a trained physician may not be feasible. Children who present with ominous signs such as inability to drink, convulsions, lethargy, and severe malnutrition are categorized as having very severe disease without further evaluation by the community health care worker, are given antibiotics, and are immediately referred to a hospital for diagnosis and management. Children who present with cough and tachypnea (the latter defined according to specific age strata) are further stratified into severity categories based on the presence or absence of lower chest wall indrawing and are managed accordingly with either antibiotics alone or antibiotics and referral to a hospital facility. Children with cough but no tachypnea are categorized as having a nonpneumonia respiratory illness.

■ CLINICAL MANIFESTATIONS

The clinical manifestations of pneumococcal disease depend on the site of infection and the duration of illness. Clinical syndromes are classified as noninvasive (e.g., otitis media and nonbacteremic pneumonia) or invasive (e.g., bacteremic pneumonia). The pathogenesis of noninvasive illness involves contiguous spread from the nasopharynx or skin; invasive disease involves infection of a normally sterile body fluid or follows bacteremia.

Pneumonia Pneumonia is the most common serious pneumococcal syndrome and is considered invasive when associated with a positive blood culture. Pneumococcal pneumonia can present as a mild community-acquired infection at one extreme and as a life-threatening disease requiring intubation and intensive support at the other.

Presenting manifestations

The presentation of pneumococcal pneumonia does not reliably distinguish it from pneumonia of other etiologies. In a subset of cases, pneumococcal pneumonia is recognized at the outset as associated with a viral upper respiratory infection and is characterized by the abrupt onset of cough and dyspnea accompanied by fever, shaking chills, and myalgias. The cough evolves from nonpurulent to productive of sputum that is purulent and sometimes tinged with blood. Patients may describe stabbing pleuritic chest pain and significant dyspnea indicating involvement of the parietal pleura. Among the elderly, the presenting clinical symptoms may be less specific, with confusion or malaise but without fever or cough. In such cases, a high index of suspicion is required because failure to treat pneumococcal pneumonia promptly in an elderly patient is likely to result in rapid evolution of the infection, with increased severity, morbidity, and risk of death.

Findings on physical examination

The clinical signs associated with pneumococcal pneumonia among adults include tachypnea (>30 breaths/min) and tachycardia, hypotension in severe cases, and fever in most cases (although not in all elderly patients). Respiratory signs are varied, including dullness to percussion in areas of the chest with significant consolidation, crackles on auscultation, reduced expansion of the chest in some cases as a result of splinting to reduce pain, bronchial breathing in a minority of cases, pleural rub in occasional cases, and cyanosis in cases with significant hypoxemia. Among infants with severe pneumonia, chest wall indrawing and nasal flaring are common. Nonrespiratory findings can include upper abdominal pain if the diaphragmatic pleura is involved as well as mental status changes, particularly confusion among elderly patients.

Differential diagnosis

The differential diagnosis of pneumococcal pneumonia includes cardiac conditions such as myocardial infarction and heart failure with atypical pulmonary edema; pulmonary conditions such as atelectasis; and pneumonia caused by viral pathogens, mycoplasmas, *Haemophilus influenzae*, *Klebsiella pneumoniae*, *Staphylococcus aureus*, *Legionella*, or (in HIV-infected and otherwise immunocompromised hosts) *Pneumocystis*. In cases including abdominal symptoms, the differential diagnosis includes cholecystitis, appendicitis, perforated peptic ulcer disease, and subphrenic abscesses. The challenge in cases with abdominal symptoms is to remember to include pneumococcal pneumonia—a nonabdominal process—in the differential diagnosis.

Diagnosis

Some authorities advocate treating uncomplicated, nonsevere, community-acquired pneumonia without determining the microbiologic etiology, given that this information is unlikely to alter clinical management. However, efforts to identify the cause of pneumonia are important when the disease is more severe and when the diagnosis of pneumonia is not clearly established. The gold standard for etiologic diagnosis of pneumococcal pneumonia is pathologic examination of lung tissue. In lieu of that procedure, evidence of an infiltrate on chest radiography warrants a diagnosis of pneumonia. However, cases of pneumonia without radiographic evidence do occur. An infiltrate can be absent either early in the course of the illness or with dehydration; upon rehydration, an infiltrate usually appears. The radiographic appearance of pneumococcal pneumonia is varied; it classically consists of lobar or segmental consolidation (Fig. 134-6) but in some cases is patchy. More than one lobe is involved in ~30%

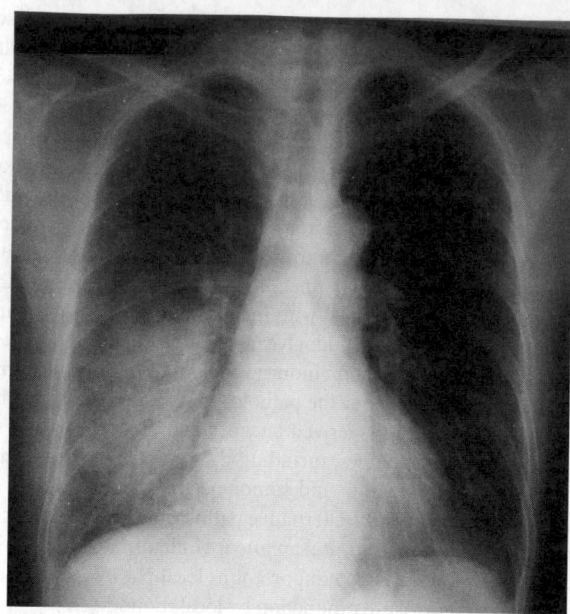

Figure 134-6   Chest radiograph depicting classic lobar pneumonia in the right lower lobe of an elderly patient's lung.

of cases. Consolidation may be associated with a small pleural effusion or empyema in complicated cases. In children, "round pneumonia," a distinctly spherical consolidation on chest radiography, is associated with a pneumococcal etiology. Round pneumonia is uncommon in adults. *S. pneumoniae* is not the only cause of such lesions; other causes, especially cancer, should be considered.

Blood drawn from patients with suspected pneumococcal pneumonia can be used for supportive or definitive diagnostic tests. Blood cultures are positive for pneumococci in a minority (<30%) of cases of pneumococcal pneumonia. Nonspecific findings include an elevated polymorphonuclear leukocyte count (>15,000/μL in most cases and upward of 40,000/μL in some), leukopenia in <10% of cases (a poor prognostic sign associated with a fatal outcome), and elevated values in liver function tests (e.g., both conjugated and unconjugated hyperbilirubinemia). Anemia, low serum albumin levels, hyponatremia, and elevated serum creatinine levels are all found in ~20–30% of patients.

Urinary pneumococcal antigen assays have facilitated etiologic diagnosis. In adults, among whom the prevalence of pneumococcal nasopharyngeal colonization is relatively low, a positive pneumococcal urinary antigen test has a high predictive value. The same is not true for children, in whom a positive urinary antigen test can reflect the mere presence of *S. pneumoniae* in the nasopharynx.

Most cases of pneumococcal pneumonia are diagnosed by Gram's staining and culture of sputum. The utility of a sputum specimen is directly related to its quality and the patient's antibiotic treatment status.

Complications

Empyema is the most common focal complication of pneumococcal pneumonia, occurring in <5% of cases. When fluid in the pleural space is accompanied by fever and leukocytosis (even low-grade) after 4–5 days of appropriate antibiotic treatment for pneumococcal pneumonia, empyema should be considered. Parapneumonic effusions are more common than empyema, representing a self-limited inflammatory response to pneumonia. Pleural fluid with frank pus, bacteria (detected by microscopic examination), or a pH of ≤7.1 indicates empyema and demands aggressive and complete drainage, usually through chest tube insertion.

Meningitis   Pneumococcal meningitis typically presents as a pyogenic condition that is clinically indistinguishable from meningitis of other bacterial etiologies. Meningitis can be the primary presenting pneumococcal syndrome or a complication of other conditions such as skull fracture, otitis media, bacteremia, or mastoiditis. Now that *H. influenzae* type b vaccine is routinely used, *S. pneumoniae* and *Neisseria meningitidis* are the most common bacterial causes of meningitis in both adults and children. Pyogenic meningitis, including that due to *S. pneumoniae*, is associated clinically with findings that include severe, generalized, gradual-onset headache, fever, and nausea as well as specific CNS manifestations such as stiff neck, photophobia, seizures, and confusion. Clinical signs include a toxic appearance, altered consciousness, bradycardia, and hypertension indicative of increased intracranial pressure. A small proportion of adult patients have Kernig's or Brudzinski's sign or cranial nerve palsies (particularly of the 3rd and 6th cranial nerves).

A definitive diagnosis of pneumococcal meningitis rests on the examination of CSF for (1) evidence of turbidity (visual inspection); (2) elevated protein level, elevated white blood cell count, and reduced glucose concentration (quantitative measurement); and (3) specific identification of the etiologic agent (culture, Gram's staining, antigen testing, or PCR). A blood culture positive for *S. pneumoniae* in conjunction with clinical manifestations of meningitis is also considered confirmatory. Among adults, detection of pneumococcal antigen in urine is considered highly specific because of the low prevalence of nasopharyngeal colonization in this age group.

The mortality rate for pneumococcal meningitis is ~20%. In addition, up to 50% of survivors experience acute or chronic complications, including deafness, hydrocephalus, and mental retardation in children and diffuse brain swelling, subarachnoid bleeding, hydrocephalus, cerebrovascular complications, and hearing loss in adults.

Other invasive syndromes *S. pneumoniae* can cause other invasive syndromes involving virtually any body site. These syndromes include primary bacteremia without other sites of infection (bacteremia without a source; occult bacteremia), osteomyelitis, septic arthritis, endocarditis, pericarditis, and peritonitis. The essential diagnostic approach is collection of fluid from the site of infection by sterile technique and examination by Gram's staining, culture, and—when relevant—capsular antigen assay or PCR. Hemolytic-uremic syndrome can complicate invasive pneumococcal disease.

Noninvasive syndromes The two major noninvasive syndromes caused by *S. pneumoniae* are sinusitis and otitis media; the latter is the most common pneumococcal syndrome and most often affects young children. The manifestations of otitis media include the acute onset of severe pain, fever, deafness, and tinnitus, most frequently in the setting of a recent upper respiratory tract infection. Clinical signs include a red, swollen, often bulging tympanic membrane with reduced movement on insufflation or tympanography. Redness of the tympanic membrane is not sufficient for the diagnosis of otitis media.

Pneumococcal sinusitis is also a complication of upper respiratory tract infections and presents with facial pain, congestion, fever, and—in many cases—persistent nighttime cough. A definitive diagnosis is made by aspiration and culture of sinus material; however, presumptive treatment is most commonly initiated after application of a strict set of clinical diagnostic criteria.

> **TREATMENT**   Pneumococcal Infections

Historically, the activity of penicillin against pneumococci made parenteral penicillin G the drug of choice for disease caused by susceptible organisms, including community-acquired pneumonia. For susceptible strains, penicillin G remains the most commonly used agent, with daily doses ranging from 50,000 U/kg for minor infections to 300,000 U/kg for meningitis. Other parenteral β-lactam drugs, such as ampicillin, cefotaxime, ceftriaxone, and cefuroxime, can be used against penicillin-susceptible strains but offer little advantage over penicillin. Macrolides and cephalosporins are alternatives for penicillin-allergic patients. While agents such as clindamycin, tetracycline, and trimethoprim-sulfamethoxazole exhibit some activity against pneumococci, resistance to these agents is frequently encountered in different parts of the world.

Penicillin-resistant pneumococci were first described in the mid-1960s, at which point tetracycline- and macrolide-resistant strains had already been reported. Multidrug-resistant strains were first described in the 1970s, but it was during the 1990s that pneumococcal drug resistance reached pandemic proportions. The use of antibiotics selects for resistant pneumococci, and strains resistant to β-lactam agents and to multiple drugs are now found all over the world. The emergence of high rates of macrolide and fluoroquinolone resistance has also been described.

The molecular basis of penicillin resistance in *S. pneumoniae* is the alteration of penicillin-binding protein (PBP) genes by transformation and horizontal transfer of DNA from related streptococcal species. Such alteration of PBPs results in lower affinity for penicillins. Depending on the specific PBP(s) and the number of PBPs altered, the level of resistance ranges from intermediate to high. For many years, penicillin susceptibility breakpoints have been defined by MICs as follows: susceptible, ≤0.06 µg/mL; intermediate, 0.12–1.0 µg/mL; and resistant, ≥2.0 µg/mL. However, in vitro results often were not predictive of the response of a patient to treatment for pneumococcal diseases other than meningitis. New recommendations have been based on the revised penicillin G breakpoints established in 2008 by the Clinical and Laboratory Standards Institute. For IV treatment of meningitis with at least 24 million units per day in 8 divided doses, the susceptibility breakpoint remains ≤0.06 µg/mL, and MICs of ≥0.12 µg/mL indicate resistance. For IV treatment of nonmeningeal infections with 12 million units per day in 6 divided doses, the breakpoints are ≤2 µg/mL for susceptible organisms, 4 µg/mL for intermediate organisms, and ≥8 µg/mL for resistant organisms; a dosage of 18–24 million units per day is recommended for strains with MICs in the intermediate category. The original breakpoints remain the same for oral treatment of nonmeningeal infections with penicillin V.

Although guidelines for antibiotic therapy should be driven in part by local patterns of resistance, guidelines from national organizations in many countries (e.g., the Infectious Diseases Society of America/American Thoracic Society, the British Thoracic Society, and the European Respiratory Society) lay out evidence-based approaches. The following guidelines for individual sepsis syndromes are based on those advocated by the American Academy of Pediatrics and published in the 2009 *Red Book*.

Meningitis Likely or Proven to Be Due to *S. pneumoniae* As a result of the increased prevalence of resistant pneumococci, first-line therapy for persons ≥1 month of age is a combination of vancomycin (adults, 30–60 mg/kg per day; infants and children, 60 mg/kg per day) and cefotaxime (adults, 8–12 g/d in 4–6 divided doses; children, 225–300 mg/kg per day in 1 dose or 2 divided doses) or ceftriaxone (adults, 4 g/d in 1 dose or 2 divided doses; children, 100 mg/kg per day in 1 dose or 2 divided doses). If children are hypersensitive to β-lactam agents (penicillins and cephalosporins), rifampin (adults, 600 mg/d; children, 20 mg/d in 1 dose or 2 divided doses) can be substituted for cefotaxime or ceftriaxone. A lumbar puncture should be considered after 48 h if the organism is not susceptible to penicillin and information on cephalosporin sensitivity is not yet available, if the patient's clinical condition does not improve or deteriorates, or if dexamethasone has been administered and may be compromising clinical evaluation. When antibiotic sensitivity data become available, treatment should be modified accordingly. If the isolate is sensitive to penicillin, vancomycin can be discontinued and penicillin can replace the cephalosporin, or cefotaxime or ceftriaxone can be continued alone. If the isolate displays any resistance to penicillin but is susceptible to the cephalosporins, vancomycin can be discontinued and cefotaxime or ceftriaxone continued. If the isolate exhibits any resistance to penicillin and is not susceptible to cefotaxime and ceftriaxone, vancomycin and high-dose cefotaxime or ceftriaxone can be continued; rifampin may be added as well if the isolate is susceptible and the patient's clinical condition is worsening, if the CSF remains positive for bacteria, or if the MIC of the cephalosporin in question against the infecting strain is high. Some physicians advocate the use of glucocorticoids in children >6 months old, but this recommendation remains controversial and is not universally considered the standard of care. Glucocorticoids significantly reduce rates of mortality, severe hearing loss, and neurologic sequelae in adults and should be administered to those with community-acquired bacterial meningitis. If dexamethasone is given to either adults or children, it should be administered before or in conjunction with the first antibiotic dose.

Invasive Infections (Excluding Meningitis) In previously well children with noncritical illness, antibiotic therapy with a recommended antibiotic should be instigated at the following dosages: penicillin G, 250,000–400,000 units/kg per day (in divided doses 4–6 h apart); cefotaxime, 75–100 mg/d (doses 8 h apart); or ceftriaxone, 50–75 mg/d (doses 12–24 h apart). For critically ill children, including those with myocarditis or multilobular pneumonia with hypoxia or hypotension, vancomycin may be added if the isolate may possibly be resistant to β-lactam drugs, with its use reviewed once susceptibility data become available. If the organism is resistant to β-lactam agents, therapy should be modified on the basis of clinical response and susceptibility to other antibiotics. Clindamycin or vancomycin can be used as a first-line agent for children with severe β-lactam hypersensitivity, but vancomycin should not be continued if the organism is shown to be sensitive to other non-β-lactam antibiotics.

For outpatient management, amoxicillin (1 g every 8 h) provides effective treatment for virtually all cases of pneumococcal pneumonia. Neither cephalosporins nor quinolones, which are far more expensive, offer any advantage over amoxicillin. Levofloxacin (500–750 mg/d as a single dose) and moxifloxacin (400 mg/d as a single dose) are also highly likely to be effective in the United States except in patients who come from closed populations where these drugs are used widely or who have themselves been treated recently with a quinolone. Clindamycin (600–1200 mg/d every 6 h) is effective in 90% of cases and azithromycin (500 mg on day 1 followed by 250–500 mg/d) or clarithromycin (500–750 mg/d as a single dose) in 80% of cases. Treatment failure resulting in bacteremic disease due to macrolide-resistant isolates has been amply documented in patients given azithromycin empirically. As noted above, rates of resistance to all these antibiotics are relatively low in some countries and much higher in others; high-dose amoxicillin remains the best option worldwide.

The optimal duration of treatment for pneumococcal pneumonia is uncertain, but its continuation for at least 5 days once the patient becomes afebrile appears to be a prudent approach. Cases with a second focus of infection (e.g., empyema or septic arthritis) require longer therapy.

Acute Otitis Media Amoxicillin (80–90 mg/kg per day) is recommended for children with acute otitis media except in situations where observation and symptom-based treatment without antibiotics are advocated. These situations include nonsevere illness and an uncertain diagnosis in children 6 months to 2 years of age and nonsevere illness (even if the diagnosis seems certain) in children >2 years of age. Although the optimal duration of therapy has not been conclusively established, a 10-day course is recommended for younger children and for children with severe disease at any age. For children >6 years old who have mild or moderate disease, a course of 5–7 days is considered adequate. Patients whose illness fails to respond should be reassessed at 48–72 h. If acute otitis media is confirmed and antibiotic treatment has not been started, administration of amoxicillin should be commenced. If antibiotic therapy fails, a change is indicated. Failure to respond to second-line antibiotics as well indicates that myringotomy or tympanocentesis may need to be undertaken in order to obtain samples for culture.

The above recommendations can also be followed for the treatment of sinusitis. Detailed information on the further management of these conditions in children has been published by the American Academy of Pediatrics and the American Academy of Family Physicians.

■ PREVENTION

Measures to prevent pneumococcal disease include vaccination against *S. pneumoniae* and influenza viruses, reduction of comorbidities that increase the risk of pneumococcal disease, and prevention of antibiotic overuse, which fuels pneumococcal resistance.

Capsular polysaccharide vaccines

The 23-valent pneumococcal polysaccharide vaccine (PPV23), containing 25 μg of each capsular polysaccharide, has been licensed for use since 1983. Recommendations for its use vary by country. The U.S. Advisory Committee on Immunization Practices recommends PPV23 for all persons ≥65 years of age and for those 2–64 years of age who have underlying medical conditions that put them at increased risk for pneumococcal disease or severity (Table 134-1; see also http://www.cdc.gov/vaccines/recs/schedules/default.htm). Revaccination 5 years after the first dose is recommended for persons >2 years of age who have underlying medical conditions but not routinely for those whose only indication is an age of ≥65 years. PPV23 does not induce an anamnestic response, and antibody concentrations wane over time; thus revaccination is particularly important for individuals with conditions resulting in loss of antibody. Concerns about repeated revaccination have focused on safety (i.e., local reactions) and the induction of immune hyporesponsiveness. Neither the clinical relevance nor the biological basis of hyporesponsiveness is clear, but, given the possibility of its occurrence, more than one revaccination has not been recommended.

The effectiveness of PPV23 against IPD, pneumococcal pneumonia, all-cause pneumonia, and death is controversial, with wide variation in observations. The many published meta-analyses of PPV efficacy have often reached opposing conclusions with regard to a given clinical entity. Generally, observational studies cite greater effectiveness than do controlled clinical trials. The consensus is that PPV is effective against IPD but is less effective or ineffective against nonbacteremic pneumococcal pneumonia. However, published trials, observational studies, and meta-analyses contradict this view. Efficacy is often lower in the elderly and in immunodeficient patients whose condition is associated with reduced antibody responses to vaccines than in younger, healthier populations. When PPV is effective, the duration of protection following a single dose of vaccine is estimated to be ~5 years.

What is not disputed is that improved pneumococcal vaccines are needed for adults. Even in the setting of routine vaccination of infants (which indirectly protects adults from vaccine-serotype strains), disease caused by serotypes not represented in the vaccine continues to be responsible for a significant burden of disease among adults.

Polysaccharide–protein conjugate vaccines

Infants and young children respond poorly to PPV, which contains T cell–independent antigens. Consequently, another class of pneumococcal vaccines, the PCVs, were developed specifically for infants and young children. The first product, a 7-valent PCV, was licensed in 2000 in the United States. As of 2010, three PCV products—containing 7, 10, and 13 serotypes, respectively—were commercially available. The serotypes included in these PCV formulations are important causes of IPD and antibiotic resistance among young children. Randomized controlled trials have demonstrated a high degree of efficacy of PCVs against vaccine-serotype IPD as well as efficacy against pneumonia, otitis media, nasopharyngeal colonization, and all-cause mortality. PCVs are recommended by the World Health Organization for inclusion in routine childhood immunization schedules worldwide, especially in countries with high infant mortality rates.

The United States was the first country to introduce PCV and therefore has the longest experience with its community-wide effects. The introduction of PCV in the United States has resulted in a >90% reduction in vaccine-serotype IPD among the whole population (Fig. 134-7). This decline has been noted not only in those age groups immunized but also in adults and is attributable to the near elimination of vaccine-serotype nasopharyngeal colonization in immunized infants, which reduces spread to adults. This protection of unimmunized community members through vaccination of a subset of the community is termed *the indirect effect*. Increases in colonization with—and concomitantly in disease due to—non-vaccine-serotype strains (i.e., replacement colonization and disease) have been seen; however, the absolute rate increases in IPD caused by non-vaccine serotypes are generally small, especially relative to decreases in vaccine-serotype IPD (see "Epidemiology," above). Since vaccine-serotype strains are more commonly resistant to antibiotics than are non-vaccine serotypes, use of PCV has also resulted in dramatic declines in the proportion and absolute rates of drug-resistant pneumococcal disease. The recommendations of the Advisory Committee on Immunization Practices for the use of conjugate vaccines can be found at *http://www.cdc.gov/MMWR/pdf/wk/mm5909.pdf*. Recently, PCV has been shown to prevent pneumococcal infection in HIV-infected adults.

Other prevention strategies Pneumococcal disease can also be averted through the prevention of illnesses that predispose individuals to pneumococcal infections. Relevant measures include influenza vaccination and improved management and control of diabetes, HIV infection, heart disease, and lung disease. Finally, the reduction of antibiotic misuse is a strategy for the prevention of pneumococcal disease in that antimicrobial resistance directly and indirectly perpetuates organism transmission and disease in the community.

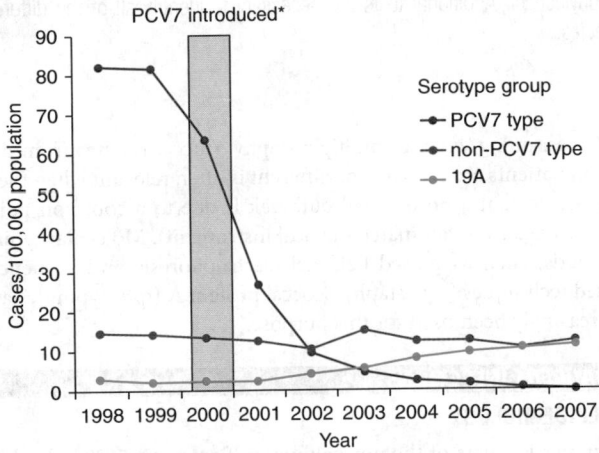

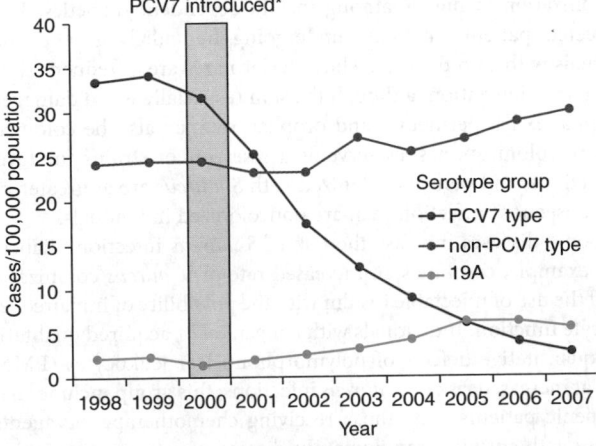

Figure 134-7 Changes in invasive pneumococcal disease (IPD) incidence, by serotype group, among children <5 years old (*top*) and adults >65 years old (*bottom*), 1998–2007. *7-Valent pneumococcal conjugate vaccine (PCV7) was introduced in the United States for routine administration to infants and young children during the second half of 2000. (*Reprinted with permission from Pilishvili et al, 2010.*)

FURTHER READINGS

FRENCH N et al: A trial of a 7-valent pneumococcal conjugate vaccine in HIV-infected adults. N Engl J Med 362:812, 2010

GOLDBLATT D et al: Antibody responses to nasopharyngeal carriage of *Streptococcus pneumoniae* in adults: A longitudinal household study. J Infect Dis 192:387, 2005

HUSS A et al: Efficacy of pneumococcal vaccination in adults: A meta-analysis. CMAJ 180:48, 2009

LUCERO MG et al: Pneumococcal conjugate vaccines for preventing vaccine-type invasive pneumococcal disease and X-ray defined pneumonia in children less than two years of age. Cochrane Database Syst Rev Oct 7(4):CD004977, 2009

MORENS DM et al: Predominant role of bacterial pneumonia as a cause of death in pandemic influenza: Implications for pandemic influenza preparedness. J Infect Dis 198:962, 2008

O'BRIEN KL et al: Burden of disease caused by *Streptococcus pneumoniae* in children younger than 5 years: Global estimates. Lancet 374:893, 2009

PILISHVILI T et al: Sustained reductions in invasive pneumococcal disease in the era of conjugate vaccine. J Infect Dis 201:32, 2010

SIBER GR et al (eds): *Pneumococcal Vaccines: The Impact of Conjugate Vaccines.* Washington, DC, ASM Press, 2008

VAN DER POLL T, OPAL SM: Pathogenesis, treatment, and prevention of pneumococcal pneumonia. Lancet 374:1543, 2009

WEB SITES

American Academy of Pediatrics RED BOOK. The report of the Committee on Infectious Diseases: *http://aapredbook. aappublications.org*

Pneumococcal Regional Serotype Distribution for Pneumococcal AMC TPP: *www.gavialliance.org/library/documents/amc/tpp-codebook/*

CHAPTER 135

Staphylococcal Infections

Franklin D. Lowy

Staphylococcus aureus, the most virulent of the many staphylococcal species, has demonstrated its versatility by remaining a major cause of morbidity and mortality despite the availability of numerous effective antistaphylococcal antibiotics. *S. aureus* is a pluripotent pathogen, causing disease through both toxin-mediated and non-toxin-mediated mechanisms. This organism is responsible for both nosocomial and community-based infections that range from relatively minor skin and soft tissue infections primarily to life-threatening systemic infections.

The "other" staphylococci, collectively designated *coagulase-negative staphylococci* (CoNS), are considerably less virulent than *S. aureus* but remain important pathogens in infections primarily associated with prosthetic devices.

MICROBIOLOGY AND TAXONOMY

Staphylococci, gram-positive cocci in the family Micrococcaceae, form grapelike clusters on Gram's stain (Fig. 135-1). These organisms are catalase-positive (unlike streptococcal species), nonmotile, aerobic, and facultatively anaerobic. They are capable of prolonged survival on environmental surfaces in varying conditions.

More than 30 staphylococcal species are pathogenic. A simple strategy for identification of the more clinically important species is outlined in Fig. 135-2. Automated diagnostic systems, kits for biochemical characterization, and DNA-based assays are available for species identification. With few exceptions, *S. aureus* is distinguished from other staphylococcal species by its production of coagulase, a surface enzyme that converts fibrinogen to fibrin. Latex kits designed to detect both protein A and clumping factor also distinguish *S. aureus* from other staphylococcal species. *S. aureus* ferments mannitol, is positive for protein A, and produces DNAse. On blood agar plates, *S. aureus* tends to form golden β-hemolytic colonies; in contrast, CoNS produce small white nonhemolytic colonies.

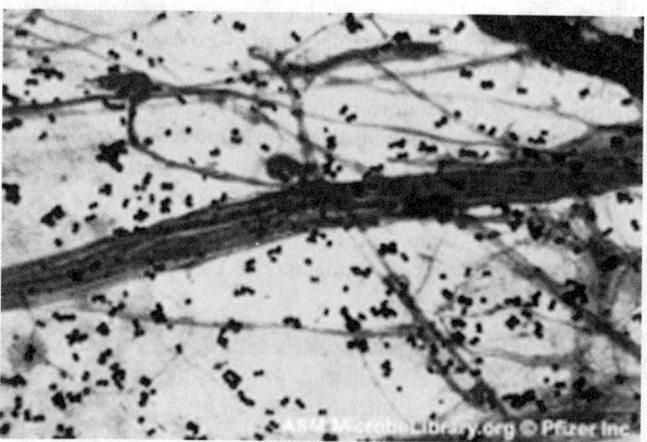

Figure 135-1 Gram's stain of *S. aureus* in a sputum sample with polymorphonuclear leukocytes. *(From ASM MicrobeLibrary.org.© Pfizer, Inc.)*

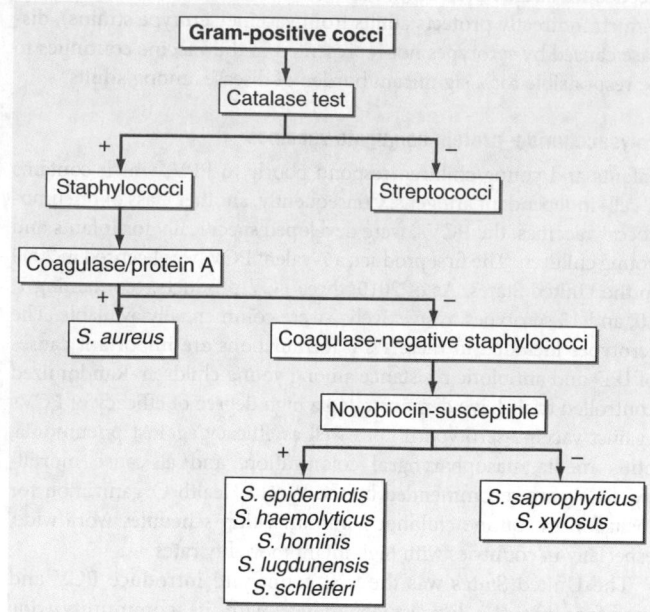

Figure 135-2 **Biochemical characterization of staphylococci:** algorithm of biochemical tests used to discriminate among the clinically important staphylococci. Additional tests are necessary to identify all of the different species.

Determining whether multiple staphylococcal isolates from different patients are the same or different is often relevant when there is concern that a nosocomial outbreak is due to a common point source (e.g., a contaminated medical instrument). Molecular typing methods, such as pulsed-field gel electrophoresis and sequence-based techniques [e.g., staphylococcal protein A (*spa*) typing], have increasingly been used for this purpose.

S. AUREUS INFECTIONS

■ EPIDEMIOLOGY

S. aureus is a part of the normal human flora; ~25–50% of healthy persons may be persistently or transiently colonized. The rate of colonization is higher among insulin-dependent diabetics, HIV-infected patients, patients undergoing hemodialysis, and individuals with skin damage. The anterior nares are a frequent site of human colonization, although the skin (especially when damaged), vagina, axilla, perineum, and oropharynx may also be colonized. These colonization sites serve as a reservoir of strains for future infections, and persons colonized with *S. aureus* are at greater risk of subsequent infection than are noncolonized individuals.

Some diseases increase the risk of *S. aureus* infection; diabetes, for example, combines an increased rate of *S. aureus* colonization and the use of injectable insulin with the possibility of impaired leukocyte function. Individuals with congenital or acquired qualitative or quantitative defects of polymorphonuclear leukocytes (PMNs) are at increased risk of *S. aureus* infections; this group includes neutropenic patients (e.g., those receiving chemotherapeutic agents), those with chronic granulomatous disease, and those with Job's or Chédiak-Higashi syndrome. Other groups at risk include individuals with skin abnormalities and those with prosthetic devices.

Overall, *S. aureus* is a leading cause of nosocomial infections. It is the most common cause of surgical wound infections and is second only to CoNS as a cause of primary bacteremia. Increasingly, nosocomial isolates are resistant to multiple antibiotics. In the community, *S. aureus* remains an important cause of skin and soft tissue infections, respiratory infections, and (among injection drug users) infective endocarditis. The increasing prevalence of home infusion therapy is another cause of community-acquired staphylococcal infections.

Most individuals who develop *S. aureus* infections are infected with their own colonizing strains. However, *S. aureus* may also be acquired from other people or from environmental exposures. Transmission most frequently results from transient colonization of the hands of hospital personnel, who then transfer strains from one patient to another. Spread of staphylococci in aerosols of respiratory or nasal secretions from heavily colonized individuals has also been reported.

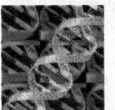 In the past 10 years, numerous outbreaks of community-based infection caused by methicillin-resistant *S. aureus* (MRSA) in individuals with no prior medical exposure have been reported. These outbreaks have taken place in both rural and urban settings in widely separated regions throughout the world. The reports document a dramatic change in the epidemiology of MRSA infections. The outbreaks have occurred among such diverse groups as children, prisoners, athletes, Native Americans, and drug users. Risk factors common to these outbreaks include poor hygienic conditions, close contact, contaminated material, and damaged skin. The community-associated infections have been caused by a limited number of MRSA strains. In the United States, strain USA300 (defined by pulsed-field gel electrophoresis) has been the predominant clone. While the majority of infections caused by this community-based clone of MRSA have involved the skin and soft tissue, 5–10% have been invasive. USA300 is also responsible for an increasing number of nosocomial infections. Of concern has been the apparent capacity of community-acquired MRSA (CA-MRSA) strains to cause serious disease in immunocompetent individuals.

■ PATHOGENESIS

General concepts

S. aureus is a pyogenic pathogen known for its capacity to induce abscess formation at sites of both local and metastatic infections. This classic pathologic response to *S. aureus* defines the framework within which the infection will progress. The bacteria elicit an inflammatory response characterized by an initial intense infiltration of PMNs and a subsequent infiltration of macrophages and fibroblasts. Either the host cellular response (including the deposition of fibrin and collagen) contains the infection, or infection spreads to the adjoining tissue or the bloodstream.

In toxin-mediated staphylococcal disease, infection is not invariably present. For example, once toxin has been elaborated into food, staphylococcal food poisoning can develop in the absence of viable bacteria. In staphylococcal toxic shock syndrome (TSS), conditions allowing toxin elaboration at colonization sites (e.g., the presence of a superabsorbent tampon) suffice for initiation of clinical illness.

The *S. aureus* genome

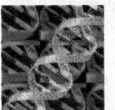 The entire genome has been sequenced for numerous strains of *S. aureus*. Among the interesting revelations are (1) a high degree of nucleotide sequence similarity among the different strains; (2) acquisition of a relatively large amount of genetic information by horizontal transfer from other bacterial species; and (3) the presence of unique "pathogenicity" or "genomic" islands—mobile genetic elements that contain clusters of enterotoxin and exotoxin genes or antimicrobial resistance determinants. Among the genes in these islands are those carrying *mecA*, the gene responsible for methicillin resistance. Methicillin resistance–containing islands have been designated

staphylococcal cassette chromosome *mecs* (SCC*mecs*) and range in size from ~20 to 60 kb. To date, eight SCC*mecs* have been identified. Types 1–3 are traditionally associated with nosocomial MRSA isolates, while types 4–6 have been associated with the epidemic CA-MRSA strains.

A limited number of MRSA clones have been responsible for most community and hospital-associated infections worldwide. A comparison of these strains with those from earlier outbreaks (e.g., the phage 80/81 strains from the 1950s) has revealed preservation of the nucleotide sequence over time. This observation suggests that these strains possess determinants that facilitate survival and spread.

Regulation of virulence gene expression

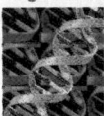 In both toxin-mediated and non-toxin-mediated diseases due to *S. aureus*, the expression of virulence determinants associated with infection depends on a series of regulatory genes [e.g., accessory gene regulator (*agr*) and staphylococcal accessory regulator (*sar*)] that coordinately control the expression of many virulence genes. The regulatory gene *agr* is part of a quorum-sensing signal transduction pathway that senses and responds to bacterial density. Staphylococcal surface proteins are synthesized during the bacterial exponential growth phase in vitro. In contrast, many secreted proteins, such as α toxin, the enterotoxins, and assorted enzymes, are released during the postexponential growth phase in response to transcription of the effector molecule of *agr*, RNAIII.

It has been hypothesized that these regulatory genes serve a similar function in vivo. Successful invasion requires the sequential expression of these different bacterial elements. Bacterial adhesins are needed to initiate colonization of host tissue surfaces. The subsequent release of various enzymes enables the colony to obtain nutritional support and permits bacteria to spread to adjacent tissues. Studies with strains in which these regulatory genes are inactivated show reduced virulence in several animal models of *S. aureus* infection.

Pathogenesis of invasive *S. aureus* infection

Staphylococci are opportunists. For these organisms to invade the host and cause infection, some or all of the following steps are necessary: contamination and colonization of tissue surfaces, establishment of a localized infection, invasion, evasion of the host response, and metastatic spread. The initiation of staphylococcal infection requires a breach in cutaneous or mucosal barriers. Colonizing strains or strains transferred from other individuals are introduced into damaged skin, a wound, or the bloodstream. Recurrences of *S. aureus* infections are common, apparently because of the capacity of these pathogens to survive, to persist in a quiescent state in various tissues, and then to cause recrudescent infections when suitable conditions arise.

***S. aureus* colonization of body surfaces**   The anterior nares are a principal site of staphylococcal colonization in humans. Colonization appears to involve the attachment of *S. aureus* to keratinized epithelial cells of the anterior nares. Other factors that may contribute to colonization include the influence of other resident nasal flora and their bacterial density, host factors, and nasal mucosal damage (e.g., that resulting from inhalational drug use). Other colonized body sites, such as damaged skin, the groin, and the oropharynx, may be particularly important reservoirs for CA-MRSA strains.

Inoculation and colonization of tissue surfaces   Staphylococci may be introduced into tissue as a result of minor abrasions, administration of medications such as insulin, or establishment of IV access with catheters. After their introduction into a tissue site, bacteria replicate and colonize the host tissue surface. A family of structurally related *S. aureus* surface proteins referred to as MSCRAMMs (microbial surface components recognizing adhesive matrix molecules) plays an important role as a mediator of adherence to these sites. By adhering to exposed matrix molecules (e.g., fibrinogen, fibronectin), MSCRAMMs such as clumping factor and collagen-binding protein enable the bacteria to colonize different tissue surfaces; these proteins contribute to the pathogenesis of invasive infections such as endocarditis and arthritis by facilitating the adherence of *S. aureus* to surfaces with exposed fibrinogen or collagen.

Although CoNS are classically known for their ability to elaborate biofilms and to colonize prosthetic devices, *S. aureus* also possesses the genes responsible for biofilm formation, such as the intercellular adhesion (*ica*) locus. Binding to these devices occurs in a stepwise fashion, involving staphylococcal adherence to serum constituents that have coated the device surface and subsequent biofilm elaboration. *S. aureus* is thus a frequent cause of biomedical-device infections.

Invasion After colonization, staphylococci replicate at the initial site of infection, elaborating enzymes that include serine proteases, hyaluronidases, thermonucleases, and lipases. These enzymes facilitate bacterial survival and local spread across tissue surfaces, although their precise role in infections is not well defined. The lipases may facilitate survival in lipid-rich areas such as the hair follicles, where *S. aureus* infections are often initiated. The *S. aureus* toxin Panton-Valentine leukocidin is cytolytic to PMNs, macrophages, and monocytes. Strains elaborating this toxin have been epidemiologically linked with cutaneous and more serious infections caused by strains of CA-MRSA.

Constitutional findings may result from either localized or systemic infections. The staphylococcal cell wall—consisting of alternating N-acetyl muramic acid and N-acetyl glucosamine units in combination with an additional cell wall component, lipoteichoic acid—can initiate an inflammatory response that includes the sepsis syndrome. Staphylococcal α toxin, which causes pore formation in various eukaryotic cells, can also initiate an inflammatory response with findings suggestive of sepsis.

Evasion of host defense mechanisms Evasion of host defense mechanisms is critical to invasion. Staphylococci possess an antiphagocytic polysaccharide microcapsule. Most human *S. aureus* infections are due to capsular types 5 and 8. The *S. aureus* capsule also plays a role in the induction of abscess formation. The capsular polysaccharides are zwitterionic: they have both negative and positive charges—a feature that is critical to abscess formation. Protein A, an MSCRAMM unique to *S. aureus*, acts as an Fc receptor, binding the Fc portion of IgG subclasses 1, 2, and 4 and preventing opsonophagocytosis by PMNs. Both chemotaxis inhibitory protein of staphylococci (CHIPS, a secreted protein) and extracellular adherence protein (EAP, a surface protein) interfere with PMN migration to sites of infection.

An additional potential mechanism of *S. aureus* evasion is its capacity for intracellular survival. Both professional and nonprofessional phagocytes internalize staphylococci. Internalization by endothelial cells may provide a sanctuary that protects bacteria against the host's defenses. It also results in cellular changes, such as the expression of integrins and Fc receptors that may contribute to systemic manifestations of disease, including sepsis and vasculitis. The intracellular environment favors the phenotypic expression of *S. aureus* small-colony variants. These menadione- and hemin-auxotrophic mutants are generally deficient in α toxin and can persist within endothelial cells. Small-colony variants are often selected after aminoglycoside therapy and are more commonly found in sites of persistent infections (e.g., chronic bone infections) and in respiratory secretions from patients with cystic fibrosis. These variants may facilitate prolonged staphylococcal survival and enhance the likelihood of recurrences. Finally, *S. aureus* can survive within PMNs and may use these cells to spread and to seed other tissue sites.

Pathogenesis of community-acquired MRSA infections A number of different virulence determinants have been identified as contributing to the pathogenesis of CA-MRSA infections. There is a strong epidemiologic association linking the presence of the gene for the Panton-Valentine leukocidin with skin and soft tissue infections as well as with invasive infections such as necrotizing pneumonia. Other determinants that may play a role in the pathogenesis of these infections include the arginine catabolic mobile element (ACME), a cluster of unique genes that may facilitate evasion of host defense mechanisms; phenol-soluble modulins, a family of cytolytic peptides; and alpha toxin.

Host response to *S. aureus* infection

The primary host response to *S. aureus* infection is the recruitment of PMNs. These cells are attracted to infection sites by bacterial components such as formylated peptides or peptidoglycan as well as by the cytokines tumor necrosis factor (TNF) and interleukins (ILs) 1 and 6, which are released by activated macrophages and endothelial cells.

Although most individuals have antistaphylococcal antibodies, it is not clear that the antibody levels are qualitatively or quantitatively sufficient to protect against infection. Although anticapsular and anti-MSCRAMM antibodies facilitate opsonization in vitro and have been protective against infection in several animal models, they have not yet successfully prevented staphylococcal infections in clinical trials.

Pathogenesis of toxin-mediated disease

S. aureus produces three types of toxin: cytotoxins, pyrogenic toxin superantigens, and exfoliative toxins. Both epidemiologic data and studies in animals suggest that antitoxin antibodies are protective against illness in TSS, staphylococcal food poisoning, and staphylococcal scalded-skin syndrome (SSSS). Illness develops after toxin synthesis and absorption and the subsequent toxin-initiated host response.

Enterotoxin and toxic shock syndrome toxin 1 (TSST-1) The pyrogenic toxin superantigens are a family of small-molecular-size, structurally similar proteins that are responsible for two diseases: TSS and food poisoning. TSS results from the ability of enterotoxins and TSST-1 to function as T cell mitogens. In the normal process of antigen presentation, the antigen is first processed within the cell, and peptides are then presented in the major histocompatibility complex (MHC) class II groove, initiating a measured T cell response. In contrast, enterotoxins bind directly to the invariant region of MHC—outside the MHC class II groove. The enterotoxins can then bind T cell receptors via the vβ chain, and this binding results in a dramatic overexpansion of T cell clones (up to 20% of the total T cell population). The consequence of this T cell expansion is a "cytokine storm," with the release of inflammatory mediators that include interferon γ, IL-1, IL-6, TNF-α, and TNF-β. The resulting multisystem disease produces a constellation of findings that mimic those in endotoxin shock; however, the pathogenic mechanisms differ. The release of endotoxin from the gastrointestinal tract may synergistically enhance the toxin's effects.

A different region of the enterotoxin molecule is responsible for the symptoms of food poisoning. The enterotoxins are heat stable and can survive conditions that kill the bacteria. Illness results from the ingestion of preformed toxin. As a result, the incubation period is short (1–6 h). The toxin stimulates the vagus nerve and the vomiting center of the brain. It also appears to stimulate intestinal peristaltic activity.

Exfoliative toxins and the staphylococcal scalded-skin syndrome The exfoliative toxins are responsible for SSSS. The toxins that produce disease in humans are of two serotypes: ETA and ETB. These toxins disrupt the desmosomes that link adjoining cells. Although the mechanism of this disruption remains uncertain, studies suggest that the toxins possess serine protease activity, which—through undefined mechanisms—triggers exfoliation. The result is a split in the epidermis at the granular level, and this event is responsible for the superficial desquamation of the skin that typifies this illness.

■ DIAGNOSIS

Staphylococcal infections are readily diagnosed by Gram's stain (Fig. 135-1) and microscopic examination of abscess contents or of infected tissue. Routine culture of infected material usually yields positive results, and blood cultures are sometimes positive even when infections are localized to extravascular sites. Polymerase chain reaction (PCR)–based assays have been applied to the rapid diagnosis of *S. aureus* infection and are increasingly used in clinical microbiology laboratories. To date, serologic assays have not proved useful for the diagnosis of staphylococcal infections. Determining whether patients with documented *S. aureus* bacteremia also have infective endocarditis or a metastatic focus of infection remains a diagnostic challenge. Uniformly positive blood cultures suggest an endovascular infection such as endocarditis (see "Bacteremia, Sepsis, and Infective Endocarditis," below).

■ CLINICAL SYNDROMES

(Table 135-1)

Skin and soft tissue infections

S. aureus causes a variety of cutaneous infections, many of which can also be caused by group A streptococci or (less commonly) other streptococcal species. Common factors predisposing to *S. aureus* cutaneous infection include chronic skin conditions (e.g., eczema), skin damage (e.g., insect bites, minor trauma), injections (e.g., in diabetes, injection drug use), and poor personal hygiene. These infections are characterized by the formation of pus-containing blisters, which often begin in hair follicles and spread to adjoining tissues. *Folliculitis* is a superficial infection that involves the hair follicle, with a central area of purulence (pus) surrounded by induration and erythema. *Furuncles* (boils) are more extensive, painful lesions that tend to occur in hairy, moist regions of the body and extend from the hair follicle to become a true abscess with an area of central purulence. *Carbuncles* are most often located in the lower neck and are even more severe and painful, resulting from the coalescence of other lesions that extend to a deeper layer of the subcutaneous tissue. In general, furuncles and carbuncles are readily apparent, with pus often expressible or discharging from the abscess.

Mastitis develops in 1–3% of nursing mothers. This infection of the breast, which generally presents within 2–3 weeks after delivery, is characterized by findings that range from cellulitis to abscess formation. Systemic signs, such as fever and chills, are often present in more severe cases. Other cutaneous *S. aureus* infections include impetigo, cellulitis, and hidradenitis suppurativa (a recurrent follicular infection in regions with apocrine glands, such as the axilla). *S. aureus* is one of the most common causes of surgical wound infection.

Musculoskeletal infections

S. aureus is among the most common causes of bone infections—both those resulting from hematogenous dissemination and those arising from contiguous spread from a soft tissue site. *Hematogenous osteomyelitis* in children most often involves the long bones. Infections present as fever and bone pain or with a child's reluctance to bear weight. The white blood cell count and erythrocyte

TABLE 135-1 Common Illnesses Caused by *Staphylococcus Aureus*

Skin and Soft Tissue Infections
- Folliculitis
- Furuncle, carbuncle
- Cellulitis
- Impetigo
- Mastitis
- Surgical wound infections
- Hidradenitis suppurativa

Musculoskeletal Infections
- Septic arthritis
- Osteomyelitis
- Pyomyositis
- Psoas abscess

Respiratory Tract Infections
- Ventilator-associated or nosocomial pneumonia
- Septic pulmonary emboli
- Postviral pneumonia (e.g., influenza)
- Empyema

Bacteremia and Its Complications
- Sepsis, septic shock
- Metastatic foci of infection (kidney, joints, bone, lung)
- Infective endocarditis

Infective Endocarditis
- Injection drug use–associated
- Native-valve
- Prosthetic-valve
- Nosocomial

Device-Related Infections (e.g., intravascular catheters, prosthetic joints)

Toxin-Mediated Illnesses
- Toxic shock syndrome
- Food poisoning
- Staphylococcal scalded-skin syndrome

Invasive Infections Associated with Community-Acquired MRSA
- Necrotizing fasciitis
- Waterhouse-Friderichsen syndrome
- Necrotizing pneumonia
- Purpura fulminans

sedimentation rate are often elevated. Blood cultures are positive in ~50% of cases. When necessary, bone biopsies for culture and histopathologic examination are usually diagnostic. Routine x-rays may be normal for up to 14 days after the onset of symptoms. ⁹⁹ᵐTc-phosphonate scanning often detects early evidence of infection. MRI is more sensitive than other techniques in establishing a radiologic diagnosis.

In adults, hematogenous osteomyelitis involving the long bones is less common. However, *vertebral osteomyelitis* is among the more common clinical presentations. Vertebral bone infections

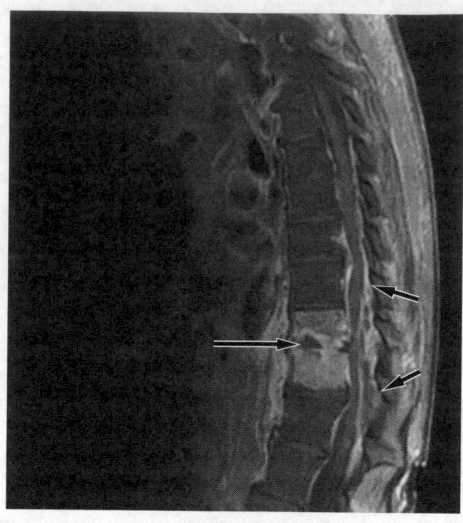

Figure 135-3 *S. aureus* vertebral osteomyelitis and epidural abscess involving the thoracic disk between T9 and T10. Sagittal postcontrast MRI of the spine illustrates destruction of the T9–T10 intervertebral space with enhancement (*arrow*). There is impingement on the thoracic cord and an epidural collection extending from T9 through T11 (*short arrows*).

are most often seen in patients with endocarditis, those undergoing hemodialysis, diabetics, and injection drug users. These infections may present as intense back pain and fever but may also be clinically occult, presenting as chronic back pain and low-grade fever. *S. aureus* is the most common cause of epidural abscess, a complication that can result in neurologic compromise. Patients complain of difficulty voiding or walking and of radicular pain in addition to the symptoms associated with their osteomyelitis. Surgical intervention in this setting often constitutes a medical emergency. MRI most reliably establishes the diagnosis (Fig. 135-3).

Bone infections that result from contiguous spread tend to develop from soft tissue infections, such as those associated with diabetic or vascular ulcers, surgery, or trauma. Exposure of bone, a draining fistulous tract, failure to heal, or continued drainage suggests involvement of underlying bone. Bone involvement is established by bone culture and histopathologic examination (revealing, for example, evidence of PMN infiltration). Contamination of culture material from adjacent tissue can make the diagnosis of osteomyelitis difficult in the absence of pathologic confirmation. In addition, it is sometimes hard to distinguish radiologically between osteomyelitis and overlying soft tissue infection with underlying osteitis.

In both children and adults, *S. aureus* is the most common cause of *septic arthritis* in native joints. This infection is rapidly progressive and may be associated with extensive joint destruction if left untreated. It presents as intense pain on motion of the affected joint, swelling, and fever. Aspiration of the joint reveals turbid fluid, with >50,000 PMNs/μL and gram-positive cocci in clusters on Gram's stain (Fig. 135-1). In adults, arthritis may result from trauma, surgery, or hematogenous dissemination. The most commonly involved joints include the knees, shoulders, hips, and phalanges. Infection frequently develops in joints previously damaged by osteoarthritis or rheumatoid arthritis. Iatrogenic infections resulting from aspiration or injection of agents into the joint also occur. In these settings, the patient experiences increased pain and swelling in the involved joint in association with fever.

Pyomyositis is an unusual infection of skeletal muscles that is seen primarily in tropical climates but also occurs in immunocompromised and HIV-infected patients. Pyomyositis presents as fever, swelling, and pain overlying the involved muscle. Aspiration of fluid from the involved tissue reveals pus. Although a history of trauma may be associated with the infection, its pathogenesis is poorly understood.

Respiratory tract infections

Respiratory tract infections caused by *S. aureus* occur in selected clinical settings. *S. aureus* is a cause of serious respiratory tract infections in newborns and infants; these infections present as shortness of breath, fever, and respiratory failure. Chest x-ray may reveal pneumatoceles (shaggy, thin-walled cavities). Pneumothorax and empyema are recognized complications of this infection.

In adults, nosocomial *S. aureus* pulmonary infections are commonly seen in intubated patients in intensive care units. Nasally colonized patients are at increased risk of these infections. The clinical presentation is no different from that encountered in pulmonary infections of other bacterial etiologies. Patients produce increased volumes of purulent sputum and develop respiratory distress, fever, and new pulmonary infiltrates. Distinguishing bacterial pneumonia from respiratory failure of other causes or new pulmonary infiltrates in critically ill patients is often difficult and relies on a constellation of clinical, radiologic, and laboratory findings.

Community-acquired respiratory tract infections due to *S. aureus* usually follow viral infections—most commonly influenza. Patients may present with fever, bloody sputum production, and midlung-field pneumatoceles or multiple, patchy pulmonary infiltrates (Fig. 135-4). Diagnosis is made by sputum Gram's stain and culture. Blood cultures, although useful, are usually negative.

Bacteremia, sepsis, and infective endocarditis

S. aureus bacteremia may be complicated by sepsis, endocarditis, vasculitis, or metastatic seeding (establishment of suppurative collections at other tissue sites). The frequency of metastatic seeding during bacteremia has been estimated to be as high as 31%. Among the more commonly seeded tissue sites are bones, joints, kidneys, and lungs.

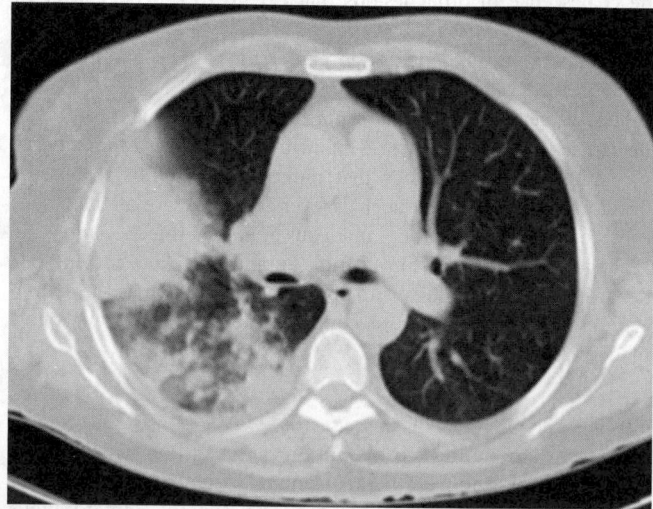

Figure 135-4 CT illustrating necrotizing pneumonia due to community-acquired **MRSA** in a diabetic woman who originally presented with a cutaneous abscess.

Recognition of these complications by clinical and laboratory diagnostic methods alone is often difficult. Comorbid conditions that are frequently seen in association with *S. aureus* bacteremia and that increase the risk of complications include diabetes, HIV infection, and renal insufficiency. Other host factors associated with an increased risk of complications include presentation with community-acquired *S. aureus* bacteremia (except in injection drug users), lack of an identifiable primary focus of infection, and the presence of prosthetic devices or material.

Clinically, *S. aureus* sepsis presents in a manner similar to that documented for sepsis due to other bacteria. The well-described progression of hemodynamic changes—beginning with respiratory alkalosis and clinical findings of hypotension and fever—is commonly seen. The microbiologic diagnosis is established by positive blood cultures.

The overall incidence of *S. aureus* endocarditis has increased over the past 20 years. *S. aureus* is now the leading cause of endocarditis worldwide, accounting for 25–35% of cases. This increase is due, at least in part, to the increased use of intravascular devices; transesophageal echocardiography studies found an infective endocarditis incidence of 25% among patients with *S. aureus* bacteremia and intravascular catheters. Other factors associated with an increased risk of endocarditis are injection drug use, hemodialysis, the presence of intravascular prosthetic devices at the time of bacteremia, and immunosuppression. Despite the availability of effective antibiotics, mortality rates from these infections continue to range from 20 to 40%, depending on both the host and the nature of the infection. Complications of *S. aureus* endocarditis include cardiac valvular insufficiency, peripheral emboli, metastatic seeding, and central nervous system (CNS) involvement (e.g., mycotic aneurysms, embolic strokes).

S. aureus endocarditis is encountered in four clinical settings: (1) right-sided endocarditis in association with injection drug use, (2) left-sided native-valve endocarditis, (3) prosthetic-valve endocarditis, and (4) nosocomial endocarditis. In each of these settings, the diagnosis is established by recognition of clinical stigmata suggestive of endocarditis. These findings include cardiac manifestations, such as new or changing cardiac valvular murmurs; cutaneous evidence, such as vasculitic lesions, Osler's nodes, or Janeway lesions; evidence of right- or left-sided embolic disease; and a history suggesting a risk for *S. aureus* bacteremia. In the absence of antecedent antibiotic therapy, blood cultures are almost uniformly positive. Transthoracic echocardiography, while less sensitive than transesophageal echocardiography, is less invasive and often establishes the presence of valvular vegetations. The Duke criteria (see Table 124-3) are now commonly used to help establish the likelihood of this diagnosis.

Acute right-sided tricuspid valvular *S. aureus* endocarditis is most often seen in injection drug users. The classic presentation includes a high fever, a toxic clinical appearance, pleuritic chest pain, and the production of purulent (sometimes bloody) sputum. Chest x-rays reveal evidence of septic pulmonary emboli (small, peripheral, circular lesions that may cavitate with time). A high percentage of affected patients have no history of antecedent valvular damage. At the outset of their illness, patients may present with fever alone, without cardiac or other localizing findings. As a result, a high index of clinical suspicion is essential for diagnosis.

Individuals with antecedent cardiac valvular damage more commonly present with left-sided native-valve endocarditis involving the previously affected valve. These patients tend to be older than those with right-sided endocarditis, their prognosis is worse, and their incidence of complications (including peripheral emboli, cardiac decompensation, and metastatic seeding) is higher.

S. aureus is one of the more common causes of prosthetic-valve endocarditis. This infection is especially fulminant in the early postoperative period and is associated with a high mortality rate. In most instances, medical therapy alone is not sufficient and urgent valve replacement is necessary. Patients are prone to develop valvular insufficiency or myocardial abscesses originating from the region of valve implantation.

The increased frequency of nosocomial endocarditis (15–30% of cases, depending on the series) reflects in part the increased use of intravascular devices. This form of endocarditis is most commonly caused by *S. aureus*. Because patients often are critically ill, are receiving antibiotics for various other indications, and have comorbid conditions, the diagnosis is often missed.

Urinary tract infections

Urinary tract infections (UTIs) are infrequently caused by *S. aureus*. In contrast with that of most other urinary pathogens, the presence of *S. aureus* in the urine suggests hematogenous dissemination. Ascending *S. aureus* infections occasionally result from instrumentation of the genitourinary tract.

Prosthetic device–related infections

S. aureus accounts for a large proportion of prosthetic device–related infections. These infections often involve intravascular catheters, prosthetic valves, orthopedic devices, peritoneal catheters, pacemakers, left-ventricular-assist devices, and vascular grafts. In contrast with the more indolent presentation of CoNS infections, *S. aureus* device-related infections often present more acutely, with both localized and systemic manifestations. The latter infections also tend to progress more rapidly. It is relatively common for a pyogenic collection to be present at the device site. Aspiration of these collections and performance of blood cultures are important components in establishing a diagnosis. *S. aureus* infections tend to occur more commonly soon after implantation unless the device is used for access (e.g., intravascular or hemodialysis catheters). In the latter instance, infections can occur at any time. As in most prosthetic-device infections, successful therapy usually involves removal of the device. Left in place, the device is a potential nidus for either persistent or recurrent infections.

Infections associated with community-acquired MRSA

While the skin and soft tissues are the most common sites of infection associated with CA-MRSA, 5–10% of these infections are invasive and can even be life-threatening. The latter infections include necrotizing fasciitis, necrotizing pneumonia, and sepsis with Waterhouse-Friderichsen syndrome or purpura fulminans. These life-threatening infections reflect the increased virulence of MRSA strains.

Toxin-mediated diseases

Food poisoning *S. aureus* is among the most common causes of foodborne outbreaks of infection in the United States. Staphylococcal food poisoning results from the inoculation of toxin-producing *S. aureus* into food by colonized food handlers. Toxin is then elaborated in such growth-promoting food as custards, potato salad, or processed meats. Even if the bacteria are killed by warming, the heat-stable toxin is not destroyed. The onset of illness is rapid, occurring within 1–6 h of ingestion. The illness is characterized by nausea and vomiting, although diarrhea, hypotension, and dehydration may also occur. The differential diagnosis includes diarrhea of other etiologies, especially that caused by similar toxins (e.g., the toxins elaborated by *Bacillus cereus*). The rapidity of onset, the absence of fever, and the epidemic nature of the presentation (without 2° spread) arouse suspicion of staphylococcal food poisoning. Symptoms generally resolve within 8–10 h. The diagnosis can be established by the demonstration of bacteria or the documentation of enterotoxin in the implicated food. Treatment is entirely supportive.

Toxic shock syndrome TSS gained attention in the early 1980s, when a nationwide outbreak occurred among young, otherwise healthy, menstruating women. Epidemiologic investigation demonstrated that these cases were associated with the use of a highly absorbent tampon that had recently been introduced to the market. Subsequent studies established the role of TSST-1 in these illnesses. Withdrawal of the tampon from the market resulted in a rapid decline in the incidence of this disease. However, menstrual and nonmenstrual cases continue to be reported.

The clinical presentation is similar in menstrual and nonmenstrual TSS, although the nature of the risk differs. Evidence of clinical *S. aureus* infection is not a prerequisite. TSS results from the elaboration of an enterotoxin or the structurally related enterotoxin-like TSST-1. More than 90% of menstrual cases are caused by TSST-1, whereas a high percentage of nonmenstrual cases are caused by enterotoxins. TSS begins with relatively nonspecific flu-like symptoms. In menstrual cases, the onset usually comes 2 or 3 days after the start of menstruation. Patients present with fever, hypotension, and erythroderma of variable intensity. Mucosal involvement is common (e.g., conjunctival hyperemia). The illness can rapidly progress to symptoms that include vomiting, diarrhea, confusion, myalgias, and abdominal pain. These symptoms reflect the multisystemic nature of the disease, with involvement of the liver, kidneys, gastrointestinal tract, and/or CNS. Desquamation of the skin occurs during convalescence, usually 1–2 weeks after the onset of illness. Laboratory findings may include azotemia, leukocytosis, hypoalbuminemia, thrombocytopenia, and liver function abnormalities.

Diagnosis of TSS still depends on a constellation of findings rather than one specific finding and on a lack of evidence of other possible infections (e.g., Rocky Mountain spotted fever; Table 135-2). Other diagnoses to be considered are drug toxicities, viral exanthems, sepsis, and Kawasaki disease. Illness occurs only in persons who lack antibody to TSST-1. Recurrences are possible if antibody fails to develop after the illness.

Staphylococcal scalded-skin syndrome SSSS most often affects newborns and children. The illness may vary from localized blister formation to exfoliation of much of the skin surface. The skin is usually fragile and often tender, with thin-walled, fluid-filled bullae. Gentle pressure results in rupture of the lesions, leaving denuded underlying skin (Nikolsky's sign; Fig. 135-5). The mucous membranes are usually spared. In more generalized infection, there are often constitutional symptoms, including fever, lethargy, and irritability with poor feeding. Significant amounts of fluid can be lost in more extensive cases. Illness usually follows localized infection at one of a number of possible sites. SSSS is much less common among adults but can follow infections caused by exfoliative toxin–producing strains.

■ PREVENTION

Prevention of the spread of *S. aureus* infections in the hospital setting involves hand washing and careful attention to appropriate isolation procedures. Through careful screening for MRSA carriage and strict isolation practices, some Scandinavian countries have been remarkably successful at preventing the introduction and dissemination of MRSA in hospitals. Other countries, such as the United States and Great Britain, have been less successful.

The use of topical antimicrobial agents (e.g., mupirocin) to eliminate nasal colonization and/or chlorhexidine to eliminate

TABLE 135-2 Case Definition of *S. aureus* Toxic Shock Syndrome

1. Fever: temperature of ≥38.9°C (≥102°F)
2. Hypotension: systolic blood pressure of ≤90 mmHg, or orthostatic hypotension (orthostatic drop in diastolic blood pressure by ≥15 mmHg, orthostatic syncope, or orthostatic dizziness)
3. Diffuse macular rash, with desquamation 1–2 weeks after onset (including the palms and soles)
4. Multisystem involvement
   a. Hepatic: bilirubin or aminotransferase levels ≥2 times normal
   b. Hematologic: platelet count ≤100,000/μL
   c. Renal: blood urea nitrogen or serum creatinine level ≥2 times the normal upper limit
   d. Mucous membranes: vaginal, oropharyngeal, or conjunctival hyperemia
   e. Gastrointestinal: vomiting or diarrhea at onset of illness
   f. Muscular: severe myalgias or serum creatine phosphokinase level ≥2 times the upper limit
   g. Central nervous system: disorientation or alteration in consciousness without focal neurologic signs and in the absence of fever and hypotension
5. Negative serologic or other tests for measles, leptospirosis, and Rocky Mountain spotted fever as well as negative blood or cerebrospinal fluid cultures for organisms other than *S. aureus*

Source: M Wharton et al: Case definitions for public health surveillance. MMWR 39:1, 1990; with permission.

cutaneous colonization with *S. aureus* and to prevent subsequent infection has been investigated in a number of clinical settings. Elimination of nasal carriage of *S. aureus* has reduced the incidence of infections among patients undergoing hemodialysis and peritoneal dialysis. Mupirocin effectively eliminates nasal colonization with *S. aureus*. An analysis of clinical trials suggests that there may also be a reduction in the incidence of postsurgical infections in those nasally colonized with *S. aureus*.

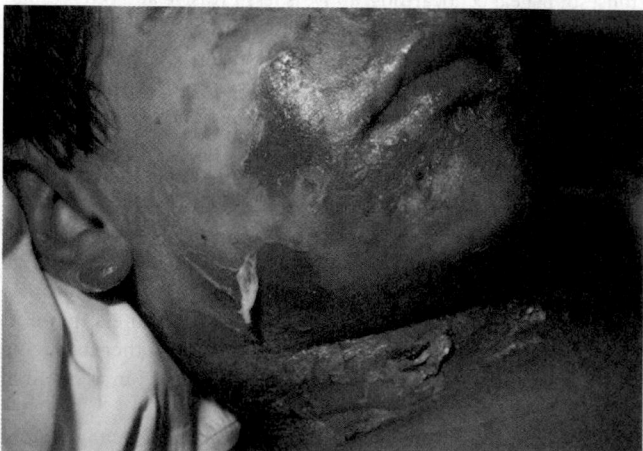

Figure 135-5 Evidence of staphylococcal scalded-skin syndrome in a 6-year-old boy. Nikolsky's sign, with separation of the superficial layer of the outer epidermal layer, is visible. *(Reprinted with permission from LA Schenfeld et al: N Engl J Med 342:1178, 2000. © 2000 Massachusetts Medical Society. All rights reserved.)*

"Bundling" (the application of selected medical interventions in a sequence of prescribed steps) has reduced rates of nosocomial infections related to such procedures as the insertion of intravenous catheters, in which staphylococci are among the most common pathogens (see Table 131-3). A number of immunization strategies to prevent *S. aureus* infections—both active (e.g., capsular polysaccharide–protein conjugate vaccine) and passive (e.g., clumping factor antibody)—have been assessed. However, none has been successful for either prophylaxis or therapy.

COAGULASE-NEGATIVE STAPHYLOCOCCAL INFECTIONS

CoNS, although considerably less virulent than *S. aureus*, are among the most common causes of prosthetic-device infections. Approximately half of the identified CoNS species have been associated with human infections. Of these species, *S. epidermidis* is the most common human pathogen. This component of the normal human flora is found on the skin (where it is the most abundant bacterial species) as well as in the oropharynx and vagina. *S. saprophyticus*, a novobiocin-resistant species, is a pathogen in UTIs.

◼ PATHOGENESIS

Among CoNS, *S. epidermidis* is the species most commonly associated with prosthetic-device infections. Infection is a two-step process, with initial adhesion to the device followed by colonization. *S. epidermidis* is uniquely adapted to colonize these devices by its capacity to elaborate the extracellular polysaccharide (glycocalyx or slime) that facilitates formation of a protective biofilm on the device surface.

Implanted prosthetic material is often coated with host serum or tissue constituents such as fibrinogen or fibronectin. These molecules serve as potential bridging ligands, facilitating initial bacterial attachment to the device surface. A number of surface-associated proteins, such as autolysin (AtlE), fibrinogen-binding protein, and accumulation-associated protein (AAP), may play a role in attachment to either modified or unmodified prosthetic surfaces. The polysaccharide intercellular adhesin facilitates subsequent staphylococcal colonization and accumulation on the device surface. In *S. epidermidis*, intercellular adhesin (*ica*) genes are more commonly found in strains associated with device infections than in strains associated with colonization of mucosal surfaces. Biofilm appears to act as a barrier protecting bacteria from host defense mechanisms as well as from antibiotics, while providing a suitable environment for bacterial survival. Poly-γ-DL-glutamic acid is secreted by *S. epidermidis* and promotes protection against neutrophil phagocytosis.

Two additional staphylococcal species, *S. lugdunensis* and *S. schleiferi*, produce more serious infections (native-valve endocarditis and osteomyelitis) than do other CoNS. The basis for this enhanced virulence is not known, although both species appear to share more virulence determinants with *S. aureus* (e.g., clumping factor and lipase) than do other CoNS.

The capacity of *S. saprophyticus* to cause UTIs in young women appears to be related to its enhanced capacity to adhere to uroepithelial cells. A 160-kDa hemagglutinin/adhesin may contribute to this affinity.

◼ DIAGNOSIS

While the detection of CoNS at sites of infection or in the bloodstream is not difficult by standard microbiologic culture methods, interpretation of these results is frequently problematic. Since these organisms are present in large numbers on the skin, they often contaminate cultures. It has been estimated that only 10–25% of blood cultures positive for CoNS reflect true bacteremia. Similar problems arise with cultures of other sites. Among the clinical findings suggestive of true bacteremia are fever, evidence of local infection (e.g., erythema or purulent drainage at the IV catheter site), leukocytosis, and systemic signs of sepsis. Laboratory findings suggestive of true bacteremia include multiple isolations of the same strain (i.e., the same species with the same antibiogram or a closely related DNA fingerprint) from separate cultures, growth of the strain within 48 h, and bacterial growth in both aerobic and anaerobic bottles.

◼ CLINICAL SYNDROMES

CoNS cause diverse prosthetic device–related infections, including those that involve prosthetic cardiac valves and joints, vascular grafts, intravascular devices, and CNS shunts. In all of these settings, the clinical presentation is similar. The signs of localized infection are often subtle, the rate of disease progression is slow, and the systemic findings are often limited. Signs of infection, such as purulent drainage, pain at the site, or loosening of prosthetic implants, are sometimes evident. Fever is frequently but not always present, and there may be mild leukocytosis. Acute-phase reactant levels, the erythrocyte sedimentation rate, and the C-reactive protein concentration may be elevated.

Infections that are not associated with prosthetic devices are infrequent, although native-valve endocarditis due to CoNS has accounted for ~5% of cases in some reviews. *S. lugdunensis* appears to be a more aggressive pathogen in this setting, causing greater mortality and rapid valvular destruction with abscess formation.

TREATMENT | Staphylococcal Infections

GENERAL PRINCIPLES OF THERAPY Surgical incision and drainage of all suppurative collections constitute the most important therapeutic intervention for staphylococcal infections. The emergence of MRSA in the community has increased the importance of culturing all collections in order to identify pathogens and to determine antimicrobial susceptibility. Prosthetic-device infections are unlikely to be successfully managed unless the device is removed. In the limited number of situations in which removal is not possible or the infection is due to CoNS, an initial attempt at medical therapy without device removal may be warranted. Because of the well-recognized risk of complications associated with *S. aureus* bacteremia (e.g., endocarditis, metastatic foci of infection), therapy is generally prolonged (4–8 weeks) unless the patient is identified as being among the small percentage of individuals who are at low risk for complications.

DURATION OF ANTIMICROBIAL THERAPY Debate continues regarding the duration of therapy for bacteremic *S. aureus* infections. Among the findings associated with an increased risk of complicated bacteremia are persistently positive blood cultures 48–96 h after institution of therapy, acquisition of the infection in the community, failure to remove a removable focus of infection (i.e., an intravascular catheter), and infection with cutaneous or embolic manifestations. For immunocompetent patients in whom short-course therapy is planned, transesophageal echocardiography to rule out endocarditis is warranted since neither clinical nor laboratory findings are adequate to detect cardiac involvement. In addition, an aggressive radiologic investigation to identify potential metastatic collections is often indicated. All symptomatic sites must be carefully evaluated.

CHOICE OF ANTIMICROBIAL AGENTS The choice of antimicrobial agents to treat both coagulase-positive and coagulase-negative staphylococcal infections has become increasingly problematic because of the prevalence of multidrug-resistant strains. Staphylococcal resistance to most antibiotic families, including β-lactams, aminoglycosides, fluoroquinolones, and (to a lesser extent) glycopeptides, has increased. This trend is more apparent with CoNS: >80% of nosocomial isolates are resistant to methicillin, and these methicillin-resistant strains are usually resistant to most other antibiotics as well. Because the selection of antimicrobial agents for *S. aureus* infections is similar to that for CoNS infections, treatment options for these pathogens are discussed together and are summarized in Table 135-3.

As a result of the widespread dissemination of plasmids containing the enzyme penicillinase, few strains of staphylococci (≤5%) remain susceptible to penicillin. However, against susceptible strains, penicillin remains the drug of choice. Penicillin-resistant isolates are treated with semisynthetic penicillinase-resistant penicillins (SPRPs), such as oxacillin or nafcillin. Methicillin, the first of the SPRPs, is now used infrequently. Cephalosporins are alternative therapeutic agents for these infections. Second- and third-generation cephalosporins do not have a therapeutic advantage over first-generation cephalosporins for the treatment of staphylococcal infections. The carbapenems have excellent activity against methicillin-sensitive *S. aureus* but not against MRSA.

The isolation of MRSA was reported within 1 year of the introduction of methicillin. The prevalence of MRSA has since increased steadily. In many hospitals, 40–50% of *S. aureus* isolates are now resistant to methicillin. Resistance to methicillin indicates resistance to all SPRPs as well as to all cephalosporins. Production of a novel penicillin-binding protein (PBP 2a or 2′) is responsible for methicillin resistance. This protein is synthesized by the *mecA* gene, which (as stated above) is part of a large mobile genetic element—a pathogenicity or genomic island—called SCC*mec*. It is hypothesized that this genetic material was acquired via horizontal transfer from a related staphylococcal species, such as *S. sciuri*. Phenotypic expression of methicillin resistance may be constitutive (i.e., expressed in all organisms in a population) or heterogeneous (i.e., displayed by only a proportion of the total organism population). Detection of methicillin resistance in the clinical microbiology laboratory can be difficult if the strain expresses heterogeneous resistance. Therefore, susceptibility studies are routinely performed at reduced temperatures (≤35°C for 24 h), with increased concentrations of salt in the medium to enhance the expression of resistance. In addition to PCR-based techniques, a number of rapid methods for the detection of methicillin resistance have been developed.

Vancomycin remains the drug of choice for the treatment of MRSA infections. Because it is less bactericidal than the β-lactams, it should be used only after careful consideration in patients with a history of β-lactam allergies. Three types of staphylococcal resistance to vancomycin have emerged. (1) Minimum inhibitory concentration (MIC) "creep" refers to the incremental increase in vancomycin MICs that has been detected in various geographic areas. Studies suggest that infections due to *S. aureus* strains with vancomycin MICs of >1 μg/mL may not respond as well to vancomycin therapy as those due to strains with MICs of <1 μg/mL. Some authorities (e.g., *The Medical Letter*) have recommended choosing an alternative agent in this setting. (2) In 1997, an *S. aureus* strain with reduced susceptibility to vancomycin (VISA) was reported from Japan. Subsequently, additional clinical isolates of VISA were reported. These strains were all resistant to methicillin and many other antimicrobial agents. The VISA strains appear to evolve (under vancomycin selective pressure) from strains that are susceptible to vancomycin but are heterogeneous, with a small proportion of the bacterial population expressing the resistance phenotype. The

mechanism of VISA resistance is due to an abnormally large cell wall. Vancomycin is trapped by the abnormal peptidoglycan cross-linking and is unable to gain access to its target site. (3) In 2002, the first clinical isolate of fully vancomycin-resistant *S. aureus* was reported. Resistance in this and six subsequently reported clinical isolates was due to the presence of *vanA*, the gene responsible for expression of vancomycin resistance in enterococci. This observation suggested that resistance was acquired as a result of horizontal conjugal transfer from a vancomycin-resistant strain of *Enterococcus faecalis*. Several patients had both MRSA and vancomycin-resistant enterococci cultured from infection sites. The *vanA* gene is responsible for the synthesis of the dipeptide D-Ala-D-Lac in place of D-Ala-D-Ala. Vancomycin cannot bind to the altered peptide.

Telavancin is a parenteral lipoglycopeptide derivative of vancomycin that was recently approved by the U.S. Food and Drug Administration for the treatment of complicated skin and soft tissue infections. This drug has two targets: the cell wall and the cell membrane. It remains active against VISA strains.

Daptomycin, a parenteral bactericidal agent with antistaphylococcal activity, is approved for the treatment of bacteremia (including right-sided endocarditis) and complicated skin infections. It is not effective in respiratory infections. This drug has a novel mechanism of action: it disrupts the cytoplasmic membrane. Staphylococcal resistance to daptomycin, sometimes developing during therapy, has been reported.

Linezolid—the first oxazolidinone—is bacteriostatic against staphylococci and offers the advantage of comparable bioavailability after oral or parenteral administration. Cross-resistance with other inhibitors of protein synthesis has not been detected. However, resistance to linezolid has been reported. Serious adverse reactions to linezolid include thrombocytopenia, occasional cases of neutropenia, and rare instances of peripheral neuropathy.

The parenteral streptogramin antibiotic quinupristin/dalfopristin displays bactericidal activity against all staphylococci, including VISA strains. This drug has been used successfully to treat serious MRSA infections. In cases of resistance to erythromycin or clindamycin, quinupristin/dalfopristin is bacteriostatic against staphylococci. There are limited data on the efficacy of either quinupristin/dalfopristin or linezolid for the treatment of infective endocarditis.

Although the quinolones are reasonably active against staphylococci in vitro, the frequency of staphylococcal resistance to these agents has increased progressively, especially among methicillin-resistant isolates. Of particular concern in MRSA is the possible emergence of quinolone resistance during therapy. Resistance to the quinolones is most commonly chromosomal and results from mutations of the topoisomerase IV or DNA gyrase genes, although multidrug efflux pumps may also contribute. While the newer quinolones exhibit increased in vitro activity against staphylococci, it is uncertain whether this increase translates into enhanced in vivo activity.

Tigecycline, a broad-spectrum minocycline analogue, has bacteriostatic activity against MRSA and is approved for use in skin and soft tissue infections as well as intraabdominal infections caused by *S. aureus*. Other antibiotics, such as minocycline and trimethoprim-sulfamethoxazole, have been used successfully to treat MRSA infections in cases of vancomycin toxicity or intolerance.

Combinations of antistaphylococcal agents are sometimes used to enhance bactericidal activity in the treatment of serious infections such as endocarditis or osteomyelitis. In selected instances (e.g., right-sided endocarditis), drug combinations are also used to shorten the duration of therapy. Among the antimicrobial agents used in combinations are

TABLE 135-3 Antimicrobial Therapy for Staphylococcal Infections[a]

Sensitivity/Resistance of Isolate	Drug of Choice	Alternative(s)	Comments
Parenteral Therapy for Serious Infections			
Sensitive to penicillin	Penicillin G (4 mU q4h)	Nafcillin or oxacillin (2 g q4h), cefazolin (2 g q8h), vancomycin (1 g q12h[b])	Fewer than 5% of isolates are sensitive to penicillin.
Sensitive to methicillin	Nafcillin or oxacillin (2 g q4h)	Cefazolin (2 g q8h[b]), vancomycin (15–20 mg/kg q8–12h[b])	Patients with penicillin allergy can be treated with a cephalosporin if the allergy does not involve an anaphylactic or accelerated reaction; desensitization to β-lactams may be indicated in selected cases of serious infection when maximal bactericidal activity is needed (e.g., prosthetic valve endocarditis[d]). Type A β-lactamase may rapidly hydrolyze cefazolin and reduce its efficacy in endocarditis. Vancomycin is a less effective option.
Resistant to methicillin	Vancomycin (15–20 mg/kg q8–12h[b])	Daptomycin (6 mg/kg q24h[b,c]) for bacteremia, endocarditis, and complicated skin infections; linezolid (600 mg q12h except: 400 mg q12h for uncomplicated skin infections); quinupristin/dalfopristin (7.5 mg/kg q8h)	Sensitivity testing is necessary before an alternative drug is used. Adjunctive drugs (those that should be used only in combination with other antimicrobial agents) include gentamicin (1 mg/kg q8h[b]), rifampin (300 mg PO q8h), and fusidic acid (500 mg q8h; not readily available in the United States). For some serious infections, higher doses of daptomycin have been used. Quinupristin/dalfopristin is bactericidal against methicillin-resistant isolates unless the strain is resistant to erythromycin or clindamycin. The efficacy of adjunctive therapy is not well established in many settings. Both linezolid and quinupristin/dalfopristin have had in vitro activity against most VISA and VRSA strains. See footnote for treatment of prosthetic-valve endocarditis.[d]
Resistant to methicillin with intermediate or complete resistance to vancomycin[e]	Uncertain	Same as for methicillin-resistant strains; check antibiotic susceptibilities	Same as for methicillin-resistant strains; check antibiotic susceptibilities
Not yet known (i.e., empirical therapy)	Vancomycin (15–20 mg/kg q8–12h[b])	–	Empirical therapy is given when the susceptibility of the isolate is not known. Vancomycin with or without an aminoglycoside is recommended for suspected community- or hospital-acquired *Staphylococcus aureus* infections because of the increased frequency of methicillin-resistant strains in the community.
Oral Therapy for Skin and Soft Tissue Infections			
Sensitive to methicillin	Dicloxacillin (500 mg qid), cephalexin (500 mg qid)	Minocycline or doxycycline (100 mg q12h[b]), TMP-SMX (1 or 2 ds tablets bid), clindamycin (300–450 mg/kg tid)	It is important to know the antibiotic susceptibility of isolates in the specific geographic region. All drainage should be cultured.
Resistant to methicillin	Clindamycin (300–450 mg/kg tid), TMP-SMX (1 or 2 ds tablets bid), minocycline or doxycycline (100 mg q12h[b]), linezolid (400–600 mg bid)		It is important to know the antibiotic susceptibility of isolates in the specific geographic region. All drainage should be cultured.

[a]Recommended dosages are for adults with normal renal and hepatic function.

[b]The dosage must be adjusted for patients with reduced creatinine clearance.

[c]Daptomycin cannot be used for pneumonia.

[d]For the treatment of prosthetic valve endocarditis, the addition of gentamicin (1 mg/kg q8h) and rifampin (300 mg PO q8h) is recommended, with adjustment of the gentamicin dosage if the creatinine clearance rate is reduced.

[e]Vancomycin-resistant *S. aureus* isolates from clinical infections have been reported.

Abbreviations: TMP-SMX, trimethoprim-sulfamethoxazole; VISA, vancomycin-intermediate *S. aureus*; VRSA, vancomycin-resistant *S. aureus*.

Source: Modified with permission from FD Lowy: N Engl J Med 339:520, 1998 (© 1998 Massachusetts Medical Society. All rights reserved.) and from DL Stevens et al: Clin Infect Dis 41:1373, 2006, and Med Lett 48:13, 2006.

rifampin, aminoglycosides (e.g., gentamicin), and fusidic acid (which is not readily available in the United States). While these agents are not effective singly because of the frequent emergence of resistance, they may be useful in combination with other agents because of their bactericidal activity against staphylococci. So far, however, clinical studies have not documented a therapeutic benefit, and recent reports have raised concern with regard to the potential nephrotoxicity of gentamicin and adverse drug reactions from the addition of rifampin.

ANTIMICROBIAL THERAPY FOR SELECTED SETTINGS When necessary, the use of oral antistaphylococcal agents for uncomplicated skin and soft tissue infections is usually successful. For other infections, parenteral therapy is indicated.

S. aureus endocarditis is usually an acute, life-threatening infection. Thus prompt collection of blood for cultures must be followed immediately by empirical antimicrobial therapy. For life-threatening *S. aureus* native-valve endocarditis, many clinicians begin therapy with a 3- to 5-day course of a β-lactam and an aminoglycoside (gentamicin, 1 mg/kg IV every 8 h), although limited clinical data support this choice. If a MRSA strain is isolated, vancomycin (15–20 mg/kg every 8–12 h, given in equal doses up to a total of 2 g) is recommended. The vancomycin dose should be adjusted on the basis of trough vancomycin levels. Patients are generally treated for 4–6 weeks, with duration depending on whether there are complications. In prosthetic-valve endocarditis, surgery in addition to antibiotic therapy is often necessary. The combination of a β-lactam agent—or, if the isolate is β-lactam-resistant, vancomycin (30 mg/kg every 24 h, given in doses up to a total of 2 g)—with an aminoglycoside (gentamicin, 1 mg/kg IV every 8 h) and rifampin (300 mg orally or IV every 8 h) is recommended. This combination is used to avoid the possible emergence of rifampin resistance during therapy if only two drugs are used.

For hematogenous osteomyelitis or septic arthritis in children, a 4-week course of therapy is usually adequate. In adults, treatment is often more prolonged. For chronic forms of osteomyelitis, surgical debridement is necessary in combination with antimicrobial therapy. For joint infections, a critical component of therapy is the repeated aspiration or arthroscopy of the affected joint to prevent damage from leukocytes. The combination of rifampin with ciprofloxacin has been used successfully to treat prosthetic-joint infections, especially when the device cannot be removed. The efficacy of this combination may reflect enhanced activity against staphylococci in biofilms as well as the attainment of effective intracellular concentrations.

The choice of empirical therapy for staphylococcal infections depends in part on susceptibility data for the local geographic area. Increasingly, vancomycin (in combination with an aminoglycoside or rifampin for serious infections) is the drug of choice for both community- and hospital-acquired infections. The increase in CA-MRSA skin and soft tissue infections has drawn attention to the need for initiation of appropriate empirical therapy. Oral agents that have been effective against these isolates include clindamycin, trimethoprim-sulfamethoxazole, doxycycline, and linezolid.

THERAPY FOR TOXIC SHOCK SYNDROME Supportive therapy with reversal of hypotension is the mainstay of therapy for TSS. Both fluids and pressors may be necessary. Tampons or other packing material should be promptly removed. The role of antibiotics is less clear. Some investigators recommend a combination of clindamycin and a semisynthetic penicillin or vancomycin (if the isolate is resistant to methicillin). Clindamycin is advocated because, as a protein synthesis inhibitor, it reduces toxin synthesis in vitro. Linezolid also appears to be effective as a toxin synthesis inhibitor. A semisynthetic penicillin or glycopeptide is suggested to eliminate any potential focus of infection as well as to eradicate persistent carriage that might increase the likelihood of recurrent illness. Anecdotal reports document the successful use of IV immunoglobulin to treat TSS. The role of glucocorticoids in the treatment of this disease is uncertain.

THERAPY FOR OTHER TOXIN-MEDIATED DISEASES Therapy for staphylococcal food poisoning is entirely supportive. For SSSS, antistaphylococcal therapy targets the primary site of infection.

FURTHER READINGS

BODE LG et al: Preventing surgical-site infections in nasal carriers of *Staphylococcus aureus*. N Engl J Med 362:9, 2010

BURTON DC et al: Methicillin-resistant *Staphylococcus aureus* central line–associated bloodstream infections in US intensive care units, 1997–2007. JAMA 301:727, 2009

DELEO FR et al: Community-associated meticillin-resistant *Staphylococcus aureus*. Lancet 375:1557, 2010

FOWLER VG JR et al: Daptomycin versus standard therapy for bacteremia and endocarditis caused by *Staphylococcus aureus*. N Engl J Med 355:653, 2006

GRUNDMANN H et al: Emergence and resurgence of meticillin-resistant *Staphylococcus aureus* as a public-health threat. Lancet 368:874, 2006

KLEVENS RM et al: Invasive methicillin-resistant *Staphylococcus aureus* infections in the United States. JAMA 298:1763, 2007

LOWY FD: Antimicrobial resistance: The example of *Staphylococcus aureus*. J Clin Invest 111:1265, 2003

MCCORMICK JK et al: Toxic shock syndrome and bacterial superantigens: An update. Annu Rev Microbiol 55:77, 2001

MORAN GJ et al: Methicillin-resistant *S. aureus* infections among patients in the emergency department. N Engl J Med 355:666, 2006

MURDOCH DR et al: Clinical presentation, etiology, and outcome of infective endocarditis in the 21st century: The International Collaboration on Endocarditis–Prospective Cohort Study. Arch Intern Med 169:463, 2009

OTTO M: *Staphylococcus epidermidis*—the 'accidental' pathogen. Nat Rev Microbiol 7:555, 2009

CHAPTER 136

Streptococcal Infections

Michael R. Wessels

Many varieties of streptococci are found as part of the normal flora colonizing the human respiratory, gastrointestinal, and genitourinary tracts. Several species are important causes of human disease. Group A *Streptococcus* (GAS, *S. pyogenes*) is responsible for streptococcal pharyngitis, one of the most common bacterial infections of school-age children, and for the postinfectious syndromes of acute rheumatic fever (ARF) and poststreptococcal glomerulonephritis (PSGN). Group B *Streptococcus* (GBS, *S. agalactiae*) is the leading cause of bacterial sepsis and meningitis in newborns and a major cause of endometritis and fever in parturient women. Viridans streptococci are the most common cause of bacterial endocarditis. Enterococci, which are morphologically similar to streptococci, are now considered a separate genus on the basis of DNA homology studies. Thus, the species previously designated as *S. faecalis* and *S. faecium* have been renamed *Enterococcus faecalis* and *E. faecium*, respectively. The enterococci are discussed in Chap. 137.

Streptococci are gram-positive, spherical to ovoid bacteria that characteristically form chains when grown in liquid media. Most streptococci that cause human infections are facultative anaerobes, although some are strict anaerobes. Streptococci are relatively fastidious organisms, requiring enriched media for growth in the laboratory. Clinicians and clinical microbiologists identify streptococci by several classification systems, including hemolytic pattern, Lancefield group, species name, and common or trivial name. Many streptococci associated with human infection produce a zone of complete (β) hemolysis around the bacterial colony when cultured on blood agar. The β-hemolytic streptococci can be classified by the Lancefield system, a serologic grouping based on the reaction of specific antisera with bacterial cell-wall carbohydrate antigens. With rare exceptions, organisms belonging to Lancefield groups A, B, C, and G are all β-hemolytic, and each is associated with characteristic patterns of human infection. Other streptococci produce a zone of partial (α) hemolysis, often imparting a greenish appearance to the agar. These α-hemolytic streptococci are further identified by biochemical testing and include *S. pneumoniae* (Chap. 134), an important cause of pneumonia, meningitis, and other infections, and the several species referred to collectively as the *viridans streptococci*, which are part of the normal oral flora and are important agents of subacute bacterial endocarditis. Finally, some streptococci are nonhemolytic, a pattern sometimes called γ hemolysis. Among the organisms classified serologically as group D streptococci, the enterococci are classified as a distinct genus (Chap. 137). The classification of the major streptococcal groups causing human infections is outlined in Table 136-1.

GROUP A STREPTOCOCCI

Lancefield's group A consists of a single species, *S. pyogenes*. As its species name implies, this organism is associated with a variety of suppurative infections. In addition, GAS can trigger the postinfectious syndromes of ARF (which is uniquely associated with *S. pyogenes* infection; Chap. 322) and PSGN (Chap. 283).

 Worldwide, GAS infections and their postinfectious sequelae (primarily ARF and rheumatic heart disease) account for an estimated 500,000 deaths per year. Although data are incomplete, the incidence of all forms of GAS infection and that of rheumatic heart disease are thought to be tenfold higher in resource-limited countries than in developed countries (Fig. 136-1).

■ PATHOGENESIS

GAS elaborates a number of cell-surface components and extracellular products important in both the pathogenesis of infection and the human immune response. The cell wall contains a carbohydrate antigen that may be released by acid treatment. The reaction of such acid extracts with group A–specific antiserum is the basis for definitive identification of a streptococcal strain as *S. pyogenes*. The major surface protein of GAS is M protein, which occurs in more than 100 antigenically distinct types and is the basis for the serotyping

TABLE 136-1 Classification of Streptococci

Lancefield Group	Representative Species	Hemolytic Pattern	Typical Infections
A	*S. pyogenes*	β	Pharyngitis, impetigo, cellulitis, scarlet fever
B	*S. agalactiae*	β	Neonatal sepsis and meningitis, puerperal infection, urinary tract infection, diabetic ulcer infection, endocarditis
C, G	*S. dysgalactiae* subsp. *equisimilis*	β	Cellulitis, bacteremia, endocarditis
D	Enterococci[a]: *E. faecalis*; *E. faecium*	Usually nonhemolytic	Urinary tract infection, nosocomial bacteremia, endocarditis
	Nonenterococci: *S. bovis*	Usually nonhemolytic	Bacteremia, endocarditis
Variable or nongroupable	Viridans streptococci: *S. sanguis*; *S. mitis*	α	Endocarditis, dental abscess, brain abscess
	Intermedius or *milleri* group: *S. intermedius, S. anginosus, S. constellatus*	Variable	Brain abscess, visceral abscess
	Anaerobic streptococci[b]: *Peptostreptococcus magnus*	Usually nonhemolytic	Sinusitis, pneumonia, empyema, brain abscess, liver abscess

[a]See Chap. 137.
[b]See Chap. 164.

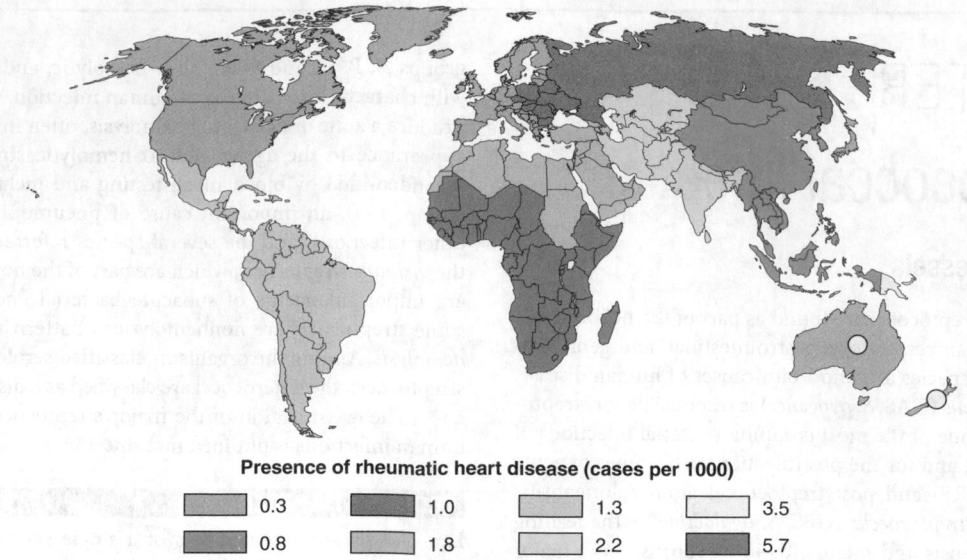

Figure 136-1 **Prevalence of rheumatic heart disease in children 5–14 years old.** The circles within Australia and New Zealand represent indigenous populations (and also Pacific Islanders in New Zealand). *(From Carapetis et al, 2005, with permission.)*

Presence of rheumatic heart disease (cases per 1000)

0.3	1.0	1.3	3.5
0.8	1.8	2.2	5.7

of strains with specific antisera. The M protein molecules are fibrillar structures anchored in the cell wall of the organism that extend as hairlike projections away from the cell surface. The amino acid sequence of the distal or amino-terminal portion of the M protein molecule is quite variable, accounting for the antigenic variation of the different M types, while more proximal regions of the protein are relatively conserved. A newer technique for assignment of M type to GAS isolates uses the polymerase chain reaction to amplify the variable region of the *emm* gene, which encodes M protein. DNA sequence analysis of the amplified gene segment can be compared with an extensive database [developed at the Centers for Disease Control and Prevention (CDC)] for assignment of *emm* type. This method eliminates the need for typing sera, which are available in only a few reference laboratories. The presence of M protein on a GAS isolate correlates with its capacity to resist phagocytic killing in fresh human blood. This phenomenon appears to be due, at least in part, to the binding of plasma fibrinogen to M protein molecules on the streptococcal surface, which interferes with complement activation and deposition of opsonic complement fragments on the bacterial cell. This resistance to phagocytosis may be overcome by M protein–specific antibodies; thus individuals with antibodies to a given M type acquired as a result of prior infection are protected against subsequent infection with organisms of the same M type but not against that with different M types.

GAS also elaborates, to varying degrees, a polysaccharide capsule composed of hyaluronic acid. The production of large amounts of capsule by certain strains imparts a characteristic mucoid appearance to the colonies. The capsular polysaccharide plays an important role in protecting GAS from ingestion and killing by phagocytes. In contrast to M protein, the hyaluronic acid capsule is a weak immunogen, and antibodies to hyaluronate have not been shown to be important in protective immunity. The presumed explanation is the apparent structural identity between streptococcal hyaluronic acid and the hyaluronic acid of mammalian connective tissues. The capsular polysaccharide may also play a role in GAS colonization of the pharynx by binding to CD44, a hyaluronic acid–binding protein expressed on human pharyngeal epithelial cells.

GAS produces a large number of extracellular products that may be important in local and systemic toxicity and in the spread of infection through tissues. These products include streptolysins S and O, toxins that damage cell membranes and account for the hemolysis produced by the organisms; streptokinase; DNAses; SpyCEP, a serine protease that cleaves and inactivates the chemoattractant cytokine interleukin 8, thereby inhibiting neutrophil recruitment to the site of infection; and several pyrogenic exotoxins. Previously known as erythrogenic toxins, the pyrogenic exotoxins cause the rash of scarlet fever. Since the mid-1980s, pyrogenic exotoxin–producing strains of GAS have been linked to unusually severe invasive infections, including necrotizing fasciitis and the streptococcal toxic shock syndrome (TSS). Several extracellular products stimulate specific antibody responses useful for serodiagnosis of recent streptococcal infection. Tests for these antibodies are used primarily for detection of preceding streptococcal infection in cases of suspected ARF or PSGN.

■ CLINICAL MANIFESTATIONS

Pharyngitis

Although seen in patients of all ages, GAS pharyngitis is one of the most common bacterial infections of childhood, accounting for 20–40% of all cases of exudative pharyngitis in children; it is rare among those under the age of 3. Younger children may manifest streptococcal infection with a syndrome of fever, malaise, and lymphadenopathy without exudative pharyngitis. Infection is acquired through contact with another individual carrying the organism. Respiratory droplets are the usual mechanism of spread, although other routes, including food-borne outbreaks, have been well described. The incubation period is 1–4 days. Symptoms include sore throat, fever and chills, malaise, and sometimes abdominal complaints and vomiting, particularly in children. Both symptoms and signs are quite variable, ranging from mild throat discomfort with minimal physical findings to high fever and severe sore throat associated with intense erythema and swelling of the pharyngeal mucosa and the presence of purulent exudate over the posterior pharyngeal wall and tonsillar pillars. Enlarged, tender anterior cervical lymph nodes commonly accompany exudative pharyngitis.

The differential diagnosis of streptococcal pharyngitis includes the many other bacterial and viral etiologies (Table 136-2).

TABLE 136-2 Infectious Etiologies of Acute Pharyngitis

Organism	Associated Clinical Syndrome(s)
Viruses	
Rhinovirus	Common cold
Coronavirus	Common cold
Adenovirus	Pharyngoconjunctival fever
Influenza virus	Influenza
Parainfluenza virus	Cold, croup
Coxsackievirus	Herpangina, hand-foot-and-mouth disease
Herpes simplex virus	Gingivostomatitis (primary infection)
Epstein-Barr virus	Infectious mononucleosis
Cytomegalovirus	Mononucleosis-like syndrome
HIV	Acute (primary) infection syndrome
Bacteria	
Group A streptococci	Pharyngitis, scarlet fever
Group C or G streptococci	Pharyngitis
Mixed anaerobes	Vincent's angina
Arcanobacterium haemolyticum	Pharyngitis, scarlatiniform rash
Neisseria gonorrhoeae	Pharyngitis
Treponema pallidum	Secondary syphilis
Francisella tularensis	Pharyngeal tularemia
Corynebacterium diphtheriae	Diphtheria
Yersinia enterocolitica	Pharyngitis, enterocolitis
Yersinia pestis	Plague
Chlamydiae	
Chlamydophila pneumoniae	Bronchitis, pneumonia
Chlamydophila psittaci	Psittacosis
Mycoplasmas	
Mycoplasma pneumoniae	Bronchitis, pneumonia

Streptococcal infection is an unlikely cause when symptoms and signs suggestive of viral infection are prominent (conjunctivitis, coryza, cough, hoarseness, or discrete ulcerative lesions of the buccal or pharyngeal mucosa). Because of the range of clinical presentations of streptococcal pharyngitis and the large number of other agents that can produce the same clinical picture, diagnosis of streptococcal pharyngitis on clinical grounds alone is not reliable. The throat culture remains the diagnostic gold standard. Culture of a throat specimen that is properly collected (i.e., by vigorous rubbing of a sterile swab over both tonsillar pillars) and properly processed is the most sensitive and specific means of definitive diagnosis. A rapid diagnostic kit for latex agglutination or enzyme immunoassay of swab specimens is a useful adjunct to throat culture. While precise figures on sensitivity and specificity vary, rapid diagnostic kits generally are >95% specific. Thus a positive result can be relied upon for definitive diagnosis and eliminates the need for throat culture. However, because rapid diagnostic tests are less sensitive than throat culture (relative sensitivity in comparative studies, 55–90%), a negative result should be confirmed by throat culture.

TREATMENT GAS Pharyngitis

In the usual course of uncomplicated streptococcal pharyngitis, symptoms resolve after 3–5 days. The course is shortened little by treatment, which is given primarily to prevent suppurative complications and ARF. Prevention of ARF depends on eradication of the organism from the pharynx, not simply on resolution of symptoms, and requires 10 days of penicillin treatment (Table 136-3). A first-generation cephalosporin, such as cephalexin or cefadroxil, may be substituted for penicillin in cases of penicillin allergy if the nature of the allergy is not an immediate hypersensitivity reaction (anaphylaxis or urticaria) or another potentially life-threatening manifestation (e.g., severe rash and fever). Alternative agents are erythromycin and azithromycin. Azithromycin is more expensive but offers the advantages of better gastrointestinal tolerability, once-daily dosing, and a 5-day treatment course at a dose of 12 mg/kg once daily (maximum, 500 mg).

Resistance to erythromycin and other macrolides is common among isolates from several countries, including Spain, Italy, Finland, Japan, and Korea. Macrolide resistance may be becoming more prevalent elsewhere with the increasing use of this class of antibiotics. In areas with resistance rates exceeding 5–10%, macrolides should be avoided unless results of susceptibility testing are known. Follow-up culture after treatment is no longer routinely recommended but may be warranted in selected cases, such as those involving patients or families with frequent streptococcal infections or those occurring in situations in which the risk of ARF is thought to be high (e.g., when cases of ARF have recently been reported in the community).

TABLE 136-3 Treatment of Group A Streptococcal Infections

Infection	Treatment[a]
Pharyngitis	Benzathine penicillin G, 1.2 mU IM; *or* penicillin V, 250 mg PO tid or 500 mg PO bid × 10 days (Children <27 kg: Benzathine penicillin G, 600,000 units IM; *or* penicillin V, 250 mg PO bid or tid × 10 days)
Impetigo	Same as pharyngitis
Erysipelas/cellulitis	Severe: Penicillin G, 1–2 mU IV q4h Mild to moderate: Procaine penicillin, 1.2 mU IM bid
Necrotizing fasciitis/myositis	Surgical debridement; *plus* penicillin G, 2–4 mU IV q4h; *plus* clindamycin,[b] 600–900 mg q8h
Pneumonia/empyema	Penicillin G, 2–4 mU IV q4h; *plus* drainage of empyema
Streptococcal toxic shock syndrome	Penicillin G, 2–4 mU IV q4h; *plus* clindamycin,[b] 600–900 mg q8h; *plus* IV immunoglobulin,[b] 2 g/kg as a single dose

[a]Penicillin allergy: A first-generation cephalosporin, such as cephalexin or cefadroxil, may be substituted for penicillin in cases of penicillin allergy if the nature of the allergy is not an immediate hypersensitivity reaction (anaphylaxis or urticaria) or another potentially life-threatening manifestation (e.g., severe rash and fever). Alternative agents for oral therapy are erythromycin (10 mg/kg PO qid, up to a maximum of 250 mg per dose) and azithromycin (a 5-day treatment course at a dose of 12 mg/kg once daily, up to a maximum of 500 mg per day). Vancomycin is an alternative for parenteral therapy.

[b]Efficacy unproven, but recommended by several experts. See text for discussion.

Complications Suppurative complications of streptococcal pharyngitis have become uncommon with the widespread use of antibiotics for most symptomatic cases. These complications result from the spread of infection from the pharyngeal mucosa to deeper tissues by direct extension or by the hematogenous or lymphatic route and may include cervical lymphadenitis, peritonsillar or retropharyngeal abscess, sinusitis, otitis media, meningitis, bacteremia, endocarditis, and pneumonia. Local complications, such as peritonsillar or parapharyngeal abscess formation, should be considered in a patient with unusually severe or prolonged symptoms or localized pain associated with high fever and a toxic appearance. Nonsuppurative complications include ARF (Chap. 322) and PSGN (Chap. 283), both of which are thought to result from immune responses to streptococcal infection. Penicillin treatment of streptococcal pharyngitis has been shown to reduce the likelihood of ARF but not that of PSGN.

Bacteriologic treatment failure and the asymptomatic carrier state

Surveillance cultures have shown that up to 20% of individuals in certain populations may have asymptomatic pharyngeal colonization with GAS. There are no definitive guidelines for management of these asymptomatic carriers or of asymptomatic patients who still have a positive throat culture after a full course of treatment for symptomatic pharyngitis. A reasonable course of action is to give a single 10-day course of penicillin for symptomatic pharyngitis and, if positive cultures persist, not to re-treat unless symptoms recur. Studies of the natural history of streptococcal carriage and infection have shown that the risk both of developing ARF and of transmitting infection to others is substantially lower among asymptomatic carriers than among individuals with symptomatic pharyngitis. Therefore, overly aggressive attempts to eradicate carriage probably are not justified under most circumstances. An exception is the situation in which an asymptomatic carrier is a potential source of infection to others. Outbreaks of food-borne infection and nosocomial puerperal infection have been traced to asymptomatic carriers who may harbor the organisms in the throat, vagina, or anus or on the skin.

| TREATMENT | Asymptomatic Pharyngeal Colonization with GAS |

When a carrier is transmitting infection to others, attempts to eradicate carriage are warranted. Data are limited on the best regimen to clear GAS after penicillin alone has failed. The combination of penicillin V (500 mg four times daily for 10 days) and rifampin (600 mg twice daily for the last 4 days) has been used to eliminate pharyngeal carriage. A 10-day course of oral vancomycin (250 mg four times daily) and rifampin (600 mg twice daily) has eradicated rectal colonization.

Scarlet fever

Scarlet fever consists of streptococcal infection, usually pharyngitis, accompanied by a characteristic rash (Fig. 136-2). The rash arises from the effects of one of three toxins, currently designated streptococcal pyrogenic exotoxins A, B, and C and previously known as erythrogenic or scarlet fever toxins. In the past, scarlet fever was thought to reflect infection of an individual lacking toxin-specific immunity with a toxin-producing strain of GAS. Susceptibility to scarlet fever was correlated with results of the Dick test, in which a small amount of erythrogenic toxin injected intradermally produced local erythema in susceptible individuals but elicited no reaction in those with specific immunity. Subsequent studies have suggested that development of the scarlet fever rash may reflect a hypersensitivity reaction requiring prior exposure to the toxin. For reasons that are not clear, scarlet fever has become less common in recent years,

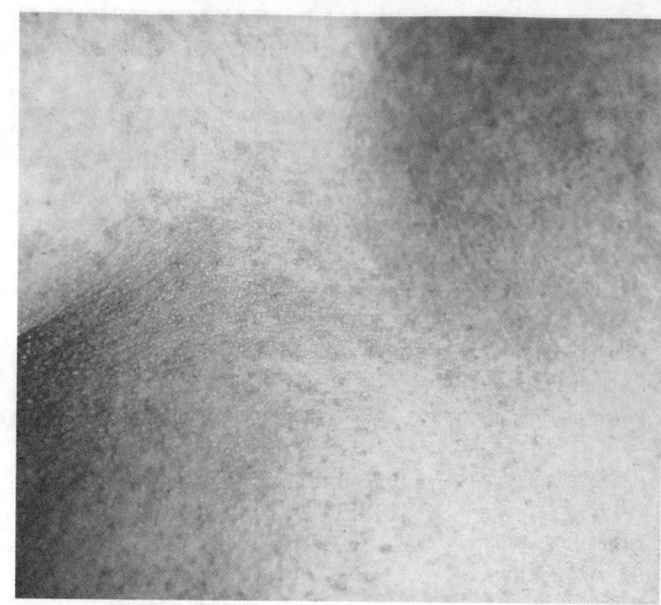

Figure 136-2   Scarlet fever exanthem. Finely punctate erythema has become confluent (scarlatiniform); petechiae can occur and have a linear configuration within the exanthem in body folds (Pastia's lines). *(From Fitzpatrick, Johnson, Wolff: Color Atlas and Synopsis of Clinical Dermatology, 4th ed, New York, McGraw-Hill, 2001, with permission.)*

although strains of GAS that produce pyrogenic exotoxins continue to be prevalent in the population. The symptoms of scarlet fever are the same as those of pharyngitis alone. The rash typically begins on the first or second day of illness over the upper trunk, spreading to involve the extremities but sparing the palms and soles. The rash is made up of minute papules, giving a characteristic "sandpaper" feel to the skin. Associated findings include circumoral pallor, "strawberry tongue" (enlarged papillae on a coated tongue, which later may become denuded), and accentuation of the rash in skinfolds (Pastia's lines). Subsidence of the rash in 6–9 days is followed after several days by desquamation of the palms and soles. The differential diagnosis of scarlet fever includes other causes of fever and generalized rash, such as measles and other viral exanthems, Kawasaki disease, toxic shock syndrome, and systemic allergic reactions (e.g., drug eruptions).

Skin and soft tissue infections

GAS—and occasionally other streptococcal species—causes a variety of infections involving the skin, subcutaneous tissues, muscles, and fascia. While several clinical syndromes offer a useful means for classification of these infections, not all cases fit exactly into one category. The classic syndromes are general guides to predicting the level of tissue involvement in a particular patient, the probable clinical course, and the likelihood that surgical intervention or aggressive life support will be required.

Impetigo (pyoderma) Impetigo, a superficial infection of the skin, is caused primarily by GAS and occasionally by other streptococci or *Staphylococcus aureus*. Impetigo is seen most often in young children, tends to occur during warmer months, and is more common in semitropical or tropical climates than in cooler regions. Infection is more common among children living under conditions of poor hygiene. Prospective studies have shown that colonization of unbroken skin with GAS precedes clinical infection. Minor trauma, such as a scratch or an insect bite, may then serve to inoculate organisms into the skin. Impetigo is best prevented, therefore, by attention to adequate hygiene. The usual sites of involvement are the face (particularly around the nose and mouth) and the legs,

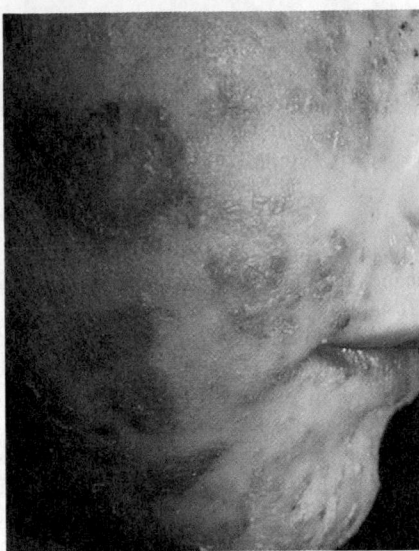

Figure 136-3 Impetigo contagiosa is a superficial streptococcal or *Staphylococcus aureus* infection consisting of honey-colored crusts and erythematous weeping erosions. Occasionally, bullous lesions may be seen. *(Courtesy of Mary Spraker, MD; with permission.)*

although lesions may occur at other locations. Individual lesions begin as red papules, which evolve quickly into vesicular and then pustular lesions that break down and coalesce to form characteristic honeycomb-like crusts (Fig. 136-3). Lesions generally are not painful, and patients do not appear ill. Fever is not a feature of impetigo and, if present, suggests either infection extending to deeper tissues or another diagnosis. The classic presentation of impetigo usually poses little diagnostic difficulty. Cultures of impetiginous lesions often yield *S. aureus* as well as GAS. In almost all cases, streptococci are isolated initially and staphylococci appear later, presumably as secondary colonizing flora. In the past, penicillin was nearly always effective against these infections. However, an increasing frequency of penicillin treatment failure suggests that *S. aureus* may have become more prominent as a cause of impetigo. *Bullous impetigo* due to *S. aureus* is distinguished from typical streptococcal infection by more extensive, bullous lesions that break down and leave thin paper-like crusts instead of the thick amber crusts of streptococcal impetigo. Other skin lesions that may be confused with impetigo include herpetic lesions—either those of orolabial herpes simplex or those of chickenpox or zoster. Herpetic lesions can generally be distinguished by their appearance as more discrete, grouped vesicles and by a positive Tzanck test. In difficult cases, cultures of vesicular fluid should yield GAS in impetigo and the responsible virus in *Herpesvirus* infections.

TREATMENT Streptococcal Impetigo

Treatment of streptococcal impetigo is the same as that for streptococcal pharyngitis. In view of evidence that *S. aureus* has become a relatively frequent cause of impetigo, empirical regimens should cover both streptococci and *S. aureus*. For example, either dicloxacillin or cephalexin can be given at a dose of 250 mg four times daily for 10 days. Topical mupirocin ointment is also effective. Culture may be indicated to rule out methicillin-resistant *S. aureus*, especially if the response to empirical treatment is unsatisfactory. ARF is not a sequela to streptococcal skin infections, although PSGN may follow either skin or throat infection.

The reason for this difference is not known. One hypothesis is that the immune response necessary for development of ARF occurs only after infection of the pharyngeal mucosa. In addition, the strains of GAS that cause pharyngitis are generally of different M protein types than those associated with skin infections; thus the strains that cause pharyngitis may have rheumatogenic potential, while the skin-infecting strains may not.

Cellulitis Inoculation of organisms into the skin may lead to *cellulitis*: infection involving the skin and subcutaneous tissues. The portal of entry may be a traumatic or surgical wound, an insect bite, or any other break in skin integrity. Often, no entry site is apparent. One form of streptococcal cellulitis, *erysipelas*, is characterized by a bright red appearance of the involved skin, which forms a plateau sharply demarcated from surrounding normal skin (Fig. 136-4). The lesion is warm to the touch, may be tender, and appears shiny and swollen. The skin often has a *peau d'orange* texture, which is thought to reflect involvement of superficial lymphatics; superficial blebs or bullae may form, usually 2–3 days after onset. The lesion typically develops over a few hours and is associated with fever and chills. Erysipelas tends to occur on the malar area of the face (often with extension over the bridge of the nose to the contralateral malar region) and the lower extremities. After one episode, recurrence at the same site—sometimes years later—is not uncommon. Classic cases of erysipelas, with typical features, are almost always due to β-hemolytic streptococci, usually GAS and occasionally group C or G. Often, however, the appearance of streptococcal cellulitis is not sufficiently distinctive to permit a specific diagnosis on clinical grounds. The area involved may not be typical for erysipelas, the lesion may be less intensely red than usual and may fade into surrounding skin, and/or the patient may appear only mildly ill. In such cases, it is prudent to broaden the spectrum of empirical antimicrobial therapy to include other pathogens, particularly *S. aureus*, that can produce cellulitis with the same appearance. Staphylococcal infection should be suspected if cellulitis develops around a wound or an ulcer.

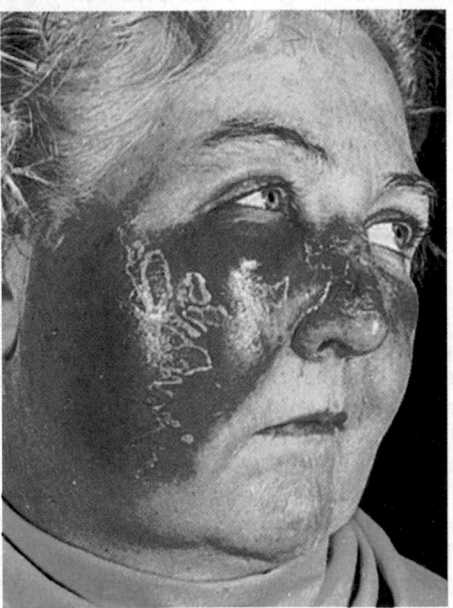

Figure 136-4 Erysipelas is a streptococcal infection of the superficial **dermis** and consists of well-demarcated, erythematous, edematous, warm plaques.

Streptococcal cellulitis tends to develop at anatomic sites in which normal lymphatic drainage has been disrupted, such as sites of prior cellulitis, the arm ipsilateral to a mastectomy and axillary lymph node dissection, a lower extremity previously involved in deep venous thrombosis or chronic lymphedema, or the leg from which a saphenous vein has been harvested for coronary artery bypass grafting. The organism may enter via a dermal breach some distance from the eventual site of clinical cellulitis. For example, some patients with recurrent leg cellulitis following saphenous vein removal stop having recurrent episodes only after treatment of tinea pedis on the affected extremity. Fissures in the skin presumably serve as a portal of entry for streptococci, which then produce infection more proximally in the leg at the site of previous injury. Streptococcal cellulitis may also involve recent surgical wounds. GAS is among the few bacterial pathogens that typically produce signs of wound infection and surrounding cellulitis within the first 24 h after surgery. These wound infections are usually associated with a thin exudate and may spread rapidly, either as cellulitis in the skin and subcutaneous tissue or as a deeper tissue infection (see below). Streptococcal wound infection or localized cellulitis may also be associated with *lymphangitis*, manifested by red streaks extending proximally along superficial lymphatics from the infection site.

TREATMENT | Streptococcal Cellulitis

See Table 136-3 and Chap. 125.

Deep soft tissue infections

Necrotizing fasciitis (*hemolytic streptococcal gangrene*) involves the superficial and/or deep fascia investing the muscles of an extremity or the trunk. The source of the infection is either the skin, with organisms introduced into tissue through trauma (sometimes trivial), or the bowel flora, with organisms released during abdominal surgery or from an occult enteric source, such as a diverticular or appendiceal abscess. The inoculation site may be inapparent and is often some distance from the site of clinical involvement; e.g., the introduction of organisms via minor trauma to the hand may be associated with clinical infection of the tissues overlying the shoulder or chest. Cases associated with the bowel flora are usually polymicrobial, involving a mixture of anaerobic bacteria (such as *Bacteroides fragilis* or anaerobic streptococci) and facultative organisms (usually gram-negative bacilli). Cases unrelated to contamination from bowel organisms are most commonly caused by GAS alone or in combination with other organisms (most often *S. aureus*). Overall, GAS is implicated in ~60% of cases of necrotizing fasciitis. The onset of symptoms is usually quite acute and is marked by severe pain at the site of involvement, malaise, fever, chills, and a toxic appearance. The physical findings, particularly early on, may not be striking, with only minimal erythema of the overlying skin. Pain and tenderness are usually severe. In contrast, in more superficial cellulitis, the skin appearance is more abnormal, but pain and tenderness are only mild or moderate. As the infection progresses (often over several hours), the severity and extent of symptoms worsen, and skin changes become more evident, with the appearance of dusky or mottled erythema and edema. The marked tenderness of the involved area may evolve into anesthesia as the spreading inflammatory process produces infarction of cutaneous nerves.

Although myositis is more commonly due to *S. aureus* infection, GAS occasionally produces abscesses in skeletal muscles (*streptococcal myositis*), with little or no involvement of the surrounding fascia or overlying skin. The presentation is usually subacute, but a fulminant form has been described in association with severe systemic toxicity,

bacteremia, and a high mortality rate. The fulminant form may reflect the same basic disease process seen in necrotizing fasciitis, but with the necrotizing inflammatory process extending into the muscles themselves rather than remaining limited to the fascial layers.

TREATMENT | Deep Soft Tissue Infections

Once necrotizing fasciitis is suspected, early surgical exploration is both diagnostically and therapeutically indicated. Surgery reveals necrosis and inflammatory fluid tracking along the fascial planes above and between muscle groups, without involvement of the muscles themselves. The process usually extends beyond the area of clinical involvement, and extensive debridement is required. Drainage and debridement are central to the management of necrotizing fasciitis; antibiotic treatment is a useful adjunct (Table 136-3), but surgery is life-saving. Treatment for streptococcal myositis consists of surgical drainage—usually by an open procedure that permits evaluation of the extent of infection and ensures adequate debridement of involved tissues—and high-dose penicillin (Table 136-3).

Pneumonia and empyema

GAS is an occasional cause of pneumonia, generally in previously healthy individuals. The onset of symptoms may be abrupt or gradual. Pleuritic chest pain, fever, chills, and dyspnea are the characteristic manifestations. Cough is usually present but may not be prominent. Approximately one-half of patients with GAS pneumonia have an accompanying pleural effusion. In contrast to the sterile parapneumonic effusions typical of pneumococcal pneumonia, those complicating streptococcal pneumonia are almost always infected. The empyema fluid is usually visible by chest radiography on initial presentation, and its volume may increase rapidly. These pleural collections should be drained early, as they tend to become loculated rapidly, resulting in a chronic fibrotic reaction that may require thoracotomy for removal.

Bacteremia, puerperal sepsis, and streptococcal toxic shock syndrome

GAS bacteremia is usually associated with an identifiable local infection. Bacteremia occurs rarely with otherwise uncomplicated pharyngitis, occasionally with cellulitis or pneumonia, and relatively frequently with necrotizing fasciitis. Bacteremia without an identified source raises the possibility of endocarditis, an occult abscess, or osteomyelitis. A variety of focal infections may arise secondarily from streptococcal bacteremia, including endocarditis, meningitis, septic arthritis, osteomyelitis, peritonitis, and visceral abscesses. GAS is occasionally implicated in infectious complications of childbirth, usually endometritis and associated bacteremia. In the preantibiotic era, puerperal sepsis was commonly caused by GAS; currently, it is more often caused by GBS. Several nosocomial outbreaks of puerperal GAS infection have been traced to an asymptomatic carrier, usually someone present at delivery. The site of carriage may be the skin, throat, anus, or vagina.

Beginning in the late 1980s, several reports described patients with GAS infections associated with shock and multisystem organ failure. This syndrome was called the streptococcal TSS because it shares certain features with staphylococcal TSS. In 1993, a case definition for streptococcal TSS was formulated (Table 136-4). The general features of the illness include fever, hypotension, renal impairment, and respiratory distress syndrome. Various types of rash have been described, but rash usually does not develop. Laboratory abnormalities include a marked shift to the left in the white blood cell differential, with many immature granulocytes; hypocalcemia; hypoalbuminemia; and thrombocytopenia, which usually becomes

TABLE 136-4 Proposed Case Definition for the Streptococcal Toxic Shock Syndrome[a]

I. Isolation of group A streptococci (*Streptococcus pyogenes*)

  A. From a normally sterile site

  B. From a nonsterile site

II. Clinical signs of severity

  A. Hypotension *and*

  B. ≥2 of the following signs

    1. Renal impairment

    2. Coagulopathy

    3. Liver function impairment

    4. Adult respiratory distress syndrome

    5. A generalized erythematous macular rash that may desquamate

    6. Soft tissue necrosis, including necrotizing fasciitis or myositis; *or* gangrene

[a] An illness fulfilling criteria IA, IIA, and IIB is defined as a *definite* case. An illness fulfilling criteria IB, IIA, and IIB is defined as a *probable* case if no other etiology for the illness is identified.

Source: Modified from Working Group on Severe Streptococcal Infections: JAMA 269:390, 1993.

more pronounced on the second or third day of illness. In contrast to patients with staphylococcal TSS, the majority with streptococcal TSS are bacteremic. The most common associated infection is a soft tissue infection—necrotizing fasciitis, myositis, or cellulitis—although a variety of other associated local infections have been described, including pneumonia, peritonitis, osteomyelitis, and myometritis. Streptococcal TSS is associated with a mortality rate of ≥30%, with most deaths secondary to shock and respiratory failure. Because of its rapidly progressive and lethal course, early recognition of the syndrome is essential. Patients should receive aggressive supportive care (fluid resuscitation, pressors, and mechanical ventilation) in addition to antimicrobial therapy and, in cases associated with necrotizing fasciitis, surgical debridement. Exactly why certain patients develop this fulminant syndrome is not known. Early studies of the streptococcal strains isolated from these patients demonstrated a strong association with the production of pyrogenic exotoxin A. This association has been inconsistent in subsequent case series. Pyrogenic exotoxin A and several other streptococcal exotoxins act as superantigens to trigger release of inflammatory cytokines from T lymphocytes. Fever, shock, and organ dysfunction in streptococcal TSS may reflect, in part, the systemic effects of superantigen-mediated cytokine release.

TREATMENT   Streptococcal Toxic Shock Syndrome

In light of the possible role of pyrogenic exotoxins or other streptococcal toxins in streptococcal TSS, treatment with clindamycin has been advocated by some authorities (Table 136-3), who argue that, through its direct action on protein synthesis, clindamycin is more effective in rapidly terminating toxin production than penicillin—a cell-wall agent. Support for this view comes from studies of an experimental model of streptococcal myositis, in which mice given clindamycin had a higher rate of survival than those given penicillin. Comparable data on the treatment of human infections are not available, although

retrospective analysis has suggested a better outcome when patients with invasive soft tissue infection are treated with clindamycin rather than with cell wall–active antibiotics. Although clindamycin resistance in GAS is uncommon (<2% among U.S. isolates), it has been documented. Thus, if clindamycin is used for initial treatment of a critically ill patient, penicillin should be given as well until the antibiotic susceptibility of the streptococcal isolate is known. IV immunoglobulin has been used as adjunctive therapy for streptococcal TSS (Table 136-3). Pooled immunoglobulin preparations contain antibodies capable of neutralizing the effects of streptococcal toxins. Anecdotal reports and case series have suggested favorable clinical responses to IV immunoglobulin, but no adequately powered, prospective, controlled trials have been reported.

Prevention

No vaccine against GAS is commercially available. A formulation that consists of recombinant peptides containing epitopes of 26 M-protein types has undergone phase 1 and 2 testing in volunteers. Early results indicate that the vaccine is well tolerated and elicits type-specific antibody responses. Vaccines based on a conserved region of M protein or on a mixture of other conserved GAS protein antigens are in earlier stages of development.

Household contacts of individuals with invasive GAS infection (e.g., bacteremia, necrotizing fasciitis, or streptococcal TSS) are at greater risk of invasive infection than the general population. Asymptomatic pharyngeal colonization with GAS has been detected in up to 25% of persons with >4 h/d of same-room exposure to an index case. However, antibiotic prophylaxis is not routinely recommended for contacts of patients with invasive disease since such an approach (if effective) would require treatment of hundreds of contacts to prevent a single case.

STREPTOCOCCI OF GROUPS C AND G

Group C and group G streptococci are β-hemolytic bacteria that occasionally cause human infections similar to those caused by GAS. Strains that form small colonies on blood agar (<0.5 mm) are generally members of the *S. milleri* (*S. intermedius, S. anginosus*) group (see "Viridans Streptococci," below). Large-colony group C and G streptococci of human origin are now considered a single species, *S. dysgalactiae* subsp. *equisimilis*. They have been associated with pharyngitis, cellulitis and soft tissue infections, pneumonia, bacteremia, endocarditis, and septic arthritis. Puerperal sepsis, meningitis, epidural abscess, intraabdominal abscess, urinary tract infection, and neonatal sepsis have also been reported. Group C or G streptococcal bacteremia most often affects elderly or chronically ill patients and, in the absence of obvious local infection, is likely to reflect endocarditis. Septic arthritis, sometimes involving multiple joints, may complicate endocarditis or develop in its absence. Distinct streptococcal species of Lancefield group C cause infections in domesticated animals, especially horses and cattle; some human infections are acquired through contact with animals or consumption of unpasteurized milk. These zoonotic organisms include *S. equi* subsp. *zooepidemicus* and *S. equi* subsp. *equi*.

TREATMENT   Group C or G Streptococcal Infection

Penicillin is the drug of choice for treatment of group C or G streptococcal infections. Antibiotic treatment is the same as for similar syndromes due to GAS (Table 136-3). Patients with bacteremia or septic arthritis should receive IV penicillin (2–4 mU every 4 h). All group C and G streptococci are sensitive to penicillin; nearly all are inhibited in vitro by concentrations of ≤0.03 μg/mL. Occasional isolates exhibit tolerance: although inhibited by low concentrations of penicillin, they are killed only by significantly higher concentrations. The clinical significance of tolerance is unknown. Because of the poor clinical response of some patients to penicillin alone, the addition of gentamicin (1 mg/kg every 8 h for patients with normal renal function) is recommended by some authorities for treatment of endocarditis or septic arthritis due to group C or G streptococci; however, combination therapy has not been shown to be superior to penicillin treatment alone. Patients with joint infections often require repeated aspiration or open drainage and debridement for cure; the response to treatment may be slow, particularly in debilitated patients and those with involvement of multiple joints. Infection of prosthetic joints almost always requires prosthesis removal in addition to antibiotic therapy.

GROUP B STREPTOCOCCI

Identified first as a cause of mastitis in cows, streptococci belonging to Lancefield's group B have since been recognized as a major cause of sepsis and meningitis in human neonates. GBS is also a frequent cause of peripartum fever in women and an occasional cause of serious infection in nonpregnant adults. Since the widespread institution of prenatal screening for GBS in the 1990s, the incidence of neonatal infection per 1000 live births has fallen from ~2–3 cases to ~0.8 case. During the same period, GBS infection in adults with underlying chronic illnesses has become more common; adults now account for a larger proportion of invasive GBS infections than do newborns. Lancefield group B consists of a single species, *S. agalactiae*, which is definitively identified with specific antiserum to the group B cell wall–associated carbohydrate antigen. A streptococcal isolate can be classified presumptively as GBS on the basis of biochemical tests, including hydrolysis of sodium hippurate (in which 99% of isolates are positive), hydrolysis of bile esculin (in which 99–100% are negative), bacitracin susceptibility (in which 92% are resistant), and production of CAMP factor (in which 98–100% are positive). CAMP factor is a phospholipase produced by GBS that causes synergistic hemolysis with β lysin produced by certain strains of *S. aureus*. Its presence can be demonstrated by cross-streaking of the test isolate and an appropriate staphylococcal strain on a blood agar plate. GBS organisms causing human infections are encapsulated by one of ten antigenically distinct polysaccharides. The capsular polysaccharide is an important virulence factor. Antibodies to the capsular polysaccharide afford protection against GBS of the same (but not of a different) capsular type.

■ INFECTION IN NEONATES

Two general types of GBS infection in infants are defined by the age of the patient at presentation. *Early-onset infections* occur within the first week of life, with a median age of 20 h at onset. Approximately half of these infants have signs of GBS disease at birth. The infection is acquired during or shortly before birth from the colonized maternal genital tract. Surveillance studies have shown that 5–40% of women are vaginal or rectal carriers of GBS. Approximately 50% of infants delivered vaginally by carrier mothers become colonized, although only 1–2% of those colonized develop clinically evident infection. Prematurity and maternal risk factors (prolonged labor, obstetric complications, and maternal fever) are often involved. The presentation of early-onset infection is the same as that of other forms of neonatal sepsis. Typical findings include respiratory distress, lethargy, and hypotension. Essentially all infants with early-onset disease are bacteremic, one-third to one-half have pneumonia and/or respiratory distress syndrome, and one-third have meningitis.

Late-onset infections occur in infants 1 week to 3 months old and, in rare instances, in older infants (mean age at onset, 3–4 weeks). The infecting organism may be acquired during delivery (as in early-onset cases) or during later contact with a colonized mother, nursery personnel, or another source. Meningitis is the most common manifestation of late-onset infection and in most cases is associated with a strain of capsular type III. Infants present with fever, lethargy or irritability, poor feeding, and seizures. The various other types of late-onset infection include bacteremia without an identified source, osteomyelitis, septic arthritis, and facial cellulitis associated with submandibular or preauricular adenitis.

TREATMENT	Group B Streptococcal Infection in Neonates

Penicillin is the agent of choice for all GBS infections. Empirical broad-spectrum therapy for suspected bacterial sepsis, consisting of ampicillin and gentamicin, is generally administered until culture results become available. If cultures yield GBS, many pediatricians continue to administer gentamicin, along with ampicillin or penicillin, for a few days until clinical improvement becomes evident. Infants with bacteremia or soft tissue infection should receive penicillin at a dosage of 200,000 units/kg per day in divided doses. For meningitis, infants ≤7 days of age should receive 250,000–450,00 units/kg per day in three divided doses; infants >7 days of age should receive 450,000–500,000 units/kg per day in four divided doses. Meningitis should be treated for at least 14 days because of the risk of relapse with shorter courses.

Prevention

The incidence of GBS infection is unusually high among infants of women with risk factors: preterm delivery, early rupture of membranes (>24 h before delivery), prolonged labor, fever, or chorioamnionitis. Because the usual source of the organisms infecting a neonate is the mother's birth canal, efforts have been made to prevent GBS infections by the identification of high-risk carrier mothers and their treatment with various forms of antibiotic or immunoprophylaxis. Prophylactic administration of ampicillin or penicillin to such patients during delivery reduces the risk of infection in the newborn. This approach has been hampered by logistical difficulties in identifying colonized women before delivery; the results of vaginal cultures early in pregnancy are poor predictors of carrier status at delivery. The CDC recommends screening for anogenital colonization at 35–37 weeks of pregnancy by a swab culture of the lower vagina and anorectum; intrapartum chemoprophylaxis is recommended for culture-positive women and for women who, regardless of culture status, have previously given birth to an infant with GBS infection or have a history of GBS bacteriuria during pregnancy. Women whose culture status is unknown and who develop premature labor (<37 weeks), prolonged rupture of membranes (>18 h), or intrapartum fever should also receive intrapartum chemoprophylaxis. The recommended regimen for chemoprophylaxis is a loading dose of 5 million units of penicillin G followed by 2.5 million units every 4 h until delivery. Cefazolin is an alternative for women with a history of penicillin allergy who are thought not to be at high risk for anaphylaxis. For women with a history of immediate hypersensitivity, clindamycin or erythromycin may be substituted, but only if the colonizing isolate has been demonstrated to be susceptible. If susceptibility testing results are not available or indicate resistance, vancomycin should be used in this situation.

Treatment of all pregnant women who are colonized or have risk factors for neonatal infection will result in exposure of up to one-third of pregnant women and newborns to antibiotics, with the attendant risks of allergic reactions and selection for resistant organisms.

Although still in the developmental stages, a GBS vaccine may ultimately offer a better solution to prevention. Because transplacental passage of maternal antibodies produces protective antibody levels in newborns, efforts are under way to develop a vaccine against GBS that can be given to childbearing-age women before or during pregnancy. Results of phase 1 clinical trials of GBS capsular polysaccharide–protein conjugate vaccines suggest that a multivalent conjugate vaccine would be safe and highly immunogenic.

◼ INFECTION IN ADULTS

The majority of GBS infections in otherwise healthy adults are related to pregnancy and parturition. Peripartum fever, the most common manifestation, is sometimes accompanied by symptoms and signs of endometritis or chorioamnionitis (abdominal distention and uterine or adnexal tenderness). Blood and vaginal swab cultures are often positive. Bacteremia is usually transitory but occasionally results in meningitis or endocarditis. Infections in adults that are not associated with the peripartum period generally involve individuals who are elderly or have an underlying chronic illness, such as diabetes mellitus or a malignancy. Among the infections that develop with some frequency in adults are cellulitis and soft tissue infection (including infected diabetic skin ulcers), urinary tract infection, pneumonia, endocarditis, and septic arthritis. Other reported infections include meningitis, osteomyelitis, and intraabdominal or pelvic abscesses. Relapse or recurrence of invasive infection weeks to months after a first episode is documented in ~4% of cases.

TREATMENT   Group B Streptococcal Infection in Adults

GBS is less sensitive to penicillin than GAS, requiring somewhat higher doses. Adults with serious localized infections (pneumonia, pyelonephritis, abscess) should receive doses of ~12 million units of penicillin G daily; patients with endocarditis or meningitis should receive 18–24 million units per day in divided doses. Vancomycin is an acceptable alternative for penicillin-allergic patients.

NONENTEROCOCCAL GROUP D STREPTOCOCCI

The main nonenterococcal group D streptococci that cause human infections belong to several species previously considered a single species, S. bovis. The organisms encompassed by S. bovis have recently been subdivided into four species: S. gallolyticus, S. pasteurianus, S. infantarius, and S. lutetiensis. S. bovis endocarditis is often associated with neoplasms of the gastrointestinal tract—most frequently, a colon carcinoma or polyp—but is also reported in association with other bowel lesions. When occult gastrointestinal lesions are carefully sought, abnormalities are found in >60% of patients with S. bovis endocarditis. In contrast to the enterococci, nonenterococcal group D streptococci like S. bovis are reliably killed by penicillin as a single agent, and penicillin is the agent of choice for S. bovis infections.

VIRIDANS AND OTHER STREPTOCOCCI

◼ VIRIDANS STREPTOCOCCI

Consisting of multiple species of α-hemolytic streptococci, the viridans streptococci are a heterogeneous group of organisms that are important agents of bacterial endocarditis (Chap. 124). Several species of viridans streptococci, including S. salivarius, S. mitis, S. sanguis, and S. mutans, are part of the normal flora of the mouth, where they live in close association with the teeth and gingiva. Some species contribute to the development of dental caries.

Previously known as S. morbillorum, Gemella morbillorum has been placed in a separate genus, along with G. haemolysans, on the basis of genetic-relatedness studies. These species resemble viridans streptococci with respect to habitat in the human host and associated infections.

The transient viridans streptococcal bacteremia induced by eating, tooth-brushing, flossing, and other sources of minor trauma, together with adherence to biologic surfaces, is thought to account for the predilection of these organisms to cause endocarditis (see Fig. 124-1). Viridans streptococci are also isolated, often as part of a mixed flora, from sites of sinusitis, brain abscess, and liver abscess.

Viridans streptococcal bacteremia occurs relatively frequently in neutropenic patients, particularly after bone marrow transplantation or high-dose chemotherapy for cancer. Some of these patients develop a sepsis syndrome with high fever and shock. Risk factors for viridans streptococcal bacteremia include chemotherapy with high-dose cytosine arabinoside, prior treatment with trimethoprim-sulfamethoxazole or a fluoroquinolone, treatment with antacids or histamine antagonists, mucositis, and profound neutropenia.

The S. milleri group (also referred to as the S. intermedius or S. anginosus group) includes three species that cause human disease: S. intermedius, S. anginosus, and S. constellatus. These organisms are often considered viridans streptococci, although they differ somewhat from other viridans streptococci in both their hemolytic pattern (they may be α-, β-, or nonhemolytic) and the disease syndromes they cause. This group commonly produces suppurative infections, particularly abscesses of brain and abdominal viscera, and infections related to the oral cavity or respiratory tract, such as peritonsillar abscess, lung abscess, and empyema.

TREATMENT   Infection with Viridans Streptococci

Isolates from neutropenic patients with bacteremia are often resistant to penicillin; thus these patients should be treated presumptively with vancomycin until the results of susceptibility testing become available. Viridans streptococci isolated in other clinical settings usually are sensitive to penicillin.

◼ ABIOTROPHIA AND GRANULICATELLA SPECIES (NUTRITIONALLY VARIANT STREPTOCOCCI)

Occasional isolates cultured from the blood of patients with endocarditis fail to grow when subcultured on solid media. These nutritionally variant streptococci require supplemental thiol compounds or active forms of vitamin B_6 (pyridoxal or pyridoxamine) for growth in the laboratory. The nutritionally variant streptococci are generally grouped with the viridans streptococci because they cause similar types of infections. However, they have been reclassified on the basis of 16S ribosomal RNA sequence comparisons into two separate genera: Abiotrophia, with a single species (A. defectivus), and Granulicatella, with three species associated with human infection (G. adjacens, G. para-adjacens, and G. elegans).

TREATMENT   Infection with Nutritionally Variant Streptococci

Treatment failure and relapse appear to be more common in cases of endocarditis due to nutritionally variant streptococci than in those due to the usual viridans streptococci. Thus the addition of gentamicin (1 mg/kg every 8 h for patients with normal renal function) to the penicillin regimen is recommended for endocarditis due to the nutritionally variant organisms.

◼ OTHER STREPTOCOCCI

S. suis is an important pathogen in swine and has been reported to cause meningitis in humans, usually in individuals with occupational exposure to pigs. Strains of *S. suis* associated with human infections have generally reacted with Lancefield group R typing serum and sometimes with group D typing serum as well. Isolates may be α- or β-hemolytic and are sensitive to penicillin. *S. iniae*, a pathogen of fish, has been associated with infections in humans who have handled live or freshly killed fish. Cellulitis of the hand is the most common form of human infection, although bacteremia and endocarditis have been reported. *Anaerobic streptococci*, or *peptostreptococci*, are part of the normal flora of the oral cavity, bowel, and vagina. Infections caused by the anaerobic streptococci are discussed in Chap. 164.

FURTHER READINGS

BISNO AL, STEVENS DL: Streptococcal infections of skin and soft tissues. N Engl J Med 334:240, 1996

BRUCKNER L, GIGLIOTTI F: Viridans group streptococcal infections among children with cancer and the importance of emerging antibiotic resistance. Semin Pediatr Infect Dis 17:153, 2006

CARAPETIS JR et al: The global burden of group A streptococcal diseases. Lancet Infect Dis 5:685, 2005

EDWARDS MS, BAKER CJ: Group B streptococcal infections in elderly adults. Clin Infect Dis 41:839, 2005

GERBER MA et al: Prevention of rheumatic fever and diagnosis and treatment of acute streptococcal pharyngitis: A scientific statement from the American Heart Association Rheumatic Fever, Endocarditis, and Kawasaki Disease Committee of the Council on Cardiovascular Disease in the Young, the Interdisciplinary Council on Functional Genomics and Translational Biology, and the Interdisciplinary Council on Quality of Care and Outcomes Research: Endorsed by the American Academy of Pediatrics. Circulation 119:1541, 2009

GIBBS RS et al: Perinatal infections due to group B streptococci. Obstet Gynecol 104:1062, 2004

KOTLOFF K: The prospect of vaccination against group A beta-hemolytic streptococci. Curr Infect Dis Rep 10:192, 2008

PHARES CR et al: Epidemiology of invasive group B streptococcal disease in the United States, 1999–2005. JAMA 299:2056, 2008

THE PREVENTION OF INVASIVE GROUP A STREPTOCOCCAL INFECTIONS WORKSHOP PARTICIPANTS: Prevention of invasive group A streptococcal disease among household contacts of case patients and among postpartum and postsurgical patients: Recommendations from the Centers for Disease Control and Prevention. Clin Infect Dis 35:950, 2002

VAN DYKE MK et al: Evaluation of universal antenatal screening for group B streptococcus. N Engl J Med 360:2626, 2009

CHAPTER 137
Enterococcal Infections

Cesar A. Arias
Barbara E. Murray

Enterococci have been recognized as potential human pathogens for more than a century, but only in recent years have these organisms acquired prominence as causes of nosocomial infections. The ability of enterococci to survive and/or disseminate in the hospital environment and to acquire antibiotic resistance determinants makes the treatment of some enterococcal infections in critically ill patients a difficult challenge. Enterococci were first mentioned in the French literature in 1899; the "entérocoque" was found in the human gastrointestinal tract and was noted to have the potential to produce significant disease. Indeed, the first pathologic description of an enterococcal infection dates to the same year. A clinical isolate recovered from a patient who died as a consequence of endocarditis was initially designated *Micrococcus zymogenes*, was later named *Streptococcus faecalis* subspecies *zymogenes*, and would now be classified as *Enterococcus faecalis*. The ability of this isolate to cause severe disease in both rabbits and mice illustrated its potential lethality in the appropriate settings.

ETIOLOGY

Enterococci are gram-positive organisms. In clinical specimens, they are usually observed as single cells, diplococci, or short chains (Fig. 137-1), although long chains are noted with some strains. Enterococci were originally classified as streptococci because organisms of the two genera share many morphologic and phenotypic characteristics, including a generally negative catalase reaction.

Only DNA hybridization studies and then 16S rRNA sequencing clearly demonstrated that enterococci should be grouped as a genus distinct from the streptococci. Nonetheless, unlike the majority of streptococci, enterococci hydrolyze esculin in the presence of 40% bile salts and grow at high salt concentrations (6.5%) and at high temperatures (46°C). Enterococci are usually reported by the clinical laboratory to be nonhemolytic on the basis of their inability

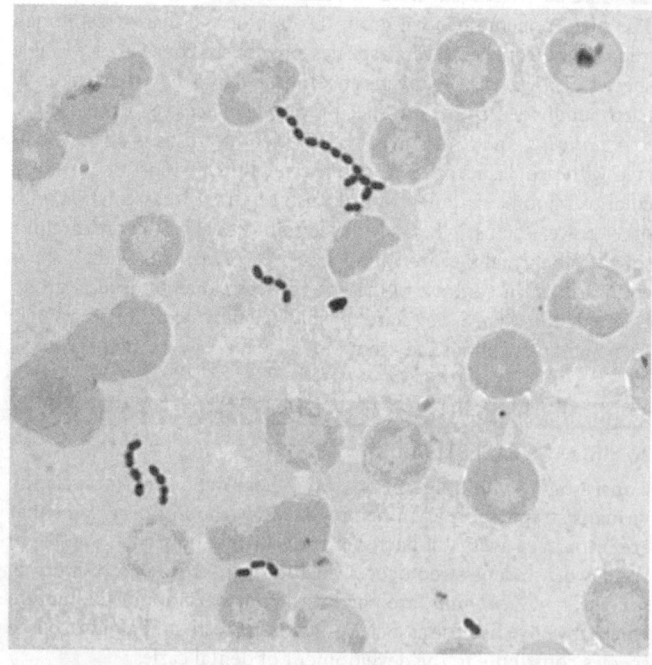

Figure 137-1 Gram's stain of cultured blood from a patient with enterococcal bacteremia. Oval gram-positive bacterial cells are arranged as diplococci and short chains. *(Courtesy of Audrey Wanger, PhD.)*

to lyse the ovine or bovine red blood cells (RBCs) commonly used in agar plates; however, some strains of *E. faecalis* do lyse RBCs from humans, horses, and rabbits. The majority of clinically relevant enterococcal species hydrolyze pyrrolidonyl-β-naphthylamide (PYR); this characteristic is helpful in differentiating enterococci from organisms of the *Streptococcus bovis* group (*S. gallolyticus* subsp. *gallolyticus*, *S. gallolyticus* subsp. *pasteurianus*, and *S. infantarius* subsp. *coli*) and from *Leuconostoc* species. Although at least 18 species of enterococci have been isolated from human infections, the overwhelming majority of cases are caused by two species: *E. faecalis* and *E. faecium*. Less frequently isolated species include *E. gallinarum*, *E. durans*, *E. hirae*, and *E. avium*.

PATHOGENESIS

Enterococci are normal inhabitants of the large bowel of human adults, although they usually make up <1% of the culturable intestinal microflora. In the healthy human gastrointestinal tract, enterococci are typically symbionts that coexist with other bacteria; in fact, the utility of certain enterococcal strains as probiotics in the treatment of diarrhea suggests their possible role in maintaining the homeostatic equilibrium of the human bowel. Enterococci are intrinsically resistant to a variety of commonly used antibiotics; thus one of the most important factors that disrupts this equilibrium and promotes increased gastrointestinal colonization by enterococci is the administration of antimicrobial agents. In particular, antibiotics that are excreted in the bile and have broad-spectrum activity (i.e., certain cephalosporins that target anaerobes and gram-negative bacteria) are associated with the recovery of higher numbers of enterococci from feces. This increased colonization appears to be due not only to simple enterococcal replacement in a given "biological niche" after the eradication of competing components of the flora but also (at least in mice) to the suppression—upon reduction of the gram-negative microflora by antibiotics—of important immunologic signals (e.g., the lectin RegIIIγ) that help keep enterococcal counts low in the normal human bowel. Several studies have shown that higher levels of gastrointestinal colonization are a critical factor in the pathogenesis of enterococcal infections. However, the mechanisms by which enterococci successfully colonize the bowel and gain access to the lymphatics and/or bloodstream remain incompletely understood.

Several vertebrate, worm, and insect models have been developed to study the role of possible pathogenic determinants of both *E. faecalis* and *E. faecium*. Three main groups of factors may increase the ability of enterococci to colonize the gastrointestinal tract and/or cause disease. The first group, *enterococcal secreted factors*, are molecules released outside the bacterial cell that contribute to the process of infection; the best-studied of these molecules include enterococcal hemolysin/cytolysin and two enterococcal proteases (gelatinase and serine protease). Enterococcal cytolysin is a heterodimeric toxin produced by some strains of *E. faecalis* that is capable of lysing human RBCs as well as polymorphonuclear leukocytes and macrophages. The *E. faecalis* proteases GelE and SprE are thought to mediate virulence by several mechanisms, including the degradation of host tissues and the modification of critical components of the immune system. Mutants lacking the genes corresponding to these proteins are highly attenuated in experimental peritonitis, endocarditis, and endophthalmitis.

The second group of virulence factors, *enterococcal surface components* (e.g., adhesins), are thought to contribute to bacterial attachment to extracellular matrix molecules in the human host. Several molecules on the surface of enterococci have been characterized and shown to play a role in the pathogenesis of enterococcal infections. Among the characterized adhesins is aggregation substance of *E. faecalis*, which mediates the attachment of cells to each other, thereby facilitating conjugative plasmid exchange. Several lines of evidence indicate that aggregation substance and enterococcal cytolysin act synergistically to increase the virulence potential of *E. faecalis* strains in experimental endocarditis. The *E. faecalis* surface protein (adhesin of collagen of *E. faecalis*, or Ace) and its *E. faecium* homologue (Acm) are microbial surface components recognizing adhesive matrix molecules (MSCRAMMs) involved in bacterial attachment to host proteins such as collagen, fibronectin, and fibrinogen; both Ace and Acm are important in the pathogenesis of experimental endocarditis. Pili of gram-positive bacteria have been shown to be important mediators of attachment to and invasion of host tissues and are considered potential targets for immunotherapy. Both *E. faecalis* and *E. faecium* have surface pili. Mutants of *E. faecalis* lacking pili are attenuated in both experimental endocarditis and urinary tract infections (UTIs). Other surface proteins that share structural homology with MSCRAMMs and appear to play a role in enterococcal attachment to the host and in virulence include the *E. faecalis* enterococcal surface protein (Esp) and its *E. faecium* homologue (Esp$_{fm}$), the second collagen adhesin of *E. faecium* (Scm), the surface proteins of *E. faecium* (Fms), SgrA (which binds to components of the basal lamina), and EcbA (which binds to collagen type V). Additional surface components apparently associated with pathogenicity include polysaccharides, which are thought to interfere with phagocytosis of the organism by host immune cells. Some *E. faecalis* strains appear to harbor at least three distinct classes of capsular polysaccharide; some of these polysaccharides play a role in virulence and are potential targets for immunotherapy.

The third group of virulence factors have not been well characterized: the *E. faecalis* stress protein Gls24, which has been associated with enterococcal resistance to bile salts and appears to be important in the pathogenesis of endocarditis, and the hyl_{Efm}-containing plasmids of *E. faecium*, which are transferable between strains and increase colonization by *E. faecium*. In a mouse model of peritonitis, acquisition of these plasmids augmented the lethality of a commensal strain of *E. faecium*.

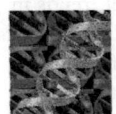

GENETICS

The sequencing of bacterial genomes has increased our understanding of bacterial diversity, evolution, pathogenesis, and antibiotic resistance mechanisms. The genome sequences of >80 enterococcal strains are currently available, and some have been entirely closed and annotated. Sequence analysis has shown that the genetic diversity of enterococci is due mainly to the acquisition of mobile DNA (e.g., plasmids, transposons, and phages) and the recombination of "core" genomes. Furthermore, analysis of *E. faecium* indicates that this species harbors a malleable genome (the *accessory* genome) into which exogenous elements (including DNA from phages) are incorporated at substantial levels. This genomic information has provided new clues about enterococcal evolution from a commensal organism into an important nosocomial pathogen.

EPIDEMIOLOGY

According to the National Healthcare Safety Network of the Centers for Disease Control and Prevention, enterococci are the second most common organisms (after staphylococci) isolated from hospital-associated infections in the United States. Although *E. faecalis* remains the predominant species recovered from nosocomial infections, the isolation of *E. faecium* has increased substantially in the past 10–15 years. In fact, *E. faecium* is now almost as common as *E. faecalis* as an etiologic agent of hospital-associated infections. This point is important, since *E. faecium* is by far the most resistant and challenging enterococcal species to treat; indeed, >80% of *E. faecium* isolates recovered in U.S. hospitals are resistant to vancomycin, and >90% are resistant to ampicillin (historically the most effective β-lactam drug against enterococci). Resistance to vancomycin and ampicillin in *E. faecalis* isolates is much less common (~7% and ~4%, respectively).

The dynamics of enterococcal transmission and dissemination in the hospital environment have been extensively studied, with a focus on vancomycin-resistant enterococci (VRE). These studies have revealed that VRE colonization of the gastrointestinal tract is a critical step in the natural history of enterococcal disease and that a substantial proportion of patients colonized with VRE remain colonized for prolonged periods (sometimes >1 year) and are more likely to develop an *Enterococcus*-related illness (e.g., bacteremia) than are patients colonized with antibiotic-susceptible strains. The most important factors associated with VRE colonization and persistence in the gut include prolonged hospitalization; long courses of antibiotic therapy; hospitalization in long-term-care facilities, surgical units, and/or intensive care units; organ transplantation; renal failure (particularly in patients undergoing hemodialysis) and/or diabetes; high APACHE scores; and physical proximity to patients infected or colonized with VRE or to these patients' rooms. Once a patient becomes colonized with VRE, several key factors are involved in the organisms' dissemination in the hospital environment. VRE can survive exposure to heat and certain disinfectants and have been found on numerous inanimate objects in the hospital, including bed rails, medical equipment, doorknobs, gloves, telephones, and computer keyboards. Thus health care workers play a pivotal role in enterococcal transmission from patient to patient, and infection control measures are crucial in breaking the chain of transmission. Moreover, two meta-analyses have found that VRE infection increases the risk of death, independent of the patient's clinical status, over that among individuals infected with a glycopeptide-susceptible enterococcal strain.

■ GLOBAL PERSPECTIVE

The epidemiology of enterococcal disease and the emergence of VRE have followed somewhat different trends in other parts of the world than in the United States. In Europe, the emergence of VRE in the mid-1980s was seen primarily in isolates recovered from animals and healthy humans rather than from hospitalized patients. The presence of VRE was associated with the use of the glycopeptide avoparcin as a growth promoter in animal feeds; this association prompted the European Union to ban the use of this compound in animal husbandry in 1996. However, after an initial decrease in the isolation of VRE from animals and humans, the prevalence of hospital-associated VRE infections has slowly increased in some European countries, with important regional differences. For example, rates of vancomycin resistance among *E. faecium* clinical isolates in Europe are highest in Greece, the United Kingdom, and Portugal (10–30%), whereas rates in Scandinavian countries and the Netherlands are <1%. These regional differences have been attributed in part to the implementation of aggressive policies of infection control in countries such as the Netherlands; these policies have kept the frequency of nosocomial methicillin-resistant *Staphylococcus aureus* (MRSA) and VRE very low. In spite of regional differences, rates of VRE continue to be much lower in most of Europe than in the United States. The reasons are not totally understood, although it has been postulated that the difference is related to the higher levels of human antibiotic use in the United States. Rates of enterococcal resistance to vancomycin in some Latin American countries are also lower (~4%) than those in the United States. Conversely, in Asia, rates of vancomycin resistance among enterococci appear to be similar to those in U.S. hospitals. Genetic analyses of vancomycin-resistant *E. faecium* in different parts of the world suggest that the nosocomial emergence and dissemination of these organisms globally is related to the success of unique clonal lineages (e.g., clonal cluster 17, or CC17) that was initially characterized by resistance to ampicillin and later acquired the genes responsible for resistance to vancomycin.

CLINICAL SYNDROMES

■ URINARY TRACT INFECTIONS AND PROSTATITIS

Enterococci are well-known agents of nosocomial UTI, the most common infection caused by these organisms (Chap. 288). Enterococcal UTIs are usually associated with indwelling catheterization, instrumentation, or anatomic abnormalities of the genitourinary tract, and it is often challenging to differentiate between true infection and colonization (particularly in patients with chronic indwelling catheters). The presence of leukocytes in the urine in conjunction with systemic manifestations (e.g., fever) or local signs and symptoms of infection with no other explanation and a positive urine culture (>10⁵ CFU) suggests the diagnosis. Moreover, enterococcal UTIs often occur in critically ill patients whose comorbidities may obscure the diagnosis. In many cases, removal of the indwelling catheter may suffice without specific antimicrobial therapy. In rare circumstances, UTIs caused by enterococci may run a complicated course, with the development of pyelonephritis and perinephric abscesses that may be a portal of entry for bloodstream infections (see below). Enterococci are also known causes of chronic prostatitis, particularly in patients in whom the urinary tract has been manipulated surgically or endoscopically. These infections can be difficult to treat since the agents most potent against enterococci (i.e., aminopenicillins and glycopeptides) penetrate prostatic tissue poorly. Chronic prostatic infection can be a source of recurrent enterococcal bacteremia.

■ BACTEREMIA AND ENDOCARDITIS

Bacteremia without endocarditis is one of the most common presentations of enterococcal disease. Intravascular catheters and other devices are commonly associated with these bacteremic episodes (Chap. 131). Other well-known sources of enterococcal bacteremia include the gastrointestinal and hepatobiliary tracts; pelvic and intraabdominal foci; and (less frequently) wound infections, UTIs, and bone infections. In the United States, enterococci rank second (after coagulase-negative staphylococci) as etiologic agents of central line–associated bacteremia. Patients with enterococcal bacteremia usually have comorbidities, have been in the hospital for prolonged periods, and/or have received several courses of antibiotics. Several studies indicate that the presence of *E. faecium* (as opposed to other enterococcal species) in the bloodstream may lead to worse outcomes and increased mortality rates; this finding may be related to the higher prevalence of vancomycin and ampicillin resistance in *E. faecium*, with the consequent reduction of therapeutic options. In many cases (usually when the gastrointestinal tract is the source), enterococcal bacteremia may be polymicrobial, with gram-negative organisms isolated at the same time. In addition, several cases have now been documented in which enterococcal bacteremia was associated with *Strongyloides stercoralis* hyperinfection syndrome in immunocompromised patients.

Enterococci are important causes of community- and health care–associated endocarditis, ranking second after staphylococci in the latter infections (Chap. 124). The presumed initial source of bacteremia leading to endocarditis is the gastrointestinal or genitourinary tract—e.g., in patients who have malignant and inflammatory conditions of the gut or have undergone procedures in which these tracts are manipulated. The affected patients tend to be male and elderly and to have other debilitating diseases and heart conditions. Both prosthetic and native valves can be involved; mitral and aortic valves are affected most often. Community-associated endocarditis (usually caused by *E. faecalis*) also occurs in patients with no apparent risk factors or cardiac abnormalities. Endocarditis in women of childbearing age has been well described. The typical presentation of enterococcal endocarditis is a subacute course with fever, weight loss, malaise, and a cardiac murmur; typical stigmata of endocarditis (e.g., petechiae, Osler's nodes, Roth's spots) are found in only a minority of patients. Some atypical manifestations include arthralgias and signs and symptoms of metastatic disease (splenic abscesses, hiccups, pain in the left flank, pleural effusion, and spondylodiscitis). Embolic complications are variable and can affect the brain. Heart failure is a common complication of enterococcal endocarditis, and valve replacement may be critical in curing this infection, particularly when multidrug-resistant organisms or major complications are involved. The duration of therapy is usually 4–6 weeks, with more prolonged courses suggested for multidrug-resistant isolates in the absence of valvular replacement or with prolonged illness prior to treatment.

▇ MENINGITIS

Enterococcal meningitis is an uncommon disease (accounting for only ~4% of meningitis cases) that is often associated with neurosurgical interventions and conditions such as shunts, central nervous system (CNS) trauma, and cerebrospinal fluid (CSF) leakage (Chap. 381). In some instances—usually in patients with a debilitating condition such as cardiovascular or congenital heart disease, chronic renal failure, malignancy, receipt of immunosuppressive therapy, or HIV/AIDS—presumed hematogenous seeding of the meninges is seen in infections such as endocarditis or bacteremia. Fever and changes in mental status are common, whereas overt meningeal signs are less so. CSF findings are consistent with bacterial infection—i.e., pleocytosis with a predominance of polymorphonuclear leukocytes (average, ~500/μL), an elevated protein level (usually >100 mg/dL), and a decreased glucose concentration (average, 28 mg/dL). Gram's staining yields a positive result in about half of cases, with a high rate of organism recovery from CSF cultures; the most common species isolated are *E. faecalis* and *E. faecium*. Complications include hydrocephalus, brain abscesses, and stroke; an association with *Strongyloides* hyperinfection has also been documented.

▇ INTRAABDOMINAL, PELVIC, AND SOFT TISSUE INFECTIONS

As mentioned earlier, enterococci are part of the commensal flora of the gastrointestinal tract and can produce spontaneous peritonitis in cirrhotic individuals and in patients undergoing chronic ambulatory peritoneal dialysis (Chap. 127). These organisms are commonly found (usually along with other bacteria, including enteric gram-negative species and anaerobes) in clinical samples from intraabdominal and pelvic collections. The presence of enterococci in intraabdominal infections is sometimes considered to be of low clinical relevance. Several studies have shown that the role of enterococci in intraabdominal infections originating in the community and involving previously healthy patients is minor, since surgery and broad-spectrum antimicrobial drugs that do not target enterococci are often sufficient in managing these infections successfully. In the last few decades, however, these organisms have become prominent as a cause of intraabdominal infections in hospitalized patients because of the emergence and spread of vancomycin resistance among enterococci and the increase in rates of nosocomial infections due to multidrug-resistant *E. faecium* isolates. In fact, several studies have now documented treatment failures due to enterococci, with consequently increased rates of postoperative complications and death in intraabdominal infections. Thus, anti-enterococcal therapy is recommended for nosocomial peritonitis in immunocompromised or severely ill patients who have had a prolonged hospital stay, have undergone multiple procedures, have persistent abdominal sepsis and collections, or have risk factors for the development of endocarditis (i.e., prosthetic or damaged heart valves). Conversely, treatment for enterococci in the first episode of intraabdominal infections originating in the community and affecting previously healthy patients with no important cardiac risk factors for endocarditis does not appear to be beneficial.

Enterococci are commonly isolated from soft tissue infections (Chap. 125), particularly those involving surgical wounds (Chap. 131). In fact, these organisms rank third as agents of nosocomial surgical-site infection, with *E. faecalis* the most frequently isolated species. The clinical relevance of enterococci in some of these infections—as in intraabdominal infections—is a matter of debate; differentiating between colonization and true infection can be challenging, although in some cases enterococci have been recovered from lung, liver, and skin abscesses. Diabetic foot and decubitus ulcers are often colonized with enterococci and may be the portal of entry for bone infections.

▇ OTHER INFECTIONS

Enterococci are well-known causes of neonatal infections including sepsis (mostly late-onset), bacteremia, meningitis, pneumonia, and UTI. Outbreaks of enterococcal sepsis in neonatal units have been well documented. Risk factors for enterococcal disease in newborns include prematurity, low birth weight, indwelling devices, and abdominal surgery. Enterococci have also been described as etiologic agents of bone and joint infections including vertebral osteomyelitis, usually in patients with underlying conditions such as diabetes or endocarditis. Similarly, enterococci have been isolated from bone infections in patients who have undergone arthroplasty or reconstruction of fractures with the placement of hardware. Since enterococci can produce a biofilm that is likely to alter the efficacy of otherwise active anti-enterococcal agents, treatment of infections that involve foreign material is challenging, and removal of the hardware may be necessary to eradicate the infection. Rare cases of enterococcal pneumonia, lung abscess, and spontaneous empyema have been reported.

TREATMENT   Enterococcal Infections

GENERAL PRINCIPLES   Enterococci are intrinsically resistant and/or tolerant to several antimicrobial agents [with *tolerance* defined as lack of killing by drug concentrations 16 times higher than the minimal inhibitory concentration (MIC)]. Monotherapy for endocarditis with a β-lactam antibiotic (to which many enterococci are tolerant) has produced disappointing results, with low cure rates at the end of therapy. However, the addition of an aminoglycoside to a cell wall–active agent (a β-lactam or a glycopeptide) increases cure rates and eradicates the organisms; moreover, this combination is synergistic and bactericidal in vitro. Therefore, combination therapy with a cell wall–active agent and an aminoglycoside is the standard of care for endovascular infections caused by enterococci. This synergistic effect can be explained, at least in part, by the increased penetration of the aminoglycoside into the bacterial cell, presumably as a result of cell wall alterations attributable to the β-lactam or glycopeptide. Nonetheless, attaining synergistic bactericidal activity in the treatment of severe enterococcal infections has become increasingly difficult because of the development of resistance to virtually all antibiotics available for this purpose.

The treatment of *E. faecalis* differs substantially from that of *E. faecium* (Tables 137-1 and 137-2), mainly because of differences

TABLE 137-1 Suggested Regimens for the Management of Infections Caused by *Enterococcus faecalis*

Clinical Syndrome	Ampicillin or Penicillin[a]	High-Level Resistance to Aminoglycosides[b]	Suggested Therapeutic Options[c]
Endovascular infections (includes endocarditis)	Susceptible	No	Ampicillin (12 g/d IV in divided doses q4h or by continuous infusion) *or* penicillin (18–30 million units/d IV in divided doses q4h or by continuous infusion) *plus* an aminoglycoside[d]
			Vancomycin (15–20 mg/kg per dose q8–12h, not to exceed 2 g per dose)[e] *plus* an aminoglycoside[d]
	Susceptible	Yes	Ampicillin (12 g/d IV in divided doses q4h) *plus* ceftriaxone (2 g q12h) *or* cefotaxime
			High-dose daptomycin[f] ± another active agent[g]
			Vancomycin (15–20 mg/kg per dose q8–12h, not to exceed 2 g per dose)[e]
			Ampicillin *plus* imipenem
Nonendovascular bacteremia[h]	Susceptible	No	Ampicillin (12 g/d IV in divided doses q4h) *or* penicillin (18 mU/d IV in divided doses q4h)[i]
			Vancomycin (15–20 mg/kg per dose q8–12h, not to exceed 2 g per dose)[e,i]
	Susceptible	Yes	Ampicillin[j] (12 g/d IV in divided doses q4h) *or* penicillin
			Vancomycin (15–20 mg/kg per dose q8–12 h, not to exceed 2 g per dose)[e]
			High-dose daptomycin[f]
Meningitis	Susceptible	No	Ampicillin (20–24 g/d IV in divided doses q4h) *or* penicillin (24 mU/d IV in divided doses q4h) *plus* an aminoglycoside[k]
			Vancomycin (500–750 mg IV q6h)[e] *plus* an aminoglycoside[k]
			Linezolid
	Susceptible	Yes	Ampicillin (20–24 g/d IV in divided doses q4h) *or* penicillin (24 mU/d IV in divided doses q4h) *plus* ceftriaxone (2 g q12h) *or* cefotaxime
			Vancomycin (500–750 mg IV q6h)[e]
			Linezolid
			High-dose daptomycin[f] (*plus* intrathecal daptomycin) ± another active agent[g]
Urinary tract infections (uncomplicated)	Not applicable	Not applicable	Ampicillin (500 mg IV or PO q6h)
			Nitrofurantoin (100 mg PO q6h)
			Fosfomycin (3-g single dose PO)[l]

[a]In rare cases, β-lactamase-producing isolates may be found. Because these isolates are not detected by conventional MIC determination, additional tests (e.g., the nitrocefin disk test) are recommended for isolates from endocarditis. The use of ampicillin/sulbactam (12–24 g/d) is suggested in these cases.

[b]Determined by the clinical microbiology laboratory only for gentamicin or streptomycin as growth of enterococci in brain-heart infusion agar containing gentamicin (500 μg/mL) and streptomycin (2000 μg/mL). Resistance to one compound does not indicate resistance to the other, and the laboratory reports high-level resistance to each compound individually. In this table, *Yes* to high-level resistance to aminoglycosides indicates that the laboratory has reported resistance to synergism with both gentamicin and streptomycin.

[c]Author's first-choice regimen is underlined for each category.

[d]Gentamicin (1–1.5 mg/kg IV q8h) or streptomycin (15 mg/kg per day IV or IM in two divided doses).

[e]Vancomycin is recommended only as an alternative to β-lactam agents in case of allergy, toxicity, or inability to desensitize. Monitoring of vancomycin levels is recommended, although no data for enterococci are available; a regimen that achieves trough serum levels of 15–20 μg/mL is suggested by some experts, although high doses may predispose to renal toxicity. CSF concentrations may also be determined. Vancomycin-resistant strains of *E. faecalis* have been reported.

[f]Consider doses of 8–12 mg/kg per day (off-label use).

[g]Active agents may include ampicillin, a fluoroquinolone (which, if the isolate is susceptible, may be favored in meningitis), and tigecycline.

[h]In selected cases of catheter-associated bacteremia, removal of the catheter and a short course of therapy (~5–7 days) may be sufficient. A single positive blood culture that is likely to be associated with a catheter in a patient who is otherwise doing well may not require therapy after removal of the catheter.

[i]The addition of an aminoglycoside may be considered in severe infections.

[j]The addition of ceftriaxone (or cefotaxime) may be considered in severe infections.

[k]The addition of intrathecal or intraventricular therapy with gentamicin (2–10 mg/d) or vancomycin (10–20 mg/d), when the isolate is susceptible, has been suggested by some authorities for recalcitrant cases.

[l]Approved by the FDA only for uncomplicated urinary tract infections caused by vancomycin-susceptible *E. faecalis*.

Clinical Syndrome	Ampicillin MIC (µg/mL)	High-Level Resistance to Aminoglycosides[a]	Suggested Therapeutic Options[b]
Endovascular infections (includes endocarditis)	≤64	No	High-dose ampicillin[c] ***plus*** an aminoglycoside[d]
			See regimens for MIC >64 µg/mL
	>64	No	High-dose daptomycin[e] ***plus*** an aminoglycoside[d] ± another active agent[f]
			Q/D[g] (22.5 mg/kg per day in divided doses q8h) ± another active agent[f]
			Linezolid[g] (600 mg IV q12h) ± another active agent[f]
	≤64	Yes	High-dose ampicillin[c] ***plus*** high-dose daptomycin[e]
			Q/D[g] (22.5 mg/kg per day in divided doses q8h) ***plus*** high-dose ampicillin[c] *or* doxycycline (100 mg IV q12h) with rifampin (300 mg PO q12h, if susceptible)
			High-dose ampicillin[c] ***plus*** imipenem-cilastatin (500 mg IV q6h)[h]
	>64	Yes	High-dose daptomycin[e] ***plus*** another active agent[f]
			Q/D[g] (22.5 mg/kg per day in divided doses q8h) ***plus*** doxycycline (100 mg IV q12h) with rifampin (300 mg PO q12h, if susceptible) Linezolid[g] (600 mg IV q12h) ± another active agent[f]
Non endovascular bacteremia[i]	≤64	No	High-dose ampicillin[c] ± an aminoglycoside[d]
			Q/D[g] ± another active agent[f]
	>64	No	Daptomycin[e] ± an aminoglycoside[d]
			Linezolid[g] ± another active agent[f]
	≤64	Yes	High-dose ampicillin[c] ± Q/D[g] (22.5 mg/kg per day in divided doses q8h)
			High-dose ampicillin[c] ± daptomycin[e]
			Linezolid[g] (600 mg IV q12h) ± another active agent[f]
			Q/D[g] (22.5 mg/kg per day in divided doses q8h) ± another active agent[f]
	>64	Yes	Daptomycin[e] ± another active agent[f]
			Linezolid[g] (600 mg IV q12h) ± another active agent[f]
Meningitis[j]	<16	No	High-dose ampicillin[c] ***plus*** gentamicin (5.1–7 mg/kg, single daily dose) *or* streptomycin (15 mg/kg, single daily dose)
	≥16	No	Linezolid ± another CSF-penetrating active agent[k]
			High-dose daptomycin[e] (plus intrathecal daptomycin[j]) ***plus*** gentamicin (5.1–7 mg/kg, single daily dose) *or* streptomycin (15 mg/kg, single daily dose)[j] ± another CSF-penetrating active agent[k]
	<16	Yes	High-dose ampicillin[c] ***plus*** high-dose daptomycin[e] (plus intrathecal daptomycin)[j]
			Linezolid ± another CSF-penetrating active agent[k]
			Q/D[j] (22.5 mg/kg per day in divided doses q8h) ***plus*** intrathecal Q/D ***plus*** high-dose ampicillin[c]
	≥16	Yes	Linezolid ± another CSF-penetrating active agent[k]
			High-dose daptomycin[e] ± another CSF-penetrating active agent[k]
			Q/D[j] (22.5 mg/kg per (plus intrathecal daptomycin) in divided doses q8h) ***plus*** intrathecal Q/D ± another CSF-penetrating active agent[k]

(continued)

TABLE 137-2 Suggested Regimens for the Management of Infections Caused by Vancomycin-Resistant *Enterococcus faecium* **(Continued)**

Clinical Syndrome	Ampicillin MIC (µg/mL)	High-level Resistance to Aminoglycosides[a]	Suggested Therapeutic Options[b]
Urinary tract infections	≤512	Not applicable	Nitrofurantoin (100 mg PO q6h)
			Fosfomycin (3 g PO, one dose)[l]
			Ampicillin or amoxicillin (2 g IV or PO q4–6h)[m]

[a]*Yes* to high-level resistance to aminoglycosides indicates resistance to both gentamicin and streptomycin (the only two aminoglycosides recommended for the treatment of enterococcal infections). Resistance to one compound does not indicate resistance to the other.

[b]Author's first-choice regimen(s) are underlined for each category.

[c]Doses up to 30 g/d IV in divided doses q4h may be considered; clinical data on safety at these high doses are not available.

[d]Gentamicin (1–1.5 mg/kg IV q8h) or streptomycin (15 mg/kg per day IV or IM in two divided doses).

[e]Daptomycin at a dosage of 8–12 mg/kg once daily is suggested (off-label); close monitoring of creatine phosphokinase levels is recommended throughout therapy because of possible rhabdomyolysis.

[f]Agents with potential activity include doxycycline with rifampin or tigecycline (50 mg IV q12h after an initial loading dose of 100 mg IV) or fluoroquinolones (if the isolate is susceptible to each agent).

[g]Quinupristin-dalfopristin (Q/D) and linezolid are listed in the American Heart Association recommendations for the treatment of endocarditis caused by vancomycin- and ampicillin-resistant *E. faecium*.

[h]If the imipenem MIC is <32 µg/mL.

[i]In selected cases of catheter-associated bacteremia, removal of the catheter and a short course of therapy (~5–7 days) may be sufficient. A single positive blood culture that is likely to be associated with a catheter in a patient who is otherwise doing well may not require therapy after removal of the catheter.

[j]Intrathecal gentamicin (if no high-level resistance is detected; 2–10 mg/d) or Q/D (1–5 mg/d) has been used in combination with systemic therapy in refractory cases of postoperative meningitis. If Q/D is chosen, simultaneous systemic and intrathecal therapy is suggested. Intraventricular daptomycin has been used in two cases of meningitis.

[k]Fluoroquinolone antibiotics (e.g., moxifloxacin) and rifampin (if the isolate is susceptible to each agent) reach therapeutic levels in CSF.

[l]Approved by the FDA only for uncomplicated urinary tract infections caused by vancomycin-susceptible *E. faecalis*.

[m]Concentrations of amoxicillin in urine far exceed those in serum and can be potentially effective even against isolates with high MICs. Doses up to 12 g/d are suggested for isolates with MICs of ≥64 µg/mL.

in resistance profiles (see below); for example, resistance to ampicillin and vancomycin is rare in *E. faecalis*, whereas these antibiotics are only infrequently useful against current isolates of *E. faecium*. Moreover, as a consequence of the challenges and therapeutic limitations posed by the emergence of drug resistance, valve replacement may need to be considered in the treatment of endocarditis caused by multidrug-resistant enterococci. Less severe infections are often related to indwelling intravascular catheters; removal of the catheter increases the likelihood of enterococcal eradication of the organism by a short course of appropriate antimicrobial therapy.

■ CHOICE OF ANTIMICROBIAL AGENTS

Among the β-lactam agents, the most active are the aminopenicillins (ampicillin, amoxicillin) and ureidopenicillins (i.e., piperacillins); next most active are penicillin G and imipenem. Against *E. faecium*, a combination of high-dose ampicillin (up to 30 g/d) and an aminoglycoside (Table 137-2) has been suggested even for ampicillin-resistant strains if the MIC is <64 µg/mL, since a plasma ampicillin concentration of >100 µg/mL can be achieved at high doses. The only two aminoglycosides recommended for synergistic therapy in severe enterococcal infections are gentamicin and streptomycin. The use of amikacin is discouraged, tobramycin should never be used against *E. faecium*, and aminoglycoside monotherapy is not effective. Vancomycin is an alternative to β-lactam drugs for the treatment of *E. faecalis* infections but is less useful against *E. faecium* because resistance is common. Cephalosporins (except ceftobiprole for *E. faecalis*) are inactive against enterococci.

Linezolid and quinupristin/dalfopristin (Q/D) are approved by the U.S. Food and Drug Administration (FDA) for the treatment of some VRE infections (Table 137-2). Linezolid is not bactericidal, and its use in severe endovascular infections has produced mixed results; therefore, it is recommended only as an alternative to other agents. In addition, linezolid may cause significant toxicities (thrombocytopenia and peripheral neuropathy) when used in regimens given for >2 weeks. Nonetheless, this drug may play a role in the treatment of enterococcal meningitis and other CNS infections, although clinical data are limited. Q/D is not active against most *E. faecalis* isolates, and its in vivo efficacy against *E. faecium* may be compromised by resistance (see below). Adverse reactions to Q/D (including pain and inflammation at the infusion site and severe arthralgias and myalgias leading to discontinuation of treatment) are common. Therefore, this drug should be used with caution and probably combined with other agents (Table 137-2). The lipopeptide daptomycin is a bactericidal antibiotic with potent in vitro activity against all enterococci. Although daptomycin is not approved by the FDA for the treatment of VRE or *E. faecium* infections, it has been used alone (at high dosage) or in combination with other agents with apparent success against multidrug-resistant enterococcal infections (Tables 137-1 and 137-2). The main adverse reactions to daptomycin are elevated creatinine phosphokinase levels and eosinophilic pneumonitis. Daptomycin is not useful against pulmonary infections because the pulmonary surfactant inhibits its antibacterial activity. Although the glycylcycline tigecycline is active in vitro against all enterococci (regardless of the isolates' vancomycin susceptibility), its use as monotherapy for endovascular or severe enterococcal infections is not recommended because of low attainable blood levels. Telavancin, a lipoglycopeptide approved by the FDA for the treatment of skin and soft tissue infections, is active against vancomycin-susceptible enterococci but less so against VRE. Oritavancin, a compound of the same class that is active against

VRE, is in the late stages of clinical development and may offer promise for the treatment of VRE infections in the future.

■ ANTIMICROBIAL RESISTANCE

As mentioned above, resistance to ampicillin continues to be observed only infrequently in *E. faecalis*, although rare outbreaks caused by β-lactamase-producing isolates have occurred in the United States and Argentina. However, ampicillin resistance is common in *E. faecium*. The mechanism of ampicillin resistance in *E. faecium* is related to a penicillin-binding protein (PBP) designated PBP5, which is the target of β-lactam antibiotics. PBP5 exhibits lower affinity for ampicillin than other PBPs and can synthesize cell wall in the presence of this antibiotic, even when other PBPs are inhibited. Two common mechanisms of high-level ampicillin resistance (MIC, >64 μg/mL) in clinical strains are (1) mutations in the PBP5-encoding gene that further decrease the affinity of PBP5 for ampicillin and (2) hyperproduction of PBP5. These factors preclude the use of all β-lactam agents in the treatment of *E. faecium* infections.

Vancomycin is a glycopeptide antibiotic that inhibits cell wall peptidoglycan synthesis in susceptible enterococci and has been widely used against enterococcal infections in clinical practice when the use of penicillins is limited by resistance, allergy, or adverse reactions. This effect is mediated by binding of the antibiotic to peptidoglycan precursors (UDP-MurNAc-pentapeptides) upon their exit from the bacterial cytoplasm. The interaction of vancomycin with the peptidoglycan is specific and involves the last two D-alanine residues of the precursor. The first isolates of VRE were documented in 1986, and vancomycin resistance (particularly in *E. faecium*) has since increased considerably around the world. The mechanism involves the replacement of the last D-alanine residue of peptidoglycan precursors with D-lactate or D-serine, with consequent high- and low-level resistance, respectively. There is significant heterogeneity among isolates, but either substitution substantially decreases the affinity of vancomycin for the peptidoglycan; with the D-lactate substitution, the MIC is increased by up to one thousand-fold. Vancomycin-resistant organisms also produce enzymes that destroy the D-alanine–D-alanine-ending

precursors, ensuring that additional binding sites for vancomycin are not available.

High-level resistance to aminoglycosides (of which gentamicin and streptomycin are the only two tested in clinical laboratories) abolishes the synergism observed between cell wall–active agents and the aminoglycoside. This important phenotype is routinely sought in isolates from serious infections (Tables 137-1 and 137-2). The laboratory reports high-level resistance as gentamicin and streptomycin MICs of >500 μg/mL and >2000 μg/mL, respectively (agar dilution method), or as "SYN-R" (resistance to synergism). Genes encoding aminoglycoside-modifying enzymes are usually the cause of high-level resistance to these compounds and are widely disseminated among enterococci, decreasing the options for the treatment of severe enterococcal infections. The aforementioned enterococcal resistance to newer antibiotics such as linezolid (usually due to mutations in the 23S rRNA genes), Q/D, daptomycin, and tigecycline further reduces therapeutic alternatives.

FURTHER READINGS

ARIAS CA, MURRAY BE: *Enterococcus* species, *Streptococcus bovis* group and *Leuconostoc* species, in *Principles and Practice of Infectious Diseases*, 7th ed, GL Mandell et al (eds). Philadelphia, Churchill Livingstone Elsevier, 2010, pp 2643–2654

———— et al: Management of multidrug-resistant enterococcal infections. Clin Microbiol Infect 16:555, 2010

BRANDL K et al: Vancomycin-resistant enterococci exploit antibiotic-induced innate immune deficits. Nature 455:804, 2008

FACKLAM RR et al: History, taxonomy, biochemical characteristics and antibiotic susceptibility testing of enterococci, in *The Enterococci: Pathogenesis, Molecular Biology and Antibiotic Resistance*, MS Gilmore (ed). Washington, DC, ASM Press, 2002, pp 1–54

NALLAPAREDDY SR et al: Endocarditis and biofilm associated pili of *Enterococcus faecalis*. J Clin Invest 116:2799, 2006

WILLEMS RJ, VAN SCHAIK W: Transition of *Enterococcus faecium* from commensal organism to nosocomial pathogen. Future Microbiol 4:1125, 2009

CHAPTER 138

Diphtheria and Other Infections Caused by Corynebacteria and Related Species

William R. Bishai

John R. Murphy

DIPHTHERIA

Diphtheria is a nasopharyngeal and skin infection caused by *Corynebacterium diphtheriae*. Toxigenic strains of *C. diphtheriae* produce a protein toxin that causes systemic toxicity, myocarditis, and polyneuropathy. The toxin is associated with the formation of pseudomembranes in the pharynx during respiratory diphtheria. While toxigenic strains most frequently cause pharyngeal diphtheria, nontoxigenic strains commonly cause cutaneous disease.

In the United States and Europe, diphtheria has been controlled in recent years with effective vaccination, although sporadic outbreaks have occurred. Diphtheria is still common in the Caribbean, Latin America, and the Indian subcontinent, where mass immunization programs are not enforced. Large epidemics have occurred in the independent states formerly encompassed by the Soviet Union. Additional outbreaks have been reported in Algeria, China, and Ecuador.

ETIOLOGY

C. diphtheriae is a gram-positive, unencapsulated, nonmotile, non-sporulating bacillus. *C. diphtheriae* organisms have a characteristic club-shaped bacillary appearance and typically form clusters of parallel rays (palisades) that are referred to as *Chinese characters*. In the specific laboratory media recommended for the cultivation of *C. diphtheriae*, tellurite, colistin, or nalidixic acid allows selective isolation of the organism in the presence of other autochthonous pharyngeal microbes. Human isolates of *C. diphtheriae* may display nontoxigenic (*tox⁻*) or toxigenic (*tox⁺*) phenotypes. Corynebacteriophage beta carries the structural gene (*tox*) encoding diphtheria toxin, and a family of closely related corynebacteriophages are responsible for toxigenic conversion of *tox⁻ C. diphtheriae* to the *tox⁺* phenotype. Moreover, lysogenic conversion from a nontoxigenic to a toxigenic phenotype has been shown to occur in situ. Growth of toxigenic strains of *C. diphtheriae* under iron-limiting conditions leads to the optimal expression of diphtheria toxin, and these conditions are believed to trigger *tox* expression and subsequent pathogenesis during human infection.

EPIDEMIOLOGY

C. diphtheriae is transmitted via the aerosol route, primarily during close contact. There are no significant reservoirs other than humans. The incubation period for respiratory diphtheria is 2–5 days; however, disease can develop as long as 10 days after exposure. Before the vaccine era, most individuals over the age of 10 were immune to *C. diphtheriae*; infants were protected by maternal IgG antibodies but became susceptible after ~6 months of age. Thus, the disease was seen primarily in children and nonimmune young adults. In temperate regions, respiratory diphtheria occurs year-round but is most common during winter months.

The development of diphtheria antitoxin and diphtheria toxoid vaccine led to the near-elimination of diphtheria in Western countries. The annual peak incidence rate was 191 cases per 100,000 population in the United States in 1921; in contrast, since 1980, the annual figure for the United States as a whole has been <5 cases. Nevertheless, pockets of colonization have persisted in North America, particularly in South Dakota, Ontario, and Washington state. Immunity induced by vaccination during childhood gradually decreases in adulthood. An estimated 30% of men 60–69 years old have antitoxin titers below the protective level. In addition to older age and lack of vaccination, risk factors for diphtheria outbreaks include alcoholism, low socioeconomic status, crowded living conditions, and Native American ethnic background. An outbreak that occurred in Seattle in 1972–1982 included 1100 cases, primarily manifesting as cutaneous disease. During the 1990s in the states of the former Soviet Union, a much larger diphtheria epidemic caused >150,000 cases and >5000 deaths. Clonally related toxigenic *C. diphtheriae* strains of the ET8 complex were associated with this outbreak. Given that the ET8 complex expressed a toxin against which the prevalent diphtheria toxoid vaccine was effective, the epidemic was attributed to failure of the public health infrastructure to effectively vaccinate the population. Beginning in 1998, the epidemic was controlled by mass vaccination programs. During the epidemic, the incidence rate was high among individuals from >15 years of age up to 50 years of age. Socioeconomic instability, migration, deteriorating public health programs, frequent vaccine shortages, delays in implementation of vaccination and of treatment in response to cases, and lack of public education and awareness were contributing factors in that outbreak.

Significant outbreaks of diphtheria and diphtheria-related mortality continue to be reported from many developing countries, particularly in Africa and Asia. Statistics collected by the World Health Organization indicate the occurrence of ~7000 reported diphtheria cases in 2008 and ~5000 diphtheria deaths in 2004. Although ~82% of the global population has been adequately vaccinated, only 26% of countries have successfully vaccinated >80% of individuals in all districts.

Cutaneous diphtheria is usually a secondary infection that follows a primary skin lesion due to trauma, allergy, or autoimmunity. Most often, isolates from cases of cutaneous disease lack the *tox* gene and therefore do not express diphtheria toxin. In tropical regions, cutaneous diphtheria is more common than respiratory diphtheria. In contrast to respiratory disease, cutaneous diphtheria is not a reportable disease in United States.

Nontoxigenic strains of *C. diphtheriae* have also been associated with bacteremia and invasive disease in the urban poor in Vancouver, Canada, and with pharyngitis in Europe. Outbreaks have occurred among homosexual men and IV drug users.

PATHOGENESIS AND IMMUNOLOGY

Diphtheria toxin, produced by toxigenic strains of *C. diphtheriae*, is the primary virulence factor in clinical disease. The toxin is synthesized in precursor form; is released as a 535-amino-acid, single-chain protein; and has an LD_{50} of ~100 ng/kg of body weight. The toxin is produced in the pseudomembranous lesion and is taken up into the bloodstream, through which it is distributed to all organ systems. Once bound to its cell surface receptor (a heparin-binding, epidermal growth factor–like precursor), the toxin is internalized by receptor-mediated endocytosis and enters the cytosol from an acidified early endosomal compartment. In vitro, the toxin may be separated into two chains after digestion with serine proteases: the N-terminal A fragment and the C-terminal B fragment. Delivery of the A fragment into the eukaryotic cell cytosol results in irreversible inhibition of protein synthesis by NAD+-dependent ADP ribosylation of elongation factor 2. The eventual result is the death of the cell.

In 1926, Ramon at the Institut Pasteur found that formalinization of diphtheria toxin resulted in the production of diphtheria toxoid, which was nontoxic but highly immunogenic. Subsequent studies showed that immunization with diphtheria toxoid elicited antibodies that neutralized the toxin and prevented most manifestations of diphtheria. In the 1930s, mass immunization of children and susceptible adults commenced in the United States and Europe.

Individuals with an antitoxin titer of >0.01 unit/mL are at low risk of diphtheria disease. In populations where a majority of individuals have protective antitoxin titers, the carrier rate for toxigenic strains of *C. diphtheriae* decreases and the overall risk of diphtheria among susceptible individuals is reduced. Nevertheless, individuals with nonprotective titers may contract diphtheria through either travel or exposure to individuals who have recently returned from regions where the disease is endemic.

Characteristic pathologic findings of diphtheria include mucosal ulcers with a pseudomembranous coating composed of an inner band of fibrin and a luminal band of neutrophils. Initially white and firmly adherent, in advanced diphtheria the pseudomembranes turn gray and even green or black as necrosis progresses. Mucosal ulcers result from toxin-induced necrosis of the epithelium accompanied by edema, hyperemia, and vascular congestion of the submucosal base. A fibrinosuppurative exudate from the ulcer develops into the pseudomembrane. Ulcers and pseudomembranes in severe respiratory diphtheria may extend from the pharynx into medium-sized bronchial airways. Expanding and sloughing membranes may result in fatal airway obstruction.

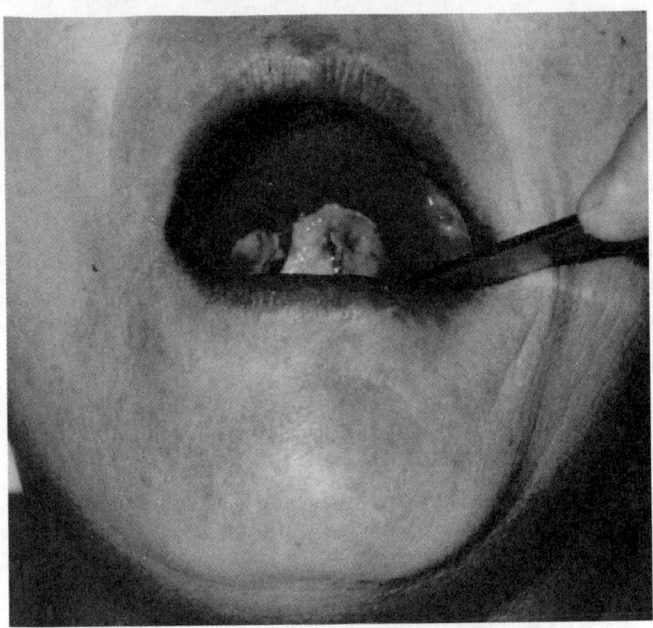

Figure 138-1 Respiratory diphtheria due to toxigenic *C. diphtheriae* producing exudative pharyngitis in a 47-year-old woman with neck edema and a pseudomembrane extending from the uvula to the pharyngeal wall. The characteristic white pseudomembrane is caused by diphtheria toxin–mediated necrosis of the respiratory epithelial layer, producing fibrinous coagulative exudate. Submucosal edema adds to airway narrowing. The pharyngitis is acute in onset, and respiratory obstruction from the pseudomembrane may occur in severe cases. Inoculation of pseudomembrane fragments or submembranous swabs onto Löffler's or tellurite selective medium reveals *C. diphtheriae*. (Photograph by P. Strebel, MD, used by permission. From Kadirova R et al: J Infect Dis 181:S110, 2000.)

APPROACH TO THE PATIENT | **Diphtheria**

Although diphtheria is rare in the United States and other developed countries, this diagnosis should be considered in patients who have severe pharyngitis, particularly with difficulty swallowing, respiratory compromise, or signs of systemic disease including myocarditis or generalized weakness. In the differential diagnosis, the leading causes of pharyngitis that should be considered are respiratory viruses (rhinoviruses, influenza viruses, parainfluenza viruses, coronaviruses, and adenoviruses; ~25% of cases), group A streptococci (15–30%), group C streptococci (~5%), atypical bacteria such as *Mycoplasma pneumoniae* and *Chlamydophila pneumoniae* (15–20% in some series), and other viruses such as herpes simplex virus (~4%) and Epstein-Barr virus (EBV; <1% in infectious mononucleosis). Less common causes are acute HIV infection, infection with *Neisseria gonorrhoeae*, fusobacterial infection (e.g., Lemierre syndrome), and thrush due to *Candida albicans* or other *Candida* species. The presence of a pharyngeal pseudomembrane or an extensive exudate should prompt consideration of diphtheria (Fig. 138-1).

■ CLINICAL MANIFESTATIONS

Respiratory diphtheria

The clinical diagnosis of diphtheria is based on the constellation of sore throat; adherent tonsillar, pharyngeal, or nasal pseudomembranous lesions; and low-grade fever. In addition, diagnosis requires the isolation of *C. diphtheriae* or the histopathologic isolation of compatible gram-positive organisms. The Centers for

Disease Control and Prevention (CDC) recognizes confirmed respiratory diphtheria (laboratory proven or epidemiologically linked to a culture-confirmed case) and probable respiratory diphtheria (clinically compatible but not laboratory proven or epidemiologically linked). Carriers are defined as individuals who have positive cultures for *C. diphtheriae* and either are asymptomatic or have symptoms but lack pseudomembranes. Most patients seek medical care for initial manifestations of sore throat and fever. Occasionally, weakness, dysphagia, headache, and voice change are the initial manifestations. Neck edema and difficulty breathing are seen in more advanced cases and carry a poor prognosis.

The systemic manifestations of diphtheria stem from the effects of diphtheria toxin and include weakness as a result of neurotoxicity and cardiac arrhythmias or congestive heart failure due to myocarditis. The pseudomembranous lesion is most often located in the tonsillopharyngeal region. Less commonly, the lesions are detected in the larynx, nares, and trachea or bronchial passages. Large pseudomembranes are associated with severe disease and a poor prognosis. A few patients develop massive swelling of the tonsils and present with "bull-neck" diphtheria, which results from massive edema of the submandibular and paratracheal region and is further characterized by foul breath, thick speech, and stridorous breathing. The diphtheritic pseudomembrane is gray or whitish and sharply demarcated. Unlike the exudative lesion associated with streptococcal pharyngitis, the pseudomembrane in diphtheria is tightly adherent to the underlying tissues. Attempts to dislodge the membrane may cause bleeding. Hoarseness suggests laryngeal diphtheria, in which laryngoscopy may be diagnostically helpful.

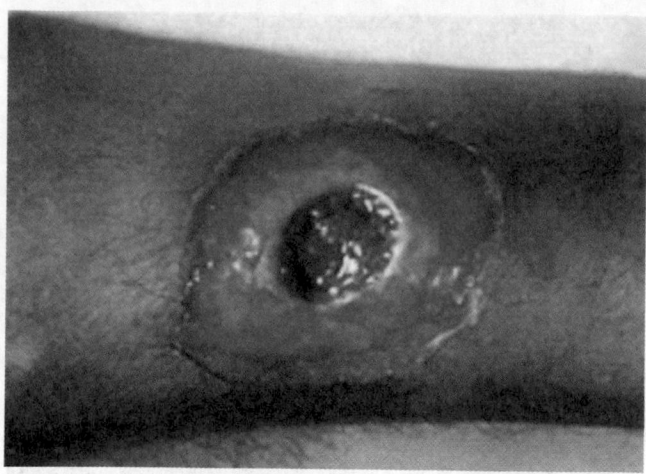

Figure 138-2 Cutaneous diphtheria due to nontoxigenic *C. diphtheriae* on the lower extremity. *(From the Centers for Disease Control and Prevention.)*

Cutaneous diphtheria

This is a variable dermatosis most often characterized by punched-out ulcerative lesions with necrotic sloughing or pseudomembrane formation (Fig. 138-2). The diagnosis requires cultivation of *C. diphtheriae* from lesions, which most commonly occur on the extremities. Patients usually seek medical attention because of nonhealing or enlarging skin ulcers, which may be associated with a preexisting wound or dermatoses such as eczema, psoriasis, and venous stasis disease. The lesions rarely exceed 5 cm.

Other clinical manifestations

C. diphtheriae causes rare cases of endocarditis and septic arthritis, most often in patients with preexisting risk factors such as cardiac valvular disease, injection drug use, or cirrhosis.

■ COMPLICATIONS

Airway obstruction poses a significant early risk in patients presenting with advanced diphtheria. Pseudomembranes may slough and obstruct the airway or may advance to the larynx or into the tracheobronchial tree. Children are particularly prone to obstruction because of their small airways.

Polyneuropathy and myocarditis are late toxic manifestations of diphtheria. During the outbreak in the Kyrgyz Republic in 1995, myocarditis was seen in 22% and neuropathy in 5% of hospitalized patients. The mortality rate was 7% among patients with myocarditis as opposed to 2% among those without myocardial manifestations. The median time to death in hospitalized patients was 4.5 days. Myocarditis is typically associated with dysrhythmia of the conduction tract and dilated cardiomyopathy.

Neurologic manifestations may appear during the first or second week of illness, typically beginning with dysphagia and nasal dysarthria and progressing to other signs of cranial nerve involvement, including weakness of the tongue and facial numbness. Ciliary paralysis, which is typical, manifests as blurred vision due to paralysis of pupillary accommodation, with a preserved light reflex. Cranial neuropathy may be followed by respiratory and abdominal muscle weakness requiring artificial ventilation. Several weeks later—sometimes as cranial neuropathy is improving—a generalized sensorimotor polyneuropathy may appear, with prominent autonomic manifestations (including hypotension) in some cases. The clinical syndrome and the findings on lumbar puncture of

raised levels of protein without pleocytosis in cerebrospinal fluid resemble Guillain-Barré syndrome (Chap. 385). Pathologically, diphtheria neuropathy is a noninflammatory demyelinating disorder mediated by the exotoxin. Gradual improvement is the rule in patients who survive the acute phase.

Other complications of diphtheria include pneumonia, renal failure, encephalitis, cerebral infarction, and pulmonary embolism. Serum sickness can result from treatment with diphtheria antitoxin (see "Diphtheria Treatment," below).

■ DIAGNOSIS

The diagnosis of diphtheria is based on clinical signs and symptoms plus laboratory confirmation. Respiratory diphtheria should be considered in patients with sore throat, pharyngeal exudates, and fever. Other symptoms may include hoarseness, stridor, or palatal paralysis. The presence of a pseudomembrane should prompt consideration of diphtheria. Once a clinical diagnosis of diphtheria is made, diphtheria antitoxin should be administered as soon as possible.

Laboratory diagnosis is based either on cultivation of *C. diphtheriae* or toxigenic *C. ulcerans* from the site of infection or on the demonstration of local lesions with characteristic histopathology. *C. pseudodiphtheriticum*, a nontoxigenic organism, is a common component of the normal throat flora and does not pose a significant risk. Throat samples should be submitted to the laboratory for culture with the notation that diphtheria is being considered. This information should prompt cultivation on special selective medium and subsequent biochemical testing to differentiate *C. diphtheriae* from other nasopharyngeal commensal corynebacteria. All laboratory isolates of *C. diphtheriae*, including nontoxigenic strains, should be submitted to the CDC.

A diagnosis of cutaneous diphtheria requires laboratory confirmation since the lesions are not characteristic and are clinically indistinguishable from other dermatoses. Diphtheritic ulcers occasionally—but not consistently—have a punched-out appearance (Fig. 138-2). Patients in whom cutaneous diphtheria is identified should have the nasopharynx cultured for *C. diphtheriae*. The laboratory media for cutaneous diphtheria are the same as those used for respiratory diphtheria: Löffler's or Tinsdale's selective medium in addition to nonselective medium such as blood agar. As has been mentioned, respiratory diphtheria remains a notifiable disease in the United States, whereas cutaneous diphtheria is not.

TREATMENT | Diphtheria

DIPHTHERIA ANTITOXIN Prompt administration of diphtheria antitoxin is critical in the management of respiratory diphtheria. The antitoxin—a horse antiserum—is effective in reducing the extent of local disease as well as the risk of complications of myocarditis and neuropathy. Rapid institution of antitoxin therapy is also associated with a significant reduction in mortality risk. Because diphtheria antitoxin cannot neutralize cell-bound toxin, prompt initiation is important. This product, which is no longer made commercially in the United States, is available from the CDC under an investigational new drug protocol and may be obtained by calling the Emergency Operations Center at 770-488-7100; the relevant Web site is *www.cdc.gov/vaccines/vpd-vac/diphtheria/dat/dat-main.htm*. The current protocol for the use of antitoxin includes a test dose to rule out immediate-type hypersensitivity. Patients who exhibit hypersensitivity require desensitization before a full therapeutic dose of antitoxin is administered.

ANTIMICROBIAL THERAPY Antibiotics are used in the management of diphtheria primarily to prevent transmission to other susceptible contacts. Recommended options for the treatment of patients with respiratory diphtheria are as follows: (1) procaine penicillin G at a dosage of 600,000 units (for children, 12,500–25,000 U/kg) IM every 12 h until the patient can swallow comfortably, after which oral penicillin V is given at 125–250 mg four times daily to complete a 14-day course; or (2) erythromycin at a dosage of 500 mg IV every 6 h (for children, 40–50 mg/kg per day IV in two or four divided doses) until the patient can swallow comfortably, after which 500 mg is given by mouth four times daily to complete a 14-day course.

A clinical study in Vietnam found that penicillin was associated with a more rapid resolution of fever and a lower rate of bacterial resistance than erythromycin; however, relapses were more common with penicillin. Erythromycin therapy targets protein synthesis and thus offers the presumed benefit of stopping toxin synthesis more quickly than a cell wall–active β-lactam agent. Alternative agents for patients who are allergic to penicillin or cannot take erythromycin include rifampin and clindamycin. Eradication of *C. diphtheriae* should be documented at least 1 day after antimicrobial therapy is complete. A repeat throat culture 2 weeks later is recommended. For patients in whom the organism is not eradicated after a 14-day course of erythromycin or penicillin, an additional 10-day course followed by repeat culture is recommended.

Cutaneous diphtheria should be treated as described above for respiratory disease. Individuals infected with toxigenic strains should receive antitoxin. It is important to treat the underlying cause of the dermatoses in addition to the superinfection with *C. diphtheriae*.

Patients who recover from respiratory or cutaneous diphtheria should have antitoxin levels measured. If diphtheria antitoxin has been administered, this test should be performed 6 months later. Patients who recover from respiratory or cutaneous diphtheria should receive the appropriate vaccine (see "Prevention," below) to ensure the development of protective antibody titers, which does not occur in all cases.

MANAGEMENT Patients in whom diphtheria is suspected should be hospitalized in respiratory isolation rooms, with close monitoring of cardiac and respiratory function. A cardiac workup is recommended to assess the possibility of myocarditis. In patients with extensive pseudomembranes, consultation with an anesthesiologist or an ear, nose, and throat specialist is recommended because of the possibility that tracheostomy or intubation will be required. In some settings, pseudomembranes can be removed surgically. Treatment with glucocorticoids has not been shown to reduce the risk of myocarditis or polyneuropathy.

■ PROGNOSIS

Fatal pseudomembranous diphtheria typically occurs in patients with nonprotective antibody titers and in unimmunized patients. The pseudomembrane may increase in size from the time it is first noted. Risk factors for death include bull-neck diphtheria; myocarditis with ventricular tachycardia; atrial fibrillation; complete heart block; an age of >60 years or <6 months; alcoholism; extensive pseudomembrane elongation; and laryngeal, tracheal, or bronchial involvement. Another important predictor of fatal outcome is the interval between local disease development and antitoxin administration. Cutaneous diphtheria has a low mortality rate and is rarely associated with myocarditis or peripheral neuropathy.

■ PREVENTION

Vaccination

Sustained campaigns for vaccination of children and adequate boosting vaccination of adults are responsible for the exceedingly low incidence of diphtheria in most developed nations. At present, diphtheria toxoid vaccine is coadministered with tetanus (with or without acellular pertussis) vaccine. DTaP (full-level diphtheria and tetanus toxoids and acellular pertussis vaccine, adsorbed) is the currently recommended vaccine for children up to the age of 7; DTaP replaced DTP (diphtheria and tetanus toxoids and whole-cell pertussis vaccine) in 1997. Tdap is a tetanus toxoid, reduced diphtheria toxoid, and acellular pertussis vaccine formulated for adolescents and adults. Tdap was licensed for use in the United States in 2005 and is the recommended booster vaccine for children 11–12 years old and the recommended catch-up vaccine for children 7–10 and 13–18 years old. As of 2006, it is recommended that (1) adults 19–64 years old receive a single dose of Tdap if their last dose of Td (tetanus and reduced-dose diphtheria toxoids, adsorbed) was >10 years earlier and (2) intervals of <10 years be implemented for Tdap vaccination of health care workers, adults anticipating contact with infants, and adults not previously vaccinated for pertussis. Adults who have received acellular pertussis vaccines should continue to receive decennial Td booster vaccinations. The vaccination schedule is detailed in Chap. 122.

Prophylaxis of contacts

Close contacts of diphtheria cases should undergo throat culture to determine whether they are carriers. After samples for throat culture are obtained, antimicrobial prophylaxis should be considered for all close contacts, even those who are culture-negative. The options are 7–10 days of oral erythromycin or one dose of IM benzathine penicillin G (1.2 million units for persons ≥6 years old or 600,000 units for children <6 years old).

Contacts of diphtheria cases who have an uncertain immunization status should receive the appropriate diphtheria toxoid–containing vaccine. Tdap (rather than Td) is now recommended as the booster vaccine of choice for adults who have not recently received an acellular pertussis–containing vaccine. Carriers of *C. diphtheriae* in the community should be treated and vaccinated when identified.

NONDIPHTHERIAL CORYNEBACTERIA AND RELATED SPECIES

Nondiphtherial corynebacteria, which are also referred to as *diphtheroids* or *coryneforms*, are a widely diverse collection of bacteria that are taxonomically lumped together on the basis of their 16S rDNA signature nucleotides. The diversity of this group is exemplified by the wide range in guanine-plus-cytosine content (45–70%). Although frequently considered colonizers or contaminants, the nondiphtherial corynebacteria have been associated with invasive disease, particularly in immunocompromised patients. Specifically, for example, these organisms have been implicated in bacteremia, endocarditis, and other serious infections, particularly in association with catheters and prosthetic devices. Patients infected with nondiphtherial corynebacteria usually have significant medical comorbidity or immunosuppression. Several of these organisms, including *C. jeikeium* and *C. urealyticum*, are associated with resistance to multiple antibiotics. The related organism *Rhodococcus equi* is associated with necrotizing pneumonia and granulomatous infection, particularly in immunocompromised individuals. Other related species that can cause infections in humans are *Actinomyces* (formerly *Corynebacterium*) *pyogenes* and *Arcanobacterium* (formerly *Corynebacterium*) *haemolyticum*.

■ MICROBIOLOGY AND LABORATORY DIAGNOSIS

These organisms are non-acid-fast, catalase-positive, aerobic or facultatively anaerobic bacilli. Their colonial morphologies vary widely; some species are small and α-hemolytic (similar to lactobacilli), whereas others form large white colonies (similar to yeasts). Many nondiphtherial coryneforms require special medium (e.g., Löffler's, Tinsdale's, or telluride medium) for growth.

■ EPIDEMIOLOGY

Humans are the natural reservoirs for several nondiphtherial coryneforms, including *C. xerosis, C. pseudodiphtheriticum, C. striatum, C. minutissimum, C. jeikeium, C. urealyticum,* and *A. haemolyticum*. Animal reservoirs are responsible for carriage of *A. pyogenes, C. ulcerans,* and *C. pseudotuberculosis*. Soil is the natural reservoir for *R. equi*.

C. pseudodiphtheriticum is part of the normal flora of the human pharynx and skin. *C. xerosis* is found on the skin, nasopharynx, and conjunctiva; *C. auris* in the external auditory canal; and *C. striatum* in the anterior nares and on the skin. *C. jeikeium* and *C. urealyticum* are found in the axilla, groin, and perineum, particularly in hospitalized patients. *C. ulcerans* and *C. pseudotuberculosis* infections have been associated with the consumption of raw milk from infected cattle.

■ SPECIFIC NONDIPHTHERIAL CORYNEFORMS

C. ulcerans

This organism causes a diphtherialike illness and produces both diphtheria toxin and a dermonecrotic toxin. *C. ulcerans* is a commensal in horses and cattle and has been isolated from cow's milk. The organism causes exudative pharyngitis, primarily during summer months, in rural areas, and among individuals exposed to cattle. In contrast to diphtheria, *C. ulcerans* infection is considered a zoonosis, and pigs have been identified as a source of human infection; person-to-person transmission has not been established. Nevertheless, treatment with antitoxin and antibiotics should be initiated when respiratory *C. ulcerans* is identified, and a contact investigation (including throat cultures to determine the need for antimicrobial prophylaxis and vaccination with the appropriate diphtheria toxoid–containing vaccine for unimmunized human contacts) should be conducted. The organism grows on Löffler's, Tinsdale's, and telluride media as well as blood agar. In addition to exudative pharyngitis, cutaneous disease due to *C. ulcerans* has been reported. *C. ulcerans* is susceptible to a wide panel of antibiotics. Erythromycin and macrolides appear to be the first-line agents.

C. pseudotuberculosis (ovis)

Infections caused by *C. pseudotuberculosis* are rare and are reported almost exclusively from Australia. *C. pseudotuberculosis* causes suppurative granulomatous lymphadenitis and an eosinophilic pneumonia syndrome among individuals who handle horses, cattle, goats, and deer or who drink unpasteurized milk. The organism is an important veterinary pathogen, causing suppurative lymphadenitis, abscesses, and pneumonia, but is rarely a human pathogen. Successful treatment with erythromycin or tetracycline has been reported, with surgery also performed when indicated.

C. jeikeium (group JK)

After a 1976 survey of diseases caused by nondiphtherial corynebacteria, CDC group JK was recognized as an important opportunistic pathogen among neutropenic patients and later emerged in HIV-infected patients as a cause of AIDS-associated opportunistic infection. Accordingly, the organism was reclassified as a separate species, *C. jeikeium*. The predominant syndrome associated with

C. jeikeium is sepsis, which can occur in conjunction with pneumonia, endocarditis, meningitis, osteomyelitis, or epidural abscess. Risk factors for *C. jeikeium* infection include hematologic malignancy, neutropenia from comorbid conditions, prolonged hospitalization, exposure to multiple antibiotics, and skin disruption. There is evidence that *C. jeikeium* is part of the normal flora of the inguinal, axillary, genital, and perirectal areas in hospitalized patients.

Broad-spectrum antimicrobial therapy appears to select for colonization. Originally described in the United States, *C. jeikeium* has also been reported in Europe. The gram-positive coccobacilli, which slightly resemble streptococci, grow as small, gray to white, glistening, nonhemolytic colonies on blood agar. *C. jeikeium* lacks urease and nitrate reductase and does not ferment most carbohydrates. It is resistant to most antibiotics tested except for vancomycin. Effective therapy involves removal of the source of infection, be it a catheter, a prosthetic joint, or a prosthetic valve. There have been efforts to prevent *C. jeikeium* infection by use of antibacterial soap in the care of high-risk patients in intensive care settings.

C. urealyticum (group D2)

Identified as a urease-positive nondiphtherial *Corynebacterium* in 1972, *C. urealyticum* is an opportunistic cause of sepsis and urinary tract infection. This organism appears to be the etiologic agent of a severe urinary tract syndrome known as *alkaline-encrusted cystitis*: a chronic inflammatory bladder infection associated with deposition of ammonium magnesium phosphate on the surface and walls of ulcerating lesions in the bladder. Obstructive uropathy due to this organism has been reported in renal transplant recipients. In addition, *C. urealyticum* has been associated with pneumonia, peritonitis, endocarditis, osteomyelitis, and wound infection. It is similar to *C. jeikeium* in its resistance to most antibiotics except vancomycin, which has been used successfully in the treatment of severe infections.

C. minutissimum

Erythrasma is a cutaneous infection producing reddish-brown, macular, scaly, pruritic intertriginous patches. The dermatologic presentation under the Wood's lamp is of coral-red fluorescence. *C. minutissimum* appears to be a common cause of erythrasma, although there is evidence for a polymicrobial etiology in certain settings. In addition, this fluorescent microbe has been associated with bacteremia in patients with hematologic malignancy. Erythrasma responds to topical erythromycin, clarithromycin, clindamycin, or fusidic acid, although more severe infections may require oral macrolide therapy.

■ OTHER NONDIPHTHERIAL CORYNEBACTERIA

C. xerosis is a human commensal found in the conjunctiva, nasopharynx, and skin. This nontoxigenic organism is occasionally identified as a source of invasive infection in immunocompromised or postoperative patients and prosthetic joint recipients. *C. striatum* is found in the anterior nares and on the skin, face, and upper torso of normal individuals. Also nontoxigenic, this organism has been associated with invasive opportunistic infections in severely ill or immunocompromised patients. *C. amycolatum* is a species isolated from human skin and is identified on the basis of a unique 16S ribosomal RNA sequence associated with opportunistic infection. *C. glucuronolyticum* is a nonlipophilic species that causes male genitourinary tract infections such as prostatitis and urethritis. These infections may be successfully treated with a wide variety of antibacterial agents, including β-lactams, rifampin, aminoglycosides, or vancomycin; however, the organism appears to be resistant to fluoroquinolones, macrolides, and tetracyclines. *C. imitans* has been identified in Eastern Europe as a nontoxigenic cause of pharyngitis. *C. auris* has been isolated from children with otitis media and is susceptible to fluoroquinolones, rifampin, tetracycline, and vancomycin but resistant to penicillin G and variably susceptible to macrolides. *C. pseudodiphtheriticum* (*C. hofmannii*) is a nontoxigenic component of the normal human flora. Human infections—particularly endocarditis of either prosthetic or native valves and invasive pneumonia—have been identified only rarely. Although *C. pseudodiphtheriticum* may be isolated from the nasopharynx of patients with suspected diphtheria, it is part of the normal flora and does not produce diphtheria toxin. *C. propinquum*, a close relative of *C. pseudodiphtheriticum*, is part of CDC group ANF-3 and is isolated from human respiratory tract specimens and blood. *C. afermentans* subspecies *lipophilum* belongs to CDC group ANF-1 and has been isolated from human blood and abscess infections. *C. accolens* has been isolated from wound drainage, throat swabs, and sputum and is typically identified as a satellite of staphylococcal organisms; it has been associated with endocarditis. *C. bovis* is a veterinary commensal that has not been clearly identified as a cause of human disease. *C. aquaticum* is a water-associated organism that is occasionally isolated from patients using medical devices (e.g., for chronic ambulatory peritoneal dialysis or venous access).

■ *RHODOCOCCUS*

Rhodococcus species are phylogenetically related to the corynebacteria. These gram-positive coccobacilli have been associated with tuberculosis-like infections in humans with granulomatous pathology. Although *R. equi* is best known, other species have been identified, including *R.* (also *Gordonia*) *bronchialis*, *R.* (also *Tsukamurella*) *aurantiacus*, *R. luteus*, *R. erythropolis*, *R. rhodochrous*, and *R. rubropertinctus*. *R. equi* has been recognized as a cause of pneumonia in horses since the 1920s; it causes related infections in cattle, sheep, and swine. *R. equi* is found in soil as an environmental microbe. The organisms vary in length; appear as spherical to long, curved, clubbed rods; and produce large, irregular mucoid colonies. *R. equi* does not ferment carbohydrates or liquefy gelatin and is often acid-fast. An intracellular pathogen of macrophages, *R. equi* can cause granulomatous necrosis and caseation. The organism has been identified most commonly in pulmonary infections, but infections of brain, bone, and skin have also been reported. Most commonly, *R. equi* disease manifests as nodular cavitary pneumonia of the upper lobe—a picture similar to that seen in tuberculosis or nocardiosis. Most patients are immunocompromised, often with HIV infection. Subcutaneous nodular lesions have also been identified. The involvement of *R. equi* should be considered in any patient presenting with a tuberculosis-like syndrome.

Infection due to *R. equi* has been treated successfully with antibiotics that penetrate intracellularly, including macrolides, clindamycin, rifampin, trimethoprim-sulfamethoxazole, tigecycline, and linezolid. β-Lactam antibiotics have not been useful. The organism is routinely susceptible to vancomycin, which is considered the drug of choice although there may be a role for oral therapies with bactericidal agents such as linezolid.

■ *ACTINOMYCES PYOGENES*

A cause of seasonal leg ulcers in humans in rural Thailand, *A. pyogenes* is a well-known pathogen of cattle, sheep, goats, and pigs. A few human cases of sepsis, endocarditis, septic arthritis, pneumonia, meningitis, and empyema have been reported. The agent is susceptible to β-lactams, tetracycline, aminoglycosides, and fluoroquinolones.

■ *ARCANOBACTERIUM HAEMOLYTICUM*

A. haemolyticum was identified as an agent of wound infections in U.S. soldiers in the South Pacific during World War II. This organism appears to be a commensal of the human nasopharynx and skin but has been implicated as a cause of pharyngitis and chronic skin ulcers. In contrast to the much more common pharyngitis caused by *Streptococcus pyogenes*, *A. haemolyticum* pharyngitis is associated with a scarlatiniform rash on the trunk and proximal extremities in about half of cases; this illness is occasionally confused with toxic shock syndrome. Because *A. haemolyticum* pharyngitis primarily affects teenagers, it has been postulated that the rash-pharyngitis syndrome may represent copathogenicity or synergy with EBV or opportunistic secondary infection complicating EBV infection. *A. haemolyticum* has also been reported as a cause of bacteremia, soft tissue infection, osteomyelitis, and cavitary pneumonia, predominantly in the setting of underlying diabetes mellitus. The organism is susceptible to β-lactams, macrolides, fluoroquinolones, clindamycin, vancomycin, and doxycycline. Penicillin resistance has been reported.

FURTHER READINGS

CENTERS FOR DISEASE CONTROL AND PREVENTION: Availability of diphtheria antitoxin through an investigational new drug protocol. MMWR Morb Mortal Wkly Rep 53:413, 2004

DITTMANN S et al: Successful control of epidemic diphtheria in the states of the former Union of Soviet Socialist Republics: Lessons learned. J Infect Dis 181(Suppl 1):S10, 2000

KRETSINGER K et al: Preventing tetanus, diphtheria, and pertussis among adults: Use of tetanus toxoid, reduced diphtheria toxoid, and acellular pertussis vaccine; recommendations of the Advisory Committee on Immunization Practices (ACIP) and recommendation of ACIP, supported by the Healthcare Infection Control Practices Advisory Committee (HICPAC), for use of Tdap among health-care personnel. MMWR Recomm Rep 55(RR-17):1, 2006

LÓPEZ-MEDRANO F et al: Urinary tract infection due to *Corynebacterium urealyticum* in kidney transplant recipients: An underdiagnosed etiology for obstructive uropathy and graft dysfunction—results of a prospective cohort study. Clin Infect Dis 46:825, 2008

MACGREGOR RR: *Corynebacterium diphtheriae*, in *Principles and Practice of Infectious Diseases*, 7th ed, GL Mandell et al (eds). Philadelphia, Elsevier Churchill Livingstone, 2010, pp 2687–2694

MEYER DK, REBOLI AC: Other coryneform bacteria and *Rhodococcus*, in *Principles and Practice of Infectious Diseases*, 7th ed, GL Mandell et al (eds). Philadelphia, Elsevier Churchill Livingstone, 2010, pp 2695–2706

MURPHY TV et al: Prevention of pertussis, tetanus, and diphtheria among pregnant and postpartum women and their infants: Recommendations of the Advisory Committee on Immunization Practices (ACIP). MMWR Recomm Rep 57(RR-4): 1, 2008

ROMNEY MG et al: Emergence of an invasive clone of nontoxigenic *Corynebacterium diphtheriae* in the urban poor population of Vancouver, Canada. J Clin Microbiol 44:1625, 2006

SCHUHEGGER R et al: Pigs as source for toxigenic *Corynebacterium ulcerans*. Emerg Infect Dis 15:1314, 2009

WAGNER KS et al: A review of the international issues surrounding the availability and demand for diphtheria antitoxin for therapeutic use. Vaccine 28:14, 2009

CHAPTER 139

Listeria monocytogenes Infections

Elizabeth L. Hohmann
Daniel A. Portnoy

Listeria monocytogenes is a food-borne pathogen that can cause serious infections, particularly in pregnant women and immuno-compromised individuals. A ubiquitous saprophytic environmental bacterium, *L. monocytogenes* is also a facultative intracellular pathogen with a broad host range. Humans are probably accidental hosts for this microorganism. *L. monocytogenes* is of interest not only to clinicians but also to basic scientists as a model intracellular pathogen that is used to study basic mechanisms of microbial pathogenesis and host immunity.

■ MICROBIOLOGY

L. monocytogenes is a facultatively anaerobic, nonsporulating, gram-positive rod that grows over a broad temperature range, including refrigeration temperatures. This organism is motile during growth at low temperatures but much less so at 37°C. The vast majority of cases of human listerial disease can be traced to serotypes 1/2a, 1/2b, and 4. *L. monocytogenes* is weakly β-hemolytic on blood agar, and (as detailed below) its β-hemolysin is an essential determinant of its pathogenicity.

■ PATHOGENESIS

Infections with *L. monocytogenes* follow ingestion of contaminated food that contains the bacteria at high concentrations. The conversion from environmental saprophyte to pathogen involves the coordinate regulation of bacterial determinants of pathogenesis that mediate entry into cells, intracellular growth, and cell-to-cell spread. Many of the organism's pathogenic strategies can be examined experimentally in tissue culture models of infection; such a model is presented in Fig. 139-1. Like other enteric pathogens, *L. monocytogenes* induces its own internalization by cells that are not normally phagocytic. Its entry into cells is mediated by host surface proteins classified as internalins. Internalin-mediated entry is important in the crossing of intestinal, blood-brain, and fetoplacental barriers, although how *L. monocytogenes* traffics from the intestine to the brain or fetus is only beginning to be investigated. In a pregnant guinea pig model of infection, *L. monocytogenes* was shown to traffic from maternal organs to the placenta; surprisingly, however, it also trafficked from the placenta back to maternal organs. These data are consistent with a model in which miscarriage can be viewed as a host defense strategy to eliminate a nidus of infection.

An essential determinant of the pathogenesis of *L. monocytogenes* is its β-hemolysin, listeriolysin O (LLO). LLO is a pore-forming, cholesterol-dependent cytolysin. (Related cytolysins include streptolysin O, pneumolysin, and perfringolysin O, all of which are produced by extracellular pathogens.) LLO is largely responsible for mediating the rupture of the phagosomal membrane that forms after phagocytosis of *L. monocytogenes*. LLO probably acts by inserting itself into an acidifying phagosome, thereby preventing the vesicle's maturation. In addition, LLO acts as a translocation pore for one or both of the *L. monocytogenes* phospholipases that

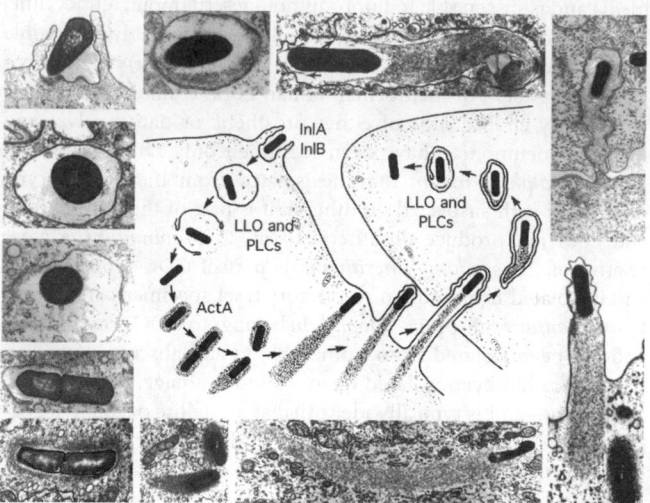

Figure 139-1 Stages in the intracellular life cycle of *Listeria monocytogenes.* The central diagram depicts cell entry, escape from a vacuole, actin nucleation, actin-based motility, and cell-to-cell spread. Surrounding the diagram are representative electron micrographs from which it was derived. ActA, surface protein mediating nucleation of host actin filaments to propel bacteria intra- and intercellularly; LLO, listeriolysin O; PLCs, phospholipases C; Inl, internalin. See text for further details. *(Adapted with permission from LG Tilney and DA Portnoy: J Cell Biol 109:1597, 1989. © Rockefeller University Press.)*

also contribute to vacuolar lysis. LLO synthesis and activity are controlled at multiple levels to ensure that its lytic activity is limited to acidic vacuoles and does not affect the cytosol. Mutations in LLO that influence its synthesis, cytosolic half-life, or pH optimum cause premature toxicity to infected cells. There is an inverse relationship between toxicity and virulence—i.e., the more cytotoxic the strain, the less virulent it is in animals. This relationship may seem paradoxical, but, as an intracellular pathogen, *L. monocytogenes* benefits from leaving its host cell unharmed.

Shortly after exposure to the mammalian-cell cytosol, *L. monocytogenes* expresses a surface protein, ActA, that mediates the nucleation of host actin filaments to propel the bacteria intra- and intercellularly. ActA mimics host proteins of the Wiskott-Aldrich syndrome protein (WASP) family by promoting the actin nucleation properties of the Arp2/3 complex. Thus, *L. monocytogenes* can enter the cytosol of almost any eukaryotic cell or cell extract and can exploit a conserved and essential actin-based motility system. Other pathogens as diverse as certain *Shigella*, *Mycobacterium*, *Rickettsia*, and *Burkholderia* spp. use a related pathogenic strategy that allows cell-to-cell spread without exposure to the extracellular milieu.

■ IMMUNE RESPONSE

The innate and acquired immune responses to *L. monocytogenes* have been studied extensively in mice. Shortly after IV injection, most bacteria are found in Kupffer cells in the liver, with some organisms in splenic dendritic cells and macrophages. Listeriae that survive the bactericidal activity of initially infected macrophages grow in the cytosol and spread from cell to cell. In the liver, the result is infection of hepatocytes. Neutrophils are crucial to host defense during the first 24 h of infection, while influx of activated macrophages from the bone marrow is critical subsequently. Mice that survive sublethal infection clear the infection within a week, with consequent sterile immunity. Studies with knockout mice have been instrumental in dissecting the roles played by chemokines and cytokines during infection. For example, interferon γ and tumor necrosis factor (TNF) are essential in controlling infection. While innate immunity is sufficient to control infection, the acquired immune response is required for sterile immunity. Immunity is cell-mediated; antibody plays no measurable role. The critical effector cells are cytotoxic (CD8+) T cells that recognize and lyse infected cells, and the resulting extracellular bacteria are killed by circulating activated phagocytes. Animals that survive challenge with sublethal doses of bacteria become immune to subsequent infection. A hallmark of the *L. monocytogenes* model is that killed vaccines do not provide protective immunity. The explanation for this fundamental observation is multifactorial, involving the generation of appropriate cytokines and the compartmentalization of bacterial proteins for antigen processing and presentation. Because the organism has the capacity to induce a robust cell-mediated immune response, attenuated strains have been engineered to express foreign antigens and are undergoing clinical studies as therapeutic vaccines for cancer and infectious disease applications.

EPIDEMIOLOGY

L. monocytogenes usually enters the body via the gastrointestinal tract in foods. Listeriosis is most often sporadic, although outbreaks do occur. Recent annual incidences in the United States range from 2 to 9 cases per 1 million population. No epidemiologic or clinical evidence supports human-to-human transmission (other than vertical transmission from mother to fetus) or waterborne infection. In line with its survival and multiplication at refrigeration temperatures, *L. monocytogenes* is commonly found in processed and unprocessed foods of animal and plant origin, especially soft cheeses, delicatessen meats, hot dogs, milk, and cold salads. Because food supplies are increasingly centralized and normal hosts tolerate the organism well, outbreaks may not be immediately apparent; pulsed-field gel electrophoresis has proved useful in linking cases to specific foods. FoodNet, an active U.S. surveillance program, documented no significant change in the estimated incidence of listeriosis from 2005 through 2008. The U.S. Food and Drug Administration has a zero-tolerance policy for *L. monocytogenes* in ready-to-eat foods.

DIAGNOSIS

Symptoms of listerial infection overlap greatly with those of other infectious diseases. Timely diagnosis requires that the illness be considered in groups at risk: pregnant women; elderly persons; neonates; individuals immunocompromised by organ transplants, cancer, or treatment with TNF antagonists or glucocorticoids; and patients with a variety of chronic medical conditions, including alcoholism, diabetes, renal disease, rheumatologic illness, and iron overload. Meningitis in older adults (especially with parenchymal brain involvement or subcortical brain abscess) should trigger consideration of *L. monocytogenes* infection. Listeriosis occasionally affects healthy, young, nonpregnant individuals. HIV-infected patients are at risk; however, listeriosis seems to be prevented by trimethoprim-sulfamethoxazole (TMP-SMX) prophylaxis targeting other AIDS-related infections. The diagnosis is typically made by culture of blood, cerebrospinal fluid (CSF), or amniotic fluid. *L. monocytogenes* may be confused with "diphtheroids" or pneumococci in gram-stained CSF or may be gram-variable and confused with *Haemophilus* spp. Serologic tests and polymerase chain reaction assays are not clinically useful diagnostic tools at present.

CLINICAL MANIFESTATIONS

Listerial infections present as several clinical syndromes, of which meningitis and septicemia are most common. Monocytosis is seen in infected rabbits but is not a hallmark of human infection.

Gastroenteritis

Appreciated only since the outbreaks of the late 1980s, listerial gastroenteritis typically develops within 48 h of ingestion of a large inoculum of bacteria in contaminated foods such as milk, deli meats, and salads. Attack rates are high (50–100%). *L. monocytogenes* is neither sought nor found in routine fecal cultures, but its involvement should be considered in outbreaks when cultures for other likely pathogens are negative. Sporadic intestinal illness appears to be uncommon. Manifestations include fever, diarrhea, headache, and constitutional symptoms. The largest reported outbreak occurred in an Italian school system and included 1566 individuals; ~20% of patients were hospitalized, but only one person had a positive blood culture. Isolated gastrointestinal illness does not require antibiotic treatment. Surveillance studies show that 0.1–5% of healthy asymptomatic adults may have stool cultures positive for the organism.

Bacteremia

L. monocytogenes septicemia presents with fever, chills, and myalgias/arthralgias and cannot be differentiated from septicemia involving other organisms. Meningeal symptoms, focal neurologic findings, or mental status changes may suggest the diagnosis. Bacteremia is documented in 70–90% of cancer patients with listeriosis. A nonspecific flulike illness with fever is a common presentation in pregnant women. Endocarditis of prosthetic and native valves is an uncommon complication, with reported fatality rates of 35–50% in case series. A lumbar puncture is often prudent, although not necessary, in pregnant women without central nervous system (CNS) symptoms.

Meningitis

L. monocytogenes causes ~5–10% of all cases of community-acquired bacterial meningitis in adults in the United States. Case-fatality rates are reported to be 15–26% and do not appear to have changed over time. This diagnosis should be considered in all older or chronically ill adults with "aseptic" meningitis. The presentation is more frequently subacute (with illness developing over several days) than in meningitis of other bacterial etiologies, and nuchal rigidity and meningeal signs are less common. Photophobia is infrequent. Focal findings and seizures are common in some but not all series. The CSF profile in listerial meningitis most often shows white blood cell (WBC) counts in the range of 100–5000/μL (rarely higher); 75% of patients have WBC counts below 1000/μL, usually with a neutrophil predominance more modest than that in other bacterial meningitides. Low glucose levels and positive results on Gram's staining are found ~30–40% of the time. Hydrocephalus can occur.

Meningoencephalitis and Focal CNS Infection

L. monocytogenes can directly invade the brain parenchyma, producing either cerebritis or focal abscess. Approximately 10% of cases of CNS infection are macroscopic abscesses resulting from bacteremic seeding; the affected patients often have positive blood cultures. Concurrent meningitis can exist, but the CSF may appear normal. Abscesses can be misdiagnosed as metastatic or primary tumors and, in rare instances, occur in the cerebellum and the spinal cord. Invasion of the brainstem results in a characteristic severe rhombencephalitis, usually in otherwise healthy older adults. The presentation may be biphasic, with a prodrome of fever and headache followed by asymmetric cranial nerve deficits, cerebellar signs, and hemiparetic and hemisensory deficits. Respiratory failure can occur. The subacute course and the often minimally abnormal CSF findings may delay the diagnosis, which may be suggested by MRI images showing ring-enhancing lesions after gadolinium contrast and hyperintense lesions on diffusion-weighted imaging. MRI is superior to CT for the diagnosis of these infections.

Infection in Pregnant Women and Neonates

Listeriosis in pregnancy is a severe and important infection. The usual presentation is a nonspecific acute or subacute febrile illness with myalgias, arthralgias, backache, and headache. Pregnant women with listeriosis are usually bacteremic. This syndrome should prompt blood cultures, especially in the absence of another reasonable explanation. Involvement of the CNS is rare in the absence of other risk factors. Preterm delivery is a common complication, and the diagnosis may be made only postpartum. As many as 70–90% of fetuses from infected women can become infected. Prepartum treatment of bacteremic women enhances the chances of delivery of a healthy infant. Women usually do well after delivery: maternal deaths are very rare, even when the diagnosis is made late in pregnancy or postpartum. Overall mortality rates for fetuses infected in utero approach 50% in some series; among live-born neonates treated with antibiotics, mortality rates are much lower (~20%). *Granulomatosis infantiseptica* is an overwhelming listerial fetal infection with miliary microabscesses and granulomas, most often in the skin, liver, and spleen. Less severe neonatal infection acquired in utero presents at birth. "Late-onset" neonatal illness typically develops ~10–30 days postpartum. Mothers of infants with late-onset disease are not ill .

| TREATMENT | Infections Caused by *Listeria monocytogenes* |

No clinical trials have compared antimicrobial agents for the treatment of *L. monocytogenes* infections. Data obtained in studies conducted in vitro and in animals as well as observational clinical data indicate that ampicillin is the drug of choice, although penicillin is also highly active. Adults should receive IV ampicillin at high doses (2 g every 4 h), and many experts recommend the addition of gentamicin for synergy (1.0–1.7 mg/kg every 8 h); retrospective uncontrolled trials are not conclusive, but one study suggests that gentamicin may not help. TMP-SMX, given IV, is the best alternative for the penicillin-allergic patient (15–20 mg of TMP/kg per day in divided doses every 6–8 h). The dosages recommended cover CNS infection and bacteremia (see below for duration) ; dosages must be reduced for patients with renal insufficiency. One small nonrandomized study supports a combination of ampicillin and TMP-SMX. Case reports document success with vancomycin, imipenem, meropenem, linezolid, tetracycline, and macrolides , although there are also reports of clinical failure or disease development with some of these agents. Cephalosporins are *not* effective and should not be used. Neonates should receive ampicillin and gentamicin at doses based on weight.

The duration of therapy depends on the syndrome: 2 weeks for bacteremia, 3 weeks for meningitis, 6–8 weeks for brain abscess/encephalitis, and 4–6 weeks for endocarditis in both neonates and adults. Early-onset neonatal disease may be more severe and should be treated for >2 weeks.

■ COMPLICATIONS AND PROGNOSIS

Many individuals who are promptly diagnosed and treated recover fully, but permanent neurologic sequelae are common in patients with brain abscess or rhombencephalitis. Focal infections of visceral organs; the eye; the pleural, peritoneal, and pericardial spaces; and the bones and joints have all been reported. Of 100 live-born treated neonates in one series, 60% recovered fully, 24% died, and 13% had long-term neurologic or other complications.

■ PREVENTION

Healthy persons should take standard precautions to prevent food-borne illness: fully cooking meats, washing fresh vegetables, carefully cleaning utensils, and avoiding unpasteurized dairy products. In addition, persons at risk for listeriosis, including pregnant women, should avoid soft cheeses (although hard cheeses and yogurt are not problematic) and should avoid or thoroughly reheat ready-to-eat and delicatessen foods, even though the absolute risk they pose is relatively low.

FURTHER READINGS

BAKARDJIEV AI ET AL: *Listeria monocytogenes* traffics from maternal organs to the placenta and back. PLoS Pathog 2:e66, 2006

BROCKSTEDT DG ET AL: Promises and challenges for the development of *Listeria monocytogenes*–based therapeutics. Expert Rev Vaccines 7:1069, 2008

CENTERS FOR DISEASE CONTROL AND PREVENTION: FoodNet— Foodborne Diseases Active Surveillance Network. Accessed at *www.cdc.gov/foodnet/*

FREITAG NE ET AL: *Listeria monocytogenes*—from saprophyte to intracellular pathogen. Nat Rev Microbiol 9:623, 2009

HAMON M ET AL: *Listeria monocytogenes*: A multifaceted model. Nat Rev Microbiol 4:423, 2006

MITJA O ET AL: Predictors of mortality and impact of aminoglycosides on outcome in listeriosis in a retrospective cohort study. J Antimicrob Chemother 64:416, 2009

MYLONAKIS E ET AL: Listeriosis during pregnancy: A case series and review of 222 cases. Medicine (Baltimore) 81:260, 2002

OOI ST, LORBER B: Gastroenteritis due to *Listeria monocytogenes*. Clin Infect Dis 40:1327, 2005

PAMER ER: Immune responses to *Listeria monocytogenes*. Nat Rev Immunol 4:812, 2004

SCHNUPF P, PORTNOY DA: Listeriolysin: A phagosome-specific lysin. Microbes Infect 10:1176, 2007

CHAPTER 140

Tetanus

C. Louise Thwaites

Lam Minh Yen

Tetanus is an acute disease manifested by skeletal muscle spasm and autonomic nervous system disturbance. It is caused by a powerful neurotoxin produced by the bacterium *Clostridium tetani* and is completely preventable by vaccination. *C. tetani* is found throughout the world, and tetanus commonly occurs where the vaccination coverage rate is low. In developed countries, the disease is seen occasionally in individuals who are incompletely vaccinated. In any setting, established tetanus is a severe disease with a high mortality rate.

■ DEFINITION

Tetanus is diagnosed on clinical grounds (sometimes with supportive laboratory confirmation of the presence of *C. tetani*; see "Diagnosis," below), and case definitions are often used to facilitate clinical and epidemiologic assessments. The Centers for Disease Control and Prevention (CDC) defines tetanus as "the acute onset of hypertonia or…painful muscular contractions (usually of the muscles of the jaw and neck) and generalized muscle spasms without other apparent medical cause." Neonatal tetanus is defined by the World Health Organization (WHO) as "an illness occurring in a child who has the normal ability to suck and cry in the first 2 days of life but who loses this ability between days 3 and 28 of life and becomes rigid and has spasms." Given the unique presentation of neonatal tetanus, the history generally permits accurate classification of the illness with a high degree of probability. Maternal tetanus is defined by the WHO as tetanus occurring during pregnancy or within 6 weeks after the conclusion of pregnancy (whether with birth, miscarriage, or abortion).

■ ETIOLOGY

C. tetani is an anaerobic, gram-positive, spore-forming rod whose spores are highly resilient and can survive readily in the environment throughout the world. Spores resist boiling and many disinfectants. In addition, *C. tetani* spores and bacilli survive in the intestinal systems of many animals, and fecal carriage is common. The spores or bacteria enter the body through abrasions, wounds, or (in the case of neonates) the umbilical stump. Once in a suitable anaerobic environment, the organisms grow, multiply, and release tetanus toxin, an exotoxin that enters the nervous system and causes disease. Very low concentrations of this highly potent toxin can result in tetanus (minimum lethal human dose, 2.5 ng/kg).

In ~20% of cases of tetanus, no puncture entry wound is found. Superficial abrasions to the limbs are the commonest infection sites in adults. Deeper infections (e.g., attributable to open fracture, abortion, or drug injection) are associated with more severe disease and worse outcomes. In neonates, infection of the umbilical stump can result from inadequate umbilical cord care; in some cultures, for example, the cord is cut with grass or animal dung is applied to the stump. Circumcision or ear-piercing can also result in neonatal tetanus.

■ EPIDEMIOLOGY

 Reliable epidemiologic data on worldwide incidence are difficult to obtain, and tetanus is notoriously underreported. Studies have shown that in much of the world only 2–10% of tetanus cases are recorded. Estimates from the early 1980s suggested that tetanus caused >1 million deaths annually. As worldwide vaccination coverage has improved, the number of cases has fallen, particularly among children and neonates, who have been predominantly targeted in recent vaccination programs. In 2006, an estimated 290,000 people died of tetanus, mostly in Southeast Asia and Africa.

The elimination of maternal and neonatal tetanus is one goal of the WHO and its Expanded Programme on Immunization (EPI). An estimated 5% of maternal mortality in the 1990s was attributed to maternal tetanus. Tetanus in pregnant women and neonates is prevented by maternal immunization during pregnancy (see "Prevention," below), which is an integral component of the EPI. Although immunization coverage continues to increase, maternal and neonatal tetanus still represents an important global health burden, causing ~180,000 deaths per year.

Tetanus is a rare disease in the developed world. In 2007, a total of 28 cases were reported to the U.S. national surveillance system. Most cases occur in incompletely vaccinated or unvaccinated individuals. Persons >60 years of age are at greater risk of tetanus because antibody levels decrease over time. Injection drug users—particularly those injecting heroin subcutaneously ("skin-popping")—are increasingly recognized as a high-risk group. Between 1995 and 2000, 15–18% of U.S. tetanus infections occurred in injection drug users. In 2004, an outbreak of tetanus occurred in the United Kingdom, which had previously reported low rates among drug users. The reasons for this outbreak remain unclear but are thought to involve a combination of heroin contamination, skin-popping, and incomplete vaccination.

■ PATHOGENESIS

C. tetani produces two exotoxins: tetanolysin and tetanospasmin. Tetanolysin, which is related to the clostridial toxins and streptolysin, plays no role in the pathogenesis of the disease. Tetanospasmin, generally referred to as "tetanus toxin," is the neurotoxin that causes the manifestations of disease.

Toxin is transported by intra-axonal transport to motor nuclei of the cranial nerves or ventral horns of the spinal cord. Tetanus toxin is produced as a single 150-kDa protein that is cleaved to produce heavy (100-kDa) and light (50-kDa) chains linked by a disulfide bond and noncovalent forces. The carboxy terminal of the heavy chain binds to specific membrane components in presynaptic α-motor nerve terminals; evidence suggests binding to both polysialogangliosides and membrane proteins. This binding results in toxin internalization and uptake into the nerves. (Botulinum toxins enter the nervous system by a similar method but remain mostly at the neuromuscular junction and thus produce different clinical features.)

Once inside the neuron, the toxin enters a retrograde transport pathway, whereby it is transported proximally to the motor neuron body in what appears to be a highly specific process. Unlike other components of the endosomal contents, which undergo acidification following internalization, tetanus toxin is transported in a carefully regulated pH-neutral environment that prevents an acid-induced conformational change that would result in light-chain expulsion into the surrounding cytosol.

The next stage in toxin trafficking is less clearly understood but involves tetanus toxin's escaping normal lysosomal degradation processes and undergoing translocation across the synapse to the GABA-ergic presynaptic inhibitory interneuron terminals. Here the light chain, which is a zinc-dependent endopeptidase, cleaves vesicle-associated membrane protein 2 (VAMP2, also known as synaptobrevin). This molecule is necessary for presynaptic binding and release of neurotransmitter; thus tetanus toxin prevents transmitter release and effectively blocks inhibitory interneuron discharge. The result is unregulated activity in the motor nervous system. Similar activity in the autonomic system accounts for the characteristic features of skeletal muscle spasm and autonomic system disturbance. The increased circulating catecholamine levels in severe tetanus are associated with cardiovascular complications.

Relatively little is known about the processes of recovery from tetanus. Recovery can take several weeks. Peripheral nerve sprouting is involved in recovery from botulism, and similar central nervous system sprouting may occur in tetanus. Other evidence suggests toxin degradation as a mechanism of recovery.

> **APPROACH TO THE PATIENT** | **Tetanus**
>
> The clinical manifestations of tetanus occur only after tetanus toxin has reached presynaptic inhibitory nerves. Once these effects become apparent, there may be little that can be done to affect disease progression. Management strategies aim to support vital functions until the effects of the toxin have worn off. Recent interest has focused on intrathecal methods of antitoxin administration to neutralize toxin within the central nervous system and limit disease progression (see "Treatment," below).

■ CLINICAL MANIFESTATIONS

Tetanus produces a wide spectrum of clinical features that are broadly divided into generalized (including neonatal) and local. In the usually mild form of local tetanus, only isolated areas of the body are affected and only small areas of local muscle spasm may be apparent. If the cranial nerves are involved in localized cephalic tetanus, the pharyngeal or laryngeal muscles may spasm, with consequent aspiration or airway obstruction, and the prognosis may be poor. In the typical progression of generalized tetanus (Fig. 140-1), muscles of the face and jaw often are affected first, presumably because of the shorter distances toxin must travel up motor nerves to reach presynaptic terminals.

In assessing prognosis, the speed at which tetanus develops is important. The incubation period (time from wound to first symptom) and the period of onset (time from first symptom to first generalized spasm) are of particular significance; shorter times are associated with worse outcome. In neonatal tetanus, the younger the infant is when symptoms occur, the worse the prognosis.

The commonest initial symptoms are trismus (lockjaw), muscle pain and stiffness, back pain, and difficulty swallowing. In neonates, difficulty in feeding is the usual presentation. As the disease progresses, muscle spasm develops. Generalized muscle spasm can be very painful. Commonly, the laryngeal muscles are involved early or even in isolation. This is a life-threatening event as complete airway obstruction may ensue. Spasm of the respiratory muscles results in respiratory failure. Without ventilatory support, respiratory failure is the commonest cause of death in tetanus. Spasms strong enough to produce tendon avulsions and crush fractures have been reported, but this outcome is rare.

Autonomic disturbance is maximal during the second week of severe tetanus, and death due to cardiovascular events becomes the major risk. Blood pressure is usually labile, with rapid fluctuations from high to low accompanied by tachycardia. Episodes of bradycardia and heart block can also occur. Autonomic involvement is evidenced by gastrointestinal stasis, sweating, increased tracheal secretions, and acute (often high-output) renal failure.

■ DIAGNOSIS

The diagnosis of tetanus is clinical; culture of *C. tetani* from a wound provides supportive evidence. The few conditions that mimic generalized tetanus include strychnine poisoning and dystonic reactions to antidopaminergic drugs. Abdominal muscle rigidity is characteristically continuous in tetanus but is episodic in the latter two conditions. Cephalic tetanus can be confused with other causes of trismus, such as oropharyngeal infection. Hypocalcemia and meningoencephalitis are included in the differential diagnosis of neonatal tetanus.

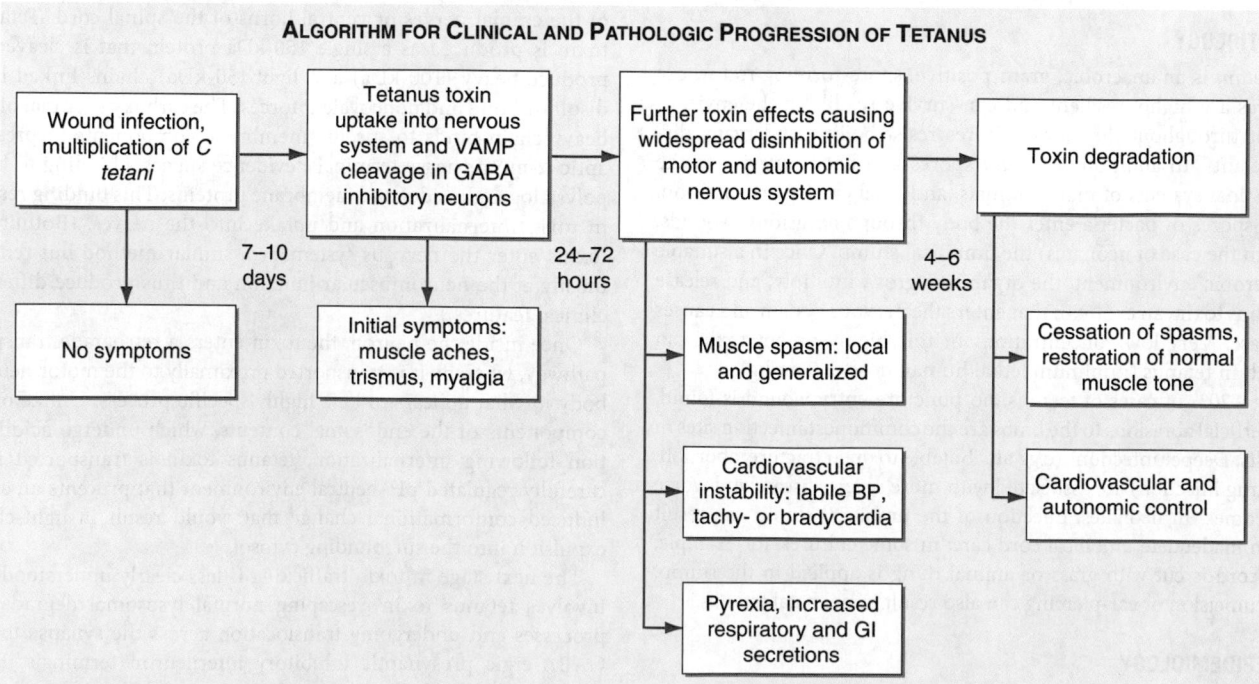

ALGORITHM FOR CLINICAL AND PATHOLOGIC PROGRESSION OF TETANUS

Figure 140-1 Clinical and pathologic progression of tetanus. BP, blood pressure; GABA, γ-aminobutyric acid; GI, gastrointestinal; VAMP, vesicle-associated monophosphate (synaptobrevin).

TREATMENT   Tetanus

If possible, the entry wound should be identified, cleaned, and debrided of necrotic material in order to remove anaerobic foci of infection and prevent further toxin production. Metronidazole (400 mg rectally or 500 mg IV every 6 h for 7 days) is the preferred antibiotic. An alternative is penicillin (100,000–200,000 IU/kg per day), although this drug theoretically may exacerbate spasms. Failure to remove pockets of ongoing infection may result in recurrent or prolonged tetanus.

Antitoxin should be given early in an attempt to deactivate any circulating tetanus toxin and prevent its uptake into the nervous system. Two preparations are available: human tetanus immune globulin (TIG) and equine antitoxin. TIG is the preparation of choice as it is less likely to be associated with anaphylactoid reactions. Standard therapy is 3000–6000 IU of TIG or 10,000–20,000 U of equine antitoxin as a single IM dose. However, there is evidence that intrathecal administration of TIG inhibits disease progression and leads to a better outcome. The results of a randomized controlled trial have been supported by a meta-analysis of trials involving both adults and neonates, with TIG doses of 50–1500 IU administered intrathecally.

Spasms are controlled by heavy sedation using benzodiazepines. Chlorpromazine or phenobarbital are commonly used worldwide, and IV magnesium sulfate has been used as a muscle relaxant. A significant problem with all these treatments is that the doses necessary to control spasms also cause respiratory depression; thus, in resource-limited settings without mechanical ventilators, controlling spasms while maintaining adequate ventilation is problematic, and respiratory failure is a common cause of death. In locations with ventilation equipment, severe spasms are best controlled with a combination of sedatives or magnesium and relatively short-acting, cardiovascularly inert, nondepolarizing neuromuscular blocking agents that allow titration against spasm intensity. Infusions of propofol have also been used successfully to control spasms and provide sedation.

It is important to establish a secure airway early in severe tetanus. Ideally, patients should be nursed in calm, quiet environments because light and noise can trigger spasms. Tracheal secretions are increased in tetanus, and dysphagia due to pharyngeal involvement combined with hyperactivity of laryngeal muscles makes endotracheal intubation difficult. Thus tracheostomy is the usual method of securing the airway in severe tetanus.

Cardiovascular instability in severe tetanus is notoriously difficult to treat. Rapid fluctuations in blood pressure and heart rate can occur. Cardiovascular stability is improved by increasing sedation with IV magnesium sulfate (plasma concentration, 2–4 mmol/L), morphine, or other sedatives. In addition, drugs acting specifically on the cardiovascular system (e.g., esmolol, calcium antagonists, and inotropes) may be required. Short-acting drugs that allow rapid titration are preferred; particular care should be taken when longer-acting β antagonists are administered, as their use has been associated with hypotensive cardiac arrest.

Complications arising from treatment are common and include thrombophlebitis associated with diazepam injection, ventilator-associated pneumonia, central-line infections, and septicemia. In some centers, prophylaxis against deep-vein thrombosis and thromboembolism is routine.

Recovery from tetanus may take 4–6 weeks. Patients must be given a full primary course of immunization as tetanus toxin is poorly immunogenic and the immune response following natural infection is inadequate.

PROGNOSIS

Rapid development of tetanus is associated with more severe disease and poorer outcome; it is important to note time of onset and length of incubation period. More sophisticated modeling based on data from adults has revealed other important predictors of prognosis (Table 140-1). Few studies have formally addressed long-term outcomes of tetanus. However, it is generally accepted that recovery is typically complete unless periods of hypoventilation have been prolonged or other complications have ensued. Studies of children and neonates have suggested that neonates who have experienced prolonged periods of hypoxia may be at increased risk of learning disabilities, behavioral problems, and cerebral palsy.

PREVENTION

Tetanus is prevented by good wound care and immunization (Chap. 122). In neonates, use of safe, clean delivery and cord-care practices as well as maternal vaccination are essential. Tetanus toxoid (TT) for vaccination is available in various preparations: single-dose TT, TT with high- or low-dose diphtheria toxoid, or TT with diphtheria toxoid in combination with whole-cell/acellular pertussis, *Haemophilus influenzae* type b, hepatitis B, or polio vaccine.

The WHO guidelines for tetanus vaccination consist of a primary course of three doses in infancy, boosters at 4–7 and 12–15 years of age, and one booster in adulthood. In the United States, the CDC suggests an additional dose at 14–16 months and boosters every 10 years. "Catch-up" schedules recommend a three-dose primary course for unimmunized adolescents followed by two further doses. For persons who have received a complete primary course in childhood but no further boosters, two doses at least 4 weeks apart are recommended.

Standard WHO recommendations for prevention of maternal and neonatal tetanus call for administration of two doses of TT at least 4 weeks apart to the previously unimmunized pregnant woman. However, in high-risk areas, a more intensive approach has been successful, with all women of childbearing age receiving a primary course along with education on safe delivery and postnatal practices.

Individuals sustaining tetanus-prone wounds should be immunized if their vaccination status is incomplete or unknown or if

TABLE 140-1   Factors Associated With a Poor Prognosis in Tetanus

Adult Tetanus	Neonatal Tetanus
Age >70 years	Younger age, premature birth
Incubation period <7 days	Incubation period <6 days
Short time from first symptom to admission	Delay in hospital admission
Puerperal, IV, postsurgery, burn entry site	Grass used to cut cord
Period of onset[a] <48 h	
Heart rate >140 bpm[b]	
Systolic blood pressure >140 mmHg[b]	
Severe disease or spasms[b]	
Temperature >38.5°C[b]	

[a]Time from first symptom to first generalized spasm.
[b]At hospital admission.

their last booster was given >10 years earlier. Patients sustaining wounds not classified as clean or minor should also undergo passive immunization with TIG.

FURTHER READINGS

ADVISORY COMMITTEE ON IMMUNIZATION PRACTICES: ACIP recommendations. MMWR Morb Mortal Wkly Rep 55:1, 2006

ATTYGALLE D, RODRIGO N: New trends in the management of tetanus. Expert Rev Anti Infect Ther 2:73, 2004

CALEO M, SCHIAVO G: Central effects of tetanus and botulinum neurotoxins. Toxicon 54:593, 2009

CENTERS FOR DISEASE CONTROL AND PREVENTION: Health Information for International Travel 2010. Atlanta, CDC, 2010 (wwwnc.cdc.gov/travel/content/yellowbook/home-2010.aspx)

GALAZKA A et al: Tetanus, in The Global Epidemiology of Infectious Diseases, CJL Murray et al (eds). Geneva, World Health Organization, 2004, pp 151–199 (whqlibdoc.who.int/publications/2004/9241592303.pdf)

KRETSINGER K, SRIVASTAVA P: Tetanus, in Manual for the Surveillance of Vaccine-Preventable Diseases, 4th ed. Atlanta, Centers for Disease Control and Prevention, 2008, Chap. 16

MIRANDA-FILHO DDE B et al: Randomised controlled trial of tetanus treatment with antitetanus immunoglobulin by the intrathecal or intramuscular route. BMJ 328:615, 2004

ROPER MH et al: Maternal and neonatal tetanus. Lancet 270:1906, 2007

THWAITES CL et al: Magnesium sulphate for treatment of severe tetanus: A randomised controlled trial. Lancet 368:1436, 2006

WORLD HEALTH ORGANIZATION: WHO-recommended standards for surveillance of selected vaccine-preventable diseases. Geneva, WHO, Vaccines and Biologicals 2003 WHO/V&B/03.01 (www.who.int/immunization_monitoring/burden/routine_surveillance/en/)

CHAPTER 141

Botulism

Jeremy Sobel
Susan Maslanka

Botulinum toxin is the most toxic substance known. Botulism, a rare disease, occurs naturally as four syndromes: (1) food-borne illness due to ingestion of toxin in contaminated food; (2) wound infection due to wound colonization by toxigenic clostridia with in situ toxin production; (3) infant botulism due to colonization of the infant intestine by toxigenic clostridia with in situ toxin production; and (4) adult intestinal toxemia, a rare form of colonization with similarities to infant botulism. In addition to these recognized natural forms, botulism has been reported in association with injections of botulinum toxin for cosmetic or therapeutic purposes and after inhalation of aerosolized botulinum toxin. Botulism is caused by the toxin's inhibition of acetylcholine release at the neuromuscular junction through an enzymatic mechanism. All forms of botulism manifest as a distinct clinical syndrome of symmetric cranial nerve palsies followed by descending symmetric flaccid paralysis of voluntary muscles, which may progress to respiratory compromise and death. The mainstays of therapy are meticulous intensive care and timely treatment with antitoxin, which may limit the extent of paralysis. Rapid clinical diagnosis is critical for decisions about treatment.

■ ETIOLOGY AND PATHOGENESIS

Botulinum toxin–producing clostridia are anaerobic gram-positive organisms that form subterminal spores and are ubiquitous in the environment. The hardy spores survive environmental conditions and ordinary cooking procedures. Toxin production, however, requires spore germination, which occurs only with a rare confluence of circumstances: an anaerobic atmosphere, a pH of >4.5, low salt and sugar concentrations, and temperatures of 4–120°C. Although commonly ingested, spores do not normally germinate in the intestine.

The various species of toxigenic clostridia—C. botulinum groups I, II, and III; C. argentinense (toxin type G); C. baratii (toxin type F); and C. butyricum (toxin type E)—can be differentiated on the basis of phenotypic characteristics, including specific biochemical properties and morphologic appearance on egg yolk agar. Strains of a given species can be distinguished by the antigenic specificity of the botulinum neurotoxin they produce; certain strains may produce more than one toxin serotype.

The seven identified toxin serotypes (A, B, C, D, E, F, and G) are antigenically distinct but structurally similar (~150-kDa zinc-endopeptidase proteins consisting of a 100-kDa heavy chain and a 50-kDa light chain). Whether ingested, inhaled, or produced in the intestine or a wound, botulinum neurotoxin enters the vascular system and is transported to peripheral cholinergic nerve terminals, including neuromuscular junctions, postganglionic parasympathetic nerve endings, and peripheral ganglia. The central nervous system probably is not involved. Steps in neurotoxin activity include (1) heavy-chain binding to nerve terminals, (2) internalization in endocytic vesicles, (3) translocation to cytosol, and (4) light-chain serotype-specific cleavage of one of several proteins involved in the release of the neurotransmitter acetylcholine. Inhibition of acetylcholine release by any of the seven toxin serotypes results in characteristic flaccid paralysis. Recovery follows sprouting of new nerve terminals.

Toxin serotypes A, B, E, and (rarely) F cause human disease. Toxin type A produces the most severe syndrome, with the greatest proportion of patients requiring mechanical ventilation. Toxin type B appears to cause milder disease than type A. Two cases of human illness due to toxin type C and one outbreak caused by toxin type D were reported more than 50 years ago. The reasons for the rarity of cases due to types C and D are not known; all four serotypes that affect humans produce botulism in experimental models. Toxin type E, most often associated with foods of aquatic origin, produces a syndrome of variable severity. The rare cases of illness caused by toxin type F are characterized by rapid progression to quadriplegia and respiratory failure but also by relatively rapid recovery.

■ EPIDEMIOLOGY

Person-to-person transmission of botulism has not been described. *Food-borne botulism* is caused by consumption of foods contaminated with botulinum toxin. Most botulism cases are sporadic; outbreaks are typically small, involving two or three cases. The wide variation in reported rates of

PART 8 Infectious Diseases

botulism by region and continent probably reflects differences both in true incidence and in diagnostic and reporting capacity. Worldwide, the highest incidence rate is reported from the Republic of Georgia and Armenia in the southern Caucasus region, where illness is associated with risky home-canning practices. In the United States during 1990–2000, the median number of food-borne cases per year was 23 (range, 17–43). The incidence rate was highest and the number of cases greatest in Alaska, with contaminated traditional Alaskan Native dishes implicated in every instance. Outside Alaska, food was implicated in 75 of 101 botulinum intoxication events. Of the 68 events caused by homemade foods, 47 (69%) involved home-canned items. Of the 7 events caused by non-homemade foods, five (affecting 10 people) were caused by commercial foods, and two (affecting 25 people) were caused by restaurant-prepared foods. Severe outbreaks traced to commercially prepared foods have occurred in more recent years. In 2006, patients in the U.S. states of Georgia and Florida as well as in the Canadian province of Ontario developed severe botulism after consuming commercially produced carrot juice contaminated with a high level of toxin type A. Very high toxin levels were recorded in some of the patients' serum samples, with toxemia persisting for a record 25 days after illness onset in one patient. Outbreaks caused by contaminated commercial chili occurred in 2001 (15 cases in Texas) and 2007 (8 cases in Ohio, Indiana, and Texas).

Wound botulism is caused by contamination of wounds with *C. botulinum* spores, subsequent spore germination, and toxin production in the anaerobic milieu of an abscess. Since the early 1990s, cases in the United States have occurred almost exclusively in injection drug users. The typical patient is a 30- to 50-year-old resident of the western United States with a long history of black-tar heroin injection.

Infant botulism results from absorption of toxin produced in situ by toxigenic clostridia colonizing the intestine of children ≤1 year of age. Colonization is believed to occur because the normal bowel flora is not yet fully established; this theory is supported by studies in animals. Infant botulism is the most common form of the disease in the United States, with ~80–100 cases reported annually. Geographic "hot spots" are located in areas around Pennsylvania and California.

Adult intestinal toxemia botulism results from absorption of toxin produced in situ after rarely occurring intestinal colonization with toxigenic clostridia. Typically, patients have some anatomic or functional bowel abnormality or have recently used antibiotics that may protect normally fastidious *Clostridium* species from competing components of the bowel flora. Despite antitoxin treatment, protracted symptoms or relapse due to ongoing intraluminal production of toxin may be observed.

Iatrogenic botulism results from injection of toxin. Paralysis of variable severity has followed injection of licensed botulinum toxin products for treatment of conditions involving hypertonicity of large muscle groups. Injection of approved doses of licensed products for cosmetic purposes has not been associated with botulism. Botulism requiring ventilator support has also resulted from illegal injection of research-grade toxin.

Botulism as a potential weapon of bioterrorism

Botulinum toxin has been "weaponized" by governments and terrorist organizations. An attack might employ aerosolization of toxin or contamination of foods or beverages ranging in scope from small-scale tampering to contamination of a widely distributed food item. Initially, it might be difficult to differentiate a naturally occurring outbreak from an intentional attack. An unnatural event may be suggested by unusual relationships between patients and atypical exposure vehicles and toxin types. Epidemiologic features consistent with aerosol dissemination may include the victims' being in a common location (e.g., a building or public area) or being exposed to a common ventilation system, along with lack of a common food exposure. Unusual epidemiologic features of an outbreak of food-borne botulism might include implication of an unlikely commercial food product. Nevertheless, an unintentional food-borne botulism outbreak can likewise have unusual features, and an intentional event may have conventional features.

■ CLINICAL MANIFESTATIONS

The distinctive clinical syndrome of botulism consists of symmetric cranial nerve palsies followed by symmetric descending flaccid paralysis that may progress to respiratory arrest and death. In *food-borne botulism*, the incubation period from ingestion of food containing botulinum toxin to onset of symptoms is usually 18–36 h but, depending on the toxin dose, can range from a few hours to several days. The extent of paralysis (from a few cranial nerves only to quadriplegia) also depends on the toxin dose. The illness ranges from a mild condition for which no medical advice is sought to severe disease that can result in death within 24 h. In *wound botulism* in injection drug users, the incubation period is difficult to establish because most patients inject drug several times daily. The clinical syndrome is indistinguishable from that of food-borne botulism except that gastrointestinal symptoms are typically absent. Often the abscess is a minor lesion, a furuncle, or cellulitic in appearance. The clinical presentation of *infant botulism* resembles that of adult forms of botulism, including inability to suck and swallow, weakened voice, ptosis, and floppy neck, sometimes with progression to generalized flaccidity and respiratory compromise.

Cranial nerve involvement, which almost always marks the onset of symptoms of botulism, usually produces diplopia, dysarthria, dysphonia, and/or dysphagia. Cranial nerve palsies are the presenting manifestations that typically cause patients to seek medical care; their absence or their onset after the appearance of other true neurologic symptoms makes botulism highly unlikely. Weakness progresses, often rapidly, from the head to involve the neck, arms, thorax, and legs; occasionally, weakness is asymmetric.

Cranial nerve palsies are characteristically followed by flaccid, descending, completely symmetric paralysis of voluntary muscles. Paresthesias have been reported and may represent secondary nerve compression from immobility due to paralysis. Paralysis of the diaphragm and accessory breathing muscles may result in respiratory compromise or arrest and death. Pharyngeal collapse secondary to cranial nerve paralysis may compromise the airway and require intubation in the absence of respiratory muscle compromise. Autonomic symptoms may include anhidrosis, with pronounced mucosal erythema and pain mimicking pharyngitis, and postural hypotension. In food-borne botulism, nausea, vomiting, and abdominal pain may precede or follow the onset of paralysis. Constipation due to paralytic ileus is nearly universal, and urinary retention is also common. Extraocular muscle paralysis manifests as blurred vision or diplopia and an inability to accommodate near vision. Ptosis and facial paralysis are frequent; the pupillary reflexes may be depressed, and fixed or dilated pupils are noted in half of patients. Dizziness, dry mouth, and very dry, occasionally sore throat are common. Vital signs are usually normal, but in some cases hypotension occurs. Patients are usually afebrile. The gag reflex may be suppressed, and deep tendon reflexes may be normal or may progressively disappear.

Patients usually exhibit no sensory or cognitive deficits. They are generally alert and oriented, but they may be drowsy, agitated, and anxious. Even when intubated, patients can respond to questions by moving their fingers or toes unless paralysis has affected the digits.

Unfortunately, in some instances the severe ptosis, expressionless facies, and weak phonation of patients with botulism have been interpreted as signs of mental status changes from alcohol intoxication, drug overdose, encephalitis, or meningitis; in such cases, the consequences can be delayed diagnosis, prolonged paralysis, and complications. Because of skeletal muscle paralysis, patients experiencing respiratory distress may appear placid and detached even as they near respiratory arrest. Death in untreated botulism is usually due to airway obstruction from pharyngeal muscle paralysis and inadequate tidal volume resulting from paralysis of diaphragmatic and accessory respiratory muscles. Death can also result from nosocomial infections and other sequelae of long-term paralysis, hospitalization, and mechanical ventilatory support.

Toxin binding is irreversible, but nerve terminals do regenerate. In the United States, 95% of patients recover fully, but this process may take many months and often requires extended outpatient rehabilitation therapy.

■ DIAGNOSIS

Differential diagnosis

In the setting of an outbreak with multiple cases, the diagnosis readily suggests itself; that is, a cluster of two or more cases with compatible symptoms is essentially pathognomonic since other illnesses that resemble botulism do not cause outbreaks. In lone (sporadic) cases, however, the diagnosis is often missed. The differential diagnosis includes Guillain-Barré syndrome (GBS), myasthenia gravis, stroke syndromes, Eaton-Lambert syndrome, and tick paralysis. Less likely are poisoning by tetrodotoxin, shellfish, or a host of rarer agents and antimicrobial drug–associated paralysis. A thorough history and meticulous physical examination can effectively eliminate most alternative diagnoses. Brain imaging may help rule out rare nonlateralizing stroke syndromes.

GBS, a rare autoimmune demyelinating polyneuropathy that often follows an acute infection, presents most often as an ascending paralysis and never causes outbreaks. Occasional GBS cases present as the Miller Fisher variant, whose characteristic triad of ophthalmoplegia, ataxia, and areflexia is easily mistaken for the early descending paralysis of botulism. Protein levels in cerebrospinal fluid (CSF) are elevated in all forms of GBS; because this increase may be delayed until several days after symptom onset, an early lumbar puncture with a negative result may need to be repeated. In contrast, CSF findings are generally normal in botulism, although marginally elevated CSF protein concentrations have been reported in some patients with wound botulism. In experienced hands, electromyography may demonstrate findings consistent with GBS but not with botulism.

The edrophonium (Tensilon) test is sometimes of value in distinguishing botulism (usually a negative result; sometimes borderline positive) from myasthenia gravis (a positive result). A strongly positive edrophonium test, in either the presence or the absence of anti–acetylcholine receptor autoantibodies, confirms the diagnosis of myasthenia gravis.

In most cerebrovascular accidents, physical examination reveals asymmetry of paralysis and upper motor neuron signs. Brain imaging can reveal the rare basilar stroke that produces symmetric bulbar palsies. Eaton-Lambert syndrome usually manifests as proximal limb weakness in a patient already debilitated by cancer. Tick paralysis is a rare flaccid condition closely resembling botulism and caused by neurotoxins of certain ticks.

History and laboratory confirmation

In suspected food-borne botulism, a 3- to 5-day food history should be obtained, with specific questions about home-canned, exotic, and unusual foods. A history of recent consumption of home-canned food substantially enhances the probability of food-borne botulism. The names of contacts who may have shared foods should be obtained early in case the patient's illness progresses to respiratory failure. In wound botulism, material from abscesses should be collected in anaerobic culture tubes for testing at public health laboratories, and serum samples should be collected. Standard blood work and radiologic studies are not useful in diagnosing botulism.

Botulism in a symptomatic patient can be confirmed in the laboratory by demonstration of toxin in clinical specimens (serum, stool, sterile water or saline enema, gastric aspirates, wound material) or in samples of ingested foods. Isolation of toxigenic clostridia from stool also constitutes evidence of botulism; the organism is rarely isolated from the stools of asymptomatic persons. Wound cultures yielding the organism are highly suggestive in symptomatic cases. In the United States, testing is conducted only in public health laboratories staffed by experienced personnel. The universally accepted method for confirmation of botulism is the mouse bioassay. Neutralization of the paralytic effects in mice by a specific antitoxin provides evidence of that toxin serotype in the clinical sample. Mouse bioassay results may not be available for up to 48 h; accordingly, all decisions about clinical management, including the administration of botulinum antitoxin, must be based on the clinical presentation, with bioassay results serving as confirmation. The sensitivity of the bioassay varies inversely with the time elapsed between symptom onset and sample collection. A test may be negative even when a patient has botulism; however, if the clinical presentation is questionable and test results are negative, additional tests may be necessary to rule out other conditions. New tests for botulism are being developed but remain experimental. At this time, no alternative to the mouse bioassay exists for laboratory confirmation of botulism. In affected muscles, findings consistent with botulism include reduced amplitude of motor potentials and potentiation with rapid repetitive stimulation.

The earliest available serum sample (e.g., that obtained at admission) should be preserved for testing. Vomit or nasogastric tube secretions should be collected immediately. A stool sample should be collected by means of a sterile water enema if the patient is constipated or otherwise unable to produce a sample. All samples, including suspect foods, should be kept refrigerated—not frozen—pending shipment directions from public health officials. In general, ingested toxin is not demonstrable in serum later than 1 week after exposure, although detection 25 days after ingestion has been documented. Toxin and toxigenic clostridia can be detected in stool later in the course of illness, and the toxin is stable indefinitely in many food matrices. Diagnosis of adult intestinal toxemia botulism requires the demonstration of protracted excretion of organisms and toxin in the stool.

TREATMENT Botulism

The cornerstones of treatment for botulism are meticulous intensive care and immediate administration of botulinum antitoxin. Persons of all ages (including infants) in whom botulism is suspected should be hospitalized immediately in an intensive care setting, with frequent monitoring of vital capacity and mechanical ventilation if required. Paralysis may last for weeks or months, and meticulous intensive care is required throughout this period of debilitation. The decision to administer botulinum antitoxin—the only specific treatment—must be based on a clinical diagnosis and cannot be postponed while laboratory confirmation is awaited. Botulinum antitoxin neutralizes only toxin molecules that have not yet bound to nerve endings; it cannot

reverse existing paralysis. Thus antitoxin should be given early in the course of illness, ideally <24 h after symptom onset. Infant botulism is treated with a licensed human-origin antitoxin; although the survival rate in infant botulism is nearly 100% with or without antitoxin therapy, this treatment halves the median hospitalization period (from 6 to 3 weeks). Other forms of botulism are treated with equine-source antitoxin. Treatment with the licensed, non-despeciated, equine-origin antitoxins long used in the United States is associated with anaphylaxis, other hypersensitivity reactions, and serum sickness. A new heptavalent despeciated equine antitoxin has replaced the previously used non-despeciated equine antitoxin in this country.

In wound botulism, suspect wounds and abscesses should be cleaned, debrided, and drained promptly. *C. botulinum* is susceptible to penicillins and various other antimicrobial agents. The effectiveness of antimicrobial therapy for wound botulism has not been established, and such treatment should be guided by clinical judgment.

Although no case of person-to-person transmission of botulism has been reported and although levels of toxin in bodily fluids (including serum and stool) are insufficient to cause serious illness, absorption of botulinum toxin through mucosal surfaces, the eye, or nonintact skin sometimes causes local paralysis. Standard precautions should be exercised when evaluating and treating patients. As a precaution, persons exposed to bodily fluids or stool of botulism patients should be advised of the early signs of botulism and instructed to report for evaluation if these signs are noted. Standard hospital decontamination procedures should be used to clean medical equipment and supplies that have come into contact with a botulism patient.

■ NOTIFICATION, EXPERT CONSULTATION, AND ANTITOXIN PROVISION

Every botulism case is a public health emergency. The clinician must report a suspected case on an emergency basis to the state health department, which will initiate an epidemiologic investigation and put the physician in contact with the Centers for Disease Control and Prevention (CDC) 24-h botulism consultancy service (Emergency Operations Center: 770-488-7100) or a locally available service. The CDC consultant will (1) review the case by telephone; (2) help arrange laboratory confirmation at appropriate testing facilities; and (3) arrange emergency shipment of antitoxin (adult cases only), which in the United States is available exclusively from the CDC. In addition, the Infant Botulism Treatment and Prevention Program of the California Department of Public Health (510-231-7600) provides 24-h consultation and distributes antitoxin (licensed BabyBIG®) for the treatment of infant botulism cases. Except in cases involving infants who reside in California, laboratory testing requests must still be authorized by the state health department where the infant is located or by the CDC.

■ PREVENTION

No prophylaxis or licensed vaccine for botulism is available. An experimental vaccine for administration to laboratory workers is available from the CDC. Persons exposed to botulinum toxin should be evaluated by a physician and carefully observed for the development of symptoms. If symptoms do appear, the patient should be treated immediately with botulinum antitoxin as described above. If antitoxin supplies are limited, treatment will most likely benefit patients with symptoms that are progressive but have not yet progressed to respiratory failure.

FURTHER READINGS

ARNON SS et al: Botulism toxin as a biological weapon: Medical and public health management. JAMA 285:1059, 2001

——— et al: Human botulism immune globulin for the treatment of infant botulism. N Engl J Med 354:462, 2006

CENTERS FOR DISEASE CONTROL AND PREVENTION: Botulism in the United States, 1899–1996: Handbook for epidemiologists, clinicians and laboratory workers. Atlanta, CDC, 1998

CHERINGTON M: Electrophysiologic methods as an aid in diagnosis of botulism: A review. Muscle Nerve 5:S28, 1982

CHERTOW DS et al: Botulism in four adults following cosmetic injections with an unlicensed, highly concentrated botulinum preparation. JAMA 296:2476, 2006

GOTTLIEB SL et al: Long-term outcomes of 217 botulism cases in the Republic of Georgia. Clin Infect Dis 45:174, 2007

GUPTA A et al: Adult botulism type F in the United States. Neurology 65:1694, 2005

PASSARO DJ et al: Wound botulism associated with black tar heroin among injecting drug users. JAMA 279:859, 1998

SIMPSON LL: Identification of the major steps in botulinum toxin action. Annu Rev Pharmacol Toxicol 44:167, 2004

SOBEL J: Diagnosis and treatment of botulism: A century later, clinical suspicion remains the cornerstone. Clin Infect Dis 48:1674, 2009

YU PA et al: Botulism, in *Bacterial Infections of Humans*, PS Brachman, E Abrutyn (eds). New York, Springer Science, 2009

CHAPTER 142

Gas Gangrene and Other Clostridial Infections

Amy E. Bryant
Dennis L. Stevens

The genus *Clostridium* encompasses more than 60 species that may be commensals of the gut microflora or may cause a variety of infections in humans and animals through the production of a plethora of proteinaceous exotoxins. *C. tetani* and *C. botulinum*, for example, cause specific clinical disease by elaborating single but highly potent toxins. In contrast, *C. perfringens* and *C. septicum* cause aggressive necrotizing infections that are attributable to multiple toxins, including bacterial proteases, phospholipases, and cytotoxins.

ETIOLOGIC AGENT

Vegetative cells of *Clostridium* species are pleomorphic, rod-shaped, and arranged singly or in short chains (Fig. 142-1); the cells have rounded or sometimes pointed ends. Although clostridia stain gram-positive in the early stages of growth, they may appear to be gram-negative or gram-variable later in the growth cycle or in infected tissue specimens. Most strains are motile by means of peritrichous flagella; *C. septicum* swarms on solid media. Nonmotile species include *C. perfringens*, *C. ramosum*, and *C. innocuum*. Most species are obligately anaerobic, although clostridial tolerance to oxygen varies widely; some species (e.g., *C. septicum*, *C. tertium*) will grow but will not sporulate in air.

Clostridia produce more protein toxins than any other bacterial genus, and more than 25 clostridial toxins lethal to mice have been identified. These proteins include neurotoxins, enterotoxins, cytotoxins, collagenases, permeases, necrotizing toxins, lipases, lecithinases, hemolysins, proteinases, hyaluronidases, DNases, ADP-ribosyltransferases, and neuraminidases. Botulinum and tetanus neurotoxins are the most potent toxins known, with lethal doses of 0.2–10 ng/kg for humans. Epsilon toxin, a 33-kDa protein produced by *C. perfringens* types B and D, causes edema and hemorrhage in the brain, heart, spinal cord, and kidneys of animals. It is among the most lethal of the clostridial toxins and is considered a potential agent of bioterrorism (Chap. 221). The genomic sequences of some pathogenic clostridia are now available and are likely to facilitate a comprehensive approach to understanding the virulence factors involved in clostridial pathogenesis.

EPIDEMIOLOGY AND TRANSMISSION

Clostridium species are widespread in nature, forming endospores that are commonly found in soil, feces, sewage, and marine sediments. The ecology of *C. perfringens* in soil is greatly influenced by the degree and duration of animal husbandry in a given location and is relevant to the incidence of gas gangrene caused by contamination of war wounds with soil. For example, the incidence of clostridial gas gangrene is higher in agricultural regions of Europe than in the Sahara Desert of Africa. Similarly, the incidences of tetanus and food-borne botulism are clearly related to the presence of clostridial spores in soil, water, and many foods. Clostridia are present in large numbers in the indigenous microbiota of the intestinal tract of humans and animals, in the female genital tract, and on the oral mucosa. It should be noted that not all commensal clostridia are toxigenic.

Clostridial infections remain a serious public health concern worldwide. In developing nations, food poisoning, necrotizing enterocolitis, and gas gangrene are common because large portions of the population are poor and have little or no immediate access to health care. These infections remain prevalent in developed countries as well. Gas gangrene commonly follows knife or gunshot wounds or vehicular accidents or develops as a complication of surgery or gastrointestinal carcinoma. Severe clostridial infections have emerged as a health threat to injection drug users and to women undergoing childbirth or abortion. Historically, clostridial gas gangrene has been the scourge of the battlefield. The global political situation portends another possible scenario involving mass casualties of war or terrorism, with extensive injuries conducive to gas gangrene. Thus there is an ongoing need to develop novel strategies to prevent or attenuate the course of clostridial infections in both civilians and military personnel. Vaccination against exotoxins important in pathogenesis would be of great benefit in developing nations and could also be used safely in at-risk populations such as the elderly, patients with diabetes who may require lower-limb surgery due to trauma or poor circulation, and those undergoing intestinal surgery. Moreover, a hyperimmune globulin would be a valuable tool for prophylaxis in victims of acute traumatic injury or for attenuation of the spread of infection in patients with established gas gangrene.

CLINICAL SYNDROMES

Life-threatening clostridial infections range from intoxications (e.g., food poisoning, tetanus) to necrotizing enteritis/colitis, bacteremia, myonecrosis, and toxic shock syndrome (TSS). Tetanus and botulism are discussed in Chaps. 140 and 141, respectively. Colitis due to *C. difficile* is discussed in Chap. 129.

■ CLOSTRIDIAL WOUND CONTAMINATION

Of open traumatic wounds, 30–80% are reportedly contaminated with clostridial species. In the absence of devitalized tissue, the presence of clostridia does not necessarily lead to infection. In traumatic

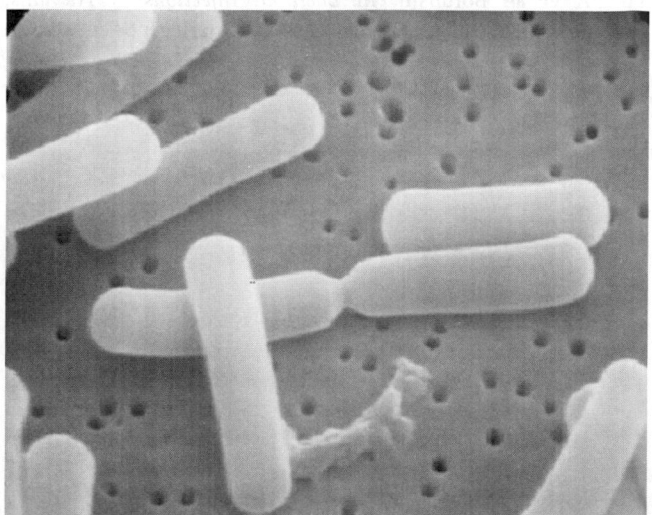

Figure 142-1 Scanning electron micrograph of *C. perfringens.*

injuries, clostridia are isolated with equal frequency from both suppurative and well-healing wounds. Thus, diagnosis and treatment of clostridial infection should be based on clinical signs and symptoms and not solely on bacteriologic findings.

■ POLYMICROBIAL INFECTIONS INVOLVING CLOSTRIDIA

Clostridial species may be found in polymicrobial infections also involving microbial components of the indigenous flora. In these infections, clostridia often appear in association with non-spore-forming anaerobes and facultative or aerobic organisms. Head and neck infections, conjunctivitis, brain abscess, sinusitis, otitis, aspiration pneumonia, lung abscess, pleural empyema, cholecystitis, septic arthritis, and bone infections all may involve clostridia. These conditions are often associated with severe local inflammation but may lack the characteristic systemic signs of toxicity and rapid progression seen in other clostridial infections. In addition, clostridia are isolated from ~66% of intraabdominal infections in which the mucosal integrity of the bowel or respiratory system has been compromised. In this setting, *C. ramosum*, *C. perfringens*, and *C. bifermentans* are the most commonly isolated species. Their presence does not invariably lead to a poor outcome. Clostridia have been isolated from suppurative infections of the female genital tract (e.g., ovarian or pelvic abscess) and from diseased gallbladders. Although the most frequently isolated species is *C. perfringens*, gangrene is not typically observed; however, gas formation in the biliary system can lead to emphysematous cholecystitis, especially in diabetic patients. *C. perfringens* in association with mixed aerobic and anaerobic microbes can cause aggressive life-threatening type I necrotizing fasciitis or Fournier's gangrene.

The treatment of mixed aerobic/anaerobic infection of the abdomen, perineum, or gynecologic organs should be based on Gram's staining, culture, and antibiotic sensitivity information.

Reasonable empirical treatment consists of ampicillin or ampicillin/sulbactam combined with either clindamycin or metronidazole (Table 142-1). Broader gram-negative coverage may be necessary if the patient has recently been hospitalized or treated with antibiotics. Such coverage can be obtained by substituting ticarcillin/clavulanic acid, piperacillin/sulbactam, or a penem antibiotic for ampicillin or by adding a fluoroquinolone or an aminoglycoside to the regimen.

■ ENTERIC CLOSTRIDIAL INFECTIONS

C. perfringens type A is one of the most common bacterial causes of food-borne illness in the United States and Canada. The foods typically implicated include improperly cooked meat and meat products (e.g., gravy) in which residual spores germinate and proliferate during slow cooling or insufficient reheating. Illness results from the ingestion of food containing at least ~10^8 viable vegetative cells, which sporulate in the alkaline environment of the small intestine, producing *C. perfringens* enterotoxin in the process. The diarrhea that develops within 7–30 h of ingestion of contaminated food is generally mild and self-limiting; however, in the very young, the elderly, and the immunocompromised, symptoms are more severe and occasionally fatal. Enterotoxin-producing *C. perfringens* has been implicated as an etiologic agent of persistent diarrhea in elderly patients in nursing homes and tertiary-care institutions and has been considered to play a role in antibiotic-associated diarrhea without pseudomembranous colitis.

C. perfringens strains associated with food poisoning possess the gene (*cpe*) coding for enterotoxin, which acts by forming pores in host cell membranes. *C. perfringens* strains isolated from non-food-borne diseases, such as antibiotic-associated and sporadic diarrhea, carry *cpe* on a plasmid that may be transmitted to other strains. Several methods have been described for the detection of

TABLE 142-1 Treatment of Clostridial Infections

Condition	Antibiotic Treatment	Penicillin Allergy	Adjunctive Treatment/Note
Wound contamination	None	—	—
Polymicrobial anaerobic infections involving clostridia (e.g., abdominal wall, gynecologic)	Ampicillin (2 g IV q4h) *plus* Clindamycin (600–900 mg IV q6–8h) *plus* Ciprofloxacin (400 mg IV q6–8 h)	Vancomycin (1 g IV q12h) *plus* Metronidazole (500 mg IV q6h) *plus* Ciprofloxacin (400 mg IV q6–8h)	Empirical therapy should be initiated. Therapy should be based on Gram's stain and culture results and on sensitivity data when available. Add gram-negative coverage if indicated (see text).
Clostridial sepsis	Penicillin, 3–4 mU IV q4–6h *plus* Clindamycin (600–900 mg IV q6–8h)	Clindamycin alone *or* Metronidazole *or* Vancomycin as for polymicrobial anaerobic infections (see above)	Transient bacteremia without signs of systemic toxicity may be clinically insignificant.
Gas gangrene	Penicillin G (4 mU IV q4–6 h) *plus* Clindamycin (600–900 mg IV q6–8h)	Cefoxitin (2 g IV q6h) *plus* Clindamycin (600–900 mg IV q6–8h)	Emergent surgical exploration and thorough debridement are extremely important. Hyperbaric oxygen therapy may be considered after surgery and antibiotics have been initiated.

C. perfringens enterotoxin in feces, including cell culture assay (Vero cells), enzyme-linked immunosorbent assay, reversed-phase latex agglutination, and polymerase chain reaction (PCR) amplification of cpe. Each method has its advantages and limitations.

Enteritis necroticans (gas gangrene of the bowel) is a fulminating clinical illness characterized by extensive necrosis of the intestinal mucosa and wall. Cases can occur sporadically in adults or as epidemics in people of all ages. Enteritis necroticans is caused by α toxin– and β toxin–producing strains of C. perfringens type C; β toxin is located on a plasmid and is mainly responsible for pathogenesis. This life-threatening infection causes ischemic necrosis of the jejunum. In Papua New Guinea during the 1960s, enteritis necroticans (known in that locale as pigbel) was found to be the most common cause of death in children; it has been associated with pig feasts and occurs both sporadically and in outbreaks. Intramuscular immunization against the β toxin resulted in a decreased incidence of the disease in Papua New Guinea. Enteritis necroticans has also been recognized in the United States, the United Kingdom, Germany ("darmbrand"), and other developed nations; especially affected are adults who are malnourished or who have diabetes, alcoholic liver disease, or neutropenia.

Necrotizing enterocolitis, a disease resembling enteritis necroticans but associated with C. perfringens type A, has been found in North America in previously healthy adults. It is also a serious gastrointestinal disease of low-birth-weight (premature) infants hospitalized in neonatal intensive care units. The etiology and pathogenesis of this disease have remained enigmatic for more than four decades. Pathologic similarities between necrotizing enterocolitis and enteritis necroticans include the pattern of small-bowel necrosis involving the submucosa, mucosa, and muscularis; the presence of gas dissecting the tissue planes; and the degree of inflammation. Enteritis necroticans most commonly involves the jejunum, whereas necrotizing enterocolitis affects the ileum and frequently the ileocecal valve. Both diseases may manifest as intestinal gas cysts, although this feature is more common in necrotizing enterocolitis. The sources of the gas, which contains hydrogen, methane, and carbon dioxide, are probably the fermentative activities of intestinal bacteria, including clostridia. Epidemiologic data support an important role for C. perfringens or other gas-producing microorganisms (e.g., C. neonatale, certain other clostridia, or Klebsiella species) in the pathogenesis of necrotizing enterocolitis.

Patients with suspected clostridial enteric infection should undergo nasogastric suction and receive IV fluids. Pyrantel is given by mouth, and the bowel is rested by fasting. Benzylpenicillin (1 mU) is given intravenously every 4 h, and the patient is observed for complications requiring surgery. Patients with mild cases recover without surgical intervention. If surgical indications are present (gas in the peritoneal cavity, absent bowel sounds, rebound tenderness, abdominal rigidity), however, the mortality rate ranges from 35% to 100%; fatal outcome is due in part to perforation of the intestine. As pigbel continues to be a common disease in Papua New Guinea, consideration should be given to the use of a C. perfringens type C toxoid vaccine in local areas. Two doses given 3–4 months apart are preventive.

■ CLOSTRIDIAL BACTEREMIA

Clostridium species are important causes of bloodstream infections. Molecular epidemiologic studies of anaerobic bacteremia have identified C. perfringens and C. tertium as the two most frequently isolated species; these organisms cause up to 79% and 5%, respectively, of clostridial bacteremias. Occasionally, C. perfringens bacteremia occurs in the absence of an identifiable infection at another site. When associated with myonecrosis, bacteremia has a grave prognosis.

C. septicum is also commonly associated with bacteremia. This species is isolated only rarely from the feces of healthy individuals but may be found in the normal appendix. More than 50% of patients whose blood cultures are positive for this organism have some gastrointestinal anomaly (e.g., diverticular disease) or underlying malignancy (e.g., carcinoma of the colon). In addition, a clinically important association of C. septicum bacteremia with neutropenia of any origin—and, more specifically, with neutropenic enterocolitis involving the terminal ileum or cecum—has been observed. Patients with diabetes mellitus, severe atherosclerotic cardiovascular disease, or anaerobic myonecrosis (gas gangrene) may also develop C. septicum bacteremia. C. septicum has been recovered from the bloodstream of cirrhotic patients, as have C. perfringens, C. bifermentans, and other clostridia. Infections of the bloodstream by C. sordellii and C. perfringens have been associated with TSS.

Bloodstream infection by C. tertium, either alone or in combination with C. septicum or C. perfringens, can be found in patients with serious underlying disease such as malignancy or acute pancreatitis, with or without neutropenic enterocolitis; the frequency has not been systematically studied. C. tertium may present special problems in terms of both identification and treatment. This organism may stain gram-negative; is aerotolerant; and is resistant to metronidazole, clindamycin, and cephalosporins.

Other clostridia from the C. clostridioforme group (including C. clostridioforme, C. hathewayi, and C. bolteae) can cause bacteremia.

The clinical importance of recognizing clostridial bacteremia—especially that due to C. septicum—and starting appropriate treatment immediately cannot be overemphasized. Patients with this condition usually are gravely ill, and infection may metastasize to distant anatomic sites, resulting in spontaneous myonecrosis (see next section). Alternative methods to identify these strains, such as PCR or other rapid diagnostic tests, are not currently available. Anaerobic blood cultures and Gram's stain interpretation remain the best diagnostic tests at this point.

■ CLOSTRIDIAL SKIN AND SOFT-TISSUE INFECTIONS

Histotoxic clostridial species such as C. perfringens, C. histolyticum, C. septicum, C. novyi, and C. sordellii cause aggressive necrotizing infections of the skin and soft tissues. These infections are attributable in part to the elaboration of bacterial proteases, phospholipases, and cytotoxins. Necrotizing clostridial soft-tissue infections are rapidly progressive and are characterized by marked tissue destruction, gas in the tissues, and shock; they frequently end in death. Severe pain, crepitus, brawny induration with rapid progression to skin sloughing, violaceous bullae, and marked tachycardia are characteristics found in the majority of patients.

Clostridial myonecrosis (gas gangrene)

Traumatic gas gangrene C. perfringens myonecrosis (gas gangrene) is one of the most fulminant gram-positive bacterial infections of humans. Even with appropriate antibiotic therapy and management in an intensive care unit, tissue destruction can progress rapidly. Gas gangrene is accompanied by bacteremia, hypotension, and multiorgan failure and is invariably fatal if untreated. Gas gangrene is a true emergency and requires immediate surgical debridement.

The development of gas gangrene requires an anaerobic environment and contamination of a wound with spores or vegetative organisms. Devitalized tissue, foreign bodies, and ischemia reduce locally available oxygen levels and favor outgrowth of vegetative cells and spores. Thus conditions predisposing to traumatic gas

gangrene include crush-type injury, laceration of large or medium-sized arteries, and open fractures of long bones that are contaminated with soil or bits of clothing containing the bacterial spores. Gas gangrene of the abdominal wall and flanks follows penetrating injuries such as knife or gunshot wounds that are sufficient to compromise intestinal integrity, with resultant leakage of the bowel contents into the soft tissues. Proximity to fecal sources of bacteria is a risk factor for cases following hip surgery, adrenaline injections into the buttocks, or amputation of the leg for ischemic vascular disease. In the last decade, cutaneous gas gangrene caused by *C. perfringens*, *C. novyi*, and *C. sordellii* has been described in the United States and northern Europe among persons injecting black-tar heroin subcutaneously.

The incubation period for traumatic gas gangrene can be as short as 6 h and is usually <4 days. The infection is characterized by the sudden onset of excruciating pain at the affected site and the rapid development of a foul-smelling wound containing a thin serosanguineous discharge and gas bubbles. Brawny edema and induration develop and give way to cutaneous blisters containing bluish to maroon-colored fluid. Such tissue later may become liquefied and slough. The margin between healthy and necrotic tissue often advances several inches per hour despite appropriate antibiotic therapy, and radical amputation remains the single best life-saving intervention. Shock and organ failure frequently accompany gas gangrene; when patients become bacteremic, the mortality rate exceeds 50%.

Diagnosis of traumatic gas gangrene is not difficult because the infection always begins at the site of significant trauma, is associated with gas in the tissue, and is rapidly progressive. Gram's staining of drainage or tissue biopsy is usually definitive, demonstrating large gram-positive (or gram-variable) rods, an absence of inflammatory cells, and widespread soft-tissue necrosis.

Spontaneous (nontraumatic) gas gangrene Spontaneous gas gangrene generally occurs via hematogenous seeding of normal muscle with histotoxic clostridia—principally *C. perfringens*, *C. septicum*, and *C. novyi* and occasionally *C. tertium*—from a gastrointestinal tract portal of entry (as in colonic malignancy, inflammatory bowel disease, diverticulitis, necrotizing enterocolitis, cecitis, or distal ileitis or after gastrointestinal surgery). These gastrointestinal pathologies permit bacterial access to the bloodstream; consequently, aerotolerant *C. septicum* can proliferate in normal tissues. Patients surviving bacteremia or spontaneous gangrene due to *C. septicum* should undergo aggressive diagnostic studies to rule out gastrointestinal pathology.

Additional predisposing host factors include leukemia, lymphoproliferative disorders, cancer chemotherapy, radiation therapy, and AIDS. Cyclic, congenital, or acquired neutropenia is also strongly associated with an increased incidence of spontaneous gas gangrene due to *C. septicum*; in such cases, necrotizing enterocolitis, cecitis, or distal ileitis is common, particularly among children.

The first symptom of spontaneous gas gangrene may be confusion followed by the abrupt onset of excruciating pain in the absence of trauma. These findings, along with fever, should heighten suspicion of spontaneous gas gangrene. However, because of the lack of an obvious portal of entry, the correct diagnosis is frequently delayed or missed. The infection is characterized by rapid progression of tissue destruction with demonstrable gas in the tissue (Fig. 142-2). Swelling increases and bullae filled with clear, cloudy, hemorrhagic, or purplish fluid appear. The surrounding skin has a purple hue, which may reflect vascular compromise resulting from the diffusion of bacterial toxins into surrounding tissues. Invasion of healthy tissue rapidly ensues, with quick progression to shock and multiple-organ failure. Mortality rates in this setting range from 67 to 100% among

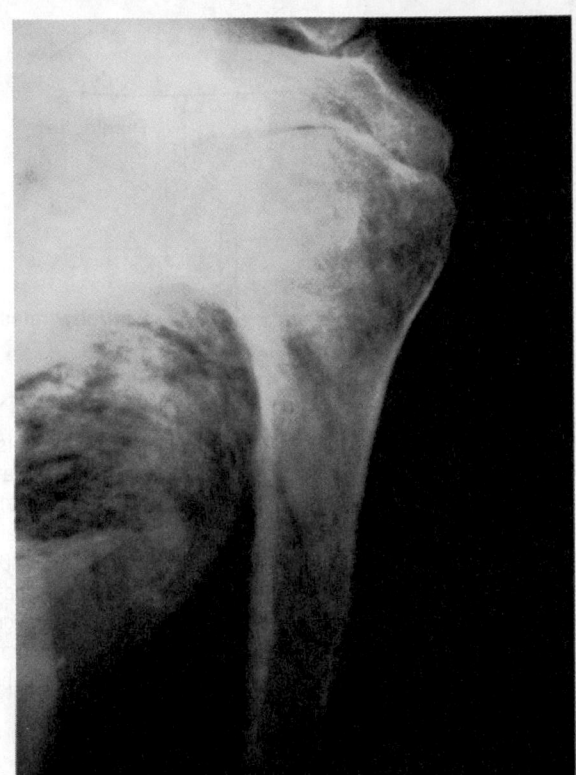

Figure 142-2 **Radiograph of patient with spontaneous gas gangrene** due to *C. septicum*, demonstrating gas in the affected arm and shoulder.

adults; among children, the mortality rate is 59%, with the majority of deaths occurring within 24 h of onset.

Pathogenesis of gas gangrene In traumatic gas gangrene, organisms are introduced into devitalized tissue. It is important to recognize that for *C. perfringens* and *C. novyi*, trauma must be sufficient to interrupt the blood supply and thereby to establish an optimal anaerobic environment for growth of these species. These conditions are not strictly required for the more aerotolerant species such as *C. septicum* and *C. tertium*, which can seed normal tissues from gastrointestinal lesions. Once introduced into an appropriate niche, the organisms proliferate locally and elaborate exotoxins.

The major *C. perfringens* extracellular toxins implicated in gas gangrene are α toxin and θ toxin. A lethal hemolysin that has both phospholipase C and sphingomyelinase activities, α toxin has been implicated as the major virulence factor of *C. perfringens*: immunization of mice with the C-terminal domain of α toxin provides protection against lethal challenge with *C. perfringens*, and isogenic α toxin–deficient mutant strains of *C. perfringens* are not lethal in a murine model of gas gangrene. It has been shown in experimental models that the severe pain, rapid progression, marked tissue destruction, and absence of neutrophils in *C. perfringens* gas gangrene are attributable in large part to α toxin–induced occlusion of blood vessels by heterotypic aggregates of platelets and neutrophils. The formation of these aggregates, which occurs within minutes, is largely mediated by α toxin's ability to activate the platelet adhesion molecule gpIIbIIIa (Fig. 142-3); the implication is that platelet glycoprotein inhibitors (e.g., eptifibatide, abciximab) may be therapeutic for maintaining tissue blood flow.

C. perfringens θ toxin (*perfringolysin*) is a member of the thiol-activated cytolysin family known as cholesterol-dependent cytolysins, which includes streptolysin O from group A *Streptococcus*,

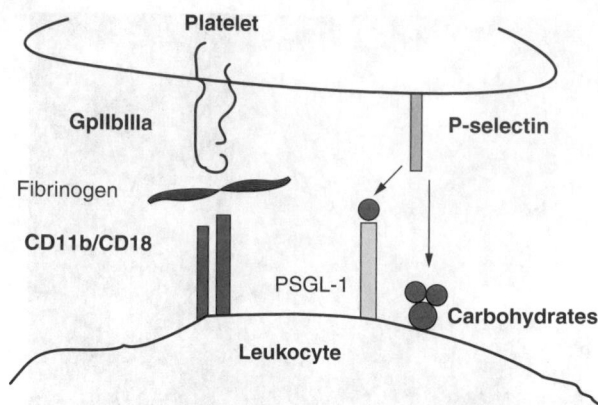

Figure 142-3 Schematic illustration of the molecular mechanisms of C. perfringens α toxin–induced platelet/neutrophil aggregates. Homotypic aggregates of platelets (not shown) and heterotypic aggregates of platelets and leukocytes are due to α toxin–induced activation of the platelet fibrinogen receptor gpIIbIIIa and upregulation of leukocyte CD11b/CD18. Binding of fibrinogen (*red*) bridges the connection between these adhesion molecules on adjacent cells. An auxiliary role for α toxin–induced upregulation of platelet P-selectin and its binding to leukocyte P-selectin glycoprotein ligand 1 (PSGL-1) or other leukocyte surface carbohydrates has also been demonstrated.

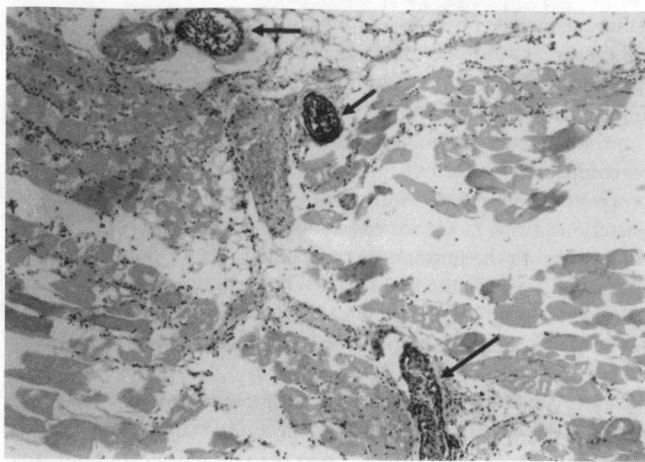

Figure 142-4 Histopathology of experimental gas gangrene due to *C. perfringens*, demonstrating widespread muscle necrosis, a paucity of leukocytes in infected tissues, and accumulation of leukocytes in adjacent vessels (*arrows*). These features are due to the effects of α and θ toxins on muscle cells, platelets, leukocytes, and endothelial cells.

pneumolysin from *Streptococcus pneumoniae*, and several other toxins. Cholesterol-dependent cytolysins bind as oligomers to cholesterol in host cell membranes. At high concentrations, these toxins form ring-like pores resulting in cell lysis. At sublytic concentrations, θ toxin hyperactivates phagocytes and vascular endothelial cells.

Cardiovascular collapse and end-organ failure occur late in the course of *C. perfringens* gas gangrene and are largely attributable to both direct and indirect effects of α and θ toxins. In experimental models, θ toxin causes markedly reduced systemic vascular resistance but increased cardiac output (e.g., "warm shock"), probably via induction of endogenous mediators (e.g., prostacyclin, platelet-activating factor) that cause vasodilation. This effect is similar to that observed in gram-negative sepsis. In sharp contrast, α toxin directly suppresses myocardial contractility; the consequence is profound hypotension due to a sudden reduction in cardiac output. The roles of other endogenous mediators, such as cytokines (e.g., tumor necrosis factor, interleukin 1, interleukin 6) and vasodilators (e.g., bradykinin) have not been fully elucidated.

C. septicum produces four main toxins—α toxin (lethal, hemolytic, necrotizing activity), β toxin (DNase), γ toxin (hyaluronidase), and Δ toxin (septicolysin, an oxygen-labile hemolysin)—as well as a protease and a neuraminidase. Unlike the α toxin of *C. perfringens*, that of *C. septicum* does not possess phospholipase activity. The mechanisms remain to be fully elucidated, but it is likely that each of these toxins contributes uniquely to *C. septicum* gas gangrene.

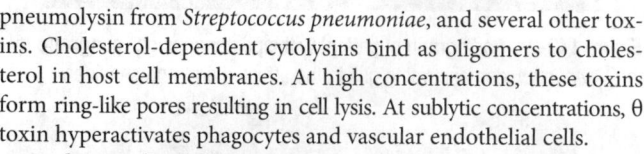

TREATMENT   Gas Gangrene

Patients with suspected gas gangrene (either traumatic or spontaneous) should undergo prompt surgical inspection of the infected site. Direct examination of a gram-stained smear of the involved tissues is of major importance. Characteristic histologic findings in clostridial gas gangrene include widespread tissue destruction, a paucity of leukocytes in infected tissues in conjunction with an accumulation of leukocytes in adjacent vessels (Fig. 142-4), and the presence of gram-positive rods (with or without spores). CT and MRI are invaluable for determining whether the infection is localized or is spreading along fascial planes, and needle aspiration or punch biopsy may provide an etiologic diagnosis in at least 20% of cases. However, these techniques should not replace surgical exploration, Gram's staining, and histopathologic examination. When spontaneous gas gangrene is suspected, blood should be cultured since bacteremia usually precedes cutaneous manifestations by several hours.

For patients with evidence of clostridial gas gangrene, thorough emergent surgical debridement is of extreme importance. All devitalized tissue should be widely resected back to healthy viable muscle and skin so as to remove conditions that allow anaerobic organisms to continue proliferating. Closure of traumatic wounds or compound fractures should be delayed for 5–6 days until it is certain that these sites are free of infection.

Antibiotic treatment of traumatic or spontaneous gas gangrene (Table 142-1) consists of the administration of penicillin and clindamycin for 10–14 days. Penicillin is recommended on the basis of in vitro sensitivity data; clindamycin is recommended because of its superior efficacy over penicillin in animal models of *C. perfringens* gas gangrene and in some clinical reports. Controlled clinical trials comparing the efficacy of these agents in humans have not been performed. In the penicillin-allergic patient, clindamycin may be used alone. The superior efficacy of clindamycin is probably due to its ability to inhibit bacterial protein toxin production, its insensitivity to the size of the bacterial load or the stage of bacterial growth, and its ability to modulate the host's immune response.

C. tertium is resistant to penicillin, cephalosporins, and clindamycin. Appropriate antibiotic therapy for *C. tertium* infection is vancomycin (1 g every 12 h IV) or metronidazole (500 mg every 8 h IV).

The value of adjunctive treatment with hyperbaric oxygen (HBO) for gas gangrene remains controversial. Basic science studies suggest that HBO can inhibit the growth of *C. perfringens* but not that of the more aerotolerant *C. septicum*. In vitro, blood and macerated muscle inhibit the bactericidal potential of HBO. Numerous studies in animals demonstrate little efficacy of HBO alone, whereas antibiotics alone—especially those that inhibit bacterial protein synthesis—confer marked benefits. Addition of HBO to the therapeutic regimen provides some additional benefit, but only if surgery and antibiotic administration precede HBO treatment.

In conclusion, gas gangrene is a rapidly progressive infection whose outcome depends on prompt recognition, emergent surgery, and timely administration of antibiotics that inhibit toxin production. Gas gangrene associated with bacteremia probably represents a later stage of illness and is associated with the worst outcomes. Emergent surgical debridement is crucial to ensure survival, and ancillary procedures (e.g., CT or MRI) or transport to HBO units should not delay this intervention. Some trauma centers associated with HBO units may have special expertise in managing these aggressive infections, but proximity and speed of transfer must be carefully weighed against the need for haste.

Prognosis of gas gangrene The prognosis for patients with gas gangrene is more favorable when the infection involves an extremity rather than the trunk or visceral organs, since debridement of the latter sites is more difficult. Gas gangrene is most likely to progress to shock and death in patients with associated bacteremia and intravascular hemolysis. Mortality rates are highest for patients in shock at the time of diagnosis. Mortality rates are relatively high among patients with spontaneous gas gangrene, especially that due to *C. septicum*. Survivors of gas gangrene may undergo multiple debridements and face long periods of hospitalization and rehabilitation.

Prevention of gas gangrene Initial aggressive debridement of devitalized tissue can reduce the risk of gas gangrene in contaminated deep wounds. Interventions to be avoided include prolonged application of tourniquets and surgical closure of traumatic wounds; patients with compound fractures are at significant risk for gas gangrene if the wound is closed surgically. Vaccination against α toxin is protective in experimental animal models of *C. perfringens* gas gangrene but has not been investigated in humans. In addition, as mentioned above, a hyperimmune globulin would represent a significant advance for prophylaxis in victims of acute traumatic injury or for attenuation of the spread of infection in patients with established gas gangrene.

Toxic shock syndrome

Clostridial infection of the endometrium, particularly that due to *C. sordellii*, can develop after gynecologic procedures, childbirth, or abortion (spontaneous or elective, surgical or medical) and, once established, proceeds rapidly to TSS and death. Systemic manifestations including edema, effusions, profound leukocytosis, and hemoconcentration are followed by the rapid onset of hypotension and multiple-organ failure. Elevation of the hematocrit to 75–80% and leukocytosis of 50,000–200,000 cells per microliter, with a left shift, are characteristic of *C. sordellii* infection. Pain may not be a prominent feature, and fever is typically absent. In one series, 18% of 45 cases of *C. sordellii* infection were associated with normal childbirth, 11% with medically induced abortion, and 0.4% with spontaneous abortion; the case-fatality rate was 100% in these groups. Of the infections in this series that were not related to gynecologic procedures or childbirth, 22% occurred in injection drug users, and 50% of these patients died. Other infections followed trauma or surgery (42%), mostly in healthy persons, and 53%

of these patients died. Overall, the mortality rate was 69% (31 of 45 cases). Of patients who succumbed, 85% died within 2–6 days of initial infection or following procedures.

Early diagnosis of *C. sordellii* infections often proves difficult for several reasons. First, the prevalence of these infections is low. Second, the initial symptoms are nonspecific and frankly misleading. Early in the course, the illness resembles any number of infectious diseases, including viral syndromes. Given these vague symptoms and an absence of fever, physicians usually do not aggressively pursue additional diagnostic tests. The absence of local evidence of infection and the lack of fever make early diagnosis of *C. sordellii* infection particularly problematic in patients who develop deep-seated infection following childbirth, therapeutic abortion, gastrointestinal surgery, or trauma. Such patients are frequently evaluated for pulmonary embolization, gastrointestinal bleeding, pyelonephritis, or cholecystitis. Unfortunately, such delays in diagnosis increase the risk of death, and, as in most necrotizing soft-tissue infections, patients are hypotensive with evidence of organ dysfunction by the time local signs and symptoms become apparent. In contrast, infection is more readily suspected in injection drug users presenting with local swelling, pain, and redness at injection sites; early recognition probably contributes to the lower mortality rates in this group.

Physicians should suspect *C. sordellii* infection in patients who present within 2–7 days after injury, surgery, drug injection, childbirth, or abortion and who complain of pain, nausea, vomiting, and diarrhea but are afebrile. There is little information regarding appropriate treatment for *C. sordellii* infections. In fact, the interval between onset of symptoms and death is often so short that there is little time to initiate empirical antimicrobial therapy. Indeed, anaerobic cultures of blood and wound aspirates are time-consuming, and many hospital laboratories do not routinely perform antimicrobial sensitivity testing on anaerobes. Antibiotic susceptibility data from older studies suggest that *C. sordellii*, like most clostridia, is susceptible to β-lactam antibiotics, clindamycin, tetracycline, and chloramphenicol but is resistant to aminoglycosides and sulfonamides. Antibiotics that suppress toxin synthesis (e.g., clindamycin) may possibly prove useful as therapeutic adjuncts since they are effective in necrotizing infections due to other toxin-producing gram-positive organisms.

Other clostridial skin and soft-tissue infections

Crepitant cellulitis (also called anaerobic cellulitis) occurs principally in diabetic patients and characteristically involves subcutaneous tissues or retroperitoneal tissues, whereas the muscle and fascia are not involved. This infection can progress to fulminant systemic disease.

Cases of *C. histolyticum* infection with cellulitis, abscess formation, or endocarditis have also been documented in injection drug users. Endophthalmitis due to *C. sordellii* or *C. perfringens* has been described. *C. ramosum* is also isolated frequently from clinical specimens, including blood and intraabdominal and soft tissues. This species may be resistant to clindamycin and multiple cephalosporins.

FURTHER READINGS

ALDAPE MJ et al: *Clostridium sordellii* infection: Epidemiology, clinical findings, and current perspectives on diagnosis and treatment. Clin Infect Dis 43:1436, 2006

BODEY GP et al: Clostridial bacteremia in cancer patients. A 12-year experience. Cancer 67:1928, 1991

BOS J et al: Fatal necrotizing colitis following a foodborne outbreak of enterotoxigenic *Clostridium perfringens* type A infection. Clin Infect Dis 40:e78, 2005

BRYANT AE et al: Clostridial gas gangrene II: Phospholipase C–induced activation of platelet gpIIb/IIIa mediates vascular occlusion and myonecrosis in *C. perfringens* gas gangrene. J Infect Dis 182:808, 2000

OBLADEN M: Necrotizing enterocolitis—150 years of fruitless search for the cause. Neonatology 96:203, 2009

SAYEED S et al: Beta toxin is essential for the intestinal virulence of *Clostridium perfringens* type C disease isolate CN3685 in a rabbit ileal loop model. Mol Microbiol 67:15, 2008

SMITH LDS, WILLIAMS BL: *The Pathogenic Anaerobic Bacteria*, 3rd ed. Springfield, IL: Charles C Thomas, 1984

STEVENS DL et al: *Clostridium*, in *American Society of Microbiology's Manual of Clinical Microbiology*, 10th ed. Washington, DC, ASM Press, 2010

———— et al: Practice guidelines for the diagnosis and management of skin and soft-tissue infections. Clin Infect Dis 41:1373, 2005

WANG C et al: Hyperbaric oxygen for treating wounds: A systematic review of the literature. Arch Surg 138:272, 2003

CHAPTER **143**

Meningococcal Infections

Andrew J. Pollard

■ DEFINITION

Infection with *Neisseria meningitidis* most commonly manifests as asymptomatic colonization in the nasopharynx of healthy adolescents and adults. Invasive disease occurs rarely, usually presenting as either bacterial meningitis or meningococcal septicemia. Patients may also present with occult bacteremia, pneumonia, septic arthritis, conjunctivitis, and chronic meningococcemia.

■ ETIOLOGY AND MICROBIOLOGY

N. meningitidis is a gram-negative aerobic diplococcus that colonizes humans only and that causes disease after transmission to a susceptible individual. Several related organisms have been recognized, including the pathogen *N. gonorrhoeae* and the commensals *N. lactamica*, *N. flavescens*, *N. mucosa*, *N. sicca*, and *N. subflava* . *N. meningitidis* is a catalase- and oxidase-positive organism that utilizes glucose and maltose to produce acid.

Meningococci associated with invasive disease are usually encapsulated with polysaccharide, and the antigenic nature of the capsule determines an organism's serogroup (Table 143-1). In total, 13 serogroups have been identified (A–D, X–Z, 29E, W135, H–J, and L), but just 5 serogroups—A, B, C, Y, and W135—account for the majority of cases of invasive disease. Acapsular meningococci are commonly isolated from the nasopharynx in studies of carriage; the lack of capsule often is a result of phase variation of capsule expression, but as many as 16% of isolates lack the genes for capsule synthesis and assembly. These "capsule-null" meningococci and those that express capsules other than A, B, C, Y, and W135 are only rarely associated with invasive disease and are most commonly identified in the nasopharynx of asymptomatic carriers.

Beneath the capsule, meningococci are surrounded by an outer phospholipid membrane containing lipopolysaccharide (LPS, endotoxin) and multiple outer-membrane proteins (Figs. 143-1 and 143-2). Antigenic variability in porins expressed in the outer

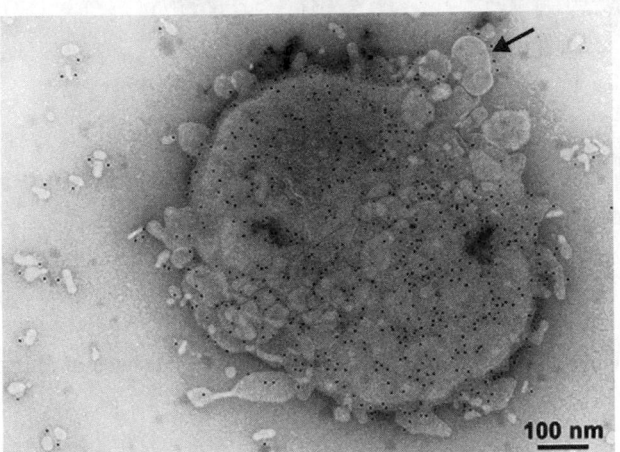

Figure 143-1 Electron micrograph of *Neisseria meningitidis*. Black dots are gold-labeled polyclonal antibodies binding surface opacity proteins. Blebs of outer membrane can be seen being released from the bacterial surface (see arrow). *(Photo courtesy of D. Ferguson, Oxford University.)*

membrane defines the serotype (PorB) and serosubtype (PorA) of the organism, and structural differences in LPS determine the immunotype. Serologic methods for typing of meningococci are restricted by the limited availability of serologic reagents that can distinguish among the organisms' highly variable surface proteins. Where available, high-throughput antigen gene sequencing has superseded serology for meningococcal typing. A large database of antigen gene sequences for the outer-membrane proteins PorA, PorB, FetA, Opa, and factor H–binding protein is available online (www.neisseria.org). The number of specialized iron-regulated proteins found in the meningococcal outer membrane (e.g., FetA and transferrin-binding proteins) highlights the organisms' dependence on iron from human sources. A thin peptidoglycan cell wall separates the outer membrane from the cytoplasmic membrane.

The structure of meningococcal populations involved in local and global spread has been studied with multilocus enzyme electrophoresis (MLEE), which characterizes isolates according to differences in the electrophoretic mobility of cytoplasmic enzymes. However, this technique has mostly been replaced by multilocus sequence typing (MLST), in which

TABLE 143-1	Structure of the Polysaccharide Capsule of Common Disease-Causing Meningococci	
Meningococcal Serogroup	Chemical Structure of Oligosaccharide	Current Disease Epidemiology
A	2-Acetamido-2-deoxy-D-mannopyranosyl phosphate	Epidemic disease mainly in sub-Saharan Africa; sporadic cases worldwide
B	α-2,8-*N*-acetylneuraminic acid	Sporadic cases worldwide; propensity to cause hyperendemic disease
C	α-2,9-O-acetylneuraminic acid	Small outbreaks and sporadic disease
Y	4-O-α-D-glucopyranosyl-*N*-acetylneuraminic acid	Sporadic disease and occasional small institutional outbreaks
W135	4-O-α-D-galactopyranosyl-*N*-acetylneuraminic acid	Sporadic disease; outbreaks of disease associated with mass gatherings; epidemics in sub-Saharan Africa

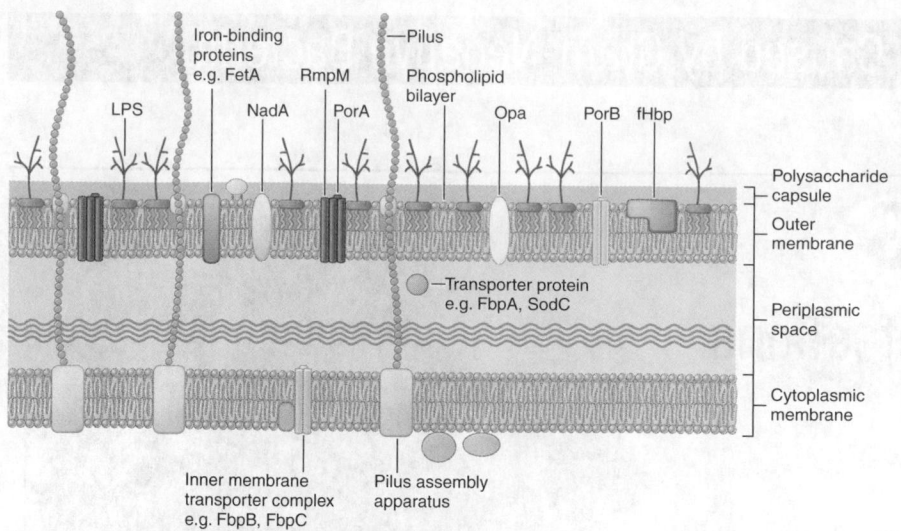

Figure 143-2 Cross-section through surface structures of *Neisseria meningitidis.* *(Reprinted with permission from Sadarangani and Pollard, 2010.)*

meningococci are characterized by sequence types assigned on the basis of sequences of internal fragments of seven housekeeping genes. The online MLST database currently includes more than 13,000 meningococcal isolates and 7600 unique sequence types *(http://pubmlst.org/neisseria/).* Seven hyperinvasive lineages of *N. meningitidis* have been identified and are responsible for the majority of cases of invasive meningococcal disease worldwide. The apparent genetic stability of these meningococcal clones over decades and during wide geographic spread indicates that they are well adapted to the nasopharyngeal environment of the host and to efficient transmission.

The group B meningococcal genome is >2 megabases in length and contains 2158 coding regions. Many genes undergo phase variation that makes it possible to control their expression; this capacity is likely to be important in meningococcal adaptation to the host environment and evasion of the immune response. Meningococci can obtain DNA from their environment and can acquire new genes—including the capsular operon—such that a switch from one serogroup to another can occur.

■ EPIDEMIOLOGY

Patterns of disease

Up to 500,000 cases of meningococcal disease are thought to occur worldwide each year, and ~10% of the individuals affected die. There are several patterns of disease: epidemic, outbreak (small clusters of cases), hyperendemic, and sporadic or endemic.

Epidemics have continued since the original descriptions of meningococcal disease, especially affecting the sub-Saharan meningitis belt of Africa, where tens to hundreds of thousands of cases (caused mainly by serogroup A but also by serogroups W135 and X) may be reported over a season and rates may be as high as 1000 cases per 100,000 population. Serogroup A epidemics took place in Europe and North America after the First and Second World Wars, and serogroup A outbreaks have been documented over the past 30 years in New Zealand, China, Nepal, Mongolia, India, Pakistan, Poland, and Russia.

Clusters of cases occur where there is an opportunity for increased transmission—i.e., in (semi-)closed communities such as schools, colleges, universities, military training centers, and refugee camps. Recently, such clusters have been especially strongly linked with a particular clone (sequence type 11) that is mainly

associated with the serogroup C capsule. Wider and more prolonged community outbreaks (hyperendemic disease) due to single clones of serogroup B meningococci account for ≥10 cases per 100,000. Regions affected in the past decade include the U.S. Pacific Northwest, New Zealand (both islands), and the province of Normandy in France.

Most countries now experience predominantly sporadic cases (0.3–5 cases per 100,000 population), with many different disease-causing clones involved and usually no clear epidemiologic link between one case and another. The disease rate and the distribution of meningococcal strains vary in different regions of the world and also in any one location over time. For example, in the United States, the rate of meningococcal disease fell from 1.2 cases per 100,000 population in 1997 to <0.4 case per 100,000 in 2007 (Fig. 143-3). Meningococcal disease in this country was previously dominated by serogroups B and C; however, serogroup Y emerged during the 1990s and became more common than serogroup C in 2007. In contrast, rates of disease in England and Wales rose to >5 cases per 100,000 during the 1990s because of an increase in cases caused by the ST11 serogroup C clone. As a result of a mass immunization program against serogroup C in 1999, almost all cases in the United Kingdom are now attributed to serogroup B (Fig. 143-4).

Factors associated with disease risk and susceptibility

The principal determinant of disease susceptibility is age, with the peak incidence in the first year of life (Fig. 143-5). The susceptibility of the very young presumably results from an absence of specific adaptive immunity in combination with very close contact with colonized individuals, including parents. Compared with other age groups, infants appear to be particularly susceptible to serogroup B disease: >30% of serogroup B cases in the United States occur during the first year of life. In the early 1990s in North America, the median ages for patients with disease due to serogroups B, C, Y, and W135 were 6, 17, 24, and 33 years, respectively.

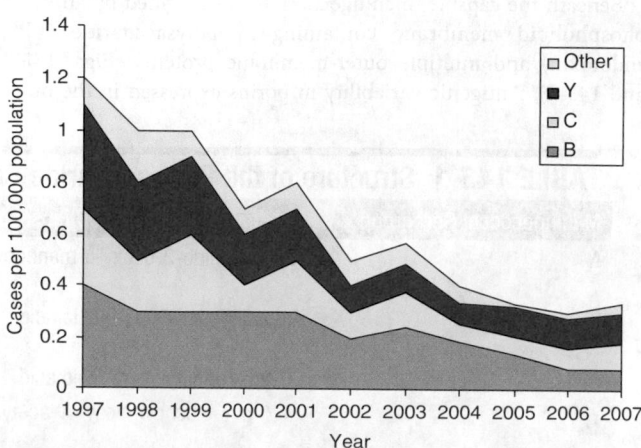

Figure 143-3 Meningococcal disease in the United States over time. *(Adapted from ABC Surveillance data, Centers for Disease Control and Prevention; www.cdc.gov.)*

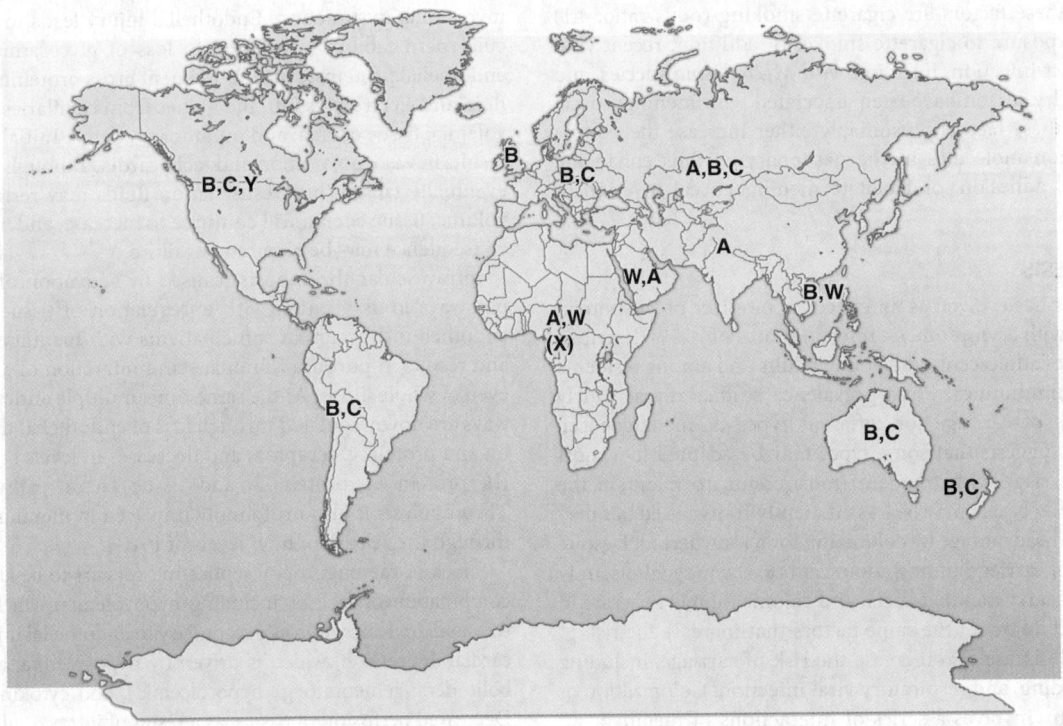

Figure 143-4 Global distribution of meningococcal serogroups, 1999–2009.

After early childhood, a second peak of disease occurs in adolescents and young adults (15–25 years of age) in Europe and North America. It is thought that this peak relates to social behaviors and environmental exposures in this age group, as discussed below. Most cases of infection with *N. meningitidis* in developed countries today are sporadic, and the rarity of the disease suggests that individual susceptibility may be important. A number of factors probably contribute to individual susceptibility, including the host's genetic constitution, environment, and contact with a carrier or a case.

The best-documented genetic association with meningococcal disease is complement deficiency, chiefly of the terminal complement components (C5–9), properdin, or factor D; such a deficiency increases the risk of disease by up to 600-fold and may result in recurrent attacks. Complement components are believed to be important for the bactericidal activity of serum, which is considered the principal mechanism of immunity against invasive meningococcal disease. However, when investigated, complement deficiency is found in only a very small proportion of individuals with meningococcal disease (0.3%). Conversely, 7–20% of persons whose disease is caused by the less common serogroups (W135, X, Y, Z, 29E) have a complement deficiency. Complement deficiency appears to be associated with serogroup B disease only rarely. Individuals with recurrences of meningococcal disease, particularly those caused by non-B serogroups, should be assessed for complement deficiency by measurement of total hemolytic complement activity. There is also limited evidence that hyposplenism (through reduction in phagocytic capacity) and hypogammaglobulinemia (through absence of specific antibody) increase the risk of meningococcal disease. Genetic studies have revealed various associations with disease susceptibility, including complement and mannose-binding lectin deficiency, single-nucleotide polymorphisms in Toll-like receptor (TLR) 4 and complement factor H, and variants of Fc gamma receptors.

Factors that increase the chance of a susceptible individual acquiring *N. meningitidis* via the respiratory route also increase the risk of meningococcal disease. Acquisition occurs through close contact with carriers as a result of overcrowding (e.g., in poor socioeconomic settings, in refugee camps, during the Hajj pilgrimage to Mecca, and during freshman-year residence in college dormitories) and certain social behaviors (e.g., attendance at bars and nightclubs, kissing). Secondary cases may occur in close contacts of an index case (e.g., household members and persons kissing the infected individual); the risk to these contacts may be as high as 1000 times the background rate in the population. Factors that damage the nasopharyngeal epithelium also increase the risk of both

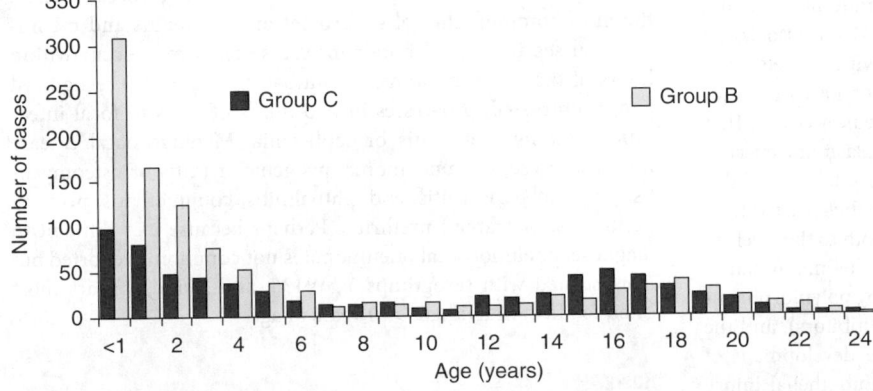

Figure 143-5 Age distribution of serogroups B and C meningococcal disease in England and Wales, 1998/1999. *(Health Protection Agency, UK; www.hpa.org.uk.)*

colonization with *N. meningitidis* and invasive disease. The most important of these factors are cigarette smoking (odds ratio, 4.1) and passive exposure to cigarette smoke. In addition, recent viral respiratory tract infection, infection with *Mycoplasma* species, and winter or the dry season have been associated with meningococcal disease; all of these factors presumably either increase the expression of adhesion molecules in the nasopharynx, thus enhancing meningococcal adhesion, or facilitate meningococcal invasion of the bloodstream.

■ PATHOGENESIS

N. meningitidis has evolved as an effective colonizer of the human nasopharynx, with asymptomatic infection rates of >25% described in some series of adolescents and young adults and among residents of crowded communities. Point-prevalence studies reveal widely divergent rates of carriage for different types of meningococci. This variation suggests that some types may be adapted to a short duration of carriage with frequent transmission to maintain the population, while others may be less efficiently transmitted but may overcome this disadvantage by colonizing for a long period. Despite the high rates of carriage among adolescents and young adults, only ~10% of adults carry meningococci, and colonization is very rare in early childhood. Many of the same factors that increase the risk of meningococcal disease also increase the risk of carriage, including smoking, crowding, and respiratory viral infection. Colonization of the nasopharynx involves a series of interactions of meningococcal adhesins (e.g., Opa proteins and pili) with their ligands on the epithelial mucosa. *N. meningitidis* produces an IgA1 protease that is likely to reduce interruption of colonization by mucosal IgA.

Colonization should be considered the normal state of meningococcal infection, with an increased risk of invasion the unfortunate consequence (for both host and organism) of adaptations of hyperinvasive meningococcal lineages. The meningococcal capsule is an important virulence factor: acapsular strains rarely cause invasive disease. The capsule provides resistance to phagocytosis and may be important in preventing desiccation during transmission between hosts. Antigenic diversity in surface structures and an ability to vary levels of their expression have probably evolved as important factors in maintaining meningococcal populations within and between individual hosts.

Invasion through the mucosa into the blood occurs rarely, usually within a few days of acquisition of an invasive strain by a susceptible individual. Only occasional cases of prolonged colonization prior to invasion have been documented. Once the organism is in the bloodstream, its growth may be limited if the individual is partially immune, although bacteremia may allow seeding of another site, such as the meninges or the joints. Alternatively, unchecked proliferation may continue, resulting in high bacterial counts in the circulation. During growth, meningococci release blebs of outer membrane (Fig. 143-1) containing outer-membrane proteins and endotoxin (LPS). Endotoxin binds cell-bound CD14 in association with TLR4 to initiate an inflammatory cascade with the release of high levels of various mediators, including tumor necrosis factor α, soluble tumor necrosis factor receptor, interleukin (IL) 1, IL-1 receptor antagonist, IL-1β, IL-6, IL-8, IL-10, plasminogen-activator inhibitor 1 (PAI-1), and leukemia inhibitory factor. Soluble CD14-bound endotoxin acts as a mediator of endothelial activation. The severity of meningococcal disease is related both to the levels of endotoxin in the blood and to the magnitude of the inflammatory response. The latter is determined to some extent by polymorphisms in the inflammatory response genes (and their inhibitors), and the release of the inflammatory cascade heralds the development of meningococcal septicemia (meningococcemia). Endothelial injury is central to many clinical features of meningococcemia, including increased vascular permeability, pathologic changes in vascular

tone, loss of thromboresistance, intravascular coagulation, and myocardial dysfunction. Endothelial injury leads to increased vascular permeability (attributed to loss of glycosaminoglycans and endothelial proteins), with subsequent gross proteinuria. Leakage of fluid and electrolytes into the tissues from capillaries leads to hypovolemia, tissue edema, and pulmonary edema. Initial compensation results in vasoconstriction and tachycardia, although cardiac output eventually falls. While resuscitation fluids may restore circulating volume, tissue edema will continue to increase, and, in the lung, the consequence may be respiratory failure.

Intravascular thrombosis (caused by activation of procoagulant pathways in association with upregulation of tissue factor on the endothelium) occurs in some patients with meningococcal disease and results in purpura fulminans and infarction of areas of skin or even of whole limbs. At the same time, multiple anticoagulant pathways are downregulated through loss of endothelial thrombomodulin and protein C receptors and decreases in levels of antithrombin III, protein C, protein S, and tissue factor pathway inhibitor. Thrombolysis is also profoundly impaired in meningococcal sepsis through the release of high levels of PAI-1.

Shock in meningococcal septicemia appears to be attributable to a combination of factors, including hypovolemia, which results from the capillary leak syndrome secondary to endothelial injury, and myocardial depression, which is driven by hypovolemia, hypoxia, metabolic derangements (e.g., hypocalcemia), and cytokines (e.g., IL-6). Decreased perfusion of tissues as a result of intravascular thrombosis, vasoconstriction, tissue edema, and reduced cardiac output in meningococcal septicemia can cause widespread organ dysfunction, including renal impairment and—later in the disease—a decreased level of consciousness due to central nervous system involvement.

Bacteria that reach the meninges cause a local inflammatory response, with release of a spectrum of cytokines similar to that seen in septicemia, that presents clinically as meningitis and is believed to determine the severity of neuronal injury. Local endothelial injury may result in cerebral edema and rapid onset of raised intracranial pressure in some cases.

■ CLINICAL MANIFESTATIONS

As discussed above, the most common form of infection with *N. meningitidis* is asymptomatic carriage of the organism in the nasopharynx. Despite the location of infection in the upper airway, meningococcal pharyngitis is rarely reported; however, upper respiratory tract symptoms are common prior to presentation with invasive disease. It is not clear whether these symptoms relate to preceding viral infection (which may promote meningococcal acquisition) or to meningococcal acquisition itself. After acquiring the organism, susceptible individuals develop disease manifestations in 1–10 days (usually <4 days, although colonization for 11 weeks has been documented).

Along the spectrum of presentations of meningococcal disease, the most common clinical syndromes are meningitis and meningococcal septicemia. In fulminant cases, death may occur within hours of the first symptoms. Occult bacteremia is also recognized and, if untreated, progresses in two-thirds of cases to focal infection including meningitis or septicemia. Meningococcal disease may also present as pneumonia, pyogenic arthritis or osteomyelitis, purulent pericarditis, endophthalmitis, conjunctivitis, primary peritonitis, or (rarely) urethritis. Perhaps because it is difficult to diagnose, pneumococcal pneumonia is not commonly reported but is associated with serogroups Y, W135, and Z and appears most often to affect individuals >10 years of age.

Rash

A nonblanching rash (petechial or purpuric) develops in >80% of cases of meningococcal disease; however, the rash is often

TABLE 143-2 Common Causes of Petechial or Purpuric Rashes

Enteroviruses

Influenza and other respiratory viruses

Measles virus

Epstein-Barr virus

Cytomegalovirus

Parvovirus

Deficiency of protein C or S (including postvaricella protein S deficiency)

Platelet disorders (e.g., idiopathic thrombocytopenic purpura, drug effects, bone marrow infiltration)

Henoch-Schönlein purpura, connective tissue disorders, trauma (including nonaccidental injuries in children)

Pneumococcal, streptococcal, staphylococcal, or gram-negative bacterial sepsis

absent early in the illness. Usually initially blanching in nature (macules, maculopapules, or urticaria) and indistinguishable from more common viral rashes, the rash of meningococcal infection becomes petechial or frankly purpuric over the hours after onset. In the most severe cases, large purpuric lesions develop (purpura fulminans). Some patients (including those with overwhelming sepsis) may have no rash. While petechial rash and fever are important signs of meningococcal disease, fewer than 10% of children (and, in some clinical settings, fewer than 1% of patients) with this presentation are found to have meningococcal disease. Most patients presenting with a petechial or purpuric rash have a viral infection (Table 143-2). The skin lesions exhibit widespread endothelial necrosis and occlusion of small vessels in the dermis and subcutaneous tissues, with a neutrophilic infiltrate.

Meningitis

Meningococcal meningitis commonly presents as nonspecific manifestations, including fever, vomiting, and (especially in infants and young children) irritability, and is indistinguishable from other forms of bacterial meningitis unless there is an associated petechial or purpuric rash, which occurs in two-thirds of cases. Headache is rarely reported in early childhood but is more common in later childhood and adulthood. When headache is present, the following features, in association with fever or a history of fever, are suggestive of bacterial meningitis: neck stiffness, photophobia, decreased level of consciousness, seizures or status epilepticus, and focal neurologic signs. Classic signs of meningitis, such as neck stiffness and photophobia, are often absent in infants and young children with bacterial meningitis.

While 30–50% of patients present with a meningitis syndrome alone, up to 40% of meningitis patients also present with some features of septicemia. Most deaths from meningococcal meningitis alone (i.e., without septicemia) are associated with raised intracranial pressure presenting as a reduced level of consciousness, relative bradycardia and hypertension, focal neurologic signs, abnormal posturing, and signs of brainstem involvement—e.g., unequal, dilated, or poorly reactive pupils; abnormal eye movement; and impaired corneal responses (Chap. 274).

Septicemia

Meningococcal septicemia alone accounts for up to 20% of cases of meningococcal disease. The condition may progress from early nonspecific symptoms to death within hours. Mortality rates among children with this syndrome have been high (25–40%), but aggressive management (as discussed below) may reduce the figure to <10%. Early symptoms are nonspecific and suggest an influenza-like illness with fever, headache, and myalgia accompanied by vomiting and abdominal pain. As discussed above, the rash, if present, may appear to be viral early in the course until petechiae or purpuric lesions develop. Purpura fulminans occurs in severe cases, with multiple large purpuric lesions and signs of peripheral ischemia. Surveys of patients have indicated that limb pain, pallor (including a mottled appearance and cyanosis), and cold hands and feet may be prominent. Shock is manifested by tachycardia, poor peripheral perfusion, tachypnea, and oliguria. Decreased cerebral perfusion leads to confusion, agitation, or decreased level of consciousness. With progressive shock, multiorgan failure ensues; hypotension is a late sign in children, who more commonly present with compensated shock. Poor outcome is associated with an absence of meningismus, hypotension, young age, coma, relatively low temperature (< 38°C), leukopenia, and thrombocytopenia. Spontaneous hemorrhage (pulmonary, gastric, or cerebral) may result from consumption of coagulation factors and thrombocytopenia.

Chronic meningococcemia

Chronic meningococcemia, which is rarely recognized, presents as repeated episodes of petechial rash associated with fever, joint pain, features of arthritis, and splenomegaly that may progress to acute meningococcal septicemia if untreated. During the relapsing course, bacteremia characteristically clears without treatment and then recurs. The differential diagnosis includes bacterial endocarditis, acute rheumatic fever, Henoch-Schönlein purpura, infectious mononucleosis, disseminated gonococcal infection, and immune-mediated vasculitis. This condition has been associated with complement deficiencies in some cases and with inadequate sulfonamide therapy in others.

Postmeningococcal reactive disease

In a small proportion of patients, an immune complex disease develops ~4–10 days after the onset of meningococcal disease, with manifestations that include a maculopapular or vasculitic rash (2% of cases), arthritis (up to 8% of cases), iritis (1%), pericarditis, and/or polyserositis associated with fever. The immune complexes involve meningococcal polysaccharide antigen and result in immunoglobulin and complement deposition with an inflammatory infiltrate. These features resolve spontaneously without sequelae. It is important to recognize this condition since a new onset of fever and rash can lead to concerns about relapse of meningococcal disease and unnecessarily prolonged antibiotic treatment.

■ DIAGNOSIS

Like other invasive bacterial infections, meningococcal disease may produce elevations of the white blood cell (WBC) count and of values for inflammatory markers (e.g., C-reactive protein and procalcitonin levels or the erythrocyte sedimentation rate). Values may be normal or low in rapidly progressive disease, and lack of these elevations does not exclude the diagnosis. However, in the presence of fever and a petechial rash, these elevations are suggestive of meningococcal disease. In patients with severe meningococcal septicemia, common laboratory findings include hypoglycemia, acidosis, hypokalemia, hypocalcemia, hypomagnesemia, hypophosphatemia, anemia, and coagulopathy.

Although meningococcal disease is often diagnosed on clinical grounds, in suspected meningococcal meningitis or meningococcemia, blood should routinely be sent for culture to confirm the diagnosis and to facilitate public health investigations; blood cultures are positive in up to 75% of cases. Culture media containing sodium polyanethol sulfonate, which may inhibit meningococcal growth, should be avoided. Meningococcal viability is reduced if there is a delay in transport of the specimen to the microbiology laboratory for culture or in plating of cerebrospinal fluid (CSF) samples. In countries where treatment with antibiotics before hospitalization is recommended for meningococcal disease, the majority of clinically suspected cases are culture negative. Real-time polymerase chain reaction (PCR) analysis of whole-blood samples increases the diagnostic yield by >40%, and results obtained with this method may remain positive for several days after administration of antibiotics. Indeed, in the United Kingdom, more than half of clinically suspected cases are currently identified by PCR.

Unless contraindications exist (raised intracranial pressure, uncorrected shock, disordered coagulation, thrombocytopenia, respiratory insufficiency, local infection, ongoing convulsions), lumbar puncture should be undertaken to identify and confirm the etiology of suspected meningococcal meningitis, whose presentation cannot be distinguished from that of meningitis of other bacterial causes. Some authorities have recommended a CT brain scan prior to lumbar puncture because of the risk of cerebral herniation in patients with raised intracranial pressure. However, a normal CT scan is not uncommon in the presence of raised intracranial pressure in meningococcal meningitis, and the decision to perform a lumbar puncture should be made on clinical grounds. CSF features of meningococcal meningitis (elevated protein level and WBC count, decreased glucose level) are indistinguishable from those of other types of bacterial meningitis unless a gram-negative diplococcus is identified. (Gram's staining is up to 80% sensitive for meningococcal meningitis.) CSF should be submitted for culture (sensitivity, 90%) and (where available) PCR analysis. CSF antigen testing with latex agglutination is insensitive and should be replaced by molecular diagnosis when possible.

Lumbar puncture should generally be avoided in meningococcal septicemia, as positioning for the procedure may critically compromise the patient's circulation in the context of hypovolemic shock. Delayed lumbar puncture may still be useful when the diagnosis is uncertain, particularly if molecular technology is available.

In other types of focal infection, culture and PCR analysis of normally sterile body fluids (e.g., synovial fluid) may aid in the diagnosis. Although some authorities have recommended cultures of scrapings or aspirates from skin lesions, this procedure adds little to the diagnostic yield when compared with a combination of blood culture and PCR analysis. Urinary antigen testing is also insensitive, and serologic testing for meningococcal infection has not been adequately studied. Because *N. meningitidis* is a component of the normal human nasopharyngeal flora, identification of the organism on throat swabs has no diagnostic value.

TREATMENT ▶ Meningococcal Infections

Death from meningococcal disease is associated most commonly with hypovolemic shock (meningococcemia) and occasionally with raised intracranial pressure (meningococcal meningitis). Therefore, management should focus on the treatment of these urgent clinical issues in addition to the administration of specific antibiotic therapy. Delayed recognition of meningococcal disease or its associated physiologic derangements, together with inadequate emergency management, is associated with poor outcome. Since the disease is rare, protocols for emergency management have been developed (see *www.meningitis.org*).

Airway patency may be compromised if the level of consciousness is depressed as a result of shock (impaired cerebral perfusion) or raised intracranial pressure; this situation may require intervention. In meningococcemia, pulmonary edema and pulmonary oligemia (presenting as hypoxia) require oxygen therapy or elective endotracheal intubation. In cases with shock, aggressive fluid resuscitation (with replacement of the circulating volume several times in severe cases) and inotropic support may be necessary to maintain cardiac output. If shock persists after volume resuscitation at 40 mL/kg, the risk of pulmonary edema is high, and elective intubation is recommended to improve oxygenation and decrease the work of breathing. Metabolic derangements including hypoglycemia, acidosis, hypokalemia, hypocalcemia, hypomagnesemia, hypophosphatemia, anemia, and coagulopathy should be anticipated and corrected. In the presence of raised intracranial pressure, management includes correction of coexistent shock and neurointensive care to maintain cerebral perfusion.

 Empirical antibiotic therapy for suspected meningococcal disease consists of a third-generation cephalosporin such as ceftriaxone [75–100 mg/kg per day (maximum, 4 g/d) in one or two divided IV doses] or cefotaxime [200 mg/kg per day (maximum, 8 g/d) in four divided IV doses] to cover the various other (potentially penicillin-resistant) bacteria that may produce an indistinguishable clinical syndrome. Although unusual in most countries, reduced meningococcal sensitivity to penicillin (a minimal inhibitory concentration of 0.12–1.0 μg/mL) has been reported from Africa, the United Kingdom, Spain, Argentina, the United States, and Canada.

Both meningococcal meningitis and meningococcal septicemia are conventionally treated for 7 days, although courses of 3–5 days may be equally effective. Furthermore, a single dose of ceftriaxone or an oily suspension of chloramphenicol has been used successfully in resource-poor settings. No data are available to guide the duration of treatment for meningococcal infection at other foci (e.g., pneumonia, arthritis); antimicrobial therapy is usually continued until clinical and laboratory evidence of infection has resolved.

The use of glucocorticoids for adjunctive treatment of meningococcal meningitis remains controversial since no relevant studies have had sufficient power to determine true efficacy. One large study in adults did indicate a trend toward benefit, and in clinical practice a decision to use glucocorticoids usually precedes a definite diagnosis. Therapeutic doses of glucocorticoids are not recommended in meningococcal septicemia, but many intensivists recommend replacement glucocorticoid doses for patients who have refractory shock in association with impaired adrenal gland responsiveness.

Various other adjunctive therapies for meningococcal disease have been considered, but few have been subjected to clinical trials and none can currently be recommended. An antibody to LPS (HA1A) failed to confer a demonstrable benefit. Recombinant bactericidal/permeability-increasing protein was tested in a study that had inadequate power to show an effect on mortality rates; however, there were trends toward lower mortality rates among patients who received a complete infusion, and this group also had fewer amputations, fewer blood-product transfusions, and a significantly improved functional outcome. Given that protein C concentrations are reduced in meningococcal disease, the use of activated protein C has been considered since a survival benefit was demonstrated in adult sepsis trials; however, trials in pediatric sepsis (of particular relevance for meningococcal disease) found no benefit and indicated a potential risk of bleeding complications with use of activated protein C.

The postmeningococcal immune-complex inflammatory syndrome has been treated with nonsteroidal anti-inflammatory agents until spontaneous resolution occurs.

COMPLICATIONS

About 10% of patients with meningococcal disease die despite the availability of antimicrobial therapy and other intensive medical interventions. The most common complication of meningococcal disease (10% of cases) is scarring after necrosis of purpuric skin lesions, for which skin grafting may be necessary. The lower limbs are most often affected; next in frequency are the upper limbs, the trunk, and the face. On average, 13% of the skin surface area is involved. Amputations are necessary in ~2% of survivors of meningococcal disease because of a loss of tissue viability after peripheral ischemia or compartment syndromes. Unless there is local infection, amputation should usually be delayed to allow the demarcation between viable and nonviable tissue to become apparent. Approximately 4% of patients with meningococcal disease suffer hearing loss, and 7% have neurologic complications. In one study, pain was reported by 21% of survivors. In some investigations, the rate of complications is higher for serogroup C disease (mostly associated with the ST11 clone) than for serogroup B disease. In patients with severe hypovolemic shock, renal perfusion may be impaired and prerenal failure is common, but permanent renal replacement therapy is rarely needed.

Several studies suggest adverse psychosocial outcomes after meningococcal disease, with reduced quality of life, lowered self-esteem, and poorer neurologic development, including increased rates of attention deficit/hyperactivity disorder and special educational needs. Other studies have not found evidence of such outcomes.

PROGNOSIS

Several prognostic scoring systems have been developed to identify patients with meningococcal disease who are least likely to survive. Factors associated with a poorer prognosis are shock; young age (infancy), old age, and adolescence; coma; purpura fulminans; disseminated intravascular coagulation; thrombocytopenia; leukopenia; absence of meningitis; metabolic acidosis; low plasma concentrations of antithrombin and proteins S and C; high blood levels of PAI-1; and a low erythrocyte sedimentation rate or C-reactive protein level. The Glasgow Meningococcal Septicaemia Prognostic Score is probably the best-performing scoring system studied so far and may be clinically useful for severity assessment in meningococcal disease. However, scoring systems do not direct the clinician to specific interventions, and the priority in management should be recognition of compromised airways, breathing, or circulation and direct, urgent intervention. Most patients improve rapidly with appropriate antibiotics and supportive therapy. Fulminant meningococcemia is more likely to result in death or ischemic skin loss than is meningitis; optimal emergency management may reduce mortality rates among the most severely affected patients.

PREVENTION

Since mortality rates in meningococcal disease remain high despite improvements in intensive care management, immunization is the only rational approach to prevention on a population level. Secondary cases are common among household and "kissing" contacts of cases, and secondary prophylaxis with antibiotic therapy is widely recommended for these contacts (see below).

Polysaccharide vaccines

Purified capsular polysaccharide has been used for immunization since the 1960s. Meningococcal polysaccharide vaccines are currently formulated as either bivalent (serogroups A and C) or quadrivalent (serogroups A, C, Y, and W135), with 50 μg of each polysaccharide per dose. Local reactions (erythema, induration, and tenderness) may occur in up to 40% of vaccinees, but serious adverse events (including febrile convulsions in young children)

are very rarely reported. In adults, the vaccines are immunogenic, but immunity appears to be relatively short-lived (with antibody levels above baseline for only 2–10 years), and booster doses do not induce a further rise in antibody concentration. Indeed, a state of immunologic hyporesponsiveness has been widely reported to follow booster doses of plain polysaccharide vaccines. The repeating units of these vaccines cross-link B cell receptors to drive specific memory B cells to become plasma cells and produce antibody. Because polysaccharides are T cell–independent antigens, no memory B cells are produced after immunization, and the memory B cell pool is depleted such that fewer polysaccharide-specific cells are available to respond to a subsequent dose of vaccine (Fig. 143-6). The clinical relevance of hyporesponsiveness is unknown. Plain polysaccharide vaccines generally are not immunogenic in early childhood, possibly because marginal-zone B cells are involved in polysaccharide responses and maturation of the splenic marginal zone is not complete until 18 months to 2 years of age. The efficacy of the meningococcal serogroup C component is >90% in young adults; no efficacy data are available for the serogroup Y and W135 polysaccharides in this age group.

Group A meningococcal polysaccharides are exceptional in that they are effective in preventing disease at all ages. Two doses administered 2–3 months apart to children 3–18 months of age or a single dose administered to older children or adults has a protective efficacy rate of >95%. The vaccine has been widely used in the control of meningococcal disease in the African meningitis belt. The duration of protection appears to be only 3–5 years.

There is no meningococcal serogroup B plain polysaccharide vaccine because α-2,8-N-acetylneuraminic acid is expressed on the surface of neural cells in the fetus such that the B polysaccharide is perceived as "self" and therefore is not immunogenic in humans.

Conjugate vaccines

The poor immunogenicity of plain polysaccharide vaccines in infancy has been overcome by chemical conjugation of the polysaccharides to a carrier protein (CRM_{197}, tetanus toxoid, or diphtheria toxoid). Conjugates that contain monovalent serogroup C polysaccharide and quadrivalent vaccines with A, C, Y, and W135 polysaccharides have been developed, as have vaccines including various other antigen combinations. After immunization, peptides from the carrier protein are conventionally believed to be presented to peptide-specific T cells in association with major histocompatibility complex (MHC) class II molecules (some recent data suggesting that carrier protein peptide may actually be presented in association with an oligosaccharide and MHCII) by polysaccharide-specific B cells; the result is a T cell–dependent immune response that allows production of antibody and generation of an expanded B cell memory pool. Unlike responses to booster doses of plain polysaccharides, responses to booster doses of conjugate vaccines have the characteristics of memory responses. Indeed, conjugate vaccines overcome the hyporesponsiveness induced by plain polysaccharides by replenishing the memory pool. The reactogenicity of conjugate vaccines is similar to that of plain polysaccharide vaccines.

The first widespread use of serogroup C meningococcal conjugate vaccine (MenC) came in 1999 in the United Kingdom after a rise in serogroup C disease. A mass vaccination campaign involving all individuals <19 years of age was undertaken, and the number of cases fell from >1000 in 1999 to just 28 in 2006. The effectiveness of the immunization program was attributed both to direct protection of immunized persons and to reduced transmission of the organism in the population as a result of decreased rates of colonization among the immunized (herd immunity). Data on immunogenicity and effectiveness have shown that the duration of protection is short when the vaccine is administered

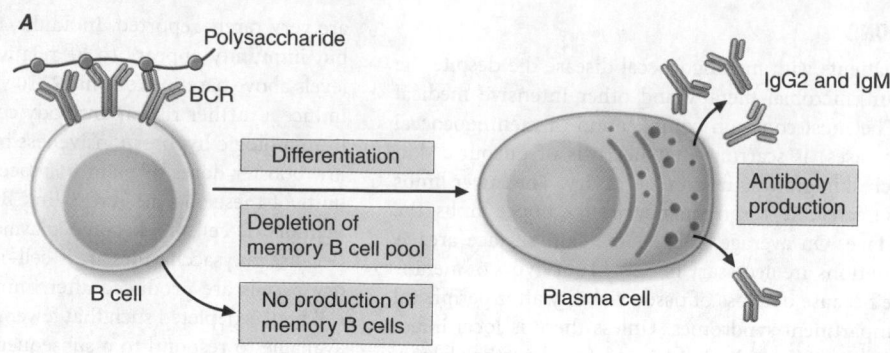

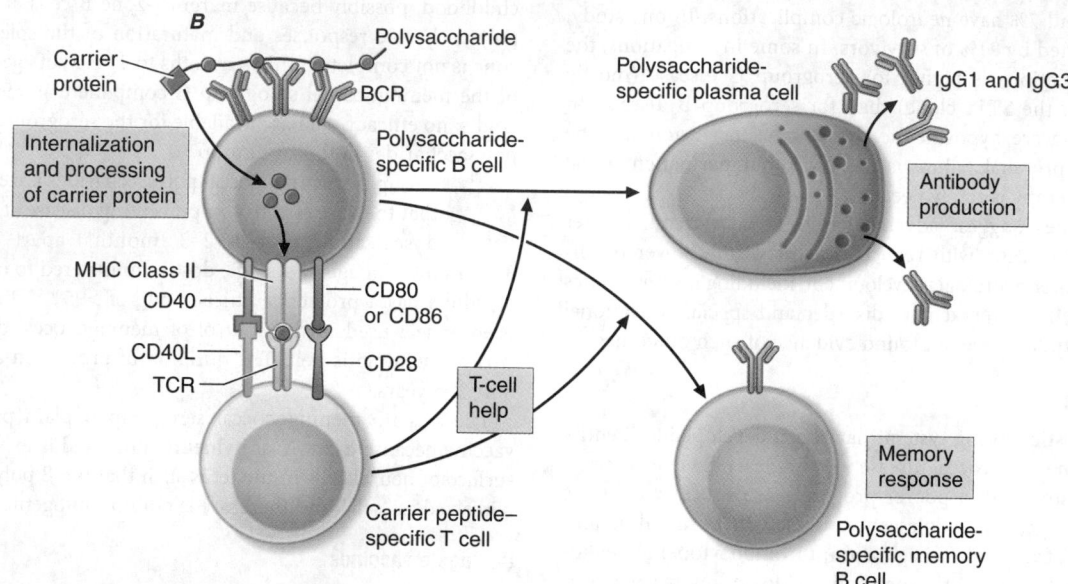

Figure 143-6 ***A.*** Polysaccharides from the encapsulated bacteria that cause disease in early childhood stimulate B cells by cross-linking the BCR and driving the production of immunoglobulins. There is no production of memory B cells, and the B cell pool may be depleted by this process such that subsequent immune responses are decreased. ***B.*** The carrier protein from protein-polysaccharide conjugate vaccines is processed by the polysaccharide-specific B cell, and peptides are presented to carrier peptide–specific T cells, with the consequent production of both plasma cells and memory B cells. BCR, B cell receptor; MHC, major histocompatibility complex; TCR, T cell receptor. *(Reprinted from Pollard et al, 2009.)*

in early childhood; thus booster doses are needed to maintain population immunity. In contrast, immunity after a dose of vaccine given in adolescence appears to be prolonged.

The first quadrivalent conjugate meningococcal vaccine containing A, C, Y, and W135 polysaccharides conjugated to diphtheria toxoid was initially recommended for all children >11 years of age in the United States in 2005. In 2007 the license was extended to high-risk children 2–10 years of age. In the same year, the vaccine was licensed in Canada for persons 2–55 years of age. Uptake was slow, but preliminary data suggest an efficacy rate of >80%. Limited data from the U.S. Vaccine Adverse Events Reporting System indicated that there might be a short-term increase in the risk of Guillain-Barré syndrome after immunization with the diphtheria conjugate vaccine; however, further investigation has not confirmed this finding. Another quadrivalent conjugate vaccine (CRM$_{197}$ carrier protein) was licensed in 2010 in both Europe and North America, and a third vaccine is in late-stage development.

A monovalent serogroup A vaccine was developed and licensed in 2010 and is being rolled out in several countries in sub-saharan Africa. The goal for this vaccine is control of epidemic meningococcal disease in the African meningitis belt.

Vaccines based on subcapsular antigens

The lack of immunogenicity of the serogroup B capsule has led to the development of vaccines based on subcapsular antigens. Various surface components have been studied in early-phase clinical trials. Outer-membrane vesicles (OMVs) containing outer-membrane proteins, phospholipid, and lipopolysaccharide can be extracted from cultures of *N. meningitidis* by detergent treatment (Fig. 143-7). OMVs prepared in this way were used in efficacy trials with a Norwegian outbreak strain and reduced the incidence of group B disease among 14- to 16-year-old schoolchildren by 53%. Similarly, OMV vaccines constructed from local outbreak strains in Cuba and New Zealand have had reported efficacy rates of >70%. These OMV vaccines appear to produce strain-specific immune responses, with only limited cross-protection, and are therefore best suited to clonal outbreaks (e.g., those in Cuba and New Zealand as well as others in Norway and the province of Normandy in France).

Several purified surface proteins have been evaluated in phase 1 clinical trials but have not yet been developed further because of variability or poor immunogenicity (e.g., transferrin-binding proteins, neisserial surface protein A). Other vaccine candidates have

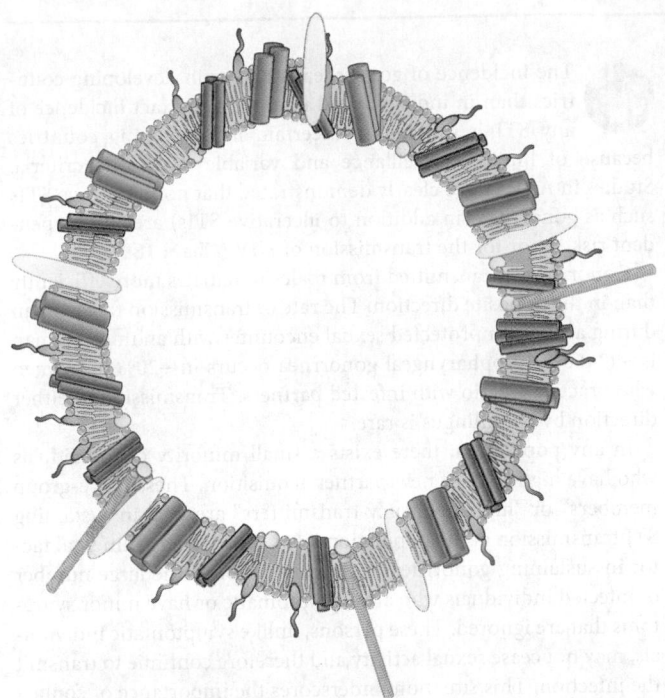

Figure 143-7 Illustration of meningococcal outer-membrane vesicle containing outer-membrane structures.

been identified since sequencing of the meningococcal genome. A combination vaccine that includes the New Zealand OMV vaccine and three proteins (neisserial adhesin A, factor H–binding protein, and neisserial heparin-binding antigen) is immunogenic in infancy and was recently submitted for licensure. Finally, a highly immunogenic vaccine based on two variants of factor H–binding protein is undergoing clinical evaluation.

■ MANAGEMENT OF CONTACTS

Close (household and kissing) contacts of individuals with meningococcal disease are at increased risk (up to 1000 times the rate for the general population) of developing secondary disease; a secondary case follows as many as 3% of sporadic cases. About one-fifth of secondary cases are actually co-primary cases—i.e., cases that occur soon after the primary case and in which transmission is presumed to have originated from the same third party. The rate of secondary cases is highest during the week after presentation of the index case. The risk falls rapidly but remains above baseline for up to 1 year after the index case; 30% of secondary cases occur in the first week, 20% in the second week, and most of the remainder over the next 6 weeks. In outbreaks of meningococcal disease, mass prophylaxis has been used; however, limited data support population intervention, and significant concerns have arisen about adverse events and the development of resistance. For these reasons, prophylaxis is usually restricted to (1) persons at greatest risk who are intimate and/or household contacts of the index case and (2) health care workers who have been directly exposed to respiratory secretions. In most cases, members of wider communities (e.g., at schools or colleges) are not offered prophylaxis.

The aim of prophylaxis is to eradicate colonization of close contacts with the strain that has caused invasive disease in the index case. Prophylaxis should be given to all contacts at the same time to avoid recolonization by meningococci transmitted from untreated contacts and should also be used as soon as possible to treat early disease in secondary cases. If the index patient is treated with an antibiotic that does not reliably clear colonization (e.g., penicillin), he or she should be given a prophylactic agent at the end of treatment to prevent relapse or onward transmission. Although rifampin has been most widely used and studied, it is not the optimal agent because it fails to eradicate carriage in 15–20% of cases, rates of adverse events have been high, compliance is affected by the need for four doses, and emerging resistance has been reported. Ceftriaxone as a single IM or IV injection is highly (97%) effective in carriage eradication and can be used at all ages and in pregnancy. Reduced susceptibility of isolates to ceftriaxone has occasionally been reported. Ciprofloxacin or ofloxacin is preferred in some countries; this agent is also highly effective and can be administered by mouth but is not recommended in pregnancy. Resistance to fluoroquinolones has been reported in some meningococci in North America, Europe, and Asia.

In documented serogroup A, C, Y, or W135 disease, contacts may be offered immunization (preferably with a conjugate vaccine) in addition to chemoprophylaxis to provide protection beyond the duration of antibiotic therapy. Mass vaccination has been used successfully to control disease during outbreaks in closed communities (educational and military establishments) as well as during epidemics in open communities.

FURTHER READINGS

CAUGANT DA, MAIDEN MC: Meningococcal carriage and disease—population biology and evolution. Vaccine 27(Suppl 2):B64, 2009

HARRISON LH et al: Global epidemiology of meningococcal disease. Vaccine 27:B51, 2009

LAFORCE FM et al: Epidemic meningitis due to group A *Neisseria meningitidis* in the African meningitis belt: A persistent problem with an imminent solution. Vaccine 27:B13, 2009

MILONOVICH LM: Meningococcemia: Epidemiology, pathophysiology, and management. J Pediatr Health Care 21:75, 2007

PACE D et al: Quadrivalent meningococcal conjugate vaccines. Vaccine 27:B30, 2009

POLLARD AJ et al: Maintaining protection against invasive bacteria in childhood with protein–polysaccharide conjugate vaccines. Nat Rev Immunol 9:213, 2009

———— et al: Early management of meningococcal disease. Arch Dis Child 80:290, 1999

SADARANGANI M, POLLARD AJ: Serogroup B meningococcal vaccines—an unfinished story. Lancet Infect Dis 10:112, 2010

STEPHENS DS et al: Epidemic meningitis, meningococcaemia, and *Neisseria meningitidis* . Lancet 369:2196, 2007

WRIGHT V et al: Genetic polymorphisms in host response to meningococcal infection: The role of susceptibility and severity genes. Vaccine 27:B90, 2009

CHAPTER 144

Gonococcal Infections

Sanjay Ram

Peter A. Rice

DEFINITION

Gonorrhea is a sexually transmitted infection (STI) of epithelium and commonly manifests as cervicitis, urethritis, proctitis, and conjunctivitis. If untreated, infections at these sites can lead to local complications such as endometritis, salpingitis, tuboovarian abscess, bartholinitis, peritonitis, and perihepatitis in female patients; periurethritis and epididymitis in male patients; and ophthalmia neonatorum in newborns. Disseminated gonococcemia is an uncommon event whose manifestations include skin lesions, tenosynovitis, arthritis, and (in rare cases) endocarditis or meningitis.

MICROBIOLOGY

Neisseria gonorrhoeae is a gram-negative, nonmotile, non-spore-forming organism that grows singly and in pairs (i.e., as monococci and diplococci, respectively). Exclusively a human pathogen, the gonococcus contains, on average, three genome copies per coccal unit; this polyploidy permits a high level of antigenic variation and the survival of the organism in its host. Gonococci, like all other *Neisseria* species, are oxidase positive. They are distinguished from other neisseriae by their ability to grow on selective media and to utilize glucose but not maltose, sucrose, or lactose.

EPIDEMIOLOGY

The incidence of gonorrhea has declined significantly in the United States, but there were still ~299,000 newly reported cases in 2008. Gonorrhea remains a major public health problem worldwide, is a significant cause of morbidity in developing countries, and may play a role in enhancing transmission of HIV.

Gonorrhea predominantly affects young, nonwhite, unmarried, less educated members of urban populations. The number of reported cases probably represents half of the true number of cases—a discrepancy resulting from underreporting, self-treatment, and nonspecific treatment without a laboratory-proven diagnosis. The number of reported cases of gonorrhea in the United States rose from ~250,000 in the early 1960s to a high of 1.01 million in 1978. The recorded incidence of gonorrhea in modern times peaked in 1975, with 468 reported cases per 100,000 population in the United States. This peak was attributable to the interaction of several variables, including improved accuracy of diagnosis, changes in patterns of contraceptive use, and changes in sexual behavior. The incidence of the disease has since declined gradually and is currently estimated at 120 cases per 100,000, a figure that is still the highest among industrialized countries. A further decline in the overall incidence of gonorrhea in the United States over the past two decades may reflect increased condom use resulting from public health efforts to curtail HIV transmission. At present, the attack rate in the United States is highest among 15- to 19-year-old women and 20- to 24-year-old men; 40% of all reported cases occur in the preceding two groups together. From the standpoint of ethnicity, rates are highest among African Americans and lowest among persons of Asian or Pacific Island descent.

The incidence of gonorrhea is higher in developing countries than in industrialized nations. The exact incidence of any STI is difficult to ascertain in developing countries because of limited surveillance and variable diagnostic criteria. Studies in Africa have clearly demonstrated that nonulcerative STIs such as gonorrhea (in addition to ulcerative STIs) are an independent risk factor for the transmission of HIV (Chap. 189).

Gonorrhea is transmitted from males to females more efficiently than in the opposite direction. The rate of transmission to a woman during a single unprotected sexual encounter with an infected man is ~40–60%. Oropharyngeal gonorrhea occurs in ~20% of women who practice fellatio with infected partners. Transmission in either direction by cunnilingus is rare.

In any population, there exists a small minority of individuals who have high rates of new-partner acquisition. These "core-group members" or "high-frequency transmitters" are vital in sustaining STI transmission at the population level. Another instrumental factor in sustaining gonorrhea in the population is the large number of infected individuals who are asymptomatic or have minor symptoms that are ignored. These persons, unlike symptomatic individuals, may not cease sexual activity and therefore continue to transmit the infection. This situation underscores the importance of contact tracing and empirical treatment of the sex partners of index cases.

PATHOGENESIS, IMMUNOLOGY, AND ANTIMICROBIAL RESISTANCE

Outer-membrane proteins

Pili Fresh clinical isolates of *N. gonorrhoeae* initially form piliated (fimbriated) colonies distinguishable on translucent agar. Pilus expression is rapidly switched off with unselected subculture because of rearrangements in pilus genes. This change is a basis for antigenic variation of gonococci. Piliated strains adhere better to cells derived from human mucosal surfaces and are more virulent in organ culture models and human inoculation experiments than nonpiliated variants. In a fallopian tube explant model, pili mediate gonococcal attachment to nonciliated columnar epithelial cells. This event initiates gonococcal phagocytosis and transport through these cells to intercellular spaces near the basement membrane or directly into the subepithelial tissue. Pili are also essential for genetic competence and transformation of *N. gonorrhoeae*, which permit horizontal transfer of genetic material between different gonococcal lineages in vivo.

Opacity-associated protein Another gonococcal surface protein that is important in adherence to epithelial cells is opacity-associated protein (Opa, formerly called protein II). Opa contributes to intergonococcal adhesion, which is responsible for the opaque nature of gonococcal colonies on translucent agar and the organism's adherence to a variety of eukaryotic cells, including polymorphonuclear leukocytes (PMNs). Certain Opa variants promote invasion of epithelial cells, and this effect has been linked with the ability of Opa to bind vitronectin, glycosaminoglycans, and several members of the carcinoembryonic antigen–related cell adhesion molecule (CEACAM) receptor family. *N. gonorrhoeae* Opa proteins that bind CEACAM 1, which is expressed by primary CD4+ T lymphocytes, suppress the activation and proliferation of these lymphocytes. This phenomenon may serve to explain the transient decrease in CD4+ T lymphocyte counts associated with gonococcal infection.

Porin Porin (previously designated protein I) is the most abundant gonococcal surface protein, accounting for >50% of the organism's total outer-membrane protein. Porin molecules exist as trimers that provide anion-transporting aqueous channels through the otherwise-hydrophobic outer membrane. Porin shows stable interstrain antigenic variation and forms the basis for gonococcal serotyping. Two main serotypes have been identified: PorB.1A strains are often associated with disseminated gonococcal infection (DGI), while PorB.1B strains usually cause local genital infections only. DGI strains are generally resistant to the killing action of normal human serum and do not incite a significant local inflammatory response; therefore, they may not cause symptoms at genital sites. These characteristics may be related to the ability of PorB.1A strains to bind to complement-inhibitory molecules, resulting in a diminished inflammatory response. Porin can translocate to the cytoplasmic membrane of host cells—a process that could initiate gonococcal endocytosis and invasion.

Other outer-membrane proteins Other notable outer-membrane proteins include H.8, a lipoprotein that is present in high concentration on the surface of all gonococcal strains and is an excellent target for antibody-based diagnostic testing. Transferrin-binding proteins (Tbp1 and Tbp2) and lactoferrin-binding protein are required for scavenging iron from transferrin and lactoferrin in vivo. Transferrin and iron have been shown to enhance the attachment of iron-deprived *N. gonorrhoeae* to human endometrial cells. IgA1 protease is produced by *N. gonorrhoeae* and may protect the organism from the action of mucosal IgA.

Lipooligosaccharide

Gonococcal lipooligosaccharide (LOS) consists of a lipid A and a core oligosaccharide that lacks the repeating O-carbohydrate antigenic side chain seen in other gram-negative bacteria (Chap. 120). Gonococcal LOS possesses marked endotoxic activity and contributes to the local cytotoxic effect in a fallopian tube model. LOS core sugars undergo a high degree of phase variation under different conditions of growth; this variation reflects genetic regulation and expression of glycotransferase genes that dictate the carbohydrate structure of LOS. These phenotypic changes may affect interactions of *N. gonorrhoeae* with elements of the humoral immune system (antibodies and complement) and may also influence direct binding of organisms to both professional phagocytes and nonprofessional phagocytes (epithelial cells). For example, gonococci that are sialylated at their LOS sites bind complement factor H and inhibit the alternative pathway of complement. LOS sialylation may also decrease nonopsonic Opa-mediated association with neutrophils and inhibit the oxidative burst in PMNs. The unsialylated terminal lactosamine residue of LOS binds to an asialoglycoprotein receptor on male epithelial cells, which facilitates binding and subsequent gonococcal invasion of these cells. Moreover, LOS oligosaccharide structures can modulate host immune responses. For example, the terminal monosaccharide expressed by LOS determines the C-type lectin receptor on dendritic cells that is targeted by the bacteria. In turn, the specific C-type lectin receptor engaged influences whether a T_H1- or T_H2-type response is elicited; the latter response may be less favorable for clearance of gonococcal infection.

Host factors

In addition to gonococcal structures that interact with epithelial cells, host factors seem to be important in mediating entry of gonococci into nonphagocytic cells. Activation of phosphatidylcholine-specific phospholipase C and acidic sphingomyelinase by *N. gonorrhoeae*, which results in the release of diacylglycerol and ceramide, is a requirement for the entry of *N. gonorrhoeae* into epithelial cells. Ceramide accumulation within cells leads to apoptosis, which may disrupt epithelial integrity and facilitate entry of gonococci into subepithelial tissue. Release of chemotactic factors as a result of complement activation contributes to inflammation, as does the toxic effect of LOS in provoking the release of inflammatory cytokines.

The importance of humoral immunity in host defenses against neisserial infections is best illustrated by the predisposition of persons deficient in terminal complement components (C5 through C9) to recurrent bacteremic gonococcal infections and to recurrent meningococcal meningitis or meningococcemia. Gonococcal porin induces T cell–proliferative responses in persons with urogenital gonococcal disease. A significant increase in porin-specific interleukin (IL) 4–producing CD4+ as well as CD8+ T lymphocytes is seen in individuals with mucosal gonococcal disease. A portion of these lymphocytes that show a porin-specific T_H2-type response could traffic to mucosal surfaces and play a role in immune protection against the disease. Few data clearly indicate that protective immunity is acquired from a previous gonococcal infection, although bactericidal and opsonophagocytic antibodies to porin and LOS may offer partial protection. On the other hand, women who are infected and acquire high levels of antibody to another outer-membrane protein, Rmp (reduction modifiable protein, formerly called protein III), may be especially likely to become reinfected with *N. gonorrhoeae* because Rmp antibodies block the effect of bactericidal antibodies to porin and LOS. Rmp shows little, if any, interstrain antigenic variation; therefore, Rmp antibodies potentially may block antibody-mediated killing of all gonococci. The mechanism of blocking has not been fully characterized, but Rmp antibodies noncompetitively inhibit binding of porin and LOS antibodies because of the proximity of these structures in the gonococcal outer membrane. In male volunteers who have no history of gonorrhea, the net effect of these events may influence the outcome of experimental challenge with *N. gonorrhoeae*. Because Rmp bears extensive homology to enterobacterial OmpA and meningococcal class 4 proteins, it is possible that these blocking antibodies result from prior exposure to cross-reacting proteins from these species and also play a role in first-time infection with *N. gonorrhoeae*.

Gonococcal resistance to antimicrobial agents

It is no surprise that *N. gonorrhoeae*, with its remarkable capacity to alter its antigenic structure and adapt to changes in the microenvironment, has become resistant to numerous antibiotics. The first effective agents against gonorrhea were the sulfonamides, which were introduced in the 1930s and became ineffective within a decade. Penicillin was then employed as the drug of choice for the treatment of gonorrhea. By 1965, 42% of gonococcal isolates had developed low-level resistance to penicillin G. Resistance due to the production of penicillinase arose later.

Gonococci become fully resistant to antibiotics either by chromosomal mutations or by acquisition of R factors (plasmids). Two types of chromosomal mutations have been described. The first type, which is drug specific, is a single-step mutation leading to high-level resistance. The second type involves mutations at several chromosomal loci that combine to determine the level as well as the pattern of resistance. Strains with mutations in chromosomal genes were first observed in the late 1950s. As recently as 2004, chromosomal mutations accounted for resistance to penicillin, tetracycline, or both in ~12% of strains surveyed in the United States.

β-Lactamase (penicillinase)–producing strains of *N. gonorrhoeae* (PPNG) carrying plasmids with the Pc^r determinant had rapidly spread worldwide by the early 1980s. *N. gonorrhoeae* strains with plasmid-borne tetracycline resistance (TRNG) can mobilize some β-lactamase plasmids, and PPNG and TRNG occur together, sometimes along with strains exhibiting chromosomally mediated resistance (CMRNG). Penicillin, ampicillin, and tetracycline are no longer reliable for the treatment of gonorrhea and should not be used.

Quinolone-containing regimens were also recommended for treatment of gonococcal infections; the fluoroquinolones offered the advantage of antichlamydial activity when administered for

7 days. However, quinolone-resistant *N. gonorrhoeae* (QRNG) appeared soon after these agents were first used to treat gonorrhea. QRNG is particularly common in the Pacific Islands (including Hawaii) and Asia, where, in certain areas, all gonococcal strains are now resistant to quinolones. At present, QRNG is also common in parts of Europe and the Middle East. In the United States, QRNG has been identified in midwestern and eastern areas as well as in states on the Pacific coast, where resistant strains were first seen. Alterations in DNA gyrase and topoisomerase IV have been implicated as mechanisms of fluoroquinolone resistance.

Resistance to spectinomycin, which has been used in the past as an alternative agent, has been reported. Since this agent usually is not associated with resistance to other antibiotics, spectinomycin can be reserved for use against multiresistant strains of *N. gonorrhoeae*. Nevertheless, outbreaks caused by strains resistant to spectinomycin have been documented in Korea and England when the drug has been used for primary treatment of gonorrhea.

Third-generation cephalosporins have remained highly effective as single-dose therapy for gonorrhea despite recent evidence that their minimal inhibitory concentrations (MICs) against strains of *N. gonorrhoeae* are increasing. Even though the MICs of ceftriaxone against certain strains may reach 0.015–0.125 μg/mL (higher than the MICs of 0.0001–0.008 μg/mL for fully susceptible strains), these levels are greatly exceeded in the blood, the urethra, and the cervix when the routinely recommended parenteral dose of ceftriaxone is administered. All *N. gonorrhoeae* strains with reduced susceptibility to ceftriaxone and cefixime (termed *cephalosporin intermediate/resistant strains*) contain (1) a mosaic *penA* allele encoding a penicillin-binding protein 2 (PBP 2) whose sequence differs in nearly 60 amino acids from that of wild-type PBP 2 and (2) additional genetic resistance determinants that are also required for high-level penicillin resistance.

■ CLINICAL MANIFESTATIONS

Gonococcal infections in males

Acute urethritis is the most common clinical manifestation of gonorrhea in males. The usual incubation period after exposure is 2–7 days, although the interval can be longer and some men remain asymptomatic. Strains of the PorB.1A serotype tend to cause a greater proportion of cases of mild and asymptomatic urethritis than do PorB.1B strains. Urethral discharge and dysuria, usually without urinary frequency or urgency, are the major symptoms. The discharge initially is scant and mucoid but becomes profuse and purulent within a day or two. Gram's stain of the urethral discharge may reveal PMNs and gram-negative intracellular monococci and diplococci (Fig. 144-1). The clinical manifestations of gonococcal urethritis are usually more severe and overt than those of

nongonococcal urethritis, including urethritis caused by *Chlamydia trachomatis* (Chap. 176); however, exceptions are common, and it is often impossible to differentiate the causes of urethritis on clinical grounds alone. The majority of cases of urethritis seen in the United States today are not caused by *N. gonorrhoeae* and/or *C. trachomatis*. Although a number of other organisms may be responsible, many cases do not have a specific etiologic agent identified.

Most symptomatic men with gonorrhea seek treatment and cease to be infectious. The remaining men, who are largely asymptomatic, accumulate in number over time and constitute about two-thirds of all infected men at any point in time. Together with men incubating the organism (who shed the organism but are asymptomatic), they serve as the source of spread of infection. Before the antibiotic era, symptoms of urethritis persisted for ~8 weeks. Epididymitis is now an uncommon complication, and gonococcal prostatitis occurs rarely, if at all. Other unusual local complications of gonococcal urethritis include edema of the penis due to dorsal lymphangitis or thrombophlebitis, submucous inflammatory "soft" infiltration of the urethral wall, periurethral abscess or fistula, inflammation or abscess of Cowper's gland, and seminal vesiculitis. Balanitis may develop in uncircumcised men.

Gonococcal infections in females

Gonococcal cervicitis Mucopurulent cervicitis is the most common STI diagnosis in American women and may be caused by *N. gonorrhoeae*, *C. trachomatis*, and other organisms. Cervicitis may coexist with candidal or trichomonal vaginitis. *N. gonorrhoeae* primarily infects the columnar epithelium of the cervical os. Bartholin's glands occasionally become infected.

Women infected with *N. gonorrhoeae* usually develop symptoms. However, the women who either remain asymptomatic or have only minor symptoms may delay in seeking medical attention. These minor symptoms may include scant vaginal discharge issuing from the inflamed cervix (without vaginitis or vaginosis per se) and dysuria (often without urgency or frequency) that may be associated with gonococcal urethritis. Although the incubation period of gonorrhea is less well defined in women than in men, symptoms usually develop within 10 days of infection and are more acute and intense than those of chlamydial cervicitis.

The physical examination may reveal a mucopurulent discharge (mucopus) issuing from the cervical os. Because Gram's stain is not sensitive for the diagnosis of gonorrhea in women, specimens should be submitted for culture or a nonculture assay (see below). Edematous and friable cervical ectopy as well as endocervical bleeding induced by gentle swabbing are more often seen in chlamydial infection. Gonococcal infection may extend deep enough to produce dyspareunia and lower abdominal or back pain. In such cases, it is imperative to consider a diagnosis of pelvic inflammatory disease (PID) and to administer treatment for that disease (Chaps. 130 and 176).

N. gonorrhoeae may be recovered from the urethra and rectum of women with cervicitis, but these are rarely the only infected sites. Urethritis in women may produce symptoms of internal dysuria, which is often attributed to "cystitis." Pyuria in the absence of bacteriuria seen on Gram's stain of unspun urine, accompanied by urine cultures that fail to yield >10² colonies of bacteria usually associated with urinary tract infection, signifies the possibility of urethritis due to *C. trachomatis*. Urethral infection with *N. gonorrhoeae* may also occur in this context, but in this instance urethral cultures are usually positive.

Gonococcal vaginitis The vaginal mucosa of healthy women is lined by stratified squamous epithelium and is rarely infected by *N. gonorrhoeae*. However, gonococcal vaginitis can occur in anestrogenic women (e.g., prepubertal girls and postmenopausal women), in

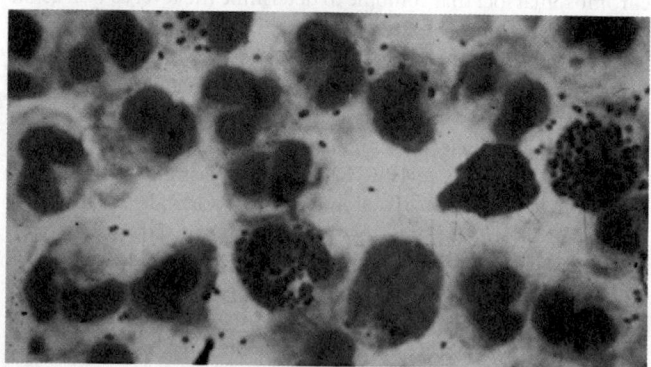

Figure 144-1 Gram's stain of urethral discharge from a male patient with gonorrhea shows gram-negative intracellular monococci and diplococci. *(From the Public Health Agency of Canada.)*

whom the vaginal stratified squamous epithelium is often thinned down to the basilar layer, which can be infected by *N. gonorrhoeae*. The intense inflammation of the vagina makes the physical (speculum and bimanual) examination extremely painful. The vaginal mucosa is red and edematous, and an abundant purulent discharge is present. Infection in the urethra and in Skene's and Bartholin's glands often accompanies gonococcal vaginitis. Inflamed cervical erosion or abscesses in nabothian cysts may also occur. Coexisting cervicitis may result in pus in the cervical os.

Anorectal gonorrhea

Because the female anatomy permits the spread of cervical exudate to the rectum, *N. gonorrhoeae* is sometimes recovered from the rectum of women with uncomplicated gonococcal cervicitis. The rectum is the sole site of infection in only 5% of women with gonorrhea. Such women are usually asymptomatic but occasionally have acute proctitis manifested by anorectal pain or pruritus, tenesmus, purulent rectal discharge, and rectal bleeding. Among men who have sex with men (MSM), the frequency of gonococcal infection, including rectal infection, fell by ≥90% throughout the United States in the early 1980s, but a resurgence of gonorrhea among MSM has been documented in several cities since the 1990s. Gonococcal isolates from the rectum of MSM tend to be more resistant to antimicrobial agents than are gonococcal isolates from other sites. Gonococcal isolates with a mutation in *mtrR* (multiple transferable resistance repressor) or in the promoter region of the gene that encodes for this transcriptional repressor develop increased resistance to antimicrobial hydrophobic agents such as bile acids and fatty acids in feces and thus are found with increased frequency in MSM. This situation may have been responsible for higher rates of failure of treatment for rectal gonorrhea with older regimens consisting of penicillin or tetracyclines.

Pharyngeal gonorrhea

Pharyngeal gonorrhea is usually mild or asymptomatic, although symptomatic pharyngitis does occasionally occur with cervical lymphadenitis. The mode of acquisition is oral-genital sexual exposure, with fellatio being a more efficient means of transmission than cunnilingus. Most cases resolve spontaneously, and transmission from the pharynx to sexual contacts is rare. Pharyngeal infection almost always coexists with genital infection. Swabs from the pharynx should be plated directly onto gonococcal selective media. Pharyngeal colonization with *Neisseria meningitidis* needs to be differentiated from that with other *Neisseria* species.

Ocular gonorrhea in adults

Ocular gonorrhea in an adult usually results from autoinoculation from an infected genital site. As in genital infection, the manifestations range from severe to occasionally mild or asymptomatic disease. The variability in clinical manifestations may be attributable to differences in the ability of the infecting strain to elicit an inflammatory response. Infection may result in a markedly swollen eyelid, severe hyperemia and chemosis, and a profuse purulent discharge. The massively inflamed conjunctiva may be draped over the cornea and limbus. Lytic enzymes from the infiltrating PMNs occasionally cause corneal ulceration and rarely cause perforation.

Prompt recognition and treatment of this condition are of paramount importance. Gram's stain and culture of the purulent discharge establish the diagnosis. Genital cultures should also be performed.

Gonorrhea in pregnant women, neonates, and children

Gonorrhea in pregnancy can have serious consequences for both the mother and the infant. Recognition of gonorrhea early in pregnancy also identifies a population at risk for other STIs, particularly chlamydial infection, syphilis, and trichomoniasis. The risks of salpingitis and PID—conditions associated with a high rate of fetal loss—are highest during the first trimester. Pharyngeal infection, most often asymptomatic, may be more common during pregnancy because of altered sexual practices. Prolonged rupture of the membranes, premature delivery, chorioamnionitis, funisitis (infection of the umbilical cord stump), and sepsis in the infant (with *N. gonorrhoeae* detected in the newborn's gastric aspirate during delivery) are common complications of maternal gonococcal infection at term. Other microorganisms and conditions, including *Mycoplasma hominis*, *Ureaplasma urealyticum*, *C. trachomatis*, and bacterial vaginosis (often accompanied by infection with *Trichomonas vaginalis*), have been associated with similar complications.

The most common form of gonorrhea in neonates is ophthalmia neonatorum, which results from exposure to infected cervical secretions during parturition. Ocular neonatal instillation of a prophylactic agent (e.g., 1% silver nitrate eyedrops or ophthalmic preparations containing erythromycin or tetracycline) prevents ophthalmia neonatorum but is not effective for its treatment, which requires systemic antibiotics. The clinical manifestations are acute and usually begin 2–5 days after birth. An initial nonspecific conjunctivitis with a serosanguineous discharge is followed by tense edema of the eyelids, chemosis, and a profuse, thick, purulent discharge. Corneal ulcerations that result in nebulae or perforation may lead to anterior synechiae, anterior staphyloma, panophthalmitis, and blindness. Infections described at other mucosal sites in infants, including vaginitis, rhinitis, and anorectal infection, are likely to be asymptomatic. Pharyngeal colonization has been demonstrated in 35% of infants with gonococcal ophthalmia, and coughing is the most prominent symptom in these cases. Septic arthritis (see below) is the most common manifestation of systemic infection or DGI in the newborn. The onset usually comes at 3–21 days of age, and polyarticular involvement is common. Sepsis, meningitis, and pneumonia are seen in rare instances.

Any STI in children beyond the neonatal period raises the possibility of sexual abuse. Gonococcal vulvovaginitis is the most common manifestation of gonococcal infection in children beyond infancy. Anorectal and pharyngeal infections are common in these children and are frequently asymptomatic. The urethra, Bartholin's and Skene's glands, and the upper genital tract are rarely involved. All children with gonococcal infection should also be evaluated for chlamydial infection, syphilis, and possibly HIV infection.

Gonococcal arthritis (DGI)

DGI (gonococcal arthritis) results from gonococcal bacteremia. In the 1970s, DGI occurred in ~0.5–3% of persons with untreated gonococcal mucosal infection. The lower incidence of DGI at present is probably attributable to a decline in the prevalence of particular strains that are likely to disseminate. DGI strains resist the bactericidal action of human serum and generally do not incite inflammation at genital sites, probably because of limited generation of chemotactic factors. Strains recovered from DGI cases in the 1970s were often of the PorB.1A serotype, were highly susceptible to penicillin, and had special growth requirements—including arginine, hypoxanthine, and uracil—that made the organism more fastidious and more difficult to isolate.

Menstruation is a risk factor for dissemination, and approximately two-thirds of cases of DGI are in women. In about half of affected women, symptoms of DGI begin within 7 days of onset of menses. Complement deficiencies, especially of the components involved in the assembly of the membrane attack complex (C5 through C9), predispose to neisserial bacteremia, and persons with more than one episode of DGI should be screened with an assay for total hemolytic complement activity.

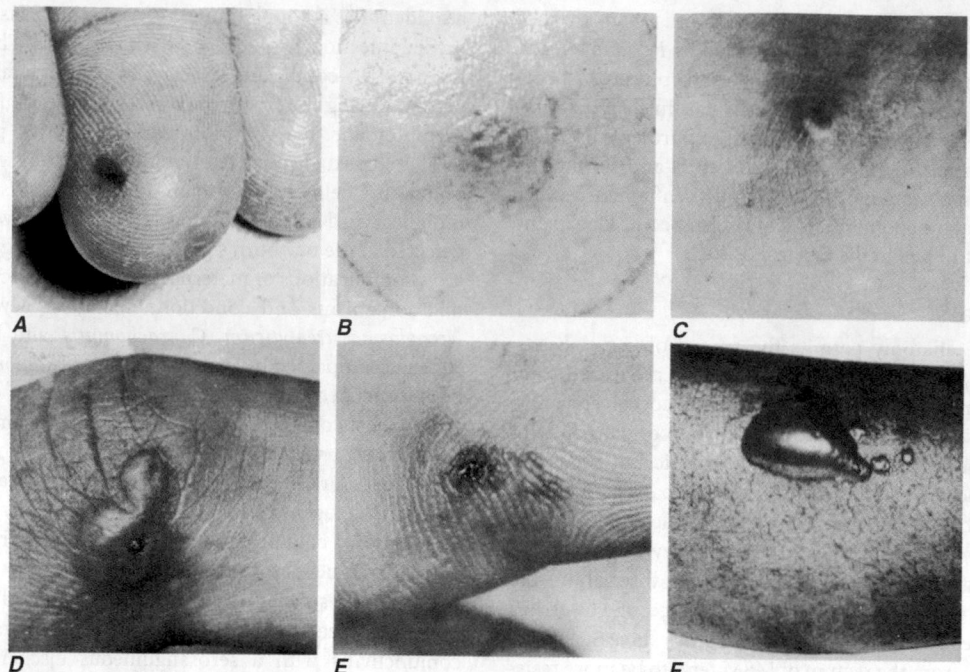

Figure 144-2 Characteristic skin lesions in patients with proven gonococcal bacteremia. The lesions are in various stages of evolution. **A.** Very early petechia on finger. **B.** Early papular lesion, 7 mm in diameter, on lower leg. **C.** Pustule with central eschar resulting from early petechial lesion. **D.** Pustular lesion on finger. **E.** Mature lesion with central necrosis (black) on hemorrhagic base. **F.** Bullae on anterior tibial surface. *(Reprinted with permission from KK Holmes et al: Disseminated gonococcal infection. Ann Intern Med 74:979, 1971.)*

The clinical manifestations of DGI have sometimes been classified into two stages: a bacteremic stage, which is less common today, and a joint-localized stage with suppurative arthritis. A clear-cut progression usually is not evident. Patients in the bacteremic stage have higher temperatures, and chills more frequently accompany their fever. Painful joints are common and often occur together with tenosynovitis and skin lesions. Polyarthralgias usually include the knees, elbows, and more distal joints; the axial skeleton is generally spared. Skin lesions are seen in ~75% of patients and include papules and pustules, often with a hemorrhagic component (Fig. 144-2; see also Fig. e7-44). Other manifestations of noninfectious dermatitis, such as nodular lesions, urticaria, and erythema multiforme, have been described. These lesions are usually on the extremities and number between 5 and 40. The differential diagnosis of the bacteremic stage of DGI includes reactive arthritis, acute rheumatoid arthritis, sarcoidosis, erythema nodosum, drug-induced arthritis, and viral infections (e.g., hepatitis B and acute HIV infection). The distribution of joint symptoms in reactive arthritis differs from that in DGI (Fig. 144-3), as do the skin and genital manifestations (Chap. 325).

Suppurative arthritis involves one or two joints, most often the knees, wrists, ankles, and elbows (in decreasing order of frequency); other joints occasionally are involved. Most patients who develop gonococcal septic arthritis do so without prior polyarthralgias or skin lesions; in the absence of symptomatic genital infection, this disease cannot be distinguished from septic arthritis caused by other pathogens. The differential diagnosis of acute arthritis in young adults is discussed in Chap. 334. Rarely, osteomyelitis complicates septic arthritis involving small joints of the hand.

Gonococcal endocarditis, although rare today, was a relatively common complication of DGI in the preantibiotic era, accounting for about one-quarter of reported cases of endocarditis. Another unusual complication of DGI is meningitis.

Gonococcal infections in HIV-infected persons

The association between gonorrhea and the acquisition of HIV has been demonstrated in several well-controlled studies, mainly in Kenya and Zaire. The nonulcerative STIs enhance the transmission of HIV by three- to fivefold, possibly because of increased viral shedding by persons with urethritis or cervicitis (Chap. 189). HIV has been detected by polymerase chain reaction (PCR) more commonly

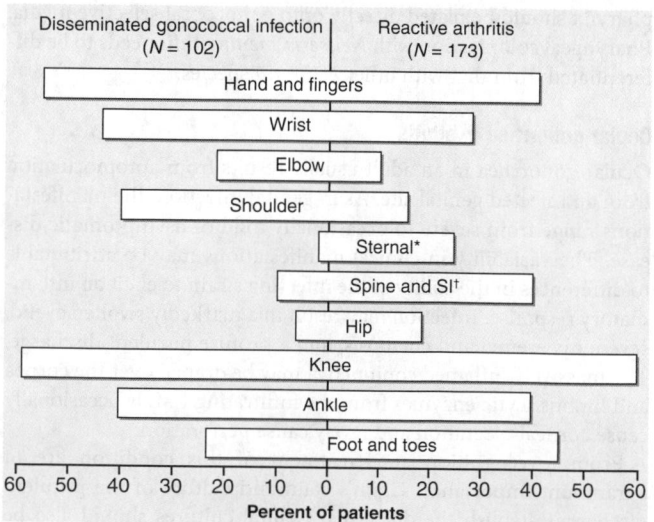

Figure 144-3 Distributions of joints with arthritis in 102 patients with disseminated gonococcal infection and 173 patients with reactive arthritis. *Includes the sternoclavicular joints. †SI, sacroiliac joint. *(Reprinted with permission from M Kousa et al: Frequent association of chlamydial infection with Reiter's syndrome. Sex Transm Dis 5:57, 1978.)*

in ejaculates from HIV-positive men with gonococcal urethritis than in those from HIV-positive men with nongonococcal urethritis. PCR positivity diminishes by twofold after appropriate therapy for urethritis. Not only does gonorrhea enhance the transmission of HIV, it may also increase the individual's risk for acquisition of HIV. A proposed mechanism is the significantly greater number of CD4+ T lymphocytes and dendritic cells that can be infected by HIV in endocervical secretions of women with nonulcerative STIs than in those of women with ulcerative STIs.

LABORATORY DIAGNOSIS

A rapid diagnosis of gonococcal infection in men may be obtained by Gram's staining of urethral exudates (Fig. 144-1). The detection of gram-negative intracellular monococci and diplococci is usually highly specific and sensitive in diagnosing gonococcal urethritis in symptomatic males but is only ~50% sensitive in diagnosing gonococcal cervicitis. Samples should be collected with Dacron or rayon swabs. Part of the sample should be inoculated onto a plate of modified Thayer-Martin or other gonococcal selective medium for culture. It is important to process all samples immediately because gonococci do not tolerate drying. If plates cannot be incubated immediately, they can be held safely for several hours at room temperature in candle extinction jars prior to incubation. If processing is to occur within 6 h, transport of specimens may be facilitated by the use of nonnutritive swab transport systems such as Stuart or Amies medium. For longer holding periods (e.g., when specimens for culture are to be mailed), culture media with self-contained CO_2-generating systems (such as the JEMBEC or Gono-Pak systems) may be used. Specimens should also be obtained for the diagnosis of chlamydial infection (Chap. 176).

PMNs are often seen in the endocervix on a Gram's stain, and an abnormally increased number (≥30 PMNs per field in five 1000× oil-immersion microscopic fields) establishes the presence of an inflammatory discharge. Unfortunately, the presence or absence of gram-negative intracellular monococci or diplococci in cervical smears does not accurately predict which patients have gonorrhea, and the diagnosis in this setting should be made by culture or another suitable nonculture diagnostic method. The sensitivity of a single endocervical culture is ~80–90%. If a history of rectal sex is elicited, a rectal wall swab (uncontaminated with feces) should be cultured. A presumptive diagnosis of gonorrhea cannot be made on the basis of gram-negative diplococci in smears from the pharynx, where other *Neisseria* species are components of the normal flora.

Increasingly, nucleic acid probe tests are being substituted for culture for the direct detection of *N. gonorrhoeae* in urogenital specimens. A common assay employs a nonisotopic chemiluminescent DNA probe that hybridizes specifically with gonococcal 16S ribosomal RNA; this assay is as sensitive as conventional culture techniques. A disadvantage of non-culture-based assays is that *N. gonorrhoeae* cannot be grown from the transport systems. Thus a culture-confirmatory test and formal antimicrobial susceptibility testing, if needed, cannot be performed. Nucleic acid amplification tests (NAATs), including Roche Amplicor, Gen-Probe APTIMA Combo2 (which also detects *Chlamydia*), and BD ProbeTec ET, offer an advantage: urine samples can be tested with a sensitivity similar to that obtained when urethral or cervical swab samples are assessed by culture and other non-NAATs.

Because of the legal implications, the preferred method for the diagnosis of gonococcal infection in children is a standardized culture. Two positive NAATs, each targeting a different nucleic acid sequence, may be substituted for culture of the cervix or the urethra as legal evidence of infection; however, cervical specimens are not recommended for prepubertal girls. Nonculture tests for gonococcal infection have not been approved by the U.S. Food and Drug Administration for use with specimens obtained from the pharynx and rectum of infected children. Cultures should be obtained from the pharynx and anus of both girls and boys, the vagina of girls, and the urethra of boys. For boys with a urethral discharge, a meatal specimen of the discharge is adequate for culture. Presumptive colonies of *N. gonorrhoeae* should be identified definitively by at least two independent methods.

Blood should be cultured in suspected cases of DGI. The use of Isolator blood culture tubes may enhance the yield. The probability of positive blood cultures decreases after 48 h of illness. Synovial fluid should be inoculated into blood culture broth medium and plated onto chocolate agar rather than selective medium because this fluid is not likely to be contaminated with commensal bacteria. Gonococci are infrequently recovered from early joint effusions containing <20,000 leukocytes/μL but may be recovered from effusions containing >80,000 leukocytes/μL. The organisms are seldom recovered from blood and synovial fluid of the same patient.

TREATMENT   Gonococcal Infections

Treatment failure can lead to continued transmission and the emergence of antibiotic resistance. The importance of adequate treatment with a regimen that the patient will adhere to cannot be overemphasized. Thus highly effective single-dose regimens have been developed for uncomplicated gonococcal infections. The 2010 treatment guidelines for gonococcal infections from the Centers for Disease Control and Prevention are summarized in Table 144-1; the recommendations for uncomplicated gonorrhea apply to HIV-infected as well as HIV-uninfected patients.

Single-dose regimens of the third-generation cephalosporins ceftriaxone (given IM) and cefixime (given orally) currently are the mainstays of therapy for uncomplicated gonococcal infection of the urethra, cervix, rectum, or pharynx and almost always result in an effective cure. Outside the United States, cefixime has been associated with rare treatment failures caused by strains of *N. gonorrhoeae* with elevated MICs of third-generation cephalosporins. Quinolone-containing regimens are no longer recommended in the United States as first-line treatment because of widespread resistance to these agents.

Because co-infection with *C. trachomatis* occurs frequently, initial treatment regimens must also incorporate an agent (e.g., azithromycin or doxycycline) that is effective against chlamydial infection. Pregnant women with gonorrhea, who should not take doxycycline, should receive concurrent treatment with a macrolide antibiotic for possible chlamydial infection. A single 1-g dose of azithromycin, which is effective therapy for uncomplicated chlamydial infections, results in an unacceptably low cure rate (93%) for gonococcal infections and should not be used alone. A single 2-g dose of azithromycin, particularly in the extended-release microsphere formulation, delivers azithromycin to the lower gastrointestinal tract, thereby improving tolerability. Azithromycin is effective against sensitive strains, but this drug is expensive, causes gastrointestinal distress, and is not recommended for routine or first-line treatment of gonorrhea. Spectinomycin has been used as an alternative regimen for the treatment of uncomplicated gonococcal infections in penicillin-allergic persons outside the United States but is not currently available in this country. Of note, the limited effectiveness of spectinomycin for the treatment of pharyngeal infection reduces its utility in populations among whom such infection is common, such as MSM.

Persons with uncomplicated infections who receive a recommended regimen do not need a test of cure. Cultures for *N. gonorrhoeae* should be performed if symptoms persist after

TABLE 144-1 Recommended Treatment for Gonococcal Infections: 2010 Guidelines of the Centers for Disease Control and Prevention

Diagnosis	Treatment of Choice[a]
Uncomplicated gonococcal infection of the cervix, urethra, pharynx[b], or rectum	
First-line regimens	Ceftriaxone (250 mg IM, single dose)
	or
	Cefixime (400 mg PO, single dose)
	plus
	Treatment for *Chlamydia* if chlamydial infection is not ruled out:
	Azithromycin (1 g PO, single dose)
	or
	Doxycycline (100 mg PO bid for 7 days)
Alternative regimens	Ceftizoxime (500 mg IM, single dose)
	or
	Cefotaxime (500 mg IM, single dose)
	or
	Spectinomycin (2 g IM, single dose)[c,d]
	or
	Cefotetan (1 g IM, single dose) plus probenecid (1 g PO, single dose)[c]
	or
	Cefoxitin (2 g IM, single dose) plus probenecid (1 g PO, single dose)[c]
Epididymitis	See Chap. 130
Pelvic inflammatory disease	See Chap. 130
Gonococcal conjunctivitis in an adult	Ceftriaxone (1 g IM, single dose)[e]
Ophthalmia neonatorum[f]	Ceftriaxone (25–50 mg/kg IV, single dose, not to exceed 125 mg)
Disseminated gonococcal infection[g]	
Initial therapy[h]	
Patient tolerant of β-lactam drugs	Ceftriaxone (1 g IM or IV q24h; recommended)
	or
	Cefotaxime (1 g IV q8h)
	or
	Ceftizoxime (1 g IV q8h)
Patients allergic to β-lactam drugs	Spectinomycin (2 g IM q12h)[d]
Continuation therapy	Cefixime (400 mg PO bid)
Meningitis or endocarditis	See text[i]

[a]True failure of treatment with a recommended regimen is rare and should prompt an evaluation for reinfection or consideration of an alternative diagnosis.

[b]Ceftriaxone is the only agent recommended for treatment of pharyngeal infection.

[c]Spectinomycin, cefotetan, and cefoxitin, which are alternative agents, currently are unavailable or in short supply in the United States.

[d]Spectinomycin may be ineffective for the treatment of pharyngeal gonorrhea.

[e]Plus lavage of the infected eye with saline solution (once).

[f]Prophylactic regimens are discussed in the text.

[g]Hospitalization is indicated if the diagnosis is uncertain, if the patient has frank arthritis with an effusion, or if the patient cannot be relied on to adhere to treatment.

[h]All initial regimens should be continued for 24–48 h after clinical improvement begins, at which time the switch may be made to one of the continuation regimens to complete a full week of antimicrobial treatment. Treatment for chlamydial infection (as above) should be given if this infection has not been ruled out. Fluoroquinolones may be an option if antimicrobial susceptibility can be documented by culture of the causative organism.

[i]Hospitalization is indicated to exclude suspected meningitis or endocarditis.

therapy with an established regimen, and any gonococci isolated should be tested for antimicrobial susceptibility.

Symptomatic gonococcal pharyngitis is more difficult to eradicate than genital infection. Persons who cannot tolerate cephalosporins and those in whom quinolones are contraindicated may be treated with spectinomycin if it is available, but this agent results in a cure rate of ≤52%. Persons given spectinomycin should have a pharyngeal sample cultured 3–5 days after treatment as a test of cure. A single 2-g dose of azithromycin may be used in areas where rates of resistance to azithromycin are low.

Treatments for gonococcal epididymitis and PID are discussed in Chap. 130. Ocular gonococcal infections in older children and adults should be managed with a single dose of ceftriaxone combined with saline irrigation of the conjunctivae (both undertaken expeditiously), and patients should undergo a careful ophthalmologic evaluation that includes a slit-lamp examination.

DGI may require higher dosages and longer durations of therapy (Table 144-1). Hospitalization is indicated if the diagnosis is uncertain, if the patient has localized joint disease that requires aspiration, or if the patient cannot be relied on to comply with treatment. Open drainage is necessary only occasionally—e.g., for management of hip infections that may be difficult to drain percutaneously. Nonsteroidal anti-inflammatory agents may be indicated to alleviate pain and hasten clinical improvement of affected joints. Gonococcal meningitis and endocarditis should be treated in the hospital with high-dose IV ceftriaxone (1–2 g every 12 h); therapy should continue for 10–14 days for meningitis and for at least 4 weeks for endocarditis. All persons who experience more than one episode of DGI should be evaluated for complement deficiency.

■ PREVENTION AND CONTROL

Condoms, if properly used, provide effective protection against the transmission and acquisition of gonorrhea as well as other infections that are transmitted to and from genital mucosal surfaces. Spermicidal preparations used with a diaphragm or cervical sponges impregnated with nonoxynol 9 offer some protection against gonorrhea and chlamydial infection. However, the frequent use of preparations that contain nonoxynol 9 is associated with mucosal disruption that paradoxically may enhance the risk of HIV infection in the event of exposure. All patients should be instructed to refer sex partners for evaluation and treatment. All sex partners of persons with gonorrhea should be evaluated and treated for *N. gonorrhoeae* and *C. trachomatis* infections if their last contact with the patient took place within 60 days before the onset of symptoms or the diagnosis of infection in the patient. If the patient's last sexual encounter was >60 days before onset of symptoms or diagnosis, the patient's most recent sex partner should be treated. Partner-delivered medications or prescriptions for medications to treat gonorrhea and chlamydial infection diminish the likelihood of reinfection (or relapse) in the infected patient. In states where it is legal, this approach is an option for partner management. Patients should be instructed to abstain from sexual intercourse until therapy is completed and until they and their sex partners no longer have symptoms. Greater emphasis must be placed on prevention by public health education, individual patient counseling, and behavior modification. Sexually active persons, especially adolescents, should be offered screening for STIs. For males, a NAAT on urine or a urethral swab may be used for screening. Preventing the spread of gonorrhea may help reduce the transmission of HIV. No effective vaccine for gonorrhea is yet available, but efforts to test several candidates are under way.

ACKNOWLEDGMENTS

The authors acknowledge the contributions of Dr. King K. Holmes and Dr. Stephen A. Morse to the chapter on this subject in earlier editions.

FURTHER READINGS

CENTERS FOR DISEASE CONTROL AND PREVENTION: Gonococcal Isolate Surveillance Project (GISP); *www.cdc.gov/std/GISP/*

———: Sexually transmitted diseases treatment guidelines, 2010. MMWR Recomm Rep 59(RR-12):49, 2010

GAYDOS CA: Nucleic acid amplification tests for gonorrhea and *Chlamydia*: Practice and applications. Infect Dis Clin North Am 19:367, 2005

GOLDEN MR et al: Effect of expedited treatment of sex partners on recurrent or persistent gonorrhea or chlamydial infections. N Engl J Med 352:676, 2005

HOOK EW III, HOLMES KK: Gonococcal infections. Ann Intern Med 102:229, 1985

LAGA M et al: Non-ulcerative sexually transmitted diseases as risk factors for HIV-1 transmission in women: Results from a cohort study. AIDS 7:95, 1993

O'BRIEN JP et al: Disseminated gonococcal infection: A prospective analysis of 49 patients and a review of pathophysiology and immune mechanisms. Medicine (Baltimore) 62:395, 1983

WORKOWSKI KA et al: Emerging antimicrobial resistance in *Neisseria gonorrhoeae*: Urgent need to strengthen prevention strategies. Ann Intern Med 148:606, 2008

ZHAO S et al: Genetics of chromosomally mediated intermediate resistance to ceftriaxone and cefixime in *Neisseria gonorrhoeae*. Antimicrob Agents Chemother 53:3744, 2009

CHAPTER 145

Haemophilus and Moraxella Infections

Timothy F. Murphy

HAEMOPHILUS INFLUENZAE

◼ MICROBIOLOGY

Haemophilus influenzae was first recognized in 1892 by Pfeiffer, who erroneously concluded that the bacterium was the cause of influenza. The bacterium is a small (1- by 0.3-μm) gram-negative organism of variable shape; hence, it is often described as a pleomorphic coccobacillus. In clinical specimens such as cerebrospinal fluid (CSF) and sputum, it frequently stains only faintly with safranin and therefore can easily be overlooked.

H. influenzae grows both aerobically and anaerobically. Its aerobic growth requires two factors: hemin (X factor) and nicotinamide adenine dinucleotide (V factor). These requirements are used in the clinical laboratory to identify the bacterium. Caution must be used to distinguish *H. influenzae* from *H. haemolyticus*, a respiratory tract commensal that has identical growth requirements. *H. haemolyticus* has classically been distinguished from *H. influenzae* by hemolysis on horse blood agar. However, a significant proportion of isolates of *H. haemolyticus* have now been recognized as nonhemolytic. Analysis of 16S ribosomal sequences is one reliable method to distinguish these two species.

Six major serotypes of *H. influenzae* have been identified; designated *a* through *f*, they are based on antigenically distinct polysaccharide capsules. In addition, some strains lack a polysaccharide capsule and are referred to as *nontypable* strains. Type b and nontypable strains are the most relevant strains clinically (Table 145-1), although encapsulated strains other than type b can cause disease. *H. influenzae* was the first free-living organism to have its entire genome sequenced.

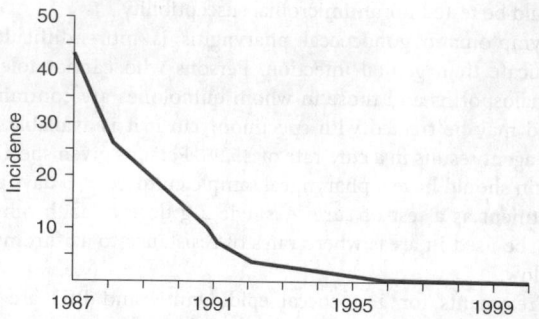

Figure 145-1   Estimated incidence (rate per 100,000) of invasive disease due to *Haemophilus influenzae* type b among children <5 years of age: 1987–2000. Fewer than 40 cases per year have been reported since 2000. *(Data from the Centers for Disease Control and Prevention.)*

The antigenically distinct type b capsule is a linear polymer composed of ribosyl-ribitol phosphate. Strains of *H. influenzae* type b (Hib) cause disease primarily in infants and children <6 years of age. Nontypable strains are primarily mucosal pathogens but occasionally cause invasive disease.

◼ EPIDEMIOLOGY AND TRANSMISSION

H. influenzae, an exclusively human pathogen, is spread by airborne droplets or by direct contact with secretions or fomites. Colonization with nontypable *H. influenzae* is a dynamic process; new strains are acquired and other strains are replaced periodically.

The widespread use of Hib conjugate vaccines in many industrialized countries has resulted in striking decreases in the rate of nasopharyngeal colonization by Hib and in the incidence of Hib infection (Fig. 145-1). However, the majority of the world's children remain unimmunized. Worldwide, invasive Hib disease occurs predominantly in unimmunized children and in those who have not completed the primary immunization series. Certain groups have a higher incidence of invasive Hib disease than the general population, including black children and Native American groups. Although this increased incidence has not yet been accounted for, several factors may be relevant, including age at exposure to the bacterium, socioeconomic conditions, and genetic differences.

◼ PATHOGENESIS

Hib strains cause systemic disease by invasion and hematogenous spread from the respiratory tract to distant sites such as the meninges, bones, and joints. The type b polysaccharide capsule is an important virulence factor affecting the bacterium's ability to avoid opsonization and cause systemic disease.

Nontypable strains cause disease by local invasion of mucosal surfaces. Otitis media results when bacteria reach the middle ear by way of the eustachian tube. Adults with chronic bronchitis experience recurrent lower respiratory tract infection due to nontypable strains. In addition, persistent nontypable *H. influenzae* colonization of the lower airways of adults with chronic obstructive pulmonary disease (COPD) contributes to the airway inflammation that is a hallmark of the disease. Nontypable strains that cause infection in adults with COPD differ in pathogenic potential and genome content from strains that cause otitis media. The incidence of invasive disease caused by nontypable strains is low. Strains that cause invasive disease are genetically and phenotypically diverse.

◼ IMMUNE RESPONSE

Antibody to the capsule is important in protection from infection by Hib strains. The level of (maternally acquired) serum antibody

TABLE 145-1   Characteristics of Type b and Nontypable Strains of *Haemophilus influenzae*

Feature	Type b Strains	Nontypable Strains
Capsule	Ribosyl-ribitol phosphate	Unencapsulated
Pathogenesis	Invasive infections due to hematogenous spread	Mucosal infections due to contiguous spread
Clinical manifestations	Meningitis and invasive infections in incompletely immunized infants and children	Otitis media in infants and children; lower respiratory tract infections in adults with chronic bronchitis
Evolutionary history	Basically clonal	Genetically diverse
Vaccine	Highly effective conjugate vaccines	None available; under development

to the capsular polysaccharide, which is a polymer of polyribitol ribose phosphate (PRP), declines from birth to 6 months of age and, in the absence of vaccination, remains low until ~2 or 3 years of age. The age at the antibody nadir correlates with that of the peak incidence of type b disease. Antibody to PRP then appears partly as a result of exposure to Hib or cross-reacting antigens. Systemic Hib disease is unusual after the age of 6 years because of the presence of protective antibody. Vaccines in which PRP is conjugated to protein carrier molecules have been developed and are now used widely. These vaccines generate an antibody response to PRP in infants and effectively prevent invasive infections in infants and children.

Since nontypable strains lack a capsule, the immune response to infection is directed at noncapsular antigens. These antigens have generated considerable interest as immune targets and potential vaccine components. The human immune response to nontypable strains appears to be strain-specific, accounting in part for the propensity of these strains to cause recurrent otitis media and recurrent exacerbations of chronic bronchitis in immunocompetent hosts.

■ CLINICAL MANIFESTATIONS

Hib

The most serious manifestation of infection with Hib is *meningitis* (Chap. 381), which primarily affects children <2 years of age. The clinical manifestations of Hib meningitis are similar to those of meningitis caused by other bacterial pathogens. Fever and altered central nervous system function are the most common features at presentation. Nuchal rigidity may or may not be evident. Subdural effusion, the most common complication, is suspected when, despite 2 or 3 days of appropriate antibiotic therapy, the infant has seizures, hemiparesis, or continued obtundation. The overall mortality rate from Hib meningitis is ~5%, and the morbidity rate is high. Of survivors, 6% have permanent sensorineural hearing loss, and about one-fourth have a significant handicap of some type. If more subtle handicaps are sought, up to half of survivors are found to have some neurologic sequelae, such as partial hearing loss and delayed language development.

Epiglottitis (Chap. 31) is a life-threatening Hib infection involving cellulitis of the epiglottis and supraglottic tissues. It can lead to acute upper airway obstruction. Its unique epidemiologic features are its occurrence in an older age group (2–7 years old) than other Hib infections and its absence among Navajo Indians and Alaskan Eskimos. Sore throat and fever rapidly progress to dysphagia, drooling, and airway obstruction. Epiglottitis also occurs in adults.

Cellulitis (Chap. 125) due to Hib occurs in young children. The most common location is on the head or neck, and the involved area sometimes takes on a characteristic bluish-red color. Most patients have bacteremia, and 10% have an additional focus of infection.

Hib causes *pneumonia* in infants. The infection is clinically indistinguishable from other types of bacterial pneumonia (e.g., pneumococcal pneumonia) except that Hib is more likely to involve the pleura.

Several less common invasive conditions can be important clinical manifestations of Hib infection in children. These include osteomyelitis, septic arthritis, pericarditis, orbital cellulitis, endophthalmitis, urinary tract infection, abscesses, and bacteremia without an identifiable focus.

Nontypable *H. influenzae*

Nontypable *H. influenzae* is the most common bacterial cause of exacerbations of COPD; these exacerbations are characterized by increased cough, sputum production, and shortness of breath. Fever is low-grade, and no infiltrates are evident on chest x-ray.

Nontypable strains also cause community-acquired bacterial pneumonia in adults, especially among patients with COPD or AIDS. The clinical features of *H. influenzae* pneumonia are similar to those of other types of bacterial pneumonia (including pneumococcal pneumonia).

Nontypable *H. influenzae* is one of the three most common causes of childhood otitis media (the other two being *Streptococcus pneumoniae* and *Moraxella catarrhalis*) (Chap. 31). Infants are febrile and irritable, while older children report ear pain. Symptoms of viral upper respiratory infection often precede otitis media. The diagnosis is made by pneumatic otoscopy. An etiologic diagnosis, although not routinely sought, can be established by tympanocentesis and culture of middle-ear fluid. Clinical features associated with *H. influenzae* otitis media include a history of recurrent episodes, treatment failure, concomitant conjunctivitis, bilateral otitis media, and recent antimicrobial therapy. The increasing use of pneumococcal polysaccharide conjugate vaccines in infants is resulting in a relative increase in the proportion of otitis media cases that are caused by *H. influenzae*.

Nontypable *H. influenzae* also causes puerperal sepsis and is an important cause of neonatal bacteremia. These nontypable strains, which are closely related to *H. haemolyticus*, tend to be of biotype IV and cause invasive disease after colonizing the female genital tract.

Nontypable *H. influenzae* causes sinusitis (Chap. 31) in adults and children. In addition, the bacterium is a less common cause of various invasive infections. These infections include empyema, adult epiglottitis, pericarditis, cellulitis, septic arthritis, osteomyelitis, endocarditis, cholecystitis, intraabdominal infections, urinary tract infections, mastoiditis, aortic graft infection, and bacteremia without a detectable focus. Most *H. influenzae* invasive infections in countries where Hib vaccines are used widely are caused by nontypable strains. Many patients with *H. influenzae* bacteremia have an underlying condition, such as HIV infection, cardiopulmonary disease, alcoholism, or cancer.

■ DIAGNOSIS

The most reliable method for establishing a diagnosis of Hib infection is recovery of the organism in culture. The presence of gram-negative coccobacilli in Gram-stained CSF is strong evidence for Hib meningitis. Recovery of the organism from CSF confirms the diagnosis. Cultures of other normally sterile body fluids, such as blood, joint fluid, pleural fluid, pericardial fluid, and subdural effusion, are confirmatory in other infections.

Detection of PRP is an important adjunct to culture in rapid diagnosis of Hib meningitis. Immunoelectrophoresis, latex agglutination, coagglutination, and enzyme-linked immunosorbent assay are effective in detecting PRP. These assays are particularly helpful when patients have received prior antimicrobial therapy and thus are especially likely to have negative cultures.

Because nontypable *H. influenzae* is primarily a mucosal pathogen, it is a component of a mixed flora; thus etiologic diagnosis is challenging. Nontypable *H. influenzae* infection is strongly suggested by the predominance of gram-negative coccobacilli among abundant polymorphonuclear leukocytes in a Gram-stained sputum specimen from a patient in whom pneumonia is suspected. Although bacteremia is detectable in a small proportion of patients with pneumonia due to nontypable *H. influenzae*, most such patients have negative blood cultures.

A diagnosis of otitis media is based on the detection by pneumatic otoscopy of fluid in the middle ear. An etiologic diagnosis requires tympanocentesis but is not routinely sought. An invasive procedure is also required to determine the etiology of sinusitis; thus, treatment is often empirical once the diagnosis is suspected in light of clinical symptoms and sinus radiographs.

Initial therapy for meningitis due to Hib should consist of a cephalosporin such as ceftriaxone or cefotaxime. For children, the dosage of ceftriaxone is 75–100 mg/kg daily given in two doses 12 h apart. The pediatric dosage of cefotaxime is 200 mg/kg daily given in four doses 6 h apart. Adult dosages are 2 g every 12 h for ceftriaxone and 2 g every 4–6 h for cefotaxime. An alternative regimen for initial therapy is ampicillin (200–300 mg/kg daily in four divided doses) plus chloramphenicol (75–100 mg/kg daily in four divided doses). Therapy should continue for a total of 1–2 weeks.

Administration of glucocorticoids to patients with Hib meningitis reduces the incidence of neurologic sequelae. The presumed mechanism is reduction of the inflammation induced by bacterial cell-wall mediators of inflammation when cells are killed by antimicrobial agents. Dexamethasone (0.6 mg/kg per day intravenously in four divided doses for 2 days) is recommended for the treatment of Hib meningitis in children >2 months of age.

Invasive infections other than meningitis are treated with the same antimicrobial agents. For epiglottitis, the dosage of ceftriaxone is 50 mg/kg daily, and the dosage of cefotaxime is 150 mg/kg daily, given in three divided doses 8 h apart. Epiglottitis constitutes a medical emergency, and maintenance of an airway is critical. The duration of therapy is determined by the clinical response. A course of 1–2 weeks is usually appropriate.

Many infections caused by nontypable strains of *H. influenzae*, such as otitis media, sinusitis, and exacerbations of COPD, can be treated with oral antimicrobial agents. Approximately 20–35% of nontypable strains produce β-lactamase (with the exact proportion depending on geographic location), and these strains are resistant to ampicillin. Several agents have excellent activity against nontypable *H. influenzae*, including amoxicillin/clavulanic acid, various extended-spectrum cephalosporins, and the macrolides azithromycin and clarithromycin. Fluoroquinolones are highly active against *H. influenzae* and are useful in adults with exacerbations of COPD. However, fluoroquinolones are not currently recommended for the treatment of children or pregnant women because of possible effects on articular cartilage.

In addition to β-lactamase production, alteration of penicillin-binding proteins—a second mechanism of ampicillin resistance—has been detected in isolates of *H. influenzae*. Although rare in the United States, these β-lactamase–negative ampicillin-resistant strains are increasing in prevalence in Europe and Japan. Continued monitoring of the evolving antimicrobial susceptibility patterns of *H. influenzae* will be important.

■ PREVENTION

Vaccination

(See also Chap. 122) Two conjugate vaccines that prevent invasive infections with Hib in infants and children are licensed in the United States. In addition to eliciting protective antibody, these vaccines prevent disease by reducing rates of pharyngeal colonization with Hib. The widespread use of conjugate vaccines has dramatically reduced the incidence of Hib disease in developed countries. Even though the manufacture of Hib vaccines is costly, vaccination is cost-effective. The Global Alliance for Vaccines and Immunizations has recognized the underuse of Hib conjugate vaccines. The disease burden has been reduced in developing countries that have implemented routine vaccination (e.g.,

The Gambia, Chile). An important obstacle to more widespread vaccination is the lack of data on the epidemiology and burden of Hib disease in many developing countries.

All children should be immunized with an Hib conjugate vaccine, receiving the first dose at ~2 months of age, the rest of the primary series at 2–6 months of age, and a booster dose at 12–15 months of age. Specific recommendations vary for the different conjugate vaccines. The reader is referred to the recommendations of the American Academy of Pediatrics (Chap. 122 and www.cispimmunize.org).

Currently, no vaccines are available for the prevention of disease caused by nontypable *H. influenzae*. However, a vaccine that contains a surface protein of *H. influenzae* conjugated to pneumococcal polysaccharides has shown partial efficacy in preventing *H. influenzae* otitis media. Additional progress in the development of vaccines against nontypable *H. influenzae* is anticipated.

Chemoprophylaxis

The risk of secondary disease is greater than normal among household contacts of patients with Hib disease. Therefore, all children and adults (except pregnant women) in households with at least one incompletely immunized contact <4 years of age should receive prophylaxis with oral rifampin. When two or more cases of invasive Hib disease have occurred within 60 days at a child-care facility attended by incompletely vaccinated children, administration of rifampin to all attendees and personnel is indicated, as is recommended for household contacts. Chemoprophylaxis is not indicated in nursery and child-care contacts of a single index case. The reader is referred to the recommendations of the American Academy of Pediatrics.

HAEMOPHILUS DUCREYI

Haemophilus ducreyi is the etiologic agent of chancroid (Chap. 130), a sexually transmitted disease characterized by genital ulceration and inguinal adenitis. *H. ducreyi* poses a significant health problem in developing countries. In addition to being a cause of morbidity in itself, chancroid is associated with HIV infection because of the role played by genital ulceration in HIV transmission. Chancroid increases both the efficiency of, transmission of, and the degree of susceptibility to HIV infection.

■ MICROBIOLOGY

H. ducreyi is a highly fastidious coccobacillary gram-negative bacterium whose growth requires X factor (hemin). Although, in light of this requirement, the bacterium has been classified in the genus *Haemophilus*, DNA homology and chemotaxonomic studies have established substantial differences between *H. ducreyi* and other *Haemophilus* species. Taxonomic reclassification of the organism is likely in the future but awaits further study. Ulcers contain predominantly T cells. The fact that patients who have had chancroid may have repeated infections indicates that infection does not confer protection.

■ EPIDEMIOLOGY AND PREVALENCE

Chancroid is a common cause of genital ulcers in developing countries. In the United States, several large outbreaks have occurred since 1981. Recurring epidemiologic themes have been apparent in these outbreaks: (1) transmission has been predominantly heterosexual; (2) males have outnumbered females by ratios of 3:1 to 25:1; (3) prostitutes have been important in transmission of the infection; and (4) chancroid has been strongly associated with illicit drug use. The annual number of cases reported in the United States has remained stable since 2000.

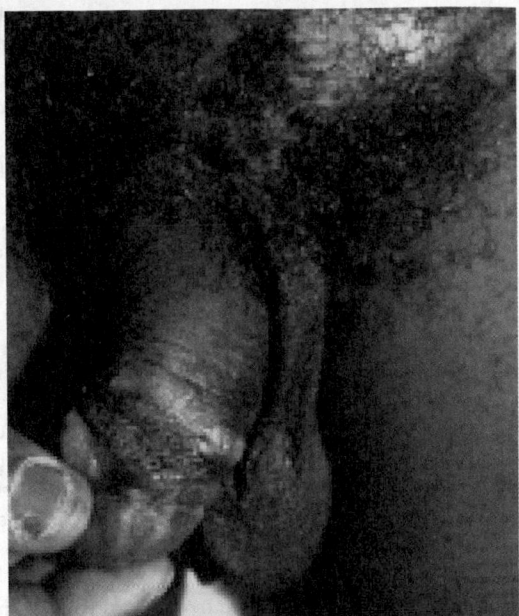

Figure 145-2 Chancroid with characteristic penile ulcers and associated left inguinal adenitis (bubo).

■ CLINICAL MANIFESTATIONS

Infection is acquired as the result of a break in the epithelium during sexual contact with an infected individual. After an incubation period of 4–7 days, the initial lesion—a papule with surrounding erythema—appears. In 2 or 3 days, the papule evolves into a pustule, which spontaneously ruptures and forms a sharply circumscribed ulcer that is generally not indurated (Fig. 145-2). The ulcers are painful and bleed easily; little or no inflammation of the surrounding skin is evident. Approximately half of patients develop enlarged, tender inguinal lymph nodes, which frequently become fluctuant and spontaneously rupture. Patients usually seek medical care after 1–3 weeks of painful symptoms.

The presentation of chancroid does not usually include all of the typical clinical features and is sometimes atypical. Multiple ulcers can coalesce to form giant ulcers. Ulcers can appear and then resolve, with inguinal adenitis (Fig. 145-2) and suppuration following 1–3 weeks later; this clinical picture can be confused with that of lymphogranuloma venereum (Chap. 176). Multiple small ulcers can resemble folliculitis. Other differential diagnostic considerations include the various infections causing genital ulceration, such as primary syphilis, secondary syphilis (condyloma latum), genital herpes, and donovanosis. In rare cases, chancroid lesions become secondarily infected with bacteria; the result is extensive inflammation.

■ DIAGNOSIS

Clinical diagnosis of chancroid is often inaccurate, and laboratory confirmation should be attempted in suspected cases. An accurate diagnosis of chancroid relies on culture of *H. ducreyi* from the lesion. In addition, aspiration and culture of suppurative lymph nodes should be considered. Since the organism can be difficult to grow, the use of selective and supplemented media is necessary. A multiplex polymerase chain reaction assay has been developed for simultaneous amplification of DNA targets from *H. ducreyi*, *Treponema pallidum*, and herpes simplex virus types 1 and 2. When this assay becomes commercially available, it will be a useful diagnostic tool with which to identify the etiology of genital ulcers.

TREATMENT   *Haemophilus ducreyi*

Treatment regimens recommended by the Centers for Disease Control and Prevention include (1) a single 1-g oral dose of azithromycin; (2) ceftriaxone (250 mg intramuscularly in a single dose); (3) ciprofloxacin (500 mg by mouth twice a day for 3 days); and (4) erythromycin base (500 mg by mouth three times a day for 7 days). Isolates from patients who do not respond promptly to treatment should be tested for antimicrobial resistance. In patients with HIV infection, healing may be slow and longer courses of treatment may be necessary. Clinical treatment failure in HIV-seropositive patients may reflect co-infection, especially with herpes simplex virus. Contacts of patients with chancroid should be identified and treated, whether or not symptoms are present, if they have had sexual contact with the patient during the 10 days preceding the patient's onset of symptoms.

MORAXELLA CATARRHALIS

■ MICROBIOLOGY

M. catarrhalis is an unencapsulated gram-negative diplococcus the ecologic of which niche is the human respiratory tract. The organism was initially designated *Micrococcus catarrhalis*, but its name was changed to *Neisseria catarrhalis* in 1970 because of phenotypic similarities to commensal *Neisseria* species. On the basis of more rigorous analysis of genetic relatedness, *Moraxella catarrhalis* is now the widely accepted name for this species.

■ EPIDEMIOLOGY

Nasopharyngeal colonization by *M. catarrhalis* is common in infancy, with colonization rates ranging between 33% and 100% and depending on geographic location. Several factors probably account for this geographic variation, including living conditions, day-care attendance, hygiene, household smoking, and population genetics. The prevalence of colonization decreases steadily with age.

The widespread use of pneumococcal conjugate vaccines in some countries has resulted in alterations in patterns of nasopharyngeal colonization in resident populations. A relative increase in colonization by nonvaccine pneumococcal serotypes, nontypable *H. influenzae*, and *M. catarrhalis* has occurred. These changes in colonization patterns may be altering the distribution of pathogens of both otitis media and sinusitis in children.

■ PATHOGENESIS

M. catarrhalis causes mucosal infections of the respiratory tract. Strains exhibit substantial genetic diversity and differences in virulence properties. The species is composed of two distinct genetic lineages; the complement-resistant lineage is more strongly associated with virulence than are complement-sensitive strains.

The expression of several adhesin molecules with differing specificities for various host cell receptors reflects the importance of adherence to the respiratory epithelial surface in the pathogenesis of infection. *M. catarrhalis* invades multiple cell types. Its intracellular residence in lymphoid tissue provides a potential reservoir for persistence in the human respiratory tract.

■ CLINICAL MANIFESTATIONS

In children, *M. catarrhalis* causes predominantly mucosal infections when the bacterium migrates from the nasopharynx to the middle ear or the sinuses (Chap. 31). The inciting event for both otitis media and sinusitis is often a preceding viral infection. Overall, cultures of middle-ear fluid obtained by tympanocentesis indicate that *M. catarrhalis* causes 15–20% of cases of acute otitis media. Acute otitis media caused by *M. catarrhalis* or nontypable *H. influenzae* is clinically milder than otitis media caused by *S. pneumoniae*, with less fever and a lower prevalence of a red bulging tympanic membrane. However, substantial overlap makes it impossible to predict etiology in an individual child on the basis of clinical features.

A small proportion of viral upper respiratory tract infections are complicated by bacterial sinusitis. Cultures of sinus puncture aspirates show that *M. catarrhalis* accounts for ~20% of cases of acute bacterial sinusitis in children and for a smaller proportion in adults.

M. catarrhalis is a common cause of exacerbations in adults with COPD. The bacterium has been overlooked in this clinical setting because it has long been considered to be a commensal and because it is easily mistaken for commensal *Neisseria* species in cultures of respiratory secretions (see "Diagnosis," below). Several independent lines of evidence have established *M. catarrhalis* as a pathogen in COPD. These include (1) the demonstration of *M. catarrhalis* in the lower airways during exacerbations, (2) the association of exacerbation with acquisition of new strains, (3) elevations of inflammatory markers in association with *M. catarrhalis*, and (4) the development of specific immune responses following infection. *M. catarrhalis* is the second most common bacterial cause of COPD exacerbations (after *H. influenzae*), as shown in a 10-year prospective study; the distribution of new-strain acquisitions is shown in Fig. 145-3. Not included are culture-negative cases or cases from which a pathogen had been previously isolated. With the application of rigorous clinical criteria for defining the etiology of exacerbations (both culture-positive and culture-negative), ~10% of all exacerbations in the same study were caused by *M. catarrhalis*. The clinical features of an exacerbation due to *M. catarrhalis* are similar to those of exacerbations due to other bacterial pathogens, including *H. influenzae* and *S. pneumoniae*. The cardinal symptoms are cough with increased sputum production, sputum purulence, and dyspnea in comparison with baseline symptoms.

Pneumonia due to *M. catarrhalis* occurs in the elderly, particularly in the setting of underlying cardiopulmonary disease, but is infrequent. Invasive infections, such as bacteremia, endocarditis, neonatal meningitis, and septic arthritis, are rare.

■ DIAGNOSIS

Tympanocentesis is required for etiologic diagnosis of otitis media, but this procedure is not performed routinely. Therefore, treatment of otitis media is generally empirical. Similarly, an etiologic diagnosis of sinusitis requires an invasive procedure and thus is usually not available to the clinician. Isolation of *M. catarrhalis* from an expectorated sputum sample from an adult experiencing clinical symptoms of an exacerbation is suggestive, but not diagnostic, of *M. catarrhalis* as the cause.

Upon culture, colonies of *M. catarrhalis* resemble commensal neisseriae that are part of the normal upper airway flora. As mentioned above, the difficulty in distinguishing colonies of *M. catarrhalis* from neisserial colonies in cultures of respiratory secretions explains in part why *M. catarrhalis* has been overlooked as a pathogen. In contrast to these *Neisseria* species, *M. catarrhalis* colonies can be slid across the agar surface without disruption (the "hockey puck sign"). In addition, after 48 h of growth, *M. catarrhalis* colonies take on a pink color and tend to be larger than neisserial colonies. A variety of biochemical tests can distinguish *M. catarrhalis* from neisseriae. Kits that rely on these biochemical reactions are commercially available.

TREATMENT	*Moraxella catarrhalis*

M. catarrhalis rapidly acquired β-lactamases during the 1970s and 1980s; antimicrobial susceptibility patterns have remained relatively stable since that time, with >90% of strains now producing β-lactamase and thus resistant to amoxicillin. Otitis media in children and exacerbations of COPD in adults are generally managed empirically with antimicrobial agents that are active against *S. pneumoniae*, *H. influenzae*, and *M. catarrhalis*. Most strains of *M. catarrhalis* are susceptible to amoxicillin/clavulanic acid, extended-spectrum cephalosporins, newer macrolides (azithromycin, clarithromycin), trimethoprim-sulfamethoxazole, and fluoroquinolones.

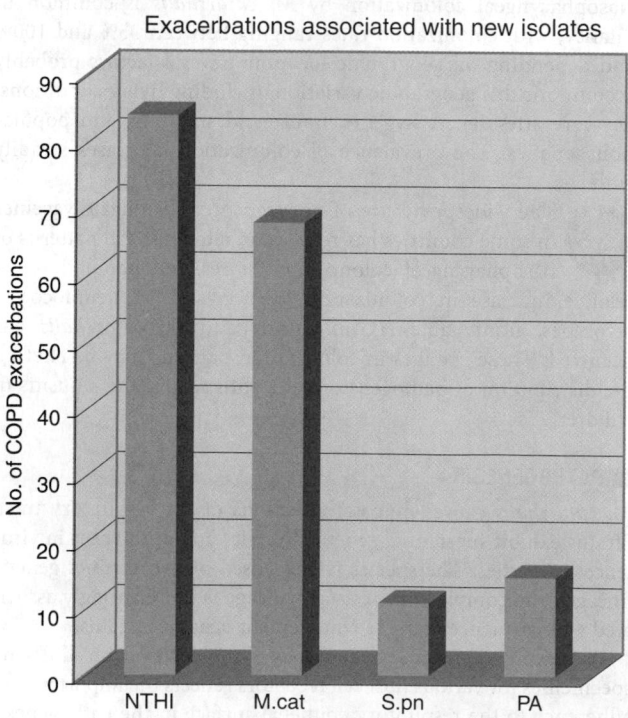

Exacerbations associated with new isolates

Figure 145-3 Cumulative results of a prospective study (1994–2004) of bacterial infection in COPD showing etiology of exacerbations. The numbers of exacerbations shown indicate the acquisition of a new strain simultaneous with clinical symptoms of an exacerbation. NTHI, nontypable *H. influenzae*; M.cat, *M. catarrhalis*; S.pn, *Streptococcus pneumoniae*; PA, *Pseudomonas aeruginosa*. (*Adapted from Murphy and Parameswaran, with permission.* © 2009 Infectious Diseases Society of America.)

FURTHER READINGS

BROIDES A et al: Acute otitis media caused by *Moraxella catarrhalis*: Epidemiologic and clinical characteristics. Clin Infect Dis 49:1641, 2009

DWORKIN MS et al: The changing epidemiology of invasive *Haemophilus influenzae* disease, especially in persons > or = 65 years old. Clin Infect Dis 44:810, 2007

MAWAS F et al: Current progress with *Moraxella catarrhalis* antigens as vaccine candidates. Expert Rev Vaccines 8:77, 2009

MOHAMMED TT, OLUMIDE YM: Chancroid and human immunodeficiency virus infection—a review. Int J Dermatol 47:1, 2008

MURPHY TF et al: Nontypeable *Haemophilus influenzae* as a pathogen in children. Pediatr Infect Dis J 28:43, 2009

—— et al: *Haemophilus haemolyticus*: A human respiratory tract commensal to be distinguished from *Haemophilus influenzae*. J Infect Dis 195:81, 2007

MURPHY TF, PARAMESWARAN GI: *Moraxella catarrhalis*, a human respiratory tract pathogen. Clin Infect Dis 49:124, 2009

PRYMULA R et al: Pneumococcal capsular polysaccharides conjugated to protein D for prevention of acute otitis media caused by both *Streptococcus pneumoniae* and non-typable *Haemophilus influenzae*: A randomised double-blind efficacy study. Lancet 367:740, 2006

SETHI S, MURPHY TF: Infection in the pathogenesis and course of chronic obstructive pulmonary disease. N Engl J Med 359:2355, 2008

WIRTH T et al: The rise and spread of a new pathogen: Seroresistant *Moraxella catarrhalis*. Genome Res 17:1647, 2007

CHAPTER 146

Infections Due to the HACEK Group and Miscellaneous Gram-Negative Bacteria

Tamar F. Barlam
Dennis L. Kasper

THE HACEK GROUP

HACEK organisms are a group of fastidious, slow-growing, gram-negative bacteria the growth of which requires an atmosphere of carbon dioxide. Species belonging to this group include several *Haemophilus* species, *Aggregatibacter* (formerly *Actinobacillus*) *actinomycetemcomitans*, *Cardiobacterium hominis*, *Eikenella corrodens*, and *Kingella kingae*. HACEK bacteria normally reside in the oral cavity and have been associated with local infections in the mouth. They are also known to cause severe systemic infections—most often bacterial endocarditis, which can develop on either native or prosthetic valves (Chap. 124).

■ HACEK ENDOCARDITIS

In large series, up to 3% of cases of infective endocarditis are attributable to HACEK organisms, most often *A. actinomycetemcomitans*, *Haemophilus* species, and *C. hominis*. Invasive infection typically occurs in patients with a history of cardiac valvular disease, often in the setting of a recent dental procedure, nasopharyngeal infection, or tongue piercing or scraping. The aortic and mitral valves are most commonly affected. The clinical course of HACEK endocarditis tends to be subacute; however, embolization is common. The overall prevalence of major emboli associated with HACEK endocarditis ranges from 28% to 71% in different series. On echocardiography, valvular vegetations are seen in up to 85% of patients. The vegetations are frequently large, although vegetation size has not been directly correlated with the risk of embolization. Cultures of blood from patients with suspected HACEK endocarditis may require up to 30 days to become positive, and the microbiology laboratory should be alerted when a HACEK organism is being considered. However, most cultures that ultimately yield a HACEK organism become positive within the first week, especially with improved culture systems such as BACTEC. In addition, polymerase chain reaction techniques (e.g., of cardiac valves) are facilitating the diagnosis of HACEK infections. Because of the organisms' slow growth, antimicrobial testing may be difficult, and β-lactamase production may not be detected. E-test methodology may increase the accuracy of susceptibility testing.

Haemophilus species

Haemophilus species are differentiated by their in vitro growth requirements for X factor (hemin) and V factor (nicotinamide adenine dinucleotide). *H. aphrophilus* requires only X factor for growth, while species designated *para-* require only V factor. *H. aphrophilus* and *H. parainfluenzae* are the *Haemophilus* species most commonly isolated from cases of HACEK endocarditis; *H. paraphrophilus* is less common. Of patients with HACEK endocarditis due to *Haemophilus* species, 60% have been ill for <2 months before presentation, and 19–50% develop congestive heart failure. Mortality rates as high as 30–50% were reported in older series; however, more recent studies have documented mortality rates of <5%. *H. aphrophilus* also causes invasive bone and joint infections, and *H. parainfluenzae* has been isolated from other infections, such as meningitis; brain, dental, and liver abscess; pneumonia; and septicemia.

Aggregatibacter actinomycetemcomitans

A. actinomycetemcomitans can be isolated from soft tissue infections and abscesses in association with *Actinomyces israelii*. Typically, patients who develop endocarditis with *A. actinomycetemcomitans* have severe periodontal disease or have recently undergone dental procedures in the setting of underlying cardiac valvular damage. The disease is insidious; patients may be sick for several months before diagnosis. Frequent complications include embolic phenomena, congestive heart failure, and renal failure. *A. actinomycetemcomitans* has been isolated from patients with brain abscess, meningitis, endophthalmitis, parotitis, osteomyelitis, urinary tract infection, pneumonia, and empyema, among other infections.

Cardiobacterium hominis

C. hominis primarily causes endocarditis in patients with underlying valvular heart disease or with prosthetic valves. This organism most frequently affects the aortic valve. Many patients have signs and symptoms of long-standing infection before diagnosis, with evidence of arterial embolization, vasculitis, cerebrovascular accidents, immune complex glomerulonephritis, or arthritis at presentation. Embolization, mycotic aneurysms, and congestive heart failure are common complications. A second species, *C. valvarum*, has now been described in association with endocarditis.

Eikenella corrodens

E. corrodens is most frequently recovered from sites of infection in conjunction with other bacterial species. Clinical sources of *E. corrodens* include sites of human bite wounds (clenched-fist injuries), endocarditis, soft tissue infections, osteomyelitis, head and neck infections, respiratory infections, chorioamnionitis, gynecologic infections associated with intrauterine devices, meningitis and brain abscesses, and visceral abscesses.

Kingella kingae

Because of improved microbiologic methodology, isolation of *K. kingae* is increasingly common. Inoculation of clinical specimens (e.g., synovial fluid) into aerobic blood culture bottles enhances recovery of this organism. Specific real-time PCR studies of joint fluid can identify *K. kingae* in culture-negative cases. Invasive *K. kingae* infections with bacteremia are associated with upper respiratory tract infections and stomatitis in 80% of cases. Rates of oropharyngeal colonization with *K. kingae* are highest in the first 3 years of life, coinciding with increased incidence of skeletal infections due to this organism. *K. kingae* bacteremia can present with a petechial rash similar to that seen in *Neisseria meningitidis* sepsis.

Infective endocarditis, unlike other infections with *K. kingae*, occurs in older children and adults. The majority of patients have preexisting valvular disease. There is a high incidence of complications, including arterial emboli, cerebrovascular accidents, tricuspid insufficiency, and congestive heart failure with cardiovascular collapse.

TREATMENT Endocarditis Caused by HACEK Organisms

See Table 146-1. Native-valve endocarditis should be treated for 4 weeks with antibiotics, whereas prosthetic-valve endocarditis requires 6 weeks of therapy. The cure rates for HACEK prosthetic-valve endocarditis appear to be high. Unlike prosthetic-valve endocarditis caused by other gram-negative organisms, HACEK endocarditis is often cured with antibiotic treatment alone—i.e., without surgical intervention.

OTHER GRAM-NEGATIVE BACTERIA

Achromobacter xylosoxidans

Achromobacter (previously *Alcaligenes*) *xylosoxidans* is probably part of the endogenous intestinal flora and has been isolated from a variety of water sources, including well water, IV fluids, and humidifiers. Immunocompromised hosts, including patients with cancer and postchemotherapy neutropenia, cirrhosis, chronic renal failure, and cystic fibrosis, are at increased risk. Nosocomial outbreaks and pseudo-outbreaks of *A. xylosoxidans* infection have been attributed to contaminated fluids, and clinical illness has been associated with isolates from many sites, including blood (often in the setting of intravascular devices). Community-acquired *A. xylosoxidans* bacteremia usually occurs in the setting of pneumonia. Metastatic skin lesions are present in one-fifth of cases. The reported mortality rate is 67%—a figure similar to rates for other bacteremic gram-negative pneumonias.

TREATMENT Achromobacter xylosoxidans Infections

Treatment is based on in vitro susceptibility testing of all clinically relevant isolates. Imipenem, piperacillin-tazobactam, and trimethoprim-sulfamethoxazole (TMP-SMX) are typically the most active agents, but multidrug-resistant isolates sensitive only to colistin have been reported.

Aeromonas species

More than 85% of *Aeromonas* infections are caused by *A. hydrophila*, *A. caviae*, and *A. veronii* biovar *sobria*. *Aeromonas* proliferates in potable water, freshwater, and soil. It remains controversial whether *Aeromonas* is a cause of bacterial gastroenteritis; asymptomatic colonization of the intestinal tract with *Aeromonas* occurs frequently. However, rare cases of hemolytic-uremic syndrome following bloody diarrhea have been shown to be secondary to the presence of *Aeromonas*.

Aeromonas causes sepsis and bacteremia in infants with multiple medical problems and in immunocompromised hosts, particularly those with cancer or hepatobiliary disease. *Aeromonas* infection and sepsis can occur in patients with trauma (including severe trauma with myonecrosis) and in burn patients exposed to *Aeromonas* by environmental (freshwater or soil) contamination of their wounds. Reported mortality rates range from 25% among immunocompromised adults with sepsis to >90% among patients with myonecrosis. *Aeromonas* can produce ecthyma gangrenosum (hemorrhagic vesicles surrounded by a rim of erythema with central necrosis and ulceration; see Fig. e7-35) resembling the lesions seen in *Pseudomonas aeruginosa* infection. *Aeromonas* causes nosocomial infections related to catheters, surgical incisions, or use of leeches.

TABLE 146-1 Treatment of Endocarditis Caused by HACEK Group Organisms[a]

Organism	Initial Therapy	Alternative Agents	Comments
Haemophilus species, *Aggregatibacter actinomycetemcomitans*	Ceftriaxone (2 g/d)	Ampicillin/sulbactam (3 g of ampicillin q6h) **or** fluoroquinolones[b]	Ampicillin ± an aminoglycoside can be used if the organism does not produce β-lactamase.[c]
Cardiobacterium hominis	Ceftriaxone (2 g/d)	Ampicillin/sulbactam (3 g of ampicillin q6h)	Penicillin (16–18 mU q4h) or ampicillin (2 g q4h) should be used if the organism is susceptible.
Eikenella corrodens	Ampicillin (2 g q4h)	Ceftriaxone (2 g/d) **or** fluoroquinolones[b]	The organism is typically resistant to clindamycin, metronidazole, and aminoglycosides.
Kingella kingae	Ceftriaxone (2 g/d) **or** ampicillin/sulbactam (3 g of ampicillin q6h)	Fluoroquinolones[b]	The prevalence of β-lactamase-producing strains is increasing. Efficacy for invasive infections is best demonstrated for first-line treatments.

[a]Susceptibility testing should be performed in all cases to guide therapy. See text for recommended durations of treatment.
[b]Fluoroquinolones are not recommended for treatment of children <18 years of age.
[c]European guidelines for endocarditis recommend the addition of gentamicin (3 mg/kg per day in 3 divided doses for 2–4 weeks).

Other manifestations include necrotizing fasciitis, meningitis, peritonitis, pneumonia, and ocular infections.

TREATMENT *Aeromonas* Infections

Aeromonas species are generally susceptible to fluoroquinolones (e.g., ciprofloxacin at a dosage of 500 mg every 12 h PO or 400 mg every 12 h IV), third-generation cephalosporins, carbapenems, and aminoglycosides. Because *Aeromonas* can produce various β-lactamases, including carbapenemases, susceptibility testing must be used to guide therapy. Antibiotic prophylaxis (e.g., with ciprofloxacin) is indicated when medicinal leeches are used.

Capnocytophaga species

This genus of fastidious, fusiform, gram-negative coccobacilli is facultatively anaerobic and requires an atmosphere enriched in carbon dioxide for optimal growth. *C. ochracea*, *C. gingivalis*, *C. haemolytica*, and *C. sputigena* have been associated with sepsis in immunocompromised hosts, particularly neutropenic patients with oral ulcerations. These species have been isolated from many other sites as well, usually as part of a polymicrobial infection. Most *Capnocytophaga* infections are contiguous with the oropharynx (e.g., periodontal disease, respiratory tract infections, cervical abscesses, and endophthalmitis).

C. canimorsus and *C. cynodegmi* are endogenous to the canine mouth (Chap. e24). Patients infected with these species frequently have a history of dog bites or of exposure to dogs without scratches or bites. Asplenia, glucocorticoid therapy, and alcohol abuse are predisposing conditions that can be associated with severe sepsis with shock and disseminated intravascular coagulation. Patients typically have a petechial rash that can progress from purpuric lesions to gangrene. Meningitis, endocarditis, cellulitis, osteomyelitis, and septic arthritis have also been associated with these organisms.

TREATMENT *Capnocytophaga* Infections

Because of increasing β-lactamase production, a penicillin derivative plus a β-lactamase inhibitor—such as ampicillin/sulbactam (1.5–3.0 g of ampicillin every 6 h)—is currently recommended for empirical treatment of infections caused by *Capnocytophaga* species. If the isolate is known to be susceptible, infections with *C. canimorsus* should be treated with penicillin (12–18 million units every 4 h). *Capnocytophaga* is also susceptible to clindamycin (600–900 mg every 6–8 h). This regimen or ampicillin/sulbactam should be given prophylactically to asplenic patients who have sustained dog-bite injuries.

Chryseobacterium species

Chryseobacterium (formerly *Flavobacterium*) *meningosepticum* is an important cause of nosocomial infections, including outbreaks due to contaminated fluids (e.g., disinfectants and aerosolized antibiotics) and sporadic infections due to indwelling devices, feeding tubes, and other fluid-associated apparatuses. Nosocomial *C. meningosepticum* infection usually involves neonates or patients with underlying immunosuppression (e.g., related to malignancy). *C. meningosepticum* has been reported to cause meningitis (primarily in neonates), pneumonia, sepsis, endocarditis, bacteremia, and soft tissue infections. *C. indologenes* has caused bacteremia, sepsis, and pneumonia, typically in immunocompromised patients with indwelling devices.

TREATMENT *Chryseobacterium* Infections

Chryseobacteria are often susceptible to fluoroquinolones and TMP-SMX. They may be susceptible to β-lactam/β-lactamase inhibitor agents such as piperacillin-tazobactam but can possess extended-spectrum β-lactamases and metallo-β-lactamases. Susceptibility testing should be performed.

Pasteurella multocida

P. multocida is a bipolar-staining, gram-negative coccobacillus that colonizes the respiratory and gastrointestinal tracts of domestic animals; oropharyngeal colonization rates are 70–90% in cats and 50–65% in dogs. *P. multocida* can be transmitted to humans through bites or scratches, via the respiratory tract from contact with contaminated dust or infectious droplets, or via deposition of the organism on injured skin or mucosal surfaces during licking. Most human infections affect skin and soft tissue; almost two-thirds of these infections are caused by cats. Patients at the extremes of age or with serious underlying disorders (e.g., cirrhosis, diabetes) are at increased risk for systemic manifestations, including meningitis, peritonitis, osteomyelitis and septic arthritis, endocarditis, and septic shock, but cases have also occurred in healthy individuals. If inhaled, *P. multocida* can cause acute respiratory tract infection, particularly in patients with underlying sinus and pulmonary disease.

TREATMENT *Pasteurella multocida* Infections

P. multocida is susceptible to penicillin, ampicillin, ampicillin/sulbactam, second- and third-generation cephalosporins, tetracyclines, and fluoroquinolones. β-lactamase-producing strains have been reported.

MISCELLANEOUS ORGANISMS

Rhizobium (formerly *Agrobacterium*) *radiobacter* has usually been associated with infection in the presence of medical devices, including intravascular catheter–related infections, prosthetic-joint and prosthetic-valve infections, and peritonitis caused by dialysis catheters. Most cases occur in immunocompromised hosts, especially individuals with malignancy or HIV infection. Strains are usually susceptible to fluoroquinolones, third- and fourth-generation cephalosporins, and carbapenems.

Shewanella putrefaciens and *S. algae* are ubiquitous organisms found primarily in seawater. Devitalized tissues can become colonized with *Shewanella* and serve as a nidus for systemic infection. *Shewanella* species cause skin and soft tissue infections, chronic ulcers of the lower extremities, ear infections, biliary tract infections, pneumonia, necrotizing fasciitis, bacteremia, and sepsis. A fulminant course is associated with cirrhosis, malignancy, or other severe underlying conditions. Organisms are often susceptible to fluoroquinolones, third- and fourth-generation cephalosporins, and aminoglycosides.

Chromobacterium violaceum has been responsible for life-threatening infections with severe sepsis and metastatic abscesses, particularly in children with defective neutrophil function (e.g., those with chronic granulomatous disease). *Ochrobactrum anthropi* causes infections related to central venous catheters in compromised hosts; other invasive infections have been described. Other organisms implicated in human infections include *Weeksella* species; various CDC groups, such as EF4 and Ve-2; *Flavimonas* species; *Sphingobacterium* species; *Protomonas* species; and *Oligella urethralis*. The reader is advised to consult subspecialty texts and references for further guidance on these organisms.

FURTHER READINGS

DAS M et al: Infective endocarditis caused by HACEK microorganisms. Annu Rev Med 48:25, 1997

DUBNOV-RAZ G et al: Invasive *Kingella kingae* infections in children: Clinical and laboratory characteristics. Pediatrics 122:1305, 2008

HUNG PP et al: *Chryseobacterium meningosepticum* infection: Antibiotic susceptibility and risk factors for mortality. J Microbiol Immunol Infect 41:137, 2008

JOLIVET-GOUGEON A et al: Antimicrobial treatment of *Capnocytophaga* infections. Int J Antimicrob Agents 29:367, 2007

KRISTINSSON G, ADAM HM: *Pasteurella multocida* infections. Pediatr Rev 28:472, 2007

LAMY B et al: Prospective nationwide study of *Aeromonas* infections in France. J Clin Microbiol 47:1234, 2009

OEHLER RL et al: Bite-related and septic syndromes caused by cats and dogs. Lancet Infect Dis 9:439, 2009

TENG SO et al: Complicated intra-abdominal infection caused by extended drug-resistant *Achromobacter xylosoxidans*. J Microbiol Immunol Infect 42:176, 2009

UDAKA T et al: *Eikenella corrodens* in head and neck infections. J Infect 54:343, 2007

YAGUPSKY P et al: Dissemination of *Kingella kingae* in the community and long-term persistence of invasive clones. Pediatr Infect Dis J 28:707, 2009

CHAPTER **147**

Legionella Infections

Miguel Sabria
Victor L. Yu

Legionellosis refers to the two clinical syndromes caused by bacteria of the genus *Legionella*. *Pontiac fever* is an acute, febrile, self-limited illness that has been serologically linked to *Legionella* species, whereas *Legionnaires' disease* is the designation for pneumonia caused by these species. Legionnaires' disease was first recognized in 1976, when an outbreak of pneumonia took place at a Philadelphia hotel during an American Legion convention.

■ MICROBIOLOGY

The family Legionellaceae comprises more than 50 species with more than 70 serogroups. The species *L. pneumophila* causes 80–90% of human infections and includes at least 16 serogroups; serogroups 1, 4, and 6 are most commonly implicated in human infections. To date, 18 species other than *L. pneumophila* have been associated with human infections, among which *L. micdadei* (Pittsburgh pneumonia agent), *L. bozemanii*, *L. dumoffii*, and *L. longbeachae* are the most common. Members of the Legionellaceae are aerobic gram-negative bacilli that do not grow on routine microbiologic media. Buffered charcoal yeast extract (BCYE) agar is the medium used to grow *Legionella*.

■ ECOLOGY AND TRANSMISSION

The natural habitats for *L. pneumophila* are aquatic bodies, including lakes and streams. *L. longbeachae* has been isolated from natural soil and commercial potting soil. Legionellae can survive under a wide range of environmental conditions; for example, the organisms can live for years in refrigerated water samples. Natural bodies of water contain only small numbers of legionellae. However, once the organisms enter human-constructed aquatic reservoirs (such as drinking-water systems), they can grow and proliferate. Factors known to enhance colonization by and amplification of legionellae include warm temperatures (25°–42°C) and scale and sediment. *L. pneumophila* can form microcolonies within biofilms; its eradication from drinking-water requires disinfectants that can penetrate the biofilm. The presence of symbiotic microorganisms, including algae, amebas, ciliated protozoa, and other water-dwelling bacteria, promotes the growth of legionellae. The organisms can invade and multiply within free-living protozoa. Rainfall and humidity have been identified as environmental risk factors.

Sporadic community-acquired Legionnaires' disease has been linked to colonization of residential, hotel, and industrial water supplies. Drinking-water systems in hospitals and extended-care facilities have been linked to health care–associated Legionnaires' disease.

Cooling towers and evaporative condensers have been overestimated as sources of *Legionella*. Early investigations that implicated cooling towers antedated the discovery that the organism could also exist in drinking water. In many outbreaks attributed to cooling towers, cases of Legionnaires' disease continued to occur despite disinfection of the cooling towers; drinking water was the actual source. Koch's postulates have never been fulfilled for cooling tower–associated outbreaks as they have been for hospital-acquired Legionnaires' disease. Nevertheless, cooling towers have occasionally been identified in community-acquired outbreaks, including an outbreak in Murcia, Spain, in which several hundred suspected cases of Legionnaires' disease occurred over a 3-week period. As mentioned above, *L. longbeachae* infections have been linked to potting soil, but the mode of transmission remains to be clarified.

Multiple modes of transmission of *Legionella* to humans exist, including aerosolization, aspiration, and direct instillation into the lungs during respiratory tract manipulations. Aspiration is now known to be the predominant mode of transmission, but it is unclear whether *Legionella* enters the lungs via oropharyngeal colonization or directly via the drinking of contaminated water. Oropharyngeal colonization has been demonstrated in patients undergoing transplantation. Nasogastric tubes have been linked to hospital-acquired Legionnaires' disease; microaspiration of contaminated water was the hypothesized mode of transmission. Surgery with general anesthesia is a known risk factor that is consistent with aspiration. Especially compelling is the reported 30% incidence of postoperative Legionnaires' disease among patients undergoing head and neck surgery at a hospital with a contaminated water supply; aspiration is a recognized sequela in such cases. Studies of patients with hospital-acquired Legionnaires' disease have shown that these individuals underwent endotracheal intubation significantly more often and for a significantly longer duration than patients with hospital-acquired pneumonia of other etiologies.

Aerosolization of *Legionella* by devices filled with tap water, including whirlpools, nebulizers, and humidifiers, has been implicated. An ultrasonic mist machine in the produce section of a grocery store was the source in a community outbreak. Pontiac fever has been linked to *Legionella*-containing aerosols from water-using machinery, a cooling tower, air-conditioners, and whirlpools.

■ EPIDEMIOLOGY

The incidence of Legionnaires' disease depends on the degree of contamination of the aquatic reservoir, the immune status of the persons exposed to water from that reservoir, the intensity of exposure, and the availability of specialized laboratory tests on which the correct diagnosis can be based. Numerous prospective studies have ranked *Legionella* among the top four microbial causes of community-acquired pneumonia, accounting for 2–9% of cases. (*Streptococcus pneumoniae*, *Haemophilus influenzae*, and *Chlamydophila pneumoniae* are usually ranked first, second, and third, respectively.) On the basis of a multihospital study of community-acquired pneumonia in Ohio, the Centers for Disease Control and Prevention (CDC) estimated that as many as 18,000 cases of sporadic community-acquired Legionnaires' disease occur annually in the United States and that only 3% of these cases are correctly diagnosed. *Legionella* is responsible for 10–50% of cases of nosocomial pneumonia when a hospital's water system is colonized with the organisms. The incidence of hospital-acquired Legionnaires' disease depends on the degree of contamination of drinking water as defined by the rate of positivity of distal water sites (not as defined quantitatively by the number of colony-forming units per milliliter).

Risk factors for Legionnaires' disease include cigarette smoking; chronic lung disease; advanced age; prior hospitalization, with discharge within 10 days before onset of pneumonia symptoms; and immunosuppression. Immunosuppressive conditions that predispose to Legionnaires' disease include transplantation, HIV infection, and treatment with glucocorticoids or tumor necrosis factor α antagonists. However, in a large prospective study of community-acquired pneumonia, 28% of patients with Legionnaires' disease did not have these classic risk factors. Surgery is a prominent predisposing factor in hospital-acquired infection, with transplant recipients at highest risk. Hospital-acquired cases are now being recognized among neonates and immunosuppressed children.

Pontiac fever occurs in epidemics. The high attack rate (>90%) reflects airborne transmission.

■ PATHOGENESIS AND IMMUNITY

Legionella enters the lungs through aspiration or direct inhalation. Attachment to host cells is mediated by bacterial type IV pili, heat-shock proteins, a major outer-membrane protein, and complement. Because the organism possesses pili that mediate adherence to respiratory tract epithelial cells, conditions that impair mucociliary clearance, including cigarette smoking, lung disease, or alcoholism, predispose to Legionnaires' disease.

Both the innate and adaptive immune responses play a role in host defense. Toll-like receptors mediate recognition of *L. pneumophila* in alveolar macrophages and enhance early neutrophil recruitment to the site of infection. Alveolar macrophages phagocytose legionellae by a conventional or a coiling mechanism. The macrophage infectivity potentiation (MIP) surface protein enhances infection of the macrophages. After phagocytosis, *L. pneumophila* evades intracellular killing by inhibiting phagosome-lysosome fusion. Although many legionellae are killed, some proliferate intracellularly until the cells rupture; the bacteria are then phagocytosed again by newly recruited phagocytes, and the cycle begins anew. The role of neutrophils in immunity appears to be minimal: neutropenic patients are not predisposed to Legionnaires' disease. Although *L. pneumophila* is susceptible to oxygen-dependent microbiologic systems in vitro,

it resists killing by neutrophils. The humoral immune system is active against *Legionella*. Type-specific IgM and IgG antibodies are measurable within weeks of infection. In vitro, antibodies promote killing of *Legionella* by phagocytes (neutrophils, monocytes, and alveolar macrophages). Immunized animals develop a specific antibody response, with subsequent resistance to *Legionella* challenge. However, antibodies neither enhance lysis by complement nor inhibit intracellular multiplication within phagocytes.

Some *L. pneumophila* strains are clearly more virulent than others, although the precise factors mediating virulence remain uncertain. For example, although multiple strains may colonize water-distribution systems, only a few cause disease in patients exposed to water from these systems. At least one surface epitope of *L. pneumophila* serogroup 1 is associated with virulence. Monoclonal antibody subtype mAb2 has been linked to virulence. *L. pneumophila* serogroup 6 is more commonly involved in hospital-acquired Legionnaires' disease and is more likely to be associated with a poor outcome.

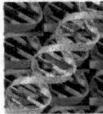 The genome of *L. pneumophila* has been sequenced. A broad range of membrane transporters within the genome are thought to optimize the use of nutrients in water and soil.

■ CLINICAL AND LABORATORY FEATURES

Pontiac fever

Pontiac fever is an acute, self-limiting, flu-like illness with an incubation period of 24–48 h. Pneumonia does not develop. Malaise, fatigue, and myalgias are the most common symptoms, occurring in 97% of cases. Fever (usually with chills) develops in 80–90% of cases and headache in 80%. Other symptoms (seen in <50% of cases) include arthralgias, nausea, cough, abdominal pain, and diarrhea. Modest leukocytosis with a neutrophilic predominance is sometimes detected. Complete recovery occurs within a few days; antibiotic therapy is unnecessary. A few patients may experience lassitude for many weeks after recovery. The diagnosis is established by antibody seroconversion.

Legionnaires' disease (pneumonia)

Legionnaires' disease is often included in the differential diagnosis of "atypical pneumonia," along with pneumonia due to *C. pneumoniae*, *Chlamydophila psittaci*, *Mycoplasma pneumoniae*, *Coxiella burnetii*, and some viruses. The clinical similarities among these types of pneumonia include a relatively nonproductive cough and a low incidence of grossly purulent sputum. However, the clinical manifestations of Legionnaires' disease are usually more severe than those of most "atypical" pneumonias, and the course and prognosis of *Legionella* pneumonia more closely resemble those of bacteremic pneumococcal pneumonia than those of pneumonia due to other "atypical" pathogens. Patients with community-acquired Legionnaires' disease are significantly more likely than patients with pneumonia of other etiologies to be admitted to an intensive care unit on presentation.

The incubation period for Legionnaires' disease is usually 2–10 days, although longer incubation periods have been documented. The symptoms and signs may range from a mild cough and a slight fever to stupor with widespread pulmonary infiltrates and multisystem failure. Nonspecific symptoms—malaise, fatigue, anorexia, and headache—are seen early in the illness. Myalgias and arthralgias are uncommon but are prominent in a few patients. Upper respiratory symptoms, including coryza, are rare.

The mild cough of Legionnaires' disease is only slightly productive. Sometimes the sputum is streaked with blood. Chest pain—either pleuritic or nonpleuritic—can be a prominent feature and, when coupled with hemoptysis, can lead to an incorrect diagnosis

TABLE 147-1 Clinical Clues Suggestive of Legionnaires' Disease

Diarrhea

High fever (>40°C; >104°F)

Numerous neutrophils but no organisms revealed by Gram's staining of respiratory secretions

Hyponatremia (serum sodium level <131 mg/dL)

Failure to respond to β-lactam drugs (penicillins or cephalosporins) and aminoglycoside antibiotics

Occurrence of illness in an environment in which the potable water supply is known to be contaminated with *Legionella*

Onset of symptoms within 10 days after discharge from the hospital

---

of pulmonary embolism. Shortness of breath is reported by one-third to one-half of patients. Gastrointestinal difficulties are often pronounced; abdominal pain, nausea, and vomiting affect 10–20% of patients. Diarrhea (watery rather than bloody) is reported in 25–50% of cases. The most common neurologic abnormalities are confusion or changes in mental status; however, the multitudinous neurologic symptoms reported range from headache and lethargy to encephalopathy.

Patients with Legionnaires' disease virtually always have fever. Temperatures in excess of 40.5°C (104.9°F) were recorded in 20% of the cases in one series. Relative bradycardia has been overemphasized as a useful diagnostic finding; it occurs primarily in older patients with severe pneumonia. Chest examination reveals rales early in the course and evidence of consolidations as the disease progresses. Abdominal examination may reveal generalized or local tenderness.

Although the clinical manifestations often considered classic for Legionnaires' disease (Table 147-1) may suggest the diagnosis, prospective comparative studies have shown that clinical manifestations are generally nonspecific and that Legionnaires' disease is not readily distinguishable from pneumonia of other etiologies. In a review of 13 studies of community-acquired pneumonia, clinical manifestations that occurred significantly more often in Legionnaires' disease included diarrhea, neurologic findings (including confusion), and a temperature of >39°C. Hyponatremia, elevated values in liver function tests, and hematuria also occurred more frequently in Legionnaires' disease. Other laboratory abnormalities include

creatine phosphokinase elevation, hypophosphatemia, serum creatinine elevation, and proteinuria.

 Sporadic cases of Legionnaires' disease appear to be more severe than outbreak-associated and hospital-acquired cases, presumably because their diagnosis is delayed. Results of the German CAPNETZ Study showed that, among cases of community-acquired *Legionella* pneumonia, ambulatory cases were as common as cases requiring hospitalization.

Extrapulmonary legionellosis

Since the portal of entry for *Legionella* is the lung in virtually all cases, extrapulmonary manifestations usually result from blood-borne dissemination from the lung. *Legionella* has been identified in lymph nodes, spleen, liver, or kidneys in autopsied cases. The most common extrapulmonary site of legionellosis is the heart; numerous reports have described myocarditis, pericarditis, postcardiotomy syndrome, and prosthetic-valve endocarditis. Most cases have been hospital-acquired. In some patients without overt evidence of pneumonia, the organisms may gain entry through a postoperative sternal wound exposed to contaminated tap water or through a mediastinal-tube insertion site. Sinusitis, peritonitis, pyelonephritis, skin and soft tissue infection, septic arthritis, and pancreatitis have been seen predominantly in immunosuppressed patients.

Chest radiography

Virtually all patients with Legionnaires' disease have abnormal chest radiographs showing pulmonary infiltrates at the time of clinical presentation. In a few cases of hospital-acquired disease, fever and respiratory tract symptoms have preceded the radiographic appearance of the infiltrate. Radiologic findings are nonspecific. Pleural effusion is evident in 28–63% of patients on hospital admission. In immunosuppressed patients, especially those receiving glucocorticoids, distinctive rounded nodular opacities may be seen; these lesions may expand and cavitate (Fig. 147-1). Likewise, abscesses can occur in immunosuppressed hosts. The progression of infiltrates and pleural effusion on chest radiography despite appropriate antibiotic therapy within the first week is common, and radiographic improvement lags behind clinical improvement by several days. Complete clearing of infiltrates requires 1–4 months.

■ DIAGNOSIS

Given the nonspecific clinical manifestations of Legionnaires' disease and the high mortality rates for untreated Legionnaires' disease, the use of *Legionella* testing—especially the *Legionella* urinary

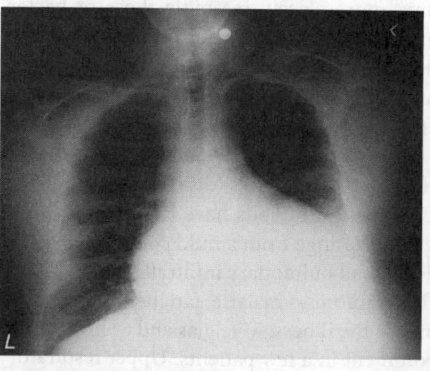
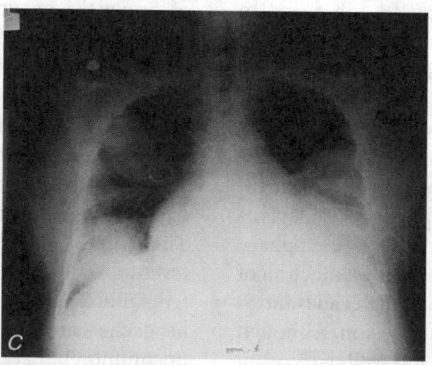
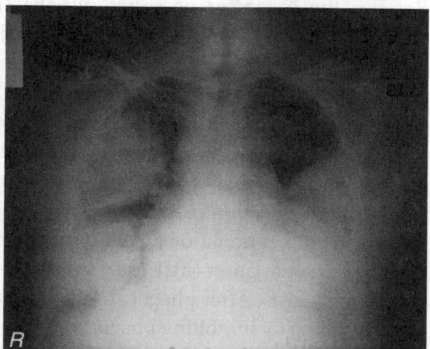

Figure 147-1   Chest radiographic findings in a 52-year-old man who presented with pneumonia subsequently diagnosed as Legionnaires' disease. The patient was a cigarette smoker with chronic obstructive pulmonary disease and alcoholic cardiomyopathy; he had received glucocorticoids. *L. pneumophila* was identified by direct fluorescent antibody staining and culture of sputum. *Left:* Baseline chest radiograph showing long-standing cardiomegaly. *Center:* Admission chest radiograph showing new rounded opacities. *Right:* Chest radiograph taken 3 days after admission, during treatment with erythromycin.

TABLE 147-2 Utility of Special Laboratory Tests for the Diagnosis of Legionnaires' Disease

Test	Sensitivity, %	Specificity, %
Culture		
Sputum[a]	80	100
Transtracheal aspirate	90	100
Direct fluorescent antibody staining of sputum	50–70	96–99
Urinary antigen testing[b]	70	100
Antibody serology[c]	40–60	96–99

[a]Use of multiple selective media with dyes.
[b]Serogroup 1 only.
[c]IgG and IgM testing of both acute- and convalescent-phase sera. A single titer of ≥1:256 is considered presumptive, while fourfold seroconversion is considered definitive.

antigen test—is recommended for all patients with community-acquired pneumonia, including patients with ambulatory pneumonia and hospitalized children. *Legionella* cultures should be made more widely available since the urinary antigen test can diagnose only *L. pneumophila* serogroup 1. Hospitals in which the drinking water is known to be colonized with *Legionella* species should have *Legionella* cultures routinely available for all patients with hospital-acquired pneumonia.

The diagnosis of Legionnaires' disease requires special microbiologic tests (Table 147-2). The sensitivity of bronchoscopy specimens is similar to that of sputum samples for culture on selective media; if sputum is not available, bronchoscopy specimens may yield the organism. Bronchoalveolar lavage fluid gives higher yields than bronchial wash specimens. Thoracentesis should be performed if pleural effusion is found, and the fluid should be evaluated by direct fluorescent antibody (DFA) staining, culture, and the antigen assay designed for use with urine.

Staining

Gram's staining of material from normally sterile sites, such as pleural fluid or lung tissue, occasionally suggests the diagnosis; efforts to detect *Legionella* in sputum by Gram's staining typically reveal numerous leukocytes but no organisms. When they are visualized, the organisms appear as small, pleomorphic, faint, gram-negative bacilli. *L. micdadei* organisms can be detected as weakly or partially acid-fast bacilli in clinical specimens.

The DFA test is rapid and highly specific but is less sensitive than culture because large numbers of organisms are required for microscopic visualization. This test is more likely to be positive in advanced than in early disease.

Culture

The definitive method for diagnosis of *Legionella* infection is isolation of the organism from respiratory secretions, although culture for 3–5 days is required. Antibiotics added to the medium suppress the growth of competing flora from nonsterile sites, and dyes color the colonies and assist in identification. The use of multiple selective BCYE media is necessary for maximal sensitivity. When culture plates are overgrown with other microflora, pretreatment of the specimen with acid or heat can markedly improve the yield. *L. pneumophila* is often isolated from sputum that is not grossly or microscopically purulent; sputum containing more than 25 epithelial cells per high-power field (a finding that classically suggests contamination) may still yield *L. pneumophila*.

Antibody detection

Antibody testing of both acute- and convalescent-phase sera is necessary. A fourfold rise in titer is diagnostic; 12 weeks are often required for the detection of an antibody response. A single titer of 1:128 in a patient with pneumonia constitutes circumstantial evidence for Legionnaires' disease. Serology is of use primarily in epidemiologic studies. The specificity of serology for *Legionella* species other than *L. pneumophila* is uncertain; there is cross-reactivity with *Legionella* species and some gram-negative bacilli.

Urinary antigen

The assay for *Legionella* soluble antigen in urine is rapid, relatively inexpensive, easy to perform, second only to culture in terms of sensitivity, and highly specific. Several enzyme immunoassays and a rapid immunochromatographic assay are commercially available. The rapid immunochromatographic assay is relatively inexpensive and easy to perform. The urinary antigen test is available only for *L. pneumophila* serogroup 1, which causes ~80% of *Legionella* infections. Cross-reactivity with other *L. pneumophila* serogroups and other *Legionella* species has been detected in up to 22% of urine samples from patients with culture-proven cases. Antigen in urine is detectable 3 days after the onset of clinical disease and disappears over 2 months; positivity can be prolonged when patients receive glucocorticoids. The test is not affected by antibiotic administration.

Molecular methods

DFA stains can identify a number of *Legionella* species. Both polyclonal and monoclonal antibody stains are commercially available. Although its application is currently limited to research investigations, polymerase chain reaction (PCR) with DNA probes is theoretically more sensitive and specific than other methods. A molecular probe is undergoing evaluation. PCR has proven somewhat useful in the identification of *Legionella* from environmental water specimens. In PCR (unlike culture), epidemiologic links cannot be made since the infecting pathogen is not available for molecular subtyping.

TREATMENT   *Legionella* Infection

Because *Legionella* is an intracellular pathogen, antibiotics that can attain high intracellular concentrations are most likely to be effective. The dosages for various drugs used in the treatment of *Legionella* infection are listed in Table 147-3.

The macrolides (especially azithromycin) and the respiratory quinolones are now the antibiotics of choice and are effective as monotherapy. Compared with erythromycin, the newer macrolides have superior in vitro activity, display greater intracellular activity, reach higher concentrations in respiratory secretions and lung tissue, and have fewer adverse effects. The pharmacokinetics of the newer macrolides and quinolones also allow once- or twice-daily dosing. Quinolones are the preferred antibiotics for transplant recipients because both macrolides and rifampin interact pharmacologically with cyclosporine and tacrolimus. Retrospective uncontrolled studies have shown that complications of pneumonia are fewer and clinical response is more rapid in patients receiving quinolones than in those receiving macrolides. Alternative agents include tetracycline and its

TABLE 147-3 Antibiotic Therapy for *Legionella* Infection

Antimicrobial Agent	Dosage[a]
Macrolides	
Azithromycin	500 mg[b] PO or IV[c] q24h
Clarithromycin	500 mg PO or IV[c] q12h
Quinolones	
Levofloxacin	750 mg IV q24h
	500 mg[b] PO q24h
Ciprofloxacin	400 mg IV q8h
	750 mg PO q12h
Moxifloxacin	400 mg[b] PO q24h
Ketolide	
Telithromycin	800 mg PO q24h
Tetracyclines	
Doxycycline	100 mg[b] PO or IV q12h
Minocycline	100 mg[b] PO or IV q12h
Tetracycline	500 mg PO or IV q6h
Tigecycline	100-mg IV load, then 50 mg IV q12h
Others	
Trimethoprim-sulfamethoxazole	160/800 mg IV q8h
Rifampin[d]	160/800 mg PO q12h
	300–600 mg PO or IV q12h

[a] Dosages are derived from clinical experience.
[b] The authors recommend doubling the first dose.
[c] The IV formulation is not available in some countries.
[d] Rifampin should be used only in combination with a macrolide or a quinolone.

analogues doxycycline and minocycline. Tigecycline is active in vitro but clinical experience is minimal. Anecdotal reports have described both successes and failures with trimethoprim-sulfamethoxazole, imipenem, and clindamycin. For severely ill patients with extensive pulmonary infiltrates, a two-drug combination of a newer macrolide or a quinolone with rifampin may be considered for initial treatment. Rifampin is highly active in vitro and in cell models, but its interaction with many other medications, including macrolides, is problematic. Initial therapy should be given by the IV route. A clinical response usually occurs within 3–5 days, after which oral therapy can be substituted. The total duration of therapy in the immunocompetent host is 10–14 days; a longer course (3 weeks) may be appropriate for immunosuppressed patients and those with advanced disease. For azithromycin, with its long half-life, a 5- to 10-day course is sufficient.

Pontiac fever requires only symptom-based treatment, not antimicrobial therapy.

■ PROGNOSIS

Mortality rates for Legionnaires' disease vary with the patient's underlying disease and its severity, the patient's immune status, the severity of pneumonia, and the timing of administration of appropriate antimicrobial therapy. Mortality rates are highest

(80%) among immunosuppressed patients who do not receive appropriate antimicrobial therapy early in the course of illness. With appropriate and timely antibiotic treatment, mortality rates from community-acquired Legionnaires' disease among immunocompetent patients range from 0 to 11%; without treatment, the figure may be as high as 31%. In a study of survivors of an outbreak of community-acquired Legionnaires' disease, sequelae of fatigue, neurologic symptoms, and weakness were found in 63–75% of patients 17 months after receipt of antibiotics.

■ PREVENTION

 Routine environmental culture of hospital water supplies is recommended as an approach to the prevention of hospital-acquired Legionnaires' disease. Guidelines mandating this proactive approach have been adopted throughout Europe and in several U.S. states. Positive cultures from the water supply mandate the use of specialized laboratory tests (especially culture on selective media and the urinary antigen test) for patients with hospital-acquired pneumonia. Studies have shown that neither a high degree of outward cleanliness of the water system nor routine application of maintenance measures decreases the frequency or intensity of *Legionella* contamination. Thus, engineering guidelines and building codes, although routinely advocated as preventive measures, have little impact on the presence of *Legionella*.

Disinfection of the drinking water supply is effective. Two methods have proved reliable and cost-effective. The superheat-and-flush method requires heating of the water so that the distal-outlet temperature is 70–80°C and flushing of the distal outlets with hot water for at least 30 min. This method is ideal for emergency situations. Commercial copper and silver ionization systems have proven effective in numerous hospitals. Chlorine dioxide is a promising modality. Tap water filters have been effective for high-risk patient areas, such as transplantation or intensive care units. Hyperchlorination is no longer recommended because of its expense, carcinogenicity, corrosive effects on piping, and unreliable efficacy.

FURTHER READINGS

CASATI S et al: Compost facilities as a reservoir of *Legionella pneumophila* and other *Legionella* species. Clin Microbiol Infect 16:945, 2010

GREENBERG D et al: Problem pathogens: Paediatric legionellosis—implications for improved diagnosis. Lancet Infect Dis 6:529, 2006

HOFMANN A et al: Fulminant legionellosis in two patients treated with infliximab for Crohn's disease: Case series and literature review. Can J Gastroenterol 23:829, 2009

PEDRO-BOTET ML, YU VL: Treatment strategies for *Legionella* infection. Expert Opin Pharmacother 10:1109, 2009

RICKETTS KD et al: Weather patterns and Legionnaires' disease: A meteorological study. Epidemiol Infect 137:1003, 2009

SHIN S, ROY CR: Host cell processes that influence the intracellular survival of *Legionella pneumophila*. Cell Microbiol 10:1209, 2008

SOPENA N et al: Sporadic and epidemic community legionellosis: Two faces of the same illness. Eur Respir J 29:138, 2007

SQUIER CL et al: A proactive approach to prevention of health-care-acquired Legionnaires' disease: The Allegheny County (Pittsburgh) experience. Am J Infect Control 33:360, 2005

Stout JE et al: Role of environmental surveillance in determining risk for hospital-acquired legionellosis: A national surveillance study with clinical correlations. Infect Control Hosp Epidemiol 28:818, 2007

Von Baum H et al: Community-acquired *Legionella* pneumonia: New insights from the German Competence Network for Community Acquired Pneumonia. Clin Infect Dis 46:1356, 2008

Yu VL, Lee TC: Neonatal legionellosis: The tip of the iceberg for pediatric hospital-acquired pneumonia. Pediatr Infect Dis 29:282, 2010

CHAPTER 148

Pertussis and Other *Bordetella* Infections

Scott A. Halperin

Pertussis is an acute infection of the respiratory tract caused by *Bordetella pertussis*. The name *pertussis* means "violent cough," which aptly describes the most consistent and prominent feature of the illness. The inspiratory sound made at the end of an episode of paroxysmal coughing gives rise to the common name for the illness, "whooping cough." However, this feature is variable: it is uncommon among infants ≤6 months of age and is frequently absent in older children and adults. The Chinese name for pertussis is "the 100-day cough," which accurately describes the clinical course of the illness. The identification of *B. pertussis* was first reported by Bordet and Gengou in 1906, and vaccines were produced over the following two decades.

■ MICROBIOLOGY

Of the 10 identified species in the genus *Bordetella*, only three are of major medical significance. *B. pertussis* infects only humans and is the most important *Bordetella* species causing human disease. *B. parapertussis* causes an illness in humans that is similar to pertussis but is typically milder; co-infections with *B. parapertussis* and *B. pertussis* have been documented. *B. bronchiseptica* is an important pathogen of domestic animals that causes kennel cough in dogs, atrophic rhinitis and pneumonia in pigs, and pneumonia in cats. Both respiratory infection and opportunistic infection due to *B. bronchiseptica* are occasionally reported in humans. Two additional species, *B. hinzii* and *B. holmesii*, are unusual causes of bacteremia; both have been isolated from patients with sepsis, most often from those who are immunocompromised.

Bordetella species are gram-negative pleomorphic aerobic bacilli that share common genotypic characteristics. *B. pertussis* and *B. parapertussis* are the most similar of the species, but *B. parapertussis* does not express the gene coding for pertussis toxin. *B. pertussis* is a slow-growing fastidious organism that requires selective medium and forms small glistening bifurcated colonies. Suspicious colonies are presumptively identified as *B. pertussis* by direct fluorescent antibody testing or by agglutination with species-specific antiserum. *B. pertussis* is further differentiated from other *Bordetella* species by biochemical and motility characteristics.

B. pertussis produces a wide array of toxins and biologically active products that are important in its pathogenesis and in immunity. Most of these virulence factors are under the control of a single genetic locus that regulates their production, resulting in antigenic modulation and phase variation. Although these processes occur both in vitro and in vivo, their importance in the pathobiology of the organism is unknown; they may play a role in intracellular persistence and person-to-person spread. The organism's most important virulence factor is *pertussis toxin*, which is composed of a B oligomer–binding subunit and an enzymatically active A protomer that ADP-ribosylates a guanine nucleotide-binding regulatory protein (G protein) in target cells, producing a variety of biologic effects. Pertussis toxin has important mitogenic activity, affects the circulation of lymphocytes, and serves as an adhesin for bacterial binding to respiratory ciliated cells. Other important virulence factors and adhesins are *filamentous hemagglutinin*, a component of the cell wall, and *pertactin*, an outer-membrane protein. *Fimbriae*, bacterial appendages that play a role in bacterial attachment, are the major antigens against which agglutinating antibodies are directed. These agglutinating antibodies have historically been the primary means of serotyping *B. pertussis* strains. Other virulence factors include tracheal cytotoxin, which causes respiratory epithelial damage; adenylate cyclase toxin, which impairs host immune-cell function; dermonecrotic toxin, which may contribute to respiratory mucosal damage; and lipooligosaccharide, which has properties similar to those of other gram-negative bacterial endotoxins.

■ EPIDEMIOLOGY

Pertussis is a highly communicable disease, with attack rates of 80–100% among unimmunized household contacts and 20% within households in well-immunized populations. The infection has a worldwide distribution, with cyclical outbreaks every 3–5 years (a pattern that has persisted despite widespread immunization). Pertussis occurs in all months; however, in North America, its activity peaks in summer and autumn.

In developing countries, pertussis remains an important cause of infant morbidity and death. The reported incidence of pertussis worldwide has decreased as a result of improved vaccine coverage. However, coverage rates are still <50% in many developing nations (Fig. 148-1); the World Health Organization (WHO) estimates that 90% of the burden of pertussis is in developing regions. In addition, overreporting of immunization coverage and underreporting of disease result in substantial underestimation of the global burden of pertussis. The WHO estimates that there were 254,000 deaths from pertussis among children in 2004.

Before the institution of widespread immunization programs in the developed world, pertussis was one of the most common infectious causes of morbidity and death. In the United States before the 1940s, between 115,000 and 270,000 cases of pertussis were reported annually, with an average yearly rate of 150 cases per 100,000 population. With universal childhood immunization, the number of reported cases fell by >95%, and mortality rates decreased even more dramatically. Only 1010 cases of pertussis

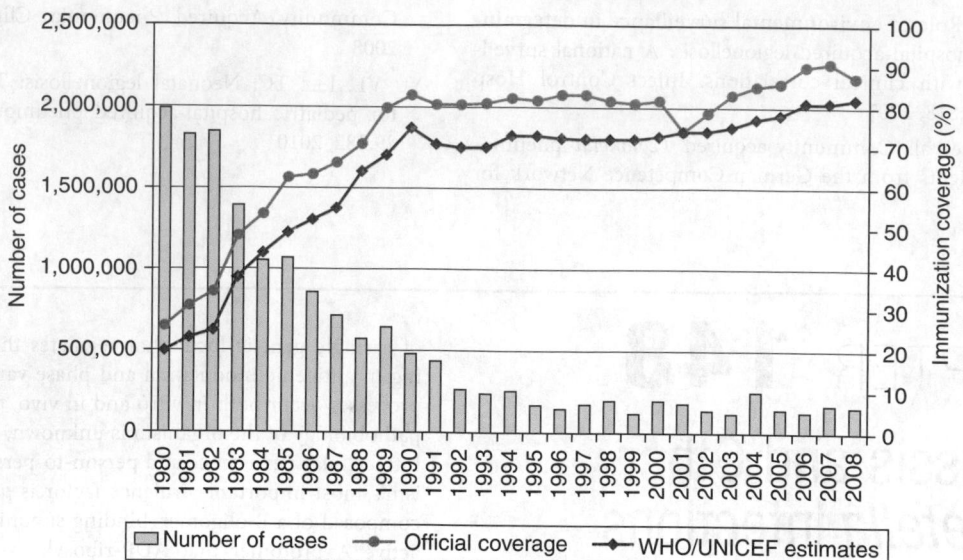

Figure 148-1 Global annual reported pertussis incidence and rate of coverage with DTP3 (diphtheria toxoid, tetanus toxoid, and pertussis vaccine; 3 doses), 1980–2008. (© World Health Organization, 2009.

Source: WHO/IVB database, 2009.)

were reported in 1976 (Fig. 148-2). After that historic low, rates of pertussis slowly increased, peaking at >25,000 cases annually in 2004 and 2005. In 2007, 10,454 cases of pertussis were reported in the United States.

Although thought of as a disease of childhood, pertussis can affect people of all ages and is increasingly being identified as a cause of prolonged coughing illness in adolescents and adults. In unimmunized populations, pertussis incidence peaks during the preschool years, and well over half of children have the disease before reaching adulthood. In highly immunized populations such as those in North America, the peak incidence is among infants <1 year of age who have not completed the three-dose primary immunization series. Recent trends, however, show an increasing incidence of pertussis among adolescents and adults. In the United States in 2007, although infants <6 months of age had the highest incidence of pertussis, most cases were reported in adolescents and adults. Moreover, the figures for adolescents

and adults are likely to be underestimates because of a greater degree of underrecognition and underreporting in these age groups. A number of studies of prolonged coughing illness suggest that pertussis may be the etiologic agent in 12–30% of adults with cough that does not improve within 2 weeks. In one study of the efficacy of an acellular pertussis vaccine in adolescents and adults, the incidence of pertussis in the placebo group was 3.7–4.5 cases per 1000 person-years. Although this prospective cohort study yielded a lower estimate than the studies of cough illness, its results still translate to 600,000–800,000 cases of pertussis annually among adults in the United States. Severe morbidity and high mortality rates, however, are restricted almost entirely to infants. In Canada, there were 16 deaths from pertussis between 1991 and 2001; all those who died were infants ≤6 months of age. Although school-age children are the source of infection for most households, adults are the likely source for high-risk infants and may serve as the reservoir of infection between epidemic years.

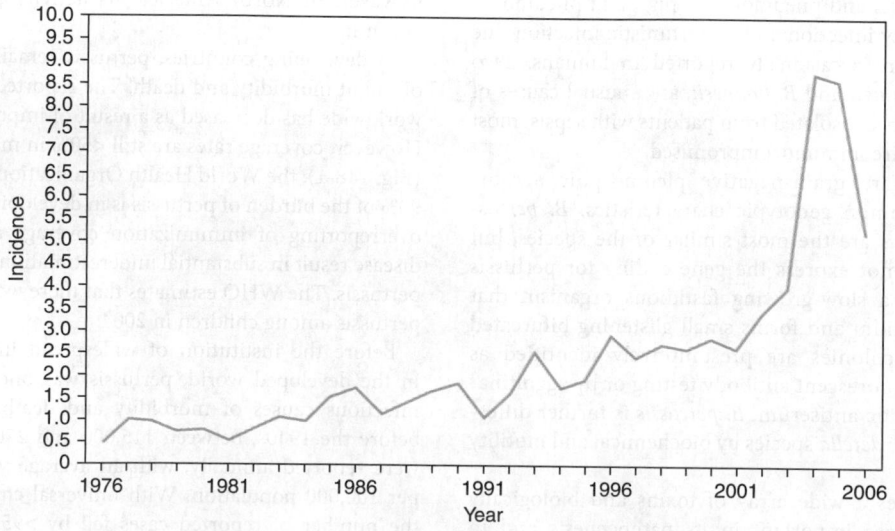

Figure 148-2 Pertussis incidence (per 100,000 population) by year—United States, 1976–2006. [From the Centers for Disease Control and Prevention, MMWR Morb Mortal Wkly Rep 55(53):60, 2008.]

PATHOGENESIS

Infection with *B. pertussis* is initiated by attachment of the organism to the ciliated epithelial cells of the nasopharynx. Attachment is mediated by surface adhesins (e.g., pertactin and filamentous hemagglutinin), which bind to the integrin family of cell-surface proteins, probably in conjunction with pertussis toxin. The role of fimbriae in adhesion and in maintenance of infection has not been fully delineated. At the site of attachment, the organism multiplies, producing a variety of other toxins that cause local mucosal damage (tracheal cytotoxin, dermonecrotic toxin). Impairment of host defense by *B. pertussis* is mediated by pertussis toxin and adenylate cyclase toxin. There is local cellular invasion, with intracellular bacterial persistence; however, systemic dissemination does not occur. Systemic manifestations (lymphocytosis) result from the effects of the toxins.

The pathogenesis of the clinical manifestations of pertussis is poorly understood. It is not known what causes the hallmark paroxysmal cough. A pivotal role for pertussis toxin has been proposed. Proponents of this position point to the efficacy of preventing clinical symptoms with a vaccine containing only pertussis toxoid. Detractors counter that pertussis toxin is not the critical factor because paroxysmal cough also occurs in patients infected with *B. parapertussis*, which does not produce pertussis toxin. It is thought that neurologic events in pertussis, such as seizures and encephalopathy, are due to hypoxia from coughing paroxysms or apnea rather than to the effects of specific bacterial products. *B. pertussis* pneumonia, which occurs in up to 10% of infants with pertussis, is usually a diffuse bilateral primary infection. In older children and adults with pertussis, pneumonia is often due to secondary bacterial infection with streptococci or staphylococci.

IMMUNITY

Both humoral and cell-mediated immunity are thought to be important in pertussis. Antibodies to pertussis toxin, filamentous hemagglutinin, pertactin, and fimbriae are all protective in animal models. Pertussis agglutinins were correlated with protection in early studies of whole-cell pertussis vaccines. Serologic correlates of protection conferred by acellular pertussis vaccines have not been established, although antibody to pertactin, fimbriae, and (to a lesser degree) pertussis toxin correlated best with protection in two efficacy trials. The duration of immunity after whole-cell pertussis vaccination is short-lived, with little protection remaining after 10–12 years. After a three-dose infant primary series of acellular pertussis vaccine, protection persists for at least 5–6 years; the duration of immunity after a four- or five-dose schedule is not yet known, but serologic and modeling studies suggest that a booster may be needed after 10 years. Although immunity after natural infection was thought to be lifelong, seroepidemiologic evidence demonstrates that it clearly is not and that subsequent episodes of clinical pertussis are prevented by intermittent subclinical infection.

CLINICAL MANIFESTATIONS

Pertussis is a prolonged coughing illness with clinical manifestations that vary by age (Table 148-1). Although not uncommon among adolescents and adults, classic pertussis is most often seen in preschool and school-age children. After an incubation period averaging 7–10 days, an illness develops that is indistinguishable from the common cold and is characterized by coryza, lacrimation, mild cough, low-grade fever, and malaise. After 1–2 weeks, this *catarrhal phase* evolves into the *paroxysmal phase*: the cough becomes more frequent and spasmodic with repetitive bursts of 5–10 coughs, often within a single expiration. Posttussive vomiting is frequent, with a mucous plug occasionally expelled at the end of an episode. The episode may be terminated by an audible whoop, which occurs upon rapid inspiration against a closed glottis at the end of a paroxysm.

TABLE 148-1 Clinical Features of Pertussis, by Age Group and Diagnostic Status

Feature	Percentage of Patients		
	Adolescents and Adults		
	Laboratory Confirmation	No Laboratory Confirmation	Children
Cough	95–100	95–100	95–100
Prolonged	60–80	60–80	60–95
Paroxysmal	60–90	50–90	80–95
Sleep-disturbing	50–80	50–80	90–100
Whoop	10–40	5–30	40–80
Posttussive vomiting	20–50	5–30	80–90

During a spasm, there may be impressive neck-vein distension, bulging eyes, tongue protrusion, and cyanosis. Paroxysms may be precipitated by noise, eating, or physical contact. Between attacks, the patient's appearance is normal but increasing fatigue is evident. The frequency of paroxysmal episodes varies widely, from several per hour to 5–10 per day. Episodes are often worse at night and interfere with sleep. Weight loss is not uncommon as a result of the illness's interference with eating. Most complications occur during the paroxysmal stage. Fever is uncommon and suggests bacterial superinfection.

After 2–4 weeks, the coughing episodes become less frequent and less severe—changes heralding the onset of the *convalescent phase*. This phase can last 1–3 months and is characterized by gradual resolution of coughing episodes. For 6–12 months, intercurrent viral infections may be associated with a recrudescence of paroxysmal cough.

Not all individuals who develop pertussis have classic disease. The clinical manifestations in adolescents and adults are more often atypical. In a German study of pertussis in adults, more than two-thirds had paroxysmal cough and more than one-third had whoop. Adult illness in North America differs from this experience: the cough may be severe and prolonged but is less frequently paroxysmal, and a whoop is uncommon. Vomiting with cough is the best predictor of pertussis as the cause of prolonged cough in adults. Other predictive features are a cough at night and exposure to other individuals with a prolonged coughing illness.

COMPLICATIONS

Complications are frequently associated with pertussis and are more common among infants than among older children or adults. Subconjunctival hemorrhages, abdominal and inguinal hernias, pneumothoraces, and facial and truncal petechiae can result from increased intrathoracic pressure generated by severe fits of coughing. Weight loss can follow decreased caloric intake. In a series of >1100 children <2 years of age who were hospitalized with pertussis, 27.1% had apnea, 9.4% had pneumonia, 2.6% had seizures, and 0.4% had encephalopathy; 10 children (0.9%) died. Pneumonia is reported in <5% of adolescents and adults and increases in frequency after 50 years of age. In contrast to the primary *B. pertussis* pneumonia that develops in infants, pneumonia in adolescents and adults with pertussis is usually caused by a secondary infection with encapsulated organisms such as *Streptococcus pneumoniae* or *Haemophilus influenzae*. Pneumothorax, severe weight loss, inguinal hernia, rib fracture, carotid artery aneurysm, and cough syncope have all been reported in adolescents and adults with pertussis.

DIAGNOSIS

If the classic symptoms of pertussis are present, clinical diagnosis is not difficult. However, particularly in older children and adults, it is difficult to differentiate infections caused by *B. pertussis* and *B. parapertussis* from other respiratory tract infections on clinical grounds. Therefore, laboratory confirmation should be attempted in all cases. Lymphocytosis—an absolute lymphocyte count of $>10^8-10^9$/L—is common among young children (in whom it is unusual with other infections) but not among adolescents and adults. Culture of nasopharyngeal secretions remains the gold standard of diagnosis, although DNA detection by polymerase chain reaction (PCR) has replaced culture in many laboratories because of increased sensitivity and quicker results. The best specimen is collected by nasopharyngeal aspiration, in which a fine flexible plastic catheter attached to a 10-mL syringe is passed into the nasopharynx and withdrawn while gentle suction is applied. Since *B. pertussis* is highly sensitive to drying, secretions for culture should be inoculated without delay onto appropriate medium (Bordet-Gengou or Regan-Lowe), or the catheter should be flushed with a phosphate-buffered saline solution for culture and/or PCR. An alternative to the aspirate is a Dacron or rayon nasopharyngeal swab; again, inoculation of culture plates should be immediate or an appropriate transport medium (e.g., Regan-Lowe charcoal medium) should be used. Results of PCR can be available within hours; cultures become positive by day 5 of incubation. *B. pertussis* and *B. parapertussis* can be differentiated by agglutination with specific antisera or by direct immunofluorescence.

Nasopharyngeal cultures in untreated pertussis remain positive for a mean of 3 weeks after the onset of illness; these cultures become negative within 5 days of the institution of appropriate antimicrobial therapy. The duration of a positive PCR in untreated pertussis or after therapy is not known but exceeds that of positive cultures. Since much of the period during which the organism can be recovered from the nasopharynx falls into the catarrhal phase, when the etiology of the infection is not suspected, there is only a small window of opportunity for culture-proven diagnosis. Cultures from infants and young children are more frequently positive than those from older children and adults; this difference may reflect earlier presentation of the former age group for medical care. Direct fluorescent antibody tests of nasopharyngeal secretions for direct diagnosis may still be available in some laboratories but should not be used because of poor sensitivity and specificity. Pseudo-outbreaks of pertussis have been reported as a result of false-positive PCR results. Greater standardization of PCR methodology can alleviate this problem.

As a result of the difficulties with laboratory diagnosis of pertussis in adolescents, adults, and patients who have been symptomatic for >4 weeks, increasing attention is being given to serologic diagnosis. Enzyme immunoassays detecting IgA and IgG antibodies to pertussis toxin, filamentous hemagglutinin, pertactin, and fimbriae have been developed and assessed for reproducibility. Two- or fourfold increases in antibody titer are suggestive of pertussis, although cross-reactivity of some antigens (such as filamentous hemagglutinin and pertactin) among *Bordetella* species makes it difficult to depend diagnostically on seroconversion involving a single type of antibody. Late presentation for medical care and prior immunization also complicate serologic diagnosis because the first sample obtained may in fact be a convalescent-phase specimen. Criteria for serologic diagnosis based on comparison of results for a single serum specimen with established population values are gaining acceptance, and serologic measurement of antibody to pertussis toxin will probably become more widely standardized and available for diagnostic purposes.

DIFFERENTIAL DIAGNOSIS

A child presenting with paroxysmal cough, posttussive vomiting, and whoop is likely to have an infection caused by *B. pertussis* or *B. parapertussis*; lymphocytosis increases the likelihood of a *B. pertussis* etiology. Viruses such as respiratory syncytial virus and adenovirus have been isolated from patients with clinical pertussis but probably represent co-infection.

In adolescents and adults, who often do not have paroxysmal cough or whoop, the differential diagnosis of a prolonged coughing illness is more extensive. Pertussis should be suspected when any patient has a cough that does not improve within 14 days, a paroxysmal cough of any duration, a cough followed by vomiting (adolescents and adults), or any respiratory symptoms after contact with a laboratory-confirmed case of pertussis. Other etiologies to consider include infections caused by *Mycoplasma pneumoniae*, *Chlamydophila pneumoniae*, adenovirus, influenza virus, and other respiratory viruses. Use of angiotensin-converting enzyme (ACE) inhibitors, reactive airway disease, and gastroesophageal reflux disease are well-described noninfectious causes of prolonged cough in adults.

TREATMENT   Pertussis

ANTIBIOTICS   The purpose of antibiotic therapy for pertussis is to eradicate the infecting bacteria from the nasopharynx; therapy does not substantially alter the clinical course unless given early in the catarrhal phase. Macrolide antibiotics are the drugs of choice for treatment of pertussis (Table 148-2); macrolide-resistant *B. pertussis* strains have been reported but are rare. Trimethoprim-sulfamethoxazole is recommended as an alternative for individuals allergic to macrolides.

SUPPORTIVE CARE   Young infants have the highest rates of complication and death from pertussis; therefore, most infants (and older children with severe disease) should be hospitalized. A quiet environment may decrease the

---

TABLE 148-2   Antimicrobial Therapy for Pertussis

Drug	Adult Daily Dose	Frequency	Duration (Days)	Comments
Erythromycin estolate	1–2 g	3 divided doses	7–14	Frequent gastrointestinal side effects
Clarithromycin	500 mg	2 divided doses	7	
Azithromycin	500 mg on day 1, 250 mg subsequently	1 daily dose	5	
Trimethoprim-sulfamethoxazole	160 mg of trimethoprim, 800 mg of sulfamethoxazole	2 divided doses	14	For patients allergic to macrolides; data on effectiveness limited

stimulation that can trigger paroxysmal episodes. Use of β-adrenergic agonists and/or glucocorticoids has been advocated by some authorities but has not been proven to be effective. Cough suppressants are not effective and play no role in the management of pertussis.

INFECTION CONTROL MEASURES Hospitalized patients with pertussis should be placed in respiratory isolation, with the use of precautions appropriate for pathogens spread by large respiratory droplets. Isolation should continue for 5 days after initiation of erythromycin therapy or for 3 weeks (i.e., until nasopharyngeal cultures are consistently negative) when the patient cannot tolerate antimicrobial therapy.

PREVENTION

Chemoprophylaxis

Because the risk of transmission of *B. pertussis* within households is high, chemoprophylaxis is widely recommended for household contacts of pertussis cases. The effectiveness of chemoprophylaxis, although unproven, is supported by several epidemiologic studies of institutional and community outbreaks. In the only randomized placebo-controlled study, erythromycin estolate (50 mg/kg per day in three divided doses; maximum dose, 1 g/d) was effective in reducing the incidence of bacteriologically confirmed pertussis by 67%; however, there was no decrease in the incidence of clinical disease. Despite these disappointing results, many authorities continue to recommend chemoprophylaxis, particularly in households with members at high risk of severe disease (children <1 year of age, pregnant women). Data are not available on use of the newer macrolides for chemoprophylaxis, but these drugs are commonly used because of their increased tolerability and their effectiveness.

Immunization

(See also Chap. 122) The mainstay of pertussis prevention is active immunization. Pertussis vaccine, now available for >80 years, became widely used in North America after 1940; the reported number of pertussis cases has since fallen by >90%. Whole-cell pertussis vaccines are prepared through the heating, chemical inactivation, and purification of whole *B. pertussis* organisms. Although effective (average efficacy estimate, 85%; range for different products, 30–100%), whole-cell pertussis vaccines are associated with adverse events—both common (fever; injection-site pain, erythema, and swelling; irritability) and uncommon (febrile seizures, hypotonic hyporesponsive episodes). Alleged associations of whole-cell pertussis vaccine with encephalopathy, sudden infant death syndrome, and autism, although not substantiated, have spawned an active anti-immunization lobby. The development of acellular pertussis vaccines, which are effective but less reactogenic, has greatly alleviated concerns about the inclusion of pertussis vaccine in the combined infant immunization series.

Although whole-cell vaccines are still used extensively in developing regions of the world, acellular pertussis vaccines are used exclusively for childhood immunization in much of the developed world. In North America, acellular pertussis vaccines for children are given as a three-dose primary series at 2, 4, and 6 months of age, with a reinforcing dose at 15–18 months of age and a booster dose at 4–6 years of age.

Although a wide variety of acellular pertussis vaccines were developed, only a few are still widely marketed; all contain pertussis toxoid and filamentous hemagglutinin. One acellular pertussis vaccine also contains pertactin, and another contains pertactin and two types of fimbriae. In light of phase 3 efficacy studies, most experts have concluded that two-component acellular pertussis vaccines are more effective than monocomponent vaccines and that the addition of pertactin increases efficacy still more. The further addition of fimbriae appears to enhance protective efficacy against milder disease. In two studies, protection conferred by pertussis vaccines correlated best with the production of antibody to pertactin, fimbriae, and pertussis toxin.

Adult formulations of acellular pertussis vaccines have been shown to be safe, immunogenic, and efficacious in clinical trials in adolescents and adults and are now recommended for routine immunization of these groups in several countries, including the United States. In this country, adolescents should receive a dose of the adult-formulation diphtheria–tetanus–acellular pertussis vaccine at the preadolescent physician's visit, and all unvaccinated adults should receive a single dose of this combined vaccine. In addition, it is recommended that all health care workers in the United States be vaccinated against pertussis. Pertussis vaccine coverage among U.S. adolescents rose from 10.8% to 30.4% from 2006 to 2007. Further improvements in adolescent and adult vaccine coverage may permit better control of pertussis across the age spectrum, with collateral protection of infants too young to be immunized.

FURTHER READINGS

DE GREEFF SC et al: Pertussis disease burden in the household: How to protect young infants. Clin Infect Dis 50:1339, 2010

DE SERRES G et al: Morbidity of pertussis in adolescents and adults. J Infect Dis 182:174, 2000

FORSYTH KD et al: Prevention of pertussis: Recommendations derived from the second Global Pertussis Initiative roundtable meeting. Vaccine 25:2634, 2007

HALPERIN SA: The control of pertussis—2007 and beyond. N Engl J Med 356:110, 2007

KRETSINGER K et al: Preventing tetanus, diphtheria, and pertussis among adults: Use of tetanus toxoid, reduced diphtheria toxoid and acellular pertussis vaccine. Recommendations of the Advisory Committee on Immunization Practices (ACIP), supported by the Healthcare Infection Control Practices Advisory Committee (HICPAC), for use of Tdap among health-care personnel. MMWR Recomm Rep 55(RR-17):1, 2006

LEE GM et al: Pertussis in adolescents and adults: Should we vaccinate? Pediatrics 115:1675, 2005

MATTOO S, CHERRY JD: Molecular pathogenesis, epidemiology, and clinical manifestations of respiratory infections due to *Bordetella pertussis* and other *Bordetella* subspecies. Clin Microbiol Rev 18:326, 2005

WARD JI et al: APERT Study Group. Efficacy of an acellular pertussis vaccine among adolescents and adults. N Engl J Med 353:1555, 2005

WATERS V et al: Outbreak of atypical pertussis detected by polymerase chain reaction in immunized preschool-aged children. Pediatr Infect Dis J 28:582, 2009

WENDELBOE AM et al: Infant Pertussis Study Group. Transmission of *Bordetella pertussis* to young infants. Pediatr Infect Dis J 26:293, 2007

CHAPTER 149

Diseases Caused by Gram-Negative Enteric Bacilli

Thomas A. Russo

James R. Johnson

GENERAL FEATURES AND PRINCIPLES

The gram-negative enteric bacilli are common causes of a wide variety of infections involving diverse anatomic sites in both healthy and compromised hosts. Some members of this group have become increasingly resistant to antimicrobial treatment, and new infectious syndromes have emerged. Therefore, a thorough knowledge of clinical presentations and appropriate therapeutic choices is necessary for optimal outcomes.

■ EPIDEMIOLOGY

Escherichia coli, *Klebsiella*, *Proteus*, *Enterobacter*, *Serratia*, *Citrobacter*, *Morganella*, *Providencia*, and *Edwardsiella* are components of the normal animal and human colonic flora and/or of the flora of a variety of environmental habitats, including long-term-care facilities (LTCFs) and hospitals. As a result, except for certain pathotypes of intestinal pathogenic *E. coli*, these genera are global pathogens. In healthy humans, *E. coli* is the predominant species of gram-negative bacilli (GNB) in the colonic flora. GNB (primarily *E. coli*, *Klebsiella*, and *Proteus*) only transiently colonize the oropharynx and skin of healthy individuals. In contrast, in LTCF and hospital settings, a variety of GNB emerge as the dominant flora of both mucosal and skin surfaces, particularly in association with antimicrobial use, severe illness, and extended length of stay.

This colonization may lead to subsequent infection; for example, oropharyngeal colonization may lead to pneumonia. In general, among adults, the incidence of infection due to these agents increases with age. Thus, as the mean age of the population increases, so will the number of these infections.

■ STRUCTURE AND FUNCTION

GNB possess an extracytoplasmic outer membrane, a feature shared generally among gram-negative bacteria. This outer membrane consists of a lipid bilayer with associated proteins, lipoproteins, and polysaccharides [capsule, lipopolysaccharide (LPS)]. The outer membrane interfaces with the bacterial environment, including the human host. A variety of components of the outer membrane are critical determinants in pathogenesis and antimicrobial resistance.

■ PATHOGENESIS

Multiple bacterial virulence factors are required for the pathogenesis of infections caused by GNB. Possession of specialized virulence genes defines pathogens and enables them to infect the host efficiently. Hosts and their cognate pathogens have been co-adapting throughout evolutionary history, and it has been speculated that infection is just one point on the spectrum of evolved relationships between microbes and hosts. At one end of this spectrum is a commensal/symbiotic interaction (e.g., mitochondria—formerly bacteria—within eukaryotic cells); at the other end is a lethal outcome, producing a dead-end relationship (e.g., Ebola virus). During the host-pathogen "chess match" over time, various and redundant strategies have emerged in both the pathogens and their hosts that enable these partners to maintain their coexistence (Table 149-1).

Extraintestinal pathogenic *E. coli* (ExPEC) strains and the other genera discussed in this chapter cause infection outside the bowel. All are primarily extracellular pathogens and therefore share certain pathogenic features. Innate immunity (including the activities of complement, antimicrobial peptides, and professional phagocytes) and humoral immunity are the principal host defense components. Both susceptibility to and severity of infection

TABLE 149-1 Interactions of Extraintestinal Pathogenic *E. coli* With the Human Host: A Paradigm for Extracellular, Extraintestinal Gram-Negative Bacterial Pathogens

Bacterial Goal	Host Obstacle	Bacterial Solution
Extraintestinal attachment	Flow of urine, mucociliary blanket	Multiple adhesins (e.g., type I, S, and F1C fimbriae; P pili)
Nutrient acquisition for growth	Nutrient sequestration (e.g., iron via intracellular storage and extracellular scavenging via lactoferrin and transferrin)	Cellular lysis (e.g., hemolysin), multiple mechanisms for competing for iron (e.g., siderophores) and other nutrients
Initial avoidance of host bactericidal activity	Complement, phagocytic cells, antimicrobial peptides	Capsular polysaccharide, lipopolysaccharide
Transmission	?	Irritant tissue damage resulting in increased excretion (e.g., toxins such as hemolysin)
Late avoidance of host bactericidal activity	Acquired immunity (e.g., specific antibodies), treatment with antibiotics	?Cell entry, acquisition of antimicrobial resistance

are increased with dysfunction or deficiencies of these components (Chap. 119). In contrast, the virulence traits of intestinal pathogenic *E. coli*—i.e., the distinctive strains that can cause diarrheal disease—are for the most part different from those of ExPEC and other GNB that cause extraintestinal infections. This distinction reflects site-specific differences in host environments and defense mechanisms.

The virulence factors of extraintestinal pathogenic GNB subserve diverse functions. A given strain usually possesses multiple adhesins for binding to a variety of host cells (e.g., in *E. coli*: type 1, S, and F1C fimbriae; P pili). Nutrient acquisition (e.g., of iron via siderophores) requires many genes that are necessary but not sufficient for pathogenesis. The ability to resist the bactericidal activity of complement and phagocytes in the absence of antibody (e.g., as conferred by capsule or O antigen of LPS) is one of the defining traits of an extracellular pathogen. Tissue damage (e.g., as mediated by hemolysin in the case of *E. coli*) may facilitate spread within the host. Without doubt, many important virulence genes await identification, and our understanding of many aspects of the pathogenesis of infections due to GNB is in its infancy (Chap. 120).

The ability to induce septic shock is another defining feature of these genera. GNB are the most common causes of this potentially lethal syndrome. The lipid A moiety of LPS (via interaction with host Toll-like receptor 4) and probably also other bacterial factors stimulate a proinflammatory host response that, if overly exuberant, results in shock (Chap. 271).

Many antigenic variants (serotypes) exist in most genera of GNB. For example, there are >150 O-specific antigens and >80 capsular antigens in *E. coli*. This antigenic variability, which permits immune evasion and allows recurrent infection by different strains of the same species, has impeded vaccine development (Chap. 122).

INFECTIOUS SYNDROMES

Although certain strains of *E. coli* have evolved to be strictly intestinal pathogens, causing gastroenteritis by a variety of unique pathogenic mechanisms, extraintestinal infections are the predominant disease presentation caused by enteric GNB generally. Depending on both the host and the pathogen, nearly every organ or body cavity can be infected with GNB. *E. coli* and—to a lesser degree— *Klebsiella* and *Proteus* account for most extraintestinal infections due to GNB and are the most virulent pathogens within this group. However, the other genera are becoming increasingly important, particularly among LTCF residents and hospitalized patients. This expanding spectrum of disease-causing genera is due in large part to the intrinsic or acquired antimicrobial resistance of these organisms and the increasing number of individuals with alterations or disruptions of host defenses. The mortality rate is substantial in many GNB infections and correlates with the severity of illness. Especially problematic are pneumonia and bacteremia (arising from any source) when complicated by organ failure (severe sepsis) and/or shock, for which the associated mortality rates are 20–50%.

DIAGNOSIS

Isolation of GNB from ordinarily sterile anatomic sites almost always implies infection, whereas their isolation from nonsterile sites, particularly from open soft-tissue wounds and the respiratory tract, requires clinical correlation to differentiate colonization from infection. Tentative laboratory identification based on lactose fermentation and indole production (described for each genus below), which usually is possible before final identification of the organism and determination of its antimicrobial susceptibilities, may guide empirical antimicrobial therapy.

<table>
<tr><td>**TREATMENT**</td><td>**Infections Caused By Gram-Negative Enteric Bacilli**</td></tr>
</table>

(See also Chap. 133) In this chapter, the Clinical Laboratory Standards Institute (CLSI) classification of cephalosporins will be used, according to which the previously designated first-, second-, third-, and fourth-generation cephalosporins will be designated cephalosporins I, II, III, and IV, respectively. Likewise, the terms *extended* or *expanded spectrum*, which have been used to describe third- and fourth-generation cephalosporins, will be avoided. Accumulating evidence indicates that initiation of appropriate empirical antimicrobial therapy early in the course of GNB infections (particularly serious infections) leads to improved outcomes. Familiarity with evolving patterns of antimicrobial resistance in enteric GNB is necessary in the selection of appropriate empirical therapy, particularly given the lag between published and real-time resistance rates and the ever-increasing prevalence of multidrug-resistant (MDR) GNB. However, if broad-spectrum treatment has been initiated and information on antimicrobial susceptibilities becomes available, it is just as important to use the most appropriate narrower-spectrum agent. Such responsible antimicrobial stewardship will avoid unnecessary selection of and potential superinfection with resistant bacteria, may decrease costs, and will maximize the useful longevity of available antimicrobial agents. Likewise, it is important not to treat patients who are colonized but not infected. The antimicrobial resistance profiles of GNB vary by species, geographic location, regional antimicrobial use, and hospital site [e.g., intensive care units (ICUs) versus wards]. At present, the most reliably active agents against enteric GNB are the carbapenems (e.g., imipenem), the aminoglycoside amikacin, the cephalosporin IV cefepime, and piperacillin-tazobactam.

β-Lactamases, which inactivate β-lactam agents, are the most important mediators of resistance to these drugs in GNB. Decreased permeability and/or active efflux of β-lactam agents, although less common, may occur alone or in combination with β-lactamase-mediated resistance. *Broad-spectrum* β-lactamases, which mediate resistance to many penicillins and cephalosporins I, are frequently expressed in enteric GNB. These enzymes are inhibited by agents such as clavulanate. *Extended-spectrum* β-lactamases (ESBLs) confer resistance to the same drugs as broad-spectrum β-lactamases as well as to cephalosporins III, aztreonam, and (in some instances) cephalosporins IV. The prevalence of acquired ESBL-encoding genes via transferable plasmids is increasing in GNB worldwide, with rates varying greatly even among hospitals in a given region. To date, ESBLs are most prevalent in *Klebsiella pneumoniae*, *K. oxytoca*, and *E. coli* but also occur (and are probably underrecognized) in *Enterobacter*, *Citrobacter*, *Proteus*, *Serratia*, and other enteric GNB. At present, the regional prevalence of ESBL-producing GNB declines in rank order as follows: Latin America > Western Pacific > Europe > United States and Canada. ESBL-producing GNB were initially described in hospitals (ICUs > wards) and LTCFs. However, over the last decade, CTX-M ESBLs have been increasingly described in community-acquired strains. Hospital outbreaks due to ESBL-producing strains have been associated with extensive use of cephalosporins III, particularly ceftazidime. The carbapenems are the most reliably active β-lactam agents against ESBL-expressing strains. GNB that express ESBLs may also possess porin mutations that result in decreased uptake of cephalosporins and β-lactam/β-lactamase inhibitor combinations. Thus, ESBL-producing isolates should be considered resistant to all penicillins, cephalosporins, and aztreonam. Ceftobiprole, which is currently under review by the U.S. Food and Drug Administration (FDA), is a first-in-class cephalosporin with activity against methicillin-resistant *Staphylococcus aureus* and most Enterobacteriaceae; however, it has poor activity in vitro against ESBL-producing GNB. Oral options for the treatment of strains expressing CTX-M ESBLs are limited (see "Treatment of Extraintestinal *E. coli* Infections," below).

AmpC β-lactamases confer resistance to the same substrates as ESBLs plus the cephamycins (e.g., cefoxitin and cefotetan). AmpC enzymes resist inhibition by β-lactamase inhibitors. The presence of constitutive chromosomal AmpC β-lactamases in nearly all strains of *Enterobacter, Serratia, Citrobacter, Proteus vulgaris, Providencia*, and *Morganella* results in resistance to aminopenicillins, cefazolin, and cefoxitin. In addition, some strains of *E. coli, K. pneumoniae*, and other Enterobacteriaceae have acquired plasmids containing AmpC β-lactamase genes. The cephalosporin IV cefepime is stable to AmpC β-lactamases and is an appropriate treatment option if the concomitant presence of an ESBL can be excluded.

Carbapenemases (e.g., the IMP, VIM, and KPC families) confer resistance to the same drugs as ESBLs plus cephamycins and carbapenems. Linked resistance to fluoroquinolones and aminoglycosides is common. Occasionally, resistance to carbapenems is due to the possession of a β-lactamase plus decreased permeability. Unfortunately, carbapenemase-producing enteric GNB are becoming increasingly common, and infection with these strains is associated with elevated mortality rates. Automated susceptibility systems may be unreliable for detection of carbapenemases, particularly those conferring resistance to imipenem and meropenem. Resistance to ertapenem is the most sensitive marker for carbapenem resistance in automated systems. An elevated carbapenem minimal inhibitory concentration should prompt additional polymerase chain reaction (PCR) testing for resistance genes or a modified Hodge test; these methods are more reliable for detection of carbapenemase-producing strains. Tigecycline and the polymyxins exhibit the greatest in vitro activity against such strains. However, tigecycline reaches only low concentrations in serum and urine, a characteristic that warrants concern about its use in the treatment of bacteremia and urinary tract infection (UTI). Furthermore, emerging resistance to both of these agents poses the risk of onset of a post-antimicrobial era with respect to GNB.

Resistance to fluoroquinolones usually is due to alterations of the target site (DNA gyrase and/or topoisomerase IV), with or without decreased permeability, active efflux, or protection of the target site. Resistance to fluoroquinolones is increasingly prevalent among GNB and is associated with resistance to other antimicrobial classes; for example, 20–80% of ESBL-producing enteric GNB are also resistant to fluoroquinolones. At present, fluoroquinolones should be considered unreliable as empirical therapy for infections due to GNB in critically ill patients.

Given the increasing prevalence of MDR GNB, it is reasonable—pending susceptibility results—to combine agents for empirical treatment of GNB infections in critically ill patients. Antimicrobial resistance may not always be identified by in vitro testing; therefore, it is important to assess the clinical response to treatment. Moreover, resistance may evolve during therapy (e.g., through stable derepression of AmpC β-lactamases). In addition, drainage of abscesses and removal of infected foreign bodies are often required for cure. GNB are commonly involved in polymicrobial infections, in which the role of each individual pathogen is uncertain (Chap. 164). Although some GNB are more pathogenic than others, it is usually prudent, if possible, to design an antimicrobial regimen active against all of the GNB

identified, since each is capable of pathogenicity in its own right. Finally, the possibility of a superinfection (e.g., *Clostridium difficile* colitis) must always be kept in mind.

■ PREVENTION

(See also Chap. 131) Diligent adherence to hand-hygiene protocols by health care personnel and avoidance of inappropriate antimicrobial use are key measures in preventing infection and the further development of antimicrobial resistance. Contact precautions should be implemented for patients colonized or infected with carbapenem-resistant (and perhaps other MDR) GNB. Likewise, avoidance of the use of indwelling devices (e.g., urinary and intravascular catheters, endotracheal tubes) and, when they are necessary, placement according to an appropriate protocol decrease infection risk. Positioning (e.g., head of bed at ≥30°) and good oral hygiene decrease the incidence of pneumonia in ventilated patients.

ESCHERICHIA COLI INFECTIONS

■ COMMENSAL STRAINS

For the most part, commensal *E. coli* variants, which constitute the bulk of the normal facultative intestinal flora in most humans, confer benefits to the host (e.g., resistance to colonization with pathogenic organisms). These strains generally lack the specialized virulence traits that enable extraintestinal and intestinal pathogenic *E. coli* strains to cause disease outside and within the gastrointestinal tract, respectively. However, even commensal *E. coli* strains can be involved in extraintestinal infections in the presence of an aggravating factor, such as a foreign body (e.g., a urinary catheter), host compromise (e.g., local anatomic or functional abnormalities such as urinary or biliary tract obstruction or systemic immunocompromise), or an inoculum that is large or contains a mixture of bacterial species (e.g., fecal contamination of the peritoneal cavity).

■ EXTRAINTESTINAL PATHOGENIC (ExPEC) STRAINS

The majority of *E. coli* isolates from symptomatic infections of the urinary tract, bloodstream, cerebrospinal fluid, respiratory tract, and peritoneum (spontaneous bacterial peritonitis) can be differentiated from commensal and intestinal pathogenic strains of *E. coli* by virtue of their distinctive virulence factor profiles (Tables 149-1 and 149-2) and phylogenetic background. ExPEC strains can also cause surgical wound infection, osteomyelitis, and myositis, but the number of cases evaluated to date is too small for a reliable assessment of proportions.

Like commensal *E. coli* (but in contrast to intestinal pathogenic *E. coli*), ExPEC strains are often found in the intestinal flora of healthy individuals and do not cause gastroenteritis in humans. Although acquisition of an ExPEC strain by the host is a prerequisite for ExPEC infection, it is not the rate-limiting step, which instead is entry of an ExPEC strain from its site of colonization (e.g., the colon, vagina, or oropharynx) into a normally sterile extraintestinal site (e.g., the urinary tract, peritoneal cavity, or lungs). ExPEC strains have acquired genes encoding diverse extraintestinal virulence factors that enable the bacteria to cause infections outside the gastrointestinal tract in both normal and compromised hosts (Table 149–1). These virulence genes are, for the most part, distinct from those that enable intestinal pathogenic strains to cause diarrheal disease. All age groups, all types of hosts, and nearly all organs and anatomic sites are susceptible to infection by ExPEC. Even previously healthy hosts can become severely ill or die when infected with ExPEC; however, adverse outcomes are more common among hosts with comorbid illnesses and host defense abnormalities. *E. coli* is the most common enteric GNB to cause extraintestinal infection

TABLE 149-2 **Intestinal Pathogenic *E. coli***

Pathotype[a]	Epidemiology	Clinical Syndrome[b]	Defining Molecular Trait	Responsible Genetic Element[c]
STEC/EHEC	Food, water, person-to-person; all ages, industrialized countries	Hemorrhagic colitis, hemolytic-uremic syndrome	Shiga toxin	Lambda-like Stx1- or Stx2-encoding bacteriophage
ETEC	Food, water; young children in and travelers to developing countries	Traveler's diarrhea	Heat-stable and -labile enterotoxins, colonization factors	Virulence plasmid(s)
EPEC	Person-to-person; young children and neonates in developing countries	Watery diarrhea, persistent diarrhea	Localized adherence, attaching and effacing lesion on intestinal epithelium	EPEC adherence factor plasmid pathogenicity island [locus for enterocyte effacement (LEE)]
EIEC	Food, water; children in and travelers to developing countries	Dysentery	Invasion of colonic epithelial cells, intracellular multiplication, cell-to-cell spread	Multiple genes contained primarily in a large virulence plasmid
EAEC	?Food, water; children in and travelers to developing countries; all ages, industrialized countries	Traveler's diarrhea, acute diarrhea, persistent diarrhea	Aggregative/diffuse adherence, virulence factors regulated by AggR	Chromosomal or plasmid-associated adherence and toxin genes

[a]EAEC, enteroadherent *E. coli*; EHEC, enterohemorrhagic *E. coli*; EIEC, enteroinvasive *E. coli*; EPEC, enteropathogenic *E. coli*; ETEC, enterotoxigenic *E. coli*; STEC, Shiga toxin–producing *E. coli*.
[b]Classic syndromes; see text for details on disease spectrum.
[c]Pathogenesis involves multiple genes, including genes in addition to those listed.

in ambulatory, LTCF, and hospital settings. The diversity and the medical and economic impact of ExPEC infections are evident from consideration of the following specific syndromes.

Extraintestinal infectious syndromes

Urinary tract infection The urinary tract is the site most frequently infected by ExPEC. An exceedingly common infection among ambulatory patients, UTI accounts for 1% of ambulatory care visits in the United States and is second only to lower respiratory tract infection among infections responsible for hospitalization. UTIs are best considered by clinical syndrome (e.g., uncomplicated cystitis, pyelonephritis, and catheter-associated UTIs) and within the context of specific hosts (e.g., premenopausal women, compromised hosts; Chap. 288). *E. coli* is the single most common pathogen for all UTI syndrome/host group combinations. Each year in the United States, *E. coli* causes 85–95% of an estimated 6–8 million episodes of uncomplicated cystitis in premenopausal women, with an estimated $1.6 billion in direct health care costs. Furthermore, 20% of women with an initial cystitis episode develop frequent recurrences (from 0.3 to >20 per year).

Uncomplicated cystitis, the most common acute UTI syndrome, is characterized by dysuria, urinary frequency, and suprapubic pain. Fever and/or back pain suggests progression to pyelonephritis. Even with appropriate treatment of pyelonephritis, fever may take 5–7 days to resolve completely. Persistently elevated or increasing fever and neutrophil counts should prompt evaluation for intrarenal or perinephric abscess and/or obstruction. Renal parenchymal damage and loss of renal function during pyelonephritis occur primarily with urinary obstruction. Pregnant women are at unusually high risk for developing pyelonephritis, which can adversely affect the outcome of pregnancy. As a result, prenatal screening for and treatment of asymptomatic bacteriuria are standard. Prostatic infection is a potential complication of UTI in men. The diagnosis and treatment of UTI, as detailed in Chap. 288, should be tailored to the individual host, the nature and site of infection, and local patterns of antimicrobial susceptibility.

Abdominal and pelvic infection The abdomen/pelvis is the second most common site of extraintestinal infection due to *E. coli*. A wide variety of clinical syndromes occur in this location, including acute peritonitis secondary to fecal contamination, spontaneous bacterial peritonitis, dialysis-associated peritonitis, diverticulitis, appendicitis, intraperitoneal or visceral abscesses (hepatic, pancreatic, splenic), infected pancreatic pseudocysts, and septic cholangitis and/or cholecystitis. In intraabdominal infections, *E. coli* can be isolated either alone or (as often occurs) in combination with other facultative and/or anaerobic members of the intestinal flora (Chap. 127).

Pneumonia *E. coli* is not usually considered a cause of pneumonia (Chap. 257). Indeed, enteric GNB account for only 2–5% of cases of community-acquired pneumonia (CAP), in part because these organisms only transiently colonize the oropharynx in a minority of healthy individuals. However, rates of oral colonization with *E. coli* and other GNB increase with severity of illness and antibiotic use. Consequently, GNB are a common cause of pneumonia among residents of LTCFs and are the most common cause (60–70% of cases) of hospital-acquired pneumonia (HAP) (Chap. 127), particularly among postoperative and ICU patients (e.g., ventilator-associated pneumonia). Pulmonary infection is usually acquired by small-volume aspiration but occasionally occurs via hematogenous spread, in which case multifocal nodular infiltrates can be seen. Tissue necrosis, probably due to cytotoxins produced by GNB, is common. Despite significant institutional variation, *E. coli* is generally the third or fourth most commonly isolated GNB in hospital-acquired pneumonia, accounting for 5–8% of episodes in both U.S.-based and European-based studies. Regardless of the host, pneumonia due to enteric GNB is a serious disease, with high crude and attributable mortality rates (20–60% and 10–20%, respectively).

Meningitis (See also Chap. 381) *E. coli* is one of the two leading causes of neonatal meningitis, the other being group B *Streptococcus*. Most *E. coli* strains that cause neonatal meningitis possess the K1 capsular antigen and derive from a limited number of familiar meningitis-associated clonal groups. After the first month of life, *E. coli* meningitis is uncommon, occurring predominantly in the setting of disruption of the meninges from craniotomy or trauma or in the presence of cirrhosis. In patients with cirrhosis who develop meningitis, the meninges are presumably seeded as a result of poor hepatic clearance of portal vein bacteremia.

Cellulitis/musculoskeletal infection *E. coli* contributes frequently to infection of decubitus ulcers and occasionally to infection of ulcers and wounds of the lower extremity in diabetic patients and other hosts with neurovascular compromise. Osteomyelitis secondary to contiguous spread can occur in these settings. *E. coli* also causes cellulitis or infections of burn sites or surgical wounds (accounting, in fact, for 10% of surgical site infections), particularly when the infection originates close to the perineum. Hematogenously acquired osteomyelitis, especially of vertebral bodies, is more commonly caused by *E. coli* than is generally appreciated; this organism accounts for up to 10% of cases in some series (Chap. 126). *E. coli* occasionally causes orthopedic device–associated infection or septic arthritis and rarely causes hematogenous myositis. Upper-leg myositis or fasciitis due to *E. coli* should prompt an evaluation for an abdominal source with contiguous spread.

Endovascular infection Despite being one of the most common causes of bacteremia, *E. coli* rarely seeds native heart valves. When the organism does seed native valves, it usually does so in the setting of prior valvular disease. *E. coli* infections of aneurysms and vascular grafts are quite uncommon.

Miscellaneous infections *E. coli* can cause infection in nearly every organ and anatomic site. It occasionally causes postoperative mediastinitis or complicated sinusitis and uncommonly causes endophthalmitis or brain abscess.

Bacteremia *E. coli* bacteremia can arise from primary infection at any extraintestinal site. In addition, primary *E. coli* bacteremia can arise from percutaneous intravascular devices or transrectal prostate biopsy or from the increased intestinal mucosal permeability seen in neonates and in the settings of neutropenia and chemotherapy-induced mucositis, trauma, and burns. Roughly equal proportions of *E. coli* bacteremia cases originate in the community and in the hospital. In most studies, *E. coli* and *S. aureus* are the two most common blood isolates of clinical significance. *E. coli*, which accounts for 17–37% of cases, is the most frequent GNB blood isolate in the ambulatory setting and in most LTCF and hospital settings. Isolation of *E. coli* from the blood is almost always clinically significant and is typically accompanied by the sepsis syndrome, severe sepsis (sepsis-induced dysfunction of at least one organ or system), or septic shock (Chap. 271). Calculations based on conservative estimates for the incidence of severe sepsis (0.76/1000), the proportional contribution of *E. coli* to severe sepsis (17%), and a sepsis-associated mortality rate of 30% translate into an estimated 265,000 deaths annually in the world (2009 census data).

The urinary tract is the most common source of *E. coli* bacteremia, accounting for one-half to two-thirds of episodes. Bacteremia from a urinary tract source is particularly common in patients with pyelonephritis, urinary tract obstruction, or urinary instrumentation in the presence of infected urine. The abdomen is the second most common source, accounting for 25% of episodes. Although biliary obstruction (stones, tumor) and overt bowel disruption, which typically are readily apparent, are responsible for many of these cases, some abdominal sources (e.g., abscesses) are remarkably silent clinically and require identification via imaging studies (e.g., CT). Therefore, the physician should be cautious in designating the urinary tract as the source of *E. coli* bacteremia in the absence of characteristic signs and symptoms of UTI. Soft tissue, bone, pulmonary, and intravascular catheter infections are other sources of *E. coli* bacteremia.

Diagnosis

Strains of *E. coli* that cause extraintestinal infections usually grow both aerobically and anaerobically within 24 h on standard diagnostic media and are easily identified by the clinical microbiology laboratory according to routine biochemical criteria. More than 90% of ExPEC strains are rapid lactose fermenters and are indole positive.

| **TREATMENT** | Extraintestinal *E. coli* Infections |

In the past, most *E. coli* isolates were highly susceptible to a broad range of antimicrobial agents. Unfortunately, this situation has changed, and, of the Enterobacteriaceae, *E. coli* is the species in which resistance is evolving most rapidly. In general, the high prevalence of resistance precludes empirical use of ampicillin and amoxicillin-clavulanate, even for community-acquired infections. The prevalence of resistance to cephalosporins I and trimethoprim-sulfamethoxazole (TMP-SMX) is increasing among community-acquired strains in the United States (with current rates of 10–40%) and is even higher outside North America. Until recently, TMP-SMX was the drug of choice for the treatment of uncomplicated cystitis in many locales. Although continued empirical use of TMP-SMX will predictably result in ever-diminishing cure rates, a wholesale switch to alternative agents (e.g., fluoroquinolones) will just as predictably accelerate the widespread emergence of resistance to these antimicrobial classes, as has already occurred in some areas. More than 90% of isolates that cause uncomplicated cystitis remain susceptible to nitrofurantoin and fosfomycin. The prevalence of resistance to fluoroquinolones has increased steadily over the last decade (e.g., from 5% to 20% in North America between 2002 and 2005 and from 8% to 25% among bacteremia isolates from the United Kingdom and Ireland between 2001 and 2006) and is even higher in other regions (Mexico, India). Prevalence figures are higher in settings where fluoroquinolone prophylaxis is used extensively (e.g., in patients with leukemia, transplant recipients, and patients with cirrhosis) and among isolates from LTCFs and hospitals. As for cephalosporin resistance, data from the U.S. National Healthcare Safety Network (NHSN) indicated that just 6% of *E. coli* device-associated/surgical site infections were due to strains resistant to cephalosporins III in 2006–2007. However, significantly higher rates have been reported outside North America; 54% of isolates assessed by the International Nosocomial Infection Control Consortium (INICC) in 2002–2007 were resistant. ESBL-containing strains are increasingly prevalent among both health care–associated (5–10%) and ambulatory isolates (region-dependent figures). An increasing number of reports describe *E. coli* strains causing community-acquired UTIs that contain CTX-M ESBLs. Data suggest that acquisition of CTX-M-containing and fluoroquinolone-resistant strains may result from consumption of meat products from food animals treated with cephalosporins III and IV and fluoroquinolones. Oral treatment options are limited with these strains; however, in vitro and limited clinical data indicate that fosfomycin and—for cystitis—nitrofurantoin appear to be viable options. Carbapenems (e.g., imipenem) and amikacin are the most predictably active agents overall, but carbapenemase-producing strains are on the rise (1–5% among health care–associated isolates). Tigecycline and polymyxin B have been used most frequently for these nearly panresistant isolates. Although this evolving antimicrobial resistance is a source of serious concern, of equal importance is the need to use the most appropriate narrower-spectrum agent whenever possible and to avoid treating colonized but uninfected patients so that the ever-escalating selection of increasingly resistant bacteria is not unnecessarily fueled.

■ INTESTINAL PATHOGENIC STRAINS

Certain strains of *E. coli* are capable of causing diarrheal disease. Other important intestinal pathogens are discussed in Chaps. 128, 142, and 153–156. At least in the industrialized world, intestinal pathogenic strains of *E. coli* are rarely encountered in the fecal flora of healthy persons and instead appear to be essentially obligate pathogens. These strains have evolved a special ability to cause enteritis, enterocolitis, and colitis when ingested in sufficient quantities by a naive host. At least five distinct pathotypes of intestinal pathogenic *E. coli* exist: (1) Shiga toxin–producing *E. coli* (STEC)/enterohemorrhagic *E. coli* (EHEC), (2) enterotoxigenic *E. coli* (ETEC), (3) enteropathogenic *E. coli* (EPEC), (4) enteroinvasive *E. coli* (EIEC), and (5) enteroaggregative *E. coli* (EAEC). Diffusely adherent *E. coli* (DAEC) and cytodetaching *E. coli* are additional putative pathotypes. Transmission occurs predominantly via contaminated food and water for ETEC, STEC/EHEC, EIEC, and EAEC and by person-to-person spread for EPEC (and occasionally STEC/EHEC). Gastric acidity confers some protection against infection; therefore, persons with decreased stomach acid levels are especially susceptible. Humans are the major reservoir (except for STEC/EHEC, with regard to which bovines are the main concern); host range appears to be dictated by species-specific attachment factors. Although there is some overlap, each pathotype possesses a unique combination of virulence traits that results in a distinctive intestinal pathogenic mechanism (Table 149-2). These strains are largely incapable of causing disease outside the intestinal tract. Except in the cases of STEC/EHEC and EAEC, disease due to this group of pathogens occurs primarily in developing countries.

■ SHIGA TOXIN–PRODUCING AND ENTEROHEMORRHAGIC *E. COLI*

STEC/EHEC strains constitute an emerging group of pathogens that can cause hemorrhagic colitis and the hemolytic-uremic syndrome (HUS). Several large outbreaks resulting from the consumption of fresh produce (e.g., lettuce, spinach, sprouts) and of undercooked ground beef have received significant attention in the media. O157:H7 is the most prominent serotype, but serogroups O6, O26, O55, O91, O103, O111, O113, and OX3 have also been associated with these syndromes. The ability of STEC/EHEC to produce Shiga toxin (Stx2 and/or Stx1) or related toxins is a critical factor in the expression of clinical disease. *Shigella dysenteriae* strains that produce the closely related Shiga toxin Stx can cause the same syndrome. Stx2 and its Stx2C variant (which may be variably present in combination with Stx2 and/or Stx1) appear to be more important than Stx1 in the development of HUS. All Shiga toxins studied to date are multimers composing one enzymatically active A subunit and five identical B subunits that mediate binding to globosyl ceramides, which are membrane-associated glycolipids expressed on certain host cells. The Stx1 A subunit cleaves an adenine from the host cell's 28S rRNA, thereby irreversibly inhibiting ribosomal function, whereas the Stx2 A subunit inactivates Bcl2, inducing apoptosis.

Additional properties, such as acid tolerance and adherence, are necessary for full pathogenicity among STEC strains. Most disease-causing isolates possess the chromosomal locus for enterocyte effacement (LEE). This pathogenicity island was first described in EPEC strains and contains genes that mediate adherence to intestinal epithelial cells. EHEC strains make up the subgroup of STEC strains that possess stx_1 and/or stx_2 as well as LEE.

Domesticated ruminant animals, particularly cattle and young calves, serve as the major reservoir for STEC/EHEC. Ground beef—the most common food source of STEC/EHEC strains—is often contaminated during processing. Furthermore, manure from cattle or other animals (including that in the form of fertilizer) can contaminate produce (potatoes, lettuce, spinach, sprouts, fallen apples), and fecal runoff from this source can contaminate water systems. Petting zoos are another source of infection. It is estimated that $<10^2$ CFU of STEC/EHEC can cause disease. Therefore, not only can low levels of food or environmental contamination (e.g., in water swallowed while swimming) result in disease, but person-to-person transmission (e.g., at day-care centers and in institutions) is an important route for secondary spread. Laboratory-associated infections also take place. Illness due to this group of pathogens occurs both as outbreaks and as sporadic cases, with a peak incidence in the summer months.

 In contrast to other intestinal pathotypes, STEC/EHEC causes infections more frequently in industrialized countries than in developing regions. O157:H7 strains are the fourth most commonly reported cause of bacterial diarrhea in the United States (after *Campylobacter*, *Salmonella*, and *Shigella*). Colonization of the colon and perhaps the ileum results in symptoms after an incubation period of 3 or 4 days. Colonic edema and an initial nonbloody secretory diarrhea may develop into the STEC/EHEC hallmark syndrome of grossly bloody diarrhea (as detected by history or examination) in >90% of cases. Significant abdominal pain and fecal leukocytes are common (70% of cases), whereas fever is not; absence of fever can incorrectly lead to consideration of noninfectious conditions (e.g., intussusception and inflammatory or ischemic bowel disease). Occasionally, infections caused by *C. difficile*, *K. oxytoca* (see "*Klebsiella* Infections," below), *Campylobacter*, and *Salmonella* present in a similar fashion. STEC/EHEC disease is usually self-limited, lasting 5–10 days. An uncommon but feared complication of this infection is HUS, which occurs 2–14 days after diarrhea in 2–8% of cases, most often affecting very young or elderly patients. It is estimated that >50% of all cases of HUS in the United States and 90% of HUS cases in children are caused by STEC/EHEC. This complication is probably mediated by the systemic translocation of Shiga toxins. Erythrocytes may serve as carriers of Stx to endothelial cells located in the small vessels of the kidney and brain. The subsequent development of thrombotic microangiopathy (perhaps with direct toxin-mediated effects on various non-endothelial cells) commonly produces some combination of fever, thrombocytopenia, renal failure, and encephalopathy. Although the mortality rate with dialysis support is <10%, residual renal and neurologic dysfunction may persist.

■ ENTEROTOXIGENIC *E. COLI*

 In tropical or developing countries, ETEC is a major cause of endemic diarrhea. After weaning, children in these locales commonly experience several episodes of ETEC infection during the first 3 years of life. The incidence of disease diminishes with age, a pattern that correlates with the development of mucosal immunity to colonization factors (i.e., adhesins). In industrialized countries, infection usually follows travel to endemic areas, although occasional foodborne outbreaks occur. ETEC is the most common agent of traveler's diarrhea, causing 25–75% of cases. The incidence of infection may be decreased by prudent avoidance of potentially contaminated fluids and foods (Chap. 123). ETEC infection is uncommon in the United States, but outbreaks secondary to consumption of food products imported from endemic areas have occurred. A large inoculum (10^6–10^{10} CFU) is needed to produce disease. After ingestion of contaminated water or food (particularly items that are poorly cooked, unpeeled, or unrefrigerated), colonization factor–mediated intestinal adherence occurs over 12–72 h.

Disease is mediated primarily by a heat-labile toxin (LT-1) and/or a heat-stable toxin (STa) that causes net fluid secretion via activation of adenylate cyclase (LT-1) and/or guanylate cyclase (STa) in the jejunum and ileum. The result is watery diarrhea accompanied by cramps. LT-1 consists of an A and a B subunit and is structurally and functionally similar to cholera toxin. Strong binding of the B subunit to the GM_1 ganglioside on intestinal epithelial cells leads to the intracellular translocation of the A subunit, which functions as an ADP-ribosyltransferase. Mature STa is an 18- or 19-amino-acid secreted peptide whose biologic activity is mediated by binding to the guanylate cyclase C found in the brush-border membrane of enterocytes; this binding results in increased intracellular concentrations of cyclic GMP. Characteristically absent in ETEC-mediated disease are histopathologic changes within the small bowel; mucus, blood, and inflammatory cells in stool; and fever. The disease spectrum ranges from a mild illness to a life-threatening cholera-like syndrome. Although symptoms are usually self-limited (typically lasting for 3 days), infection may result in significant morbidity and mortality (mostly from profound volume depletion) when access to health care or suitable rehydration fluids is limited and when small and/or undernourished children are affected.

ENTEROPATHOGENIC E. COLI

EPEC causes disease primarily in young children, including neonates. The first *E. coli* pathotype recognized as an agent of diarrheal disease, EPEC was responsible for outbreaks of infantile diarrhea (including some outbreaks in hospital nurseries) in industrialized countries in the 1940s and 1950s. At present, EPEC infection is an uncommon cause of diarrhea in developed countries but is an important cause of diarrhea (both sporadic and epidemic) among infants in developing countries. Breast-feeding diminishes the incidence of EPEC infection. Rapid person-to-person spread may occur. Upon colonization of the small bowel, symptoms develop after a brief incubation period (1 or 2 days). Initial localized adherence leads to a characteristic effacement of microvilli, with the formation of cuplike, actin-rich pedestals. The actual mechanisms of diarrhea production are an area of ongoing investigation. Diarrheal stool often contains mucus but not blood. Although usually self-limited (lasting 5–15 days), EPEC diarrhea may persist for weeks.

ENTEROINVASIVE E. COLI

EIEC, a relatively uncommon cause of diarrhea, is rarely identified in the United States, although a few food-related outbreaks have been described. In developing countries, sporadic disease is infrequently recognized in children and travelers. EIEC shares many genetic and clinical features with *Shigella*; however, unlike *Shigella*, EIEC produces disease only at a large

inoculum (10^8–10^{10} CFU), with onset generally following an incubation period of 1–3 days. Initially, enterotoxins are believed to induce secretory small-bowel diarrhea. Subsequently, colonization and invasion of the colonic mucosa, followed by replication therein and cell-to-cell spread, result in the development of inflammatory colitis characterized by fever, abdominal pain, tenesmus, and scant stool containing mucus, blood, and inflammatory cells. Symptoms are usually self-limited (7–10 days).

ENTEROAGGREGATIVE AND DIFFUSELY ADHERENT E. COLI

EAEC has been described primarily in developing countries and in young children. However, recent studies indicate that it may be a relatively common cause of diarrhea in all age groups in industrialized countries. EAEC has also been recognized increasingly as an important cause of traveler's diarrhea. A large inoculum is required for infection, which manifests as watery and sometimes persistent diarrhea in both healthy and HIV-infected hosts. In vitro, the organisms exhibit a diffuse or "stacked-brick" pattern of adherence to epithelial cells. Virulence factors that probably are necessary for disease are regulated in part by the transcriptional activator AggR and include the aggregative adherence fimbriae (AAF/I-III); the Hda adhesin; surface protein dispersion; and the enterotoxins Pet, EAST-1, ShET1, and ShET2. Some strains of DAEC are capable of causing diarrheal disease, primarily in children 2–6 years of age in some developing countries, and may perhaps cause traveler's diarrhea. The Afa/Dr adhesins may contribute to the pathogenesis of infection.

DIAGNOSIS

A practical approach to the evaluation of diarrhea is to distinguish noninflammatory from inflammatory cases (Chap. 128). ETEC, EPEC, and DAEC are uncommon causes of noninflammatory diarrhea in the United States; the incidence of EAEC infection in this country may be underrecognized. The diagnosis of these infections requires specialized assays (e.g., PCR-based tests for pathotype-specific genes) that are not routinely available and are rarely needed since the diseases are self-limited. ETEC causes the majority and EAEC a minority of cases of noninflammatory traveler's diarrhea. Definitive diagnosis generally is not necessary. Empirical antimicrobial (or symptom-based) treatment, along with rehydration therapy, is a reasonable approach. If diarrhea persists despite treatment, *Giardia* or *Cryptosporidium* (or, in immunocompromised hosts, certain other microbial agents) should be sought. The diagnosis of infection with EIEC, a rare cause of inflammatory diarrhea in the United States, also requires specialized assays. However, evaluation for STEC/EHEC infection, particularly when bloody diarrhea is reported or observed, is appropriate. Although the most common method currently used to detect STEC/EHEC is to screen for *E. coli* strains that do not ferment sorbitol, with subsequent serotyping for O157, testing for Shiga toxins or toxin genes is more sensitive, specific, and rapid. The latter approach offers the added advantage of detecting both non-O157 STEC/EHEC strains and sorbitol-fermenting strains of O157:H7, which otherwise are difficult to identify. DNA-based, enzyme-linked immunosorbent, and cytotoxicity assays are in various stages of development and are emerging as the diagnostic methods of choice.

TREATMENT — Intestinal *E. coli* Infections

(See also Chap. 128) The mainstay of treatment for all diarrheal syndromes is replacement of water and electrolytes. The use of prophylactic antibiotics to prevent traveler's diarrhea generally should be discouraged, especially in light of high rates of antimicrobial resistance. However, in selected patients (e.g., those who cannot afford a brief illness or have an increased susceptibility to infection), the use of rifaximin, which is non-absorbable and is well tolerated, is reasonable. When stools are free of mucus and blood, early patient-initiated treatment of traveler's diarrhea with a fluoroquinolone or azithromycin decreases the duration of illness, and the use of loperamide may halt symptoms within a few hours. Although dysentery caused by EIEC is self-limited, treatment hastens the resolution of symptoms, particularly in severe cases. In contrast, antimicrobial therapy for STEC/EHEC infection (the presence of which is suggested by grossly bloody diarrhea without fever) should be avoided, since antibiotics may increase the incidence of HUS (possibly via increased production/release of Stx).

KLEBSIELLA INFECTIONS

K. pneumoniae is the most important *Klebsiella* species from a medical standpoint, causing community-acquired, LTCF-acquired, and nosocomial infections. *K. oxytoca* is primarily a pathogen in LTCF and hospital settings. *Klebsiella* species are broadly prevalent in the environment and colonize mucosal surfaces of mammals. In healthy humans, the prevalence of *K. pneumoniae* colonization is 5–35% in the colon and 1–5% in the oropharynx; the skin is usually colonized only transiently. In LTCFs and hospitals, colonization with *K. oxytoca* also occurs, and carriage rates are substantial among both staff and patients. Person-to-person spread is the predominant mode of acquisition. Most *Klebsiella* infections due to "classic" *K. pneumoniae* (cKP) now occur in hospitals and LTCFs. The most common clinical syndromes due to cKP are pneumonia, UTI, abdominal infection, intravascular device infection, surgical site infection, soft tissue infection, and subsequent bacteremia. A critical feature of cKP as a successful health care–associated pathogen has been its evolution into an MDR gram-negative bacillus. MDR strains of cKP have caused a number of nosocomial infection outbreaks in ICUs and neonatal nurseries. Historically, cKP caused severe community-acquired pneumonia, primarily in alcoholics; this syndrome is still observed with some frequency in Africa and Asia but has become increasingly uncommon in the United States and Europe. cKP strains appear to be genomically distinct from hypervirulent *K. pneumoniae* (hvKP), an emerging pathogen that has been recognized increasingly over the past two decades (see "Abdominal Infection," below); it is possible, however, that cKP and hvKP strains have virulence factors in common. *K. pneumoniae* subspecies *rhinoscleromatis* is the causative agent of rhinoscleroma, a granulomatous mucosal upper respiratory infection that progresses slowly (over months or years) and causes necrosis and occasionally obstruction of the nasal passages. *K. pneumoniae* subspecies *ozaenae* has been implicated as a cause of chronic atrophic rhinitis and rarely of invasive disease in compromised hosts. These two *K. pneumoniae* subspecies are usually isolated from patients in tropical climates and are genomically distinct from both cKP and hvKP.

■ INFECTIOUS SYNDROMES
Pneumonia

K. pneumoniae accounts for only a small proportion of cases of CAP (Chap. 257); however, CAP due to *K. pneumoniae* is more common in Africa and Asia than in Europe and the United States. This infection occurs primarily in hosts with underlying conditions (e.g., alcoholism, diabetes, or chronic lung disease). Pulmonary infection is especially common among residents of LTCFs and hospitalized patients because of increased rates of oropharyngeal colonization. Mechanical ventilation is an important risk factor. As in all pneumonias

due to enteric GNB, production of purulent sputum and evidence of airspace disease are typical. Presentation with earlier, less extensive infection is more common than the classically described lobar infiltrate with a bulging fissure. Pulmonary necrosis, pleural effusion, and empyema can occur with disease progression.

UTI

K. pneumoniae accounts for only 1–2% of UTI episodes among otherwise healthy adults but for 5–17% of episodes of complicated UTI, including infections associated with indwelling urinary catheters.

Abdominal infection

Klebsiella causes a spectrum of abdominal infections similar to that caused by *E. coli* but is less frequently isolated from these infections. The new hypervirulent variant of *K. pneumoniae* (hvKP) that has emerged over the past decade was initially reported from the Pacific Rim but was later described in the United States, Canada, Europe, and elsewhere. At first, hvKP infection was characterized and distinguished from traditional infections due to cKP by (1) presentation as community-acquired hepatic abscess, (2) occurrence in patients lacking a history of hepatobiliary disease, and (3) a propensity for metastatic spread to distant sites (e.g., eyes, central nervous system, lungs) in 11–80% of cases (Fig. 149-1, left). More recently, this variant has been identified as the cause of a variety of serious extrahepatic abscesses/infections as well. The affected individuals often have diabetes mellitus and are of Asian extraction; however, nondiabetics and all ethnic groups can be affected. Not uncommonly, hosts are young and healthy. Survivors with metastatic spread often suffer catastrophic morbidity, such as loss of vision and neurologic sequelae.

Other infections

Klebsiella cellulitis or soft tissue infection most frequently affects devitalized tissue (e.g., decubitus and diabetic ulcers, burn sites) and immunocompromised hosts. *Klebsiella* causes some cases of surgical site infection, hematogenously derived endophthalmitis (especially in association with hepatic abscess), and nosocomial sinusitis in addition to occasional cases of osteomyelitis contiguous to soft tissue infection, nontropical myositis, and meningitis (both during the neonatal period and after neurosurgery). Cytotoxin-producing strains of *K. oxytoca* have been implicated as a cause of hemorrhagic (but *not* nonhemorrhagic) antibiotic-associated non–*C. difficile* colitis.

Bacteremia

Klebsiella infection at any site can produce bacteremia. Infections of the urinary tract, respiratory tract, and abdomen (especially hepatic abscess) each account for 15–30% of episodes of *Klebsiella* bacteremia. Intravascular device–related infections account for another 5–15% of episodes, and surgical site and miscellaneous infections account for the rest. *Klebsiella* is a cause of sepsis in neonates and of bacteremia in neutropenic patients. Like enteric GNB in general, *Klebsiella* rarely causes endocarditis or endovascular infection.

■ DIAGNOSIS

Klebsiellae are readily isolated and identified in the laboratory. These organisms usually ferment lactose, although the subspecies *rhinoscleromatis* and *ozaenae* are nonfermenters and are indole negative. The new hypervirulent clinical variant most commonly is capsular serotype K1 or K2 and possesses a hypermucoviscous phenotype (Fig. 149-1, right).

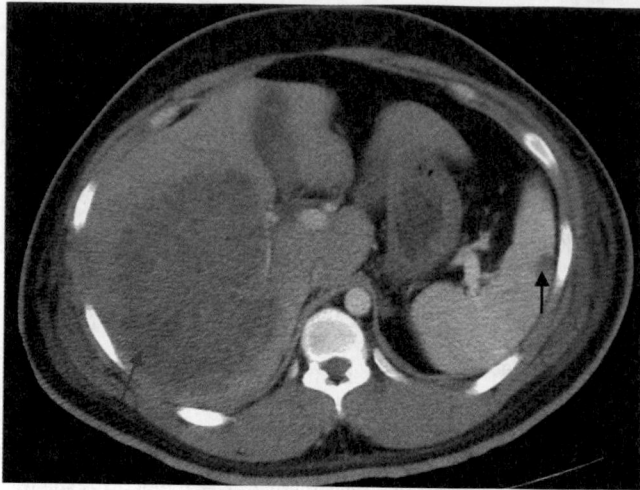
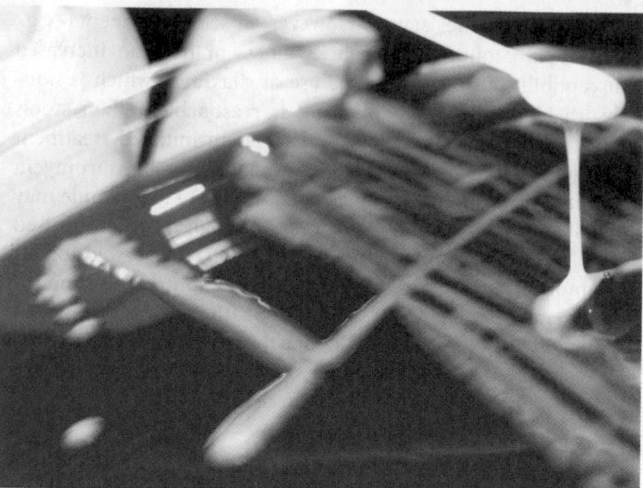

Figure 149-1   New hypervirulent variant of *K. pneumoniae* (hvKP).
Left: An image from an abdominal CT scan of a previously healthy 24-year-old Vietnamese man shows a primary liver abscess (*red arrow*) with metastatic spread to the spleen (*black arrow*). *(Courtesy of Drs. Chiu-Bin Hsaio and Diana Pomakova.) Right*: A culture of the responsible hvKP strain was grown from the patient's blood and the abscess. A hypermucoviscous phenotype has been associated with hvKP strains that cause community-acquired primary liver abscess. This phenotype has been semiquantitatively defined by a positive "string test" (formation of a viscous string >5 mm long when bacterial colonies on an agar plate are stretched by an inoculation loop).

TREATMENT   *Klebsiella* Infections

K. pneumoniae and *K. oxytoca* have largely similar antibiotic resistance profiles. These species are intrinsically resistant to ampicillin and ticarcillin, and nitrofurantoin is only poorly active against them. Data from the NHSN indicated that 24% of *K. pneumoniae* device-associated infections were due to strains resistant to cephalosporins III in 2006–2007. Even higher rates have been reported outside North America, with 68% of isolates from the INICC resistant in 2002–2007. This increasing resistance is mediated primarily by plasmid-encoded ESBLs. In addition, such plasmids usually encode resistance to aminoglycosides, tetracyclines, and TMP-SMX. Furthermore, isolates of *K. pneumoniae* that contain CTX-M ESBLs have been obtained from ambulatory patients with no recent health care contact (see *E. coli* for treatment options). Resistance to β-lactam/β-lactamase inhibitor combinations and cephamycins independent of ESBL-encoding plasmids has also been described with increasing frequency, particularly in Latin America. The prevalence of fluoroquinolone resistance is 15–20% overall and is 50% among ESBL-containing strains. Given both the undesirability of treating the latter strains with penicillins or cephalosporins and the fluoroquinolone resistance often associated with ESBLs, empirical treatment of serious or health care–associated *Klebsiella* infections with amikacin or carbapenems is prudent. Predictably, however, the ESBL-driven use of carbapenems has selected for strains of *Klebsiella* that possess carbapenemases, which confer resistance to the substrates of ESBLs as well as to cephamycins and carbapenems. In the United States, some strains of *Klebsiella* possess KPC-family carbapenemases on transferable plasmids and also exhibit resistance to fluoroquinolones and aminoglycosides. Treatment of infections due to strains that possess carbapenemases is highly challenging, and these strains are increasingly nearly panresistant. The optimal choice for therapy is unclear. Tigecycline, polymyxin B, and polymyxin E (colistin) are the most active agents in vitro and are used most frequently. However, resistance to these agents is already emerging, and strains of *Klebsiella* resistant to all known antimicrobial agents have been described in the United States

and globally. At present, there are no treatment options for these strains. In treating isolates that are more "antimicrobial friendly," it is critical to use the most appropriate narrower-spectrum agent whenever possible.

PROTEUS INFECTIONS

P. mirabilis causes 90% of *Proteus* infections, which occur in the community, LTCFs, and hospitals. *P. vulgaris* and *P. penneri* are associated primarily with infections acquired in LTCFs or hospitals. *Proteus* species are part of the colonic flora of a wide variety of mammals, birds, fish, and reptiles. The ability of these GNB to generate histamine from contaminated fish has implicated them in the pathogenesis of scombroid (fish) poisoning (Chap. 396). *P. mirabilis* colonizes healthy humans (prevalence, 50%), whereas *P. vulgaris* and *P. penneri* are isolated primarily from individuals with underlying disease. The urinary tract is by far the most common site of *Proteus* infection, with adhesins, flagella, IgA protease, and urease representing the principal known urovirulence factors. *Proteus* less commonly causes infection at a variety of other extraintestinal sites.

■ INFECTIOUS SYNDROMES

UTI

Most *Proteus* infections arise from the urinary tract. *P. mirabilis* causes only 1–2% of cases of UTI in healthy women, and *Proteus* species collectively cause only 5% of cases of hospital-acquired UTI. However, *Proteus* is responsible for 10–15% of cases of complicated UTI, primarily those associated with catheterization; indeed, among UTI isolates from chronically catheterized patients, the prevalence of *Proteus* is 20–45%. This high prevalence is due in part to bacterial production of urease, which hydrolyzes urea to ammonia and results in alkalization of the urine. Alkalization of urine, in turn, leads to precipitation of organic and inorganic compounds, which contributes to formation of struvite and carbonate-apatite crystals, formation of biofilms on catheters, and/or development of frank calculi. *Proteus* becomes associated with the stones and biofilms; thereafter, it usually can be eradicated only by removal of the stones or the catheter. Over time, staghorn calculi may form within the renal pelvis and lead to obstruction and renal failure. Thus, urine samples with unexplained alkalinity should be cultured for *Proteus*, and identification of a *Proteus* species in urine should prompt consideration of an evaluation for urolithiasis.

Other infections

Proteus occasionally causes pneumonia (primarily in LTCF residents or hospitalized patients), nosocomial sinusitis, intraabdominal abscesses, biliary tract infection, surgical site infection, soft tissue infection (especially decubitus and diabetic ulcers), and osteomyelitis (primarily contiguous); in rare cases, it causes nontropical myositis. In addition, *Proteus* uncommonly causes neonatal meningitis, with the umbilicus commonly implicated as the source; this disease is often complicated by development of a cerebral abscess. Otogenic brain abscess also occurs.

Bacteremia

The majority of *Proteus* bacteremia episodes originate from the urinary tract; however, any of the less common sites of infection as well as intravascular devices are also potential sources. Endovascular infection is rare. *Proteus* species are occasional agents of sepsis in neonates and of bacteremia in neutropenic patients.

■ DIAGNOSIS

Proteus is readily isolated and identified in the laboratory. Most strains are lactose negative, produce H_2S, and demonstrate characteristic swarming motility on agar plates. *P. mirabilis* is indole negative, whereas *P. vulgaris* and *P. penneri* are indole positive.

TREATMENT *Proteus* Infections

P. mirabilis is usually susceptible to most antimicrobial agents except tetracycline, nitrofurantoin, polymyxin B, and tigecycline. Resistance to ampicillin and cephalosporins I has been acquired by 10–50% of strains. Overall, 10–15% of *P. mirabilis* isolates are resistant to fluoroquinolones; 5% of isolates in the United States now produce ESBLs. Furthermore, isolates of *P. mirabilis* that contain CTX-M ESBLs have been obtained from ambulatory patients with no recent health care contact (see *E. coli* for treatment options). *P. vulgaris* and *P. penneri* exhibit more extensive drug resistance than does *P. mirabilis*. Resistance to ampicillin and cephalosporins I is the rule, and 30–40% of isolates are resistant to fluoroquinolones. Derepression of an inducible chromosomal AmpC β-lactamase (not present in *P. mirabilis*) occurs in up to 30% of *P. vulgaris* isolates. Imipenem, cephalosporins IV (e.g., cefepime), amikacin, and TMP-SMX display excellent activity against *Proteus* species (90–100% of isolates susceptible).

ENTEROBACTER INFECTIONS

E. cloacae and *E. aerogenes* are responsible for most *Enterobacter* infections (65–75% and 15–25%, respectively); *E. sakazakii* (recently renamed *Cronobacter sakazakii*) and *E. gergoviae* are less commonly isolated (1% and <1% of *Enterobacter* isolates, respectively). *Enterobacter* species cause primarily hospital-acquired and other health care–related infections. The organisms are widely prevalent in foods, environmental sources (including equipment at health care facilities), and a variety of animals. Few healthy humans are colonized, but the percentage increases significantly with LTCF residence or hospitalization. Although colonization is an important prelude to infection, direct introduction via IV lines (e.g., contaminated IV fluids or pressure monitors) also occurs. Extensive antibiotic resistance has developed in *Enterobacter* species and probably has contributed to the emergence of the organisms as prominent nosocomial pathogens. Individuals who have previously received antibiotic treatment, have comorbid disease, and are being treated in ICUs are at greatest risk for infection. *Enterobacter* causes a spectrum of extraintestinal infections similar to that described for other GNB.

■ INFECTIOUS SYNDROMES

Pneumonia, UTI (particularly catheter-related), intravascular device–related infection, surgical site infection, and abdominal infection (primarily postoperative or related to devices such as biliary stents) are the most common syndromes encountered. Nosocomial sinusitis, meningitis related to neurosurgical procedures (including use of intracranial pressure monitors), osteomyelitis, and endophthalmitis after eye surgery are less frequent. *E. (C.) sakazakii* is associated with neonatal meningitis/sepsis (particularly in premature infants); contaminated formula has been implicated as a source of this infection, which is often complicated by brain abscess or ventriculitis. Bacteremia can result from infection at any anatomic site. In *Enterobacter* bacteremia of unclear origin, the contamination of IV fluids or medications, blood components or plasma derivatives, catheter-flushing fluids, pressure monitors, and dialysis equipment should be considered, particularly in an outbreak setting. *Enterobacter* can also cause bacteremia in neutropenic patients. *Enterobacter* endocarditis is rare, occurring primarily in association with illicit IV drug use or prosthetic valves.

■ DIAGNOSIS

Enterobacter is readily isolated and identified in the laboratory. Most strains are lactose positive and indole negative.

TREATMENT *Enterobacter* Infections

Significant antimicrobial resistance exists among *Enterobacter* strains. Ampicillin and cephalosporins I and II have little or no activity. The extensive use of cephalosporins III has resulted in the selection of strains that are derepressed for production of AmpC β-lactamase, which confers resistance to cephalosporins III, monobactams (e.g., aztreonam), and—in many cases—β-lactam/β-lactamase inhibitor combinations. Resistance may emerge during therapy; in one study, emergence of resistance was documented in 20% of patients. De novo resistance should be considered when clinical deterioration follows initial improvement, and cephalosporins III should be avoided in the treatment of serious *Enterobacter* infections. National Nosocomial Infections Surveillance System data for 2003 identified resistance to cephalosporins III in 31% of ICU isolates, and INICC data for 2002–2007 reported such resistance in 57% of isolates. Cefepime is stable in the presence of AmpC β-lactamases; thus, it is a suitable option for treatment of *Enterobacter* infections so long as no coexistent ESBL is present. However, the prevalence of ESBL production in *Enterobacter* species (particularly *E. cloacae*) has been increasing and is now 5–30%. Such strains, which are also resistant to cefepime, can be challenging to treat. Fortunately, in the United States, carbapenems, amikacin, and fluoroquinolones have generally retained excellent activity (90–99% of isolates susceptible). Although clinical experience is limited, tigecycline is highly active in vitro. Once again, it is critical to use the most appropriate narrower-spectrum agent whenever possible.

SERRATIA INFECTIONS

S. marcescens causes the majority (>90%) of *Serratia* infections; *S. liquefaciens*, *S. rubidaea*, *S. fonticola*, and *S. odorifera* are isolated occasionally. Serratiae are found primarily in the environment (including in health care institutions), particularly in moist settings. Although serratiae have been isolated from a variety of animals, healthy humans are rarely colonized. In LTCFs or hospitals, reservoirs for the organisms include the hands and fingernails of health care personnel, food, milk (on neonatal units), sinks, respiratory equipment, pressure monitors, IV solutions or parenteral medications (particularly those generated by compounding pharmacies), multiply accessed medication vials, blood products (e.g., platelets), hand soaps and lotions, irrigation solutions, and even disinfectants. Infection results from either direct inoculation (e.g., via IV fluid) or colonization (primarily of the respiratory tract) and subsequent infection. Sporadic infection is most common, but epidemics (often involving MDR strains in adult and neonatal ICUs) and common-source outbreaks occasionally occur. The spectrum of extraintestinal infections caused by *Serratia* is similar to that for other GNB. *Serratia* species are usually considered as causative agents of health care–associated infection and account for 1–3% of hospital-acquired infections. However, population-based laboratory surveillance studies in Canada and Australia demonstrated that community-acquired infections occur more commonly than was previously appreciated.

■ INFECTIOUS SYNDROMES

The respiratory tract, the genitourinary tract, intravascular devices, and surgical wounds are the most common sites of *Serratia* infection and sources of *Serratia* bacteremia. Soft tissue infections (including myositis), osteomyelitis, abdominal and biliary tract infection (postprocedural), contact lens–associated keratitis, endophthalmitis, septic arthritis (primarily from intraarticular injections), and infusion-related bacteremias occur less commonly. Serratiae are uncommon causes of neonatal or postsurgical meningitis and of bacteremia in neutropenic patients. Endocarditis is rare.

■ DIAGNOSIS

Serratiae are readily cultured and identified by the laboratory and are usually lactose and indole negative. Some *S. marcescens* strains and *S. rubidaea* are red-pigmented.

TREATMENT   *Serratia* Infections

Most *Serratia* strains (>80%) are resistant to ampicillin, cephalosporins I, nitrofurantoin, and polymyxin B. In general, >90% of *Serratia* isolates are susceptible to other antibiotics appropriate for use against GNB. Stable derepression of inducible chromosomal AmpC β-lactamases may be preexistent or may develop during therapy. Both in the United States and globally, the prevalence of ESBL-producing isolates is <5%.

CITROBACTER INFECTIONS

C. freundii and *C. koseri* cause most human *Citrobacter* infections, which are epidemiologically and clinically similar to *Enterobacter* infections. *Citrobacter* species are commonly present in water, food, soil, and certain animals. *Citrobacter* is part of the normal fecal flora in a minority of healthy humans, but colonization rates increase in LTCFs and hospitals—the settings in which nearly all *Citrobacter* infections occur. *Citrobacter* species account for 1–2% of nosocomial infections. The affected hosts are usually immunocompromised or have comorbid disease. *Citrobacter* causes extraintestinal infections similar to those described for other GNB.

■ INFECTIOUS SYNDROMES

The urinary tract accounts for 40–50% of *Citrobacter* infections. Less commonly involved sites include the biliary tree (particularly with stones or obstruction), the respiratory tract, surgical sites, soft tissue (e.g., decubitus ulcers), the peritoneum, and intravascular devices. Osteomyelitis (usually from a contiguous focus), neurosurgery-related infection, and myositis occur rarely. *Citrobacter* (particularly *C. koseri*) also uncommonly causes neonatal meningitis, with brain abscess complicating 50–80% of cases. Bacteremia is most often due to UTI, biliary or abdominal infection, or intravascular device infection. *Citrobacter* occasionally causes bacteremia in neutropenic patients. Endocarditis and endovascular infections are rare.

■ DIAGNOSIS

Citrobacter species are readily isolated and identified; 35–50% of isolates are lactose positive, and 100% are oxidase negative. *C. freundii* is indole negative, whereas *C. koseri* is indole positive.

TREATMENT   *Citrobacter* Infections

C. freundii is more extensively resistant to antibiotics than is *C. koseri*. Ampicillin and the cephalosporins I and II display poor activity. *Citrobacter* species possess inducible AmpC β-lactamases; stable derepression may be preexistent or may develop during therapy. Resistance to antipseudomonal penicillins, aztreonam, fluoroquinolones, gentamicin, and cephalosporins III is variable but increasing. The prevalence of ESBL-producing isolates is <5%. Carbapenems, amikacin, cefepime, tigecycline (with which there is limited clinical experience), ceftobiprole (FDA approval pending), fosfomycin (available in the United States only as an oral formulation), and polymyxins (the agents of last resort because of potential toxicities) are most active, with >90% of strains susceptible.

MORGANELLA AND PROVIDENCIA INFECTIONS

M. morganii, *P. stuartii*, and (less frequently) *P. rettgeri* are the members of their respective genera that cause human infections. In terms of epidemiologic associations, pathogenic properties, and clinical manifestations, these organisms are largely similar to *Proteus* species; however, *Morganella* and *Providencia* occur more commonly among LTCF residents; to a lesser degree, they affect hospitalized patients.

■ INFECTIOUS SYNDROMES

These species are primarily urinary tract pathogens, causing UTIs that are most often associated with long-term (>30-day) catheterization. Such infections commonly lead to biofilm formation and catheter encrustation (sometimes causing catheter obstruction) or the development of struvite bladder or renal stones (sometimes causing renal obstruction and serving as foci for relapse). Other, less common infectious syndromes include surgical site infection, soft tissue infection (primarily involving decubitus and diabetic ulcers), burn site infection, pneumonia (particularly ventilator-associated), intravascular device infection, and intraabdominal infection. Rarely, the other extraintestinal infections described for GNB also occur. Bacteremia is uncommon; although any infected site can serve as the source, the urinary tract accounts for most cases, and the next most common sources are surgical, soft tissue, and hepatobiliary sites.

■ DIAGNOSIS

M. morganii and *Providencia* are readily isolated and identified. Nearly all isolates are lactose negative and indole positive.

TREATMENT   *Morganella* and *Providencia* Infections

Morganella and *Providencia* may be extensively resistant to antibiotics. Most isolates are resistant to ampicillin, cephalosporins I, nitrofurantoin, fosfomycin, tigecycline, and polymyxin B; 40% are resistant to quinolones. *Morganella* and *Providencia* possess inducible AmpC β-lactamases; stable derepression may be preexistent or may develop during therapy. Resistance to antipseudomonal penicillins, aztreonam, gentamicin, TMP-SMX, and cephalosporins II and III is emerging but still variably prevalent. The β-lactamase inhibitor tazobactam increases susceptibility to β-lactam agents, but sulbactam and clavulanic acid do not. Imipenem, amikacin, and cefepime are the most active agents (>90% of isolates susceptible). Removal of a colonized catheter or stone is critical for eradication of UTI.

EDWARDSIELLA INFECTIONS

E. tarda is the only member of the genus *Edwardsiella* that is associated with human disease. This organism is found predominantly in freshwater and marine environments and the associated animal species. Human acquisition occurs primarily during interaction with these reservoirs. *E. tarda* infection is rare in the United States; recently reported cases are mostly from Southeast Asia. This pathogen shares clinical features with both *Salmonella* species (as a diarrheal pathogen; Chap. 153) and *Vibrio vulnificus* (as an extraintestinal pathogen; Chap. 156).

■ INFECTIOUS SYNDROMES

Gastroenteritis is the predominant infectious syndrome (50–80% of infections). Self-limiting watery diarrhea is most common, but severe colitis also occurs. The most common extraintestinal infection is wound infection due to direct inoculation, which is often associated with freshwater-, marine-, or snake-related injuries. Other infectious syndromes result from invasion of the gastrointestinal tract and subsequent bacteremia. Most afflicted hosts have comorbidities (e.g., hepatobiliary disease, iron overload, cancer, or diabetes mellitus). A primary bacteremic syndrome, sometimes complicated by meningitis, has a 40% case-fatality rate. Visceral (primarily hepatic) and intraperitoneal abscesses also occur.

■ DIAGNOSIS

Although *E. tarda* can readily be isolated and identified, most laboratories do not routinely seek to identify it in stool samples. Production of hydrogen sulfide is a characteristic biochemical property.

TREATMENT   *Edwardsiella* Infections

E. tarda is susceptible to most antimicrobial agents appropriate for use against GNB. Gastroenteritis is generally self-limiting, but treatment with a fluoroquinolone may hasten resolution. In the setting of severe sepsis, fluoroquinolones, cephalosporins III and IV, carbapenems, and amikacin—either alone or in combination—are the safest choices pending susceptibility information.

INFECTIONS CAUSED BY MISCELLANEOUS GENERA

Species of *Hafnia*, *Kluyvera*, *Cedecea*, *Pantoea*, *Ewingella*, *Leclercia*, and *Photorhabdus* are occasionally isolated from diverse clinical specimens, including blood, sputum, cerebrospinal fluid, joint fluid, bile, and wounds. These organisms are rare and usually cause infection in a compromised host or in the setting of an invasive procedure or a foreign body.

FURTHER READINGS

ENGEL HJ et al: *Serratia* sp. bacteremia in Canberra, Australia: A population-based study over 10 years. Eur J Clin Microbiol Infect Dis 28:821, 2009

FALAGAS ME et al: Fosfomycin: Use beyond urinary tract and gastrointestinal infections. Clin Infect Dis 46:1069, 2008

FLORES J, OKHUYSEN PC: Enteroaggregative *Escherichia coli* infection. Curr Opin Gastroenterol 25:8, 2009

FREEMAN JT et al: Emergence of extended-spectrum beta-lactamase-producing *Escherichia coli* in community hospitals throughout North Carolina: A harbinger of a wider problem in the United States? Clin Infect Dis 49:e30, 2009

HIDRON AI et al: NHSN annual update: Antimicrobial-resistant pathogens associated with healthcare-associated infections: Annual summary of data reported to the National Healthcare Safety Network at the Centers for Disease Control and Prevention, 2006–2007. Infect Control Hosp Epidemiol 29:996, 2008

HOGENAUER C et al: *Klebsiella oxytoca* as a causative organism of antibiotic-associated hemorrhagic colitis. N Engl J Med 355:2418, 2006

JOHNSON JR et al: Molecular analysis of *Escherichia coli* from retail meats (2002–2004) from the United States National Antimicrobial Resistance Monitoring System. Clin Infect Dis 49:195, 2009

RODRIGUEZ-BANO J et al: Community-onset bacteremia due to extended-spectrum β-lactamase-producing *Escherichia coli*: Risk factors and prognosis. Clin Infect Dis 50:40, 2010

SAMONIS G et al: *Citrobacter* infections in a general hospital: Characteristics and outcomes. Eur J Clin Microbiol Infect Dis 28:61, 200

SOULI M et al: An outbreak of infection due to β-lactamase *Klebsiella pneumoniae* carbapenemase 2-producing *K. pneumoniae* in a Greek university hospital: Molecular characterization, epidemiology, and outcomes. Clin Infect Dis 50:364, 2010

CHAPTER 150

Acinetobacter Infections

David L. Paterson
Anton Y. Peleg

Infections with bacteria of the genus *Acinetobacter* have become a significant problem worldwide. *Acinetobacter baumannii* is particularly formidable because of its propensity to acquire antibiotic resistance determinants. Outbreaks of infection caused by strains of *A. baumannii* resistant to multiple antibiotic classes, including carbapenems, are a serious concern in many specialized hospital units, including intensive care units (ICUs). The foremost implication of infection with carbapenem-resistant *A. baumannii* is the need to use "last-line" antibiotics such as colistin, polymyxin B, or tigecycline; these options have the potential to render these bacteria resistant to all available antibiotics.

■ DEFINITION

Acinetobacter species are oxidase-negative, nonmotile, nonfermenting, short gram-negative bacilli that grow well at 37° C in aerobic conditions on a range of laboratory media (e.g., blood agar). Some species may not grow on MacConkey agar. Differentiation of *Acinetobacter* species is difficult with the means typically available to most clinical microbiology laboratories, including commercial semiautomated identification systems. DNA-DNA hybridization is a method used for speciation in reference laboratories. Identification of the most clinically relevant species, *A. baumannii*, by detection of the bla_{OXA-51}-like carbapenemase gene intrinsic to this species has been described.

■ ETIOLOGY

Widely distributed in nature, *Acinetobacter* species can be found in water, in soil, and on vegetables. *Acinetobacter* is a component of the human skin flora and is sometimes identified as a contaminant in blood samples collected for culture. Fecal carriage can be detected in both healthy and hospitalized individuals. Despite the ubiquity of some *Acinetobacter* species, the natural habitat of *A. baumannii* remains to be fully defined.

■ EPIDEMIOLOGY

A. baumannii infections have been diagnosed in patients on all inhabited continents. The vast majority of infections occur in hospitalized patients and other patients with significant health care contact. Outbreaks of carbapenem-resistant *A. baumannii* are particularly problematic. A significant issue is the introduction of carbapenem-resistant *A. baumannii* into hospitals as a result of medical transfers, especially from hospitals where the organism is highly endemic.

The Americas

In 1991 and 1992, outbreaks of carbapenem-resistant *A. baumannii* infection occurred in a hospital in New York City. Subsequently, numerous other hospitals in the United States and South America have had outbreaks of carbapenem-resistant *A. baumannii*. The incidence of infections with *A. baumannii* among military personnel from the United States and Canada has increased since 2002; 102 patients had bloodstream infections at facilities treating U.S.

military personnel injured in Iraq or Afghanistan from January 1, 2002, through August 31, 2004. An epidemiologic investigation revealed that *A. baumannii* could be grown from environmental sites in field hospitals and that the environmental strains were closely related genotypically to clinical isolates. *A. baumannii* strains from injured military personnel from the United States and the United Kingdom were also genotypically related; this finding provided further evidence that *A. baumannii* was being acquired in field hospitals.

Europe

A. baumannii infections have posed a substantial clinical challenge in many parts of Europe since the early 1980s. Three clones (European clones I, II, and III) have been the predominant causes of *A. baumannii* infection in hospitals in Europe. Carbapenem resistance in *A. baumannii* is a significant issue in many European countries, most notably the United Kingdom, Greece, Italy, Spain, and Turkey.

Asia, Australia, the Middle East, and Africa

Although surveillance data are sparse from many countries in these regions, problems with carbapenem-resistant *A. baumannii* abound. Community-acquired infections are well described in northern Australia and some parts of Asia. These infections may be more likely in men >45 years of age who have histories of cigarette smoking, alcoholism, diabetes mellitus, or chronic obstructive airway disease. Community-acquired strains are more susceptible to antimicrobial agents than are hospital-acquired strains.

■ PATHOGENESIS

A. baumannii colonizes patients exposed to heavily contaminated hospital environments or to the hands of health care workers in these locations. Colonization of the upper airways in mechanically ventilated patients may lead to nosocomial pneumonia. Colonization of the skin may lead to central line–associated bloodstream infection, catheter-associated urinary tract infection (UTI), wound infection, or postneurosurgical meningitis. Throat carriage and microaspiration may be involved in the pathogenesis of community-acquired pneumonia due to *A. baumannii*.

Much less is known about the virulence mechanisms of and host responses to *A. baumannii* than about these aspects of other pathogenic gram-negative bacteria. Because of the emergence of multidrug-resistant strains, including those resistant to all available antibiotics, the impetus to study *A. baumannii* pathogenesis has grown. Novel targets for antibacterial drug development are desperately required, and drugs that have antivirulence mechanisms may provide new therapeutic options. Specific virulence mechanisms in *A. baumannii* include iron acquisition and transport systems; outer-membrane protein A (OmpA), which mediates mammalian cell adhesion, invasion, and cytotoxicity through mitochondrial damage and initiation of caspase-dependent apoptosis; lipopolysaccharide (LPS); and the ability to form biofilm on abiotic and biotic surfaces. Biofilm formation on abiotic surfaces is dependent on a pilus assembly system, which in turn is controlled by a traditional two-component regulatory system mediated by *bfmR*. Also important in biofilm formation are biofilm-associated protein; OmpA; the quorum-sensing gene *abaI*, which controls the secretion of 3-hydroxy-C_{12}-homoserine lactone; and the *pga* locus, which is essential for the production of the polysaccharide poly-β-1,6-*N*-acetylglucosamine.

New model systems for the study of *A. baumannii* infection, including both nonmammalian (invertebrate) and mammalian models, have been described. Furthermore, the use of *A. baumannii* transposon-generated mutant libraries to screen for mutants with attenuated growth in human biological fluids (serum and ascites fluid) has allowed the identification of new virulence mechanisms. These include phospholipase D; capsule production mediated by *ptk* and *epsA*; penicillin-binding protein 7/8 encoded by the *pbpG* gene; and a glycosyltransferase important for LPS biosynthesis encoded by the *lpsB* gene.

The LPS of *A. baumannii* appears to play a significant role in eliciting host responses. In studies with knockout mice, Toll-like receptor 4 and CD14 were shown to be important in host recognition, signaling, and cytokine production in response to *A. baumannii*. Humoral responses targeting iron-regulated outer-membrane proteins and the O-polysaccharide component of LPS have also been described.

APPROACH TO THE PATIENT: *Acinetobacter* Infection

Acinetobacter must be considered in the differential diagnosis of hospital-acquired pneumonia, central line–associated bloodstream infection, posttraumatic wound infection in military personnel returning from Iraq and Afghanistan, and postneurosurgical meningitis.

■ CLINICAL MANIFESTATIONS

Pneumonia

It may be difficult to distinguish between upper-airway colonization with *A. baumannii* and hospital-acquired pneumonia. An estimated 5–10% of cases of ventilator-associated pneumonia are due to *A. baumannii*, although much regional variation exists. Typically, patients with *A. baumannii* ventilator-associated pneumonia have had a prolonged stay in ICUs; in outbreak situations, however, patients may acquire the infection within days of arrival in an ICU.

Community-acquired pneumonia due to *A. baumannii* has been described in tropical regions of Australia and Asia. The disease typically occurs during the "wet" season among people with a history of alcohol abuse. Infection may result in fulminant pneumonia requiring admission to an ICU, with a mortality rate of ~50%.

Bloodstream infection

Although *A. baumannii* accounts for only ~1–2% of nosocomial bloodstream infections, crude mortality rates from these infections may be as high as 40%. Sources of bloodstream infection are typically a central line or underlying pneumonia, UTI, or wound infection.

Traumatic battlefield and other wounds

A. baumannii is a well-known pathogen in burn units. This organism is commonly isolated from wounds of combat casualties from Iraq or Afghanistan; it was the most commonly isolated organism in one assessment of combat victims with open tibial fractures but did not appear to contribute directly to persistent nonunion or the need for amputation.

Meningitis

A. baumannii may cause meningitis following neurosurgical procedures. Patients typically have an external ventricular drain in situ.

Urinary tract infection

A. baumannii is an occasional cause of catheter-associated UTI. It is highly unusual for this organism to cause uncomplicated UTI in healthy women.

Other clinical manifestations

A small number of case reports describe *Acinetobacter* prosthetic-valve endocarditis and endophthalmitis/keratitis. The latter is sometimes related to contact lens use or eye surgery.

■ DIAGNOSIS

Acinetobacter infection should be suspected when plump coccobacilli are seen in Gram's-stained respiratory tract secretions, blood cultures, or cerebrospinal fluid. Sometimes the organisms are difficult to de-stain. Given their small size, they may be misidentified as either gram-negative or gram-positive cocci.

TREATMENT: *Acinetobacter* Infection (Table 150-1)

Treatment is hampered by the remarkable ability of *A. baumannii* to upregulate or acquire antibiotic resistance determinants. The most prominent example is that of β-lactamases, including those capable of inactivating carbapenems, cephalosporins, and penicillins. These enzymes, which include the OXA-type β-lactamases (e.g., OXA-23) and the metallo-β-lactamases, are typically resistant to β-lactamase inhibitors such as clavulanate or tazobactam. Plasmids harboring genes encoding these β-lactamases may also harbor genes encoding resistance to aminoglycosides and sulfur antibiotics. The end result is that carbapenem-resistant *A. baumannii* may become truly multidrug resistant.

Selection of empirical antibiotic therapy when *A. baumannii* is suspected is challenging and must rely on a knowledge of local epidemiology. The interval from onset of infection to initiation of effective empirical therapy clearly influences outcome. Given the diversity of resistance mechanisms in *A. baumannii*, definitive therapy should be based on the results of antimicrobial susceptibility testing. Carbapenems (imipenem, meropenem, and doripenem but not ertapenem) have long been thought of as the agents of choice for serious *A. baumannii* infections. However, the clinical utility of carbapenems is increasingly jeopardized by the production of carbapenemases, as described above. Sulbactam may be an alternative to carbapenems. Unlike other β-lactamase inhibitors (e.g., clavulanic acid and tazobactam),

TABLE 150-1 Treatment Options for *Acinetobacter* Infections

Antibiotic	Comments
Sulbactam	Intrinsic activity against *Acinetobacter*, not linked to β-lactamase inhibition
Trimethoprim-sulfamethoxazole	May be an option for urinary tract infection or wound infection
Meropenem	Widely used in ventilator-associated pneumonia, but carbapenem resistance is widespread
Amikacin	May be an option for carbapenem-resistant strains
Tigecycline	May be an option for carbapenem-resistant strains but inappropriate for urinary tract infection, bloodstream infection, or meningitis
Colistin or polymyxin B	May be an option for carbapenem-resistant strains, but pharmacokinetics not yet well understood

sulbactam has intrinsic activity against *Acinetobacter*; this activity is mediated by the drug's binding to penicillin-binding protein 2 rather than its ability to inhibit β-lactamases. Sulbactam is commercially available in a combined formulation with either ampicillin or cefoperazone and may also be available as a single agent in some countries. Despite the absence of randomized clinical trials, sulbactam seems to be equivalent to carbapenems in clinical effectiveness against susceptible strains.

Therapy for carbapenem-resistant *A. baumannii* is particularly problematic. The only currently available choices are polymyxins (colistin and polymyxin B) or tigecycline. Neither option is perfect. Polymyxins may be nephrotoxic and neurotoxic. The optimal dose and schedule for administration of polymyxins to patients in vulnerable groups (e.g., those requiring renal replacement therapy) are unknown. Conventional doses of tigecycline may not result in serum concentrations adequate to treat bloodstream infections. Resistance of *A. baumannii* to tigecycline may develop during treatment with this drug. Clearly, new treatment options are needed for serious *A. baumannii* infections.

■ COMPLICATIONS AND PROGNOSIS

Given the propensity of *A. baumannii* to cause infections in seriously ill patients in ICUs, it is not surprising that *A. baumannii* infections are associated with high mortality rates. Thus a pertinent question is whether *A. baumannii* infections are associated with high attributable mortality rates after the severity of illness is controlled for. A number of studies have addressed this issue but have had disparate results. Whether the discrepant results can be explained purely by methodologic differences is unknown at present.

■ PREVENTION

Multidrug-resistant *A. baumannii* clearly causes outbreaks of infection. In many outbreaks, just one or two strain types are found by molecular epidemiologic analysis. Even in endemic situations, a small number of strain types predominate. In the outbreaks in New York City, for example, two strain types accounted for >80% of carbapenem-resistant isolates. This "oligoclonality" plainly demonstrates the potential importance of infection control interventions in response to outbreaks of multidrug-resistant *A. baumannii* infection.

The hospital environment is an important reservoir of organisms capable of colonizing patients and causing infection. Environmental sources of *A. baumannii* include computer keyboards, glucometers, multidose medication vials, IV nutrition, inadequately sterilized reusable arterial pressure transducers, ventilator tubing, suction catheters, humidifiers, containers of distilled water, urine collection jugs, and moist bedding articles. Pulsatile-lavage wound treatment—a high-pressure irrigation system used to debride wounds—has been associated with an outbreak of *A. baumannii* infection.

Contaminated inanimate objects should be removed from the patient-care environment or subjected to enhanced environmental cleaning. Although contact-isolation procedures (use of gloves and gowns when dealing with colonized patients or their environment), accommodation of patients in single rooms, and improved hand hygiene are critical, attention to the patient-care environment may be the only measure that leads to control of outbreaks of *A. baumannii* infection.

FURTHER READINGS

CHOI CH et al: Outer membrane protein 38 of *Acinetobacter baumannii* localizes to the mitochondria and induces apoptosis of epithelial cells. Cell Microbiol 7:1127, 2005

DOI Y et al: Extensively drug-resistant *Acinetobacter baumannii*. Emerg Infect Dis 15:980, 2009

GADDY JA et al: Regulation of *Acinetobacter baumannii* biofilm formation. Future Microbiol 4:273, 2009

GUERRERO DM et al: *Acinetobacter baumannii*–associated skin and soft tissue infections: Recognizing a broadening spectrum of disease. Surg Infect 11:49, 2010

JACOBS AC et al: Inactivation of phospholipase D diminishes *Acinetobacter baumannii* pathogenesis. Infect Immun 78:1952, 2010

KIM BN et al: Management of meningitis due to antibiotic-resistant *Acinetobacter* species. Lancet Infect Dis 9:245, 2009

KNAPP S et al: Differential roles of CD14 and Toll-like receptors 4 and 2 in murine *Acinetobacter* pneumonia. Am J Respir Crit Care Med 173:122, 2006

MUNOZ-PRICE LS, WEINSTEIN RA: *Acinetobacter* infection. N Engl J Med 358:1271, 2008

PELEG AY et al: *Acinetobacter baumannii*: Emergence of a successful pathogen. Clin Microbiol Rev 21:538, 2008

PEREZ F et al: Antibiotic resistance determinants in *Acinetobacter* spp and clinical outcomes in patients from a major military treatment facility. Am J Infect Control 38:63, 2010

RODRIGUEZ-BANO J et al: Long-term control of hospital-wide, endemic multidrug-resistant *Acinetobacter baumannii* through a comprehensive "bundle" approach. Am J Infect Control 37:715, 2009

SMITH MG et al: New insights into *Acinetobacter baumannii* pathogenesis revealed by high-density pyrosequencing and transposon mutagenesis. Genes Dev 21:601, 2007

PART 8

Infectious Diseases

CHAPTER 151

Helicobacter pylori Infections

John C. Atherton

Martin J. Blaser

DEFINITION

Helicobacter pylori colonizes the stomachs of ~50% of the world's human population throughout their lifetimes. Colonization with this organism is the main risk factor for peptic ulceration (Chap. 293) as well as for gastric adenocarcinoma and gastric MALT (mucosa-associated lymphoid tissue) lymphoma (Chap. 91). Treatment for *H. pylori* has revolutionized the management of peptic ulcer disease, providing a permanent cure in most cases. Such treatment also represents first-line therapy for patients with low-grade gastric MALT lymphoma. Treatment of *H. pylori* is of no benefit in the treatment of gastric adenocarcinoma, but prevention of *H. pylori* colonization could potentially prevent gastric malignancy and peptic ulceration. In contrast, increasing evidence indicates that lifelong *H. pylori* colonization may offer some protection against complications of gastroesophageal reflux disease (GERD), including esophageal adenocarcinoma. Recent research has focused on whether *H. pylori* colonization is a risk factor for some extragastric diseases and whether it is protective against some recently emergent medical problems, such as asthma and obesity.

ETIOLOGIC AGENT

H. pylori is a gram-negative bacillus that has naturally colonized humans for at least 50,000 years—and probably throughout human evolution. It lives in gastric mucus, with a small proportion of the bacteria adherent to the mucosa and possibly a very small number of the organisms entering cells or penetrating the mucosa; its distribution is never systemic. Its spiral shape and flagella render *H. pylori* motile in the mucus environment. The organism has several acid-resistance mechanisms, most notably a highly expressed urease that catalyzes urea hydrolysis to produce buffering ammonia. *H. pylori* is microaerophilic (requiring low levels of oxygen), is slow-growing, and requires complex growth media in vitro. Publication of several complete genomic sequences of *H. pylori* since 1997 has led to significant advances in the understanding of the organism's biology.

A very small proportion of gastric *Helicobacter* infections are due to species other than *H. pylori*, possibly acquired as zoonoses. Whether these non-*pylori* gastric helicobacters cause disease remains controversial. In immunocompromised hosts, several nongastric (intestinal) *Helicobacter* species can cause disease with clinical features resembling those of *Campylobacter* infections; these species are covered in Chap. 155.

EPIDEMIOLOGY

The prevalence of *H. pylori* among adults is ~30% in the United States and other developed countries as opposed to >80% in most developing countries. In the United States, prevalence varies with age: ~50% of 60-year-old persons, ~20% of 30-year-old persons, and <10% of children are colonized. *H. pylori* is usually acquired in childhood. The age association is due mostly to a birth-cohort effect whereby current 60-year-olds were more commonly colonized as children than are current children. Spontaneous acquisition or loss of *H. pylori* in adulthood is uncommon. Other strong risk factors for *H. pylori* colonization are markers of crowding and maternal colonization. The low incidence among children in developed countries at present is due, at least in part, to decreased maternal colonization and increased use of antibiotics.

Humans are the only important reservoir of *H. pylori*. Children may acquire the organism from their parents (more often from the mother) or from other children. Whether transmission takes place more often by the fecal-oral or the oral-oral route is unknown, but *H. pylori* is easily cultured from vomitus and gastroesophageal refluxate and is less easily cultured from stool.

PATHOLOGY AND PATHOGENESIS

H. pylori colonization induces a tissue response in the stomach, *chronic superficial gastritis*, which includes infiltration of the mucosa by both mononuclear and polymorphonuclear cells. (The term *gastritis* should be used specifically to describe histologic features; it has also been used to describe endoscopic appearances and even symptoms, which do not correlate with microscopic findings or even with the presence of *H. pylori*.) Although *H. pylori* is capable of numerous adaptations that prevent excessive stimulation of the immune system, colonization is accompanied by a considerable persistent immune response, including the production of both local and systemic antibodies as well as cell-mediated responses. However, these responses are ineffective in clearing the bacterium. This inefficient clearing appears to be due in part to *H. pylori*'s downregulation of the immune system, which fosters its own persistence.

Most *H. pylori*–colonized persons do not develop clinical sequelae. That some persons develop overt disease whereas others do not is related to a combination of factors: bacterial strain differences, host susceptibility to disease, and environmental factors.

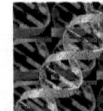 Several *H. pylori* virulence factors are more common among strains that are associated with disease than among those that are not. The *cag* island is a group of genes that encodes a bacterial secretion system through which a specific protein, CagA, is translocated into epithelial cells. CagA affects host cell signal transduction, inducing proliferative, cytoskeletal, and inflammatory changes; a proportion of transgenic mice expressing CagA in the stomach develop gastric adenocarcinoma. The secretion system also translocates soluble components of the peptidoglycan cell wall into the gastric epithelial cell; these components are recognized by the intracellular emergency bacterial receptor Nod1, which stimulates a proinflammatory cytokine response resulting in enhanced gastric inflammation. Patients with peptic ulcer disease or gastric adenocarcinoma are more likely than persons without these conditions to be colonized by *cag*-positive strains. The secreted *H. pylori* protein VacA occurs in several forms. Strains with the more active forms are more commonly isolated from patients with peptic ulcer disease or gastric carcinoma than from persons without these conditions. Other bacterial factors that are associated with increased disease risk include adhesins, such as BabA and SabA, and incompletely characterized genes, such as *dupA*.

The best-characterized host determinants of disease are genetic polymorphisms leading to enhanced activation of the innate immune response, such as polymorphisms in cytokine genes or genes encoding bacterial recognition proteins such as Toll-like receptors (TLRs). For example, colonized people with polymorphisms in the interleukin (IL) 1 gene that cause the production of large quantities of this cytokine in response to *H. pylori* infection are at increased risk of gastric adenocarcinoma. In addition, environmental cofactors are important in pathogenesis. Smoking increases the risks of ulcers and cancer in *H. pylori*–positive individuals. Diets high in salt and preserved foods increase cancer risk, whereas diets high in antioxidants and vitamin C are protective.

The pattern of gastric inflammation is associated with disease risk: antral-predominant gastritis is most closely linked with duodenal ulceration, whereas pangastritis is linked with gastric ulceration and adenocarcinoma. This difference probably explains why patients with duodenal ulceration are not at high risk of developing gastric adenocarcinoma later in life, despite being colonized by *H. pylori*.

How gastric colonization causes duodenal ulceration is now becoming clearer. *H. pylori*–induced inflammation diminishes the number of somatostatin-producing D cells. Since somatostatin inhibits gastrin release, gastrin levels are higher than in *H. pylori*–negative persons, and these higher levels lead to increased meal-stimulated acid secretion in the gastric corpus, which is only mildly inflamed in antral-predominant gastritis. How this increases duodenal ulcer risk remains controversial, but the increased acid secretion may contribute to the formation of the potentially protective gastric metaplasia found in the duodenum of duodenal ulcer patients. Gastric metaplasia in the duodenum may become colonized by *H. pylori* and subsequently inflamed and ulcerated.

The pathogenesis of gastric ulceration and that of gastric adenocarcinoma are less well understood, although both conditions arise in association with pan- or corpus-predominant gastritis. The hormonal changes described above still occur, but the inflammation in the gastric corpus means that it produces less acid (hypochlorhydria) despite hypergastrinemia. Gastric ulcers usually occur at the junction of antral and corpus-type mucosa, and this region is particularly inflamed. Gastric cancer probably stems from progressive DNA damage and the survival of abnormal epithelial cell clones. The DNA damage is thought to be due principally to reactive oxygen and nitrogen species arising from inflammatory cells and perhaps in relation to other bacteria that survive in a hypochlorhydric stomach. Longitudinal analyses of gastric biopsy specimens taken years apart from the same patient show that the common *intestinal* type of gastric adenocarcinoma follows stepwise changes from simple gastritis to gastric atrophy, intestinal metaplasia, and dysplasia. A second, *diffuse* type of gastric adenocarcinoma may arise directly from chronic gastritis alone.

CLINICAL MANIFESTATIONS

Essentially all *H. pylori*–colonized persons have gastric tissue responses, but fewer than 15% develop associated illnesses such as peptic ulceration, gastric adenocarcinoma, or gastric lymphoma (Fig. 151-1).

Worldwide, >80% of duodenal ulcers and >60% of gastric ulcers are related to *H. pylori* colonization (Chap. 293), although the proportion of ulcers due to aspirin and nonsteroidal anti-inflammatory drugs (NSAIDs) is increasing, especially in developed countries. The main lines of evidence for an ulcer-promoting role for *H. pylori* are that (1) the presence of the organism is a risk factor for the development of ulcers, (2) non-NSAID-induced ulcers rarely develop in the absence of *H. pylori*, (3) eradication of *H. pylori* markedly reduces rates of ulcer relapse, and (4) experimental *H. pylori* infection of gerbils causes gastric ulceration.

Prospective nested case-control studies have shown that *H. pylori* colonization is a risk factor for adenocarcinomas of the distal (noncardia) stomach (Chap. 91). Long-term experimental infection of gerbils also may result in gastric adenocarcinoma. Moreover, the presence of *H. pylori* is strongly associated with primary gastric lymphoma, although this condition is much less common. Many low-grade gastric B cell lymphomas arising from MALT are driven by T cell proliferation, which in turn is driven by *H. pylori* antigen stimulation; *H. pylori* antigen–driven tumors may regress either fully or partially after *H. pylori* eradication but require careful long-term monitoring.

Many patients have upper gastrointestinal symptoms but have normal results in upper gastrointestinal endoscopy (so-called functional or nonulcer dyspepsia; Chap. 293). Because *H. pylori* is common, some of these patients will be colonized with the organism. *H. pylori* eradication leads to symptom resolution a little (7%) more commonly than does placebo treatment. Whether such patients have peptic ulcers in remission at the time of endoscopy or whether a small subgroup of patients with true functional dyspepsia respond to *H. pylori* treatment is unclear.

Much interest has focused on a possible protective role for *H. pylori* against GERD (Chap. 292), Barrett's esophagus (Chap. 292), and adenocarcinoma of the esophagus and gastric cardia (Chap. 91). The main lines of evidence for this role are (1) that there is a temporal relationship between a falling prevalence of gastric *H. pylori* colonization and a rising incidence of these conditions and (2) that, in most studies, the prevalence of *H. pylori* colonization (especially with proinflammatory *cagA*+ strains) is significantly lower among patients with these esophageal diseases than among control subjects. The mechanism underlying this protective effect appears to include *H. pylori*–induced hypochlorhydria. Since, at the individual level, GERD symptoms may decrease, worsen, or remain unchanged after treatment targeting *H. pylori*, concerns about GERD should not affect decisions about *H. pylori* treatment when an indication exists.

H. pylori has an increasingly recognized role in other gastric pathologies. It may be one initial precipitant of autoimmune gastritis and pernicious

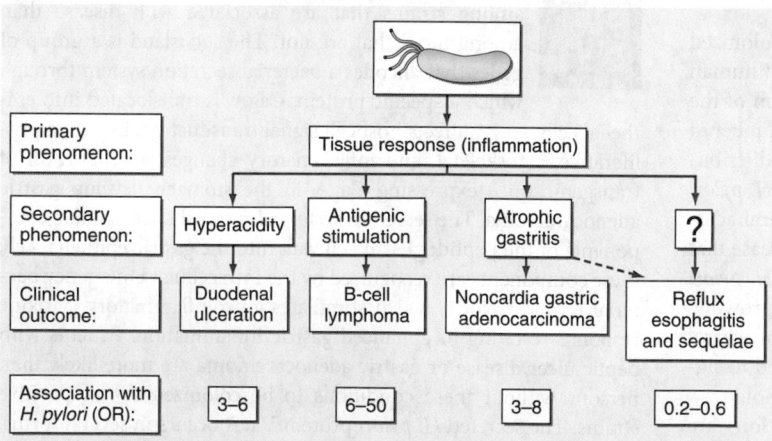

Figure 151-1 **Schematic of the relationships between colonization with *Helicobacter pylori* and diseases of the upper gastrointestinal tract among persons in developed countries.** Essentially all persons colonized with *H. pylori* develop a host response, which is generally termed chronic gastritis. The nature of the interaction of the host with the particular bacterial population determines the clinical outcome. *H. pylori* colonization increases the lifetime risk of peptic ulcer disease, noncardia gastric cancer, and B cell non-Hodgkin's gastric lymphoma [odds ratios (ORs) for all, >3]. In contrast, a growing body of evidence indicates that *H. pylori* colonization (especially with *cagA*+ strains) protects against adenocarcinoma of the esophagus (and the sometimes related gastric cardia) and premalignant lesions such as Barrett's esophagus (OR, <1). While the incidences of peptic ulcer disease (cases not due to nonsteroidal anti-inflammatory drugs) and noncardia gastric cancer are declining in developed countries, the incidence of adenocarcinoma of the esophagus is rapidly increasing. *(Adapted from MJ Blaser: Hypothesis: The changing relationships of Helicobacter pylori and humans: Implications for health and disease. J Infect Dis 179:1523, 1999, with permission.)*

anemia and also may predispose some patients to iron deficiency through occult blood loss and/or hypochlorhydria and reduced iron absorption. In addition, several extragastrointestinal pathologies have been linked with *H. pylori* colonization, although evidence of causality is less strong. Several small studies of *H. pylori* treatment in idiopathic thrombocytopenic purpura have described improvement in or even normalization of platelet counts. Potentially important but even more controversial associations are with ischemic heart disease and cerebrovascular disease. However, the strength of these latter associations is reduced if confounding factors are taken into account, and most authorities consider the associations to be noncausal. Recent studies have shown an inverse association of *cagA*+ *H. pylori* with childhood-onset asthma, hay fever, and atopic disorders. Whether *H. pylori* status is merely a marker or is causally associated with protection against these diseases remains to be determined.

■ DIAGNOSIS

Tests for the presence of *H. pylori* can be divided into two groups: invasive tests, which require upper gastrointestinal endoscopy and are based on the analysis of gastric biopsy specimens, and noninvasive tests (Table 151-1). Endoscopy often is not performed in the initial management of young dyspeptic patients without "alarm" symptoms but is commonly used to exclude malignancy in older patients. If endoscopy is performed, the most convenient biopsy-based test is the biopsy urease test, in which one large or two small antral biopsy specimens are placed into a gel containing urea and an indicator. The presence of *H. pylori* urease leads to a pH alteration and therefore to a color change, which often occurs within minutes but can require up to 24 h. Histologic examination of biopsy specimens for *H. pylori* also is accurate, provided that a special stain (e.g., a modified Giemsa or silver stain) permitting optimal visualization of the organism is used. If biopsy specimens are obtained from both antrum and corpus, histologic study yields additional information, including the degree and pattern of inflammation, atrophy, metaplasia, and dysplasia. Microbiologic culture is most specific but may be insensitive because of difficulty with *H. pylori* isolation. Once the organism is cultured, its identity as *H. pylori* can be confirmed by its typical appearance on Gram's stain and its positive reactions in oxidase, catalase, and urease tests. Moreover, the organism's susceptibility to antibiotics can be determined, and this information can be clinically useful in difficult cases. The occasional biopsy specimens containing the less common non-*pylori* gastric helicobacters give only weakly positive results in the biopsy urease test. Positive identification of these bacteria requires visualization of the characteristic long, tight spirals in histologic sections.

Noninvasive *H. pylori* testing is the norm if gastric cancer does not need to be excluded by endoscopy. The most consistently accurate test is the urea breath test. In this simple test, the patient drinks a solution of urea labeled with the nonradioactive isotope ¹³C and then blows into a tube. If *H. pylori* urease is present, the urea is hydrolyzed and labeled carbon dioxide is detected in breath samples. The stool antigen test, another simple assay, is more convenient and potentially less expensive than the urea breath test but has been slightly less accurate in some comparative studies. The simplest tests for ascertaining *H. pylori* status are serologic assays measuring specific IgG levels in serum by enzyme-linked immunosorbent assay or immunoblot. The best of these tests are as accurate as other diagnostic methods, but many commercial tests—especially rapid office tests—do not perform well.

The urea breath test, the stool antigen test, and biopsy-based tests can all be used to assess the success of treatment (Fig. 151-2). However, because these tests are dependent on *H. pylori* load, their use <4 weeks after treatment may yield false-negative results. Furthermore, these tests are unreliable if performed within 4 weeks of intercurrent treatment with antibiotics or bismuth compounds or within 2 weeks of the discontinuation of proton pump inhibitor (PPI) treatment. In the assessment of treatment success, noninvasive tests are normally preferred; however, after gastric ulceration, endoscopy should be repeated to ensure healing and to exclude gastric carcinoma by further histologic sampling.

Serologic tests are not used to monitor treatment success, as the gradual drop in titer of *H. pylori*–specific antibodies is too slow to be of practical use.

TABLE 151-1 Tests Commonly Used to Detect *Helicobacter pylori*

Test	Advantages	Disadvantages
Invasive (Based on Endoscopic Biopsy)		
Biopsy urease test	Quick, simple	Some commercial tests not fully sensitive before 24 h
Histology	May give additional histologic information	Sensitivity dependent on experience and use of special stains
Culture	Permits determination of antibiotic susceptibility	Sensitivity dependent on experience
Noninvasive		
Serology	Inexpensive and convenient; not affected by recent antibiotics or proton pump inhibitors to the same extent as breath and stool tests	Cannot be used for early follow-up after treatment; some commercial kits inaccurate, and all less accurate than breath test
¹³C urea breath test	Inexpensive and simpler than endoscopy; useful for follow-up after treatment	Requires fasting; not as convenient as blood or stool tests
Stool antigen test	Inexpensive and convenient; useful for follow-up after treatment; may be useful in children	May be disliked by people from some cultures; may be slightly less accurate than urea breath test, particularly when used to assess treatment success

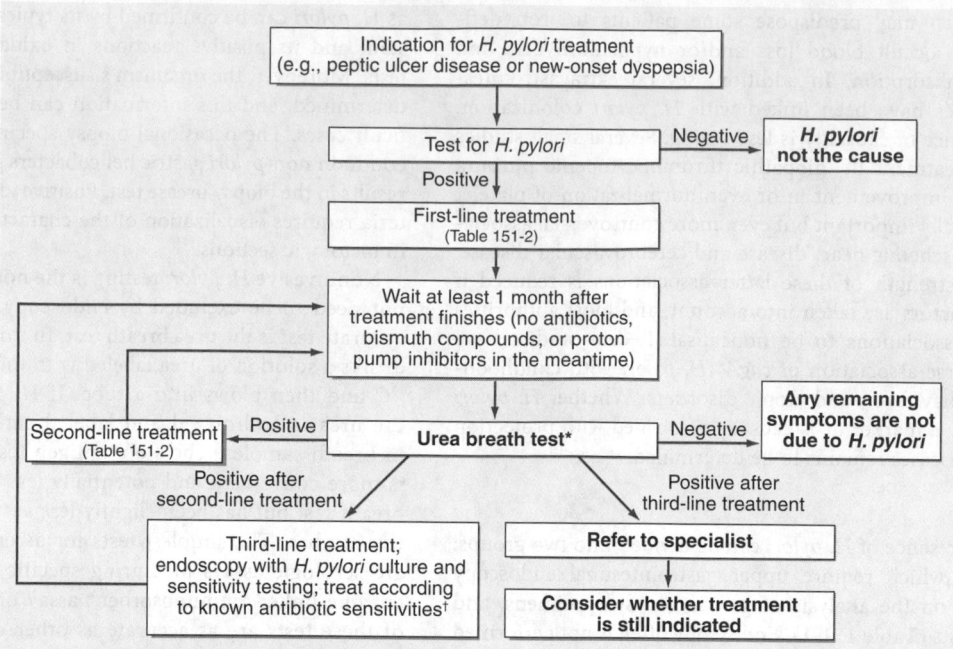

Figure 151-2 Algorithm for the management of *Helicobacter pylori* infection. *Occasionally, an endoscopy and a biopsy-based test are used instead of a urea breath test in follow-up after treatment. The main indication for these invasive tests is gastric ulceration; in this condition, as opposed to duodenal ulceration, it is important to check healing and to exclude underlying gastric adenocarcinoma. †Some authorities now use empirical third-line regimens, several of which have been described.

TREATMENT   *H. pylori* Infections

The most clear-cut indications for treatment are *H. pylori*–related duodenal or gastric ulceration or low-grade gastric B cell lymphoma. *H. pylori* should be eradicated in patients with documented ulcer disease, whether or not the ulcers are currently active, to reduce the likelihood of relapse (Fig. 151-2). Many guidelines now recommend *H. pylori* eradication in uninvestigated simple dyspepsia following noninvasive diagnosis; others also recommend treatment in functional dyspepsia, in case the patient is one of the perhaps 7% (beyond placebo effects) to benefit from such treatment. Individuals with a strong family history of gastric cancer should be treated to eradicate *H. pylori* in the hope that their cancer risk will be reduced. Currently, widespread community screening for and treatment of *H. pylori* as primary prophylaxis for gastric cancer and peptic ulcers are not recommended, mainly because it is unclear whether treatment for *H. pylori* reduces the risk of cancer to that in persons who have never acquired the organism. The largest randomized controlled study to date (performed in China) showed no cancer risk reduction during the 7 years of follow-up, although a post hoc subgroup analysis documented improvement in the group of participants who did not already have gastric atrophy or intestinal metaplasia. Other studies have found a reduced cancer risk after treatment, but the size of this effect in different populations remains unclear, and the results of further large-scale prospective interventional studies must be awaited. Other reasons for not treating *H. pylori* in asymptomatic populations at present include (1) the adverse side effects of the multiple-antibiotic regimens used (which are common and can be severe in rare cases); (2) antibiotic resistance, which may arise in *H. pylori* or other incidentally carried bacteria; (3) the anxiety that may arise in otherwise healthy people, especially if treatment is unsuccessful; and (4) the apparent existence of a subset of people who will develop GERD symptoms after treatment, although on average *H. pylori* treatment does not affect GERD symptoms or severity.

Although *H. pylori* is susceptible to a wide range of antibiotics in vitro, monotherapy is not usually successful, probably because of inadequate antibiotic delivery to the colonization niche. Failure of monotherapy has prompted the development of multidrug regimens, the most successful of which are triple and quadruple combinations. Initially these regimens produced *H. pylori* eradication rates of >90% in many trials; in recent years, however, resistance to key antibiotics has become more common, a trend leading to *H. pylori* eradication rates of only 75–80% for the most commonly used regimens. Current regimens consist of a PPI or ranitidine bismuth citrate and two or three antimicrobial agents given for 7–14 days (Table 151-2). Research on optimizing drug combinations to increase efficacy continues, and it is likely that guidelines will change as the field develops and as countries increasingly individualize treatment to suit local antibiotic resistance patterns and economic needs.

The two most important factors in successful *H. pylori* treatment are the patient's close compliance with the regimen and the use of drugs to which the patient's strain of *H. pylori* has not acquired resistance. Treatment failure following minor lapses in compliance is common and often leads to acquired resistance to metronidazole or clarithromycin. To stress the importance of compliance, written instructions should be given to the patient, and minor side effects of the regimen should be explained. Resistance to clarithromycin and, to a lesser extent, to metronidazole are of growing concern. Clarithromycin resistance is less prevalent but, if present, usually results in treatment failure. Strains of *H. pylori* that are apparently resistant to metronidazole are more common but still may be cleared by metronidazole-containing regimens, which have only slightly reduced efficacy. Assessment of antibiotic susceptibilities before treatment would be optimal but is not usually undertaken because endoscopy and mucosal biopsy are necessary to obtain

TABLE 151-2 Recommended Treatment Regimens for *Helicobacter pylori*

Regimen (Duration)	Drug 1	Drug 2	Drug 3	Drug 4
Regimen 1: OCM (7–14 days)[a]	Omeprazole[b] (20 mg bid)	Clarithromycin (500 mg bid)	Metronidazole (500 mg bid)	—
Regimen 2: OCA (7–14 days)[a]	Omeprazole[b] (20 mg bid)	Clarithromycin (500 mg bid)	Amoxicillin (1 g bid)	—
Regimen 3: OBTM (14 days)[c]	Omeprazole[b] (20 mg bid)	Bismuth subsalicylate (2 tabs qid)	Tetracycline HCl (500 mg qid)	Metronidazole (500 mg tid)
Regimen 4[d]: sequential (5 days + 5 days)	Omeprazole[b] (20 mg bid)	Amoxicillin 1 g bid		
	Omeprazole[b] (20 mg bid)	Clarithromycin (500 mg bid)	Tinidazole (500 mg bid)	
Regimen 5[e]: OAL (10 days)	Omeprazole[b] (20 mg bid)	Amoxicillin (1 g bid)	Levofloxacin (500 mg qid)	

[a]Meta-analyses show that a 14-day course of therapy is slightly superior to a 7-day course. However, in populations where 7-day treatment is known to have very high success rates, this shorter course is still often used.

[b]Omeprazole may be replaced with any proton pump inhibitor at an equivalent dosage or, in regimens 1 and 2, with ranitidine bismuth citrate (400 mg).

[c]Data supporting this regimen come mainly from Europe and are based on the use of bismuth subcitrate and metronidazole (400 mg tid). This is the most commonly used second-line regimen.

[d]Data supporting this regimen come from Europe. Although the two 5-day courses of different drugs have usually been given sequentially, recent evidence suggests no added benefit from this approach. Thus 10 days of the four drugs combined may be as good and may aid compliance.

[e]Data supporting this second- or third-line regimen come from Europe. This regimen may be less effective where rates of quinolone use are high. Theoretically, it may also be wise to avoid it in populations where *Clostridium difficile* infection is common after broad-spectrum antibiotic use.

H. pylori for culture and because most microbiology laboratories are inexperienced in *H. pylori* culture. In the absence of susceptibility information, a history of the patient's (even distant) antibiotic use for other conditions should be obtained; use of the agent should then be avoided if possible, particularly in the case of clarithromycin (e.g., previous use for upper respiratory infection). If initial *H. pylori* treatment fails, one of two strategies may be used (Fig. 151-2). The more common approach is empirical re-treatment with another drug regimen, usually quadruple therapy (Table 151-2). The second approach is endoscopy, biopsy, and culture plus treatment based on documented antibiotic sensitivities. If re-treatment fails, susceptibility testing should ideally be performed, although empirical third-line therapies are often used.

Clearance of non-*pylori* gastric helicobacters can follow the use of bismuth compounds alone or of triple-drug regimens. However, in the absence of trials, it is unclear whether this outcome represents successful treatment or natural clearance of the bacterium.

■ PREVENTION

Carriage of *H. pylori* has considerable public health significance in developed countries, where it is associated with peptic ulcer disease and gastric adenocarcinoma, and in developing countries, where gastric adenocarcinoma may be an even more common cause of cancer death late in life. If mass prevention were contemplated, vaccination would be the most obvious method, and experimental immunization of animals has given promising results. However, given that *H. pylori* has co-evolved with its human host over millennia, preventing or eliminating colonization on a population basis may have distinct disadvantages. For example, lifelong absence of *H. pylori* is a risk factor for GERD complications, including esophageal adenocarcinoma. We have

speculated that the disappearance of *H. pylori* may be associated with an increased risk of other emerging diseases reflecting aspects of the current Western lifestyle, such as asthma, obesity, and conceivably even type 2 diabetes mellitus.

FURTHER READINGS

ATHERTON JC, BLASER MJ: Co-adaptation of *Helicobacter pylori* and humans: Ancient history and modern implications. J Clin Invest 119:2475, 2009

BACKERT S, SELBACH M: The role of type IV secretion in *Helicobacter pylori* pathogenesis. Cell Microbiol 10:1573, 2008

CHEY WD et al: American College of Gastroenterology guidelines on the management of *Helicobacter pylori* infection. Am J Gastroenterol 102:1808, 2007

EL-OMAR EM et al: Interleukin-1 polymorphisms associated with increased risk of gastric cancer. Nature 404:398, 2000

LINZ B et al: An African origin for the intimate association between humans and *Helicobacter pylori*. Nature 445:915, 2007

MARSHALL BJ, WARREN JR: Unidentified curved bacilli in the stomach of patients with gastritis and peptic ulceration. Lancet 1:1311, 1984

OHNISHI N et al: Transgenic expression of *Helicobacter pylori* CagA induces gastrointestinal and hematopoietic neoplasms in mouse. Proc Natl Acad Sci USA 105:1003, 2008

POLK DB, PEEK RM JR: *Helicobacter pylori*: Gastric cancer and beyond. Nat Rev Cancer 10:403, 2010

WONG BC et al: *Helicobacter pylori* eradication to prevent gastric cancer in a high-risk region of China: A randomized controlled trial. JAMA 291:187, 2004

WU C-Y et al: Early *Helicobacter pylori* eradication decreases risk of gastric cancer in patients with peptic ulcer disease. Gastroenterology 137:1641, 2009

CHAPTER 152

Infections Due to *Pseudomonas* Species and Related Organisms

Reuben Ramphal

The pseudomonads are a heterogeneous group of gram-negative bacteria that have in common an inability to ferment lactose. Formerly classified in the genus *Pseudomonas*, the members of this group are now assigned to three medically important genera—*Pseudomonas*, *Burkholderia*, and *Stenotrophomonas*—whose biologic behaviors encompass both similarities and marked differences and whose genetic repertoires differ in many respects. The pathogenicity of most pseudomonads is based on opportunism; the exceptions are the organisms that cause melioidosis (*B. pseudomallei*) and glanders (*B. mallei*), which can be considered primary pathogens.

P. aeruginosa, the major pathogen of the group, is a significant cause of infections in hospitalized patients and in patients with cystic fibrosis (CF; Chap. 259). Cytotoxic chemotherapy, mechanical ventilation, and broad-spectrum antibiotic therapy probably paved the way for increasing numbers of patients colonized and infected by this organism. Since the implementation of these advances in medical therapy, most conditions predisposing to *P. aeruginosa* infections have involved host compromise and/or broad-spectrum antibiotic use. The other members of the genus *Pseudomonas*—*P. putida*, *P. fluorescens*, and *P. stutzeri*—infect humans infrequently.

The genus *Burkholderia* comprises >40 species, of which *B. cepacia* is most frequently encountered in Western countries. Like *P. aeruginosa*, *B. cepacia* is both a nosocomial pathogen and a cause of infection in CF. The other medically important members of this genus are *B. pseudomallei* and *B. mallei,* which, as stated above, cause melioidosis and glanders, respectively.

The genus *Stenotrophomonas* contains one species of medical significance, *S. maltophilia* (previously classified in the genera *Pseudomonas* and *Xanthomonas*). This organism is strictly an opportunist that "overgrows" in the setting of potent broad-spectrum antibiotic use.

PSEUDOMONAS AERUGINOSA

■ EPIDEMIOLOGY

P. aeruginosa is found in most moist environments. Soil, plants, vegetables, tap water, and countertops can all be reservoirs for this microbe, as it has simple nutritional needs. Given the ubiquity of *P. aeruginosa*, contact with the organism obviously is not sufficient for colonization or infection. Clinical and experimental observations suggest that *P. aeruginosa* infection often occurs concomitantly with host defense compromise, mucosal trauma, physiologic derangement, and antibiotic-mediated suppression of normal flora. Thus, it comes as no surprise that the majority of *P. aeruginosa* infections occur in intensive care units (ICUs), where these factors frequently converge. It is believed that the organism is initially acquired from environmental sources, but patient-to-patient spread also occurs in clinics and families.

Burn patients once appeared to be unusually susceptible to *P. aeruginosa*. For example, in 1959–1963, *Pseudomonas* burn-wound sepsis was the principal cause of death in 60% of burned patients dying at the U.S. Army Institute of Surgical Research. For reasons that are unclear, *P. aeruginosa* infection in burns is no longer the major problem that it was during the 1950s and 1960s. Similarly, in the 1960s, *P. aeruginosa* appeared as a common pathogen in patients receiving cytotoxic chemotherapy at many institutions in the United States, but it subsequently diminished in importance. Despite this subsidence, *P. aeruginosa* remains one of the most feared pathogens in this population because of its high attributable mortality rate.

In some parts of Asia and Latin America, *P. aeruginosa* continues to be the most common cause of gram-negative bacteremia in neutropenic patients.

In contrast to the trends for burn patients and neutropenic patients in the United States, the incidence of *P. aeruginosa* infections among patients with CF has not changed. *P. aeruginosa* remains the most common contributing factor to respiratory failure in CF and is responsible for the majority of deaths among CF patients.

■ LABORATORY FEATURES

P. aeruginosa is a nonfastidious, motile, gram-negative rod that grows on most common laboratory media, including blood and MacConkey agars. It is easily identified in the laboratory on primary-isolation agar plates by pigment production that confers a yellow to dark green or even bluish appearance. Colonies have a shiny "gun-metal" appearance and a characteristic fruity odor. Two of the identifying biochemical characteristics of *P. aeruginosa* are an inability to ferment lactose on MacConkey agar and a positive reaction in the oxidase test. Most strains are identified on the basis of these readily detectable laboratory features even before extensive biochemical testing is done. Some isolates from CF patients are easily identified by their mucoid appearance, which is due to the production of large amounts of the mucoid exopolysaccharide or alginate.

■ PATHOGENESIS

Unraveling the mechanisms underlying disease caused by *P. aeruginosa* has proved challenging. Of the common gram-negative bacteria, no other species produces such a large number of putative virulence factors (Table 152-1). Yet *P. aeruginosa* rarely initiates an infectious process in the absence of host injury or compromise, and

TABLE 152-1 Main Putative Virulence Factors of *Pseudomonas aeruginosa*

Substance/ Organelle	Function	Virulence in Animal Disease
Pili	Adhesion to cells	?
Flagella	Adhesion, motility, inflammation	Yes
Lipopolysaccharide	Antiphagocytic activity, inflammation	Yes
Type III secretion system	Cytotoxic activity (ExoU)	Yes
Proteases	Proteolytic activity, cytotoxicity	?
Phospholipases	Cytotoxicity	?
Exotoxin A	Cytotoxicity	?

few of its putative virulence factors have been shown definitively to be involved in disease in humans. Despite its metabolic versatility and possession of multiple colonizing factors, *P. aeruginosa* exhibits no competitive advantage over enteric bacteria in the human gut; neither is it a normal inhabitant of the human gastrointestinal tract, despite the host's continuous environmental exposure to the organism.

Virulence attributes involved in acute *P. aeruginosa* infections

Motility and colonization A general tenet of bacterial pathogenesis is that most bacteria must adhere to surfaces or colonize a host niche in order to initiate disease. Most pathogens examined thus far possess adherence factors called *adhesins*. *P. aeruginosa* is no exception. Among its many adhesins are its pili, which demonstrate adhesive properties for a variety of cells and adhere best to injured cell surfaces. In the organism's flagellum, the flagellin molecule binds to cells, and the flagellar cap attaches to mucins through the recognition of glycan chains. Nonflagellated *P. aeruginosa* mutants are less virulent or avirulent in some but not all animal models; however, it is unclear whether this decreased virulence is due to the loss of adhesion or to the loss of other flagellar functions. Other *P. aeruginosa* adhesins include the outer core of the lipopolysaccharide (LPS) molecule, which binds to the cystic fibrosis transmembrane conductance regulator (CFTR) and aids in internalization of the organism, and the alginate coat of mucoid strains, which enhances adhesion to cells and mucins. In addition, membrane proteins and lectins have been proposed as colonization factors. It appears that the deletion of any given adhesin is not sufficient to abrogate the ability of *P. aeruginosa* to colonize surfaces.

Evasion of host defenses The transition from bacterial colonization to disease requires the evasion of host defenses by a substantial number of bacteria. *P. aeruginosa* appears to be well equipped for evasion. Attached bacteria inject four known toxins (ExoS, ExoU, ExoT, and ExoY) via a type III secretion system that allows the bacteria to evade phagocytic cells either by cytotoxicity or by inhibition of phagocytosis. Mutants with defects in this system fail to disseminate in some animal models of infection. Secreted toxins such as exotoxin A and leukocidin have the potential to kill phagocytic cells, and multiple secreted proteases may degrade host effector molecules such as cytokines and chemokines that are released in response to infection.

Tissue injury Among gram-negative bacteria, *P. aeruginosa* probably produces the largest number of substances that are toxic to cells and thus may injure tissues. The toxins secreted by its type III secretion system are capable of tissue injury. However, their delivery requires the adherence of the organism to cells. Thus, the effects of these toxins are likely to be local or to depend on the presence of vast numbers of bacteria. On the other hand, diffusible toxins, secreted by the organism's type II secretion system, can act freely wherever they come into contact with cells. Exotoxin A, four different proteases, at least two phospholipases, rhamnolipids, pyocyanin, and hydrocyanic acid are all produced by *P. aeruginosa* and are all capable of inducing host injury.

Inflammatory components The inflammatory components of *P. aeruginosa* [e.g., the inflammatory responses to the lipid A component of LPSs and to flagellin, mediated through the Toll-like receptor (TLR) system (principally TLR4 and TLR5)] have been thought to represent the most important factor in disease causation. Although these inflammatory responses are required for successful defense against *P. aeruginosa* (i.e., in their absence, animals are defenseless against *P. aeruginosa* infection), florid responses are likely to result in disease. When the sepsis syndrome and septic shock develop in *P. aeruginosa* infection, they are probably the result of the host response to one or both of these substances, but

injury to the lung by *Pseudomonas* toxins may also result in sepsis syndromes, possibly by causing cell death and the release of cellular components (e.g., heat-shock proteins) that may activate the TLR or another proinflammatory system.

Chronic *P. aeruginosa* infections

Chronic infection due to *P. aeruginosa* occurs mainly in the lungs in the setting of structural pulmonary diseases. The classic example is CF; others include bronchiectasis and chronic relapsing panbronchiolitis, a disease seen in Japan and some Pacific Islands. Hallmarks of these illnesses are altered mucociliary clearance leading to mucus stasis and mucus accumulation in the lungs. There is probably a common factor that selects for *P. aeruginosa* colonization in these lung diseases—perhaps the adhesiveness of *P. aeruginosa* for mucus, a phenomenon that is not noted for most other common gram-negative bacteria, and/or the ability of *P. aeruginosa* to evade host defenses in mucus. Furthermore, *P. aeruginosa* seems to evolve in ways that allow its prolonged survival in the lung without an early fatal outcome for the host. The strains found in CF patients exhibit minimal production of virulence factors. Some strains even lose the ability to produce pili and flagella, and most become complement-sensitive because of the loss of the O side chain of their LPS molecules. An example of the impact of these changes is found in the organism's discontinuation of the production of flagellin (probably its most strongly proinflammatory molecule) when it encounters purulent mucus. This response probably dampens the host's response, allowing the organism to survive in mucus. *P. aeruginosa* is also believed to lose the ability to secrete many of its injectable toxins during growth in mucus. Although the alginate coat is thought to play a role in the organism's survival, alginate is not essential, as nonmucoid strains may also predominate for long periods. In short, virulence in chronic infections may be mediated mainly by the attenuated host inflammatory response, which injures the lungs over decades.

■ CLINICAL MANIFESTATIONS

P. aeruginosa causes infections at almost all sites in the body but shows a rather strong predilection for the lungs. The infections encountered most commonly in hospitalized patients are described below.

Bacteremia

Crude mortality rates exceeding 50% have been reported among patients with *P. aeruginosa* bacteremia. Consequently, this clinical entity has been much feared, and its management has been attempted with the use of multiple antibiotics. Recent publications report attributable mortality rates of 28–44%, with the precise figure depending on the adequacy of treatment and the seriousness of the underlying disease. In the past, the patient with *P. aeruginosa* bacteremia classically was neutropenic or had a burn injury. Today, however, a minority of such patients have bacteremic *P. aeruginosa* infections. Rather, *P. aeruginosa* bacteremia is seen most often in patients on ICUs.

The clinical presentation of *P. aeruginosa* bacteremia rarely differs from that of sepsis in general (Chap. 270). Patients are usually febrile, but those who are most severely ill may be in shock or even hypothermic. The only point differentiating this entity from gram-negative sepsis of other causes may be the distinctive skin lesions (ecthyma gangrenosum) of *Pseudomonas* infection, which occur almost exclusively in markedly neutropenic patients and patients with AIDS. These small or large, painful, reddish, maculopapular lesions have a geographic margin; they are initially pink, then darken to purple, and finally become black and necrotic (Fig. 152-1). Histopathologic studies indicate that the lesions are due to vascular invasion and are teeming with bacteria. Although

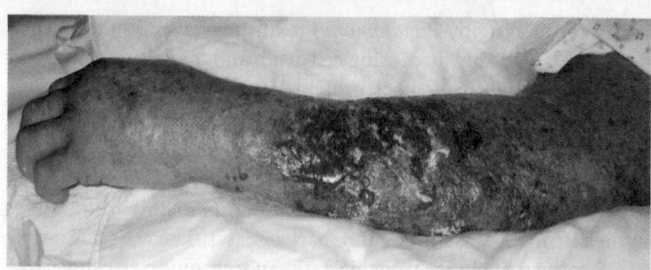

Figure 152-1 Ecthyma gangrenosum in a neutropenic patient 3 days after onset.

similar lesions may occur in aspergillosis and mucormycosis, their presence suggests *P. aeruginosa* bacteremia as the most likely diagnosis.

TREATMENT   Bacteremia

(Table 152-2) Antimicrobial treatment of *P. aeruginosa* bacteremia has been controversial. Before 1971, the outcome of *Pseudomonas* bacteremia in febrile neutropenic patients treated with the available agents—gentamicin and the polymyxins—was dismal. Studies published around that time indicated that treatment with carbenicillin, with or without an aminoglycoside, significantly improved outcomes. Concurrently, several retrospective analyses suggested that the use of two agents that were synergistic against gram-negative pathogens in vitro resulted in better outcomes in neutropenic patients. Thus, combination therapy became the standard of care—first for *P. aeruginosa* bacteremia in febrile neutropenic patients and then for all *P. aeruginosa* infections in neutropenic or nonneutropenic patients.

With the introduction of newer antipseudomonal drugs, a number of studies have revisited the choice between combination treatment and monotherapy for *Pseudomonas* bacteremia. Although the majority of experts still favor combination therapy, most of these observational studies indicate that a single modern antipseudomonal β-lactam agent to which the isolate is sensitive is as efficacious as a combination. Even in patients at greatest risk of early death from *P. aeruginosa* bacteremia (i.e., those with fever and neutropenia), empirical antipseudomonal monotherapy is deemed to be as efficacious as empirical combination therapy by the practice guidelines of the Infectious Diseases Society of America. One firm conclusion is that monotherapy with an aminoglycoside is not optimal.

There are, of course, institutions and countries where rates of susceptibility of *P. aeruginosa* to first-line antibiotics are <80%. Thus, when a septic patient with a high probability of *P. aeruginosa* infection is encountered in such settings, empirical combination therapy should be administered until the pathogen is identified and susceptibility data become available. Thereafter, whether one or two agents should be continued remains a matter of individual preference.

Acute pneumonia

Respiratory infections are the most common of all infections caused by *P. aeruginosa*. This organism appears first or second on most lists of the causes of ventilator-associated pneumonia (VAP). However, much debate centers on the actual role of *P. aeruginosa* in VAP. Many

of the relevant data are based on cultures of sputum or endotracheal tube aspirates and may represent nonpathogenic colonization of the tracheobronchial tree, biofilms on the endotracheal tube, or simple tracheobronchitis.

Older reports of *P. aeruginosa* pneumonia described patients with an acute clinical syndrome of fever, chills, cough, and necrotizing pneumonia indistinguishable from other gram-negative bacterial pneumonias. The traditional accounts described a fulminant infection, with cyanosis, tachypnea, copious sputum, and systemic toxicity. Chest radiographs demonstrated bilateral pneumonia, often with nodular densities with or without cavities. This picture is now remarkably rare. Today, the typical patient is using a ventilator, has a slowly progressive infiltrate, and has been colonized with *P. aeruginosa* for days. While some cases may progress rapidly over 48–72 h, they are the exceptions. Nodular densities are not commonly seen. However, infiltrates may go on to necrosis. Necrotizing pneumonia has also been seen in the community (e.g., after inhalation of hot-tub water contaminated with *P. aeruginosa*). The typical patient has fever, leukocytosis, and purulent sputum, and the chest radiograph shows a new infiltrate or the expansion of a preexisting infiltrate. Chest examination generally detects rales or dullness. Of course, such findings are quite common among ventilated patients in the ICU. A sputum Gram's stain showing mainly polymorphonuclear leukocytes (PMNs) in conjunction with a culture positive for *P. aeruginosa* in this setting suggests a diagnosis of acute *P. aeruginosa* pneumonia. There is no consensus about whether an invasive procedure (e.g., bronchoalveolar lavage or protected-brush sampling of the distal airways) is superior to tracheal aspiration to obtain samples for lung cultures in order to substantiate the occurrence of *P. aeruginosa* pneumonia and prevent antibiotic overuse.

TREATMENT   Acute Pneumonia

(Table 152-2) The results of therapy for *P. aeruginosa* pneumonia have been unsatisfactory. Reports suggest mortality rates of 40–80%, but how many of these deaths are attributable to underlying disease remains unknown. The drugs of choice for *P. aeruginosa* pneumonia are similar to those given for bacteremia. A potent antipseudomonal β-lactam drug is the mainstay of therapy. Failure rates were high when aminoglycosides were used as single agents, possibly because of their poor penetration into the airways and their binding to airway secretions. Thus a strong case cannot be made for the inclusion of the aminoglycoside component in regimens used against fully susceptible organisms, especially given the evidence that aminoglycosides are not optimally active in the lungs at concentrations normally reached after IV administration. Nonetheless, aminoglycosides are commonly used in clinical practice. Some experts suggest the combination of a β-lactam agent and an antipseudomonal fluoroquinolone instead when combination therapy is desired.

Chronic respiratory tract infections

P. aeruginosa is responsible for chronic infections of the airways associated with a number of underlying or predisposing conditions—most commonly CF in Caucasian populations (Chap. 259). A state of chronic colonization beginning early in childhood is seen in some Asian populations with chronic or diffuse panbronchiolitis, a disease of unknown etiology. *P. aeruginosa* is one of the organisms that colonizes damaged bronchi in bronchiectasis, a disease secondary to multiple causes in which profound structural abnormalities of the airways result in mucus stasis.

TABLE 152-2 Antibiotic Treatment of Infections Due to *Pseudomonas aeruginosa* and Related Species

Infection	Antibiotics and Dosages	Other Considerations
Bacteremia Nonneutropenic host	Monotherapy: Ceftazidime (2 g q8h IV) or cefepime (2 g q12h IV) Combination therapy: Piperacillin/tazobactam (3.375 g q4h IV) or imipenem (500 mg q6h IV) or meropenem (1 g q8h IV) or doripenem (500 mg q8h IV) *plus* Amikacin (7.5 mg/kg q12h or 15 mg/kg q24h IV)	Add an aminoglycoside for patients in shock and in regions or hospitals where rates of resistance to the primary β-lactam agents are high. Tobramycin may be used instead of amikacin (susceptibility permitting).
Neutropenic host	Cefepime (2 g q8h IV) or all other agents (except doripenem) in above dosages	
Endocarditis	Antibiotic regimens as for bacteremia for 6–8 weeks	Resistance during therapy is common. Surgery is required for relapse.
Pneumonia	Drugs and dosages as for bacteremia, except that the available carbapenems should not be the sole primary drugs because of high rates of resistance during therapy	IDSA guidelines recommend the addition of an aminoglycoside or ciprofloxacin. The duration of therapy is 10–14 days.
Bone infection, malignant otitis externa	Cefepime or ceftazidime at the same dosages as for bacteremia; aminoglycosides not a necessary component of therapy; ciprofloxacin (500–750 mg q12h PO) may be used	Duration of therapy varies with the drug used (e.g., 6 weeks for a β-lactam agent; at least 3 months for oral therapy except in puncture-wound osteomyelitis, for which the duration should be 2–4 weeks).
Central nervous system infection	Ceftazidime or cefepime (2 g q8h IV) or meropenem (1 g q8h IV)	Abscesses or other closed-space infections may require drainage. The duration of therapy is ≥2 weeks.
Eye infection Keratitis/ulcer	Topical therapy with tobramycin/ciprofloxacin/levofloxacin eyedrops	Use maximal strengths available or compounded by pharmacy.
Endophthalmitis	Ceftazidime or cefepime as for central nervous system infection *plus* Topical therapy	
Urinary tract infection	Ciprofloxacin (500 mg q12h PO) or levofloxacin (750 mg q24h) or any aminoglycoside (total daily dose given once daily)	Relapse may occur if an obstruction or a foreign body is present.
Multidrug-resistant *P. aeruginosa* infection	Colistin (100 mg q12h IV) for the shortest possible period to obtain a clinical response	Doses used have varied. Dosage adjustment is required in renal failure. Inhaled colistin may be added for pneumonia (100 mg q12h).
Stenotrophomonas maltophilia infection	TMP-SMX (1600/320 mg q12h IV for 14 days) Ticarcillin/clavulanate (3.1 g q4h IV for 14 days)	Resistance to all agents is increasing. Levofloxacin may be an alternative, but there is little published clinical experience with this agent.
Burkholderia cepacia infection	Meropenem (1 g q8h IV for 14 days) TMP-SMX (1600/320 mg q12h IV for 14 days)	Resistance to both agents is increasing. Do not use them in combination because of possible antagonism.
Melioidosis, glanders	Ceftazidime (2 g q6h for 2 weeks) or meropenem (1 g q8h for 2 weeks) or imipenem (500 mg q6h for 2 weeks) *followed by* TMP-SMX (1600/320 mg q12h PO for 3 months)	See "Further Readings" for more details on therapy and alternative agents.

Abbreviations: IDSA, Infectious Diseases Society of America; TMP-SMX, trimethoprim-sulfamethoxazole.

TREATMENT ▸ Chronic Respiratory Tract Infections

Optimal management of chronic *P. aeruginosa* lung infection has not been determined. Patients respond clinically to antipseudomonal therapy, but the organism is rarely eradicated. Since eradication is unlikely, the aim of treatment for chronic infection is to quell exacerbations of inflammation. The regimens used are similar to those used for pneumonia, but an aminoglycoside is almost always added because resistance is common in chronic disease. However, it may be appropriate to use an inhaled aminoglycoside preparation in order to maximize airway drug levels.

Endovascular infections

Infective endocarditis due to *P. aeruginosa* is a disease of IV drug users whose native valves are involved. This organism has also been reported to cause prosthetic valve endocarditis. Sites of prior native-valve injury due to the injection of foreign material such as talc or fibers probably serve as niduses for bacterial attachment to the heart valve. The manifestations of *P. aeruginosa* endocarditis resemble those of other forms of acute endocarditis in IV drug users except that the disease is more indolent than *Staphylococcus aureus* endocarditis. While most disease involves the right side of the heart, left-sided involvement is not rare and multivalvular disease is common. Fever is a common manifestation, as is pulmonary involvement (due to septic emboli to the lungs). Hence, patients may also experience chest pain and hemoptysis. Involvement of the left side of the heart may lead to signs of cardiac failure, systemic emboli, and local cardiac involvement with sinus of Valsalva abscesses and conduction defects. Skin manifestations are rare in this disease, and ecthyma gangrenosum is not seen. The diagnosis is based on positive blood cultures along with clinical signs of endocarditis.

TREATMENT   Endovascular Infections

(Table 152-2) It has been customary to use synergistic antibiotic combinations in treating *P. aeruginosa* endocarditis because of the development of resistance during therapy with a single antipseudomonal β-lactam agent. Which combination therapy is preferable is unclear, as all combinations have failed. Cases of *P. aeruginosa* endocarditis that relapse during or fail to respond to therapy are often caused by resistant organisms and may require surgical therapy. Other considerations for valve replacement are similar to those in other forms of endocarditis (Chap. 124).

Bone and joint infections

Although *P. aeruginosa* is an infrequent cause of bone and joint infections, *Pseudomonas* bacteremia or infective endocarditis caused by the injection of contaminated illicit drugs has been well documented to result in vertebral osteomyelitis and sternoclavicular joint arthritis. The clinical presentation of vertebral *P. aeruginosa* osteomyelitis is more indolent than that of staphylococcal osteomyelitis. The duration of symptoms in IV drug users with vertebral osteomyelitis due to *P. aeruginosa* varies from weeks to months. Fever is not uniformly present; when present, it tends to be low grade. There may be mild tenderness at the site of involvement. Blood cultures are usually negative unless there is concomitant endocarditis. The erythrocyte sedimentation rate (ESR) is generally elevated. Vertebral osteomyelitis due to *P. aeruginosa* has also been reported in the elderly, in whom it originates from urinary tract infections (UTIs). The infection generally involves the lumbosacral area because of a shared venous drainage (Batson's plexus) between the lumbosacral spine and the pelvis. Sternoclavicular septic arthritis due to *P. aeruginosa* is seen almost exclusively in IV drug users. This disease may occur with or without endocarditis, and a primary site of infection often is not found. Plain radiographs show joint or bone involvement. Treatment of these forms of disease is generally successful.

Pseudomonas osteomyelitis of the foot most often follows puncture wounds through sneakers and mostly affects children. The main manifestation is pain in the foot, sometimes with superficial cellulitis around the puncture wound and tenderness on deep palpation of the wound. Multiple joints or bones of the foot may be involved. Systemic symptoms are generally absent, and blood cultures are usually negative. Radiographs may or may not be abnormal, but the bone scan is usually positive, as are MRI studies. Needle aspiration usually yields a diagnosis. Prompt surgery, with exploration of the nail puncture tract and debridement of the involved bones and cartilage, is generally recommended in addition to antibiotic therapy.

Central nervous system (CNS) infections

CNS infections due to *P. aeruginosa* are relatively rare. Involvement of the CNS is almost always secondary to a surgical procedure or head trauma. The entity seen most often is postoperative or post-traumatic meningitis. Subdural or epidural infection occasionally results from contamination of these areas. Embolic disease arising from endocarditis in IV drug users and leading to brain abscesses has also been described. The cerebrospinal fluid (CSF) profile of *P. aeruginosa* meningitis is no different from that of pyogenic meningitis of any other etiology.

TREATMENT   Central Nervous System Infections

(Table 152-2) Treatment of *Pseudomonas* meningitis is difficult; little information has been published, and no controlled trials in humans have been undertaken. However, the general principles involved in the treatment of meningitis apply, including the need for high doses of bactericidal antibiotics to attain high drug levels in the CSF. The agent with which there is the most published experience in *P. aeruginosa* meningitis is ceftazidime, but other antipseudomonal β-lactam drugs that reach high CSF concentrations, such as cefepime and meropenem, have also been used successfully. Other forms of *P. aeruginosa* CNS infection, such as brain abscesses and epidural and subdural empyema, generally require surgical drainage in addition to antibiotic therapy.

Eye infections

Eye infections due to *P. aeruginosa* occur mainly as a result of direct inoculation into the tissue during trauma or surface injury by contact lenses. Keratitis and corneal ulcers are the most common types of eye disease and are often associated with contact lenses (especially the extended-wear variety). Keratitis can be slowly or rapidly progressive, but the classic description is disease progressing over 48 h to involve the entire cornea, with opacification and sometimes perforation. *P. aeruginosa* keratitis should be considered a medical emergency because of the rapidity with which it can progress to loss of sight. *P. aeruginosa* endophthalmitis secondary to bacteremia is the most devastating of *P. aeruginosa* eye infections. The disease is fulminant, with severe pain, chemosis, decreased visual acuity, anterior uveitis, vitreous involvement, and panophthalmitis.

TREATMENT   Eye Infections

(Table 152-2) The usual therapy for keratitis is the administration of topical antibiotics. Therapy for endophthalmitis includes the use of high-dose local and systemic antibiotics (to achieve higher drug concentrations in the eye) and vitrectomy.

Ear infections

P. aeruginosa infections of the ears vary from mild swimmer's ear to serious life-threatening infections with neurologic sequelae. Swimmer's ear is common among children and results from infection of moist macerated skin of the external ear canal. Most cases resolve with treatment, but some patients develop chronic drainage. Swimmer's ear is managed with topical antibiotic agents (otic solutions). The most serious form of *Pseudomonas* infection involving the ear has been given various names: two of these designations, malignant otitis externa and necrotizing otitis externa, are now used for the same entity. This disease was originally described in elderly diabetic patients, in whom the majority of cases still occur. However, it has also been described in patients with AIDS and in elderly patients without underlying diabetes or immunocompromise. The usual presenting symptoms are decreased hearing and ear pain, which may be severe and lancinating. The pinna is usually painful, and the external canal may be tender. The ear canal almost always shows signs of inflammation, with granulation tissue and exudate. Tenderness anterior to the tragus may extend as far as the temporomandibular joint and mastoid process. A small minority of patients have systemic symptoms. Patients in whom the diagnosis is made late may present with cranial nerve palsies or even with cavernous venous sinus thrombosis. The ESR is invariably elevated (≥100 mm/h). The diagnosis is made on clinical grounds in severe cases; however, the "gold standard" is a positive technetium-99 bone scan in a patient with otitis externa due to *P. aeruginosa*. In diabetic patients, a positive bone scan constitutes presumptive evidence for this diagnosis and should prompt biopsy or empirical therapy.

TREATMENT   Ear Infections

(Table 152-2) Given the infection of the ear cartilage, sometimes with mastoid or petrous ridge involvement, patients with malignant (necrotizing) otitis externa are treated as for osteomyelitis.

Urinary tract infections

UTIs due to *P. aeruginosa* generally occur as a complication of a foreign body in the urinary tract, an obstruction in the genitourinary system, or urinary tract instrumentation or surgery. However, UTIs caused by *P. aeruginosa* have been described in pediatric outpatients without stones or evident obstruction.

TREATMENT   Urinary Tract Infections

(Table 152-2) Most *P. aeruginosa* UTIs are considered complicated infections that must be treated longer than uncomplicated cystitis. In general, a 7- to 10-day course of treatment suffices, with up to 2 weeks of therapy in cases of pyelonephritis. Urinary catheters, stents, or stones should be removed to prevent relapse, which is common and may be due not to resistance but rather to factors such as a foreign body that has been left in place or an ongoing obstruction.

Skin and soft tissue infections

Besides pyoderma gangrenosum in neutropenic patients, folliculitis and other papular or vesicular lesions due to *P. aeruginosa* have been extensively described and are collectively referred to as *dermatitis*. Multiple outbreaks have been linked to whirlpools, spas, and swimming pools. To prevent such outbreaks, the growth of *P. aeruginosa* in the home and in recreational environments must be controlled by proper chlorination of water. Most cases of hot-tub folliculitis are self-limited, requiring only the avoidance of exposure to the contaminated source of water.

Toe-web infections occur especially often in the tropics, and the "green nail syndrome" is caused by *P. aeruginosa* paronychia, which results from frequent submersion of the hands in water. In the latter entity, the green discoloration results from diffusion of pyocyanin into the nail bed. *P. aeruginosa*

remains a prominent cause of burn wound infections in some parts of the world. The management of these infections is best left to specialists in burn wound care.

Infections in febrile neutropenic patients

In febrile neutropenia, *P. aeruginosa* has historically been the organism against which empirical coverage is always essential. In the 1960s and early 1970s, *P. aeruginosa* infection occurred commonly in febrile neutropenic patients, with high associated mortality rates. Although in Western countries these infections are now less common, their importance has not been diminished because of persistently high mortality rates. In other parts of the world as well, *P. aeruginosa* continues to be a significant problem in febrile neutropenia, causing a larger proportion of infections in febrile neutropenic patients than any other single organism. For example, *P. aeruginosa* was responsible for 28% of documented infections in 499 febrile neutropenic patients in one study from the Indian subcontinent and for 31% of such infections in another. In a large study of infections in leukemia patients from Japan, *P. aeruginosa* was the most frequently documented cause of bacterial infection. In studies performed in North America, northern Europe, and Australia, the incidence of *P. aeruginosa* bacteremia in febrile neutropenia was quite variable. In a review of 97 reports published in 1987–1994, the incidence was reported to be 1–2.5% among febrile neutropenic patients given empirical therapy and 5–12% among microbiologically documented infections. The most common clinical syndromes encountered were bacteremia, pneumonia, and soft tissue infections manifesting mainly as ecthyma gangrenosum.

TREATMENT   Infections in Febrile Neutropenic Patients

(Table 152-2) Compared with rates three decades ago, improved rates of response to antibiotic therapy have been reported in many studies. A study of 127 patients demonstrated a reduction in the mortality rate from 71% to 25% with the introduction of ceftazidime and imipenem. Since neutrophils—the normal host defenses against this organism—are absent in febrile neutropenic patients, maximal doses of antipseudomonal β-lactam antibiotics should be used for the management of *P. aeruginosa* bacteremia in this setting.

Infections in patients with AIDS

Both community- and hospital-acquired *P. aeruginosa* infections were documented in patients with AIDS before the advent of antiretroviral therapy. Since the introduction of protease inhibitors, *P. aeruginosa* infections in AIDS patients have been seen less frequently but still occur, particularly in the form of sinusitis. The clinical presentation of *Pseudomonas* infection (especially pneumonia and bacteremia) in AIDS patients is remarkable in that, although the illness may appear not to be severe, the infection may nonetheless be fatal. Patients with bacteremia may have only a low-grade fever and may present with ecthyma gangrenosum. Bacteremia may herald underlying disease at another site (often pneumonia or sinusitis). Pneumonia, with or without bacteremia, is perhaps the most common type of *P. aeruginosa* infection in AIDS patients. Patients with AIDS and *P. aeruginosa* pneumonia exhibit the classic clinical signs and symptoms of pneumonia, such as fever, productive cough, and chest pain. The infection may be lobar or multilobar and shows no predisposition for any particular location. The most striking feature is the high frequency of cavitary disease.

TREATMENT Infections in Patients with AIDS

Therapy for any of these conditions in AIDS patients is no different from that in other patients. However, relapse is the rule unless the patient's CD4+ T cell count rises to >50/μL or suppressive antibiotic therapy is given. In attempts to achieve cures and prevent relapses, therapy tends to be more prolonged than in the case of an immunocompetent patient.

Multidrug-resistant infections

(Table 152-2) *P. aeruginosa* is notorious for antibiotic resistance. During three decades, the impact of resistance was minimized by the rapid development of potent antipseudomonal agents. However, the situation has recently changed, with the worldwide selection of strains carrying determinants that mediate resistance to β-lactams, fluoroquinolones, and aminoglycosides. This situation has been compounded by the lack of development of new classes of antipseudomonal drugs for nearly two decades. Physicians now resort to drugs such as colistin and polymyxin, which were discarded decades ago. These alternative approaches to the management of multiresistant *P. aeruginosa* infections were first used some time ago in CF patients, who receive colistin (polymyxin E) IV and by aerosol despite its renal toxicity. Colistin is rapidly becoming the last-resort agent of choice, even in non-CF patients infected with multiresistant *P. aeruginosa*.

The clinical outcome of multidrug-resistant *P. aeruginosa* infections treated with colistin is difficult to judge from case reports, especially given the many drugs used in the complicated management of these patients. Although earlier reports described marginal efficacy and serious nephrotoxicity and neurotoxicity, recent reports have been more encouraging. Because colistin shows synergy with other antimicrobial agents in vitro, it may be possible to reduce the dosage—and thus the toxicity—of this drug when it is combined with drugs such as rifampin and β-lactams; however, no studies in humans or animals support this approach at this time.

OTHER PSEUDOMONADS

■ STENOTROPHOMONAS MALTOPHILIA

S. maltophilia is the only potential human pathogen among a genus of ubiquitous organisms found in the rhizosphere (i.e., the soil that surrounds the roots of plants). The organism is an opportunist that is acquired from the environment but is even more limited than *P. aeruginosa* in its ability to colonize patients or cause infections. Immunocompromise is not sufficient to permit these events; rather, major perturbations of the human flora are usually necessary for the establishment of *S. maltophilia*. Accordingly, most cases of human infection occur in the setting of very broad-spectrum antibiotic therapy with agents such as advanced cephalosporins and carbapenems, which eradicate the normal flora and other pathogens. The remarkable ability of *S. maltophilia* to resist virtually all classes of antibiotics is attributable to the possession of antibiotic efflux pumps and of two β-lactamases (L1 and L2) that mediate β-lactam resistance, including that to carbapenems. It is fortunate that the virulence of *S. maltophilia* appears to be limited. Although a serine protease is present in some strains, virulence is probably a result of the host's inflammatory response to components of the organism such as LPS and flagellin. *S. maltophilia* is most commonly found in the respiratory tract of ventilated patients, where the distinction between its roles as a colonizer and as a pathogen is often difficult to make. However, *S. maltophilia* does cause pneumonia and bacteremia in such patients, and these infections have led to septic shock. Also common is central venous line–associated infection (with or without bacteremia), which has been reported most often in patients with cancer. *S. maltophilia* is a rare cause of ecthyma gangrenosum in neutropenic patients. It has been isolated from ~5% of CF patients but is not believed to be a significant pathogen in this setting.

TREATMENT *S. maltophilia* Infections

The intrinsic resistance of *S. maltophilia* to most antibiotics renders infection difficult to treat. The antibiotics to which it is most often (although not uniformly) susceptible are trimethoprim-sulfamethoxazole (TMP-SMX), ticarcillin/clavulanate, and levofloxacin (Table 152-2). Consequently, a combination of TMP-SMX and ticarcillin/clavulanate is recommended for initial therapy. Catheters must be removed in the treatment of bacteremia to hasten cure and prevent relapses. The treatment of VAP due to *S. maltophilia* is much more difficult than that of bacteremia, with the frequent development of resistance during therapy.

■ BURKHOLDERIA CEPACIA

B. cepacia gained notoriety as the cause of a rapidly fatal syndrome of respiratory distress and septicemia (the "cepacia syndrome") in CF patients. Previously, it had been recognized as an antibiotic-resistant nosocomial pathogen (then designated *P. cepacia*) in ICU patients. Patients with chronic granulomatous disease are also predisposed to *B. cepacia* lung disease. The organism has been reclassified into nine subgroups, only some of which are common in CF. *B. cepacia* is an environmental organism that inhabits moist environments and is found in the rhizosphere. This organism possesses multiple virulence factors that may play roles in disease as well as colonizing factors that are capable of binding to lung mucus—an ability that may explain the predilection of *B. cepacia* for the lungs in CF. *B. cepacia* secretes elastase and possesses components of an injectable toxin-secretion system like that of *P. aeruginosa*; its LPS is among the most potent of all LPSs in stimulating an inflammatory response in the lungs. Inflammation may be the major cause of the lung disease seen in the cepacia syndrome. The organism can penetrate epithelial surfaces by virtue of motility and inhibition of host innate immune defenses. Besides infecting the lungs in CF, *B. cepacia* appears as an airway colonizer during broad-spectrum antibiotic therapy and is a cause of VAP, catheter-associated infections, and wound infections.

TREATMENT *B. cepacia* Infections

B. cepacia is intrinsically resistant to many antibiotics. Therefore, treatment must be tailored according to sensitivities. TMP-SMX, meropenem, and doxycycline are the most effective agents in vitro and may be started as first-line agents (Table 152-2). Some strains are susceptible to third-generation cephalosporins and fluoroquinolones, and these agents may be used against isolates known to be susceptible. Combination therapy for serious pulmonary infection (e.g., in CF) is suggested for multidrug-resistant strains; the combination of meropenem and TMP-SMX may be antagonistic, however. Resistance to all agents used has been reported during therapy.

■ BURKHOLDERIA PSEUDOMALLEI

B. pseudomallei is the causative agent of melioidosis, a disease of humans and animals that is geographically restricted to Southeast Asia and northern Australia, with occasional cases in countries such as India and China. This organism may be isolated from individuals returning directly from these endemic regions and from military personnel who have served in endemic regions and then returned home after stops in Europe. Symptoms of this illness may develop only at a later date because of the organism's ability to cause latent infections. *B. pseudomallei* is found in soil and water. Humans and animals are infected by inoculation, inhalation, or ingestion; only rarely is the organism transmitted from person to person. Humans are not colonized without being infected. Among the pseudomonads, *B. pseudomallei* is perhaps the most virulent. Host compromise is not an essential prerequisite for disease, although many patients have common underlying medical diseases (e.g., diabetes or renal failure). *B. pseudomallei* is a facultative intracellular organism whose replication in PMNs and macrophages may be aided by the possession of a polysaccharide capsule. The organism also possesses elements of a type III secretion system that plays a role in its intracellular survival. During infection, there is a florid inflammatory response whose role in disease is unclear.

B. pseudomallei causes a wide spectrum of disease, ranging from asymptomatic infection to abscesses, pneumonia, and disseminated disease. It is a significant cause of fatal community-acquired pneumonia and septicemia in endemic areas, with mortality rates as high as 44% reported in Thailand. Acute pulmonary infections are the most commonly diagnosed form of melioidosis. Pneumonia may be asymptomatic (with routine chest radiographs showing mainly upper-lobe infiltrates) or may present as severe necrotizing disease. *B. pseudomallei* also causes chronic pulmonary infections with systemic manifestations that mimic those of tuberculosis, including chronic cough, fever, hemoptysis, night sweats, and cavitary lung disease. Besides pneumonia, the other principal form of *B. pseudomallei* disease is skin ulceration with associated lymphangitis and regional lymphadenopathy. Spread from the lungs or skin, which is most often documented in debilitated individuals, gives rise to septicemic forms of melioidosis that carry a high mortality rate.

TREATMENT   *B. pseudomallei* Infections

B. pseudomallei is susceptible to advanced penicillins and cephalosporins and to carbapenems (Table 152-2). Treatment is divided into two stages: an intensive 2-week phase of therapy with ceftazidime or a carbapenem followed by at least 12 weeks of oral TMP-SMX to eradicate the organism and prevent relapse. The recognition of this bacterium as a potential agent of biologic warfare has stimulated interest in the development of a vaccine.

■ BURKHOLDERIA MALLEI

B. mallei causes the equine disease glanders in Africa, Asia, and South America. The organism was eradicated from Europe and North America decades ago. The last case seen in the United States occurred in 2001 in a laboratory worker; before that, *B. mallei* had last been seen in this country in 1949. In contrast to the other organisms discussed in this chapter, *B. mallei* is not an environmental organism and does not persist outside its equine hosts. Consequently, *B. mallei* infection is an occupational risk for handlers of horses, equine butchers, and veterinarians in areas

of the world where it still exists. The polysaccharide capsule is a critical virulence determinant; diabetics are thought to be more susceptible to infection by this organism. The organism is transmitted from animals to humans by inoculation into the skin, where it causes local infection with nodules and lymphadenitis. Regional lymphadenopathy is common. Respiratory secretions from infected horses are extremely infectious. Inhalation results in clinical signs of typical pneumonia but may also cause an acute febrile illness with ulceration of the trachea. The organism may disseminate from the skin or lungs to cause septicemia with signs of sepsis. The septicemic form is frequently associated with shock and a high mortality rate. The infection may also enter a chronic phase and present as disseminated abscesses. *B. mallei* infection may present as early as 1–2 days after inhalation or (in cutaneous disease) may not become evident for months.

TREATMENT   *B. mallei* Infections

The antibiotic susceptibility pattern of *B. mallei* is similar to that of *B. pseudomallei*; in addition, the organism is susceptible to the newer macrolides azithromycin and clarithromycin. *B. mallei* infection should be treated with the same drugs and for the same duration as melioidosis.

FURTHER READINGS

CHASTRE J et al: Comparison of 8 vs 15 days of antibiotic therapy for ventilator-associated pneumonia in adults: A randomized trial. JAMA 290:2588, 2003

CURRIE BJ: *Burkholderia pseudomallei* and *Burkholderia mallei*: Melioidosis and glanders, in *Principles and Practice of Infectious Diseases*, 7th ed, GL Mandell et al (eds). Philadelphia, Elsevier Churchill Livingstone, 2010, pp 2869–2879

JOHNSON MP, RAMPHAL R: Malignant external otitis: Report on therapy with ceftazidime and review of therapy and prognosis. Rev Infect Dis 12:173, 1990

KALLEL H et al: Colistin as a salvage therapy for nosocomial infections caused by multidrug-resistant bacteria in the ICU. Int J Antimicrob Agents 28:366, 2006

LODISE TP JR et al: Predictors of 30-day mortality among patients with *Pseudomonas aeruginosa* bloodstream infections: Impact of delayed appropriate antibiotic selection. Antimicrob Agents Chemother 51:3510, 2007

MASCHMEYER G, GÖBEL UB: *Stenotrophomonas maltophilia* and *Burkholderia cepacia* complex, in *Principles and Practice of Infectious Diseases*, 7th ed, GL Mandell et al (eds). Philadelphia, Elsevier Churchill Livingstone, 2010, pp 2861–2868

MENDELSON MH et al: *Pseudomonas aeruginosa* bacteremia in AIDS. Clin Infect Dis 18:886, 1994

MICEK ST et al: *Pseudomonas aeruginosa* bloodstream infection: Importance of appropriate antibiotic therapy. Antimicrob Agents Chemother 49:1306, 2005

OBRITSCH MD et al: Nosocomial infections due to multidrug resistant *Pseudomonas aeruginosa*: Epidemiology and treatment options. Pharmacotherapy 25:1353, 2006

PIER GB, RAMPHAL R: *Pseudomonas aeruginosa*, in *Principles and Practice of Infectious Diseases*, 7th ed, GL Mandell et al (eds). Philadelphia, Elsevier Churchill Livingstone, 2010, pp 2835–2860

CHAPTER 153

Salmonellosis

David A. Pegues
Samuel I. Miller

Bacteria of the genus *Salmonella* are highly adapted for growth in both humans and animals and cause a wide spectrum of disease. The growth of serotypes *S. typhi* and *S. paratyphi* is restricted to human hosts, in whom these organisms cause enteric (typhoid) fever. The remaining serotypes (nontyphoidal *Salmonella*, or NTS) can colonize the gastrointestinal tracts of a broad range of animals, including mammals, reptiles, birds, and insects. More than 200 serotypes are pathogenic to humans, in whom they often cause gastroenteritis and can be associated with localized infections and/or bacteremia.

■ ETIOLOGY

This large genus of gram-negative bacilli within the family Enterobacteriaceae consists of two species: *S. enterica*, which contains six subspecies, and *S. bongori*. *S. enterica* subspecies I includes almost all the serotypes pathogenic for humans. According to the current *Salmonella* nomenclature system, the full taxonomic designation *S. enterica* subspecies *enterica* serotype *typhimurium* can be shortened to *Salmonella* serotype *typhimurium* or simply *S. typhimurium*.

Members of the seven *Salmonella* subspecies are classified into >2500 serotypes (serovars) according to the somatic O antigen [lipopolysaccharide (LPS) cell-wall components], the surface Vi antigen (restricted to *S. typhi* and *S. paratyphi* C), and the flagellar H antigen. For simplicity, most *Salmonella* serotypes are named for the city where they were identified, and the serotype is often used as the species designation.

Salmonellae are gram-negative, non-spore-forming, facultatively anaerobic bacilli that measure 2–3 by 0.4–0.6 μm. The initial identification of salmonellae in the clinical microbiology laboratory is based on growth characteristics. Salmonellae, like other Enterobacteriaceae, produce acid on glucose fermentation, reduce nitrates, and do not produce cytochrome oxidase. In addition, all salmonellae except *S. gallinarum-pullorum* are motile by means of peritrichous flagella, and all but *S. typhi* produce gas (H_2S) on sugar fermentation. Notably, only 1% of clinical isolates ferment lactose; a high level of suspicion must be maintained to detect these rare clinical lactose-fermenting isolates.

Although serotyping of all surface antigens can be used for formal identification, most laboratories perform a few simple agglutination reactions that define specific O-antigen serogroups, designated A, B, C_1, C_2, D, and E. Strains in these six serogroups cause ~99% of *Salmonella* infections in humans and other warm-blooded animals. Molecular typing methods, including pulsed-field gel electrophoresis and polymerase chain reaction (PCR) fingerprinting, are used in epidemiologic investigations to differentiate *Salmonella* strains of a common serotype.

■ PATHOGENESIS

All *Salmonella* infections begin with ingestion of organisms, most commonly in contaminated food or water. The infectious dose is 10^3–10^6 colony-forming units. Conditions that decrease either stomach acidity (an age of <1 year, antacid ingestion, or achlorhydric disease) or intestinal integrity (inflammatory bowel disease, prior gastrointestinal surgery, or alteration of the intestinal flora by antibiotic administration) increase susceptibility to *Salmonella* infection.

Once *S. typhi* and *S. paratyphi* reach the small intestine, they penetrate the mucus layer of the gut and traverse the intestinal layer through phagocytic microfold (M) cells that reside within Peyer's patches. Salmonellae can trigger the formation of membrane ruffles in normally nonphagocytic epithelial cells. These ruffles reach out and enclose adherent bacteria within large vesicles by a process referred to as *bacteria-mediated endocytosis* (BME). BME is dependent on the direct delivery of *Salmonella* proteins into the cytoplasm of epithelial cells by a specialized bacterial secretion system (*type III secretion*). These bacterial proteins mediate alterations in the actin cytoskeleton that are required for *Salmonella* uptake.

After crossing the epithelial layer of the small intestine, *S. typhi* and *S. paratyphi*, which cause enteric (typhoid) fever, are phagocytosed by macrophages. These salmonellae survive the antimicrobial environment of the macrophage by sensing environmental signals that trigger alterations in regulatory systems of the phagocytosed bacteria. For example, PhoP/PhoQ (the best-characterized regulatory system) triggers the expression of outer-membrane proteins and mediates modifications in LPS so that the altered bacterial surface can resist microbicidal activities and potentially alter host cell signaling. In addition, salmonellae encode a second type III secretion system that directly delivers bacterial proteins across the phagosome membrane into the macrophage cytoplasm. This secretion system functions to remodel the *Salmonella*-containing vacuole, promoting bacterial survival and replication.

Once phagocytosed, typhoidal salmonellae disseminate throughout the body in macrophages via the lymphatics and colonize reticuloendothelial tissues (liver, spleen, lymph nodes, and bone marrow). Patients have relatively few or no signs and symptoms during this initial incubation stage. Signs and symptoms, including fever and abdominal pain, probably result from secretion of cytokines by macrophages and epithelial cells in response to bacterial products that are recognized by innate immune receptors when a critical number of organisms have replicated. Over time, the development of hepatosplenomegaly is likely to be related to the recruitment of mononuclear cells and the development of a specific acquired cell-mediated immune response to *S. typhi* colonization. The recruitment of additional mononuclear cells and lymphocytes to Peyer's patches during the several weeks after initial colonization/ infection can result in marked enlargement and necrosis of the Peyer's patches, which may be mediated by bacterial products that promote cell death as well as the inflammatory response.

In contrast to enteric fever, which is characterized by an infiltration of mononuclear cells into the small-bowel mucosa, NTS gastroenteritis is characterized by massive polymorphonuclear leukocyte (PMN) infiltration into both the large- and small-bowel mucosa. This response appears to depend on the induction of interleukin (IL) 8, a strong neutrophil chemotactic factor, which is secreted by intestinal cells as a result of *Salmonella* colonization and translocation of bacterial proteins into host cell cytoplasm. The degranulation and release of toxic substances by neutrophils may result in damage to the intestinal mucosa, causing the inflammatory diarrhea observed with nontyphoidal gastroenteritis.

ENTERIC (TYPHOID) FEVER

Enteric (typhoid) fever is a systemic disease characterized by fever and abdominal pain and caused by dissemination of *S. typhi* or *S. paratyphi*. The disease was initially called *typhoid fever* because of its clinical similarity to typhus. However, in the early 1800s, typhoid fever was clearly defined pathologically as a unique illness on the basis of its association with enlarged Peyer's patches and mesenteric lymph nodes. In 1869, given the anatomic site of infection, the term *enteric fever* was proposed as an alternative designation to distinguish typhoid fever from typhus. However, to this day, the two designations are used interchangeably.

■ EPIDEMIOLOGY

In contrast to other *Salmonella* serotypes, the etiologic agents of enteric fever—*S. typhi* and *S. paratyphi* serotypes A, B, and C—have no known hosts other than humans. Most commonly, food-borne or waterborne transmission results from fecal contamination by ill or asymptomatic chronic carriers. Sexual transmission between male partners has been described. Health care workers occasionally acquire enteric fever after exposure to infected patients or during processing of clinical specimens and cultures.

With improvements in food handling and water/sewage treatment, enteric fever has become rare in developed nations. Worldwide, however, there are an estimated 22 million cases of enteric fever, with 200,000 deaths annually. The incidence is highest (>100 cases per 100,000 population per year) in south central and Southeast Asia; medium (10–100 cases per 100,000) in the rest of Asia, Africa, Latin America, and Oceania (excluding Australia and New Zealand); and low in other parts of the world (Fig. 153-1). A high incidence of enteric fever correlates with poor sanitation and lack of access to clean drinking water. In endemic regions, enteric fever is more common in urban than rural areas and among young children and adolescents. Risk factors include contaminated water or ice, flooding, food and drinks purchased from street vendors, raw fruits and vegetables grown in fields fertilized with sewage, ill household contacts, lack of hand washing and toilet access, and evidence of prior *Helicobacter pylori* infection (an association probably related to chronically reduced gastric acidity). It is estimated that there is one case of paratyphoid fever for every four cases of typhoid fever, but the incidence of infection associated with *S. paratyphi* A appears to be increasing, especially in India; this increase may be a result of vaccination for *S. typhi*.

Multidrug-resistant (MDR) strains of *S. typhi* emerged in 1989 in China and Southeast Asia and have since disseminated widely. These strains contain plasmids encoding resistance to chloramphenicol, ampicillin, and trimethoprim—antibiotics long used to treat enteric fever. With the increased use of fluoroquinolones to treat MDR enteric fever in the 1990s, strains of *S. typhi* and *S. paratyphi* with reduced susceptibility to ciprofloxacin [minimal inhibitory concentration (MIC), 0.125–1 μg/mL] have emerged in the Indian subcontinent, southern Asia, and (most recently) sub-Saharan Africa and have been associated with clinical treatment failure. Testing of isolates for resistance to the first-generation quinolone nalidixic acid detects most but not all strains with reduced susceptibility to ciprofloxacin.

The incidence of enteric fever among U.S. travelers is estimated at 3–30 cases per 100,000. Of 1902 cases of *S. typhi*–associated enteric fever reported to the Centers for Disease Control and Prevention (CDC) in 1999–2006, 79% were associated with recent international travel, most commonly to India (47%), Pakistan (10%), Bangladesh (10%), Mexico (7%), and the Philippines (4%). Only 5% of travelers diagnosed with enteric fever had received *S. typhi* vaccine. Overall, 13% of *S. typhi* isolates in the United States were resistant to ampicillin, chloramphenicol, and trimethoprim-sulfamethoxazole (TMP-SMX), and the proportion of isolates resistant to nalidixic acid increased from 19% in 1999 to 58% in 2006. Infection with nalidixic acid-resistant (NAR) *S. typhi* was associated with travel to the Indian subcontinent. Of the 25–30% of reported cases of enteric fever in the United States that are domestically acquired, the majority are sporadic, but outbreaks linked to contaminated food products and previously unrecognized chronic carriers continue to occur.

■ CLINICAL COURSE

Enteric fever is a misnomer, in that the hallmark features of this disease—fever and abdominal pain—are variable. While fever is documented at presentation in >75% of cases, abdominal pain is reported in only 30–40%. Thus, a high index of suspicion for this potentially fatal systemic illness is necessary when a person presents with fever and a history of recent travel to a developing country.

The incubation period for *S. typhi* averages 10–14 days but ranges from 3–21 days, depending on the inoculum size and the host's health and immune status. The most prominent symptom is prolonged fever (38.8°–40.5°C; 101.8°–104.9°F), which can continue for up to 4 weeks if untreated. *S. paratyphi* A is

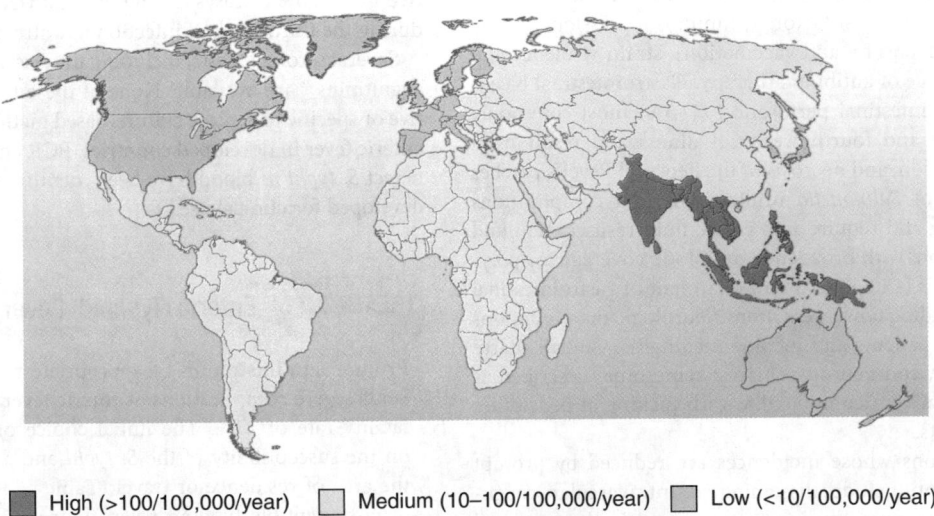

■ High (>100/100,000/year)   ■ Medium (10–100/100,000/year)   ■ Low (<10/100,000/year)

Figure 153-1   **Annual incidence of typhoid fever per 100,000 population.** *(Adapted from Crump JA et al. The global burden of typhoid fever. Bull World Health Organ 82:346, 2004.)*

Figure 153-2 "Rose spots," the rash of enteric fever due to *S. typhi* or *S. paratyphi.*

thought to cause milder disease than *S. typhi*, with predominantly gastrointestinal symptoms. However, a prospective study of 669 consecutive cases of enteric fever in Kathmandu, Nepal, found that the infections were clinically indistinguishable. In this series, symptoms reported on initial medical evaluation included headache (80%), chills (35–45%), cough (30%), sweating (20–25%), myalgias (20%), malaise (10%), and arthralgia (2–4%). Gastrointestinal symptoms included anorexia (55%), abdominal pain (30–40%), nausea (18–24%), vomiting (18%), and diarrhea (22–28%) more commonly than constipation (13–16%). Physical findings included coated tongue (51–56%), splenomegaly (5–6%), and abdominal tenderness (4–5%).

Early physical findings of enteric fever include rash ("rose spots"; 30%), hepatosplenomegaly (3–6%), epistaxis, and relative bradycardia at the peak of high fever (<50%). Rose spots (Fig. 153-2; see also Fig. e7-9) make up a faint, salmon-colored, blanching, maculopapular rash located primarily on the trunk and chest. The rash is evident in ~30% of patients at the end of the first week and resolves without a trace after 2–5 days. Patients can have two or three crops of lesions, and *Salmonella* can be cultured from punch biopsies of these lesions. The faintness of the rash makes it difficult to detect in highly pigmented patients.

The development of severe disease (which occurs in ~10–15% of patients) depends on host factors (immunosuppression, antacid therapy, previous exposure, and vaccination), strain virulence and inoculum, and choice of antibiotic therapy. Gastrointestinal bleeding (10–20%) and intestinal perforation (1–3%) most commonly occur in the third and fourth weeks of illness and result from hyperplasia, ulceration, and necrosis of the ileocecal Peyer's patches at the initial site of *Salmonella* infiltration. Both complications are life-threatening and require immediate fluid resuscitation and surgical intervention, with broadened antibiotic coverage for polymicrobial peritonitis (Chap. 127) and treatment of gastrointestinal hemorrhages, including bowel resection. Neurologic manifestations occur in 2–40% of patients and include meningitis, Guillain-Barré syndrome, neuritis, and neuropsychiatric symptoms (described as "muttering delirium" or "coma vigil"), with picking at bedclothes or imaginary objects.

Rare complications whose incidences are reduced by prompt antibiotic treatment include disseminated intravascular coagulation, hematophagocytic syndrome, pancreatitis, hepatic and splenic abscesses and granulomas, endocarditis, pericarditis, myocarditis, orchitis, hepatitis, glomerulonephritis, pyelonephritis and hemolytic-uremic syndrome, severe pneumonia, arthritis, osteomyelitis, and parotitis. Up to 10% of patients develop mild relapse, usually within 2–3 weeks of fever resolution and in association with the same strain type and susceptibility profile.

Up to 10% of untreated patients with typhoid fever excrete *S. typhi* in the feces for up to 3 months, and 1–4% develop chronic asymptomatic carriage, shedding *S. typhi* in either urine or stool for >1 year. Chronic carriage is more common among women, infants, and persons who have biliary abnormalities or concurrent bladder infection with *Schistosoma haematobium*. The anatomic abnormalities associated with the latter conditions presumably allow prolonged colonization.

■ DIAGNOSIS

Since the clinical presentation of enteric fever is relatively nonspecific, the diagnosis needs to be considered in any febrile traveler returning from a developing region, especially the Indian subcontinent, the Philippines, or Latin America. Other diagnoses that should be considered in these travelers include malaria, hepatitis, bacterial enteritis, dengue fever, rickettsial infections, leptospirosis, amebic liver abscesses, and acute HIV infection (Chap. 123). Other than a positive culture, no specific laboratory test is diagnostic for enteric fever. In 15–25% of cases, leukopenia and neutropenia are detectable. Leukocytosis is more common among children, during the first 10 days of illness, and in cases complicated by intestinal perforation or secondary infection. Other nonspecific laboratory findings include moderately elevated liver function tests and muscle enzyme levels.

The definitive diagnosis of enteric fever requires the isolation of *S. typhi* or *S. paratyphi* from blood, bone marrow, other sterile sites, rose spots, stool, or intestinal secretions. The sensitivity of blood culture is only 40–80%, probably because of high rates of antibiotic use in endemic areas and the small quantities of *S. typhi* (i.e., <15 organisms/mL) typically present in the blood. Since almost all *S. typhi* organisms in blood are associated with the mononuclear-cell/platelet fraction, centrifugation of blood and culture of the buffy coat can substantially reduce the time to isolation of the organism but do not increase sensitivity.

Bone marrow culture is 55–90% sensitive, and, unlike that of blood culture, its yield is not reduced by up to 5 days of prior antibiotic therapy. Culture of intestinal secretions (best obtained by a noninvasive duodenal string test) can be positive despite a negative bone marrow culture. If blood, bone marrow, and intestinal secretions are all cultured, the yield is >90%. Stool cultures, while negative in 60–70% of cases during the first week, can become positive during the third week of infection in untreated patients.

Several serologic tests, including the classic Widal test for "febrile agglutinins," are available. None of these tests is sufficiently sensitive or specific to replace culture-based methods for the diagnosis of enteric fever in developed countries. PCR and DNA probe assays to detect *S. typhi* in blood have been identified but have not yet been developed for clinical use.

TREATMENT   Enteric (Typhoid) Fever

Prompt administration of appropriate antibiotic therapy prevents severe complications of enteric fever and results in a case-fatality rate of <1%. The initial choice of antibiotics depends on the susceptibility of the *S. typhi* and *S. paratyphi* strains in the area of residence or travel (Table 153-1). For treatment of drug-susceptible typhoid fever, fluoroquinolones are the most effective class of agents, with cure rates of ~98% and relapse and fecal carriage rates of <2%. Experience is most extensive

TABLE 153-1 Antibiotic Therapy for Enteric Fever in Adults

Indication	Agent	Dosage (Route)	Duration, Days
Empirical Treatment			
	Ceftriaxone[a]	1–2 g/d (IV)	7–14
	Azithromycin	1 g/d (PO)	5
Fully Susceptible			
	Ciprofloxacin[b] (first line)	500 mg bid (PO) or 400 mg q12h (IV)	5–7
	Amoxicillin (second line)	1 g tid (PO) or 2 g q6h (IV)	14
	Chloramphenicol	25 mg/kg tid (PO or IV)	14–21
	Trimethoprim-sulfamethoxazole	160/800 mg bid (PO)	7–14
Multidrug-Resistant			
	Ciprofloxacin	500 mg bid (PO) or 400 mg q12h (IV)	5–7
	Ceftriaxone	2–3 g/d (IV)	7–14
	Azithromycin	1 g/d (PO)[c]	5
Nalidixic Acid–Resistant			
	Ceftriaxone	2–3 g/d (IV)	7–14
	Azithromycin	1 g/d (PO)	5
	High-dose ciprofloxacin	750 mg bid (PO) or 400 mg q8h (IV)	10–14

[a] Or another third-generation cephalosporin [e.g., cefotaxime, 2 g q8h (IV); or cefixime, 400 mg bid (PO)].
[b] Or ofloxacin, 400 mg bid (PO) for 2–5 days.
[c] Or 1 g on day 1 followed by 500 mg/d PO for 6 days.

with ciprofloxacin. Short-course ofloxacin therapy is similarly successful against infection caused by nalidixic acid–susceptible strains. However, the increased incidence of NAR *S. typhi* in Asia, which is probably related to the widespread availability of fluoroquinolones over the counter, is now limiting the use of this drug class for empirical therapy. Patients infected with NAR *S. typhi* strains should be treated with ceftriaxone, azithromycin, or high-dose ciprofloxacin. High-dose fluoroquinolone therapy for 7 days for NAR enteric fever has been associated with delayed resolution of fever and high rates of fecal carriage during convalescence. For NAR strains, 10–14 days of high-dose ciprofloxacin is preferred.

Ceftriaxone, cefotaxime, and (oral) cefixime are effective for treatment of MDR enteric fever, including NAR and fluoroquinolone-resistant strains. These agents clear fever in ~1 week, with failure rates of ~5–10%, fecal carriage rates of <3%, and relapse rates of 3–6%. Oral azithromycin results in defervescence in 4–6 days, with rates of relapse and convalescent stool carriage of <3%. Against NAR strains, azithromycin is associated with lower rates of treatment failure and shorter durations of hospitalization than are fluoroquinolones. Despite efficient in vitro killing of *Salmonella*, first- and second-generation cephalosporins as well as aminoglycosides are ineffective in the treatment of clinical infections.

Most patients with uncomplicated enteric fever can be managed at home with oral antibiotics and antipyretics. Patients with persistent vomiting, diarrhea, and/or abdominal distension should be hospitalized and given supportive therapy as well as a parenteral third-generation cephalosporin or fluoroquinolone, depending on the susceptibility profile. Therapy should be administered for at least 10 days or for 5 days after fever resolution.

In a randomized, prospective, double-blind study of critically ill patients with enteric fever (i.e., those with shock and obtundation) in Indonesia in the early 1980s, the administration of dexamethasone (an initial dose of 3 mg/kg followed by eight doses of 1 mg/kg every 6 h) with chloramphenicol was associated with a substantially lower mortality rate than was treatment with chloramphenicol alone (10% vs 55%). Although this study has not been repeated in the "post-chloramphenicol era," severe enteric fever remains one of the few indications for glucocorticoid treatment of an acute bacterial infection.

The 1–5% of patients who develop chronic carriage of *Salmonella* can be treated for 4–6 weeks with an appropriate oral antibiotic. Treatment with oral amoxicillin, TMP-SMX, ciprofloxacin, or norfloxacin is ~80% effective in eradicating chronic carriage of susceptible organisms. However, in cases of anatomic abnormality (e.g., biliary or kidney stones), eradication often requires both antibiotic therapy and surgical correction.

■ PREVENTION AND CONTROL

Theoretically, it is possible to eliminate the salmonellae that cause enteric fever since they survive only in human hosts and are spread by contaminated food and water. However, given the high prevalence of the disease in developing countries that lack adequate sewage disposal and water treatment, this goal is currently unrealistic. Thus, travelers to developing countries should be advised to monitor their food and water intake carefully and to consider vaccination.

Two typhoid vaccines are commercially available: (1) Ty21a, an oral live attenuated *S. typhi* vaccine (given on days 1, 3, 5, and 7, with a booster every 5 years); and (2) Vi CPS, a parenteral vaccine consisting of purified Vi polysaccharide from the bacterial capsule (given in 1 dose, with a booster every 2 years). The old parenteral whole-cell typhoid/paratyphoid A and B vaccine is no longer licensed, largely because of significant side effects (see below). An acetone-killed whole-cell vaccine is available only for use by the U.S. military. The minimal age for vaccination is 6 years for Ty21a and 2 years for Vi CPS. Currently, there is no licensed vaccine for paratyphoid fever.

A large-scale meta-analysis of vaccine trials comparing whole-cell vaccine, Ty21a, and Vi CPS in populations in endemic areas indicates that, while all three vaccines are similarly effective for the first year, the 3-year cumulative efficacy of the whole-cell vaccine (73%) exceeds that of both Ty21a (51%) and Vi CPS (55%). In addition, the heat-killed whole-cell vaccine maintains its efficacy for 5 years, whereas Ty21a and Vi CPS maintain their efficacy for 4 and 2 years, respectively. However, the whole-cell vaccine is associated with a much higher incidence of side effects (especially fever: 16% vs 1–2%) than the other two vaccines.

Vi CPS typhoid vaccine is poorly immunogenic in children <5 years of age because of T cell–independent properties. In the recently developed Vi-rEPA vaccine, Vi is bound to a nontoxic recombinant protein that is identical to *Pseudomonas aeruginosa* exotoxin A. In 2- to 4-year-olds, two injections of Vi-rEPA induced higher T cell responses and higher levels of serum IgG antibody to Vi than did Vi CPS in 5- to 14-year-olds. In a two-dose trial in 2- to 5-year-old children in Vietnam, Vi-rEPA provided 91% efficacy at 27 months and 88% efficacy at 43 months and was very well tolerated. This vaccine is not yet commercially available in the United States. At least three new live vaccines are in clinical development and may prove more efficacious and longer-lasting than previous live vaccines.

Typhoid vaccine is not required for international travel, but it is recommended for travelers to areas where there is a moderate to high risk of exposure to *S. typhi*, especially those who are traveling to southern Asia and other developing regions of Asia, Africa, the Caribbean, and Central and South America and who will be exposed to potentially contaminated food and drink. Typhoid vaccine should be considered even for persons planning <2 weeks of travel to high-risk areas. In addition, laboratory workers who deal with *S. typhi* and household contacts of known *S. typhi* carriers should be vaccinated. Because the protective efficacy of vaccine can be overcome by the high inocula that are commonly encountered in food-borne exposures, immunization is an adjunct and not a substitute for avoiding high-risk foods and beverages. Immunization is not recommended for adults residing in typhoid-endemic areas or for the management of persons who may have been exposed in a common-source outbreak.

Enteric fever is a notifiable disease in the United States. Individual health departments have their own guidelines for allowing ill or colonized food handlers or health care workers to return to their jobs. The reporting system enables public health departments to identify potential source patients and to treat chronic carriers in order to prevent further outbreaks. In addition, since 1–4% of patients with *S. typhi* infection become chronic carriers, it is important to monitor patients (especially child-care providers and food handlers) for chronic carriage and to treat this condition if indicated.

NONTYPHOIDAL SALMONELLOSIS

■ EPIDEMIOLOGY

In the United States, the incidence of NTS infection has doubled in the past 2 decades; the 2009 figure is ~14 million cases annually. In 2007, the incidence of NTS infection in this country was 14.9 per 100,000 persons—the highest rate among the 11 food-borne enteric pathogens under active surveillance. Five serotypes accounted for one-half of U.S. infections in 2007: *typhimurium* (19%), *enteritidis* (14%), Newport (9%), Javiana (5%), and Heidelberg (4%).

The incidence of nontyphoidal salmonellosis is highest during the rainy season in tropical climates and during the warmer months in temperate climates, coinciding with the peak in food-borne outbreaks. Rates of morbidity and mortality associated with NTS are highest among the elderly, infants, and immunocompromised individuals, including those with hemoglobinopathies, HIV infection, or infections that cause blockade of the reticuloendothelial system (e.g., bartonellosis, malaria, schistosomiasis, and histoplasmosis).

Unlike *S. typhi* and *S. paratyphi*, whose only reservoir is humans, NTS can be acquired from multiple animal reservoirs. Transmission is most commonly associated with animal food products, especially eggs, poultry, undercooked ground meat, dairy products, and fresh produce contaminated with animal waste.

S. enteritidis infection associated with chicken eggs emerged as a major cause of food-borne disease during the 1980s and 1990s. *S. enteritidis* infection of the ovaries and upper oviduct tissue of hens results in contamination of egg contents before shell deposition. Infection is spread to egg-laying hens from breeding flocks and through contact with rodents and manure. Of the 997 outbreaks of *S. enteritidis* with a confirmed source that were reported to the CDC in 1985–2003, 75% were associated with raw or undercooked eggs. After peaking at 3.9 cases per 100,000 U.S. population in 1995, the incidence of *S. enteritidis* infection declined substantially to 1.7 per 100,000 in 2003; this decrease probably reflected improved on-farm control measures, refrigeration, and education of consumers and food-service workers. Transmission via contaminated eggs can be prevented by cooking eggs until the yolk is solidified and through pasteurization of egg products.

Centralization of food processing and widespread food distribution have contributed to the increased incidence of NTS in developed countries. Manufactured foods to which recent *Salmonella* outbreaks have been traced include peanut butter; milk products, including infant formula; and various processed foods, including packaged breakfast cereal, salsa, frozen prepared meals, and snack foods. Large outbreaks have also been linked to fresh produce, including alfalfa sprouts, cantaloupe, fresh-squeezed orange juice, and tomatoes; these items become contaminated by manure or water at a single site and then are widely distributed.

An estimated 6% of sporadic *Salmonella* infections in the United States are attributed to contact with reptiles and amphibians, especially iguanas, snakes, turtles, and lizards. Reptile-associated *Salmonella* infection more commonly leads to hospitalization and more frequently involves infants than do other *Salmonella* infections. Other pets, including African hedgehogs, snakes, birds, rodents, baby chicks, ducklings, dogs, and cats, are also potential sources of NTS.

Increasing antibiotic resistance in NTS species is a global problem and has been linked to the widespread use of antimicrobial agents in food animals and especially in animal feed. In the early 1990s, *S. typhimurium* definitive phage type 104 (DT104), characterized by resistance to ≥5 antibiotics (ampicillin, chloramphenicol, streptomycin, sulfonamides, and tetracyclines; R-type ACSSuT), emerged worldwide. In 2005, resistance to at least ACSSuT was the most common MDR phenotype among NTS isolates in the United States. Acquisition is associated with exposure to ill farm animals and to various meat products, including uncooked or undercooked ground beef. Although probably no more virulent than susceptible *S. typhimurium* strains, DT104 strains are associated with an increased risk of bloodstream infection and hospitalization. NAR and trimethoprim-resistant DT104 strains are emerging, especially in the United Kingdom.

Because of increased resistance to conventional antibiotics such as ampicillin and TMP-SMX, extended-spectrum cephalosporins and fluoroquinolones have emerged as the agents of choice for the treatment of MDR NTS infections. In 2005, 2% of all NTS strains and 12.6% of *S. Newport* strains were resistant to ceftriaxone. Most ceftriaxone-resistant isolates were from children <18 years of age, in whom ceftriaxone is the antibiotic of choice for treatment of invasive NTS infection. These strains contained plasmid-encoded AmpC β-lactamases that were probably acquired by horizontal genetic transfer from *Escherichia coli* strains in food-producing animals—an event linked to the widespread use of the veterinary cephalosporin ceftiofur.

Resistance to nalidixic acid and fluoroquinolones also has begun to emerge and is most commonly associated with point mutations in the DNA gyrase genes *gyr*A and *gyr*B. Nalidixic acid resistance is a good predictor of reduced susceptibility to clinically useful fluoroquinolones. From 1996–2005, the rate of NAR NTS isolates in the United States increased fivefold (from 0.5–2.4%). In Denmark, infection with NAR *S. typhimurium* DT104 has been linked to swine and associated with a threefold higher risk of invasive disease or death within 90 days. In Taiwan in 2000, a strain of ciprofloxacin-resistant (MIC, ≥4 mcg/mL) *S. choleraesuis* caused a large outbreak of invasive infections that was linked to the use of enrofloxacin in swine feed.

■ CLINICAL MANIFESTATIONS

Gastroenteritis

Infection with NTS most often results in gastroenteritis indistinguishable from that caused by other enteric pathogens. Nausea, vomiting, and diarrhea occur 6–48 h after the ingestion of contaminated food or water. Patients often experience abdominal cramping and fever (38–39°C; 100.5–102.2°F). Diarrheal stools are usually loose, nonbloody, and of moderate volume. However, large-volume watery stools, bloody stools, or symptoms of dysentery may occur. Rarely, NTS causes pseudoappendicitis or an illness that mimics inflammatory bowel disease.

Gastroenteritis caused by NTS is usually self-limited. Diarrhea resolves within 3–7 days and fever within 72 h. Stool cultures remain positive for 4–5 weeks after infection and—in rare cases of chronic carriage (<1%)—for >1 year. Antibiotic treatment usually is not recommended and may prolong fecal carriage. Neonates, the elderly, and immunosuppressed patients (e.g., transplant recipients, HIV-infected persons) with NTS gastroenteritis are especially susceptible to dehydration and dissemination and may require hospitalization and antibiotic therapy. Acute NTS gastroenteritis was associated with a threefold increased risk of dyspepsia and irritable bowel syndrome at 1 year in a recent study from Spain.

Bacteremia and endovascular infections

Up to 8% of patients with NTS gastroenteritis develop bacteremia; of these, 5–10% develop localized infections. Bacteremia and metastatic infection are most common with *S. choleraesuis* and *S. Dublin* and among infants, the elderly, and immunocompromised patients. NTS endovascular infection should be suspected in high-grade or persistent bacteremia, especially with preexisting valvular heart disease, atherosclerotic vascular disease, prosthetic vascular graft, or aortic aneurysm. Arteritis should be suspected in elderly patients with prolonged fever and back, chest, or abdominal pain developing after an episode of gastroenteritis. Endocarditis and arteritis are rare (<1% of cases) but are associated with potentially fatal complications, including valve perforation, endomyocardial abscess, infected mural thrombus, pericarditis, mycotic aneurysms, aneurysm rupture, aortoenteric fistula, and vertebral osteomyelitis. In some areas of sub-Saharan Africa, NTS may be among the most common causes—or even the most common cause—of bacteremia in children. NTS bacteremia among these children is not associated with diarrhea and has been associated with nutritional status and HIV infection.

Localized infections

Intraabdominal infections   Intraabdominal infections due to NTS are rare and usually manifest as hepatic or splenic abscesses or as cholecystitis. Risk factors include hepatobiliary anatomic abnormalities (e.g., gallstones), abdominal malignancy, and sickle cell disease (especially with splenic abscesses). Eradication of the infection often requires surgical correction of abnormalities and percutaneous drainage of abscesses.

Central nervous system infections   NTS meningitis most commonly develops in infants 1–4 months of age. It often results in severe sequelae (including seizures, hydrocephalus, brain infarction, and mental retardation) with death in up to 60% of cases. Other rare central nervous system infections include ventriculitis, subdural empyema, and brain abscesses.

Pulmonary infections   NTS pulmonary infections usually present as lobar pneumonia, and complications include lung abscess, empyema, and bronchopleural fistula formation. The majority of cases occur in patients with lung cancer, structural lung disease, sickle cell disease, or glucocorticoid use.

Urinary and genital tract infections   Urinary tract infections caused by NTS present as either cystitis or pyelonephritis. Risk factors include malignancy, urolithiasis, structural abnormalities, HIV infection, and renal transplantation. NTS genital infections are rare and include ovarian and testicular abscesses, prostatitis, and epididymitis. Like other focal infections, both genital and urinary tract infections can be complicated by abscess formation.

Bone, joint, and soft tissue infections   *Salmonella* osteomyelitis most commonly affects the femur, tibia, humerus, or lumbar vertebrae and is most often seen in association with sickle cell disease, hemoglobinopathies, or preexisting bone disease (e.g., fractures). Prolonged antibiotic treatment is recommended to decrease the risk of relapse and chronic osteomyelitis. Septic arthritis occurs in the same patient population as osteomyelitis and usually involves the knee, hip, or shoulder joints. Reactive arthritis (Reiter's syndrome) can follow NTS gastroenteritis and is seen most frequently in persons with the HLA-B27 histocompatibility antigen. NTS rarely can cause soft tissue infections, usually at sites of local trauma in immunosuppressed patients.

■ DIAGNOSIS

The diagnosis of NTS infection is based on isolation of the organism from freshly passed stool or from blood or another ordinarily sterile body fluid. All salmonellae isolated in clinical laboratories should be sent to local public health departments for serotyping. Blood cultures should be done whenever a patient has prolonged or recurrent fever. Endovascular infection should be suspected if there is high-grade bacteremia (>50% of three or more positive blood cultures). Echocardiography, CT, and indium-labeled white cell scanning are used to identify localized infection. When another localized infection is suspected, joint fluid, abscess drainage, or cerebrospinal fluid should be cultured, as clinically indicated.

TREATMENT   Nontyphoidal Salmonellosis

Antibiotics should not be used routinely to treat uncomplicated NTS gastroenteritis. The symptoms are usually self-limited, and the duration of fever and diarrhea is not significantly decreased by antibiotic therapy. In addition, antibiotic treatment has been

CHAPTER 153 Salmonellosis

associated with increased rates of relapse, prolonged gastro-intestinal carriage, and adverse drug reactions. Dehydration secondary to diarrhea should be treated with fluid and electrolyte replacement.

Preemptive antibiotic treatment (Table 153-2) should be considered for patients at increased risk for invasive NTS infection, including neonates (probably up to 3 months of age); persons >50 years of age with suspected atherosclerosis; and patients with immunosuppression, cardiac valvular or endovascular abnormalities, or significant joint disease. Treatment should consist of an oral or IV antibiotic administered for 48–72 h or until the patient becomes afebrile. Immunocompromised persons may require up to 7–14 days of therapy. The <1% of persons who develop chronic carriage of NTS should receive a prolonged antibiotic course, as described above for chronic carriage of *S. typhi*.

Because of the increasing prevalence of antibiotic resistance, empirical therapy for life-threatening NTS bacteremia or focal NTS infection should include a third-generation cephalosporin or a fluoroquinolone (Table 153-2). If the bacteremia is low-grade (<50% of positive blood cultures), the patient should be treated for 7–14 days. Patients with HIV/AIDS and NTS bacteremia should receive 1–2 weeks of IV antibiotic therapy followed

by 4 weeks of oral therapy with a fluoroquinolone. Patients whose infections relapse after this regimen should receive long-term suppressive therapy with a fluoroquinolone or TMP-SMX, as indicated by bacterial sensitivities.

If the patient has endocarditis or arteritis, treatment for 6 weeks with an IV β-lactam antibiotic (such as ceftriaxone or ampicillin) is indicated. IV ciprofloxacin followed by prolonged oral therapy is an option, but published experience is limited. Early surgical resection of infected aneurysms or other infected endovascular sites is recommended. Patients with infected prosthetic vascular grafts that cannot be resected have been maintained successfully on chronic suppressive oral therapy. For extraintestinal non-vascular infections, a 2- to 4-week course of antibiotic therapy (depending on the infection site) is usually recommended. In chronic osteomyelitis, abscess, or urinary or hepatobiliary infection associated with anatomic abnormalities, surgical resection or drainage may be required in addition to prolonged antibiotic therapy for eradication of infection.

PREVENTION AND CONTROL

Despite widespread efforts to prevent or reduce bacterial contamination of animal-derived food products and to improve food-safety

TABLE 153-2 Antibiotic Therapy for Nontyphoidal *Salmonella* Infection in Adults

Indication	Agent	Dosage (Route)	Duration, Days
Preemptive Treatment[a]			
	Ciprofloxacin[b]	500 mg bid (PO)	2–3
Severe Gastroenteritis[c]			
	Ciprofloxacin	500 mg bid (PO) or 400 mg q12h (IV)	3–7
	Trimethoprim-sulfamethoxazole	160/800 mg bid (PO)	
	Amoxicillin	1 g tid (PO)	
	Ceftriaxone	1–2 g/d (IV)	
Bacteremia			
	Ceftriaxone[d]	2 g/d (IV)	7–14
	Ciprofloxacin	400 mg q12h (IV), then 500 mg bid (PO)	
Endocarditis or Arteritis			
	Ceftriaxone	2 g/d (IV)	42
	Ciprofloxacin	400 mg q8h (IV), then 750 mg bid (PO)	
	Ampicillin	2 g q4h (IV)	
Meningitis			
	Ceftriaxone	2 g q12 h (IV)	14–21
	Ampicillin	2 g q4h (IV)	
Other Localized Infection			
	Ceftriaxone	2 g/d (IV)	14–28
	Ciprofloxacin	500 mg bid (PO) or 400 mg q12h (IV)	
	Ampicillin	2 g q6h (IV)	

[a]Consider for neonates; persons >50 years of age with possible atherosclerotic vascular disease; and patients with immunosuppression, endovascular graft, or joint prosthesis.
[b]Or ofloxacin, 400 mg bid (PO).
[c]Consider on an individualized basis for patients with severe diarrhea and high fever who require hospitalization.
[d]Or cefotaxime, 2 g q8h (IV).

education and training, recent declines in the incidence of NTS in the United States have been modest compared with those of other food-borne pathogens. This observation probably reflects the complex epidemiology of NTS. Identifying effective risk-reduction strategies requires monitoring of every step of food production, from handling of raw animal or plant products to preparation of finished foods. Contaminated food can be made safe for consumption by pasteurization, irradiation, or proper cooking. All cases of NTS infection should be reported to local public health departments, since tracking and monitoring of these cases can identify the source(s) of infection and help authorities anticipate large outbreaks. Lastly, the prudent use of antimicrobial agents in both humans and animals is needed to limit the emergence of MDR *Salmonella*.

FURTHER READINGS

COHEN JI et al: Extra-intestinal manifestations of *Salmonella* infections. Medicine 66:349, 1987

GLYNN MK et al: Emergence of multidrug-resistant *Salmonella enterica* serotype *typhimurium* DT104 infections in the United States. N Engl J Med 338:1333, 1998

HARAGA A et al: *Salmonella* interplay with host cells. Nat Rev Micobiol 6:53, 2008

LIN FY et al: The efficacy of a *Salmonella typhi* Vi conjugate vaccine in two- to five-year-old children. N Engl J Med 344:1263, 2001

LYNCH MF et al: Typhoid fever in the United States, 1990–2006. JAMA 302:859, 2009

MASKEY AP et al: *Salmonella* enteric serovar Paratyphi A and *S. enterica* serovar Typhi cause indistinguishable clinical syndromes in Kathmandu, Nepal. Clin Infect Dis 42:1247, 2006

STEINBERG EB et al: Typhoid fever in travelers: Who should be targeted for prevention? Clin Infect Dis 39:186, 2004

SU LH et al: Antimicrobial resistance in nontyphoid *Salmonella* serotypes: A global challenge. Clin Infect Dis 39:546, 2004

THAVER D et al: Fluoroquinolones for treating typhoid and paratyphoid fever (enteric fever). Cochrane Database Syst Rev CD004530, 2008

VARMA JK et al: Antimicrobial-resistant nontyphoidal *Salmonella* is associated with excess bloodstream infections and hospitalizations. J Infect Dis 191:554, 2005

CHAPTER **154**

Shigellosis

Philippe Sansonetti
Jean Bergounioux

The discovery of *Shigella* as the etiologic agent of dysentery—a clinical syndrome of fever, intestinal cramps, and frequent passage of small, bloody, mucopurulent stools—is attributed to the Japanese microbiologist Kiyoshi Shiga, who isolated the Shiga bacillus (now known as *Shigella dysenteriae* type 1) from patients' stools in 1897 during a large and devastating dysentery epidemic. *Shigella* cannot be distinguished from *Escherichia coli* by DNA hybridization and remains a separate species only on historical and clinical grounds.

■ DEFINITION

Shigella is a nonspore-forming, gram-negative bacterium that, unlike *E. coli*, is nonmotile and does not produce gas from sugars, decarboxylate lysine, or hydrolyze arginine. Some serovars produce indole, and occasional strains utilize sodium acetate. *S. dysenteriae*, *S. flexneri*, *S. boydii*, and *S. sonnei* (serogroups A, B, C, and D, respectively) can be differentiated on the basis of biochemical and serologic characteristics. Genome sequencing of *E. coli* K12, *S. flexneri* 2a, *S. sonnei*, *S. dysenteriae* type 1, and *S. boydii* has revealed that these species have ~93% of genes in common. The three major genomic "signatures" of *Shigella* are (1) a 215-kb virulence plasmid that carries most of the genes required for pathogenicity (particularly invasive capacity); (2) the lack or alteration of genetic sequences encoding products (e.g., lysine decarboxylase) that, if expressed, would attenuate pathogenicity; and (3) in *S. dysenteriae* type 1, the presence of genes encoding Shiga toxin, a potent cytotoxin.

■ EPIDEMIOLOGY

The human intestinal tract represents the major reservoir of *Shigella*, which is also found (albeit rarely) in the higher primates. Because excretion of shigellae is greatest in the acute phase of disease, the bacteria are transmitted most efficiently by the fecal-oral route via hand carriage; however, some outbreaks reflect food-borne or waterborne transmission. In impoverished areas, *Shigella* can be transmitted by flies. The high-level infectivity of *Shigella* is reflected by the very small inoculum required for experimental infection of volunteers [100 colony-forming units (CFU)], by the very high attack rates during outbreaks in day-care centers (33–73%), and by the high rates of secondary cases among family members of sick children (26–33%). Shigellosis can also be transmitted sexually.

Throughout history, *Shigella* epidemics have often occurred in settings of human crowding under conditions of poor hygiene—e.g., among soldiers in campaigning armies, inhabitants of besieged cities, groups on pilgrimages, and refugees in camps. Epidemics follow a cyclical pattern in areas such as the Indian subcontinent and sub-Saharan Africa. These devastating epidemics, which are most often caused by *S. dysenteriae* type 1, are characterized by high attack and mortality rates. In Bangladesh, for instance, an epidemic caused by *S. dysenteriae* type 1 was associated with a 42% increase in mortality rate among children 1–4 years of age. Apart from these epidemics, shigellosis is mostly an endemic disease, with 99% of cases occurring in the developing world and the highest prevalences in the most impoverished areas, where personal and general hygiene is below standard. *S. flexneri* isolates predominate in the least developed areas, whereas *S. sonnei* is more prevalent in economically emerging countries and in the industrialized world.

Prevalence in the developing world

In a review published under the auspices of the World Health Organization (WHO), the total annual number of cases in 1966–1997 was estimated at 165 million, and 69% of these cases occurred in children <5 years of age. In this review, the annual number of deaths was calculated to range between 500,000 and 1.1 million.

More recent data (2000–2004) from six Asian countries indicate that even though the incidence of shigellosis remains stable, mortality rates associated with this disease may have decreased significantly, possibly as a result of improved nutritional status. However, extensive and essentially uncontrolled use of antibiotics, which may also account for declining mortality rates, has increased the rate of emergence of multidrug-resistant *Shigella* strains. An often-overlooked complication of shigellosis is the short- and long-term impairment of the nutritional status of infected children in endemic areas. Combined with anorexia, the exudative enteropathy resulting from mucosal abrasions contributes to rapid deterioration of the patient's nutritional status. Shigellosis is thus a major contributor to stunted growth among children in developing countries.

Peaking in incidence in the pediatric population, endemic shigellosis is rare in young and middle-aged adults, probably because of naturally acquired immunity. Incidence then increases again in the elderly population.

Prevalence in the industrialized world

In pediatric populations, local outbreaks occur when proper and adapted hygiene policies are not implemented in group facilities like day-care centers and institutions for the mentally retarded. In adults, as in children, sporadic cases occur among travelers returning from endemic areas, and rare outbreaks of varying size can follow waterborne or food-borne infections.

■ PATHOGENESIS AND PATHOLOGY

Shigella infection occurs essentially through oral contamination via direct fecal-oral transmission, the organism being poorly adapted to survive in the environment. Resistance to low-pH conditions allows shigellae to survive passage through the gastric barrier, an ability that may explain in part why a small inoculum (as few as 100 CFU) is sufficient to cause infection.

The watery diarrhea that usually precedes the dysenteric syndrome is attributable to active secretion and abnormal water reabsorption—a secretory effect at the jejunal level described in experimentally infected rhesus monkeys. This initial purge is probably due to the combined action of an enterotoxin (ShET-1) and

mucosal inflammation. The dysenteric syndrome, manifested by bloody and mucopurulent stools, reflects invasion of the mucosa.

The pathogenesis of *Shigella* is essentially determined by a large virulence plasmid of 214 kb comprising ~100 genes, of which 25 encode a type III secretion system that inserts into the membrane of the host cell to allow effectors to transit from the bacterial cytoplasm to the host cell cytoplasm (Fig. 154-1). Bacteria are thereby able to invade intestinal epithelial cells by inducing their own uptake after the initial crossing of the epithelial barrier through M cells (the specialized translocating epithelial cells in the follicle-associated epithelium that covers mucosal lymphoid nodules). The organisms induce apoptosis of subepithelial resident macrophages. Once inside the cytoplasm of intestinal epithelial cells, *Shigella* effectors trigger the cytoskeletal rearrangements necessary to direct uptake of the organism into the epithelial cell. The *Shigella*-containing vacuole is then quickly lysed, releasing bacteria into the cytosol.

Intracellular shigellae next use cytoskeletal components to propel themselves inside the infected cell; when the moving organism and the host cell membrane come into contact, cellular protrusions form and are engulfed by neighboring cells. This series of events permits bacterial cell-to-cell spread.

Cytokines released by a growing number of infected intestinal epithelial cells attract increased numbers of immune cells [particularly polymorphonuclear leukocytes (PMNs)] to the infected site, thus further destabilizing the epithelial barrier, exacerbating inflammation, and leading to the acute colitis that characterizes shigellosis. Evidence indicates that some type III secretion system–injected effectors can control the extent of inflammation, thus facilitating bacterial survival.

Shiga toxin produced by *S. dysenteriae* type 1 increases disease severity. This toxin belongs to a group of A1-B5 protein toxins whose B subunit binds to the receptor globotriaosylceramide on the target cell surface and whose catalytic A subunit is internalized by receptor-mediated endocytosis and interacts with the subcellular machinery to inhibit protein synthesis by expressing RNA N-glycosidase activity on 28S ribosomal RNA. This process leads to inhibition of binding of the amino-acyl-tRNA to the 60S ribosomal subunit and thus to a general shutoff of cell protein

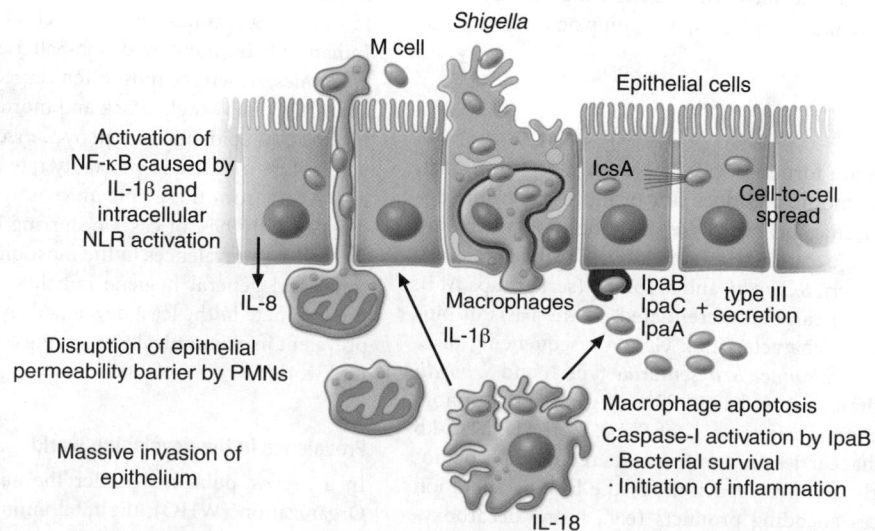

Figure 154-1 **Invasive strategy of *Shigella flexneri*.** IL, interleukin; NF-κB, nuclear factor κB; NLR, NOD-like receptor; PMN, polymorphonuclear leukocyte.

biosynthesis. Shiga toxins are translocated from the bowel into the circulation. After binding of the toxins to target cells in the kidney, pathophysiologic alterations may result in hemolytic-uremic syndrome (HUS; see below).

■ CLINICAL MANIFESTATIONS

The presentation and severity of shigellosis depend to some extent on the infecting serotype but even more on the age and the immunologic and nutritional status of the host. Poverty and poor standards of hygiene are strongly related to the number and severity of diarrheal episodes, especially in children <5 years old who have been weaned.

Shigellosis typically evolves through four phases: incubation, watery diarrhea, dysentery, and the postinfectious phase. The incubation period usually lasts 1–4 days but may be as long as 8 days. Typical initial manifestations are transient fever, limited watery diarrhea, malaise, and anorexia. Signs and symptoms may range from mild abdominal discomfort to severe cramps, diarrhea, fever, vomiting, and tenesmus. The manifestations are usually exacerbated in children, with temperatures up to 40°–41°C (104.0°–105.8°F) and more severe anorexia and watery diarrhea. This initial phase may represent the only clinical manifestation of shigellosis, especially in developed countries. Otherwise, dysentery follows within hours or days and is characterized by uninterrupted excretion of small volumes of bloody mucopurulent stools with increased tenesmus and abdominal cramps. At this stage, *Shigella* produces acute colitis involving mainly the distal colon and the rectum. Unlike most diarrheal syndromes, dysenteric syndromes rarely present with dehydration as a major feature. Endoscopy shows an edematous and hemorrhagic mucosa, with ulcerations and possibly overlying exudates resembling pseudomembranes. The extent of the lesions correlates with the number and frequency of stools and with the degree of protein loss by exudative mechanisms. Most episodes are self-limited and resolve without treatment in 1 week. With appropriate treatment, recovery takes place within a few days to a week, with no sequelae.

Acute life-threatening complications are seen most often in children <5 years of age (particularly those who are malnourished) and in elderly patients. Risk factors for death in a clinically severe case include nonbloody diarrhea, moderate to severe dehydration, bacteremia, absence of fever, abdominal tenderness, and rectal prolapse. Major complications are predominantly intestinal (e.g., toxic megacolon, intestinal perforations, rectal prolapse) or metabolic (e.g., hypoglycemia, hyponatremia, dehydration). Bacteremia is rare and is reported most frequently in severely malnourished and HIV-infected patients. Alterations of consciousness, including seizures, delirium, and coma, may occur, especially in children <5 years old, and are associated with a poor prognosis; fever and severe metabolic alterations are more often the major causes of altered consciousness than is meningitis or the Ekiri syndrome (toxic encephalopathy associated with bizarre posturing, cerebral edema, and fatty degeneration of viscera), which has been reported mostly in Japanese children. Pneumonia, vaginitis, and keratoconjunctivitis due to *Shigella* are rarely reported. In the absence of serious malnutrition, severe and very unusual clinical manifestations, such as meningitis, may be linked to genetic defects in innate immune functions [i.e., deficiency in interleukin 1 receptor–associated kinase 4 (IRAK-4)] and may require genetic investigation.

Two complications of particular importance are toxic megacolon and HUS. Toxic megacolon is a consequence of severe inflammation extending to the colonic smooth-muscle layer and causing paralysis and dilatation. The patient presents with abdominal distention and tenderness, with or without signs of localized or generalized peritonitis. The abdominal x-ray characteristically shows marked dilatation of the transverse colon (with the greatest distention in the ascending and descending segments); thumbprinting caused by mucosal inflammatory edema; and loss of the normal haustral pattern associated with pseudopolyps, often extending into the lumen. Pneumatosis coli is an occasional finding. If perforation occurs, radiographic signs of pneumoperitoneum may be apparent. Predisposing factors (e.g., hypokalemia and use of opioids, anticholinergics, loperamide, psyllium seeds, and antidepressants) should be investigated.

Shiga toxin produced by *S. dysenteriae* type 1 has been linked to HUS in developing countries but rarely in industrialized countries, where enterohemorrhagic *E. coli* (EHEC) predominates as the etiologic agent of this syndrome. HUS is an early complication that most often develops after several days of diarrhea. Clinical examination shows pallor, asthenia, and irritability and, in some cases, bleeding of the nose and gums, oliguria, and increasing edema. HUS is a nonimmune (Coombs test–negative) hemolytic anemia defined by a diagnostic triad: microangiopathic hemolytic anemia [hemoglobin level typically <80 g/L (<8 g/dL)], thrombocytopenia (mild to moderate in severity; typically <60,000 platelets/μL), and acute renal failure due to thrombosis of the glomerular capillaries (with markedly elevated creatinine levels). Anemia is severe, with fragmented red blood cells (schizocytes) in the peripheral smear, high serum concentrations of lactate dehydrogenase and free circulating hemoglobin, and elevated reticulocyte counts. Acute renal failure occurs in 55–70% of cases; however, renal function recovers in most of these cases (up to 70% in various series). Leukemoid reactions, with leukocyte counts of 50,000/μL, are sometimes noted in association with HUS.

The postinfectious immunologic complication known as reactive arthritis can develop weeks or months after shigellosis, especially in patients expressing the histocompatibility antigen HLA-B27. About 3% of patients infected with *S. flexneri* later develop this syndrome, with arthritis, ocular inflammation, and urethritis—a condition that can last for months or years and can progress to difficult-to-treat chronic arthritis. Postinfectious arthropathy occurs only after infection with *S. flexneri* and not after infection with the other *Shigella* serotypes.

■ LABORATORY DIAGNOSIS

The differential diagnosis in patients with a dysenteric syndrome depends on the clinical and environmental context. In developing areas, infectious diarrhea caused by other invasive pathogenic bacteria (*Salmonella, Campylobacter jejuni, Clostridium difficile, Yersinia enterocolitica*) or parasites (*Entamoeba histolytica*) should be considered. Only bacteriologic and parasitologic examinations of stool can truly differentiate among these pathogens. A first flare of inflammatory bowel disease, such as Crohn's disease or ulcerative colitis (Chap. 295), should be considered in patients in industrialized countries. Despite similar symptoms, anamnesis discriminates between shigellosis, which usually follows recent travel in an endemic zone, and these other conditions.

Microscopic examination of stool smears shows the presence of erythrophagocytic trophozoites with very few PMNs in *E. histolytica* infection, whereas bacterial enteroinvasive infections (particularly shigellosis) are characterized by high PMN counts in each microscopic field. However, because shigellosis often manifests only as watery diarrhea, systematic attempts to isolate *Shigella* are necessary.

The "gold standard" for the diagnosis of *Shigella* infection remains the isolation and identification of the pathogen from fecal material. One major difficulty, particularly in endemic areas where laboratory facilities are not immediately available, is the fragility of *Shigella* and its common disappearance during transport, especially with rapid changes in temperature and pH. In the absence of a reliable enrichment medium, buffered glycerol saline or Cary-Blair medium can be used as a holding medium, but prompt inoculation onto isolation medium is essential. The probability of isolation is higher if the portion of stools that contains bloody and/or mucopurulent material is directly sampled. Rectal swabs can be used, as they offer the highest rate of successful isolation during the acute phase of disease. Blood cultures are positive in <5% of cases but should be done when a patient presents with a clinical picture of severe sepsis.

In addition to quick processing, the use of several media increases the likelihood of successful isolation: a nonselective medium such as bromocresol-purple agar lactose; a low-selectivity medium such as MacConkey or eosin-methylene blue; and a high-selectivity medium such as Hektoen, *Salmonella-Shigella*, or xylose-lysine-deoxycholate agar. After incubation on these media for 12–18 h at 37°C (98.6°F), shigellae appear as nonlactose-fermenting colonies that measure 0.5–1 mm in diameter and have a convex, translucent, smooth surface. Suspected colonies on nonselective or low-selectivity medium can be subcultured on a high-selectivity medium before being specifically identified or can be identified directly by standard commercial systems on the basis of four major characteristics: glucose positivity (usually without production of gas), lactose negativity, H_2S negativity, and lack of motility. The four *Shigella* serogroups (A–D) can then be differentiated by additional characteristics. This approach adds time and difficulty to the identification process; however, after presumptive diagnosis, the use of serologic methods (e.g., slide agglutination, with group- and then type-specific antisera) should be considered. Group-specific antisera are widely available; in contrast, because of the large number of serotypes and sub-serotypes, type-specific antisera are rare and more expensive and thus are often restricted to reference laboratories.

TREATMENT ▶ Shigellosis

ANTIBIOTIC SUSCEPTIBILITY OF *SHIGELLA* As an enteroinvasive disease, shigellosis requires antibiotic treatment. Since the mid-1960s, however, increasing resistance to multiple drugs has been a dominant factor in treatment decisions. Resistance rates are highly dependent on the geographic area. Clonal spread of particular strains and horizontal transfer of resistance determinants, particularly via plasmids and transposons, contribute to multidrug resistance. The current global status—i.e., high rates of resistance to classic first-line antibiotics such as amoxicillin—has led to a rapid switch to quinolones such as nalidixic acid. However, resistance to such early-generation quinolones has also emerged and spread quickly as a result of chromosomal mutations affecting DNA gyrase and topoisomerase IV; this resistance has necessitated the use of later-generation quinolones as first-line antibiotics in many areas. For instance, a review of the antibiotic resistance history of *Shigella* in India found that, after their introduction in the late 1980s, the second-generation quinolones norfloxacin, ciprofloxacin, and ofloxacin were highly effective in the treatment of shigellosis, including cases caused by multidrug-resistant strains of *S. dysenteriae* type 1. However, investigations of subsequent outbreaks in India and Bangladesh detected resistance to norfloxacin, ciprofloxacin, and ofloxacin in 5% of isolates. The incidence of multidrug resistance parallels the widespread, uncontrolled use of antibiotics and calls for the rational use of effective drugs.

TABLE 154-1 Recommended Antimicrobial Therapy for Shigellosis

Antimicrobial Agent	Treatment Schedule Children	Treatment Schedule Adults	Limitations
First line			
Ciprofloxacin	15 mg/kg	500 mg	
	2 times per day for 3 days, PO		
Second line			
Pivmecillinam	20 mg/kg	100 mg	Cost
	4 times per day for 5 days, PO		No pediatric formulation
			Frequent administration
			Resistance emerging
Ceftriaxone	50–100 mg/kg	–	Efficacy not validated
	Once a day IM for 2–5 days		Must be injected
Azithromycin	6–20 mg/kg	1–1.5 g	Cost
	Once a day for 1–5 days, PO		Efficacy not validated
			MIC near serum concentration
			Rapid emergence of resistance and spread to other bacteria

Source: WHO Library Cataloguing-in-Publication Data: Guidelines for the control of shigellosis, including epidemics due to *Shigella dysenteriae* type 1 (*www.searo. who.int/LinkFiles/CAH_Publications_shigella.pdf*).

ANTIBIOTIC TREATMENT OF SHIGELLOSIS (Table 154-1) Because of the ready transmissibility of *Shigella*, current public health recommendations in the United States are that every case be treated with antibiotics. Ciprofloxacin is recommended as first-line treatment. A number of other drugs have been tested and shown to be effective, including ceftriaxone, azithromycin, pivmecillinam, and some fifth-generation quinolones. While infections caused by non-*dysenteriae Shigella* in immunocompetent individuals are routinely treated with a 3-day course of antibiotics, it is recommended that *S. dysenteriae* type 1 infections be treated for 5 days and that *Shigella* infections in immunocompromised patients be treated for 7–10 days.

Treatment for shigellosis must be adapted to the clinical context, with the recognition that the most fragile patients are children <5 years old, who represent two-thirds of all cases worldwide. There are few data on the use of quinolones in children, but *Shigella*-induced dysentery is a well-recognized indication for their use. The half-life of ciprofloxacin is longer in infants than in older individuals. The ciprofloxacin dose generally recommended for children is 30 mg/kg per d in two divided doses. Adults living in areas with high standards of hygiene are likely to develop milder, shorter-duration disease, whereas infants in endemic areas can develop severe, sometimes fatal dysentery. In the former setting, treatment will remain minimal and bacteriologic proof of infection will often come after symptoms have resolved; in the latter setting, antibiotic treatment and more aggressive measures, possibly including resuscitation, are often required.

REHYDRATION AND NUTRITION *Shigella* infection rarely causes significant dehydration. Cases requiring aggressive rehydration (particularly in industrialized countries) are uncommon. In developing countries, malnutrition remains the primary indicator for diarrhea-related death, highlighting the importance of nutrition in early management. Rehydration should be oral unless the patient is comatose or presents in shock. Because of the improved effectiveness of reduced-osmolarity oral rehydration solution (especially for children with acute noncholera diarrhea), the WHO and UNICEF now recommend a standard solution of 245 mOsm/L (sodium, 75 mmol/L; chloride, 65 mmol/L; glucose (anhydrous), 75 mmol/L; potassium, 20 mmol/L; citrate, 10 mmol/L). In shigellosis, the coupled transport of sodium to glucose may be variably affected, but oral rehydration therapy remains the easiest and most efficient form of rehydration, especially in severe cases.

Nutrition should be started as soon as possible after completion of initial rehydration. Early refeeding is safe, well tolerated, and clinically beneficial. Because breast-feeding reduces diarrheal losses and the need for oral rehydration in infants, it should be maintained in the absence of contraindications (e.g., maternal HIV infection).

NONSPECIFIC, SYMPTOM-BASED THERAPY Antimotility agents have been implicated in prolonged fever in volunteers with shigellosis. These agents are suspected of increasing the risk of toxic megacolon and are thought to have been responsible for HUS in children infected by EHEC strains. For safety reasons, it is better to avoid antimotility agents in bloody diarrhea.

TREATMENT OF COMPLICATIONS There is no consensus regarding the best treatment for toxic megacolon. The patient should be assessed frequently by both medical and surgical teams. Anemia, dehydration, and electrolyte deficits (particularly hypokalemia) may aggravate colonic atony and should be actively treated. Nasogastric aspiration helps to deflate the colon. Parenteral nutrition has not been proven to be beneficial. Fever persisting beyond 48–72 h raises the possibility of local perforation or abscess. Most studies recommend colectomy if, after 48–72 h, colonic distention persists. However, some physicians recommend continuation of medical therapy for up to 7 days if the patient seems to be improving clinically despite persistent megacolon without free perforation. Intestinal perforation, either isolated or complicating toxic megacolon, requires surgical treatment and intensive medical support.

Rectal prolapse must be treated as soon as possible. With the health care provider using surgical gloves or a soft warm wet cloth and the patient in the knee-chest position, the prolapsed rectum is gently pushed back into place. If edema of the rectal mucosa is evident (rendering reintegration difficult), it can be osmotically reduced by applying gauze impregnated with a warm solution of saturated magnesium sulfate. Rectal prolapse often relapses but usually resolves along with the resolution of dysentery.

HUS must be treated by water restriction, including discontinuation of oral rehydration solution and potassium-rich alimentation. Hemofiltration is usually required.

■ PREVENTION

Hand washing after defecation or handling of children's feces and before handling of food is recommended. Stool decontamination (e.g., with sodium hypochlorite), together with a cleaning protocol for medical staff as well as for patients, has proven useful in limiting the spread of infection during *Shigella* outbreaks. Ideally, patients should have a negative stool culture before their infection is considered cured. Recurrences are rare if therapeutic and preventive measures are correctly implemented.

Although several live attenuated oral and subunit parenteral vaccine candidates have been produced and are undergoing clinical trials, no vaccine against shigellosis is currently available. Especially given the rapid progression of antibiotic resistance in *Shigella*, a vaccine is urgently needed.

FURTHER READINGS

BENNISH ML, WOJTYNIAK BJ: Mortality due to shigellosis: Community and hospital data. Rev Infect Dis 13(Suppl 4):S245, 1991

COSSART P, SANSONETTI PJ: Bacterial invasion: The paradigms of enteroinvasive pathogens. Science 304:242, 2004

KOTLOFF KL ET AL: Overview of live vaccine strategies against *Shigella*, in *New Generation Vaccines*, 3d ed, MM Levine et al (eds). London, Informa Healthcare, 2004, pp 723–735

—— et al: Global burden of *Shigella* infections: Implications for vaccine development and implementation of control strategies. Bull World Health Organ 77:651, 1999

NIYOGI SK: Shigellosis. J Microbiol 43:133, 2005

PHALIPON A, SANSONETTI PJ: Shigella's ways of manipulating the host intestinal innate and adaptive immune system: A tool box for survival? Immunol Cell Biol 85:119, 2007

TRAA BS et al: Antibiotics for the treatment of dysentery in children. Int J Epidemiol 39 (Suppl 1):i70, 2010

VON SEIDLEIN L ET AL: A multicentre study of *Shigella* diarrhoea in six Asian countries: Disease burden, clinical manifestations, and microbiology. PLoS Med 3:e353, 2006

WORLD HEALTH ORGANIZATION: Guidelines for the control of shigellosis, including epidemics due to *Shigella dysenteriae* type 1. WHO Library Cataloguing-in-Publication Data (*www.searo. who.int/LinkFiles/CAH_Publications_shigella.pdf*)

CHAPTER 155

Infections Due to *Campylobacter* and Related Organisms

Martin J. Blaser

◼ DEFINITION

Bacteria of the genus *Campylobacter* and of the related genera *Arcobacter* and *Helicobacter* (Chap. 151) cause a variety of inflammatory conditions. Although acute diarrheal illnesses are most common, these organisms may cause infections in virtually all parts of the body, especially in compromised hosts, and these infections may have late nonsuppurative sequelae. The designation *Campylobacter* comes from the Greek for "curved rod" and refers to the organism's vibrio-like morphology.

◼ ETIOLOGY

Campylobacters are motile, non-spore-forming, curved, gram-negative rods. Originally known as *Vibrio fetus*, these bacilli were reclassified as a new genus in 1973, after their dissimilarity to other vibrios was recognized. More than 15 species have since been identified. These species are currently divided into three genera: *Campylobacter*, *Arcobacter*, and *Helicobacter*. Not all of the species are pathogens of humans. The human pathogens fall into two major groups: those that primarily cause diarrheal disease and those that cause extraintestinal infection. The principal diarrheal pathogen is *C. jejuni*, which accounts for 80–90% of all cases of recognized illness due to campylobacters and related genera. Other organisms that cause diarrheal disease include *C. coli*, *C. upsaliensis*, *C. lari*, *C. hyointestinalis*, *C. fetus*, *A. butzleri*, *A. cryaerophilus*, *H. cinaedi*, and *H. fennelliae*. The two *Helicobacter* species causing diarrheal disease, *H. cinaedi* and *H. fennelliae*, are intestinal rather than gastric organisms; in terms of the clinical features of the illnesses they cause, these species most closely resemble *Campylobacter* rather than *H. pylori* (Chap. 151) and thus are considered in this chapter.

The major species causing extraintestinal illnesses is *C. fetus*. However, any of the diarrheal agents listed above may cause systemic or localized infection as well, especially in compromised hosts. Neither aerobes nor strict anaerobes, these microaerophilic organisms are adapted for survival in the gastrointestinal mucous layer. This chapter focuses on *C. jejuni* and *C. fetus* as the major pathogens in and prototypes for their groups. The key features of infection are listed by species (excluding *C. jejuni*, described in detail in the text below) in Table 155-1.

◼ EPIDEMIOLOGY

Campylobacters are found in the gastrointestinal tract of many animals used for food (including poultry, cattle, sheep, and swine) and many household pets (including birds, dogs, and cats). These microorganisms usually do not cause illness in their animal hosts. In most cases, campylobacters are transmitted to humans in raw or undercooked food products or through direct contact with infected animals. In the United States and other developed countries, ingestion of contaminated poultry that has not been sufficiently cooked is the most common mode of acquisition (30–70% of cases). Other modes include ingestion of raw (unpasteurized) milk or untreated water, contact with infected household pets, travel to developing countries (campylobacters being among the leading causes of traveler's diarrhea; Chaps. 123 and 128), oral-anal sexual contact, and (occasionally) contact with an index case who is incontinent of stool (e.g., a baby).

Campylobacter infections are common. Several studies indicate that, in the United States, diarrheal disease due to campylobacters is more common than that due to *Salmonella* and *Shigella* combined. Infections occur throughout the year, but their incidence peaks during summer and early autumn. Persons of all ages are affected; however, attack rates for *C. jejuni* are highest among young children and young adults, while those for *C. fetus* are highest at the extremes of age. Systemic infections due to *C. fetus* (and to other *Campylobacter* and related species) are most common among compromised hosts. Persons at increased risk include those with AIDS, hypogammaglobulinemia, neoplasia, liver disease, diabetes mellitus, and generalized atherosclerosis as well as neonates and pregnant women. However, apparently healthy nonpregnant persons occasionally develop transient *Campylobacter* bacteremia as part of a gastrointestinal illness.

In contrast, in many developing countries, *C. jejuni* infections are hyperendemic, with the highest rates among children <2 years old. Infection rates fall with age, as does the illness-to-infection ratio. These observations suggest that frequent exposure to *C. jejuni* leads to the acquisition of immunity.

◼ PATHOLOGY AND PATHOGENESIS

C. jejuni infections may be subclinical, especially in hosts in developing countries who have had multiple prior infections and thus are partially immune. Symptomatic infections mostly occur within 2–4 days (range, 1–7 days) of exposure to the organism in food or water. The sites of tissue injury include the jejunum, ileum, and colon. Biopsies show an acute nonspecific inflammatory reaction, with neutrophils, monocytes, and eosinophils in the lamina propria, as well as damage to the epithelium, including loss of mucus, glandular degeneration, and crypt abscesses. Biopsy findings may be consistent with Crohn's disease or ulcerative colitis, but these "idiopathic" chronic inflammatory diseases should not be diagnosed unless infectious colitis, *specifically including* that due to infection with *Campylobacter* species and related organisms, has been ruled out.

The high frequency of *C. jejuni* infections and their severity and recurrence among hypogammaglobulinemic patients suggest that antibodies are important in protective immunity. The pathogenesis of infection is uncertain. Both the motility of the strain and its capacity to adhere to host tissues appear to favor disease, but classic enterotoxins and cytotoxins (although described and including cytolethal distending toxin, or CDT) appear not to play substantial roles in tissue injury or disease production. The organisms have been visualized within the epithelium, albeit in low numbers. The documentation of a significant tissue response and occasionally of *C. jejuni* bacteremia further suggests that tissue invasion is clinically significant, and in vitro studies are consistent with this pathogenetic feature.

The pathogenesis of *C. fetus* infections is better defined. Virtually all clinical isolates of *C. fetus* possess a proteinaceous capsule-like structure (an S-layer) that renders the organisms resistant to complement-mediated killing and opsonization. As a result, *C. fetus* can cause bacteremia and can seed sites beyond the intestinal tract. The ability of the organism to switch the S-layer proteins expressed—a phenomenon that results in antigenic variability—may contribute

TABLE 155-1 Clinical Features Associated With Infection Due to "Atypical" *Campylobacter* and Related Species Implicated as Causes of Human Illness

Species	Common Clinical Features	Less Common Clinical Features	Additional Information
Campylobacter coli	Fever, diarrhea, abdominal pain	Bacteremia[a]	Clinically indistinguishable from *C. jejuni*
Campylobacter fetus	Bacteremia,[a] sepsis, meningitis, vascular infections	Diarrhea, relapsing fevers	Not usually isolated from media containing cephalothin or incubated at 42°C
Campylobacter upsaliensis	Watery diarrhea, low-grade fever, abdominal pain	Bacteremia, abscesses	Difficult to isolate because of cephalothin susceptibility
Campylobacter lari	Abdominal pain, diarrhea	Colitis, appendicitis	Seagulls frequently colonized; organism often transmitted to humans via contaminated water
Campylobacter hyointestinalis	Watery or bloody diarrhea, vomiting, abdominal pain	Bacteremia	Causes proliferative enteritis in swine
Helicobacter fennelliae	Chronic mild diarrhea, abdominal cramps, proctitis	Bacteremia[a]	Best treated with fluoroquinolones
Helicobacter cinaedi	Chronic mild diarrhea, abdominal cramps, proctitis	Bacteremia[a]	Best treated with fluoroquinolones; identified in healthy hamsters
Campylobacter jejuni subspecies **doylei**	Diarrhea	Chronic gastritis, bacteremia[b]	Uncertain role as human pathogen
Arcobacter cryaerophilus	Diarrhea	Bacteremia	Cultured under aerobic conditions
Arcobacter butzleri	Fever, diarrhea, abdominal pain, nausea	Bacteremia, appendicitis	Cultured under aerobic conditions; enzootic in nonhuman primates
Campylobacter sputorum	Pulmonary, perianal, groin, and axillary abscesses; diarrhea	Bacteremia	Three clinically relevant biovars: *sputorum, fecalis,* and *paraureolyticus*

[a]In immunocompromised hosts, especially HIV-infected persons.
[b]In children.
Source: Adapted from BM Allos, MJ Blaser: Clin Infect Dis 20:1092, 1995.

to the chronicity and high rate of recurrence of *C. fetus* infections in compromised hosts.

CLINICAL MANIFESTATIONS

The clinical features of infections due to *Campylobacter* and the related *Arcobacter* and intestinal *Helicobacter* species causing enteric disease appear to be highly similar. *C. jejuni* can be considered the prototype, in part because it is by far the most common enteric pathogen in the group. A prodrome of fever, headache, myalgia, and/or malaise often occurs 12–48 h before the onset of diarrheal symptoms. The most common signs and symptoms of the intestinal phase are diarrhea, abdominal pain, and fever. The degree of diarrhea varies from several loose stools to grossly bloody stools; most patients presenting for medical attention have ≥10 bowel movements on the worst day of illness. Abdominal pain usually consists of cramping and may be the most prominent symptom. Pain is usually generalized but may become localized; *C. jejuni* infection may cause pseudoappendicitis. Fever may be the only initial manifestation of *C. jejuni* infection, a situation mimicking the early stages of typhoid fever. Febrile young children may develop convulsions. *Campylobacter* enteritis is generally self-limited; however, symptoms persist for >1 week in 10–20% of patients seeking medical attention, and clinical relapses occur in 5–10% of such untreated patients. Studies of common-source epidemics indicate that milder illnesses or asymptomatic infections may commonly occur.

C. fetus may cause a diarrheal illness similar to that due to *C. jejuni*, especially in normal hosts. This organism also may cause either intermittent diarrhea or nonspecific abdominal pain without localizing signs. Sequelae are uncommon, and the outcome is benign. *C. fetus* may also cause a prolonged relapsing systemic illness (with fever, chills, and myalgias) that has no obvious primary source; this manifestation is especially common among compromised hosts. Secondary seeding of an organ (e.g., meninges, brain, bone, urinary tract, or soft tissue) complicates the course, which may be fulminant. *C. fetus* infections have a tropism for vascular sites: endocarditis, mycotic aneurysm, and septic thrombophlebitis may all occur. Infection during pregnancy often leads to fetal death. A variety of *Campylobacter* species and *H. cinaedi* can cause recurrent cellulitis with fever and bacteremia in immunocompromised hosts.

COMPLICATIONS

Except in infection with *C. fetus*, bacteremia is uncommon, developing most often in immunocompromised hosts and at the extremes of age. Three patterns of extraintestinal infection have been noted: (1) transient bacteremia in a normal host with enteritis (benign course, no specific treatment needed); (2) sustained bacteremia or focal infection in a normal host (bacteremia originating from enteritis, with patients responding well to antimicrobial therapy); and (3) sustained bacteremia or focal infection in a compromised host. Enteritis may not be clinically apparent. Antimicrobial therapy, possibly prolonged, is necessary for suppression or cure of the infection.

Campylobacter, Arcobacter, and intestinal *Helicobacter* infections in patients with AIDS or hypogammaglobulinemia may be severe, persistent, and extraintestinal; relapse after cessation of therapy is common. Hypogammaglobulinemic patients also may develop osteomyelitis and an erysipelas-like rash or cellulitis.

Local suppurative complications of infection include cholecystitis, pancreatitis, and cystitis; distant complications include meningitis, endocarditis, arthritis, peritonitis, cellulitis, and septic abortion. All these complications are rare, except in immunocompromised hosts. Hepatitis, interstitial nephritis, and the hemolytic-uremic syndrome occasionally complicate acute infection. Reactive arthritis and other rheumatologic complaints may develop several weeks after infection, especially in persons with the HLA-B27 phenotype. Guillain-Barré syndrome or its Miller Fisher (cranial polyneuropathy) variant follows *Campylobacter* infections uncommonly—i.e., in 1 of every 1000–2000 cases or, for certain *C. jejuni* serotypes (such as O19), in 1 of every 100–200 cases. Despite the low frequency of this complication, it is now estimated that *Campylobacter* infections, because of their high incidence, may trigger 20–40% of all cases of Guillain-Barré syndrome. Asymptomatic *Campylobacter* infection also may trigger this syndrome. Immunoproliferative small-intestinal disease (*alpha chain disease*), a form of lymphoma that originates in small-intestinal mucosa-associated lymphoid tissue, has been associated with *C. jejuni*; antimicrobial therapy has led to marked clinical improvement.

■ DIAGNOSIS

In patients with *Campylobacter* enteritis, peripheral leukocyte counts reflect the severity of the inflammatory process. However, stools from nearly all *Campylobacter*-infected patients presenting for medical attention in the United States contain leukocytes or erythrocytes. Gram- or Wright-stained fecal smears should be examined in all suspected cases. When the diagnosis of *Campylobacter* enteritis is suspected on the basis of findings indicating inflammatory diarrhea (fever, fecal leukocytes), clinicians can ask the microbiology laboratory to attempt the visualization of organisms with characteristic vibrioid morphology by direct microscopic examination of stools with Gram's staining or to use phase-contrast or dark-field microscopy to identify the organisms' characteristic "darting" motility. Confirmation of the diagnosis of *Campylobacter* infection is based on identification of an isolate from cultures of stool, blood, or another site. *Campylobacter*-specific media should be used to culture stools from all patients with inflammatory or bloody diarrhea. Since all *Campylobacter* species are fastidious, they will not be isolated unless selective media or other selective techniques are used. Not all media are equally useful for isolation of the broad array of campylobacters; therefore, failure to isolate campylobacters from stool does not entirely rule out their presence. The detection of the organisms in stool almost always implies infection; there is a brief period of postconvalescent fecal carriage and no obvious commensalism in humans. In contrast, *C. sputorum* and related organisms found in the oral cavity are commensals that only rarely have pathogenic significance. Because of the low levels of metabolic activity of *Campylobacter* species in standard blood culture media, *Campylobacter* bacteremia may be difficult to detect unless laboratorians check for low-positive results in quantitative assays.

■ DIFFERENTIAL DIAGNOSIS

The symptoms of *Campylobacter* enteritis are not sufficiently unusual to distinguish this illness from that due to *Salmonella*, *Shigella*, *Yersinia*, and other pathogens. The combination of fever and fecal leukocytes or erythrocytes is indicative of inflammatory diarrhea, and definitive diagnosis is based on culture or demonstration of the characteristic organisms on stained fecal smears.

Similarly, extraintestinal *Campylobacter* illness is diagnosed by culture. Infection due to *Campylobacter* should be suspected in the setting of septic abortion, and that due to *C. fetus* should be suspected specifically in the setting of septic thrombophlebitis. It is important to reiterate that (1) the presentation of *Campylobacter* enteritis may mimic that of ulcerative colitis or Crohn's disease, (2) *Campylobacter* enteritis is much more common than either of the latter (especially among young adults), and (3) biopsy may not distinguish among these entities. Thus a diagnosis of inflammatory bowel disease should not be made until *Campylobacter* infection has been ruled out, especially in persons with a history of foreign travel, significant animal contact, immunodeficiency, or exposure incurring a high risk of transmission.

TREATMENT   *Campylobacter* Infection

Fluid and electrolyte replacement is central to the treatment of diarrheal illnesses (Chap. 128). Even among patients presenting for medical attention with *Campylobacter* enteritis, not all clearly benefit from specific antimicrobial therapy. Indications for therapy include high fever, bloody diarrhea, severe diarrhea, persistence for >1 week, and worsening of symptoms. A 5- to 7-day course of erythromycin (250 mg orally four times daily or—for children—30–50 mg/kg per day, in divided doses) is the regimen of choice. Both clinical trials and in vitro susceptibility testing indicate that other macrolides, including azithromycin (a 1- or 3-day regimen), also are useful therapeutic agents. An alternative regimen for adults is ciprofloxacin (500 mg orally twice daily) or another fluoroquinolone for 5–7 days, but resistance to this class of agents as well as to tetracyclines has been increasing. Patients infected with antibiotic-resistant strains are at increased risk of adverse outcomes. Use of antimotility agents, which may prolong the duration of symptoms and have been associated with toxic megacolon and with death, is not recommended.

For systemic infections, treatment with gentamicin (1.7 mg/kg IV every 8 h after a loading dose of 2 mg/kg), imipenem (500 mg IV every 6 h), or chloramphenicol (50 mg/kg IV each day in three or four divided doses) should be started empirically, but susceptibility testing should then be performed. Ciprofloxacin and amoxicillin/clavulanate are alternative agents for susceptible strains. In the absence of immunocompromise or endovascular infections, therapy should be administered for 14 days. For immunocompromised patients with systemic infections due to *C. fetus* and for patients with endovascular infections, prolonged therapy (for up to 4 weeks) is usually necessary. For recurrent infections in immunocompromised hosts, lifelong therapy/ prophylaxis is sometimes necessary.

■ PROGNOSIS

Nearly all patients recover fully from *Campylobacter* enteritis, either spontaneously or after antimicrobial therapy. Volume depletion probably contributes to the few deaths that are reported. As stated above, occasional patients develop reactive arthritis or Guillain-Barré syndrome or its variants. Systemic infection with *C. fetus* is much more often fatal than that due to related species; this higher mortality rate reflects in part the population affected. Prognosis depends on the rapidity with which appropriate therapy is begun. Otherwise-healthy hosts usually survive *C. fetus* infections without sequelae. Compromised hosts often have recurrent and/or life-threatening infections due to a variety of *Campylobacter* species.

FURTHER READINGS

GRADEL KO et al: Increased short- and long-term risk of inflammatory bowel disease after *Salmonella* or *Campylobacter* gastroenteritis. Gastroenterology 137:495, 2009

——— et al: Increased risk of zoonotic *Salmonella* and *Campylobacter* gastroenteritis in patients with haematological malignancies: A population-based study. Ann Hematol 88:761, 2009

HELMS M et al: Adverse health events associated with antimicrobial drug resistance in *Campylobacter* species: A registry-based cohort study. J Infect Dis 191:1050, 2005

LANG DR et al (eds): Development of Guillain-Barré syndrome following *Campylobacter* infection. J Infect Dis 176:S91, 1997

LECUIT M et al: Immunoproliferative small intestinal disease associated with *Campylobacter jejuni*. N Engl J Med 350:239, 2004

MEAD PS et al: Food-related illness and death in the United States. Emerg Infect Dis 5:607, 1999

NACHAMKIN I et al (eds): *Campylobacter jejuni*, 3rd ed. Washington, American Society for Microbiology, 2008

NYLUND CM et al: Bacterial enteritis as a risk factor for childhood intussusception: A retrospective cohort study. J Pediatr 156:761, 2010

SMITH KE et al: Quinolone-resistant *Campylobacter jejuni* infections in Minnesota, 1992–1998. Investigation Team. N Engl J Med 340:1525, 1999

TRIBBLE DR et al: Traveler's diarrhea in Thailand: Randomized, double-blind trial comparing single-dose and 3-day azithromycin-based regimens with a 3-day levofloxacin regimen. Clin Infect Dis 44:338, 2007

CHAPTER **156**

Cholera and Other Vibrioses

Matthew K. Waldor
Edward T. Ryan

Members of the genus *Vibrio* cause a number of important infectious syndromes. Classic among them is cholera, a devastating diarrheal disease caused by *V. cholerae* that has been responsible for seven global pandemics and much suffering over the past two centuries. Epidemic cholera remains a significant public health concern in the developing world today. Other vibrioses caused by other *Vibrio* species include syndromes of diarrhea, soft tissue infection, or primary sepsis. All *Vibrio* species are highly motile, facultatively anaerobic, curved gram-negative rods with one or more flagella. In nature, vibrios most commonly reside in tidal rivers and bays under conditions of moderate salinity. They proliferate in the summer months when water temperatures exceed 20°C. As might be expected, the illnesses they cause also increase in frequency during the warm months.

CHOLERA

■ DEFINITION

Cholera is an acute diarrheal disease that can, in a matter of hours, result in profound, rapidly progressive dehydration and death. Accordingly, cholera gravis (the severe form of cholera) is a much-feared disease, particularly in its epidemic presentation. Fortunately, prompt aggressive fluid repletion and supportive care can obviate the high mortality that cholera has historically wrought. While the term *cholera* has occasionally been applied to any severely dehydrating secretory diarrheal illness, whether infectious in etiology or not, it now refers to disease caused by *V. cholerae* serogroup O1 or O139— i.e., the serogroups with epidemic potential.

■ MICROBIOLOGY AND EPIDEMIOLOGY

The species *V. cholerae* is classified into more than 200 serogroups based on the carbohydrate determinants of their lipopolysaccharide (LPS) O antigens. Although some non-O1 *V. cholerae* serogroups (strains that do not agglutinate in antisera to the O1 group antigen) have occasionally caused sporadic outbreaks of diarrhea, serogroup O1 was, until the emergence of serogroup O139 in 1992, the exclusive cause of epidemic cholera. Two biotypes of *V. cholerae* O1, classical and El Tor, are distinguished. Each biotype is further subdivided into two serotypes, termed *Inaba* and *Ogawa*.

The natural habitat of *V. cholerae* is coastal salt water and brackish estuaries, where the organism lives in close relation to plankton. Humans become infected incidentally but, once infected, can act as vehicles for spread. Ingestion of water contaminated by human feces is the most common means of acquisition of *V. cholerae*. Consumption of contaminated food also can contribute to spread. There is no known animal reservoir. While the infectious dose is relatively high, it is markedly reduced in hypochlorhydric persons, in those using antacids, and when gastric acidity is buffered by a meal. Cholera is predominantly a pediatric disease in endemic areas, but it affects adults and children equally when newly introduced into a population. In endemic areas, the burden of disease is often greatest during "cholera seasons" associated with high temperatures, heavy rainfall, and flooding, but cholera can occur year-round. For unexplained reasons, susceptibility to cholera is significantly influenced by ABO blood group status; persons with type O blood are at greatest risk of severe disease if infected, while those with type AB are at least risk.

Cholera is native to the Ganges delta in the Indian subcontinent. Since 1817, seven global pandemics have occurred. The current (seventh) pandemic—the first due to the El Tor biotype—began in Indonesia in 1961 and spread throughout Asia as *V. cholerae* El Tor displaced the endemic classical biotype. In the early 1970s, El Tor cholera erupted in Africa, causing major epidemics before becoming a persistent endemic problem. Currently, >90% of cholera cases reported annually to the World Health Organization (WHO) are from Africa (Fig. 156-1), but the true burden in Africa as well as in Asia is unknown since diagnosis is often syndromic and since many countries with endemic cholera do not report cholera to the WHO. It is possible that >3 million cases of cholera occur yearly (of which only ~200,000 are reported to the WHO), resulting in >100,000 deaths annually (of which <5000 are reported to the WHO).

The recent history of cholera has been punctuated by severe outbreaks, especially among impoverished or displaced persons. Such outbreaks are often precipitated by war or other circumstances that lead to the breakdown of public health measures. Such was the case in the camps for Rwandan refugees set up in 1994 around Goma, Zaire; in 2008–2009 in Zimbabwe; and in 2010 in Haiti. Since 1973, sporadic endemic infections due to *V. cholerae* O1 strains related to

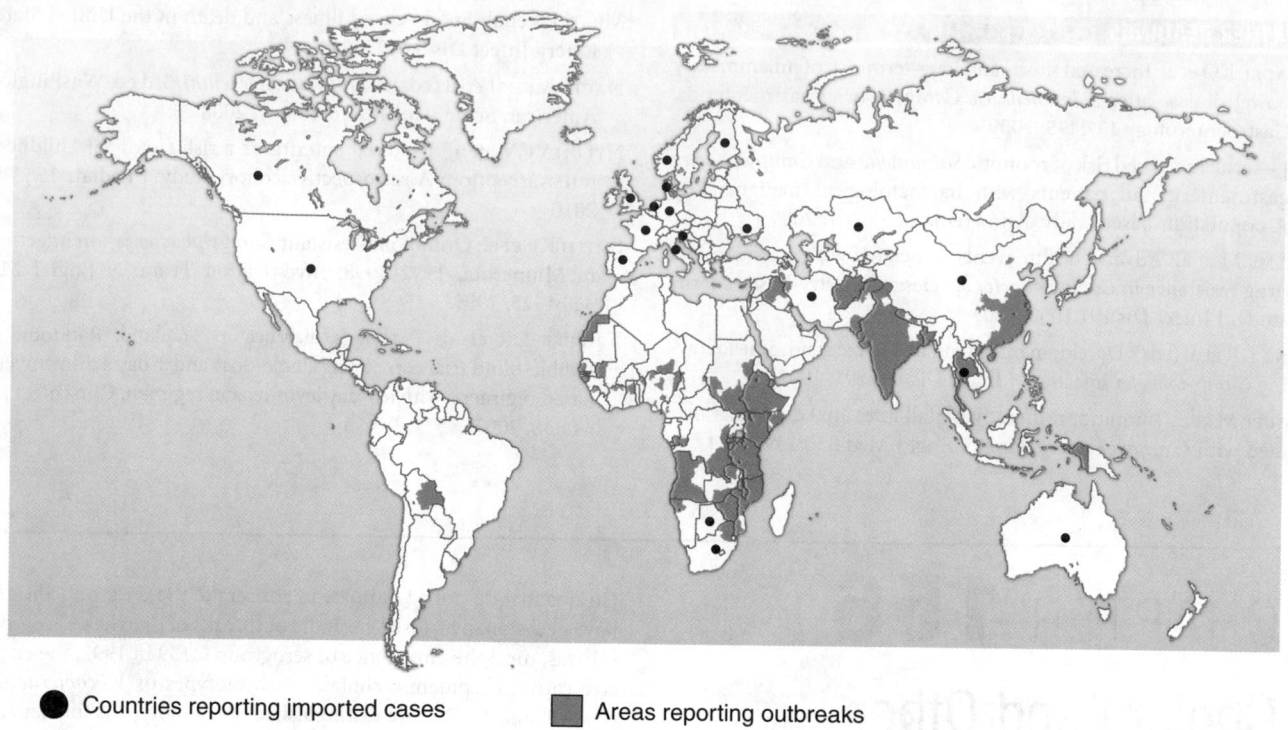

● Countries reporting imported cases   ▮ Areas reporting outbreaks

Figure 156-1 **World distribution of cholera in 2009.** *(Adapted from WHO: Cholera, 2009.)*

the seventh-pandemic strain have been recognized along the U.S. Gulf Coast of Louisiana and Texas. These infections are typically associated with the consumption of contaminated, locally harvested shellfish. Occasionally, cases in U.S. locations remote from the Gulf Coast have been linked to shipped-in Gulf Coast seafood.

After a century without cholera in Latin America, the current cholera pandemic reached Central and South America in 1991. Following an initial explosive spread that affected millions (Fig. 156-2), the burden of disease has markedly decreased in Latin America, although, as it did in Africa two decades earlier, the epidemic El Tor strain proved capable of establishing itself in inland fresh waters rather than in its classic niche of coastal salt waters. In 2010, cholera reappeared in Haiti after a century-long absence.

In October 1992, a large-scale outbreak of clinical cholera caused by a new serogroup, O139, occurred in southeastern India. The organism appears to be a derivative of El Tor O1 but has a distinct LPS and an immunologically related O-antigen polysaccharide capsule. (O1 organisms are not encapsulated.) After an initial spread across 11 Asian countries (Fig. 156-3), *V. cholerae* O139 has once again been largely replaced by O1, although O139 still causes a minority of cases in some Asian countries. The clinical manifestations of disease caused by *V. cholerae* O139 are indistinguishable from those of O1 cholera. Immunity to one, however, is not protective against the other.

■ PATHOGENESIS

In the final analysis, cholera is a toxin-mediated disease. The watery diarrhea characteristic of cholera is due to the action of cholera toxin, a potent protein enterotoxin elaborated by the organism in the small intestine. The toxin-coregulated pilus (TCP), so named because its synthesis is regulated in parallel with that of cholera toxin, is essential for *V. cholerae* to survive and multiply in (colonize) the small intestine. Cholera toxin, TCP, and several other virulence factors are coordinately regulated by ToxR. This protein modulates the expression of genes coding for virulence factors in response to environmental signals via a cascade of regulatory proteins.

Additional regulatory processes, including bacterial responses to the density of the bacterial population (in a phenomenon known as *quorum sensing*), control the virulence of *V. cholerae*.

Once established in the human small bowel, the organism produces cholera toxin, which consists of a monomeric enzymatic

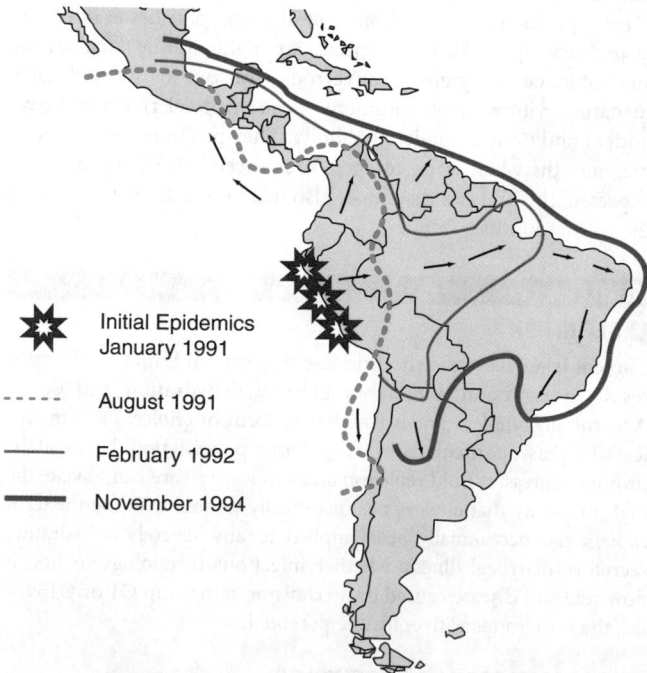

✦ Initial Epidemics January 1991

- - - - August 1991

──── February 1992

━━━━ November 1994

Figure 156-2 **Spread of *Vibrio cholerae* O1 in the Americas, 1991–1994.** *(Courtesy of Dr. Robert V. Tauxe, Centers for Disease Control and Prevention, Atlanta; with permission.)*

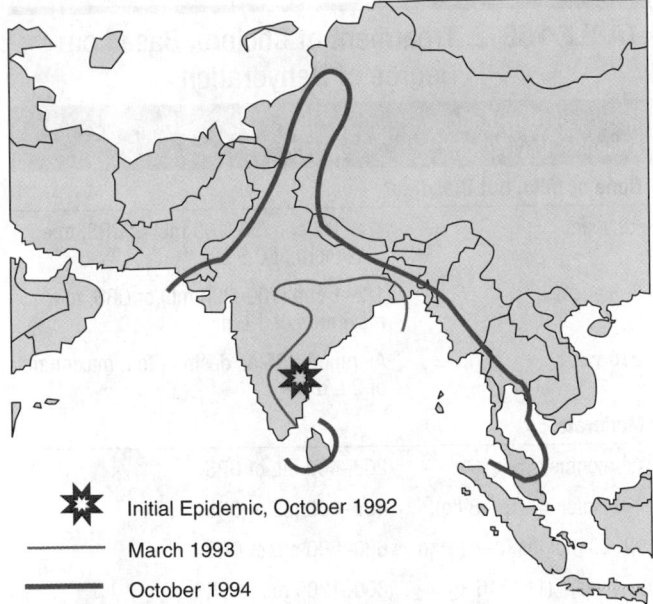

Figure 156-3 Spread of *Vibrio cholerae* O139 in the Indian subcontinent and elsewhere in Asia, 1992–1994. *(Courtesy of Dr. Robert V. Tauxe, CDC, Atlanta; with permission.)*

✴ Initial Epidemic, October 1992

—— March 1993

—— October 1994

moiety (the A subunit) and a pentameric binding moiety (the B subunit). The B pentamer binds to GM_1 ganglioside, a glycolipid on the surface of epithelial cells that serves as the toxin receptor and makes possible the delivery of the A subunit to its cytosolic target. The activated A subunit (A_1) irreversibly transfers ADP-ribose from nicotinamide adenine dinucleotide to its specific target protein, the GTP-binding regulatory component of adenylate cyclase. The ADP-ribosylated G protein upregulates the activity of adenylate cyclase; the result is the intracellular accumulation of high levels of cyclic AMP. In intestinal epithelial cells, cyclic AMP inhibits the absorptive sodium transport system in villus cells and activates the secretory chloride transport system in crypt cells, and these events lead to the accumulation of sodium chloride in the intestinal lumen. Since water moves passively to maintain osmolality, isotonic fluid accumulates in the lumen. When the volume of that fluid exceeds the capacity of the rest of the gut to resorb it, watery diarrhea results. Unless the wasted fluid and electrolytes are adequately replaced, shock (due to profound dehydration) and acidosis (due to loss of bicarbonate) follow. Although perturbation of the adenylate cyclase pathway is the primary mechanism by which cholera toxin causes excess fluid secretion, cholera toxin also enhances intestinal secretion via prostaglandins and/or neural histamine receptors.

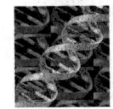
The *V. cholerae* genome comprises two circular chromosomes. Lateral gene transfer has played a key role in the evolution of epidemic *V. cholerae*. The genes encoding cholera toxin (*ctxAB*) are part of the genome of a bacteriophage, CTXΦ. The receptor for this phage on the *V. cholerae* surface is the intestinal colonization factor TCP. Since *ctxAB* is part of a mobile genetic element (CTXΦ), horizontal transfer of this bacteriophage may account for the emergence of new toxigenic *V. cholerae* serogroups. Many of the other genes important for *V. cholerae* pathogenicity, including the genes encoding the biosynthesis of TCP, those encoding accessory colonization factors, and those regulating virulence gene expression, are clustered together in the *V. cholerae* pathogenicity island. Similar clustering of virulence genes is found in other bacterial pathogens. It is believed that pathogenicity islands are acquired by horizontal gene

transfer. *V. cholerae* O139 is probably derived from an El Tor O1 strain that acquired the genes for O139 O-antigen synthesis by horizontal gene transfer.

■ CLINICAL MANIFESTATIONS

Individuals infected with *V. cholerae* O1 or O139 exhibit a range of clinical manifestations. Some individuals are asymptomatic or have only mild diarrhea; others present with the sudden onset of explosive and life-threatening diarrhea (*cholera gravis*). The reasons for the range in signs and symptoms of disease are incompletely understood but include the level of preexisting immunity, blood type, and nutritional status. In a nonimmune individual, after a 24- to 48-h incubation period, cholera characteristically begins with the sudden onset of painless watery diarrhea that may quickly become voluminous. Patients often vomit. In severe cases, volume loss can exceed 250 mL/kg in the first 24 h. If fluids and electrolytes are not replaced, hypovolemic shock and death may ensue. Fever is usually absent. Muscle cramps due to electrolyte disturbances are common. The stool has a characteristic appearance: a nonbilious, gray, slightly cloudy fluid with flecks of mucus, no blood, and a somewhat fishy, inoffensive odor. It has been called "rice-water" stool because of its resemblance to the water in which rice has been washed (Fig. 156-4). Clinical symptoms parallel volume contraction: At losses of <5% of normal body weight, thirst develops; at 5–10%, postural hypotension, weakness, tachycardia, and decreased skin turgor are documented; and at >10%, oliguria, weak or absent pulses, sunken eyes (and, in infants, sunken fontanelles), wrinkled ("washerwoman") skin, somnolence, and coma are characteristic. Complications derive exclusively from the effects of volume and electrolyte depletion and include renal failure due to acute tubular

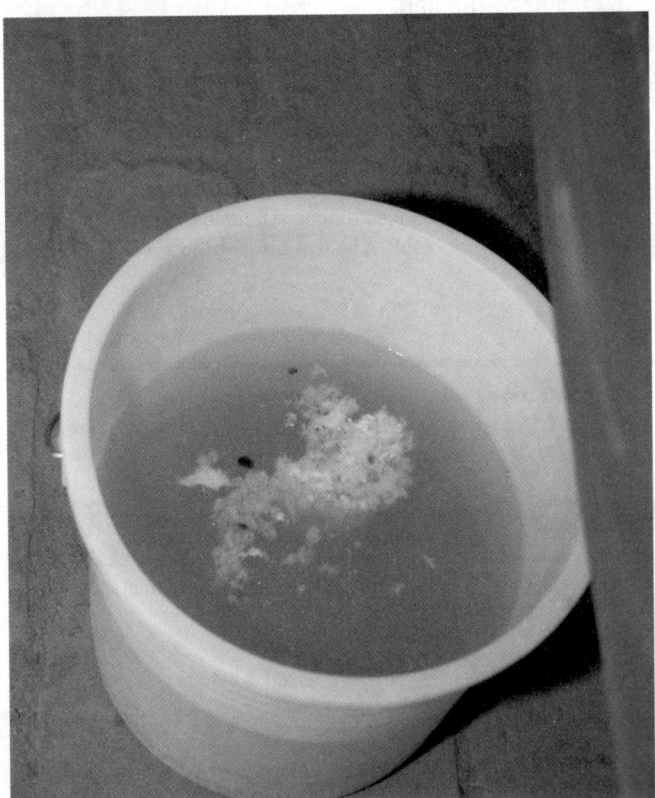

Figure 156-4 **Rice water cholera stool.** Note floating mucus and gray watery appearance. *(Courtesy of Dr. ASG Faruque, International Centre for Diarrhoeal Disease Research, Dhaka; with permission.)*

necrosis. Thus, if the patient is adequately treated with fluid and electrolytes, complications are averted and the process is self-limited, resolving in a few days.

Laboratory data usually reveal an elevated hematocrit (due to hemoconcentration) in nonanemic patients; mild neutrophilic leukocytosis; elevated levels of blood urea nitrogen and creatinine consistent with prerenal azotemia; normal sodium, potassium, and chloride levels; a markedly reduced bicarbonate level (<15 mmol/L); and an elevated anion gap (due to increases in serum lactate, protein, and phosphate). Arterial pH is usually low (~7.2).

■ DIAGNOSIS

The clinical suspicion of cholera can be confirmed by the identification of *V. cholerae* in stool; however, the organism must be specifically sought. With experience, it can be detected directly by dark-field microscopy on a wet mount of fresh stool, and its serotype can be discerned by immobilization with specific antiserum. Laboratory isolation of the organism requires the use of a selective medium such as taurocholate-tellurite-gelatin (TTG) agar or thiosulfate–citrate–bile salts–sucrose (TCBS) agar. If a delay in sample processing is expected, Carey-Blair transport medium and/or alkaline-peptone water-enrichment medium may be used as well. In endemic areas, there is little need for biochemical confirmation and characterization, although these tasks may be worthwhile in places where *V. cholerae* is an uncommon isolate. Standard microbiologic biochemical testing for Enterobacteriaceae will suffice for identification of *V. cholerae*. All vibrios are oxidase-positive. A point-of-care antigen-detection cholera dipstick assay is now commercially available for use in the field or where laboratory facilities are lacking.

TREATMENT   Cholera

Death from cholera is due to hypovolemic shock; thus treatment of individuals with cholera first and foremost requires fluid resuscitation and management. In light of the level of dehydration (Table 156-1) and the patient's age and weight, euvolemia should first be rapidly restored, and adequate hydration should then be maintained to replace ongoing fluid losses (Table 156-2). Administration of oral rehydration solution (ORS) takes

TABLE 156-1 Assessing the Degree of Dehydration in Patients With Cholera

Degree of Dehydration	Clinical Findings
None or mild, but diarrhea	Thirst in some cases; <5% loss of total body weight
Moderate	Thirst, postural hypotension, weakness, tachycardia, decreased skin turgor, dry mouth/tongue, no tears; 5–10% loss of total body weight
Severe	Unconsciousness, lethargy, or "floppiness"; weak or absent pulse; inability to drink; sunken eyes (and, in infants, sunken fontanelles); >10% loss of total body weight

TABLE 156-2 Treatment of Cholera, Based on Degree of Dehydration[a]

Degree of Dehydration, Patient's Age (Weight)	Treatment
None or Mild, but Diarrhea[b]	
<2 years	1/4–1/2 cup (50–100 mL) of ORS, to a maximum of 0.5 L/d
2–9 years	1/2–1 cup (100–200 mL) of ORS, to a maximum of 1 L/d
≥10 years	As much ORS as desired, to a maximum of 2 L/d
Moderate[b,c]	
<4 months (<5 kg)	200–400 mL of ORS
4–11 months (5–<8 kg)	400–600 mL of ORS
12–23 months (8–<11 kg)	600–800 mL of ORS
2–4 years (11–<16 kg)	800–1200 mL of ORS
5–14 years (16–<30 kg)	1200–2200 mL of ORS
≥15 years (≥30 kg)	2200–4000 mL of ORS
Severe[b]	
All ages and weights	IV fluid replacement with Ringer's lactate (or, if not available, normal saline): 100 mL/kg in first 3-h period (or first 6-h period for children <12 months old); start rapidly, then slow down; total of 200 mL/kg in first 24 h; continue until patient is awake, can ingest ORS, and no longer has a weak pulse

Note: Continue normal feeding during treatment.
[a]Adapted from World Health Organization: First steps for managing an outbreak of acute diarrhoea. Global Task Force on Cholera Control, 2009 (www.who.int/topics/cholera). ORS, oral rehydration solution.
[b]Reassess regularly; monitor stool and vomit output.
[c]Amounts of ORS listed should be given within the first 4 h.

advantage of the hexose-Na+ co-transport mechanism to move Na+ across the gut mucosa together with an actively transported molecule such as glucose (or galactose). Cl− and water follow. This transport mechanism remains intact even when cholera toxin is active. ORS may be made by adding safe water to pre-packaged sachets containing salts and sugar or by adding 0.5 teaspoon of table salt (NaCl; 3.5 g) and 4 tablespoons of table sugar (glucose; 40 g) to 1 L of safe water. Potassium intake in bananas or green coconut water should be encouraged. A number of ORS formulations are available, and the WHO now recommends "low-osmolarity" ORS for treatment of individuals with dehydrating diarrhea of any cause (Table 156-3). If available, rice-based ORS is considered superior to standard ORS in the treatment of cholera. ORS can be administered via a nasogastric tube to individuals who cannot ingest fluid; however, optimal management of individuals with severe dehydration includes the administration of IV fluid and electrolytes. Because profound acidosis (pH < 7.2) is common in this group, Ringer's lactate is the best choice among commercial products (Table 156-4). It must be used with additional potassium supplements, preferably given by mouth. The total fluid deficit in severely dehydrated patients (>10% of body weight) can be replaced safely within

TABLE 156-3 Composition of World Health Organization Reduced-Osmolarity Oral Rehydration Solution (ORS)[a,b]

Constituent	Concentration, mmol/L
Na+	75
K+	20
Cl−	65
Citrate[c]	10
Glucose	75
Total osmolarity	245

[a]Contains (per package, to be added to 1 L of drinking water): NaCl, 2.6 g; Na₃C₆H₅O₇·2H₂O, 2.9 g; KCl, 1.5 g; and glucose (anhydrous), 13.5 g.

[b]If prepackaged ORS is unavailable, a simple homemade alternative can be prepared by combining 3.5 g (~1/2 teaspoon) of NaCl with either 50 g of precooked rice cereal or 40 g (4 tablespoons) of table sugar (sucrose) in 1 L of drinking water. In that case, potassium must be supplied separately (e.g., in orange juice or coconut water).

[c]10 mmol citrate per liter, which supplies 30 mmol HCO₃/L.

the first 3–6 h of therapy, half within the first hour. Transient muscle cramps and tetany are common. Thereafter, oral therapy can usually be initiated, with the goal of maintaining fluid intake equal to fluid output. However, patients with continued large-volume diarrhea may require prolonged IV treatment to match gastrointestinal fluid losses. Severe hypokalemia can develop but will respond to potassium given either IV or orally. In the absence of adequate staff to monitor the patient's progress, the oral route of rehydration and potassium replacement is safer than the IV route.

Although not necessary for cure, the use of an antibiotic to which the organism is susceptible diminishes the duration and volume of fluid loss and hastens clearance of the organism from the stool. The WHO recommends administration of antibiotics to cholera patients only if they are severely dehydrated, although wider use is often justifiable. Doxycycline (a single dose of 300 mg) or tetracycline (12.5 mg/kg four times a day for 3 days) may be effective in adults but is not recommended for children <8 years of age because of possible deposition in bone and developing teeth. Emerging drug resistance is an ever-present concern. For nonpregnant adults with cholera

TABLE 156-4 Electrolyte Composition of Cholera Stool and of Intravenous Rehydration Solution

Substance	Concentration, mmol/L			
	Na+	K+	Cl−	Base
Stool				
Adult	135	15	100	45
Child	100	25	90	30
Ringer's lactate	130	4[a]	109	28

[a]Potassium supplements, preferably administered by mouth, are required to replace the usual potassium losses from stool.

in areas where tetracycline resistance is prevalent, ciprofloxacin [either in a single dose (30 mg/kg, not to exceed a total dose of 1 g) or in a short course (15 mg/kg bid for 3 days, not to exceed a total daily dose of 1 g)], erythromycin (40–50 mg/kg daily in three divided doses for 3 days), or azithromycin (a single 1-g dose) may be a clinically effective substitute. Pregnant women and children are usually treated with erythromycin or azithromycin (10 mg/kg in children).

■ PREVENTION

Provision of safe water and facilities for sanitary disposal of feces, improved nutrition, and attention to food preparation and storage in the household can significantly reduce the incidence of cholera.

Much effort has been devoted to the development of an effective cholera vaccine over the past few decades, with a particular focus on oral vaccine strains. Traditional killed cholera vaccine given intramuscularly provides little protection to nonimmune subjects and predictably causes adverse effects, including pain at the injection site, malaise, and fever. The vaccine's limited efficacy is due, at least in part, to its failure to induce a local immune response at the intestinal mucosal surface.

Two types of oral cholera vaccines have been developed. The first is a killed whole-cell (WC) vaccine. Two formulations of the killed WC vaccine have been prepared: one that also contains the nontoxic B subunit of cholera toxin (WC/BS) and one composed solely of killed bacteria. In placebo-controlled field trials in Bangladesh, both of the killed vaccines offered significant protection from cholera for the first 6 months after vaccination, with protection rates of ~58% for WC vaccine and 85% for WC/BS vaccine. Protective efficacy rates for both vaccines declined to ~50% by 3 years after vaccine administration. Immunity was relatively sustained in persons vaccinated at an age of >5 years but was not well sustained in younger vaccinees. The WC/BS vaccine proved effective in a trial conducted in a sub-Saharan African population with a high prevalence of HIV infection. Trials of locally produced killed WC vaccines have yielded promising results in Vietnam and in Kolkata (Calcutta), India. Killed oral vaccines also confer herd protection to unvaccinated individuals living in proximity to vaccinated individuals. The WHO now recommends that vaccination against cholera be part of a larger response plan for populations at risk for epidemic cholera. The oral killed vaccines are available in Europe and Asia but (like other cholera vaccines) are not available in the United States.

The second type of cholera vaccine under development involves the use of oral live attenuated vaccine strains developed, for example, by the isolation or creation of mutants lacking the genes encoding cholera toxin. One such vaccine, CVD 103-HgR, was safe and immunogenic in phase 1 and 2 studies but afforded minimal protection in a large field trial in Indonesia. Other live attenuated vaccine candidate strains have been prepared from El Tor and O139 *V. cholerae* and are now undergoing clinical trials. The development of effective and safe cholera vaccines and strategies that provide long-lasting protective mucosal immunity, especially among malnourished, impoverished, and potentially HIV-infected adults and children (the individuals most at risk for cholera), is a priority. As mentioned above, no cholera vaccine is commercially available in the United States.

OTHER *VIBRIO* SPECIES

 The genus *Vibrio* includes several human pathogens that do not cause cholera. Abundant in coastal waters throughout the world, noncholera vibrios can reach high concentrations in the tissues of filter-feeding mollusks. As a result, human infection commonly follows the ingestion of seawater or of raw or undercooked shellfish (Table 156-5). Most noncholera vibrios can be

TABLE 156-5 Features of Selected Noncholera Vibrioses

Organism	Vehicle or Activity	Host at Risk	Syndrome
V. parahaemolyticus	Shellfish, seawater	Normal	Gastroenteritis
	Seawater	Normal	Wound infection
Non-O1/O139 V. cholerae	Shellfish, travel	Normal	Gastroenteritis
	Seawater	Normal	Wound infection, otitis media
V. vulnificus	Shellfish	Immunosuppressed[a]	Sepsis, secondary cellulitis
	Seawater	Normal, immunosuppressed[a]	Wound infection, cellulitis
V. alginolyticus	Seawater	Normal	Wound infection, cellulitis, otitis
	Seawater	Burned, other immunosuppressed	Sepsis

[a]Especially with liver disease or hemochromatosis.

Source: Table 161-3 in *Harrisons Principles of Internal Medicine*, 14th edition.

cultured on blood or MacConkey agar, which contains enough salt to support the growth of these halophilic species. In the microbiology laboratory, the species of noncholera vibrios are distinguished by standard biochemical tests. The most important of these organisms are *V. parahaemolyticus* and *V. vulnificus*.

The two major types of syndromes for which these species are responsible are gastrointestinal illness (due to *V. parahaemolyticus*, non-O1/O139 *V. cholerae*, *V. mimicus*, *V. fluvialis*, *V. hollisae*, and *V. furnissii*) and soft tissue infections (due to *V. vulnificus*, *V. alginolyticus*, and *V. damselae*). *V. vulnificus* is also a cause of primary sepsis in some compromised individuals.

■ SPECIES ASSOCIATED PRIMARILY WITH GASTROINTESTINAL ILLNESS

V. parahaemolyticus

Widespread in marine environments, the halophilic *V. parahaemolyticus* causes food-borne enteritis worldwide. This species was originally implicated in enteritis in Japan in 1953, accounting for 24% of reported cases in one study—a rate that presumably was due to the common practice of eating raw seafood in that country. In the United States, common-source outbreaks of diarrhea caused by this organism have been linked to the consumption of undercooked or improperly handled seafood or of other foods contaminated by seawater. Since the mid-1990s, the incidence of *V. parahaemolyticus* infections has increased in several countries, including the United States. Serotypes O3:K6, O4:K68, and O1:K-untypable, which are genetically related to one another, account for this increase. The enteropathogenicity of *V. parahaemolyticus* is linked to its ability to cause hemolysis on Wagatsuma agar (i.e., the *Kanagawa phenomenon*). Although the mechanism by which the organism causes diarrhea remains unclear, the genome sequence of *V. parahaemolyticus* contains two type III secretion systems, which directly inject toxic bacterial proteins into host cells. *V. parahaemolyticus* should be considered a possible etiologic agent in all cases of diarrhea that can be linked epidemiologically to seafood consumption or to the sea itself.

Infections with *V. parahaemolyticus* can result in two distinct gastrointestinal presentations. The more common of the two presentations (including nearly all cases in North America) is characterized by watery diarrhea, usually occurring in conjunction with abdominal cramps, nausea, and vomiting and accompanied in ~25% of cases by fever and chills. After an incubation period of 4 h to 4 days, symptoms develop and persist for a median of 3 days.

Dysentery, the less common presentation, is characterized by severe abdominal cramps, nausea, vomiting, and bloody or mucoid stools. *V. parahaemolyticus* also causes rare cases of wound infection and otitis and very rare cases of sepsis.

Most cases of *V. parahaemolyticus*–associated gastrointestinal illness, regardless of the presentation, are self-limited and require neither antimicrobial treatment nor hospitalization. Deaths are extremely rare among immunocompetent individuals. Severe infections are associated with underlying diseases, including diabetes, preexisting liver disease, iron-overload states, or immunosuppression. The occasional severe case should be treated with fluid replacement and antibiotics, as described above for cholera.

Non-O1/O139 (noncholera) *V. cholerae*

The heterogeneous non-O1/O139 *V. cholerae* organisms cannot be distinguished from *V. cholerae* O1 or O139 by routine biochemical tests but do not agglutinate in O1 or O139 antiserum. Non-O1/O139 strains have caused several well-studied food-borne outbreaks of gastroenteritis and have also been responsible for sporadic cases of otitis media, wound infection, and bacteremia; although gastroenteritis outbreaks can occur, non-O1/O139 *V. cholerae* strains do not cause epidemics of cholera. Like other vibrios, non-O1/O139 *V. cholerae* organisms are widely distributed in marine environments. In most instances, recognized cases in the United States have been associated with the consumption of raw oysters or with recent travel, typically to Mexico. The broad clinical spectrum of diarrheal illness caused by these organisms is probably due to the group's heterogeneous virulence attributes.

In the United States, about half of all non-O1/O139 *V. cholerae* isolates are from stool samples. The typical incubation period for gastroenteritis due to these organisms is <2 days, and the illness lasts for ~2–7 days. Patients' stools may be copious and watery or may be partly formed, less voluminous, and bloody or mucoid. Diarrhea can result in severe dehydration. Many cases include abdominal cramps, nausea, vomiting, and fever. Like those with cholera, patients who are seriously dehydrated should receive oral or IV fluids; the value of antibiotics is not clear.

Extraintestinal infections due to non-O1/O139 *V. cholerae* commonly follow occupational or recreational exposure to seawater. Around 10% of non-O1/O139 *V. cholerae* isolates come from cases of wound infection, 10% from cases of otitis media, and 20% from cases of bacteremia (which is particularly likely to develop in patients with liver disease). Extraintestinal infections should be treated with antibiotics. Information to guide antibiotic selection and dosing is limited, but most strains are sensitive in vitro to tetracycline, ciprofloxacin, and third-generation cephalosporins.

■ SPECIES ASSOCIATED PRIMARILY WITH SOFT TISSUE INFECTION OR BACTEREMIA

(See also Chap. 125)

V. vulnificus

Infection with *V. vulnificus* is rare, but this organism is the most common cause of severe *Vibrio* infections in the United States. Like most vibrios, *V. vulnificus* proliferates in the warm summer months and requires a saline environment for growth. In this country, infections in humans typically occur in coastal states between May and October and most commonly affect men >40 years of age. *V. vulnificus* has been linked to two distinct syndromes: primary sepsis, which usually occurs in patients with underlying liver disease, and primary wound infection, which generally affects people without underlying disease. (*Vulnificus* is Latin for "wound maker.") Some authors have suggested that *V. vulnificus* also causes gastroenteritis independent of other clinical manifestations. *V. vulnificus* is endowed with a number of virulence attributes, including a capsule that confers resistance to phagocytosis and to the bactericidal activity of human serum as well as a cytolysin. Measured as the 50% lethal dose in mice, the organism's virulence is considerably increased under conditions of iron overload; this observation is consistent with the propensity of *V. vulnificus* to infect patients who have hemochromatosis.

Primary sepsis most often develops in patients who have cirrhosis or hemochromatosis. However, *V. vulnificus* bacteremia can also affect individuals who have hematopoietic disorders or chronic renal insufficiency, those who are using immunosuppressive medications or alcohol, or (in rare instances) those who have no known underlying disease. After a median incubation period of 16 h, the patient develops malaise, chills, fever, and prostration. One-third of patients develop hypotension, which is often apparent at admission. Cutaneous manifestations develop in most cases (usually within 36 h of onset) and characteristically involve the extremities (the lower more often than the upper). In a common sequence, erythematous patches are followed by ecchymoses, vesicles, and bullae. In fact, sepsis and hemorrhagic bullous skin lesions suggest the diagnosis in appropriate settings. Necrosis and sloughing may also be evident. Laboratory studies reveal leukopenia more often than leukocytosis, thrombocytopenia, or elevated levels of fibrin split products. *V. vulnificus* can be cultured from blood or cutaneous lesions. The mortality rate approaches 50%, with most deaths due to uncontrolled sepsis. Accordingly, prompt treatment is critical and should include empirical antibiotic administration, aggressive debridement, and general supportive care. *V. vulnificus* is sensitive in vitro to a number of antibiotics, including tetracycline, fluoroquinolones, and third-generation cephalosporins. Data from animal models suggest that either a fluoroquinolone or the combination of minocycline and cefotaxime should be used in the treatment of *V. vulnificus* septicemia.

V. vulnificus can infect either a fresh or an old wound that comes into contact with seawater; the patient may or may not have underlying disease. After a short incubation period (4 h to 4 days; mean, 12 h), the disease begins with swelling, erythema, and (in many cases) intense pain around the wound. These signs and symptoms are followed by cellulitis, which spreads rapidly and is sometimes accompanied by vesicular, bullous, or necrotic lesions. Metastatic events are uncommon. Most patients have a fever and leukocytosis. *V. vulnificus* can be cultured from skin lesions and occasionally from the blood. Prompt antibiotic therapy and debridement are usually curative.

V. alginolyticus

First identified as a pathogen of humans in 1973, *V. alginolyticus* occasionally causes eye, ear, and wound infections. This species is the most salt-tolerant of the vibrios and can grow in salt concentrations of >10%. Most clinical isolates come from superinfected wounds that presumably become contaminated at the beach. Although its severity varies, *V. alginolyticus* infection tends not to be serious and generally responds well to antibiotic therapy and drainage. A few cases of otitis externa, otitis media, and conjunctivitis due to this pathogen have been described. Tetracycline treatment usually results in cure. *V. alginolyticus* is a rare cause of bacteremia in immunocompromised hosts.

ACKNOWLEDGMENT
The authors gratefully acknowledge the valuable contributions of Drs. Robert Deresiewicz and Gerald T. Keusch, coauthors of this chapter for previous editions.

FURTHER READINGS

CENTERS FOR DISEASE CONTROL AND PREVENTION: Update on cholera—Haiti, Dominican Republic, and Florida, 2010. MMWR Morb Mortal Wkly Rep 59:1637, 2010

CHIN CS et al: The origin of the Haitian cholera outbreak strain. N Engl J Med 364:33, 2011

LUCAS MES et al: Effectiveness of mass oral cholera vaccination in Beira, Mozambique. N Engl J Med 352:757, 2005

RYAN ET: The cholera pandemic, still with us after half a century: Time to rethink. PLoS Negl Trop Dis 5:e1003, 2011

SACK DA et al: Cholera. Lancet 363:223, 2004

SAHA D et al: Single-dose azithromycin for the treatment of cholera in adults. N Engl J Med 354:2452, 2006

SUR D et al: Efficacy and safety of a modified killed-whole-cell oral cholera vaccine in India: An interim analysis of a cluster-randomised, double-blind, placebo-controlled trial. Lancet 374:1694, 2009

VACCINE RESOURCE LIBRARY: Cholera Outbred Strains and Shigellosis (COTS) Program (*http://www.path.org/vaccineresources/details.php?i=736*)

WORLD HEALTH ORGANIZATION: Cholera vaccines: WHO position paper. Wkly Epidemiol Rec 85:117, 2010

———: *The Treatment of Diarrhoea: A Manual for Physicians and Other Senior Health Workers.* Geneva, World Health Organization, 2005 (*http://www.who.int/child_adolescent_health/documents/9241593180/en/index.html*)

———: Cholera: global surveillance summary 2008. Wkly Epidemiol Rec 84:309, 2009 (*http://www.who.int/wer/2009/wer8431/en/index.html*)

———: "Cholera" and "First steps for managing an outbreak of acute diarrhoea" (*www.who.int/topics/cholera/en/*)

CHAPTER 157

Brucellosis

Michael J. Corbel

Nicholas J. Beeching

■ DEFINITION

Brucellosis is a bacterial zoonosis transmitted directly or indirectly to humans from infected animals, predominantly domesticated ruminants and swine. The disease is known colloquially as *undulant fever* because of its remittent character. Its distribution is worldwide apart from the few countries where it has been eradicated from the animal reservoir. Although brucellosis commonly presents as an acute febrile illness, its clinical manifestations vary widely, and definitive signs indicative of the diagnosis may be lacking. Thus the clinical diagnosis usually must be supported by the results of bacteriologic and/or serologic tests.

■ ETIOLOGIC AGENTS

Human brucellosis is caused by strains of *Brucella*, a bacterial genus that was previously suggested, on genetic grounds, to comprise a single species, *B. melitensis,* with a number of biologic variants exhibiting particular host preferences. This view was challenged on the basis of detailed differences in chromosomal structure and host preference. The traditional classification into nomen species is now favored both because of these differences and because this classification scheme closely reflects the epidemiologic patterns of the infection. The nomen system recognizes *B. melitensis*, which is the most common cause of symptomatic disease in humans and for which the main sources are sheep, goats, and camels; *B. abortus,* which is usually acquired from cattle or buffalo: *B. suis,* which generally is acquired from swine but has one variant enzootic in reindeer and caribou and another in rodents; and *B. canis*, which is acquired most often from dogs. *B. ovis,* which causes reproductive disease in sheep, and *B. neotomae,* which is specific for desert rodents, have not been clearly implicated in human disease. Other brucellae have been isolated from marine mammals, and two new nomen species, *B. ceti* sp. nov. and *B. pinnipedialis* sp. nov., have been proposed for these isolates; at least one case of laboratory-acquired human disease due to one of these proposed species has been described, and apparent cases of natural human infection have been reported. As infections in marine mammals seem widespread, more cases of zoonotic infection may be identified. Other newly proposed species include *B. microti* sp. nov. isolated from field voles and *B. inopinata* sp. nov. isolated from a patient with a breast implant. Moreover, it has become apparent that *Brucella* is closely related to the genus *Ochrobactrum,* which includes environmental bacteria sometimes associated with opportunistic infections.

All brucellae are small, gram-negative, unencapsulated, nonsporulating, nonmotile rods or coccobacilli. They grow aerobically on peptone-based medium incubated at 37°C; the growth of some types is improved by supplementary CO_2. In vivo, brucellae behave as facultative intracellular parasites. The organisms are sensitive to sunlight, ionizing radiation, and moderate heat; they are killed by boiling and pasteurization but are resistant to freezing and drying. Their resistance to drying renders brucellae stable in aerosol form, facilitating airborne transmission. The organisms can survive for up to 2 months in soft cheeses made from goat's or sheep's milk; for at least 6 weeks in dry soil contaminated with infected urine, vaginal discharge, or placental or fetal tissues; and for at least 6 months in damp soil or liquid manure kept under cool dark conditions. Brucellae are easily killed by a wide range of common disinfectants used under optimal conditions but are likely to be much more resistant at low temperatures or in the presence of heavy organic contamination.

■ EPIDEMIOLOGY

Brucellosis is a zoonosis whose occurrence is closely related to its prevalence in domesticated animals. The true global prevalence of human brucellosis is unknown because of the imprecision of diagnosis and the inadequacy of reporting and surveillance systems in many countries. Even in developed countries, the true incidence may be 10–20 times higher than the reported figures. Bovine brucellosis has been the target of control programs in many parts of the world and has been eradicated from the cattle populations of Australia, New Zealand, Bulgaria, Canada, Cyprus, Great Britain (including the Channel Islands), Japan, Luxembourg, Romania, the Scandinavian countries, Switzerland, and the Czech and Slovak Republics, among other nations. Its incidence has been reduced to a low level in the United States and most Western European countries, with a varied picture in other parts of the world. There is evidence of a resurgence in Eastern Europe following economic changes in recent years, and outbreaks have also occurred in Ireland. Efforts to eradicate *B. melitensis* infection from sheep and goat populations have been much less successful. These efforts have relied heavily on vaccination programs, which have tended to fluctuate with changing economic and political conditions. In some countries (e.g., Israel), *B. melitensis* has caused serious outbreaks in cattle. Infections with *B. melitensis* still pose a major public health problem in Mediterranean countries; in western, central, and southern Asia; and in parts of Africa and South and Central America.

Human brucellosis is usually associated with occupational or domestic exposure to infected animals or their products. Farmers, shepherds, goatherds, veterinarians, and employees in slaughterhouses and meat-processing plants in endemic areas are occupationally exposed to infection. Family members of individuals involved in animal husbandry may be at risk, although it is often difficult to differentiate food-borne infection from environmental contamination under these circumstances. Laboratory workers who handle cultures or infected samples are also at risk. Travelers and urban residents usually acquire the infection through consumption of contaminated foods. In countries that have eradicated the disease, new cases are most commonly acquired abroad. Dairy products, especially soft cheeses, unpasteurized milk, and ice cream, are the most frequently implicated sources of infection; raw meat and bone marrow may be sources under exceptional circumstances. Infections acquired through cosmetic treatments using materials of fetal origin have been reported. Person-to-person transmission is extremely rare, as is transfer of infection by blood or tissue donation. Although brucellosis is a chronic intracellular infection, there is no evidence for increased prevalence or severity among individuals with HIV infection or with immunodeficiency or immunosuppression of other etiologies.

Brucellosis may be acquired by ingestion, inhalation, or mucosal or percutaneous exposure. Accidental injection of the live vaccine strains of *B. abortus* (19 and RB51) and *B. melitensis* (Rev 1) can cause disease. *B. melitensis* and *B. suis* have been developed as biological weapons by several countries and could be exploited for bioterrorism (Chap. 221). This possibility should be borne in mind in the event of sudden unexplained outbreaks.

■ IMMUNITY AND PATHOGENESIS

Exposure to brucellosis elicits both humoral and cell-mediated immune responses. The mechanisms of protective immunity against human brucellosis are presumed to be similar to those documented in laboratory animals. The response to infection and its outcome are influenced by the virulence, phase, and species of the infecting strain. Differences have been reported between *B. abortus* and *B. suis* in modes of cellular entry and subsequent compartmentalization and processing. Antibodies promote clearance of extracellular brucellae by bactericidal action and by facilitation of phagocytosis by polymorphonuclear and mononuclear phagocytes; however, antibodies alone cannot eradicate infection. Organisms taken up by macrophages and other cells can establish persistent intracellular infections. The key target cell is the macrophage, and bacterial mechanisms for suppressing intracellular killing and apoptosis result in very large intracellular populations. Opsonized bacteria are actively phagocytosed by neutrophilic granulocytes and by monocytes. In these and other cells, initial attachment takes place via specific receptors, including Fc, C3, fibronectin, and mannose-binding proteins. Opsonized—but not unopsonized—bacteria trigger an oxidative burst inside phagocytes. Unopsonized bacteria are internalized via similar receptors but at much lower efficiency. Smooth strains enter host cells via lipid rafts. Smooth lipopolysaccharide (LPS), β-cyclic glucan, and possibly an invasion-attachment protein (IalB) are involved in this process. Tumor necrosis factor α (TNF-α) produced early in the course of infection stimulates cytotoxic lymphocytes and activates macrophages, which can kill intracellular brucellae (probably mainly through production of reactive oxygen and nitrogen intermediates) and may clear infection. However, virulent *Brucella* cells can suppress the TNF-α response, and control of infection in this situation depends on macrophage activation and interferon γ (IFN-γ) responses. Cytokines such as interleukin (IL) 12 promote production of IFN-γ, which drives T_H1-type responses and stimulates macrophage activation. Inflammatory cytokines, including IL-4, IL-6, and IL-10, downregulate the protective response. As in other types of intracellular infection, it is assumed that initial replication of brucellae takes place within cells of the lymph nodes draining the point of entry. Subsequent hematogenous spread may result in chronic localizing infection at almost any site, although the reticuloendothelial system, musculoskeletal tissues, and genitourinary system are most frequently targeted. Both acute and chronic inflammatory responses develop in brucellosis, and the local tissue response may include granuloma formation with or without necrosis and caseation. Abscesses may also develop, especially in chronic localized infection.

The determinants of pathogenicity of *Brucella* have not been fully characterized, and the mechanisms underlying the manifestations of brucellosis are incompletely understood. The organism is a "stealth" pathogen whose survival strategy is centered on processes that avoid triggering innate immune responses and that permit survival within monocytic cells. The smooth *Brucella* LPS, which has an unusual O-chain and core-lipid composition, has relatively low endotoxin activity and plays a key role in pyrogenicity and in resistance to phagocytosis and serum killing in the nonimmune host. In addition, LPS is believed to play a key role in suppressing phagosome-lysosome fusion and diverting the internalized bacteria into vacuoles located in endoplasmic reticulum, where intracellular replication takes place. Specific exotoxins have not been isolated, but a type IV secretion system (VirB) that regulates intracellular survival and trafficking has been identified. In *B. abortus* this system can be activated extracellularly, but in *B. suis* it is activated (by low pH) only during intracellular growth. Brucellae then produce acid-stable proteins that facilitate the organisms' survival in phagosomes and may enhance their resistance to reactive oxygen intermediates.

A type III secretion system based on modified flagellar structures has also been identified. Virulent brucellae are resistant to defensins and produce a Cu-Zn superoxide dismutase that increases their resistance to reactive oxygen intermediates. A hemolysin-like protein may trigger the release of brucellae from infected cells.

■ CLINICAL FEATURES

Brucellosis almost invariably causes fever, which may be associated with profuse sweats, especially at night. In endemic areas, brucellosis may be difficult to distinguish from the many other causes of fever. However, two features recognized in the nineteenth century distinguish brucellosis from other tropical fevers, such as typhoid and malaria: (1) Left untreated, the fever of brucellosis shows an undulating pattern that persists for weeks before the commencement of an afebrile period that may be followed by relapse. (2) The fever of brucellosis is associated with musculoskeletal symptoms and signs in about one-half of all patients.

The clinical syndromes caused by the different nomen species are similar, although *B. melitensis* tends to be associated with a more acute and aggressive presentation and *B. suis* with focal abscess induction. *B. abortus* infections may be more insidious in onset and more likely to become chronic. *B. canis* infections are reported to present frequently with acute gastrointestinal symptoms.

The incubation period varies from 1 week to several months, and the onset of fever and other symptoms may be abrupt or insidious. In addition to experiencing fever and sweats, patients become increasingly apathetic and fatigued; lose appetite and weight; and have nonspecific myalgia, headache, and chills. Overall, the presentation of brucellosis often fits one of three patterns: febrile illness that resembles typhoid but is less severe; fever and acute monoarthritis, typically of the hip or knee, in a young child; and long-lasting fever, misery, and low-back or hip pain in an older man. In an endemic area (e.g., much of the Middle East), a patient with fever and difficulty walking into the clinic would be regarded as having brucellosis until it was proved otherwise.

Diagnostic clues in the patient's history include travel to an endemic area, employment in a diagnostic microbiology laboratory, consumption of unpasteurized milk products (including soft cheeses), contact with animals, accidental inoculation with veterinary *Brucella* vaccines, and—in an endemic setting—a history of similar illness in the family (documented in almost 50% of cases). Focal features are present in the majority of patients. The most common are musculoskeletal pain and physical findings in the peripheral and axial skeleton (~40% of cases). Osteomyelitis more commonly involves the lumbar and low thoracic vertebrae than the cervical and high thoracic spine. Individual joints that are most commonly affected by septic arthritis are the knee, hip, sacroiliac, shoulder, and sternoclavicular joints; the pattern may be one of monoarthritis or polyarthritis. Osteomyelitis may also accompany septic arthritis.

In addition to the usual causes of vertebral osteomyelitis or septic arthritis, the most important differential diagnosis is tuberculosis. This point influences the therapeutic approach as well as the prognosis, given that several antimicrobial agents used to treat brucellosis are also used to treat tuberculosis. Septic arthritis in brucellosis progresses slowly, starting with small pericapsular erosions. In the vertebrae, anterior erosions of the superior end plate are typically the first features to become evident, with eventual involvement and sclerosis of the whole vertebra. Anterior osteophytes eventually develop, but vertebral destruction or impingement on the spinal cord is rare and usually suggests tuberculosis (Table 157-1).

Other systems may be involved in a manner that resembles typhoid. About one-quarter of patients have a dry cough, usually with few changes visible on the chest x-ray, although pneumonia,

TABLE 157-1 Radiology of the Spine: Differentiation of Brucellosis From Tuberculosis

	Brucellosis	Tuberculosis
Site	Lumbar and others	Dorsolumbar
Vertebrae	Multiple or contiguous	Contiguous
Diskitis	Late	Early
Body	Intact until late	Morphology lost early
Canal compression	Rare	Common
Epiphysitis	Anterosuperior (Pom's sign)	General: upper and lower disk regions, central, subperiosteal
Osteophyte	Anterolateral (parrot beak)	Unusual
Deformity	Wedging uncommon	Anterior wedge, gibbus
Recovery	Sclerosis, whole body	Variable
Paravertebral abscess	Small, well-localized	Common and discrete loss, transverse process
Psoas abscess	Rare	More likely

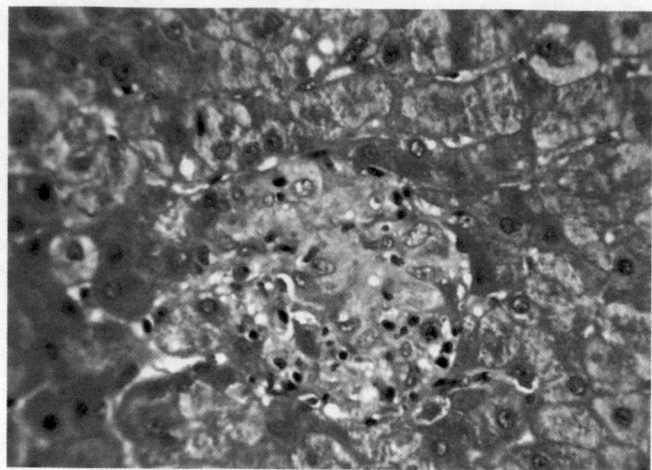

Figure 157-1 Liver biopsy specimen from a patient with brucellosis shows a noncaseating granuloma. *[From Mandell's Atlas of Infectious Diseases, Vol II, in DL Stevens (ed): Skin, Soft Tissue, Bone and Joint Infections, Fig. 5-9; with permission.]*

empyema, intrathoracic adenopathy, or lung abscess can occur. One-quarter of patients have hepatosplenomegaly, and 10–20% have significant lymphadenopathy; the differential diagnosis includes glandular fever–like illness such as that caused by Epstein-Barr virus, *Toxoplasma*, cytomegalovirus, HIV, or *Mycobacterium tuberculosis*. Up to 10% of men have acute epididymoorchitis, which must be distinguished from mumps and from surgical problems such as torsion. Prostatitis, inflammation of the seminal vesicles, salpingitis, and pyelonephritis all occur. There is an increased incidence of fetal loss among infected pregnant women, although teratogenicity has not been described and the tendency toward abortions is much less pronounced in humans than in farm animals.

Neurologic involvement is common, with depression and lethargy whose severity may not be fully appreciated by either the patient or the physician until after treatment. A small proportion of patients develop lymphocytic meningoencephalitis that mimics neurotuberculosis, atypical leptospirosis, or noninfectious conditions and that may be complicated by intracerebral abscess, a variety of cranial nerve deficits, or ruptured mycotic aneurysms.

Endocarditis occurs in ~1% of cases, most often affecting the aortic valve (natural or prosthetic). Any site in the body may be involved in metastatic abscess formation or inflammation; the female breast and the thyroid gland are affected particularly often. Nonspecific maculopapular rashes and other skin manifestations are uncommon and are rarely noticed by the patient even if they develop.

■ DIAGNOSIS

Because the clinical picture of brucellosis is not distinctive, the diagnosis must be based on a history of potential exposure, a presentation consistent with the disease, and supporting laboratory findings. Results of routine biochemical assays are usually within normal limits, although serum levels of hepatic enzymes and bilirubin may be elevated. Peripheral leukocyte counts are usually normal or low, with relative lymphocytosis. Mild anemia may be documented. Thrombocytopenia and disseminated intravascular coagulation with raised levels of fibrinogen degradation products can develop.

The erythrocyte sedimentation rate and C-reactive protein levels are often normal but may be raised.

In body fluids such as cerebrospinal fluid (CSF) or joint fluid, lymphocytosis and low glucose levels are the norm. Elevated CSF levels of adenosine deaminase cannot be used to distinguish tubercular meningitis, as they may also be found in brucellosis. Biopsied samples of tissues such as lymph node or liver may show noncaseating granulomas (Fig. 157-1) without acid/alcohol-fast bacilli. The radiologic features of bony disease develop late and are much more subtle than those of tuberculosis or septic arthritis of other etiologies, with less bone and joint destruction. Isotope scanning is more sensitive than plain x-ray and continues to give positive results long after successful treatment.

Isolation of brucellae from blood, CSF, bone marrow, or joint fluid or from a tissue aspirate or biopsy sample is definitive, and attempts at isolation are usually successful in 50–70% of cases. Duplicate cultures should be incubated for up to 6 weeks (in air and 10% CO_2, respectively). Concentration and lysis of buffy coat cells before culture may increase the isolation rate. Cultures in modern nonradiometric or similar signaling systems (e.g., Bactec) usually become positive within 7–10 days but should be maintained for at least 3 weeks before the results are declared negative. All cultures should be handled under containment conditions appropriate for dangerous pathogens. *Brucella* species may be misidentified as *Agrobacterium*, *Ochrobactrum*, or *Psychrobacter (Moraxella) phenylpyruvicus* by the gallery identification strips commonly used in the diagnostic laboratory.

The peripheral blood–based polymerase chain reaction has enormous potential to detect bacteremia, to predict relapse, and to exclude "chronic brucellosis." This method is probably more sensitive and is certainly quicker than blood culture, and it does not carry the attendant biohazard risk posed by culture. Nucleic acid amplification techniques are now quite widely used, although no single standardized procedure has been adopted. Primers for the spacer region between the genes encoding the 16S and 23S ribosomal RNAs (*rrs-rrl*), the outer-membrane protein Omp2, the insertion sequence *IS711*, and the protein BCSP31 are sensitive and specific. Blood and other tissues are the most suitable samples for analysis.

Serologic examination often provides the only positive laboratory findings in brucellosis. In acute infection, IgM antibodies appear early and are followed by IgG and IgA. All these antibodies are active in agglutination tests, whether performed by tube, plate, or microagglutination methods. The majority of patients have detectable agglutinins at this stage. As the disease progresses, IgM levels decline, and the avidity and subclass distribution of IgG and IgA change. The result is reduced or undetectable agglutinin titers. However, the antibodies are detectable by alternative tests, including the complement fixation test, Coomb's antiglobulin test, and enzyme-linked immunosorbent assay. There is no clear cutoff value for a diagnostic titer. Rather, serology results must be interpreted in the context of exposure history and clinical presentation. In endemic areas or in settings of potential occupational exposure, agglutinin titers of 1:320–1:640 or higher are considered diagnostic; in nonendemic areas, a titer of ≥1:160 is considered significant. Repetition of tests after 2–4 weeks may demonstrate a rising titer.

In most centers, the standard agglutination test (SAT) is still the mainstay of serologic diagnosis, although some investigators rely on the rose bengal test, which has not been fully validated for human diagnostic use. Dipstick assays for anti-*Brucella* IgM are useful for the diagnosis of acute infection but are less sensitive for infection with symptoms of several months' duration. In an endemic setting, >90% of patients with acute bacteremia have SAT titers of at least 1:320. Other screening tests are used in some centers.

Antibody to the *Brucella* LPS O chain—the dominant antigen—is detected by all the conventional tests that employ smooth *B. abortus* cells as antigen. Since *B. abortus* cross-reacts with *B. melitensis* and *B. suis*, there is no advantage in replicating the tests with these antigens. Cross-reactions also occur with the O chains of some other gram-negative bacteria, including *Escherichia coli* O157, *Francisella tularensis*, *Salmonella enterica* group N, *Stenotrophomonas maltophilia*, and *Vibrio cholerae*. Cross-reactions do not occur with the cell-surface antigens of rough *Brucella* strains such as *B. canis* or *B. ovis*; serologic tests for these nomen species must employ an antigen prepared from either one. The live *B. abortus* vaccine strain RB51 does not elicit responses in standard serologic testing. Most protein antigens are shared by all *Brucella* strains, and some are also common to *Ochrobactrum* species. Immunoblotting against protein extracts has been advocated as a differential test, but no validated procedure is yet available.

TREATMENT ▶ Brucellosis

The broad aims of antimicrobial therapy are to treat and relieve the symptoms of current infection and to prevent relapse. Focal disease presentations may require specific intervention in addition to more prolonged and tailored antibiotic therapy. In addition, tuberculosis must always be excluded, or—to prevent the emergence of resistance—therapy must be tailored to specifically exclude drugs active against tuberculosis (e.g., rifampin used alone) or to include a full antituberculous regimen.

Early experience with streptomycin monotherapy showed that relapse was common; thus dual therapy with tetracyclines became the norm. This is still the most effective combination, but alternatives may be used, with the options depending on local or national policy about the use of rifampin for the treatment of nonmycobacterial infection. For the several antimicrobial agents that are active in vivo, efficacy can usually be predicted by in vitro testing. However, numerous *Brucella* strains show in vitro sensitivity to a whole range of antimicrobials that are therapeutically ineffective, including assorted β-lactams. Moreover, the use of fluoroquinolones remains controversial despite the good in vitro activity and white-cell penetration of most agents of this class. Low intravacuolar pH is probably a factor in the poor performance of these drugs.

For adults with acute nonfocal brucellosis (duration, <1 month), a 6-week course of therapy incorporating at least two antimicrobial agents is required. Complex or focal disease necessitates ≥3 months of therapy. Adherence to the therapeutic regimen is very important, and poor adherence underlies almost all cases of apparent treatment failure; such failure is rarely due to the emergence of drug resistance, although increasing resistance to trimethoprim-sulfamethoxazole (TMP-SMX) has been reported at one center. There is good retrospective evidence that a 3-week course of two agents is as effective as a 6-week course for treatment and prevention of relapse in children, but this point has not yet been proven in prospective studies.

The gold standard for the treatment of brucellosis in adults is IM streptomycin (0.75–1 g daily for 14–21 days) together with doxycycline (100 mg twice daily for 6 weeks). In both clinical trials and observational studies, relapse follows such treatment in 5–10% of cases. The usual alternative regimen (and the current World Health Organization recommendation) is rifampin (600–900 mg/d) plus doxycycline (100 mg twice daily) for 6 weeks. The relapse/failure rate is ~10% in trial conditions but rises to >20% in many non-trial situations, possibly because doxycycline levels are reduced and clearance rates increased by concomitant rifampin administration. Patients who cannot tolerate or receive tetracyclines (children, pregnant women) can be given high-dose TMP-SMX instead (two or three standard-strength tablets twice daily for adults, depending on weight).

Increasing evidence supports the use of an aminoglycoside such as gentamicin (5–6 mg/kg per day for at least 2 weeks) instead of streptomycin. Shorter courses have been associated with high failure rates in adults. A 5- to 7-day course of therapy with gentamicin and a 3-week course of TMP-SMX may be adequate for children with uncomplicated disease, but prospective trials are still needed to support this recommendation. Early experience with fluoroquinolone monotherapy was disappointing, although it was suggested that ofloxacin or ciprofloxacin, given together with rifampin for 6 weeks, might be an acceptable alternative to the other 6-week regimens for adults. However, a meta-analysis did not support the use of fluoroquinolones in first-line treatment regimens, and these drugs are not recommended by an expert consensus group (the Ioannina Group) except in the context of well-designed clinical trials. A triple-drug regimen—doxycycline and rifampin combined with an initial course of an aminoglycoside—was superior to double-drug regimens in a meta-analysis. The triple-drug regimen should be considered for all patients with complicated disease and for those for whom treatment adherence is likely to be a problem.

Significant neurologic disease due to *Brucella* species requires prolonged treatment (i.e., for 3–6 months), usually with ceftriaxone supplementation of a standard regimen. *Brucella* endocarditis is treated with at least three drugs (an aminoglycoside, a tetracycline, and rifampin), and many experts add ceftriaxone and/or a fluoroquinolone to reduce the need for valve replacement. Treatment is usually given for at least 6 months, and clinical endpoints for its discontinuation are often difficult to define. Surgery is still required for the majority of cases of infection of prosthetic heart valves and prosthetic joints.

There is no evidence base to guide prophylaxis after exposure to *Brucella* organisms (e.g., in the laboratory), inadvertent immunization with live vaccine intended for use in animals, or exposure to deliberately released brucellae. Most authorities have recommended the administration of rifampin plus doxycycline for 3 weeks after a low-risk exposure (e.g., a nonspecific laboratory accident) and for 6 weeks after a major exposure to aerosol or injected material. However, such regimens are poorly tolerated, and doxycycline monotherapy of the same duration may be substituted. Rifampin should be omitted after exposure to vaccine strain RB51, which is resistant to rifampin but sensitive to doxycycline. After significant brucellosis exposure, expert consultation is advised for women who are (or may be) pregnant.

■ PROGNOSIS AND FOLLOW-UP

Relapse occurs in up to 30% of poorly compliant patients. Thus patients should ideally be followed clinically for up to 2 years to detect relapse, which responds to a prolonged course of the same therapy used originally. The general well-being and the body weight of the patient are more useful guides than serology to lack of relapse. IgG antibody levels detected by the SAT and its variants can remain in the diagnostic range for >2 years after successful treatment. Complement fixation titers usually fall to normal within 1 year of cure. Immunity is not solid; patients can be reinfected after repeated exposures. Fewer than 1% of patients die of brucellosis. When the outcome is fatal, death is usually a consequence of cardiac involvement; more rarely, it results from severe neurologic disease. Despite the low mortality rate, recovery from brucellosis is slow, and the illness can cause prolonged inactivity, with domestic and economic consequences.

The existence of a prolonged chronic brucellosis state after successful treatment remains controversial. Evaluation of patients in whom this state is considered (often those with work-related exposure to brucellae) includes careful exclusion of malingering, nonspecific chronic fatigue syndromes, and other causes of excessive sweating, such as alcohol abuse and obesity. In the future, the availability of more sensitive assays to detect *Brucella* antigen or DNA may help to identify patients with ongoing infection.

■ PREVENTION

Vaccines based on live attenuated *Brucella* strains, such as *B. abortus* strain 19BA or 104M, have been used in some countries to protect high-risk populations but have displayed only short-term efficacy and high reactogenicity. Subunit vaccines have been developed but are of uncertain value and cannot be recommended at present. Research in this area has been stimulated by interest in biodefense (Chap. 221) and may eventually yield new products, some of which may be based on the live attenuated WR 201 variant of *B. melitensis* strain 16M. The mainstay of veterinary prevention is a national commitment to testing and slaughter of infected herds/flocks (with compensation for owners), control of animal movement, and active immunization of animals. These measures are usually sufficient to control human disease as well. In their absence, pasteurization of all milk products before consumption is sufficient to prevent non-occupational animal-to-human transmission. All cases of brucellosis in animals and humans should be reported to the appropriate public health authorities.

FURTHER READINGS

Ariza J et al: Perspectives for the treatment of brucellosis in the 21st century: The Ioannina recommendations. PLoS Med 4:e317, 2007

Ashford DA et al: Adverse events in humans associated with accidental exposure to the livestock brucellosis vaccine RB51. Vaccine 22:3435, 2004

Barquero-Calvo E et al: *Brucella abortus* uses a stealth strategy to avoid activation of the innate immune system during the onset of infection. PLoS ONE 2:e631, 2007

Centers for Disease Control and Prevention: Laboratory-acquired brucellosis, Indiana and Minnesota, 2006. MMWR Morb Mortal Wkly Rep 57:39, 2008

Corbel MJ (ed): Brucellosis in humans and animals. Geneva, World Health Organization in collaboration with Food and Agriculture Organization and World Organization for Animal Health, 2006

———, Banai M: Genus *Brucella* Meyer and Shaw 1920,173AL, in *Bergey's Manual of Systematic Bacteriology*, 2nd ed, vol 2: *The Proteobacteria*, DJ Brenner et al (eds). New York, Springer, 2006, pp 370–386

Franco MP et al: Human brucellosis. Lancet Infect Dis 7:775, 2007

Pappas G et al: The new global map of human brucellosis. Lancet Infect Dis 6:91, 2006

Queipo-Ortuno MI et al: Usefulness of a quantitative real-time PCR assay using serum samples to discriminate between inactive, serologically positive and active human brucellosis. Clin Microbiol Infect 14:1128, 2008

Skalsky K et al: Treatment of human brucellosis: Systematic review and meta-analysis of randomised controlled trials. Br Med J 336:701, 2008

Whatmore AM: Current understanding of the genetic diversity of *Brucella*, an expanding genus of zoonotic pathogens. Infect Genet Evol 9:1168, 2009

CHAPTER **158**

Tularemia

Richard F. Jacobs
Gordon E. Schutze

Tularemia is a zoonosis caused by *Francisella tularensis*. Humans of any age, sex, or race are universally susceptible to this systemic infection. Tularemia is primarily a disease of wild animals and persists in contaminated environments, ectoparasites, and animal carriers. Human infection is incidental and usually results from interaction with biting or blood-sucking insects, contact with wild or domestic animals, ingestion of contaminated water or food, or inhalation of infective aerosols. The illness is characterized by various clinical syndromes, the most common of which consists of an ulcerative lesion at the site of inoculation, with regional lymphadenopathy and lymphadenitis. Systemic manifestations, including pneumonia, typhoidal tularemia, meningitis, and fever without localizing findings, pose a greater diagnostic challenge.

■ ETIOLOGY AND EPIDEMIOLOGY

Tularemia is common in Arkansas, Oklahoma, Missouri, and South Dakota; these states account for more than half of all reported cases in the United States. Small outbreaks in higher-risk populations (e.g., professional landscapers cutting up brush, mowing, and using a leaf blower) have been reported from the island of Martha's Vineyard in Massachusetts. Although the irregular distribution of cases of tularemia makes worldwide estimates difficult, increasing numbers of cases have been reported from the Scandinavian countries, Eastern Europe, and Siberia.

With rare exceptions, tularemia is the only disease produced by *F. tularensis*—a small (0.2 µm by 0.2–0.7 µm), gram-negative, pleomorphic, nonmotile, non-spore-forming bacillus. Bipolar staining results in a coccoid appearance. The organism is a thinly encapsulated, nonpiliated strict aerobe that invades host cells. In nature, *F. tularensis* is a hardy organism that persists for weeks or months in mud, water, and decaying animal carcasses. Dozens of biting and blood-sucking insects, especially ticks and tabanid flies, serve as vectors. Ticks and wild rabbits are the source for most human cases in endemic areas of the southeastern and Rocky Mountain states. In Utah, Nevada, and California, tabanid flies are the most common vectors. Animal reservoirs include wild rabbits, squirrels, birds, sheep, beavers, muskrats, and domestic dogs and cats. Person-to-person transmission is rare or nonexistent. Tularemia is more common among men than among women.

The four subspecies of *F. tularensis* are *tularensis, holarctica, novicida,* and *mediasiatica*. The first three of these subspecies are found in North America; in fact, subspecies *tularensis* has been isolated only in North America, where it accounts for >70% of cases of tularemia and produces more serious human disease than other subspecies (although, with treatment, the associated fatality rate is <2%). The progression of illness depends on the infecting strain's virulence, the inoculum size, the portal of entry, and the host's immune status. *F. tularensis* is a class A bioterrorism agent.

Ticks pass *F. tularensis* to their offspring transovarially. The organism is found in tick feces but not in large quantities in tick salivary glands. In the United States, the disease is carried by *Dermacentor andersoni* (Rocky Mountain wood tick), *D. variabilis*

(American dog tick), *D. occidentalis* (Pacific Coast dog tick), and *Amblyomma americanum* (Lone Star tick). *F. tularensis* is transmitted frequently during blood meals taken by embedded ticks after hours of attachment. It is the taking of a blood meal through a fecally contaminated field that transmits the organism. Transmission by ticks and tabanid flies takes place mainly in the spring and summer. However, continued transmission in the winter by trapped or hunted animals has been documented.

■ PATHOGENESIS AND PATHOLOGY

The most common portal of entry for human infection is through skin or mucous membranes, either directly—through the bite of ticks, other arthropods, or other animals—or via inapparent abrasions. Inhalation or ingestion of *F. tularensis* also can result in infection. *F. tularensis* is extremely infectious: Although >10^8 organisms are usually required to produce infection via the oral route (oropharyngeal or gastrointestinal tularemia), as few as 10 organisms can result in infection when injected into the skin (ulceroglandular/glandular tularemia) or inhaled (pulmonary tularemia). After inoculation into the skin, the organism multiplies locally; within 2–5 days (range, 1–10 days), it produces an erythematous, tender, or pruritic papule. The papule rapidly enlarges and forms an ulcer with a black base (chancriform lesion). The bacteria spread to regional lymph nodes, producing lymphadenopathy (buboes). All forms can lead to bacteremia with spread to distant organs, including the central nervous system.

Tularemia is characterized by mononuclear cell infiltration with pyogranulomatous pathology. The histopathologic findings can be quite similar to those in tuberculosis, although tularemia develops more rapidly. As a facultatively intracellular bacterium, *F. tularensis* can parasitize both phagocytic and nonphagocytic host cells and can survive intracellularly for prolonged periods. In the acute phase of infection, the primary organs affected (skin, lymph nodes, liver, and spleen) include areas of focal necrosis, which are initially surrounded by polymorphonuclear leukocytes (PMNs). Subsequently, granulomas form, with epithelioid cells, lymphocytes, and multinucleated giant cells surrounded by areas of necrosis. These areas may resemble caseation necrosis but later coalesce to form abscesses.

Conjunctival inoculation can result in infection of the eye, with regional lymph node enlargement (preauricular lymphadenopathy, Parinaud's complex). Aerosolization and inhalation or hematogenous spread of organisms can result in pneumonia. In the lung, an inflammatory reaction develops, including foci of alveolar necrosis and cell infiltration (initially polymorphonuclear and later mononuclear) with granulomas. Chest roentgenograms usually reveal bilateral patchy infiltrates rather than large areas of consolidation. Pleural effusions are common and may contain blood. Lymphadenopathy occurs in regions draining infected organs. Therefore, in pulmonary infection, mediastinal adenopathy may be evident, whereas patients with oropharyngeal tularemia develop cervical lymphadenopathy. In gastrointestinal or typhoidal tularemia, mesenteric lymphadenopathy may follow the ingestion of large numbers of organisms. (The term *typhoidal tularemia* may be used to describe severe bacteremic disease, irrespective of the mode of transmission or portal of entry.) Meningitis has been reported as a primary or secondary manifestation of bacteremia. Patients may also present with fever and no localizing signs.

■ IMMUNOLOGY

Although a complete and widely accepted understanding of the protective immune response to *F. tularensis* is lacking, significant advances in the study of natural and protective immunity have been made in recent years and may ultimately result in a vaccine candidate.

The availability of attenuated *F. tularensis* strains developed through genetic manipulation is facilitating research that will expand our knowledge in this area.

A number of investigators have studied various models and proposed various hypotheses regarding the induction of protective immunity to *F. tularensis*. Although further research is needed, a synergy between humoral and cell-mediated immune (CMI) responses appears to be critical in inducing effective immune protection. Elucidation of the molecular mechanisms for the organism's evasion of the host response, pathogen-associated molecular patterns, and effective host immune protection has led to novel vaccination strategies tested in animal models. Antibodies to Fc receptors on antigen-presenting cells have been shown to be protective in animal models of pulmonary tularemia, resulting in both mucosal and CMI responses. This enhanced understanding of mucosal and serum antibodies in combination with a targeted CMI response holds great promise for future vaccine development.

■ CLINICAL MANIFESTATIONS

Tularemia often starts with a sudden onset of fever, chills, headache, and generalized myalgias and arthralgias (Table 158-1). This onset takes place when the organism penetrates the skin, is ingested, or is inhaled. An incubation period of 2–10 days is followed by the formation of an ulcer at the site of penetration, with local inflammation. The ulcer may persist for several months as organisms are transported via the lymphatics to the regional lymph nodes. These nodes enlarge and may become necrotic and suppurative. If the organism enters the bloodstream, widespread dissemination can result.

In the United States, most patients with tularemia (75–85%) acquire the infection by inoculation of the skin. In adults, the most common localized form is inguinal/femoral lymphadenopathy; in children, it is cervical lymphadenopathy. About 20% of patients develop a generalized maculopapular rash, which occasionally becomes pustular. Erythema nodosum occurs infrequently. The clinical manifestations of tularemia have been divided into various syndromes, which are listed in Table 158-2.

Ulceroglandular/glandular tularemia

These two forms of tularemia account for ~75–85% of cases. The predominant form in children involves cervical or posterior auricular lymphadenopathy and is usually related to tick bites on the head and neck. In adults, the most common form is inguinal/

TABLE 158-1 Clinical Presentation of Tularemia

Sign or Symptom	Rate of Occurrence, %	
	Children	Adults
Lymphadenopathy	96	65
Fever (≥38.3°C or ≥101°F)	87	21
Ulcer/eschar/papule	45	51
Myalgias/arthralgias	39	2
Headache	9	5
Cough	9	5
Pharyngitis	43	—
Diarrhea	43	—

Source: Adapted from RF Jacobs, JP Narain: Pediatrics 76:818, 1985; with permission.

TABLE 158-2 Clinical Syndromes of Tularemia

Syndrome	Rate of Occurrence, %	
	Children	Adults
Ulceroglandular	45	51
Glandular	25	12
Pulmonary (pneumonia)	14	18
Oropharyngeal	4	—
Oculoglandular	2	—
Typhoidal	2	12
Unclassified	6	11

Source: Adapted from RF Jacobs, JP Narain: Pediatrics 76:818, 1985; with permission.

femoral lymphadenopathy resulting from insect and tick exposures on the lower limbs. In cases related to wild game, the usual portal of entry for *F. tularensis* is either an injury sustained while skinning or cleaning an animal carcass or a bite (usually on the hand). Epitrochlear lymphadenopathy/lymphadenitis is common in patients with bite-related injuries.

In ulceroglandular tularemia, the ulcer is erythematous, indurated, and nonhealing, with a punched-out appearance that lasts 1–3 weeks. The papule may begin as an erythematous lesion that is tender or pruritic; it evolves over several days into an ulcer with sharply demarcated edges and a yellow exudate. The ulcer gradually develops a black base, and simultaneously the regional lymph nodes become tender and severely enlarged (Fig. 158-1). The affected lymph nodes may become fluctuant and drain spontaneously, but the condition usually resolves with effective treatment. Late suppuration of lymph nodes has been described in up to 25% of patients with ulceroglandular/glandular tularemia. Examination of material taken from these late fluctuant nodes after successful antimicrobial treatment reveals sterile necrotic tissue. In 5–10% of patients, the skin lesion may be inapparent, with lymphadenopathy plus systemic signs and symptoms the only physical findings (*glandular tularemia*). Conversely, a tick or deerfly bite on the trunk may result in an ulcer without evident lymphadenopathy.

Oculoglandular tularemia

In ~1% of patients, the portal of entry for *F. tularensis* is the conjunctiva, which the organism usually reaches through contact with contaminated fingers. The inflamed conjunctiva is painful,

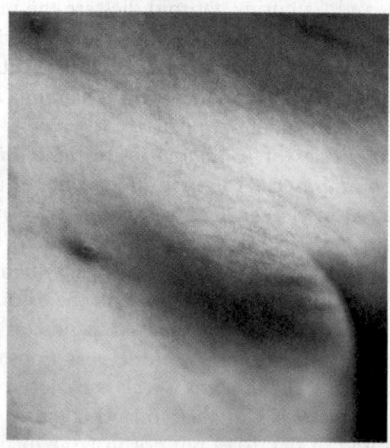

Figure 158-1 An 8-year-old boy with inguinal lymphadenitis and associated tick-bite site characteristic of ulceroglandular tularemia.

with numerous yellowish nodules and pinpoint ulcers. Purulent conjunctivitis with regional lymphadenopathy (preauricular, submandibular, or cervical) is evident. Because of debilitating pain, the patient may seek medical attention before regional lymphadenopathy develops. Painful preauricular lymphadenopathy is unique to tularemia and distinguishes it from tuberculosis, sporotrichosis, and syphilis. Corneal perforation may occur.

Oropharyngeal and gastrointestinal tularemia

Rarely, tularemia follows ingestion of contaminated undercooked meat, oral inoculation of *F. tularensis* from the hands in association with the skinning and cleaning of animal carcasses, or consumption of contaminated food or water. Oral inoculation may result in acute, exudative, or membranous pharyngitis associated with cervical lymphadenopathy or in ulcerative intestinal lesions associated with mesenteric lymphadenopathy, diarrhea, abdominal pain, nausea, vomiting, and gastrointestinal bleeding. Infected tonsils become enlarged and develop a yellowish-white pseudomembrane, which can be confused with that of diphtheria. The clinical severity of gastrointestinal tularemia varies from mild, unexplained, persistent diarrhea with no other symptoms to a fulminant, fatal disease. In fatal cases, the extensive intestinal ulceration found at autopsy suggests an enormous inoculum.

Pulmonary tularemia

Pneumonia due to *F. tularensis* presents as variable parenchymal infiltrates that are unresponsive to treatment with β-lactam antibiotics. Tularemia must be considered in the differential diagnosis of atypical pneumonia in a patient with a history of travel to an endemic area. The disease can result from inhalation of an infectious aerosol or can spread to the lungs and pleura via bacteremia. Inhalation-related pneumonia has been described in laboratory workers after exposure to contaminated materials and, if untreated, can be associated with a relatively high mortality rate. Exposure to *F. tularensis* in aerosols from live domestic animals or dead wildlife (including birds) has been reported to cause pneumonia. Hematogenous dissemination to the lungs occurs in 10–15% of cases of ulceroglandular tularemia and in about half of cases of typhoidal tularemia. Previously, tularemia pneumonia was thought to be a disease of older patients, but as many as 10–15% of children with clinical manifestations of tularemia have parenchymal infiltrates detected by chest roentgenography. Patients with pneumonia usually have a nonproductive cough and may have dyspnea or pleuritic chest pain. Roentgenograms of the chest usually reveal bilateral patchy infiltrates (described as ovoid or lobar densities), lobar parenchymal infiltrates, and cavitary lesions. Pleural effusions may have a predominance of mononuclear leukocytes or PMNs and sometimes red blood cells. Empyema may develop. Blood cultures may be positive for *F. tularensis*.

Typhoidal tularemia

The typhoidal presentation is now considered rare in the United States. The source of infection in typhoidal tularemia is usually associated with pharyngeal and/or gastrointestinal inoculation or bacteremic disease. Fever usually develops without apparent skin lesions or lymphadenopathy. Some patients have cervical and mesenteric lymphadenopathy. In the absence of a history of possible contact with a vector, diagnosis can be extremely difficult. Blood cultures may be positive and patients may present with classic sepsis or septic shock in this acute systemic form of the infection. Typhoidal tularemia is usually associated with a huge inoculum or with a preexisting compromising condition. High continuous fevers, signs of sepsis, and severe headache are common. The patient may be delirious and may develop prostration and shock. If presumptive antibiotic therapy in culture-negative cases does not include an aminoglycoside, the estimated mortality rate is relatively high.

Other manifestations

F. tularensis infection has been associated with meningitis, pericarditis, hepatitis, peritonitis, endocarditis, osteomyelitis, and sepsis and septic shock with rhabdomyolysis and acute renal failure. In cases of tularemia meningitis, a mean white blood cell count of 1788/μL, a predominantly mononuclear cell response (70–100%), a depressed glucose level, an elevated protein concentration, and a negative Gram's stain are typically found on examination of cerebrospinal fluid.

■ DIFFERENTIAL DIAGNOSIS

When patients in endemic areas present with fever, chronic ulcerative skin lesions, and large tender lymph nodes (Fig. 158-1), a diagnosis of tularemia should be made presumptively, and confirmatory diagnostic testing and appropriate therapy should be undertaken. When the possibility of tularemia is considered in a nonendemic area, an attempt should be made to identify contact with a potential animal vector. The level of suspicion should be especially high in hunters, trappers, game wardens, professional landscapers, veterinarians, laboratory workers, and individuals exposed to an insect or another animal vector. However, up to 40% of patients with tularemia have no known history of epidemiologic contact with an animal vector.

The characteristic presentation of ulceroglandular tularemia does not pose a diagnostic problem, but a less classic progression of regional lymphadenopathy or glandular tularemia must be differentiated from other diseases (Table 158-3). The skin lesion of tularemia may resemble those seen in various other diseases but is generally accompanied by more impressive regional lymphadenopathy. In children, the differentiation of tularemia from cat-scratch disease is made more difficult by the chronic papulovesicular lesion associated with *Bartonella henselae* infection (Chap. 160). Oropharyngeal tularemia can resemble and must be differentiated from pharyngitis due to other bacteria or viruses. Pulmonary tularemia may resemble any atypical pneumonia. Typhoidal tularemia and tularemia meningitis may resemble a variety of other infections.

■ LABORATORY DIAGNOSIS

The diagnosis of tularemia is most frequently confirmed by agglutination testing. Microagglutination and tube agglutination are the techniques most commonly used to detect antibody to *F. tularensis*. In the standard tube agglutination test, a single titer of ≥1:160 is interpreted as a presumptive positive result. A fourfold increase in titer between paired serum samples collected 2–3 weeks apart is considered diagnostic. False-negative serologic responses are obtained early in infection; up to 30% of patients infected for 3 weeks have sera that test negative. Late in infection, titers into the thousands are common, and titers of 1:20–1:80 may persist for years. Enzyme-linked immunosorbent assays have proved useful for the detection of both antibodies and antigens.

Culture and isolation of *F. tularensis* are difficult. In one study, the organism was isolated in only 10% of more than 1000 human cases, 84% of which were confirmed by serology. The medium of choice is cysteine-glucose-blood agar. *F. tularensis* can be isolated directly from infected ulcer scrapings, lymph-node biopsy specimens, gastric washings, sputum, and blood cultures. Colonies are blue-gray, round, smooth, and slightly mucoid. On media containing blood, a small zone of α hemolysis usually surrounds the colony. Slide agglutination tests or direct fluorescent antibody tests with commercially available antisera can be applied directly to culture suspensions for identification. Most clinical laboratories will not attempt to culture *F. tularensis* because of the infectivity of the organism from the culture media and the consequent risk of a laboratory-acquired infection. Although tularemia is not spread from person to person, the organism can be inhaled from culture

TABLE 158-3 Tularemia: Differential Diagnosis, by Clinical Disease Category

Glandular	Oropharyngeal	Typhoidal	Pulmonary
Pyogenic bacterial infection[a]	Group A streptococcal pharyngitis	Typhoid fever	Mycoplasma pneumoniae pneumonia
Nontuberculous mycobacterial infection	Arcanobacterium haemolyticum pharyngitis	Other Salmonella bacteremias	Chlamydia pneumoniae pneumonia
Sporotrichosis	Diphtheria	Rocky Mountain spotted fever	
Tuberculosis	Infectious mononucleosis	Human monocytotropic ehrlichiosis	Psittacosis
Syphilis	Various viral infections[b]	Human granulocytotropic anaplasmosis	Legionella pneumophila pneumonia
Anthrax		Infectious mononucleosis	Q fever
Rat-bite fever		Brucellosis	Histoplasmosis
Scrub typhus		Toxoplasmosis	Blastomycosis
Plague		Tuberculosis	Coccidioidomycosis
Lymphogranuloma venereum		Sarcoidosis	Various viral infections[d]
Cat-scratch disease		Malignancy[c]	

[a] Staphylococcus aureus, Streptococcus pyogenes.
[b] Adenovirus, enteroviruses, parainfluenza virus, influenza virus A and B, respiratory syncytial virus.
[c] Hematologic and reticuloendothelial malignancies.
[d] Influenza virus A and B, parainfluenza virus, respiratory syncytial virus, adenovirus, enteroviruses, hantavirus.

plates and infect unsuspecting laboratory workers. In most clinical laboratories, biosafety level 2 practices are recommended to handle clinical specimens thought to contain *F. tularensis*; however, biosafety level 3 conditions are required for procedures that produce aerosols or droplets during manipulation of cultures containing or possibly containing this organism.

A variety of polymerase chain reaction (PCR) methods have been used to detect *F. tularensis* DNA in many clinical specimens but mostly in ulceroglandular disease.. The majority of these methods target the genes encoding the outer-membrane proteins (e.g., *fopA* or *tul4*). A 16S rDNA sequence identification PCR may be helpful when the patient's clinical information does not lead the clinician to suspect a diagnosis of tularemia.

TREATMENT   Tularemia

Only aminoglycosides, tetracyclines, chloramphenicol, and rifampin are currently approved by the U.S. Food and Drug Administration for the treatment of tularemia. Gentamicin is considered the drug of choice for both adults and children. The dosage for adults is 5 mg/kg daily in two divided doses. The dosage for children is 2.5 mg/kg three times daily or 5 mg/kg twice daily. Gentamicin therapy is typically continued for 7–10 days; however, in mild to moderate cases of tularemia in which the patient becomes afebrile within the first 48–72 h of gentamicin treatment, a 5- to 7-day course has been successful.

If available, streptomycin given intramuscularly is also effective. The dosage for adults is 2 g/d in two divided doses. For children, the dosage is 30 mg/kg daily in two divided doses (maximal daily dose, 2 g). After a clinical response is demonstrated at 3–5 days, the dosage for children can be reduced to 10–15 mg/kg daily in two divided doses. The total duration of streptomycin therapy in both adults and children is usually 10 days. Unlike streptomycin and gentamicin, tobramycin is ineffective in the treatment of tularemia and should not be used.

Since doxycycline is bacteriostatic against *F. tularensis*, there is a risk of relapse if the patient is not treated for a long enough period. Therefore, if doxycycline is used, it should be given for at least 14 days. The lack of availability of chloramphenicol limits the utility of this agent as a viable treatment option. Fluoroquinolones—specifically, ciprofloxacin and levofloxacin—have been used with good outcomes to treat infections caused by subspecies *holarctica*, which is most often found in Europe. The lack of data on the efficacy of these agents against subspecies *tularensis* limits their use in North America at this time.

F. tularensis cannot be subjected to standardized antimicrobial susceptibility testing because the organism will not grow on the media used. A wide variety of antibiotics, including all β-lactam antibiotics and the newer cephalosporins, are ineffective for the treatment of tularemia. Several studies indicated that third-generation cephalosporins were active against *F. tularensis* in vitro, but clinical case reports suggested a nearly universal failure rate of ceftriaxone in pediatric patients with tularemia. Although in vitro data indicate that imipenem may be active, therapy with imipenem, sulfanilamides, and macrolides is not presently recommended because of the lack of relevant clinical data.

Virtually all strains of *F. tularensis* are susceptible to streptomycin and gentamicin. In successfully treated patients, defervescence usually occurs within 2 days, but skin lesions and lymph nodes may take 1–2 weeks to heal. When therapy is not initiated within the first several days of illness, defervescence may be delayed. Relapses are uncommon with streptomycin or gentamicin therapy. Late lymph-node suppuration, however, occurs in ~40% of children, regardless of the treatment received. These nodes have typically been found to contain sterile necrotic tissue without evidence of active infection. Patients with fluctuant nodes should receive several days of antibiotic therapy before drainage to minimize the risk to hospital personnel.

■ PROGNOSIS

If tularemia goes untreated, symptoms usually last 1–4 weeks but may continue for months. The mortality rate from severe untreated infection (including all cases of untreated pulmonary and typhoidal tularemia) can be as high as 30%. However, the overall mortality rate for untreated tularemia is <8%. With appropriate treatment, the mortality rate is <1%. Poor outcomes are often associated with long delays in diagnosis and treatment. Lifelong immunity usually follows tularemia.

■ PREVENTION

The prevention of tularemia is based on avoidance of exposure to biting and blood-sucking insects, especially ticks and deerflies. A wide range of approaches to vaccine development are being evaluated, but no vaccine against tularemia is yet licensed. Prophylaxis of tularemia has not proved effective in patients with embedded ticks or insect bites. However, in patients who are known to have been exposed to large quantities of organisms (e.g., in the laboratory) and who have incubating infection with *F. tularensis*, early treatment can prevent the development of significant clinical disease.

FURTHER READINGS

BARNS SM et al: Detection of diverse new *Francisella*-like bacteria in environmental samples. Appl Environ Microbiol 71:5494, 2005

CENTERS FOR DISEASE CONTROL AND PREVENTION: Tularemia—Missouri, 2000–2007. MMWR Morb Mortal Wkly Rep 58:744, 2009

ELIASSON H et al: The 2000 tularemia outbreak: A case-control study of risk factors in disease-endemic and emergent areas, Sweden. Emerg Infect Dis 8:956, 2002

HOFINGER DM et al: Tularemic meningitis in the United States. Arch Neurol 66:523, 2009

IKÄHEIMO I et al: In vitro antibiotic susceptibility of *Francisella tularensis* isolated from humans and animals. J Antimicrob Chemother 46:287, 2000

JOHANSSON A et al: In vitro susceptibility to quinolones of *Francisella tularensis* subspecies *tularensis*. Scand J Infect Dis 34:327, 2002

JOUNIO U et al: An outbreak of holarctica-type tularemia in pediatric patients. Pediatr Infect Dis J 29:160, 2010

KIRIMANJESWARA GS et al: Humoral and cell-mediated immunity to the intracellular pathogen *Francisella tularensis*. Immunol Rev 225:244, 2008

OYSTON PCF et al: Tularaemia: Bioterrorism defense renews interest in *Francisella tularensis*. Nat Rev Microbiol 2:967, 2004

SJOSTEDT A: Tularemia: History, epidemiology, pathogen physiology, and clinical manifestations. Ann NY Acad Sci 1105:1, 2007

STAPLES JE et al: Epidemiology and molecular analysis of human tularemia, United States, 1964–2004. Emerg Infect Dis 12:1113, 2006

TÄRVNIK A et al: New approaches to diagnosis and therapy of tularemia. Ann NY Acad Sci 1105:378, 2007

CHAPTER 159

Plague and Other *Yersinia* Infections

Michael B. Prentice

PLAGUE

Plague is a systemic zoonosis caused by *Yersinia pestis*. It predominantly affects small rodents in rural areas of Africa, Asia, and the Americas and is usually transmitted to humans by an arthropod vector (the flea). Less often, infection follows contact with animal tissues or respiratory droplets. Plague is an acute febrile illness that is treatable with antimicrobial agents, but mortality rates among untreated patients are high. Patients can present with the bubonic, septicemic, or pneumonic form of the disease. Although there is concern among the general public about epidemic spread of plague by the respiratory route, this is not the usual route of plague transmission, and established infection-control measures for respiratory plague exist. However, the fatalities associated with plague and the capacity for infection via the respiratory tract mean that *Y. pestis* fits the profile of a potential agent of bioterrorism. Consequently, measures have been taken to restrict access to the organism, including legislation affecting diagnostic and research procedures in some countries (e.g., the United States).

■ ETIOLOGY

The genus *Yersinia* comprises gram-negative bacteria of the family Enterobacteriaceae (gamma proteobacteria). Overwhelming taxonomic evidence showing *Y. pestis* strains as a clonal group within *Y. pseudotuberculosis* suggests recent evolution from the latter organism—an enteric pathogen of mammals that is spread by the fecal-oral route and thus has a phenotype distinctly different from that of *Y. pestis*. When grown in vivo or at 37°C, *Y. pestis* forms an amorphous capsule made from a plasmid-specified fimbrial protein, Caf or fraction 1 (F1) antigen, which is an immunodiagnostic marker of infection.

■ EPIDEMIOLOGY

Human plague generally follows an outbreak in a host rodent population (epizootic). Mass deaths among the rodent primary hosts lead to a search by fleas for new hosts, with consequent incidental infection of other mammals. The precipitating cause for an epizootic may ultimately be related to climate or other environmental factors. The reservoir for *Y. pestis* causing enzootic plague in natural endemic foci between epizootics (i.e., when the organism may be difficult to detect in rodents or fleas) is a topic of ongoing research and may not be the same in all regions. The enzootic/epizootic pattern may be the result of complex dynamic interactions of host rodents that have different plague susceptibilities and different flea vectors; alternatively, an environmental reservoir may be important.

■ GLOBAL FEATURES

In general, the enzootic areas for plague are lightly populated regions of Asia, Africa, and the Americas (Fig. 159-1). Between 1989 and 2003, 38,359 cases of plague were reported to the World Health Organization (WHO) under the International Health Regulations then in force, which required national authorities to report all cases of plague in their jurisdiction and according to which plague was one of just three infectious diseases to be so reported. More than 80% of these cases were in Africa, and the percentage of all cases in Africa increased over this period; the majority of cases were reported from East Africa and the island of Madagascar. In 2007, the second edition of the International Health Regulations came into force, widening reporting to any disease event that could have a serious public health impact or could rapidly spread internationally. For plague, this requirement entails specific reporting of pneumonic plague or any suspected case of plague in an area not known to be endemic for plague. Recent

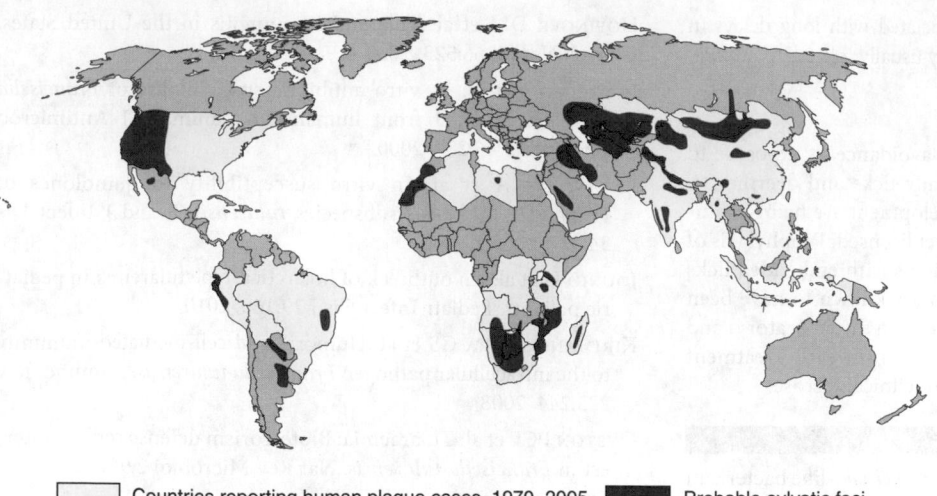

Countries reporting human plague cases, 1970–2005 ▮ Probable sylvatic foci

Figure 159-1   Approximate global distribution of *Yersinia pestis*. *(Compiled from WHO, CDC, and country sources. Reprinted with permission from DT Dennis, GL Campbell: Plague and other Yersinia infections, in Harrison's Principles of Internal Medicine, 17th ed, AS Fauci et al (eds). New York, McGraw-Hill, Chap. 152, 2008.)*

outbreaks of pneumonic plague have been recorded in Uganda, the Democratic Republic of the Congo, and China.

Plague was introduced into North America via the port of San Francisco in 1900 as part of the Third Pandemic, which spread around the world from Hong Kong. The disease is presently enzootic on the western side of the continent from southwestern Canada to Mexico. Most human cases in the United States occur in two regions: "Four Corners" (the junction point of New Mexico, Arizona, Colorado, and Utah), especially northern New Mexico, northern Arizona, and southern Colorado; and further west in California, southern Oregon, and western Nevada *(http://www.cdc. gov/ncidod/dvbid/plague/epi.htm)*. From 1990 to 2005, 107 cases of plague were reported in the United States, with a median of seven cases per year. Most cases occurred from May to October—the time of year when people are outdoors and rodents and their fleas are most plentiful. Infection is most often acquired by fleabite in peridomestic environments. Infection can also occur through the handling of living or dead small mammals (e.g., rabbits, hares, and prairie dogs) or wild carnivores (e.g., wildcats, coyotes, or mountain lions). Dogs and cats may bring plague-infected fleas into the home, and infected cats may transmit plague directly to humans by the respiratory route. The last recorded case of person-to-person transmission in the United States occurred in 1925.

Plague most often develops in areas with poor sanitary conditions and infestations of rats—in particular, the widely distributed roof rat *Rattus rattus* and the brown rat *R. norvegicus* (which serves as a laboratory model of plague). Rat control in warehouses and shipping facilities has been recognized as important in preventing the spread of plague since the early twentieth century and features in the current WHO International Health Regulations. Urban rodents acquire infection from wild rodents, and the proximity of the former to humans increases the risk of transmission. The oriental rat flea *Xenopsylla cheopis* is the most efficient vector for transmission of plague among rats and onward to humans in Asia, Africa, and South America.

Worldwide, bubonic plague is the predominant form reported (80–95% of suspected cases), with mortality rates of 10–20%. The mortality rate is higher (22%) in the small proportion of patients (10–20%) with primary septicemic plague (i.e., systemic *Y. pestis* sepsis with no bubo; see "Clinical Manifestations," below) and is highest with primary pulmonary plague; in this, the least common of the main plague presentations, mortality rate approaches 100% without antimicrobial treatment and is >50% even with such

treatment. Rare outbreaks of pharyngeal plague following consumption of raw or undercooked camel or goat meat have been reported.

A total of 81 (76%) of the 107 plague cases reported in the United States from 1990 to 2005 were primary bubonic disease, 19 (18%) were primary septicemic disease, and 5 (5%) were primary pneumonic disease; 2 cases (2%) were not classified. Eleven cases (10%) were fatal.

■ PATHOGENESIS

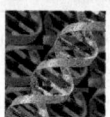

As mentioned earlier, genetic evidence suggests that *Y. pestis* is a clone derived from the enteric pathogen *Y. pseudotuberculosis* in the recent evolutionary past (9000–40,000 years ago). The change from infection by the fecal-oral route to a two-stage life cycle, with alternate parasitization of arthropod and mammalian hosts, followed the acquisition of two plasmids—pFra and pPst—in conjunction with some adaptation of preexisting properties of the *Y. pseudotuberculosis* ancestor, including the presence of a third plasmid, pYV. In the arthropod-parasitizing portion of its life cycle, *Y. pestis* multiplies and forms biofilm-embedded aggregates in the flea midgut after ingestion of a blood meal containing bacteria. In some fleas, biofilm-embedded bacteria eventually fill the proventriculus (a valve connecting the esophagus to the midgut) and block normal blood feeding. "Blocked" fleas die within a few days but in the interim make persistent efforts to feed, regurgitating esophageal contents and inoculating *Y. pestis* into each bite site. The ability of *Y. pestis* to colonize and multiply in the flea requires phospholipase D encoded by the *ymt* gene on the pFra plasmid, and biofilm synthesis requires the chromosomal *hms* locus shared with *Y. pseudotuberculosis*. Blockage takes days or weeks to come about after initial infection of the flea and is followed by the flea's death. Historically, blockage was thought to be required for efficient transmission, but many flea vectors (including *X. cheopis*) are, in fact, able to transmit plague in an early unblocked state or without blockage.

Y. pestis disseminates from the site of inoculation in the mammalian host in a process initially dependent on plasminogen activator Pla, which is encoded by the small pPst plasmid. This surface protease activates mammalian plasminogen, degrades complement, and adheres to the extracellular matrix component laminin. Pla is essential for the high-level virulence of *Y. pestis* in mice given an inoculum by subcutaneous or intradermal injection (laboratory proxies for fleabites) and for the development of primary pneumonic plague. When actual fleabite inoculation is used in mouse models, the fimbrial capsule-forming protein (Ca1 or fraction 1; F1 antigen) encoded on pFra increases the efficiency of transmission, and plasminogen activator is required for the formation of buboes. Because the antiphagocytic systems in *Y. pestis* are not fully operational at the time of inoculation into the mammalian host, the organism is taken up by macrophages from the inoculation site and transported to regional lymph nodes. After intracellular replication, *Y. pestis* switches to extracellular replication with full expression of its antiphagocytic systems: the type III secretion machines and their effectors encoded by pYV as well as the F1 capsule. Overproduction of the type III secretion substrate and translocation protein LcrV exerts an anti-inflammatory effect, reducing host immune responses.

Likewise, *Y. pestis* lipopolysaccharide is modified to minimize stimulation of host Toll-like receptor 4, thereby reducing protective host inflammatory responses during peripheral infection and prolonging host survival with high-grade bacteremia—an effect that probably enhances the pathogen's subsequent transmission by fleabite.

Replication of *Y. pestis* in a regional lymph node results in the local swelling of the lymph node and periglandular region known as a *bubo*. On histology, the node is found to be hemorrhagic or necrotic, with thrombosed blood vessels, and the lymphoid cells and normal architecture are replaced by large numbers of bacteria and fibrin. Periglandular tissues are inflamed and also contain large numbers of bacteria in a serosanguineous, gelatinous exudate.

Continued spread through the lymphatic vessels to contiguous lymph nodes produces second-order primary buboes. Infection is initially contained in the infected regional lymph nodes, although transient bacteremia can be detected. As the infection progresses, spread via efferent lymphatics to the thoracic duct produces high-grade bacteremia. Hematogenous spread to the spleen, liver, and secondary buboes follows, with subsequent uncontrolled septicemia, endotoxic shock, and disseminated intravascular coagulation leading to death. In some patients, this septicemic phase occurs without obvious prior bubo development or lung disease (septicemic plague). Hematogenous spread to the lungs results in secondary plague pneumonia, with bacteria initially more prominent in the interstitium than in the air spaces (the reverse being the case in primary plague pneumonia). Hematogenous spread to other organs, including the meninges, can occur.

CLINICAL MANIFESTATIONS

Bubonic plague

After an incubation period of 2–6 days, the onset of bubonic plague is sudden and is characterized by fever (>38°C), malaise, myalgia, dizziness, and increasing pain due to progressive lymphadenitis in the regional lymph nodes near the fleabite or other inoculation site. Lymphadenitis manifests as a tense, tender swelling (bubo) that, when palpated, has a boggy consistency with an underlying hard core. Generally, there is one painful and erythematous bubo with surrounding periganglionic edema. The bubo is most commonly inguinal but can also be crural, axillary (Fig. 159-2), cervical, or submaxillary, depending on the site of the bite. Abdominal pain from intraabdominal node involvement can occur without other visible signs. Children are most likely to present with cervical or axillary buboes.

The differential diagnosis includes acute focal lymphadenopathy of other etiologies, such as streptococcal or staphylococcal infection, tularemia, cat-scratch disease, tick typhus, infectious mononucleosis, or lymphatic filariasis. These infections do not progress as rapidly, are not as painful, and are associated with visible cellulitis or ascending lymphangitis—both of which are absent in plague.

Without treatment, *Y. pestis* dissemination occurs and causes serious illness, including pneumonia (secondary pneumonic plague) and meningitis. Secondary pneumonic plague can be the source of person-to-person transmission of respiratory infection by productive cough (droplet infection), with the consequent development of primary plague pneumonia. Appropriate treatment of bubonic plague results in fever resolution within 2–5 days, but buboes may remain enlarged for >1 week after initial treatment and can become fluctuant.

Primary septicemic plague

A minority (10–25%) of infections with *Y. pestis* present as gram-negative septicemia (hypotension, shock) without preceding lymphadenopathy. Septicemic plague occurs in all age groups, but persons older than age 40 years are at elevated risk. The term *septicemic plague* can be confusing since most patients with buboes have

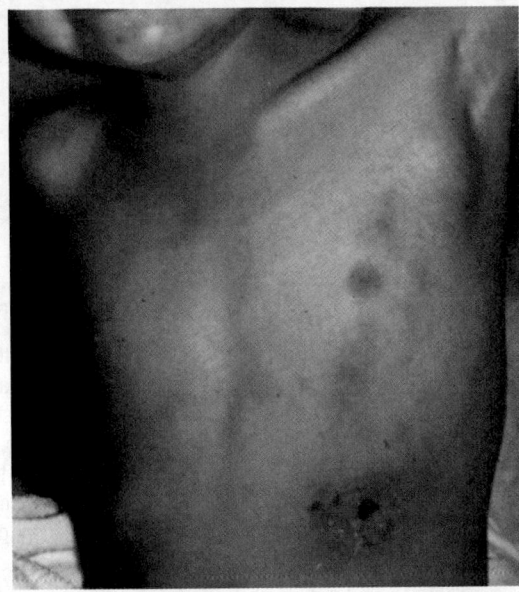

Figure 159-2   Plague patient in the southwestern United States with a left axillary bubo and an unusual plague ulcer and eschar at the site of the infective flea bite. *(Reprinted with permission from DT Dennis, GL Campbell: Plague and other Yersinia infections, in Harrison's Principles of Internal Medicine, 17th ed, AS Fauci et al (eds). New York, McGraw-Hill, Chap. 152, 2008.)*

detectable bacteremia at some stage, with or without systemic signs of sepsis. In laboratory experiments, however, septicemic disease without histologic changes in lymph nodes is seen in a minority of mice infected via fleabites.

Pneumonic plague

Primary pneumonic plague results from inhalation of infectious bacteria in droplets expelled from another person or an animal with primary or secondary plague pneumonia. This syndrome has a short incubation period, averaging from a few hours to 2–3 days (range, 1–7 days), and is characterized by a sudden onset of fever, headache, myalgia, weakness, nausea, vomiting, and dizziness. Respiratory signs—cough, dyspnea, chest pain, and sputum production with hemoptysis—typically arise after 24 h. Progression of initial segmental pneumonitis to lobar pneumonia and then to bilateral lung involvement may occur (Fig. 159-3). The possible release of aerosolized *Y. pestis* bacteria in a bioterrorist attack, manifesting as an outbreak of primary pneumonic plague in nonendemic regions or in an urban setting where plague is rarely seen, has been a source of public health concern. Secondary pneumonic plague is a consequence of bacteremia occurring in ~10–15% of patients with bubonic plague. Bilateral alveolar infiltrates are seen on chest X-ray, and diffuse interstitial pneumonitis with scanty sputum production is typical.

Meningitis

Meningeal plague is uncommon, occurring in ≤6% of plague cases reported in the United States. Presentation with headache and fever typically occurs >1 week after the onset of bubonic or septicemic plague and may be associated with suboptimal antimicrobial therapy (delayed therapy, penicillin administration, or low-dose tetracycline treatment) and cervical or axillary buboes.

Pharyngitis

Symptomatic plague pharyngitis can follow the consumption of contaminated meat from an animal dying of plague or contact with persons or animals with pneumonic plague. This condition can resemble tonsillitis, with peritonsillar abscess and cervical lymphadenopathy.

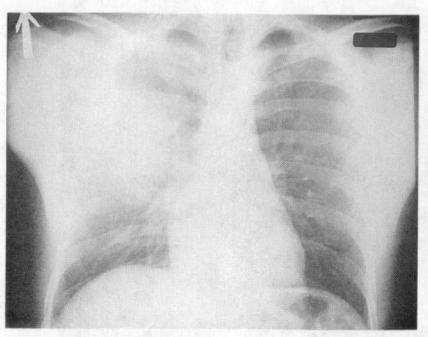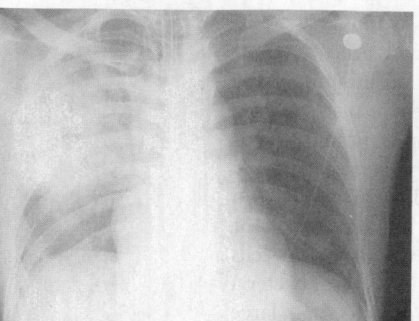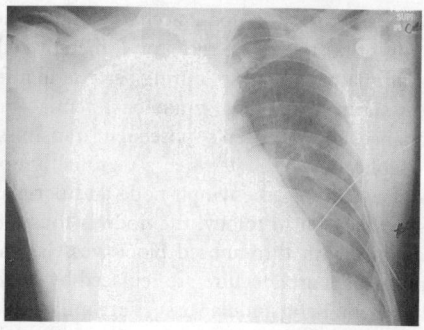

Figure 159-3 Sequential chest radiographs of a patient with fatal primary plague pneumonia. *Left:* Upright posteroanterior film taken at admission to hospital emergency department on third day of illness, showing segmental consolidation of right upper lobe. ***Center:*** Portable anteroposterior film taken 8 h after admission, showing extension of pneumonia to right middle and right lower lobes. ***Right:*** Portable anteroposterior film taken 13 h after admission (when patient had clinical adult respiratory distress syndrome), showing diffuse infiltration throughout right lung and patchy infiltration of left lower lung. A cavity later developed at the site of initial right-upper-lobe consolidation. *(Reprinted with permission from DT Dennis, GL Campbell: Plague and other Yersinia infections, in Harrison's Principles of Internal Medicine, 17th ed. AS Fauci et al (eds). New York, McGraw-Hill, Chap. 152, 2008.)*

Asymptomatic pharyngeal carriage of *Y. pestis* can also occur in close contacts of patients with pneumonic plague.

■ LABORATORY DIAGNOSIS

Because of the scarcity of laboratory facilities in regions where human *Y. pestis* infection is most common, and because of the potential significance of *Y. pestis* isolation in a nonendemic area or an area from which human plague has been absent for many years, the WHO recommends an initial presumptive diagnosis followed by reference laboratory confirmation (Table 159-1). In the United States, comprehensive national diagnostic facilities for plague have been in place since a federal Laboratory Response Network (LRN; *www.bt.cdc.gov/lrn/*) was set up in 1999 to detect possible use of biological terrorism agents, including *Y. pestis*. Routine diagnostic clinical microbiology laboratories that are included in this network as sentinel-level laboratories use joint protocols from the Centers for Disease Control and Prevention (CDC) and the American Society for Microbiology to identify suspected *Y. pestis* isolates and to refer these specimens to LRN reference laboratories for confirmatory tests. *Y. pestis* is designated a "select agent" under the Public Health Security and Bioterrorism Preparedness and Response Act of 2002; the provisions of this act and of the Patriot Act of 2001 apply to all U.S. laboratories and individuals working with *Y. pestis*. Details of the applicable regulations are available from the CDC.

Yersinia species are gram-negative coccobacilli (short rods with rounded ends) 1–3 μm in length and 0.5–0.8 μm in diameter. *Y. pestis* in particular appears bipolar (with a "closed safety pin" appearance) and pleomorphic when stained with a polychromatic stain (Wayson or Wright-Giemsa; Fig. 159-4). Its lack of motility distinguishes *Y. pestis* from other *Yersinia* species, which are motile at 25°C and nonmotile at 37°C. Transport medium (e.g., Cary-Blair medium) preserves the viability of *Y. pestis* if transport is delayed.

The appropriate specimens for diagnosis of bubonic, pneumonic, and septicemic plague are bubo aspirate, bronchoalveolar lavage fluid or sputum, and blood, respectively. Culture of postmortem organ biopsy samples can also be diagnostic. A bubo aspirate is obtained by injection of 1 mL of sterile normal saline into a bubo under local anesthetic and aspiration of a small amount of (usually blood-stained) fluid. Gram's staining of these specimens may reveal gram-negative rods, which are shown by Wayson or Wright-Giemsa staining to be bipolar. These bacteria may even be visible in direct blood smears in septicemic plague (Fig. 159-4); this finding indicates very high numbers of circulating bacteria and a poor prognosis.

Y. pestis grows on nutrient agar and other standard laboratory media but forms smaller colonies than do other Enterobacteriaceae. Specimens should be inoculated onto nutrient-rich media such as sheep blood agar (SBA), into nutrient-rich broth such as brain-heart infusion broth, and onto selective agar such as MacConkey or eosin methylene blue (EMB) agar. *Yersinia*-specific CIN [cefsulodin, triclosan (Irgasan), novobiocin] agar can be useful for culture of contaminated specimens, such as sputum. Blood should be cultured in a standard blood culture system. The optimal growth temperature is <37°C (25–29°C), with pinpoint colonies only on SBA at 24 h. Slower growth occurs at 37°C. *Y. pestis* is oxidase-negative, catalase-positive, urea-negative, indole-negative, and lactose-negative. Automated biochemical identification systems can misidentify *Y. pestis* as *Y. pseudotuberculosis* or other bacterial species.

Reference laboratory tests for definitive identification of isolates include direct immunofluorescence for F1 antigen; specific polymerase chain reaction (PCR) for targets such as F1 antigen, the pesticin gene, and the plasminogen activator gene; and specific bacteriophage lysis. PCR can also be applied to diagnostic specimens, as can direct immunofluorescence for F1 antigen (produced in large amounts by *Y. pestis*) by slide microscopy. An immunochromatographic test strip for F1 antigen detection by monoclonal antibodies in clinical specimens has been devised in Madagascar. This method is effective for both laboratory and near-patient use but is not yet commercially available. Several other rapid diagnostic kits for possible bioterrorism pathogens, including *Y. pestis*, have been described in recent years, but none is widely used for primary or reference laboratory identification.

In the absence of other positive laboratory diagnostic tests, a retrospective serologic diagnosis may be made on the basis of rising titers of hemagglutinating antibody to F1 antigen. Enzyme-linked immunosorbent assays (ELISAs) for IgG and IgM antibodies to F1 antigen are also available.

The white blood cell (WBC) count is generally raised (to 10,000–20,000/μL) in plague, with neutrophilic leukocytosis and a left shift (numerous immature neutrophils); in some cases, however, the WBC count is normal or leukopenia develops. WBC counts are occasionally very high, especially in children (>100,000/μL). Levels of fibrinogen degradation products are elevated in a majority of patients, but platelet counts are usually normal or low-normal. However, disseminated intravascular coagulation, with low platelet counts, prolonged prothrombin times, reduced fibrinogen, and elevated fibrinogen degradation product levels, occurs in a significant minority of patients.

TABLE 159-1 World Health Organization Case Definitions of Plague

Suspected case	Compatible clinical presentation *and* Consistent epidemiologic features, such as exposure to infected animals or humans and/or evidence of fleabites and/or residence in or travel to a known endemic focus within the previous 10 days
Presumptive case	Meeting the definition of a suspected case *plus*: **Putative new or reemerging focus**: ≥2 of the following tests positive • Microscopy: gram-negative coccobacilli in material from bubo, blood, or sputum; bipolar appearance on Wayson or Wright-Giemsa staining • F1 antigen detected in bubo aspirate, blood, or sputum • A single anti-F1 serology without evidence of previous *Y. pestis* infection or immunization • PCR detection of *Y. pestis* in bubo aspirate, blood, or sputum **Known endemic focus**: ≥1 of the following tests positive • Microscopic evidence of gram-negative or bipolar (Wayson, Wright-Giemsa) coccobacilli from bubo, blood, or sputum sample • A single anti-F1 serology without evidence of previous plague infection or immunization • F1 antigen detected in bubo aspirate, blood, or sputum • PCR detection of *Y. pestis* in bubo aspirate, blood, or sputum
Confirmed case	Meeting the definition of a suspected case *plus*: • Identification of an isolate from a clinical sample as *Y. pestis* (colonial morphology and 2 of the 4 following tests positive: phage lysis of cultures at 20–25°C and 37°C; F1 antigen detection; PCR; *Y. pestis* biochemical profile) *or* • A fourfold rise in anti-F1 antibody titer in paired serum samples *or* • In endemic areas when no other confirmatory test can be performed, a positive rapid diagnostic test with immunochromatography to detect F1 antigen

Source: Interregional Meeting on Prevention and Control of Plague, Antananarivo, Madagascar, 7–11 April 2006 *(www.who.int/entity/csr/resources/publications/WHO_HSE_EPR_2008_3w.pdf).*

TREATMENT ▶ **Plague**

Guidelines for the treatment of plague are given in Table 159-2. A 10-day course of antimicrobial therapy is recommended. Streptomycin has historically been the parenteral treatment of choice for plague and is approved for this indication by the U.S. Food and Drug Administration (FDA). Although not yet approved by the FDA for plague, gentamicin has proven safe

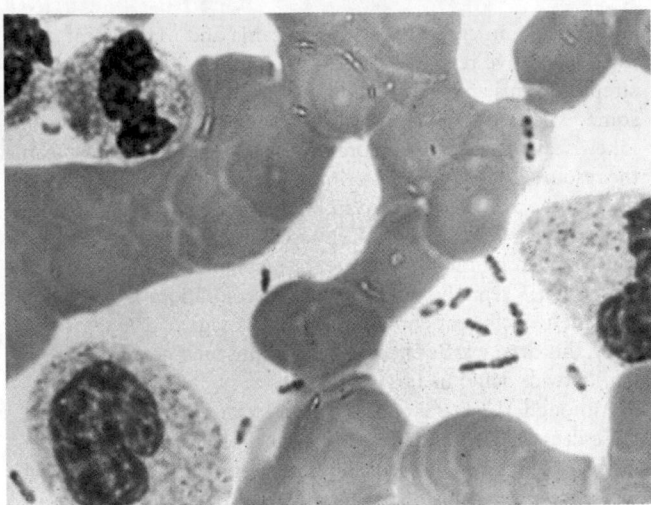

Figure 159-4 Peripheral blood smear from a patient with fatal plague septicemia and shock, showing characteristic bipolar-staining *Yersinia pestis* bacilli (Wright's stain, oil immersion). *(Reprinted with permission from DT Dennis, GL Campbell: Plague and other Yersinia infections, in Harrison's Principles of Internal Medicine, 17th ed, AS Fauci et al (eds). New York, McGraw-Hill, Chap. 152, 2008.)*

TABLE 159-2 Guidelines for the Treatment of Plague

Drug	Daily Dose	Interval, h	Route
Gentamicin			
Adult	5 mg/kg[a]	24	IM/IV
	3–5 mg/kg	8 (2-mg/kg loading dose followed by 1.7 mg/kg tid, then by 1 mg/kg tid as soon as clinically indicated)	IM/IV
Child	5 mg/kg[a]	24	IM/IV
	7.5 mg/kg	8 (2.5 mg/kg tid)	IM/IV
Streptomycin			
Adult	2 g	12	IM
Child	30 mg/kg	12	IM
Doxycycline			
Adult	200 mg	12 or 24	PO/IV
Child ≥8 years	4.4 mg/kg	12 or 24	PO/IV
Tetracycline			
Adult	2 g	6	PO/IV
Child ≥8 years	25–50 mg/kg	6	PO/IV
Chloramphenicol			
Adult	50 mg/kg	6	PO/IV
Child ≥1 year	50 mg/kg	6	PO/IV

[a]The dose must be adjusted in cases of reduced renal function. There are no published trial data for once-daily gentamicin as therapy for plague in adults or children, but this regimen is efficacious in sepsis of other gram-negative etiologies and has been successful in a recent outbreak of pneumonic plague in the Democratic Republic of the Congo. Neonates up to 1 week of age and premature infants should receive 2.5 mg/kg IV bid.
Source: Inglesby et al, 2000.

and effective in clinical trials in Tanzania and Madagascar and in retrospective reviewed cases in the United States. In view of streptomycin's adverse-reaction profile and limited availability, some experts now recommend gentamicin over streptomycin. Likewise, while systemic chloramphenicol therapy is available in the resource-poor countries primarily affected by plague, it is less likely to be available or used in high-income countries because of its adverse-effect profile. Tetracyclines are also effective and can be given by mouth but are not recommended for children under age 7 years because of tooth discoloration. Doxycycline is the tetracycline of choice; at an oral dosage of 100 mg twice daily, this drug was as effective as intramuscular gentamicin (2.5 mg/kg twice daily) in a trial in Tanzania.

Although *Y. pestis* is sensitive to β-lactam drugs in vitro and these drugs have been efficacious against plague in some animal models, the response to penicillins has been poor in some clinical cases; thus β-lactams and macrolides are not generally recommended as first-line therapy. Chloramphenicol, alone or in combination, is recommended for some focal complications of plague (e.g., meningitis, endophthalmitis, myocarditis) because of its tissue penetration properties. Fluoroquinolones, which have been effective in vitro and in animal models, are recommended in guidelines for possible bioterrorism-associated pneumonic plague and are increasingly used in therapy, although the only human efficacy data available so far are from a case report. Animal and in vitro studies suggest that fluoroquinolones at doses used in systemic gram-negative sepsis should be effective as therapy for plague: e.g., ciprofloxacin (400 mg twice daily IV, 500 mg twice daily by mouth), levofloxacin (500 mg/d IV or by mouth), ofloxacin (400 mg twice daily IV or by mouth), or moxifloxacin (400 mg/d IV or by mouth).

■ PREVENTION

In endemic areas, the control of plague in humans is based on reduction of the likelihood of being bitten by infected fleas or exposed to infected droplets from either humans or animals with plague pneumonia. In the United States, residence and outdoor activity in rural areas of western states where epizootics occur are the main risk factors for infection. To assess potential risks to humans in specific areas, surveillance for *Y. pestis* infection among animal plague hosts and vectors is carried out regularly as well as in response to observed animal die-offs. Personal protective measures include avoidance of areas where a plague epizootic has been identified and publicized (e.g., by warning signs or closure of campsites). Sick or dead animals should not be handled by the general public. Hunters and zoologists should wear gloves when handling wild animal carcasses in endemic areas. General measures to avoid rodent fleabite during outdoor activity are appropriate and include the use of insect repellant, insecticide, and protective clothing. General measures to reduce peridomestic and occupational human contact with rodents are advised and include rodent-proofing of buildings and food waste stores and removal of potential rodent habitats (e.g., woodpiles and junk heaps). Flea control by insecticide treatment of wild rodents is an effective means of minimizing human contact with plague if an epizootic is identified in an area close to human habitation. Any attempt to reduce rodent numbers must be preceded by flea suppression to reduce the migration of infected fleas to human hosts.

Patients in whom pneumonic plague is suspected should be managed in isolation, with droplet precautions observed until pneumonia is excluded or effective antimicrobial therapy has been given for 48 h. Review of the literature published before the advent of antimicrobial agents suggests that the main infective risk is posed by patients in the final stages of disease who are coughing up sputum with plentiful visible blood and/or pus. Cotton and

TABLE 159-3 Guidelines for Plague Prophylaxis

Drug	Daily Dose	Interval, h	Route
Doxycycline			
Adult	200 mg	12 or 24	PO
Child ≥8 y	If weight is ≥45 kg, give adult dosage; if <45 kg, give 2.2 mg/kg PO bid (maximum, 200 mg/d)	12	PO
Tetracycline			
Adult	1–2 g	6 or 12	PO
Child ≥8 y	25–50 mg/kg	6 or 12	PO
Ciprofloxacin			
Adult	1 g	12	PO
Child	40 mg/kg	12	PO
Trimethoprim-sulfamethoxazole			
Adult	320 mg[a]	12	PO
Child ≥2 months	8 mg/kg[a]	12	PO

[a]Trimethoprim component.

Source: DT Dennis, GL Campbell: Plague and other *Yersinia* infections, in *Harrison's Principles of Internal Medicine*, 17th ed, AS Fauci et al (eds). New York, McGraw-Hill, Chap. 152, 2008.

gauze masks were protective in these circumstances. Current surgical masks capable of barrier protection against droplets, including large respiratory particles, are considered protective; a particulate respirator (e.g., N95 or greater) is not required.

Antimicrobial prophylaxis

Postexposure antimicrobial prophylaxis lasting 7 days is recommended following household, hospital, or other close contact with persons with untreated pneumonic plague. (*Close contact* is defined as contact with a patient at <2 m.) Doxycycline is probably the first choice for prophylaxis (Table 159-3).

Immunization

Studies with candidate plague vaccines in animal models show that neutralizing antibody provides protection against exposure but that cell-mediated immunity is critical for protection and clearance of *Y. pestis* from the host. A killed whole-cell vaccine used in humans required multiple doses, caused significant local and systemic reactions, and was not protective against pneumonic plague; this vaccine is not currently available in the United States. A live attenuated vaccine based on strain EV76 is still used in countries of the former Soviet Union but has significant side effects. Most research to date has focused on a subunit vaccine of recombinant F1 (rF1) and V (rV) proteins produced in *Escherichia coli*, combined either as a fusion protein or as a mixture, purified, and adsorbed to aluminum hydroxide for injection. This combination protects mice against both bubonic and pneumonic plague and has been evaluated in phase 2 clinical trials. Phase 3 trials are planned, but special ethical considerations with controlled clinical studies involving plague in humans make field efficacy studies unlikely. In the United States, the FDA is therefore prepared to assess this vaccine for human use under the Animal Rule, using efficacy data and other results from animal studies (*www.fda.gov/BiologicsBloodVaccines/*

Future developments may include noninvasive vaccines (with intranasal administration or inhalation of dry powder incorporating these or other antigens) and mucosal delivery of microencapsulated proteins. Other antigens that could be added to this type of subunit vaccine are being investigated. Providing impetus for exploration of these antigens are (1) the recovery of F1-negative *Y. pestis* strains from natural sources and (2) the observation that F1 antigen is not required for virulence in primate models of pneumonic plague.

YERSINIOSIS

Yersiniosis is a zoonotic infection with an enteropathogenic *Yersinia* species, usually *Y. enterocolitica* or *Y. pseudotuberculosis*. The usual hosts for these organisms are pigs and other wild and domestic animals; humans are usually infected by the oral route, and outbreaks from contaminated food occur. Yersiniosis is most common in childhood and in colder climates. Patients present with abdominal pain and sometimes with diarrhea (which may not occur in up to 50% of cases). *Y. enterocolitica* is more closely associated with terminal ileitis and *Y. pseudotuberculosis* with mesenteric adenitis, but both organisms may cause mesenteric adenitis and symptoms of abdominal pain and tenderness that result in pseudoappendicitis, with the surgical removal of a normal appendix. Diagnosis is based on culture of the organism or convalescent serology. *Y. pseudotuberculosis* and some rarer strains of *Y. enterocolitica* are especially likely to cause systemic infection, which is also more likely in patients with diabetes or iron overload. Systemic sepsis is treatable with antimicrobial agents, but postinfective arthropathy responds poorly to such therapy. Ten other *Yersinia* species are now recognized, but all lack the virulence plasmid pYV common to *Y. pestis*, *Y. pseudotuberculosis*, and *Y. enterocolitica* and are generally considered to be, at most, opportunistic pathogens of humans (*Y. aldovae*, *Y. bercovieri*, *Y. frederiksenii*, *Y. intermedia*, *Y. kristensenii*, *Y. massiliensis*, *Y. mollaretii*, *Y. rohdei*, *Y. similis*, and *Y. ruckeri*).

■ EPIDEMIOLOGY

Y. enterocolitica

Y. enterocolitica is found worldwide and has been isolated from a wide variety of wild and domestic animals and environmental samples, including samples of food and water. Strains are differentiated by combined biochemical reactions (biovar) and serogroup. Most clinical infections are associated with serogroups O:3, O:9, and O:5,27, with a declining number of O:8 infections in North America. Yersiniosis, mostly due to *Y. enterocolitica*, is the third commonest zoonosis reported in Europe; most reports come from northern Europe, especially Germany and Scandinavia. The incidence is highest among children; children under the age of 4 years are more likely to present with diarrhea than are older children. Abdominal pain with mesenteric adenitis and terminal ileitis is more prominent among older children and adults. Septicemia is more likely in patients with preexisting conditions such as diabetes mellitus, liver disease, any condition involving iron overload (including thalassemia and hemochromatosis), advanced age, malignancy, or HIV/AIDS. As in enteritis of other bacterial etiologies, postinfective complications such as reactive arthritis occur mainly in individuals who are HLA-B27 positive. Erythema nodosum (Fig. e7-40) following *Yersinia* infection is not associated with HLA-B27 and is more common among women than among men.

Consumption or preparation of raw pork products (such as chitterlings) and some processed pork products is strongly linked with infection because a high percentage of pigs carry pathogenic *Y. enterocolitica* strains. Outbreaks of *Y. enterocolitica* infection have been associated with consumption of milk (pasteurized, unpasteurized, and chocolate-flavored) and various foods contaminated with

springwater. Person-to-person transmission is suspected in a few cases (e.g., in nosocomial and familial outbreaks) but is much less likely with *Y. enterocolitica* than with other causes of gastrointestinal infection, such as *Salmonella*. A multivariate analysis indicates that contact with companion animals is a risk factor for *Y. enterocolitica* infection among children in Sweden, and low-level colonization of dogs and cats with *Y. enterocolitica* has been reported. Transfusion-associated septicemia due to *Y. enterocolitica*, while recognized as a rare but frequently fatal event for nearly 30 years, has been difficult to eradicate.

Y. pseudotuberculosis

Y. pseudotuberculosis is less frequently reported as a cause of human disease than *Y. enterocolitica*, and infection with *Y. pseudotuberculosis* is more likely to present as fever and abdominal pain due to mesenteric lymphadenitis. This organism is associated with wild mammals (rodents, rabbits, and deer), birds, and domestic pigs. Strains are differentiated by combined biochemical reactions (biovar) and serogroup. Although outbreaks are generally rare, several have recently occurred in Finland and have been associated with lettuce and raw carrots.

■ PATHOGENESIS

The usual route of infection is oral. Studies with both *Y. enterocolitica* and *Y. pseudotuberculosis* in animal models suggest that initial replication in the small intestine is followed by invasion of Peyer's patches of the distal ileum via M cells, with onward spread to mesenteric lymph nodes. The liver and spleen can also be involved after oral infection. The characteristic histologic appearance of enteropathogenic *Yersinia* after invasion of host tissues is as extracellular microabscesses surrounded by an epithelioid granulomatous lesion.

Experiments involving oral infection of mice with tagged *Y. enterocolitica* show that only a very small proportion of bacteria in the gut invade tissues. Individual bacterial clones from an orally inoculated pool give rise to each microabscess in a Peyer's patch, and the host restricts the invasion of previously infected Peyer's patches. A prior model positing progressive bacterial spread from Peyer's patches and mesenteric lymph nodes to the liver and spleen appears to be inaccurate: spread of individually tagged clones of *Y. pseudotuberculosis* to the liver and spleen of mice occurs independently of regional lymph node colonization and in mice lacking Peyer's patches.

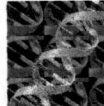 Invasion requires the expression of several nonfimbrial adhesins, such as invasin (Inv) and—in *Y. pseudotuberculosis*—*Yersinia* adhesin A (YadA). Inv interacts directly with $\beta 1$ integrins, which are expressed on the apical surfaces of M cells but not enterocytes. YadA of *Y. pseudotuberculosis* interacts with extracellular matrix proteins such as collagen and fibronectin to facilitate host cell integrin association and invasion. YadA of *Y. enterocolitica* lacks a crucial N-terminal region and binds collagen and laminin but not fibronectin and does not cause invasion. Inv is chromosomally encoded, whereas YadA is encoded on the virulence plasmid pYV. YadA helps to confer serum resistance by binding host complement regulators such as factor H and C4-binding protein. Another chromosomal gene, *ail* (attachment and invasion locus), encodes the extracellular protein Ail, which also confers serum resistance by binding these complement regulators.

By binding to host cell surfaces, YadA allows targeting of immune effector cells by the pYV plasmid–encoded type III secretion system (injectisome). As a consequence, the host's innate immune response is altered; toxins (*Yersinia* outer proteins, or Yops) are injected into host macrophages, neutrophils, and dendritic cells, affecting signal transduction pathways, resulting in reduced phagocytosis and inhibited production of reactive oxygen species by neutrophils, and triggering apoptosis of macrophages. Other factors functional in invasive disease include yersiniabactin (Ybt), a siderophore produced by some strains of *Y. pseudotuberculosis* and *Y. enterocolitica* as well as other Enterobacteriaceae. Yersiniabactin allows bacteria to access iron from saturated lactoferrin during infection and reduces production of reactive oxygen species by innate immune effector cells, thereby decreasing bacterial killing.

■ CLINICAL MANIFESTATIONS

Self-limiting diarrhea is the most common reported presentation in infection with pathogenic *Y. enterocolitica*, especially in children under the age of 4, who form the single largest group in most case series. Blood may be detected in diarrheal stool. Older children and adults are more likely than younger children to present with abdominal pain, which can be localized to the right iliac fossa—a situation that often leads to laparotomy for presumed appendicitis (pseudoappendicitis). Appendectomy is not indicated for *Yersinia* infection causing pseudoappendicitis. Thickening of the terminal ileum and cecum is seen on endoscopy and ultrasound, with elevated round or oval lesions that may overlie Peyer's patches. Mesenteric lymph nodes are enlarged. Ulcerations of the mucosa are noted on endoscopy. Gastrointestinal complications include granulomatous appendicitis, a chronic inflammatory condition affecting the appendix that is responsible for ≤2% of cases of appendicitis; *Yersinia* is involved in a minority of cases. *Y. enterocolitica* infection can present as acute pharyngitis with or without other gastrointestinal symptoms. Fatal *Y. enterocolitica* pharyngitis has been recorded. Mycotic aneurysm can follow *Y. enterocolitica* bacteremia, as can focal infection (abscess) in many other sites and body compartments (liver, spleen, kidney, bone, meninges, endocardium).

In all age groups, *Y. pseudotuberculosis* is more likely to present as abdominal pain and fever than as diarrhea. A superantigenic toxin—*Y. pseudotuberculosis* mitogen (YPM)—is produced by strains seen in eastern Russia in association with Far Eastern scarlet-like fever, a childhood illness with desquamating rash, arthralgia, and toxic shock. A similar illness is recognized in Japan (Izumi fever) and Korea. Similarities have been noted with Kawasaki's disease, the idiopathic acute systematic vasculitis of childhood. There is an epidemiologic link between exposure of populations to superantigen-positive *Y. pseudotuberculosis* and an elevated incidence of Kawasaki's disease.

Y. enterocolitica or *Y. pseudotuberculosis* septicemia presents as a severe illness with fever and leukocytosis, often without localizing features, and is significantly associated with predisposing conditions such as diabetes mellitus, liver disease, and iron overload. Hemochromatosis combines several of these risk factors. Administration of iron chelators like desferrioxamine, which provide iron accessible to *Yersinia* (and have an inhibitory effect on neutrophil function), may result in *Yersinia* septicemia in patients with iron overload who presumably have an otherwise mild gastrointestinal infection. HIV/AIDS has been associated with *Y. pseudotuberculosis* septicemia. The unusual phenomenon of transfusion-associated septicemia is linked to the ability of *Y. enterocolitica* to multiply at refrigerator temperature (psychrotrophy). Typically, the transfused unit has been stored for >20 days, and it is believed that small numbers of yersiniae from an apparently healthy donor with subclinical bacteremia are amplified to very high numbers by growth inside the bag at ≤4°C, with consequent septic shock after transfusion. A method for preventing this very rare event (i.e., a range of 1 case in 500,000 to 1 case in several million transfused units in countries such as the United States and France) without unacceptable restriction in the blood supply has not yet been devised.

■ POSTINFECTIVE PHENOMENA

As in other invasive intestinal infections (salmonellosis, shigellosis), reactive arthritis (articular arthritis of multiple joints developing within 2–4 weeks of a preceding infection) occurs as a result of autoimmune activity initiated by the deposition of bacterial components (not viable bacteria) in joints in combination with the immune response to invading bacteria. The majority of individuals affected by reactive arthritis due to *Yersinia* are HLA-B27 positive. Myocarditis with electrocardiographic ST-segment abnormalities may occur with *Yersinia*-associated reactive arthritis. Most *Yersinia*-associated cases follow *Y. enterocolitica* infection (presumably because it is more common than infection with other species), but *Y. pseudotuberculosis*–associated reactive arthritis is also well documented in Finland, where sporadic and outbreak infections with *Y. pseudotuberculosis* are more common than in other countries. Of infected individuals identified in a recent *Y. pseudotuberculosis* serotype O:3 outbreak in Finland, 12% developed reactive arthritis affecting the small joints of the hands and feet, knees, ankles, and shoulders and lasting >6 months in most cases. Erythema nodosum (Fig. e7-40) occurs after *Yersinia* infection (more commonly in women) with no evidence of HLA-B27 linkage.

There is a long-standing association between antithyroid and anti-*Yersinia* antibodies. Antibody evidence of prior *Y. enterocolitica* infection in Graves' disease and increased levels of antithyroid antibody in patients with *Y. enterocolitica* antibodies were first noted in the 1970s. *Y. enterocolitica* contains a thyroid-stimulating hormone (TSH)–binding site that is recognized by anti-TSH antibodies from Graves' disease patients. Raised titers of antibodies to *Y. enterocolitica* whole cells and Yops have been found in some series of Graves' disease patients but not in others. One Danish study of twins found no evidence of an association between asymptomatic *Yersinia* infection (as evidenced by anti-Yop antibody titers) and antithyroid antibodies in euthyroid individuals, while another Danish study of twins with and without Graves' disease found that increased anti-Yop antibody titers were associated with Graves' disease. It remains unclear whether this cross-reactivity is significant in the etiology of Graves' disease.

■ LABORATORY DIAGNOSIS

Standard laboratory culture methods can be used to isolate enteropathogenic *Yersinia* species from sterile samples, including blood and cerebrospinal fluid. Culture on specific selective media (CIN agar), with or without preenrichment in broth or phosphate-buffered saline at either 4°C or 16°C, is the basis of most schema for isolation of yersiniae from stool or other nonsterile samples. Outside known high-incidence areas, specific culture may be carried out by laboratories only upon request. Virulence plasmid–negative strains of *Y. enterocolitica* can be isolated from cultures of stool from asymptomatic individuals, especially after cold enrichment. These strains usually differ in biotype (typically biovar 1a) from virulence plasmid–possessing strains; although some display apparent pathogenicity in a mouse model, virulence plasmid–negative strains are not commonly accepted as human pathogens. Because of the frequency with which the virulence plasmid is lost on laboratory subculture, combined biochemical identification (with biotyping according to a standard schema) and serologic identification are usually required to interpret the significance of an isolate of *Y. enterocolitica* from a nonsterile site. Most pathogenic *Y. enterocolitica* strains currently isolated from humans are of serogroup O:3/biovar 4 or serogroup O:9/biovar 2; this pattern holds even in the United States, where serogroup O:8/biovar 1B strains were previously predominant. Many self-validated multiplex PCR screens for detection of *Y. enterocolitica* in clinical samples—and rather more for its detection in food—have been described, but none of these assays is widely used outside its originating laboratory. A standard for PCR detection in food samples is being prepared by the International Organization for Standardization.

Agglutinating or ELISA antibody titers to specific O-antigen types are used in the retrospective diagnosis of both *Y. enterocolitica* and *Y. pseudotuberculosis* infections. IgA and IgG antibodies persist in patients with reactive arthritis. Serologic cross-reactions between *Y. enterocolitica* serogroup O:9 and *Brucella* are due to the similarity of their lipopolysaccharide structures. Multiple assays are required to cover even the predominant serogroups (*Y. enterocolitica* O:3, O5,27, and O:9; *Y. pseudotuberculosis* O:1a, O:1b, and O:3), and these assays are generally available only in reference laboratories. ELISA and western blot tests for antibodies to Yops, which are expressed by all pathogenic strains of *Y. enterocolitica* and *Y. pseudotuberculosis*, are also available; most of the positivity in these assays probably relates to previous infection with *Y. enterocolitica*.

| TREATMENT | Yersiniosis |

Most cases of diarrhea caused by enteropathogenic *Yersinia* are self-limiting. Data from clinical trials do not support antimicrobial treatment for adults or children with *Y. enterocolitica* diarrhea. Systemic infections with bacteremia or focal infections outside the gastrointestinal tract generally require antimicrobial therapy. Infants <3 months of age with documented *Y. enterocolitica* infection may require antimicrobial treatment because of the increased likelihood of bacteremia in this age group. *Y. enterocolitica* strains nearly always express β-lactamases. Because of the relative rarity of systemic *Y. enterocolitica* infection, there are no clinical trial data to guide antimicrobial choice or to suggest the optimal dose and duration of therapy. On the basis of retrospective case series and in vitro sensitivity data, fluoroquinolone therapy is effective for bacteremia in adults; for example, ciprofloxacin is given at a typical dose of 500 mg twice daily by mouth or 400 mg twice daily IV for at least 2 weeks (longer if positive blood cultures persist). A third-generation cephalosporin is an alternative—e.g., cefotaxime (typical dose, 6–8 g/d in 3 or 4 divided doses). In children, third-generation cephalosporins are effective; for example, cefotaxime is given to children ≥1month of age at a typical dose of 75–100 mg/kg per day in 3 or 4 divided doses, with an increase to 150–200 mg/kg per day in severe cases (maximal daily dose, 8–10 g). Amoxicillin and amoxicillin/clavulanate have shown poor efficacy in case series. Trimethoprim-sulfamethoxazole, gentamicin, and imipenem are all active in vitro. *Y. pseudotuberculosis* strains do not express β-lactamase but are intrinsically resistant to polymyxin. Because human infection with *Y. pseudotuberculosis* is less common than that with *Y. enterocolitica*, less case information is available; however, studies in mice suggest that ampicillin is ineffective. Drugs similar to those used against *Y. enterocolitica* should be used. The best results have been obtained with a quinolone.

Some trials of treatment for reactive arthritis (with a large proportion of cases due to *Yersinia*) found that 3 months of oral ciprofloxacin therapy did not affect outcome. One trial in which the same therapy was given specifically for *Y. enterocolitica*–reactive arthritis found that, while outcome indeed was not affected, there was a trend toward faster remission of symptoms in the treated group. Follow-up 4–7 years after initial antibiotic treatment of reactive arthritis (predominantly following *Salmonella* and *Yersinia* infections) demonstrated apparent efficacy in the prevention of chronic arthritis in HLA-B27-positive individuals. A trial showing that azithromycin therapy did not affect outcome in reactive arthritis included cases believed to follow yersiniosis, although no breakdown of cases was provided. A Cochrane review evaluating the use of antibiotics for reactive arthritis is in progress.

PREVENTION AND CONTROL

Current control measures are similar to those used against other enteric pathogens like *Salmonella* and *Campylobacter*, which colonize the intestine of food animals. The focus is on safe handling and processing of food. No vaccine is effective in preventing intestinal colonization of food animals by enteropathogenic *Yersinia*. Consumption of food made from raw pork (which is popular in Germany and Belgium) should be discouraged at present because it is not possible to eliminate contamination with the enteropathogenic *Yersinia* strains found worldwide in pigs. Exposure of infants to raw pig intestine during domestic preparation of chitterlings is inadvisable. Modification of abattoir technique in Scandinavian countries from the 1990s onward included the removal of pig intestines in a closed plastic bag; levels of carcass contamination with *Y. enterocolitica* were reduced, but such contamination was not eliminated. Experimental pig herds free of pathogenic *Y. enterocolitica* O:3 (and also of *Salmonella*, *Toxoplasma*, and *Trichinella*) have been established in Norway and may be commercialized in the future because of their enhanced safety. In the food industry, vigilance is required because of the potential for large outbreaks if small numbers of enteropathogenic yersiniae contaminate any ready-to-eat food whose safe preservation is based on refrigeration before consumption.

The rare phenomenon of contamination of blood for transfusion has proved impossible to eradicate. However, leukodepletion is now practiced in most blood transfusion centers, primarily to prevent nonhemolytic febrile transfusion reactions and alloimmunization against HLA antigens. This measure reduces but does not eliminate the risk of *Yersinia* blood contamination.

Notification of yersiniosis is now obligatory in some countries.

FURTHER READINGS

ABDEL-HAQ NM et al: *Yersinia enterocolitica* infection in children. Pediatr Infect Dis J 19:954, 2000

BOQVIST S et al: Sources of sporadic *Yersinia enterocolitica* infection in children in Sweden, 2004: A case-control study. Epidemiol Infect 137:897, 2009

GAGE KL, KOSOY MY: Natural history of plague: Perspectives from more than a century of research. Annu Rev Entomol 50:505, 2005

INGLESBY TV et al: Plague as a biological weapon: Medical and public health management. Working Group on Civilian Biodefense. JAMA 283:2281, 2000

KOOL JL: Risk of person-to-person transmission of pneumonic plague. Clin Infect Dis 40:1166, 2005

LONG C et al: *Yersinia pseudotuberculosis* and *Y. enterocolitica* infections, FoodNet, 1996–2007. Emerg Infect Dis 16:566, 2010

PERDIKOGIANNI C et al: *Yersinia enterocolitica* infection mimicking surgical conditions. Pediatr Surg Int 22:589, 2006

PRENTICE MB, RAHALISON L: Plague. Lancet 369:1196, 2007

WILLIAMSON ED: Plague. Vaccine 27(Suppl 4):D56, 2009

WORLD HEALTH ORGANIZATION: International Meeting on Preventing and Controlling Plague: The old calamity still has a future. Wkly Epidemiol Rec 28:278, 2006

CHAPTER 160

Bartonella Infections, Including Cat-Scratch Disease

Michael Giladi

Moshe Ephros

Bartonella species are fastidious, facultative intracellular, slow-growing, gram-negative bacteria that cause a broad spectrum of diseases in humans. This genus includes at least 27 distinct species or subspecies, of which at least 13 have been recognized as confirmed or potential human pathogens; *B. bacilliformis, B. quintana,* and *B. henselae* are most commonly identified (Table 160-1). Most *Bartonella* species have successfully adapted to survival in specific domestic or wild mammals. Prolonged intraerythrocytic infection in these animals creates a reservoir for human infections. *B. bacilliformis* and *B. quintana,* which are not zoonotic, are exceptions to this rule. Arthropod vectors are often involved. Isolation and characterization of *Bartonella* species are difficult and require special techniques. Clinical presentation generally depends on both the infecting *Bartonella* species and the immune status of the infected individual. *Bartonella* species are susceptible to many antibiotics in vitro; however, clinical responses to therapy and studies in animal models suggest that the minimal inhibitory concentrations of many antimicrobial agents correlate poorly with the drugs' in vivo efficacies in patients with *Bartonella* infections.

CAT-SCRATCH DISEASE

■ DEFINITION AND ETIOLOGY

Usually a self-limited illness, cat-scratch disease (CSD) has two general clinical presentations. *Typical* CSD, the more common, is characterized by subacute regional lymphadenopathy; *atypical* CSD is the collective designation for numerous extranodal manifestations involving various organs. *B. henselae* is the principal etiologic agent of CSD. Rare cases have been associated with *Afipia felis* and *B. quintana; B. clarridgeiae* may occasionally be involved as well.

■ EPIDEMIOLOGY

CSD occurs worldwide, favoring warm and humid climates. In temperate climates, incidence peaks during fall and winter; in the tropics, disease occurs year-round. Adults are affected nearly as frequently as children. Intrafamilial clustering is rare, and person-to-person transmission does not occur. Apparently healthy cats constitute the major reservoir of *B. henselae,* and cat fleas (*Ctenocephalides felis*) may be responsible for cat-to-cat transmission. CSD usually follows contact with cats (especially kittens), but other animals (e.g., dogs) have been implicated as possible reservoirs in rare instances. In the United States, the estimated disease incidence is ~10 cases per 100,000 population. About 10% of patients are hospitalized.

■ PATHOGENESIS

Inoculation of *B. henselae,* possibly via contaminated flea feces, usually results from a cat scratch or bite. Exposure to mucous membranes or conjunctivae via droplets or licking may possibly be

TABLE 160-1 *Bartonella* Species Known or Suspected to Be Human Pathogens

Bartonella Species[a]	Disease	Reservoir Host[b]	Arthropod Vector
B. henselae	Cat-scratch disease, bacillary angiomatosis, bacillary peliosis, bacteremia, endocarditis	Cats, other felines	Cat fleas (*Ctenocephalides felis*): associated with cat-to-cat, but not with cat-to-human, transmission
B. quintana	Trench fever, chronic bacteremia, bacillary angiomatosis, endocarditis	Humans	Human body lice (*Pediculus humanus corporis*)
B. bacilliformis	Bartonellosis (Carrion's disease)	Humans	Sandflies (*Lutzomyia verrucarum*)
B. elizabethae	Endocarditis	Rats, dogs	Unknown
B. grahamii	Retinitis	Mice, voles	Fleas
B. vinsonii subsp. *arupensis*	Endocarditis	Mice	Ticks
B. vinsonii subsp. *berkhoffii*	Endocarditis	Domestic dogs, coyotes, gray foxes	Ticks
B. washoensis	Myocarditis, meningitis	Squirrels, possibly other rodents	Fleas
B. alsatica	Endocarditis	Rabbits	Unknown
B. koehlerae	Endocarditis	Cats	Unknown
B. clarridgeiae	Possibly cat-scratch disease	Cats	Unknown
B. rochalimae	Bacteremia, fever, splenomegaly	Unknown	Possibly fleas
B. tamiae	Bacteremia, fever, myalgia, rash	Unknown	Unknown

[a]Many other *Bartonella* species exist but are not recognized as human pathogens.
[b]Animals are implicated when existing evidence supports their infection with *Bartonella* species. Data supporting animal-to-human transmission may be lacking.

involved as well. With lymphatic drainage to one or more regional lymph nodes in immunocompetent hosts, a T_H1 response can result in necrotizing granulomatous lymphadenitis. Dendritic cells, along with their associated chemokines, play a role in the host inflammatory response and granuloma formation.

■ CLINICAL MANIFESTATIONS AND PROGNOSIS

Of patients with CSD, 85–90% have typical disease. The primary lesion, a small (0.3- to 1-cm) painless erythematous papule or pustule, develops at the inoculation site (usually the site of a scratch or a bite) within days to 2 weeks in about two-thirds of patients (Fig. 160-1 A, B). Lymphadenopathy develops ≥1–3 weeks after cat contact. The affected lymph node(s) are enlarged and usually painful, sometimes have overlying erythema, and suppurate in 10–15% of cases (Fig. 160-1 C, D, and E). Axillary/epitrochlear nodes are most commonly involved; next in frequency are head/neck nodes and then inguinal/femoral nodes. Approximately 50% of patients have fever, malaise, and anorexia. A smaller proportion experience weight loss and night sweats mimicking the presentation of lymphoma. Fever is usually low-grade but infrequently rises to ≥39°C. Resolution is slow, requiring weeks (for fever, pain, and accompanying signs and symptoms) to months (for node shrinkage).

Atypical CSD occurs in 10–15% of patients as extranodal or complicated disease in the absence or presence of lymphadenopathy. Atypical disease includes Parinaud's oculoglandular syndrome (granulomatous conjunctivitis with ipsilateral preauricular lymphadenitis; Fig. 160-1, E), granulomatous hepatitis/splenitis, neuroretinitis (often presenting as unilateral deterioration of vision; Fig. 160-1F), and other ophthalmologic manifestations. In addition, neurologic involvement (encephalopathy, seizures, myelitis, radiculitis, cerebellitis, facial and other cranial or peripheral palsies), fever of unknown origin (FUO), debilitating myalgia, arthritis or arthralgia (affecting mostly women >20 years old), osteomyelitis (including multifocal disease), tendinitis, neuralgia, and dermatologic manifestations [including erythema nodosum (see Fig. e7-40), sometimes accompanying arthropathy] occur. Other manifestations and syndromes [pneumonitis, pleural effusion, idiopathic thrombocytopenic purpura, Henoch-Schönlein purpura, erythema multiforme (see Fig. e7-25), hypercalcemia, glomerulonephritis, myocarditis] have also been associated with CSD. In elderly patients (>60 years old), lymphadenopathy is most often absent, but encephalitis and FUO are more common than in younger patients. In immunocompetent individuals, CSD—whether typical or atypical—usually resolves without treatment and without sequelae. Lifelong immunity is the rule.

■ DIAGNOSIS

Routine laboratory tests usually yield normal or nonspecific results. Histopathology initially shows lymphoid hyperplasia and later demonstrates stellate granulomata with necrosis, coalescing microabscesses, and occasional multinucleated giant cells, findings which, although nonspecific, may narrow the differential diagnosis. Serologic testing (immunofluorescence or enzyme immunoassay) is the most commonly used laboratory diagnostic approach, with variable sensitivity and specificity. Seroconversion may take a few weeks. Other tests are of low sensitivity (culture, Warthin-Starry silver staining), of low specificity (cytology, histopathology), or of limited availability in routine diagnostic laboratories (PCR, immunohistochemistry). PCR of lymph node tissue, pus, or the primary

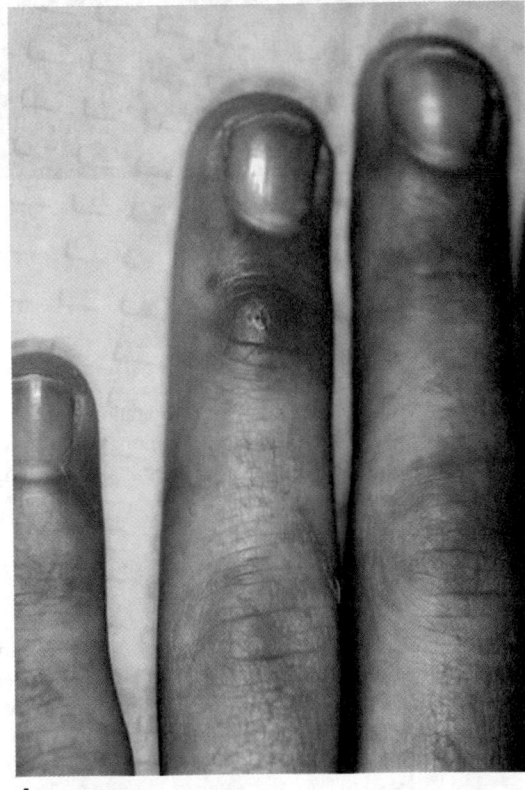

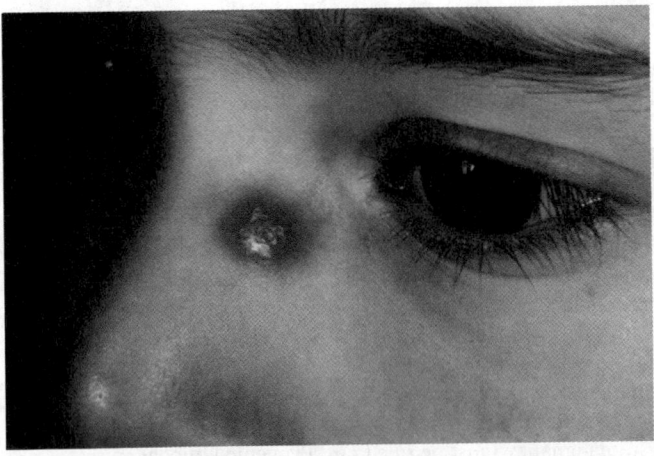

**Figure 160-1 Manifestations of cat-scratch disease. *A:* Primary inoculation lesion. Axillary and epitrochlear lymphadenitis appeared 2 weeks later. *B:* Primary inoculation lesion. Submental lymphadenitis appeared 10 days later. *C:* Axillary lymphadenopathy of 2 weeks' duration. The overlying skin appears normal. *D:* Cervical lymphadenopathy of 6 weeks' duration. The overlying skin is red. Thick, odorless pus (12 mL) was aspirated. *E:* Preauricular lymphadenopathy. *F:* Left-eye neuroretinitis. Note papilledema and stellate macular exudates ("macular star").

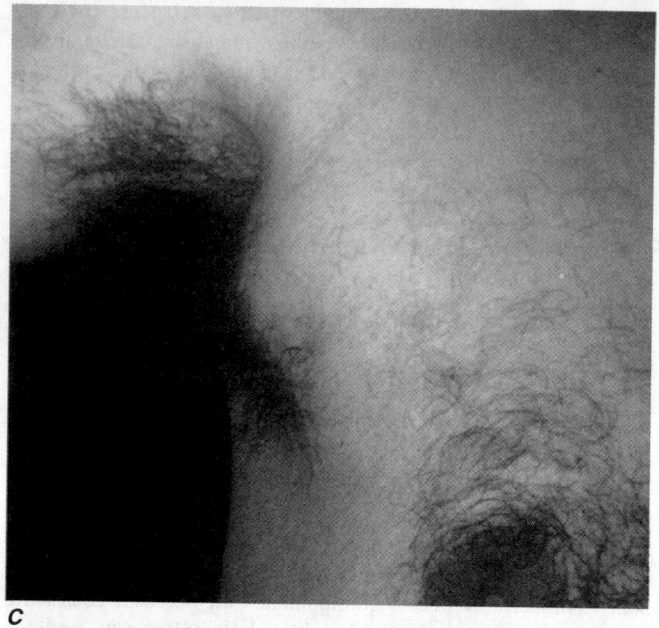

C

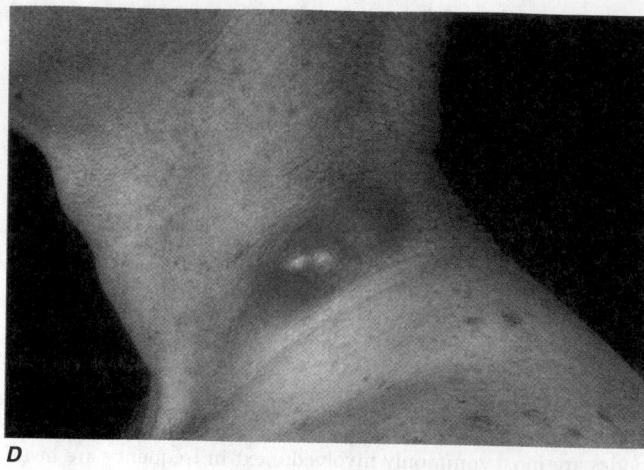

D

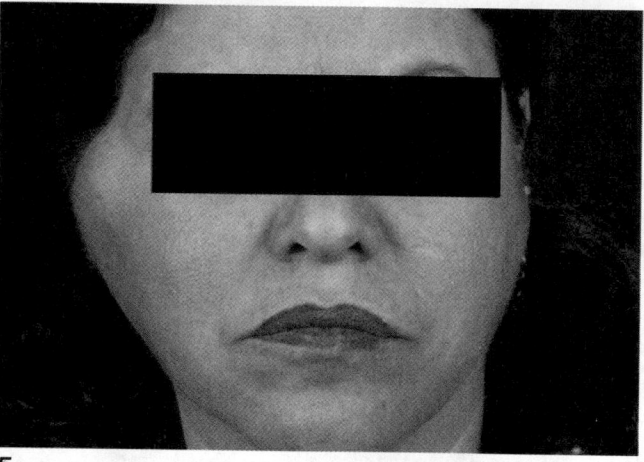

E

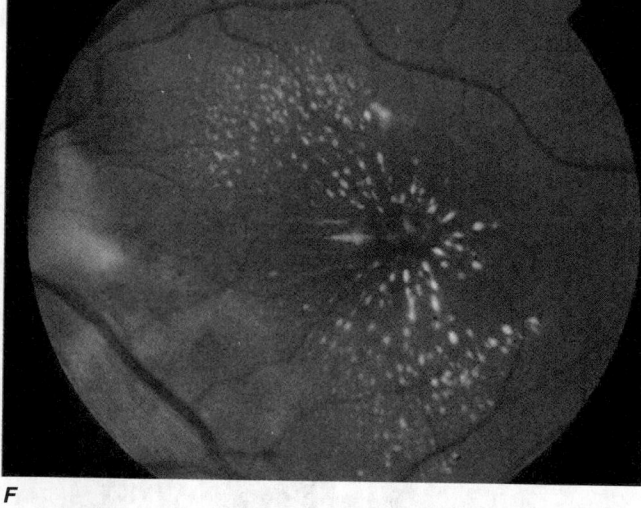

F

Figure 160-1 *(Continued)*

inoculation lesion is highly sensitive and specific and is particularly useful for definitive and rapid diagnosis in seronegative patients.

APPROACH TO THE PATIENT: Cat-Scratch Disease

A history of cat contact, a primary inoculation lesion, and regional lymphadenopathy are highly suggestive of CSD. A characteristic clinical course and corroborative laboratory tests make the diagnosis very likely. Conversely, when acute- and convalescent-phase sera are negative (as is the case in 10–20% of CSD patients), when spontaneous regression of lymph node size does not occur, and particularly when constitutional symptoms persist, malignancy must be ruled out. Pyogenic lymphadenitis, mycobacterial infection, brucellosis, syphilis, tularemia, plague, toxoplasmosis, sporotrichosis, and histoplasmosis should also be considered. In clinically suspected CSD in a seronegative individual, fine-needle aspiration may be adequate and PCR can confirm the diagnosis. When data are less supportive of CSD, lymph node biopsy rather than fine-needle aspiration is preferred. In seronegative CSD patients with lymphadenopathy and severe complications (e.g., encephalitis or neuroretinitis), early biopsy is important to establish a specific diagnosis.

TREATMENT: Cat-Scratch Disease

(Table 160-2) Treatment regimens are based on only minimal data. Suppurative nodes should be drained by large-bore needle aspiration and not by incision and drainage in order to avoid chronic draining tracts. Immunocompromised patients must always be treated with systemic antimicrobials.

■ PREVENTION

Avoiding cats (especially kittens) and instituting flea control are options for immunocompromised patients and for patients with valvular heart disease.

TABLE 160-2 Antimicrobial Therapy for Disease Caused by *Bartonella* Species in Adults

Disease	Antimicrobial Therapy
Typical cat-scratch disease	Not routinely indicated; for patients with extensive lymphadenopathy, consider azithromycin (500 mg PO on day 1, then 250 mg PO qd for 4 days)
Cat-scratch disease retinitis	Doxycycline (100 mg PO bid) *plus* rifampin (300 mg PO bid) for 4–6 weeks
Other atypical cat-scratch disease manifestations[a]	As per retinitis; treatment duration should be individualized
Trench fever or chronic bacteremia with *B. quintana*	Gentamicin (3 mg/kg IV qd for 14 days) *plus* doxycycline (200 mg PO qd or 100 mg PO bid for 6 weeks)
Suspected *Bartonella* endocarditis	Gentamicin[b] (1 mg/kg IV q8h for ≥14 days) *plus* doxycycline (100 mg PO/IV bid for 6 weeks[c]) *plus* ceftriaxone (2 g IV qd for 6 weeks)
Confirmed *Bartonella* endocarditis	As for suspected *Bartonella* endocarditis *minus* ceftriaxone
Bacillary angiomatosis	Erythromycin[d] (500 mg PO qid for 3 months) *or* Doxycycline (100 mg PO bid for 3 months)
Bacillary peliosis	Erythromycin[d] (500 mg PO qid for 4 months) *or* Doxycycline (100 mg PO bid for 4 months)
Bartonellosis (Carrion's disease)	
Oroya fever	Chloramphenicol (500 mg PO/IV qid for 14 days) *plus* another antibiotic (β-lactam preferred) *or* Ciprofloxacin (500 mg PO bid for 10 days)
Verruga peruana	Rifampin (10 mg/kg PO qd, to a maximum of 600 mg, for 14 days) *or* Streptomycin (15–20 mg/kg IM qd for 10 days)

[a]Data on treatment efficacy for encephalitis and hepatosplenic CSD are lacking. Therapy similar to that given for retinitis is reasonable.
[b]Some experts recommend gentamicin at 3 mg/kg IV qd. If gentamicin is contraindicated, rifampin (300 mg PO bid) can be added to doxycycline for documented *Bartonella* endocarditis.
[c]Some experts recommend extending oral doxycycline therapy for 3–6 months.
[d]Other macrolides are probably effective and may be substituted for erythromycin or doxycycline.
Source: Recommendations are modified from Rolain et al, 2004.

TRENCH FEVER AND CHRONIC BACTEREMIA

■ DEFINITION AND ETIOLOGY

Trench fever, also known as *5-day fever* or *quintan fever*, is a febrile illness caused by *B. quintana*. It was first described as an epidemic in the trenches of World War I and recently reemerged as chronic bacteremia seen most often in homeless people (also referred to as *urban* or *contemporary trench fever*).

■ EPIDEMIOLOGY

In addition to epidemics during World Wars I and II, sporadic outbreaks of trench fever have been reported in many regions of the world. The human body louse (*Pediculus humanus corporis*) has been identified as the vector and humans as the only known reservoir. After a hiatus of several decades during which trench fever was almost forgotten, small clusters of cases of *B. quintana* chronic bacteremia were reported sporadically, primarily from the United States and France, in HIV-uninfected homeless people. Alcoholism and louse infestation were identified as risk factors.

■ CLINICAL MANIFESTATIONS

The typical incubation period is 15–25 days (range, 3–38 days). "Classical" trench fever, as described in 1919, ranges from a mild febrile illness to a recurrent or protracted and debilitating disease. Onset may be abrupt or preceded by a prodrome of several days. Fever is often periodic, lasting 4–5 days with 5-day (range, 3- to 8-day) intervals between episodes. Other symptoms and signs include headache, back and limb pain, profuse sweating, shivering, myalgia, arthralgia, splenomegaly, a maculopapular rash in occasional cases, and nuchal rigidity in some cases. Untreated, the disease usually lasts 4–6 weeks. Death is rare. The clinical spectrum of *B. quintana* bacteremia in homeless people ranges from asymptomatic infection to a febrile illness with headache, severe leg pain, and thrombocytopenia. Endocarditis sometimes develops.

■ DIAGNOSIS

Definitive diagnosis requires isolation of *B. quintana* by blood culture. Some patients have positive blood cultures for several weeks. Patients with acute trench fever typically develop significant titers of antibody to *Bartonella*, whereas those with chronic *B. quintana* bacteremia may be seronegative. Patients with high titers of IgG antibodies should be evaluated for endocarditis. In epidemics, trench fever should be differentiated from epidemic louse-borne typhus and relapsing fever, which occur under similar conditions and share many features.

TREATMENT   Bacteremia

(Table 160-2) In a small, randomized, placebo-controlled trial involving homeless people with *B. quintana* bacteremia, therapy with gentamicin and doxycycline was superior to administration of placebo in eradicating bacteremia. Treatment of bacteremia is important even in clinically mild cases to prevent endocarditis. Optimal therapy for trench fever without documented bacteremia is uncertain.

BARTONELLA ENDOCARDITIS

■ DEFINITION AND ETIOLOGY

Coxiella burnetii (Chap. 174) and *Bartonella* species are the most common pathogens in culture-negative endocarditis (Chap. 124). In France, for example, *Bartonella* species were identified as the etiologic agents in 28% of 348 cases of culture-negative endocarditis. Prevalence, however, varies by geographic location and epidemiologic setting. In addition to *B. quintana* and *B. henselae* (the most common *Bartonella* species implicated in endocarditis, with the former more commonly involved than the latter), other *Bartonella* species have reportedly caused rare cases (Table 160-1).

■ EPIDEMIOLOGY

Bartonella endocarditis has been reported worldwide. Most patients are adults; more are male than female. Risk factors associated with *B. quintana* endocarditis include homelessness, alcoholism, and body louse infestation; however, individuals with no risk factors have had *Bartonella* endocarditis diagnosed as well. *B. henselae* endocarditis is associated with exposure to cats. Most cases involve native rather than prosthetic valves; the aortic valve accounts for ~60% of cases. Patients with *B. henselae* endocarditis usually have preexisting valvulopathy, whereas *B. quintana* often infects normal valves.

■ CLINICAL MANIFESTATIONS

Clinical manifestations are usually characteristic of subacute endocarditis of any etiology. However, a substantial number of patients have a prolonged, minimally febrile or even afebrile indolent illness, with mild nonspecific symptoms lasting weeks or months before the diagnosis is made. Initial echocardiography may not show vegetations. Acute, aggressive disease is rare.

■ DIAGNOSIS

Blood cultures, even with use of special techniques (lysis centrifugation or EDTA-containing tubes), are positive in only ~25% of cases—mostly those caused by *B. quintana* and only rarely those caused by *B. henselae*. Prolonged incubation of cultures (up to 6 weeks) is required. Serologic tests—either immunofluorescence or enzyme immunoassay—usually demonstrate high-titer IgG antibodies to *Bartonella*. Because of cross-antigenicity, serology does not distinguish between *B. quintana* and *B. henselae* and may also be low-titer cross-reactive with other pathogens, such as *C. burnetii* and *Chlamydophila* species. Identification of *Bartonella* to the species level is usually accomplished by application of PCR-based methods to valve tissue.

TREATMENT   *Bartonella* Endocarditis

(Table 160-2) For patients with culture-negative endocarditis suspected to be due to *Bartonella* species, empirical treatment consists of gentamicin, doxycycline, and ceftriaxone; the major role of ceftriaxone in this regimen is to adequately treat other potential causes of culture-negative endocarditis, including members of the HACEK group. Once a diagnosis of *Bartonella* endocarditis has been established, ceftriaxone is discontinued. Aminoglycosides, the only antibiotics known to be bactericidal against *Bartonella*, should be included in the regimen for ≥2 weeks. Indications for valvular surgery are the same as in subacute endocarditis due to other pathogens; however, the proportion of patients who undergo surgery (~60%) is high, probably as a consequence of delayed diagnosis.

BACILLARY ANGIOMATOSIS AND PELIOSIS

■ DEFINITION AND ETIOLOGY

Bacillary angiomatosis (sometimes called *bacillary epithelioid angiomatosis* or *epithelioid angiomatosis*) is a disease of severely immunocompromised patients, is caused by *B. henselae* or *B. quintana*, and is characterized by neovascular proliferative lesions involving the skin and other organs. Both species cause cutaneous lesions; hepatosplenic lesions are caused only by *B. henselae*, while subcutaneous and lytic bone lesions are more frequently associated with *B. quintana*. Bacillary peliosis is a closely related angioproliferative disorder caused by *B. henselae* and involving primarily the liver (peliosis hepatis) but also the spleen and lymph nodes. Bacillary peliosis is characterized by blood-filled cystic structures whose size ranges from microscopic to several millimeters.

■ EPIDEMIOLOGY

Bacillary angiomatosis and bacillary peliosis occur primarily in HIV-infected persons (Chap. 189) with CD4+ T cell counts <100/μL but also affect other immunosuppressed patients and, in rare instances, immunocompetent patients. The previously reported incidence of ~1 case per 1000 HIV-infected persons is now lower; the recent decrease is most likely attributable to effective antiretroviral therapy and the routine use of rifabutin and macrolides to prevent *Mycobacterium avium* complex infection in AIDS patients. Contact with cats or cat fleas elevates the risk of *B. henselae* infection. Risk factors for *B. quintana* infection are low income, homelessness, and body louse infestation.

■ CLINICAL MANIFESTATIONS

Bacillary angiomatosis presents most commonly as one or more cutaneous lesions that are not painful and that may be tan, red, or purple in color. Subcutaneous masses or nodules, superficial ulcerated plaques (Fig. 160-2), and verrucous growths are also seen. Nodular forms resemble those seen in fungal or mycobacterial infections. Subcutaneous nodules are often tender. Painful osseous lesions, most often involving long bones, may underlie cutaneous lesions and occasionally develop in their absence. In rare cases, other organs are involved in bacillary angiomatosis. Patients usually have constitutional symptoms, including fever, chills, malaise, headache, anorexia, weight loss, and night sweats. In osseous disease, lytic lesions are generally seen on radiography, and technetium scan shows focal uptake. The differential diagnosis of cutaneous bacillary angiomatosis includes Kaposi's sarcoma, pyogenic granuloma, subcutaneous tumors, and verruga peruana. In bacillary peliosis, hypodense hepatic areas are usually evident on imaging. In patients with advanced immunodeficiency, *B. henselae* and *B. quintana* are important causes of FUO. Intermittent bacteremia with positive blood cultures can occur with or without endocarditis.

■ PATHOLOGY

Bacillary angiomatosis consists of lobular proliferations of small blood vessels lined by enlarged endothelial cells interspersed with mixed infiltrates of neutrophils and lymphocytes, with predominance of the former. Histologic examination of organs with bacillary

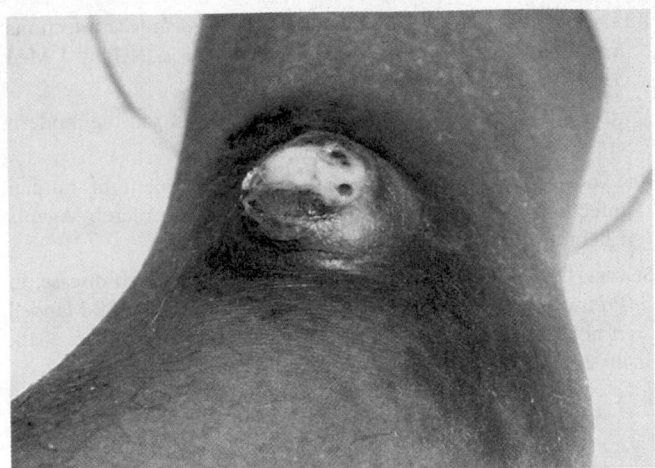

Figure 160-2 Nodular lesion of bacillary angiomatosis with superficial ulceration in an AIDS patient with advanced immunodeficiency. *[Reprinted with permission from DH Spach and E Darby: Bartonella Infections, Including Cat-Scratch Disease, in Harrison's Principles of Internal Medicine, 17th ed, AF Fauci et al (eds). New York, McGraw-Hill, 2008, p 989.]*

peliosis reveals small blood-filled cystic lesions partially lined by endothelial cells that can be several millimeters in size. Peliotic lesions are surrounded by fibromyxoid stroma containing inflammatory cells, dilated capillaries, and clumps of granular material. Warthin-Starry silver staining of bacillary angiomatosis and peliosis lesions reveals clusters of bacilli. Cultures are usually negative.

◼ DIAGNOSIS

Bacillary angiomatosis and bacillary peliosis are diagnosed on histologic grounds. Blood cultures may be positive.

TREATMENT   Bacillary Angiomatosis and Peliosis

(Table 160-2) Prolonged therapy with a macrolide or doxycycline is recommended for both bacillary angiomatosis and bacillary peliosis.

◼ PREVENTION

Control of cat-flea infestation and avoidance of cat scratches (for prevention of *B. henselae*) and avoidance and treatment of body louse infestation (for prevention of *B. quintana*) are reasonable strategies for HIV-infected persons. Primary prophylaxis is not recommended, but suppressive therapy with a macrolide or doxycycline is indicated in HIV-infected patients with bacillary angiomatosis or bacillary peliosis until CD4+ T cell counts are >200/μL. Relapse may necessitate lifelong suppressive therapy in individual cases.

BARTONELLOSIS (CARRIÓN'S DISEASE)

◼ DEFINITION AND ETIOLOGY

Bartonellosis is a biphasic disease caused by *B. bacilliformis*. *Oroya fever* is the initial, bacteremic, systemic form, and *verruga peruana* is its late-onset, eruptive manifestation.

◼ EPIDEMIOLOGY AND PREVENTION

 Infection is endemic to the geographically restricted Andes valleys of Peru, Ecuador, and Colombia (~500–3200 m above sea level). Sporadic epidemics occur. The disease is

transmitted by the phlebotomine sandfly *Lutzomyia verrucarum*. Humans are the only known reservoir of *B. bacilliformis*. Sandfly control measures (e.g., insecticides) as well as personal protection measures (e.g., repellents, screening, bednets) may decrease the risk of infection.

◼ PATHOGENESIS

After inoculation by the sandfly, bacteria invade the blood vessel endothelium and proliferate; the reticuloendothelial system and various organs may also be involved. Upon re-entry into blood vessels, *B. bacilliformis* invades, replicates, and ultimately destroys erythrocytes, with consequent massive hemolysis and sudden, severe anemia. Microvascular thrombosis results in end-organ ischemia. Survivors sometimes develop cutaneous hemangiomatous lesions characterized by various inflammatory cells, endothelial proliferation, and the presence of *B. bacilliformis*.

◼ CLINICAL MANIFESTATIONS

The incubation period is 3 weeks (range, 2–14 weeks). Oroya fever may present as a nonspecific bacteremic febrile illness without anemia or as an acute, severe hemolytic anemia with hepatomegaly and jaundice of rapid onset leading to vascular collapse and clouded sensorium. Myalgia, arthralgia, lymphadenopathy, and abdominal pain may develop. Temperature is elevated but not extremely so; high fever may suggest intercurrent infection. Subclinical asymptomatic infection also occurs. In verruga peruana, red, hemangioma-like, cutaneous vascular lesions of various sizes appear either weeks to months after systemic illness or with no previous suggestive history. These lesions persist for months up to 1 year. Mucosal and internal lesions may also develop.

◼ DIAGNOSIS AND APPROACH TO THE PATIENT

Systemic illness (with or without anemia) or the development of cutaneous lesions in a person who has been to an endemic area raises the possibility of *B. bacilliformis* infection. Severe anemia with exuberant reticulocytosis—and sometimes thrombocytopenia—can occur. In systemic illness, Giemsa-stained blood films show typical intraerythrocytic bacilli, and blood and bone marrow cultures are positive. Serologic assays may be helpful. Biopsy may be required to confirm the diagnosis of verruga peruana. Differential diagnosis includes the spectrum of coendemic systemic febrile illnesses (e.g., typhoid fever, malaria, brucellosis) as well as diseases producing cutaneous vascular lesions (e.g., hemangiomata, bacillary angiomatosis, Kaposi's sarcoma).

TREATMENT   Bartonellosis

(Table 160-2) Antibiotic therapy for systemic *B. bacilliformis* infection usually results in rapid defervescence. Additional antibiotic treatment of intercurrent infection (particularly salmonellosis) is often required. Blood transfusion may be necessary. Treatment of verruga peruana usually is not required, although large lesions or those interfering with function may require excision. Patients with numerous lesions, especially lesions that have been present for only a short period, may respond well to antibiotic therapy.

◼ COMPLICATIONS AND PROGNOSIS

Mortality rates associated with Oroya fever have been reported to be as high as 40% without treatment but are considerably lower (~10%) with treatment. Complications such as bacterial superinfection and neurologic and cardiac manifestations occur frequently.

Generalized massive edema (anasarca) and petechiae are associated with poor outcome. Permanent immunity usually develops.

FURTHER READINGS

CENTERS FOR DISEASE CONTROL AND PREVENTION: Guidelines for prevention and treatment of opportunistic infections in HIV-infected adults and adolescents. MMWR Recomm Rep 58:1, 2009

FLORIN TA et al: Beyond cat scratch disease: Widening spectrum of *Bartonella henselae* infection. Pediatrics 121:e1413, 2008

FOURNIER PE et al: Epidemiologic and clinical characteristics of *Bartonella quintana* and *Bartonella henselae* endocarditis: A study of 48 patients. Medicine (Baltimore) 80:245, 2001

KOEHLER JE et al: Molecular epidemiology of *Bartonella* infections in patients with bacillary angiomatosis-peliosis. N Engl J Med 337:1876, 1997

MAGUINA C et al: Bartonellosis (Carrión's disease) in the modern era. Clin Infect Dis 33:772, 2001

ROLAIN JM et al: Recommendations for treatment of human infections caused by *Bartonella* species. Antimicrob Agents Chemother 48:1921, 2004

SLATER LN, Welch DF: *Bartonella* including cat scratch disease, in *Principles and Practice of Infectious Diseases*, 7th ed, GL Mandell et al (eds). Philadelphia, Elsevier Churchill Livingstone, 2010, pp 2995–3009

CHAPTER 161

Donovanosis

Nigel O'Farrell

Donovanosis is a chronic, progressive bacterial infection that usually involves the genital region. The condition is generally regarded as a sexually transmitted infection of low infectivity. This infection has been known by many other names, the most common being *granuloma inguinale*.

ETIOLOGY

The causative organism has been reclassified as *Klebsiella granulomatis comb nov* on the basis of phylogenetic analysis, although there is ongoing debate about this decision. Some authorities consider the original nomenclature (*Calymmatobacterium granulomatis*), which is based on analysis of 16S rRNA gene sequences, to be more appropriate.

Donovanosis was first described in Calcutta in 1882, and the causative organism was recognized by Charles Donovan in Madras in 1905. He identified the characteristic Donovan bodies, measuring 1.5×0.7 μm, in macrophages and the stratum Malpighii. The organism was not reproducibly cultured until the mid-1990s, when its isolation in peripheral blood monocytes and human epithelial cell lines was reported.

EPIDEMIOLOGY

Donovanosis has an unusual geographic distribution that includes Papua New Guinea, parts of southern Africa, India, French Guyana, Brazil, and aboriginal communities in Australia. In Australia, donovanosis has virtually been eliminated through a sustained program backed by strong political commitment and resources at the primary health care level. Although few cases are now reported in the United States, donovanosis was once prevalent in this country, with 5000–10,000 cases recorded in 1947. The largest epidemic recorded was in Dutch South Guinea, where 10,000 cases were identified in a population of 15,000 (the Marind-anim people) between 1922 and 1952.

Donovanosis is associated with poor hygiene and is more common in lower socioeconomic groups than in those who are better off and in men than in women. Infection in sexual partners of index cases occurs to a limited extent. Donovanosis is a risk factor for HIV infection (Chap. 189).

Globally, the incidence of donovanosis has decreased significantly in recent times. This decline probably reflects a greater focus on effective management of genital ulcers because of their role in facilitating HIV transmission.

CLINICAL FEATURES

A lesion starts as a papule or subcutaneous nodule that later ulcerates after trauma. The incubation period is uncertain, but experimental infections in humans indicate that it lasts ~50 days. Four types of lesions have been described: (1) the classic ulcerogranulomatous lesion (Fig. 161-1), a beefy red ulcer that bleeds readily when touched; (2) a hypertrophic or verrucous ulcer with a raised irregular edge; (3) a necrotic, offensive-smelling ulcer causing tissue destruction; and (4) a sclerotic or cicatricial lesion with fibrous and scar tissue.

The genitals are affected in 90% of patients and the inguinal region in 10%. The most common sites of infection are the prepuce, coronal sulcus, frenum, and glans in men and the labia minora and fourchette in women. Cervical lesions may mimic cervical carcinoma. In men, lesions are associated with lack of circumcision. Lymphadenitis is uncommon. Extragenital lesions occur in 6% of cases and may involve the lip, gums, cheek, palate, pharynx, larynx, and chest. Hematogenous spread of *K. granulomatis comb nov* to liver and bone has been reported. During pregnancy, lesions tend to develop more quickly and respond more slowly to treatment. Polyarthritis and osteomyelitis are rare complications. In newborn infants, donovanosis may present with ear infection. Cases in children have been attributed to sitting on the laps of infected adults. As

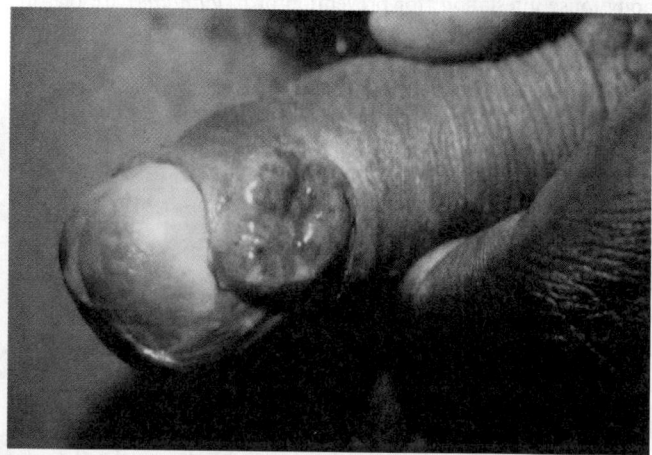

Figure 161-1 Ulcerogranulomatous penile lesion of donovanosis, with some hypertrophic features.

the incidence of donovanosis has decreased, the number of unusual case reports has appeared to be increasing.

Complications include neoplastic changes, pseudo-elephantiasis, and stenosis of the urethra, vagina, or anus.

■ DIAGNOSIS

A clinical diagnosis of donovanosis is made by an experienced practitioner on the basis of the lesion's appearance and usually has a high positive predictive value. The diagnosis is confirmed by microscopic identification of Donovan bodies (Fig. 161-2) in tissue smears. Preparation of a good-quality smear is important. If donovanosis is suspected on clinical grounds, the smear for Donovan bodies should be taken before swab samples to be tested for other causes of genital ulceration so that enough material can be collected from the ulcer. A swab should be rolled firmly over an ulcer previously cleaned with a dry swab to remove debris. Smears can be examined in a clinical setting by direct microscopy with a rapid Giemsa or Wright's stain. Alternatively, a piece of granulation tissue crushed and spread between two slides can be used. Donovan bodies can be seen in large, mononuclear (Pund) cells as gram-negative intracytoplasmic cysts filled with deeply staining bodies that may have a safety-pin appearance. These cysts eventually rupture and release the infective organisms. Histologic changes include chronic inflammation with infiltration of plasma cells and neutrophils. Epithelial changes include ulceration, microabscesses, and elongation of rete ridges.

A diagnostic polymerase chain reaction (PCR) test was developed in light of the observation that two unique base changes in the *phoE* gene eliminate Hae111 restriction sites, enabling differentiation of *K. granulomatis comb nov* from related *Klebsiella* species. PCR analysis with a colorimetric detection system can now be used in routine diagnostic laboratories. A genital ulcer multiplex PCR that includes *K. granulomatis* has been developed. Serologic tests are only poorly specific and are not used currently.

The differential diagnosis includes primary syphilitic chancres, secondary syphilis (condylomata lata), chancroid, lymphogranuloma venereum, genital herpes, neoplasm, and amebiasis. Mixed infections

TABLE 161-1 Effective Antibiotics for the Treatment of Donovanosis

Antibiotic	Oral Dose
Azithromycin	1 g on day 1, then 500 mg daily for 7 days or 1 g weekly for 4 weeks
Trimethoprim-sulfamethoxazole	960 mg bid for 14 days
Doxycycline	100 mg bid for 14 days
Erythromycin	500 mg qid for 14 days (in pregnant women)
Tetracycline	500 mg qid for 14 days

are common. Histologic appearances should be distinguished from those of rhinoscleroma, leishmaniasis, and histoplasmosis.

TREATMENT   Donovanosis

Many patients with donovanosis present quite late with extensive ulceration. They may be embarrassed and have low self-esteem related to their disease. Reassurance that they have a treatable condition is important, as is the need to administer antibiotics and monitor patients for an adequate interval (see below). Epidemiologic treatment of sexual partners and advice about how to improve genital hygiene are recommended.

The recommended drug regimens for donovanosis are shown in Table 161-1. Gentamicin can be added if the response is slow. Ceftriaxone, chloramphenicol, and norfloxacin are also effective. Patients treated for 14 days should be monitored until lesions have healed completely. Those treated with azithromycin probably do not need such rigorous follow-up.

Surgery may be indicated for very advanced lesions.

■ CONTROL AND PREVENTION

Donovanosis is probably the cause of genital ulceration that is most readily recognizable clinically. Donovanosis is now limited to a few specific locations, and its global eradication is a distinct possibility.

FURTHER READINGS

Bowden FJ: Donovanosis in Australia: Going, going.... Sex Transm Infect 81:365, 2005

Carter J et al: Phylogenetic evidence for reclassification of *Calymmatobacterium granulomatis* as *Klebsiella granulomatis comb nov*. Int J Syst Bacteriol 49:1695, 1999

Kharsany AB et al: Phylogenetic analysis of *Calymmatobacterium granulomatis* based on 16S sequences. J Med Microbiol 48:841, 1999

Mackay IM et al: Detection and discrimination of herpes simplex viruses, *Haemophilus ducreyi*, *Treponema pallidum*, and *Calymmatobacterium (Klebsiella) granulomatis* from genital ulcers. Clin Infect Dis 42:1431, 2006

O'Farrell N: Donovanosis, in *Sexually Transmitted Diseases*, 4th ed, KK Holmes et al (eds). New York, McGraw-Hill, 2008, pp 700–708

——— et al: Risk factors for HIV-1 in heterosexual attenders at a sexually transmitted diseases clinic in Durban, South Africa. S Afr Med J 80:17, 1991

Rajam RV, Rangiah PN: Donovanosis, granuloma inguinale, granuloma venereum. Geneva, World Health Organization, 1954, pp 1–72

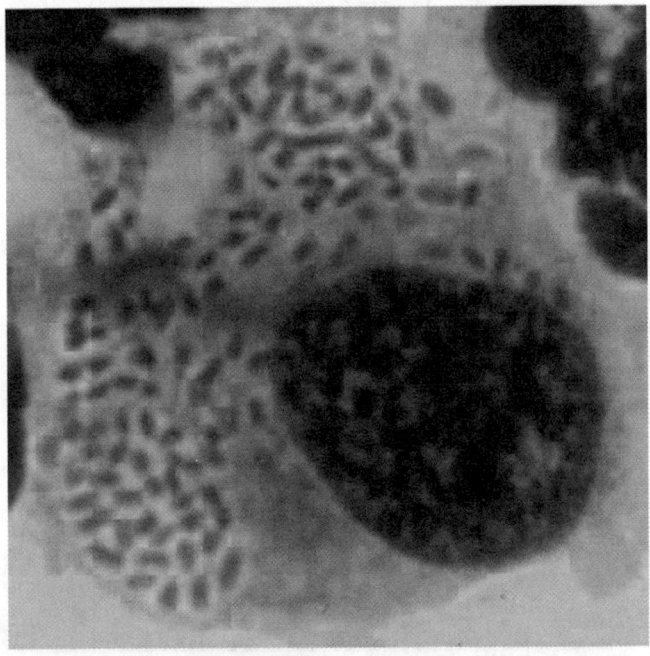

Figure 161-2   Pund cell stained by rapid Giemsa (RapiDiff) technique showing numerous Donovan bodies.

CHAPTER 162

Nocardiosis

Gregory A. Filice

Nocardia species are saprophytic aerobic actinomycetes and are common worldwide in soil, where they contribute to the decay of organic matter. More than 50 species have been identified, mostly on the basis of 16S rRNA gene sequences. More than 30 species have been associated with human disease. Until recently, isolates from the majority of cases of pneumonia and systemic disease were identified as *Nocardia asteroides*, but human disease involving *N. asteroides* proper is actually rare. Nocardiae are relatively inactive in standard biochemical tests, and speciation is difficult or impossible without molecular phylogenetic techniques. Most clinical laboratories cannot speciate isolates accurately and may identify them simply as *N. asteroides* or *Nocardia* species.

Nine species or species complexes are most commonly associated with human disease (Table 162-1). Most systemic disease involves

N. cyriacigeorgica, N. farcinica, N. pseudobrasiliensis, and species in the *N. transvalensis* and *N. nova* complexes. *N. brasiliensis* is usually associated with disease limited to the skin. Actinomycetoma—an indolent, slowly progressive disease of skin and underlying tissues with nodular swellings and draining sinuses—is often associated with *N. brasiliensis, N. otitidiscaviarum, N. transvalensis* complex strains, or other actinomycetes.

■ EPIDEMIOLOGY

Nocardiosis occurs worldwide. The annual incidence has been estimated on three continents (North America, Europe, and Australia) and is ~0.375 cases per 100,000 persons. The disease is more common among adults than among children and among males than among females. Nearly all cases are sporadic, but outbreaks have been associated with contamination of the hospital environment, solutions, or drug injection equipment. Person-to-person spread is not well documented. There is no known seasonality.

More than 90% of cases of pulmonary or disseminated disease occur in people with a host defense defect. Most have deficient cell-mediated immunity, especially that associated with lymphoma, transplantation, glucocorticoid therapy, or AIDS. The incidence is ~140-fold greater among patients with AIDS and ~340-fold greater among bone marrow transplant recipients

TABLE 162-1 *Nocardia* Species Most Commonly Associated With Human Disease and Their In Vitro Susceptibility Patterns

Species	Susceptible to	Resistant to
N. abscessus	Amikacin, amoxicillin/clavulanic acid, ampicillin, cefotaxime, ceftriaxone, gentamicin, linezolid, minocycline, sulfamethoxazole	Ciprofloxacin, clarithromycin, erythromycin, imipenem (v)[a]
N. brevicatena/paucivorans complex (*N. brevicatena, N. paucivorans, N. carnea,* others)	Amikacin, amoxicillin/clavulanic acid, ampicillin, cefotaxime, ceftriaxone, ciprofloxacin, linezolid, minocycline, tobramycin, sulfamethoxazole	Ciprofloxacin, clarithromycin, erythromycin, gentamicin, imipenem (v)
N. nova complex (*N. nova, N. veterana, N. africana, N. kruczakiae, N. elegans,* others)	Amikacin, ampicillin, ceftriaxone, clarithromycin, erythromycin, imipenem, linezolid, minocycline, sulfamethoxazole	Amoxicillin/clavulanic acid, ciprofloxacin, gentamicin
N. transvalensis complex (*N. blacklockiae, N. wallacei,* others)	Cefotaxime (v), ceftriaxone (v), ciprofloxacin, imipenem, linezolid, sulfamethoxazole	Amikacin, ampicillin, clarithromycin, erythromycin, gentamicin
N. farcinica	Amikacin, ciprofloxacin, imipenem, linezolid, sulfamethoxazole	Ampicillin, cefotaxime, ceftriaxone, clarithromycin, erythromycin, gentamicin, tobramycin
N. cyriacigeorgica	Amikacin, cefotaxime, ceftriaxone, imipenem, linezolid, minocycline (v), sulfamethoxazole	Amoxicillin/clavulanic acid, ampicillin (v), ciprofloxacin, erythromycin, gentamicin
N. brasiliensis	Amikacin, amoxicillin/clavulanic acid, cefotaxime, ceftriaxone, minocycline, sulfamethoxazole	Ampicillin, ciprofloxacin, clarithromycin, imipenem
N. pseudobrasiliensis	Amikacin, cefotaxime (v), ceftriaxone (v), ciprofloxacin, clarithromycin, sulfamethoxazole	Amoxicillin/clavulanic acid, ampicillin, imipenem, minocycline
N. otitidiscaviarum complex	Amikacin, ciprofloxacin, gentamicin, sulfamethoxazole	Amoxicillin/clavulanic acid, ampicillin, ceftriaxone, imipenem

[a](v), variable.
Source: Adapted from Brown-Elliott et al, 2006.

than in general populations. In AIDS, nocardiosis usually affects persons with <250 CD4+ T lymphocytes/μL. Nocardiosis has also been associated with pulmonary alveolar proteinosis, tuberculosis and other mycobacterial diseases, chronic granulomatous disease, interleukin 12 deficiency, and treatment with monoclonal antibodies to tumor necrosis factor. Any child with nocardiosis and no known cause of immunosuppression should undergo tests to determine the adequacy of the phagocytic respiratory burst.

Cases of actinomycetoma occur mainly in tropical and subtropical regions, especially those of Mexico, Central and South America, Africa, and India. The most important risk factor is frequent contact with soil or vegetable matter, especially in laborers.

■ PATHOLOGY AND PATHOGENESIS

Pneumonia and disseminated disease are both thought to follow inhalation of fragmented bacterial mycelia. The characteristic histologic feature of nocardiosis is an abscess with extensive neutrophil infiltration and prominent necrosis. Granulation tissue usually surrounds the lesions, but extensive fibrosis or encapsulation is uncommon.

Actinomycetoma is characterized by suppurative inflammation with sinus tract formation. Granules—microcolonies composed of dense masses of bacterial filaments extending radially from a central core—are occasionally observed in histologic preparations. They are frequently found in discharges from lesions of actinomycetoma but almost never in discharges from lesions in other forms of nocardiosis. Infrequently, nocardiae and other indolent pathogens, including fungi or mycobacteria, are isolated from the same patient.

Nocardiae have evolved a number of properties that enable them to survive within phagocytes, including neutralization of oxidants, prevention of phagosome-lysosome fusion, and prevention of phagosome acidification. Neutrophils phagocytose the organisms and limit their growth but do not kill them efficiently. Cell-mediated immunity is important for definitive control and elimination of nocardiae.

■ CLINICAL MANIFESTATIONS

Respiratory tract disease

Pneumonia, the most common form of nocardial disease in the respiratory tract, is typically subacute; symptoms have usually been present for days or weeks at presentation. The onset is occasionally more acute in immunosuppressed patients. Cough is prominent and produces small amounts of thick, purulent sputum that is not malodorous. Fever, anorexia, weight loss, and malaise are common; dyspnea, pleuritic pain, and hemoptysis are less common. Remissions and exacerbations over several weeks are frequent. Roentgenographic patterns vary, but some are highly suggestive of nocardial pneumonia. Infiltrates vary in size and are typically dense. Single or multiple nodules are common (Figs. 162-1 and 162-2), sometimes suggesting tumors or metastases. Infiltrates and nodules tend to cavitate (Fig. 162-2). Empyema is present in one-quarter of cases.

Nocardiosis may spread directly from the lungs to adjacent tissues. Pericarditis, mediastinitis, and the superior vena cava syndrome have all been reported. Nocardial laryngitis, tracheitis, bronchitis, and sinusitis are much less common than pneumonia. In the major airways, disease often presents as a nodular or granulomatous mass. Nocardiae are sometimes isolated from respiratory secretions of persons without apparent nocardial disease, usually individuals who have underlying lung or airway abnormalities.

Extrapulmonary disease

In half of all cases of pulmonary nocardiosis, disease appears outside the lungs. In one-fifth of cases of disseminated disease, lung

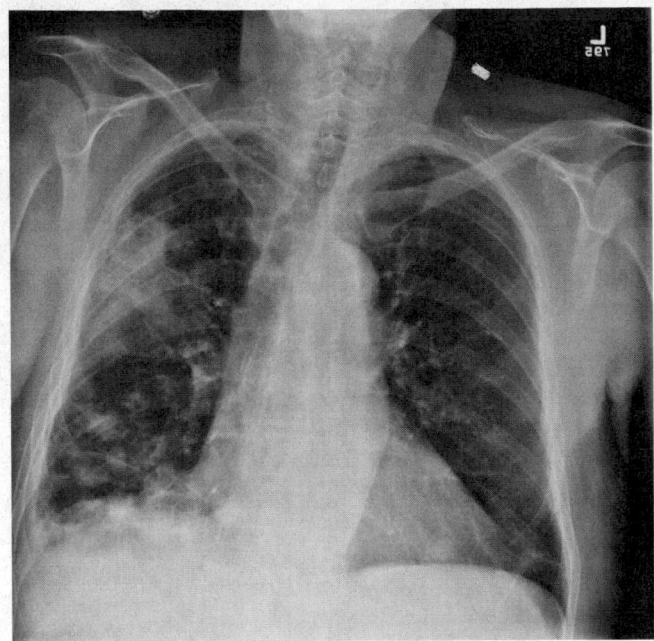

Figure 162-1   Nocardial pneumonia. A dense infiltrate with a possible cavity and several nodules are apparent in the right lung.

disease is not apparent. The most common site of dissemination is the brain. Other common sites include the skin and supporting structures, kidneys, bone, and muscle, but almost any organ can be involved. Peritonitis has been reported in patients undergoing peritoneal dialysis. Nocardiae have been recovered from blood in a few cases of pneumonia, disseminated disease, or central venous catheter infection. Nocardial endocarditis occurs rarely and can affect either native or prosthetic valves.

The typical manifestation of extrapulmonary dissemination is a subacute abscess. A minority of abscesses outside the lungs or central nervous system (CNS) form fistulas and discharge small amounts of pus. In CNS infections, brain abscesses are usually supratentorial, are often multiloculated, and may be single or

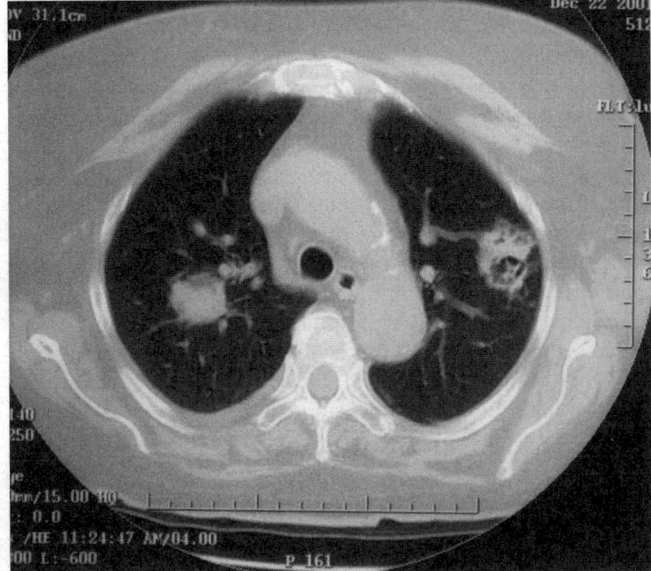

Figure 162-2   Nocardial pneumonia. A CT scan shows bilateral nodules, with cavitation in the nodule in the left lung.

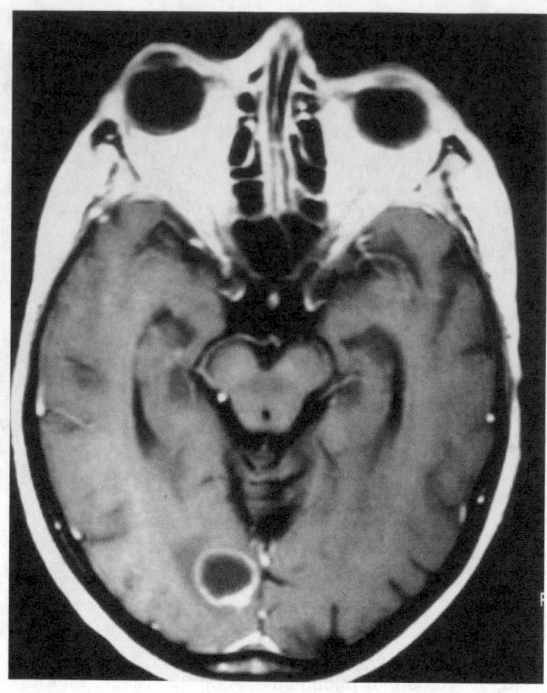

Figure 162-3 **Nocardial abscesses** in the right occipital lobe.

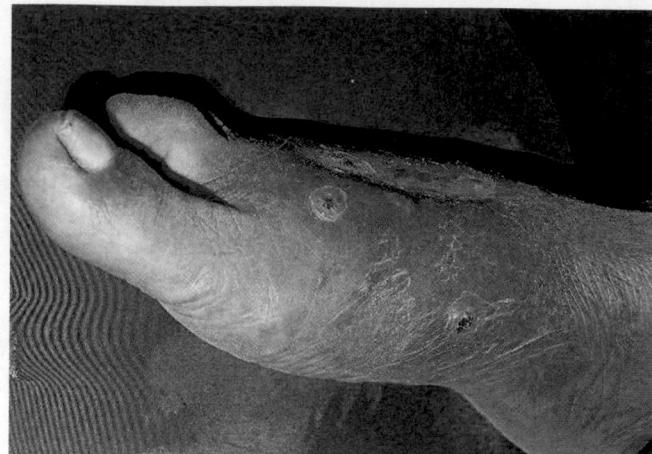

Figure 162-4 **Common features of nocardial actinomycetoma** include swelling, multiple sinus tracts, and involvement of the foot. *(Image provided by Amor Khachemoune and Ronald O. Perelman, New York University School of Medicine.)*

multiple (Fig. 162-3). Brain abscesses tend to burrow into the ventricles or extend out into the subarachnoid space. The symptoms and signs are somewhat more indolent than those of other types of bacterial brain abscess. Meningitis is uncommon and is usually due to spread from a nearby brain abscess. Nocardiae are not easily recovered from cerebrospinal fluid (CSF).

Disease following transcutaneous inoculation

Disease that follows transcutaneous nocardial inoculation usually takes one of three forms: cellulitis, lymphocutaneous syndrome, or actinomycetoma.

Cellulitis generally begins 1–3 weeks after a recognized breach of the skin, often with soil contamination. Subacute cellulitis, with pain, swelling, erythema, and warmth, develops over days to weeks. The lesions are usually firm and not fluctuant. Disease may progress to involve underlying muscles, tendons, bones, or joints. Dissemination is rare. *N. brasiliensis* and species in the *N. otitidis-caviarum* complex are most common in cellulitis cases.

Lymphocutaneous disease usually begins as a pyodermatous nodule at the site of inoculation, with central ulceration and purulent or honey-colored drainage. Subcutaneous nodules often appear along lymphatics that drain the primary lesion. Most cases of nocardial lymphocutaneous syndrome are associated with *N. brasiliensis*. Similar disease occurs with other pathogens, most notably *Sporothrix schenckii* (sporotrichosis, Chap. 206).

Actinomycetoma (Fig. 162-4) usually begins with a nodular swelling, sometimes at a site of local trauma. Lesions typically develop on the feet or hands but may involve the posterior part of the neck, the upper back, the head, and other sites. The nodule eventually breaks down, and a fistula appears, typically followed by others. The fistulas tend to come and go, with new ones forming as old ones disappear. The discharge is serous or purulent, may be bloody, and often contains 0.1- to 2-mm white granules consisting of masses of mycelia. The lesions spread slowly along fascial planes to involve adjacent areas of skin, subcutaneous tissue, and bone. Over months or years, there may be extensive deformation of the affected part. Lesions involving soft tissues are only mildly painful; those affecting bones

or joints are more so. Systemic symptoms are absent or minimal. Infection rarely disseminates from actinomycetoma, and lesions on the hands and feet usually cause only local disability. Lesions on the head, neck, and trunk can invade locally to involve deep organs, with consequent severe disability or death.

Eye infections

Nocardia species are uncommon causes of subacute keratitis, usually following eye trauma. Nocardial endophthalmitis can develop after eye surgery. In one series, nocardiae accounted for more than half of culture-proved cases of endophthalmitis after cataract surgery. Endophthalmitis can also occur during disseminated disease. Nocardial infection of lachrymal glands has been reported.

■ DIAGNOSIS

The first step in diagnosis is examination of sputum or pus for crooked, branching, beaded, gram-positive filaments 1 μm wide and up to 50 μm long (Fig. 162-5). Most nocardiae are acid-fast in direct

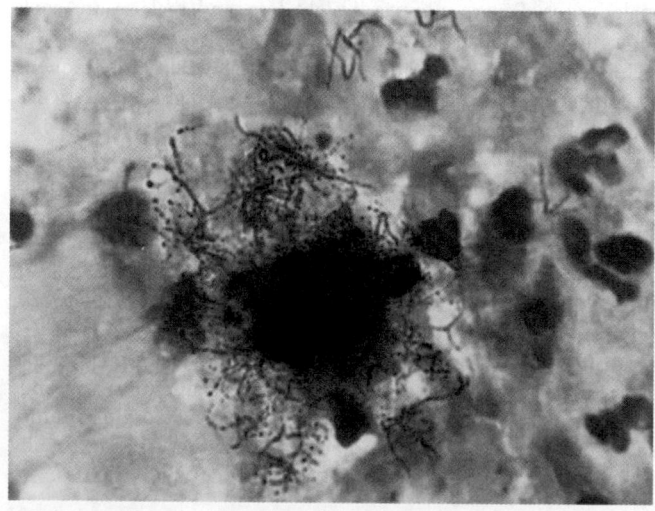

Figure 162-5 **Gram-stained sputum** from a patient with nocardial pneumonia. *(Image provided by Charles Cartwright and Susan Nelson, Hennepin County Medical Center, Minneapolis, MN.)*

smears if a weak acid is used for decolorization (e.g., in the modified Kinyoun, Ziehl-Neelsen, and Fite-Faraco methods). The organisms often take up silver stains. Recovery from specimens containing a mixed flora can be improved with selective media (colistin–nalidixic acid agar, modified Thayer-Martin agar, or buffered charcoal–yeast extract agar). Nocardiae grow well on most fungal and mycobacterial media, but procedures used for decontamination of specimens for mycobacterial culture can kill nocardiae and thus should not be used when these organisms are suspected. Nocardiae grow relatively slowly; colonies may take up to 2 weeks to appear and may not develop their characteristic appearance—white, yellow, or orange, with aerial mycelia and delicate, dichotomously branched substrate mycelia—for up to 4 weeks. Several blood culture systems support nocardial growth, although nocardiae may not be detected for up to 2 weeks. The growth of nocardiae is so different from that of more common pathogens that the laboratory should be alerted when nocardiosis is suspected in order to maximize the likelihood of isolation.

In nocardial pneumonia, sputum smears are often negative. Unless the diagnosis can be made in smear-negative cases by sampling lesions in more accessible sites, bronchoscopy or lung aspiration is usually necessary. To evaluate the possibility of dissemination in patients with nocardial pneumonia, a careful history should be obtained and a thorough physical examination performed. Suggestive symptoms or signs should be pursued with further diagnostic tests. CT or MRI of the head, with and without contrast material, should be undertaken if signs or symptoms suggest brain involvement. Some authorities recommend brain imaging in all cases of pulmonary or disseminated disease. When clinically indicated, CSF or urine should be concentrated and then cultured. Actinomycetoma, eumycetoma (cases involving fungi, Chap. 206), and botryomycosis (cases involving cocci or bacilli, often *Staphylococcus aureus*) are difficult to distinguish clinically but are readily distinguished with microbiologic testing. Granules should be sought in any discharge. Suspect particles should be washed in saline, examined microscopically, and cultured. Granules in actinomycetoma cases are usually white, pale yellow, pink, or red. Viewed microscopically, they consist of tight masses of fine filaments (0.5–1 μm wide) radiating outward from a central core. Granules from eumycetoma cases are white, yellow, brown, black, or green. Under the microscope, they appear as masses of broader filaments (2–5 μm wide) encased in a matrix. Granules of botryomycosis consist of loose masses of cocci or bacilli. Organisms can also be seen in wound discharge or histologic specimens. The most reliable way to differentiate among the various organisms associated with mycetoma is by culture.

Isolation of nocardiae from sputum or blood occasionally represents colonization, transient infection, or contamination. In typical cases of respiratory tract colonization, Gram-stained specimens are negative and cultures are only intermittently positive. A positive sputum culture in an immunosuppressed patient usually reflects disease. When nocardiae are isolated from sputum of an immunocompetent patient without apparent nocardial disease, the patient should be observed carefully without treatment. A patient with a host-defense defect that increases the risk of nocardiosis should usually receive antimicrobial treatment.

TREATMENT Nocardiosis

The Clinical Laboratory Standards Institute has approved a broth dilution antimicrobial susceptibility test protocol for use with human nocardial isolates. Procedures differ from those used with common human bacterial pathogens, and most clinical laboratories will not be sufficiently experienced with *Nocardia* to produce reliable results. Because nocardiosis is uncommon, data on the relation between susceptibility test results for specific drugs and clinical outcomes in patients treated with these drugs are meager. Empirical therapy with the drugs discussed below is recommended for newly diagnosed cases. When possible, and especially in severe cases or cases that do not improve promptly with empirical therapy, clinicians should arrange for susceptibility tests at a laboratory with experience in nocardial microbiology, such as the Mycobacteria/Nocardia Laboratory at the University of Texas Health Science Center (11937 US Highway 271, Tyler, TX 75708-3154; phone, 903-877-7685; fax, 903-877-7652).

Sulfonamides are the drugs of choice (Tables 162-1 and 162-2). The combination of sulfamethoxazole (SMX) and trimethoprim (TMP) is probably equivalent to a sulfonamide alone; some authorities believe that the combination may in fact be more effective, but it also poses a modestly greater risk of hematologic toxicity. At the outset, 10–20 mg of TMP per kg and 50–100 mg of SMX per kg are given each day in two divided doses. Later, daily doses can be decreased to as little as 5 mg/kg and 25 mg/kg, respectively. In persons with sulfonamide allergies, desensitization usually allows continuation of therapy with these effective and inexpensive drugs.

Clinical experience with other oral drugs is limited. Minocycline (100–200 mg twice a day) is often effective; other tetracyclines are usually less effective. Linezolid is active against all species in vitro and has been effective in a few clinical cases, but adverse effects are common with long-term use. Tigecycline appears to be active in vitro against some species, but no relevant clinical experience has been reported. Amoxicillin (875 mg) combined with clavulanic acid (125 mg), given twice a day, has been effective in some cases but should be avoided in cases involving strains of the N. nova complex, in which clavulanate induces β-lactamase production. Among quinolones, ciprofloxacin has been studied most often, but moxifloxacin and gemifloxacin now appear to be more active.

TABLE 162-2 Treatment Duration for Nocardiosis

Disease	Duration
Pulmonary or systemic	
Intact host defenses	6–12 months
Deficient host defenses	12 months[a]
CNS disease	12 months[b]
Cellulitis, lymphocutaneous syndrome	2 months
Osteomyelitis, arthritis, laryngitis, sinusitis	4 months
Actinomycetoma	6–12 months after clinical cure
Keratitis	Topical: until apparent cure
	Systemic: until 2–4 months after apparent cure

[a]In some patients with AIDS and CD4+ T lymphocyte counts of <200/µL or with chronic granulomatous disease, therapy for pulmonary or systemic disease must be continued indefinitely.

[b]If all apparent CNS disease has been excised, the duration of therapy may be reduced to 6 months.

Amikacin, the best-established parenteral drug except in cases involving the *N. transvalensis* complex, is given in doses of 5–7.5 mg/kg every 12 h or 15 mg/kg every 24 h. Serum drug levels should be monitored during prolonged therapy in patients with diminished renal function and in the elderly. Cefotaxime, ceftriaxone, and imipenem are usually effective except as indicated in Table 162-1.

Patients with severe disease are initially treated with a combination including TMP-SMX, amikacin, and ceftriaxone or imipenem. Clinical improvement is usually noticeable after 1–2 weeks of therapy but may take longer, especially with CNS disease. After definite clinical improvement, therapy can be continued with a single drug (usually one that can be taken by mouth) in most cases. Some experts use two or more drugs for the entire course of therapy in some cases, but whether multiple drugs are better than a single agent is not known, and additional drugs increase the risk of toxicity. In patients with nocardiosis who need immunosuppressive therapy for an underlying disease or prevention of transplant rejection, immunosuppressive therapy should be continued.

Use of SMX and TMP in high-risk populations to prevent *Pneumocystis* disease or urinary tract infections appears to reduce but not eliminate the risk of nocardiosis. The incidence of nocardiosis is low enough that prophylaxis solely to prevent this disease is not recommended.

Surgical management of nocardial disease is similar to that of other bacterial diseases. Brain abscesses should be aspirated, drained, or excised if the diagnosis is unclear, if an abscess is large and accessible, or if an abscess fails to respond to chemotherapy. Small or inaccessible brain abscesses should be treated medically; clinical improvement should be noticeable within 1–2 weeks. Brain imaging should be repeated to document the resolution of lesions, although abatement on images often lags behind clinical improvement.

Antimicrobial therapy usually suffices for nocardial actinomycetoma. In deep or extensive cases, drainage or excision of heavily involved tissue may facilitate healing, but structure and function should be preserved whenever possible. Keratitis is treated with topical sulfonamide or amikacin drops plus a sulfonamide or an alternative drug given by mouth.

Nocardial infections tend to relapse (particularly in patients with chronic granulomatous disease), and long courses of antimicrobial therapy are necessary (Table 162-2). If disease is unusually extensive or if the response to therapy is slow, the recommendations in Table 162-2 should be exceeded.

With appropriate treatment, the mortality rate for pulmonary or disseminated nocardiosis outside the CNS should be <5%. CNS disease carries a higher mortality rate. Patients should be followed carefully for at least 6 months after therapy has ended.

FURTHER READINGS

AMEEN M, ARENAS R: Developments in the management of mycetomas. Clin Exp Dermatol 34:1, 2009

BROWN-ELLIOTT BA et al: Clinical and laboratory features of the *Nocardia* spp. based on current molecular taxonomy. Clin Microbiol Rev 19:259, 2006

FILICE GA: Nocardiosis in persons with human immunodeficiency virus infection, transplant recipients, and large, geographically defined populations. J Lab Clin Med 145:156, 2005

HEARNE CB et al: The gardener's cellulitis. Am J Med 122:27, 2009

JODLOWSKI TZ et al: Linezolid for the treatment of *Nocardia* spp. infections. Ann Pharmacother 41:1694, 2007

KHAN BA et al: *Nocardia* infection in lung transplant recipients. Clin Transplant 22:562, 2008

MARAKI S et al: Nocardial infection in Crete, Greece: Review of fifteen cases from 2003 to 2007. Scand J Infect Dis 41:122, 2009

MINERO MV et al: Nocardiosis at the turn of the century. Medicine (Baltimore) 88:250, 2009

PINTADO V et al: Infection with *Nocardia* species: Clinical spectrum of disease and species distribution in Madrid, Spain, 1978–2001. Infection 30:338, 2002

POONYAGARIYAGORN HK et al: Challenges in the diagnosis and management of *Nocardia* infections in lung transplant recipients. Transpl Infect Dis 10:403, 2008

CHAPTER 163

Actinomycosis

Thomas A. Russo

Actinomycosis is an indolent, slowly progressive infection caused by anaerobic or microaerophilic bacteria, primarily of the genus *Actinomyces*, that colonize the mouth, colon, and vagina. Mucosal disruption may lead to infection at virtually any site in the body. In vivo growth of actinomycetes usually results in the formation of characteristic clumps called *grains* or *sulfur granules*. The clinical presentations of actinomycosis are myriad. Common in the preantibiotic era, actinomycosis has diminished in incidence, as has its timely recognition. Actinomycosis has been called the most misdiagnosed disease, and it has been said that no disease is so often missed by experienced clinicians. Thus this entity remains a diagnostic challenge.

Three clinical presentations that should prompt consideration of this unique infection are (1) the combination of chronicity, progression across tissue boundaries, and mass-like features (mimicking malignancy, with which it is often confused); (2) the development of a sinus tract, which may spontaneously resolve and recur; and (3) a refractory or relapsing infection after a short course of therapy, since cure of established actinomycosis requires prolonged treatment. An awareness of the full spectrum of the disease, prompting clinical suspicion, will expedite its diagnosis and treatment and will minimize the unnecessary surgical interventions, morbidity, and mortality that are reported all too often.

■ ETIOLOGIC AGENTS

Actinomycosis is most commonly caused by *A. israelii*. *A. naeslundii*, *A. odontolyticus*, *A. viscosus*, *A. meyeri*, and *A. gerencseriae* are established but less common causes. Most if not all actinomycotic infections are polymicrobial. *Aggregatibacter (Actinobacillus) actinomycetemcomitans*, *Eikenella corrodens*, Enterobacteriaceae, and species of *Fusobacterium*, *Bacteroides*, *Capnocytophaga*,

Staphylococcus, and Streptococcus are commonly isolated with actinomycetes in various combinations, depending on the site of infection. The contribution of these other species to the pathogenesis of actinomycosis is uncertain.

Comparative 16S rRNA gene sequencing has led to the identification of an ever-expanding list of *Actinomyces* species and to the reclassification of some actinomycetes as *Arcanobacterium*. Increasing data support the *Actinomyces* species *A. europaeus*, *A. neuii*, *A. radingae*, *A. graevenitzii*, *A. turicensis*, *A. cardiffensis*, *A. houstonensis*, *A. hongkongensis*, *A. lingnae*, and *A. funkei* as well as two former *Actinomyces* species now classified as *Arcanobacterium* (*A. pyogenes* and *A. bernardiae*) as additional causes of human actinomycosis.

■ EPIDEMIOLOGY

Actinomycosis has no geographic boundaries and occurs throughout life, with a peak incidence in the middle decades. Males have a threefold higher incidence than females, possibly because of poorer dental hygiene and/or more frequent trauma. Factors that have probably contributed to the decrease in actinomycosis incidence since the advent of antibiotics include improved dental hygiene and the initiation of antimicrobial treatment before the disease develops fully. Individuals who do not seek or have access to health care, those who have an intrauterine contraceptive device (IUCD) in place for a prolonged period (see "Pelvic Disease," below), and those who receive bisphosphonate treatment (see "Oral-Cervicofacial Disease," below) are probably at higher risk.

■ PATHOGENESIS AND PATHOLOGY

The etiologic agents of actinomycosis are members of the normal oral flora and are often cultured from the bronchi, the gastrointestinal tract, and the female genital tract. The critical step in the development of actinomycosis is disruption of the mucosal barrier. Local infection may ensue. Once established, actinomycosis spreads contiguously in a slow progressive manner, ignoring tissue planes. Although acute inflammation may initially develop at the infection site, the hallmark of actinomycosis is the characteristic chronic, indolent phase manifested by lesions that usually appear as single or multiple indurations. Central necrosis consisting of neutrophils and sulfur granules develops and is virtually diagnostic. The fibrotic walls of the mass are typically described as "wooden." The responsible bacterial and/or host factors have not been identified. Over time, sinus tracts to the skin, adjacent organs, or bone may develop. In rare instances, distant hematogenous seeding may occur. As mentioned above, these unique features of actinomycosis mimic malignancy, with which it is often confused.

Foreign bodies appear to facilitate infection. This association most frequently involves IUCDs. Reports have described an association of actinomycosis with HIV infection; transplantation; treatment with infliximab, glucocorticoids, or bisphosphonates; and radio- or chemotherapy. Ulcerative mucosal infections (e.g., by herpes simplex virus or cytomegalovirus) may facilitate the development of actinomycosis.

■ CLINICAL MANIFESTATIONS

Oral-cervicofacial disease

Actinomycosis occurs most frequently at an oral, cervical, or facial site, usually as a soft tissue swelling, abscess, or mass lesion that is often mistaken for a neoplasm. The angle of the jaw is generally involved, but a diagnosis of actinomycosis should be considered with any mass lesion or relapsing infection in the head and neck (Chap. 31). Radiation therapy and especially

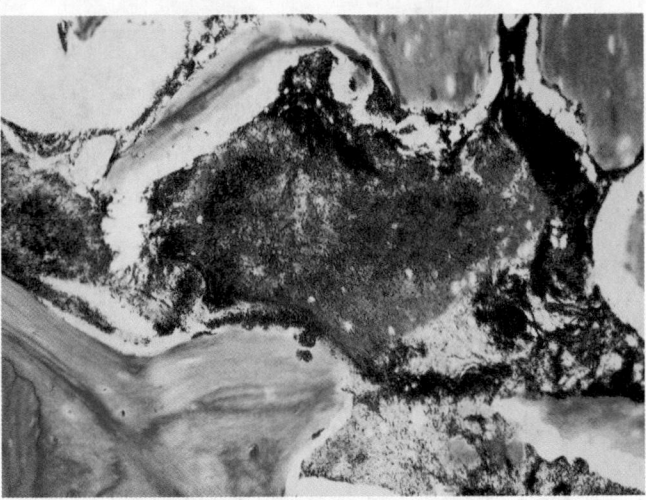

Figure 163-1 Bisphosphonate-associated maxillary osteomyelitis due to *A. viscosus*. A sulfur granule is seen within the bone. *(Reprinted with permission from NH Naik and TA Russo. © 2009 University of Chicago Press.)*

bisphosphonate treatment have been recognized as contributing to an increasing incidence of actinomycotic infection of the mandible and maxilla (Fig. 163-1). Otitis, sinusitis, and canaliculitis (most commonly due to *Propionibacterium propionicum*) also can develop. Pain, fever, and leukocytosis are variably reported. Contiguous extension to the cranium, cervical spine, or thorax is a potential sequela.

Thoracic disease

Thoracic actinomycosis usually follows an indolent progressive course, with involvement of the pulmonary parenchyma and/or the pleural space. Chest pain, fever, and weight loss are common. A cough, when present, is variably productive. The usual radiographic finding is either a mass lesion or pneumonia. On CT, central areas of low attenuation and ringlike rim enhancement may be seen. Cavitary disease or hilar adenopathy may develop. More than 50% of cases include pleural thickening, effusion, or empyema (Fig. 163-2). Rarely, pulmonary nodules or endobronchial lesions occur. Pulmonary lesions suggestive of actinomycosis may cross fissures or pleura; may involve the mediastinum, contiguous bone, or chest wall; or may be associated with a sinus tract. In the absence of these findings, thoracic actinomycosis is usually mistaken for a neoplasm or for pneumonia due to more usual causes.

Mediastinal infection is uncommon, usually arising from thoracic extension but rarely resulting from perforation of the esophagus, from trauma, or from head and neck or abdominal disease. The structures within the mediastinum and the heart can be involved in various combinations; consequently, the possible presentations are diverse. Primary endocarditis and isolated disease of the breast have been described.

Abdominal disease

Abdominal actinomycosis poses a great diagnostic challenge. Months or years usually pass from the inciting event (e.g., appendicitis, diverticulitis, peptic ulcer disease, spillage of gall stones or bile during laparoscopic cholecystectomy, foreign-body perforation, bowel surgery, or ascension from IUCD-associated pelvic disease) to clinical recognition. Because of the flow of peritoneal fluid and/or the direct extension of primary disease,

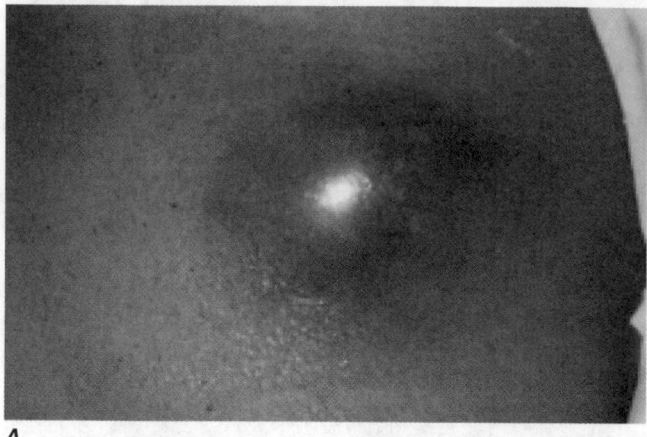

A

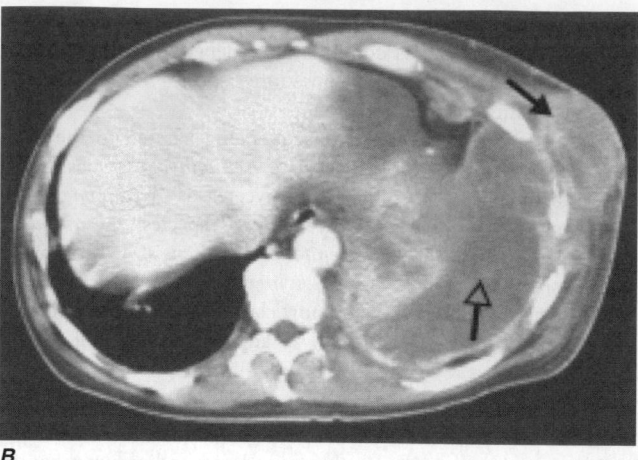

B

Figure 163-2 Thoracic actinomycosis. *A.* A chest wall mass from extension of pulmonary infection. *B.* Pulmonary infection is complicated by empyema (*open arrow*) and extension to the chest wall (*closed arrow*).

(Courtesy of Dr. C. B. Hsiao, Division of Infectious Diseases, Department of Medicine, State University of New York at Buffalo.)

virtually any abdominal organ, region, or space can be involved. The disease usually presents as an abscess, a mass, or a mixed lesion that is often fixed to underlying tissue and mistaken for a tumor. On CT, enhancement is most often heterogeneous and adjacent bowel is thickened. Sinus tracts to the abdominal wall, to the perianal region, or between the bowel and other organs may develop and mimic inflammatory bowel disease (Chap. 295). Recurrent disease or a wound or fistula that fails to heal suggests actinomycosis.

Hepatic infection usually presents as one or more abscesses or masses (Fig. 163-3). Isolated disease presumably develops via hematogenous seeding from cryptic foci. Imaging and percutaneous techniques have resulted in improved diagnosis and treatment.

All levels of the urogenital tract can be infected. Renal disease usually presents as pyelonephritis and/or renal and perinephric abscess. Bladder involvement, usually due to extension of pelvic disease, may result in ureteral obstruction or fistulas to bowel, skin, or uterus. *Actinomyces* can be detected in urine with appropriate stains and cultures.

Pelvic disease

Actinomycotic involvement of the pelvis occurs most commonly in association with an IUCD. When an IUCD is in place or has recently been removed, pelvic symptoms should prompt consideration of actinomycosis. The risk, although not quantified, appears small. The disease rarely develops when the IUCD has been in place for <1 year, but the risk increases with time. Actinomycosis can also present months after IUCD removal. Symptoms are typically indolent; fever, weight loss, abdominal pain, and abnormal vaginal bleeding or discharge are the most common. The earliest stage of disease—often endometritis—commonly progresses to pelvic masses or a tuboovarian abscess (Fig. 163-4). Unfortunately, because the diagnosis is often delayed, a "frozen pelvis" mimicking malignancy or endometriosis can develop by the time of recognition.

Identification of *Actinomyces*-like organisms (ALOs) on Papanicolaou-stained specimens, which occurs on average in 7% of women using an IUCD, has a low positive predictive value for a diagnosis of pelvic infection. Although the risk appears small, the

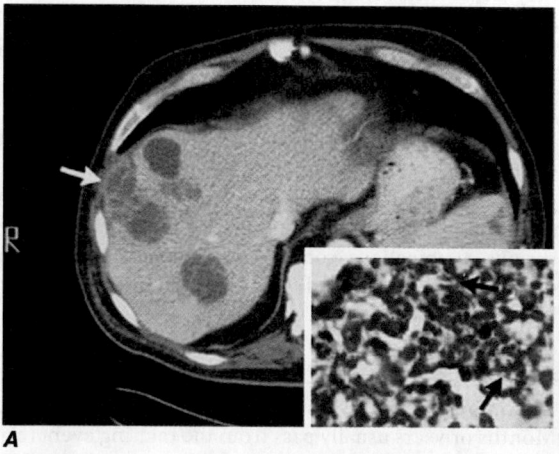

A

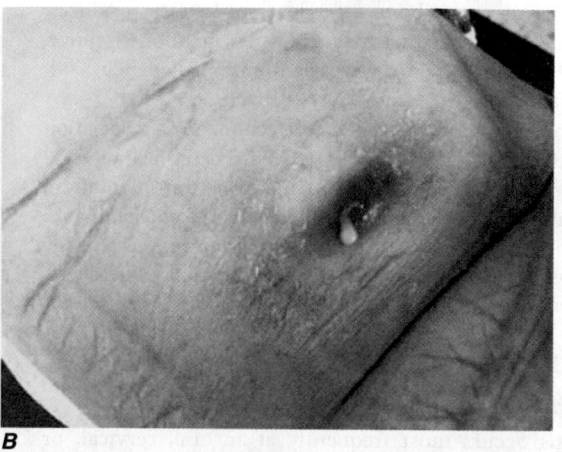

B

Figure 163-3 Hepatic-splenic actinomycosis. *A.* Computed tomogram showing multiple hepatic abscesses and a small splenic lesion due to *A. israelii*. Arrow indicates extension outside the liver. *Inset:* Gram's stain of abscess fluid demonstrating beaded filamentous gram-positive rods).

B. Subsequent formation of a sinus tract. (*Reprinted with permission from Saad M: Actinomyces hepatic abscess with cutaneous fistula. N Engl J Med 353:e16, 2005. © 2005 Massachusetts Medical Society. All rights reserved.*)

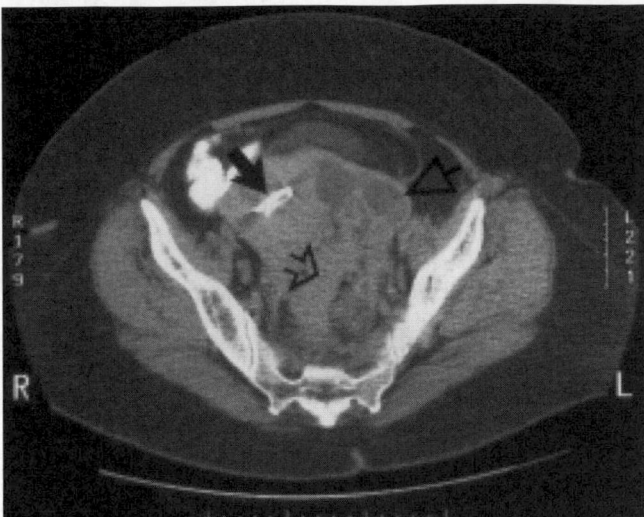

Figure 163-4 Computed tomogram showing pelvic actinomycosis associated with an intrauterine contraceptive device. The device is encased by endometrial fibrosis (*solid arrow*); also visible are paraendometrial fibrosis (*open triangular arrowhead*) and an area of suppuration (*open arrow*).

consequences of infection are significant. Therefore, until more quantitative data become available, it seems prudent to remove the IUCD in the presence of symptoms that cannot be accounted for, regardless of whether ALOs are detected, and—if advanced disease is excluded—to initiate a 14-day course of empirical treatment for possible early pelvic actinomycosis. The detection of ALOs in the absence of symptoms warrants education of the patient and close follow-up but not removal of the IUCD unless a suitable contraceptive alternative is agreed on.

Central nervous system disease

Actinomycosis of the central nervous system (CNS) is rare. Single or multiple brain abscesses are most common. An abscess usually appears on CT as a ring-enhancing lesion with a thick wall that may be irregular or nodular. Magnetic resonance perfusion and spectroscopy findings have also been described, as have meningitis, epidural or subdural space infection, and cavernous sinus syndrome.

Musculoskeletal and soft tissue infection

Actinomycotic infection of bone is usually due to adjacent soft-tissue infection but may be associated with trauma (e.g., fracture of the mandible), osteoradionecrosis and bisphosphonate osteonecrosis (limited to mandibular and maxillary bones), or hematogenous spread. Because of slow disease progression, new bone formation and bone destruction are seen concomitantly. Infection of an extremity is uncommon and is usually a result of trauma. Skin, subcutaneous tissue, muscle, and bone (with periostitis or acute or chronic osteomyelitis) are involved alone or in various combinations. Cutaneous sinus tracts frequently develop.

Disseminated disease

Hematogenous dissemination of disease from any location rarely results in multiple-organ involvement. The lungs and liver are most commonly affected, with the presentation of multiple nodules mimicking disseminated malignancy. The clinical presentation may be surprisingly indolent given the extent of disease.

■ DIAGNOSIS

The diagnosis of actinomycosis is rarely considered. All too often, the first mention of actinomycosis is by the pathologist after extensive surgery. Since medical therapy alone is frequently sufficient for cure, the challenge for the clinician is to consider the possibility of actinomycosis, to diagnose it in the least invasive fashion, and to avoid unnecessary surgery. The clinical and radiographic presentations that suggest actinomycosis are discussed above. Of note, hypermetabolism has been demonstrated by positive emission tomography in actinomycotic disease. Aspirations and biopsies (with or without CT or ultrasound guidance) are being used successfully to obtain clinical material for diagnosis, although surgery may be required. The diagnosis is most commonly made by microscopic identification of sulfur granules (an in vivo matrix of bacteria, calcium phosphate, and host material) in pus or tissues. Occasionally, these granules are identified grossly from draining sinus tracts or pus. Although sulfur granules are a defining characteristic of actinomycosis, granules are also found in mycetoma (Chaps. 162 and 206) and botryomycosis (a chronic suppurative bacterial infection of soft tissue or, in rare cases, visceral tissue that produces clumps of bacteria resembling granules). These entities can easily be differentiated from actinomycosis with appropriate histopathologic and microbiologic studies. Microbiologic identification of actinomycetes is often precluded by prior antimicrobial therapy or failure to perform appropriate microbiologic cultures. For optimal yield, the avoidance of even a single dose of antibiotics is mandatory. Primary isolation usually requires 5–7 days but may take as long as 2–4 weeks. Although not routinely used, 16S rRNA gene amplification and sequencing have been successfully applied to increase diagnostic sensitivity. Because actinomycetes are components of the normal oral and genital-tract flora, their identification in the absence of sulfur granules in sputum, bronchial washings, and cervicovaginal secretions is of little significance.

| TREATMENT | Actinomycosis |

Decisions about treatment are based on the collective clinical experience of the past 50 years. Actinomycosis requires prolonged treatment with high doses of antimicrobial agents. The need for intensive treatment is presumably due to the drugs' poor penetration of the thick-walled masses common in this infection and/or the sulfur granules themselves, which may represent a biofilm. Although therapy must be individualized, the IV administration of 18–24 million units of penicillin daily for 2–6 weeks, followed by oral therapy with penicillin or amoxicillin (total duration, 6–12 months), is a reasonable guideline for serious infections and bulky disease. Less extensive disease, particularly that involving the oral-cervicofacial region, may be cured with a shorter course. If therapy is extended beyond the resolution of measurable disease, the risk of relapse—a clinical hallmark of this infection—will be minimized; CT and MRI are generally the most sensitive and objective techniques by which to accomplish this goal. A similar approach is reasonable for immunocompromised patients, although refractory disease has been described in HIV-infected individuals. Suitable alternative antimicrobial agents and those deemed unreliable are listed in Table 163-1. Although the role played by "companion" microbes in actinomycosis is unclear, many isolates are pathogens in their own right, and a regimen covering these organisms during the initial treatment course is reasonable.

TABLE 163-1 Appropriate and Inappropriate Antibiotic Therapy for Actinomycosis[a]

Category	Agent
Extensive successful clinical experience[b]	Penicillin: 3–4 million units IV q4h
	Amoxicillin: 500 mg PO q6h
	Erythromycin: 500–1000 mg IV q6h or 500 mg PO q6h
	Tetracycline: 500 mg PO q6h
	Doxycycline: 100 mg IV or PO q12h
	Minocycline: 100 mg IV or PO q12h
	Clindamycin: 900 mg IV q8h or 300–450 mg PO q6h
Anecdotal successful clinical experience	Ceftriaxone[c]
	Ceftizoxime
	Imipenem-cilastatin
	Piperacillin-tazobactam
Agents that should be avoided	Metronidazole
	Aminoglycosides
	Oxacillin
	Dicloxacillin
	Cephalexin
Agents predicted to be efficacious on the basis of in vitro activity	Moxifloxacin
	Vancomycin
	Linezolid
	Quinupristin-dalfopristin
	Ertapenem[c]
	Azithromycin[c]

[a]Additional coverage for concomitant "companion" bacteria may be required.

[b]Controlled evaluations have not been performed. Dose and duration require individualization depending on the host, site, and extent of infection. As a general rule, a maximal parenteral antimicrobial dose for 2–6 weeks followed by oral therapy, for a total duration of 6–12 months, is required for serious infections and bulky disease, whereas a shorter course may suffice for less extensive disease, particularly in the oral-cervicofacial region. Monitoring the impact of therapy with CT or MRI is advisable when appropriate.

[c]This agent can be considered for at-home parenteral therapy.

Combined medical-surgical therapy is still advocated in some reports. However, an increasing body of literature now supports an initial attempt at cure with medical therapy alone, even in extensive disease. CT and MRI should be used to monitor the response to therapy. In most cases, either surgery can be avoided or a less extensive procedure can be used. This approach is particularly valuable in sparing critical organs, such as the bladder or the reproductive organs in women of child-bearing age. For a well-defined abscess, percutaneous drainage in combination with medical therapy is a reasonable approach. When a critical location is involved (e.g., the epidural space, the CNS) or when suitable medical therapy fails, surgical intervention may be appropriate.

FURTHER READINGS

COHEN RD et al: Pulmonary actinomycosis complicating infliximab therapy for Crohn's disease. Thorax 62:1013, 2007

HO L et al: Actinomycosis mimicking anastomotic recurrent esophageal cancer on PET-CT. Clin Nucl Med 31:646, 2006

JOSHI C et al: Pelvic actinomycosis: A rare entity presenting as a tubo-ovarian abscess. Arch Gynecol Obstet 281:305, 2010

NAIK NH, RUSSO TA: Bisphosphonate related osteonecrosis of the jaw: The role of *Actinomyces*. Clin Infect Dis 49:1729, 2009

RUSSO TA: Agents of actinomycosis, in *Principles and Practice of Infectious Diseases*, 7th ed, GL Mandell et al (eds). New York, Churchill Livingstone, 2010, pp 3209–3219

VYAS JM et al: Abdominal abscesses due to actinomycosis after laparoscopic cholecystectomy: Case reports and review. Clin Infect Dis 44:e1, 2007

WANG S et al: Actinomycotic brain infection: Registered diffusion, perfusion MR imaging and MR spectroscopy. Neuroradiology 48:346, 2006

WESTHOFF C: IUDs and colonization or infection with *Actinomyces*. Contraception 75:S48, 2007

PART 8

Infectious Diseases

CHAPTER **164**

Infections Due to Mixed Anaerobic Organisms

Dennis L. Kasper

Ronit Cohen-Poradosu

■ DEFINITIONS

Anaerobic bacteria are organisms that require reduced oxygen tension for growth, failing to grow on the surface of solid media in 10% CO_2 in air. (In contrast, *microaerophilic bacteria* can grow in an atmosphere of 10% CO_2 in air or under anaerobic or aerobic conditions, although they grow best in the presence of only a small amount of atmospheric oxygen, and *facultative bacteria* can grow in the presence or absence of air.) This chapter describes infections caused by nonsporulating anaerobic bacteria. Most clinically relevant anaerobes, such as *Bacteroides fragilis*, *Prevotella melaninogenica*, and *Fusobacterium nucleatum*, are relatively aerotolerant. Although they can survive for sustained periods in the presence of up to 2–8% oxygen, generally they do not multiply in this environment. A far smaller number of pathogenic anaerobic bacteria (which are also part of the normal flora) die after brief contact with oxygen, even in low concentrations.

Most human mucocutaneous surfaces harbor a rich indigenous flora composed of aerobic and anaerobic bacteria. These surfaces are dominated by anaerobic bacteria, which often account for 99.0–99.9% of the culturable flora and range in concentration from 10^9/mL in saliva to 10^{12}/mL in gingival scrapings and the colon. Most of the normal anaerobic flora cannot be grown or characterized by current laboratory methods. The major reservoirs of these bacteria are the mouth, lower gastrointestinal tract, skin, and female genital tract (Table 164-1). In the oral cavity, the ratio of anaerobic to aerobic bacteria ranges from 1:1 on the surface of a tooth to 1000:1 in the gingival crevices. Anaerobic bacteria are not found in appreciable numbers in the normal upper intestine until the distal ileum. In the colon, the proportion of anaerobes increases

significantly, as does the overall bacterial count; for example, there are 10^{11}–10^{12} organisms per gram of stool, and >99% of these organisms are anaerobic, with an anaerobe-to-aerobe ratio of ~1000:1. In the female genital tract, there are ~10^9 organisms per milliliter of secretions, with an anaerobe-to-aerobe ratio of ~10:1.

Commensal anaerobes have been implicated as crucial mediators of physiologic, metabolic, and immunologic functions of the mammalian host. One of the most important roles that anaerobes serve as components of the normal colonic flora is colonization resistance, in which their presence effectively interferes with colonization by potentially pathogenic bacterial species through the depletion of oxygen and nutrients, the production of enzymes and toxic end products, and the modulation of the host's intestinal innate immune response. *Bacteroides* and other intestinal bacteria ferment carbohydrates and produce volatile fatty acids that are reabsorbed and used by the host as an energy source. The anaerobic intestinal microflora is also responsible for the production of secreted products that promote human health (e.g., vitamin K and bile acids).

The anaerobic intestinal flora influences the development of an intact mucosa and of mucosa-associated lymphoid tissue. Colonization of germ-free mice with a single species, *Bacteroides thetaiotaomicron*, affects the expression of various host genes and corrects deficiencies of nutrient uptake, metabolism, angiogenesis, mucosal barrier function, and enteric nervous system development. The symbiosis factor polysaccharide A of *B. fragilis* influences the normal development and function of the mammalian immune system and protects mice against colitis in a model of inflammatory bowel disease.

Hundreds of species of anaerobic bacteria have been identified as part of the normal flora of humans. Despite the complex array of bacteria in the normal flora, relatively few species are isolated commonly from human infection. Anaerobic infections occur when the harmonious relationship between the host and the bacteria is disrupted. Any site in the body is susceptible to infection with these indigenous organisms when a mucosal barrier or the skin is compromised by surgery, trauma, tumor, ischemia, or necrosis, all of which can reduce local tissue redox potentials. Because the sites that are colonized by anaerobes contain many species of bacteria, disruption of anatomic barriers allows the penetration of many organisms, resulting in mixed infections involving multiple species of anaerobes combined with facultative or microaerophilic

TABLE 164-1 Anaerobic Human Flora: An Overview

Anatomic Site	Total Bacteria[a]	Anaerobic/ Aerobic Ratio	Potential Pathogens
Oral cavity			
Saliva	10^8–10^9	1:1	*Fusobacterium nucleatum*, *Prevotella melaninogenica*, *Prevotella oralis* group, *Bacteroides ureolyticus* group, *Peptostreptococcus* spp.
Tooth surface	10^{10}–10^{11}	1:1	
Gingival crevices	10^{11}–10^{12}	10^3:1	
Gastrointestinal tract			
Stomach	0–10^5	1:1	*Bacteroides* spp. (principally members of the *B. fragilis* group), *Prevotella* spp., *Clostridium* spp., *Peptostreptococcus* spp.
Jejunum/ileum	10^4–10^7	1:1	
Terminal ileum and colon	10^{11}–10^{12}	10^3:1	
Female genital tract	10^7–10^9	10:1	*Peptostreptococcus* spp., *Bacteroides* spp., *Prevotella bivia*

[a]Per gram or milliliter.

organisms. Such mixed infections are seen in the head and neck (chronic sinusitis, chronic otitis media, Ludwig's angina, and periodontal abscesses). Brain abscesses and subdural empyema are the most common anaerobic infections of the central nervous system (CNS). Anaerobes are responsible for pleuropulmonary diseases such as aspiration pneumonia, necrotizing pneumonia, lung abscess, and empyema. These organisms also play an important role in various intraabdominal infections, such as peritonitis and intraabdominal and hepatic abscesses (Chap. 127). They are isolated frequently in female genital tract infections, such as salpingitis, pelvic peritonitis, tuboovarian abscess, vulvovaginal abscess, septic abortion, and endometritis (Chap. 130). Anaerobic bacteria are also found often in bacteremia and in infections of the skin, soft tissues, and bones.

■ ETIOLOGY

The taxonomic classification of anaerobes is rapidly evolving, with frequent changes in nomenclature based on newly discovered relationships among bacterial species. Infections caused by anaerobic bacteria most frequently are due to more than one organism. These polymicrobial infections may be caused by one or several anaerobic species or by a combination of anaerobic organisms and microaerophilic or facultative bacteria acting synergistically. The major anaerobic gram-positive cocci that produce disease are *Peptostreptococcus* species; the major species of this genus that are involved in infections are *P. micros*, *P. magnus*, *P. asaccharolyticus*, *P. anaerobius*, and *P. prevotii*. Clostridia (Chap. 142) are spore-forming gram-positive rods that are isolated from wounds, abscesses, sites of abdominal infection, and blood. Gram-positive anaerobic non-spore-forming bacilli are uncommon as etiologic agents of human infection. *Propionibacterium acnes*, a component of the skin flora and a rare cause of foreign-body infections, is one of the few nonclostridial gram-positive rods associated with infections. The principal anaerobic gram-negative bacilli found in human infections are the *B. fragilis* group as well as *Fusobacterium*, *Prevotella*, and *Porphyromonas* species.

The most important potential anaerobic pathogens found in the upper airways and isolated from clinical specimens of oral and pleuropulmonary infections are the *Fusobacterium* species *F. necrophorum*, *F. nucleatum*, and *F. varium*; *P. melaninogenica*; the *Prevotella oralis* group; *Porphyromonas gingivalis*; *Porphyromonas asaccharolytica*; *Peptostreptococcus* species; and the *Bacteroides ureolyticus* group.

The *B. fragilis* group contains the anaerobic pathogens most frequently isolated from clinical infections. Members of this group are part of the normal bowel flora; they include several distinct species, such as *B. fragilis*, *B. thetaiotaomicron*, *B. vulgatus*, *B. uniformis*, *B. ovatus*, and *Parabacteroides distasonis*. *B. fragilis* is the most important clinical isolate, although it is isolated in lower numbers than some other *Bacteroides* species from cultures of commensal fecal flora.

In female genital tract infections, organisms normally colonizing the vagina (e.g., *Prevotella bivia* and *Prevotella disiens*) are the most common isolates. However, *B. fragilis* is not uncommon.

■ PATHOGENESIS

Anaerobic bacterial infections usually occur when an anatomic barrier is disrupted and constituents of the local flora enter a site that was previously sterile. Because of the specific growth requirements of anaerobic organisms and their presence as commensals on mucosal surfaces, conditions must arise that allow these organisms to penetrate mucosal barriers and enter tissue with a lowered oxidation-reduction potential. Therefore, tissue ischemia, trauma, surgery, perforated viscus, shock, and aspiration

provide environments conducive to the proliferation of anaerobes. The introduction of many bacterial species into otherwise-sterile sites leads to a polymicrobial infection in which certain organisms predominate. Three major factors are involved in the pathogenesis of anaerobic infections: bacterial synergy, bacterial virulence factors, and mechanisms of abscess formation. The ability of different anaerobic bacteria to act synergistically during polymicrobial infection contributes to the pathogenesis of anaerobic infections. It has been postulated that facultative organisms function in part to lower the oxidation-reduction potential in the microenvironment, allowing the propagation of obligate anaerobes. Anaerobes can produce compounds such as succinic acid and short-chain fatty acids that inhibit the ability of phagocytes to clear facultative organisms. In experimental models, facultative and obligate anaerobes synergistically potentiate abscess formation. Virulence factors associated with anaerobes typically confer the ability to evade host defenses, adhere to cell surfaces, produce toxins and/or enzymes, or display surface structures such as capsular polysaccharides and lipopolysaccharide (LPS) that contribute to pathogenic potential. The ability of an organism to adhere to host tissues is important to the establishment of infection. Some oral species adhere to the epithelium in the oral cavity. *P. melaninogenica* actually attaches to other microorganisms. *P. gingivalis*, a common isolate in periodontal disease, has fimbriae that facilitate attachment. Some *Bacteroides* strains appear to be piliated, a characteristic that may account for their ability to adhere.

The most extensively studied virulence factor of the nonsporulating anaerobes is the capsular polysaccharide complex of *B. fragilis*. This organism is unique among anaerobes in its potential for virulence during growth at normally sterile sites. Although it constitutes only 0.5–1% of the normal colonic flora, *B. fragilis* is the anaerobe most commonly isolated from intraabdominal infections and bacteremia. One polysaccharide of *B. fragilis*, polysaccharide A, has a unique zwitterionic motif of charged sugars that confers distinct biologic properties, such as the ability to promote abscess formation. Intraabdominal abscess induction is related to the capacity of this polysaccharide to stimulate the release of cytokines and chemokines—in particular, interleukin (IL) 8, IL-17, and tumor necrosis factor α (TNF-α)—from resident peritoneal cells. The release of cytokines and chemokines results in the chemotaxis of polymorphonuclear neutrophils (PMNs) into the peritoneum, where they adhere to mesothelial cells induced by TNF-α to upregulate their expression of intercellular adhesion molecule 1 (ICAM-1). PMNs adherent to ICAM-1-expressing cells probably represent the nidus for an abscess. Polysaccharide A also activates T cells to produce certain cytokines, including IL-17 and interferon γ, that are necessary for abscess formation. Furthermore, when the same polysaccharide is administered to experimental animals prophylactically or therapeutically, it confers protection against abscess induction after challenge with microorganisms capable of inducing abscesses. This protection is mediated by IL-10-producing T cells.

Anaerobic bacteria produce a number of exoproteins that can enhance the organisms' virulence. The collagenase produced by *P. gingivalis* may enhance tissue destruction. An enterotoxin has been identified in *B. fragilis* strains associated with diarrheal disease in animals and young children. Exotoxins produced by clostridial species, including botulinum toxins, tetanus toxin, *C. difficile* toxins A and B, and five toxins produced by *C. perfringens*, are among the most virulent bacterial toxins in mouse lethality assays. Anaerobic gram-negative bacteria such as *B. fragilis* possess LPSs (endotoxins) that are 100–1000 times less biologically potent than endotoxins associated with aerobic gram-negative bacteria. This relative biologic inactivity may account for the lower frequency of disseminated intravascular coagulation and purpura in *Bacteroides* bacteremia than in facultative and aerobic gram-negative bacillary bacteremia. An exception is the LPS from *Fusobacterium*, which may account for the severity of Lemierre's syndrome.

APPROACH TO THE PATIENT	Infections Due to Mixed Anaerobic Organisms

The physician must consider several points when approaching the patient with presumptive infection due to anaerobic bacteria.

1. Most of the organisms colonizing mucosal sites are harmless commensals; very few cause disease. When these organisms do cause disease, it often occurs in proximity to the mucosal site they colonize.

2. For anaerobes to cause tissue infection, they must spread beyond the normal mucosal barriers.

3. Conditions favoring the propagation of these bacteria, particularly a lowered oxidation-reduction potential, are necessary. These conditions exist at sites of trauma, tissue destruction, compromised vascular supply, and complications of preexisting infection, which produce necrosis.

4. There is a complex array of infecting flora. For example, as many as 12 types of organisms can be isolated from a suppurative site.

5. Anaerobic organisms tend to be found in abscess cavities or in necrotic tissue. The failure of an abscess to yield organisms on routine culture is a clue that the abscess is likely to contain anaerobic bacteria. Often smears of this "sterile pus" are found to be teeming with bacteria when Gram's stain is applied. Although some facultative organisms (e.g., *Staphylococcus aureus*) are also capable of causing abscesses, abscesses in organs or deeper body tissues should call to mind anaerobic infection.

6. Gas is found in many anaerobic infections of deep tissues but is not diagnostic because it can be produced by aerobic bacteria as well.

7. Although a putrid-smelling infection site or discharge is considered diagnostic for anaerobic infection, this manifestation usually develops late in the course and is present in only 30–50% of cases.

8. Some species (the best example being the *B. fragilis* group) require specific therapy. However, many synergistic infections can be cured with antibiotics directed at some but not all of the organisms involved. Antibiotic therapy, combined with debridement and drainage, disrupts the interdependent relationship among the bacteria, and some species that are resistant to the antibiotic do not survive without the co-infecting organisms.

9. Manifestations of severe sepsis and disseminated intravascular coagulation are unusual in patients with purely anaerobic infection.

◼ EPIDEMIOLOGY

Difficulties in the performance of appropriate cultures, contamination of cultures by components of the normal flora, and the lack of readily available, reliable culture techniques have made it impossible to obtain accurate data on incidence or prevalence. However, anaerobic infections are encountered frequently in hospitals with active surgical, trauma, and obstetric and gynecologic services. Depending on the institution, anaerobic bacteria account for 0.5–12% of all cases of bacteremia.

◼ CLINICAL MANIFESTATIONS

Anaerobic infections of the mouth, head, and neck

(See also Chap. 31) Anaerobic bacteria are commonly involved in infections of the mouth, head, and neck. The predominant isolates are components of the normal flora of the upper airways—mainly the *Bacteroides oralis* group, pigmented *Prevotella* species, *P. asaccharolytica*, *Fusobacterium* species, peptostreptococci, and microaerophilic streptococci.

Soft tissue infections of the oral-facial area may or may not be odontogenic. Odontogenic infections—primarily dental caries and periodontal disease (gingivitis and periodontitis)—are common and have both local consequences (especially tooth loss) and the potential for life-threatening spread to the deep fascial spaces of the head and neck. Infections of the mouth can arise from either a supragingival or a subgingival dental plaque composed of bacteria colonizing the tooth surface. Supragingival plaque formation begins with the adherence of gram-positive bacteria to the tooth surface. This form of plaque is influenced by salivary and dietary components, oral hygiene, and local host factors. Supragingival plaque can lead to dental caries and, with further invasion, to pulpitis (endodontic infection) that can further perforate the alveolar bone, causing periapical abscess. Subgingival plaque is associated with periodontal infections (e.g., gingivitis, periodontitis, and periodontal abscess) that can further disseminate to adjacent structures such as the mandible, causing osteomyelitis of the maxillary sinuses. Periodontitis may also result in spreading infection that can involve adjacent bone or soft tissues. In the healthy periodontium, the sparse microflora consists mainly of gram-positive organisms such as *Streptococcus sanguinis* and *Actinomyces* species. In the presence of gingivitis, there is a shift to a greater proportion of anaerobic gram-negative bacilli in the subgingival flora, with predominance of *Prevotella intermedia*. In well-established periodontitis, the complexity of the flora increases further. The predominant isolates are *P. gingivalis*, *P. intermedia*, *Aggregatibacter* (formerly *Actinobacillus*) *actinomycetemcomitans*, *Treponema denticola*, and *Tannerella forsythensis*.

Necrotizing ulcerative gingivitis

Gingivitis may become a necrotizing infection (trench mouth, Vincent's stomatitis). The onset of disease is usually sudden and is associated with tender bleeding gums, foul breath, and a bad taste. The gingival mucosa, especially the papillae between the teeth, becomes ulcerated and may be covered by a gray exudate, which is removable with gentle pressure. Patients may become systemically ill, developing fever, cervical lymphadenopathy, and leukocytosis. Occasionally, ulcerative gingivitis can spread to the buccal mucosa, the teeth, and the mandible or maxilla, resulting in widespread destruction of bone and soft tissue. This infection is termed acute necrotizing ulcerative mucositis (cancrum oris, noma). It destroys tissue rapidly, causing the teeth to fall out and large areas of bone—or even the whole mandible—to be sloughed. A strong putrid odor is frequently detected, although the lesions are not painful. The gangrenous lesions eventually heal, leaving large disfiguring defects. This infection most commonly follows a debilitating illness or affects severely malnourished children. It has been known to complicate leukemia or to develop in individuals with a genetic deficiency of catalase.

Acute necrotizing infections of the pharynx

These infections usually occur in association with ulcerative gingivitis. Symptoms include an extremely sore throat, foul breath, and a bad taste accompanied by fever and a sensation of choking. Examination of the pharynx demonstrates that the tonsillar pillars are swollen, red, ulcerated, and covered with a grayish membrane that peels easily. Lymphadenopathy and leukocytosis are common. The disease may last for only a few days or, if not treated, may persist for weeks. Lesions begin unilaterally but may spread to the other side of the pharynx or the larynx. Aspiration of the infected material by the patient can result in lung abscesses.

Peripharyngeal space infections

These infections arise from the spread of organisms from the upper airways to potential spaces formed by the fascial planes of the head and neck. The etiology is typically polymicrobial and represents the normal flora of the mucosa of the originating site.

Peritonsillar abscess (*quinsy*) is a complication of acute tonsillitis caused mainly by a mixed flora containing anaerobes and group A *Streptococcus*. In submandibular space infection (*Ludwig's angina*), 80% of cases are caused by infection of the tissues surrounding the second and third molar teeth. This infection results in marked local swelling of tissues, with pain, trismus, and superior and posterior displacement of the tongue. Submandibular swelling of the neck can impair swallowing and cause respiratory obstruction. In some cases, tracheotomy may be life-saving. Cervicofacial actinomycosis (Chap. 163) is caused by a branching, gram-positive, non-spore-forming, strict/facultative anaerobe that is a part of the normal oral flora. This chronic disease is characterized by abscesses, draining sinus tracts, fistula, bone destruction, and fibrosis. It can easily be mistaken for malignancy or granulomatous disease. Actinomycosis less frequently involves the thorax, abdomen, pelvis, and CNS.

Sinusitis and otitis

Anaerobic bacteria have been implicated in chronic sinusitis but play little role in acute sinusitis. In several studies on chronic sinusitis, anaerobic bacteria were found in 12–93% of cases, depending on the method used to collect specimens. Predominant isolates were pigmented *Prevotella, Fusobacterium,* and *Peptostreptococcus* species. Aerobic gram-negative bacilli and *S. aureus* have also been implicated in chronic sinusitis. Polymicrobial infection is common and may be synergistic.

Anaerobic bacteria are much more easily implicated in chronic suppurative otitis media than in acute otitis media. Purulent exudate from chronically draining ears has been found to contain anaerobes, particularly *Bacteroides* species, in up to 50% of cases. *B. fragilis* has been isolated from up to 28% of patients with chronic otitis media.

Complications of anaerobic head and neck infections

Contiguous cranial spread of these infections may result in osteomyelitis of the skull or mandible or in intracranial infections such as brain abscess and subdural empyema. Caudal spread can produce mediastinitis or pleuropulmonary infection. Hematogenous complications may also result from anaerobic infections of the head and neck. Bacteremia, which occasionally is polymicrobial, can lead to endocarditis or other distant infections. Lemierre's syndrome, which has been uncommon in the antimicrobial era, is an acute oropharyngeal infection with secondary septic thrombophlebitis of the internal jugular vein and frequent metastasis, most commonly to the lung. *F. necrophorum* is the usual cause. This infection typically begins with pharyngitis, which is followed by local invasion in the lateral pharyngeal space with resultant internal jugular vein thrombophlebitis. A typical clinical triad seen in recent series is pharyngitis, a tender/swollen neck, and noncavitating pulmonary infiltrates.

CNS infections

CNS infections associated with anaerobic bacteria are brain abscess (Chap. 381), epidural abscess, and subdural empyema. Anaerobic meningitis is rare and is usually related to parameningeal collection or shunt infection. If optimal bacteriologic techniques are employed, as many as 85% of brain abscesses yield anaerobic bacteria, which usually originate from otorhinolaryngeal infection. However, intraabdominal or pelvic infections can occasionally lead to bacteremia with an anaerobic organism that seeds the cerebral cortex. Commonly isolated are *Peptostreptococcus, Fusobacterium, Bacteroides, Prevotella, Propionibacterium, Eubacterium, Veillonella,* and *Actinomyces* species. Facultative or microaerophilic streptococci and coliforms are often part of a mixed infecting flora in brain abscesses.

Pleuropulmonary infections

Anaerobic pleuropulmonary infections result from the aspiration of oropharyngeal contents, often in the context of an altered state of consciousness or an absent gag reflex. Four clinical syndromes are associated with anaerobic pleuropulmonary infection produced by aspiration: simple aspiration pneumonia, necrotizing pneumonia, lung abscess, and empyema. Many of these infections have an indolent course that may serve as a clinical clue differentiating them, for example, from pneumococcal pneumonia, which often presents with abrupt onset, shaking chills, and rapid progression.

Aspiration pneumonitis Bacterial aspiration pneumonitis must be distinguished from two other clinical syndromes associated with aspiration that are not of bacterial etiology. One syndrome results from aspiration of solids, usually food. Obstruction of major airways typically results in atelectasis and moderate nonspecific inflammation. Therapy consists of removal of the foreign body.

The second aspiration syndrome is more easily confused with bacterial aspiration. *Mendelson's syndrome*, a chemical pneumonitis, results from regurgitation of stomach contents and aspiration of chemical material, usually acidic gastric juices. Pulmonary inflammation—including the destruction of the alveolar lining, with transudation of fluid into the alveolar space—occurs with remarkable rapidity. Typically this syndrome develops within hours, often following anesthesia when the gag reflex is depressed. The patient becomes tachypneic, hypoxic, and febrile. The leukocyte count may rise, and the chest x-ray may evolve suddenly from normal to a complete bilateral "whiteout" within 8–24 h. Sputum production is minimal. The pulmonary signs and symptoms can resolve quickly with symptom-based therapy or can culminate in respiratory failure, with the subsequent development of bacterial superinfection over a period of days. Antibiotic therapy is not indicated unless bacterial infection supervenes.

In contrast to these syndromes, bacterial aspiration pneumonia develops over a period of several days or weeks rather than hours. It is seen in patients who are hospitalized and have a depressed gag reflex, impaired swallowing, or a tracheal or nasogastric tube; elderly patients; and patients with transiently impaired consciousness in the wake of seizures, cerebrovascular accidents, or alcoholic blackouts. Patients who enter the hospital with this syndrome typically have been ill for several days and generally report low-grade fever, malaise, and sputum production. In some patients, weight loss and anemia reflect a more chronic process. Usually the history reveals factors predisposing to aspiration, such as alcohol overdose or residence in a nursing home. Examination sometimes yields evidence of periodontal disease. Sputum characteristically is not malodorous unless the process has been under way for at least a week. A mixed bacterial flora with many PMNs is evident on Gram's staining of sputum. Expectorated sputum is unreliable for anaerobic cultures because of inevitable contamination by normal oral flora. Reliable specimens for culture can be obtained by transtracheal or transthoracic aspiration—techniques that are rarely used at present. Culture of protected-brush specimens or bronchoalveolar lavage fluid obtained by bronchoscopy is controversial.

Chest x-rays show consolidation in dependent pulmonary segments: in the basilar segments of the lower lobes if the patient has aspirated while upright and in either the posterior segment of the upper lobe (usually on the right side) or the superior segment of the lower lobe if the patient has aspirated while supine. The organisms isolated from the lungs reflect the pharyngeal flora; pigmented and nonpigmented *Prevotella* species, *Peptostreptococcus* species, *Bacteroides* species, *Fusobacterium* species, and anaerobic cocci are the most common isolates. While most patients with aspiration pneumonia acquired in the community have a mixed infection caused by anaerobes and aerobic or microaerophilic streptococci, the patient who aspirates in the hospital may also have a mixed infection involving enteric gram-negative rods. In a study on the microbiology of severe aspiration pneumonia in institutionalized elderly patients, gram-negative bacilli were cultured in 49% of cases (with an anaerobe also recovered in 14% of this group), anaerobes in 16%, and *S. aureus* in 12%.

Necrotizing pneumonitis This form of anaerobic pneumonitis is characterized by numerous small abscesses that spread to involve several pulmonary segments. The process can be indolent or fulminating. This syndrome is less common than either aspiration pneumonia or lung abscess and includes features of both types of infection.

Anaerobic lung abscesses These abscesses result from subacute anaerobic pulmonary infection. The clinical syndrome typically involves a history of constitutional signs and symptoms (including malaise, weight loss, fever, night sweats, and foul-smelling sputum), perhaps over a period of weeks (Chap. 257). Patients who develop lung abscesses characteristically have dental infection and periodontitis, but lung abscesses in edentulous patients have been reported. Abscess cavities may be single or multiple and generally occur in dependent pulmonary segments (Fig. 164-1). Anaerobic abscesses must be distinguished from lesions associated with tuberculosis, neoplasia, and other conditions. Oral anaerobes predominate and are found in 60–80% of cases. There is also an important role for microaerophilic streptococci such as *S. milleri*. *S. aureus* and enteric

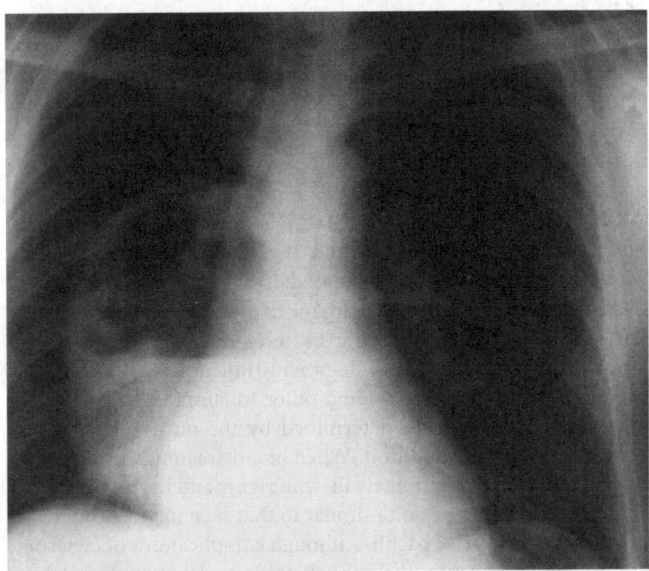

Figure 164-1   Chest radiograph of right-lower-lobe lung abscess in a 60-year-old alcoholic patient. *[From GL Mandell (ed): Atlas of Infectious Diseases, Vol VI. Philadelphia, Current Medicine Inc, Churchill Livingstone, 1996; with permission.]*

gram-negative bacilli may be found as well. Septic pulmonary emboli may originate from intraabdominal or female genital tract infections and can produce anaerobic pneumonia and abscess.

Empyema Empyema is a manifestation of long-standing anaerobic pulmonary infection. The clinical presentation, which includes foul-smelling sputum, resembles that of other anaerobic pulmonary infections. Patients may report pleuritic chest pain and marked chest-wall tenderness.

Empyema may be masked by overlying pneumonitis and should be considered especially in cases of persistent fever despite antibiotic therapy. Diligent physical examination and the use of ultrasound to localize a loculated empyema are important diagnostic tools. The collection of a foul-smelling exudate by thoracentesis is typical. Cultures of infected pleural fluid yield an average of 3.5 anaerobic and 0.6 facultative or aerobic bacterial species. Drainage is required. Defervescence, a return to a feeling of well-being, and resolution of the process may require several months.

Extension from a subdiaphragmatic infection may also result in anaerobic empyema.

Intraabdominal infections

Intraabdominal infections—mainly peritonitis and abscesses—are usually polymicrobial and represent the normal intestinal (especially colonic) flora. These infections usually follow a breach in the mucosal barrier resulting from appendicitis, diverticulitis, neoplasm, inflammatory bowel disease, surgery, or trauma. On average, four to six bacterial species are isolated per specimen submitted to the microbiology laboratory, with a predominance of enteric aerobic/facultative gram-negative bacilli, anaerobes, and streptococci/enterococci. The most common isolates are *Escherichia coli* (found in ≥50% of patients) and *B. fragilis* (30–50%). Disease originating from proximal-bowel perforation reflects the flora of this site, with a predominance of aerobic and anaerobic gram-positive bacteria and *Candida*.

Enterotoxigenic *B. fragilis* has been associated with watery diarrhea in a few young children and adults. In case-control studies of children with undiagnosed diarrheal disease, enterotoxigenic *B. fragilis* was isolated from significantly more children with diarrhea than children in the control group. Neutropenic enterocolitis (typhlitis) has been associated with anaerobic infection of the cecum but—in the setting of neutropenia (Chap. 86)—may involve the entire bowel. Patients usually present with fever; abdominal pain, tenderness, and distention; and watery diarrhea. The bowel wall is edematous with hemorrhage and necrosis. The primary pathogen is thought by some authorities to be *Clostridium septicum*, but other clostridia and mixed anaerobes have also been implicated. More than 50% of patients developing early clinical signs can benefit from antibiotic therapy and bowel rest. Surgery is sometimes required to remove gangrenous bowel. See Chap. 127 for a complete discussion of intraabdominal infections.

Pelvic infections

The vagina of a healthy woman is a major reservoir of anaerobic and aerobic bacteria. In the normal flora of the female genital tract, anaerobes outnumber aerobes by a ratio of ~10:1 and include anaerobic gram-positive cocci and *Bacteroides* species (Table 164-1). Anaerobes are isolated from most women with genital tract infections that are not caused by a sexually transmitted pathogen. The major anaerobic pathogens are *B. fragilis*, *P. bivia*, *P. disiens*, *P. melaninogenica*, anaerobic cocci, and *Clostridium* species. Anaerobes are frequently encountered in Bartholin gland abscess, salpingitis, tuboovarian abscess, septic abortion, pyometra, endometritis, and postoperative wound infection, particularly following hysterectomy. These infections are often of mixed etiology, involving both anaerobes and coliforms; pure anaerobic infections without coliform or other facultative bacterial species occur more often in pelvic than in intraabdominal sites. Suppurative thrombophlebitis of the pelvic veins may complicate the infections and lead to repeated episodes of septic pulmonary emboli. See Chap. 130 for a complete discussion of pelvic inflammatory disease.

Anaerobic bacteria have been thought to be contributing factors in the etiology of bacterial vaginosis. This syndrome of unknown etiology is characterized by a profuse malodorous discharge and a change in the bacterial ecology that results in replacement of the *Lactobacillus*-dominated normal flora with an overgrowth of bacterial species including *Gardnerella vaginalis*, *Prevotella* species, *Mobiluncus* species, peptostreptococci, and genital mycoplasmas. A study based on 16S rRNA identification found other anaerobes that were predominant in cases but not in controls: *Atopobium*, *Leptotrichia*, *Megasphaera*, and *Eggerthella*. Pelvic infections due to *Actinomyces* species have been associated with the use of intrauterine devices (Chap. 163).

Skin and soft tissue infections

Injury to skin, bone, or soft tissue by trauma, ischemia, or surgery creates a suitable environment for anaerobic infections. These infections are most frequently found in sites prone to contamination with feces or with upper airway secretions—e.g., wounds associated with intestinal surgery, decubitus ulcers, or human bites. Moreover, anaerobes have been isolated from cutaneous abscesses, rectal abscesses, and axillary sweat gland infections (hidradenitis suppurativa). Anaerobes are also frequently cultured from foot ulcers of diabetic patients. The deep soft-tissue infections associated with anaerobic bacteria are crepitant cellulitis, synergistic cellulitis, gangrene, and necrotizing fasciitis (Chaps. 125 and 142).

These soft tissue or skin infections are usually polymicrobial. A mean of 4.8 bacterial species are isolated, with an anaerobe-to-aerobe ratio of ~3:2. The most frequently isolated organisms include *Bacteroides*, *Peptostreptococcus*, *Clostridium*, *Enterococcus*, and *Proteus* species. The involvement of anaerobes in these types of infections is associated with a higher frequency of fever, foul-smelling lesions, gas in the tissues, and visible foot ulcer.

Anaerobic bacterial synergistic gangrene (*Meleney's gangrene*), a rare infection of the superficial fascia, is characterized by exquisite pain, redness, and swelling followed by induration. Erythema surrounds a central zone of necrosis. A granulating ulcer forms at the original center as necrosis and erythema extend outward. Symptoms are limited to pain; fever is not typical. These infections usually involve a combination of *Peptostreptococcus* species and *S. aureus*; the usual site of infection is an abdominal surgical wound or the area surrounding an ulcer on an extremity. Treatment includes surgical removal of necrotic tissue and antimicrobial administration.

Necrotizing fasciitis, a rapidly spreading destructive disease of the fascia, is usually attributed to group A streptococci (Chap. 136) but can also be a mixed infection involving anaerobes and aerobes, usually after surgeries and in patients with diabetes or peripheral vascular disease. The most frequently isolated anaerobes in these infections are *Peptostreptococcus* and *Bacteroides* species. Gas may be found in the tissues. Similarly, myonecrosis can be associated with mixed anaerobic infection. *Fournier's gangrene* consists of cellulitis involving the scrotum, perineum, and anterior abdominal wall, with mixed anaerobic organisms spreading along deep external fascial planes and causing extensive loss of skin.

Bone and joint infections

Although actinomycosis (Chap. 163) accounts on a worldwide basis for most anaerobic infections in bone, organisms including peptostreptococci or microaerophilic cocci, *Bacteroides* species, *Fusobacterium* species, and *Clostridium* species can also be involved. These infections frequently arise adjacent to soft tissue infections. Hematogenous seeding of bone is uncommon. *Prevotella* and *Porphyromonas* species are detected in infections involving the maxilla and mandible, whereas *Clostridium* species have been reported as anaerobic pathogens in cases of osteomyelitis of the long bones following fracture or trauma. Fusobacteria have been isolated in pure culture from sites of osteomyelitis adjacent to the perinasal sinuses. Peptostreptococci and microaerophilic cocci have been reported as significant pathogens in infections involving the skull, mastoid, and prosthetic implants placed in bone. In patients with osteomyelitis (Chap. 126), the most reliable culture specimen is a bone biopsy sample free of normal uninfected skin and subcutaneous tissue. In patients with anaerobic osteomyelitis, a mixed flora is frequently isolated from a bone biopsy specimen.

In cases of anaerobic septic arthritis, the most common isolates are *Fusobacterium* species. Most of the patients involved have uncontrolled peritonsillar infections progressing to septic cervical venous thrombophlebitis (Lemierre's syndrome) and resulting in hematogenous dissemination with a predilection for the joints. Unlike anaerobic osteomyelitis, anaerobic pyoarthritis in most cases is not polymicrobial and may be acquired hematogenously. Anaerobes are important pathogens in infections involving prosthetic joints; in these infections, the causative organisms (such as *Peptostreptococcus* species and *P. acnes*) are part of the normal skin flora.

Bacteremia

Transient bacteremia is a well-known event in healthy individuals whose anatomic mucosal barriers have been injured (e.g., during dental extractions or dental scaling). These bacteremic episodes, which are often due to anaerobes, have no pathologic consequences. However, anaerobic bacteria are found in cultures of blood from clinically ill patients when proper culture techniques are used. Anaerobes have accounted for 2–5% of all bacteremias, depending on the institution. *B. fragilis* is the single most common anaerobic isolate from the bloodstream, accounting for 35–80% of anaerobic bacteremias. The rate decreased from the 1970s through the early 1990s. This change may be related to the administration of antibiotic prophylaxis before intestinal surgery, the earlier recognition of localized infections, and the empirical use of broad-spectrum antibiotics for presumed infection. However, anaerobic bacteremia may be reemerging. Comparing two periods (1993–1996 and 2001–2004), investigators at the Mayo Clinics found a 74% increase in the incidence of anaerobic bacteremias per 100,000 patient-days; this finding contrasts with a 45% decrease in incidence from 1977 to 1988 at the same institution.

Once the organism in the blood has been identified, both the portal of bloodstream entry and the underlying problem that probably led to seeding of the bloodstream can often be deduced from an understanding of the organism's normal site of residence. For example, mixed anaerobic bacteremia including *B. fragilis* usually implies colonic pathology with mucosal disruption from neoplasia, diverticulitis, or some other inflammatory lesion. The initial manifestations are determined by the portal of entry and reflect the localized condition. When bloodstream invasion occurs, patients can become extremely ill, with rigors and hectic fevers. The clinical picture may be quite similar to that seen in sepsis involving aerobic gram-negative bacilli. Although complications of anaerobic bacteremia (e.g., septic thrombophlebitis and septic shock) have been reported, their incidence in association with anaerobic bacteremia is low. Anaerobic bacteremia is potentially fatal and requires rapid diagnosis and appropriate therapy. The mortality rate appears to increase with the age of the patient (with reported rates of >66%

among patients >60 years old), with the isolation of multiple species from the bloodstream, and with the failure to surgically remove a focus of infection. The attributable mortality rate for bacteremia associated with the *B. fragilis* group was examined in a matched case-control study. Patients with *B. fragilis*–group bacteremia had a significantly higher mortality rate (28% vs 8%), with an attributable mortality rate of 19.3% and a mortality risk ratio of 3.2.

Endocarditis and pericarditis

(See also Chap. 124) Endocarditis due to anaerobes is uncommon. However, anaerobic streptococci, which are often classified incorrectly, are responsible for this disease more frequently than is generally appreciated. Gram-negative anaerobes are unusual causes of endocarditis. Signs and symptoms of anaerobic endocarditis are similar to those of endocarditis due to facultative organisms. Mortality rates of 21–43% have been reported for anaerobic endocarditis.

Anaerobes, particularly *B. fragilis* and *Peptostreptococcus* species, are uncommonly found in infected pericardial fluids. Anaerobic pericarditis is associated with a mortality rate of >50%. Anaerobes can reach the pericardial space by hematogenous spread, by spread from a contiguous site of infection (e.g., heart or esophagus), or by direct inoculation arising from trauma or surgery.

■ DIAGNOSIS

There are three critical steps in the diagnosis of anaerobic infection: (1) proper specimen collection; (2) rapid transport of the specimens to the microbiology laboratory, preferably in anaerobic transport media; and (3) proper handling of the specimens by the laboratory. Specimens must be collected by meticulous sampling of infected sites, with avoidance of contamination by the normal flora. When such contamination is likely, the specimen is unacceptable. Examples of specimens unacceptable for anaerobic culture include sputum collected by expectoration or nasal tracheal suction, bronchoscopy specimens, samples collected directly through the vaginal vault, urine collected by voiding, and feces. Specimens appropriate for anaerobic culture include sterile body fluids such as blood, pleural fluid, peritoneal fluid, cerebrospinal fluid, and aspirates or biopsies from normally sterile sites. As a general rule, liquid or tissue specimens are preferred; swab specimens should be avoided.

Because even brief exposure to oxygen may kill some anaerobic organisms and result in failure to isolate them in the laboratory, air must be expelled from the syringe used to aspirate the abscess cavity, and the needle must be capped with a sterile rubber stopper. It is also important to remember that prior antibiotic therapy reduces cultivability of these bacteria. Specimens can be injected into transport bottles containing a reduced medium or taken immediately in syringes to the laboratory for direct culture on anaerobic media. Delays in transport may lead to a failure to isolate anaerobes due to exposure to oxygen or overgrowth of facultative organisms, which may eliminate or obscure any anaerobes that are present. All clinical specimens from suspected anaerobic infections should be Gram-stained and examined for organisms with characteristic morphology. It is not unusual for organisms to be observed on Gram's staining but not isolated in culture.

Because of the time and difficulty involved in the isolation of anaerobic bacteria, diagnosis of anaerobic infections must frequently be based on presumptive evidence. There are few clinical clues to the probable presence of anaerobic bacteria at infected sites. The involvement of certain sites with lowered oxidation-reduction potential (e.g., avascular necrotic tissues) and the presence of an abscess favor the diagnosis of an anaerobic infection. When infections occur in proximity to mucosal surfaces normally harboring an anaerobic flora, such as the gastrointestinal tract, female genital tract, or oropharynx, anaerobes should be considered as potential etiologic agents. A foul odor is often indicative of anaerobes, which produce certain organic acids as they proliferate in necrotic tissue. Although these odors are nearly pathognomonic for anaerobic infection, the absence of odor does not exclude an anaerobic etiology. Because anaerobes often coexist with other bacteria to cause mixed or synergistic infection, Gram's staining of exudate frequently reveals multiple morphotypes suggestive of anaerobes. Sometimes these organisms have morphologic characteristics associated with specific species.

The presence of gas in tissues is highly suggestive, but not diagnostic, of anaerobic infection. When cultures of obviously infected sites or purulent material yield no growth, streptococci only, or a single aerobic species (such as *E. coli*) and Gram's staining reveals a mixed flora, the involvement of anaerobes should be suspected; the implication is that the anaerobic microorganisms failed to grow because of inadequate transport and/or culture techniques. Failure of an infection to respond to antibiotics that are not active against anaerobes (e.g., aminoglycosides and—in some circumstances—penicillin, cephalosporins, or tetracyclines) suggests an anaerobic etiology.

TREATMENT   Anaerobic Infections

Successful therapy for anaerobic infections requires the administration of a combination of appropriate antibiotics, surgical resection, debridement of devitalized tissues, and drainage either surgically or percutaneously (guided by an imaging technique such as CT, MRI, or ultrasound). Any anatomic breach must be closed promptly, closed spaces drained, tissue compartments decompressed, and an adequate blood supply established. Abscess cavities should be drained as soon as fluctuation or localization occurs.

ANTIBIOTIC THERAPY AND RESISTANCE Decisions about the treatment of anaerobic infections with antibiotics are usually based on known resistance patterns in certain species, on the likelihood of encountering a given species in the case at hand, and on Gram's stain findings. Antibiotics active against clinically relevant anaerobes can be grouped into four categories on the basis of their predicted activity (Table 164-2). (Nearly all the drugs listed have toxic side effects, which are described in detail in Chap. 133.) In many infections, anaerobes are mixed with coliforms and other facultative organisms. The best therapeutic regimens, therefore, are usually those active against both aerobic and anaerobic bacteria. The choice of empirical antibiotics for the anaerobes in mixed infections can nearly always be made reliably, since patterns of antimicrobial susceptibility are usually predictable (Chap. 133 and Table 164-2).

Antibiotic susceptibility testing of anaerobic bacteria has been difficult and controversial. Owing to the slow growth rate of many anaerobes, the lack of standardized testing methods and of clinically relevant standards for resistance, and the generally good results obtained with empirical therapy, there has been limited interest in testing these organisms for antibiotic susceptibility. However, one study of antibiotic-treated patients with *Bacteroides* isolates from blood found mortality rates of 45% among those whose isolates were deemed resistant to the agent used and 16% among those whose isolates were deemed sensitive. These figures suggest that in vitro susceptibility testing should be performed for *Bacteroides* isolates from hospitalized patients with bacteremia and that the results of this testing should guide treatment. In general, cure rates of >80% can be attained among *Bacteroides*-infected patients with appropriate

TABLE 164-2 Antimicrobial Therapy for Infections Involving Commonly Encountered Anaerobic Gram-Negative Rods

Category 1 (<2% Resistance)	Category 2 (<15% Resistance)	Category 3 (Variable Resistance)	Category 4 (Resistance)
Carbapenems (imipenem, meropenem, doripenem) Metronidazole[a] β-Lactam/β-lactamase inhibitor combination (ampicillin/sulbactam, ticarcillin/clavulanic acid, piperacillin/tazobactam) Chloramphenicol[b]	Tigecycline High-dose antipseudomonal penicillins	Cephamycins Clindamycin Penicillin Cephalosporins Tetracycline Vancomycin Erythromycin Moxifloxacin	Aminoglycosides Monobactams Trimethoprim-sulfamethoxazole

[a]Usually needs to be given in combination with aerobic bacterial coverage. For infections originating below the diaphragm, aerobic gram-negative coverage is essential. For infections from an oral source, aerobic gram-positive coverage is added. Metronidazole also is not active against *Actinomyces*, *Propionibacterium*, or other gram-positive non-spore-forming bacilli (e.g., *Eubacterium*, *Bifidobacterium*) and is unreliable against peptostreptococci.

[b]Chloramphenicol is probably not as effective as other category 1 antimicrobial agents in treating anaerobic infections.

antimicrobial therapy and drainage. Of the drugs active against most clinically relevant anaerobes, metronidazole, β-lactam/β-lactamase inhibitor combinations, and carbapenems are preferred.

Antibiotic resistance in anaerobic bacteria is an increasing problem. Resistance rates vary with the institution and the geographic region. In recent years, the activity of clindamycin, cefoxitin, cefotetan, and moxifloxacin has decreased against *B. fragilis* and related strains (*B. distasonis*, *B. ovatus*, *B. thetaiotaomicron*, *B. uniformis*, *B. vulgatus*). Nearly all organisms in the *B. fragilis* group (>97%) are resistant to penicillin G. Rates of resistance to β-lactam agents among anaerobes other than *Bacteroides* are lower but highly variable. β-Lactam/β-lactamase inhibitor combinations such as ampicillin/sulbactam, ticarcillin/clavulanic acid, and piperacillin/tazobactam are usually a good therapeutic option, but decreased susceptibility in up to 10% of *B. fragilis*–group isolates has been observed in a study from Belgium. Rates of resistance to the cephamycins (cefoxitin and cefotetan) have varied between 8% and 33% in different surveys. Metronidazole is active against gram-negative anaerobes, including the *B. fragilis* group; resistance is rare but has been reported. Resistance to metronidazole is more common among gram-positive anaerobes, including *P. acnes*, *Actinomyces* species, lactobacilli, and anaerobic streptococci. In the United States, rates of clindamycin resistance among isolates of the *B. fragilis* group increased from 3% in 1982 to 16% in 1996 and 26% in 2000, with figures as high as 44% in some series. Rates of resistance to clindamycin among non-*Bacteroides* anaerobes are much lower (<10%). Carbapenems (ertapenem, doripenem, meropenem, and imipenem) are equally active against anaerobes, with <1% of *B. fragilis* strains showing resistance. Tigecycline is active against some anaerobic bacteria, including *Peptostreptococcus*, *Propionibacterium*, *Prevotella*, *Fusobacterium*, and most *Bacteroides* species. Its efficacy for treatment of intraabdominal infections was comparable to that of imipenem in two phase 2 clinical trials. Low resistance rates (~4%) have been observed. High rates of resistance to moxifloxacin among *Bacteroides* and *Prevotella* species have been reported, ranging up to 32% in a recent survey from Greece.

If a patient fails to respond to one of the category 1 or category 2 drugs (Table 164-2), consideration should be given to alternative therapy and to determination of the resistance patterns among *Bacteroides* isolates. Although in vitro resistance of *Bacteroides* species to chloramphenicol has not been reported, this drug may not be as effective as other category 1 drugs.

INFECTIONS AT SPECIFIC SITES In clinical situations, specific regimens must be tailored to the initial site of infection. The duration of therapy also depends on the infection site; the reader is referred to specific chapters on sites of infection for recommendations.

Infections above the diaphragm usually reflect the orodental flora, which does not include the *B. fragilis* group. β-Lactamase production has been reported in anaerobic strains that are usually isolated from infections originating above the diaphragm. Up to 60% of clinical isolates classified as *Prevotella* or *Porphyromonas* species, non–*B. fragilis* species of *Bacteroides*, or *Fusobacterium* species reportedly produce β-lactamase; thus all β-lactam drugs (penicillins and cephalosporins) are poor options. Because most of these infections have a mixed etiology that includes microaerophilic and aerobic streptococci, antibiotics that cover both aerobic and anaerobic bacteria are recommended. The recommended regimens include clindamycin, a β-lactam/β-lactamase inhibitor combination, or metronidazole in combination with a drug active against microaerophilic and aerobic streptococci.

Although many oral anaerobic infections and most cases of anaerobic pneumonia still respond to penicillin therapy, some infections due to oral organisms fail to respond to this drug, and in these cases the use of a drug that is effective against penicillin-resistant anaerobes is recommended (Table 164-2). Life-threatening infections involving the anaerobic flora of the mouth, such as space infections of the head and neck, should be treated empirically as if penicillin-resistant anaerobes are involved. Less serious infections involving the oral microflora can be treated with penicillin alone; metronidazole can be added (or clindamycin can be substituted) if the patient responds poorly to penicillin therapy. Bronchoscopy in lung abscess is indicated only to rule out airway obstruction and does not enhance drainage; in any event, it should be delayed until the antimicrobial regimen has begun to affect the disease process so that the procedure does not spread the infection. Surgery is almost never indicated because of the danger of spilling the abscess contents into the lungs.

Chloramphenicol has been used successfully against anaerobic CNS infections at doses of 30–60 mg/kg per day, with the exact dose depending on the severity of illness. However, penicillin G and metronidazole also cross the blood-brain barrier and are bactericidal for many anaerobic organisms (Chap. 381).

Anaerobic infections arising below the diaphragm (e.g., colonic and intraabdominal infections) must be treated specifically with agents active against *Bacteroides* species (Table 164-2). In intraabdominal sepsis (Chap. 127), the use of antibiotics effective against penicillin-resistant anaerobes has clearly reduced the incidence of postoperative infections and serious infectious complications. Specifically, a drug from category 1 (Table 164-2) must be included for broad-spectrum coverage. Recommended doses for commonly used category 1 drugs are given in Table 164-3. Therapy for intraabdominal sepsis must also include drugs active against the gram-negative aerobic flora of the bowel. If the involvement of gram-positive bacteria such as enterococci is suspected, either ampicillin or vancomycin should be added. A meta-analysis of 40 randomized or quasi-randomized controlled trials of 16 antibiotic regimens for secondary peritonitis showed equivalent clinical success for all regimens.

Cases of anaerobic osteomyelitis in which a mixed flora is isolated from a bone biopsy specimen should be treated with a regimen that covers all the isolates. When an anaerobic organism is recognized as a major or sole pathogen infecting a joint, the duration of treatment should be similar to that used for arthritis caused by aerobic bacteria (Chap. 334). Therapy includes the management of underlying disease states, the administration of appropriate antimicrobial agents, temporary joint immobilization, percutaneous drainage of effusions, and (usually) the removal of infected prostheses or internal fixation devices. Surgical drainage and debridement procedures such as sequestrectomy are essential for the removal of necrotic tissue that can sustain anaerobic infections.

The outcome of anaerobic bacteremia is significantly better in patients either initially given or switched to appropriate therapy based on known antibiotic susceptibilities.

FAILURE OF THERAPY Anaerobic infections that fail to respond to treatment or that relapse should be reassessed. Consideration should be given to additional surgical drainage or debridement. Superinfections with resistant gram-negative facultative or aerobic bacteria should be ruled out. The possibility of drug resistance must be entertained; if resistance is involved, repeated cultures may yield the pathogenic organism.

SUPPORTIVE MEASURES Other supportive measures in the management of anaerobic infections include careful attention to fluid and electrolyte balance (since extensive local edema may lead to hypoalbuminemia), hemodynamic support for septic shock, immobilization of infected extremities, maintenance of adequate nutrition during chronic infections by parenteral hyperalimentation, relief of pain, and anticoagulation with heparin for thrombophlebitis. For patients with severe anaerobic infections of soft tissues, hyperbaric oxygen therapy is advocated by some experts, but its value has not been proven in controlled trials.

FURTHER READINGS

CHUNG H, KASPER DL: Microbiota-stimulated immune mechanisms to maintain gut homeostasis. Curr Opin Immunol 22:455, 2010

COHEN-PORADOSU R et al: Anaerobic infections: General concepts, in *Principles and Practice of Infectious Diseases*, 7th ed, GL Mandell et al (eds). Philadelphia, Elsevier Churchill Livingstone, 2010, p 3083

LASSMAN B et al: Reemergence of anaerobic bacteremia. Clin Infect Dis 44:895, 2007

MAZMANIAN SK et al: The love-hate relationship between bacterial polysaccharides and the immune system. Nat Rev Immunol 6:849, 2006

SNYDMAN DR et al: Lessons learned from the anaerobe survey: Historical perspective and review of the most recent data (2005-2007). Clin Infect Dis 50:S26, 2010

SOLOMKIN JS et al: Diagnosis and management of complicated intra-abdominal infections in adults and children: Guidelines by the Surgical Infection Society and the Infectious Diseases Society of America. Clin Infect Dis 50:133, 2010

WEXLER HM: *Bacteroides*: The good, the bad, and the nitty-gritty. Clin Microbiol Rev 20:593, 2007

TABLE 164-3 Doses and Schedules for Treatment of Serious Infections Due to Commonly Encountered Anaerobic Gram-Negative Rods

First-Line Therapy	Dose	Schedule[a]
Metronidazole[b]	500 mg	q6h
Ticarcillin/clavulanic acid	3.1 g	q4h
Piperacillin/tazobactam	3.375 g	q6h
Imipenem	0.5 g	q6h
Meropenem	1.0 g	q8h

[a]See disease-specific chapters for recommendations on duration of therapy.

[b]Should generally be used in conjunction with drugs active against aerobic or facultative organisms.

Note: All drugs are given by the IV route.

CHAPTER 165

Tuberculosis

Mario C. Raviglione
Richard J. O'Brien

Tuberculosis (TB), which is one of the oldest diseases known to affect humans and is likely to have existed in prehominids, is a major cause of death worldwide. This disease is caused by bacteria of the *Mycobacterium tuberculosis* complex and usually affects the lungs, although other organs are involved in up to one-third of cases. If properly treated, TB caused by drug-susceptible strains is curable in virtually all cases. If untreated, the disease may be fatal within 5 years in 50–65% of cases. Transmission usually takes place through the airborne spread of droplet nuclei produced by patients with infectious pulmonary TB.

ETIOLOGIC AGENT

Mycobacteria belong to the family Mycobacteriaceae and the order Actinomycetales. Of the pathogenic species belonging to the *M. tuberculosis* complex, the most common and important agent of human disease is *M. tuberculosis*. The complex includes *M. bovis* (the bovine tubercle bacillus—characteristically resistant to pyrazinamide, once an important cause of TB transmitted by unpasteurized milk, and currently the cause of a small percentage of cases worldwide), *M. caprae* (related to *M. bovis*), *M. africanum* (isolated from cases in West, Central, and East Africa), *M. microti* (the "vole" bacillus, a less virulent and rarely encountered organism), *M. pinnipedii* (a bacillus infecting seals and sea lions in the Southern Hemisphere and recently isolated from humans), and *M. canetti* (a rare isolate from East African cases that produces unusual smooth colonies on solid media and is considered closely related to a supposed progenitor type).

M. tuberculosis is a rod-shaped, nonspore-forming, thin aerobic bacterium measuring 0.5 μm by 3 μm. Mycobacteria, including *M. tuberculosis*, are often neutral on Gram's staining. However, once stained, the bacilli cannot be decolorized by acid alcohol; this characteristic justifies their classification as acid-fast bacilli (AFB; Fig. 165-1). Acid fastness is due mainly to the organisms' high content of mycolic acids, long-chain cross-linked fatty acids, and other cell-wall lipids. Microorganisms other than mycobacteria that display some acid fastness include species of *Nocardia* and *Rhodococcus*, *Legionella micdadei*, and the protozoa *Isospora* and *Cryptosporidium*. In the mycobacterial cell wall, lipids (e.g., mycolic acids) are linked to underlying arabinogalactan and peptidoglycan. This structure confers very low permeability of the cell wall, thus reducing the effectiveness of most antibiotics. Another molecule in the mycobacterial cell wall, lipoarabinomannan, is involved in the pathogen-host interaction and facilitates the survival of *M. tuberculosis* within macrophages. The complete genome sequence of *M. tuberculosis* comprises 4043 genes encoding 3993 proteins and 50 genes encoding RNAs; its high guanine-plus-cytosine content (65.6%) is indicative of an aerobic "lifestyle." A large proportion of genes are devoted to the production of enzymes involved in cell wall metabolism.

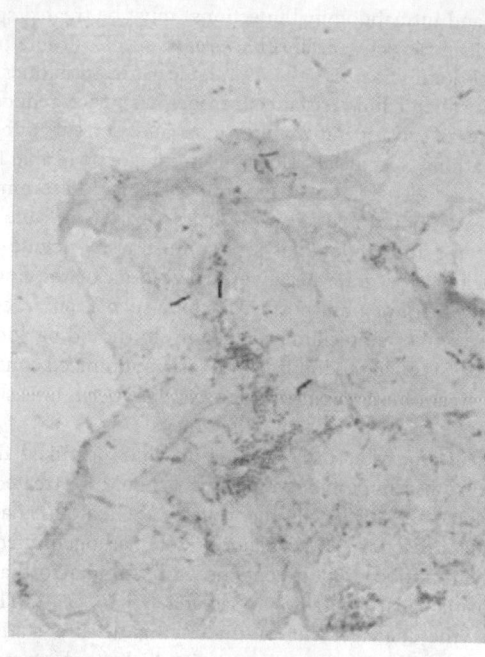

Figure 165-1   Acid-fast bacillus smear showing *M. tuberculosis* bacilli. *(Courtesy of the CDC, Atlanta.)*

EPIDEMIOLOGY

More than 5.8 million new cases of TB (all forms, both pulmonary and extrapulmonary) were reported to the World Health Organization (WHO) in 2009; 95% of cases were reported from developing countries. However, because of insufficient case detection and incomplete notification, reported cases represent only ~63% (range, 60–67%) of total estimated cases. The WHO estimated that 9.4 million (range, 8.9–9.9 million) new cases of TB occurred worldwide in 2009, 95% of them in developing countries of Asia (5.2 million), Africa (2.8 million), the Middle East (0.7 million), and Latin America (0.3 million). It is further estimated that 1.7 million (range, 1.5–1.9 million) deaths from TB, including 0.4 million among people living with HIV infection, occurred in 2008, 96% of them in developing countries. Estimates of TB incidence rates (per 100,000 population) and numbers of TB-related deaths in 2008 are depicted in Figs. 165-2 and 165-3, respectively. During the late 1980s and early 1990s, numbers of reported cases of TB increased in industrialized countries. These increases were related largely to immigration from countries with a high prevalence of TB; infection with HIV; social problems, such as increased urban poverty, homelessness, and drug abuse; and dismantling of TB services. During the past few years, numbers of reported cases have begun to decline again or stabilized in industrialized nations. In the United States, with the implementation of stronger control programs, the decrease resumed in 1993. In 2009, 11,540 cases of TB (3.8 cases per 100,000 population) were reported to the Centers for Disease Control and Prevention (CDC).

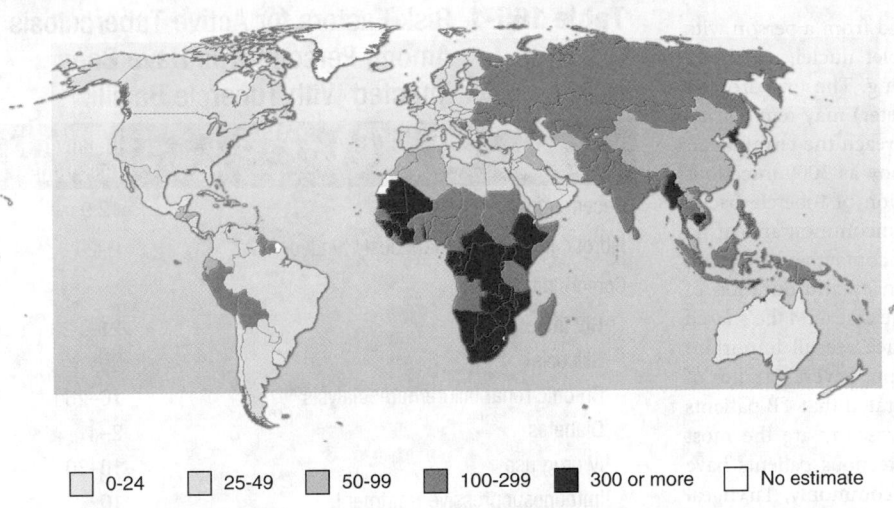

□ 0-24   □ 25-49   □ 50-99   ■ 100-299   ■ 300 or more   □ No estimate

Figure 165-2   Estimated tuberculosis incidence rates (per 100,000 population) in 2008. The designations employed and the presentation of material on this map do not imply the expression of any opinion whatsoever on the part of the WHO concerning the legal status of any country, territory, city, or area or of its authorities or concerning the delimitation of its frontiers or boundaries. White lines on maps represent approximate border lines for which there may not yet be full agreement. *(Courtesy of the Stop TB Department, WHO; with permission.)*

In the United States, TB is uncommon among young adults of European descent, who have only rarely been exposed to *M. tuberculosis* infection during recent decades. In contrast, because of a high risk of transmission in the past, the prevalence of *M. tuberculosis* infection is relatively high among elderly whites. Blacks, however, account for the highest proportion of cases (41.4% of 4499) among U.S.-born persons. TB in the United States is also a disease of adult members of the HIV-infected population, the foreign-born population (60% of all cases in 2009), and

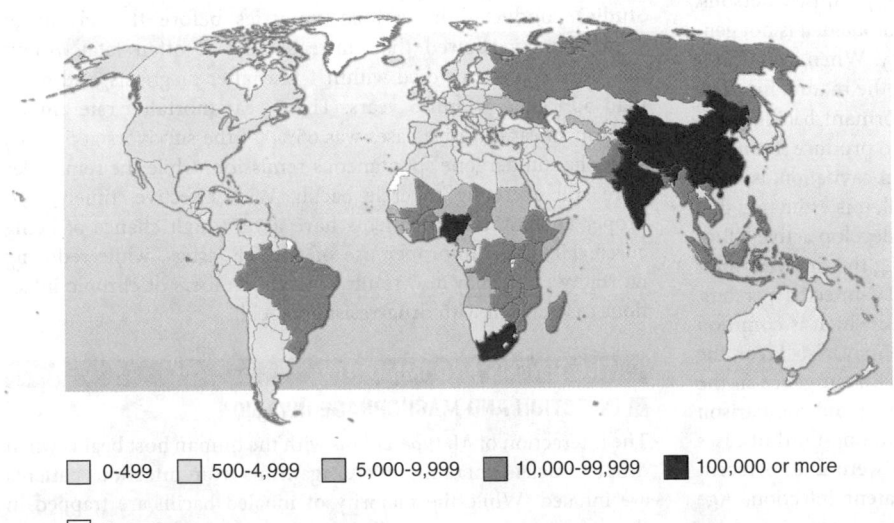

□ 0-499   □ 500-4,999   □ 5,000-9,999   ■ 10,000-99,999   ■ 100,000 or more

□ No estimate

Figure 165-3   Estimated numbers of tuberculosis-related deaths in 2008. *(See disclaimer in Fig. 165-2. Courtesy of the Stop TB Department, WHO; with permission.)*

disadvantaged/marginalized populations. Overall, more TB cases were reported among Hispanics than among other ethnic groups; next in frequency were cases among Asians and blacks, with the highest rates per capita among Asians. Similarly, in Europe, TB has reemerged as an important public health problem, mainly as a result of cases among immigrants from high-prevalence countries and among marginalized populations. In many western European countries, there are currently more cases among foreign-born than native populations.

Recent data on global trends indicate that in 2009 TB incidence was stable or falling in most regions; this trend began in 2004 and appears to continue, with an average annual decline of <1% globally. This global decrease is due largely to a reduction (after a peak in 2004) in sub-Saharan Africa, where incidence had risen steeply since the 1980s as a result of the HIV epidemic and the weakness of health systems and services. In eastern Europe, incidence increased during the 1990s because of deterioration in socioeconomic conditions and the health care infrastructure; however, after peaking in 2001, incidence has since declined slowly.

Of the 9.4 million new cases estimated for 2009, 12% (1.1 million) were associated with HIV, and 80% of these HIV-associated cases occurred in Africa. An estimated 0.4 million deaths due to HIV-associated TB occurred in 2008. Furthermore, an estimated 440,000 cases of multidrug-resistant TB (MDR-TB), a form of disease caused by bacilli resistant at least to isoniazid and rifampin, may have emerged in 2008. At present, >90% of these cases are not identified because of a lack of culture and drug-susceptibility testing capacity in most settings worldwide. The independent states of the former Soviet Union have reported the highest rates of MDR-TB among new cases (up to 20% or even higher); several provinces of China follow, with peaks of 10%. Overall, 60% of all MDR-TB cases are in India, China, and the Russian Federation. Starting in 2006, 58 countries, including the United States, reported cases of extensively drug-resistant TB (XDR-TB), in which MDR-TB is compounded by additional resistance to the most powerful second-line anti-TB drugs (fluoroquinolones and at least one of the injectable drugs amikacin, kanamycin, and capreomycin). Probably ~10% of the MDR-TB cases worldwide are XDR-TB, but the vast majority of XDR cases remain undiagnosed.

■ FROM EXPOSURE TO INFECTION

M. tuberculosis is most commonly transmitted from a person with infectious pulmonary TB to others by droplet nuclei, which are aerosolized by coughing, sneezing, or speaking. The tiny droplets dry rapidly; the smallest (<5–10 μm in diameter) may remain suspended in the air for several hours and may reach the terminal air passages when inhaled. There may be as many as 3000 infectious nuclei per cough. Other routes of transmission of tubercle bacilli (e.g., through the skin or the placenta) are uncommon and of no epidemiologic significance. The probability of contact with a person who has an infectious form of TB, the intimacy and duration of that contact, the degree of infectiousness of the case, and the shared environment in which the contact takes place are all important determinants of the likelihood of transmission. Several studies of close-contact situations have clearly demonstrated that TB patients whose sputum contains AFB visible by microscopy are the most likely to transmit the infection. The most infectious patients have cavitary pulmonary disease or, much less commonly, laryngeal TB and produce sputum containing as many as 10^5–10^7 AFB/mL. Patients with sputum smear–negative/culture-positive TB are less infectious, although they have been responsible for up to 20% of transmission in some studies in the United States, and those with culture-negative pulmonary TB and extrapulmonary TB are essentially noninfectious. Because persons with both HIV infection and TB are less likely to have cavitations, they may be less infectious than persons without HIV co-infection. Crowding in poorly ventilated rooms is one of the most important factors in the transmission of tubercle bacilli, since it increases the intensity of contact with a case.

In short, the risk of acquiring *M. tuberculosis* infection is determined mainly by exogenous factors. Because of delays in seeking care and in making a diagnosis, it is generally believed that, in high-prevalence settings, up to 20 contacts may be infected by each AFB-positive case before the index case is found to have TB.

■ FROM INFECTION TO DISEASE

Unlike the risk of acquiring infection with *M. tuberculosis*, the risk of developing disease after being infected depends largely on endogenous factors, such as the individual's innate immunologic and nonimmunologic defenses and level of function of cell-mediated immunity (CMI). Clinical illness directly following infection is classified as *primary TB* and is common among children in the first few years of life and among immunocompromised persons. Although primary TB may be severe and disseminated, it is not generally associated with high-level transmissibility. When infection is acquired later in life, the chance is greater that the mature immune system will contain it at least temporarily. Dormant bacilli, however, may persist for years before reactivating to produce *secondary* (or *postprimary) TB*, which, because of frequent cavitation, is more often infectious than is primary disease. Overall, it is estimated that up to 10% of infected persons will eventually develop active TB in their lifetime, with half of them doing so during the first year after infection. The risk is much higher among HIV-infected persons. Reinfection of a previously infected individual, which is common in areas with high rates of TB transmission, may also favor the development of disease. At the height of the TB resurgence in the United States in the early 1990s, molecular typing and comparison of strains of *M. tuberculosis* suggested that up to one-third of cases of active TB in some inner-city communities were due to recent transmission rather than to reactivation of latent infection. Age is an important determinant of the risk of disease after infection. Among infected persons, the incidence of TB is highest during late adolescence and early adulthood; the reasons are unclear. The incidence among women peaks at 25–34 years of age. In this age group

Table 165-1 Risk Factors for Active Tuberculosis Among Persons Who Have Been Infected With Tubercle Bacilli

Factor	Relative Risk/Odds[a]
Recent infection (<1 year)	12.9
Fibrotic lesions (spontaneously healed)	2–20
Comorbidity	
HIV infection	21–>30
Silicosis	30
Chronic renal failure/hemodialysis	10–25
Diabetes	2–4
IV drug use	10–30
Immunosuppressive treatment	10
Gastrectomy	2–5
Jejunoileal bypass	30–60
Posttransplantation period (renal, cardiac)	20–70
Tobacco smoking	2–3
Malnutrition and severe underweight	2

[a]Old infection = 1.

rates among women may be higher than those among men, while at older ages the opposite is true. The risk increases in the elderly, possibly because of waning immunity and comorbidity.

A variety of diseases and conditions favor the development of active TB (Table 165-1). In absolute terms, the most potent risk factor for TB among infected individuals is clearly HIV co-infection, which suppresses cellular immunity. The risk that latent *M. tuberculosis* infection will proceed to active disease is directly related to the patient's degree of immunosuppression. In a study of HIV-infected, tuberculin skin test (TST)–positive persons, this risk varied from 2.6 to 13.3 cases per 100 person-years and increased as the CD4+ T cell count decreased.

■ NATURAL HISTORY OF DISEASE

Studies conducted in various countries before the advent of chemotherapy showed that untreated TB is often fatal. About one-third of patients died within 1 year after diagnosis, and more than 50% died within 5 years. The 5-year mortality rate among sputum smear–positive cases was 65%. Of the survivors at 5 years, ~60% had undergone spontaneous remission, while the remainder were still excreting tubercle bacilli. With effective, timely, and proper chemotherapy, patients have a very high chance of being cured. However, improper use of anti-TB drugs, while reducing mortality rates, may also result in large numbers of chronic infectious cases, often with drug-resistant bacilli.

PATHOGENESIS AND IMMUNITY

■ INFECTION AND MACROPHAGE INVASION

The interaction of *M. tuberculosis* with the human host begins when droplet nuclei containing microorganisms from infectious patients are inhaled. While the majority of inhaled bacilli are trapped in the upper airways and expelled by ciliated mucosal cells, a fraction (usually <10%) reach the alveoli. There, alveolar macrophages that have not yet been activated phagocytize the bacilli. Adhesion of mycobacteria to macrophages results largely from binding of the bacterial cell wall with a variety of macrophage cell-surface molecules, including complement receptors, the mannose receptor, the immunoglobulin GFcγ receptor, and type A scavenger receptors. Phagocytosis is enhanced by complement activation leading to opsonization of bacilli with C3 activation products such as C3b. After a phagosome forms, the survival of *M. tuberculosis* within it seems to depend on reduced acidification due to lack of accumulation of vesicular proton-adenosine triphosphatase. A complex series of events is probably generated by the bacterial cell-wall glycolipid lipoarabinomannan. This glycolipid inhibits the intracellular increase of Ca^{2+}. Thus the Ca^{2+}/calmodulin pathway (leading to phagosome-lysosome fusion) is impaired, and the bacilli may survive within the phagosomes. The *M. tuberculosis* phagosome has been found to inhibit the production of phosphatidylinositol 3-phosphate (PI3P). Normally, PI3P earmarks phagosomes for membrane sorting and maturation including phagolysosome formation, which would destroy the bacteria. Bacterial factors have also been found to block the newly identified host defense of autophagy, in which the cell sequesters the phagosome in a double-membrane vesicle (*autophagosome*) that is destined to fuse with lysosomes. If the bacilli are successful in arresting phagosome maturation, then replication begins and the macrophage eventually ruptures and releases its bacillary contents. Other uninfected phagocytic cells are then recruited to continue the infection cycle by ingesting dying macrophages and their bacillary content, thus in turn becoming infected themselves and expanding the infection.

■ VIRULENCE OF TUBERCLE BACILLI

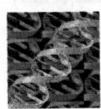 Since the elucidation of the *M. tuberculosis* genome in 1998, large mutant collections have been generated, and many bacterial genes that contribute to *M. tuberculosis* virulence have been found. Different patterns of virulence defects have been defined in various animal models, predominantly mice but also guinea pigs, rabbits, and nonhuman primates. The *katG* gene encodes for a catalase/peroxidase enzyme that protects against oxidative stress and is required for isoniazid activation and subsequent bactericidal activity. Region of difference 1 (RD1) is a 9.5-kb locus that encodes two key small protein antigens—early secretory antigen-6 (ESAT-6) and culture filtrate protein-10 (CFP-10)—as well as a putative secretion apparatus that may facilitate their egress; the absence of this locus in the vaccine strain *M. bovis* bacille Calmette-Guérin (BCG) has been shown to be a key attenuating mutation. A recent observation in *Mycobacterium marinum*, the validity of which needs to be confirmed in *M. tuberculosis*, showed that a mutation in the RD1 virulence locus encoding the ESX1 secretion system impairs the capacity of apoptotic macrophages to recruit uninfected cells for further rounds of infection. The results are less replication and fewer new granulomas. Mutants lacking key enzymes of bacterial biosynthesis become auxotrophic for the missing substrate and are often totally unable to proliferate in animals; these include the *leuD* and *panCD* mutants, which require leucine and pantothenic acid, respectively. The isocitrate lyase gene *icl1* encodes a key step in the glyoxylate shunt that facilitates bacterial growth on fatty acid substrates; this gene is required for long-term persistence of *M. tuberculosis* infection in mice with chronic TB. *M. tuberculosis* mutants in regulatory genes such as sigma factor C and sigma factor H (*sigC* and *sigH*) are associated with normal bacterial growth in mice, but they fail to elicit full tissue pathology. Finally, the recently identified mycobacterial protein CarD (expressed by the *carD* gene) seems essential for the control of rRNA transcription that is required for replication and persistence in the host cell. Its loss exposes mycobacteria to oxidative stress, starvation, DNA damage, and ultimately sensitivity to killing by a variety of host mutagens and defensive mechanisms.

■ INNATE RESISTANCE TO INFECTION

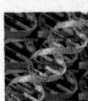 Several observations suggest that genetic factors play a key role in innate nonimmune resistance to infection with *M. tuberculosis* and the development of disease. The existence of this resistance, which is polygenic in nature, is suggested by the differing degrees of susceptibility to TB in different populations. In mice, a gene called *Nramp1* (natural resistance–associated macrophage protein 1) plays a regulatory role in resistance/susceptibility to mycobacteria. The human homologue NRAMP1, which maps to chromosome 2q, may play a role in determining susceptibility to TB, as is suggested by a study among West Africans. Recent studies of mouse genetics identified a novel host resistance gene, *ipr1*, that is encoded within the *sst1* locus; *ipr1* encodes an interferon (IFN)-inducible nuclear protein that interacts with other nuclear proteins in macrophages primed with IFNs or infected by *M. tuberculosis*. In addition, polymorphisms in multiple genes, such as those encoding for various histocompatibility leukocyte antigen (HLA) alleles, IFN-γ, T cell growth factor β, interleukin (IL) 10, mannose-binding protein, IFN-γ receptor, Toll-like receptor 2, vitamin D receptor, and IL-1, have been associated with susceptibility to TB.

■ THE HOST RESPONSE AND GRANULOMA FORMATION

In the initial stage of host-bacterium interaction, prior to the onset of an acquired CMI response, *M. tuberculosis* undergoes a period of extensive growth within naïve unactivated macrophages, and additional naïve macrophages are recruited to the early granuloma. Studies suggest that *M. tuberculosis* uses a specific virulence mechanism to subvert host cellular signaling and to elicit an early proinflammatory response that promotes granuloma expansion and bacterial growth during this key early phase. A recent study of *M. marinum* infection in zebrafish has delineated the likely molecular mechanism by which mycobacteria induce granuloma formation. The mycobacterial protein ESAT-6 induces secretion of matrix metalloproteinase 9 (MMP9) by nearby epithelial cells that are in contact with infected macrophages. MMP9 in turn stimulates recruitment of naïve macrophages, thus inducing granuloma maturation and bacterial growth. Disruption of MMP9 function results in reduced bacterial growth. Another study has shown that *M. tuberculosis*–derived cyclic AMP is secreted from the phagosome into host macrophages, subverting the cell's signal transduction pathways and stimulating an elevation in the secretion of tumor necrosis factor α (TNF-α) and further proinflammatory cell recruitment. Ultimately, the chemoattractants and bacterial products released during the repeated rounds of cell lysis and infection of newly arriving macrophages enable dendritic cells to access bacilli; these cells migrate to the draining lymph nodes and present mycobacterial antigens to T lymphocytes. At this point, the development of CMI and humoral immunity begins. These initial stages of infection are usually asymptomatic.

About 2–4 weeks after infection, two host responses to *M. tuberculosis* develop: a macrophage-activating CMI response and a tissue-damaging response. The *macrophage-activating response* is a T cell–mediated phenomenon resulting in the activation of macrophages that are capable of killing and digesting tubercle bacilli. The *tissue-damaging response* is the result of a delayed-type hypersensitivity (DTH) reaction to various bacillary antigens; it destroys unactivated macrophages that contain multiplying bacilli but also causes caseous necrosis of the involved tissues (see below). Although both of these responses can inhibit mycobacterial growth, it is the balance between the two that determines the form of TB that will develop subsequently.

With the development of specific immunity and the accumulation of large numbers of activated macrophages at the site of the primary lesion, granulomatous lesions (tubercles) are formed. These lesions consist of accumulations of lymphocytes and activated macrophages that evolve toward epithelioid and giant cell morphologies. Initially, the tissue-damaging response can limit mycobacterial growth within macrophages. As stated above, this response, mediated by various bacterial products, not only destroys macrophages but also produces early solid necrosis in the center of the tubercle. Although *M. tuberculosis* can survive, its growth is inhibited within this necrotic environment by low oxygen tension and low pH. At this point, some lesions may heal by fibrosis, with subsequent calcification, whereas inflammation and necrosis occur in other lesions. Some observations have challenged the traditional view that any encounter between mycobacteria and macrophages results in chronic infection. It is possible that an immune response capable of eradicating early infection may sometimes develop as a consequence, for instance, of disabling mutations in mycobacterial genomes rendering their replication ineffective.

■ MACROPHAGE-ACTIVATING RESPONSE

CMI is critical at this early stage. In the majority of infected individuals, local macrophages are activated when bacillary antigens processed by macrophages stimulate T lymphocytes to release a variety of lymphokines. These activated macrophages aggregate around the lesion's center and effectively neutralize tubercle bacilli without causing further tissue destruction. In the central part of the lesion, the necrotic material resembles soft cheese (*caseous necrosis*)—a phenomenon that may also be observed in other conditions, such as neoplasms. Even when healing takes place, viable bacilli may remain dormant within macrophages or in the necrotic material for many years. These "healed" lesions in the lung parenchyma and hilar lymph nodes may later undergo calcification.

■ DELAYED-TYPE HYPERSENSITIVITY

In a minority of cases, the macrophage-activating response is weak, and mycobacterial growth can be inhibited only by intensified DTH reactions, which lead to lung tissue destruction. The lesion tends to enlarge further, and the surrounding tissue is progressively damaged. At the center of the lesion, the caseous material liquefies. Bronchial walls as well as blood vessels are invaded and destroyed, and cavities are formed. The liquefied caseous material, containing large numbers of bacilli, is drained through bronchi. Within the cavity, tubercle bacilli multiply, spill into the airways, and are discharged into the environment through expiratory maneuvers such as coughing and talking. In the early stages of infection, bacilli are usually transported by macrophages to regional lymph nodes, from which they gain access to the central venous return; from there they reseed the lungs and may also disseminate beyond the pulmonary vasculature throughout the body via the systemic circulation. The resulting extrapulmonary lesions may undergo the same evolution as those in the lungs, although most tend to heal. In young children with poor natural immunity, hematogenous dissemination may result in fatal miliary TB or tuberculous meningitis.

■ ROLE OF MACROPHAGES AND MONOCYTES

While CMI confers partial protection against *M. tuberculosis*, humoral immunity plays a less well-defined role in protection (although evidence is accumulating on the existence of antibodies to lipoarabinomannan, which may prevent dissemination of infection in children). In the case of CMI, two types of cells are essential: macrophages, which directly phagocytize tubercle bacilli, and T cells (mainly CD4+ T lymphocytes), which induce protection through the production of cytokines, especially IFN-γ. After infection with *M. tuberculosis*, alveolar macrophages secrete various cytokines responsible for a number of events (e.g., the formation

of granulomas) as well as systemic effects (e.g., fever and weight loss). Monocytes and macrophages attracted to the site are key components of the immune response. Their primary mechanism is probably related to production of nitric oxide, which has antimycobacterial activity and increases the synthesis of cytokines such as TNF-α and IL-1, which in turn regulate the release of reactive nitrogen intermediates. In addition, macrophages can undergo apoptosis—a defensive mechanism to prevent release of cytokines and bacilli via their sequestration in the apoptotic cell.

■ ROLE OF T LYMPHOCYTES

Alveolar macrophages, monocytes, and dendritic cells are also critical in processing and presenting antigens to T lymphocytes, primarily CD4+ and CD8+ T cells; the result is the activation and proliferation of CD4+ T lymphocytes, which are crucial to the host's defense against *M. tuberculosis*. Qualitative and quantitative defects of CD4+ T cells explain the inability of HIV-infected individuals to contain mycobacterial proliferation. Activated CD4+ T lymphocytes can differentiate into cytokine-producing T_H1 or T_H2 cells. T_H1 cells produce IFN-γ—an activator of macrophages and monocytes—and IL-2. T_H2 cells produce IL-4, IL-5, IL-10, and IL-13 and may also promote humoral immunity. The interplay of these various cytokines and their cross-regulation determine the host's response. The role of cytokines in promoting intracellular killing of mycobacteria, however, has not been entirely elucidated. IFN-γ may induce the generation of reactive nitrogen intermediates and regulate genes involved in bactericidal effects. TNF-α also seems to be important. Observations made originally in transgenic knockout mice and more recently in humans suggest that other T cell subsets, especially CD8+ T cells, may play an important role. CD8+ T cells have been associated with protective activities via cytotoxic responses and lysis of infected cells as well as with production of IFN-γ and TNF-α. Finally, natural killer cells act as co-regulators of CD8+ T cell lytic activities, and γδ T cells are increasingly thought to be involved in protective responses in humans.

■ MYCOBACTERIAL LIPIDS AND PROTEINS

Lipids have been involved in mycobacterial recognition by the innate immune system, and lipoproteins (such as 19-kDa lipoprotein) have been proven to trigger potent signals through Toll-like receptors present in blood dendritic cells. *M. tuberculosis* possesses various protein antigens. Some are present in the cytoplasm and cell wall; others are secreted. That the latter are more important in eliciting a T lymphocyte response is suggested by experiments documenting the appearance of protective immunity in animals after immunization with live, protein-secreting mycobacteria. Among the antigens that may play a protective role are the 30-kDa (or 85B) and ESAT-6 antigens. Protective immunity is probably the result of reactivity to many different mycobacterial antigens.

■ SKIN TEST REACTIVITY

Coincident with the appearance of immunity, DTH to *M. tuberculosis* develops. This reactivity is the basis of the TST, which is used primarily for the detection of *M. tuberculosis* infection in persons without symptoms. The cellular mechanisms responsible for TST reactivity are related mainly to previously sensitized CD4+ T lymphocytes, which are attracted to the skin-test site. There, they proliferate and produce cytokines. While DTH is associated with protective immunity (TST-positive persons being less susceptible to a new *M. tuberculosis* infection than TST-negative persons), it by no means guarantees protection against reactivation. In fact, cases of active TB are often accompanied by strongly positive skin-test reactions. There is also evidence of reinfection with a new strain of *M. tuberculosis* in patients previously treated for active disease. This evidence underscores the fact that previous latent or active TB may not confer fully protective immunity.

CLINICAL MANIFESTATIONS

TB is classified as pulmonary, extrapulmonary, or both. Before the advent of HIV infection, ~80% of all new cases of TB were limited to the lungs. However, up to two-thirds of HIV-infected patients with TB may have both pulmonary and extrapulmonary TB or extrapulmonary TB alone.

■ PULMONARY TB

Pulmonary TB can be conventionally categorized as primary or postprimary (adult-type, secondary). This distinction has been challenged by molecular evidence from TB-endemic areas indicating that a large percentage of cases of adult pulmonary TB result from recent infection (either primary infection or reinfection) and not from reactivation.

Primary disease

Primary pulmonary TB occurs soon after the initial infection with tubercle bacilli. It may be asymptomatic or present with fever and occasionally pleuritic chest pain. In areas of high TB transmission, this form of disease is often seen in children. Because most inspired air is distributed to the middle and lower lung zones, these areas of the lungs are most commonly involved in primary TB. The lesion forming after initial infection (the Ghon focus) is usually peripheral and accompanied by transient hilar or paratracheal lymphadenopathy, which may not be visible on standard chest radiography. Some patients develop erythema nodosum in the legs or phlyctenular conjunctivitis. In the majority of cases, the lesion heals spontaneously and only becomes evident as a small calcified nodule. Pleural reaction overlying a subpleural focus is also common. The Ghon focus, with or without overlying pleural reaction, thickening, and regional lymphadenopathy, is referred to as the *Ghon complex*.

In young children with immature CMI and in persons with impaired immunity (e.g., those with malnutrition or HIV infection), primary pulmonary TB may progress rapidly to clinical illness. The initial lesion increases in size and can evolve in different ways. Pleural effusion, which is found in up to two-thirds of cases, results from the penetration of bacilli into the pleural space from an adjacent subpleural focus. In severe cases, the primary site rapidly enlarges, its central portion undergoes necrosis, and cavitation develops (*progressive primary TB*). TB in young children is almost invariably accompanied by hilar or paratracheal lymphadenopathy due to the spread of bacilli from the lung parenchyma through lymphatic vessels. Enlarged lymph nodes may compress bronchi, causing total obstruction with distal collapse, partial obstruction with large-airway wheezing, or a ball-valve effect with segmental/lobar hyperinflation. Lymph nodes may also rupture into the airway with development of pneumonia, often including areas of necrosis and cavitation, distal to the obstruction. Bronchiectasis may develop in any segment/lobe damaged by progressive caseating pneumonia. Occult hematogenous dissemination commonly follows primary infection. However, in the absence of a sufficient acquired immune response, which usually contains the infection, disseminated or miliary disease may result (Fig. 165-4). Small granulomatous lesions develop in multiple organs and may cause locally progressive disease or result in tuberculous meningitis; this is a particular concern in very young children and immunocompromised persons (e.g., patients with HIV infection).

Postprimary (adult-type) disease

Also referred to as *reactivation* or *secondary TB*, postprimary TB is probably most accurately termed *adult-type TB*, since it may result

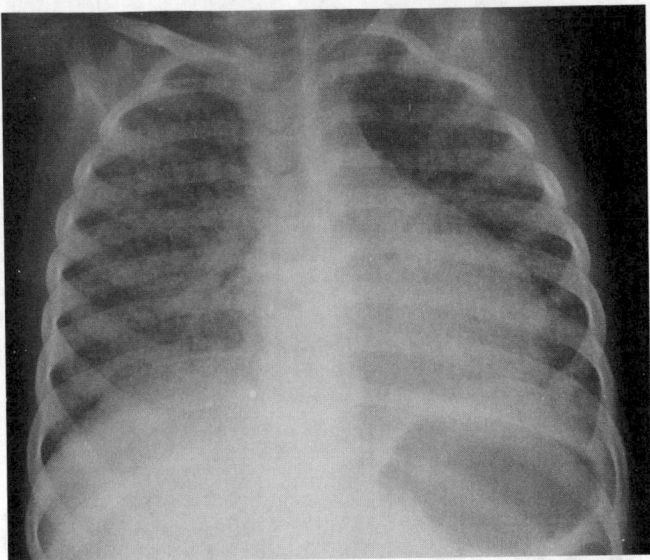

Figure 165-4 Chest radiograph showing bilateral miliary (millet-sized) infiltrates in a child. *(Courtesy of Prof. Robert Gie, Department of Paediatrics and Child Health, Stellenbosch University, South Africa; with permission.)*

from endogenous reactivation of distant latent infection or recent infection (primary infection or reinfection). It is usually localized to the apical and posterior segments of the upper lobes, where the substantially higher mean oxygen tension (compared with that in the lower zones) favors mycobacterial growth. The superior segments of the lower lobes are also more frequently involved. The extent of lung parenchymal involvement varies greatly, from small infiltrates to extensive cavitary disease. With cavity formation, liquefied necrotic contents are ultimately discharged into the airways and may undergo bronchogenic spread, resulting in satellite lesions within the lungs that may in turn undergo cavitation (Figs. 165-5 and 165-6). Massive involvement of pulmonary segments or lobes, with coalescence of lesions, produces caseating pneumonia. While up to one-third of untreated patients reportedly succumb to severe pulmonary TB within a few months after onset (the classic "galloping consumption" of the past), others may undergo a process of spontaneous remission or proceed along a chronic, progressively debilitating course ("consumption" or *phthisis*). Under these circumstances, some pulmonary lesions become fibrotic and may later calcify, but cavities persist in other parts of the lungs. Individuals with such chronic disease continue to discharge tubercle bacilli into the environment. Most patients respond to treatment, with defervescence, decreasing cough, weight gain, and a general improvement in well-being within several weeks.

Early in the course of disease, symptoms and signs are often nonspecific and insidious, consisting mainly of diurnal fever and night sweats due to defervescence, weight loss, anorexia, general malaise, and weakness. However, in up to 90% of cases, cough eventually develops—often initially nonproductive and limited to the morning and subsequently accompanied by the production of purulent sputum, sometimes with blood streaking. Hemoptysis develops in 20–30% of cases, and massive hemoptysis may ensue as a consequence of the erosion of a blood vessel in the wall of a cavity. Hemoptysis, however, may also result from rupture of a dilated vessel in a cavity (*Rasmussen's aneurysm*) or from aspergilloma formation in an old cavity. Pleuritic chest pain sometimes develops in patients with subpleural parenchymal lesions or pleural disease. Extensive disease may produce dyspnea and, in rare instances, adult

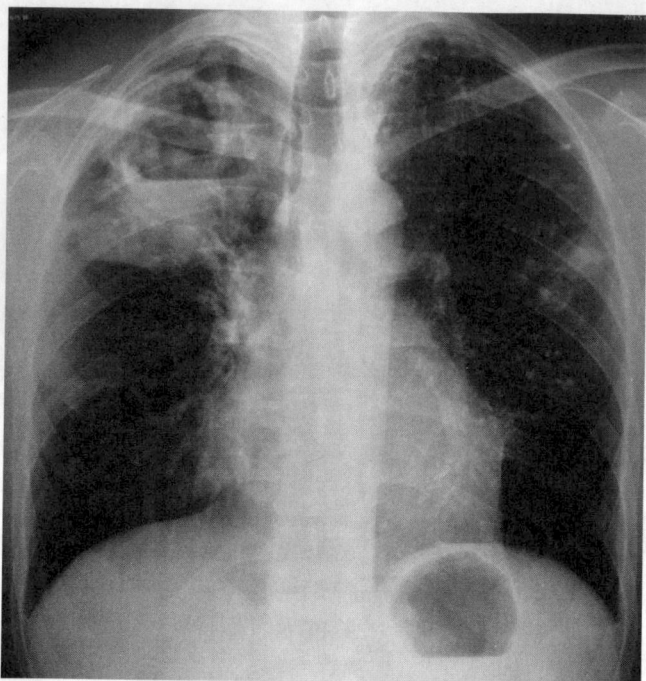

Figure 165-5 Chest radiograph showing a right-upper-lobe infiltrate and a cavity with an air-fluid level in a patient with active tuberculosis. *(Courtesy of Dr. Andrea Gori, Department of Infectious Diseases, S. Paolo University Hospital, Milan, Italy; with permission.)*

respiratory distress syndrome. Physical findings are of limited use in pulmonary TB. Many patients have no abnormalities detectable by chest examination, whereas others have detectable rales in the involved areas during inspiration, especially after coughing. Occasionally, rhonchi due to partial bronchial obstruction and classic amphoric breath sounds in areas with large cavities may be heard. Systemic features include fever (often low grade and intermittent) in up to 80% of cases and wasting. Absence of fever, however, does not exclude TB. In some cases, pallor and finger clubbing

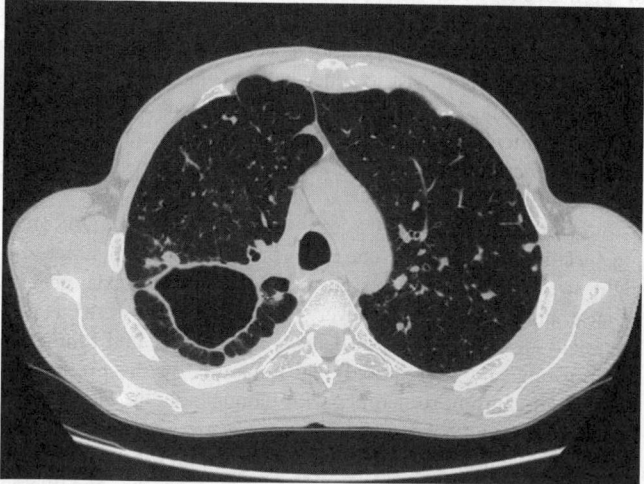

Figure 165-6 CT scan showing a large cavity in the right lung of a patient with active tuberculosis. *(Courtesy of Dr. Enrico Girardi, National Institute for Infectious Diseases, Spallanzani Hospital, Rome, Italy; with permission.)*

develop. The most common hematologic findings are mild anemia, leukocytosis, and thrombocytosis with a slightly elevated erythrocyte sedimentation rate and/or C-reactive protein level. None of these findings is consistent or sufficiently accurate for diagnostic purposes. Hyponatremia due to the syndrome of inappropriate secretion of antidiuretic hormone has also been reported.

■ EXTRAPULMONARY TB

In order of frequency, the extrapulmonary sites most commonly involved in TB are the lymph nodes, pleura, genitourinary tract, bones and joints, meninges, peritoneum, and pericardium. However, virtually all organ systems may be affected. As a result of hematogenous dissemination in HIV-infected individuals, extrapulmonary TB is seen more commonly today than in the past.

Lymph node TB (tuberculous lymphadenitis)

The most common presentation of extrapulmonary TB in both HIV-seronegative and HIV-infected patients (35% in general and >40% of cases in the United States in recent series), lymph node disease is particularly frequent among HIV-infected patients and in children. In the United States, besides children, women (particularly non-Caucasians) seem to be especially susceptible. Once caused mainly by *M. bovis*, tuberculous lymphadenitis is today due largely to *M. tuberculosis*. Lymph node TB presents as painless swelling of the lymph nodes, most commonly at posterior cervical and supraclavicular sites (a condition historically referred to as *scrofula*). Lymph nodes are usually discrete in early disease but develop into a matted nontender mass over time and may result in a fistulous tract draining caseous material. Associated pulmonary disease is present in <50% of cases, and systemic symptoms are uncommon except in HIV-infected patients. The diagnosis is established by fine-needle aspiration biopsy (with a yield of up to 80%) or surgical excision biopsy. Bacteriologic confirmation is achieved in the vast majority of cases, granulomatous lesions with or without visible AFBs are typically seen, and cultures are positive in 70–80% of cases. Among HIV-infected patients, granulomas are less well organized and are frequently absent entirely, but bacterial loads are heavier than in HIV-seronegative patients, with higher yields from microscopy and culture. Differential diagnosis includes a variety of infectious conditions, neoplastic diseases such as lymphomas or metastatic carcinomas, and rare disorders like Kikuchi's disease (necrotizing histiocytic lymphadenitis), Kimura's disease, and Castleman's disease.

Pleural TB

Involvement of the pleura accounts for ~20% of extrapulmonary cases in the United States and elsewhere. Isolated pleural effusion usually reflects recent primary infection, and the collection of fluid in the pleural space represents a hypersensitivity response to mycobacterial antigens. Pleural disease may also result from contiguous parenchymal spread, as in many cases of pleurisy accompanying postprimary disease. Depending on the extent of reactivity, the effusion may be small, remain unnoticed, and resolve spontaneously or may be sufficiently large to cause symptoms such as fever, pleuritic chest pain, and dyspnea. Physical findings are those of pleural effusion: dullness to percussion and absence of breath sounds. A chest radiograph reveals the effusion and, in up to one-third of cases, also shows a parenchymal lesion. Thoracentesis is required to ascertain the nature of the effusion and to differentiate it from manifestations of other etiologies. The fluid is straw colored and at times hemorrhagic; it is an exudate with a protein concentration >50% of that in serum (usually ~4–6 g/dL), a normal to low glucose concentration, a pH of ~7.3 (occasionally <7.2), and detectable white blood cells (usually 500–6000/μL). Neutrophils may predominate in the early stage, but lymphocyte predominance is the typical finding later.

Mesothelial cells are generally rare or absent. AFB are seen on direct smear in only 10–25% of cases, but cultures may be positive for *M. tuberculosis* in 25–75% of cases; positive cultures are more common among postprimary cases. Determination of the pleural concentration of adenosine deaminase (ADA) is a useful screening test: tuberculosis is virtually excluded if the value is very low. Lysozyme is also present in the pleural effusion. Measurement of IFN-γ, either directly or through stimulation of sensitized T cells with mycobacterial antigens, can be helpful. Needle biopsy of the pleura is often required for diagnosis and reveals granulomas and/or yields a positive culture in up to 80% of cases. This form of pleural TB responds rapidly to chemotherapy and may resolve spontaneously. Concurrent glucocorticoid administration may reduce the duration of fever and/or chest pain but is of not proven benefit.

Tuberculous empyema is a less common complication of pulmonary TB. It is usually the result of the rupture of a cavity, with spillage of a large number of organisms into the pleural space. This process may create a bronchopleural fistula with evident air in the pleural space. A chest radiograph shows hydropneumothorax with an air-fluid level. The pleural fluid is purulent and thick and contains large numbers of lymphocytes. Acid-fast smears and mycobacterial cultures are often positive. Surgical drainage is usually required as an adjunct to chemotherapy. Tuberculous empyema may result in severe pleural fibrosis and restrictive lung disease. Removal of the thickened visceral pleura (decortication) is occasionally necessary to improve lung function.

TB of the upper airways

Nearly always a complication of advanced cavitary pulmonary TB, TB of the upper airways may involve the larynx, pharynx, and epiglottis. Symptoms include hoarseness, dysphonia, and dysphagia in addition to chronic productive cough. Findings depend on the site of involvement, and ulcerations may be seen on laryngoscopy. Acid-fast smear of the sputum is often positive, but biopsy may be necessary in some cases to establish the diagnosis. Carcinoma of the larynx may have similar features but is usually painless.

Genitourinary TB

Genitourinary TB, which accounts for ~10–15% of all extrapulmonary cases in the United States and elsewhere, may involve any portion of the genitourinary tract. Local symptoms predominate, and up to 75% of patients have chest radiographic abnormalities suggesting previous or concomitant pulmonary disease. Urinary frequency, dysuria, nocturia, hematuria, and flank or abdominal pain are common presentations. However, patients may be asymptomatic and the disease discovered only after severe destructive lesions of the kidneys have developed. Urinalysis gives abnormal results in 90% of cases, revealing pyuria and hematuria. The documentation of culture-negative pyuria in acidic urine raises the suspicion of TB. IV pyelography, abdominal CT, or MRI (Fig. 165-7) may show deformities and obstructions, and calcifications and ureteral strictures are suggestive findings. Culture of three morning urine specimens yields a definitive diagnosis in nearly 90% of cases. Severe ureteral strictures may lead to hydronephrosis and renal damage. Genital TB is diagnosed more commonly in female than in male patients. In female patients, it affects the fallopian tubes and the endometrium and may cause infertility, pelvic pain, and menstrual abnormalities. Diagnosis requires biopsy or culture of specimens obtained by dilatation and curettage. In male patients, genital TB preferentially affects the epididymis, producing a slightly tender mass that may drain externally through a fistulous tract; orchitis and prostatitis may also develop. In almost half of cases of genitourinary TB, urinary tract disease is also present. Genitourinary TB responds well to chemotherapy.

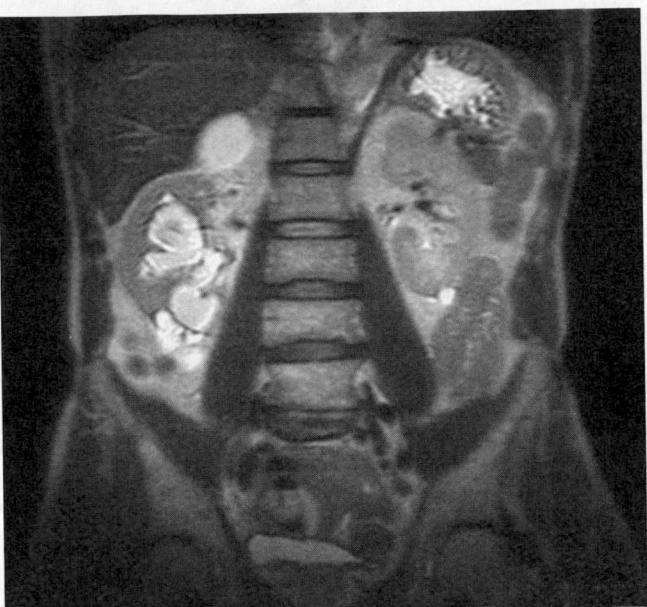

Figure 165-7   MRI of culture-confirmed renal tuberculosis. T2-weighted coronary plane: coronal sections showing several renal lesions in both the cortical and the medullary tissues of the right kidney. *(Courtesy of Dr. Alberto Matteelli, Department of Infectious Diseases, University of Brescia, Italy; with permission.)*

Skeletal TB

In the United States, TB of the bones and joints is responsible for ~10% of extrapulmonary cases. In bone and joint disease, pathogenesis is related to reactivation of hematogenous foci or to spread from adjacent paravertebral lymph nodes. Weight-bearing joints (the spine in 40% of cases, the hips in 13%, and the knees in 10%) are most commonly affected. Spinal TB (Pott's disease or tuberculous spondylitis; Fig. 165-8) often involves two or more adjacent vertebral bodies. While the upper thoracic spine is the most common

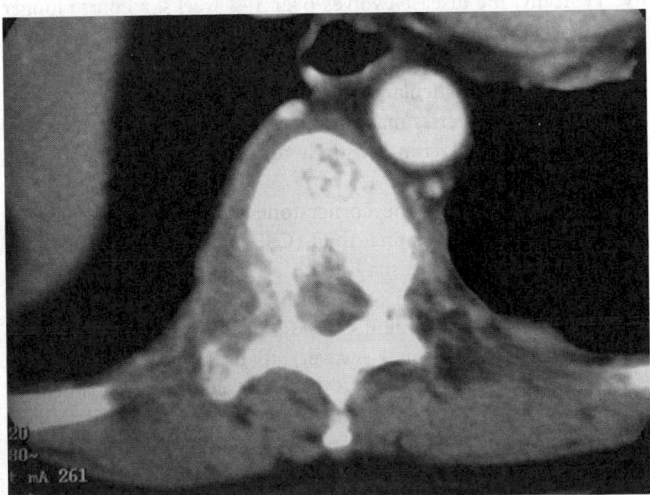

Figure 165-8   CT scan demonstrating destruction of the right pedicle of T10 due to Pott's disease. The patient, a 70-year-old Asian woman, presented with back pain and weight loss and had biopsy-proven tuberculosis. *(Courtesy of Charles L. Daley, MD, University of California, San Francisco; with permission.)*

site of spinal TB in children, the lower thoracic and upper lumbar vertebrae are usually affected in adults. From the anterior superior or inferior angle of the vertebral body, the lesion slowly reaches the adjacent body, later affecting the intervertebral disk. With advanced disease, collapse of vertebral bodies results in kyphosis (*gibbus*). A paravertebral "cold" abscess may also form. In the upper spine, this abscess may track to and penetrate the chest wall, presenting as a soft tissue mass; in the lower spine, it may reach the inguinal ligaments or present as a psoas abscess. CT or MRI reveals the characteristic lesion and suggests its etiology. The differential diagnosis includes tumors and other infections. Pyogenic bacterial osteomyelitis, in particular, involves the disk very early and produces rapid sclerosis. Aspiration of the abscess or bone biopsy confirms the tuberculous etiology, as cultures are usually positive and histologic findings highly typical. A catastrophic complication of Pott's disease is paraplegia, which is usually due to an abscess or a lesion compressing the spinal cord. Paraparesis due to a large abscess is a medical emergency and requires rapid drainage. TB of the hip joints, usually involving the head of the femur, causes pain; TB of the knee produces pain and swelling. If the disease goes unrecognized, the joints may be destroyed. Diagnosis requires examination of the synovial fluid, which is thick in appearance, with a high protein concentration and a variable cell count. Although synovial fluid culture is positive in a high percentage of cases, synovial biopsy and tissue culture may be necessary to establish the diagnosis. Skeletal TB responds to chemotherapy, but severe cases may require surgery.

Tuberculous meningitis and tuberculoma

TB of the central nervous system accounts for ~5% of extrapulmonary cases in the United States. It is seen most often in young children but also develops in adults, especially those infected with HIV. Tuberculous meningitis results from the hematogenous spread of primary or postprimary pulmonary TB or from the rupture of a subependymal tubercle into the subarachnoid space. In more than half of cases, evidence of old pulmonary lesions or a miliary pattern is found on chest radiography. The disease often presents subtly as headache and slight mental changes after a prodrome of weeks of low-grade fever, malaise, anorexia, and irritability. If not recognized, tuberculous meningitis may evolve acutely with severe headache, confusion, lethargy, altered sensorium, and neck rigidity. Typically, the disease evolves over 1–2 weeks, a course longer than that of bacterial meningitis. Since meningeal involvement is pronounced at the base of the brain, paresis of cranial nerves (ocular nerves in particular) is a frequent finding, and the involvement of cerebral arteries may produce focal ischemia. The ultimate evolution is toward coma, with hydrocephalus and intracranial hypertension.

Lumbar puncture is the cornerstone of diagnosis. In general, examination of cerebrospinal fluid (CSF) reveals a high leukocyte count (up to 1000/μL), usually with a predominance of lymphocytes but sometimes with a predominance of neutrophils in the early stage; a protein content of 1–8 g/L (100–800 mg/dL); and a low glucose concentration. However, any of these three parameters can be within the normal range. AFB are seen on direct smear of CSF sediment in up to one-third of cases, but repeated lumbar punctures increase the yield. Culture of CSF is diagnostic in up to 80% of cases and remains the gold standard. Polymerase chain reaction (PCR) has a sensitivity of up to 80%, but rates of false-positivity reach 10%. Imaging studies (CT and MRI) may show hydrocephalus and abnormal enhancement of basal cisterns or ependyma. If unrecognized, tuberculous meningitis is uniformly fatal. This disease responds to chemotherapy; however, neurologic sequelae are documented in 25% of treated cases, in most of which

the diagnosis has been delayed. Clinical trials have demonstrated that patients given adjunctive glucocorticoids may experience faster resolution of CSF abnormalities and elevated CSF pressure. In one study, adjunctive dexamethasone (0.4 mg/kg per day given IV and tapering by 0.1 mg/kg per week until the fourth week, when 0.1 mg/kg per day was administered; followed by 4 mg/d given by mouth and tapering by 1 mg per week until the fourth week, when 1 mg/d was administered) significantly enhanced the chances of survival among persons >14 years of age but did not reduce the frequency of neurologic sequelae.

Tuberculoma, an uncommon manifestation of central nervous system TB, presents as one or more space-occupying lesions and usually causes seizures and focal signs. CT or MRI reveals contrast-enhanced ring lesions, but biopsy is necessary to establish the diagnosis.

Gastrointestinal TB

Gastrointestinal TB is uncommon, making up 3.5% of extrapulmonary cases in the United States. Various pathogenetic mechanisms are involved: swallowing of sputum with direct seeding, hematogenous spread, or (largely in developing areas) ingestion of milk from cows affected by bovine TB. Although any portion of the gastrointestinal tract may be affected, the terminal ileum and the cecum are the sites most commonly involved. Abdominal pain (at times similar to that associated with appendicitis) and swelling, obstruction, hematochezia, and a palpable mass in the abdomen are common findings at presentation. Fever, weight loss, anorexia, and night sweats are also common. With intestinal-wall involvement, ulcerations and fistulae may simulate Crohn's disease; the differential diagnosis with this entity is always difficult. Anal fistulae should prompt an evaluation for rectal TB. As surgery is required in most cases, the diagnosis can be established by histologic examination and culture of specimens obtained intraoperatively.

Tuberculous peritonitis follows either the direct spread of tubercle bacilli from ruptured lymph nodes and intraabdominal organs (e.g., genital TB in women) or hematogenous seeding. Nonspecific abdominal pain, fever, and ascites should raise the suspicion of tuberculous peritonitis. The coexistence of cirrhosis (Chap. 307) in patients with tuberculous peritonitis complicates the diagnosis. In tuberculous peritonitis, paracentesis reveals an exudative fluid with a high protein content and leukocytosis that is usually lymphocytic (although neutrophils occasionally predominate). The yield of direct smear and culture is relatively low; culture of a large volume of ascitic fluid can increase the yield, but peritoneal biopsy (with a specimen best obtained by laparoscopy) is often needed to establish the diagnosis.

Pericardial TB (tuberculous pericarditis)

Due either to direct extension from adjacent mediastinal or hilar lymph nodes or to hematogenous spread, pericardial TB has often been a disease of the elderly in countries with low TB prevalence. However, it also develops frequently in HIV-infected patients. Case-fatality rates are as high as 40% in some series. The onset may be subacute, although an acute presentation, with dyspnea, fever, dull retrosternal pain, and a pericardial friction rub, is possible. An effusion eventually develops in many cases; cardiovascular symptoms and signs of cardiac tamponade may ultimately appear (Chap. 239). In the presence of effusion, TB must be suspected if the patient belongs to a high-risk population (HIV-infected, originating in a high-prevalence country); if there is evidence of previous TB in other organs; or if echocardiography, CT, or MRI shows effusion and thickness across the pericardial space. A definitive diagnosis can be obtained by pericardiocentesis under echocardiographic guidance. The pericardial fluid must be submitted for biochemical, cytologic, and microbiologic study. The effusion is exudative in nature, with a high count of lymphocytes and monocytes. Hemorrhagic effusion is common. Direct smear examination is very rarely positive. Culture of pericardial fluid reveals *M. tuberculosis* in up to two-thirds of cases, while pericardial biopsy has a higher yield. High levels of ADA, lysozyme, and IFN-γ may suggest a tuberculous etiology. PCR may also be useful.

Without treatment, pericardial TB is usually fatal. Even with treatment, complications may develop, including chronic constrictive pericarditis with thickening of the pericardium, fibrosis, and sometimes calcification, which may be visible on a chest radiograph. Systematic reviews and meta-analyses show that adjunctive glucocorticoid treatment remains controversial with no conclusive evidence of benefits for all principal outcomes of pericarditis—i.e., no significant impact on resolution of effusion, no significant difference in functional status after treatment, and no significant reduction in the frequency of development of constriction or death. However, in HIV-infected patients, glucocorticoids do improve functional status after treatment.

Caused by direct extension from the pericardium or through retrograde lymphatic extension from affected mediastinal lymph nodes, tuberculous myocarditis is an extremely rare disease. Usually it is fatal and is diagnosed post-mortem.

Miliary or disseminated TB

Miliary TB is due to hematogenous spread of tubercle bacilli. Although in children it is often the consequence of primary infection, in adults it may be due to either recent infection or reactivation of old disseminated foci. The lesions are usually yellowish granulomas 1–2 mm in diameter that resemble millet seeds (thus the term *miliary*, coined by nineteenth-century pathologists). Clinical manifestations are nonspecific and protean, depending on the predominant site of involvement. Fever, night sweats, anorexia, weakness, and weight loss are presenting symptoms in the majority of cases. At times, patients have a cough and other respiratory symptoms due to pulmonary involvement as well as abdominal symptoms. Physical findings include hepatomegaly, splenomegaly, and lymphadenopathy. Eye examination may reveal choroidal tubercles, which are pathognomonic of miliary TB, in up to 30% of cases. Meningismus occurs in <10% of cases. A high index of suspicion is required for the diagnosis of miliary TB. Frequently, chest radiography (Fig. 165-4) reveals a miliary reticulonodular pattern (more easily seen on underpenetrated film), although no radiographic abnormality may be evident early in the course and among HIV-infected patients. Other radiologic findings include large infiltrates, interstitial infiltrates (especially in HIV-infected patients), and pleural effusion. Sputum smear microscopy is negative in 80% of cases. Various hematologic abnormalities may be seen, including anemia with leukopenia, lymphopenia, neutrophilic leukocytosis and leukemoid reactions, and polycythemia. Disseminated intravascular coagulation has been reported. Elevation of alkaline phosphatase levels and other abnormal values in liver function tests are detected in patients with severe hepatic involvement. The TST may be negative in up to half of cases, but reactivity may be restored during chemotherapy. Bronchoalveolar lavage and transbronchial biopsy are more likely to provide bacteriologic confirmation, and granulomas are evident in liver or bone-marrow biopsy specimens from many patients. If it goes unrecognized, miliary TB is lethal; with proper early treatment, however, it is amenable to cure. Glucocorticoid therapy has not proved beneficial.

A rare presentation seen in the elderly is *cryptic miliary TB* that has a chronic course characterized by mild intermittent fever, anemia, and—ultimately—meningeal involvement preceding death. An acute septicemic form, *nonreactive miliary TB*, occurs very rarely and is due to massive hematogenous dissemination of tubercle

bacilli. Pancytopenia is common in this form of disease, which is rapidly fatal. At postmortem examination, multiple necrotic but nongranulomatous ("nonreactive") lesions are detected.

Less common extrapulmonary forms

TB may cause chorioretinitis, uveitis, panophthalmitis, and painful hypersensitivity-related phlyctenular conjunctivitis. Tuberculous otitis is rare and presents as hearing loss, otorrhea, and tympanic membrane perforation. In the nasopharynx, TB may simulate granulomatosis with polyangiitis (Wegener's). Cutaneous manifestations of TB include primary infection due to direct inoculation, abscesses and chronic ulcers, scrofuloderma, lupus vulgaris (a smoldering disease with nodules, plaques, and fissures), miliary lesions, and erythema nodosum. Tuberculous mastitis results from retrograde lymphatic spread, often from the axillary lymph nodes. Adrenal TB is a manifestation of disseminated disease presenting rarely as adrenal insufficiency. Finally, congenital TB results from transplacental spread of tubercle bacilli to the fetus or from ingestion of contaminated amniotic fluid. This rare disease affects the liver, spleen, lymph nodes, and various other organs.

HIV-associated TB

(See also Chap. 189) TB is one of the most common diseases among HIV-infected persons worldwide and a major cause of death. In some African countries, the rate of HIV infection among TB patients reaches 70–80% in certain urban settings. A person with a positive TST who acquires HIV infection has a 3–13% annual risk of developing active TB. A new TB infection acquired by an HIV-infected individual may evolve to active disease in a matter of weeks rather than months or years. TB can appear at any stage of HIV infection, and its presentation varies with the stage. When CMI is only partially compromised, pulmonary TB presents in a typical manner (Figs. 165-4 and 165-5), with upper-lobe infiltrates and cavitation and without significant lymphadenopathy or pleural effusion. In late stages of HIV infection, a primary TB–like pattern, with diffuse interstitial or miliary infiltrates, little or no cavitation, and intrathoracic lymphadenopathy, is more common. However, these forms are becoming less common because of the expanded use of antiretroviral treatment (ART). Overall, sputum smears may be positive less frequently among TB patients with HIV infection than among those without; thus, the diagnosis of TB may be unusually difficult, especially in view of the variety of HIV-related pulmonary conditions mimicking TB. Extrapulmonary TB is common among HIV-infected patients. In various series, extrapulmonary TB—alone or in association with pulmonary disease—has been documented in 40–60% of all cases in HIV-co-infected individuals. The most common forms are lymphatic, disseminated, pleural, and pericardial. Mycobacteremia and meningitis are also frequent, particularly in advanced HIV disease. The diagnosis of TB in HIV-infected patients may be difficult not only because of the increased frequency of sputum-smear negativity (up to 40% in culture-proven pulmonary cases) but also because of atypical radiographic findings, a lack of classic granuloma formation in the late stages, and a negative TST. Delays in treatment may prove fatal.

Exacerbations in systemic or respiratory symptoms, signs, and laboratory or radiographic manifestations of TB—termed the *immune reconstitution inflammatory syndrome* (IRIS)—have been associated with the administration of ART. Usually occurring 1–3 months after initiation of ART, IRIS is more common among patients with advanced immunosuppression and extrapulmonary TB. "Unmasking IRIS" may also develop after the initiation of ART in patients with undiagnosed subclinical TB. The presumed pathogenesis of IRIS is an immune response that is elicited by antigens released as bacilli are killed during effective chemotherapy and that is temporally associated with improving immune function. The first priority in the management of a possible case of IRIS is to ensure that the clinical syndrome does not represent a failure of TB treatment or the development of another infection. Mild paradoxical reactions can be managed with symptom-based treatment. Glucocorticoids have been used for more severe reactions, although their use in this setting has not been formally evaluated in clinical trials.

Recommendations for the prevention and treatment of TB in HIV-infected individuals are provided below.

DIAGNOSIS

The key to the diagnosis of TB is a high index of suspicion. Diagnosis is not difficult with a high-risk patient—e.g., a homeless alcoholic who presents with typical symptoms and a classic chest radiograph showing upper-lobe infiltrates with cavities (Fig. 165-5). On the other hand, the diagnosis can easily be missed in an elderly nursing home resident or a teenager with a focal infiltrate. Often, the diagnosis is first entertained when the chest radiograph of a patient being evaluated for respiratory symptoms is abnormal. If the patient has no complicating medical conditions that cause immunosuppression, the chest radiograph may show typical upper-lobe infiltrates with cavitation (Fig. 165-5). The longer the delay between the onset of symptoms and the diagnosis, the more likely is the finding of cavitary disease. In contrast, immunosuppressed patients, including those with HIV infection, may have "atypical" findings on chest radiography—e.g., lower-zone infiltrates without cavity formation.

■ AFB MICROSCOPY

A presumptive diagnosis is commonly based on the finding of AFB on microscopic examination of a diagnostic specimen, such as a smear of expectorated sputum or of tissue (e.g., a lymph node biopsy). Although inexpensive, AFB microscopy has relatively low sensitivity (40–60%) in culture-confirmed cases of pulmonary TB. The traditional method—light microscopy of specimens stained with Ziehl-Neelsen basic fuchsin dyes—is nevertheless satisfactory, although time-consuming. Most modern laboratories processing large numbers of diagnostic specimens use auramine-rhodamine staining and fluorescence microscopy. Less expensive light-emitting diode (LED) fluorescence microscopes are now available and should, over time, replace conventional light and fluorescence microscopes, especially facilitating the use of this technology in developing countries. For patients with suspected pulmonary TB, it has been recommended that two or three sputum specimens, preferably collected early in the morning, should be submitted to the laboratory for AFB smear and mycobacterial culture. Recent reviews have emphasized that two specimens collected on the same visit may be as effective as three. If tissue is obtained, it is critical that the portion of the specimen intended for culture not be put in formaldehyde. The use of AFB microscopy on urine or gastric lavage fluid is limited by the presence of commensal mycobacteria that can cause false-positive results.

■ MYCOBACTERIAL CULTURE

Definitive diagnosis depends on the isolation and identification of *M. tuberculosis* from a clinical specimen or the identification of specific sequences of DNA in a nucleic acid amplification test (see below). Specimens may be inoculated onto egg- or agar-based medium (e.g., Löwenstein-Jensen or Middlebrook 7H10) and incubated at 37°C (under 5% CO_2 for Middlebrook medium). Because most species of mycobacteria, including *M. tuberculosis*, grow slowly, 4–8 weeks may be required before growth is detected. Although *M. tuberculosis* may be identified presumptively on the

basis of growth time and colony pigmentation and morphology, a variety of biochemical tests have traditionally been used to speciate mycobacterial isolates. In modern, well-equipped laboratories, the use of liquid culture for isolation and species identification by molecular methods or high-pressure liquid chromatography of mycolic acids has replaced isolation on solid media and identification by biochemical tests. A low-cost, rapid immunochromatographic lateral flow assay based on detection of MTP64 antigen may also be used for species identification of *M. tuberculosis* complex in culture isolates. These new methods, which should be introduced rapidly in developing countries, have decreased the time required for bacteriologic confirmation of TB to 2–3 weeks.

■ NUCLEIC ACID AMPLIFICATION

Several test systems based on amplification of mycobacterial nucleic acid are available. These systems permit the diagnosis of TB in as little as several hours, with high specificity and sensitivity approaching that of culture. These tests are most useful for the rapid confirmation of TB in persons with AFB-positive specimens but also have utility for the diagnosis of AFB-negative pulmonary and extrapulmonary TB. In settings where these tests are available, nucleic acid amplification testing should be performed on at least one respiratory specimen from patients being evaluated for suspected pulmonary TB.

■ DRUG SUSCEPTIBILITY TESTING

The initial isolate of *M. tuberculosis* should be tested for susceptibility to isoniazid and rifampin to detect MDR-TB, particularly if one or more risk factors for drug resistance are identified or the patient either fails to respond to initial therapy or has a relapse after the completion of treatment (see "Treatment Failure and Relapse," below). In addition, expanded susceptibility testing for second-line anti-TB drugs (especially the fluoroquinolones and the injectable drugs) is mandatory when MDR-TB is found. Susceptibility testing may be conducted directly (with the clinical specimen) or indirectly (with mycobacterial cultures) on solid or liquid medium. Results are obtained rapidly by direct susceptibility testing on liquid medium, with an average reporting time of 3 weeks. With indirect testing on solid medium, results may be unavailable for ≥8 weeks. Molecular methods for the rapid identification of genetic mutations known to be associated with resistance to rifampin and isoniazid (such as the line probe assays) have been developed and are being widely implemented for screening patients at increased risk of drug-resistant TB. Until the capacity for molecular testing is developed, a few noncommercial culture and drug-susceptibility testing methods (e.g., microscopically observed drug susceptibility, nitrate reductase assays, and colorimetric redox indicator assays) may be useful in resource-limited settings. Their use is limited to national reference laboratories with proven proficiency and adequate external quality control.

■ RADIOGRAPHIC PROCEDURES

As noted above, the initial suspicion of pulmonary TB is often based on abnormal chest radiographic findings in a patient with respiratory symptoms. Although the "classic" picture is that of upper-lobe disease with infiltrates and cavities (Fig. 165-5), virtually any radiographic pattern—from a normal film or a solitary pulmonary nodule to diffuse alveolar infiltrates in a patient with adult respiratory distress syndrome—may be seen. In the era of AIDS, no radiographic pattern can be considered pathognomonic. CT (Fig. 165-6) may be useful in interpreting questionable findings on plain chest radiography and may be helpful in diagnosing some forms of extrapulmonary TB (e.g., Pott's disease; Fig. 165-8). MRI is useful in the diagnosis of intracranial TB.

ADDITIONAL DIAGNOSTIC PROCEDURES

Other diagnostic tests may be used when pulmonary TB is suspected. Sputum induction by ultrasonic nebulization of hypertonic saline may be useful for patients who cannot produce a sputum specimen spontaneously. Frequently, patients with radiographic abnormalities that are consistent with other diagnoses (e.g., bronchogenic carcinoma) undergo fiberoptic bronchoscopy with bronchial brushings and endobronchial or transbronchial biopsy of the lesion. Bronchoalveolar lavage of a lung segment containing an abnormality may also be performed. In all cases, it is essential that specimens be submitted for AFB smear and mycobacterial culture. For the diagnosis of primary pulmonary TB in children, who often do not expectorate sputum, induced sputum specimens and specimens from early-morning gastric lavage may yield positive cultures.

Invasive diagnostic procedures are indicated for patients with suspected extrapulmonary TB. In addition to testing of specimens from involved sites (e.g., CSF for tuberculous meningitis, pleural fluid and biopsy samples for pleural disease), biopsy and culture of bone marrow and liver tissue have a good diagnostic yield in disseminated (miliary) TB, particularly in HIV-infected patients, who also have a high frequency of positive blood cultures. In some cases, cultures are negative but a clinical diagnosis of TB is supported by consistent epidemiologic evidence (e.g., a history of close contact with an infectious patient), a positive TST or IFN-γ release assay (IGRA; see below), and a compatible clinical and radiographic response to treatment. In the United States and other industrialized countries with low rates of TB, some patients with limited abnormalities on chest radiographs and sputum positive for AFB are infected with nontuberculous mycobacteria, most commonly organisms of the *M. avium* complex or *M. kansasii* (Chap. 167). Factors favoring the diagnosis of nontuberculous mycobacterial disease over TB include an absence of risk factors for TB, a negative TST or IGRA, and underlying chronic pulmonary disease.

Patients with HIV-associated TB pose several diagnostic problems (see "HIV-associated TB," above). Moreover, HIV-infected patients with sputum culture–positive, AFB-positive TB may present with a normal chest radiograph. With the advent of ART, the occurrence of disseminated *M. avium* complex disease that can be confused with TB has become much less common.

SEROLOGIC AND OTHER DIAGNOSTIC TESTS FOR ACTIVE TB

A number of serologic tests based on detection of antibodies to a variety of mycobacterial antigens are marketed in developing countries but not in the United States. Careful independent assessments of these tests suggest that they are not useful as diagnostic aids, especially in persons with a low probability of TB. Various methods aimed at detection of mycobacterial antigens in diagnostic specimens are being investigated but are limited at present by low sensitivity. Determinations of ADA and IFN-γ levels in pleural fluid may be useful as adjunct tests in the diagnosis of pleural TB; the utility of these tests in the diagnosis of other forms of extrapulmonary TB (e.g., pericardial, peritoneal, and meningeal) is less clear.

DIAGNOSIS OF LATENT *M. TUBERCULOSIS* INFECTION

Tuberculin skin testing

In 1891, Robert Koch discovered that components of *M. tuberculosis* in a concentrated liquid culture medium, subsequently named "old tuberculin," were capable of eliciting a skin reaction when injected subcutaneously into patients with TB. In 1932, Seibert and Munday purified this product by ammonium sulfate precipitation to produce an active protein fraction known as *tuberculin purified protein derivative* (PPD). In 1941, PPD-S, developed by Seibert and

Glenn, was chosen as the international standard. Later, the WHO and UNICEF sponsored large-scale production of a master batch of PPD (RT23) and made it available for general use. The greatest limitation of PPD is its lack of mycobacterial species specificity, a property due to the large number of proteins in this product that are highly conserved in the various species. In addition, subjectivity of the skin-reaction interpretation, deterioration of the product, and batch-to-batch variations limit the usefulness of PPD.

Skin testing with tuberculin-PPD (TST) is most widely used in screening for latent *M. tuberculosis* infection (LTBI). The test is of limited value in the diagnosis of active TB because of its relatively low sensitivity and specificity and its inability to discriminate between latent infection and active disease. False-negative reactions are common in immunosuppressed patients and in those with overwhelming TB. False-positive reactions may be caused by infections with nontuberculous mycobacteria (Chap. 167) and by BCG vaccination.

IFN-γ release assays

Two in vitro assays that measure T cell release of IFN-γ in response to stimulation with the highly TB-specific antigens ESAT-6 and CFP-10 are available. The T-SPOT.TB® (Oxford Immunotec, Oxford, UK) is an enzyme-linked immunospot (ELISpot) assay, and the QuantiFERON-TB Gold® (Cellestis Ltd., Carnegie, Australia) is a whole-blood enzyme-linked immunosorbent assay (ELISA) for measurement of IFN-γ. The QuantiFERON-TB Gold In-Tube assay, which facilitates blood collection and initial incubation, also contains another specific antigen, TB7.7.

IGRAs are more specific than the TST as a result of less cross-reactivity due to BCG vaccination and sensitization by nontuberculous mycobacteria. Although diagnostic sensitivity for LTBI cannot be directly estimated because of the lack of a gold standard, these tests have shown better correlation than the TST with exposure to *M. tuberculosis* in contact investigations in low-incidence settings. However, their performance in high TB- and/or HIV-burden settings has been much more varied. Although limited, direct comparative studies of the two assays in routine practice suggest that the ELISpot has a lower rate of indeterminate results and probably has a higher degree of diagnostic sensitivity than whole-blood ELISA. Other potential advantages of IGRAs include logistical convenience, the need for fewer patient visits to complete testing, the avoidance of somewhat subjective measurements such as skin induration, and the ability to perform serial testing without inducing the boosting phenomenon (a spurious TST conversion due to boosting of reactivity on subsequent TSTs among BCG-vaccinated persons and those infected with other mycobacteria). IGRAs require that blood be drawn from patients and delivered to the laboratory in a timely fashion. Because of high specificity and other potential advantages, IGRAs may replace the TST for LTBI diagnosis in low-incidence, high-income settings where cross-reactivity due to BCG might adversely impact the interpretation and utility of the TST.

A number of national guidelines on the use of IGRAs for LTBI testing have been issued. In the United States, an IGRA is preferred over the TST for most persons over the age of 5 years who are being screened for LTBI. However, for those at high risk of progression to active TB (e.g., HIV-infected persons), either test may be used, or both may be used to optimize sensitivity. Because of the paucity of data on IGRA testing in children, the TST is preferred for LTBI testing of children under age 5. In Canada and some European countries, a two-step approach for those with positive TSTs—i.e., initial TST followed by an IGRA—is recommended. However, a TST may boost an IGRA response if the interval between the two tests exceeds 3 days.

The two aims of TB treatment are (1) to interrupt transmission by rendering patients noninfectious and (2) to prevent morbidity and death by curing patients with TB while preventing the emergence of drug resistance. Chemotherapy for TB became possible with the discovery of streptomycin in 1943. Randomized clinical trials clearly indicated that the administration of streptomycin to patients with chronic TB reduced mortality rates and led to cure in the majority of cases. However, monotherapy with streptomycin was frequently associated with the development of resistance to this drug and the attendant failure of treatment. With the introduction into clinical practice of para-aminosalicylic acid (PAS) and isoniazid, it became axiomatic in the early 1950s that cure of TB required the concomitant administration of at least two agents to which the organism was susceptible. Furthermore, early clinical trials demonstrated that a long period of treatment— i.e., 12–24 months—was required to prevent recurrence. The introduction of rifampin (rifampicin) in the early 1970s heralded the era of effective short-course chemotherapy, with a treatment duration of <12 months. The discovery that pyrazinamide, which was first used in the 1950s, augmented the potency of isoniazid/rifampin regimens led to the use of a 6-month course of this triple-drug regimen as standard therapy.

DRUGS Four major drugs are considered the first-line agents for the treatment of TB: isoniazid, rifampin, pyrazinamide, and ethambutol (Table 165-2). These drugs are well absorbed after oral administration, with peak serum levels at 2–4 h and nearly complete elimination within 24 h. These agents are recommended on the basis of their bactericidal activity (i.e., their ability to rapidly reduce the number of viable organisms and render patients noninfectious), their sterilizing activity (i.e., their ability

to kill all bacilli and thus sterilize the affected tissues, measured in terms of the ability to prevent relapses), and their low rate of induction of drug resistance. Rifapentine and rifabutin, two drugs related to rifampin, are also available in the United States and are useful for selected patients. For a detailed discussion of the drugs used for the treatment of TB, see Chap. 168.

Because of a lower degree of efficacy and a higher degree of intolerability and toxicity, six classes of second-line drugs are generally used only for the treatment of patients with TB resistant to first-line drugs. Included in this group are the injectable aminoglycosides streptomycin (formerly a first-line agent), kanamycin, and amikacin; the injectable polypeptide capreomycin; the oral agents ethionamide, cycloserine, and PAS; and the fluoroquinolone antibiotics. Of the quinolones, third-generation agents are preferred: levofloxacin, gatifloxacin (no longer marketed in the United States because of its severe toxicity), and moxifloxacin. Today amithiozone (thiacetazone) is used very rarely (mainly for MDR-TB) since it is associated with severe and sometimes even fatal skin reactions among HIV-infected patients. Other drugs of unproven efficacy that have been used in the treatment of patients with resistance to most of the first- and second-line agents include clofazimine, amoxicillin/clavulanic acid, clarithromycin, imipenem, and linezolid. Two novel drugs currently under clinical development— OPC-67683, a nitroimidazole; and TMC207, a diarylquinoline— are active against MDR-TB and offer promise in shortening the course of treatment required for drug-susceptible TB as well. Moxifloxacin and gatifloxacin (see above) are in late-phase clinical development as 4-month treatment-shortening regimens for drug-susceptible TB.

REGIMENS Standard short-course regimens are divided into an initial, or bactericidal, phase and a continuation, or sterilizing, phase. During the initial phase, the majority of the tubercle bacilli are killed, symptoms resolve, and usually the patient becomes noninfectious. The continuation phase is required to eliminate persisting mycobacteria and prevent relapse. The treatment regimen of choice for virtually all forms of TB in adults consists of a 2-month initial phase of isoniazid, rifampin, pyrazinamide, and ethambutol followed by a 4-month continuation phase of isoniazid and rifampin (Table 165-3). In children, most forms can be safely treated without ethambutol in the intensive phase. Treatment may be given daily throughout the course or intermittently (either three times weekly throughout the course or twice weekly after an initial phase of daily therapy, although the twice-weekly option is not recommended by the WHO). However, HIV-infected patients should receive their initial-phase regimen daily. A continuation phase of once-weekly rifapentine and isoniazid is equally effective for HIV-seronegative patients with noncavitary pulmonary TB who have negative sputum cultures at 2 months. Intermittent treatment is especially useful for patients whose therapy can be directly observed (see below). Patients with cavitary pulmonary TB and delayed sputum-culture conversion (i.e., those who remain culture-positive at 2 months) should have the continuation phase extended by 3 months, for a total course of 9 months. For patients with sputum culture–negative pulmonary TB, the duration of treatment may be reduced to a total of 4 months. To prevent isoniazid-related neuropathy, pyridoxine (10–25 mg/d) should be added to the regimen given to persons at high risk of vitamin B6 deficiency (e.g., alcoholics; malnourished persons; pregnant and lactating women; and patients with conditions such as chronic renal failure, diabetes, and HIV infection, which are also associated with neuropathy). A full course of therapy

TABLE 165-2 Recommended Dosage[a] for Initial Treatment of Tuberculosis in Adults[b]

Drug	Dosage	
	Daily Dose	Thrice-Weekly Dose[c]
Isoniazid	5 mg/kg, max 300 mg	10 mg/kg, max 900 mg
Rifampin	10 mg/kg, max 600 mg	10 mg/kg, max 600 mg
Pyrazinamide	25 mg/kg, max 2 g	35 mg/kg, max 3 g
Ethambutol[d]	15 mg/kg	30 mg/kg

[a]The duration of treatment with individual drugs varies by regimen, as detailed in Table 165-3.

[b]Dosages for children are similar, except that some authorities recommend higher doses of isoniazid (10–15 mg/kg daily; 20–30 mg/kg intermittent) and rifampin (10–20 mg/kg).

[c]Dosages for twice-weekly administration are the same for isoniazid and rifampin but are higher for pyrazinamide (50 mg/kg, with a maximum of 4 g/d) and ethambutol (40–50 mg/d).

[d]In certain settings, streptomycin (15 mg/kg daily, with a maximum dose of 1 g; or 25–30 mg/kg thrice weekly, with a maximum dose of 1.5 g) can replace ethambutol in the initial phase of treatment. However, streptomycin is no longer considered a first-line drug by the ATS, the IDSA, or the CDC.

Source: Based on recommendations of the American Thoracic Society, the Infectious Diseases Society of America, and the Centers for Disease Control and Prevention and of the World Health Organization.

TABLE 165-3 Recommended Antituberculosis Treatment Regimens

Indication	Initial Phase Duration, Months	Initial Phase Drugs	Continuation Phase Duration, Months	Continuation Phase Drugs
New smear- or culture-positive cases	2	HRZE[a,b]	4	HR[a,c,d]
New culture-negative cases	2	HRZE[a]	4	HR[a]
Pregnancy	2	HRE[e]	7	HR
Relapses and treatment default (pending susceptibility testing)	3	HRZES[f]	5	HRE
Failures[g]	—	—	—	—
Resistance (or intolerance) to H	Throughout (6)	RZE[h]		
Resistance (or intolerance) to R	Throughout (12–18)	HZEQ[i]		
Resistance to H + R	Throughout (at least 20 months)	ZEQ + S (or another injectable agent[j])		
Resistance to all first-line drugs	Throughout (at least 20 months)	1 injectable agent[j] + 3 of these 4: ethionamide, cycloserine, Q, PAS		
Intolerance to Z	2	HRE	7	HR

[a]All drugs can be given daily or intermittently (three times weekly throughout). A twice-weekly regimen after 2–8 weeks of daily therapy during the initial phase is sometimes used, although it is not recommended by the WHO.

[b]Streptomycin can be used in place of ethambutol but is no longer considered to be a first-line drug by the ATS/IDSA/CDC.

[c]The continuation phase should be extended to 7 months for patients with cavitary pulmonary tuberculosis who remain sputum culture–positive after the initial phase of treatment.

[d]HIV-negative patients with noncavitary pulmonary tuberculosis who have negative sputum AFB smears after the initial phase of treatment can be given once-weekly rifapentine/isoniazid in the continuation phase.

[e]The 6-month regimen with pyrazinamide can probably be used safely during pregnancy and is recommended by the WHO and the International Union Against Tuberculosis and Lung Disease. If pyrazinamide is not included in the initial treatment regimen, the minimum duration of therapy is 9 months.

[f]Streptomycin should be discontinued after 2 months. Drug susceptibility results will determine the best regimen option.

[g]The regimen is tailored according to the results of drug susceptibility tests. The availability of rapid molecular methods to identify drug resistance allows initiation of a proper regimen at the start of treatment.

[h]A fluoroquinolone may strengthen the regimen for patients with extensive disease.

[i]Streptomycin for the initial 2 months may strengthen the regimen for patients with extensive disease.

[j]Amikacin, kanamycin, or capreomycin. All these agents should be used for at least 6 months and for 4 months after culture conversion. If susceptibility is confirmed, streptomycin could be used as the injectable agent.

Abbreviations: E, ethambutol; H, isoniazid; PAS, para-aminosalicylic acid; Q, a quinolone antibiotic; R, rifampin; S, streptomycin; Z, pyrazinamide.

(completion of treatment) is defined more accurately by the total number of doses taken than by the duration of treatment. Specific recommendations on the required numbers of doses for each of the various treatment regimens have been published jointly by the American Thoracic Society, the Infectious Diseases Society of America, and the CDC. In some developing countries where the ability to ensure compliance with treatment is limited, a continuation-phase regimen of daily isoniazid and ethambutol for 6 months has been used. However, this regimen is associated with a higher rate of relapse and failure, especially among HIV-infected patients, and is no longer recommended by the WHO.

Lack of adherence to treatment is recognized worldwide as the most important impediment to cure. Moreover, the tubercle bacilli infecting patients who do not adhere to the prescribed regimen are likely to become drug resistant. Both patient- and provider-related factors may affect compliance. Patient-related factors include a lack of belief that the illness is significant and/or that treatment will have a beneficial effect; the existence of concomitant medical conditions (notably substance abuse); lack of social support; and poverty, with attendant joblessness and homelessness. Provider-related factors that may promote compliance include the education and encouragement of patients,

the offering of convenient clinic hours, and the provision of incentives and enablers such as meals and travel vouchers. In addition to specific measures addressing noncompliance, two other strategic approaches are used: direct observation of treatment and provision of fixed-drug-combination products. Because it is difficult to predict which patients will adhere to the recommended treatment, all patients should have their therapy directly supervised, especially during the initial phase. In the United States, personnel to supervise therapy are usually available through TB control programs of local public health departments. Supervision increases the proportion of patients completing treatment and greatly lessens the chances of relapse and acquired drug resistance. Fixed-drug-combination products (e.g., isoniazid/rifampin, isoniazid/rifampin/pyrazinamide, and isoniazid/rifampin/pyrazinamide/ethambutol) are available (except, in the United States, for the four-drug fixed drug combination) and are strongly recommended as a means of minimizing the likelihood of prescription error and of the development of drug resistance as the result of monotherapy. In some formulations of these combination products, the bioavailability of rifampin has been found to be substandard. In North America and Europe, regulatory authorities ensure that combination products are of good quality; however, this type of quality assurance cannot be assumed to be operative in less affluent countries. Alternative regimens for patients who exhibit drug intolerance or adverse reactions are listed in Table 165-3. However, severe side effects prompting discontinuation of any of the first-line drugs and use of these alternative regimens are uncommon.

MONITORING TREATMENT RESPONSE AND DRUG TOXICITY

Bacteriologic evaluation is essential in monitoring the response to treatment for TB. Patients with pulmonary disease should have their sputum examined monthly until cultures become negative. With the recommended regimen, >80% of patients will have negative sputum cultures at the end of the second month of treatment. By the end of the third month, virtually all patients should be culture-negative. In some patients, especially those with extensive cavitary disease and large numbers of organisms, AFB smear conversion may lag behind culture conversion. This phenomenon is presumably due to the expectoration and microscopic visualization of dead bacilli. As noted above, patients with cavitary disease in whom sputum culture conversion does not occur by 2 months require extended treatment. When a patient's sputum cultures remain positive at ≥3 months, treatment failure and drug resistance or poor adherence to the regimen should be suspected (see below). A sputum specimen should be collected by the end of treatment to document cure. If mycobacterial cultures are not practical, then monitoring by AFB smear examination should be undertaken at 2, 5, and 6 months. Patients whose smears remain positive at 2 months should undergo a repeat examination at 3 months. Smears that are positive after 3 months of treatment when the patient is known to be adherent are indicative of treatment failure and possible drug resistance. Therefore, drug susceptibility testing should be done. Bacteriologic monitoring of patients with extrapulmonary TB is more difficult and often is not feasible. In these cases, the response to treatment must be assessed clinically and radiographically.

Monitoring of the response during chemotherapy by serial chest radiographs is not recommended, as radiographic changes may lag behind bacteriologic response and are not highly sensitive. After the completion of treatment, neither sputum examination nor chest radiography is recommended for routine follow-up purposes. However, a chest radiograph obtained at the end of treatment may be useful for comparative purposes should the patient develop symptoms of recurrent TB months or years later. Patients should be instructed to report promptly for medical assessment should they develop any such symptoms.

During treatment, patients should be monitored for drug toxicity (Table 165-3). The most common adverse reaction of significance is hepatitis. Patients should be carefully educated about the signs and symptoms of drug-induced hepatitis (e.g., dark urine, loss of appetite) and should be instructed to discontinue treatment promptly and see their health care provider should these symptoms occur. Although biochemical monitoring is not routinely recommended, all adult patients should undergo baseline assessment of liver function (e.g., measurement of serum levels of hepatic aminotransferases and serum bilirubin). Older patients, those with concomitant diseases, those with a history of hepatic disease (especially hepatitis C), and those using alcohol daily should be monitored especially closely (i.e., monthly), with repeated measurements of aminotransferases, during the initial phase of treatment. Up to 20% of patients have small increases in aspartate aminotransferase (up to three times the upper limit of normal) that are not accompanied by symptoms and are of no consequence. For patients with symptomatic hepatitis and

those with marked (five- to sixfold) elevations in serum levels of aspartate aminotransferase, treatment should be stopped and drugs reintroduced one at a time after liver function has returned to normal. Hypersensitivity reactions usually require the discontinuation of all drugs and rechallenge to determine which agent is the culprit. Because of the variety of regimens available, it is usually not necessary—although it is possible—to desensitize patients. Hyperuricemia and arthralgia caused by pyrazinamide can usually be managed by the administration of acetylsalicylic acid; however, pyrazinamide treatment should be stopped if the patient develops gouty arthritis. Individuals who develop autoimmune thrombocytopenia secondary to rifampin therapy should not receive the drug thereafter. Similarly, the occurrence of optic neuritis with ethambutol is an indication for permanent discontinuation of this drug. Other common manifestations of drug intolerance, such as pruritus and gastrointestinal upset, can generally be managed without the interruption of therapy.

TREATMENT FAILURE AND RELAPSE   As stated above, treatment failure should be suspected when a patient's sputum smears and/or cultures remain positive after 3 months of treatment. In the management of such patients, it is imperative that the current isolate be tested for susceptibility to first- and second-line agents. Initial molecular testing for rifampin resistance should also be done if the technology is available. When the results of susceptibility testing are expected to become available within a few weeks, changes in the regimen can be postponed until that time. However, if the patient's clinical condition is deteriorating, an earlier change in regimen may be indicated. A cardinal rule in the latter situation is always to add more than one drug at a time to a failing regimen: at least two and preferably three drugs that have never been used and to which the bacilli are likely to be susceptible should be added. The patient may continue to take isoniazid and rifampin along with these new agents pending the results of susceptibility tests.

Patients who experience a recurrence after apparently successful treatment (relapses) are less likely to harbor drug-resistant strains (see below) than are patients in whom treatment has failed. However, if the regimen administered initially does not contain rifampin, the probability of isoniazid resistance is high. Acquired resistance is uncommon among strains from patients who relapse after completing a standard short-course regimen. However, it is prudent to begin the treatment of all patients who have relapsed with all four first-line drugs plus streptomycin, pending the results of susceptibility testing. In less affluent countries and other settings where facilities for culture and drug susceptibility testing are not yet routinely available, the WHO recommends that a standard regimen with all four first-line drugs plus streptomycin be used in all instances of relapse and treatment default. Patients with treatment failure should receive an empirical regimen, including second-line agents, based on their history of anti-TB treatment and the drug resistance patterns in the population (Table 165-3). Once drug susceptibility testing results are available, the regimen should be adjusted accordingly.

DRUG-RESISTANT TB   Strains of *M. tuberculosis* resistant to individual drugs arise by spontaneous point mutations in the mycobacterial genome that occur at low but predictable rates (10^{-7}–10^{-10} for the key drugs). Because there is no cross-resistance among the commonly used drugs, the probability that a strain will be resistant to two drugs is the product of the probabilities of resistance to each drug and thus is low. The development of drug-resistant TB is invariably the result of monotherapy—i.e., the failure of the health care provider to prescribe at least two

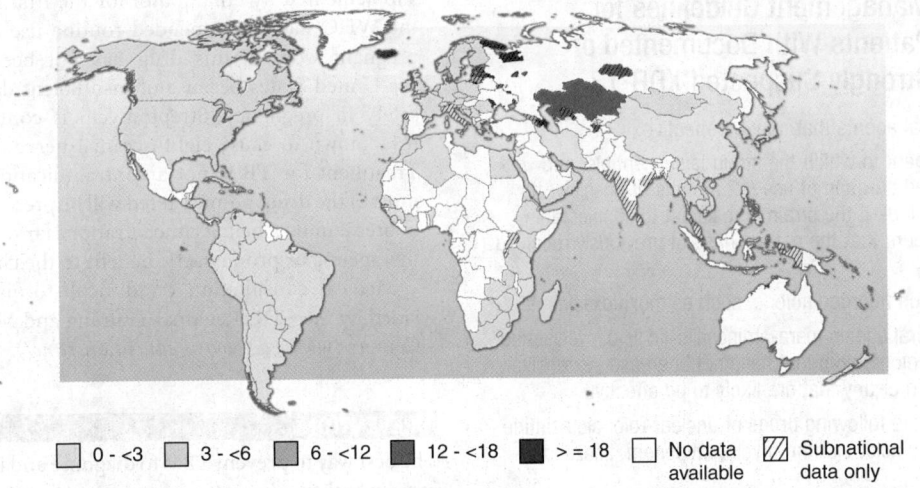

Figure 165-9 **Percentage of new tuberculosis cases with multidrug resistance** in all countries surveyed by the WHO/Union Global Drug Resistance Surveillance Project during 1994–2008. *(See disclaimer in Fig. 165-2. Courtesy of the Stop TB Department, WHO; with permission.)*

drugs to which tubercle bacilli are susceptible or of the patient to take properly prescribed therapy. Drug-resistant TB may be either primary or acquired. Primary drug resistance is that which develops in a strain infecting a patient who has not previously been treated. Acquired resistance develops during treatment with an inappropriate regimen. In North America and western Europe, rates of primary resistance are generally low, and isoniazid resistance is most common. In the United States, while rates of primary isoniazid resistance have been stable at ~7–8%, the rate of primary MDR-TB has declined from 2.5% in 1993 to 1% since 2000. Resistance rates are higher among foreign-born and HIV-infected patients. As described above, worldwide, MDR-TB is an increasingly serious problem in some regions, especially in the states of the former Soviet Union and in other parts of Asia (Fig. 165-9). Even more serious is the recently described occurrence of virtually untreatable XDR-TB due to MDR strains that are resistant to all fluoroquinolones and to at least one of three second-line injectable agents (amikacin, kanamycin, and capreomycin). Drug-resistant TB can be prevented by adherence to the principles of sound therapy: the inclusion of at least two bactericidal drugs to which the organism is susceptible, the use of fixed-drug-combination products, and the verification that patients complete the prescribed course.

Although the 6-month regimen described in Table 165-3 is generally effective for patients with initial isoniazid-resistant disease, it is prudent to include at least ethambutol and possibly pyrazinamide for the full 6 months. In such cases, isoniazid probably does not contribute to a successful outcome and could be omitted. For patients with extensive disease, a fluoroquinolone may be added. Patients whose isolates exhibit monoresistance to rifampin should receive a regimen containing isoniazid, pyrazinamide, ethambutol, and a fluoroquinolone for 12–18 months. MDR-TB is more difficult to manage than is disease caused by drug-susceptible organisms, especially because resistance to other first-line drugs besides isoniazid and rifampin is common. For treatment of TB due to strains resistant to isoniazid and rifampin, combinations of a fluoroquinolone, ethambutol, pyrazinamide, and streptomycin or, for strains resistant to streptomycin as well, another injectable agent (amikacin, kanamycin, or capreomycin) should be used. For patients with bacilli resistant to all of the first-line agents, cure may be attained with a combination of four second-line drugs, including one injectable agent (Table 165-3). Although the optimal duration of treatment is not known, a course of at least 20 months, is recommended. Patients with XDR-TB have fewer treatment options and a much poorer prognosis. However, observational studies have shown that aggressive management of cases comprising early drug-susceptibility testing, rational combination of at least five drugs, readjustment of the regimen, strict directly observed therapy, bacteriologic monitoring, and intensive patient support may result in cure rates of up to 60% and may avert deaths. Table 165-4 describes how to manage patients with XDR-TB. For patients with localized disease and sufficient pulmonary reserve, lobectomy or pneumonectomy may be considered. Because the management of patients with MDR- and XDR-TB is complicated by both social and medical factors, care of these patients is ideally provided in specialized centers or, in their absence, in the context of programs with adequate resources and capacity.

HIV-ASSOCIATED TB In general, the standard treatment regimens are equally efficacious in HIV-negative and HIV-positive patients. However, adverse drug effects may be more pronounced in HIV-infected patients. Three important considerations are relevant to TB treatment in HIV-infected patients: an increased frequency of paradoxical reactions, drug interactions between ART and rifamycins, and development of rifampin monoresistance with widely spaced intermittent treatment. IRIS—i.e., the exacerbation of symptoms and signs of TB—has been described above. All HIV-infected TB patients are candidates for ART, and the optimal timing for its initiation is as soon as possible and within the first 8 weeks of anti-TB therapy. Rifampin, a potent inducer of enzymes of the cytochrome P450 system, lowers serum levels of many HIV protease inhibitors and some non-nucleoside reverse transcriptase inhibitors—essential drugs used in ART. In such cases, rifabutin, which has much less enzyme-inducing activity, has been recommended in place of rifampin. However, dosage adjustment for rifabutin and/or the antiretroviral drugs may be necessary. Because recommendations are frequently updated, consultation of the CDC website is advised (*www.cdc.gov/tb*). Several clinical trials have found that patients with HIV-associated TB whose immunosuppression is advanced (CD4+ T cell counts of <100/μL) are prone to treatment failure

TABLE 165-4 Management Guidelines for Patients With Documented or Strongly Suspected XDR-TB

1. Use any first-line oral agents that may be effective.

2. Use an injectable agent to which the strain is susceptible, and consider an extended duration of use (12 months or possibly the whole treatment period). If the strain is resistant to all injectable agents, use of an agent that the patient has not previously received is recommended.[a]

3. Use a later-generation fluoroquinolone, such as moxifloxacin.

4. Use all second-line oral agents (para-aminosalicylic acid, cycloserine, ethionamide, or prothionamide) that have not been used extensively in a previous regimen or any that are likely to be effective.

5. Use two or more of the following drugs of unclear role: clofazimine, amoxicillin/clavulanic acid, clarithromycin, imipenem, linezolid, thiacetazone.

6. Consider treatment with high-dose isoniazid if low-level resistance to this drug is documented.

7. Consider adjuvant surgery if there is localized disease.

8. Enforce strong infection-control measures.

9. Implement strict directly observed therapy and full adherence support as well as comprehensive bacteriologic and clinical monitoring.

[a]This recommendation is made because, while the reproducibility and reliability of susceptibility testing with injectable agents are good, there are few data on the correlation of clinical efficacy with test results. Options with XDR-TB are very limited, and some strains may be affected in vivo by an injectable agent even though they test resistant in vitro.

Source: Adapted from the World Health Organization, 2008.

and relapse with rifampin-resistant organisms when treated with "highly intermittent" (i.e., once- or twice-weekly) rifamycin-containing regimens. Consequently, it is recommended that these patients receive daily therapy for at least the initial phase.

SPECIAL CLINICAL SITUATIONS Although comparative clinical trials of treatment for extrapulmonary TB are limited, the available evidence indicates that most forms of disease can be treated with the 6-month regimen recommended for patients with pulmonary disease. The American Academy of Pediatrics recommends that children with bone and joint TB, tuberculous meningitis, or miliary TB receive 9–12 months of treatment. Treatment for TB may be complicated by underlying medical problems that require special consideration. As a rule, patients with chronic renal failure should not receive aminoglycosides and should receive ethambutol only if serum drug levels can be monitored. Isoniazid, rifampin, and pyrazinamide may be given in the usual doses in cases of mild to moderate renal failure, but the dosages of isoniazid and pyrazinamide should be reduced for all patients with severe renal failure except those undergoing hemodialysis. Patients with hepatic disease pose a special problem because of the hepatotoxicity of isoniazid, rifampin, and pyrazinamide. Patients with severe hepatic disease may be treated with ethambutol, streptomycin, and possibly another drug (e.g., a fluoroquinolone); if required, isoniazid and rifampin may be administered under close supervision. The use of pyrazinamide by patients with liver failure should be avoided. Silicotuberculosis necessitates the extension of therapy by at least 2 months.

The regimen of choice for pregnant women (Table 165-3) is 9 months of treatment with isoniazid and rifampin supplemented by ethambutol for the first 2 months. Although the WHO has recommended routine use of pyrazinamide for pregnant women, this drug has not been recommended in the United States because of insufficient data documenting its safety in pregnancy. Streptomycin is contraindicated because it is known to cause eighth-cranial-nerve damage in the fetus. Treatment for TB is not a contraindication to breast-feeding; most of the drugs administered will be present in small quantities in breast milk, albeit at concentrations far too low to provide any therapeutic or prophylactic benefit to the child.

Medical consultation on difficult-to-manage cases is provided by the CDC Regional Training and Medical Consultation Centers (www.cdc.gov/tb/education/rtmc/).

PREVENTION

The best way to prevent TB is to diagnose and isolate infectious cases rapidly and to administer appropriate treatment until patients are rendered noninfectious (usually 2–4 weeks after the start of proper treatment) and the disease is cured. Additional strategies include BCG vaccination and treatment of persons with latent tuberculosis infection who are at high risk of developing active disease.

■ BCG VACCINATION

BCG was derived from an attenuated strain of *M. bovis* and was first administered to humans in 1921. Many BCG vaccines are available worldwide; all are derived from the original strain, but the vaccines vary in efficacy, ranging from 80% to nil in randomized, placebo-controlled trials. A similar range of efficacy was found in recent observational studies (case-control, historic cohort, and cross-sectional) in areas where infants are vaccinated at birth. These studies also found higher rates of efficacy in the protection of infants and young children from relatively serious forms of TB, such as tuberculous meningitis and miliary TB. BCG vaccine is safe and rarely causes serious complications. The local tissue response begins 2–3 weeks after vaccination, with scar formation and healing within 3 months. Side effects—most commonly, ulceration at the vaccination site and regional lymphadenitis—occur in 1–10% of vaccinated persons. Some vaccine strains have caused osteomyelitis in ~1 case per million doses administered. Disseminated BCG infection ("BCGitis") and death have occurred in 1–10 cases per 10 million doses administered, although this problem is restricted almost exclusively to persons with impaired immunity, such as children with severe combined immunodeficiency syndrome or adults with HIV infection. BCG vaccination induces TST reactivity, which tends to wane with time. The presence or size of TST reactions after vaccination does not predict the degree of protection afforded.

BCG vaccine is recommended for routine use at birth in countries with high TB prevalence. However, because of the low risk of transmission of TB in the United States, the unreliable protection afforded by BCG, and its impact on the TST, the vaccine has never been recommended for general use in the United States. HIV-infected adults and children should not receive BCG vaccine. Moreover, infants whose HIV status is unknown but who have signs and symptoms consistent with HIV infection or who are born to HIV-infected mothers should not receive BCG.

TREATMENT   Latent Tuberculosis Infection

Treatment of selected persons with LTBI aims at preventing active disease. This intervention (also called *preventive chemotherapy* or *chemoprophylaxis*) is based on the results of a

TABLE 165-5 Tuberculin Reaction Size and Treatment of Latent _Mycobacterium tuberculosis_ Infection

Risk Group	Tuberculin Reaction Size, mm
HIV-infected persons or persons receiving immuno-suppressive therapy	≥5
Close contacts of tuberculosis patients	≥5[a]
Persons with fibrotic lesions on chest radiography	≥5
Recently infected persons (≤2 years)	≥10
Persons with high-risk medical conditions[b]	≥10
Low-risk persons[c]	≥15

[a]Tuberculin-negative contacts, especially children, should receive prophylaxis for 2–3 months after contact ends and should then undergo repeat TST. Those whose results remain negative should discontinue prophylaxis. HIV-infected contacts should receive a full course of treatment regardless of TST results.
[b]Includes diabetes mellitus, some hematologic and reticuloendothelial diseases, injection drug use (with HIV seronegativity), end-stage renal disease, and clinical situations associated with rapid weight loss.
[c]Except for employment purposes where longitudinal TST screening is anticipated, TST is not indicated for these low-risk persons. A decision to treat should be based on individual risk/benefit considerations.

large number of randomized, placebo-controlled clinical trials demonstrating that a 6- to 12-month course of isoniazid reduces the risk of active TB in infected people by up to 90%. Analysis of available data indicates that the optimal duration of treatment is 9–10 months. In the absence of reinfection, the protective effect is believed to be lifelong. Clinical trials have shown that isoniazid reduces rates of TB among TST-positive persons with HIV infection. Studies in HIV-infected patients have also demonstrated the effectiveness of shorter courses of rifampin-based treatment.

Candidates for treatment of LTBI (Table 165-5) are identified by TST or IGRA of persons in defined high-risk groups. For skin testing, 5 tuberculin units of polysorbate-stabilized PPD should be injected intradermally into the volar surface of the forearm (Mantoux method). Multipuncture tests are not recommended. Reactions are read at 48–72 h as the transverse diameter (in millimeters) of induration; the diameter of erythema is not considered. In some persons, TST reactivity wanes with time but can be recalled by a second skin test administered ≥1 week after the first (i.e., two-step testing). For persons periodically undergoing the TST, such as health care workers and individuals admitted to long-term-care institutions, initial two-step testing may preclude subsequent misclassification of persons with boosted reactions as TST converters. The cutoff for a positive TST (and thus for treatment) is related both to the probability that the reaction represents true infection and to the likelihood that the individual, if truly infected, will develop TB (Table 165-5). Thus, positive reactions for close contacts of infectious cases, persons with HIV infection, persons receiving drugs that suppress the immune system, and previously untreated persons whose chest radiograph is consistent with healed TB are defined as an area of induration ≥5 mm in diameter. A 10-mm cutoff is used to define positive reactions in most other at-risk persons. For persons with a very low risk of developing TB if infected, a cutoff of 15 mm is used. (Except for employment purposes where longitudinal screening is anticipated, the TST is not indicated for these low-risk persons.) Treatment should be considered for persons from TB-endemic countries who have a history of BCG vaccination. A positive IGRA is based on the manufacturers' recommendations. For the ELISpot assay, there is an uncertainty zone (5–7 spots) for which epidemiologic and clinical factors guide the decision to implement treatment for LTBI. This approach has also been suggested for interpretation of results in the whole-blood assay that are close to the recommended cutoff for a positive test (0.35 IU of IFN-γ). Some TST- and IGRA-negative individuals are also candidates for treatment. Infants and children who have come into contact with infectious cases should be treated and should have a repeat skin test 2 or 3 months after contact ends. Those whose test results remain negative should discontinue treatment. HIV-infected persons who have been exposed to an infectious TB patient should receive treatment regardless of the TST result. Any HIV-infected candidate for LTBI treatment must be screened carefully to exclude active TB, which would necessitate full treatment.

Isoniazid is administered at a daily dose of 5 mg/kg (up to 300 mg/d) for 9 months (Table 165-6). On the basis of cost-benefit analyses, a 6-month period of treatment has been recommended in the past and may be considered for HIV-negative adults with normal chest radiographs when financial considerations are important. When supervised treatment is desirable and feasible, isoniazid may be given at a dose of 15 mg/kg (up to 900 mg) twice weekly. An alternative regimen for adults is 4 months of daily rifampin. A 3-month regimen of isoniazid and rifampin is recommended in the United Kingdom for both adults and children. A previously recommended regimen of 2 months of rifampin and pyrazinamide has been associated with serious and fatal hepatotoxicity and now is generally not recommended. The rifampin regimen should be considered for persons who are likely to have been infected with an isoniazid-resistant strain. Pending the results of a large-scale study of LTBI treatment conducted by the CDC, it is possible that a regimen of isoniazid and rifapentine given once weekly for 12 weeks will also become an option. Furthermore, clinical trials are under way to assess the efficacy of long-term isoniazid administration (i.e., for at least 3 years). Isoniazid should not be given to persons with active liver disease. All persons at increased risk of hepatotoxicity (e.g., those abusing alcohol daily and those with a history of liver disease) should undergo baseline and then monthly assessment of liver function. All patients should be carefully educated about hepatitis and instructed to discontinue use of the drug immediately should any symptoms develop. Moreover, patients should be seen and questioned monthly during therapy about adverse reactions and should be given no more than 1 month's supply of drug at each visit.

It may be more difficult to ensure compliance when treating persons with latent infection than when treating those with active TB. If family members of active cases are being treated, compliance and monitoring may be easier. When feasible, twice-weekly supervised therapy may increase the likelihood of completion. As in active cases, the provision of incentives may also be helpful.

PRINCIPLES OF TB CONTROL

The highest priority in any TB control program is the prompt detection of cases and the provision of short-course chemotherapy to all TB patients under proper case-management

TABLE 165-6 Revised Drug Regimens for Treatment of Latent Tuberculosis Infection (LTBI) in Adults

Drug	Interval and Duration	Comments[a]	Rating[b] (Evidence[c]) HIV-Negative	Rating[b] (Evidence[c]) HIV-Infected
Isoniazid	Daily for 9 months[d,e]	In HIV-infected persons, isoniazid may be administered concurrently with nucleoside reverse transcriptase inhibitors, protease inhibitors, or NNRTIs.	A (II)	A (II)
	Twice weekly for 9 months[d,e]	DOT must be used with twice-weekly dosing.	B (II)	B (II)
	Daily for 6 months[e]	Regimen is not indicated for HIV-infected persons, those with fibrotic lesions on chest radiographs, or children.	B (I)	C (I)
	Twice weekly for 6 months[e]	DOT must be used with twice-weekly dosing.	B (II)	C (I)
Rifampin[f]	Daily for 4 months	Regimen is used for contacts of patients with isoniazid-resistant, rifampin-susceptible tuberculosis. In HIV-infected persons, most protease inhibitors and delavirdine should not be administered concurrently with rifampin. Rifabutin, with appropriate dose adjustments, can be used with protease inhibitors (saquinavir should be augmented with ritonavir) and NNRTIs (except delavirdine). Clinicians should consult web-based updates for the latest specific recommendations.	B (II)	B (III)
Rifampin plus pyrazinamide	Daily for 2 months	Regimen generally should not be offered for treatment of LTBI in either HIV-infected or HIV-negative persons.	D (II)	D (II)
	Twice weekly for 2–3 months		D (III)	D (III)

[a] Interactions with HIV-related drugs are updated frequently and are available at www.aidsinfo.nih.gov/guidelines.
[b] Strength of the recommendation: A. Both strong evidence of efficacy and substantial clinical benefit support recommendation for use. Should always be offered. B. Moderate evidence for efficacy or strong evidence for efficacy but only limited clinical benefit supports recommendation for use. Should generally be offered. C. Evidence for efficacy is insufficient to support a recommendation for or against use, or evidence for efficacy might not outweigh adverse consequences (e.g., drug toxicity, drug interactions) or cost of the treatment or alternative approaches. Optional. D. Moderate evidence for lack of efficacy or for adverse outcome supports a recommendation against use. Should generally not be offered. E. Good evidence for lack of efficacy or for adverse outcome supports a recommendation against use. Should never be offered.
[c] Quality of evidence supporting the recommendation: I. Evidence from at least one properly randomized controlled trial. II. Evidence from at least one well-designed clinical trial without randomization, from cohort or case-controlled analytic studies (preferably from more than one center), from multiple time-series studies, or from dramatic results in uncontrolled experiments. III. Evidence from opinions of respected authorities based on clinical experience, descriptive studies, or reports of expert committees.
[d] Recommended regimen for persons aged <18 years.
[e] Recommended regimen for pregnant women.
[f] The substitution of rifapentine for rifampin is not recommended because rifapentine's safety and effectiveness have not been established for patients with LTBI.
Abbreviations: DOT, directly observed therapy; NNRTIs, nonnucleoside reverse transcriptase inhibitors.
Source: Adapted from CDC: Targeted tuberculin testing and treatment of latent tuberculosis infection. MMWR Recomm Rep 49:RR-6, 2000

conditions, including directly observed therapy. In addition, in low-prevalence countries with adequate resources (and increasingly in developing countries as well), screening of high-risk groups, such as immigrants from high-prevalence countries, migratory workers, prisoners, homeless individuals, substance abusers, and HIV-seropositive persons, is recommended. TST-positive high-risk persons should be treated for latent infection. Contact investigation is an important component of efficient TB control. In the United States and other countries worldwide, a great deal of attention has been given to the transmission of TB (particularly in association with HIV infection) in institutional settings such as hospitals, homeless shelters, and prisons. Measures to limit such transmission include respiratory isolation of persons with suspected TB until they are proven to be noninfectious (i.e., at least by sputum AFB smear negativity), proper ventilation in rooms of patients with infectious TB, use of ultraviolet irradiation in areas of increased risk of TB transmission, and periodic screening of personnel who may come into contact with known or unsuspected cases of TB. In the past, radiographic surveys, especially those conducted with portable equipment and miniature films, were advocated for case finding. Today, however, the prevalence of TB in industrialized countries is sufficiently low that "mass miniature radiography" is not cost-effective.

In high-prevalence countries, most TB control programs have made remarkable progress in reducing morbidity and mortality during the past 15 years by adopting and implementing the DOTS strategy promoted by the WHO. Between 1995 and 2008, 36 million TB cases were cured and more than 6 million deaths averted compared with the pre-DOTS period. The DOTS approach consists of: (1) political commitment with increased and sustained financing; (2) case detection through quality-assured bacteriology (starting with microscopic examination of sputum from patients with cough of >2–3 weeks' duration, culture, and possibly drug susceptibility testing); (3) administration of standardized short-course chemotherapy, with direct supervision and patient support; (4) an effective drug supply and management system; and (5) a monitoring and evaluation system, with impact measurement (including assessment of treatment outcomes—e.g., cure, completion of treatment without bacteriologic proof of cure, death, treatment failure, and default—in all cases registered and notified). In 2006, the WHO indicated that, while DOTS remains the essential component of any control strategy, additional steps must be undertaken to reach the 2015 TB control targets set within the United Nations Millennium Development Goals. Thus, a new "Stop TB Strategy" with six components has been promoted: (1) Pursue high-quality DOTS expansion and enhancement. (2) Address HIV-associated TB, MDR-TB, and the needs of poor and vulnerable populations. (3) Contribute to health system strengthening. (4) Engage all care providers. (5) Empower people with TB and [their] communities. (6) Enable and promote research. As part of the fourth component, evidence-based International Standards for Tuberculosis Care, focused on diagnosis, treatment, and public health responsibilities, have recently been introduced for wide adoption by medical and professional societies, academic institutions, and all practitioners worldwide. Care and control of HIV-associated TB is particularly challenging in developing countries, since existing interventions require collaboration between HIV/AIDS and TB programs as well as standard services. While TB programs must test every patient for HIV in order to provide access to trimethoprim-sulfamethoxazole prophylaxis against common infections and ART, HIV/AIDS programs must regularly screen persons living with HIV/AIDS for active TB and provide treatment for LTBI. Early and active case detection is considered an important intervention not only among persons living with HIV/AIDS but also among other vulnerable populations, as it reduces transmission in a community and provides early effective care. For TB control efforts to succeed, programs must optimize their performance and include additional interventions as described. However, bold public health policies must be enforced to support work on TB control and care. These policies include free access to diagnosis and treatment, at least for the poorest patients; sound regulations to ensure drug quality; rational use of drugs by all care providers; laboratory networks equipped with the latest technology for rapid diagnosis; and airborne infection control in all facilities and congregate settings attended by TB patients, especially where HIV prevalence is high. Finally, elimination of TB will require control and attenuation of the multitude of risk factors (e.g., HIV, smoking, and diabetes) and socioeconomic determinants (e.g., extreme poverty, inadequate living conditions and bad housing, alcoholism, malnutrition, and indoor air pollution) with clear policies within the health sector and other sectors linked to human development and welfare.

FURTHER READINGS

CENTERS FOR DISEASE CONTROL AND PREVENTION: Control of tuberculosis in the United States: Recommendations from the American Thoracic Society, CDC, and the Infectious Diseases Society of America. MMWR Recomm Rep 54:RR-12, 2005

LIENHARDT C et al: New drugs and new regimens for the treatment of tuberculosis: Review of the drug development pipeline and implications for national programmes. Curr Opin Pulmon Med 16:186, 2010

LÖNNROTH K et al: Tuberculosis control and elimination 2010–50: Cure, care, and social development. Lancet 375:1814, 2010

MENZIES D et al: Effect of duration and intermittency of rifampin on tuberculosis treatment outcomes: A systematic review and meta-analysis. PLoS Medicine 6:e1000146, 2009

PAI M et al: Evidence-based tuberculosis diagnosis. PLoS Medicine 5:e156, 2008

RAVIGLIONE MC (ed): *Tuberculosis, The Essentials. Lung Biology in Health and Disease*, vol 237, 4th ed. New York, Informa Health Care USA, 2009

TUBERCULOSIS COALITION FOR TECHNICAL ASSISTANCE: International standards for tuberculosis care (ISTC), 2d ed. The Hague, 2009

WORLD HEALTH ORGANIZATION: Treatment of tuberculosis: Guidelines, 4th ed. Geneva, WHO, 2009 (*www.who.int/tb/publications/2009/who_htm_tb_2009_420_beforeprint.pdf*)

———: Guidelines for the programmatic management of drug-resistant tuberculosis. Emergency update 2008. Geneva, WHO, 2008

WRIGHT A: Epidemiology of anti-tuberculosis drug resistance 2002–2007: An updated analysis of the Global Project on Anti-Tuberculosis Drug Resistance Surveillance. Lancet 373:1861, 2009

CHAPTER **166**

Leprosy

Robert H. Gelber

Leprosy, first described in ancient Indian texts from the sixth century B.C., is a nonfatal, chronic infectious disease caused by *Mycobacterium leprae,* the clinical manifestations of which are largely confined to the skin, peripheral nervous system, upper respiratory tract, eyes, and testes. The unique tropism of *M. leprae* for peripheral nerves (from large nerve trunks to microscopic dermal nerves) and certain immunologically mediated reactional states are the major causes of morbidity in leprosy. The propensity of the disease, when untreated, to result in characteristic deformities and the recognition in most cultures that the disease is communicable from person to person have resulted historically in a profound social stigma. Today, with early diagnosis and the institution of appropriate and effective antimicrobial therapy, patients can lead productive lives in the community, and deformities and other visible manifestations can largely be prevented.

■ ETIOLOGY

M. leprae is an obligate intracellular bacillus (0.3–1 μm wide and 1–8 μm long) that is confined to humans, armadillos in certain locales, and sphagnum moss. The organism is acid-fast, indistinguishable microscopically from other mycobacteria, and ideally detected in tissue sections by a modified Fite stain. Strain variability has been documented in this organism. *M. leprae* produces no known toxins and is well adapted to penetrate and reside within macrophages, yet it may survive outside the body for months. In untreated patients, only ~1% of *M. leprae* organisms are viable. The morphologic index (MI), a measure of the number of acid-fast bacilli (AFB) in skin scrapings that stain uniformly bright, correlates with viability. The bacteriologic index (BI), a logarithmic-scaled measure of the density of *M. leprae* in the dermis, may be as high as 4–6+ in untreated patients and falls by 1 unit per year during effective antimicrobial therapy; the rate of decrease is independent of the relative potency of therapy. A rising MI or BI suggests relapse and perhaps—if the patient is being treated—drug resistance. Drug resistance can be confirmed or excluded in the mouse model of leprosy, and resistance to dapsone and rifampin can be documented by the recognition of mutant genes. However, the availability of these technologies is extremely limited.

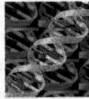

As a result of reductive evolution, almost half of the *M. leprae* genome contains nonfunctional genes; only 1605 genes encode for proteins, and 1439 genes are shared with *Mycobacterium tuberculosis.* In contrast, *M. tuberculosis* uses 91% of its genome to encode for 4000 proteins. Among the lost genes in *M. leprae* are those for catabolic and respiratory pathways; transport systems; purine, methionine, and glutamine synthesis; and nitrogen regulation. The genome of *M. leprae*

provides a metabolic rationale for its obligate intracellular existence and reliance on host biochemical support, a template for targets of drug development, and ultimately a pathway to cultivation. The finding of strain variability among *M. leprae* isolates has provided a powerful tool with which to address anew the organism's epidemiology and pathobiology and to determine whether relapse represents reactivation or reinfection. The bacterium's complex cell wall contains large amounts of an *M. leprae*–specific phenolic glycolipid (PGL-1), which is detected in serologic tests. The unique trisaccharide of *M. leprae* binds to the basal lamina of Schwann cells; this interaction is probably relevant to the fact that *M. leprae* is the only bacterium to invade peripheral nerves.

Although it was the first bacterium to be etiologically associated with human disease, *M. leprae* remains one of the few bacterial species that still has not been cultivated on artificial medium or tissue culture. The multiplication of *M. leprae* in mouse footpads (albeit limited, with a doubling time of ~2 weeks) has provided a means to evaluate antimicrobial agents, monitor clinical trials, and screen vaccines. *M. leprae* grows best in cooler tissues (the skin, peripheral nerves, anterior chamber of the eye, upper respiratory tract, and testes), sparing warmer areas of the skin (the axilla, groin, scalp, and midline of the back).

EPIDEMIOLOGY

Demographics

Leprosy is almost exclusively a disease of the developing world, affecting areas of Asia, Africa, Latin America, and the Pacific (Fig. 166-1). While Africa has the highest disease prevalence, Asia has the most cases. More than 80% of the world's cases occur in a few countries: India, China, Myanmar, Indonesia, Brazil, Nigeria, Madagascar, and Nepal. Within endemic locales, the distribution of leprosy is quite uneven, with areas of high prevalence bordering on areas with little or no disease. In Brazil the majority of cases occur in the Amazon basin and two western states, while in Mexico leprosy is mostly confined to the Pacific coast. Except as imported cases, leprosy is largely absent from the United States, Canada, and northwestern Europe. In the United States, ~4000 persons have leprosy and 100–200 new cases are reported annually, most of them in California, Texas, New York, and Hawaii among immigrants from Mexico, Southeast Asia, the Philippines, and the Caribbean. The comparative genomics of single-nucleotide polymorphisms support the likelihood that four distinct strains exist, having originated in East Africa or Central Asia. A mutation spread to Europe and subsequently underwent two separate mutations that were then followed by spread to West Africa and the Americas.

The global prevalence of leprosy is difficult to assess, given that many of the locales with high prevalence lack a significant medical or public health infrastructure. Estimates range from 0.6 to 8 million affected individuals. The lower estimate includes only persons who have not completed chemotherapy, excluding those who may be physically or psychologically damaged from leprosy and who may yet relapse or develop immune-mediated reactions. The higher figure includes patients whose infections probably are already cured and many who have no leprosy-related deformity or disability. Although the figures on the worldwide prevalence of leprosy are debatable, it is not falling; there are an estimated 600,000 new cases annually, 60% of them in India.

Leprosy is associated with poverty and rural residence. It appears not to be associated with AIDS, perhaps because of leprosy's long incubation period. Most individuals appear to be naturally immune to leprosy and do not develop disease manifestations after exposure. The time of peak onset is in the second and third decades of life. The most severe lepromatous form of leprosy is twice as common among men as among women and is rarely encountered in children. The frequency of the polar forms of leprosy in different countries varies widely and may in part be genetically determined; certain human leukocyte antigen (HLA) associations are known for both polar forms of leprosy (see below). Furthermore, variations in immunoregulatory genes are associated with an increased susceptibility to leprosy, particularly the multibacillary form. In India and Africa, 90% of cases are tuberculoid; in Southeast Asia, 50% are tuberculoid and 50% lepromatous; and in Mexico, 90% are lepromatous. (For definitions of disease types, see Table 166-1 and "Clinical, Histologic, and Immunologic Spectrum," below.)

Transmission

The route of transmission of leprosy remains uncertain, and transmission routes may in fact be multiple. Nasal droplet infection,

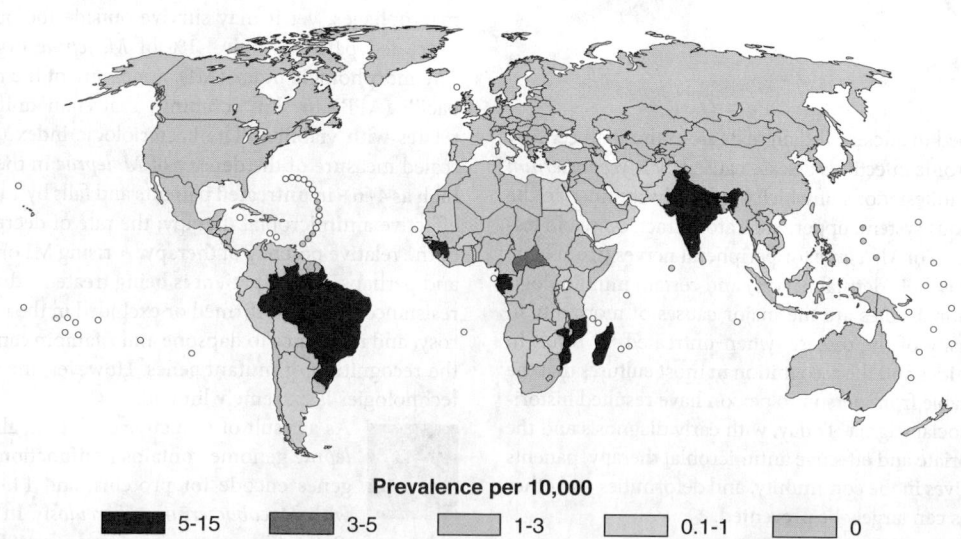

Prevalence per 10,000

| ■ 5-15 | ■ 3-5 | ■ 1-3 | □ 0.1-1 | □ 0 |

Figure 166-1 Estimated prevalence of leprosy at the turn of the millennium. Because data on leprosy prevalence in many endemic countries are unreliable, global prevalence is difficult to assess with any great degree of accuracy; however, it is not falling (see text). (*Courtesy of Patrick J. Brennan, PhD, with permission.*)

TABLE 166-1 Clinical, Bacteriologic, Pathologic, and Immunologic Spectrum of Leprosy

Feature	Tuberculoid (TT, BT) Leprosy	Borderline (BB, BL) Leprosy	Lepromatous (LL) Leprosy
Skin lesions	One or a few sharply defined annular asymmetric macules or plaques with a tendency toward central clearing, elevated borders	Intermediate between BT- and LL-type lesions; ill-defined plaques with an occasional sharp margin; few or many in number	Symmetric, poorly marginated, multiple infiltrated nodules and plaques or diffuse infiltration; xanthoma-like or dermatofibroma papules; leonine facies and eyebrow alopecia
Nerve lesions	Skin lesions anesthetic early; nerve near lesions sometimes enlarged; nerve abscesses most common in BT	Hypesthetic or anesthetic skin lesions; nerve trunk palsies, at times symmetric	Hypesthesia a late sign; nerve palsies variable; acral, distal, symmetric anesthesia common
Acid-fast bacilli (BI^a)	0–1+	3–5+	4–6+
Lymphocytes	2+	1+	0–1+
Macrophage differentiation	Epithelioid	Epithelioid in BB; usually undifferentiated, but may have foamy changes in BL	Foamy change the rule; may be undifferentiated in early lesions
Langhans giant cells	1–3+	—	—
Lepromin skin test	+++	—	—
Lymphocyte transformation test	Generally positive	1–10%	1–2%
CD4+/CD8+ T cell ratio in lesions	1.2	BB (NT); BL: 0.48	0.50
M. leprae PGL-1 antibodies	60%	85%	95%

^{a}See text.

Abbreviations: BB, mid-borderline; BL, borderline lepromatous; BT, borderline tuberculoid; TT, polar tuberculoid; LL, polar lepromatous; BI, bacteriologic index; NT, not tested; PGL-1, phenolic glycolipid 1.

contact with infected soil, and even insect vectors have been considered the prime candidates. Aerosolized *M. leprae* can cause infection in immunosuppressed mice, and a sneeze from an untreated lepromatous patient may contain >10^{10} AFB. Furthermore, both IgA antibody to *M. leprae* and genes of *M. leprae*—demonstrable by polymerase chain reaction (PCR)—have been found in the nose of individuals without signs of leprosy from endemic areas and in 19% of occupational contacts of lepromatous patients. Several lines of evidence implicate soil transmission. (1) In endemic countries such as India, leprosy is primarily a rural and not an urban disease. (2) *M. leprae* products reside in soil in endemic locales. (3) Direct dermal inoculation (e.g., during tattooing) may transmit *M. leprae*, and common sites of leprosy in children are the buttocks and thighs, suggesting that microinoculation of infected soil may transmit the disease. Evidence for insect vectors of leprosy includes the demonstration that bedbugs and mosquitoes in the vicinity of leprosaria regularly harbor *M. leprae* and that experimentally infected mosquitoes can transmit infection to mice. Skin-to-skin contact is generally not considered an important route of transmission.

In endemic countries, ~50% of leprosy patients have a history of intimate contact with an infected person (often a household member), while, for unknown reasons, leprosy patients in nonendemic locales can identify such contact only 10% of the time. Moreover, household contact with an infected lepromatous case carries an eventual risk of disease acquisition of ~10% in endemic areas as opposed to only 1% in nonendemic locales. Contact with a tuberculoid case carries a very low risk. Physicians and nurses caring for leprosy patients and the co-workers of these patients are not at risk for leprosy.

Although multilocus variable-number short-nucleotide tandem-repeat (VNTR) analyses have generally demonstrated considerable variability among isolates, highly similar and even identical VNTR results have been obtained with isolates from a limited number of families with multiple cases. Moreover, VNTR results have been similar for isolates within certain geographic locales and divergent for isolates within others. These findings suggest that genomic analyses may prove useful in the future for defining *M. leprae* transmission patterns.

M. leprae causes disease primarily in humans. However, in Texas and Louisiana, 15% of nine-banded armadillos are infected, and armadillo contact occasionally results in human disease. Armadillos develop disseminated infection after IV inoculation of live *M. leprae*.

■ CLINICAL, HISTOLOGIC, AND IMMUNOLOGIC SPECTRUM

The incubation period prior to manifestation of clinical disease can vary between 2 and 40 years, although it is generally 5–7 years in duration. This long incubation period is probably, at least in part, a consequence of the extremely long doubling time for *M. leprae* (14 days in mice versus in vitro doubling times of 1 day and 20 min for *M. tuberculosis* and *Escherichia coli*, respectively). Leprosy presents as a spectrum of clinical manifestations that have bacteriologic, pathologic, and immunologic counterparts. The spectrum from polar tuberculoid (TT) to borderline tuberculoid (BT) to mid-borderline (BB, which is rarely encountered) to borderline lepromatous (BL) to polar lepromatous (LL) disease is associated with an evolution from asymmetric localized macules and plaques to nodular and indurated symmetric generalized skin manifestations, an increasing bacterial load, and loss of *M. leprae*–specific cellular immunity (Table 166-1). Distinguishing dermatopathologic characteristics include the number of lymphocytes, giant cells, and AFB as well as the nature of epithelioid cell differentiation. Where a patient presents on the clinical spectrum largely determines prognosis, complications, reactional states, and the intensity of antimicrobial therapy required.

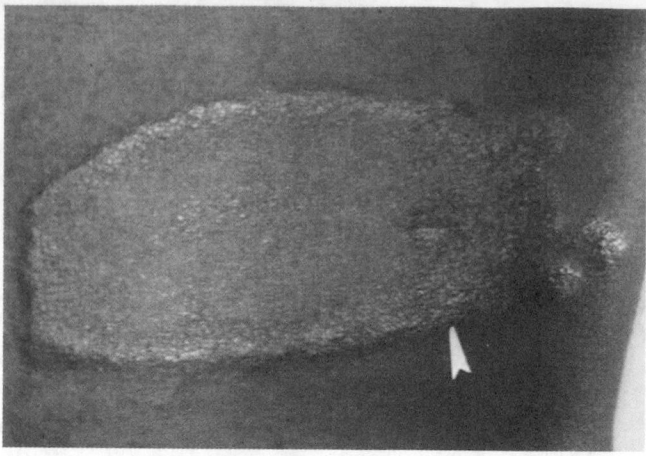

Figure 166-2 Tuberculoid (TT) leprosy: a well-defined, hypopigmented, anesthetic macule with anhidrosis and a raised granular margin *(arrowhead)*.

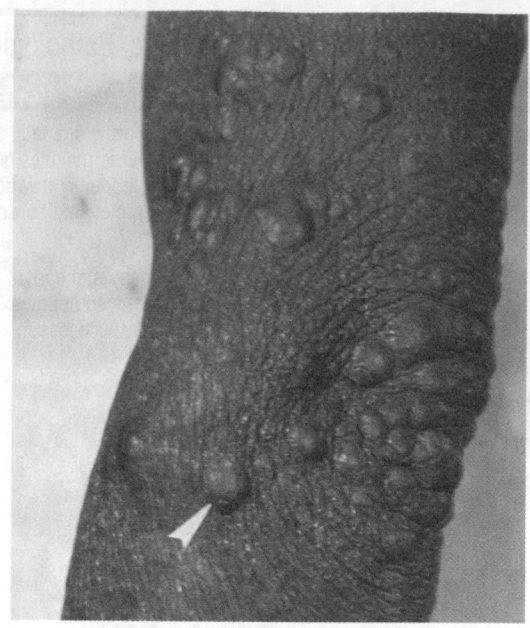

Figure 166-3 Lepromatous (LL) leprosy: advanced nodular lesions.

Tuberculoid leprosy

At the less severe end of the spectrum is tuberculoid leprosy, which encompasses TT and BT disease. In general, these forms of leprosy result in symptoms confined to the skin and peripheral nerves. The skin lesions of tuberculoid leprosy consist of one or a few hypopigmented macules or plaques (Fig. 166-2) that are sharply demarcated and hypesthetic, often have erythematous or raised borders, and are devoid of the normal skin organs (sweat glands and hair follicles) and thus are dry, scaly, and anhidrotic. AFB are generally absent or few in number. Tuberculoid leprosy patients may have asymmetric enlargement of one or a few peripheral nerves. Indeed, leprosy and certain rare hereditary neuropathies are the only human diseases associated with peripheral-nerve enlargement. Although any peripheral nerve may be enlarged (including small digital and supraclavicular nerves), those most commonly affected are the ulnar, posterior auricular, peroneal, and posterior tibial nerves, with associated hypesthesia and myopathy. TT leprosy is the most common form of the disease encountered in India and Africa but is virtually absent in Southeast Asia, where BT leprosy is frequent.

In tuberculoid leprosy, T cells breach the perineurium, and destruction of Schwann cells and axons may be evident, resulting in fibrosis of the epineurium, replacement of the endoneurium with epithelial granulomas, and occasionally caseous necrosis. Such invasion and destruction of nerves in the dermis by T cells are pathognomonic for leprosy.

Circulating lymphocytes from patients with tuberculoid leprosy readily recognize *M. leprae* and its constituent proteins, patients have positive lepromin skin tests (see "Diagnosis," below), and—owing to a type 1 cytokine pattern in tuberculoid tissues—strong T cell and macrophage activation results in a localized infection. In tuberculoid leprosy tissue, there is a 2:1 predominance of helper CD4+ over CD8+ T lymphocytes. Tuberculoid tissues are rich in the mRNAs of the proinflammatory T_H1 family of cytokines: interleukin (IL) 2, interferon γ (IFN-γ), and IL-12; in contrast, IL-4, IL-5, and IL-10 mRNAs are scarce.

Lepromatous leprosy

Lepromatous leprosy patients present with symmetrically distributed skin nodules (Fig. 166-3), raised plaques, or diffuse dermal infiltration, which, when on the face, results in leonine facies. Late manifestations include loss of eyebrows (initially the lateral margins only) and eyelashes, pendulous earlobes, and dry scaling

skin, particularly on the feet. In LL leprosy, bacilli are numerous in the skin (as many as 10^9/g), where they are often found in large clumps (*globi*), and in peripheral nerves, where they initially invade Schwann cells, resulting in foamy degenerative myelination and axonal degeneration and later in Wallerian degeneration. In addition, bacilli are plentiful in circulating blood and in all organ systems except the lungs and the central nervous system. Nevertheless, patients are afebrile, and there is no evidence of major organ system dysfunction. Found almost exclusively in western Mexico and the Caribbean is a form of lepromatous leprosy without visible skin lesions but with diffuse dermal infiltration and a demonstrably thickened dermis, termed *diffuse lepromatosis*. In lepromatous leprosy, nerve enlargement and damage tend to be symmetric, result from actual bacillary invasion, and are more insidious but ultimately more extensive than in tuberculoid leprosy. Patients with LL leprosy have acral, distal, symmetric peripheral neuropathy and a tendency toward symmetric nerve-trunk enlargement. They may also have signs and symptoms related to involvement of the upper respiratory tract, the anterior chamber of the eye, and the testes.

In untreated LL patients, lymphocytes regularly fail to recognize either *M. leprae* or its protein constituents, and lepromin skin tests are negative (see "Diagnosis," below). This loss of protective cellular immunity appears to be antigen-specific, as patients are not unusually susceptible to opportunistic infections, cancer, or AIDS and maintain delayed-type hypersensitivity to *Candida*, *Trichophyton*, mumps, tetanus toxoid, and even purified protein derivative of tuberculin. At times, *M. leprae*–specific anergy is reversible with effective chemotherapy. In LL tissues, there is a 2:1 ratio of CD8+ to CD4+ T lymphocytes. LL patients have a predominant T_H2 response and hyperglobulinemia, and LL tissues demonstrate a T_H2 cytokine profile, being rich in mRNAs for IL-4, IL-5, and IL-10 and poor in those for IL-2, IFN-γ, and IL-12. It appears that cytokines mediate a protective tissue response in leprosy, as injection of IFN-γ or IL-2 into lepromatous lesions causes a loss of AFB and histopathologic conversion toward a tuberculoid pattern. Macrophages of lepromatous leprosy patients appear to be functionally intact; circulating monocytes exhibit normal microbicidal function and responsiveness to IFN-γ.

Reactional states

Lepra reactions comprise several common immunologically mediated inflammatory states that cause considerable morbidity. Some of these reactions precede diagnosis and the institution of effective antimicrobial therapy; indeed, these reactions may precipitate presentation for medical attention and diagnosis. Other reactions occur after the initiation of appropriate chemotherapy and may cause patients to perceive that their leprosy is worsening and to lose confidence in conventional therapy. Only by warning patients of the potential for these reactions and describing their manifestations can physicians treating leprosy patients ensure continued credibility.

Type 1 lepra reactions (downgrading and reversal reactions) Type 1 lepra reactions occur in almost half of patients with borderline forms of leprosy but not in patients with pure lepromatous disease. Manifestations include classic signs of inflammation within previously involved macules, papules, and plaques and, on occasion, the appearance of new skin lesions, neuritis, and (less commonly) fever—generally low-grade. The nerve trunk most commonly involved in this process is the ulnar nerve at the elbow, which may be painful and exquisitely tender. If patients with affected nerves are not treated promptly with glucocorticoids (see below), irreversible nerve damage may result in as little as 24 h. The most dramatic manifestation is footdrop, which occurs when the peroneal nerve is involved.

When type 1 lepra reactions precede the initiation of appropriate antimicrobial therapy, they are termed *downgrading reactions*, and the case becomes histologically more lepromatous; when they occur after the initiation of therapy, they are termed *reversal reactions*, and the case becomes more tuberculoid. Reversal reactions often occur in the first months or years after the initiation of therapy but may also develop several years thereafter.

Edema is the most characteristic microscopic feature of type 1 lepra lesions, whose diagnosis is primarily clinical. Reversal reactions are typified by a T_H1 cytokine profile, with an influx of CD4+ T helper cells and increased levels of IFN-γ and IL-2. In addition, type 1 reactions are associated with large numbers of T cells bearing γ/δ receptors—a unique feature of leprosy.

Type 2 lepra reactions: erythema nodosum leprosum Erythema nodosum leprosum (ENL) (Fig. 166-4) occurs exclusively in patients near the lepromatous end of the leprosy spectrum (BL-LL), affecting nearly 50% of this group. Although ENL may precede leprosy diagnosis and initiation of therapy (sometimes, in fact, prompting the diagnosis), in 90% of cases it follows the institution of chemotherapy, generally within 2 years. The most common features of ENL are crops of painful erythematous papules that resolve spontaneously in a few days to a week but may recur; malaise; and fever that can be profound. However, patients may also experience symptoms of neuritis, lymphadenitis, uveitis, orchitis, and glomerulonephritis and may develop anemia, leukocytosis, and abnormal liver function tests (particularly increased aminotransferase levels). Individual patients may have either a single bout of ENL or chronic recurrent manifestations. Bouts may be either mild or severe and generalized; in rare instances, ENL results in death. Skin biopsy of ENL papules reveals vasculitis or panniculitis, sometimes with many lymphocytes but characteristically with polymorphonuclear leukocytes as well.

Elevated levels of circulating tumor necrosis factor (TNF) have been demonstrated in ENL; thus, TNF may play a central role in the pathobiology of this syndrome. ENL is thought to be a consequence of immune complex deposition, given its T_H2 cytokine profile and its high levels of IL-6 and IL-8. However, in ENL tissue, the presence of HLA-DR framework antigen of epidermal cells—considered a marker for a delayed-type hypersensitivity response—and evidence of higher levels of IL-2 and IFN-γ than are usually seen in polar lepromatous disease suggest an alternative mechanism.

Lucio's phenomenon Lucio's phenomenon is an unusual reaction seen exclusively in patients from the Caribbean and Mexico who have the diffuse lepromatosis form of lepromatous leprosy, most often those who are untreated. Patients with this reaction develop recurrent crops of large, sharply marginated, ulcerative lesions—particularly on the lower extremities—that may be generalized and, when so, are frequently fatal as a result of secondary infection and consequent septic bacteremia. Histologically, the lesions are characterized by ischemic necrosis of the epidermis and superficial dermis, heavy parasitism of endothelial cells with AFB, and endothelial proliferation and thrombus formation in the larger vessels of the deeper dermis. Like ENL, the Lucio phenomenon is probably mediated by immune complexes.

Complications

The extremities Complications of the extremities in leprosy patients are primarily a consequence of neuropathy leading to insensitivity and myopathy. Insensitivity affects fine touch, pain, and heat receptors but generally spares position and vibration appreciation. The most commonly affected nerve trunk is the ulnar nerve at the elbow, whose involvement results in clawing of the fourth and fifth fingers, loss of dorsal interosseous musculature in the affected hand, and loss of sensation in these distributions. Median nerve involvement in leprosy impairs thumb opposition and grasp; radial nerve dysfunction, although rare in leprosy, leads to wristdrop. Tendon transfers can restore hand function but should not be performed until 6 months after the initiation of antimicrobial therapy and the conclusion of episodes of acute neuritis.

Plantar ulceration, particularly at the metatarsal heads, is probably the most frequent complication of leprous neuropathy. Therapy requires careful debridement; administration of appropriate antibiotics; avoidance of weight-bearing until ulcerations are healed, with slowly progressive ambulation thereafter; and wearing of special shoes to prevent recurrence.

Footdrop as a result of peroneal nerve palsy should be treated with a simple nonmetallic brace within the shoe or with surgical correction attained by tendon transfers. Although uncommon, Charcot's joints, particularly of the foot and ankle, may result from leprosy.

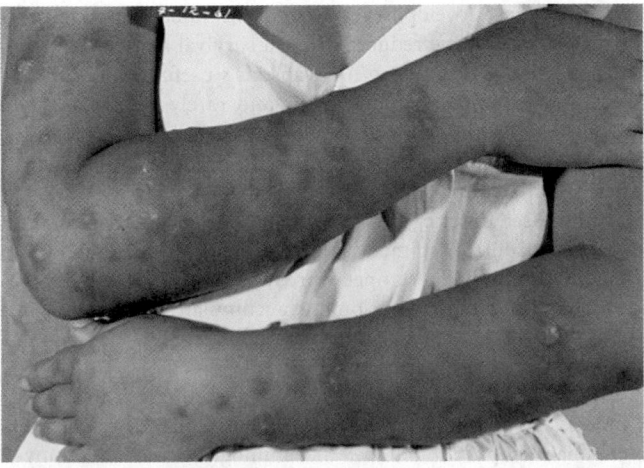

Figure 166-4 Moderately severe skin lesions of erythema nodosum leprosum (ENL), some with pustulation and ulceration.

The loss of distal digits in leprosy is a consequence of insensitivity, trauma, secondary infection, and—in lepromatous patients—a poorly understood and sometimes profound osteolytic process. Conscientious protection of the extremities during cooking and work and the early institution of therapy have substantially reduced the frequency and severity of distal digit loss in recent times.

The nose In lepromatous leprosy, bacillary invasion of the nasal mucosa can result in chronic nasal congestion and epistaxis. Saline nose drops may relieve these symptoms. Long-untreated LL leprosy may further result in destruction of the nasal cartilage, with consequent saddle-nose deformity or anosmia (more common in the preantibiotic era than at present). Nasal reconstructive procedures can ameliorate significant cosmetic defects.

The eye Owing to cranial nerve palsies, lagophthalmos and corneal insensitivity may complicate leprosy, resulting in trauma, secondary infection, and (without treatment) corneal ulcerations and opacities. For patients with these conditions, eyedrops during the day and ointments at night provide some protection from such consequences. Furthermore, in LL leprosy, the anterior chamber of the eye is invaded by bacilli, and ENL may result in uveitis, with consequent cataracts and glaucoma. Thus leprosy is a major cause of blindness in the developing world. Slit-lamp evaluation of LL patients often reveals "corneal beading," representing globi of *M. leprae*.

The testes *M. leprae* invades the testes, while ENL may cause orchitis. Thus males with lepromatous leprosy often manifest mild to severe testicular dysfunction, with an elevation of luteinizing and follicle-stimulating hormones, decreased testosterone, and aspermia or hypospermia in 85% of LL patients but in only 25% of BL patients. LL patients may become impotent and infertile. Impotence is sometimes responsive to testosterone replacement.

Amyloidosis Secondary amyloidosis is a complication of LL leprosy and ENL that is encountered infrequently in the antibiotic era. This complication may result in abnormalities of hepatic and particularly renal function.

Nerve abscesses Patients with various forms of leprosy, but particularly those with the BT form, may develop abscesses of nerves (most commonly the ulnar) with an adjacent cellulitic appearance of the skin. In such conditions, the affected nerve is swollen and exquisitely tender. Although glucocorticoids may reduce signs of inflammation, rapid surgical decompression is necessary to prevent irreversible sequelae.

■ DIAGNOSIS

Leprosy most commonly presents with both characteristic skin lesions and skin histopathology. Thus the disease should be suspected when a patient from an endemic area has suggestive skin lesions or peripheral neuropathy. The diagnosis should be confirmed by histopathology. In tuberculoid leprosy, lesional areas—preferably the advancing edge—must be biopsied because normal-appearing skin does not have pathologic features. In lepromatous leprosy, nodules, plaques, and indurated areas are optimal biopsy sites, but biopsies of normal-appearing skin are also generally diagnostic. Lepromatous leprosy is associated with diffuse hyperglobulinemia, which may result in false-positive serologic tests (e.g., Venereal Disease Research Laboratory, rheumatoid arthritis, and antinuclear antibody tests) and therefore may cause diagnostic confusion. On occasion, tuberculoid lesions may not (1) appear typical, (2) be hypesthetic, and (3) contain granulomas but only nonspecific lymphocytic infiltrates. In such instances, two of these three characteristics are considered sufficient for a diagnosis. It is preferable to overdiagnose leprosy rather than to allow a patient to remain untreated.

IgM antibodies to PGL-1 are found in 95% of patients with untreated lepromatous leprosy; the titer decreases with effective therapy. However, in tuberculoid leprosy—the form of disease most often associated with diagnostic uncertainty owing to the absence or paucity of AFB—patients have significant antibodies to PGL-1 only 60% of the time; moreover, in endemic locales, exposed individuals without clinical leprosy may harbor antibodies to PGL-1. Thus PGL-1 serology is of little diagnostic utility in tuberculoid leprosy. Heat-killed *M. leprae* (lepromin) has been used as a skin test reagent. It generally elicits a reaction in tuberculoid leprosy patients, may do so in individuals without leprosy, and gives negative results in lepromatous leprosy patients; consequently, it is likewise of little diagnostic value. Unfortunately, PCR of the skin for *M. leprae*, although positive in LL and BL leprosy, yields negative results in 50% of tuberculoid leprosy cases, again offering little diagnostic assistance.

Included in the differential diagnosis of lesions that resemble leprosy are sarcoidosis, leishmaniasis, lupus vulgaris, dermatofibroma, histiocytoma, lymphoma, syphilis, yaws, granuloma annulare, and various other disorders causing hypopigmentation (notably pityriasis alba, tinea, and vitiligo). Sarcoidosis may result in perineural inflammation, but actual granuloma formation within dermal nerves is pathognomonic for leprosy. In lepromatous leprosy, sputum specimens may be loaded with AFB—a finding that can be inappropriately interpreted as representing pulmonary tuberculosis.

TREATMENT   Leprosy

ANTIMICROBIAL THERAPY

Active Agents Established agents used to treat leprosy include dapsone (50–100 mg/d), clofazimine (50–100 mg/d, 100 mg three times weekly, or 300 mg monthly), and rifampin (600 mg daily or monthly; see "Choice of Regimens," below). Of these drugs, only rifampin is bactericidal. The sulfones (folate antagonists), the foremost of which is dapsone, were the first antimicrobial agents found to be effective for the treatment of leprosy and are still the mainstay of therapy. With sulfone treatment, skin lesions resolve and numbers of viable bacilli in the skin are reduced. Although primarily bacteriostatic, dapsone monotherapy results in only a 2.5% resistance-related relapse rate; after ≥18 years of therapy and subsequent discontinuation, only another 10% of patients relapse, developing new, usually asymptomatic, shiny, "histoid" nodules. Dapsone is generally safe and inexpensive. Individuals with glucose-6-phosphate dehydrogenase deficiency who are treated with dapsone may develop severe hemolysis; those without this deficiency also have reduced red cell survival and a hemoglobin decrease averaging 1 g/dL. Dapsone's usefulness is limited occasionally by allergic dermatitis and rarely by the sulfone syndrome (including high fever, anemia, exfoliative dermatitis, and a mononucleosis-type blood picture). It must be remembered that rifampin induces microsomal enzymes, necessitating increased doses of medications such as glucocorticoids and oral birth control regimens. Clofazimine is often cosmetically unacceptable to light-skinned leprosy patients because it causes a red-black skin discoloration that accumulates, particularly in lesional areas, and makes the patient's diagnosis obvious to members of the community.

Other antimicrobial agents active against *M. leprae* in animal models and at the usual daily doses used in clinical trials include ethionamide/prothionamide; the aminoglycosides streptomycin, kanamycin, and amikacin (but not gentamicin or tobramycin); minocycline; clarithromycin; and several fluoroquinolones, particularly ofloxacin. Next to rifampin, minocycline, clarithromycin, and ofloxacin appear to be most bactericidal for *M. leprae*, but these drugs have not been used extensively in leprosy control programs. Most recently, rifapentine and moxifloxacin have been found to be especially potent against *M. leprae* in mice. In a clinical trial in lepromatous leprosy, moxifloxacin was profoundly bactericidal, matched in potency only by rifampin.

Choice of Regimens   Antimicrobial therapy for leprosy must be individualized, depending on the clinical/pathologic form of the disease encountered. Tuberculoid leprosy, which is associated with a low bacterial burden and a protective cellular immune response, is the easiest form to treat and can be cured reliably with a finite course of chemotherapy. In contrast, lepromatous leprosy may have a higher bacillary load than any other human bacterial disease, and the absence of a salutary T cell repertoire requires prolonged or even lifelong chemotherapy. Hence, careful classification of disease prior to therapy is important.

In developed countries, clinical experience with leprosy classification is limited; fortunately, however, the resources needed for skin biopsy are highly accessible and pathologic interpretation is readily available. In developing countries, clinical expertise is greater but is now waning substantially as the care of leprosy patients is integrated into general health services. In addition, access to dermatopathology services is often limited. In such instances, skin smears may prove useful, but in many locales access to the resources needed for their preparation and interpretation may also be unavailable. Use of skin smears is no longer encouraged by the World Health Organization (WHO) and is often replaced by mere counting of lesions, which, together with the lack of histopathology, may negatively affect decisions about chemotherapy, increase the potential for reactions, and worsen the ultimate prognosis. A reasoned approach to the treatment of leprosy is confounded by these and several other issues:

1. Even without therapy, TT leprosy may heal spontaneously, and prolonged dapsone monotherapy (even for LL leprosy) is generally curative in 80% of cases.
2. In tuberculoid disease, it is common for no bacilli to be found in the skin prior to therapy, and thus there is no objective measure of therapeutic success. Furthermore, despite adequate treatment, TT and particularly BT lesions often resolve little or incompletely, while relapse and late type 1 lepra reactions can be difficult to distinguish.
3. LL leprosy patients commonly harbor viable persistent *M. leprae* organisms after prolonged intensive therapy; the propensity of these organisms to initiate clinical relapse is unclear. Because relapse in LL patients after discontinuation of rifampin-containing regimens usually begins only after

7–10 years, follow-up over the very long term is necessary to assess ultimate clinical outcomes.
4. Even though primary dapsone resistance is exceedingly rare and multidrug therapy is generally recommended (at least for lepromatous leprosy), there is a paucity of information from experimental animals and clinical trials on the optimal combination of antimicrobial agents, dosing schedule, or duration of therapy.

In 1982, the WHO made recommendations for "the chemotherapy of leprosy for control programs." These recommendations came on the heels of the demonstration of the relative success of long-term dapsone monotherapy and in the context of concerns about dapsone resistance. Other complicating considerations included the limited resources available for leprosy care in the very areas where it is most prevalent and the frustration and discouragement of patients and program managers with the previous requirement for lifelong therapy for many leprosy patients. Thus, for the first time, the WHO delineated a finite duration of therapy for all forms of leprosy and—given the prohibitive cost of daily rifampin treatment in developing countries—encouraged the monthly administration of this agent as part of a multidrug regimen. Over the ensuing years, the WHO recommendations have been broadly implemented, and the duration of therapy required, particularly for lepromatous leprosy, has been progressively shortened. For treatment purposes, the WHO classifies patients as *paucibacillary* or *multibacillary*. Previously, patients without demonstrable AFB in the dermis were classified as paucibacillary and those with AFB as multibacillary. Currently, in light of the perceived unreliability of skin smears in the field, patients are classified as multibacillary if they have six or more skin lesions and as paucibacillary if they have fewer. (Unfortunately, this classification method has been found wanting, as some patients near the lepromatous pole have only one or a few skin lesions.) The WHO recommends that paucibacillary adults be treated with 100 mg of dapsone daily and 600 mg of rifampin monthly (supervised) for 6 months (Table 166-2). For patients with single-lesion paucibacillary leprosy, the WHO recommends as an alternative a single dose of rifampin (600 mg), ofloxacin (400 mg), and minocycline (100 mg). Multibacillary adults should be treated with 100 mg of dapsone plus 50 mg of clofazimine daily (unsupervised) and with 600 mg of rifampin plus 300 mg of clofazimine monthly (supervised). Originally, the WHO recommended that lepromatous patients be treated for 2 years or until smears became negative (generally in ~5 years); subsequently, the acceptable course was reduced to 1 year—a change that remains especially controversial in the absence of supporting clinical trials.

TABLE 166-2   Antimicrobial Regimens Recommended for the Treatment of Leprosy in Adults

Form of Leprosy	More Intensive Regimen	WHO Recommended Regimen (1982)
Tuberculoid (paucibacillary)	Dapsone (100 mg/d) for 5 years	Dapsone (100 mg/d, unsupervised) *plus* rifampin (600 mg/month, supervised) for 6 months
Lepromatous (multibacillary)	Rifampin (600 mg/d) for 3 years *plus* dapsone (100 mg/d) indefinitely	Dapsone (100 mg/d) *plus* clofazimine (50 mg/d), unsupervised; *and* rifampin (600 mg) *plus* clofazimine (300 mg) monthly (supervised) for 1–2 years

Note: See text for discussion and comparison of WHO recommendations and more intensive approach as well as alternative WHO regimen for single-lesion paucibacillary leprosy.

Several factors have caused many authorities to question the WHO recommendations and to favor a more intensive approach. Among these factors are—for multibacillary patients—a high (double-digit) relapse rate in three locales (reaching 20–40% in one locale, with the rate directly related to the initial bacterial burden) and—for paucibacillary patients—demonstrable lesional activity for years in fully half of patients after the completion of therapy. The more intensive approach (Table 166-2) calls for tuberculoid leprosy to be treated with dapsone (100 mg/d) for 5 years and for lepromatous leprosy to be treated with rifampin (600 mg/d) for 3 years and with dapsone (100 mg/d) throughout life.

With effective antimicrobial therapy, new skin lesions and signs and symptoms of peripheral neuropathy cease appearing. Nodules and plaques of lepromatous leprosy noticeably flatten in 1–2 months and resolve in 1 year or a few years, while tuberculoid skin lesions may disappear, improve, or remain relatively unchanged. Although the peripheral neuropathy of leprosy may improve somewhat in the first few months of therapy, rarely is it significantly alleviated by treatment.

Given the recent findings that moxifloxacin, like rifampin, is profoundly bactericidal in leprosy patients and that short-course chemotherapy for tuberculosis is possible only when two or more bactericidal agents are used, a moxifloxacin/rifampin-based regimen including either minocycline or clarithromycin appears promising; such a regimen may prove to be more reliably curative than WHO-recommended multidrug therapy for lepromatous leprosy and may allow a considerably shorter course of treatment.

THERAPY FOR REACTIONS

Type 1 Type 1 lepra reactions are best treated with glucocorticoids (e.g., prednisone, initially at doses of 40–60 mg/d). As the inflammation subsides, the glucocorticoid dose can be tapered, but steroid therapy must be continued for at least 3–6 months lest recurrence supervene. Because of the myriad toxicities of prolonged glucocorticoid therapy, the indications for its initiation are strictly limited to lesions whose intense inflammation poses a threat of ulceration; lesions at cosmetically important sites, such as the face; and cases in which neuritis is present. Mild to moderate lepra reactions that do not meet these criteria should be tolerated and glucocorticoid treatment withheld. Thalidomide is ineffective against type 1 lepra reactions. Clofazimine (200–300 mg/d) is of questionable benefit but in any event is far less efficacious than glucocorticoids.

Type 2 Treatment of ENL must be individualized. If ENL is mild (i.e., without fever or other organ involvement, with occasional crops of only a few skin papules), it may be treated with antipyretics alone. However, in cases with many skin lesions, fever, malaise, and other tissue involvement, brief courses (1–2 weeks) of glucocorticoids (initially 40–60 mg/d) are often effective. With or without therapy, individual inflamed papules last for >1 week. Successful therapy is defined by the cessation of skin lesion development and the disappearance of other systemic signs and symptoms. If, despite two courses of glucocorticoid therapy, ENL appears to be recurring and persisting, treatment with thalidomide (100–300 mg nightly) should be initiated, with the dose depending on the initial severity of the reaction. Because even a single dose of thalidomide administered early in pregnancy may result in severe birth defects, including phocomelia, the use of this drug in the United States for the treatment of fertile female patients is tightly regulated and requires informed consent, prior pregnancy testing, and

maintenance of birth control measures. Although the mechanism of thalidomide's dramatic action against ENL is not entirely clear, the drug's efficacy is probably attributable to its reduction of TNF levels and IgM synthesis and its slowing of polymorphonuclear leukocyte migration. After the reaction is controlled, lower doses of thalidomide (50–200 mg nightly) are effective in preventing relapses of ENL. Clofazimine in high doses (300 mg nightly) has some efficacy against ENL, but its use permits only a modest reduction of the glucocorticoid dose necessary for ENL control.

Lucio's Phenomenon Neither glucocorticoids nor thalidomide is effective against this syndrome. Optimal wound care and therapy for bacteremia are indicated. Ulcers tend to be chronic and heal poorly. In severe cases, exchange transfusion may prove useful.

◼ PREVENTION AND CONTROL

Vaccination at birth with bacille Calmette-Guérin (BCG) has proved variably effective in preventing leprosy: the results have ranged from total inefficacy to 80% efficacy. The addition of heat-killed *M. leprae* to BCG does not increase the effectiveness of vaccine. Because whole mycobacteria contain large amounts of lipids and carbohydrates that have proved in vitro to be immunosuppressive for lymphocytes and macrophages, *M. leprae* proteins may prove to be superior vaccines. Data from a mouse model support this possibility.

Chemoprophylaxis with dapsone may reduce the number of cases of tuberculoid leprosy but not of lepromatous leprosy and hence is not recommended, even for household contacts. Because leprosy transmission appears to require close prolonged household contact, hospitalized patients need not be isolated.

In 1992, the WHO—on the basis of that organization's treatment recommendations—launched a landmark campaign to eliminate leprosy as a public health problem by the year 2000 (goal, <1 case per 10,000 population). The campaign mobilized and energized nongovernmental organizations and national health services to treat leprosy with multiple drugs and to clean up outdated registries. In these respects, the effort has proven hugely successful, with >6 million patients completing therapy. However, the target of leprosy elimination has not yet been reached. In fact, the success of the WHO campaign in reducing the number of cases worldwide has been largely attributable to the redefinition of what constitutes a case of leprosy. Formerly calculated by disease prevalence, the case count is now limited to those not yet treated with multiple drugs. In each of the 23 countries with the largest number of leprosy cases, the annual incidence of leprosy is stable or actually rising. Furthermore, after the completion of therapy, when a patient is no longer considered to represent a "case," half of all patients continue to manifest disease activity for years; relapse rates (at least for multibacillary patients) are unacceptably high; disabilities and deformities go unchecked; and the social stigma of the disease persists.

During most of the twentieth century, nongovernmental organizations, particularly Christian missionaries, provided a medical infrastructure devoted to the care and treatment of leprosy patients—the envy of those with other medical priorities in the developing world. With the public perception that leprosy is near eradication, resources for patient care are rapidly being diverted, and the burden of patient care is being transferred to nonexistent or overloaded national health services and to health workers who lack the tools and skills needed for disease diagnosis, classification, and nuanced therapy (particularly in cases of reactional neuritis). Thus the prerequisites for a salutary outcome increasingly go unmet.

FURTHER READINGS

COLE ST et al: Massive gene decay in the leprosy bacillus. Nature 409:1007, 2001

FAJARDO TT et al: A comparative clinical trial in multibacillary leprosy with long-term relapse rates of four different multidrug regimens. Am J Trop Med Hyg 81:330, 2009

GELBER RH et al: The relapse rate in MB leprosy patients treated with 2-years of WHO-MDT is not low. Int J Lepr Other Mycobact Dis 72:493, 2004

LOCKWOOD D: Leprosy elimination—a virtual phenomenon or a reality? BMJ 324:1516, 2002

MODLIN RL, REA TH: Immunology of leprosy granulomas. Springer Semin Immunopathol 10:359, 1998

MONET M et al: On the origin of leprosy. Science 308:1040, 2005

PARDILLO FE et al: Powerful bactericidal activity of moxifloxacin in human leprosy. Antimicrob Agents Chemother 52:3113, 2008

RIDLEY DS: Histological classification and the immunological spectrum of leprosy. Bull World Health Organ 51:451, 1974

WHO EXPERT COMMITTEE ON LEPROSY: Seventh Report. WHO Tech Rep Ser No. 874. Geneva, World Health Organization, 1998

ZHANG FR et al: Genomewide association study of leprosy. N Engl J Med 361:2609, 2010

CHAPTER 167

Nontuberculous Mycobacterial Infections

Steven M. Holland

Several terms—nontuberculous mycobacteria (NTM), atypical mycobacteria, mycobacteria other than tuberculosis, and environmental mycobacteria—all refer to mycobacteria other than *Mycobacterium tuberculosis*, its close relatives (*M. bovis, M. caprae, M. africanum, M. pinnipedii, M. canetti*), and *M. leprae*. The number of identified species of NTM is growing and will continue to do so because of the use of DNA sequence typing for speciation. The number of known species currently exceeds 150. NTM are highly adaptable and can inhabit hostile environments, including industrial solvents.

■ EPIDEMIOLOGY

NTM are ubiquitous in soil and water. Specific organisms have recurring niches, such as *M. simiae* in certain aquifers, *M. fortuitum* in pedicure baths, and *M. immunogenum* in metalworking fluids. Most NTM cause disease in humans only rarely unless some aspect of host defense is impaired, as in bronchiectasis, or breached, as by inoculation (e.g., liposuction, trauma). There are no known instances of human-to-human transmission of NTM. Because infections due to NTM are rarely reported to health agencies and because their identification is sometimes problematic, reliable data on incidence and prevalence are lacking. Disseminated disease denotes significant immune dysfunction (e.g., advanced HIV infection), whereas pulmonary disease, which is much more common, is highly associated with pulmonary epithelial defects but not with systemic immunodeficiency.

In the United States, the incidence and prevalence of pulmonary infection with NTM, mostly in association with bronchiectasis (Chap. 258), have for many years been several-fold higher than the corresponding figures for tuberculosis, and rates of the former are increasing among the elderly. Among patients with cystic fibrosis, who often have bronchiectasis, rates of clinical infection with NTM range from 3% to 15%, with even higher rates among older patients. Although NTM may be recovered from the sputa of many individuals, it is critical to differentiate active disease from commensal harboring of the organisms. A scheme to help with the proper diagnosis of pulmonary infection caused by NTM has been developed by the American Thoracic Society and is widely used. The bulk of nontuberculous mycobacterial disease in North America is due to *M. kansasii*, organisms of the *M. avium* complex (MAC), and *M. abscessus*.

In Europe, Asia, and Australia, the distribution of NTM in clinical specimens is roughly similar to that in North America, with MAC species and rapidly growing organisms such as *M. abscessus* encountered frequently. *M. xenopi* and *M. malmoense* are especially prominent in northern Europe. *M. ulcerans* causes the distinct clinical entity Buruli ulcer, which occurs throughout tropical zones, especially in western Africa. *M. marinum* is a common cause of cutaneous and tendon infections in coastal regions and among individuals exposed to fish tanks or swimming pools.

The true international epidemiology of infections due to NTM is hard to determine since the isolation of these organisms often is not reported and speciation often is not performed. The increasing ease of identification and speciation of these organisms should have a major impact on the description of their international epidemiology in the next few years.

■ PATHOBIOLOGY

Because exposure to NTM is essentially universal and disease is rare, it can be assumed that normal host defenses against these organisms must be strong and that otherwise healthy individuals in whom significant disease develops are highly likely to have specific susceptibility factors that permit NTM to become established, multiply, and cause disease. At the advent of HIV infection, CD4+ T lymphocytes were recognized as key effector cells against NTM; the development of disseminated MAC disease was highly correlated with a decline in CD4+ T lymphocyte numbers. Such a decrease has also been implicated in disseminated MAC infection in patients with idiopathic CD4+ T lymphocytopenia. Potent inhibitors of tumor necrosis factor α (TNF-α), such as infliximab, adalimumab, certolizumab, and etanercept, can neutralize this critical cytokine. The occasional result is severe mycobacterial or fungal infection; these associations indicate that TNF-α is a crucial element in mycobacterial control. However, in cases without the above risk factors, much of the genetic basis of susceptibility to disseminated infection with NTM is accounted for by specific mutations in the interferon γ (IFN-γ)/interleukin 12 (IL-12) synthesis and response pathways.

Mycobacteria are typically phagocytosed by macrophages, which respond with the production of IL-12, a heterodimer composed of IL-12p35 and IL-12p40 moieties that together make up IL-12p70. IL-12 activates T lymphocytes and natural killer cells through binding to its receptor (composed of IL-12Rβ1 and IL-12Rβ2/IL-23R), with consequent phosphorylation of STAT4. IL-12 stimulation of STAT4 leads to secretion of IFN-γ, which activates neutrophils and macrophages to produce reactive oxidants, increase expression of the major histocompatibility complex and Fc receptors, and concentrate certain antibiotics intracellularly. Signaling by IFN-γ through its receptor (composed of IFN-γR1 and IFN-γR2) leads to phosphorylation of STAT1, which in turn regulates IFN-γ-responsive genes, such as those coding for IL-12 and TNF-α. TNF-α signals through its own receptor via a downstream complex containing the nuclear factor κB (NFκB) essential modulator (NEMO). Therefore, the positive feedback loop between IFN-γ and IL-12/IL-23 drives the immune response to mycobacteria and other intracellular infections. These genes are known to be the critical ones in the pathway of mycobacterial control: specific Mendelian mutations have been identified in IFN-γR1, IFN-γR2, STAT1, IL-12A, IL-12Rβ1, and NEMO (Fig. 167-1). Despite the identification of genes associated with disseminated disease, only ~50% of cases of disseminated nontuberculous mycobacterial infections that are not associated with HIV infection have a genetic diagnosis; the implication is that more mycobacterial susceptibility genes and pathways remain to be identified.

In contrast to the recognized genes and mechanisms associated with disseminated nontuberculous mycobacterial infection, the best-recognized underlying condition for pulmonary infection with NTM is bronchiectasis (Chap. 258). Most of the well-characterized forms of bronchiectasis, including cystic fibrosis, primary ciliary dyskinesia, STAT3-deficient hyper-IgE syndrome, and idiopathic bronchiectasis, have high rates of association with nontuberculous mycobacterial infection. The precise mechanism by which bronchiectasis predisposes to locally destructive but not systemic involvement is unknown.

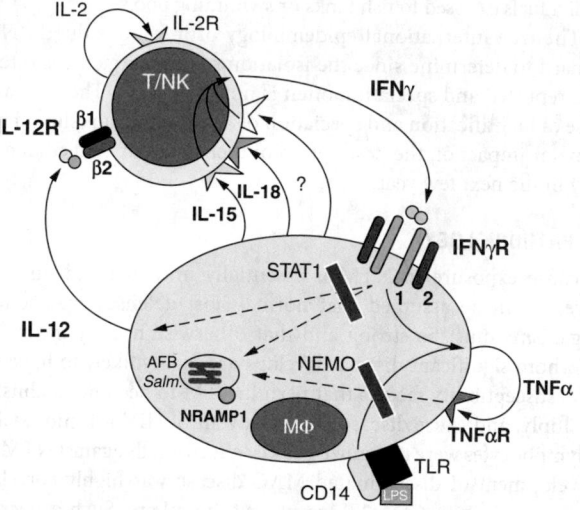

Figure 167-1 Cytokine interactions of infected macrophages (Mφ) with T and natural killer (NK) lymphocytes. Infection of macrophages by mycobacteria (AFB) leads to the release of heterodimeric interleukin 12 (IL-12). IL-12 acts on its receptor complex, with consequent STAT4 activation and production of homodimeric interferon γ (IFNγ). IFNγ acts through its receptor to activate STAT1, to stimulate the production of tumor necrosis factor α (TNFα), and to kill intracellular organisms such as mycobacteria, salmonellae, and some fungi. Homotrimeric TNFα acts through its receptor and requires nuclear factor κB essential modulator (NEMO) to activate nuclear factor κB, which also contributes to the killing of intracellular bacteria. Both IFNγ and TNFα lead to upregulation of IL-12. TNFα-blocking antibodies work either by blocking the ligand (infliximab, adalimumab, certolizumab) or by providing soluble receptor (etanercept). Mutations in IFNγR1, IFNγR2, IL-12p40, IL-12Rβ1, STAT1, and NEMO have been associated with a predisposition to mycobacterial infections. Other cytokines, such as IL-15 and IL-18, also contribute to IFNγ production. Signaling through the Toll-like receptor (TLR) complex and CD14 also upregulates TNFα production. LPS, lipopolysaccharide; NRAMP1, natural resistance-associated macrophage protein 1.

Unlike disseminated or pulmonary infection, "hot-tub lung" represents pulmonary hypersensitivity to NTM—most commonly MAC organisms—growing in underchlorinated, often indoor hot tubs.

■ CLINICAL MANIFESTATIONS

Disseminated disease

Disseminated MAC or *M. kansasii* infections in patients with advanced HIV infection are now uncommon in North America because of effective antimycobacterial prophylaxis and improved treatment of HIV infection. When such mycobacterial disease was common, the portal of entry was the bowel, with spread to bone marrow and the bloodstream. Surprisingly, disseminated infections with rapidly growing NTM (e.g., *M. abscessus*, *M. fortuitum*) are very rare in HIV-infected patients, even those with very advanced HIV infection. Because these organisms are of low intrinsic virulence and disseminate only in conjunction with impaired immunity, disseminated disease can be indolent and progressive over weeks to months. Typical manifestations of malaise, fever, and weight loss are often accompanied by organomegaly, lymphadenopathy, and anemia. Since special cultures or stains are required to identify the organisms, the most critical step in diagnosis is to suspect infection with NTM. Blood cultures may be negative, but involved organs typically have significant organism burdens, sometimes with a grossly impaired granulomatous response. In a child, disseminated involvement (i.e., involvement of two or more organs) without an underlying iatrogenic cause should prompt an investigation of the IFN-γ/IL-12 pathway. Recessive mutations in IFN-γR1 and IFN-γR2 typically lead to severe infection with NTM. In contrast, dominant negative mutations in IFN-γR1, which lead to overaccumulation of a defective interfering mutant receptor on the cell surface, inhibit normal IFN-γ signaling and thus lead to nontuberculous mycobacterial osteomyelitis. Dominant negative mutations in STAT1 and recessive mutations in IL-12Rβ1 can have variable phenotypes consistent with their residual capacities for IFN-γ synthesis and response. Male patients who have disseminated nontuberculous mycobacterial infections along with conical, peg, or missing teeth and an abnormal hair pattern should be evaluated for defects in the pathway that activates NFκB through NEMO. These patients may have associated immune globulin defects as well. A recently recognized group of patients that often develops disseminated infections with rapidly growing NTM (predominantly *M. abscessus*) as well as other opportunistic infections has high-titer neutralizing autoantibodies to IFN-γ. Thus far, this syndrome has been reported most frequently in East Asian female patients.

IV catheters can become infected with NTM, usually as a consequence of contaminated water. *M. abscessus* and *M. fortuitum* sometimes infect deep indwelling lines as well as fluids used in eye surgery, subcutaneous injections, and local anesthetics. Infected catheters should be removed.

Pulmonary disease

Lung disease is by far the most common form of nontuberculous mycobacterial infection in North America and the rest of the industrialized world. The clinical presentation typically consists of months or years of throat clearing, nagging cough, and slowly progressive fatigue. Patients will often have seen physicians multiple times and received symptom-based or transient therapy before the diagnosis is entertained and samples are sent for mycobacterial stains and cultures. Because not all patients can produce sputum, bronchoscopy may be required for diagnosis. The typical lag between onset of symptoms and diagnosis is ~5 years in older women. Predisposing factors include underlying lung diseases such as bronchiectasis (Chap. 258), pneumoconiosis (Chap. 256), chronic obstructive pulmonary disease (Chap. 260), primary ciliary dyskinesia (Chap. 258), alpha-1 antitrypsin deficiency (Chap. 309), and cystic fibrosis (Chap. 259). Bronchiectasis and nontuberculous mycobacterial infection often coexist and progress in tandem. This situation makes causality difficult to determine in a given index case, but bronchiectasis is certainly among the most critical predisposing factors that are exacerbated by infection.

MAC organisms are the most common causes of pulmonary nontuberculous mycobacterial infection in North America, but rates vary somewhat by region. MAC infection most commonly develops during the sixth or seventh decade of life in women who have had months or years of nagging intermittent cough and fatigue, with or without sputum production or chest pain. The constellation of pulmonary disease due to NTM in a tall and thin woman who may have chest wall abnormalities is often referred to as Lady Windermere's syndrome, after an Oscar Wilde character of the same name. In fact, pulmonary MAC infection does afflict older nonsmoking white women more than men, with onset at ~60 years. Patients tend to be taller and thinner than the general population, with high rates of scoliosis, mitral valve prolapse, and pectus anomalies. Whereas male smokers with upper-lobe cavitary disease tend to carry the same single strain of MAC indefinitely, nonsmoking females with nodular bronchiectasis tend to carry several strains of MAC simultaneously, with changes over the course of their disease.

M. kansasii can cause a clinical syndrome that strongly resembles tuberculosis, consisting of hemoptysis, chest pain, and cavitary lung disease. The rapidly growing NTM, such as *M. abscessus*, have been associated with esophageal motility disorders such as achalasia. Patients with pulmonary alveolar proteinosis are prone to pulmonary nontuberculous mycobacterial and *Nocardia* infections; the underlying mechanism may be inhibition of alveolar macrophage function due to the autoantibodies to granulocyte-macrophage colony-stimulating factor found in these patients.

Cervical lymph nodes

The most common form of nontuberculous mycobacterial infection among young children in North America is isolated cervical lymphadenopathy, most frequently caused by MAC organisms but also by other NTM. The cervical swelling is typically firm and relatively painless, with a paucity of systemic signs. Since the differential diagnosis of painless adenopathy includes malignancy, many children have infection with NTM diagnosed inadvertently at biopsy; cultures and special stains may not have been requested because mycobacterial disease was not ranked high in the differential. Local fistulae usually resolve completely with resection and/or antibiotic therapy. Likewise, the entity of isolated pediatric intrathoracic nontuberculous mycobacterial infection, which is probably related to cervical lymph node infection, is usually mistaken for cancer. In neither isolated cervical nor isolated intrathoracic infections with NTM have children with underlying immune defects been identified, nor do the affected children go on to develop other opportunistic infections.

Skin and soft tissue disease

Cutaneous involvement with NTM usually requires a break in the skin for introduction of the bacteria. Pedicure bath–associated infection with *M. fortuitum* is more likely if skin abrasion (e.g., during leg shaving) has occurred just before the pedicure. Outbreaks of skin infection are often caused by rapidly growing NTM (especially *M. abscessus*, *M. fortuitum*, and *M. chelonae*) acquired via skin contamination from surgical instruments (especially in cosmetic surgery), injections, and other procedures. These infections are typically accompanied by painful, erythematous, draining subcutaneous nodules, usually without associated fever or systemic symptoms.

M. marinum lives in many water sources and can be acquired from fish tanks, swimming pools, barnacles, and fish scales. This organism typically causes papules or ulcers ("fish-tank granuloma"), but the infection can progress to tendonitis with significant impairment of manual dexterity. Lesions appear days to weeks after inoculation of organisms by a typically minor trauma (e.g., incurred during the cleaning of boats or the handling of fish). Tender nodules due to *M. marinum* can advance up the arm in a pattern also seen with *Sporothrix schenckii* (*sporotricoid spread*). The typical carpal tendon involvement may be the first presenting manifestation and may lead to surgical exploration or steroid injection. The index of suspicion must be high for *M. marinum* infections to ensure that proper specimens obtained during procedures are sent for culture.

M. ulcerans, another waterborne skin pathogen, is found mainly in the tropics, especially in tropical areas of Africa. Infection follows skin trauma or insect bites that allow admission to contaminated water. The skin lesions are typically painless, clean ulcers that slough and can cause osteomyelitis. The toxin mycolactone accounts for the modest host inflammatory response and the painless ulcerations.

■ DIAGNOSIS

NTM can be detected on acid-fast or fluorochrome smears of sputum or other body fluids. When the organism burden is high, the organisms may appear as gram-positive beaded rods, but this finding is unreliable. (In contrast, nocardiae may appear as gram-positive and beaded but filamentous bacteria.) Again, the requisite and most sensitive step in the diagnosis of any mycobacterial disease is to think of including it in the differential. In almost all laboratories, mycobacterial sample processing, staining, and culture are conducted separately from routine bacteriologic tests; thus many infections go undiagnosed because of the physician's failure to request the appropriate test. In addition, mycobacteria usually require separate blood culture media. NTM are broadly differentiated into rapidly growing (<7 days) and slowly growing (≥7 days) forms. Because *M. tuberculosis* typically takes ≥2 weeks to grow, many laboratories refuse to consider culture results final until 6 weeks have elapsed. Newer techniques using liquid culture media permit more rapid isolation of mycobacteria from specimens than is possible with traditional media. Species more readily detected with incubation at 30°C include *M. marinum*, *M. haemophilum*, and *M. ulcerans*. *M. haemophilum* prefers iron supplementation or blood, while *M. genavense* requires supplemented medium with the additive mycobactin J. Bacterial formation of pigment in light conditions (photochromogenicity) or dark conditions (scotochromogenicity) or a lack of bacterial pigment formation (nonchromogenicity) has been used to help categorize NTM. In contrast to NTM, *M. tuberculosis* is beige, rough, dry, and flat. Current identification schemes can reliably use biochemical, nucleic acid, or cell wall composition, as assessed by high-performance liquid chromatography or mass spectrometry, for speciation. With the remarkable decline in U.S. cases of tuberculosis over recent decades, NTM have become the mycobacteria most commonly isolated from humans in North America. However, not all isolations of NTM, especially from the lung, reflect pathology and require treatment. Whereas identification of an organism in a blood or organ biopsy specimen in a compatible clinical setting is diagnostic, the American Thoracic Society recommends that pulmonary infection due to NTM be diagnosed only when disease is clearly demonstrable—i.e., in an appropriate clinical and radiographic setting (nodules, bronchiectasis, cavities) and with repeated isolation of NTM from expectorated sputum or recovery of NTM from bronchoscopy or biopsy specimens. Given the large number of species of NTM and the importance of accurate diagnosis for the implementation of proper therapy, identification of these organisms is ideally taken to the species level.

The purified protein derivative (PPD) of tuberculin is delivered intradermally to evoke a memory T cell response to mycobacterial antigens. This test is variously referred to as the PPD test, the tuberculin skin test, and the Mantoux test, among other designations. Unfortunately, the cutaneous immune response to these tuberculosis-derived filtrate proteins does not differentiate well between infection with NTM and that with *M. tuberculosis*. Since intermediate reactions (~10 mm) to PPD in latent tuberculosis and nontuberculous mycobacterial infections can overlap significantly, the progressive decline in active tuberculosis in the United States means that NTM probably account for increasing proportions of PPD reactivity. In addition, bacille Calmette-Guérin (BCG) can cause some degree of cross-reactivity, posing problems of interpretation for patients who have received BCG vaccine. Assays to measure the elaboration of IFN-γ in response to the relatively tuberculosis-specific proteins ESAT6 and CFP10 form the basis for IFN-γ-release assays (IGRAs). These assays can be performed with whole blood or on membranes. It is important to note that *M. marinum*, *M. kansasii*, and *M. szulgai* also have ESAT6 and CFP10 and may cause false-positive reactions in IGRAs. Despite cross-reactivity with NTM, large PPD reactions (>15 mm) most commonly signify tuberculosis.

Isolation of NTM from blood specimens is clear evidence of disease. Whereas rapidly growing mycobacteria may proliferate in routine blood culture media, slow-growing NTM typically do not; thus it is imperative to suspect the diagnosis and to use the correct bottles for cultures. Isolation of NTM from a biopsy specimen constitutes strong evidence for infection, but cases of laboratory contamination do occur. Identification of organisms on stained sections of biopsy material confirms the authenticity of the culture. Certain NTM require lower incubation temperatures (*M. genavense*) or special additives (*M. haemophilum*) for growth. Some NTM (e.g., *M. tilburgii*) remain noncultivable but can be identified molecularly in clinical samples.

The radiographic appearance of nontuberculous mycobacterial disease in the lung depends on the underlying disease, the severity of the infection, and the imaging modality used. The advent and increase in the use of CT has allowed the identification of characteristic changes that are highly consistent with nontuberculous mycobacterial infection, such as the "tree-in-bud" pattern of bronchiolar inflammation (Fig. 167-2). Involvement of the lingual and right-middle lobes is commonly seen on chest CT but is difficult to appreciate on plain film. Severe bronchiectasis and cavity formation

are common in more advanced disease. Isolation of NTM from respiratory samples can be confusing. *M. gordonae* is often recovered from respiratory samples but is not usually seen on smear and is almost never a pathogen. Patients with bronchiectasis occasionally have NTM recovered from sputum culture with a negative smear. The American Thoracic Society has developed guidelines for the diagnosis of infection with MAC, *M. abscessus*, and *M. kansasii*. A positive diagnosis requires the growth of NTM from two of three sputum samples, regardless of smear findings; a positive bronchoscopic alveolar sample, regardless of smear findings; or a pulmonary parenchyma biopsy sample with granulomatous inflammation or mycobacteria found on section and NTM on culture. These guidelines probably apply to other NTM as well.

While many laboratories use DNA probes to identify *M. tuberculosis*, MAC, *M. gordonae*, and *M. kansasii*, speciation of NTM helps determine the antimycobacterial therapy to be used. Only testing of MAC organisms for susceptibility to clarithromycin and of *M. kansasii* for susceptibility to rifampin is indicated; few data support other in vitro susceptibility tests, attractive though they appear. MAC isolates that have not been exposed to macrolides are almost always susceptible. NTM that have persisted beyond a course of antimicrobial therapy are often tested for antibiotic susceptibility, but the value and meaning of these tests are undetermined.

■ PREVENTION

Prophylaxis of MAC disease in patients infected with HIV is started when the CD4+ T lymphocyte count falls to <50/μL. Azithromycin (1200 mg weekly), clarithromycin (1000 mg daily), or rifabutin (300 mg daily) is effective. Macrolide prophylaxis in immunodeficient patients who are susceptible to NTM (e.g., those with defects in the IFN-γ/IL-12 axis) has not been prospectively validated but seems prudent.

| TREATMENT | Nontuberculous Mycobacteria |

NTM cause chronic infections that evolve relatively slowly over a period of weeks to years. Therefore, it is rarely necessary to initiate treatment on an emergent basis before the diagnosis is clear and the infecting species is known. Treatment of NTM is complex, often poorly tolerated, and potentially toxic. Just as in tuberculosis, inadequate single-drug therapy is almost always associated with the emergence of antimicrobial resistance and relapse.

MAC infection often requires multidrug therapy, the foundation of which is a macrolide (clarithromycin or azithromycin), ethambutol, and a rifamycin (rifampin or rifabutin). For disseminated nontuberculous mycobacterial disease in HIV-infected patients, the use of rifamycins poses special problems—i.e., rifamycin interactions with protease inhibitors. For pulmonary MAC disease, thrice-weekly administration of a macrolide, a rifamycin, and ethambutol has been successful. Therapy is prolonged, generally continuing for 12 months after culture conversion; typically, a course lasts for at least 18 months. Other drugs with activity against MAC organisms include IV and aerosolized aminoglycosides, fluoroquinolones, and clofazimine. In elderly patients, rifabutin can exert significant toxicity. However, with only modest efforts, most antimycobacterial regimens are well tolerated by most patients. Resection of cavitary lesions or severely bronchiectatic segments has been advocated for some patients, especially those with macrolide-resistant infections. The success of therapy for pulmonary MAC infections depends on whether disease is nodular or cavitary and on whether it is early or advanced, ranging from 20% to 80%.

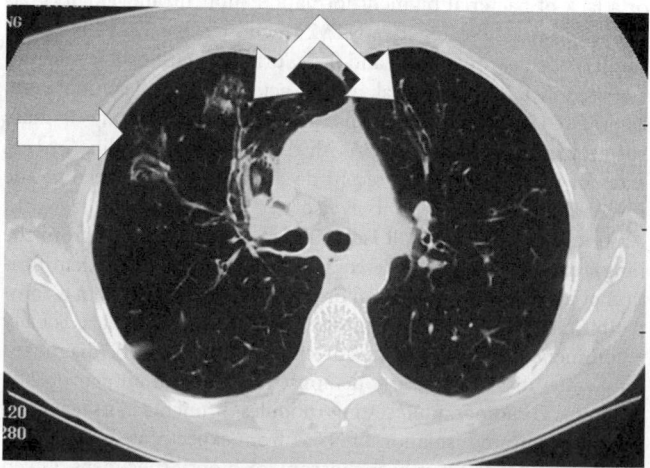

Figure 167-2 Chest CT of a patient with pulmonary MAC infection. Arrows indicate the "tree-in-bud" pattern of bronchiolar inflammation (peripheral right lung) and bronchiectasis (central right and left lungs).

M. kansasii lung disease is similar to tuberculosis in many ways and is also effectively treated with isoniazid (300 mg/d), rifampin (600 mg/d), and ethambutol (15 mg/kg per day). Other drugs with very high-level activity against *M. kansasii* include clarithromycin, fluoroquinolones, and aminoglycosides. Treatment should continue until cultures have been negative for at least 1 year. In most instances, *M. kansasii* infection is easily cured.

Rapidly growing mycobacteria pose special therapeutic problems. Extrapulmonary disease in an immunocompetent host is usually due to inoculation (e.g., via surgery, injections, or trauma) or to line infection and is often treated successfully with a macrolide and another drug (with the choice based on in vitro susceptibility), along with removal of the offending focus. In contrast, pulmonary disease, especially that caused by *M. abscessus*, is extremely difficult to cure. Repeated courses of treatment are usually effective in reducing the infectious burden and symptoms. Therapy generally includes a macrolide along with an IV-administered agent such as amikacin, a carbapenem, cefoxitin, or tigecycline. Other oral agents (used according to in vitro susceptibility testing and tolerance) include fluoroquinolones, doxycycline, and linezolid. Because nontuberculous mycobacterial infections are chronic, care must be taken in the long-term use of drugs with neurotoxicities, such as linezolid and ethambutol. Prophylactic pyridoxine has been suggested in these cases. Durations of therapy for *M. abscessus* lung disease are difficult to predict since so many cases are chronic and require intermittent therapy. Expert consultation and management are strongly recommended.

Once recognized, *M. marinum* infection is highly responsive to antimicrobial therapy and is cured relatively easily with any combination of a macrolide, ethambutol, and a rifamycin. Therapy should be continued for 1–2 months after clinical resolution of isolated soft tissue disease; tendon and bone involvement may require longer courses in light of clinical evolution. Other drugs with activity against *M. marinum* include sulfonamides, trimethoprim-sulfamethoxazole, doxycycline, and minocycline.

Treatment of the other NTM is less well defined, but macrolides and aminoglycosides are usually effective, with other agents added as indicated. Expert consultation is strongly encouraged for difficult or unusual infections due to NTM.

◼ PROGNOSIS

The outcomes of nontuberculous mycobacterial infections are closely tied to the underlying condition (e.g., IFN-γ/IL-12 pathway defect, cystic fibrosis) and can range from recovery to death. With no or inadequate treatment, symptoms and signs can be debilitating, including persistent cough, fever, anorexia, and severe lung destruction. With treatment, patients typically regain strength and energy. The optimal duration of therapy when NTM persist in sputum is unknown, but treatment in this situation can be prolonged.

FURTHER READINGS

BROWNE SK, HOLLAND SM: Anticytokine autoantibodies in infectious diseases: Pathogenesis and mechanisms. Lancet Infect Dis 10:875, 2010

DALEY CL, GRIFFITH DE: Pulmonary non-tuberculous mycobacterial infections. Int J Tuberc Lung Dis 14:665, 2010

FALKINHAM JO III: Surrounded by mycobacteria: Nontuberculous mycobacteria in the human environment. J Appl Microbiol 107:356, 2009

GRIFFITH DE et al: American Thoracic Society: Diagnosis, treatment and prevention of nontuberculous mycobacterial diseases. Am J Respir Crit Care Med 175:367, 2007

KIM RD et al: Pulmonary nontuberculous mycobacterial disease: Prospective study of a distinct preexisting syndrome. Am J Respir Crit Care Med 178:1066, 2008

PREVOTS DR et al: Nontuberculous mycobacterial lung disease prevalence at four integrated health care delivery systems. Am J Respir Crit Care Med 182:970, 2010

SOLOGUREN I et al: Partial recessive IFN-γR1 deficiency: Genetic, immunological and clinical features of 14 patients from 11 kindreds. Hum Mol Genet 20:1509, 2011

Changing epidemiology of pulmonary nontuberculous mycobacteria infections. Emerg Infect Dis 16:1576, 2010

VAN DE VOSSE E et al: Genetic deficiencies of innate immune signalling in human infectious disease. Lancet Infect Dis 9:688, 2009

WALLIS RS: Infectious complications of tumor necrosis factor blockade. Curr Opin Infect Dis 22:403, 2009

CHAPTER 168
Antimycobacterial Agents

Max R. O'Donnell
Jussi J. Saukkonen

Agents used for the treatment of mycobacterial infections, including tuberculosis (TB), leprosy (Hansen's disease), and infections due to nontuberculous mycobacteria (NTM), are administered in multiple-drug regimens for prolonged courses. Currently, more than 150 species of mycobacteria have been identified, the majority of which do not cause disease in humans. While the incidence of disease caused by *M. tuberculosis* has been declining in the United States, TB remains a leading cause of morbidity and mortality in developing countries—particularly in sub-Saharan Africa, where the HIV epidemic rages. Not only effective drug regimens are needed; without a well-organized infrastructure for diagnosis and treatment of TB, therapeutic and control efforts are severely hampered. Infections with NTM have gained in clinical prominence in the United States and other developed countries. These largely environmental organisms often establish infection in immunocompromised patients or in persons with structural lung disease.

TUBERCULOSIS

◼ GENERAL PRINCIPLES

The earliest recorded human case of TB dates back 9000 years. Early treatment modalities, such as bloodletting, were replaced by sanatorium regimens in the late 19th century. The discovery of streptomycin in 1943 launched the era of antibiotic treatment for TB. Over subsequent decades, the discovery of additional agents and the use of multiple-drug regimens allowed progressive shortening of the treatment course from years to as little as 6 months with

TABLE 168-1 Regimens for the Treatment of Latent Tuberculosis Infection (LTBI) in Adults

Regimen	Schedule	Duration	Comments
Isoniazid	300 mg daily (5 mg/kg) Alternative: 900 mg twice weekly (15 mg/kg)	9 months	Supplement with pyridoxine (25–50 mg daily). Twice-weekly regimens require directly observed therapy.
Rifampin	600 mg daily (10 mg/kg)	4 months	Broader efficacy studies are needed.
Isoniazid plus rifapentine[a]	900 mg weekly + 900 mg weekly (15 mg/kg)	4 months	Weekly regimens require directly observed therapy. Supplement with pyridoxine (25–50 mg daily).

[a]Under investigation.

the regimen for drug-susceptible TB. Latent TB infection (LTBI) and active TB disease are diagnosed by history, physical examination, tuberculin skin test, interferon γ release assay, radiographic imaging, and/or mycobacterial cultures. LTBI is treated with either isoniazid (9 months) or rifampin (4 months) (Table 168-1).

For active or suspected TB disease, clinical factors, including HIV co-infection, symptom duration, radiographic appearance, and public health concerns about TB transmission, drive diagnostic testing and treatment initiation. Multiple-drug regimens are used for the treatment of TB disease (Table 168-2). Initially, an intensive phase consisting of four drugs—isoniazid, rifampin, pyrazinamide, and ethambutol given for 2 months—is followed by a continuation phase of isoniazid and rifampin for 4 months, for a total treatment duration of 6 months. The continuation phase is extended to 7 months (for a total treatment duration of 9 months) if the 2-month course of pyrazinamide is not completed or, for patients with cavitary pulmonary TB, if sputum cultures remain positive beyond 2 months of treatment (delayed culture conversion).

Treatment of TB in individuals co-infected with HIV poses significant challenges, but some progress is being made. Recent data show improved survival when antiretroviral therapy (ART) is initiated early in TB therapy. Interactions of rifampin with protease inhibitors or nonnucleotide reverse transcriptase inhibitors are significant and require close monitoring and dose adjustments. The TB immune reconstitution inflammatory syndrome (IRIS) may appear as early as 1 week after initiation of ART and manifests as paradoxical worsening or unmasking of existing TB infection.

Conservative management consists of continued administration of ART and TB medications; however, severe or debilitating IRIS has been anecdotally treated with varying doses of glucocorticoids. Intermittent therapy in patients co-infected with HIV and M. tuberculosis has been associated with low plasma levels of several key TB drugs and with higher rates of treatment failure or relapse; therefore, intermittent twice-weekly therapy for TB in HIV-co-infected individuals is not recommended.

Adherence to medications is critical in achieving a cure with antimycobacterial therapy. Consequently, directly observed therapy (DOT) by trained staff, either in the clinic or at home, is recommended to ensure adherence. In addition, monthly dispensing of TB medicines is recommended, since monthly clinical monitoring for hepatotoxicity due to these medications is essential for all patients. Discontinuation of suspected offending agents at the onset of hepatitis symptoms reduces the risk of progression to fatal hepatitis. Clinical monitoring includes at least monthly assessment for symptoms and signs (nausea, vomiting, abdominal discomfort, and unexplained fatigue) and signs (jaundice, dark urine, light stools, diffuse pruritus) of hepatotoxicity, although the latter represent comparatively late manifestations (Table 168-3). The presence of such symptoms and signs mandates provisional discontinuation of potentially hepatotoxic agents. Biochemical testing of at least serum alanine aminotransferase and total bilirubin levels and exclusion of other causes of these abnormalities are also indicated. For patients with active TB, monthly mycobacterial cultures of sputum are recommended until it is certain that the organisms have been cleared and the patient has responded to therapy or until no sputum is available for culture.

TABLE 168-2 Simplified Approach to Treatment of Active Tuberculosis in Adults

Culture Results	Intensive Phase	Continuation Phase	Extension of Total Treatment
Culture positive	HRZE for 2 months, daily or intermittent (with dose adjustment)	HR for 4 months, daily or 5 d/wk or HR for 4 months, intermittent (with dose adjustment)	To 9 months, if 2 months of Z is not completed or culture conversion is prolonged[a] and/or cavitation is documented
Culture negative	HRZE for 2 months	2 months	To 6 months, if patient is infected with HIV
Resistant to H	RZE or S (Q[b]) for 6 months	. . .	Prolonged culture conversion, cavitation
Resistant to R	HZEQ[b] (IA[c]) for 2 months	HEQ(S) for 10–16 months	Prolonged culture conversion, delayed response
Resistant to HR[d]	ZEQ[b](IA[c]) ± alternative agents[e] for 18–24 months	. . .	Prolonged culture conversion

[a]Beyond 2 months.
[b]Moxifloxacin and levofloxacin are the preferred fluoroquinolones; ciprofloxacin should be avoided.
[c]Injectable agents: streptomycin, amikacin, kanamycin, and capreomycin.
[d]Management of multidrug-resistant TB should be performed by or in close consultation with an expert TB clinician. Surgical management should be considered.
[e]Alternative agents: cycloserine, ethionamide, para-aminosalicylic acid, clarithromycin, linezolid, and amoxicillin-clavulanate.
Abbreviations: E, ethambutol; H, isoniazid; IA, injectable agent; Q, fluoroquinolone; R, rifampin; S, streptomycin; Z, pyrazinamide.

TABLE 168-3 Monitoring and Clinical Management of Tuberculosis Treatment in Adults[a]

Drug	Assessment	Management
LTBI Treatment		
With hepatic risk factors[b], check ALT and bilirubin at baseline. If ALT is ≥3 × ULN or total bilirubin is >2, defer treatment and reevaluate.		
Isoniazid	Determine whether hepatic risk factors are present. If so, obtain baseline and periodic ALT and bilirubin values.	If ALT is 5 × ULN (or 3 × ULN with symptoms)[c] or if bilirubin reaches jaundice levels (usually >2 × ULN), interrupt treatment. With normalization, consider an alternative agent.
Rifampin	Same	Same
TB Treatment		
Check ALT, bilirubin, platelets, creatinine, and hepatitis panel on all patients at baseline. If hepatic risk factors are present, check ALT and bilirubin monthly.		
Isoniazid	If ALT is >5 × ULN (or >3 × ULN with hepatitis symptoms)[c]	Obtain history of alcohol consumption and concomitant drugs. In most instances, discontinue H, Z, R, and other hepatotoxic drugs. Consider alternative agents. Obtain viral hepatitis serologies. Rechallenge: With normalization of liver enzymes, sequentially reintroduce R and then H. With no recurrence of hepatotoxicity, do not resume Z. Alternative rechallenge protocols have been proposed.
Rifampin	If primary elevation is in bilirubin and alkaline phosphatase, more likely rifampin	Discontinue R if bilirubin reaches jaundice levels (usually >2 × ULN). May try to reintroduce. If not tolerated, may substitute Q.
Ethambutol	Decrease in visual acuity or color vision or appearance on monthly screening	Discontinue ethambutol and repeat ocular exam. Peripheral neuropathy may be a precursor of ocular toxicity; if it occurs, consider repeat ocular exam.
Pyrazinamide	If ALT is >5 × ULN (or >3 × ULN with symptoms)[c]	Same as for H
Fluoroquinolone	If QT$_c$ prolongation is discovered incidentally on ECG	Check audiometry and at least BUN and creatinine monthly.
Aminoglycoside	Abnormal results on audiometry testing, BUN, creatinine, electrolytes at baseline or on monthly check	Discontinue aminoglycoside if not MDR-TB. As appropriate, assess renal function, correct electrolytes, or seek ENT consultation.

[a]All regimens require monthly clinical monitoring.
[b]Hepatic risk factors: chronic alcohol use, viral hepatitis, preexisting liver disease, pregnancy or 3 months postpartum, hepatotoxic medications.
[c]Relevant manifestations include nausea, vomiting, abdominal pain, jaundice, or unexplained fatigue.
Abbreviations: ALT, alanine aminotransferase; BUN, blood urea nitrogen; H, isoniazid; Q, fluoroquinolone; R, rifampin; Z, pyrazinamide; Q, fluoroquinolone; ULN, upper limit of normal; MDR-TB, multidrug-resistant tuberculosis; ENT, ear, nose, and throat.

If significant clinical improvement does not occur or the patient's condition deteriorates over the course of therapy, possibilities include treatment failure due to nonadherence to therapy, poor medication absorption, or the development of resistance. For patients co-infected with HIV and *M. tuberculosis*, immune reconstitution inflammatory syndrome (IRIS) is a possibility and is a diagnosis of exclusion. or mycobacterial resistance should be suspected. Drug susceptibility testing should be repeated at this point. If resistance is documented or strongly suspected, at least two efficacious drugs to which the isolate is susceptible or which the patient has not already taken should be added to the therapeutic regimen.

Multidrug-resistant tuberculosis (MDR-TB) is defined as disease caused by a strain of *M. tuberculosis* that is resistant to both isoniazid and rifampin—the most efficacious of the first-line TB drugs. The risk of MDR-TB is elevated in patients presenting from geographic areas in which ≥5% of incident TB is MDR-TB and in patients previously treated for TB. Treatment regimens for MDR-TB generally include a late-generation fluoroquinolone and an injectable second-line agent (such as capreomycin, amikacin, or kanamycin). Regimens of at least five drugs are recommended for the treatment of MDR-TB. Both standardized and optimized/customized regimens are in use around the world. Extensively drug-resistant tuberculosis (XDR-TB) is defined as MDR-TB with additional resistance to any fluoroquinolone and at least one of the second-line injectable agents. Treatment of XDR-TB is individualized on the basis of extended antimicrobial susceptibility testing. Therapeutic regimens for either MDR-TB or XDR-TB should be constructed with input from clinicians experienced in the management of TB.

■ FIRST-LINE ANTITUBERCULOSIS DRUGS

Isoniazid

Isoniazid is a critical drug for treatment of both TB disease and LTBI. Isoniazid has excellent bactericidal activity against both intracellular and extracellular, actively dividing *M. tuberculosis*. This drug is bacteriostatic against slowly dividing organisms. In treatment of LTBI, isoniazid is considered the first-line agent because it is generally well tolerated, has well-established efficacy, and is inexpensive. In this setting, the drug is taken daily or intermittently (i.e., twice weekly) as DOT for 9 months. The 9-month course is more efficacious than the 6-month course (75–90% vs. ≤65%), but extension of treatment to 12 months is not likely to provide further protection. A 6-month course of daily or intermittent isoniazid is considered second-line, but acceptable, therapy.

For treatment of TB, isoniazid is used in combination with other agents to ensure killing of both actively dividing *M. tuberculosis* and slowly growing "persister" organisms. Unless the organism is resistant, the standard regimen includes isoniazid, rifampin, ethambutol, and pyrazinamide (Table 168-2). Isoniazid is often given together with 25–50 mg of pyridoxine daily to prevent drug-related peripheral neuropathy.

Mechanism of action Isoniazid is a prodrug activated by the mycobacterial KatG catalase/peroxidase; isoniazid is coupled with reduced nicotinamide adenine dinucleotide (NADH). The resulting isonicotinic acyl-NADH complex blocks the mycobacterial ketoenoylreductase known as InhA, binding to its substrate and inhibiting fatty acid synthase and ultimately mycolic acid synthesis. Mycolic acids are essential requirements for the mycobacterial cell wall. KatG activation of isoniazid also results in the release of free radicals that have antimycobacterial activity, including nitric oxide.

The minimal inhibitory concentrations (MICs) of isoniazid for wild-type (untreated) susceptible strains are <0.1 µg/mL for *M. tuberculosis* and 0.5–2 µg/mL for *M. kansasii*.

Pharmacology Isoniazid is the hydrazide of isonicotinic acid, a small, water-soluble molecule. The usual adult oral daily dose of 300 mg results in peak serum levels of 3–5 µg/mL within 30 min to 2 h after ingestion—well in excess of the MICs for most susceptible strains of *M. tuberculosis*. Both oral and IM preparations of isoniazid achieve good levels in the body, although antacids and high-carbohydrate meals may interfere with oral absorption. Isoniazid diffuses well throughout the body, reaching therapeutic concentrations in body cavities and fluids, with concentrations in cerebrospinal fluid (CSF) comparable to those in serum.

Isoniazid is metabolized in the liver via acetylation by *N*-acetyltransferase 2 (NAT2) and hydrolysis. Both fast- and slow-acetylation phenotypes occur; patients who are "fast acetylators" may have lower serum levels of isoniazid, whereas slow acetylators may have higher levels and experience more toxicity. Satisfactory isoniazid levels are attained in the majority of homozygous fast NAT2 acetylators given a dose of 6 mg/kg and in the majority of homozygous slow acetylators given only 3 mg/kg. Genotyping is increasingly being used to characterize isoniazid-related pharmacogenomic responses.

Isoniazid's interactions with other drugs are due primarily to its inhibition of the cytochrome P450 system. Among the drugs with significant isoniazid interactions are warfarin, carbamazepine, benzodiazepines, acetaminophen, clopidogrel, maraviroc, dronedarone, salmeterol, tamoxifen, eplerenone, and phenytoin.

Dosing The recommended daily dose for the treatment of TB in the United States is 5 mg/kg for adults and 10–20 mg/kg for children, with a maximal daily dose of 300 mg for both. For intermittent therapy in adults (usually twice per week), the dose is 15 mg/kg with a maximal daily dose of 900 mg. Isoniazid does not require dosage adjustment in patients with renal disease.

Resistance Although isoniazid is, along with rifampin, the mainstay of TB treatment regimens, ~7% of clinical *M. tuberculosis* isolates in the United States are resistant. Rates of primary isoniazid resistance among untreated patients are significantly higher in many populations born outside the United States. Four separate pathways for isoniazid resistance have been elucidated. Most strains have amino acid changes in either the catalase-peroxidase gene (*katG*) or the mycobacterial ketoenoylreductase gene (*inhA*). Less frequently, alterations in *kasA*, the gene for an enzyme involved in mycolic acid elongation, and loss of NADH dehydrogenase 2 activity confer isoniazid resistance.

Adverse effects Although isoniazid is generally well tolerated, drug-induced liver injury and peripheral neuropathy are significant adverse effects associated with this agent. Isoniazid may cause asymptomatic transient elevation of aminotransferase levels (often termed *hepatic adaptation*) in up to 20% of recipients. Other adverse reactions include rash (2%), fever (1.2%), anemia, acne, arthritic symptoms, a systemic lupus erythematosus–like syndrome,

optic atrophy, seizures, and psychiatric symptoms. Symptomatic hepatitis occurs in fewer than 0.1% of persons treated with isoniazid alone for LTBI, and fulminant hepatitis with hepatic failure occurs in fewer than 0.01%. Isoniazid-associated hepatitis is idiosyncratic, but its incidence increases with age, with daily alcohol consumption, and in women who are within 3 months postpartum.

In patients who have liver disorders or HIV infection, who are pregnant or in the 3-month postpartum period, who have a history of liver disease (e.g., hepatitis B or C, alcoholic hepatitis, or cirrhosis), who use alcohol regularly, who have multiple medical problems, or who have other risk factors for chronic liver disease, the risks and benefits of treatment for LTBI should be weighed. If treatment is undertaken, these patients should have serum concentrations of alanine aminotransferase (ALT) determined at baseline. Routine baseline hepatic ALT testing based solely on an age of >35 years is optional and depends on individual concerns. Monthly biochemical monitoring during isoniazid treatment is indicated for patients whose baseline liver function tests yield abnormal results and for persons at risk for hepatic disease, including the groups just mentioned. Guidelines recommend that isoniazid be discontinued in the presence of hepatitis symptoms or jaundice and an ALT level three times the upper limit of normal or in the absence of symptoms with an ALT level five times the upper limit of normal (Table 168-3).

Peripheral neuropathy associated with isoniazid occurs in up to 2% of patients given 5 mg/kg. Isoniazid appears to interfere with pyridoxine (vitamin B_6) metabolism. The risk of isoniazid-related neurotoxicity is greatest for patients with preexisting disorders that also pose a risk of neuropathy, such as HIV infection; for those with diabetes mellitus, alcohol abuse, or malnutrition; and for those simultaneously receiving other potentially neuropathic medications, such as stavudine. These patients should be given prophylactic pyridoxine (25–50 mg/d).

Rifampin

Rifampin is a semisynthetic derivative of *Amycolatopsis rifamycinica* (formerly known as *Streptomyces mediterranei*). The most active antimycobacterial agent available, rifampin is the keystone of first-line treatment for TB. Introduced in 1968, this drug eventually permitted dramatic shortening of TB treatment. Rifampin has bactericidal activity against both dividing and nondividing *M. tuberculosis*, with sterilizing activity. The drug is also active against an array of other organisms, including some gram-positive and gram-negative bacteria, *Legionella*, *M. kansasii*, and *M. marinum*.

Rifampin, administered for 4 months, is also an alternative agent to isoniazid for the treatment of LTBI, although efficacy data are scant at this time. A 3-month course of rifampin alone has been found to be similar in efficacy to a 6-month course of isoniazid. Although the 4-month regimen of rifampin has not yet been compared with 9 months of isoniazid, randomized safety and tolerability studies indicate that rates of discontinuation, hepatotoxicity, and adverse reaction are lower with the former than with the latter. The rates of treatment completion are also higher for the 4-month rifampin regimen.

Mechanism of action Rifampin exerts both intracellular and extracellular bactericidal activity. Like other rifamycins, rifampin specifically binds to and inhibits mycobacterial DNA-dependent RNA polymerase, blocking RNA synthesis. Susceptible strains of *M. tuberculosis* as well as *M. kansasii* and *M. marinum* are inhibited by rifampin concentrations of 1 µg/mL.

Pharmacology Rifampin is a fat-soluble, complex macrocyclic molecule readily absorbed after oral administration. Serum levels of 10–20 µg/mL are achieved 2.5 h after the usual adult oral dose of 10 mg/kg (given without food). Rifampin has a half-life of 1.5–5 h.

The drug distributes well throughout most body tissues, including CSF. Rifampin turns body fluids such as urine, saliva, sputum, and tears a reddish-orange color—an effect that offers a simple means of assessing patients' adherence to this medication. Rifampin is excreted primarily through the bile and enters the enterohepatic circulation; <30% of a dose is renally excreted.

As a potent inducer of the hepatic cytochrome P450 system, rifampin can decrease the half-life of some drugs, such as digoxin, warfarin, phenytoin, prednisone, cyclosporine, methadone, oral contraceptives, clarithromycin, azole antifungal agents, quinidine, and antiretroviral protease inhibitors and nonnucleoside reverse transcriptase inhibitors. The Centers for Disease Control and Prevention has issued guidelines for the management of drug interactions during treatment of HIV and *M. tuberculosis* co-infection (*www.cdc.gov/tb/*).

Dosing The daily dosage of rifampin is 10 mg/kg for adults and 10–20 mg/kg for children, with a maximum of 600 mg/d for both. The drug is given once daily, twice weekly, or three times weekly. No adjustments of dose or frequency are necessary in patients with renal insufficiency.

Resistance Resistance to rifampin in *M. tuberculosis*, *M. leprae*, and other organisms is the consequence of spontaneous, mostly missense point mutations in a core region of the bacterial gene coding for the β subunit of RNA polymerase (*rpoB*). RNA polymerase altered in this manner is no longer subject to inhibition by rifampin. Most rapidly and slowly growing NTM harbor intrinsic resistance to rifampin, for which the mechanism has yet to be determined.

Adverse effects Adverse events associated with rifampin are infrequent and generally mild. Hepatotoxicity due to rifampin alone is uncommon in the absence of preexisting liver disease and often consists of isolated hyperbilirubinemia rather than aminotransferase elevation. Other adverse reactions include rash, pruritus, gastrointestinal symptoms, and pancytopenia. Rarely, a hypersensitivity reaction may occur with intermittent therapy, manifesting as fever, chills, malaise, rash, and—in some instances—renal and hepatic failure.

Ethambutol

Ethambutol is a bacteriostatic antimycobacterial agent first synthesized in 1961. A component of the standard first-line regimen, ethambutol provides synergy with the other drugs in the regimen and is generally well tolerated. Susceptible species include *M. tuberculosis*, *M. marinum*, *M. kansasii*, and organisms of the *M. avium* complex (MAC); however, among first-line drugs, ethambutol is the least potent against *M. tuberculosis*. This agent is also used in combination with other agents in the continuation phase of treatment in patients who cannot tolerate isoniazid or rifampin or who are infected with organisms resistant to either of the latter drugs.

Mechanism of action Ethambutol is bacteriostatic against *M. tuberculosis*. Its primary mechanism of action is the inhibition of the arabinosyltransferases involved in cell wall synthesis, which probably inhibits the formation of arabinogalactan and lipoarabinomannan.

Pharmacology and dosing From a single dose of ethambutol, 75–80% is absorbed within 2–4 h of administration. Serum levels peak at 2–4 μg/mL after the standard adult daily dose of 15 mg/kg. Ethambutol is well distributed throughout the body except in the CSF; a dosage of 25 mg/kg is necessary for attainment of a CSF level half of that in serum. For intermittent therapy, the dosage is 50 mg/kg twice weekly. To prevent toxicity, the dosage must be lowered and the frequency of administration reduced for patients with renal insufficiency.

Adverse effects Ethambutol is usually well tolerated and has no significant interactions with other drugs. Optic neuritis, the most serious adverse effect reported, typically presents as reduced visual acuity, central scotoma, and loss of the ability to see green (or, less commonly, red). The cause of this neuritis is unknown, but it may be due to an effect of ethambutol on the amacrine and bipolar cells of the retina. Symptoms typically develop several months after initiation of therapy, but ocular toxicity soon after initiation of ethambutol has been described. The risk of ocular toxicity is dose dependent, with occurrence in 1–5% of patients, and can be increased by renal insufficiency. The routine use of ethambutol in younger children is not recommended, as monitoring for visual complications can be difficult. If drug-resistant TB is suspected, ethambutol can be used in children.

All patients starting therapy with ethambutol should have a baseline test for visual acuity, visual fields, and color vision and should undergo an examination of the optic fundus. Visual acuity and color vision should be monitored monthly or less often as needed. Cessation of ethambutol in response to early symptoms of ocular toxicity usually results in reversal of the deficit within several months. Recovery of all visual function may take up to 1 year. In the elderly and in patients in whom symptoms are not recognized early, deficits may be permanent. Some experts think that supplementation with hydroxycobalamin (vitamin B$_{12}$) is beneficial for patients with ethambutol-related ocular toxicity.

Other adverse effects of ethambutol are rare. Peripheral sensory neuropathy occurs in rare instances.

Resistance Ethambutol resistance in *M. tuberculosis* and NTM is associated primarily with missense mutations in the *embB* gene that encodes for arabinosyltransferase. Mutations have been found in resistant strains at codon 306 in 50–70% of cases. Mutations at *embB*306 can cause significantly increased MICs of ethambutol, resulting in clinical resistance.

Pyrazinamide

A nicotinamide analog, pyrazinamide is an important bactericidal drug used in the initial phase of TB treatment. Its administration for the first 2 months of therapy with rifampin and isoniazid allows treatment duration to be shortened from 9 months to 6 months and decreases rates of relapse.

Mechanism of action Pyrazinamide's antimycobacterial activity is essentially limited to *M. tuberculosis*. The drug is more active against slowly replicating organisms than against actively replicating organisms. Pyrazinamide is a prodrug that is converted by the mycobacterial pyrimidase to the active form, pyrazinoic acid (POA). This agent is active only in acidic environments (pH <6.0), as are found within phagocytes or granulomas. The exact mechanism of action of POA is unclear, but fatty acid synthetase I may be the primary target in *M. tuberculosis*.

Pharmacology and dosing Pyrazinamide is well absorbed after oral administration, with peak serum concentrations of 20–60 μg/mL at 1–2 h after ingestion of the recommended adult daily dose of 15–30 mg/kg (maximum, 2 g/d). It distributes well to various body compartments, including CSF, and is an important component of treatment for tuberculous meningitis. The serum half-life of the drug is 9–11 h with normal renal and hepatic function. Pyrazinamide is metabolized in the liver to POA, 5-hydroxypyrazinamide, and 5-hydroxy-POA. A high proportion of pyrazinamide and its metabolites (~70%) is excreted in the urine. The dosage must be adjusted according to the level of renal function in patients with reduced creatinine clearance.

Adverse effects At the higher dosages used previously, hepatotoxicity was seen in as many as 15% of patients treated with pyrazinamide. However, at the currently recommended dosages, hepatotoxicity now occurs less commonly when this drug is administered with isoniazid and rifampin during the treatment of TB. Older age, active liver disease, HIV infection, and low albumin levels may increase the risk of hepatotoxicity. The use of pyrazinamide with rifampin for the treatment of LTBI is no longer recommended because of unacceptable rates of hepatotoxicity and death in this setting. Hyperuricemia is a common adverse effect of pyrazinamide therapy that usually can be managed conservatively. Clinical gout is rare.

Although pyrazinamide is recommended by international tuberculosis organizations for routine use in pregnancy, it is not recommended in the United States because of inadequate teratogenicity data.

Resistance The basis of pyrazinamide resistance in *M. tuberculosis* is a mutation in the *pncA* gene coding for pyrazinamidase, the enzyme that converts the prodrug to active POA. Resistance to pyrazinamide is associated with loss of pyrazinamidase activity, which prevents conversion of pyrazinamide to POA. Of pyrazinamide-resistant *M. tuberculosis* isolates, 72–98% have mutations in *pncA*. Conventional methods of testing for susceptibility to pyrazinamide may produce both false-negative and false-positive results because the high-acidity environment required for the drug's activation also inhibits the growth of *M. tuberculosis*. There is some controversy as to the clinical significance of in vitro pyrazinamide resistance.

■ FIRST-LINE SUPPLEMENTAL DRUGS

Rifabutin

Rifabutin, a semisynthetic derivative of rifamycin S, inhibits mycobacterial DNA-dependent RNA polymerase. Although rifabutin is active in vitro against some strains of rifampin-resistant *M. tuberculosis*, its clinical utility in this situation is not clear. Rifabutin is more active than rifampin against MAC organisms and other NTM in vitro.

Rifabutin is recommended in place of rifampin for the treatment of HIV-co-infected individuals who are taking protease inhibitors or nonnucleoside reverse transcriptase inhibitors, particularly nevirapine. Rifabutin's effect on hepatic enzyme induction is less pronounced than that of rifampin. Protease inhibitors may cause significant increases in rifabutin levels through inhibition of hepatic metabolism.

Pharmacology Like rifampin, rifabutin is lipophilic and is absorbed rapidly after oral administration, reaching peak serum levels 2–4 h after ingestion. Rifabutin distributes best to tissues, reaching levels 5–10 times higher than those in plasma. Unlike rifampin, rifabutin and its metabolites are partially cleared by the hepatic microsomal system. Rifabutin's slow clearance results in a mean serum half-life of 45 h—much longer than the 3- to 5-h half-life of rifampin. Clarithromycin (but not azithromycin) and fluconazole appear to increase rifabutin levels by inhibiting hepatic metabolism.

Adverse effects Rifabutin is generally well tolerated, with adverse effects occurring at higher doses. The most common adverse events are gastrointestinal; other reactions include rash, headache, asthenia, chest pain, myalgia, and insomnia. Less common adverse reactions include fever, chills, a flulike syndrome, anterior uveitis, hepatitis, *Clostridium difficile*–associated diarrhea, a diffuse polymyalgia syndrome, and yellow skin discoloration ("pseudo-jaundice"). Laboratory abnormalities include neutropenia, leukopenia, thrombocytopenia, and increased levels of liver enzymes.

Resistance Resistance to rifabutin is mediated by some mutations in *rpoB*.

Rifapentine

Rifapentine is a semisynthetic cyclopentyl rifamycin, sharing a mechanism of action with rifampin. Rifapentine is lipophilic and has a prolonged half-life that permits weekly or twice-weekly dosing (although dosing and frequency of administration are still being actively studied). Because of higher rates of relapse, rifapentine is not approved for administration to patients with HIV disease. It is being studied for treatment of LTBI in a weekly combination regimen with isoniazid given for 3 months (versus the standard 9-month regimen).

Pharmacology Rifapentine's good absorption is improved when the drug is taken with food. After oral administration, rifapentine reaches peak serum concentrations in 5–6 h and achieves a steady state in 10 days. The half-life of rifapentine and its active metabolite, 25-desacetyl rifapentine, is ~13 h. The administered dose is excreted via the liver (70%).

Adverse effects The adverse-effects profile of rifapentine is similar to that of other rifamycins. Rifapentine is teratogenic in animal models and is relatively contraindicated in pregnancy.

Resistance Rifapentine resistance is mediated by mutations in *rpoB*. Mutations that cause resistance to rifampin also cause resistance to rifapentine.

Streptomycin

Streptomycin was the first antimycobacterial agent used for the treatment of TB. Derived from *Streptomyces griseus*, streptomycin is bactericidal against dividing *M. tuberculosis* organisms but has only low-level early bactericidal activity. This drug is administered only by the IM and IV routes. In developed nations, streptomycin is used infrequently because of its toxicity, the inconvenience of injections, and drug resistance. In developing countries, however, streptomycin is used because of its low cost.

Mechanism of action Streptomycin inhibits protein synthesis by binding at a site on the 30S mycobacterial ribosome.

Pharmacology and dosing Serum levels of streptomycin peak at 25–45 µg/mL after a 1-g dose. This agent penetrates poorly into the CSF, reaching levels that are only 20% of serum levels. The usual daily dose of streptomycin (given IM either daily or 5 days per week) is 15 mg/kg for adults and 20–40 mg/kg for children, with a maximum of 1 g/d for both. For patients ≥60 years of age, 10 mg/kg is the recommended daily dose, with a maximum of 750 mg/d. Because streptomycin is eliminated almost exclusively by the kidneys, its use in patients with renal impairment should be avoided or implemented with caution, with lower doses and less frequent administration.

Adverse effects Adverse reactions occur frequently with streptomycin (10–20% of patients). Ototoxicity (primarily vestibulotoxicity), neuropathy, and renal toxicity are the most common and the most serious. Renal toxicity, usually manifested as nonoliguric renal failure, is less common with streptomycin than with other frequently used aminoglycosides, such as gentamicin. Manifestations of vestibular toxicity include loss of balance, vertigo, and tinnitus. Patients receiving streptomycin must be monitored carefully for these adverse effects, undergoing audiometry at baseline and monthly thereafter.

Resistance Spontaneous mutations conferring resistance to streptomycin are relatively common, occurring in 1 in 10⁶ organisms. In the two-thirds of streptomycin-resistant *M. tuberculosis* strains exhibiting high-level resistance, mutations have been identified in one of two genes: a 16S rRNA gene (*rrs*) or the gene encoding ribosomal protein S12 (*rpsL*). Both targets are believed to be involved in streptomycin ribosomal binding. However, low-level resistance, which is seen in about one-third of resistant isolates, has no associated resistance mutation. A gene (*gidB*) that confers low-level resistance to streptomycin has recently been identified. Strains of *M. tuberculosis* resistant to streptomycin generally are not cross-resistant to capreomycin or amikacin.

■ SECOND-LINE ANTITUBERCULOSIS DRUGS

Second-line antituberculosis agents are indicated for treatment of drug-resistant TB, for patients who are intolerant or allergic to first-line agents, and when first-line supplemental agents are unavailable.

Fluoroquinolones

Fluoroquinolones inhibit mycobacterial DNA gyrase and topoisomerase IV, preventing cell replication and protein synthesis, and are bactericidal. The later-generation fluoroquinolones moxifloxacin and levofloxacin are the most active against *M. tuberculosis* and are being investigated for their potential to shorten the course of treatment for TB. Gatifloxacin, although also being assessed for shortening of treatment duration, causes significant dysglycemia. Ciprofloxacin is no longer recommended for the treatment of TB because of poor efficacy.

The fluoroquinolones are well absorbed orally, achieve high serum levels, and distribute well into body tissues and fluids. Their absorption is decreased by co-ingestion with products containing multivalent cations, such as antacids. Adverse effects are relatively infrequent (0.5–10% of patients) and include gastrointestinal intolerance, rashes, dizziness, and headache. Most studies of fluoroquinolone side effects have been based on relatively short-term administration for bacterial infections, but trials have now shown the relative safety and tolerability of fluoroquinolones administered for months during TB treatment in adults. The potential to prolong the QT_c interval leading to cardiac arrhythmias has been a source of concern with fluoroquinolones. QT_c prolongation requiring cessation of treatment is rare. There is increasing interest in the use of fluoroquinolones in children, which has traditionally been avoided because of the risks of tendon rupture and cartilage damage, as the benefits in treatment of drug-resistant TB may outweigh the risks.

Mycobacterial resistance can develop rapidly when a fluoroquinolone is inadvertently administered alone. Empirical fluoroquinolone therapy for presumed community-acquired pneumonia is associated with increased resistance in *M. tuberculosis*. Mutations in the genes encoding for DNA gyrase (*gyrA* and *gyrB*) are implicated in many but not all cases of clinical resistance to fluoroquinolones.

Capreomycin

Capreomycin, a cyclic peptide antibiotic derived from *Streptomyces capreolus*, is an important second-line agent used for treatment of MDR-TB, particularly when additional resistance to aminoglycosides is documented. Capreomycin is administered by the IM route; an inhaled preparation is under study. A dose of 15 mg/kg per day is given five to seven times per week (maximal daily dose, 1 g) and results in peak blood levels of 20–40 μg/mL. The dosage may be reduced to 1 g two or three times per week 2–4 months after mycobacterial cultures become negative. For individuals ≥60 years of age, the dose should be reduced to 10 mg/kg per day (maximal daily dose, 750 mg). For patients with renal insufficiency, the drug should be given intermittently and at lower dosage (12–15 mg/kg two or three times per week). A minimal duration of 3 months is recommended for MDR-TB treatment. Penetration of capreomycin into the CSF is believed to be poor.

The mechanism of capreomycin's action is not well understood but involves interference with the mycobacterial ribosome and inhibition of protein synthesis. Resistance to capreomycin is associated

with mutations that inactivate a ribosomal methylase (TlyA) or that encode genes for the 16S ribosomal subunit (*rrs*). Cross-resistance to kanamycin and amikacin is common. However, some strains that are resistant to streptomycin, kanamycin, and amikacin generally remain susceptible to capreomycin.

Adverse effects of capreomycin are relatively common. Significant hypokalemia and hypomagnesemia as well as oto- and renal toxicity have been reported.

Amikacin and kanamycin

Amikacin and kanamycin are aminoglycosides that exert mycobactericidal activity by binding to the 16S ribosomal subunit. The spectrum of antibiotic activity for amikacin and kanamycin includes *M. tuberculosis*, several NTM species, and aerobic gram-negative and gram-positive bacteria. Although amikacin is highly active against *M. tuberculosis*, it is used only infrequently because of its significant side effects. The usual daily adult dosage of both amikacin and kanamycin is 15–30 mg/kg given IM or IV (maximal daily dose, 1 g), with a reduction to 10 mg/kg for patients ≥60 years old. For patients with renal insufficiency, the dose and frequency should be reduced (12–15 mg/kg two or three times per week). Mycobacterial resistance is due to mutations in the genes encoding the 16S ribosomal RNA gene. Cross-resistance among kanamycin, amikacin, and capreomycin is common. Isolates resistant to streptomycin are frequently susceptible to amikacin or kanamycin. Adverse effects of amikacin include ototoxicity (in up to 10% of recipients, with auditory dysfunction occurring more commonly than vestibulotoxicity), nephrotoxicity, and neurotoxicity. Kanamycin has a similar side-effects profile, but adverse reactions are thought to be less frequent and less severe.

Ethionamide

Ethionamide is a derivative of isonicotinic acid. Its mechanism of action is through inhibition of the *inhA* gene product enoyl–acyl carrier protein (acp) reductase, which is involved in mycolic acid synthesis. Ethionamide is bacteriostatic against metabolically active *M. tuberculosis* and some NTM. It is used in the treatment of drug-resistant TB, but its use is limited by severe gastrointestinal reactions (including abdominal pain, nausea, and vomiting) as well as significant central and peripheral neurologic side effects, reversible hepatitis (in ~5% of recipients), hypersensitivity reactions, and hypothyroidism. Ethionamide should be taken with food to reduce gastrointestinal effects and with pyridoxine (50–100 mg/d) to limit neuropathic side effects.

Para-aminosalicylic acid

Para-aminosalicylic acid (PAS, 4-aminosalicylic acid) is an oral agent used in the treatment of MDR- and XDR-TB. Its bacteriostatic activity is due to inhibition of folate synthesis and of iron uptake. PAS has relatively little activity as an anti-tuberculous agent, with a high level nausea, vomiting, and diarrhea. PAS may cause hemolysis in patients with glucose-6-phosphate dehydrogenase deficiency. The drug should be taken with acidic foods to improve absorption. Enteric-coated PAS granules (4 g orally every 8 h) appear to be better tolerated than other formulations and produce higher therapeutic blood levels. PAS has a short half-life (1 h), and 80% of the dose is excreted in the urine.

Cycloserine

Cycloserine is an analog of the amino acid D-alanine and prevents cell wall synthesis. It inhibits the action of enzymes, including alanine racemase, that are involved in the production of peptidoglycans. Cycloserine is active against a range of bacteria, including *M. tuberculosis*. Mechanisms of mycobacterial resistance are not well understood, but overexpression of alanine racemase can confer resistance in *M. smegmatis*. Cycloserine is well absorbed after oral administration and is widely distributed throughout body fluids, including CSF. The usual adult dosage is 250 mg two or three times per day. Serious potential side effects include seizures and psychosis (with suicide in some cases), peripheral neuropathy, headache, somnolence, and allergic reactions. Drug levels are monitored to achieve optimal dosing and to reduce the risk of adverse effects, especially in patients with renal failure. Cycloserine should be administered as DOT only with caution and with support from experienced TB physicians to patients with epilepsy, active alcohol abuse, severe renal insufficiency, or a history of depression or psychosis.

■ NEWER ANTITUBERCULOSIS DRUGS IN CLINICAL TRIALS

Linezolid

Linezolid is an oxazolidinone used primarily for the treatment of drug-resistant gram-positive infections. However, this drug is active in vitro against *M. tuberculosis* and NTM. Several case series have suggested that linezolid may help clear organisms relatively rapidly when included in a regimen for the treatment of complex MDR- and XDR-TB. Linezolid's mechanism of action is disruption of protein synthesis by binding to the 50S bacterial ribosome. Linezolid has nearly 100% oral bioavailability, with good penetration into tissues and fluids, including CSF. Clinical drug resistance to linezolid has been reported, but the mechanism is unclear. Adverse effects may include optic and peripheral neuropathy, pancytopenia, and lactic acidosis. Linezolid is a weak MAO inhibitor and can be associated with the serotonin syndrome when given concomitantly with serotonergic drugs (primarily antidepressants such as selective serotonin reuptake inhibitors). Prolonged administration for TB and other mycobacterial infections may be associated with an increased rate of side effects.

TMC207

TMC207 is a new diarylquinoline with a novel mechanism of action: inhibition of the mycobacterial ATP synthetase proton pump. TMC207 is bactericidal for drug-susceptible and MDR strains of *M. tuberculosis*. Resistance has been reported and is due to point mutations in the gene coding for the ATP synthetase proton pump. A phase 2 randomized controlled clinical trial demonstrated substantial improvement in rates of 2-month culture conversion, with improved clearance of mycobacterial cultures, for MDR-TB patients. This drug is metabolized by the hepatic cytochrome CYP3A4. Rifampin lowers TMC207 levels by 50%, and protease inhibitors also interact significantly with this drug. The oral bioavailability of TMC207 appears to be excellent. The dosage is 400 mg/d for the first 2 weeks and then 200 mg thrice weekly. The elimination half-life is long (>14 days). Adverse effects are reported to be minimal, with nausea and slight prolongation of the QT_c interval.

OPC-67683 and PA 824

The prodrugs OPC-67683 and PA 824 are novel nitro-dihydro-imidazooxazole derivatives whose antimycobacterial activity is attributable to inhibition of mycolic acid biosynthesis. Early clinical trials of these compounds are ongoing.

NONTUBERCULOUS MYCOBACTERIA

More than 150 species of NTM have been identified. Only a minority of these environmental organisms, which extensive are found in soil and water, are important human pathogens. NTM cause extensive disease primarily in persons with preexisting

pulmonary disease or immunocompromise but can cause nodular/bronchiectatic disease in otherwise seemingly normal hosts. They are also important causes of infections in surgical settings. Two major classes of NTM are the slow-growing and rapidly growing species. Subcultures of the latter grow within 1 week. The growth characteristics of NTM have diagnostic, thapeutic, and prognostic implications. The rate of growth can provide useful preliminary information within a specific clinical context, in that growth within 2 -3 weeks is much more likely to indicate an NTM than *M. tuberculosis*. When NTM do grow from cultures, colonization should be distinguished from active disease in order to optimize the risk and benefit of prolonged treatment with multiple medications. Significant clinical manifestations and/or sputum radiographic evidence of progressive disease consistent with NTM as well as either reproducible sputum culture results or a single positive culture are required to diagnose NTM pulmonary disease, according to the recommendations of the American Thoracic Society and the Infectious Diseases Society of America. Isolation of NTM from blood or from an infected-appearing extrapulmonary site, such as soft tissue or bone, is usually indicative of disseminated or local NTM infection (see Chap. 167). Treatment of NTM disease is prolonged and requires multiple medications. Side effects of the regimens employed are common, and intermittent therapy is often used to mitigate these adverse events. Treatment regimens depend on the NTM species, the extent or type of disease, and—to some degree—drug susceptibility test results. The nodular bronchiectatic form of MAC infection is generally treated three times per week, whereas fibrocavitary or disseminated MAC infection is treated daily.

■ THERAPEUTIC CONSIDERATIONS FOR SPECIFIC NTM

M. avium complex

Among the NTM, MAC organisms most commonly cause human disease. In immunocompetent hosts, MAC species are most often found in conjunction with underlying significant lung disease, such as chronic obstructive pulmonary disease or bronchiectasis. For patients with nodular or bronchiectatic MAC lung disease, a initial regimen consisting of clarithromycin or azithromycin, is testing or rifabutin, and ethambutol is (i.e., with cultures persistently positive for NTM). given three times per week. Routine initial testing for macrolide resistance is recommended, as is testing at 6 months in a failing regimens (i.e., with cultures persistently positive for NTM).

In immunocompromised individuals, disseminated MAC infection is generally treated with clarithromycin, ethambutol, and rifabutin. Azithromycin may be substituted in patients unable to tolerate clarithromycin. Amikacin and fluoroquinolones are often used in salvage regimens. Treatment for disseminated MAC infection in AIDS patients may be lifelong in the absence of immune reconstitution. At least 12 months of MAC therapy and 6 months of effective immune reconstitution may be adequate.

Mycobacterium kansasii

M. kansasii is the second most common NTM causing human disease. It is also the second most common cause of NTM pulmonary disease in the United States, where most commonly reported in southeast region. *M. kansasii* infection can be treated with isoniazid, rifampin, and ethambutol; therapy continues for 12 months after culture conversion. Rifampin-resistant *M. kansasii* has been treated with clarithromycin, trimethoprim-sulfamethoxazole, and streptomycin.

Rapidly growing mycobacteria

Rapidly growing mycobacteria causing human disease include *M. abscessus*, *M. fortuitum*, and *M. chelonae*. Treatment of these mycobacteria is complex and should be undertaken with input from experienced clinicians. Testing for macrolide resistance is recommended. However, in rapidly growing mycobacteria, an inducible *erm* gene may confer in vivo macrolide resistance to isolates that are susceptible in vitro.

Mycobacterium marinum

M. marinum is an NTM found in salt water and freshwater, including swimming pools and fish tanks. It is a cause of localized soft tissue infections, which may require surgical management. Combination regimens include clarithromycin and either ethambutol or rifampin. Other agents with activity against *M. marinum* include doxycycline, minocycline, and trimethoprim-sulfamethoxazole.

■ DRUGS FOR THE TREATMENT OF NTM

Clarithromycin

Clarithromycin is a macrolide antibiotic with broad activity against many gram-positive and gram-negative bacteria as well as NTM. This drug is active against MAC organisms and many other NTM species, inhibiting protein synthesis by binding to the 50S mycobacterial ribosomal subunit. NTM resistance to macrolides is probably caused by overexpression of the gene *ermB*, with consequent methylation of the binding site. Clarithromycin is well absorbed orally and distributes well to tissues. It is cleared both hepatically and renally; the dosage should be reduced in renal insufficiency. Clarithromycin is a substrate for and inhibits cytochrome 3A4 and should not be administered with cisapride, pimozide, or terfenadine, as cardiac arrhythmias may occur. Numerous drugs interact with clarithromycin through the CYP3A4 metabolic pathway. Rifampin lowers clarithromycin levels; conversely, rifampin levels are increased by clarithromycin. However, the clinical relevance of this interaction does not appear to be prominent.

For patients with nodular/bronchiectatic MAC infection, the dosage of clarithromycin is 500 mg, given morning and evening, three times a week. For the treatment of fibrocavitary or severe nodular/bronchiectatic MAC infection, a dose of 500–1000 mg is given daily. Disseminated MAC infection is treated with 1000 mg daily. Clarithromycin is used in combination regimens that typically include ethambutol and a rifamycin in order to avoid the development of macrolide resistance. Adverse effects include frequent gastrointestinal intolerance, hepatotoxicity, headache, rash, and rare instances of hypoglycemia. Clarithromycin is contraindicated during pregnancy because of its teratogenicity in animal models.

Azithromycin

Azithromycin is a derivative of erythromycin. Although technically an azalide and not a macrolide, it works similarly to macrolides, inhibiting protein synthesis through binding to the 50S ribosomal subunit. Resistance to azithromycin is almost always associated with complete cross-resistance to clarithromycin. Azithromycin is well absorbed orally, with good tissue penetration and a prolonged half-life (~48 h). The usual dosage for treatment of MAC infection is 250 mg daily or 500 mg three times per week. Azithromycin is used in combination with other agents to avoid development of resistance.

For prophylaxis against disseminated MAC infection in immuno-compromised individuals, a dose of 1200 mg once per week is given. Because azithromycin is not metabolized by cytochrome P450, it interacts with few drugs. Adjustment of the dosage on the basis of renal function is not necessary.

Cefoxitin

Cefoxitin is a second-generation parenteral cephalosporin with activity against rapidly growing NTM, particularly *M. abscessus, M. marinum,* and *M. chelonae*. Its mechanism of action against NTM is unknown but may involve inactivation of cell wall synthesis enzymes. High doses are used for treatment of NTM: 200 mg/kg IV three or four times per day, with a maximal daily dose of 12 g. The half-life of cefoxitin is ~1 h, with primarily renal clearance that requires adjustment in renal insufficiency. Adverse effects are uncommon but include gastrointestinal manifestations, rash, eosinophilia, fever, and neutropenia.

CONCLUSION

Treatment of mycobacterial infections requires multiple-drug regimens that often exert significant side effects with the potential to limit tolerability. The prolonged duration of treatment has vastly improved results over those obtained in decades past, but drugs and regimens that will shorten treatment duration and limit adverse drug effects and interactions are needed.

FURTHER READINGS

ABDOOL KARIM SS et al: Timing of initiation of antiretroviral drugs during tuberculosis therapy. N Engl J Med 372:697, 2010

AMERICAN THORACIC SOCIETY/CENTERS FOR DISEASE CONTROL AND PREVENTION/INFECTIOUS DISEASES SOCIETY OF AMERICA: Treatment of tuberculosis. Am J Respir Crit Care Med 167:603, 2003

CROFTON J, MITCHISON DA: Streptomycin resistance in pulmonary tuberculosis. BMJ 2:1009, 1948

DIACON AH et al: The diarylquinoline TMC207 for multidrug-resistant tuberculosis. N Engl J Med 360:2397, 2009

GRIFFITH D et al: An official ATS/IDSA statement: Diagnosis, treatment, and prevention of non-tuberculous mycobacterial diseases. Am J Respir Crit Care Med 175:367, 2007

MENZIES D et al: Adverse events with 4 months of rifampin therapy or 9 months of isoniazid therapy for latent tuberculosis infection: A randomized trial. Ann Intern Med 149:689, 2008

MITNICK C et al: Comprehensive treatment of extensively drug-resistant tuberculosis. N Engl J Med 359:563, 2008

SAUKKONEN JJ et al: An official ATS statement: Hepatotoxicity of antituberculosis therapy. Am J Respir Crit Care Med 174:935, 2006

WORLD HEALTH ORGANIZATION: Anti-tuberculosis drug resistance in the world. Report No. 4. Geneva, WHO, 2008

YEW WW et al: Outcomes of patients with multidrug-resistant pulmonary tuberculosis treated with ofloxacin/levofloxacin-containing regimens. Chest 117:744, 2000

CHAPTER 169

Syphilis

Sheila A. Lukehart

DEFINITION

Syphilis, a chronic systemic infection caused by *Treponema pallidum* subspecies *pallidum*, is usually sexually transmitted and is characterized by episodes of active disease interrupted by periods of latency. After an incubation period averaging 2–6 weeks, a primary lesion appears, often associated with regional lymphadenopathy. The secondary stage, associated with generalized mucocutaneous lesions and generalized lymphadenopathy, is followed by a latent period of subclinical infection lasting years or decades. Central nervous system (CNS) involvement may occur early in infection and may be symptomatic or asymptomatic. In about one-third of untreated cases, the tertiary stage appears, characterized by progressive destructive mucocutaneous, musculoskeletal, or parenchymal lesions; aortitis; or late CNS manifestations.

ETIOLOGY

The Spirochaetales include four genera that are pathogenic for humans and for a variety of other animals: *Leptospira* species, which cause leptospirosis (Chap. 171); *Borrelia* species, which cause relapsing fever and Lyme disease (Chaps. 172 and 173); *Brachyspira* species, which cause intestinal infections; and *Treponema* species, which cause the diseases known collectively as treponematoses (see also Chap. 170). The *Treponema* species include *T. pallidum* subspecies *pallidum*, which causes venereal syphilis; *T. pallidum* subspecies *pertenue*, which causes yaws; *T. pallidum* subspecies *endemicum*, which causes endemic syphilis or bejel; and *T. carateum*, which causes pinta. Until recently, the subspecies were distinguished primarily by the clinical syndromes they produce. Researchers have now identified molecular signatures that can differentiate the three subspecies of *T. pallidum* by culture-independent methods based on polymerase chain reaction (PCR). Other *Treponema* species found in the human mouth, genital mucosa, and gastrointestinal tract have been associated with disease (e.g., periodontitis), but their role as primary etiologic agents is unclear.

T. pallidum subspecies *pallidum* (referred to hereafter as *T. pallidum*), a thin spiral organism, has a cell body surrounded by a trilaminar cytoplasmic membrane, a delicate peptidoglycan layer providing some structural rigidity, and a lipid-rich outer membrane containing relatively few integral membrane proteins. Endoflagella wind around the cell body in the periplasmic space and are responsible for motility.

T. pallidum cannot be cultured in vitro, and little was known about its metabolism until the genome was sequenced in 1998. This spirochete possesses severely limited metabolic capabilities, lacking the genes required for de novo synthesis of most amino acids, nucleotides, and lipids. In addition, *T. pallidum* lacks genes encoding the enzymes of the Krebs cycle and oxidative phosphorylation. To compensate, the organism contains numerous genes predicted to encode transporters of amino acids, carbohydrates, and cations. In addition, genome analyses and other studies have revealed the existence of a 12-member gene family (*tpr*) that bears similarities to variable outer-membrane antigens of other spirochetes. One member, TprK, has discrete variable (V) regions that undergo antigenic variation during infection, probably as a mechanism for immune evasion.

The only known natural host for *T. pallidum* is the human. *T. pallidum* can infect many mammals, but only humans, higher apes, and a few laboratory animals regularly develop syphilitic lesions. Virulent strains of *T. pallidum* are grown in rabbits.

TRANSMISSION AND EPIDEMIOLOGY

Nearly all cases of syphilis are acquired by sexual contact with infectious lesions [i.e., the chancre, mucous patch, skin rash, or condylomata lata (see Fig. e7-20)]. Less common modes of transmission include nonsexual personal contact, infection in utero, blood transfusion, and organ transplantation.

■ SYPHILIS IN THE UNITED STATES

With the advent of penicillin therapy, the total number of cases of syphilis reported annually in the United States declined significantly to a low of 31,575 in 2000—a 95% decrease from 1943—with <6000 reported cases of primary and secondary syphilis. Since 2000, the number of cases of infectious primary and secondary syphilis (a better indicator of disease activity) has more than doubled, with 13,500 cases reported in 2008. These cases have particularly affected men who have sex with men (MSM), many of whom are co-infected with HIV. This outbreak among MSM is occurring throughout North America. Increases in the number of cases among women in the United States in recent years indicate that heterosexual transmission is becoming more common. Surveillance of the number of new cases of primary and secondary syphilis has revealed multiple cycles of 7–10 years, which have been attributed to herd immunity in at-risk populations. A recent re-analysis of the data, however, fails to support this conclusion and proposes alternative explanations for the periodic rise and fall of infectious syphilis cases, including changing sexual behaviors and control efforts.

The populations at highest risk for acquiring syphilis have changed over time, with outbreaks among MSM in the late 1970s and early 1980s as well as at present. The epidemic that peaked in 1990 predominantly involved African-American heterosexual men and women and occurred largely in urban areas, where infectious syphilis was correlated significantly with the exchange of sex for crack cocaine. Although the rate of primary and secandary syphilis among African Americans declined from 1996 through 2003, the rate has nearly doubled since then and remains higher than rates for other racial/ethnic groups.

The incidence of congenital syphilis roughly parallels that of infectious syphilis in females. In 2008, 431 cases in infants <1 year of age were reported. The case definition for congenital syphilis was broadened in 1989 and now includes all live or stillborn infants delivered to women with untreated or inadequately treated syphilis.

One-third to one-half of individuals named as sexual contacts of persons with infectious syphilis become infected. Many will have already developed manifestations of syphilis when they are first seen, and ~30% of asymptomatic contacts examined within 30 days

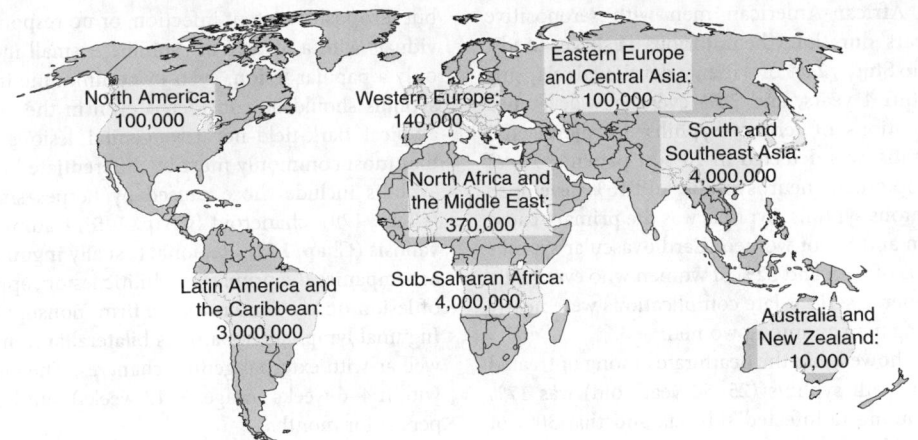

Figure 169-1 Estimated annual new cases of syphilis among adults, 1999. *(Courtesy of the World Health Organization.)*

of exposure actually have incubating infection and will later develop infectious syphilis if not treated. Thus, identification and treatment of all recently exposed sexual contacts continue to be important aspects of syphilis control.

■ GLOBAL SYPHILIS

Syphilis remains a significant health problem globally; the number of new infections is estimated at nearly 12 million per year. The regions that are most affected include sub-Saharan Africa, South America, China, and Southeast Asia (Fig. 169-1). During the past decade, the number of reported cases in China has increased 10-fold, and higher rates have been reported among MSM in many European countries. Worldwide, congenital syphilis has been reported to account for up to 50% of stillbirths, and between 500,000 and 1.5 million cases of congenital syphilis are estimated to occur annually.

NATURAL COURSE AND PATHOGENESIS OF UNTREATED SYPHILIS

T. pallidum rapidly penetrates intact mucous membranes or microscopic abrasions in skin and, within a few hours, enters the lymphatics and blood to produce systemic infection and metastatic foci long before the appearance of a primary lesion. Blood from a patient with incubating or early syphilis is infectious. The generation time of *T. pallidum* during early active disease in vivo is estimated to be ~30 h, and the incubation period of syphilis is inversely proportional to the number of organisms inoculated. The 50% infectious dose for intradermal inoculation in humans has been calculated to be 57 organisms, and the treponeme concentration generally reaches 10^7/g of tissue before a clinical lesion appears. The median incubation period in humans (~21 days) suggests an average inoculum of 500–1000 infectious organisms for naturally acquired disease; the incubation period rarely exceeds 6 weeks.

The primary lesion appears at the site of inoculation, usually persists for 4–6 weeks, and then heals spontaneously. Histopathologic examination shows perivascular infiltration, chiefly by CD4+ and CD8+ T lymphocytes, plasma cells, and macrophages, with capillary endothelial proliferation and subsequent obliteration of small blood vessels. The cellular infiltration displays a T_H1-type cytokine profile consistent with the activation of macrophages. Phagocytosis of opsonized organisms by activated macrophages ultimately causes their destruction, resulting in spontaneous resolution of the chancre.

The generalized parenchymal, constitutional, and mucocutaneous manifestations of secondary syphilis usually appear ~6–8 weeks after the chancre heals. Approximately 15% of patients with secondary syphilis still have persisting or healing chancres, and the stages may overlap more frequently in persons with concurrent HIV infection. In other patients, secondary lesions may appear several months after the chancre has healed, and some patients may enter the latent stage without ever recognizing secondary lesions. The histopathologic features of secondary maculopapular skin lesions include hyperkeratosis of the epidermis, capillary proliferation with endothelial swelling in the superficial corium, dermal papillae with transmigration of polymorphonuclear leukocytes, and—in the deeper corium—perivascular infiltration by CD8+ T lymphocytes, CD4+ T lymphocytes, macrophages, and plasma cells. Treponemes are found in many tissues, including the aqueous humor of the eye and the cerebrospinal fluid (CSF). Invasion of the CNS by *T. pallidum* occurs during the first weeks or months of infection, and CSF abnormalities are detected in as many as 40% of patients during the secondary stage. Clinical hepatitis and immune complex–induced glomerulonephritis are relatively rare but recognized manifestations of secondary syphilis; liver function tests may yield abnormal results in up to one-quarter of patients with early syphilis. Generalized nontender lymphadenopathy is noted in 85% of patients with secondary syphilis. The paradoxical appearance of secondary manifestations despite high titers of antibody (including immobilizing antibody) to *T. pallidum* may result from antigenic variation or changes in expression of surface antigens. Secondary lesions subside within 2–6 weeks, and the infection enters the latent stage, which is detectable only by serologic testing. In the preantibiotic era, up to 25% of untreated patients experienced at least one generalized or localized mucocutaneous relapse, usually during the first year. Therefore, identification and examination of sexual contacts are most important for patients with syphilis of <1 year's duration.

About one-third of patients with untreated latent syphilis developed clinically apparent tertiary disease in the preantibiotic era. In industrialized countries today, specific treatment for early and latent syphilis and coincidental therapy have nearly eliminated tertiary disease except for cases of neurosyphilis in HIV-infected persons. In the past, the most common types of tertiary disease were the gumma (a usually benign granulomatous lesion), cardiovascular syphilis (usually involving the vasa vasorum of the ascending aorta and resulting in aneurysm), and late symptomatic neurosyphilis (tabes dorsalis and paresis). Asymptomatic CNS involvement, however, is still demonstrable in up to 25% of patients with late latent syphilis. The factors that contribute to the development and progression of tertiary disease are unknown.

The course of untreated syphilis was studied retrospectively in a group of nearly 2000 patients with primary or secondary disease diagnosed clinically (the Oslo Study, 1891–1951) and was assessed prospectively in 431 African-American men with seropositive latent syphilis of ≥3 years' duration (the notorious Tuskegee Study, 1932–1972). In the Oslo Study, 24% of patients developed relapsing secondary lesions within 4 years, and 28% eventually developed one or more manifestations of tertiary syphilis. Cardiovascular syphilis, including aortitis, was detected in 10% of patients; 7% of patients developed symptomatic neurosyphilis, and 16% developed benign tertiary gummatous syphilis. Syphilis was the primary cause of death in 15% of men and 8% of women. Cardiovascular syphilis was documented in 35% of men and 22% of women who eventually came to autopsy. In general, serious late complications were nearly twice as common among men as among women.

The Tuskegee Study showed that the death rate among untreated African-American men with syphilis (25–50 years old) was 17% higher than the rate among uninfected subjects and that 30% of all deaths were attributable to cardiovascular or, to a lesser extent, CNS syphilis. Anatomic evidence of aortitis was found in 40–60% of autopsied subjects with syphilis (vs. 15% of control subjects), whereas CNS syphilis was found in only 4%. Rates of hypertension were also higher among the infected subjects. The ethical issues eventually raised by this study, begun in the preantibiotic era but continuing into the early 1970s, had a major influence on the development of current guidelines for human medical experimentation, and the history of the study may still contribute to a reluctance of some African Americans to participate as subjects in clinical research.

CLINICAL MANIFESTATIONS

Primary syphilis

The typical primary chancre usually begins as a single painless papule that rapidly becomes eroded and usually becomes indurated, with a characteristic cartilaginous consistency on palpation of the edge and base of the ulcer. Multiple primary lesions are seen in a minority of patients. In heterosexual men the chancre is usually located on the penis (Fig. 169-2), whereas in homosexual men it may be found in the anal canal or rectum, in the mouth, or on the external genitalia. In women, common primary sites are the cervix and labia. Consequently, primary syphilis goes unrecognized in women and homosexual men more often than in heterosexual men.

Atypical primary lesions are common. The clinical appearance depends on the number of treponemes inoculated and on the immunologic status of the patient. A large inoculum produces a dark-field-positive ulcerative lesion in nonimmune volunteers but may produce a small dark-field-negative papule, an asymptomatic

but seropositive latent infection, or no response at all in some individuals with a history of syphilis. A small inoculum may produce only a papular lesion, even in nonimmune individuals. Therefore, syphilis should be considered even in the evaluation of trivial or atypical dark-field-negative genital lesions. The genital lesions that most commonly must be differentiated from those of primary syphilis include those caused by herpes simplex virus infection (Chap. 179), chancroid (Chap. 145), traumatic injury, and donovanosis (Chap. 161). Regional (usually inguinal) lymphadenopathy accompanies the primary syphilitic lesion, appearing within 1 week of lesion onset. The nodes are firm, nonsuppurative, and painless. Inguinal lymphadenopathy is bilateral and may occur with anal as well as with external genital chancres. The chancre generally heals within 4–6 weeks (range, 2–12 weeks), but lymphadenopathy may persist for months.

Secondary syphilis

The protean manifestations of the secondary stage usually include mucocutaneous lesions and generalized nontender lymphadenopathy. The healing primary chancre may still be present in ~15% of cases, and the stages may overlap more frequently in persons with concurrent HIV infection. The skin rash consists of macular, papular, papulosquamous, and occasionally pustular syphilides; often more than one form is present simultaneously. The eruption may be very subtle, and 25% of patients with a discernible rash may be unaware that they have dermatologic manifestations. Initial lesions are pale red or pink, nonpruritic, discrete macules distributed on the trunk and proximal extremities; these macules progress to papular lesions that are distributed widely and that frequently involve the palms and soles (Fig. 169-3; see also Figs. e7-18 and e7-19). Rarely, severe necrotic lesions (lues maligna) may appear; they are more commonly reported in HIV-infected individuals. Involvement of the hair follicles may result in patchy alopecia of the scalp hair, eyebrows, or beard in up to 5% of cases.

In warm, moist, intertriginous areas (commonly the perianal region, vulva, and scrotum), papules can enlarge to produce broad, moist, pink or gray-white, highly infectious lesions [condylomata lata (see Fig. e7-20)] in 10% of patients with secondary syphilis. Superficial mucosal erosions (mucous patches) occur in 10–15% of patients and commonly involve the oral or genital mucosa. The typical mucous patch is a painless silver-gray erosion surrounded by a red periphery.

Constitutional symptoms that may accompany or precede secondary syphilis include sore throat (15–30%), fever (5–8%), weight loss (2–20%), malaise (25%), anorexia (2–10%), headache (10%), and meningismus (5%). Acute meningitis occurs in only 1–2% of cases, but CSF cell and protein concentrations are increased in up to 40% of cases, and T. pallidum has been recovered from CSF during primary and secondary syphilis in 30% of cases; the latter finding is often but not always associated with other CSF abnormalities.

Less common complications of secondary syphilis include hepatitis, nephropathy, gastrointestinal involvement (hypertrophic gastritis, patchy proctitis, or a rectosigmoid mass), arthritis, and periostitis. Ocular findings that suggest secondary syphilis include pupillary abnormalities and optic neuritis as well as the classic iritis or uveitis. The diagnosis of secondary syphilis is often considered in affected patients only after they fail to respond to steroid therapy. Anterior uveitis has been reported in 5–10% of patients with secondary syphilis, and T. pallidum has been demonstrated in aqueous humor from such patients. Hepatic involvement is common in syphilis; although usually asymptomatic, up to 25% of patients may have abnormal liver function tests. Frank syphilitic hepatitis may be seen. Renal involvement usually results from immune complex deposition and produces proteinuria associated with an acute

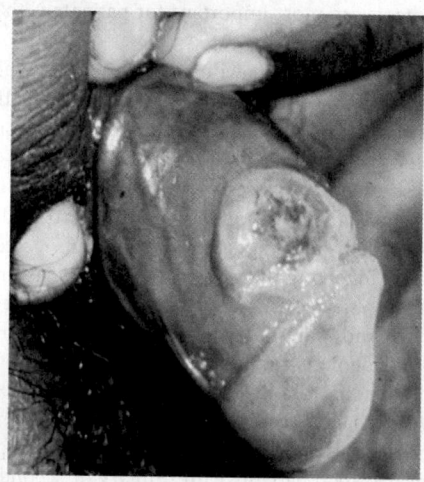

Figure 169-2 Primary syphilis with a firm, nontender chancre.

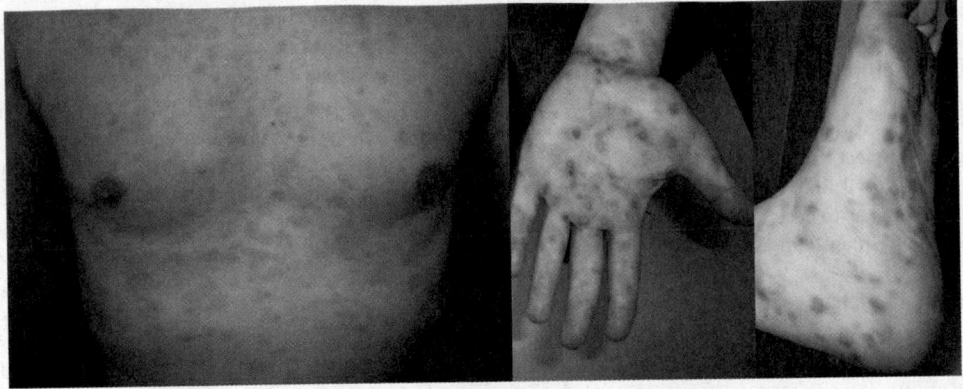

Figure 169-3   Secondary syphilis. *Left:* Maculopapular truncal eruption. *Middle:* Papules on the palms. *Right:* Papules on the soles. *(Courtesy of Jill McKenzie and Christina Marra.)*

nephrotic syndrome. Like those of primary syphilis, the manifestations of the secondary stage resolve spontaneously, usually within 1–6 months.

Latent syphilis

Positive serologic tests for syphilis, together with a normal CSF examination and the absence of clinical manifestations of syphilis, indicate a diagnosis of latent syphilis in an untreated person. The diagnosis is often suspected on the basis of a history of primary or secondary lesions, a history of exposure to syphilis, or the delivery of an infant with congenital syphilis. A previous negative serologic test or a history of lesions or exposure may help establish the duration of latent infection, which is an important factor in the selection of appropriate therapy. *Early latent* syphilis is limited to the first year after infection, whereas *late latent* syphilis is defined as that of ≥1 year's (or unknown) duration. *T. pallidum* may still seed the bloodstream intermittently during the latent stage, and pregnant women with latent syphilis may infect the fetus in utero. Moreover, syphilis has been transmitted through blood transfusion or organ donation from patients with latent syphilis. It was previously thought that untreated late latent syphilis had three possible outcomes: (1) persistent lifelong infection; (2) development of late syphilis; or (3) spontaneous cure, with reversion of serologic tests to negative. It is now apparent, however, that the more sensitive treponemal antibody tests rarely, if ever, become negative without treatment. Although progression to clinically evident late syphilis is very rare today, the occurrence of spontaneous cure is in doubt.

Involvement of the CNS

Traditionally, neurosyphilis has been considered a late manifestation of syphilis, but this view is inaccurate. CNS syphilis represents a continuum encompassing early invasion (usually within the first weeks or months of infection), months to years of asymptomatic involvement, and, in some cases, development of early or late neurologic manifestations.

Asymptomatic neurosyphilis   The diagnosis of asymptomatic neurosyphilis is made in patients who lack neurologic symptoms and signs but who have CSF abnormalities including mononuclear pleocytosis, increased protein concentrations, or CSF reactivity in the Venereal Disease Research Laboratory test. CSF abnormalities are demonstrated in up to 40% of cases of primary or secondary syphilis and in 25% of cases of latent syphilis. *T. pallidum* has been recovered by CSF inoculation into rabbits from up to 30% of patients with primary or secondary syphilis but rarely from those with latent syphilis. The presence of *T. pallidum* in CSF is often associated with other CSF abnormalities, but organisms can be recovered from patients

with otherwise-normal CSF. Although the prognostic implications of these findings in early syphilis are uncertain, it may be appropriate to conclude that even patients with early syphilis who have such findings do indeed have asymptomatic neurosyphilis and should be treated for neurosyphilis; such treatment is particularly important in patients with concurrent HIV infection. Before the advent of penicillin, the risk of development of clinical neurosyphilis in untreated asymptomatic persons was roughly proportional to the intensity of CSF changes, with the overall cumulative probability of progression to clinical neurosyphilis ~20% in the first 10 years but increasing with time. Most experts agree that neurosyphilis is more common in HIV-infected persons, while immunocompetent patients with untreated latent syphilis and normal CSF probably run a very low risk of subsequent neurosyphilis. In several recent studies, neurosyphilis was associated with a rapid plasma reagin titer of ≥1:32, regardless of clinical stage or HIV infection status.

Symptomatic neurosyphilis   The major clinical categories of symptomatic neurosyphilis include meningeal, meningovascular, and parenchymatous syphilis. The last category includes general paresis and tabes dorsalis. The onset of symptoms usually occurs <1 year after infection for meningeal syphilis, up to 10 years after infection for meningovascular syphilis, at ~20 years for general paresis, and at 25–30 years for tabes dorsalis. However, symptomatic neurosyphilis, particularly in the antibiotic era, often presents not as a classic picture but rather as mixed and subtle or incomplete syndromes.

Meningeal syphilis may present as headache, nausea, vomiting, neck stiffness, cranial nerve involvement, seizures, and changes in mental status. This condition may be concurrent with or may follow the secondary stage. Patients presenting with uveitis, iritis, or hearing loss often have meningeal syphilis, but these clinical findings can also be seen in patients with normal CSF.

Meningovascular syphilis reflects meningitis together with inflammatory vasculitis of small, medium, or large vessels. The most common presentation is a stroke syndrome involving the middle cerebral artery of a relatively young adult. However, unlike the usual thrombotic or embolic stroke syndrome of sudden onset, meningovascular syphilis often becomes manifest after a subacute encephalitic prodrome (with headaches, vertigo, insomnia, and psychological abnormalities), which is followed by a gradually progressive vascular syndrome.

The manifestations of *general paresis* reflect widespread late parenchymal damage and include abnormalities corresponding to the mnemonic *paresis:* personality, affect, reflexes (hyperactive), eye (e.g., Argyll Robertson pupils), sensorium (illusions, delusions, hallucinations), intellect (a decrease in recent memory and in the capacity for orientation, calculations, judgment, and insight), and speech. *Tabes dorsalis* is a late manifestation of syphilis that presents as symptoms and signs of demyelination of the posterior columns, dorsal roots, and dorsal root ganglia. Symptoms include ataxic wide-based gait and foot drop; paresthesia; bladder disturbances; impotence; areflexia; and loss of positional, deep-pain, and temperature sensations. Trophic joint degeneration (Charcot's joints) and perforating ulceration of the feet can result from loss of pain sensation. The small, irregular Argyll Robertson pupil, a feature of both tabes dorsalis and paresis, reacts to accommodation but not to light. *Optic atrophy* also occurs frequently in association with tabes.

Other manifestations of late syphilis

The slowly progressive inflammatory disease leading to tertiary disease begins early during infection, although these manifestations may not become clinically apparent for years or decades. Early syphilitic aortitis becomes evident soon after secondary lesions subside, and treponemes that trigger the development of gummas may have seeded the tissue years earlier.

Cardiovascular syphilis Cardiovascular manifestations, usually appearing 10–40 years after infection, are attributable to endarteritis obliterans of the vasa vasorum, which provide the blood supply to large vessels; *T. pallidum* DNA has been detected by PCR in aortic tissue. Cardiovascular involvement results in uncomplicated aortitis, aortic regurgitation, saccular aneurysm (usually of the ascending aorta), or coronary ostial stenosis. In the preantibiotic era, symptomatic cardiovascular complications developed in ~10% of persons with late untreated syphilis, although syphilitic aortitis was demonstrated at autopsy in about one-half of African-American men with untreated syphilis. Today, this form of late syphilis is rarely seen in the developed world. Linear calcification of the ascending aorta on chest x-ray films suggests asymptomatic syphilitic aortitis, as arteriosclerosis seldom produces this sign. Syphilitic aneurysms—usually saccular, occasionally fusiform—do not lead to dissection. Only 1 in 10 aortic aneurysms of syphilitic origin involves the abdominal aorta.

Late benign syphilis (gumma) Gummas are usually solitary lesions ranging from microscopic to several centimeters in diameter. Histologic examination shows a granulomatous inflammation, with a central area of necrosis due to endarteritis obliterans. Although rarely demonstrated microscopically, *T. pallidum* has been detected by PCR or recovered from these lesions, and penicillin treatment results in rapid resolution, confirming the treponemal stimulus for the inflammation. Common sites include the skin and skeletal system; however, any organ (including the brain) may be involved. Gummas of the skin produce indolent, painless, indurated nodular or ulcerative lesions that may resemble other chronic granulomatous conditions, including tuberculosis, sarcoidosis, leprosy, and deep fungal infections. Skeletal gummas most frequently involve the long bones, although any bone may be affected. Upper respiratory gummas can lead to perforation of the nasal septum or palate.

Congenital syphilis

Transmission of *T. pallidum* across the placenta from a syphilitic woman to her fetus may occur at any stage of pregnancy, but fetal damage generally does not occur until after the fourth month of gestation, when fetal immunologic competence begins to develop. This timing suggests that the pathogenesis of congenital syphilis, like that of adult syphilis, depends on the host immune response rather than on a direct toxic effect of *T. pallidum*. The risk of fetal infection during untreated early maternal syphilis is ~75–95%, decreasing to ~35% for maternal syphilis of >2 years' duration. Adequate treatment of the woman before the 16th week of pregnancy should prevent fetal damage, and treatment before the third trimester should adequately treat the infected fetus. Untreated maternal infection may result in a rate of fetal loss of up to 40% (with stillbirth more common than abortion because of the late

onset of fetal pathology), prematurity, neonatal death, or nonfatal congenital syphilis. Among infants born alive, only fulminant congenital syphilis is clinically apparent at birth, and these babies have a very poor prognosis. The most common clinical problem is the healthy-appearing baby born to a mother with a positive serologic test. Routine serologic testing in early pregnancy is considered cost-effective in virtually all populations, even in areas with a low prenatal prevalence of syphilis. Low-tech point-of-care tests are being developed to facilitate antenatal testing in resource-poor settings. Where the prevalence of syphilis is high or when the patient is at high risk of re-infection, serologic testing should be repeated in the third trimester and at delivery. Neonatal congenital syphilis must be differentiated from other generalized congenital infections, including rubella, cytomegalovirus or herpes simplex virus infection, and toxoplasmosis, as well as from erythroblastosis fetalis.

The manifestations of congenital syphilis include (1) early manifestations, which appear within the first 2 years of life (often at 2–10 weeks of age), are infectious, and resemble the manifestations of secondary syphilis in the adult; (2) late manifestations, which appear after 2 years and are noninfectious; and (3) residual stigmata. The earliest manifestations of congenital syphilis (appearing 2–6 weeks after birth) include rhinitis, or "snuffles" (23%); mucocutaneous lesions (35–41%); bone changes (61%), including osteochondritis, osteitis, and periostitis detectable by x-ray examination of long bones; hepatosplenomegaly (50%); lymphadenopathy (32%); anemia (34%); jaundice (30%); thrombocytopenia; and leukocytosis. CNS invasion by *T. pallidum* is detectable in 22% of infected neonates. Neonatal death is usually due to pulmonary hemorrhage, secondary bacterial infection, or severe hepatitis.

Late congenital syphilis (untreated after 2 years of age) is subclinical in 60% of cases; the clinical spectrum in the remainder of cases may include interstitial keratitis (which occurs at 5–25 years of age), eighth-nerve deafness, and recurrent arthropathy. Bilateral knee effusions are known as *Clutton's joints*. Asymptomatic neurosyphilis is present in about one-third of untreated patients, and clinical neurosyphilis occurs in one-quarter of untreated individuals >6 years old. Gummatous periostitis occurs at 5–20 years of age and, as in nonvenereal endemic syphilis, tends to cause destructive lesions of the palate and nasal septum.

Classic stigmata include *Hutchinson's teeth* (centrally notched, widely spaced, peg-shaped upper central incisors), "mulberry" molars (sixth-year molars with multiple, poorly developed cusps), saddle nose, and saber shins.

LABORATORY EXAMINATIONS

Demonstration of the organism

T. pallidum cannot be detected by culture. Historically, dark-field microscopy and immunofluorescence antibody staining have been used to identify this spirochete in samples from moist lesions such as chancres or condylomata lata, but these tests are rarely available today outside of research laboratories. More sensitive PCR tests have been developed but are not commercially available, although some laboratories perform in-house PCR testing.

T. pallidum can be found in tissue with appropriate silver stains, but these results should be interpreted with caution because artifacts resembling *T. pallidum* are often seen. Tissue treponemes can be demonstrated more reliably in research laboratories by PCR or by immunofluorescence or immunohistochemical methods using specific monoclonal or polyclonal antibodies to *T. pallidum*.

Serologic tests for syphilis

There are two types of serologic test for syphilis: nontreponemal and treponemal. Both are reactive in persons with any treponemal infection, including yaws, pinta, and endemic syphilis.

The most widely used nontreponemal antibody tests for syphilis are the rapid plasma reagin (RPR) and Venereal Disease Research Laboratory (VDRL) tests, which measure IgG and IgM directed against a cardiolipin-lecithin-cholesterol antigen complex. The RPR test is easier to perform and uses unheated serum; it is the test of choice for rapid serologic diagnosis in a clinical setting and can be automated. The VDRL test remains the standard for examining CSF. The RPR and VDRL tests are recommended for screening or for quantitation of serum antibody. The titer reflects disease activity, rising during the evolution of early syphilis and often exceeding 1:32 in secondary syphilis. After therapy for early syphilis, a persistent fall by fourfold or more (e.g., a decline from 1:32 to 1:8) is considered an adequate response. VDRL titers do not correspond directly to RPR titers, and sequential quantitative testing (as for response to therapy) must employ a single test. As will be discussed (see "Evaluation for Neurosyphilis," below), the RPR titer may be useful in determining which patients will benefit from CSF examination.

Treponemal tests measure antibodies to native or recombinant *T. pallidum* antigens and include the fluorescent treponemal antibody–absorbed (FTA-ABS) test and the *T. pallidum* particle agglutination (TPPA) test, both of which are more sensitive for primary syphilis than the previously used hemagglutination tests. The *T. pallidum* hemagglutination (TPHA) test is widely used in Europe but is not available in the United States. When used to confirm positive nontreponemal test results, treponemal tests have a very high positive predictive value for diagnosis of syphilis. In a screening setting, however, these tests give false-positive results at rates as high as 1–2%. Treponemal tests are likely to remain reactive even after adequate treatment and cannot differentiate past from current *T. pallidum* infection.

Treponemal immunochromatographic strip (ICS) tests and enzyme immunoassays (EIAs), based largely on reactivity to recombinant antigens, have also been developed. Treponemal EIAs have been approved as confirmatory tests and, because of their ease of automation, are now used for screening purposes by some large laboratories. Because treponemal tests cannot distinguish between current and treated syphilis or may be falsely reactive, clinicians may be uncertain about how to interpret reactive EIA screening results. Figure 169-4 provides a suggested algorithm for management of such cases.

Considerable interest has recently been focused on point-of-care ICS tests that can be used in the field or in resource-poor settings. These treponemal tests are not yet approved for use in the United States but have been assessed in antenatal clinics in a number of developing countries.

Both nontreponemal and treponemal tests may be nonreactive in early primary syphilis, although treponemal tests are slightly more sensitive (85–90%) during this stage than nontreponemal tests (~80%). All tests are reactive during secondary syphilis. (Fewer than 1% of patients with high titers have a nontreponemal test that is nonreactive or weakly reactive with undiluted serum but is reactive with diluted serum—the *prozone phenomenon*.) VDRL and RPR sensitivity and titers may decline in untreated persons with late latent or late syphilis, but treponemal tests remain sensitive in these stages. Whereas nontreponemal test titers will decline or the tests will become nonreactive after therapy for early syphilis, treponemal tests often remain reactive after therapy and are not helpful in determining the infection status of persons with past syphilis.

For practical purposes, most clinicians need to be familiar with three uses of serologic tests for syphilis: (1) screening or diagnosis (RPR or VDRL), (2) quantitative measurement of antibody to assess clinical syphilis activity or to monitor response to therapy (RPR or VDRL), and (3) confirmation of a syphilis diagnosis in a patient with a reactive RPR or VDRL test (FTA-ABS, TPPA, EIA). Studies have

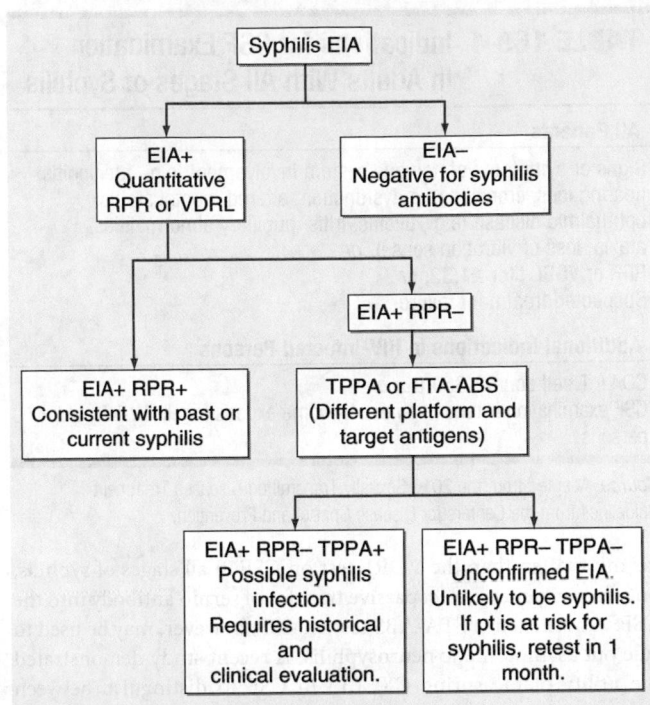

Figure 169-4 Algorithm for interpretation of results from syphilis enzyme immunoassays (EIAs) used for screening. RPR, rapid plasma reagin; VDRL, Venereal Disease Research Laboratory; TPPA, *T. pallidum* particle agglutination; FTA-ABS, fluorescent treponemal antibody–absorbed. (*Based on the 2010 Sexually Transmitted Diseases Treatment Guidelines from the Centers for Disease Control and Prevention.*)

not demonstrated the utility of IgM testing for adult syphilis. While IgM titers appear to decline after therapy, the presence or absence of specific IgM does not strictly correlate with *T. pallidum* infection. Moreover, no commercially available IgM test is recommended for evaluation of infants with suspected congenital syphilis.

False-positive serologic tests for syphilis

The lipid antigens of nontreponemal tests are similar to those found in human tissues, and the tests may be reactive (usually with titers ≤1:8) in persons without treponemal infection. Among patients being screened for syphilis because of risk factors, clinical suspicion, or history of exposure, ~1% of reactive tests are falsely positive. Modern VDRL and RPR tests are highly specific, and false-positive reactions are largely limited to persons with autoimmune conditions or injection drug use. The prevalence of false-positive results increases with advancing age, approaching 10% among persons >70 years old. In a patient with a false-positive nontreponemal test, syphilis is excluded by a nonreactive treponemal test.

Evaluation for neurosyphilis

Involvement of the CNS is detected by examination of CSF for pleocytosis (>5 white blood cells/μL), increased protein concentration (>45 mg/dL), or VDRL reactivity. Elevated CSF cell counts and protein concentrations are not specific for neurosyphilis and may be confounded by HIV co-infection. Because CSF pleocytosis may also be due to HIV, some studies have suggested using a CSF white-cell cutoff of 20 cells/μL as diagnostic of neurosyphilis in HIV-infected patients with syphilis. The CSF VDRL test is highly specific and, when reactive, is considered diagnostic of neurosyphilis; however, this test is insensitive and may be nonreactive even in cases of symptomatic neurosyphilis. The FTA-ABS test on CSF is reactive

TABLE 169-1 Indications for CSF Examination in Adults With All Stages of Syphilis

All Patients

Signs or symptoms of nervous system involvement [e.g., meningitis, hearing loss, cranial nerve dysfunction, altered mental status, ophthalmic disease (e.g., uveitis, iritis, pupillary abnormalities), ataxia, loss of vibration sense], *or*
RPR or VDRL titer ≥1:32, *or*
Suspected treatment failure

Additional Indications in HIV-Infected Persons

CD4+ T cell count ≤350/μL, *or*
CSF examination is recommended by some experts for all HIV-infected persons.

Source: Adapted from the 2010 Sexually Transmitted Diseases Treatment Guidelines from the Centers for Disease Control and Prevention.

far more often than the VDRL test on CSF in all stages of syphilis, but reactivity may reflect passive transfer of serum antibody into the CSF. A nonreactive FTA-ABS test on CSF, however, may be used to rule out asymptomatic neurosyphilis. A recent study demonstrated the utility of measuring CXCL13 in CSF to distinguish between neurosyphilis and HIV-related CSF abnormalities.

Clearly, all *T. pallidum*–infected patients who have signs or symptoms consistent with neurologic disease (e.g., meningitis, hearing loss) or ophthalmic disease (e.g., uveitis, iritis) should have a CSF examination, regardless of disease stage. The appropriate management of asymptomatic persons is less clear. Lumbar puncture on all asymptomatic patients with untreated syphilis is impractical and unnecessary. Because standard therapy with penicillin G benzathine fails to result in treponemicidal drug levels in CSF, it is important to identify those persons at higher risk for having or developing neurosyphilis so that appropriate therapy may be given. Large-scale prospective studies have now provided evidence-based guidelines for determining which syphilis patients may benefit most from CSF examination for evidence of neurosyphilis. Specifically, patients with RPR titers of ≥1:32 are at higher risk of having neurosyphilis (11-fold and 6-fold higher in HIV-infected and HIV-uninfected persons, respectively), as are HIV-infected patients with CD4+ T cell counts of ≤350/μL. Current recommendations for CSF examination are shown in Table 169-1.

Evaluation of HIV-infected patients for syphilis

Because persons at highest risk for syphilis are also at increased risk for HIV infection, these two infections frequently coexist. There is evidence that syphilis and other genital ulcer diseases may be important risk factors in the acquisition and transmission of HIV infection. Some manifestations of syphilis may be altered in patients with concurrent HIV infection, and multiple cases of neurologic relapse after standard therapy have been reported in these patients. *T. pallidum* has been isolated from the CSF of several patients (with and without concurrent HIV infection) after penicillin G benzathine therapy for early syphilis.

Persons with newly diagnosed HIV infection should be tested for syphilis; conversely, all patients with newly diagnosed syphilis should be tested for HIV infection. Some authorities, persuaded by reports of persistent *T. pallidum* in CSF of HIV-infected persons after standard therapy for early syphilis, recommend CSF examination for evidence of neurosyphilis for all co-infected patients, regardless of the stage of syphilis, with treatment for neurosyphilis if CSF abnormalities are found. Others, on the basis of their own clinical experience, believe that standard therapy—without CSF examination—is sufficient for all cases of early syphilis in HIV-infected

patients without neurologic signs or symptoms. As described above, RPR titer and CD4+ T cell count can be used to identify patients at higher risk of neurosyphilis for lumbar puncture, although some cases of neurosyphilis will not be identified by these criteria. Table 169-1 summarizes guidelines suggested by published studies. Serologic testing after treatment is important for all patients with syphilis, particularly for those also infected with HIV.

TREATMENT   Syphilis

TREATMENT OF ACQUIRED SYPHILIS   The CDC's 2010 guidelines for the treatment of syphilis are summarized in Table 169-2 and are discussed below. Penicillin G is the drug of choice for all stages of syphilis. *T. pallidum* is killed by very low concentrations of penicillin G, although a long period of exposure to penicillin is required because of the unusually slow rate of multiplication of the organism. The efficacy of penicillin against syphilis remains undiminished after 60 years of use, and there is no evidence of penicillin resistance in *T. pallidum*. Other antibiotics effective in syphilis include the tetracyclines and the cephalosporins. Aminoglycosides and spectinomycin inhibit *T. pallidum* only in very large doses, and the sulfonamides and the quinolones are inactive. Azithromycin has shown significant promise as an effective oral agent against *T. pallidum*; however, strains harboring 23S rRNA mutations that confer macrolide resistance are widespread; such strains represent >50% of recent isolates from Seattle and San Francisco and have now been identified in multiple North American and European sites. Macrolide resistance mutations have been identified in nearly all samples reported from China. In contrast, three studies conducted in Africa (Uganda, Tanzania, and Madagascar) have documented the clinical efficacy of azithromycin and, for the subset of samples examined, have found no molecular evidence of the mutation. In short, the prevalence of resistant strains varies widely by geographic location, and routine treatment of syphilis with azithromycin is not recommended. In all cases, careful follow-up of any patient treated for syphilis with azithromycin must be ensured.

Early Syphilis Patients and Their Contacts   Penicillin G benzathine is the most widely used agent for the treatment of early syphilis; a single dose of 2.4 million units is recommended. Preventive treatment is also recommended for individuals who have been exposed to infectious syphilis within the previous 3 months. *The regimens recommended for prevention are the same as those recommended for early syphilis.* Penicillin G benzathine cures >95% of cases of early syphilis, although clinical relapse can follow treatment, particularly in patients with concurrent HIV infection. Because the risk of neurologic relapse may be higher in HIV-infected patients, CSF examination is recommended in HIV-seropositive individuals with syphilis of any stage, particularly those with a serum RPR titer of ≥1:32 or a CD4+ T cell count of ≤350/μL. Therapy appropriate for neurosyphilis should be given if there is any evidence of CNS disease.

Late Latent and Late Syphilis   If CSF abnormalities are found, the patient should be treated for neurosyphilis. If CSF is normal, the recommended treatment is penicillin G benzathine (7.2 million units total; Table 169-2). The clinical response to treatment for benign tertiary syphilis is usually impressive. However, responses to therapy for cardiovascular syphilis are not dramatic because aortic aneurysm and aortic regurgitation cannot be reversed by antibiotics.

TABLE 169-2 Recommendations for the Treatment of Syphilis[a]

Stage of Syphilis	Patients without Penicillin Allergy	Patients with Confirmed Penicillin Allergy[b]
Primary, secondary, or early latent	*CSF normal or not examined:* Penicillin G benzathine (single dose of 2.4 mU IM) *CSF abnormal:* Treat as neurosyphilis	*CSF normal or not examined:* Tetracycline HCl (500 mg PO qid) or doxycycline (100 mg PO bid) for 2 weeks CSF abnormal: Treat as neurosyphilis
Late latent (or latent of uncertain duration), cardiovascular, or benign tertiary	*CSF normal or not examined:* Penicillin G benzathine (2.4 mU IM weekly for 3 weeks) *CSF abnormal:* Treat as neurosyphilis	*CSF normal and patient not infected with HIV:* Tetracycline HCl (500 mg PO qid) or doxycycline (100 mg PO bid) for 4 weeks *CSF normal and patient infected with HIV:* Desensitization and treatment with penicillin if compliance cannot be ensured CSF abnormal: Treat as neurosyphilis
Neurosyphilis (asymptomatic or symptomatic)	Aqueous crystalline penicillin G (18–24 mU/d IV, given as 3–4 mU q4h or continuous infusion) for 10–14 days *or* Aqueous procaine penicillin G (2.4 mU/d IM) plus oral probenecid (500 mg qid), both for 10–14 days	Desensitization and treatment with penicillin[c]
Syphilis in pregnancy	According to stage	Desensitization and treatment with penicillin

[a]See Table 169-1 and text for indications for CSF examination.
[b]Because of the documented presence of macrolide resistance in many *T. pallidum* strains in North America, Europe, and China, azithromycin should be used with caution only when treatment with penicillin or doxycycline is not feasible. Azithromycin should not be used for men who have sex with men or for pregnant women.
[c]Limited data suggest that ceftriaxone (2 g/d either IM or IV for 10–14 days) can be used; however, cross-reactivity between penicillin and ceftriaxone is possible.
Abbreviations: CSF, cerebrospinal fluid; mU, million units.
Source: Based on the 2010 Sexually Transmitted Diseases Treatment Guidelines from the Centers for Disease Control and Prevention.

Penicillin-Allergic Patients For penicillin-allergic patients with syphilis, a 2-week (early syphilis) or 4-week (late or late latent syphilis) course of therapy with doxycycline or tetracycline is recommended. These regimens appear to be effective in early syphilis but have not been tested for late or late latent syphilis, and compliance may be problematic. Limited studies suggest that ceftriaxone (1 g/d, given IM or IV, for 8–10 days) is effective for early syphilis. These nonpenicillin regimens have not been carefully evaluated in HIV-infected individuals and should be used with caution. If compliance and follow-up cannot be ensured, penicillin-allergic HIV-infected persons with late latent or late syphilis should be desensitized and treated with penicillin.

Neurosyphilis Penicillin G benzathine, given in total doses of up to 7.2 million units, does not produce detectable concentrations of penicillin G in CSF and should not be used for treatment of neurosyphilis. Asymptomatic neurosyphilis may relapse into symptomatic disease following treatment with benzathine penicillin, and the risk of relapse may be higher in HIV-infected patients. Both symptomatic and asymptomatic neurosyphilis should be treated with aqueous penicillin. Administration either of IV aqueous crystalline penicillin G or of aqueous procaine penicillin G plus probenecid in recommended doses is thought to ensure treponemicidal concentrations of penicillin G in CSF. The clinical response to penicillin therapy for meningeal syphilis is dramatic, but treatment of neurosyphilis with existing parenchymal damage may only arrest disease progression. Neurologic relapse has been reported after high-dose IV penicillin therapy for neurosyphilis in an HIV-infected patient. No alternative therapies have been studied, but careful follow-up is essential, and re-treatment is warranted in such patients. No data suggest that additional therapy (e.g., penicillin G benzathine for 3 weeks) is beneficial after treatment for neurosyphilis.

The use of antibiotics other than penicillin G for the treatment of neurosyphilis has not been studied, although very limited data suggest that ceftriaxone may be used. In patients with penicillin allergy demonstrated by skin testing, desensitization and treatment with penicillin are recommended.

Management of Syphilis in Pregnancy Every pregnant woman should undergo a nontreponemal test at her first prenatal visit and, if at high risk of exposure, again in the third trimester and at delivery. In the untreated pregnant patient with presumed syphilis, expeditious treatment appropriate to the stage of the disease is essential. Patients should be warned of the risk of a Jarisch-Herxheimer reaction, which may be associated with mild premature contractions but rarely results in premature delivery.

Penicillin is the only recommended agent for the treatment of syphilis in pregnancy. If the patient has a documented penicillin allergy, desensitization and penicillin therapy should be undertaken according to the CDC's 2010 guidelines. After treatment, a quantitative nontreponemal test should be repeated monthly throughout pregnancy to assess therapeutic efficacy. Treated women whose antibody titers rise by fourfold or whose titers do not decrease by fourfold over a 3-month period should be re-treated.

EVALUATION AND MANAGEMENT OF CONGENITAL SYPHILIS
Whether or not they are infected, newborn infants of mothers with reactive serologic tests may themselves have reactive tests because of transplacental transfer of maternal IgG antibody. For asymptomatic infants born to women treated adequately with penicillin during the first or second trimester of pregnancy, monthly quantitative nontreponemal tests may be performed to monitor for appropriate reduction in antibody titers. Rising or persistent titers indicate infection, and the

infant should be treated. Detection of neonatal IgM antibody may be useful, but no commercially available test is currently recommended.

An infant should be treated at birth if the treatment status of the seropositive mother is unknown; if the mother has received inadequate or nonpenicillin therapy or has received penicillin therapy in the third trimester; or if the infant may be difficult to follow. The CSF should be examined to obtain baseline values before treatment. Penicillin is the only recommended drug for the treatment of syphilis in infants. Specific recommendations for the treatment of infants and older children are included in the CDC's 2010 treatment guidelines.

JARISCH-HERXHEIMER REACTION A dramatic though usually mild reaction consisting of fever, chills, myalgias, headache, tachycardia, increased respiratory rate, increased circulating neutrophil count, and vasodilation with mild hypotension may follow the initiation of treatment for syphilis. This reaction is thought to be a response to lipoproteins released by dying *T. pallidum* organisms. The Jarisch-Herxheimer reaction occurs in ~50% of patients with primary syphilis, 90% of those with secondary syphilis, and a lower proportion of persons with later-stage disease. Defervescence takes place within 12–24 h. In patients with secondary syphilis, erythema and edema of the mucocutaneous lesions may increase. Patients should be warned to expect such symptoms, which can be managed with symptom-based treatment. Steroid and other anti-inflammatory therapy is not required for this mild transient reaction.

FOLLOW-UP EVALUATION OF RESPONSES TO THERAPY Efficacy of treatment should be assessed by clinical evaluation and monitoring of the quantitative VDRL or RPR titer for a four-fold decline (e.g., from 1:32 to 1:8). Patients with primary or secondary syphilis should be examined 6 and 12 months after treatment and persons with latent or late syphilis at 6, 12, and 24 months. More frequent clinical and serologic examination (3, 6, 9, 12, and 24 months) is recommended for patients concurrently infected with HIV, regardless of the stage of syphilis.

After successful treatment of seropositive first-episode primary or secondary syphilis, the VDRL or RPR titer progressively declines, becoming negative by 12 months in 40–75% of seropositive primary cases and in 20–40% of secondary cases. Patients with HIV infection or a history of prior syphilis are less likely to become nonreactive in the VDRL or RPR test. Rates of decline of serologic titers appear to be slower and serologically defined treatment failures more common among HIV-infected patients than among those without HIV co-infection; however, effective antiretroviral therapy may reduce these differences. Re-treatment should be considered if serologic responses are not adequate or if clinical signs persist or recur. Because it is difficult to differentiate treatment failure from reinfection, the CSF should be examined, with treatment for neurosyphilis if CSF is abnormal and treatment for late latent syphilis if CSF is normal. Patients treated for late latent syphilis frequently have low initial VDRL or RPR titers and may not have a fourfold decline after therapy with penicillin. In such patients, re-treatment is not warranted unless the titer rises or signs and symptoms of syphilis appear. Because treponemal tests may remain positive despite treatment for seropositive syphilis, these tests are not useful in following the response to therapy.

The activity of neurosyphilis (symptomatic or asymptomatic) correlates best with CSF pleocytosis, and this measure provides the most sensitive index of response to treatment. Repeat CSF examinations should be performed every 6 months until the cell count is normal. An elevated CSF cell count falls to normal in 3–12 months in adequately treated HIV-uninfected patients. The persistence of mild pleocytosis in HIV-infected patients may be due to the presence of HIV in CSF; this scenario may be difficult to distinguish from treatment failure. Elevated levels of CSF protein fall more slowly, and the CSF VDRL titer declines gradually over several years. In patients treated for neurosyphilis, a fourfold reduction in serum RPR titer has been positively correlated with normalization of CSF abnormalities; this correlation is stronger in HIV-uninfected patients and in HIV-infected patients receiving effective antiretroviral therapy.

IMMUNITY TO SYPHILIS

The rate of development of acquired resistance to *T. pallidum* after natural or experimental infection is related to the size of the antigenic stimulus, which depends on both the size of the infecting inoculum and the duration of infection before treatment. Both humoral and cellular responses are considered to be of major importance in immunity and in the healing of early lesions. Cellular infiltration, predominantly by T lymphocytes and macrophages, produces a T_H1 cytokine milieu consistent with the clearance of organisms by activated macrophages. Specific antibody enhances phagocytosis and is required for macrophage-mediated killing of *T. pallidum*. Recent studies demonstrate antigenic variation of the TprK protein, which may lead to persistence of infection and determine susceptibility to reinfection with another strain. Comparative genomic studies have revealed some sequence variations among *T. pallidum* strains. Strains can be differentiated by molecular typing methods, and a possible correlation between molecular type and clinical manifestations is being examined.

FURTHER READINGS

BREBAN R et al: Is there any evidence that syphilis epidemics cycle? Lancet Infect Dis 8:577, 2008

CENTERS FOR DISEASE CONTROL AND PREVENTION: Sexually transmitted diseases treatment guidelines, 2010. MMWR Recommend Rep 59(RR-12): 1–110, 2010

GHANEM KG et al: Lumbar puncture in HIV-infected patients with syphilis and no neurologic symptoms. Clin Infect Dis 48:816, 2009

LAFOND RE, LUKEHART SA: Biological basis for syphilis. Clin Microbiol Rev 19:29, 2006

MARRA CM et al: Cerebrospinal fluid abnormalities in patients with syphilis: Association with clinical and laboratory features. J Infect Dis 189:369, 2004

—— et al: Normalization of serum rapid plasma reagin titer predicts normalization of cerebrospinal fluid and clinical abnormalities after treatment of neurosyphilis. Clin Infect Dis 47:893, 2008

—— et al: CXCL13 as a cerebrospinal fluid marker for neurosyphilis in HIV-infected patients with syphilis. Sex Transm Dis 37:283, 2010

STAMM LV: Global challenge of antibiotic-resistant *Treponema pallidum*. Antimicrob Agents Chemother 54:583, 2010

TUCKER JD et al: Lues maligna in early HIV infection: Case report and review of the literature. Sex Transm Dis 36:512, 2009

CHAPTER **170**

Endemic Treponematoses

Sheila A. Lukehart

The endemic, or nonvenereal, treponematoses are bacterial infections caused by close relatives of *Treponema pallidum* subspecies *pallidum*, the etiologic agent of venereal syphilis (Chap. 169). Yaws, pinta, and endemic syphilis are traditionally distinguished from venereal syphilis by mode of transmission, age of acquisition, geographic distribution, and clinical features. These infections are limited to rural areas of developing nations and are seen in developed countries only among recent immigrants from endemic regions. Our "knowledge" about the endemic treponematoses is based on observations by health care workers who have visited endemic areas; virtually no well-designed studies of the natural history, diagnosis, or treatment of these infections have been conducted. The treponemal infections are compared and contrasted in Table 170-1.

■ EPIDEMIOLOGY

The endemic treponematoses are chronic diseases transmitted by direct contact during childhood and, like syphilis, can cause severe late manifestations years after initial infection. In a World Health Organization (WHO)–sponsored mass eradication campaign from 1952 to 1969, more than 160 million people in Africa, Asia, and South America were examined for treponemal infections, and more than 50 million cases, contacts, and latent infections were treated. This campaign reduced the prevalence of active yaws from >20% to <1% in many areas. In recent decades, lack of focused surveillance and diversion of resources have resulted in documented resurgence of these infections in some

regions. The estimated geographic distribution of the endemic treponematoses in the 1990s is shown in Fig. 170-1. The most recent WHO estimate (1997) suggested that there are 460,000 new cases per year and a prevalence of 2.5 million infected persons; during the subsequent decade, an increased incidence was documented in some countries. Areas of resurgent yaws morbidity include West Africa (Ivory Coast, Ghana, Togo, Benin), the Central African Republic, Nigeria, and rural Democratic Republic of Congo. The prevalence of endemic syphilis is estimated to be >10% in some regions of Ghana, Mali, Niger, Burkina Faso, and Senegal. In Asia and the Pacific Islands, reports suggest active outbreaks of yaws in Indonesia, Papua New Guinea, East Timor, Vanuatu, Laos, and Kampuchea. India actively renewed its focus on yaws eradication in 1996 and has reported no new cases since 2003. In the Americas, foci of yaws are thought to persist in Haiti and other Caribbean islands, Peru, Colombia, Ecuador, Brazil, Guyana, and Surinam. Pinta is limited to Central America and northern South America, where it is found rarely and only in remote villages. Evidence of yaws-like disease and seroreactivity in wild gorillas and baboons in Africa has led to speculation that there may be an animal reservoir for yaws, although strains recently obtained from humans and nonhuman primates have not been subjected to molecular comparison. A single strain isolated from a baboon in 1966 contains several identified genetic differences from available yaws isolates from humans.

■ MICROBIOLOGY

The etiologic agents of the endemic treponematoses are *T. pallidum* subspecies *pertenue* (yaws), *T. pallidum* subspecies *endemicum* (endemic syphilis), and *T. carateum* (pinta). These little-studied organisms are morphologically identical to *T. pallidum* subspecies *pallidum*, and no definitive antigenic differences among them have been identified to date. A controversy has existed about whether the pathogenic treponemes are truly different organisms. Three of the four organisms are classified as subspecies of *T. pallidum*; the fourth (*T. carateum*) remains a separate species simply because no

TABLE 170-1 Comparison of the Treponemes and Associated Diseases

Feature	Venereal Syphilis	Yaws	Endemic Syphilis	Pinta
Organism	*T. pallidum* subsp. *pallidum*	*T. pallidum* subsp. *pertenue*	*T. pallidum* subsp. *endemicum*	*T. carateum*
Modes of transmission	Sexual, transplacental	Skin-to-skin	Household contacts: mouth-to-mouth or via shared drinking/eating utensils	Skin-to-skin
Usual age of acquisition	Adulthood or in utero	Early childhood	Early childhood	Late childhood
Primary lesion	Cutaneous ulcer (chancre)	Papilloma, often ulcerative	Rarely seen	Nonulcerating papule with satellites, pruritic
Location	Genital, oral, anal	Extremities	Oral	Extremities, face
Secondary lesions	Mucocutaneous lesions; condylomata lata	Cutaneous papulosquamous lesions; osteoperiostitis	Florid mucocutaneous lesions (mucous patch, split papule, condyloma latum); osteoperiostitis	Pintides, pigmented, pruritic
Infectious relapses	~25%	Common	Unknown	None
Late complications	Gummas, cardiovascular and CNS involvement[a]	Destructive gummas of skin, bone, cartilage	Destructive gummas of skin, bone, cartilage	Nondestructive, dyschromic, achromic macules

[a]CNS involvement in the endemic treponematoses has been postulated by some investigators (see text).

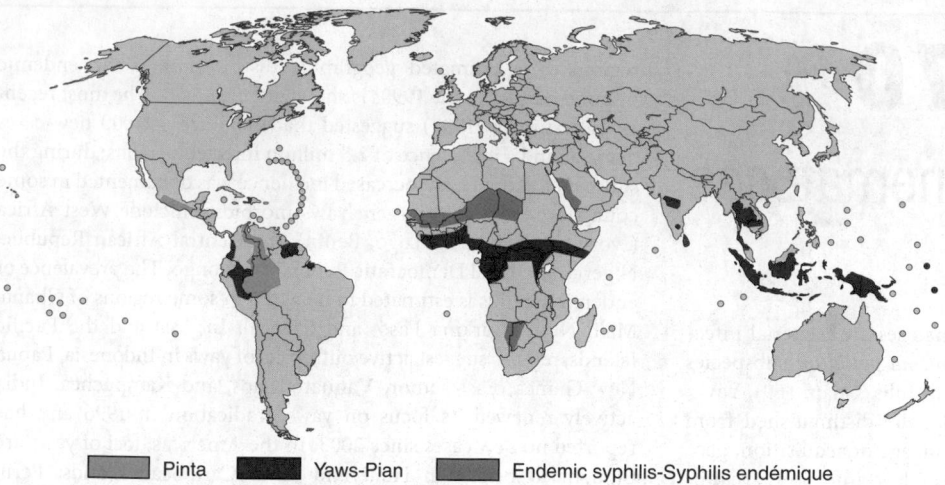

Figure 170-1 **Geographic distribution of endemic treponematoses in the 1990s.** *(Courtesy of the World Health Organization; www.who.int/yaws/epidemiology/Map_yaws_90s.jpg.)*

Pinta   Yaws-Pian   Endemic syphilis-Syphilis endémique

organisms have been available for genetic studies. A number of genetic loci distinguish the agents of venereal and nonvenereal treponemal infections, and molecular signatures (assessed by polymerase chain reaction amplification of *tpr* genes and restriction digestion) can differentiate the individual agents of venereal syphilis, yaws, and bejel. Whether these genetic differences are related to the distinct clinical courses of these diseases has not been determined.

■ CLINICAL FEATURES

All of the treponemal infections are chronic and are characterized by defined disease stages, with a localized primary lesion, disseminated secondary lesions, periods of latency, and possible late lesions. Primary and secondary stages are more frequently overlapping in yaws and endemic syphilis than in venereal syphilis, and the late manifestations of pinta are very mild relative to the destructive lesions of the other treponematoses. The current preference is to divide the clinical course of the endemic treponematoses into "early" and "late" stages.

The major clinical distinctions made between venereal syphilis and the nonvenereal infections are the apparent lack of congenital transmission and of central nervous system (CNS) involvement in the nonvenereal infections. It is not known whether these distinctions are entirely accurate. Because of the high degree of genetic relatedness among the organisms, there is little biological reason to think that *T. pallidum* subspecies *endemicum* and *T. pallidum* subspecies *pertenue* would be unable to cross the blood-brain barrier or to invade the placenta. These organisms are like *T. pallidum* subspecies *pallidum* in that they can disseminate from the site of primary infection and can persist for decades. The lack of recognized congenital infection may be due to the fact that childhood infections are often in the latent stage (low bacterial load) before girls reach sexual maturity. Neurologic involvement may go unrecognized because of the lack of trained medical personnel in endemic regions, the delay of many years between infection and possible CNS manifestations, or a low rate of symptomatic CNS disease. Some published evidence supports congenital transmission as well as cardiovascular, ophthalmologic, and CNS involvement in yaws. Although the reported studies have been small, have failed to control for other causes of CNS abnormalities, have not included specific treponemal serologic tests, and have not analyzed the response to therapy, it may be erroneous to accept unquestioningly the frequently repeated belief that these organisms fail to cause such manifestations.

Yaws

Also known as *pian*, *framboesia*, or *bouba*, yaws is characterized by the development of one or several primary lesions ("mother yaw") followed by multiple disseminated skin lesions. All early skin lesions are infectious and may persist for many months; cutaneous relapses are common during the first 5 years. Late manifestations, affecting 10% of untreated persons, are destructive and can involve skin, bone, and joints.

The infection is transmitted by direct contact with infectious lesions, often during play or group sleeping, and may be enhanced by disruption of the skin by insect bites or abrasions. After an average of 3–4 weeks, the first lesion begins as a papule—usually on an extremity—and then enlarges (particularly during moist warm weather) to become papillomatous or "raspberry-like" (thus the name "framboesia") (Fig. 170-2, left). Regional lymphadenopathy develops, and the lesion usually heals within 6 months; dissemination is thought to occur during the early weeks of infection. A generalized secondary eruption, accompanied by generalized lymphadenopathy, appears either concurrent with or following the primary lesion, may take several forms (macular, papular, or papillomatous), and may become secondarily infected with other bacteria. Painful papillomatous lesions on the soles of the feet result in a crablike gait ("crab yaws"), and periostitis may result in nocturnal bone pain and polydactylitis. Late yaws is manifested by gummas of the skin and long bone, hyperkeratoses of the palms and soles, osteitis and periostitis, and hydrarthrosis. The late gummatous lesions are characteristically extensive. Destruction of the nose, maxilla, palate, and pharynx is termed *gangosa* and is similar to the destructive lesions seen in leprosy and leishmaniasis.

Endemic syphilis

The early lesions of endemic syphilis (*bejel*, *siti*, *dichuchwa*, *njovera*, *skerljevo*) are localized primarily to mucocutaneous and mucosal surfaces. The infection is reported to be transmitted by direct contact, by kissing, or by sharing drinking and eating utensils. A role for insects in transmission has been suggested but is unproven. The initial lesion, usually an intraoral papule (Fig. 170-2, center), often goes unrecognized and is followed by mucous patches on the oral mucosa and mucocutaneous lesions resembling the condylomata lata of secondary syphilis. This eruption may last for months or even years, and treponemes can readily be demonstrated in early lesions. Periostitis and regional lymphadenopathy are common. After a variable period of latency, late manifestations may appear, including osseous and cutaneous gummas. Destructive gummas, osteitis, and gangosa are more common in endemic syphilis than in late yaws.

Pinta

Pinta (*mal del pinto, carate, azul, purupuru*) is the most benign of the treponemal infections. This disease has three stages that are characterized by marked changes in skin color (Fig. 170-2, right), but pinta does not appear to cause destructive lesions or to involve other tissues. The initial papule is most often located on the extremities or

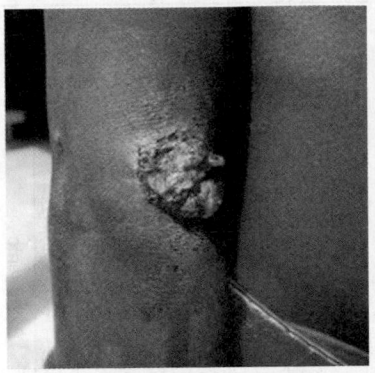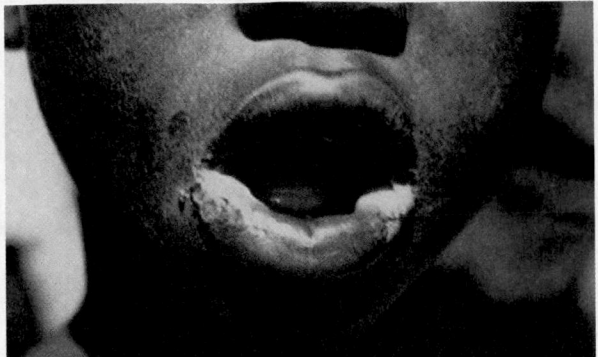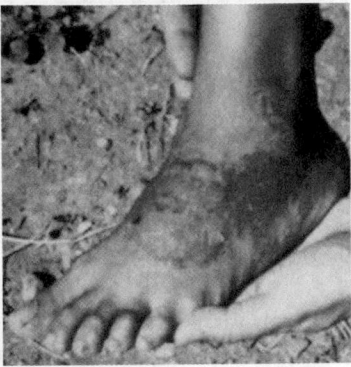

Figure 170-2 Clinical manifestations of endemic treponematoses. *Left:* Papillomatous primary lesion of yaws. ***Center:*** Split papules of early endemic syphilis. ***Right:*** Pigmented macules of pinta. *[Photos published with permission from Professor H. Assé, Côte d'Ivoire (left) and from PL Perine et al: Handbook of Endemic Treponematoses, Geneva, World Health Organization, 1984 (center and right).]*

face and is pruritic. After one to many months of infection, numerous disseminated secondary lesions (*pintides*) appear. These lesions are initially red but become deeply pigmented, ultimately turning a dark slate blue. The secondary lesions are infectious and highly pruritic and may persist for years. Late pigmented lesions are called *dyschromic macules* and contain treponemes. Over time, most pigmented lesions show varying degrees of depigmentation, becoming brown and eventually white and giving the skin a mottled appearance. White achromic lesions are characteristic of the late stage.

DIAGNOSIS

Diagnosis of the endemic treponematoses is based on clinical manifestations and, when available, dark-field microscopy and serologic testing. The same serologic tests that are used for venereal syphilis (Chap. 169) become reactive during all treponemal infections. Although several targets have been evaluated for specific serodiagnosis, to date there is no test that can discriminate among the different infections. The nonvenereal treponemal infections should be considered in the evaluation of a reactive syphilis serology in any person who has emigrated from an endemic area.

TREATMENT   Endemic Treponematoses

The WHO-recommended therapy for patients and their contacts is benzathine penicillin (1.2 million units IM for adults; 600,000 units for children <10 years old). This dose is half of that recommended for early venereal syphilis, and no controlled efficacy studies have been conducted. Definitive evidence of resistance to penicillin is lacking, although relapsing lesions have been reported after penicillin treatment in Papua New Guinea. Limited data suggest the efficacy of tetracycline for treatment of yaws, but no data exist for other endemic treponematoses. Solely on the basis of experience with venereal syphilis, it is thought that doxycycline or tetracycline (at doses appropriate

for syphilis; Chap. 169) are alternatives for patients allergic to penicillin. Macrolide resistance mutations have been identified in *T. pallidum* subspecies *pallidum*, but no data are available on possible mutations in the nonvenereal treponemes. A Jarisch-Herxheimer reaction (Chap. 169) may follow treatment of endemic treponematoses. Nontreponemal serologic titers [in the Venereal Disease Research Laboratory (VDRL) slide test or the rapid plasma reagin (RPR) test] usually decline after effective therapy, but patients may not become seronegative.

CONTROL

Because of lack of ongoing surveillance for the endemic treponematoses, these potentially destructive diseases are not recognized by public health decision-makers and control efforts are rarely undertaken, even though penicillin therapy is inexpensive and effective. There is concern that, as HIV spreads throughout developing countries, it may markedly affect the manifestations and transmission of the endemic treponematoses.

FURTHER READINGS

Antal GM et al: The endemic treponematoses. Microbes Infect 4:83, 2002

Aseidu K et al: Yaws eradication: Past efforts and future perspectives. Bull WHO 86:499, 2008

Centurion-Lara A et al: Molecular differentiation of *Treponema pallidum* subspecies. J Clin Microbiol 44:3377, 2006

Gerstl S et al: Prevalence study of yaws in the Democratic Republic of Congo using the lot quality assurance sampling method. PLoS ONE 4:e6338, 2009

Rinaldi A: Yaws: A second (and maybe last?) chance for eradication. PLoS Negl Trop Dis 2:e275, 2008

Satter E, Tokarz VA: Secondary yaws: An endemic treponemal infection. Ped Dermatol 27:364, 2010

CHAPTER 171

Leptospirosis

Joseph M. Vinetz

Leptospirosis is a globally important zoonotic disease caused by spirochetes of the genus *Leptospira* (Fig. 171-1). In 1885, Adolf Weil described the clinical hallmarks of this disease as an acute process characterized by splenomegaly, jaundice, and nephritis. With time, the designation *Weil's disease* came to signify severe leptospirosis characterized by diverse clinical findings, particularly fever, jaundice, acute renal injury, refractory shock, and hemorrhage (especially pulmonary hemorrhage). The global burden of leptospirosis is hard to quantify because of the difficulties encountered in its clinical diagnosis and the lack of efficient confirmatory laboratory testing, which limits public health reporting.

■ ETIOLOGIC AGENT

The genus *Leptospira* (order Spirochetales, family Leptospiraceae) constitutes the most ancient lineage of spirochetes pathogenic for humans and the only spirochetes that can live both in animals and free in the environment. This genus includes 20 named species, 9 of which are classified as pathogenic, 5 as intermediately pathogenic, and 6 as nonpathogenic (saprophytic) based on molecular phylogenetic analysis (Fig. 171-2). Of the pathogenic and intermediate *Leptospira* species, more than 250 serovars—classified on the basis of agglutination testing with specific antisera—cause disease in humans and animals. New species and serovars continue to be

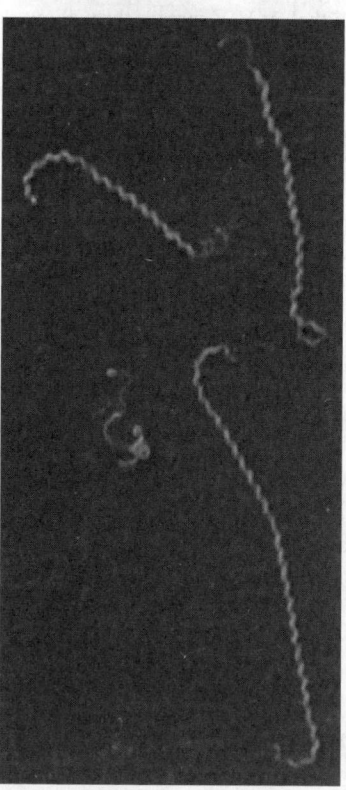

Figure 171-1 Transmission electron micrograph of *Leptospira interrogans* serovar Icterohaemorrhagiae.

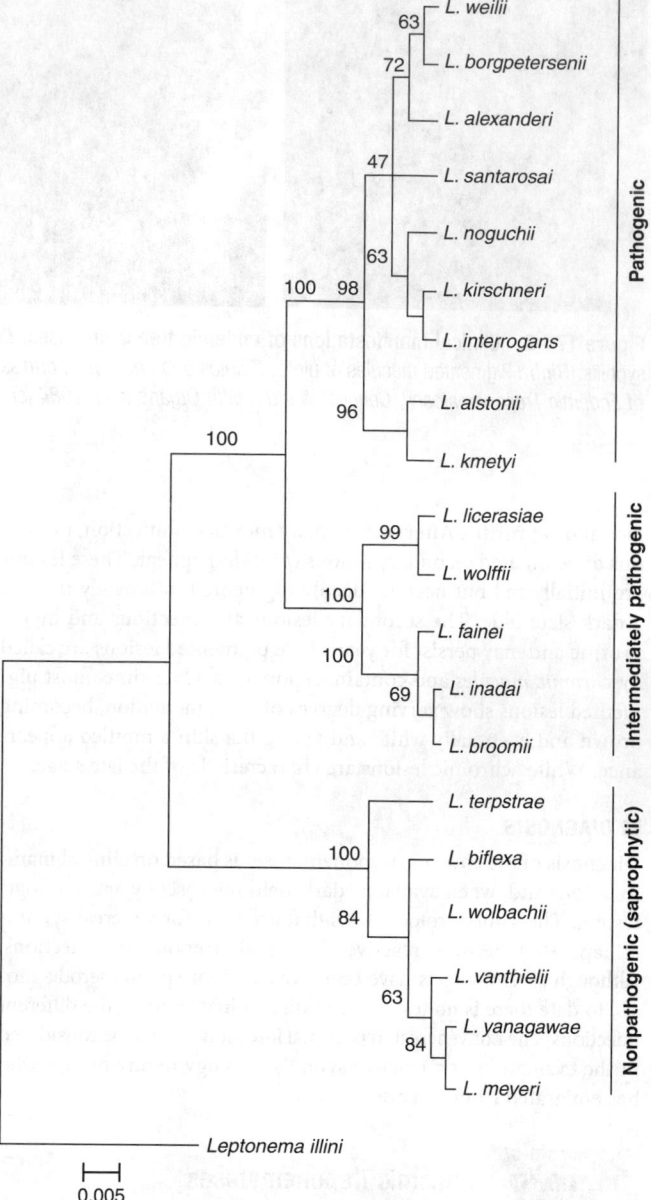

Figure 171-2 Differentiation of pathogenic, intermediately pathogenic, and nonpathogenic (saprophytic) *Leptospira* species based on molecular phylogenetic analysis using the 16S rRNA gene. Scale bar indicates rate of nucleotide substitution per base pair.

discovered. Although all species, serovars, and strains are morphologically identical, leptospires are described by serovar for clinical and epidemiologic reasons.

The dimensions and motility of leptospires (~0.1 × 6–20 μm) allow them to pass through filters used to sterilize culture medium. Leptospires are tightly and regularly coiled, with characteristic hooked ends (hence the species name *interrogans*), and are highly motile, spinning around their longitudinal axis and darting back and forth. The organisms cannot be seen by direct light microscopy. To visualize the spirochetes directly in culture or in clinical specimens, dark-field or phase-contrast microscopy must be used. Small protein strands that appear motile by Brownian movement can easily be confused with leptospires. In tissues, leptospires can be visualized by silver impregnation (i.e., Warthin-Starry staining), immunohistochemistry, or immunofluorescence microscopy.

Leptospires are difficult to isolate in pure culture from clinical specimens such as blood, urine, and cerebrospinal fluid (CSF), although certain species and serovars (e.g., *L. interrogans* serovar Copenhageni) are grown more easily than others. The organisms have peculiar nutritional requirements, particularly their inability to ferment glucose and their apparently exclusive use of long-chain fatty acids to generate energy and metabolites for cell division and growth. Standard leptospiral culture medium [Ellinghausen–McCullough–Johnson–Harris (EMJH)] contains oleic acid polymers (Tween60 and Tween40) as fatty acid sources. These spirochetes do not grow in medium typically used in automated blood culture systems but can be recovered if specimens are subcultured within ~1 week onto EMJH, Stuart, Fletcher's, or Korthoff's medium. EMJH, the standard for isolation of *Leptospira* from clinical specimens, is a liquid polysorbate-Tween medium to which 0.1% agar is added (sometimes supplemented with antibiotics to prevent growth of contaminants). The primary isolation of *Leptospira* requires the presence of a solid phase in the medium, which is provided by the agar particles. Cultures are maintained in the dark at 28–30°C and are examined at weekly intervals by dark-field microscopy for up to 3 months. After some weeks, florid growth sometimes produces a dense ring of organisms—Dinger's ring—just under the surface of the medium.

■ EPIDEMIOLOGY

Leptospirosis is a zoonotic disease. Human-to-human transmission does not occur. Although more than 100 different mammals can be infected, the most important sources of transmission to humans are rats, dogs, cattle, and pigs. Rats do not become ill from leptospiral infection, but dogs often develop severe disease similar to that in humans; infection can cause reproductive failure in cattle and pigs. Even when vaccinated, asymptomatic dogs, cattle, and pigs can be leptospiruric and thus transmit infection to humans. Classic (but not exclusive) serovar-animal associations include Icterohaemorrhagiae and Copenhageni in domestic rats (*Rattus norvegicus, R. rattus*), Grippotyphosa in opossums and raccoons (emerging in the United States and Canada in the absence of a vaccine that covers this serovar), Canicola in dogs, Hardjo in cattle and buffalo, and Pomona in pigs.

Patterns of leptospirosis transmission are characterized as epidemic, endemic, and sporadic. Factors that facilitate human infection are those that bring susceptible persons into indirect contact with contaminated animal urine through surface waters, moist soil, or other wet environments or into direct contact with urine and other excreta (e.g., products of parturition, placenta) of infected animals. In recent years, fewer occupation-related cases and more cases related to environmental exposure have been seen. Seasonal rains and seasonal flooding are the most important factors in the occurrence of epidemic leptospirosis. Tropical humid environments, poor sanitation leading to rodent infestation, and uncontrolled dog populations are important for endemic transmission. Sporadic leptospirosis is associated with human contact with contaminated environments in various settings: on the job (veterinary, sewer, and slaughterhouse workers), in poorly hygienic inner-city alleys and slums, during adventure travel and other non-work-related outdoor activities, and during military training exercises in endemic regions.

Reliable data on the incidence of leptospirosis and on rates of associated morbidity and mortality remain scant and are generally drawn from biased hospital-based series or from governmental registries including passively reported serologic results. In the United States, leptospirosis was removed from the list of notifiable diseases in the 1990s. The ~50–100 cases passively reported annually to the Centers for Disease Control and Prevention (CDC) clearly represent an underestimate; the majority of these cases are from Hawaii, and others are sporadically acquired in inner-city settings or in association with environments such as farms, lakes, and adventure-sport locales. In large urban centers in Brazil that are subject to seasonal flooding (e.g., São Paulo, Rio de Janeiro, and Salvador), tens of thousands of cases are estimated to occur annually. Prospective, population-based cohort studies in Salvador indicate that 5% of slum dwellers are infected annually and that some people are reinfected. Case-fatality rates among hospitalized patients in São Paulo can be as high as ~20% despite state-of-the-art intensive care unit and supportive care. In the Peruvian Amazon, ~30–50% of patients with acute undifferentiated fever have been identified as having leptospirosis; the disease is severe in a small minority of such cases (<2%), and these severe cases are often associated with urban acquisition of infection. Men are affected more often by clinical disease than are women.

Infection by *Leptospira* does not occur via inhalation, and leptospirosis is a rare cause of laboratory-acquired infection. Laboratory strains usually used for serologic diagnosis have been serially passaged for long periods and usually have lost their virulence.

Global features

Leptospirosis affects urban and rural populations in industrialized and developing countries alike. The highest burden of disease falls upon those at lower socioeconomic levels whose activities of daily living bring them into contact with surface waters contaminated with the urine of animals carrying the infection. High rates of endemic leptospirosis, associated with both mild and severe disease, are found throughout tropical regions. Torrential seasonal flooding in areas of high population density (e.g., in urban slums in Brazil, India, and Thailand) is the major risk factor for epidemic severe disease. In 2009, outbreaks after typhoons in the Philippines affected large populations, prompting the Ministry of Health to provide antimicrobial chemoprophylaxis to millions of people; the efficacy of this intervention remains unknown.

Military training, outdoor athletic activities, and adventure travel have led to recognized outbreaks and sporadic cases of leptospirosis. Now-classic examples include the frequent occurrence of leptospirosis in U.S. soldiers undergoing jungle training in Panama (in which context the first clinical trial of antibiotic prophylaxis was carried out), whitewater rafters in Costa Rica, and almost half of the participants in Eco-Challenge Sabah in Borneo, Malaysia, in 2000.

Sporadic leptospirosis, which is likely to be common but underrecognized in urban and rural settings, is generally identified when the manifestations of disease are severe and the index of suspicion is high.

■ PATHOGENESIS

Leptospires infect humans through the mucosa (usually conjunctival and possibly oral or tonsillar) or through macerated, punctured, or abraded skin. The organisms resist innate immune defenses (e.g., complement), proliferate in the bloodstream or extracellularly within organs, and then disseminate hematogenously to all organs. The incubation period averages 5–14 days (range, 2–30 days); leptospires can be isolated from blood during the first 3–10 days of clinical illness (Fig. 171-3). As antibodies develop, leptospires disappear from the blood but persist in various organs, including brain (the meninges and possibly other sites), liver, lung, heart, and kidney. The life cycle is completed as leptospires traverse the interstitial spaces of the kidney, penetrate the basement membrane of the proximal renal tubules, cross through proximal renal tubule epithelial cells, and become adherent to the proximal renal tubular brush border, whence they are excreted in the urine. In humans, as in other mammalian hosts, chronic and persistent renal colonization can last for weeks or years, with unknown pathophysiologic consequences.

Although severe human disease due to a wide variety of leptospires has been reported, some of the leptospires involved are thought to be more intrinsically pathogenic than others. Rat-associated *L. interrogans* serovars Icterohaemorrhagiae and Copenhageni are mostly commonly associated with Weil's disease; jaundice, renal

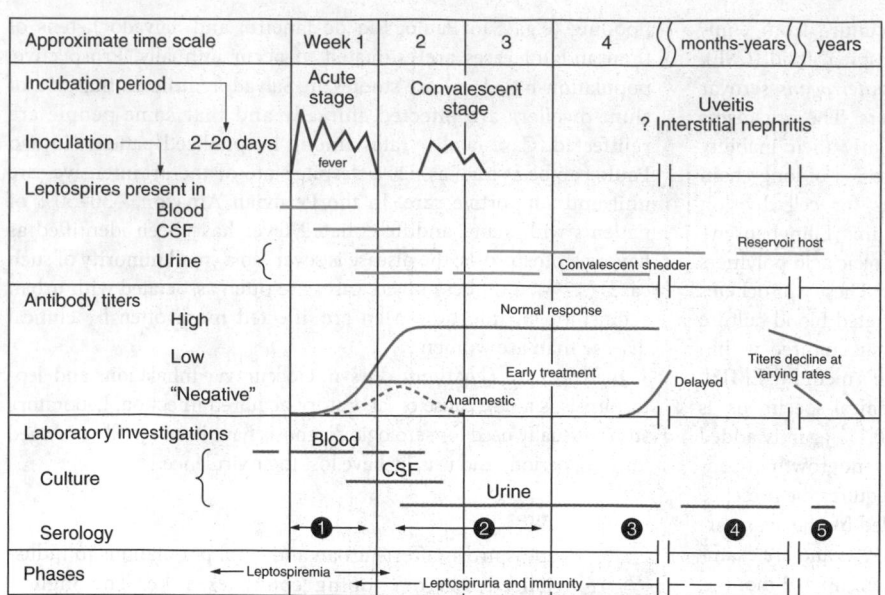

Figure 171-3 Biphasic nature of leptospirosis and relevant investigations at different stages of disease. Specimens 1 and 2 for serology are acute-phase serum samples; specimen 3 is a convalescent-phase serum sample that may facilitate detection of a delayed immune response; and specimens 4 and 5 are follow-up serum samples that can provide epidemiologic information, such as the presumptive infecting serogroup. *[Reprinted as adapted by Levitt (from Turner LH: Leptospirosis. BMJ 1:231, 1969) with permission from the American Society for Microbiology and the BMJ Publishing Group.]*

failure, shock, and hemorrhage due to other species and serovars have been reported as well. Specific molecular determinants and virulence mechanisms responsible for disease manifestations have not been identified. An unusual lipid A structure renders the leptospiral lipopolysaccharide of low endotoxic potential in experimental systems. Multiple in vitro studies have shown that leptospires and their extracts cause cellular toxicity; however, the biochemical nature of damage to host cells and the underlying mechanisms remain unclear.

Pathologic findings are organ specific. Acute and chronic inflammation within the kidney is associated with acute tubular necrosis and interstitial nephritis. Autopsy studies have revealed abnormal regulation of fluid and electrolyte transporters—including the endogenous sodium/hydrogen exchanger isoform 3 (NHE 3), aquaporins 1 and 2, α-Na+K+ATPase, and sodium–potassium–chloride cotransporter (NKCC2 isoform)—in both the presence and the absence of acute tubular necrosis. Primary injury of the proximal convoluted tubules is the primary renal pathophysiologic lesion in acute leptospirosis, with secondary increased distal tubular potassium excretion, hypokalemia, and polyuria.

Hepatic histopathology in fatal cases is associated with disruption of cellular cohesion, plugging of bile canaliculi, occasional acute inflammatory infiltrates, and focal periportal cellular necrosis and steatosis; widespread hepatocellular necrosis is not found. Cases of severe pulmonary hemorrhage syndrome that come to autopsy are characterized by the absence of inflammation, the paucity of organisms visible by silver or immunohistochemical staining, and grossly obvious frank hemorrhage (Fig. 171-4). Ultrastructural features of the lung in the few fatal cases reported include swelling, increased pinocytotic vesicles, and giant dense bodies in the cytoplasm of epithelial cells; these abnormalities are limited to hemorrhagic areas, and the intercellular junctions are preserved. Platelets are adherent to activated but abnormal-appearing endothelial cells. Septal capillary lesions seem to be causally related to death, leading to pulmonary hemorrhage; in both animal models and human cases, immunoglobulin and complement deposition have been demonstrated in lung tissue involved in leptospiral pulmonary hemorrhage.

The relation of disseminated intravascular coagulation to leptospirosis has long been debated. The prothrombin and activated partial thromboplastin times are not necessarily elevated in severe leptospirosis, and fibrinogen levels are typically elevated. Thrombocytopenia is characteristic, probably reflecting platelet consumption in the activated endothelial surface; platelet counts are lower in severe than in mild leptospirosis. Nonetheless, proteolytic products of fibrinogen (e.g., D-dimers), thrombin–antithrombin III complexes, and prothrombin fragment 1,2 have been found to be elevated in cases of leptospirosis in Thailand (but with no difference between severe and nonsevere cases), a finding indicating pathologic activation of the coagulation system in leptospirosis.

In the heart, pericardial and endocardial hemorrhage, disruption of myocardial fiber organization, and scattered myocyte necrosis (accompanied, grossly, by dilation of both right and left ventricles) are pathological lesions associated with severe leptospirosis.

Despite the traditional view that leptospirosis is characterized by vasculitis, formal demonstration of inflammatory infiltrates within any blood vessel has not been shown to be involved in the pathogenesis of this disease. A more likely possibility is that leptospires induce endothelial cell dysfunction with organ dysfunction and systemic disease, but this hypothesis remains to be validated.

◼ CLINICAL MANIFESTATIONS

The clinical expression of infection by *Leptospira*, which is related to diverse focal organ dysfunction, includes subclinical infection, an undifferentiated febrile illness, and Weil's disease—the most severe form. Leptospirosis is classically described as biphasic (Fig. 171-3). Acute fever in the initial leptospiremic phase lasts for 3–10 days, during which period the organism may be cultured from blood. In a later immune phase, fever is not responsive to antibiotic therapy but leptospires can be isolated from urine. Unlike milder forms, Weil's disease may also be monophasic and fulminant.

Physical examination may include any of the following findings, none of which is pathognomonic for leptospirosis: conjunctival suffusion (dilated conjunctival blood vessels in the absence of discharge); pharyngeal erythema without exudate; muscle tenderness; rales on lung auscultation or dullness on chest percussion over areas of pleural hemorrhage; rash (which may be macular, maculopapular, erythematous, petechial, or ecchymotic); jaundice; meningismus; and hypo- or areflexia, particularly in the legs.

The natural course of mild uncomplicated leptospirosis usually ends in spontaneous resolution within 7–10 days without sequelae, but the difficulties of rapid diagnosis do not permit the initiation of specific antimicrobial therapy. Biomarkers to predict progression to severe disease are not available. Some patients experience a return of fever, headache, and other systemic symptoms after 3–10 days (the immune phase) in association with the clearance of leptospires from the blood and the appearance of antibodies; this phase of illness does not respond to antibiotic therapy.

Weil's disease is characterized by variable combinations of jaundice, acute kidney injury, hypotension, and hemorrhage—most commonly involving the lungs (Fig. 171-4) but also potentially affecting the gastrointestinal tract, retroperitoneum, pericardium, and brain. Other syndromes include aseptic meningitis, uveitis, cholecystitis,

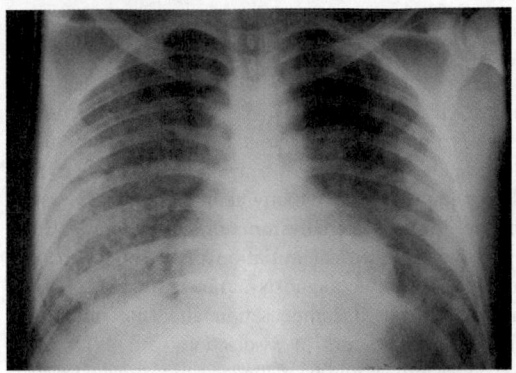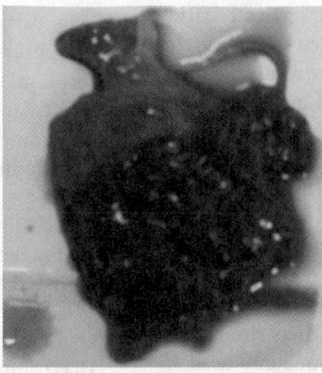

Figure 171-4 Severe pulmonary hemorrhage in leptospirosis. *Left:* Chest x-ray. *Right:* Gross appearance of right lower lobe of lung at autopsy. This patient, a 15-year-old in the Peruvian Amazonian city of Iquitos, died several days after presentation with acute illness, jaundice, and hemoptysis. Blood culture yielded *Leptospira interrogans* serovar Copenhageni/Icterohaemorrhagiae. *(Adapted with permission from Segura et al, 2005. ©2005 by the Infectious Diseases Society of America.)*

acute abdomen, and pancreatitis (with hypo- or hyperglycemia). Jaundice is not associated with fulminant hepatic necrosis or hepatocellular damage, but rather with abnormal laboratory values (see "Diagnosis," below). The liver can be enlarged and tender; splenomegaly is reported in a minority of cases. Acute kidney injury manifests after several days of illness and can be nonoliguric or oliguric, with serum electrolyte abnormalities reflecting proximal renal tubular dysfunction. Hypokalemia and hypomagnesemia are common in nonoliguric renal failure; hypomagnesemia can cause severe muscle weakness. Hypotension is associated with acute tubular necrosis and oliguria, requiring fluid resuscitation, sometimes pressors, and hemodialysis. Renal function typically returns to normal in survivors of severe disease. Severe pulmonary hemorrhage in leptospirosis is a clinical problem wherever the disease is endemic, manifesting with cough, chest pain, and hemoptysis but without purulent sputum.

Cardiac involvement is commonly reflected on the electrocardiogram as nonspecific ST and T wave changes but also as right-bundle-branch block and right- and/or left-sided ventricular dilation indicating myocarditis. Skeletal muscle involvement manifests as severe myalgia, typically of the legs (especially the calves) but also of the abdominal muscles (mimicking acute abdomen); these symptoms are associated with a moderately elevated serum concentration of creatine kinase that, by itself, is not sufficient to result in acute kidney injury. Skin abnormalities include petechiae and ecchymosis as well as macular and maculopapular rash. Neurologic findings include aseptic meningitis (in which CSF pleocytosis can range from a few cells to >1000 cells/μL, with a polymorphonuclear cell predominance) and hypo- or areflexia, especially of the legs.

■ DIAGNOSIS

Leptospirosis should be suspected on the basis of an appropriate exposure history combined with any of the infection's protean manifestations. A high index of suspicion prompting elicitation of a detailed exposure history is critical and guides confirmatory testing (see below). Leptospiral infection is usually associated with obvious exposure events that go beyond casual activities such as simply having been on a farm or in an urban alley. An infected person usually has been immersed in or has had mucosal or percutaneous exposure to contaminated animal urine. Leptospiral infection resulting from the bite of a rat or another animal is rare.

Biochemical, hematologic, and urinalysis findings in acute leptospirosis are not specific, but certain patterns suggest the diagnosis. In the context of an appropriate exposure history and in the absence of a more likely explanation, classic Weil's disease is suggested by

elevated levels of blood urea nitrogen and serum creatinine in conjunction with mixed conjugated and unconjugated hyperbilirubinemia with aminotransferase elevation to less than five times the upper limit of normal. In all forms of leptospirosis (not just Weil's disease), a variety of abnormalities can occur. Urinalysis may show abnormalities of the sediment (leukocytes, erythrocytes, hyaline and granular cases). Elevation of the noncardiac isoform of creatine kinase may indicate skeletal muscle damage. Troponin levels indicative of myocarditis have not been adequately studied in leptospirosis. Hematologic abnormalities are variable but common: leukocytosis (typical in severe disease), leukopenia, hemolytic anemia, mild to moderate anemia, and thrombocytopenia.

On chest radiography, the appearance of the lungs varies. Alveolar infiltrates predominate and are associated with hemoptysis but not with purulent sputum. Other findings include diffuse interstitial infiltrate patterns corresponding to hyaline membrane disease (acute respiratory distress syndrome) and small nodular infiltrates and pleural-based densities representing hemorrhage.

The confirmation of leptospirosis requires laboratory testing. Definitive diagnosis rests on demonstrating the presence of the organism by culture isolation, detection of nucleic acids or antigen in body fluids, or immunohistochemical visualization in tissue. Direct examination of urine or blood by dark-field microscopy has the potential to provide a rapid diagnosis but is not recommended because of complicating artifacts. Leptospiral cultures do not become positive for weeks and therefore cannot guide clinical care. Polymerase chain reaction–based assays have been used in research laboratories to detect leptospiral DNA but are not clinically available. Moreover, a negative result does not rule out the diagnosis: the assays' sensitivity is insufficient when the level of bacteremia is below a detectable threshold, and inhibitors in blood and urine can interfere with these tests.

Serologic assays are the diagnostic mainstay in leptospirosis. In the United States, the gold standard—the microscopic agglutination test (MAT)—is performed only at the CDC; likewise, in other countries, performance of the MAT is generally limited to reference laboratories. The MAT entails growth of a battery of serovars representing the 26 leptospiral serogroups, incubation of a standard quantity of leptospires with the patient's serum on a microtiter plate, and detection of agglutination by dark-field microscopy. The highest dilution of serum that yields significant (50%) agglutination is reported as the titer. Although antibody titers are reported by serovar, a positive MAT result reflects the presence only of *Leptospira*-specific antibodies and cannot be used to precisely identify the infecting serovar because one serovar may induce antibodies that cross-react with other serovars. When patients have a high pretest probability of leptospirosis, a single antibody titer >1:200 is considered strong evidence of infection; however, in regions where leptospirosis transmission and subclinical disease are common, higher titers are generally required for a confident diagnosis because of long-lasting antibodies after a previous infection. Because the MAT is generally negative in the first 7–10 days after the onset of infection, paired acute- and convalescent-phase serum samples are preferred to document seroconversion or a fourfold rise in titer.

Other serologic tests for leptospirosis (e.g., enzyme-linked immunosorbent assay, indirect hemagglutination, dot-blot, and lateral flow) are based on solid-phase assays; some of these tests are commercially available. Such assays use the saprophytic (non-disease-associated) leptospire *L. biflexa* as antigen. *L. biflexa* has lipopolysaccharide epitopes in common with pathogenic *Leptospira* species. While useful in some regions of the world, *L. biflexa*-based tests are relatively insensitive (because of regional variation of leptospires) and nonspecific (because of previous exposure) and must be interpreted with caution.

Leptospires can be cultured from blood and CSF during the first 7–10 days of illness and from urine beginning in the second week. Cultures usually become positive after 2–4 weeks (range, 1 week to 6 months). Urine cultures can remain positive for months or years despite antibiotic therapy. Because leptospires can remain viable for as long as ~10 days at room temperature, specimens can be shipped to reference laboratories in anticoagulated blood (heparin, citrate, EDTA). Although leptospires do not grow in medium used in automated blood culture detection systems, inoculated bottles can be subcultured into leptospiral culture medium within 1 week after inoculation for attempted isolation.

■ DIFFERENTIAL DIAGNOSIS

The differential diagnosis of acute leptospirosis is broad, reflecting its diverse clinical presentations and depending on the patient's travel and exposure history and geographic region of presentation. When fever and severe myalgia predominate, influenza is often considered, although the absence of coryza, sore throat, and cough is not consistent with this diagnosis. Other important possibilities include malaria, rickettsial diseases, arboviral infections (e.g., dengue and chikungunya), typhoid fever, hantavirus infection (hemorrhagic fever with renal syndrome or hantavirus cardiopulmonary syndrome), and viral hepatitis.

TREATMENT ▶ Leptospirosis

Although the value of antimicrobial treatment (Table 171-1) has not been proven in clinical trials, its prompt initiation probably shortens the course of severe leptospirosis and prevents the progression of mild disease. Despite debates about efficacy, antimicrobial drugs (typically penicillin, ceftriaxone, or cefotaxime) should be used to treat severe later-stage leptospirosis. Mild leptospirosis often is not specifically identified and typically resolves without antibiotic treatment. If clinical suspicion is high or the

TABLE 171-1 Treatment and Chemoprophylaxis of Leptospirosis in Adults[a]

Indication	Regimen
Treatment	
Mild leptospirosis	Doxycycline (100 mg PO bid) *or*
	Amoxicillin (500 mg PO tid) *or*
	Ampicillin (500 mg PO tid)
Moderate/severe leptospirosis	Penicillin (1.5 million units IV or IM q6h) *or*
	Ceftriaxone (1 g/d IV) *or*
	Cefotaxime (1 g IV q6h)
Chemoprophylaxis[b]	
	Doxycycline (200 mg PO once a week) *or*
	Azithromycin (250 mg PO once or twice a week)

[a]All regimens are given for 7 days.
[b]The efficacy of doxycycline prophylaxis in endemic or epidemic settings remains unclear. Experiments in animal models and a cost-effectiveness model indicate that azithromycin has a number of characteristics that may make it efficacious in treatment and prophylaxis, but clinical trials have not been performed.

diagnosis is suggested or confirmed by laboratory findings in an appropriate context (e.g., clinical presentation, exposure history), mild disease should be treated with oral antibiotics—in particular, doxycycline, especially where rickettsial infections (including scrub typhus) are coendemic. Solid data from studies of animals indicate that oral azithromycin is also likely to be useful in mild leptospirosis. Like many acute bacterial diseases manifesting as multiorgan system dysfunction, severe leptospirosis frequently requires empirical initiation of broad-spectrum parenteral therapy before the diagnosis can be confirmed.

In rare instances, acute decompensation after the initiation of antimicrobial therapy occurs in association with a Jarisch-Herxheimer response and should be managed supportively. Fresh-frozen plasma, plasmapheresis, glucocorticoids, and activated protein C have no demonstrated role in the treatment of leptospirosis. Anecdotal reports in which inhaled nitric oxide was successfully used by leptospirosis patients with severe pulmonary involvement must be confirmed before such treatment can be recommended.

■ PROGNOSIS

The severity of illness in terms of pulmonary and renal dysfunction is the most important determinant of prognosis. Advanced age, clinically evident pulmonary involvement, elevated serum creatinine level, oliguria, and thrombocytopenia are associated with a poor prognosis; liver dysfunction in acute leptospirosis has not been confirmed to be an independent risk factor for death. Chronic alcoholism seems to be associated with severe disease. Reported mortality rates among hospitalized patients have varied from <5% to >20%.

Leptospirosis is generally considered to leave no permanent sequelae, although renal dysfunction, as manifested by electrolyte imbalances, may persist for days or weeks after acute illness resolves. Severe pulmonary hemorrhage and liver disease are not known to lead to persistent or progressive organ dysfunction. Some authorities have suggested that neuropsychiatric disturbance may follow severe disease; such conclusions must be assessed in a prospective clinical investigation.

■ PREVENTION

No vaccine is available for human leptospirosis. Preventive strategies, including prophylaxis with doxycycline, have been variably effective in different settings. Antibiotic prophylaxis can be considered for anticipated short-term, well-defined exposures, such as those incurred during military training or specific adventure travel (with, for example, fresh-water swimming). Long-term antibiotic prophylaxis has not been shown to be effective in preventing infection in high-transmission endemic settings. General sanitation approaches (e.g., rodent control) and avoidance of swimming in potentially contaminated places (e.g., for recreational use) are recommended, but these measures are difficult to apply consistently.

FURTHER READINGS

Araujo ER et al: Acute kidney injury in human leptospirosis: An immunohistochemical study with pathophysiological correlation. Virchows Arch 456:367, 2010

Bharti AR et al: Leptospirosis: A zoonotic disease of global importance. Lancet Infect Dis 3:757, 2003

Faine S et al (eds): *Leptospira and Leptospirosis.* Melbourne, MedScience, 1999

Ganoza CA et al: Determining risk for severe leptospirosis by molecular analysis of environmental surface waters for pathogenic *Leptospira*. PLoS Med 3:E308, 2006

Gouveia EL et al: Leptospirosis-associated severe pulmonary hemorrhagic syndrome, Salvador, Brazil. Emerg Infect Dis 14:505, 2008

Ko AI et al: *Leptospira*: The dawn of the molecular genetics era for an emerging zoonotic pathogen. Nat Rev Microbiol 7:736, 2009

——— et al: Urban epidemic of severe leptospirosis in Brazil. Lancet 354:820, 1999

Medeiros FD et al: Leptospirosis-associated disturbances of blood vessels, lungs and hemostasis. Acta Trop 115:155, 2010

Segura E et al: Clinical spectrum of pulmonary involvement in leptospirosis in an endemic region, with quantification of leptospiral burden. Clin Infect Dis 40:343, 2005

Vinetz JM et al: Sporadic urban leptospirosis. Ann Intern Med 125:794, 1996

CHAPTER **172**

Relapsing Fever

Mark S. Dworkin

Relapsing fever is an illness characterized by recurring episodes of fever and nonspecific symptoms (e.g., headache, myalgia, arthralgia, shaking chills, and abdominal symptoms) after infection with one of several species of *Borrelia*.

■ GLOBAL FEATURES

In North America, relapsing fever (a zoonosis) is transmitted by the bite of an *Ornithodoros* tick. In many other parts of the world, including Africa and Asia, relapsing fever is endemic and occurs after the bite of a tick or the human body louse (*Pediculus humanus*). Tick-borne relapsing fever (TBRF) is also reported from countries in the Middle East, including Israel, Iran, and Jordan. Louse-borne relapsing fever (LBRF) is occasionally imported into the United States by a traveler. TBRF is rarely fatal in North America, where it is most often sporadic; in some African countries (e.g., Senegal and Tanzania), TBRF is a more significant bacterial infection, causing morbidity and death. Conditions that favor infestation with *P. humanus*, such as living in refugee camps or other stressful situations in which many people are crowded together without access to good hygiene and nutrition, have led to large outbreaks of LBRF with substantial rates of morbidity and death; thus, LBRF is also known as *epidemic relapsing fever*.

■ ETIOLOGY AND PATHOGENESIS

The borreliae are helical or wavy motile spirochetes whose length ranges from 3 to 25 μm and whose width is usually 0.2–0.3 μm. In fixed Wright-stained differential smears, the organisms appear as loose coils (Fig. 172-1). Borreliae are transmitted to humans by exposure to the bite of an infected *Ornithodoros* tick (TBRF) or to the hemolymph of an infected human body louse, which may be found on clothing (LBRF). For louse-borne disease, it is not the louse's bite that causes transmission; rather, spirochetes are introduced when the louse is crushed (e.g., by scratching) and the insect's infected hemolymph is released and contaminates abraded or normal skin and mucous membranes. Relapsing fever results when variation in borrelial surface antigens leads to repeated bacteremia and stimulation of the immune system by each new antigen. Each time the organism changes its surface antigens, thus evading the immune system, another febrile response occurs. LBRF is caused by *Borrelia recurrentis*, whereas TBRF is caused by a variety of *Borrelia* species whose names sometimes correspond to their tick vectors. For example, *B. hermsii* is transmitted by the tick *O. hermsi*, and *B. turicatae* is transmitted by *O. turicata* (Fig. 172-2).

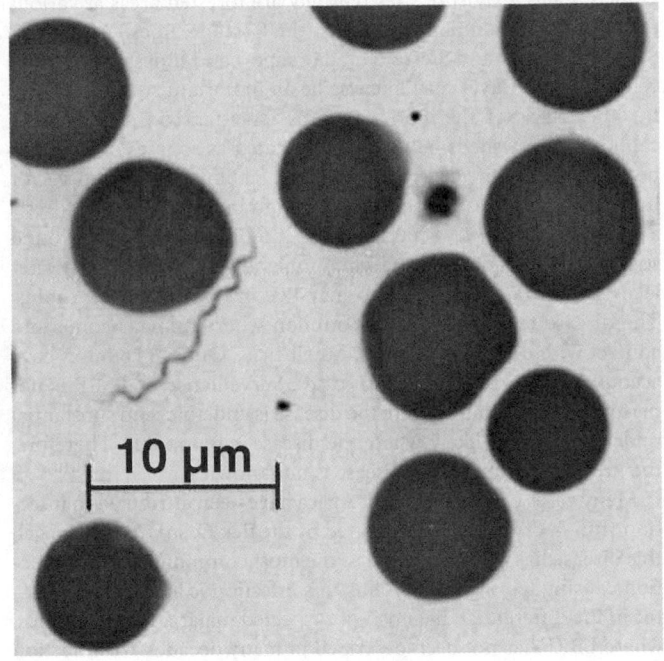

Figure 172-1 Photomicrograph of tick-borne relapsing fever spirochete (*Borrelia hermsii*) in a Wright-Giemsa–stained peripheral blood film. *[Reprinted with permission from Dennis DT: Relapsing fever, in Harrison's Principles of Internal Medicine, 17th ed, AF Fauci et al (eds). New York, McGraw-Hill, 2008, p 1054.]*

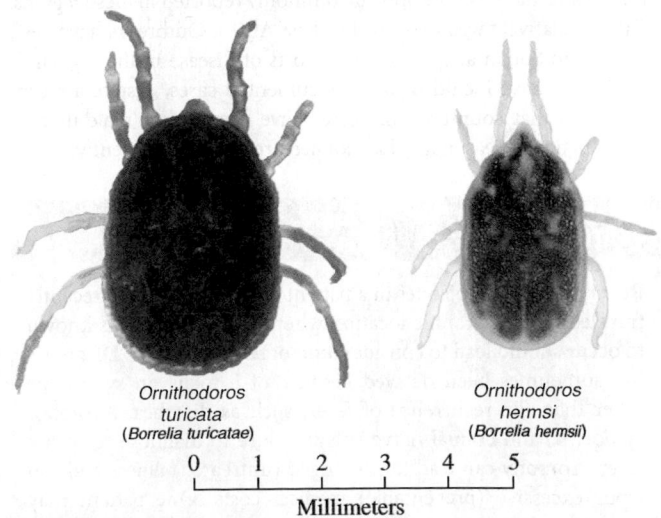

Figure 172-2 *Ornithodoros turicata* and *O. hermsi,* two of the many species of blood-feeding soft ticks responsible for transmitting tick-borne relapsing fever. *(Reprinted from Dworkin et al., 2008, with permission from Elsevier.)*

EPIDEMIOLOGY

TBRF is endemic in the western United States, southern British Columbia, the plateau regions of Mexico, Central and South America, the Mediterranean, Central Asia, and throughout much of Africa. In the United States, it typically is not reported farther east than Montana, Colorado, New Mexico, and Texas, although cases have been acquired in Oklahoma, Kansas, and Ohio and one case has been reported from Wyoming. A relapsing fever spirochete has been described as far east as Florida, although human infections have not yet been reported in that state. In the United States, exposure sites typically are forested areas at various elevations in mountainous regions (the Cascade, Rocky Mountain, San Bernardino, and Sierra Nevada ranges) and limestone caves in central Texas. Caves may likewise be an important source of TBRF in other areas of the world, such as Israel and Jordan. Houses, cabins, and cowsheds have been implicated as sources of infection because of tick-infested rodent nesting. The most common vector in the United States, *O. hermsi*, is often found in coniferous forests at elevations of 1500–8000 ft, where it feeds primarily on ground squirrels, tree squirrels, and chipmunks dwelling near freshwater lakes that attract humans who may live in or rent nearby cabins. The disease tends to be most common where humans come into contact with diurnal rodents and their ticks. Only 13 counties have accounted for ~50% of all U.S. cases. Surveillance of TBRF is not performed in all states where the disease is endemic, and substantial underreporting is likely where the disease is reportable. Therefore, the precise distribution of disease is not known.

Many cases of TBRF in West Africa have been attributed to infection with *B. crocidurae* transmitted by the tick *O. sonrai*. In Senegal, this disease has been identified as the most common bacterial infection causing febrile illness. Thus this infection is an important factor in the differential diagnosis of suspected malaria in West Africa, where LBRF has not been described in many decades. Co-infection with *Plasmodium* species was reported in more than one-third of blood films from Senegalese TBRF patients. In eastern sub-Saharan Africa, *B. duttonii* is more prevalent. TBRF has been detected (albeit less commonly) in northern Africa (e.g., in Morocco), where *B. hispanica* and *B. crocidurae* have been identified.

The epidemiology of LBRF is not as well characterized as that of TBRF, probably in part because of the higher prevalence of the former in regions with relatively few resources for communicable disease surveillance. Historically, LBRF has been described in North America and Europe, but it is now only uncommonly reported in these regions. LBRF is relatively well described in East Africa. Outbreaks have been reported in Sudan and Ethiopia. Reports of disease in the highlands of Ethiopia have included many documented cases, despite a recent decline; in that country, more cases have occurred in male than in female patients. Seasonality has not been reported consistently.

APPROACH TO THE PATIENT | **Relapsing Fever**

Recurring febrile episodes in a patient who lives in or has recently traveled to a geographic location where relapsing fever is known to occur should lead to consideration of relapsing fever. Diagnosis has sometimes been delayed because of a focus on symptoms other than the recurrence of fever, such as diarrhea, thrombocytopenia, and cranial nerve palsy. Failure to diagnose relapsing fever promptly can lead to prolonged (untreated) illness and can incur excessive (preventable) medical costs. One patient may present with illness resembling meningitis, another with illness resembling influenza, and others with a febrile gastrointestinal illness or no physical findings. In all these instances, the patient may undergo a variety of unnecessary invasive and noninvasive tests.

In addition, some patients may have more than one diagnosis (e.g., LBRF and typhus); therefore, other local tick-borne or louse-borne diseases should be kept in mind during evaluation.

CLINICAL MANIFESTATIONS

The mean incubation period is 7 days for TBRF (range, 4–18 days or longer) and 8 days for LBRF (range, 5–15 days; sometimes a shorter period in North Africa). Regardless of the tick or louse vector, the clinical manifestations of relapsing fever are similar, although not identical. The signs and symptoms documented in a large series of cases of TBRF are listed with their frequencies in Table 172-1. Alteration of sensorium, abdominal pain, and vomiting are common. Diarrhea may develop in 25% of cases. Jaundice; central nervous system (CNS) involvement; petechiae on the trunk, extremities, and mucous membranes; epistaxis; and blood-tinged sputum are more likely in LBRF. Uncommon manifestations of relapsing fever include iritis, acute respiratory distress syndrome, uveitis, iridocyclitis, myocarditis, and splenic rupture. Cranial nerve palsy and other neurologic manifestations are often reversible. Neurologic findings may occur in 10–30% of cases and are more common in LBRF. These findings may include signs of meningitis with or without cerebrospinal fluid abnormalities, seizure, focal deficits, hemiplegia, paraplegia, paresthesias, psychosis, hallucinations, and delirium. Certain species of tick-borne *Borrelia* have been reported with particular frequency in cases with neurologic complications (*B. duttonii* and *B. turicatae*).

The average duration of the first episode of TBRF is 3 days (range, 12 h to 17 days), and the episode terminates in a crisis. In contrast, the average duration of the first episode of LBRF is 5.5 days (range, 4–10 days). Subsequent relapsing febrile episodes are typically of shorter duration. The average time between the first episode and the first relapse is 7 days for TBRF and 9 days for LBRF. During afebrile intervals, the patient may have symptoms (e.g., malaise) or may feel well.

The differential diagnosis of infectious diseases causing fevers that may relapse or have biphasic patterns includes but is not

---

TABLE 172-1 Manifestations of Tick-Borne Relapsing Fever Acquired in the Northwestern United States and Southwestern British Columbia

Sign or Symptom	%	Sign or Symptom	%
Headache	94	Photophobia	25
Myalgia	92	Neck pain	24
Chills	88	Rash	18
Nausea	76	Dysuria	13
Arthralgia	73	Jaundice	10
Vomiting	71	Hepatomegaly	10
Abdominal pain	44	Splenomegaly	6
Confusion	38	Conjunctival injection	5
Dry cough	27	Eschar	2
Eye pain	26	Meningitis	2
Diarrhea	25	Nuchal rigidity	2
Dizziness	25		

Source: From a review of 182 cases reported during 1980–1995 (Dworkin et al. ©1998 Clinical Infectious Diseases).

limited to Colorado tick fever, yellow fever, dengue fever, lymphocytic choriomeningitis, brucellosis, malaria, leptospirosis, chronic meningococcemia, rat-bite fever, and infection with echovirus 9 or *Bartonella* species. The many other diagnoses that may overlap with relapsing fever in terms of other manifestations include typhus and typhoid fever. A history of travel, place of residence, and animal exposures is useful when patients have these fever patterns.

■ DIAGNOSIS

Detection and isolation of spirochetes

During asymptomatic intervals, relapsing fever borreliae are undetectable in the bloodstream by microscopy. Laboratory confirmation is made by the detection or isolation of spirochetes from blood during a febrile episode. Spirochetal counts may be high in the blood. Typically, an average of five organisms per oil-immersion field are observed in routine differential fixed smears of blood obtained from patients during the acute febrile phase of illness. A thin smear or a thick drop of blood is applied to a standard glass microscope slide, stained with Wright or Giemsa, and examined with a bright-field microscope at 1000x with oil immersion. Spirochetes also may be visualized by direct or indirect immunofluorescent staining and fluorescence microscopy. A dark-field microscope may be used to observe spirochetes in the blood. However, microscopic observation of spirochetes is relatively insensitive. Quantitative buffy coat analysis is an alternative method. Other available methods are most often used in research settings. Polymerase chain reaction (PCR)

and monoclonal antibody can be used to determine the species of *Borrelia*. For laboratories with PCR technology and expertise, this method is more sensitive than microscopy.

Serology

Serologic confirmation of TBRF is demonstrated by a fourfold rise in antibody titer between acute- and convalescent-phase serum samples or by the diagnostic reactivity of a single convalescent-phase serum sample. However, serology may not be reliable because of lack of standardization. Patients infected previously with other species of spirochetes may have false-positive reactions in the enzyme-linked immunosorbent assay (ELISA) and the indirect fluorescence antibody (IFA) assay. The most reliable method—the recombinant GlpQ assay—is not widely available. Therefore, blood samples are often screened with ELISA or IFA, and, if the result is positive (e.g., an IFA titer of 1:128–1:256 or higher), an immunoblot can be performed to determine the pattern of reactivity. This procedure has led to recognition of patients erroneously diagnosed with Lyme disease who actually have TBRF.

TREATMENT | **Relapsing Fever**

Treatment options for adults with relapsing fever are summarized in Fig. 172-3. Relapsing fever spirochetes are commonly sensitive to antibiotics such as doxycycline and erythromycin.

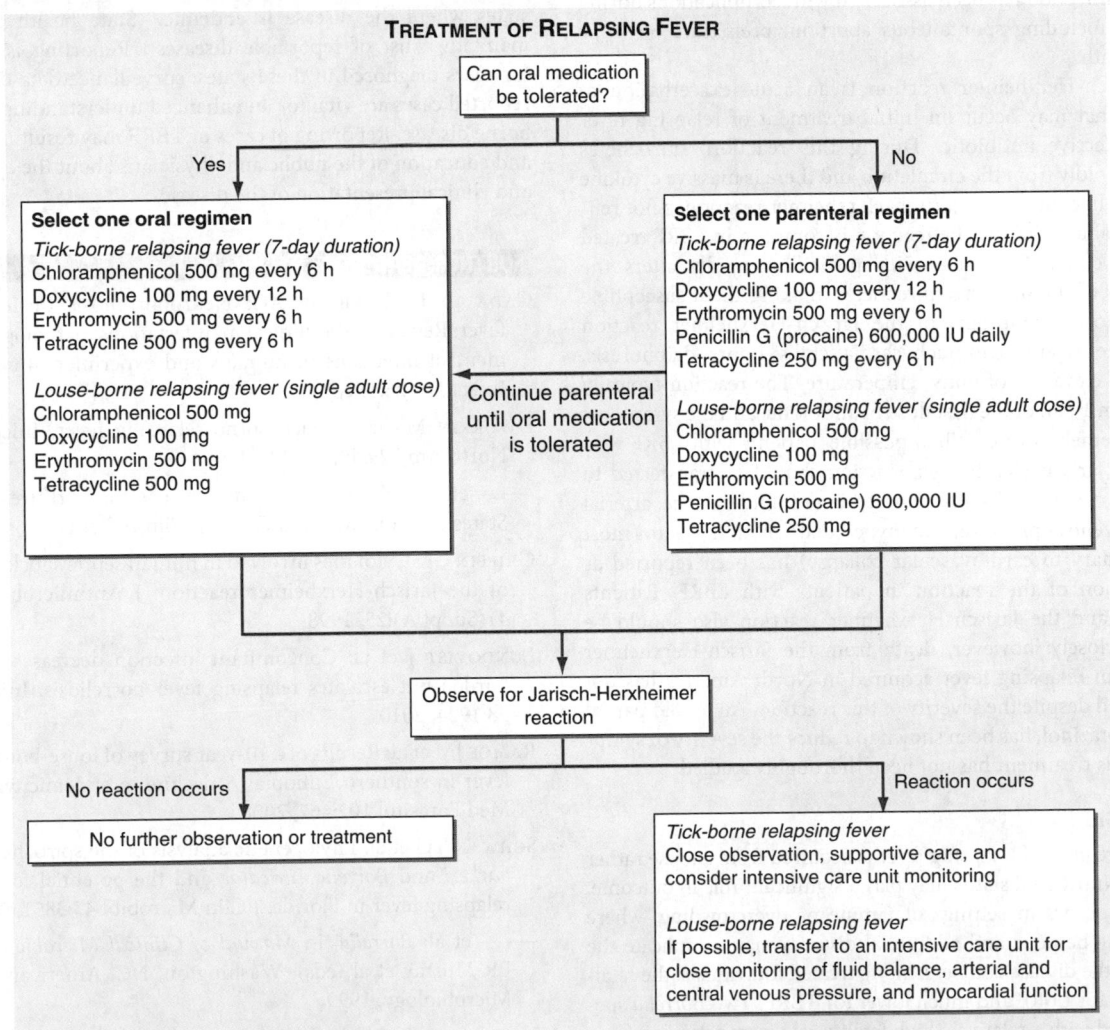

TREATMENT OF RELAPSING FEVER

Can oral medication be tolerated?

Yes → **Select one oral regimen**

Tick-borne relapsing fever (7-day duration)
Chloramphenicol 500 mg every 6 h
Doxycycline 100 mg every 12 h
Erythromycin 500 mg every 6 h
Tetracycline 500 mg every 6 h

Louse-borne relapsing fever (single adult dose)
Chloramphenicol 500 mg
Doxycycline 100 mg
Erythromycin 500 mg
Tetracycline 500 mg

No → **Select one parenteral regimen**

Tick-borne relapsing fever (7-day duration)
Chloramphenicol 500 mg every 6 h
Doxycycline 100 mg every 12 h
Erythromycin 500 mg every 6 h
Penicillin G (procaine) 600,000 IU daily
Tetracycline 250 mg every 6 h

Louse-borne relapsing fever (single adult dose)
Chloramphenicol 500 mg
Doxycycline 100 mg
Erythromycin 500 mg
Penicillin G (procaine) 600,000 IU
Tetracycline 250 mg

Continue parenteral until oral medication is tolerated

Observe for Jarisch-Herxheimer reaction

No reaction occurs → No further observation or treatment

Reaction occurs →
Tick-borne relapsing fever
Close observation, supportive care, and consider intensive care unit monitoring

Louse-borne relapsing fever
If possible, transfer to an intensive care unit for close monitoring of fluid balance, arterial and central venous pressure, and myocardial function

Figure 172-3 Treatment of relapsing fever and approach to the Jarisch-Herxheimer reaction.

Single-dose therapy is generally recommended for LBRF, while a 7-day (or 10-day) course is usually used for TBRF. Insufficient information is available on the efficacy of single-dose therapy for TBRF.

Lumbar puncture should be considered when signs of meningitis or encephalitis are present; cerebrospinal fluid evidence of these neurologic conditions suggests the need for treatment with an IV antibiotic regimen. This issue is especially relevant in TBRF due to certain species such as *B. duttonii* in Africa and *B. turicatae* in the southwestern United States because these species are more prone to invade the CNS and can reenter the bloodstream after antibiotic treatment if a regimen with good CNS penetration is not used.

Children <8 years of age and pregnant women with relapsing fever should be treated with penicillin or erythromycin. When a Jarisch-Herxheimer reaction occurs (and its occurrence is unpredictable), it may be milder in children than in adults. Monitoring of patients for this reaction for the first 12 h after the first dose of antibiotic is recommended (see below).

■ COMPLICATIONS

Moderate to severe thrombocytopenia, although not associated with a fatal outcome, is a typical finding in acute TBRF. Bleeding complications, such as epistaxis, purpura, hemoptysis, hematemesis, bloody diarrhea, hematuria, subarachnoid and cerebral hemorrhages, splenic rupture, and retinal hemorrhage, are more common with LBRF. Although death from TBRF in North America is rare, this infection has been associated with complications during pregnancy, including spontaneous abortion, premature birth, or neonatal death.

The Jarisch-Herxheimer reaction is an acute exacerbation of symptoms that may occur on initial treatment of relapsing fever with an effective antibiotic. During this reaction, spirochetes disappear rapidly from the circulation and there is massive cytokine release. The likelihood of a Jarisch-Herxheimer reaction is not reliably predictable in TBRF; the reaction is common in LBRF treated with tetracycline. Treatment with penicillin rapidly alters the morphology of the dividing spirochetes, making them susceptible to phagocytosis. Symptoms of the Jarisch-Herxheimer reaction often include hypotension, tachycardia, chills, rigors, diaphoresis, and marked elevation of body temperature. The reaction typically begins within 1–4 h of the first dose of antibiotic, and the symptoms may be extremely severe. When possible, patients with LBRF who develop the Jarisch-Herxheimer reaction should be transferred to an intensive care unit for close monitoring of fluid balance, arterial and central venous pressure, and myocardial function. Death (most often secondary to cardiovascular collapse) has been reported as a complication of the reaction in patients with LBRF. Patients with TBRF and the Jarisch-Herxheimer reaction also should be monitored closely; however, death from the Jarisch-Herxheimer reaction from relapsing fever acquired in North America has not been reported despite the severity of this reaction. An opioid partial agonist, meptazinol, has been shown to reduce the severity of symptoms, but this treatment has not been thoroughly studied.

■ PROGNOSIS

Death is more likely if relapsing fever is acquired from a louse rather than a tick. Nutritional status may play a significant role in outcome. LBRF often occurs in settings of famine or overcrowding, where nutrition may be poor and additional diseases may complicate the diagnosis or the disease course. Among treated individuals, the fatality rate is 5% for LBRF and much lower for TBRF. Two *Borrelia* species associated with a relatively high fatality rate from relapsing fever are *B. recurrentis* (louse-borne) and *B. duttonii* (tick-borne).

■ PREVENTION

Prevention of TBRF includes the avoidance of rodent- and tick-infested dwellings as well as infested natural sites, such as animal burrows or caves. Environmental health specialists from local health departments and pest removal services may be consulted about rodent-proofing of homes and vacation cabins and reduction of rodent habitat around homes (e.g., by removal of rodent nesting material from walls, ceilings, and floors). Chemical treatment of rodent-infested areas should be undertaken only by pest control specialists. Contact with ticks and potential animal hosts should occur only while gloves are worn, given that TBRF has been contracted through skin contact with contaminated blood (e.g., in laboratory accidents and blood transfusions). Wearing clothing that protects the skin (e.g., long pants and long-sleeved shirts) and applying insect repellents such as DEET and permethrin to exposed skin and clothing, respectively, can prevent transmission of disease by hard ticks and possibly by soft ticks in some settings (e.g., in caves or—as a partial measure of protection—during sleep). Protection while sleeping in a potentially infested dwelling may best be provided by topical repellents. Sleeping on the floor or on a bed positioned directly against a wall should be avoided.

To prevent LBRF, it is necessary to prevent louse infestation by promoting personal hygiene (e.g., bathing) and systematic delousing (e.g., application of permethrin to clothing). Laundering or disposal of infested clothing and bedding is another important measure. Control of epidemics may involve widespread antibiotic use.

TBRF is reportable through local health departments in some states where the disease is endemic. (State health departments maintain a list of reportable diseases.) Reporting is encouraged for cases diagnosed in these states; surveillance data derived from reported cases are vital for an enhanced understanding of this tick-borne disease. Reporting of cases of TBRF may result in prevention and education of the public and physicians about the epidemiology and clinical presentation of the disease.

FURTHER READINGS

CADAVID D, BARBOUR AG: Neuroborreliosis during relapsing fever: Review of the clinical manifestations, pathology, and treatment of infections in humans and experimental animals. Clin Infect Dis 26:151, 1998

DWORKIN MS et al: Tick-borne relapsing fever. Infect Dis Clin North Am 22:449, 2008

——— et al: Tick-borne relapsing fever in the northwestern United States and southwestern Canada. Clin Infect Dis 26:122, 1998

GRIFFIN GE: Cytokines involved in human septic shock—the model of the Jarisch-Herxheimer reaction. J Antimicrob Chemother 41(Suppl A):25, 1998

LUNDQVIST J et al: Concomitant infection decreases the malaria burden but escalates relapsing fever borreliosis. Infect Immun 78:1924, 2010

RAMOS JM et al: Results of a 10-year survey of louse-borne relapsing fever in southern Ethiopia: A decline in endemicity. Ann Trop Med Parasitol 102:467, 2008

SCHWAN TG et al: Phylogenetic analysis of the spirochetes *Borrelia parkeri* and *Borrelia turicatae* and the potential for tick-borne relapsing fever in Florida. J Clin Microbiol 43:3851, 2005

——— et al: *Borrelia*, in *Manual of Clinical Microbiology*, 7th ed, PR Murray et al (eds). Washington, DC, American Society for Microbiology, 1999

VIAL L et al: Incidence of tick-borne relapsing fever in west Africa: Longitudinal study. Lancet 368:37, 2006

CHAPTER 173

Lyme Borreliosis

Allen C. Steere

DEFINITION

Lyme borreliosis is caused by a spirochete, *Borrelia burgdorferi sensu lato*, that is transmitted by ticks of the *Ixodes ricinus* complex. The infection usually begins with a characteristic expanding skin lesion, erythema migrans (EM; stage 1, localized infection). After several days or weeks, the spirochete may spread to many different sites (stage 2, disseminated infection). Possible manifestations of disseminated infection include secondary annular skin lesions, meningitis, cranial neuritis, radiculoneuritis, peripheral neuritis, carditis, atrioventricular nodal block, or migratory musculoskeletal pain. Months or years later (usually after periods of latent infection), intermittent or persistent arthritis, chronic encephalopathy or polyneuropathy, or acrodermatitis may develop (stage 3, persistent infection). Most patients experience early symptoms of the illness during the summer, but the infection may not become symptomatic until it progresses to stage 2 or 3.

Lyme disease was recognized as a separate entity in 1976 because of geographic clustering of children in Lyme, Connecticut, who were thought to have juvenile rheumatoid arthritis. It became apparent that Lyme disease was a multisystemic illness that affected primarily the skin, nervous system, heart, and joints. Epidemiologic studies of patients with EM implicated certain *Ixodes* ticks as vectors of the disease. Early in the twentieth century, EM had been described in Europe and attributed to *I. ricinus* tick bites. In 1982, a previously unrecognized spirochete, now called *Borrelia burgdorferi*, was recovered from *Ixodes scapularis* ticks and then from patients with Lyme disease. The entity is now called Lyme disease or Lyme borreliosis.

ETIOLOGIC AGENT

B. burgdorferi, the causative agent of Lyme disease, is a fastidious microaerophilic bacterium. The spirochete's genome is quite small (~1.5 Mb) and consists of a highly unusual linear chromosome of 950 kb as well as 17–21 linear and circular plasmids. The most remarkable aspect of the *B. burgdorferi* genome is that there are sequences for more than 100 known or predicted lipoproteins—a larger number than in any other organism. The spirochete has few proteins with biosynthetic activity and depends on its host for most of its nutritional requirements. It has no sequences for recognizable toxins.

Currently, 13 closely related borrelial species are collectively referred to as *Borrelia burgdorferi sensu lato* (i.e., *B. burgdorferi* in the general sense). The human infection Lyme borreliosis is caused primarily by three pathogenic genospecies: *B. burgdorferi sensu stricto* (*B. burgdorferi* in the strict sense, hereafter referred to as *B. burgdorferi*), *Borrelia garinii*, and *Borrelia afzelii*. *B. burgdorferi* is the sole cause of the infection in the United States; all three genospecies are found in Europe, and the latter two species occur in Asia.

Strains of *B. burgdorferi* have been subdivided according to several typing schemes, including one based on sequence variation of outer-surface protein C (OspC) and a second based on differences in the 16S–23S rRNA intergenic spacer region (RST or IGS). From these typing systems, it is apparent that strains of *B. burgdorferi* differ in pathogenicity. OspC type A (RST1) strains seem to be particularly virulent and may have played a role in the emergence of Lyme disease in epidemic form in the late twentieth century.

EPIDEMIOLOGY

The 13 known genospecies of *B. burgdorferi sensu lato* live in nature in enzootic cycles involving 14 species of ticks that are part of the *I. ricinus* complex. *I. scapularis* (Fig. 397-1) is the principal vector in the eastern United States from Maine to Georgia and in the midwestern states of Wisconsin, Minnesota, and Michigan. *I. pacificus* is the vector in the western states of California and Oregon. The disease is acquired throughout Europe (from Great Britain to Scandinavia to European Russia), where *I. ricinus* is the vector, and in Asian Russia, China, and Japan, where *I. persulcatus* is the vector. These ticks may transmit other diseases as well. In the United States, *I. scapularis* also transmits babesiosis and human anaplasmosis; in Europe and Asia, *I. ricinus* and *I. persulcatus* also transmit tick-borne encephalitis.

Ticks of the *I. ricinus* complex have larval, nymphal, and adult stages. They require a blood meal at each stage. The risk of infection in a given area depends largely on the density of these ticks as well as their feeding habits and animal hosts, which have evolved differently in different locations. For *I. scapularis* in the northeastern United States, the white-footed mouse and certain other rodents are the preferred hosts of the immature larvae and nymphs. It is critical that both of the tick's immature stages feed on the same host because the life cycle of the spirochete depends on horizontal transmission: in early summer from infected nymphs to mice and in late summer from infected mice to larvae, which then molt to become the infected nymphs that will begin the cycle again the following year. It is the tiny nymphal tick that is primarily responsible for transmission of the disease to humans during the early summer months. White-tailed deer, which are not involved in the life cycle of the spirochete, are the preferred host for the adult stage of *I. scapularis* and seem to be critical to the tick's survival.

Lyme disease is now the most common vector-borne infection in the United States and Europe. Since surveillance was begun by the Centers for Disease Control and Prevention (CDC) in 1982, the number of cases in the United States has increased dramatically. More than 25,000 new cases are now reported each summer. In Europe, the highest reported frequencies of the disease are in the middle of the continent and in Scandinavia.

PATHOGENESIS AND IMMUNITY

To maintain its complex enzootic cycle, *B. burgdorferi* must adapt to two markedly different environments: the tick and the mammalian host. The spirochete expresses outer-surface protein A (OspA) in the midgut of the tick, whereas OspC is upregulated as the organism travels to the tick's salivary gland. There, OspC binds a tick salivary-gland protein (Salp15), which is required for infection of the mammalian host. The tick must usually be attached for at least 24 h for transmission of *B. burgdorferi*.

After injection into the human skin, *B. burgdorferi* may migrate outward, producing EM, and may spread hematogenously or in the lymph to other organs. The only known virulence factors of *B. burgdorferi* are surface proteins that allow the spirochete to attach to mammalian proteins, integrins, glycosaminoglycans, or glycoproteins. For example, spread through the skin and other tissue matrices may be facilitated by the binding of human plasminogen and its activators to the surface of the spirochete. Some *Borrelia* strains bind complement regulator–acquiring surface proteins (FHL-1/reconectin, or factor H), which help to protect spirochetes from complement-mediated lysis. Dissemination of the organism in the blood is facilitated by binding to the fibrinogen receptor on activated platelets ($\alpha_{IIb}\beta_3$) and the vitronectin receptor ($\alpha_v\beta_3$) on endothelial cells. As the name indicates, spirochetal decorin-binding proteins A and B bind decorin, a glycosaminoglycan on collagen fibrils; this binding may explain why the organism is commonly aligned with collagen fibrils in the extracellular matrix in the heart, nervous system, or joints.

To control and eradicate *B. burgdorferi*, the host mounts both innate and adaptive immune responses, resulting in macrophage- and antibody-mediated killing of the spirochete. As part of the innate immune response, complement may lyse the spirochete in the skin. Chemokines released by constituent cells in the skin lead to the recruitment of neutrophils and macrophages; the latter release potent proinflammatory cytokines. The purpose of the adaptive immune response appears to be the production of specific antibodies, which opsonize the organism—a step necessary for optimal spirochetal killing. Studies with protein arrays expressing ~1400 *B. burgdorferi* proteins detected antibody responses to a total of 89 spirochetal proteins (primarily outer-surface lipoproteins) in a population of patients with Lyme arthritis. Histologic examination of all affected tissues reveals an infiltration of lymphocytes, macrophages, and plasma cells with some degree of vascular damage (including mild vasculitis or hypervascular occlusion). These findings suggest that the spirochete may have been present in or around blood vessels.

In enzootic infection, *B. burgdorferi* spirochetes must survive this immune assault only during the summer months before returning to larval ticks to begin the cycle again the following year. In contrast, infection of humans is a dead-end event for the spirochete. Within several weeks or months, innate and adaptive immune mechanisms—even without antibiotic treatment—control widely disseminated infection, and generalized systemic symptoms wane. However, without antibiotic therapy, spirochetes may survive in localized niches for several more years. For example, *B. burgdorferi* infection in the United States may cause persistent arthritis or, in rare cases, subtle encephalopathy or polyneuropathy. Thus, immune mechanisms seem to succeed eventually in the near or total eradication of *B. burgdorferi* from selected niches, including the joints or nervous system.

■ CLINICAL MANIFESTATIONS

Early infection: stage 1 (localized infection)

Because of the small size of nymphal ixodid ticks, most patients do not remember the preceding tick bite. After an incubation period of 3–32 days, EM, which occurs at the site of the tick bite, usually begins as a red macule or papule that expands slowly to form a large annular lesion (Fig. 173-1). As the lesion increases in size, it often develops a bright red outer border and partial central clearing. The center of the lesion sometimes becomes intensely erythematous and indurated, vesicular, or necrotic. In other instances, the expanding lesion remains an even, intense red; several red rings are found within an outside ring; or the central area turns blue before the lesion clears. Although EM can be located anywhere, the thigh, groin, and axilla are particularly common sites. The lesion is warm but not often painful. Approximately 20% of patients do not exhibit this characteristic skin manifestation.

Early infection: stage 2 (disseminated infection)

In cases in the United States, *B. burgdorferi* often spreads hematogenously to many sites within days or weeks after the onset of EM. In these cases, patients may develop secondary annular skin lesions similar in appearance to the initial lesion. Skin involvement is commonly accompanied by severe headache, mild stiffness of the

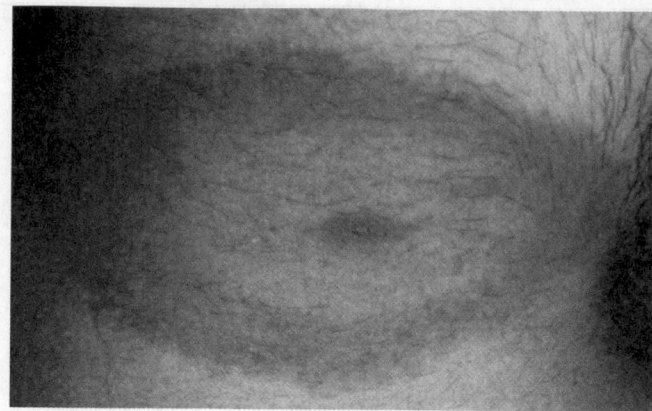

Figure 173-1 A classic erythema migrans lesion (9 cm in diameter) is shown near the right axilla. The lesion has partial central clearing, a bright red outer border, and a target center. *(Courtesy of Vijay K. Sikand, MD; with permission.)*

neck, fever, chills, migratory musculoskeletal pain, arthralgias, and profound malaise and fatigue. Less common manifestations include generalized lymphadenopathy or splenomegaly, hepatitis, sore throat, nonproductive cough, conjunctivitis, iritis, or testicular swelling. Except for fatigue and lethargy, which are often constant, the early signs and symptoms of Lyme disease are typically intermittent and changing. Even in untreated patients, the early symptoms usually become less severe or disappear within several weeks. In ~15% of patients, the infection presents with these nonspecific systemic symptoms.

Symptoms suggestive of meningeal irritation may develop early in Lyme disease when EM is present but usually are not associated with cerebrospinal fluid (CSF) pleocytosis or an objective neurologic deficit. After several weeks or months, ~15% of untreated patients develop frank neurologic abnormalities, including meningitis, subtle encephalitic signs, cranial neuritis (including bilateral facial palsy), motor or sensory radiculoneuropathy, peripheral neuropathy, mononeuritis multiplex, cerebellar ataxia, or myelitis—alone or in various combinations. In the United States, the usual pattern consists of fluctuating symptoms of meningitis accompanied by facial palsy and peripheral radiculoneuropathy. Lymphocytic pleocytosis (~100 cells/µL) is found in CSF, often along with elevated protein levels and normal or slightly low glucose concentrations. In Europe and Asia, the first neurologic sign is characteristically radicular pain, which is followed by the development of CSF pleocytosis (called meningopolyneuritis, or *Bannwarth's syndrome*); meningeal or encephalitic signs are frequently absent. In children, the optic nerve may be affected because of inflammation or increased intracranial pressure, which may lead to blindness. These early neurologic abnormalities usually resolve completely within months, but in rare cases chronic neurologic disease may occur later.

Within several weeks after the onset of illness, ~8% of patients develop cardiac involvement. The most common abnormality is a fluctuating degree of atrioventricular block (first-degree, Wenckebach, or complete heart block). Some patients have more diffuse cardiac involvement, including electrocardiographic changes indicative of acute myopericarditis, left ventricular dysfunction evident on radionuclide scans, or (in rare cases) cardiomegaly or pancarditis. Cardiac involvement usually lasts for only a few weeks but may recur. Chronic cardiomyopathy caused by *B. burgdorferi* has been reported in Europe.

During this stage, musculoskeletal pain is common. The typical pattern consists of migratory pain in joints, tendons, bursae, muscles, or bones (usually without joint swelling) lasting for hours or days and affecting one or two locations at a time.

Late infection: stage 3 (persistent infection)

Months after the onset of infection, ~60% of patients in the United States who have received no antibiotic treatment develop frank arthritis. The typical pattern comprises intermittent attacks of oligoarticular arthritis in large joints (especially the knees), lasting for weeks or months in a given joint. A few small joints or periarticular sites may also be affected, primarily during early attacks. The number of patients who continue to have recurrent attacks decreases each year. However, in a small percentage of cases, involvement of large joints—usually one or both knees—is persistent and may lead to erosion of cartilage and bone.

White cell counts in joint fluid range from 500 to 110,000/μL (average, 25,000/μL); most of these cells are polymorphonuclear leukocytes. Tests for rheumatoid factor or antinuclear antibodies usually give negative results. Examination of synovial biopsy samples reveals fibrin deposits, villous hypertrophy, vascular proliferation, microangiopathic lesions, and a heavy infiltration of lymphocytes and plasma cells.

Although most patients with Lyme arthritis respond well to antibiotic therapy, a small percentage in the northeastern United States have persistent arthritis for months or even for several years after the near or total eradication of spirochetes from the joints by antibiotic therapy. Compared with antibiotic-responsive patients, those with antibiotic-refractory arthritis are more often infected with RST1 strains of *B. burgdorferi*; have a higher frequency of certain class II major histocompatibility complex molecules (particularly HLA-DRBI*0401 or -*0101 molecules) that bind an epitope of OspA (OspA$_{163-175}$); and often exhibit T cell recognition of this epitope. In addition, these patients have significantly higher levels of proinflammatory chemokines and cytokines in joint fluid (especially CXCL9 and interferon γ) than do antibiotic-responsive patients; these higher levels persist during the postantibiotic period, when polymerase chain reaction (PCR) results for *B. burgdorferi* DNA are uniformly negative. It has been postulated that, in these genetically susceptible individuals, *B. burgdorferi* may trigger localized, tissue-specific autoimmunity within the proinflammatory milieu of the joints.

Although rare, chronic neurologic involvement may also become apparent from months to several years after the onset of infection, sometimes following long periods of latent infection. The most common form of chronic central nervous system involvement is subtle encephalopathy affecting memory, mood, or sleep, and the most common form of peripheral neuropathy is an axonal polyneuropathy manifested as either distal paresthesia or spinal radicular pain. Patients with encephalopathy frequently have evidence of memory impairment in neuropsychological tests and abnormal results in CSF analyses. In cases of polyneuropathy, electromyography generally shows extensive abnormalities of proximal and distal nerve segments. Encephalomyelitis or leukoencephalitis, a rare manifestation of Lyme borreliosis associated primarily with *B. garinii* infection in Europe, is a severe neurologic disorder that may include spastic paraparesis, upper motor-neuron bladder dysfunction, and, rarely, lesions in the periventricular white matter.

Acrodermatitis chronica atrophicans, the late skin manifestation of Lyme borreliosis, has been associated primarily with *B. afzelii* infection in Europe and Asia. It has been observed especially often in elderly women. The skin lesions, which are usually found on the acral surface of an arm or leg, begin insidiously with reddish-violaceous discoloration; they become sclerotic or atrophic over a period of years.

The basic patterns of Lyme borreliosis are similar worldwide, but there are regional variations, primarily between the illness found in North America, which is caused exclusively by *B. burgdorferi*, and that found in Europe, which is caused primarily by *B. afzelii* and *B. garinii*. With each of the *Borrelia* species, the infection usually begins with EM. However, *B. burgdorferi* often disseminates widely; it is particularly arthritogenic, and it may cause antibiotic-refractory arthritis. *B. garinii* typically disseminates less widely, but it is especially neurotropic and may cause borrelial encephalomyelitis. *B. afzelii* often infects only the skin but may persist in that site, where it may cause several different dermatoborrelioses, including acrodermatitis chronica atrophicans.

Post–Lyme syndrome (chronic Lyme disease)

Despite resolution of the objective manifestations of the infection with antibiotic therapy, a small percentage of patients have pain, neurocognitive manifestations, or fatigue symptoms for months or years afterward. This syndrome is similar to or indistinguishable from chronic fatigue syndrome (Chap. 389) and fibromyalgia (Chap. 335). Compared with symptoms of active Lyme disease, post-Lyme symptoms tend to be more generalized or disabling. They include marked fatigue, severe headache, diffuse musculoskeletal pain, multiple symmetric tender points in characteristic locations, pain and stiffness in many joints, diffuse paresthesias, difficulty with concentration, and sleep disturbances. Patients with this condition lack evidence of joint inflammation, have normal neurologic test results, and may exhibit anxiety and depression. In contrast, late manifestations of Lyme disease, including arthritis, encephalopathy, and neuropathy, are usually associated with minimal systemic symptoms. Currently, no evidence indicates that persistent subjective symptoms after recommended courses of antibiotic therapy are caused by active infection.

■ DIAGNOSIS

The culture of *B. burgdorferi* in Barbour-Stoenner-Kelly (BSK) medium permits definitive diagnosis, but this method has been used primarily in research studies. Moreover, with a few exceptions, positive cultures have been obtained only early in the illness—particularly from biopsy samples of EM skin lesions, less often from plasma samples, and occasionally from CSF samples. Later in the infection, PCR is greatly superior to culture for the detection of *B. burgdorferi* DNA in joint fluid—the major use for PCR testing in Lyme disease. However, the sensitivity of PCR determinations in CSF from patients with neuroborreliosis has been much lower. There seems to be little if any role for PCR in the detection of *B. burgdorferi* DNA in blood or urine samples. Moreover, this procedure must be carefully controlled to prevent contamination.

Because of the problems associated with direct detection of *B. burgdorferi*, Lyme disease is usually diagnosed by the recognition of a characteristic clinical picture with serologic confirmation. Although serologic testing may yield negative results during the first several weeks of infection, most patients have a positive antibody response to *B. burgdorferi* after that time. The limitation of serologic tests is that they do not clearly distinguish between active and inactive infection. Patients with previous Lyme disease—particularly in cases progressing to late stages—often remain seropositive for years, even after adequate antibiotic treatment. In addition, ~10% of patients are seropositive because of asymptomatic infection. If these individuals subsequently develop another illness, the positive serologic test for Lyme disease may cause diagnostic confusion. According to an algorithm published by the American College of Physicians (Table 173-1), serologic testing for Lyme disease is recommended only for patients with at least an intermediate pretest probability of Lyme disease, such as those with oligoarticular arthritis. It should not be used as a screening procedure in patients with pain or fatigue syndromes. In such patients, the probability of a false-positive serologic result is higher than that of a true-positive result.

TABLE 173-1 Algorithm for Testing for and Treating Lyme Disease

Pretest Probability	Example	Recommendation
High	Patients with erythema migrans	Empirical antibiotic treatment without serologic testing
Intermediate	Patients with oligoarticular arthritis	Serologic testing and antibiotic treatment if test results are positive
Low	Patients with nonspecific symptoms (myalgias, arthralgias, fatigue)	Neither serologic testing nor antibiotic treatment

Source: Adapted from the recommendations of the American College of Physicians (G Nichol et al: Ann Intern Med 128:37, 1998, with permission).

For serologic analysis of Lyme disease in the United States, the CDC recommends a two-step approach in which samples are first tested by enzyme-linked immunosorbent assay (ELISA) and equivocal or positive results are then tested by western blotting. During the first month of infection, both IgM and IgG responses to the spirochete should be determined, preferably in both acute- and convalescent-phase serum samples. Approximately 20–30% of patients have a positive response detectable in acute-phase samples, whereas ~70–80% have a positive response during convalescence (2–4 weeks later). After 4–8 weeks of infection (by which time most patients with active Lyme disease have disseminated infection), the sensitivity and specificity of the IgG response to the spirochete are both very high—in the range of 99%—as determined by the two-test approach of ELISA and western blot. At this point and thereafter, a single test (that for IgG) is usually sufficient. In persons with illness of >2 months' duration, a positive IgM test result alone is likely to be false-positive and therefore should not be used to support the diagnosis.

According to current criteria adopted by the CDC, an IgM western blot is considered positive if two of the following three bands are present: 23, 39, and 41 kDa. However, the combination of the 23- and 41-kDa bands may still represent a false-positive result. Misuse or misinterpretation of IgM blots has been a factor in the incorrect diagnosis of Lyme disease in patients with other illnesses. An IgG blot is considered positive if 5 of the following 10 bands are present: 18, 23, 28, 30, 39, 41, 45, 58, 66, and 93 kDa. In European cases, there is less expansion of the antibody response, and no single set of criteria for the interpretation of immunoblots results in high levels of sensitivity and specificity in all countries.

The most promising second-generation serologic test is the C6 peptide IgG ELISA, which employs a 26-mer of the sixth invariant region of the VlsE lipoprotein of *B. burgdorferi*. The results achieved with this test are similar to those obtained with the standard two-test approach (sonicate IgM and IgG ELISA and western blot). The principal advantage of the C6 peptide ELISA is the early detection of an IgG response, which renders an IgM test unnecessary. However, not all patients with late Lyme disease have a response to the C6 peptide, and this test is not quite as specific as sonicate western blot. Thus, at present, a two-test approach that includes western blot is still recommended. Like sonicate test responses, the response to the VlsE peptide may persist for months or years after successful antibiotic treatment; therefore, persistence of antibody to VlsE cannot be equated with spirochetal persistence in Lyme disease.

■ DIFFERENTIAL DIAGNOSIS

Classic EM is a slowly expanding erythema, often with partial central clearing. If the lesion expands little, it may represent the red papule of an uninfected tick bite. If the lesion expands rapidly, it may represent cellulitis (e.g., streptococcal cellulitis) or an allergic reaction, perhaps to tick saliva. Patients with secondary annular lesions may be thought to have erythema multiforme, but neither the development of blistering mucosal lesions nor the involvement of the palms or soles is a feature of *B. burgdorferi* infection. In the southeastern United States, an EM-like skin lesion, sometimes with mild systemic symptoms, may be associated with *Amblyomma americanum* tick bites. However, the cause of this Southern tick-associated rash illness (STARI) has not yet been identified.

In the United States, *I. scapularis* ticks may transmit not only *B. burgdorferi* but also *Babesia microti*, a red blood cell parasite (Chap. 211), or *Anaplasma phagocytophilum*, the agent of human granulocytotropic anaplasmosis (formerly human granulocytotropic ehrlichiosis; Chap. 174). Although babesiosis and anaplasmosis are most often asymptomatic, infection with any of these three agents may cause nonspecific systemic symptoms, and co-infected patients may have more severe or persistent symptoms than patients infected with a single agent. Standard blood counts may yield clues regarding the presence of co-infection. Anaplasmosis may cause leukopenia or thrombocytopenia, and babesiosis may cause thrombocytopenia or (in severe cases) hemolytic anemia. IgM serologic responses may confuse the diagnosis. For example, *A. phagocytophilum* may elicit a positive IgM response to *B. burgdorferi*. The frequency of co-infection in different studies has been variable. In one prospective study, 4% of patients with EM had evidence of co-infection.

Facial palsy caused by *B. burgdorferi*, which occurs in the early disseminated phase of the infection (often in July, August, or September), is usually recognized by its association with EM. However, in rare cases, facial palsy without EM may be the presenting manifestation of Lyme disease. In such cases, both the IgM and the IgG responses to the spirochete are usually positive. The most common infectious agents that cause facial palsy are herpes simplex virus type 1 (Bell's palsy; Chap. 179) and varicella-zoster virus (Ramsay Hunt syndrome; Chap. 180).

Later in the infection, oligoarticular Lyme arthritis most resembles reactive arthritis in an adult or the pauciarticular form of juvenile idiopathic arthritis in a child. Patients with Lyme arthritis usually have the strongest IgG antibody responses seen in Lyme borreliosis, with reactivity to many spirochetal proteins.

The most common problem in diagnosis is to mistake Lyme disease for chronic fatigue syndrome (Chap. 389) or fibromyalgia (Chap. 335). This difficulty is compounded by the fact that a small percentage of patients do in fact develop these chronic pain or fatigue syndromes in association with or soon after Lyme disease. Moreover, a counterculture has emerged that ascribes pain and fatigue syndromes to chronic Lyme disease when there is little or no evidence of *B. burgdorferi* infection. In such cases, the term *chronic Lyme disease*, which is equated with chronic *B. burgdorferi* infection, is a misnomer, and the use of prolonged, dangerous, and expensive antibiotic treatment is not warranted.

TREATMENT Lyme Borreliosis

ANTIBIOTIC TREATMENT As outlined in the algorithm in Fig. 173-2, the various manifestations of Lyme disease can usually be treated successfully with orally administered antibiotics; the exceptions are objective neurologic abnormalities and third-degree atrioventricular heart block, which are generally treated with IV antibiotics. For early Lyme disease, doxycycline is

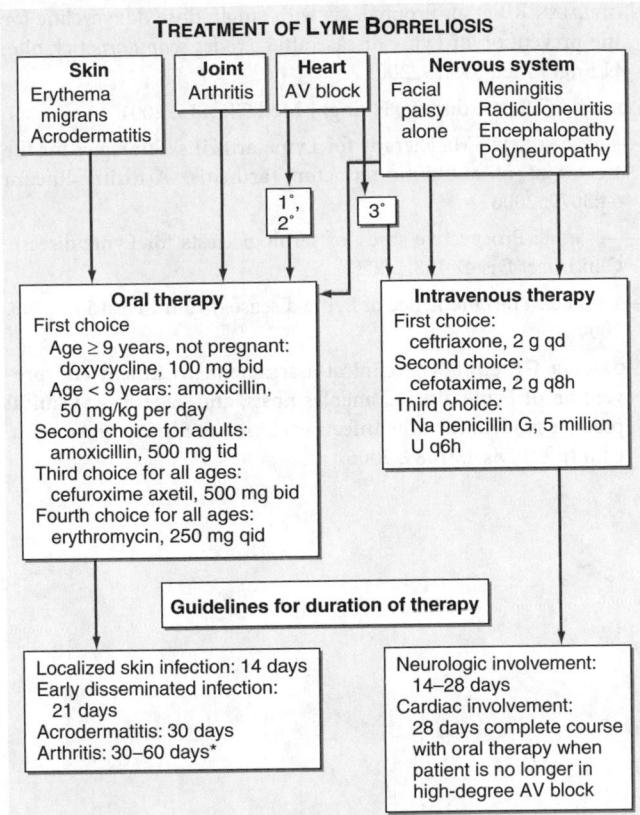

TREATMENT OF LYME BORRELIOSIS

Skin	Joint	Heart	Nervous system
Erythema migrans Acrodermatitis	Arthritis	AV block	Facial palsy alone / Meningitis Radiculoneuritis Encephalopathy Polyneuropathy

1° 2° 3°

Oral therapy

First choice
  Age ≥ 9 years, not pregnant:
    doxycycline, 100 mg bid
  Age < 9 years: amoxicillin,
    50 mg/kg per day
Second choice for adults:
  amoxicillin, 500 mg tid
Third choice for all ages:
  cefuroxime axetil, 500 mg bid
Fourth choice for all ages:
  erythromycin, 250 mg qid

Intravenous therapy

First choice:
  ceftriaxone, 2 g qd
Second choice:
  cefotaxime, 2 g q8h
Third choice:
  Na penicillin G, 5 million
  U q6h

Guidelines for duration of therapy

Localized skin infection: 14 days
Early disseminated infection:
  21 days
Acrodermatitis: 30 days
Arthritis: 30–60 days*

Neurologic involvement:
  14–28 days
Cardiac involvement:
  28 days complete course
  with oral therapy when
  patient is no longer in
  high-degree AV block

Figure 173-2 Algorithm for the treatment of the various acute or chronic manifestations of Lyme borreliosis. AV, atrioventricular. *For Lyme arthritis, IV ceftriaxone (2 g given once a day for 14–28 days) is also effective and is necessary for a small percentage of patients; however, compared with oral treatment, this regimen is less convenient to administer, has more side effects, and is more expensive.

effective and can be administered to men and nonpregnant women. An advantage of this regimen is that it is also effective against *A. phagocytophilum*, which is transmitted by the same tick that transmits the Lyme disease agent. Amoxicillin, cefuroxime axetil, and erythromycin or its congeners are second-, third-, and fourth-choice alternatives, respectively. In children, amoxicillin is effective (not more than 2 g/d); in cases of penicillin allergy, cefuroxime axetil or erythromycin may be used. In contrast to second- or third-generation cephalosporin antibiotics, first-generation cephalosporins, such as cephalexin, are not effective. For patients with infection localized to the skin, a 14-day course of therapy is generally sufficient; in contrast, for patients with disseminated infection, a 21-day course is recommended. Approximately 15% of patients experience a Jarisch-Herxheimer-like reaction during the first 24 h of therapy. In multicenter studies, >90% of patients whose early Lyme disease was treated with these regimens had satisfactory outcomes. Although some patients reported symptoms after treatment, objective evidence of persistent infection or relapse was rare, and re-treatment was usually unnecessary.

Oral administration of doxycycline or amoxicillin for 30 days is recommended for the initial treatment of Lyme arthritis in patients who do not have concomitant neurologic involvement. Among patients with arthritis who do not respond to oral antibiotics, re-treatment with IV ceftriaxone for 28 days is appropriate. In patients with arthritis in whom—despite a negative PCR result for *B. burgdorferi* DNA in joint fluid—joint inflammation persists for months or even several years after both oral and IV antibiotics, treatment with anti-inflammatory agents or synovectomy may be successful.

In the United States, parenteral antibiotic therapy is usually used for objective neurologic abnormalities (with the possible exception of facial palsy alone). Patients with neurologic involvement are most commonly treated with IV ceftriaxone for 14–28 days, but IV cefotaxime or IV penicillin G for the same duration may also be effective. In Europe, similar results have been achieved with oral doxycycline and IV antibiotics in the treatment of acute neuroborreliosis. In patients with high-degree atrioventricular block or a PR interval of >0.3 s, IV therapy for at least part of the course and cardiac monitoring are recommended, but the insertion of a permanent pacemaker is not necessary.

It is unclear how and whether asymptomatic infection should be treated, but patients with such infection are often given a course of oral antibiotics. Because maternal-fetal transmission of *B. burgdorferi* seems to occur rarely (if at all), standard therapy for the manifestations of the illness is recommended for pregnant women. Long-term persistence of *B. burgdorferi* has not been documented in any large series of patients after treatment with currently recommended regimens. Although an occasional patient requires a second course of antibiotics, there is no indication for multiple, repeated antibiotic courses in the treatment of Lyme disease.

CHRONIC LYME DISEASE After appropriately treated Lyme disease, a small percentage of patients continue to have subjective symptoms, primarily musculoskeletal pain, neurocognitive difficulties, or fatigue. This *chronic Lyme disease* or *post–Lyme syndrome* is a disabling condition that is similar to chronic fatigue syndrome or fibromyalgia. In a large study, one group of patients with post–Lyme syndrome received IV ceftriaxone for 30 days followed by oral doxycycline for 60 days, while another group received IV and oral placebo preparations for the same durations. No significant differences were found between groups in the numbers of patients reporting that their symptoms had improved, become worse, or stayed the same. Such patients are best treated for the relief of symptoms rather than with prolonged courses of antibiotics.

PROPHYLAXIS AFTER A TICK BITE The risk of infection with *B. burgdorferi* after a recognized tick bite is so low that antibiotic prophylaxis is not routinely indicated. However, if an attached, engorged *I. scapularis* nymph is found or if follow-up is anticipated to be difficult, a single 200-mg dose of doxycycline, which usually prevents Lyme disease when given within 72 h after the tick bite, may be administered.

■ **PROGNOSIS**

The response to treatment is best early in the disease. Later treatment of Lyme borreliosis is still effective, but the period of convalescence may be longer. Eventually, most patients recover with minimal or no residual deficits.

■ **REINFECTION**

Reinfection may occur after EM when patients are treated with antimicrobial agents. In such cases, the immune response is not adequate to provide protection from subsequent infection. However, patients who develop an expanded immune response to the spirochete over a period of months (e.g., those with Lyme arthritis) have protective immunity for a period of years and do not acquire the infection again.

■ PREVENTION

Protective measures for the prevention of Lyme disease may include the avoidance of tick-infested areas, the use of repellents and acaricides, tick checks, and modification of landscapes in or near residential areas. Although a vaccine for Lyme disease used to be available, the manufacturer has discontinued its production. Therefore, no vaccine is now commercially available for the prevention of this infection.

FURTHER READINGS

Feder HM Jr et al: A critical appraisal of "chronic Lyme disease." N Engl J Med 357:1422, 2007

Klempner MS et al: Two controlled trials of antibiotic treatment in patients with persistent symptoms and a history of Lyme disease. N Engl J Med 345:85, 2001

Nadelman RB et al: Prophylaxis with single-dose doxycycline for the prevention of Lyme disease after *Ixodes scapularis* tick bite. N Engl J Med 345:79, 2001

Steere AC: Lyme disease. N Engl J Med 345:115, 2001

——, Angelis SM: Therapy for Lyme arthritis: Strategies for the treatment of antibiotic-refractory arthritis. Arthritis Rheum 54:3079, 2006

—— et al: Prospective study of serologic tests for Lyme disease. Clin Infect Dis 47:188, 2008

—— et al: The emergence of Lyme disease. J Clin Invest 113:1093, 2004

Wormser GP et al: The clinical assessment, treatment and prevention of Lyme disease, anaplasmosis, and babesiosis: Clinical practice guidelines of the Infectious Diseases Society of America. Clin Infect Dis 43:1089, 2006

CHAPTER 174

Rickettsial Diseases

David H. Walker

J. Stephen Dumler

Thomas Marrie

The rickettsiae are a heterogeneous group of small, obligately intracellular, gram-negative coccobacilli and short bacilli, most of which are transmitted by a tick, mite, flea, or louse vector. Except in the case of louse-borne typhus, humans are incidental hosts. Among rickettsiae, *Coxiella burnetii*, *Rickettsia prowazekii*, and *R. typhi* have the well-documented ability to survive for an extended period outside the reservoir or vector and to be extremely infectious: inhalation of a single *Coxiella* microorganism can cause pneumonia. High infectivity and severe illness after inhalation make *R. prowazekii*, *R. rickettsii*, *R. typhi*, *R. conorii*, and *C. burnetii* bioterrorism threats.

Clinical infections with rickettsiae can be classified according to (1) the taxonomy and diverse microbial characteristics of the agents, which belong to six genera (*Rickettsia*, *Orientia*, *Ehrlichia*, *Anaplasma*, *Neorickettsia*, and *Coxiella*); (2) epidemiology; or (3) clinical manifestations. The clinical manifestations of all the acute presentations are similar during the first 5 days: fever, headache, and myalgias with or without nausea, vomiting, and cough. As the course progresses, clinical manifestations—including occurrence of a macular, maculopapular, or vesicular rash; eschar; pneumonitis; and meningoencephalitis—vary from one disease to another. Given the 14 etiologic agents with varied mechanisms of transmission, geographic distributions, and associated disease manifestations, the consideration of rickettsial diseases as a single entity poses complex challenges (Table 174-1).

Establishing the etiologic diagnosis of rickettsioses is very difficult during the acute stage of illness, and definitive diagnosis usually requires the examination of paired serum samples after convalescence. Heightened clinical suspicion is based on epidemiologic data, history of exposure to vectors or reservoir animals, travel to endemic locations, clinical manifestations (sometimes including rash or eschar), and characteristic laboratory findings [including thrombocytopenia, normal or low white blood cell (WBC) counts, elevated hepatic enzyme levels, and hyponatremia]. Such suspicion should prompt empirical treatment. Doxycycline is the drug of choice for most of these infections. Only one agent, *C. burnetii*, has been documented to cause chronic illness. One other, *R. prowazekii*, causes recrudescent illness (Brill-Zinsser disease) when latent infection is reactivated years after resolution of the acute illness.

Rickettsial infections dominated by fever may resolve without further clinical evolution. However, after nonspecific early manifestations, the illnesses can also evolve along one or more of several principal clinical lines: (1) development of a macular or maculopapular rash; (2) development of an eschar at the site of tick or mite feeding; (3) development of a vesicular rash (often in rickettsialpox and African tick-bite fever); (4) development of pneumonitis with chest radiographic opacities and/or rales [Q fever and severe

cases of Rocky Mountain spotted fever (RMSF), Mediterranean spotted fever (MSF), louse-borne typhus, human monocytotropic ehrlichiosis (HME), human granulocytotropic anaplasmosis (HGA), scrub typhus, and murine typhus]; (5) development of meningoencephalitis [louse-borne typhus and severe cases of RMSF, scrub typhus, HME, murine typhus, MSF, and (rarely) Q fever]; and (6) progressive hypotension and multiorgan failure as seen with sepsis or toxic shock syndrome (RMSF, MSF, louse-borne typhus, murine typhus, scrub typhus, HME, and HGA).

Epidemiologic clues to the transmission of a particular pathogen include (1) environmental exposure to ticks, fleas, or mites during the season of activity of the vector species for the disease in the appropriate geographic region (spotted fever and typhus rickettsioses, scrub typhus, ehrlichioses, anaplasmosis); (2) travel to or residence in an endemic geographic region during the incubation period (Table 174-1); (3) exposure to parturient ruminants, cats, and dogs (Q fever); (4) exposure to flying squirrels (*R. prowazekii* infection); and (5) history of previous louse-borne typhus (recrudescent typhus).

Clinical laboratory findings, such as thrombocytopenia (particularly in spotted fever and typhus rickettsioses, ehrlichioses, anaplasmosis, and scrub typhus), normal or low WBC counts, mild to moderate serum elevations of hepatic aminotransferases, and hyponatremia suggest some common pathophysiologic mechanisms.

Application of these clinical, epidemiologic, and laboratory principles requires consideration of a rickettsial diagnosis and knowledge of the individual diseases.

TICK-, MITE-, LOUSE-, AND FLEA-BORNE RICKETTSIOSES

These diseases, caused by organisms of the genera *Rickettsia* and *Orientia* in the family Rickettsiaceae, result from endothelial infection and increased vascular permeability. Pathogenic rickettsial species are very closely related, have small genomes (as a result of reductive evolution, which eliminated many genes for biosynthesis of intracellularly available molecules), and are traditionally separated into typhus and spotted fever groups on the basis of lipopolysaccharide antigens. Some diseases and their agents (e.g., *R. africae*, *R. parkeri*, and *R. sibirica*) are too similar to require separate descriptions. Indeed, the similarities among MSF [*R. conorii* (all strains)] and *R. massiliae*, North Asian tick typhus (*R. sibirica*), Japanese spotted fever (*R. japonica*), and Flinders Island spotted fever (*R. honei*) far outweigh the minor variations. The Rickettsiaceae that cause life-threatening infections are, in order of decreasing case-fatality rate, *R. rickettsii* (RMSF); *R. prowazekii* (louse-borne typhus); *Orientia tsutsugamushi* (scrub typhus); *R. conorii* (MSF); *R. typhi* (murine typhus); and, in rare cases, other spotted fever–group organisms. Some agents (e.g., *R. parkeri*, *R. africae*, *R. akari*, *R. slovaca*, *R. honei*, *R. felis*, *R. massiliae*, *R. helvetica*, *R. heilongjiangensis*, *R. aeschlimannii*, and *R. monacensis*) have never been documented to cause a fatal illness.

ROCKY MOUNTAIN SPOTTED FEVER

RMSF occurs in 47 states (with the highest prevalence in the south-central and southeastern states) as well as in Canada, Mexico, and Central and South America. The infection is transmitted by *Dermacentor variabilis*, the American dog tick, in the eastern two-thirds of the United States and

TABLE 174-1 Features of Selected Rickettsial Infections

Disease	Organism	Transmission	Geographic Range	Incubation Period, Days	Duration, Days	Rash, %	Eschar, %	Lymphade-nopathy[a]
Rocky Mountain spotted fever	*Rickettsia rickettsii*	Tick bite: *Dermacentor andersoni, D. variabilis*	United States	2–14	10–20	90	<1	+
		Amblyomma cajennense, A. aureolatum	Central/South America					
		Rhipicephalus sanguineus	Mexico, Brazil, United States					
Mediterranean spotted fever	*R. conorii*	Tick bite: *R. sanguineus, R. pumilio*	Southern Europe, Africa, Middle East, Central Asia	5–7	7–14	97	50	+
African tick-bite fever	*R. africae*	Tick bite: *A. hebraeum, A. variegatum*	Sub-Saharan Africa, West Indies	4–10	?	50	90	++++
Maculatum disease	*R. parkeri*	*A. maculatum*	United States, South America	2–10	?	88	94	++
Rickettsialpox	*R. akari*	Mite bite: *Liponyssoides sanguineus*	United States, Ukraine, Turkey, Mexico, Croatia	10–17	3–11	100	90	+++
Tick-borne lymphadenopathy	*R. slovaca*	Tick bite: *Dermacentor marginatus, D. reticularis*	Europe	7–9	17–180	5	100	++++
Flea-borne spotted fever	*R. felis*	Flea (mechanism undetermined): *Ctenocephalides felis*	Worldwide	8–16	8–16	80	15	—
Epidemic typhus	*R. prowazekii*	Louse feces: *Pediculus humanus corporis,* fleas and lice of flying squirrels, or recrudescence	Worldwide	7–14	10–18	80	None	—
Murine typhus	*R. typhi*	Flea feces: *Xenopsylla cheopis, C. felis,* others	Worldwide	8–16	9–18	80	None	—
Human monocytotropic ehrlichiosis	*Ehrlichia chaffeensis*	Tick bite: *Amblyomma americanum, D. variabilis*	United States	1–21	3–21	26	None	++
Ewingii ehrlichiosis	*E. ewingii*	Tick bite: *A. americanum*	United States				None	
Human granulocytotropic anaplasmosis	*Anaplasma phagocytophilum*	Tick bite: *Ixodes scapularis, I. ricinus, I. pacificus, I. persulcatus*	United States, Europe, Asia	4–8	3–14	Rare	None	—
Scrub typhus	*Orientia tsutsugamushi*	Mite bite: *Leptotrombidium deliense,* others	Asia, Australia, New Guinea, Pacific Islands	9–18	6–21	50	35	+++
Q fever	*Coxiella burnetii*	Inhalation of aerosols of infected parturition material (sheep, dogs, others), ingestion of infected milk or milk products	Worldwide	3–30	5–57	<1	None	—

[a]++++, severe; +++, marked; ++, moderate; +, present in a small portion of cases; —, not a noted feature.

California; by *D. andersoni*, the Rocky Mountain wood tick, in the western United States; by *Rhipicephalus sanguineus* in Mexico, Arizona, and probably Brazil; and by *Amblyomma cajennense* in Central and South America. Maintained principally by transovarian transmission from one generation of ticks to the next, *R. rickettsii* can be acquired by uninfected ticks through the ingestion of a blood meal from rickettsemic small mammals.

Humans become infected during tick season (in the Northern Hemisphere, from May to September), although some cases occur in winter. The mortality rate was 20–25% in the preantibiotic era

and remains at ~3–5% principally because of delayed diagnosis and treatment. The case-fatality ratio increases with each decade of life above age 20.

Pathogenesis

R. rickettsii organisms are inoculated into the dermis along with secretions of the tick's salivary glands after ≥6 h of feeding. The rickettsiae spread lymphohematogenously throughout the body and infect numerous foci of contiguous endothelial cells. The dose-dependent incubation period is ~1 week (range, 2–14 days). Occlusive thrombosis and ischemic necrosis are not the fundamental pathologic basis for tissue and organ injury. Instead, increased vascular permeability, with resulting edema, hypovolemia, and ischemia, is responsible. Consumption of platelets results in thrombocytopenia in 32–52% of patients, but disseminated intravascular coagulation with hypofibrinogenemia is rare. Activation of platelets, generation of thrombin, and activation of the fibrinolytic system all appear to be homeostatic physiologic responses to endothelial injury.

Clinical manifestations

Early in the illness, when medical attention usually is first sought, RMSF is difficult to distinguish from many self-limiting viral illnesses. Fever, headache, malaise, myalgia, nausea, vomiting, and anorexia are the most common symptoms during the first 3 days. The patient becomes progressively more ill as vascular infection and injury advance. In one large series, only one-third of patients were diagnosed with presumptive RMSF early in the clinical course and treated appropriately as outpatients. In the tertiary-care setting, RMSF is all too often recognized only when late severe manifestations, developing at the end of the first week or during the second week of illness in patients without appropriate treatment, prompt return to a physician or hospital and admission to an intensive care unit.

The progressive nature of the infection is clearly manifested in the skin. Rash is evident in only 14% of patients on the first day of illness and in only 49% during the first 3 days. Macules (1–5 mm) appear first on the wrists and ankles and then on the remainder of the extremities and the trunk. Later, more severe vascular damage results in frank hemorrhage at the center of the maculopapule, producing a petechia that does not disappear upon compression (Fig. 174-1). This sequence of events is sometimes delayed or aborted by effective treatment. However, the rash is a variable manifestation, appearing on day 6 or later in 20% of cases and not appearing at all in 9–16% of cases. Petechiae occur in 41–59% of cases, appearing on or after day 6 in 74% of cases that manifest a rash. Involvement of the palms and soles, often considered diagnostically important, usually develops relatively late in the course (after day 5 in 43% of cases) and does not develop at all in 18–64% of cases.

Hypovolemia leads to prerenal azotemia and (in 17% of cases) hypotension. Infection of the pulmonary microcirculation leads to noncardiogenic pulmonary edema; 12% of patients have severe respiratory disease, and 8% require mechanical ventilation. Cardiac involvement manifests as dysrhythmia in 7–16% of cases.

Besides respiratory failure, central nervous system (CNS) involvement is the other important determinant of the outcome of RMSF. Encephalitis, presenting as confusion or lethargy, is apparent in 26–28% of cases. Progressively severe encephalitis manifests as stupor or delirium in 21–26% of cases, ataxia in 18%, coma in 10%, and seizures in 8%. Numerous focal neurologic deficits have been reported. Meningoencephalitis results in cerebrospinal fluid (CSF) pleocytosis in 34–38% of cases; usually there are 10–100 cells/μL and a mononuclear predominance, but occasionally there are >100 cells/μL and a polymorphonuclear predominance. The CSF protein concentration is increased in 30–35% of cases, but the CSF glucose concentration is usually normal.

Renal failure, often reversible with rehydration, is caused by acute tubular necrosis in severe cases with shock. Hepatic injury with increased serum aminotransferase concentrations (38% of cases) is due to focal death of individual hepatocytes without hepatic failure. Jaundice is recognized in 9% of cases and an elevated serum bilirubin concentration in 18–30%.

Life-threatening bleeding is rare. Anemia develops in 30% of cases and is severe enough to require transfusions in 11%. Blood is detected in the stools or vomitus of 10% of patients, and death has followed massive upper gastrointestinal hemorrhage.

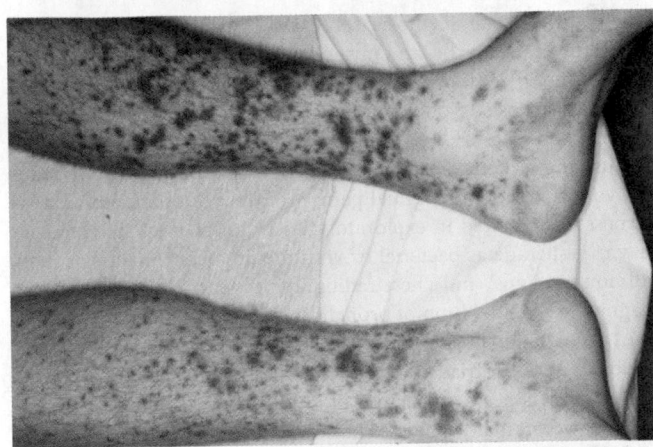

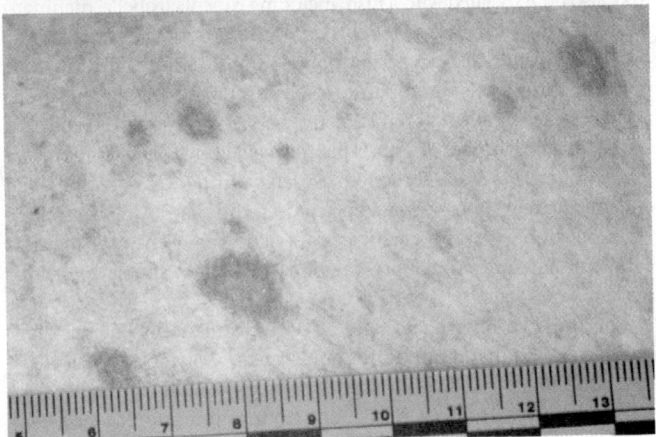

Figure 174-1 *Top:* Petechial lesions of Rocky Mountain spotted fever on the lower legs and soles of a young, previously healthy patient. *Bottom:* **Close-up of lesions** from the same patient. *(Photos courtesy of Dr. Lindsey Baden; with permission.)*

Other characteristic clinical laboratory findings include increased plasma levels of proteins of the acute-phase response (C-reactive protein, fibrinogen, ferritin, and others), hypoalbuminemia, and hyponatremia (in 56% of cases) due to the appropriate secretion of antidiuretic hormone in response to the hypovolemic state. Myositis occurs occasionally, with marked elevations in serum creatine kinase levels and multifocal rhabdomyonecrosis. Ocular involvement includes conjunctivitis in 30% of cases and retinal vein engorgement, flame hemorrhages, arterial occlusion, and papilledema with normal CSF pressure in some instances.

In untreated cases, the patient usually dies 8–15 days after onset. A rare presentation, fulminant RMSF, is fatal within 5 days after onset. This fulminant presentation is seen most often in male black patients with glucose-6-phosphate dehydrogenase (G6PD) deficiency and may be related to an undefined effect of hemolysis on the rickettsial infection. Although survivors of RMSF usually return to their previous state of health, permanent sequelae, including neurologic deficits and gangrene necessitating amputation of extremities, may follow severe illness.

Diagnosis

The diagnosis of RMSF during the acute stage is more difficult than is generally appreciated. The most important epidemiologic factor is a history of exposure to a potentially tick-infested environment within the 12 days preceding disease onset during a season of possible tick activity. However, only 60% of patients actually recall being bitten by a tick during the incubation period.

The differential diagnosis for early clinical manifestations of RMSF (fever, headache, and myalgia without a rash) includes influenza, enteroviral infection, infectious mononucleosis, viral hepatitis, leptospirosis, typhoid fever, gram-negative or gram-positive bacterial sepsis, HME, HGA, murine typhus, sylvatic flying-squirrel typhus, and rickettsialpox. Enterocolitis may be suggested by nausea, vomiting, and abdominal pain; prominence of abdominal tenderness has resulted in exploratory laparotomy. CNS involvement may masquerade as bacterial or viral meningoencephalitis. Cough, pulmonary signs, and chest radiographic opacities may lead to a diagnostic consideration of bronchitis or pneumonia.

At presentation during the first 3 days of illness, only 3% of patients exhibit the classic triad of fever, rash, and history of tick exposure. When a rash appears, a diagnosis of RMSF should certainly be considered. However, many illnesses considered in the differential diagnosis may also be associated with a rash, including rubeola, rubella, meningococcemia, disseminated gonococcal infection, secondary syphilis, toxic shock syndrome, drug hypersensitivity, idiopathic thrombocytopenic purpura, thrombotic thrombocytopenic purpura, Kawasaki syndrome, and immune complex vasculitis. Conversely, any person in an endemic area with a provisional diagnosis of one of the above illnesses may have RMSF. Thus, if a viral infection is suspected during RMSF season in an endemic area, it should always be kept in mind that RMSF can mimic viral infection early in the course; if the illness worsens over the next couple of days after initial presentation, the patient should return for reevaluation.

The most common serologic test for confirmation of the diagnosis is the indirect immunofluorescence assay. Not until 7–10 days after onset is a diagnostic titer of ≥1:64 usually detectable. The sensitivity and specificity of the indirect immunofluorescence assay are 94–100% and 100%, respectively. It is important to understand that serologic tests for RMSF are usually negative at the time of presentation for medical care and that treatment should not be delayed while a positive serologic result is awaited.

The only diagnostic test that is useful during the acute illness is immunohistologic examination of a cutaneous biopsy sample from a rash lesion for *R. rickettsii*. Examination of a 3-mm punch biopsy from such a lesion is 70% sensitive and 100% specific. The sensitivity of polymerase chain reaction (PCR) amplification and detection of *R. rickettsii* DNA in peripheral blood is improving. However, although rickettsiae are present in large quantities in heavily infected foci of endothelial cells, there are relatively low quantities in the circulation. Cultivation of rickettsiae in cell culture is feasible but is seldom undertaken because of biohazard concerns. The recent dramatic increase in the reported incidence of RMSF correlates with the use of single-titer spotted fever–group cross-reactive enzyme immunoassay serology, with which few cases are specifically determined to be caused by *R. rickettsii*.

TREATMENT   Rocky Mountain Spotted Fever

The drug of choice for the treatment of both children and adults with RMSF is doxycycline, except when the patient is pregnant or allergic to this drug (see below). Because of the severity of RMSF, immediate empirical administration of doxycycline should be strongly considered for any patient with a consistent clinical presentation in the appropriate epidemiologic setting. Doxycycline is administered orally (or, in the presence of coma or vomiting, intravenously) at 200 mg/d in two divided doses. For children with suspected RMSF, up to five courses of doxycycline may be administered with minimal risk of dental staining. Other regimens include oral tetracycline (25–50 mg/kg per day) in four divided doses. Treatment with chloramphenicol, a less

effective drug, is advised only for patients who are pregnant or allergic to doxycycline. The antirickettsial drug should be administered until the patient has been afebrile and improving clinically for 2–3 days. β-Lactam antibiotics, erythromycin, and aminoglycosides have no role in the treatment of RMSF, and sulfa-containing drugs are likely to exacerbate this infection. There is little clinical experience with fluoroquinolones, clarithromycin, and azithromycin, which are not recommended. The most seriously ill patients are managed in intensive care units, with careful administration of fluids to achieve optimal tissue perfusion without precipitating noncardiogenic pulmonary edema. In some severely ill patients, hypoxemia requires intubation and mechanical ventilation; oliguric or anuric acute renal failure requires hemodialysis; seizures necessitate the use of antiseizure medication; anemia or severe hemorrhage necessitates transfusions of packed red blood cells; or bleeding with severe thrombocytopenia requires platelet transfusions. Heparin is not a useful component of treatment, and there is no evidence that glucocorticoids affect outcome.

Prevention

Avoidance of tick bites is the only available preventive approach. Use of protective clothing and tick repellents, inspection of the body once or twice a day, and removal of ticks before they inoculate rickettsiae reduce the risk of infection.

■ MEDITERRANEAN SPOTTED FEVER (BOUTONNEUSE FEVER), AFRICAN TICK-BITE FEVER, AND OTHER TICK-BORNE SPOTTED FEVERS

R. conorii is prevalent in southern Europe, Africa, and southwestern and south-central Asia. Regional names for the disease caused by this organism include Mediterranean spotted fever, Kenya tick typhus, Indian tick typhus, Israeli spotted fever, and Astrakhan spotted fever. The disease is characterized by high fever, rash, and—in most geographic locales—an inoculation eschar (*tâche noire*) at the site of the tick bite. A severe form of the disease (mortality rate, 50%) occurs in patients with diabetes, alcoholism, or heart failure.

African tick-bite fever, caused by *R. africae*, occurs in rural areas of sub-Saharan Africa and in the Caribbean islands and is transmitted by *Amblyomma hebraeum* and *A. variegatum* ticks. The average incubation period is 4–10 days. The mild illness consists of headache, fever, eschar, and regional lymphadenopathy. *Amblyomma* ticks often feed in groups, with the consequent development of multiple eschars. Rash may be vesicular, sparse, or absent altogether. Because of tourism in sub-Saharan Africa, African tick-bite fever is the most frequently imported rickettsiosis in Europe and North America. A similar disease caused by the very closely related *R. parkeri* is transmitted by *A. maculatum* in the United States and *A. triste* in South America.

R. japonica causes Japanese spotted fever, which also occurs in Korea. Similar diseases in northern Asia are caused by *R. sibirica* and *R. heilongjiangensis*. Queensland tick typhus due to *R. australis* is transmitted by *Ixodes holocyclus*. Flinders Island spotted fever, found on the island for which it is named as well as in Tasmania, mainland Australia, and southeastern Asia, is caused by *R. honei*. In Europe, patients infected with *R. slovaca* after a wintertime *Dermacentor* tick bite manifest an afebrile illness with an eschar (usually on the scalp) and painful regional lymphadenopathy.

Diagnosis

Diagnosis of these tick-borne spotted fevers is based on clinical and epidemiologic findings and is confirmed by serology, immunohistochemical demonstration of rickettsiae in skin biopsy specimens, cell-culture isolation of rickettsiae, or PCR of skin biopsy or blood samples. The serologic identification of the etiologic species requires knowledge of all the potential agents as well as expensive, laborious cross-adsorption of the patient's serum. In an endemic area, a possible diagnosis of one of these rickettsial spotted fevers should be considered when patients present with fever, rash, and/or a skin lesion consisting of a black necrotic area or a crust surrounded by erythema.

TREATMENT | **Tick-Borne Spotted Fevers**

Successful therapeutic agents include doxycycline (100 mg bid orally for 1–5 days), ciprofloxacin (750 mg bid orally for 5 days), and chloramphenicol (500 mg qid orally for 7–10 days). Pregnant patients may be treated with josamycin (3 g/d orally for 5 days). Data on the efficacy of treatment of mildly ill children with clarithromycin or azithromycin should not be extrapolated to adults or to patients with moderate or severe illness.

■ RICKETTSIALPOX

R. akari infects mice and their mites (*Liponyssoides sanguineus*), which maintain the organisms by transovarian transmission.

Epidemiology

Rickettsialpox is recognized principally in New York City, but cases have also been reported in other urban and rural locations in the United States and in Ukraine, Croatia, Mexico, and Turkey. Investigation of eschars suspected of representing bioterrorism-associated cutaneous anthrax revealed that rickettsialpox occurs more frequently than previously realized.

Clinical manifestations

A papule forms at the site of the mite's feeding, develops a central vesicle, and becomes a 1- to 2.5-cm painless black crusted eschar surrounded by an erythematous halo (Fig. 174-2). Enlargement of the regional lymph nodes draining the eschar suggests initial lymphogenous spread. After an incubation period of 10–17 days, during which the eschar and regional lymphadenopathy frequently go unnoticed, onset is marked by malaise, chills, fever, headache, and

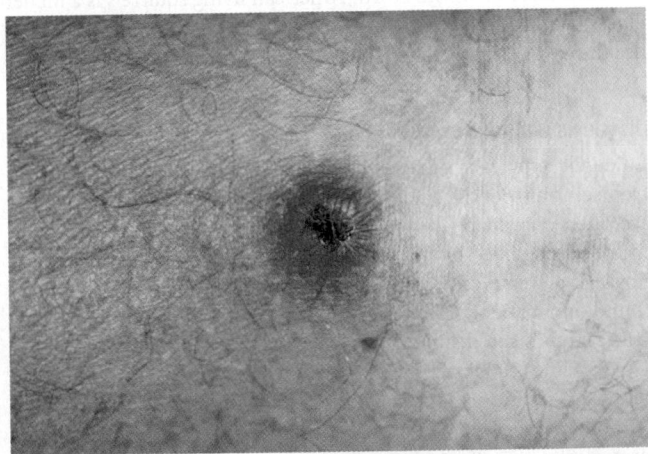

Figure 174-2 Eschar at the site of the mite bite in a patient with rickettsialpox. *(Reprinted from A Krusell et al: Emerg Infect Dis 8:727, 2002. Photo obtained by Dr. Kenneth Kaye.)*

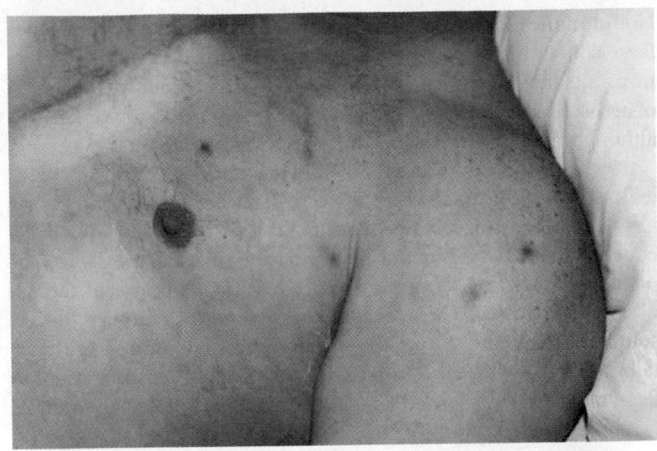

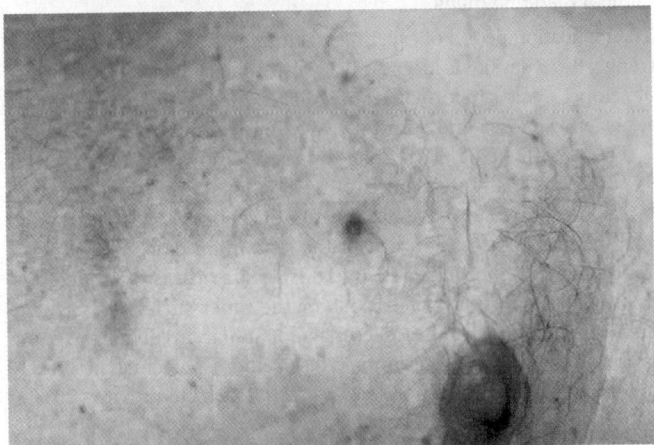

Figure 174-3 *Top:* **Papulovesicular lesions on the trunk of the patient with rickettsialpox** shown in Fig. 174-2. *Bottom:* **Close-up of lesions** from the same patient. *(Reprinted from A Krusell et al: Emerg Infect Dis 8:727, 2002. Photos obtained by Dr. Kenneth Kaye.)*

myalgia. A macular rash appears 2–6 days after onset and evolves sequentially into papules, vesicles, and crusts that heal without scarring (Fig. 174-3). The rash may remain macular or maculopapular. Some patients develop nausea, vomiting, abdominal pain, cough, conjunctivitis, or photophobia. If untreated, fever lasts 6–10 days.

Diagnosis and treatment

Clinical, epidemiologic, and convalescent serologic data establish the diagnosis of a spotted fever–group rickettsiosis that is seldom pursued further. Doxycycline is the drug of choice for treatment.

■ FLEA-BORNE SPOTTED FEVER

An emerging rickettsiosis caused by *R. felis* occurs worldwide. Maintained transovarially in the geographically widespread cat flea *Ctenocephalides felis*, the infection has been described as moderately severe, with fever, rash, headache, and CNS, gastrointestinal, and pulmonary symptoms.

■ ENDEMIC MURINE TYPHUS

Epidemiology

R. typhi is maintained in mammalian host/flea cycles, with rats (*Rattus rattus* and *R. norvegicus*) and the Oriental rat flea (*Xenopsylla cheopis*) as the classic zoonotic niche. Fleas acquire *R. typhi* from rickettsemic rats and carry the organism throughout their life span.

Nonimmune rats and humans are infected when rickettsia-laden flea feces contaminates pruritic bite lesions; less frequently, the flea bite transmits the organisms. Transmission also may occur via inhalation of aerosolized rickettsiae from flea feces. Infected rats appear healthy, although they are rickettsemic for ~2 weeks.

Murine typhus occurs mainly in southern Texas and southern California, where the classic rat/flea cycle is absent and an opossum/cat flea (*C. felis*) cycle is prominent. Globally, endemic typhus occurs mainly in warm (often coastal) areas throughout the tropics and subtropics, where it is highly prevalent though often unrecognized. The incidence peaks from April through June in southern Texas and during the warm months of summer and early fall in other geographic locations. Patients seldom recall exposure to fleas, although exposure to animals such as cats, opossums, and rats is reported in nearly 40% of cases.

Clinical manifestations

The incubation period of experimental murine typhus averages 11 days (range, 8–16 days). Headache, myalgia, arthralgia, nausea, and malaise develop 1–3 days before onset of chills and fever. Nearly all patients experience nausea and vomiting early in the illness.

The duration of untreated illness averages 12 days (range, 9–18 days). Rash is present in only 13% of patients at presentation for medical care (usually ~4 days after onset of fever), appearing an average of 2 days later in half of the remaining patients and never appearing in the others. The initial macular rash is often detected by careful inspection of the axilla or the inner surface of the arm. Subsequently, the rash becomes maculopapular, involving the trunk more often than the extremities; it is seldom petechial and rarely involves the face, palms, or soles. A rash is detected in only 20% of patients with darkly pigmented skin.

Pulmonary involvement is frequently prominent; 35% of patients have a hacking, nonproductive cough, and 23% of patients who undergo chest radiography have pulmonary densities due to interstitial pneumonia, pulmonary edema, and pleural effusions. Bibasilar rales are the most common pulmonary sign. Less common clinical manifestations include abdominal pain, confusion, stupor, seizures, ataxia, coma, and jaundice. Clinical laboratory studies frequently reveal anemia and leukopenia early in the course, leukocytosis late in the course, thrombocytopenia, hyponatremia, hypoalbuminemia, mildly increased serum hepatic aminotransferases, and prerenal azotemia. Complications may include respiratory failure, hematemesis, cerebral hemorrhage, and hemolysis. Severe illness necessitates the admission of 10% of hospitalized patients to an intensive care unit. Greater severity is generally associated with old age, underlying disease, and treatment with a sulfonamide; the case-fatality rate is 1%. In a study of children with murine typhus, 50% suffered only nocturnal fevers, feeling well enough for active daytime play.

Diagnosis and treatment

Cultivation, PCR, or cross-adsorption serologic studies of acute- and convalescent-phase sera can provide a specific diagnosis, and an immunohistochemical method for identification of typhus group-specific antigens has been developed. Nevertheless, most patients are treated empirically with doxycycline (100 mg bid orally for 7–15 days) on the basis of clinical suspicion. Ciprofloxacin provides an alternative if doxycycline is contraindicated. Serologic methods are usually used when laboratory confirmation of the diagnosis is sought.

■ EPIDEMIC (LOUSE-BORNE) TYPHUS

The human body louse (*Pediculus humanus corporis*) lives in clothing under poor hygienic conditions and usually in impoverished cold areas. Lice acquire *R. prowazekii* when they ingest blood from a rickettsemic patient. The rickettsiae multiply in the midgut epithelial cells of the louse and are shed in the louse's feces. The infected louse leaves a febrile person and deposits infected feces on its subsequent host during its blood meal; the patient autoinoculates the organisms by scratching. The louse is killed by the rickettsiae and does not pass *R. prowazekii* to its offspring.

Epidemic typhus haunts regions afflicted by wars and disasters. An outbreak involved 100,000 people in refugee camps in Burundi in 1997. A small focus occurred in Russia in 1998; sporadic cases have been reported from Algeria, and frequent outbreaks have occurred in Peru. Eastern flying squirrels (*Glaucomys volans*) and their lice and fleas maintain *R. prowazekii* in a zoonotic cycle. The fleas transmit the infection sporadically to humans.

Brill-Zinsser disease is a recrudescent illness occurring years after acute epidemic typhus, probably as a result of waning immunity. *R. prowazekii* remains latent for years; its reactivation results in sporadic cases of disease in louse-free populations or in epidemics in louse-infested populations.

Rickettsiae are potential agents of bioterrorism (Chap. 221). Infections with *R. prowazekii* and *R. rickettsii* have high case-fatality ratios. These organisms cause difficult-to-diagnose diseases, are highly infectious when inhaled as aerosols, and have been selected for resistance to tetracycline or chloramphenicol in the laboratory.

Clinical manifestations

After an incubation period of ~1–2 weeks, the onset of illness is abrupt, with prostration, severe headache, and fever rising rapidly to 38.8°–40.0°C (102°–104°F). Cough is prominent, occurring in 70% of patients. Myalgias are usually severe. In the outbreak in Burundi, the disease was referred to as sutama ("crouching"), a designation reflecting the posture of patients attempting to alleviate the pain. A rash begins on the upper trunk, usually on the fifth day, and then becomes generalized, involving the entire body except the face, palms, and soles. Initially, this rash is macular; without treatment, it becomes maculopapular, petechial, and confluent. The rash often is not detected in black skin; 60% of African patients have spotless epidemic typhus. Photophobia, with considerable conjunctival injection and eye pain, is common. The tongue may be dry, brown, and furred. Confusion and coma are common. Skin necrosis and gangrene of the digits as well as interstitial pneumonia may occur in severe cases. Untreated disease is fatal in 7–40% of cases, with outcome depending primarily on the condition of the host. Patients with untreated infections develop renal insufficiency and multiorgan involvement in which neurologic manifestations are frequently prominent. Overall, 12% of patients with epidemic typhus have neurologic involvement. Infection associated with North American flying squirrels is a milder illness; whether this milder disease is due to host factors (e.g., better health status) or attenuated virulence is unknown.

Diagnosis and treatment

Epidemic typhus is sometimes misdiagnosed as typhoid fever in tropical countries (Chap. 153). The means even for serologic studies are often unavailable in settings of louse-borne typhus. Epidemics may be recognized by the serologic or immunohistochemical diagnosis of a single case or by detection of *R. prowazekii* in a louse found on a patient. Cross-adsorption indirect fluorescent antibody (IFA) studies can distinguish *R. prowazekii* and *R. typhi* infections. Doxycycline (200 mg/d, given in two divided doses) is administered orally or—if the patient is comatose or vomiting—intravenously. Although under epidemic conditions a single 200-mg dose has proved effective, treatment is generally continued until 2–3 days after defervescence. Pregnant patients should be evaluated individually and treated with either chloramphenicol early in pregnancy or, if necessary, doxycycline late in pregnancy.

Prevention

Prevention of epidemic typhus involves control of body lice. Clothes should be changed regularly, and insecticides should be used every 6 weeks to control the louse population.

SCRUB TYPHUS

O. tsutsugamushi differs substantially from *Rickettsia* species both genetically and in terms of cell wall composition (i.e., it lacks lipopolysaccharide). *O. tsutsugamushi* is maintained by transovarian transmission in trombiculid mites. After hatching, infected larval mites (chiggers, the only stage that feeds on a host) inoculate organisms into the skin. Infected chiggers are found particularly in areas of heavy scrub vegetation during the wet season, when mites lay eggs.

Scrub typhus is endemic and reemerging in eastern and southern Asia, northern Australia, and islands of the western Pacific and Indian Oceans. Infections are prevalent in these regions; in some areas, >3% of the population is infected or reinfected each month. Immunity wanes over 1–3 years, and the organism exhibits remarkable antigenic diversity.

Clinical manifestations

Illness varies from mild and self-limiting to fatal. After an incubation period of 6–21 days, onset is characterized by fever, headache, myalgia, cough, and gastrointestinal symptoms. Some patients recover spontaneously after a few days. The classic case description includes an eschar where the chigger has fed, regional lymphadenopathy, and a maculopapular rash—signs that are seldom seen in indigenous patients. Fewer than 50% of Westerners develop an eschar, and fewer than 40% develop a rash (on day 4–6 of illness). Severe cases typically include encephalitis and interstitial pneumonia due to vascular injury. The case-fatality rate for untreated classic cases is 7% but would probably be lower if all mild cases were diagnosed.

Diagnosis and treatment

Serologic assays (IFA, indirect immunoperoxidase, and enzyme immunoassays) are the mainstays of laboratory diagnosis, and PCR amplification of *Orientia* genes from eschars and blood is also effective. Patients are treated with doxycycline (100 mg bid orally for 7–15 days), azithromycin (500 mg orally for 3 days), or chloramphenicol (500 mg qid orally for 7–15 days). Some cases of scrub typhus in Thailand are caused by doxycycline- or chloramphenicol-resistant strains that are susceptible to azithromycin and rifampin.

EHRLICHIOSES AND ANAPLASMOSIS

Ehrlichioses are acute febrile infections caused by members of the family Anaplasmataceae, which is made up of obligately intracellular organisms comprised by four genera: *Ehrlichia*, *Anaplasma*, *Wolbachia*, and *Neorickettsia*. The bacteria reside in vertebrate reservoirs and target vacuoles of hematopoietic cells (Fig. 174-4). Two *Ehrlichia* species and one *Anaplasma* species are transmitted by ticks to humans and cause infection that can be severe and prevalent. *E. chaffeensis*, the agent of HME, infects predominantly mononuclear phagocytes; *E. ewingii* and *A. phagocytophilum* infect neutrophils.

Ehrlichia and *Anaplasma* are maintained by horizontal tick-mammal-tick transmission, and humans are only inadvertently infected. Wolbachiae are associated with human filariasis, since they are important for filarial viability and pathogenicity; antibiotic treatment targeting wolbachiae is a strategy for filariasis control. Neorickettsiae parasitize flukes that in turn parasitize aquatic snails, fish, and insects. Only a single human neorickettsiosis has been described: sennetsu fever, an infectious mononucleosis–like

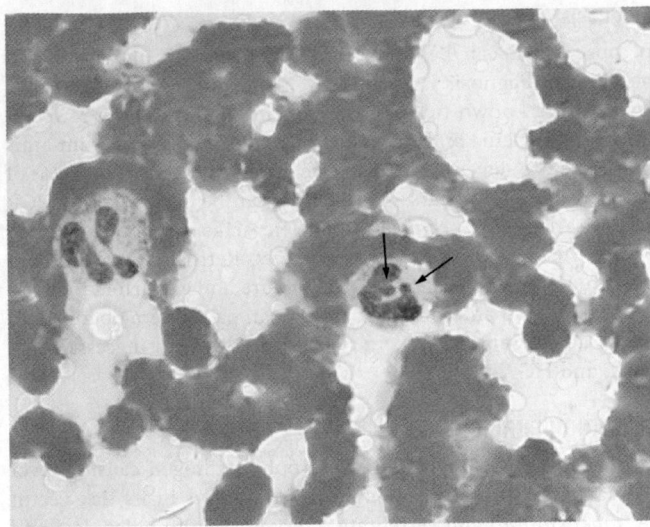

Figure 174-4 Peripheral blood smear from a patient with human granulocytotropic anaplasmosis. A neutrophil contains two morulae (vacuoles filled with *A. phagocytophilum*). *(Photo courtesy of Dr. J. Stephen Dumler.)*

illness that was first identified in 1953 and is probably due to the ingestion of raw fish containing *N. sennetsu*–infected flukes.

■ HUMAN MONOCYTOTROPIC EHRLICHIOSIS

Epidemiology

More than 5496 cases of *E. chaffeensis* infection had been reported to the Centers for Disease Control and Prevention (CDC) as of November 2009. However, active prospective surveillance has demonstrated an incidence as high as 414 cases per 100,000 population in some U.S. regions. Most *E. chaffeensis* infections are identified in the south-central, southeastern, and mid-Atlantic states, but cases have also been recognized in California, New York, and Minnesota. All stages of the Lone Star tick (*A. americanum*) feed on white-tailed deer—a major reservoir. Dogs and coyotes also serve as reservoirs and often lack clinical signs. Tick bites and exposures are frequently reported by patients in rural areas especially in May through July. The median age of HME patients is 53 years; however, severe and fatal infections in children are also well recognized. Of patients with HME, 61% are male.

Clinical manifestations

E. chaffeensis disseminates hematogenously from the dermal blood pool created by the feeding tick. After a median incubation period of 8 days, illness develops. Clinical manifestations are undifferentiated and include fever (96% of cases), headache (72%), myalgia (68%), and malaise (77%). Less frequently observed are nausea, vomiting, and diarrhea (25–57%); cough (28%); rash (26% overall, 6% at presentation); and confusion (20%). HME can be severe: 62% of patients with documented cases are hospitalized, and ~3% die. Severe manifestations include toxic shock–like or septic shock–like syndrome, adult respiratory distress syndrome, cardiac failure, hepatitis, meningoencephalitis, hemorrhage, and—in immunocompromised patients—overwhelming ehrlichial infection. Laboratory findings are valuable in the differential diagnosis of HME; 61% of patients have leukopenia (initially lymphopenia, later neutropenia), 73% have thrombocytopenia, and 84% have elevated serum levels of hepatic aminotransferases. Despite low blood cell counts, the bone marrow is hypercellular, and noncaseating granulomas may be present. Vasculitis is not a component of HME.

Diagnosis

Because HME can be fatal, empirical antibiotic therapy based on clinical diagnosis is required. This diagnosis is suggested by fever with a known tick exposure during the preceding 3 weeks, thrombocytopenia and/or leukopenia, and increased serum aminotransferase levels. Morulae are demonstrated on <10% of peripheral-blood smears. Acute HME can be confirmed by PCR amplification of *E. chaffeensis* nucleic acids in blood obtained before the start of doxycycline therapy. Retrospective serodiagnosis requires a consistent clinical picture and a fourfold increase in *E. chaffeensis* antibody titer to ≥1:64 in paired sera obtained ~3 weeks apart. Separate specific diagnostic tests are necessary for HME and HGA.

■ EWINGII EHRLICHIOSIS

Ehrlichia ewingii, originally a neutrophil pathogen causing fever and lameness in dogs, resembles *E. chaffeensis* in its tick vector (*A. americanum*) and vertebrate reservoirs (white-tailed deer and dogs). *E. ewingii* illness is similar to but less severe than HME. The majority of cases have occurred in immunocompromised patients. No specific diagnostic test for ewingii ehrlichiosis is readily available.

TREATMENT   Ehrlichioses

Doxycycline is effective for HME and ewingii ehrlichiosis. Therapy with doxycycline (100 mg given orally or intravenously twice daily) or tetracycline (250–500 mg given orally every 6 h) lowers hospitalization rates and shortens fever duration. *E. chaffeensis* is not susceptible to chloramphenicol in vitro, and the use of this drug is controversial. While a few reports document *E. chaffeensis* persistence in humans, this finding is rare; most infections are cured by short courses of doxycycline (continuing for 3–5 days after defervescence). Although poorly studied, rifampin may be suitable when doxycycline is contraindicated.

Prevention

HME and ewingii ehrlichiosis are prevented by the avoidance of ticks in endemic areas. The use of protective clothing and tick repellents, careful postexposure tick searches, and prompt removal of attached ticks probably diminish infection risk.

■ HUMAN GRANULOCYTOTROPIC ANAPLASMOSIS

Epidemiology

As of November 2009, 6218 cases of HGA had been reported to the CDC, most in the upper midwestern and northeastern United States; the geographic distribution is similar to that for Lyme disease because of the shared *I. scapularis* tick vector. White-footed mice, squirrels, and white-tailed deer in the United States and red deer in Europe are natural reservoirs for *A. phagocytophilum*. HGA incidence peaks in May through July, but the disease can occur throughout the year with exposure to *Ixodes* ticks. HGA often affects males (57%) and older persons (median age, 51 years).

Clinical manifestations

Seroprevalence rates are high in endemic regions; thus it seems likely that most individuals develop subclinical infections. The incubation period for HGA is 4–8 days, after which the disease manifests as fever (91% of cases), myalgia (77%), headache (77%), and malaise (94%). A minority of patients develop nausea, vomiting, or diarrhea (16–38%); cough (21%); or confusion (17%). Rash (6%) is almost invariably concurrent erythema migrans attributable to Lyme disease. Most patients develop thrombocytopenia (69%) and/or leukopenia (48%) with increased serum hepatic aminotransferase levels (71%).

Severe complications occur most often in the elderly and include adult respiratory distress syndrome, toxic shock–like syndrome, and life-threatening opportunistic infections. Meningoencephalitis has not been conclusively documented with HGA, but brachial plexopathy and demyelinating polyneuropathy are reported. For HGA, 7% of patients require intensive care, and the case-fatality rate is 0.5%. Neither vasculitis nor granulomas are components of HGA. While co-infections with *Borrelia burgdorferi* and *Babesia microti* [transmitted by the same tick vector(s)] occur, there is little evidence of comorbidity or persistence.

Diagnosis

HGA should be included in the differential diagnosis of influenza-like illnesses during seasons with *Ixodes* tick activity (May through December), especially with tick bite or exposure. Concurrent thrombocytopenia, leukopenia, or elevation in serum alanine or aspartate aminotransferase further increases the likelihood of HGA. Many HGA patients develop Lyme disease antibodies in the absence of clinical findings consistent with that diagnosis. Thus, HGA should be considered in the differential diagnosis of atypical severe Lyme disease presentations. Peripheral-blood film examination for neutrophil morulae can yield a diagnosis in 20–75% of infections. PCR testing of blood from patients with active disease before doxycycline therapy is sensitive and specific. Serodiagnosis is retrospective, requiring a fourfold increase in *A. phagocytophilum* antibody titer (to ≥1:80) in paired serum samples obtained 1 month apart. Since seroprevalence is high in some regions, a single acute-phase titer should not be used for diagnosis.

TREATMENT   Human Granulocytotropic Anaplasmosis

No prospective studies of therapy for HGA have been conducted. However, doxycycline (100 mg by mouth twice daily) is effective. Rifampin therapy is associated with improvement of HGA in pregnant women and children. Most treated patients defervesce within 24–48 h.

Prevention

HGA prevention requires tick avoidance. Transmission can be documented as few as 4 h after a tick bite.

Q FEVER

The agent of Q fever is *C. burnetii*, a small intracellular microorganism that only recently was grown in cell-free medium. *C. burnetii*, a pleomorphic coccobacillus with a gram-negative cell wall, survives in harsh environments; it escapes intracellular killing in macrophages by inhibiting the final phagosome maturation step (cathepsin fusion) and has adapted to the acidic phagolysosome by producing superoxide dismutase. Infection with *C. burnetii* induces a range of immunomodulatory responses, from immunosuppression in chronic Q fever to the production of autoantibodies, particularly those to smooth muscle and cardiac muscle.

Q fever encompasses two broad clinical syndromes: acute and chronic infection. The host's immune response (rather than the particular strain) most likely determines whether chronic Q fever develops. *C. burnetii* survives in monocytes from patients with chronic Q fever but not in monocytes from patients with acute Q fever or from uninfected subjects. Impairment of the bactericidal activity of the *C. burnetii*–infected monocyte is associated with overproduction of interleukin 10. The CD4+/CD8+ ratio is decreased in Q fever endocarditis. Very few organisms and a strong cellular response are observed in patients with acute Q fever, while many organisms and a moderate cellular response occur in chronic Q fever. Immune control of *C. burnetii* is T cell–dependent, but 80–90% of bone marrow aspirates obtained years after recovery from Q fever contain *C. burnetii* DNA.

Epidemiology

Q fever is a zoonosis. The primary sources of human infection are infected cattle, sheep, and goats. However, cats, rabbits, pigeons, and dogs have also served as sources for transmission of *C. burnetii* to humans. The wildlife reservoir is extensive and includes ticks, coyotes, gray foxes, skunks, raccoons, rabbits, deer, mice, bears, birds, and opossums. In female animals *C. burnetii* localizes to the uterus and mammary glands. Infection is reactivated during pregnancy and following radiotherapy in mouse models. High concentrations of *C. burnetii* are found in the placenta. At the time of parturition, the bacteria are released into the air, and infection follows inhalation of aerosolized organisms by a susceptible host. Windstorms can generate *C. burnetii* aerosols months after soil contamination during parturition. Individuals up to 18 km from the source have been infected. Because it is easily dispersed as an aerosol, *C. burnetii* is a potential agent of bioterrorism, with a high infectivity rate and pneumonia as the major manifestation.

Determining the source of an outbreak of Q fever can be challenging. An outbreak of Q fever at a horse-boarding ranch in Colorado in 2005 was due to spread of infection from two herds of goats that had been acquired by the owners. PCR testing confirmed the presence of *C. burnetii* in the soil and among the goats. Of 138 persons who lived within 1 mile of the ranch and who were also tested, 11 (8%) had evidence of *C. burnetii* infection, and 8 of these 11 individuals had had no direct contact with the ranch.

Persons at risk for Q fever include abattoir workers, veterinarians, farmers, and other individuals who have contact with infected animals, particularly newborn animals, or products of conception. The organism is shed in milk for weeks to months after parturition. The ingestion of contaminated milk in some geographic areas probably represents a major route of transmission to humans, although experimental evidence on this point is contradictory. In rare instances, human-to-human transmission has followed labor and childbirth in an infected woman, autopsy of an infected individual, or blood transfusion. Some evidence suggests that *C. burnetii* can be sexually transmitted among humans. Crushing an infected tick between the fingers has resulted in Q fever; the implication is that percutaneous transmission can occur.

Infections due to *C. burnetii* occur in most geographic locations except New Zealand and Antarctica. Thus Q fever can be associated with travel. The number of reported cases of Q fever in the United States ranges from 28 to 54 per year. More than 70% of these cases occur in males, and April through June is the most common time for acquisition. Q fever continues to be common in Australia, with 30 cases per 1 million population per year. Cases among abattoir workers in Australia declined dramatically due to a vaccination program. An outbreak of Q fever began in the Netherlands in 2007, and by August 2009 more than 2000 cases had been reported. Pneumonia was a common manifestation in this outbreak, which appeared to be primarily due to transmission from infected goats.

The primary manifestations of acute Q fever differ geographically (e.g., pneumonia in Nova Scotia and granulomatous hepatitis in Marseille). These differences may reflect the route of infection (i.e., ingestion of contaminated milk for hepatitis and inhalation of contaminated aerosols for pneumonia).

Young age seems to be protective against infection with *C. burnetii*. In a large outbreak in Switzerland, symptomatic infection occurred five times more often among persons >15 years of age than among younger individuals. In many outbreaks, men are affected more commonly than women; the proposed explanation is that female hormones are partially protective.

Clinical manifestations

Acute Q fever After an incubation period of 3–30 days, 1070 patients with acute Q fever in southern France presented with hepatitis (40%), both pneumonia and hepatitis (20%), pneumonia (17%), isolated fever (14%), CNS involvement (2%), and pericarditis or myocarditis (1%). Acalculous cholecystitis, pancreatitis, lymphadenopathy, spontaneous rupture of the spleen, transient hypoplastic anemia, bone marrow necrosis, hemolytic anemia, histiocytic hemophagocytosis, optic neuritis, and erythema nodosum are less common manifestations.

The symptoms of acute Q fever are nonspecific; common among them are fever, extreme fatigue, photophobia, and severe headache that is frequently retro-orbital. Other symptoms include chills, sweats, nausea, vomiting, and diarrhea, each occurring in 5–20% of cases. Cough develops in about half of patients with Q fever pneumonia. Neurologic manifestations of acute Q fever are uncommon; however, in one outbreak in the United Kingdom, 23% of 102 patients had neurologic signs and symptoms as the major manifestation. A nonspecific rash may be evident in 4–18% of patients. The WBC count is usually normal. Thrombocytopenia occurs in ~25% of patients, and reactive thrombocytosis (with platelet counts exceeding $10^6/\mu L$) frequently develops during recovery. Chest radiography may show opacities similar to those seen in pneumonia caused by other pathogens, but multiple rounded opacities in patients in endemic areas suggest a diagnosis of Q fever pneumonia.

Acute Q fever occasionally complicates pregnancy. In one series, it resulted in premature birth in 35% of cases and in abortion or neonatal death in 43%. Neonatal death (previous or current) and lower infant birth weight are three times more likely among women seropositive for *C. burnetii*.

Post–Q fever fatigue syndrome Prolonged fatigue can follow Q fever and can be accompanied by a constellation of symptoms including headaches, sweats, arthralgia, myalgias, blurred vision, muscle fasciculations, and enlarged and painful lymph nodes. Long-term persistence of a noninfective, nonbiodegraded complex of *Coxiella* cell components with its antigens and specific lipopolysaccharide has been detected in the affected persons. Patients who develop this syndrome have a higher frequency of carriage of HLA-DRB1*11 and of the 2/2 genotype of the interferon γ intron 1 microsatellite.

Chronic Q fever Chronic Q fever almost always implies endocarditis and usually occurs in patients with previous valvular heart disease, immunosuppression, or chronic renal insufficiency. Fever is usually absent or low grade. Valvular vegetations are detected in only 12% of patients by transthoracic echocardiography, but the rate of detection is higher with transesophageal echocardiography. The vegetations in chronic Q fever endocarditis differ from those in bacterial endocarditis, manifesting as endothelium-covered nodules on the valves. A high index of suspicion is necessary for timely diagnosis. Patients with chronic Q fever are often ill for >1 year before the diagnosis is made. The disease should be suspected in all patients with culture-negative endocarditis. In addition, all patients with valvular heart disease and an unexplained purpuric eruption, renal insufficiency, stroke, and/or progressive heart failure should be tested for *C. burnetii* infection. Patients with chronic Q fever have hepatomegaly and/or splenomegaly, which, in combination with rheumatoid factor, elevated erythrocyte sedimentation rate, high C-reactive protein level, and/or increased γ-globulin concentrations (up to 60–70 g/L), suggests this diagnosis. Other manifestations of chronic Q fever include infection of vascular prostheses, aneurysms, and bone as well as chronic sternal wound infection. Unusual manifestations include chronic thrombocytopenia, mixed cryoglobulinemia, and livedo reticularis.

Diagnosis

Isolation of *C. burnetii* from buffy-coat blood samples or tissue specimens by a shell-vial technique is easy but requires a biosafety level 3 laboratory. PCR detects *C. burnetii* DNA in tissue specimens, including paraffin-embedded samples. Serology is the most commonly used diagnostic tool. Indirect immunofluorescence is sensitive and specific and is the method of choice. Rheumatoid factor should be adsorbed from the specimen before testing. An IgG antibody titer of ≥1:800 to phase I antigen (i.e., naturally occurring *C. burnetii* with intact lipopolysaccharide) is suggestive of chronic Q fever; in chronic infection, the titer to phase I antigen is usually much higher than that to phase II antigen (i.e., *C. burnetii* that has truncated lipopolysaccharide associated with gene deletions during laboratory passages). The reverse is true in acute Q fever, in which a fourfold rise in titer may be demonstrated between acute- and convalescent-phase serum samples.

TREATMENT Q Fever

Treatment of acute Q fever with doxycycline (100 mg twice daily for 14 days) is usually successful. Quinolones are also effective. When Q fever is diagnosed during pregnancy, treatment with trimethoprim-sulfamethoxazole (TMP-SMX) is recommended for the duration of the pregnancy. One study showed no intrauterine fetal deaths and substantial reduction of obstetric complications in a group of Q fever patients treated with TMP-SMX.

The treatment of chronic Q fever is difficult and requires careful follow-up. Addition of hydroxychloroquine (to alkalinize the phagolysosome) renders doxycycline bactericidal against *C. burnetii,* and this combination is currently the favored regimen. Treatment with doxycycline (100 mg bid) and hydroxychloroquine (200 mg tid; plasma concentration maintained at 0.8–1.2 μg/mL) for 18 months is superior to a regimen of doxycycline and ofloxacin. Among 21 patients who received doxycycline and hydroxychloroquine, 1 died of a surgical complication, 2 were still being treated at the end of the study, 1 was still being evaluated, and 17 were cured. The mean duration of treatment was 31 months. In the ofloxacin and doxycycline group of 14 patients, 1 had died, 1 was still being treated, 7 had relapsed, and 5 had been cured by the end of the study. Optimal management of Q fever endocarditis entails determining the minimal inhibitory concentration (MIC) of doxycycline for the patient's isolate and measuring serum doxycycline levels. A serum level–to–doxycycline MIC ratio of ≥1 is associated with a rapid decline in phase I antibodies with the doxycycline-hydroxychloroquine regimen. Patients treated with this regimen must be advised about photosensitivity and retinal toxicity risks. The doxycycline-hydroxychloroquine regimen was successful in one patient with HIV infection and Q fever endocarditis. The Jarisch-Herxheimer reaction occasionally complicates the treatment of chronic Q fever. Treatment of *C. burnetii*–infected aortic aneurysms is the same as that for Q fever endocarditis. Surgical intervention is often required.

If doxycycline-hydroxychloroquine cannot be used, the regimen chosen should include at least two antibiotics active against *C. burnetii*. Rifampin (300 mg once daily) combined with doxycycline (100 mg twice daily) or ciprofloxacin (750 mg twice daily) has been used successfully. The optimal duration of antibiotic therapy for chronic Q fever remains undetermined. At least 3 years of treatment, with discontinuation only if the phase I IgA antibody titer is ≤1:50 and the phase I IgG titer is ≤1:200, is recommended.

Patients with acute Q fever and lesions of native heart valves (e.g., bicuspid aortic valve), prosthetic valves, or prosthetic intravascular material should undergo serologic monitoring every 4 months for 2 years. If the phase I IgG titer is >1:800, further investigation is warranted. Some authorities recommend that patients with valvulopathy and acute Q fever receive doxycycline and hydroxychloroquine to prevent chronic Q fever. For women who exhibit a serologic profile of chronic Q fever after childbirth, hydroxychloroquine and doxycycline should be given for 1 year.

THERAPY WITH BIOLOGIC MODIFYING AGENTS Interferon γ was successful in the treatment of a 3-year-old boy with prolonged fever, abdominal pain, and thrombocytopenia due to *C. burnetii* that had not been eradicated with conventional antibiotic therapy. Many patients with granulomatous hepatitis due to Q fever have a prolonged febrile illness that is unresponsive to antibiotics. For these individuals, treatment with prednisone (0.5 mg/kg) has resulted in defervescence within 2–15 days. After defervescence, the glucocorticoid dose is tapered over the next month.

Prevention

A whole-cell vaccine (Q-Vax) licensed in Australia effectively prevents Q fever in abattoir workers. Before administration of the vaccine, skin testing with intradermal diluted *C. burnetii* vaccine is performed, serologic testing is undertaken, and a history of possible Q fever is sought. Vaccine is given only to patients with no history of Q fever and negative results in serologic and skin testing.

Good animal-husbandry practices are important in preventing widespread contamination of the environment by *C. burnetii*. These practices include isolating aborting animals for up to 14 days, raising feed bunks to prevent contamination of feed by excreta, destroying aborted materials (by burning and burying fetal membranes and stillborn animals), and wearing masks and gloves when handling aborted materials. Only seronegative pregnant animals should be used in research settings, and only seronegative animals should be permitted in petting zoos.

During an outbreak of Q fever and for 4 weeks after it ceases, blood donations should not be accepted from individuals who live in the affected area.

ACKNOWLEDGMENT
The contributions of Didier Raoult, MD, to this chapter in previous editions are gratefully acknowledged.

FURTHER READINGS

Bakken JS, Dumler S: Human granulocytic anaplasmosis. Infect Dis Clin North Am 22:433, 2008

Bechah Y et al: Epidemic typhus. Lancet Infect Dis 8:417, 2008

Chapman AS et al: Cluster of sylvatic epidemic typhus cases associated with flying squirrels, 2004–2006. Emerg Infect Dis 15:1005, 2009

——— et al: Diagnosis and management of tickborne rickettsial diseases: Rocky Mountain spotted fever, ehrlichioses, and anaplasmosis—United States. MMWR Recomm Rep 55:1, 2006

De Sousa R et al: Host- and microbe-related risk factors for and pathophysiology of fatal *Rickettsia conorii* infection in Portuguese patients. J Infect Dis 198:576, 2008

Harris RJ et al: Long-term persistence of *Coxiella burnetii* in the host after primary Q fever. Epidemiol Infect 124:543, 2000

Hechemy KE et al (eds): *Century of Rickettsiology: Emerging, Reemerging Rickettsioses, Molecular Diagnostics, and Emerging Veterinary Rickettsioses.* Malden, MA, Blackwell Scientific, 2006

Holman RC et al: Analysis of risk factors for fatal Rocky Mountain spotted fever: Evidence for superiority of tetracyclines for therapy. J Infect Dis 184:1437, 2001

McQuiston JH et al: National surveillance and the epidemiology of Q fever in the United States, 1978–2004. Am J Trop Med Hyg 75:36, 2006

Paddock CD et al: *Rickettsia parkeri* rickettsiosis and its clinical distinction from Rocky Mountain spotted fever. Clin Infect Dis 47:1188, 2008

Raoult D et al: Q fever 1985–1998. Clinical and epidemiologic features of 1,383 infections. Medicine (Baltimore) 79:109, 2000

Walker DH: Rickettsiae and rickettsial infections: The current state of knowledge. Clin Infect Dis 45(Suppl1):539, 2007

——— et al: Emerging and re-emerging tick-transmitted rickettsial and ehrlichial infections. Med Clin North Am 92:1345, 2008

CHAPTER **175**

Infections Due to Mycoplasmas

R. Doug Hardy

Mycoplasmas are prokaryotes of the class Mollicutes. Their size (150–350 nm) is closer to that of viruses than to that of bacteria. Unlike viruses, however, mycoplasmas grow in cell-free culture media; in fact, they are the smallest organisms capable of independent replication.

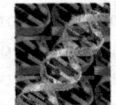 The entire genomes of many *Mycoplasma* species have been sequenced and have been found to be among the smallest of all prokaryotic genomes. Sequencing information for these genomes has helped define the minimal set of genes necessary for cellular life. The absence of genes related to the synthesis of amino acids, fatty acid metabolism, and cholesterol dictates the mycoplasmas' parasitic or saprophytic dependence on a host for exogenous nutrients and necessitates the use of complex fastidious media to culture these organisms. Mycoplasmas lack a cell wall and are bound only by a cell membrane. The absence of a cell wall explains the inactivity of β-lactam antibiotics (penicillins and cephalosporins) against infections caused by these organisms.

At least 13 *Mycoplasma* species, two *Acholeplasma* species, and two *Ureaplasma* species have been isolated from humans. Most of these species are thought to be normal inhabitants of oral and urogenital mucous membranes. Only four species—*M. pneumoniae, M. hominis, U. urealyticum,* and *U. parvum*—have been shown conclusively to be pathogenic in immunocompetent humans. *M. pneumoniae* primarily infects the respiratory tract, while *M. hominis, U. urealyticum,* and *U. parvum* are associated with a variety of genitourinary tract disorders and neonatal infections. Some data indicate that *M. genitalium* may be a cause of disease in humans. Other mycoplasmas may cause disease in immunocompromised persons.

MYCOPLASMA PNEUMONIAE

■ PATHOGENICITY

M. pneumoniae is generally thought to act as an extracellular pathogen. Although the organism has been shown to exist and replicate within human cells, it is not known whether these intracellular events contribute to the pathogenesis of disease. *M. pneumoniae* attaches to ciliated respiratory epithelial cells by means of a complex terminal organelle at the tip of one end of the organism. Cytoadherence is mediated by interactive adhesins and accessory proteins clustered on this organelle. After extracellular attachment, *M. pneumoniae* causes injury to host respiratory tissue. The mechanism of injury is thought to be mediated by the production of hydrogen peroxide and of a recently identified ADP-ribosylating and vacuolating cytotoxin of *M. pneumoniae* that has many similarities to pertussis toxin. Because mycoplasmas lack a cell wall, they also lack cell wall–derived stimulators of the innate immune system, such as lipopolysaccharide, lipoteichoic acid, and murein (peptidoglycan) fragments. However, lipoproteins from the mycoplasmal cell membrane appear to have inflammatory properties, probably acting through Toll-like receptors (primarily TLR2) on macrophages and other cells. Lung biopsy specimens from patients with *M. pneumoniae* respiratory tract infection reveal an inflammatory process involving the trachea, bronchioles, and peribronchial tissue, with a monocytic infiltrate coinciding with a luminal exudate of polymorphonuclear leukocytes.

Experimental evidence indicates that innate immunity provides most of the host's defense against mycoplasmal infection in the lungs, whereas cellular immunity may actually play an immunopathogenic role, exacerbating mycoplasmal lung disease. Humoral immunity appears to provide protection against dissemination of *M. pneumoniae* infection; patients with humoral immunodeficiencies do not have more severe lung disease than do immunocompetent patients in the early stages of infection but more often develop disseminated infection resulting in syndromes such as arthritis, meningitis, and osteomyelitis. The immunity that follows severe *M. pneumoniae* infections is more protective and longer-lasting than that following mild infections. Genuine second attacks of *M. pneumoniae* pneumonia have been reported infrequently.

■ EPIDEMIOLOGY

M. pneumoniae infection occurs worldwide. It is likely that the incidence of upper respiratory illness due to *M. pneumoniae* is up to 20 times that of pneumonia caused by this organism. Infection is spread from one person to another by respiratory droplets expectorated during coughing and results in clinically apparent disease in an estimated 80% of cases. The incubation period for *M. pneumoniae* is 2–4 weeks; therefore, the time-course of infection in a specific population may be several weeks long. Intrafamilial attack rates are as high as 84% among children and

41% among adults. Outbreaks of *M. pneumoniae* illness often occur in institutional settings such as military bases, boarding schools, and summer camps. Infections tend to be endemic, with sporadic epidemics every 4–7 years. There is no seasonal pattern.

Most significantly, *M. pneumoniae* is a major cause of community-acquired respiratory illness in both children and adults and is often grouped with *Chlamydophila pneumoniae* and *Legionella* species as being among the most important bacterial causes of "atypical" community-acquired pneumonia. For community-acquired pneumonia in adults, *M. pneumoniae* is the most frequently detected "atypical" organism. Analysis of 13 studies of community-acquired pneumonia published since 1995 (which included 6207 ambulatory and hospitalized adults) showed that the overall prevalence of *M. pneumoniae* was 22.7%; by comparison, the prevalence of *C. pneumoniae* was 11.7%, and that of *Legionella* species was 4.6%. *M. pneumoniae* pneumonia is also referred to as Eaton agent pneumonia (the organism having first been isolated in the early 1940s by Monroe Eaton), primary atypical pneumonia, and "walking" pneumonia.

CLINICAL MANIFESTATIONS

Upper respiratory tract infections and pneumonia

Acute *M. pneumoniae* infections generally manifest as pharyngitis, tracheobronchitis, reactive airway disease/wheezing, or a nonspecific upper respiratory syndrome. Little evidence supports the commonly held belief that this organism is an important cause of otitis media, with or without bullous myringitis. Pneumonia develops in 3–13% of infected individuals; its onset is usually gradual, occurring over several days, but may be more abrupt. Although *Mycoplasma* pneumonia may begin with a sore throat, the most common presenting symptom is cough. The cough is typically nonproductive, but some patients produce sputum. Headache, malaise, chills, and fever are noted in the majority of patients.

On physical examination, wheezes or rales are detected in ~80% of patients with *M. pneumoniae* pneumonia. In many patients, however, pneumonia can be diagnosed only by chest radiography. The most common radiographic pattern is that of peribronchial pneumonia with thickened bronchial markings, streaks of interstitial infiltration, and areas of subsegmental atelectasis. Segmental or lobar consolidation is not uncommon. While clinically evident pleural effusions are uncommon, lateral decubitus views reveal that up to 20% of patients have pleural effusions.

Overall, the clinical presentation of pneumonia in an individual patient is not useful for differentiating *M. pneumoniae* pneumonia from other types of community-acquired pneumonia. The possibility of *M. pneumoniae* infection deserves particular consideration when community-acquired pneumonia fails to respond to treatment with a penicillin or a cephalosporin—antibiotics that are ineffective against mycoplasmas. Symptoms usually resolve within 2–3 weeks after the onset of illness. Although *M. pneumoniae* pneumonia is generally self-limited, appropriate antimicrobial therapy significantly shortens the duration of clinical illness. Infection uncommonly results in critical illness and only rarely in death. In some patients, long-term recurrent wheezing may follow the resolution of acute pneumonia. The significance of chronic infection, especially as it relates to asthma, is an area of active investigation.

Extrapulmonary manifestations

An array of extrapulmonary manifestations may develop during *M. pneumoniae* infection. The most significant are neurologic, dermatologic, cardiac, rheumatologic, and hematologic in nature. Extrapulmonary manifestations can be a result of active infection (e.g., septic arthritis) or postinfectious autoimmune phenomena (e.g., Guillain-Barré syndrome). Overall, these manifestations are uncommon, given the frequency of *M. pneumoniae* infection.

Notably, many patients with extrapulmonary *M. pneumoniae* disease do not have respiratory disease.

Skin eruptions described with *M. pneumoniae* infection include erythematous (macular or maculopapular), vesicular, bullous, petechial, and urticarial rashes. In some reports, 17% of patients with *M. pneumoniae* pneumonia have had an exanthem. Erythema multiforme major (Stevens-Johnson syndrome) is the most clinically significant skin eruption associated with *M. pneumoniae* infection; it appears to occur more commonly with *M. pneumoniae* than with other infectious agents.

A wide spectrum of neurologic manifestations has been reported with *M. pneumoniae* infection. The most common are meningoencephalitis, encephalitis, Guillain-Barré syndrome, and aseptic meningitis. *M. pneumoniae* has been implicated as a likely etiologic agent in 5–7% of cases of encephalitis. Other neurologic manifestations may include cranial neuropathy, acute psychosis, cerebellar ataxia, acute demyelinating encephalomyelitis, cerebrovascular thromboembolic events, and transverse myelitis. The roles of antimicrobial drugs, glucocorticoids, and IV immunoglobulin in the treatment of neurologic disease due to *M. pneumoniae* remain unknown.

Hematologic manifestations of *M. pneumoniae* infection include hemolytic anemia, aplastic anemia, cold agglutinins, disseminated intravascular coagulation, and hypercoagulopathy. When anemia does occur, it generally develops in the second or third week of illness.

In addition, hepatitis, glomerulonephritis, pancreatitis, myocarditis, pericarditis, rhabdomyolysis, and arthritis (septic and reactive) have been convincingly ascribed to *M. pneumoniae* infection. Septic arthritis has been described most commonly in hypogammaglobulinemic patients.

DIAGNOSIS (TABLE 175-1)

Clinical findings, nonmicrobiologic laboratory tests, and chest radiography are not useful for differentiating *M. pneumoniae* pneumonia from other types of community-acquired pneumonia. In addition, since *M. pneumoniae* lacks a cell wall, it is not visible on Gram's stain. Although of historical interest, the measurement of cold agglutinin titers is no longer recommended for the diagnosis of *M. pneumoniae* infection because the findings are nonspecific and assays specific for *M. pneumoniae* are now available.

Acute *M. pneumoniae* infection can be diagnosed by polymerase chain reaction (PCR) detection of the organism in respiratory tract secretions or by isolation of the organism in culture.

TABLE 175-1 Diagnostic Tests for Respiratory *Mycoplasma pneumoniae* Infection[a]

Test	Sensitivity, %	Specificity, %	Comment
Respiratory culture	≤60	100	—
Respiratory PCR	65–90	90–100	—
Serologic studies	55–100	55–100	Acute- and convalescent-phase serum samples are recommended.

[a]A combination of PCR and serology is suggested for routine diagnosis. If macrolide resistance is suspected, *M. pneumoniae* culture may prove useful, providing an isolate for susceptibility testing.

Abbreviation: PCR, polymerase chain reaction.

Oropharyngeal, nasopharyngeal, and pulmonary specimens are all acceptable for diagnosing *M. pneumoniae* pneumonia. Other bodily fluids, such cerebrospinal fluid, are acceptable for extrapulmonary infection. *M. pneumoniae* culture (which requires special media) is not recommended for routine diagnosis because the organism may take weeks to grow and is often difficult to isolate from clinical specimens. In contrast, PCR allows rapid, specific diagnosis earlier in the course of clinical illness.

The diagnosis can also be established by serologic tests for IgM and IgG antibodies to *M. pneumoniae* in paired (acute- and convalescent-phase) serum samples; enzyme-linked immunoassay is the recommended serologic method. An acute-phase sample alone is not adequate for diagnosis, as antibodies to *M. pneumoniae* may not develop until 2 weeks into the illness; therefore, it is important to test paired samples. In addition, IgM antibody to *M. pneumoniae* can persist for up to 1 year after acute infection. Thus its presence may indicate recent rather than acute infection.

The combination of PCR of respiratory tract secretions and serologic testing constitutes the most sensitive and rapid approach to the diagnosis of *M. pneumoniae* infection.

TREATMENT	*Mycoplasma pneumoniae* Infections (Table 175-2)

Although in the majority of untreated cases symptoms resolve within 2–3 weeks without significant associated morbidity, *M. pneumoniae* pneumonia can be a serious illness that responds to appropriate antimicrobial therapy. Randomized, double-blind, placebo-controlled trials have demonstrated that antimicrobial treatment significantly decreases the duration of fever, cough, malaise, hospitalization, and radiologic abnormalities in *M. pneumoniae* pneumonia. Treatment options for acute *M. pneumoniae* infection include macrolides (e.g., oral azithromycin, 500 mg on day 1, then 250 mg/d on days 2–5), tetracyclines (e.g., oral doxycycline, 100 mg twice daily for 10–14 days), and respiratory fluoroquinolones. However, ciprofloxacin and ofloxacin are *not* recommended because of their high minimal inhibitory concentrations against *M. pneumoniae* isolates and their poor performance in experimental studies. A 10- to 14-day course of therapy appears adequate.

In Japan and China, high levels of *M. pneumoniae* resistance to macrolides have been reported. In Europe and to a lesser degree in the United States, macrolide-resistant *M. pneumoniae* is emerging. If macrolide resistance is prominent in a geographic locale or is suspected, then a non-macrolide antibiotic should be considered for treatment; in addition, culture of *M. pneumoniae* may prove useful in these instances, providing an isolate for susceptibility testing.

Clinical observations and experimental data suggest that the addition of glucocorticoids to an antibiotic regimen may be of value for the treatment of severe or refractory *M. pneumoniae* pneumonia. However, relevant clinical experience is still limited. Even though appropriate antibiotic therapy significantly reduces the duration of respiratory illness, it does not appear to shorten the duration of detection of *M. pneumoniae* by culture or PCR; therefore, a test of cure or eradication is not suggested.

UROGENITAL MYCOPLASMAS (SEE ALSO CHAP. 130)

■ EPIDEMIOLOGY

M. hominis, *M. genitalium*, *U. urealyticum*, and *U. parvum* can cause urogenital tract disease. The significance of isolation of these organisms in a variety of other syndromes is unknown and in some cases is being investigated. *M. fermentans* has not been shown convincingly to cause human disease.

While urogenital mycoplasmas may be transmitted to a fetus during passage through a colonized birth canal, sexual contact is the major mode of transmission, and the risk of colonization increases dramatically with increasing numbers of sexual partners. In asymptomatic women, these mycoplasmas may be found throughout the lower urogenital tract. The vagina yields the largest number of organisms; next most densely colonized are the periurethral area and the cervix. Ureaplasmas are isolated less often from urine than from the cervix, but *M. hominis* is found with approximately the same frequency at these two sites. Ureaplasmas are isolated from the vagina of 40–80% of sexually active, asymptomatic women and *M. hominis* from 21–70%. The two microorganisms are found concurrently in 31–60% of women. In men, colonization with each organism is less prevalent. Mycoplasmas have been isolated from urine, semen, and the distal urethra of asymptomatic men.

■ CLINICAL MANIFESTATIONS

Urethritis, pyelonephritis, and urinary calculi

In many episodes of *Chlamydophila*-negative nongonococcal urethritis, ureaplasmas may be the causative agent. These organisms may also cause chronic voiding symptoms in women. The common presence of ureaplasmas in the urethra of asymptomatic men suggests either that only certain serovars are pathogenic or that predisposing factors, such as lack of immunity, must exist in persons who develop symptomatic infection. Alternatively, disease may develop only upon initial exposure to ureaplasmas. Ureaplasmas have been implicated in epididymitis. *M. genitalium* also appears to cause urethritis. *M. genitalium* and ureaplasmas do not have a known role in prostatitis. *M. hominis* does not appear to have a primary etiologic role in urethritis, epididymitis, or prostatitis.

Evidence suggests that *M. hominis* causes up to 5% of cases of acute pyelonephritis. Ureaplasmas have not been associated with this disease.

Ureaplasmas play a limited role in the production of urinary calculi. The frequency with which ureaplasmas reach the kidney, the predisposing factors that allow them to do so, and the relative frequency of urinary tract calculi induced by this organism (as compared with other organisms) are not known.

Pelvic inflammatory disease

M. hominis can cause pelvic inflammatory disease. In most episodes, *M. hominis* occurs as part of a polymicrobial infection, but

TABLE 175-2 Antimicrobial Agents of Choice for Mycoplasma Infections[a]

Organism	Drug(s)
M. pneumoniae	Azithromycin, clarithromycin, erythromycin, doxycycline, levofloxacin, moxifloxacin, gemifloxacin (*not* ciprofloxacin)
U. urealyticum, *U. parvum*	Azithromycin, clarithromycin, erythromycin, doxycycline
M. hominis	Doxycycline, clindamycin
M. genitalium	Azithromycin

[a]Antimicrobial resistance has been reported for mycoplasmas, as described in the text.

the organism may play an independent role in a limited number of cases. Some data also support an association of *M. genitalium* with pelvic inflammatory disease. Ureaplasmas are not thought to cause pelvic inflammatory disease.

Postpartum and postabortal infection

Studies implicate *M. hominis* as the primary pathogen in ~5–10% of women who have postpartum or postabortal fever; ureaplasmas have been implicated to a lesser degree. These infections are generally self-limited; however, if symptoms persist, specific antimicrobial therapy should be given. Ureaplasmas also appear to play a role in occasional postcesarean wound infections.

Nonurogenital infection

M. hominis rarely causes nonurogenital infections, such as brain abscess, wound infection, poststernotomy mediastinitis, endocarditis, and neonatal meningitis. These infections are most common among immunocompromised and hypogammaglobulinemic patients. Ureaplasmas and *M. hominis* can cause septic arthritis in immunodeficient patients. Ureaplasmas probably cause neonatal pneumonitis; their significant role in the development of bronchopulmonary dysplasia, the chronic lung disease of premature infants, has been documented in a number of studies. It is unclear whether ureaplasmas and *M. hominis* cause infertility, spontaneous abortion, premature labor, low birth weight, or chorioamnionitis.

■ DIAGNOSIS

Culture and PCR are both appropriate methods for the isolation of urogenital mycoplasmas. Culture of these organisms, however, requires special techniques and media that generally are available only at larger medical centers and reference laboratories. Serologic testing is not recommended for the clinical diagnosis of urogenital mycoplasma infections.

TREATMENT | Urogenital Mycoplasma Infections (Table 175-2)

Because colonization with urogenital mycoplasmas is common, it appears at present that their isolation from the urogenital tract in the absence of disease generally does not warrant treatment. Macrolides and doxycycline are considered the antimicrobial agents of choice for *Ureaplasma* infections. *Ureaplasma* resistance to macrolides, doxycycline, quinolones, and chloramphenicol has been reported. *M. hominis* is resistant to macrolides. Doxycycline is generally the drug of choice for *M. hominis* infections, although resistance has been reported. Clindamycin is also generally active against *M. hominis*. Quinolones are active in vitro against *M. hominis*. For *M. genitalium,* the agent of choice appears to be azithromycin; treatment failures have been reported with other macrolides as well as with quinolones.

FURTHER READINGS

BAKA S et al: Prevalence of *Ureaplasma urealyticum* and *Mycoplasma hominis* in women with chronic urinary symptoms. Urology 74:62, 2009

CHRISTIE LJ et al: Pediatric encephalitis: What is the role of *Mycoplasma pneumoniae*? Pediatrics 120:305, 2007

HARDY RD et al: Analysis of pulmonary inflammation and function in the mouse and baboon after exposure to *Mycoplasma pneumoniae* CARDS toxin. PLoS One 4:e7562, 2009

KANNAN TR, BASEMAN JB: ADP-ribosylating and vacuolating cytotoxin of *Mycoplasma pneumoniae* represents unique virulence determinant among bacterial pathogens. Proc Natl Acad Sci USA 103:6724, 2006

LI X et al: Emerging macrolide resistance in *Mycoplasma pneumoniae* in children: Detection and characterization of resistant isolates. Pediatr Infect Dis J 28:693, 2009

McCRACKEN GH: Current status of antibiotic treatment for *Mycoplasma pneumoniae* infections. Pediatr Infect Dis 5:167, 1986

MENA LA et al: A randomized comparison of azithromycin and doxycycline for the treatment of *Mycoplasma genitalium*-positive urethritis in men. Clin Infect Dis 48:1649, 2009

SUZUKI S et al: Clinical evaluation of macrolide-resistant *Mycoplasma pneumoniae*. Antimicrob Agents Chemother 50:709, 2006

TAGLIABUE C et al: The impact of steroids given with macrolide therapy on experimental *Mycoplasma pneumoniae* respiratory infection. J Infect Dis 198:1180, 2008

WAITES KB et al: New insights into the pathogenesis and detection of *Mycoplasma pneumoniae* infections. Future Microbiol 3:635, 2008

CHAPTER 176

Chlamydial Infections

Charlotte A. Gaydos
Thomas C. Quinn

Chlamydiae are obligate intracellular bacteria that cause a wide variety of diseases in humans and animals.

ETIOLOGIC AGENTS

The chlamydiae were originally classified as four species in the genus *Chlamydia*: *C. trachomatis*, *C. pneumoniae*, *C. psittaci*, and *C. pecorum* (the last species being found in ruminants). The *C. psittaci* group has been separated into three species: *C. psittaci*, *C. felis*, and *C. abortus*. The mouse pneumonitis strain (MoPn) is now classified as *C. muridarum*, and the guinea pig inclusion conjunctivitis strain (GPIC) is now designated *C. caviae*.

C. trachomatis is divided into two biovars: trachoma and LGV (lymphogranuloma venereum). The trachoma biovar causes two major types of disease in humans: ocular trachoma, the leading infectious cause of preventable blindness in the developing world; and urogenital infections, which are sexually or neonatally transmitted. The 18 serovars of *C. trachomatis* fall into three groups: the trachoma serovars A, B, Ba, and C; the oculogenital serovars D–K; and the LGV serovars L_1–L_3. Serovars can be distinguished by serologic typing with monoclonal antibodies or by molecular gene typing. However, serovar identification usually is not important clinically, since the antibiotic susceptibility pattern is the same for all three groups. The one exception applies when LGV is suspected on clinical grounds; in this situation, serovar determination is important because a longer treatment duration is required for LGV strains.

BIOLOGY, GROWTH CYCLE, AND PATHOGENESIS

■ BIOLOGY

During their intracellular growth, chlamydiae produce characteristic intracytoplasmic inclusions that can be visualized by direct fluorescent antibody (DFA) or Giemsa staining of infected clinical material, such as conjunctival scrapings or cervical or urethral epithelial cells. Chlamydiae are nonmotile, gram-negative, obligate intracellular bacteria that replicate within the cytoplasm of host cells, forming the characteristic membrane-bound inclusions that are the basis for some diagnostic tests. Originally considered to be large viruses, chlamydiae differ from viruses in possessing RNA and DNA as well as a cell wall that is quite similar in structure to the cell wall of typical gram-negative bacteria. However, chlamydiae lack peptidoglycan; their structural integrity depends on disulfide binding of outer-membrane proteins.

■ GROWTH CYCLE

Among the defining characteristics of chlamydiae is a unique growth cycle that involves alternation between two highly specialized morphologic forms (Figs. 176-1 and 176-2): the elementary body (EB), which is the infectious form and is specifically adapted for extracellular survival, and the metabolically active and replicating reticulate body (RB), which is not infectious, is adapted for an intracellular environment, and does not survive well outside

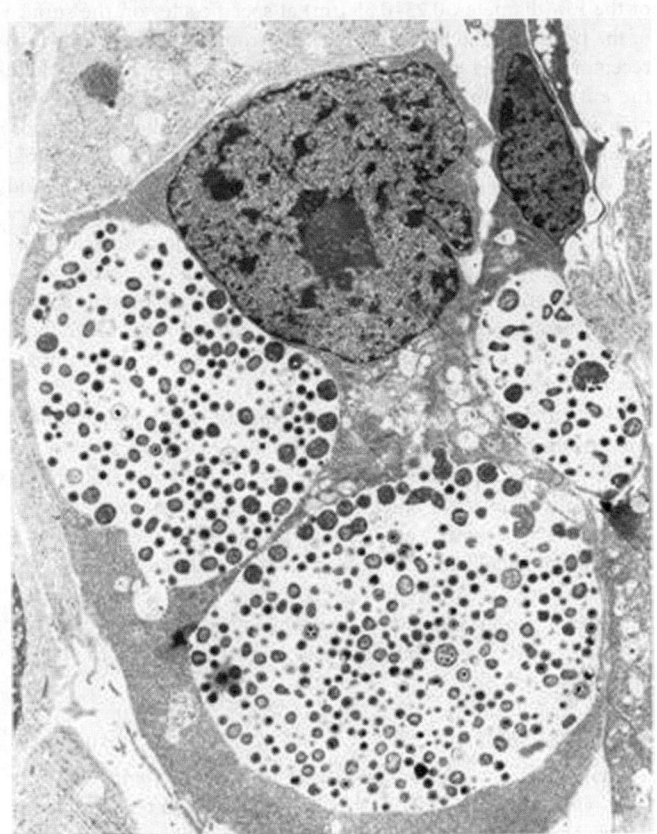

Figure 176-1   Chlamydial intracellular inclusions filled with smaller dense elementary bodies and larger reticulate bodies. *[Reprinted with permission from WE Stamm: Chlamydial infections, in Harrison's Principles of Internal Medicine, 17th ed, AS Fauci et al (eds). New York, McGraw-Hill, 2008, p 1070.]*

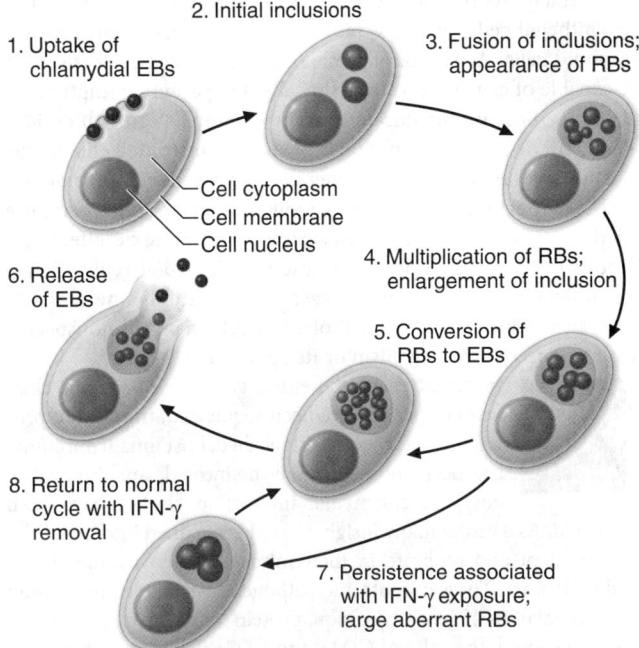

Figure 176-2   Chlamydial life cycle. EBs, elementary bodies; RBs, reticulate bodies; IFN-γ, interferon γ. *[Reprinted with permission from WE Stamm: Chlamydial infections, in Harrison's Principles of Internal Medicine, 17th ed, AS Fauci et al (eds). New York, McGraw-Hill, 2008, p 1071.]*

the host cell. The biphasic growth cycle begins with attachment of the EB (diameter, 0.25–0.35 μm) at specific sites on the surface of the host cell. The EB enters the cell through a process similar to receptor-mediated endocytosis and resides in an inclusion, where the entire growth cycle is completed. The chlamydiae prevent phagosome-lysosome fusion. The inclusion membrane is modified by insertion of chlamydial antigens. Once the EB has entered the cell, it reorganizes into an RB, which is larger (0.5–1 μm) and contains more RNA. After ~8 h, the RB starts to divide by binary fission. The intracytoplasmic, membrane-bound inclusion body containing the RBs increases in size as the RBs multiply. Approximately 18–24 h after infection of the cell, these RBs begin to become EBs by a reorganization or condensation process that is poorly understood. After rupture of the inclusion body, the EBs are released to initiate another cycle of infection.

Chlamydiae are susceptible to many broad-spectrum antibiotics and possess a number of enzymes, but they have a very restricted metabolic capacity. None of these metabolic reactions results in the production of energy. Chlamydiae have thus been considered to be energy parasites that use the ATP produced by the host cell for their own metabolic functions. Many aspects of chlamydial molecular biology are not well understood, but the sequencing of several chlamydial genomes and new proteomics research have provided researchers with many relevant tools for elucidating the biology of the life cycle.

■ PATHOGENESIS

Genital infections are mostly caused by *C. trachomatis* serovars D–K, with serovars D, E, and F involved most often. Molecular typing of the major outer-membrane protein gene (*omp1*) from which serovar differences arise has been used to demonstrate that polymorphisms can occur in isolates from patients who are exposed frequently to multiple infections, while less variation is observed in isolates from less sexually active populations. Polymorphisms in the major outer-membrane protein may provide antigenic variation, and the different forms allow persistence in the community because immunity to one is not protective against the others.

The trachoma biovar is essentially a parasite of squamocolumnar epithelial cells; the LGV biovar is more invasive and involves lymphoid cells. As is typical of chlamydiae, *C. trachomatis* strains are capable of causing chronic, clinically inapparent, asymptomatic infections. Because the duration of the chlamydial growth cycle is ~48–72 h, the incubation period of sexually transmitted chlamydial infections is relatively long—generally 1–3 weeks. *C. trachomatis* causes cell death as a result of its replicative cycle and can induce cell damage whenever it persists. However, few toxic effects are demonstrated, and cell death because of chlamydial replication is not sufficient to account for disease manifestations, the majority of which are due to immunopathologic mechanisms or nonspecific host responses to the organism or its byproducts.

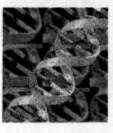 In recent years, the entire genomes of various chlamydial species have been sequenced, the field of proteomics has become established, host innate immunity has been more precisely delineated, and innovative host cell–chlamydial interaction studies have been conducted. As a result, many insights have been gained into how chlamydiae adapt and replicate in their intracellular environment and produce disease. These insights into pathogenesis include information on the regulation of gene expression, protein localization, the type III secretion system, the roles of CD4+ and CD8+ T lymphocytes in the host response, and T lymphocyte trafficking.

The chlamydial heat-shock protein, which shares antigenic epitopes with similar proteins of other bacteria and with human heat-shock protein, may sensitize the host, and repeated infections may cause host cell damage. Persistent or recurrent chlamydial infections are associated with fibrosis, scarring, and complications following simple epithelial infections. A common endpoint of these late consequences is scarring of mucous membranes. Genital complications can lead to pelvic inflammatory disease (PID) and its late consequences of infertility, ectopic pregnancy, and chronic pelvic pain, while ocular infections may lead to blinding trachoma. High levels of antibody to human heat-shock protein have been associated with tubal factor infertility and ectopic pregnancy. Without adequate therapy, chlamydial infections may persist for several years, although symptoms—if present—usually abate.

Pathogenic mechanisms of *C. pneumoniae* have yet to be completely elucidated. The same is true for *C. psittaci,* except that this agent infects cells very efficiently and causes disease that may reflect direct cytopathic effects.

CHLAMYDIA TRACHOMATIS INFECTIONS

■ GENITAL INFECTIONS

Spectrum

Although chlamydiae cause a number of human diseases, localized lower genital tract infections caused by *C. trachomatis* and the sequelae of such infections are the most important in terms of medical and economic impact. Oculogenital infections due to *C. trachomatis* serovars D–K are transmitted during sexual contact or from mother to baby during childbirth and are associated with many syndromes, including cervicitis, salpingitis, acute urethral syndrome, endometritis, ectopic pregnancy, infertility, and PID in female patients; urethritis, proctitis, and epididymitis in male patients; and conjunctivitis and pneumonia in infants. Women bear the greatest burden of morbidity because of the serious sequelae of these infections. Untreated infections lead to PID, and multiple episodes of PID can lead to tubal factor infertility and chronic pelvic pain. Studies estimate that up to 80–90% of women and >50% of men with *C. trachomatis* genital infections lack symptoms; other patients have very mild symptoms. Thus a large reservoir of infected persons continues to transmit infection to sexual partners.

As their designations reflect, the LGV serovars (L_1, L_2, and L_3) cause LGV, an invasive sexually transmitted disease (STD) characterized by acute lymphadenitis with bubo formation and/or acute hemorrhagic proctitis (see "Lymphogranuloma Venereum," below).

Epidemiology

C. trachomatis genital infections are global in distribution. The World Health Organization (WHO) estimates that >89 million cases occur annually worldwide. In the United States, these infections are the most commonly reported of all infectious diseases. In 2009, 1.24 million cases were reported to the U.S. Centers for Disease Control and Prevention (CDC); however, the CDC estimates that 2–3 million new cases occur per year, with substantial underreporting due to lack of screening in some populations. Rates of infection increase every year; higher rates among women than among men reflect the focus on expansion of screening programs in women during the past 20 years, the use of increasingly sensitive diagnostic tests, an increased emphasis on case reporting, and improvements in the information systems used for reporting. The CDC and other professional organizations recommend annual screening of all sexually active women ≤25 years of age as well as rescreening of previously infected individuals at 3 months. Young women have the highest infection rates; in 2008, the figures were 3275.8 and 3179.9 cases per 100,000 population at 15–19 and 20–24 years of age, respectively. Age-specific rates among men, while much lower than those among women, were highest in the 20- to 24-year-old age group, at 1056.1 cases per 100,000. In 2008, rates increased for all racial and ethnic groups; however, the rate among blacks was more than eight times higher than that among whites, with 1519.3 and 173.6 cases per 100,000, respectively. The rates among American Indian/Alaska Natives (808.8) and Latinos (510.4) were 4.7 and 2.9 times higher, respectively, than that among whites. These disparities are important reflections of health inequities in the United States.

The above statistics are based on case reporting. Studies based on screening surveys estimate that the U.S. prevalence of *C. trachomatis* cervical infection is 5% among asymptomatic female college students and prenatal patients, >10% for women seen in family planning clinics, and >20% for women seen in STD clinics. The prevalence of genital *C. trachomatis* infections varies substantially by geographic locale, with the highest rates in the southeastern United States. However, asymptomatic infections have been detected in >8–10% of young female military recruits from all parts of the country. The prevalence of *C. trachomatis* in the cervix of pregnant women is 5–10 times higher than that of *Neisseria gonorrhoeae*. The prevalence of genital infection with either agent is highest among women who are between the ages of 18 and 24, single, and non-Caucasian (e.g., African-American, Latina, Asian, Pacific Islander). Recurrent infections occur frequently in these same risk groups and are often acquired from untreated sexual partners. The use of oral contraception and the presence of cervical ectopy also confer an increased risk. The proportion of infections that are asymptomatic appears to be higher for *C. trachomatis* than for *N. gonorrhoeae*, and symptomatic *C. trachomatis* infections are clinically less severe. Mild or asymptomatic *C. trachomatis* infections of the fallopian tubes nonetheless cause ongoing tubal damage and infertility. The costs of *C. trachomatis* infections and their complications to the U.S. health care system are projected to be >$2.4 billion annually.

Clinical manifestations

Nongonococcal and postgonococcal urethritis *C. trachomatis* is the most common cause of nongonococcal urethritis (NGU) and postgonococcal urethritis (PGU). The designation *PGU* refers to NGU developing in men 2–3 weeks after treatment of gonococcal urethritis with single doses of agents such as penicillin or cephalosporins, which lack antimicrobial activity against chlamydiae. Since current treatment regimens for gonorrhea have evolved and now include combination therapy with tetracycline, doxycycline, or azithromycin—all of which are effective against concomitant chlamydial infection—both the incidence of PGU and the causative role of *C. trachomatis* in this syndrome have declined.

In the United States, most of the estimated 2 million cases of acute urethritis are NGU, and *C. trachomatis* is implicated in 30–50% of these cases. The cause of most of the remaining cases of NGU is uncertain, but recent evidence suggests that *Ureaplasma urealyticum*, *Mycoplasma genitalium*, *Trichomonas vaginalis*, and herpes simplex virus (HSV) cause some cases. The rate of involvement of *C. trachomatis* in urethral infection ranges from 3–7% among asymptomatic men to 15–20% among symptomatic men attending STD clinics. One recent multisite study of men in Baltimore, Seattle, Denver, and San Francisco reported an overall chlamydial prevalence of 7% in urine samples assessed by nucleic acid amplification tests (NAATs). As in women, infection in men is age related, with young age as the greatest risk factor for chlamydial urethritis. The prevalence among men is highest at 20–24 years of age. In STD clinics, urethritis is usually less prevalent among men who have sex with men (MSM) than among heterosexual men and is almost always much more common among black men than among white men. One study reported prevalences of 19% and 9% among nonwhite and white heterosexual men, respectively.

NGU is diagnosed by documentation of a leukocytic urethral exudate and by exclusion of gonorrhea by Gram's staining or culture.

C. trachomatis urethritis is generally less severe than gonococcal urethritis, although in any individual patient these two forms of urethritis cannot reliably be differentiated solely on clinical grounds. Symptoms include urethral discharge (often whitish and mucoid rather than frankly purulent), dysuria, and urethral itching. Physical examination may reveal meatal erythema and tenderness as well as a urethral exudate that is often demonstrable only by stripping of the urethra.

At least one-third of male patients with *C. trachomatis* urethral infection have no evident signs or symptoms of urethritis. The availability of NAATs for first-void urine specimens has facilitated broader-based testing for asymptomatic infection in male patients. As a result, asymptomatic chlamydial urethritis has been demonstrated in 5–10% of sexually active male adolescents screened at school-based clinics or community centers. Such patients generally have pyuria (≥15 leukocytes per 400× microscopic field in the sediment of first-void urine), a positive leukocyte esterase test, or an increased number of leukocytes on a Gram-stained smear prepared from a urogenital swab inserted 1–2 cm into the anterior urethra. To differentiate between true urethritis and functional symptoms in symptomatic patients or to make a presumptive diagnosis of *C. trachomatis* infection in high-risk but asymptomatic men (e.g., male patients in STD clinics, sex partners of women with nongonococcal salpingitis or mucopurulent cervicitis, fathers of children with inclusion conjunctivitis), the examination of an endourethral specimen for increased leukocytes is useful if specific diagnostic tests for chlamydiae are not available. Alternatively, urethritis can be assayed noninvasively by examination of a first-void urine sample for pyuria, either by microscopy or by the leukocyte esterase test. Urine (or a urethral swab) can also be tested directly for chlamydiae by DNA amplification methods, as described below (see "Detection Methods").

Epididymitis Chlamydial urethritis may be followed by acute epididymitis, but this condition is rare, generally occurring in sexually active patients <35 years of age; in older men, epididymitis is usually associated with gram-negative bacterial infection and/or instrumentation procedures. It is estimated that 50–70% of cases of acute epididymitis are caused by *C. trachomatis*. The condition usually presents as unilateral scrotal pain with tenderness, swelling, and fever in a young man, often occurring in association with chlamydial urethritis. The illness may be mild enough to treat with oral antibiotics on an outpatient basis or severe enough to require hospitalization and parenteral therapy. Testicular torsion should be excluded promptly by radionuclide scan, Doppler flow study, or surgical exploration in a teenager or young adult who presents with acute unilateral testicular pain without urethritis. The possibility of testicular tumor or chronic infection (e.g., tuberculosis) should be excluded when a patient with unilateral intrascrotal pain and swelling does not respond to appropriate antimicrobial therapy.

Reactive arthritis Reactive arthritis (formerly known as Reiter's syndrome) consists of conjunctivitis, urethritis (or, in female patients, cervicitis), arthritis, and characteristic mucocutaneous lesions. It may develop in 1–2% of cases of NGU and is thought to be the most common type of peripheral inflammatory arthritis in young men. *C. trachomatis* has been recovered from the urethra of 16–44% of patients with reactive arthritis and from 69% of men who have signs of urogenital inflammation at the time of examination. Antibodies to *C. trachomatis* have also been detected in 46–67% of patients with reactive arthritis, and *Chlamydia*-specific cell-mediated immunity has been documented in 72%. In addition, *C. trachomatis* has been isolated from synovial biopsy samples from 15 of 29 patients in a number of small series and from a smaller proportion of synovial fluid specimens. Chlamydial nucleic acids have been identified in synovial membranes and chlamydial EBs in joint fluid. The pathogenesis of reactive arthritis is unclear, but this condition probably represents an abnormal host response to a number of infectious agents, including those associated with bacterial gastroenteritis (e.g., *Salmonella*, *Shigella*, *Yersinia*, or *Campylobacter*) or to infection with *C. trachomatis* or *N. gonorrhoeae*. Since >80% of affected patients have the HLA-B27 phenotype and since other mucosal infections produce an identical syndrome, chlamydial infection is thought to initiate an aberrant hyperactive immune response that produces inflammation of the involved target organs in these genetically predisposed individuals. Evidence of exaggerated cell-mediated and humoral immune responses to chlamydial antigens in reactive arthritis supports this hypothesis. The finding of chlamydial EBs and DNA in joint fluid and synovial tissue from patients with reactive arthritis suggests that chlamydiae may actually spread from genital to joint tissues in these patients—perhaps in macrophages.

NGU is the initial manifestation of reactive arthritis in 80% of patients, typically occurring within 14 days after sexual exposure. The urethritis may be mild and may even go unnoticed by the patient. Similarly, gonococcal urethritis may precede reactive arthritis, but co-infection with an agent of NGU is difficult to rule out. The urethral discharge may be purulent or mucopurulent, and patients may or may not report dysuria. Accompanying prostatitis, usually asymptomatic, has been described. Arthritis usually begins ~4 weeks after the onset of urethritis but may develop sooner or, in a small percentage of cases, may actually precede urethritis. The knees are most frequently involved; next most commonly affected are the ankles and small joints of the feet. Sacroiliitis, either symmetrical or asymmetrical, is documented in two-thirds of patients. Mild bilateral conjunctivitis, iritis, keratitis, or uveitis is sometimes present but lasts for only a few days. Finally, dermatologic manifestations occur in up to 50% of patients. The initial lesions—usually papules with a central yellow spot—most often involve the soles and palms and, in ~25% of patients, eventually epithelialize and thicken to produce keratoderma blenorrhagicum. Circinate balanitis is usually painless and occurs in fewer than half of patients. The initial episode of reactive arthritis usually lasts 2–6 months.

Proctitis Primary anal or rectal infections with *C. trachomatis* have been described in women and MSM who practice anal intercourse. In these infections, rectal involvement is initially characterized by severe anorectal pain, a bloody mucopurulent discharge, and tenesmus. Oculogenital serovars D–K and LGV serovars L$_1$, L$_2$, and L$_3$ have been found to cause proctitis. The LGV serovars are far more invasive and cause much more severely symptomatic disease, including severe ulcerative proctocolitis that can be clinically confused with HSV proctitis. Histologically, LGV proctitis may resemble Crohn's disease in that giant cell formation and granulomas are detected. In the United States and Europe, cases of LGV proctitis occur almost exclusively in MSM, many of whom are positive for HIV infection.

The less invasive non-LGV serovars of *C. trachomatis* cause mild proctitis. Many infected individuals are asymptomatic, and in these cases infection is diagnosed only by routine culture or NAAT of rectal swabs. The number of fecal leukocytes is usually abnormal in both asymptomatic and symptomatic cases. Sigmoidoscopy may yield normal findings or may reveal mild inflammatory changes or small erosions or follicles in the lower 10 cm of the rectum. Histologic examination of rectal biopsies generally shows anal crypts and prominent follicles as well as neutrophilic infiltration of the lamina propria. Chlamydial proctitis is best diagnosed by isolation of *C. trachomatis* from the rectum and documentation of a response to appropriate therapy. NAATs are reportedly more sensitive than culture for diagnosis and are also specific.

Mucopurulent cervicitis Although many women with chlamydial infections of the cervix have no symptoms, almost half generally have local signs of infection on examination. Cervicitis is usually characterized by the presence of a mucopurulent discharge, with >20 neutrophils per microscopic field visible in strands of cervical mucus in a thinly smeared, gram-stained preparation of endocervical exudate. Hypertrophic ectopy of the cervix may also be evident as an edematous area near the cervical os that is congested and bleeds easily on minor trauma (e.g., when a specimen is collected with a swab). A Papanicolaou smear shows increased numbers of neutrophils as well as a characteristic pattern of mononuclear inflammatory cells including plasma cells, transformed lymphocytes, and histiocytes. Cervical biopsy shows a predominantly mononuclear cell infiltrate of the subepithelial stroma. Clinical experience and collaborative studies indicate that a cutoff of >30 polymorphonuclear leukocytes (PMNs)/1000× field in a gram-stained smear of cervical mucus correlates best with chlamydial or gonococcal cervicitis.

Clinical recognition of chlamydial cervicitis depends on a high index of suspicion and careful cervical examination. No genital symptoms are specifically correlated with chlamydial cervical infection. The differential diagnosis of a mucopurulent discharge from the endocervical canal in a young, sexually active woman includes gonococcal endocervicitis, salpingitis, endometritis, and intrauterine contraceptive device–induced inflammation. Diagnosis of cervicitis is based on the presence of PMNs on a cervical swab as noted above; the presence of chlamydiae is confirmed by either culture or NAAT.

Pelvic inflammatory disease Inflammation of sections of the fallopian tube is often referred to as salpingitis or PID. The proportion of acute salpingitis cases caused by *C. trachomatis* varies geographically and with the population studied. It has been estimated that *C. trachomatis* causes up to 50% of PID cases in the United States. PID occurs via ascending intraluminal spread of *C. trachomatis* or *N. gonorrhoeae* from the lower genital tract. Mucopurulent cervicitis is often followed by endometritis, endosalpingitis, and finally pelvic peritonitis. Evidence of mucopurulent cervicitis is often found in women with laparoscopically verified salpingitis. Similarly, endometritis, demonstrated by an endometrial biopsy showing plasma cell infiltration of the endometrial epithelium, is documented in most women with laparoscopy-verified chlamydial (or gonococcal) salpingitis. Chlamydial endometritis can also occur in the absence of clinical evidence of salpingitis. Histologic evidence of endometritis has been correlated with a syndrome consisting of vaginal bleeding, lower abdominal pain, and uterine tenderness in the absence of adnexal tenderness. Chlamydial salpingitis produces milder symptoms than gonococcal salpingitis and may be associated with less marked adnexal tenderness. Thus, mild adnexal or uterine tenderness in a sexually active woman with cervicitis suggests chlamydial PID.

Chronic untreated endometrial and tubal inflammation can result in tubal scarring, impaired tubal function, tubal occlusion, and infertility even among women who report no prior treatment for PID. *C. trachomatis* has been particularly implicated in "subclinical" PID on the basis of a lack of history of PID among *Chlamydia*-seropositive women with tubal damage and detection of chlamydial DNA or antigen among asymptomatic women with tubal infertility. These data suggest that the best method to prevent PID and its sequelae is surveillance and control of lower genital tract infections along with diagnosis and treatment of sex partners and prevention of reinfections. Promotion of early symptom recognition and health care presentation may reduce the frequency and severity of sequelae of PID.

Perihepatitis The Fitz-Hugh–Curtis syndrome was originally described as a complication of gonococcal PID. However, studies over the past several decades have suggested that chlamydial infection is more commonly associated with perihepatitis than is *N. gonorrhoeae*. Perihepatitis should be suspected in young, sexually active women who develop right-upper-quadrant pain, fever, or nausea. Evidence of salpingitis may or may not be found on examination. Frequently, perihepatitis is strongly associated with extensive tubal scarring, adhesions, and inflammation observed at laparoscopy, and high titers of antibody to the 57-kDa chlamydial heat-shock protein have been documented. Culture and/or serologic evidence of *C. trachomatis* is found in three-fourths of women with this syndrome.

Urethral syndrome in women In the absence of infection with uropathogens such as coliforms or *Staphylococcus saprophyticus*, *C. trachomatis* is the pathogen most commonly isolated from college women with dysuria, frequency, and pyuria. Screening studies can recover *C. trachomatis* at both the cervix and the urethra; in up to 25% of infected women, the organism is isolated only from the urethra. The urethral syndrome in women consists of dysuria and frequency in conjunction with chlamydial urethritis, pyuria, and no bacteriuria or urinary pathogens. Although symptoms of the urethral syndrome may develop in some women with chlamydial infection, the majority of women attending STD clinics for urethral chlamydial infection do not have dysuria or frequency. Even in women with chlamydial urethritis causing the acute urethral syndrome, signs of urethritis such as urethral discharge, meatal redness, and swelling are uncommon. However, mucopurulent cervicitis in a woman presenting with dysuria and frequency strongly suggests *C. trachomatis* urethritis. Other correlates of chlamydial urethral syndrome include a duration of dysuria of >7–10 days, lack of hematuria, and lack of suprapubic tenderness. Abnormal urethral Gram's stains showing >10 PMNs/1000x field in women with dysuria but without coliform bacteriuria support the diagnosis of chlamydial urethritis. Other possible diagnoses include gonococcal or trichomonal infection of the urethra.

Infection in pregnancy and the neonatal period Infections during pregnancy can be transmitted to infants during delivery. Approximately 20–30% of infants exposed to *C. trachomatis* in the birth canal develop conjunctivitis, and 10–15% subsequently develop pneumonia. Consequently, all newborn infants receive ocular prophylaxis at birth to prevent ophthalmia neonatorum. Without treatment, conjunctivitis usually develops at 5–19 days of life and often results in a profuse mucopurulent discharge. Roughly half of infected infants develop clinical evidence of inclusion conjunctivitis. However, it is impossible to differentiate chlamydial conjunctivitis from other forms of neonatal conjunctivitis (e.g., that due to *N. gonorrhoeae*, *Haemophilus influenzae*, *Streptococcus pneumoniae*, or HSV) on clinical grounds; thus laboratory diagnosis is required. Inclusions within epithelial cells are often detected in Giemsa-stained conjunctival smears, but these smears are considerably less sensitive than cultures or NAATs for chlamydiae. Gram-stained smears may show gonococci or occasional small gram-negative coccobacilli in *Haemophilus* conjunctivitis, but smears should be accompanied by cultures or NAATs for these agents.

C. trachomatis has also been isolated frequently and persistently from the nasopharynx, rectum, and vagina of infected infants—occasionally for >1 year in the absence of treatment. In some cases, otitis media results from perinatally acquired chlamydial infection. Pneumonia may develop in infants from 2 weeks to 4 months of age. *C. trachomatis* is estimated to cause 20–30% of pneumonia cases in infants <6 months of age. Epidemiologic studies have linked chlamydial pulmonary infection in infants with increased occurrence of subacute lung disease (bronchitis, asthma, wheezing) in later childhood.

 Lymphogranuloma venereum *C. trachomatis* serovars L$_1$, L$_2$, and L$_3$ cause LGV, an invasive systemic STD. The peak incidence of LGV corresponds with the age of greatest sexual activity: the second and third decades of life. The worldwide incidence of LGV is falling, but the disease is still endemic and a major cause of morbidity in parts of Asia, Africa, South America, and the Caribbean. LGV is rare in industrialized countries; for more than a decade, the reported incidence in the United States has been only 0.1 case per 100,000 population. In the Bahamas, an apparent outbreak of LGV was described in association with a concurrent increase in heterosexual infection with HIV. Reports of outbreaks with the newly identified variant L$_{2b}$ in Europe, Australia, and the United States indicate that LGV is becoming more prevalent among MSM. These cases have usually presented as hemorrhagic proctocolitis in HIV-positive men. More widespread use of NAATs for identification of rectal infections may have enhanced case recognition.

The frequency of infection following exposure is believed to be much lower for LGV than for gonorrhea and syphilis. Early manifestations are recognized more often in men than in women, who usually present with late complications. In the United States, where the reported male-to-female ratio of cases is 3.4:1, most cases involve MSM and persons returning from abroad (travelers, sailors, and military personnel).

LGV begins as a small painless papule that tends to ulcerate at the site of inoculation, often escaping attention. This primary lesion heals in a few days without scarring and, even when noticed, is usually recognized as LGV only in retrospect. LGV strains of *C. trachomatis* have occasionally been recovered from genital ulcers and from the urethra of men and the endocervix of women who present with inguinal adenopathy; these areas may be the primary sites of infection in some cases. Proctitis is more common among people who practice receptive anal intercourse, and an elevated white blood cell count in anorectal smears may predict LGV in these patients. Ulcer formation may facilitate transmission of HIV infection and other sexually transmitted and blood-borne diseases.

As NAATs for *C. trachomatis* are being used more often, increasing numbers of cases of LGV proctitis are being recognized in MSM. Such patients present with anorectal pain and mucopurulent, bloody rectal discharge. Although these patients may report diarrhea, they are often referring not to diarrhea but rather to frequent, painful, unsuccessful attempts at defecation (tenesmus). Sigmoidoscopy reveals ulcerative proctitis or proctocolitis, with purulent exudate and mucosal bleeding. Histopathologic findings in the rectal mucosa include granulomas with giant cells, crypt abscesses, and extensive inflammation. These clinical, sigmoidoscopic, and histopathologic findings may closely resemble those of Crohn's disease of the rectum.

The most common presenting picture in heterosexual men and women is the *inguinal syndrome*, which is characterized by painful inguinal lymphadenopathy beginning 2–6 weeks after presumed exposure; in rare instances, the onset comes after a few months. The inguinal adenopathy is unilateral in two-thirds of cases, and palpable enlargement of the iliac and femoral nodes is often evident on the same side as the enlarged inguinal nodes. The nodes are initially discrete, but progressive periadenitis results in a matted mass of nodes that becomes fluctuant and suppurative. The overlying skin becomes fixed, inflamed, and thin, and multiple draining fistulas finally develop. Extensive enlargement of chains of inguinal nodes above and below the inguinal ligament ("the sign of the groove") is not specific and, although not uncommon, is documented in only a minority of cases. On histologic examination, infected nodes are initially found to have characteristic small stellate abscesses surrounded by histiocytes. These abscesses coalesce to form large, necrotic, suppurative foci. Spontaneous healing usually takes place after several months; inguinal scars or granulomatous masses of various sizes persist for life. Massive pelvic lymphadenopathy may lead to exploratory laparotomy.

Constitutional symptoms are common during the stage of regional lymphadenopathy and, in cases of proctitis, may include fever, chills, headache, meningismus, anorexia, myalgias, and arthralgias. These findings in the presence of lymphadenopathy are sometimes mistakenly interpreted as malignant lymphoma. Other systemic complications are infrequent but include arthritis with sterile effusion, aseptic meningitis, meningoencephalitis, conjunctivitis, hepatitis, and erythema nodosum (Fig. e7-40). *C. trachomatis* has been recovered from the cerebrospinal fluid and in one case was isolated from the blood of a patient with severe constitutional symptoms—a result indicating dissemination of infection. Laboratory-acquired infections suspected of being due to the inhalation of aerosols have been associated with mediastinal lymphadenitis, pneumonitis, and pleural effusion.

Complications of untreated anorectal infection include perirectal abscess; anal fistulas; and rectovaginal, rectovesical, and ischiorectal fistulas. Secondary bacterial infection probably contributes to these complications. Rectal stricture is a late complication of anorectal infection and usually develops 2–6 cm from the anal orifice—i.e., at a site within reach on digital rectal examination. Proximal extension of the stricture for several centimeters may lead to a mistaken clinical and radiographic diagnosis of carcinoma. A small percentage of cases of LGV in men present as chronic progressive infiltrative, ulcerative, or fistular lesions of the penis, urethra, or scrotum. Associated lymphatic obstruction may produce elephantiasis. When urethral stricture occurs, it usually involves the posterior urethra and causes incontinence or difficulty with urination.

Diagnosis

Detection methods   Historically, chlamydiae were cultivated in the yolk sac of embryonated eggs. The organisms can be grown more easily in tissue culture, but cell culture—once considered the diagnostic gold standard—has been replaced by nonculture assays (Table 176-1). In general, culture for chlamydiae in clinical specimens is now performed only in specialized laboratories. The first nonculture assays, such as DFA staining of clinical material and enzyme immunoassay (EIA), have been replaced by molecular tests that amplify the nucleic acids in clinical specimens. These NAATS are currently recommended by the CDC as the diagnostic assays of choice.

Choice of specimen   Cervical and urethral swabs have traditionally been used for the diagnosis of STDs in female and male patients, respectively. However, given the greatly increased sensitivity and specificity of NAATs, less invasive samples (e.g., urine for both sexes and vaginal swabs for women) can be used. For screening of asymptomatic women, the CDC now recommends that self-collected vaginal swabs, which are slightly more sensitive than urine, be used. Urine screening tests are often used in outreach screening programs, however. For symptomatic women undergoing a pelvic examination, cervical swab samples are desirable because they have slightly higher chlamydial counts. For male patients, a urine specimen is the sample of choice.

Alternative specimen types   Ocular samples from babies and adults can be assessed by NAATs. However, since commercial NAATs for this purpose have not yet been approved by the U.S. Food and Drug Administration (FDA), laboratories must perform their own verification studies. Samples from rectal and pharyngeal sites have been used successfully to detect chlamydiae, but again, laboratories must verify test performance.

Other diagnostic issues   Because NAATs measure nucleic acids instead of live organisms, they should be used with caution as test-of-cure assays. Residual nucleic acid from cells rendered noninfective by antibiotics may continue to yield a positive result in NAATs until as long as 3 weeks after therapy, when viable organisms have actually been eradicated. Therefore, clinicians should not use NAATs for test of cure until after 3 weeks. The CDC currently does not recommend a test of cure after treatment for infection with *C. trachomatis*. However, because incidence studies have demonstrated that previous chlamydial infection increases the probability of becoming reinfected, the CDC does recommend that previously infected individuals be rescreened 3 months after treatment.

Serology   Serologic testing may be helpful in the diagnosis of LGV and neonatal pneumonia caused by *C. trachomatis*. The serologic test of choice is the microimmunofluorescence (MIF) test, in which high-titer purified EBs mixed with embryonated chicken yolk sac material are affixed to a glass microscope slide to which dilutions of sera are applied. After incubation and washing, fluorescein-conjugated IgG or IgM antibody is applied. The test is read with an epifluorescence microscope, with the highest dilution of serum producing visible fluorescence designated as the titer. The MIF test is not widely available and is highly labor intensive. Although the complement fixation (CF) test can also be used, it employs only lipopolysaccharide (LPS) as the antigen and therefore identifies the pathogen only to the genus level. Single-point titers of >1:64 support a diagnosis of LGV, in which it is difficult to demonstrate rising antibody titers—i.e., paired serum samples are difficult to obtain since, by its very nature, the disease results in the patient's being seen by the physician after the acute stage. Any antibody titer of >1:16 is considered significant evidence of exposure to chlamydiae. However, serologic testing is not recommended for diagnosis of uncomplicated genital infections of the cervix, urethra, and lower genital tract or for *C. trachomatis* screening of asymptomatic individuals.

TREATMENT   *C. trachomatis* Genital Infections

A 7-day course of tetracycline (500 mg four times daily), doxycycline (100 mg twice daily), erythromycin (500 mg four times daily), or a fluoroquinolone (ofloxacin, 300 mg twice daily; or levofloxacin, 500 mg/d) can be used for treatment of uncomplicated chlamydial infections. A single 1-g oral dose of azithromycin is as effective as a 7-day course of doxycycline for the treatment of uncomplicated genital *C. trachomatis* infections in adults. Azithromycin causes fewer adverse gastrointestinal reactions than do older macrolides such as erythromycin. The single-dose regimen of azithromycin has great appeal for the treatment of patients with uncomplicated chlamydial infection (especially those without symptoms and those with a likelihood of poor compliance) and of the sexual partners of infected patients. These advantages must be weighed against the considerably greater cost of azithromycin. Whenever possible, the single 1-g dose should be given as directly observed therapy. Although not approved by the FDA for use in pregnancy, this regimen appears to be safe and effective for this purpose. However, amoxicillin (500 mg three times daily for 7 days) can also be given to pregnant women. The fluoroquinolones are contraindicated in pregnancy. A 2-week course of treatment is recommended for complicated chlamydial infections (e.g., PID, epididymitis) and at least a 3-week course of doxycycline (100 mg orally twice daily) or erythromycin base (500 mg orally four times daily) for LGV. Failure of treatment with a tetracycline in genital infections usually indicates poor compliance or reinfection rather than involvement of a drug-resistant strain. To date, clinically significant drug resistance has not been observed in *C. trachomatis*.

TABLE 176-1 Diagnostic Tests for Sexually Transmitted and Perinatal *Chlamydia trachomatis* Infection

Infection	Suggestive Signs/Symptoms	Presumptive Diagnosis[a]	Confirmatory Test of Choice
Men			
NGU, PGU	Discharge, dysuria	Gram's stain with >4 neutrophils per oil-immersion field; no gonococci	Urine or urethral NAAT for *C. trachomatis*
Epididymitis	Unilateral intrascrotal swelling, pain, tenderness; fever; NGU	Gram's stain with >4 neutrophils per oil-immersion field; no gonococci; urinalysis with pyuria	Urine or urethral NAAT for *C. trachomatis*
Women			
Cervicitis	Mucopurulent cervical discharge, bleeding and edema of the zone of cervical ectopy	Cervical Gram's stain with ≥20 neutrophils per oil-immersion field in cervical mucus	Urine, cervical, or vaginal NAAT for *C. trachomatis*
Salpingitis	Lower abdominal pain, cervical motion tenderness, adnexal tenderness or masses	*C. trachomatis* always potentially present in salpingitis	Urine, cervical, or vaginal NAAT for *C. trachomatis*
Urethritis	Dysuria and frequency without hematuria	MPC; sterile pyuria; negative routine urine culture	Urine or urethral NAAT for *C. trachomatis*
Adults of Either Sex			
Proctitis	Rectal pain, discharge, tenesmus, bleeding; history of receptive anorectal intercourse	Negative gonococcal culture and Gram's stain; at least 1 neutrophil per oil-immersion field in rectal Gram's stain	Rectal NAAT for *C. trachomatis* or culture
Reactive arthritis	NGU, arthritis, conjunctivitis, typical skin lesions	Gram's stain with >4 neutrophils per oil-immersion field; lack of gonococci indicative of NGU	Urine or urethral NAAT for *C. trachomatis*
LGV	Regional adenopathy, primary lesion, proctitis, systemic symptoms	None	Culture of LGV strain from node or rectum, occasionally from urethra or cervix; NAAT for *C. trachomatis* from these sites; LGV CF titer, ≥1:64; micro-IF titer, ≥1:512
Neonates			
Conjunctivitis	Purulent conjunctival discharge 6–18 days after delivery	Negative culture and Gram's stain for gonococci, *Haemophilus* spp., pneumococci, staphylococci	Conjunctival NAAT for *C. trachomatis*; FA-stained scraping of conjunctival material
Infant pneumonia	Afebrile, staccato cough, diffuse rales, bilateral hyperinflation, interstitial infiltrates	None	Chlamydial culture or NAAT of sputum, pharynx, eye, rectum; micro-IF antibody to *C. trachomatis*—fourfold change in IgG or IgM antibody titer

[a]A presumptive diagnosis of chlamydial infection is often made in the syndromes listed when gonococci are not found. A positive test for *Neisseria gonorrhoeae* does not exclude the involvement of *C. trachomatis*, which often is present in patients with gonorrhea.

Abbreviations: CF, complement-fixing; FA, fluorescent antibody; LGV, lymphogranuloma venereum; micro-IF, microimmunofluorescence; MPC, mucopurulent cervicitis; NAAT, nucleic acid amplification test; NGU, nongonococcal urethritis; PGU, postgonococcal urethritis.

Source: Reprinted with permission from WE Stamm: Chlamydial infections, in *Harrison's Principles of Internal Medicine*, 17th ed, AS Fauci et al (eds). New York, McGraw-Hill, 2008, p 1075.

Treatment or testing for chlamydiae should be considered among *N. gonorrhoeae*–infected patients because of the frequency of co-infection. Systemic treatment with erythromycin has been recommended for ophthalmia neonatorum and for *C. trachomatis* pneumonia in infants. For the treatment of adult inclusion conjunctivitis, a single 1-g dose of azithromycin was as effective as standard 10-day treatment with doxycycline. Recommended treatment regimens for both bubonic and anogenital LGV include tetracycline, doxycycline, or erythromycin for 21 days.

SEX PARTNERS The continued high prevalence of chlamydial infections in most parts of the United States is due primarily to the failure to diagnose—and therefore treat—patients with symptomatic or asymptomatic infection and their sex partners. Urethral or cervical infection with *C. trachomatis* has been well documented in a high proportion of the sex partners of patients with NGU, epididymitis, reactive arthritis, salpingitis, and endocervicitis. If possible, confirmatory laboratory tests for chlamydiae should be undertaken in these individuals, but even those without positive tests or evidence of clinical disease who have recently been exposed to proven or possible chlamydial infection (e.g., NGU) should be offered therapy. A novel approach is partner-delivered therapy, in which infected patients receive treatment and are also provided with single-dose azithromycin to give to their sex partner(s).

NEONATES AND INFANTS In neonates with conjunctivitis or infants with pneumonia, erythromycin ethylsuccinate or estolate can be given orally at a dosage of 50 mg/kg per day, preferably in four divided doses, for 2 weeks. Careful attention must be given to compliance with therapy—a frequent problem. Relapses of eye infection are common after topical treatment with erythromycin or tetracycline ophthalmic ointment and may also follow oral erythromycin therapy. Thus follow-up cultures should be performed after treatment. Both parents should be examined for *C. trachomatis* infection and, if diagnostic testing is not readily available, should be treated with doxycycline or azithromycin.

Prevention

Since many chlamydial infections are asymptomatic, effective control and prevention must involve periodic screening of individuals at risk. Selective cost-effective screening criteria have been developed. Among women, young age (generally <25 years) is a critical risk factor for chlamydial infections in nearly all studies. Other risk factors include mucopurulent cervicitis; multiple, new, or symptomatic male sex partners; and lack of barrier contraceptive use. In some settings, screening based on young age may be as sensitive as criteria that incorporate behavioral and clinical measures. Another strategy is universal testing of all patients in high-prevalence clinic populations (e.g., STD clinics, juvenile detention facilities, and family planning clinics).

The effectiveness of selective screening in reducing the prevalence of chlamydial infection among women has been demonstrated in several studies. In the Pacific Northwest, where extensive screening began in family planning clinics in 1998 and in STD clinics in 1993, the prevalence declined from 10% in the 1980s to <5% in 2000. Similar trends have occurred in association with screening programs elsewhere. In addition, screening can effect a reduction in upper genital tract disease. In Seattle, women at a large health maintenance organization who were screened for chlamydial infection on a routine basis had a lower incidence of symptomatic PID than did women who received standard care and underwent more selective screening.

In settings with low to moderate prevalence, the prevalence at which selective screening becomes more cost-effective than universal screening must be defined. Most studies have concluded that universal screening is preferable in settings with a chlamydial prevalence of >3–7%. Depending on the criteria used, selective screening is likely to be more cost-effective when prevalence falls below 3%. Nearly all regions of the United States have now initiated screening programs, particularly in family planning and STD clinics. Along with single-dose therapy, the availability of highly sensitive and specific diagnostic NAATs using urine specimens and self-obtained vaginal swabs makes it feasible to mount an effective nationwide *Chlamydia* control program, with screening of high-risk individuals in traditional health-care settings and in novel outreach and community-based settings.

■ TRACHOMA

Epidemiology

Trachoma—a sequela of ocular disease in developing countries—continues to be a leading cause of preventable infectious blindness worldwide. The WHO estimates that ~6 million people have been blinded by trachoma and that ~1.3 million people in developing countries still suffer from preventable blindness due to trachoma; certainly hundreds of millions live in trachoma-endemic areas. Foci of trachoma persist in Australia, the South Pacific, and Latin America. Serovars A, B, Ba, and C are isolated from patients with clinical trachoma in areas of endemicity in developing countries in Africa, the Middle East, Asia, and South America.

The trachoma-hyperendemic areas of the world are in northern and sub-Saharan Africa, the Middle East, drier regions of the Indian subcontinent, and Southeast Asia. In hyperendemic areas, the prevalence of trachoma is essentially 100% by the second or third year of life. Active disease is most common among young children, who are the reservoir for trachoma. By adulthood, active infection is infrequent but sequelae result in blindness. In such areas, trachoma constitutes the major cause of blindness.

Trachoma is transmitted through contact with discharges from the eyes of infected patients. Transmission is most common under poor hygienic conditions and most often takes place between family members or between families with shared facilities. Flies can also transfer the mucopurulent ocular discharges, carrying the organisms on their legs from one person to another. The International Trachoma Initiative founded by the WHO in 1998 aims to eliminate blinding trachoma globally by 2020.

Clinical manifestations

Both endemic trachoma and adult inclusion conjunctivitis present initially as conjunctivitis characterized by small lymphoid follicles in the conjunctiva. In regions with hyperendemic classic blinding trachoma, the disease usually starts insidiously before the age of 2 years. Reinfection is common and probably contributes to the pathogenesis of trachoma. Studies using polymerase chain reaction (PCR) or other NAATs indicate that chlamydial DNA is often present in the ocular secretions of patients with trachoma, even in the absence of positive cultures. Thus persistent infection may be more common than was previously thought.

The cornea becomes involved, with inflammatory leukocytic infiltrations and superficial vascularization (pannus formation). As the inflammation continues, conjunctival scarring eventually distorts the eyelids, causing them to turn inward so that the lashes constantly abrade the eyeball (trichiasis and entropion); eventually the corneal epithelium is abraded and may ulcerate, with subsequent corneal scarring and blindness. Destruction of the conjunctival goblet cells, lacrimal ducts, and lacrimal gland may produce a "dry-eye" syndrome, with resultant corneal opacity due to drying (xerosis) or secondary bacterial corneal ulcers.

Communities with blinding trachoma often experience seasonal epidemics of conjunctivitis due to *H. influenzae* that contribute to the intensity of the inflammatory process. In such areas, the active infectious process usually resolves spontaneously in affected persons at 10–15 years of age, but conjunctival scars continue to shrink, producing trichiasis and entropion with subsequent corneal scarring in adults. In areas with milder and less prevalent disease, the process may be much slower, with active disease continuing into adulthood; blindness is rare in these cases.

Eye infection with oculogenital *C. trachomatis* strains in sexually active young adults presents as an acute onset of unilateral follicular conjunctivitis and preauricular lymphadenopathy similar to that seen in acute conjunctivitis caused by adenovirus or HSV. If untreated, the disease may persist for 6 weeks to 2 years. It is frequently associated with corneal inflammation in the form of discrete opacities ("infiltrates"), punctate epithelial erosions, and minor degrees of superficial corneal vascularization. Very rarely, conjunctival scarring and eyelid distortion occur, particularly in patients treated for many months with topical glucocorticoids. Recurrent eye infections develop most often in patients whose sexual partners are not treated with antimicrobial agents.

Diagnosis

The clinical diagnosis of classic trachoma can be made if two of the following signs are present: (1) lymphoid follicles on the upper tarsal conjunctiva; (2) typical conjunctival scarring; (3) vascular pannus; or (4) limbal follicles or their sequelae, Herbert's pits. The clinical diagnosis of endemic trachoma should be confirmed by laboratory tests in children with relatively marked degrees of inflammation. Intracytoplasmic chlamydial inclusions are found in 10–60% of Giemsa-stained conjunctival smears in such populations, but chlamydial NAATs are more sensitive and are often positive when smears or cultures are negative. Follicular conjunctivitis in European or American adults living in trachomatous regions is rarely due to trachoma.

TREATMENT   Trachoma

Adult inclusion conjunctivitis responds well to treatment with the same regimens used in uncomplicated genital infections—namely, azithromycin (a 1-g single oral dose) or doxycycline (100 mg twice daily for 7 days). Simultaneous treatment of all sexual partners is necessary to prevent ocular reinfection and chlamydial genital disease. Topical antibiotic treatment is not required for patients who receive systemic antibiotics.

PSITTACOSIS

Psittacine birds and many other avian species act as natural reservoirs for *C. psittaci*–type organisms, common pathogens in domestic mammals and birds. The species *C. psittaci,* which now includes only avian strains, affects humans only as a zoonosis. (The other strains previously included in this species have been placed into different species that reflect the animals they infect: *C. abortus, C. muridarum, C. suis, C. felis,* and *C. caviae.*) Although all birds are susceptible, pet birds (parrots, parakeets, macaws, and cockatiels) and poultry (turkeys and ducks) are most frequently involved in transmission of *C. psittaci* to humans. Exposure is greatest in poultry-processing workers and in owners of pet birds. Infectious forms of the organisms are shed from both symptomatic and apparently healthy birds and may remain viable for several months. *C. psittaci* can be transmitted to humans by direct contact with infected birds or by inhalation of aerosols from avian nasal discharges and from infectious avian fecal or feather dust. Transmission from person to person has never been demonstrated.

The diagnosis is usually established serologically. Psittacosis in humans may present as acute primary atypical pneumonia (which can be fatal in up to 10% of untreated cases); as severe chronic pneumonia; or as a mild illness or asymptomatic infection in persons exposed to infected birds.

■ EPIDEMIOLOGY

Fewer than 50 confirmed cases of psittacosis are reported in the United States each year, although many more cases probably occur than are reported. Control of psittacosis depends on control of avian sources of infection. A pandemic of psittacosis was once stopped by banning shipment or importation of psittacine birds. Birds can receive prophylaxis in the form of a tetracycline-containing feed. Imported birds are currently quarantined for 30 days of treatment.

■ CLINICAL MANIFESTATIONS

Typical symptoms include fever, chills, muscular aches and pains, severe headache, hepato- and/or splenomegaly, and gastrointestinal symptoms. Cardiac complications may involve endocarditis

and myocarditis. Fatal cases were common in the preantibiotic era. As a result of quarantine of imported birds and improved veterinary-hygienic measures, outbreaks and sporadic cases of psittacosis are now rare. Severe pneumonia requiring management in an intensive care unit may develop. Endocarditis, hepatitis, and neurologic complications may occur, and fatal cases have been reported. The incubation period is usually 5–19 days but can last as long as 28 days.

■ DIAGNOSIS

Previously, the most widely used serologic test for diagnosing chlamydial infections was the genus-specific CF test, in which assay of paired serum specimens often shows fourfold or greater increases in antibody titer. The CF test remains useful, but the gold standard of serologic tests is now the MIF test, which is not widely available (see section on diagnosis of *C. trachomatis* genital infection, above). Any antibody titer above 1:16 is considered significant evidence of exposure to chlamydiae, and a fourfold titer rise in paired sera in combination with a clinically compatible syndrome can be used to diagnose psittacosis. Some commercially available serologic tests based on measurement of antibodies to LPS can be useful when the clinical diagnosis is consistent with bird exposure; however, since these tests are reactive for all chlamydiae (i.e., all chlamydiae contain LPS), caution must be used in their interpretation.

TREATMENT   Psittacosis

The antibiotic of choice is tetracycline; the dosage for adults is 250 mg four times a day, continued for at least 3 weeks to avoid relapse. Severely ill patients may need cardiovascular and respiratory support. Erythromycin (500 mg four times a day by mouth) is an alternative therapy.

CHLAMYDIA PNEUMONIAE INFECTIONS

C. pneumoniae is a common cause of human respiratory diseases, such as pneumonia and bronchitis. This organism has been reported to account for as many as 10% of cases of community-acquired pneumonia, most of which are diagnosed by serology. Serologic studies have linked *C. pneumoniae* to atherosclerosis; isolation and PCR detection in cardiovascular tissues have also been reported. These findings suggest an expanded range of diseases and syndromes for *C. pneumoniae*. The role of *C. pneumoniae* in the etiology of atherosclerosis has been discussed since 1988, when Finnish researchers presented serologic evidence of an association of this organism with coronary heart disease and acute myocardial infarction. Subsequently, the organism was identified in atherosclerotic lesions by culture, PCR, immunohistochemistry, and transmission electron microscopy; however, discrepant study results (including those of animal studies) and failure of large-scale treatment studies have raised doubts as to the etiologic role of *C. pneumoniae* in atherosclerosis. Large-scale case-cohort studies have recently demonstrated some association of *C. pneumoniae* with lung cancer, as evaluated by serology.

■ EPIDEMIOLOGY

Primary infection occurs mainly in school-aged children and reinfection in adults. Seroprevalence rates of 40–70% show that *C. pneumoniae* is widespread in both industrialized and developing countries. Seropositivity usually is first detected at school age, and rates generally increase by ~10% per decade. About 50% of individuals have detectable antibody at 30 years of age, and most have detectable antibody by the eighth decade of life. Although serologic evidence suggests that *C. pneumoniae* may be associated with up to 10% of cases of community-acquired pneumonia, most of this evidence is based not on paired serum samples but rather on a single high IgG titer. Some doubt exists about the true prevalence and etiologic role of *C. pneumoniae* in atypical pneumonia, especially since reports of cross-reactivity have raised questions about the specificity of serology when only a single serum sample is used for diagnosis.

■ PATHOGENESIS

Little is known about the pathogenesis of *C. pneumoniae* infection. It begins in the upper respiratory tract and, in many persons, persists as a prolonged asymptomatic condition of the upper respiratory mucosal surfaces. However, evidence of replication within vascular endothelium and synovial membranes of joints shows that, in at least some individuals, the organism is transported to distant sites, perhaps within macrophages. A *C. pneumoniae* outer-membrane protein may induce host immune responses whose cross-reactivity with human proteins results in an autoimmune reaction.

As mentioned above, epidemiologic studies have demonstrated an association between serologic evidence of *C. pneumoniae* infection and atherosclerotic disease of the coronary and other arteries. In addition, *C. pneumoniae* has been identified in atherosclerotic plaques by electron microscopy, DNA hybridization, and immunocytochemistry. The organism has been recovered in culture from atheromatous plaque—a result indicating the presence of viable replicating bacteria in vessels. Evidence from animal models supports the hypothesis that *C. pneumoniae* infection of the upper respiratory tract is followed by recovery of the organism from atheromatous lesions in the aorta and that the infection accelerates the process of atherosclerosis, especially in hypercholesterolemic animals. Antimicrobial treatment of the infected animals reverses the increased risk of atherosclerosis. In humans, two small trials in patients with unstable angina or recent myocardial infarction suggested that antibiotics reduce the likelihood of subsequent untoward cardiac events. However, larger-scale trials have not documented an effect of various antichlamydial regimens on the risk of these events.

■ CLINICAL MANIFESTATIONS

C. pneumoniae was first reported as the etiologic agent of mild atypical pneumonia in military recruits and college students. The clinical spectrum of *C. pneumoniae* infection includes acute pharyngitis, sinusitis, bronchitis, and pneumonitis, primarily in young adults. The clinical manifestations of primary infection appear to be more severe and prolonged than those of reinfection. The pneumonitis of *C. pneumoniae* pneumonia resembles that of *Mycoplasma* pneumonia in that leukocytosis is frequently lacking and patients often have prominent antecedent upper respiratory tract symptoms, fever, nonproductive cough, mild to moderate illness, minimal findings on chest auscultation, and small segmental infiltrates on chest x-ray. In elderly patients, pneumonia due to *C. pneumoniae* can be especially severe and may necessitate hospitalization and respiratory support.

Chronic infection with *C. pneumoniae* has been reported among patients with chronic obstructive pulmonary disease and may also play a role in the natural history of asthma, including exacerbations. The clinical symptoms of respiratory infections caused by *C. pneumoniae* are nonspecific and do not differ from those caused by other agents of atypical pneumonia, such as *Mycoplasma pneumoniae*.

■ DIAGNOSIS

Serology, PCR amplification, and culture can be used to diagnose *C. pneumoniae* infection. Serology has been the traditional method of diagnosing infection by *C. pneumoniae*. The gold standard serologic test is the MIF test (see section on diagnosis of *C. trachomatis* genital infection, above). Any antibody titer above 1:16 is considered significant evidence of exposure to chlamydiae. According to a CDC-sponsored expert working group, the diagnosis of acute *C. pneumoniae* infection requires demonstration of a fourfold rise in titer in paired serum samples. There are no official recommendations for diagnosis of chronic infections, although many research studies have used high titers of IgA as an indicator. The older CF tests and EIAs for LPS are not recommended, as they are not specific for *C. pneumoniae* but identify the chlamydiae only to the genus level. The organism is very difficult to grow in tissue culture but has been cultivated in HeLa cells, HEp-2 cells, and HL cells. Although NAATs are commercially available for *C. trachomatis*, only research-based PCR assays are available for *C. pneumoniae*.

TREATMENT   *C. pneumoniae* Infections

Although few controlled trials of treatment have been reported, *C. pneumoniae* is inhibited in vitro by erythromycin, tetracycline, azithromycin, clarithromycin, gatifloxacin, and gemifloxacin. Recommended therapy consists of 2 g/d of either tetracycline or erythromycin for 10–14 days. Other macrolides (e.g., azithromycin) and some fluoroquinolones (e.g., levofloxacin and gatifloxacin) also appear to be effective.

ACKNOWLEDGMENT
The authors wish to acknowledge the late Walter E. Stamm, MD, for his significant contributions to the field of Chlamydia research. Dr. Stamm wrote the chapters on chlamydiae for previous editions of Harrison's Principles of Internal Medicine, and we thank the editors for permission to reproduce Figs. 176-1 and 176-2 as well as Table 176-1 from his chapter in the 17th edition. Dr. Stamm died on December 14, 2009, and this chapter is dedicated to him.

FURTHER READINGS

ASSOCIATION OF PUBLIC HEALTH LABORATORIES: *Guidelines for the Laboratory Testing of STDs, 2009.* Silver Spring, MD, Association of Public Health Laboratories, 2009 (*www.aphl.org/aphlprograms/infectious/std/Pages/stdtestingguidelines.aspx*)

BAVOIL PM, WYRICK PB: *Chlamydia: Genomics and Pathogenesis.* Norfolk, UK, Horizon Bioscience, 2006, 542 pp

CAMPBELL LA et al: Chlamydial infections, in *Manual of Molecular and Clinical Laboratory Immunology*, 7th ed, B Detrick et al (eds). Washington, DC, ASM Press, 2006, pp 518–525

CENTERS FOR DISEASE CONTROL AND PREVENTION: *Sexually Transmitted Disease Surveillance, 2009.* Atlanta, U.S. Department of Health and Human Services, 2010 (*www.cdc.gov/std/stats09/default.htm*)

——— : Sexually transmitted diseases treatment guidelines, 2010. MMWR Recomm Rep 59(RR-12):1–110, 2010

GAYDOS CA: Chlamydiae, in *Clinical Virology Manual*, 4th ed, S Spector et al (eds). Washington, DC, ASM Press, 2009, pp 630–640

Kuypers J et al: Principles of laboratory diagnosis of STIs, in *Sexually Transmitted Diseases*, 4th ed, KK Holmes et al (eds). New York, McGraw-Hill, 2008, pp 937–948

Schachter J, Stephens RS: Biology of *Chlamydia trachomatis*, in *Sexually Transmitted Diseases*, 4th ed, KK Holmes et al (eds). New York, McGraw-Hill, 2008, pp 555–574

Scholes D et al: Prevention of pelvic inflammatory disease by screening for cervical chlamydial infection. N Engl J Med 334:1362, 1996

Taylor HR: *Trachoma: A Blinding Scourge from the Bronze Age to the Twenty-First Century*. East Melbourne, Victoria, Australia, Centre for Eye Research Australia/Haddington Press, 2008, 282 pp

CHAPTER **177**

Medical Virology

Fred Wang

Elliott Kieff

DEFINING A VIRUS

Viruses consist of a nucleic acid surrounded by one or more proteins. Some viruses also have an outer-membrane envelope. Viruses are obligate intracellular parasites: they can replicate only within cells since their nucleic acids do not encode the many enzymes necessary for protein, carbohydrate, or lipid metabolism and for the generation of high-energy phosphates. Typically, viral nucleic acids encode proteins necessary for replicating and packaging the nucleic acids within the biochemical milieu of host cells.

Viruses differ from virusoids, viroids, and prions. *Virusoids* are nucleic acids that depend on helper viruses to package their nucleic acids into virus-like particles. *Viroids* are naked, cyclical, mostly double-strand, small RNAs that appear to be restricted to plants, spread from cell to cell, and are replicated by cellular RNA polymerase II. *Prions* (Chap. 383) are abnormal protein molecules that can spread, reproducing by changing the structure of their normal cellular protein counterparts. Prions have been implicated in neurodegenerative conditions such as Creutzfeldt-Jakob disease, Gerstmann-Sträussler disease, kuru, and human bovine spongiform encephalopathy ("mad cow disease").

VIRAL STRUCTURE

Viral genomes consist of (1) a single-strand or double-strand DNA, (2) a single-strand sense RNA, (3) a single-strand or segmented antisense RNA, or (4) a double-strand segmented RNA genome. The viral nucleic acid may encode only a few genes or more than 100. Sense-strand RNA genomes can be translated directly into protein, whereas antisense RNAs must be copied into translatable RNA. Sense and antisense genomes are also referred to as *positive-strand* and *negative-strand genomes*, respectively. Viral nucleic acid is usually associated with one or more virus-encoded nucleoproteins in the core of the viral particle. The viral nucleic acid and nucleoproteins are almost always enclosed in a protein shell called a *capsid*. Because of the limited genetic complexity of viruses, their capsids are usually composed of multimers of identical capsomeres. Capsomeres are in turn composed of one or a few proteins. Capsids have icosahedral or helical symmetry. Icosahedral structures approximate spheres but have two-, three-, and fivefold axes of symmetry, while helical structures have only a twofold axis of symmetry. The entire structural unit of nucleic acid, nucleoprotein(s), and capsid is called a *nucleocapsid*.

Many human viruses are composed simply of a core and a capsid. For these viruses, the outer surface of the capsid mediates contact with uninfected cells. Other viruses are more complex and have an outer lipid-containing envelope derived from virus-modified membranes of the infected cell. The piece of infected-cell membrane that becomes the viral envelope has usually been modified

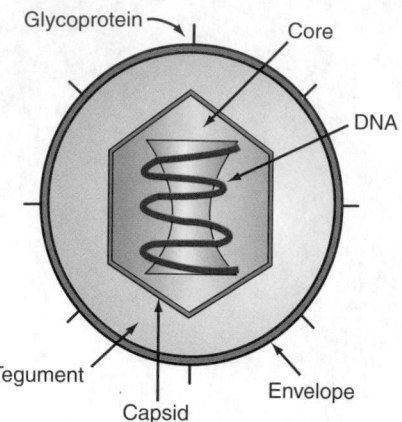

Figure 177-1 **Schematic diagram of an enveloped herpesvirus with an icosahedral nucleocapsid.** The approximate respective dimensions of the nucleocapsid and the enveloped particles are 110 and 180 nm. The capsid is composed of 162 capsomeres: 150 with sixfold and 12 with fivefold axes of symmetry.

during infection by the insertion of virus-encoded glycoproteins, which mediate contact of enveloped viruses with uninfected cells. Matrix or tegument proteins fill the space between the nucleocapsid and the envelope in many enveloped viruses. In general, enveloped viruses are sensitive to lipid solvents and nonionic detergents that can dissolve the envelope, while viruses that consist only of nucleocapsids are somewhat resistant. A schematic diagram for large and complex herpesviruses is shown in Fig. 177-1. Prototypical pathogenic human viruses are listed in Table 177-1. The relative sizes and structures of typical pathogenic human viruses are shown in Fig. 177-2.

TAXONOMY OF PATHOGENIC HUMAN VIRUSES

As is apparent from Table 177-1 and Fig. 177-2, the classification of viruses into orders and families is based on nucleic acid composition, nucleocapsid size and symmetry, and presence or absence of an envelope. Viruses of a single family have similar types of genomes and are often morphologically indistinguishable in electron micrographs. Further subclassification into genera depends on similarities in epidemiology, biologic effects, and nucleic acid sequence.

Most human viruses have a common name related to their pathologic effects or the circumstances of their discovery. Formal species names have been assigned by the International Committee on Taxonomy of Viruses. The formal designation consists of the name of the host followed by the family or genus of the virus and a number. This dual terminology can cause confusion when viruses are referred to and referenced by either name—e.g., varicella-zoster virus (VZV) or human herpesvirus (HHV) 3.

VIRAL INFECTION IN VITRO

■ STAGES OF VIRAL INFECTION AT THE CELLULAR LEVEL

Viral interactions with the cell surface and cell entry

All viruses must overcome the barrier posed by the cell's plasma membrane in order to deliver their payload of nucleic acid into the

TABLE 177-1 Virus Families Pathogenic for Humans

Family	Representative Viruses	Type of RNA/DNA	Lipid Envelope
RNA Viruses			
Picornaviridae	Poliovirus Coxsackievirus Echovirus Enterovirus Rhinovirus Hepatitis A virus	(+) RNA	No
Caliciviridae	Norwalk agent Hepatitis E virus	(+) RNA	No
Togaviridae	Rubella virus Eastern equine encephalitis virus Western equine encephalitis virus	(+) RNA	Yes
Flaviviridae	Yellow fever virus Dengue virus St. Louis encephalitis virus West Nile virus Hepatitis C virus Hepatitis G virus	(+) RNA	Yes
Coronaviridae	Coronaviruses[a]	(+) RNA	Yes
Rhabdoviridae	Rabies virus Vesicular stomatitis virus	(−) RNA	Yes
Filoviridae	Marburg virus Ebola virus	(−) RNA	Yes
Paramyxoviridae	Parainfluenza virus Respiratory syncytial virus Newcastle disease virus Mumps virus Rubeola (measles) virus	(−) RNA	Yes
Orthomyxoviridae	Influenza A, B, and C viruses	(−) RNA, 8 segments	Yes
Bunyaviridae	Hantavirus California encephalitis virus Sandfly fever virus	(−) RNA, 3 circular segments	Yes
Arenaviridae	Lymphocytic choriomeningitis virus Lassa fever virus South American hemorrhagic fever virus	(−) RNA, 2 circular segments	Yes
Reoviridae	Rotavirus Reovirus Colorado tick fever virus	ds RNA, 10–12 segments	No
Retroviridae	Human T lymphotropic virus types I and II Human immunodeficiency virus types 1 and 2	(+) RNA, 2 identical segments	Yes
DNA Viruses			
Hepadnaviridae	Hepatitis B virus	ds DNA with ss portions	Yes
Parvoviridae	Parvovirus B19	ss DNA	No
Papovaviridae	Human papillomaviruses JC virus BK virus	ds DNA	No
Adenoviridae	Human adenoviruses	ds DNA	No

(*continued*)

TABLE 177-1 Virus Families Pathogenic for Humans (*Continued*)

Family	Representative Viruses	Type of RNA/DNA	Lipid Envelope
Herpesviridae	Herpes simplex virus types 1 and 2[b] Varicella-zoster virus[c] Epstein-Barr virus[d] Cytomegalovirus[e] Human herpesvirus 6 Human herpesvirus 7 Kaposi's sarcoma–associated herpesvirus[f]	ds DNA	Yes
Poxviridae	Variola (smallpox) virus Orf virus Molluscum contagiosum virus	ds DNA	Yes

[a]Including the coronavirus causing severe acute respiratory syndrome (SARS).

[b]Also called human herpesvirus (HHV) 1 and 2, respectively.

[c]Also called HHV-3.

[d]Also called HHV-4.

[e]Also called HHV-5.

[f]Also called HHV-8.

Abbreviations: ds, double-strand; ss, single-strand.

Positive-strand RNA viruses

	Picornaviridae	Caliciviridae	Togaviridae	Flaviviridae	Coronaviridae
Genome size (kb)	7.2-8.4	8	12	10	16-21
Envelope	No	No	Yes	Yes	Yes
Capsid symmetry	Icosahedral	Icosahedral	Icosahedral	Icosahedral	Helical

Negative-strand RNA viruses

	Rhabdoviridae	Filoviridae	Paramyxoviridae
Genome size (kb)	13-16	13	16-20
Envelope	Yes	Yes	Yes
Capsid symmetry	Helical	Helical	Helical

Segmented negative-strand RNA viruses   **Segmented double-strand RNA viruses**

	Orthomyxoviridae	Bunyaviridae	Arenaviridae	Reoviridae
Genome size (kb)	14	13-21	10-14	16-27
Envelope	Yes	Yes	Yes	No
Capsid symmetry	Helical	Helical	Helical	Icosahedral

Retroviruses

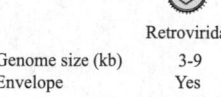

	Retroviridae
Genome size (kb)	3-9
Envelope	Yes
Capsid symmetry	Icosahedral

DNA viruses

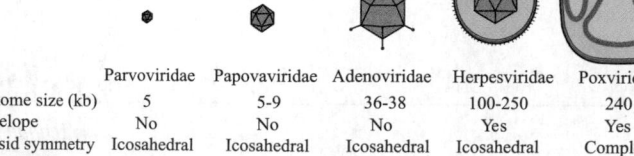

	Parvoviridae	Papovaviridae	Adenoviridae	Herpesviridae	Poxviridae
Genome size (kb)	5	5-9	36-38	100-250	240
Envelope	No	No	No	Yes	Yes
Capsid symmetry	Icosahedral	Icosahedral	Icosahedral	Icosahedral	Complex

├──────┤
100 nm

Figure 177-2   Schematic diagrams of the major virus families including species that infect humans. The viruses are grouped by genome type and are drawn approximately to scale. Prototype viruses of each family that cause human disease are listed in Table 177-1.

cell. Infection is initiated by attachment of the virus to the cell surface. Various cellular proteins, carbohydrates, and lipids (e.g., heparan sulfate proteoglycans, sialic acids, and lectins) can act as attachment factors that concentrate viruses at the cell surface through relatively weak or nonspecific interactions with viral surface proteins. Higher-affinity binding of viral surface proteins to specific cell-surface proteins, or receptors (see Table 120-1), is more critical for viral infection. Receptor binding is often augmented by interaction of viral surface proteins with other cell-surface proteins, or co-receptors, important for various aspects of virus entry. Receptors and co-receptors are important determinants of the cell types and species that a virus can infect. For example, the HIV envelope glycoprotein binds to the T cell surface protein CD4 and then engages one of several chemokine receptors that are co-receptors for the virus. Epstein-Barr virus (EBV) glycoprotein gp350 binds to the B lymphocyte complement receptor CD21 and then uses major histocompatibility complex (MHC) class II molecules as a co-receptor.

Viruses use different strategies to penetrate the cell membrane. Some enveloped viruses use membrane fusion to deliver their contents into the cytoplasm. In general, a trigger (e.g., receptor binding) induces a conformational change that allows the viral surface protein to extend into the cell membrane, bringing the virus and cell membrane into close proximity and thereby enabling fusion and formation of a pore through which the viral nucleocapsid can be delivered into the cytoplasm. Nonenveloped viruses and some enveloped viruses cannot use direct membrane fusion at the plasma membrane and are internalized by endocytosis. The low pH in endosomes can trigger viral membrane or capsid fusion with the endocytic membrane. Conformational changes in nonenveloped capsids can lead to endosomal membrane penetration and release of viral nucleic acid into the cytoplasm.

Influenza virus provides a well-studied example of the effect of low pH on viral penetration. Influenza hemagglutinin mediates adsorption, receptor aggregation, and endocytosis. In low-pH endosomes, changes in conformation of the hemagglutinin expose amphipathic domains that interact chemically with the cell membrane and initiate fusion of the virus and cell membranes. For influenza virus, the M2 membrane protein plays a key role in the uncoating of the viral envelope by providing an ion channel in the envelope.

The fusion of viral proteins with cell membranes is a crucial step in viral infection. The hydrophobic interactions required for fusion can be susceptible to chemical inhibition or blockade. The HIV envelope glycoprotein gp120 is associated with gp41 on the viral surface. Binding of HIV gp120 to CD4 and chemokine receptors results in a conformational change, allowing gp41 to initiate cell membrane fusion. Enfuvirtide is a small-peptide drug derived from gp41 that binds to gp41 and prevents the conformational change required for fusion. Maraviroc prevents virus entry by binding to CCR5, blocking interaction with gp120, and preventing fusion triggering.

Viral gene expression and replication

After uncoating and release of viral nucleoprotein into the cytoplasm, the viral genome is transported to a site for expression and replication. In order to produce infectious progeny, viruses must (1) produce proteins necessary to replicate their nucleic acid, (2) produce structural proteins, and (3) assemble the nucleic acid and proteins into progeny virions. Different viruses use different strategies and gene repertoires to accomplish these goals. DNA viruses, except for poxviruses, replicate their nucleic acid and assemble into nucleocapsid complexes in the cell nucleus. RNA viruses, except for influenza viruses, transcribe and replicate their nucleic acid and assemble entirely in the cytoplasm. Thus, the replication strategies of DNA and RNA viruses are presented separately below. Positive-strand and negative-strand RNA viruses are discussed separately. Medically important viruses of each group are used for illustrative purposes.

Positive-strand RNA viruses Medically important positive-strand RNA viruses include picornaviruses, flaviviruses, togaviruses, caliciviruses, and coronaviruses. Genomic RNA from positive-strand RNA viruses is released into the cytoplasm without associated enzymes. Cell ribosomes recognize and associate with an internal ribosome entry sequence in the viral RNA and translate a polyprotein. Protease components of the polyprotein cleave out the viral RNA polymerase and other viral proteins necessary for replication. Antigenomic RNA is then transcribed from the genomic RNA template. Positive-strand genomes and mRNAs are next transcribed from the antigenomic RNA by the viral RNA polymerase and are translated into capsid proteins. Genomic RNA is encapsidated in the cytoplasm as the infected cell undergoes lysis.

Negative-strand RNA viruses Medically important negative-strand RNA viruses include rhabdoviruses, filoviruses, paramyxoviruses, orthomyxoviruses, and bunyaviruses. The genomes of negative-strand viruses are frequently segmented. Negative-strand RNA virus genomes are released into the cytoplasm with an associated RNA polymerase and one or more polymerase accessory proteins. The viral RNA polymerase transcribes messenger RNAs (mRNAs) as well as full-length antigenomic RNA, which is the template for genomic RNA replication. Viral mRNAs encode the viral RNA polymerase and accessory factors as well as viral structural proteins. Except for influenza virus, which transcribes its mRNAs and antigenomic RNAs in the cell's nucleus, negative-strand RNA viruses replicate entirely in the cytoplasm. All negative-strand RNA viruses, including influenza viruses, assemble in the cytoplasm.

Double-strand segmented RNA viruses Double-strand RNA viruses are taxonomically grouped in the family Reoviridae. The medically important viruses in this group are rotaviruses and Colorado tick fever virus. Reovirus genomes have 10–12 RNA segments. Reovirus particles contain an RNA polymerase complex. These viruses replicate and assemble in the cytoplasm.

DNA viruses Medically important DNA viruses include parvoviruses, papovaviruses [e.g., human papillomaviruses (HPVs) and polyomaviruses], adenoviruses, herpesviruses, and poxviruses. Most DNA virus genomes enter the cell's nucleus and are transcribed by cellular RNA polymerase II. For example, after receptor binding and fusion with plasma membranes or endocytic vesicle membranes, herpesvirus nucleocapsids are released into the cytoplasm along with tegument proteins. The nucleocapsid is transported along microtubules to a nuclear pore. Capsids then release DNA into the nucleus.

DNA virus transcription and mRNA processing depend on both viral and cellular proteins. For herpes simplex virus (HSV), a viral tegument protein enters the nucleus and activates immediate-early genes, the first genes expressed after infection. Transcription of immediate-early genes requires the viral tegument protein and cell transcription factors. HSV becomes nonreplicating, or latent, in neurons because essential cell transcription factors for viral immediate-early gene expression are docked in the cytoplasm in neurons. Heat shock or other cell stresses can cause these cell factors to enter the nucleus, activate viral gene expression, and initiate replication. This information explains HSV-1 latency in neurons and activation of lytic infection.

For adenoviruses and herpesviruses, immediate-early gene transcription results in expression of early proteins necessary for viral DNA replication. Viral DNA synthesis is required to turn on late gene expression and production of viral structural components. The HPVs, polyomaviruses, and parvoviruses are not dependent on transactivators encoded from the viral genome for early-gene transcription. Instead, their early genes have upstream enhancing elements that bind cell transcription factors. The early genes encode proteins that are necessary for viral DNA synthesis and late-gene transcription. DNA virus late genes encode structural proteins necessary for viral assembly and for viral egress from the infected cell. Late-gene transcription is continuously dependent on DNA replication. Therefore, inhibitors of DNA replication also stop late-gene transcription.

Each DNA virus family uses unique mechanisms for replicating its DNA. Adenovirus and herpesvirus DNAs are linear in the virion. Adenovirus DNA remains linear in infected cells and replicates as a linear genome, using an initiator protein-DNA complex. In contrast, herpesvirus DNA circularizes in the infected cell, and genomes replicate into linear concatemers through a "rolling-circle" mechanism. Full-length DNA genomes are cleaved and packaged into virus. Herpesviruses encode a DNA polymerase and at least six other viral proteins necessary for viral DNA replication. These viruses also encode enzymes that increase the deoxynucleotide triphosphate pools. HPV and polyomavirus DNAs are circular both within the virus and in infected cells. These genomes are reproduced by cellular DNA replication enzymes and remain circular through replication and packaging. HPV and polyomavirus early proteins are necessary for latent and lytic viral DNA replication. Early viral proteins stimulate cells to remain in cycle, facilitating viral DNA replication.

Parvoviruses have negative single-strand DNA genomes and are the smallest DNA viruses. Their genomes are half the size of the papovavirus genomes and include only two genes. The replication of autonomous parvoviruses, such as B19, depends on cellular DNA replication and requires the virus-encoded Rep protein. Other parvoviruses, such as adeno-associated virus (AAV), are not autonomous and require helper viruses of the adenovirus or herpesvirus family for their replication. AAV is being used as a potentially safe human gene therapy vector because its replication protein causes integration at a single chromosome site. The small genome size limits the range of proteins that can be expressed from AAV vectors.

Poxviruses are the largest DNA viruses. They are unique among DNA viruses in replicating and assembling in the cytoplasm. To accomplish cytoplasmic replication, poxviruses encode transcription factors, an RNA polymerase II orthologue, enzymes for RNA capping, enzymes for RNA polyadenylation, and enzymes for viral DNA synthesis. Poxvirus DNA also has a unique structure. The double-strand linear DNA is covalently linked at the ends; the packaged genome is therefore a covalently closed single-strand circle. In addition, there are inverted repeats at the ends of the linear DNA. During DNA replication, the genome is cleaved within the terminal inverted repeat, and the inverted repeats self-prime complementary-strand synthesis by the virus-encoded DNA polymerase. Like herpesviruses, poxviruses encode several enzymes that increase deoxynucleotide triphosphate precursor levels and thus facilitate viral DNA synthesis.

Viruses that use both RNA and DNA genomes in their life cycle
Retroviruses, including HIV, are RNA viruses that use a DNA intermediate to replicate their genomes; hepatitis B virus (HBV) is a DNA virus that uses an RNA intermediate to replicate its genome. Thus these viruses are not purely RNA or DNA viruses. Retroviruses are enveloped RNA viruses with two identical sense-strand genomes and associated reverse transcriptase and integrase enzymes. Retroviruses differ from all other viruses in that they reverse-transcribe themselves into partially duplicated double-strand DNA copies and then routinely integrate into the host genome as part of their replication strategy. The fact that remnants and even complete copies of simple retroviral DNA are integrated into the human genome raises the possibility of replication-competent simple human retroviruses. However, replication has not been documented or associated with any disease. Integrated, replication-competent retroviral DNAs are also present in many animal species, such as pigs. These porcine retroviruses are a potential cause for concern in xenotransplantation because retroviral replication could cause disease in humans.

Cellular RNA polymerase II and transcription factors regulate transcription from the integrated provirus DNA genome. Some retroviruses also encode for regulators of transcription and RNA processing, such as Tax and Rex in human T lymphotropic virus (HTLV) types I and II. HIV-1 and HIV-2 have orthologous Tat and Rev genes as well as the additional accessory proteins Vpr, Vpu, and Vif, which are important for efficient infection and immune escape. Full-length proviral transcripts are made from a promoter in the viral terminal repeat and serve as both genomic RNAs that will be packaged in the nucleocapsids and differentially spliced mRNAs that encode for the viral Gag protein, polymerase/integrase protein, and envelope glycoprotein. The Gag protein includes a protease that cleaves it into several components, including a viral matrix protein that coats the viral RNA. Viral RNA polymerase/integrase, matrix protein, and cellular tRNA are key components of the viral nucleocapsid. The HIV reverse transcriptase, integrase, and Gag protease are important targets for inhibition of HIV replication.

HBV replication is unique in several respects. HBV has a partially double-strand DNA genome that is repaired to a fully double-strand circular DNA by the virion polymerase upon entry into an infected cell. Viral mRNAs are transcribed from the closed circular viral episome by cellular RNA polymerase II and are translated to produce viral proteins including core protein, surface antigen, and polymerase. In addition, a full-genome-length mRNA is packaged

into viral core particles in the cytoplasm of infected cells as an intermediate for viral DNA replication. This RNA associates with the viral polymerase, which also has reverse transcriptase activity, to convert the full-length encapsidated RNA genome into partially double-strand DNA. HBV is believed to mature by budding through the cell's plasma membrane, which has been modified by the insertion of viral surface antigen protein.

Viral assembly and egress
For most viruses, nucleic acid and structural protein synthesis is accompanied by the assembly of protein and nucleic acid complexes. The assembly and egress of mature infectious virus mark the end of the eclipse phase of infection, during which infectious virus cannot be recovered from the infected cell. Nucleic acids from RNA viruses and poxviruses assemble into nucleocapsids in the cytoplasm. For all DNA viruses except poxviruses, viral DNA assembles into nucleocapsids in the nucleus. In general, the capsid proteins of viruses with icosahedral nucleocapsids can self-assemble into densely packed and highly ordered capsid structures. Herpesviruses require an assemblin protein as a scaffold for capsid assembly. Viral nucleic acid then spools into the assembled capsid. For herpesviruses, a full unit of the viral DNA genome is packaged into the capsid, and a capsid-associated nuclease cleaves the viral DNA at both ends. In the case of viruses with helical nucleocapsids, the protein component appears to assemble around the nucleic acid, which contributes to capsid organization.

Viruses must egress from the infected cell and not bind back to their receptor(s) on the outer surface of the plasma membrane. Viruses can acquire envelopes from cytoplasmic membranes or by budding through the cell's plasma membrane. Excess viral membrane glycoproteins are synthesized to saturate cell receptors and facilitate separation of the virus from the infected cell. Some viruses encode membrane proteins with enzymatic activity for receptor destruction. Influenza virus, for example, encodes a glycoprotein with neuraminidase activity. Neuraminidase destroys sialic acid on the infected cell's plasma membrane so that newly released virus does not get stuck to the dying cell. Herpesvirus nucleocapsids acquire an initial envelope by assembling in the nucleus and then budding through the nuclear membrane into the endoplasmic reticular space. The initially enveloped herpesvirus is then de-enveloped and released from the cell either by exocytosis or by re-envelopment at the plasma membrane. Nonenveloped viruses depend on the death and dissolution of the infected cell for their release.

■ FIDELITY OF VIRAL REPLICATION
Hundreds or thousands of progeny may be produced from a single virus-infected cell. Many particles partially assemble and never mature into virions. Many mature-appearing virions are imperfect and have only incomplete or nonfunctional genomes. Despite the inefficiency of assembly, a typical virus-infected cell releases 10–1000 infectious progeny. Some of these progeny may contain genomes that differ from those of the virus that infected the cell. Smaller, "defective" viral genomes have been noted with the replication of many RNA and DNA viruses. Virions with defective genomes can be produced in large numbers through packaging of incompletely synthesized nucleic acid. Adenovirus packaging is notoriously inefficient, and a high ratio of particle to infectious virus may limit the amount of recombinant adenovirus that can be administered for gene therapy since the immunogenicity of defective particles may contribute to adverse effects.

Changes in viral genomes can lead to mutant viruses of medical significance. In general, viral nucleic acid replication is more error-prone than cellular nucleic acid replication. RNA polymerases and reverse transcriptases are significantly more error-prone than

DNA polymerases. Mutations can also be introduced into the HIV genome by APOBEC3G, a cellular protein that is packaged in the virion. APOBEC3G deaminates cytidine in the virion RNA to uridine. When reverse transcriptase subsequently uses the altered virion RNA as a template in the infected cell, a guanosine-to-adenosine mutation is introduced into the proviral DNA. Mutations resulting in less efficient viral growth, or fitness, may be detrimental to the virus. HIV-encoded Vif blocks APOBEC3G activity in the virion, inhibiting the debilitating effects of hypermutation on genetic integrity. Nevertheless, mutations resulting in evasion of the host immune response or resistance to antiviral drugs are preferentially selected in patients, with the consequent perpetuation of infection. Viral genomes can also be altered by recombination or reassortment between two related viruses in a single infected cell. While this occurrence is unusual under most circumstances of natural infection, the genome changes can be substantial and can significantly alter virulence or epidemiology. Reassortment of the avian or mammalian influenza A hemagglutinin gene into a human influenza background can result in the emergence of new epidemic or pandemic influenza A strains.

VIRAL GENES NOT REQUIRED FOR VIRAL REPLICATION

Viruses frequently have genes encoding proteins that are not directly involved in replication or packaging of the viral nucleic acid, in virion assembly, or in regulation of the transcription of viral genes involved in those processes. Most of these proteins fall into five classes: (1) proteins that directly or indirectly alter cell growth; (2) proteins that inhibit cellular RNA or protein synthesis so that viral mRNA can be efficiently transcribed or translated; (3) proteins that promote cell survival or inhibit apoptosis so that progeny virus can mature and escape from the infected cell; (4) proteins that inhibit the host interferon response; and (5) proteins that downregulate host inflammatory or immune responses so that viral infection can proceed in an infected person to the extent consistent with the survival of the virus and its efficient transmission to a new host. More complex viruses of the poxvirus or herpesvirus family encode many proteins that serve these functions. Some of these viral proteins have motifs similar to those of cellular proteins, while others are quite novel. Virology has increasingly focused on these more sophisticated strategies evolved by viruses to permit the establishment of long-term infection in humans and other animals. These strategies often provide unique insights into the control of cell growth, cell survival, macromolecular synthesis, proteolytic processing, immune or inflammatory suppression, immune resistance, cytokine mimicry, or cytokine blockade.

MicroRNAs (miRNAs) are small noncoding RNAs that can regulate gene expression at the posttranscriptional level by targeting—and usually silencing—mRNAs. MiRNAs were initially discovered in plants and plant viruses, where they alter expression of cell defensins. Herpesviruses are especially rich in miRNAs; for example, at least 23 miRNAs have been identified in EBV and 11 in cytomegalovirus (CMV). Adenovirus and polyomavirus miRNAs have also been described. Increasing data indicate that animal viruses encode miRNAs to alter the growth and survival of host cells and the innate and acquired immune responses.

HOST RANGE

The concept of host range was originally based on the cell types in which a virus replicates in tissue culture. For the most part, the host range is limited by specific cell-surface proteins required for viral adsorption or penetration—i.e., to the cell types that express receptors or co-receptors for a specific virus. Another common basis for host-range limitation is the degree of transcriptional activity from viral promoters in different cell types. Most DNA viruses depend not only on cellular RNA polymerase II and the basal components of the cellular transcription complex but also on activated components and transcriptional accessory factors, both of which differ among differentiated tissues, among cells at various phases of the cell cycle, and between resting and cycling cells. APOBEC3G, an important cell restriction factor for HIV infection, hypermutates viral RNA. The balance between HIV Vif and APOBEC3G is an important determinant of HIV-1 infection.

The importance of host range factors is illustrated by the effects of specific host determinants that limit the replication of influenza virus with avian or porcine hemagglutinins in humans. These viral proteins have adapted to bind avian or porcine sialic acids, and spread of avian or porcine influenza viruses in human populations is limited by their ability to infect human cells.

VIRAL CYTOPATHIC EFFECTS AND INHIBITORS OF APOPTOSIS

The replication of almost all viruses has adverse effects on the infected cell, inhibiting cellular synthesis of DNA, RNA, or proteins through efficient competition for key substrates and enzymatic processes. These general inhibitory effects enable viruses to nonspecifically limit components of innate host resistance, such as interferon (IFN) production. Viruses can specifically inhibit host protein synthesis by attacking a component of the translational initiation complex—frequently, a component that is not required for efficient translation of viral RNAs. Poliovirus protease 2A, for example, cleaves a cellular component of the complex that ordinarily facilitates translation of cellular mRNAs by interacting with their cap structure. Poliovirus RNA is efficiently translated without a cap since it has an internal ribosome entry sequence. Influenza virus inhibits the processing of mRNA by snatching cap structures from nascent cellular RNAs and using them as primers in the synthesis of viral mRNA. HSV has a virion tegument protein that inhibits cellular mRNA translation.

Apoptosis is the expected consequence of virus-induced inhibition of cellular macromolecular synthesis and viral nucleic acid replication. While the induction of apoptosis may be important for the release of some viruses (particularly nonenveloped viruses), many viruses have acquired genes or parts of genes that enable them to forestall infected-cell death. This delay increases the yield from viral replication. Adenoviruses and herpesviruses encode analogues of the cellular Bc12 protein, which blocks mitochondrial enhancement of proapoptotic stimuli. Poxviruses and some herpesviruses also encode caspase inhibitors. Many viruses, including HPVs and adenoviruses, encode proteins that inhibit p53 or its downstream proapoptotic effects.

VIRAL INFECTION IN VIVO

TRANSMISSION

The capsid and envelope of a virus protect the genome and enable efficient transmission of the virus from cell to cell and to new prospective hosts. Most common viral infections are spread by direct contact, by ingestion of contaminated water or food, or by inhalation of aerosolized particles. In all these situations, infection begins on an epithelial or mucosal surface and spreads along the mucosa and into deeper tissues. Infection may spread to cells that can enter blood vessels, lymphatics, or neural circuits. HBV, hepatitis C virus (HCV), HTLV, and HIV are dependent on transmission by parenteral inoculation. Insect vectors can mediate parenteral transfer of viruses that reach high titers in animal or human hosts.

Some viruses are transmitted only between humans. The dependence of smallpox and poliovirus infections on interhuman transmission makes it feasible to eliminate these viruses from human circulation by mass vaccination. Herpesviruses also survive by interhuman transmission but may be more difficult to eliminate because they establish persistent latent infection in humans and continuously reactivate to infect new and naïve generations.

Animals are also important reservoirs and vectors for transmission of viruses causing human disease. Arboviruses are parenterally transmitted from mammalian species to humans by mosquito vectors. Herpes B, monkeypox, rabies, and viral hemorrhagic fevers are other examples of zoonotic infections caused by direct contact with animals, animal tissues, or arthropod vectors.

■ PRIMARY INFECTION

Initial viral infections usually last for several days or weeks. During this period, the concentration of virus at sites of infection rises and then falls, usually to unmeasurable levels. The rise and fall of viral replication at a given site depend on local innate immune responses and the access of systemic antibody and cell immune effectors to the virus. Typically, primary infections with enteroviruses, mumps virus, measles virus, rubella virus, rotavirus, influenza virus, AAV, adenovirus, HSV, and VZV are cleared from almost all sites within 3–4 weeks. Some viruses are especially proficient in altering or evading innate and acquired immune responses. Primary infection with AAV, EBV, or CMV can last for several months. Characteristically, primary infections due to HBV, HCV, hepatitis D virus (HDV), HIV, HPV, and molluscum contagiosum virus (MCV) extend beyond several weeks. For some of these viruses (e.g., HPV, HBV, HCV, HDV, and MCV), the manifestations of primary infection are almost indistinguishable from the persistent phase.

Disease manifestations usually arise as a consequence of viral replication, infected cell injury or death, and local inflammatory and innate immune responses. Disease severity may not necessarily correlate with the level of viral replication alone. For example, the clinical manifestations of intense primary infection with poliovirus, enterovirus, rabies virus, measles virus, mumps virus, or HSV at mucosal surfaces may be inapparent or relatively mild, whereas limited replication in neural cells can have dramatic consequences. Similarly, rubella virus or CMV infections in utero or neonatal HSV infections may have much more devastating effects than infections in adults.

Primary infections are cleared by nonspecific innate and specific adaptive immune responses. Thereafter, an immunocompetent host is usually immune to the disease manifestations of reinfection by the same virus. Immunity frequently does not prevent transient surface colonization on re-exposure, persistent colonization, or even limited deeper infection.

■ PERSISTENT AND LATENT INFECTIONS

Relatively few viruses cause persistent or latent infections. HBV, HCV, rabies virus, measles virus, HIV, HTLV, HPV, HHVs, and MCV are notable exceptions. The mechanisms for persistent infection vary. HCV RNA polymerase and HIV reverse transcriptase are error prone and generate variant genomes. Genome variation can be sufficient to permit evasion of host immune responses, thereby allowing persistent infection. HIV is also directly immunosuppressive, depleting CD4+ T lymphocytes and compromising CD8+ cytotoxic T cell immune responsiveness. Moreover, HIV encodes the Nef protein, which downmodulates MHC class I expression, rendering HIV-infected cells partially resistant to immune CD8+ T cell lysis.

DNA viruses have low mutation rates. Their persistence in human populations usually depends on their ability to establish latent infection in some cells, to reactivate from latency, and then to replicate at epithelial surfaces. *Latency* is defined as a state of infection in which virus is not replicating, viral genes associated with lytic infection are not expressed, and infectious virus is not made. The complete viral genome is present and may be replicated by cellular DNA polymerase in conjunction with replication of the cell's genome. HPVs establish latent infection in basal epithelial cells. The latently infected basal cell replicates, along with the HPV episome, by using cellular DNA polymerase. Some of the progeny cells provide new latently infected basal cells, while others go on to squamous differentiation. Infected cells that differentiate to squamous cells become permissive for lytic viral infection. Herpesviruses establish latent infection in nonreplicating neural cells (HSV and VZV) or in replicating cells of hematopoietic lineages [EBV, CMV, HHV-6, HHV-7, and Kaposi's sarcoma–associated herpesvirus (KSHV, also known as HHV-8)]. In their latent stage, HPV and herpesvirus genomes are largely hidden from the normal immune response. Reactivated HPV and herpesvirus infections escape immediate and effective immune responses in highly immune hosts by inhibiting host innate immune and inflammatory responses. In addition, HPV, HSV, and VZV are somewhat protected because they replicate in the middle and upper layers of the squamous epithelium—sites not routinely visited by cells that mediate or amplify immune and inflammatory responses. HSV and CMV are also known to encode proteins that downregulate MHC class I expression and antigenic peptide presentation, enabling infected cells to escape recognition by and cytotoxic effects of CD8+ T lymphocytes.

Like other poxviruses, MCV cannot establish latent infection. This virus causes persistent infection in hypertrophic skin lesions that last for months or years. MCV encodes a chemokine homologue that probably blocks inflammatory responses, an MHC class I analogue that blocks cytotoxic T lymphocyte attack, and inhibitors of cell death that prolong infected cell viability.

■ PERSISTENT VIRAL INFECTIONS AND CANCER

Persistent viral infection is estimated to be the root cause of as many as 20% of human malignancies. Cancer is an accidental and highly unusual or long-term effect of oncogenic human virus infection. With most "oncogenic viruses," infection is a critical and ultimately determinative early step in carcinogenesis. Latent HPV infection can block cell death and cause cervical cells to proliferate. A virus-infected cell with an integrated HPV genome overexpressing E6 and E7 undergoes subsequent cellular genetic changes that enhance autonomous malignant cell growth.

Most hepatocellular carcinoma is believed to be caused by chronic inflammatory, immune, and regenerative responses to HBV or HCV infection. Epidemiologic data firmly link HBV and HCV infections to hepatocellular carcinoma. These infections elicit repetitive cycles of virus-induced liver injury followed by tissue repair and regeneration. Over decades, chronic virus infection, repetitive tissue regeneration, and acquired chromosomal changes can result in proliferative nodules. Further chromosomal mutations can lead to the degeneration of cells in a proliferating nodule into hepatocellular carcinoma. In rare instances, HBV DNA integrates into cellular DNA, promoting overexpression of a cell gene that can also contribute to oncogenesis.

Most cervical carcinoma is caused by persistent infection with "high-risk" HPV type 16 or 18. In contrast to HBV and HCV infections, which stimulate cell growth as a consequence of virus-induced cell death, HPV type 16 or 18 proteins E6 and E7 destroy p53 and pRB, respectively. Elimination of these key tumor-suppressive cell proteins increases cell growth, cell survival, and cell genome instability. However, like HBV and HCV infections, HPV infection alone is not sufficient for carcinogenesis. Cervical carcinoma is inevitably associated with persistent HPV infection and integration of the HPV genome into chromosomal DNA. Integrations that result in overexpression of E6 and E7 from HPV type 16 or 18 cause more profound changes in cell growth and survival and enable subsequent chromosomal changes that result in cervical carcinoma.

EBV is the most unusual oncogenic virus in that normal B cell infection results in latency with expression of viral proteins that can cause endless B lymphocyte growth. In almost all humans, strong CD4+ and CD8+ T cell immune responses to the antigenic EBV latent-infection nuclear proteins prevent uncontrolled B cell lymphoproliferation. However, when humans are severely immunosuppressed by transplantation-associated medication, HIV infection, or genetic immunodeficiencies, EBV-induced B cell malignancies can emerge.

EBV infection also plays a role in the long-term development of B lymphocyte and epithelial cell malignancies. Persistent EBV infection with expression of an EBV latency-associated integral membrane protein (LMP1) in latently infected epithelial cells appears to be a critical early step in the evolution of anaplastic nasopharyngeal carcinoma, a common malignancy in populations in southern China and northern Africa. Genomic instability and chromosomal abnormalities also contribute to the development of EBV-associated nasopharyngeal carcinomas. EBV is an important cause of Hodgkin's lymphoma. High-level expression of LMP1 or LMP2 in Reed-Sternberg cells is a hallmark in up to 50% of Hodgkin's lymphoma cases. LMP1-induced nuclear factor κB (NF-κB) activity may prolong the survival of defective B cells that are normally eliminated by apoptosis, thereby allowing the acquisition of other genetic changes leading to malignant Reed-Sternberg cells.

The HTLV-I Tax and Rex proteins are critical to the initiation of cutaneous adult T cell lymphoma/leukemias that occur long after primary HTLV-I infection. Tax-induced NF-κB activation may contribute to cytokine production, infected cell survival, and eventual outgrowth of malignant cells.

Molecular data confirm the presence of KSHV DNA in all Kaposi's tumors, including those associated with HIV infection, transplantation, and familial transmission. KSHV infection is also etiologically implicated in pleural-effusion lymphomas and multicentric Castleman's disease, which are more common among HIV-infected than among HIV-uninfected people. KSHV can express a virus-encoded cyclin, an IFN regulatory factor, and a latency-associated nuclear antigen that are implicated in increased cell proliferation and survival.

Evidence supporting a causal role for virus infection in all of these malignancies includes (1) epidemiologic data, (2) the presence of viral DNA in all tumor cells, (3) the ability of the viruses to transform human cells in culture, (4) the results of in vitro cell culture–based assays that reveal transforming effects of specific viral genes on cell growth or survival, (5) pathologic data indicating the expression of transforming viral genes in premalignant or malignant cells in vivo, (6) the demonstration in animal models that these viral genes can cause malignant cell growth, and (7) the ability of virus-specific vaccines to reduce the incidence of virus-associated malignancy. Virus-related malignancies provide an opportunity to expand our understanding of the biologic mechanisms important in the development of cancer. They also offer unique opportunities to develop diagnostics, vaccines, or therapeutics that could prevent or specifically treat cancers associated with virus infection. Widespread immunization against hepatitis B has resulted in a decreased prevalence of HBV-associated hepatitis and will probably prevent most HBV-related liver cancers. An HPV vaccine can reduce rates of colonization with high-risk HPV strains and thereby decrease the risk of cervical cancer. The successful use of in vitro–expanded EBV-specific T cell populations to treat or prevent EBV-associated posttransplantation lymphoproliferative disease demonstrates the potential of immunoprevention or immunotherapy against virus-associated cancers.

■ RESISTANCE TO VIRAL INFECTIONS

Resistance to viral infections is initially provided by factors that are not virus-specific. Physical protection is afforded by the cornified layers of the skin and by mucous secretions that continuously sweep over mucosal surfaces. Once the first cell is infected, IFNs are induced and confer resistance to viral replication. Viral infection may also trigger the release of other cytokines from infected cells. These cytokines may be chemotactic to inflammatory and immune cells. Viral protein epitopes expressed on the cell surface in the context of MHC class I and II proteins can stimulate the expansion of T cell populations with receptors that can recognize the virus-encoded peptides. Cytokines and antigens released by virus-induced cell death further attract inflammatory cells, dendritic cells, granulocytes, natural killer (NK) cells, and B lymphocytes to sites of infection and to draining lymph nodes. IFNs and NK cells are particularly important in containing viral infection for the first several days. Granulocytes and macrophages are also important in the phagocytosis and degradation of viruses, especially after an initial antibody response.

By 7–10 days after infection, virus-specific antibody responses, virus-specific HLA class II–restricted CD4+ helper T lymphocyte responses, and virus-specific HLA class I–restricted CD8+ cytotoxic T lymphocyte responses develop. These responses, whose magnitude typically increases over the second and third weeks of infection, are important for rapid recovery. Also between the second and third weeks, the antibody type usually changes from IgM to IgG; IgG or IgA antibody can then be detected at infected mucosal surfaces. Antibody may directly neutralize virus by binding to its surface and preventing cell attachment or penetration. Complement can significantly enhance antibody-mediated virus neutralization. Antibody and complement can also lyse virus-infected cells that express viral membrane proteins on the cell surface. Cells infected with a replicating enveloped virus usually express the virus-envelope glycoproteins on the cell plasma membrane. Specific antibodies can bind to the glycoproteins, fix complement, and lyse the infected cell.

Antibody and CD4+/CD8+ T lymphocyte responses to virus infection can persist at high levels for several months after primary infection. Antibody-producing B lymphocytes and CD4+ or CD8+ T lymphocyte responses can persist in small numbers as memory cells and begin to proliferate rapidly in response to a second infection, providing an early barrier to reinfection with the same virus. Redevelopment of T cell immunity may take longer than secondary antibody responses, particularly when many years have elapsed between primary infection and re-exposure. However, persistent infections or frequent reactivations from latency can result in sustained high-level T cell responses. EBV and CMV typically induce high-level CD4+ and CD8+ T cell responses that are maintained for decades after primary infection.

Some viruses have genes that alter innate and acquired host defenses. Adenoviruses encode small RNAs that inhibit IFN-induced, protein kinase R (PKR)–mediated shutoff of infected-cell protein synthesis. Adenovirus E1A can also directly inhibit IFN-mediated changes in cell gene transcription. Moreover, adenovirus E3 proteins prevent tumor necrosis factor (TNF)–induced cytolysis and block HLA class I antigen synthesis by the infected cell. HSV ICP47 and CMV US11 also block class I antigen presentation. EBV encodes an interleukin (IL) 10 homologue that inhibits NK and T cell responses. Vaccinia virus encodes a soluble receptor for IFN-α and binding proteins for IFN-γ, IL-1, IL-18, and TNF, which inhibit host innate and adaptive immune responses. Vaccinia virus also encodes a caspase inhibitor that inhibits the ability of CD8+ cytotoxic T cells to kill virus-infected cells. Some poxviruses and herpesviruses encode chemokine-binding proteins that inhibit cell inflammatory responses. The adoption of these strategies by viruses highlights the importance of the corresponding host resistance factors in containing viral infection and the importance of redundancy in host resistance.

The host inflammatory and immune responses to viral infection do not come without a price. These responses contribute to the symptoms, signs, and other pathophysiologic manifestations of viral infection. Inflammation at sites of viral infection can subvert an effective immune response and induce tissue death and dysfunction. Moreover, immune responses to viral infection could, in principle, result in immune attack upon cross-reactive epitopes on normal cells, with consequent autoimmunity.

■ INTERFERONS

All human cells can synthesize IFN-α or IFN-β in response to viral infection. These IFN responses are usually induced by the presence of double-strand viral RNA, which can be made by both RNA and DNA viruses and sensed by double-strand RNA binding proteins (e.g., PKR and RIG-I) in the cell cytoplasm. IFN-γ is not closely related to IFN-α or IFN-β and is produced mainly by NK cells and by immune T lymphocytes responding to IL-12. IFN-α and -β bind to the IFN-α receptor, while IFN-γ binds to a different but related receptor. Both receptors signal through receptor-associated JAK kinases and other cytoplasmic proteins, including "STAT" proteins, which are tyrosine-phosphorylated by JAK kinases, translocate to the nucleus, and activate promoters for specific cell genes. Three types of antiviral effects are induced by IFN at the transcriptional level. The first effect is attributable to the induction of 2′-5′ oligo(A) synthetases, which require double-strand RNA for their activation. Activated synthetase polymerizes oligo(A) and thereby activates RNAse L, which in turn degrades single-strand RNA. A second effect results from the induction of PKR, a serine and threonine kinase that is also activated by double-strand RNA. PKR phosphorylates and negatively regulates the translational initiation factor eIF2α, shutting down protein synthesis in the infected cell. A third effect is initiated through the induction of Mx proteins, a family of GTPases that is particularly important in inhibiting the replication of influenza virus and vesicular stomatitis virus. These IFN effects are mostly directed against the infected cell, causing virus and cell dysfunction and thereby limiting viral replication.

■ DIAGNOSTIC VIROLOGY

A wide variety of methods are used to diagnose viral infection. Serology and virus isolation in tissue culture remain important standards. Acute- and convalescent-phase sera with rising titers of antibody to virus-specific antigens and a shift from IgM to IgG antibodies are generally accepted as diagnostic of acute viral infection. Serologic diagnosis is based on a >4-fold rise in IgG antibody concentration when acute- and convalescent-phase serum samples are analyzed at the same time.

Immunofluorescence, hemadsorption, and hemagglutination assays for antiviral antibodies are labor-intensive and have been replaced by enzyme-linked immunosorbent assays (ELISAs), which generally use the specific viral proteins most frequently targeted by the antibody response. The proteins are purified from virus-infected cells or produced by recombinant DNA technology and are attached to a solid phase, where they can be incubated with serum, washed to eliminate nonspecific antibodies, and allowed to react with an enzyme-linked reagent to detect human IgG or IgM antibody specifically adhering to the viral antigen. The amount of antibody can then be quantitated by the intensity of a color reaction mediated by the linked enzyme. ELISAs can be sensitive and automated. Western blots can simultaneously confirm the presence of antibody to multiple specific viral proteins. The proteins are separated by size and transferred to an inert membrane, where they are incubated with serum antibodies. Western blots have an internal specificity control, since the level of reactivity for viral proteins can be compared with that for cellular proteins in the same sample. Western blots require individual evaluation and are inherently difficult to quantitate or automate.

Isolation of virus in tissue culture depends on infection and replication in susceptible cells. Growth of virus in cell cultures can frequently be identified by effects on cell morphology under light microscopy. For example, HSV produces a typical cytopathic effect in rabbit kidney cells within 3 days. Other viral cytopathic effects may not be as diagnostically distinctive. Identification usually requires confirmation by staining with virus-specific monoclonal antibodies. The efficiency and speed of virus identification can be enhanced by combining short-term culture with immune detection. In assays with "shell vials" of tissue culture cells growing on a coverslip, viral infection can be detected by staining with a monoclonal antibody to a specific viral protein expressed early in viral replication. Thus, virus-infected cells can be detected within hours or days of inoculation, whereas several rounds of infection would be required to produce visible cytopathic effects.

Isolation of virus in tissue culture also depends on the collection of specimens from appropriate sites and the rapid transport of these specimens in appropriate medium to the virology laboratory (Chap. e22). Rapid transport maintains viral viability and limits bacterial and fungal overgrowth. Enveloped viruses are generally more sensitive to freezing and thawing than nonenveloped viruses. The most appropriate site for culture depends on the pathogenesis of the virus in question. Nasopharyngeal, tracheal, or endobronchial aspirates are most appropriate for the identification of respiratory viruses. Sputum cultures generally are less appropriate since bacterial contamination and viscosity threaten tissue-culture cell viability. Aspirates of vesicular fluid are useful for isolation of HSV and VZV. Nasopharyngeal aspirates and stool specimens may be useful when the patient has fever and a rash and an enteroviral infection is suspected. Adenoviruses can be cultured from the urine of patients with hemorrhagic cystitis. CMV can frequently be isolated from cultures of urine or buffy coat. Biopsy material can be effectively cultured when viruses infect major organs, as in HSV encephalitis or adenovirus pneumonia.

The isolation of a virus does not necessarily establish disease causality. Viruses can persistently or intermittently colonize normal human mucosal surfaces. Saliva can be positive for herpesviruses, and normal urine samples can be positive for CMV. Isolations from blood, cerebrospinal fluid (CSF), or tissue are more often diagnostic of significant viral infection.

Another method aimed at increasing the speed of viral diagnosis is direct testing for antigen or cytopathic effects. Virus-infected cells from the patient may be detected by staining with virus-specific monoclonal antibodies. For example, epithelial cells obtained by nasopharyngeal aspiration can be stained with a variety of specific monoclonal antibodies to identify the specific infecting respiratory virus.

Nucleic acid amplification techniques bring speed, sensitivity, and specificity to diagnostic virology. The ability to directly amplify minute amounts of viral nucleic acids in specimens means that detection no longer depends on viable virus and its replication. For example, amplification and detection of HSV nucleic acids in the CSF of patients with HSV encephalitis is a more sensitive detection method than culture of virus from CSF. The extreme sensitivity of these tests can be a problem, since subclinical infection or contamination can lead to false-positive results. Detection of viral nucleic acids does not necessarily indicate virus-induced disease.

Measurement of the amount of viral RNA or DNA in peripheral blood is an important means for determining whether a patient is at increased risk for virus-induced disease and for evaluating clinical responses to antiviral chemotherapy. Nucleic acid technologies for RNA quantification are routinely used in AIDS patients to evaluate responses to antiviral agents and to detect viral resistance or noncompliance with therapy. Viral-load measurements are also useful for evaluating the treatment of patients with HBV and HCV infections. Nucleic acid testing or direct staining with CMV-specific monoclonal antibodies to quantitate virus-infected cells in the peripheral blood (CMV antigenemia) is useful for identifying immunosuppressed patients who may be at risk for CMV-induced disease.

■ DRUG TREATMENT FOR VIRAL INFECTIONS

Multiple steps in the life cycles of viruses can be effectively targeted by antiviral drugs (see also Chaps. 178 and 189). Nucleoside and nonnucleoside reverse transcriptase inhibitors prevent HIV provirus synthesis, while protease inhibitors block maturation of the HIV polyprotein after infection of the cell. Enfuvirtide is a small peptide derived from HIV gp41 that acts before cell infection by preventing a conformational change required for initial fusion of the virus with the cell membrane. Raltegravir is an integrase inhibitor that is approved for use with other anti-HIV drugs. Amantadine and rimantadine inhibit the influenza M2 protein, preventing release of viral RNA early during infection, whereas zanamivir and oseltamivir inhibit the influenza neuraminidase, which is necessary for the efficient release of mature virions from infected cells.

Viral genomes can evolve resistance to drugs by mutation and selection, by recombination with a drug-resistant virus, or (in the case of influenza virus and other segmented RNA viral genomes) by reassortment. The emergence of drug-resistant strains can limit the efficacy of antiviral therapy. As in antibacterial therapy, excessive and inappropriate use of antiviral therapy can select for the emergence of drug-resistant strains. HIV genotyping is a rapid method for identifying drug-resistant viruses. Resistance to reverse transcriptase or protease inhibitors has been associated with specific mutations in the reverse transcriptase or protease genes. Identification of these mutations by polymerase chain reaction amplification and nucleic acid sequencing can be clinically useful for determining which antiviral agents may still be effective. Drug resistance also can arise in herpesviruses but is a less common clinical problem.

■ IMMUNIZATION FOR THE PREVENTION OF VIRAL INFECTIONS

Viral vaccines are among the outstanding accomplishments of medical science. Smallpox has been eradicated except as a potential weapon of biological warfare or bioterrorism (Chap. 221). Poliovirus eradication may soon follow. Measles can be contained or eliminated. Excess mortality due to influenza virus epidemics can be prevented, and the threat of influenza pandemics can be decreased by contemporary killed or live attenuated influenza vaccines. Mumps, rubella, and chickenpox are well controlled by childhood vaccination in the developed world. Reimmunization of mature adults can be used to control herpes zoster. New rotavirus vaccines can have a major impact on this leading cause of gastroenteritis and prominent cause of childhood death worldwide. Widespread HBV vaccination has dramatically lowered the frequency of acute and chronic hepatitis and is expected to lead to a dramatic decrease in the incidence of hepatocellular carcinoma. The HPV vaccine was the first vaccine specifically licensed to prevent virus-induced cancer. Use of purified proteins, genetically engineered live-virus vaccines, and recombinant DNA–based strategies will make it possible to immunize against severe infections with other viruses. The development of effective HIV and HCV vaccines is complicated by the high mutation rate of viral RNA polymerase and reverse transcriptase, the population-based and individual divergence of HIV or HCV genomes, and repeated high-level exposure in some populations. Concerns about the use of smallpox and other viruses as weapons necessitate maintenance of immunity to agents that are not encountered naturally.

■ VIRUSES AS NOVEL THERAPEUTIC TOOLS OR AGENTS

Viruses are being used experimentally to deliver biotherapeutic agents or novel vaccines. Foreign genes can be inserted into viral nucleic acids, and the recombinant virus vectors can be used to infect the patient or the patient's cells ex vivo. Retrovirus integration into the cell genome has been used to functionally replace the abnormal gene in T cells of patients with severe combined immunodeficiency, thereby restoring immune function. Recombinant adenovirus, AAV, and retroviruses are being explored for use in diseases due to single-gene defects, such as cystic fibrosis and hemophilia. Recombinant poxviruses, adenoviruses, and influenza viruses are also being used experimentally as vaccine vectors. Viral vectors are being tested experimentally for the expression of cytokines that can enhance immunity against tumor cells or for the expression of proteins that can increase the sensitivity of tumor cells to chemotherapy. HSV deficient for replication in resting cells is being used to selectively kill proliferating glioblastoma cells after injections into CNS tumors. For improved safety, nonreplicating viruses are frequently employed in clinical trials. Potential adverse events associated with virus-mediated gene transfer include the induction of inflammatory and antiviral immune responses. Instances of retrovirus-induced human malignances have raised concerns about the safety of retroviral gene therapy vectors.

FURTHER READINGS

Cullen BR: Viral and cellular messenger RNA targets of viral microRNAs. Nature 457:421, 2009

Future II Study Group: Quadrivalent vaccine against human papillomavirus to prevent high-grade cervical lesions. N Engl J Med 356:1915, 2007

Harrison SC: Viral membrane fusion. Nat Struct Mol Biol 15:690, 2008

Knipe DM et al (eds): *Fields Virology*, 5th ed. New York, Lippincott Williams & Wilkins, 2006

Malim MH: APOBEC proteins and intrinsic resistance to HIV-1 infection. Philos Trans R Soc Lond B Biol Sci 364:675, 2009

CHAPTER 178

Antiviral Chemotherapy, Excluding Antiretroviral Drugs

Lindsey R. Baden

Raphael Dolin

The field of antiviral therapy—both the number of antiviral drugs and our understanding of their optimal use—historically has lagged behind that of antibacterial drug treatment, but significant progress has been made in recent years on new drugs for several viral infections. The development of antiviral drugs poses several challenges. Viruses replicate intracellularly and often employ host cell enzymes, macromolecules, and organelles for synthesis of viral particles. Therefore, useful antiviral compounds must discriminate between host and viral functions with a high degree of specificity; agents without such selectivity are likely to be too toxic for clinical use.

Significant progress has also been made in the development of laboratory assays to assist clinicians in the appropriate use of antiviral drugs. Phenotypic and genotypic assays for resistance to antiviral drugs are becoming more widely available, and correlations of laboratory results with clinical outcomes are being better defined. Of particular note has been the development of highly sensitive and specific methods that measure the concentration of virus in blood (*virus load*) and permit direct assessment of the antiviral effect of a given drug regimen in that host site. Virus load measurements have been useful in recognizing the risk of disease progression in patients with certain viral infections and in identifying patients for whom antiviral chemotherapy might be of greatest benefit. As with any in vitro laboratory test, results are highly dependent on (and likely to vary with) the laboratory techniques employed.

Information regarding the pharmacokinetics of some antiviral drugs, particularly in diverse clinical settings, is limited. Assays to measure the concentrations of these drugs, especially of their active moieties within cells, are primarily research procedures and are not widely available to clinicians. Thus, there are relatively few guidelines for adjusting dosages of antiviral agents to maximize antiviral activity and minimize toxicity. Consequently, clinical use of antiviral drugs must be accompanied by particular vigilance with regard to unanticipated adverse effects.

Like that of other infections, the course of viral infections is profoundly affected by an interplay of the pathogen with a complex set of host defenses. The presence or absence of preexisting immunity, the ability to mount humoral and/or cell-mediated immune responses, and the stimulation of innate immunity are important determinants of the outcome of viral infections. The state of the host's defenses needs to be considered when antiviral agents are used or evaluated.

As with any therapy, the optimal use of antiviral compounds requires a specific and timely diagnosis. For some viral infections, such as herpes zoster, the clinical manifestations are so characteristic that a diagnosis can be made on clinical grounds alone. For other viral infections, such as influenza A, epidemiologic information (e.g., the documentation of a community-wide outbreak) can be used to make a presumptive diagnosis with a high degree of accuracy. However, for most of the remaining viral infections, including herpes simplex encephalitis, cytomegaloviral infections other than retinitis, and enteroviral infections, diagnosis on clinical grounds alone cannot be accomplished with certainty. For such infections, rapid viral diagnostic techniques are of great importance. Considerable progress has also been made in recent years in the development of such tests, which are now widely available for a number of viral infections.

Despite these complexities, the efficacy of a number of antiviral compounds has been clearly established in rigorously conducted and controlled studies. As summarized in Table 178-1, this chapter reviews the antiviral drugs that are currently approved or are likely to be considered for approval in the near future for use against viral infections other than those caused by HIV. Antiretroviral drugs are reviewed in Chap. 189.

ANTIVIRAL DRUGS ACTIVE AGAINST RESPIRATORY INFECTIONS (ALSO SEE CHAP. 187)

■ ZANAMIVIR, OSELTAMIVIR, AND PERAMIVIR

Zanamivir and oseltamivir are inhibitors of the influenza viral neuraminidase enzyme, which is essential for release of the virus from infected cells and for its subsequent spread throughout the respiratory tract of the infected host. The enzyme cleaves terminal sialic acid residues and thus destroys the cellular receptors to which the viral hemagglutinin attaches. Zanamivir and oseltamivir are sialic acid transition-state analogues and are highly active and specific inhibitors of the neuraminidases of both influenza A and B viruses. The antineuraminidase activity of the two drugs is similar, although zanamivir has somewhat greater in vitro activity against influenza B. Both zanamivir and oseltamivir act through competitive and reversible inhibition of the active site of influenza A and B viral neuraminidases and have relatively little effect on mammalian cell enzymes.

Oseltamivir phosphate is an ethyl ester prodrug that is converted to oseltamivir carboxylate by esterases in the liver. Orally administered oseltamivir has a bioavailability of >60% and a plasma half-life of 7–9 h. The drug is excreted unmetabolized, primarily by the kidneys. Zanamivir has low oral bioavailability and is administered orally via a hand-held inhaler. By this route, ~15% of the dose is deposited in the lower respiratory tract, and low plasma levels of the drug are detected.

Orally inhaled zanamivir is generally well tolerated, although exacerbations of asthma may occur. The toxicities most frequently encountered with orally administered oseltamivir are nausea, gastrointestinal discomfort, and (less commonly) vomiting. Gastrointestinal discomfort is usually transient and is less likely if the drug is administered with food. Neuropsychiatric events (delirium, self-injury) have been reported in children who have been taking oseltamivir, primarily in Japan. An IV formulation of zanamivir is under development and is available from GlaxoSmith Kline as part of clinical trials.

Inhaled zanamivir and orally administered oseltamivir have been effective in the treatment of naturally occurring, uncomplicated influenza A or B in otherwise healthy adults. In placebo-controlled studies, illness has been shortened by 1.0–1.5 days of therapy with either of these drugs when treatment is administered within 2 days of onset. Pooled analyses of clinical studies of oseltamivir suggest that treatment may reduce the likelihood of hospitalizations and of certain respiratory tract complications associated with influenza (Chap. 187). Once-daily inhaled zanamivir or once-daily orally administered oseltamivir can provide prophylaxis against laboratory-documented influenza A– and influenza B–associated illness.

TABLE 178-1 Antiviral Chemotherapy and Chemoprophylaxis

Infection	Drug	Route	Dosage	Comment
Influenza A and B: Treatment	Oseltamivir	Oral	Adults: 75 mg bid × 5 d Children 1–12 years: 30–75 mg bid, depending on weight,^{a} × 5 d	When started within 2 days of onset in uncomplicated disease, zanamivir and oseltamivir reduce symptom duration by 1.0–1.5 and 1.3 d, respectively. Their effectiveness in prevention or treatment of complications is unclear, although some analyses suggest that oseltamivir may reduce the frequency of respiratory tract complications and hospitalizations. Oseltamivir's side effects of nausea and vomiting can be reduced in frequency by drug administration with food. Zanamivir may exacerbate bronchospasm in patients with asthma. Amantadine and rimantadine are not recommended for routine use unless antiviral susceptibilities are known because of widespread resistance in A/H3N2 viruses since 2005–2006 and in pandemic A/H1N1 viruses in 2009–2010. Their efficacy in treatment of uncomplicated disease caused by sensitive viruses has been similar to that of neuraminidase inhibitors.
	Zanamivir	Inhaled orally	Adults and children ≥7 years: 10 mg bid × 5 d	
	Amantadine^b	Oral	Adults: 100 mg qd or bid × 5–7 d Children 1–9 years: 5 mg/kg per day (maximum, 150 mg/d) × 5–7 d	
	Rimantadine^b	Oral	100 mg qd or bid × 5–7 d in adults	
Influenza A and B: Prophylaxis	Oseltamivir	Oral	Adults: 75 mg/d Children ≥1 year: 30–75 mg/d, depending on weight^a	Prophylaxis must be continued for the duration of exposure and can be administered simultaneously with inactivated vaccine. Unless the sensitivity of isolates is known, neither amantadine nor rimantadine is currently recommended for prophylaxis or therapy.
	Zanamivir	Inhaled orally	Adults and children ≥5 years: 10 mg/d	
	Amantadine^b or rimantadine^b	Oral	Adults: 200 mg/d Children 1–9 years: 5 mg/kg per day (maximum, 150 mg/d)	
RSV infection	Ribavirin	Small-particle aerosol	Administered 12–18 h/d from reservoir containing 20 mg/mL × 3–6 d	Use of ribavirin is to be "considered" for treatment of infants and young children hospitalized with RSV pneumonia and bronchiolitis, according to the American Academy of Pediatrics.
CMV disease	Ganciclovir	IV	5 mg/kg bid × 14–21 d; then 5 mg/kg per day as maintenance dose	Ganciclovir, valganciclovir, foscarnet, and cidofovir are approved for treatment of CMV retinitis in patients with AIDS. They are also used for colitis, pneumonia, or "wasting" syndrome associated with CMV and for prevention of CMV disease in transplant recipients.
	Valganciclovir	Oral	900 mg bid × 21 d; then 900 mg/d as maintenance dose	Valganciclovir has largely supplanted oral ganciclovir and is frequently used in place of IV ganciclovir.
	Foscarnet	IV	60 mg/kg q8h × 14–21 d; then 90–120 mg/kg per day as maintenance dose	Foscarnet is not myelosuppressive and is active against acyclovir- and ganciclovir-resistant herpesviruses.
	Cidofovir	IV	5 mg/kg once weekly × 2 weeks, then once every other week; given with probenecid and hydration	
	Fomivirsen	Intravitreal	330 mg on days 1 and 15 followed by 330 mg monthly as maintenance	Fomivirsen has reduced the rate of progression of CMV retinitis in patients in whom other regimens have failed or have not been well tolerated. The major form of toxicity is ocular inflammation.
Varicella: Immunocompetent host	Acyclovir	Oral	20 mg/kg (maximum, 800 mg) 4 or 5 times daily × 5 d	Treatment confers modest clinical benefit when administered within 24 h of rash onset.
	Valacyclovir	Oral	Children 2–18 years: 20 mg/kg tid, not to exceed 1 g tid, × 5 d	
Varicella: Immunocompromised host	Acyclovir	IV	10 mg/kg q8h × 7 d	A change to oral valacyclovir can be considered once fever has subsided if there is no evidence of visceral involvement.
Herpes simplex encephalitis	Acyclovir	IV	10 mg/kg q8h × 14–21 d	Results are optimal when therapy is initiated early. Some authorities recommend treatment for 21 d to prevent relapses.

(continued)

TABLE 178-1 Antiviral Chemotherapy and Chemoprophylaxis (*Continued*)

Infection	Drug	Route	Dosage	Comment
Neonatal herpes simplex	Acyclovir	IV	20 mg/kg q8h × 14–21 d	Serious morbidity is common despite therapy. Prolonged oral administration after initial IV therapy has been suggested because of long-term sequelae associated with cutaneous recurrences of HSV infection.
Genital herpes simplex: Primary (treatment)	Acyclovir	IV	5 mg/kg q8h × 5–10 d	The IV route is preferred for infections severe enough to warrant hospitalization or with neurologic complications.
		Oral	400 mg tid or 200 mg 5 times daily × 7–10 d or 800 mg tid × 2 d	The oral route is preferred for patients whose condition does not warrant hospitalization. Adequate hydration must be maintained.
		Topical	5% ointment; 4–6 applications daily × 7–10 d	Topical use—largely supplemented by oral therapy—may obviate systemic administration to pregnant women. Systemic symptoms and untreated areas are not affected.
	Valacyclovir	Oral	1 g bid × 7–10 d	Valacyclovir appears to be as effective as acyclovir but can be administered less frequently.
	Famciclovir	Oral	250 mg tid × 7–10 d[c]	Famciclovir appears to be similar in effectiveness to acyclovir.
Genital herpes simplex: Recurrent (treatment)	Acyclovir	Oral	400 mg tid or 800 mg bid × 5 d	The clinical effect is modest and is enhanced if therapy is initiated early. Treatment does not affect recurrence rates.
	Famciclovir	Oral	125 mg bid × 5 d or 1000 mg bid × 1 d	
	Valacyclovir	Oral	500 mg bid × 3 d or 1 g once a day × 5 d	
Genital herpes simplex: Recurrent (suppression)	Acyclovir	Oral	400 mg bid	Suppressive therapy is recommended only for patients with at least 6–10 recurrences per year. "Breakthrough" occasionally takes place, and asymptomatic shedding of virus occurs. The need for suppressive therapy should be reevaluated after 1 year. Suppression with valacyclovir reduces transmission of genital HSV among discordant couples.
	Valacyclovir	Oral	500–1000 mg/d	
	Famciclovir	Oral	250 mg bid	
Mucocutaneous herpes simplex in immunocompromised host: Treatment	Acyclovir	IV	5 mg/kg q8h × 7–14 d	The choice of the IV or oral route and the duration of therapy depend on the severity of infection and the patient's ability to take oral medication. Oral or IV treatment has supplanted topical therapy except for small, easily accessible lesions. Foscarnet is used for acyclovir-resistant viruses.
		Oral	400 mg 5 times daily × 10–14 d	
		Topical	5% ointment; 4–6 applications daily × 7 d or until healed	
	Valacyclovir	Oral	1 g tid × 7–10 d[c]	
	Famciclovir	Oral	500 mg bid × 7–10 d[d]	
Mucocutaneous herpes simplex in immunocompromised host: Prevention of recurrence during intense immunosuppression	Acyclovir	Oral	400 mg 2–5 times daily or 800 mg bid	Treatment is administered during periods when intense immunosuppression is expected—e.g., during antitumor chemotherapy or after transplantation—and is usually continued for 2–3 months.
		IV	5 mg/kg q12h	
	Valacyclovir	Oral	500 mg to 1 g bid or tid	
	Famciclovir	Oral	500 mg bid[c]	
Herpes simplex orolabialis (recurrent)[e]	Penciclovir	Topical	1.0% cream applied q2h during waking hours × 4 d	Treatment shortens healing time and symptom duration by 0.5–1.0 d (compared with placebo).
	Valacyclovir	Oral	2 g q12h × 1 d	Therapy begun at the earliest symptom reduces disease duration by 1 d.
	Famciclovir[c]	Oral	1500 mg once or 750 bid × 1 d	Therapy begun within 1 h of prodrome decreased time to healing by 1.8–2.2 d.
	Docosanol[f]	Topical	10% cream 5 times daily until healed	Application at initial symptoms reduces healing time by 1 d.

(*continued*)

TABLE 178-1 Antiviral Chemotherapy and Chemoprophylaxis (*Continued*)

Infection	Drug	Route	Dosage	Comment
Herpes simplex keratitis	Trifluridine	Topical	1 drop of 1% ophthalmic solution q2h while awake (maximum, 9 drops daily)	Therapy should be undertaken in consultation with an ophthalmologist.
	Vidarabine	Topical	0.5-in. ribbon of 3% ophthalmic ointment 5 times daily	
Herpes zoster: Immunocompetent host	Valacyclovir	Oral	1 g tid × 7 d	Valacyclovir may be more effective than acyclovir for pain relief; otherwise, it has a similar effect on cutaneous lesions and should be given within 72 h of rash onset.
	Famciclovir	Oral	500 mg q8h × 7 d	The duration of postherpetic neuralgia is shorter than with placebo. Famciclovir showed overall efficacy similar to that of acyclovir in a comparative trial. It should be given ≤72 h after rash onset.
	Acyclovir	Oral	800 mg 5 times daily × 7–10 d	Acyclovir causes faster resolution of skin lesions than placebo and provides some relief of acute symptoms if given within 72 h of rash onset. Combined with tapering doses of prednisone, acyclovir improves quality-of-life outcomes.
Herpes zoster: Immunocompromised host	Acyclovir	IV	10 mg/kg q8h × 7 d	Effectiveness in localized zoster is most marked when treatment is given early. Foscarnet may be used for acyclovir-resistant VZV infections.
		Oral	800 mg 5 times daily × 7 d	
	Famciclovir	Oral	500 mg tid × 10 d^c	
Herpes zoster ophthalmicus	Acyclovir	Oral	600–800 mg 5 times daily × 10 d	Treatment reduces ocular complications, including ocular keratitis and uveitis.
	Valacyclovir	Oral	1 g tid × 7 d	
	Famciclovir	Oral	500 mg tid × 7 d	
Condyloma acuminatum	IFN-α2b	Intralesional	1 million units per wart (maximum of 5) thrice weekly × 3 weeks	Intralesional treatment frequently results in regression of warts, but lesions often recur. Parenteral administration may be useful if lesions are numerous.
	IFN-αn3	Intralesional	250,000 units per wart (maximum of 10) twice weekly × up to 8 weeks	
Chronic hepatitis B	IFN-α2b	SC	5 million units daily or 10 million units thrice weekly × 16–24 weeks	HBeAg and DNA are eliminated in 33–37% of cases. Histopathologic improvement is also seen.
	Pegylated IFN-α2a	SC	180 μg weekly × 48 weeks	ALT levels return to normal in 39% of patients, and histologic improvement occurs in 38%.
	Lamivudine	Oral	100 mg/d × 12–18 months; 150 mg bid as part of therapy for HIV infection	Lamivudine monotherapy is well tolerated and effective in reduction of HBV DNA levels, normalization of ALT levels, and improvement in histopathology. However, resistance develops in 24% of recipients when lamivudine is used as monotherapy for 1 year.
	Adefovir dipivoxil	Oral	10 mg/d × 48 weeks	A return of ALT levels to normal is documented in 48–72% of recipients and improved liver histopathology in 53–64%. Adefovir is effective in lamivudine-resistant hepatitis B. Renal function should be monitored.
	Entecavir	Oral	0.5 mg/d × 48 weeks (1 mg/d if HBV is resistant to lamivudine)	Normalization of ALT is seen in 68–78% of recipients and loss of HBeAg in 21%. Entecavir is active against lamivudine-resistant HBV.
	Telbivudine	Oral	600 mg/d × 52 weeks	HBV DNA is reduced by >5 log$_{10}$ copies/mL along with normalization of ALT levels in 74–77% of patients and improved histopathology in 65–67%. Resistance develops in 9–22% of patients after 2 years of therapy. Elevated CPK levels and myopathy may occur.
	Tenofovir	Oral	300 mg/d × 48 weeks	ALT levels return to normal in 68–76% of patients, and liver histopathology improves in 72–74%. Resistance is uncommon with up to 2 years of therapy.

(*continued*)

TABLE 178-1 Antiviral Chemotherapy and Chemoprophylaxis (*Continued*)

Infection	Drug	Route	Dosage	Comment
Chronic hepatitis C	IFN-α2a or IFN-α2b	SC	3 million units thrice weekly × 12–24 months	SVRs are noted in 20–30% of patients. Normalization of ALT levels and improvements in liver histopathology are also seen.
	IFN-α2b/ ribavirin	SC (IFN)/oral (ribavirin)	3 million units thrice weekly (IFN)/1000–1200 mg daily (ribavirin) × 6–12 months	Combination therapy results in SVR in up to 40–50% of recipients.
	Pegylated IFN-α2b	SC	1.5 µg weekly × 48 weeks	The slower clearance of pegylated IFNs than of standard IFNs permits once-weekly administration. Pegylated formulations appear to be superior to standard IFNs in efficacy, both as monotherapy and in combination with ribavirin, and have largely supplanted standard IFNs in treatment of hepatitis C. SVRs were seen in 42–51% of patients infected with genotype 1 and in 76–82% of those infected with genotype 2 or 3.
	Pegylated IFN-α2a	SC	180 µg weekly × 48 weeks	
	Pegylated IFN-α2b/ ribavirin	SC (IFN)/oral (ribavirin)	1.5 µg/kg weekly (IFN)/800–1400 mg daily (ribavirin) × 24–48 weeks	
	Pegylated IFN-α2a/ ribavirin	SC (IFN)/oral (ribavirin)	180 µg weekly (IFN)/800–1200 mg daily (ribavirin) × 24–48 weeks	
	IFN-alfacon	SC	9–15 µg thrice weekly × 6–12 months	Doses of 9 and 15 µg are equivalent to IFN-α2a and IFN-α2b doses of 3 million and 5 million units, respectively.
Chronic hepatitis D	IFN-α2a or IFN-α2b	SC	9 million units thrice weekly × 12 months	The overall efficacy and the optimal regimen and duration of therapy have not been established. Response rates have varied among studies.
	Pegylated IFN-α2b	SC	1.5 µg weekly × 48 weeks	
	Pegylated IFN-α2a	SC	180 µg weekly × 48 weeks	

^aFor detailed weight recommendations and for children <1 year of age, see *www.cdc.gov/flu/professionals/antivirals/summary-clinicians.htm*.
^bAmantadine and rimantadine are not recommended for routine use because of widespread resistance in A/H3N2 and pandemic A/H1N1 viruses in 2009–2010. Their use may be considered if sensitivities become reestablished.
^cNot approved for this indication by the U.S. Food and Drug Administration (FDA).
^dApproved by the FDA for treatment of HIV-infected individuals.
^eAcyclovir suspension (15 mg/kg PO to a maximum of 200 mg per dose) given for 7 d has been reported to be effective in treatment of primary herpetic gingivostomatitis in children.
^fActive ingredient: benzyl alcohol. Available without prescription.
Abbreviations: ALT, alanine aminotransferase; CMV, cytomegalovirus; CPK, creatine phosphokinase; HBeAg, hepatitis B e antigen; HBV, hepatitis B virus; HSV, herpes simplex virus; IFN, interferon; RSV, respiratory syncytial virus; SVR, sustained virologic response; UV, ultraviolet; VZV, varicella-zoster virus.

Resistance to the neuraminidase inhibitors may develop by changes in the viral neuraminidase enzyme, by changes in the hemagglutinin that make it more resistant to the actions of the neuraminidase, or by both mechanisms. Isolates that are resistant to oseltamivir—most commonly through the H275Y mutation, which leads to a change from histidine to tyrosine at that residue in the neuraminidase—remain sensitive to zanamivir. Certain mutations impart resistance to both oseltamivir and zanamivir (e.g., I223R, which leads to a change from isoleucine to arginine). Since the mechanisms of action of the neuraminidase inhibitors differ from those of the adamantanes (see below), zanamivir and oseltamivir are active against strains of influenza A virus that are resistant to amantadine and rimantadine.

Appropriate use of antiviral agents against influenza viruses depends on a knowledge of the resistance patterns of circulating viruses. For example, in the 2008–2009 influenza season, the circulating influenza A/H3N2 viruses were sensitive to both oseltamivir and zanamivir, whereas the seasonal A/H1N1 viruses, although also sensitive to zanamivir, were resistant to oseltamivir. Moreover, the pandemic A/H1N1 viruses that circulated in 2009–2010 remained sensitive to zanamivir and oseltamivir, with a few exceptions in the latter case. Up-to-date information on resistance patterns to antiviral drugs is available from the Centers for Disease Control and Prevention (CDC) at *www.cdc.gov/flu*.

Zanamivir and oseltamivir have been approved by the U.S. Food and Drug Administration (FDA) for treatment of influenza in adults and in children (those ≥7 years old for zanamivir and those ≥1 year old for oseltamivir) who have been symptomatic for ≤2 days. Oseltamivir is approved for prophylaxis of influenza in individuals ≥1 year of age and zanamivir for those ≥5 years of age (Table 178-1). Guidelines for use of oseltamivir in children <1 year of age can be accessed through the CDC website, as noted in the footnote to Table 178-1.

Peramivir, an investigational neuraminidase inhibitor that can be administered intravenously to patients for whom such an intervention is considered necessary, is available as part of clinical trials through BioCryst Pharmaceuticals. Oseltamivir-resistant viruses generally exhibit reduced sensitivity to peramivir.

■ AMANTADINE AND RIMANTADINE

Amantadine and the closely related compound rimantadine are primary symmetric amines that have antiviral activity limited to influenza A viruses. Amantadine and rimantadine have been shown to be efficacious in the prophylaxis and treatment of influenza A infections in humans for >45 years. High frequencies of resistance to these drugs were noted among influenza A/H3N2 viruses in the 2005–2006 influenza season and continued to be seen in 2008–2009. The pandemic A/H1N1 viruses that circulated in 2009–2010 were also resistant to amantadine and rimantadine. Therefore, these agents are no longer recommended for use unless the sensitivity of the individual influenza A isolate is known, in which case their use may be considered. Amantadine and rimantadine act through inhibition of the ion channel function of the influenza A M2 matrix protein, on which uncoating of the virus depends. A substitution of a single amino acid at critical sites in the M2 protein can result in a virus that is resistant to amantadine and rimantadine.

Amantadine and rimantadine have been shown to be effective in the prophylaxis of influenza A in large-scale studies of young adults and in less extensive studies of children and elderly persons. In such studies, efficacy rates of 55–80% in the prevention of influenza-like illness were noted, and even higher rates were reported when virus-specific attack rates were calculated. Amantadine and rimantadine have also been found to be effective in the treatment of influenza A infection in studies involving predominantly young adults and, to a lesser extent, children. Administration of these compounds within 24–72 h after the onset of illness has resulted in a reduction of the duration of signs and symptoms by ~50% compared to that in placebo recipients. The effect on signs and symptoms of illness is superior to that of commonly used antipyretic-analgesic agents. Only anecdotal reports are available concerning the efficacy of amantadine or rimantadine in the prevention or treatment of complications of influenza (e.g., pneumonia).

Amantadine and rimantadine are available only in oral formulations and are ordinarily administered to adults once or twice daily, with a dosage of 100–200 mg/d. Despite their structural similarities, the two compounds have different pharmacokinetics. Amantadine is not metabolized and is excreted almost entirely by the kidneys, with a half-life of 12–17 h and peak plasma concentrations of 0.4 μg/mL. In contrast, rimantadine is extensively metabolized to hydroxylated derivatives and has a half-life of 30 h. Only 30–40% of an orally administered dose of rimantadine is recovered in the urine. The peak plasma levels of rimantadine are approximately half those of amantadine, but rimantadine is concentrated in respiratory secretions to a greater extent than amantadine. For prophylaxis, the compounds must be administered daily for the period at risk (i.e., duration of the exposure). For therapy, amantadine or rimantadine is generally administered for 5–7 days.

Although these compounds are generally well tolerated, 5–10% of amantadine recipients experience mild central nervous system side effects consisting primarily of dizziness, anxiety, insomnia, and difficulty in concentrating. These effects are rapidly reversible upon cessation of the drug's administration. At a dose of 200 mg/d, rimantadine is better tolerated than amantadine; in a large-scale study of young adults, adverse effects were no more frequent among rimantadine recipients than among placebo recipients. Seizures and worsening of congestive heart failure have also been reported in patients treated with amantadine, although a causal relationship has not been established. The dosage of amantadine should be reduced to 100 mg/d in patients with renal insufficiency [i.e., a creatinine clearance rate (Cr_{Cl}) of <50 mL/min] and in the elderly. A rimantadine dose of 100 mg/d should be used for patients with a Cr_{Cl} of <10 mL/min and for the elderly.

■ RIBAVIRIN

Ribavirin is a synthetic nucleoside analogue that inhibits a wide range of RNA and DNA viruses. The mechanism of action of ribavirin is not completely defined and may be different for different groups of viruses. Ribavirin-5′-monophosphate blocks the conversion of inosine-5′-monophosphate to xanthosine-5′-monophosphate and interferes with the synthesis of guanine nucleotides as well as that of both RNA and DNA. Ribavirin-5′-monophosphate also inhibits capping of virus-specific messenger RNA in certain viral systems.

Ribavirin administered as a small-particle aerosol to young children hospitalized with RSV infection has been clinically beneficial and has improved oxygenation in some studies (7 of 11). Although ribavirin has been approved for treatment of infants hospitalized with respiratory syncytial virus (RSV) infection, the American Academy of Pediatrics has recommended that it be considered on an individual basis rather than used routinely in that setting. Aerosolized ribavirin has also been administered to older children and adults (including immunosuppressed patients) with severe RSV and parainfluenza virus infections and to older children and adults with influenza A or B infection, but the benefit of this treatment, if any, is unclear. In RSV infections in immunosuppressed patients, ribavirin is often given in combination with anti-RSV immunoglobulins.

Orally administered ribavirin has not been effective in the treatment of influenza A virus infections. IV or oral ribavirin has reduced mortality rates among patients with Lassa fever; it has been particularly effective in this regard when given within the first 6 days of illness. IV ribavirin has been reported to be of clinical benefit in the treatment of hemorrhagic fever with renal syndrome caused by Hantaan virus and as therapy for Argentinean hemorrhagic fever. Oral ribavirin has also been recommended for the treatment and prophylaxis of Congo-Crimean hemorrhagic fever. An open-label trial suggested that oral ribavirin may be beneficial in the treatment of Nipah virus encephalitis. Use of IV ribavirin in patients with hantavirus pulmonary syndrome in the United States has not been associated with clear-cut benefits. Oral administration of ribavirin reduces serum aminotransferase levels in patients with chronic hepatitis C virus (HCV) infection; since it appears not to reduce serum HCV RNA levels, the mechanism of this effect is unclear. The drug provides added benefit when given by mouth in doses of 800–1200 mg/d in combination with interferon (IFN) α2b or α2a (see below), and the ribavirin/IFN combination has been approved for the treatment of patients with chronic HCV infection. Large oral doses of ribavirin (800–1000 mg/d) have been associated with reversible hematopoietic toxicity. This effect has not been observed with aerosolized ribavirin, apparently because little drug is absorbed systemically. Aerosolized administration of ribavirin is generally well tolerated but occasionally is associated with bronchospasm, rash, or conjunctival irritation. It should be administered under close supervision—particularly in the setting of mechanical ventilation, where precipitation of the drug is possible. Health care workers exposed to the drug have experienced minor toxicity, including eye and respiratory tract irritation. Because ribavirin is mutagenic, teratogenic, and embryotoxic, its use is generally contraindicated in pregnancy. Its administration as an aerosol poses a risk to pregnant health care workers. Because clearance of ribavirin is primarily renal, dose reduction is required in the setting of significant renal dysfunction.

ANTIVIRAL DRUGS ACTIVE AGAINST HERPESVIRUS INFECTIONS

■ ACYCLOVIR AND VALACYCLOVIR

Acyclovir is a highly potent and selective inhibitor of the replication of certain herpesviruses, including herpes simplex virus (HSV) types 1 and 2, varicella-zoster virus (VZV), and Epstein-Barr virus (EBV). It is relatively ineffective in the treatment of human cytomegalovirus (CMV) infections; however, some studies have indicated effectiveness in the prevention of CMV-associated disease in immunosuppressed patients. Valacyclovir, the L-valyl ester of acyclovir, is converted almost entirely to acyclovir by intestinal and hepatic hydrolysis after oral administration. Valacyclovir has pharmacokinetic advantages over orally administered acyclovir: it exhibits significantly greater oral bioavailability, results in higher blood levels, and can be given less frequently than acyclovir (two or three rather than five times daily).

The high degree of selectivity of acyclovir is related to its mechanism of action, which requires that the compound first be phosphorylated to acyclovir monophosphate. This phosphorylation occurs efficiently in herpesvirus-infected cells by means of a virus-coded thymidine kinase. In uninfected mammalian cells, little phosphorylation of acyclovir occurs, and the drug is therefore concentrated in herpesvirus-infected cells. Acyclovir monophosphate is subsequently converted by host cell kinases to a triphosphate that is a potent inhibitor of virus-induced DNA polymerase but has relatively little effect on host cell DNA polymerase. Acyclovir triphosphate can also be incorporated into viral DNA, with early chain termination.

Acyclovir is available in IV, oral, and topical forms, while valacyclovir is available in an oral formulation. IV acyclovir is effective in the treatment of mucocutaneous HSV infections in immunocompromised hosts, in whom it reduces time to healing, duration of pain, and virus shedding. When administered prophylactically during periods of intense immunosuppression (e.g., related to chemotherapy for leukemia or transplantation) and before the development of lesions, IV acyclovir reduces the frequency of HSV-associated disease. After prophylaxis is discontinued, HSV lesions recur. IV acyclovir is also effective in the treatment of HSV encephalitis.

Because VZV is generally less sensitive to acyclovir than is HSV, higher doses of acyclovir must be used to treat VZV infections. In immunocompromised patients with herpes zoster, IV acyclovir reduces the frequency of cutaneous dissemination and visceral complications and—in one comparative trial—was more effective than vidarabine. Acyclovir, administered at oral doses of 800 mg five times a day, had a modest beneficial effect on localized herpes zoster lesions in both immunocompromised and immunocompetent patients. Combination of acyclovir with a tapering regimen of prednisone appeared to be more effective than acyclovir alone in terms of quality-of-life outcomes in immunocompetent patients over age 50 with herpes zoster. A comparative study of acyclovir (800 mg PO five times daily) and valacyclovir (1 g PO three times daily) in immunocompetent patients with herpes zoster indicated that the latter drug may be more effective in eliciting the resolution of zoster-associated pain. Orally administered acyclovir (600 mg five times a day) reduced complications of herpes zoster ophthalmicus in a placebo-controlled trial.

In chickenpox, a modest overall clinical benefit is attained when oral acyclovir therapy is begun within 24 h of the onset of rash in otherwise healthy children (20 mg/kg, up to a maximum of 800 mg, four times a day) or adults (800 mg five times a day). IV acyclovir has also been reported to be effective in the treatment of immunocompromised children with chickenpox.

The most widespread use of acyclovir is in the treatment of genital HSV infections. IV or oral acyclovir or oral valacyclovir has shortened the duration of symptoms, reduced virus shedding, and accelerated healing when employed for the treatment of primary genital HSV infections. Oral acyclovir and valacyclovir have also had a modest effect in treatment of recurrent genital HSV infections. However, the failure of treatment of either primary or recurrent disease to reduce the frequency of subsequent recurrences has indicated that acyclovir is ineffective in eliminating latent infection. Chronic oral administration of acyclovir for ≥1–6 years or of valacyclovir for ≥1 year has reduced the frequency of recurrences markedly during therapy; once the drug is discontinued, lesions recur. In one study, suppressive therapy with valacyclovir (500 mg once daily for 8 months) reduced transmission of HSV-2 genital infections among discordant couples by 50%. A modest effect on herpes labialis (i.e., a reduction of disease duration by 1 day) was seen when valacyclovir was administered upon detection of the first symptom of a lesion at a dose of 2 g every 12 h for 1 day. In

AIDS patients, chronic or intermittent administration of acyclovir has been associated with the development of HSV and VZV strains resistant to the action of the drug and with clinical failures. The most common mechanism of resistance is a deficiency of the virus-induced thymidine kinase. Patients with HSV or VZV infections resistant to acyclovir have frequently responded to foscarnet.

With the availability of the oral and IV forms, there are few indications for topical acyclovir, although treatment with this formulation has been modestly beneficial in primary genital HSV infections and in mucocutaneous HSV infections in immunocompromised hosts.

Overall, acyclovir is remarkably well tolerated and is generally free of toxicity. The most frequently encountered form of toxicity is renal dysfunction because of drug crystallization, particularly after rapid IV administration or with inadequate hydration. Central nervous system changes, including lethargy and tremors, are occasionally reported, primarily in immunosuppressed patients. However, whether these changes are related to acyclovir, to concurrent administration of other therapy, or to underlying infection remains unclear. Acyclovir is excreted primarily unmetabolized by the kidneys via both glomerular filtration and tubular secretion. Approximately 15% of a dose of acyclovir is metabolized to 9-[(carboxymethoxy)methyl]guanine or other minor metabolites. Reduction in dosage is indicated in patients with a Cr_{Cl} of <50 mL/min. The half-life of acyclovir is ~3 h in normal adults, and the peak plasma concentration after a 1-h infusion of a dose of 5 mg/kg is 9.8 μg/mL. Approximately 22% of an orally administered acyclovir dose is absorbed, and peak plasma concentrations of 0.3–0.9 μg/mL are attained after administration of a 200-mg dose. Acyclovir penetrates relatively well into the cerebrospinal fluid (CSF), with concentrations approaching half of those found in plasma.

Acyclovir causes chromosomal breakage at high doses, but its administration to pregnant women has not been associated with fetal abnormalities. Nonetheless, the potential risks and benefits of acyclovir should be carefully assessed before the drug is used in pregnancy.

Valacyclovir exhibits three to five times greater bioavailability than acyclovir. The concentration-time curve for valacyclovir, given as 1 g PO three times daily, is similar to that for acyclovir, given as 5 mg/kg IV every 8 h. The safety profiles of valacyclovir and acyclovir are similar, although thrombotic thrombocytopenic purpura/hemolytic-uremic syndrome has been reported in immunocompromised patients who have received high doses of valacyclovir (8 g/d). Valacyclovir is approved for the treatment of herpes zoster, of initial and recurrent episodes of genital HSV infection, and of herpes labialis in immunocompetent adults as well as for suppressive treatment of genital herpes. Although it has not been extensively studied in other clinical settings involving HSV or VZV infections, many consultants use valacyclovir rather than oral acyclovir in settings where only the latter has been approved because of valacyclovir's superior pharmacokinetics and more convenient dosing schedule.

■ CIDOFOVIR

Cidofovir is a phosphonate nucleotide analogue of cytosine. Its major use is in CMV infections, particularly retinitis, but it is active against a broad range of herpesviruses, including HSV, human herpesvirus (HHV) type 6, HHV-8, and certain other DNA viruses such as polyomaviruses, papillomaviruses, adenoviruses, and poxviruses, including variola (smallpox) and vaccinia. Cidofovir does not require initial phosphorylation by virus-induced kinases; the drug is phosphorylated by host cell enzymes to cidofovir diphosphate, which is a competitive inhibitor of viral DNA polymerases and, to a lesser extent, of host cell DNA polymerases. Incorporation of cidofovir diphosphate slows or terminates nascent DNA chain elongation. Cidofovir is active against HSV isolates that are resistant to acyclovir because of absent or altered thymidine kinase and against CMV isolates that are resistant to ganciclovir because of UL97 phosphotransferase mutations. CMV isolates resistant to ganciclovir on the basis of UL54 mutations are usually resistant to cidofovir as well. Cidofovir is usually active against foscarnet-resistant CMV, although cross-resistance to foscarnet has also been described.

Cidofovir has poor oral availability and is administered intravenously. It is excreted primarily by the kidney and has a plasma half-life of 2.6 h. Cidofovir diphosphate's intracellular half-life of >48 h is the basis for the recommended dosing regimen of 5 mg/kg once a week for the initial 2 weeks and then 5 mg/kg every other week. The major toxic effect of cidofovir is proximal renal tubular injury, as manifested by elevated serum creatinine levels and proteinuria. The risk of nephrotoxicity can be reduced by vigorous saline hydration and by concomitant oral administration of probenecid. Neutropenia, rashes, and gastrointestinal tolerance may also occur.

IV cidofovir has been approved for the treatment of CMV retinitis in AIDS patients who are intolerant of ganciclovir or foscarnet or in whom those drugs have failed. In a controlled study, a maintenance dosage of 5 mg/kg per week administered to AIDS patients reduced the progression of CMV retinitis from that seen at 3 mg/kg. Intravitreal cidofovir has been used to treat CMV retinitis but has been associated with significant toxicity. IV cidofovir has been reported anecdotally to be effective for treatment of acyclovir-resistant mucocutaneous HSV infections. Likewise, topically administered cidofovir is reportedly beneficial against mucocutaneous HSV infections in HIV-infected patients. Anecdotal use of IV cidofovir has been described in disseminated adenoviral infections in immunosuppressed patients and in genitourinary infections with BK virus in renal transplant recipients; however, its efficacy, if any, in these circumstances is not established.

■ FOMIVIRSEN

Fomivirsen is the first antisense oligonucleotide approved by the FDA for therapy in humans. This phosphorothioate oligonucleotide, 21 nucleotides in length, inhibits CMV replication through interaction with CMV messenger RNA. Fomivirsen is complementary to messenger transcripts of the major immediate early region 2 (IE2) of CMV, which codes for proteins regulating viral gene expression. In addition to its antisense mechanism of action, fomivirsen may exert activity against CMV through inhibition of viral adsorption to cells as well as direct inhibition of viral replication. Because of its different mechanism of action, fomivirsen is active against CMV isolates that are resistant to nucleoside or nucleotide analogues, such as ganciclovir, foscarnet, or cidofovir.

Fomivirsen has been approved for intravitreal administration in the treatment of CMV retinitis in AIDS patients who have failed to respond to other treatments or cannot tolerate them. Injections of 330 mg for two doses 2 weeks apart, followed by maintenance doses of 330 mg monthly, significantly reduce the rate of progression of CMV retinitis. The major toxicity is ocular inflammation, including vitritis and iritis, which usually responds to topically administered glucocorticoids.

■ GANCICLOVIR AND VALGANCICLOVIR

An analogue of acyclovir, ganciclovir is active against HSV and VZV and is markedly more active than acyclovir against CMV. Ganciclovir triphosphate inhibits CMV DNA polymerase and can be incorporated into CMV DNA, whose elongation it eventually terminates. In HSV- and VZV-infected cells, ganciclovir is phosphorylated by virus-encoded thymidine kinases; in CMV-infected cells, it is phosphorylated by a viral kinase encoded by the UL97 gene. Ganciclovir triphosphate is present in tenfold higher concentrations in CMV-infected cells than in uninfected

cells. Ganciclovir is approved for the treatment of CMV retinitis in immunosuppressed patients and for the prevention of CMV disease in transplant recipients. It is widely used for the treatment of other CMV-associated syndromes, including pneumonia, esophagogastrointestinal infections, hepatitis, and "wasting" illness.

Ganciclovir is available for IV or oral administration. Because its oral bioavailability is low (5–9%), relatively large doses (1 g three times daily) must be administered by this route. Oral ganciclovir has largely been supplanted by valganciclovir, which is the L-valyl ester of ganciclovir. Valganciclovir is well absorbed orally, with a bioavailability of 60%, and is rapidly hydrolyzed to ganciclovir in the intestine and liver. The area under the curve for a 900-mg dose of valganciclovir is equivalent to that for 5 mg/kg of IV ganciclovir, although peak serum concentrations are ~40% lower for valganciclovir. The serum half-life is 3.5 h after IV administration of ganciclovir and 4.0 h after PO administration of valganciclovir. Ganciclovir is excreted primarily by the kidneys in an unmetabolized form, and its dosage should be reduced in cases of renal failure. Ganciclovir therapy at the most commonly employed initial IV dosage—i.e., 5 mg/kg every 12 h for 14–21 days—can be changed to valganciclovir (900 mg PO twice daily) when the patient can tolerate oral therapy. The maintenance dose is 5 mg/kg IV daily or five times per week for ganciclovir and 900 mg by mouth once a day for valganciclovir. Dose adjustment in patients with renal dysfunction is required. Intraocular ganciclovir, given by either intravitreal injection or intraocular implantation, has also been used to treat CMV retinitis.

Ganciclovir is effective as prophylaxis against CMV-associated disease in organ and bone marrow transplant recipients. Oral ganciclovir administered prophylactically to AIDS patients with CD4+ T cell counts of <100/μL has provided protection against the development of CMV retinitis. However, the long-term benefits of this approach to prophylaxis in AIDS patients have not been established, and most experts do not recommend the use of oral ganciclovir for this purpose. As already mentioned, valganciclovir has supplanted oral ganciclovir in settings where oral prophylaxis or therapy is considered.

The administration of ganciclovir has been associated with profound bone marrow suppression, particularly neutropenia, which significantly limits the drug's use in many patients. Bone marrow toxicity is potentiated in the setting of renal dysfunction and when other bone marrow suppressants, such as zidovudine or mycophenolate mofetil, are used concomitantly.

Resistance has been noted in CMV isolates obtained after therapy with ganciclovir, especially in patients with AIDS. Such resistance may develop through a mutation in either the viral UL97 gene or the viral DNA polymerase. Ganciclovir-resistant isolates are usually sensitive to foscarnet (see below) or cidofovir (see above).

■ FAMCICLOVIR AND PENCICLOVIR

Famciclovir is the diacetyl 6-deoxyester of the guanosine analogue penciclovir. Famciclovir is well absorbed orally, has a bioavailability of 77%, and is rapidly converted to penciclovir by deacetylation and oxidation in the intestine and liver. Penciclovir's spectrum of activity and mechanism of action are similar to those of acyclovir. Thus, penciclovir usually is not active against acyclovir-resistant viruses. However, some acyclovir-resistant viruses with altered thymidine kinase or DNA polymerase substrate specificity may be sensitive to penciclovir. This drug is phosphorylated initially by a virus-encoded thymidine kinase and subsequently by cellular kinases to penciclovir triphosphate, which inhibits HSV-1, HSV-2, VZV, and EBV as well as hepatitis B virus (HBV). The serum half-life of penciclovir is 2 h, but the intracellular half-life of penciclovir triphosphate is 7–20 h—markedly longer than that of acyclovir triphosphate. The latter is the basis for the less frequent (twice-daily) dosing schedule for famciclovir than for acyclovir. Penciclovir is eliminated primarily in the urine by both glomerular filtration and tubular secretion. The usually recommended dosage interval should be adjusted for renal insufficiency.

Clinical trials involving immunocompetent adults with herpes zoster showed that famciclovir was superior to placebo in eliciting the resolution of skin lesions and virus shedding and in shortening the duration of postherpetic neuralgia; moreover, administered at 500 mg every 8 h, famciclovir was at least as effective as acyclovir administered at an oral dose of 800 mg five times daily. Famciclovir was also effective in the treatment of herpes zoster in immunosuppressed patients. Clinical trials have demonstrated its effectiveness in the suppression of genital HSV infections for up to 1 year and in the treatment of initial and recurrent episodes of genital herpes. Famciclovir is effective as therapy for mucocutaneous HSV infections in HIV-infected patients. Application of a 1% penciclovir cream reduces the duration of signs and symptoms of herpes labialis in immunocompetent patients (by 0.5–1 day) and has been approved for that purpose by the FDA. Famciclovir is generally well tolerated, with occasional headache, nausea, and diarrhea reported in frequencies similar to those among placebo recipients. The administration of high doses of famciclovir for 2 years was associated with an increased incidence of mammary adenocarcinomas in female rats, but the clinical significance of this effect is unknown.

◼ FOSCARNET

Foscarnet (phosphonoformic acid) is a pyrophosphate-containing compound that potently inhibits herpesviruses, including CMV. This drug inhibits DNA polymerases at the pyrophosphate binding site at concentrations that have relatively little effect on cellular polymerases. Foscarnet does not require phosphorylation to exert its antiviral activity and is therefore active against HSV and VZV isolates that are resistant to acyclovir because of deficiencies in thymidine kinase as well as against most ganciclovir-resistant strains of CMV. Foscarnet also inhibits the reverse transcriptase of HIV and is active against HIV in vivo.

Foscarnet is poorly soluble and must be administered intravenously via an infusion pump in a dilute solution over 1–2 h. The plasma half-life of foscarnet is 3–5 h and increases with decreasing renal function, since the drug is eliminated primarily by the kidneys. It has been estimated that 10–28% of a dose may be deposited in bone, where it can persist for months. The most common initial dosage of foscarnet—60 mg/kg every 8 h for 14–21 days—is followed by a maintenance dose of 90–120 mg/kg once a day.

Foscarnet is approved for the treatment of CMV retinitis in patients with AIDS and of acyclovir-resistant mucocutaneous HSV infections. In a comparative clinical trial, the drug appeared to be about as efficacious as ganciclovir against CMV retinitis but was associated with a longer survival period, possibly because of its activity against HIV. Intraocular foscarnet has been used to treat CMV retinitis. Foscarnet has also been employed to treat acyclovir-resistant HSV and VZV infections as well as ganciclovir-resistant CMV infections, although resistance to foscarnet has been reported in CMV isolates obtained during therapy. Foscarnet has also been used to treat HHV-6 infections in immunosuppressed patients.

The major form of toxicity associated with foscarnet is renal impairment. Thus renal function should be monitored closely, particularly during the initial phase of therapy. Since foscarnet binds divalent metal ions, hypocalcemia, hypomagnesemia, hypokalemia, and hypo- or hyperphosphatemia can develop. Saline hydration and slow infusion appear to protect the patient against nephrotoxicity and electrolyte disturbances. Although hematologic abnormalities have been documented (most commonly anemia), foscarnet is not

generally myelosuppressive and can be administered concomitantly with myelosuppressive medications such as zidovudine.

◼ TRIFLURIDINE

Trifluridine is a pyrimidine nucleoside active against HSV-1, HSV-2, and CMV. Trifluridine monophosphate irreversibly inhibits thymidylate synthetase, and trifluridine triphosphate inhibits viral and, to a lesser extent, cellular DNA polymerases. Because of systemic toxicity, its use is limited to topical therapy. Trifluridine is approved for treatment of HSV keratitis, against which trials have shown that it is more effective than topical idoxuridine but similar in efficacy to topical vidarabine. The drug has benefited some patients with HSV keratitis who have failed to respond to idoxuridine or vidarabine. Topical application of trifluridine to sites of acyclovir-resistant HSV mucocutaneous infections has also been beneficial in some cases.

◼ VIDARABINE

Vidarabine is a purine nucleoside analogue with activity against HSV-1, HSV-2, VZV, and EBV. Vidarabine inhibits viral DNA synthesis through its 5′-triphosphorylated metabolite, although its precise molecular mechanisms of action are not completely understood. IV-administered vidarabine has been shown to be effective in the treatment of herpes simplex encephalitis, mucocutaneous HSV infections, herpes zoster in immunocompromised patients, and neonatal HSV infections. Its use has been supplanted by that of IV acyclovir, which is more effective and easier to administer. Production of the IV preparation has been discontinued by the manufacturer, but vidarabine is available as an ophthalmic ointment, which is effective in the treatment of HSV keratitis.

ANTIVIRAL DRUGS ACTIVE AGAINST HEPATITIS VIRUSES

◼ LAMIVUDINE

Lamivudine is a pyrimidine nucleoside analogue that is used primarily in combination therapy against HIV infection (Chap. 189). Its activity against hepatitis B virus (HBV) is attributable to inhibition of the viral DNA polymerase. This drug has also been approved for the treatment of chronic HBV infection. At doses of 100 mg/d given for 1 year to patients positive for hepatitis B e antigen (HBeAg), lamivudine is well tolerated and results in suppression of HBV DNA levels, normalization of serum aminotransferase levels in 40–75% of patients, and reduction of hepatic inflammation and fibrosis in 50–60% of patients. Loss of HBeAg occurs in 30% of patients. Lamivudine also appears to be useful in the prevention or suppression of HBV infection associated with liver transplantation. Resistance to lamivudine develops in 24% of patients treated for 1 year and is associated with changes in the YMDD motif of HBV DNA polymerase. Because of the frequency of development of resistance, lamivudine has been largely supplanted by less-resistance-prone drugs for the treatment of HBV infection.

◼ ADEFOVIR DIPIVOXIL

Adefovir dipivoxil is the oral prodrug of adefovir, an acyclic nucleotide analogue of adenosine monophosphate that has activity against HBV, HIV, HSV, CMV, and poxviruses. It is phosphorylated by cellular kinases to the active triphosphate moiety, which is a competitive inhibitor of HBV DNA polymerase and results in chain termination after incorporation into nascent viral DNA. Adefovir is administered orally and is eliminated primarily by the kidneys, with a plasma half-life of 5–7.5 h. In clinical studies, therapy with adefovir at a dose of 10 mg/d for 48 weeks resulted in normalization of serum alanine aminotransferase (ALT) levels in 48–72% of patients and improved liver histology in 53–64%; it also resulted in a 3.5- to 3.9-$\log_{10}$ reduction in the number of HBV DNA copies per milliliter of plasma. Adefovir was effective in treatment-naïve patients as well as in those infected with lamivudine-resistant HBV. Resistance to adefovir appears to develop less readily than that to lamivudine, but adefovir resistance rates of 15–18% have been reported after 192 weeks of treatment and may reach 30% after 5 years. This agent is generally well tolerated. Significant nephrotoxicity attributable to adefovir is uncommon at the dose employed in the treatment of HBV infections (10 mg/d) but is a treatment-limiting adverse effect at the higher doses used in therapy for HIV infections (30–120 mg/d). In any case, renal function should be monitored in patients taking adefovir, even at the lower dose. Adefovir is approved only for treatment of chronic HBV infection.

TENOFOVIR

Tenofovir disoproxil fumarate is a prodrug of tenofovir, a nucleotide analogue of adenosine monophosphate with activity against both retroviruses and hepadnaviruses. In both immunocompetent and immunocompromised patients (including those co-infected with HIV and HBV), tenofovir given at a dose of 300 mg/d for 48 weeks reduced HBV replication by 4.6–6 $\log_{10}$, normalized ALT levels in 68–76% of patients, and improved liver histopathology in 72–74% of patients. Resistance develops uncommonly during ≥2 years of therapy, and tenofovir is active against lamivudine-resistant HBV. The safety profile of tenofovir is similar to that of adefovir, but nephrotoxicity has not been encountered at the dose used for HBV therapy. Tenofovir is approved for the treatment of HIV and chronic HBV infections. For a more detailed discussion of tenofovir, see Chap. 189.

ENTECAVIR

Entecavir is a cyclopentyl 2′-deoxyguanosine analogue that inhibits HBV through interaction of entecavir triphosphate with several HBV DNA polymerase functions. At a dose of 0.5 mg/d given for 48 weeks, entecavir reduced HBV DNA copies by 5.0–6.9 $\log_{10}$, normalized serum aminotransferase levels in 68–78% of patients, and improved histopathology in 70–72% of patients. Entecavir inhibits lamivudine-resistant viruses that have M550I or M550V/L526M mutations but only at serum concentrations 20- or 30-fold higher than those obtained with the 0.5-mg/d dose. Thus, higher doses of entecavir (1 mg/d) are recommended for the treatment of patients infected with lamivudine-resistant HBV. Development of resistance to entecavir is uncommon in treatment-naïve patients but does occur at unacceptably high rates (43% after 4 years) in patients previously infected with lamivudine-resistant virus. Entecavir-resistant strains appear to be sensitive to adefovir and tenofovir.

Entecavir is highly bioavailable but should be taken on an empty stomach since food interferes with its absorption. The drug is eliminated primarily in unchanged form by the kidneys, and its dosage should be adjusted for patients with Cr_{Cl} values of <50 mL/min. Overall, entecavir is well tolerated, with a safety profile similar to that of lamivudine. As with other anti-HBV treatments, exacerbation of hepatitis may occur when entecavir therapy is stopped. Entecavir is approved for treatment of chronic hepatitis B, including infection with lamivudine-resistant viruses, in adults. Entecavir has some activity against HIV-1 (median effective concentration, 0.026 to >10 μM) but should not be used as monotherapy in HIV-positive patients because of the potential for development of HIV resistance due to the M184V mutation.

TELBIVUDINE

Telbivudine is a β-L enantiomer of thymidine and is a potent, selective inhibitor of HBV. Its active form is telbivudine triphosphate, which inhibits HBV DNA polymerase and causes chain termination but has little or no activity against human DNA polymerase. Administration of telbivudine at an oral dose of 600 mg/d for 52 weeks to patients with chronic hepatitis B resulted in reduction of HBV DNA by 5.2–6.4 $\log_{10}$ copies/mL along with normalization of ALT levels in 74–77% of recipients and improved histopathology in 65–67% of patients. Telbivudine-resistant HBV is generally cross-resistant with lamivudine-resistant virus but is usually susceptible to adefovir. After 2 years of therapy, resistance to telbivudine was noted in isolates from 22% of HBeAg-positive patients and in those from 9% of HBeAg-negative patients.

Orally administered telbivudine is rapidly absorbed; because it is eliminated primarily by the kidneys, its dosage should be reduced in patients with a Cr_{Cl} value of <50 mL/min. Telbivudine is generally well tolerated, but increases in serum levels of creatinine kinases as well as fatigue and myalgias have been observed. As with other anti-HBV drugs, hepatitis may be exacerbated in patients who discontinue telbivudine therapy. Telbivudine has been approved for the treatment of adults with chronic hepatitis B who have evidence of viral replication and either persistently elevated serum aminotransferase levels or histopathologically active disease, but it has not been widely used because of the frequency of development of resistance noted above.

INTERFERONS

IFNs are cytokines that exhibit a broad spectrum of antiviral activities as well as immunomodulating and antiproliferative properties. IFNs are not available for oral administration but must be given IM, SC, or IV. Early studies with human leukocyte IFN demonstrated an effect in the prophylaxis of experimentally induced rhinovirus infections in humans and in the treatment of VZV infections in immunosuppressed patients. DNA recombinant technology has made available highly purified α, β, and γ IFNs that have been evaluated in a variety of viral infections. Results of such trials have confirmed the effectiveness of intranasally administered IFN in the prophylaxis of rhinovirus infections, although its use has been associated with nasal mucosal irritation. Studies have also demonstrated a beneficial effect of intralesionally or systemically administered IFNs on genital warts. The effect of systemic administration consists primarily of a reduction in the size of the warts, and this mode of therapy may be useful in persons who have numerous warts that cannot easily be treated by individual intralesional injections. However, lesions frequently recur after either intralesional or systemic IFN therapy is discontinued.

IFNs have undergone extensive study in the treatment of chronic HBV infection. The administration of standard IFN-α2b (5 million units daily or 10 million units three times a week for 16–24 weeks) to patients with stable chronic HBV infection resulted in loss of markers of HBV replication, such as HBeAg and HBV DNA, in 33–37% of cases; 8% of patients also became negative for hepatitis B surface antigen. In most patients who lose HBeAg and HBV DNA markers, serum aminotransferases return to normal levels, and both short- and long-term improvements in liver histopathology have been described. Predictors of a favorable response to standard IFN therapy include low pretherapy levels of HBV DNA, high pretherapy serum levels of ALT, a short duration of chronic HBV infection, and active inflammation in liver histopathology. Poor responses are seen in immunosuppressed patients, including those with HIV infection.

In pegylated IFNs, IFN alphas are linked to polyethylene glycol. This linkage results in slower absorption, decreased clearance, and more sustained serum concentrations, thereby permitting a more convenient, once-weekly dosing schedule; in many instances, pegylated IFN has supplanted standard IFN. After 48 weeks of treatment with 180 μg of pegylated IFN-α2a, HBV DNA was reduced by 4.1–4.5 $\log_{10}$ copies/mL, with normalization of serum ALT levels in 39% of patients and improved histology in 38%. Response rates were somewhat higher when lamivudine was administered with pegylated IFN-α2a. Adverse effects of IFN are common and include fever, chills, myalgia, fatigue, neurotoxicity (manifested primarily as somnolence, depression, anxiety, and confusion), and leukopenia. Autoantibodies (e.g., antithyroid antibodies) can also develop. IFN-α2b and pegylated IFN-α2a are approved for the treatment of patients with chronic hepatitis B. Data supporting the therapeutic efficacy of pegylated interferon-α2b in HBV infection have been published; the drug has not been approved for this indication in the United States but has been approved for treatment of chronic HBV infection in other countries.

Several IFN preparations, including IFN-α2a, IFN-α2b, IFN-alfacon-1, and IFN-αm1 (lymphoblastoid), have been studied as therapy for chronic HCV infections. A variety of monotherapy regimens have been studied, of which the most common for standard IFN is IFN-α2b or -α2a at 3 million units three times per week for 12–18 months. The addition of oral ribavirin to IFN-α2b—either as initial therapy or after failure of IFN therapy alone—results in significantly higher rates of sustained virologic and/or serum ALT responses (40–50%) than are obtained with monotherapy. Comparative studies indicate that pegylated IFN-α2b or -α2a therapy is more effective than standard IFN treatment against chronic HCV infection. The combination of SC pegylated IFN and oral ribavirin is more convenient and appears to be the most effective regimen for treatment of chronic hepatitis C. With this combination regimen, sustained virologic responses (SVRs) were seen in 42–51% of patients with genotype 1 infection and in 76–82% of patients with genotype 2 or 3 infection. Ribavirin appears to have a small antiviral effect in HCV infection but may also be working through an immunomodulatory effect in combination with IFN. Optimal results with ribavirin appear to be associated with weight-based dosing. Prognostic factors for a favorable response include an age of <40 years, a short duration of infection, low levels of HCV RNA, a lesser degree of liver histopathology, and infection with HCV genotypes other than 1. IFN-alfacon, a synthetic "consensus" α interferon, appears to produce response rates similar to those elicited by standard IFN-α2a or -α2b alone and is also approved in the United States for the treatment of chronic hepatitis C.

The efficacy of IFN-α treatment for chronic hepatitis D remains unestablished. Anecdotal reports suggested that doses ranging from 5 million units daily to 9 million units three times per week for 12 months elicit biochemical and virologic responses. Results from small controlled trials have been inconsistent, and observed responses have not generally been sustained. Limited experience has been published with the use of pegylated IFN-α2a or -α2b for treatment of hepatitis D, but some consultants prefer these agents for this indication because of their pharmacologic advantages over standard IFN.

PROTEASE INHIBITORS

This drug class is specifically designed to inhibit the 3/4A (NS3/4A) HCV protease. These agents resemble the HCV polypeptide and, when processed by the viral protease, form a covalent bond with the catalytic serine residues and block further activity. The most clinically advanced compound in this class is telaprevir. In initial phase 1 and 2 clinical studies, telaprevir monotherapy decreased the HCV load by 2–5 $\log_{10}$. Telaprevir in combination with IFN and ribavirin increased the SVR rate from ~40% to 60% when used

as primary therapy for genotype 1 infections. For re-treatment of HCV-infected patients in whom prior IFN/ribavirin therapy had failed, the addition of telaprevir plus pegylated IFN/ribavirin increased the SVR rate to 51–53%. The combination of telaprevir/pegylated IFN and ribavirin is superior to this combination without ribavirin. Typically, an oral loading dose of 1125 mg is followed by 750 mg every 8 h orally for 12–24 weeks. Monotherapy is associated with the rapid emergence of antiviral resistance; substitutions are found in the NS3 protease, especially double variants at positions V35M and R155K. Telaprevir therapy is associated with rashes in ~50% of patients; these eruptions are severe in ~5% of cases and often develop weeks after therapy has begun. Data suggest that telaprevir has the potential to increase the SVR rate and may shorten the overall duration of HCV therapy from 48 to 24 weeks when used in conjunction with pegylated IFN and ribavirin. As of this writing (February 2011), protease inhibitors have not been approved for treatment of HCV.

FURTHER READINGS

AOKI F et al: Antiviral drugs (other than antiretrovirals), in *Principles and Practice of Infectious Diseases*, 7th ed, GL Mandell et al (eds). Philadelphia, Elsevier Churchill Livingstone, 2010, pp 565–610

COUCH RB: Drug therapy: Prevention and treatment of influenza. N Engl J Med 343:1778, 2000

CRUMPACKER CS: Ganciclovir. N Engl J Med 335:721, 1996

DOLIN R et al: A controlled trial of amantadine and rimantadine in the prophylaxis of influenza A infection. N Engl J Med 307:580, 1982

FIELD JJ, HOOFNAGLE JH: Mechanism of action of interferon and ribavirin in treatment of hepatitis C. Nature 436:967, 2005

GISH RG et al: Safety and antiviral activity of emtricitabine (FTC) for the treatment of chronic hepatitis B infection: A two-year study. J Hepatol 43:60, 2005

HALL CB et al: Aerosolized ribavirin treatment of infants with respiratory syncytial viral infection: A randomized double-blind study. N Engl J Med 308:1443, 1983

LAI CL et al: Entecavir versus lamivudine for patients with HBeAg-negative chronic hepatitis B. N Engl J Med 354:186, 2006

LALEZARI JP et al: Randomized controlled study of the safety and efficacy of IV cidofovir for the treatment of relapsing cytomegalovirus retinitis in patients with AIDS. J AIDS 17:339, 1998

LOK AS et al: Management of hepatitis B: 2000—summary of a workshop. Gastroenterology 120:1828, 2001

MARTIN DF et al: A controlled trial of valganciclovir as induction therapy for cytomegalovirus retinitis. N Engl J Med 346:1119, 2002

NATIONAL INSTITUTES OF HEALTH CONSENSUS DEVELOPMENT CONFERENCE STATEMENT: Management of hepatitis C. September 12, 2002 (available at *www.niaid.nih.gov*)

PIRET J, BOIVIN G: Resistance of herpes simplex viruses to nucleoside analogues: Mechanisms, prevalence, and management. Antimicrob Agents Chemother 55:459, 2011

TREANOR JJ et al: Efficacy and safety in treating acute influenza: A randomized controlled trial. U.S. Oral Neuraminidase Study Group. JAMA 283:1016, 2000

CHAPTER **179**

Herpes Simplex Virus Infections

Lawrence Corey

■ DEFINITION

Herpes simplex viruses (HSV-1, HSV-2; *Herpesvirus hominis*) produce a variety of infections involving mucocutaneous surfaces, the central nervous system (CNS), and—on occasion—visceral organs. Prompt recognition and treatment reduce the morbidity and mortality rates associated with HSV infections.

■ ETIOLOGIC AGENT

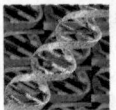
The genome of HSV is a linear, double-strand DNA molecule (molecular weight, ~100 × 10^6) that encodes >90 transcription units with 84 identified proteins. The genomic structures of the two HSV subtypes are similar. The overall genomic sequence homology between HSV-1 and HSV-2 is ~50%, while the proteome homology is >80%. The homologous sequences are distributed over the entire genome map, and most of the polypeptides specified by one viral type are antigenically related to polypeptides of the other viral type. Many type-specific regions unique to HSV-1 and HSV-2 proteins do exist, however, and a number of them appear to be important in host immunity. These type-specific regions have been used to develop serologic assays that distinguish between the two viral subtypes. Either restriction endonuclease analysis or sequencing of viral DNA can be used to distinguish between the two subtypes and among strains of each subtype. The variability of nucleotide sequences from clinical strains of HSV-1 and HSV-2 is such that HSV isolates obtained from two individuals can be differentiated by restriction enzyme patterns or genomic sequences. Moreover, epidemiologically related sources, such as sexual partners, mother-infant pairs, or persons involved in a common-source outbreak, can be inferred from such patterns.

The viral genome is packaged in a regular icosahedral protein shell (capsid) composed of 162 capsomeres (see Fig. 177-1). The outer covering of the virus is a lipid-containing membrane (envelope) acquired as the DNA-containing capsid buds through the inner nuclear membrane of the host cell. Between the capsid and lipid bilayer of the envelope is the tegument. Viral replication has both nuclear and cytoplasmic phases. Initial attachment to the cell membrane involves interactions of viral glycoproteins C and B with several cellular heparan sulfate–like surface receptors. Subsequently, viral glycoprotein D binds to cellular co-receptors that belong to the tumor necrosis factor receptor family of proteins, the immunoglobulin superfamily (nectin family), or both. The ubiquity of these receptors contributes to the wide host range of herpesviruses. Replication is highly regulated. After fusion and entry, the nucleocapsid enters the cytoplasm and several viral proteins are released from the virion. Some of these viral proteins shut off host protein synthesis (by increasing cellular RNA degradation), while others "turn on" the transcription of early genes of HSV replication. These early gene products, designated α *genes*, are required for synthesis of the subsequent polypeptide group, the β polypeptides, many of which are regulatory proteins and enzymes required for DNA replication. Most current antiviral drugs interfere with β proteins, such as viral DNA polymerase. The third (γ) class of HSV genes requires viral DNA replication for expression and constitutes most structural proteins specified by the virus.

After viral genome replication and structural protein synthesis, nucleocapsids are assembled in the cell's nucleus. Envelopment occurs as the nucleocapsids bud through the inner nuclear membrane into the perinuclear space. In some cells, viral replication in the nucleus forms two types of inclusion bodies: type A basophilic Feulgen-positive bodies that contain viral DNA and eosinophilic inclusion bodies that are devoid of viral nucleic acid or protein and represent a "scar" of viral infection. Enveloped virions are then transported via the endoplasmic reticulum and the Golgi apparatus to the cell surface.

Viral genomes are maintained by some neuronal cells in a repressed state called *latency*. Latency, which is associated with transcription of only a limited number of virus-encoded RNAs, accounts for the presence of viral DNA and RNA in neural tissue at times when infectious virus cannot be isolated. Maintenance and growth of neural cells from latently infected ganglia in tissue culture result in production of infectious virions (explantation) and in subsequent permissive infection of susceptible cells (cocultivation). Activation of the viral genome may then occur, resulting in *reactivation*, the normal pattern of regulated viral gene expression, replication, and release of HSV. The release of virions from the neuron follows a complex process of anterograde transport down the length of neuronal axons. In experimental animals, ultraviolet light, systemic and local immunosuppression, and trauma to the skin or ganglia are associated with reactivation.

To date, three noncoding RNA latency-associated transcripts (LATs) are the only abundant transcripts in the nuclei of latently infected neurons. Deletion mutants of the genomic region that can become latent have been made, and the efficiency of their later reactivation is reduced. In addition, substitution of HSV-1 LATs for HSV-2 LATs induces an HSV-1 reactivation pattern. Thus, LATs appear to maintain—rather than establish—latency. HSV-1 LATs promote the survival of acutely infected neurons, perhaps by inhibiting apoptotic pathways. Highly expressed during latency, LAT-derived micro-RNA appears to silence expression of the key neurovirulence factor infected-cell protein 34.5 (ICP34.5) and to bind in an antisense configuration to ICP0 messenger RNA to prevent expression of this immediate-early protein, which is vital to HSV reactivation. Studies of individual neurons from cadaveric trigeminal ganglionic explants by microdissection and real-time polymerase chain reaction (PCR) revealed that many more neurons (2–11%) harbor HSV than would be predicted by in situ hybridization studies for LAT and that DNA copy number is similar in LAT-positive and LAT-negative neurons. These findings make it less clear what role LATs play in preventing reactivation. At present, the molecular mechanisms of HSV latency are not completely understood; CD8+ T cells have been found in ganglia of experimental animals and humans and appear to influence the process of reactivation, possibly by inducing antiviral factors such as interferon (IFN) γ. Strategies to interrupt or maintain latency in neurons are not available.

■ PATHOGENESIS

Exposure to HSV at mucosal surfaces or abraded skin sites permits entry of the virus into cells of the epidermis and dermis and initiation of viral replication therein. HSV infections are usually acquired subclinically. Whether clinical or subclinical, HSV acquisition is associated with sufficient viral replication to permit infection of either sensory or autonomic nerve endings. On entry into the neuronal cell, the virus—or, more likely, the nucleocapsid—is transported intra-axonally to the nerve cell bodies in ganglia. In humans, the transit interval from inoculation of virus in peripheral tissue to spread to the ganglia is unknown. During the initial phase of infection, viral replication occurs in ganglia and contiguous neural tissue. Virus then spreads to other mucocutaneous surfaces through centrifugal migration of infectious virions via peripheral sensory nerves. This mode of spread helps explain the large surface area involved, the high frequency of new lesions distant from the initial crop of vesicles that is characteristic in patients with primary genital or oral-labial HSV infection, and the ability to recover virus from neural tissue distant from neurons innervating the inoculation site. Contiguous spread of locally inoculated virus also may take place and allow further mucosal extension of disease. Recent studies have demonstrated HSV viremia—another mechanism for extension of infection throughout the body—in ~30–40% of persons with primary HSV-2 infection. Latent infection with both viral subtypes in both sensory and autonomic ganglia has been demonstrated. For HSV-1 infection, trigeminal ganglia are most commonly infected, although extension to the inferior and superior cervical ganglia also occurs. With genital infection, sacral nerve root ganglia (S2–S5) are most commonly affected.

After resolution of primary disease, infectious HSV can no longer be cultured from the ganglia; however, latent infection, as defined by the presence of viral DNA, persists in 2–11% of ganglionic cells in the anatomic region of the initial infection. The mechanism of reactivation from latency is unknown. Increasingly, studies indicate that host T cell responses at the ganglionic and peripheral mucosal level influence the frequency and severity of HSV reactivation. HSV-specific T cells have been recovered from peripheral nerve root ganglia. Many of these resident CD8+ T cells are juxtaposed with latently HSV-1-infected neurons in the trigeminal ganglia and can block reactivation with both IFN-γ release and granzyme B degradation of the immediate-early protein ICP4. In addition, there appears to be a latent viral load in the ganglia that correlates positively with the number of neurons infected and the rate of reactivation but inversely with the number of CD8+ cells present. It is not known whether reactivating stimuli transiently suppress these immune cells, independently upregulate transcription of lytic genes, or both. However, once virus reaches the dermal-epidermal junction, there are two possible outcomes: subclinical shedding or recurrence (the latter defined clinically by a skin blister and ulceration). Histologically, herpetic lesions involve a thin-walled vesicle or ulceration in the basal region, multinucleated cells that may include intranuclear inclusions, necrosis, and an acute inflammatory infection. Re-epithelialization occurs once viral replication is restricted, almost always in the absence of a scar.

Analysis of the DNA from sequential isolates of HSV or from isolates from multiple infected ganglia in any one individual has revealed similar, if not identical, restriction endonuclease or DNA sequence patterns in most persons. The finding of individual neurons infected with multiple strains of drug-susceptible and drug-resistant virus in severely immunosuppressed patients indicates that ganglia can be reseeded during chronic infection. As exposure to

mucosal shedding is relatively common during a person's lifetime, current data suggest that exogenous infection with different strains of the same subtype, while possible, is uncommon.

■ IMMUNITY

Host responses influence the acquisition of HSV disease, the severity of infection, resistance to the development of latency, the maintenance of latency, and the frequency of recurrences. Both antibody-mediated and cell-mediated reactions are clinically important. Immunocompromised patients with defects in cell-mediated immunity experience more severe and more extensive HSV infections than those with deficits in humoral immunity, such as agammaglobulinemia. Experimental ablation of lymphocytes indicates that T cells play a major role in preventing lethal disseminated disease, although antibodies help reduce titers of virus in neural tissue. Some clinical manifestations of HSV appear to be related to the host immune response (e.g., stromal opacities associated with recurrent herpetic keratitis). The surface viral glycoproteins have been shown to be targets of antibodies that mediate neutralization and immune-mediated cytolysis (antibody-dependent cell-mediated cytotoxicity). Monoclonal antibodies specific for each of the known viral glycoproteins have, in experimental infections, conferred protection against subsequent neurologic disease or ganglionic latency. In humans, however, subunit glycoprotein vaccines have been only partially successful in reducing acquisition of infection. Multiple cell populations, including natural killer cells, macrophages, and a variety of T lymphocytes, play a role in host defenses against HSV infections, as do lymphokines generated by T lymphocytes. In animals, passive transfer of primed lymphocytes confers protection from subsequent challenge. Maximal protection usually requires the activation of multiple T cell subpopulations, including cytotoxic T cells and T cells responsible for delayed hypersensitivity. The latter cells may confer protection by the antigen-stimulated release of lymphokines (e.g., IFNs), which in turn have a direct antiviral effect and both activate and enhance a variety of specific and nonspecific effector cells. Increasing evidence suggests that HSV-specific CD8+ T cell responses are critical for clearance of virus from lesions. In addition, immunosuppressed patients with frequent and prolonged HSV lesions have fewer functional CD8+ T cells directed at HSV. The HSV virion contains a variety of genes that are directed at the inhibition of host responses. These include gene no. 12 (US-12), which can bind to the cellular transporter-activating protein TAP-1 and reduce the ability of this protein to bind HSV peptides to human leukocyte antigen (HLA) class I, thereby reducing recognition of viral proteins by cytotoxic T cells of the host. This effect can be overcome by the addition of IFN-γ, but this reversal requires 24–48 h; thus, the virus has time to replicate and invade other host cells. Entry of infectious HSV-1 and HSV-2 inhibits several signaling pathways of both CD4+ and CD8+ T cells, leading to their functional impairment in killing and influencing the spectrum of their cytokine secretion.

Recent studies suggest that the rate of HSV reactivation is far more frequent than previously recognized. PCR analysis of daily anogenital swab samples has shown that the virus is shed on a median of 25% of days by the 95% of patients who are positive for antibody to HSV-2 and who shed virus, with a wide range of interpatient variability (range, 2–75%). In studies with sampling performed every 6 h, 49% of genital reactivation episodes lasted <12 h and 29% lasted <6 h. Many of these short bursts of reactivation were associated with copy numbers thought to be high enough to cause transmission to susceptible sexual partners. These data suggest that peripheral immune control may dictate the likelihood and severity of recurrences as well as the frequency of subclinical shedding. There is a strong association between the magnitude of the CD8+ T lymphocyte response and the clearance of virus from genital lesions. The lack of this response, rather than a low CD4+ T lymphocyte count, also predicts frequent and severe HSV-2 recurrences in untreated as well as treated HIV-1-infected patients. HSV-2-specific CD8+ and CD4+ T cells appear to persist for prolonged periods (months) in genital skin previously involved in an HSV-2 reactivation. The location, effectiveness, and longevity of the T lymphocytes (and perhaps of other immune effector cells) may be important in the expression of disease and the likelihood of transmission over time.

■ EPIDEMIOLOGY

Seroepidemiologic studies have documented HSV infections worldwide. Serologic assays with whole-virus antigen preparations, such as complement fixation, neutralization, indirect immunofluorescence, passive hemagglutination, radioimmunoassay, and enzyme-linked immunosorbent assay, are useful for differentiating uninfected (seronegative) persons from those with past HSV-1 or HSV-2 infection, but they do not reliably distinguish between the two viral subtypes. Serologic assays that identify antibodies to type-specific surface proteins (epitopes) of the two viral subtypes have been developed and can distinguish reliably between the human antibody responses to HSV-1 and HSV-2. The most commonly used assays are those that measure antibodies to glycoprotein G of HSV-1 (gG1) and HSV-2 (gG2). A western blot assay that can detect several HSV type-specific proteins can also be used.

Infection with HSV-1 is acquired more frequently and earlier than infection with HSV-2. More than 90% of adults have antibodies to HSV-1 by the fifth decade of life. In populations of low socioeconomic status, most persons acquire HSV-1 infection before the third decade of life. Antibodies to HSV-2 are not detected routinely until puberty. Antibody prevalence rates correlate with past sexual activity and vary greatly among different population groups. There is some evidence that the prevalence of HSV-2 has decreased slightly over the past decade in the United States. Serosurveys indicate that 15–20% of the U.S. population has antibodies to HSV-2. In most routine obstetric and family planning clinics, 25% of women have HSV-2 antibodies, although only 10% of those who are seropositive for HSV-2 report a history of genital lesions. As many as 50% of heterosexual adults attending sexually transmitted disease clinics have antibodies to HSV-2.

A wide variety of serologic surveys have indicated a similar or even higher seroprevalence of HSV-2 in most parts of Central America, South America, and Africa. There is an epidemiologic synergy between HSV-2 and HIV-1. HSV-2 infection is associated with a two- to fourfold increase in HIV-1 acquisition. In addition, HSV-2 is reactivated and transmitted more frequently in persons co-infected with HIV-1 and HSV-2 than in persons not infected with HIV-1. Thus, most areas of the world with a high HIV-1 prevalence also have a high HSV-2 prevalence. In Africa, HSV-2 seroprevalence has ranged from 40% to 70% in obstetric and other sexually experienced populations. Antibody prevalence rates average ~5–10% higher among women than among men.

Several studies suggest that many cases of "asymptomatic" genital HSV-2 infection are, in fact, simply unrecognized: when "asymptomatic" seropositive persons are shown pictures of genital lesions, >60% subsequently identify episodes of symptomatic reactivation. Most important, these asymptomatic seropositive persons with reactivation shed virus on mucosal surfaces almost as frequently as do those with symptomatic disease. The large reservoir of unidentified carriers of HSV-2 and the frequent asymptomatic reactivation of the virus from the genital tract have fostered the continued spread of genital herpes throughout the world. HSV-2 infection is an independent risk factor for the acquisition and transmission of infection

with HIV-1. Among co-infected persons, HIV-1 virions can be shed from herpetic lesions of the genital region. This shedding may facilitate the spread of HIV through sexual contact. HSV-2 reactivation is associated with a localized persistent inflammatory response consisting of high concentrations of CCR5-enriched CD4+ T cells as well as inflammatory dendritic cells in the submucosa of the genital skin. These cells can support HIV infection and replication and hence are likely to account for the two- to threefold increase in HIV acquisition among persons with genital herpes. Unfortunately, antiviral therapy does not reduce this subclinical postreactivation inflammation, probably because of the inability of current antiviral agents to prevent the release of small amounts of HSV antigen into the genital mucosa.

HSV infections occur throughout the year. Transmission can result from contact with persons who have active ulcerative lesions or with persons who have no clinical manifestations of infection but who are shedding HSV from mucocutaneous surfaces. HSV reactivation on genital skin and mucosal surfaces is common. With once-daily sampling of immunocompetent adults, HSV-2 can be cultured from the genital tract on 2–10% of days tested, and HSV DNA can be detected on 20–30% of days by PCR. Corresponding figures for HSV-1 in oral secretions are similar. Rates of shedding are highest during the initial years after acquisition, with viral shedding occurring on as many as 30–50% of days during this period. Immunosuppressed patients shed HSV from mucosal sites at an even higher frequency (20–80% of days). With increased sampling frequency (e.g., four times daily), the rates of reactivation are two- to fourfold higher, with many episodes lasting <12 h. These high rates of mucocutaneous reactivation suggest that exposure to HSV from sexual or other close contact (kissing, sharing of glasses or silverware) is common and help explain the continuing spread and high seroprevalence of HSV infections worldwide. Reactivation rates vary widely among individuals. Among HIV-positive patients, a low CD4+ T cell count and a heavy viral load are associated with increased rates of HSV reactivation. Daily antiviral chemotherapy for HSV-2 infection can reduce shedding rates but does not eliminate shedding, as measured by PCR or culture.

■ CLINICAL SPECTRUM

HSV has been isolated from nearly all visceral and mucocutaneous sites. The clinical manifestations and course of HSV infection depend on the anatomic site involved, the age and immune status of the host, and the antigenic type of the virus. Primary HSV infections (i.e., first infections with either HSV-1 or HSV-2 in which the host lacks HSV antibodies in acute-phase serum) are frequently accompanied by systemic signs and symptoms. Compared with recurrent episodes, primary infections, which involve both mucosal and extramucosal sites, are characterized by a longer duration of symptoms and virus isolation from lesions. The incubation period ranges from 1 to 26 days (median, 6–8 days). Both viral subtypes can cause genital and oral-facial infections, and the infections caused by the two subtypes are clinically indistinguishable. However, the frequency of reactivation of infection is influenced by anatomic site and virus type. Genital HSV-2 infection is twice as likely to reactivate and recurs 8–10 times more frequently than genital HSV-1 infection. Conversely, oral-labial HSV-1 infection recurs more frequently than oral-labial HSV-2 infection. Asymptomatic shedding rates follow the same pattern.

Oral-facial infections

Gingivostomatitis and pharyngitis are the most common clinical manifestations of first-episode HSV-1 infection, while recurrent herpes labialis is the most common clinical manifestation of reactivation HSV-1 infection. HSV pharyngitis and gingivostomatitis usually result from primary infection and are most commonly seen among children and young adults. Clinical symptoms and signs, which include fever, malaise, myalgias, inability to eat, irritability, and cervical adenopathy, may last 3–14 days. Lesions may involve the hard and soft palate, gingiva, tongue, lip, and facial area. HSV-1 or HSV-2 infection of the pharynx usually results in exudative or ulcerative lesions of the posterior pharynx and/or tonsillar pillars. Lesions of the tongue, buccal mucosa, or gingiva may occur later in the course in one-third of cases. Fever lasting 2–7 days and cervical adenopathy are common. It can be difficult to differentiate HSV pharyngitis clinically from bacterial pharyngitis, *Mycoplasma pneumoniae* infections, and pharyngeal ulcerations of noninfectious etiologies (e.g., Stevens-Johnson syndrome). No substantial evidence suggests that reactivation of oral-labial HSV infection is associated with symptomatic recurrent pharyngitis.

Reactivation of HSV from the trigeminal ganglia may be associated with asymptomatic virus excretion in the saliva, development of intraoral mucosal ulcerations, or herpetic ulcerations on the vermilion border of the lip or external facial skin. About 50–70% of seropositive patients undergoing trigeminal nerve-root decompression and 10–15% of those undergoing dental extraction develop oral-labial HSV infection a median of 3 days after these procedures. Clinical differentiation of intraoral mucosal ulcerations due to HSV from aphthous, traumatic, or drug-induced ulcerations is difficult.

In immunosuppressed patients, HSV infection may extend into mucosal and deep cutaneous layers. Friability, necrosis, bleeding, severe pain, and inability to eat or drink may result. The lesions of HSV mucositis are clinically similar to mucosal lesions caused by cytotoxic drug therapy, trauma, or fungal or bacterial infections. Persistent ulcerative HSV infections are among the most common infections in patients with AIDS. HSV and *Candida* infections often occur concurrently. Systemic antiviral therapy speeds the rate of healing and relieves the pain of mucosal HSV infections in immunosuppressed patients. The frequency of HSV reactivation during the early phases of transplantation or induction chemotherapy is high (50–90%), and prophylactic systemic antiviral agents such as IV acyclovir and penciclovir or the oral congeners of these drugs are used to reduce reactivation rates. Patients with atopic eczema may also develop severe oral-facial HSV infections (*eczema herpeticum*), which may rapidly involve extensive areas of skin and occasionally disseminate to visceral organs. Extensive eczema herpeticum has resolved promptly with the administration of IV acyclovir. Erythema multiforme may also be associated with HSV infections (see Figs. 51-9 and e7-25); some evidence suggests that HSV infection is the precipitating event in ~75% of cases of cutaneous erythema multiforme. HSV antigen has been demonstrated both in circulatory immune complexes and in skin lesion biopsy samples from these cases. Patients with severe HSV-associated erythema multiforme are candidates for chronic suppressive oral antiviral therapy.

HSV-1 and varicella-zoster virus (VZV) have been implicated in the etiology of Bell's palsy (flaccid paralysis of the mandibular portion of the facial nerve). Some but not all trials have documented quicker resolution of facial paralysis with the prompt initiation of antiviral therapy, with or without glucocorticoids. However, other trials have shown little benefit. Thus there is no consensus on the relative value of antiviral drugs alone, glucocorticoids alone, and the two modalities combined for the treatment of Bell's palsy.

Genital infections

First-episode primary genital herpes is characterized by fever, headache, malaise, and myalgias. Pain, itching, dysuria, vaginal and urethral discharge, and tender inguinal lymphadenopathy are the predominant local symptoms. Widely spaced bilateral lesions of

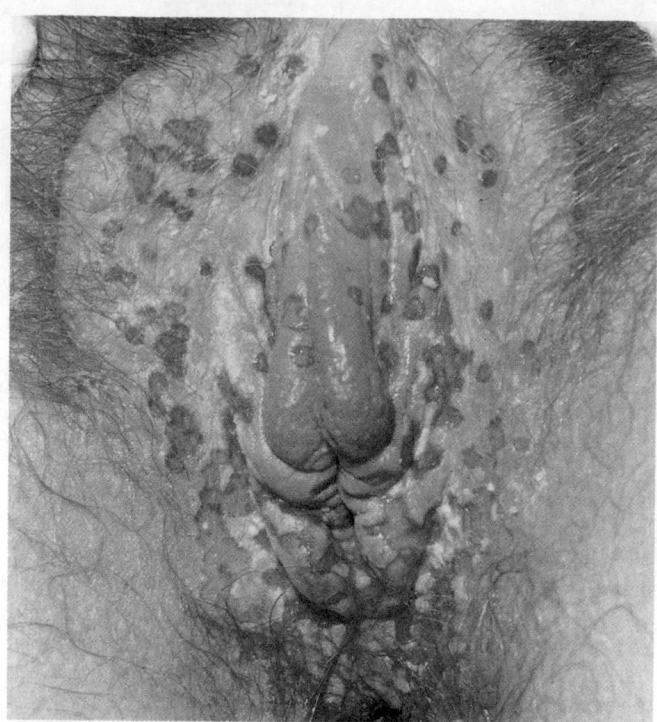

Figure 179-1 Genital herpes: primary vulvar infection. Multiple, extremely painful, punched-out, confluent, shallow ulcers on the edematous vulva and perineum. Micturition is often very painful. Associated inguinal lymphadenopathy is common. *(Reprinted with permission from K Wolff, RA Johnson, D Summond: Fitzpatrick's Color Atlas and Synopsis of Clinical Dermatology, 5th ed, New York, McGraw-Hill, 2005.)*

the external genitalia are characteristic (Fig. 179-1). Lesions may be present in varying stages, including vesicles, pustules, or painful erythematous ulcers. The cervix and urethra are involved in >80% of women with first-episode infections. First episodes of genital herpes in patients who have had prior HSV-1 infection are associated with systemic symptoms in a few patients and with faster healing than primary genital herpes. Subclinical DNAemia has been found in ~30% of cases of true primary genital herpes. The clinical courses of acute first-episode genital herpes are similar for HSV-1 and HSV-2 infection. However, the recurrence rates of genital disease differ with the viral subtype: the 12-month recurrence rates among patients with first-episode HSV-2 and HSV-1 infections are ~90% and ~55%, respectively (median number of recurrences, 4 and <1, respectively). Recurrence rates for genital HSV-2 infections vary greatly among individuals and over time within the same individual. HSV has been isolated from the urethra and urine of men and women without external genital lesions. A clear mucoid discharge and dysuria are characteristics of symptomatic HSV urethritis. HSV has been isolated from the urethra of 5% of women with the dysuria-frequency syndrome. Occasionally, HSV genital tract disease is manifested by endometritis and salpingitis in women and by prostatitis in men. About 15% of cases of HSV-2 acquisition are associated with nonlesional clinical syndromes, such as aseptic meningitis, cervicitis, or urethritis. A more complete discussion of the differential diagnosis of genital herpes is presented in Chap. 130.

Both HSV-1 and HSV-2 can cause symptomatic or asymptomatic rectal and perianal infections. HSV proctitis is usually associated with rectal intercourse. However, subclinical perianal shedding of HSV is detected in women and men who report no rectal intercourse. This phenomenon is due to the establishment of latency in the sacral dermatome from prior genital tract infection, with subsequent reactivation in epithelial cells in the perianal region. Such reactivations are often subclinical. Symptoms of HSV proctitis include anorectal pain, anorectal discharge, tenesmus, and constipation. Sigmoidoscopy reveals ulcerative lesions of the distal 10 cm of the rectal mucosa. Rectal biopsies show mucosal ulceration, necrosis, polymorphonuclear and lymphocytic infiltration of the lamina propria, and (in occasional cases) multinucleated intranuclear inclusion–bearing cells. Perianal herpetic lesions are also found in immunosuppressed patients receiving cytotoxic therapy. Extensive perianal herpetic lesions and/or HSV proctitis is common among patients with HIV infection.

Herpetic whitlow

Herpetic whitlow—HSV infection of the finger—may occur as a complication of primary oral or genital herpes by inoculation of virus through a break in the epidermal surface or by direct introduction of virus into the hand through occupational or some other type of exposure. Clinical signs and symptoms include abrupt-onset edema, erythema, and localized tenderness of the infected finger. Vesicular or pustular lesions of the fingertip that are indistinguishable from lesions of pyogenic bacterial infection are seen. Fever, lymphadenitis, and epitrochlear and axillary lymphadenopathy are common. The infection may recur. Prompt diagnosis (to avoid unnecessary and potentially exacerbating surgical therapy and/or transmission) is essential. Antiviral chemotherapy is usually recommended (see below).

Herpes gladiatorum

HSV may infect almost any area of skin. Mucocutaneous HSV infections of the thorax, ears, face, and hands have been described among wrestlers. Transmission of these infections is facilitated by trauma to the skin sustained during wrestling. Several recent outbreaks have illustrated the importance of prompt diagnosis and therapy to contain the spread of this infection.

Eye infections

HSV infection of the eye is the most common cause of corneal blindness in the United States. HSV keratitis presents as an acute onset of pain, blurred vision, chemosis, conjunctivitis, and characteristic dendritic lesions of the cornea. Use of topical glucocorticoids may exacerbate symptoms and lead to involvement of deep structures of the eye. Debridement, topical antiviral treatment, and/or IFN therapy hastens healing. However, recurrences are common, and the deeper structures of the eye may sustain immunopathologic injury. Stromal keratitis due to HSV appears to be related to T cell–dependent destruction of deep corneal tissue. An HSV-1 epitope that is autoreactive with T cell–targeting corneal antigens has been postulated to be a factor in this infection. Chorioretinitis, usually a manifestation of disseminated HSV infection, may occur in neonates or in patients with HIV infection. HSV and VZV can cause acute necrotizing retinitis as an uncommon but severe manifestation.

Central and peripheral nervous system infections

HSV accounts for 10–20% of all cases of sporadic viral encephalitis in the United States. The estimated incidence is ~2.3 cases per 1 million persons per year. Cases are distributed throughout the year, and the age distribution appears to be biphasic, with peaks at 5–30 and >50 years of age. HSV-1 causes >95% of cases.

The pathogenesis of HSV encephalitis varies. In children and young adults, primary HSV infection may result in encephalitis; presumably, exogenously acquired virus enters the CNS by neurotropic spread from the periphery via the olfactory bulb. However, most adults with HSV encephalitis have clinical or serologic evidence of mucocutaneous HSV-1 infection before the onset of CNS symptoms. In ~25% of the cases examined, the HSV-1 strains from the oropharynx and brain tissue of the same patient differ; thus some cases may result from reinfection with another strain of HSV-1 that reaches the CNS. Two theories have been proposed to explain the development of actively replicating HSV in localized areas of the CNS in persons whose ganglionic and CNS isolates are similar. Reactivation of latent HSV-1 infection in trigeminal or autonomic nerve roots may be associated with extension of virus into the CNS via nerves innervating the middle cranial fossa. HSV DNA has been demonstrated by DNA hybridization in brain tissue obtained at autopsy—even from healthy adults. Thus, reactivation of long-standing latent CNS infection may be another mechanism for the development of HSV encephalitis.

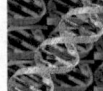 Recent studies have identified genetic polymorphisms in two separate genes among families with a high frequency of HSV encephalitis. Peripheral-blood mononuclear cells from these patients (predominantly children) appear to secrete reduced levels of IFN in response to HSV. These observations suggest that some cases of sporadic HSV encephalitis may be related to host genetic determinants.

The clinical hallmark of HSV encephalitis has been the acute onset of fever and focal neurologic symptoms and signs, especially in the temporal lobe (Fig. 179-2). Clinical differentiation of HSV encephalitis from other viral encephalitides, focal infections, or noninfectious processes is difficult. Elevated cerebrospinal fluid

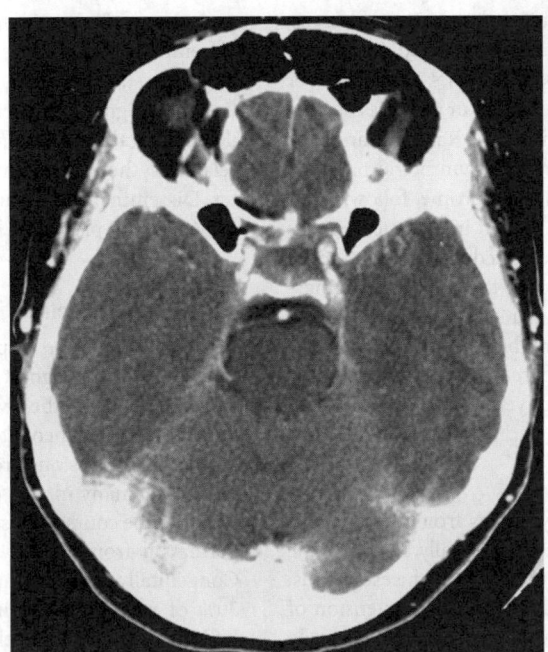
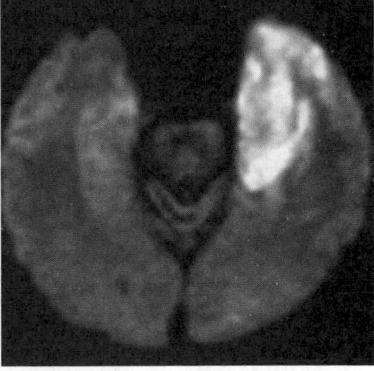

Figure 179-2 **CT and diffusion-weighted MRI scans** of the brain of a patient with left-temporal-lobe HSV encephalitis.

(CSF) protein levels, leukocytosis (predominantly lymphocytes), and red blood cell counts due to hemorrhagic necrosis are common. While brain biopsy has been the gold standard for defining HSV encephalitis, a highly sensitive and specific PCR for detection of HSV DNA in CSF has largely replaced biopsy for defining CNS infection. Although titers of antibody to HSV in CSF and serum increase in most cases of HSV encephalitis, they rarely do so earlier than 10 days into the illness and therefore, while useful retrospectively, are generally not helpful in establishing an early clinical diagnosis. Demonstration of HSV antigen, HSV DNA, or HSV replication in brain tissue obtained by biopsy is highly sensitive and has a low complication rate; examination of such tissue also provides the best opportunity to identify alternative, potentially treatable causes of encephalitis. Antiviral chemotherapy with acyclovir reduces the rate of death from HSV encephalitis. Even with therapy, however, neurologic sequelae are common, especially among persons >50 years of age. Most authorities recommend the administration of IV acyclovir to patients with presumed HSV encephalitis until the diagnosis is confirmed or an alternative diagnosis is made. All confirmed cases should be treated with IV acyclovir (30 mg/kg per day in three divided doses for 14–21 days). After the completion of therapy, the clinical recurrence of encephalitis requiring more treatment has been reported. For this reason, some authorities prefer to treat initially for 21 days, and many continue therapy until HSV DNA has been eliminated from the CSF. Even with therapy, neurologic sequelae are common, especially among persons >35 years of age.

HSV DNA has been detected in CSF from 3–15% of persons presenting to the hospital with aseptic meningitis. HSV meningitis, which is usually seen in association with primary genital HSV infection, is an acute, self-limited disease manifested by headache, fever, and mild photophobia and lasting 2–7 days. Lymphocytic pleocytosis in the CSF is characteristic. Neurologic sequelae of HSV meningitis are rare. HSV is the most commonly identified cause of recurrent lymphocytic meningitis (Mollaret's meningitis). Demonstration of HSV antibodies in CSF or persistence of HSV DNA in CSF can establish the diagnosis. For persons with frequent recurrences of HSV meningitis, daily antiviral therapy has reduced the occurrence of such episodes.

Autonomic nervous system dysfunction, especially of the sacral region, has been reported in association with both HSV and VZV infections. Numbness, tingling of the buttocks or perineal areas, urinary retention, constipation, CSF pleocytosis, and (in males) impotence may occur. Symptoms appear to resolve slowly over days or weeks. Occasionally, hypoesthesia and/or weakness of the lower extremities persists for many months. Rarely, transverse myelitis, manifested by a rapidly progressive symmetric paralysis of the lower extremities or Guillain-Barré syndrome, follows HSV infection. Similarly, peripheral nervous system involvement (Bell's palsy) or cranial polyneuritis may be related to reactivation of HSV-1 infection. Transitory hypoesthesia of the area of skin innervated by the trigeminal nerve and vestibular system dysfunction (as measured by electronystagmography) are the predominant signs of disease. Whether antiviral chemotherapy can abort these signs or reduce their frequency and severity is not yet known.

Visceral infections

HSV infection of visceral organs usually results from viremia, and multiple-organ involvement is common. Occasionally, however, the clinical manifestations of HSV infection involve only the esophagus, lung, or liver. HSV esophagitis may result from direct extension of oral-pharyngeal HSV infection into the esophagus or may occur de novo by reactivation and spread of HSV to the esophageal mucosa via the vagus nerve. The predominant symptoms of HSV esophagitis are odynophagia, dysphagia, substernal pain, and weight loss.

Multiple oval ulcerations appear on an erythematous base with or without a patchy white pseudomembrane. The distal esophagus is most commonly involved. With extensive disease, diffuse friability may spread to the entire esophagus. Neither endoscopic nor barium examination can reliably differentiate HSV esophagitis from *Candida* esophagitis or from esophageal ulcerations due to thermal injury, radiation, or corrosives. Endoscopically obtained secretions for cytologic examination and culture or DNA detection by PCR provide the most useful material for diagnosis. Systemic antiviral chemotherapy usually reduces the severity and duration of symptoms and heals esophageal ulcerations.

HSV pneumonitis is uncommon except in severely immunosuppressed patients and may result from extension of herpetic tracheobronchitis into lung parenchyma. Focal necrotizing pneumonitis usually ensues. Hematogenous dissemination of virus from sites of oral or genital mucocutaneous disease may also occur, producing bilateral interstitial pneumonitis. Bacterial, fungal, and parasitic pathogens are commonly present in HSV pneumonitis. The mortality rate from untreated HSV pneumonia in immunosuppressed patients is high (>80%). HSV has also been isolated from the lower respiratory tract of persons with adult respiratory distress syndrome and prolonged intubation. Most authorities believe that the presence of HSV in tracheal aspirates in such settings is due to reactivation of HSV in the tracheal region and localized tracheitis in persons with long-standing intubation. Such patients should be evaluated for extension of HSV infection into the lung parenchyma. Controlled trials evaluating the role of antiviral agents used against HSV in morbidity and mortality associated with acute respiratory distress syndrome have not been conducted. The role of lower respiratory tract HSV infection in overall rates of morbidity and mortality associated with these conditions is unclear. HSV is an uncommon cause of hepatitis in immunocompetent patients. HSV infection of the liver is associated with fever, abrupt elevations of bilirubin and serum aminotransferase levels, and leukopenia (<4000 white blood cells/μL). Disseminated intravascular coagulation may also develop.

Other reported complications of HSV infection include monarticular arthritis, adrenal necrosis, idiopathic thrombocytopenia, and glomerulonephritis. Disseminated HSV infection in immunocompetent patients is rare. In immunocompromised, burned, or malnourished patients, HSV occasionally disseminates to other visceral organs, such as the adrenal glands, pancreas, small and large intestines, and bone marrow. Rarely, primary HSV infection in pregnancy disseminates and may be associated with the death of both mother and fetus. This uncommon event is usually related to the acquisition of primary infection in the third trimester. Disseminated HSV infection is best detected by the presence of HSV DNA in plasma or blood.

Neonatal HSV infections

Of all HSV-infected populations, neonates (infants younger than 6 weeks) have the highest frequency of visceral and/or CNS infection. Without therapy, the overall rate of death from neonatal herpes is 65%; <10% of neonates with CNS infection develop normally. Although skin lesions are the most commonly recognized features of disease, many infants do not develop lesions at all or do so only well into the course of disease. Neonatal infection is usually acquired perinatally from contact with infected genital secretions at delivery. Congenitally infected infants have been reported. In most series, 30% of neonatal HSV infections are due to HSV-1 and 70% to HSV-2. The risk of developing neonatal HSV infection is 10 times higher for an infant born to a mother who has recently acquired HSV than for other infants. Neonatal HSV-1 infections may also be acquired through postnatal contact with immediate family members who have symptomatic or asymptomatic oral-labial HSV-1 infection or through nosocomial transmission within the hospital. All neonates with presumed herpes should be treated with IV acyclovir. Antiviral chemotherapy with high-dose IV acyclovir (60 mg/kg per day) has reduced the mortality rate from neonatal herpes to ~15%. However, rates of morbidity, especially among infants with HSV-2 infection involving the CNS, are still very high.

HSV in Pregnancy

In the United States, 22% of all pregnant women and 55% of non-Hispanic black pregnant women are seropositive for HSV-2. However, the risk of mother-to-child transmission of HSV in the perinatal period is highest when the infection is acquired near the time of labor—that is, in previously HSV-seronegative women. The clinical manifestations of recurrent genital herpes—including the frequency of subclinical versus clinical infection, duration of lesions, pain, and constitutional symptoms—are similar in pregnant and nonpregnant women. Recurrences increase in frequency over the course of pregnancy. However, when women are seropositive for HSV-2 at the outset of pregnancy, no effect on neonatal outcomes (including birth weight and gestational age) is seen. First-episode infections in pregnancy have more severe consequences for mother and infant. Maternal visceral dissemination during the third trimester occasionally occurs, as does premature birth or intrauterine growth retardation. The acquisition of primary disease in pregnancy, whether related to HSV-1 or HSV-2, carries the risk of transplacental transmission of virus to the neonate and can result in spontaneous abortion, although this outcome is relatively uncommon. Most authorities recommend antiviral treatment for newly acquired genital HSV infection during pregnancy with acyclovir (400 mg three times daily) or valacyclovir (500–1000 mg twice daily) administered for 7–10 days. However, the impact of this intervention on transmission is unknown. The high HSV-2 prevalence rate in pregnancy and the low incidence of neonatal disease (1 case per 6000–20,000 live births) indicate that only a few infants are at risk of acquiring HSV. Therefore, cesarean section is not warranted for all women with recurrent genital disease. Because intrapartum transmission of infection accounts for the majority of cases, only women who are shedding HSV at delivery need be considered for abdominal delivery. Several studies have shown no correlation between recurrence of viral shedding before delivery and viral shedding at term. Hence, weekly virologic monitoring and amniocentesis are not recommended.

The frequency of transmission from mother to infant is markedly higher among women who acquire HSV near term (30–50%) than among those in whom HSV-2 infection is reactivated at delivery (<1%). Although maternal antibody to HSV-2 is protective, antibody to HSV-1 offers little or no protection against neonatal HSV-2 infection. Primary genital infection with HSV-1 leads to a particularly high risk of transmission during pregnancy and accounts for an increasing proportion of neonatal HSV cases. Moreover, during reactivation, HSV-1 appears more transmissible to the neonate than HSV-2. Only 2% of women who are seropositive for HSV-2 have HSV-2 isolated from cervical secretions at delivery, and only 1% of infants exposed in this manner develop infection, presumably because of the protective effects of maternally transferred antibodies and perhaps lower viral titers during reactivation. Despite the low frequency of transmission of HSV in this setting, 30–50% of infants with neonatal HSV are born to mothers with established genital herpes.

Isolation of HSV by cervicovaginal swab at the time of delivery is the greatest risk factor for intrapartum HSV transmission (relative risk = 346); however, culture-negative, PCR-positive cases of intrapartum transmission are well described. New acquisition of HSV [odds ratio (OR) = 49], isolation of HSV-1 versus HSV-2 (OR = 35), cervical versus vulvar HSV detection (OR = 15), use of fetal scalp electrodes (OR = 3.5), and young age confer further risk of transmission, whereas abdominal delivery is protective (OR = 0.14). Physical examination poorly predicts the absence of shedding, and PCR far exceeds culture in terms of sensitivity and speed. Therefore, PCR detection at the onset of labor should be used to aid clinical decision-making for women with HSV-2 antibody. Because cesarean section appears to be an effective means of reducing maternal-fetal transmission, patients with recurrent genital herpes should be encouraged to come to the hospital early at the time of delivery for careful examination of the external genitalia and cervix as well as collection of a swab sample for viral isolation. Women who have no evidence of lesions should have a vaginal delivery. The presence of active lesions on the cervix or external genitalia is an indication for abdominal delivery.

If first-episode exposure has occurred (e.g., if HSV serologies show that the mother is seronegative or if the mother is HSV-1-seropositive and the isolate at delivery is found to be HSV-2), many authorities would initiate antiviral therapy for the infant with IV acyclovir. At a minimum, samples for viral cultures and PCR should be obtained from the throat, nasopharynx, eyes, and rectum of these infants immediately and at 5- to 10-day intervals. Lethargy, skin lesions, or fever should be evaluated promptly. All infants from whom HSV is isolated 24 h after delivery should be treated with IV acyclovir at recommended doses.

■ DIAGNOSIS

Both clinical and laboratory criteria are useful for diagnosing HSV infections. A clinical diagnosis can be made accurately when characteristic multiple vesicular lesions on an erythematous base are present. However, herpetic ulcerations may resemble skin ulcerations of other etiologies. Mucosal HSV infections may also present as urethritis or pharyngitis without cutaneous lesions. Thus, laboratory studies to confirm the diagnosis and to guide therapy are recommended. While staining of scrapings from the base of the lesions with Wright's, Giemsa's (Tzanck preparation), or Papanicolaou's stain to detect giant cells or intranuclear inclusions of *Herpesvirus* infection is a well-described procedure, few clinicians are skilled in these techniques, the sensitivity of staining is low (<30% for mucosal swabs), and these cytologic methods do not differentiate between HSV and VZV infections.

HSV infection is best confirmed in the laboratory by detection of virus, viral antigen, or viral DNA in scrapings from lesions. HSV DNA detection by PCR is the most sensitive laboratory technique for detecting mucosal or visceral HSV infections and should be utilized when available. HSV causes a discernible cytopathic effect in a variety of cell culture systems, and this effect can be identified within 48–96 h after inoculation. Spin-amplified culture with subsequent staining for HSV antigen has shortened the time needed to identify HSV to <24 h. The sensitivity of all detection methods depends on the stage of the lesions (with higher sensitivity for vesicular than for ulcerative lesions), on whether the patient has a first or a recurrent episode of the disease (with higher sensitivity in first than in recurrent episodes), and on whether the sample is from an immunosuppressed or an immunocompetent patient (with more antigen or DNA in immunosuppressed patients). Laboratory confirmation permits subtyping of the virus; information on subtype may be useful epidemiologically and may help to predict the frequency of reactivation after first-episode oral-labial or genital HSV infection.

Acute- and convalescent-phase serum can be useful in demonstrating seroconversion during primary HSV-1 or HSV-2 infection. However, few available tests report titers, and increases in index values do not reflect first episodes in all patients. Serologic assays based on type-specific proteins should be used to identify asymptomatic carriers of HSV-1 or HSV-2. No reliable IgM method for defining acute HSV infection is available.

Several studies have shown that persons with previously unrecognized HSV-2 infection can be taught to identify symptomatic reactivations. Individuals seropositive for HSV-2 should be told about the high frequency of subclinical reactivation in mucosal surfaces that are not visible to the eye (e.g., cervix, urethra, perianal skin) or in microscopic ulcerations that may not be clinically symptomatic. Transmission of infection during such episodes is well established. HSV-2-seropositive persons should be educated about the high likelihood of subclinical shedding and the role condoms (male or female) may play in reducing transmission. Antiviral therapy with valacyclovir (500 mg once daily) has been shown to reduce the transmission of HSV-2 between sexual partners.

TREATMENT   Herpes Simplex Virus Infections

Many aspects of mucocutaneous and visceral HSV infections are amenable to antiviral chemotherapy. For mucocutaneous infections, acyclovir and its congeners famciclovir and valacyclovir have been the mainstays of therapy. Several antiviral agents are available for topical use in HSV eye infections: idoxuridine, trifluorothymidine, topical vidarabine, and cidofovir. For HSV encephalitis and neonatal herpes, IV acyclovir is the treatment of choice.

All licensed antiviral agents for use against HSV inhibit the viral DNA polymerase. One class of drugs, typified by the drug acyclovir, is made up of substrates for the HSV enzyme thymidine kinase (TK). Acyclovir, ganciclovir, famciclovir, and valacyclovir are all selectively phosphorylated to the monophosphate form in virus-infected cells. Cellular enzymes convert the monophosphate form of the drug to the triphosphate, which is then incorporated into the viral DNA chain. Acyclovir is the agent most frequently used for the treatment of HSV infections and is available in IV, oral, and topical formulations. Valacyclovir, the valyl ester of acyclovir, offers greater bioavailability than acyclovir and thus can be administered less frequently. Famciclovir, the oral formulation of penciclovir, is clinically effective in the treatment of a variety of HSV-1 and HSV-2 infections. Ganciclovir is active against both HSV-1 and HSV-2; however, it is more toxic than acyclovir, valacyclovir, and famciclovir and generally is not recommended for the treatment of HSV infections. Anecdotal case reports suggest that ganciclovir may also be less effective than acyclovir for treatment of HSV infections. All three recommended compounds—acyclovir, valacyclovir, and famciclovir—have proved effective in shortening the duration of symptoms and lesions of mucocutaneous HSV infections in both immunocompromised and immunocompetent patients (Table 179-1). IV and oral formulations prevent reactivation of HSV in seropositive immunocompromised patients during induction chemotherapy or in the period immediately after bone marrow or solid organ transplantation. Chronic daily suppressive therapy reduces the frequency of reactivation disease among patients with frequent genital or oral-labial herpes. Only valacyclovir has been subjected to clinical trials that demonstrated reduced transmission of HSV-2 infection between sexual partners. IV acyclovir (30 mg/kg per day, given as a 10-mg/kg infusion over 1 h at 8-h intervals) is effective in reducing rates of death and morbidity from HSV encephalitis. Early initiation of therapy is a critical factor in outcome. The major side effect associated with IV acyclovir is transient renal insufficiency,

usually due to crystallization of the compound in the renal parenchyma. This adverse reaction can be avoided if the medication is given slowly over 1 h and the patient is well hydrated. Because CSF levels of acyclovir average only 30–50% of plasma levels, the dosage of acyclovir used for treatment of CNS infection (30 mg/kg per day) is double that used for treatment of mucocutaneous or visceral disease (15 mg/kg per day). Even higher doses of IV acyclovir are used for neonatal HSV infection (60 mg/kg per day in three divided doses).

Increasingly, shorter courses of therapy are being used for treatment of recurrent mucocutaneous infection with HSV-1 or HSV-2 in immunocompetent patients. One-day courses of famciclovir and valacyclovir are clinically effective, more convenient, and generally less costly than longer courses of therapy (Table 179-1). These short-course regimens should be reserved for immunocompetent hosts.

SUPPRESSION OF MUCOCUTANEOUS HERPES   Recognition of the high frequency of subclinical reactivation provides a well-accepted rationale for the use of daily antiviral therapy to suppress reactivations of HSV, especially in persons with frequent clinical reactivations (e.g., those with recently acquired genital HSV infection). Immunosuppressed persons, including those with HIV infection, may also benefit from daily antiviral therapy. Recent studies have shown the efficacy of daily acyclovir and valacyclovir in reducing the frequency of HSV reactivations among HIV-positive persons. Regimens used include acyclovir (400–800 mg twice daily), famciclovir (500 mg twice daily), and valacyclovir (500 mg twice daily); valacyclovir at a dose of 4 g daily was associated with thrombotic thrombocytopenic purpura in one study of HIV-infected persons. In addition, daily treatment of HSV-2 reduces the titer of HIV RNA in plasma (0.5-log reduction) and in genital mucosa (0.33-log reduction).

REDUCED HSV TRANSMISSION TO SEXUAL PARTNERS   Once-daily valacyclovir (500 mg) has been shown to reduce transmission of HSV-2 between sexual partners. Transmission rates are higher from males to females and among persons with frequent HSV-2 reactivation. Serologic screening can be used to identify at-risk couples. Daily valacyclovir appears to be more effective at reducing subclinical shedding than daily famciclovir.

ACYCLOVIR RESISTANCE   Acyclovir-resistant strains of HSV have been identified. Most of these strains have an altered substrate specificity for phosphorylating acyclovir. Thus, cross-resistance to famciclovir and valacyclovir is usually found. Occasionally, an isolate with altered TK specificity arises and is sensitive to famciclovir but not to acyclovir. In some patients infected with TK-deficient virus, higher doses of acyclovir are associated with clearing of lesions. In others, clinical disease progresses despite high-dose therapy. Almost all clinically significant acyclovir resistance has been seen in immunocompromised patients, and HSV-2 isolates are more often resistant than HSV-1 strains. A study by the Centers for Disease Control and Prevention indicated that ~5% of HSV-2 isolates from HIV-positive persons exhibit some degree of in vitro resistance to acyclovir. Of HSV-2 isolates from immunocompetent patients attending sexually transmitted disease clinics, <0.5% show reduced in vitro sensitivity to acyclovir. The lack of appreciable change in the frequency of detection of such isolates in the past 20 years probably reflects the reduced transmission of TK-deficient mutants. Isolation of HSV from lesions persisting despite adequate dosages and blood levels of acyclovir should raise the suspicion of acyclovir resistance. Therapy with the antiviral drug foscarnet is useful in acyclovir-resistant cases

TABLE 179-1 Antiviral Chemotherapy for HSV Infection

I. Mucocutaneous HSV infections

A. Infections in immunosuppressed patients

1. *Acute symptomatic first or recurrent episodes:* IV acyclovir (5 mg/kg q8h) or oral acyclovir (400 mg qid), famciclovir (500 mg bid or tid), or valacyclovir (500 mg bid) is effective. Treatment duration may vary from 7 to 14 days.

2. *Suppression of reactivation disease (genital or oral-labial):* IV acyclovir (5 mg/kg q8h) or oral valacyclovir (500 mg bid) or acyclovir (400–800 mg 3–5 times per day) prevents recurrences during the 30-day period immediately after transplantation. Longer-term HSV suppression is often used for persons with continued immunosuppression. In bone marrow and renal transplant recipients, oral valacyclovir (2 g/d) is also effective in reducing cytomegalovirus infection. Oral valacyclovir at a dose of 4 g/d has been associated with thrombotic thrombocytopenic purpura after extended use in HIV-positive persons. In HIV-infected persons, oral acyclovir (400–800 mg bid), valacyclovir (500 mg bid), or famciclovir (500 mg bid) is effective in reducing clinical and subclinical reactivations of HSV-1 and HSV-2.

B. Infections in immunocompetent patients

1. *Genital herpes*

   a. *First episodes:* Oral acyclovir (200 mg 5 times per day or 400 mg tid), valacyclovir (1 g bid), or famciclovir (250 mg bid) for 7–14 days is effective. IV acyclovir (5 mg/kg q8h for 5 days) is given for severe disease or neurologic complications such as aseptic meningitis.

   b. *Symptomatic recurrent genital herpes:* Short-course (1- to 3-day) regimens are preferred because of low cost, likelihood of adherence, and convenience. Oral acyclovir (800 mg tid for 2 days), valacyclovir (500 mg bid for 3 days), or famciclovir (750 or 1000 mg bid for 1 day, a 1500-mg single dose, or 500 mg stat followed by 250 mg q12h for 3 days) effectively shortens lesion duration. Other options include oral acyclovir (200 mg 5 times per day), valacyclovir (500 mg bid), and famciclovir (125 mg bid for 5 days).

   c. *Suppression of recurrent genital herpes:* Oral acyclovir (400–800 mg bid) or valacyclovir (500 mg daily) is given. Patients with >9 episodes per year should take oral valacyclovir (1 g daily or 500 mg bid) or famciclovir (250 mg bid or 500 mg bid).

2. *Oral-labial HSV infections*

   a. *First episode:* Oral acyclovir (200 mg) is given 4 or 5 times per day; an oral acyclovir suspension can be used (600 mg/m² qid). Oral famciclovir (250 mg bid) or valacyclovir (1 g bid) has been used clinically.

   b. *Recurrent episodes:* If initiated at the onset of the prodrome, single-dose or 1-day therapy effectively reduces pain and speeds healing. Regimens include oral famciclovir (a 1500-mg single dose or 750 mg bid for 1 day) or valacyclovir (a 2-g single dose or 2 g bid for 1 day). Self-initiated therapy with 6-times-daily topical penciclovir cream effectively speeds healing of oral-labial HSV. Topical acyclovir cream has also been shown to speed healing.

   c. *Suppression of reactivation of oral-labial HSV:* If started before exposure and continued for the duration of exposure (usually 5–10 days), oral acyclovir (400 mg bid) prevents reactivation of recurrent oral-labial HSV infection associated with severe sun exposure.

3. *Surgical prophylaxis of oral or genital HSV infection:* Several surgical procedures, such as laser skin resurfacing, trigeminal nerve-root decompression, and lumbar disk surgery, have been associated with HSV reactivation. IV acyclovir (3–5 mg/kg q8h) or oral acyclovir (800 mg bid), valacyclovir (500 mg bid), or famciclovir (250 mg bid) effectively reduces reactivation. Therapy should be initiated 48 h before surgery and continued for 3–7 days.

4. *Herpetic whitlow:* Oral acyclovir (200 mg; alternative: 400 mg tid) is given 5 times daily for 7–10 days.

5. *HSV proctitis:* Oral acyclovir (400 mg 5 times per day) is useful in shortening the course of infection. In immunosuppressed patients or in patients with severe infection, IV acyclovir (5 mg/kg q8h) may be useful.

6. *Herpetic eye infections:* In acute keratitis, topical trifluorothymidine, vidarabine, idoxuridine, acyclovir, penciclovir, and interferon are all beneficial. Debridement may be required. Topical steroids may worsen disease.

II. CNS HSV infections

A. *HSV encephalitis:* IV acyclovir (10 mg/kg q8h; 30 mg/kg per day) is given for 10 days or until HSV DNA is no longer detected in CSF.

B. *HSV aseptic meningitis:* No studies of systemic antiviral chemotherapy exist. If therapy is to be given, IV acyclovir (15–30 mg/kg per day) should be used.

C. *Autonomic radiculopathy:* No studies are available. Most authorities recommend a trial of IV acyclovir.

III. Neonatal HSV infections:
Oral acyclovir (60 mg/kg per day, divided into 3 doses) is given. The recommended duration of treatment is 21 days. Monitoring for relapse should be undertaken, and some authorities recommend continued suppression with oral acyclovir suspension for 3–4 months.

IV. Visceral HSV infections

A. *HSV esophagitis:* IV acyclovir (15 mg/kg per day). In some patients with milder forms of immunosuppression, oral therapy with valacyclovir or famciclovir is effective.

B. *HSV pneumonitis:* No controlled studies exist. IV acyclovir (15 mg/kg per day) should be considered.

V. Disseminated HSV infections:
No controlled studies exist. IV acyclovir (5 mg/kg q8h) should be tried. Adjustments for renal insufficiency may be needed. No definite evidence indicates that therapy will decrease the risk of death.

VI. Erythema multiforme associated with HSV:
Anecdotal observations suggest that oral acyclovir (400 mg bid or tid) or valacyclovir (500 mg bid) will suppress erythema multiforme.

VII. Infections due to acyclovir-resistant HSV:
IV foscarnet (40 mg/kg IV q8h) should be given until lesions heal. The optimal duration of therapy and the usefulness of its continuation to suppress lesions are unclear. Some patients may benefit from cutaneous application of trifluorothymidine or 5% cidofovir gel.

(Chap. 178). Because of its toxicity and cost, this drug is usually reserved for patients with extensive mucocutaneous infections. Cidofovir is a nucleotide analogue and exists as a phosphonate or monophosphate form. Most TK-deficient strains of HSV are sensitive to cidofovir. Cidofovir ointment speeds healing of acyclovir-resistant lesions. No well-controlled trials of systemic cidofovir have been reported. True TK-negative variants of HSV appear to have a reduced capacity to spread because of altered neurovirulence—a feature important in the relatively infrequent presence of such strains in immunocompetent populations, even with increasing use of antiviral drugs.

PREVENTION

The success of efforts to control HSV disease on a population basis through suppressive antiviral chemotherapy and/or educational programs will be limited. Barrier forms of contraception (especially condoms) decrease the likelihood of transmission of HSV infection, particularly during periods of asymptomatic viral excretion. When lesions are present, HSV infection may be transmitted by skin-to-skin contact despite the use of a condom. Nevertheless, the available data suggest that consistent condom use is an effective means of reducing the risk of genital HSV-2 transmission. Chronic daily antiviral therapy with valacyclovir can also be partially effective in reducing acquisition of HSV-2, especially among susceptible women. There are no comparative efficacy studies of valacyclovir versus condom use. Most authorities suggest both approaches. The need for a vaccine to prevent acquisition of HSV infection is great, especially in light of the role HSV-2 plays in enhancing the acquisition and transmission of HIV-1.

A substantial portion of neonatal HSV cases could be prevented by reducing the acquisition of HSV by women in the third trimester of pregnancy. Neonatal HSV infection can result from either the acquisition of maternal infection near term or the reactivation of infection at delivery in the already-infected mother. Thus strategies for reducing neonatal HSV are complex. Some authorities have recommended that antiviral therapy with acyclovir or valacyclovir be given to HSV-2-infected women in late pregnancy as a means of reducing reactivation of HSV-2 at term. Data are not available to support the efficacy of this approach. Moreover, the high treatment-to-prevention ratio makes this a dubious public health approach, even though it can reduce the frequency of HSV-associated cesarean delivery.

FURTHER READINGS

ABU-RADDAD LJ et al: Genital herpes has played a more important role than any other sexually transmitted infection in driving HIV prevalence in Africa. PLoS ONE 3:e2230, 2008

CHILUKURI S, ROSEN T: Management of acyclovir-resistant herpes simplex virus. Dermatol Clin 21:311, 2003

COREY L, WALD A: Maternal and neonatal herpes simplex virus infections. N Engl J Med 361:1376, 2009

JAMES SH et al: Antiviral therapy for herpesvirus central nervous system infections: Neonatal herpes simplex virus infection, herpes simplex encephalitis, and congenital cytomegalovirus infection. Antiviral Res 83:207, 2009

MARK KE et al: Rapidly cleared episodes of herpes simplex virus reactivation in immunocompetent adults. J Infect Dis 198:1141, 2008

ZHU J et al: Persistence of HIV-1 receptor-positive cells after HSV-2 reactivation is a potential mechanism for increased HIV-1 acquisition. Nat Med 15:886: 2009

CHAPTER 180

Varicella-Zoster Virus Infections

Richard J. Whitley

DEFINITION

Varicella-zoster virus (VZV) causes two distinct clinical entities: varicella (chickenpox) and herpes zoster (shingles). Chickenpox, a ubiquitous and extremely contagious infection, is usually a benign illness of childhood characterized by an exanthematous vesicular rash. With reactivation of latent VZV (which is most common after the sixth decade of life), herpes zoster presents as a dermatomal vesicular rash, usually associated with severe pain.

ETIOLOGY

A clinical association between varicella and herpes zoster has been recognized for nearly 100 years. Early in the twentieth century, similarities in the histopathologic features of skin lesions resulting from varicella and herpes zoster were demonstrated. Viral isolates from patients with chickenpox and herpes zoster produced similar alterations in tissue culture—specifically, the appearance of eosinophilic intranuclear inclusions and multinucleated giant cells. These results suggested that the viruses were biologically similar. Restriction endonuclease analyses of viral DNA from a patient with chickenpox who subsequently developed herpes zoster verified the molecular identity of the two viruses responsible for these different clinical presentations.

VZV is a member of the family Herpesviridae, sharing with other members such structural characteristics as a lipid envelope surrounding a nucleocapsid with icosahedral symmetry, a total diameter of ~180–200 nm, and centrally located double-stranded DNA that is ~125,000 bp in length.

PATHOGENESIS AND PATHOLOGY

Primary infection

Transmission occurs readily by the respiratory route; the subsequent localized replication of the virus at an undefined site (presumably the nasopharynx) leads to seeding of the reticuloendothelial system and ultimately to the development of viremia. Viremia in patients with chickenpox is reflected in the diffuse and scattered nature of the skin lesions and can be verified in selected cases by the recovery of VZV from the blood or routinely by the detection of viral DNA in either blood or lesions by polymerase chain reaction (PCR). Vesicles involve the corium and dermis, with degenerative changes characterized by ballooning, the presence of multinucleated giant cells, and eosinophilic intranuclear inclusions. Infection may involve localized blood vessels of the skin, resulting in necrosis and epidermal hemorrhage. With the evolution of disease, the vesicular fluid becomes cloudy because of the recruitment of polymorpho-nuclear leukocytes and the presence of degenerated cells and fibrin. Ultimately, the vesicles either rupture and release their fluid (which includes infectious virus) or are gradually reabsorbed.

Recurrent infection

The mechanism of reactivation of VZV that results in herpes zoster is unknown. Presumably, the virus infects dorsal root ganglia during chickenpox, where it remains latent until reactivated. Histopathologic examination of representative dorsal root ganglia during active herpes zoster demonstrates hemorrhage, edema, and lymphocytic infiltration.

Active replication of VZV in other organs, such as the lung or the brain, can occur during either chickenpox or herpes zoster but is uncommon in the immunocompetent host. Pulmonary involvement is characterized by interstitial pneumonitis, multinucleated giant cell formation, intranuclear inclusions, and pulmonary hemorrhage. Central nervous system (CNS) infection leads to histopathologic evidence of perivascular cuffing similar to that encountered in measles and other viral encephalitides. Focal hemorrhagic necrosis of the brain, characteristic of herpes simplex virus (HSV) encephalitis, is uncommon in VZV infection.

■ EPIDEMIOLOGY AND CLINICAL MANIFESTATIONS

Chickenpox

Humans are the only known reservoir for VZV. Chickenpox is highly contagious, with an attack rate of at least 90% among susceptible (seronegative) individuals. Persons of both sexes and all races are infected equally. The virus is endemic in the population at large; however, it becomes epidemic among susceptible individuals during seasonal peaks—namely, late winter and early spring in the temperate zone. Much of our knowledge of the disease's natural history and incidence predates the licensure of the chickenpox vaccine in 1995. Historically, children 5–9 years old are most commonly affected and account for 50% of all cases. Most other cases involve children 1–4 and 10–14 years old. Approximately 10% of the population of the United States over the age of 15 is susceptible to infection. VZV vaccination during the second year of life has dramatically changed the epidemiology of infection, causing a significant decrease in the annualized incidence of chickenpox.

The incubation period of chickenpox ranges from 10–21 days but is usually 14–17 days. Secondary attack rates in susceptible siblings within a household are 70–90%. Patients are infectious ~48 h before onset of the vesicular rash, during the period of vesicle formation (which generally lasts 4–5 days), and until all vesicles are crusted.

Clinically, chickenpox presents with a rash, low-grade fever, and malaise, although a few patients develop a prodrome 1–2 days before onset of the exanthem. In the immunocompetent patient, chickenpox is usually a benign illness associated with lassitude and with body temperatures of 37.8°–39.4°C (100°–103°F) of 3–5 days' duration. The skin lesions—the hallmark of the infection—include maculopapules, vesicles, and scabs in various stages of evolution (Fig. 180-1). These lesions, which evolve from maculopapules to vesicles over hours to days, appear on the trunk and face and rapidly spread to involve other areas of the body. Most are small and have an erythematous base with a diameter of 5–10 mm. Successive crops appear over a 2- to 4-day period. Lesions can also be found on the mucosa of the pharynx and/or the vagina. Their severity varies from one person to another. Some individuals have very few lesions, while others have as many as 2000. Younger children tend to have fewer vesicles than older individuals. Secondary and tertiary cases within families are associated with a relatively large number of vesicles. Immunocompromised patients—both children and

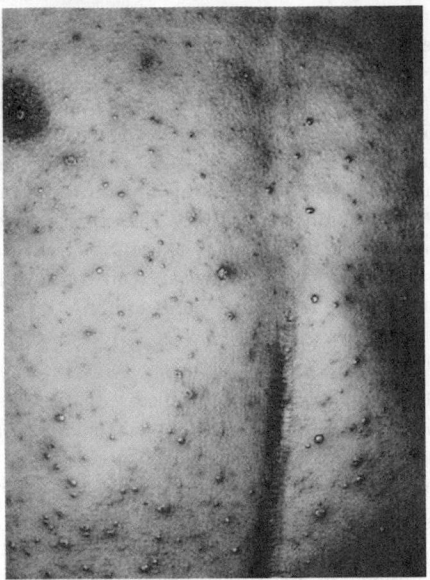

Figure 180-1   Varicella lesions at various stages of evolution: vesicles on an erythematous base, umbilical vesicles, and crusts.

adults, particularly those with leukemia—have lesions (often with a hemorrhagic base) that are more numerous and take longer to heal than those of immunocompetent patients. Immunocompromised individuals are also at greater risk for visceral complications, which occur in 30–50% of cases and are fatal 15% of the time in the absence of antiviral therapy.

The most common infectious complication of varicella is secondary bacterial superinfection of the skin, which is usually caused by *Streptococcus pyogenes* or *Staphylococcus aureus,* including strains that are methicillin-resistant. Skin infection results from excoriation of lesions after scratching. Gram's staining of skin lesions should help clarify the etiology of unusually erythematous and pustulated lesions.

The most common extracutaneous site of involvement in children is the CNS. The syndrome of acute cerebellar ataxia and meningeal inflammation generally appears ~21 days after onset of the rash and rarely develops in the preeruptive phase. The cerebrospinal fluid (CSF) contains lymphocytes and elevated levels of protein. CNS involvement is a benign complication of VZV infection in children and generally does not require hospitalization. Aseptic meningitis, encephalitis, transverse myelitis, and Guillain-Barré syndrome can also occur. Reye's syndrome has been reported in children concomitantly treated with aspirin. Encephalitis is reported in 0.1–0.2% of children with chickenpox. Other than supportive care, no specific therapy (e.g., acyclovir administration) has proved efficacious for patients with CNS involvement.

Varicella pneumonia, the most serious complication following chickenpox, develops more commonly in adults (up to 20% of cases) than in children and is particularly severe in pregnant women. Pneumonia due to VZV usually has its onset 3–5 days into the illness and is associated with tachypnea, cough, dyspnea, and fever. Cyanosis, pleuritic chest pain, and hemoptysis are common. Roentgenographic evidence of disease consists of nodular infiltrates and interstitial pneumonitis. Resolution of pneumonitis parallels improvement of the skin rash; however, patients may have persistent fever and compromised pulmonary function for weeks.

Other complications of chickenpox include myocarditis, corneal lesions, nephritis, arthritis, bleeding diatheses, acute glomerulonephritis, and hepatitis. Hepatic involvement, distinct from Reye's syndrome and usually asymptomatic, is common in chickenpox and is generally characterized by elevated levels of liver enzymes, particularly aspartate and alanine aminotransferases.

Perinatal varicella is associated with a high mortality rate when maternal disease develops within 5 days before delivery or within 48 h thereafter. Because the newborn does not receive protective transplacental antibodies and has an immature immune system, the illness may be unusually severe. The reported mortality rate is as high as 30% in this group. *Congenital varicella*, with clinical manifestations of limb hypoplasia, cicatricial skin lesions, and microcephaly at birth, is extremely uncommon.

Herpes zoster

Herpes zoster (shingles) is a sporadic disease that results from reactivation of latent VZV from dorsal root ganglia. Most patients with shingles have no history of recent exposure to other individuals with VZV infection. Herpes zoster occurs at all ages, but its incidence is highest (5–10 cases per 1000 persons) among individuals in the sixth decade of life and beyond. Data suggest that 1.2 million cases occur annually in the United States. Recurrent herpes zoster is exceedingly rare except in immunocompromised hosts, especially those with AIDS.

Herpes zoster is characterized by a unilateral vesicular dermatomal eruption, often associated with severe pain. The dermatomes from T3 to L3 are most frequently involved. If the ophthalmic branch of the trigeminal nerve is involved, *zoster ophthalmicus* results. The factors responsible for the reactivation of VZV are not known. In children, reactivation is usually benign; in adults, it can be debilitating because of pain. The onset of disease is heralded by pain within the dermatome, which may precede lesions by 48–72 h; an erythematous maculopapular rash evolves rapidly into vesicular lesions (Fig. 180-2). In the normal host, these lesions may remain few in number and continue to form for only 3–5 days. The total duration of disease is generally 7–10 days; however, it may take as long as 2–4 weeks for the skin to return to normal. Patients with herpes zoster can transmit infection to seronegative individuals, with consequent chickenpox. In a few patients, characteristic localization of pain to a dermatome with serologic evidence of herpes

zoster has been reported in the absence of skin lesions, an entity known as *zoster sine herpetica*. When branches of the trigeminal nerve are involved, lesions may appear on the face, in the mouth, in the eye, or on the tongue. *Zoster ophthalmicus* is usually a debilitating condition that can result in blindness in the absence of antiviral therapy. In the *Ramsay Hunt syndrome*, pain and vesicles appear in the external auditory canal, and patients lose their sense of taste in the anterior two-thirds of the tongue while developing ipsilateral facial palsy. The geniculate ganglion of the sensory branch of the facial nerve is involved.

In both normal and immunocompromised hosts, the most debilitating complication of herpes zoster is pain associated with acute neuritis and postherpetic neuralgia. Postherpetic neuralgia is uncommon in young individuals; however, at least 50% of zoster patients over age 50 report some degree of pain in the involved dermatome months after the resolution of cutaneous disease. Changes in sensation in the dermatome, resulting in either hypo- or hyperesthesia, are common.

CNS involvement may follow localized herpes zoster. Many patients without signs of meningeal irritation have CSF pleocytosis and moderately elevated levels of CSF protein. Symptomatic meningoencephalitis is characterized by headache, fever, photophobia, meningitis, and vomiting. A rare manifestation of CNS involvement is granulomatous angiitis with contralateral hemiplegia, which can be diagnosed by cerebral arteriography. Other neurologic manifestations include transverse myelitis with or without motor paralysis.

Like chickenpox, herpes zoster is more severe in immunocompromised than immunocompetent individuals. Lesions continue to form for >1 week, and scabbing is not complete in most cases until 3 weeks into the illness. Patients with Hodgkin's disease and non-Hodgkin's lymphoma are at greatest risk for progressive herpes zoster. Cutaneous dissemination (Fig. 180-3) develops in ~40% of these patients. Among patients with cutaneous dissemination, the risk of pneumonitis, meningoencephalitis, hepatitis, and other serious complications is increased by 5–10%. However, even in immunocompromised patients, disseminated zoster is rarely fatal.

Recipients of hematopoietic stem cell transplants are at particularly high risk of VZV infection. Of all cases of posttransplantation VZV infection, 30% occur within 1 year (50% of these within 9 months); 45% of the patients involved have cutaneous or

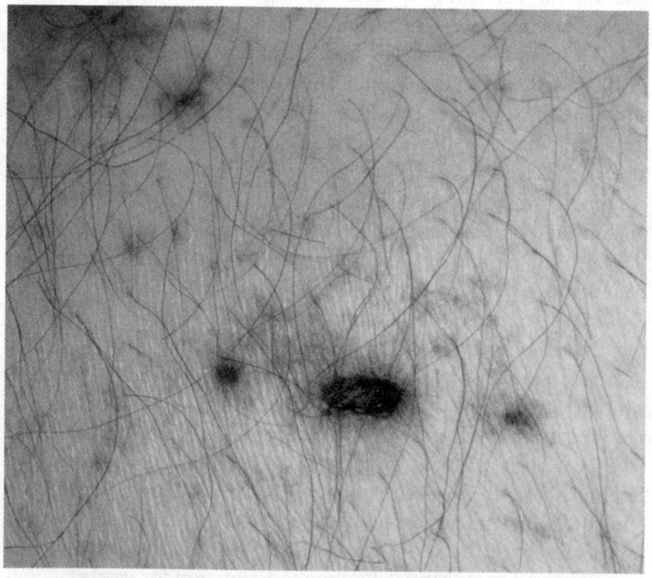

Figure 180-2 Close-up of lesions of disseminated zoster. Note lesions at different stages of evolution, including pustules and crusting. *(Photo courtesy of Lindsey Baden; with permission.)*

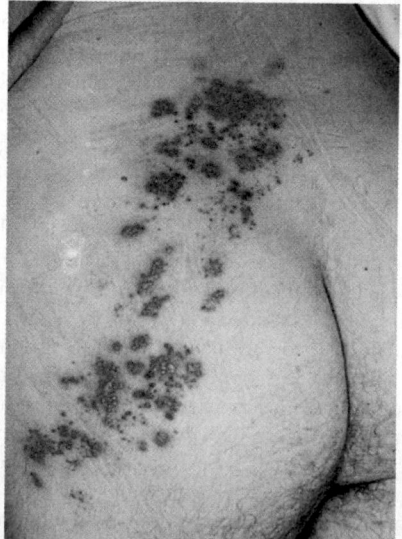

Figure 180-3 Herpes zoster in an HIV-infected patient is seen as hemorrhagic vesicles and pustules on an erythematous base grouped in a dermatomal distribution.

visceral dissemination. The mortality rate in this situation is 10%. Postherpetic neuralgia, scarring, and bacterial superinfection are especially common in VZV infections occurring within 9 months of transplantation. Among infected patients, concomitant graft-versus-host disease increases the chance of dissemination and/or death.

DIFFERENTIAL DIAGNOSIS

(See also Chap. e7) The diagnosis of chickenpox is not difficult. The characteristic rash and a history of recent exposure should lead to a prompt diagnosis. Other viral infections that can mimic chickenpox include disseminated HSV infection in patients with atopic dermatitis and the disseminated vesiculopapular lesions sometimes associated with coxsackievirus infection, echovirus infection, or atypical measles. However, these rashes are more commonly morbilliform with a hemorrhagic component rather than vesicular or vesiculopustular. Rickettsialpox (Chap. 174) can be confused with chickenpox; however, rickettsialpox can be distinguished easily by detection of the "herald spot" at the site of the mite bite and the development of a more pronounced headache. Serologic testing is also useful in differentiating rickettsialpox from varicella and can confirm susceptibility in adults unsure of their chickenpox history. Concern about smallpox has recently increased because of the threat of bioterrorism (Chap. 221). The lesions of smallpox are larger than those of chickenpox and are all at the same stage of evolution at any given time.

Unilateral vesicular lesions in a dermatomal pattern should lead rapidly to the diagnosis of herpes zoster, although the occurrence of shingles without a rash has been reported. Both HSV and coxsackievirus infections can cause dermatomal vesicular lesions. Supportive diagnostic virology and fluorescent staining of skin scrapings with monoclonal antibodies are helpful in ensuring the proper diagnosis. In the prodromal stage of herpes zoster, the diagnosis can be exceedingly difficult and may be made only after lesions have appeared or by retrospective serologic assessment.

LABORATORY FINDINGS

Unequivocal confirmation of the diagnosis is possible only through the isolation of VZV in susceptible tissue-culture cell lines, the demonstration of either seroconversion or a fourfold or greater rise in antibody titer between acute-phase and convalescent-phase serum specimens, or the detection of VZV DNA by PCR. A rapid impression can be obtained by a Tzanck smear, with scraping of the base of the lesions in an attempt to demonstrate multinucleated giant cells; however, the sensitivity of this method is low (~60%). PCR technology for the detection of viral DNA in vesicular fluid is available in a limited number of diagnostic laboratories. Direct immunofluorescent staining of cells from the lesion base or detection of viral antigens by other assays (such as the immunoperoxidase assay) is also useful, although these tests are not commercially available. The most frequently employed serologic tools for assessing host response are the immunofluorescent detection of antibodies to VZV membrane antigens, the fluorescent antibody to membrane antigen (FAMA) test, immune adherence hemagglutination, and enzyme-linked immunosorbent assay (ELISA). The FAMA test and the ELISA appear to be most sensitive.

TREATMENT   Varicella-Zoster Virus Infections

Medical management of chickenpox in the immunologically normal host is directed toward the prevention of avoidable complications. Obviously, good hygiene includes daily bathing and

soaks. Secondary bacterial infection of the skin can be avoided by meticulous skin care, particularly with close cropping of fingernails. Pruritus can be decreased with topical dressings or the administration of antipruritic drugs. Tepid water baths and wet compresses are better than drying lotions for the relief of itching. Administration of aspirin to children with chickenpox should be avoided because of the association of aspirin derivatives with the development of Reye's syndrome. Acyclovir (800 mg by mouth five times daily), valacyclovir (1 g three times daily), or famciclovir (250 mg three times daily) for 5–7 days is recommended for adolescents and adults with chickenpox of ≤24 h duration. (Valacyclovir is licensed for use in children and adolescents. Famciclovir is recommended but not licensed for varicella.) Likewise, acyclovir therapy may be of benefit to children <12 years of age if initiated early in the disease (<24 h) at a dose of 20 mg/kg every 6 h. The advantages (i.e., pharmacokinetics) of the second-generation agents valacyclovir and famciclovir are described in Chap. 178.

Aluminum acetate soaks for the management of herpes zoster can be both soothing and cleansing. Patients with herpes zoster benefit from oral antiviral therapy, as evidenced by accelerated healing of lesions and resolution of zoster-associated pain with acyclovir, valacyclovir, or famciclovir. Acyclovir, now off patent, is administered at a dosage of 800 mg five times daily for 7–10 days. Famciclovir, the prodrug of penciclovir, is at least as effective as acyclovir and perhaps more so; the dose is 500 mg by mouth three times daily for 7 days. Valacyclovir, the prodrug of acyclovir that is now off patent, accelerates healing and resolution of zoster-associated pain more promptly than acyclovir. The dose is 1 g by mouth three times daily for 5–7 days. Compared with acyclovir, both famciclovir and valacyclovir offer the advantage of less frequent administration.

In severely immunocompromised hosts (e.g., transplant recipients, patients with lymphoproliferative malignancies), both chickenpox and herpes zoster (including disseminated disease) should be treated, at least at the outset, with IV acyclovir, which reduces the occurrence of visceral complications but has no effect on healing of skin lesions or pain. The dose is 10 mg/kg every 8 h for 7 days. For low-risk immunocompromised hosts, oral therapy with valacyclovir or famciclovir appears beneficial. If medically feasible, it is desirable to decrease immunosuppressive treatment concomitant with the administration of IV acyclovir.

Patients with varicella pneumonia often require ventilatory support. Persons with zoster ophthalmicus should be referred immediately to an ophthalmologist. Therapy for this condition consists of the administration of analgesics for severe pain and the use of atropine. Acyclovir, valacyclovir, and famciclovir all accelerate healing. Decisions about the use of glucocorticoids should be made by the ophthalmologist.

The management of acute neuritis and/or postherpetic neuralgia can be particularly difficult. In addition to the judicious use of analgesics, ranging from nonnarcotics to narcotic derivatives, drugs such as gabapentin, pregabalin, amitriptyline hydrochloride, lidocaine (patches), and fluphenazine hydrochloride are reportedly beneficial for pain relief. In one study, glucocorticoid therapy administered early in the course of localized herpes zoster significantly accelerated such quality-of-life improvements as a return to usual activity and termination of analgesic medications. The dose of prednisone administered orally was 60 mg/d on days 1–7, 30 mg/d on days 8–14, and 15 mg/d on days 15–21. This regimen is appropriate only for relatively healthy elderly persons with moderate or severe pain at presentation. Patients with osteoporosis, diabetes mellitus, glycosuria, or hypertension may not be appropriate candidates. Glucocorticoids should not be used without concomitant anti-viral therapy.

■ PREVENTION

Three methods are used for the prevention of VZV infections. First, a live attenuated varicella vaccine (Oka) is recommended for all children >1 year of age (up to 12 years of age) who have not had chickenpox and for adults known to be seronegative for VZV. Two doses are recommended for all children: the first at 12–15 months of age and the second at ~4–6 years of age. VZV-seronegative persons >13 years of age should receive two doses of vaccine at least 1 month apart. The vaccine is both safe and efficacious. Breakthrough cases are mild and may result in spread of the vaccine virus to susceptible contacts. The universal vaccination of children is resulting in a decreased incidence of chickenpox in sentinel communities. Furthermore, inactivation of the vaccine virus significantly decreases the occurrence of herpes zoster after hematopoietic stem-cell transplantation. In individuals >60 years of age, a VZV vaccine with 18 times the viral content of the Oka vaccine decreased the incidence of shingles by 51%, the burden of illness by 61%, and the incidence of postherpetic neuralgia by 66%. The Advisory Committee on Immunization Practices has therefore recommended that persons in this age group be offered this vaccine in order to reduce the frequency of shingles and the severity of postherpetic neuralgia.

A second approach is to administer varicella-zoster immune globulin (VZIG) to individuals who are susceptible, are at high risk for developing complications of varicella, and have had a significant exposure. This product should be given within 96 h (preferably within 72 h) of the exposure. Indications for administration of VZIG appear in Table 180-1. VZIG is available under an investigational new drug protocol from FFF Enterprises (800-843-7477).

Lastly, antiviral therapy can be given as prophylaxis to individuals at high risk who are ineligible for vaccine or who are beyond the 96-h window after direct contact. While the initial studies have used acyclovir, similar benefit can be anticipated with either valacyclovir or famciclovir. Therapy is instituted 7 days after intense exposure. At this time, the host is midway into the incubation period. This approach significantly decreases disease severity, if not totally preventing disease.

TABLE 180-1 Recommendations for VZIG Administration

Exposure Criteria

1. Exposure to person with chickenpox or zoster
   a. Household: residence in the same household
   b. Playmate: face-to-face indoor play
   c. Hospital
      Varicella: same 2- to 4-bed room or adjacent beds in large ward, face-to-face contact with infectious staff member or patient, visit by a person deemed contagious
      Zoster: intimate contact (e.g., touching or hugging) with a person deemed contagious
   d. Newborn infant: onset of varicella in the mother ≤5 days before delivery or ≤48 h after delivery; VZIG not indicated if the mother has zoster
2. Patient should receive VZIG as soon as possible but not >96 h after exposure

Candidates (Provided They Have Significant Exposure) Include:

1. Immunocompromised susceptible children without a history of varicella or varicella immunization
2. Susceptible pregnant women
3. Newborn infants whose mother had onset of chickenpox within 5 days before or within 48 h after delivery
4. Hospitalized premature infant (≥28 weeks of gestation) whose mother lacks a reliable history of chickenpox or serologic evidence of protection against varicella
5. Hospitalized premature infant (<28 weeks of gestation or ≤1000-g birth weight), regardless of maternal history of varicella or varicella-zoster virus serologic status

---

FURTHER READINGS

ARVIN A: Aging, immunity, and the varicella-zoster virus. N Engl J Med 352:2266, 2005

GERSHON AA, GERSHON MD: Perspectives on vaccines against varicella-zoster virus infections. Curr Top Microbiol Immuno 342:359, 2010

———: Varicella vaccine. N Engl J Med 356:2648, 2007

GNANN JW, WHITLEY RJ: Herpes zoster. N Engl J Med 347:340, 2002

KIMBERLIN DW, WHITLEY RJ: Varicella-zoster vaccine for the prevention of herpes zoster. N Engl J Med 356:1338, 2007

NGUYEN HQ et al: Decline in mortality due to varicella after implementation of varicella vaccination in the United States. N Engl J Med 352:450, 2005

OXMAN MN et al: A vaccine to prevent herpes zoster and postherpetic neuralgia in older adults. N Engl J Med 352:2271, 2005

SEWARD JF et al: Contagiousness of varicella in vaccinated cases: A household contact study. JAMA 292:704, 2004

——— et al: Varicella disease after introduction of varicella vaccine in the United States, 1995–2000. JAMA 28:606, 2002

CHAPTER 181

Epstein-Barr Virus Infections, Including Infectious Mononucleosis

Jeffrey I. Cohen

■ DEFINITION

Epstein-Barr virus (EBV) is the cause of heterophile-positive infectious mononucleosis (IM), which is characterized by fever, sore throat, lymphadenopathy, and atypical lymphocytosis. EBV is also associated with several human tumors, including nasopharyngeal carcinoma, Burkitt's lymphoma, Hodgkin's disease, and (in patients with immunodeficiencies) B cell lymphoma. The virus is a member of the family Herpesviridae. The two types of EBV that are widely prevalent in nature are not distinguishable by conventional serologic tests.

■ EPIDEMIOLOGY

EBV infections occur worldwide. These infections are most common in early childhood, with a second peak during late adolescence. By adulthood, more than 90% of individuals have been infected and have antibodies to the virus. IM is usually a disease of young adults. In lower socioeconomic groups and in areas of the world with deficient standards of hygiene (e.g., developing regions), EBV tends to infect children at an early age, and IM is uncommon. In areas with higher standards of hygiene, infection with EBV is often delayed until adulthood, and IM is more prevalent.

EBV is spread by contact with oral secretions. The virus is frequently transmitted from asymptomatic adults to infants and among young adults by transfer of saliva during kissing. Transmission by less intimate contact is rare. EBV has been transmitted by blood transfusion and by bone marrow transplantation. More than 90% of asymptomatic seropositive individuals shed the virus in oropharyngeal secretions. Shedding is increased in immunocompromised patients and those with IM.

■ PATHOGENESIS

EBV is transmitted by salivary secretions. The virus infects the epithelium of the oropharynx and the salivary glands and is shed from these cells. While B cells may become infected after contact with epithelial cells, studies suggest that lymphocytes in the tonsillar crypts can be infected directly. The virus then spreads through the bloodstream. The proliferation and expansion of EBV-infected B cells along with reactive T cells during IM result in enlargement of lymphoid tissue. Polyclonal activation of B cells leads to the production of antibodies to host-cell and viral proteins. During the acute phase of IM, up to 1 in every 100 B cells in the peripheral blood is infected by EBV; after recovery, 1–50 in every 1 million B cells is infected. During IM, there is an inverted CD4+/CD8+ T cell ratio. The percentage of CD4+ T cells decreases, while there are large clonal expansions of CD8+ T cells; up to 40% of CD8+ T cells are directed against EBV antigens during acute infection. Memory B cells, not epithelial cells, are the reservoir for EBV in the body. When patients are treated with acyclovir, shedding of EBV from the oropharynx stops but the virus persists in B cells.

The EBV receptor (CD21) on the surface of B cells is also the receptor for the C3d component of complement. EBV infection of epithelial cells results in viral replication and production of virions. When B cells are infected by EBV in vitro, they become transformed and can proliferate indefinitely. During latent infection of B cells, only the EBV nuclear antigens (EBNAs), latent membrane proteins (LMPs), and small EBV RNAs are expressed in vitro. EBV-transformed B cells secrete immunoglobulin; only a small fraction of cells produce virus.

Cellular immunity is more important than humoral immunity in controlling EBV infection. In the initial phase of infection, suppressor T cells, natural killer cells, and nonspecific cytotoxic T cells are important in controlling the proliferation of EBV-infected B cells. Levels of markers of T cell activation and serum interferon (IFN) γ are elevated. Later in infection, human leukocyte antigen–restricted cytotoxic T cells that recognize EBNAs and LMPs and destroy EBV-infected cells are generated. Studies have shown that one of the late proteins expressed during EBV replication, BCRF1, is a homologue of interleukin 10 and can inhibit the production of IFN-γ by mononuclear cells in vitro.

If T cell immunity is compromised, EBV-infected B cells may begin to proliferate. When EBV is associated with lymphoma, virus-induced proliferation is but one step in a multistep process of neoplastic transformation. In many EBV-containing tumors, LMP-1 mimics members of the tumor necrosis factor receptor family (e.g., CD40), transmitting growth-proliferating signals.

■ CLINICAL MANIFESTATIONS

Signs and symptoms

Most EBV infections in infants and young children either are asymptomatic or present as mild pharyngitis with or without tonsillitis. In contrast, up to 75% of infections in adolescents present as IM. IM in the elderly presents relatively often as nonspecific symptoms, including prolonged fever, fatigue, myalgia, and malaise. In contrast, pharyngitis, lymphadenopathy, splenomegaly, and atypical lymphocytes are relatively rare in elderly patients.

The incubation period for IM in young adults is ~4–6 weeks. A prodrome of fatigue, malaise, and myalgia may last for 1–2 weeks before the onset of fever, sore throat, and lymphadenopathy. Fever is usually low-grade and is most common in the first 2 weeks of the illness; however, it may persist for >1 month. Common signs and symptoms are listed along with their frequencies in Table 181-1. Lymphadenopathy and pharyngitis are most prominent during the first 2 weeks of the illness, while splenomegaly is more prominent during the second and third weeks. Lymphadenopathy most often affects the posterior cervical nodes but may be generalized. Enlarged lymph nodes are frequently tender and symmetric but are not fixed in place. Pharyngitis, often the most prominent sign, can be accompanied by enlargement of the tonsils with an exudate resembling that of streptococcal pharyngitis. A morbilliform or papular rash, usually on the arms or trunk, develops in ~5% of cases (Fig. 181-1). Most patients treated with ampicillin develop a macular rash; this rash is not predictive of future adverse reactions to penicillins. Erythema nodosum and erythema multiforme have also been described (Chap. 53). Most patients have symptoms for 2–4 weeks, but malaise and difficulty concentrating can persist for months.

Laboratory findings

The white blood cell count is usually elevated and peaks at 10,000–20,000/μL during the second or third week of illness. Lymphocytosis is usually demonstrable, with >10% atypical lymphocytes. The latter cells are enlarged lymphocytes that have abundant cytoplasm,

TABLE 181-1 Signs and Symptoms of Infectious Mononucleosis

Manifestation	Median Percentage of Patients (Range)
Symptoms	
Sore throat	75 (50–87)
Malaise	47 (42–76)
Headache	38 (22–67)
Abdominal pain, nausea, or vomiting	17 (5–25)
Chills	10 (9–11)
Signs	
Lymphadenopathy	95 (83–100)
Fever	93 (60–100)
Pharyngitis or tonsillitis	82 (68–90)
Splenomegaly	51 (43–64)
Hepatomegaly	11 (6–15)
Rash	10 (0–25)
Periorbital edema	13 (2–34)
Palatal enanthem	7 (3–13)
Jaundice	5 (2–10)

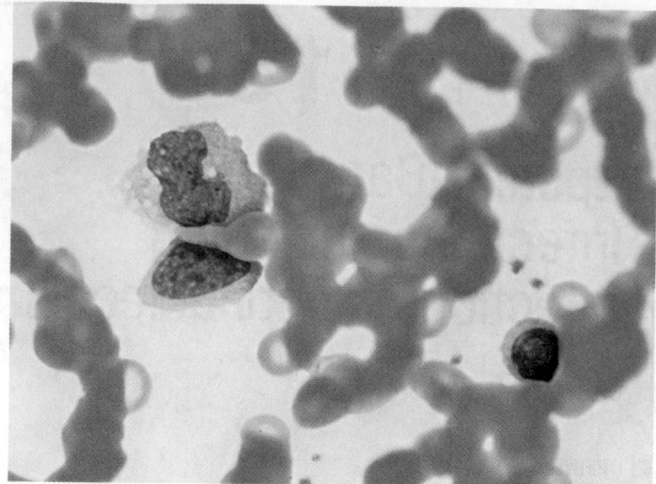

Figure 181-2   Atypical lymphocytes from a patient with infectious mononucleosis due to Epstein-Barr virus.

vacuoles, and indentations of the cell membrane (Fig. 181-2). CD8+ cells predominate among the atypical lymphocytes. Low-grade neutropenia and thrombocytopenia are common during the first month of illness. Liver function is abnormal in >90% of cases. Serum levels of aminotransferases and alkaline phosphatase are usually mildly elevated. The serum concentration of bilirubin is elevated in ~40% of cases.

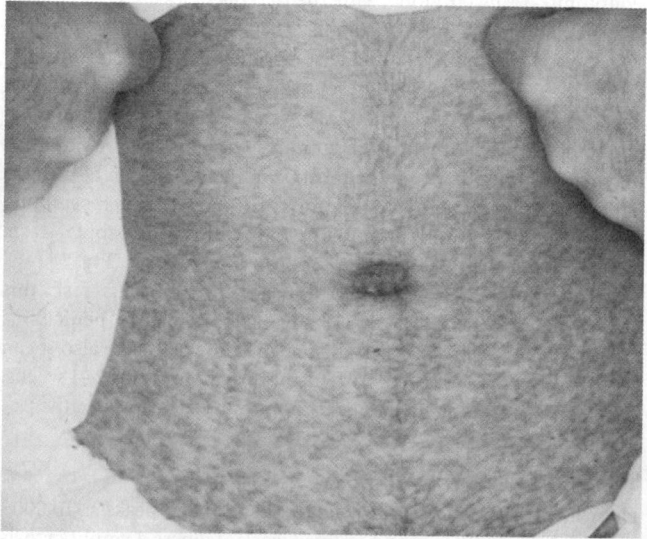

Figure 181-1   Rash in a patient with infectious mononucleosis due to Epstein-Barr virus. *(Courtesy of Maria Turner, MD; with permission.)*

Complications

Most cases of IM are self-limited. Deaths are very rare and most often are due to central nervous system (CNS) complications, splenic rupture, upper airway obstruction, or bacterial superinfection.

When CNS complications develop, they usually do so during the first 2 weeks of EBV infection; in some patients, especially children, they are the only clinical manifestations of IM. Heterophile antibodies and atypical lymphocytes may be absent. Meningitis and encephalitis are the most common neurologic abnormalities, and patients may present with headache, meningismus, or cerebellar ataxia. Acute hemiplegia and psychosis have also been described. The cerebrospinal fluid (CSF) contains mainly lymphocytes, with occasional atypical lymphocytes. Most cases resolve without neurologic sequelae. Acute EBV infection has also been associated with cranial nerve palsies (especially those involving cranial nerve VII), Guillain-Barré syndrome, acute transverse myelitis, and peripheral neuritis.

Autoimmune hemolytic anemia occurs in ~2% of cases during the first 2 weeks. In most cases, the anemia is Coombs-positive, with cold agglutinins directed against the red blood cell antigen. Most patients with hemolysis have mild anemia that lasts for 1–2 months, but some patients have severe disease with hemoglobinuria and jaundice. Nonspecific antibody responses may also include rheumatoid factor, antinuclear antibodies, anti–smooth muscle antibodies, antiplatelet antibodies, and cryoglobulins. IM has been associated with red-cell aplasia, severe granulocytopenia, thrombocytopenia, pancytopenia, and hemophagocytic lymphohistiocytosis. The spleen ruptures in <0.5% of cases. Splenic rupture is more common among male than female patients and may manifest as abdominal pain, referred shoulder pain, or hemodynamic compromise.

Hypertrophy of lymphoid tissue in the tonsils or adenoids can result in upper airway obstruction, as can inflammation and edema of the epiglottis, pharynx, or uvula. About 10% of patients with IM develop streptococcal pharyngitis after their initial sore throat resolves.

Other rare complications associated with acute EBV infection include hepatitis (which can be fulminant), myocarditis or pericarditis with electrocardiographic changes, pneumonia with pleural effusion, interstitial nephritis, genital ulcerations, and vasculitis.

EBV-associated diseases other than IM

EBV-associated lymphoproliferative disease has been described in patients with congenital or acquired immunodeficiency, including

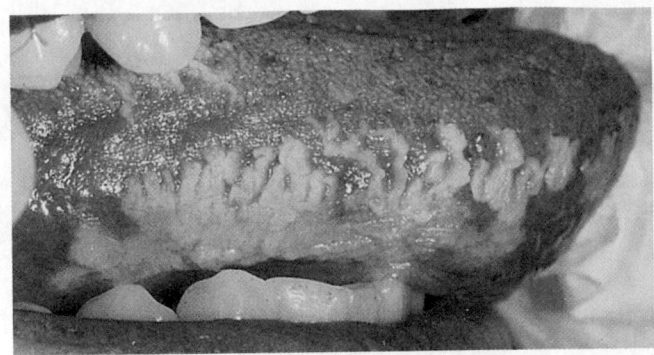

Figure 181-3   Oral hairy leukoplakia often presents as white plaques on the lateral surface of the tongue and is associated with Epstein-Barr virus infection.

those with severe combined immunodeficiency, patients with AIDS, and recipients of bone marrow or organ transplants who are receiving immunosuppressive drugs (especially cyclosporine). Proliferating EBV-infected B cells infiltrate lymph nodes and multiple organs, and patients present with fever and lymphadenopathy or gastrointestinal symptoms. Pathologic studies show B cell hyperplasia or poly- or monoclonal lymphoma. X-linked lymphoproliferative disease (XLPD) is a recessive disorder of young boys who have a normal response to childhood infections but develop fatal lymphoproliferative disorders after infection with EBV. The protein associated with most cases of this syndrome (SAP) binds to a protein that mediates interactions of B and T cells. Most patients with this syndrome die of acute IM. Others develop hypogammaglobulinemia, malignant B cell lymphomas, aplastic anemia, or agranulocytosis. Disease resembling XLPD has also been associated with mutations in the XIAP or ITK proteins. Moreover, IM has proved fatal to some patients with no obvious preexisting immune abnormality.

Oral hairy leukoplakia (Fig. 181-3) is an early manifestation of infection with HIV in adults (Chap. 189). Most patients present with raised, white corrugated lesions on the tongue (and occasionally on the buccal mucosa) that contain EBV DNA. Children infected with HIV can develop lymphoid interstitial pneumonitis; EBV DNA is often found in lung tissue from these patients.

Patients with chronic fatigue syndrome may have titers of antibody to EBV that are elevated but are not significantly different from those in healthy EBV-seropositive adults. While some patients have malaise and fatigue that persist for weeks or months after IM, persistent EBV infection is not a cause of chronic fatigue syndrome. Chronic active EBV infection is very rare and is distinct from chronic fatigue syndrome. The affected patients have an illness lasting >6 months, with elevated levels of EBV DNA in the blood, very high titers of antibody to EBV, and evidence of organ involvement, including hepatosplenomegaly, lymphadenopathy, and pneumonitis, uveitis, or neurologic disease.

EBV is associated with several malignancies. About 15% of cases of Burkitt's lymphoma in the United States and ~90% of those in Africa are associated with EBV (Chap. 110). African patients with Burkitt's lymphoma have high levels of antibody to EBV, and their tumor tissue usually contains viral DNA. Malaria infection in Africa may impair cellular immunity to EBV and induce polyclonal B cell activation with an expansion of EBV-infected B cells. These changes may enhance the proliferation of B cells with elevated EBV DNA in the bloodstream, thereby increasing the likelihood of a *c-myc* translocation—the hallmark of Burkitt's lymphoma. EBV-containing Burkitt's lymphoma also occurs in patients with AIDS.

Anaplastic nasopharyngeal carcinoma is common in southern China and is uniformly associated with EBV; the affected tissues contain viral DNA and antigens. Patients with nasopharyngeal carcinoma often have elevated titers of antibody to EBV (Chap. 88). High levels of EBV plasma DNA before treatment or detectable levels of EBV DNA after radiation therapy correlate with lower rates of overall survival and relapse-free survival among patients with nasopharyngeal carcinoma.

EBV has been associated with Hodgkin's disease, especially the mixed-cellularity type (Chap. 110). Patients with Hodgkin's disease often have elevated titers of antibody to EBV. In about half of cases in the United States, viral DNA and antigens are found in Reed-Sternberg cells. The risk of EBV-positive Hodgkin's disease is significantly increased in young adults after EBV-seropositive IM. About 50% of non-Hodgkin's lymphomas in patients with AIDS are EBV-positive.

EBV is present in B cells of lesions from patients with lymphomatoid granulomatosis. In some cases, EBV DNA has been detected in tumors from immunocompetent patients with angiocentric nasal NK/T cell lymphoma, T cell lymphoma, gastric carcinoma, and CNS lymphoma. Studies have demonstrated viral DNA in leiomyosarcomas from AIDS patients and in smooth-muscle tumors from organ transplant recipients. Virtually all CNS lymphomas in AIDS patients are associated with EBV. Studies have found that a history of IM and higher levels of antibodies to EBV before the onset of disease is more common in persons with multiple sclerosis than in the general population, and additional research on a possible causal relationship is needed.

■ DIAGNOSIS

Serologic testing

The heterophile test is used for the diagnosis of IM in children and adults (Table 181-2). In the test for this antibody, human serum is absorbed with guinea pig kidney, and the heterophile titer is defined as the greatest serum dilution that agglutinates sheep, horse, or cow erythrocytes. The heterophile antibody does not interact with EBV proteins. A titer of ≥forty-fold is diagnostic of acute EBV infection in a patient who has symptoms compatible with IM and atypical lymphocytes. Tests for heterophile antibodies are positive in 40% of patients with IM during the first week of illness and in 80–90% during the third week. Therefore, repeated testing may be necessary, especially if the initial test is performed early. Tests usually remain positive for 3 months after the onset of illness, but heterophile antibodies can persist for up to 1 year. These antibodies usually are not detectable in children <5 years of age, in the elderly, or in patients presenting with symptoms not typical of IM. The commercially available monospot test for heterophile antibodies is somewhat more sensitive than the classic heterophile test. The monospot test is ~75% sensitive and ~90% specific compared with EBV-specific serologies. False-positive monospot results are more common among persons with connective tissue disease, lymphoma, viral hepatitis, and malaria.

EBV-specific antibody testing is used for patients with suspected acute EBV infection who lack heterophile antibodies and for patients with atypical infections (Table 181-2). Titers of IgM and IgG antibodies to viral capsid antigen (VCA) are elevated in the serum of more than 90% of patients at the onset of disease. IgM antibody to VCA is most useful for the diagnosis of acute IM because it is present at elevated titers only during the first 2–3 months of the disease; in contrast, IgG antibody to VCA is usually not useful for diagnosis of IM but is often used to assess past exposure to EBV because it persists for life. Seroconversion to EBNA positivity is also useful for the diagnosis of acute infection with EBV. Antibodies to EBNA become detectable relatively late

TABLE 181-2 Serologic Features of EBV-Associated Diseases

Condition	Heterophile	Anti-VCA IgM	Anti-VCA IgG	Anti-EA EA-D	Anti-EA EA-R	Anti-EBNA
Acute infectious mononucleosis	+	+	++	+	−	−
Convalescence	±	−	+	−	±	+
Past infection	−	−	+	−	−	+
Reactivation with immunodeficiency	−	−	++	+	+	±
Burkitt's lymphoma	−	−	+++	±	++	+
Nasopharyngeal carcinoma	−	−	+++	++	±	+

Abbreviations: EA, early antigen; EA-D antibody, antibody to early antigen in diffuse pattern in nucleus and cytoplasm of infected cells; EA-R antibody, antibody to early antigen restricted to the cytoplasm; EBNA, Epstein-Barr nuclear antigen; VCA, viral capsid antigen.

Source: Adapted from Okano M et al: Clin Microbiol Rev 1:300, 1988.

(3–6 weeks after the onset of symptoms) in nearly all cases of acute EBV infection and persist for the lifetime of the patient. These antibodies may be lacking in immunodeficient patients and in those with chronic active EBV infection.

Titers of other antibodies may also be elevated in IM; however, these elevations are less useful for diagnosis. Antibodies to early antigens (EAs) are detectable 3–4 weeks after the onset of symptoms in patients with IM. About 70% of individuals with IM have EA-D antibodies during the illness; the presence of EA-D antibodies is especially likely in patients with relatively severe disease. These antibodies usually persist for only 3–6 months. Levels of EA-D antibodies are also elevated in patients with nasopharyngeal carcinoma or chronic active EBV infection. EA-R antibodies are only occasionally detected in patients with IM but are often found at elevated titers in patients with African Burkitt's lymphoma or chronic active EBV infection. IgA antibodies to EBV antigens have proved useful for the identification of patients with nasopharyngeal carcinoma and of persons at high risk for the disease.

Other studies

Detection of EBV DNA, RNA, or proteins has been valuable in demonstrating the association of the virus with various malignancies. The polymerase chain reaction has been used to detect EBV DNA in the CSF of some AIDS patients with lymphomas and to monitor the amount of EBV DNA in the blood of patients with lymphoproliferative disease. Detection of high levels of EBV DNA in blood during the first few weeks of IM may be useful if serologic studies yield equivocal results. Culture of EBV from throat washings or blood is not helpful in the diagnosis of acute infection, since EBV commonly persists in the oropharynx and in B cells for the lifetime of the infected individual.

Differential diagnosis

Whereas ~90% of cases of IM are due to EBV, 5–10% of cases are due to cytomegalovirus (CMV). CMV is the most common cause of heterophile-negative mononucleosis; less common causes of IM and differences from IM due to EBV are shown in Table 181-3.

TABLE 181-3 Differential Diagnosis of Infectious Mononucleosis

Etiology	Fever	Adenopathy	Sore Throat	Atypical Lymphocytes	Differences from EBV Mononucleosis
EBV	+	+	+	+	—
CMV	+	±	±	+	Older age at presentation, longer duration of fever
HIV	+	+	+	±	Diffuse rash, oral/genital ulcers, aseptic meningitis
Toxoplasmosis	+	+	±	±	Less splenomegaly, exposure to cats or raw meat
HHV-6	+	+	+	+	Older age at presentation
Streptococcal pharyngitis	+	+	+	−	No splenomegaly, less fatigue
Viral hepatitis	+	±	−	±	Higher aminotransferase levels
Rubella	+	+	±	±	Maculopapular rash, no splenomegaly
Lymphoma	+	+	+	+	Fixed, nontender lymph nodes
Drugs[a]	+	+	−	±	Occurs at any age

[a]Most commonly phenytoin, carbamazepine, sulfonamides, or minocycline. CMV, cytomegalovirus; EBV, Epstein-Barr virus; HHV, human herpesvirus.

TREATMENT   EBV-Associated Disease

Therapy for IM consists of supportive measures, with rest and analgesia. Excessive physical activity during the first month should be avoided to reduce the possibility of splenic rupture, which necessitates splenectomy. Glucocorticoid therapy is not indicated for uncomplicated IM and in fact may predispose to bacterial superinfection. Prednisone (40–60 mg/d for 2–3 days, with subsequent tapering of the dose over 1–2 weeks) has been used for the prevention of airway obstruction in patients with severe tonsillar hypertrophy, for autoimmune hemolytic anemia, for hemophagocytic lymphohistiocytosis, and for severe thrombocytopenia. Glucocorticoids have also been administered to a few selected patients with severe malaise and fever and to patients with severe CNS or cardiac disease.

Acyclovir has had no significant clinical impact on IM in controlled trials. In one study, the combination of acyclovir and prednisolone had no significant effect on the duration of symptoms of IM.

Acyclovir, at a dosage of 400–800 mg five times daily, has been effective for the treatment of oral hairy leukoplakia (despite common relapses). The posttransplantation EBV lymphoproliferative syndrome (Chap. 132) generally does not respond to antiviral therapy. When possible, therapy should be directed toward reduction of immunosuppression. Antibody to CD20 (rituximab) has been effective in some cases. Infusions of donor lymphocytes are often effective for stem cell transplant recipients, although graft-versus-host disease can occur. Infusions of EBV-specific cytotoxic T cells have been used to prevent EBV lymphoproliferative disease in high-risk settings as well as to treat the disease. IFN-α administration, cytotoxic chemotherapy, and radiation therapy (especially for CNS lesions) have also been used. Infusion of autologous EBV-specific cytotoxic T lymphocytes has shown promise in small studies of patients with nasopharyngeal carcinoma and Hodgkin's disease. Treatment of several cases of XLPD with antibody to CD20 resulted in a successful outcome of what otherwise would probably have been fatal acute EBV infection.

■ PREVENTION

The isolation of patients with IM is unnecessary. A vaccine directed against the major EBV glycoprotein reduced the frequency of IM but did not affect the rate of asymptomatic infection.

FURTHER READINGS

CHOQUET S et al: Efficacy and safety of rituximab in B-cell post-transplant lymphoproliferative disorders: Results of a prospective multicenter phase 2 study. Blood 107:3053, 2006

COHEN JI et al: Current understanding of the role of Epstein-Barr virus in lymphomagenesis and therapeutic approaches to EBV-associated lymphomas. Leuk Lymphoma 49(Suppl 1):27, 2008

———: Epstein-Barr virus infection. N Engl J Med 343:481, 2000

GULLEY ML, TANG W: Using Epstein-Barr viral load assays to diagnose, monitor, and prevent posttransplant lymphoproliferative disorder. Clin Microbiol Rev 23:350, 2010

HAQUE T et al: Allogeneic cytotoxic T-cell therapy for EBV-positive posttransplantation lymphoproliferative disease: Results of a phase 2 multicenter clinical trial. Blood 110:1123, 2007

LANDGREN O et al: Risk factors for lymphoproliferative disorders after allogeneic hematopoietic cell transplantation. Blood 113:4992, 2009

LUZURIAGA K, SULLIVAN JL: Infectious mononucleosis. N Engl J Med 362:1993, 2010

MILNONE MC et al: Treatment of primary Epstein-Barr virus infection in patients with X-linked lymphoproliferative disease using B-cell-directed therapy. Blood 105:994, 2005

NJIE R et al: The effects of acute malaria on Epstein-Barr virus (EBV) load and EBV-specific T cell immunity in Gambian children. J Infect Dis 199:31, 2009

TORRE D, TAMBINI R: Acyclovir for treatment of infectious mononucleosis: A meta-analysis. Scand J Infect Dis 31:543, 1999

CHAPTER 182

Cytomegalovirus and Human Herpesvirus Types 6, 7, and 8

Martin S. Hirsch

CYTOMEGALOVIRUS

■ DEFINITION

Cytomegalovirus (CMV), which was initially isolated from patients with congenital cytomegalic inclusion disease, is now recognized as an important pathogen in all age groups. In addition to inducing severe birth defects, CMV causes a wide spectrum of disorders in older children and adults, ranging from an asymptomatic subclinical infection to a mononucleosis syndrome in healthy individuals to disseminated disease in immunocompromised patients. Human CMV is one of several related species-specific viruses that cause similar diseases in various animals. All are associated with the production of characteristic enlarged cells—hence the name *cytomegalovirus*.

CMV, a β-herpesvirus, has double-strand DNA, four species of mRNA, a protein capsid, and a lipoprotein envelope. Like other herpesviruses, CMV demonstrates icosahedral symmetry, replicates in the cell nucleus, and can cause either a lytic and productive or a latent infection. CMV can be distinguished from other herpesviruses by certain biologic properties, such as host range and type of cytopathology. Viral replication is associated with the production of large intranuclear inclusions and smaller cytoplasmic inclusions. CMV appears to replicate in a variety of cell types in vivo; in tissue culture it grows preferentially in fibroblasts. Although there is little evidence that CMV is oncogenic in vivo, it does transform fibroblasts in rare instances, and genomic transforming fragments have been identified.

■ EPIDEMIOLOGY

 CMV has a worldwide distribution. Of newborns in the United States, ~1% are infected with CMV; the percentages are higher in many less-developed countries. Communal living and poor personal hygiene facilitate early spread. Perinatal and early childhood infections are common. CMV may be present in breast milk, saliva, feces, and urine. Transmission has occurred among young children in day-care centers and has been traced from infected toddler to pregnant mother to developing fetus. When an infected child introduces CMV into a household, 50% of susceptible family members seroconvert within 6 months.

CMV is not readily spread by casual contact but rather requires repeated or prolonged intimate exposure for transmission. In late adolescence and young adulthood, CMV is often transmitted sexually, and asymptomatic carriage in semen or cervical secretions is common. Antibody to CMV is present at detectable levels in a high proportion of sexually active men and women, who may harbor several strains simultaneously. Transfusion of whole blood or certain blood products containing viable leukocytes may transmit CMV, with a frequency of 0.14–10% per unit transfused.

Once infected, an individual generally carries CMV for life. The infection usually remains silent. However, CMV reactivation syndromes develop frequently when T lymphocyte–mediated immunity is compromised—for example, after organ transplantation, in association with lymphoid neoplasms and certain acquired immunodeficiencies (in particular, HIV infection; Chap. 189), or in critically ill patients on intensive care units. Most primary CMV infections in organ transplant recipients (Chap. 132) result from transmission in the graft itself. In CMV-seropositive transplant recipients, infection results from reactivation of latent virus or, less commonly, from reinfection by a new strain. CMV infection may also be associated with diseases as diverse as coronary artery stenosis and malignant gliomas, but these associations require further validation.

■ PATHOGENESIS

Congenital CMV infection can result from either primary or reactivation infection of the mother. However, clinical disease in the fetus or newborn is related almost exclusively to primary maternal infection (Table 182-1). The factors determining the severity of congenital infection are unknown; a deficient capacity to produce precipitating antibodies and to mount T cell responses to CMV is associated with relatively severe disease.

Primary infection with CMV in late childhood or adulthood is often associated with a vigorous T lymphocyte response that may contribute to the development of a mononucleosis syndrome similar to that observed after infection with Epstein-Barr virus (Chap. 181). The hallmark of such infection is the appearance of atypical lymphocytes in the peripheral blood; these cells are predominantly activated CD8+ T lymphocytes. Polyclonal activation of B cells by CMV contributes to the development of rheumatoid factors and other autoantibodies during mononucleosis.

Once acquired, CMV persists indefinitely in host tissues. The sites of persistent infection probably include multiple cell types and various organs. Transmission via blood transfusion or organ transplantation is due to silent infections in these tissues. Autopsy studies suggest that salivary glands and bowel may be sites of latent infection.

If the host's T cell responses become compromised by disease or by iatrogenic immunosuppression, latent virus can be reactivated to cause a variety of syndromes. Chronic antigenic stimulation in the presence of immunosuppression (for example, after tissue transplantation) appears to be an ideal setting for CMV activation and CMV-induced disease. Certain particularly potent suppressants of T cell immunity (e.g., antithymocyte globulin) are associated with a high rate of clinical CMV syndromes, which may follow either primary or reactivation infection. CMV may itself contribute to further T lymphocyte hyporesponsiveness, which often precedes superinfection with other opportunistic pathogens, such as *Pneumocystis*. CMV and *Pneumocystis* are frequently found together in immunosuppressed patients with severe interstitial pneumonia.

■ PATHOLOGY

Cytomegalic cells in vivo (presumed to be infected epithelial cells) are two to four times larger than surrounding cells and often contain an 8- to 10-μm intranuclear inclusion that is eccentrically placed and is surrounded by a clear halo, producing an "owl's eye" appearance. Smaller granular cytoplasmic inclusions are demonstrated occasionally. Cytomegalic cells are found in a wide variety of organs, including the salivary gland, lung, liver, kidney, intestine, pancreas, adrenal gland, and central nervous system.

The cellular inflammatory response to infection consists of plasma cells, lymphocytes, and monocyte-macrophages. Granulomatous reactions occasionally develop, particularly in the liver. Immunopathologic reactions may contribute to CMV disease. Immune complexes have been detected in infected infants, sometimes in association with CMV-related glomerulopathies. Immune-complex glomerulopathy has also been observed in some CMV-infected patients after renal transplantation.

TABLE 182-1 CMV Disease in the Immunocompromised Host

Population	Risk Factors	Principal Syndromes	Treatment	Prevention
Fetus	Primary maternal infection/early pregnancy	Cytomegalic inclusion disease	Ganciclovir for symptomatic neonates	Avoidance of exposure; possibly, maternal treatment with CMV immunoglobulin during pregnancy
Organ transplant recipient	Seropositivity of donor and/or recipient; immunosuppressive regimen; high degree of rejection	Febrile leukopenia; pneumonia; gastrointestinal disease	Ganciclovir or valganciclovir	Donor matching; prophylaxis or preemptive therapy with ganciclovir or valganciclovir
Bone marrow transplant recipient	Graft-vs.-host disease; older age of recipient; seropositive recipient; viremia	Pneumonia; gastrointestinal disease	Ganciclovir plus CMV immunoglobulin	Donor matching; prophylaxis or preemptive therapy with ganciclovir or valganciclovir
Person with AIDS	<100 CD4+ T cells/μL; CMV seropositivity	Retinitis; gastrointestinal disease; neurologic disease	Ganciclovir, valganciclovir, foscarnet, or cidofovir	Oral valganciclovir

CLINICAL MANIFESTATIONS

Congenital CMV infection

Fetal infections range from inapparent to severe and disseminated. Cytomegalic inclusion disease develops in ~5% of infected fetuses and is seen almost exclusively in infants born to mothers who develop primary infections during pregnancy. Petechiae, hepatosplenomegaly, and jaundice are the most common presenting features (60–80% of cases). Microcephaly with or without cerebral calcifications, intrauterine growth retardation, and prematurity are reported in 30–50% of cases. Inguinal hernias and chorioretinitis are less common. Laboratory abnormalities include elevated alanine aminotransferase levels in serum, thrombocytopenia, conjugated hyperbilirubinemia, hemolysis, and elevated protein levels in cerebrospinal fluid. The prognosis for severely infected infants is poor; the mortality rate is 20–30%, and few survivors escape intellectual or hearing difficulties later in childhood. The differential diagnosis of cytomegalic inclusion disease in infants includes syphilis, rubella, toxoplasmosis, infection with herpes simplex virus or enterovirus, and bacterial sepsis.

Most congenital CMV infections are clinically inapparent at birth. Of asymptomatically infected infants, 5–25% develop significant psychomotor, hearing, ocular, or dental abnormalities over the next several years.

Perinatal CMV infection

The newborn may acquire CMV at delivery by passage through an infected birth canal or by postnatal contact with infected breast milk or other maternal secretions. Of infants who are breast-fed for >1 month by seropositive mothers, 40–60% become infected. Iatrogenic transmission can result from neonatal blood transfusion; screening of blood products before transfusion into low-birth-weight seronegative infants or seronegative pregnant women decreases risk.

The great majority of infants infected at or after delivery remain asymptomatic. However, protracted interstitial pneumonitis has been associated with perinatally acquired CMV infection, particularly in premature infants, and occasionally has been accompanied by infection with *Chlamydia trachomatis*, *Pneumocystis*, or *Ureaplasma urealyticum*. Poor weight gain, adenopathy, rash, hepatitis, anemia, and atypical lymphocytosis may also be found, and CMV excretion often persists for months or years.

CMV mononucleosis

The most common clinical manifestation of CMV infection in immunocompetent hosts beyond the neonatal period is a heterophile antibody–negative mononucleosis syndrome, which may develop spontaneously or follow transfusion of leukocyte-containing blood products. Although the syndrome occurs at all ages, it most often involves sexually active young adults. With incubation periods of 20–60 days, the illness generally lasts for 2–6 weeks. Prolonged high fevers, sometimes with chills, profound fatigue, and malaise, characterize this disorder. Myalgias, headache, and splenomegaly are common, but in CMV (as opposed to Epstein-Barr virus) mononucleosis, exudative pharyngitis, and cervical lymphadenopathy are rare. Occasional patients develop rubelliform rashes, often after exposure to ampicillin or certain other antibiotics. Less common are interstitial or segmental pneumonia, myocarditis, pleuritis, arthritis, and encephalitis. In rare cases, Guillain-Barré syndrome complicates CMV mononucleosis. The characteristic laboratory abnormality is relative lymphocytosis in peripheral blood, with >10% atypical lymphocytes. Total leukocyte counts may be low, normal, or markedly elevated. Although significant jaundice is uncommon, serum aminotransferase and alkaline phosphatase levels are often moderately elevated. Heterophile antibodies are absent; however, transient immunologic abnormalities are common

and may include the presence of cryoglobulins, rheumatoid factors, cold agglutinins, and antinuclear antibodies. Hemolytic anemia, thrombocytopenia, and granulocytopenia complicate recovery in rare instances.

Most patients recover without sequelae, although postviral asthenia may persist for months. The excretion of CMV in urine, genital secretions, and/or saliva often continues for months or years. Rarely, CMV infection is fatal in immunocompetent hosts; survivors can have recurrent episodes of fever and malaise, sometimes associated with autonomic nervous system dysfunction (e.g., attacks of sweating or flushing).

CMV infection in the immunocompromised host

(Table 182-1) CMV appears to be the most common and important viral pathogen complicating organ transplantation (Chap. 132). In recipients of kidney, heart, lung, and liver transplants, CMV induces a variety of syndromes, including fever and leukopenia, hepatitis, pneumonitis, esophagitis, gastritis, colitis, and retinitis. CMV disease may be an independent risk factor for both graft loss and death. The period of maximal risk is between 1 and 4 months after transplantation, although retinitis may be a later complication. Disease likelihood and viral replication levels generally are greater after primary infection than after reactivation. In addition, molecular studies indicate that seropositive transplant recipients are susceptible to reinfection with donor-derived, genotypically variant CMV, and such infection often results in disease. Reactivation infection, although common, is less likely than primary infection to be important clinically. The risk of clinical disease is related to various factors, such as degree of immunosuppression; use of antibodies to T cell receptors; lack of utilization of anti-CMV prophylaxis; and co-infection with other pathogens. The transplanted organ is particularly vulnerable as a target for CMV infection; thus, there is a tendency for CMV hepatitis to follow liver transplantation and for CMV pneumonitis to follow lung transplantation.

CMV pneumonia occurs in 15–20% of bone marrow transplant recipients; the case-fatality rate is 84–88%, although the risk of severe disease may be reduced by prophylaxis or preemptive therapy with antiviral drugs. The risk is greatest 5–13 weeks after transplantation, and identified risk factors include certain types of immunosuppressive therapy, acute graft-versus-host disease, older age, viremia, and pretransplantation seropositivity.

CMV is an important pathogen in patients with advanced HIV infection (Chap. 189), in whom it may cause retinitis or disseminated disease, particularly when peripheral-blood CD4+ T cell counts fall below 50–100/μL. As treatment for underlying HIV infection has improved, the incidence of serious CMV infections (e.g., retinitis) has decreased. However, during the first few weeks after institution of highly active antiretroviral therapy, acute flareups of CMV retinitis may occur secondary to an immune reconstitution inflammatory syndrome.

Syndromes produced by CMV in immunocompromised hosts often begin with prolonged fever, malaise, anorexia, fatigue, night sweats, and arthralgias or myalgias. Liver function abnormalities, leukopenia, thrombocytopenia, and atypical lymphocytosis may be observed during these episodes. The development of tachypnea, hypoxemia, and unproductive cough signals respiratory involvement. Radiologic examination of the lung often shows bilateral interstitial or reticulonodular infiltrates that begin in the periphery of the lower lobes and spread centrally and superiorly; localized segmental, nodular, or alveolar patterns are less common. The differential diagnosis includes *Pneumocystis* infection; other viral, bacterial, or fungal infections; pulmonary hemorrhage; and injury secondary to irradiation or to treatment with cytotoxic drugs.

Gastrointestinal CMV involvement may be localized or extensive and almost exclusively affects compromised hosts. Ulcers of the

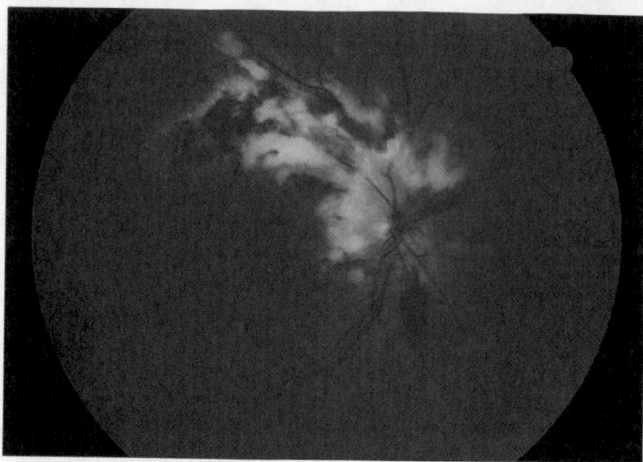

Figure 182-1 Cytomegalovirus infection in a patient with AIDS may appear as an arcuate zone of retinitis with hemorrhages and optic disk swelling. Often CMV is confined to the retinal periphery, beyond view of the direct ophthalmoscope.

esophagus, stomach, small intestine, or colon may result in bleeding or perforation. CMV infection may lead to exacerbations of underlying ulcerative colitis. Hepatitis occurs frequently, particularly after liver transplantation, and acalculous cholecystitis and adrenalitis have been described.

CMV rarely causes meningoencephalitis in otherwise-healthy individuals. Two forms of CMV encephalitis are seen in patients with AIDS. One resembles HIV encephalitis and presents as progressive dementia; the other is a ventriculoencephalitis characterized by cranial-nerve deficits, nystagmus, disorientation, lethargy, and ventriculomegaly. In immunocompromised patients, CMV can also cause subacute progressive polyradiculopathy, which is often reversible if recognized and treated promptly.

CMV retinitis is an important cause of blindness in immunocompromised patients, particularly patients with advanced AIDS (Chap. 189). Early lesions consist of small, opaque, white areas of granular retinal necrosis that spread in a centrifugal manner and are later accompanied by hemorrhages, vessel sheathing, and retinal edema (Fig. 182-1). CMV retinopathy must be distinguished from that due to other conditions, including toxoplasmosis, candidiasis, and herpes simplex virus infection.

Fatal CMV infections are often associated with persistent viremia and the involvement of multiple organ systems. Progressive pulmonary infiltrates, pancytopenia, hyperamylasemia, and hypotension are characteristic features that are frequently found in conjunction with a terminal bacterial, fungal, or protozoan superinfection. Extensive adrenal necrosis with CMV inclusions is often documented at autopsy, as is CMV involvement of many other organs.

■ DIAGNOSIS

The diagnosis of CMV infection usually cannot be made reliably on clinical grounds alone. Isolation of CMV or detection of its antigens or DNA in appropriate clinical specimens is the preferred approach. Virus excretion or viremia is readily detected by culture of appropriate specimens on human fibroblast monolayers. If CMV titers are high, as is common in congenital disseminated infection and in patients with AIDS, characteristic cytopathic effects may be detected within a few days. However, in some situations (e.g., CMV mononucleosis), viral titers are low, and cytopathic effects may take several weeks to appear. Many laboratories expedite diagnosis with an overnight tissue-culture method (shell vial assay) involving centrifugation and an immunocytochemical detection technique employing monoclonal antibodies to an immediate-early CMV antigen. Isolation of virus from urine or saliva does not, by itself, constitute proof of acute infection, since excretion from these sites may continue for months or years after illness. Detection of viremia is a better predictor of acute infection.

Detection of CMV antigens (pp65) in peripheral-blood leukocytes or of CMV DNA in blood or tissues may hasten diagnosis. Such assays may yield a positive result several days earlier than culture methods. The most sensitive way to detect CMV in blood or other fluids may be by amplifying CMV DNA by polymerase chain reaction (PCR). PCR detection of CMV DNA in blood may predict the risk for disease progression, particularly in immunocompromised hosts, and PCR detection of CMV DNA in cerebrospinal fluid is useful in the diagnosis of CMV encephalitis or polyradiculopathy. However, considerable variation among different assays and different laboratories has been observed.

A variety of serologic assays detect increases in titers of antibody to CMV antigens. An increased antibody level may not be detectable for up to 4 weeks after primary infection, and titers often remain high for years after infection. For this reason, single-sample antibody determinations are of no value in assessing the acuteness of infection. Detection of CMV-specific IgM is sometimes useful in the diagnosis of recent or active infection; however, circulating rheumatoid factors may result in occasional false-positive IgM tests.

TREATMENT   Cytomegalovirus Infection

Several measures are useful for the prevention of CMV infection in high-risk patients. The use of blood from seronegative donors or of blood that has been frozen, thawed, and deglycerolized greatly decreases the rate of transfusion-associated transmission. Matching of organ or bone marrow transplants by CMV serology, with exclusive use of organs from seronegative donors in seronegative recipients, reduces rates of primary infection after transplantation. A CMV glycoprotein B vaccine reduced infections in a placebo-controlled trial among 464 CMV-seronegative women; this outcome raises the possibility that this experimental vaccine will reduce congenital infections, but further studies must validate this approach.

CMV immune or hyperimmune globulin has been reported (1) to reduce rates of CMV-associated syndromes and of fungal or parasitic superinfections among seronegative renal transplant recipients and (2) to prevent congenital CMV infection in infants of women with primary infection during pregnancy. Studies in bone marrow transplant recipients have produced conflicting results. Prophylactic acyclovir or valacyclovir may reduce rates of CMV infection and disease in certain seronegative renal transplant recipients, although neither drug is effective in the treatment of active CMV disease.

Ganciclovir is a guanosine derivative that has considerably more activity against CMV than its congener acyclovir. After intracellular conversion by a viral phosphotransferase encoded by CMV gene region UL97, ganciclovir triphosphate is a selective inhibitor of CMV DNA polymerase. Several clinical studies have indicated response rates of 70–90% among patients with AIDS who are given ganciclovir for the treatment of CMV retinitis or colitis. In severe infections (e.g., CMV pneumonia in bone marrow transplant recipients), ganciclovir is often combined with CMV immune globulin. Prophylactic or suppressive (preemptive) ganciclovir may be useful in high-risk bone marrow or organ transplant recipients (e.g., those who are CMV-seropositive before transplantation or who are CMV culture–positive afterward). In many patients with AIDS, persistently low CD4+ T cell counts, and CMV disease, clinical and virologic relapses occur promptly if treatment with ganciclovir is discontinued. Therefore, prolonged maintenance regimens are recommended for such patients. Resistance to ganciclovir is common among patients treated for >3 months and is usually related to mutations in the CMV UL97 gene.

Valganciclovir is an orally bioavailable prodrug that is rapidly metabolized to ganciclovir in intestinal tissues and the liver. Approximately 60–70% of an oral dose of valganciclovir is absorbed. An oral valganciclovir dose of 900 mg results in ganciclovir blood levels similar to those obtained with an IV ganciclovir dose of 5 mg/kg. Oral valganciclovir appears to be as effective as IV ganciclovir for both CMV induction and maintenance regimens. Furthermore, the adverse-event profiles and rates of resistance development for the two drugs are similar.

Ganciclovir or valganciclovir therapy for CMV retinitis consists of a 14- to 21-day induction course (5 mg/kg IV twice daily for ganciclovir or 900 mg twice daily for valganciclovir) followed by prolonged maintenance therapy. For parenteral maintenance, the ganciclovir dose is 5 mg/kg daily or 6 mg/kg 5 days per week; for oral maintenance, 900 mg of valganciclovir once daily is recommended. Peripheral-blood neutropenia develops in 16–29% of treated patients but may be ameliorated by granulocyte colony-stimulating factor or granulocyte-macrophage colony-stimulating factor. Discontinuation of maintenance therapy should be considered in patients with AIDS who, while receiving antiretroviral therapy, have a sustained (3- to 6-month) increase in CD4+ T cell counts to >100/μL.

For treatment of CMV retinitis, ganciclovir may also be administered via a slow-release pellet sutured into the eye. Although this intraocular device provides good local protection, contralateral eye disease and disseminated disease are not affected, and early retinal detachment is possible. A combination of intraocular and systemic therapy may be better than the intraocular implant alone.

Foscarnet (sodium phosphonoformate) inhibits CMV DNA polymerase. Because this agent does not require phosphorylation to be active, it is also effective against most ganciclovir-resistant isolates. Foscarnet is less well tolerated than ganciclovir and causes considerable toxicity, including renal dysfunction, hypomagnesemia, hypokalemia, hypocalcemia, genital ulcers, dysuria, nausea, and paresthesia. Moreover, foscarnet administration requires the use of an infusion pump and close clinical monitoring. With aggressive hydration and dose adjustments for renal dysfunction, the toxicity of foscarnet can be reduced. The use of foscarnet should be avoided when a saline load cannot be tolerated (e.g., in cardiomyopathy). The approved induction regimen is 60 mg/kg every 8 h for 2 weeks, although 90 mg/kg every 12 h is equally effective and no more toxic. Maintenance infusions should deliver 90–120 mg/kg once daily. No oral preparation is available. Foscarnet-resistant virus may emerge during extended therapy.

Cidofovir is a nucleotide analogue with a long intracellular half-life that allows intermittent IV administration. Induction regimens of 5 mg/kg weekly for 2 weeks are followed by maintenance regimens of 3–5 mg/kg every 2 weeks. Cidofovir can cause severe nephrotoxicity through dose-dependent proximal tubular cell injury; however, this adverse effect can be tempered somewhat by saline hydration and probenecid.

It is not clear whether universal prophylaxis or preemptive therapy is the preferable approach in CMV-seropositive immunocompromised hosts. Both ganciclovir and valganciclovir have been used successfully for prophylaxis and preemptive therapy in transplant recipients. For patients with advanced HIV infection (CD4+ T cell counts of <50/μL), some authorities have advocated prophylaxis with oral ganciclovir or valganciclovir. However, side effects, lack of proven benefit, possible induction of viral resistance, and high cost have precluded the wide acceptance of this practice. Preemptive ganciclovir or valganciclovir therapy based on detection of CMV viremia by either antigenemia or PCR techniques is under study.

HUMAN HERPESVIRUS TYPES 6, 7, AND 8

Human herpesvirus (HHV) type 6 was first isolated in 1986 from peripheral-blood leukocytes of six persons with various lymphoproliferative disorders. The virus has a worldwide distribution, and two genetically distinct variants (HHV-6A and HHV-6B) are now recognized. HHV-6 appears to be transmitted by saliva and possibly by genital secretions.

Infection with HHV-6 frequently occurs during infancy as maternal antibody wanes. The peak age of acquisition is 9–21 months; by 24 months, seropositivity rates approach 80%. Older siblings appear to serve as a source of transmission. Congenital infection may also occur, and ~1% of newborns are infected with HHV-6; placental infection with HHV-6 has been described. Most postnatally infected children develop symptoms (fever, fussiness, and diarrhea). A minority develop exanthem subitum (roseola infantum; see Fig. e7-5), a common illness characterized by fever with subsequent rash. In addition, ~10–20% of febrile seizures without rash during infancy are caused by HHV-6. After initial infection, HHV-6 persists in peripheral-blood mononuclear cells as well as in the central nervous system, salivary glands, and female genital tract.

In older age groups, HHV-6 has been associated with mononucleosis syndromes; focal encephalitis; and (in immunocompromised hosts) pneumonitis, syncytial giant-cell hepatitis, and disseminated disease. In transplant recipients, HHV-6 infection may be associated with similar syndromes and with graft dysfunction. Acute HHV-6-associated limbic encephalitis has been reported in transplant recipients and is characterized by memory loss, confusion, seizures, hyponatremia, and abnormal electroencephalographic and magnetic resonance imaging results. High plasma loads of HHV-6 DNA in stem cell transplant recipients are associated with allelic-mismatched donors, use of glucocorticoids, delayed monocyte and platelet engraftment, development of limbic encephalitis, and increased all-cause mortality rates. Like many other viruses, HHV-6 has been implicated in the pathogenesis of multiple sclerosis, although further study is needed to distinguish between association and etiology.

HHV-7 was isolated in 1990 from T lymphocytes from the peripheral blood of a healthy 26-year-old man. The virus is frequently acquired during childhood, albeit at a later age than HHV-6. HHV-7 is commonly present in saliva, which is presumed to be the principal source of infection; breast milk can also carry the virus. Viremia can be associated with either primary or reactivation infection. The most common clinical manifestations of childhood HHV-7 infections are fever and seizures. Some children present with respiratory or gastrointestinal signs and symptoms. An association has been made between HHV-7 and pityriasis rosea, but evidence is insufficient to indicate a causal relationship.

HHV-6, HHV-7, and CMV infections may cluster in transplant recipients, making it difficult to sort out the roles of the various agents in individual clinical syndromes. HHV-6 and HHV-7 appear to be susceptible to ganciclovir and foscarnet, although definitive evidence of clinical response is lacking.

Unique herpesvirus-like DNA sequences were reported during 1994 and 1995 in tissues derived from Kaposi's sarcoma (KS) and body cavity–based lymphoma occurring in patients with AIDS. The virus from which these sequences were derived is designated HHV-8 or Kaposi's sarcoma–associated herpesvirus (KSHV). HHV-8, which infects B lymphocytes, macrophages, and both endothelial and epithelial cells, appears to be causally related not only to KS but also to a subgroup of AIDS-related B cell body cavity–based lymphomas (primary effusion lymphomas) and to multicentric Castleman's disease, a lymphoproliferative disorder of B cells. The association of HHV-8 with several other diseases has been reported but not confirmed.

Unlike other herpesvirus infections, HHV-8 infection is much more common in some geographic areas (e.g., central and southern Africa) than in others (North America, Asia, northern Europe). In high-prevalence areas, infection occurs in childhood, seropositivity is associated with having a seropositive mother or (to a lesser extent) older sibling, and HHV-8 may be transmitted in saliva. In low-prevalence areas, infections typically occur in adults, probably with sexual transmission. Concurrent epidemics of HIV-1 and HHV-8 infections among certain populations (e.g., men who have sex with men) in the late 1970s and early 1980s appear to have resulted in the frequent association of AIDS and KS. Transmission of HHV-8 may also be associated with organ transplantation, injection drug use, and blood transfusion; however, transmission via blood transfusion in the United States appears to be rare or nonexistent.

Primary HHV-8 infection in immunocompetent children may manifest as fever and maculopapular rash. Among individuals with intact immunity, chronic asymptomatic infection is the rule, and neoplastic disorders generally develop only after subsequent immunocompromise. Immunocompromised persons with primary infection may present with fever, splenomegaly, lymphoid hyperplasia, pancytopenia, or rapid-onset KS. Quantitative analysis of HHV-8 DNA suggests a predominance of latently infected cells in KS lesions and frequent lytic replication in multicentric Castleman's disease.

Effective antiretroviral therapy for HIV-infected individuals has led to a marked reduction in rates of KS among persons dually infected with HHV-8 and HIV in resource-rich areas.

HHV-8 itself is susceptible in vitro to ganciclovir, foscarnet, and cidofovir. A small randomized, double-blind, placebo-controlled, crossover trial suggested that oral valganciclovir administered once daily reduced HHV-8 replication. However, clinical benefits of valganciclovir or other drugs in HHV-8 infection have not yet been demonstrated.

FURTHER READINGS

ASAHI-OZAKI Y et al: Quantitative analysis of Kaposi sarcoma–associated herpesvirus (KSHV) in KSHV-associated diseases. J Infect Dis 193:773, 2006

CANNON MJ et al: Lack of evidence for human herpesvirus-8 transmission via blood transfusion in a historical US cohort. J Infect Dis 199:1592, 2009

CASERTA MT et al: Human herpesviruses (HHV)-6 and HHV-7 infections in pregnant women. J Infect Dis 196:1296, 2007

CASPER C et al: Valganciclovir for suppression of human herpesvirus-8 replication: A randomized, double-blind, placebo-controlled, crossover trial. J Infect Dis 198:23, 2008

—— et al: Frequent and asymptomatic oropharyngeal shedding of human herpesvirus 8 among immunocompetent men. J Infect Dis 195:30, 2007

MBULAITEYE S et al: Molecular evidence for mother-to-child transmission of Kaposi sarcoma–associated herpesvirus in Uganda and K1 gene evolution within the host. J Infect Dis 193:1250, 2006

NIGRO G et al: Passive immunization during pregnancy for congenital cytomegalovirus infection. N Engl J Med 353:1350, 2005

PANG XL et al: Interlaboratory comparison of cytomegalovirus viral load assays. Am J Transplant 9:258, 2009

TORRES-MADRIZ G, BOUCHER HW: Perspectives in the treatment and prophylaxis of cytomegalovirus disease in solid-organ transplant recipients. Clin Infect Dis 47:702, 2008

YAO K et al: Detection of human herpesvirus-6 in cerebrospinal fluid of patients with encephalitis. Ann Neurol 65:235, 2009

CHAPTER 183

Molluscum Contagiosum, Monkeypox, and Other Poxvirus Infections

Fred Wang

The poxvirus family includes a large number of related DNA viruses that infect various vertebrate hosts. The poxviruses responsible for infections in humans, along with the main manifestations of these infections, are listed in Table 183-1. Infections with orthopoxviruses—e.g., smallpox (variola major) virus (Chap. 221) or the zoonotic monkeypox virus—can result in systemic, potentially lethal human disease. Other poxvirus infections cause primarily localized skin disease in humans.

MOLLUSCUM CONTAGIOSUM

Molluscum contagiosum virus is an obligate human pathogen that causes distinctive proliferative skin lesions. These lesions measure 2–5 mm in diameter and are pearly, flesh-colored, and umbilicated, with a characteristic dimple at the center (Fig. 183-1). A relative lack of inflammation and necrosis distinguishes these proliferative lesions from other poxvirus lesions. Lesions may be found—singly or in clusters—anywhere on the body except on the palms and soles and may be associated with an eczematous rash.

Molluscum contagiosum is highly prevalent in children and is the most common human disease resulting from poxvirus infection. Swimming pools are a common vector for transmission. Atopy and compromise of skin integrity increase the risk of infection. Genital lesions are more frequent in adults, to whom the virus may be transmitted by sexual contact. The incubation period ranges from 2 weeks to 6 months, with an average of 2–7 weeks. In most cases, the disease is self-limited and regresses spontaneously after 3–4 months in immunocompetent hosts. There are no systemic complications, but skin lesions may persist for 3–5 years. Molluscum contagiosum can be associated with immunosuppression and is frequently seen among HIV-infected patients (Chap. 189). The disease can be more

TABLE 183-1 Poxviruses and Human Infections

Genus	Species	Geographic Location	Host Reservoir	Human Disease
Orthopoxvirus	Variola[a]	Extinct	Humans	Smallpox, systemic
	Monkeypox	Africa	Rodents	Smallpox-like, systemic
	Cowpox	Europe	Rodents	Local pox lesion, occasionally systemic
	Buffalopox	Indian subcontinent	Water buffalo	Local pox lesion, mild illness
	Cantagalo and Araçatuba	South America	Cattle	Local pox lesion, mild illness
	Vaccinia	—	—	Smallpox vaccine
Molluscipoxvirus	Molluscum contagiosum	Worldwide	Humans	Multiple cutaneous lesions (molluscum contagiosum)
Parapoxvirus	Orf	Worldwide	Sheep, goats	Local pox lesions (contagious pustular dermatitis)
	Pseudocowpox (paravaccinia)	Worldwide	Cattle	Local pox lesions (milker's nodule)
	Bovine papular stomatitis	Worldwide	Cattle	Local pox lesions
	Deerpox	Deer herds	Deer	Local pox lesions
	Sealpox	Seal colonies	Seals	Local pox lesions
Yatapoxvirus	Tanapox	Africa	Monkeys	Local pox lesions

[a]See Chap. 221.

generalized, severe, and persistent in AIDS patients than in other groups. Moreover, molluscum contagiosum can be exacerbated in the immune reconstitution inflammatory syndrome (IRIS) associated with the initiation of antiretroviral therapy.

The diagnosis of molluscum contagiosum is typically based on its clinical presentation and can be confirmed by histologic demonstration of the cytoplasmic eosinophilic inclusions (*molluscum bodies*) that are characteristic of poxvirus replication. Molluscum contagiosum virus cannot be propagated in vitro, but electron microscopy and molecular studies can be used for its identification.

There is no specific systemic treatment for molluscum contagiosum, but a variety of techniques for physical ablation have been used. Cidofovir displays in vitro activity against many poxviruses, and case reports suggest that parenteral or topical cidofovir may have some efficacy in the treatment of recalcitrant molluscum contagiosum in immunosuppressed hosts.

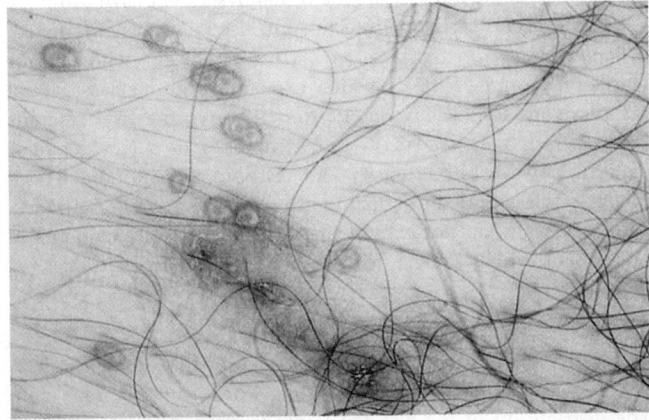

Figure 183-1 Molluscum contagiosum is a cutaneous poxvirus infection characterized by multiple umbilicated flesh-colored or hypopigmented papules.

MONKEYPOX

  Although monkeypox virus was named after the animal from which it was originally isolated, rodents are the primary viral reservoir. Human infections with monkeypox virus typically occur in Africa when humans come into direct contact with infected animals. Human-to-human propagation of monkeypox infection is rare. Human disease is characterized by a systemic illness and vesicular rash similar to those of variola. The clinical presentation of monkeypox can be confused with that of the more common varicella-zoster virus infection (Chap. 180). Compared with the lesions of this herpesvirus infection, monkeypox lesions tend to be more uniform (i.e., in the same stage of development), diffuse, and peripheral in distribution. Lymphadenopathy is a prominent feature of monkeypox infection.

The first outbreak of human monkeypox infection in the Western Hemisphere occurred during 2003, when more than 70 cases were reported in the midwestern United States. The outbreak was linked to contact with pet prairie dogs that had become infected while being housed with rodents imported from Ghana. Patients presented most frequently with fever, rash, and lymphadenopathy ~12 days after exposure. Nine patients were hospitalized, but there were no deaths. Smallpox vaccination can provide cross-reactive immunity to monkeypox infection; studies of people exposed in the outbreak detected subclinical infection in a few vaccinated individuals—an observation suggesting the possibility of long-term vaccine protection. The risk of human disease from animal orthopoxvirus infections may increase as smallpox immunity wanes in the general population and the popularity of exotic animals as household pets grows.

OTHER ZOONOTIC POXVIRUS INFECTIONS

  Cowpox and buffalopox are rare zoonotic infections characterized by cutaneous poxlike lesions and mild systemic illness. Outbreaks of similar poxlike lesions among cattle and farm workers in Brazil have been due to Cantagalo and Araçatuba viruses, which are virtually identical to vaccinia virus and may have become established in cattle during smallpox vaccination programs.

Parapoxviruses are widely scattered among animal species, but only a few are known to cause human disease via direct contact with infected animals. Parapoxviruses are antigenically distinct from orthopoxviruses and share no cross-immunity. *Tanapox* virus belongs to a separate, antigenically distinct genus and usually causes a single nodular lesion on the exposed area after contact with infected monkeys.

FURTHER READINGS

GUR I: The epidemiology of molluscum contagiosum in HIV-seropositive patients: A unique entity or insignificant finding? Int J STD AIDS 19:503, 2008

HAMMARLUND E et al: Multiple diagnostic techniques identify previously vaccinated individuals with protective immunity against monkeypox. Nat Med 11:1005, 2005

LEWIS-JONES S: Zoonotic poxvirus infections in humans. Curr Opin Infect Dis 2:81, 2004

VAN DER WOUDEN JC et al: Interventions for cutaneous molluscum contagiosum. Cochrane Database Syst Rev 4:CD004767, 2009

CHAPTER 184
Parvovirus Infections

Kevin E. Brown

Parvoviruses, members of the family Parvoviridae, are small (diameter, ~22 nm), nonenveloped, icosahedral-shaped viruses with a linear single-strand DNA genome of ~5000 nucleotides. These viruses are dependent on either rapidly dividing host cells or helper viruses for replication. At least four groups of parvoviruses infect humans: parvovirus B19 (B19V), dependoviruses (adeno-associated viruses; AAVs), PARV4/5 virus, and human bocaviruses (HBoVs). Human dependoviruses are nonpathogenic and will not be considered further in this chapter.

PARVOVIRUS B19

■ DEFINITION

B19V is the type member of the genus *Erythrovirus*. On the basis of viral sequence, B19V is divided into three genotypes (designated 1, 2, and 3), but only a single B19V antigenic type has been described. Genotype 1 is predominant in most parts of the world; genotype 2 is rarely associated with active infection; and genotype 3 appears to predominate in parts of western Africa.

■ EPIDEMIOLOGY

B19V exclusively infects humans, and infection is endemic in virtually all parts of the world. Transmission occurs predominantly via the respiratory route and is followed by the onset of rash and arthralgia. By the age of 15 years, ~50% of children have detectable IgG; this figure rises to >90% among the elderly. In pregnant women, the estimated annual seroconversion rate is ~1%. Within households, secondary infection rates approach 50%.

Detection of high-titer B19V in blood is not unusual (see "Pathogenesis," below). Transmission can occur as a result of transfusion, most commonly of pooled components. To reduce the risk of transmission, plasma pools are screened by nucleic acid amplification technology, and high-titer pools are discarded. B19V is resistant to both heat and solvent-detergent inactivation.

■ PATHOGENESIS

B19V replicates primarily in erythroid progenitors. This specificity is due in part to the limited tissue distribution of the primary B19V receptor, blood group P antigen (globoside). Infection leads to high-titer viremia, with >10^{12} virus particles (or IU)/mL detectable in the blood at the apex (Fig. 184-1), and virus-induced cytotoxicity results in cessation of red cell production. In immunocompetent individuals, viremia and arrest of erythropoiesis are transient and resolve as the IgM and IgG antibody response is mounted. In individuals with normal erythropoiesis, there is only a minimal drop in hemoglobin levels; however, in those with increased erythropoiesis (especially with hemolytic anemia), this cessation of red cell production can induce a transient crisis with severe anemia (Fig. 184-1). Similarly, if an individual (or, after maternal infection, a fetus) does not mount a neutralizing antibody response and halt the lytic infection, erythroid production is compromised and chronic anemia develops (Fig. 184-1).

The immune-mediated phase of illness, which begins 2–3 weeks after infection as the IgM response peaks, manifests as the rash of fifth disease together with arthralgia and/or frank arthritis. Low-level B19V DNA can be detected by polymerase chain reaction (PCR) in blood and tissues for months to years after acute infection. The B19V receptor is found in a variety of other cells and tissues, including megakaryocytes, endothelial cells, placenta, myocardium, and liver. Infection of these tissues by B19V may be responsible for some of the more unusual presentations of the infection. Rare individuals who lack P antigen are naturally resistant to B19V infection.

■ CLINICAL MANIFESTATIONS

Erythema infectiosum

Most B19V infections are asymptomatic or are associated with only a mild nonspecific illness. The main manifestation of symptomatic B19V infection is erythema infectiosum, also known as *fifth disease* or *slapped-cheek disease* (Fig. 184-2). Infection begins with a minor febrile prodrome ~7–10 days after exposure, and the classic facial rash develops several days later; after 2–3 days, the erythematous macular rash may spread to the extremities in a lacy reticular pattern. However, its intensity and distribution vary, and B19V-induced rash is difficult to distinguish from other viral exanthems. Adults typically do not exhibit the "slapped-cheek" phenomenon but present with arthralgia, with or without the macular rash.

Polyarthropathy syndrome

Although uncommon among children, arthropathy occurs in ~50% of adults and is more common among women than among men. The distribution of the affected joints is often symmetrical, with arthralgia affecting the small joints of the hands and occasionally the ankles, knees, and wrists. Resolution usually occurs within a few weeks, but recurring symptoms can continue for months. The

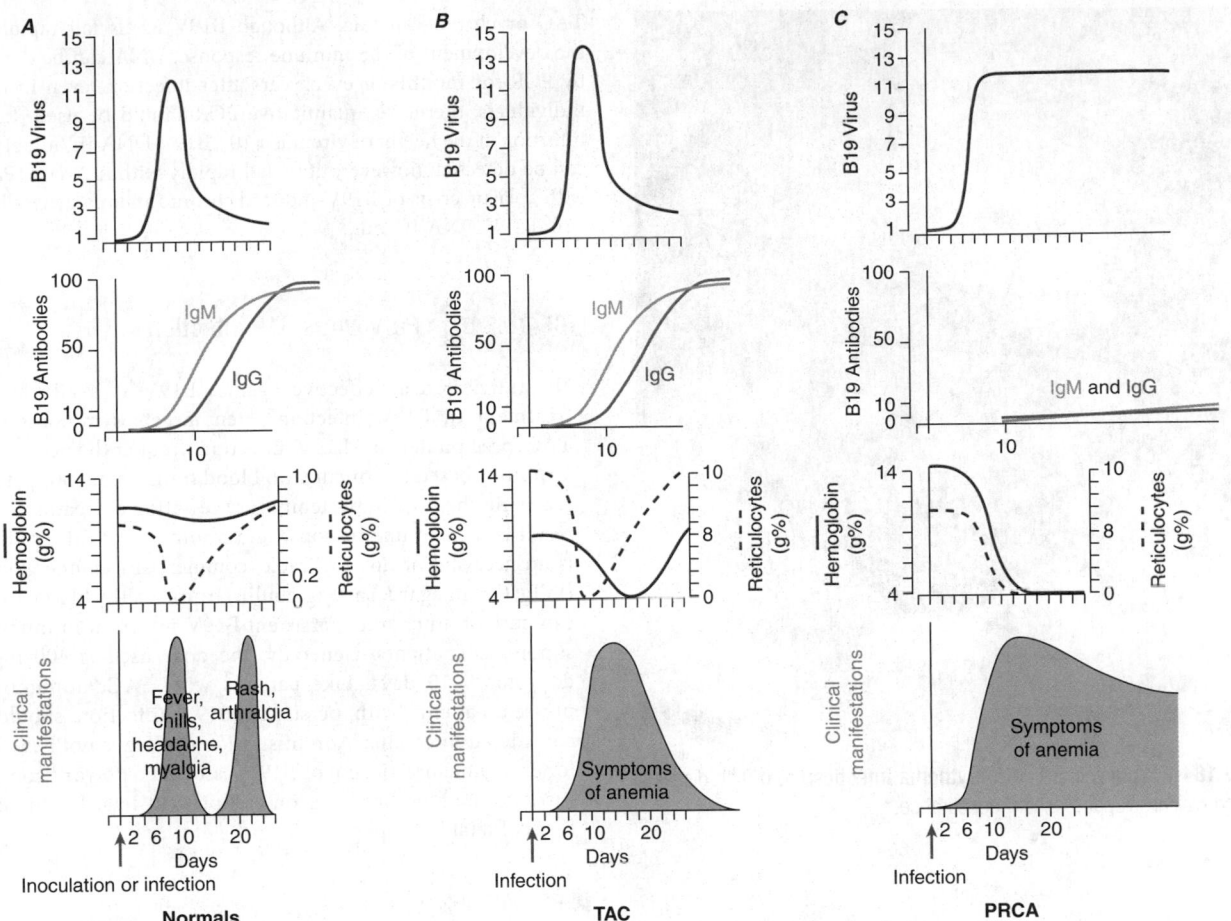

Figure 184-1 Schematic of the time course of parvovirus B19V infection in (**A**) normals (erythema infectiosum), (**B**) transient aplastic crisis (TAC), and (**C**) chronic anemia/pure red-cell aplasia (PRCA). *(Reprinted with* *permission from Young and Brown, 2004. © 2004 Massachusetts Medical Society. All rights reserved.)*

illness may mimic rheumatoid arthritis, and rheumatoid factor can often be detected in serum. B19V infection may trigger rheumatoid disease in some patients and has been associated with juvenile idiopathic arthritis.

Transient aplastic crisis

Asymptomatic transient reticulocytopenia occurs in most individuals with B19V infection. However, in patients who depend on continual rapid production of red cells, infection can cause transient aplastic crisis (TAC). Affected individuals include those with hemolytic disorders, hemoglobinopathies, red cell enzymopathies, and autoimmune hemolytic anemias. Patients present with symptoms of severe anemia (sometimes life-threatening) and a low reticulocyte count, and bone marrow examination reveals an absence of erythroid precursors and characteristic giant pronormoblasts. As its name indicates, the illness is transient, and anemia resolves with the cessation of cytopathic infection in the erythroid progenitors.

Pure red-cell aplasia/chronic anemia

Chronic B19V infection has been reported in a wide range of immunosuppressed patients, including those with congenital immunodeficiency, AIDS (Chap. 189), lymphoproliferative disorders (especially acute lymphocytic leukemia), and transplantation (Chap. 132). Patients have persistent anemia with reticulocytopenia, absent or low levels of B19V IgG, high titers of B19V DNA

in serum, and—in many cases—scattered giant pronormoblasts in bone marrow. Rarely, nonerythroid hematologic lineages are also affected. Transient neutropenia, lymphopenia, and thrombocytopenia (including idiopathic thrombocytopenic purpura) have been observed. B19V occasionally causes a hemophagocytic syndrome.

 A recent study in Papua New Guinea, where malaria is endemic, suggested that B19V infection plays a major role in the development of severe anemia. Further studies must determine whether B19V infection contributes to severe anemia in other malarial regions.

Hydrops fetalis

B19V infection during pregnancy can lead to hydrops fetalis and/or fetal loss. The risk of transplacental fetal infection is ~30%, and the risk of fetal loss (predominantly early in the second trimester) is ~9%. The risk of congenital infection is <1%. Although B19V does not appear to be teratogenic, anecdotal cases of eye damage and central nervous system (CNS) abnormalities have been reported. Cases of congenital anemia have also been described. B19V probably causes 10–20% of all cases of nonimmune hydrops.

Unusual manifestations

B19V infection may rarely cause hepatitis, vasculitis, myocarditis, glomerulosclerosis, or meningitis. A variety of other cardiac manifestations, CNS diseases, and autoimmune infections have also been

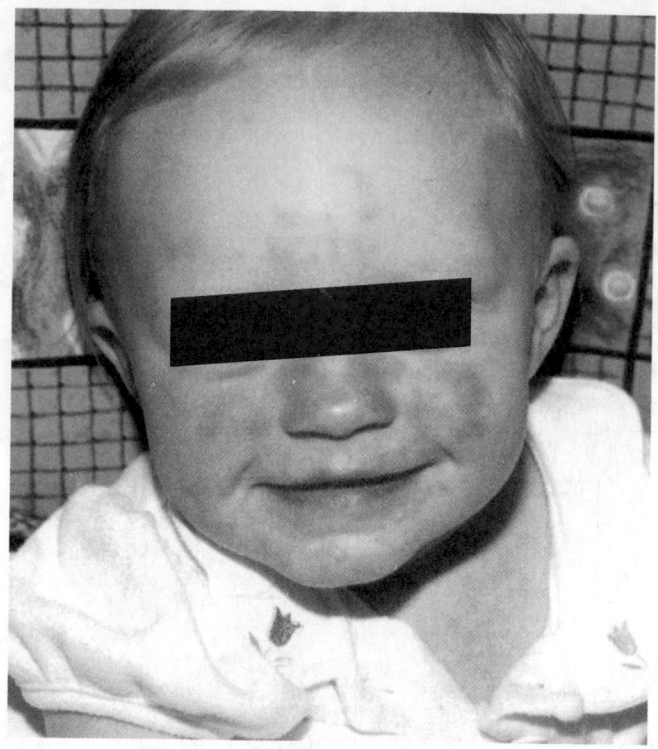

Figure 184-2 Young child with erythema infectiosum, or fifth disease, showing typical "slapped-cheek" appearance.

reported. However, B19V DNA can be detected by PCR for years in many tissues; this finding is of no known clinical significance, but its interpretation may cause confusion regarding B19V disease association.

■ DIAGNOSIS

Diagnosis of B19V infection in immunocompetent individuals is generally based on detection of B19V IgM antibodies (Table 184-1). IgM can be detected at the time of rash in erythema infectiosum and by the third day of TAC in patients with hematologic disorders; these antibodies remain detectable for ~3 months. B19V IgG is detectable by the seventh day of illness and persists throughout life. Detection of B19V DNA should be used for the diagnosis of early

TAC or chronic anemia. Although B19V levels fall rapidly with the development of the immune response, DNA can be detectable by PCR for months or even years after infection, even in healthy individuals; therefore, quantitative PCR should be used. In acute infection at the height of viremia, $>10^{12}$ B19V DNA IU/mL of serum can be detected; however, titers fall rapidly within 2 days. Patients with aplastic crisis or B19V-induced chronic anemia generally have $>10^5$ B19V DNA IU/mL.

> **TREATMENT** Parvovirus B19 Infection

No antiviral drug effective against B19V is available, and treatment of B19V infection often targets symptoms only. TAC precipitated by B19V infection frequently necessitates symptom-based treatment with blood transfusions. In patients receiving chemotherapy, temporary cessation of treatment may result in an immune response and resolution. If this approach is unsuccessful or not applicable, commercial immune globulin (IVIg; Gammagard, Sandoglobulin) from healthy blood donors can cure or ameliorate persistent B19V infection in immunosuppressed patients. Generally, the dose used is 400 mg/kg daily for 5–10 days. Like patients with TAC, immunosuppressed patients with persistent B19V infection should be considered infectious. Administration of IVIg is not beneficial for erythema infectiosum or B19V-associated polyarthropathy. Intrauterine blood transfusion can prevent fetal loss in some cases of fetal hydrops.

■ PREVENTION

No vaccine has been approved for the prevention of B19V infection. A vaccine based on virus-like particles expressed in insect cells is under development; the results of phase 1 trials were promising.

PARV4/5

■ DEFINITION

The PARV4 viral sequence was initially detected in a patient with an acute viral syndrome. Similar sequences, including the related PARV5 sequence, have been detected in pooled plasma collections. The DNA sequence of PARV4/5 is distinctly different from that of all other parvoviruses, and this virus cannot be classified within the current genera of Parvoviridae.

TABLE 184-1 Diseases Associated With Human Parvovirus B19 Infection and Methods of Diagnosis

Disease	Host(s)	IgM	IgG	PCR	Quantitative PCR
Fifth disease	Healthy children	Positive	Positive	Positive	$>10^3$ IU/mL
Polyarthropathy syndrome	Healthy adults (more often women)	Positive within 3 months of onset	Positive	Positive	$>10^3$ IU/mL
Transient aplastic crisis	Patients with increased erythropoiesis	Negative/positive	Negative/ positive	Positive	Often $>10^{12}$ IU/mL, but rapidly decreases
Persistent anemia/pure red-cell aplasia	Immunodeficient or immunocompetent patients	Negative/weakly positive	Negative/ weakly positive	Positive	Often $>10^{12}$ IU/mL, but should be $>10^6$ in the absence of treatment
Hydrops fetalis/congenital anemia	Fetus (<20 weeks)	Negative/positive	Positive	Positive amniotic fluid or tissue	n/a

Abbreviations: IU, international units (1 IU equals ~1 genome); n/a, not applicable; PCR, polymerase chain reaction.

EPIDEMIOLOGY

Parv4 DNA is commonly found in plasma pools but at lower titers than those of B19V found before plasma pool screening. The higher levels of Parv4 DNA and IgG antibody in tissues (bone marrow and lymphoid tissue) and sera from IV drug users than in the corresponding specimens from control patients suggest that the virus is transmitted predominantly by parenteral means.

CLINICAL MANIFESTATIONS

Parv4/5 infection has not been associated with any clinical disease to date.

HUMAN BOCAVIRUSES

DEFINITION

Animal bocaviruses are associated with mild respiratory symptoms and enteritis in young animals. HBoV was originally identified in the respiratory tract of young children with lower respiratory tract infections. More recently, HBoV and the related viruses HBoV2 and HBoV3 have all been identified in human fecal samples.

EPIDEMIOLOGY

Seroepidemiologic studies with HBoV virus-like particles suggest that human bocavirus infection is common. Worldwide, most individuals are infected before the age of 5 years.

CLINICAL MANIFESTATIONS

Although HBoV DNA is commonly found in respiratory secretions from children with acute respiratory infection, the role of this finding in pathogenesis is unknown, and HBoV sequences are often found in the presence of other pathogens. However, increasing evidence indicates that the virus is associated with wheezing in young children. The role of human bocaviruses in childhood gastroenteritis remains to be established.

FURTHER READINGS

ALLANDER T et al: Cloning of a human parvovirus by molecular screening of respiratory tract samples. Proc Natl Acad Sci USA 102:12891, 2005

ARTHUR JL et al: A novel bocavirus associated with acute gastroenteritis in Australian children. PLoS Pathog 5:e1000391, 2009

BROWN KE et al: Resistance to parvovirus B19 infection due to lack of virus receptor (erythrocyte P antigen). N Engl J Med 330:1192, 1994

——— et al: Erythrocyte P antigen: Cellular receptor for B19 parvovirus. Science 262:114, 1993

FRYER JF et al: Novel parvovirus and related variant in human plasma. Emerg Infect Dis 12:151, 2006

KERR JR et al: *Parvoviruses.* London, Hodder Arnold, 2006

KURTZMAN GJ et al: Chronic bone marrow failure due to persistent B19 parvovirus infection. N Engl J Med 317:287, 1987

SCHILDGEN O et al: Human bocavirus: Passenger or pathogen in acute respiratory tract infections? Clin Microbiol Rev 21:291, 2008

YOUNG NS, BROWN KE: Parvovirus B19. N Engl J Med 350:586, 2004

CHAPTER 185

Human Papillomavirus Infections

Richard C. Reichman

DEFINITION

Human papillomaviruses (HPVs) selectively infect the epithelium of skin and mucous membranes. These infections may be asymptomatic, produce warts, or be associated with a variety of both benign and malignant neoplasias.

ETIOLOGIC AGENT

Papillomaviruses constitute the *Papillomavirus* genus of the family Papillomaviridae. They are nonenveloped, measure 50–55 nm in diameter, have icosahedral capsids composed of 72 capsomeres, and contain a double-strand circular DNA genome of ~7900 base pairs. The genomic organization of all papillomaviruses is similar and consists of an early (E) region, a late (L) region, and a noncoding upstream regulatory region (URR). Oncogenic HPV types can immortalize human keratinocytes, and this activity has been mapped to products of early genes E6 and E7. E6 protein facilitates the degradation of the p53 tumor-suppressor protein, and E7 protein binds the retinoblastoma gene product and related proteins. The E1 and E2 proteins modulate viral DNA replication and regulate gene expression. The L1 gene codes for the major capsid protein, which makes up 80% of the virion mass. L2 codes for a minor capsid protein. Type-specific conformational antigenic determinants are located on the virion surface. Papillomavirus types are distinguished from one another by the degree of nucleic acid sequence homology. Distinct types share <90% of their DNA sequences in L1. More than 100 HPV types are recognized, and individual types are associated with specific clinical manifestations. For example, HPV-1 causes plantar warts, HPV-6 causes anogenital warts, and HPV-16 infection can produce cervical dysplasia and invasive cervical cancer. HPVs are species-specific and have not been propagated in routine tissue culture or in common experimental animals. However, some HPV types have been propagated in organotypic culture systems, and some have been produced in human tissues implanted in immunodeficient mice.

EPIDEMIOLOGY

There are few good studies of the incidence or prevalence of human warts in well-defined populations. Common warts (*verruca vulgaris*) are found in as many as 25% of some groups and are most prevalent among young children. Plantar warts (*verruca plantaris*) are also widely prevalent; they occur most often among adolescents and young adults. Anogenital warts (*condyloma acuminatum*) represent one of the most common sexually transmitted diseases in the United States. HPV infection of the uterine cervix produces the squamous cell abnormalities most frequently detected on Papanicolaou smears.

Most anogenital HPV infections are transmitted through direct contact with infectious lesions. However, lesion characteristics that are associated with transmission, including appearance, have not been defined, and individuals without obvious disease may transmit infection. Close personal contact is also assumed to play a role in the transmission of most cutaneous warts; the importance of fomites in this setting is not clear. Minor trauma at the site of inoculation may facilitate transmission. Recurrent respiratory papillomatosis in young children is an uncommon disease that is acquired from the infected maternal genital tract. In adults, orogenital sexual contact may transmit the disease.

A large body of epidemiologic and biologic data has established that some HPV infections cause cervical cancer. For example, >95% of cervical cancers contain HPV DNA of oncogenic (high-risk) types, such as 16, 18, 31, 33, and 45. HPV DNA is also present in the precursor lesions of cervical cancer (cervical intraepithelial neoplasias). Such lesions containing DNA of oncogenic types are more likely to progress than those associated with low-risk HPV types, such as 6 and 11. HPV DNA is transcribed in tumor tissues, and many epidemiologic studies have confirmed a strong relationship between HPV infection (with or without cofactors) and the development of cervical cancer. Definitive proof of the causative role of high-risk HPV types in the pathogenesis of high-grade cervical dysplasia has been provided by the results of recently conducted trials of HPV vaccines. However, it is important to realize that most cervical HPV infections, including those caused by high-risk types, are self-limited. Infection with high-risk HPV types has also been associated with squamous cell carcinomas and dysplasias of the penis, anus, vagina, and vulva. HPV infection may play a role in squamous cell carcinomas of the head and neck. In patients with *epidermodysplasia verruciformis* (see "Clinical Manifestations," below), squamous cell cancers develop frequently at sites infected with specific HPV types, including 5 and 8.

■ CLINICAL MANIFESTATIONS

The clinical manifestations of HPV infection depend on the location of lesions and the type of virus. Common warts usually occur on the hands as flesh-colored to brown, exophytic, and hyperkeratotic papules. Plantar warts may be quite painful; they can be differentiated from calluses by paring of the surface to reveal thrombosed capillaries. Flat warts (*verruca plana*) are most common among children and occur on the face, neck, chest, and flexor surfaces of the forearms and legs.

Anogenital warts develop on the skin and mucosal surfaces of external genitalia and perianal areas (Fig. 185-1). Among circumcised men, warts are most commonly found on the penile shaft. Lesions frequently occur at the urethral meatus and may extend proximally. Receptive anal intercourse predisposes both men and women to the development of perianal warts, but such lesions occasionally develop without such a history. In women, warts appear first at the posterior introitus and on the adjacent labia. They then spread to other parts of the vulva and commonly involve the vagina and cervix. In both sexes, external warts suggest the presence of internal lesions; however, internal lesions may be present without external warts, particularly in women. The differential diagnosis of anogenital warts includes condylomata lata of secondary syphilis, molluscum contagiosum, hirsutoid papillomatosis (pearly penile papules), fibroepitheliomas, and a variety of benign and malignant mucocutaneous neoplasms. Respiratory papillomatosis in young children, which may be life-threatening, presents as hoarseness, stridor, or respiratory distress. The disease in adults is usually milder.

Immunosuppressed patients, particularly those undergoing organ transplantation, often develop pityriasis versicolor–like lesions, from which DNA of several HPV types has been extracted. Occasionally, such lesions appear to undergo malignant transformation. Patients

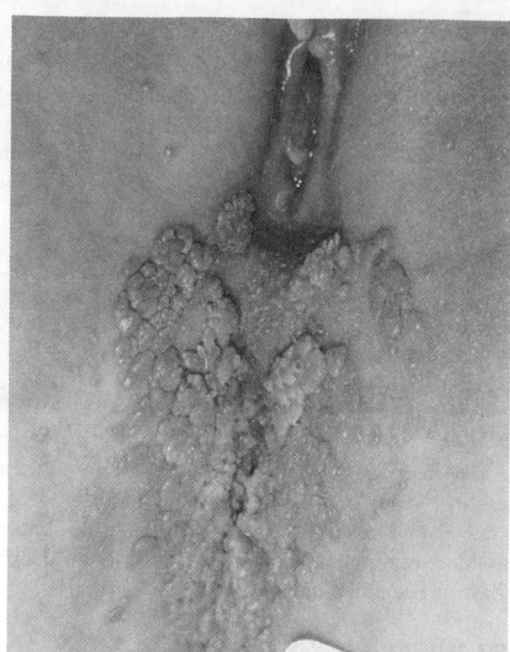

Figure 185-1   Anogenital warts are lesions produced by human papillomavirus and in this patient are seen as multiple verrucous papules coalescing into plaques.

infected with HIV are often infected with uncommon HPV types, frequently have severe clinical manifestations of HPV infection, and are at high risk for cervical and anal dysplasia as well as for invasive cancer. HPV disease in patients with HIV infection may be associated with multiple HPV types, is difficult to treat, and often recurs (Chap. 189).

Epidermodysplasia verruciformis is a rare autosomal recessive disease characterized by an inability to control HPV infection. Patients are often infected with unique HPV types (i.e., types that affect only this group) and frequently develop cutaneous squamous cell malignancies, particularly in sun-exposed areas. The lesions resemble flat warts or macules similar to those of pityriasis versicolor.

The complications of warts include itching and occasionally bleeding. In rare cases, warts become secondarily infected with bacteria or fungi. Large masses of warts may cause mechanical problems, such as obstruction of the birth canal or the urinary tract. Dysplasias of the uterine cervix are generally asymptomatic until frank carcinoma develops. Patients with anogenital HPV disease may develop serious psychological symptoms due to anxiety and depression over this condition.

■ PATHOGENESIS

The incubation period of HPV disease is usually 3–4 months (range, 1 month to 2 years). All types of squamous epithelium can be infected by HPV, and the gross and histologic appearances of individual lesions vary with the site of infection and the type of virus. The replication of HPV begins with infection of basal cells. As cellular differentiation proceeds, HPV DNA replicates and is transcribed. Ultimately, virions are assembled in the nucleus and released when keratinocytes are shed. This process is associated with proliferation of all epidermal layers except the basal layer and produces acanthosis, parakeratosis, and hyperkeratosis. Koilocytes—large round cells with pyknotic nuclei—appear in the granular layer. Histologically normal epithelium may contain HPV

DNA, and residual DNA after treatment can be associated with recurrent disease.

Episomal HPV DNA is present in the nuclei of infected cells in benign lesions caused by HPV. However, in severe dysplasias and cancers, HPV DNA is generally integrated, with disruption of the E1/E2 open reading frames. This disruption leads to upregulation of E6 and E7 and subsequent interference with cellular tumor-suppressor proteins. Expression of E6 and E7 proteins of oncogenic HPV types is necessary for the development and maintenance of the transformed state in both cervical cancers and cell lines derived from these tumors.

Host defense responses to HPV infection remain incompletely understood. However, several studies of recently developed HPV vaccines have demonstrated that production of high titers of type-specific neutralizing antibodies by vaccinated individuals is associated with type-specific protection from HPV infection and disease. Because patients with defects in cell-mediated immune responses (including transplant recipients and patients with HIV infection) frequently develop severe HPV disease, such responses are probably important for the control of established virus replication and disease. Histologic studies demonstrating an epidermal lymphomonocytic infiltrate in resolving warts suggest that local immunity may be of particular importance in the resolution of disease. HPV infection also elicits a detectable serologic response in many patients. Using HPV virus-like particles (VLPs) as antigens, type-specific antibodies can be found in sera of about two-thirds of patients with anogenital infection. Antibodies to E-region proteins, most notably E7, have been detected among patients with cervical carcinoma.

■ DIAGNOSIS

Most warts that are visible to the naked eye can be diagnosed correctly by history and physical examination alone. The use of a colposcope is invaluable in assessing vaginal and cervical lesions and is helpful in the diagnosis of oral and cutaneous HPV disease as well. Application of 3–5% solutions of acetic acid may aid in the visualization of lesions, although the sensitivity and specificity of this procedure are unknown. Papanicolaou smears prepared from cervical or anal scrapings often show cytologic evidence of HPV infection. Persistent or atypical lesions should be biopsied and examined by routine histologic methods. The most sensitive and specific methods of virologic diagnosis use techniques such as the polymerase chain reaction or the hybrid capture assay to detect HPV nucleic acids and to identify specific virus types. Such tests may be useful in the diagnosis and management of cervical HPV disease, although their utility may vary according to the prevalence of disease and the availability of traditional cytologic and histologic testing. Serologic techniques to diagnose HPV infection are not helpful in individual cases and are not widely available.

TREATMENT · Human Papillomavirus Infections

(Table 185-1) Decisions regarding the initiation of therapy should be made with the recognition that currently available modes of treatment are not completely effective and some have significant side effects. In addition, treatment may be expensive, and many HPV lesions resolve spontaneously. Frequently used therapies include cryosurgery, application of caustic agents, electrodesiccation, surgical excision, and ablation with a laser. Topical antimetabolites such as 5-fluorouracil have also been used. Both failure and recurrence have been well documented with all of these methods of treatment. Cryosurgery is the initial treatment of choice for condyloma acuminatum. Topically

TABLE 185-1 Treatment of External, Exophytic Anogenital Warts

I. Administered by provider
  A. Cryotherapy with liquid nitrogen or cryoprobe weekly
  B. Podophyllin resin, 10–25% weekly for up to 4 weeks
  C. Trichloroacetic acid or bichloroacetic acid, 80–90% weekly
  D. Surgical excision
  E. Other regimens
    1. Intralesionally administered interferon
    2. Laser surgery

II. Administered by patient
  A. Podofilox, 0.5% solution or gel twice daily for 3 days, followed by 4 days without therapy. This cycle may be repeated four times.
  B. Imiquimod, 5% cream 3 times per week for up to 16 weeks

Source: Modified from Centers for Disease Control and Prevention: MMWR Recomm Rep 55(RR-11):1, 2006 (www.cdc.gov/mmwr/preview/mmwrhtml/rr5511a1/htm).

applied podophyllum preparations as well as podofilox may also be used. Various interferon preparations have been employed with modest success in the treatment of respiratory papillomatosis and condyloma acuminatum. A topically applied interferon inducer, imiquimod, is also of benefit in the treatment of condyloma acuminatum. The diagnosis and management of anogenital dysplasias and of internal anogenital warts require special skills and resources, and patients with such lesions should be referred to a qualified specialist.

■ PREVENTION

Recently developed HPV VLP vaccines dramatically reduce rates of infection and disease produced by the HPV types in the vaccines. These products are directed against virus types that cause anogenital tract disease and are derived from expression of the major capsid protein (L1) gene in tissue culture. When expressed using appropriate vectors and tissue culture systems, L1 self-assembles into a VLP that cannot be distinguished morphologically or antigenically from its wild-type counterpart (Fig. 185-2) but that contains no viral nucleic acid. To date, one quadrivalent product (Gardasil, Merck) containing HPV types 6, 11, 16, and 18 and one bivalent product (Cervarix, GlaxoSmithKline) containing HPV types 16 and 18 have been licensed in the United States. HPV types 6 and 11 cause 90% of anogenital warts, whereas types 16 and 18 are responsible for 70% of cervical cancers. Both vaccines are highly immunogenic, as measured by serum antibody titers after vaccination. Vaccine efficacy has varied according to the immunologic and virologic characteristics of study populations at baseline and according to the endpoints evaluated. Among study participants who are shown at baseline not to be infected with a specific virus type contained in the vaccine and who adhere to the study protocol, rates of vaccine efficacy regularly exceed 90%, as measured by both infection and disease caused by that specific virus type. Study participants who are already infected at baseline with a specific virus type contained in the vaccine do not benefit from vaccination against that type but may benefit from vaccination against other virus types contained in the vaccine preparation. Thus available HPV vaccines have potent prophylactic effects but no therapeutic effects. The Advisory Committee on Immunization Practices (ACIP) of the Centers for Disease Control and Prevention has recommended that HPV vaccination be routinely offered to

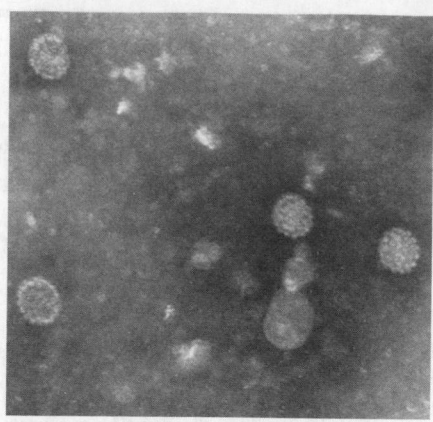

HPV-11 virus particles

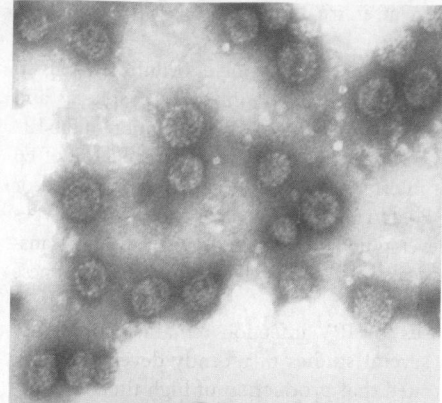

HPV-11 virus-like particles

Figure 185-2   HPV-11 virus-like particles produced in insect cells (**right**) are morphologically and antigenically indistinguishable from wild-type HPV-11 particles (**left**). *(Images courtesy of Drs. William Bonnez and Robert C. Rose; with permission.)*

girls and young women 9–26 years of age. The quadrivalent vaccine has also been licensed in the United States for use in males; the ACIP has stated that this product may be used to prevent anogenital warts in boys and young men 9–26 years of age. Because 30% of cervical cancers are caused by HPV types not contained in the vaccines, no changes in cervical cancer screening programs are currently recommended. Barrier methods of contraception may also be helpful in preventing transmission of condyloma acuminatum and other anogenital HPV-associated diseases. Methods to prevent other HPV infections are limited to avoidance of contact with infectious lesions.

FURTHER READINGS

ADVISORY COMMITTEE ON IMMUNIZATION PRACTICES: Recommended adult immunization schedule: United States, 2010. Ann Intern Med 152:36, 2010

BONNEZ W, REICHMAN RC: Papillomaviruses, in *Principles and Practice of Infectious Diseases*, 7th ed, GL Mandell et al (eds). Churchill Livingstone, Philadelphia, 2010, pp 2035–2049

CENTERS FOR DISEASE CONTROL AND PREVENTION: Sexually transmitted diseases treatment guidelines, 2006. MMWR Recomm Rep 55:1, 2006 (*www.cdc.gov/mmwr/preview/mmwrhtml/rr5511a1.htm*)

D'SOUZA G et al: Case-control study of human papillomavirus and oropharyngeal cancer. N Engl J Med 356:1944, 2007

FUTURE II STUDY GROUP: Quadrivalent vaccine against human papillomavirus to prevent high-grade cervical lesions. N Engl J Med 356:1915, 2007

GARLAND SM et al: Quadrivalent vaccine against human papillomavirus to prevent anogenital diseases. N Engl J Med 356:1928, 2007

MARKOWITZ LE et al: Seroprevalence of human papillomavirus types 6, 11, 16, and 18 in the United States: National Health and Nutrition Examination Survey 2003–2004. J Infect Dis 200:1059, 2009

PAAVONEN J et al: Efficacy of human papillomavirus (HPV)-16/18 AS04-adjuvanted vaccine against cervical infection and precancer caused by oncogenic HPV types (PATRICIA): Final analysis of a double-blind, randomised study in young women. Lancet 374:301, 2009

SCHIFFMAN M et al: Human papillomavirus and cervical cancer. Lancet 370:890, 2007

SYCURO LK et al: Persistence of genital human papillomavirus infection in a long-term follow-up study of female university students. J Infect Dis 198:971, 2008

PART 8

Infectious Diseases

CHAPTER 186

Common Viral Respiratory Infections

Raphael Dolin

■ GENERAL CONSIDERATIONS

Acute viral respiratory illnesses are among the most common of human diseases, accounting for one-half or more of all acute illnesses. The incidence of acute respiratory disease in the United States is 3–5.6 cases per person per year. The rates are highest among children <1 year old (6.1–8.3 cases per year) and remain high until age 6, when a progressive decrease begins. Adults have 3–4 cases per person per year. Morbidity from acute respiratory illnesses accounts for 30–50% of time lost from work by adults and for 60–80% of time lost from school by children. The use of antibacterial agents to treat viral respiratory infections represents a major source of abuse of that category of drugs.

It has been estimated that two-thirds to three-fourths of cases of acute respiratory illnesses are caused by viruses. More than 200 antigenically distinct viruses from 10 genera have been reported to cause acute respiratory illness, and it is likely that additional agents will be described in the future. The vast majority of these viral infections involve the upper respiratory tract, but lower respiratory tract disease can also develop, particularly in younger age groups, in the elderly, and in certain epidemiologic settings.

The illnesses caused by respiratory viruses traditionally have been divided into multiple distinct syndromes, such as the "common cold," pharyngitis, croup (laryngotracheobronchitis), tracheitis, bronchiolitis, bronchitis, and pneumonia. Each of these general categories of illness has a certain epidemiologic and clinical profile; for example, croup occurs exclusively in very young children and has a characteristic clinical course. Some types of respiratory illness are more likely to be associated with certain viruses (e.g., the common cold with rhinoviruses), while others occupy characteristic epidemiologic niches (e.g., adenovirus infections in military recruits). The syndromes most commonly associated with infections with the major respiratory virus groups are summarized in Table 186-1. Most respiratory viruses clearly have the potential to cause more than one type of respiratory illness, and features of several types of illness may be found in the same patient. Moreover, the clinical illnesses induced by these viruses are rarely sufficiently distinctive to permit an etiologic diagnosis on clinical grounds alone, although the epidemiologic setting increases the likelihood that one group of viruses rather than another is involved. In general, laboratory methods must be relied on to establish a specific viral diagnosis.

This chapter reviews viral infections caused by six of the major groups of respiratory viruses: rhinoviruses, coronaviruses, respiratory syncytial viruses, metapneumoviruses, parainfluenza viruses, and adenoviruses. The extraordinary outbreaks of lower respiratory tract disease associated with coronaviruses (severe acute respiratory syndrome, or SARS) in 2002–2003 are also discussed. Influenza viruses, which are a major cause of death as well as morbidity, are reviewed in Chap. 187. Herpesviruses, which occasionally cause pharyngitis and which also cause lower respiratory tract disease in immunosuppressed patients, are reviewed in Chap. 179. Enteroviruses, which account for occasional respiratory illnesses during the summer months, are reviewed in Chap. 191.

RHINOVIRUS INFECTIONS

■ ETIOLOGIC AGENT

Rhinoviruses are members of the Picornaviridae family, small (15- to 30-nm) nonenveloped viruses that contain a single-stranded RNA genome and have been divided into three genetic species: HRV-A, HRV-B, and HRV-C. In contrast to other members of the picornavirus family, such as enteroviruses, rhinoviruses are acid-labile and are almost completely inactivated at pH ≤ 3. Rhinoviruses grow preferentially at 33°–34°C (the temperature of the human nasal passages) rather than at 37°C (the temperature of the lower respiratory tract). Of the 102 recognized serotypes of rhinovirus, 91 use intercellular adhesion molecule 1 (ICAM-1) as a cellular receptor and constitute the "major" receptor group, 10 use the low-density lipoprotein receptor (LDLR) and constitute the "minor" receptor group, and 1 uses decay-accelerating factor.

■ EPIDEMIOLOGY

Rhinoviruses are a prominent cause of the common cold and have been detected in up to 50% of common cold–like illnesses by tissue culture and polymerase chain reaction (PCR) techniques. Overall rates of rhinovirus infection are higher among infants and young children and decrease with increasing age. Rhinovirus infections occur throughout the year, with seasonal peaks in early fall and spring in temperate climates. These infections are most often introduced into families by preschool or grade-school children <6 years old. Of initial illnesses in family settings, 25–70% are followed by secondary cases, with the highest attack rates among the youngest siblings at home. Attack rates also increase with family size.

Rhinoviruses appear to spread through direct contact with infected secretions, usually respiratory droplets. In some studies of volunteers, transmission was most efficient by hand-to-hand contact, with subsequent self-inoculation of the conjunctival or nasal mucosa. Other studies demonstrated transmission by large- or small-particle aerosol. Virus can be recovered from plastic surfaces inoculated 1–3 h previously; this observation suggests that environmental surfaces contribute to transmission. In studies of married couples in which neither partner had detectable serum antibody, transmission was associated with prolonged contact (≥122 h) during a 7-day period. Transmission was infrequent unless (1) virus was recoverable from the donor's hands and nasal mucosa, (2) at least 1000 $TCID_{50}$ of virus was present in nasal washes from the donor, and (3) the donor was at least moderately symptomatic with the "cold." Despite anecdotal observations, exposure to cold temperatures, fatigue, and sleep deprivation have not been associated with increased rates of rhinovirus-induced illness in volunteers, although some studies have suggested that psychologically defined "stress" may contribute to development of symptoms.

Infection with rhinoviruses is worldwide in distribution. By adulthood, nearly all individuals have neutralizing antibodies to multiple serotypes, although the prevalence of antibody to any one serotype varies widely. Multiple serotypes circulate simultaneously, and generally no single serotype or group of serotypes has been more prevalent than the others.

TABLE 186-1 Illnesses Associated With Respiratory Viruses

Virus	Frequency of Respiratory Syndromes		
	Most Frequent	Occasional	Infrequent
Rhinoviruses	Common cold	Exacerbation of chronic bronchitis and asthma	Pneumonia in children
Coronaviruses[a]	Common cold	Exacerbation of chronic bronchitis and asthma	Pneumonia and bronchiolitis
Human respiratory syncytial virus	Pneumonia and bronchiolitis in young children	Common cold in adults	Pneumonia in elderly and immunosuppressed patients
Parainfluenza viruses	Croup and lower respiratory tract disease in young children	Pharyngitis and common cold	Tracheobronchitis in adults; lower respiratory tract disease in immunosuppressed patients
Adenoviruses	Common cold and pharyngitis in children	Outbreaks of acute respiratory disease in military recruits[b]	Pneumonia in children; lower respiratory tract and disseminated disease in immunosuppressed patients
Influenza A viruses	Influenza[c]	Pneumonia and excess mortality in high-risk patients	Pneumonia in healthy individuals
Influenza B viruses	Influenza[c]	Rhinitis or pharyngitis alone	Pneumonia
Enteroviruses	Acute undifferentiated febrile illnesses[d]	Rhinitis or pharyngitis alone	Pneumonia
Herpes simplex viruses	Gingivostomatitis in children; pharyngotonsillitis in adults	Tracheitis and pneumonia in immunocompromised patients	Disseminated infection in immunocompromised patients
Human metapneumoviruses	Upper and lower respiratory tract disease in children	Upper respiratory tract illness in adults	Pneumonia in elderly and immunosuppressed patients

[a]SARS-associated coronavirus (SARS-CoV) caused epidemics of pneumonia from November 2002 to July 2003 (see text).
[b]Serotypes 4 and 7.
[c]Fever, cough, myalgia, malaise.
[d]May or may not have a respiratory component.

■ PATHOGENESIS

Rhinoviruses infect cells through attachment to specific cellular receptors; as mentioned above, most serotypes attach to ICAM-1, while a few use LDLR. Relatively limited information is available on the histopathology and pathogenesis of acute rhinovirus infections in humans. Examination of biopsy specimens obtained during experimentally induced and naturally occurring illness indicates that the nasal mucosa is edematous, is often hyperemic, and—during acute illness—is covered by a mucoid discharge. There is a mild infiltrate with inflammatory cells, including neutrophils, lymphocytes, plasma cells, and eosinophils. Mucus-secreting glands in the submucosa appear hyperactive; the nasal turbinates are engorged, a condition that may lead to obstruction of nearby openings of sinus cavities. Several mediators—e.g., bradykinin; lysylbradykinin; prostaglandins; histamine; interleukins 1β, 6, and 8; and tumor necrosis factor α—have been linked to the development of signs and symptoms in rhinovirus-induced colds.

The incubation period for rhinovirus illness is short, generally 1–2 days. Virus shedding coincides with the onset of illness or may begin shortly before symptoms develop. The mechanisms of immunity to rhinovirus infection are not well worked out. In some studies, the presence of homotypic antibody has been associated with significantly reduced rates of subsequent infection and illness, but data conflict regarding the relative importance of serum and local antibody in protection from rhinovirus infection.

■ CLINICAL MANIFESTATIONS

The most common clinical manifestations of rhinovirus infections are those of the common cold. Illness usually begins with rhinorrhea and sneezing accompanied by nasal congestion. The throat is frequently sore, and in some cases sore throat is the initial complaint. Systemic signs and symptoms, such as malaise and headache, are mild or absent, and fever is unusual. Illness generally lasts for 4–9 days and resolves spontaneously without sequelae. In children, bronchitis, bronchiolitis, and bronchopneumonia have been reported; nevertheless, it appears that rhinoviruses are not major causes of lower respiratory tract disease in children. Rhinoviruses may cause exacerbations of asthma and chronic pulmonary disease in adults. The vast majority of rhinovirus infections resolve without sequelae, but complications related to obstruction of the eustachian tubes or sinus ostia, including otitis media or acute sinusitis, can develop. In immunosuppressed patients, particularly bone marrow transplant recipients, severe and even fatal pneumonias have been associated with rhinovirus infections.

■ DIAGNOSIS

Although rhinoviruses are the most frequently recognized cause of the common cold, similar illnesses are caused by a variety of other viruses, and a specific viral etiologic diagnosis cannot be made on clinical grounds alone. Rather, rhinovirus infection is diagnosed by isolation of the virus from nasal washes or nasal secretions in tissue culture. In practice, this procedure is rarely undertaken because of the benign, self-limited nature of the illness. In most settings, detection of rhinovirus RNA by PCR is more sensitive than that by tissue culture; however, PCR for rhinoviruses is largely a research procedure. Given the many serotypes of rhinovirus, diagnosis by serum antibody tests is currently impractical. Likewise, common laboratory tests, such as white blood cell count and erythrocyte sedimentation rate, are not helpful.

TREATMENT   Rhinovirus Infections

Because rhinovirus infections are generally mild and self-limited, treatment is not usually necessary. Therapy in the form of first-generation antihistamines and nonsteroidal anti-inflammatory drugs may be beneficial in patients with particularly pronounced symptoms, and an oral decongestant may be added if nasal obstruction is particularly troublesome. Reduction of activity is prudent in instances of significant discomfort or fatigability. Antibacterial agents should be used only if bacterial complications such as otitis media or sinusitis develop. Specific antiviral therapy is not available.

■ PREVENTION

Intranasal application of interferon sprays has been effective in the prophylaxis of rhinovirus infections but is also associated with local irritation of the nasal mucosa. Studies of prevention of rhinovirus infection by blocking of ICAM-1 or by drug binding to parts of the viral capsid (pleconaril) have yielded mixed results. Experimental vaccines to certain rhinovirus serotypes have been generated, but their usefulness is questionable because of the myriad serotypes and the uncertainty about mechanisms of immunity. Thorough hand washing, environmental decontamination, and protection against autoinoculation may help to reduce rates of transmission of infection.

CORONAVIRUS INFECTIONS

■ ETIOLOGIC AGENT

Coronaviruses are pleomorphic, single-stranded RNA viruses that measure 100–160 nm in diameter. The name derives from the crownlike appearance produced by the club-shaped projections that stud the viral envelope. Coronaviruses infect a wide variety of animal species and have been divided into three antigenic and genetic groups. Before the emergence of the coronavirus associated with SARS (SARS-CoV), coronaviruses recognized as causes of infection in humans fell into groups 1 and 2, which include human isolates HCoV-229E and HCoV-OC43, respectively. SARS-CoV was at first believed to represent a novel group but now is considered to be a distantly related member of group 2. The SARS-CoV strains that have been fully sequenced have shown only minimal variation.

In general, human coronaviruses have been difficult to cultivate in vitro, and some strains grow only in human tracheal organ cultures rather than in tissue culture. SARS-CoV is an exception whose ready growth in African green monkey kidney (Vero E6) cells greatly facilitates its study.

■ EPIDEMIOLOGY

Generally, human coronavirus infections are present throughout the world. Seroprevalence studies of strains HCoV-229E and HCoV-OC43 have demonstrated that serum antibodies are acquired early in life and increase in prevalence with advancing age, so that >80% of adult populations have antibodies as measured by enzyme-linked immunosorbent assay (ELISA). Overall, coronaviruses account for 10–35% of common colds, depending on the season. Coronavirus infections appear to be particularly prevalent in late fall, winter, and early spring—times when rhinovirus infections are less common.

An extraordinary outbreak of the coronavirus-associated illness known as SARS occurred in 2002–2003. The outbreak apparently began in southern China and eventually resulted in 8096 recognized cases in 28 countries in Asia, Europe, and North and South America; ~90% of cases occurred in China and Hong Kong. The natural reservoir of SARS-CoV appeared to be the horseshoe bat, and the outbreak may have originated from human contact with infected semidomesticated animals such as the palm civet. In most cases, however, the infection was transmitted from human to human. Case-fatality rates varied among outbreaks, with an overall figure of ~9.5%. The disease appeared to be somewhat milder in cases in the United States and was clearly less severe among children. The outbreak ceased in 2003; 17 cases were detected in 2004, mostly in laboratory-associated settings, and no cases were reported in 2005–2009.

The mechanisms of transmission of SARS are incompletely understood. Clusters of cases suggest that spread may occur by both large and small aerosols and perhaps by the fecal-oral route as well. The outbreak of illness in a large apartment complex in Hong Kong suggested that environmental sources, such as sewage or water, may also play a role in transmission. Some ill individuals ("superspreaders") appeared to be hyperinfectious and were capable of transmitting infection to 10–40 contacts, although most infections resulted in spread either to no one or to three or fewer individuals.

■ PATHOGENESIS

Coronaviruses that cause the common cold (e.g., strains HCoV-229E and HCoV-OC43) infect ciliated epithelial cells in the nasopharynx via the aminopeptidase N receptor (group 1) or a sialic acid receptor (group 2). Viral replication leads to damage of ciliated cells and induction of chemokines and interleukins, with consequent common-cold symptoms similar to those induced by rhinoviruses.

SARS-CoV infects cells of the respiratory tract via the angiotensin-converting enzyme 2 receptor. The result is a systemic illness in which virus is also found in the bloodstream, in the urine, and (for up to 2 months) in the stool. Virus persists in the respiratory tract for 2–3 weeks, and titers peak ~10 days after the onset of systemic illness. Pulmonary pathology consists of hyaline membrane formation, desquamation of pneumocytes in alveolar spaces, and an interstitial infiltrate made up of lymphocytes and mononuclear cells. Giant cells are frequently seen, and coronavirus particles have been detected in type II pneumocytes. Elevated levels of proinflammatory cytokines and chemokines have been detected in sera from patients with SARS.

■ CLINICAL MANIFESTATIONS

After an incubation period that generally lasts 2–7 days (range, 1–14 days), SARS usually begins as a systemic illness marked by the onset of fever, which is often accompanied by malaise, headache, and myalgias and is followed in 1–2 days by a nonproductive cough and dyspnea. Approximately 25% of patients have diarrhea. Chest x-rays can show a variety of infiltrates, including patchy areas of consolidation—most frequently in peripheral and lower lung fields—or interstitial infiltrates, which can progress to diffuse involvement.

In severe cases, respiratory function may worsen during the second week of illness and progress to frank adult respiratory distress syndrome accompanied by multiorgan dysfunction. Risk factors for severe disease include an age of >50 years and comorbidities such as cardiovascular disease, diabetes, or hepatitis. Illness in pregnant women may be particularly severe, but SARS-CoV infection appears to be milder in children than in adults.

The clinical features of common colds caused by human coronaviruses are similar to those of illness caused by rhinoviruses. In studies of volunteers, the mean incubation period of colds induced by coronaviruses (3 days) is somewhat longer than that of illness caused by rhinoviruses, and the duration of illness is somewhat shorter (mean, 6–7 days). In some studies, the amount of nasal discharge was greater in colds induced by coronaviruses than in those induced by rhinoviruses. Coronaviruses other than SARS-CoV have been recovered occasionally from infants with pneumonia and from military recruits with lower respiratory tract disease and have been associated with worsening of chronic bronchitis. Two novel coronaviruses, HCoV-NL63 (group 1) and HCoV-HKU1 (group 2), have been isolated from patients hospitalized with acute respiratory illness. Their overall role as causes of human respiratory disease remains to be determined.

◼ LABORATORY FINDINGS AND DIAGNOSIS

Laboratory abnormalities in SARS include lymphopenia, which is present in ~50% of cases and which mostly affects CD4+ T cells but also involves CD8+ T cells and natural killer cells. Total white blood cell counts are normal or slightly low, and thrombocytopenia may develop as the illness progresses. Elevated serum levels of aminotransferases, creatine kinase, and lactate dehydrogenase have been reported.

A rapid diagnosis of SARS-CoV infection can be made by reverse-transcription PCR (RT-PCR) of respiratory tract samples and plasma early in illness and of urine and stool later on. SARS-CoV can also be grown from respiratory tract samples by inoculation into Vero E6 tissue culture cells, in which a cytopathic effect is seen within days. RT-PCR appears to be more sensitive than tissue culture, but only around one-third of cases are positive by PCR at initial presentation. Serum antibodies can be detected by ELISA or immunofluorescence, and nearly all patients develop detectable serum antibodies within 28 days after the onset of illness.

Laboratory diagnosis of coronavirus-induced colds is rarely required. Coronaviruses that cause those illnesses are frequently difficult to cultivate in vitro but can be detected in clinical samples by ELISA or immunofluorescence assays or by RT-PCR for viral RNA. These research procedures can be used to detect coronaviruses in unusual clinical settings.

TREATMENT	Coronavirus Infections

There is no specific therapy of established efficacy for SARS. Although ribavirin has frequently been used, it has little if any activity against SARS-CoV in vitro, and no beneficial effect on the course of illness has been demonstrated. Because of suggestions that immunopathology may contribute to the disease, glucocorticoids have also been widely used, but their benefit, if any, is likewise unestablished. Supportive care to maintain pulmonary and other organ-system functions remains the mainstay of therapy.

The approach to the treatment of common colds caused by coronaviruses is similar to that discussed above for rhinovirus-induced illnesses.

◼ PREVENTION

The recognition of SARS led to a worldwide mobilization of public health resources to apply infection control practices to contain the disease. Case definitions were established, travel advisories were proposed, and quarantines were imposed in certain locales. As of this writing, no additional cases of SARS have been reported since 2004. However, it remains unknown whether the disappearance of cases is a result of control measures, whether it is part of a seasonal or otherwise unexplained epidemiologic pattern of SARS, or when or whether SARS might reemerge. The U.S. Centers for Disease Control and Prevention and the World Health Organization maintain recommendations for surveillance and assessment of potential cases of SARS (*www.cdc.gov/ncidod/sars/*).

The frequent transmission of the disease to health care workers makes it mandatory that strict infection-control practices be employed by health care facilities to prevent airborne, droplet, and contact transmission from any suspected cases of SARS. Health care workers who enter areas in which patients with SARS may be present should don gowns, gloves, and eye and respiratory protective equipment (e.g., an N95 filtering facepiece respirator certified by the National Institute for Occupational Safety and Health).

Vaccines have been developed against several animal coronaviruses but not against known human coronaviruses. The emergence of SARS-CoV has stimulated interest in the development of vaccines against such agents.

HUMAN RESPIRATORY SYNCYTIAL VIRUS INFECTIONS

◼ ETIOLOGIC AGENT

Human respiratory syncytial virus (HRSV) is a member of the Paramyxoviridae family (genus *Pneumovirus*). An enveloped virus ~150–350 nm in diameter, HRSV is so named because its replication in vitro leads to the fusion of neighboring cells into large multinucleated syncytia. The single-stranded RNA genome codes for 11 virus-specific proteins. Viral RNA is contained in a helical nucleocapsid surrounded by a lipid envelope bearing two glycoproteins: the G protein, by which the virus attaches to cells, and the F (fusion) protein, which facilitates entry of the virus into the cell by fusing host and viral membranes. HRSV is considered to be of a single antigenic type, but two distinct subgroups (A and B) and multiple subtypes within each subgroup have now been described. Antigenic diversity is reflected by differences in the G protein, while the F protein is highly conserved. Both antigenic groups can circulate simultaneously in outbreaks, although there are typically alternating patterns in which one subgroup predominates over 1- to 2-year periods.

◼ EPIDEMIOLOGY

HRSV is a major respiratory pathogen of young children and the foremost cause of lower respiratory disease in infants. Infection with HRSV is seen throughout the world in annual epidemics that occur in late fall, winter, or spring and last up to 5 months. The virus is rarely encountered during the summer. Rates of illness are highest among infants 1–6 months of age, peaking at 2–3 months of age. The attack rates among susceptible infants and children are extraordinarily high, approaching 100% in settings such as day-care centers where large numbers of susceptible infants are present. By age 2, virtually all children will have been infected with HRSV. HRSV accounts for 20–25% of hospital admissions of young infants and children for pneumonia and for up to 75% of cases of bronchiolitis in this age group. It has been estimated that more than half of infants who are at risk will become infected during an HRSV epidemic.

In older children and adults, reinfection with HRSV is frequent but disease is milder than in infancy. A common cold–like syndrome is the illness most commonly associated with HRSV infection in adults. Severe lower respiratory tract disease with pneumonitis can occur in elderly (often institutionalized) adults and in patients with immunocompromising disorders or treatment, including recipients of stem cell and solid-organ transplants. HRSV is also an important nosocomial pathogen; during an outbreak, it can infect pediatric patients and up to 25–50% of the staff on pediatric wards. The spread of HRSV among families is efficient: up to 40% of siblings may become infected when the virus is introduced into the family setting.

HRSV is transmitted primarily by close contact with contaminated fingers or fomites and by self-inoculation of the conjunctiva or anterior nares. Virus may also be spread by coarse aerosols produced by coughing or sneezing, but it is inefficiently spread by fine-particle aerosols. The incubation period is ~4–6 days, and virus shedding may last for ≥2 weeks in children and for shorter periods in adults. In immunosuppressed patients, shedding can continue for weeks.

PATHOGENESIS

Little is known about the histopathology of minor HRSV infection. Severe bronchiolitis or pneumonia is characterized by necrosis of the bronchiolar epithelium and a peribronchiolar infiltrate of lymphocytes and mononuclear cells. Interalveolar thickening and filling of alveolar spaces with fluid can also be found. The correlates of protective immunity to HRSV are incompletely understood. Because reinfection occurs frequently and is often associated with illness, the immunity that develops after single episodes of infection clearly is not complete or long-lasting. However, the cumulative effect of multiple reinfections is to temper subsequent disease and to provide some temporary measure of protection against infection. Studies of experimentally induced disease in healthy volunteers indicate that the presence of nasal IgA neutralizing antibody correlates more closely with protection than does the presence of serum antibody. Studies in infants, however, suggest that maternally acquired antibody provides some protection from lower respiratory tract disease, although illness can be severe even in infants who have moderate levels of maternally derived serum antibody. The relatively severe disease observed in immunosuppressed patients and experimental animal models indicates that cell-mediated immunity is an important mechanism of host defense against HRSV. Evidence suggests that major histocompatibility class I–restricted cytotoxic T cells may be particularly important in this regard.

CLINICAL MANIFESTATIONS

HRSV infection leads to a wide spectrum of respiratory illnesses. In infants, 25–40% of infections result in lower respiratory tract involvement, including pneumonia, bronchiolitis, and tracheobronchitis. In this age group, illness begins most frequently with rhinorrhea, low-grade fever, and mild systemic symptoms, often accompanied by cough and wheezing. Most patients recover gradually over 1–2 weeks. In more severe illness, tachypnea and dyspnea develop, and eventually frank hypoxia, cyanosis, and apnea can ensue. Physical examination may reveal diffuse wheezing, rhonchi, and rales. Chest radiography shows hyperexpansion, peribronchial thickening, and variable infiltrates ranging from diffuse interstitial infiltrates to segmental or lobar consolidation. Illness may be particularly severe in children born prematurely and in those with congenital cardiac disease, bronchopulmonary dysplasia, nephrotic syndrome, or immunosuppression. One study documented a 37% mortality rate among infants with HRSV pneumonia and congenital cardiac disease.

In adults, the most common symptoms of HRSV infection are those of the common cold, with rhinorrhea, sore throat, and cough. Illness is occasionally associated with moderate systemic symptoms such as malaise, headache, and fever. HRSV has also been reported to cause lower respiratory tract disease with fever in adults, including severe pneumonia in the elderly—particularly in nursing-home residents, among whom its impact can rival that of influenza. HRSV pneumonia can be a significant cause of morbidity and death among patients undergoing stem cell and solid-organ transplantation, in whom case-fatality rates of 20–80% have been reported. Sinusitis, otitis media, and worsening of chronic obstructive and reactive airway disease have also been associated with HRSV infection.

LABORATORY FINDINGS AND DIAGNOSIS

The diagnosis of HRSV infection can be suspected on the basis of a suggestive epidemiologic setting—that is, severe illness among infants during an outbreak of HRSV in the community. Infections in older children and adults cannot be differentiated with certainty from those caused by other respiratory viruses. The specific diagnosis is established by detection of HRSV in respiratory secretions, such as sputum, throat swabs, or nasopharyngeal washes. Virus can be isolated in tissue culture, but this method has been largely supplanted by rapid viral diagnostic techniques consisting of immunofluorescence or ELISA of nasopharyngeal washes, aspirates, and (less satisfactorily) nasopharyngeal swabs. With specimens from children, these techniques have sensitivities and specificities of 80–95%; they are somewhat less sensitive with specimens from adults. RT-PCR detection techniques have shown even higher rates of sensitivity and specificity, particularly in adults. Serologic diagnosis may be made by comparison of acute- and convalescent-phase serum specimens by ELISA or by neutralization or complement-fixation tests. These tests may be useful in older children and adults but are less sensitive in children <4 months of age.

| TREATMENT | Human Respiratory Syncytial Virus Infections |

Treatment of upper respiratory tract HRSV infection is aimed primarily at the alleviation of symptoms and is similar to that for other viral infections of the upper respiratory tract. For lower respiratory tract infections, respiratory therapy, including hydration, suctioning of secretions, and administration of humidified oxygen and antibronchospastic agents, is given as needed. In severe hypoxia, intubation and ventilatory assistance may be required. Studies of infants with HRSV infection who were given aerosolized ribavirin, a nucleoside analogue active in vitro against HRSV, demonstrated a modest beneficial effect on the resolution of lower respiratory tract illness, including alleviation of blood-gas abnormalities, in some studies. The American Academy of Pediatrics recommends that treatment with aerosolized ribavirin "may be considered" for infants who are severely ill or who are at high risk for complications of HRSV infection; included are premature infants and those with bronchopulmonary dysplasia, congenital heart disease, or immunosuppression. The efficacy of ribavirin against HRSV pneumonia in older children and adults, including those with immunosuppression, has not been established. No benefit has been found in the treatment of HRSV pneumonia with standard immunoglobulin; immunoglobulin with high titers of antibody to HRSV (RSVIg), which is no longer available; or chimeric mouse-human monoclonal IgG antibody to HRSV (palivizumab). Combined therapy with aerosolized ribavirin and palivizumab is being evaluated in immunosuppressed patients with HRSV pneumonia.

PREVENTION

Monthly administration of RSVIg (no longer available) or palivizumab has been approved as prophylaxis against HRSV for children <2 years of age who have bronchopulmonary dysplasia or cyanotic heart disease or who were born prematurely. Considerable interest exists in the development of vaccines against HRSV. Inactivated whole-virus vaccines have been ineffective; in one study, they actually potentiated disease in infants. Other approaches include immunization with purified F and G surface glycoproteins of HRSV or generation of stable, live attenuated virus vaccines. In settings such as pediatric wards where rates of transmission are high, barrier methods for the protection of hands and conjunctivae may be useful in reducing the spread of virus.

HUMAN METAPNEUMOVIRUS INFECTIONS

■ ETIOLOGIC AGENT

Human metapneumovirus (HMPV) is a viral respiratory pathogen that has been assigned to the Paramyxoviridae family (genus *Metapneumovirus*). Its morphology and genomic organization are similar to those of avian metapneumoviruses, which are recognized respiratory pathogens of turkeys. HMPV particles may be spherical, filamentous, or pleomorphic in shape and measure 150–600 nm in diameter. Particles contain 15-nm projections from the surface that are similar in appearance to those of other Paramyxoviridae. The single-stranded RNA genome codes for nine proteins that, except for the absence of nonstructural proteins, generally correspond to those of HRSV. HMPV is of only one antigenic type; two closely related genotypes (A and B), four subgroups, and two sublineages have been described.

■ EPIDEMIOLOGY

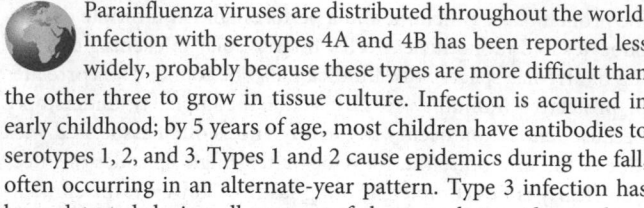

HMPV infections are worldwide in distribution, are most frequent during the winter, and occur early in life, so that serum antibodies to the virus are present in nearly all children by the age of 5. HMPV infections have been detected in older age groups, including elderly adults, and in both immunocompetent and immunosuppressed hosts. This virus accounts for 1–5% of childhood upper respiratory tract infections and for 10–15% of respiratory tract illnesses requiring hospitalization of children. In addition, HMPV causes 2–4% of acute respiratory illnesses in ambulatory adults and elderly patients. HMPV has been detected in a few cases of SARS, but its role (if any) in these illnesses has not been established.

■ CLINICAL MANIFESTATIONS

The spectrum of clinical illnesses associated with HMPV is similar to that associated with HRSV and includes both upper and lower respiratory tract illnesses, such as bronchiolitis, croup, and pneumonia. Reinfection with HMPV is common among older children and adults and has manifestations ranging from subclinical infections to common cold syndromes and occasionally pneumonia, which is seen primarily in elderly patients and those with cardiopulmonary diseases. Serious HMPV infections occur in immunocompromised patients, including those with neoplasia and hematopoietic stem cell transplants.

■ DIAGNOSIS

HMPV can be detected in nasal aspirates and respiratory secretions by immunofluorescence, by PCR, or by growth in rhesus monkey kidney (LLC-MK2) tissue cultures. A serologic diagnosis can be made by ELISA, which uses HMPV-infected tissue culture lysates as sources of antigens.

TREATMENT   Human Metapneumovirus Infections

Treatment for HMPV infections is primarily supportive and symptom-based. Ribavirin is active against HMPV in vitro, but its efficacy in vivo is unknown.

■ PREVENTION

Vaccines against HMPV are in the early stages of development.

PARAINFLUENZA VIRUS INFECTIONS

■ ETIOLOGIC AGENT

Parainfluenza viruses belong to the Paramyxoviridae family (genera *Respirovirus* and *Rubulavirus*). They are 150–200 nm in diameter,

are enveloped, and contain a single-stranded RNA genome. The envelope is studded with two glycoproteins: one possesses both hemagglutinin and neuraminidase activity, and the other contains fusion activity. The viral RNA genome is enclosed in a helical nucleocapsid and codes for six structural and several accessory proteins. All five serotypes of parainfluenza virus (1, 2, 3, 4A, and 4B) share certain antigens with other members of the Paramyxoviridae family, including mumps and Newcastle disease viruses.

■ EPIDEMIOLOGY

Parainfluenza viruses are distributed throughout the world; infection with serotypes 4A and 4B has been reported less widely, probably because these types are more difficult than the other three to grow in tissue culture. Infection is acquired in early childhood; by 5 years of age, most children have antibodies to serotypes 1, 2, and 3. Types 1 and 2 cause epidemics during the fall, often occurring in an alternate-year pattern. Type 3 infection has been detected during all seasons of the year, but epidemics have occurred annually in the spring.

The contribution of parainfluenza infections to respiratory disease varies with both the location and the year. In studies conducted in the United States, parainfluenza virus infections have accounted for 4.3–22% of respiratory illnesses in children. In adults, parainfluenza infections are generally mild and account for <10% of respiratory illnesses. The major importance of parainfluenza viruses is as a cause of respiratory illness in young children, in whom they rank second only to HRSV as causes of lower respiratory tract illness. Parainfluenza virus type 1 is the most frequent cause of croup (laryngotracheobronchitis) in children, while serotype 2 causes similar, although generally less severe, disease. Type 3 is an important cause of bronchiolitis and pneumonia in infants, while illnesses associated with types 4A and 4B have generally been mild. Unlike types 1 and 2, type 3 frequently causes illness during the first month of life, when passively acquired maternal antibody is still present. Parainfluenza viruses are spread through infected respiratory secretions, primarily by person-to-person contact and/or by large droplets. The incubation period has varied from 3 to 6 days in experimental infections but may be somewhat shorter for naturally occurring disease in children.

■ PATHOGENESIS

Immunity to parainfluenza viruses is incompletely understood, but evidence suggests that immunity to infections with serotypes 1 and 2 is mediated by local IgA antibodies in the respiratory tract. Passively acquired serum neutralizing antibodies also confer some protection against infection with types 1, 2, and (to a lesser degree) 3. Studies in experimental animal models and in immunosuppressed patients suggest that T cell–mediated immunity may also be important in parainfluenza virus infections.

■ CLINICAL MANIFESTATIONS

Parainfluenza virus infections occur most frequently among children, in whom initial infection with serotype 1, 2, or 3 is associated with an acute febrile illness in 50–80% of cases. Children may present with coryza, sore throat, hoarseness, and cough that may or may not be croupy. In severe croup, fever persists, with worsening coryza and sore throat. A brassy or barking cough may progress to frank stridor. Most children recover over the next 1 or 2 days, although progressive airway obstruction and hypoxia ensue occasionally. If bronchiolitis or pneumonia develops, progressive cough accompanied by wheezing, tachypnea, and intercostal retractions may occur. In this setting, sputum production increases modestly. Physical examination shows nasopharyngeal discharge and oropharyngeal injection, along with rhonchi, wheezes, or coarse breath sounds. Chest x-rays can show air trapping and occasionally interstitial infiltrates.

In older children and adults, parainfluenza infections tend to be milder, presenting most frequently as a common cold or as hoarseness, with or without cough. Lower respiratory tract involvement in older children and adults is uncommon, but tracheobronchitis in adults has been reported. Severe, prolonged, and even fatal parainfluenza infection has been reported in children and adults with severe immunosuppression, including hematopoietic stem cell and solid-organ transplant recipients.

LABORATORY FINDINGS AND DIAGNOSIS

The clinical syndromes caused by parainfluenza viruses (with the possible exception of croup in young children) are not sufficiently distinctive to be diagnosed on clinical grounds alone. A specific diagnosis is established by detection of virus in respiratory tract secretions, throat swabs, or nasopharyngeal washings. Viral growth in tissue culture is detected either by hemagglutination or by a cytopathic effect. Rapid viral diagnosis may be made by identification of parainfluenza antigens in exfoliated cells from the respiratory tract with immunofluorescence or ELISA, although these techniques appear to be less sensitive than tissue culture. Highly specific and sensitive PCR assays have also been developed. Serologic diagnosis can be established by hemagglutination inhibition, complement-fixation, or neutralization tests of acute- and convalescent-phase specimens. However, since frequent heterotypic responses occur among the parainfluenza serotypes, the serotype causing illness often cannot be identified by serologic techniques alone.

Acute epiglottitis caused by *Haemophilus influenzae* type b must be differentiated from viral croup. Influenza A virus is also a common cause of croup during epidemic periods.

TREATMENT Parainfluenza Virus Infections

For upper respiratory tract illness, symptoms can be treated as discussed for other viral respiratory tract illnesses. If complications such as sinusitis, otitis, or superimposed bacterial bronchitis develop, appropriate antibacterial antibiotics should be administered. Mild cases of croup should be treated with bed rest and moist air generated by vaporizers. More severe cases require hospitalization and close observation for the development of respiratory distress. If acute respiratory distress develops, humidified oxygen and intermittent racemic epinephrine are usually administered. Aerosolized or systemically administered glucocorticoids are beneficial; the latter have a more profound effect. No specific antiviral therapy is available, although ribavirin is active against parainfluenza viruses in vitro and anecdotal reports describe its use clinically, particularly in immunosuppressed patients.

PREVENTION

Vaccines against parainfluenza viruses are under development.

ADENOVIRUS INFECTIONS

ETIOLOGIC AGENT

Adenoviruses are complex DNA viruses that measure 70–80 nm in diameter. Human adenoviruses belong to the genus *Mastadenovirus*, which includes 51 serotypes. Adenoviruses have a characteristic morphology consisting of an icosahedral shell composed of 20 equilateral triangular faces and 12 vertices. The protein coat (capsid) consists of hexon subunits with group-specific and type-specific antigenic determinants and penton subunits at each vertex primarily containing group-specific antigens. A fiber with a knob at the end projects from each penton; this fiber contains type-specific and some group-specific antigens. Human adenoviruses have been divided into six subgroups (A through F) on the basis of the homology of DNA genomes and other properties. The adenovirus genome is a linear double-stranded DNA that codes for structural and nonstructural polypeptides. The replicative cycle of adenovirus may result either in lytic infection of cells or in the establishment of a latent infection (primarily involving lymphoid cells). Some adenovirus types can induce oncogenic transformation, and tumor formation has been observed in rodents; however, despite intensive investigation, adenoviruses have not been associated with tumors in humans.

EPIDEMIOLOGY

Adenovirus infections most frequently affect infants and children. Infections occur throughout the year but are most common from fall to spring. Adenoviruses account for ~10% of acute respiratory infections in children but for <2% of respiratory illnesses in civilian adults. Nearly 100% of adults have serum antibody to multiple serotypes—a finding indicating that infection is common in childhood. Types 1, 2, 3, and 5 are the most common isolates from children. Certain adenovirus serotypes—particularly 4 and 7 but also 3, 14, and 21—are associated with outbreaks of acute respiratory disease in military recruits in winter and spring. Adenovirus infection can be transmitted by inhalation of aerosolized virus, by inoculation of virus into conjunctival sacs, and probably by the fecal-oral route as well. Type-specific antibody generally develops after infection and is associated with protection, albeit incomplete, against infection with the same serotype.

CLINICAL MANIFESTATIONS

In children, adenoviruses cause a variety of clinical syndromes. The most common is an acute upper respiratory tract infection, with prominent rhinitis. On occasion, lower respiratory tract disease, including bronchiolitis and pneumonia, also develops. Adenoviruses, particularly types 3 and 7, cause pharyngoconjunctival fever, a characteristic acute febrile illness of children that occurs in outbreaks, most often in summer camps. The syndrome is marked by bilateral conjunctivitis in which the bulbar and palpebral conjunctivae have a granular appearance. Low-grade fever is frequently present for the first 3–5 days, and rhinitis, sore throat, and cervical adenopathy develop. The illness generally lasts for 1–2 weeks and resolves spontaneously. Febrile pharyngitis without conjunctivitis has also been associated with adenovirus infection. Adenoviruses have been isolated from cases of whooping cough with or without *Bordetella pertussis*; the significance of adenovirus in that disease is unknown.

In adults, the most frequently reported illness has been acute respiratory disease caused by adenovirus types 4 and 7 in military recruits. This illness is marked by a prominent sore throat and the gradual onset of fever, which often reaches 39°C (102.2°F) on the second or third day of illness. Cough is almost always present, and coryza and regional lymphadenopathy are frequently seen. Physical examination may show pharyngeal edema, injection, and tonsillar enlargement with little or no exudate. If pneumonia has developed, auscultation and x-ray of the chest may indicate areas of patchy infiltration.

Adenoviruses have been associated with a number of non–respiratory tract diseases, including acute diarrheal illness caused by types 40 and 41 in young children and hemorrhagic cystitis caused by types 11 and 21. Epidemic keratoconjunctivitis, caused most frequently by types 8, 19, and 37, has been associated with contaminated common sources such as ophthalmic solutions and roller towels. Adenoviruses have also been implicated in disseminated disease and pneumonia in immunosuppressed patients, including recipients of solid-organ or hematopoietic stem cell transplants. In hematopoietic stem cell transplant recipients, adenovirus infections have been manifested as pneumonia, hepatitis, nephritis, colitis, encephalitis, and hemorrhagic cystitis. In solid-organ transplant recipients, adenovirus infection may involve the organ transplanted (e.g., hepatitis in liver transplants, nephritis in renal transplants) but can disseminate to other organs as well. In patients with AIDS, high-numbered and intermediate adenovirus serotypes have been isolated, usually in the setting of low CD4+ T cell counts, but their isolation often has not been clearly linked to disease manifestations. Adenovirus nucleic acids have been detected in myocardial cells from patients with "idiopathic" myocardiopathies, and adenoviruses have been suggested as causative agents in some cases.

■ LABORATORY FINDINGS AND DIAGNOSIS

Adenovirus infection should be suspected in the epidemiologic setting of acute respiratory disease in military recruits and in certain of the clinical syndromes (such as pharyngoconjunctival fever or epidemic keratoconjunctivitis) in which outbreaks of characteristic illnesses occur. In most cases, however, illnesses caused by adenovirus infection cannot be differentiated from those caused by a number of other viral respiratory agents and *Mycoplasma pneumoniae*. A definitive diagnosis of adenovirus infection is established by detection of the virus in tissue culture (as evidenced by cytopathic changes) and by specific identification with immunofluorescence or other immunologic techniques. Rapid viral diagnosis can be established by immunofluorescence or ELISA of nasopharyngeal aspirates, conjunctival or respiratory secretions, urine, or stool. Highly sensitive and specific PCR assays and nucleic acid hybridization are also available. Adenovirus types 40 and 41, which have been associated with diarrheal disease in children, require special tissue-culture cells for isolation, and these serotypes are most commonly detected by direct ELISA of stool. Serum antibody rises can be demonstrated by complement-fixation or neutralization tests, ELISA, radioimmunoassay, or (for those adenoviruses that hemagglutinate red cells) hemagglutination inhibition tests.

TREATMENT   Adenovirus Infections

Only symptom-based treatment and supportive therapy are available for adenovirus infections, and clinically useful antiviral therapy has not been established. Ribavirin and cidofovir are active in vitro against certain adenoviruses. Retrospective studies and anecdotes describe the use of these agents in disseminated adenovirus infections, but definitive efficacy data from controlled studies are not available.

■ PREVENTION

Live vaccines have been developed against adenovirus types 4 and 7 and have been used to control illness among military recruits. These vaccines consist of live, unattenuated virus administered in enteric-coated capsules. Infection of the gastrointestinal tract with types 4 and 7 does not cause disease but stimulates local and systemic antibodies that are protective against subsequent acute respiratory disease due to those serotypes. This vaccine has not been produced since 1999, and outbreaks of acute respiratory illness caused by adenovirus types 4 and 7 have again emerged among military recruits. Therefore, a program to redevelop type 4 and 7 vaccines is under way. Adenoviruses are also being studied as live-virus vectors for the delivery of vaccine antigens and for gene therapy.

FURTHER READINGS

AMERICAN ACADEMY OF PEDIATRICS: Diagnosis and management of bronchiolitis. Pediatrics 118:1774, 2006

ECHAVARRÍA M: Adenoviruses in immunocompromised hosts. Clin Microbiol Rev 21:704, 2008

GRAHAM BS et al: Respiratory syncytial virus immunobiology and pathogenesis. Virology 297:1, 2002

NAIR H et al: Global burden of acute lower respiratory infections due to respiratory syncytial virus in young children: A systematic review and meta-analysis. Lancet 375:545, 2010

PEIRIS JS et al: Severe acute respiratory syndrome. Nat Med 10:S88, 2004

PERET T et al: Characterization of human metapneumoviruses isolated from patients in North America. J Infect Dis 185:1660, 2002

PYRC K et al: Identification of new human coronaviruses. Expert Rev Anti Infect Ther 2:245, 2007

TURNER RB: Rhinoviruses, in *Principles and Practice of Infectious Diseases*, 7th ed, GF Mandell et al (eds). Philadelphia, Elsevier, 2010, pp 2389–2398

WALSH EE et al: Human metapneumovirus infections in adults: Another piece of the puzzle. Arch Intern Med 168:2489, 2008

WRIGHT PF: Parainfluenza viruses, in *Viral Infections of the Respiratory Tract*, R Dolin, PF Wright (eds). New York, Marcel Dekker, 1999

CHAPTER **187**

Influenza

Raphael Dolin

■ DEFINITION

Influenza is an acute respiratory illness caused by infection with influenza viruses. The illness affects the upper and/or lower respiratory tract and is often accompanied by systemic signs and symptoms such as fever, headache, myalgia, and weakness. Outbreaks of illness of variable extent and severity occur nearly every year. Such outbreaks result in significant morbidity rates in the general population and in increased mortality rates among certain high-risk patients, mainly as a result of pulmonary complications.

■ ETIOLOGIC AGENT

Influenza viruses are members of the Orthomyxoviridae family, of which influenza A, B, and C viruses constitute three separate genera. The designation of influenza viruses as type A, B, or C is based on antigenic characteristics of the nucleoprotein (NP) and matrix (M) protein antigens. Influenza A viruses are further subdivided (subtyped) on the basis of the surface hemagglutinin (H) and neuraminidase (N) antigens (see below); individual strains are designated according to the site of origin, isolate number, year of isolation, and subtype—for example, influenza A/California/07/2009 (H1N1). Influenza A has 16 distinct H subtypes and 9 distinct N subtypes, of which only H1, H2, H3, N1, and N2 have been associated with epidemics of disease in humans. Influenza B and C viruses are similarly designated, but H and N antigens from these viruses do not receive subtype designations, since intratypic variations in influenza B antigens are less extensive than those in influenza A viruses and may not occur with influenza C virus.

Influenza A and B viruses are major human pathogens and the most extensively studied of the Orthomyxoviridae. Type A and type B viruses are morphologically similar. The virions are irregularly shaped spherical particles, measure 80–120 nm in diameter, and have a lipid envelope from the surface of which the H and N glycoproteins project (Fig. 187-1). The hemagglutinin is the site by which the virus binds to sialic acid cell receptors, whereas the neuraminidase degrades the receptor and plays a role in the release of the virus from infected cells after replication has taken place. Influenza viruses enter cells by receptor-mediated endocytosis, forming a virus-containing endosome. The viral hemagglutinin mediates fusion of the endosomal membrane with the virus envelope, and viral nucleocapsids are subsequently released into the cytoplasm. Immune responses to the H antigen are the major determinants of protection against infection with influenza virus, while those to the N antigen limit viral spread and contribute to reduction of the infection. The lipid envelope of influenza A virus also contains the M proteins M1 and M2, which are involved in stabilization of the lipid envelope and in virus assembly. The virion also contains the NP antigen, which is associated with the viral genome, as well as three polymerase (P) proteins that are essential for transcription and synthesis of viral RNA. Two nonstructural proteins function as an interferon antagonist and posttranscriptional regulator (NS1) and a nuclear export factor (NS2 or NEP).

The genomes of influenza A and B viruses consist of eight single-strand RNA segments, which code for the structural and nonstructural proteins. Because the genome is segmented, the opportunity for gene reassortment during infection is high; reassortment often occurs during infection of cells with more than one influenza A virus.

■ EPIDEMIOLOGY

Influenza outbreaks are recorded virtually every year, although their extent and severity vary widely. Localized outbreaks take place at variable intervals, usually every 1–3 years. Global pandemics have occurred at variable intervals, but much less frequently than interpandemic outbreaks (Table 187-1). The most recent pandemic emerged in March of 2009 and was caused by an influenza A/H1N1 virus that rapidly spread worldwide over the next several months.

Influenza A virus

Antigenic variation and influenza outbreaks and pandemics The most extensive and severe outbreaks of influenza are caused by influenza A viruses, in part because of the remarkable propensity of the H and N antigens of these viruses to undergo periodic antigenic variation. Major antigenic variations, called *antigenic shifts*, are seen only

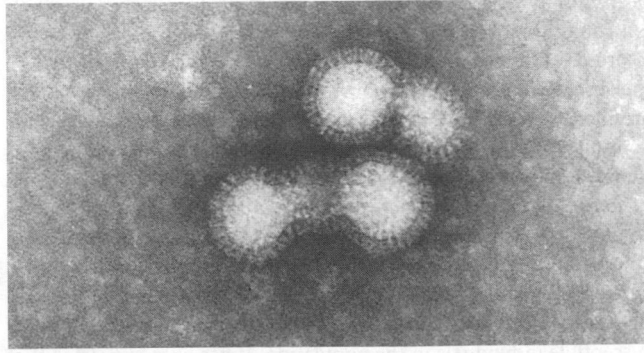

Figure 187-1 An electron micrograph of influenza A virus (×40,000).

TABLE 187-1 Emergence of Antigenic Subtypes of Influenza A Virus Associated With Pandemic or Epidemic Disease

Years	Subtype	Extent of Outbreak
1889–1890	H2N8[a]	Severe pandemic
1900–1903	H3N8[a]	?Moderate epidemic
1918–1919	H1N1[b] (formerly HswN1)	Severe pandemic
1933–1935	H1N1[b] (formerly H0N1)	Mild epidemic
1946–1947	H1N1	Mild epidemic
1957–1958	H2N2	Severe pandemic
1968–1969	H3N2	Moderate pandemic
1977–1978[c]	H1N1	Mild pandemic
2009–2010[d]	H1N1	Pandemic

[a]As determined by retrospective serologic survey of individuals alive during those years ("seroarchaeology").

[b]Hemagglutinins formerly designated as Hsw and H0 are now classified as variants of H1.

[c]From this time until 2008–2009, viruses of the H1N1 and H3N2 subtypes circulated either in alternating years or concurrently.

[d]Novel influenza A/H1N1 emerged to cause this pandemic.

with influenza A viruses and may be associated with pandemics. Minor variations are called *antigenic drifts*. Antigenic variation may involve the hemagglutinin alone or both the hemagglutinin and the neuraminidase. An example of an antigenic shift involving both the hemagglutinin and the neuraminidase is that of 1957, when the predominant influenza A virus subtype shifted from H1N1 to H2N2; this shift resulted in a severe pandemic, with an estimated 70,000 excess deaths (i.e., deaths in excess of the number expected without an influenza epidemic) in the United States alone. In 1968, an antigenic shift involving only the hemagglutinin occurred (H2N2 to H3N2); the subsequent pandemic was less severe than that of 1957. In 1977, an H1N1 virus emerged and caused a pandemic that primarily affected younger individuals (i.e., those born after 1957). As can be seen in Table 187-1, H1N1 viruses circulated from 1918 to 1956; thus, individuals born prior to 1957 would be expected to have some degree of immunity to H1N1 viruses. The pandemic of 2009–2010 was caused by an A/H1N1 virus against which little immunity was present in the general population, although approximately one-third of individuals born before 1950 had some apparent immunity to related H1N1 strains.

During most outbreaks of influenza A, a single subtype has circulated at a time. However, since 1977, H1N1 and H3N2 viruses have circulated simultaneously, resulting in outbreaks of varying severity. In some outbreaks, influenza B viruses have also circulated simultaneously with influenza A viruses. In 2009–2010, the pandemic A/H1N1 virus appeared to circulate nearly exclusively.

Avian influenza A viruses In 1997, human cases of influenza caused by avian influenza viruses (A/H5N1) were detected in Hong Kong during an extensive outbreak of influenza in poultry. Between that time and February 2010, 478 cases of avian influenza in humans were reported in Asia and the Middle East. Nearly all of these cases were associated with contact with infected poultry. Efficient person-to-person transmission has not been observed to date. Mortality rates have been high (60%), and clinical manifestations have differed somewhat from those associated with "typical" outbreaks of influenza (see below). Transmission of avian influenza A/H7N7 viruses from infected poultry to humans has been observed, including outbreaks in the Netherlands, which resulted predominantly in cases of conjunctivitis and some respiratory illnesses. Infection with avian A/H9N2 viruses along with mild respiratory illness has been reported in children in Hong Kong. Because of the absence of widespread immunity to the H5, H7, and H9 viruses, concern persists that avian-to-human transmission might also contribute to the emergence of pandemic strains.

The origin of actual pandemic influenza A virus strains has been partially elucidated with molecular virologic techniques. It appears that the pandemic strains of 1957 and 1968 resulted from a genetic reassortment between human viruses and avian viruses with novel surface glycoproteins (H2N2, H3). The pandemic A/H1N1 virus of 2009–2010 was a quadruple reassortant among swine influenza viruses that circulated in North America and Eurasia, an avian virus, and a human influenza virus. The influenza A/H1N1 virus responsible for the most severe pandemic of modern times (1918–1919) appears to have represented an adaptation of an avian virus to efficient infection of humans.

Features of pandemic and interpandemic influenza A Pandemics provide the most dramatic evidence of the impact of influenza A. However, illnesses occurring between pandemics (interpandemic disease) also account for extensive mortality and morbidity rates, albeit over a longer period. In the United States, influenza was associated with at least 19,000 excess deaths per season in 1976–1990 and with 36,000 excess deaths per season in 1990–1999. On average, there were 226,000 influenza-associated hospitalizations per year in this country in 1979–2001.

Influenza A viruses that circulate between pandemics demonstrate antigenic drifts in the H antigen. These antigenic drifts result from point mutations involving the RNA segment that codes for the hemagglutinin, which occur most frequently in five hypervariable regions. Epidemiologically significant strains—that is, those with the potential to cause widespread outbreaks—exhibit changes in amino acids in at least two of the major antigenic sites in the hemagglutinin molecule. Since two point mutations are unlikely to occur simultaneously, it is believed that antigenic drifts result from point mutations occurring sequentially during the spread of virus from person to person. Antigenic drifts have been reported nearly annually since 1977 for H1N1 viruses and since 1968 for H3N2 viruses.

Interpandemic influenza A outbreaks usually begin abruptly, peak over a 2- to 3-week period, generally last for 2–3 months, and often subside almost as rapidly as they began. In contrast, pandemic influenza may begin with rapid transmission at multiple locations, have high attack rates, and extend beyond the usual seasonality, with multiple waves of attack before or after the main outbreak. In interpandemic outbreaks, the first indication of influenza activity is an increase in the number of children with febrile respiratory illnesses who present for medical attention. This increase is followed by increases in rates of influenza-like illnesses among adults and eventually by an increase in hospital admissions for patients with pneumonia, worsening of congestive heart failure, and exacerbations of chronic pulmonary disease. Rates of absence from work and school also rise at this time. An increase in the number of deaths caused by pneumonia and influenza is generally a late observation in an outbreak. Attack rates have been highly variable from outbreak to outbreak in interpandemic influenza but most commonly are in the range of 10–20% of the general population.

While pandemic influenza may occur throughout the year, interpandemic influenza occurs almost exclusively during the winter months in the temperate zones of the Northern and Southern hemispheres. In those locations, it is highly unusual to detect influenza A virus at other times, although rises in serum antibody titer or even outbreaks have been noted rarely during warm-weather months. In contrast, influenza virus infections occur throughout the year in the tropics. Where or how influenza A viruses persist between outbreaks in temperate zones is unknown. It is possible that the viruses are maintained in the human population on a worldwide basis by person-to-person transmission and that large population clusters support a low level of interepidemic transmission. Alternatively, human strains may persist in animal reservoirs. Convincing evidence to support either explanation is not available. In the modern era, rapid transportation may contribute to the transmission of viruses among widespread geographic locales.

The factors that result in the inception and termination of outbreaks of influenza A are incompletely understood. A major determinant of the extent and severity of an outbreak is the level of immunity in the population at risk. With the emergence of an antigenically novel influenza virus to which little or no immunity is present in a community, extensive outbreaks may occur. When the absence of immunity is worldwide, epidemic disease may spread around the globe, resulting in a pandemic. Such pandemic waves can continue for several years, until immunity in the population reaches a high level. In the years following pandemic influenza, antigenic drifts among influenza viruses result in outbreaks of variable severity in populations with high levels of immunity to the pandemic strain that circulated earlier. This situation persists until another antigenically novel pandemic strain emerges. On the other hand, outbreaks sometimes end despite the persistence of a large pool of susceptible individuals in the population. It has been suggested that certain influenza A viruses may be intrinsically less virulent and cause less severe disease than other variants, even in immunologically virgin subjects. If so, then other (undefined) factors besides the level of preexisting immunity must play a role in the epidemiology of influenza.

Influenza B and C viruses

Influenza B virus causes outbreaks that are generally less extensive and are associated with less severe disease than those caused by influenza A virus. The hemagglutinin and neuraminidase of influenza B virus undergo less frequent and less extensive variation than those of influenza A viruses; this characteristic may account, in part, for the lesser extent of disease. Influenza B outbreaks are seen most frequently in schools and military camps, although outbreaks in institutions in which elderly individuals reside have also been noted on occasion. The most serious complication of influenza B virus infection is Reye's syndrome.

In contrast to influenza A and B viruses, influenza C virus appears to be a relatively minor cause of disease in humans. It has been associated with common cold–like symptoms and occasionally with lower respiratory tract illness. The widespread prevalence of serum antibody to this virus indicates that asymptomatic infection may be common.

Influenza-associated morbidity and mortality rates

The morbidity and mortality rates caused by influenza outbreaks continue to be substantial. Most individuals who die in this setting have underlying diseases that place them at high risk for complications of influenza (Table 187-2). Excess annual hospitalizations for groups of adults and children with high-risk medical conditions ranged from 40 to 1900 per 100,000 during outbreaks of influenza in 1973–2004. The most prominent high-risk conditions are chronic cardiac and pulmonary diseases and old age. Mortality rates among individuals with chronic metabolic or renal diseases or certain immunosuppressive diseases have also been elevated, albeit lower than those among patients with chronic cardiopulmonary diseases. In the pandemic of 2009–2010, increased risk for severe disease was noted in children from birth to 4 years of age and in pregnant women. The morbidity rate attributable to influenza in the general population is considerable. It is estimated that interpandemic outbreaks of influenza currently incur annual economic

---

TABLE 187-2 Persons at Higher Risk for Complications of Influenza

Children from birth to 4 years old

Pregnant women

Persons ≥65 years old

Children and adolescents (6 months to 18 years old) who are receiving long-term aspirin therapy and therefore may be at risk for developing Reye's syndrome after influenza

Adults and children who have chronic disorders of the pulmonary or cardiovascular system, including asthma

Adults and children who have chronic metabolic diseases (including diabetes mellitus), renal dysfunction, hemoglobinopathies, or immunodeficiency (including immunodeficiency caused by medications or by HIV)

Adults and children who have any condition that can compromise respiratory function or compromise the handling of respiratory secretions or can increase the risk of aspiration

Residents of nursing homes and other chronic-care facilities that house persons of any age who have chronic medical conditions

---

costs of more than $87 billion in the United States. For pandemics, it is estimated that annual economic costs would range from $89.7 to $209.4 billion for attack rates of 15–35%.

■ PATHOGENESIS AND IMMUNITY

The initial event in influenza is infection of the respiratory epithelium with influenza virus acquired from respiratory secretions of acutely infected individuals. In all likelihood, the virus is transmitted via aerosols generated by coughs and sneezes, although hand-to-hand contact, other personal contact, and even fomite transmission may take place. Experimental evidence suggests that infection by a small-particle aerosol (particle diameter, <10 μm) is more efficient than that by larger droplets. Initially, viral infection involves the ciliated columnar epithelial cells, but it may also involve other respiratory tract cells, including alveolar cells, mucous gland cells, and macrophages. In infected cells, virus replicates within 4–6 h, after which infectious virus is released to infect adjacent or nearby cells. In this way, infection spreads from a few foci to a large number of respiratory cells over several hours. In experimentally induced infection, the incubation period of illness has ranged from 18 to 72 h, depending on the size of the viral inoculum. Histopathologic study reveals degenerative changes, including granulation, vacuolization, swelling, and pyknotic nuclei, in infected ciliated cells. The cells eventually become necrotic and desquamate; in some areas, previously columnar epithelium is replaced by flattened and metaplastic epithelial cells. The severity of illness is correlated with the quantity of virus shed in secretions; thus, the degree of viral replication itself may be an important factor in pathogenesis. Despite the frequent development of systemic signs and symptoms such as fever, headache, and myalgias, influenza virus has only rarely been detected in extrapulmonary sites (including the bloodstream). Evidence suggests that the pathogenesis of systemic symptoms in influenza may be related to the induction of certain cytokines, particularly tumor necrosis factor α, interferon α, interleukin 6, and interleukin 8, in respiratory secretions and in the bloodstream.

The host response to influenza infections involves a complex interplay of humoral antibody, local antibody, cell-mediated immunity, interferon, and other host defenses. Serum antibody responses, which can be detected by the second week after primary infection, are measured by a variety of techniques: hemagglutination inhibition (HI), complement fixation (CF), neutralization, enzyme-linked immunosorbent assay (ELISA), and antineuraminidase antibody assay. Antibodies to the hemagglutinin appear to be the most important mediators of immunity; in several studies, HI titers of ≥40 have been associated with protection from infection. Secretory antibodies produced in the respiratory tract are predominantly of the IgA class and also play a major role in protection against infection. Secretory antibody neutralization titers of ≥4 have also been associated with protection. A variety of cell-mediated immune responses, both antigen-specific and antigen-nonspecific, can be detected early after infection and depend on the prior immune status of the host. These responses include T cell proliferative, T cell cytotoxic, and natural killer cell activity. In humans, CD8+ human leukocyte antigen class I–restricted cytotoxic T lymphocytes (CTLs) are directed at conserved regions of internal proteins (NP, M, and P) as well as at the surface proteins H and N. Interferons can be detected in respiratory secretions shortly after the shedding of virus has begun, and rises in interferon titers coincide with decreases in virus shedding.

The host defense factors responsible for cessation of virus shedding and resolution of illness have not been defined specifically. Virus shedding generally stops within 2–5 days after symptoms first appear, at a time when serum and local antibody responses often are not detectable by conventional techniques (although antibody rises may be detected earlier by use of highly sensitive techniques, particularly in individuals with previous immunity to the virus). It has been suggested that interferon, cell-mediated immune responses, and/or nonspecific inflammatory responses all contribute to the resolution of illness. CTL responses may be particularly important in this regard.

CLINICAL MANIFESTATIONS

Influenza has most frequently been described as an illness characterized by the abrupt onset of systemic symptoms, such as headache, feverishness, chills, myalgia, and malaise, as well as accompanying respiratory tract signs, particularly cough and sore throat. In many cases, the onset is so abrupt that patients can recall the precise time they became ill. However, the spectrum of clinical presentations is wide, ranging from a mild, afebrile respiratory illness similar to the common cold (with either a gradual or an abrupt onset) to severe prostration with relatively few respiratory signs and symptoms. In most of the cases that come to a physician's attention, the patient has a fever, with temperatures of 38°–41°C (100.4°–105.8°F). A rapid temperature rise within the first 24 h of illness is generally followed by gradual defervescence over 2–3 days, although, on occasion, fever may last as long as 1 week. Patients report a feverish feeling and chilliness, but true rigors are rare. Headache, either generalized or frontal, is often particularly troublesome. Myalgias may involve any part of the body but are most common in the legs and lumbosacral area. Arthralgias may also develop.

Respiratory symptoms often become more prominent as systemic symptoms subside. Many patients have a sore throat or persistent cough, which may last for ≥1 week and which is often accompanied by substernal discomfort. Ocular signs and symptoms include pain on motion of the eyes, photophobia, and burning of the eyes.

Physical findings are usually minimal in uncomplicated influenza. Early in the illness, the patient appears flushed and the skin is hot and dry, although diaphoresis and mottled extremities are sometimes evident, particularly in older patients. Examination of the pharynx may yield surprisingly unremarkable results despite a severe sore throat, but injection of the mucous membranes and postnasal discharge are apparent in some cases. Mild cervical lymphadenopathy may be noted, especially in younger individuals. The results of chest examination are largely negative in uncomplicated influenza, although rhonchi, wheezes, and scattered rales have been reported with variable frequency in different outbreaks. Frank dyspnea, hyperpnea, cyanosis, diffuse rales, and signs of consolidation are indicative of pulmonary complications. Patients with apparently uncomplicated influenza have been reported to have a variety of mild ventilatory defects and increased alveolar-capillary diffusion gradients; thus, subclinical pulmonary involvement may be more common than is appreciated.

In uncomplicated influenza, the acute illness generally resolves over 2–5 days, and most patients have largely recovered in 1 week, although cough may persist 1–2 weeks longer. In a significant minority (particularly the elderly), however, symptoms of weakness or lassitude (postinfluenza asthenia) may persist for several weeks and may prove troublesome for persons who wish to resume their full level of activity promptly. The pathogenetic basis for this asthenia is unknown, although pulmonary function abnormalities may persist for several weeks after uncomplicated influenza.

COMPLICATIONS

Complications of influenza (Table 187-2) occur most frequently in patients >65 years old and in those with certain chronic disorders, including cardiac or pulmonary diseases, diabetes mellitus, hemoglobinopathies, renal dysfunction, and immunosuppression. Pregnancy in the second or third trimester predisposes to complications with influenza. Children <5 years old (especially infants) are also at high risk for complications.

Pulmonary complications

Pneumonia The most significant complication of influenza is pneumonia: "primary" influenza viral pneumonia, secondary bacterial pneumonia, or mixed viral and bacterial pneumonia.

Primary influenza viral pneumonia Primary influenza viral pneumonia is the least common but most severe of the pneumonic complications. It presents as acute influenza that does not resolve but instead progresses relentlessly, with persistent fever, dyspnea, and eventual cyanosis. Sputum production is generally scanty, but the sputum can contain blood. Few physical signs may be evident early in the illness. In more advanced cases, diffuse rales may be noted, and chest x-ray findings consistent with diffuse interstitial infiltrates and/or acute respiratory distress syndrome may be present. In such cases, arterial blood-gas determinations show marked hypoxia. Viral cultures of respiratory secretions and lung parenchyma, especially if samples are taken early in illness, yield high titers of virus. In fatal cases of primary viral pneumonia, histopathologic examination reveals a marked inflammatory reaction in the alveolar septa, with edema and infiltration by lymphocytes, macrophages, occasional plasma cells, and variable numbers of neutrophils. Fibrin thrombi in alveolar capillaries, along with necrosis and hemorrhage, have also been noted. Eosinophilic hyaline membranes can be found lining alveoli and alveolar ducts.

Primary influenza viral pneumonia has a predilection for individuals with cardiac disease, particularly those with mitral stenosis, but has also been reported in otherwise-healthy young adults as well as in older individuals with chronic pulmonary disorders. In some pandemics of influenza (notably those of 1918 and 1957), pregnancy increased the risk of primary influenza pneumonia. Subsequent epidemics of influenza have been associated with increased rates of hospitalization among pregnant women, which were also noted in the pandemic of 2009–2010.

Secondary bacterial pneumonia Secondary bacterial pneumonia follows acute influenza. Improvement of the patient's condition over 2–3 days is followed by a reappearance of fever along with clinical signs and symptoms of bacterial pneumonia, including cough, production of purulent sputum, and physical and x-ray signs of consolidation. The most common bacterial pathogens in this setting are *Streptococcus pneumoniae*, *Staphylococcus aureus*, and *Haemophilus influenzae*—organisms that can colonize the nasopharynx and that cause infection in the wake of changes in bronchopulmonary defenses. The etiology can often be determined by Gram's staining and culture of an appropriately obtained sputum specimen. Secondary bacterial pneumonia occurs most frequently in high-risk individuals with chronic pulmonary and cardiac disease and in elderly individuals. Patients with secondary bacterial pneumonia often respond to antibiotic therapy when it is instituted promptly.

Mixed viral and bacterial pneumonia Perhaps the most common pneumonic complications during outbreaks of influenza have mixed features of viral and bacterial pneumonia. Patients may experience a gradual progression of their acute illness or may show transient improvement followed by clinical exacerbation, with eventual manifestation of the clinical features of bacterial pneumonia. Sputum cultures may contain both influenza A virus and one of the bacterial pathogens described above. Patchy infiltrates or areas of consolidation may be detected by physical examination and chest x-ray. Patients with mixed viral and bacterial pneumonia generally have less widespread involvement of the lung than those with primary viral pneumonia, and their bacterial infections may respond to appropriate antibacterial drugs. Mixed viral and bacterial pneumonia occurs primarily in patients with chronic cardiovascular and pulmonary diseases.

Other pulmonary complications Other pulmonary complications associated with influenza include worsening of chronic obstructive pulmonary disease and exacerbation of chronic bronchitis and asthma. In children, influenza infection may present as croup. Sinusitis as well as otitis media (the latter occurring particularly often in children) may also be associated with influenza.

Extrapulmonary complications

In addition to the pulmonary complications of influenza, a number of extrapulmonary complications may occur. These include *Reye's syndrome*, a serious complication in children that is associated with influenza B and to a lesser extent with influenza A virus infection as well as with varicella-zoster virus infection. An epidemiologic association between Reye's syndrome and aspirin therapy for the antecedent viral infection has been noted, and the syndrome's incidence has decreased markedly with widespread warnings regarding aspirin use by children with acute viral respiratory infections.

Myositis, rhabdomyolysis, and myoglobinuria are occasional complications of influenza infection. Although myalgias are exceedingly common in influenza, true myositis is rare. Patients with acute myositis have exquisite tenderness of the affected muscles, most commonly in the legs, and may not be able to tolerate even the slightest pressure, such as the touch of bedsheets. In the most severe cases, there is frank swelling and bogginess of muscles. Serum levels of creatine phosphokinase and aldolase are markedly elevated, and an occasional patient develops renal failure from myoglobinuria. The pathogenesis of influenza-associated myositis is also unclear, although the presence of influenza virus in affected muscles has been reported.

Myocarditis and pericarditis were reported in association with influenza virus infection during the 1918–1919 pandemic; these reports were based largely on histopathologic findings, and these complications have been reported only infrequently since that time. Electrocardiographic changes during acute influenza are common among patients who have cardiac disease but have been ascribed most often to exacerbations of the underlying cardiac disease rather than to direct involvement of the myocardium with influenza virus.

Central nervous system (CNS) diseases, including encephalitis, transverse myelitis, and Guillain-Barré syndrome, have been reported during influenza. The etiologic relationship of influenza virus to such CNS illnesses remains uncertain. Toxic shock syndrome associated with *S. aureus* or group A streptococcal infection following acute influenza infection has also been reported (Chaps. 135 and 136).

In addition to complications involving the specific organ systems described above, influenza outbreaks include a number of cases in which elderly and other high-risk individuals develop influenza and subsequently experience a gradual deterioration of underlying cardiovascular, pulmonary, or renal function—changes that occasionally are irreversible and lead to death. These deaths contribute to the overall excess mortality rate associated with influenza A outbreaks.

Complications of avian influenza

Cases of influenza caused by avian A/H5N1 virus are reportedly associated with high rates of pneumonia (>50%) and extrapulmonary manifestations such as diarrhea and CNS involvement. Deaths have been associated with multisystem dysfunction, including cardiac and renal failure.

■ LABORATORY FINDINGS AND DIAGNOSIS

During acute influenza, virus may be detected in throat swabs, nasopharyngeal swabs or washes, or sputum. The virus can be isolated by use of tissue culture—or, less commonly, chick embryos—within 48–72 h after inoculation. Most commonly, the laboratory diagnosis is established with rapid tests that detect viral antigens by means of immunologic or enzymatic techniques. The tests are relatively specific but are of variable sensitivity depending on the technique and the virus to be detected. Some rapid tests can distinguish between influenza A and B viruses, but detection of differences in hemagglutinin subtypes requires additional subtype-specific immunologic techniques. The most sensitive and specific in vitro test for influenza virus is reverse-transcriptase polymerase chain reaction; this test proved particularly important in detecting the 2009–2010 pandemic A/H1N1 viruses, for which some rapid antigen detection tests were poorly sensitive. Serologic methods for diagnosis require comparison of antibody titers in sera obtained during the acute illness with those in sera obtained 10–14 days after the onset of illness and are useful primarily in retrospect. Fourfold or greater titer rises as detected by HI or CF or significant rises as measured by ELISA are diagnostic of acute infection. Other laboratory tests generally are not helpful in the specific diagnosis of influenza virus infection. Leukocyte counts are variable, frequently being low early in illness and normal or slightly elevated later. Severe leukopenia has been described in overwhelming viral or bacterial infection, while leukocytosis with >15,000 cells/µL raises the suspicion of secondary bacterial infection.

■ DIFFERENTIAL DIAGNOSIS

During a community-wide outbreak, a clinical diagnosis of influenza can be made with a high degree of certainty in patients who present to a physician's office with the typical febrile respiratory illness described above. In the absence of an outbreak (i.e., in sporadic or isolated cases), influenza may be difficult to differentiate on clinical grounds alone from an acute respiratory illness caused by any of a variety of respiratory viruses or by *Mycoplasma pneumoniae*. Severe streptococcal pharyngitis or early bacterial pneumonia may mimic acute influenza, although bacterial pneumonias generally do not run a self-limited course. Purulent sputum in which a bacterial pathogen can be detected by Gram's staining is an important diagnostic feature in bacterial pneumonia.

TREATMENT   Influenza

Specific antiviral therapy is available for influenza (Table 187-3): the neuraminidase inhibitors zanamivir, oseltamivir, and peramivir for both influenza A and influenza B and the adamantane agents amantadine and rimantadine for influenza A (Chap. 178). A 5-day course of oseltamivir or zanamivir reduces the duration of signs and symptoms of uncomplicated influenza by 1–1.5 days if treatment is started within 2 days of the onset of illness. Zanamivir may exacerbate bronchospasm in asthmatic patients, and oseltamivir has been associated with nausea and vomiting, whose frequency can be reduced by administration of the drug with food. Oseltamivir has also been associated with neuropsychiatric side effects in children. Peramivir, an investigational neuraminidase inhibitor that can be administered intravenously, is being evaluated in clinical trials, as is an intravenous form of zanamivir. Access to these medications can be sought through the FDA's Emergency Investigational New Drug (E-IND) application procedures.

Amantadine or rimantadine treatment of illness caused by sensitive strains of influenza A virus similarly reduces the duration of symptoms of uncomplicated influenza by ~50% if begun within 48 h of onset of illness. Five to 10% of amantadine recipients experience mild CNS side effects, primarily jitteriness, anxiety, insomnia, or difficulty concentrating. These side effects

TABLE 187-3 Antiviral Medications for Treatment and Prophylaxis of Influenza

Antiviral Drug	Age Group (Years)		
	Children (≤12)	13–64	≥65
Oseltamivir			
Treatment, influenza A and B	Age 1–12, dose varies by weight[a]	75 mg PO bid	75 mg PO bid
Prophylaxis, influenza A and B	Age 1–12, dose varies by weight[b]	75 PO qd	75 mg PO qd
Zanamivir			
Treatment, influenza A and B	Age 7–12, 10 mg bid by inhalation	10 mg bid by inhalation	10 mg bid by inhalation
Prophylaxis, influenza A and B	Age 5–12, 10 mg qd by inhalation	10 mg qd by inhalation	10 mg qd by inhalation
Amantadine[c]			
Treatment, influenza A	Age 1–9, 5 mg/kg in 2 divided doses, up to 150 mg/d	Age ≥10, 100 mg PO bid	≤100 mg/d
Prophylaxis, influenza A	Age 1–9, 5 mg/kg in 2 divided doses, up to 150 mg/d	Age ≥10, 100 mg PO bid	≤100 mg/d
Rimantadine[c]			
Treatment, influenza A	Not approved	100 mg PO bid	100–200 mg/d
Prophylaxis, influenza A	Age 1–9, 5 mg/kg in 2 divided doses, up to 150 mg/d	Age ≥10, 100 mg PO bid	100–200 mg/d

[a]<15 kg: 30 mg bid; >15–23 kg: 45 mg bid; >23–40 kg: 60 mg bid; >40 kg: 75 mg bid. For children <1 year of age, see *www.cdc.gov/h1n1flu/recommendations.htm*.
[b]<15 kg: 30 mg qd; >15–23 kg: 45 mg qd; >23–40 kg: 60 mg qd; >40 kg: 75 mg qd. For children <1 year of age, see *www.cdc.gov/h1n1flu/recommendations.htm*.
[c]Amantadine and rimantadine are not currently recommended (2009–2010) because of widespread resistance in influenza A viruses. Their use may be reconsidered if viral susceptibility is reestablished.

disappear promptly upon cessation of therapy. Rimantadine appears to be equally efficacious and is associated with less frequent CNS side effects than is amantadine. In adults, the usual dose of amantadine or rimantadine is 200 mg/d for 3–7 days. Since both drugs are excreted via the kidney, the dose should be reduced to ≤100 mg/d in elderly patients and in patients with renal insufficiency.

The epidemiologic patterns of resistance to the influenza antiviral drugs are crucial elements in agent selection. Since 2005–2006, the vast majority of A/H3N2 viruses, including >90% of U.S. isolates, have been resistant to the adamantanes but have remained sensitive to neuraminidase inhibitors. In contrast, the seasonal A/H1N1 viruses that circulated in 2008–2009 remained sensitive to the adamantanes but were resistant to oseltamivir (although still sensitive to zanamivir). The pandemic A/H1N1 viruses that circulated in 2009–2010 were resistant to the adamantanes but sensitive to zanamivir and usually to oseltamivir; a few oseltamivir-resistant isolates were identified. Up-to-date information on patterns of resistance to influenza antiviral drugs is available through *www.cdc.gov/flu*.

Ribavirin is a nucleoside analogue with activity against influenza A and B viruses in vitro. It has been reported to be variably effective against influenza when administered as an aerosol but ineffective when administered orally. Its efficacy in the treatment of influenza A or B has not been established.

The therapeutic efficacy of antiviral compounds in influenza has been demonstrated primarily in studies of young adults with uncomplicated disease. The effectiveness of these drugs in the treatment or prevention of complications of influenza is unclear. Pooled analyses of observational investigations and some efficacy studies have suggested that treatment with oseltamivir may reduce the frequency of lower respiratory complications and hospitalization. Therapy for primary influenza pneumonia is directed at maintaining oxygenation and is most appropriately undertaken in an intensive care unit, with aggressive respiratory and hemodynamic support as needed.

Antibacterial drugs should be reserved for the treatment of bacterial complications of acute influenza, such as secondary bacterial pneumonia. The choice of antibiotics should be guided by Gram's staining and culture of appropriate specimens of respiratory secretions, such as sputum. If the etiology of a case of bacterial pneumonia is unclear from an examination of respiratory secretions, empirical antibiotics effective against the most common bacterial pathogens in this setting (*S. pneumoniae*, *S. aureus*, and *H. influenzae*) should be selected (Chaps. 134, 135, and 145).

For uncomplicated influenza in individuals at low risk for complications, symptom-based rather than antiviral therapy may be considered. Acetaminophen or nonsteroidal anti-inflammatory agents can be used for relief of headache, myalgia, and fever, but salicylates should be avoided in children <18 years of age because of the possible association with Reye's syndrome. Since cough is ordinarily self-limited, treatment with cough suppressants generally is not indicated; codeine-containing compounds may be employed if the cough is particularly troublesome. Patients should be advised to rest and maintain hydration during acute illness and to return to full activity only gradually after illness has resolved, especially if it has been severe.

■ PROPHYLAXIS

The major public health measure for prevention of influenza is vaccination. Both inactivated (killed) and live attenuated vaccines are available and are generated from influenza A and B virus isolates that circulated in the previous influenza seasons and are anticipated to circulate in the upcoming season. For inactivated vaccines, 50–80% protection against influenza is expected if the vaccine virus and the currently circulating viruses are closely related. Available inactivated vaccines have been highly purified and are associated with few reactions. Up to 5% of individuals experience low-grade fever and mild systemic symptoms 8–24 h after vaccination, and up to one-third develop mild redness or tenderness at the vaccination site. Since the vaccine used in the United States and many other countries is produced in eggs, individuals with true hypersensitivity to egg products either should be desensitized or should not be vaccinated. Although the 1976 swine influenza vaccine appears to have been associated with an increased frequency of Guillain-Barré syndrome, influenza vaccines administered since 1976 generally have not been. Possible exceptions were noted during the 1992–1993 and 1993–1994 influenza seasons, when there may have been an excess risk of Guillain-Barré syndrome of slightly more than 1 case per million vaccine recipients. However, the overall health risk following influenza outweighs the potential risk associated with vaccination.

A live attenuated influenza vaccine administered by intranasal spray is available. The vaccine is generated by reassortment between currently circulating strains of influenza A and B virus and a cold-adapted, attenuated master strain. The cold-adapted vaccine is well tolerated and highly efficacious (>90% protective) in young children; in one study, it provided protection against a circulating influenza virus that had drifted antigenically away from the vaccine strain. Live attenuated vaccine is approved for use in healthy nonpregnant persons 2–49 years of age.

Historically, the U.S. Public Health Service has recommended influenza vaccination for certain groups at high risk for complications of influenza on the basis of age or underlying disease or for their close contacts (Table 187-2). While such individuals will continue to be the focus of vaccination programs, the recommendations have been progressively expanded. In 2009–2010, immunization of all children 6 months to 18 years of age was recommended; for 2010–2011, recommendations are for immunization of the entire population above the age of 6 months, including adults. This expanded recommendation reflects increased recognition of previously unappreciated risk factors, including obesity, postpartum conditions, and racial or ethnic influences, as well as an appreciation that more widespread use of vaccine is required for influenza control. Inactivated vaccines may be administered safely to immunocompromised patients. Influenza vaccination is not associated with exacerbations of chronic nervous-system diseases such as multiple sclerosis. Vaccine should be administered early in the autumn before influenza outbreaks occur and should then be given annually to maintain immunity against the most current influenza virus strains.

Although antiviral drugs provide chemoprophylaxis against influenza, their use for that purpose has been limited because of concern about current patterns and further development of resistance. Chemoprophylaxis with oseltamivir or zanamivir has been 84–89% efficacious against influenza A and B (Table 187-3).

Chemoprophylaxis with amantadine or rimantadine is no longer recommended because of widespread resistance to these drugs. In earlier studies with sensitive viruses, prophylaxis with amantadine or rimantadine (100–200 mg/d) was 70–100% effective against illness associated with influenza A.

Chemoprophylaxis for healthy persons after community exposure generally is not recommended but may be considered for individuals at high risk of complications who have had close contact with an acutely ill person with influenza. During an outbreak, antiviral chemoprophylaxis can be administered simultaneously with inactivated vaccine, since the drugs do not interfere with an immune response to the vaccine. However, concurrent administration of chemoprophylaxis and live attenuated vaccine may interfere with the immune response to the latter. Antiviral drugs should not be administered until at least 2 weeks after administration of live vaccine, and administration of live vaccine should not begin until at least 48 h after antiviral drug administration has been stopped. Chemoprophylaxis may also be considered to control nosocomial outbreaks of influenza. For that purpose, prophylaxis should be instituted promptly when influenza activity is detected and must be continued daily for the duration of the outbreak.

FURTHER READINGS

BEIGEL JH et al: Avian influenza A (H5N1) infection in humans. N Engl J Med 353:1374, 2005

BELSHE RB et al: The efficacy of live attenuated, cold adapted trivalent, intranasal influenza vaccine in children. N Engl J Med 38:1405, 1998

DAWOOD FS et al: Emergence of a novel swine-origin influenza A (H1N1) virus in humans. N Engl J Med 360:2605, 2009

DOLIN R: Interpandemic as well as pandemic disease. N Engl J Med 353:2535, 2005

FIORE AE et al: Prevention and control of influenza with vaccines. Recommendations of the Advisory Committee on Immunization Practices (ACIP), 2010. MMWR Rec Rep 59:1, 2010

GARTEN RJ et al: Antigenic and genetic characteristics of swine-origin 2009 A(H1N1) influenza viruses circulating in humans. Science 325:197, 2009

JEFFERSON T et al: Neuraminidase inhibitors for preventing and treating influenza in healthy adults: Systematic review and meta-analyses. Br Med J 339:b5106, 2009

MELTZER MI et al: The economic impact of pandemic influenza in the United States: Priorities for intervention. Emerg Infect Dis 5:659, 1999

MIST [MANAGEMENT OF INFLUENZA IN THE SOUTHERN HEMISPHERE TRIALISTS] STUDY GROUP: Randomized trial of efficacy and safety of inhaled zanamivir in treatment of influenza A and B infections. Lancet 352:1871, 1998

TREANOR JJ: Influenza virus, in *Principles and Practice of Infectious Diseases*, 7th ed, GL Mandell et al (eds). Philadelphia, Elsevier, 2010, pp 2265–2288

CHAPTER 188

The Human Retroviruses

Dan L. Longo

Anthony S. Fauci

The retroviruses, which make up a large family (Retroviridae), infect mainly vertebrates. These viruses have a unique replication cycle whereby their genetic information is encoded by RNA rather than DNA. Retroviruses contain an RNA-dependent DNA polymerase (a reverse transcriptase) that directs the synthesis of a DNA form of the viral genome after infection of a host cell. The designation *retrovirus* denotes that information in the form of RNA is transcribed into DNA in the host cell—a sequence that overturned a central dogma of molecular biology: that information passes unidirectionally from DNA to RNA to protein. The observation that RNA was the source of genetic information in the causative agents of certain animal tumors led to a number of paradigm-shifting biologic insights regarding not only the direction of genetic information passage but also the viral etiology of certain cancers and the concept of oncogenes as normal host genes scavenged and altered by a viral vector.

The family Retroviridae includes seven subfamilies (Table 188-1). Members of two of the families infect humans with pathologic consequences: the deltaretroviruses, of which human T cell lymphotropic virus (HTLV) type I is the most important in humans; and lentiviruses, of which HIV is the most important in humans.

TABLE 188-1 Classification of Retroviruses: the Family Retroviridae

Genus	Example(s)	Feature
Alpharetrovirus	Rous sarcoma virus	Contains *src* oncogene
Betaretrovirus	Mouse mammary tumor virus	Exogenous or endogenous
Gammaretrovirus	Abelson murine leukemia virus	Contains *abl* oncogene
Deltaretrovirus	HTLV-I	Causes T cell lymphoma and neurologic disease
Epsilonretrovirus	Walleye dermal sarcoma virus	
Lentivirus	HIV-1, 2	Causes AIDS
Spumavirus	Simian foamy virus	Not known to be pathogenic in humans

The wide variety of interactions of a retrovirus with its host range from completely benign events (e.g., silent carriage of endogenous retroviral sequences in the germ-line genome of many animal species) to rapidly fatal infections (e.g., exogenous infection with an oncogenic virus such as Rous sarcoma virus in chickens). The ability of retroviruses to acquire and alter the structure and function of host cell sequences has revolutionized our understanding of molecular carcinogenesis. The viruses can insert into the germ-line genome of the host cell and behave as a transposable or movable genetic element. They can activate or inactivate genes near the site of integration into the genome. They can rapidly alter their own genome by recombination and mutation under selective environmental stimuli.

Most human viral diseases occur as a consequence of tissue destruction either directly by the virus itself or indirectly by the host's response to the virus. Although these mechanisms are operative in retroviral infections, retroviruses have additional mechanisms of inducing disease, including the malignant transformation of an infected cell and the induction of an immunodeficiency state that renders the host susceptible to opportunistic diseases (infections and neoplasms; Chap. 189).

■ STRUCTURE AND LIFE CYCLE

All retroviruses are similar in structure, genome organization, and mode of replication. Retroviruses are 70–130 nm in diameter and have a lipid-containing envelope surrounding an icosahedral capsid with a dense inner core. The core contains two identical copies of the single-strand RNA genome. The RNA molecules are 8–10 kb long and are complexed with reverse transcriptase and tRNA. Other viral proteins, such as integrase, are also components of the virion particle. The RNA has features usually found in mRNA: a cap site at the 5′ end of the molecule, which is important in the initiation of mRNA translation, and a polyadenylation site at the 3′ end, which influences mRNA turnover (i.e., messages with shorter polyA tails turn over faster than messages with longer polyA tails). However, the retroviral RNA is not translated; instead it is transcribed into DNA. The DNA form of the retroviral genome is called a *provirus*.

The replication cycle of retroviruses proceeds in two phases (Fig. 188-1). In the first phase, the virus enters the cytoplasm after binding to one or more specific cell-surface receptors; the viral RNA and reverse transcriptase synthesize a double-strand DNA version of the RNA template; and the provirus moves into the nucleus and integrates into the host cell genome. This proviral integration is permanent. Although some animal retroviruses integrate into a single specific site of the host genome in every infected cell, the human retroviruses integrate randomly. This first phase of replication depends entirely on gene products in the virus. The second phase includes the synthesis and processing of viral genomes, mRNAs, and proteins using host cell machinery, often under the influence of viral gene products. Virions are assembled and released from the cell by budding from the membrane; host cell membrane proteins are frequently incorporated into the envelope of the virus. Proviral integration occurs during the S-phase of the cell cycle; thus, in general, nondividing cells are resistant to retroviral infection. Only the lentiviruses are able to infect nondividing cells. Once a host cell is infected, it is infected for the life of the cell.

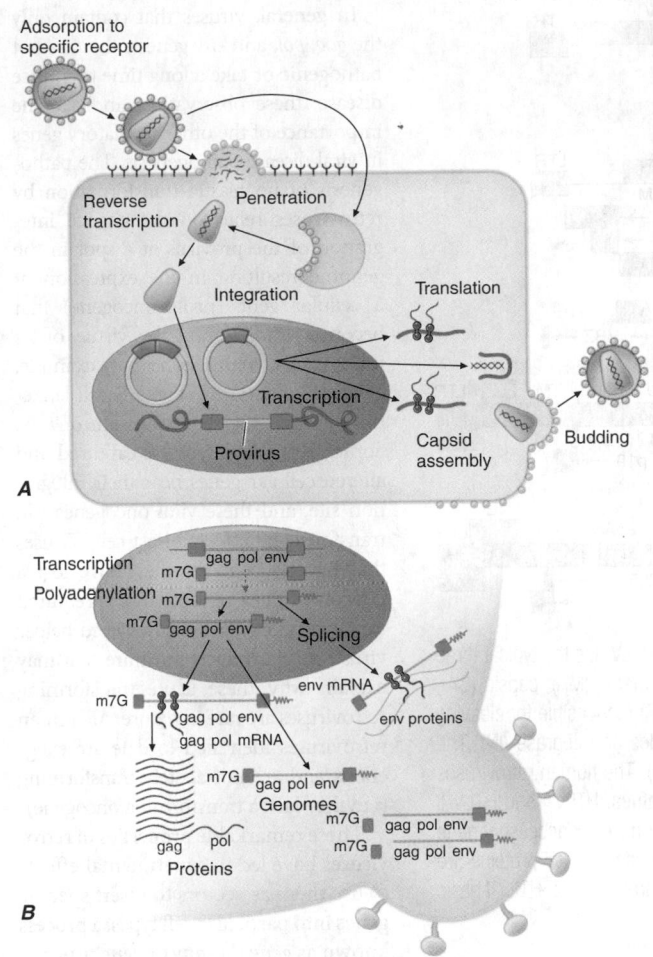

A

B

Figure 188-1 **The life cycle of retroviruses. *A.*** Overview of virus replication. The retrovirus enters a target cell by binding to a specific cell-surface receptor; once the virus is internalized, its RNA is released from the nucleocapsid and is reverse-transcribed into proviral DNA. The provirus is inserted into the genome and then transcribed into RNA; the RNA is translated; and virions assemble and are extruded from the cell membrane by budding. ***B.*** Overview of retroviral gene expression. The provirus is transcribed, capped, and polyadenylated. Viral RNA molecules then have one of three fates: they are exported to the cytoplasm, where they are packaged as the viral RNA in infectious viral particles; they are spliced to form the message for the envelope polyprotein; or they are translated into Gag and Pol proteins. Most of the messages for the Pol protein fail to initiate Pol translation because of a stop codon before its initiation; however, in a fraction of the messages, the stop codon is missed and the Pol proteins are translated. *[Modified from JM Coffin, in BN Fields, DM Knipe (eds): Fields Virology. New York, Raven, 1990; with permission.]*

Retroviral genomes include both coding and noncoding sequences (Fig. 188-2). In general, noncoding sequences are important recognition signals for DNA or RNA synthesis or processing events and are located in the 5′ and 3′ terminal regions of the genome. All retroviral genomes are terminally redundant, containing identical sequences called *long terminal repeats* (LTRs). The ends of the retroviral RNA genome differ slightly in sequence from the integrated retroviral DNA. In the latter, the LTR sequences are repeated in both the 5′ and the 3′ terminus of the virus. The LTRs contain sequences involved in initiating the expression of the viral proteins, the integration of the provirus, and the polyadenylation of viral RNAs. The primer binding site, which is critical for the initiation of reverse transcription, and the

viral packaging sequences are located outside the LTR sequences. The coding regions include the *gag* (group-specific antigen, core protein), *pol* (RNA-dependent DNA polymerase), and *env* (envelope) genes. The *gag* gene encodes a precursor polyprotein that is cleaved to form three to five capsid proteins; a fraction of the Gag precursor proteins also contain a protease responsible for cleaving the Gag and Pol polyproteins. A Gag-Pol polyprotein gives rise to the protease that is responsible for cleaving the Gag-Pol polyprotein. The *pol* gene encodes three proteins: the reverse transcriptase, the integrase, and the protease. The reverse transcriptase copies the viral RNA into the double-strand DNA provirus, which inserts itself into the host cell DNA via the action of integrase. The protease cleaves the Gag-Pol polyprotein into smaller protein products. The *env* gene encodes the envelope glycoproteins: one protein that binds to specific surface receptors and determines what cell types can be infected and a smaller transmembrane protein that anchors the complex to the envelope. Fig. 188-3 shows how the retroviral gene products make up the virus structure.

HTLVs have a region between *env* and the 3′ LTR that encodes several proteins and transcripts in overlapping reading frames (Fig. 188-2). Tax is a 40-kDa protein that does not bind to DNA but induces the expression of host cell transcription factors that alter host cell gene expression and is capable of inducing cell transformation under certain circumstances. Rex is a 27-kDa protein that regulates the expression of viral mRNAs. Other transcripts from this region (p12, p13, p30) tend to restrict expression of viral genes and diminish the immunogenicity of infected cells. HBZ is a product of the complementary proviral DNA strand, and its protein interacts with many cellular transcription factors and signaling proteins. It stimulates proliferation of infected cells and is the only viral product universally expressed in HTLV-I-infected tumor cells. These proteins are produced from messages that are similar but that are spliced differently from overlapping but distinct exons.

The lentiviruses in general, and HIV-1 and -2 in particular, contain a larger genome than other pathogenic retroviruses. They contain an untranslated region between *pol* and *env* that encodes portions of several proteins, varying with the reading frame into which the mRNA is spliced. Tat is a 14-kDa protein that augments the expression of virus from the LTR. The Rev protein of HIV-1, similar to the Rex protein of HTLV, regulates RNA splicing and/or RNA transport. The Nef protein downregulates CD4, the cellular receptor for HIV; alters host T cell activation pathways; and enhances viral infectivity. The Vif protein is necessary for the proper assembly of the HIV nucleoprotein core in many types of cells; without Vif, proviral DNA is not efficiently produced in these infected cells. In addition, the Vif protein targets APOBEC (apolipoprotein B mRNA-editing enzyme catalytic polypeptide, a cytidine deaminase that mutates the viral sequence) for proteasomal degradation, thus blocking its virus-suppressing effect. Vpr, Vpu (HIV-1 only), and Vpx (HIV-2 only) are viral proteins encoded by translation of the same message in different reading frames. As noted above, oncogenic retroviruses depend on cell proliferation for their replication; lentiviruses can infect nondividing cells, largely through effects mediated by Vpr. Vpr facilitates transport of the provirus into the nucleus and can induce other cellular changes, such as G_2 growth arrest and differentiation of some target cells. Vpx is structurally related to Vpr, but its functions are not fully defined. Vpu promotes the degradation of CD4 in the endoplasmic reticulum and stimulates the release of virions from infected cells.

Retroviruses can be either exogenously acquired (by infection with an infected cell or a free virion capable of replication) or transmitted in the germ line as endogenous virus. Endogenous retroviruses are often replication defective. The human genome contains endogenous retroviral sequences, but there are no known replication-competent endogenous retroviruses in humans.

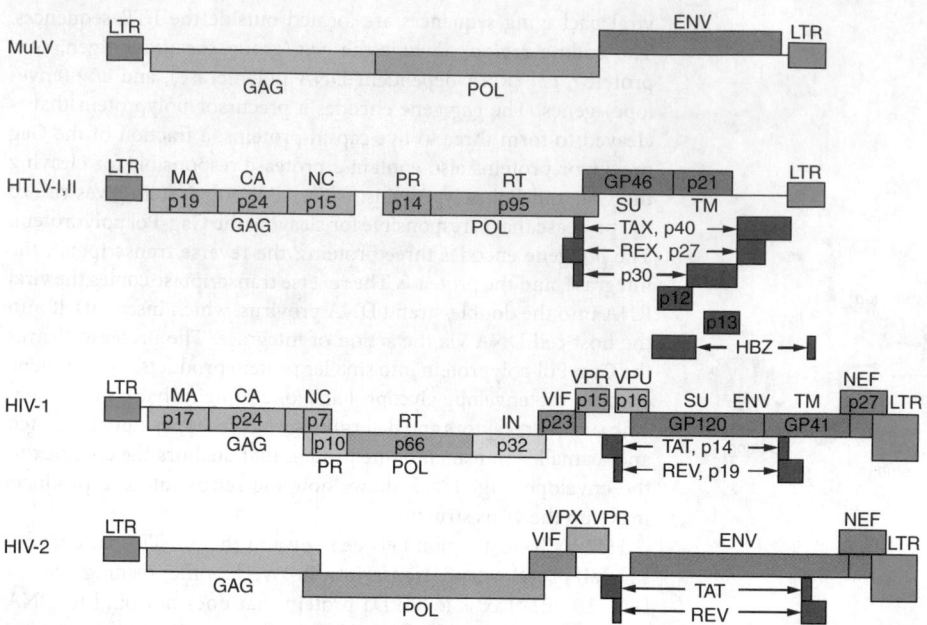

Figure 188-2 Genomic structure of retroviruses. The murine leukemia virus MuLV has the typical three structural genes: *gag*, *pol*, and *env*. The *gag* region gives rise to three proteins: matrix (MA), capsid (CA), and nucleic acid–binding (NC) proteins. The *pol* region encodes both a protease (PR) responsible for cleaving the viral polyproteins and a reverse transcriptase (RT). In addition, HIV *pol* encodes an integrase (IN). The *env* region encodes a surface protein (SU) and a small transmembrane protein (TM). The human retroviruses have additional gene products translated in each of the three possible reading frames. HTLV-I and HTLV-II have *tax* and *rex* genes with exons on either side of the *env* gene. HIV-1 and HIV-2 have six accessory gene products: *tat*, *rev*, *vif*, *nef*, *vpr*, and either *vpu* (in HIV-1) or *vpx* (in HIV-2). The genes for these proteins are located mainly between the *pol* and *env* genes. LTR, long terminal repeat; GP, glycoprotein; HBZ, HTLV-I basic leucine zipper domain-containing protein.

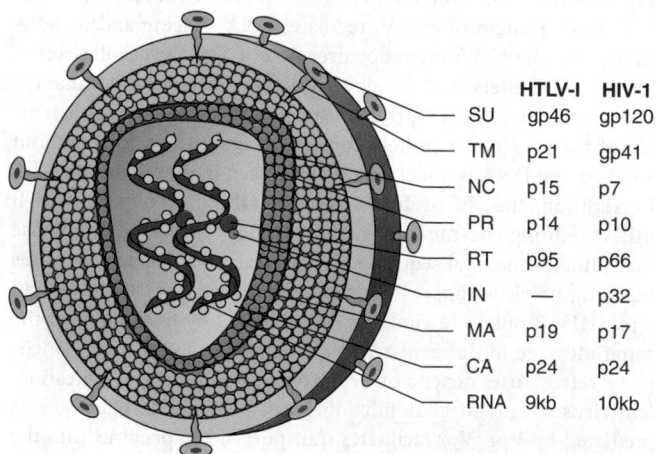

	HTLV-I	HIV-1
SU	gp46	gp120
TM	p21	gp41
NC	p15	p7
PR	p14	p10
RT	p95	p66
IN	—	p32
MA	p19	p17
CA	p24	p24
RNA	9kb	10kb

Figure 188-3 Schematic structure of human retroviruses. The surface glycoprotein (SU) is responsible for binding to receptors of host cells. The transmembrane protein (TM) anchors SU to the virus. NC is a nucleic acid–binding protein found in association with the viral RNA. A protease (PR) cleaves the polyproteins encoded by the *gag*, *pol*, and *env* genes into their functional components. RT is reverse transcriptase, and IN is an integrase present in some retroviruses (e.g., HIV-1) that facilitates insertion of the provirus into the host genome. The matrix protein (MA) is a Gag protein closely associated with the lipid of the envelope. The capsid protein (CA) forms the major internal structure of the virus, the core shell.

In general, viruses that contain only the *gag*, *pol*, and *env* genes either are not pathogenic or take a long time to induce disease; these observations indicate the importance of the other regulatory genes in viral disease pathogenesis. The pathogenesis of neoplastic transformation by retroviruses relies on the chance integration of the provirus at a spot in the genome resulting in the expression of a cellular gene (proto-oncogene) that becomes transforming by virtue of its unregulated expression. For example, avian leukosis virus causes B cell leukemia by inducing the expression of *myc*. Some retroviruses possess captured and altered cellular genes near their integration site, and these viral oncogenes can transform the infected host cell. Viruses that have oncogenes often have lost a portion of their genome that is required for replication. Such viruses need helper viruses to reproduce, a feature that may explain why these acute transforming retroviruses are rare in nature. All human retroviruses identified to date are exogenous and are not acutely transforming (i.e., they lack a transforming oncogene).

These remarkable properties of retroviruses have led to experimental efforts to use them as vectors to insert specific genes into particular cell types, a process known as *gene therapy* or *gene transfer*. The process could be used to repair a genetic defect or to introduce a new property that could be used therapeutically; for example, a gene (e.g., thymidine kinase) that would make a tumor cell susceptible to killing by a drug (e.g., ganciclovir) could be inserted. One source of concern about the use of retroviral vectors in humans is that replication-competent viruses might rescue endogenous retroviral replication, with unpredictable results. This concern is not merely hypothetical: the detection of proteins encoded by endogenous retroviral sequences on the surface of cancer cells implies that the genetic events leading to the cancer were able to activate the synthesis of these usually silent genes.

HUMAN T CELL LYMPHOTROPIC VIRUS

HTLV-I was isolated in 1980 from a T cell lymphoma cell line from a patient originally thought to have cutaneous T cell lymphoma. Later it became clear that the patient had a distinct form of lymphoma (originally reported in Japan) called *adult T cell leukemia/lymphoma* (ATL). Serologic data have determined that HTLV-I is the cause of at least two important diseases: ATL and tropical spastic paraparesis, also called *HTLV-I-associated myelopathy* (HAM). HTLV-I may also play a role in infective dermatitis, arthritis, uveitis, and Sjögren's syndrome.

Two years after the isolation of HTLV-I, HTLV-II was isolated from a patient with an unusual form of hairy cell leukemia that affected T cells. Epidemiologic studies of HTLV-II failed to reveal a consistent disease association.

■ BIOLOGY AND MOLECULAR BIOLOGY

Because the biology of HTLV-I and that of HTLV-II are similar, the following discussion will focus on HTLV-I.

Human glucose transporter protein 1 (GLUT-1) functions as a receptor for HTLV-1, probably acting together with neuropilin-1

(NRP1) and heparan sulfate proteoglycans. Generally, only T cells are productively infected, but infection of B cells and other cell types is occasionally detected. The most common outcome of HTLV-I infection is latent carriage of randomly integrated provirus in CD4+ T cells. HTLV-I does not contain an oncogene and does not insert into a unique site in the genome. Indeed, most infected cells express no viral gene products. The only viral gene product that is routinely expressed in tumor cells transformed by HTLV-I in vivo is *hbz*. The *tax* gene is thought to be critical to the transformation process but is not expressed in the tumor cells of many ATL patients, possibly because of the immunogenicity of *tax*-expressing cells. Cells transformed in vitro, by contrast, actively transcribe HTLV-I RNA and produce infectious virions. Most HTLV-I-transformed cell lines are the result of the infection of a normal host T cell in vitro. It is difficult to establish cell lines derived from authentic ATL cells.

Although *tax* does not itself bind to DNA, it does induce the expression of a wide range of host cell gene products, including transcription factors (especially c-rel/NF-κB, ets-1 and -2, and members of the fos/jun family), cytokines [e.g., interleukin (IL) 2, granulocyte-macrophage colony-stimulating factor, and tumor necrosis factor], and membrane proteins and receptors [major histocompatibility (MHC) molecules and IL-2 receptor α]. The genes activated by *tax* are generally controlled by transcription factors of the c-rel/NF-κB and cyclic AMP response element binding (CREB) protein families. It is unclear how this induction of host gene expression leads to neoplastic transformation; *tax* can interfere with G₁ and mitotic cell-cycle checkpoints, block apoptosis, inhibit DNA repair, and promote antigen-independent T cell proliferation. Induction of a cytokine-autocrine loop has been proposed; however, IL-2 is not the crucial cytokine. The involvement of IL-4, IL-7, and IL-15 has been proposed.

In light of the irregular expression of *tax* in ATL cells, it has been suggested that *tax* is important in the early phases of transformation but is not essential for the maintenance of the transformed state. The maintenance role is thought to be due to *hbz* expression. As is clear from the epidemiology of HTLV-I infection, transformation of an infected cell is a rare event and may depend on heterogeneous second, third, or fourth genetic hits. No consistent chromosomal abnormalities have been described in ATL; however, aneuploidy is common and individual cases with p53 mutations and translocations involving the T cell receptor genes on chromosome 14 have been reported. *Tax* may repress certain DNA repair enzymes, permitting the accumulation of genetic damage that would normally be repaired. However, the molecular pathogenesis of HTLV-I-induced neoplasia is not fully understood.

■ FEATURES OF HTLV-I INFECTION

Epidemiology

HTLV-I infection is transmitted in at least three ways: from mother to child, especially via breast milk; through sexual activity, more commonly from men to women; and through the blood—via contaminated transfusions or contaminated needles. The virus is most commonly transmitted perinatally. Compared with HIV, which can be transmitted in cell-free form, HTLV-I is less infectious, and its transmission usually requires cell-to-cell contact.

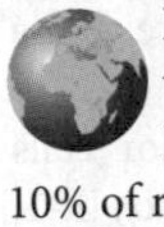

HTLV-I is endemic in southwestern Japan and Okinawa, where >1 million persons are infected. Antibodies to HTLV-I are present in the serum of up to 35% of Okinawans, 10% of residents of the Japanese island of Kyushu, and <1% of persons in nonendemic regions of Japan. Despite this high prevalence of infection, only ~500 cases of ATL are diagnosed in this area each year. Clusters of infection have been noted in other areas of the Orient, such as Taiwan; in the Caribbean basin, including northeastern South America; in northwestern South America; in central and southern Africa; in Italy, Israel, Iran, and Papua New Guinea; in the Arctic; and in the southeastern part of the United States (Fig. 188-4). An estimated 15–20 million persons have HTLV-I infection worldwide.

Progressive spastic or ataxic myelopathy developing in an individual who is HTLV-I positive (i.e., who has serum antibodies to HTLV-I) may be due to direct infection of the nervous system with the virus, but destruction of the pyramidal tracts appears to involve HTLV-I-infected CD4+ T cells; a similar disorder may result from infection with HIV or HTLV-II. In rare instances, patients with HAM are seronegative but have detectable antibody to HTLV-I in the cerebrospinal fluid (CSF).

The cumulative lifetime risk of developing ATL is 3% among HTLV-I-infected patients, with a threefold greater risk among men than among women; a similar cumulative risk is projected for HAM (4%), but with women more commonly affected than men. The distribution of the two diseases overlaps the distribution of HTLV-I, with >95% of affected patients showing serologic evidence of HTLV-I infection. The latency period between infection and the emergence of disease is 20–30 years for ATL. For HAM, the median latency period is ~3.3 years (range, 4 months to 30 years). The development of ATL is rare among persons infected by blood products; however, ~20% of patients with HAM acquire HTLV-I from contaminated blood. ATL is more common among perinatally infected individuals, whereas HAM is more common among persons infected via sexual transmission.

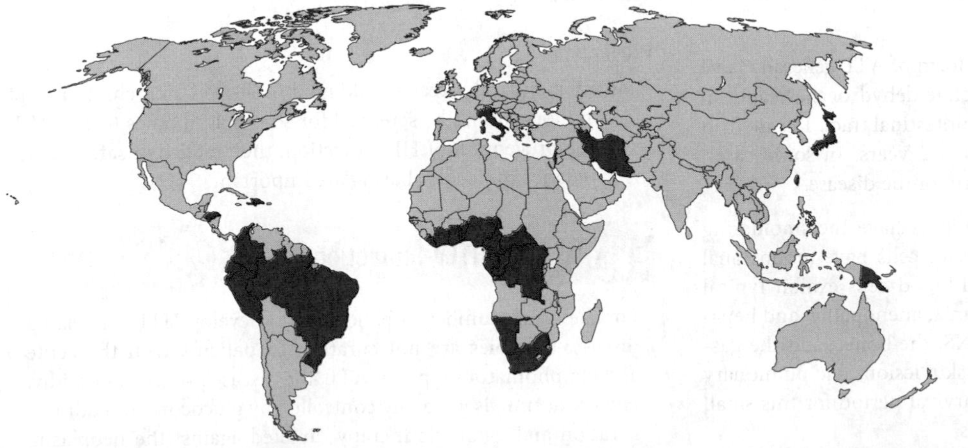

Associated diseases

ATL Four clinical types of HTLV-I-induced neoplasia have been described: acute, lymphomatous, chronic, and smoldering. All of these tumors are monoclonal proliferations of CD4+ postthymic T cells with clonal proviral integrations and clonal T cell receptor gene rearrangements.

Figure 188-4   Global distribution of HTLV-I infection. Countries with a prevalence of HTLV-I infection of 1–5% are shaded darkly. Note that the distribution of infected patients is not uniform in endemic countries. For example, the people of southwestern Japan and northeastern Brazil are more commonly affected than those in other regions of those countries.

Acute ATL   About 60% of patients who develop malignancy have classic acute ATL, which is characterized by a short clinical prodrome (~2 weeks between the first symptoms and the diagnosis) and an aggressive natural history (median survival period, 6 months). The clinical picture is dominated by rapidly progressive skin lesions, pulmonary involvement, hypercalcemia, and lymphocytosis with cells containing lobulated or "flower-shaped" nuclei (see Fig. 110-10). The malignant cells have monoclonal proviral integrations and express CD4, CD3, and CD25 (low-affinity IL-2 receptors) on their surface. Serum levels of CD25 can be used as a tumor marker. Anemia and thrombocytopenia are rare. The skin lesions may be difficult to distinguish from those in mycosis fungoides. Lytic bone lesions, which are common, do not contain tumor cells but rather are composed of osteolytic cells, usually without osteoblastic activity. Despite the leukemic picture, bone marrow involvement is patchy in most cases.

The hypercalcemia of ATL is multifactorial; the tumor cells produce osteoclast-activating factors (tumor necrosis factor α, IL-1, lymphotoxin) and can also produce a parathyroid hormone–like molecule. Affected patients have an underlying immunodeficiency that makes them susceptible to opportunistic infections similar to those seen in patients with AIDS (Chap. 189). The pathogenesis of the immunodeficiency is unclear. Pulmonary infiltrates in ATL patients reflect leukemic infiltration half the time and opportunistic infections with organisms such as *Pneumocystis* and other fungi the other half. Gastrointestinal symptoms are nearly always related to opportunistic infection. *Strongyloides stercoralis* is a gastrointestinal parasite that has a pattern of endemic distribution similar to that of HTLV-I. HTLV-I–infected persons also infected with this parasite may develop ATL more often or more rapidly than those without *Strongyloides* infections. Serum concentrations of lactate dehydrogenase and alkaline phosphatase are often elevated in ATL. About 10% of patients have leptomeningeal involvement leading to weakness, altered mental status, paresthesia, and/or headache. Unlike other forms of central nervous system (CNS) lymphoma, ATL may be accompanied by normal CSF protein levels. The diagnosis depends on finding ATL cells in the CSF (Chap. 110).

Lymphomatous ATL   The lymphomatous type of ATL occurs in ~20% of patients and is similar to the acute form in its natural history and clinical course, except that circulating abnormal cells are rare and lymphadenopathy is evident. The histology of the lymphoma is variable but does not influence the natural history. In general, the diagnosis is suspected on the basis of the patient's birthplace (see "Epidemiology," above) and the presence of skin lesions and hypercalcemia. The diagnosis is confirmed by the detection of antibodies to HTLV-I in serum.

Chronic ATL   Patients with the chronic form of ATL generally have normal serum levels of calcium and lactate dehydrogenase and no involvement of the CNS, bone, or gastrointestinal tract. The median duration of survival for these patients is 2 years. In some cases, chronic ATL progresses to the acute form of the disease.

Smoldering ATL   Fewer than 5% of patients have the smoldering form of ATL. In this form, the malignant cells have monoclonal proviral integration; <5% of peripheral blood cells exhibit typical morphologic abnormalities; hypercalcemia, adenopathy, and hepatosplenomegaly do not develop; the CNS, the bones, and the gastrointestinal tract are not involved; and skin lesions and pulmonary lesions may be present. The median survival period for this small subset of patients appears to be ≥5 years.

HAM (tropical spastic paraparesis)   In contrast to ATL, in which there is a slight predominance of male patients, HAM affects female patients disproportionately. HAM resembles multiple sclerosis in certain ways (Chap. 380). The onset is insidious. Symptoms include weakness or stiffness in one or both legs, back pain, and urinary incontinence. Sensory changes are usually mild, but peripheral neuropathy may develop. The disease generally takes the form of slowly progressive and unremitting thoracic myelopathy; one-third of patients are bedridden within 10 years of diagnosis, and one-half are unable to walk unassisted by this point. Patients display spastic paraparesis or paraplegia with hyperreflexia, ankle clonus, and extensor plantar responses. Cognitive function is usually spared; cranial nerve abnormalities are unusual.

MRI reveals lesions in both the white matter and the paraventricular regions of the brain as well as in the spinal cord. Pathologic examination of the spinal cord shows symmetric degeneration of the lateral columns, including the corticospinal tracts; some cases involve the posterior columns as well. The spinal meninges and cord parenchyma contain an inflammatory infiltrate with myelin destruction.

HTLV-I is not usually found in cells of the CNS but may be detected in a small population of lymphocytes present in the CSF. In general, HTLV-I replication is greater in HAM than in ATL, and patients with HAM have a stronger immune response to the virus. Antibodies to HTLV-I are present in the serum and appear to be produced in the CSF of HAM patients, where titers are often higher than in the serum. The pathophysiology of HAM may involve the induction of autoimmune destruction of neural cells by T cells with specificity for viral components such as Tax or Env proteins. One theory is that susceptibility to HAM may be related to the presence of human leukocyte antigen (HLA) alleles capable of presenting viral antigens in a fashion that leads to autoimmunity. Insufficient data are available to confirm an HLA association. However, antibodies in the sera of HAM patients have been shown to bind a neuron-specific antigen [heteronuclear ribonuclear protein A1 (hnRNP A1)] and to interfere with neurotransmission in vitro.

It is unclear what factors influence whether HTLV-I infection will cause disease and, if it does, whether it will induce a neoplasm (ATL) or an autoimmune disorder (HAM). Differences in viral strains, the susceptibility of particular MHC haplotypes, the route of HTLV-I infection, the viral load, and the nature of the HTLV-I–related immune response are putative factors, but few definitive data are available.

Other putative HTLV-I–related diseases   In areas where HTLV-I is endemic, diverse inflammatory and autoimmune diseases have been attributed to the virus, including uveitis, dermatitis, pneumonitis, rheumatoid arthritis, and polymyositis. However, a causal relationship between HTLV-I and these illnesses has not been established.

Prevention

Women in endemic areas should not breast-feed their children, and blood donors should be screened for serum antibodies to HTLV-I. As in the prevention of HIV infection, the practice of safe sex and the avoidance of needle sharing are important.

TREATMENT   **HTLV-I Infection**

For the small number of patients who develop HTLV-I–related disease, therapies are not curative. In patients with the acute and lymphomatous types of ATL, the disease progresses rapidly. Hypercalcemia is generally controlled by glucocorticoid administration and cytotoxic therapy directed against the neoplasm. The tumor is highly responsive to combination chemotherapy that is employed against other forms of lymphoma; however, patients are susceptible to overwhelming bacterial and opportunistic infections, and ATL relapses within 4–10 months after remission in most cases. The combination of interferon α and zidovudine may extend survival. Because viral replication is not clearly associated with ATL progression, zidovudine is probably effective through its cytotoxic effects (as a chain-terminating thymidine analogue) rather than its antiviral effects. An experimental approach using an yttrium 90–labeled or toxin-conjugated antibody to the IL-2 receptor appears promising but is not widely available. Patients with the chronic or smoldering form of ATL may be managed with an expectant approach: treat any infections, and watch and wait for signs of progression to acute disease.

Patients with HAM may obtain some benefit from the use of glucocorticoids to reduce inflammation. Antiretroviral regimens have not been effective. In one study, danazol (200 mg three times daily) produced significant neurologic improvement in five of six treated patients, with resolution of urinary incontinence in two cases, decreased spasticity in three, and restoration of the ability to walk after confinement to a wheelchair in two. Physical therapy and rehabilitation are important components of management.

■ FEATURES OF HTLV-II INFECTION

Epidemiology

HTLV-II is endemic in certain Native American tribes and in Africa. It is generally considered to be a New World virus that was brought from Asia to the Americas 10,000–40,000 years ago during the migration of infected populations across the Bering land bridge. The mode of transmission of HTLV-II is probably the same as that of HTLV-I (see above). HTLV-II may be less readily transmitted sexually than HTLV-I.

Studies of large cohorts of injection drug users with serologic assays that reliably distinguish HTLV-I from HTLV-II indicated that the vast majority of HTLV-positive cohort members were infected with HTLV-II. The seroprevalence of HTLV in a cohort of 7841 injection drug users from drug treatment centers in Baltimore, Chicago, Los Angeles, New Jersey (Asbury Park and Trenton), New York City (Brooklyn and Harlem), Philadelphia, and San Antonio was 20.9%, with >97% of cases due to HTLV-II. The seroprevalence of HTLV-II was higher in the Southwest and the Midwest than in the Northeast. In contrast, the seroprevalence of HIV-1 was higher in the Northeast than in the Southwest or the Midwest. Approximately 3% of the cohort members were infected with both HTLV-II and HIV-1. The seroprevalence of HTLV-II increased linearly with age. Women were significantly more likely to be infected with HTLV-II than were men; the virus is thought to be more efficiently transmitted from male to female than from female to male.

Associated diseases

Although HTLV-II was isolated from a patient with a T cell variant of hairy cell leukemia, this virus has not been consistently associated with a particular disease and in fact has been thought of as "a virus searching for a disease." However, evidence is accumulating that HTLV-II may play a role in certain neurologic, hematologic, and dermatologic diseases. These data require confirmation, particularly in light of the previous confusion regarding the relative prevalences of HTLV-I and HTLV-II among injection drug users.

Prevention

Avoidance of needle sharing, adherence to safe-sex practices, screening of blood (by assays for HTLV-I, which also detect HTLV-II), and avoidance of breast-feeding by infected women are important principles in the prevention of spread of HTLV-II.

HUMAN IMMUNODEFICIENCY VIRUS

HIV-1 and HIV-2 are members of the lentivirus subfamily of Retroviridae and are the only lentiviruses known to infect humans. The lentiviruses are slow-acting by comparison with viruses that cause acute infection (e.g., influenza virus) but not by comparison with other retroviruses. The features of acute primary infection with HIV resemble those of more classic acute infections. The characteristic chronicity of HIV disease is consistent with the designation *lentivirus*. For a detailed discussion of HIV, see Chap. 189.

FURTHER READINGS

Boxus M, Willems L: Mechanisms of HTLV-1 persistence and transformation. Br J Cancer 101:1497, 2009

Lee SM et al: HTLV-1 induced molecular mimicry in neurological disease. Curr Top Microbiol Immunol 296:125, 2005

Legros S et al: Protein-protein interactions and gene expression regulation in HTLV-1-infected cells. Front Biosci 14:4138, 2009

Matsuoka M, Jeang KT: Human T-cell leukaemia virus type 1 (HTLV-1) infectivity and cellular transformation. Nat Rev Cancer 7:270, 2007

Mori N: Cell signaling modifiers for molecular targeted therapy in ATLL. Front Biosci 14:1479, 2009

Nyborg JK et al: The HTLV-1 Tax protein: Revealing mechanisms of transcriptional activation through histone acetylation and nucleosome disassembly. Biochim Biophys Acta 1799:266, 2010

Proietti FA et al: Global epidemiology of HTLV-I infection and associated diseases. Oncogene 24:6058, 2005

Tsukasaki K et al: Definition, prognostic factors, treatment, and response criteria of adult-T-cell leukemia-lymphoma: A proposal from an international consensus meeting. J Clin Oncol 27:453, 2008

CHAPTER 189

Human Immunodeficiency Virus Disease: AIDS and Related Disorders

Anthony S. Fauci
H. Clifford Lane

AIDS was first recognized in the United States in the summer of 1981, when the U.S. Centers for Disease Control and Prevention (CDC) reported the unexplained occurrence of *Pneumocystis jiroveci* (formerly *P. carinii*) pneumonia in five previously healthy homosexual men in Los Angeles and of Kaposi's sarcoma (KS) with or without *P. jiroveci* pneumonia in 26 previously healthy homosexual men in New York and Los Angeles. The disease was soon recognized in male and female injection drug users; in hemophiliacs and blood transfusion recipients; among female sexual partners of men with AIDS; and among infants born to mothers with AIDS or with a history of injection drug use. In 1983, human immunodeficiency virus (HIV) was isolated from a patient with lymphadenopathy, and by 1984 it was demonstrated clearly to be the causative agent of AIDS. In 1985, a sensitive enzyme-linked immunosorbent assay (ELISA) was developed; this led to an appreciation of the scope and evolution of the HIV epidemic at first in the United States and other developed nations and ultimately among developing nations throughout the world (see "HIV infection and AIDS Worldwide" below). The staggering worldwide evolution of the HIV pandemic has been matched by an explosion of information in the areas of HIV virology, pathogenesis (both immunologic and virologic), treatment of HIV disease, treatment and prophylaxis of the opportunistic diseases associated with HIV infection, prevention of infection, and vaccine development. The information flow related to HIV disease is enormous and continues to expand, and it has become almost impossible for the health care generalist to stay abreast of the literature. The purpose of this chapter is to present the most current information available on the scope of the epidemic; on its pathogenesis, treatment, and prevention; and on prospects for vaccine development. Above all, the aim is to provide a solid scientific basis and practical clinical guidelines for a state-of-the-art approach to the HIV-infected patient.

■ DEFINITION

The current CDC classification system for HIV-infected adolescents and adults categorizes persons on the basis of clinical conditions associated with HIV infection and CD4+ T lymphocyte counts. The system is based on three ranges of CD4+ T lymphocyte counts and three clinical categories and is represented by a matrix of nine mutually exclusive categories (Tables 189-1 and 189-2). Using this system, any HIV-infected individual with a CD4+ T cell count of <200/μL has AIDS by definition, regardless of the presence of symptoms or opportunistic diseases (Table 189-1). Once individuals have had a clinical condition in category B, their disease classification cannot be reverted back to category A, even if the condition resolves; the same holds true for category C in relation to category B.

The definition of AIDS is indeed complex and comprehensive and was established not for the practical care of patients, but

TABLE 189-1   1993 Revised Classification System for HIV Infection and Expanded AIDS Surveillance Case Definition for Adolescents and Adults

CD4+ T Cell Categories	Clinical Categories		
	A Asymptomatic, Acute (Primary) HIV or PGL	B Symptomatic, Not A or C Conditions	C AIDS-Indicator Conditions
>500/μL	A1	B1	C1
200–499/μL	A2	B2	C2
<200/μL	A3	B3	C3

Abbreviation: PGL, progressive generalized lymphadenopathy.
Source: MMWR 42(No. RR-17), December 18, 1992.

for surveillance purposes. Thus, the clinician should not focus on whether the patient fulfills the strict definition of AIDS but should view HIV disease as a spectrum ranging from primary infection, with or without the acute syndrome, to the asymptomatic stage, to advanced stages associated with opportunistic diseases (see "Pathophysiology and Pathogenesis," below).

ETIOLOGIC AGENT

HIV is the etiologic agent of AIDS; it belongs to the family of human retroviruses (Retroviridae) and the subfamily of lentiviruses (Chap. 188). Nononcogenic lentiviruses cause disease in other animal species, including sheep, horses, goats, cattle, cats, and monkeys. The four retroviruses known to cause human disease belong to two distinct groups: the human T lymphotropic viruses (HTLV)-I and HTLV-II, which are transforming retroviruses; and the human immunodeficiency viruses, HIV-1 and HIV-2, which cause cytopathic effects either directly or indirectly (Chap. 188). The most common cause of HIV disease throughout the world, and certainly in the United States, is HIV-1, which comprises several subtypes with different geographic distributions (see "Molecular Heterogeneity of HIV-1," below). HIV-2 was first identified in 1986 in West African patients and was originally confined to West Africa. However, a number of cases that generally can be traced to West Africa or to sexual contacts with West Africans have been identified throughout the world. The currently defined groups of HIV-1 (M, N, O, P) and the HIV-2 groups A through G each are likely derived from a separate transfer to humans from a nonhuman primate reservoir. HIV-1 viruses likely came from chimpanzees and/or gorillas, and HIV-2 from sooty mangabeys. The AIDS pandemic is primarily caused by the HIV-1 M group viruses. Although HIV-1 group O and HIV-2 viruses have been found in numerous countries, including those in the developed world, they have caused much more localized epidemics. The taxonomic relationship between primate lentiviruses is shown in Fig. 189-1.

■ MORPHOLOGY OF HIV

Electron microscopy shows that the HIV virion is an icosahedral structure (Fig. 189-2) containing numerous external spikes formed by the two major envelope proteins, the external gp120 and the transmembrane gp41. The virion buds from the surface of the infected cell and incorporates a variety of host proteins, including major histocompatibility complex (MHC) class I and II antigens (Chap. 315), into its lipid bilayer. The structure of HIV-1 is schematically diagrammed in Fig. 189-2*B* (Chap. 188).

TABLE 189-2 Clinical Categories of HIV Infection

Category A: Consists of one or more of the conditions listed below in an adolescent or adult (>13 years) with documented HIV infection. Conditions listed in categories B and C must not have occurred.

    Asymptomatic HIV infection

    Persistent generalized lymphadenopathy

    Acute (primary) HIV infection with accompanying illness or history of acute HIV infection

Category B: Consists of symptomatic conditions in an HIV-infected adolescent or adult that are not included among conditions listed in clinical category C and that meet at least one of the following criteria: (1) The conditions are attributed to HIV infection or are indicative of a defect in cell-mediated immunity; or (2) the conditions are considered by physicians to have a clinical course or to require management that is complicated by HIV infection. Examples include, but are not limited to, the following:

    Bacillary angiomatosis

    Candidiasis, oropharyngeal (thrush)

    Candidiasis, vulvovaginal; persistent, frequent, or poorly responsive to therapy

    Cervical dysplasia (moderate or severe)/cervical carcinoma in situ

    Constitutional symptoms, such as fever (38.5°C) or diarrhea lasting >1 month

    Hairy leukoplakia, oral

    Herpes zoster (shingles), involving at least two distinct episodes or more than one dermatome

    Idiopathic thrombocytopenic purpura

    Listeriosis

    Pelvic inflammatory disease, particularly if complicated by tuboovarian abscess

    Peripheral neuropathy

Category C: Conditions listed in the AIDS surveillance case definition.

    Candidiasis of bronchi, trachea, or lungs

    Candidiasis, esophageal

    Cervical cancer, invasive[a]

    Coccidioidomycosis, disseminated or extrapulmonary

    Cryptococcosis, extrapulmonary

    Cryptosporidiosis, chronic intestinal (>1 month's duration)

    Cytomegalovirus disease (other than liver, spleen, or nodes)

    Cytomegalovirus retinitis (with loss of vision)

    Encephalopathy, HIV-related

    Herpes simplex: chronic ulcer(s) (>1 month's duration); or bronchitis, pneumonia, or esophagitis

    Histoplasmosis, disseminated or extrapulmonary

    Isosporiasis, chronic intestinal (>1 month's duration)

    Kaposi's sarcoma

    Lymphoma, Burkitt's (or equivalent term)

    Lymphoma, primary, of brain

    Mycobacterium avium complex or *M. kansasii*, disseminated or extrapulmonary

    Mycobacterium tuberculosis, any site (pulmonary[a] or extrapulmonary)

    Mycobacterium, other species or unidentified species, disseminated or extrapulmonary

    Pneumocystis jiroveci pneumonia

    Pneumonia, recurrent[a]

    Progressive multifocal leukoencephalopathy

    Salmonella septicemia, recurrent

    Toxoplasmosis of brain

    Wasting syndrome due to HIV

[a]Added in the 1993 expansion of the AIDS surveillance case definition.
Source: MMWR 42(No. RR-17), December 18, 1992.

■ REPLICATION CYCLE OF HIV

HIV is an RNA virus whose hallmark is the reverse transcription of its genomic RNA to DNA by the enzyme *reverse transcriptase*. The replication cycle of HIV begins with the high-affinity binding of the gp120 protein via a portion of its V1 region near the N terminus to its receptor on the host cell surface, the CD4 molecule (Fig. 189-3). The CD4 molecule is a 55-kDa protein found predominantly on a subset of T lymphocytes that are responsible for helper function in the immune system (Chap. 314). It is also expressed on the surface of monocytes/macrophages and dendritic/Langerhans cells. Once gp120 binds to CD4, the gp120 undergoes a conformational change that facilitates binding to one of two major co-receptors. The two major co-receptors for HIV-1 are CCR5 and CXCR4. Both receptors belong to the family of seven-transmembrane-domain G protein–coupled cellular receptors, and the use of one or the other or both receptors by the virus for entry into the cell is an important determinant of the cellular tropism of the virus. Certain dendritic cells express a diversity of C-type lectin receptors on their surface, one of which is called *DC-SIGN*, that also bind with high affinity to the HIV gp120 envelope protein, allowing the dendritic cell to facilitate the binding of virus to the CD4+ T cell upon engagement of dendritic cells with CD4+ T cells. Following binding of the envelope protein to the CD4 molecule associated with the above-mentioned conformational change in the viral envelope gp120, fusion with the host cell membrane occurs via the newly exposed gp41 molecule penetrating the plasma membrane of the target cell and then coiling upon itself to bring the virion and target cell together. Following fusion, the preintegration complex, composed of viral RNA and viral enzymes and surrounded by a capsid protein coat, is released into the cytoplasm of the target cell (Fig. 189-4). As the preintegration complex traverses the cytoplasm to reach the nucleus (Fig. 189-3), the viral reverse transcriptase enzyme catalyzes the reverse transcription of the genomic RNA into DNA, and the protein coat opens to release the resulting double-strand proviral HIV-DNA. At this point in the replication cycle, the viral genome is vulnerable to cellular factors that can block the progression of infection. In particular, the cytoplasmic TRIM5-α protein in rhesus macaque cells blocks simian immunodeficiency virus (SIV) replication at a point shortly after the virus fuses with the host cell. Although the exact mechanisms of action of TRIM5-α remain unclear, the human form is inhibited by cyclophilin A and is not effective in restricting HIV replication in human cells. The recently described APOBEC family of cellular proteins also inhibits progression of virus infection after virus has entered the cell. APOBEC proteins bind to nascent reverse transcripts and deaminate viral cytidine, causing hypermutation of HIV genomes. It is still not clear whether viral replication is inhibited by: (1) the binding of APOBEC to the virus genome with subsequent accumulation of reverse transcripts, or (2) the hypermutations caused by the enzymatic deaminase activity of APOBEC proteins. HIV has evolved a powerful strategy to protect itself from APOBEC. The viral protein Vif targets APOBEC for proteasomal degradation.

With activation of the cell, the viral DNA accesses the nuclear pore and is exported from the cytoplasm to the nucleus, where it is integrated into the host cell chromosomes through the action of another virally encoded enzyme, *integrase*. HIV provirus (DNA) integrates into the nuclear DNA preferentially within introns of active genes and regional hotspots. This provirus may remain transcriptionally inactive (latent) or it may manifest varying levels of gene expression, up to active production of virus.

Cellular activation plays an important role in the replication cycle of HIV and is critical to the pathogenesis of HIV disease (see "Pathogenesis and Pathophysiology," below). Following initial binding and internalization of virions into the target cell, incompletely reverse-transcribed DNA intermediates are labile

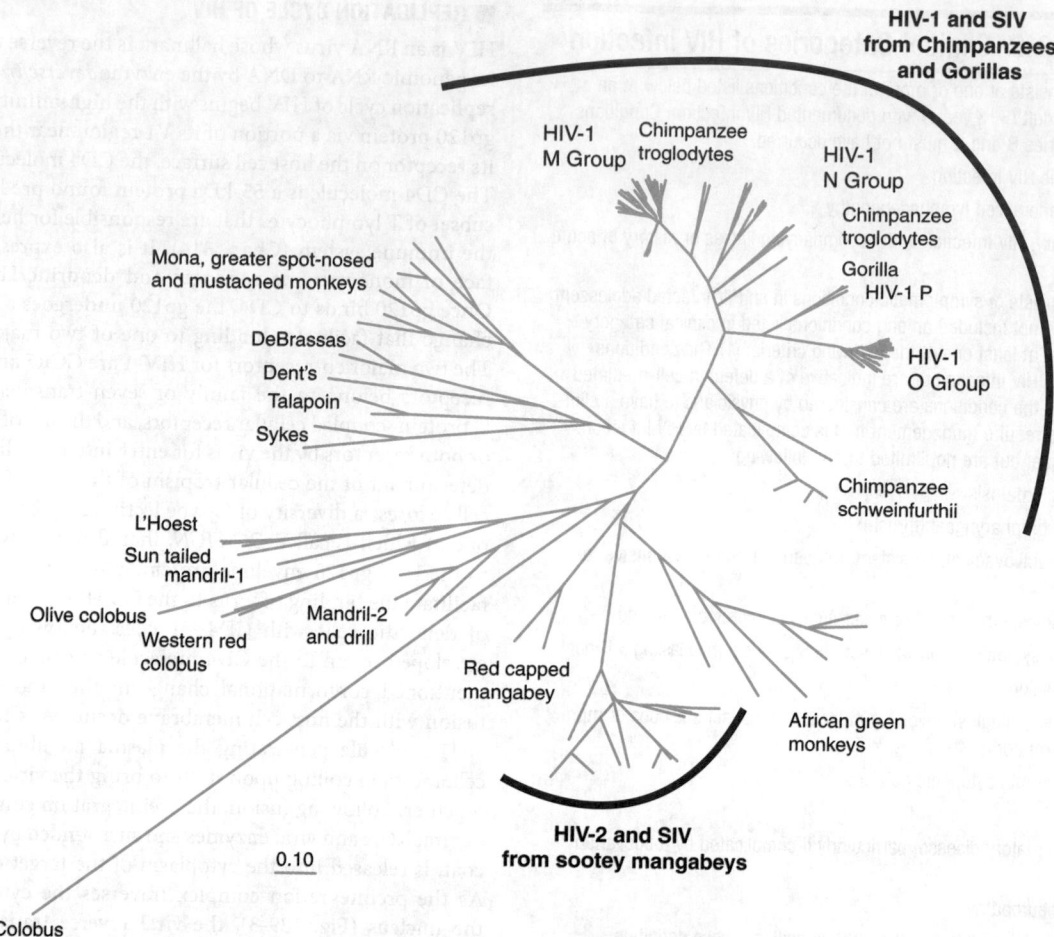

Figure 189-1   A phylogenetic tree based on the complete genomes of primate immunodeficiency viruses. The scale (0.10) indicates a 10% difference at the nucleotide level. *(Prepared by Brian Foley, PhD, of the HIV Sequence Database, Theoretical Biology and Biophysics Group, Los Alamos National Laboratory; additional information at www.hiv.lanl.gov/content/sequence/HelpDocs/subtypes.html.)*

In the tree (labels): HIV-1 and SIV from Chimpanzees and Gorillas; HIV-1 M Group; Chimpanzee troglodytes; HIV-1 N Group; Chimpanzee troglodytes; Gorilla HIV-1 P; HIV-1 O Group; Mona, greater spot-nosed and mustached monkeys; DeBrassas; Dent's; Talapoin; Sykes; Chimpanzee schweinfurthii; L'Hoest; Sun tailed mandril-1; Olive colobus; Mandril-2 and drill; Western red colobus; Red capped mangabey; African green monkeys; 0.10; HIV-2 and SIV from sootey mangabeys; Colobus

in quiescent cells and do not integrate efficiently into the host cell genome unless cellular activation occurs shortly after infection. Furthermore, some degree of activation of the host cell is required for the initiation of transcription of the integrated proviral DNA into either genomic RNA or mRNA. This latter process may not necessarily be associated with the detectable expression of the classic cell-surface markers of activation. In this regard, activation of HIV expression from the latent state depends on the interaction of a number of cellular and viral factors. Following transcription, HIV mRNA is translated into proteins that undergo modification through glycosylation, myristoylation, phosphorylation, and cleavage. The viral particle is formed by the assembly of HIV proteins, enzymes, and genomic RNA at the plasma membrane of the cells. Budding of the progeny virion occurs through specialized regions in the lipid bilayer of the host cell membrane known as *lipid rafts*, where the core acquires its external envelope (Chap. 188). The virally encoded protease then catalyzes the cleavage of the gag-pol precursor to yield the mature virion. Progression through the virus replication cycle is profoundly influenced by a variety of viral regulatory gene products. Likewise, each point in the replication cycle of HIV is a real or potential target for therapeutic intervention. Thus far, the reverse transcriptase, protease, and integrase enzymes as well as the process of virus–target cell binding and fusion have proved clinically to be susceptible to pharmacologic disruption.

■ HIV GENOME

Figure 189-5 illustrates schematically the arrangement of the HIV genome. Like other retroviruses, HIV-1 has genes that encode the structural proteins of the virus: *gag* encodes the proteins that form the core of the virion (including p24 antigen); *pol* encodes the enzymes responsible for protease processing of viral proteins, reverse transcription, and integration; and *env* encodes the envelope glycoproteins. However, HIV-1 is more complex than other retroviruses, particularly those of the nonprimate group, in that it also contains at least six other genes (*tat, rev, nef, vif, vpr,* and *vpu*), which code for proteins involved in the modification of the host cell to enhance virus growth and the regulation of viral gene expression (Chap. 188). Several of these proteins are thought to play a role in the pathogenesis of HIV disease; their various functions are listed in Fig. 189-5. Flanking these genes are the long terminal repeats (LTRs), which contain regulatory elements involved in gene expression (Fig. 189-5). The major difference between the genomes of HIV-1 and HIV-2 is the fact that HIV-2 lacks the *vpu* gene and has a *vpx* gene not contained in HIV-1.

■ MOLECULAR HETEROGENEITY OF HIV-1

Molecular analyses of HIV isolates reveal varying levels of sequence diversity over all regions of the viral genome. For example, the degree of difference in the coding sequences of the viral envelope protein ranges from a few percent (very close, among isolates from the same infected individual) to 50% (extreme

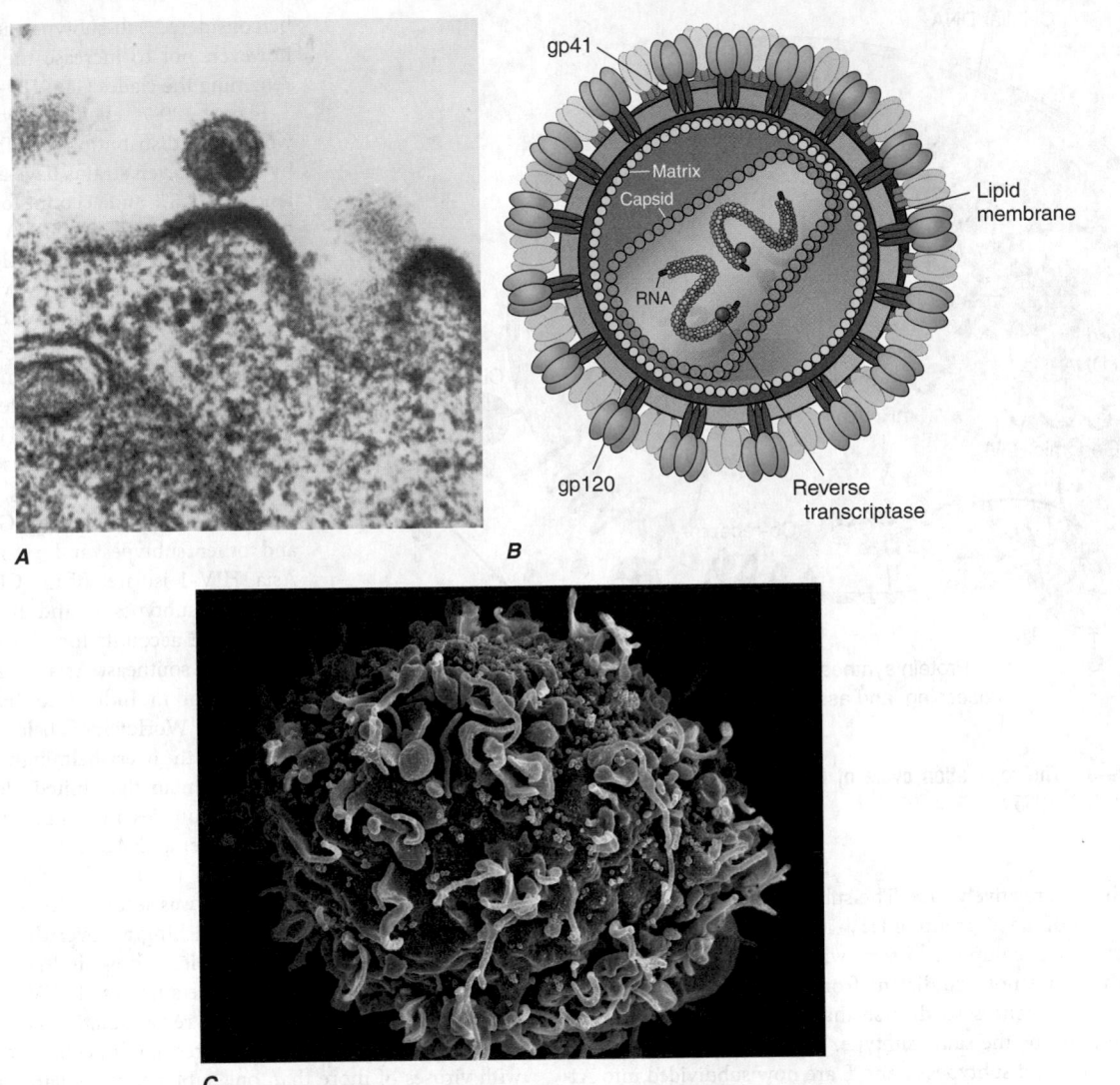

Figure 189-2   A. Electron micrograph of HIV. Figure illustrates a typical virion following budding from the surface of a CD4+ T lymphocyte, together with two additional incomplete virions in the process of budding from the cell membrane. **B.** Structure of HIV-1, including the gp120 envelope, gp41 transmembrane components of the envelope, genomic RNA, enzyme reverse transcriptase, p18(17) inner membrane (matrix), and p24 core protein (capsid). *(Copyright by George V. Kelvin). (Adapted from RC Gallo: Sci Am 256:46, 1987.)* **C.** Scanning electron micrograph of HIV-1 virions infecting a human CD4+ T lymphocyte. The original photograph was imaged at 8000× magnification. *(Courtesy of Elizabeth R. Fischer, Rocky Mountain Laboratories, National Institute of Allergy and Infectious Diseases; with permission.)*

diversity, among isolates from the different groups of HIV-1, M, N, O, and P). The changes tend to cluster in hypervariable regions. HIV can evolve by several means, including simple base substitution, insertions and deletions, recombination, and gain and loss of glycosylation sites. HIV sequence diversity arises directly from the limited fidelity of the reverse transcriptase. The balance of immune pressure and functional constraints on proteins influences the regional level of variation within proteins. For example, Envelope, which is exposed on the surface of the virion and is under immune selective pressure from both antibodies and cytolytic T lymphocytes, is extremely variable, with clusters of mutations in hypervariable domains. In contrast, reverse transcriptase, with important enzymatic functions, is relatively conserved, particularly around the active site. The extraordinary variability of HIV-1 is in marked contrast to the relative stability of HTLV-I and -II.

Four groups of HIV-1 have been defined. Group M (major) is responsible for most of the infections in the world. Group O (outlier) is a relatively rare viral form found originally in Cameroon, Gabon, and France. Group N was first identified in a Cameroonian

woman with AIDS; very few group N isolates have been identified and sequenced. An additional human immunodeficiency virus, related to gorilla SIV and distinct from other HIV-1 groups, was identified in a Cameroonian woman in 2009 and proposed as group P.

Among primate lentiviruses, HIV-1 is most closely related to viruses isolated from chimpanzees and gorillas. The chimpanzee subspecies *Pan troglodytes troglodytes* has been established to be the natural reservoir of the HIV-1 M and N groups. The HIV-1 O group is most closely related to viruses found in Cameroonian gorillas. The M group comprises nine subtypes, or *clades*, designated A, B, C, D, F, G, H, J, and K, as well as a growing number of major and minor circulating recombinant forms (CRFs). CRFs are generated by infection of an individual with two subtypes that then recombine and create a virus with a selective advantage. These CRFs range from highly prevalent forms such as the AE virus, CRF01_AE, which is predominant in southeast Asia and often referred to simply as E, despite the fact that the parental E virus has never been found, and CRF02_AG from west and central Africa, to a large number

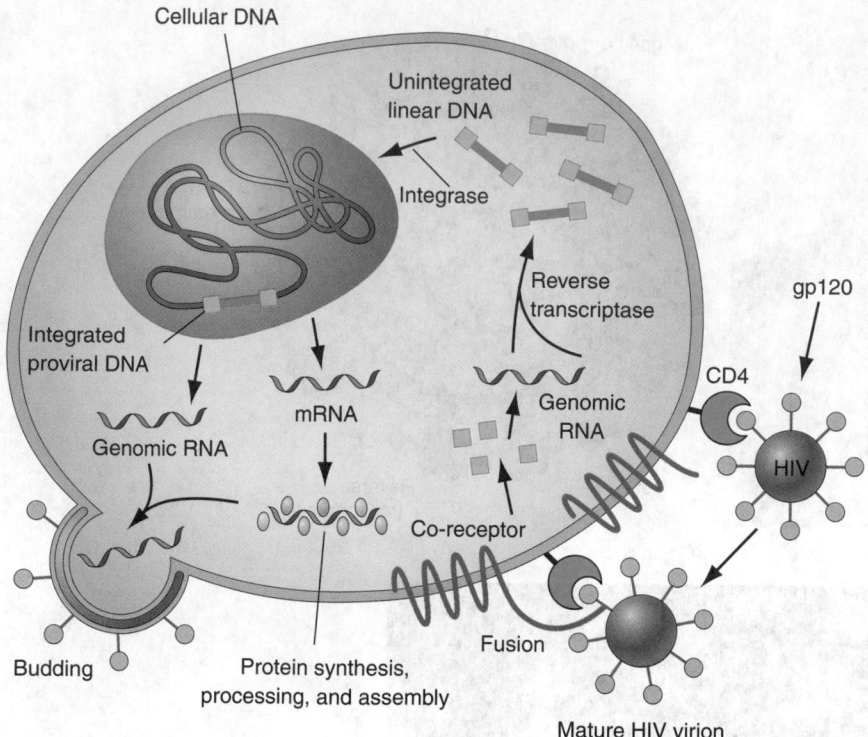

Figure 189-3 The replication cycle of HIV. See text for description. *(Adapted from AS Fauci: Nature 384:529, 1996.)*

of CRFs that are relatively rare. The subtypes and CRFs create the major lineages of the M group of HIV-1.

The picture was complicated somewhat when it was found that some subtypes are not equidistant from one another, while others contained sequences so diverse that they could not properly be considered to be the same subtype. Thus the term *sub-subtype* was introduced, and subtypes A and F are now subdivided into A1 and A2, and F1 and F2, respectively. It has also been argued that subtypes B and D are too close to be separate subtypes and should

be considered sub-subtypes; it was decided, however, not to increase the confusion by renaming the clades (Fig. 189-6).

Figure 189-7 schematically diagrams the worldwide distribution of HIV-1 subtypes by region. Seven strains have a global prevalence of >2.5% and account for the majority of HIV infections globally: HIV-1 subtypes A, B, C, D, G and two of the CRFs, CRF01_AE and CRF02_AG. Subtype C viruses (of the M group) are by far the most common form worldwide, accounting for ~50% of prevalent infections worldwide. In sub-Saharan Africa, home to approximately two-thirds of all individuals living with HIV/AIDS, the majority of infections are caused by subtype C, with smaller proportions of infections caused by subtype A, subtype G, CRF02_AG, and other subtypes and recombinants. In Asia, HIV-1 isolates of the CRF01_AE lineage and subtypes C and B predominate. CRF01_AE accounts for most infections in south and southeast Asia, while subtype C is prevalent in India (see "HIV Infection and AIDS Worldwide," below). Subtype B viruses are the overwhelmingly predominant viruses seen in the United States, Canada, certain countries in South America, western Europe, and Australia and account for 12–13% of global infections. It is thought that, purely by chance, subtype B was seeded into the United States in the late 1970s, thereby establishing an overwhelming founder effect. Many countries have co-circulating viral subtypes that are giving rise to new CRFs. Sequence analyses of HIV-1 isolates from infected individuals indicate that recombination among viruses of different clades likely occurs as a result of infection of an individual with viruses of more than one subtype, particularly in geographic areas where subtypes overlap.

The extraordinary diversity of HIV, reflected by the presence of multiple subtypes, circulating recombinant forms, and continuous viral evolution, has implications for possible differential rates of disease progression, responses to therapy, and the development of resistance to antiretroviral drugs. This diversity is also a formidable obstacle to HIV vaccine development, as a broadly useful vaccine would need to induce protective responses against a wide range of viral strains.

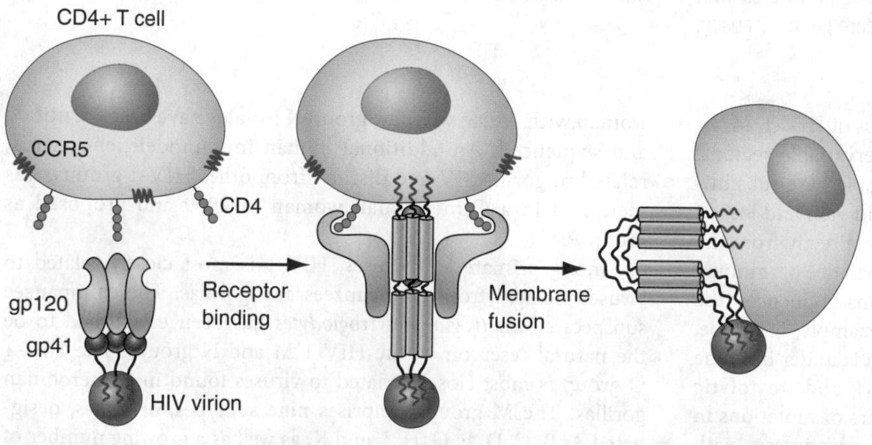

TRANSMISSION

HIV is transmitted primarily by sexual contact (both heterosexual and male to male); by blood and blood products; and by infected mothers to infants intrapartum, perinatally, or via breast milk. After ~30 years of scrutiny, there is no evidence that HIV is transmitted by casual contact or that the virus can be spread by insects, such as by a mosquito bite.

■ SEXUAL TRANSMISSION

HIV infection is predominantly a sexually transmitted disease (STD) worldwide. By far the most common mode of infection, particularly in developing countries, is heterosexual

Figure 189-4 Binding and fusion of HIV-1 with its target cell. HIV-1 binds to its target cell via the CD4 molecule, leading to a conformational change in the gp120 molecule that allows it to bind to the co-receptor CCR5 (for R5-using viruses). The virus then firmly attaches to the host cell membrane in a coiled-spring fashion via the newly exposed gp41 molecule. Virus-cell fusion occurs as the transitional intermediate of gp41 undergoes further changes to form a hairpin structure that draws the two membranes into close proximity (see text for details). *(Adapted from D Montefiori, JP Moore: Science 283:336, 1999; with permission.)*

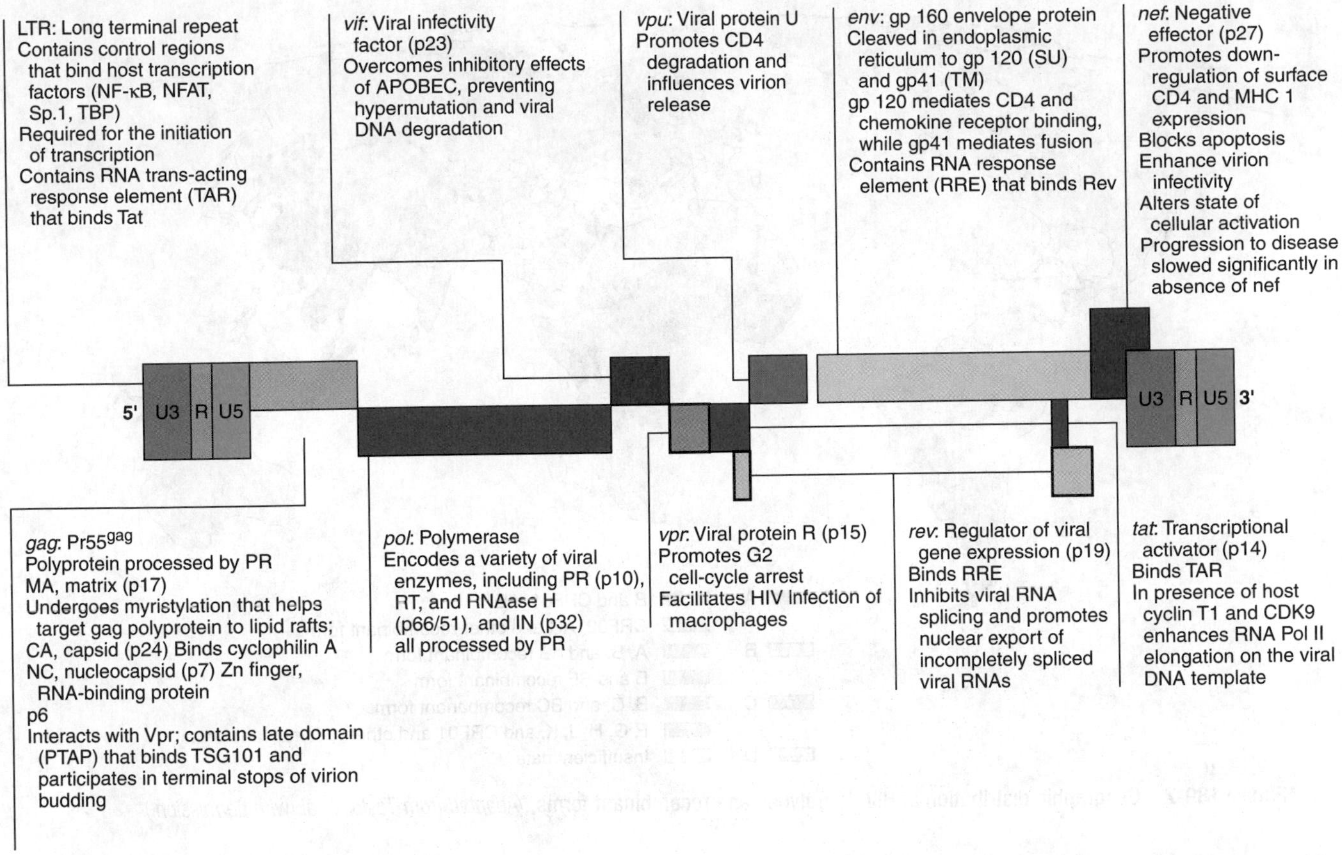

LTR: Long terminal repeat
Contains control regions that bind host transcription factors (NF-κB, NFAT, Sp.1, TBP)
Required for the initiation of transcription
Contains RNA trans-acting response element (TAR) that binds Tat
vif: Viral infectivity factor (p23)
Overcomes inhibitory effects of APOBEC, preventing hypermutation and viral DNA degradation
vpu: Viral protein U
Promotes CD4 degradation and influences virion release
env: gp 160 envelope protein
Cleaved in endoplasmic reticulum to gp 120 (SU) and gp41 (TM)
gp 120 mediates CD4 and chemokine receptor binding, while gp41 mediates fusion
Contains RNA response element (RRE) that binds Rev
nef: Negative effector (p27)
Promotes down-regulation of surface CD4 and MHC 1 expression
Blocks apoptosis
Enhance virion infectivity
Alters state of cellular activation
Progression to disease slowed significantly in absence of nef
5'
U3
R
U5
U3
R
U5
3'
gag: Pr55[gag]
Polyprotein processed by PR
MA, matrix (p17)
Undergoes myristylation that helps target gag polyprotein to lipid rafts;
CA, capsid (p24) Binds cyclophilin A
NC, nucleocapsid (p7) Zn finger, RNA-binding protein
p6
Interacts with Vpr; contains late domain (PTAP) that binds TSG101 and participates in terminal stops of virion budding
pol: Polymerase
Encodes a variety of viral enzymes, including PR (p10), RT, and RNAase H (p66/51), and IN (p32) all processed by PR
vpr: Viral protein R (p15)
Promotes G2 cell-cycle arrest
Facilitates HIV infection of macrophages
rev: Regulator of viral gene expression (p19)
Binds RRE
Inhibits viral RNA splicing and promotes nuclear export of incompletely spliced viral RNAs
tat: Transcriptional activator (p14)
Binds TAR
In presence of host cyclin T1 and CDK9 enhances RNA Pol II elongation on the viral DNA template

Figure 189-5 Organization of the genome of the HIV provirus together with a summary description of its 9 genes encoding 15 proteins. *(Adapted from Greene and Peterlin.)*

HIV-1 M Group
CPZpttMB89
CPZpttMB66
CPZpttLB7
HIV-1 N
CPZpttEK50
CPZpttDP94
CPZpttCAM3
CPZpttCAM5
CPZpttGAB2
.10
CPZpttUS
CPZpttMT14
CPZpttGAB1
CPZpttCAM1
CPZptsTAN2
CPZptsTAN3
CPZptsTAN1
GORCP684
GORCP2135
GOR2139_28
HIV-1 P
CPZptsANT
HIV-1 O Group

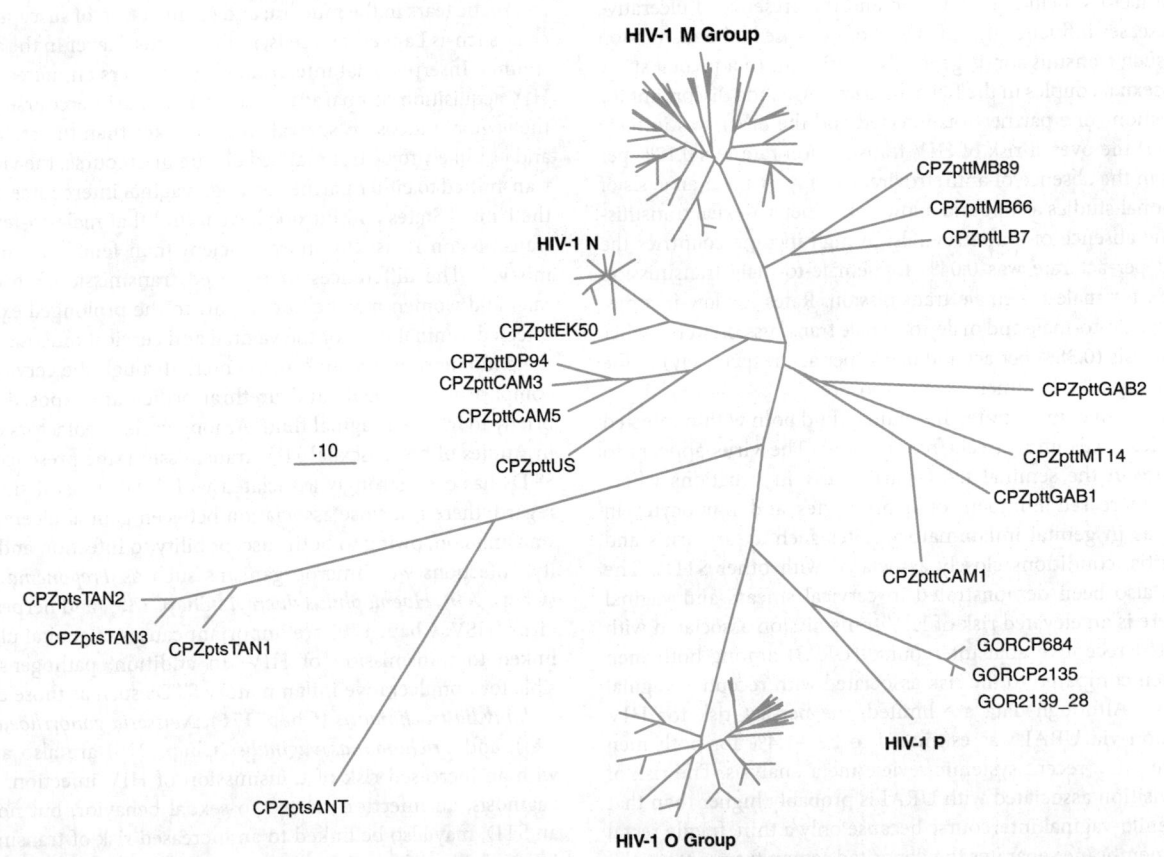

Figure 189-6 Phylogenetic tree constructed from representative viral envelope sequences of the subtypes and CRF01 in HIV-1 group M, some isolates from groups N, O, and P (also human HIV-1), CPZ (chimpanzee), and gorilla (GOR). The scale bar indicates the genetic distances between the sequences. *(Prepared by Brian Foley, PhD, of the HIV Sequence Database, Theoretical Biology and Biophysics Group, Los Alamos National Laboratory.)*

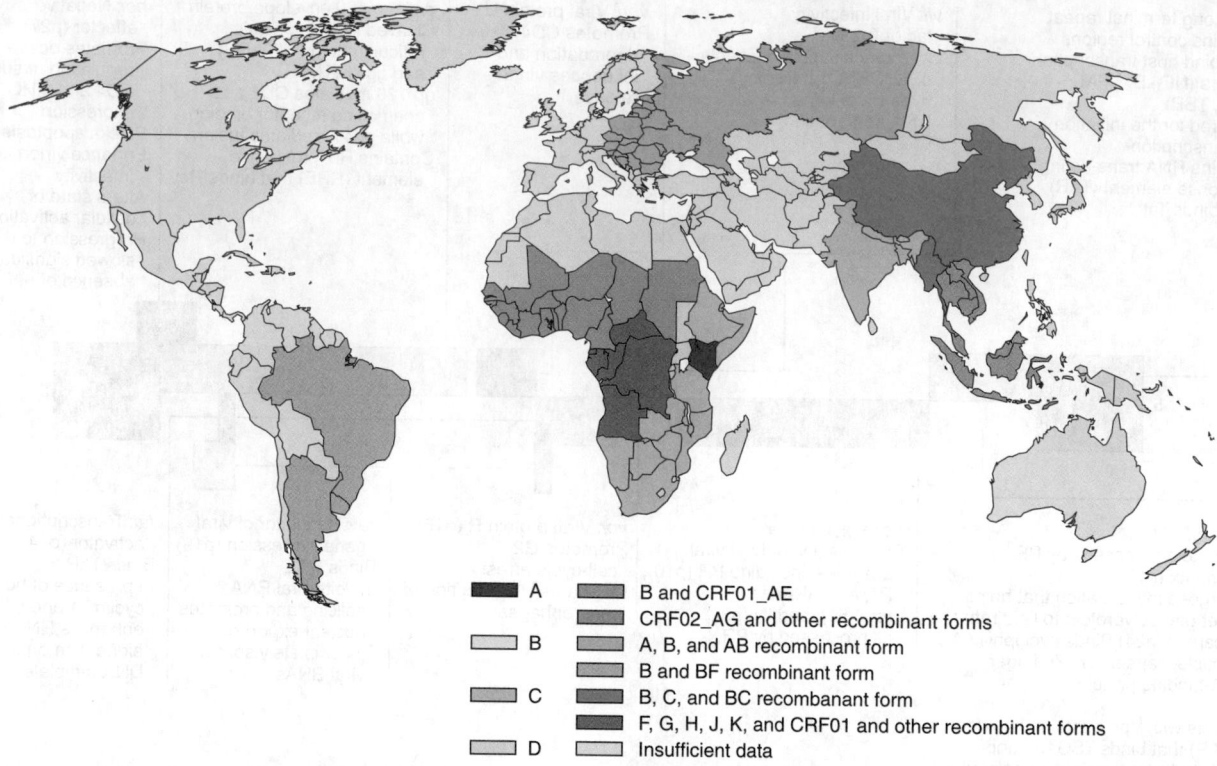

Figure 189-7 Geographic distribution of HIV-1 subtypes and recombinant forms. *(Adapted from Taylor et al; with permission.)*

Legend:
- A
- B
- C
- D
- B and CRF01_AE
- CRF02_AG and other recombinant forms
- A, B, and AB recombinant form
- B and BF recombinant form
- B, C, and BC recombinant form
- F, G, H, J, K, and CRF01 and other recombinant forms
- Insufficient data

PART 8
Infectious Diseases

transmission, although in many western countries a resurgence of male-to-male sexual transmission has occurred. Although a wide variety of factors including viral load and the presence of ulcerative genital diseases influence the efficiency of heterosexual transmission of HIV, such transmission is generally inefficient. In a pivotal study of heterosexual couples in the Rakai district of Uganda discordant for HIV infection (one partner was infected and the other was initially uninfected) the overall risk of HIV transmission rate was 0.12% per coital act in the absence of antiretroviral therapy. A meta-analysis of observational studies also found a low risk of heterosexual transmission in the absence of antiretrovirals: in high-income countries the estimated per-act rate was 0.04% for female-to-male transmission and 0.08% for male-to-female transmission. Rates for low-income-country female-to-male and male-to-female transmission were higher in this analysis (0.38% per act and 0.30% per act, respectively) in the absence of reported commercial sex exposure.

HIV has been demonstrated in seminal fluid both within infected mononuclear cells and in cell-free material. The virus appears to concentrate in the seminal fluid, particularly in situations where there are increased numbers of lymphocytes and monocytes in the fluid, as in genital inflammatory states such as urethritis and epididymitis, conditions closely associated with other STDs. The virus has also been demonstrated in cervical smears and vaginal fluid. There is an elevated risk of HIV transmission associated with unprotected receptive anal intercourse (URAI) among both men and women compared to the risk associated with receptive vaginal intercourse. Although data are limited, the per-act risk for HIV transmission via URAI was estimated to be ~1.4% for both men and women in a recent systemic review/meta-analysis. The risk of HIV acquisition associated with URAI is probably higher than that seen in penile-vaginal intercourse because only a thin, fragile rectal mucosal membrane separates the deposited semen from potentially susceptible cells in and beneath the mucosa, and trauma may be associated with anal intercourse. Anal douching and sexual practices that traumatize the rectal mucosa also increase the likelihood

of infection. It is likely that anal intercourse provides at least two modalities of infection: (1) direct inoculation into blood in cases of traumatic tears in the mucosa; and (2) infection of susceptible target cells, such as Langerhans cells, in the mucosal layer in the absence of trauma. Insertive anal intercourse also confers an increased risk of HIV acquisition compared to insertive vaginal intercourse. Although the vaginal mucosa is several layers thicker than the rectal mucosa and less likely to be traumatized during intercourse, the virus can be transmitted to either partner through vaginal intercourse. Studies in the United States and Europe have found that male-to-female HIV transmission is usually more efficient than female-to-male transmission. The differences in reported transmission rates between men and women may be due in part to the prolonged exposure to infected seminal fluid of the vaginal and cervical mucosa, as well as the endometrium (when semen enters through the cervical os). By comparison, the penis and urethral orifice are exposed relatively briefly to infected vaginal fluid. Among various cofactors examined in studies of heterosexual HIV transmission, the presence of other STDs has been strongly associated with HIV transmission. In this regard, there is a close association between genital ulcerations and transmission, owing to both susceptibility to infection and infectivity. Infections with microorganisms such as *Treponema pallidum* (Chap. 169), *Haemophilus ducreyi* (Chap. 145), and herpes simplex virus (HSV; Chap. 179) are important causes of genital ulcerations linked to transmission of HIV. In addition, pathogens responsible for nonulcerative inflammatory STDs such as those caused by *Chlamydia trachomatis* (Chap. 176), *Neisseria gonorrhoeae* (Chap. 144), and *Trichomonas vaginalis* (Chap. 215) are also associated with an increased risk of transmission of HIV infection. Bacterial vaginosis, an infection related to sexual behavior, but not strictly an STD, may also be linked to an increased risk of transmission of HIV infection. Several studies suggest that treating other STDs and genital tract syndromes may help prevent transmission of HIV. This effect is most prominent in populations in which the prevalence of HIV infection is relatively low.

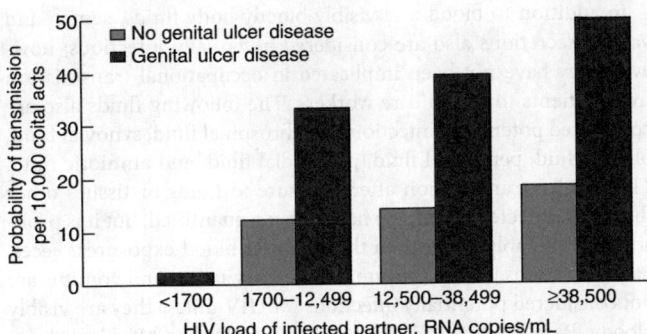

Figure 189-8 Probability of HIV transmission per coital act among monogamous, heterosexual, HIV-serodiscordant couples in Uganda. *(From RH Gray et al.)*

The quantity of HIV-1 in plasma is a primary determinant of the risk of HIV-1 transmission. In a cohort of heterosexual couples in Uganda discordant for HIV infection and not receiving antiretroviral therapy, the mean serum HIV RNA level was significantly higher among HIV-infected subjects whose partners seroconverted than among those whose partners did not seroconvert. In fact, transmission was rare when the infected partner had a plasma level of <1700 copies of HIV RNA per milliliter, even when genital ulcer disease was present (Fig 189-8). The rate of HIV transmission per coital act was highest during the early stage of HIV infection when plasma HIV RNA levels were high and in advanced disease as the viral set point increased.

Antiretroviral therapy dramatically reduces plasma viremia in most HIV-infected individuals (see "Treatment," below) and is associated with a reduction in risk of transmission. For example, in an analysis of ~3400 HIV serodiscordant heterosexual couples from 7 African countries, use of antiretroviral therapy by the infected person was accompanied by a 92% reduction in risk of HIV-1 transmission to the uninfected partner. Several studies also have suggested a beneficial effect of antiretroviral treatment at the community level.

A number of studies including large, randomized, controlled trials clearly have indicated that male *circumcision* is associated with a lower risk of HIV infection for heterosexual men. Studies are conflicting as to whether circumcision protects against HIV acquisition among men who have sex with men. The benefit of circumcision may be due to increased susceptibility of uncircumcised men to ulcerative STDs, as well as to other factors such as microtrauma to the foreskin and glans penis. In addition, the highly vascularized inner foreskin tissue contains a high density of Langerhans cells as well as increased numbers of CD4+ T cells, macrophages, and other cellular targets for HIV. Finally, the moist environment under the foreskin may promote the presence or persistence of microbial flora that, via inflammatory changes, may lead to even higher concentrations of target cells for HIV in the foreskin. In some studies the use of oral contraceptives was associated with an increase in incidence of HIV infection over and above that which might be expected by not using a condom for birth control. This phenomenon may be due to drug-induced changes in the cervical mucosa, rendering it more vulnerable to penetration by the virus. Adolescent girls might also be more susceptible to infection upon exposure due to the properties of an immature genital tract with increased cervical ectopy or exposed columnar epithelium.

Oral sex is a much less efficient mode of transmission of HIV than is anal intercourse or vaginal intercourse. A number of studies have reported that the incidence of transmission of infection by oral sex among couples discordant for HIV was extremely low. However, there have been reports of documented HIV transmission resulting solely from receptive fellatio and insertive cunnilingus. Therefore, the assumption that oral sex is completely safe is not warranted.

The association of alcohol consumption and illicit drug use with unsafe sexual behavior, both homosexual and heterosexual, leads to an increased risk of sexual transmission of HIV. Methamphetamine and other so-called club drugs (e.g., ecstasy, ketamine, and gamma hydroxybutyrate), sometimes taken in conjunction with PDE-5 inhibitors such as sildenafil (Viagra), tadalafil (Cialis), or vardenafil (Levitra), have been associated with risky sexual practices and increased risk of HIV infection, particularly among men who have sex with men.

◼ TRANSMISSION BY BLOOD AND BLOOD PRODUCTS

HIV can be transmitted to individuals who receive HIV-tainted blood transfusions, blood products, or transplanted tissue as well as to IDUs who are exposed to HIV while sharing injection paraphernalia such as needles, syringes, the water in which drugs are mixed, or the cotton through which drugs are filtered. Parenteral transmission of HIV during injection drug use does not require IV puncture; SC ("skin popping") or IM ("muscling") injections can transmit HIV as well, even though these behaviors are sometimes erroneously perceived as low-risk. Among IDUs, the risk of HIV infection increases with the duration of injection drug use; the frequency of needle sharing; the number of partners with whom paraphernalia are shared, particularly in the setting of "shooting galleries" where drugs are sold and large numbers of IDUs may share a limited number of "works"; comorbid psychiatric conditions such as antisocial personality disorder; the use of cocaine in injectable form or smoked as "crack"; and the use of injection drugs in a geographic location with a high prevalence of HIV infection, such as certain inner-city areas in the United States.

The first cases of AIDS among transfusion recipients and individuals with hemophilia or other clotting disorders were reported in 1982. The vast majority of HIV infections acquired via contaminated blood transfusions, blood components, or transplanted tissue in resource-rich countries occurred prior to the spring of 1985, when mandatory testing of donated blood for HIV-1 was initiated. It is estimated that >90% of individuals exposed to HIV-contaminated blood products become infected; unfortunately, in resource-poor countries, HIV continues to be transmitted by blood, blood products, and tissues due to the large number of blood donations that are inadequately screened for HIV. Transfusions of whole blood, packed red blood cells, platelets, leukocytes, and plasma are all capable of transmitting HIV infection. In contrast, hyperimmune gamma globulin, hepatitis B immune globulin, plasma-derived hepatitis B vaccine, and Rh$_o$ immune globulin have not been associated with transmission of HIV infection. The procedures involved in processing these products either inactivate or remove the virus.

Currently, in the United States and in most developed countries, the following measures have made the risk of transmission of HIV infection by transfused blood or blood products extremely small: the screening of blood donations for HIV antibodies, HIV p24 antigen, and HIV nucleic acid; the careful selection of potential blood donors with health history questionnaires to exclude individuals with risk behavior; and opportunities for self-deferral and the screening out of HIV-negative individuals with serologic testing for infections that have shared risk factors with HIV, such as hepatitis B and C. The chance of infection of a hemophiliac via clotting factor concentrates has essentially been eliminated because of the added layer of safety resulting from heat treatment of the concentrates.

It is currently estimated that the risk of infection with HIV in the United States via transfused screened blood is approximately 1 in 1.5 million units. Therefore, among the ~16 million donations collected in the United States each year, there are about 11 infectious donations leading to approximately 20 HIV-positive blood components being released each year that could potentially infect recipients. Thus, despite the best efforts of science, one cannot completely eliminate the risk of transfusion-related transmission of HIV since current technology cannot detect HIV RNA for the first 10–15 days following infection due to the low levels of viremia. In this regard, 4 cases of transfusion-associated HIV infection attributable to infected blood that tested negative for HIV were reported in the United States in the period 2000–2008.

In other countries, there have been reports of sporadic breakdowns in routinely available screening procedures in which contaminated blood was allowed to be transfused, resulting in small clusters of patients becoming infected. For example, in China in the 1990s, a disturbingly large number of persons became infected by selling blood in situations where the collectors reused needles that were contaminated and, in some instances, mixed blood products from a number of individuals, separated the plasma, and reinfused mixed red blood cells back into the individual donors.

There have been no reported cases of transmission of HIV-2 in the United States via donated blood or tissues, and, currently, donated blood is screened for both HIV-1 and HIV-2. Transmission of HIV (both HIV-1 and HIV-2) by blood or blood products is still an ongoing threat in certain developing countries, particularly in sub-Saharan Africa, where routine screening of blood is not universally practiced.

Prior to the screening of donors, a small number of cases of transmission of HIV via semen used in artificial insemination and tissues used in organ transplantation were documented. At present, donors of such tissues are prescreened for HIV infection. With regard to HIV-serodiscordant couples (male, HIV-infected; female, HIV-uninfected) who wish to conceive a child, assisted reproductive techniques using sperm-washing to reduce the risk of HIV transmission have been successfully employed, with only one well-documented seroconversion in the uninfected female partner, reported in 1990.

■ OCCUPATIONAL TRANSMISSION OF HIV: HEALTH CARE WORKERS, LABORATORY WORKERS, AND THE HEALTH CARE SETTING

There is a small but definite occupational risk of HIV transmission to health care workers and laboratory personnel and potentially others who work with HIV-containing materials, particularly when sharp objects are used. An estimated 600,000 to 800,000 health care workers are stuck with needles or other sharp medical instruments in the United States each year.

Exposures that place a health care worker at potential risk of HIV infection are percutaneous injuries (e.g., a needle stick or cut with a sharp object) or contact of mucous membrane or nonintact skin (e.g., exposed skin that is chapped, abraded, or afflicted with dermatitis) with blood, tissue, or other potentially infectious body fluids. Large, multi-institutional studies have indicated that the risk of HIV transmission following skin puncture from a needle or a sharp object that was contaminated with blood from a person with documented HIV infection is ~0.3% and after a mucous membrane exposure it is 0.09% (see "HIV and the Health Care Worker," below) if the injured and/or exposed person is not treated within 24 h with antiretroviral drugs. HIV transmission after nonintact skin exposure has been documented, but the average risk for transmission by this route has not been precisely determined; however, it is estimated to be less than the risk for mucous membrane exposure. Transmission of HIV through intact skin has not been documented. Currently, virtually all puncture wounds and mucous membrane exposures in health care workers involving blood from a patient with documented HIV infection are treated prophylactically with combination antiretroviral therapy (cART). This practice has dramatically reduced the occurrence of puncture-related transmissions of HIV to health care workers.

In addition to blood and visibly bloody body fluids, semen and vaginal secretions also are considered potentially infectious; however, they have not been implicated in occupational transmission from patients to health care workers. The following fluids also are considered potentially infectious: cerebrospinal fluid, synovial fluid, pleural fluid, peritoneal fluid, pericardial fluid, and amniotic fluid. The risk for transmission after exposure to fluids or tissues other than HIV-infected blood also has not been quantified, but it is probably considerably lower than the risk after blood exposures. Feces, nasal secretions, saliva, sputum, sweat, tears, urine, and vomitus are not considered potentially infectious for HIV unless they are visibly bloody. Rare cases of HIV transmission via human bites have been reported, but not in the setting of occupational exposure.

An increased risk for HIV infection following percutaneous exposures to HIV-infected blood is associated with exposures involving a relatively large quantity of blood, as in the case of a device visibly contaminated with the patient's blood, a procedure that involves a hollow-bore needle placed directly in a vein or artery, or a deep injury. Factors that might be associated with mucocutaneous transmission of HIV include exposure to an unusually large volume of blood, prolonged contact, and a potential portal of entry. In addition, the risk increases for exposures to blood from patients with advanced-stage disease or those patients in the acute stage of HIV infection, owing to the higher levels of HIV in the blood under those circumstances. The use of antiretroviral drugs as postexposure prophylaxis decreases the risk of infection compared with historic controls in occupationally exposed health care workers (see "HIV and the Health Care Worker," below). The risk of hepatitis B virus (HBV) infection following a similar type of exposure is ~6–30% in nonimmune individuals; if a susceptible worker is exposed to HBV, postexposure prophylaxis with hepatitis B immune globulin and initiation of HBV vaccine is >90% effective in preventing HBV infection. The risk of hepatitis C virus (HCV) infection following percutaneous injury is ~1.8% (Chap. 304).

Since the beginning of the HIV epidemic, there have been rare instances where transmission of infection from a health care worker to patients seemed highly probable. One notable cluster of infections involved an HIV-infected dentist in Florida who apparently infected as many as six of his patients, most likely through contaminated instruments. Despite these small number of documented cases, the risk of HIV transmission involving health care workers (infected or not) to patients is extremely low in developed countries—in fact, too low to be measured accurately. In this regard, several epidemiologic studies have been performed tracing thousands of patients of HIV-infected dentists, physicians, surgeons, obstetricians, and gynecologists, and no other cases of HIV transmission that could be linked to the health care providers were identified.

Breaches in infection control and the reuse of contaminated syringes have also resulted in the transmission of HIV from patient to patient in hospitals, nursing homes, and outpatient settings. For example, in the only report of HIV transmission from patient to patient during a surgical procedure, several patients in Australia apparently were infected by an HIV-negative general surgeon during routine outpatient surgery. Although the mechanism of transmission was not definitively identified, a failure on the part of the surgeon to sterilize instruments properly following prior surgery on an HIV-infected patient was considered a likely explanation for this outbreak. Three patients (two in hospitals in the United States and one in the Netherlands) undergoing nuclear medicine procedures were reported to have inadvertently received IV injections of blood or other material from patients infected with HIV. Hemodialysis centers have also been implicated in several reported HIV transmission incidents.

The most dramatic reports of HIV infection in the health care setting involved transmission of HIV to 8000–10,000 children in

Romanian orphanages in the 1980s. Other large incidents occurred in hospitals in Russia and Libya in the late 1980s and late 1990s, respectively. Each of these incidents received considerable attention and likely was related to reuse of contaminated needles and/or administration of contaminated blood products. Finally, these very rare occurrences of transmission of HIV as well as HBV and HCV to and from health care workers in the workplace underscore the importance of the use of universal precautions when caring for all patients (see below and Chap. 131).

■ MATERNAL-FETAL/INFANT TRANSMISSION

HIV infection can be transmitted from an infected mother to her fetus during pregnancy, during delivery, or by breast-feeding. This remains an important form of transmission of HIV infection in certain developing countries, where the proportion of infected women to infected men is ~1:1. Virologic analyses of aborted fetuses indicate that HIV can be transmitted to the fetus during the first or second trimesters of pregnancy. However, maternal transmission to the fetus occurs most commonly in the perinatal period. Two studies performed in Rwanda and the former Zaire indicated that the relative proportions of mother-to-child transmissions were 23–30% before birth, 50–65% during birth, and 12–20% via breast-feeding.

In the absence of prophylactic antiretroviral therapy to the mother during pregnancy, labor, and delivery, and to the fetus following birth, the probability of transmission of HIV from mother to infant/fetus ranges from 15 to 25% in industrialized countries and from 25 to 35% in developing countries. These differences may relate to the adequacy of prenatal care as well as to the stage of HIV disease and the general health of the mother during pregnancy. Higher rates of transmission have been reported to be associated with many factors, the best documented of which is the presence of high maternal levels of plasma viremia. In one study of 552 singleton pregnancies in the United States, the rate of mother-to-baby transmission was 0% among women with <1000 copies of HIV RNA per milliliter of blood, 16.6% among women with 1000–10,000 copies/mL, 21.3% among women with 10,001–50,000 copies/mL, 30.9% among women with 50,001–100,000 copies/mL, and 40.6% among women with >100,000 copies/mL. However, there may not be a lower "threshold" below which transmission never occurs, since other studies have reported transmission by women with viral RNA levels <50 copies/mL. Low maternal CD4+ T cell counts also have been associated with higher rates of transmission; however, since low CD4+ T cell counts are often associated with high levels of plasma viremia, in one study using multivariate analysis including plasma viral load and CD4+ T cell count, only the level of plasma HIV RNA was significant. Increased mother-to-child transmission is also correlated with closer human leukocyte antigen (HLA) match between mother and child. A prolonged interval between membrane rupture and delivery is another well-documented risk factor for transmission. Other conditions that are potential risk factors, but that have not been consistently demonstrated, are the presence of chorioamnionitis at delivery; STDs during pregnancy; hard drug use during pregnancy; cigarette smoking; preterm delivery; and obstetric procedures such as amniocentesis, amnioscopy, fetal scalp electrodes, and episiotomy. In a seminal study conducted in the United States and France in the 1990s, zidovudine treatment of HIV-infected pregnant women from the beginning of the second trimester through delivery and of the infant for 6 weeks following birth dramatically decreased the rate of intrapartum and perinatal transmission of HIV infection from 22.6% in the untreated group to <5%. Today, the rate of mother-to-child transmission has fallen to 1% or less in pregnant women who are receiving combination antiretroviral therapy for their HIV infection. Such treatment, combined with cesarean section delivery, has rendered mother-to-child

transmission of HIV an unusual event in the United States and other developed nations. In developed countries, current recommendations to reduce perinatal transmission of HIV include universal voluntary HIV testing and counseling of pregnant women, antiretroviral prophylaxis with one or more drugs in cases in which the mother does not require therapy for her HIV infection, combination therapy for women who do require therapy, obstetric management that attempts to minimize exposure of the infant to maternal blood and genital secretions, and avoidance of breast-feeding. It is recommended that the choice of antiretroviral therapy for pregnant women be based on the same considerations used for women who are not pregnant, with discussion of the recognized and unknown risks and benefits of such therapy during pregnancy (see below under "Treatment").

Certain studies have demonstrated that truncated regimens of zidovudine alone or in combination with lamivudine given to the mother during the last few weeks of pregnancy or even only during labor and delivery, and to the infant for a week or less, significantly reduced transmission to the infant compared with placebo. Short-course prophylactic antiretroviral regimens, such as a single dose of nevirapine given to the mother at the onset of labor and a single dose to the infant within 72 h of birth, are of particular relevance to low- to mid-income nations because of the low cost and the fact that in these regions perinatal care is often not available and pregnant women are often seen by a health care provider for the first time at or near the time of delivery. Given that cART is now increasingly available to individuals in developing countries due to the lower cost of drugs and programs that are making drugs available to these regions of the world, combinations of drugs are being used more frequently, where available, to treat HIV-infected pregnant women. This has had the effect of benefitting the women, blocking HIV transmission to the fetus, and protecting against subsequent transmission by breast-feeding.

Breast-feeding is an important modality of transmission of HIV infection in developing countries, particularly where mothers continue to breast-feed for prolonged periods. The risk factors for mother-to-child transmission of HIV via breast-feeding are not fully understood; factors that increase the likelihood of transmission include detectable levels of HIV in breast milk, the presence of mastitis, low maternal CD4+ T cell counts, and maternal vitamin A deficiency. The risk of HIV infection via breast-feeding is highest in the early months of breast-feeding. In addition, exclusive breast-feeding has been reported to carry a lower risk of HIV transmission than mixed feeding. Certainly in developed countries, breast-feeding by an infected mother should be avoided. However, there is disagreement regarding recommendations for breast-feeding in certain developing countries, where breast milk is the only source of adequate nutrition as well as immunity against potentially serious non-HIV infections for the infant. The optimal approach to prevent transmission by infected mothers who choose to breast-feed would be to provide continual treatment to the infected mother. This approach has become more feasible as cART becomes more widely available in developing countries. Despite progress in this regard, such therapy is currently available to only ~30–40% of persons in developing nations who require it.

■ TRANSMISSION BY OTHER BODY FLUIDS

Although HIV can be isolated typically in low titers from saliva of a small proportion of infected individuals, there is no convincing evidence that saliva can transmit HIV infection, either through kissing or through other exposures, such as occupationally to health care workers. Saliva contains endogenous antiviral factors; among these factors, HIV-specific immunoglobulins of IgA, IgG, and IgM isotypes are detected readily in salivary secretions of infected individuals. It has been suggested that large glycoproteins such as mucins and thrombospondin 1 sequester HIV into aggregates for clearance by the host. In addition, a number of soluble salivary factors inhibit HIV to various degrees in vitro, probably by targeting host cell receptors rather than the virus itself. Perhaps the best studied of these, secretory leukocyte protease inhibitor (SLPI), blocks HIV infection in several cell culture systems, and it is found in saliva at levels that approximate those required for inhibition of HIV in vitro. In this regard, higher salivary levels of SLPI in breast-fed infants were associated with a decreased risk of HIV transmission through breast milk. It has also been suggested that submandibular saliva reduces HIV infectivity by stripping gp120 from the surface of virions, and that saliva-mediated disruption and lysis of HIV-infected cells occurs because of the hypotonicity of oral secretions. There have been outlier cases of suspected transmission by saliva, but these have probably been blood-to-blood transmissions. Transmission of HIV by a human bite can occur but is a rare event. In addition, a most unusual form of HIV transmission from infected children to mothers in the former Soviet Union has been identified. In those cases, the children (infected through transfusion) were said to have bleeding sores in the mouth, and the mothers were said to have lacerations and abrasions on and around the nipples of the breast resulting from trauma from the children's teeth. Breast-feeding had been continued until the children were older than is usual in other developed countries.

Although virus can be identified, if not isolated, from virtually any body fluid, there is no evidence that HIV transmission can occur as a result of exposure to tears, sweat, or urine. However, there have been isolated cases of transmission of HIV infection by body fluids that may or may not have been contaminated with blood. Most of these situations occurred in the setting of a close relative providing intensive nursing care for an HIV-infected person without observing universal precautions, underscoring the importance of adhering to such precautions in the handling of body fluids and wastes from HIV-infected individuals.

EPIDEMIOLOGY

■ HIV INFECTION AND AIDS WORLDWIDE

HIV infection/AIDS is a global pandemic, with cases reported from virtually every country. At the end of 2009, an estimated 33.3 million individuals were living with HIV infection according to the Joint United Nations Programme on HIV/AIDS (UNAIDS). More than 95% of people living with HIV/AIDS reside in low- and middle-income countries; ~50% are female, and 2.5 million are children <15 years. The global distribution of these cases is illustrated in Fig. 189-9. As illustrated in Fig. 189-10A, the estimated number of people living with HIV—i.e., the global prevalence—has increased approximately fourfold since 1990, reflecting the combined effects of continued high rates of new HIV infections and the beneficial (life-prolonging) impact of antiretroviral therapy.

In 2009, there were an estimated 2.6 million new cases of HIV infection worldwide, including 370,000 in children <15 years. UNAIDS estimates that the global spread of HIV peaked in 1997, when ~3.2 million new HIV infections occurred. In 2009, the estimated number of new HIV infections globally was approximately 21% lower than at the peak of the pandemic (Fig. 189-10B). Recent reductions in global HIV incidence likely reflect natural trends in the pandemic as well as the results of prevention programs resulting in behavior change. In 2009, global AIDS deaths totaled 1.8 million (including 260,000 children <15 years). A rapid expansion of access to antiretroviral therapy likely has helped lower AIDS-related death rates in recent years (Fig. 189-10C). Since the beginning of the pandemic the cumulative total of AIDS deaths globally exceeds 25 million.

The HIV epidemic has occurred in "waves" in different regions of the world, each wave having somewhat different characteristics depending on the demographics of the country and region in question and the timing of the introduction of HIV into the population. Although the AIDS epidemic was first recognized in the United States and shortly thereafter in Western Europe, it very likely began

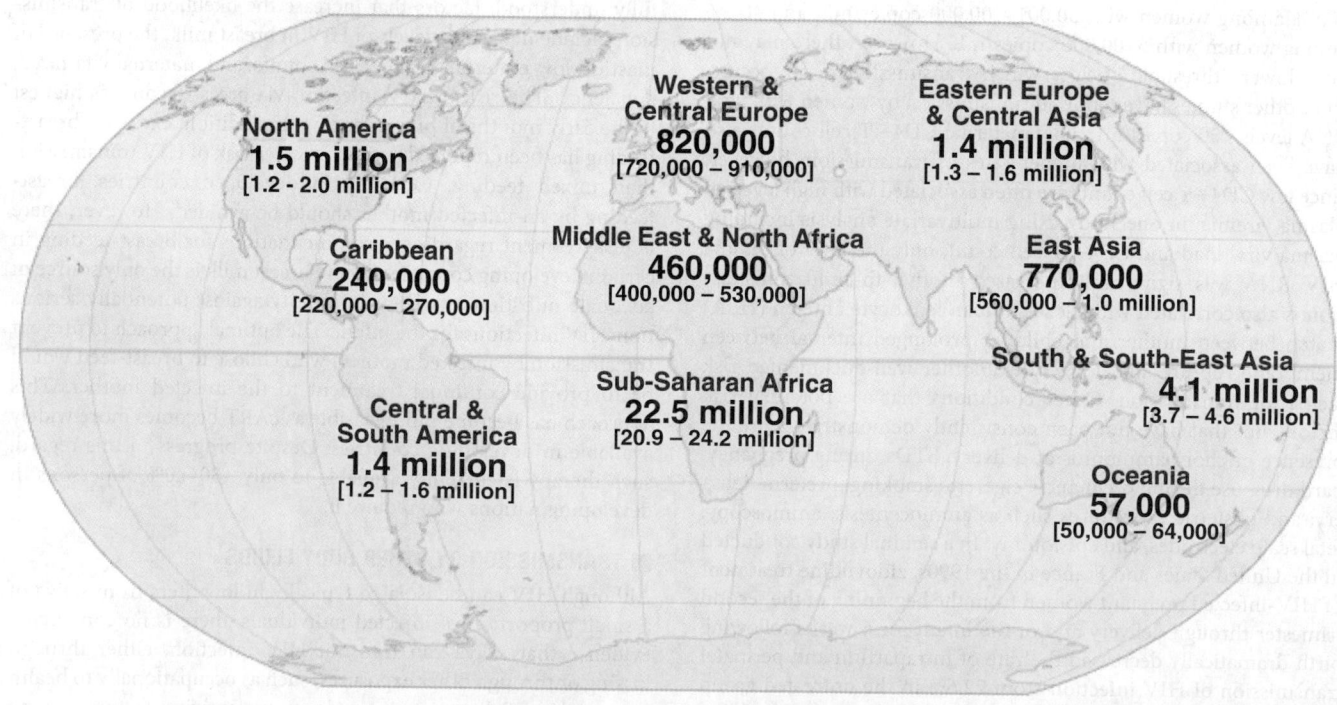

Total: 33.3 (31.4 - 35.3) million

Figure 189-9 Estimated number of adults and children living with HIV infection as of December, 2009. Total: 33.3 (31.4–35.3) (31.1–35.8) million. [From Joint United Nations Programme on HIV/AIDS (UNAIDS).]

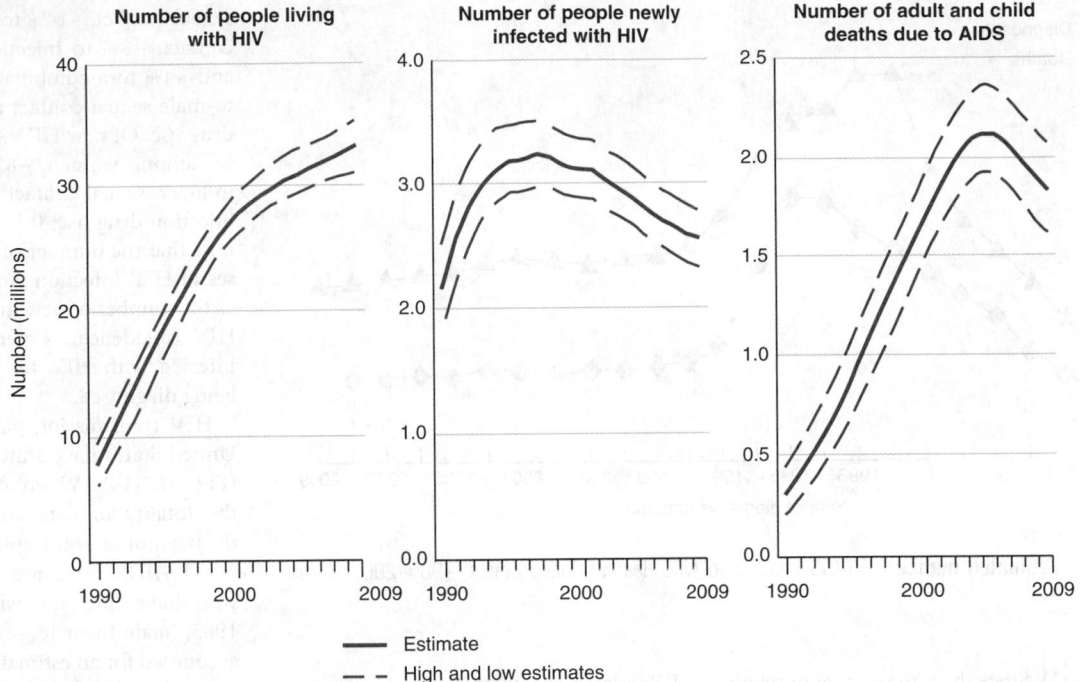

Number of people living with HIV

Number of people newly infected with HIV

Number of adult and child deaths due to AIDS

— Estimate

- - High and low estimates

Figure 189-10 **Global HIV/AIDS epidemiologic estimates, 1990–2009.** ***A.*** Number of people living with HIV. ***B.*** Number of people newly infected with HIV globally. ***C.*** Number of adult and child deaths due to AIDS. *(From UNAIDS.)*

in sub-Saharan Africa (see above), which has been particularly devastated by the epidemic. More than two-thirds of all people with HIV infection (~22.5 million) live in that region, even though sub-Saharan Africa is home to just 10–11% of the world's population (Fig. 189-9). Within the region, southern Africa is worst-affected. In each of the nine southern African countries, available seroprevalence data indicate that >10% of the adult population age 15–49 is HIV-infected. In addition, among high-risk individuals (e.g., commercial sex workers, patients attending STD clinics) who live in urban areas of sub-Saharan Africa, seroprevalence is now >50% in some countries. Sub-Saharan Africa's HIV regional epidemics vary significantly, with most appearing to have stabilized, although frequently at very high levels. Heterosexual exposure is the primary mode of HIV transmission in sub-Saharan Africa, with women and girls disproportionately affected, accounting for ~60 percent of all HIV infections in that region. In 2009, an estimated 460,000 people were living with HIV in the Middle East/North Africa region. Cases are largely concentrated among IDUs, men who have sex with men, and sex workers and their clients.

In east, south, and southeast Asia, an estimated 4.9 million people were living with HIV at the end of 2009. In this region of the world, national HIV prevalence is highest in southeast Asian countries, with wide variation in trends between different countries. Among countries in Asia, only Thailand has an adult seroprevalence rate of >1%. However, the populations of many Asian nations are so large (especially India and China) that even low infection and seroprevalence rates result in large numbers of people living with HIV. Although Asia's epidemic has been concentrated for some time among specific populations—sex workers and their clients, men who have sex with men, and IDUs—it is expanding to the heterosexual partners of those most at risk. While the regional epidemic appears to be stable overall, HIV prevalence has increased in certain countries such as Bangladesh and Pakistan.

The epidemic is expanding in Eastern Europe and Central Asia, where ~1.4 million people were living with HIV at the end of 2009.

The Russian Federation and Ukraine account for the majority of HIV cases in the region; the Ukraine has an adult seroprevalence rate of 1.1%, the highest in all of Europe. Driven initially by injection drug use and increasingly by heterosexual transmission, the number of new infections in this region has increased dramatically over the past decade.

Approximately 1.6 million people are living with HIV/AIDS in Central and South America and the Caribbean. Brazil is home to the largest number of HIV-infected people in the region. However, the epidemic has been slowed in that country due to successful treatment and prevention efforts. Men who have sex with men account for the largest proportion of HIV infections in Central and South America. The Caribbean region has the highest regional adult seroprevalence rate after Africa, due in large part to the huge case load in Haiti. Heterosexual transmission, often tied to sex work, is the main driver of transmission in the region.

Approximately 2.4 million people are living with HIV/AIDS in North America, western and central Europe, and Oceania. The number of new infections among men who have sex with men has increased over the past decade in these mostly high-income areas, while rates of new infections among heterosexuals have stabilized and infections among IDUs have fallen.

■ AIDS IN THE UNITED STATES

HIV/AIDS continues to have an extraordinary public health impact in the United States. As of January 1, 2010, an estimated 1,108,611 cases of AIDS had been diagnosed in the United States. Approximately 1.1 million individuals in the United States were living with HIV infection, ~21 percent of whom are unaware of their infection, according to recent analysis. Approximately two-thirds of those living with HIV/AIDS were nonwhite and nearly half (48%) were men who have sex with men. The estimated HIV seroprevalence rate among individuals age 13 years or older in the United States is ~0.5%.

The number of AIDS cases and deaths in the United States rose steadily through the 1980s; AIDS cases peaked in 1993 and deaths in

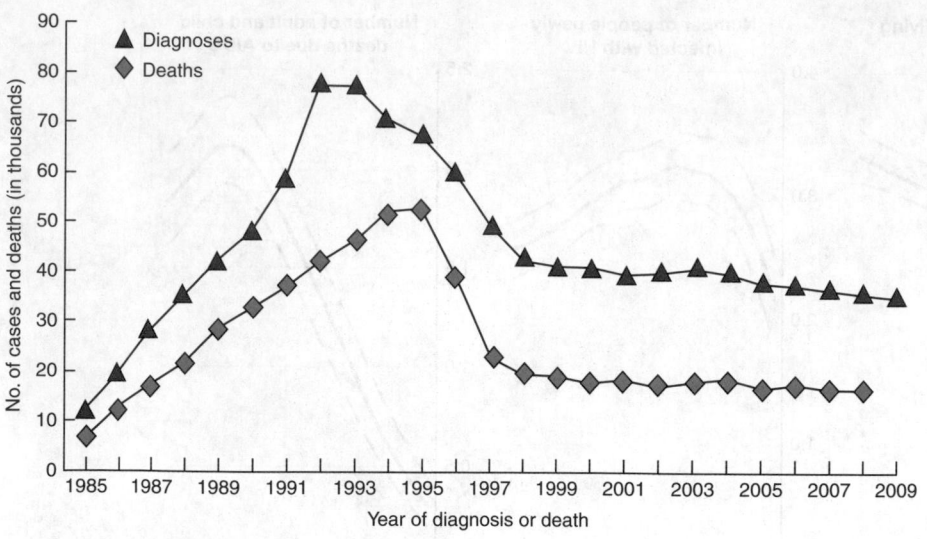

Figure 189-11 **Estimated number of AIDS cases** and AIDS deaths, United States, 1985–2009. *(From CDC.)*

sexual contact, ~14% to heterosexual contact, ~8% to injection drug use, and ~4% to a combination of male-to-male sexual contact and injection drug use. Of new HIV/AIDS diagnoses among women, ~85% were due to heterosexual contact and ~15% to injection drug use. It is important to note that the number of new diagnoses of HIV infection is not the same as the number of new infections with HIV (incidence): a person may be infected with HIV for years before being diagnosed.

HIV transmission patterns in the United States have shifted over time (Fig. 189-14). When one looks at the totality of data collected from the beginning of the epidemic, ~48% of all AIDS cases are among men who have had sex with men. In 1985, male-to-male sexual contact accounted for an estimated 65% of all AIDS diagnoses; this proportion reached its lowest point in 1999 at ~40% of diagnoses. Since then, the percentage of AIDS diagnoses attributed to male-to-male sexual contact has increased; in 2009 this transmission category accounted for 48% of all AIDS diagnoses. The estimated percentage of AIDS diagnoses attributed to injection drug use increased from 20% to 31% during 1985–1994 and decreased since that time, accounting for 15% of diagnoses in 2009. The estimated percentage of AIDS diagnoses attributed to heterosexual contact increased from 3% in 1985 to 31% in 2009.

HIV infection and AIDS have disproportionately affected minority populations in the United States. Among those diagnosed with HIV (regardless of AIDS status) in 2009, 52% percent were blacks/African Americans, a group that constitutes only 12% of the U.S. population (Fig. 189-15A). The estimated rate of new HIV diagnoses in 2009 by race/ethnicity per 100,000 population is shown in Fig. 189-15B.

1995 (Fig. 189-11). Since then, the annual numbers of AIDS-related deaths in the United States have fallen ~70%. This trend is due to several factors, including the improved prophylaxis and treatment of opportunistic infections, the growing experience among the health professions in caring for HIV-infected individuals, improved access to health care, and a decrease in new infections due to saturational effects and prevention efforts. However, the most influential factor clearly has been the increased use of potent antiretroviral drugs, generally administered in a combination of three or four agents.

An estimated 56,000 individuals are newly infected each year in the United States. This *HIV incidence* figure has remained stable for at least 15 years (Fig. 189-12). Among adults and adolescents newly diagnosed with HIV infection (regardless of AIDS status) in 2009, ~76% were men and ~24% were women (Fig. 189-13). Of new HIV/AIDS *diagnoses* among men, ~75% were due to male-to-male

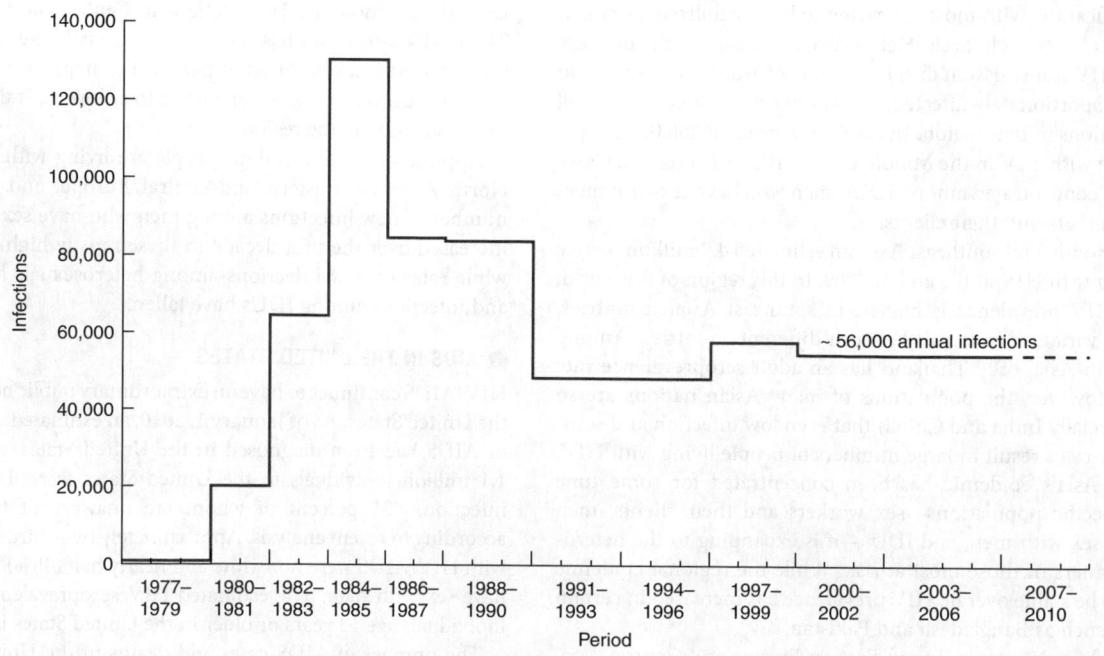

Figure 189-12 **Estimated number of new HIV infections, United States.** *(From Hall et al.)*

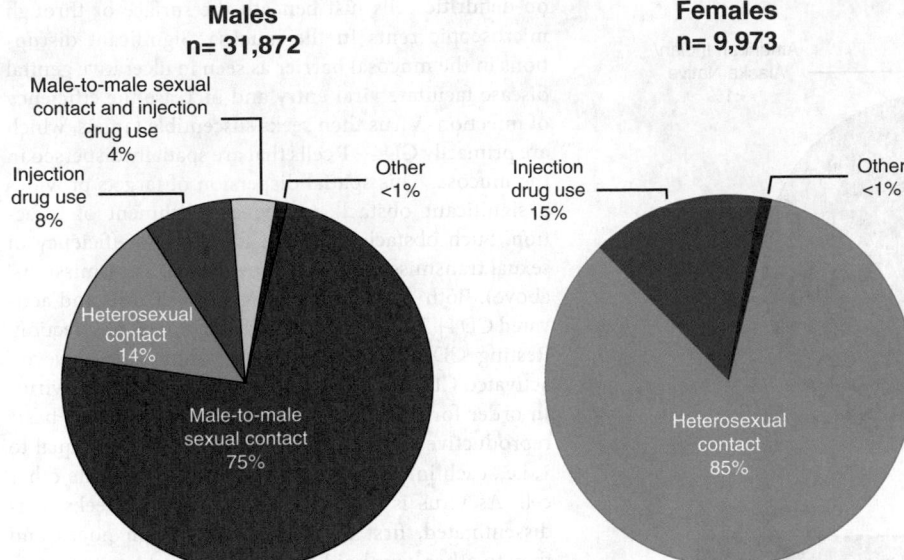

Males
n= 31,872

Male-to-male sexual contact and injection drug use 4%

Injection drug use 8%

Heterosexual contact 14%

Male-to-male sexual contact 75%

Other <1%

Females
n= 9,973

Injection drug use 15%

Heterosexual contact 85%

Other <1%

Figure 189-13 **Transmission categories of adults and adolescents with HIV/AIDS** diagnosed during 2009 in the United States. Estimates from 40 states with confidential, name-based HIV infection reporting. Data include persons with a diagnosis of HIV infection regardless of AIDS status at diagnosis. *(From CDC.)*

Although the HIV/AIDS epidemic on the whole is plateauing in the United States, it is spreading rapidly among certain populations, stabilizing in others, and decreasing in others. Similar to other STDs, HIV infection will not spread homogeneously throughout the population of the United States. However, it is clear that anyone who practices high-risk behavior is at risk for HIV infection. In addition, recent increases in infections and AIDS cases among young men who have sex with men as well as the spread in pockets of poverty in both urban and rural regions (particularly among underserved minority populations in the southern United States with inadequate access to health care) testify that the epidemic of HIV infection in the United States remains a public health problem of major proportions.

PATHOPHYSIOLOGY AND PATHOGENESIS

The hallmark of HIV disease is a profound immunodeficiency resulting primarily from a progressive quantitative and qualitative deficiency of the subset of T lymphocytes referred to as *helper T cells* occurring in a setting of polyclonal immune activation. The *helper* subset of T cells is defined phenotypically by the presence on its surface of the CD4 molecule (Chap. 314), which serves as the primary cellular receptor for HIV. A co-receptor must also be present together with CD4 for efficient binding, fusion, and entry of HIV-1 into its target cells (Figs. 189-3 and 189-4). HIV uses two major co-receptors, CCR5 and CXCR4, for fusion and entry; these co-receptors are also the primary receptors for certain chemoattractive cytokines termed *chemokines* and belong to the seven-transmembrane-domain G protein–coupled family of receptors. A number of mechanisms responsible for cellular depletion and/or immune dysfunction of CD4+ T cells have been demonstrated in vitro; these include direct infection and destruction of these cells by HIV, as well as indirect effects such as immune clearance of infected cells, immune exhaustion due to aberrant cellular activation, and activation-induced cell death. Patients with CD4+ T cell levels below certain thresholds are at high risk of developing a variety of opportunistic diseases, particularly the infections and neoplasms that are AIDS-defining illnesses. Some features of AIDS, such as Kaposi's sarcoma and certain neurologic abnormalities, cannot be explained completely by the immunodeficiency caused by HIV infection, since these complications may occur prior to the development of severe immunologic impairment.

The combination of viral pathogenic and immunopathogenic events that occurs during the course of HIV disease from the moment of initial (primary) infection through the development of advanced-stage disease is complex and varied. It is important to appreciate that the pathogenic mechanisms of HIV disease are multifactorial and

As of January 1, 2010, an estimated 9448 cases of AIDS in children <13 years old had been diagnosed in the Unites States, and ~59% of these individuals have died. Approximately 91% of these children were born to mothers who were HIV-infected or who were at risk for HIV infection; in the majority of those cases, the mother was either an IDU or the heterosexual partner of an IDU. The estimated number of AIDS cases diagnosed among children perinatally exposed to HIV peaked in 1992 and has decreased in recent years (Fig. 189-16). The decline of these cases is likely associated with the implementation of guidelines for the universal counseling and voluntary HIV testing of pregnant women and the use of cART for pregnant women and newborn infants in order to prevent infection. Another contributing factor is the effective treatment of HIV infection in children who have become infected.

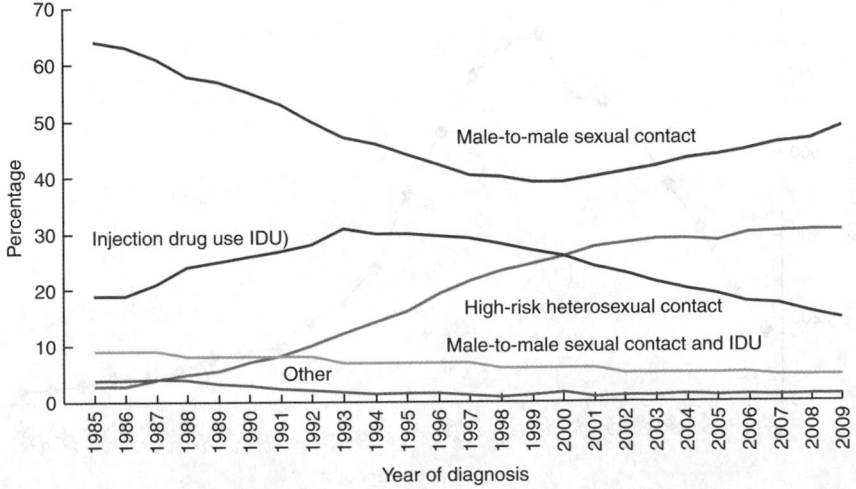

Figure 189-14 **Estimated AIDS diagnoses among adults and adolescents,** by transmission category and year of diagnosis, United States, 1985–2009. *(From CDC.)*

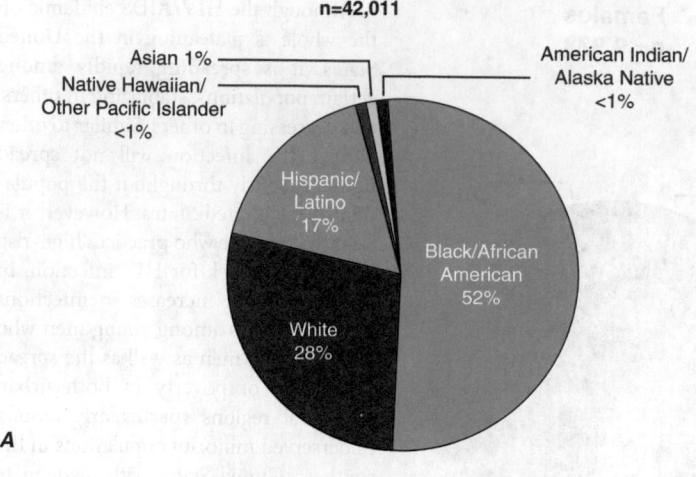

n=42,011

Asian 1%
Native Hawaiian/
Other Pacific Islander
<1%

American Indian/
Alaska Native
<1%

Hispanic/
Latino
17%

Black/African
American
52%

White
28%

A

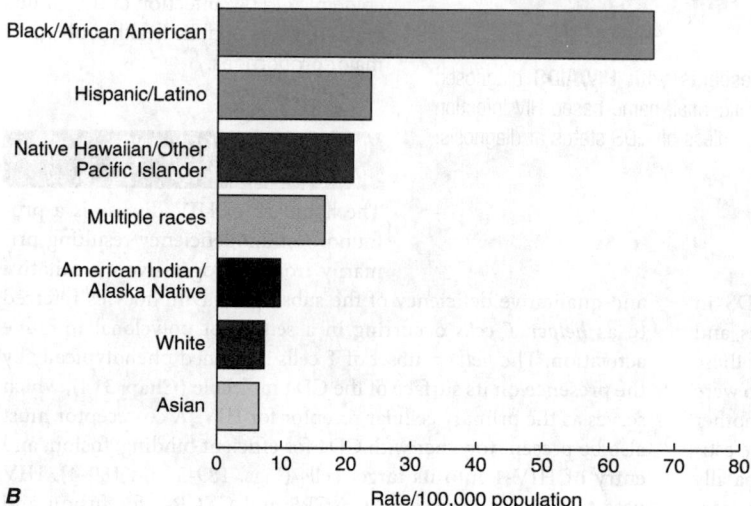

B   Rate/100,000 population

Figure 189-15 Race/ethnicity of persons (including children) with HIV/AIDS diagnosed during 2009 in the United States. *A.* Proportion of new infections by race/ethnicity. *B.* Rate of new infections by race/ethnicity (per 100,000 population). Estimates from 40 states with confidential, name-based HIV infection reporting. Data include persons with a diagnosis of HIV infection regardless of AIDS status at diagnosis. *(From CDC.)*

on dendritic cells just beneath the surface or through microscopic rents in the mucosa. Significant disruptions in the mucosal barrier as seen in ulcerative genital disease facilitate viral entry and increase the efficiency of infection. Virus then seeks susceptible targets, which are primarily CD4+ T cells that are spatially dispersed in the mucosa. This spatial dispersion of targets provides a significant obstacle to the establishment of infection. Such obstacles account for the low efficiency of sexual transmission of HIV (see "Sexual Transmission," above). Both "partially" resting CD4+ T cells and activated CD4+ T cells serve as early amplifiers of infection. Resting CD4+ T cells are more abundant; however, activated CD4+ T cells produce larger amounts of virus. In order for infection to become established, the basic reproductive rate (R_0) must become greater or equal to 1, i.e., each infected cell would infect at least one other cell. As virus is produced within days to weeks, it is disseminated, first to the draining lymph nodes and then to other lymphoid compartments where it has easy access to dense concentrations of CD4+ T cell targets, allowing for a burst of high-level viremia (Fig. 189-18). An important lymphoid organ, the gut-associated lymphoid tissue (GALT), is a major target of HIV infection and the location where large numbers of CD4+ T cells (usually memory cells) are infected and depleted, both by direct viral effects and by activation-associated apoptosis. Once virus replication reaches this threshold and virus is widely disseminated, infection is firmly established and the process is irreversible. It is important to point out that the initial infection of susceptible cells may vary somewhat with the route of infection. Virus that enters directly into the bloodstream via infected blood or blood products (i.e., transfusions, use of contaminated needles for injection drugs, sharp-object injuries, maternal-to-fetal transmission either intrapartum or perinatally, or sexual intercourse where there is enough trauma to cause bleeding) is likely cleared from the circulation to the spleen and other lymphoid organs, where primary focal infections begin, followed by wider dissemination throughout other lymphoid tissues as described above.

multiphasic and are different at different stages of the disease. Therefore, it is essential to consider the typical clinical course of an untreated HIV-infected individual in order to more fully appreciate these pathogenic events (Fig. 189-17).

■ EARLY EVENTS IN HIV INFECTION: PRIMARY INFECTION AND INITIAL DISSEMINATION OF VIRUS

Using mucosal transmission as a model, the earliest events (within hours) that occur following exposure of HIV to the mucosal surface determine whether an infection will be established as well as the subsequent course of events following infection. Although the mucosal barrier is relatively effective in limiting access of HIV to susceptible targets in the lamina propria, the virus can cross the barrier by transport

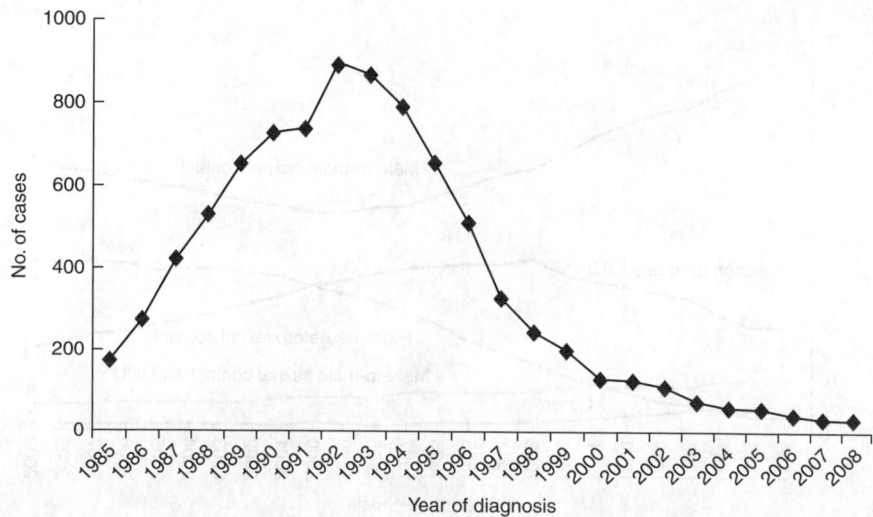

Figure 189-16 Estimated numbers of perinatally acquired AIDS cases in children by year of diagnosis, 1985–2009, United States *(From CDC.)*

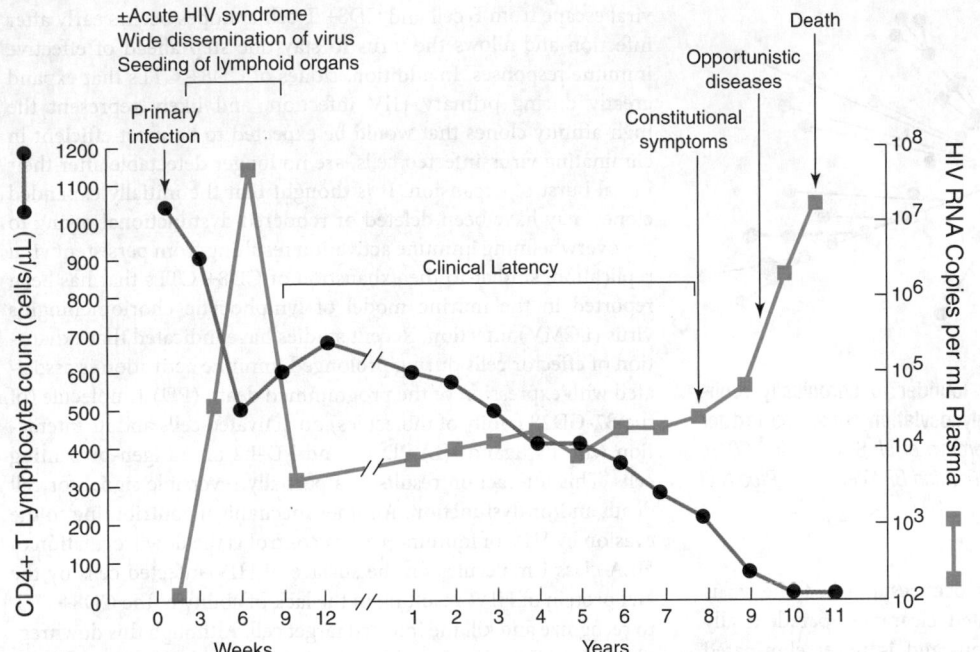

Figure 189-17 **Typical course of an untreated HIV-infected individual.** See text for detailed description. *(From G Pantaleo et al: N Engl J Med 328:327, 1993. Copyright 1993 Massachusetts Medical Society. All rights reserved.)*

It has been demonstrated that sexual transmission of HIV is the result of a single infectious event and that a viral genetic bottleneck exists for transmission. In this regard, certain characteristics of the HIV envelope glycoprotein have a major influence on transmission, at least in subtype A and C viruses. Transmitting viruses, often referred to as "founder viruses," are usually underrepresented in the circulating viremia of the transmitting partner and are less-diverged viruses with signature sequences including shorter V1–V2 loop sequences and fewer predicted N-linked glycosylation sites relative to the major circulating variants. These viruses are usually sensitive to neutralization by antibody from the transmitting partner. Once

replication proceeds in the newly infected partner, the founder virus diverges and accumulates glycosylation sites, becoming progressively more resistant to neutralization (Fig. 189-19).

The acute burst of viremia and wide dissemination of virus in primary HIV infection may be associated with an *acute HIV syndrome*, which occurs to varying degrees in ~50% of individuals with primary infection. This syndrome is usually associated with high levels of viremia measured in millions of copies of HIV RNA per milliliter of plasma that last for several weeks. Acute mononucleosis-like symptoms are well correlated with the presence of viremia. Virtually all patients develop some degree of viremia during primary infection, which contributes to virus dissemination throughout the lymphoid tissue, even though they may remain asymptomatic or not recall experiencing symptoms. It appears that the initial level of plasma viremia in primary HIV infection does not necessarily determine the rate of disease progression; however, the set point of the level of steady-state plasma viremia after ~1 year does seem to correlate with the slope of disease progression in the untreated patient.

ESTABLISHMENT OF CHRONIC AND PERSISTENT INFECTION

Persistent virus replication

HIV infection is unique among human viral infections. Despite the robust cellular and humoral immune responses that are mounted following primary infection (see "Immune Response

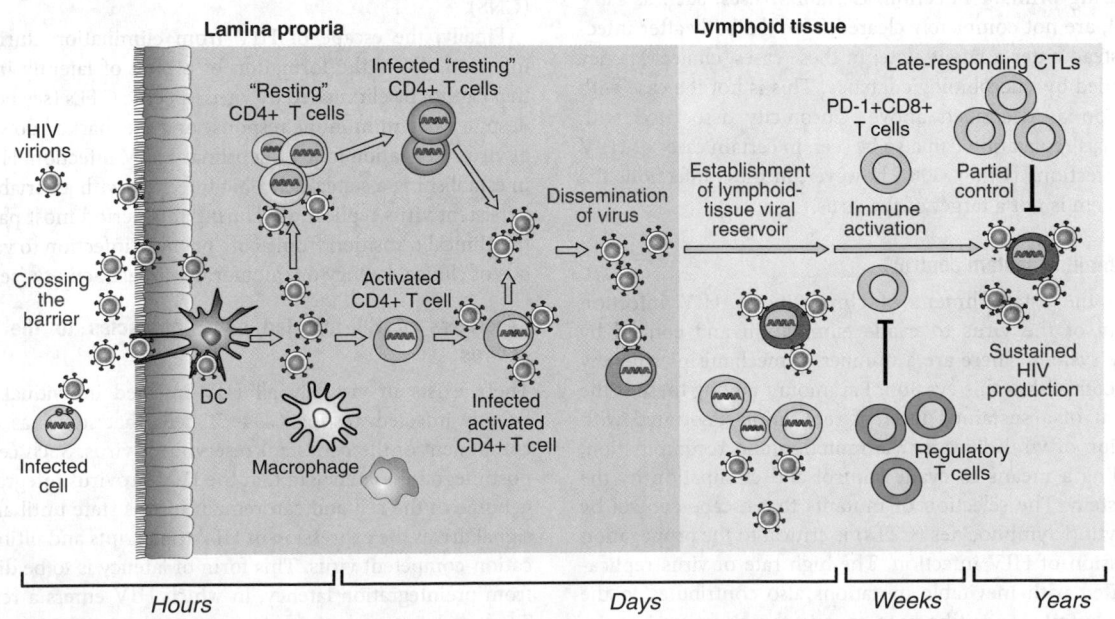

Figure 189-18 **Summary of early events in HIV infection.** See text for detailed description. CTLs, cytolytic T lymphocytes; HIV, human immunodeficiency virus. *(Adapted from Haase, 2005.)*

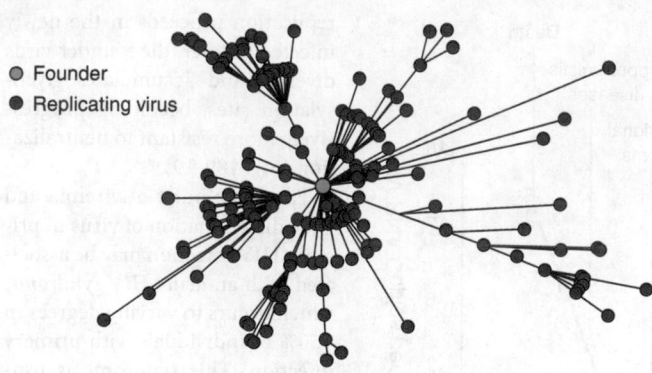

● Founder
● Replicating virus

Figure 189-19 As HIV diverges from founder to chronically replicating virus, it accumulates N-linked glycosylation sites. See text for detailed description. *(Adapted from CA Derdeyn et al: Science 303:2019, 2004; B Chohan et al: J Virol 79:6528, 2005; and BF Keele et al: Proc Natl Acad Sci USA 105:7552, 2008.)*

to HIV," below), once infection has been established the virus succeeds in escaping immune-mediated clearance, paradoxically seems to thrive on immune activation, and is never eliminated completely from the body. Rather, a chronic infection develops and persists with varying degrees of continual virus replication in the untreated patient for a median of ~10 years before the patient becomes clinically ill (see "Advanced HIV Disease" below). It is this establishment of a chronic, persistent infection that is the hallmark of HIV disease. Throughout the often protracted course of chronic infection, virus replication can invariably be detected in untreated patients, both by highly sensitive assays for plasma viremia as well as by demonstration of cell-associated HIV RNA in immunocompetent cells (predominantly CD4+ T cells and macrophages) in the circulation and in lymphoid tissue. Recent studies using highly sensitive molecular techniques have demonstrated that even in certain patients in whom plasma viremia is suppressed to below 50 copies of HIV RNA/mL by cART, there is a continual low level of virus replication. In other human viral infections, with very few exceptions, if the host survives, the virus is completely cleared from the body and a state of immunity against subsequent infection develops. HIV infection very rarely kills the host during primary infection. Certain viruses, such as HSV (Chap. 179), are not completely cleared from the body after infection but instead enter a latent state; in these cases, clinical latency is accompanied by microbiologic latency. This is not the case with HIV infection as described above. Chronicity associated with persistent virus replication can also be seen in certain cases of HBV and HCV infections (Chap. 306); however, in these infections the immune system is not a target of the virus.

Evasion of immune system control

Inherent to the establishment of chronicity of HIV infection is the ability of the virus to evade elimination and control by the immune system. There are a number of mechanisms whereby the virus accomplishes this evasion. Paramount among these is the establishment of a sustained level of replication associated with the generation of viral diversity via mutation and recombination, thus providing a means to evade control and elimination by the immune system. The selection of mutants that escape control by CD8+ cytolytic T lymphocytes (CTLs) is critical to the propagation and progression of HIV infection. The high rate of virus replication associated with inevitable mutations also contributes to the inability of neutralizing antibody to contain the virus quasispecies present in an individual at any given time. Extensive analyses of sequential HIV isolates and host responses have demonstrated that

viral escape from B cell and CD8+ T cell epitopes occurs early after infection and allows the virus to stay one step ahead of effective immune responses. In addition, clones of CD8+ CTLs that expand greatly during primary HIV infection, and likely represent the high-affinity clones that would be expected to be most efficient in eliminating virus-infected cells, are no longer detectable after their initial burst of expansion. It is thought that the initially expanded clones may have been deleted or rendered dysfunctional owing to the overwhelming immune activation resulting from persistent viral replication, similar to the exhaustion of CD8+ CTLs that has been reported in the murine model of lymphocytic choriomeningitis virus (LCMV) infection. Recent studies have indicated that exhaustion of effector cells during prolonged immune activation is associated with expression of the programmed death (PD) 1 molecule (of the B7-CD28 family of molecules) on activated cells and its interaction with its ligands (L) PD-L1 and PD-L2 on antigen-presenting cells. This interaction results in a partially reversible signal for cell death and/or dysfunction. Another mechanism contributing to the evasion by HIV of immune system control is the downregulation of HLA class I molecules on the surface of HIV-infected cells by the Nef protein of HIV, resulting in the lack of ability of the CD8+ CTL to recognize and kill the infected target cell. Although this downregulation of HLA class I molecules would favor elimination of HIV-infected cells by natural killer (NK) cells, this latter mechanism does not seem to remove HIV-infected cells effectively (see below). The principal targets of neutralizing antibodies against HIV are the envelope proteins gp120 and gp41. HIV employs at least three mechanisms to evade neutralizing responses: hypervariability in the primary sequence of the envelope, extensive glycosylation of the envelope, and conformational masking of neutralizing epitopes.

CD4+ T cell help is essential for the integrity of antigen-specific immune responses, both humoral and cell-mediated. HIV preferentially infects activated CD4+ T cells including HIV-specific CD4+ T cells, and so this loss of viral-specific helper T cell responses has profound negative consequences for the immunologic control of HIV replication. Furthermore, this loss occurs early in the course of infection, and animal studies indicate that 40–70% of all memory CD4+ T cells in the GALT are eliminated during acute infection. Another potential means of escape of HIV-infected cells from elimination by CD8+ CTLs is the sequestration of infected cells in immunologically privileged sites such as the central nervous system (CNS).

Finally, the escape of HIV from elimination during primary infection allows the formation of a pool of latently infected cells that cannot be eliminated by virus-specific CTLs (see below). Thus, despite a potent immune response and the marked downregulation of virus replication following primary HIV infection, HIV succeeds in establishing a state of chronic infection with a variable degree of persistent virus replication. During this period most patients make the clinical transition from acute primary infection to variable periods of clinical latency or smoldering disease activity (see below).

Reservoirs of HIV-infected cells: obstacles to the eradication of virus

There exists in virtually all HIV-infected individuals a pool of latently infected, resting CD4+ T cells that serves as at least one component of the persistent reservoir of virus. Such cells manifest postintegration latency in that the HIV provirus integrates into the genome of the cell and can remain in this state until an activation signal drives the expression of HIV transcripts and ultimately replication-competent virus. This form of latency is to be distinguished from preintegration latency, in which HIV enters a resting CD4+ T cell and, in the absence of an activation signal, reverse transcription of the HIV genome occurs to a certain extent but the resulting proviral DNA fails to integrate into the host genome. This period of

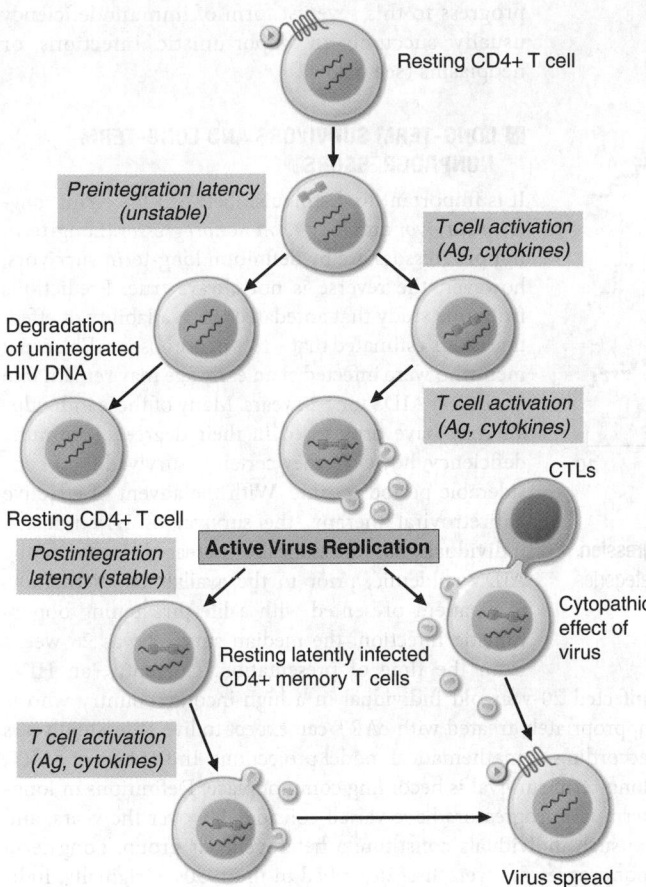

Figure 189-20 Generation of latently infected, resting CD4+ T cells in HIV-infected individuals. See text for details. Ag, antigen; CTLs, cytolytic T lymphocytes. *(Courtesy of TW Chun; with permission.)*

preintegration latency may last hours to days, and if no activation signal is delivered to the cell, the proviral DNA loses its capacity to initiate a productive infection. If these cells do become activated, reverse transcription proceeds to completion and the virus continues along its replication cycle (see above and Fig. 189-20). The pool of cells that are in the postintegration state of latency is established early during the course of primary HIV infection. Despite the suppression of plasma viremia to <50 copies of HIV RNA per milliliter by potent combinations of several antiretroviral drugs administered over several years, this pool of latently infected cells persists and can give rise to replication-competent virus. Modeling studies built on projections of decay curves have estimated that in such a setting of prolonged suppression, it would require 7–70 years for the pool of latently infected cells to be completely eliminated. Furthermore, the reservoir of latently infected cells is replenished during minor detectable rebounds or "blips" of virus replication that may occur intermittently, superimposed on the low levels of persistent virus replication that may remain below the limits of detection of current assays (see below) (Fig. 189-20), even in patients who for the most part are treated successfully. Reservoirs of HIV-infected cells, latent or otherwise, can exist in a number of compartments including the lymphoid tissue, peripheral blood, and the CNS (likely in cells of the monocyte/macrophage lineage) as well as in

other unidentified locations. Over the past several years attempts have been made to eliminate HIV in the latent viral reservoir using agents that stimulate resting CD4+ T cells during the course of antiretroviral therapy; however, such attempts have been unsuccessful. Thus, this persistent reservoir of infected cells at various stages of latency and/or low levels of persistent virus replication are major obstacles to any goal of eradication of virus from infected individuals, despite the favorable clinical outcomes that have resulted from cART.

Viral dynamics

The dynamics of viral production and turnover have been quantified using mathematical modeling in the setting of the administration of reverse transcriptase and protease inhibitors to HIV-infected individuals in clinical studies. Treatment with these drugs resulted in a precipitous decline in the level of plasma viremia, which typically fell by well over 90% within 2 weeks. The number of CD4+ T cells in the blood increased concurrently, which suggested that the killing of CD4+ T cells was linked directly to the levels of replicating virus. However, a significant component of the early rise in CD4+ T cell numbers following the initiation of therapy may be due to the redistribution of cells into the peripheral blood from other body compartments as a consequence of therapy-related diminution in viremia-associated immune system activation. It was determined on the basis of modeling the kinetics of viral decline and the emergence of resistant mutants during therapy that 93–99% of the circulating virus originated from recently infected, rapidly turning over CD4+ T cells and that ~1–7% of circulating virus originated from longer-lived cells, likely monocytes/macrophages. A negligible amount of circulating virus originated from the pool of latently infected cells (Fig. 189-21). It was also determined that the half-life of a circulating virion was ~30–60 min and that of productively infected cells was 1 day. Given the relatively steady level of plasma viremia and of infected cells, it appears that extremely large amounts of virus (~10^{10}–10^{11} virions) are produced and cleared from the circulation each day. In addition, data suggest that the minimal duration of the HIV-1 replication cycle in vivo is ~2 days. Other studies have demonstrated that the decrease in plasma viremia that results from cART correlates closely with a decrease in virus replication in lymph nodes, further confirming that lymphoid tissue is the main site of HIV replication and the main source of plasma viremia.

The level of steady-state viremia, called the viral *set point*, at ~1 year has important prognostic implications for the progression

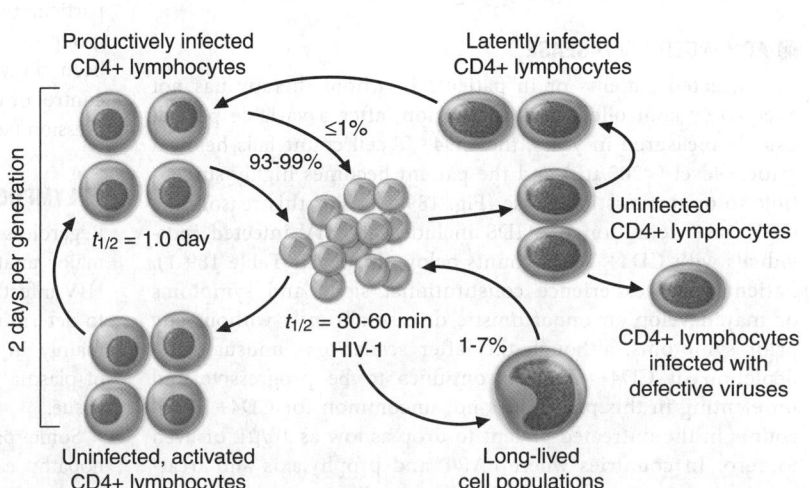

Figure 189-21 Dynamics of HIV infection in vivo. See text for detailed description. *(From AS Perelson et al: Science 271:1582, 1996.)*

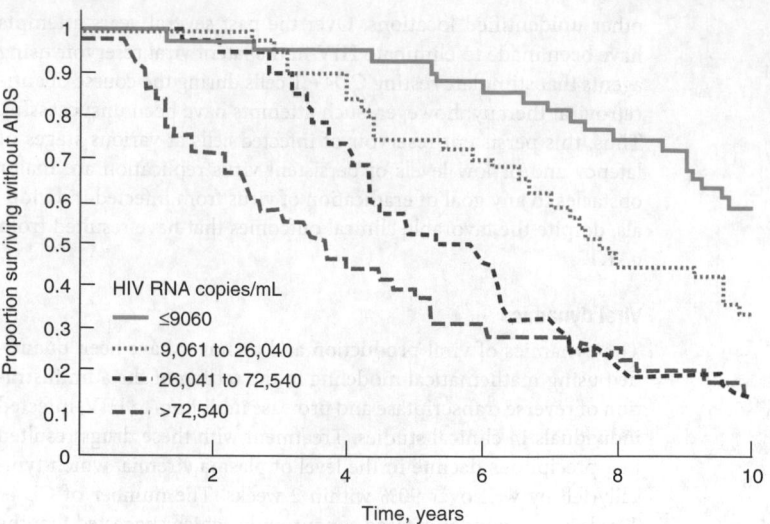

Figure 189-22 Relationship between levels of virus and rates of disease progression. Kaplan-Meier curves for AIDS-free survival stratified by baseline HIV-1 RNA categories (copies per milliliter). *(From Mellors et al.)*

of HIV disease in the untreated patient. It has been demonstrated that as a group untreated HIV-infected individuals who have a low set point at 6 months to 1 year following infection progress to AIDS much more slowly than individuals whose set point is very high at that time (Fig. 189-22).

Clinical latency versus microbiologic latency

With the exception of long-term nonprogressors (see "Long-Term Survivors and Long-Term Nonprogressors," below), the level of CD4+ T cells in the blood decreases progressively in HIV-infected individuals. The decline in CD4+ T cells may be gradual or abrupt, the latter usually reflecting a significant spike in the level of plasma viremia. Most patients are relatively asymptomatic while this progressive decline is taking place (see below) and are often described as being in a state of *clinical latency*. However, this term is misleading; it does not mean disease latency, since progression, although slow in many cases, is generally relentless during this period. Furthermore, clinical latency should not be confused with microbiologic latency, since varying levels of virus replication inevitably occur during this period of clinical latency. Even in those rare patients who have <50 copies of HIV RNA per milliliter in the absence of therapy, there is virtually always some degree of ongoing virus replication.

■ ADVANCED HIV DISEASE

In untreated patients or in patients in whom therapy has not adequately controlled virus replication, after a variable period, usually measured in years, the CD4+ T cell count falls below a critical level (<200/μL) and the patient becomes highly susceptible to opportunistic disease (Fig. 189-17). For this reason, the CDC case definition of AIDS includes all HIV-infected individuals with CD4+ T cell counts below this level (Table 189-1). Patients may experience constitutional signs and symptoms or may develop an opportunistic disease abruptly without any prior symptoms, although the latter scenario is unusual. The depletion of CD4+ T cells continues to be progressive and unrelenting in this phase. It is not uncommon for CD4+ T cell counts in the untreated patient to drop as low as 10/μL or even to zero. In countries where cART and prophylaxis and treatment for opportunistic infections are readily accessible to such patients, survival is increased dramatically even in those patients with advanced HIV disease. In contrast, untreated patients who

progress to this severest form of immunodeficiency usually succumb to opportunistic infections or neoplasms (see below).

■ LONG-TERM SURVIVORS AND LONG-TERM NONPROGRESSORS

It is important to distinguish between the terms *long-term survivor* and *long-term nonprogressor*. Long-term nonprogressors are by definition long-term survivors; however, the reverse is not always true. Predictions from one study that antedated the availability of effective cART estimated that ~13% of homosexual/bisexual men who were infected at an early age may remain free of clinical AIDS for >20 years. Many of these individuals may have progressed in their degree of immune deficiency; however, they certainly survived for a considerable period of time. With the advent of effective antiretroviral therapy, the survival of HIV-infected individuals has dramatically increased. Early in the AIDS epidemic, prior to the availability of therapy, if a patient presented with a life-threatening opportunistic infection, the median survival was 26 weeks from the time of presentation. Currently, an HIV-infected 20-year-old individual in a high-income country who is appropriately treated with cART can expect to live at least 50 years according to mathematical model projections. In the face of cART, long-term survival is becoming commonplace. Definitions of long-term nonprogressors have varied considerably over the years, and so such individuals constitute a heterogeneous group. Long-term nonprogressors were first described in the 1990s. Originally, individuals were considered to be long-term nonprogressors if they had been infected with HIV for a long period (≥10 years), their CD4+ T cell counts were in the normal range, and they remained stable over years without receiving cART. Approximately 5–15% of HIV-infected individuals fell into this broader nonprogressor category. However, this group was rather heterogenous and over time a significant proportion of these individuals progressed and ultimately required therapy. From this broader group, a much smaller subgroup of "elite" controllers or nonprogressors was identified, and they constituted less than 1% of HIV-infected individuals. These elite controllers, by definition, have extremely low levels of plasma viremia and normal CD4+ T cell counts. It is noteworthy that certain of their HIV-specific immune responses are robust and clearly superior to those of HIV-infected progressors. In this group of elite controllers certain HLA class I haplotypes are overrepresented, particularly HLA-B57-01 and HLA-B27-05. Outside of the subgroup of elite controllers, a number of other genetic factors have been shown to be involved to a greater or lesser degree in the control of virus replication and thus in the rate of HIV disease progression (see "Genetic Factors in HIV Pathogenesis," below).

■ LYMPHOID ORGANS AND HIV PATHOGENESIS

Regardless of the portal of entry of HIV, lymphoid tissues are the major anatomic sites for the establishment and propagation of HIV infection. Despite the use of measurements of plasma viremia to determine the level of disease activity, virus replication occurs mainly in lymphoid tissue and not in blood; indeed, the level of plasma viremia directly reflects virus production in lymphoid tissue.

Some patients experience progressive generalized lymphadenopathy early in the course of the infection; others experience varying degrees of transient lymphadenopathy. Lymphadenopathy reflects the cellular activation and immune response to the virus in the lymphoid tissue, which is generally characterized by follicular or germinal center hyperplasia. Lymphoid tissue involvement is a common denominator of virtually all patients with HIV infection, even those without easily detectable lymphadenopathy.

Simultaneous examinations of lymph tissue and peripheral blood in patients and monkeys during various stages of HIV and SIV infection, respectively, have led to substantial insight into the pathogenesis of HIV disease. In most of the original human studies, peripheral lymph nodes have been used predominantly as the source of lymphoid tissue. More recent studies in monkeys and humans have focused on the GALT, where the earliest burst of virus replication occurs associated with marked depletion of CD4+ T cells. In detailed studies of peripheral lymph node tissue, using a combination of polymerase chain reaction (PCR) techniques for HIV DNA and HIV RNA in tissue and HIV RNA in plasma, in situ hybridization for HIV RNA, and light and electron microscopy, the following picture has emerged. During acute HIV infection resulting from mucosal transmission, virus replication progressively amplifies from scattered lymphoid cells in the lamina propria to draining lymphoid tissue, leading to high levels of plasma viremia. The GALT plays a major role in the amplification of virus replication, and virus is disseminated from replication in the GALT to peripheral lymphoid tissue. A profound degree of cellular activation occurs (see below) and is reflected in follicular or germinal center hyperplasia. At this time copious amounts of extracellular virions (both infectious and defective) are trapped on the processes of the follicular dendritic cells (FDCs) in the germinal centers of the lymph nodes. Virions that have bound complement components on their surfaces attach to the surface of FDCs via interactions with complement receptors and likely via Fc receptors that bind to antibodies that are attached to the virions. In situ hybridization reveals expression of virus in individual cells of the paracortical area and, to a lesser extent, the germinal center (Fig. 189-23). The persistence of trapped virus after the transition from acute to chronic infection likely reflects a steady state whereby trapped virus turns over and is replaced by fresh virions that are continually produced. The trapped virus, either as whole virion or shed envelope, serves as a continual activator of CD4+ T cells, thus driving further virus replication.

During early-stage HIV disease, the architecture of the germinal centers is generally preserved and may even be hyperplastic owing to in situ proliferation of cells (mostly B lymphocytes) and recruitment to the lymph nodes of a number of cell types (B cells, CD4+ and CD8+ T cells). Electron-microscopic studies have demonstrated a fine network of FDCs with many long, fingerlike processes that envelop virtually every lymphocyte in the germinal center. Extracellular virions can be seen attached to the processes, yet the FDCs appear to be relatively healthy. The trapping of antigen is a physiologically normal function for the FDCs, which present antigen to B cells and contribute to the generation of B cell memory. However, in the case of HIV, the trapped virions serve as a persistent source of cellular activation, resulting in the secretion of proinflammatory cytokines such as interleukin (IL) 1β, tumor necrosis factor (TNF) α, and IL-6, which can upregulate virus replication in infected cells (see below). Furthermore, although trapped virus is coated by neutralizing antibodies, it has been demonstrated that certain of these virions remain infectious for CD4+ T cells while attached to the processes of the FDCs. CD4+ T cells that migrate into the germinal center to provide help to B cells in the generation of an HIV-specific immune response are susceptible to infection by these trapped virions. Thus, in HIV infection, a normal physiologic function of the immune system that contributes to the clearance of virus, as well as to the generation of a specific immune response, can also have deleterious consequences.

As the disease progresses, the architecture of the germinal centers begins to show disruption. Electron microscopy reveals swollen organelles, and the FDCs begin to undergo cell death. The mechanisms of FDC death remain unclear; there is no indication by electron microscopy of copious virus replication or budding of virions off the cell in great quantities. This process of FDC death is accompanied by the deposition of collagen, leading to irreparable damage to the germinal centers. As the disease progresses to an advanced stage, there is complete disruption of the architecture of the germinal centers, accompanied by dissolution of the FDC network and massive dropout of FDCs. At this point, the lymph nodes are "burnt out." This destruction of lymphoid tissue compounds the immunodeficiency of HIV disease and contributes both to the inability to control HIV replication (leading usually to high levels of plasma viremia in the untreated or inadequately treated patient) and to the inability to mount adequate immune responses against opportunistic pathogens. The events from primary infection to the ultimate destruction of the immune system are illustrated in Fig. 189-24. Recently, nonhuman primate studies and some human studies have examined GALT at various stages of HIV disease. Within the GALT, the basal level of activation combined with virus-mediated cellular activation results in the infection and elimination of an estimated 50–90% of CD4+ T cells in the gut. The extent of this early damage to GALT, which constitutes a major component of lymphoid tissue in the body, may play a role in determining the potential for immunologic recovery of the memory cell subset.

■ IMMUNE ACTIVATION, INFLAMMATION, AND HIV PATHOGENESIS

Activation of the immune system and variable degrees of inflammation are essential components of any appropriate immune response to a foreign antigen. However, immune activation and inflammation, which can be considered aberrant in HIV-infected individuals, play a critical role in the pathogenesis of HIV disease and other chronic conditions associated with HIV disease. Immune activation and inflammation in the HIV-infected individual contribute substantially to (1) the replication of HIV, (2) the induction of immune dysfunction, and (3) the increased incidence of chronic conditions associated with persistent immune activation and inflammation (Table 189-3).

Induction of HIV replication by aberrant immune activation
The immune system is normally in a state of homeostasis, awaiting perturbation by foreign antigenic stimuli. Once the immune

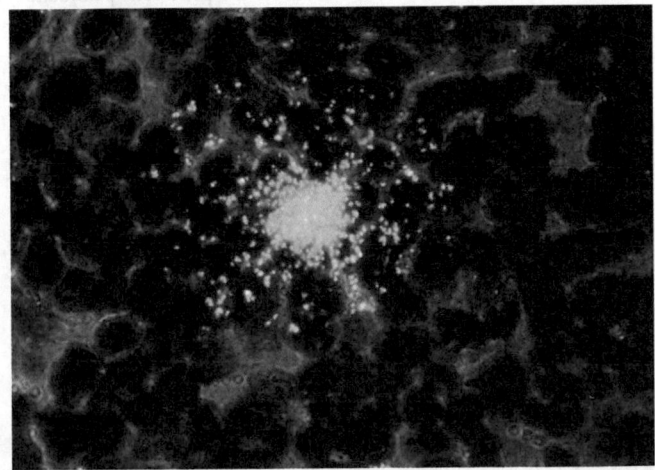

Figure 189-23 HIV in the lymph node of an HIV-infected individual. An individual cell infected with HIV shown expressing HIV RNA by in situ hybridization using a radiolabeled molecular probe. Original ×500. *(Adapted from G Pantaleo, AS Fauci.)*

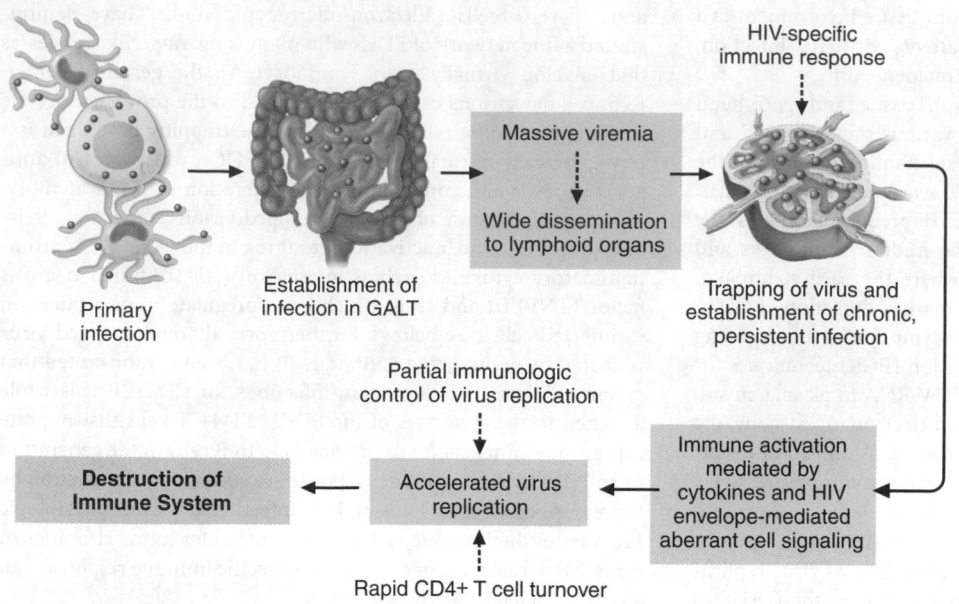

Figure 189-24 Events that transpire from primary HIV infection through the establishment of chronic persistent infection to the ultimate destruction of the immune system. See text for details. CTLs, cytolytic T lymphocytes; GALT, gut-associated lymphoid tissue.

response deals with and clears the antigen, the system returns to relative quiescence (Chap. 314). This is generally not the case in HIV infection where, in the untreated patient, virus replication is invariably persistent with very few exceptions and immune activation is persistent. HIV replicates most efficiently in activated CD4+ T cells; in HIV infection, chronic activation provides the cell substrates necessary for persistent virus replication throughout the course of HIV disease, particularly in the untreated patient and to variable degrees even in certain patients receiving cART whose levels of plasma viremia are suppressed to below the level of detection by standard assays. From a virologic standpoint, although quiescent CD4+ T cells can be infected with HIV, reverse transcription, integration, and virus spread are much more efficient in activated cells. Furthermore, cellular activation induces expression of virus in cells latently infected with HIV. In essence, immune activation and inflammation provide the engine that drives HIV replication. In addition to endogenous factors such as cytokines, a number of exogenous factors such as other microbes that are associated with heightened cellular activation can enhance HIV replication and thus may have important effects on HIV pathogenesis. Co-infection in vivo or in vitro with a range of viruses, such as HSV types 1 and 2, cytomegalovirus (CMV), human herpesvirus (HHV) 6, Epstein-Barr virus (EBV), HBV, adenovirus, and HTLV-I have been shown to upregulate HIV expression. In addition, infestation with nematodes has been shown to be associated with a heightened state of immune activation that facilitates HIV replication; in certain studies deworming of the infected host has resulted in a decrease in plasma viremia. Two diseases of extraordinary global health significance, malaria and tuberculosis (TB), have been shown to increase HIV viral load in dually infected individuals. Globally, *Mycobacterium tuberculosis* is the most common opportunistic infection globally in HIV-infected individuals (Chap. 165). In addition to the fact that HIV-infected individuals are more likely to develop active TB after exposure, it has been demonstrated that active TB can accelerate the course of HIV infection. It has also been shown that levels of plasma viremia are greatly elevated in HIV-infected individuals with active TB who are not on cART, compared with pre-TB levels and levels of viremia after successful treatment of the active TB. The situation is similar in the interaction between HIV and malaria parasites (Chap. 210). Acute infection of HIV-infected individuals with *Plasmodium falciparum* increases HIV viral load, and the increased viral load is reversed by effective malaria treatment.

Microbial translocation and persistent immune activation
One proposed mechanism of persistent immune activation involves the disruption of the mucosal barrier in the gut due to HIV replication in and disruption of submucosal lymphoid tissue. As a result of this disruption, there is an increase in the products, particularly lipopolysaccharide (LPS), of bacteria that translocate from the bowel lumen through the damaged mucosa to the circulation, leading to persistent systemic immune activation and inflammation. This effect can persist even after the HIV viral load is brought to <50 copies/mL by cART. Depletion in the GALT of IL-17–producing T cells, which are responsible for defense against extracellular bacteria and fungi, is also thought to contribute to HIV pathogenesis.

Persistent immune activation and inflammation induce immune dysfunction The activated state in HIV infection is reflected by hyperactivation of B cells leading to hypergammaglobulinemia; increased lymphocyte turnover; activation of monocytes; expression of activation markers on CD4+ and CD8+ T cells; increased activation-associated cellular apoptosis; lymph node hyperplasia, particularly early in the course of disease; increased secretion of proinflammatory cytokines, particularly IL-6; elevated levels of high-sensitivity C-reactive protein, fibrinogen, D-dimer, neopterin, β_2-microglobulin, acid-labile interferon, soluble (s) IL-2 receptors (R), sTNFR, sCD27, and sCD40L; and autoimmune phenomena (see "Autoimmune Phenomena," below). Even in the absence of direct infection of a target cell, HIV envelope proteins

TABLE 189-3 Conditions Associated With Persistent Immune Activation and Inflammation in Patients With HIV Infection

- Accelerated aging syndrome
- Bone fragility
- Cancers
- Cardiovascular disease
- Diabetes
- Kidney disease
- Liver disease
- Neurocognitive dysfunction

can interact with cellular receptors (CD4 molecules and chemokine receptors) to deliver potent activation signals resulting in calcium flux, the phosphorylation of certain proteins involved in signal transduction, co-localization of cytoplasmic proteins including those involved in cell trafficking, immune dysfunction, and, under certain circumstances, apoptosis. From an immunologic standpoint, chronic exposure of the immune system to a particular antigen over an extended period may ultimately lead to an inability to sustain an adequate immune response to the antigen in question. In many chronic viral infections, including HIV infection, persistent viremia is associated with "functional exhaustion" and apoptosis of virus-specific T cells. It has been demonstrated that this phenomenon may be mediated, at least in part, by the engagement of PD-1, which is highly expressed on the majority of HIV-specific T cells, with its ligands (PD-L1 and PD-L2) on antigen-presenting cells and epithelial cells, resulting in either T cell death or anergy. Furthermore, the ability of the immune system to respond to a broad spectrum of antigens may be compromised if immunocompetent cells are maintained in a state of chronic activation.

The deleterious effects of chronic immune activation on the progression of HIV disease are well established. As in most conditions of persistent antigen exposure, the host must maintain sufficient activation of antigen (HIV)-specific responses but must also prevent excessive activation and potential immune-mediated damage to tissues. Certain studies suggest that normal immunosuppressive mechanisms that act to keep hyperimmune activation in check, particularly CD4+, FoxP3+, CD25+ regulatory T cells (T-regs), may be dysfunctional or depleted in the context of advanced HIV disease.

Medical conditions associated with persistent immune activation and inflammation in HIV disease It has become clear as the survival of HIV-infected individuals has increased that a number of previously unrecognized medical complications are associated with HIV disease and that these complications relate to chronic immune activation and inflammation (Table 189-3). These complications can appear even after patients have experienced years of adequate control of viral replication (plasma viremia below detectable levels) for several years. Of particular note are endothelial cell dysfunction and its relationship to cardiovascular disease. Other chronic conditions that have been reported include bone fragility, certain cancers, persistent immune dysfunction, diabetes, kidney and liver disease, and neurocognitive dysfunction, thus presenting an overall picture of accelerated aging.

Apoptosis

Apoptosis is a form of programmed cell death that is a normal mechanism for the elimination of effete cells in organogenesis as well as in the cellular proliferation that occurs during a normal immune response (Chap. 314). Apoptosis is largely dependent on cellular activation, and the aberrant cellular activation associated with HIV disease is correlated with a heightened state of apoptosis. HIV can trigger both Fas-dependent and Fas-independent pathways of apoptosis. Mechanisms involved in this process include upregulation of Fas and Fas ligand, upregulation of caspase-1 and caspase-6, downregulation of the antiapoptotic Bcl-2 protein, and activation of cyclin-dependent kinases. Certain viral gene products have been associated with enhanced susceptibility to apoptosis; these include Env, Tat, and Vpr. In contrast, Nef has been shown to possess antiapoptotic properties. A number of studies, including those examining lymphoid tissue, have demonstrated that the rate of apoptosis is elevated in HIV infection and that apoptosis is seen in "bystander" cells such as CD8+ T cells and B cells as well as in uninfected CD4+ T cells. The intensity of apoptosis correlates with the general state of activation of the immune system and not with the stage of disease or with viral burden. It is likely that nonspecific apoptosis of immunocompetent cells related to immune activation contributes to the immune abnormalities in HIV disease.

Autoimmune phenomena

The autoimmune phenomena that are common in HIV-infected individuals reflect, at least in part, chronic immune system activation as well as molecular mimicry by viral components. Although these phenomena usually occur in the absence of autoimmune disease, a wide spectrum of clinical manifestations that may be associated with autoimmunity have been described (see "Immunologic and Rheumatologic Diseases," below). Autoimmune phenomena include antibodies to lymphocytes and, less commonly, to platelets and neutrophils. Antiplatelet antibodies have some clinical relevance, in that they may contribute to the thrombocytopenia of HIV disease (see below). Antibodies to nuclear and cytoplasmic components of cells have been reported, as have antibodies to cardiolipin; CD4 molecules; CD43 molecules; C1q-A; variable regions of the T cell receptor α, β, and γ chains; Fas; denatured collagen; and IL-2. In addition, autoantibodies to a range of serum proteins, including albumin, immunoglobulin, and thyroglobulin, have been reported. There is antigenic cross-reactivity between HIV viral proteins (gp120 and gp41) and MHC class II determinants, and anti-MHC class II antibodies have been reported in HIV infection. These antibodies could potentially lead to the elimination of MHC class II–bearing cells via antibody-dependent cellular cytotoxicity (ADCC), although this has not been clearly demonstrated to occur (Chap. 314). In addition, regions of homology exist between HIV envelope glycoproteins and IL-2 as well as MHC class I molecules. The increased occurrence and/or exacerbation of certain autoimmune diseases have been reported in HIV infection; these diseases include psoriasis, idiopathic thrombocytopenic purpura, Graves' disease, antiphospholipid antibody syndrome, and primary biliary cirrhosis. With the widespread use of effective antiretroviral therapy, an *immune reconstitution inflammatory syndrome* (IRIS) has become increasingly common. IRIS is an autoimmune-like phenomenon characterized by a paradoxical deterioration of clinical condition, which is usually compartmentalized to a particular organ system, in individuals in whom cART has recently been initiated. It is associated with a decrease in viral load and at least partial recovery of immune competence, which is usually associated with increases in CD4+ T cell counts. The immunopathogenesis is felt to be related to an increase in immune response against the presence of residual antigens that are usually microbial and is commonly seen with underlying *Mycobacterium tuberculosis* and cryptococcosis. This syndrome is discussed in more detail below.

■ THE CYTOKINE NETWORK IN HIV PATHOGENESIS

The immune system is homeostatically regulated by a complex network of immunoregulatory cytokines, which are pleiotropic and redundant and operate in an autocrine and paracrine manner. They are expressed continuously, even during periods of apparent quiescence of the immune system. On perturbation of the immune system by antigenic challenge, the expression of cytokines increases to varying degrees (Chap. 314). Cytokines that are important components of this immunoregulatory network have been demonstrated to play a major role in the regulation of HIV expression in vitro. Potent modulation of HIV expression has been demonstrated either by manipulating endogenous cytokines or by adding exogenous cytokines to culture. Cytokines that induce or enhance HIV expression in one or more of these systems include IL-1, IL-2, IL-3, IL-6, IL-12, IL-18, TNF-α, TNF-β, macrophage colony-stimulating factor (M-CSF), and granulocyte-macrophage colony-stimulating factor (GM-CSF). IL-18 has also been shown to play a role in the development of the HIV-associated lipodystrophy syndrome. Among these cytokines, the most consistent and potent inducers of HIV expression are the *proinflammatory cytokines* TNF-α, IL-1β, and IL-6. Interferon (IFN) α and β as well as IL-32 suppress HIV replication, whereas transforming growth factor (TGF) β, IL-4, IL-10, and IFN-γ can either induce or suppress HIV expression, depending on the system involved. IL-27 suppresses HIV replication by inducing IFN-associated genes. The *CC-chemokines* RANTES (CCL5), macrophage inflammatory protein (MIP) 1α (CCL3), and MIP-1β (CCL4) (Chap. 314) inhibit infection by and spread of R5 HIV-1 strains, while *stromal cell–derived factor* (SDF) 1 inhibits infection by and spread of X4 strains (see below). The alpha defensin family of cytokines has been shown to inhibit both R5 and X4 viruses, and other soluble factors that have not yet been fully characterized have also been shown to suppress HIV replication.

The molecular mechanisms of HIV regulation are best understood for TNF-α, which activates NF-κB proteins that function as transcriptional activators of HIV expression. The HIV-inducing effect of IL-1β is thought to occur at the level of viral transcription in an NF-κB-independent manner. IL-6, GM-CSF, and IFN-γ regulate HIV expression mainly by posttranscriptional mechanisms. Elevated levels of TNF-α and IL-6 have been demonstrated in plasma and cerebrospinal fluid (CSF), and increased expression of TNF-α, IL-1β, IFN-γ, and IL-6 has been demonstrated in the lymph nodes of HIV-infected individuals. The mechanisms whereby the CC-chemokines RANTES (CCL5), MIP-1α (CCL3), and MIP-1β (CCL4) inhibit infection of R5 strains of HIV or SDF-1 blocks X4 strains of HIV involve blocking of the binding of the virus to its co-receptors, the CC-chemokine receptor CCR5 and the CXC-chemokine receptor CXCR4, respectively. However, several CC-chemokines, including but not limited to CCL3, -4, and -5, induce intracellular signals that actually enhance infection by X4 strains of virus at both the entry and postentry levels. The mechanisms whereby other less well characterized factors inhibit HIV replication are not completely understood.

Blocking of endogenous HIV-inducing cytokines or addition of inhibitors of HIV-suppressor cytokines in cultures of peripheral blood and lymph node mononuclear cells from HIV-infected individuals has demonstrated that HIV replication is controlled tightly by endogenous cytokines that act synergistically and in an autocrine and paracrine manner, similar to their physiologic function in the regulation of the immune system. Indeed, the net level of virus replication in an HIV-infected individual reflects at least in part a balance between inductive and suppressive host factors, mediated mainly by cytokines. Finally, the secretion of certain proinflammatory and immunoregulatory cytokines is both a consequence of the aberrant immune activation associated with HIV infection and a mechanism of propagation of the process of aberrant cellular activation (see "Immune Activation, Inflammation, and HIV Pathogenesis," above).

■ LYMPHOCYTE TURNOVER IN HIV INFECTION

The immune systems of patients with HIV infection are characterized by a profound increase in lymphocyte turnover that is immediately reduced with effective cART. Studies utilizing in vivo or in vitro labeling of lymphocytes in the S-phase of the cell cycle have demonstrated a tight correlation between the degree of lymphocyte turnover and plasma levels of HIV RNA. This increase in turnover is seen in CD4+ and CD8+ T lymphocytes as well as B lymphocytes and can be observed in peripheral blood and lymphoid tissue. Mathematical models derived from these data suggest that one can view the lymphoid pool as consisting of dynamically distinct subpopulations of cells that are differentially affected by HIV infection. A major consequence of HIV infection appears to be a shift in cells from a more quiescent pool to a pool with a higher turnover rate. It is likely that a consequence of a higher rate of turnover is a higher rate of cell death. The role of the thymus in adult human T cell

homeostasis and HIV pathogenesis is an area of controversy. While some data point to an important role for the thymus in maintaining T cell numbers and suggest that impairment of thymic function may be responsible for the declines in CD4+ T cells seen in the setting of HIV infection, other studies have concluded that the thymus plays a minor role in HIV pathogenesis. Among the data supporting an important role for the thymus are those that demonstrate an increase in the levels of T cell receptor excision circles (TRECs) following initiation of cART. TRECs are a byproduct of T cell development and represent episomal fragments of DNA that are excised during T cell receptor gene rearrangement (Chap. 314). Levels of TRECs will be the net result of changes in thymic output together with changes in T cell turnover. An increase in thymic output and/or a decrease in T cell turnover will lead to an increase in levels of TRECs. While it is clear that levels of TRECs increase following initiation of cART, it is not clear whether this is a consequence of increased thymic output or decreased T cell turnover.

■ THE ROLE OF VIRAL RECEPTORS AND CO-RECEPTORS IN HIV PATHOGENESIS

As mentioned above, HIV-1 utilizes two major co-receptors along with CD4 to bind to, fuse with, and enter target cells; these co-receptors are CCR5 and CXCR4, which are also receptors for certain endogenous chemokines. Strains of HIV that utilize CCR5 as a co-receptor are referred to as *R5 viruses*. Strains of HIV that utilize CXCR4 are referred to as *X4 viruses*. Many virus strains are *dual tropic* in that they utilize both CCR5 and CXCR4; these are referred to as *R5X4 viruses*.

The natural chemokine ligands for the major HIV co-receptors can readily block entry of HIV. For example, the CC-chemokines RANTES (CCL5), MIP-1α (CCL3), and MIP-1β (CCL4), which are the natural ligands for CCR5, block entry of R5 viruses, whereas SDF-1, the natural ligand for CXCR4, blocks entry of X4 viruses. The mechanism of inhibition of viral entry is a steric inhibition of binding that is not dependent on signal transduction (Fig. 189-25).

The transmitting virus is almost invariably an R5 virus that predominates during the early stages of HIV disease. In ~40% of HIV-infected individuals, there is a transition to a predominantly X4 virus that is associated with a relatively rapid progression of disease. However, at least 60% of infected individuals progress in their disease while maintaining predominance of an R5 virus. It should be pointed out that clade C viruses, unlike other subgroups, almost never switch from CCR5 tropism to CXCR4 tropism; the reason for this difference is unclear.

The basis for the tropism of different envelope glycoproteins for either CCR5 or CXCR4 relates to the ability of the HIV envelope, including the third variable region (V3 loop) of gp120, to interact with these co-receptors. In this regard, binding of gp120 to CD4 induces a conformational change in gp120 that increases its affinity for CCR5 (see above). Finally, R5 viruses are more efficient in infecting monocytes/macrophages and microglial cells of the brain (see "Neuropathogenesis," below).

The integrin α4β7 and mucosal transmission of HIV A recently identified receptor for HIV has been reported; this receptor is not necessary for virus binding and fusion to its target CD4+ T cell or for virus replication, but it likely plays an important role in the transmission of HIV at mucosal surfaces such as the genital tract and gut. The integrin α4β7, which is the gut homing receptor for peripheral T cells, binds in its activated form to a specific tripeptide in the V2 loop of gp120 resulting in rapid activation of leukocyte function-associated antigen 1 (LFA-1), the central integrin in the establishment of virologic synapses, which facilitate efficient cell-to-cell spread of HIV. It has been demonstrated that α4β7^{high} CD4+ T cells are more susceptible to

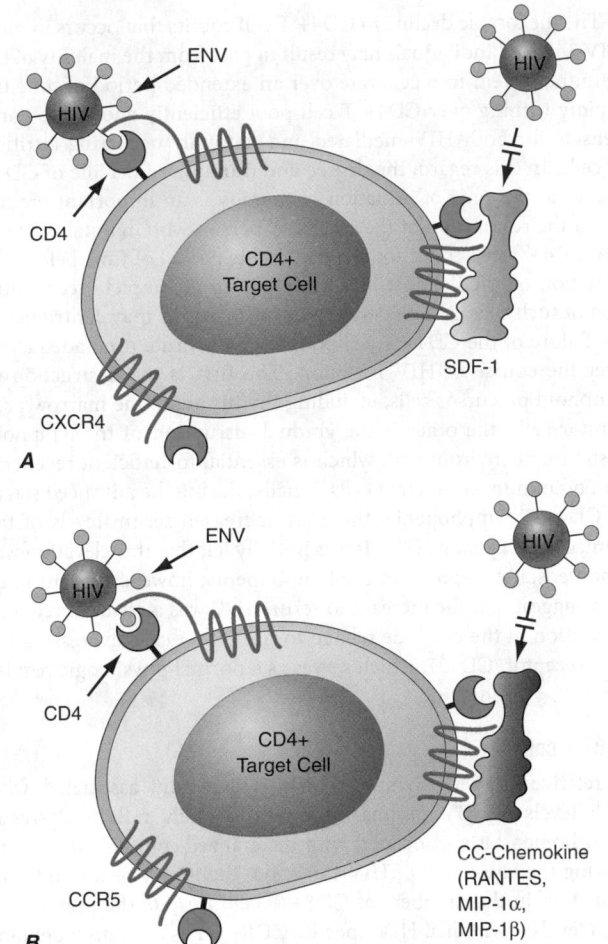

Figure 189-25   Model for the role of co-receptors CXCR4 and CCR5 in the efficient binding and entry of X4 (***A***) and R5 (***B***) strains of HIV-1, respectively, into CD4+ target cells. Blocking of this initial event in the virus life cycle can be accomplished by inhibition of binding to the co-receptor by the normal ligand for the receptor in question. The ligand for CXCR4 is stromal cell–derived factor (SDF-1); the ligands for CCR5 are RANTES, MIP-1α, and MIP-1β.

productive infection than are α4β7$^{low–neg}$ CD4+ T cells because this cellular subset is enriched with metabolically active CD4+ T cells that are CCR5^{high}. These cells are present at the gut and genital tract mucosal surfaces. Importantly, it has been demonstrated that the virus that is transmitted during sexual exposure binds much more efficiently to α4β7 than does the virus that diversifies from the transmitting virus over time by mutation, particularly involving the accumulation of glycosylation sites (see "Early Events in HIV Infection: Primary Infection and Initial Dissemination of Virus," above).

CELLULAR TARGETS OF HIV

Although the CD4+ T lymphocytes and to a lesser extent CD4+ cells of monocyte lineage are the principal targets of HIV, virtually any cell that expresses the CD4 molecule together with co-receptor molecules (see above and below) can potentially be infected with HIV. Circulating dendritic cells have been reported to express low levels of CD4, and, depending on their stage of maturation, these cells can be infected with HIV. Epidermal Langerhans cells express CD4 and have been infected by HIV in vivo, although as has been shown in vivo for dendritic cells, FDCs, and B cells, these cells are more likely to bind and transfer virus to activated CD4+ T cells than to themselves be productively infected.

In vitro, HIV has been reported also to infect a wide range of cells and cell lines that express low levels of CD4, no detectable CD4, or only CD4 mRNA. However, since the only cells that have been shown unequivocally to be infected with HIV and to support replication of the virus are CD4+ T lymphocytes and cells of monocyte/macrophage lineage, the relevance of the in vitro infection of these other cell types is questionable.

Of potentially important clinical relevance is the demonstration that thymic precursor cells, which were assumed to be negative for CD3, CD4, and CD8 molecules, actually do express low levels of CD4 and can be infected with HIV in vitro. In addition, human thymic epithelial cells transplanted into an immunodeficient mouse can be infected with HIV by direct inoculation of virus into the thymus. Since these cells may play a role in the normal regeneration of CD4+ T cells, it is possible that their infection and depletion contribute, at least in part, to the impaired ability of the CD4+ T cell pool to completely reconstitute itself in certain infected individuals in whom cART has suppressed viral replication to <50 copies of HIV RNA per milliliter (see below). In addition, CD34+ monocyte precursor cells have been shown to be infected in vivo in patients with advanced HIV disease. It is likely that these cells express low levels of CD4, and therefore it is not essential to invoke CD4-independent mechanisms to explain the infection.

ABNORMALITIES OF MONONUCLEAR CELLS

CD4+ T cells

The primary immunopathogenic lesion in HIV infection involves CD4+ T cells, and the range of CD4+ T cell abnormalities in advanced HIV infection is broad. The defects are both quantitative and qualitative and ultimately impact virtually every limb of the immune system, indicating the critical dependence of the integrity of the immune system on the inducer/helper function of CD4+ T cells. In advanced HIV disease, most of the observed immune defects can ultimately be explained by the quantitative depletion of CD4+ T cells. However, T cell dysfunction can be demonstrated in patients early in the course of infection, even when the CD4+ T cell count is in the low-normal range. The degree and spectrum of dysfunctions increase as the disease progresses. One of the first abnormalities to be detected is a defect in response to remote recall antigens, such as tetanus toxoid and influenza, at a time when mononuclear cells can still respond normally to mitogenic stimulation. Indeed, defects of central memory cells are a critical component of HIV immunopathogenesis. The progressive loss of antigen-specific CD4+ T cells has important implications for the control of HIV infection. In this regard, there is a correlation between the maintenance of HIV-specific CD4+ T cell proliferative responses and improved control of infection. Essentially every T cell function has been reported to be abnormal at some stage of HIV infection. Loss of polyfunctional HIV-specific CD4+ T cells, especially those that produce IL-2, occurs early in disease, whereas IFN-producing CD4+ T cells are maintained longer and do not correlate with control of HIV viremia. Loss of IL-2-producing polyfunctional CD4+ T cells is also associated with decreased capacity to upregulate CD40 ligand, which may contribute to the dysregulation of B cell function observed in HIV disease. Other abnormalities include impaired expression of IL-2 receptors, defective IL-2 production, reduced expression of the IL-7 receptor (CD127), and decreased proportion of CD4+ T cells that express CD28, a major co-stimulatory molecule necessary for the normal activation of T cells. Cells lacking expression of CD28 do not respond normally to activation signals and may express markers of terminal activation including HLA-DR, CD38, and CD45RO. As mentioned above ("Immune Activation, Inflammation, and HIV Pathogenesis"), a subset of CD4+ T cells referred to as *T regulatory cells*, or T-regs, may be involved in

TABLE 189-4 Mechanisms of CD4+ T Cell Dysfunction and Depletion

Direct Mechanisms	Indirect Mechanisms
Loss of plasma membrane integrity due to viral budding	Aberrant intracellular signaling events
	Autoimmunity
Accumulation of unintegrated viral DNA	Innocent bystander killing of viral antigen–coated cells
Interference with cellular RNA processing	Apoptosis
	Inhibition of lymphopoiesis
Intracellular gp120-CD4 autofusion events	Activation-induced cell death
Syncytia formation	Elimination of HIV-infected cells by virus-specific immune responses

damping aberrant immune activation that propagates HIV replication. The presence of these T-reg cells correlates with lower viral loads and higher CD4+/CD8+ T cell ratios. A loss of this T-reg capability with advanced disease may be detrimental to the control of virus replication.

It is difficult to explain completely the profound immunodeficiency noted in HIV-infected individuals solely on the basis of direct infection and quantitative depletion of CD4+ T cells. This is particularly apparent during the early stages of HIV disease, when CD4+ T cell numbers may be only marginally decreased. In this regard, it is likely that CD4+ T cell dysfunction results from a combination of depletion of cells due to direct infection of the cell and a number of virus-related but indirect effects on the cell (Table 189-4). Certain of these effects have been demonstrated by exposure of cells to virus in vitro and so their clinical relevance is not completely clear. However, it has been clearly demonstrated that patients with high levels of plasma viremia have a variety of subtle abnormalities of CD4+ T cell function, particularly involving aberrancies in signal transduction pathways. These abnormalities could be due either to aberrant activation induced by the cascade of cytokines that are expressed in viremic patients or to the direct effect of virus on the cell. In this regard, certain of these abnormalities can be reproduced by exposing CD4+ T cells of normal individuals to oligomeric HIV envelope proteins in vitro.

Humoral and cellular immune responses to HIV may contribute to protective immunity by eliminating virus and virus-infected cells (see "Immune Response to HIV," below). However, since the main targets of HIV infection are immunocompetent cells, these responses may contribute to immune cell depletion and immunologic dysfunction by eliminating both infected cells and "innocent bystander" cells. Soluble viral proteins, particularly gp120, can bind with high affinity to the CD4 molecules on uninfected T cells and monocytes; in addition, virus and/or viral proteins can bind to dendritic cells or FDCs. HIV-specific antibody can recognize these bound molecules and potentially collaborate in the elimination of the cells by ADCC.

HIV envelope glycoproteins gp120 and gp160 manifest high-affinity binding to CD4 as well as to various chemokine receptors. Intracellular signals transduced by gp120 through both CD4 and CCR5/CXCR4 have been associated with a number of immunopathogenic processes including anergy, apoptosis, and abnormalities of cell trafficking. The molecular mechanisms responsible for these abnormalities include dysregulation of the T cell receptor–phosphoinositide pathway, p56lck activation, phosphorylation of focal adhesion kinase, activation of the MAP kinase and ras signaling pathways, and downregulation of the co-stimulatory molecules CD40 ligand and CD80.

The inexorable decline in CD4+ T cell counts that occurs in most HIV-infected individuals may result in part from the inability of the immune system to regenerate over an extended period of time the rapidly turning over CD4+ T cell pool efficiently enough to compensate for both HIV-mediated and naturally occurring attrition of cells. In this regard, the degree and duration of decline of CD4+ T cells at the time of initiation of therapy is an important predictor of the restoration of these cells. A person who maintains a very low CD4+ T cell count for a considerable period of time before the initiation of ART almost invariably has an incomplete reconstitution of such cells. At least two major mechanisms may contribute to the failure of the CD4+ T cell pool to reconstitute itself adequately over the course of HIV infection. The first is the destruction of lymphoid precursor cells, including thymic and bone marrow progenitor cells; the other is the gradual disruption of the lymphoid tissue microenvironment, which is essential for efficient regeneration of immunocompetent cells. Finally, during the advanced stages of CD4+ T lymphopenia, there are increased serum levels of the homeostatic cytokine IL-7. It was initially felt that this elevation was a homeostatic response to the lymphopenia; however, recent findings suggest that the increase in serum IL-7 was a result of reduced utilization of the cytokine related to the loss of cells expressing the IL-7 receptor, CD127, which serves as a normal physiologic regulator of IL-7 production.

CD8+ T cells

A relative CD8+ T lymphocytosis is generally associated with high levels of HIV plasma viremia and likely reflects dysregulated homeostasis associated with generalized immune activation. During the late stages of HIV infection, there may be a significant reduction in the numbers of CD8+ T cells despite the presence of high levels of viremia. HIV-specific CD8+ CTLs have been demonstrated in HIV-infected individuals early in the course of disease. The emergence of HIV escape mutants may ultimately evade these HIV-specific CD8+ T cells. However, as the disease progresses, the functional capability of these cells gradually decreases and may be lost entirely. The cause of this loss of cytolytic activity is unclear, although functional impairment is thought to be associated with the persistent nature of HIV infection and disease progression. In this regard, as chronic immune activation persists, CD8+ T cells assume an abnormal phenotype characterized by expression of activation markers such as HLA-DR and CD38 with an absence of expression of the IL-2 receptor (CD25), and a reduced expression of the IL-7 receptor (CD127). In addition, CD8+ T cells lacking CD28 expression are increased in HIV disease, reflecting a skewed expansion of a less differentiated CD8+ T cell subset. This skewing of subsets is also associated with diminished polyfunctionality, a qualitative difference that distinguishes nonprogressors from progressors. It has been reported that nonprogressors can also be distinguished from progressors by the maintenance in the former of a high proliferative capacity of their HIV-specific CD8+ T cells coupled to increases in perforin expression, characteristics that are markedly diminished in advanced HIV disease. It has been reported that the phenotype of CD8+ T cells in HIV-infected individuals may be of prognostic significance. Those individuals whose CD8+ T cells developed a phenotype of HLA-DR+/CD38– following seroconversion had stabilization of their CD4+ T cell counts, whereas those whose CD8+ T cells developed a phenotype of HLA-DR+/CD38+ had a more aggressive course and a poorer prognosis. In addition to the defects in HIV-specific CD8+ CTLs, functional defects in other MHC-restricted CTLs, such as those directed against influenza and CMV, have been demonstrated. CD8+ T cells secrete a variety of soluble factors that inhibit HIV replication including the CC-chemokines RANTES (CCL5), MIP-1α (CCL3), and MIP-1β (CCL4) as well as one or more as yet poorly identified factors. The presence of high levels of HIV viremia in vivo as well as exposure of CD8+ T cells in vitro to HIV envelope, both of which are associated with aberrant immune activation, have been shown to be associated with a variety of cellular functional abnormalities. Furthermore, since the integrity of CD8+ T cell function depends in part on adequate inductive signals from CD4+ T cells, the defect in CD8+ CTLs is likely compounded by the quantitative loss and qualitative dysfunction of CD4+ T cells. Finally, certain cell surface negative regulatory molecules such as CTLA-4 and PD-1 are upregulated on activated T cells, and engagement of these molecules with their ligands may play a role in the exhaustion and death of CD8+, HIV-specific T cells.

B cells

The predominant defect in B cells from HIV-infected individuals is one of aberrant cellular activation, which is reflected by spontaneous proliferation and immunoglobulin secretion and by increased spontaneous secretion of TNF-α and IL-6. In addition, B cells from HIV viremic patients manifest a decreased capacity to mount a proliferative response to ligation of the B cell antigen receptor and other B cell stimuli in vitro, yet at the same time they are capable of robust differentiation in vivo as a result of HIV-induced immune activation. B cells from HIV-infected individuals manifest enhanced spontaneous secretion of immunoglobulins in vitro, a process that reflects their highly differentiated state in vivo. There is also an increased incidence of EBV-related B cell lymphomas in HIV-infected individuals that are likely due to combined effects of defective T cell immune surveillance and increased turnover that increases the risk of oncogenesis. Untransformed B cells cannot be infected with HIV, although HIV or its products can activate B cells directly. B cells from patients with high levels of viremia bind virions to their surface via the CD21 complement receptor. It is likely that in vivo activation of B cells by replication-competent or -defective virus as well as viral products during the viremic state accounts at least in part for the spontaneous activation of these cells noted ex vivo. B cell subpopulations from HIV-infected individuals undergo a number of changes over the course of HIV disease, including the attrition of resting memory B cells and replacement with several aberrant memory and differentiated B cell subpopulations that collectively express reduced levels of CD21 and either increased expression of activation markers or inhibitory receptors associated with functional exhaustion. The more activated and differentiated B cells are also responsible for increased secretion of immunoglobulins and increased susceptibility to Fas-mediated apoptosis. In more advanced disease, there is also the appearance of immature B cells associated with CD4+ T cell lymphopenia. Cognate B cell–CD4+ T cell interactions are abnormal in viremic HIV-infected individuals in that B cells respond poorly to CD4+ T cell help and CD4+ T cells receive inadequate co-stimulatory signals from activated B cells. In vivo, the aberrant activated state of B cells manifests itself by hypergammaglobulinemia and by the presence of circulating immune complexes and autoantibodies. HIV-infected individuals respond poorly to primary and secondary immunizations with protein and polysaccharide antigens. Using immunization with influenza vaccine, it has been demonstrated that there is a memory B cell defect in HIV-infected individuals, particularly those with high levels of HIV viremia. Taken together, these B cell defects are likely responsible in part for the decreased response to vaccinations and the increase in certain bacterial infections seen in advanced HIV disease in adults, as well as for the important role of bacterial infections in the morbidity and mortality rates of HIV-infected children, who cannot mount an adequate humoral response to common bacterial pathogens. The absolute number of circulating B cells may be depressed in HIV infection; this phenomenon likely reflects increased activation-induced apoptosis as well as a redistribution of cells out of the circulation and into the lymphoid tissue—phenomena that are associated with ongoing viral replication.

Monocytes/macrophages

Circulating monocytes are generally normal in number in HIV-infected individuals. Monocytes express the CD4 molecule and several co-receptors for HIV on their surface, including CCR5, CXCR4, and CCR3, and thus are targets of HIV infection. The degree of cytopathicity of HIV for cells of the monocyte lineage is low, and HIV can replicate extensively in cells of the monocyte lineage with relatively little cytopathic effect. Hence, monocyte-lineage cells may play a role in the dissemination of HIV in the body and can serve as reservoirs of HIV infection, thus representing an obstacle to the eradication of HIV by antiretroviral drugs. In vivo infection of circulating monocytes is difficult to demonstrate; however, infection of tissue macrophages and macrophage-lineage cells in the brain (infiltrating macrophages or resident microglial cells) and lung (pulmonary alveolar macrophages) can be demonstrated easily. Tissue macrophages are an important source of HIV during the inflammatory response associated with opportunistic infections. Infection of monocyte precursors in the bone marrow may directly or indirectly be responsible for certain of the hematologic abnormalities in HIV-infected individuals. A number of abnormalities of circulating monocytes have been reported in HIV-infected individuals, many of which may be related directly or indirectly to aberrant in vivo immune activation. In this regard, increased levels of lipopolysaccharide (LPS) are found in the sera of HIV-infected individuals due, at least in part, to translocation across the gut mucosal barrier (see above). LPS is a highly inflammatory bacterial product that preferentially binds to macrophages through CD14 and Toll-like receptors, resulting in cellular activation. Increased levels of soluble CD14 in plasma are associated with poor overall clinical outcomes. Monocyte/macrophage functional abnormalities in HIV disease include decreased secretion of IL-1 and IL-12; increased secretion of IL-10; defects in antigen presentation and induction of T cell responses due to decreased MHC class II expression; and abnormalities of Fc receptor function, C3 receptor–mediated clearance, oxidative burst responses, and certain cytotoxic functions such as ADCC, possibly related to low levels of expression of Fc and complement receptors. Exposure of monocytes in vitro to viral proteins such as gp120 and Tat, as well as to certain cytokines, can cause abnormal activation, and this may play a role in cellular dysfunction.

Dendritic and Langerhans cells

Dendritic cells (DCs) may play an important role in the initiation of HIV infection by virtue of the ability of HIV to bind to cell-surface C-type lectin receptors, particularly DC-SIGN (see above). This allows efficient presentation of virus to CD4+ T cell targets that become infected; complexes of infected CD4+ T cells and DCs provide an optimal microenvironment for virus replication. There has been considerable disagreement regarding the HIV infectibility and hence the depletion as well as the dysfunction of DCs themselves. The situation has recently been clarified by the recognition that DCs can be classified into myeloid (mDC) and plasmacytoid (pDC) subsets, leading to an appreciation of specific DC dysfunction in HIV disease. pDCs are an important component of the innate immune system and secrete large amounts of IFN-α in response to viral infections. The numbers of circulating pDCs are decreased in HIV infection through mechanisms that remain unclear. It has recently been demonstrated that HIV gp120 interacts directly with pDCs and interferes with TLR9 activation, resulting in a decreased ability of pDCs to secrete antiviral and inflammatory factors that play a role in immune responses against invading pathogens.

Natural killer cells

The role of NK cells is to provide immunosurveillance against virus-infected cells, certain tumor cells, and allogeneic cells (Chap. 314). There are no convincing data that HIV productively infects NK cells in vivo; however, functional abnormalities in NK cells have been observed throughout the course of HIV disease, and the severity of these abnormalities increases as disease progresses. In addition, it has been reported that HIV envelope induces aberrant signaling in NK cells that increases their susceptibility to apoptosis. HIV infection of target cells downregulates HLA-A and -B, but not HLA-C and -D molecules; this may explain in part the relative inability of NK cells to kill HIV-infected target cells. Most studies report that NK cells are normal in number; however, patients with high levels of virus replication manifest an abnormal representation of a functionally defective CD56–/CD16+ NK cell subset. This abnormal subset of NK cells manifests an increased expression of inhibitory NK cell receptors (iNKRs) and a substantial decrease in expression of natural cytotoxicity receptors (NCRs) and shows a markedly impaired lytic activity. The overrepresentation of this abnormal subset of NK cells may explain in part the observed defects in NK cell function in HIV-infected individuals. NK cells also serve as important sources of HIV-inhibitory CC-chemokines. NK cells isolated from HIV-infected individuals constitutively produce high levels of MIP-1α (CCL3), MIP-1β (CCL4), and RANTES (CCL5). In addition, high levels of these chemokines are seen when NK cells are stimulated with IL-2 or IL-15 or when CD16 is cross-linked or during the process of lytic killing of target cells. HIV-infected patients with high levels of plasma viremia manifest a decreased ability, compared with HIV-infected individuals who are aviremic, of their NK cells to block HIV replication in vitro in assays of both cell contact and supernatant-mediated suppression of virus. Finally, NK cell–dendritic cell interactions are important for normal immune function. NK cells and dendritic cells reciprocally modulate each other's activation and maturation. These interactions are markedly impaired in HIV-infected individuals with high levels of plasma viremia.

■ GENETIC FACTORS IN HIV PATHOGENESIS

Genetic association studies have served as a powerful means to identify host factors that influence HIV-AIDS pathogenesis in vivo. Polymorphisms in several genes have now been identified that influence several phenotypes relevant to HIV infection: risk of acquiring HIV, rates of disease progression, long-term nonprogression, spontaneous virologic control, and immunologic responses following initiation of ART. These include polymorphisms in genes in the MHC locus, chemokine receptors and chemokines, cytokines, and other host factors (Table 189-5). Recent studies have capitalized on genome-wide association studies to identify novel genetic factors that influence HIV disease progression rates, and rapid progress is anticipated in this area. Moreover, in vitro genome-wide functional scanning using RNA interference techniques suggests that up to hundreds of host factors may be involved in the HIV replication life cycle. Theoretically, variations in all these genes could impact HIV susceptibility and/or disease progression. Below is a discussion of some representative genes.

Researchers recently employed a genome-wide association strategy and identified polymorphisms within HLA-B (e.g., HCP-5 gene) and HLA-C that explained approximately 15% of the variation in viral load among individuals during the asymptomatic period of infection. A number of mechanisms have been proposed whereby MHC-encoded molecules might predispose an individual either to rapid progression or to nonprogression to AIDS. These proposed mechanisms include the ability to present certain immunodominant HIV T helper or CTL epitopes, leading to a relatively protective immune response against HIV and hence to a slower rate of disease progression. In contrast, certain MHC class I or class II alleles might predispose an individual to an immunopathogenic response against viral epitopes in certain tissues, such as the CNS or lungs, or against certain HIV-infected cell types, such as macrophages or dendritic cells/Langerhans cells. In addition, certain rare MHC class I and class II alleles might facilitate rapid recognition of HIV-infected cells from the infecting partner in primary HIV infection and promote rejection of these cells by alloreactive responses. Similarly, common MHC alleles could lead to less effective removal of HIV-infected allogeneic cells. In this regard, it has been demonstrated that allele sharing at HLA-B locus is associated with increased risk of transmission of HIV infection between heterosexual Zambian couples discordant for HIV. It has also been demonstrated that HLA heterozygosity for class I loci (A, B, and C) is associated with a delayed onset of AIDS among HIV-infected individuals, whereas homozygosity for these loci is associated with a more rapid progression to AIDS and death. This observation is likely due to the fact that individuals who are heterozygous at HLA loci are able to present a greater variety of antigenic peptides to cytotoxic T lymphocytes than are homozygotes, resulting in a more effective immune response against a number of pathogens including HIV. Of particular note is the fact that the HLA class I alleles B*35 and Cw*04 were consistently associated with rapid development of AIDS. Other data have indicated that transporter associated with antigen-processing (TAP) genes play a role in determining the outcome of HIV infection. HLA profiles that reflect certain combinations of MHC-encoded TAP and class I and class II genes are strongly associated with different rates of progression to AIDS. It is noteworthy that the extended HLA haplotype 8.1 (A1-B8-DR3) has also been consistently correlated with a rapid decline in CD4+ T cells and development of HIV-related symptoms.

Recent genetic association studies have also highlighted the role for NK cells in HIV disease. A single nucleotide polymorphism (SNP) in the killer immunoglobulin-like receptor (KIR) gene was shown to be strongly associated with rapid progression to AIDS. However, when KIR3DS1 was present with HLA-Bw4-80I, the resultant phenotype was delayed progression to AIDS, even though this HLA-B allele alone has no effect on HIV disease progression. Furthermore, KIR3DS1/HLA-Bw4-80I-carrying individuals had a significantly reduced viral load, beginning early in the course of infection, and protection against opportunistic infections during the later stages of the disease. This observation points to the potential role of NK cells in the maintenance of the viral set point and strongly suggests that HLA-Bw4-80I serves as the ligand activating the KIR, resulting in the death of the target cell. These gene-gene interactions between KIR and MHC genes are illustrated in Table 189-5.

The most dramatic example of a genetic factor influencing HIV infection and/or pathogenesis relates to the gene that encodes for CC chemokine receptor 5 (CCR5), the major HIV co-receptor for cell entry. There are reports of rare individuals who have remained uninfected despite repetitive sexual exposure to HIV in high-risk situations (e.g., commercial sex workers). The peripheral blood mononuclear cells of two such individuals were found to be highly resistant to infection in vitro with R5 strains of HIV-1 but were readily infected with X4 strains. Genetic analysis revealed that these two individuals inherited a homozygous defect in the gene that encodes for CCR5. The defective CCR5 allele contained a 32-bp deletion corresponding to the second extracellular loop of the receptor (Δ32 allele). The encoded protein is severely truncated and is not expressed on the cell surface; it is therefore nonfunctional, explaining the refractoriness to infection with R5 strains of HIV-1. Population studies revealed that ~1% of the Caucasian population of western European ancestry possessed the homozygous defect for the CCR5 Δ32 allele, and subjects with this genotype are highly

Gene[a]	Genetic Variation	Mechanisms[b]	Genetic Effect on HIV-AIDS[c]
Genes in MHC Locus			
HLA-B	B*27 and B*57	Presentation of specific immunogenic HIV antigens	Slow progression to AIDS; low viral load
	B*35Px	Restriction of specific immunogenic HIV peptide presentation	Fast progression to AIDS; high viral load
	HLA-Bw4	Providing ligands for activating KIR	Slow progression to AIDS
HLA class I allele	Homozygosity of HLA-A, B, C alleles	Reduced epitope recognition repertoire	Faster progression to AIDS; increased risk of mother-to-child transmission
	Shared donor-recipient HLA alleles	Preadaptation of HIV strains	Faster disease progression
	Rare HLA alleles	Limited adaptation of HIV strains; less frequent escape mutants	Protection against HIV infection
HLA extended haplotype	A1-B8-DR3-DQ2 (8.1)	Unknown; may influence immunologic hyperresponsiveness	Faster progression to AIDS
HLA-C	rs9264942-C	Increased expression of HLA-C; association may be due to linkage disequilibrium with HLA-B57	Decreased viral load set point
HCP5	rs2395029-G	Linkage disequilibrium with HLA-B*5701	Reduced viremia
ZNRD1	rs9261174-C	Possible interference in processing of HIV transcripts; influences ZNRD1 expression; linkage disequilibrium with *HLA-A10*	AIDS disease retardation
Chemokine Receptors			
CCR5	32-bp deletion in the ORF (Δ32)	Truncated CCR5 protein	Δ32/Δ32: resistance to acquiring HIV infection
			Δ32/wt: Delays AIDS onset; improves immune reconstitution during ART
	Promoter SNPs/ haplotypes (HHA to HHG*2)	Altered CCR5 expression, e.g., HHE allele correlates with high CCR5 expression	HHE/HHE genotype associates with increased HIV/AIDS susceptibility
CCR2	Valine to isoleucine change (64 V→I)	Possibly due to linkage with polymorphism in *CCR5* promoter	Delayed AIDS onset
CX3CR1	SNPs in ORF (*249 V→I, 280 T→M*)	280M reduces receptor expression and binding of fractalkine, the CX3CR1 ligand	249I and 280M are associated with faster AIDS onset in some Caucasian cohorts; inconsistent effects were detected in other cohorts
DARC	African-specific promoter SNP (*46T→C*)	−46C/C associates with low neutrophil counts; influences circulating chemokine levels; alters HIV binding to RBCs and transinfection of HIV-1	−46C/C: increased risk of acquiring HIV but slow HIV disease progression; the disease-retarding effects associated with −46C/C occur mainly in those HIV+ African Americans who are also leukopenic
Chemokines			
CCL3L, CCL4L	Gene copy number of *CCL3L* and *CCL4L*	High gene copies correlate with high CCL3L and CCL4L levels	Gene copy number lower than population median associates with increased HIV/AIDS susceptibility and reduced immune reconstitution during ART
CCL5	Promoter SNPs	Altered gene expression	Altered HIV-AIDS susceptibility
CCL2	Promoter SNP (−2578 T→G)	*−2578G allele:* increased CCL2 expression and monocyte recruitment	−2578G/G associates with increased risk of developing HIV-1-associated dementia and a rapid AIDS onset
Cytokines			
IL-6	Promoter SNP (−174 G→C)	−174C associates with altered IL-6 and CRP levels	Altered risk of KS development and variable recovery of CD4 cells during ART
IL-10	Promoter SNP	−592A results in decreased IL-10 levels	Increased HIV-AIDS susceptibility
Innate Immunity Genes			
MBL	Coding alleles (O)	Low plasma concentration and structural damage of MBL	Slow progression to AIDS in heterozygous subjects (A/O)
	X allele (promoter SNP −221)	Decreased levels of MBL	Faster progression to AIDS in homozygous X/X subjects
Apobec-3G	ORF SNP (186 H→R)	Reduced anti-HIV-1 activity	186R associates with rapid AIDS onset in African Americans

(continued)

Gene[a]	Genetic Variation	Mechanisms[b]	Genetic Effect on HIV-AIDS[c]
Others			
ApoE	E4, E3, E2 allele	E4 enhances HIV cell entry in vitro	ApoE4/E4 associates with rapid AIDS onset and dementia
Gene–Gene Interaction			
KIR+HLA	KIR3DS1 with HLA Bw4-80I + or 80I −	Altered NK cell activity required to kill HIV-infected cells	KIR3DS1 with HLA Bw4-80I +: delayed AIDS onset KIR3DS1 with HLA Bw4-80I −: rapid AIDS onset
CCL3L1 + CCR5	Low CCL3L1 gene copies + detrimental CCR5 genotypes	Low CCL3L1 and high CCR5 expression	Increased HIV/AIDS susceptibility and reduced immune reconstitution during ART

[a]Representative genes and polymorphisms and [b]possible mechanisms are listed. [c]Some of the associations are population specific and may display cohort-specific effects.

Note: Apobec, apolipoprotein B mRNA editing enzyme, catalytic polypeptide-like; ApoE, apolipoprotein E; ART, antiretroviral therapy; CCL, CC ligand; CCL3L, CCL3-like; CCR5, CC chemokine receptor 5; CRP, C-reactive protein; DARC, Duffy antigen receptor for chemokines; HCP5, HLA class I histocompatibility antigen protein P5; HHE, human haplogroup E; HLA, human leukocyte antigen; IL, interleukin; KIR, killer cell immunoglobulin-like receptors; KS, Kaposi's sarcoma; MBL, mannose-binding lectin; MHC, major histocompatibility complex; ORF, open reading frame; SNP, single nucleotide polymorphism; VL, viral load; wt, wild-type; ZNRD1, zinc ribbon domain containing 1; +, present; −, absent.

Sources: Sunil K. Ahuja, MD, Weijing He, MD, and *www.hiv-pharmacogenomics.org*. Reviews for additional information: P An et al: Trends Genet 26:119, 2010; J Fellay: Antivir Ther 14:731, 2009; RA Kaslow et al: J Infect Dis 191:S68, 2005.

resistant to HIV infection. A number of studies have found that the frequency of *CCR5 Δ32* allele was enriched in exposed, uninfected individuals of European descent. It is noteworthy that several individuals have been identified as homozygous for the *CCR5 Δ32* defect and in fact did become infected with HIV. These individuals were found to have an X4 strain of HIV that was associated in some cases with an accelerated disease course. X4 strain uses CXCR4 as the co-receptor for cell entry instead of CCR5. Up to 20% of individuals of European descent are heterozygous for the *CCR5 Δ32* allele and display partial resistance to acquiring HIV and a delayed disease course. Cohort studies of hundreds of DNA samples originating from western and central Africa and Far East Asia indicate that the *CCR5 Δ32* allele is either absent or extremely rare in these populations.

A number of SNPs in the *CCR5* promoter have been associated with varied rates of disease progression and altered risk of acquiring HIV. The promoter SNPs along the *CCR5 Δ32* and CCR2-V64I alleles define nine *CCR5* human haplogroups (HH) designated as HHA through HHE, HHF*1, HHF*2, HHG*1 and HHG*2 (Table 189-5). Studies have shown that homozygosity for the *CCR5* HHE haplotype is associated with an increased risk of acquiring HIV and progressing rapidly to AIDS. Pairing of the HHC and the *CCR5 Δ32*-containing HHG*2 haplotype is associated with a slower rate of disease progression and reduced risk of acquiring HIV. Heterozygosity for the *CCR2-64I* polymorphism associates with a slow rate of HIV disease course. This *CCR2-64I* allele–associated effect could be due to its linkage with SNPs in the *CCR5* promoter that are known to influence disease progression rates and/or due to dimerization of CXCR4 with the mutated *CCR2-64I*, resulting in a decreased expression of CXCR4 on the cell surface. Variations in the ligands of CCR5 (e.g., copy number of *CCL3L* genes) and CCR2 (e.g., *CCL2*) may also influence HIV-AIDS susceptibility.

NEUROPATHOGENESIS

While there has been a remarkable decrease in the incidence of HIV encephalopathy among those with access to treatment in the era of effective cART, HIV-infected individuals can still experience a variety of neurologic abnormalities due either to opportunistic infections and neoplasms or to direct effects of HIV or its products. With regard to the latter, HIV has been demonstrated in the brain and CSF of infected individuals with and without neuropsychiatric abnormalities. The main cell types that are infected in the brain in vivo are the perivascular macrophages and the microglial cells; monocytes that have already been infected in the blood can migrate into the brain, where they then reside as macrophages, or macrophages can be directly infected within the brain. The precise mechanisms whereby HIV enters the brain are unclear; however, they are thought to relate, at least in part, to the ability of virus-infected and immune-activated macrophages to induce adhesion molecules such as E-selectin and vascular cell adhesion molecule 1 (VCAM-1) on brain endothelium. Other studies have demonstrated that HIV gp120 enhances the expression of intercellular adhesion molecule 1 (ICAM-1) in glial cells; this effect may facilitate entry of HIV-infected cells into the CNS. Virus isolates from the brain are preferentially R5 strains as opposed to X4 strains; in this regard, HIV-infected individuals who are heterozygous for *CCR5-Δ32* appear to be relatively protected against the development of HIV encephalopathy compared with wild-type individuals. Distinct HIV envelope sequences are associated with the clinical expression of the AIDS dementia complex (see below). There is no convincing evidence that brain cells other than those of monocyte/macrophage lineage can be productively infected in vivo.

HIV-infected individuals may manifest white matter lesions as well as neuronal loss. Given the absence of evidence of HIV infection of neurons either in vivo or in vitro, it is highly unlikely that direct infection of these cells accounts for their loss. Rather, the HIV-mediated effects on neurons and oligodendrocytes are thought to involve indirect pathways whereby viral proteins, particularly gp120 and Tat, trigger the release of endogenous neurotoxins from macrophages and to a lesser extent from astrocytes. In addition, it has been demonstrated that both HIV-1 Nef and Tat can induce chemotaxis of leukocytes, including monocytes, into the CNS. Neurotoxins can be released from monocytes as a consequence of infection and/or immune activation. Monocyte-derived neurotoxic factors have been reported to kill neurons via the N-methyl-D-aspartate (NMDA) receptor. In addition, HIV gp120 shed by virus-infected monocytes could cause neurotoxicity by antagonizing the function of vasoactive intestinal peptide (VIP), by elevating intracellular calcium levels, and by decreasing nerve growth factor levels in the cerebral cortex. A variety of monocyte-derived cytokines can contribute directly or indirectly to the neurotoxic effects in HIV infection; these include TNF-α, IL-1, IL-6, TGF-β, IFN-γ, platelet-activating factor, and endothelin. Furthermore, among the CC-chemokines, elevated levels of monocyte chemotactic protein (MCP) 1 in the brain and CSF have been shown to correlate best with the presence and degree of HIV encephalopathy. In addition, infection and/or activation of monocyte-lineage cells can result in increased production of eicosanoids, quinolinic acid, nitric oxide, excitatory amino acids such as L-cysteine and glutamate, arachidonic acid, platelet activating factor, free radicals, TNF-α, and TGF-β, which may contribute to neurotoxicity. Astrocytes may play diverse roles in HIV neuropathogenesis. Reactive gliosis or astrocytosis has been demonstrated in the brains of HIV-infected individuals, and TNF-α and IL-6 have been shown to induce astrocyte proliferation. In addition, astrocyte-derived IL-6 can induce HIV expression in infected cells in vitro. Furthermore, it has been suggested that astrocytes may downregulate macrophage-produced neurotoxins. It has been reported that HIV-infected individuals with the E4 allele for apolipoprotein E (apo E) are at increased risk for AIDS encephalopathy and peripheral neuropathy. The likelihood that HIV or its products are involved in neuropathogenesis is supported by the observation that neuropsychiatric abnormalities may undergo remarkable and rapid improvement upon the initiation of cART.

It has also been suggested that the CNS may serve as a relatively sequestered site for a reservoir of latently infected cells that might be a barrier for the eradication of virus by cART (see "Reservoirs of HIV-Infected Cells: Obstacles to the Eradication of Virus," above).

■ PATHOGENESIS OF KAPOSI'S SARCOMA

There are at least four distinct epidemiologic forms of KS: (1) the classic form that occurs in older men of predominantly Mediterranean or eastern European Jewish backgrounds with no recognized contributing factors; (2) the equatorial African form that occurs in all ages, also without any recognized precipitating factors; (3) the form associated with organ transplantation and its attendant iatrogenic immunosuppressed state; and (4) the form associated with HIV-1 infection. In the latter two forms, KS is an opportunistic disease; in HIV-infected individuals, unlike typical opportunistic infections, its occurrence is not strictly related to the level of depression of CD4+ T cell counts. The pathogenesis of KS is complex; fundamentally, it is an angioproliferative disease that is not a true neoplastic sarcoma, at least not in its early stages. It is a manifestation of excessive proliferation of spindle cells that are believed to be of vascular origin and have features in common with endothelial and smooth-muscle cells. In HIV disease the development of KS is dependent on the interplay of a variety of factors including HIV-1 itself, human herpes virus 8 (HHV-8), immune activation, and cytokine secretion. A number of epidemiologic and virologic studies have clearly linked HHV-8, which is also referred to as Kaposi's sarcoma–associated herpesvirus (KSHV), to KS not only in HIV-infected individuals but also in individuals with the other forms of KS. HHV-8 is a γ-herpesvirus related to EBV and herpesvirus saimiri. It encodes a homologue to human IL-6 and, in addition to KS, has been implicated in the pathogenesis of body cavity lymphoma, multiple myeloma, and monoclonal gammopathy of undetermined significance. Sequences of HHV-8 are found universally in the lesions of KS, and patients with KS are virtually

all seropositive for HHV-8. HHV-8 DNA sequences can be found in the B cells of 30–50% of patients with KS and 7% of patients with AIDS without clinically apparent KS.

Between 1 and 2% of eligible blood donors are positive for antibodies to HHV-8, while the prevalence of HHV-8 seropositivity in HIV-infected men is 30–35%. The prevalence of HHV-8 seropositivity in HIV-infected women is ~4%. This finding is reflective of the lower incidence of KS in women. It has been debated whether HHV-8 is actually the transforming agent in KS; the bulk of the cells in the tumor lesions of KS are not neoplastic cells. However, it has been demonstrated that endothelial cells can be transformed in vitro by HHV-8. In this regard, HHV-8 possesses a number of genes, including homologues of the IL-8 receptor, Bcl-2, and cyclin D, that can potentially transform the host cell. Despite the complexity of the pathogenic events associated with the development of KS in HIV-infected individuals, HHV-8 is the etiologic agent of this disease. The initiation and/or propagation of KS requires an activated state and is mediated, at least in part, by cytokines. A number of factors, including TNF-α, IL-1β, IL-6, GM-CSF, basic fibroblast growth factor, and oncostatin M, function in an autocrine and paracrine manner to sustain the growth and chemotaxis of the KS spindle cells. In this regard, KSHV-derived IL-6 has been demonstrated to induce proliferation of lymphoma cells and to inhibit the cytostatic effects of INF-α on KSHV-infected lymphoma cells.

IMMUNE RESPONSE TO HIV

As detailed above and below, following the initial burst of viremia during primary infection, HIV-infected individuals mount robust immune responses that in most cases substantially curtail the levels of plasma viremia and likely contribute to delaying the ultimate development of clinically apparent disease for a median of 10 years in untreated individuals. This immune response contains elements of both humoral and cell-mediated immunity involving both innate and adaptive immune responses (Table 189-6; Fig. 189-26). It is directed against multiple antigenic determinants of the HIV virion as well as against viral proteins expressed on the surface of infected cells. Ironically, those CD4+ T cells with T cell receptors specific for HIV are theoretically those CD4+ T cells most likely to be

TABLE 189-6 Elements of the Immune Response to HIV

Humoral immunity
  Binding antibodies
  Neutralizing antibodies
    Type specific
    Group specific
  Antibodies participating in antibody-dependent cellular cytotoxicity (ADCC)
    Protective
    Pathogenic (bystander killing)
  Enhancing antibodies
  Complement
Cell-mediated immunity
  Helper CD4+ T lymphocytes
  Class I MHC–restricted cytotoxic CD8+ T lymphocytes
  CD8+ T cell–mediated inhibition (noncytolytic)
  ADCC
  Natural killer cells

Abbreviation: MHC, major histocompatibility complex.

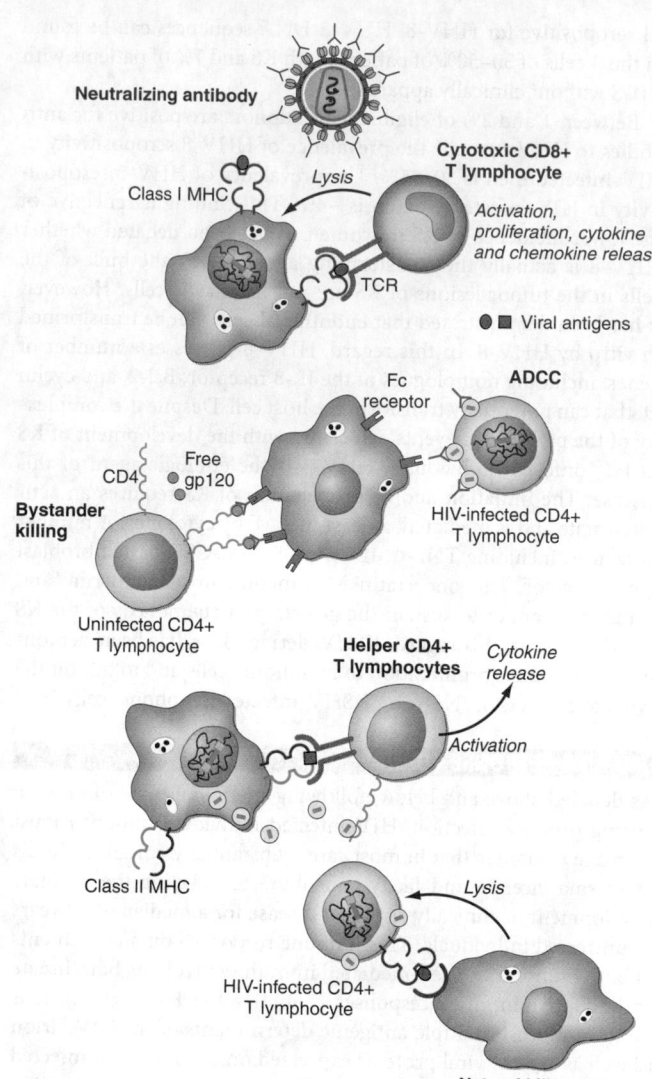

Figure 189-26 **Schematic representation of the different immunologic effector mechanisms** thought to be active in the setting of HIV infection. Detailed descriptions are given in the text. ADCC, antibody-dependent cellular cytotoxicity; MHC, major histocompatibility complex; TCR, T cell receptor.

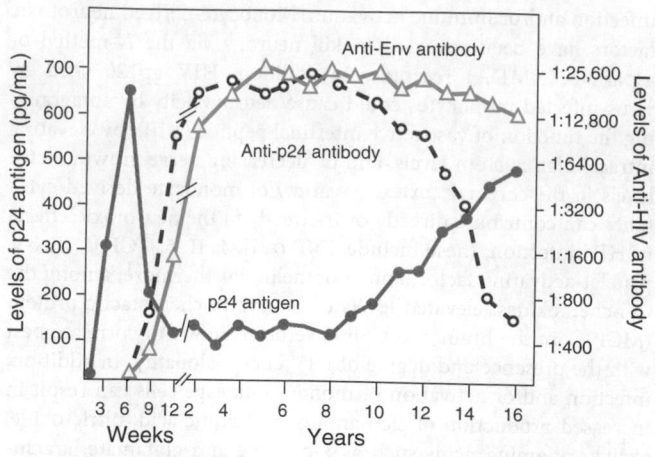

Figure 189-27 **Relationship between antigenemia and the development of antibodies to HIV.** Antibodies to HIV proteins are generally seen 6–12 weeks following infection and 3–6 weeks after the development of plasma viremia. Late in the course of illness, antibody levels to p24 decline, generally in association with a rising titer of p24 antigen.

activated—and thus to serve as early targets for productive HIV infection and the cell death or dysfunction associated with infection. Thus, an early consequence of HIV infection is interference with and decrease of the helper T cell population needed to generate an effective immune response.

Although a great deal of investigation has been directed toward delineating and better understanding the components of this immune response, it remains unclear which immunologic effector mechanisms are most important in delaying progression of infection and which, if any, play a role in the pathogenesis of HIV disease. This lack of knowledge has also hampered the ability to develop an effective vaccine for HIV disease.

■ HUMORAL IMMUNE RESPONSE

Antibodies to HIV usually appear within 3–6 weeks and almost invariably within 12 weeks of primary infection (Fig. 189-27); rare exceptions are individuals who have defects in the ability to produce HIV-specific antibodies. Detection of these antibodies forms the basis of most diagnostic screening tests for HIV infection. The appearance of HIV-binding antibodies detected by ELISA and

Western blot assays occurs prior to the appearance of neutralizing antibodies; the latter generally appear following the initial decreases in plasma viremia, which is more closely related to the appearance of HIV-specific CD8+ T lymphocytes. The first antibodies detected are those directed against the immunodominant region of the envelope gp41, followed by the appearance of antibodies to the structural or gag protein p24 and the gag precursor p55. Antibodies to p24 gag are followed by the appearance of antibodies to the outer envelope glycoprotein (gp120), the gag protein p17, and the products of the *pol* gene (p31 and p66). In addition, one may see antibodies to the low-molecular-weight regulatory proteins encoded by the HIV genes *vpr, vpu, vif, rev, tat,* and *nef.* On rare occasion, levels of HIV-specific antibodies may decline during treatment of acute HIV infection.

While antibodies to multiple antigens of HIV are produced, the precise functional significance of these different antibodies is unclear. The only viral proteins that elicit neutralizing antibodies are the envelope proteins gp120 and gp41. Antibodies directed toward the envelope proteins of HIV have been characterized both as being protective and as possibly contributing to the pathogenesis of HIV disease. Among the protective antibodies are those that function to neutralize HIV directly and prevent the spread of infection to additional cells, as well as those that participate in ADCC. Within the first 6 months of infection, neutralizing antibodies appear; however, the virus quickly escapes these neutralizing antibodies. One of the principal mechanisms of immune escape is the addition of N-linked glycosylation sites. The added carbohydrate moieties interfere with envelope recognition by these initial antibodies. The hyperglycosylation of the envelope protein has been termed the *glycan shield.* Neutralizing antibodies appear to be of two forms, type-specific and group-specific. *Type-specific neutralizing antibodies* are generally directed to the V3 loop region. These antibodies appear early after infection and are generally directed toward linear epitopes within the V2 and V3 variable regions of gp120. They neutralize only viruses of a given strain and are present in low titer in most infected individuals. *Group-specific neutralizing antibodies* appear later in infection and are capable of neutralizing a wide variety of HIV isolates. At least two forms of group-specific antibodies have been identified: those directed toward the CD4 binding site (CD4bs) of gp120, and those binding to the membrane-proximal region of gp41 (Fig. 189-28). The other major class of protective antibodies are those that participate in ADCC, which is actually a form of

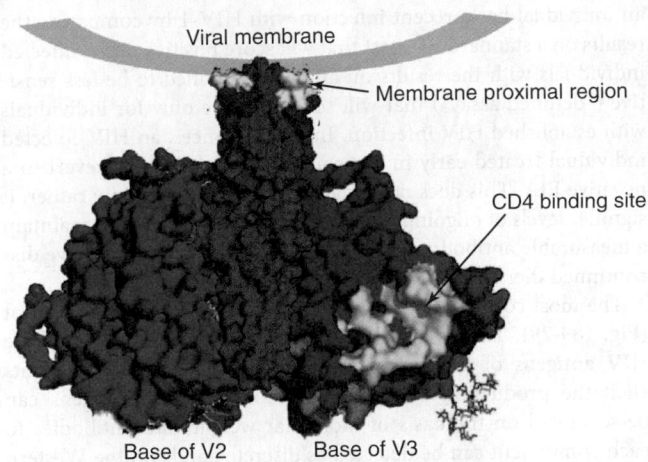

Figure 189-28 Known targets of neutralizing antibodies against HIV-1. Group-specific antibody-binding regions include the membrane proximal region and the CD4 binding site. Type-specific antibody-binding regions include V2 and V3 loops. *(Adapted from DR Burton et al: Nat Immunol 5:233, 2004.)*

cell-mediated immunity (Chap. 314) in which NK cells that bear Fc receptors are armed with specific anti-HIV antibodies that bind to the NK cells via their Fc portion. These armed NK cells then bind to and destroy cells expressing HIV antigens. Antibodies to both gp120 and gp41 have been shown to participate in ADCC-mediated killing of HIV-infected cells. The levels of antienvelope antibodies capable of mediating ADCC are highest in the earlier stages of HIV infection. In vitro, IL-2 can augment ADCC-mediated killing.

In addition to playing a role in host defense, HIV-specific antibodies have also been implicated in disease pathogenesis. Antibodies directed to gp41, when present in low titer, have been shown in vitro to be capable of facilitating infection of cells through an Fc receptor–mediated mechanism known as *antibody enhancement*. Thus, the same regions of the envelope protein of HIV that give rise to antibodies capable of mediating ADCC also elicit the production of antibodies that can facilitate infection of cells in vitro. In addition, it has been postulated that anti-gp120 antibodies that participate in the ADCC killing of HIV-infected cells might also kill uninfected CD4+ T cells if the uninfected cells had bound free gp120, a phenomenon referred to as *bystander killing*. One of the most primitive components of the humoral immune system is the complement system (Chap. 314). This element of innate immunity consists of ~30 proteins that are found circulating in blood or associated with cell membranes. While HIV alone is capable of directly activating the complement cascade, the resulting lysis is weak due to the presence of host cell regulatory proteins captured in the virion envelope during budding. It is possible that complement-opsonized HIV virions have increased infectivity in a manner analogous to antibody-mediated enhancement.

■ CELLULAR IMMUNE RESPONSE

Given the fact that T cell–mediated immunity is known to play a major role in host defense against most viral infections (Chap. 314), it is generally thought to be an important component of the host immune response to HIV. T cell immunity can be divided into two major categories: that mediated by *helper/inducer CD4+ T cells* and that mediated by *cytotoxic/immunoregulatory CD8+ T cells*.

HIV-specific CD4+ T cells can be detected in the majority of HIV-infected patients through the use of flow cytometry to measure intracellular cytokine production in response to MHC class II tetramers pulsed with HIV peptides or through lymphocyte proliferation assays utilizing HIV antigens such as p24. These cells likely play a critical role in the orchestration of the immune response to HIV by providing help to HIV-specific B cells and CD8+ T cells. They may also be capable of directly killing HIV-infected cells. HIV-specific CD4+ T cells may be preferential targets of HIV infection by HIV-infected antigen-presenting cells during the generation of an immune response to HIV (Fig. 189-26). However, they also are likely to undergo clonal expansions in response to HIV antigens and thus survive as a population of cells. No clear correlations exist between levels of HIV-specific CD4+ T lymphocytes and plasma HIV RNA levels; however, in the setting of high viral loads, CD4+ T cell responses to HIV antigens appear to shift from one of proliferation and IL-2 production to one of IFN-γ production. Thus, while a reverse correlation exists between the level of p24-specific proliferation and levels of plasma HIV viremia, the nature of the causal relationship between these parameters is unclear.

MHC class I–restricted, HIV-specific CD8+ T cells have been identified in the peripheral blood of patients with HIV-1 infection. These cells include CTLs that produce perforins and T cells that can be induced by HIV antigens to express an array of cytokines such as IFN-γ, IL-2, and TNF-α. CTLs have been identified in the peripheral blood of patients within weeks of HIV infection and prior to the appearance of plasma virus. The selective pressure they exert on the evolution of the population of circulating viruses reflects their potential role in control of HIV infection. These CD8+ T lymphocytes, through their HIV-specific antigen receptors, bind to and cause the lytic destruction of target cells bearing autologous MHC class I molecules presenting HIV antigens. Two types of CTL activity can be demonstrated in the peripheral blood or lymph node mononuclear cells of HIV-infected individuals. The first type directly lyses appropriate target cells in culture without prior in vitro stimulation (*spontaneous CTL activity*). The other type of CTL activity reflects the *precursor frequency of CTLs* (CTLp); this type of CTL activity can be demonstrated by stimulation of CD8+ T cells in vitro with a mitogen such as phytohemagglutinin or anti-CD3 antibody.

In addition to CTLs, CD8+ T cells capable of being induced by HIV antigens to express cytokines such as IFN-γ also appear in the setting of HIV-1 infection. It is not clear whether these are the same or different effector pools compared with those cells mediating cytotoxicity; in addition, the relative roles of each in host defense against HIV are not fully understood. It does appear that these CD8+ T cells are driven to in vivo expansion by HIV antigen. There is a direct correlation between levels of CD8+ T cells capable of producing IFN-γ in response to HIV antigens and plasma levels of HIV-1 RNA. Thus, while these cells are clearly induced by HIV-1 infection, their overall ability to control infection remains unclear. Multiple HIV antigens, including Gag, Env, Pol, Tat, Rev, and Nef, can elicit CD8+ T cell responses. Among patients who control viral replication in the absence of antiretroviral drugs are a subset of patients referred to as elite nonprogressors (see "Long-Term Survivors and Long-Term Nonprogressors," above) whose peripheral blood contains a population of CD8+ T cells that undergo substantial proliferation and perforin expression in response to HIV antigens. It is possible that these cells play an important role in HIV-specific host defense.

At least three other forms of cell-mediated immunity to HIV have been described: CD8+ T cell–mediated suppression of HIV replication, ADCC, and NK cell activity. *CD8+ T cell–mediated suppression of HIV replication* refers to the ability of CD8+ T cells from an HIV-infected patient to inhibit the replication of HIV in tissue culture in a noncytolytic manner. There is no requirement for HLA compatibility between the CD8+ T cells and the HIV-infected cells. This effector mechanism is thus nonspecific and appears to be mediated by soluble factor(s) including the CC-chemokines

RANTES (CCL5), MIP-1α (CCL3), and MIP-1β (CCL4). These CC-chemokines are potent suppressors of HIV replication and operate at least in part via blockade of the HIV co-receptor (*CCR5*) for R5 (macrophage-tropic) strains of HIV-1 (see above). *ADCC*, as described above in relation to humoral immunity, involves the killing of HIV-expressing cells by NK cells armed with specific antibodies directed against HIV antigens. Finally, *NK cells* alone have been shown to be capable of killing HIV-infected target cells in tissue culture. This primitive cytotoxic mechanism of host defense is directed toward nonspecific surveillance for neoplastic transformation and viral infection through recognition of altered class I MHC molecules.

DIAGNOSIS AND LABORATORY MONITORING OF HIV INFECTION

The establishment of HIV as the causative agent of AIDS and related syndromes early in 1984 was followed by the rapid development of sensitive screening tests for HIV infection. By March 1985, blood donors in the United States were routinely screened for antibodies to HIV. In 1996, blood banks in the United States added the p24 antigen capture assay to the screening process to help identify the rare infected individuals who were donating blood in the time (up to 3 months) between infection and the development of antibodies. In 2002, the ability to detect early infection with HIV was further enhanced by the licensure of nucleic acid testing (NAT) as a routine part of blood donor screening. These refinements decreased the interval between infection and detection (window period) from 22 days for antibody testing to 16 days with p24 antigen testing and subsequently to 12 days with nucleic acid testing. The development of sensitive assays for monitoring levels of plasma viremia ushered in a new era of being able to monitor the progression of HIV disease more closely. Utilization of these tests, coupled with the measurement of levels of CD4+ T lymphocytes in peripheral blood, is essential in the management of patients with HIV infection.

■ DIAGNOSIS OF HIV INFECTION

The CDC has recommended that screening for HIV infection be performed as a matter of routine health care. The diagnosis of HIV infection depends on the demonstration of antibodies to HIV and/or the direct detection of HIV or one of its components. As noted above, antibodies to HIV generally appear in the circulation 3–12 weeks following infection.

The standard blood screening test for HIV infection is the ELISA, also referred to as an *enzyme immunoassay* (EIA). This solid-phase assay is an extremely good screening test with a sensitivity of >99.5%. Most diagnostic laboratories use a commercial EIA kit that contains antigens from both HIV-1 and HIV-2 and thus are able to detect either. These kits use both natural and recombinant antigens and are continuously updated to increase their sensitivity to newly discovered species, such as group O viruses (Fig. 189-6). The fourth-generation EIA tests combine detection of antibodies to HIV with detection of the p24 antigen of HIV. EIA tests are generally scored as positive (highly reactive), negative (nonreactive), or indeterminate (partially reactive). While the EIA is an extremely sensitive test, it is not optimal with regard to specificity. This is particularly true in studies of low-risk individuals, such as volunteer blood donors. In this latter population, only 10% of EIA-positive individuals are subsequently confirmed to have HIV infection. Among the factors associated with false-positive EIA tests are antibodies to class II antigens (such as may be seen following pregnancy, blood transfusion, or transplantation), autoantibodies, hepatic disease, recent influenza vaccination, and acute viral infections. For these reasons, anyone suspected of having HIV infection based on a positive or inconclusive EIA result must have the result confirmed with a more specific assay such as the Western blot. One can estimate whether an individual has a recent infection with HIV-1 by comparing the results on a standard EIA test that will score positive for all infected individuals with the results on an assay modified to be less sensitive ("detuned assay") that will score positive only for individuals with established HIV infection. In rare instances, an HIV-infected individual treated early in the course of infection may revert to a negative EIA. This does *not* indicate clearing of infection; rather, it signifies levels of ongoing exposure to virus insufficient to maintain a measurable antibody response. When these individuals have discontinued therapy, viruses and antibodies have reappeared.

The most commonly used confirmatory test is the Western blot (Fig. 189-29). This assay takes advantage of the fact that multiple HIV antigens of different, well-characterized molecular weights elicit the production of specific antibodies. These antigens can be separated on the basis of molecular weight, and antibodies to each component can be detected as discrete bands on the Western blot. A negative Western blot is one in which no bands are present at molecular weights corresponding to HIV gene products. In a patient with a positive or indeterminate EIA and a negative Western blot, one can conclude with certainty that the EIA reactivity was a false positive. On the other hand, a Western blot demonstrating antibodies to products of all three of the major genes of HIV (*gag*, *pol*, and *env*) is conclusive evidence of infection with HIV. Criteria established by the U.S. Food and Drug Administration (FDA) in 1993 for a positive Western blot state that a result is considered positive if antibodies exist to two of the three HIV proteins: p24, gp41, and gp120/160. Using these criteria, ~10% of all blood donors deemed positive for HIV-1 infection lacked an antibody band to the *pol* gene product p31. Some 50% of these blood donors were subsequently found to be false positives. Thus, the absence of the p31 band should increase the suspicion that one may be dealing with a false-positive test result. In this setting it is prudent to obtain additional confirmation with an RNA-based test for HIV-1 and/or a follow-up Western blot. By definition, Western blot patterns of reactivity that do not fall into the positive or negative categories are considered "indeterminate." There are two possible explanations for an indeterminate Western blot result. The most likely explanation in a low-risk individual is that the patient being tested has antibodies that cross-react with one of the proteins of HIV. The most common patterns of cross-reactivity are antibodies that react with p24 and/or p55. The least likely explanation in this setting is that the individual is infected with HIV and is in the process of mounting a classic antibody response. In either instance, the Western blot should be repeated in 1 month to determine whether the indeterminate pattern is a pattern in evolution. In addition, one may attempt to confirm a diagnosis of HIV infection with the p24 antigen capture assay or one of the tests for HIV RNA (discussed below). While the Western blot is an excellent confirmatory test for HIV infection in patients with a positive or indeterminate EIA, it is a poor screening test. Among individuals with a negative EIA and PCR for HIV, 20–30% may show one or more bands on Western blot. While these bands are usually faint and represent cross-reactivity, their presence creates a situation in which other diagnostic modalities (such as DNA PCR, RNA PCR, the bDNA assay, or p24 antigen capture) must be employed to ensure that the bands do not indicate early HIV infection.

A guideline for the use of these serologic tests in attempting to make a diagnosis of HIV infection is depicted in Fig. 189-30. In patients in whom HIV infection is suspected, the appropriate initial test is the EIA. If the result is negative, unless there is strong reason to suspect early HIV infection (as in a patient exposed within the previous 3 months), the diagnosis is ruled out and retesting should be performed only as clinically indicated. If the EIA is indeterminate or positive, the test should be repeated. If the repeat is negative on two occasions, one can assume that the initial positive reading

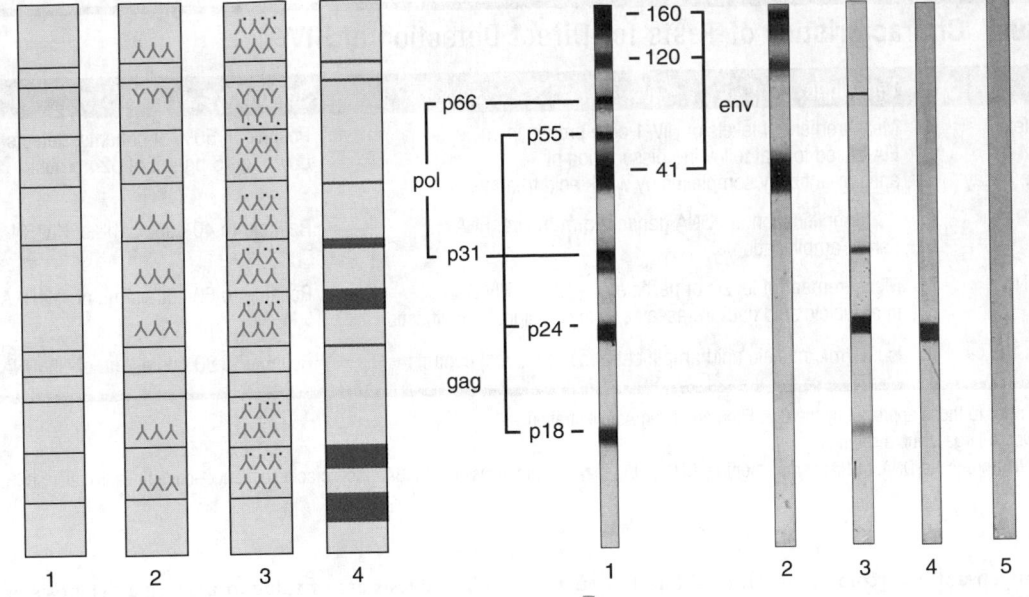

A
1. Virus digested: digest separated into components by molecular weight
2. Proteins transferred to filter paper: reaction with test serum
3. Enzyme-conjugated antihuman antibody added
4. Substrate added and color noted

B
1. Positive HIV-1 infection
2. gp 160 immunization
3. Indeterminate (HIV-2 infection)
4. Indeterminate (cross-reacting antibody to p24)
5. Negative

Figure 189-29 Western blot assay for detection of antibodies to HIV. *A.* Schematic representation of how a Western blot is performed. *B.* Examples of patterns of Western blot reactivity. In each instance the Western blot strip contains antigens to HIV-1. The serum from the patient

immunized to the HIV-1 envelope gp160 contains only antibodies to the HIV-1 envelope proteins. The serum from the patient with HIV-2 infection cross-reacts with both *reverse transcriptase* and *gag* gene products of HIV-1.

was due to a technical error in the performance of the assay and that the patient is negative. If the repeat is indeterminate or positive, one should proceed to the HIV-1 Western blot. If the Western blot is positive, the diagnosis is HIV-1 infection. If the Western blot is negative, the EIA can be assumed to have been a false positive for HIV-1 and the diagnosis of HIV-1 infection is ruled out. It would also be prudent at this point to perform specific serologic testing for

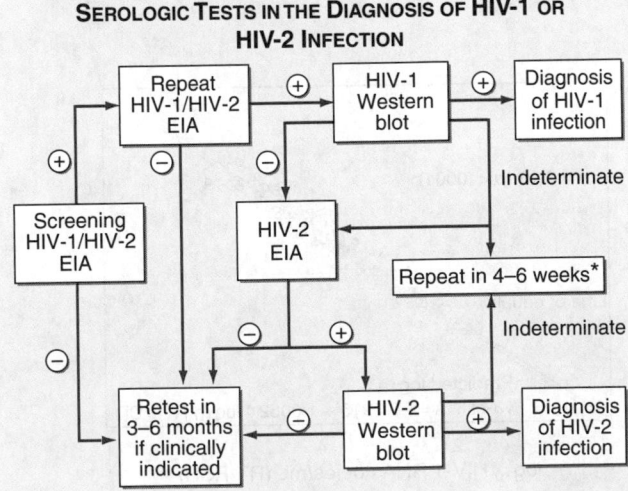

SEROLOGIC TESTS IN THE DIAGNOSIS OF HIV-1 OR HIV-2 INFECTION

Figure 189-30 Algorithm for the use of serologic tests in the diagnosis of HIV-1 or HIV-2 infection. *Stable indeterminate Western blot 4–6 weeks later makes HIV infection unlikely. However, it should be repeated twice at 3-month intervals to rule out HIV infection. Alternatively, one may test for HIV-1 p24 antigen or HIV RNA. EIA, enzyme immunoassay.

HIV-2 following the same type of algorithm. If the Western blot for HIV-1 is indeterminate, it should be repeated in 4–6 weeks; in addition, one may proceed to a p24 antigen capture assay, HIV-1 RNA assay, or HIV-1 DNA PCR and specific serologic testing for HIV-2. If the p24 and HIV RNA assays are negative and there is no progression in the Western blot, a diagnosis of HIV-1 is ruled out. If either the p24 or HIV-1 RNA assay is positive and/or the HIV-1 Western blot shows progression, a tentative diagnosis of HIV-1 infection can be made and later confirmed with a follow-up Western blot demonstrating a positive pattern. In addition to these standard laboratory-based assays for detecting antibodies to HIV, a series of point-of-care tests are also available that can provide results in 1–60 minutes. Among the most popular of these is the OraQuick Rapid HIV-1 antibody test that can be run on blood, plasma, or saliva. The sensitivity and specificity of this test are each ~99%. While negative results from this test are adequate to rule out a diagnosis of HIV infection, a positive finding should be considered preliminary and confirmed with standard serologic testing, as described above.

A variety of laboratory tests are available for the direct detection of HIV or its components (Table 189-7; Fig. 189-31). These tests may be of considerable help in making a diagnosis of HIV infection when the Western blot results are indeterminate. In addition, the tests detecting levels of HIV RNA can be used to determine prognosis and to assess the response to antiretroviral therapies. The simplest of the direct detection tests is the *p24 antigen capture assay*. This is an EIA-type assay in which the solid phase consists of antibodies to the p24 antigen of HIV. It detects the viral protein p24 in the blood of HIV-infected individuals where it exists either as free antigen or complexed to anti-p24 antibodies. Overall, ~30% of individuals with untreated HIV infection have detectable levels of free p24 antigen. This increases to ~50% when samples are treated with a weak acid

TABLE 189-7 **Characteristics of Tests for Direct Detection of HIV**

Test	Technique	Sensitivity[a]	Cost/Test[b]
Immune complex–dissociated p24 antigen capture assay	Measurement of levels of HIV-1 core protein in an EIA-based format following dissociation of antigen-antibody complexes by weak acid treatment	Positive in 50% of patients; detects down to 15 pg/mL of p24 protein	$1–2
HIV RNA by PCR	PCR amplification of cDNA generated from viral RNA (target amplification)	Reliable to 40 copies/mL of HIV RNA	$75–150
HIV RNA by bDNA	Measurement of levels of particle-associated HIV RNA in a nucleic acid capture assay employing signal amplification	Reliable to 50 copies/mL of HIV RNA	$75–150
HIV RNA by NASBA	Isothermic nucleic acid amplification with internal controls	Reliable to 80 copies/mL of HIV RNA	$75–150

[a]Sensitivity figures refer to those approved by the U.S. Food and Drug Administration.
[b]Prices may be lower in large-volume settings.
Abbreviations: bDNA, branched DNA; cDNA; complementary DNA;. EIA, enzyme immunoassay; NASBA, nucleic acid sequence–based amplification; PCR, polymerase chain reaction.

to dissociate antigen-antibody complexes. Throughout the course of HIV infection, an equilibrium exists between p24 antigen and anti-p24 antibodies. During the first few weeks of infection, before an immune response develops, there is a brisk rise in p24 antigen levels (Fig. 189-27). After the development of anti-p24 antibodies, these levels decline. Late in the course of infection, when circulating levels of virus are high, p24 antigen levels also increase, particularly when detected by techniques involving dissociation of antigen-antibody complexes. The p24 antigen capture assay has its greatest use as a screening test for HIV infection in patients suspected of having the acute HIV syndrome, as high levels of p24 antigen are present prior to the development of antibodies. Its use for routine blood donor screening for HIV infection has been replaced by use of nucleic acid testing. The ability to measure and monitor levels of HIV RNA in the plasma of patients with HIV infection has been of extraordinary value in furthering our understanding of the pathogenesis of HIV infection and in providing a diagnostic tool in settings where measurements of anti-HIV antibodies may be misleading, such as in acute infection and neonatal infection. Three assays are predominantly used for this purpose. They are reverse transcriptase PCR (*RT-PCR*; Amplicor); branched DNA (*bDNA*; VERSANT); and nucleic acid sequence–based amplification (*NASBA*; NucliSens).

These tests are of value in making a diagnosis of HIV infection, in establishing initial prognosis, in determining the need for therapy, and for monitoring the effects of therapy. In addition to these three commercially available tests, the *DNA PCR* is also employed by research laboratories for making a diagnosis of HIV infection by amplifying HIV proviral DNA from peripheral blood mononuclear cells. The commercially available RNA detection tests have a sensitivity of 40–80 copies of HIV RNA per milliliter of plasma. Research laboratory–based RNA assays can detect as few as one HIV RNA copy per milliliter, while the DNA PCR tests can detect proviral DNA at a frequency of one copy per 10,000–100,000 cells. Thus, these tests are extremely sensitive. One frequent consequence of a high degree of sensitivity is some loss of specificity, and false-positive results have been reported with each of these techniques. For this reason, a positive EIA with a confirmatory Western blot remains the "gold standard" for a diagnosis of HIV infection, and the interpretation of other test results must be done with this in mind.

In the RT-PCR technique, following DNAse treatment, a cDNA copy is made of all RNA species present in plasma. Insofar as HIV is an RNA virus, this will result in the production of DNA copies of the HIV genome in amounts proportional to the amount of HIV RNA present in plasma. This cDNA is then amplified and

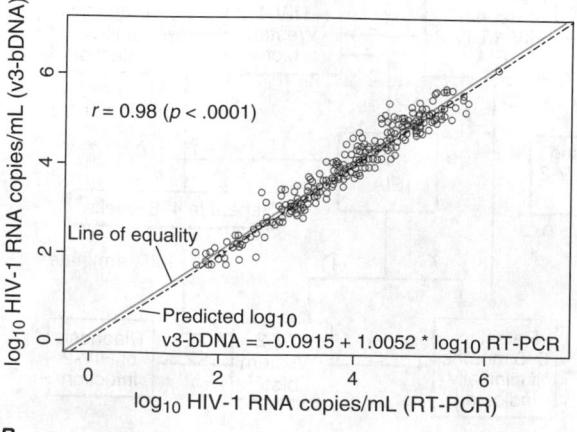

Figure 189-31 **Comparison of RT-PCR and bDNA assays. *A.*** Schematic representation of reverse transcriptase–polymerase chain reaction (RT-PCR) and bDNA assays. See text for detailed description. ***B.*** Scatter plot of $\log_{10}$ v3-bDNA versus $\log_{10}$ RT-PCR with the line of equity (solid) and the fitted regression line (hatched). The equation for the fitted regression line is given in the lower-right-hand corner. There is good agreement between the two assays. v3, version 3 of the bDNA assay. *(Adapted from HC Highbarger et al: J Clin Microbiol 37:3612, 1999.)*

PART 8 Infectious Diseases

characterized using standard PCR techniques, employing primer pairs that can distinguish genomic cDNA from messenger cDNA. The bDNA assay involves the use of a solid-phase nucleic acid capture system and signal amplification through successive nucleic acid hybridizations to detect small quantities of HIV RNA. Both tests can achieve a tenfold increase in sensitivity to 40–50 copies of HIV RNA per milliliter with a preconcentration step in which plasma undergoes ultracentrifugation to pellet the viral particles. The NASBA technique involves the isothermal amplification of a sequence within the gag region of HIV in the presence of internal standards and employs the production of multiple RNA copies through the action of T7-RNA polymerase. The resulting RNA species are quantitated through hybridization with a molecular beacon DNA probe that is quenched in the absence of hybridization. The lower limit of detection for the NucliSens assay is 80 copies/mL.

In addition to being a diagnostic and prognostic tool, RT-PCR and DNA-PCR are also useful for amplifying defined areas of the HIV genome for sequence analysis and have become an important technique for studies of sequence diversity and microbial resistance to antiretroviral agents. In patients with a positive or indeterminate EIA test and an indeterminate Western blot, and in patients in whom serologic testing may be unreliable (such as patients with hypogammaglobulinemia or advanced HIV disease), these tests for quantitating HIV RNA in plasma or detecting proviral DNA in peripheral blood mononuclear cells are valuable tools for making a diagnosis of HIV infection; however, they should be used for diagnosis only when standard serologic testing has failed to provide a definitive result.

■ LABORATORY MONITORING OF PATIENTS WITH HIV INFECTION

The epidemic of HIV infection and AIDS has provided the clinician with new challenges for integrating clinical and laboratory data to effect optimal patient management. The close relationship between clinical manifestations of HIV infection and CD4+ T cell count has made measurement of CD4+ T cell numbers a routine part of the evaluation of HIV-infected individuals. The discovery of HIV as the cause of AIDS led to the development of sensitive tests that allow one to monitor the levels of HIV in the blood. Determinations of peripheral blood CD4+ T cell counts and measurements of the plasma levels of HIV RNA plasma provide a powerful set of tools for determining prognosis and monitoring response to therapy.

CD4+ T cell counts

The CD4+ T cell count is the laboratory test generally accepted as the best indicator of the immediate state of immunologic competence of the patient with HIV infection. This measurement, which can be made directly or calculated as the product of the percent of CD4+ T cells (determined by flow cytometry) and the total lymphocyte count [determined by the white blood cell count (WBC) multiplied by the lymphocyte differential percent], has been shown to correlate very well with the level of immunologic

competence. Patients with CD4+ T cell counts <200/μL are at high risk of disease from *P. jiroveci*, while patients with CD4+ T cell counts <50/μL are at high risk of disease from CMV, mycobacteria of the *M. avium* complex (MAC), and/or *T. gondii* (Fig. 189-32). Patients with HIV infection should have CD4+ T cell measurements performed at the time of diagnosis and every 3–6 months thereafter. More frequent measurements should be made if a declining trend is noted. According to U.S. Department of Health and Human Services Guidelines, a CD4+ T cell count <500/μL is an indication for initiating cART, and a decline in CD4+ T cell count of >25% is an indication for considering a change in therapy. Once the CD4+ T cell count is <200/μL, patients should be placed on a regimen for *P. jiroveci* prophylaxis, and once the count is <50/μL, primary prophylaxis for MAC infection is indicated. As with any laboratory measurement, one may wish to obtain two determinations prior to any significant changes in patient management based on CD4+ T cell count alone. There are a handful of clinical situations in which the CD4+ T cell count may be misleading. Patients with HTLV-1/HIV co-infection may have elevated CD4+ T cell counts that do not accurately reflect their degree of immune competence. In patients with hypersplenism or those who have undergone splenectomy, and in patients receiving medications that suppress the bone marrow such as IFN-α, the CD4+ T cell percentage may be a more reliable indication of immune function than the CD4+ T cell count. A CD4+ T cell percent of 15 is comparable to a CD4+ T cell count of 200/μL.

HIV RNA determinations

Facilitated by highly sensitive techniques for the precise quantitation of small amounts of nucleic acids, the measurement of serum or plasma levels of HIV RNA has become an essential component in the monitoring of patients with HIV infection. As discussed under "Diagnosis of HIV Infection," above, the two most commonly used techniques are the RT-PCR assay and the bDNA assay. Both assays generate data in the form of number of copies of HIV RNA per milliliter of serum or plasma. Standard assays can detect as few as 40–50 copies of HIV RNA per milliliter of plasma, while research-based

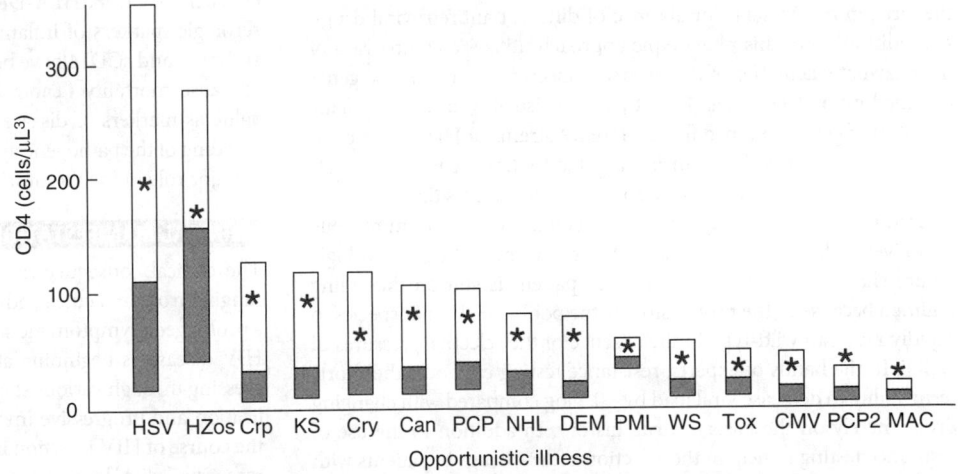

Figure 189-32 Relationship between CD4+ T cell counts and the development of opportunistic diseases. Boxplot of the median (line inside the box), first quartile (bottom of the box), third quartile (top of the box), and mean (asterisk) CD4+ lymphocyte count at the time of the development of opportunistic disease. Can, candidal esophagitis; CMV, cytomegalovirus infection; Crp, cryptosporidiosis; Cry, cryptococcal meningitis; DEM, AIDS dementia complex; HSV, herpes simplex virus infection; HZos, herpes zoster; KS, Kaposi's sarcoma; MAC, *Mycobacterium avium* complex bacteremia; NHL, non-Hodgkin's lymphoma; PCP, primary *Pneumocystis jiroveci* pneumonia; PCP2, secondary *P. jiroveci* pneumonia; PML, progressive multifocal leukoencephalopathy; Tox, *Toxoplasma gondii* encephalitis; WS, wasting syndrome. *(From RD Moore, RE Chaisson: Ann Intern Med 124:633, 1996.)*

assays can detect down to one copy per milliliter. While it is common practice to describe levels of HIV RNA below these cut-offs as "undetectable," this is a term that should be avoided as it is imprecise and leaves the false impression that the level of virus is 0. By utilizing more sensitive, nested PCR techniques and by studying tissue levels of virus as well as plasma levels, HIV RNA can be detected in virtually every patient with HIV infection. One notable exception to this is a patient who underwent cytoreducion therapy followed by a bone marrow transplant from a CCR5Δ32 homozygous donor. Measurements of changes in HIV RNA levels over time have been of great value in delineating the relationship between levels of virus and rates of disease progression (Fig. 189-22), the rates of viral turnover, the relationship between immune system activation and viral replication, and the time to development of drug resistance. HIV RNA measurements are greatly influenced by the state of activation of the immune system and may fluctuate greatly in the setting of secondary infections or immunization. For these reasons, decisions based on HIV RNA levels should never be made on a single determination. Measurements of plasma HIV RNA levels should be made at the time of HIV diagnosis and every 3–6 months thereafter in the untreated patient. Following the initiation of therapy or any change in therapy, plasma HIV RNA levels should be monitored approximately every 4 weeks until the effectiveness of the therapeutic regimen is determined by the development of a new steady-state level of HIV RNA. In most instances of effective antiretroviral therapy the plasma level of HIV RNA will drop to <50 copies per milliliter within 6 months of the initiation of treatment. During therapy, levels of HIV RNA should be monitored every 3–4 months to evaluate the continuing effectiveness of therapy.

HIV resistance testing

The availability of multiple antiretroviral drugs as treatment options has generated a great deal of interest in the potential for measuring the sensitivity of an individual's HIV virus(es) to different antiretroviral agents. HIV resistance testing can be done through either genotypic or phenotypic measurements. In the genotypic assays, sequence analyses of the HIV genomes obtained from patients are compared with sequences of viruses with known antiretroviral resistance profiles. In the phenotypic assays, the in vivo growth of viral isolates obtained from the patient is compared to the growth of reference strains of the virus in the presence or absence of different antiretroviral drugs. A modification of this phenotypic approach utilizes a comparison of the enzymatic activities of the reverse transcriptase or protease genes obtained by molecular cloning of patients' isolates to the enzymatic activities of genes obtained from reference strains of HIV in the presence or absence of different drugs targeted to these genes. These tests are quite good in identifying those antiretroviral agents that have been utilized in the past and suggesting agents that may be of future value in a given patient. Drug resistance testing in the setting of virologic failure should be performed while the patient is still on the failing regimen because of the propensity for the pool of HIV quasispecies to rapidly revert to wild-type in the absence of the selective pressures of cART. In the hands of experts, resistance testing enhances the short-term ability to decrease viral load by ~0.5 log compared with changing drugs merely on the basis of drug history. In addition to the use of resistance testing to help in the selection of new drugs in patients with virologic failure, it may also be of value in selecting an initial regimen for treatment of therapy-naïve individuals. This is particularly true in geographic areas with a high level of background resistance.

Co-receptor tropism assays

Following the licensure of maraviroc as the first CCR5 antagonist for the treatment of HIV infection (see below), it became necessary to be able to determine whether a patient's virus was likely to respond to this treatment. Patients tend to have CCR5-tropic virus

TABLE 189-8 Association Between High-Sensitivity CRP, IL-6, and D-Dimer With All-Cause Mortality in Patients With HIV Infection

Marker	Unadjusted		Adjusted	
	Odds Ratio (Fourth/First)	p	Odds Ratio (Fourth/First)	p
Hs-CRP	2.0	.05	2.8	.03
IL-6	8.3	<.0001	11.8	<.0001
D-dimer	12.4	<.0001	26.5	<.0001

Note: Hs-CRP, high-sensitivity C-reactive protein; IL-6, interleukin 6.
Source: From Kuller et al.

early in the course of infection with a trend toward CXCR4 viruses later in disease. The antiretroviral agent maraviroc is effective only against CCR5-tropic viruses. Because the genotypic determinants of cellular tropism are poorly defined, a phenotypic assay is necessary to determine this property of HIV. Two commercial assays, the Trofile assay (Monogram Biosciences) and the Phenoscript assay (VIRalliance), are available to make this determination. These assays clone the envelope regions of the patient's virus into an indicator virus that is then used to infect target cells expressing either CCR5 or CXCR4 as their co-receptor. These assays take weeks to perform and are expensive. Although commercial genotypic assays of proviral DNA are available, their role as predictors of response to CCR5 inhibitor therapy is unclear.

Other tests

A variety of other laboratory tests have been studied as potential markers of HIV disease activity. Among these are quantitative culture of replication-competent HIV from plasma, peripheral blood mononuclear cells, or resting CD4+ T cells; circulating levels of β_2-microglobulin, soluble IL-2 receptor, IgA, acid-labile endogenous IFN, or TNF-α; and the presence or absence of activation markers such as CD38, HLA-DR, or PD-1 on CD8+ T cells. Nonspecific serologic markers of inflammation and/or coagulation such as IL-6, D-dimer, and sCD14 have been shown to have a high correlation with all-cause mortality (Table 189-8). While these measurements have value as markers of disease activity and help to increase our understanding of the pathogenesis of HIV disease, they do not currently play a major role in the monitoring of patients with HIV infection.

CLINICAL MANIFESTATIONS

The clinical consequences of HIV infection encompass a spectrum ranging from an acute syndrome associated with primary infection to a prolonged asymptomatic state to advanced disease. It is best to regard HIV disease as beginning at the time of primary infection and progressing through various stages. As mentioned above, active virus replication and progressive immunologic impairment occur throughout the course of HIV infection in most patients. With the exception of the rare, true, "elite" long-term nonprogressors (see "Long-Term Survivors and Long-Term Nonprogressors," above), HIV disease in untreated patients inexorably progresses even during the clinically latent stage. Since the mid-1990s, cART has had a major impact on preventing and reversing the progression of disease over extended periods of time in a substantial proportion of adequately treated patients.

■ THE ACUTE HIV SYNDROME

It is estimated that 50–70% of individuals with HIV infection experience an acute clinical syndrome ~3–6 weeks after primary

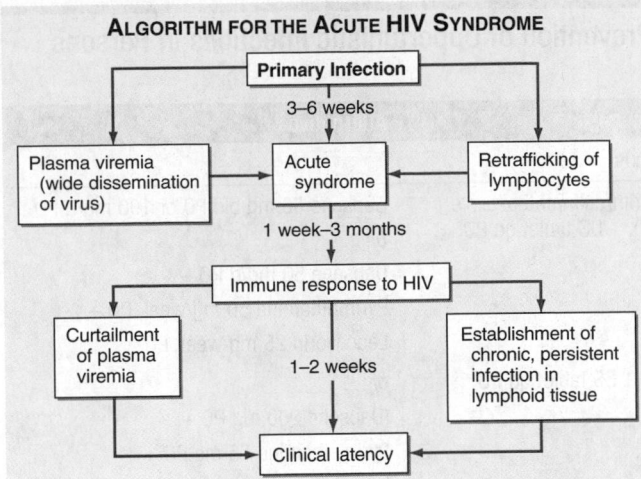

ALGORITHM FOR THE ACUTE HIV SYNDROME

Figure 189-33 The acute HIV syndrome. See text for detailed description. *(Adapted from G Pantaleo et al: N Engl J Med 328:327, 1993. Copyright 1993 Massachusetts Medical Society. All rights reserved.)*

infection (Fig. 189-33). Varying degrees of clinical severity have been reported, and although it has been suggested that symptomatic seroconversion leading to the seeking of medical attention indicates an increased risk for an accelerated course of disease, there does not appear to be a correlation between the level of the initial burst of viremia in acute HIV infection and the subsequent course of disease. The typical clinical findings in the acute HIV syndrome are listed in Table 189-9; they occur along with a burst of plasma viremia. It has been reported that several symptoms of the acute HIV syndrome (fever, skin rash, pharyngitis, and myalgia) occur less frequently in those infected by injection drug use compared with those infected by sexual contact. The syndrome is typical of an acute viral syndrome and has been likened to acute infectious mononucleosis. Symptoms usually persist for one to several weeks and gradually subside as an immune response to HIV develops and the levels of plasma viremia decrease. Opportunistic infections have been reported during this stage of infection, reflecting the immunodeficiency that results from reduced numbers of CD4+ T cells and likely also from the dysfunction of CD4+ T cells owing to viral protein and endogenous cytokine-induced perturbations of cells (Table 189-4) associated with the extremely high levels of plasma viremia. A number of immunologic abnormalities accompany the acute HIV syndrome, including multiphasic perturbations of the numbers of circulating lymphocyte subsets. The number of total lymphocytes and T cell subsets (CD4+ and CD8+) are initially reduced. An inversion of the CD4+/CD8+ T cell ratio occurs later because of a rise in the number of CD8+ T cells. In fact, there may be a selective and transient expansion of CD8+ T cell subsets, as determined by T cell receptor analysis (see above). The total circulating CD8+ T cell count may remain elevated or return to normal; however, CD4+ T cell levels usually remain somewhat depressed, although there may be a slight rebound toward normal. Lymphadenopathy occurs in ~70% of individuals with primary HIV infection. Most patients recover spontaneously from this syndrome and many are left with only a mildly depressed CD4+ T cell count that remains stable for a variable period before beginning its progressive decline; in some individuals, the CD4+ T cell count returns to the normal range. Approximately 10% of patients manifest a fulminant course of immunologic and clinical deterioration after primary infection, even after the disappearance of initial symptoms. In most patients, primary infection with or without the acute syndrome is followed by a prolonged period of clinical latency or smoldering low disease activity. A small percentage of HIV-infected individuals treated with antiretroviral drugs during acute infection may revert to a negative EIA test during the time they remain on therapy. They rapidly re-seroconvert with the discontinuation of treatment.

■ THE ASYMPTOMATIC STAGE—CLINICAL LATENCY

Although the length of time from initial infection to the development of clinical disease varies greatly, the median time for untreated patients is ~10 years. As emphasized above, HIV disease with active virus replication is ongoing and progressive during this asymptomatic period. The rate of disease progression is directly correlated with HIV RNA levels. Patients with high levels of HIV RNA in plasma progress to symptomatic disease faster than do patients with low levels of HIV RNA (Fig. 189-22). Some patients referred to as *long-term nonprogressors* show little if any decline in CD4+ T cell counts over extended periods of time. These patients generally have extremely low levels of HIV RNA; a subset, referred to as *elite nonprogressors*, exhibits HIV RNA levels <50 copies per milliliter. Certain other patients remain entirely asymptomatic despite the fact that their CD4+ T cell counts show a steady progressive decline to extremely low levels. In these patients, the appearance of an opportunistic disease may be the first manifestation of HIV infection. During the asymptomatic period of HIV infection, the average rate of CD4+ T cell decline is ~50/μL per year. When the CD4+ T cell count falls to <200/μL, the resulting state of immunodeficiency is severe enough to place the patient at high risk for opportunistic infection and neoplasms and, hence, for clinically apparent disease.

■ SYMPTOMATIC DISEASE

Symptoms of HIV disease can appear at any time during the course of HIV infection. Generally speaking, the spectrum of illnesses that one observes changes as the CD4+ T cell count declines. The more severe and life-threatening complications of HIV infection occur in patients with CD4+ T cell counts <200/μL. A diagnosis of AIDS is made in anyone with HIV infection and a CD4+ T cell count <200/μL and in anyone with HIV infection who develops one of the HIV-associated diseases considered to be indicative of a severe defect in cell-mediated immunity (category C, Table 189-2). While the causative agents of the secondary infections are characteristically opportunistic organisms such as *P. jiroveci*, atypical mycobacteria, CMV, and other organisms that do not ordinarily cause disease in the absence of a compromised immune system, they also include common bacterial and mycobacterial pathogens. Following the widespread use of cART and implementation of guidelines for the prevention of opportunistic infections (Table 189-10), the

TABLE 189-9 Clinical Findings in the Acute HIV Syndrome

General	Neurologic
Fever	Meningitis
Pharyngitis	Encephalitis
Lymphadenopathy	Peripheral neuropathy
Headache/retroorbital pain	Myelopathy
Arthralgias/myalgias	Dermatologic
Lethargy/malaise	Erythematous maculopapular rash
Anorexia/weight loss	Mucocutaneous ulceration
Nausea/vomiting/diarrhea	

Source: From B Tindall, DA Cooper: AIDS 5:1, 1991.

TABLE 189-10 NIH/CDC/IDSA 2009 Guidelines for the Prevention of Opportunistic Infections in Persons Infected With HIV

Pathogen	Indications	First Choice(s)	Alternatives
Recommended as Standard of Care for Primary and Secondary Prophylaxis			
Pneumocystis jiroveci	CD4+ T cell count <200/μL *or* Oropharyngeal candidiasis *or* Prior bout of PCP	Trimethoprim/sulfamethoxazole (TMP/SMX), 1 DS tablet qd PO *or*	Dapsone 50 mg bid PO or 100 mg/d PO *or* Dapsone 50 mg/d PO + Pyrimethamine 50 mg/week PO + Leucovorin 25 mg/week PO
	May stop prophylaxis if CD4+ T cell count >200/μL for ≥3 months	TMP/SMX, 1 SS tablet qd PO	*or* (Dapsone 200 mg PO + Pyrimethamine 75 mg PO + Leucovorin 25 mg) weekly PO *or* Aerosolized pentamidine, 300 mg via Respirgard II nebulizer every month *or* Atovaquone 1500 mg/d PO *or* TMP/SMX 1 DS tablet 3×/week PO
Mycobacterium tuberculosis			
Isoniazid sensitive	Skin test >5 mm *or* Prior positive test without treatment *or* Close contact with case of active pulmonary TB	(Isoniazid 300 mg PO + Pyridoxine 50 mg PO) qd × 9 months *or* Isoniazid 900 mg PO twice weekly + Pyridoxine 50 mg PO daily × 9 months	Rifabutin 300 mg or rifampin 600 mg PO qd × 4 months
Isoniazid resistant	Same with high probability of exposure to isoniazid-resistant TB	(Rifabutin 300 mg or Rifampin 600 mg) PO qd ×4 months	
Multidrug resistant	Same with high probability of exposure to multidrug-resistant TB	Consult local public health authorities	
Mycobacterium-avium complex	CD4+ T cell count <50/μL	Azithromycin 1200 mg weekly PO *or* Clarithromycin 500 mg bid PO	Rifabutin 300 mg/d PO *or* Azithromycin 600 mg twice weekly PO
	Prior documented disseminated disease May stop prophylaxis if CD4+ T cell count >100/μL for ≥3 months	Clarithromycin 500 mg bid PO + Ethambutol 15 (mg/kg)/d PO ± Rifabutin 300 mg/d PO	Azithromycin 500 mg/d PO + Ethambutol 15 (mg/kg)/d PO ± Rifabutin 300 mg/d PO
Toxoplasma gondii	TOXO IgG antibody positive and CD4+ T cell count <100/μL	TMP/SMX 1 DS tablet PO qd	TMP/SMX 1 DS 3× weekly PO *or* TMP/SMX, 1 SS PO daily *or* Dapsone 50 mg/d PO + Pyrimethamine 50 mg weekly PO + Leucovorin 25 mg weekly PO *or* (Dapsone 200 mg PO + Pyrimethamine 75 mg PO + Leucovorin 25 mg PO) weekly *or* (Atovaquone 1500 mg PO ± Pyrimethamine 25 mg PO + Leucovorin 10 mg PO) daily

(continued)

Pathogen	Indications	First Choice(s)	Alternatives
	Prior toxoplasmic encephalitis and CD4+ T cell count <200/μL	Sulfadiazine 500–1000 mg qid PO + Pyrimethamine 25–50 mg/d PO + Leucovorin 10–25 mg/d PO	Clindamycin 600 mg q8h PO + Pyrimethamine 25–50 mg/d PO + Leucovorin 10–25 mg/d PO
	May stop prophylaxis if CD4+ T cell count >200/μL for ≥3 months		Atovaquone 750 mg PO q6–12 h ± Pyrimethamine 25 mg/d PO + Leucovorin 10 mg/d PO
Varicella zoster virus	Significant exposure to chickenpox or shingles in a patient with no history of immunization or prior exposure to either	Varicella zoster immune globulin, IM, within 96 h of exposure (1-800-843-74+77)	Acyclovir 800 mg PO 5 × 1 day for 5 days
Cryptococcus neoformans	Prior documented disease	Fluconazole 200 mg/d PO	Itraconazole 200 mg/d PO
	May stop prophylaxis if CD4+ T cell count >200/μL for 6 months and no evidence of active infection		
Histoplasma capsulatum	Prior documented disease or CD4+ T cell count <150μL and high risk (endemic area or occupational exposure)	Itraconazole 200 mg bid PO	Fluconazole 800 mg/d PO
	May stop prophylaxis after 1 year if CD4+ T cell count >150/μL and patient on ARV therapy for ≥6 months		
Coccidioides immitis	Prior documented disease *or* positive serology and CD4+ T cell count <250/μL if from a disease endemic area. (For this indication prophylaxis can be stopped if CD4+ T cell count ≥250 for 6 months.)	Fluconazole 400 mg/d PO	Itraconazole 200 mg bid PO
Penicillium marneffei	Prior documented disease	Itraconazole 200 mg/d PO	
	May stop secondary prophylaxis in patients on ARV therapy with CD4+ T cell count >100/μL for ≥6 months		
Salmonella species	Prior reament bacteremia	Ciprofloxacin 500 mg bid PO for ≥6 months	
Bartonella	Prior infection	Doxycycline 200 mg/d *or* Azithromycin 1200 mg weekly PO *or* Clarithromycin 500 mg bid PO	
	May stop if CD4+ T cell count >200/μL for >3 months		
Cytomegalovirus	Prior end-organ disease	Valganciclovir 900 mg bid PO *or* Ganciclovir sustained-release implant q6–9 months + Valganciclovir 900 mg bid PO	Cidofovir 5 mg/kg every other week IV + Probenecid *or* Fomivirsen 330 μg intravitreal q2–4 week *or* Foscarnet 90–120 (mg/kg)/d IV
	May stop prophylaxis if CD4+ T cell count >100/μL for 6 months and no evidence of active CMV disease		
	Restart if prior retinitis and CD4+ T cells <100/μL		

Immunizations Generally Recommended

Hepatitis B virus	All susceptible (anti-HBc-and anti-HBs-negative) patients	Hepatitis B vaccine: 3 doses	
Hepatitis A virus	All susceptible (anti-HAV-negative) patients	Hepatitis A vaccine: 2 doses	
Influenza virus	All patients annually	Inactivated trivalent influenza virus vaccine 1 dose yearly	Oseltamivir 75 mg PO qd *or* Rimantadine or amantadine 100 mg PO bid (influenza A only)

(continued)

TABLE 189-10 NIH/CDC/IDSA 2009 Guidelines for the Prevention of Opportunistic Infections in Persons Infected With HIV (Continued)

Pathogen	Indications	First Choice(s)	Alternatives
Streptococcus pneumoniae	All patients, preferably before CD4+ T cell count ≤200/μL	Pneumococcal vaccine 0.5 mL IM ×1 if CD4+ T cell count >200/μL	
		Reimmunize patients initially immunized at a CD4+ T cell count <100/μL whose CD4+ T cell count then increases to >200/μL	
Human papillomavirus	All patients 9–26 years of age	HPV vaccine; 3 doses	

Recommended for Prevention of Severe or Frequent Recurrences

Herpes simplex	Frequent/severe recurrences	Valacyclovir 500 mg bid PO *or* Acyclovir 400 mg bid PO *or* Famciclovir 500 mg bid PO	
Candida	Frequent/severe recurrences	Fluconazole 100–200 mg/d PO	Itraconazole solution 200 mg/d PO posacomagole 400 mg bid PO

Abbreviations: ARV, antiretroviral; bid, twice daily; DS, double-strength; PCP, *Pneumocystis jiroveci* pneumonia; PO, by mouth; SS, single-strength; TB, tuberculosis.

incidence of these secondary infections has decreased dramatically (Fig. 189-34). Overall, the clinical spectrum of HIV disease is constantly changing as patients live longer and new and better approaches to treatment and prophylaxis are developed. In addition to the classic AIDS-defining illnesses, patients with HIV infection also have an increase in serious non-AIDS illnesses, including non-AIDS related cancers and, cardiovascular, renal and hepatic disease. Non-AIDS events dominate the disease burden for patients with HIV infection receiving cART (Table 189-3). Fewer than 50% of deaths among AIDS patients are as a direct result of an AIDS-defining illness. The physician providing care to a patient with HIV infection must be well versed in general internal medicine as well as HIV-related opportunistic diseases. In general, it should be stressed that a key element of treatment of symptomatic complications of HIV disease, whether they are primary or secondary, is achieving good control of HIV replication through the use of cART and instituting primary and secondary prophylaxis for opportunistic infections as indicated.

Diseases of the respiratory system

Acute bronchitis and sinusitis are prevalent during all stages of HIV infection. The most severe cases tend to occur in patients with lower CD4+ T cell counts. Sinusitis presents as fever, nasal congestion, and headache. The diagnosis is made by CT or MRI. The maxillary sinuses are most commonly involved; however, disease is also frequently seen in the ethmoid, sphenoid, and frontal sinuses. While some patients may improve without antibiotic therapy, radiographic improvement is quicker and more pronounced in patients who have received antimicrobial therapy. It is postulated that this high incidence of sinusitis results from an increased frequency of infection with encapsulated organisms such as *H. influenzae* and *Streptococcus pneumoniae*. In patients with low CD4+ T cell counts one may see mucormycosis infections of the sinuses. In contrast to the course of this infection in other patient populations, mucormycosis of the sinuses in patients with HIV infection may progress more slowly. In this setting aggressive, frequent local debridement in addition to local and systemic amphotericin B may result in effective treatment.

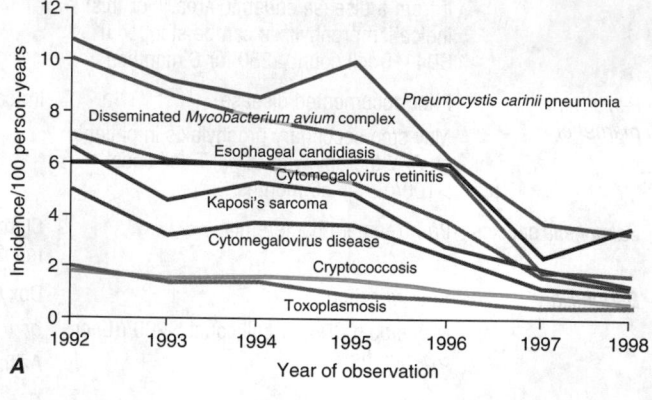

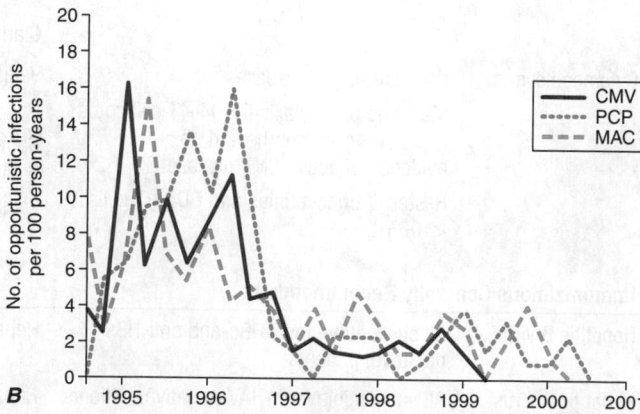

Figure 189-34 A. Decrease in the incidence of opportunistic infections and Kaposi's sarcoma in HIV-infected individuals with CD4+ T cell counts <100/μL from 1992 through 1998. [*Adapted and updated from FJ Palella et al: N Engl J Med 338:853, 1998, and JE Kaplan et al: Clin Infect Dis 30(S1):S5, 2000, with permission.*] **B.** Quarterly incidence rates of cytomegalovirus (CMV), *Pneumocystis jiroveci* pneumonia (PCP), and *Mycobacterium avium* complex (MAC) from 1995 to 2001. (*From FJ Palella et al: AIDS 16:1617, 2002.*)

Pulmonary disease is one of the most frequent complications of HIV infection. The most common manifestation of pulmonary disease is pneumonia. Three of the 10 most common AIDS-defining illnesses are recurrent bacterial pneumonia, tuberculosis, and pneumonia due to the unicellular fungus *P. jiroveci*. Other major causes of pulmonary infiltrates include other mycobacterial infections, other fungal infections, nonspecific interstitial pneumonitis, KS, and lymphoma.

Bacterial pneumonia is seen with an increased frequency in patients with HIV infection, with 0.8–2.0 cases per 100 person-years. Patients with HIV infection are particularly prone to infections with encapsulated organisms. *S. pneumoniae* (Chap. 134) and *H. influenzae* (Chap. 145) are responsible for most cases of bacterial pneumonia in patients with AIDS. This may be a consequence of altered B cell function and/or defects in neutrophil function that may be secondary to HIV disease (see above). Pneumonias due to *S. aureus* (Chap. 135) and *P. aeruginosa* (Chap. 152) are also reported to occur with an increased frequency in patients with HIV infection. *S. pneumoniae* (pneumococcal) infection may be the earliest serious infection to occur in patients with HIV disease. This can present as pneumonia, sinusitis, and/or bacteremia. Patients with untreated HIV infection have a sixfold increase in the incidence of pneumococcal pneumonia and a 100-fold increase in the incidence of pneumococcal bacteremia. Pneumococcal disease may be seen in patients with relatively intact immune systems. In one study, the baseline CD4+ T cell count at the time of a first episode of pneumococcal pneumonia was ~300/μL. Of interest is the fact that the inflammatory response to pneumococcal infection appears proportional to the CD4+ T cell count. Due to this high risk of pneumococcal disease, immunization with pneumococcal polysaccharide is one of the generally recommended prophylactic measures for patients with HIV infection. This is likely most effective if given while the CD4+ T cell count is >200/μL and, if given to patients with lower CD4+ T cell counts, should be repeated once the count has been above 200 for 6 months. Although clear guidelines do not exist, it also makes sense to repeat immunization every 5 years. The incidence of bacterial pneumonia is cut in half when patients quit smoking.

Pneumocystis pneumonia (PCP), once the hallmark of AIDS, has dramatically declined in incidence following the development of effective prophylactic regimens and the widespread use of cART. It is, however, still the single most common cause of pneumonia in patients with HIV infection in the United States and can be identified as a likely etiologic agent in 25% of cases of pneumonia in patients with HIV infection, with an incidence in the range of 2–3 cases per 100 person-years. Approximately 50% of cases of HIV-associated PCP occur in patients who are unaware of their HIV status. The risk of PCP is greatest among those who have experienced a previous bout of PCP and those who have CD4+ T cell counts of <200/μL. Overall, 79% of patients with PCP have CD4+ T cell counts <100/μL and 95% of patients have CD4+ T cell counts <200/μL. Recurrent fever, night sweats, thrush, and unexplained weight loss are also associated with an increased incidence of PCP. For these reasons, it is strongly recommended that all patients with CD4+ T cell counts <200/μL (or a CD4 percentage <15) receive some form of PCP prophylaxis. The incidence of PCP is approaching zero in patients with known HIV infection receiving appropriate cART and prophylaxis. In the United States, primary PCP is now occurring at a median CD4+ T cell count of 36/μL, while secondary PCP is occurring at a median CD4+ T cell count of 10/μL. Patients with PCP generally present with fever and a cough that is usually nonproductive or productive of only scant amounts of white sputum. They may complain of a characteristic retrosternal chest pain that is worse on inspiration and is described as sharp or burning. HIV-associated PCP may have an indolent course characterized by weeks of vague symptoms and should be included

in the differential diagnosis of fever, pulmonary complaints, or unexplained weight loss in any patient with HIV infection and <200 CD4+ T cells/μL. The most common finding on chest x-ray is either a normal film, if the disease is suspected early, or a faint bilateral interstitial infiltrate. The classic finding of a dense perihilar infiltrate is unusual in patients with AIDS. In patients with PCP who have been receiving aerosolized pentamidine for prophylaxis, one may see an x-ray picture of upper lobe cavitary disease, reminiscent of TB. Other less common findings on chest x-ray include lobar infiltrates and pleural effusions. Thin-section CT may demonstrate a patchy ground-glass appearance. Routine laboratory evaluation is usually of little help in the differential diagnosis of PCP. A mild leukocytosis is common, although this may not be obvious in patients with prior neutropenia. Elevation of lactate dehydrogenase is common. Arterial blood-gases may indicate hypoxemia with a decline in Pa_{O_2} and an increase in the arterial-alveolar (a–A) gradient. Arterial blood-gas measurements not only aid in making the diagnosis of PCP but also provide important information for staging the severity of the disease and directing treatment (see below). A definitive diagnosis of PCP requires demonstration of the organism in samples obtained from induced sputum, bronchoalveolar lavage, transbronchial biopsy, or open-lung biopsy. PCR has been used to detect specific DNA sequences for *P. jiroveci* in clinical specimens where histologic examinations have failed to make a diagnosis.

In addition to pneumonia, a number of other clinical problems have been reported in HIV-infected patients as a result of infection with *P. jiroveci*. Otic involvement may be seen as a primary infection, presenting as a polypoid mass involving the external auditory canal. In patients receiving aerosolized pentamidine for prophylaxis against PCP, one may see a variety of extrapulmonary manifestations of *P. jiroveci*. These include ophthalmic lesions of the choroid, a necrotizing vasculitis that resembles Burger's disease, bone marrow hypoplasia, and intestinal obstruction. Other organs that have been involved include lymph nodes, spleen, liver, kidney, pancreas, pericardium, heart, thyroid, and adrenals. Organ infection may be associated with cystic lesions that may appear calcified on CT or ultrasound.

The standard treatment for PCP or disseminated pneumocystosis is trimethoprim/sulfamethoxazole (TMP/SMX). A high (20–85%) incidence of side effects, particularly skin rash and bone marrow suppression, is seen with TMP/SMX in patients with HIV infection. Alternative treatments for mild to moderate PCP include dapsone/trimethoprim, clindamycin/primaquine, and atovaquone. IV pentamidine is the treatment of choice for severe disease in the patient unable to tolerate TMP/SMX. For patients with a Pa_{O_2} <70 mmHg or with an a–A gradient >35 mmHg, adjunct glucocorticoid therapy should be used in addition to specific antimicrobials. Overall, treatment should be continued for 21 days and followed by secondary prophylaxis. Prophylaxis for PCP is indicated for any HIV-infected individual who has experienced a prior bout of PCP, any patient with a CD4+ T cell count of <200/μL or a CD4 percentage <15, any patient with unexplained fever for >2 weeks, and any patient with a history of oropharyngeal candidiasis. The preferred regimen for prophylaxis is TMP/SMX, one double-strength tablet daily. This regimen also provides protection against toxoplasmosis and some bacterial respiratory pathogens. For patients who cannot tolerate TMP/SMX, alternatives for prophylaxis include dapsone plus pyrimethamine plus leucovorin, aerosolized pentamidine administered by the Respirgard II nebulizer, and atovaquone. Primary or secondary prophylaxis for PCP can be discontinued in those patients treated with cART who maintain good suppression of HIV (<50 copies per milliliter) and CD4+ T cell counts >200/μL for 3–6 months.

M. tuberculosis, once thought to be on its way to extinction in the United States, experienced a resurgence associated with the

HIV epidemic (Chap. 165). Worldwide, approximately one-third of all AIDS-related deaths are associated with TB, and TB is the primary cause of death for 10–15% of patients with HIV infection. In the United States ~5% of AIDS patients have active TB. Patients with HIV infection are more likely to have active TB by a factor of 100 when compared with an HIV-negative population. For an asymptomatic HIV-negative person with a positive purified protein derivative (PPD) skin test, the risk of reactivation TB is around 1% per year. For the patient with untreated HIV infection, a positive PPD skin test, and no signs or symptoms of TB, the rate of reactivation TB is 7–10% per year. Untreated TB can accelerate the course of HIV infection. Levels of plasma HIV RNA increase in the setting of active TB and decline in the setting of successful TB treatment. Active TB is most common in patients 25–44 years of age, in African Americans and Hispanics, in patients in New York City and Miami, and in patients in developing countries. In these demographic groups, 20–70% of the new cases of active TB are in patients with HIV infection. The epidemic of TB embedded in the epidemic of HIV infection probably represents the greatest health risk to the general public and the health care profession associated with the HIV epidemic. In contrast to infection with atypical mycobacteria such as MAC, active TB often develops relatively early in the course of HIV infection and may be an early clinical sign of HIV disease. In one study, the median CD4+ T cell count at presentation of TB was 326/μL. The clinical manifestations of TB in HIV-infected patients are quite varied and generally show different patterns as a function of the CD4+ T cell count. In patients with relatively high CD4+ T cell counts, the typical pattern of pulmonary reactivation occurs: patients present with fever, cough, dyspnea on exertion, weight loss, night sweats, and a chest x-ray revealing cavitary apical disease of the upper lobes. In patients with lower CD4+ T cell counts, disseminated disease is more common. In these patients the chest x-ray may reveal diffuse or lower lobe bilateral reticulonodular infiltrates consistent with miliary spread, pleural effusions, and hilar and/or mediastinal adenopathy. Infection may be present in bone, brain, meninges, GI tract, lymph nodes (particularly cervical lymph nodes), and viscera. Some patients with advanced HIV infection and active TB may have no symptoms of illness, and thus screening for TB should be part of the initial evaluation of every patient with HIV infection. Approximately 60–80% of HIV-infected patients with TB have pulmonary disease, and 30–40% have extrapulmonary disease. Respiratory isolation and a negative-pressure room should be used for patients in whom a diagnosis of pulmonary TB is being considered. This approach is critical to limit nosocomial and community spread of infection. Culture of the organism from an involved site provides a definitive diagnosis. Blood cultures are positive in 15% of patients. This figure is higher in patients with lower CD4 +T cell counts. In the setting of fulminant disease one cannot rely on the accuracy of a negative PPD skin test to rule out a diagnosis of TB. TB is one of the conditions associated with HIV infection for which cure is possible with appropriate therapy. Therapy for TB is generally the same in the HIV-infected patient as in the HIV-negative patient (Chap. 165). Due to the possibility of multidrug-resistant or extensively drug-resistant TB, drug susceptibility testing should be performed to guide therapy. Due to pharmacokinetic interactions, adjusted doses of rifabutin should be substituted for rifampin in patients receiving the HIV protease inhibitors or nonnucleoside reverse transcriptase inhibitors. Treatment is most effective in programs that involve directly observed therapy. Initiation of cART and/or anti-TB therapy may be associated with clinical deterioration due to immune reconstitution inflammatory syndrome (IRIS) reactions. These are most common in patients initiating both treatments at the same time, may occur as early as 1 week after initiation of therapy, and are seen more frequently in patients with advanced HIV disease. For these reasons it is often

recommended that initiation of cART be delayed in antiretroviral-naïve patients until 2–8 weeks following the initiation of treatment for TB. Effective prevention of active TB can be a reality if the health care professional is aggressive in looking for evidence of latent or active TB by making sure that all patients with HIV infection receive a PPD skin test or evaluation with an IFN-γ release assay. Anergy testing is not of value in this setting. Since these tests rely on the host mounting an immune response to *M. tuberculosis*, patients with CD4+ T cell counts <200 cells/μL should be retested if their CD4+ T cell counts rise to persistently above 200. Patients at risk of continued exposure to TB should be tested annually. HIV-infected individuals with a skin-test reaction of >5 mm, those with a positive IFN-γ release assay, or those who are close household contacts of persons with active TB should receive treatment with 9 months of isoniazid and pyridoxine.

Atypical mycobacterial infections are also seen with an increased frequency in patients with HIV infection. Infections with at least 12 different mycobacteria have been reported, including *M. bovis* and representatives of all four Runyon groups. The most common atypical mycobacterial infection is with *M. avium* or *M. intracellulare* species—the *Mycobacterium avium* complex (MAC). Infections with MAC are seen mainly in patients in the United States and are rare in Africa. It has been suggested that prior infection with *M. tuberculosis* decreases the risk of MAC infection. MAC infections probably arise from organisms that are ubiquitous in the environment, including both soil and water. There is little evidence for person-to-person transmission of MAC infection. The presumed portals of entry are the respiratory and GI tract. MAC infection is a late complication of HIV infection, occurring predominantly in patients with CD4+ T cell counts of <50/μL. The average CD4+ T cell count at the time of diagnosis is 10/μL. The most common presentation is disseminated disease with fever, weight loss, and night sweats. At least 85% of patients with MAC infection are mycobacteremic, and large numbers of organisms can often be demonstrated on bone marrow biopsy. The chest x-ray is abnormal in ~25% of patients, with the most common pattern being that of a bilateral, lower lobe infiltrate suggestive of miliary spread. Alveolar or nodular infiltrates and hilar and/or mediastinal adenopathy can also occur. Other clinical findings include endobronchial lesions, abdominal pain, diarrhea, and lymphadenopathy. Anemia and elevated liver alkaline phosphatase are common. The diagnosis is made by the culture of blood or involved tissue. The finding of two consecutive sputum samples positive for MAC is highly suggestive of pulmonary infection. Cultures may take 2 weeks to turn positive. Therapy consists of a macrolide, usually clarithromycin, with ethambutol. Some physicians elect to add a third drug from among rifabutin, ciprofloxacin, or amikacin in patients with extensive disease. Therapy was generally for life; however, with the use of cART it is possible to discontinue therapy in patients with sustained suppression of HIV replication and CD4+ T cell counts >100/μL for 3–6 months. Primary prophylaxis for MAC is indicated in patients with HIV infection and CD4+ T cell counts <50/μL (Table 189-10). This may be discontinued in patients in whom cART induces a sustained suppression of viral replication and increases in CD4+ T cell counts to >100/μL for ≥3 months.

Rhodococcus equi is a gram-positive, pleomorphic, acid-fast, non-spore-forming bacillus that can cause pulmonary and/or disseminated infection in patients with advanced HIV infection. Fever and cough are the most common presenting signs. Radiographically one may see cavitary lesions and consolidation. Blood cultures are often positive. Treatment is based on antimicrobial sensitivity testing.

Fungal infections of the lung, in addition to PCP, can be seen in patients with AIDS. Patients with pulmonary cryptococcal disease present with fever, cough, dyspnea, and, in some cases, hemoptysis. A focal or diffuse interstitial infiltrate is seen on chest x-ray in >90%

of patients. In addition, one may see lobar disease, cavitary disease, pleural effusions, and hilar or mediastinal adenopathy. More than half of patients are fungemic, and 90% of patients have concomitant CNS infection. *Coccidioides immitis* is a mold that is endemic in the southwest United States. It can cause a reactivation pulmonary syndrome in patients with HIV infection. Most patients with this condition will have CD4+ T cell counts <250/μL. Patients present with fever, weight loss, cough, and extensive, diffuse reticulonodular infiltrates on chest x-ray. One may also see nodules, cavities, pleural effusions, and hilar adenopathy. While serologic testing is of value in the immunocompetent host, serologies are negative in 25% of HIV-infected patients with coccidioidal infection. Invasive aspergillosis is not an AIDS-defining illness and is generally not seen in patients with AIDS in the absence of neutropenia or administration of glucocorticoids. When it does occur, *Aspergillus* infection may have an unusual presentation in the respiratory tract of patients with AIDS, where it gives the appearance of a pseudomembranous tracheobronchitis. Primary pulmonary infection of the lung may be seen with *histoplasmosis*. The most common pulmonary manifestation of histoplasmosis, however, is in the setting of disseminated disease, presumably due to reactivation. In this setting respiratory symptoms are usually minimal, with cough and dyspnea occurring in 10–30% of patients. The chest x-ray is abnormal in ~50% of patients, showing either a diffuse interstitial infiltrate or diffuse small nodules.

Two forms of *idiopathic interstitial pneumonia* have been identified in patients with HIV infection: lymphoid interstitial pneumonitis (LIP) and nonspecific interstitial pneumonitis (NIP). LIP, a common finding in children, is seen in about 1% of adult patients with untreated HIV infection. This disorder is characterized by a benign infiltrate of the lung and is thought to be part of the polyclonal activation of lymphocytes seen in the context of HIV and EBV infections. Transbronchial biopsy is diagnostic in 50% of the cases, with an open-lung biopsy required for diagnosis in the remainder of cases. This condition is generally self-limited and no specific treatment is necessary. Severe cases have been managed with brief courses of glucocorticoids. Although rarely a clinical problem since the use of cART, evidence of NIP may be seen in up to half of all patients with untreated HIV infection. Histologically, interstitial infiltrates of lymphocytes and plasma cells in a perivascular and peribronchial distribution are present. When symptomatic, patients present with fever and nonproductive cough occasionally accompanied by mild chest discomfort. Chest x-ray is usually normal or may reveal a faint interstitial pattern. Similar to LIP, NIP is a self-limited process for which no therapy is indicated other than appropriate management of the underlying HIV infection. HIV-related pulmonary arterial hypertension (HIV-PAH) is seen in ~0.5% of HIV-infected individuals. Patients may present with an array of symptoms including shortness of breath, fatigue, syncope, chest pain, and signs of right-sided heart failure. Chest x-ray reveals dilated pulmonary vessels and right-sided cardiomegaly with right ventricular hypertrophy seen on electrocardiogram. cART does not appear to be of clear benefit, and the prognosis is quite poor with a median survival in the range of 2 years.

Neoplastic diseases of the lung including KS and lymphoma are discussed below in the section on neoplastic diseases.

Diseases of the cardiovascular system

Heart disease is a relatively common postmortem finding in HIV-infected patients (25–75% in autopsy series). The most common form of heart disease is coronary heart disease. In one large series the overall rate of myocardial infarction (MI) was 3.5/1000 patient-years, 28% of these events were fatal, and MI was responsible for 7% of all deaths in the cohort. In patients with HIV infection, cardiovascular disease may be associated with classic risk factors such as

smoking, a direct consequence of HIV infection, or a complication of cART. Patients with HIV infection have higher levels of triglycerides, lower levels of high-density lipoprotein cholesterol, and a higher prevalence of smoking than cohorts of individuals without HIV infection. The finding that the rate of cardiovascular disease events was lower in patients on antiretroviral therapy than in those randomized to undergo a treatment interruption identified a clear association between HIV replication and risk of cardiovascular disease. In one study, a baseline CD4+ T cell count of <500/μL was found to be an independent risk factor for cardiovascular disease comparable in magnitude to that attributable to smoking. While the precise pathogenesis of this association remains unclear, it is likely related to the immune activation and increased propensity for coagulation seen as a consequence of HIV replication. Exposure to HIV protease inhibitors and certain reverse transcriptase inhibitors has been associated with increases in total cholesterol and/or risk of MI. Any increases in the risk of death from MI resulting from the use of certain antiretrovirals must be balanced against the marked increases in overall survival brought about by these drugs.

Another form of heart disease associated with HIV infection is a dilated cardiomyopathy associated with congestive heart failure (CHF) referred to as *HIV-associated cardiomyopathy*. This generally occurs as a late complication of HIV infection and, histologically, displays elements of myocarditis. For this reason some have advocated treatment with IV immunoglobulin (IVIg). HIV can be directly demonstrated in cardiac tissue in this setting, and there is debate over whether it plays a direct role in this condition. Patients present with typical findings of CHF including edema and shortness of breath. Patients with HIV infection may also develop cardiomyopathy as side effects of IFN-α or nucleoside analogue therapy. These are reversible once therapy is stopped. KS, cryptococcosis, Chagas' disease, and toxoplasmosis can involve the myocardium, leading to cardiomyopathy. In one series, most patients with HIV infection and a treatable myocarditis were found to have myocarditis associated with toxoplasmosis. Most of these patients also had evidence of CNS toxoplasmosis. Thus, MRI or double-dose contrast CT scan of the brain should be included in the workup of any patient with advanced HIV infection and cardiomyopathy.

A variety of other cardiovascular problems are found in patients with HIV infection. Pericardial effusions may be seen in the setting of advanced HIV infection. Predisposing factors include TB, CHF, mycobacterial infection, cryptococcal infection, pulmonary infection, lymphoma, and KS. While pericarditis is quite rare, in one series 5% of patients with HIV disease had pericardial effusions that were considered to be moderate or severe. Tamponade and death have occurred in association with pericardial KS, presumably owing to acute hemorrhage. Nonbacterial thrombotic endocarditis has been reported and should be considered in patients with unexplained embolic phenomena. Intravenous pentamidine, when given rapidly, can result in hypotension as a consequence of cardiovascular collapse.

Diseases of the oropharynx and gastrointestinal system

Oropharyngeal and GI diseases are common features of HIV infection. They are most frequently due to secondary infections. In addition, oral and GI lesions may occur with KS and lymphoma.

Oral lesions, including *thrush*, *hairy leukoplakia*, and *aphthous ulcers* (Fig. 189-35), are particularly common in patients with untreated HIV infection. Thrush, due to *Candida* infection, and oral hairy leukoplakia, presumed due to EBV, are usually indicative of fairly advanced immunologic decline; they generally occur in patients with CD4+ T cell counts of <300/μL. In one study, 59% of patients with oral candidiasis went on to develop AIDS in the next year. Thrush appears as a white, cheesy exudate, often on an erythematous mucosa in the posterior oropharynx. While most commonly seen on the soft palate, early lesions are often found along the gingival

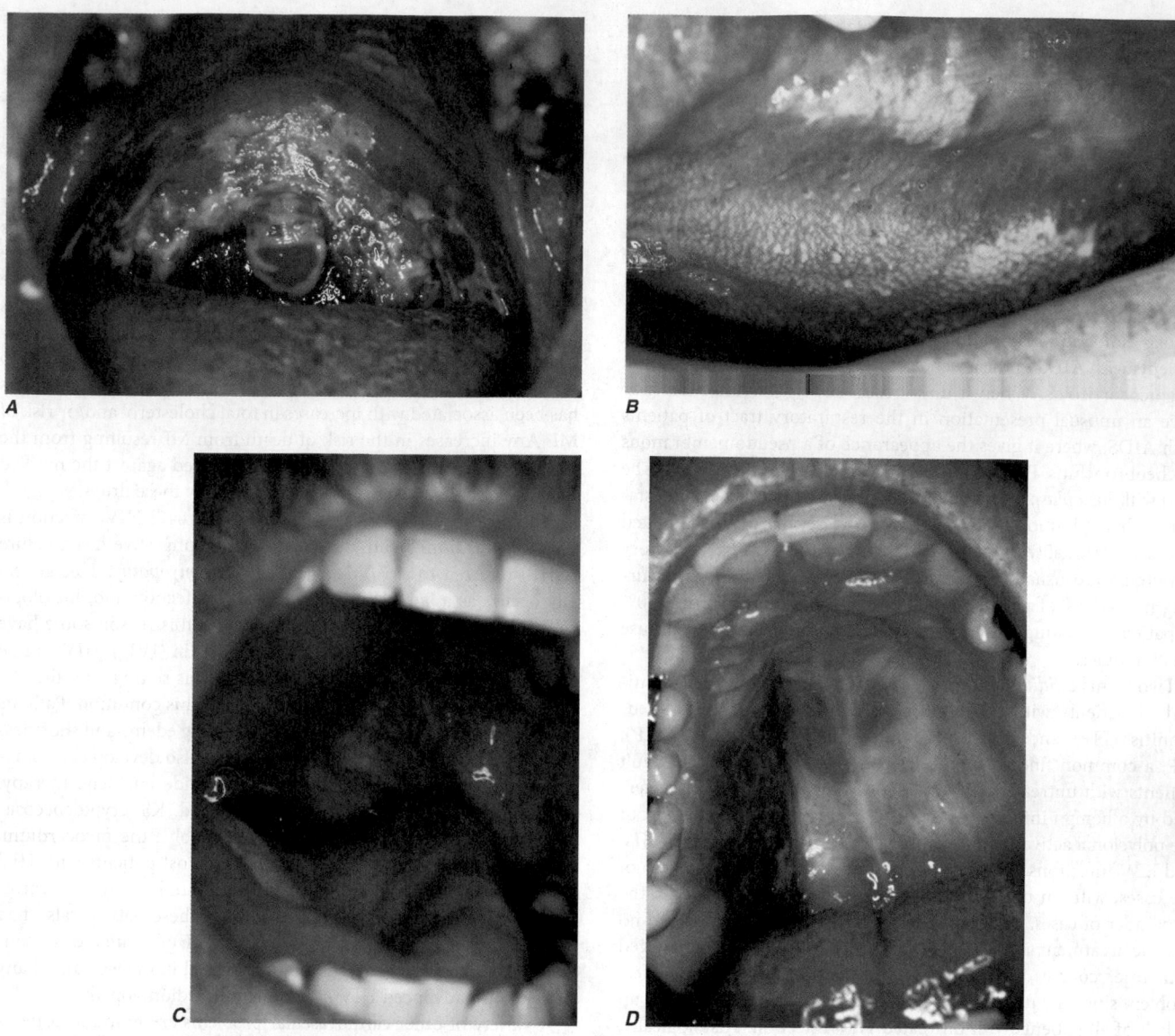

Figure 189-35 **Various oral lesions in HIV-infected individuals.** *A.* Thrush. *B.* Hairy leukoplakia. *C.* Aphthous ulcer. *D.* Kaposi's sarcoma.

border. The diagnosis is made by direct examination of a scraping for pseudohyphal elements. Culturing is of no diagnostic value, as patients with HIV infection may have a positive throat culture for *Candida* in the absence of thrush. Oral hairy leukoplakia presents as white, frondlike lesions, generally along the lateral borders of the tongue and sometimes on the adjacent buccal mucosa (Fig. 189-35). Despite its name, oral hairy leukoplakia is not considered a premalignant condition. Lesions are associated with florid replication of EBV. While usually more disconcerting as a sign of HIV-associated immunodeficiency than a clinical problem in need of treatment, severe cases have been reported to respond to topical podophyllin or systemic therapy with anti-herpesvirus agents. Aphthous ulcers of the posterior oropharynx are also seen with regularity in patients with HIV infection (Fig. 189-35). These lesions are of unknown etiology and can be quite painful and interfere with swallowing. Topical anesthetics provide immediate symptomatic relief of short duration. The fact that thalidomide is an effective treatment for this condition suggests that the pathogenesis may involve the action of tissue-destructive cytokines. Palatal, glossal, or gingival ulcers may also result from cryptococcal disease or histoplasmosis.

Esophagitis (Fig. 189-36) may present with odynophagia and retrosternal pain. Upper endoscopy is generally required to make

an accurate diagnosis. Esophagitis may be due to *Candida*, CMV, or HSV. While CMV tends to be associated with a single large ulcer, HSV infection is more often associated with multiple small ulcers. The esophagus may also be the site of KS and lymphoma. Like the oral mucosa, the esophageal mucosa may have large, painful ulcers of unclear etiology that may respond to thalidomide. While achlorhydria is a common problem in patients with HIV infection, other gastric problems are generally rare. Among the neoplastic conditions involving the stomach are KS and lymphoma.

Infections of the small and large intestine leading to diarrhea, abdominal pain, and occasionally fever are among the most significant GI problems in HIV-infected patients. They include infections with bacteria, protozoa, and viruses.

Bacteria may be responsible for secondary infections of the GI tract. Infections with enteric pathogens such as *Salmonella*, *Shigella*, and *Campylobacter* are more common in homosexual men and are often more severe and more apt to relapse in patients with HIV infection. Patients with untreated HIV have approximately a 20-fold increased risk of infection with *S. typhimurium*. They may present with a variety of nonspecific symptoms including fever, anorexia, fatigue, and malaise of several weeks' duration. Diarrhea is common but may be absent. Diagnosis is made by

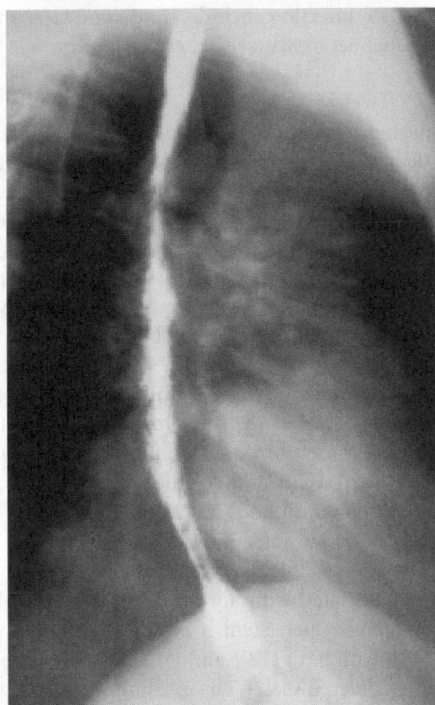

Figure 189-36 Barium swallow of a patient with *Candida* esophagitis. The flow of barium along the mucosal surface is grossly irregular.

culture of blood and stool. Long-term therapy with ciprofloxacin is the recommended treatment. HIV-infected patients also have an increased incidence of *S. typhi* infection in areas of the world where typhoid is a problem. *Shigella* spp., particularly *S. flexneri*, can cause severe intestinal disease in HIV-infected individuals. Up to 50% of patients will develop bacteremia. *Campylobacter* infections occur with an increased frequency in patients with HIV infection. While *C. jejuni* is the strain most frequently isolated, infections with many other strains have been reported. Patients usually present with crampy abdominal pain, fever, and bloody diarrhea. Infection may also present as proctitis. Stool examination reveals the presence of fecal leukocytes. Systemic infection can occur, with up to 10% of infected patients exhibiting bacteremia. Most strains are sensitive to erythromycin. Abdominal pain and diarrhea may be seen with MAC infection.

Fungal infections may also be a cause of diarrhea in patients with HIV infection. Histoplasmosis, coccidioidomycosis, and penicilliosis have all been identified as a cause of fever and diarrhea in patients with HIV infection. Peritonitis has been seen with *C. immitis*.

Cryptosporidia, microsporidia, and *Isospora belli* (Chap. 215) are the most common opportunistic protozoa that infect the GI tract and cause diarrhea in HIV-infected patients. Cryptosporidial infection may present in a variety of ways, ranging from a self-limited or intermittent diarrheal illness in patients in the early stages of HIV infection to a severe, life-threatening diarrhea in severely immunodeficient individuals. In patients with untreated HIV infection and CD4+ T cell counts of <300/μL, the incidence of cryptosporidiosis is ~1% per year. In 75% of cases the diarrhea is accompanied by crampy abdominal pain, and 25% of patients have nausea and/or vomiting. Cryptosporidia may also cause biliary tract disease in the HIV-infected patient, leading to cholecystitis with or without accompanying cholangitis and pancreatitis secondary to papillary stenosis. The diagnosis of cryptosporidial diarrhea is made by stool examination or biopsy of the small intestine. The diarrhea is non-inflammatory, and the characteristic finding is the presence of oocysts that stain with acid-fast dyes. Therapy is predominantly supportive,

and marked improvements have been reported in the setting of effective cART. Treatment with up to 2000 mg/d of nitazoxanide (NTZ) is associated with improvement in symptoms or a decrease in shedding of organisms in about half of patients. Its overall role in the management of this condition remains unclear. Patients can minimize their risk of developing cryptosporidiosis by avoiding contact with human and animal feces, by not drinking untreated water from lakes or rivers, and by not eating raw shellfish.

Microsporidia are small, unicellular, obligate intracellular parasites that reside in the cytoplasm of enteric cells (Chap. 215). The main species causing disease in humans is *Enterocytozoon bieneusi*. The clinical manifestations are similar to those described for cryptosporidia and include abdominal pain, malabsorption, diarrhea, and cholangitis. The small size of the organism may make it difficult to detect; however, with the use of chromotrope-based stains, organisms can be identified in stool samples by light microscopy. Definitive diagnosis generally depends on electron-microscopic examination of a stool specimen, intestinal aspirate, or intestinal biopsy specimen. In contrast to cryptosporidia, microsporidia have been noted in a variety of extraintestinal locations, including the eye, brain, sinuses, muscle, and liver, and they have been associated with conjunctivitis and hepatitis. The most effective way to deal with microsporia in a patient with HIV infection is to restore the immune system by treating the HIV infection with cART. Albendazole, 400 mg bid, has been reported to be of benefit in some patients.

I. belli is a coccidian parasite (Chap. 215) most commonly found as a cause of diarrhea in patients from tropical and subtropical regions. Its cysts appear in the stool as large, acid-fast structures that can be differentiated from those of cryptosporidia on the basis of size, shape, and number of sporocysts. The clinical syndromes of *Isospora* infection are identical to those caused by cryptosporidia. The important distinction is that infection with *Isospora* is generally relatively easy to treat with TMP/SMX. While relapses are common, a thrice-weekly regimen of TMP/SMX appears adequate to prevent recurrence.

CMV colitis was once seen as a consequence of advanced immunodeficiency in 5–10% of patients with AIDS. It is much less common with the advent of cART. CMV colitis presents as diarrhea, abdominal pain, weight loss, and anorexia. The diarrhea is usually nonbloody, and the diagnosis is achieved through endoscopy and biopsy. Multiple mucosal ulcerations are seen at endoscopy, and biopsies reveal characteristic intranuclear and cytoplasmic inclusion bodies. Secondary bacteremias may result as a consequence of thinning of the bowel wall. Treatment is with either ganciclovir or foscarnet for 3–6 weeks. Relapses are common, and maintenance therapy is typically necessary in patients whose HIV infection is poorly controlled. Patients with CMV disease of the GI tract should be carefully monitored for evidence of CMV retinitis.

In addition to disease caused by specific secondary infections, patients with HIV infection may also experience a chronic diarrheal syndrome for which no etiologic agent other than HIV can be identified. This entity is referred to as *AIDS enteropathy* or *HIV enteropathy*. It is most likely a direct result of HIV infection in the GI tract. Histologic examination of the small bowel in these patients reveals low-grade mucosal atrophy with a decrease in mitotic figures, suggesting a hyporegenerative state. Patients often have decreased or absent small-bowel lactase and malabsorption with accompanying weight loss.

The initial evaluation of a patient with HIV infection and diarrhea should include a set of stool examinations, including culture, examination for ova and parasites, and examination for *Clostridium difficile* toxin. Approximately 50% of the time this workup will demonstrate infection with pathogenic bacteria, mycobacteria, or protozoa. If the initial stool examinations are negative, additional

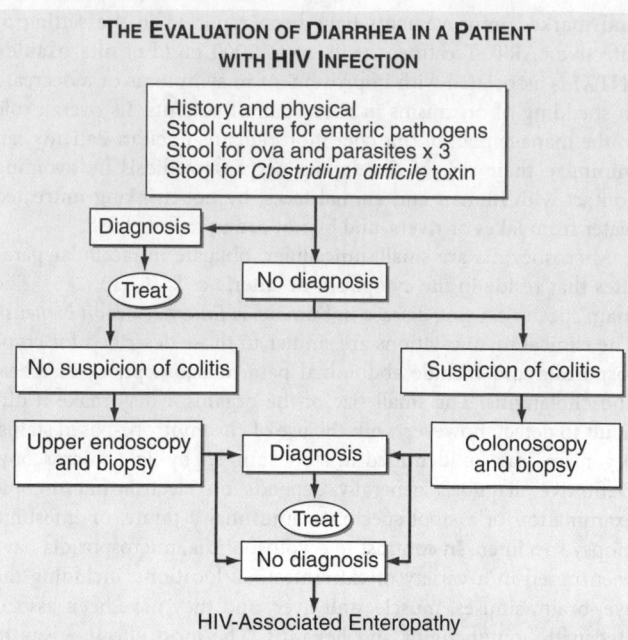

THE EVALUATION OF DIARRHEA IN A PATIENT WITH HIV INFECTION

Figure 189-37 Algorithm for the evaluation of diarrhea in a patient with HIV infection. HIV-associated enteropathy is a diagnosis of exclusion and can be made only after other, generally treatable, forms of diarrheal illness have been ruled out.

evaluation, including upper and/or lower endoscopy with biopsy, will yield a diagnosis of microsporidial or mycobacterial infection of the small intestine ~30% of the time. In patients for whom this diagnostic evaluation is nonrevealing, a presumptive diagnosis of HIV enteropathy can be made if the diarrhea has persisted for >1 month. An algorithm for the evaluation of diarrhea in patients with HIV infection is given in Fig. 189-37.

Rectal lesions are common in HIV-infected patients, particularly the perirectal ulcers and erosions due to the reactivation of HSV (Fig. 189-38). These lesions may appear quite atypical, as denuded skin without vesicles, and they respond well to treatment with acyclovir, famciclovir, or foscarnet. Other rectal lesions encountered in

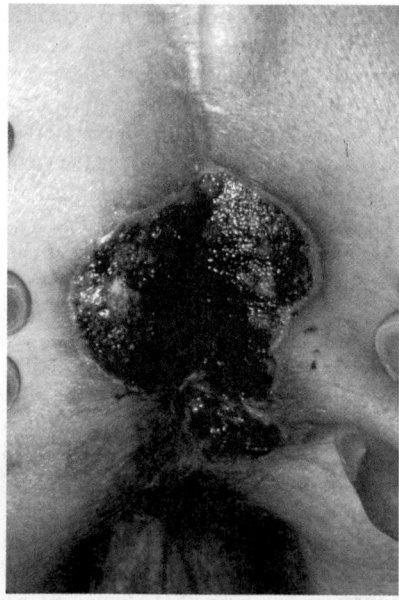

Figure 189-38 Severe, erosive perirectal herpes simplex in a patient with AIDS.

patients with HIV infection include condylomata acuminata, KS, and intraepithelial neoplasia (see below).

Hepatobiliary diseases

Diseases of the hepatobiliary system are a major problem in patients with HIV infection. It has been estimated that approximately one-third of the deaths of patients with HIV infection are in some way related to liver disease. While this is predominantly a reflection of the problems encountered in the setting of co-infection with hepatitis B or C, it is also a reflection of the hepatic injury, ranging from hepatic steatosis to hypersensitivity reactions to immune reconstitution, that can be seen in the context of cART.

The prevalence of co-infection with HIV and hepatitis viruses varies by geographic region. In the United States, ~90% of HIV-infected individuals have evidence of infection with HBV; 6–14% have chronic HBV infection; 5–50% of current or past patients are co-infected with HCV; and co-infection with hepatitis D, E, and/or G viruses is common. Among IV drug users with HIV infection, rates of HCV infection range from 70 to 95%. HIV infection has a significant impact on the course of hepatitis virus infection. It is associated with approximately a threefold increase in the development of persistent hepatitis B surface antigenemia. Patients infected with both HBV and HIV have decreased evidence of inflammatory liver disease. The presumption that this is due to the immunosuppressive effects of HIV infection is supported by the observations that this situation can be reversed, and one may see the development of more severe hepatitis following the initiation of effective cART. In studies of the impact of HIV on HBV infection, four- to tenfold increases in liver-related mortality rates have been noted in patients with HIV and active HBV infection compared to rates in patients with either infection alone. There is, however, only a slight increase in overall mortality rate in HIV-infected individuals who are also hepatitis B surface antigen (HBsAg)–positive. IFN-α is less successful as a treatment of HBV in patients with HIV co-infection. Lamivudine, emtricitabine, adefovir/tenofovir/entecavir, and telbivudine alone or in combination are useful in the treatment of hepatitis B in patients with HIV infection. It is important to remember that all the above-mentioned drugs also have activity against HIV and should not be used alone in patients with HIV infection, in order to avoid the emergence quasispecies of HIV resistant to these drugs. For this reason, the need to treat hepatitis B infection in a patient with HIV infection is an indication to treat HIV infection in that same patient, regardless of CD4+ T cell count. HCV infection is more severe in the patient with HIV infection; it does not appear to affect overall mortality rate in HIV-infected individuals when other variables such as age, baseline CD4+ T cell count, and use of cART are taken into account. In the setting of HIV and HCV co-infection, levels of HCV are approximately tenfold higher than in the HIV-negative patient with HCV infection and there is a tenfold increased risk of death due to liver disease in co-infected patients. Treatment for HCV infection consists of pegylated IFN-α and ribavirin with an array of experimental therapies currently in clinical trials. If a 2-log drop in levels of HCV RNA is not seen within 12 weeks, it is unlikely that therapy will be of value. Hepatitis A virus infection is not seen with an increased frequency in patients with HIV infection. It is recommended that all patients with HIV infection who have not experienced natural infection be immunized with hepatitis A and/or hepatitis B vaccines. Infection with hepatitis G virus, also known as GB virus C, is seen in ~50% of patients with HIV infection. For reasons that are currently unclear, there are data to suggest that patients with HIV infection co-infected with this virus have a decreased rate of progression to AIDS.

A variety of other infections may also involve the liver. Granulomatous hepatitis may be seen as a consequence of mycobacterial or fungal infections, particularly MAC infection. Hepatic masses may be seen in the context of TB, peliosis hepatis, or fungal infection. Among the fungal opportunistic infections, *C. immitis* and *Histoplasma capsulatum* are those most likely to involve the liver. Biliary tract disease in the form of papillary stenosis or sclerosing cholangitis has been reported in the context of cryptosporidiosis, CMV infection, and KS.

Many of the drugs used to treat HIV infection are metabolized by the liver and can cause liver injury. Fatal hepatic reactions have been reported with a wide array of antiretrovirals including nucleoside analogues, nonnucleoside analogues, and protease inhibitors. Nucleoside analogues work by inhibiting DNA synthesis. This can result in toxicity to mitochondria, which can lead to disturbances in oxidative metabolism. This may manifest as hepatic steatosis and, in severe cases, lactic acidosis and fulminant liver failure. It is important to be aware of this condition and to watch for it in patients with HIV infection receiving nucleoside analogues. It is reversible if diagnosed early and the offending agent(s) discontinued. Nevirapine has been associated with at times fatal fulminant and cholestatic hepatitis, hepatic necrosis, and hepatic failure. Indinavir may cause mild to moderate elevations in serum bilirubin in 10–15% of patients in a syndrome similar to Gilbert's syndrome. A similar pattern of hepatic injury may be seen with atazanavir. In the patient receiving cART with an unexplained increase in hepatic transaminases, strong consideration should be given to drug toxicity. *Pancreatic injury* is most commonly a consequence of drug toxicity, notably that secondary to pentamidine or dideoxynucleosides. While up to half of patients in some series have biochemical evidence of pancreatic injury, <5% of patients show any clinical evidence of pancreatitis that is not linked to a drug toxicity.

Diseases of the kidney and genitourinary tract

Diseases of the kidney or genitourinary tract may be a direct consequence of HIV infection, due to an opportunistic infection or neoplasm, or related to drug toxicity. Overall, microalbuminuria is seen in ~20% of untreated HIV-infected patients; significant proteinuria is seen in closer to 2%. The presence of microalbuminuria has been associated with an increase in all-cause mortality rate. *HIV-associated nephropathy* (HIVAN) was first described in IDUs and was initially thought to be IDU nephropathy in patients with HIV infection; it is now recognized as a true direct complication of HIV infection. Although the majority of patients have CD4+ T cell counts <200/μL, HIV-associated nephropathy can be an early manifestation of HIV infection and is also seen in children. Over 90% of reported cases have been in African-American or Hispanic individuals; the disease is not only more prevalent in these populations but also more severe and is the third leading cause of end-stage renal failure among African Americans age 20–64 in the United States. Proteinuria is the hallmark of this disorder. Edema and hypertension are rare. Ultrasound examination reveals enlarged, hyperechogenic kidneys. A definitive diagnosis is obtained through renal biopsy. Histologically, focal segmental glomerulosclerosis is present in 80%, and mesangial proliferation in 10–15% of cases. Prior to effective antiretroviral therapy, this disease was characterized by relatively rapid progression to end-stage renal disease. Patients with HIV-associated nephropathy should be treated for their HIV infection regardless of CD4+ T cell count. Treatment with angiotensin-converting enzyme (ACE) inhibitors and/or prednisone, 60 mg/d, has also been reported to be of benefit in some cases. The incidence of this disease in patients receiving adequate cART has not been well defined; however, the impression is that it has decreased in frequency and severity. It is the leading cause of end-stage renal disease in patients with HIV infection.

Among the drugs commonly associated with renal damage in patients with HIV disease are pentamidine, amphotericin, adefovir, cidofovir, tenofovir, and foscarnet. TMP/SMX may compete for tubular secretion with creatinine and cause an increase in the serum creatinine level. Sulfadiazine may crystallize in the kidney and result in an easily reversible form of renal shutdown, while indinavir may form renal calculi. Adequate hydration is the mainstay of treatment and prevention for these latter two conditions.

Genitourinary tract infections are seen with a high frequency in patients with HIV infection; they present with skin lesions, dysuria, hematuria, and/or pyuria and are managed in the same fashion as in patients without HIV infection. Infections with HSV are covered below ("Dermatologic Diseases"). Infections with *T. pallidum*, the etiologic agent of *syphilis*, play an important role in the HIV epidemic. In HIV-negative individuals, genital syphilitic ulcers as well as the ulcers of chancroid are major predisposing factors for heterosexual transmission of HIV infection. While most HIV-infected individuals with syphilis have a typical presentation, a variety of formerly rare clinical problems may be encountered in the setting of dual infection. Among them are *lues maligna*, an ulcerating lesion of the skin due to a necrotizing vasculitis; unexplained fever; nephrotic syndrome; and neurosyphilis. The most common presentation of syphilis in the HIV-infected patient is that of *condylomata lata*, a form of secondary syphilis. Neurosyphilis may be asymptomatic or may present as acute meningitis, neuroretinitis, deafness, or stroke. The rate of neurosyphilis may be as high as 1% in patients with HIV infection, and one should consider a lumbar puncture to look for neurosyphilis in all patients with HIV infection and secondary syphilis. As a consequence of the immunologic abnormalities seen in the setting of HIV infection, diagnosis of syphilis through standard serologic testing may be challenging. On the one hand, a significant number of patients have false-positive Venereal Disease Research Laboratory (VDRL) tests due to polyclonal B cell activation. On the other hand, the development of a new positive VDRL may be delayed in patients with new infections, and the anti–fluorescent treponemal antibody (anti-FTA) test may be negative due to immunodeficiency. Thus, dark-field examination of appropriate specimens should be performed in any patient in whom syphilis is suspected, even if the patient has a negative VDRL. Similarly, any patient with a positive serum VDRL test, neurologic findings, and an abnormal spinal fluid examination should be considered to have neurosyphilis and treated accordingly, regardless of the CSF VDRL result. In any setting, patients treated for syphilis need to be carefully monitored to ensure adequate therapy. Approximately one-third of patients with HIV infection will experience a Jarisch-Herxheimer reaction upon initiation of therapy for syphilis.

Vulvovaginal candidiasis is a common problem in women with HIV infection. Symptoms include pruritus, discomfort, dyspareunia, and dysuria. Vulvar infection may present as a morbilliform rash that may extend to the thighs. Vaginal infection is usually associated with a white discharge, and plaques may be seen along an erythematous vaginal wall. Diagnosis is made by microscopic examination of the discharge for pseudohyphal elements in a 10% potassium hydroxide solution. Mild disease can be treated with topical therapy. More serious disease can be treated with fluconazole. Other causes of vaginitis include *Trichomonas* and mixed bacteria.

Diseases of the endocrine system and metabolic disorders

A variety of endocrine and metabolic disorders are seen in the context of HIV infection. These may be a direct consequence of HIV infection, secondary to opportunistic infections or neoplasms, or related to medication side effects. Between 33 and 75% of patients with HIV infection receiving cART develop a syndrome often referred to as *lipodystrophy*, consisting of elevations in plasma triglycerides, total cholesterol, and apolipoprotein B, as well as hyperinsulinemia and hyperglycemia. Many of the patients have been noted to have a characteristic set of body habitus changes associated with fat redistribution, consisting of truncal obesity coupled with peripheral wasting (Fig. 189-39). Truncal obesity is apparent as an increase in

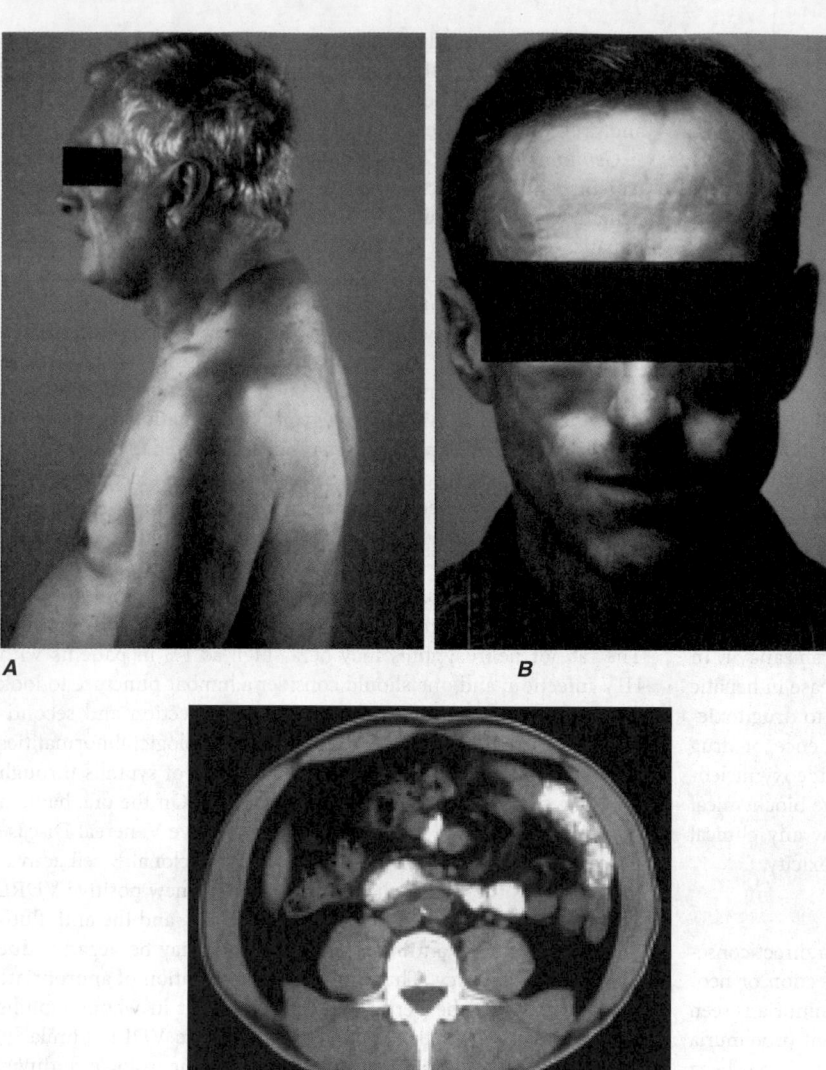

Figure 189-39   Characteristics of lipodystrophy. *A.* Truncal obesity and buffalo hump. *B.* Facial wasting. *C.* Accumulation of intraabdominal fat on CT scan.

incidence of osteonecrosis or avascular necrosis of the hip and shoulders. In a study of asymptomatic patients, 4.4% were found to have evidence of osteonecrosis on MRI. This complication has been associated with the use of lipid-lowering agents, systemic glucocorticoids, or testosterone; bodybuilding exercise; alcohol consumption; and the presence of anticardiolipin antibodies. Osteoporosis has been reported in 7% of women with HIV infection, with 41% of women demonstrating some degree of osteopenia. In addition, lactic acidosis is associated with cART. This is most commonly seen with nucleoside analogue reverse transcriptase inhibitors and can be fatal (see below).

Patients with advanced HIV disease may develop hyponatremia due to the syndrome of inappropriate antidiuretic hormone (vasopressin) secretion (SIADH) as a consequence of increased free-water intake and decreased free-water excretion. SIADH is usually seen in conjunction with pulmonary or CNS disease. Low serum sodium may also be due to adrenal insufficiency; a concomitant high serum potassium should alert one to this possibility. Hyperkalemia may be secondary to adrenal insufficiency; HIV nephropathy; or medications, particularly trimethoprim and pentamidine. Hypokalemia may be seen in the setting of tenofovir therapy. Adrenal gland disease may be due to mycobacterial infections, CMV disease, cryptococcal disease, histoplasmosis, or ketoconazole toxicity. Iatrogenic Cushing's syndrome with suppression of the hypothalamic-pituitary-adrenal axis may be seen with the use of local glucocorticoids (injected or inhaled) in patients receiving ritonavir. This is due to inhibition of the hepatic enzyme CYP3A4 by ritonavir leading to prolongation of the glucocorticoid half-life.

abdominal girth related to increases in mesenteric fat, a dorsocervical fat pad ("buffalo hump") reminiscent of patients with Cushing's syndrome, and enlargement of the breasts. The peripheral wasting, or lipoatrophy, is particularly noticeable in the face and buttocks and by the prominence of the veins in the legs. These changes may develop at any time ranging from ~6 weeks to several years following the initiation of cART. Approximately 20% of the patients with HIV-associated lipodystrophy meet the criteria for the *metabolic syndrome* as defined by The International Diabetes Federation or The U.S. National Cholesterol Education Program Adult Treatment Panel III. The lipodystrophy syndrome has been reported in association with regimens containing a variety of different drugs, and while initially reported in the setting of protease inhibitor therapy, it appears that similar changes can also be induced by potent protease-sparing regimens. It has been suggested that the lipoatrophy changes are particularly severe in patients receiving the thymidine analogues stavudine and zidovudine. National Cholesterol Education Program (NCEP) guidelines should be followed in the management of these lipid abnormalities (Chap. 241). Due to concerns regarding drug interactions, the most commonly utilized lipid-lowering agents in this setting are gemfibrozil and atorvastatin.

In addition to these abnormalities, patients with HIV infection treated with cART have been found to have an increased

Thyroid function may be altered in 10–15% of patients with HIV infection. Both hypo- and hyperthyroidism may be seen. The predominant abnormality is subclinical hypothyroidism. In the setting of cART, up to 10% of patients have been noted to have elevated thyroid-stimulating hormone levels, suggesting that this may be a manifestation of immune reconstitution. Immune-reconstitution Graves' disease may occur as a late (9–48 months) complication of cART. In advanced HIV disease, infection of the thyroid gland may occur with opportunistic pathogens, including *P. jiroveci*, CMV, mycobacteria, *Toxoplasma gondii*, and *Cryptococcus neoformans*. These infections are generally associated with a nontender, diffuse enlargement of the thyroid gland. Thyroid function is usually normal. Diagnosis is made by fine-needle aspirate or open biopsy.

Depending on the severity of disease, HIV infection is associated with *hypogonadism* in 20–50% of men. While this is generally a complication of underlying illness, testicular dysfunction may also be a side effect of ganciclovir therapy. In some surveys, up to two-thirds of patients report decreased libido and one-third complain of erectile dysfunction. Androgen-replacement therapy should be considered in patients with symptomatic hypogonadism. HIV infection does not seem to have a significant effect on the menstrual cycle outside the setting of advanced disease.

Immunologic and rheumatologic diseases

Immunologic and rheumatologic disorders are common in patients with HIV infection and range from excessive immediate-type hypersensitivity reactions (Chap. 317) to an increase in the incidence of reactive arthritis (Chap. 325) to conditions characterized by a diffuse infiltrative lymphocytosis. The occurrence of these phenomena is an apparent paradox in the setting of the profound immunodeficiency and immunosuppression that characterizes HIV infection and reflects the complex nature of the immune system and its regulatory mechanisms.

Drug allergies are the most significant allergic reactions occurring in HIV-infected patients and appear to become more common as the disease progresses. They occur in up to 65% of patients who receive therapy with TMP/SMX for PCP. In general, these drug reactions are characterized by erythematous, morbilliform eruptions that are pruritic, tend to coalesce, and are often associated with fever. Nonetheless, ~33% of patients can be maintained on the offending therapy, and thus these reactions are not an immediate indication to stop the drug. Anaphylaxis is extremely rare in patients with HIV infection, and patients who have a cutaneous reaction during a single course of therapy can still be considered candidates for future treatment or prophylaxis with the same agent. The one exception to this is the nucleoside analogue abacavir, where fatal hypersensitivity reactions have been reported with rechallenge. This hypersensitivity is strongly associated with the HLA-B5701 haplotype, and a hypersensitivity reaction to abacavir is an absolute contraindication to future therapy. For other agents, including TMP/SMX, desensitization regimens are moderately successful. While the mechanisms underlying these allergic-type reactions remain unknown, patients with HIV infection have been noted to have elevated IgE levels that increase as the CD4+ T cell count declines. The numerous examples of patients with multiple drug reactions suggest that a common pathway is involved.

HIV infection shares many similarities with a variety of autoimmune diseases, including a substantial polyclonal B cell activation that is associated with a high incidence of antiphospholipid antibodies, such as anticardiolipin antibodies, VDRL antibodies, and lupus-like anticoagulants. In addition, HIV-infected individuals have an increased incidence of antinuclear antibodies. Despite these serologic findings, there is no evidence that HIV-infected individuals have an increase in two of the more common autoimmune diseases, i.e., systemic lupus erythematosus and rheumatoid arthritis. In fact, it has been observed that these diseases may be somewhat ameliorated by the concomitant presence of HIV infection, suggesting that an intact CD4+ T cell limb of the immune response plays an integral role in the pathogenesis of these conditions. Similarly, there are anecdotal reports of patients with common variable immunodeficiency (Chap. 316), characterized by hypogammaglobulinemia, who have had a normalization of Ig levels following the development of HIV infection, suggesting a possible role for overactive CD4+ T cell immunity in certain forms of that syndrome. The one autoimmune disease that may occur with an increased frequency in patients with HIV infection is a variant of primary Sjögren's syndrome (Chap. 324). Patients with HIV infection may develop a syndrome consisting of parotid gland enlargement, dry eyes, and dry mouth that is associated with lymphocytic infiltrates of the salivary gland and lung. One also can see peripheral neuropathy, polymyositis, renal tubular acidosis, and hepatitis. In contrast to Sjögren's syndrome, in which the lymphocytic infiltrates are composed predominantly of CD4+ T cells, in patients with HIV infection the infiltrates are composed predominantly of CD8+ T cells. In addition, while patients with Sjögren's syndrome

are mainly women who have autoantibodies to Ro and La and who frequently have HLA-DR3 or -B8 MHC haplotypes, HIV-infected individuals with this syndrome are usually African-American men who do not have anti-Ro or anti-La and who most often are HLA-DR5. This syndrome appears to be less common with the increased use of effective cART. The term *diffuse infiltrative lymphocytosis syndrome* (DILS) is used to describe this entity and to distinguish it from Sjögren's syndrome.

Approximately one-third of HIV-infected individuals experience arthralgias; furthermore, 5–10% are diagnosed as having some form of reactive arthritis, such as Reiter's syndrome or psoriatic arthritis as well as undifferentiated spondyloarthropathy (Chap. 325). These syndromes occur with increasing frequency as the competency of the immune system declines. This association may be related to an increase in the number of infections with organisms that may trigger a reactive arthritis with progressive immunodeficiency or to a loss of important regulatory T cells. Reactive arthritides in HIV-infected individuals generally respond well to standard treatment; however, therapy with methotrexate has been associated with an increase in the incidence of opportunistic infections and should be used with caution and only in severe cases.

HIV-infected individuals also experience a variety of joint problems without obvious cause that are referred to generically as *HIV-* or *AIDS-associated arthropathy*. This syndrome is characterized by subacute oligoarticular arthritis developing over a period of 1–6 weeks and lasting 6 weeks to 6 months. It generally involves the large joints, predominantly the knees and ankles, and is nonerosive with only a mild inflammatory response. X-rays of the joint are nonrevealing. Nonsteroidal anti-inflammatory drugs are only marginally helpful; however, relief has been noted with the use of intraarticular glucocorticoids. A second form of arthritis also thought to be secondary to HIV infection is called *painful articular syndrome*. This condition, reported as occurring in as many as 10% of AIDS patients, presents as an acute, severe, sharp pain in the affected joint. It affects primarily the knees, elbows, and shoulders; lasts 2–24 h; and may be severe enough to require narcotic analgesics. The cause of this arthropathy is unclear; however, it is thought to result from a direct effect of HIV on the joint. This condition is reminiscent of the fact that other lentiviruses, in particular the caprine arthritis-encephalitis virus, are capable of directly causing arthritis.

A variety of other immunologic or rheumatologic diseases have been reported in HIV-infected individuals, either de novo or in association with opportunistic infections or drugs. Using the criteria of widespread musculoskeletal pain of at least 3 months' duration and the presence of at least 11 of 18 possible tender points by digital palpation, 11% of an HIV-infected cohort containing 55% IDUs were diagnosed as having *fibromyalgia* (Chap. 335). While the incidence of frank arthritis was less in this population than in other studied populations that consisted predominantly of men who have sex with men, these data support the concept that there are musculoskeletal problems that occur as a direct result of HIV infection. In addition there have been reports of leukocytoclastic vasculitis in the setting of zidovudine therapy. CNS angiitis and polymyositis have also been reported in HIV-infected individuals. Septic arthritis is surprisingly rare, especially given the increased incidence of staphylococcal bacteremias seen in this population. When septic arthritis has been reported, it has usually been due to *Staphylococcus aureus*, systemic fungal infection with *C. neoformans*, *Sporothrix schenckii*, or *H. capsulatum* or to systemic mycobacterial infection with *M. tuberculosis*, *M. haemophilum*, *M. avium*, or *M. kansasii*.

As noted above, 4.4% of patients with HIV infection were found to have some evidence of osteonecrosis by MRI during systematic screening of asymptomatic patients. The percentage of patients with symptomatic osteonecrosis has been estimated to be as high

TABLE 189-11 Characteristics of Immune Reconstitution Inflammatory Syndrome (IRIS)

- Paradoxical worsening of clinical condition is seen following the initiation of antiretroviral therapy
- Occurs weeks to months following the initiation of antiretroviral therapy
- Is most common in patients starting therapy with a CD4+ T cell count under 50/μL who experience a precipitous drop in viral load
- Is frequently seen in the setting of tuberculosis
- Can be fatal

TABLE 189-12 Causes of Bone Marrow Suppression in Patients With HIV Infection

HIV infection	Medications
Mycobacterial infections	Zidovudine
Fungal infections	Dapsone
B19 parvovirus infection	Trimethoprim/sulfamethoxazole
Lymphoma	Pyrimethamine
	5-Flucytosine
	Ganciclovir
	Interferon α
	Trimetrexate
	Foscarnet

as 1%. While this problem was first recognized in the setting of cART, it has been difficult to establish a cause-and-effect relationship. Alcohol consumption and a history of glucocorticoid use have been particularly associated with this condition in patients with HIV infection.

Immune reconstitution inflammatory syndrome (IRIS)

Following the initiation of effective cART, a paradoxical worsening of preexisting, untreated, or partially treated opportunistic infections may be noted. One may also see exacerbations of pre-existing or the development of new autoimmune conditions following the initiation of antiretrovirals (Table 189-11). IRIS related to a pre-existing infection is often referred to as immune reconstitution disease (IRD) to distinguish it from the autoimmune manifestations of IRIS. IRD is particularly common in patients with underlying untreated mycobacterial or fungal infections. IRIS is seen in anywhere from 10 to 30% of patients, depending on the clinical setting, and is most common in patients starting therapy with CD4+ T cell counts <50 cells/μL who have a precipitous drop in HIV RNA levels following the initiation of cART. Signs and symptoms may appear anywhere from 2 weeks to 2 years after the initiation of cART and can include localized lymphadenitis, prolonged fever, pulmonary infiltrates, increased intracranial pressure, uveitis, sarcoidosis, and Graves' disease. The clinical course can be protracted and severe cases can be fatal. The underlying mechanism appears to be related to a phenomenon similar to type IV hypersensitivity reactions and reflects the immediate improvements in immune function that occur as levels of HIV RNA drop and the immunosuppressive effects of HIV infection are controlled. In severe cases, the use of immunosuppressive drugs such as glucocorticoids may be required to blunt the inflammatory component of these reactions while specific antimicrobial therapy takes effect.

Diseases of the hematopoietic system

Disorders of the hematopoietic system including lymphadenopathy, anemia, leukopenia, and/or thrombocytopenia are common throughout the course of HIV infection and may be the direct result of HIV, manifestations of secondary infections and neoplasms, or side effects of therapy (Table 189-12). Direct histologic examination and culture of lymph node or bone marrow tissue are often diagnostic. A significant percentage of bone marrow aspirates from patients with HIV infection have been reported to contain lymphoid aggregates, the precise significance of which is unknown. Initiation of cART will lead to reversal of most hematologic complications that are the direct result of HIV infection.

Some patients, otherwise asymptomatic, may develop *persistent generalized lymphadenopathy* as an early clinical manifestation of HIV infection. This condition is defined as the presence of enlarged lymph nodes (>1 cm) in two or more extrainguinal sites for >3 months without an obvious cause. The lymphadenopathy is due to marked follicular hyperplasia in the node in response to HIV infection. The nodes are generally discrete and freely movable. This feature of HIV disease may be seen at any point in the spectrum of immune dysfunction and is not associated with an increased likelihood of developing AIDS. Paradoxically, a loss in lymphadenopathy or a decrease in lymph node size outside the setting of cART may be a prognostic marker of disease progression. In patients with CD4+ T cell counts >200/μL, the differential diagnosis of lymphadenopathy includes KS, TB, Castleman's disease, and lymphoma. In patients with more advanced disease, lymphadenopathy may also be due to atypical mycobacterial infection, toxoplasmosis, systemic fungal infection, or bacillary angiomatosis. While indicated in patients with CD4+ T cell counts <200/μL, lymph node biopsy is not indicated in patients with early-stage disease unless there are signs and symptoms of systemic illness, such as fever and weight loss, or unless the nodes begin to enlarge, become fixed, or coalesce. Monoclonal gammopathy of unknown significance (MGUS) (Chap. 111), defined as the presence of a serum monoclonal IgG, IgA, or IgM in the absence of a clear cause, has been reported in 3% of patients with HIV infection. The overall clinical significance of this finding in patients with HIV infection is unclear, although it has been associated with other viral infections, non-Hodgkin's lymphoma, and plasma cell malignancy.

Anemia is the most common hematologic abnormality in HIV-infected patients and, in the absence of a specific treatable cause, is independently associated with a poor prognosis. While generally mild, anemia can be quite severe and require chronic blood transfusions. Among the specific reversible causes of anemia in the setting of HIV infection are drug toxicity, systemic fungal and mycobacterial infections, nutritional deficiencies, and parvovirus B19 infections. Zidovudine may block erythroid maturation prior to its effects on other marrow elements. A characteristic feature of zidovudine therapy is an elevated mean corpuscular volume (MCV). Another drug used in patients with HIV infection that has a selective effect on the erythroid series is dapsone. This drug can cause a serious hemolytic anemia in patients who are deficient in glucose-6-phosphate dehydrogenase and can create a functional anemia in others through induction of methemoglobinemia. Folate levels are usually normal in HIV-infected individuals; however, vitamin B$_{12}$ levels may be depressed as a consequence of achlorhydria or malabsorption. True autoimmune hemolytic anemia is rare, although ~20% of patients with HIV infection may have a positive direct antiglobulin test as a consequence of polyclonal B cell activation. Infection with parvovirus B19 may also cause anemia. It is important to recognize this possibility given the fact that it responds well to treatment with IVIg. Erythropoietin levels in patients with HIV infection and anemia are generally lower than expected given the degree of anemia. Treatment with erythropoietin may result in an increase in hemoglobin levels. An exception to this is a subset of patients with zidovudine-associated anemia in whom erythropoietin levels may be quite high.

During the course of HIV infection, neutropenia may be seen in approximately half of patients. In most instances it is mild; however, it can be severe and can put patients at risk of spontaneous bacterial infections. This is most frequently seen in patients with severely advanced HIV disease and in patients receiving any of a number of potentially myelosuppressive therapies. In the setting of neutropenia, diseases that are not commonly seen in HIV-infected patients, such as aspergillosis or mucormycosis, may occur. Both granulocyte colony-stimulating factor (G-CSF) and GM-CSF increase neutrophil counts in patients with HIV infection regardless of the cause of the neutropenia. Earlier concerns about the potential of these agents to also increase levels of HIV were not confirmed in controlled clinical trials.

Thrombocytopenia may be an early consequence of HIV infection. Approximately 3% of patients with untreated HIV infection and CD4+ T cell counts ≥400/μL have platelet counts <150,000/μL. For untreated patients with CD4+ T cell counts <400/μL, this incidence increases to 10%. In patients receiving antiretrovirals, thrombocytopenia is associated with hepatitis C, cirrhosis, and ongoing high-level HIV replication. Thrombocytopenia is rarely a serious clinical problem in patients with HIV infection and generally responds well to successful cART. Clinically, it resembles the thrombocytopenia seen in patients with idiopathic thrombocytopenic purpura (Chap. 115). Immune complexes containing anti-gp120 antibodies and anti-anti-gp120 antibodies have been noted in the circulation and on the surface of platelets in patients with HIV infection. Patients with HIV infection have also been noted to have a platelet-specific antibody directed toward a 25-kDa component of the surface of the platelet. Other data suggest that the thrombocytopenia in patients with HIV infection may be due to a direct effect of HIV on megakaryocytes. Whatever the cause, it is very clear that the most effective medical approach to this problem has been the use of cART. For patients with platelet counts <20,000/μL a more aggressive approach combining IVIg or anti-Rh Ig for an immediate response with cART for a more lasting response is appropriate. Rituximab has been used with some success in otherwise refractory cases. Splenectomy is a rarely needed option and is reserved for patients refractory to medical management. Because of the risk of serious infection with encapsulated organisms, all patients with HIV infection about to undergo splenectomy should be immunized with pneumococcal polysaccharide. It should be noted that, in addition to causing an increase in the platelet count, removal of the spleen will result in an increase in the peripheral blood lymphocyte count, making CD4+ T cell counts unreliable markers of immunocompetence. In this setting, the clinician should rely on the CD4+ T cell percent for making diagnostic decisions with respect to the likelihood of opportunistic infections. A CD4+ T cell percent of 15 is approximately equivalent to a CD4+ T cell count of 200/μL. In patients with early HIV infection, thrombocytopenia has also been reported as a consequence of classic thrombotic thrombocytopenic purpura (Chap. 115). This clinical syndrome, consisting of fever, thrombocytopenia, hemolytic anemia, and neurologic and renal dysfunction, is a rare complication of early HIV infection. As in other settings, the appropriate management is the use of salicylates and plasma exchange. Other causes of thrombocytopenia include lymphoma, mycobacterial infections, and fungal infections.

The incidence of venous thromboembolic disease such as deep-vein thrombosis or pulmonary embolus is approximately 1% per year in patients with HIV infection. This is approximately 10 times higher than that seen in an age-matched population. Among the factors associated with clinical thrombosis are age over 45, history of an opportunistic infection, lower CD4 count, and estrogen use. Abnormalities of the coagulation cascade including decreased protein S activity, increases in factor VIII, anticardiolipin antibodies, or lupus-like anticoagulant have been reported in more than 50% of patients with HIV infection. The clinical significance of this increased propensity toward thromboembolic disease is likely reflected in the observation that elevations in D-dimer are strongly associated with all-cause mortality in patients with HIV infection (Table 189-8).

Dermatologic diseases

Dermatologic problems occur in >90% of patients with HIV infection. From the macular, roseola-like rash seen with the acute seroconversion syndrome to extensive end-stage KS, cutaneous manifestations of HIV disease can be seen throughout the course of HIV infection. Among the more common nonneoplastic problems are seborrheic dermatitis, folliculitis, and opportunistic infections. Extrapulmonary pneumocystosis may cause a necrotizing vasculitis. Neoplastic conditions are covered below.

Seborrheic dermatitis occurs in 3% of the general population and in up to 50% of patients with HIV infection. Seborrheic dermatitis increases in prevalence and severity as the CD4+ T cell count declines. In HIV-infected patients, seborrheic dermatitis may be aggravated by concomitant infection with *Pityrosporum*, a yeastlike fungus; use of topical antifungal agents has been recommended in cases refractory to standard topical treatment.

Folliculitis is among the most prevalent dermatologic disorders in patients with HIV infection and is seen in ~20% of patients. It is more common in patients with CD4+ T cell counts <200 cells/μL. Pruritic papular eruption is one of the most common pruritic rashes in patients with HIV infection. It appears as multiple papules on the face, trunk, and extensor surfaces and may improve with cART. *Eosinophilic pustular folliculitis* is a rare form of folliculitis that is seen with increased frequency in patients with HIV infection. It presents as multiple, urticarial perifollicular papules that may coalesce into plaquelike lesions. Skin biopsy reveals an eosinophilic infiltrate of the hair follicle, which in certain cases has been associated with the presence of a mite. Patients typically have an elevated serum IgE level and may respond to treatment with topical anthelmintics. Pruritus is a common symptom in patients with HIV infection and can lead to prurigo nodularis. Patients with HIV infection have also been reported to develop a severe form of *Norwegian scabies* with hyperkeratotic psoriasiform lesions.

Both *psoriasis* and *ichthyosis*, although they are not reported to be increased in frequency, may be particularly severe when they occur in patients with HIV infection. Preexisting psoriasis may become guttate in appearance and more refractory to treatment in the setting of HIV infection.

Reactivation herpes zoster (shingles) is seen in 10–20% of patients with HIV infection. This reactivation syndrome of varicella-zoster virus indicates a modest decline in immune function and may be the first indication of clinical immunodeficiency. In one series, patients who developed shingles did so an average of 5 years after HIV infection. In a cohort of patients with HIV infection and localized zoster, the subsequent rate of the development of AIDS was 1% per month. In that study, AIDS was more likely to develop if the outbreak of zoster was associated with severe pain, extensive skin involvement, or involvement of cranial or cervical dermatomes. The clinical manifestations of reactivation zoster in HIV-infected patients, although indicative of immunologic compromise, are not as severe as those seen in other immunodeficient conditions. Thus, while lesions may extend over several dermatomes, involve the spinal cord, and/or be associated with frank cutaneous dissemination, visceral involvement has not been reported. In contrast to patients without a known underlying immunodeficiency state, patients with HIV infection tend to have recurrences of zoster with a relapse rate of ~20%. Valacyclovir, acyclovir or famciclovir is the treatment of choice. Foscarnet may be of value in patients with acyclovir-resistant virus.

Infection with *herpes simplex virus* in HIV-infected individuals is associated with recurrent orolabial, genital, and perianal lesions as part of recurrent reactivation syndromes (Chap. 179). As HIV disease progresses and the CD4+ T cell count declines, these infections become more frequent and severe. Lesions often appear as beefy red, are exquisitely painful, and have a tendency to occur high in the gluteal cleft (Fig. 189-38). Perirectal HSV may be associated with proctitis and anal fissures. HSV should be high in the differential diagnosis of any HIV-infected patient with a poorly healing, painful perirectal lesion. In addition to recurrent mucosal ulcers, recurrent HSV infection in the form of *herpetic whitlow* can be a problem in patients with HIV infection, presenting with painful vesicles or extensive cutaneous erosion. Valacyclovir, acyclovir or famciclovir is the treatment of choice in these settings. Of note is the fact that even subclinical reactivation of herpes simplex may be associated with increases in plasma HIV RNA levels.

Diffuse skin eruptions due to *Molluscum contagiosum* may be seen in patients with advanced HIV infection. These flesh-colored, umbilicated lesions may be treated with local therapy. They tend to regress with effective cART. Similarly, *condyloma acuminatum* lesions may be more severe and more widely distributed in patients with low CD4+ T cell counts. Imiquimod cream may be helpful in some cases. Atypical mycobacterial infections may present as erythematous cutaneous nodules, as may fungal infections, *Bartonella, Acanthamoeba*, and KS.

The skin of patients with HIV infection is often a target organ for drug reactions (Chap. 55). Although most skin reactions are mild and not necessarily an indication to discontinue therapy, patients may have particularly severe cutaneous reactions, including erythroderma, *Stevens-Johnson syndrome*, and toxic epidermal necrolysis, as a reaction to drugs—particularly sulfa drugs, the nonnucleoside reverse transcriptase inhibitors, abacavir, amprenavir, darunavir, fosamprenavir, and tipranavir. Similarly, patients with HIV infection are often quite photosensitive and burn easily following exposure to sunlight or as a side effect of radiation therapy (Chap. 56).

HIV infection and its treatment may be accompanied by cosmetic changes of the skin that are not of great clinical importance but may be troubling to patients. Yellowing of the nails and straightening of the hair, particularly in African-American patients, have been reported as a consequence of HIV infection. Zidovudine therapy has been associated with elongation of the eyelashes and the development of a bluish discoloration to the nails, again more common in African-American patients. Therapy with clofazimine may cause a yellow-orange discoloration of the skin and urine.

Neurologic diseases

Clinical disease of the nervous system accounts for a significant degree of morbidity in a high percentage of patients with HIV infection (Table 189-13). The neurologic problems that occur in HIV-infected individuals may be either primary to the pathogenic processes of HIV infection or secondary to opportunistic infections or neoplasms (see above). Among the more frequent opportunistic diseases that involve the CNS are toxoplasmosis, cryptococcosis, progressive multifocal leukoencephalopathy, and primary CNS lymphoma. Other less common problems include mycobacterial infections; syphilis; and infection with CMV, HTLV-I,

TABLE 189-13 Neurologic Diseases in Patients With HIV Infection

Opportunistic infections	Result of HIV-1 infection (con't)
Toxoplasmosis	Myelopathy
Cryptococcosis	Vacuolar myelopathy
Progressive multifocal leukoencephalopathy	Pure sensory ataxia
Cytomegalovirus	Paresthesia/dysesthesia
Syphilis	Peripheral neuropathy
Mycobacterium tuberculosis	Acute inflammatory demyelinating polyneuropathy (Guillain-Barré syndrome)
HTLV-I infection	
Amebiasis	
Neoplasms	Chronic inflammatory demyelinating polyneuropathy (CIDP)
Primary CNS lymphoma	
Kaposi's sarcoma	Mononeuritis multiplex
Result of HIV-1 infection	Distal symmetric polyneuropathy
Aseptic meningitis	
HIV-associated neurocognitive disorders, including HIV encephalopathy/AIDS dementia complex	Myopathy

Trypanosoma cruzi, or *Acanthamoeba*. Overall, secondary diseases of the CNS have been reported to occur in approximately one-third of patients with AIDS. These data antedate the widespread use of cART, and this frequency is considerably lower in patients receiving effective antiretroviral drugs. Primary processes related to HIV infection of the nervous system are reminiscent of those seen with other lentiviruses, such as the Visna-Maedi virus of sheep.

Neurologic problems directly attributable to HIV occur throughout the course of infection and may be inflammatory, demyelinating, or degenerative in nature. The term *HIV-associated neurocognitive disorders* (HAND) is used to describe a spectrum of disorders that range from asymptomatic neurocognitive impairment (ANI) to minor neurocognitive disorder (MND) to clinically severe dementia. The most severe form, *HIV-associated dementia* (HAD), also referred to as the *AIDS dementia complex*, or *HIV encephalopathy*, is considered an AIDS-defining illness. Most HIV-infected patients have some neurologic problem during the course of their disease. Even in the setting of suppressive cART, approximately 50% of HIV-infected individuals can be shown to have mild to moderate neurocognitive impairment using sensitive neuropsychiatric testing. As noted in the section on pathogenesis, damage to the CNS may be a direct result of viral infection of the CNS macrophages or glial cells or may be secondary to the release of neurotoxins and potentially toxic cytokines such as IL-1β, TNF-α, IL-6, and TGF-β. It has been reported that HIV-infected individuals with the E4 allele for apo E are at increased risk for AIDS encephalopathy and peripheral neuropathy. Virtually all patients with HIV infection have some degree of nervous system involvement with the virus. This is evidenced by the fact that CSF findings are abnormal in ~90% of patients, even during the asymptomatic phase of HIV infection. CSF abnormalities include pleocytosis (50–65% of patients), detection of viral RNA (~75%), elevated CSF protein (35%), and evidence of intrathecal synthesis of anti-HIV antibodies (90%). It is important to point out that evidence of infection of the CNS with HIV does not imply impairment of cognitive function. The neurologic function of an HIV-infected individual should be considered normal unless clinical signs and symptoms suggest otherwise.

Aseptic meningitis may be seen in any but the very late stages of HIV infection. In the setting of acute primary infection, patients may experience a syndrome of headache, photophobia, and meningismus. Rarely, an acute encephalopathy due to encephalitis may occur. Cranial nerve involvement may be seen, predominantly cranial nerve VII but occasionally V and/or VIII. CSF findings include a lymphocytic pleocytosis, elevated protein level, and normal glucose level. This syndrome, which cannot be clinically differentiated from other viral meningitides (Chap. 382), usually resolves spontaneously within 2–4 weeks; however, in some patients, signs and symptoms may become chronic. Aseptic meningitis may occur any time in the course of HIV infection; however, it is rare following the development of AIDS. This fact suggests that clinical aseptic meningitis in the context of HIV infection is an immune-mediated disease.

C. neoformans is the leading infectious cause of meningitis in patients with AIDS (Chap. 202). It is the initial AIDS-defining illness in ~2% of patients and generally occurs in patients with CD4+ T cell counts <100/μL. Cryptococcal meningitis is particularly common in untreated patients with AIDS in Africa, occurring in ~5% of patients. Most patients present with a picture of subacute meningoencephalitis with fever, nausea, vomiting, altered mental status, headache, and meningeal signs. The incidence of seizures and focal neurologic deficits is low. The CSF profile may be normal or may show only modest elevations in WBC or protein levels and decreases in glucose. The opening pressure in the CSF is usually elevated. In addition to meningitis, patients may develop cryptococcomas and cranial nerve involvement. Approximately one-third of patients also have pulmonary disease. Uncommon manifestations of cryptococcal infection include skin lesions that resemble *molluscum contagiosum*, lymphadenopathy, palatal and glossal ulcers, arthritis, gastroenteritis, myocarditis, and prostatitis. The prostate gland may serve as a reservoir for smoldering cryptococcal infection. The diagnosis of cryptococcal meningitis is made by identification of organisms in spinal fluid with india ink examination or by the detection of cryptococcal antigen. Blood cultures for fungus are often positive. A biopsy may be needed to make a diagnosis of CNS cryptococcoma. Treatment is with IV amphotericin B 0.7 mg/kg daily, or liposomal amphotericin 4–6 mg/kg daily, with flucytosine 25 mg/kg qid for at least 2 weeks and, if possible, until the CSF culture turns negative. This is followed by fluconazole 400 mg/d PO for 8 weeks, and then fluconazole 200 mg/d until the CD4+ T cell count has increased to >200 cells/μL for 6 months in response to cART. Repeated lumbar puncture may be required to manage increased intracranial pressure. Symptoms may recur with initiation of cART

as an immune reconstitution syndrome (see above). Other fungi that may cause meningitis in patients with HIV infection are *C. immitis* and *H. capsulatum*. Meningoencephalitis has also been reported due to *Acanthamoeba* or *Naegleria*.

HIV-associated dementia consists of a constellation of signs and symptoms of CNS disease. While this is generally a late complication of HIV infection that progresses slowly over months, it can be seen in patients with CD4+ T cell counts >350 cells/μL. A major feature of this entity is the development of dementia, defined as a decline in cognitive ability from a previous level. It may present as impaired ability to concentrate, increased forgetfulness, difficulty reading, or increased difficulty performing complex tasks. Initially these symptoms may be indistinguishable from findings of situational depression or fatigue. In contrast to "cortical" dementia (such as Alzheimer's disease), aphasia, apraxia, and agnosia are uncommon, leading some investigators to classify HIV encephalopathy as a "subcortical dementia" characterized by defects in short-term memory and executive function (see below). In addition to dementia, patients with HIV encephalopathy may also have motor and behavioral abnormalities. Among the motor problems are unsteady gait, poor balance, tremor, and difficulty with rapid alternating movements. Increased tone and deep tendon reflexes may be found in patients with spinal cord involvement. Late stages may be complicated by bowel and/or bladder incontinence. Behavioral problems include apathy, irritability, and lack of initiative, with progression to a vegetative state in some instances. Some patients develop a state of agitation or mild mania. These changes usually occur without significant changes in level of alertness. This is in contrast to the finding of somnolence in patients with dementia due to toxic/metabolic encephalopathies.

HIV-associated dementia is the initial AIDS-defining illness in ~3% of patients with HIV infection and thus only rarely precedes clinical evidence of immunodeficiency. Clinically significant encephalopathy eventually develops in ~25% of untreated patients with AIDS. As immunologic function declines, the risk and severity of HIV-associated dementia increases. Autopsy series suggest that 80–90% of patients with HIV infection have histologic evidence of CNS involvement. Several classification schemes have been developed for grading HIV encephalopathy; a commonly used clinical staging system is outlined in Table 189-14.

The precise cause of HIV-associated dementia remains unclear, although the condition is thought to be a result of a combination of direct effects of HIV on the CNS and associated immune

TABLE 189-14 Clinical Staging of HIV Encephalopathy (AIDS Dementia Complex)

Stage	Definition
0 (Normal)	Normal mental and motor function.
0.5 (Equivocal/ subclinical)	Absent, minimal, or equivocal symptoms without impairment of work or capacity to perform activities of daily living. Mild signs (snout response, slowed ocular or extremity movements) may be present. Gait and strength are normal.
1 (Mild)	Able to perform all but the more demanding aspects of work or activities of daily living but with unequivocal evidence (signs or symptoms that may include performance on neuropsychological testing) of functional, intellectual, or motor impairment. Can walk without assistance.
2 (Moderate)	Able to perform basic activities of self-care but cannot work or maintain the more demanding aspects of daily life. Ambulatory, but may require a single prop.
3 (Severe)	Major intellectual incapacity (cannot follow news or personal events, cannot sustain complex conversation, considerable slowing of all output) or motor disability (cannot walk unassisted, usually with slowing and clumsiness of arms as well).
4 (End-stage)	Nearly vegetative. Intellectual and social comprehension and output are at a rudimentary level. Nearly or absolutely mute. Paraparetic or paraplegic with urinary and fecal incontinence.

Source: Adapted from JJ Sidtis, RW Price: Neurology 40:197, 1990.

activation. HIV has been found in the brains of patients with HIV encephalopathy by Southern blot, in situ hybridization, PCR, and electron microscopy. Multinucleated giant cells, macrophages, and microglial cells appear to be the main cell types harboring virus in the CNS. Histologically, the major changes are seen in the subcortical areas of the brain and include pallor and gliosis, multinucleated giant cell encephalitis, and vacuolar myelopathy. Less commonly, diffuse or focal spongiform changes occur in the white matter. Areas of the brain involved in motor, language, and judgment are most severely affected.

There are no specific criteria for a diagnosis of HIV-associated dementia, and this syndrome must be differentiated from a number of other diseases that affect the CNS of HIV-infected patients (Table 189-13). The diagnosis of dementia depends on demonstrating a decline in cognitive function. This can be accomplished objectively with the use of a Mini-Mental Status Examination (MMSE) in patients for whom prior scores are available. For this reason, it is advisable for all patients with a diagnosis of HIV infection to have a baseline MMSE. However, changes in MMSE scores may be absent in patients with mild HIV encephalopathy. Imaging studies of the CNS, by either MRI or CT, often demonstrate evidence of cerebral atrophy (Fig. 189-40). MRI may also reveal small areas of increased density on T2-weighted images. Lumbar puncture is an important element of the evaluation of patients with HIV infection and neurologic abnormalities. It is generally most helpful in ruling out or making a diagnosis of opportunistic infections. In HIV encephalopathy, patients may have the nonspecific findings of an increase in CSF cells and protein level. While HIV RNA can often be detected in the spinal fluid and HIV can be cultured from the CSF, this finding is not specific for HIV encephalopathy. There appears to be no correlation between the presence of HIV in the CSF and the presence of HIV encephalopathy. Elevated levels of macrophage chemoattractant protein (MCP-1), β_2-microglobulin, neopterin, and quinolinic acid (a metabolite of tryptophan reported to cause CNS injury) have been noted in the CSF of patients with HIV encephalopathy. These findings suggest that these factors as well as inflammatory cytokines may be involved in the pathogenesis of this syndrome.

Combination antiretroviral therapy is of benefit in patients with HIV-associated dementia. Improvement in neuropsychiatric test scores has been noted for both adult and pediatric patients treated with antiretrovirals. The rapid improvement in cognitive function noted with the initiation of cART suggests that at least some component of this problem is quickly reversible, again supporting at least a partial role of soluble mediators in the pathogenesis. It should also be noted that these patients have an increased sensitivity to the side effects of neuroleptic drugs. The use of these drugs for symptomatic treatment is associated with an increased risk of extrapyramidal side effects; therefore, patients with HIV encephalopathy who receive these agents must be monitored carefully. It is felt by many physicians that the decrease in the prevalence of severe cases of HAND brought about by cART has resulted in an increase in the prevalence of milder forms of this disorder.

Seizures may be a consequence of opportunistic infections, neoplasms, or HIV encephalopathy (Table 189-15). The seizure threshold is often lower than normal in patients with advanced HIV infection due to the frequent presence of electrolyte abnormalities. Seizures are seen in 15–40% of patients with cerebral toxoplasmosis, 15–35% of patients with primary CNS lymphoma, 8% of patients with cryptococcal meningitis, and 7–50% of patients with HIV encephalopathy. Seizures may also be seen in patients with CNS tuberculosis, aseptic meningitis, and progressive multifocal leukoencephalopathy. Seizures may be the presenting clinical symptom of HIV disease. In one study of 100 patients with HIV infection presenting with a first seizure, cerebral mass lesions were the most common cause, responsible for 32 of the 100 new-onset seizures. Of these 32 cases, 28 were due to toxoplasmosis and 4 to lymphoma. HIV encephalopathy accounted for an additional 24 new-onset seizures. Cryptococcal meningitis was the third most common diagnosis, responsible for 13 of the 100 seizures. In 23 cases, no cause could be found, and it is possible that these cases represent a subcategory of HIV encephalopathy. Of these 23 cases, 16 (70%) had two or more seizures, suggesting that anticonvulsant therapy is indicated in all patients with HIV infection and seizures unless a rapidly correctable cause is found. While phenytoin remains the initial treatment of choice, hypersensitivity reactions to this drug have been reported in >10% of patients with AIDS, and therefore the use of phenobarbital or valproic acid must be considered as alternatives. Due to a variety of drug-drug interactions between antiseizure medications and antiretrovirals, drug levels need to be monitored carefully.

Patients with HIV infection may present with *focal neurologic deficits* from a variety of causes. The most common causes are

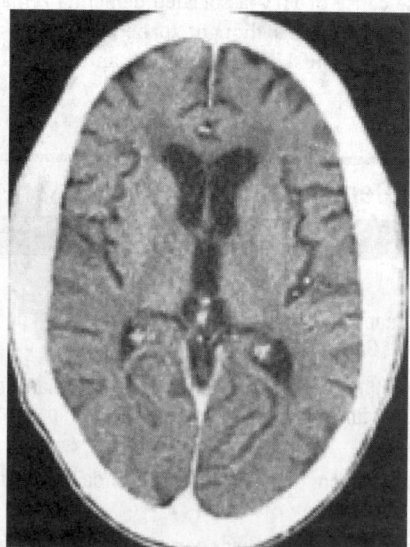

Figure 189-40 AIDS dementia complex. Postcontrast CT scan through the lateral ventricles of a 47-year-old man with AIDS, altered mental status, and dementia. The lateral and third ventricles and the cerebral sulci are abnormally prominent. Mild white matter hypodensity is also seen adjacent to the frontal horns of the lateral ventricles.

TABLE 189-15 Causes of Seizures in Patients With HIV Infection

Disease	Overall Contribution to First Seizure, %	Fraction of Patients Who Have Seizures, %
HIV encephalopathy	24–47	7–50
Cerebral toxoplasmosis	28	15–40
Cryptococcal meningitis	13	8
Primary central nervous system lymphoma	4	15–30
Progressive multifocal leukoencephalopathy	1	

Source: From DM Holtzman et al: Am J Med 87:173, 1989.

toxoplasmosis, progressive multifocal leukoencephalopathy, and CNS lymphoma. Other causes include cryptococcal infections (discussed above; also Chap. 202), stroke, and reactivation of Chagas' disease.

Toxoplasmosis has been one of the most common causes of secondary CNS infections in patients with AIDS, but its incidence is decreasing in the era of cART. It is most common in patients from the Caribbean and from France, where the seroprevalence of *T. gondii* is around 50%. This figure is closer to 15% in the United States. Toxoplasmosis is generally a late complication of HIV infection and usually occurs in patients with CD4+ T cell counts <200/μL. Cerebral toxoplasmosis is thought to represent a reactivation of latent tissue cysts. It is 10 times more common in patients with antibodies to the organism than in patients who are seronegative. Patients diagnosed with HIV infection should be screened for IgG antibodies to *T. gondii* during the time of their initial workup. Those who are seronegative should be counseled about ways to minimize the risk of primary infection including avoiding the consumption of undercooked meat and careful hand washing after contact with soil or changing the cat litter box. The most common clinical presentation of cerebral toxoplasmosis in patients with HIV infection is fever, headache, and focal neurologic deficits. Patients may present with seizure, hemiparesis, or aphasia as a manifestation of these focal deficits or with a picture more influenced by the accompanying cerebral edema and characterized by confusion, dementia, and lethargy, which can progress to coma. The diagnosis is usually suspected on the basis of MRI findings of multiple lesions in multiple locations, although in some cases only a single lesion is seen. Pathologically, these lesions generally exhibit inflammation and central necrosis and, as a result, demonstrate ring enhancement on contrast MRI (Fig. 189-41) or, if MRI is unavailable or contraindicated, on double-dose contrast CT. There is usually evidence of surrounding edema. In addition to toxoplasmosis, the differential diagnosis of single or multiple enhancing mass lesions in the HIV-infected patient includes primary CNS lymphoma and, less commonly, TB or fungal or bacterial abscesses. The definitive diagnostic procedure is brain biopsy. However, given the morbidity rate that can accompany this procedure, it is usually reserved for the patient who has failed 2–4 weeks of empiric therapy. If the patient is seronegative for *T. gondii*, the likelihood that a mass lesion is due to toxoplasmosis is <10%. In that setting, one may choose to be more aggressive and perform a brain biopsy sooner. Standard treatment is sulfadiazine and pyrimethamine with leucovorin as needed for a minimum of 4–6 weeks. Alternative therapeutic regimens include clindamycin in combination with pyrimethamine; atovaquone plus pyrimethamine; and azithromycin plus pyrimethamine plus rifabutin. Relapses are common, and it is recommended that patients with a history of prior toxoplasmic encephalitis receive maintenance therapy with sulfadiazine, pyrimethamine, and leucovorin as long as their CD4+ T cell counts remain <200 cells/μL. Patients with CD4+ T cell counts <100/μL and IgG antibody to *Toxoplasma* should receive primary prophylaxis for toxoplasmosis. Fortunately, the same daily regimen of a single double-strength tablet of TMP/SMX used for *P. jiroveci* prophylaxis provides adequate primary protection against toxoplasmosis. Secondary prophylaxis/maintenance therapy for toxoplasmosis may be discontinued in the setting of effective cART and increases in CD4+ T cell counts to >200/μL for 6 months.

JC virus, a human polyomavirus that is the etiologic agent of *progressive multifocal leukoencephalopathy* (PML), is an important opportunistic pathogen in patients with AIDS (Chap. 381). While ~80% of the general adult population has antibodies to JC virus, indicative of prior infection, <10% of healthy adults show any evidence of ongoing viral replication. PML is the only known clinical manifestation of JC virus infection. It is a late manifestation of AIDS and is seen in ~4% of patients with AIDS. The lesions of PML begin as small foci of demyelination in subcortical white matter that eventually coalesce. The cerebral hemispheres, cerebellum, and brainstem may all be involved. Patients typically have a protracted course with multifocal neurologic deficits, with or without changes in mental status. Approximately 20% of patients experience seizures. Ataxia, hemiparesis, visual field defects, aphasia, and sensory defects may occur. Headache, fever, nausea, and vomiting are rarely seen. Their presence should suggest another diagnosis. MRI typically reveals multiple, nonenhancing white matter lesions that may coalesce and have a predilection for the occipital and parietal lobes. The lesions show signal hyperintensity on T2-weighted images and diminished signal on T1-weighted images. The measurement of JC virus DNA levels in CSF has a diagnostic sensitivity of 76% and a specificity of close to 100%. Prior to the availability of cART, the majority of patients with PML died within 3–6 months of the onset of symptoms. Paradoxical worsening of PML has been seen with initiation of cART as an immune reconstitution syndrome. There is no specific treatment for PML; however, a median survival of 2 years and survival of >15 years have been reported in patients with PML treated with cART for their HIV disease. Despite having a significant impact on survival, only ~50% of patients with HIV infection and PML show neurologic improvement with cART. Studies with other antiviral agents such as cidofovir have failed to show clear benefit. Factors influencing a favorable prognosis for PML in the setting of HIV infection include a CD4+ T cell count >100/μL at baseline and the ability to maintain an HIV viral load of <500 copies per milliliter. Baseline HIV-1 viral load does not have independent predictive value of survival. PML is one of the few opportunistic infections that continues to occur with some frequency despite the widespread use of cART.

Reactivation American trypanosomiasis may present as acute meningoencephalitis with focal neurologic signs, fever, headache, vomiting, and seizures. Accompanying cardiac disease in the form of arrhythmias or heart failure should increase the index of suspicion. The presence of antibodies to *T. cruzi* supports the diagnosis. In South America, reactivation of *Chagas' disease* is considered to be an AIDS-defining condition and may be the initial AIDS-defining condition. The majority of cases occur in patients with CD4+ T cell counts <200 cells/μL. Lesions appear radiographically as single or multiple hypodense areas, typically with ring enhancement and

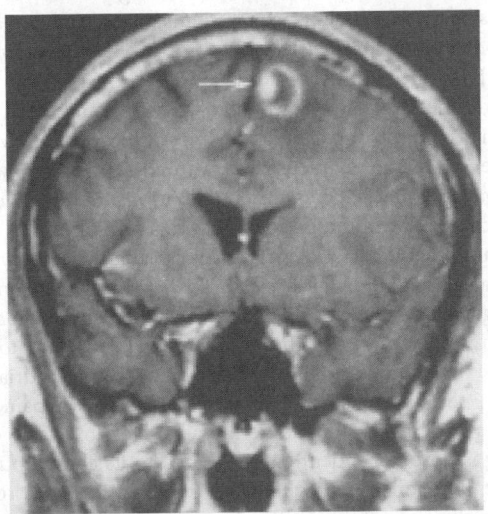

Figure 189-41   Central nervous system toxoplasmosis. A coronal postcontrast T1-weighted MRI scan demonstrates a peripheral enhancing lesion in the left frontal lobe, associated with an eccentric nodular area of enhancement (*arrow*); this so-called eccentric target sign is typical of toxoplasmosis.

edema. They are found predominantly in the subcortical areas, a feature that differentiates them from the deeper lesions of toxoplasmosis. *T. cruzi* amastigotes, or trypanosomes, can be identified from biopsy specimens or CSF. Other CSF findings include elevated protein and a mild (<100 cells/μL) lymphocytic pleocytosis. Organisms can also be identified by direct examination of the blood. Treatment consists of benzimidazole (2.5 mg/kg bid) or nifurtimox (2 mg/kg qid) for at least 60 days, followed by maintenance therapy for the duration of immunodeficiency with either drug at a dose of 5 mg/kg three times a week. As is the case with cerebral toxoplasmosis, successful therapy with antiretrovirals may allow discontinuation of therapy for Chagas' disease.

Stroke may occur in patients with HIV infection. In contrast to the other causes of focal neurologic deficits in patients with HIV infection, the symptoms of a stroke are sudden in onset. Patients with HIV infection have an increased prevalence of many classic risk factors associated with stroke, including smoking and diabetes. It also appears that HIV infection itself can lead to an increase in carotid artery stiffness. Among the secondary infectious diseases in patients with HIV infection that may be associated with stroke are vasculitis due to cerebral varicella zoster or neurosyphilis and septic embolism in association with fungal infection. Other elements of the differential diagnosis of stroke in the patient with HIV infection include atherosclerotic cerebral vascular disease, thrombotic thrombocytopenic purpura, and cocaine or amphetamine use.

Primary CNS lymphoma is discussed below in the section on neoplastic diseases.

Spinal cord disease, or myelopathy, is present in ~20% of patients with AIDS, often as part of HIV-associated neurocognitive disorder. In fact, 90% of the patients with HIV-associated myelopathy have some evidence of dementia, suggesting that similar pathologic processes may be responsible for both conditions. Three main types of spinal cord disease are seen in patients with AIDS. The first of these is a vacuolar myelopathy, as mentioned above. This condition is pathologically similar to subacute combined degeneration of the cord, such as that occurring with pernicious anemia. Although vitamin B₁₂ deficiency can be seen in patients with AIDS as a primary complication of HIV infection, it does not appear to be responsible for the myelopathy seen in the majority of patients. Vacuolar myelopathy is characterized by a subacute onset and often presents with gait disturbances, predominantly ataxia and spasticity; it may progress to include bladder and bowel dysfunction. Physical findings include evidence of increased deep tendon reflexes and extensor plantar responses. The second form of spinal cord disease involves the dorsal columns and presents as a pure sensory ataxia. The third form is also sensory in nature and presents with paresthesias and dysesthesias of the lower extremities. In contrast to the cognitive problems seen in patients with HIV encephalopathy, these spinal cord syndromes do not respond well to antiretroviral drugs, and therapy is mainly supportive.

One important disease of the spinal cord that also involves the peripheral nerves is a *myelopathy* and *polyradiculopathy* seen in association with CMV infection. This entity is generally seen late in the course of HIV infection and is fulminant in onset, with lower extremity and sacral paresthesias, difficulty in walking, areflexia, ascending sensory loss, and urinary retention. The clinical course is rapidly progressive over a period of weeks. CSF examination reveals a predominantly neutrophilic pleocytosis, and CMV DNA can be detected by CSF PCR. Therapy with ganciclovir or foscarnet can lead to rapid improvement, and prompt initiation of foscarnet or ganciclovir therapy is important in minimizing the degree of permanent neurologic damage. Combination therapy with both drugs should be considered in patients who have been previously treated for CMV disease. Other diseases involving the spinal cord in patients with HIV infection include HTLV-I-associated myelopathy (HAM) (Chap. 188), neurosyphilis (Chap. 169), infection

with herpes simplex (Chap. 179) or varicella-zoster (Chap. 180), TB (Chap. 165), and lymphoma (Chap. 110).

Peripheral neuropathies are common in patients with HIV infection. They occur at all stages of illness and take a variety of forms. Early in the course of HIV infection, an acute inflammatory demyelinating polyneuropathy resembling Guillain-Barré syndrome may occur (Chap. 385). In other patients, a progressive or relapsing-remitting inflammatory neuropathy resembling chronic inflammatory demyelinating polyneuropathy (CIDP) has been noted. Patients commonly present with progressive weakness, areflexia, and minimal sensory changes. CSF examination often reveals a mononuclear pleocytosis, and peripheral nerve biopsy demonstrates a perivascular infiltrate suggesting an autoimmune etiology. Plasma exchange or IVIg has been tried with variable success. Because of the immunosuppressive effects of glucocorticoids, they should be reserved for severe cases of CIDP refractory to other measures. Another autoimmune peripheral neuropathy seen in patients with AIDS is mononeuritis multiplex (Chaps. 385 and 326) due to a necrotizing arteritis of peripheral nerves. The most common peripheral neuropathy in patients with HIV infection is a *distal sensory polyneuropathy* (DSPN) also referred to as painful sensory neuropathy (HIV-SN), predominantly sensory neuropathy, or distal symmetric peripheral neuropathy. This condition may be a direct consequence of HIV infection or a side effect of dideoxynucleoside therapy. It is more common in taller individuals, older individuals, and those with lower CD4 counts. Two-thirds of patients with AIDS may be shown by electrophysiologic studies to have some evidence of peripheral nerve disease. Presenting symptoms are usually painful burning sensations in the feet and lower extremities. Findings on examination include a stocking-type sensory loss to pinprick, temperature, and touch sensation and a loss of ankle reflexes. Motor changes are mild and are usually limited to weakness of the intrinsic foot muscles. Response of this condition to antiretrovirals has been variable, perhaps because antiretrovirals are responsible for the problem in some instances. When due to dideoxynucleoside therapy, patients with lower extremity peripheral neuropathy may complain of a sensation that they are walking on ice. Other entities in the differential diagnosis of peripheral neuropathy include diabetes mellitus, vitamin B₁₂ deficiency, and side effects from metronidazole or dapsone. For distal symmetric polyneuropathy that fails to resolve following the discontinuation of dideoxynucleosides, therapy is symptomatic; gabapentin, carbamazepine, tricyclics, or analgesics may be effective for dysesthesias. Treatment-naïve patients may respond to cART.

Myopathy may complicate the course of HIV infection; causes include HIV infection itself, zidovudine, and the generalized wasting syndrome. HIV-associated myopathy may range in severity from an asymptomatic elevation in creatine kinase levels to a subacute syndrome characterized by proximal muscle weakness and myalgias. Quite pronounced elevations in creatine kinase may occur in asymptomatic patients, particularly after exercise. The clinical significance of this as an isolated laboratory finding is unclear. A variety of both inflammatory and noninflammatory pathologic processes have been noted in patients with more severe myopathy, including myofiber necrosis with inflammatory cells, nemaline rod bodies, cytoplasmic bodies, and mitochondrial abnormalities. Profound muscle wasting, often with muscle pain, may be seen after prolonged zidovudine therapy. This toxic side effect of the drug is dose-dependent and is related to its ability to interfere with the function of mitochondrial polymerases. It is reversible following discontinuation of the drug. Red ragged fibers are a histologic hallmark of zidovudine-induced myopathy.

Ophthalmologic diseases

Ophthalmologic problems occur in ~50% of patients with advanced HIV infection. The most common abnormal findings on funduscopic examination are cotton-wool spots. These are hard white spots that appear on the surface of the retina and often have an irregular edge. They represent areas of retinal ischemia secondary to microvascular disease. At times they are associated with small areas of hemorrhage and thus can be difficult to distinguish from CMV retinitis. In contrast to CMV retinitis, however, these lesions are not associated with visual loss and tend to remain stable or improve over time.

One of the most devastating consequences of HIV infection is CMV retinitis. Patients at high risk of CMV retinitis (CD4+ T cell count <100/μL) should undergo an ophthalmologic examination every 3–6 months. The majority of cases of CMV retinitis occur in patients with a CD4+ T cell count <50/μL. Prior to the availability of cART, this CMV reactivation syndrome was seen in 25–30% of patients with AIDS. CMV retinitis usually presents as a painless, progressive loss of vision. Patients may also complain of blurred vision, "floaters," and scintillations. The disease is usually bilateral, although typically it affects one eye more than the other. The diagnosis is made on clinical grounds by an experienced ophthalmologist. The characteristic retinal appearance is that of perivascular hemorrhage and exudate. In situations where the diagnosis is in doubt due to an atypical presentation or an unexpected lack of response to therapy, vitreous or aqueous humor sampling with molecular diagnostic techniques may be of value. CMV infection of the retina results in a necrotic inflammatory process, and the visual loss that develops is irreversible. CMV retinitis may be complicated by rhegmatogenous retinal detachment as a consequence of retinal atrophy in areas of prior inflammation. Therapy for CMV retinitis consists of oral valganciclovir, IV ganciclovir, or IV foscarnet, with cidofovir as an alternative. Combination therapy with ganciclovir and foscarnet has been shown to be slightly more effective than either ganciclovir or foscarnet alone in the patient with relapsed CMV retinitis. A 3-week induction course is followed by maintenance therapy with oral valganciclovir. If CMV disease is limited to the eye, a ganciclovir-releasing intraocular implant, periodic injections of the antisense nucleic acid preparation fomivirsen (no longer available in the United States), or intravitreal injections of ganciclovir or foscarnet may be considered; some choose to combine intraocular implants with oral valganciclovir. Intravitreal injections of cidofovir are generally avoided due to the increased risk of uveitis and hypotony. Maintenance therapy is continued until the CD4+ T cell count remains >100–150/μL for >6 months. The majority of patients with HIV infection and CMV disease develop some degree of uveitis with the initiation of cART. The etiology of this is unknown; however, it has been suggested that this may be due to the generation of an enhanced immune response to CMV as an IRIS (see above). In some instances this has required the use of topical glucocorticoids.

Both HSV and varicella zoster virus can cause a rapidly progressing, bilateral necrotizing retinitis referred to as the *acute retinal necrosis syndrome*, or *progressive outer retinal necrosis* (PORN). This syndrome, in contrast to CMV retinitis, is associated with pain, keratitis, and iritis. It is often associated with orolabial HSV or trigeminal zoster. Ophthalmologic examination reveals widespread pale gray peripheral lesions. This condition is often complicated by retinal detachment. It is important to recognize and treat this condition with IV acyclovir as quickly as possible to minimize the loss of vision.

Several other secondary infections may cause ocular problems in HIV-infected patients. *P. jiroveci* can cause a lesion of the choroid that may be detected as an incidental finding on ophthalmologic examination. These lesions are typically bilateral, are from half to twice the disc diameter in size, and appear as slightly elevated yellow-white plaques. They are usually asymptomatic and may be confused with cotton-wool spots. Chorioretinitis due to toxoplasmosis can be

seen alone or, more commonly, in association with CNS toxoplasmosis. KS may involve the eyelid or conjunctiva, while lymphoma may involve the retina. Syphilis may lead to a uveitis that is highly associated with the presence of neurosyphilis.

Additional disseminated infections and wasting syndrome

Infections with species of the small, gram-negative, *Rickettsia*-like organism *Bartonella* (Chap. 160) are seen with increased frequency in patients with HIV infection. While it is not considered an AIDS-defining illness by the CDC, many experts view infection with *Bartonella* as indicative of a severe defect in cell-mediated immunity. It is usually seen in patients with CD4+ T cell counts <100/μL and is a significant cause of unexplained fever in patients with advanced HIV infection. Among the clinical manifestations of *Bartonella* infection are bacillary angiomatosis, cat-scratch disease, and trench fever. *Bacillary angiomatosis* is usually due to infection with *B. henselae* and is linked to exposure to flea-infested cats. It is characterized by a vascular proliferation that leads to a variety of skin lesions that have been confused with the skin lesions of KS. In contrast to the lesions of KS, the lesions of bacillary angiomatosis generally blanch, are painful, and typically occur in the setting of systemic symptoms. Infection can extend to the lymph nodes, liver (peliosis hepatis), spleen, bone, heart, CNS, respiratory tract, and GI tract. *Cat-scratch disease* is also due to *B. henselae* and generally begins with a papule at the site of inoculation. This is followed several weeks later by the development of regional adenopathy and malaise. Infection with *B. quintana* is transmitted by lice and has been associated with case reports of trench fever, endocarditis, adenopathy, and bacillary angiomatosis. The organism is quite difficult to culture, and diagnosis often relies on identifying the organism in biopsy specimens using the Warthin-Starry or similar stains. Treatment is with either doxycycline or erythromycin for at least 3 months.

Histoplasmosis is an opportunistic infection that is seen most frequently in patients in the Mississippi and Ohio River valleys, Puerto Rico, the Dominican Republic, and South America. These are all areas in which infection with *H. capsulatum* is endemic (Chap. 199). Because of this limited geographic distribution, the percentage of AIDS cases in the United States with histoplasmosis is only ~0.5. Histoplasmosis is generally a late manifestation of HIV infection; however, it may be the initial AIDS-defining condition. In one study, the median CD4+ T cell count for patients with histoplasmosis and AIDS was 33/μL. While disease due to *H. capsulatum* may present as a primary infection of the lung, disseminated disease, presumably due to reactivation, is the most common presentation in HIV-infected patients. Patients usually present with a 4- to 8-week history of fever and weight loss. Hepatosplenomegaly and lymphadenopathy are each seen in about 25% of patients. CNS disease, either meningitis or a mass lesion, is seen in 15% of patients. Bone marrow involvement is common, with thrombocytopenia, neutropenia, and anemia occurring in 33% of patients. Approximately 7% of patients have mucocutaneous lesions consisting of a maculopapular rash and skin or oral ulcers. Respiratory symptoms are usually mild, with chest x-ray showing a diffuse infiltrate or diffuse small nodules in ~50% of cases. Diagnosis is made by culturing the organisms from blood, bone marrow, or tissue or by detecting antigen in blood or urine. Treatment is typically with liposomal amphotericin B followed by maintenance therapy with oral itraconazole until the serum histoplasma antigen is <2 units, the patient has been on antiretrovirals for at least 6 months, and the CD4 count is >150 cells/μL. In the setting of mild infection, it may be appropriate to initiate therapy with itraconazole alone.

Following the spread of HIV infection to southeast Asia, disseminated infection with the fungus *Penicillium marneffei* was recognized as a complication of HIV infection and is considered an AIDS-defining condition in those parts of the world where it occurs. *P. marneffei* is the third most common AIDS-defining illness in Thailand, following TB and cryptococcosis. It is more frequently diagnosed in the rainy than the dry season. Clinical features include fever, generalized lymphadenopathy, hepatosplenomegaly, anemia, thrombocytopenia, and papular skin lesions with central umbilication. Treatment is with amphotericin B followed by itraconazole until the CD4+ T cell count is >100 cells/μL for at least 6 months.

Visceral leishmaniasis (Chap. 212) is recognized with increasing frequency in patients with HIV infection who live in or travel to areas endemic for this protozoal infection transmitted by sandflies. The clinical presentation is one of hepatosplenomegaly, fever, and hematologic abnormalities. Lymphadenopathy and other constitutional symptoms may be present. A chronic, relapsing course is seen in two-thirds of co-infected patients. Organisms can be isolated from cultures of bone marrow aspirates. Histologic stains may be negative, and antibody titers are of little help. Patients with HIV infection usually respond well initially to standard therapy with amphotericin B or pentavalent antimony compounds. Eradication of the organism is difficult, however, and relapses are common.

Patients with HIV infection are at a slightly increased risk of clinical malaria. This is particularly true for patients from nonendemic areas with presumed primary infection and in patients with lower CD4+ T cell counts. HIV-positive individuals with CD4+ T cell counts <300 cells/μL have a poorer response to malaria treatment than others. Co-infection with malaria is associated with a modest increase in HIV viral load. The risk of malaria may be decreased with TMP/SMX prophylaxis.

Generalized wasting is an AIDS-defining condition; it is defined as involuntary weight loss of >10% associated with intermittent or constant fever and chronic diarrhea or fatigue lasting >30 days in the absence of a defined cause other than HIV infection. Prior to the widespread use of cART it was the initial AIDS-defining condition in ~10% of patients with AIDS in the United States and is an indication for initiation of cART. Generalized wasting is rarely seen today with the earlier initiation of antiretrovirals. A constant feature of this syndrome is severe muscle wasting with scattered myofiber degeneration and occasional evidence of myositis. Glucocorticoids may be of some benefit; however, this approach must be carefully weighed against the risk of compounding the immunodeficiency of HIV infection. Androgenic steroids, growth hormone, and total parenteral nutrition have been used as therapeutic interventions with variable success.

Neoplastic diseases

The neoplastic diseases considered to be AIDS-defining conditions are Kaposi's sarcoma, non-Hodgkin's lymphoma, and invasive cervical carcinoma. In addition, there is also an increase in the incidence of a variety of non-AIDS-defining malignancies including Hodgkin's disease; multiple myeloma; leukemia; melanoma; and cervical, brain, testicular, oral, lung, gastric, liver, renal, and anal cancers. Since the introduction of potent cART, there has been a marked reduction in the incidence of KS (Fig. 189-34) and CNS lymphoma, such that the non-AIDS-defining malignancies now account for more morbidity and mortality in patients with HIV infection than the AIDS-defining malignancies. Rates of non-Hodgkin's lymphoma have declined as well; however, this decline has not been as dramatic as the decline in rates of KS. In contrast, cART has had little effect on human papillomavirus (HPV)-associated malignancies. As patients with HIV infection live longer, a wider array of cancers is seen in this population. While some may only reflect known risk factors (e.g., smoking, alcohol consumption, co-infection with other viruses such as hepatitis B) that are increased in patients with HIV infection, some may be a direct consequence of HIV and are clearly increased in patients with lower CD4+ T cell counts.

Kaposi's sarcoma is a multicentric neoplasm consisting of multiple vascular nodules appearing in the skin, mucous membranes, and viscera. The course ranges from indolent, with only minor skin or lymph node involvement, to fulminant, with extensive cutaneous and visceral involvement. In the initial period of the AIDS epidemic, KS was a prominent clinical feature of the first cases of AIDS, occurring in 79% of the patients diagnosed in 1981. By 1989 it was seen in only 25% of cases, by 1992 the number had decreased to 9%, and by 1997 the number was <1%. HHV-8 or KSHV has been strongly implicated as a viral cofactor in the pathogenesis of KS.

Clinically, KS has varied presentations and may be seen at any stage of HIV infection, even in the presence of a normal CD4+ T cell count. The initial lesion may be a small, raised reddish-purple nodule on the skin (Fig. 189-42), a discoloration on the oral mucosa (Fig. 189-35*D*), or a swollen lymph node. Lesions often appear in sun-exposed areas, particularly the tip of the nose, and have a propensity to occur in areas of trauma (Koebner phenomenon). Because of the vascular nature of the tumors and the presence of extravasated red blood cells in the lesions, their colors range from reddish to purple to brown and often take the appearance of a bruise, with yellowish discoloration and tattooing. Lesions range in size from a few millimeters to several centimeters in diameter and may be either discrete or confluent. KS lesions most commonly appear as raised macules; however, they can also be papular, particularly in patients with higher CD4+ T cell counts. Confluent lesions may give rise to surrounding lymphedema and may be disfiguring when they involve the face and disabling when they involve the lower extremities or the surfaces of joints. Apart from skin, the lymph nodes, GI tract, and lung are the organ systems most commonly affected by KS. Lesions have been reported in virtually every organ, including the heart and the CNS. In contrast to most malignancies, in which lymph node involvement implies metastatic

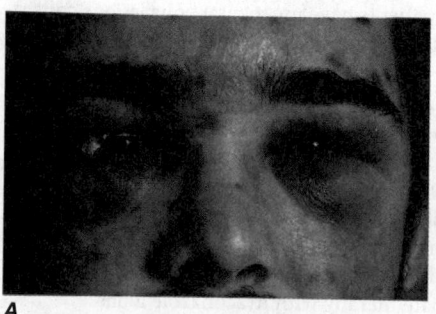 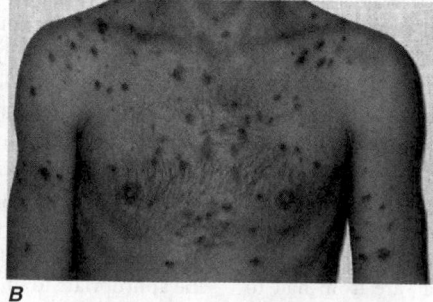 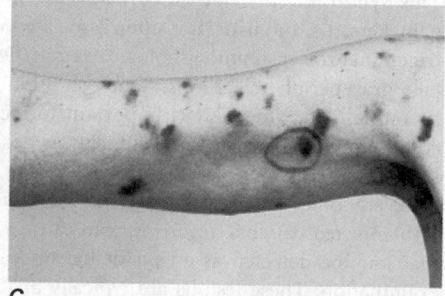

Figure 189-42   Kaposi's sarcoma in three patients with AIDS demonstrating *(A)* periorbital edema and bruising; *(B)* classic truncal distribution of lesions; and *(C)* upper extremity lesions.

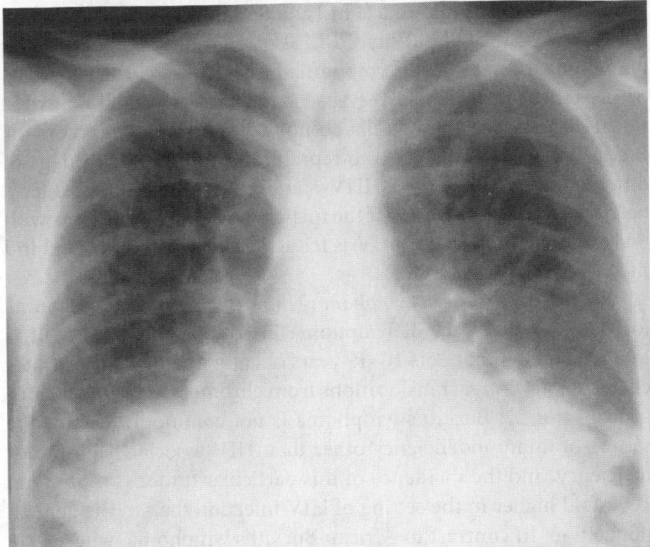

Figure 189-43 Chest x-ray of a patient with AIDS and pulmonary Kaposi's sarcoma. The characteristic findings include dense bilateral lower lobe infiltrates obscuring the heart borders and pleural effusions.

spread and a poor prognosis, lymph node involvement may be seen very early in KS and is of no special clinical significance. In fact, some patients may present with disease limited to the lymph nodes. These are generally patients with relatively intact immune function and thus the patients with the best prognosis. Pulmonary involvement with KS generally presents with shortness of breath. Some 80% of patients with pulmonary KS also have cutaneous lesions. The chest x-ray characteristically shows bilateral lower lobe infiltrates that obscure the margins of the mediastinum and diaphragm (Fig. 189-43). Pleural effusions are seen in 70% of cases of pulmonary KS, a fact that is often helpful in the differential diagnosis. GI involvement is seen in 50% of patients with KS and usually takes one of two forms: (1) mucosal involvement, which may lead to bleeding that can be severe; these patients sometimes also develop symptoms of GI obstruction if lesions become large; and (2) biliary tract involvement. KS lesions may infiltrate the gallbladder and biliary tree, leading to a clinical picture of obstructive jaundice similar to that seen with sclerosing cholangitis. Several staging systems have been proposed for KS. One in common use was developed by the National Institute of Allergy and Infectious Diseases AIDS Clinical Trials Group; it distinguishes patients on the basis of tumor extent, immunologic function, and presence or absence of systemic disease (Table 189-16).

A diagnosis of KS is based on biopsy of a suspicious lesion. Histologically one sees a proliferation of spindle cells and endothelial cells, extravasation of red blood cells, hemosiderin-laden macrophages, and, in early cases, an inflammatory cell infiltrate. Included in the differential diagnosis are lymphoma (particularly for oral lesions), bacillary angiomatosis, and cutaneous mycobacterial infections.

Management of KS (Table 189-17) should be carried out in consultation with an expert since definitive treatment guidelines do not exist. In the majority of cases, effective cART will go a long way in achieving control. Antiretroviral therapy has been associated with the spontaneous regression of KS lesions. Paradoxically, it has also been associated with the initial appearance of KS as a form of IRIS. For patients in whom tumor persists or in whom control of HIV replication is not possible, a variety of options exist. In some cases, lesions remain quite indolent, and many of these patients can be managed with no specific treatment. Fewer than 10% of AIDS patients with KS die as a consequence of their malignancy, and death from secondary infections is considerably more common. Thus, whenever possible one should avoid treatment regimens that may further suppress the immune system and increase susceptibility to opportunistic infections. Treatment is indicated under two main circumstances. The first is when a single lesion or a limited number of lesions are causing significant discomfort or cosmetic problems, such as with prominent facial lesions, lesions overlying a joint, or lesions in the oropharynx that interfere with swallowing or breathing. Under these circumstances, treatment with localized radiation, intralesional vinblastine, topical 9-*cis*-retinoic acid, or cryotherapy may be helpful. It should be noted that patients with HIV infection are particularly sensitive to the side effects of radiation therapy. This is especially true with respect to the development of radiation-induced mucositis; doses of radiation directed at mucosal surfaces, particularly in the head and neck region, should be adjusted accordingly. The use of systemic therapy, either IFN-α or chemotherapy, should be considered in patients with a large number of lesions or in patients with visceral involvement. The single most important determinant of response appears to be the CD4+ T cell count. This relationship between response rate and baseline CD4+ T cell count is particularly true for IFN-α. The response rate for patients with CD4+ T cell counts >600/μL is ~80%, while the response rate for patients with counts <150/μL is <10%. In contrast to the other systemic therapies, IFN-α provides an added advantage of having antiretroviral activity; thus, it may be the appropriate first choice for single-agent systemic therapy for early patients with disseminated disease. A variety of chemotherapeutic agents have also been shown to have activity against KS. Three of them, liposomal daunorubicin, liposomal doxorubicin, and paclitaxel, have been approved by the FDA for this indication. Liposomal daunorubicin is approved as first-line therapy for patients with advanced KS. It has fewer side effects than conventional chemotherapy. In contrast, liposomal doxorubicin and paclitaxel are approved only for KS patients who have failed standard

TABLE 189-16 National Institute of Allergy and Infectious Diseases AIDS Clinical Trials Group TIS Staging System for Kaposi's Sarcoma

Parameter	Good Risk (Stage 0): All of the Following	Poor Risk (Stage 1): Any of the Following
Tumor (T)	Confined to skin and/or lymph nodes and/or minimal oral disease	Tumor-associated edema or ulceration Extensive oral lesions GI lesions Nonnodal visceral lesions
Immune system (I)	CD4+ T cell count ≥200/μL	CD4+ T cell count <200/μL
Systemic illness (S)	No B symptoms[a] Karnofsky performance status ≥70 No history of opportunistic infection, neurologic disease, lymphoma, or thrush	B symptoms[a] present Karnofsky performance status <70 History of opportunistic infection, neurologic disease, lymphoma, or thrush

[a]Defined as unexplained fever, night sweats, >10% involuntary weight loss, or diarrhea persisting for more than 2 weeks.

TABLE 189-17 Management of AIDS-Associated Kaposi's Sarcoma

Observation and optimization of antiretroviral therapy
Single or limited number of lesions
   Radiation
   Intralesional vinblastine
   Cryotherapy
Extensive disease
   Initial therapy
      Interferon α (if CD4+ T cells >150/μL)
      Liposomal daunorubicin
   Subsequent therapy
      Liposomal doxorubicin
      Paclitaxel
Combination chemotherapy with low-dose doxorubicin, bleomycin, and vinblastine (ABV)
Targeted radiation

chemotherapy. Response rates vary from 23 to 88%, appear to be comparable to what had been achieved earlier with combination chemotherapy regimens, and are greatly influenced by CD4+ T cell count.

Lymphomas occur with an increased frequency in patients with congenital or acquired T cell immunodeficiencies (Chap. 316). AIDS is no exception; at least 6% of all patients with AIDS develop lymphoma at some time during the course of their illness. This is a 120-fold increase in incidence compared with the general population. In comparison to the situation with KS, primary CNS lymphoma, and most opportunistic infections, the incidence of AIDS-associated systemic lymphomas has not experienced as dramatic a decrease as a consequence of the widespread use of effective cART. Lymphoma occurs in all risk groups, with the highest incidence in patients with hemophilia and the lowest incidence in patients from the Caribbean or Africa with heterosexually acquired infection. Lymphoma is a late manifestation of HIV infection, generally occurring in patients with CD4+ T cell counts <200/μL. As HIV disease progresses, the risk of lymphoma increases. The attack rate for lymphoma increases exponentially with increasing duration of HIV infection and decreasing level of immunologic function. At 3 years following a diagnosis of HIV infection, the risk of lymphoma is 0.8% per year; by 8 years after infection, it is 2.6% per year. As individuals with HIV infection live longer as a consequence of improved cART and better treatment and prophylaxis of opportunistic infections, it is anticipated that the incidence of lymphomas may increase.

Three main categories of lymphoma are seen in patients with HIV infection: grade III or IV immunoblastic lymphoma, Burkitt's lymphoma, and primary CNS lymphoma. Approximately 90% of these lymphomas are B cell in phenotype; more than half contain EBV DNA. Some are associated with KSHV. These tumors may be either monoclonal or oligoclonal in nature and are probably in some way related to the pronounced polyclonal B cell activation seen in patients with AIDS.

Immunoblastic lymphomas account for ~60% of the cases of lymphoma in patients with AIDS. The majority of these are diffuse large B cell lymphomas (DLBCL). They are generally high grade and would have been classified as diffuse histiocytic lymphomas in earlier classification schemes. This tumor is more common in older patients, increasing in incidence from 0% in HIV-infected individuals <1 year old to >3% in those >50. Two variants of immunoblastic lymphoma that are seen primarily in HIV-infected patients are

primary effusion lymphoma (PEL) and its solid variant, plasmacytic lymphoma of the oral cavity. PEL, also referred to as body cavity lymphoma, presents with lymphomatous pleural, pericardial, and/or peritoneal effusions in the absence of discrete nodal or extranodal masses. The tumor cells do not express surface markers for B cells or T cells and are felt to represent a preplasmacytic stage of differentiation. While both HHV-8 and EBV DNA sequences have been found in the genomes of the malignant cells from patients with body cavity lymphoma, KSHV is felt to be the driving force behind the oncogenesis (see above).

Small noncleaved cell lymphoma (*Burkitt's lymphoma*) accounts for ~20% of the cases of lymphoma in patients with AIDS. It is most frequent in patients 10–19 years old and usually demonstrates characteristic c-*myc* translocations from chromosome 8 to chromosomes 14 or 22. Burkitt's lymphoma is not commonly seen in the setting of immunodeficiency other than HIV-associated immunodeficiency, and the incidence of this particular tumor is more than 1000-fold higher in the setting of HIV infection than in the general population. In contrast to African Burkitt's lymphoma, where 97% of the cases contain EBV genome, only 50% of HIV-associated Burkitt's lymphomas are EBV-positive.

Primary CNS lymphoma accounts for ~20% of the cases of lymphoma in patients with HIV infection. In contrast to HIV-associated Burkitt's lymphoma, primary CNS lymphomas are usually positive for EBV. In one study, the incidence of Epstein-Barr positivity was 100%. This malignancy does not have a predilection for any particular age group. The median CD4+ T cell count at the time of diagnosis is ~50/μL. Thus, CNS lymphoma generally presents at a later stage of HIV infection than does systemic lymphoma. This may explain, at least in part, the poorer prognosis for this subset of patients.

The clinical presentation of lymphoma in patients with HIV infection is quite varied, ranging from focal seizures to rapidly growing mass lesions in the oral mucosa (Fig. 189-44) to persistent unexplained fever. At least 80% of patients present with extranodal disease, and a similar percentage have B-type symptoms of fever, night sweats, or weight loss. Virtually any site in the body may be involved. The most common extranodal site is the CNS, which is involved in approximately one-third of all patients with lymphoma. Approximately 60% of these cases are primary CNS lymphoma. Primary CNS lymphoma generally presents with focal neurologic deficits, including cranial nerve findings, headaches, and/or seizures. MRI or CT generally reveals a limited number (one to three) of 3- to 5-cm lesions (Fig. 189-45). The lesions often show ring enhancement on contrast administration and may occur in any

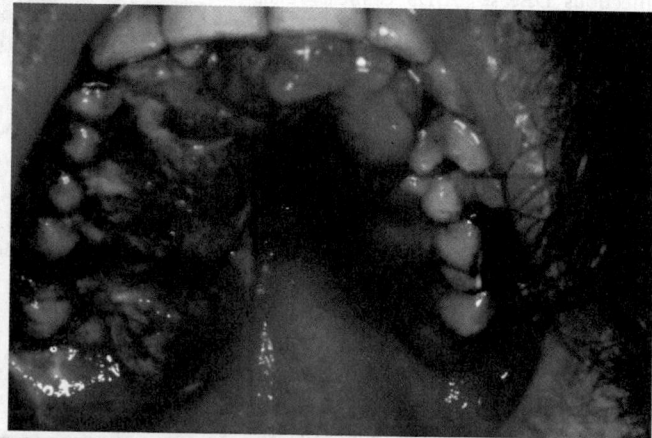

Figure 189-44 Immunoblastic lymphoma involving the hard palate of a patient with AIDS.

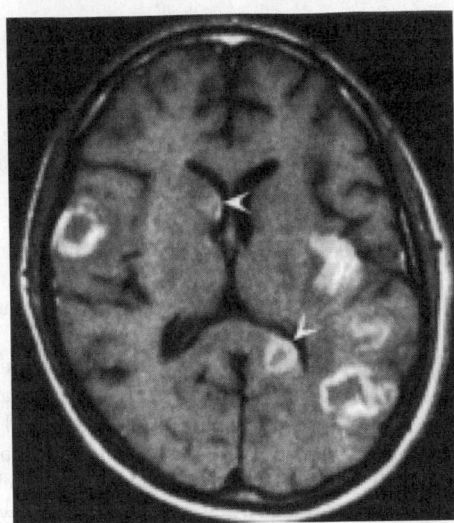

Figure 189-45 Central nervous system lymphoma. Postcontrast T1-weighted MRI scan in a patient with AIDS, an altered mental status, and hemiparesis. Multiple enhancing lesions, some ring-enhancing, are present. The left sylvian lesion shows gyral and subcortical enhancement, and the lesions in the caudate and splenium (*arrowheads*) show enhancement of adjacent ependymal surfaces.

location. Contrast enhancement is usually less pronounced than that seen with toxoplasmosis. Locations that are most commonly involved with CNS lymphoma are deep in the white matter. The main diseases in the differential diagnosis are cerebral toxoplasmosis and cerebral Chagas' disease. In addition to the 20% of lymphomas in HIV-infected individuals that are primary CNS lymphomas, CNS disease is also seen in HIV-infected patients with systemic lymphoma. Approximately 20% of patients with systemic lymphoma have CNS disease in the form of leptomeningeal involvement. This fact underscores the importance of lumbar puncture in the staging evaluation of patients with systemic lymphoma.

Systemic lymphoma is seen at earlier stages of HIV infection than primary CNS lymphoma. In one series the mean CD4+ T cell count was 189/μL. In addition to lymph node involvement, systemic lymphoma may commonly involve the GI tract, bone marrow, liver, and lung. GI tract involvement is seen in ~25% of patients. Any site in the GI tract may be involved, and patients may complain of difficulty swallowing or abdominal pain. The diagnosis is usually suspected on the basis of CT or MRI of the abdomen. Bone marrow involvement is seen in ~20% of patients and may lead to pancytopenia. Liver and lung involvement are each seen in ~10% of patients. Pulmonary disease may present as a mass lesion, multiple nodules, or an interstitial infiltrate.

Both conventional and unconventional approaches have been employed in an attempt to treat HIV-related lymphomas. Systemic lymphoma is generally treated by the oncologist with combination chemotherapy. Earlier disappointing figures are being replaced with more optimistic results for the treatment of systemic lymphoma following the availability of more effective cART and the use of rituximab in CD20+ tumors. While there is controversy regarding the use of antiretrovirals during chemotherapy, there is no question that their use overall in patients with HIV lymphoma has improved survival. As in most situations in patients with HIV disease, those with the higher CD4+ T cell counts tend to fare better. Response rates as high as 72% with a median survival of 33 months and disease-free intervals up to 9 years have been reported. Treatment of primary CNS lymphoma remains a significant challenge. Treatment is complicated by the fact that this illness usually occurs in patients with advanced HIV disease. Palliative measures such as radiation

therapy provide some relief. The prognosis remains poor in this group, with a 2-year survival of 29%.

Multicentric Castleman's disease is a KSHV-associated lymphoproliferative disorder that is seen with an increased frequency in patients with HIV infection. While not a true malignancy, it shares many features with lymphoma including generalized lymphadenopathy, hepatosplenomegaly, and systemic symptoms of fever, fatigue, and weight loss. Pulmonary symptoms may be seen in ~50% of patients. KS is present in 75–82% of cases. Lymph node biopsies reveal a predominance of interfollicular plasma cells and/or germinal centers with vascularization and an "onionskin" (hyaline vascular) appearance. Prior to the availability of cART, HIV-infected patients with multicentric Castleman's disease had a 15-fold increased risk of developing non-Hodgkin's lymphoma compared with HIV-infected patients in general. Treatment typically involves chemotherapy. Anecdotal reports of success with rituximab suggest that more specific treatment may be successful, although in one series treatment with rituximab was associated with worsening of coexisting KS. The median survival of patients with treated multicentric Castleman's disease pre-cART was 14 months. This has increased to a 2-year survival of more than 90% in the era of cART.

Evidence of infection with *human papillomavirus* (HPV), associated with *intraepithelial dysplasia of the cervix* or *anus*, is approximately twice as common in HIV-infected individuals as in the general population and can lead to intraepithelial neoplasia and eventually invasive cancer. In a series of studies, HIV-infected men were examined for evidence of anal dysplasia, and Papanicolaou (Pap) smears were found to be abnormal in 20–80%. These changes tend to persist and are generally not affected by cART, raising the possibility of a subsequent transition to a more malignant condition. While the incidence of an abnormal Pap smear of the cervix is ~5% in otherwise healthy women, the incidence of abnormal cervical smears in women with HIV infection is 30–60%, and *invasive cervical cancer* is included as an AIDS-defining condition. Thus far, however, only small increases in the incidence of cervical or anal cancer have been seen as a consequence of HIV infection. However, given this high rate of dysplasia, a comprehensive gynecologic and rectal examination, including Pap smear, is indicated at the initial evaluation and 6 months later for all patients with HIV infection. If these examinations are negative at both time points, the patient should be followed with yearly evaluations. If an initial or repeat Pap smear shows evidence of severe inflammation with reactive squamous changes, the next Pap smear should be performed at 3 months. If, at any time, a Pap smear shows evidence of squamous intraepithelial lesions, colposcopic examination with biopsies as indicated should be performed. The 2-year survival rate for HIV-infected patients with invasive cervical cancer is 64% compared with 79% in non-HIV-infected patients. The most common HPV genotypes in the general population and the genotypes upon which current HPV vaccines are based are 16 and 18. This is not the case in the HIV-infected population, where other genotypes such as 56 and 53 predominate. This raises concerns as to the potential effectiveness of the current HPV vaccines for HIV-infected patients.

IDIOPATHIC CD4+ T LYMPHOCYTOPENIA

A syndrome was recognized in 1992 that was characterized by an absolute CD4+ T cell count of <300/μL or <20% of total T cells on a minimum of two occasions at least 6 weeks apart; no evidence of HIV-1, HIV-2, HTLV-I, or HTLV-II on testing; and the absence of any defined immunodeficiency or therapy associated with decreased levels of CD4+ T cells. By mid-1993, ~100 patients had been described. After extensive multicenter investigations, a series of reports were published in early 1993, which together allowed a number of conclusions. Idiopathic CD4+ lymphocytopenia (ICL) is a very rare syndrome, as determined by studies of blood donors and cohorts of HIV-seronegative men who have sex with men. Cases were clearly identified as early as 1983 and were remarkably similar to the clinical features of ICL that had been identified decades earlier. The definition of ICL based on CD4+ T cell counts coincided with the ready availability of testing for CD4+ T cells in patients suspected of being immunodeficient. Although, as a result of immune deficiency, certain patients with ICL develop some of the opportunistic diseases (particularly cryptococcosis, nontuberculous mycobacterial infections, and cervical dysplasia) seen in HIV-infected patients, the syndrome is demographically, clinically, and immunologically unlike HIV infection and AIDS. Fewer than half of the reported ICL patients had risk factors for HIV infection, and there were wide geographic and age distributions. The fact that a significant proportion of patients did have risk factors probably reflects a selection bias, in that physicians who take care of HIV-infected patients are more likely to monitor CD4+ T cells. Approximately half of the patients are women, compared with approximately one-third among HIV-infected individuals in the United States. Many patients with ICL remained clinically stable, and their condition did not deteriorate progressively as is common with seriously immunodeficient HIV-infected patients. Approximately 15% of patients with ICL experience spontaneous reversal of the CD4+ T lymphocytopenia. Immunologic abnormalities in ICL are somewhat different from those of HIV infection. ICL patients often have increases in CD4+ T cell activation with decreases in CD8+ T cells and B cells. Furthermore, immunoglobulin levels are either normal or, more commonly, decreased in patients with ICL, compared with the usual hypergammaglobulinemia of HIV-infected individuals. Virologic studies of these patients have revealed no evidence of HIV-1, HIV-2, HTLV-I, or HTLV-II or of any other mononuclear cell–tropic virus. Furthermore, there has been no epidemiologic evidence to suggest that a transmissible microbe was involved. The cases of ICL have been widely dispersed, with no clustering. Close contacts and sexual partners who were studied were clinically well and were serologically, immunologically, and virologically negative for HIV. ICL is a heterogeneous syndrome, and it is highly likely that there is no common cause; however, there may be common causes among subgroups of patients that are currently unrecognized.

Patients who present with laboratory data consistent with ICL should be worked up for underlying diseases that could be responsible for the immune deficiency. If no underlying cause is detected, no specific therapy should be initiated. However, if opportunistic diseases occur, they should be treated appropriately (see above). Depending on the level of the CD4+ T cell count, patients should receive prophylaxis for the commonly encountered opportunistic infections.

TREATMENT   **AIDS and Related Disorders**

GENERAL PRINCIPLES OF PATIENT MANAGEMENT The CDC guidelines call for the testing for HIV infection to be a part of routine medical care. It is recommended that the patient be informed of the intention to test, as is the case with other routine laboratory determinations, and be given the opportunity to "opt out." Such an approach is critical to the goal of identifying as many infected individuals as possible since ~21% of the >1 million individuals in the United States who are HIV-infected are not aware of their status. Under these circumstances of routine testing, although it is desirable, pretest counseling may not always be built into the testing process. However, no matter how well prepared a patient is for adversity, the discovery of a diagnosis of HIV infection is a devastating event. Thus, physicians should be sensitive to this fact and, where possible, execute some degree of pretest counseling to at least partially prepare the patient should the results demonstrate the presence of HIV infection. Following a diagnosis of HIV infection, the health care provider should be prepared to immediately activate support systems for the newly diagnosed patient. These should include an experienced social worker or nurse who can spend time talking to the person and ensuring that he or she is emotionally stable. Most communities have HIV support centers that can be of great help in these difficult situations.

The treatment of patients with HIV infection requires not only a comprehensive knowledge of the possible disease processes that may occur and up-to-date knowledge of and experience with cART, but also the ability to deal with the problems of a chronic, potentially life-threatening illness. A comprehensive knowledge of internal medicine is required to deal with the changing spectrum of illness associated with HIV infection. Great advances have been made in the treatment of patients with HIV infection. The appropriate use of potent cART and other treatment and prophylactic interventions are of critical importance in providing each patient with the best opportunity to live a long and healthy life despite the presence of HIV infection. In contrast to the earlier days of this epidemic, a diagnosis of HIV infection need no longer be equated with having an inevitably fatal disease. In addition to medical interventions, the health care provider has a responsibility to provide each patient with appropriate counseling and education concerning their disease as part of a comprehensive care plan. Patients must be educated about the potential transmissibility of their infection and about the fact that while health care providers may refer to levels of the virus as "undetectable," this is more a reflection of the sensitivity of the assay being used to measure the virus than a comment on the presence or absence of the virus. It is important for patients to be aware that the virus is still present and capable of being transmitted at all stages of HIV disease. Thus, there must be frank discussions concerning sexual practices and the sharing of syringes and other paraphernalia used in illicit drug use. The treating physician not only must be aware of the latest medications available for patients with HIV infection but also must educate patients concerning the natural history of their illness and listen and be sensitive to their fears and concerns. As with other diseases, therapeutic decisions should be made in consultation with the patient, when possible, and with the patient's proxy if the patient is incapable of making decisions. In this regard, it is recommended that all patients with HIV infection, and in particular those with CD4+ T cell counts <200/μL, designate a trusted individual with durable power of attorney to make medical decisions on their behalf, if necessary.

Following a diagnosis of HIV infection, there are several examinations and laboratory studies that should be performed to help determine the extent of disease and provide baseline standards for future reference (Table 189-18). In addition to routine chemistry, fasting lipid profile, aspartate aminotransferase, alanine aminotransferase, total and direct bilirubin, fasting glucose and hematology screening panels, Pap smear, urinalysis, and chest x-ray, one should also obtain a CD4+ T cell count, two separate plasma HIV RNA levels, an HIV resistance test, a rapid plasma reagin or VDRL test, an anti-*Toxoplasma* antibody titer, and serologies for hepatitis A, B, and C. A PPD test should be done and an MMSE performed and recorded. A pregnancy test should be done in women in whom the drug efavirenz is being considered, and HLA-B5701 testing should be done in all patients in whom the drug abacavir is being

TABLE 189-18 Initial Evaluation of the Patient With HIV Infection

History and physical examination

Routine chemistry and hematology

AST, ALT, direct and indirect bilirubin

Lipid profile and fasting glucose

CD4+ T lymphocyte count

Two plasma HIV RNA levels

HIV resistance testing

HLA-B5701 screening

RPR or VDRL test

Anti-*Toxoplasma* antibody titer

PPD skin test

Mini-Mental Status Examination

Serologies for hepatitis A, hepatitis B, and hepatitis C

Immunization with pneumococcal polysaccharide; influenza as indicated

Immunization with hepatitis A and hepatitis B if seronegative

Counseling regarding natural history and transmission

Help contacting others who might be infected

Abbreviations: ALT, alanine aminotransferase; AST, aspartate aminotransferase; PPD, purified protein derivative; RPR, rapid plasma reagin; VDRL, Venereal Disease Research Laboratory.

considered. Patients should be immunized with pneumococcal polysaccharide, with annual influenza shots, and, if seronegative for these viruses, with hepatitis A and hepatitis B vaccines. The status of hepatitis C infection should be determined. In addition, patients should be counseled with regard to sexual practices and needle sharing, and counseling should be offered to those whom the patient knows or suspects may also be infected. Once these baseline activities are performed, short- and long-term medical management strategies should be developed based on the most recent information available and modified as new information becomes available. The field of HIV medicine is changing rapidly, and it is difficult to remain fully up to date. Fortunately there are a series of excellent sites on the Internet that are frequently updated, and they provide the most recent information on a variety of topics, including consensus panel reports on treatment (Table 189-19).

ANTIRETROVIRAL THERAPY Combination antiretroviral therapy (cART), also referred to as highly active antiretroviral therapy (HAART), is the cornerstone of management of patients with HIV infection. Following the initiation of widespread use of cART in the United States in 1995–1996, marked declines

TABLE 189-19 Resources Available on the World Wide Web on HIV Disease

aidsinfo.nih.gov	AIDSinfo, a service of the U.S. Department of Health and Human Services, posts federally approved treatment guidelines for HIV and AIDS; provides information on federally funded and privately funded clinical trials and CDC publications and data
www.cdcnpin.org	Updates on epidemiologic data and prevention information from the CDC

Note: CDC, Centers for Disease Control and Prevention.

were noted in the incidence of most AIDS-defining conditions (Fig. 189-34). Suppression of HIV replication is an important component in prolonging life as well as in improving the quality of life in patients with HIV infection. Adequate suppression requires strict adherence to prescribed regimens of antiretroviral drugs. This has been facilitated by the coformulations of antiretrovirals and the development of once-daily regimens. Unfortunately, many of the most important questions related to the treatment of HIV disease currently lack definitive answers. Among them are the questions of when therapy should be started, what the best initial regimen is, when a given regimen should be changed, and what it should be changed to when a change is made. Notwithstanding these uncertainties, the physician and patient must come to a mutually agreeable plan based on the best available data. In an effort to facilitate this process, the U.S. Department of Health and Human Services makes available on the Internet (*www.aidsinfo.nih.gov*) a series of periodically updated guidelines, including "*Principles of Therapy of HIV Infection,*" "*Guidelines for the Use of Antiretroviral Agents in HIV-Infected Adults and Adolescents,*" and "*Guidelines for the Prevention of Opportunistic Infections in Persons Infected with Human Immunodeficiency Virus.*" At present, an extensive clinical trials network, involving both clinical investigators and patient advocates, is in place attempting to develop improved approaches to therapy. Consortia comprising representatives of academia, industry, independent foundations, and the federal government are involved in the process of drug development, including a wide-ranging series of clinical trials. As a result, new therapies and new therapeutic strategies are continually emerging. New drugs are often available through expanded access programs prior to official licensure. Given the complexity of this field, decisions regarding cART are best made in consultation with experts.

Currently available drugs for the treatment of HIV infection fall into four categories: those that inhibit the viral reverse transcriptase enzyme (nucleoside and nucleotide reverse transcriptase inhibitors; nonnucleoside reverse transcriptase inhibitors), those that inhibit the viral protease enzyme (protease inhibitors), those that inhibit the viral integrase enzyme (integrase inhibitors), and those that interfere with viral entry (fusion inhibitors; CCR5 antagonists) (Table 189-20; Fig. 189-46).

The FDA-approved reverse transcriptase inhibitors include the *nucleoside analogues* zidovudine, didanosine, zalcitabine, stavudine, lamivudine, abacavir, and emtricitabine; the *nucleotide analogue* tenofovir; and the *nonnucleoside reverse transcriptase inhibitors* nevirapine, delavirdine, efavirenz, and etravirine (Fig. 189-46; Table 189-20). These represent the first class of drugs licensed for the treatment of HIV infection. They are indicated for this use as part of combination regimens. It should be stressed that none of these drugs should be used as monotherapy for HIV infection due to the relative ease with which drug resistance may develop under such circumstances. Thus, when lamivudine, emtricitabine, or tenofovir is used to treat hepatitis B infection in the setting of HIV infection, one should ensure that the patient is also on additional antiretroviral medication. The reverse transcriptase inhibitors block the HIV replication cycle at the point of RNA-dependent DNA synthesis, the reverse transcription step. While the nonnucleoside reverse transcriptase inhibitors are quite selective for the HIV-1 reverse transcriptase, the nucleoside and nucleotide analogues inhibit a variety of DNA polymerases in addition to those of the HIV-1 reverse transcriptase. For this reason, serious side effects are more varied with the nucleoside analogues and include mitochondrial damage that can lead to hepatic steatosis and lactic acidosis as

TABLE 189-20 Antiretroviral Drugs Used in the Treatment of HIV Infection

Drug	Status	Indication	Dose in Combination	Supporting Data	Toxicity
Nucleoside or Neucleotide Reverse Transcriptase Inhibitors					
Zidovudine (AZT, azidothymidine, Retrovir, 3'azido-3'-deoxythymidine)	Licensed	Treatment of HIV infection in combination with other antiretroviral agents	200 mg q8h or 300 mg bid	19 vs 1 death in original placebo-controlled trial in 281 patients with AIDS or ARC	Anemia, granulocytopenia, myopathy, lactic acidosis, hepatomegaly with steatosis, headache, nausea, nail pigmentation, lipid abnormalities, lipoatrophy, hyperglycemia
		Prevention of maternal-fetal HIV transmission		In pregnant women with CD4+ T cell count ≥200/μL, AZT PO beginning at weeks 14–34 of gestation plus IV drug during labor and delivery plus PO AZT to infant for 6 weeks decreased transmission of HIV by 67.5% (from 25.5% to 8.3%), $n = 363$	
Didanosine (Videx, Videx EC, ddI, dideoxyinosine, 2',3'-dideoxyinosine)	Licensed	For treatment of HIV infection in combination with other antiretroviral agents	Buffered: Requires 2 tablets to achieve adequate buffering of stomach acid; should be administered on an empty stomach ≥60 kg: 200 mg bid <60 kg: 125 mg bid Enteric coated: ≥60 kg: 400 mg qd < 60 kg: 250 mg qd	Clinically superior to AZT as monotherapy in 913 patients with prior AZT therapy; clinically superior to AZT and comparable to AZT + ddI and AZT + ddC in 1067 AZT-naïve patients with CD4+ T cell counts of 200–500/μL	Pancreatitis, peripheral neuropathy, abnormalities on liver function tests, lactic acidosis, hepatomegaly with steatosis, optic neuritis, nausea, hyperglycemia
Zalcitabine (ddC, HIVID, 2'3'-dideoxycytidine)	Licensed Discontinued in 2006	In combination with other antiretroviral agents for the treatment of HIV infection	0.75 mg tid	Clinically inferior to AZT monotherapy as initial treatment; clinically as good as ddI in advanced patients intolerant to AZT; in combination with AZT, was clinically superior to AZT alone in patients with AIDS or CD4+ T cell count <350/μL	Peripheral neuropathy, pancreatitis, lactic acidosis, hepatomegaly with steatosis, oral ulcers
Stavudine (d4T, Zerit, 2'3'-didehydro-3'-dideoxythymidine)	Licensed	Treatment of HIV-infected patients in combination with other antiretroviral agents	≥60 kg: 40 mg bid <60 kg: 30 mg bid	Superior to AZT with respect to changes in CD4+ T cell counts in 359 patients who had received ≥24 weeks of AZT; following 12 weeks of randomization, the CD4+ T cell count had decreased in AZT-treated controls by a mean of 22/μL, while in stavudine-treated patients, it had increased by a mean of 22/μL	Peripheral neuropathy, pancreatitis, lactic acidosis, hepatomegaly with steatosis, ascending neuromuscular weakness, lipodystrophy, lipid abnormalities, hyperglycemia
Lamivudine (Epivir, 2'3'-dideoxy-3'-thiacytidine, 3TC)	Licensed	In combination with other antiretroviral agents for the treatment of HIV infection	150 mg bid 300 mg qd	In combination with AZT superior to AZT alone with respect to changes in CD4+ T cell counts in 495 patients who were zidovudine-naïve and 477 patients who were zidovudine-experienced; overall CD4+ T cell counts for the zidovudine group were at baseline by 24 weeks, while in the group treated with zidovudine plus lamivudine, they were 10–50 cells/μL above baseline; 54% decrease in progression to AIDS/death compared with AZT alone	Flare of hepatitis in HBV-coinfected patients who discontinue drug

(continued)

Drug	Status	Indication	Dose in Combination	Supporting Data	Toxicity
Emtricitabine (FTC, Emtriva)	Licensed	In combination with other antiretroviral agents for the treatment of HIV infection	200 mg qd	Comparable to d4T in combination with ddI and efavirenz in 571 treatment-naïve patients; similar to 3TC in combination with AZT or d4T + NNRTI or PI in 440 patients doing well for ≥12 weeks on a 3TC regimen	Hepatotoxicity in HBV-coinfected patients who discontinue drug, skin discoloration
Abacavir (Ziagen)	Licensed	For treatment of HIV infection in combination with other antiretroviral agents	300 mg bid	Abacavir + AZT + 3TC equivalent to indinavir + AZT + 3TC with regard to viral load suppression (~60% in each group with <400 HIV RNA copies/mL plasma) and CD4+ T cell increase (~100/µL in each group) at 24 weeks	Hypersensitivity reaction In HLA-B5701+ individuals (can be fatal); fever, rash, nausea, vomiting, malaise or fatigue, and loss of appetite
Tenofovir (Viread)	Licensed	For use In combination with other antiretroviral agents when treatment is indicated	300 mg qd	Reduction of ~0.6 log in HIV-1 RNA levels when added to background regimen in treatment-experienced patients	Renal osteomalacia, flare of hepatitis in HBV-coinfected patients who discontinue drug

Non-Nucleoside Reverse Transcriptase Inhibitors

Drug	Status	Indication	Dose in Combination	Supporting Data	Toxicity
Delavirdine (Rescriptor)	Licensed	For use in combination with appropriate antiretrovirals when treatment is warranted	400 mg tid	Delavirdine + AZT superior to AZT alone with regard to viral load suppression at 52 weeks	Skin rash, abnormalities in liver function tests
Nevirapine (Viramune)	Licensed	In combination with other antiretroviral agents for treatment of progressive HIV infection	200 mg/d × 14 days then 200 mg bid *or* 400 mg extended release qd	Increase in CD4+ T cell count, decrease in HIV RNA when used in combination with nucleosides	Skin rash, hepatotoxicity
Efavirenz (Sustiva)	Licensed	For treatment of HIV infection in combination with other antiretroviral agents	600 mg qhs	Efavirenz + AZT + 3TC comparable to indinavir + AZT + 3TC with regard to viral load suppression (a higher percentage of the efavirenz group achieved viral load <50 copies/mL, but the discontinuation rate in the indinavir group was unexpectedly high, accounting for most treatment "failures"); CD4 cell increase (~140/µL in each group) at 24 weeks	Rash, dysphoria, elevated liver function tests, drowsiness, abnormal dreams, depression, lipid abnormalities, potentially teratogenic
Etravirine (Intelence)	Licensed	In combination with other antiretroviral agents in treatment-experienced patients whose HIV is resistant to non-nucleoside reverse transcriptase inhibitors and other antiretroviral medications	200 mg bid	Higher rates of HIV RNA suppression to <50 copies/mL (56% vs 39%); greater increases in CD4+ T cell count (89 vs 64 cells) compared to placebo when given in combination with an optimized background regimen	Rash, nausea, hypersensitivity reactions
Rilpivirine (Edurant)	Licensed	In combination with other drugs in previously untreated patients when treatment is indicated.	25 mg qd	Non-inferior to Efavirenz with respect to suppression at week 48 in 1368 treatment-naive individuals	Nausea, dizziness, somnolence, vertigo, less CNS toxicity and rash than Efavirenz

(*continued*)

Drug	Status	Indication	Dose in Combination	Supporting Data	Toxicity
Protease Inhibitors					
Saquinavir mesylate (Invirase—hard-gel capsule)	Licensed	In combination with other antiretroviral agents when therapy is warranted	1000 mg + 100 mg ritonavir bid	Increases in CD4+ T cell counts, reduction in HIV RNA most pronounced in combination therapy with ddC; 50% reduction in first AIDS-defining event or death in combination with ddC compared with either agent alone	Diarrhea, nausea, headaches, hyperglycemia, fat redistribution, lipid abnormalities, PR and QT interval prolongation
(Fortovase—soft-gel capsule)	Licensed Discontinued 2006	For use in combination with other antiretroviral agents when treatment is warranted	1200 mg tid	Reduction in the mortality rate and AIDS-defining events for patients who received hard-gel formulation in combination with ddC	Diarrhea, nausea, abdominal pain, headaches, hyperglycemia, fat redistribution, lipid abnormalities
Ritonavir (Norvir)	Licensed	In combination with other antiretroviral agents for treatment of HIV infection when treatment is warranted	600 mg bid (also used in lower doses as pharmacokinetic booster)	Reduction in the cumulative incidence of clinical progression or death from 34 to 17% in patients with CD4+ T cell count <100/μL treated for a median of 6 months	Nausea, abdominal pain, hyperglycemia, fat redistribution, lipid abnormalities, may alter levels of many other drugs, including saquinavir, paresthesias, hepatitis
Indinavir sulfate (Crixivan)	Licensed	For treatment of HIV infection in combination with other antiretroviral agents when antiretroviral treatment is warranted	800 mg q8h or 800 mg + 100 mg ritonavir bid or 1000 mg q8h when used with efavirenz or nevirapine	Increase in CD4+ T cell count by 100/μL and 2-log decrease in HIV RNA levels when given in combination with zidovudine and lamivudine; decrease of 50% in risk of progression to AIDS or death when given with zidovudine and lamivudine compared with zidovudine and lamivudine alone	Nephrolithiasis, indirect hyperbilirubinemia, hyperglycemia, fat redistribution, lipid abnormalities, nausea, transaminase elevations, headache
Nelfinavir mesylate (Viracept)	Licensed	For treatment of HIV infection in combination with other antiretroviral agents when antiretroviral therapy is warranted	750 mg tid or 1250 mg bid	2.0-log decline in HIV RNA when given in combination with stavudine	Diarrhea, loose stools, hyperglycemia, fat redistribution, lipid abnormalities, transaminase elevations
Amprenavir (Agenerase)	Licensed	In combination with other antiretroviral agents for treatment of HIV infection	Amprenavir: 1200 mg bid or 600 mg + 100 mg ritonavir bid or 1200 mg + 200 mg ritonavir qd	In treatment-naïve patients, amprenavir + AZT + 3TC superior to AZT + 3TC with regard to viral load suppression (53% vs 11% with <400 HIV RNA copies/mL plasma at 24 weeks); CD4+ T cell responses similar between treatment groups; in treatment-experienced patients, amprenavir + NRTIs similar to indinavir + NRTIs with regard to viral load suppression (43% vs 53% with <400 HIV RNA copies/mL plasma at 24 weeks); CD4+ T cell responses superior in the indinavir + NRTIs group	Nausea, vomiting, diarrhea, rash, oral paresthesias, elevated liver function tests, hyperglycemia, fat redistribution, lipid abnormalities, headache, nephrolithiasis
Fosamprenavir (Lexiva)	Licensed		Fosamprenavir: 1400 mg bid or 700 mg + 100 mg ritonavir bid or 1400 mg + 200 mg ritonavir qd		
Lopinavir/ritonavir (Kaletra)	Licensed	For treatment of HIV infection in combination with other antiretroviral agents	400 mg/100 mg bid	In treatment-naïve patients, lopinavir/ritonavir + d4T + 3TC superior to nelfinavir + d4T + 3TC with regard to viral load suppression (79% vs 64% with <400 HIV RNA copies/mL at 40 weeks); CD4+ T cell increases similar in both groups	Diarrhea, hyperglycemia, fat redistribution, lipid abnormalities, nausea, pancreatitis, elevated liver function tests, PR and QT interval prolongations

(*continued*)

TABLE 189-20 Antiretroviral Drugs Used in the Treatment of HIV Infection (*Continued*)

Drug	Status	Indication	Dose in Combination	Supporting Data	Toxicity
Atazanavir (Reyataz)	Licensed	For treatment of HIV infection in combination with other antiretroviral agents	400 mg qd or 300 mg qd + ritonavir 100 mg qd when given with efavirenz	Comparable to efavirenz when given in combination with AZT + 3TC in a study of 810 treatment-naïve patients; comparable to nelfinavir when given in combination with d4T + 3TC in a study of 467 treatment-naïve patients	Hyperbilirubinemia, PR prolongation, nausea, vomiting, hyperglycemia, fat maldistribution, rash transaminase elevations
Tipranavir (Aptivus)	Licensed	In combination with 200 mg ritonavir for combination therapy in treatment-experienced adults	500 mg + 200 mg ritonavir twice daily	At 24 weeks, patients with prior extensive exposure to ARV therapy showed a −0.8 log change in HIV RNA levels and a 34-cell increase in CD4+ T cells compared with −0.25 log and 4 cells in the control arm; inferior to lopinavir/ritonavir in a randomized, controlled trial in naïve patients	Diarrhea, nausea, fatigue, headache, skin rash, hepatotoxicity, intracranial hemorrhage, hyperglycemia, lipid abnormalities, fat redistribution
Darunavir (Prezista)	Licensed	In combination with 100 mg ritonavir for combination therapy in treatment-experienced adults	600 mg + 100 mg ritonavir twice daily with food	At 24 weeks, patients with prior extensive exposure to antiretrovirals treated with a new combination including darunavir showed a −1.89 log change in HIV RNA levels and a 92-cell increase in CD4+ T cells compared with −0.48 log and 17 cells in the control arm	Diarrhea, nausea, headache, skin rash, hepatoxicity, hyperlipidemia, hyperglycemia
Entry Inhibitors					
Enfuvirtide (Fuzeon)	Licensed	In combination with other agents in treatment-experienced patients with evidence of HIV-1 replication despite ongoing antiretroviral therapy	90 mg SC bid	In treatment of experienced patients, superior to placebo when added to new optimized background (37% vs 16% with <400 HIV RNA copies/mL at 24 weeks; + 71 vs + 35 CD4+ T cells at 24 weeks)	Local injection reactions, hypersensitivity reactions, increased rate of bacterial pneumonia
Maraviroc (Selzentry)	Licensed	In combination with other antiretroviral agents in adults infected with only CCR5-tropic HIV-1	150–600 mg bid depending on concomitant medications (see text)	At 24 weeks, among 635 patients with CCR5-tropic virus and HIV-1 RNA >5000 copies/mL despite at least 6 months of prior therapy with at least 1 agent from 3 of the 4 antiretroviral drug classes, 61% of patients randomized to maraviroc achieved HIV RNA levels <400 copies/mL compared with 28% of patients randomized to placebo	Hepatotoxicity, nasopharyngitis, fever, cough, rash, abdominal pain, dizziness, musculoskeletal symptoms
Integrase Inhibitor					
Raltegravir (Isentress)	Licensed	In combination with other antiretroviral agents	400 mg bid	At 24 weeks, among 436 patients with 3-class drug resistance, 76% of patients randomized to receive raltegravir achieved HIV RNA levels <400 copies/mL compared with 41% of patients randomized to receive placebo	Nausea, headache, diarrhea, CPK elevation, muscle weakness and rhabdomyolysis
Elvitegravir	Investigational	In combination	150 mg qdt pharmacoenhancing agent cobicistat	Non-inferior to raltegravir in treatment-experienced patients	

Abbreviations: ARC, AIDS-related complex; NRTIs, nonnucleoside reverse transcriptase inhibitors.

well as peripheral neuropathy and pancreatitis. The use of either of the thymidine analogues zidovudine and stavudine has been associated with a syndrome of hyperlipidemia, glucose intolerance/insulin resistance, and fat redistribution often referred to as *lipodystrophy syndrome* (discussed in "Diseases of the Endocrine System and Metabolic Disorders," above).

Zidovudine (AZT; 3'-azido-2',3'-dideoxythymidine) was the first drug approved for the treatment of HIV infection and is the prototype nucleoside analogue. These compounds, in which the hydroxyl group in the 3' position of the ribose moiety is substituted with a hydrogen or other chemical group, act as DNA chain terminators owing to their inability to form a 3'–5' phosphodiester linkage with another nucleoside. They bind much more avidly to the active site of the RNA-dependent DNA polymerase of HIV (reverse transcriptase) than to the active site of mammalian cell DNA polymerases; this explains their selective effect on HIV replication. Zidovudine also has a relatively high avidity for the DNA polymerase γ of human mitochondria. This may contribute to the development of the fatty liver and myopathy sometimes observed in patients taking zidovudine. As with all the nucleoside analogues, the active form of zidovudine is the triphosphate, and the rate of phosphorylation, a thymidine kinase–dependent pathway, may be different in different cells. This may explain why zidovudine is more effective at inhibiting HIV replication in some cells than in others. The clinical benefit of zidovudine was clearly established in 1986 in a phase II, randomized, placebo-controlled trial in patients with advanced HIV disease. However, while treatment of patients with early stages of HIV infection with zidovudine monotherapy was associated with increases in CD4+ T cell count, it was not associated with a better overall outcome than waiting until later to treat. Subsequent trials established the ability of this drug to dramatically decrease the incidence of perinatal transmission of HIV from infected mother to infant. Eventually a series of studies demonstrated the superiority of cART regimens over zidovudine alone, and combination therapy (discussed below) remains the standard of treatment today. Among the side effects of zidovudine at the initiation of therapy are fatigue, malaise,

nausea, and headache. These side effects often subside over time. Patients on zidovudine may develop a macrocytic anemia, neutropenia, myopathy, cardiomyopathy, and lactic acidosis associated with fatty infiltration of the liver. As with every antiretroviral drug, HIV has the ability to develop resistance to zidovudine. Zidovudine resistance has been reported to occur ~6 months following the initiation of zidovudine monotherapy. More recently, zidovudine-resistant viruses have been noted in patients with acute infection prior to the initiation of therapy, implying that zidovudine-resistant viruses can be transmitted from person to person. Resistance emerges more rapidly in late-stage patients, presumably as a consequence of a greater degree of viral replication and thus a greater opportunity for mutation. A variety of amino acid changes including substitutions, insertions, and deletions have been reported to confer zidovudine resistance (Fig. 189-47). One combination preparation, Combivir, consists of zidovudine and lamivudine, while another, Trizivir, consists of zidovudine, lamivudine, and abacavir.

Didanosine (ddI; 2',3'-dideoxyinosine) was the second drug licensed for the treatment of HIV infection, followed shortly thereafter by zalcitabine. Didanosine is metabolized to dideoxyadenosine in vivo. It is best absorbed on an empty stomach at a high pH. The toxicity profile of didanosine is quite different from that of zidovudine. The most common toxicity is a painful sensory peripheral neuropathy that occurs in ~30% of patients receiving >400 mg/d. It generally resolves with discontinuation of the drug and may not recur if the drug is resumed at a reduced dose. At higher doses than are currently used, one may see pancreatitis in ~10% of patients. Pancreatitis associated with didanosine therapy can be fatal. Didanosine should be discontinued if a patient experiences abdominal pain consistent with pancreatitis or if an elevated serum amylase or lipase level is found in association with an edematous pancreas on ultrasound. Didanosine is contraindicated in patients with a prior history of pancreatitis, regardless of etiology. A higher incidence of didanosine-associated toxicities has been seen when it is used in combination with stavudine, hydroxyurea, ribavirin, or tenofovir.

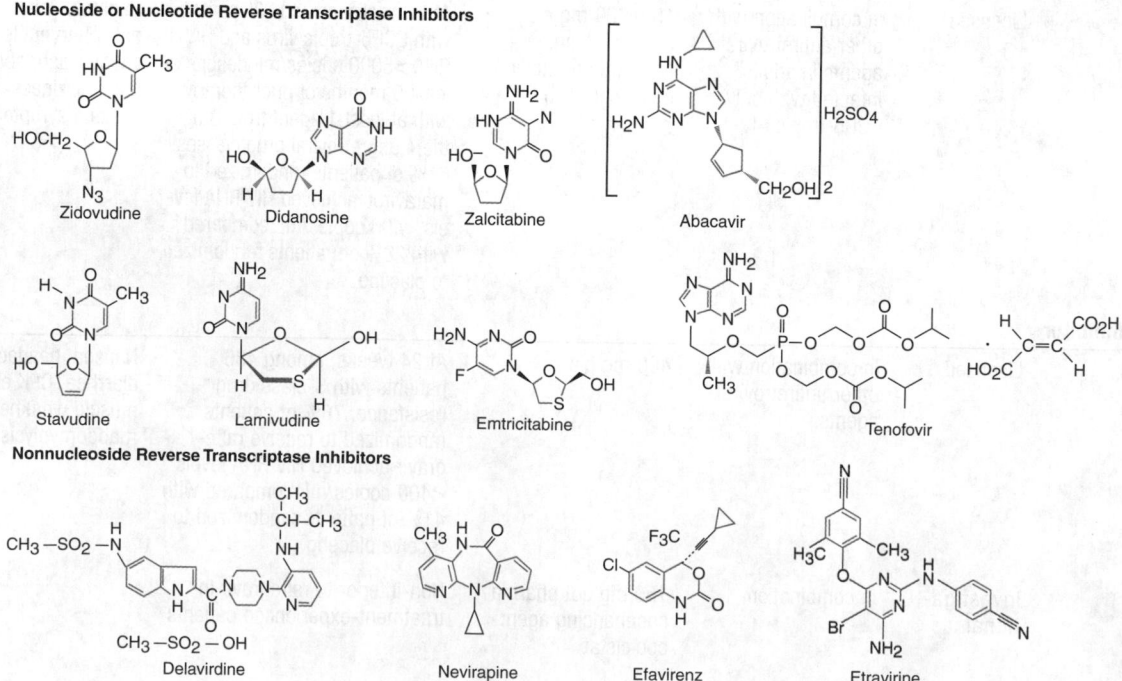

Figure 189-46 Molecular structures of antiretroviral agents.

Protease Inhibitors

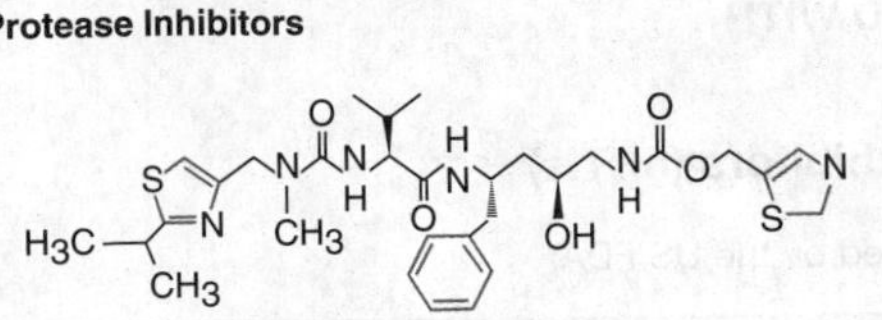

Ritonavir

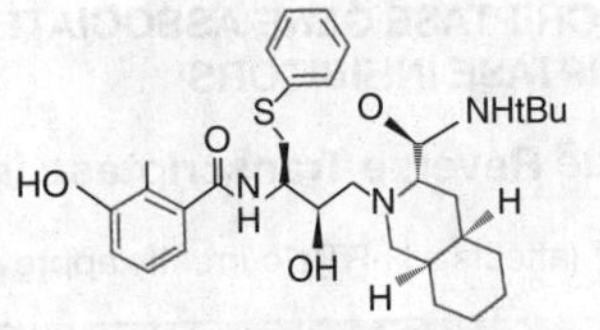

Nelfinavir mesylate

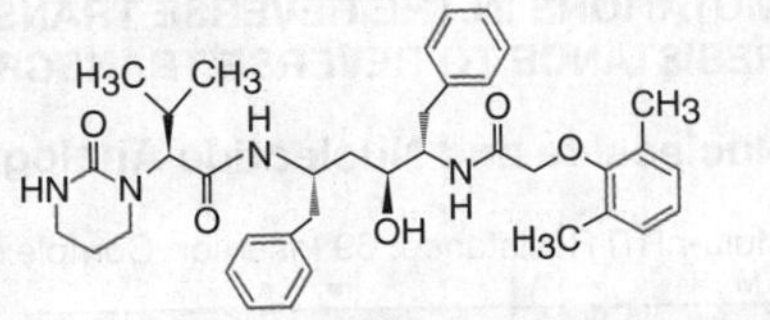

Lopinavir

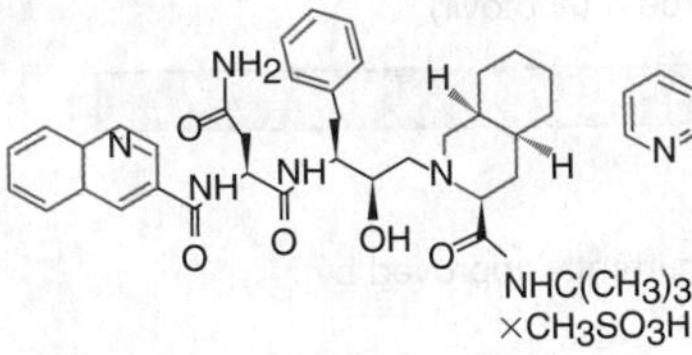

Saquinavir mesylate

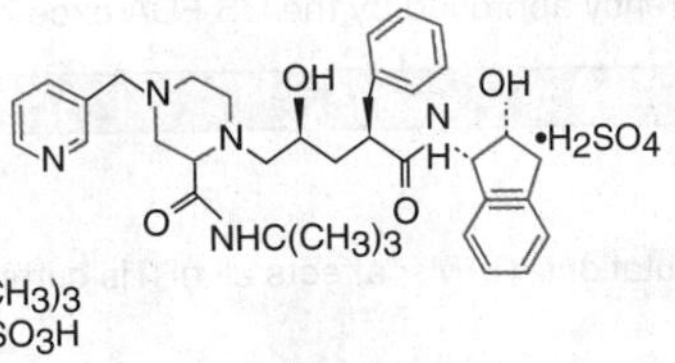

Indinavir sulfate

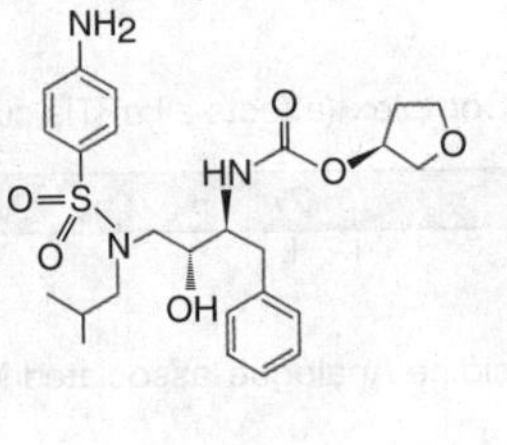

Amprenavir

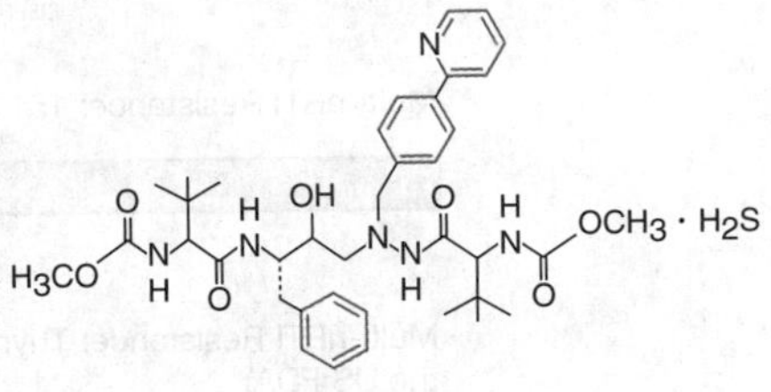

Atazanavir

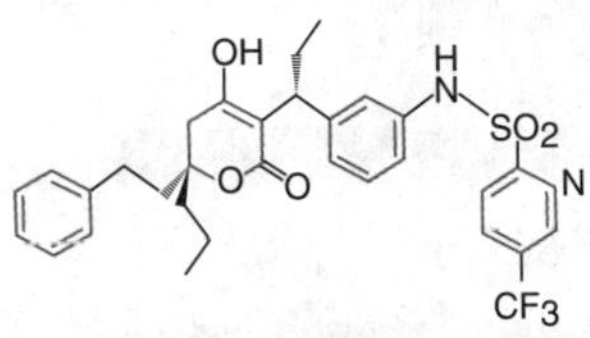

Tipranavir

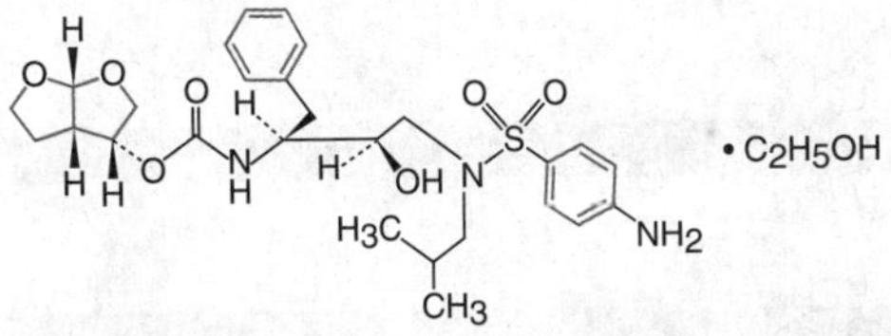

Darunavir

Entry Inhibitors

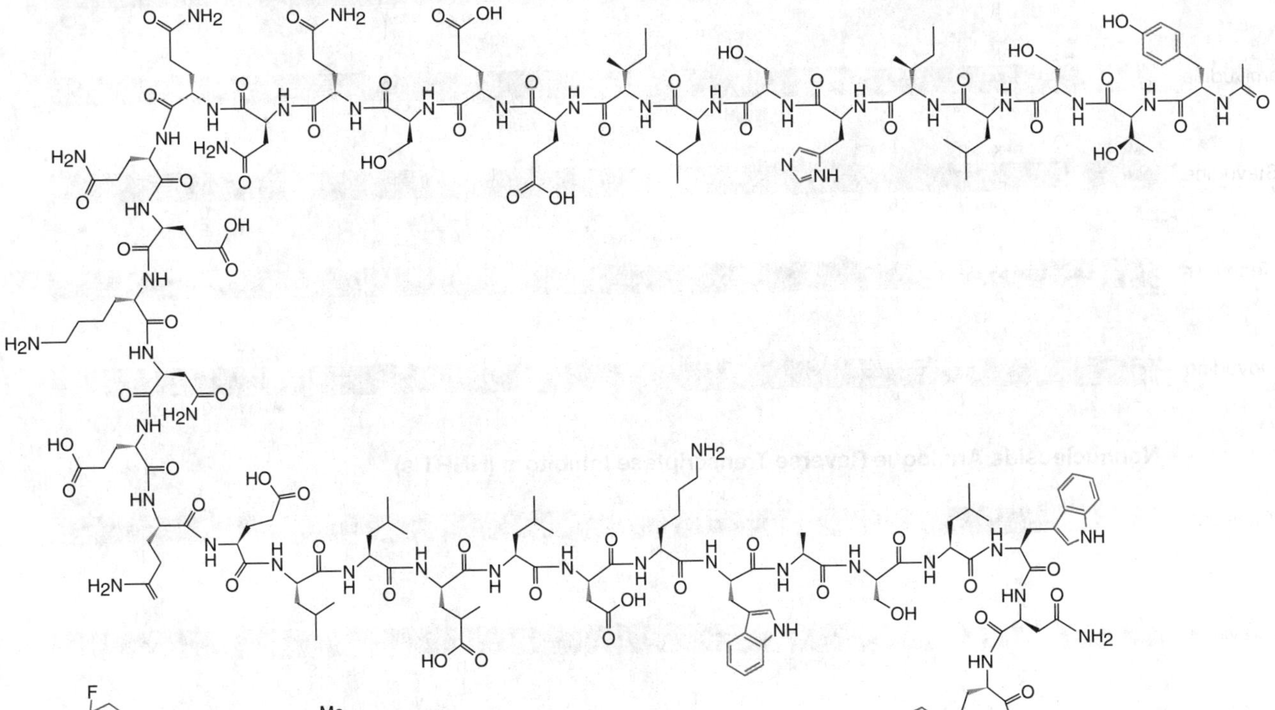

Enfuvirtide

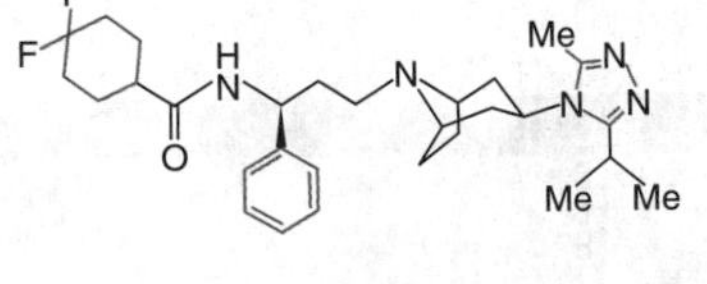

Maraviroc

Integrase Inhibitor

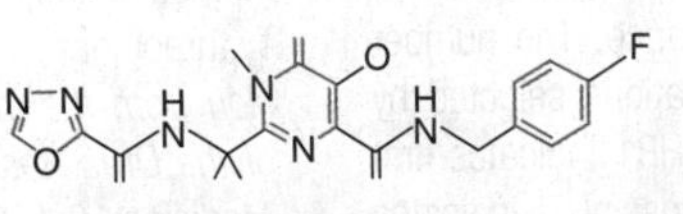

Raltegravir

Figure 189-46   *(continued)*

MUTATIONS IN THE REVERSE TRANSCRIPTASE GENE ASSOCIATED WITH RESISTANCE TO REVERSE TRANSCRIPTASE INHIBITORS

Nucleoside and Nucleotide Analogue Reverse Transcriptase Inhibitors (nRTIs)

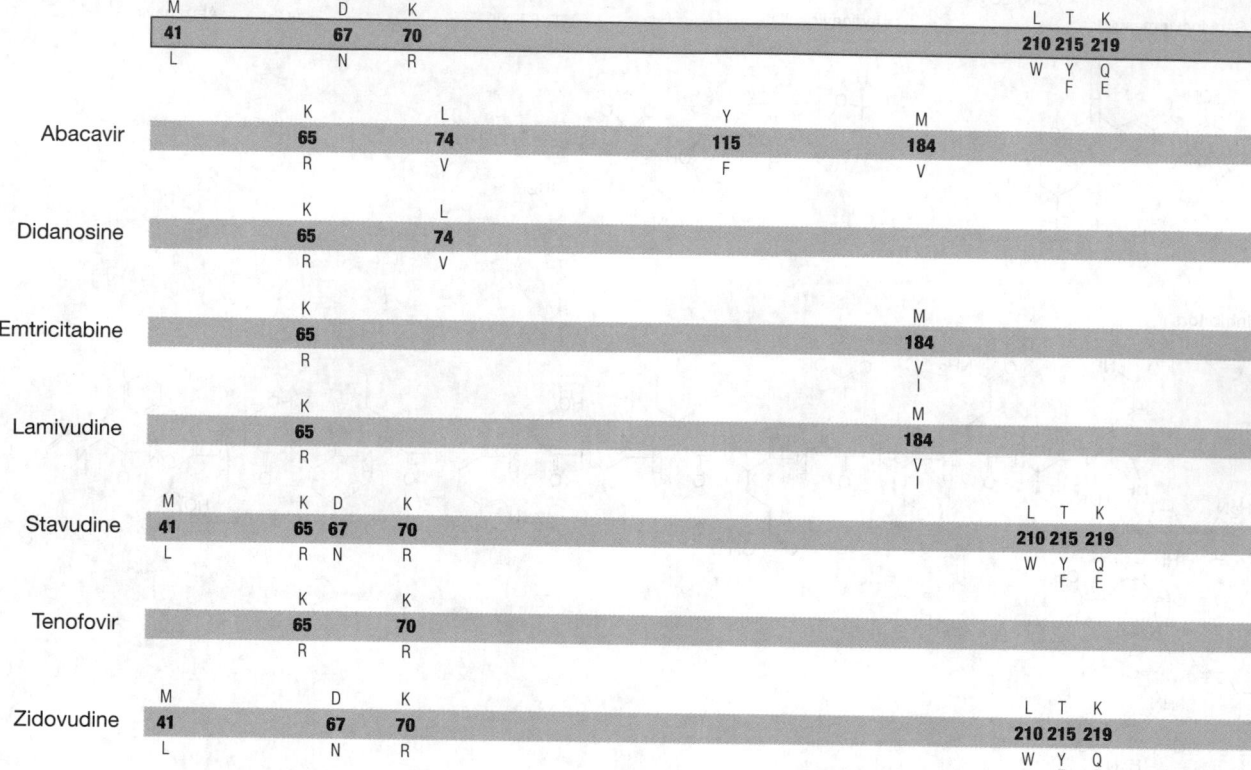

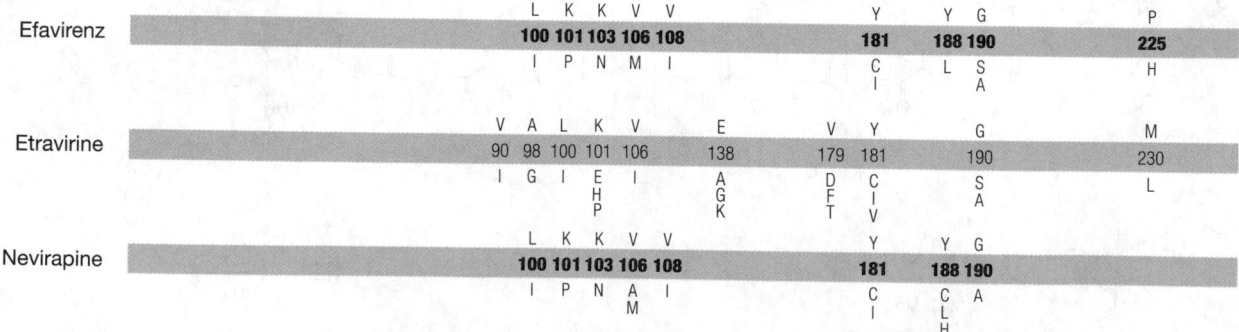

Figure 189-47 Amino acid substitutions conferring resistance to antiretroviral drugs. For each amino acid residue, the letter above the bar indicates the amino acid associated with wild-type virus and the letter(s) below indicate the substitution(s) that confer viral resistance. The number shows the position of the mutation in the protein. Mutations selected by protease inhibitors in Gag cleavage sites are not listed. HR1 indicates first heptad repeat; NAMs indicates nRTI-associated mutations; nRTI indicates nucleoside reverse transcriptase inhibitor; NNRTI indicates nonnucleoside reverse transcriptase inhibitor; PI indicates protease inhibitor. Amino acid abbreviations: A, alanine; C, cysteine; D, aspartate; E, glutamic acid; F, phenylalanine; G, glycine; H, histidine; I, isoleucine; K, lysine; L, leucine; M, methionine; N, asparagine; P, proline; Q, glutamine; R, arginine; S, serine; T, threonine; V, valine; W, tryptophan; Y, tyrosine. *[Reprinted with permission from the International AIDS Society—USA. VA Johnson et al: Update of the Drug Resistance Mutations in HIV-1: December 2010. Topics in HIV Medicine 18:156–163, 2010. Updated information (and thorough explanatory notes) is available at www.iasusa.org.]*

MUTATIONS IN THE PROTEASE GENE ASSOCIATED WITH RESISTANCE TO PROTEASE INHIBITORS

Atazanavir +/– ritonavir

L 10	G 16	K 20	L 24		V 32	L 33	E 34	M 36		M 46		G 48	I 50	F 53	I 54	D 60	I 62	I 64	A 71	G 73		V 82	I 84	I 85	N 88	L 90	I 93
I F V C	E	R M I T V	I		I F V	I Q L V		L		L		V	L Y		L V M T A	E	V L M	V I T L	V I C S T A	T		A T F I	V V	V	S M	M L	L M

Fosamprenavir/ ritonavir

L 10					V 32					M 46	I 47		I 50		I 54					T 73	L 76		V 82	I 84			L 90
F I R V					I					I L	V		V		L V M					S V	S	A F S T	V			M

Darunavir/ ritonavir

V 11					V 32	L 33				I 47			I 50		I 54					T 74	L 76		I 84	L 89
I					I	F				V			V		M L					P V	V		V	V

Indinavir/ ritonavir

L 10	K 20	L 24		V 32		M 36		M 46			I 54			A 71	G 73	L 76	V 77	V 82	I 84		L 90
I R V	M R	I		I		I		I L			V			V S	S A	V	I	A F T	V		M

Lopinavir/ ritonavir

L 10	K 20	L 24	V 32	L 33		M 46	I 47		I 50	F 53	I 54	L 63	A 71	G 73	L 76	V 82	I 84		L 90
F I R V	M R	I	I	F		I L	V A		V	L	V L A M T S	P	V T	S V	V	A F T S	V		M

Nelfinavir

L 10	D 30		M 36		M 46		A 71		V 77	V 82	I 84	N 88	L 90
F I	N		I		I L		V T		I	A F T S	V	D S	M

Saquinavir/ ritonavir

L 10	L 24		G 48		I 54	A 62	G 71	G 73	V 77	V 82	I 84	L 90
I R V	I		V		V L	V	V T	S	I	A F T S	V	M

Tipranavir/ ritonavir

L 10		L 33	M 36		K 43	M 46	I 47		I 54	Q 58		H 69	T 74	V 82	N 83	I 84		L 89
V		F	I L V		T	L	V	A M V	E		K R	P	L T	D	V		M

MUTATIONS IN THE ENVELOPE GENE ASSOCIATED WITH RESISTANCE TO ENTRY INHIBITORS

Enfuvirtide

G 36	I 37	V 38	Q 39	Q 40		N 42	N 43
D S	V	A M E	R	H		T	D

Maraviroc

ACTIVITY LIMITED TO PATIENTS WITH R5 VIRUSES

MUTATIONS IN THE INTEGRASE GENE ASSOCIATED WITH RESISTANCE TO INTEGRASE INHIBITORS

Raltegravir

E 92	Y 143	Q 148	N 155
Q	R H C	H K R	H

MUTATIONS

Insertion

Amino acid, wild-type — L

Amino acid position — **90** / 54

Major (boldface type; protease only)[15] — M

Amino acid substitution conferring resistance

Minor (lightface type; protease only)[15]

Figure 189-47 (continued)

Zalcitabine (ddC; 2′,3′-dideoxycytidine) is rarely used today in the management of patients with HIV infection and was discontinued from the U.S. market in 2006. Among the nucleoside analogues licensed for the treatment of HIV infection, it is probably the weakest. The main toxicities of ddC are peripheral neuropathy and pancreatitis.

Stavudine (d4T; 2′,3′-didehydro-3′-deoxythymidine) was the fourth drug licensed for the treatment of HIV infection. Like zidovudine, stavudine is a thymidine analogue. These two drugs are antagonistic in vitro and in vivo and should not be given together. Stavudine has been associated with a higher incidence of mitochondrial toxicity than the other licensed nucleoside analogues. Peripheral neuropathy, lipoatrophy, lactic acidosis, and hepatic steatosis are the main toxicities of stavudine.

Lamivudine (3TC; 2′,3′-dideoxy-3′-thiacytidine) is the fifth of the nucleoside analogues to be licensed in the United States. It is the negative enantiomer of a dideoxy analogue of cytidine. In actual practice, lamivudine or the closely related drug emtricitabine (see below) is a frequent element of many different combination regimens currently in use. These two drugs and the nucleotide reverse transcriptase inhibitor tenofovir (see below) also have activity against hepatitis B virus. For this reason flares of hepatitis may be seen in co-infected patients starting and/or or stopping any of these three agents due to the confounding issues of direct effects on hepatitis B, direct effects on HIV, and immune reconstitution (see above). To prevent the development of resistant strains of HIV, these drugs should never be used on their own for the treatment of hepatitis B in the patient with HIV infection. Lamivudine is available either alone or in coformulations including zidovudine and/or abacavir (Table 189-21). One reason behind the excellent synergy seen between lamivudine and the other nucleoside analogues may be that strains of HIV resistant to lamivudine (M184V substitution) appear to have enhanced sensitivity to other nucleosides, and thus development of dual resistance is more difficult. In addition, there is a suggestion that 3TC-resistant strains of HIV may be less virulent and are less able to generate new mutants than are strains of HIV that are 3TC-sensitive. Lamivudine is among the best tolerated and least toxic of the nucleoside analogues.

Emtricitabine (FTC; 5-fluoro-1-(2R,5S)-[2-(hydroxymethyl)-1,3-oxathiolan-5-yl]cytosine) is the negative enantiomer of a thio analogue of cytidine with a fluorine in the 5 position. It is licensed for use in combination with other antiretroviral agents for treatment of HIV-1 infection in adults. Compared with lamivudine, it is similar in activity and has a longer half-life. It is available either alone or coformulated with tenofovir or tenofovir and efavirenz (Table 189-21). As with lamivudine,

resistance to emtricitabine is associated with the M184V mutation in reverse transcriptase. Viruses showing the K65R mutation in reverse transcriptase may have reduced susceptibility to emtricitabine.

Abacavir {(1S,cis)-4-[2-amino-6-(cyclopropylamino)-9H-purin-9-yl]-2-cyclopentene-1-methanol sulfate (salt)(2:1)} is a synthetic carbocyclic analogue of the nucleoside guanosine. It is licensed to be used in combination with other antiretroviral agents for the treatment of HIV-1 infection. Hypersensitivity reactions that may occur with initial therapy or rechallenge have been reported in ~4% of patients treated with this drug, and patients developing signs or symptoms of hypersensitivity such as fever, skin rash, fatigue, and GI symptoms should discontinue the drug and not restart it. Fatal hypersensitivity reactions have been reported with rechallenge. Abacavir hypersensitivity occurs with a higher frequency in patients who are HLA-B5701-positive. It is recommended that patients be screened for HLA-B5701 prior to initiation of abacavir and that abacavir only be used as a last resort and with close monitoring in patients who are HLA-B5701-positive. Abacavir-resistant strains of HIV are typically also resistant to lamivudine, emtricitabine, didanosine, and zalcitabine. Abacavir is formulated alone as well as in combination with lamivudine or zidovudine and lamivudine.

Tenofovir disoproxil fumarate (9-[(R)-2-[[bis[[(isopropoxy-carbonyl)oxy]methoxy]phosphinyl]methoxy]propyl]adenine fumarate (1:1)) is an acyclic nucleoside phosphonate diester analogue of adenosine monophosphate. It undergoes diester hydrolysis to form the nucleoside monophosphate tenofovir and is the first nucleotide analogue to be licensed for treatment of HIV infection. It is indicated in combination with other antiretroviral agents for the treatment of HIV-1 infection. HIV isolates with increased resistance typically express a K65R mutation in reverse transcriptase and a three- to fourfold reduction in sensitivity to tenofovir. Tenofovir is primarily eliminated by the kidneys, and renal impairment including a Fanconi-like syndrome with hypophosphatemia may occur. Tenofovir is contraindicated in patients with renal impairment. Coadministration with didanosine leads to a 60% increase in didanosine levels, and thus doses of didanosine need to be adjusted and patients monitored carefully if these two drugs are used in combination. In addition CD4+ T cell increases may be blunted in patients on this combination. Coadministration of tenofovir with atazanavir leads to a decrease in atazanavir levels, and thus low-dose ritonavir (see below) needs to be added when these drugs are used in combination. Tenofovir is available alone and coformulated with emtricitabine or emtricitabine and efavirenz.

Nevirapine, delavirdine, efavirenz, etravirine, and *rilpivirine* are nonnucleoside inhibitors of the HIV-1 reverse transcriptase and are licensed for use in combination with nucleoside analogues for the treatment of HIV-infected adults. Coformulations that include efavirenz or nevirapine are available (Table 189-21). These agents inhibit reverse transcriptase by binding to regions of the enzyme outside the active site and causing conformational changes in the enzyme that render it inactive. Although these agents are active in the nanomolar range, they are also very selective for the reverse transcriptase of HIV-1, have no activity against HIV-2, and, when used as monotherapy, are associated with the rapid emergence of drug-resistant mutants (Table 189-20; Fig. 189-47). Efavirenz and rilpivirine are administered once a day, nevirapine and etravirine twice a day, and delavirdine three times a day. All are associated with the development of a maculopapular rash, generally seen within the first few weeks of therapy. While it is possible to treat through this rash, it is important to be sure that one is not dealing with a more

TABLE 189-21 Combination Formulations of Antiretroviral Drugs

Name	Combination
Combivir	Zidovudine + lamivudine
Epzicom	Zidovudine + abacavir
Trizivir	Zidovudine + lamivudine + abacavir
Truvada	Tenofovir + emtricitabine
Atripla	Tenofovir + emtricitabine + efavirenz
Triomune[a]	Stavudine + lamivudine + nevirapine

[a]Not licensed in the United States.

severe eruption such as Stevens-Johnson syndrome by looking carefully for signs of mucosal involvement, significant fever, or painful lesions with desquamation. Severe, life-threatening, and in some cases fatal hepatotoxicity, including fulminant and cholestatic hepatitis, hepatic necrosis, and hepatic failure, have been reported in patients treated with nevirapine. There is a suggestion that this is more common in women with higher CD4+ T cell counts. Many patients treated with efavirenz note a feeling of light-headedness, dizziness, or out of sorts following the initiation of therapy. Some complain of vivid dreams. These symptoms tend to disappear after several weeks of therapy. Aside from difficulties with dreams, taking efavirenz at bedtime may minimize the side effects. Efavirenz may cause fetal harm when administered during the first trimester to a pregnant woman. Women of childbearing potential should undergo pregnancy testing prior to initiation of efavirenz. Efavirenz is commonly used in combination with two nucleoside analogues as part of initial treatment regimens. Etravirine is a diarylpyrimidine derivative currently licensed for treatment of HIV infection in combination with other agents. In contrast to the other nonnucleoside reverse transcriptase inhibitors, which all exhibit cross-resistance, etravirine may be active against strains of HIV that are resistant to other nonnucleoside reverse transcriptase inhibitors. Among its side effects are rash, headache, nausea, and diarrhea. Rilpivirine is effective across a broad range of NNRTI resistant viruses and shares cross-resistance with etravirine. It is better tolerated and a has higher rate of virologic failure than efavirenz, particularly in those with HIV RNA >100,000.

The HIV-1 protease inhibitors (saquinavir, indinavir, ritonavir, nelfinavir, amprenavir, fosamprenavir, lopinavir/ritonavir, atazanavir, tipranavir, and darunavir) are a major part of the therapeutic armamentarium of antiretrovirals. When used as part of initial regimens in combination with reverse transcriptase inhibitors, these agents have been shown to be capable of suppressing levels of HIV replication to under 50 copies per milliliter in the majority of patients for a minimum of 5 years. As in the case of reverse transcriptase inhibitors, resistance to protease inhibitors can develop rapidly in the setting of monotherapy, and thus these agents should be used only as part of combination therapeutic regimens. A summary of known resistance mutations for protease inhibitors is shown in Fig. 189-47.

Saquinavir was the first of the HIV-1 protease inhibitors to be licensed. It is typically given with low doses of ritonavir to obtain therapeutic levels. Saquinavir is metabolized by the cytochrome P450 system in both the GI tract and the liver. Low-dose ritonavir results in inhibition of cytochrome P450. Thus, when both drugs are administered together there is an increase in saquinavir levels. This use of low doses of ritonavir to provide pharmacodynamic boosting of other agents is a common strategy in HIV therapy. Saquinavir is among the best-tolerated protease inhibitors.

Ritonavir was the first protease inhibitor for which clinical efficacy was demonstrated. In a study of 1090 patients with CD4+ T cell counts <100/µL who were randomized to receive either placebo or ritonavir in addition to any other licensed medications, patients receiving ritonavir had a reduction in the cumulative incidence of clinical progression or death from 34% to 17%. Mortality decreased from 10.1 to 5.8%. At full doses, ritonavir is poorly tolerated. Among the main side effects are nausea, diarrhea, abdominal pain, hyperlipidemia, and circumoral paresthesia. Ritonavir has a high affinity for several isoforms of cytochrome P450 (3A4, 2D6), and its use can result in large increases in the plasma concentrations of drugs metabolized by these pathways. Among the agents affected in this manner

are most other protease inhibitors, macrolide antibiotics, *R*-warfarin, ondansetron, rifabutin, most calcium channel blockers, glucocorticoids, and some of the chemotherapeutic agents used to treat KS and/or lymphomas. In addition, ritonavir may increase the activity of glucuronyltransferases, thus decreasing the levels of drugs metabolized by this pathway. Overall, great care must be taken when prescribing additional drugs to patients taking protease inhibitors in general and ritonavir in particular. As mentioned above, the pharmacodynamic boosting property of ritonavir, seen with doses as low as 100–200 mg once or twice a day, is often used in the setting of cART for HIV infection to derive more convenient regimens. For example, when given with low-dose ritonavir, saquinavir and indinavir can be given on twice-a-day schedules and taken with food.

Indinavir was the first protease inhibitor used in combination with dual nucleoside therapy. The combination of zidovudine, lamivudine, and indinavir was the first "triple combination" shown to have a profound effect on HIV replication. The main side effects of indinavir are nephrolithiasis (seen in 4% of patients) and asymptomatic indirect hyperbilirubinemia (seen in 10%). Indinavir is predominantly metabolized by the liver. The dose should be lowered in patients with cirrhosis. Levels of indinavir are decreased during concurrent therapy with rifabutin, efavirenz, or nevirapine and increased during concurrent therapy with ketoconazole, delavirdine, or ritonavir. Dosages should be modified appropriately in these circumstances. (Table 189-20).

Nelfinavir was approved in 1997 and *amprenavir* was approved in 1999 for the treatment of adult or pediatric HIV infection when cART is warranted. As with most of the antiretroviral agents licensed since 1999, these approvals were based on randomized, controlled trials that demonstrated decreases in plasma HIV RNA levels and increases in CD4+ T cell counts rather than clinical endpoints. Both nelfinavir and amprenavir have unique resistance profiles. Nelfinavir resistance is associated with a D30N substitution in the protease gene. Viruses harboring this single mutation retain sensitivity to other protease inhibitors. While it has been suggested that for this reason nelfinavir is a good initial protease inhibitor, enthusiasm for its use waned following 48-week clinical trials data demonstrating the virologic inferiority of nelfinavir to lopinavir/ritonavir, fosamprenavir, and efavirenz. Protease inhibitor resistance typically involves multiple amino acid substitutions and reduced susceptibility across the class. Amprenavir resistance is associated with a unique substitution at amino acid 50 (I50V). Nelfinavir and amprenavir are both associated with GI side effects. About 1% of patients receiving amprenavir have experienced severe and life-threatening skin reactions. An additional disadvantage of amprenavir is that the original formulation requires the patient to take 8 large capsules twice a day. Amprenavir has largely been replaced by fosamprenavir (see below).

Fosamprenavir was licensed in 2003 for the treatment of HIV infection in combination with other antiretroviral agents in adults. It is a prodrug of amprenavir that is rapidly converted to amprenavir by cellular phosphatases. It is supplied as a 700-mg tablet. The recommended dosage regimens are as follows: 1400 mg twice a day; 700 mg twice a day with ritonavir, 100 mg twice a day; or 1400 mg once a day with ritonavir, 200 mg once a day. As noted above, ritonavir-boosted fosamprenavir has been shown to have efficacy comparable to lopinavir/ritonavir and to efavirenz in combination regimens.

Lopinavir/ritonavir (Kaletra) is a fixed-dose combination of the protease inhibitors lopinavir (200 mg) and ritonavir (50 mg). It was licensed in 2000 for treatment of HIV-1 infection in adults and children in combination with other agents. A main advantage of this pill is that it combines the pharmacologic enhancement of low-dose ritonavir with a second protease inhibitor in a single capsule. In a randomized, controlled trial, this combination capsule was found to be superior to nelfinavir. Its main complications are GI upset and hyperlipidemia.

Atazanavir is an azapeptide inhibitor of the HIV-1 protease that was licensed in 2003. An advantage of atazanavir is that total cholesterol and triglyceride levels do not increase as much with atazanavir as with other protease inhibitors. This coupled with the fact that it can be given on a once-daily schedule has made atazanavir a popular component of initial treatment regimens. Atazanavir is associated with increases in serum bilirubin and prolongations of the ECG PR interval. Atazanavir-resistant isolates emerging in previously treatment-naïve individuals frequently harbor an I50L substitution. This mutation in some instances is associated with increased sensitivity to other protease inhibitors. Atazanavir requires an acidic gastric pH for absorption, and its use in combination with a proton pump inhibitor is contraindicated due to concerns about absorption. Atazanavir is an inhibitor of cytochrome P3A, and its use may be associated with increased levels of calcium channel blockers, macrolide antibiotics, HMG-CoA reductase inhibitors, and sildenafil. Levels of atazanavir are lower in the presence of tenofovir or efavirenz. In these settings, levels of atazanavir should be boosted with the use of low-dose ritonavir.

Tipranavir is a nonpeptidic HIV protease inhibitor licensed in 2005. It is licensed for use in combination with 200 mg ritonavir and is indicated for cART of HIV-1 infection in treatment-experienced adults or in adults with evidence of HIV-1 strains resistant to multiple protease inhibitors. Tipranavir was found to be inferior to lopinavir/ritonavir in a randomized controlled trial in naïve patients. In that study, at lower doses it was virologically inferior, while at higher doses it exhibited a greater degree of hepatotoxicity. The main side effects of tipranavir are GI intolerance and skin rash; the latter is seen in ~10% of patients and may be related to the sulfonamide moiety in the molecule. Tipranavir coadministered with ritonavir has also been associated with reports of intracranial hemorrhage as well as reports of clinical hepatitis and hepatic decompensation, including some fatalities in both settings. The risk of hepatotoxicity is increased in patients with hepatitis B or C co-infection.

Darunavir is a nonpeptidic HIV protease inhibitor initially licensed in 2006. It is indicated for coadministration with 100 mg of ritonavir and other antiretroviral agents for the treatment of HIV infection. In initial studies in treatment-experienced subjects, 46% of patients achieved a reduction in HIV RNA viral loads to <50 copies per milliliter. Studies in treatment-naïve patients demonstrated efficacy comparable to lopinavir/ritonavir-containing regimens. Skin rash, which may be severe, is seen in 7% of patients and may be related to the sulfonamide moiety contained in the molecule. GI intolerance and headache are the other most frequent side effects.

Entry inhibitors act by interfering with the binding of HIV to its receptor or co-receptor or by interfering with the process of fusion (see above). The first drug in this class to be licensed was the fusion inhibitor *enfuvirtide*, or T-20, followed by the CCR5 antagonist *maraviroc*. A variety of additional small molecules that bind to HIV-1 co-receptors are currently in clinical trials.

Enfuvirtide is a linear 36-amino-acid synthetic peptide with the N terminus acetylated and the C terminus a carboxamide. It is composed of naturally occurring L-amino acid residues and interferes with the fusion of the viral and cellular membranes by binding to the HR1 region in the gp41 subunit of the HIV-1 envelope. This binding interferes with the coil-coil interaction required to approximate the viral envelope and the host cell membrane during the process of viral fusion. Enfuvirtide was licensed in 2003 for treatment of HIV-1 infection in combination with other antiretroviral agents in treatment-experienced patients with ongoing viral replication despite antiretroviral therapy. Enfuvirtide is not active against HIV-2. Enfuvirtide resistant isolates of HIV exhibit amino acid changes in positions 36–45 of gp41. In two independent studies, patients who had persistent viremia despite prior treatment with agents from all three available classes of drugs were randomized to receive an individualized regimen (based on prior treatment history and resistance profile) with or without enfuvirtide. The change in plasma HIV-1 RNA from baseline was ~1 log greater (−1.53 vs. −0.68) in patients randomized to receive enfuvirtide. Among the drawbacks of this agent are the requirement for twice-a-day injection, the occurrence of injection site reactions in close to 100% of patients, and an increase in bacterial pneumonia in the enfuvirtide-treated patients compared with the control patients (4.68 vs 0.61 events per 100 patient-years) in the phase III studies.

Maraviroc is a CCR5 antagonist that interferes with HIV binding at the stage of co-receptor engagement. It was licensed in 2007 for treatment of HIV infection in combination with other agents in treatment-experienced patients infected with only CCR5-tropic (R5) virus resistant to multiple agents. The license was extended in 2009 to include treatment-naïve patients with R5 virus. A co-receptor tropism assay should be performed if one is considering the use of maraviroc to ensure that the potential patient is harboring R5 virus. In phase III trials of treatment-experienced patients randomized to receive optimal therapy plus maraviroc or placebo, 61% of patients randomized to maraviroc achieved HIV RNA levels <400 copies/mL compared with 28% of patients randomized to placebo. An allergic reaction–associated hepatotoxicity has been reported with maraviroc. Among the most common side effects of maraviroc are dizziness due to postural hypotension, cough, fever, colds, rash, muscle and joint pain, and stomach pain. Maraviroc is a substrate of CYP3A and Pgp, and the recommend dose varies depending on concomitant medications. In combination with nucleoside analogues, tipranavir/ritonavir, enfuvirtide, and/or nevirapine, the dose is 300 mg twice daily. In the presence of CYP3A inhibitors, such as most protease inhibitors, the dose is 150 mg twice daily. In the presence of CYP3A inducers such as efavirenz, the dose is 600 mg twice daily.

The newest class of antiretroviral compounds is the *integrase inhibitors*. *Raltegravir* is an inhibitor of the viral enzyme integrase and the first of this class to be approved. Elvitegravir is currently in clinical trials. Raltegravir was approved in 2007 for treatment of HIV infection in combination with other agents in treatment-experienced patients, and the approval was extended in 2009 to include treatment-naïve patients. Raltegravir exhibits a wide range of activity against HIV-1 and HIV-2, including viruses with multiple resistance mutations to other classes of drugs. As with several other compounds, resistance to raltegravir comes at the expense of replicative fitness. In two phase III studies in which 436 patients with 3-class antiretroviral drug resistance were randomized to an optimized background regimen with raltegravir or placebo, 76% of patients receiving raltegravir achieved HIV RNA levels <400 copies/mL compared with 41% of patients randomized to the placebo arm. In contrast to many other antiretroviral drugs the side-effect profile of raltegravir is minimal, with similar side-effect profiles noted for the raltegravir and placebo groups.

PRINCIPLES OF THERAPY The principles of therapy for HIV infection have been articulated by a panel sponsored by the U.S. Department of Health and Human Services as a working group of the NIH Office of AIDS Research Advisory Council. These principles are summarized in Table 189-22. As noted in these guidelines, cART of HIV infection does not lead to eradication or cure of HIV. Treatment decisions must take into account the fact that one is dealing with a chronic infection. While early therapy is generally the rule in infectious diseases, immediate treatment of every HIV-infected individual upon diagnosis may not be prudent, and therapeutic decisions must take into account the balance between risks and benefits. Patients initiating antiretroviral therapy must be willing to commit to life-long treatment and understand the importance of adherence to their prescribed regimen. The importance of adherence is illustrated by the observation that treatment interruption is associated with rapid increases in HIV RNA levels, rapid declines in CD4+ T cell counts, and an increased risk of clinical progression. While it seems reasonable to assume that the complications associated with cART could be minimized by regimens designed to minimize exposure to the drugs in question, all efforts to do so have paradoxically been associated with an increase in serious adverse events in the patients randomized to intermittent therapy, suggesting that some "non-AIDS-associated" serious adverse events such as heart attack and stroke may be linked to HIV replication. Thus, unless contraindicated for reasons of toxicity, patients started on cART should remain on cART.

TABLE 189-22 Principles of Therapy of HIV Infection

1. Ongoing HIV replication leads to immune system damage and progression to AIDS.

2. Plasma HIV RNA levels indicate the magnitude of HIV replication and the rate of CD4+ T cell destruction. CD4+ T cell counts indicate the current level of competence of the immune system.

3. Rates of disease progression differ among individuals, and treatment decisions should be individualized based on plasma HIV RNA levels and CD4+ T cell counts.

4. Maximal suppression of viral replication is a goal of therapy; the greater the suppression the less likely the appearance of drug-resistant quasispecies.

5. The most effective therapeutic strategies involve the simultaneous initiation of combinations of effective anti-HIV drugs with which the patient has not been previously treated and that are not cross-resistant with antiretroviral agents that the patient has already received.

6. The antiretroviral drugs used in combination regimens should be used according to optimum schedules and dosages.

7. The number of available drugs is limited. Any decisions on antiretroviral therapy have a long-term impact on future options for the patient.

8. Women should receive optimal antiretroviral therapy regardless of pregnancy status.

9. The same principles apply to children and adults. The treatment of HIV-infected children involves unique pharmacologic, virologic, and immunologic considerations.

10. Compliance is an important part of ensuring maximal effect from a given regimen. The simpler the regimen, the easier it is for the patient to be compliant.

Source: Modified from *Principles of Therapy of HIV Infection*, USPHS, and the Henry J. Kaiser Family Foundation.

TABLE 189-23 Indications for the Initiation of Antiretroviral Therapy in Patients With HIV Infection

I. Acute infection syndrome

II. Chronic infection

  A. Symptomatic disease (including HIV-associated nephropathy)

  B. Asymptomatic disease

    1. CD4+ T cell count <500/μL[a]

    2. Pregnancy

III. Postexposure prophylaxis

[a]This is an area of controversy. Some experts would treat everyone regardless of CD4+ T cell count.

Source: *Guidelines for the Use of Antiretroviral Agents in HIV-Infected Adults and Adolescents,* USPHS.

At present, a reasonable course of action is to initiate cART in anyone with the acute HIV syndrome; all pregnant women; patients with an AIDS-defining illness; patients with HIV-associated nephropathy; patients with hepatitis B infection when treatment for hepatitis B is indicated, and patients with asymptomatic disease with CD4+ T cell counts <500/μL (Table 189-23). Clinical trials are underway to determine the value of even earlier intervention, and some experts would place everyone with HIV infection on antiretroviral therapy. In addition, one may wish to administer a 6-week course of therapy to uninfected individuals immediately following a high-risk exposure to HIV. Studies are underway to define the role of pre-exposure prophylaxis. For patients diagnosed with an opportunistic infection and HIV infection at the same time, one may consider a 2- to 4-week delay in the initiation of antiretroviral therapy during which time treatment is focused on the opportunistic infection. While not proven, it is postulated that this delay may decrease the severity of any subsequent immune reconstitution inflammatory syndrome by lowering the antigenic burden of the opportunistic infection.

Once the decision has been made to initiate therapy, the health care provider must decide which drugs to use as the first regimen. The decision regarding choice of drugs not only will affect the immediate response to therapy but also will have implications regarding options for future therapeutic regimens. The initial regimen is usually the most effective insofar as the virus has yet to develop significant resistance. Given that patients can be infected with viruses that harbor drug resistance mutations, it is recommended that a viral genotype be done prior to the initiation of therapy to optimize the selection of antiretroviral agents. The three options for initial therapy most commonly in use today are three different three-drug regimens. The first regimen utilizes a nucleotide and a nucleoside analogue (tenofovir and emtricitabine) and a nonnucleoside reverse transcriptase inhibitor (efavirenz). The second regimen utilizes a ritonavir-boosted protease inhibitor (atazanavir or darunavir) in place of the nonnucleoside reverse transcriptase inhibitor. The third regimen utilizes an integrase inhibitor (raltegravir) in place of the nonnucleoside reverse transcriptase inhibitor. Unfortunately there are no clear data at present on which to base distinctions between these three approaches. Following the initiation of therapy one should expect a rapid, at least 1-log (tenfold) reduction in plasma HIV RNA levels within 1–2 months and then a slower decline in plasma HIV RNA levels to <50 copies per

TABLE 189-24 Indications for Changing Antiretroviral Therapy in Patients With HIV Infection[a]

Less than a 1-log drop in plasma HIV RNA by 4 weeks following the initiation of therapy

A reproducible significant increase (defined as threefold or greater) from the nadir of plasma HIV RNA level not attributable to intercurrent infection, vaccination, or test methodology

Persistently declining CD4+ T cell numbers

Clinical deterioration

Side effects

[a]Generally speaking, a change should involve the initiation of at least two drugs felt to be effective in the given patient. The exception to this is when change is being made to manage toxicity, in which case a single substitution is reasonable.

Source: *Guidelines for the Use of Antiretroviral Agents in HIV-Infected Adults and Adolescents,* USPHS.

milliliter within 6 months. During this same time there should be a rise in the CD4+ T cell count of 100–150/μL that is also particularly brisk during the first month of therapy. Subsequently, one should anticipate a CD4+ T cell count increase of 50–100 cells/year until numbers approach normal. Many clinicians feel that failure to achieve these endpoints is an indication for a change in therapy. Other reasons for a change in therapy include a persistently declining CD4+ T cell count, a consistent increase in HIV RNA levels to >1000 copies/mL, clinical deterioration, or drug toxicity (Table 189-24). As in the case of initiating therapy, changing therapy may have a lasting impact on future therapeutic options. When changing therapy because of treatment failure (clinical progression or worsening laboratory parameters), it is important to attempt to provide a regimen with at least two new active drugs. This decision can be guided by resistance testing (see below). In the patient in whom a change is made for reasons of drug toxicity, a simple replacement of one drug is reasonable. It should be stressed that in attempting to sort out a drug toxicity it may be advisable to hold all therapy for a period of time to distinguish between drug toxicity and disease progression. Drug toxicity will usually begin to show signs of reversal within 1–2 weeks. Prior to changing a treatment regimen because of drug failure, it is important to ensure that the patient has been adherent to the prescribed regimen. As in the case of initial therapy, the simpler the new therapeutic regimen, the easier it is for the patient to be compliant. Plasma HIV RNA levels and CD4+ T lymphocyte counts should be monitored every 3–6 months during therapy and more frequently if one is contemplating a change in regimen or immediately following a change in regimen.

In an attempt to determine an optimal therapeutic regimen for initial therapy or for a patient on a failing regimen, one may attempt to measure antiretroviral drug susceptibility through genotyping or phenotyping of HIV quasispecies and to determine adequacy of dosing through measurement of drug levels. Genotyping may be done through dideoxynucleotide sequencing, DNA chip hybridization, or line probe assays. Phenotypic assays typically measure the enzymatic activity of viral enzymes in the presence or absence of different concentrations of different drugs and have also been used to determine co-receptor tropism. These assays will generally detect quasispecies present at a frequency of ≥10%. It is generally recommended that resistance testing be used in selecting initial therapy in settings where the risk of transmission of resistant virus is high (such as the United States and Europe) and in determining new regimens for patients experiencing virologic failure while on therapy. Resistance testing may be of particular value in distinguishing drug-resistant virus from poor patient compliance. Due to the rapid rate at which drug-resistant viruses revert to wild-type, it is recommended that resistance testing performed in the setting of drug failure be carried out while the patient is still on the failing regimen. Measurement of plasma drug levels can also be used to tailor an individual treatment. The inhibitory quotient, defined as the trough blood level/IC_{50} of the patient's virus, is used by some to determine the adequacy of dosing of a given treatment regimen. Despite the best of efforts there will still be patients with ongoing high levels of HIV replication while receiving the best available therapy. These patients will receive benefit from remaining on antiretroviral therapy even though it is not fully suppressive.

In addition to the licensed medications discussed above, a large number of experimental agents are being evaluated as possible therapies for HIV infection. Therapeutic strategies are being developed that interfere with virtually every step of the replication cycle of the virus (Fig. 189-3). In addition, as more is discovered about the role of the immune system in controlling viral replication, additional strategies, generically referred to as "immune-based therapies," are being developed as a complement to antiviral therapy. Among the antiviral agents in early clinical trials are additional nucleoside and nucleotide analogues, protease inhibitors, fusion inhibitors, receptor and co-receptor antagonists, and integrase inhibitors as well as new antiviral strategies including antisense nucleic acids and maturation inhibitors. Among the immune-based therapies being evaluated are IFN-α, bone marrow transplantation, adoptive transfer of lymphocytes genetically modified to resist infection or enhance HIV-specific immunity, active immunotherapy with inactivated HIV or its components, IL-7, and IL-15.

HIV AND THE HEALTH CARE WORKER

Health care workers, especially those who deal with large numbers of HIV-infected patients, have a small but definite risk of becoming infected with HIV as a result of professional activities (see "Occupational Transmission of HIV: Health Care Workers, Laboratory Workers, and the Health Care Setting," above). The first case of HIV transmission from a patient to health care worker was reported in 1984. Occupational transmission of HIV has been reported in most countries, but the global surveillance data required to estimate the true frequency of this problem are not available.

In the United States between 1981 and 2006 , 57 health care workers for whom case investigations were completed had documented seroconversions to HIV following occupational exposures. The routes of exposure resulting in infection were as follows: 48 percutaneous (puncture/cut injury); 5 mucocutaneous (mucous membrane and/or skin); 2 both percutaneous and mucocutaneous; and 2 of unknown route. Of the 57 health care personnel, 49 were exposed to HIV-infected blood; 3 to concentrated virus in a laboratory; 1 to visibly bloody fluid; and 4 to an unspecified fluid. The individuals with documented seroconversions included 19 laboratory workers (16 of whom were clinical laboratory workers), 24 nurses, 6 physicians, 2 surgical technicians, 1 dialysis technician, 1 respiratory therapist, 1 health aide, 1 embalmer/morgue technician, and 2 housekeeper/maintenance workers. In addition, at least 140 possible cases of occupationally acquired HIV infection have been reported among health care personnel in the United States. The number of these workers who actually acquired their infection through occupational exposures is not known. Taken together, data from several large studies suggest that the risk of HIV infection following a percutaneous exposure to HIV-contaminated blood is ~0.3%, and after a mucous membrane exposure, ~0.09%. Although episodes of HIV transmission after nonintact skin exposure have been documented, the average risk for transmission by this route has not been precisely quantified but is estimated to be less than the risk for mucous membrane exposures. The risk for transmission after exposure to fluids or tissues other than HIV-infected blood also has not been quantified but is probably considerably lower than for blood exposures. A seroprevalence survey of 3420 orthopedic surgeons, 75% of whom practiced in an area with a relatively high prevalence of HIV infection and 39% of whom reported percutaneous exposure to patient blood, usually through an accident involving a suture needle, failed to reveal any cases of possible occupational infection, suggesting that the risk of infection with a suture needle may be considerably less than that with a blood-drawing (hollow-bore) needle.

Most cases of health care worker seroconversion occur as a result of needle-stick injuries. When one considers the circumstances that result in needle-stick injuries, it is immediately obvious that adhering to the standard guidelines for dealing with sharp objects would result in a significant decrease in this type of accident. In one study, 27% of needle-stick injuries resulted from improper disposal of the needle (over half of these were due to recapping the needle), 23% occurred during attempts to start an IV line, 22% occurred during blood drawing, 16% were associated with an IM or SC injection, and 12% were associated with giving an IV infusion.

Clinicians should consider potential occupational exposures to HIV as urgent medical concerns to ensure timely postexposure management and possible administration of postexposure antiretroviral prophylaxis (PEP). Recommendations regarding PEP must take into account that a variety of circumstances determine the risk of transmission of HIV following occupational exposure. In this regard, several factors have been associated with an increased risk for occupational transmission of HIV infection, including deep injury, the presence of visible blood on the instrument causing the exposure, injury with a device that had been placed in the vein or artery of the source patient, terminal illness in the source patient, and lack of postexposure cART in the exposed health care worker. Other important considerations when considering PEP in the health care worker include known or suspected pregnancy or breast-feeding, the possibility of exposure to drug-resistant virus, and toxicities of PEP regimens. Regardless of the decision to use PEP, the wound should be cleansed immediately and antiseptic applied. If a decision is made to offer PEP, U.S. Public Health Service guidelines recommend (1) a combination of two nucleoside analogue reverse transcriptase inhibitors given for 4 weeks for less severe exposures, or (2) a combination of two nucleoside analogue reverse transcriptase inhibitors plus a third drug given for 4 weeks for more severe exposures. Most clinicians administer the latter regimen in all cases in which a decision is made to treat. Detailed guidelines are available from the *Updated U.S. Public Health Service Guidelines for the Management of Occupational Exposures to HIV and Recommendations for Postexposure Prophylaxis* (CDC, 2005). The report emphasizes the importance of adherence to PEP when it is indicated, follow-up of exposed workers to improve PEP adherences, monitoring for adverse events (including seroconversion), and expert consultation in the management of exposures.

For consultation on the treatment of occupational exposures to HIV and other bloodborne pathogens, the clinician managing the exposed patient can call the National Clinicians' Post-Exposure Prophylaxis Hotline (PEPline) at 888-448-4911. This service is available 24 hours a day at no charge. (Additional information on the Internet is available at *www.nccc.ucsf.edu*.) PEPline support may be especially useful in challenging situations, such as when drug-resistant HIV strains are suspected or the health care worker is pregnant.

Health care workers can minimize their risk of occupational HIV infection by following the CDC guidelines of July 1991, which include adherence to universal precautions, refraining from direct patient care if one has exudative lesions or weeping dermatitis, and disinfecting and sterilizing reusable devices employed in invasive procedures. The premise of universal precautions is that every specimen should be handled as if it came from someone infected with a bloodborne pathogen. All samples should be double-bagged, gloves should be worn when drawing blood, and spills should be immediately disinfected with bleach.

In attempting to put this small but definite risk to the health care worker in perspective, it is important to point out that ~200 health care workers die each year as a result of occupationally acquired hepatitis B infection. The tragedy in this instance is that these infections and deaths due to HBV could be greatly decreased by more extended use of the HBV vaccine. The risk of HBV infection following a needle-stick injury from a hepatitis antigen–positive patient is much higher than the risk of HIV infection (see "Transmission," above). There are multiple examples of needle-stick injuries where the patient was positive for both HBV and HIV and the health care worker became infected only with HBV. For these reasons, it is advisable, given the high prevalence of HBV infection in HIV-infected individuals, that all health care workers dealing with HIV-infected patients be immunized with the HBV vaccine.

TB is another infection common to HIV-infected patients that can be transmitted to the health care worker. For this reason, all health care workers should know their PPD status, have it checked yearly, and receive 6 months of isoniazid treatment if their skin test converts to positive. In addition, all patients in whom a diagnosis of TB is being entertained should be placed immediately in respiratory isolation, pending results of the diagnostic evaluation. The emergence of drug-resistant organisms, including the extensively drug-resistant TB strains that have been identified in Africa, has made TB an increasing problem for health care workers. This is particularly true for the health care worker with preexisting HIV infection.

One of the most charged issues ever to come between health care workers and patients is that of transmission of infection from HIV-infected health care workers to their patients. This is discussed under "Occupational Transmission of HIV: Health Care Workers, Laboratory Workers, and the Health Care Setting," above. Theoretically, the same universal precautions that are used to protect the health care worker from the HIV-infected patient will also protect the patient from the HIV-infected health care worker.

A PREVENTIVE VACCINE AGAINST HIV INFECTION

Given that human behavior, especially human sexual behavior, is extremely difficult to change, a critical modality for preventing the spread of HIV infection is the development of a safe and effective vaccine. Historically, vaccines have provided a safe, cost-effective, and efficient means of preventing illness, disability, and death from infectious diseases. Successful vaccines for the most part are predicated on the assumptions that the body can mount an adequate immune response to the microbe or virus in question during natural infection and that the vaccine will mimic the natural response to infection. Even with serious diseases, such as smallpox, poliomyelitis, measles, and influenza among others, the body in the vast majority of cases clears the infectious agent and provides protection, which is usually life-long against future exposure. Unfortunately, this is not the case with HIV infection since the natural immune response to HIV infection is unable to clear the virus from the body and cases of superinfection have been reported. Some of the factors that contribute to the problematic nature of development of a preventive HIV vaccine are the high mutability of the virus, the fact that the infection can be transmitted by cell-free or cell-associated virus, the fact that the HIV provirus integrates itself into the genome of the target cell and may remain in a latent form unexposed to the immune system, the likely need for the development of effective mucosal immunity, and the fact that it has been difficult to establish the precise correlates of protective immunity to HIV infection. Some HIV-infected individuals are long-term nonprogressors, and a number of individuals have been exposed to HIV multiple times but remain uninfected; these facts suggest that there are elements of host defense or an HIV-specific immune response that have the potential to be protective. Early attempts to develop a vaccine with the envelope protein gp120 aimed at inducing neutralizing antibodies in humans were performed based on the induction of neutralizing antibodies in nonhuman primates. The significance of the laboratory assays were unknown at the time, and the elicited antisera failed to neutralize primary isolates of HIV cultured and tested in fresh peripheral blood mononuclear cells. In this regard, two phase 3 trials were undertaken in the United States and Thailand using soluble gp120, and the vaccines failed to protect human volunteers from HIV infection. A number of studies in monkeys using vaccines that induce predominantly cellular (T cell) immune responses have not protected the animals against infection but have lowered the initial burst of viremia following acute infection as well as decreased temporarily the viral set point. Since most sexually transmitted HIV infections occur when the transmitting partner is experiencing high levels of viremia such as during the acute phase of HIV infection or during the advanced stage of disease when the viral load is high, such a vaccine, which might limit the initial burst of viremia in primary infection and decrease the established viral set point, could have benefits for the individual as well as for their sexual partners. However, such a "T cell vaccine" failed in human clinical trials to lower either the initial burst of viremia or the viral set point after acquisition of infection. Recently, a vaccine using a poxvirus vector prime expressing various viral proteins followed by an envelope protein boost was tested in a 16,000-person clinical trial conducted in Thailand among predominantly low-prevalence heterosexuals. The vaccine provided the first positive, albeit very modest, signal ever reported in an HIV vaccine trial, showing 31% protection against acquisition of infection. Such a result is certainly not sufficient justification for clinical use of the vaccine, but it serves as an important first step in the direction of the development of a safe and effective vaccine against HIV infection. The next important step is to determine the correlate or correlates of immunity that provided the modest protection against infection.

PREVENTION

Education, counseling, and behavior modification are the cornerstones of an HIV prevention strategy. A major problem in the United States and elsewhere is that many infections are passed on by those who do not know that they are infected. Of the ~1.1 million persons in the United States who are HIV-infected, it is estimated that ~21% do not know their HIV status and thus may be putting others at risk by their own behavior. In this regard, the CDC has recently recommended that HIV testing become part of routine medical care and that all individuals between the ages of 13 and 64 years be informed of the testing and be tested without the need for written informed consent. The individual could "opt out" of testing, but if not, testing would be routinely administered. In addition to identifying individuals who might benefit from cART, information gathered from such an approach should serve as the basis for behavior-modification programs, both for infected individuals who may be unaware of their HIV status and who could infect others and for uninfected individuals practicing high-risk behavior. The practice of "safer sex" is the most effective way for sexually active

uninfected individuals to avoid contracting HIV infection and for infected individuals to avoid spreading infection. Abstinence from sexual relations is the only absolute way to prevent sexual transmission of HIV infection. However, for many individuals this may not be feasible, and there are a number of relatively safe practices that can markedly decrease the chances of transmission of HIV infection. Partners engaged in monogamous sexual relationships who wish to be assured of safety should both be tested for HIV antibody. If both are negative, it must be understood that any divergence from monogamy puts both partners at risk; open discussion of the importance of honesty in such relationships should be encouraged. When the HIV status of either partner is not known, or when one partner is positive, there are a number of options. Use of condoms can markedly decrease the chance of HIV transmission. It should be remembered that condoms are not 100% effective in preventing transmission of HIV infection, and there is a ~10% failure rate of condoms used for contraceptive purposes. Most condom failures result from breakage or improper usage, such as not wearing the condom for the entire period of intercourse. Latex condoms are preferable, since virus has been shown to leak through natural skin condoms. Petroleum-based gels should never be used for lubrication of the condom, since they increase the likelihood of condom rupture. Some men who have sex with men practice fellatio as a "minimal risk" activity compared to anal intercourse. It should be emphasized that receptive fellatio is definitely not safe sex, and although the incidence of transmission via fellatio is considerably less than that of rectal or vaginal intercourse, there has been documentation of transmission of HIV where receptive fellatio was the only sexual act performed (see "Transmission," above). Topical microbicides for vaginal and anal use are being pursued actively as a means by which individuals could avoid infection when the insertive partner cannot be relied on to use a condom. In 2010, a topical microbicide composed of 1% tenofovir in a gel was demonstrated in a clinical trial in South Africa to be 39% effective in preventing acquisition of HIV infection in women engaging in vaginal intercourse. Three clinical trials of heterosexual men in South Africa, Uganda, and Kenya have shown that adult male circumcision results in a 50% to 65% reduction in HIV acquisition in the circumcised subject. Clearly, this approach has considerable potential as a preventive strategy for HIV infection and is currently being pursued, particularly in developing nations, as a component of HIV prevention. In 2010, a study of pre-exposure prophylaxis using two drugs (tenofovir plus emtricitabine; see "Treatment", above) on a daily basis in uninfected men who have sex with men and transgender women demonstrated a 44% efficacy. When participants had a high level of adherence to the regimen, the level of protection rose to 73%. Also in 2010, a study demonstrated that treatment of the infected partner in an HIV-discordant relationship with antiretroviral therapy provided a 92% protection to the uninfected partner.

The most effective way to prevent transmission of HIV infection among IDUs is to stop the use of injectable drugs. Unfortunately, that is extremely difficult to accomplish unless the individual enters a treatment program. For those who will not or cannot participate in a drug treatment program and who will continue to inject drugs, the avoidance of sharing of needles and other paraphernalia ("works") is the next best way to avoid transmission of infection. However, the cultural and social factors that contribute to the sharing of paraphernalia are complex and difficult to overcome. In addition, needles and syringes may be in short supply. Under these circumstances, paraphernalia should be cleaned after each usage with a virucidal solution, such as undiluted sodium hypochlorite (household bleach). Data from a number of studies have indicated that programs that provide sterile needles to addicts in exchange for used needles have resulted in a decrease in HIV transmission without increasing the use of injection drugs. It is important for

IDUs to be tested for HIV infection and counseled to avoid transmission to their sexual partners. Secondary and tertiary spread of HIV infection by the heterosexual route within settings of a high level of injection drug use has increased greatly in the United States, particularly among African Americans. Studies are underway to determine the safety and efficacy of preexposure administration of antiretroviral drugs for the prevention of HIV infection.

Transmission of HIV via transfused blood or blood products has been decreased dramatically by a combination of screening of all blood donors for HIV infection by assays for both HIV antibody and nucleic acid and self-deferral of individuals at risk for HIV infection. In addition, clotting factor concentrates are heat-treated, essentially eliminating the risk to hemophiliacs who require these products. Autologous transfusions are preferable to transfusions from another individual. However, logistic constraints as well as the unpredictability of the need for most transfusions limit the feasibility of this approach. At present the risk of becoming HIV-infected from a contaminated blood transfusion is approximately 1 in 1.5 million donations in the United States.

Treatment of an HIV-infected mother with antiretroviral therapy during pregnancy and the infant during the first weeks following birth has proved very effective in dramatically decreasing mother-to-child transmission of HIV. In situations such as that seen in certain developing countries where pregnant women frequently present to a health care system during labor, administration of a short course (as little as a single dose of one drug) of antiretroviral therapy to the mother during labor and to the infant within 48 h of birth has also been successful in decreasing the incidence of mother-to-child transmission of HIV.

HIV can be transmitted via breast milk and colostrum. The avoidance of breast-feeding may not be practical in developing countries, where nutritional concerns override the risk of HIV transmission. However, it is becoming appreciated that 5–15% of infants who were born of HIV-infected mothers and who were fortunate enough not to have been infected intrapartum or peripartum become infected via breast-feeding. Therefore, in developing countries, breast-feeding from an infected mother should be avoided if at all possible. Unfortunately, this is rarely the case, and given the disadvantages of withholding breast-feeding in developing countries, health authorities in most developing countries continue to recommend breast-feeding despite the potential for HIV transmission. In this regard, the most effective way to avoid mother-to-child transmission of HIV is to treat the infected mother throughout the entire pregnancy and to continue therapy during breast-feeding and beyond if the mother's clinical status warrants such treatment. Such an approach has become more feasible over the past few years as the availability of antiretroviral therapy in the developing world has increased as a result of various programs such as the President's Emergency Plan for AIDS Relief (PEPFAR) and the Global Fund to Fight AIDS, Tuberculosis and Malaria, among others. In developed countries such as the United States, where bottled formula and milk are readily accessible, breast-feeding is contraindicated when a mother is HIV-positive, even if she is receiving antiretroviral therapy.

It is clear that in order to control and ultimately end the AIDS pandemic, effective prevention is essential. There are a number of HIV preventive modalities that have been demonstrated to be effective in various target populations if properly implemented and adhered to, and several others that are showing promise in clinical trials. It is unlikely that major successes in HIV prevention will be achieved with a uni-dimensional approach. What will almost certainly be required are various versions of combination prevention strategies, depending on the target population.

FURTHER READINGS

ABDOOL KARIM Q et al: Effectiveness and safety of tenofovir gel, an antiretroviral microbicide, for the prevention of HIV infection in women. Science 329:1168, 2010

THE ANTIRETROVIRAL THERAPY COHORT COLLABORATION: Life expectancy of individuals on combination antiretroviral therapy in high-income countries: A collaborative analysis of 14 cohort studies. Lancet 372:293, 2008

ARTHOS J et al: HIV-1 envelope protein binds to and signals through integrin $\alpha4\beta7$, the gut mucosal homing receptor for peripheral T cells. Nat Immunol 9:301, 2008

ATTIA S et al: Sexual transmission of HIV according to viral load and antiretroviral therapy: Systematic review and meta-analysis. AIDS 23:1397, 2009

BAGGALEY RF et al: HIV transmission risk through anal intercourse: Systematic review, meta-analysis and implications for HIV prevention. Int J Epidemiol. 39:1048, 2010

——— et al: Systematic review of orogenital HIV-1 transmission probabilities. Int J Epidemiol 37:1255, 2008

BAILEY RC et al: Male circumcision for HIV prevention in young men in Casuum, Kenya: A randomised controlled trial. Lancet 369:643, 2007

BOILY MC et al: Heterosexual risk of HIV-1 infection per sexual act: Systematic review and meta-analysis of observational studies. Lancet Infect Dis. 9:118, 2009

BRANSON BM et al: Revised recommendations for HIV testing of adults, adolescents, and pregnant women in health-care settings. MMWR Recomm Rep 55:1, 2006

BRENCHLEY JM et al: Microbial translocation is a cause of systemic immune activation in chronic HIV infection. Nat Med 12:1365, 2006

BRENNER BG et al: High rates of forward transmission events after acute/early HIV-1 infection. J Infect Dis 195:951, 2007

BUCHACZ K et al: AIDS-defining opportunistic illnesses in US patients, 1994–2007: A cohort study. AIDS 24:1549, 2010

CARBONE A et al: HIV-associated lymphomas and gamma-herpesviruses. Blood 113:1213, 2009

CENTERS FOR DISEASE CONTROL AND PREVENTION: HIV transmission through transfusion—Missouri and Colorado, 2008. MMWR Recomm Rep 59:1335, 2010

———: HIV/AIDS Surveillance Report, 2009, 2011. Available at www.cdc.gov/hiv/topics/surveillance/resources/reports/

———: HIV prevalence estimates—United States, 2006. MMWR Recomm Rep 57:1073, 2008

———, HEALTH RESOURCES AND SERVICES ADMINISTRATION, NATIONAL INSTITUTES OF HEALTH, HIV MEDICINE ASSOCIATION OF THE INFECTIOUS DISEASES SOCIETY OF AMERICA: Incorporating HIV prevention into the medical care of persons living with HIV. MMWR Recomm Rep 52:1, 2003

CHOHAN B et al: Selection for human immunodeficiency virus type 1 envelope glycosylation variants with shorter V1-V2 loop sequences occurs during transmission of certain genetic subtypes and may impact viral RNA levels. J Virol 79:6528, 2005

CHUN TW et al: Rebound of plasma viremia following cessation of antiretroviral therapy despite profoundly low levels of HIV reservoir: implications for eradication. AIDS 24:2803, 2010

CLERICI M: Beyond IL-17: New cytokines in the pathogenesis of HIV infection. Curr Opin HIV AIDS 5:184, 2010

COREY L: Synergistic copathogens—HIV-1 and HSV-2. N Engl J Med 356:854, 2007

DAS M et al: Decreases in community viral load are accompanied by reductions in new HIV infections in San Francisco. PLoS One 5:e11068, 2010

DEPARTMENT OF HEALTH AND HUMAN SERVICES PANEL ON ANTIRETROVIRAL GUIDELINES FOR ADULTS AND ADOLESCENTS: *Guidelines for the Use of Antiretroviral Agents in HIV-1-Infected Adults and Adolescents,* January, 2011. Updates available at *www.aidsinfo.nih.gov*

DERDEYN CA et al: Envelope-constrained neutralization-sensitive HIV-1 after heterosexual transmission. Science 303:2019, 2004

DONNELL D et al: Heterosexual HIV-1 transmission after initiation of antiretroviral therapy: A prospective cohort analysis. Lancet 375:2092, 2010

DORAK MT et al: Transmission of HIV-1 and HLA-B allele-sharing within serodiscordant heterosexual Zambian couples. Lancet 363:2137, 2004

DUBE MP, SATTLER FR: Inflammation and complications of HIV disease. J Infect Dis 201:1783, 2010

EPSTEIN JS, HOLMBERG JA: Progress in monitoring blood safety. Transfusion 50:1408, 2010

ESTE JA, TELENTI A: HIV entry inhibitors. Lancet 370:81, 2007

FAUCI AS: The AIDS epidemic—considerations for the 21st century. N Engl J Med 341:1046, 1999

———, FOLKERS GK: Investing to meet the scientific challenges of HIV/AIDS. Health Aff (Millwood) 28:1629, 2009

FELLAY J et al: Host genetics and HIV-1: The final phase? PLoS Pathog 6:e1001033, 2010

FOLKERS GK, FAUCI AS: Controlling and ultimately ending the HIV/AIDS pandemic: A feasible goal. JAMA 304:350, 2010

FREIBERG M et al: The association between hepatitis C infection and prevalent cardiovascular disease among HIV-infected individuals. AIDS 21:193, 2007

FRENCH MA et al: Serum immune activation markers are persistently increased in patients with HIV infection after 6 years of antiretroviral therapy despite suppression of viral replication and reconstitution of CD4+ T cells. J Infect Dis 200:1212, 2009

GANCZAK M, BARSS P: Nosocomial HIV infection: Epidemiology and prevention—a global perspective. AIDS Rev 10:47, 2008

GERETTI AM: Epidemiology of antiretroviral drug resistance in drug-naive persons. Curr Opin Infect Dis 20:22, 2007

GETAHUN H et al: HIV infection-associated tuberculosis: The epidemiology and the response. Clin Infect Dis 50:S201, 2010

GRANT PM et al: Risk factor analyses for immune reconstitution inflammatory syndrome in a randomized study of early vs. deferred ART during an opportunistic infection. PLoS One 5:e11416, 2010

GRANT RM et al: Preexposure chemoprophylaxis for HIV prevention in men who have sex with men. N Engl J Med 363:2587, 2010

GRAY RH et al: Male circumcision for HIV prevention in men in Rakai, Uganda: A randomised trial. Lancet 369:657, 2007

——— et al: Probability of HIV-1 transmission per coital act in monogamous, heterosexual, HIV-1-discordant couples in Rakai, Uganda. Lancet 357:1149, 2001

GREENE WC, PETERLIN BM: Charting HIV's remarkable voyage through the cell: Basic science as a passport to future therapy. Nat Med 8:673, 2002

GRULICH AE: Cancer: The effects of HIV and antiretroviral therapy, and implications for early antiretroviral therapy initiation. Curr Opin HIV AIDS 4:183, 2009

GUTIERREZ F et al: Osteonecrosis in patients infected with HIV: Clinical epidemiology and natural history in a large case series from Spain. J AIDS 42:286, 2006

HAASE AT: Targeting early infection to prevent HIV-1 mucosal transmission. Nature 464:217, 2010

———: Perils at mucosal front lines for HIV and SIV and their hosts. Nat Rev Immunol 5:783, 2005

HALL HI et al: Estimation of HIV incidence in the United States. JAMA 300:520, 2008

HO DD et al: Rapid turnover of plasma virions and CD4 lymphocytes in HIV infection. Nature 373:123, 1995

JOINT UNITED NATIONS PROGRAMME ON HIV/AIDS (UNAIDS): Report on the global AIDS epidemic, 2008.

———: AIDS epidemic update, 2009.

KAPLAN JE et al: Guidelines for prevention and treatment of opportunistic infections in HIV-infected adults and adolescents. Recommendations from the CDC, the National Institutes of Health, and the HIV Medicine Association of the Infectious Diseases Society of America. MMWR Recomm Rep 58:1, 2009. Updates available at *www.aidsinfo.nih.gov*

KEELE BF et al: Chimpanzee reservoirs of pandemic and nonpandemic HIV-1. Science 313:523, 2006

KITAHATA MM et al: Effect of early versus deferred antiretroviral therapy for HIV on survival. N Engl J Med 360:1815, 2009

KULLER LH et al: Inflammatory and coagulation biomarkers and mortality in patients with HIV infection. PLoS Med 5:e203, 2008

MALVESTUTTO CD, ABERG JA: Coronary heart disease in people infected with HIV. Cleve Clin J Med 77:547, 2010

MAYER KH, VENKATESH KK: Antiretroviral therapy as HIV prevention: Status and prospects. Am J Public Health 100:1867, 2010

MELLORS JW et al: Prognosis in HIV-1 infection predicted by the quantity of virus in plasma. Science 272:1167, 1996

MIGUELES SA, CONNORS M: Long-term nonprogressive disease among untreated HIV-infected individuals: Clinical implications of understanding immune control of HIV. JAMA 304:194, 2010

MOFENSON LM: Protecting the next generation—eliminating perinatal HIV-1 infection. N Engl J Med 362:2316, 2010

——— et al: Guidelines for the prevention and treatment of opportunistic infections among HIV-exposed and HIV-infected children: Recommendations from CDC, the National Institutes of Health, the HIV Medicine Association of the Infectious Diseases Society of America, the Pediatric Infectious Diseases Society, and the American Academy of Pediatrics. MMWR Recomm Rep 58:1, 2009. Updates available at *aidsinfo.nih.gov*

MOIR S, FAUCI AS: B cells in HIV infection and disease. Nat Rev Immunol 9:235, 2009

MONTANER JS et al: Association of highly active antiretroviral therapy coverage, population viral load, and yearly new HIV diagnoses in British Columbia, Canada: A population-based study. Lancet 376: 532, 2010

NEUHAUS J et al: Markers of inflammation, coagulation, and renal function are elevated in adults with HIV infection. J Infect Dis 201:1788, 2010

Office of National AIDS Policy: National HIV/AIDS Strategy. Washington, DC, Office of National AIDS Policy, 2010. Available at *www.whitehouse.gov/onap*

Padian NS et al: Weighing the gold in the gold standard: Challenges in HIV prevention research. AIDS 24:621, 2010

Panel on Antiretroviral Therapy and Medical Management of HIV-Infected Children: Guidelines for the Use of Antiretroviral Agents in Pediatric HIV Infection. August 16, 2010. Updates available at *aidsinfo.nih.gov*

Panel on Treatment of HIV-Infected Pregnant Women and Prevention of Perinatal Transmission: Recommendations for Use of Antiretroviral Drugs in Pregnant HIV-1-Infected Women for Maternal Health and Interventions to Reduce Perinatal HIV Transmission in the United States, May, 2010. Updates available at *aidsinfo.nih.gov*

Panlilio AL et al: Updated U.S. Public Health Service guidelines for the management of occupational exposures to HIV and recommendations for postexposure prophylaxis. MMWR Recomm Rep 54:1, 2005

Pantaleo G, Fauci AS: HIV infection is active and progressive in lymphoid tissue during the clinically latent stage of disease. Nature 362:355, 1993

Phillips AN et al: The role of HIV in serious diseases other than AIDS. AIDS 22:2409, 2008

Price JC, Thio CL: Liver disease in the human immunodeficiency virus-1-infected individual. Clin Gastroenterol Hepatol 8:1002, 2010

Rerks-Ngarm S et al: Vaccination with ALVAC and AIDSVAX to prevent HIV-1 infection in Thailand. N Engl J Med 361:2209, 2009

Silvestri G et al: Understanding the benign nature of SIV infection in natural hosts. J Clin Invest 11:3148, 2007

Smith DK et al: Antiretroviral postexposure prophylaxis after sexual, injection-drug use, or other nonoccupational exposure to HIV in the United States: Recommendations from the U.S. Department of Health and Human Services. MMWR Recomm Rep. 54:1, 2005

Sterling TR et al: HIV infection-related tuberculosis: Clinical manifestations and treatment. Clin Infect Dis 50:S223, 2010

The Strategies for Management of Antiretroviral Therapy (SMART) Study Group: CD4+ count-guided interruption of antiretroviral treatment. N Engl J Med 355:2283, 2006

Taylor BS et al: The challenge of HIV-1 subtype diversity. N Engl J Med 358:1590, 2008

Thompson MA et al: Antiretroviral treatment of adult HIV infection: 2010 recommendations of the International AIDS Society-USA panel. JAMA 304:321, 2010

Trono D et al: HIV persistence and the prospect of long-term drug-free remissions for HIV-infected individuals. Science 329:174, 2010

U.S. Public Health Service: Updated U.S. Public Health Service Guidelines for the Management of Occupational Exposures to HBV, HCV, and HIV and Recommendations for Postexposure Prophylaxis. MMWR Recomm Rep 50:1, 2001. Updates available at *aidsinfo.nih.gov*

Van Sighem AI et al: Life expectancy of recently diagnosed asymptomatic HIV-infected patients approaches that of uninfected individuals. AIDS 24:1527, 2010

Wawer MJ et al: Rates of HIV-1 transmission per coital act, by stage of HIV-1 infection, in Rakai, Uganda. J Infect Dis 191:1403, 2005

Wei X et al: Viral dynamics in human immunodeficiency virus type 1 infection. Nature 373:117, 1995

World Health Organization (WHO): Antiretroviral drugs for treating pregnant women and preventing HIV infection in infants: Towards universal access. Recommendations for a public health approach, 2010

———: Antiretroviral therapy for HIV infection in adults and adolescents. Recommendations for a public health approach, 2010

———: Antiretroviral therapy for HIV infection in infants and children: Towards universal access. Recommendations for a public health approach, 2010

———: Priority interventions. HIV/AIDS prevention, treatment and care in the health sector, 2010

———, United Nations Children's Fund (UNICEF), UNAIDS: Towards universal access: Scaling up priority HIV/AIDS interventions in the health sector—progress report 2010

Zancanaro PCQ et al: Cutaneous manifestations of HIV in the era of highly active antiretroviral therapy: An institutional urban clinic experience. J Am Acad Dermatol 54:581, 2006

Zhou T et al: Structural basis for broad and potent neutralization of HIV-1 by antibody VRC01. Science 329:811, 2010

Zonios DI et al: Idiopathic CD4+ lymphocytopenia: Natural history and prognostic factors. Blood 112:287, 2010

CHAPTER 189

Human Immunodeficiency Virus Disease: AIDS and Related Disorders

CHAPTER **190**

Viral Gastroenteritis

Umesh D. Parashar
Roger I. Glass

PART 8

Infectious Diseases

Acute infectious gastroenteritis is a common illness that affects persons of all ages worldwide. It is a leading cause of mortality among children in developing countries, accounting for an estimated 1.8 million deaths each year, and is responsible for up to 10–12% of all hospitalizations among children in industrialized countries, including the United States. Elderly persons, especially those with debilitating health conditions, are also at risk of severe complications and death from acute gastroenteritis. Among healthy young adults, acute gastroenteritis is rarely fatal but incurs substantial medical and social costs, including those of time lost from work.

Several enteric viruses have been recognized as important etiologic agents of acute infectious gastroenteritis (Table 190-1, Fig. 190-1). Although most viral gastroenteritis is caused by RNA viruses, the DNA viruses that are occasionally involved (e.g., adenovirus types 40 and 41) are included in this chapter. Illness caused by these viruses is characterized by the acute onset of vomiting and/or diarrhea, which may be accompanied by fever, nausea, abdominal cramps, anorexia, and malaise. As shown in Table 190-2, several features can help distinguish gastroenteritis caused by viruses from that caused by bacterial agents. However, the distinction based on clinical and epidemiologic parameters alone is often difficult, and laboratory tests may be required to confirm the diagnosis.

■ HUMAN CALICIVIRUSES

Etiologic agent

The Norwalk virus is the prototype strain of a group of nonenveloped, small (27–40 nm), round, icosahedral viruses with relatively amorphous surface features on visualization by electron microscopy. These viruses have been difficult to classify because they have not been adapted to cell culture, they often are shed in low titers for only a few days, and no animal models are available. Molecular cloning and characterization have demonstrated that the viruses have a single, positive-strand RNA genome ~7.5 kb in length and that they possess a single virion-associated protein—similar to that of typical caliciviruses—with a molecular mass of 60 kDa. On the basis of these molecular characteristics, these viruses are presently classified in two genera belonging to the family Caliciviridae: the *noroviruses* and the *sapoviruses* (previously called Norwalk-like viruses and Sapporo-like viruses, respectively).

Epidemiology

Infections with the Norwalk and related human caliciviruses are common worldwide, and most adults have antibodies to these viruses. Antibody is acquired at an earlier age in developing countries—a pattern consistent with the presumed fecal-oral mode of transmission. Infections occur year-round, although, in temperate climates, a distinct increase has been noted in cold-weather months. Noroviruses may be the most common infectious agents of mild gastroenteritis in the community and affect all age groups, whereas sapoviruses primarily cause gastroenteritis in children. Noroviruses also cause traveler's diarrhea, and outbreaks have occurred among military personnel deployed to various parts of the world. The limited data available indicate that norovirus may be the second most common viral agent (after rotavirus) among young children and the most common agent among older children and adults. For example, in a comprehensive evaluation of eight enteric pathogens in patients with gastroenteritis in England, three-fourths of patients had at least one pathogen detected in fecal specimens, and noroviruses were the most prevalent, detected in 36% of patients and 18% of healthy controls. Noroviruses are also recognized as the major cause of epidemics of gastroenteritis worldwide. In the United States, >90% of outbreaks of nonbacterial gastroenteritis are caused by noroviruses.

Virus is transmitted predominantly by the fecal-oral route but is also present in vomitus. Because an inoculum with very few viruses can be infectious, transmission can occur by aerosolization, by contact with contaminated fomites, and by person-to-person contact. Viral shedding and infectivity are greatest during the acute illness, but challenge studies with Norwalk virus in volunteers indicate that viral antigen may be shed by asymptomatically infected persons and also by symptomatic persons before the onset of symptoms and for several weeks after the resolution of illness.

TABLE 190-1 Viral Causes of Gastroenteritis Among Humans

Virus	Family	Genome	Primary Age Group at Risk	Clinical Severity	Detection Assays
Group A rotavirus	Reoviridae	Double-strand segmented RNA	Children <5 years	+++	EM, EIA (commercial), PAGE, RT-PCR
Norovirus	Caliciviridae	Positive-sense single-strand RNA	All ages	++	EM, EIA, RT-PCR
Sapovirus	Caliciviridae	Positive-sense single-strand RNA	Children <5 years	+	EM, EIA, RT-PCR
Astrovirus	Astroviridae	Positive-sense single-strand RNA	Children <5 years	+	EM, EIA, RT-PCR
Adenovirus (types 40 and 41)	Adenoviridae	Double-strand DNA	Children <5 years	+/++	EM, EIA (commercial), PCR

Abbreviations: EIA, enzyme immunoassay; EM, electron microscopy; PAGE, polyacrylamide gel electrophoresis; PCR, polymerase chain reaction; RT-PCR, reverse-transcription PCR.

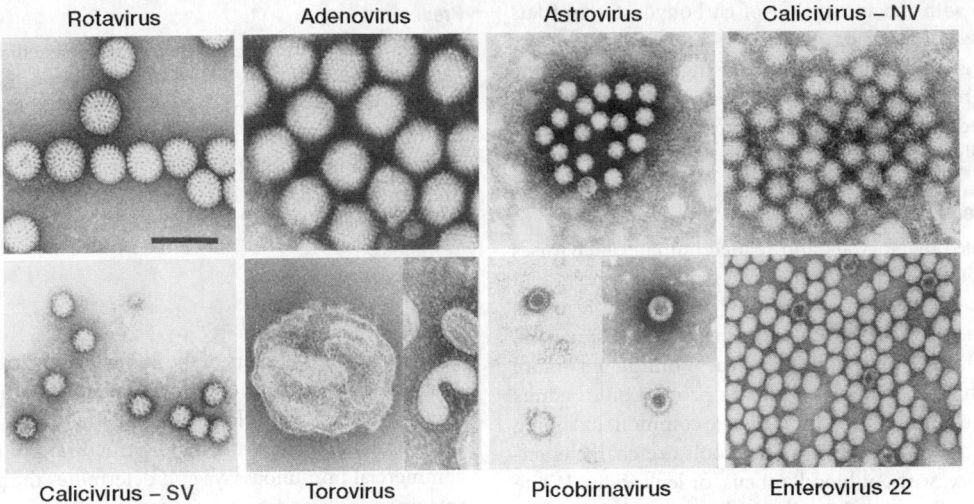

Figure 190-1 Viral agents of gastroenteritis. NV, norovirus; SV, sapovirus.

Pathogenesis

The exact sites and cellular receptors for attachment of viral particles have not been determined. Data suggest that carbohydrates that are similar to human histo-blood group antigens and are present on the gastroduodenal epithelium of individuals with the secretor phenotype may serve as ligands for the attachment of Norwalk virus. Additional studies must more fully elucidate norovirus-carbohydrate interactions, including potential strain-specific variations. After the infection of volunteers, reversible lesions are noted in the upper jejunum, with broadening and blunting of the villi, shortening of the microvilli, vacuolization of the lining epithelium, crypt hyperplasia, and infiltration of the lamina propria by polymorphonuclear neutrophils and lymphocytes. The lesions persist for at least 4 days after the resolution of symptoms

TABLE 190-2 Characteristics of Gastroenteritis Caused by Viral and Bacterial Agents

Feature	Viral Gastroenteritis	Bacterial Gastroenteritis
Setting	Incidence similar in developing and developed countries	More common in settings with poor hygiene and sanitation
Infectious dose	Low (10–100 viral particles) for most agents	High (>10^5 bacteria) for *Escherichia coli, Salmonella, Vibrio;* medium (10^2–10^5 bacteria) for *Campylobacter jejuni;* low (10–100 bacteria) for *Shigella*
Seasonality	In temperate climates, winter seasonality for most agents; year-round occurrence in tropical areas	More common in summer or rainy months, particularly in developing countries with a high disease burden
Incubation period	1–3 days for most agents; can be shorter for norovirus	1–7 days for common agents (e.g., *Campylobacter, E. coli, Shigella, Salmonella);* a few hours for bacteria producing preformed toxins (e.g., *Staphylococcus aureus, Bacillus cereus*)
Reservoir	Primarily humans	Depending on species, human (e.g., *Shigella, Salmonella*), animal (e.g., *Campylobacter, Salmonella, E. coli*), and water (e.g., *Vibrio*) reservoirs exist.
Fever	Common with rotavirus and norovirus; uncommon with other agents	Common with agents causing inflammatory diarrhea (e.g., *Salmonella, Shigella*)
Vomiting	Prominent and can be the only presenting feature, especially in children	Common with bacteria producing preformed toxins; less prominent in diarrhea due to other agents
Diarrhea	Common; nonbloody in almost all cases	Prominent and frequently bloody with agents causing inflammatory diarrhea
Duration	1–3 days for norovirus and sapovirus; 2–8 days for other viruses	1–2 days for bacteria producing preformed toxins; 2–8 days for most other bacteria
Diagnosis	This is often a diagnosis of exclusion in clinical practice. Commercial enzyme immunoassays are available for detection of rotavirus and adenovirus, but identification of other agents is limited to research and public health laboratories.	Fecal examination for leukocytes and blood is helpful in differential diagnosis. Culture of stool specimens, sometimes on special media, can identify several pathogens. Molecular techniques are useful epidemiologic tools but are not routinely used in most laboratories.
Treatment	Supportive therapy to maintain adequate hydration and nutrition should be given. Antibiotics and antimotility agents are contraindicated.	Supportive hydration therapy is adequate for most patients. Antibiotics are recommended for patients with dysentery caused by *Shigella* or *Vibrio cholerae* and for some patients with *Clostridium difficile* colitis.

and are associated with malabsorption of carbohydrates and fats and a decreased level of brush-border enzymes. Adenylate cyclase activity is not altered. No histopathologic changes are seen in the stomach or colon, but gastric motor function is delayed, and this alteration is believed to contribute to the nausea and vomiting that are typical of this illness.

Clinical manifestations

Gastroenteritis caused by Norwalk and related human caliciviruses has a sudden onset, following an average incubation period of 24 h (range, 12–72 h). The illness generally lasts 12–60 h and is characterized by one or more of the following symptoms: nausea, vomiting, abdominal cramps, and diarrhea. Vomiting is more prevalent among children, whereas a greater proportion of adults develop diarrhea. Constitutional symptoms are common, including headache, fever, chills, and myalgias. The stools are characteristically loose and watery, without blood, mucus, or leukocytes. White cell counts are generally normal; rarely, leukocytosis with relative lymphopenia may be observed. Death is a rare outcome and usually results from severe dehydration in vulnerable persons (e.g., elderly patients with debilitating health conditions).

Immunity

Approximately 50% of persons challenged with Norwalk virus become ill and acquire short-term immunity against the infecting strain. Immunity to Norwalk virus appears to correlate inversely with level of antibody; i.e., persons with higher levels of preexisting antibody to Norwalk virus are more susceptible to illness. This observation suggests that some individuals have a genetic predisposition to illness. Specific ABO, Lewis, and secretor blood group phenotypes may influence susceptibility to norovirus infection.

Diagnosis

Cloning and sequencing of the genomes of Norwalk and several other human caliciviruses have allowed the development of assays based on polymerase chain reaction (PCR) for detection of virus in stool and vomitus. Virus-like particles produced by expression of capsid proteins in a recombinant baculovirus vector have been used to develop enzyme immunoassays (EIAs) for detection of virus in stool or a serologic response to a specific viral antigen. These newer diagnostic techniques are considerably more sensitive than previous detection methods, such as electron microscopy, immune electron microscopy, and EIAs based on reagents derived from humans. However, no currently available single assay can detect all human caliciviruses because of their great genetic and antigenic diversity. In addition, the assays are still cumbersome and are available primarily in research laboratories, although they are increasingly being adopted by public health laboratories for routine screening of fecal specimens from patients affected by outbreaks of gastroenteritis. Commercial EIA kits, which are available in some European countries and in Japan but not yet in the United States, have limited sensitivity and usefulness in clinical practice and are of greatest utility in outbreaks, in which many specimens are tested and only a few need be positive to identify norovirus as the cause.

TREATMENT	Infections with Norwalk and Related Human Caliciviruses

The disease is self-limited, and oral rehydration therapy is generally adequate. If severe dehydration develops, IV fluid therapy is indicated. No specific antiviral therapy is available.

Prevention

Epidemic prevention relies on situation-specific measures, such as control of contamination of food and water, exclusion of ill food handlers, and reduction of person-to-person spread through good personal hygiene and disinfection of contaminated fomites. The role of immunoprophylaxis is not clear, given the lack of long-term immunity from natural disease, but efforts to develop norovirus vaccines are ongoing.

■ ROTAVIRUS

Etiologic agent

Rotaviruses are members of the family Reoviridae. The viral genome consists of 11 segments of double-strand RNA that are enclosed in a triple-layered, nonenveloped, icosahedral capsid 75 nm in diameter. Viral protein 6 (VP6), the major structural protein, is the target of commercial immunoassays and determines the group specificity of rotaviruses. There are seven major groups of rotavirus (A through G); human illness is caused primarily by group A and, to a much lesser extent, by groups B and C. Two outer-capsid proteins, VP7 (G-protein) and VP4 (P-protein), determine serotype specificity, induce neutralizing antibodies, and form the basis for binary classification of rotaviruses (G and P types). The segmented genome of rotavirus allows genetic reassortment (i.e., exchange of genome segments between viruses) during co-infection—a property that may play a role in viral evolution and has been utilized in the development of reassortant animal-human rotavirus–based vaccines.

Epidemiology

Worldwide, nearly all children are infected with rotavirus by 3–5 years of age. Neonatal infections are common but are often asymptomatic or mild, presumably because of protection from maternal antibody or breast-feeding. First infections after 3 months of age are likely to be symptomatic, and the incidence of disease peaks among children 4–23 months of age. Reinfections are common, but the severity of disease decreases with each repeat infection. Therefore, severe rotavirus infections are relatively uncommon among older children and adults. Nevertheless, rotavirus can cause illness in parents and caretakers of children with rotavirus diarrhea, immunocompromised persons, travelers, and elderly individuals and should be considered in the differential diagnosis of gastroenteritis among adults.

In tropical settings, rotavirus disease occurs year-round, with less pronounced seasonal peaks than in temperate settings, where rotavirus disease occurs predominantly during the cooler fall and winter months. Before the introduction of rotavirus vaccine in the United States, the rotavirus season each year began in the Southwest during the autumn and early winter (October through December) and migrated across the continent, peaking in the Northeast during late winter and spring (March through May). The reasons for this characteristic pattern are not clear, but a recent study suggested a correlation with state-specific differences in birth rates, which could influence the rate of accumulation of susceptible infants after each rotavirus season. After the implementation of routine vaccination of U.S. infants against rotavirus in 2006, the onset of the 2007–2008 and 2008–2009 rotavirus seasons was delayed by 11 weeks and 6 weeks, respectively, and the seasons were shorter, lasting 14 and 17 weeks, respectively, in comparison with a median of 26 weeks in 2000–2006 (Fig. 190-2). These changes in seasonal patterns of rotavirus activity were accompanied by declines in the number of detections of rotavirus by 64% and 60% in 2007–2008 and 2008–2009, respectively, from the figures for 2000–2006, as collected by a national network of sentinel laboratories.

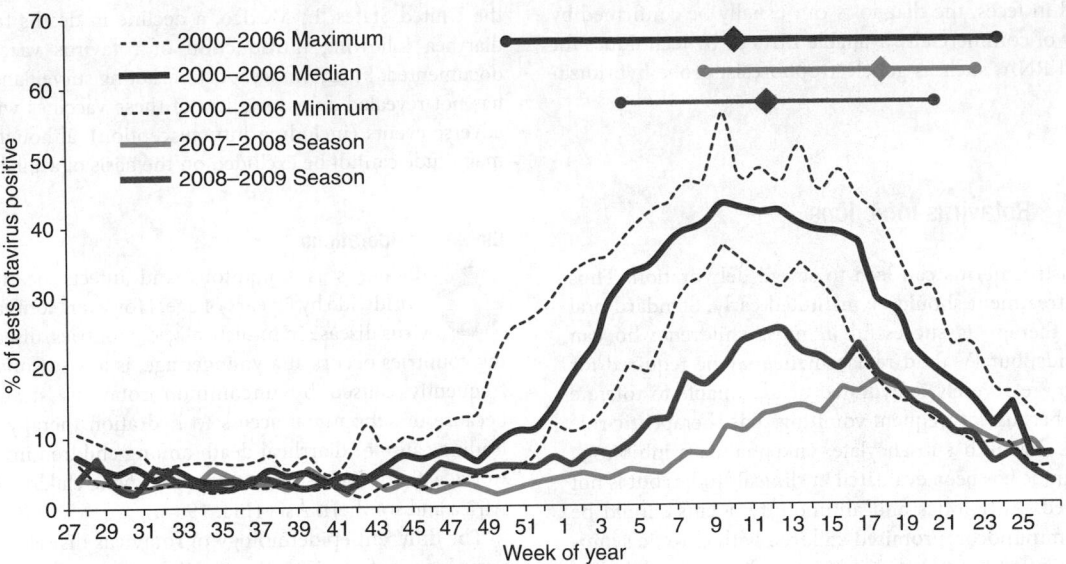

Figure 190-2 The maximal or minimal percentage of rotavirus-positive tests for 2000–2006 may have occurred during any of the six baseline seasons. The onset of rotavirus season was defined as the first of two consecutive weeks during which the percentage of stool specimens testing positive for rotavirus was ≥10%, and the end of the season was defined as the last of two consecutive weeks during which the percentage of stool specimens testing positive for rotavirus was ≥10%. At the top right, the dots bracket the rotavirus season from onset to end, and the diamond indicates the peak week during each period. (*Adapted from Centers for Disease Control and Prevention, 2009.*)

During episodes of rotavirus-associated diarrhea, virus is shed in large quantities in stool (10^7–10^{12}/g). Viral shedding detectable by EIA usually subsides within 1 week but may persist for >30 days in immunocompromised individuals. Viral shedding may be detected for longer periods by sensitive molecular assays, such as PCR. The virus is transmitted predominantly through the fecal-oral route. Spread through respiratory secretions, person-to-person contact, or contaminated environmental surfaces has also been postulated to explain the rapid acquisition of antibody in the first 3 years of life, regardless of sanitary conditions.

At least 10 different G serotypes of group A rotavirus have been identified in humans, but only five types (G1 through G4 and G9) are common. While human rotavirus strains that possess a high degree of genetic homology with animal strains have been identified, animal-to-human transmission appears to be uncommon.

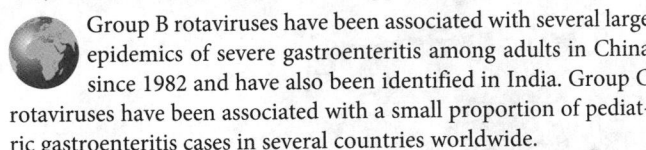 Group B rotaviruses have been associated with several large epidemics of severe gastroenteritis among adults in China since 1982 and have also been identified in India. Group C rotaviruses have been associated with a small proportion of pediatric gastroenteritis cases in several countries worldwide.

Pathogenesis

Rotaviruses infect and ultimately destroy mature enterocytes in the villous epithelium of the proximal small intestine. The loss of absorptive villous epithelium, coupled with the proliferation of secretory crypt cells, results in secretory diarrhea. Brush-border enzymes characteristic of differentiated cells are reduced, and this change leads to the accumulation of unmetabolized disaccharides and consequent osmotic diarrhea. Studies in mice indicate that a nonstructural rotavirus protein, NSP4, functions as an enterotoxin and contributes to secretory diarrhea by altering epithelial cell function and permeability. In addition, rotavirus may evoke fluid secretion through activation of the enteric nervous system in the intestinal wall. Recent data indicate that rotavirus antigenemia and viremia are common among children with acute rotavirus infection, although the antigen and RNA levels in serum are substantially lower than those in stool.

Clinical manifestations

The clinical spectrum of rotavirus infection ranges from subclinical infection to severe gastroenteritis leading to life-threatening dehydration. After an incubation period of 1–3 days, the illness has an abrupt onset, with vomiting frequently preceding the onset of diarrhea. Up to one-third of patients may have a temperature of >39°C. The stools are characteristically loose and watery and only infrequently contain red or white cells. Gastrointestinal symptoms generally resolve in 3–7 days.

Respiratory and neurologic features in children with rotavirus infection have been reported, but causal associations have not been proven. Moreover, rotavirus infection has been associated with a variety of other clinical conditions (e.g., sudden infant death syndrome, necrotizing enterocolitis, intussusception, Kawasaki's disease, and type 1 diabetes), but no causal relationship has been confirmed with any of these syndromes.

Rotavirus does not appear to be a major opportunistic pathogen in children with HIV infection. In severely immunodeficient children, rotavirus can cause protracted diarrhea with prolonged viral excretion and, in rare instances, can disseminate systemically. Persons who are immunosuppressed for bone marrow transplantation are also at risk for severe or even fatal rotavirus disease.

Immunity

Protection against rotavirus disease is correlated with the presence of virus-specific secretory IgA antibodies in the intestine and, to some extent, the serum. Because virus-specific IgA production at the intestinal surface is short lived, complete protection against disease is only temporary. However, each infection and subsequent reinfection confers progressively greater immunity; thus severe disease is most common among young children with first or second infections. Immunologic memory is believed to be important in the attenuation of disease severity upon reinfection.

Diagnosis

Illness caused by rotavirus is difficult to distinguish clinically from that caused by other enteric viruses. Because large quantities of virus are shed in feces, the diagnosis can usually be confirmed by a wide variety of commercially available EIAs or by techniques for detecting viral RNA, such as gel electrophoresis, probe hybridization, or PCR.

TREATMENT Rotavirus Infections

Rotavirus gastroenteritis can lead to severe dehydration. Thus appropriate treatment should be instituted early. Standard oral rehydration therapy is successful in most children who can take oral fluids, but IV fluid replacement may be required for patients who are severely dehydrated or are unable to tolerate oral therapy because of frequent vomiting. The therapeutic role of probiotics, bismuth subsalicylate, enkephalinase inhibitors, and nitazoxanide has been evaluated in clinical studies but is not clearly defined. Antibiotics and antimotility agents should be avoided. In immunocompromised children with chronic symptomatic rotavirus disease, orally administered immunoglobulins or colostrum may result in the resolution of symptoms, but the best choices regarding agents and their doses have not been well studied, and treatment decisions are often empirical.

Prevention

Efforts to develop rotavirus vaccines were pursued because it was apparent—given the similar rates in less-developed and industrialized nations—that improvements in hygiene and sanitation were unlikely to reduce disease incidence. The first rotavirus vaccine licensed in the United States in 1998 was withdrawn from the market within 1 year because it was linked with intussusception, a severe bowel obstruction.

In 2006, promising safety and efficacy results for two new rotavirus vaccines were reported from large clinical trials conducted in North America, Europe, and Latin America. Both vaccines are now recommended for routine immunization of all U.S. infants, and their use has rapidly led to a decline in rotavirus hospitalizations and emergency department visits at hospitals across the United States. In Mexico, a decline in deaths from childhood diarrhea following introduction of rotavirus vaccines has been documented. Furthermore, postmarketing surveillance information has not revealed an association of these vaccines with any serious adverse events (including intussusception), although a risk of low magnitude cannot be excluded on the basis of available data.

Global considerations

Rotavirus is ubiquitous and infects nearly all children worldwide by 5 years of age. However, compared with rotavirus disease in industrialized countries, disease in developing countries occurs at a younger age, is less seasonal, and is more frequently caused by uncommon rotavirus strains. Moreover, because of suboptimal access to hydration therapy, rotavirus is a leading cause of diarrheal death among children in the developing world, with the highest mortality rates among children in sub-Saharan Africa and southern Asia (Fig. 190-3).

The different epidemiology of rotavirus disease and the greater prevalence of co-infection with other enteric pathogens, of comorbidities, and of malnutrition in developing countries may adversely affect the performance of oral rotavirus vaccines, as is the case with oral vaccines against poliomyelitis, cholera, and typhoid in these regions. Therefore, evaluation of the efficacy of rotavirus vaccines in resource-poor settings of Africa and Asia was specifically recommended, and these trials have now been completed. As anticipated, the efficacy of rotavirus vaccines was moderate (50–75%) in these settings when compared with that in industrialized countries. Nevertheless, even a moderately efficacious rotavirus vaccine would be likely to have substantial public health benefits in these areas with a high disease burden. Given these considerations, in April 2009 the World Health Organization recommended the use of rotavirus vaccines in all countries worldwide.

■ OTHER VIRAL AGENTS OF GASTROENTERITIS

Enteric *adenoviruses* of serotypes 40 and 41 belonging to subgroup F are 70- to 80-nm viruses with double-strand DNA that cause ~2–12%

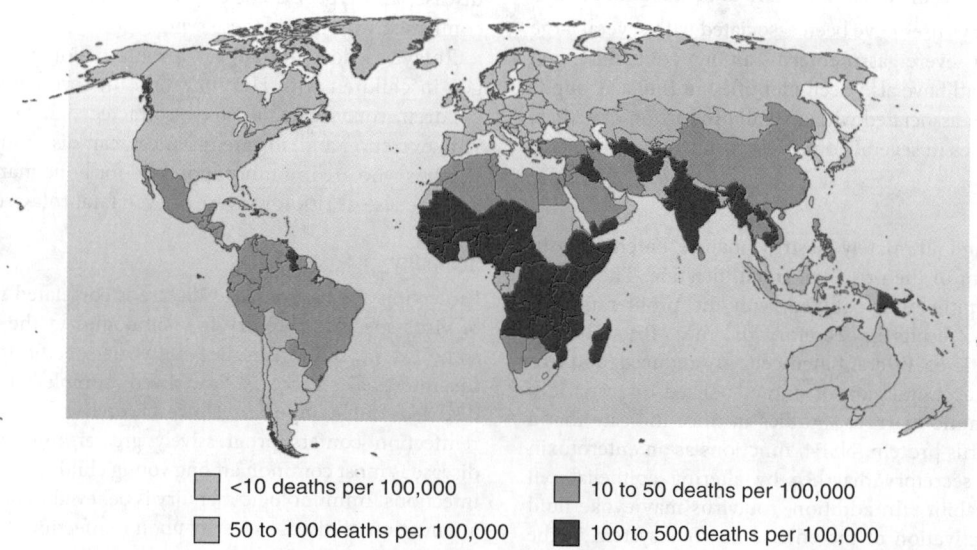

Figure 190-3 Rotavirus mortality rates by country, per 100,000 children <5 years of age. *(Reproduced with permission from UD Parashar et al: J Infect Dis 200:S9, 2009.)*

□ <10 deaths per 100,000   □ 10 to 50 deaths per 100,000
□ 50 to 100 deaths per 100,000   ■ 100 to 500 deaths per 100,000

of all diarrhea episodes in young children. Unlike adenoviruses that cause respiratory illness, enteric adenoviruses are difficult to cultivate in cell lines, but they can be detected with commercially available EIAs.

Astroviruses, 28- to 30-nm viruses with a characteristic icosahedral structure, contain a positive-sense, single-strand RNA. At least seven serotypes have been identified, of which serotype 1 is most common. Astroviruses are primarily pediatric pathogens, causing ~2–10% of cases of mild to moderate gastroenteritis in children. The availability of simple immunoassays to detect virus in fecal specimens and of molecular methods to confirm and characterize strains will permit more comprehensive assessment of the etiologic role of these agents.

Toroviruses are 100- to 140-nm, enveloped, positive-strand RNA viruses that are recognized as causes of gastroenteritis in horses (Berne virus) and cattle (Breda virus). Their role as a cause of diarrhea in humans is still unclear, but studies from Canada have demonstrated associations between torovirus excretion and both nosocomial gastroenteritis and necrotizing enterocolitis in neonates. These associations require further evaluation.

Picobirnaviruses are small, bisegmented, double-strand RNA viruses that cause gastroenteritis in a variety of animals. Their role as primary causes of gastroenteritis in humans remains unclear, but several studies have found an association between picobirnaviruses and gastroenteritis in HIV-infected adults.

Several other viruses (e.g., enteroviruses, reoviruses, pestiviruses, and parvovirus B) have been identified in the feces of patients with diarrhea, but their etiologic role in gastroenteritis has not been proven. Diarrhea has also been noted as a manifestation of infection with recently recognized viruses that primarily cause severe respiratory illness: the severe acute respiratory syndrome–associated coronavirus (SARS-CoV), influenza A/H5N1 virus, and the current pandemic strain of influenza A/H1N1 virus.

FURTHER READINGS

AMAR CF et al: Detection by PCR of eight groups of enteric pathogens in 4,627 fecal specimens: Re-examination of the English case-control Infectious Intestinal Disease Study (1993–1996). Eur J Clin Microbiol Infect Dis 26:311, 2007

CENTERS FOR DISEASE CONTROL AND PREVENTION: Reduction in rotavirus after vaccine introduction—United States, 2000–2009. MMWR Morb Mortal Wkly Rep 58:1146, 2009

CURNS AT et al: Reduction in acute gastroenteritis hospitalizations among U.S. children after introduction of rotavirus vaccine: Analysis of hospital discharge data from 18 U.S. states. J Infect Dis 201:1617, 2010

GLASS RI et al: Norovirus gastroenteritis. N Engl J Med 361:1776, 2009

MADHI SA et al: Effect of human rotavirus vaccine on severe diarrhea in African infants. N Engl J Med 362:289, 2010

PATEL MM et al: Systematic literature review of role of noroviruses in sporadic gastroenteritis. Emerg Infect Dis 14:1224, 2008

RICHARDSON V et al: Effect of rotavirus vaccination on death from childhood diarrhea in Mexico. N Engl J Med 362:299, 2010

PITZER VE et al: Demographic variability, vaccination, and the spatiotemporal dynamics of rotavirus epidemics. Science 325:274, 2009

RUIZ-PALACIOS G et al: Safety and efficacy of an attenuated vaccine against severe rotavirus gastroenteritis. N Engl J Med 354:11, 2006

VESIKARI T et al: Safety and efficacy of a pentavalent human-bovine (WC3) reassortant rotavirus vaccine. N Engl J Med 354:23, 2006

CHAPTER 191

Enteroviruses and Reoviruses

Jeffrey I. Cohen

ENTEROVIRUSES

◼ CLASSIFICATION AND CHARACTERIZATION

Enteroviruses are so named because of their ability to multiply in the gastrointestinal tract. Despite their name, these viruses are not a prominent cause of gastroenteritis. Enteroviruses encompass 96 human serotypes: 3 serotypes of poliovirus, 21 serotypes of coxsackievirus A, 6 serotypes of coxsackievirus B, 28 serotypes of echovirus, enteroviruses 68–71, and 34 new enteroviruses (beginning with enterovirus 73) that have been identified by molecular techniques. Echoviruses 22 and 23 have been reclassified as parechoviruses 1 and 2; 12 additional human parechoviruses have been identified. These viruses cause disease similar to that caused by echoviruses. Enterovirus surveillance conducted in the United States by the Centers for Disease Control and Prevention (CDC) in 2007–2008 showed that the most common serotype, coxsackievirus B1, was followed in frequency by echoviruses 18, 9, and 6; together, these four viruses accounted for 52% of all isolates.

Human enteroviruses contain a single-stranded RNA genome surrounded by an icosahedral capsid comprising four viral proteins. These viruses have no lipid envelope and are stable in acidic environments, including the stomach. They are susceptible to chlorine-containing cleansers but resistant to inactivation by standard disinfectants (e.g., alcohol, detergents) and can persist for days at room temperature.

◼ PATHOGENESIS AND IMMUNITY

Much of what is known about the pathogenesis of enteroviruses has been derived from studies of poliovirus infection. After ingestion, poliovirus is thought to infect epithelial cells in the mucosa of the gastrointestinal tract and then to spread to and replicate in the submucosal lymphoid tissue of the tonsils and Peyer's patches. The virus next spreads to the regional lymph nodes, a viremic phase ensues, and the virus replicates in organs of the reticuloendothelial system. In some cases, a second viremia occurs and the virus replicates further in various tissues, sometimes causing symptomatic disease.

It is uncertain whether poliovirus reaches the central nervous system (CNS) during viremia or whether it also spreads via peripheral nerves. Since viremia precedes the onset of neurologic disease in humans, it has been assumed that the virus enters the CNS via the bloodstream. The poliovirus receptor is a member of the immunoglobulin superfamily. Poliovirus infection is limited to primates, largely because their cells express the viral receptor. Studies demonstrating the poliovirus receptor in the end-plate region of muscle at the neuromuscular junction suggest that, if the virus enters the muscle during viremia, it could travel across the neuromuscular junction up the axon to the anterior horn cells. Studies of monkeys and of transgenic mice expressing the poliovirus receptor show that, after IM injection, poliovirus does not reach the spinal cord if the sciatic nerve is cut. Taken together, these findings suggest that poliovirus can spread directly from muscle to the CNS by neural pathways. Intercellular adhesion molecule 1 (ICAM-1) is a receptor for coxsackieviruses A13, A18, and A21; CAR for coxsackievirus B; VLA-2 integrin for echovirus types 1 and 8; CD55 for enterovirus 70 and some serotypes of coxsackievirus A and B and echovirus; and P-selectin glycoprotein ligand-1 and scavenger receptor B2 for enterovirus 71.

Poliovirus can usually be cultured from the blood 3–5 days after infection, before the development of neutralizing antibodies. While viral replication at secondary sites begins to slow 1 week after infection, it continues in the gastrointestinal tract. Poliovirus is shed from the oropharynx for up to 3 weeks after infection and from the gastrointestinal tract for as long as 12 weeks; hypogammaglobulinemic patients can shed poliovirus for >20 years. During replication in the gastrointestinal tract, attenuated oral poliovirus can mutate, reverting to a more neurovirulent phenotype within a few days; however, additional mutations are probably required for full neurovirulence.

Humoral and secretory immunity in the gastrointestinal tract is important for the control of enterovirus infections. Enteroviruses induce specific IgM, which usually persists for <6 months, and specific IgG, which persists for life. Capsid protein VP1 is the predominant target of neutralizing antibody, which generally confers lifelong protection against subsequent disease caused by the same serotype but does not prevent infection or virus shedding. Enteroviruses also induce cellular immunity whose significance is uncertain. Patients with impaired cellular immunity are not known to develop unusually severe disease when infected with enteroviruses. In contrast, the severe infections in patients with agammaglobulinemia emphasize the importance of humoral immunity in controlling enterovirus infections. Disseminated enterovirus infections have occurred in hematopoietic cell transplant recipients. IgA antibodies are instrumental in reducing poliovirus replication in and shedding from the gastrointestinal tract. Breast milk contains IgA specific for enteroviruses and can protect humans from infection.

■ EPIDEMIOLOGY

Enteroviruses have a worldwide distribution. More than 50% of nonpoliovirus enterovirus infections and more than 90% of poliovirus infections are subclinical. When symptoms do develop, they are usually nonspecific and occur in conjunction with fever; only a minority of infections are associated with specific clinical syndromes. The incubation period for most enterovirus infections ranges from 2 to 14 days but usually is <1 week.

Enterovirus infection is more common in socioeconomically disadvantaged areas, especially in those where conditions are crowded and in tropical areas where hygiene is poor. Infection is most common among infants and young children; serious illness develops most often during the first few days of life and in older children and adults. In developing countries, where children are infected at an early age, poliovirus infection has less often been associated with paralysis; in countries with better hygiene, older children and adults are more likely to be seronegative, become infected, and develop paralysis. Passively acquired maternal antibody reduces the risk of symptomatic infection in neonates. Young children are the most frequent shedders of enteroviruses and are usually the index cases in family outbreaks. In temperate climates, enterovirus infections occur most often in the summer and fall; no seasonal pattern is apparent in the tropics.

Most enteroviruses are transmitted primarily by the fecal-oral or oral-oral route. Patients are most infectious shortly before and after the onset of symptomatic disease, when virus is present in the stool and throat. The ingestion of virus-contaminated food or water can also cause disease. Certain enteroviruses (such as enterovirus 70, which causes acute hemorrhagic conjunctivitis) can be transmitted by direct inoculation from the fingers to the eye. Airborne transmission is important for some viruses that cause respiratory tract disease, such as coxsackievirus A21. Enteroviruses can be transmitted across the placenta from mother to fetus, causing severe disease in the newborn. The transmission of enteroviruses through blood transfusions or insect bites has not been documented. Nosocomial spread of coxsackievirus and echovirus has taken place in hospital nurseries.

■ CLINICAL FEATURES

Poliovirus infection

Most infections with poliovirus are asymptomatic. After an incubation period of 3–6 days, ~5% of patients present with a minor illness (abortive poliomyelitis) manifested by fever, malaise, sore throat, anorexia, myalgias, and headache. This condition usually resolves in 3 days. About 1% of patients present with aseptic meningitis (nonparalytic poliomyelitis). Examination of cerebrospinal fluid (CSF) reveals lymphocytic pleocytosis, a normal glucose level, and a normal or slightly elevated protein level; CSF polymorphonuclear leukocytes may be present early. In some patients, especially children, malaise and fever precede the onset of aseptic meningitis.

Paralytic poliomyelitis The least common presentation is that of paralytic disease. After one or several days, signs of aseptic meningitis are followed by severe back, neck, and muscle pain and by the rapid or gradual development of motor weakness. In some cases the disease appears to be biphasic, with aseptic meningitis followed first by apparent recovery but then (1–2 days later) by the return of fever and the development of paralysis; this form is more common among children than among adults. Weakness is generally asymmetric, is proximal more than distal, and may involve the legs (most commonly); the arms; or the abdominal, thoracic, or bulbar muscles. Paralysis develops during the febrile phase of the illness and usually does not progress after defervescence. Urinary retention may also occur. Examination reveals weakness, fasciculations, decreased muscle tone, and reduced or absent reflexes in affected areas. Transient hyperreflexia sometimes precedes the loss of reflexes. Patients frequently report sensory symptoms, but objective sensory testing usually yields normal results. Bulbar paralysis may lead to dysphagia, difficulty in handling secretions, or dysphonia. Respiratory insufficiency due to aspiration, involvement of the respiratory center in the medulla, or paralysis of the phrenic or intercostal nerves may develop, and severe medullary involvement may lead to circulatory collapse. Most patients with paralysis recover some function weeks to months after infection. About two-thirds of patients have residual neurologic sequelae.

Paralytic disease is more common among older individuals, pregnant women, and persons exercising strenuously or undergoing trauma at the time of CNS symptoms. Tonsillectomy predisposes to bulbar poliomyelitis, and IM injections increase the risk of paralysis in the involved limb(s).

Vaccine-associated poliomyelitis Until recently, poliomyelitis due to live poliovirus vaccine occurred in the United States. The risk of developing poliomyelitis after oral vaccination is estimated at 1 case per 2.5 million doses. The risk is ~2000 times higher among immunodeficient persons, especially in persons with hypo- or agammaglobulinemia. Before 1997, an average of eight cases of vaccine-associated poliomyelitis occurred—in both vaccinees and their contacts—in the United States each year. With the change in recommendations first to a sequential regimen of inactivated poliovirus vaccine (IPV) and oral poliovirus vaccine (OPV) in 1997 and then to an all-IPV regimen in 2000, the number of cases of vaccine-associated polio declined. From 1997 to 1999, six such cases were reported in the United States; no cases have been reported since 1999.

Postpolio syndrome The *postpolio syndrome* presents as a new onset of weakness, fatigue, fasciculations, and pain with additional atrophy of the muscle group involved during the initial paralytic disease 20–40 years earlier. The syndrome is more common among women and with increasing time after acute disease. The onset is usually insidious, and weakness occasionally extends to muscles that were not involved during the initial illness. The prognosis is generally good; progression to further weakness is usually slow, with plateau periods of 1–10 years. The postpolio syndrome is thought to be due to progressive dysfunction and loss of motor neurons that compensated for the neurons lost during the original infection and not to persistent or reactivated poliovirus infection.

Other enteroviruses

An estimated 5–10 million cases of symptomatic disease due to enteroviruses other than poliovirus occur in the United States each year. Among neonates, enteroviruses are the most common cause of aseptic meningitis and nonspecific febrile illnesses. Certain clinical syndromes are more likely to be caused by certain serotypes (Table 191-1).

Nonspecific febrile illness (summer grippe) The most common clinical manifestation of enterovirus infection is a nonspecific febrile illness. After an incubation period of 3–6 days, patients present with an acute onset of fever, malaise, and headache. Occasional cases are associated with upper respiratory symptoms, and some cases include nausea and vomiting. Symptoms often last for 3–4 days, and most cases resolve in a week. While infections with other respiratory viruses occur more often from late fall to early spring, enterovirus febrile illness frequently occurs in the summer and early fall.

Generalized disease of the newborn Most serious enterovirus infections in infants develop during the first week of life, although severe disease can occur up to 3 months of age. Neonates often present with an illness resembling bacterial sepsis, with fever, irritability, and lethargy. Laboratory abnormalities include leukocytosis with a left shift, thrombocytopenia, elevated values in liver function tests, and CSF pleocytosis. The illness can be complicated by myocarditis and hypotension, fulminant hepatitis and disseminated intravascular coagulation, meningitis or meningoencephalitis, or pneumonia. It may be difficult to distinguish neonatal enterovirus infection from bacterial sepsis, although a history of a recent virus-like illness in the mother provides a clue.

Aseptic meningitis and encephalitis In children and young adults, enteroviruses are the cause of up to 90% of cases of aseptic meningitis in which an etiologic agent can be identified. Patients with aseptic meningitis typically present with an acute onset of fever, chills, headache, photophobia, and pain on eye movement. Nausea and vomiting are also common. Examination reveals meningismus without localizing neurologic signs; drowsiness or irritability may

TABLE 191-1 Manifestations Commonly Associated With Enterovirus Serotypes

Manifestation	Serotype(s) of Indicated Virus	
	Coxsackievirus	Echovirus (E) and Enterovirus (Ent)
Acute hemorrhagic conjunctivitis	A24	E70
Aseptic meningitis	A2, 4, 7, 9, 10; B1–5	E4, 6, 7, 9, 11, 13, 16, 18, 19, 30, 33; Ent70, 71
Encephalitis	A9; B1–5	E3, 4, 6, 7, 9, 11, 18, 25, 30; Ent71
Exanthem	A4, 5, 9, 10, 16; B1, 3–5	E4–7, 9, 11, 16–19, 25, 30; Ent71
Generalized disease of the newborn	B1–5	E4–6, 7, 9, 11, 14, 16, 18, 19
Hand-foot-and-mouth disease	A5, 7, 9, 10, 16; B1, 2, 5	Ent71
Herpangina	A1–10, 16, 22; B1–5	E6, 9, 11, 16, 17, 25, 30; Ent71
Myocarditis, pericarditis	A4, 9, 16; B1–5	E6, 9, 11, 22
Paralysis	A4, 7, 9; B1–5	E2–4, 6, 7, 9, 11, 18, 30; Ent70, 71
Pleurodynia	A1, 2, 4, 6, 9, 10, 16; B1–6	E1–3, 6, 7, 9, 11, 12, 14, 16, 19, 24, 25, 30
Pneumonia	A9, 16; B1–5	E6, 7, 9, 11, 12, 19, 20, 30; Ent68, 71

also be apparent. In some cases, a febrile illness may be reported that remits but returns several days later in conjunction with signs of meningitis. Other systemic manifestations may provide clues to an enteroviral cause, including diarrhea, myalgias, rash, pleurodynia, myocarditis, and herpangina. Examination of the CSF invariably reveals pleocytosis; the CSF cell count shows a shift from neutrophil to lymphocyte predominance within 1 day of presentation, and the total cell count does not exceed 1000/μL. The CSF glucose level is usually normal (in contrast to the low CSF glucose level in mumps) with a normal or slightly elevated protein concentration. Partially treated bacterial meningitis may be particularly difficult to exclude in some instances. Enteroviral meningitis is more frequent in summer and fall in temperate climates, while viral meningitis of other etiologies is more common in winter and spring. Symptoms ordinarily resolve within a week, although CSF abnormalities can persist for several weeks. Enteroviral meningitis is often more severe in adults than in children. Neurologic sequelae are rare, and most patients have an excellent prognosis.

Enteroviral encephalitis is much less common than enteroviral aseptic meningitis. Occasional highly inflammatory cases of enteroviral meningitis may be complicated by a mild form of encephalitis that is recognized on the basis of progressive lethargy, disorientation, and sometimes seizures. Less commonly, severe primary encephalitis may develop. An estimated 10–35% of cases of viral encephalitis are due to enteroviruses. Immunocompetent patients generally have a good prognosis.

Patients with hypogammaglobulinemia or agammaglobulinemia or severe combined immunodeficiency may develop chronic meningitis or encephalitis; about half of these patients have a dermatomyositis-like syndrome, with peripheral edema, rash, and myositis. They may also have chronic hepatitis. Patients may develop neurologic disease while receiving immunoglobulin replacement therapy. Echoviruses (especially echovirus 11) are the most common pathogens in this situation.

Paralytic disease due to enteroviruses other than poliovirus occurs sporadically and is usually less severe than poliomyelitis. Most cases are due to enterovirus 70 or 71 or to coxsackievirus A7 or A9. Guillain-Barré syndrome is also associated with enterovirus infection. While some studies have suggested a link between enteroviruses and the chronic fatigue syndrome, most recent studies have not demonstrated such an association.

Pleurodynia (Bornholm disease)   Patients with pleurodynia present with an acute onset of fever and spasms of pleuritic chest or upper abdominal pain. Chest pain is more common in adults, and abdominal pain is more common in children. Paroxysms of severe, knife-like pain usually last 15–30 min and are associated with diaphoresis and tachypnea. Fever peaks within an hour after the onset of paroxysms and subsides when pain resolves. The involved muscles are tender to palpation, and a pleural rub may be detected. The white blood cell count and chest x-ray are usually normal. Most cases are due to coxsackievirus B and occur during epidemics. Symptoms resolve in a few days, and recurrences are rare. Treatment includes the administration of nonsteroidal anti-inflammatory agents or the application of heat to the affected muscles.

Myocarditis and pericarditis   Enteroviruses are estimated to cause up to one-third of cases of acute myocarditis. Coxsackievirus B and its RNA have been detected in pericardial fluid and myocardial tissue in some cases of acute myocarditis and pericarditis. Most cases of enteroviral myocarditis or pericarditis occur in newborns, adolescents, or young adults. More than two-thirds of patients are male. Patients often present with an upper respiratory tract infection that is followed by fever, chest pain, dyspnea, arrhythmias, and occasionally heart failure. A pericardial friction rub is documented in half of cases, and the electrocardiogram shows ST-segment elevations or ST- and T-wave abnormalities. Serum levels of myocardial enzymes are often elevated. Neonates commonly have severe disease, while most older children and adults recover completely. Up to 10% of cases progress to chronic dilated cardiomyopathy. Chronic constrictive pericarditis may also be a sequela.

Exanthems   Enterovirus infection is the leading cause of exanthems in children in the summer and fall. While exanthems are associated with many enteroviruses, certain types have been linked to specific syndromes. Echoviruses 9 and 16 have frequently been associated with exanthem and fever. Rashes may be discrete or confluent, beginning on the face and spreading to the trunk and extremities. Echovirus 9 is the most common cause of a rubelliform (discrete) rash. Unlike the rash of rubella, the enteroviral rash occurs in the summer and is not associated with lymphadenopathy. Roseola-like rashes develop after defervescence, with macules and papules on the face and trunk. The Boston exanthem, caused by echovirus 16, is a roseola-like rash. A variety of other rashes have been associated with enteroviruses, including erythema multiforme (see Fig. e7-25) and vesicular, urticarial, petechial, or purpuric lesions. Enanthems also occur, including lesions that resemble the Koplik's spots seen with measles (see Fig. e7-2).

Hand-foot-and-mouth disease   After an incubation period of 4–6 days, patients with hand-foot-and-mouth disease present with fever, anorexia, and malaise; these manifestations are followed by the development of sore throat and vesicles (Fig. 191-1A; see also Fig. e7-23) on the buccal mucosa and often on the tongue and then by the appearance of tender vesicular lesions on the dorsum of the hands, sometimes with involvement of the palms. The vesicles may form bullae and quickly ulcerate. About one-third of patients also have lesions on the palate, uvula, or tonsillar pillars, and one-third have a rash on the feet (including the soles) or on the buttocks (Fig. 191-1B). The disease is highly infectious, with attack rates of close to 100% among young children. The lesions usually resolve in 1 week. Most cases are due to coxsackievirus A16 or enterovirus 71.

An epidemic of enterovirus 71 infection in Taiwan in 1998 resulted in thousands of cases of hand-foot-and-mouth disease or herpangina. Severe complications included CNS disease, myocarditis, and pulmonary hemorrhage. About 90% of those who died were children ≤5 years old, and death was associated with pulmonary edema or pulmonary hemorrhage. CNS disease included aseptic meningitis, flaccid paralysis (similar to that seen in poliomyelitis), or rhombencephalitis with myoclonus and tremor or ataxia. The mean age of patients with CNS complications was 2.5 years, and MRI in cases with encephalitis usually showed brain-stem lesions. Follow-up of children at 6 months showed persistent dysphagia, cranial nerve palsies, hypoventilation, limb weakness, and atrophy; at 3 years, persistent neurologic sequelae were documented, with delayed development and impaired cognitive function.

Herpangina   Herpangina is usually caused by coxsackievirus A and presents as acute-onset fever, sore throat, odynophagia, and grayish-white papulovesicular lesions on an erythematous base that ulcerate (Fig. 191-1C). The lesions can persist for weeks; are present on the soft palate, anterior pillars of the tonsils, and uvula; and are concentrated in the posterior portion of the mouth. In contrast to herpes stomatitis, enteroviral herpangina is not associated with gingivitis. Acute lymphonodular pharyngitis associated with coxsackievirus A10 presents as white or yellow nodules surrounded by erythema in the posterior oropharynx. The lesions do not ulcerate.

Acute hemorrhagic conjunctivitis   Patients with acute hemorrhagic conjunctivitis present with an acute onset of severe eye pain, blurred vision, photophobia, and watery discharge from the eye. Examination reveals edema, chemosis, and subconjunctival hemorrhage and often shows punctate keratitis and conjunctival follicles as well (Fig. 191-1D). Preauricular adenopathy is often found. Epidemics and nosocomial spread have been associated with enterovirus 70 and coxsackievirus A24. Systemic symptoms, including headache and fever, develop in 20% of cases, and recovery is usually complete in 10 days. The sudden onset and short duration of the illness help to distinguish acute hemorrhagic conjunctivitis from other ocular infections, such as those due to adenovirus and *Chlamydia trachomatis*. Paralysis has been associated with some cases of acute hemorrhagic conjunctivitis due to enterovirus 70 during epidemics.

Other manifestations   Enteroviruses are an infrequent cause of childhood pneumonia and the common cold. Coxsackievirus B has been isolated at autopsy from the pancreas of a few children presenting with type 1 diabetes mellitus; however, most attempts to isolate the virus have been unsuccessful. Other diseases that have been associated with enterovirus infection include parotitis, bronchitis, bronchiolitis, croup, infectious lymphocytosis, polymyositis, acute arthritis, and acute nephritis.

■ DIAGNOSIS

Isolation of enterovirus in cell culture is the traditional diagnostic procedure. While cultures of stool, nasopharyngeal, or throat samples from patients with enterovirus diseases are often positive, isolation of the virus from these sites does not prove that it is directly associated with disease because these sites are frequently colonized

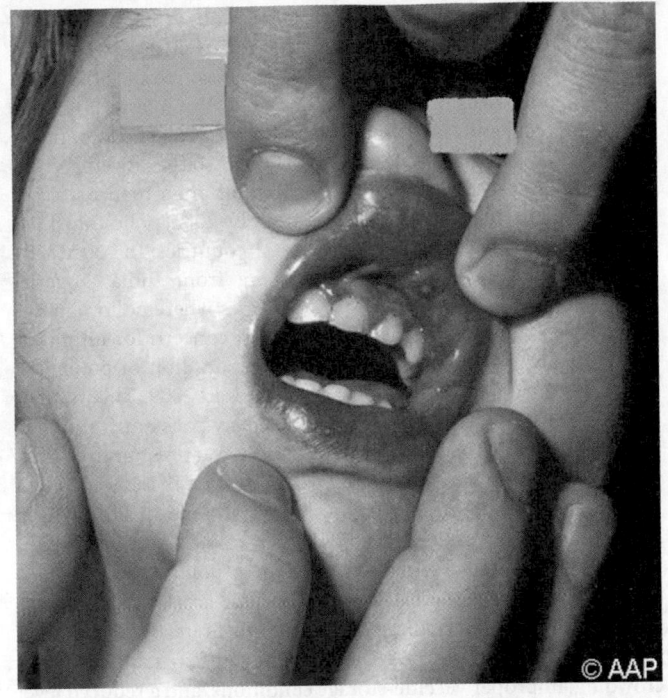

A

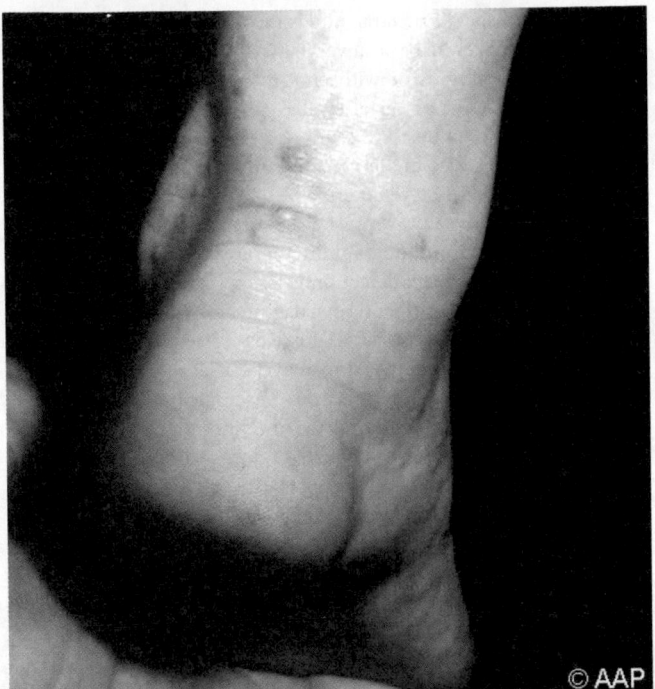

B

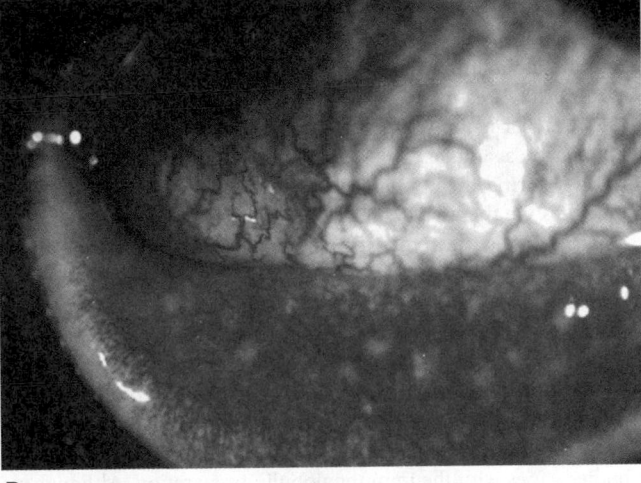

C

D

Figure 191-1 *A.* Tender vesicles in the mouth of a patient with hand-foot-and-mouth disease. *B.* Vesicles over the Achilles tendon in a patient with hand-foot-and-mouth disease. *C.* Soft-palate lesions of herpangina due to coxsackievirus. *D.* Acute hemorrhagic conjunctivitis due to enterovirus 71.

(Images are reprinted with permission from Red Book 2009: Committee on Infectious Diseases, 28th ed. Used with permission of the American Academy of Pediatrics.)

for weeks in patients with subclinical infections. Isolation of virus from the throat is more likely to be associated with disease than isolation from the stool since virus is shed for shorter periods from the throat. Cultures of CSF, serum, fluid from body cavities, or tissues are positive less frequently, but a positive result is indicative of disease caused by enterovirus. In some cases, the virus is isolated only from the blood or only from the CSF; therefore, it is important to culture multiple sites. Cultures are more likely to be positive earlier than later in the course of infection. Most human enteroviruses can be detected within a week after inoculation of cell cultures. Cultures may be negative because of the presence of neutralizing antibody, lack of susceptibility of the cells used, or inappropriate handling of the specimen. Coxsackievirus A may require inoculation into special cell-culture lines or into suckling mice.

Identification of the enterovirus serotype is useful primarily for epidemiologic studies and, with a few exceptions, has little clinical utility.

It is important to identify serious infections with enterovirus during epidemics and to distinguish the vaccine strain of poliovirus from the other enteroviruses in the throat or in the feces. Stool and throat samples for culture as well as acute- and convalescent-phase serum specimens should be obtained from all patients with suspected poliomyelitis. In the absence of a positive CSF culture, a positive culture of stool obtained within the first 2 weeks after the onset of symptoms is most often used to confirm the diagnosis of poliomyelitis. If poliovirus infection is suspected, two or more fecal and throat swab samples should be obtained at least 1 day apart and cultured for enterovirus as soon as possible. If poliovirus is isolated, it should be sent to the CDC for identification as either wild-type or vaccine virus.

The polymerase chain reaction (PCR) has been used to amplify viral nucleic acid from CSF, serum, urine, throat swabs, and tissues. A pan-enterovirus PCR assay can detect all human enteroviruses. With the proper controls, PCR of the CSF is highly sensitive

(70–100%) and specific (>80%) and is more rapid than culture. PCR of the CSF is less likely to be positive when patients present ≥3 days after the onset of meningitis or with enterovirus 71 infection; in these cases, PCR of throat or rectal swabs—although less specific than PCR of CSF—should be considered.

PCR of serum is also highly sensitive and specific in the diagnosis of disseminated disease. PCR may be particularly helpful for the diagnosis and follow-up of enterovirus disease in immunodeficient patients receiving immunoglobulin therapy, whose viral cultures may be negative. Antigen detection is less sensitive than PCR.

Serologic diagnosis of enterovirus infection is limited by the large number of serotypes and the lack of a common antigen. Demonstration of seroconversion may be useful in rare cases for confirmation of culture results, but serologic testing is usually limited to epidemiologic studies. Serum should be collected and frozen soon after the onset of disease and again ~4 weeks later. Measurement of neutralizing titers is the most accurate method for antibody determination; measurement of complement-fixation titers is usually less sensitive. Titers of virus-specific IgM are elevated in both acute and chronic infection.

TREATMENT   Enterovirus Infections

Most enterovirus infections are mild and resolve spontaneously; however, intensive supportive care may be needed for cardiac, hepatic, or CNS disease. IV, intrathecal, or intraventricular immunoglobulin has been used with apparent success in some cases for the treatment of chronic enterovirus meningoencephalitis and dermatomyositis in patients with hypogammaglobulinemia or agammaglobulinemia. The disease may stabilize or resolve during therapy; however, some patients decline inexorably despite therapy. IV immunoglobulin often prevents severe enterovirus disease in these patients. IV administration of immunoglobulin with high titers of antibody to the infecting virus has been used in some cases of life-threatening infection in neonates, who may not have maternally acquired antibody. In one trial involving neonates with enterovirus infections, immunoglobulin containing very high titers of antibody to the infecting virus reduced rates of viremia; however, the study was too small to show a substantial clinical benefit. The level of enteroviral antibodies varies with the immunoglobulin preparation. Although a phase 2 trial of pleconaril for severe neonatal enterovirus disease is in progress, the drug is no longer available on a compassionate-use basis. Glucocorticoids are contraindicated.

Good hand-washing practices and the use of gowns and gloves are important in limiting nosocomial transmission of enteroviruses during epidemics. Enteric precautions are indicated for 7 days after the onset of enterovirus infections.

■ PREVENTION AND ERADICATION OF POLIOVIRUS

(See also Chap. 122) After a peak of 57,879 cases of poliomyelitis in the United States in 1952, the introduction of inactivated vaccine in 1955 and of oral vaccine in 1961 ultimately eradicated disease due to wild-type poliovirus in the Western Hemisphere. Such disease has not been documented in the United States since 1979, when cases occurred among religious groups who had declined immunization. In the Western Hemisphere, paralysis due to wild-type poliovirus was last documented in 1991.

In 1988, the World Health Organization adopted a resolution to eradicate poliomyelitis by the year 2000. From 1988 to 2001, the number of cases worldwide decreased by >99%, with fewer than 1000 confirmed cases reported in 2001. In 2002,

however, there were ~1900 cases of polio, with ~1500 reported in India. Wild-type poliovirus type 2 has not been detected in the world since 1999. The Americas were certified free of indigenous wild-type poliovirus transmission in 1994, the Western Pacific Region in 2000, and the European Region in 2002. The total number of cases worldwide fell to a nadir of 498 in 2001. However, from 2002 to 2005, 21 countries previously free of polio reported cases imported from 6 polio-endemic countries. By 2006, polio transmission had been reduced in most of these 21 countries. In 2009, 1781 cases of polio were reported; 80% were from India, Nigeria, Pakistan, and Afghanistan, the only countries where polio remains endemic (Table 191-2). Polio is a source of concern for unimmunized or partially immunized travelers. Importation of poliovirus into 20 countries accounted for 20% of cases in 2009. The number of cases of wild-type polio remained relatively constant from 2005 through 2009, with 1315–1997 cases per year. Countries that reported cases of wild-type polio in 2010 but not in 2009 included Tajikistan, Senegal, and Nepal. Outbreaks of polio in Europe and North America have been traced to cases imported from the Indian subcontinent. Clearly, global eradication of polio is necessary to eliminate the risk of importation of wild-type virus. Outbreaks are thought to have been facilitated by suboptimal rates of vaccination, isolated pockets of unvaccinated children, poor sanitation and crowding, improper vaccine-storage conditions, and a reduced level of response to one of the serotypes in the vaccine. While the global eradication campaign has markedly reduced the number of cases of endemic polio, doubts have been raised as to whether eradication is a realistic goal given the large number of asymptomatic infections and the political instability in developing countries.

The occurrence of outbreaks of poliomyelitis due to circulating vaccine-derived poliovirus of all three types has been increasing, especially in areas with low vaccination rates. In Egypt, 32 cases of

---

TABLE 191-2   Laboratory-Confirmed Cases of Poliomyelitis in 2009

Country	Type of Transmission	No. of Cases
India	Endemic	752[a]
Nigeria	Endemic	541[b]
Pakistan	Endemic	89
Chad	Imported	66
Sudan	Imported	45
Guinea	Imported	43[c]
Afghanistan	Endemic	38
Angola	Imported	29
Cote d'Ivoire	Imported	26
Others[d]	Imported	142
Others[e]	Vaccine-derived	10
Total		**1781**

[a]Of these cases, 11 were vaccine-derived.
[b]Of these cases, 153 were vaccine-derived.
[c]Of these cases, 1 was vaccine-derived.
[d]Benin, 20; Kenya, 19; Burkina Faso, 15; Niger, 15; Central African Republic, 14; Mauritania, 13; Liberia, 11; Sierra Leone, 11; Uganda, 8; Togo, 6; Cameroon, 3; Democratic Republic of the Congo, 3; Burundi, 2; Mali, 2.
[e]Democratic Republic of the Congo, 4; Somalia, 4; Ethiopia, 2.

Source: World Health Organization.

vaccine-derived polio occurred in 1983–1993; in the Dominican Republic and Haiti, 22 cases occurred in 2000–2001; in Indonesia, 46 cases were reported in 2005; in Nigeria, 292 cases occurred in 2005–2009; in the Democratic Republic of the Congo, 20 cases were reported in 2005–2009; and fewer cases have occurred in other countries. These OPV-derived viruses reverted to a more neurovirulent phenotype after undetected circulation (probably for >2 years). The epidemic in Hispaniola was rapidly terminated after intensive vaccination with OPV. In 2005, a case of vaccine-derived polio occurred in an unvaccinated U.S. woman returning from a visit to Central and South America. In the same year, an unvaccinated immunocompromised infant in Minnesota was found to be shedding vaccine-derived poliovirus; further investigation identified 4 of 22 infants in the same community who were shedding the virus. All 5 infants were asymptomatic. These outbreaks emphasize the need for maintaining high levels of vaccine coverage and continued surveillance for circulating virus.

IPV is used in most industrialized countries and OPV in most developing countries, including those in which polio still is or recently was endemic. After several doses of OPV alone, the seropositivity rate for individual poliovirus serotypes may still be suboptimal for children in developing countries; one or more supplemental doses of IPV can increase the rate of seropositivity for these serotypes. Against a given serotype, monovalent OPV containing only that serotype is more immunogenic than trivalent vaccine because of a lack of interference from other serotypes. While IM injections of other vaccines (live or attenuated) can be given concurrently with OPV, unnecessary IM injections should be avoided during the first month after vaccination because they increase the risk of vaccine-associated paralysis. Since 1988, an enhanced-potency inactivated poliovirus vaccine has been available in the United States.

OPV and IPV induce antibodies that persist for at least 5 years. Both vaccines induce IgG and IgA antibodies. Compared with recipients of IPV, recipients of OPV shed less virus and less frequently develop reinfection with wild-type virus after exposure to poliovirus. Although IPV is safe and efficacious, OPV offers the advantages of ease of administration, lower cost, and induction of intestinal immunity resulting in a reduction in the risk of community transmission of wild-type virus. Because of progress toward global eradication of polio (with a reduced risk of imported cases) and the continued occurrence of cases of vaccine-associated polio, an all-IPV regimen was recommended in 2000 for childhood poliovirus vaccination in the United States, with vaccine administration at 2, 4, and 6–18 months and 4–6 years of age. The risk of vaccine-associated polio should be discussed before OPV is administered. Recommendations for vaccination of adults are listed in Table 191-3.

There are concerns about discontinuing vaccination in the event that endemic spread of poliovirus is eliminated. Among the reasons for these concerns are that poliovirus is shed from some immunocompromised persons for >10 years, that vaccine-derived poliovirus can circulate and cause disease, and that wild-type poliovirus is present in a large number of laboratories. A national survey began in October 2002 to encourage laboratories to dispose of all unneeded wild-type poliovirus materials and to identify laboratories that have wild-type poliovirus or specimens that may contain virus.

REOVIRUSES

Reoviruses are double-stranded RNA viruses encompassing three serotypes. Serologic studies indicate that most humans are infected with reoviruses during childhood. Most infections either are asymptomatic or cause very mild disease. One outbreak of reovirus infection in children resulted in minor upper respiratory tract symptoms. Reovirus is considered a rare cause of mild gastroenteritis in infants and children. Speculation regarding an association of reovirus type 3 with idiopathic neonatal hepatitis and extrahepatic

TABLE 191-3 Recommendations for Poliovirus Vaccination of Adults

1. Most adults in the United States have been vaccinated during childhood and have little risk of exposure to wild-type virus in the United States. Immunization is recommended for those with a higher risk of exposure than the general population, including:

   a. travelers to areas where poliovirus is or may be epidemic or endemic;

   b. members of communities or population groups with disease caused by wild-type polioviruses;

   c. laboratory workers handling specimens that may contain wild-type polioviruses; and

   d. health care workers in close contact with patients who may be excreting wild-type polioviruses.

2. Three doses of IPV are recommended for adults who need to be immunized. The second dose should be given 1–2 months after the first dose; the third dose should be given 6–12 months after the second dose.

3. Adults who are at increased risk of exposure to wild-type poliovirus and who have previously completed primary immunization should receive a single dose of IPV. Adults who did not complete primary immunization should receive the remaining vaccinations with IPV.

Abbreviation: IPV, inactivated poliovirus vaccine.

Source: Modified from Pickering LK, ed. Red Book 2009: Committee on Infectious Diseases, 28th ed. Used with permission of the American Academy of Pediatrics.

biliary atresia is based on an elevated prevalence of antibody to reovirus among some of these patients and the detection of viral RNA by PCR in hepatobiliary tissues in some studies. Two new orthoreoviruses (Melaka and Kampar viruses) have been associated with fever and acute respiratory disease in Malaysia.

FURTHER READINGS

ALEXANDER JP et al: Transmission of imported vaccine-derived poliovirus in an undervaccinated community in Minnesota. J Infect Dis 199:391, 2009

ARITA I et al: Is polio eradication realistic? Science 312:852, 2006

CENTERS FOR DISEASE CONTROL AND PREVENTION: Progress toward interruption of wild poliovirus transmission worldwide, 2009. MMWR Morb Mortal Wkly Rep 59:545, 2010

———: Update on vaccine-derived polioviruses—worldwide, January 2008–June 2009. MMWR Morb Mortal Wkly Rep 58:1002, 2009

EL-SAYED N et al: Monovalent type 1 oral poliovirus vaccine in newborns. N Engl J Med 359:1655, 2008

KEW O et al: Vaccine-derived polioviruses and the endgame strategy for global polio eradication. Annu Rev Microbiol 59:587, 2005

KUPILIA L et al: Diagnosis of enteroviral meningitis by use of polymerase chain reaction of cerebrospinal fluid, stool, and serum specimens. Clin Infect Dis 40:982, 2005

LEE TC et al: Diseases caused by enterovirus 71 infection. Pediatr Infect Dis J 28:904, 2009

PEREZ-VELEZ CM et al: Outbreak of neurologic enterovirus type 71 disease: A diagnostic challenge. Clin Infect Dis 45:950, 2007

WIKSWO MW: Increased activity of coxsackievirus B1 strains associated with severe disease among young infants in the United States, 2007–2008. Clin Infect Dis 49:e44, 2009

CHAPTER 192
Measles (Rubeola)

William J. Moss

■ DEFINITION

Measles is a highly contagious viral disease that is characterized by a prodromal illness of fever, cough, coryza, and conjunctivitis followed by the appearance of a generalized maculopapular rash. Before the widespread use of measles vaccines, it was estimated that measles caused between 5 million and 8 million deaths worldwide each year.

■ GLOBAL CONSIDERATIONS

Remarkable progress has been made in reducing global measles incidence and mortality rates through measles vaccination. In the Americas, intensive vaccination and surveillance efforts—based in part on the successful Pan American Health Organization strategy of periodic nationwide measles vaccination campaigns (supplementary immunization activities, or SIAs)—and high routine measles vaccine coverage have interrupted endemic transmission of measles virus. In the United States, high coverage with two doses of measles vaccine eliminated endemic measles virus transmission in 2000. More recently, progress has been made in reducing measles incidence and mortality rates in sub-Saharan Africa as a consequence of increasing routine measles vaccine coverage and provision of a second opportunity for measles vaccination through mass measles vaccination campaigns.

In 2003, the World Health Assembly endorsed a resolution urging member countries to reduce the number of deaths attributed to measles by 50% (compared with 1999 estimates) by the end of 2005. This target was met. Global measles mortality rates were further reduced in 2008; during that year, there were an estimated 164,000 deaths due to measles (uncertainty bounds: 115,000 and 222,000 deaths). These achievements attest to the enormous public-health significance of measles vaccination. The revised global goal, as stated in the Global Immunization Vision and Strategy 2006–2015 of the World Health Organization and United Nations Children's Fund, is to reduce global measles deaths by 90% (compared with the estimated 757,000 deaths in 2000) by 2010.

■ ETIOLOGY

Measles virus is a spherical, nonsegmented, single-stranded, negative-sense RNA virus and a member of the *Morbillivirus* genus in the family of Paramyxoviridae. Measles was originally a zoonotic infection, arising from cross-species transmission from animals to humans by an ancestral morbillivirus ~10,000 years ago, when human populations attained sufficient size to sustain virus transmission. Although RNA viruses typically have high mutation rates, measles virus is considered to be an antigenically monotypic virus; i.e., the surface proteins responsible for inducing protective immunity have retained their antigenic structure across time and space. The public health significance of this stability is that measles vaccines developed decades ago from a single strain of measles virus remain protective worldwide. Measles virus is killed by ultraviolet light and heat, and attenuated measles vaccine viruses retain these characteristics, necessitating a cold chain for vaccine transport and storage.

■ EPIDEMIOLOGY

Measles virus is one of the most highly contagious directly transmitted pathogens. Outbreaks can occur in populations in which <10% of persons are susceptible. Chains of transmission are common among household contacts, school-age children, and health care workers. There are no latent or persistent measles virus infections that result in prolonged contagiousness, nor are there animal reservoirs for the virus. Thus, measles virus can be maintained in human populations only by an unbroken chain of acute infections, which requires a continuous supply of susceptible individuals. Newborns become susceptible to measles virus infection when passively acquired maternal antibody is lost and, when not vaccinated, account for the bulk of new susceptible individuals.

Endemic measles has a typical temporal pattern characterized by yearly seasonal epidemics superimposed on longer epidemic cycles of 2–5 years or more. In temperate climates, annual measles outbreaks typically occur in the late winter and early spring. These annual outbreaks are probably attributable to social networks facilitating transmission (e.g., congregation of children at school) and environmental factors favoring the viability and transmission of measles virus. Measles cases continue to occur during interepidemic periods in large populations, but at low incidence. The longer cycles occurring every several years result from the accumulation of susceptible persons over successive birth cohorts and the subsequent decline in the number of susceptibles following an outbreak.

Secondary attack rates in susceptible household and institutional contacts generally exceed 90%. The average age at which measles occurs depends on rates of contact with infected persons, protective maternal antibody decline, and vaccine coverage. In densely populated urban settings with low vaccination coverage, measles is a disease of infants and young children. The cumulative distribution can reach 50% by 1 year of age, with a significant proportion of children acquiring measles before 9 months—the age of routine vaccination in many countries, in line with the schedule recommended by the Expanded Programme on Immunization. As measles vaccine coverage increases or population density decreases, the age distribution shifts toward older children. In such situations, measles cases predominate in school-age children. Infants and young children, although susceptible if not protected by vaccination, are not exposed to measles virus at a rate sufficient to cause a large disease burden in this age group. As vaccination coverage increases further, the age distribution of cases may be shifted into adolescence and adulthood; this distribution is seen in measles outbreaks in the United States and necessitates targeted measles vaccination programs for these older age groups.

Persons with measles are infectious for several days before and after the onset of rash, when levels of measles virus in blood and body fluids are highest and when cough, coryza, and sneezing, which facilitate virus spread, are most severe. The contagiousness of measles before the onset of recognizable disease hinders the effectiveness of quarantine measures. Measles virus can be isolated from urine as late as 1 week after rash onset, and viral shedding by children with impaired cell-mediated immunity can be prolonged.

Medical settings are well-recognized sites of measles virus transmission. Children may present to health care facilities during the prodrome, when the diagnosis is not obvious although the child is infectious and is likely to infect susceptible contacts. Health care workers can acquire measles from infected children and transmit measles virus to others. Nosocomial transmission can be reduced by maintenance of a high index of clinical suspicion, use of appropriate isolation precautions when measles is suspected, administration of measles vaccine to susceptible children and health care workers, and documentation of health care workers' immunity to measles (i.e., proof of receipt of two doses of measles vaccine or detection of antibodies to measles virus).

As efforts at measles control are increasingly successful, public perceptions of the risk of measles as a disease diminish and are replaced by concerns about possible adverse events associated with measles vaccine. As a consequence, numerous measles outbreaks have occurred because of opposition to vaccination on religious or philosophical grounds or unfounded fears of serious adverse events (see "Active Immunization," below).

■ PATHOGENESIS

Measles virus is transmitted primarily by respiratory droplets over short distances and, less commonly, by small-particle aerosols that remain suspended in the air for long periods. Airborne transmission appears to be important in certain settings, including schools, physicians' offices, hospitals, and enclosed public places. The virus can be transmitted by direct contact with infected secretions but does not survive for long on fomites.

The incubation period for measles is ~10 days to fever onset and 14 days to rash onset. This period may be shorter in infants and longer (up to 3 weeks) in adults. Infection is initiated when measles virus is deposited on epithelial cells in the respiratory tract, oropharynx, or conjunctivae (Fig. 192-1A). During the first 2–4 days after infection, measles virus proliferates locally in the respiratory mucosa and spreads to draining lymph nodes. Virus then enters the bloodstream in infected leukocytes (primarily monocytes), producing the primary viremia that disseminates infection throughout the reticuloendothelial system. Further replication results in secondary viremia that begins 5–7 days after infection and disseminates measles virus throughout the body. Replication of measles virus in these target organs, together with the host's immune response, is responsible for the signs and symptoms of measles that occur 8–12 days after infection and mark the end of the incubation period.

■ IMMUNE RESPONSES

Host immune responses to measles virus are essential for viral clearance, clinical recovery, and the establishment of long-term immunity (Fig. 192-1C). Early nonspecific (innate) immune responses during the prodromal phase include activation of natural killer (NK) cells and increased production of the antiviral proteins interferon (IFN) α and IFN-γ. The adaptive immune responses consist of measles virus–specific antibody and cellular responses. The protective efficacy of antibodies to measles virus is illustrated by the immunity conferred to infants from passively acquired maternal antibodies and the protection of exposed, susceptible individuals after administration of anti–measles virus immunoglobulin. The first measles virus–specific antibodies produced after infection are of the IgM subtype, with a subsequent switch to predominantly IgG1 and IgG4 isotypes. The IgM antibody response is typically absent following reexposure or revaccination and serves as a marker of primary infection.

The importance of cellular immunity to measles virus is demonstrated by the ability of children with agammaglobulinemia (congenital inability to produce antibodies) to recover fully from measles and the contrasting picture for children with severe defects in T lymphocyte function, who often develop severe or fatal disease (Chap. 316). The initial predominant T$_H$1 response (characterized by IFN-γ) is essential for viral clearance, and the later T$_H$2 response (characterized by interleukin 4) promotes the development of measles virus–specific antibodies that are critical for protection against reinfection.

The duration of protective immunity following wild-type measles virus infection is generally thought to be lifelong. Immunologic memory to measles virus includes both continued production of

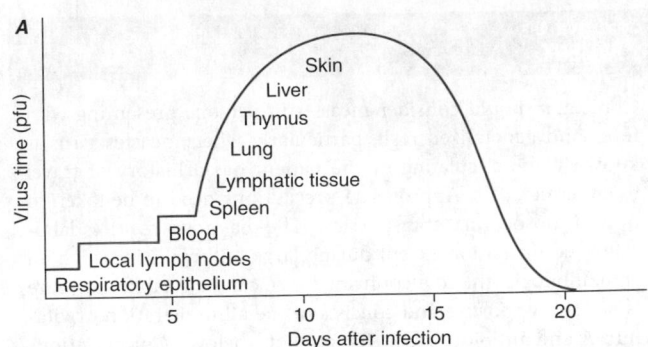

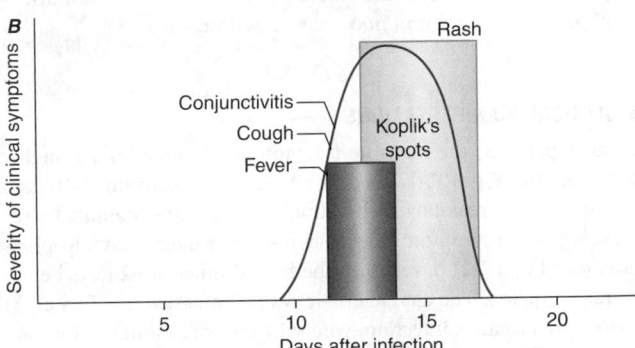

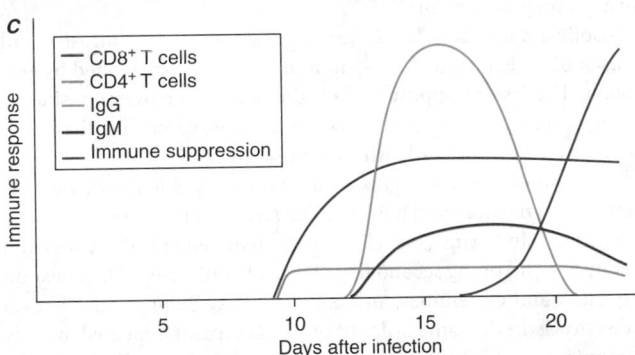

Figure 192-1 Measles virus infection: pathogenesis, clinical features, and immune responses. *A*: Spread of measles virus, from initial infection of the respiratory tract through dissemination to the skin. *B*: Appearance of clinical signs and symptoms, including Koplik's spots and rash. *C*: Antibody and T cell responses to measles virus. The signs and symptoms of measles arise coincident with the host immune response. *(Source: WJ Moss, DE Griffin: Nat Rev Microbiol 4:900, 2006.)*

measles virus–specific antibodies and circulation of measles virus–specific CD4$^+$ and CD8$^+$ T lymphocytes.

However, the intense immune responses induced by measles virus infection are paradoxically associated with depressed responses to unrelated (nonmeasles virus) antigens, which persist for several weeks to months beyond resolution of the acute illness. This state of immune suppression enhances susceptibility to secondary infections with bacteria and viruses that cause pneumonia and diarrhea and is responsible for a substantial proportion of measles-related morbidity and deaths. Delayed-type hypersensitivity responses to recall antigens, such as tuberculin, are suppressed, and cellular and humoral responses to new antigens are impaired. Reactivation of tuberculosis and remission of autoimmune diseases after measles have been described and are attributed to this state of immune suppression.

Clinicians should consider measles in persons presenting with fever and generalized rash, particularly when measles virus is known to be circulating or the patient has a history of travel to endemic areas. Appropriate precautions need to be taken to prevent nosocomial transmission. The diagnosis requires laboratory confirmation except during large outbreaks in which an epidemiologic link to a confirmed case can be established. Care is largely supportive and consists of the administration of vitamin A and antibiotics (see "Treatment," below). Complications of measles, including secondary bacterial infections and encephalitis, may occur after acute illness and require careful monitoring, particularly in immunocompromised persons.

CLINICAL MANIFESTATIONS

In most persons, the signs and symptoms of measles are highly characteristic (Fig. 192-1B). Fever and malaise beginning ~10 days after exposure are followed by cough, coryza, and conjunctivitis. These signs and symptoms increase in severity over 4 days. Koplik's spots (see Fig. e7-2) develop on the buccal mucosa ~2 days before the rash appears. The characteristic rash of measles (see Fig. e7-3) begins 2 weeks after infection, when the clinical manifestations are most severe, and signal the host's immune response to the replicating virus. Headache, abdominal pain, vomiting, diarrhea, and myalgia may be present.

Koplik's spots (Fig. e7-2) are pathognomonic of measles and consist of bluish white dots ~1 mm in diameter surrounded by erythema. The lesions appear first on the buccal mucosa opposite the lower molars but rapidly increase in number to involve the entire buccal mucosa. They fade with the onset of rash.

The rash of measles begins as erythematous macules behind the ears and on the neck and hairline. The rash progresses to involve the face, trunk, and arms (Fig. e7-3), with involvement of the legs and feet by the end of the second day. Areas of confluent rash appear on the trunk and extremities, and petechiae may be present. The rash fades slowly in the same order of progression as it appeared, usually beginning on the third or fourth day after onset. Resolution of the rash may be followed by desquamation.

Because the characteristic rash of measles is a consequence of the cellular immune response, it may not develop in persons with impaired cellular immunity (e.g., those with AIDS; Chap. 189). These persons have a high case-fatality rate and frequently develop giant-cell pneumonitis caused by measles virus. T lymphocyte defects due to causes other than HIV-1 infection (e.g., cancer chemotherapy) also are associated with increased severity of measles.

A severe atypical measles syndrome was observed in recipients of a formalin-inactivated measles vaccine (used in the United States from 1963 to 1967 and in Canada until 1970) who were subsequently exposed to wild-type measles virus. The atypical rash began on the palms and soles and spread centripetally to the proximal extremities and trunk, sparing the face. The rash was initially erythematous and maculopapular but frequently progressed to vesicular, petechial, or purpuric lesions (see Fig. e7-22).

DIFFERENTIAL DIAGNOSIS

The differential diagnosis of measles includes other causes of fever, rash, and conjunctivitis, including rubella, Kawasaki disease, infectious mononucleosis, roseola, scarlet fever, Rocky Mountain spotted fever, enterovirus or adenovirus infection, and drug sensitivity. Rubella is a milder illness without cough and with distinctive lymphadenopathy. The rash of roseola (exanthem subitum) appears after fever has subsided. The atypical lymphocytosis in infectious mononucleosis contrasts with the leukopenia commonly observed in children with measles.

DIAGNOSIS

Measles is readily diagnosed on clinical grounds by clinicians familiar with the disease, particularly during outbreaks. Koplik's spots (Fig. e7-2) are especially helpful because they appear early and are pathognomonic. Clinical diagnosis is more difficult (1) during the prodromal illness; (2) when the rash is attenuated by passively acquired antibodies or prior immunization; (3) when the rash is absent or delayed in immunocompromised or severely malnourished children with impaired cellular immunity; and (4) in regions where the incidence of measles is low and other pathogens are responsible for the majority of illnesses with fever and rash. The Centers for Disease Control and Prevention case definition for measles requires (1) a generalized maculopapular rash of at least 3 days' duration; (2) fever of at least 38.3°C (101°F); and (3) cough, coryza, or conjunctivitis.

Serology is the most common method of laboratory diagnosis. The detection of measles virus–specific IgM in a single specimen of serum or oral fluid is considered diagnostic of acute infection, as is a fourfold or greater increase in measles virus–specific IgG antibody levels between acute- and convalescent-phase serum specimens. Primary infection in the immunocompetent host results in antibodies that are detectable within 1–3 days of rash onset and reach peak levels in 2–4 weeks. Measles virus–specific IgM antibodies may not be detectable until 4–5 days or more after rash onset and usually fall to undetectable levels within 4–8 weeks of rash onset.

Several methods for measurement of antibodies to measles virus are available. Neutralization tests are sensitive and specific, and the results are highly correlated with protective immunity; however, these tests require propagation of measles virus in cell culture and thus are expensive and laborious. Commercially available enzyme immunoassays are most frequently used. Measles also can be diagnosed by isolation of the virus in cell culture from respiratory secretions, nasopharyngeal or conjunctival swabs, blood, or urine. Direct detection of giant cells in respiratory secretions, urine, or tissue obtained by biopsy provides another method of diagnosis.

For detection of measles virus RNA by reverse-transcriptase polymerase chain reaction (RT-PCR) amplification of RNA extracted from clinical specimens, primers targeted to highly conserved regions of measles virus genes are used. Extremely sensitive and specific, RT-PCR assays may also permit identification and characterization of measles virus genotypes for molecular epidemiologic studies and can distinguish wild-type from vaccine virus strains.

TREATMENT Measles

There is no specific antiviral therapy for measles. Treatment consists of general supportive measures, such as hydration and administration of antipyretic agents. Because secondary bacterial infections are a major cause of morbidity and death following measles, effective case management involves prompt antibiotic treatment for patients who have clinical evidence of bacterial infection, including pneumonia and otitis media. *Streptococcus pneumoniae* and *Haemophilus influenzae* type b are common causes of bacterial pneumonia following measles; vaccines against these pathogens probably lower the incidence of secondary bacterial infections following measles.

Vitamin A is effective for the treatment of measles and can markedly reduce rates of morbidity and mortality. The World Health Organization recommends administration of once-daily doses of 200,000 IU of vitamin A for 2 consecutive days to all children with measles who are ≥12 months of age. Lower doses are recommended for younger children: 100,000 IU per day for children 6–12 months of age and 50,000 IU per day for children <6 months old. A third dose is recommended 2–4 weeks later for children with evidence of vitamin A deficiency. While such deficiency is not a widely recognized problem in the United States, many American children with measles do, in fact, have low serum levels of vitamin A, and these children experience increased morbidity following measles. The Committee on Infectious Diseases of the American Academy of Pediatrics recommends that the administration of two consecutive daily doses of vitamin A be considered for children hospitalized with measles and its complications as well as for children with measles who are immunodeficient; who have ophthalmologic evidence of vitamin A deficiency, impaired intestinal absorption, or moderate to severe malnutrition; or who have recently immigrated from areas with high measles mortality rates. Parenteral and oral formulations of vitamin A are available.

Anecdotal reports have described the recovery of previously healthy pregnant and immunocompromised patients with measles pneumonia and of immunocompromised patients with measles encephalitis after treatment with aerosolized and IV ribavirin. However, the clinical benefits of ribavirin in persons with measles have not been conclusively demonstrated in clinical trials.

■ COMPLICATIONS

Most complications of measles involve the respiratory tract and include the effects of measles virus replication itself and secondary bacterial infections. Acute laryngotracheobronchitis (croup) can occur during measles and may result in airway obstruction, particularly in young children. Giant-cell pneumonitis due to replication of measles virus in the lungs can develop in immunocompromised children, including those with HIV-1 infection. Many children with measles develop diarrhea, which contributes to malnutrition.

Most complications of measles result from secondary bacterial infections of the respiratory tract that are attributable to a state of immune suppression lasting for several weeks to months after acute measles. Otitis media and bronchopneumonia are most common and may be caused by *S. pneumoniae*, *H. influenzae* type b, or staphylococci. Recurrence of fever or failure of fever to subside with the rash suggests secondary bacterial infection.

Rare but serious complications of measles involve the central nervous system (CNS). Postmeasles encephalomyelitis complicates ~1 in 1000 cases, affecting mainly older children and adults. Encephalomyelitis occurs within 2 weeks of rash onset and is characterized by fever, seizures, and a variety of neurologic abnormalities. The finding of periventricular demyelination, the induction of immune responses to myelin basic protein, and the absence of measles virus in the brain suggest that postmeasles encephalomyelitis is an autoimmune disorder triggered by measles virus infection. Other CNS complications that occur months to years after acute infection are measles inclusion body encephalitis (MIBE) and subacute sclerosing panencephalitis (SSPE). In contrast to postmeasles encephalomyelitis, MIBE and SSPE are caused by persistent measles virus infection. MIBE is a rare but fatal complication that affects individuals with defective cellular immunity and typically occurs months after infection. SSPE is a slowly progressive disease characterized by seizures and progressive deterioration of cognitive and motor functions, with death occurring 5–15 years after measles

virus infection. SSPE most often develops in persons infected with measles virus at <2 years of age.

■ PROGNOSIS

Most persons with measles recover and develop long-term protective immunity to reinfection. Measles case-fatality proportions vary with the average age of infection, the nutritional and immunologic status of the population, measles vaccine coverage, and access to health care. Among previously vaccinated persons who do become infected, disease is less severe and mortality rates are significantly lower. In developed countries, <1 in 1000 children with measles die. In endemic areas of sub-Saharan Africa, the measles case-fatality proportion may be 5–10% or even higher. Measles is a major cause of childhood deaths in refugee camps and in internally displaced populations, where case-fatality proportions have been as high as 20–30%.

■ PREVENTION

Passive immunization

Human immunoglobulin given shortly after exposure can attenuate the clinical course of measles. In immunocompetent persons, administration of immunoglobulin within 72 h of exposure usually prevents measles virus infection and almost always prevents clinical measles. Administered up to 6 days after exposure, immunoglobulin will still prevent or modify the disease. Prophylaxis with immunoglobulin is recommended for susceptible household and nosocomial contacts who are at risk of developing severe measles, particularly children <1 year of age, immunocompromised persons (including HIV-infected persons previously immunized with live attenuated measles vaccine), and pregnant women. Except for premature infants, children <6 months of age usually will be partially or completely protected by passively acquired maternal antibody. If measles is diagnosed in a mother, all unimmunized children in the household should receive immunoglobulin. The recommended dose is 0.25 mL/kg given intramuscularly. Immunocompromised persons should receive 0.5 mL/kg. The maximum total dose is 15 mL. IV immunoglobulin contains antibodies to measles virus; the usual dose of 100–400 mg/kg generally provides adequate prophylaxis for measles exposures occurring as long as 3 weeks or more after IV immunoglobulin administration.

Active immunization

The first live attenuated measles vaccine was developed by passage of the Edmonston strain in chick embryo fibroblasts to produce the Edmonston B virus, which was licensed in 1963 in the United States. Further passage of Edmonston B virus produced the more attenuated Schwarz vaccine that currently serves as the standard in much of the world. The Moraten ("more attenuated") strain, which was licensed in 1968 and is used in the United States, is genetically closely related to the Schwarz strain.

Lyophilized measles vaccines are relatively stable, but reconstituted vaccine rapidly loses potency. Live attenuated measles vaccines are inactivated by light and heat and lose about half their potency at 20°C and almost all their potency at 37°C within 1 h after reconstitution. Therefore, a cold chain must be maintained before and after reconstitution. Antibodies first appear 12–15 days after vaccination and peak at 1–3 months. Measles vaccines are often combined with other live attenuated virus vaccines, such as those for mumps and rubella (MMR) and for mumps, rubella, and varicella (MMR-V).

The recommended age of first vaccination varies from 6 to 15 months and represents a balance between the optimal age for seroconversion and the probability of acquiring measles before that age. The proportions of children who develop protective levels of antibody after measles vaccination approximate 85% at 9 months of age and 95% at 12 months. Common childhood illnesses concomitant with vaccination may reduce the level of immune response, but such illness is not a valid reason to withhold vaccination. Measles vaccines have been well tolerated and immunogenic in HIV-1-infected children and adults, although antibody levels may wane. Because of the potential severity of wild-type measles virus infection in HIV-1-infected children, routine measles vaccination is recommended except for those who are severely immunocompromised. Measles vaccination is contraindicated in individuals with other severe deficiencies of cellular immunity because of the possibility of disease due to progressive pulmonary or CNS infection with the vaccine virus.

The duration of vaccine-induced immunity is at least several decades if not longer. Rates of secondary vaccine failure 10–15 years after immunization have been estimated at ~5% but are probably lower when the vaccination is given after 12 months of age. Decreasing antibody concentrations do not necessarily imply a complete loss of protective immunity: a secondary immune response usually develops after reexposure to measles virus, with a rapid rise in antibody titers in the absence of overt clinical disease.

Standard doses of currently licensed measles vaccines are safe for immunocompetent children and adults. Fever to 39.4°C (103°F) occurs in ~5% of seronegative vaccine recipients, and 2% of vaccine recipients develop a transient rash. Mild transient thrombocytopenia has been reported, with an incidence of ~1 case per 40,000 doses of MMR vaccine.

Since the publication of a report in 1998 hypothesizing that MMR vaccine may cause a syndrome of autism and intestinal inflammation, much public attention has focused on this purported association. The events that followed publication of this report led to diminished vaccine coverage in the United Kingdom and provide important lessons in the misinterpretation of epidemiologic evidence and the communication of scientific results to the public. The publication that incited the concern was a case series describing 12 children with a regressive developmental disorder and chronic enterocolitis; 9 of these children had autism. In 8 of the 12 cases, the parents associated onset of the developmental delay with MMR vaccination. This simple temporal association was misinterpreted and misrepresented as a possible causal relationship, first by the lead author of the study and then by elements of the media and the public. Subsequently, several comprehensive reviews and additional epidemiologic studies refuted evidence of a causal relationship between MMR vaccination and autism.

PROSPECTS FOR MEASLES ERADICATION

Progress in global measles control has renewed discussion of measles eradication. In contrast to poliovirus eradication, the eradication of measles virus will not entail challenges posed by prolonged shedding of potentially virulent vaccine viruses and environmental viral reservoirs. However, in comparison with smallpox eradication, higher levels of population immunity will be necessary to interrupt measles virus transmission, more highly skilled health care workers will be required to administer measles vaccines, and containment through case detection and ring vaccination will be more difficult for measles virus because of infectivity before rash onset. New tools, such as aerosol administration of measles vaccines, will facilitate mass vaccination campaigns. Despite enormous progress, measles remains a leading vaccine-preventable cause of childhood mortality worldwide and continues to cause outbreaks in communities with low vaccination coverage rates in industrialized nations.

FURTHER READINGS

AMERICAN ACADEMY OF PEDIATRICS: Measles, in *Red Book: 2009 Report of the Committee on Infectious Diseases*, 28th ed, LK Pickering et al (eds). Elk Grove Village, IL, American Academy of Pediatrics, 2009, pp 444–455

DESTEFANO F, THOMPSON WW: MMR vaccine and autism: An update of the scientific evidence. Expert Rev Vaccines 3:19, 2004

DUKE T, MGONE CS: Measles: Not just another viral exanthem. Lancet 361:763, 2003

FEIKIN DR et al: Individual and community risks of measles and pertussis associated with personal exemptions to immunization. JAMA 284:3145, 2000

GERBER JS, OFFIT PA: Vaccines and autism: A tale of shifting hypotheses. Clin Infect Dis 48:456, 2009

GRIFFIN DE et al: Measles vaccines. Front Biosci 13:1352, 2008

MOSS WJ: Measles control and the prospect of eradication. Curr Top Microbiol Immunol 330:173, 2009

OMER SB et al: Vaccine refusal, mandatory immunization, and the risks of vaccine-preventable diseases. N Engl J Med 360:1981, 2009

WOLFSON LJ et al: Has the 2005 measles mortality reduction goal been achieved? A natural history modelling study. Lancet 369:191, 2007

WORLD HEALTH ORGANIZATION: Measles vaccines. Wkly Epidemiol Rec 84:349, 2009

CHAPTER **193**

Rubella (German Measles)

Laura A. Zimmerman
Susan E. Reef

Rubella was historically viewed as a variant of measles or scarlet fever. Not until the mid-1900s was a separate viral agent for rubella isolated. After an epidemic of rubella in Australia in the early 1940s, the ophthalmologist Norman Gregg noticed the occurrence of congenital cataracts among infants whose mothers had reported rubella infection during early pregnancy, and congenital rubella syndrome (CRS) was first described.

■ ETIOLOGY

Rubella virus is a member of the Togaviridae family and the only member of the genus *Rubivirus*. This single-stranded RNA enveloped virus measures 50–70 nm in diameter. Its core protein is surrounded by a single-layer lipoprotein envelope with spike-like projections containing two glycoproteins, E1 and E2. There is only one antigenic type of rubella virus, and humans are its only known reservoir.

■ PATHOGENESIS AND PATHOLOGY

Although the pathogenesis of postnatal (acquired) rubella has been well documented, data on pathology are limited because of the mildness of the disease. Rubella virus is spread from person to person via respiratory droplets. Primary implantation and replication in the nasopharynx are followed by spread to the lymph nodes. Subsequent viremia occurs, which in pregnant women often results in infection of the placenta. Placental virus replication may lead to infection of fetal organs. The pathology of CRS in the infected fetus is well defined, with almost all organs found to be infected; however, the pathogenesis of CRS is only poorly delineated. In tissue, infections with rubella virus have diverse effects, ranging from no obvious impact to cell destruction. The hallmark of fetal infection is chronicity, with persistence throughout fetal development in utero and for up to 1 year after birth.

Individuals with acquired rubella may shed virus from 7 days before rash onset to ~5–7 days thereafter. Both clinical and subclinical infections are considered contagious. Infants with CRS may shed large quantities of virus from bodily secretions, particularly from the throat and in the urine, up to 1 year of age. Outbreaks of rubella, including some in nosocomial settings, have originated with index cases of CRS. Thus only individuals immune to rubella should have contact with infants who have CRS or who are congenitally infected with rubella virus but are not showing signs of CRS.

■ EPIDEMIOLOGY

The largest recent rubella epidemic in the United States took place in 1964–1965, when an estimated 12.5 million cases occurred, resulting in ~20,000 cases of CRS. Since the introduction of the routine rubella vaccination program in the United States in 1969, the number of rubella cases reported each year has dropped by

>99%; the rate of vaccination coverage with rubella-containing vaccine has been >90% among children 19–35 months old since 1995 and >95% for kindergarten and first-grade entrants since 1980. In 1989 a goal for the elimination of rubella and CRS in the United States was set, and in 2004 a panel of experts agreed unanimously that rubella was no longer an endemic disease in this country. The criteria used to document lack of endemic transmission included low disease incidence, high nationwide rubella antibody seroprevalence, outbreaks that were few and contained (i.e., small numbers of cases), and lack of endemic virus transmission (as assessed by genetic sequencing). In the United States, interruption of endemic transmission of rubella virus has been sustained since 2001.

Although rubella and CRS are no longer endemic in the United States, they remain important public health problems globally. The number of rubella cases reported worldwide in 1999 was ~900,000; this figure declined steadily to 165,000 in 2007. However, numbers of rubella cases are substantially underestimated because cases in many countries are identified through measles surveillance systems that are not specific for rubella. In developing countries, an estimated 110,000 cases of CRS occur during nonepidemic years.

■ CLINICAL FEATURES

Acquired rubella

Acquired rubella is characterized by a generalized maculopapular rash that usually lasts for up to 3 days (Fig. 193-1). Up to 50% of rubella virus infections may be subclinical or inapparent. The rash is usually mild and may be difficult to detect in persons with darker skin. In children, rash is usually the first sign of illness. However, in older children and adults, a 1- to 5-day prodrome often precedes the rash and may include low-grade fever, malaise, and upper respiratory symptoms. The incubation period is 14 days (range, 12–23 days).

Lymphadenopathy, particularly occipital and postauricular, may be noted during the second week after exposure. Although

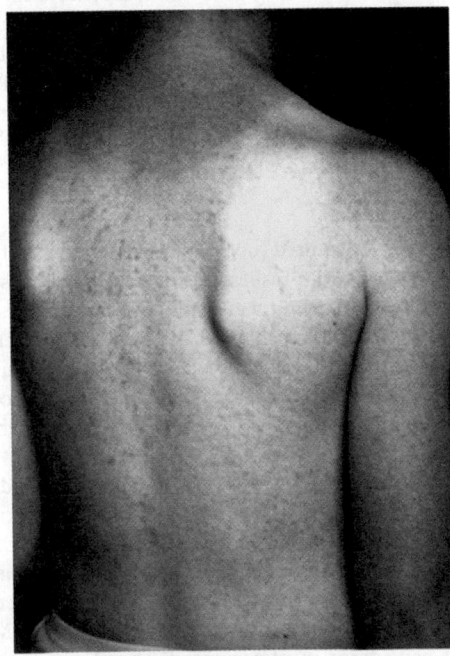

Figure 193-1   Mild maculopapular rash of rubella in a child.

TABLE 193-1 Common Transient and Permanent Manifestations in Infants With Congenital Rubella Syndrome

Transient Manifestations	Permanent Manifestations
Hepatosplenomegaly	Hearing impairment/deafness
Interstitial pneumonitis	Congenital heart defects (patent ductus arteriosus, pulmonary arterial stenosis)
Thrombocytopenia with purpura/petechiae (e.g., dermal erythropoiesis, or "blueberry muffin syndrome")	Eye defects (cataracts, cloudy cornea, microphthalmos, pigmentary retinopathy, congenital glaucoma)
Hemolytic anemia	
Bony radiolucencies	
Intrauterine growth retardation	Microcephaly
Adenopathy	
Meningoencephalitis	Central nervous system sequelae (mental and motor delay, autism)

acquired rubella is usually thought of as a benign disease, arthralgia and arthritis are common in infected adults, particularly women. Thrombocytopenia and encephalitis are less common complications.

Congenital rubella syndrome

The most serious consequence of rubella virus infection can develop when a woman becomes infected during pregnancy, particularly during the first trimester. The resulting complications may include miscarriage, fetal death, premature delivery, or live birth with congenital defects. Infants infected with rubella virus in utero may have a myriad of physical defects (Table 193-1), which most commonly relate to the eyes, ears, and heart. This constellation of severe birth defects is known as *congenital rubella syndrome*. In addition to permanent manifestations, there are a host of transient physical manifestations, including thrombocytopenia with purpura/petechiae (e.g., dermal erythropoiesis, "blueberry muffin syndrome"). Some infants may be born with congenital rubella virus infection but have no apparent signs or symptoms of CRS and are referred to as infants with congenital rubella infection only.

■ DIAGNOSIS

Acquired rubella

Clinical diagnosis of acquired rubella is difficult because of the mimicry of many illnesses with rashes, the varied clinical presentations, and the high rates of subclinical and mild disease. Illnesses that may be similar to rubella in presentation include scarlet fever, roseola, toxoplasmosis, fifth disease, measles, and illnesses with suboccipital and postauricular lymphadenopathy. Thus laboratory documentation of rubella virus infection is considered the only reliable way to confirm acute disease.

Laboratory assessment of rubella infection is conducted by serologic and virologic methods. For acquired rubella, serologic diagnosis is most common and depends on the demonstration of IgM antibodies in an acute-phase serum specimen or a fourfold rise in IgG antibody titer between acute- and convalescent-phase specimens. The enzyme-linked immunosorbent assay IgM capture technique is considered most accurate for serologic diagnosis, but the indirect IgM assay is also acceptable. After rubella virus infection,

IgM antibody may be detectable for up to 6 weeks. In case of a negative result for IgM in specimens taken earlier than day 5 after rash onset, serologic testing should be repeated. Although uncommon, reinfection with rubella virus is possible, and IgM antibodies may be present. To detect a rise in IgG antibody titer indicative of acute disease, the acute-phase serum specimen should be collected within 7–10 days after onset of illness and the convalescent-phase specimen ~14–21 days after the first specimen.

IgG avidity testing is used in conjunction with IgG testing. Low-avidity antibodies indicate recent infection. Mature (high-avidity) IgG antibodies most likely indicate an infection occurring at least 2 months previously. This test helps distinguish primary infection from reinfection.

Rubella virus can be isolated from the blood and nasopharynx during the prodromal period and for as long as 2 weeks after rash onset. However, as the secretion of virus in individuals with acquired rubella is maximal just before or up to 4 days after rash onset, this is the optimal time frame for collecting specimens for viral cultures. Rubella RNA detection by reverse-transcriptase polymerase chain reaction (RT-PCR) is a more recently developed technique for rubella diagnosis.

Congenital rubella syndrome

A clinical diagnosis of CRS is reasonable when an infant presents with a combination of cataracts, hearing impairment, and heart defects; this pattern is seen in ~10% of infants with CRS. However, as with acquired rubella, laboratory diagnosis of congenital infection is highly recommended, particularly because most features of the clinical presentation are nonspecific and may be associated with other intrauterine infections. Early diagnosis of CRS facilitates appropriate medical intervention for specific disabilities and prompts implementation of infection control measures.

Diagnostic tests used to confirm CRS include serologic assays and virus isolation. In an infant with congenital infection, serum IgM antibodies may be present for up to 1 year after birth. In some instances, IgM may not be detectable until 1 month of age; thus infants who have symptoms consistent with CRS but who test negative shortly after birth should be retested at 1 month. A rubella serum IgG titer persisting beyond the time expected after passive transfer of maternal IgG antibody (i.e., a rubella titer that does not decline at the expected rate of a twofold dilution per month) is another serologic criterion used to confirm CRS.

In congenital infection, rubella virus is isolated most commonly from throat swabs and less commonly from urine and cerebrospinal fluid. Infants with congenital rubella may excrete virus for up to 1 year, but specimens for virus isolation are most likely to be positive if obtained within the first 6 months after birth. Rubella virus in infants with CRS can also be detected by RT-PCR.

Rubella diagnosis in pregnant women

In the United States, screening for rubella IgG antibodies is recommended as part of routine prenatal care. Pregnant women with a positive IgG antibody serologic test are considered immune. Susceptible pregnant women should be vaccinated postpartum.

A susceptible pregnant woman exposed to rubella virus should be tested for IgM antibodies and a fourfold rise in IgG antibody titer between acute- and convalescent-phase serum specimens to determine whether she was infected during pregnancy. Pregnant women with evidence of acute infection must be clinically monitored, and gestational age at the time of maternal infection must be determined to assess the possibility of risk to the fetus. Of women infected with rubella virus during the first 11 weeks of gestation, up to 90% deliver an infant with CRS; for maternal infection during the first 20 weeks of pregnancy, the CRS rate is 20%.

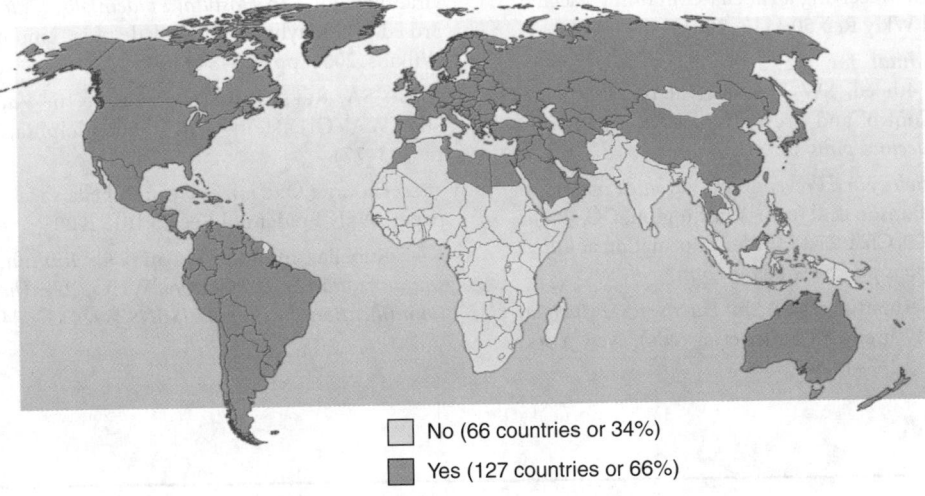

Figure 193-2 **Countries using rubella vaccine** in National Immunization Schedule, 2008. *(From the World Health Organization.)*

No (66 countries or 34%)

Yes (127 countries or 66%)

| TREATMENT | Rubella |

No specific therapy is available for rubella virus infection. Symptom-based treatment for various manifestations, such as fever and arthralgia, is appropriate. Immunoglobulin does not prevent rubella virus infection after exposure and therefore is not recommended as routine postexposure prophylaxis. Although immunoglobulin may modify or suppress symptoms, it can create an unwarranted sense of security: infants with congenital rubella have been born to women who received immunoglobulin shortly after exposure. Administration of immunoglobulin should be considered only if a pregnant woman who has been exposed to rubella will not consider termination of pregnancy under any circumstances. In such cases, IM administration of 20 mL of immunoglobulin within 72 h of rubella exposure may reduce—but does not eliminate—the risk of rubella.

▪ PREVENTION

After the isolation of rubella virus in the early 1960s and the occurrence of a devastating pandemic, a vaccine for rubella was developed and licensed in 1969. Currently, the majority of rubella-containing vaccines (RCVs) used worldwide are combined measles and rubella (MR) or measles, mumps, and rubella (MMR) formulations. A tetravalent measles, mumps, rubella, and varicella (MMRV) vaccine is available but is not widely used.

The public health burden of rubella infection is measured primarily through the resulting CRS cases. The 1964–1965 rubella epidemic in the United States encompassed >30,000 infections during pregnancy. CRS occurred in ~20,000 infants born alive, including >11,000 infants who were deaf, >3500 infants who were blind, and almost 2000 infants who were mentally retarded. The cost of the epidemic exceeded $1.5 billion. In 1982, it was estimated that the cost per child with CRS exceeded $200,000.

In most countries, there is little documented evidence to illuminate the epidemiology of CRS. Clusters of CRS cases have been reported in developing countries, and modeling studies have shown that, before the introduction of an immunization program, the incidence of CRS is 0.1–0.2 per 1000

live births during endemic periods and 1–4 per 1000 live births during epidemic periods. Where rubella virus is circulating and women of childbearing age are susceptible, CRS cases will continue to occur.

The most effective method of preventing acquired rubella and CRS is through vaccination with an RCV. One dose induces seroconversion in ≥95% of persons >1 year of age. Immunity is considered long-term and is probably lifelong. The most commonly used vaccine globally is derived from the RA27/3 virus strain. The current recommendation for routine rubella vaccination in the United States is a first dose of MMR vaccine at 12–15 months of age and a second dose at 4–6 years. Target groups for rubella vaccine in all countries include children >1 year of age, adolescents and adults without documented evidence of immunity, individuals in congregate settings (e.g., college students, military personnel, child care and health care workers), and susceptible women before and after pregnancy.

Because of the theoretical risk of transmission of live attenuated rubella vaccine virus to the developing fetus, women known to be pregnant should not receive an RCV. In addition, pregnancy should be avoided for 28 days after receipt of an RCV. In follow-up studies of 680 unknowingly pregnant women who received rubella vaccine, no infant was born with CRS. Receipt of an RCV during pregnancy is not ordinarily a reason to consider termination of the pregnancy.

As of 2008, 127 (66%) of the 193 WHO member countries recommended inclusion of an RCV in the routine childhood vaccination schedule (Fig. 193-2). Vaccination coverage varies widely among the member countries, with the European and American Regions reporting coverage of >90%. Goals for control or elimination of rubella and CRS have been established in the American Region, the European Region, and the Western Pacific Region. The other three regions (Eastern Mediterranean, South East Asian, and African) have not yet set such goals.

FURTHER READINGS

CENTERS FOR DISEASE CONTROL AND PREVENTION: Control and prevention of rubella: Evaluation and management of suspected outbreaks, rubella in pregnant women, and surveillance for congenital rubella syndrome. MMWR Morb Mortal Wkly Rep 50:1, 2001

———: Notice to readers: Revised ACIP recommendation for avoiding pregnancy after receiving a rubella-containing vaccine. MMWR Morb Mortal Wkly Rep 50:1117, 2001

———: Rubella, in *Manual for the Surveillance of Vaccine-Preventable Diseases*, 4th ed, SW Roush et al (eds). Atlanta, Centers for Disease Control and Prevention, 2008, Chapter 14 (*http://www.cdc.gov/vaccines/pubs/surv-manual/*)

———: Rubella, in *Epidemiology and Prevention of Vaccine Preventable Diseases*, 11th ed, W Atkinson et al (eds). Washington, DC, Public Health Foundation, 2009, Chapter 18 (order information at *http://www.cdc.gov/vaccines/pubs/pinkbook/default.htm*)

GERSHON A: Rubella (German measles), in *Harrison's Principles of Internal Medicine*, 17th ed, AS Fauci et al (eds). New York, McGraw Hill, 2009, pp 1217–1220

PAPANIA M et al: Nosocomial measles, mumps, rubella, and other viral infections, in *Hospital Epidemiology and Infection Control*, 3rd ed, CG Mayhall (ed). Philadelphia, Lippincott Williams and Wilkins, 2004, pp 828–849

PLOTKIN SA, REEF S: Rubella vaccine, in *Vaccines*, SA Plotkin and WA Orenstein (eds). Philadelphia, Saunders, 2008, pp 733–771

WORLD HEALTH ORGANIZATION: Rubella vaccines: WHO position paper. Wkly Epidemiol Rec 75:161, 2000

———: Rubella, module 11, in *The Immunological Basis for Immunization Series*. Geneva, WHO, 2009 (*http://www.who.int/immunization/documents/ISBN9789241596848/en/index.html*)

CHAPTER 194

Mumps

Steven Rubin
Kathryn M. Carbone

■ DEFINITION

Mumps is an acute, systemic viral infection classically associated with swelling of one or both parotid glands.

■ ETIOLOGIC AGENT

Mumps is caused by a paramyxovirus with a negative-strand non-segmented RNA genome of 15,384 bases encoding nine proteins. The nucleoprotein, phosphoprotein, and polymerase protein participate in viral replication and, together with genomic RNA, form the ribonucleocapsid. The ribonucleocapsid is surrounded by a host-derived lipid bilayer envelope containing the viral hemagglutinin-neuraminidase (HN) and fusion (F) proteins, which are responsible for cell binding by and entry of the virus and are major targets of virus-neutralizing antibodies. The functions of the other virus proteins (small-hydrophobic, matrix, V, and I) are less well understood. The small-hydrophobic gene sequence is highly variable and forms the basis for the 13 genotypes (A through M) used mainly for molecular epidemiologic purposes.

■ EPIDEMIOLOGY

Mumps is endemic worldwide, with epidemics occurring every 3–5 years in unvaccinated populations. The estimated annual global incidence is 100–1000 cases per 100,000 population in countries without national mumps vaccination programs, where virtually the entire population has been infected by adulthood. Following the 1967 introduction of mumps vaccine in the United States, the reported number of cases declined; by 2001, this number had decreased from >150,000 to <300—a 99.8% reduction from prevaccine levels. In 2006, the United States experienced its largest mumps outbreak in more than 20 years, with 6584 reported cases. This outbreak was preceded by outbreaks in the United Kingdom (2004–2005) and followed by outbreaks in Canada. Compelling epidemiologic evidence links the genotype G virus to the outbreaks in all three countries. The majority of cases occurred in college students 18–23 years of age, most of whom had been vaccinated in early childhood. These outbreaks are probably the result of several coincident circumstances, including (1) situations promoting the spread of respiratory viruses among young adults (e.g., residence in college dormitories), (2) waning of vaccine immunity with time, (3) lack of endemically circulating wild-type virus to periodically boost vaccine-induced immune responses, and (4) continuing global epidemics of mumps (due either to lack of mumps vaccination programs or to low rates of mumps vaccination where such programs do exist). Whereas in the pre- and early postvaccine era mumps was historically a disease of childhood, the majority of U.S. cases now occur in previously vaccinated young adults.

■ PATHOGENESIS

Humans are the only natural hosts for mumps virus infection. The incubation period of mumps is ~19 days (range, 7–23 days). The virus is transmitted by the respiratory route via droplets, saliva, and fomites. Mumps virus is typically shed from 1 week before to 1 week after symptom onset, although this window appears to be narrower in vaccinated individuals. Persons are most contagious 1–2 days before onset of clinical symptoms. Primary replication occurs in the nasal mucosa or upper respiratory mucosal epithelium. Mononuclear cells and cells within regional lymph nodes can become infected; such infection facilitates the development of viremia and poses a risk for a wide array of acute inflammatory reactions. Classic sites of mumps virus replication include the salivary glands, testes, pancreas, ovaries, mammary glands, and central nervous system (CNS).

Little is known of the pathology of mumps since the disease is rarely fatal. The virus replicates well in glandular epithelium, but classic parotitis is not a necessary component of mumps infection. Affected glands contain perivascular and interstitial mononuclear cell infiltrates and exhibit hemorrhage with prominent edema. Necrosis of acinar and epithelial duct cells is evident in the salivary glands and in the germinal epithelium of the seminiferous tubules of the testes. The virus probably enters cerebrospinal fluid (CSF) through the choroid plexus or via transiting mononuclear cells during plasma viremia. Although relevant data are limited, typical mumps encephalitis appears to be secondary to respiratory spread and is probably a parainfectious process, as suggested by perivenous demyelination, perivascular mononuclear cell inflammation, and relative sparing of neurons. Although rare, presumed primary encephalitis has been associated with mumps virus isolation from brain tissue. Evidence of placental and intrauterine spread in pregnancy has been found in both early and late gestation.

■ CLINICAL MANIFESTATIONS

Up to half of mumps virus infections are asymptomatic or lead to nonspecific respiratory symptoms. Inapparent infections are more common in adults than in children. The prodrome of mumps consists of low-grade fever, malaise, myalgia, headache, and anorexia. Mumps parotitis—acute-onset unilateral or bilateral swelling of the parotid or other salivary glands lasting >2 days without another apparent cause—develops in 70–90% of symptomatic infections, usually within 24 h of prodromal symptoms but sometimes as long as 1 week thereafter. Parotitis is generally bilateral, although the two sides may not be involved synchronously. Unilateral involvement is documented in about one-third of cases. Swelling of the parotid is accompanied by tenderness and obliteration of the space between the earlobe and the angle of the mandible (Figs. 194-1 and 194-2). The patient frequently reports an earache and finds it difficult to eat, swallow, or talk. The orifice of Stensen's duct is commonly red and swollen. The submaxillary and sublingual glands are involved less often than the parotid gland and are almost never involved alone. Glandular swelling increases for a few days and then gradually subsides, disappearing within 1 week. Recurrent sialadenitis is a rare sequela of mumps parotitis. In ~6% of mumps cases, obstruction of lymphatic drainage secondary to bilateral salivary gland swelling may lead to presternal pitting edema, associated often with submandibular adenitis and rarely with the more life-threatening supraglottic edema.

Epididymo-orchitis is the next most common manifestation of mumps, developing in 15–30% of cases in postpubertal males, with bilateral involvement in 10–30% of those cases. Orchitis, accompanied by fever, typically occurs during the first week of parotitis but can develop up to 6 weeks after parotitis or in its absence. The testis is painful and tender and can be enlarged to several times its normal size; this condition usually resolves within 1 week. Testicular atrophy develops in one-half of affected men. Sterility after mumps is rare, although subfertility is estimated to occur in 13% of cases of unilateral orchitis and in 30–87% of cases of bilateral orchitis. Oophoritis occurs in ~5% of women with mumps and may be associated with lower abdominal pain and vomiting but has only rarely been associated with sterility or premature menopause. Mumps infection in postpubertal women may also present with mastitis.

Documented CSF pleocytosis indicates that mumps virus invades the CNS in ~50% of cases; however, symptomatic CNS disease,

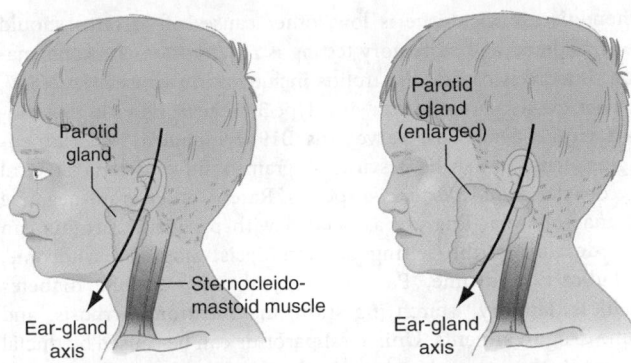

Figure 194-2 Schematic drawing of a parotid gland infected with mumps virus (*right*) compared with a normal gland (*left*). An enlarged cervical lymph node is usually posterior to the imaginary line. *(Reprinted with permission from Gershon A et al: Mumps, in* Krugman's Infectious Diseases of Children, *11th ed. Philadelphia, Elsevier, 2004, p 392.)*

typically in the form of aseptic meningitis, occurs in <10% of cases, with a male predominance. CNS symptoms of aseptic meningitis (e.g., stiff neck, headache, and drowsiness) appear ~5 days after parotitis and also occur often in the absence of parotid involvement. Within the first 24 h polymorphonuclear leukocytes may predominate in CSF (1000–2000 cells/μL), but by the second day nearly all the cells are lymphocytes. The glucose level in CSF may be low and the protein concentration high, a pattern reminiscent of bacterial meningitis. Mumps meningitis is a self-limited manifestation without significant risk of death or long-term sequelae. Cranial nerve palsies have occasionally led to permanent sequelae, particularly deafness. The reported incidence of mumps-associated hearing loss varies between 1 in 1000 and 1 in 100,000. In ~0.1% of infections, mumps virus may cause encephalitis, which presents as high fever with marked changes in the level of consciousness, seizures, and focal neurologic symptoms. Electroencephalographic abnormalities may be seen. Permanent sequelae are sometimes identified in survivors, and adult infections more commonly have poor outcomes than do pediatric infections. The mortality rate associated with mumps encephalitis is ~1.5%. Other CNS problems occasionally associated with mumps include cerebellar ataxia, facial palsy, transverse myelitis, hydrocephalus, Guillain-Barré syndrome, flaccid paralysis, and behavioral changes.

Mumps pancreatitis, which may present as abdominal pain, occurs in ~4% of infections but is difficult to diagnose because an elevated serum amylase level can be associated with either parotitis or pancreatitis. An etiologic association of mumps virus and juvenile diabetes mellitus remains controversial. Myocarditis and endocardial fibroelastosis are rare and self-limited but may represent severe complications of mumps infection; however, mumps-associated electrocardiographic abnormalities have been reported in up to 15% of cases. Other unusual complications include thyroiditis, nephritis, arthritis, hepatic disease, keratouveitis, and thrombocytopenic purpura. Abnormal renal function is common, but severe, life-threatening nephritis is rare. It remains at issue whether an excessive number of spontaneous abortions are associated with gestational mumps. Mumps in pregnancy does not appear to lead to premature birth, low birth weight, or fetal malformations.

■ DIFFERENTIAL DIAGNOSIS

During a mumps outbreak, the diagnosis is made easily in patients with parotitis and a history of recent exposure; however,

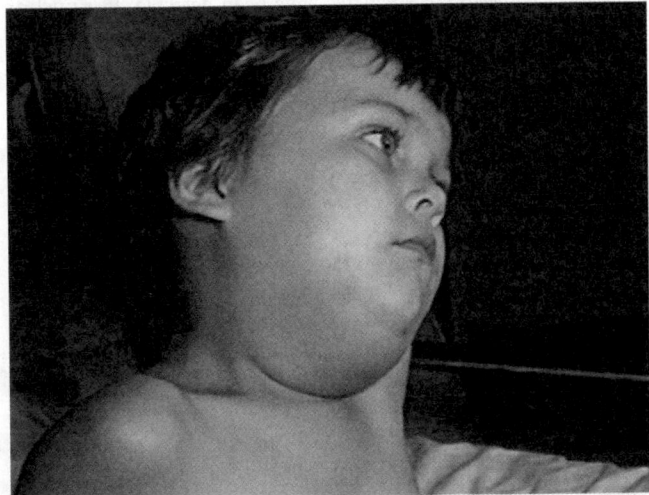

Figure 194-1 Child with mumps. Note the classic submandibular and preauricular enlargement of the parotid gland. *(From the Centers for Disease Control and Prevention.)*

when disease incidence is low, other causes of parotitis should be considered and laboratory testing is required for case confirmation. Infectious causes of parotitis include other viruses (e.g., HIV, coxsackievirus, parainfluenza virus type 3, influenza A virus, Epstein-Barr virus, adenovirus, parvovirus B19, lymphocytic choriomeningitis virus, human herpesvirus 6), gram-positive bacteria, atypical mycobacteria, and *Bartonella* species. Rarely, other gram-negative or anaerobic bacteria are associated with parotitis. Parotitis can also develop in the setting of sarcoidosis, Sjögren's syndrome, Mikulicz's syndrome, Parinaud's syndrome, uremia, diabetes mellitus, laundry starch ingestion, malnutrition, cirrhosis, and some drug treatments. Unilateral parotitis can be caused by ductal obstruction, cysts, and tumors. In the absence of parotitis or other salivary gland enlargement, symptoms of other visceral organ and/or CNS involvement may predominate, and a laboratory diagnosis is required. Other entities should be considered when manifestations consistent with mumps appear in organs other than the parotid. Testicular torsion may produce a painful scrotal mass resembling that seen in mumps orchitis. Other viruses (e.g., enteroviruses) may cause aseptic meningitis that is clinically indistinguishable from that due to mumps virus.

■ LABORATORY DIAGNOSIS

Laboratory diagnosis is based on detection of viral antigens or RNA or on serology. Viral antigens may be detected by mumps-specific immunofluorescent staining of clinical specimens either directly or, more commonly, after incubation of clinical samples with cell cultures. Most commonly, mumps virus is detected as viral RNA by reverse-transcription polymerase chain reaction (PCR), which is believed to be more rapid, sensitive, and specific than detection of live virus by immunofluorescence assays; however, false-negative results are not uncommon with either method. Virus is typically assayed in material obtained by throat swab, although it has been detected in CSF, urine, and seminal fluid. Despite the apparent frequency of viremia, mumps virus has only rarely been isolated from blood, possibly because of the presence of specific antibodies. In urine samples, presumed PCR inhibitors reduce the relative value of RNA testing methods.

Serologic diagnosis of mumps (i.e., a positive IgM response or a significant increase in IgG titer in paired acute- and convalescent-phase sera) is typically obtained by enzyme-linked immunosorbent assay (ELISA). Serologic diagnoses are now of limited value: IgM is detected in <20% of cases in immunized individuals, and IgG titers in convalescent-phase sera may be only nominally greater than those in acute-phase sera. Thus, at present, the capacity of RNA or viral antigen detection to confirm cases is much greater than that of serology. Traditional and labor-intensive serologic tests such as complement fixation, hemagglutination inhibition, and virus neutralization are now performed only rarely. The main downside to replacement of these functional serologic assays with the more rapid ELISA method is the latter's detection of all virus-specific antibodies, including those that are nonneutralizing (i.e., nonprotective). Thus, an individual may be seropositive by ELISA but may lack protective levels of antibody. While there is a strong association between the presence of mumps virus neutralizing antibody and protection from disease, an absolute antibody titer predictive of serologic protection is lacking; in this respect, mumps differs from other respiratory infections, such as measles.

■ PREVENTION

Vaccination is the only practical control measure; in the United States, the cost-benefit ratios for mumps vaccination alone are >13 for direct costs (e.g., medical expenses) and >24 for societal costs (including productivity losses for patients and caregivers). Several mumps virus vaccines are used throughout the world; in the United States, only the live attenuated Jeryl Lynn strain is used. Current recommendations are that mumps vaccine be administered as part of the combined trivalent measles-mumps-rubella vaccine (MMR-II®) or the quadrivalent measles-mumps-rubella-varicella vaccine (ProQuad®). Monovalent vaccine (MumpsVax®) is not generally available.

Before administering mumps-containing vaccine, physicians should always consult the latest recommendations from the Advisory Committee on Immunization Practices (ACIP). Current recommendations for children specify two doses of mumps-containing vaccine: the first dose on or after the first birthday and the second dose administered no earlier than 1 month after the first. In the United States, children often receive the second dose between the ages of 4 and 6 years.

In 2009, the ACIP revised its recommendations for evidence of mumps immunity in health care personnel to include (1) documented administration of two doses of a preparation containing live mumps vaccine, (2) laboratory evidence of immunity or laboratory confirmation of disease, or (3) birth date before 1957. For unvaccinated health care personnel born before 1957 who lack laboratory evidence of mumps immunity or laboratory confirmation of mumps, health care facilities should consider two doses of MMR vaccine at the appropriate interval; during a mumps outbreak, vaccination of these individuals is recommended.

Mumps vaccine contains live attenuated virus. It is not recommended for pregnant women, for individuals who have had a life-threatening allergic reaction to components of the vaccine, or for people in settings of clinically significant primary or secondary immunosuppression. (For details, see the ACIP guidelines on the website of the Centers for Disease Control and Prevention.) Occasionally, febrile reactions and parotitis have been reported soon after mumps vaccination. Allergic reactions after vaccination (e.g., rash and pruritus) are uncommon and are usually mild and self-limited. More serious complications, such as aseptic meningitis, have been causally associated with certain vaccine strains but not with the Jeryl Lynn strain.

Immunity to mumps is associated with the development of neutralizing antibody, although a specific correlate of protection has not been established. Seroconversion occurs in ~95% of recipients of the Jeryl Lynn strain; however, vaccine efficacy is ~80% for one dose and 90% for two doses. Recent data indicate declining seropositivity rates with time since vaccination. Although it is generally accepted that mumps virus is serologically monotypic, antigenic differences between virus isolates have been detected. It is unclear whether such differences can lead to immune escape. The role of the cellular arm of the immune response is unclear, but there is evidence that it may help limit virus spread and complications.

TREATMENT   Mumps

Mumps is generally a benign, self-resolving illness. Therapy for parotitis and other clinical manifestations is symptom based and supportive. The administration of analgesics and the application of warm or cold compresses to the parotid area may be helpful. Testicular pain may be minimized by the local application of cold compresses and gentle support for the scrotum. Anesthetic blocks may also be used. Neither the administration of glucocorticoids nor incision of the tunica albuginea is of proven value in severe orchitis. Anecdotal information on a small number of patients with orchitis suggests that subcutaneous administration of interferon α2b may help preserve the organ and fertility. Lumbar puncture is occasionally performed to relieve headache associated with meningitis. Mumps immune globulin has not been consistently shown to be effective in preventing mumps and is not recommended for treatment or postexposure prophylaxis.

ACKNOWLEDGMENT
The authors thank and acknowledge Dr. Anne Gershon, the author of this chapter in earlier editions of this book.

FURTHER READINGS

DAVIDKIN I et al: Etiology of mumps-like illnesses in children and adolescents vaccinated for measles, mumps, and rubella. J Infect Dis 191:719, 2005

HUANG AS et al: Risk factors for mumps at a university with a large mumps outbreak. Public Health Rep 124:419, 2009

HVIID A et al: Mumps. Lancet 371:932, 2008

KUTTY PK et al: Guidance for isolation precautions for mumps in the United States: A review of the scientific basis of policy change. Clin Infect Dis 50:1619, 2010

LEBARON CW et al: Persistence of mumps antibodies after 2 doses of measles-mumps-rubella vaccine. J Infect Dis 199:552, 2009

MARIN M et al: Use of combination measles, mumps, rubella, and varicella vaccine: Recommendations of the Advisory Committee on Immunization Practices (ACIP). MMWR Recomm Rep 59:1, 2010

MASARANI M et al: Mumps orchitis. J R Soc Med 99:573, 2006

POLGREEN PM et al: The duration of mumps virus shedding after the onset of symptoms. Clin Infect Dis 46:1447, 2008

REID F et al: Epidemiologic and diagnostic evaluation of a recent mumps outbreak using oral fluid samples. J Clin Virol 41:134, 2008

ROTA JS et al: Investigation of a mumps outbreak among university students with two measles-mumps-rubella (MMR) vaccinations, Virginia, September–December 2006. J Med Virol 81:1819, 2009

CHAPTER **195**

Rabies and Other Rhabdovirus Infections

Alan C. Jackson

RABIES

Rabies is a rapidly progressive, acute infectious disease of the central nervous system (CNS) in humans and animals that is caused by infection with rabies virus. The infection is normally transmitted from animal vectors. Rabies has encephalitic and paralytic forms that progress to death.

■ ETIOLOGIC AGENT

Rabies virus is a member of the family Rhabdoviridae. Two genera in this family, *Lyssavirus* and *Vesiculovirus*, contain species that cause human disease. Rabies virus is a lyssavirus that infects a broad range of animals and causes serious neurologic disease when transmitted to humans. This single-strand RNA virus has a nonsegmented, negative-sense (antisense) genome that consists of 11,932 nucleotides and encodes five proteins: nucleocapsid protein, phosphoprotein, matrix protein, glycoprotein, and a large polymerase protein. Rabies virus variants, which can be characterized by distinctive nucleotide sequences, are associated with specific animal reservoirs. Five other nonrabies virus species in the *Lyssavirus* genus have been reported to cause a clinical picture similar to rabies. Vesicular stomatitis virus, a vesiculovirus, causes vesiculation and ulceration in cattle, horses, and other animals and causes a self-limited, mild, systemic illness in humans (see "Other Rhabdoviruses," below).

■ EPIDEMIOLOGY

 Rabies is a zoonotic infection that occurs in a variety of mammals throughout the world except in Antarctica and on some islands. Rabies virus is usually transmitted to humans by the bite of an infected animal. Canine rabies is endemic in many resource-poor and resource-limited countries and continues to be a threat to humans, particularly in Asia and Africa (see "Global Considerations," below); endemic canine rabies has been eliminated from the United States and most other resource-rich countries. Rabies is endemic in wildlife species, and a variety of animal reservoirs have been identified in different countries. Surveillance data from 2008 identified 6841 confirmed animal cases of rabies in the United States (including Puerto Rico). Only 7% of these cases were in domestic animals, including 294 cases in cats, 75 in dogs, and 59 in cattle. North American wildlife reservoirs, including bats, raccoons, skunks, and foxes, have endemic infection, with involvement of one or more rabies virus variants in each species (Fig. 195-1). "Spillover" of rabies to other wildlife species and to domestic animals occurs. Bat rabies virus variants are present in every state except Hawaii and are responsible for most indigenously acquired human rabies cases in the United States. Raccoon rabies is endemic along the entire eastern coast of the United States. Skunk rabies is present in the midwestern states, with another focus in California. Rabies in foxes occurs in Texas, New Mexico, Arizona, and Alaska.

Rabies virus variants isolated from humans or other mammalian species can be identified by reverse-transcription polymerase chain reaction (RT-PCR) amplification and sequencing or by characterization with monoclonal antibodies. These techniques are helpful in human cases with no known history of an exposure. Worldwide, most human rabies is transmitted from dogs in countries with endemic canine rabies and dog-to-dog transmission, and human cases can be imported by travelers returning from these regions. In North America, human disease is usually associated with transmission from bats; there may be no known history of bat bite or other bat exposure in these cases. Most human cases are due to a bat rabies virus variant associated with silver-haired and eastern pipistrelle bats. These are small bats whose bite may not be recognized, and the virus has adapted for replication at skin temperature and in cell types that are present in the skin.

Transmission from nonbite exposures is relatively uncommon. Aerosols generated in the laboratory or in caves containing millions of Brazilian free-tail bats have rarely caused human rabies. Transmission has resulted from corneal transplantation and recently from solid organ transplantation and from a vascular

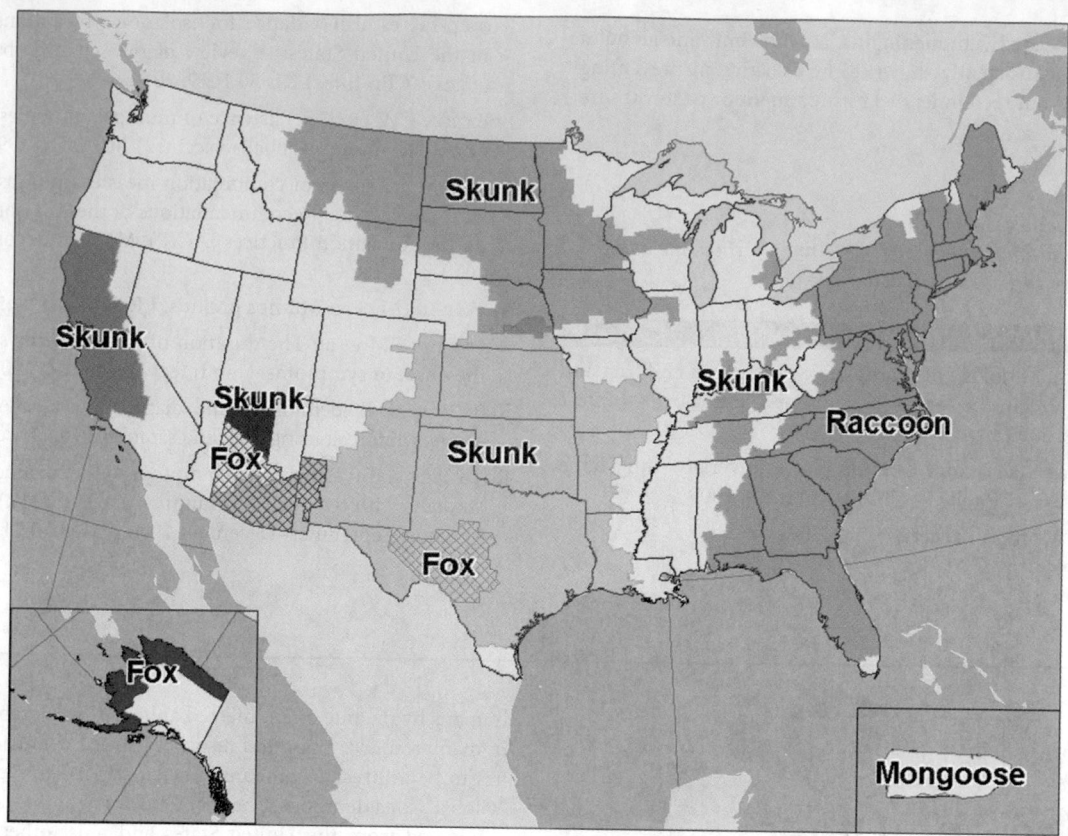

Figure 195-1 Distribution of the major rabies virus variants among wild terrestrial reservoirs in the United States and Puerto Rico, 2008. *(From JD Blanton et al: J Am Vet Med Assoc 235:676, 2009, Centers for Disease Control and Prevention.)*

conduit (for a liver transplant) from undiagnosed donors with rabies in Texas and Germany. Human-to-human transmission is extremely rare, although theoretical concern about transmission to health care workers has prompted the implementation of barrier techniques to prevent exposures.

■ PATHOGENESIS

The incubation period of rabies (defined as the interval between exposure and the onset of clinical disease) is usually 20–90 days but in rare cases is as short as a few days or is >1 year. During most of the incubation period, rabies virus is thought to be present at or close to the site of inoculation (Fig. 195-2). In muscles, the virus is known to bind to nicotinic acetylcholine receptors on postsynaptic membranes at neuromuscular junctions, but the exact details of viral entry into the skin and subcutaneous tissues have not yet been clarified. Rabies virus spreads centripetally along peripheral nerves toward the CNS at a rate up to ~250 mm/d via retrograde fast axonal transport to the spinal cord or brainstem. There is no well-documented evidence for hematogenous spread of rabies virus. Once the virus enters the CNS, it rapidly disseminates to other regions of the CNS via fast axonal transport along neuroanatomic connections. Neurons are prominently infected in rabies; infection of astrocytes is unusual. After CNS infection becomes established, there is centrifugal spread along sensory and autonomic nerves to other tissues, including the salivary glands, heart, adrenal glands, and skin. Rabies virus replicates in acinar cells of the salivary glands and is secreted in the saliva of rabid animals that serve as vectors of the disease.

Pathologic studies show mild inflammatory changes in the CNS in rabies, with mononuclear inflammatory infiltration in the leptomeninges, perivascular regions, and parenchyma, including microglial nodules called *Babes nodules*. Degenerative neuronal changes usually are not prominent, and there is little

evidence of neuronal death; neuronophagia is observed occasionally. The pathologic changes are surprisingly mild in light of the clinical severity and fatal outcome of the disease. The most characteristic pathologic finding in rabies is the *Negri body* (Fig. 195-3). Negri bodies are eosinophilic cytoplasmic inclusions in brain neurons that are composed of rabies virus proteins and viral RNA. These inclusions occur in a minority of infected neurons, are commonly observed in Purkinje cells of the cerebellum and in pyramidal neurons of the hippocampus, and are less frequently seen in cortical and brainstem neurons. Negri bodies are not observed in all cases of rabies. The lack of prominent degenerative neuronal changes has led to the concept that neuronal dysfunction—rather than neuronal death—is responsible for clinical disease in rabies. The basis for behavioral changes, including the aggressive behavior of rabid animals, is not well understood.

■ CLINICAL MANIFESTATIONS

In rabies, the emphasis must be on postexposure prophylaxis initiated before any symptoms or signs develop. Rabies should usually be suspected on the basis of the clinical presentation. The disease usually presents as an atypical encephalitis with relative preservation of consciousness. Rabies may be difficult to recognize late in the clinical course when progression to coma has occurred. A minority of patients present with acute flaccid paralysis. There are prodromal, acute neurologic, and comatose phases that usually progress to death despite aggressive therapy (Table 195-1).

Prodromal features

The earliest clinical features of rabies begin with nonspecific prodromal manifestations, including fever, malaise, headache, nausea, and vomiting. Anxiety or agitation may also occur. The earliest

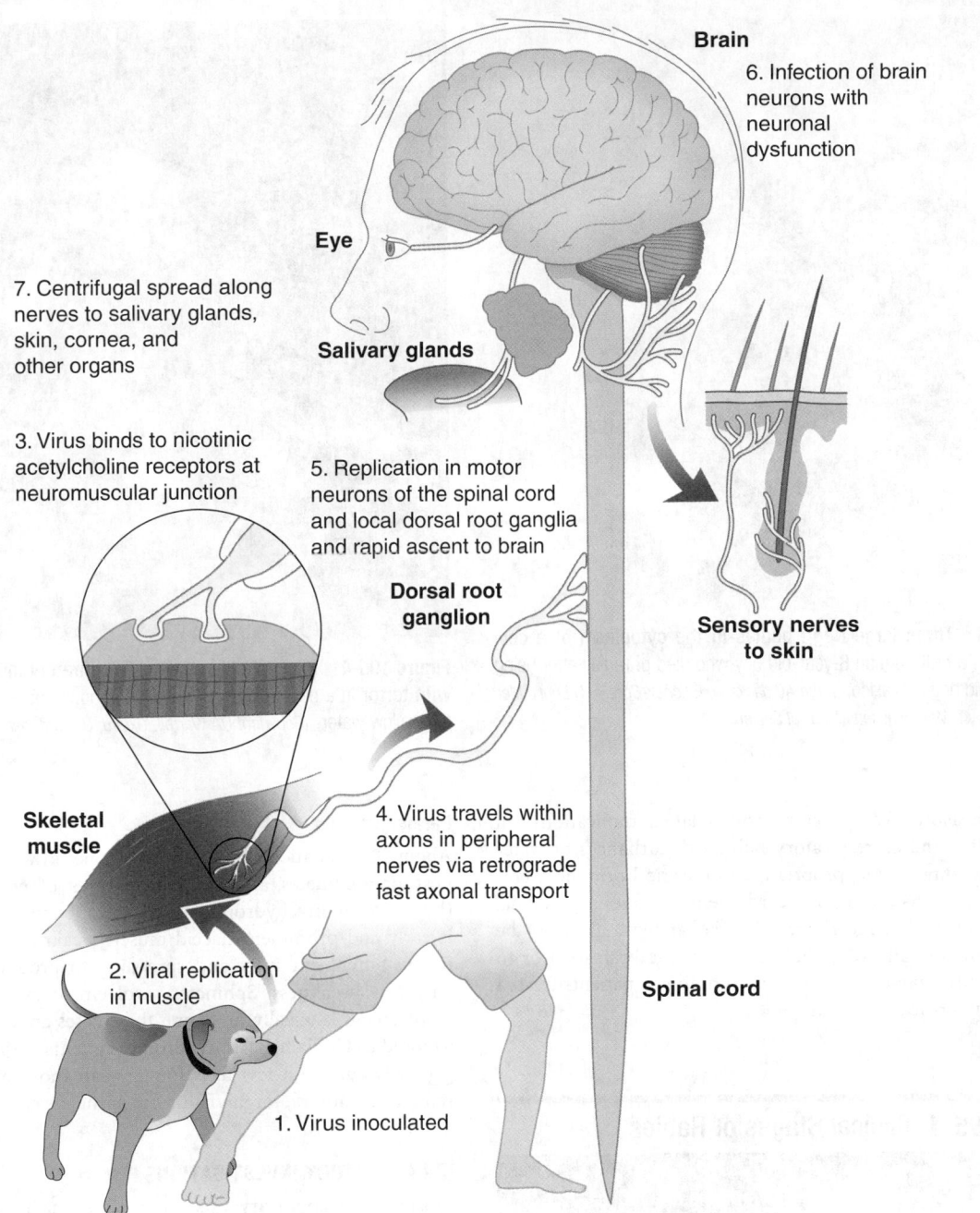

Figure 195-2 **Schematic representation of the pathogenetic events** following peripheral inoculation of rabies virus. *(Adapted from Jackson AC: Human disease, in Rabies, AC Jackson, WH Wunner (eds), San Diego, Academic Press, 2002, pp 219–244; with permission.)*

The figure includes the following labeled steps:

- **Brain** — 6. Infection of brain neurons with neuronal dysfunction
- **Eye**
- 7. Centrifugal spread along nerves to salivary glands, skin, cornea, and other organs
- **Salivary glands**
- 3. Virus binds to nicotinic acetylcholine receptors at neuromuscular junction
- 5. Replication in motor neurons of the spinal cord and local dorsal root ganglia and rapid ascent to brain
- **Dorsal root ganglion**
- **Sensory nerves to skin**
- **Skeletal muscle**
- 4. Virus travels within axons in peripheral nerves via retrograde fast axonal transport
- 2. Viral replication in muscle
- **Spinal cord**
- 1. Virus inoculated

specific neurologic symptoms of rabies include paresthesias, pain, or pruritus near the site of the exposure, which occurs in 50–80% of patients and strongly suggests rabies. The wound has usually healed by this point, and these symptoms probably reflect infection with associated inflammatory changes in local dorsal root or cranial sensory ganglia.

Encephalitic rabies

Two acute neurologic forms of rabies are seen in humans: encephalitic (furious) in 80% and paralytic in 20%. Some of the manifestations of encephalitic rabies may be seen in other viral encephalitides as well. These features include fever, confusion, hallucinations, combativeness, and seizures. Autonomic dysfunction is common and may result in hypersalivation, gooseflesh, cardiac arrhythmia, and priapism. In encephalitic rabies, episodes of hyperexcitability are typically followed by periods of complete lucidity that become shorter as the disease progresses. Rabies encephalitis is distinguished by early brainstem involvement, which results in the classic features of hydrophobia (involuntary, painful contraction of the diaphragm and accessory respiratory, laryngeal, and pharyngeal muscles in response to swallowing liquids) and aerophobia (the same features caused by stimulation from a draft of air). These symptoms are probably due to dysfunction of infected brainstem neurons that normally inhibit inspiratory neurons near the nucleus ambiguus, resulting in exaggerated defense reflexes that protect the respiratory tract. The combination of hypersalivation and pharyngeal dysfunction is also responsible for the classic appearance of "foaming at the mouth" (Fig. 195-4). Brainstem dysfunction progresses rapidly, and coma followed within days by death is the rule unless the course is prolonged by

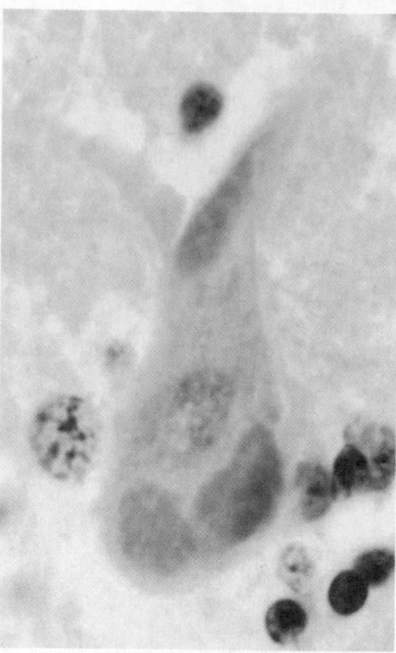

Figure 195-3 **Three large Negri bodies in the cytoplasm of a cerebellar Purkinje cell** from an 8-year-old boy who died of rabies after being bitten by a rabid dog in Mexico. *(From AC Jackson, E Lopez-Corella: N Engl J Med 335:568, 1996. © Massachusetts Medical Society.)*

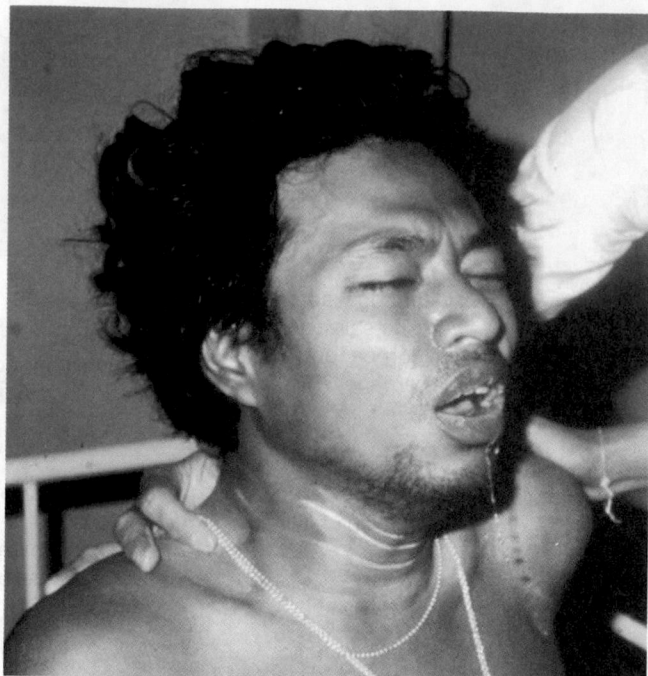

Figure 195-4 **Hydrophobic spasm of inspiratory muscles associated with terror** in a patient with encephalitic (furious) rabies who is attempting to swallow water. *(Copyright DA Warrell, Oxford, UK; with permission.)*

supportive measures. With such measures, late complications can include cardiac and/or respiratory failure, disturbances of water balance (syndrome of inappropriate antidiuretic hormone secretion or diabetes insipidus), noncardiogenic pulmonary edema, and gastrointestinal hemorrhage. Cardiac arrhythmias may be due to dysfunction affecting vital centers in the brainstem or to myocarditis. Multiple-organ failure is common in patients treated aggressively in critical care units.

TABLE 195-1 Clinical Stages of Rabies

Phase	Typical Duration	Symptoms and Signs
Incubation period	20–90 days	None
Prodrome	2–10 days	Fever, malaise, anorexia, nausea, vomiting, paresthesias, pain, or pruritus at the wound site
Acute neurologic disease		
Encephalitic (80%)	2–7 days	Anxiety, agitation, hyperactivity, bizarre behavior, hallucinations, autonomic dysfunction, hydrophobia
Paralytic (20%)	2–10 days	Flaccid paralysis in limb(s) progressing to quadriparesis with facial paralysis
Coma, death[a]	0–14 days	

[a]Recovery is rare.

Source: MAW Hattwick: Rabies virus, in *Principles and Practice of Infectious Diseases*, GL Mandell et al (eds). New York, Wiley, 1979, pp 1217–1228. Adapted with permission from Elsevier.

Paralytic rabies

About 20% of patients have paralytic rabies in which muscle weakness predominates and cardinal features of encephalitic rabies (hyperexcitability, hydrophobia, and aerophobia) are lacking. There is early and prominent flaccid muscle weakness, often beginning in the bitten extremity and spreading to produce quadriparesis and facial weakness. Sphincter involvement is common, sensory involvement is usually mild, and these cases are commonly misdiagnosed as Guillain-Barré syndrome. Patients with paralytic rabies generally survive a few days longer than those with encephalitic rabies, but multiple-organ failure nevertheless ensues.

■ LABORATORY INVESTIGATIONS

Most routine laboratory tests in rabies yield normal results or show nonspecific abnormalities. Complete blood counts are usually normal. Examination of cerebrospinal fluid (CSF) often reveals mild mononuclear cell pleocytosis with a mildly elevated protein level. Severe pleocytosis (>1000 white cells/μL) is unusual and should prompt a search for an alternative diagnosis. CT head scans are usually normal in rabies. MRI brain scans may show signal abnormalities in the brainstem or other gray-matter areas, but these findings are variable and nonspecific. Electroencephalograms show only nonspecific abnormalities. Of course, important tests in suspected cases of rabies include those that may identify an alternative, potentially treatable diagnosis (see "Differential Diagnosis," below).

■ DIAGNOSIS

In North America, a diagnosis of rabies often is not considered until relatively late in the clinical course, even with a typical clinical presentation. This diagnosis should be considered in patients presenting with acute atypical encephalitis or acute flaccid paralysis, including those in whom Guillain-Barré syndrome is suspected. The absence of an animal-bite history is common in North

America. The lack of hydrophobia is not unusual in rabies. Once rabies is suspected, rabies-specific laboratory tests should be performed to confirm the diagnosis. Diagnostically useful specimens include serum, CSF, fresh saliva, skin biopsy samples from the neck, and brain tissue (rarely obtained before death). Because skin biopsy relies on the demonstration of rabies virus antigen in cutaneous nerves at the base of hair follicles, samples are usually taken from hairy skin at the nape of the neck. Corneal impression smears are of low diagnostic yield and are generally not performed. Negative antemortem rabies-specific laboratory tests never exclude a diagnosis of rabies, and tests may need to be repeated after an interval for diagnostic confirmation.

Rabies virus–specific antibodies

In a previously unimmunized patient, serum neutralizing antibodies to rabies virus are diagnostic. However, because rabies virus infects immunologically privileged neuronal tissues, serum antibodies may not develop until late in the disease. Antibodies may be detected within a few days after the onset of symptoms, but some patients die without detectable antibodies. The presence of rabies virus–specific antibodies in the CSF suggests rabies encephalitis, regardless of immunization status.

RT-PCR amplification

Detection of rabies virus RNA by RT-PCR is highly sensitive and specific. This technique can detect virus in fresh saliva samples, CSF, and skin and brain tissues. In addition, RT-PCR with genetic sequencing can distinguish among rabies virus variants, permitting identification of the probable source of an infection.

Direct fluorescent antibody testing

Direct fluorescent antibody (DFA) testing with rabies virus antibodies conjugated to fluorescent dyes is highly sensitive and specific and can be performed quickly and applied to skin biopsies and brain tissue. In skin biopsies, rabies virus antigen may be detected in cutaneous nerves at the base of hair follicles.

■ DIFFERENTIAL DIAGNOSIS

The diagnosis of rabies may be difficult without a history of animal exposure, and no exposure to an animal (e.g., a bat) may be recalled. The presentation of rabies is usually quite different from that of acute viral encephalitis due to most other causes, including herpes simplex encephalitis and arboviral (e.g., West Nile) encephalitis. Early neurologic symptoms may occur at the site of the bite, and there may be early features of brainstem involvement with preservation of consciousness. Postinfectious (immune-mediated) encephalomyelitis may follow influenza, measles, mumps, and other infections; it may also occur as a sequela of immunization with rabies vaccine derived from neural tissues, which are used only in resource-limited and resource-poor countries. Rabies may present with unusual neuropsychiatric symptoms and may be misdiagnosed as a psychiatric disorder. Rabies hysteria may occur as a psychological response to the fear of rabies and is often characterized by a shorter incubation period than rabies, aggressive behavior, inability to communicate, and a long course with recovery.

As previously mentioned, paralytic rabies may mimic Guillain-Barré syndrome. In these cases, fever, bladder dysfunction, a normal sensory examination, and CSF pleocytosis favor a diagnosis of rabies. Conversely, Guillain-Barré syndrome may occur as a complication of rabies vaccination with a neural tissue–derived product (e.g., suckling mouse brain vaccine) and may be mistaken for paralytic rabies (i.e., vaccine failure).

TREATMENT Rabies

There is no established treatment for rabies. There have been several recent treatment failures with the combination of antiviral drugs, ketamine, and therapeutic (induced) coma—measures that were used in a healthy survivor in whom antibodies to rabies virus were detected at presentation. Expert opinion should be sought before a course of experimental therapy is embarked upon. A palliative approach may be appropriate for some patients.

■ PROGNOSIS

Rabies is an almost uniformly fatal disease but is almost always preventable with appropriate postexposure therapy during the early incubation period (see below). There are seven well-documented cases of survival from rabies. All but one of these patients had received rabies vaccine before disease onset. The single survivor who had not received vaccine had neutralizing antibodies to rabies virus in serum and CSF at clinical presentation. Most patients with rabies die within several days of illness, despite aggressive care in a critical care unit.

■ PREVENTION

Postexposure prophylaxis

Since there is no effective therapy for rabies, it is extremely important to prevent the disease after an animal exposure. Figure 195-5 shows

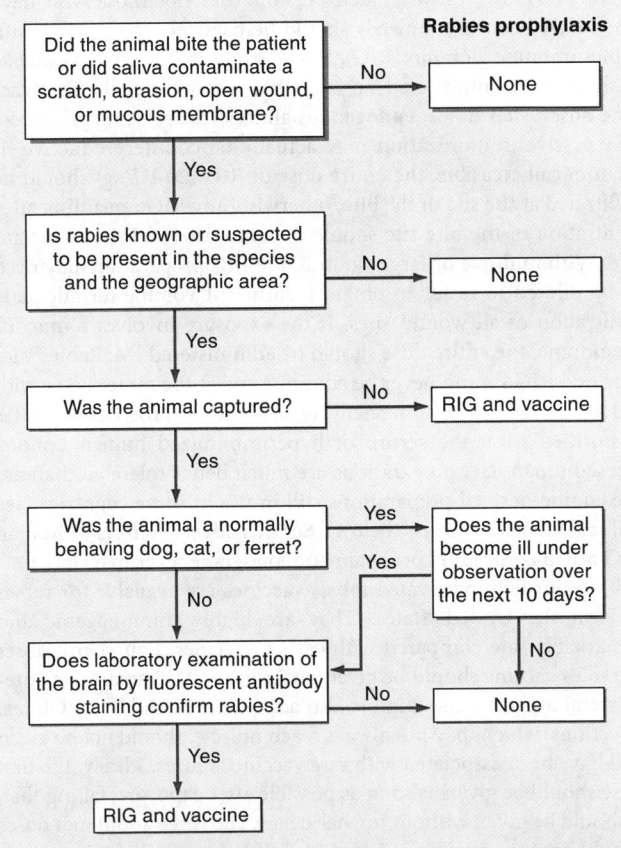

Figure 195-5 Algorithm for rabies postexposure prophylaxis. RIG, rabies immune globulin. *[From L Corey, in Harrison's Principles of Internal Medicine, 15th ed. E Braunwald et al (eds): New York, McGraw-Hill, 2001; adapted with permission.]*

the steps involved in making decisions about rabies postexposure prophylaxis (PEP). On the basis of the history of the exposure and local epidemiologic information, the physician must decide whether initiation of PEP is warranted. Healthy dogs, cats, or ferrets may be confined and observed for 10 days. PEP is not necessary if the animal remains healthy. If the animal develops signs of rabies during the observation period, it should be euthanized immediately, and the head should be transported to the laboratory under refrigeration and examined for the presence of rabies virus by DFA testing and viral isolation using cell culture and/or mouse inoculation. Any animal other than a dog, cat, or ferret should be euthanized immediately and the head submitted for laboratory examination. In high-risk exposures and in areas where canine rabies is endemic, rabies prophylaxis should be initiated without waiting for laboratory results. If the laboratory results prove to be negative, it may safely be concluded that the animal's saliva did not contain rabies virus, and immunization should be discontinued. If an animal escapes after an exposure, it must be considered rabid, and PEP must be initiated unless information from public health officials indicates otherwise (i.e., there is no endemic rabies in the area). PEP may be warranted in situations where a person (e.g., a small child or a sleeping adult) is present in the same space as a bat and an unrecognized bite cannot be reliably excluded.

PEP includes local wound care and both active and passive immunization. Local wound care is essential and may greatly decrease the risk of rabies virus infection. Wound care should not be delayed, even if the initiation of immunization is postponed pending the results of the 10-day observation period. All bite wounds and scratches should be washed thoroughly with soap and water. Devitalized tissues should be debrided, tetanus prophylaxis given, and antibiotic treatment initiated whenever indicated.

All previously unvaccinated persons (but not those who have previously been immunized) should be passively immunized with rabies immune globulin (RIG). If RIG is not immediately available, it should be administered no later than 7 days after the first vaccine dose. After day 7, endogenous antibodies are being produced, and passive immunization may actually be counterproductive. If anatomically feasible, the entire dose of RIG (20 IU/kg) should be infiltrated at the site of the bite; otherwise, any RIG remaining after infiltration of the bite site should be administered IM at a distant site. With multiple or large wounds, the RIG preparation may need to be diluted in order to obtain a sufficient volume for adequate infiltration of all wound sites. If the exposure involves a mucous membrane, the entire dose should be administered IM. Rabies vaccine and RIG should never be administered at the same site or with the same syringe. Commercially available RIG in the United States is purified from the serum of hyperimmunized human donors. These human RIG preparations are much better tolerated than are the equine-derived preparations still in use in some countries (see "Global Considerations," below). Serious adverse effects of human RIG are uncommon. Local pain and low-grade fever may occur.

Two purified inactivated rabies vaccines are available for rabies PEP in the United States. They are highly immunogenic and remarkably safe compared with earlier vaccines. Four 1-mL doses of rabies vaccine should be given IM in the deltoid area. (The anterolateral aspect of the thigh is also acceptable in children.) Gluteal injections, which may not always reach muscle, should not be given and have been associated with rare vaccine failures. Ideally, the first dose should be given as soon as possible after exposure; failing that, it should be given without further delay. The three additional doses should be given on days 3, 7, and 14; a fifth dose on day 28 is no longer recommended. Pregnancy is not a contraindication for immunization. Glucocorticoids and other immunosuppressive medications may interfere with the development of active immunity and should not be administered during PEP unless they are essential. Routine measurement of serum neutralizing antibody titers is not required, but titers should be measured 2–4 weeks after immunization in immunocompromised persons. Local reactions (pain, erythema, edema, and pruritus) and mild systemic reactions (fever, myalgias, headache, and nausea) are common; anti-inflammatory and antipyretic medications may be used, but immunization should not be discontinued. Systemic allergic reactions are uncommon, but anaphylaxis does occur rarely and can be treated with epinephrine and antihistamines. The risk of rabies development should be carefully considered before the decision is made to discontinue vaccination because of an adverse reaction.

Preexposure rabies vaccination

Preexposure rabies prophylaxis should be considered for people with an occupational or recreational risk of rabies exposures, including certain travelers to rabies-endemic areas. This primary schedule consists of three doses of rabies vaccine given on days 0, 7, and 21 or 28. Serum neutralizing antibody tests help determine the need for subsequent booster doses. When a previously immunized individual is exposed to rabies, two booster doses of vaccine should be administered on days 0 and 3. Wound care remains essential. As stated above, RIG should not be administered to previously vaccinated persons.

■ GLOBAL CONSIDERATIONS

Worldwide, endemic canine rabies is estimated to cause 55,000 human deaths annually. Most of these deaths occur in Asia and Africa, with rural populations and children most frequently affected. Most of the burden of rabies PEP is borne by people with the least resources. In Latin America, rabies control efforts in dogs have been quite successful in recent years. In Canada and Europe, epizootics of rabies in red foxes have been well controlled with the use of baits containing rabies vaccine. A similar approach is used in Canada to control raccoon rabies.

In addition to the rabies vaccines discussed above, vaccines grown in either primary cell lines (hamster or dog kidney) or continuous cell lines (Vero cells) are satisfactory and are available in many countries outside the United States. Less expensive vaccines derived from neural tissues have been used in developing countries; however, these vaccines are associated with serious neuroparalytic complications, including postinfectious encephalomyelitis and Guillain-Barré syndrome. The use of these vaccines should be discontinued as soon as possible, and progress has been made in this regard. Worldwide, >10 million individuals receive postexposure vaccination against rabies each year.

If human RIG is unavailable, purified equine RIG can be used in the same manner at a dose of 40 IU/kg. Before the administration of equine RIG, hypersensitivity should be assessed by intradermal testing with a 1:10 dilution. The incidence of anaphylactic reactions and serum sickness has been low with recent equine RIG products.

OTHER RHABDOVIRUSES

■ OTHER LYSSAVIRUSES

A growing number of lyssaviruses other than rabies virus have been discovered to infect bat populations in Africa, Europe, and Australia. Four of these viruses have produced a very small number of cases of a human disease indistinguishable from rabies: European bat lyssaviruses 1 and 2, Australian bat lyssavirus, and the Duvenhage virus (in Africa). Mokola virus, a lyssavirus that has been isolated from shrews with an unknown reservoir species in Africa, may also produce human disease indistinguishable from rabies.

VESICULAR STOMATITIS VIRUS (VSV)

Vesicular stomatitis is a viral disease of cattle, horses, pigs, and some wild mammals. VSV is a member of the genus *Vesiculovirus* in the family Rhabdoviridae. Outbreaks of vesicular stomatitis in horses and cattle occur sporadically in the southwestern United States. The animal infection is associated with severe vesiculation and ulceration of oral tissues, teats, and feet and may be clinically indistinguishable from the more dangerous foot-and-mouth disease. Epidemics are usually seasonal, typically beginning in the late spring, and are probably due to arthropod vectors. Direct animal-to-animal spread can also occur, although the virus cannot penetrate intact skin. Transmission to humans usually results from direct contact with infected animals (particularly cattle) and occasionally follows laboratory exposure. In human disease, early conjunctivitis is followed by an acute influenza-like illness with fever, chills, nausea, vomiting, headache, retrobulbar pain, myalgias, substernal pain, malaise, pharyngitis, and lymphadenitis. Small vesicular lesions may be present on the buccal mucosa or on the fingers. Encephalitis is very rare. The illness usually lasts 3–6 days, with complete recovery. Subclinical infections are common. A serologic diagnosis can be made on the basis of a rise in titer of complement-fixing or neutralizing antibodies. Therapy is symptom-based.

FURTHER READINGS

Baer GM (ed): *The Natural History of Rabies*, 2nd ed. Boca Raton, CRC Press, 1991

Jackson AC: Update on rabies diagnosis and treatment. Curr Infect Dis Rep 11:296, 2009

——, Wunner WH (eds): *Rabies*, 2nd ed. London, Elsevier, 2007

—— et al: Management of rabies in humans. Clin Infect Dis 36:60, 2003

Letchworth GJ et al: Vesicular stomatitis. Vet J 157:239, 1999

Manning SE et al: Human rabies prevention—United States, 2008: Recommendations of the Advisory Committee on Immunization Practices. MMWR Recomm Rep 57(RR-3):1, 2008

Warrell MJ, Warrell DA: Rabies and other lyssavirus diseases. Lancet 363:959, 2004

Willoughby RE Jr et al: Survival after treatment of rabies with induction of coma. N Engl J Med 352:2508, 2005

World Health Organization: *WHO Expert Consultation on Rabies: First Report*. First Report ed. Geneva, WHO, 2005

CHAPTER 196

Infections Caused by Arthropod- and Rodent-Borne Viruses

Clarence J. Peters

Some zoonotic viruses are transmitted in nature without regard to humans and only incidentally infect and produce disease in humans; in addition, a few agents are regularly spread among humans by arthropods. Most of these viruses either are maintained by arthropods or chronically infect rodents. Obviously, the mode of transmission is not a rational basis for taxonomic classification. Indeed, zoonotic viruses from at least seven families act as significant human pathogens (Table 196-1). The virus families differ fundamentally from one another in terms of morphology, replication mechanisms, and genetics. Information on a virus's membership in a family or genus is enlightening with regard to maintenance strategies, sensitivity to antiviral agents, and some aspects of pathogenesis but does not necessarily predict which clinical syndromes (if any) the virus will cause in humans.

FAMILIES OF ARTHROPOD- AND RODENT-BORNE VIRUSES (TABLE 196-1)

The Arenaviridae

The Arenaviridae are spherical, 110- to 130-nm particles that bud from the cell's plasma membrane and utilize ambisense RNA genomes with two segments for replication. There are two main phylogenetic branches of Arenaviridae: the Old World viruses, such as Lassa fever and lymphocytic choriomeningitis (LCM) viruses, and the New World viruses, including those causing the South American hemorrhagic fevers (HFs). Arenaviruses persist in nature by chronically infecting rodents with a striking one-virus–one-rodent species relationship. These rodent infections result in long-term virus excretion and perhaps in lifelong viremia; vertical infection is common with some arenaviruses. Humans become infected through the inhalation of aerosols containing arenaviruses, which are then deposited in the terminal air passages, and probably also through close contact with rodents and their excreta, which results in the contamination of mucous membranes or breaks in the skin.

The Bunyaviridae

The family Bunyaviridae includes four medically significant genera. All of these spherical viruses have three negative-sense RNA segments maturing into 90- to 120-nm particles in the Golgi complex and exiting the cell by exocytosis. Viruses of the genus *Bunyavirus* are largely mosquito-borne and have a viremic vertebrate intermediate host; many are also transovarially transmitted in their specific mosquito host. One serologic group also uses biting midges as vectors. Sandflies or mosquitoes are the vectors for the genus *Phlebovirus* (named after phlebotomus fever or sandfly fever, the best-known disease associated with the genus), while ticks serve as vectors for the genus *Nairovirus*. Viruses of both of these genera are also associated with vertical transmission in the arthropod host and with horizontal spread through viremic vertebrate hosts. The genus *Hantavirus* is unique among the Bunyaviridae in that it is not transmitted by arthropods but is maintained in nature by rodent hosts that chronically shed virus. Like the arenaviruses, the hantaviruses usually display striking virus–rodent species specificity. Hantaviruses do not cause chronic viremia in their rodent hosts and are transmitted only horizontally from rodent to rodent.

Other families

The Flaviviridae are positive-sense, single-strand RNA viruses that form particles of 40–50 nm in the endoplasmic reticulum. The flaviviruses discussed here are from the genus *Flavivirus* and make up two phylogenetically and antigenically distinct divisions transmitted among vertebrates by mosquitoes and ticks, respectively. The mosquito-borne viruses fall into phylogenetic groups that include

TABLE 196-1 Major Zoonotic Virus Families and Some Characteristics of Typical Members

Family	Genus or Group	Syndrome(s): Typical Viruses	Maintenance Strategy
Arenaviridae	Old World complex	FM, E: Lymphocytic choriomeningitis virus HF: Lassa fever virus	Chronic infection of rodents, often with persistent viremia; vertical transmission common
	New World or Tacaribe complex	HF: South American HF viruses (Machupo, Junin, Guanarito, Sabia)	Chronic infection of rodents, sometimes with persistent viremia; vertical infection may occur
Bunyaviridae	*Bunyavirus*	E: California serogroup viruses (La Crosse, Jamestown Canyon, California encephalitis) FM: Bunyamwera, group C, Tahyna viruses	Mosquito-vertebrate cycle; transovarial transmission in mosquito common
		FM: Oropouche virus	Transmitted by *Culicoides*
	Phlebovirus	FM: Sandfly fever, Toscana viruses FM: Punta Toro virus	Sandfly transmission between vertebrates, with prominent transovarial component in sandfly
		HF, FM, E: Rift Valley fever virus	Mosquito-vertebrate transmission, with transovarial component in mosquito
	Nairovirus	HF: Crimean-Congo HF virus	Tick-vertebrate, with transovarial transmission in tick
	Hantavirus	HF: Hantaan, Dobrava, Puumala viruses	Rodent reservoir; chronic virus shedding, but chronic viremia unknown
		HF: Sin Nombre and related hantaviruses	Sigmodontine rodent reservoir
Filoviridae[a]	*Ebolavirus, Marburgvirus*	HF: Marburg viruses, Ebola viruses (4 species)	Unknown
Flaviviridae	*Flavivirus* (mosquito-borne)	HF: Yellow fever virus FM, HF: Dengue viruses (4 serotypes) E: St. Louis, Japanese, West Nile, and Murray Valley encephalitis viruses; Rocio viruses	Mosquito-vertebrate; transovarial rare
	Flavivirus (tick-borne)	E: Central European tick-borne encephalitis, Russian spring-summer encephalitis, Powassan viruses	Tick-vertebrate
		HF: Omsk HF, Kyasanur Forest; Alkhurma disease viruses	
Reoviridae	*Coltivirus*	FM, E: Colorado tick fever virus	Tick-vertebrate
	Orbivirus	FM, E: Orungo, Kemerovo viruses	Arthropod-vertebrate
Rhabdoviridae[b]	*Vesiculovirus*	FM: Vesicular stomatitis virus (Indiana, New Jersey); Chandipura, Piry viruses	Sandfly-vertebrate, with prominent transovarial component in sandfly
Togaviridae	*Alphavirus*	AR: Sindbis, chikungunya, Mayaro, Ross River, Barmah Forest viruses	Mosquito-vertebrate
		E: Eastern, western, and Venezuelan equine encephalitis viruses	

[a]The Filoviridae are discussed in Chap. 197.
[b]The Rhabdoviridae are discussed in Chap. 195.
Note: Abbreviations refer to the disease syndrome most commonly associated with the virus: AR, arthritis, rash; E, encephalitis; FM, fever, myalgia; HF, hemorrhagic fever.

yellow fever virus, the four dengue viruses, and encephalitis viruses, while the tick-borne group encompasses a geographically varied spectrum of species, some of which are responsible for encephalitis or for hemorrhagic disease with encephalitis. The Reoviridae are double-strand RNA viruses with multisegmented genomes. These 80-nm particles are the only viruses discussed in this chapter that do not have a lipid envelope and thus are insensitive to detergents. The Togaviridae have a single positive-strand RNA genome and bud particles of ~60–70 nm from the plasma membrane. The toga-viruses discussed here are all members of the genus *Alphavirus* and are transmitted among vertebrates by mosquitoes in their natural cycle. The Filoviridae and the Rhabdoviridae are discussed in Chaps. 197 and 195, respectively.

■ PROMINENT FEATURES OF ARTHROPOD- AND RODENT-BORNE VIRUSES

Although this chapter discusses the major features of selected arthropod- and rodent-borne viruses, it does not deal with >500 other distinct recognized zoonotic viruses, about one-fourth of which infect humans. Zoonotic viruses are undergoing genetic evolution, "new" zoonotic viruses are being discovered, and the epidemiology of zoonotic viruses is continuing to evolve through environmental changes affecting vectors, reservoirs, and humans. These zoonotic viruses are most numerous in the tropics but are also found in temperate and frigid climates. Their distribution and seasonal activity may be variable and often depend largely on ecologic conditions such as rainfall and temperature, which in turn affect the density of vectors and reservoirs and the development of infection therein.

Maintenance and transmission

Arthropod-borne viruses infect their vectors after the ingestion of a blood meal from a viremic vertebrate. The vectors then develop chronic, systemic infection as the viruses penetrate the gut and spread throughout the body. The viruses eventually reach the salivary glands during a period that is referred to as *extrinsic incubation* and that typically lasts 1–3 weeks in mosquitoes. At this point, an arthropod is competent to continue the chain of transmission by infecting another vertebrate when a subsequent blood meal is taken. The arthropod generally is unharmed by the infection, and the natural vertebrate partner usually has only transient viremia with no overt disease. An alternative mechanism for virus maintenance in its arthropod host is transovarial transmission, which is common among members of the family Bunyaviridae.

Rodent-borne viruses such as the hantaviruses and arenaviruses are maintained in nature by chronic infection transmitted between rodents. As in arthropod-borne virus cycles, there is usually a high degree of rodent–virus specificity, and there is no overt disease in the reservoir/vector.

Epidemiology

The distribution of arthropod- and rodent-borne viruses is restricted by the areas inhabited by their reservoir/vectors and provides an important clue in the differential diagnosis. Table 196-2 shows the approximate geographic distribution of the most important of these viruses. Members of each family, each genus, and even each serologically related group usually occur in each area but may not be pathogenic in all areas or may not be a commonly recognized cause of disease in all areas and so may not be included in the table.

Most of these diseases are acquired in a rural setting; a few have urban vectors. Seoul, sandfly fever, and Oropouche viruses are examples of urban viruses, but the most notable are yellow fever, dengue, and chikungunya viruses. A history of mosquito bite has little diagnostic significance in the individual; a history of tick bite is more diagnostically specific. Rodent exposure is often reported by persons infected with an arenavirus or a hantavirus but again has little specificity. Indeed, aerosols may infect persons who have no recollection of having even seen rodents.

Syndromes

Human disease caused by arthropod- and rodent-borne viruses is often subclinical. The spectrum of possible responses to infection is wide, and our knowledge of the outcome of most of these infections is limited. The usual disease syndromes associated with these viruses have been grouped into four categories: fever and myalgia, arthritis and rash, encephalitis, and hemorrhagic fever. Although for the purposes of this discussion most viruses have been placed in a single group, the categories often overlap. For example, West Nile and Venezuelan equine encephalitis viruses are discussed as encephalitis viruses, but during epidemics many cases of milder febrile syndromes are recognized relative to less common cases of

TABLE 196-2 Geographic Distribution of Some Important and Commonly Encountered Human Zoonotic Viral Diseases

Area	Arenaviridae	Bunyaviridae	Flaviviridae	Rhabdoviridae	Togaviridae
North America	Lymphocytic choriomeningitis	La Crosse, Jamestown Canyon, California encephalitis; hantavirus pulmonary syndrome	St. Louis, Powassan, West Nile encephalitis; dengue	Vesicular stomatitis	Eastern, western equine encephalitis
South America	Bolivian (Machupo, Chapare), Argentine, Venezuelan, and Brazilian HF; lymphocytic choriomeningitis	Oropouche, group C, Punta Toro infection; hantavirus pulmonary syndrome	Yellow fever, dengue, Rocio virus infection	Vesicular stomatitis, Piry virus infection	Mayaro virus infection, Venezuelan equine encephalitis
Europe	Lymphocytic choriomeningitis	Tahyna, Toscana, sandfly fever; HF with renal syndrome	West Nile, Central European tick-borne, Russian spring-summer encephalitis	—	Sindbis virus infection
Middle East	Alkhurma HF virus infection	Sandfly fever, Crimean-Congo HF	West Nile encephalitis, dengue	—	—
Eastern Asia	—	Sandfly fever; Hantaan, Seoul virus infection	Dengue; Japanese, Russian spring-summer encephalitis; Omsk HF	Chandipura virus infection	—
Southwestern Asia	—	Sandfly fever, Crimean-Congo HF	West Nile, Japanese encephalitis; dengue; Kyasanur Forest disease	—	Chikungunya virus infection
Southeast Asia	—	Seoul virus infection	Japanese encephalitis, dengue	—	Chikungunya virus infection
Africa	Lassa fever; Lujo virus infection	Bunyamwera virus infection, Rift Valley fever	Yellow fever, dengue	—	Sindbis, chikungunya virus infection
Australia	—	—	Murray Valley encephalitis, dengue	—	Ross River, Barmah Forest virus infection

Abbreviation: HF, hemorrhagic fever.

encephalitis. Similarly, Rift Valley fever virus is best known as a cause of HF, but the attack rates for febrile disease are far higher, and encephalitis is occasionally seen as well. LCM virus is classified as a cause of fever and myalgia because this syndrome is its most common disease manifestation and because, even when central nervous system (CNS) disease occurs, it is usually mild and is preceded by fever and myalgia. Dengue virus infection is considered as a cause of fever and myalgia (dengue fever) because this is by far the most common manifestation worldwide and is the syndrome most likely to be seen in the United States; however, dengue HF is also discussed in the HF section because of its complicated pathogenesis and importance in pediatric practice in certain areas of the world.

Diagnosis

Laboratory diagnosis is required in any given case, although epidemics occasionally provide clinical and epidemiologic clues on which an educated guess as to etiology can be based. For most arthropod- and rodent-borne viruses, acute-phase serum samples (collected within 3 or 4 days of onset) have yielded isolates, and paired sera have been used to demonstrate rising antibody titers by a variety of tests. Intensive efforts to develop rapid tests for HF have resulted in an antigen-detection enzyme-linked immunosorbent assay (ELISA) and an IgM-capture ELISA that can provide a diagnosis based on a single serum sample within a few hours and are particularly useful in severe cases. More sensitive reverse-transcription polymerase chain reaction (RT-PCR) tests may yield diagnoses based on samples without detectable antigen and may also provide useful genetic information about the virus. Hantavirus infections differ from others discussed here in that severe acute disease is immunopathologic; patients present with serum IgM that serves as the basis for a sensitive and specific test.

At diagnosis, patients with encephalitis are generally no longer viremic or antigenemic and usually do not have virus in cerebrospinal fluid (CSF). In this situation, the value of serologic methods for IgM determination and RT-PCR is high. IgM capture is increasingly being used for the simultaneous testing of serum and CSF. IgG ELISA or classic serology is useful in the evaluation of past exposure to the viruses, many of which circulate in areas with a minimal medical infrastructure and sometimes cause mild or subclinical infection.

The remainder of this chapter offers general descriptions of the broad syndromes caused by arthropod- and rodent-borne viruses. Most of the diseases under consideration have not been studied in detail with modern medical approaches; thus available data may be incomplete or biased.

FEVER AND MYALGIA

Fever and myalgia constitute the syndrome most commonly associated with zoonotic virus infection. Many of the numerous viruses belonging to the families listed in Table 196-1 probably cause this syndrome, but several viruses have been selected for inclusion in the table because of their prominent associations with the syndrome and their biomedical importance.

The syndrome typically begins with the abrupt onset of fever, chills, intense myalgia, and malaise. Patients may also report joint or muscle pains, but no true arthritis is detectable. Anorexia is characteristic and may be accompanied by nausea or even vomiting. Headache is common and may be severe, with photophobia and retroorbital pain. Physical findings are minimal and are usually confined to conjunctival injection with pain on palpation of muscles or the epigastrium. The duration of symptoms is quite variable but generally is 2–5 days, with a biphasic course in some instances. The spectrum of disease varies from subclinical to temporarily incapacitating.

Less constant findings include a maculopapular rash. Epistaxis may occur but does not necessarily indicate a bleeding diathesis. A minority of the cases caused by some viruses are known or suspected to include aseptic meningitis, but this diagnosis is difficult to make in remote areas, given the patients' photophobia and myalgia as well as the lack of opportunity to examine the CSF. Although pharyngitis may be noted or radiographic evidence of pulmonary infiltrates found in some cases, these viruses are not primary respiratory pathogens. The differential diagnosis includes anicteric leptospirosis, rickettsial diseases, and the early stages of other syndromes discussed in this chapter. These diseases are often described as "flulike," but the usual absence of cough and coryza makes influenza an unlikely confounder except at the earliest stages.

Complete recovery is generally the outcome in this syndrome, although prolonged asthenia and nonspecific symptoms have been described in some cases, particularly after infection with LCM or dengue virus. Treatment is supportive, with aspirin avoided because of the potential for exacerbated bleeding and Reye's syndrome. Efforts at prevention are best based on vector control, which, however, may be expensive or impossible. For mosquito control, destruction of breeding sites is generally the most economically and environmentally sound approach. Emerging technologies include mosquito genetic transformation and introduction of *Wolbachia* to limit multiplication rates. Measures taken by the individual to avoid the vector can be valuable. Avoiding the vector's habitat and times of peak activity, using screens or other barriers (e.g., permethrin-impregnated bed nets) to prevent the vector from entering dwellings, judiciously applying arthropod repellents such as diethyltoluamide (DEET) to the skin, and wearing permethrin-impregnated clothing are all possible approaches, depending on the vector and its habits.

■ LYMPHOCYTIC CHORIOMENINGITIS

LCM is transmitted from the common house mouse (*Mus musculus*) to humans by aerosols of excreta and secreta. LCM virus, an arenavirus, is maintained in the mouse mainly by vertical transmission from infected dams. The vertically infected mouse remains viremic for life, with high concentrations of virus in all tissues. Infected colonies of pet hamsters have also served as a link to humans. LCM virus is widely used in immunology laboratories as a model of T cell function and can silently infect cell cultures and passaged tumor lines, resulting in infections among scientists and animal caretakers. Patients with LCM may have a history of residence in rodent-infested housing or other exposure to rodents. An antibody prevalence of ~5–10% has been reported among adults from the United States, Argentina, and endemic areas of Germany.

LCM differs from the general syndrome of fever and myalgia in that its onset is gradual. Among the conditions occasionally associated with LCM are orchitis, transient alopecia, arthritis, pharyngitis, cough, and maculopapular rash. An estimated one-fourth of patients or fewer experience a febrile phase of 3–6 days and then, after a brief remission, develop renewed fever accompanied by severe headache, nausea and vomiting, and meningeal signs lasting for ~1 week. These patients virtually always recover fully, as do the uncommon patients with clear-cut signs of encephalitis. Recovery may be delayed by transient hydrocephalus.

During the initial febrile phase, leukopenia and thrombocytopenia are common and virus can usually be isolated from blood. During the CNS phase, virus may be found in the CSF, but antibodies are present in blood. The pathogenesis of LCM is thought to resemble that following direct intracranial inoculation of the virus into adult mice; the onset of the immune response leads to T cell–mediated immunopathologic meningitis. During the meningeal phase, CSF mononuclear-cell counts range from the hundreds to the low thousands per microliter, and hypoglycorrhachia is found in one-third of cases. The IgM-capture ELISA of serum and CSF is usually positive; RT-PCR assays have been developed for application to CSF. Recent infections transmitted by organ transplantation did not include evidence of an immune response, followed a fulminant course (not unlike that of Lassa fever), and required immunohistochemistry or RT-PCR for diagnosis.

Infection with LCM virus should be suspected in acutely ill febrile patients with marked leukopenia and thrombocytopenia. In cases of aseptic meningitis, any of the following should suggest LCM: well-marked febrile prodrome, adult age, autumn seasonality, low CSF glucose levels, or CSF mononuclear cell counts of >1000/μL.

In pregnant women, LCM virus infection may lead to fetal invasion with consequent congenital hydrocephalus and chorioretinitis. Since the maternal infection may be mild, consisting of only a short febrile illness, antibodies to the virus should be sought in both the mother and the fetus in suspicious circumstances, particularly TORCH-negative neonatal hydrocephalus. [TORCH is a battery of tests encompassing *t*oxoplasmosis, *o*ther conditions (congenital syphilis and viral infection), *r*ubella, *c*ytomegalovirus infection, and *h*erpes simplex virus infection.]

■ BUNYAMWERA VIRUS INFECTION

The mosquito-transmitted Bunyamwera serogroup viruses are found on every continent except Australia and Antarctica. Bunyamwera virus and its close relative Ilesha virus commonly cause febrile disease in Africa. Ngari virus, a reassortant of Bunyamwera virus, has recently been identified as an important human pathogen in Africa. Other related viruses are implicated in such disease in Southeast Asia (Batai virus), Europe (Calovo virus), and South America (Wyeomyia virus). In North America, Cache Valley virus has been implicated in febrile human disease and in rare instances of more serious systemic illness; the presence of serum antibodies to this virus may be associated with congenital malformations. In Central America, the closely related Fort Sherman virus causes the fever-myalgia syndrome.

■ GROUP C VIRUS INFECTION

The group C viruses include at least 11 agents transmitted by mosquitoes in neotropical forests. These agents are among the most common causes of arboviral infection in humans entering American jungles and cause acute febrile disease.

■ TAHYNA VIRUS INFECTION

This California serogroup virus (see discussion of California encephalitis, below) occurs in central and western Europe, and related viruses are emerging in Russia. The significance of Tahyna virus in human health has been well studied only in the Czech and Slovak Republics; there, the virus was found to be a prominent cause of febrile disease, in some cases causing pharyngitis, pulmonary syndromes, and aseptic meningitis. The potential for arboviruses to be unexpectedly involved in such cases in areas of high mosquito prevalence needs to be kept in mind.

■ OROPOUCHE FEVER

Oropouche virus is transmitted in Central and South America by a biting midge, *Culicoides paraensis*, which often breeds to high density in cacao husks and other vegetable detritus found in towns and cities. Explosive epidemics involving thousands of cases have been reported from several towns in Brazil and Peru. Rash and aseptic meningitis have been detected in a number of cases.

■ SANDFLY FEVER

The sandfly *Phlebotomus papatasi* transmits sandfly fever. Female sandflies may be infected by the oral route as they take a blood meal and may transmit the virus to offspring when they lay their eggs after a second blood meal. This prominent transovarial pattern was the first to be recognized among dipterans and complicates virus control. A previous designation for sandfly fever, "3-day fever," instructively describes the brief, debilitating course associated with this essentially benign infection. There is neither a rash nor CNS involvement, and complete recovery is the rule.

Sandfly fever is found in the circum-Mediterranean area, extending to the east through the Balkans into parts of China as well as into the Middle East and southwestern Asia. The vector is found in both rural and urban settings and is known for its small size, which enables it to penetrate standard mosquito screens and netting, and for its short flight range. Epidemics have been described in the wake of natural disasters and wars. In parts of Europe, sandfly populations and virus transmission were greatly reduced by the extensive residual spraying conducted after World War II to control malaria, and the incidence continues to be low. A common pattern of disease in endemic areas consists of high attack rates among travelers and military personnel and little or no disease in the local population, who are protected after childhood infection. More than 30 related phleboviruses are transmitted by sandflies and mosquitoes, but most are of unknown significance in terms of human health.

■ TOSCANA VIRUS DISEASE

Toscana virus is a *Phlebovirus* (family Bunyaviridae) transmitted primarily by the circum-Mediterranean sandfly *P. perniciosus*. The vertebrate amplifying host, if one exists, is unknown. Toscana virus infection is common during the summer among rural residents and vacationers, particularly in Italy, Spain, and Portugal; a number of cases have been identified in travelers returning to Germany and Scandinavia. The disease may manifest as an uncomplicated febrile illness but is often associated with aseptic meningitis, with virus isolated from the CSF.

■ PUNTA TORO VIRUS DISEASE

Of the several phleboviruses that are associated with New World sandflies and infect humans, Punta Toro virus is the best known. The disease caused by this virus is clinically similar to but epidemiologically different from that caused by the Naples or Sicilian sandfly fever viruses. Punta Toro virus infections are sporadic and are acquired in the tropical forest, where the vectors rest on tree buttresses. Epidemics have not been reported, but antibody prevalences among inhabitants of villages in the endemic areas indicate a cumulative lifetime exposure rate of >50%.

■ DENGUE FEVER

All four distinct dengue viruses (dengue 1–4) have *Aedes aegypti* as their principal vector, and all cause a similar clinical syndrome. In rare cases, second infection with a serotype of dengue virus different from that involved in the primary infection leads to dengue HF with severe shock (see below). Sporadic cases are seen in the settings of endemic transmission and epidemic disease. Year-round transmission between latitudes 25°N and 25°S has been established, and seasonal forays of the viruses to points as far north as Philadelphia are thought to have taken place in the United States. Dengue fever is seen in the Caribbean region, including Puerto Rico. With increasing spread of the vector mosquito throughout the tropics and subtropics, large areas of the world have become vulnerable to the introduction of dengue viruses, particularly through air travel by infected humans, and both dengue fever and the related dengue HF are becoming increasingly common. Conditions favorable to dengue transmission exist in Hawaii and the southern United States, and bursts of dengue fever activity are to be expected in this region, particularly along the Mexican border, where water may be stored in containers and *A. aegypti* numbers may therefore be greatest. This mosquito, which is also an efficient vector of the yellow fever and chikungunya viruses, typically breeds near human habitation, using relatively fresh water from sources such as water jars, vases, discarded containers, coconut husks, and old tires. *A. aegypti* usually inhabits dwellings and bites during the day. Closed habitations with air-conditioning inhibit transmission of many arboviruses, as has been particularly well illustrated by studies along the Texas-Mexico border. *Aedes albopictus* has now extended its range from Asia to the United States, the Indian Ocean, and parts of Europe. For example, *A. albopictus* has transmitted dengue virus in Hawaii, chikungunya virus in Italy, and chikungunya virus in the Indian Ocean (see below).

After an incubation period of 2–7 days, the typical patient experiences the sudden onset of fever, headache, retroorbital pain, and back pain along with the severe myalgia that gave rise to the colloquial designation "break-bone fever." There is often a macular rash on the first day as well as adenopathy, palatal vesicles, and scleral injection. The illness may last a week, with additional symptoms usually including anorexia, nausea or vomiting, marked cutaneous hypersensitivity, and—near the time of defervescence—a maculopapular rash beginning on the trunk and spreading to the extremities and the face. Epistaxis and scattered petechiae are often noted in uncomplicated dengue, and preexisting gastrointestinal lesions may bleed during the acute illness.

Laboratory findings include leukopenia, thrombocytopenia, and, in many cases, serum aminotransferase elevations. The diagnosis is made by IgM ELISA or paired serology during recovery or by antigen-detection ELISA or RT-PCR during the acute phase. Virus is readily isolated from blood in the acute phase if mosquito inoculation or mosquito cell culture is used.

■ COLORADO TICK FEVER

Several hundred cases of Colorado tick fever are reported annually in the United States. The infection is acquired between March and November through the bite of an infected *Dermacentor andersoni* tick in mountainous western regions at altitudes of 1200–3000 m (4000–10,000 ft). Small mammals serve as the amplifying host. The most common presentation consists of fever and myalgia; meningoencephalitis is not uncommon, and hemorrhagic disease, pericarditis, myocarditis, orchitis, and pulmonary presentations are also reported. Rash develops in a substantial minority of cases. The disease usually lasts 7–10 days and is often biphasic. The most important differential diagnostic considerations since the beginning of the twentieth century have been Rocky Mountain spotted fever and tularemia. In Colorado, Colorado tick fever is much more common than Rocky Mountain spotted fever.

Infection of erythroblasts and other marrow cells by Colorado tick fever virus results in the appearance and persistence (for several weeks) of erythrocytes containing the virus. This feature, detected in smears stained by immunofluorescence, can be diagnostically helpful. The clinical laboratory detects leukopenia and thrombocytopenia.

■ *ORBIVIRUS* INFECTION

The orbiviruses encompass many human and veterinary pathogens. For example, Orungo virus is widely transmitted by mosquitoes in tropical Africa and causes febrile disease in humans. The Kemerovo complex includes the Kemerovo, Lipovnik, and Tribec viruses of

Russia and central Europe; these viruses are transmitted by ticks and are associated with febrile and neurologic disease.

ENCEPHALITIS

Arboviral encephalitis is a seasonal disease, commonly occurring in the warmer months. Its incidence varies markedly with time and place, depending on ecologic factors. The causative viruses differ substantially in terms of case-infection ratio (i.e., the ratio of clinical to subclinical infections), mortality rate, and residua (Table 196-3). Humans are not an important amplifier of these viruses.

All the viral encephalitides discussed in this section have a similar pathogenesis as far as is known. An infected arthropod ingests a blood meal from a human and infects the host. The initial period of viremia is thought to originate most commonly from the lymphoid system. Viremia leads to CNS invasion, presumably through infection of olfactory neuroepithelium with passage through the cribriform plate or through infection of brain capillaries and multifocal entry into the CNS. During the viremic phase, there may be little or no recognized disease except in the case of tick-borne flaviviral encephalitis, in which there may be a clearly delineated phase of fever and systemic illness. The disease process in the CNS arises partly from direct neuronal infection and subsequent damage and partly from edema, inflammation, and other indirect effects. The usual pathologic picture is one of focal necrosis of neurons, inflammatory glial nodules, and perivascular lymphoid cuffing; the severity and distribution of these abnormalities vary with the infecting virus. Involved areas display the "luxury perfusion" phenomenon, with normal or increased total blood flow and low oxygen extraction.

The typical patient presents with a prodrome of nonspecific constitutional symptoms, including fever, abdominal pain, vertigo, sore throat, and respiratory symptoms. Headache, meningeal signs, photophobia, and vomiting follow quickly. Involvement of deeper structures may be signaled by lethargy, somnolence, and intellectual deficit (as disclosed by the mental status examination or failure at serial 7 subtraction); more severely affected patients are obviously disoriented and may be comatose. Tremors, loss of abdominal reflexes, cranial nerve palsies, hemiparesis, monoparesis, difficulty in swallowing, and frontal lobe signs are all common. Spinal and motor neuron diseases are documented with West Nile and Japanese encephalitis viruses. Convulsions and focal signs may be evident early or may appear during the course of the disease. Some patients present with an abrupt onset of fever, convulsions, and other signs of CNS involvement. The results of human infection range from no significant symptoms through febrile headache to aseptic meningitis and finally to full-blown encephalitis; the proportions and severity of these manifestations vary with the infecting virus.

The acute encephalitis usually lasts from a few days to as long as 2–3 weeks, but recovery may be slow, with weeks or months required for the return of maximal recoupable function. Difficulty concentrating, fatigability, tremors, and personality changes are common during recovery. The acute illness requires management of a comatose patient who may have intracranial pressure elevations, inappropriate secretion of antidiuretic hormone, respiratory failure, and convulsions. There is no specific therapy for these viral encephalitides. The only practical preventive measures are vector management and personal protection against the arthropod transmitting the virus; for Japanese encephalitis or tick-borne encephalitis, vaccination should be considered in certain circumstances (see relevant sections below).

The diagnosis of arboviral encephalitis depends on the careful evaluation of a febrile patient with CNS disease, with rapid identification of treatable herpes simplex encephalitis, ruling out of brain abscess, exclusion of bacterial meningitis by serial CSF examination,

TABLE 196-3 Prominent Features of Arboviral Encephalitis

Virus	Natural Cycle	Incubation Period, Days	Annual No. of Cases	Case-to-Infection Ratio	Age of Cases	Case-Fatality Rate, %	Residua
La Crosse	*Aedes triseriatus*–chipmunk (transovarial component in mosquito also important)	~3–7	70 (U.S.)	<1:1000	<15 years	<0.5	Recurrent seizures in ~10%; severe deficits in rare cases; decreased school performance and behavioral change suspected in small proportion
St. Louis	*Culex tarsalis, C. pipiens, C. quinquefasciatus*–birds	4–21	85, with hundreds to thousands in epidemic years (U.S.)	<1:200	Milder cases in the young; more severe cases in adults >40 years old, particularly the elderly	7	Common in the elderly
Japanese	*Culex tritaeniorhynchus*–birds	5–15	>25,000	1:200–300	All ages; children in highly endemic areas	20–50	Common (approximately half of cases); may be severe
West Nile	*Culex* mosquitoes–birds	3–6	?	Very low	Mainly the elderly	5–10	Uncommon
Central European	*Ixodes ricinus*–rodents, insectivores	7–14	Thousands	1:12	All ages; milder in children	1–5	20%
Russian spring-summer	*I. persulcatus*–rodents, insectivores	7–14	Hundreds	—	All ages; milder in children	20	Approximately half of cases; often severe; limb-girdle paralysis
Powassan	*I. cookei*–wild mammals	~10	~1 (U.S.)	—	All ages; some predilection for children	~10	Common (approximately half of cases)
Eastern equine	*Culiseta melanura*–birds	~5–10	5 (U.S.)	1:40 (adult) 1:17 (child)	All ages; predilection for children	50–75	Common
Western equine	*Culex tarsalis*–birds	~5–10	~20 (U.S.)	1:1000 (adult) 1:50 (child) 1:1 (infant)	All ages; predilection for children <2 years old (increased mortality among elderly)	3–7	Common only among infants <1 year old
Venezuelan equine (epidemic)	Unknown (multiple mosquito species and horses in epidemics)	1–5	?	1:250 (adult) ~1:25 (child)	All ages; predilection for children	~10	—

and performance of laboratory studies to define the viral etiology. Leptospirosis, neurosyphilis, Lyme disease, cat-scratch fever, and newer viral encephalitides such as Nipah virus infection from Malaysia and southwestern Asia should be considered. The CSF examination usually shows a modest cell count—in the tens or hundreds or perhaps a few thousand. Early in the process, a significant proportion of these cells may be polymorphonuclear leukocytes, but usually there is a mononuclear cell predominance. CSF glucose levels are generally normal. There are exceptions to this pattern of findings. In eastern equine encephalitis, for example, polymorphonuclear leukocytes may predominate during the first 72 h of disease and hypoglycorrhachia may be detected. In LCM, lymphocyte counts may be in the thousands, and the glucose concentration may be diminished. Experience with imaging studies is still evolving; clearly, however, both CT and MRI may be normal, except for evidence of preexisting conditions, or sometimes may suggest diffuse edema. Several patients with eastern equine encephalitis have had focal abnormalities, and

individuals with severe Japanese encephalitis have presented with bilateral thalamic lesions that have often been hemorrhagic. Electroencephalography usually shows diffuse abnormalities and is not directly helpful.

A humoral immune response is usually detectable at or near the onset of disease. Both serum and CSF should be examined for IgM antibodies. Virus generally cannot be isolated from blood or CSF, although Japanese encephalitis virus has been recovered from CSF in severe cases. RT-PCR analysis of CSF may yield positive results. Virus can be obtained from and viral antigen is present in brain tissue, although its distribution may be focal.

■ CALIFORNIA, LA CROSSE, AND JAMESTOWN CANYON VIRUS ENCEPHALITIS

The isolation of California encephalitis virus established the California serogroup of viruses as a cause of encephalitis, and its use as a diagnostic antigen led to the description of many cases of "California encephalitis." In fact, however, this virus has been implicated in only a few cases of encephalitis, and the serologically related La Crosse virus is the major cause of encephalitis among viruses in the California serogroup. "California encephalitis" due to La Crosse virus infection is most commonly reported from the upper Midwest but is also found in other areas of the central and eastern United States, most often in West Virginia, Tennessee, North Carolina, and Georgia. The serogroup includes 13 other viruses, some of which may also be involved in human disease that is misattributed because of the complexity of the group's serology; these viruses include the Jamestown Canyon, snowshoe hare, Inkoo, and Trivittatus viruses, all of which have *Aedes* mosquitoes as their vector and all of which have a strong element of transovarial transmission in their natural cycles.

The mosquito vector of La Crosse virus is *A. triseriatus*. In addition to a prominent transovarial component of transmission, a mosquito can become infected through feeding on viremic chipmunks and other mammals as well as through venereal transmission from another mosquito. The mosquito breeds in sites such as tree holes and abandoned tires and bites during daylight hours. These habits correlate with the risk factors for human cases: recreation in forested areas, residence at the forest's edge, and the presence of abandoned tires around the home. Intensive environmental modification based on these findings has reduced the incidence of disease in a highly endemic area in the Midwest. Most cases occur from July through September. The Asian tiger mosquito, *A. albopictus*, efficiently transmits the virus to mice and also transmits the agent transovarially in the laboratory; this aggressive anthropophilic mosquito has the capacity to urbanize, and its possible impact on transmission to humans is of concern.

An antibody prevalence of ≥20% in endemic areas indicates that infection is common, but CNS disease has been recognized primarily in children <15 years of age. The illness varies from a picture of aseptic meningitis accompanied by confusion to severe and occasionally fatal encephalitis. Although there may be prodromal symptoms, the onset of CNS disease is sudden, with fever, headache, and lethargy often joined by nausea and vomiting, convulsions (in one-half of patients), and coma (in one-third of patients). Focal seizures, hemiparesis, tremor, aphasia, chorea, Babinski signs, and other evidence of significant neurologic dysfunction are common, but residua are not. Perhaps 10% of patients have recurrent seizures in the succeeding months. Other serious sequelae are rare, although a decrease in scholastic standing has been reported and mild personality change has occasionally been suggested. Treatment is supportive over a 1- to 2-week acute phase during which status epilepticus, cerebral edema, and inappropriate secretion of antidiuretic hormone are important concerns. Ribavirin has been used in severe cases, and a clinical trial of this drug is under way.

The blood leukocyte count is commonly elevated, sometimes reaching levels of 20,000/μL, and there is usually a left shift. CSF cell counts are typically 30–500/μL with a mononuclear cell predominance (although 25–90% of cells are polymorphonuclear in some cases). The protein level is normal or slightly increased, and the glucose level is normal. Specific virologic diagnosis based on IgM-capture assays of serum and CSF is efficient. The only human anatomic site from which virus has been isolated is the brain.

Jamestown Canyon virus has been implicated in several cases of encephalitis in adults; in these cases, the disease was usually associated with a significant respiratory illness at onset. Human infection with this virus has been documented in New York, Wisconsin, Ohio, Michigan, Ontario, and other areas of North America where the vector mosquito, *A. stimulans*, feeds on its main host, the white-tailed deer.

ST. LOUIS ENCEPHALITIS

St. Louis encephalitis virus is transmitted between *Culex* mosquitoes and birds. This virus causes low-level endemic infection among rural residents of the western and central United States, where *C. tarsalis* is the vector (see "Western Equine Encephalitis," below), but the more urbanized mosquito species *C. pipiens* and *C. quinquefasciatus* have been responsible for epidemics resulting in hundreds or even thousands of cases in cities of the central and eastern United States. Most cases occur in June through October. The urban mosquitoes breed in accumulations of stagnant water and sewage with high organic content and readily bite humans in and around houses at dusk. The elimination of open sewers and trash-filled drainage systems is expensive and may not be possible, but screening of houses and implementation of personal protective measures may be an effective approach for individuals. The rural vector is most active at dusk and outdoors; its bites can be avoided by modification of activities and use of repellents.

Disease severity increases with age: infections that result in aseptic meningitis or mild encephalitis are concentrated in children and young adults, while severe and fatal cases primarily affect the elderly. Infection rates are similar in all age groups; thus the greater susceptibility of older persons to disease is a biologic consequence of aging. The disease has an abrupt onset, sometimes following a prodrome, and begins with fever, lethargy, confusion, and headache. In addition, nuchal rigidity, hypotonia, hyperreflexia, myoclonus, and tremor are common. Severe cases can include cranial nerve palsies, hemiparesis, and convulsions. Patients often report dysuria and may have viral antigen in urine as well as pyuria. The overall mortality rate is generally ~7% but may reach 20% among patients over the age of 60. Recovery is slow. Emotional lability, difficulties in concentration and memory, asthenia, and tremor are commonly prolonged in older patients.

The CSF of patients with St. Louis encephalitis usually contains tens to hundreds of cells, with a lymphocytic predominance and a normal glucose level. Leukocytosis with a left shift is often documented.

JAPANESE ENCEPHALITIS

Japanese encephalitis virus is found throughout Asia, including far eastern Russia, Japan, China, India, Pakistan, and Southeast Asia, and causes occasional epidemics on western Pacific islands. The virus has been detected in the Torres Strait islands, and a human encephalitis case has been identified on the nearby Australian mainland. This flavivirus is particularly common in areas where irrigated rice fields attract the natural avian vertebrate hosts and provide abundant breeding sites for mosquitoes such as *C. tritaeniorhynchus*, which transmit the virus to humans. Additional amplification by pigs, which suffer abortion, and horses, which develop encephalitis, may be significant as well. Vaccination of these additional amplifying hosts may reduce the transmission of the virus. An effective, formalin-inactivated vaccine purified from mouse brain is produced in Japan and licensed for human use in the United States. It is given on days 0, 7, and 30 or—with some sacrifice in serum neutralizing titer—on days 0, 7, and 14. Vaccination is indicated for summer travelers to rural Asia, where the risk of clinical disease may be 0.05–2.1/10,000 per week. The severe and often fatal disease reported in expatriates must be balanced against the 0.1–1% chance of a late systemic or cutaneous allergic reaction. These reactions are rarely fatal but may be severe and have been known to begin 1–9 days after vaccination, with associated pruritus, urticaria, and angioedema. Live attenuated vaccines are being used in China but are not recommended in the United States at this time.

■ WEST NILE VIRUS INFECTION

West Nile virus was initially described as being transmitted among wild birds by *Culex* mosquitoes in Africa, the Middle East, southern Europe, and Asia. It is a common cause of febrile disease without CNS involvement, but it occasionally causes aseptic meningitis and severe encephalitis; these serious infections are particularly common among the elderly. The febrile-myalgic syndrome caused by West Nile virus differs from many others by the frequent appearance of a maculopapular rash concentrated on the trunk and lymphadenopathy. Headache, ocular pain, sore throat, nausea and vomiting, and arthralgia (but not arthritis) are common accompaniments. In addition, the virus has been implicated in severe and fatal hepatic necrosis in Africa.

West Nile virus was introduced into New York City in 1999 and subsequently spread to other areas of the northeastern United States, causing >60 cases of aseptic meningitis or encephalitis among humans as well as die-offs among crows, exotic zoo birds, and other birds. The virus has continued to spread and is now found in almost all states as well as in Canada, Mexico, South America, and the Caribbean. *C. pipiens* remains the major vector in the northeastern United States, but several other *Culex* species are also involved, and blue jays compete with crows as amplifiers and lethal targets in other areas of the country. Annually, ~1000–3000 cases of encephalitis with ~100–300 deaths are reported in the United States. The ratio of CNS involvement to infection is thought to be ~1:100; the remainder of patients have subclinical infection or West Nile fever. Encephalitis, sequelae, and death are all more common among elderly, diabetic, and hypertensive patients and among patients with previous CNS insults. In addition to the more severe motor and cognitive sequelae, milder findings may include tremor, slight abnormalities in motor skills, and loss of executive functions. Intense clinical interest and the availability of laboratory diagnostic methods have made it possible to define a number of unusual clinical features, including chorioretinitis, flaccid paralysis with histologic lesions resembling poliomyelitis, and initial presentation with fever and focal neurologic deficits in the absence of diffuse encephalitis. Immunosuppressed patients may have fulminant courses or develop persistent CNS infection. Virus transmission through both transplantation and blood transfusion has necessitated screening of blood and organ donors by nucleic acid–based tests. Pregnant women may occasionally infect the fetus. All these "new" findings, particularly transfusion-transmitted disease and severe disease associated with transplantation, show what could be expected in the United States should other arboviruses be transmitted in North America with a high frequency or should surveillance in other areas of the world be more efficient and deeper.

West Nile virus falls into the same phylogenetic group of flaviviruses as St. Louis and Japanese encephalitis viruses, as do Murray Valley and Rocio viruses. The latter two viruses are both maintained in mosquitoes and birds and produce a clinical picture resembling that of Japanese encephalitis. Murray Valley virus has caused occasional epidemics and sporadic cases in Australia. Rocio virus caused recurrent epidemics in a focal area of Brazil in 1975–1977 and then virtually disappeared.

■ CENTRAL EUROPEAN TICK-BORNE ENCEPHALITIS AND RUSSIAN SPRING-SUMMER ENCEPHALITIS

A spectrum of tick-borne flaviviruses has been identified across the Eurasian land mass. Many are known mainly as agricultural pathogens (e.g., louping ill virus in the United Kingdom). From Scandinavia to the Urals, central European tick-borne encephalitis is transmitted by *Ixodes ricinus*. Human cases occur between April and October, with a peak in June and July. A related and more virulent virus is that of Russian spring-summer encephalitis, which

is associated with *I. persulcatus* and is distributed from Europe across the Urals to the Pacific Ocean. The ticks transmit the disease primarily in the spring and early summer, with a lower rate of transmission later in summer. Small mammals are the vertebrate amplifiers for both viruses. The risk varies by geographic area and can be highly localized within a given area; human cases usually follow outdoor activities or consumption of raw milk from infected goats or other infected animals.

After an incubation period of 7–14 days or perhaps longer, the central European viruses classically result in a febrile-myalgic phase that lasts for 2–4 days and is thought to correlate with viremia. A subsequent remission for several days is followed by the recurrence of fever and the onset of meningeal signs. The CNS phase varies from mild aseptic meningitis, which is more common among younger patients, to severe encephalitis with coma, convulsions, tremors, and motor signs lasting for 7–10 days before improvement begins. Spinal and medullary involvement can lead to typical limb-girdle paralysis and to respiratory paralysis. Most patients recover, only a minority with significant deficits. Infections with the Far Eastern viruses generally run a more abrupt course. The encephalitic syndrome caused by these viruses sometimes begins without a remission and has more severe manifestations than the European syndrome. The mortality rate is high, and major sequelae—most notably, lower motor neuron paralyses of the proximal muscles of the extremities, trunk, and neck—are common.

In the early stage of the illness, virus may be isolated from the blood. In the CNS phase, IgM antibodies are detectable in serum and/or CSF. Thrombocytopenia sometimes develops during the initial febrile illness, which resembles the early hemorrhagic phase of some other tick-borne flaviviral infections, such as Kyasanur Forest disease. Other tick-borne flaviviruses are less common causes of encephalitis, including louping ill virus in the United Kingdom and Powassan virus.

There is no specific therapy for infection with these viruses. However, effective alum-adjuvanted, formalin-inactivated vaccines are produced in Austria, Germany, and Russia. Two doses of the Austrian vaccine separated by an interval of 1–3 months appear to be effective in the field, and antibody responses are similar when vaccine is given on days 0 and 14. Other vaccines have elicited similar neutralizing antibody titers. Since rare cases of postvaccination Guillain-Barré syndrome have been reported, vaccination should be reserved for persons likely to experience rural exposure in an endemic area during the season of transmission. Cross-neutralization for the central European and Far Eastern strains has been established, but there are no published field studies on cross-protection of formalin-inactivated vaccines. Because 0.2–4% of ticks in endemic areas may be infected, tick bites raise the issue of immunoglobulin prophylaxis. Prompt administration of high-titered specific preparations should probably be undertaken, although no controlled data are available to prove the efficacy of this measure. Immunoglobulin should not be administered late because of the risk of antibody-mediated enhancement.

■ POWASSAN ENCEPHALITIS

Powassan virus is a member of the tick-borne encephalitis virus complex and is transmitted by *I. cookei* among small mammals in eastern Canada and the United States, where it has been responsible for 20 recognized cases of human disease. Other ticks may transmit the virus in a wider geographic area, and there is some concern that *I. scapularis* (also called *I. dammini*), a competent vector in the laboratory, may become involved as it becomes more prominent in the United States. Patients with Powassan encephalitis (many of whom are children) present in May through December after outdoor exposure and an incubation period thought to be ~1 week. Powassan encephalitis is severe, and sequelae are common.

EASTERN EQUINE ENCEPHALITIS

Eastern equine encephalitis is found primarily within endemic swampy foci along the eastern coast of the United States, with a few inland foci as far removed as Michigan. Human cases present from June through October, when the bird–*Culiseta* mosquito cycle spills over into other mosquito species such as *A. sollicitans* or *A. vexans*, which are more likely to bite mammals. There is concern over the potential role of the introduced anthropophilic mosquito species *A. albopictus*, which has been found to be naturally infected and is an effective vector in the laboratory. Horses are a common target for the virus; contact with unvaccinated horses may be associated with human disease, but horses probably do not play a significant role in amplification of the virus.

Eastern equine encephalitis is one of the most destructive of the arboviral conditions, with a brusque onset, rapid progression, high mortality rate, and frequent residua. This severity is reflected in the extensive necrotic lesions and polymorphonuclear infiltrates found at postmortem examination of the brain and the acute polymorphonuclear CSF pleocytosis often occurring during the first 1–3 days of disease. In addition, leukocytosis with a left shift is a common feature. A formalin-inactivated vaccine has been used to protect laboratory workers but is not generally available or applicable.

WESTERN EQUINE ENCEPHALITIS

The primary maintenance cycle for western equine encephalitis virus in the United States is between *C. tarsalis* and birds, principally sparrows and finches. Equines and humans become infected, and both species suffer encephalitis without amplifying the virus in nature. St. Louis encephalitis is transmitted in a similar cycle in the same region but causes human disease about a month earlier than the period (July through October) in which western equine encephalitis virus is active. Large epidemics of western equine encephalitis took place in the western and central United States and Canada during the 1930s to 1950s, but in recent years the disease has been uncommon. There were 41 reported cases in the United States in 1987 but only 5 reported cases from 1988 to 2001. This decline in incidence may reflect in part the integrated approach to mosquito management that has been employed in irrigation projects and the increasing use of agricultural pesticides; it almost certainly reflects the increased tendency for humans to be indoors behind closed windows at dusk—the peak period of biting by the major vector.

Western equine encephalitis virus causes a typical diffuse viral encephalitis with an increased attack rate and increased morbidity rate among the young, particularly children <2 years old. In addition, mortality rates are high among the young and the very elderly. One-third of individuals who have convulsions during the acute illness have subsequent seizure activity. Infants <1 year old—particularly those in the first months of life—are at serious risk of motor and intellectual damage. Twice as many males as females develop clinical encephalitis after 5–9 years of age; this difference may be related to greater outdoor exposure of boys to the vector but is also likely to be due in part to biologic differences. A formalin-inactivated vaccine has been used to protect laboratory workers but is not generally available or applicable.

VENEZUELAN EQUINE ENCEPHALITIS

There are six known types of virus in the Venezuelan equine encephalitis complex. An important distinction is between the *epizootic* viruses (subtypes IAB and IC) and the *enzootic* viruses (subtypes ID to IF and types II to VI). The epizootic viruses have an unknown natural cycle but periodically cause extensive epidemics in equines and humans in the Americas. These epidemics rely on the high-level viremia in horses and mules that results in the infection of several species of mosquitoes, which in turn infect humans

and perpetuate virus transmission. Humans also have high-level viremia but probably are not important in virus transmission. Enzootic viruses are found primarily in humid tropical forest habitats and are maintained between *Culex* mosquitoes and rodents; these viruses cause human disease but are not pathogenic for horses and do not cause epizootics.

Epizootics of Venezuelan equine encephalitis occurred repeatedly in Venezuela, Colombia, Ecuador, Peru, and other South American countries at intervals of ≤10 years from the 1930s until 1969, when a massive epizootic spread throughout Central America and Mexico, reaching southern Texas in 1972. Genetic sequencing of the virus from the 1969–1972 outbreak suggested that it originated from residual "un-inactivated" virus in veterinary vaccines. The outbreak was terminated in Texas with the use of a live attenuated vaccine (TC-83) originally developed for human use by the U.S. Army; the epizootic virus was then used for further production of inactivated veterinary vaccines. No further epizootic disease was identified until 1995 and subsequently, when additional epizootics took place in Colombia, Venezuela, and Mexico. The viruses involved in these epizootics as well as previously epizootic subtype IC viruses have been shown to be close phylogenetic relatives of known enzootic subtype ID viruses. This finding suggests that active evolution and selection of epizootic viruses are under way in northern South America.

During epizootics, extensive human infection is the rule, with clinical disease in 10–60% of infected individuals. Most infections result in notable acute febrile disease, while relatively few result in encephalitis. A low rate of CNS invasion is supported by the absence of encephalitis among the many infections resulting from exposure to aerosols in the laboratory or from vaccine accidents. The most recent large epizootic of Venezuelan equine encephalitis occurred in Colombia and Venezuela in 1995; of the >85,000 clinical cases, 4% (with a higher proportion among children than adults) included neurologic symptoms and 300 ended in death.

Enzootic strains of Venezuelan equine encephalitis virus are common causes of acute febrile disease, particularly in areas such as the Florida Everglades and the humid Atlantic coast of Central America. Encephalitis has been documented only in the Florida infections; the three cases were caused by type II enzootic virus, also called *Everglades virus*. All three patients had preexisting cerebral disease. Extrapolation from the rate of genetic change suggests that Everglades virus may have been introduced into Florida <200 years ago and that it is most closely related to the ID subtypes that appear to have given evolutionary rise to the epizootic strains active in South America.

The prevention of epizootic Venezuelan equine encephalitis depends on vaccination of horses with the attenuated TC-83 vaccine or with an inactivated vaccine prepared from that strain. Humans can be protected with similar vaccines, but the use of such products is restricted to laboratory personnel because of reactogenicity and limited availability. In addition, wild-type virus and perhaps TC-83 vaccine may have some degree of fetal pathogenicity. Enzootic viruses are genetically and antigenically different from epizootic viruses, and protection against the former with vaccines prepared from the latter is relatively ineffective.

ARTHRITIS AND RASH

True arthritis is a common accompaniment of several viral diseases, such as rubella (caused by a non-alphavirus togavirus), parvovirus B19 infection, and hepatitis B; it is an occasional accompaniment of infection due to mumps virus, enteroviruses, herpesviruses, and adenoviruses. It is not generally appreciated that the alphaviruses are also common causes of arthritis. In fact, the alphaviruses discussed below all cause acute febrile diseases accompanied by the development of true arthritis and a maculopapular rash. Rheumatic involvement includes arthralgia alone, periarticular swelling, and (less commonly) joint effusions. Most of these diseases are less severe and have fewer articular manifestations in children than in adults. In temperate climates, these are summer diseases. No specific therapy or licensed vaccines exist.

SINDBIS VIRUS INFECTION

Sindbis virus is transmitted among birds by mosquitoes. Infections with the northern European strains of this virus (which cause, for example, Pogosta disease in Finland, Karelian fever in the independent states of the former Soviet Union, and Ockelbo disease in Sweden) and with the genetically related southern African strains are particularly likely to result in the arthritis-rash syndrome. Exposure to a rural environment is commonly associated with this infection, which has an incubation period of <1 week.

The disease begins with rash and arthralgia. Constitutional symptoms are not marked, and fever is modest or lacking altogether. The rash, which lasts ~1 week, begins on the trunk, spreads to the extremities, and evolves from macules to papules that often vesiculate. The arthritis of this condition is multiarticular, migratory, and incapacitating, with resolution of the acute phase in a few days. Wrists, ankles, phalangeal joints, knees, elbows, and—to a much lesser extent—proximal and axial joints are involved. Persistence of joint pains and occasionally of arthritis is a major problem and may go on for months or even years despite a lack of deformity.

CHIKUNGUNYA VIRUS INFECTION

It is likely that chikungunya virus ("that which bends up") is of African origin and is maintained among nonhuman primates on that continent by *Aedes* mosquitoes of the subgenus *Stegomyia* in a fashion similar to yellow fever virus. Like yellow fever virus, chikungunya virus is readily transmitted among humans in urban areas by *A. aegypti*. The *A. aegypti*–chikungunya virus transmission cycle has also been introduced into Asia, where it poses a prominent health problem. The disease is endemic in rural areas of Africa, and intermittent epidemics take place in towns and cities of Africa and Asia. In 2004, a massive epidemic in the Indian Ocean region began; it now appears to have been spread by travelers. *A. albopictus* was identified as the major vector, and there were multiple exportations to temperate zones and to areas where *A. aegypti* is present. Chikungunya is one more reason (in addition to dengue and yellow fever) that *A. aegypti* and *A. albopictus* must be controlled.

Full-blown disease is most common among adults, in whom the clinical picture may be dramatic. The abrupt onset follows an incubation period of 2–3 days. Fever and severe arthralgia are accompanied by chills and constitutional symptoms such as headache, photophobia, conjunctival injection, anorexia, nausea, and abdominal pain. Migratory polyarthritis mainly affects the small joints of the hands, wrists, ankles, and feet, with lesser involvement of the larger joints. Rash may appear at the outset or several days into the illness; its development often coincides with defervescence, which takes place around day 2 or 3 of disease. The rash is most intense on the trunk and limbs and may desquamate. Petechiae are occasionally seen, and epistaxis is not uncommon, but this virus is not a regular cause of the HF syndrome, even in children. A few patients develop leukopenia. Elevated levels of aspartate aminotransferase (AST) and C-reactive protein have been described, as have mildly decreased platelet counts. Recovery may require weeks. Some older patients continue to experience stiffness, joint pain, and recurrent effusions for several years; this persistence may be especially common in HLA-B27 patients. An investigational live attenuated vaccine has been developed but requires additional testing. It appears to be headed for further development and commercial manufacture stimulated by the Indian Ocean outbreak.

A related virus, O'nyong-nyong, caused a major epidemic of arthritis and rash involving at least 2 million people as it moved across eastern and central Africa in the 1960s. After its mysterious emergence, the virus virtually disappeared, leaving only occasional evidence of its persistence in Kenya until a transient resurgence of epidemic activity in 1997.

MAYARO FEVER

Mayaro virus is maintained in the forests of the Americas by *Haemagogus* mosquitoes and nonhuman primates. It causes a frequently endemic and sometimes epidemic infection of humans and appears to produce a syndrome resembling chikungunya virus infection.

EPIDEMIC POLYARTHRITIS (ROSS RIVER VIRUS INFECTION)

Ross River virus has caused epidemics of distinctive clinical disease in Australia since the beginning of the twentieth century and continues to be responsible for thousands of cases in rural and suburban areas annually. The virus is transmitted by *A. vigilax* and other mosquitoes, and its persistence is thought to involve transovarial transmission. No definitive vertebrate host has been identified, but several mammalian species, including wallabies, have been suggested. Endemic transmission has also been documented in New Guinea, and in 1979 the virus swept through the eastern Pacific Islands, causing hundreds of thousands of illnesses. The virus was carried from island to island by infected humans and was believed to have been transmitted among humans by *A. polynesiensis* and *A. aegypti*.

The incubation period is 7–11 days long, and the onset of illness is sudden, with joint pain usually ushering in the disease. The rash generally develops coincidentally or follows shortly but in some cases precedes joint pains by several days. Constitutional symptoms such as low-grade fever, asthenia, myalgia, headache, and nausea are not prominent and indeed are absent in many cases. Most patients are incapacitated for considerable periods by joint involvement, which interferes with sleeping, walking, and grasping. Wrist, ankle, metacarpophalangeal, interphalangeal, and knee joints are the most commonly involved, although toes, shoulders, and elbows may be affected with some frequency. Periarticular swelling and tenosynovitis are common, and one-third of patients have true arthritis. Only half of all arthritis patients can resume normal activities within 4 weeks, and 10% still must limit their activity at 3 months. Occasional patients are symptomatic for 1–3 years but without progressive arthropathy. Aspirin and nonsteroidal anti-inflammatory drugs are effective for the treatment of symptoms.

Clinical laboratory values are normal or variable in Ross River virus infection. Tests for rheumatoid factor and antinuclear antibodies are negative, and the erythrocyte sedimentation rate is acutely elevated. Joint fluid contains 1000–60,000 mononuclear cells/μL, and Ross River virus antigen is demonstrable in macrophages. IgM antibodies are valuable in the diagnosis of this infection, although they occasionally persist for years. The isolation of the virus from blood by mosquito inoculation or mosquito cell culture is possible early in the illness. Because of the great economic impact of annual epidemics in Australia, an inactivated vaccine is being developed and has been found to be protective in mice.

Perhaps because of the local interest in arboviruses in general and in Ross River virus in particular, other arthritogenic arboviruses have been identified in Australia, including Gan Gan virus, a member of the family Bunyaviridae; Kokobera virus, a flavivirus; and Barmah Forest virus, an alphavirus. The last virus is a common cause of infection and must be differentiated from Ross River virus by specific testing.

The viral HF syndrome is a constellation of findings based on vascular instability and decreased vascular integrity. An assault, direct or indirect, on the microvasculature leads to increased permeability and (particularly when platelet function is decreased) to actual disruption and local hemorrhage. Blood pressure is decreased, and in severe cases shock supervenes. Cutaneous flushing and conjunctival suffusion are examples of common, observable abnormalities in the control of local circulation. The hemorrhage is inconstant and is in most cases an indication of widespread vascular damage rather than a life-threatening loss of blood volume. Disseminated intravascular coagulation (DIC) is occasionally found in any severely ill patient with HF but is thought to occur regularly only in the early phases of HF with renal syndrome, Crimean-Congo HF, and perhaps some cases of filovirus HF. In some viral HF syndromes, specific organs may be particularly impaired, such as the kidney in HF with renal syndrome, the lung in hantavirus pulmonary syndrome, or the liver in yellow fever, but in all these diseases the generalized circulatory disturbance is critically important.

The pathogenesis of HF is poorly understood and varies among the viruses regularly implicated in the syndrome, which number more than a dozen. In some cases direct damage to the vascular system or even to parenchymal cells of target organs is important, whereas in others soluble mediators are thought to play the major role. The acute phase in most cases of HF is associated with ongoing virus replication and viremia. Exceptions are the hantavirus diseases and dengue HF/dengue shock syndrome (DHF/DSS), in which the immune response plays a major pathogenic role.

The HF syndromes all begin with fever and myalgia, usually of abrupt onset. Within a few days the patient presents for medical attention because of increasing prostration that is often accompanied by severe headache, dizziness, photophobia, hyperesthesia, abdominal or chest pain, anorexia, nausea or vomiting, and other gastrointestinal disturbances. Initial examination often reveals only an acutely ill patient with conjunctival suffusion, tenderness to palpation of muscles or abdomen, and borderline hypotension or postural hypotension, perhaps with tachycardia. Petechiae (often best visualized in the axillae), flushing of the head and thorax, periorbital edema, and proteinuria are common. Levels of AST are usually elevated at presentation or within a day or two thereafter. Hemoconcentration from vascular leakage, which is usually evident, is most marked in hantavirus diseases and in DHF/DSS. The seriously ill patient progresses to more severe symptoms and develops shock and other findings typical of the causative virus. Shock, multifocal bleeding, and CNS involvement (encephalopathy, coma, convulsions) are all poor prognostic signs.

One of the major diagnostic clues is travel to an endemic area within the incubation period for a given syndrome (Table 196-4). Except for Seoul, dengue, and yellow fever virus infections, which have urban vectors, travel to a rural setting is especially suggestive of a diagnosis of HF.

Early recognition is important because of the need for virus-specific therapy and supportive measures, including prompt, atraumatic hospitalization; judicious fluid therapy that takes into account the patient's increased capillary permeability; administration of cardiotonic drugs; use of pressors to maintain blood pressure at levels that will support renal perfusion; treatment of the relatively common secondary bacterial infections; replacement of clotting factors and platelets as indicated; and the usual precautionary measures used in the treatment of patients with hemorrhagic diatheses. DIC should be treated only if clear laboratory evidence of its existence is found and if laboratory monitoring of therapy is feasible; there is no proven benefit of such therapy. The available evidence suggests that HF patients have a decreased cardiac output and will respond poorly to fluid loading as it is often practiced in the treatment of shock associated with bacterial sepsis. Specific therapy is available for several of the HF syndromes. In addition, several diseases considered in the differential diagnosis—malaria, shigellosis, typhoid fever, leptospirosis, relapsing fever, and rickettsial diseases—are treatable and potentially lethal. Strict barrier nursing and other precautions against infection of medical staff and visitors are indicated in HF except that due to hantaviruses, yellow fever, Rift Valley fever, and dengue.

LASSA FEVER

Lassa virus is known to cause endemic and epidemic disease in Nigeria, Sierra Leone, Guinea, and Liberia, although it is probably more widely distributed in West Africa. This virus and its relatives exist elsewhere in Africa, but their health significance is unknown. Like other arenaviruses, Lassa virus is spread to humans by small-particle aerosols from chronically infected rodents and may also be acquired during the capture or eating of these animals. It can be transmitted by close person-to-person contact. The virus is often present in urine during convalescence and is suspected to be present in seminal fluid early in recovery. Nosocomial spread has occurred but is uncommon if proper sterile parenteral techniques are used. Individuals of all ages and both sexes are affected; the incidence of disease is highest in the dry season, but transmission takes place year-round. In countries where Lassa virus is endemic, Lassa fever can be a prominent cause of febrile disease. For example, in one hospital in Sierra Leone, laboratory-confirmed Lassa fever is consistently responsible for one-fifth of admissions to the medical wards. There are probably tens of thousands of Lassa fever cases annually in West Africa alone. New arenaviruses continue to be discovered, often without being thoroughly characterized. These arenaviruses include Chapare virus in Bolivia (distinct from Machupo virus) and Lujo virus in Zambia.

Among the HF agents, only the arenaviruses are typically associated with a gradual onset of illness. The average case of Lassa fever has a gradual onset that gives way to more severe constitutional symptoms and prostration. Bleeding is seen in only ~15–30% of cases. A maculopapular rash is often noted in light-skinned Lassa patients. Effusions are common, and male-dominant pericarditis may develop late. The fetal death rate is 92% in the last trimester, when the maternal mortality rate is also increased from the usual 15–30%; these figures suggest that interruption of the pregnancy of infected women should be considered. White blood cell counts are normal or slightly elevated, and platelet counts are normal or somewhat low. Deafness coincides with clinical improvement in ~20% of cases and is permanent and bilateral in some. Reinfection may occur but has not been associated with severe disease.

High-level viremia or a high serum concentration of AST statistically predicts a fatal outcome. Thus patients with an AST level of >150 IU/mL should be treated with IV ribavirin. This antiviral nucleoside analogue appears to be effective in reducing mortality rates from the levels documented among retrospective controls, and its only major side effect is reversible anemia that usually does not require transfusion. The drug should be given by slow IV infusion in a dose of 32 mg/kg; this dose should be followed by 16 mg/kg every 6 h for 4 days and then by 8 mg/kg every 8 h for 6 days.

SOUTH AMERICAN HF SYNDROMES (ARGENTINE, BOLIVIAN, VENEZUELAN, AND BRAZILIAN)

These diseases are similar to one another clinically, but their epidemiology differs with the habits of their rodent reservoirs and the interactions of these animals with humans. Person-to-person or nosocomial transmission is rare but has occurred.

TABLE 196-4 Viral Hemorrhagic Fever (HF) Syndromes and Their Distribution

Disease	Incubation Period, Days	Case-Infection Ratio	Case-Fatality Rate, %	Geographic Range	Target Population
Lassa fever	5–16	Mild infections probably common	15	West Africa	All ages, both sexes
South American HF	7–14	Most infections (more than half) result in disease	15–30	Selected rural areas of Bolivia, Argentina, Venezuela, and Brazil	Bolivia: Men in countryside; all ages, both sexes in villages Argentina: All ages, both sexes; excess exposure and disease in men Venezuela: All ages, both sexes
Rift Valley fever	2–5	~1:100[a]	~50	Sub-Saharan Africa, Madagascar, Egypt	All ages, both sexes; more often diagnosed in men; preexisting liver disease may predispose
Crimean-Congo HF	3–12	≥1:5	15–30	Africa, Middle East, Turkey, Balkans, southern region of former Soviet Union, western China	All ages, both sexes; men more exposed in some settings
HF with renal syndrome	9–35	Hantaan, >1:1.25; Puumala, 1:20	Hantaan, 5–15; Puumala, <1	Worldwide, depending on rodent reservoir	Excess of male patients (partially due to greater exposure); mainly adults
Hantavirus pulmonary syndrome	~7–28	Very high	40–50	Americas	Excess of male patients due to some occupational exposure; mainly adults
Marburg or Ebola HF	3–16	High	25–90	Sub-Saharan Africa	All ages, both sexes; children less exposed
Yellow fever	3–6	1:2–1:20	20	Africa, South America	All ages, both sexes; adults more exposed in jungle setting; preexisting flavivirus immunity may cross-protect
Dengue HF/dengue shock syndrome	2–7	Nonimmune, 1:10,000; heterologous immune, 1:100	<1 with supportive treatment	Tropics and subtropics worldwide	Predominantly children; previous heterologous dengue infection predisposes to HF
Kyasanur Forest/ Omsk HF	3–8	Variable	0.5–10	Mysore State, India/western Siberia	Variable

[a]Figure is for HF cases only. Most infections with Rift Valley fever virus result in fever and myalgia rather than HF.

The basic disease resembles Lassa fever, with two marked differences. First, thrombocytopenia—often marked—is the rule, and bleeding is quite common. Second, CNS dysfunction is much more common than in Lassa fever and is often manifested by marked confusion, tremors of the upper extremities and tongue, and cerebellar signs. Some cases follow a predominantly neurologic course, with a poor prognosis. The clinical laboratory is helpful in diagnosis since thrombocytopenia, leukopenia, and proteinuria are typical findings.

Argentine HF is readily treated with convalescent-phase plasma given within the first 8 days of illness. In the absence of passive antibody therapy, IV ribavirin in the dose recommended for Lassa fever is likely to be effective in all the South American HF syndromes. The transmission of the disease from men convalescing from Argentine HF to their wives suggests the need for counseling of arenavirus HF patients concerning the avoidance of intimate contacts for several weeks after recovery. A safe, effective, live attenuated vaccine exists for Argentine HF; after vaccination of >250,000 high-risk persons in the endemic area, incidence

decreased markedly. In experimental animals, this vaccine is cross-protective against the Bolivian HF virus.

■ RIFT VALLEY FEVER

The mosquito-borne Rift Valley fever virus is also a pathogen of domestic animals such as sheep, cattle, and goats. It is maintained in nature by transovarial transmission in floodwater *Aedes* mosquitoes and presumably also has a vertebrate amplifier. Epizootics and epidemics occur when sheep or cattle become infected during particularly heavy rains; developing high-level viremia, these animals infect many species of mosquitoes. Remote sensing via satellite can detect the ecologic changes associated with high rainfall that predict the likelihood of Rift Valley fever transmission; it can also detect the special depressions from which the floodwater *Aedes* mosquito vectors emerge. In addition, the virus is infectious when transmitted by contact with blood or aerosols from domestic animals or their abortuses. The slaughtered meat is not infectious; anaerobic glycolysis in postmortem tissues results in an acidic environment that rapidly inactivates Bunyaviridae such as Rift Valley fever virus and Crimean-Congo HF virus. The natural range of Rift Valley fever virus is confined to sub-Saharan Africa, where its circulation is markedly enhanced by substantial rainfall such as that which occurred during the El Niño phenomenon of 1997; subsequent spread to the Arabian Peninsula caused epidemic disease in 2000. The virus has also been found in Madagascar and has been introduced into Egypt, where it caused major epidemics in 1977–1979, 1993, and subsequently. Neither person-to-person nor nosocomial transmission has been documented.

Rift Valley fever virus is unusual in that it causes several clinical syndromes. Most infections are manifested as the febrile-myalgic syndrome. A small proportion of infections result in HF with especially prominent liver involvement. Renal failure and probably DIC are also common features. Perhaps 10% of otherwise mild infections lead to retinal vasculitis; funduscopic examination reveals edema, hemorrhages, and infarction, and some patients have permanently impaired vision. A small proportion of cases (<1 in 200) are followed by typical viral encephalitis. One of the complicated syndromes does not appear to predispose to another.

There is no proven therapy for any of the syndromes described above. Both retinal disease and encephalitis occur after the acute febrile syndrome has ended and serum neutralizing antibody has developed—events suggesting that only supportive care need be given. Epidemic disease is best prevented by vaccination of livestock. The established ability of this virus to propagate after an introduction into Egypt suggests that other potentially receptive areas, including the United States, should have a response ready for such an eventuality. It seems likely that this disease, like Venezuelan equine encephalitis, can be controlled only with adequate stocks of an effective live attenuated vaccine, and there are no such global stocks. A formalin-inactivated vaccine confers immunity to humans, but quantities are limited and three injections are required; this vaccine is recommended for exposed laboratory workers and for veterinarians working in sub-Saharan Africa. A new live attenuated vaccine, MP-12, is being tested in humans and may soon become available for general use.

CRIMEAN-CONGO HF

This severe HF syndrome has a wide geographic distribution, potentially being found wherever ticks of the genus *Hyalomma* occur. The propensity of these ticks to feed on domestic livestock and certain wild mammals means that veterinary serosurveys are the most effective mechanism for the surveillance of virus circulation in a region. Human infection is acquired via a tick bite or during the crushing of infected ticks. Domestic animals do not become ill but do develop viremia; thus, there is danger of infection at the time of slaughter and for a brief interval thereafter (through contact with hides or carcasses). Cases have followed sheep shearing. An epidemic in South Africa was associated with slaughter of tick-infested ostriches. Nosocomial epidemics are common and are usually related to extensive blood exposure or needle sticks.

Although generally similar to other HF syndromes, Crimean-Congo HF causes extensive liver damage, resulting in jaundice in some cases. Clinical laboratory values indicate DIC and show elevations in AST, creatine phosphokinase, and bilirubin. Patients with fatal cases generally have more marked changes, even in the early days of illness, and also develop leukocytosis rather than leukopenia. In addition, thrombocytopenia is more marked and develops earlier in cases with a fatal outcome.

No controlled trials have been performed with IV ribavirin, but clinical experience and retrospective comparison of patients with ominous clinical laboratory values suggest that ribavirin is efficacious and should be given. No human or veterinary vaccines are recommended.

HF WITH RENAL SYNDROME

This disease, the first to be identified as an HF, is widely distributed over Europe and Asia; the major causative viruses and their rodent reservoirs on these two continents are Puumala virus (bank vole, *Clethrionomys glareolus*) and Hantaan virus (striped field mouse, *Apodemus agrarius*), respectively. Other potential causative viruses exist, including Dobrava virus (yellow-necked field mouse, *A. flavicollis*), which causes severe HF with renal syndrome in the Balkans. Seoul virus is associated with the Norway or sewer rat, *Rattus norvegicus*, and has a worldwide distribution through the migration of the rodent; it is associated with mild or moderate HF with renal syndrome in Asia, but in many areas of the world the human disease has been difficult to identify. Most cases occur in rural residents or vacationers; the exception is Seoul virus disease, which may be acquired in an urban or rural setting or from contaminated laboratory rat colonies. Classic Hantaan disease in Korea (Korean HF) and in rural China (epidemic HF) is most common in spring and fall and is related to rodent density and agricultural practices. Human infection is acquired primarily through aerosols of rodent urine, although virus is also present in saliva and feces. Patients with hantavirus diseases are not infectious. HF with renal syndrome is the most important form of HF today, with >100,000 cases of severe disease in Asia annually and milder Puumala infections numbering in the thousands as well.

Severe cases of HF with renal syndrome caused by Hantaan virus evolve in identifiable stages: the febrile stage with myalgia, lasting 3 or 4 days; the hypotensive stage, often associated with shock and lasting from a few hours to 48 h; the oliguric stage with renal failure, lasting 3–10 days; and the polyuric stage with diuresis and hyposthenuria.

The *febrile stage* is initiated by the abrupt onset of fever, headache, severe myalgia, thirst, anorexia, and often nausea and vomiting. Photophobia, retroorbital pain, and pain on ocular movement are common, and the vision may become blurred with ciliary body inflammation. Flushing over the face, the V area of the neck, and the back is characteristic, as are pharyngeal injection, periorbital edema, and conjunctival suffusion. Petechiae often develop in areas of pressure, the conjunctivae, and the axillae. Back pain and tenderness to percussion at the costovertebral angle reflect massive retroperitoneal edema. Laboratory evidence of mild to moderate DIC is present. Other laboratory findings include proteinuria and an active urinary sediment.

The *hypotensive stage* is ushered in by falling blood pressure and sometimes by shock. The relative bradycardia typical of the febrile phase is replaced by tachycardia. Kinin activation is marked. The rising hematocrit reflects increasing vascular leakage. Leukocytosis with a left shift develops, and thrombocytopenia continues. Atypical lymphocytes—which in fact are activated CD8+ (and, to a lesser extent, CD4+) T cells—circulate. Proteinuria is marked, and the urine's specific gravity falls to 1.010. The renal circulation is congested and compromised from local and systemic circulatory changes resulting in necrosis of tubules, particularly at the corticomedullary junction, and oliguria.

During the *oliguric stage*, hemorrhagic tendencies continue, probably in large part because of uremic bleeding defects. The oliguria persists for 3–10 days before the return of renal function marks the onset of the *polyuric stage*, which carries the danger of dehydration and electrolyte abnormalities.

Mild cases of HF with renal syndrome may be much less stereotypical. The presentation may include only fever, gastrointestinal abnormalities, and transient oliguria followed by hyposthenuria.

HF with renal syndrome should be suspected in patients with rural exposure in an endemic area. Prompt recognition of the disease permits rapid hospitalization and expectant management of shock and renal failure. Useful clinical laboratory parameters include leukocytosis, which may be leukemoid and is associated with a left shift; thrombocytopenia; and proteinuria. Mainstays of therapy are the management of shock, reliance on pressors, modest crystalloid infusion, IV use of human serum albumin, and treatment of renal failure with prompt dialysis for the usual indications. Hydration may result in pulmonary edema, and hypertension should be avoided because of the possibility of intracranial hemorrhage. Use of IV ribavirin has reduced mortality and morbidity rates in severe cases provided treatment is begun within the first 4 days of illness. The case-fatality ratio may be as high as 15% but with proper therapy should be <5%. Sequelae have not been definitively established, but there is a correlation in the United States between chronic hypertensive renal failure and the presence of antibodies to Seoul virus.

Infections with Puumala virus, the most common cause of HF with renal syndrome in Europe, result in a much attenuated picture but the same general presentation. The syndrome may be referred to by its former name, *nephropathia epidemica*. Bleeding manifestations are found in only 10% of cases, hypotension rather than shock is usually seen, and oliguria is present in only about half of patients. The dominant features may be fever, abdominal pain, proteinuria, mild oliguria, and sometimes blurred vision or glaucoma followed by polyuria and hyposthenuria in recovery. The mortality rate is <1%.

The diagnosis is readily made by IgM-capture ELISA, which should be positive at admission or within 24–48 h thereafter. The isolation of virus is difficult, but RT-PCR of a blood clot collected early in the clinical course or of tissues obtained postmortem will give positive results. Such testing is usually undertaken only if definitive identification of the infecting viral species is required or if molecular epidemiologic questions exist.

■ HANTAVIRUS PULMONARY SYNDROME

Hantavirus pulmonary syndrome was discovered in 1993, but retrospective identification of cases by immunohistochemistry (1978) and serology (1959) support the idea that it is a recently discovered rather than a truly new disease. The causative agents are hantaviruses of a distinct phylogenetic lineage that is associated with the rodent subfamily Sigmodontinae. Sin Nombre virus, which chronically infects the deer mouse (*Peromyscus maniculatus*), is the most important agent of hantavirus pulmonary syndrome in the United States. The disease is also caused by a Sin Nombre virus variant from the white-footed mouse (*P. leucopus*), by Black Creek Canal virus (*Sigmodon hispidus*, the cotton rat), and by Bayou virus (*Oryzomys palustris*, the rice rat). Several other related viruses cause the disease in South America, but Andes virus is unusual in that it, alone among hantaviruses, has been implicated in human-to-human transmission. The disease is linked to rodent exposure and particularly affects rural residents living in dwellings permeable to rodent entry or working at occupations that pose a risk of rodent exposure. Each rodent species has its own particular habits; in the case of the deer mouse, these behaviors include living in and around human habitation.

The disease begins with a prodrome of ~3–4 days (range, 1–11 days) comprising fever, myalgia, malaise, and often gastrointestinal disturbances such as nausea, vomiting, and abdominal pain. Dizziness is common and vertigo occasional. Severe prodromal symptoms bring some individuals to medical attention, but patients are usually recognized as the cardiopulmonary phase begins. Typically, there is slightly lowered blood pressure, tachycardia, tachypnea, mild hypoxemia, and early radiographic signs of pulmonary edema. Physical findings in the chest are often surprisingly scant. The conjunctival and cutaneous signs of vascular involvement seen in other types of HF are absent. During the next few hours, decompensation may progress rapidly to severe hypoxemia and respiratory failure. Most patients surviving the first 48 h of hospitalization are extubated and discharged within a few days, with no apparent residua.

Management during the first few hours after presentation is critical. The goal is to prevent severe hypoxemia by oxygen therapy, with intubation and intensive respiratory management if needed. During this period, hypotension and shock with increasing hematocrit invite aggressive fluid administration, but this intervention should be undertaken with great caution. Because of low cardiac output with myocardial depression and increased pulmonary vascular permeability, shock should be managed expectantly with pressors and modest infusion of fluid guided by the pulmonary capillary wedge pressure. Mild cases can be managed by frequent monitoring and oxygen administration without intubation. Many patients require intubation to manage hypoxemia and also develop shock. Mortality rates remain at ~30–40% even with good management. The antiviral drug ribavirin inhibits the virus in vitro but did not have a marked effect on patients treated in an open-label study.

During the prodrome, the differential diagnosis of hantavirus pulmonary syndrome is difficult, but by the time of presentation or within 24 h thereafter, a number of diagnostically helpful clinical features become apparent. Cough is not usually present at the outset but may develop later. Interstitial edema is evident on the chest x-ray. Later, bilateral alveolar edema with a central distribution develops in the setting of a normal-sized heart; occasionally, the edema is initially unilateral. Pleural effusions are often seen. Thrombocytopenia, circulating atypical lymphocytes, and a left shift (often with leukocytosis) are almost always evident; thrombocytopenia is a particularly important early clue. Hemoconcentration, proteinuria, and hypoalbuminemia should also be sought. Although thrombocytopenia virtually always develops and prolongation of the partial thromboplastin time is the rule, clinical evidence for coagulopathy or laboratory indications of DIC are found in only a minority of cases, usually in severely ill patients. Patients with severe illness also have acidosis and elevated serum levels of lactate. Mildly increased values in renal function tests are common, but patients with severe cases often have markedly elevated concentrations of serum creatinine; some of the viruses other than Sin Nombre virus have been associated with more kidney involvement, but few such cases have been studied. The differential diagnosis includes abdominal surgical conditions and pyelonephritis as well as rickettsial disease, sepsis, meningococcemia, plague, tularemia, influenza, and relapsing fever.

A specific diagnosis is best made by IgM testing of acute-phase serum, which has yielded positive results even in the prodrome. Tests using a Sin Nombre virus antigen detect the related hantaviruses causing the pulmonary syndrome in the Americas. Occasionally, heterologous viruses will react only in the IgG ELISA, but this finding is highly suspicious given the very low seroprevalence of these viruses in normal populations. RT-PCR is usually positive when used to test blood clots obtained in the first 7–9 days of illness as well as tissues; this test is useful in identifying the infecting virus in areas outside the home range of the deer mouse and in atypical cases.

■ YELLOW FEVER

Yellow fever virus caused major epidemics in the Americas, Africa, and Europe before the discovery of mosquito transmission in 1900 led to its control through attacks on its urban vector, *A. aegypti*. Only then was it found that a jungle cycle also existed in Africa, involving other *Aedes* mosquitoes and monkeys, and that colonization of the New World with *A. aegypti*, originally an African species, had established urban yellow fever as well as an independent sylvatic yellow fever cycle involving *Haemagogus* mosquitoes and New World monkeys in American jungles. Today, urban yellow fever transmission occurs only in some African cities, but the threat exists in the great cities of South America, where reinfestation by *A. aegypti* has taken place and dengue transmission by the same mosquito is common. As late as 1905, New Orleans suffered >3000 cases with 452 deaths from "yellow jack." Despite the existence of a highly effective and safe vaccine, several hundred jungle yellow fever cases occur annually in South America, and thousands of jungle and urban cases occur each year in Africa.

Yellow fever is a typical HF accompanied by prominent hepatic necrosis. A period of viremia, typically lasting 3 or 4 days, is followed by a period of "intoxication." During the latter phase in severe cases, the characteristic jaundice, hemorrhages, black vomit, anuria, and terminal delirium occur, perhaps related in part to extensive hepatic involvement. Blood leukocyte counts may be normal or reduced and are often high in terminal stages. Albuminuria is usually noted and may be marked; as renal function fails in terminal or severe cases, the level of blood urea nitrogen rises proportionately. Abnormalities detected in liver function tests range from modest elevations of AST levels in mild cases to severe derangement.

Urban yellow fever can be prevented by the control of *A. aegypti*. The continuing sylvatic cycle requires vaccination of all visitors to areas of potential transmission. With few exceptions, reactions to vaccine are minimal; immunity is provided within 10 days and lasts for at least 10 years. An egg allergy dictates caution in vaccine administration. Although there are no documented harmful effects of the vaccine on the fetus, pregnant women should be immunized only if they are definitely at risk of yellow fever exposure. Since vaccination has been associated with several cases of encephalitis in children <6 months of age, it should be delayed until after 12 months of age unless the risk of exposure is very high. Rare, serious, multisystemic adverse reactions (occasionally fatal) have been reported, particularly affecting the elderly; nevertheless, the number of deaths of unvaccinated travelers with yellow fever exceeds the number of deaths from vaccination, and a liberal vaccination policy for travelers to involved areas should be pursued. Timely information on changes in yellow fever distribution and yellow fever vaccine requirements can be obtained from the Centers for Disease Control and Prevention (*wwwnc.cdc.gov/travel*).

■ DENGUE HEMORRHAGIC FEVER/DENGUE SHOCK SYNDROME

A syndrome of HF noted in the 1950s among children in the Philippines and Southeast Asia was soon associated with dengue virus infections, particularly those occurring against a background of previous exposure to another dengue-virus serotype. The transient heterotypic protection after dengue virus infection is replaced within several weeks by the potential for heterotypic infection resulting in typical dengue fever (see above) or—uncommonly—in enhanced disease (secondary DHF/DSS). In rare instances, primary dengue infections lead to an HF syndrome, but much less is known about pathogenesis in this situation. In the past 20 years, *A. aegypti* has progressively reinvaded Latin America and other areas, and frequent travel by infected individuals has introduced multiple strains of dengue virus from many geographic areas. Thus the pattern of hyperendemic transmission of multiple dengue serotypes has now been established in the Americas and the Caribbean and has led to the emergence of DHF/DSS as a major problem there as well. Millions of dengue infections, including many thousands of cases of DHF/DSS, occur annually. The severe syndrome is unlikely to be seen in U.S. citizens since few children have the dengue antibodies that can trigger the pathogenetic cascade when a second infection is acquired.

Macrophage/monocyte infection is central to the pathogenesis of dengue fever and to the origin of DHF/DSS. Previous infection with a heterologous dengue-virus serotype may result in the production of nonprotective antiviral antibodies that nevertheless bind to the virion's surface and through interaction with the Fc receptor focus secondary dengue viruses on the target cell, the result being enhanced infection. The host is also primed for a secondary antibody response when viral antigens are released and immune complexes lead to activation of the classic complement pathway, with consequent phlogistic effects. Cross-reactivity at the T cell level results in the release of physiologically active cytokines, including interferon γ and tumor necrosis factor α. The induction of vascular permeability and shock depends on multiple factors, including the following:

1. *Presence of enhancing and nonneutralizing antibodies*—Transplacental maternal antibody may be present in infants <9 months old, or antibody elicited by previous heterologous dengue infection may be present in older individuals. T cell reactivity is also intimately involved.

2. *Age*—Susceptibility to DHF/DSS drops considerably after 12 years of age.

3. *Sex*—Females are more often affected than males.

4. *Race*—Whites are more often affected than blacks.

5. *Nutritional status*—Malnutrition is protective.

6. *Sequence of infection*—For example, serotype 1 followed by serotype 2 seems to be more dangerous than serotype 4 followed by serotype 2.

7. *Infecting serotype*—Type 2 is apparently more dangerous than other serotypes.

In addition, there is considerable variation among strains of a given serotype, with Southeast Asian serotype 2 strains having more potential to cause DHF/DSS than others.

Dengue HF is identified by the detection of bleeding tendencies (tourniquet test, petechiae) or overt bleeding in the absence of underlying causes such as preexisting gastrointestinal lesions. Dengue shock syndrome, usually accompanied by hemorrhagic signs, is much more serious and results from increased vascular permeability leading to shock. In mild DHF/DSS, restlessness, lethargy, thrombocytopenia (<100,000/μL), and hemoconcentration are detected 2–5 days after the onset of typical dengue fever, usually at the time of defervescence. The maculopapular rash that often develops in dengue fever may also appear in DHF/DSS. In more severe cases, frank shock is apparent, with low pulse pressure, cyanosis, hepatomegaly, pleural effusions, ascites, and in some cases severe ecchymoses and gastrointestinal bleeding. The period of shock lasts only 1 or 2 days, and most patients respond promptly to close monitoring, oxygen administration, and infusion of crystalloid or—in severe cases—colloid. The case-fatality rates reported vary greatly with case ascertainment and the quality of treatment; however, most DHF/DSS patients respond well to supportive therapy, and the overall mortality rate at an experienced center in the tropics is probably as low as 1%.

A virologic diagnosis can be made by the usual means, although multiple flavivirus infections lead to a broad immune response to several members of the group, and this situation may result in a lack of virus specificity of the IgM and IgG immune responses. A secondary antibody response can be sought with tests against several flavivirus antigens to demonstrate the characteristic wide spectrum of reactivity.

The key to control of both dengue fever and DHF/DSS is the control of *A. aegypti*, which also reduces the risk of urban yellow fever and chikungunya virus circulation. Control efforts have been handicapped by the presence of nondegradable tires and long-lived plastic containers in trash repositories, insecticide resistance, urban poverty, and an inability of the public health community to mobilize the populace to respond to the need to eliminate mosquito breeding sites. Live attenuated dengue vaccines are in the late stages of development and have produced promising results in early tests. Whether vaccines can provide safe, durable immunity to an immunopathologic disease such as DHF/DSS in endemic areas is an issue that will have to be tested, but it is hoped that vaccination will reduce transmission to negligible levels.

KYASANUR FOREST DISEASE AND OMSK HEMORRHAGIC FEVER

Kyasanur Forest virus and Omsk HF virus are geographically restricted, tick-borne flaviviruses that cause a syndrome of viral HF during a wave of viremia and that may also enter the CNS to cause subsequent viral encephalitis (see discussion of tick-borne encephalitis, above). There is no therapy for these infections, but an inactivated vaccine has been used in India against Kyasanur Forest disease. A new and related virus isolate has been obtained from butchers with HF in the Middle East; the implication is that there are more agents in this group.

FILOVIRUS HEMORRHAGIC FEVER

See Chap. 197.

FURTHER READINGS

BRACKNEY MM et al: Epidemiology of Colorado tick fever in Montana, Utah, and Wyoming, 1995–2003. Vector Borne Zoonotic Dis 10:381, 2010

BRUNO P et al: The protean manifestations of hemorrhagic fever with renal syndrome. A retrospective review of 26 cases from Korea. Ann Intern Med 113:385, 1990

CALISHER CH: Medically important arboviruses of the United States and Canada. Clin Microbiol Rev 7:89, 1994

CENTERS FOR DISEASE CONTROL AND PREVENTION: Update: Management of patients with suspected viral hemorrhagic fever—United States. MMWR Morb Mortal Wkly Rep 44:475, 1995 (www.cdc.gov/mmwr/preview/mmwrhtml/00038033.htm)

DAVIS LE et al: North American encephalitis arboviruses. Neurol Clin 26:727, 2008

DEPAQUIT J et al: Arthropod-borne viruses transmitted by phlebotomine sandflies in Europe: A review. Euro Surveill 15:19507, 2010

DERESIEWICZ RL et al: Clinical and neuroradiographic manifestations of eastern equine encephalitis. N Engl J Med 336:1867, 1997

ENRIA D et al: Arenaviruses, in Tropical Infectious Diseases: Principles, Pathogens, & Practice, RL Guerrant et al (eds). New York, Saunders, 1999, pp 1189–1212

JONSSON CB et al: A global perspective on hantavirus ecology, epidemiology, and disease. Clin Microbiol Rev 23:412, 2010

PETERS CJ, KHAN AS: Hantavirus pulmonary syndrome: The new American hemorrhagic fever. Clin Infect Dis 34:1224, 2002

PETERSON LR, HAYES EB: West Nile virus in the Americas. Med Clin North Am 92:1307, 2008

RIVAS F et al: Epidemic Venezuelan equine encephalitis in La Guajira, Colombia, 1995. J Infect Dis 175:828, 1997

SIMPSON SQ et al: Hantavirus pulmonary syndrome. Infect Dis Clin North Am 24:159, 2010

SOLOMON SR, VAUGHN DW: Pathogenesis and clinical features of Japanese encephalitis and West Nile virus infections. Curr Top Microbiol Immunol 267:171, 2002

WURTZ R, PALEOLOGOS N: La Crosse encephalitis presenting like herpes simplex encephalitis in an immunocompromised adult. Clin Infect Dis 31:1113, 2000

CHAPTER 197

Ebola and Marburg Viruses

Clarence J. Peters

DEFINITION

Both Marburg virus and Ebola virus cause an acute febrile illness associated with a high mortality rate. This illness is characterized by multisystem involvement that begins with the abrupt onset of headache, myalgias, and fever and proceeds to prostration, rash, and shock and often to bleeding manifestations. Epidemics usually begin with a single case acquired from an unknown reservoir in nature (bats are suspected; see "Epidemiology," below) and spread mainly through close contact with sick persons or their body fluids, either at home or in the hospital.

ETIOLOGY

The family Filoviridae (Fig. 197-1) comprises two antigenically and genetically distinct genera: Marburgvirus and Ebolavirus. Ebolavirus has five readily distinguishable species named for their original sites of recognition: Zaire, Sudan, Côte d'Ivoire, Bundibugyo, and Reston. Except for the Reston virus, all the Filoviridae are African viruses that cause severe and often fatal disease in humans (Figs. 197-2 and 197-3). The Reston virus, which has been exported from the Philippines on several occasions, has caused fatal infections in monkeys but only subclinical infections in humans. Different strains of the five Ebola species, isolated over time and space, exhibit remarkable sequence conservation, indicating marked genetic stability in their selective niche.

Typical filovirus particles contain a single linear, negative-sense, single-stranded RNA arranged in a helical nucleocapsid. The virions are 790–970 nm in length; they may also appear in elongated, contorted forms (Fig. 197-4). The lipid envelope confers sensitivity to lipid solvents and common detergents. The viruses are largely destroyed by heat (60°C, 30 min) and by acidity but may persist for weeks in blood at room temperature. The glycoprotein self-associates to form the virion surface spikes, which presumably mediate attachment to cells and fusion. The glycoprotein's high sugar content may contribute to its low capacity to elicit effective neutralizing antibodies. A smaller form of the glycoprotein, bearing many of its antigenic determinants, is produced by in vitro–infected cells and is found in the circulation in human disease; it has been speculated that this circulating soluble protein may suppress the immune response to the virion surface protein or block antiviral effector mechanisms. Both Marburg virus and Ebola virus are biosafety level 4 pathogens because of their high associated mortality rate and aerosol infectivity.

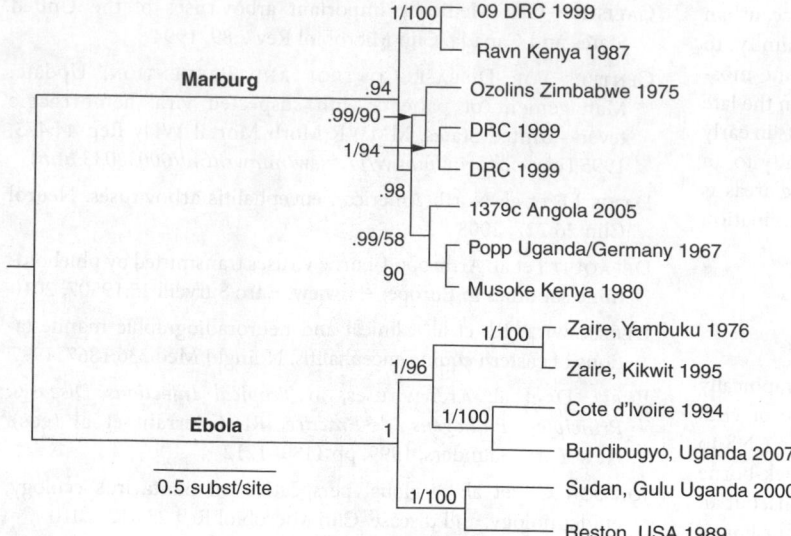

Figure 197-1 Phylogenetic tree of filoviruses. *Marburgvirus* and *Ebolavirus* are seen to be two different genera. The genus *Ebolavirus* includes five distinct species. Note that the Yambuku and Kikwit Zaire viruses are virtually identical even though the epidemics for which they were responsible are separated by two decades and hundreds of kilometers. Virtually every virus sequenced from each of those two epidemics is identical over the part of the genome examined. This pattern is typical of that seen with single introductions followed by human-to-human passage via needle or close contact in an African hospital. In the *Marburgvirus* branch of the tree, there is one major clade with a slightly divergent group characterized by the Ravn 1987 Kenya isolate. All the viruses from the major Angola 2005 outbreak are represented by a single virus because the sequences in this human-to-human epidemic are virtually identical. However, in the outbreak occurring in the Democratic Republic of the Congo (DRC) in 1999 and resulting from multiple independent infections after cave entry, two viruses with slightly different phylogenies are represented within the major group, and there is even another virus within the Ravn subgroup. These sequences were selected from hundreds determined at the U.S. Centers for Disease Control and Prevention and elsewhere. *(Adapted from Peters, 2010.)*

■ EPIDEMIOLOGY

Marburg virus was first identified in Germany in 1967, when infected African green monkeys (*Cercopithecus aethiops*) imported from Uganda transmitted the agent to workers in a vaccine laboratory. Of the 25 human cases acquired from monkeys, seven ended in death. The six secondary cases were associated with close contact or parenteral exposure. Secondary spread to the wife of one patient was documented, and virus was isolated from the husband's semen despite the presence of circulating serum antibodies. Isolated cases of Marburg virus infection were reported from eastern and southern Africa, with limited spread. Then, in 1999, repeated transmission of Marburg virus to workers in a gold mine in eastern Democratic Republic of the Congo (DRC; formerly Zaire) was studied. The secondary spread of the virus among patients' families was more extensive than previously noted, resembling that of Ebola virus and suggesting the importance of hygiene and proper barrier nursing in the epidemiology of these viruses in Africa. Finally, in 2004–2005, an alarming, massive Marburg virus epidemic, with >250 cases, occurred in Angola. The epidemiologic features resembled those of the Ebola virus epidemics described below, and the case-fatality rate was 90%. This high figure may have been due in part to poor conditions in African hospitals; however, the virus isolated in this epidemic was slightly different phylogenetically from other known strains and exhibited increased virulence in nonhuman primates.

Ebola virus first appeared in 1976, causing simultaneous epidemics of severe hemorrhagic fever

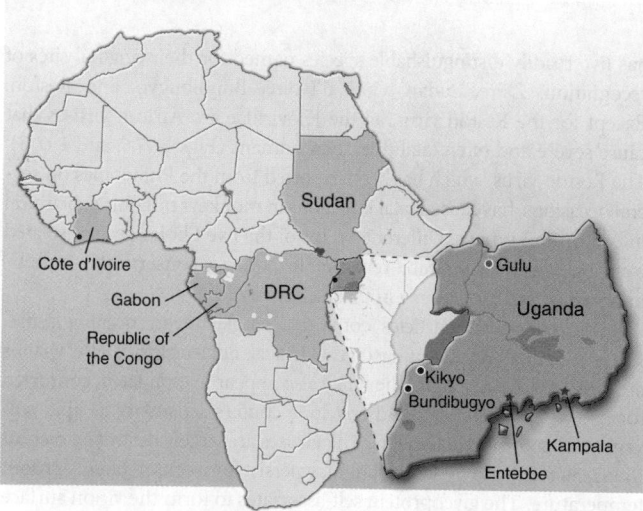

Figure 197-2 *Left:* **Geographic sites of *Ebolavirus* species identification,** as represented by dots (yellow, Zaire; green, Sudan; red, Côte d'Ivoire; black, Bundibugyo), in or adjacent to the Central African primary or secondary forest. Even *Ebolavirus* Côte d'Ivoire was isolated in the Tai forest reserve. *Right:* **Amplified map of Uganda** shows the zone along the border of the Democratic Republic of the Congo (DRC, formerly Zaire) where the newest *Ebolavirus* species, Bundibugyo, was identified. Bundibugyo and the nearby town of Kikyo, which was also affected by this epidemic, are tourist destinations close to the Ugandan capital of Kampala. *(Adapted from Peters, 2010.)*

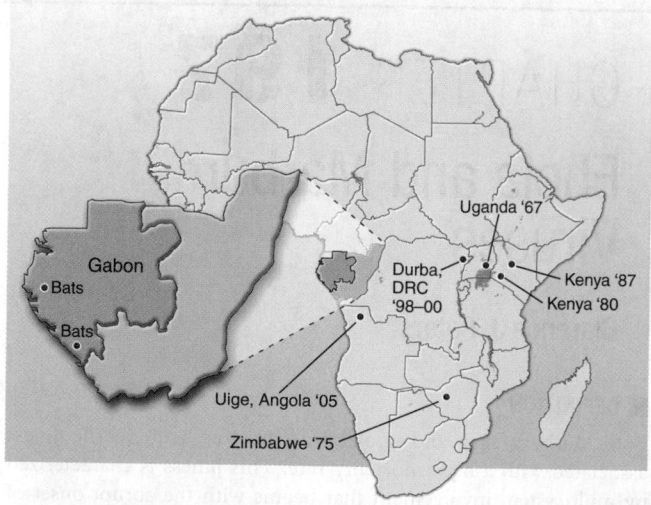

Figure 197-3 Maps of the African continent and the country of Gabon (with adjacent Republic of the Congo) show the geographic distribution of *Marburgvirus* identification. Red dots indicate a case or an epidemic. Uige, Angola, is the site of the largest Marburg epidemic (252 cases, 90% mortality rate). The Angolan strains differ by only 0–0.07% at the nucleotide level (Fig. 197-1). The Durba outbreak lasted 3 years and was characterized by multiple introductions of virus into men entering a subterranean mine. Nine distinct lineages were detected, of which one was in the rather distant (21%) Ravn lineage. Red dots on the Gabon map indicate detection of virus in bats by PCR. *(Adapted from Peters, 2010.)*

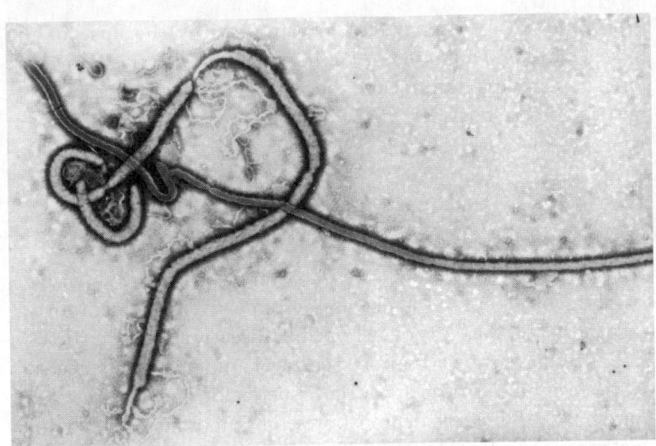

Figure 197-4 Ebola virions: diagnostic specimen from the first passage in Vero cells of a blood sample from a patient. Some of the filamentous (negatively stained) virions were fused together, end-to-end, giving the appearance of a "bowl of spaghetti." This image was from the first isolation and visualization of Ebola virus in 1970. *(Courtesy of Fredrick A. Murphy, MD, University of Texas Medical Branch, Galveston, Texas; with permission.)*

(550 human cases) in Zaire and Sudan. Later, it was shown that different species of virus (with associated mortality rates of 90% and 50%, respectively) had caused the two epidemics. Both epidemics were associated with interhuman spread (particularly in the hospital setting) and the use of unsterilized needles and syringes—a common practice in developing-country hospitals. The epidemics dwindled as the clinics were closed and as persons in the endemic area increasingly shunned affected persons and avoided traditional burial practices.

After an interval of apparent inactivity of almost 20 years, the Zaire Ebola virus recurred in a major epidemic (317 cases) in the DRC in 1995 and in smaller epidemics in Gabon in 1994–1996. Mortality rates were high (88% in the DRC), transmission to caregivers and others who had direct contact with body fluids was common, and poor hygiene in hospitals exacerbated spread. In the DRC epidemic, an index case was infected in Kikwit in January 1995. The epidemic smoldered until April, when intense nosocomial transmission forced closure of the hospitals; samples were finally sent to the laboratory for Ebola testing, which yielded positive results within a few hours. International assistance, with barrier nursing instruction and materials, was provided; nosocomial transmission ceased, hospitals reopened, and patients were segregated to prevent intrafamilial spread. The last case was reported in June 1995.

Separate emergences of Ebola virus (Zaire) were detected in Gabon in 1994–2003, usually in association with deep-forest exposure and subsequent familial and nosocomial transmission. Die-offs of nonhuman primates were sometimes documented, and Ebola infection was confirmed in at least some animals. In a 1996 episode, a physician exposed to Ebola-infected patients traveled to South Africa with a fever; a nurse who assisted in a cutdown on the physician developed Ebola hemorrhagic fever and died despite intensive care. The index patient was identified retrospectively on the basis of serum antibodies and virus isolation from semen. No additional cases arising from care of the primary or secondary case were detected, nor did any secondary cases follow care of an unsuspected Côte d'Ivoire Ebola case in Switzerland. Thus, distant transport of Ebola virus is an established risk, but limited nosocomial spread occurs under proper hygienic conditions.

After its first documented activity in 1976, the Sudan Ebola species returned in epidemic form to cause an indolent outbreak in Uganda in 2000–2001. This outbreak claimed the lives of 224 (53%) of 425 patients.

Reston Ebola virus was first seen in the United States in 1989, when it caused a fatal, highly transmissible disease among cynomolgus macaques imported from the Philippines and quarantined in Reston, Virginia, pending distribution to biomedical researchers. This and other appearances of the Reston virus have been traced to a single export facility in the Philippines, but no source in nature had been established until the discovery of this viral species in Philippine pigs. Occasional serologic evidence of human infection was found, but no cases of human disease were identified.

Epidemiologic studies (including a specific search in the Kikwit epidemic) have failed to yield evidence for an important role of airborne particles in human disease. This lack of epidemiologic evidence is surprising and seems to conflict with the viruses' classification as biosafety level 4 pathogens (which is based in large part on aerosol infectivity) and with formal laboratory assessments showing a high degree of aerosol infectivity for monkeys. Sick humans apparently do not usually generate sufficient amounts of infectious aerosols to pose a significant hazard to those around them.

Although numerous die-offs have been reported among chimpanzees and gorillas (some even threatening the viability of these endangered species), these animals (like humans) appear to be sentinels for virus activity. Speculation about the true reservoirs has centered on bats, and preliminary evidence indicates that bats may indeed be the reservoirs of filoviruses. This evidence includes the detection of antibodies and reverse-transcriptase polymerase chain reaction (RT-PCR) products in bats, the epidemiologic findings in subterranean gold mines in Durba (DRC) where Marburg transmission has occurred, and reported associations of human antibody production with the handling of bats. Recent isolation of Marburg virus from Egyptian fruit bats (*Rousettus aegyptiacus*) captured in Uganda in proximity to cases of human disease further supports bats as reservoirs, but the exact biologic relation and the natural cycle remain to be elucidated.

■ PATHOLOGY AND PATHOGENESIS

In humans and in animal models, Ebola and Marburg viruses replicate well in virtually all cell types, including endothelial cells, macrophages, and parenchymal cells of multiple organs. In macaques, the earliest involvement—that of the mononuclear phagocyte system—is responsible for initiation of the disease process. In human disease and macaque models, upregulation of tissue factor and disseminated intravascular coagulation (DIC) are the inciting mechanisms. Viral replication is associated with cellular necrosis both in vivo and in vitro. Significant findings at the light-microscopic level include liver necrosis with Councilman bodies, intracellular inclusions that correlate with extensive collections of viral nucleocapsids, interstitial pneumonitis, cerebral glial nodules, and small infarcts. Antigen and virions are abundant in fibroblasts, interstitium, and (to a lesser extent) the appendages of the subcutaneous tissues in fatal cases; escape through small breaks in the skin or possibly through sweat glands may occur and, if so, may be correlated with the established epidemiologic risk of close contact with patients and the touching of the deceased. Inflammatory cells are not prominent, even in necrotic areas.

In addition to sustaining direct damage from viral infection, patients infected with Ebola virus (Zaire) have high circulating levels of proinflammatory cytokines, which presumably contribute to the severity of the illness. In fact, the virus interacts intimately with the cellular cytokine system. It is resistant to the antiviral effects of interferon α, although this mediator is amply induced. Viral infection of endothelial cells selectively inhibits the expression of major histocompatibility complex class I molecules and blocks the induction of several genes by the interferons. In addition, glycoprotein expression inhibits αV integrin expression, an effect that leads to detachment and subsequent death of endothelial cells in vitro and that correlates with the limited inflammatory response evident in lesions.

Acute infection is associated with high levels of circulating virus and viral antigen. Clinical improvement takes place when viral titers decrease concomitant with the onset of a virus-specific immune response, as detected by enzyme-linked immunosorbent assay (ELISA) or fluorescent antibody testing. In fatal cases, there is usually little evidence of an antibody response, and there is extensive depletion of spleen and lymph nodes. Ebola Sudan virus amplification by PCR shows a correlation between serum viral RNA concentration and the likelihood of death. Recovery is apparently mediated by the cellular immune response: convalescent-phase plasma has little in vitro virus-neutralizing capacity and is not protective in humans or in passive transfer experiments in monkey and guinea pig models.

■ CLINICAL MANIFESTATIONS

After an incubation period of ~7–10 days (range, 3–16 days), the patient abruptly develops fever, severe headache, malaise, myalgia, nausea, and vomiting. Continued fever is joined by diarrhea (often severe), chest pain (accompanied by cough), prostration, and depressed mentation. In light-skinned patients (and less often in dark-skinned individuals), a maculopapular rash appears around day 5–7 and is followed by desquamation. Bleeding may begin about this time and is apparent from any mucosal site and into the skin. In some epidemics, fewer than half of patients have had overt bleeding, and this manifestation has been absent even in some fatal cases. Additional findings include edema of the face, neck, and/or scrotum; hepatomegaly; flushing; conjunctival injection; and pharyngitis. Around 10–12 days after the onset of disease, the sustained fever may break, with improvement and eventual recovery of the patient. Recrudescence of fever may be associated with secondary bacterial infections or possibly with localized virus persistence. Late hepatitis, uveitis, and orchitis have been reported, with isolation of virus from semen or detection of PCR products in vaginal secretions for several weeks.

■ LABORATORY FINDINGS

Leukopenia is common early on; neutrophilia has its onset later. Platelet counts fall below (sometimes much below) 50,000/μL. Laboratory evidence of DIC is found, but its clinical significance and the need for therapy are controversial. Serum levels of alanine and aspartate aminotransferases (particularly the latter) rise progressively, and jaundice develops in some cases. The serum amylase level may be elevated, and this elevation may be associated with abdominal pain, suggesting pancreatitis. Proteinuria is usual; decreased kidney function is proportional to shock.

■ DIAGNOSIS

Most patients acutely ill as a result of infection with Ebola or Marburg virus have high concentrations of virus in blood. Antigen-detection ELISA is a sensitive, robust diagnostic modality. Virus isolation and reverse-transcription PCR are also effective and provide additional sensitivity needed in some cases. Recovering patients develop IgM and IgG antibodies that are readily detected by ELISA. The indirect fluorescent antibody test with paired sera is an effective diagnostic tool in most acute cases but is extremely misleading in population-based serologic surveys for Ebola virus activity. Real-time PCR is extremely useful in detecting the need for quarantine or geographic spread. Skin biopsies are an extremely useful adjunct in postmortem diagnosis of infection with Ebola

virus (and, to a lesser extent, Marburg virus) because of the presence of large amounts of viral antigen, the relatively low risk posed by sample collection, and the lack of cold-chain requirements for formalin-fixed tissues.

TREATMENT   Marburg and Ebola Virus Infections

No virus-specific therapy is available, and—given the extensive viral involvement in fatal cases—supportive treatment may not be as useful as was once hoped. However, studies in rhesus monkeys have shown improved survival among animals treated with an inhibitor of factor VIIa/tissue factor or with activated protein C; this effect demonstrates the importance of DIC in pathogenesis. In addition, direct intervention against viral replication with small interfering RNA (siRNA) is effective in postexposure prophylaxis against the highly virulent Zaire species in macaques. Vigorous treatment of shock should take into account the likelihood of vascular leak in the pulmonary and systemic circulation and of myocardial functional compromise. The membrane fusion mechanism of Ebola virus resembles that of retroviruses, and the identification of "fusogenic" sequences suggests that inhibitors of cell entry may be developed. Despite the poor neutralizing capacity of polyclonal convalescent-phase sera, phage display of immunoglobulin mRNA from convalescent-phase bone marrow has yielded monoclonal antibodies that have in vitro neutralizing capacity and mediate protection in guinea pig models (but, unfortunately, not in the more sensitive monkey models).

■ PREVENTION

No vaccine or antiviral drug is currently available, but barrier nursing precautions in African hospitals can greatly decrease the spread of filoviruses beyond the index case and thus prevent epidemics of infection with these viruses and other agents as well. An adenovirus-vectored Ebola glycoprotein gene has proved protective in nonhuman primates and is undergoing phase 1 trials in humans. An experimental vesicular stomatitis virus–based vaccine has protected macaques when given both before and after infection with the Zaire Ebola virus.

FURTHER READINGS

FELDMANN H et al: Proceedings of an international symposium on filoviruses. J Infect Dis 196(Suppl 2), 2007 [whole issue]

GEISBERT TW et al: Treatment of Ebola virus infection with a recombinant inhibitor of factor VIIa/tissue factor: A study in rhesus monkeys. Lancet 362:1953, 2003

PETERS CJ: Filoviridae: Marburg and Ebola virus hemorrhagic fevers, in GL Mandell et al (eds): Principles and Practice of Infectious Diseases, 7th ed. Philadelphia, Churchill Livingstone, 2010, pp 2259–2262

———, LeDuc JW: An introduction to Ebola: The virus and the disease. J Infect Dis 179(Suppl 1):ix, 1999

SANCHEZ A et al: Analysis of human peripheral blood samples from fatal and nonfatal cases of Ebola (Sudan) hemorrhagic fever: Cellular responses, virus load, and nitric oxide levels. J Virol 78:10370, 2004

TOWNER JS et al: Marburgvirus genomics and association with a large hemorrhagic fever outbreak in Angola. J Virol 80:6497, 2006

CHAPTER 198

Diagnosis and Treatment of Fungal Infections

John E. Edwards, Jr.

■ TERMINOLOGY AND MICROBIOLOGY

Traditionally, fungal infections have been classified into specific categories based on both anatomic location and epidemiology. The most common general anatomic categories are mucocutaneous and deep organ infection; the most common general epidemiologic categories are endemic and opportunistic. Although *mucocutaneous infections* can cause serious morbidity, they are rarely fatal. *Deep organ infections* also cause severe illness in many cases and, in contrast to mucocutaneous infections, are often fatal. The *endemic mycoses* (e.g., coccidioidomycosis) are infections caused by fungal organisms that are not part of the normal human microbial flora and are acquired from environmental sources. In contrast, *opportunistic mycoses* are caused by organisms (e.g., *Candida* and *Aspergillus*) that commonly are components of the normal human flora and whose ubiquity in nature renders them easily acquired by the immunocompromised host. Opportunistic fungi cause serious infections when the immunologic response of the host becomes ineffective, allowing the organisms to transition from harmless commensals to invasive pathogens. Frequently, the diminished effectiveness of the immune system is a result of advanced modern therapies that coincidentally either unbalance the host's microflora or directly interfere with immunologic responses. Endemic mycoses cause more severe illness in immunocompromised patients than in immunocompetent individuals.

Patients acquire deep organ infection with endemic fungi almost exclusively by inhalation. Cutaneous infections result either from hematogenous dissemination or, more often, from direct contact with soil—the natural reservoir for the vast majority of endemic mycoses. The dermatophytic fungi may be acquired by human-to-human transmission, but the majority of infections result from environmental contact. In contrast, the opportunistic fungus *Candida* invades the host from normal sites of colonization, usually the mucous membranes of the gastrointestinal tract. In general, innate immunity is the primary defense mechanism against fungi. Although antibodies are formed during many fungal infections (and even during commensalism), they generally do not constitute the primary mode of defense. Nevertheless, in selected infections, as discussed below, measurement of antibody titers may be a useful diagnostic test.

Three other terms frequently used in clinical discussions of fungal infections are *yeast*, *mold*, and *dimorphic fungus*. Yeasts are seen as rounded single cells or as budding organisms. *Candida* and *Cryptococcus* are traditionally classified as yeasts. *Molds* grow as filamentous forms called *hyphae* both at room temperature and in invaded tissue. *Aspergillus*, *Rhizopus* [the species that causes mucormycosis (zygomycosis)], and fungi commonly infecting the skin to cause ringworm and related cutaneous conditions are classified as molds. Variations occur within this classification of yeasts and molds. For instance, when *Candida* infects tissue, both yeasts and filamentous forms may occur (except with *C. glabrata*, which forms only yeasts in tissue); in contrast, *Cryptococcus* exists only in yeast form. *Dimorphic* is the term used to describe fungi that grow as yeasts or large spherical structures in tissue but as filamentous forms at room temperature in the environment. Classified in this group are the organisms causing blastomycosis, paracoccidioidomycosis, coccidioidomycosis, histoplasmosis, and sporotrichosis.

The incidence of nearly all fungal infections has risen substantially. Opportunistic infections have increased in frequency as a consequence of intentional immunosuppression in organ and stem cell transplantation and other diseases, the administration of cytotoxic chemotherapy for cancers, and the liberal use of antibacterial agents. The incidence of endemic mycoses has increased in geographic locations where there has been substantial population growth.

■ DIAGNOSIS

The definitive diagnosis of any fungal infection requires histopathologic identification of the fungus invading tissue, accompanied by evidence of an inflammatory response. The identification of an inflammatory response has been especially important with regard to *Aspergillus* infection. *Aspergillus* is ubiquitous and can float from the air onto biopsy material. Therefore, in rare but important instances, this fungus is an ex vivo contaminant during processing of a specimen for microscopy, with a consequent incorrect diagnosis. The stains most commonly used to identify fungi are periodic acid–Schiff and Gomori methenamine silver. *Candida*, unlike other fungi, is visible on gram-stained tissue smears. Hematoxylin and eosin stain is not sufficient to identify *Candida* in tissue specimens. When positive, an India ink preparation of cerebrospinal fluid (CSF) is diagnostic for cryptococcosis. Most laboratories now use calcofluor white staining coupled with fluorescent microscopy to identify fungi in fluid specimens.

Extensive investigations of the diagnosis of deep organ fungal infections have yielded a variety of tests with different degrees of specificity and sensitivity. The most reliable tests are the detection of antibody to *Coccidioides immitis* in serum and CSF; of *Histoplasma capsulatum* antigen in urine, serum, and CSF; and of cryptococcal polysaccharide antigen in serum and CSF. These tests have a general sensitivity and specificity of 90%; however, because there is variability among laboratories, testing on multiple occasions is advisable. The test for galactomannan has been used extensively in Europe and is now approved in the United States for diagnosis of aspergillosis. Sources of concern regarding galactomannan are the incidence of false-negative results and the need for multiple serial tests to reduce this incidence. The β-glucan test for *Candida* is also under evaluation but, like the galactomannan test, requires additional validation; this test has a negative predictive value of ~90%. Numerous polymerase chain reaction assays to detect antigens are in the developmental stages, as are nucleic acid hybridization techniques.

Of the fungal organisms, *Candida* is by far the most frequently recovered from blood. Although *Candida* species can be detected with any of the automated blood culture systems widely used at present, the lysis-centrifugation technique increases the sensitivity of blood cultures for *Candida* and for less common organisms (e.g., *H. capsulatum*). Lysis-centrifugation should be used when disseminated fungal infection is suspected.

Except in the cases of coccidioidomycosis, cryptococcosis, and histoplasmosis, there are no fully validated and widely used tests for serodiagnosis of disseminated fungal infection. Skin tests for the endemic mycoses are no longer available.

TREATMENT Fungal Infections

This discussion is intended as a brief overview of general strategies for the use of antifungal agents in the treatment of fungal infections. Regimens, schedules, and strategies are detailed in the chapters on specific mycoses that follow in this section.

Since fungal organisms are eukaryotic cells that contain most of the same organelles (with many of the same physiologic functions) as human cells, the identification of drugs that selectively kill or inhibit fungi but are not toxic to human cells has been highly problematic. Far fewer antifungal than antibacterial agents have been introduced into clinical medicine.

AMPHOTERICIN B The introduction of amphotericin B (AmB) in the late 1950s revolutionized the treatment of fungal infections in deep organs. Before AmB became available, cryptococcal meningitis and other disseminated fungal infections were nearly always fatal. For nearly a decade after AmB was introduced, it was the only effective agent for the treatment of life-threatening fungal infections. AmB remains the broadest-spectrum antifungal agent but carries several disadvantages, including significant nephrotoxicity, lack of an oral preparation, and unpleasant side effects (fever, chills, and nausea) during treatment. To circumvent nephrotoxicity and infusion side effects, lipid formulations of AmB were developed and have virtually replaced the original colloidal deoxycholate formulation in clinical use (although the older formulation is still available). The lipid formulations include liposomal AmB (L-AmB; 3–5 mg/kg per day) and AmB lipid complex (ABLC; 5 mg/kg per day). A third preparation, AmB colloidal dispersion (ABCD; 3–4 mg/kg per day), is rarely used because of the high incidence of side effects associated with infusion. (The doses listed are standard doses for adults with invasive infection.)

The lipid formulations of AmB have the disadvantage of being considerably more expensive than the deoxycholate formulation. Experience is still accumulating on the comparative efficacy, toxicity, and advantages of the different formulations for specific clinical fungal infections [e.g., central nervous system (CNS) infection]. Whether there is a clinically significant difference in these drugs with respect to CNS penetration or nephrotoxicity remains controversial. Despite these issues and despite the expense, the lipid formulations are now much more commonly used than AmB deoxycholate in developed countries. In developing countries, AmB deoxycholate is still preferred because of the expense of the lipid formulations.

AZOLES This class of antifungal drugs offers important advantages over AmB: the azoles cause little or no nephrotoxicity and are available in oral preparations. Early azoles included ketoconazole and miconazole, which have been replaced by newer agents for the treatment of deep organ fungal infections. The azoles' mechanism of action is inhibition of ergosterol synthesis in the fungal cell wall. Unlike AmB, these drugs are considered fungistatic, not fungicidal.

Fluconazole Since its introduction, fluconazole has played an extremely important role in the treatment of a wide variety of serious fungal infections. Its major advantages are the availability of both oral and IV formulations, a long half-life, satisfactory penetration of most body fluids (including ocular fluid and CSF), and minimal toxicity (especially relative to that of AmB). Its disadvantages include (usually reversible) hepatotoxicity and—at high doses—alopecia, muscle weakness, and dry mouth with a metallic taste. Fluconazole is not effective for the treatment of aspergillosis, mucormycosis, or *Scedosporium apiospermum* infections. It is less effective than the newer azoles against *C. glabrata* and *C. krusei*.

Fluconazole has become the agent of choice for the treatment of coccidioidal meningitis, although relapses have followed therapy with this drug. In addition, fluconazole is useful for both consolidation and maintenance therapy for cryptococcal meningitis. This agent has been shown to be as efficacious as AmB in the treatment of candidemia. The effectiveness of fluconazole in candidemia and the drug's relatively minimal toxicity, in conjunction with the inadequacy of diagnostic tests for widespread hematogenously disseminated candidiasis, have led to a change in the paradigm for candidemia management. The standard of care is now to treat all candidemic patients with an antifungal agent and to change all their intravascular lines, if feasible, rather than merely to remove a singular suspect intravascular line and then observe the patient. The usual fluconazole regimen for treatment of candidemia is 400 mg/d given until 2 weeks after the last positive blood culture.

Fluconazole is considered effective as fungal prophylaxis in bone marrow transplant recipients and high-risk liver transplant patients. Its general use for prophylaxis in patients with leukemia, in AIDS patients with low CD4+ T cell counts, and in patients on surgical intensive care units remains controversial.

Voriconazole Voriconazole, which is available in both oral and IV formulations, has a broader spectrum than fluconazole against *Candida* species (including *C. glabrata* and *C. krusei*) and is active against *Aspergillus*, *Scedosporium*, and *Fusarium*. It is generally considered the first-line drug of choice for treatment of aspergillosis. A few case reports have shown voriconazole to be effective in individual patients with coccidioidomycosis, blastomycosis, and histoplasmosis, but because of limited data this agent is not recommended for treatment of the endemic mycoses. Among the disadvantages of voriconazole (compared with fluconazole) are its more numerous interactions with many of the drugs used in patients predisposed to fungal infections. Hepatotoxicity, skin rashes (including photosensitivity), and visual disturbances are relatively common. Skin cancer surveillance is now recommended for patients taking voriconazole. Voriconazole is also considerably more expensive than fluconazole. Moreover, it is advisable to monitor voriconazole levels in certain patients since (1) this drug is completely metabolized in the liver by CYP2C9, CYP3A4, and CYP2C19; and (2) human genetic variability in CYP2C19 activity exists. Dosages should be reduced accordingly in those patients with liver failure. Dose adjustments for renal insufficiency are not necessary; however, because the IV formulation is prepared in cyclodextrin, it should not be given to patients with severe renal insufficiency.

Itraconazole Itraconazole is available in IV and oral (capsule and suspension) formulations. Varying blood levels among patients taking oral itraconazole reflect a disadvantage compared with the other azoles. Itraconazole is the drug of choice for mild to moderate histoplasmosis and blastomycosis and has often been used for chronic mucocutaneous candidiasis. It has been approved by the U.S. Food and Drug Administration (FDA) for use in febrile neutropenic patients. Itraconazole has also proved useful for the treatment of chronic coccidioidomycosis, sporotrichosis, and *S. apiospermum* infection. The mucocutaneous and cutaneous fungal infections that have been treated successfully with itraconazole include oropharyngeal candidiasis (especially in AIDS patients), tinea versicolor, tinea capitis, and onychomycosis. Disadvantages of itraconazole include its poor penetration into CSF, the use of cyclodextrin in both the oral suspension and the IV preparation, the variable absorption of the drug in capsule form, and the need for monitoring of blood levels in patients taking capsules for disseminated mycoses. Reported cases of severe congestive heart failure in patients taking itraconazole have been a source of concern. Like the other azoles, itraconazole can cause hepatic toxicity.

Posaconazole Posaconazole is approved by the FDA for prophylaxis of aspergillosis and candidiasis in patients at high risk for developing these infections because of severe immunocompromise. It has also been approved for the treatment of oropharyngeal candidiasis and has been evaluated for the treatment of zygomycosis, fusariosis, aspergillosis, cryptococcosis, and various other forms of candidal infection. The relevant studies of posaconazole in zygomycosis, fusariosis, and aspergillosis have examined salvage therapy. A study of >90 patients whose zygomycosis was refractory to other therapy yielded encouraging results. No trials of posaconazole for the treatment of candidemia have yet been reported. Case reports have described the drug's efficacy in coccidioidomycosis and histoplasmosis. Controlled trials have shown its effectiveness as a prophylactic agent in patients with acute leukemia and in bone marrow transplant recipients. In addition, posaconazole has been found to be effective against fluconazole-resistant *Candida* species. The results of a large-scale study of the use of posaconazole as salvage therapy for aspergillosis indicated that it is an alternative to other agents for salvage therapy; however, that study predated the use of voriconazole and the echinocandins.

ECHINOCANDINS The echinocandins, including the FDA-approved drugs caspofungin, anidulafungin, and micafungin, have added considerably to the antifungal armamentarium. All three of these agents inhibit β-1,3-glucan synthase, which is necessary for cell wall synthesis in fungi and is not a component of human cells. None of these agents is currently available in an oral formulation. The echinocandins are considered fungicidal for *Candida* and fungistatic for *Aspergillus*. Their greatest use to date is against candidal infections. They offer two advantages: broad-spectrum activity against all *Candida* species and relatively low toxicity. The minimal inhibitory concentrations (MICs) of all the echinocandins are highest against *C. parapsilosis*; it is not clear whether these higher MIC values represent less clinical effectiveness against this species. The echinocandins are among the safest antifungal agents.

In controlled trials, *caspofungin* has been at least as efficacious as AmB for the treatment of candidemia and invasive candidiasis and as efficacious as fluconazole for the treatment of candidal esophagitis. In addition, caspofungin has been efficacious as salvage therapy for aspergillosis. *Anidulafungin* has been approved by the FDA as therapy for candidemia in nonneutropenic patients and for *Candida* esophagitis, intraabdominal infection, and peritonitis. In controlled trials, anidulafungin has been shown to be noninferior and possibly superior to fluconazole against candidemia and invasive candidiasis. It is as efficacious as fluconazole against candidal esophagitis. When anidulafungin is used with cyclosporine, tacrolimus, or voriconazole, no dosage adjustment is required for either

drug in the combination. *Micafungin* has been approved for the treatment of esophageal candidiasis and candidemia and for prophylaxis in patients receiving stem cell transplants. In a head-to-head trial, micafungin was noninferior to caspofungin for the treatment of candidemia. Studies thus far have shown that coadministration of micafungin and cyclosporine does not require dose adjustments for either drug. When micafungin is given with sirolimus, the AUC rises for sirolimus, usually necessitating a reduction in its dose. In open-label trials, favorable results have been obtained with micafungin for the treatment of deep-seated *Aspergillus* and *Candida* infections.

FLUCYTOSINE (5-FLUOROCYTOSINE) The use of flucytosine has diminished as newer antifungal drugs have been developed. Flucytosine has a unique mechanism of action based on intrafungal conversion to 5-fluorouracil, which is toxic to the fungal cell. Development of resistance to the compound has limited its use as a single agent. Flucytosine is nearly always used in combination with AmB. Its good penetration into the CSF makes it attractive for use with AmB for treatment of cryptococcal meningitis. Flucytosine has also been recommended for the treatment of candidal meningitis in combination with AmB; comparative trials with AmB alone have not been done. Significant and frequent bone marrow depression is seen with flucytosine when this drug is used with AmB.

GRISEOFULVIN AND TERBINAFINE Historically, griseofulvin has been useful primarily for ringworm infection. This agent is usually given for relatively long periods. Terbinafine has been used primarily for onychomycosis but also for ringworm. In comparative studies, terbinafine has been as effective as itraconazole and more effective than griseofulvin for both conditions.

TOPICAL ANTIFUNGAL AGENTS A detailed discussion of the agents used for the treatment of cutaneous fungal infections and onychomycosis is beyond the scope of this chapter; the reader is referred to the dermatology literature. Many classes of compounds have been used to treat the common fungal infections of the skin. Among the azoles used are clotrimazole, econazole, miconazole, oxiconazole, sulconazole, ketoconazole, tioconazole, butoconazole, and terconazole. In general, topical treatment of vaginal candidiasis has been successful. Since there is considered to be little difference in the efficacy of the various vaginal preparations, the choice of agent is made by the physician and/or the patient on the basis of preference and availability. Fluconazole given orally at 150 mg has the advantage of not requiring repeated intravaginal application. Nystatin is a polyene that has been used for both oropharyngeal thrush and vaginal candidiasis. Useful agents in other classes include ciclopirox olamine, haloprogin, terbinafine, naftifine, tolnaftate, and undecylenic acid.

FURTHER READINGS

CHEN SC et al: Antifungal therapy in invasive fungal infections. Curr Opin Pharmacol 10:522, 2010

CORNELY OA et al: Treatment outcome of invasive mould disease after sequential exposure to azoles and liposomal amphotericin B. J Antimicrob Chemother 65:114, 2010

CRONIN S, CHANDRASEKAR PH: Safety of triazole antifungal drugs in patients with cancer. J Antimicrob Chemother 65:410, 2010

KOO S et al: Prognostic features of galactomannan antigenemia in galactomannan-positive invasive aspergillosis. J Clin Microbiol 48:1255, 2010

LEVENTAKOS K et al: Fungal infections in leukemia patients: How do we prevent and treat them? Clin Infect Dis 50:405, 2010

MAERTENS J et al: Bronchoalveolar lavage fluid galactomannan for the diagnosis of invasive pulmonary aspergillosis in patients with hematologic diseases. Clin Infect Dis 49:1688, 2009

MANDELL GL et al (eds): Mycoses, in *Principles and Practice of Infectious Diseases*, 7th ed. Elsevier Churchill Livingstone, Philadelphia, 2010, pp 3221–3391

PAPPAS G et al: Clinical practice guidelines for the management of candidiasis: 2009 update by the Infectious Diseases Society of America. Clin Infect Dis 48:503, 2009

PERFECT JR et al: Clinical practice guidelines for the management of cryptococcal disease: 2010 update by the Infectious Diseases Society of America. Clin Infect Dis 50:291, 2010

RACIL Z et al: Difficulties in using 1,3-beta-D glucan as the screening test for the early diagnosis of invasive fungal diseases in patients with hematological malignancies—high frequency of false positive results and their analysis. J Med Microbol 59:1016, 2010

VYAS KS et al: Treatment of endemic mycoses. Expert Rev Respir Med 4:85, 2010

CHAPTER **199**

Histoplasmosis

Chadi A. Hage
L. Joseph Wheat

◼ ETIOLOGY

Histoplasma capsulatum, a thermal dimorphic fungus, is the etiologic agent of histoplasmosis. In most endemic areas, *H. capsulatum* var. *capsulatum* is the causative agent; in Africa, *H. capsulatum* var. *duboisii* is also found. Mycelia—the naturally infectious form of *Histoplasma*—have a characteristic appearance, with microconidial and macroconidial forms. Microconidia are oval and are small enough (2–4 μm) to reach the terminal bronchioles and alveoli. Shortly after infecting the host, mycelia transform into the yeasts that are found inside macrophages and other phagocytes. The yeast forms are characteristically small (2–5 μm), with occasional narrow budding. In the laboratory, mycelia are best grown at room temperature, whereas yeasts are grown at 37°C on enriched media.

◼ EPIDEMIOLOGY

Histoplasmosis is the most prevalent endemic mycosis in North America. Although this fungal disease has been reported throughout the world, its endemicity is particularly notable in certain parts of North, Central, and South America; Africa; and Asia. In the United States, the endemic areas spread over the Ohio and Mississippi river valleys. This pattern is related to the humid and acidic nature of the soil in these areas. Soil enriched with bird or bat droppings promotes the growth and sporulation of *Histoplasma*. Disruption of soil containing the organism leads to aerosolization of the microconidia and exposure of humans nearby. Activities associated with high-level exposure include spelunking, excavation, cleaning of chicken coops, demolition and remodeling of old buildings, and cutting of dead trees. Most cases seen outside of highly endemic areas represent imported disease—e.g., cases reported in Europe after travel to the Americas, Africa, or Asia.

◼ PATHOGENESIS AND PATHOLOGY

Infection follows inhalation of microconidia (Fig. 199-1). Once they reach the alveolar spaces, microconidia are rapidly recognized and engulfed by alveolar macrophages. At this point, the microconidia transform into budding yeasts (Fig. 199-2), a process that is integral to the pathogenesis of histoplasmosis and is dependent on the availability of calcium and iron inside the phagocytes. The yeasts

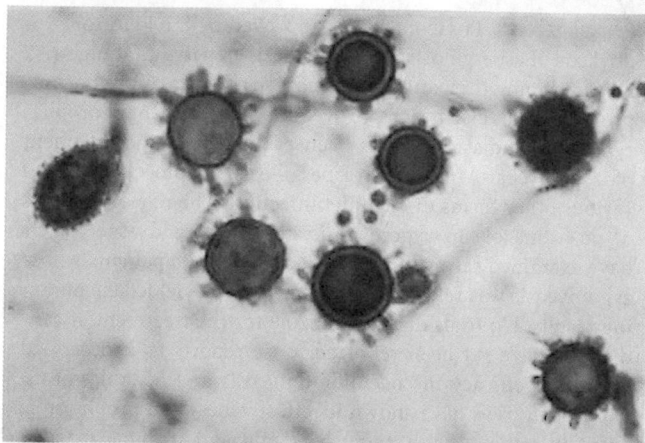

Figure 199-1   Spiked spherical conidia of *H. capsulatum* (lacto-phenol cotton blue stain).

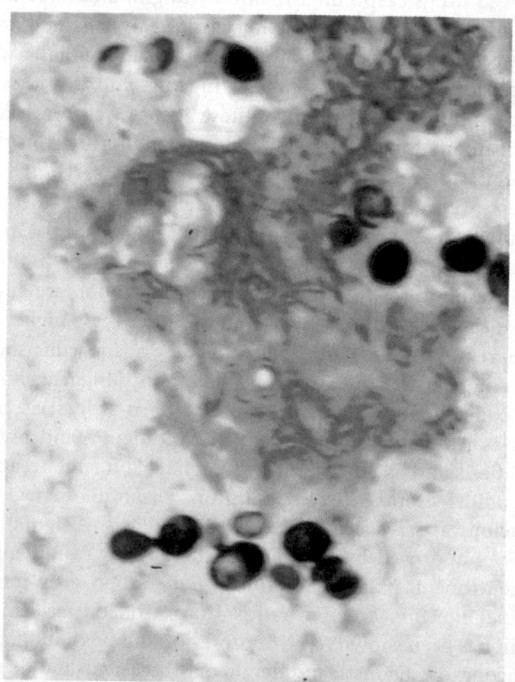

Figure 199-2   Small (2–5 μm) narrow budding yeasts of *H. capsulatum* from bronchoalveolar lavage fluid (Grocott's methenamine silver stain).

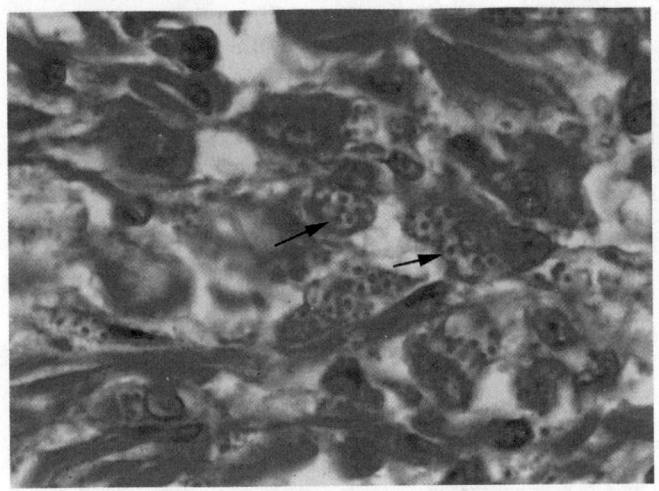

Figure 199-3 **Intracellular yeasts** (*arrows*) of *H. capsulatum* in a liver biopsy specimen (hematoxylin and eosin stain).

are capable of growing and multiplying inside resting macrophages. Neutrophils and then lymphocytes are attracted to the site of infection. Before the development of cellular immunity, yeasts use the phagosomes as a vehicle for translocation to local draining lymph nodes, whence they spread hematogenously throughout the reticuloendothelial system. Adequate cellular immunity develops ~2 weeks after infection. T cells produce interferon γ to assist the macrophages in killing the organism and controlling the progression of disease. Interleukin 12 and tumor necrosis factor α (TNF-α) play an essential role in cellular immunity to *H. capsulatum*. In the immunocompetent host, macrophages, lymphocytes, and epithelial cells eventually organize and form granulomas that contain the organisms. These granulomas typically fibrose and calcify; calcified mediastinal lymph nodes and hepatosplenic calcifications are frequently found in healthy individuals from endemic areas. In immunocompetent hosts, infection with *H. capsulatum* confers some immunity to reinfection. In patients with impaired cellular immunity, the infection is not contained and can disseminate. Progressive disseminated histoplasmosis (PDH) can involve multiple organs, most commonly the bone marrow, spleen, liver (Fig. 199-3), adrenal glands, and mucocutaneous membranes. Unlike latent tuberculosis, latent histoplasmosis rarely reactivates.

Structural lung disease (e.g., emphysema) impairs the clearance of pulmonary histoplasmosis, and chronic pulmonary disease can result. This chronic process is characterized by progressive inflammation, tissue necrosis, and fibrosis mimicking cavitary tuberculosis.

■ CLINICAL MANIFESTATIONS

The clinical spectrum of histoplasmosis ranges from asymptomatic infection to life-threatening illness. The attack rate and the extent and severity of the disease depend on the intensity of exposure, the immune status of the exposed individual, and the underlying lung architecture of the host.

In immunocompetent individuals with low-level exposure, most *Histoplasma* infections are either asymptomatic or mild and self-limited. Of adults residing in endemic areas, 50–80% have skin-test and/or radiographic evidence of previous infection without clinical manifestations. When symptoms do develop, they usually appear 1–4 weeks after exposure. Heavy exposure leads to a flulike illness with fever, chills, sweats, headache, myalgia, anorexia, cough, dyspnea, and chest pain. Chest radiographs usually show signs of pneumonitis with hilar or mediastinal adenopathy. Pulmonary

infiltrates may be focal with light exposure or diffuse with heavy exposure. Rheumatologic symptoms of arthralgia or arthritis, often associated with erythema nodosum, occur in 5–10% of patients with acute histoplasmosis. Pericarditis may also develop. These manifestations represent inflammatory responses to the acute infection rather than its direct effects. Hilar or mediastinal lymph nodes may undergo necrosis and coalesce to form large mediastinal masses that can cause compression of great vessels, proximal airways, and the esophagus. These necrotic lymph nodes may also rupture and create fistulas between mediastinal structures (e.g., bronchoesophageal fistulas).

PDH is typically seen in immunocompromised individuals, who account for ~70% of cases. Common risk factors include AIDS (CD4+ T cell count, <200/μL), extremes of age, and the use of immunosuppressive medications such as prednisone, methotrexate, and anti-TNF-α agents. The spectrum of PDH ranges from an acute, rapidly fatal course—with diffuse interstitial or reticulonodular lung infiltrates causing respiratory failure, shock, coagulopathy, and multiorgan failure—to a more subacute course with a focal organ distribution. Common manifestations include fever and weight loss. Hepatosplenomegaly is also common. Other findings may include meningitis or focal brain lesions, ulcerations of the oral mucosa, gastrointestinal ulcerations, and adrenal insufficiency. Prompt recognition of this devastating illness is of paramount importance in patients with more severe manifestations or with underlying immunosuppression, especially AIDS (Chap. 189).

Chronic cavitary histoplasmosis is seen in smokers who have structural lung disease (e.g., bullous emphysema). This chronic illness is characterized by productive cough, dyspnea, low-grade fever, night sweats, and weight loss. Chest radiographs usually show upper-lobe infiltrates, cavitation, and pleural thickening—findings resembling those of tuberculosis. Without treatment, the course is slowly progressive.

Fibrosing mediastinitis is an uncommon and serious complication of histoplasmosis. In certain patients, acute infection is followed for unknown reasons by progressive fibrosis around the hilar and mediastinal lymph nodes. Involvement may be unilateral or bilateral; bilateral involvement carries a worse prognosis. Major manifestations include superior vena cava syndrome, obstruction of pulmonary vessels, and airway obstruction. Patients may experience recurrent pneumonia, hemoptysis, or respiratory failure. Fibrosing mediastinitis is fatal in up to one-third of cases.

In healed histoplasmosis, calcified mediastinal nodes or lung parenchyma may erode through the walls of the airways and cause hemoptysis. This condition is called *broncholithiasis*.

African histoplasmosis caused by *H. capsulatum* var. *duboisii* is clinically distinct and is characterized by frequent skin and bone involvement.

■ DIAGNOSIS

Fungal culture remains the gold standard diagnostic test for histoplasmosis. However, culture results may not be known for up to 1 month, and cultures are often negative in less severe cases. Cultures are positive in ~75% of cases of PDH and chronic pulmonary histoplasmosis. Cultures of bronchoalveolar lavage (BAL) fluid are positive in about half of patients with acute pulmonary histoplasmosis causing diffuse infiltrates with hypoxemia. In PDH, the culture yield is highest for BAL fluid, bone marrow aspirate, and blood. Cultures of sputum or bronchial washings are usually positive in chronic pulmonary histoplasmosis. Cultures are typically negative, however, in other forms of histoplasmosis.

Fungal stains of cytopathology or biopsy materials showing structures resembling *Histoplasma* yeasts are helpful in the diagnosis of PDH, yielding positive results in about half of cases. Yeasts can be seen in BAL fluid (Fig. 199-2) from patients with diffuse pulmonary infiltrates, in bone marrow biopsy samples, and in biopsy specimens of other involved organs (e.g., the adrenal glands). Occasionally, yeasts are seen in blood smears from patients with severe PDH. However, staining artifacts and other fungal elements may be mis-identified as *Histoplasma* yeasts.

The detection of *Histoplasma* antigen in body fluids is extremely useful in the diagnosis of PDH and acute diffuse pulmonary histoplasmosis. The sensitivity of this technique is >95% in patients with PDH and ~80% in patients with acute pulmonary histoplasmosis if both urine and serum are tested. Antigen can be detected in cerebrospinal fluid from patients with meningitis and in BAL fluid from those with pneumonia. Cross-reactivity occurs with African histoplasmosis, blastomycosis, coccidioidomycosis, paracoccid-ioidomycosis, and *Penicillium marneffei* infection.

Serologic tests, including immunodiffusion and complement fixation, are especially useful for the diagnosis of self-limited pulmonary histoplasmosis; however, at least 1 month is required for the production of antibodies after acute infection. A fourfold rise in antibody titer may be seen in patients with acute histoplasmosis. Serologic tests are also useful for the diagnosis of chronic pulmonary histoplasmosis. Limitations of serology, however, include insensitivity early in the course of infection and in immunosuppressed patients and the persistence of detectable antibody for several years after infection. Positive results from past infection may lead to a misdiagnosis of active histoplasmosis in a patient with another disease process.

TREATMENT   Histoplasmosis

Treatment recommendations for histoplasmosis are summarized in Table 199-1. Treatment is indicated for all patients with PDH or chronic pulmonary histoplasmosis as well as for symptomatic patients with acute pulmonary histoplasmosis causing diffuse infiltrates, especially with hypoxemia. In most cases of pulmonary histoplasmosis, treatment is not recommended because the degree of exposure is not heavy; the infection is asymptomatic or symptoms are mild, subacute, and not progressive; and the illness resolves without therapy.

The preferred treatments for histoplasmosis include the lipid formulations of amphotericin B in more severe cases and itraconazole in others. Liposomal amphotericin B has been more effective than the deoxycholate formulation for treatment of PDH in patients with AIDS. The deoxycholate formulation of amphotericin B is an alternative to a lipid formulation for patients at low risk for nephrotoxicity. Posaconazole, voriconazole, and fluconazole are alternatives for patients who cannot take itraconazole.

In severe cases requiring hospitalization, a lipid formulation of amphotericin B is followed by itraconazole. In patients with meningitis, a lipid formulation of amphotericin B should be given for 4–6 weeks before the switch to itraconazole. In immunosuppressed patients, the degree of immunosuppression should be reduced if possible, although immune reconstitution inflammatory syndrome (IRIS) may ensue. Antiretroviral treatment improves the outcome of PDH in patients with AIDS and is recommended; however, whether antiretroviral treatment should be delayed to avoid IRIS is unknown.

Blood levels of itraconazole should be monitored to ensure adequate drug exposure, with target concentrations of 2–10 μg/mL. Drug interactions should be carefully assessed: itraconazole not only is cleared by cytochrome P450 metabolism but also inhibits cytochrome P450. This profile causes interactions with many other medications.

TABLE 199-1 Recommendations for the Treatment of Histoplasmosis

Type of Histoplasmosis	Treatment Recommendations	Comments
Acute pulmonary, moderate to severe illness with diffuse infiltrates and/or hypoxemia	Lipid AmB (3–5 mg/kg per day) ± glucocorticoids for 1–2 weeks; then itraconazole (200 mg bid) for 12 weeks. Monitor renal and hepatic function.	Patients with mild cases usually recover without therapy, but itraconazole should be considered if the patient's condition has not improved after 1 month.
Chronic/cavitary pulmonary	Itraconazole (200 mg qd or bid) for at least 12 months. Monitor hepatic function.	Continue treatment until radiographic findings show no further improvement. Monitor for relapse after treatment is stopped.
Progressive disseminated	Lipid AmB (3–5 mg/kg per day) for 1–2 weeks; then itraconazole (200 mg bid) for at least 12 months. Monitor renal and hepatic function.	Liposomal AmB is preferred, but the AmB lipid complex may be used because of cost. Chronic maintenance therapy may be necessary if the degree of immunosuppression cannot be reduced.
Central nervous system	Liposomal AmB (5 mg/kg per day) for 4–6 weeks; then itraconazole (200 mg bid or tid) for at least 12 months. Monitor renal and hepatic function.	A longer course of lipid AmB is recommended because of the high risk of relapse. Itraconazole should be continued until cerebrospinal fluid or CT abnormalities clear.

Abbreviation: AmB, amphotericin B.

The duration of treatment for acute pulmonary histoplasmosis is 6–12 weeks, while that for PDH and chronic pulmonary histoplasmosis is ≥1 year. Antigen levels in urine and serum should be monitored during and for at least 1 year after therapy for PDH. Stable or rising antigen levels suggest treatment failure or relapse.

Previously, lifelong itraconazole maintenance therapy was recommended for patients with AIDS once histoplasmosis was diagnosed. Today, however, maintenance therapy is not required for patients who respond well to antiretroviral therapy, with CD4+ T cell counts of at least 150/μL (preferably >250/μL); who complete at least 1 year of itraconazole therapy; and who exhibit neither clinical evidence of active histoplasmosis nor an antigenuria level of >4 ng/mL. Maintenance therapy also appears to be unnecessary in patients receiving immunosuppressive treatment if the degree of immunosuppression can be reduced through an approach similar to that used for patients with AIDS.

Fibrosing mediastinitis, which represents a chronic fibrotic reaction to past mediastinal histoplasmosis rather than an active infection, does not respond to antifungal therapy. While treatment is often prescribed for patients with pulmonary histoplasmosis who have not recovered within 1 month and for those with persistent mediastinal lymphadenopathy, the effectiveness of antifungal therapy in these situations is unknown.

FURTHER READINGS

GOLDMAN M et al: Safety of discontinuation of maintenance therapy for disseminated histoplasmosis after immunologic response to antiretroviral therapy. Clin Infect Dis 38:1485, 2004

GOODWIN RA JR, DES PREZ RM: Histoplasmosis. Am Rev Respir Dis 117:929, 1978

HAGE CA et al: Recognition, diagnosis, and treatment of histoplasmosis complicating tumor necrosis factor blocker therapy. Clin Infect Dis 50:85, 2010

—— et al: Diagnosis of histoplasmosis by antigen detection in BAL fluid Chest 137:623, 2010

—— et al: Pulmonary histoplasmosis. Semin Respir Crit Care Med 29:151, 2008

KAUFFMAN CA: Histoplasmosis: A clinical and laboratory update. Clin Microbiol Rev 20:115, 2007

SWARTZENTRUBER S et al: Diagnosis of acute pulmonary histoplasmosis by antigen detection Clin Infect Dis 49: 1878, 2009

WHEAT LJ: Approach to the diagnosis of the endemic mycoses. Clin Chest Med 30:379, 2009

CHAPTER 200

Coccidioidomycosis

Neil M. Ampel

■ DEFINITION AND ETIOLOGY

Coccidioidomycosis, commonly known as Valley Fever, is caused by dimorphic soil-dwelling fungi of the genus *Coccidioides*. Genetic analysis has demonstrated the existence of two species, *C. immitis* and *C. posadasii*. These species are indistinguishable with regard to the clinical disease they cause and their appearance on routine laboratory media. Thus, the organisms will be referred to simply as *Coccidioides* for the remainder of this chapter.

■ EPIDEMIOLOGY

Coccidioidomycosis is confined to the Western Hemisphere between the latitudes of 40°N and 40°S. In the United States, areas of high endemicity include the southern portion of the San Joaquin Valley of California and the south-central region of Arizona. However, infection may be acquired in other areas of the southwestern United States, including the southern coastal counties in California, southern Nevada, southwestern Utah, southern New Mexico, and western Texas, including the Rio Grande Valley. Outside the United States, coccidioidomycosis is endemic to northern Mexico as well as to localized regions of Central America. In South America, there are endemic foci in Colombia, Venezuela, northeastern Brazil, Paraguay, Bolivia, and north-central Argentina.

The risk of infection is increased by direct exposure to soil harboring *Coccidioides*. Because of difficulty in isolating *Coccidioides* from the soil, the precise characteristics of potentially infectious soil are not known. Several outbreaks of coccidioidomycosis have been associated with soil from archaeologic excavations of Amerindian sites both within and outside of the recognized endemic region. These cases often involved alluvial soils in regions of relative aridity with moderate temperature ranges. *Coccidioides* was isolated at depths of 2–20 cm below the surface.

In endemic areas, many cases of *Coccidioides* infection occur without obvious soil or dust exposure. Climatic factors appear to increase the infection rate in these regions. In particular, periods of aridity following rainy seasons have been associated with marked increases in the number of symptomatic cases. The number of cases of symptomatic coccidioidomycosis has increased dramatically in south-central Arizona, where most of the state's population resides. The factors causing this increase have not been fully elucidated; however, an influx of older individuals without prior coccidioidal infection into the region appears to be involved. Other variables, such as climate change, construction activity, and increased awareness and reporting, may also be factors. A similar increase in the incidence of symptomatic cases has recently been observed in the southern San Joaquin Valley of California.

■ PATHOGENESIS, PATHOLOGY, AND IMMUNE RESPONSE

On agar media and in the soil, *Coccidioides* organisms exist as filamentous molds. Within this mycelial structure, individual filaments (*hyphae*) elongate and branch, some growing upward. Alternating cells within the hyphae degenerate, leaving barrel-shaped viable elements called *arthroconidia*. Measuring ~2 by 5 μm, arthroconidia may become airborne for extended periods. Their small size allows them to evade initial mechanical mucosal defenses and reach deep into the bronchial tree, where infection is initiated in the nonimmune host.

Once in a susceptible host, the arthroconidia enlarge, become rounded, and develop internal septations. The resulting structures, called *spherules* (Fig. 200-1), may attain sizes of 200 μm and are unique to *Coccidioides*. The septations encompass uninuclear elements called *endospores*. Spherules may rupture and release packets of endospores that can themselves develop into spherules, thus propagating infection locally. If returned to artificial media or the soil, the fungus reverts to its mycelial stage.

Clinical observations and data from studies of animals strongly support the critical role of a robust cellular immune response in the host's control of coccidioidomycosis. Necrotizing granulomas containing spherules are typically identified in patients with resolved pulmonary infection. In disseminated disease, granulomas are generally poorly formed or do not develop at all, and a polymorphonuclear leukocyte response occurs frequently. In patients who are asymptomatic or in whom the initial pulmonary infection resolves, delayed-type hypersensitivity to coccidioidal antigens is routinely documented.

■ CLINICAL AND LABORATORY MANIFESTATIONS

Coccidioidomycosis is protean in its manifestations. Among infected individuals, 60% are completely asymptomatic, and the remaining 40% have symptoms that are related principally to pulmonary infection, including fever, cough, and pleuritic chest pain. The risk of symptomatic illness increases with age. Coccidioidomycosis is commonly misdiagnosed as community-acquired bacterial pneumonia.

There are several cutaneous manifestations of primary pulmonary coccidioidomycosis. Toxic erythema consisting of a maculopapular rash has been noted in some cases. Erythema nodosum (see Fig. e7-40)—typically over the lower extremities—or erythema multiforme (see Fig. e7-25)—usually in a necklace distribution—may occur;

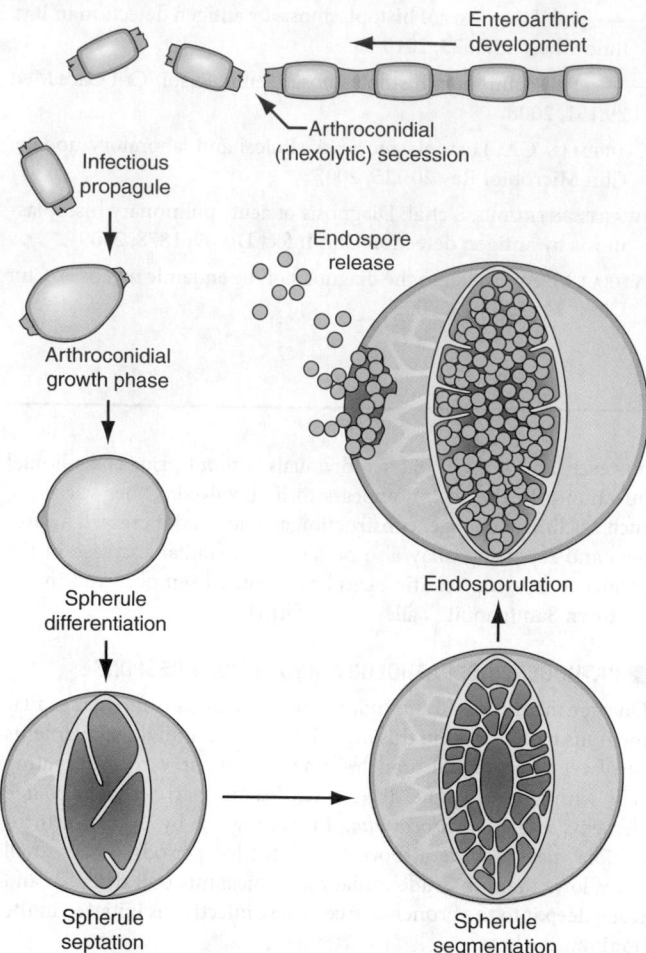

Figure 200-1 Life cycle of *Coccidioides*. *(From TN Kirkland, J Fierer: Emerg Infect Dis 2:192, 1996.)*

these manifestations are seen particularly often in women. Arthralgias and arthritis may develop. The diagnosis of primary pulmonary coccidioidomycosis is suggested by a history of night sweats or profound fatigue as well as by peripheral-blood eosinophilia and hilar or mediastinal lymphadenopathy on chest radiography. While pleuritic chest pain is common, pleural effusions occur in fewer than 10% of cases. Such effusions are invariably associated with a pulmonary infiltrate on the same side. The cellular content of these effusions is mononuclear in nature; *Coccidioides* is rarely grown from effusions.

In most patients, primary pulmonary coccidioidomycosis usually resolves without sequelae in several weeks. However, a variety of pneumonic complications may ensue. Pulmonary nodules are residua of primary pneumonia. Generally single, frequently located in the upper lobes, and ≤4 cm in diameter, nodules are often discovered on a routine chest radiograph in an asymptomatic patient. Calcification is uncommon. Coccidioidal pulmonary nodules can be difficult to distinguish radiographically from pulmonary malignancies. Like malignancies, coccidioidal nodules often enhance on positron emission tomography. However, routine CT often demonstrates multiple nodules in coccidioidomycosis. Biopsy is often required to distinguish between these two conditions.

Pulmonary cavities occur when a nodule extrudes its contents into the bronchus, resulting in a thin-walled shell. These cavities can be associated with persistent cough, hemoptysis, and pleuritic chest pain. Rarely, a cavity may rupture into the pleural space, causing pyopneumothorax. In such cases, patients present with acute dyspnea, and the chest radiograph reveals a collapsed lung with a pleural

air-fluid level. Chronic or persistent pulmonary coccidioidomycosis manifests with prolonged symptoms of fever, cough, and weight loss and is radiographically associated with pulmonary scarring, fibrosis, and cavities. It occurs in fewer than 1% of patients, many of whom already have chronic lung disease of other etiologies.

In some cases, primary pneumonia presents as a diffuse reticulonodular pulmonary process (detected by plain chest radiography) in association with dyspnea and fever. Primary diffuse coccidioidal pneumonia may occur in settings of intense environmental exposure or profoundly suppressed cellular immunity (e.g., in patients with AIDS), with unrestrained fungal growth that is frequently associated with fungemia.

Clinical dissemination outside the thoracic cavity occurs in fewer than 1% of infected individuals. Dissemination is more likely to occur in male patients, particularly those of African-American or Filipino ancestry, and in persons with depressed cellular immunity, including patients with HIV infection and peripheral-blood CD4+ T cell counts of <250/μL; those receiving chronic glucocorticoid therapy; those with allogeneic solid-organ transplants; and those being treated with tumor necrosis factor α (TNF-α) antagonists. Women who acquire infection during the second or third trimester of pregnancy are also at risk for disseminated disease. Common sites for dissemination include the skin, bone, joints, soft tissues, and meninges. Dissemination may follow symptomatic or asymptomatic pulmonary infection and may involve only one site or multiple anatomic foci. When it occurs, clinical dissemination is usually evident within the first few months after primary pulmonary infection.

Meningitis, if untreated, is uniformly fatal. Patients usually present with a persistent headache, which is occasionally accompanied by lethargy and confusion. Nuchal rigidity, if present, is not severe. Examination of cerebrospinal fluid (CSF) demonstrates lymphocytic pleocytosis with profound hypoglycorrhachia and elevated protein levels. CSF eosinophilia is occasionally documented. With or without appropriate therapy, patients may develop hydrocephalus, which presents clinically as a marked decline in mental status, often with gait disturbances.

■ DIAGNOSIS

As mentioned above, coccidioidomycosis is often misdiagnosed as community-acquired bacterial pneumonia. Serology plays an important role in establishing the diagnosis of coccidioidomycosis. Several techniques are available, including the traditional tube-precipitin (TP) and complement-fixation (CF) assays, immunodiffusion (IDTP and IDCF), and enzyme immunoassay (EIA) to detect IgM and IgG antibodies. TP and IgM antibodies are found in serum soon after infection and persist for weeks. They are not useful for gauging disease progression and are not found in the CSF. The CF and IgG antibodies occur later in the course of the disease and persist longer than TP and IgM antibodies. Rising CF titers are associated with clinical progression, and the presence of CF antibody in CSF is an indicator for coccidioidal meningitis. Antibodies disappear over time in persons whose clinical illness resolves.

Because of its commercial availability, the coccidioidal EIA is frequently used as a screening tool for coccidioidal serology. There has been concern that the IgM EIA is occasionally falsely positive. In addition, while the sensitivity and specificity of the IgG EIA appear to be high when compared with those of the CF and IDCF assays, the optical density obtained in the EIA does not correlate with the serologic titer of either of the latter tests.

Coccidioides grows within 3–7 days at 37°C on a variety of artificial media, including blood agar. Therefore, it is always useful to obtain samples of sputum or other respiratory fluids and tissues for culture in suspected cases of coccidioidomycosis. The clinical laboratory should be alerted to the possibility of this diagnosis, since

Coccidioides can pose a significant hazard to laboratory workers if it is inadvertently inhaled. The organism can also be identified directly. While treatment of samples with potassium hydroxide is rarely fruitful in establishing the diagnosis, examination of sputum or other respiratory fluids after Papanicolaou or Gomori methenamine silver staining reveals spherules in a significant proportion of patients with pulmonary coccidioidomycosis. For fixed tissues (e.g., those obtained from biopsy specimens), spherules with surrounding inflammation can be demonstrated with hematoxylin-eosin or Gomori methenamine silver staining.

A commercially available test for coccidioidal antigenuria and antigenemia that appears to be useful for the diagnosis of coccidioidomycosis, particularly in immunosuppressed patients with severe or disseminated disease, has been developed. However, this test can yield false-positive results, especially in cases of histoplasmosis and blastomycosis. Some laboratories offer genomic detection by polymerase chain reaction.

TREATMENT ▶ Coccidioidomycosis

Currently, two main classes of antifungal agents are useful for the treatment of coccidioidomycosis (Table 200-1). While once routinely prescribed, amphotericin B in all its formulations is now reserved for only the most severe cases of dissemination

TABLE 200-1 Clinical Presentations of Coccidioidomycosis, Their Frequency, and Recommended Initial Therapy for the Immunocompetent Host

Clinical Presentation	Frequency, %	Recommended Therapy
Asymptomatic	60	None
Primary pneumonia (focal)	40	In most cases, none[a]
Diffuse pneumonia	<1	Amphotericin B followed by prolonged oral triazole therapy
Pulmonary sequelae	5	
Nodule	—	None
Cavity	—	In most cases, none[b]
Chronic pneumonia	—	Prolonged triazole therapy
Disseminated disease	≤1	
Skin, bone, joint, soft tissue	—	Prolonged triazole therapy[c]
Meningitis	—	Life-long triazole therapy[d]

[a]Treatment is indicated for hosts with depressed cellular immunity as well as for those with prolonged symptoms and signs of increased severity, including night sweats for >3 weeks, weight loss of >10%, a complement-fixation titer of >1:16, and extensive pulmonary involvement on chest radiography.
[b]Treatment (usually with the oral triazoles fluconazole and itraconazole) is recommended for persistent symptoms.
[c]In severe cases, some clinicians would use amphotericin B as initial therapy.
[d]Intraventricular or intrathecal amphotericin B is recommended in cases of triazole failure. Hydrocephalus may occur, requiring a CSF shunt.
Note: See text for dosages and durations.

and for intrathecal or intraventricular administration to patients with coccidioidal meningitis in whom triazole therapy has failed. The original formulation of amphotericin B, which is dispersed with deoxycholate, is usually administered intravenously in doses of 0.7–1.0 mg/kg either daily or three times per week. The newer lipid-based formulations—amphotericin B lipid complex (ABLC), amphotericin B colloidal dispersion (ABCD), and amphotericin B liposomal complex—appear to offer no therapeutic advantage over the deoxycholate formulation for the treatment of coccidioidomycosis but are associated with less renal toxicity. The lipid dispersions are administered intravenously at doses of 5 mg/kg daily or three times per week.

Triazole antifungals are the principal drugs now used to treat most cases of coccidioidomycosis. Clinical trials have demonstrated the usefulness of both fluconazole and itraconazole, and evidence indicates that itraconazole may be more efficacious against bone and joint disease. Because of its demonstrated penetration into CSF, fluconazole is the azole of choice for the treatment of coccidioidal meningitis, but itraconazole is also effective. For both drugs, a minimal oral adult dosage of 400 mg/d should be used. The maximal dose of itraconazole is 200 mg three times daily, but higher doses of fluconazole may be given. Two newer triazole antifungals, posaconazole and voriconazole, are now available. However, given the relative paucity of clinical data, the high cost, and (particularly for voriconazole) the potential toxicity, these agents should be reserved for cases that remain recalcitrant when treated with fluconazole or itraconazole. High-dose triazole therapy may be teratogenic, particularly during the first trimester; thus, amphotericin B should be considered as therapy for coccidioidomycosis in pregnant women.

Most patients with focal primary pulmonary coccidioidomycosis require no therapy. Patients for whom antifungal therapy should be considered include those with underlying cellular immunodeficiencies and those with prolonged symptoms and signs of extensive disease. Specific criteria include symptoms persisting for ≥2 months, night sweats occurring for >3 weeks, weight loss of >10%, a serum CF antibody titer of >1:16, and extensive pulmonary involvement apparent on chest radiography.

Diffuse pulmonary coccidioidomycosis represents a special situation. Because most patients with this form of disease are profoundly hypoxemic and critically ill, many clinicians favor beginning therapy with amphotericin B and switching to an oral triazole once clinical improvement occurs.

The nodules that may follow primary pulmonary coccidioidomycosis do not require treatment. As noted above, these nodules are not easily distinguished from pulmonary malignancies by means of radiographic imaging. Close clinical follow-up and biopsy may be required to distinguish between these two entities. Most pulmonary cavities do not require therapy. Antifungal treatment should be considered in patients with persistent cough, pleuritic chest pain, and hemoptysis. Occasionally, pulmonary coccidioidal cavities become secondarily infected. This development is usually manifested by an air-fluid level within the cavity. Bacterial flora or *Aspergillus* species are commonly involved, and therapy directed at these organisms should be considered. Surgery is rarely required except in cases of persistent hemoptysis or pyopneumothorax. For chronic pulmonary coccidioidomycosis, prolonged antifungal therapy—lasting for at least 1 year—is usually required, with monitoring of symptoms, radiographic changes, sputum cultures, and serologic titers.

Most cases of disseminated coccidioidomycosis require prolonged antifungal therapy. Duration of treatment is based on resolution of the signs and symptoms of the lesion in conjunction with a significant decline in serum CF antibody titer. Such therapy routinely is continued for at least several years. Relapse occurs in 15–30% of individuals once therapy is discontinued.

Coccidioidal meningitis poses a special challenge. While most patients with this form of disease respond to treatment with oral triazoles, 80% experience relapse when therapy is stopped. Thus, life-long therapy is recommended. In cases of triazole failure, intrathecal or intraventricular amphotericin B may be used. Installation requires considerable expertise and should be performed only by an experienced health care provider. Shunting of CSF in addition to appropriate antifungal therapy is required in cases of meningitis complicated by hydrocephalus. It is prudent to obtain expert consultation in all cases of coccidioidal meningitis.

■ PREVENTION

There are no proven methods to reduce the risk of acquiring coccidioidomycosis among residents of an endemic region. Avoidance of direct contact with uncultivated soil or with visible dust containing soil presumably reduces the risk. Targeted prophylactic antifungal therapy is appropriate in patients who have evidence of active or recent coccidioidomycosis and are about to undergo allogeneic solid-organ transplantation. Data on the use of antifungal agents for prophylaxis in other situations are scanty. However, most experts would administer triazole antifungal therapy to patients with a history of active coccidioidomycosis or a positive coccidioidal serology in whom therapy with TNF–α antagonists is being initiated.

FURTHER READINGS

BINNICKER MJ et al: Detection of *Coccidioides* species in clinical specimens by real-time PCR. J Clin Microbiol 45:173, 2007

BLAIR JE: Approach to the solid organ transplantation patient with latent infection and disease caused by *Coccidioides* species. Curr Opinion Infect Dis 21:415, 2008

DURKIN M et al: Detection of *Coccidioides* antigenemia following dissociation of immune complexes. Clin Vaccine Immunol 16:1453, 2009

DRUTZ DJ, CATANZARO A: Coccidioidomycosis (parts I and II). Am Rev Respir Dis 117:559 and 727, 1978

FISHER MC et al: Molecular and phenotypic description of *Coccidioides posadasii* sp. nov., previously recognized as the non-California population of *Coccidioides immitis*. Mycologia 94:73, 2002

GALGIANI JN et al: Coccidioidomycosis. Clin Infect Dis 41:1217, 2005

——— et al: Comparison of oral fluconazole and itraconazole for progressive, nonmeningeal coccidioidomycosis. A randomized, double-blind trial. Mycoses Study Group. Ann Intern Med 133:676, 2000

KUBERSKI T et al: False-positive IgM serology in coccidioidomycosis. J Clin Microbiol 48:2047, 2010

MASSANANT FY, AMPEL NM: Coccidioidomycosis in patients with HIV-1 infection in the era of potent antiretroviral therapy. Clin Infect Dis 50:1, 2010

VALDIVIA L et al: Coccidioidomycosis as a common cause of community-acquired pneumonia. Emerg Infect Dis 12:958, 2006

CHAPTER 201

Blastomycosis

Stanley W. Chapman
Donna C. Sullivan

Blastomycosis is a systemic pyogranulomatous infection, involving primarily the lungs, that arises after inhalation of the conidia of *Blastomyces dermatitidis*. Pulmonary blastomycosis varies from an asymptomatic infection to acute or chronic pneumonia. Hematogenous dissemination occurs frequently. Extrapulmonary disease of the skin, bones, and genitourinary system is common, but almost any organ can be infected.

■ ETIOLOGIC AGENT

B. dermatitidis is the asexual state of *Ajellomyces dermatitidis*. Two serotypes have been identified on the basis of the presence or absence of the A antigen. *B. dermatitidis* exhibits thermal dimorphism, growing as the mycelial phase at room temperature and as the yeast phase at 37°C. Primary isolation is most dependable for the mycelial phase incubated at 30°C. Definitive identification usually requires conversion to the yeast phase at 37°C or, more commonly, the use of nucleic acid amplification techniques (e.g., AccuProbe, Gen-Probe, San Diego, CA) that detect mycelial-phase growth. Yeast cells are usually 8–15 μm in diameter, have thick

refractile cell walls, are multinucleate, and reproduce by a single, large, broad-based bud.

■ EPIDEMIOLOGY

Most cases of blastomycosis have been reported in North America. Endemic areas include the southeastern and south-central states bordering the Mississippi and Ohio river basins, the midwestern states and Canadian provinces bordering the Great Lakes, and a small area in New York and Canada along the St. Lawrence River. Outside North America, blastomycosis has been reported most frequently in Africa.

Early studies of endemic cases indicated that middle-aged men with outdoor occupations were at greatest risk. Reported outbreaks, however, do not suggest a predilection according to sex, age, race, occupation, or season. *B. dermatitidis* probably grows as microfoci in the warm, moist soil of wooded areas rich in organic debris. Exposure to soil, whether related to work or recreation, appears to be the common factor associated with infection.

■ PATHOGENESIS

After inhalation, the conidia of *B. dermatitidis* are susceptible to phagocytosis and killing in the lungs by polymorphonuclear leukocytes, monocytes, and alveolar macrophages. This phagocytic response represents innate immunity and probably explains the high frequency of asymptomatic infections in outbreaks. Conidia that escape phagocytosis rapidly convert to the yeast phase in tissue. The greater resistance of the thick-walled yeast form to phagocytosis and killing probably contributes to infection. This yeast-phase conversion also induces the expression of the 120-kDa glycoprotein BAD-1, which is an adhesin, an essential virulence factor, and the major epitope for humoral and cellular immunity. The primary acquired host defense against *B. dermatitidis* is cellular immunity mediated by antigen-specific T cells and lymphokine-activated macrophages.

APPROACH TO THE PATIENT **Blastomycosis**

Whether acute or chronic, blastomycosis mimics many other disease processes. For example, acute pulmonary blastomycosis may present with signs and symptoms indistinguishable from those of bacterial pneumonia or influenza. Chronic pulmonary blastomycosis most commonly mimics malignancy or tuberculosis. Skin lesions are often misdiagnosed as basal cell or squamous cell carcinoma, pyoderma gangrenosum, or keratoacanthoma. Laryngeal lesions are frequently mistaken for squamous cell carcinoma. Thus, the clinician must maintain a high index of suspicion and perform a careful histologic evaluation of secretions or biopsy material from patients who live in or have visited regions endemic for blastomycosis.

CLINICAL MANIFESTATIONS

Acute pulmonary infection is usually diagnosed in association with point-source outbreaks and is accompanied by the abrupt onset of fever, chills, pleuritic chest pain, arthralgias, and myalgias. Cough is initially nonproductive but frequently becomes purulent as disease progresses. Chest radiographs usually reveal alveolar infiltrates with consolidation. Pleural effusions and hilar adenopathy are uncommon. Most patients diagnosed with pulmonary blastomycosis have chronic indolent pneumonia with signs and symptoms of fever, weight loss, productive cough, and hemoptysis. The most common radiologic findings are alveolar infiltrates with or without cavitation, mass lesions that mimic bronchogenic carcinoma, and fibronodular infiltrates. Respiratory failure (adult respiratory distress syndrome) associated with miliary disease or diffuse pulmonary infiltrates is more common among immunocompromised patients, especially those in the late stages of AIDS (Chap. 189). Mortality rates are ≥50% among these patients, and most deaths occur within the first few days of therapy.

Skin disease is the most common extrapulmonary manifestation of blastomycosis. Two types of skin lesions occur: verrucous (more common) and ulcerative. Osteomyelitis is associated with as many as one-fourth of *B. dermatitidis* infections. The vertebrae, pelvis, sacrum, skull, ribs, or long bones are most frequently involved. Patients with *B. dermatitidis* osteomyelitis often present with contiguous soft-tissue abscesses or chronic draining sinuses. In men, blastomycosis may involve the prostate and epididymis. Central nervous system (CNS) disease occurs in <5% of immunocompetent patients with blastomycosis. In AIDS patients, however, CNS disease has been reported in ~40% of cases, usually presenting as a brain abscess. Less common forms of CNS disease are cranial or spinal epidural abscess and meningitis.

DIAGNOSIS

Definitive diagnosis of blastomycosis requires growth of the organism from sputum, pus, or biopsy material. A presumptive diagnosis is made by visualization of the characteristic broad-based budding yeast in clinical specimens. Serologic diagnosis of blastomycosis is of limited usefulness because of cross-reactivity with other fungal antigens.

A *Blastomyces* antigen assay that detects antigen in urine and serum is commercially available (Mira Vista Diagnostics, Indianapolis, IN). Antigen detection in urine appears to be more sensitive than serum antigen detection. This antigen test may be useful for monitoring of patients during therapy or for early detection of relapse. Molecular identification techniques, including DNA probe hybridization, are commercially available but are currently used only to supplement traditional methods of diagnosis.

TREATMENT **Blastomycosis**

The Infectious Diseases Society of America has published guidelines for the treatment of blastomycosis. Selection of an appropriate therapeutic regimen must be based on the clinical form and severity of the disease, the immune status of the patient, and the toxicity of the antifungal agent (Table 201-1).

TABLE 201-1 Treatment of Blastomycosis

Disease	Primary Therapy	Alternative Therapy
Immunocompetent Patient/Life-Threatening Disease		
Pulmonary	Lipid AmB, 3–5 mg/kg qd, *or* Deoxycholate AmB, 0.7–1.0 mg/kg qd (total dose: 1.5–2.5 g)	Itraconazole, 200–400 mg/d (once patient's condition has stabilized)
Disseminated		
CNS	Lipid AmB, 3–5 mg/kg qd, *or* Deoxycholate AmB, 0.7–1.0 mg/kg qd (total dose: at least 2 g)	Fluconazole, 800 mg/d (if patient is intolerant to full course of AmB)
Non-CNS	Lipid AmB, 3–5 mg/kg qd, *or* Deoxycholate AmB, 0.7–1.0 mg/kg qd (total dose: 1.5–2.5 g)	Itraconazole, 200–400 mg/d (once patient's condition has stabilized)
Immunocompetent Patient/Non-Life-Threatening Disease		
Pulmonary or disseminated (non-CNS)	Itraconazole, 200–400 mg/d, *or* Lipid AmB, 3–5 mg/kg qd, *or* Deoxycholate AmB, 0.5–0.7 mg/kg qd (in patients intolerant to itraconazole or whose disease progresses despite therapy)	Fluconazole, 400–800 mg/d, *or* Ketoconazole, 400–800 mg/d
Immunocompromised Patient[a]		
All infections	Lipid AmB, 3–5 mg/kg qd, *or* Deoxycholate AmB, 0.7–1.0 mg/kg qd (total dose: 1.5–2.5 g)	Itraconazole, 200–400 mg/d (non-CNS disease, once clinically improved)

[a]Suppressive therapy with itraconazole may be considered for patients whose immunocompromised state continues. Fluconazole (800 mg/d) may be useful for patients who have CNS disease or cannot tolerate itraconazole.
Abbreviations: AmB, amphotericin B; CNS, central nervous system.

Although spontaneous cures of acute pulmonary infection have been well documented, there are no criteria by which to distinguish patients whose disease will progress or disseminate. Thus, almost all patients with blastomycosis should be treated.

Itraconazole is the agent of choice for immunocompetent patients with mild to moderate pulmonary or non-CNS extrapulmonary disease. Therapy is continued for 6–12 months. Amphotericin B is the preferred initial treatment for patients who are severely immunocompromised, who have life-threatening disease or CNS disease, or whose disease progresses during treatment with itraconazole. Although not rigorously studied, lipid formulations of amphotericin B can provide an alternative for patients who cannot tolerate amphotericin B deoxycholate. Most patients with non-CNS disease whose clinical condition improves after an initial course of amphotericin B (usually 2 weeks in duration) can be switched to itraconazole to complete 6–12 months of therapy. Fluconazole, because of its excellent penetration of the CNS, may have a role in the treatment of patients with brain abscess or meningitis after an initial course of amphotericin B.

Voriconazole has been used successfully to treat refractory blastomycosis, blastomycosis in immunosuppressed patients, and—given its good CSF penetration—CNS blastomycosis. There are no data to support the use of posaconazole in human cases of blastomycosis. The echinocandins have variable activity against *B. dermatitidis* and have no place in the treatment of blastomycosis.

■ PROGNOSIS

Clinical and mycologic response rates are 90–95% among compliant immunocompetent patients given itraconazole for mild to moderate pulmonary and extrapulmonary disease without CNS involvement. Bone and joint disease usually requires 12 months of therapy. The <5% of infections that relapse after an initial course of itraconazole usually respond well to a second treatment course.

FURTHER READINGS

Bradsher RW: Blastomycosis, in *Clinical Mycology*, WE Dismukes et al (eds). New York, Oxford University Press, 2003, pp 299–310

Chapman SW et al: Blastomycosis. Infect Dis Clin North Am 17:21, 2003

——, Sullivan DC: *Blastomyces dermatitidis*, in *Principles and Practice of Infectious Diseases*, 7th ed, GL Mandell et al (eds). New York, Churchill Livingstone, 2010, pp 3319–3332

——, Sullivan DC: Diagnosis and treatment of blastomycosis, in *Diagnosis and Treatment of Human Mycoses*, D Hospental, M Rinaldi (eds). Totowa, NJ, Humana Press, 2007

—— et al: Clinical practice guidelines for the management of blastomycosis: 2008 update by the Infectious Diseases Society of America. Clin Infect Dis 46:1801, 2008 (updates: *www.idsociety.org*)

Deepe GS et al: Progress in vaccination for histoplasmosis and blastomycosis: Coping with cellular immunity. Med Mycol 43:381, 2005

Light RB et al: Seasonal variations in the clinical presentation of pulmonary and extrapulmonary blastomycosis. Med Mycol 46:835, 2008

Mason AR et al: Cutaneous blastomycosis: A diagnostic challenge. Int J Dermatol 47:824, 2008

CHAPTER **202**

Cryptococcosis

Arturo Casadevall

■ DEFINITION AND ETIOLOGY

Cryptococcus, a genus of yeast-like fungi, is the etiologic agent of cryptococcosis. There are two species, *C. neoformans* and *C. gattii*, each of which can cause cryptococcosis in humans. *C. neoformans* occurs in two varieties known as *grubii* and *neoformans*, which correlate with serotypes A and D, respectively. *C. gattii* has not been divided into varieties but is also antigenically diverse, consisting of serotypes B and C. Most clinical microbiology laboratories do not routinely distinguish between *C. neoformans* and *C. gattii* or among varieties, but rather identify and report all isolates simply as *C. neoformans*.

■ EPIDEMIOLOGY

Cryptococcosis was first described in the 1890s but remained relatively rare until the mid-twentieth century, when advances in diagnosis and increases in the number of immunosuppressed individuals markedly raised its reported prevalence. The spectrum of disease caused by *Cryptococcus* species consists predominantly of meningoencephalitis and pneumonia, but skin and soft tissue infections also occur. Serologic studies have shown that, although evidence for cryptococcal *infection* is common among immunocompetent individuals, cryptococcal *disease* (cryptococcosis) is relatively rare in the absence of impaired immunity. Individuals at high risk for cryptococcosis include patients with hematologic malignancies, recipients of solid organ transplants who require ongoing immunosuppressive therapy, persons whose medical conditions necessitate glucocorticoid therapy, and patients with advanced HIV infection and CD4+ T lymphocyte counts of <200/μL.

Since the onset of the HIV pandemic in the early 1980s, the overwhelming majority of cryptococcosis cases have occurred in patients with AIDS (Chap. 189). To understand the impact of HIV infection on the epidemiology of cryptococcosis, it is instructive to note that in the early 1990s there were >1000 cases of cryptococcal meningitis each year in New York City—a figure far exceeding that for all cases of bacterial meningitis. With the advent of effective antiretroviral therapy, the incidence of AIDS-related cryptococcosis has been sharply reduced among treated individuals; however, the disease remains distressingly common in regions where antiretroviral therapy is not readily available, such as Africa and Asia, where up to one-third of patients with AIDS have cryptococcosis. The global burden of cryptococcosis was recently estimated at ~1 million cases, with >600,000 deaths annually. Thus cryptococci are major human pathogens.

Cryptococcal infection is acquired from the environment. *C. neoformans* and *C. gattii* inhabit different ecologic niches. *C. neoformans* is frequently found in soils contaminated with avian excreta and can easily be recovered from shaded and humid soils contaminated with pigeon droppings. In contrast, *C. gattii* is not found in bird feces. Instead, it inhabits a variety of arboreal species, including several types of eucalyptus tree. *C. neoformans* strains are found throughout the world; however, var. *grubii* (serotype A) strains are far more common than var. *neoformans* (serotype D) strains among both clinical and environmental isolates. The geographic distribution of *C. gattii* was thought to be largely limited to tropical regions until an outbreak of cryptococcosis caused by a new serotype B strain began in Vancouver in 1999. This outbreak has extended into the United States, and *C. gattii* is now being encountered in several states in the Pacific Northwest. In addition to the different geographic distributions of the two cryptococcal species, individual susceptibility to these species affects epidemiology. Cryptococcosis caused by the *C. neoformans* varieties occurs mostly in individuals with AIDS (Chap. 189) and other forms of impaired immunity. In contrast, *C. gattii*–related disease is not associated with specific immune deficits and often occurs in immunocompetent individuals.

■ PATHOGENESIS

Cryptococcal infection is acquired by inhalation of aerosolized infectious particles. The exact nature of these particles is not known; the two leading candidate forms are small desiccated yeast cells and basidiospores. Little is known about the pathogenesis of initial infection. Serologic studies have shown that cryptococcal infection is acquired in childhood, but it is not known whether the initial infection is symptomatic. Given that cryptococcal infection is common while disease is rare, the consensus is that pulmonary defense mechanisms in immunologically intact individuals are highly effective at containing this fungus. It is not clear whether initial infection leads to a state of immunity or whether most individuals are subject throughout life to frequent and recurrent infections that resolve without clinical disease. However, evidence indicates that some human cryptococcal infections lead to a state of latency in which viable organisms are harbored for prolonged periods, possibly in granulomas. Thus the inhalation of cryptococcal cells and/or spores can be followed by either clearance or establishment of the latent state. The consequences of prolonged harboring of cryptococcal cells in the lung are not known, but evidence from animal studies indicates that the organisms' prolonged presence could alter the immunologic milieu in the lung and predispose to allergic airway disease.

Cryptococcosis usually presents clinically as chronic meningoencephalitis. The mechanisms by which the fungus undergoes extrapulmonary dissemination and enters the central nervous system (CNS) remain poorly understood. The mechanism by which cryptococcal cells cross the blood-brain barrier is a subject of intensive study. Current evidence suggests either direct fungal-cell migration across the endothelium or fungal-cell carriage inside macrophages as "Trojan horse" invaders. *Cryptococcus* species have well-defined virulence factors that include the polysaccharide capsule, the ability to make melanin, and the elaboration of enzymes (e.g., phospholipase and urease) that enhance the survival of fungal cells in tissue. Among these virulence factors, the capsule and melanin production have been most extensively studied. The cryptococcal capsule is antiphagocytic, and the capsular polysaccharide has been associated with numerous deleterious effects on host immune function. Cryptococcal infections can elicit little or no tissue inflammatory response. The immune dysfunction seen in cryptococcosis has been attributed to the release of copious amounts of capsular polysaccharide into tissues, where it probably interferes with local immune responses (Fig. 202-1). In clinical practice, the capsular polysaccharide is the antigen that is measured as a diagnostic marker of cryptococcal infection.

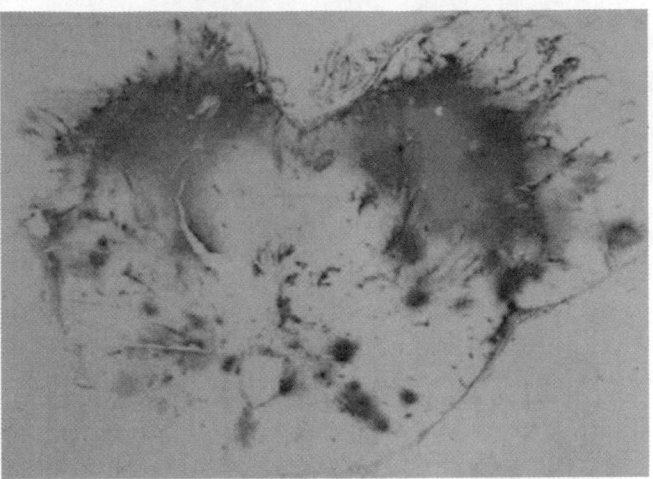

Figure 202-1 Cryptococcal antigen in human brain tissue, as revealed by immunohistochemical staining. Brown areas show polysaccharide deposits in the midbrain of a patient who died of cryptococcal meningitis. (*Reprinted with permission from SC Lee et al: Hum Pathol 27:839, 1996.*)

APPROACH TO THE PATIENT   Cryptococcosis

Cryptococcosis should be included in the differential diagnosis when any patient presents with findings suggestive of chronic meningitis. Concern about cryptococcosis is heightened by a history of headache and neurologic symptoms in a patient with an underlying immunosuppressive disorder or state that is associated with an increased incidence of cryptococcosis, such as advanced HIV infection or solid organ transplantation.

■ CLINICAL MANIFESTATIONS

The clinical manifestations of cryptococcosis reflect the site of fungal infection. Although infection can affect any tissue or organ, the majority of cases that come to clinical attention involve the CNS and/or the lungs. CNS involvement usually presents as signs and symptoms of chronic meningitis, such as headache, fever, lethargy, sensory deficits, memory deficits, cranial nerve paresis, vision deficits, and meningismus. Cryptococcal meningitis differs from bacterial meningitis in that many *Cryptococcus*-infected patients present with symptoms of several weeks' duration. In addition, classic characteristics of meningeal irritation, such as meningismus, may be absent in cryptococcal meningitis. Indolent cases can present as subacute dementia. Meningeal cryptococcosis can lead to sudden catastrophic vision loss.

Pulmonary cryptococcosis usually presents as cough, increased sputum production, and chest pain. Patients infected with *C. gattii* can present with granulomatous pulmonary masses known as *cryptococcomas*. Fever develops in a minority of cases. Like CNS disease, pulmonary cryptococcosis can follow an indolent course, and the majority of cases probably do not come to clinical attention. In fact, many cases are discovered incidentally during the workup of an abnormal chest radiograph obtained for other diagnostic purposes. Pulmonary cryptococcosis can be associated with antecedent diseases such as malignancy, diabetes, and tuberculosis.

Skin lesions are common in patients with disseminated cryptococcosis and can be highly variable, including papules, plaques, purpura, vesicles, tumor-like lesions, and rashes. The spectrum of cryptococcosis in HIV-infected patients is so varied and has changed so much since the advent of antiretroviral therapy that a distinction

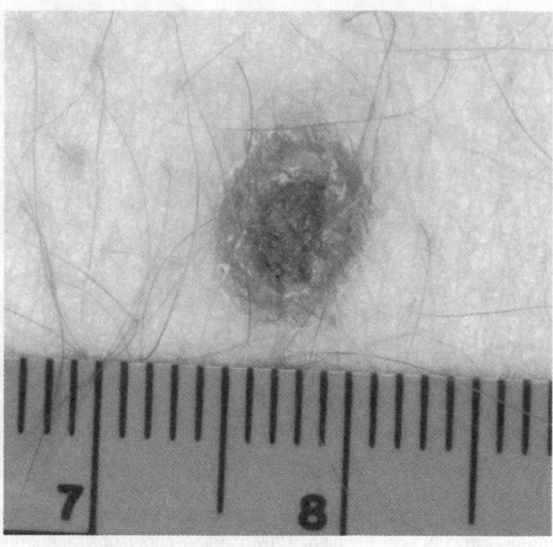

Figure 202-2 Disseminated fungal infection. A liver transplant recipient developed six cutaneous lesions similar to the one shown. Biopsy and serum antigen testing demonstrated *Cryptococcus*. Important features of the lesion include a benign-appearing fleshy papule with central umbilication resembling molluscum contagiosum. (*Photo courtesy of Dr. Lindsey Baden; with permission.*)

between HIV-related and HIV-unrelated cryptococcosis is no longer pertinent. In patients with AIDS and solid organ transplant recipients, the lesions of cutaneous cryptococcosis often resemble those of molluscum contagiosum (Fig. 202-2; Chap. 183).

◼ DIAGNOSIS

A diagnosis of cryptococcosis requires the demonstration of yeast cells in normally sterile tissues. Visualization of the capsule of fungal cells in cerebrospinal fluid (CSF) mixed with india ink is a useful rapid diagnostic technique. Cryptococcal cells in india ink have a distinctive appearance because their capsules exclude ink particles. However, the CSF india ink examination may yield negative results in patients with a low fungal burden. This examination should be performed by a trained individual, since leukocytes and fat globules can sometimes be mistaken for fungal cells. Cultures of CSF and blood that are positive for cryptococcal cells are diagnostic for cryptococcosis. In cryptococcal meningitis, CSF examination usually reveals evidence of chronic meningitis with mononuclear cell pleocytosis and increased protein levels. A particularly useful test is cryptococcal antigen (CRAg) detection in CSF and blood. The assay is based on serologic detection of cryptococcal polysaccharide and is both sensitive and specific. A positive cryptococcal antigen test provides strong presumptive evidence for cryptococcosis; however, because the result is often negative in pulmonary cryptococcosis, the test is less useful in the diagnosis of pulmonary disease.

TREATMENT	Cryptococcosis

Both the site of infection and the immune status of the host must be considered in the selection of therapy for cryptococcosis. The disease has two general patterns of manifestation: (1) pulmonary cryptococcosis, with no evidence of extrapulmonary dissemination; and (2) extrapulmonary (systemic) cryptococcosis, with or without meningoencephalitis. Pulmonary cryptococcosis in an immunocompetent host sometimes resolves without therapy. However, given the propensity of *Cryptococcus* species

to disseminate from the lung, the inability to gauge the host's immune status precisely, and the availability of low-toxicity therapy in the form of fluconazole, the current recommendation is for pulmonary cryptococcosis in an immunocompetent individual to be treated with fluconazole (200–400 mg/d for 3–6 months). Extrapulmonary cryptococcosis without CNS involvement in an immunocompetent host can be treated with the same regimen, although amphotericin B (AmB; 0.5–1 mg/kg daily for 4–6 weeks) may be required for more severe cases. In general, extrapulmonary cryptococcosis without CNS involvement requires less intensive therapy—with the caveat that morbidity and death in cryptococcosis are associated with meningeal involvement. Thus the decision to categorize cryptococcosis as "extrapulmonary without CNS involvement" should be made only after careful evaluation of the CSF reveals no evidence of cryptococcal infection. For CNS involvement in a host without AIDS or obvious immune impairment, most authorities recommend initial therapy with AmB (0.5–1 mg/kg daily) during an induction phase, which is followed by prolonged therapy with fluconazole (400 mg/d) during a consolidation phase. For cryptococcal meningoencephalitis without a concomitant immunosuppressive condition, the recommended regimen is AmB (0.5–1 mg/kg) plus flucytosine (100 mg/kg) daily for 6–10 weeks. Alternatively, patients can be treated with AmB (0.5–1 mg/kg) plus flucytosine (100 mg/kg) daily for 2 weeks and then with fluconazole (400 mg/d) for at least 10 weeks. Patients with immunosuppression are treated with the same initial regimens except that consolidation therapy with fluconazole is given for a prolonged period to prevent relapse.

Cryptococcosis in patients with HIV infection always requires aggressive therapy and is considered incurable unless immune function improves. Consequently, therapy for cryptococcosis in the setting of AIDS has two phases: induction therapy (intended to reduce the fungal burden and alleviate symptoms) and lifelong maintenance therapy (to prevent a symptomatic clinical relapse). Pulmonary and extrapulmonary cryptococcosis without evidence of CNS involvement can be treated with fluconazole (200–400 mg/d). In patients who have more extensive disease, flucytosine (100 mg/kg per day) may be added to the fluconazole regimen for 10 weeks, with lifelong fluconazole maintenance therapy thereafter. For HIV-infected patients with evidence of CNS involvement, most authorities recommend induction therapy with AmB. An acceptable regimen is AmB (0.7–1 mg/kg) plus flucytosine (100 mg/kg) daily for 2 weeks followed by fluconazole (400 mg/d) for at least 10 weeks and then by lifelong maintenance therapy with fluconazole (200 mg/d). Fluconazole (400–800 mg/d) plus flucytosine (100 mg/kg per day) for 6–10 weeks followed by fluconazole (200 mg/d) as maintenance therapy can be used as an alternative. Newer triazoles like voriconazole are highly active against cryptococcal strains, but clinical experience with these agents in the treatment of cryptococcosis is limited. Lipid formulations of AmB can be substituted for AmB deoxycholate in patients with renal impairment. Neither caspofungin nor micafungin is effective against *Cryptococcus* species; consequently, neither drug has a role in the treatment of cryptococcosis. Cryptococcal meningoencephalitis is often associated with increased intracranial pressure, which is believed to be responsible for damage to the brain and cranial nerves. Appropriate management of CNS cryptococcosis requires careful attention to the management of intracranial pressure, including the reduction of pressure by repeated therapeutic lumbar puncture and the placement of shunts.

In HIV-infected patients with previously treated cryptococcosis who are receiving fluconazole maintenance therapy, it may be possible to discontinue antifungal drug treatment if antiretroviral therapy results in immunologic improvement. However, certain recipients of maintenance therapy who have a history of successfully treated cryptococcosis can develop a troublesome immune reconstitution syndrome when antiretroviral therapy produces a rebound in immunologic function.

■ PROGNOSIS AND COMPLICATIONS

Even with antifungal therapy, cryptococcosis is associated with high rates of morbidity and death. For the majority of patients with cryptococcosis, the most important prognostic factor is the extent and the duration of the underlying immunologic deficits that predisposed them to develop the disease. Therefore, cryptococcosis is often curable with antifungal therapy in individuals with no apparent immunologic dysfunction, but, in patients with severe immunosuppression (e.g., those with AIDS), the best that can be hoped for is that antifungal therapy will induce remission, which can then be maintained with lifelong suppressive therapy. Before the advent of antiretroviral therapy, the median overall survival period for AIDS patients with cryptococcosis was <1 year. Cryptococcosis in patients with underlying neoplastic disease has a particularly poor prognosis. For CNS cryptococcosis, poor prognostic markers are a positive CSF assay for yeast cells by initial india ink examination (evidence of a heavy fungal burden), high CSF pressure, low CSF glucose levels, low CSF pleocytosis (<2/μL), recovery of yeast cells from extraneural sites, absence of antibody to capsular polysaccharide, a CSF or serum cryptococcal antigen level of ≥1:32, and concomitant glucocorticoid therapy or hematologic malignancy. A response to treatment does not guarantee cure since relapse of cryptococcosis is common even among patients with relatively intact immune systems. Complications of CNS cryptococcosis include cranial nerve deficits, vision loss, and cognitive impairment.

■ PREVENTION

No vaccine is available for cryptococcosis. In patients at high risk (e.g., those with advanced HIV infection and CD4+ T lymphocyte counts of <200/μL), primary prophylaxis with fluconazole (200 mg/d) is effective in reducing the prevalence of disease. Since antiretroviral therapy raises the CD4+ T lymphocyte count, it constitutes an immunologic form of prophylaxis. However, cryptococcosis in the setting of immune reconstitution has been reported in patients with HIV infection and recipients of solid organ transplants.

FURTHER READINGS

DATTA K et al: Spread of *Cryptococcus gattii* into the Pacific Northwest region of the United States. Emerg Infect Dis 15:1185, 2009

LILIANG P et al: Use of ventriculoperitoneal shunts to treat uncontrollable intracranial hypertension in patients who have cryptococcal meningitis without hydrocephalus. Clin Infect Dis 34:E64, 2002

LORTHOLARY O et al: Incidence and risk factors of immune reconstitution inflammatory syndrome complicating HIV-associated cryptococcosis in France. AIDS 19:1043, 2005

MASUR H et al: Guidelines for preventing opportunistic infections among HIV-infected persons—2002. Ann Intern Med 137:435, 2002

PARK BJ et al: Estimation of the global burden of cryptococcal meningitis among persons living with HIV/AIDS. AIDS 23:525, 2009

PERFECT JR et al: Clinical practice guidelines for the management of cryptococcal disease: 2010 update by the Infectious Diseases Society of America. Clin Infect Dis 50:291, 2010

SAAG MS et al: Practice guidelines for the management of cryptococcal disease. Clin Infect Dis 30:710, 2000

CHAPTER **203**

Candidiasis

John E. Edwards, Jr.

The genus *Candida* encompasses more than 150 species, only a few of which cause disease in humans. With rare exceptions, the human pathogens are *C. albicans, C. guilliermondii, C. krusei, C. parapsilosis, C. tropicalis, C. kefyr, C. lusitaniae, C. dubliniensis,* and *C. glabrata.* Ubiquitous in nature, these organisms are found on inanimate objects, in foods, and on animals and are normal commensals of humans. They inhabit the gastrointestinal tract (including the mouth and oropharynx), the female genital tract, and the skin. Although cases of candidiasis have been described since antiquity in debilitated patients, the advent of *Candida* species as common human pathogens dates to the introduction of modern therapeutic approaches that suppress normal host defense mechanisms. Of these relatively recent advances, the most important is the use of antibacterial agents that alter the normal human microbial flora and allow nonbacterial species to become more prevalent in the commensal flora. With the introduction of antifungal agents, the causes of *Candida* infections shifted from an almost complete dominance

of *C. albicans* to the common involvement of *C. glabrata* and the other species listed above. The non-*albicans* species now account for approximately half of all cases of candidemia and hematogenously disseminated candidiasis. Recognition of this change is clinically important, since the various species differ in susceptibility to the newer antifungal agents. In developed countries, where medical therapeutics are commonly used, *Candida* species are now among the most common nosocomial pathogens. In the United States, these species are the fourth most common isolates from the blood of hospitalized patients.

Candida is a small, thin-walled, ovoid yeast that measures 4–6 μm in diameter and reproduces by budding. Organisms of this genus occur in three forms in tissue: blastospores, pseudohyphae, and hyphae. *Candida* grows readily on simple medium; lysis centrifugation enhances its recovery from blood. Species are identified by biochemical testing (currently with automated devices) or on special agar.

■ PATHOGENESIS

In the most serious form of *Candida* infection, the organisms disseminate hematogenously and form microabscesses and small macroabscesses in major organs. Although the exact mechanism is not known, *Candida* probably enters the bloodstream from mucosal surfaces after growing to large numbers as a consequence of bacterial suppression by antibacterial drugs; alternatively, in some instances, the organism may enter from the skin. A change from the blastospore stage to the pseudohyphal and hyphal stages is generally considered integral to the organism's penetration into tissue. However, *C. glabrata* can cause extensive infection even though it does not transform into pseudohyphae or hyphae. Numerous reviews of cases of hematogenously disseminated candidiasis have identified the following predisposing factors or conditions: antibacterial agents, indwelling intravascular catheters, hyperalimentation fluids, indwelling urinary catheters, parenteral glucocorticoids, respirators, neutropenia, abdominal and thoracic surgery, cytotoxic chemotherapy, and immunosuppressive agents for organ transplantation. Patients with severe burns, low-birth-weight neonates, and persons using illicit IV drugs are also susceptible. HIV-infected patients with low CD4+ T cell counts and patients with diabetes are susceptible to mucocutaneous infection, which may eventually develop into the disseminated form when other predisposing factors are encountered. Women who receive antibacterial agents may develop vaginal candidiasis.

Innate immunity is the most important defense mechanism against hematogenously disseminated candidiasis, and the neutrophil is the most important component of this defense. Although many immunocompetent individuals have antibodies to *Candida*, the role of these antibodies in defense against the organism is not clear.

■ CLINICAL MANIFESTATIONS

Mucocutaneous candidiasis

Thrush is characterized by white, adherent, painless, discrete or confluent patches in the mouth, tongue, or esophagus, occasionally with fissuring at the corners of the mouth. This form of *Candida* disease may also occur at points of contact with dentures. Organisms are identifiable in gram-stained scrapings from lesions. The occurrence of thrush in a young, otherwise healthy-appearing person should prompt an investigation for underlying HIV infection. More commonly, thrush is seen as a nonspecific manifestation of severe debilitating illness. Vulvovaginal candidiasis is accompanied by pruritus, pain, and vaginal discharge that is usually thin but may contain whitish "curds" in severe cases.

Other *Candida* skin infections include *paronychia*, a painful swelling at the nail-skin interface; *onychomycosis*, a fungal nail infection rarely caused by this genus; *intertrigo*, an erythematous irritation with redness and pustules in the skin folds; *balanitis*, an erythematous-pustular infection of the glans penis; *erosio interdigitalis blastomycetica*, an infection between the digits of the hands or toes; *folliculitis*, with pustules developing most frequently in the area of the beard; *perianal candidiasis*, a pruritic, erythematous, pustular infection surrounding the anus; and *diaper rash*, a common erythematous-pustular perineal infection in infants. *Generalized disseminated cutaneous candidiasis*, another form of infection that occurs primarily in infants, is characterized by widespread eruptions over the trunk, thorax, and extremities. The diagnostic macronodular lesions of hematogenously disseminated candidiasis (Fig. 203-1) indicate a high probability of dissemination to multiple organs as well as the skin. While the lesions are seen predominantly in immunocompromised patients treated with cytotoxic drugs, they may also develop in patients without neutropenia.

Chronic mucocutaneous candidiasis is a heterogeneous infection of the hair, nails, skin, and mucous membranes that persists despite intermittent therapy. The onset of disease usually comes in infancy or within the first two decades of life but in rare cases can come in later life. The condition may be mild and limited to a specific area of the skin or nails, or it may take a severely disfiguring form (*Candida* granuloma) characterized by exophytic outgrowths on the skin. The condition is usually associated with specific

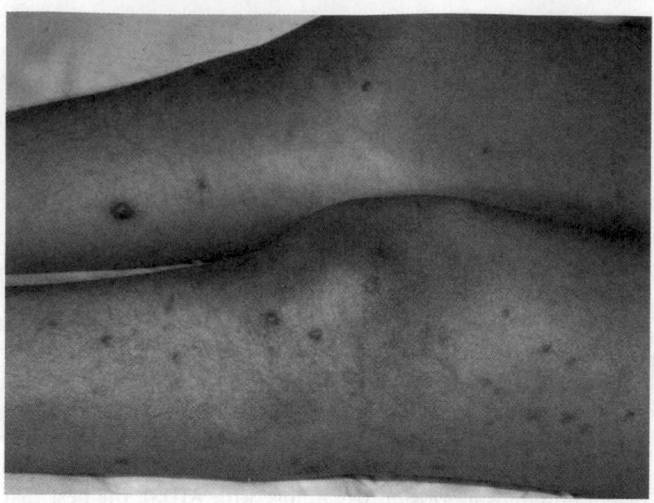

Figure 203-1 Macronodular skin lesions associated with hematogenously disseminated candidiasis. *Candida* organisms are usually but not always visible on histopathologic examination. The fungi grow when a portion of the biopsied specimen is cultured. Therefore, for optimal identification, both histopathology and culture should be performed. (*Image courtesy of Dr. Noah Craft and the Victor Newcomer collection at UCLA, archived by Logical Images, Inc.; with permission.*)

immunologic dysfunction; most frequently reported is a failure of T lymphocytes to proliferate or to stimulate cytokines in response to stimulation by *Candida* antigens in vitro. Approximately half of patients have associated endocrine abnormalities that together are designated the *autoimmune polyendocrinopathy–candidiasis–ectodermal dystrophy* (APECED) syndrome. This syndrome is due to mutations in the autoimmune regulator (*AIRE*) gene and is most prevalent among Finns, Iranian Jews, Sardinians, northern Italians, and Swedes. Conditions that usually follow the onset of the disease include hypoparathyroidism, adrenal insufficiency, autoimmune thyroiditis, Graves' disease, chronic active hepatitis, alopecia, juvenile-onset pernicious anemia, malabsorption, and primary hypogonadism. In addition, dental enamel dysplasia, vitiligo, pitted nail dystrophy, and calcification of the tympanic membranes may occur. Patients with chronic mucocutaneous candidiasis rarely develop hematogenously disseminated candidiasis, probably because their neutrophil function remains intact.

Deeply invasive candidiasis

Deeply invasive *Candida* infections may or may not be due to hematogenous seeding. Deep esophageal infection may result from penetration by organisms from superficial esophageal erosions; joint or deep wound infection from contiguous spread of organisms from the skin; kidney infection from catheter-initiated spread of organisms through the urinary tract; infection of intraabdominal organs and the peritoneum from perforation of the gastrointestinal tract; and gallbladder infection from retrograde migration of organisms from the gastrointestinal tract into the biliary drainage system.

However, far more commonly, deeply invasive candidiasis is a result of hematogenous seeding of various organs as a complication of candidemia. Once the organism gains access to the intravascular compartment (either from the gastrointestinal tract or, less often, from the skin through the site of an indwelling intravascular catheter), it may spread hematogenously to a variety of deep organs. The brain, chorioretina (Fig. 203-2), heart, and kidneys are most commonly infected and the liver and spleen less commonly so (most often in neutropenic patients). In fact, nearly any organ can

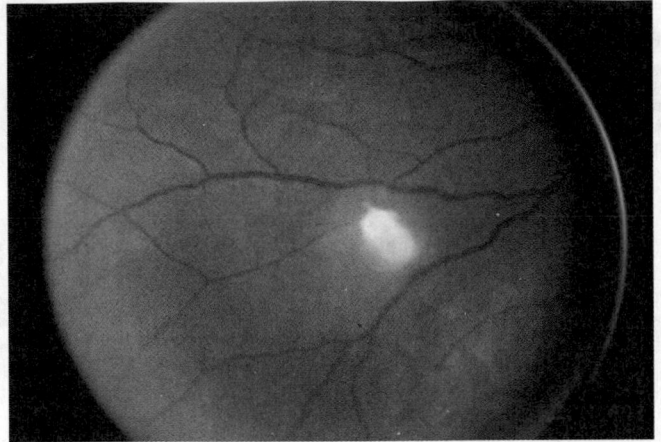

Figure 203-2 Hematogenous *Candida* endophthalmitis. A classic off-white lesion projecting from the chorioretina into the vitreous causes the surrounding haze. The lesion is composed primarily of inflammatory cells rather than organisms. Lesions of this type may progress to cause extensive vitreal inflammation and eventual loss of the eye. Partial vitrectomy, combined with IV and possibly intravitreal antifungal therapy, may be helpful in controlling the lesions. (*Image courtesy of Dr. Gary Holland; with permission.*)

TABLE 203-1 Treatment of Mucocutaneous Candidal Infections

Disease	Preferred Treatment	Alternatives
Cutaneous	Topical azole	Topical nystatin
Vulvovaginal	Oral fluconazole (150 mg) or azole cream or suppository	Nystatin suppository
Thrush	Clotrimazole troches	Nystatin
Esophageal	Fluconazole tablets (100–200 mg/d) or itraconazole solution (200 mg/d)	Caspofungin, micafungin, or amphotericin B

become involved, including the endocrine glands, pancreas, heart valves (native or prosthetic), skeletal muscle, joints (native or prosthetic), bone, and meninges. *Candida* organisms may also spread hematogenously to the skin and cause classic macronodular lesions (Fig. 203-1). Frequently, painful muscular involvement is also evident beneath the area of affected skin. Chorioretinal involvement and skin involvement are highly significant, since both findings are associated with a very high probability of abscess formation in multiple deep organs as a result of generalized hematogenous seeding. Ocular involvement (Fig. 203-2) may require specific treatment (e.g., partial vitrectomy or intraocular injection of antifungal agents) to prevent permanent blindness. An ocular examination is indicated for all patients with candidemia, whether or not they have ocular manifestations.

DIAGNOSIS

The diagnosis of *Candida* infection is established by visualization of pseudohyphae or hyphae on wet mount (saline and 10% KOH), tissue Gram's stain, periodic acid–Schiff stain, or methenamine silver stain in the presence of inflammation. Absence of organisms on hematoxylin-eosin staining does not reliably exclude *Candida* infection. The most challenging aspect of diagnosis is determining which patients with *Candida* isolates have hematogenously disseminated candidiasis. For instance, recovery of *Candida* from sputum, urine, or peritoneal catheters may indicate mere colonization rather than deep-seated infection, and *Candida* isolation from the blood of patients with indwelling intravascular catheters may reflect inconsequential seeding of the blood from or growth of the organisms on the catheter. Despite extensive research into both antigen and antibody detection systems, there is currently no widely available and validated diagnostic test to distinguish patients with inconsequential seeding of the blood from those whose positive blood cultures represent hematogenous dissemination to multiple organs. Many studies are under way to establish the utility of the β-glucan test; at present, its greatest utility is its negative predictive value (~90%). Meanwhile, the presence of ocular or macronodular skin lesions is highly suggestive of widespread infection of multiple deep organs.

TREATMENT   *Candida* Infections

MUCOCUTANEOUS CANDIDA INFECTION The treatment of mucocutaneous candidiasis is summarized in Table 203-1.

CANDIDEMIA AND SUSPECTED HEMATOGENOUSLY DISSEMINATED CANDIDIASIS All patients with candidemia are now treated with a systemic antifungal agent. A certain percentage of patients, including many of those who have candidemia associated with an indwelling intravascular catheter, probably have "benign" candidemia rather than deep-organ seeding. However, because there is no reliable way to distinguish benign candidemia from deep-organ infection, and because antifungal drugs less toxic than amphotericin B are available, it has become the standard of practice to treat all patients with candidemia, whether or not there is clinical evidence of deep-organ involvement. In addition, if an indwelling intravascular catheter may be involved, it is best to remove or replace the device whenever possible.

The drugs used for the treatment of candidemia and suspected disseminated candidiasis are listed in Table 203-2. Various lipid formulations of amphotericin B, three echinocandins, and the azoles fluconazole and voriconazole are used; no agent within a given class has been clearly identified as superior to the others. Most institutions choose an agent from each class on the basis of their own specific microbial epidemiology, strategies to minimize toxicities, and cost considerations. Unless azole resistance is considered likely, fluconazole is the agent of choice for the treatment of candidemia and suspected disseminated candidiasis in nonneutropenic, hemodynamically stable patients. Initial treatment in the context of likely azole resistance depends, as mentioned above, on the epidemiology of the individual hospital. For example, certain hospitals have a high rate of recovery of *C. glabrata*, while others do not. At institutions where non-*albicans Candida* spp. are frequently recovered, therapy with an echinocandin is typically started while the results of sensitivity testing are awaited. For hemodynamically unstable or neutropenic patients, initial treatment with broader-spectrum agents is desirable; these drugs include polyenes, echinocandins, or later-generation azoles such as voriconazole. Once the clinical response has been assessed and the pathogen specifically identified, the regimen can be altered accordingly. At present, the vast majority of *C. albicans* isolates are sensitive to fluconazole. Isolates of *C. glabrata* and *C. krusei* are less sensitive to fluconazole and more sensitive to polyenes and echinocandins. *C. parapsilosis* is less sensitive to echinocandins in vitro, although the clinical significance of this finding is not known.

TABLE 203-2 Agents for the Treatment of Disseminated Candidiasis

Agent	Route of Administration	Dose[a]	Comment
Amphotericin B deoxycholate	IV only	0.5–1.0 mg/kg daily	Being replaced by lipid formulations
Amphotericin B lipid formulations			Not FDA approved as primary therapy, but used commonly because less toxic than amphotericin B deoxycholate
Liposomal (AmBiSome, Abelcet)	IV only	3.0–5.0 mg/kg daily	
Lipid complex (ABLC)	IV only	3.0–5.0 mg/kg daily	
Colloidal dispersion (ABCD)	IV only	3.0–5.0 mg/kg daily	Associated with frequent infusion reactions
Azoles			
Fluconazole	IV and oral	400 mg/d	Most commonly used
Voriconazole	IV and oral	400 mg/d	Multiple drug interactions
			Approved for candidemia in nonneutropenic patients
Echinocandins			Broad spectrum against *Candida* species; approved for disseminated candidiasis
Caspofungin	IV only	50 mg/d	
Anidulafungin	IV only	100 mg/d	
Micafungin	IV only	100 mg/d	

[a]See Pappas et al. (2009) for loading doses and adjustments in renal failure. The recommended duration of therapy is 2 weeks beyond the last positive blood cultures and resolution of signs and symptoms of infection.

Note: Although ketoconazole is approved for the treatment of disseminated candidiasis, it has been replaced by the newer agents listed in this table. Posaconazole has been approved for prophylaxis in neutropenic patients and for oropharyngeal candidiasis. FDA, U.S. Food and Drug Administration.

Some generalizations about the management of specific *Candida* infections are possible. Recovery of *Candida* from sputum is almost never indicative of underlying pulmonary candidiasis and does not by itself warrant antifungal treatment. Similarly, *Candida* in the urine of a patient with an indwelling bladder catheter may represent colonization only rather than bladder or kidney infection; however, the threshold for systemic treatment is lower in severely ill patients in this category since it is not possible to distinguish colonization from lower or upper urinary tract infection. If the isolate is *C. albicans*, most clinicians use oral fluconazole rather than a bladder washout with amphotericin, which was more commonly used in the past. Caspofungin has been used with success; although they are poorly excreted into the urine, echinocandins may be an option, especially for non-*albicans* isolates. The doses and duration are the same as for disseminated candidiasis. The significance of the recovery of *Candida* from abdominal drains in postoperative patients is also unclear, but again the threshold for treatment is generally low because most of the affected patients have been subjected to factors predisposing to disseminated candidiasis.

Removal of the infected valve and long-term antifungal therapy constitute appropriate treatment for *Candida* endocarditis. Although definitive studies are not available, patients usually are treated for weeks with a systemic antifungal agent (Table 203-2) and then given chronic suppressive therapy for months or years (and sometimes indefinitely) with an oral azole (usually fluconazole at 400–800 mg/d).

Hematogenous *Candida* endophthalmitis is a special problem requiring ophthalmologic consultation. In lesions that are expanding or that threaten the macula, an IV polyene combined with flucytosine (25 mg/kg four times daily) has been the regimen of choice. However, as more data on the azoles and echinocandins become available, new strategies involving these agents are developing. Of paramount importance is the decision to perform a partial vitrectomy. This procedure debulks the infection and can preserve sight, which may otherwise be lost as a result of vitreal scarring. All patients with candidemia should undergo ophthalmologic examination because of the relatively high frequency of this ocular complication. Not only can this examination detect a developing eye lesion early in its course; in addition, identification of a lesion signifies a probability of ~90% of deep-organ abscesses and may prompt prolongation of therapy for candidemia beyond the recommended 2 weeks after the last positive blood culture.

Although the basis for the consensus is a very small data set, the recommended treatment for *Candida* meningitis is a polyene (Table 203-2) plus flucytosine (25 mg/kg four times daily). Successful treatment of *Candida*-infected prosthetic material (e.g., an artificial joint) nearly always requires removal of the infected material followed by long-term administration of an antifungal agent selected on the basis of the isolate's sensitivity and the logistics of administration.

PROPHYLAXIS

The use of antifungal agents to prevent *Candida* infections has been controversial, but some general principles have emerged. Most centers administer prophylactic fluconazole (400 mg/d) to recipients of allogeneic stem cell transplants. High-risk liver transplant recipients are also given fluconazole prophylaxis in most centers. The use of prophylaxis for neutropenic patients has varied considerably from center to center;

most centers that elect to give prophylaxis to this population use either fluconazole (200–400 mg/d) or a lipid formulation of amphotericin B (AmBisome, 1–2 mg/d). Caspofungin (50 mg/d) has also been recommended. Some centers have used itraconazole suspension (200 mg/d). Posaconazole (200 mg three times daily) has also been approved by the FDA for prophylaxis in neutropenic patients.

Prophylaxis is sometimes given to surgical patients at very high risk. The widespread use of prophylaxis for nearly all patients in general surgical or medical intensive care units is not—and should not be—a common practice for three reasons: (1) the incidence of disseminated candidiasis is relatively low, (2) the cost-benefit ratio is suboptimal, and (3) increased resistance with widespread prophylaxis is a valid concern.

Prophylaxis for oropharyngeal or esophageal candidiasis in HIV-infected patients is not recommended unless there are frequent recurrences.

FURTHER READINGS

Anaissie EJ et al (eds): *Clinical Mycology*, 2nd ed. Elsevier Churchill Livingstone, Philadelphia, 2009

Edwards JE Jr: Candidiasis, in *Principles and Practice of Infectious Diseases*, 7th ed, GL Mandell et al (eds). Philadelphia, Elsevier Churchill Livingstone, 2010, pp 3225–3240

Hassan I et al: Excess mortality, length of stay and cost attributable to candidaemia. J Infect 59:360, 2009

Kauffman CA: Clinical efficacy of new antifungal agents. Curr Opin Microbiol 9:1, 2006

Magill SS: The epidemiology of *Candida* colonization and invasive candidiasis in a surgical intensive care unit where fluconazole prophylaxis is utilized: Follow-up to a randomized clinical trial. Ann Surg 249:657, 2009

Maschmeyer G: The changing epidemiology of invasive fungal infections: New threats. Int J Antimicrob Agents 27:3, 2006

Moudgal V, Sobel JL: Antifungals to treat *Candida albicans*. Expert Opin Pharmacother 11:2037, 2010

Ostrosky-Zeichner L et al: Multicenter clinical evaluation of the (1→3) beta-D-glucan assay as an aid to diagnosis of fungal infections in humans. Clin Infect Dis 41:654, 2005

Pappas PG et al: Clinical practice guidelines for the management of candidiasis: 2009 update by the Infectious Diseases Society of America. Clin Infect Dis 48:503, 2009

Ruhnke M: Epidemiology of *Candida albicans* infections and role of non-*Candida-albicans* yeasts. Curr Drug Targets 7:495, 2006

Sobel JD et al: Caspofungin in the treatment of symptomatic candiduria. Clin Infect Dis 44:e46, 2007

———: *Candida* urinary tract infections—epidemiology. Clin Infect Dis 52(Suppl 6);S433, 2011 [additional relevant articles appear in this issue]

CHAPTER 204

Aspergillosis

David W. Denning

Aspergillosis is the collective term used to describe all disease entities caused by any one of ~35 pathogenic and allergenic species of *Aspergillus*. Only those species that grow at 37°C can cause invasive infection, although some species without this capability can cause allergic syndromes. *A. fumigatus* is responsible for most cases of invasive aspergillosis, almost all cases of chronic aspergillosis, and most allergic syndromes. *A. flavus* is more prevalent in some hospitals and causes a higher proportion of cases of sinus and cutaneous infections and keratitis than *A. fumigatus*. *A. niger* can cause invasive infection but more commonly colonizes the respiratory tract and causes external otitis. *A. terreus* causes only invasive disease, usually with a poor prognosis. *A. nidulans* occasionally causes invasive infection, primarily in patients with chronic granulomatous disease.

◼ EPIDEMIOLOGY AND ECOLOGY

Aspergillus has a worldwide distribution, most commonly growing in decomposing plant materials (i.e., compost) and in bedding. This hyaline (nonpigmented), septate, branching mold produces vast numbers of conidia (spores) on stalks above the surface of mycelial growth. Aspergilli are found in indoor and outdoor air, on surfaces, and in water from surface reservoirs. Daily exposures vary from a few to many millions of conidia; the latter high numbers of conidia are encountered in hay barns and other very dusty environments. The required size of the infecting inoculum is uncertain; however, only intense exposures (e.g., during construction work, handling of moldy bark or hay, or composting) are sufficient to cause disease in healthy immunocompetent individuals. Allergic syndromes may be exacerbated by continuous antigenic exposure arising from sinus or airway colonization or from nail infection. High-efficiency particulate air (HEPA) filtration is often protective against infection; thus HEPA filters should be installed and monitored for efficiency in operating rooms and in hospital environments that house high-risk patients.

The incubation period of invasive aspergillosis after exposure is highly variable, extending in documented cases from 2 to 90 days. Thus community-acquired acquisition of an infecting strain frequently manifests as invasive infection during hospitalization, although nosocomial acquisition is also common. Outbreaks usually are directly related to a contaminated air source in the hospital.

◼ RISK FACTORS AND PATHOGENESIS

The primary risk factors for invasive aspergillosis are profound neutropenia and glucocorticoid use; risk increases with longer duration of these conditions. Higher doses of glucocorticoids increase the risk of both acquisition of invasive aspergillosis and death from the infection. Neutrophil and/or phagocyte dysfunction is also an important risk factor, as evidenced by aspergillosis in chronic granulomatous disease, advanced HIV infection, and relapsed leukemia. An increasing incidence of invasive aspergillosis in medical intensive care units suggests that, in patients who are not immunocompromised, temporary abrogation of protective responses as a result of glucocorticoid use or a general anti-inflammatory state is a significant risk factor. Many patients have some evidence of prior pulmonary disease—typically, a history of pneumonia or chronic obstructive pulmonary disease. Glucocorticoid use does not appear to predispose to invasive

Aspergillus sinusitis but probably increases the risk of dissemination after pulmonary infection. Anti–tumor necrosis factor therapy also carries an increased risk of infection.

Patients with chronic pulmonary aspergillosis have a wide spectrum of underlying pulmonary disease, often tuberculosis or sarcoidosis. Patients are immunocompetent except for some cytokine regulation defects, most of which are consistent with an inability to mount an inflammatory immune (T_H1-like) response. Glucocorticoids accelerate disease progression.

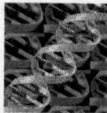 Allergic bronchopulmonary aspergillosis (ABPA) is associated with polymorphisms of interleukin (IL) 4Ra, IL-10, and SPA2 genes (and others) and with heterozygosity of the cystic fibrosis transmembrane conductance regulator (*CFTR*) gene. These associations suggest a strong genetic basis for the development of a T_H2-like and "allergic" response to *A. fumigatus*.

CD4+CD25+ T (T_{reg}) cells also appear to be pivotal in determining the disease phenotype. Remarkably, high-dose glucocorticoid treatment for exacerbations of ABPA almost never leads to invasive aspergillosis.

■ CLINICAL FEATURES AND APPROACH TO THE PATIENT
(Table 204-1)

Invasive pulmonary aspergillosis

Both the frequency of invasive disease and the pace of its progression increase with greater degrees of immunocompromise (Fig. 204-1). Invasive aspergillosis is arbitrarily divided into acute and subacute forms that have courses of ≤1 month and 1–3 months, respectively. More than 80% of cases of invasive aspergillosis involve the lungs. The most common clinical features are no symptoms at all, fever, cough (sometimes productive), nondescript chest discomfort, trivial hemoptysis, and shortness of breath. Although the fever often responds to glucocorticoids, the disease progresses. The keys to early diagnosis in at-risk patients are a high index of suspicion, screening for circulating antigen (in leukemia), and urgent CT of the thorax.

Invasive sinusitis

The sinuses are involved in 5–10% of cases of invasive aspergillosis, especially in patients with leukemia and recipients of hematopoietic stem cell transplants. In addition to fever, the most common features are nasal or facial discomfort, blocked nose, and nasal discharge (sometimes bloody). Endoscopic examination of the nose reveals pale, dusky or necrotic-looking tissue in any location. CT or MRI of the sinuses is essential but does not distinguish invasive *Aspergillus* sinusitis from preexisting allergic or bacterial sinusitis early in the disease process.

Tracheobronchitis

Occasionally, only the airways are infected by *Aspergillus*. The resulting manifestations range from acute or chronic bronchitis to ulcerative or pseudomembranous tracheobronchitis. These entities are particularly common among lung transplant recipients. Obstruction with mucous plugs occurs in normal individuals, persons with ABPA, and immunocompromised patients.

Disseminated aspergillosis

In the most severely immunocompromised patients, *Aspergillus* disseminates from the lungs to multiple organs—most often to the brain but also to the skin, thyroid, bone, kidney, liver, gastrointestinal tract, eye (endophthalmitis), and heart valve. Aside from cutaneous lesions, the most common features are gradual clinical deterioration over 1–3 days, with low-grade fever and features of mild sepsis, and nonspecific abnormalities in laboratory tests. In most cases, at least one localization becomes apparent before death occurs. Blood cultures are almost always negative.

Cerebral aspergillosis

Hematogenous dissemination to the brain is a devastating complication of invasive aspergillosis. Single or multiple lesions may develop. In acute disease, hemorrhagic infarction is most typical, and cerebral abscess is common. Rarer manifestations include meningitis, mycotic aneurysm, and cerebral granuloma. Local

TABLE 204-1 Major Manifestations of Aspergillosis

| Organ | Type of Disease | | | |
	Invasive (Acute and Subacute)	Chronic	Saprophytic	Allergic
Lung	Angioinvasive in neutropenia, non-angioinvasive, granulomatous	Chronic cavitary, chronic fibrosing	Aspergilloma (single), airway colonization	Allergic bronchopulmonary, severe asthma with fungal sensitization, extrinsic allergic alveolitis
Sinus	Acute invasive	Chronic invasive, chronic granulomatous	Maxillary fungal ball	Allergic fungal sinusitis, eosinophilic fungal rhinosinusitis
Brain	Abscess, hemorrhagic infarction, meningitis	Granulomatous, meningitis	None	None
Skin	Acute disseminated, locally invasive (trauma, burns, IV access)	External otitis, onychomycosis	None	None
Heart	Endocarditis (native or prosthetic), pericarditis	None	None	None
Eye	Keratitis, endophthalmitis	None	None	None described

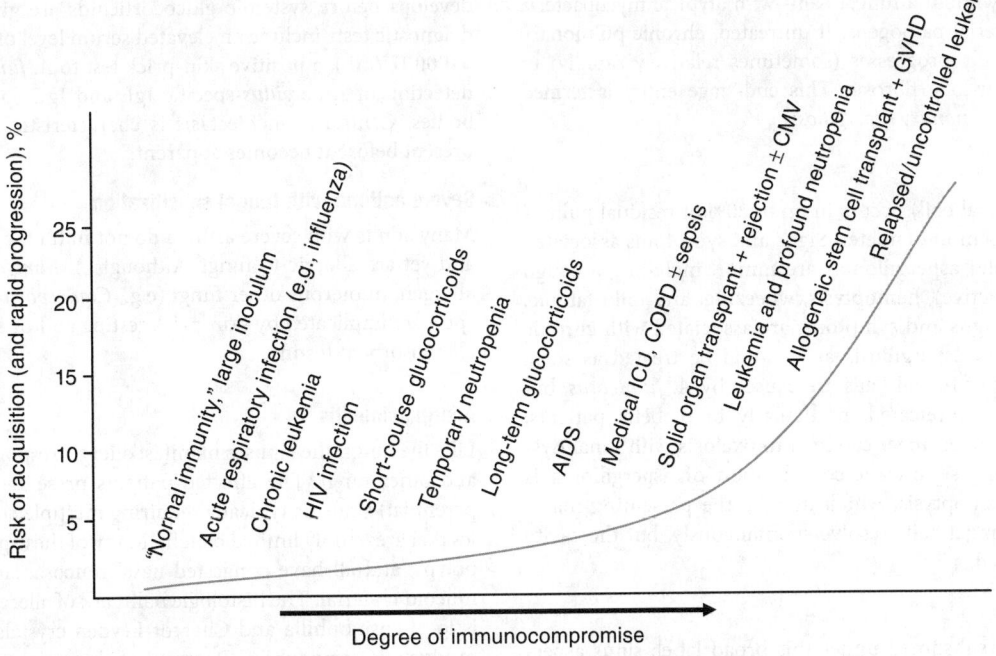

Figure 204-1 Invasive aspergillosis: conditions placing patients at elevated risk of acquisition and relatively rapid progression. CMV, cytomegalovirus; COPD, chronic obstructive pulmonary disease; GVHD, graft-versus-host disease; ICU, intensive care unit.

spread from cranial sinuses also occurs. Postoperative infection occurs rarely and is exacerbated by glucocorticoids, which are often given after neurosurgery. The presentation can be either acute or subacute, with mood changes, focal signs, seizures, and decline in mental status. Cerebral granuloma can mimic a primary or secondary tumor. MRI is the most useful immediate investigation; unenhanced CT of the brain is usually nonspecific, and contrast is often contraindicated because of poor renal function.

Endocarditis

Most cases of *Aspergillus* endocarditis are prosthetic valve infections resulting from contamination during surgery. Native valve disease is reported, especially as a feature of disseminated infection and in persons using illicit IV drugs. Culture-negative endocarditis with large vegetations is the most common presentation, but embolectomy reveals the diagnosis in a few cases.

Cutaneous aspergillosis

Dissemination of *Aspergillus* occasionally results in cutaneous features, usually an erythematous or purplish nontender area that progresses to a necrotic eschar. Direct invasion of the skin occurs in neutropenic patients at the site of IV catheter insertion and in burn patients. Rapidly progressive local aspergillosis of the skin and underlying tissue may follow trauma, and wounds may become infected with *Aspergillus* (especially *A. flavus*) after surgery.

Chronic pulmonary aspergillosis

The hallmark of chronic cavitary pulmonary aspergillosis (also called semi-invasive aspergillosis, chronic necrotizing aspergillosis, or complex aspergilloma) (Fig. 204-2) is one or more pulmonary cavities expanding over a period of months or years in association with pulmonary symptoms and systemic manifestations such as fatigue and weight loss. (Pulmonary aspergillosis developing over <3 months is better classified as subacute invasive aspergillosis.) Often mistaken initially for tuberculosis, almost all cases occur in patients

with prior pulmonary disease (e.g., tuberculosis, atypical mycobacterial infection, sarcoidosis, rheumatoid lung disease, pneumothorax, bullae) or lung surgery. The onset is insidious, and systemic features may be more prominent than pulmonary symptoms. Cavities may have a fluid level or a well-formed fungal ball, but pericavitary infiltrates and multiple cavities—with or without pleural thickening—are typical. IgG antibodies (usually precipitating) to *Aspergillus* are

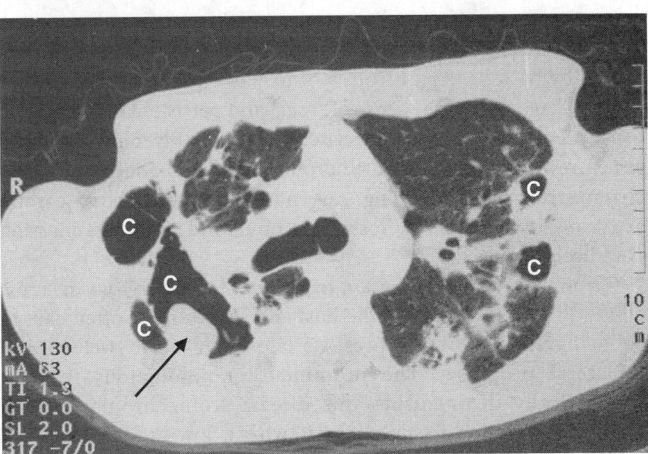

Figure 204-2 CT scan image of the chest in a patient with longstanding bilateral chronic cavitary pulmonary aspergillosis. He had a prior history of several bilateral pneumothoraces and required bilateral pleurodesis (1990). CT scan then demonstrated multiple bullae, and sputum cultures grew *A. fumigatus*. The patient had initially weakly and later strongly positive serum *Aspergillus* antibody tests (precipitins). This scan (2003) shows a mixture of thick- and thin-walled cavities in both lungs (each marked with *C*), with a probable fungal ball (*black arrow*) protruding into the large cavity on the patient's right side (*R*). There is also considerable pleural thickening bilaterally.

almost always detectable in blood. Some patients have concurrent infections—even without a fungal ball—with atypical mycobacteria and/or other bacterial pathogens. If untreated, chronic pulmonary aspergillosis typically progresses (sometimes relatively rapidly) to unilateral or upper-lobe fibrosis. This end-stage entity is termed *chronic fibrosing pulmonary aspergillosis*.

Aspergilloma

Aspergilloma (fungal ball) occurs in up to 20% of residual pulmonary cavities ≥2.5 cm in diameter. Signs and symptoms associated with single (simple) aspergillomas are minor, including a cough (sometimes productive), hemoptysis, wheezing, and mild fatigue. More significant signs and symptoms are associated with chronic cavitary pulmonary aspergillosis and should be treated as such. The vast majority of fungal balls are caused by *A. fumigatus*, but *A. niger* has been implicated, particularly in diabetic patients; aspergillomas due to *A. niger* can lead to oxalosis with renal dysfunction. The most significant complication of aspergilloma is life-threatening hemoptysis, which may be the presenting manifestation. Some fungal balls resolve spontaneously, but the cavity may still be infected.

Chronic sinusitis

Three entities are subsumed under this broad label: sinus aspergilloma, chronic invasive sinusitis, and chronic granulomatous sinusitis. *Sinus aspergilloma* is limited to the maxillary sinus and consists of a chronic saprophytic entity in which the sinus cavity is filled with a fungal ball. This form of disease is associated with prior upper-jaw root canal work and chronic (bacterial) sinusitis. About 90% of CT scans show focal hyperattenuation related to concretions; on MRI scans, the T2-weighted signal is decreased, whereas it is increased in bacterial sinusitis. Removal of the fungal ball is curative. No tissue invasion is demonstrable histologically or radiologically.

In contrast, *chronic invasive sinusitis* is a slowly destructive process that most commonly affects the ethmoid and sphenoid sinuses but can involve any sinus. Patients are usually but not always immunocompromised to some degree (e.g., as a result of diabetes or HIV infection). Imaging of the cranial sinuses shows opacification of one or more sinuses, local bone destruction, and invasion of local structures. The differential diagnosis is wide, as numerous other fungi may cause a similar disease and sphenoid sinusitis is often caused by bacteria. Apart from a history of chronic nasal discharge and blockage, loss of the sense of smell, and persistent headache, the usual presenting features are related to local involvement of critical structures. The orbital apex syndrome (blindness and proptosis) is characteristic. Facial swelling, cavernous sinus thrombosis, carotid artery occlusion, pituitary fossa, and brain and skull base invasion have been described.

Chronic granulomatous sinusitis due to *Aspergillus* is most commonly seen in the Middle East and India and is often caused by *A. flavus*. It typically presents late, with facial swelling and unilateral proptosis. The prominent granulomatous reaction histologically distinguishes this disease from chronic invasive sinusitis, in which tissue necrosis with a low-grade mixed-cell infiltrate is typical.

Allergic bronchopulmonary aspergillosis

In almost all cases, ABPA represents a hypersensitivity reaction to *A. fumigatus*; rare cases are due to other aspergilli and other fungi. ABPA occurs in ~1% of patients with asthma and in up to 15% of adults with cystic fibrosis; occasional cases are reported in patients with neither of the latter. Episodes of bronchial obstruction with mucous plugs leading to coughing fits, "pneumonia," consolidation, and breathlessness are typical. Many patients report coughing up thick sputum casts, usually brown or clear. Eosinophilia commonly develops before systemic glucocorticoids are given. The cardinal diagnostic tests include an elevated serum level of total IgE (usually >1000 IU/mL), a positive skin-prick test to *A. fumigatus* extract, or detection of *Aspergillus*-specific IgE and IgG (precipitating) antibodies. Central bronchiectasis is characteristic, but patients may present before it becomes apparent.

Severe asthma with fungal sensitization

Many adults with severe asthma do not fulfill the criteria for ABPA and yet are allergic to fungi. Although *A. fumigatus* is a common allergen, numerous other fungi (e.g., *Cladosporium* and *Alternaria* spp.) are implicated by skin-prick testing and/or specific IgE radio-allergosorbent testing.

Allergic sinusitis

Like the lungs, the sinuses manifest allergic responses to *Aspergillus* and other fungi. The affected patients present with chronic (i.e., perennial) sinusitis typically requiring multiple courses of antibiotics that are of only limited benefit. Many of these patients have nasal polyps, and all have congested nasal mucosae and sinuses full of mucoid material. The histologic hallmark of allergic fungal sinusitis is local eosinophilia and Charcot-Leyden crystals (the breakdown products of eosinophils). Removal of abnormal mucus and polyps, with local and occasionally systemic administration of glucocorticoids, usually leads to resolution. Persistent or recurrent signs and symptoms may require more extensive surgery (ethmoidectomy) and possibly local antifungal therapy.

Superficial aspergillosis

Aspergillus can cause keratitis and otitis externa. The former may be difficult to diagnose early enough to save the patient's sight. Treatment requires local surgical debridement as well as both systemic and topical antifungal therapy. Otitis externa usually resolves with debridement and local application of antifungal agents.

◼ DIAGNOSIS

Several techniques are required to establish the diagnosis of any form of aspergillosis with confidence. Patients with acute invasive aspergillosis have a relatively heavy load of fungus in the affected organ; thus culture, molecular diagnosis, antigen detection, and histopathology usually confirm the diagnosis. However, the pace of progression leaves only a narrow window for making the diagnosis without losing the patient, and some invasive procedures are not possible because of coagulopathy, respiratory compromise, and other factors. Currently, ~40% of cases of invasive aspergillosis are missed clinically and are diagnosed only at autopsy. Histologic examination of affected tissue reveals either infarction, with invasion of blood vessels by many fungal hyphae, or acute necrosis, with limited inflammation and hyphae. *Aspergillus* hyphae are hyaline, narrow, and septate, with branching at 45°; no yeast forms are present in infected tissue. Hyphae can be seen in cytology or microscopy preparations, which therefore provide a rapid means of presumptive diagnosis.

Culture is important in confirming the diagnosis, given that multiple other (rarer) fungi can mimic *Aspergillus* spp. histologically. Bacterial agar is less sensitive than fungal media for culture. Thus, if physicians do not request fungal culture, the diagnosis may be missed. Culture may be falsely positive (e.g., in patients whose airways are colonized by *Aspergillus*) or falsely negative. Only 10–30% of patients with invasive aspergillosis have a positive culture at any time. Molecular diagnostic techniques are faster and much more sensitive than culture of respiratory samples and blood.

The *Aspergillus* antigen test relies on detection of galactomannan release from *Aspergillus* spp. during growth. Antigen testing in high-risk patients is best done prospectively, as positive results usually precede clinical or radiologic features by several days. Antigen testing may be falsely positive in patients receiving certain β-lactam/β-lactamase inhibitor antibiotic combinations. Antigen and molecular testing on bronchoalveolar lavage fluid and cerebrospinal fluid are useful if performed before antifungal therapy has been given for more than a few days. The sensitivity of antigen detection is reduced by antifungal prophylaxis.

Definitive confirmation of the diagnosis requires (1) a positive culture of a sample taken directly from an ordinarily sterile site (e.g., a brain abscess) or (2) positive results of both histologic testing and culture of a sample taken from an affected organ (e.g., sinuses or skin). Most diagnoses of invasive aspergillosis are inferred from fewer data, including the presence of the *halo sign* on a high-resolution thoracic CT scan, in which a localized ground-glass appearance representing hemorrhagic infarction surrounds a nodule. While a halo sign may be produced by other fungi, *Aspergillus* spp. are by far the most common cause. Halo signs are present for ~7 days early in the course of infection in neutropenic patients and are a good prognostic feature. Thick CT sections can give the false appearance of a halo sign, as can other technical factors. Other common radiologic features of invasive pulmonary aspergillosis include pleural-based infarction or cavitation.

For chronic invasive aspergillosis, *Aspergillus* antibody testing is invaluable although relatively imprecise. Titers fall with successful therapy. Cultures are infrequently positive. Some patients with chronic pulmonary aspergillosis also have elevated titers of total serum IgE and *Aspergillus*-specific IgE.

ABPA and severe asthma with fungal sensitization are diagnosed serologically with elevated total and specific serum IgE levels and with skin-prick tests. Allergic *Aspergillus* sinusitis is usually diagnosed histologically, although precipitating antibodies in blood may also be useful.

TREATMENT   Aspergillosis

Antifungal drugs active against *Aspergillus* include voriconazole, itraconazole, posaconazole, caspofungin, micafungin, and amphotericin B. Initial IV administration is preferred for acute invasive aspergillosis and oral administration for all other disease that requires antifungal therapy. Current recommendations are shown in Table 204-2. Voriconazole is the preferred agent for invasive aspergillosis; caspofungin, posaconazole, and lipid-associated amphotericin B are second-line agents. Amphotericin B is not active against *A. terreus* or *A. nidulans*. An infectious disease consultation is advised for patients with invasive disease, given the complexity of management. It is not clear whether combination therapy for acute invasive aspergillosis is beneficial, but it is widely used for very ill patients and for those with a poor prognosis. Commonly used combinations

TABLE 204-2 Treatment of Aspergillosis

Indication	Primary Treatment	Evidence Level[a]	Precautions	Secondary Treatment	Comments
Invasive[b]	Voriconazole	AI	Drug interactions (especially with rifampin), renal failure (IV only)	AmB, caspofungin, posaconazole, micafungin	As primary therapy, voriconazole carries 20% more responses than AmB. If azole prophylaxis fails, it is unclear whether a class change is required for therapy.
Prophylaxis	Posaconazole, itraconazole solution	AI	Diarrhea and vomiting with itraconazole, vincristine interaction	Micafungin, aerosolized AmB	Some centers monitor plasma levels of itraconazole and posaconazole.
ABPA	Itraconazole	AI	Some glucocorticoid interactions, including with inhaled formulations	Voriconazole, posaconazole	Long-term therapy is helpful in most patients. No evidence indicates whether therapy modifies progression to bronchiectasis/fibrosis.
Single aspergilloma	Surgery	BII	Multicavity disease: poor outcome of surgery; medical therapy preferable	Itraconazole, voriconazole, intracavity AmB	Single large cavities with an aspergilloma are best resected.
Chronic pulmonary[b]	Itraconazole, voriconazole	BII	Poor absorption of capsules with proton pump inhibitors or H₂ blockers	Posaconazole, IV AmB, IV micafungin	Resistance may emerge during treatment, especially if plasma drug levels are subtherapeutic.

[a]Evidence levels are those used in treatment guidelines [Walsh TJ et al: Treatment of aspergillosis: Clinical practice guidelines of the Infectious Diseases Society of America (IDSA). Clin Infect Dis 46:327, 2008].

[b]An infectious disease consultation is appropriate for these patients.

Note: The oral dose is usually 200 mg bid for voriconazole and itraconazole and 400 mg bid for posaconazole. The IV dose of voriconazole is 6 mg/kg twice at 12-h intervals (loading doses) followed by 4 mg/kg q12h. Plasma monitoring is helpful in optimizing the dosage. Caspofungin is given as a single loading dose of 70 mg and then at 50 mg/d; some authorities use 70 mg/d for patients weighing >80 kg, and lower doses are required with hepatic dysfunction. Micafungin is given as 50 mg/d for prophylaxis and as at least 150 mg/d for treatment; this drug is not yet approved by the U.S. Food and Drug Administration (FDA) for this indication. AmB deoxycholate is given at a daily dose of 1 mg/kg if tolerated. Several strategies are available for minimizing renal dysfunction. Lipid-associated AmB is given at 3 mg/kg (AmBisome) or 5 mg/kg (Abelcet). Different regimens are available for aerosolized AmB, but none is FDA approved. Other considerations that may alter dose selection or route include age; concomitant medications; renal, hepatic, or intestinal dysfunction; and drug tolerability. AmB, amphotericin B.

include an azole with either caspofungin or micafungin. The interactions of voriconazole and itraconazole with many drugs must be considered before these agents are prescribed. In addition, the plasma concentrations of both drugs vary substantially from one patient to another, and many authorities recommend monitoring to ensure that drug concentrations are adequate but not excessive. The duration of therapy for invasive aspergillosis varies from ~3 months to several years, depending on the patient's immune status and response to therapy. Relapse occurs if the response is suboptimal and immune reconstitution is not complete.

Itraconazole is the preferred oral agent for chronic and allergic forms of aspergillosis. Voriconazole or posaconazole can be substituted when failure, emergence of resistance, or adverse events occur. An itraconazole dose of 200 mg twice daily is recommended, with monitoring of drug concentrations in the blood. Chronic cavitary pulmonary aspergillosis probably requires life-long therapy, whereas the duration of treatment for other forms of chronic and allergic aspergillosis requires case-by-case evaluation.

Resistance to one or more azoles, although uncommon, may develop during long-term treatment, and a positive culture during antifungal therapy is an indication for susceptibility testing. Glucocorticoids should be used with caution in chronic cavitary pulmonary aspergillosis.

Surgical treatment is important in several forms of aspergillosis, including maxillary fungal ball and single aspergillomas, in which surgery is curative; invasive aspergillosis involving bone, heart valve, sinuses, and proximal areas of the lung; brain abscess; keratitis; and endophthalmitis. In allergic fungal sinusitis, removal of abnormal mucus and polyps, with local and occasionally systemic glucocorticoid treatment, usually leads to resolution. Persistent or recurrent signs and symptoms may require more extensive surgery (ethmoidectomy) and possibly local antifungal therapy. Surgery is problematic in chronic pulmonary aspergillosis, usually resulting in serious complications. Bronchial artery embolization is preferred for problematic hemoptysis.

■ PROPHYLAXIS

In situations in which moderate or high risk is predicted (e.g., after induction therapy for acute myeloid leukemia), the need for antifungal prophylaxis for superficial and systemic candidiasis and for invasive aspergillosis is generally accepted. Fluconazole is commonly used in these situations but has no activity against *Aspergillus* spp. Itraconazole capsules are ineffective, and itraconazole solution offers only modest efficacy. Posaconazole solution is more effective. Some data support the use of IV micafungin. No prophylactic regimen is completely successful.

■ OUTCOME

Invasive aspergillosis is curable if immune reconstitution occurs, whereas allergic and chronic forms are not. The mortality rate for invasive aspergillosis is ~50% if the infection is treated but is 100% if the diagnosis is missed. Cerebral aspergillosis, *Aspergillus* endocarditis, and bilateral extensive invasive pulmonary aspergillosis have very poor outcomes, as does invasive infection in persons with late-stage AIDS or relapsed uncontrolled leukemia and in recipients of allogeneic hematopoietic stem cell transplants.

FURTHER READINGS

AGARWAL R et al: *Aspergillus* hypersensitivity and allergic bronchopulmonary aspergillosis in patients with bronchial asthma: Systematic review and meta-analysis. Int J Tuberc Lung Dis 13:936, 2009

DENNING DW et al: Randomized controlled trial of oral antifungal treatment for severe asthma with fungal sensitization (SAFS), the FAST study. Am J Respir Crit Care Med 179:11, 2009

GUINEA J et al: Pulmonary aspergillosis in patients with chronic obstructive pulmonary disease: Incidence, risk factors, and outcome. Clin Microbiol Infect 16:870, 2010

HERBRECHT R et al: Voriconazole versus amphotericin B for primary therapy of invasive aspergillosis. N Engl J Med 347:408, 2002

HOPE WW et al: Laboratory diagnosis of invasive aspergillosis. Lancet Infect Dis 9:609, 2005

—— et al: The invasive and saprophytic syndromes due to *Aspergillus* spp. Med Mycol 43:S207, 2005

MEERSSEMAN W et al: Invasive aspergillosis in the intensive care unit. Clin Infect Dis 45:205, 2007

O'GORMAN CM et al: Discovery of a sexual cycle in the opportunistic fungal pathogen *Aspergillus fumigatus*. Nature 457:471, 2009

VERWEIJ PE et al: Azole-resistance in *Aspergillus*: Proposed nomenclature and breakpoints. Drug Resist Updates 12:141, 2009

VISCOLI C et al: An EORTC phase II study of caspofungin as first-line therapy of invasive aspergillosis in haematological patients. J Antimicrob Chemother 64:1274, 2009

WALSH TJ et al: Treatment of aspergillosis: Clinical practice guidelines of the Infectious Diseases Society of America (IDSA). Clin Infect Dis 46:327, 2008

CHAPTER 205

Mucormycosis

Brad Spellberg
Ashraf S. Ibrahim

Mucormycosis represents a group of life-threatening infections caused by fungi of the order Mucorales. Recent reclassification has abolished the class Zygomycetes and placed the order Mucorales in the subphylum Mucoromycotina. Therefore, infection caused by the Mucorales is most accurately referred to as mucormycosis, although the term *zygomycosis* may still be used by some sources. Mucormycosis is highly invasive and relentlessly progressive, resulting in higher rates of morbidity and mortality (>40%) than many other infections. A high index of suspicion is critical for diagnosis, and early initiation of therapy—often before confirmation of the diagnosis—is necessary to optimize outcomes.

ETIOLOGY

Fungi of the order Mucorales belong to six families, all of which can cause mucormycosis. Among the Mucorales, *Rhizopus oryzae* (in the family Mucoraceae) is by far the most common cause of infection. Less frequently isolated species of the Mucoraceae family that cause a similar spectrum of infections include *Rhizopus microsporus*, *Rhizomucor pusillus*, *Mycocladus corymbifer* (formerly *Absidia corymbifera*), *Apophysomyces elegans*, and *Mucor* species (which, despite its name, is a rare cause of mucormycosis). Increasing numbers of cases of mucormycosis due to infection with *Cunninghamella* species (family Cunninghamellaceae) have also been reported. Rare case reports have demonstrated the ability of fungi in the remaining families of the Mucorales to cause mucormycosis.

PATHOGENESIS

The Mucorales are ubiquitous environmental fungi to which humans are constantly exposed. These fungi cause infection primarily in patients with diabetes or defects in phagocytic function (e.g., associated with neutropenia or glucocorticoid treatment). Patients with elevated levels of free iron, which supports fungal growth in serum and tissues, are likewise at increased risk for mucormycosis. In iron-overloaded patients with end-stage renal failure, treatment with deferoxamine predisposes to the development of rapidly fatal disseminated mucormycosis; this agent, an iron chelator for the human host, serves as a fungal siderophore, directly delivering iron to the Mucorales. Furthermore, patients with diabetic ketoacidosis (DKA) are at high risk of developing rhinocerebral mucormycosis. The acidosis causes dissociation of iron from sequestering proteins in serum, resulting in enhanced fungal survival and virulence. It is likely that hyperglycemia during DKA also contributes to the risk of mucormycosis through its association with poorly characterized defects in phagocytic function.

EPIDEMIOLOGY

Mucormycosis typically occurs in patients with diabetes mellitus, solid organ or hematopoietic stem cell transplantation (HSCT), prolonged neutropenia, or malignancy. In patients undergoing HSCT, mucormycosis develops at least as commonly during non-neutropenic as during neutropenic periods, probably because of glucocorticoid treatment of graft-versus-host disease. Mucormycosis

can occur as isolated cutaneous or subcutaneous infection in immunologically normal individuals after traumatic implantation of soil or vegetation, after maceration of the skin by a moist surface, or in nosocomial settings via direct access through intravenous catheters or subcutaneous injections.

Patients receiving antifungal prophylaxis with either itraconazole or voriconazole may be at increased risk of mucormycosis. These patients typically present with disseminated mucormycosis, the most lethal form of disease. Breakthrough mucormycosis has been described repeatedly in patients receiving posaconazole or echinocandin prophylaxis.

CLINICAL MANIFESTATIONS

Mucormycosis can be divided into at least six clinical categories based on clinical presentation and the involvement of a particular anatomic site: rhinocerebral, pulmonary, cutaneous, gastrointestinal, disseminated, and miscellaneous. These categories of invasive mucormycosis tend to affect patients with specific defects in host defense. For example, patients with DKA typically develop the rhinocerebral form and much more rarely develop pulmonary or disseminated disease. In contrast, pulmonary mucormycosis occurs most commonly in leukemic patients who are receiving chemotherapy and in patients undergoing HSCT.

Rhinocerebral mucormycosis continues to be the most common form of the disease. Most cases occur in patients with diabetes, although such cases (probably due to glucocorticoid use) are increasingly being described in the transplantation setting. The initial symptoms of rhinocerebral mucormycosis are nonspecific and include eye or facial pain and facial numbness followed by the onset of conjunctival suffusion, blurry vision, and soft tissue swelling. Fever may be absent in up to half of cases, while white blood cell counts are typically elevated as long as the patient has functioning bone marrow. If untreated, infection usually spreads from the ethmoid sinus to the orbit, resulting in compromise of extraocular muscle function and proptosis, typically with chemosis. Onset of signs and symptoms in the contralateral eye, with resulting bilateral proptosis, chemosis, vision loss, and ophthalmoplegia, is ominous and suggests the development of cavernous sinus thrombosis.

Upon visual inspection, infected tissue may appear to be normal during the earliest stages of fungal spread and then progresses through an erythematous phase, with or without edema, before the onset of a violaceous appearance and finally the development of a black necrotic eschar. Infection can sometimes extend from the sinuses into the mouth and produce painful necrotic ulcerations of the hard palate, but this is a late finding that suggests extensive, well-established infection.

Pulmonary mucormycosis is the second most common manifestation. Symptoms include dyspnea, cough, and chest pain; fever is often but not invariably present. Angioinvasion results in necrosis, cavitation, and/or hemoptysis. Lobar consolidation, isolated masses, nodular disease, cavities, or wedge-shaped infarcts may be seen on chest radiography. High-resolution chest CT is the best method for determining the extent of pulmonary mucormycosis and may demonstrate evidence of infection before it is seen on the chest x-ray. In the setting of cancer, where mucormycosis may be difficult to differentiate from aspergillosis, the presence of ≥10 pulmonary nodules, pleural effusion, or concomitant sinusitis makes mucormycosis more likely. It is critical to distinguish mucormycosis from aspergillosis as rapidly as possible, as treatments for these infections differ. Indeed, voriconazole—the first-line treatment for aspergillosis—exacerbates mucormycosis in mouse and fly models.

Cutaneous mucormycosis may result from external implantation of the fungus or conversely from hematogenous dissemination.

External implantation–related infection has been described in the setting of soil exposure from trauma (e.g., in a motor vehicle accident), penetrating injury with plant material (e.g., a thorn), injections of medications (e.g., insulin), catheter insertion, contaminated surgical dressings, and use of tape to secure endotracheal tubes. Cutaneous disease can be highly invasive, penetrating into muscle, fascia, and even bone. In mucormycosis, necrotizing fasciitis carries a mortality rate approaching 80%. Necrotic cutaneous lesions in the setting of hematogenous dissemination are also associated with an extremely high mortality rate. However, with prompt, aggressive surgical debridement, isolated cutaneous mucormycosis has a favorable prognosis and a low mortality rate.

Gastrointestinal mucormycosis has occurred in premature neonates in association with disseminated disease and necrotizing enterocolitis; more rarely, it has been described in adults with neutropenia or other immunocompromising conditions. In addition, gastrointestinal disease has been reported as a nosocomial process following administration of medications mixed with contaminated wooden applicator sticks. Nonspecific abdominal pain and distention associated with nausea and vomiting are the most common symptoms. Gastrointestinal bleeding is common, and fungating masses may be seen in the stomach at endoscopy. The disease may progress to visceral perforation, with extremely high mortality rates.

Hematogenously disseminated mucormycosis may originate from any primary site of infection. The most common site of dissemination is the brain, but metastatic lesions may also be found in any other organ. The mortality rate associated with dissemination to the brain approaches 100%. Even without central nervous system (CNS) involvement, mortality rates for disseminated mucormycosis exceed 90%. Miscellaneous forms of mucormycosis may affect any body site, including bones, mediastinum, trachea, kidneys, and (in association with dialysis) peritoneum.

DIAGNOSIS

A high index of suspicion is required for diagnosis of mucormycosis. Unfortunately, autopsy series have shown that up to half of cases are diagnosed only post-mortem. Because the Mucorales are environmental isolates, definitive diagnosis requires a positive culture from a sterile site (e.g., a needle aspirate, a tissue biopsy specimen, or pleural fluid) or histopathologic evidence of invasive mucormycosis. A probable diagnosis of mucormycosis can be established by culture from a nonsterile site (e.g., sputum or bronchoalveolar lavage) when a patient has appropriate risk factors as well as clinical and radiographic evidence of disease. However, given the urgency of administering therapy early, the patient should be treated while confirmation of the diagnosis is awaited.

Biopsy with histopathologic examination remains the most sensitive and specific modality for definitive diagnosis (Fig. 205-1). Biopsy reveals characteristic wide (≥6- to 30-μm), thick-walled, ribbon-like, aseptate hyphal elements that branch at right angles. Other fungi, including *Aspergillus*, *Fusarium*, and *Scedosporium* species, have septae, are thinner, and branch at acute angles. Because artificial septae may result from folding of tissue during processing (which may also alter the appearance of the angle of branching), the width and the ribbon-like form of the fungus are the most reliable features distinguishing mucormycosis. The Mucorales are visualized most effectively with periodic acid–Schiff or methenamine silver stain or, if the organism burden is high, with hematoxylin and eosin. While histopathology can identify the Mucorales, species can be identified only by culture.

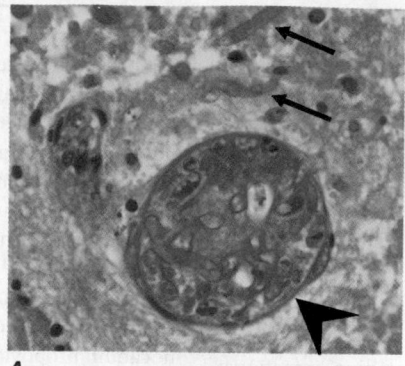 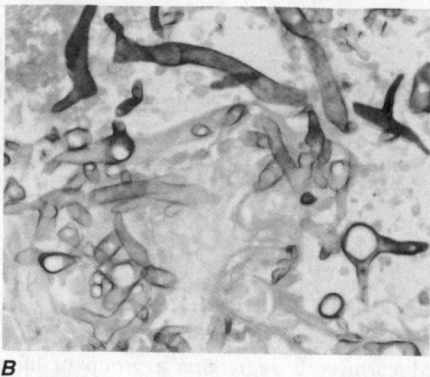

Figure 205-1 Histopathology sections of *Rhizopus oryzae* in infected brain. **A.** Broad, ribbon-like, nonseptate hyphae in the parenchyma (*arrows*) and a thrombosed blood vessel with extensive intravascular hyphae (*arrowhead*) (hematoxylin and eosin). **B.** Extensive, broad, ribbon-like hyphae invading the parenchyma (Gomori methenamine silver).

PCR is being investigated as a diagnostic tool for mucormycosis but is not yet approved by the U.S. Food and Drug Administration (FDA) for this purpose and is not generally available.

Unfortunately, cultures are positive in fewer than half of cases of mucormycosis. Nevertheless, the Mucorales are not fastidious organisms and tend to grow quickly (i.e., within 48 h) on culture media. The likely explanation for the low sensitivity of culture is that the Mucorales form long filamentous structures that are killed by tissue homogenization—the standard method for preparing tissue cultures in the clinical microbiology laboratory. Thus the laboratory should be advised when a diagnosis of mucormycosis is suspected, and the tissue should be cut into sections and placed in the center of culture dishes rather than homogenized.

Imaging techniques often yield subtle findings that underestimate the extent of disease. For example, the most common finding on CT or MRI of the head or sinuses of a patient with rhino-orbital mucormycosis is sinusitis that is indistinguishable from bacterial sinusitis. It is also common to detect no abnormalities in sinus bones despite clinical evidence of progressive disease. MRI is more sensitive (~80%) for detecting orbital and CNS disease than is CT. High-risk patients should always undergo endoscopy and/or surgical exploration, with biopsy of the areas of suspected infection. If mucormycosis is suspected, initial empirical therapy with a polyene antifungal agent should be initiated while the diagnosis is being confirmed.

DIFFERENTIAL DIAGNOSIS

Other mold infections, including aspergillosis, scedosporiosis, fusariosis, and infections caused by the dematiaceous fungi (brown-pigmented soil organisms), can cause clinical syndromes identical to mucormycosis. Histopathologic examination usually allows distinction of the Mucorales from these other organisms, and a positive culture permits definitive species identification. It is important to distinguish the Mucorales from these other fungi, as the preferred antifungal treatments differ (i.e., polyenes for the Mucorales vs. expanded-spectrum triazoles for most septate molds). The entomophthoromycoses caused by *Basidiobolus* and *Conidiobolus* (fungi formerly grouped with the Mucorales in the class Zygomycetes) can also cause identical clinical syndromes. These fungi may appear similar to the Mucorales on histopathology and can be reliably distinguished from the latter only by culture.

In a patient with sinusitis and proptosis, orbital cellulitis and cavernous sinus thrombosis caused by bacterial pathogens (most commonly *Staphylococcus aureus*, but also streptococcal and gram-negative species) must be excluded. *Klebsiella rhinoscleromatis* is a rare cause of an indolent facial rhinoscleroma syndrome that may appear similar to mucormycosis. Finally, the Tolosa-Hunt syndrome causes painful ophthalmoplegia, ptosis, headache, and cavernous sinus inflammation; biopsies and clinical follow-up may be needed to distinguish the Tolosa-Hunt syndrome from mucormycosis by the lack of progression of the former entity.

GENERAL PRINCIPLES The successful treatment of mucormycosis requires four steps: (1) early diagnosis; (2) reversal of underlying predisposing risk factors, if possible; (3) surgical debridement; and (4) prompt antifungal therapy. Early diagnosis of mucormycosis is critical, since early initiation of therapy is associated with improved outcomes. It is also crucial to reverse (or prevent) underlying defects in host defense during treatment (e.g., by stopping or reducing the dosage of immunosuppressive medications or by rapidly restoring euglycemia and normal acid-base status). Finally, it is advisable to avoid administration of iron to patients with active mucormycosis, as iron exacerbates infection in animal models.

Blood vessel thrombosis and resulting tissue necrosis during mucormycosis can result in poor penetration of antifungal agents to the site of infection. Therefore, debridement of necrotic tissues may be critical for complete eradication of disease. Surgery has been found (by logistic regression and in multiple case series) to be an independent variable for favorable outcome in patients with mucormycosis. The extent and timing of surgical debridement necessary to optimize outcomes of mucormycosis have not been defined. Limited data from a retrospective study support the use of intraoperative frozen sections to delineate the margins of infected tissues, with sparing of tissues lacking evidence of infection. A multidisciplinary team, including an internist, an infectious disease specialist, and surgical specialists relevant to the sites of infection, is typically required for the management of mucormycosis.

ANTIFUNGAL THERAPY Primary antifungal therapy for mucormycosis should be based on a polyene antibiotic (Table 205-1), except perhaps for mild localized infection (e.g., isolated suprafascial cutaneous infection) in immunocompetent

TABLE 205-1 First-Line Antifungal Options for the Treatment of Mucormycosis[a]

Drug	Recommended Dosage	Advantages and Supporting Studies	Disadvantages
Primary Antifungal Therapy			
AmB deoxycholate	• 1.0–1.5 mg/kg qd	• >5 decades of clinical experience • Inexpensive • Only licensed agent for treatment of mucormycosis	• Highly toxic • Poor CNS penetration
LAmB	• 5–10 mg/kg qd	• Less nephrotoxic than AmB deoxycholate • Better CNS penetration than AmB deoxycholate or ABLC • Better outcomes than with AmB deoxycholate in murine models and a retrospective clinical review	• Expensive
ABLC	• 5–7.5 mg/kg qd	• Less nephrotoxic than AmB deoxycholate • Murine and retrospective clinical data suggest benefit of combination therapy with echinocandins.	• Expensive • Possibly less efficacious than LAmB for CNS infection
Primary Combination Therapy[b]			
Caspofungin plus Lipid polyene	• 70-mg IV loading dose, then 50 mg/d for ≥2 weeks • 50 mg/m2 IV in children	• Favorable toxicity profile • Synergistic in murine disseminated mucormycosis • Retrospective clinical data suggest superior outcomes for rhino-orbital-cerebral mucormycosis.	• Very limited clinical data on combination therapy
Micafungin or anidulafungin *plus* Lipid polyene	• 100 mg/d for ≥2 weeks • Micafungin: 4 mg/kg qd in children • Micafungin: 10 mg/kg qd in low-birth-weight infants • Anidulafungin: 1.5 mg/kg qd in children	• Favorable toxicity profile • Synergistic with LAmB in murine model of disseminated mucormycosis	• No clinical data
Deferasirox *plus* Lipid polyene	• 20 mg/kg PO qd for 2–4 weeks	• Highly fungicidal against Mucorales in vitro • Synergistic with LAmB in murine model of disseminated mucormycosis	• Only available for enteral administration • No clinical data; phase II clinical trial completed

[a]Primary therapy should generally include a polyene. Non-polyene-based regimens may be appropriate for patients who refuse polyene therapy or for relatively immunocompetent patients with mild disease (e.g., isolated suprafascial cutaneous infection) that can be surgically eradicated.
[b]Prospective randomized trials are necessary to confirm the suggested benefit (from animal and small retrospective human studies) of combination therapy for mucormycosis. Dose escalation of any echinocandin is not recommended because of a paradoxical loss of benefit of combination therapy at echinocandin doses of ≥3 mg/kg qd.
Abbreviations: ABLC, AmB lipid complex; AmB, amphotericin B; CNS, central nervous system; LAmB, liposomal AmB.
Source: Reprinted from Spellberg et al, 2009.

patients, which has been eradicated surgically. Amphotericin B (AmB) deoxycholate remains the only licensed antifungal agent for the treatment of mucormycosis. However, lipid formulations of AmB are significantly less nephrotoxic, can be administered at higher doses, and may be more efficacious than AmB deoxycholate for this purpose.

The optimal dosages for antifungal treatment of mucormycosis are not known. Starting dosages of 1 mg/kg per day for AmB deoxycholate and 5–7.5 mg/kg per day for liposomal AmB (LAmB) and amphotericin B lipid complex (ABLC) are commonly given to adults and children. Whether higher dosages provide any additional benefit is unclear. However, dose escalation of LAmB to 10 mg/kg per day for CNS mucormycosis may be considered in light of the limited penetration of polyenes into the brain. ABLC dose escalation above 7.5 mg/kg per day is not advisable given the lack of relevant data.

Echinocandin–lipid polyene combinations improved survival rates among mice with disseminated mucormycosis (including CNS disease) and were associated with significantly better outcomes than polyene monotherapy in a small retrospective study involving primarily diabetic patients with rhino-orbital-cerebral mucormycosis. Although combination therapy may be considered on the basis of these limited data sets, definitive clinical trials are needed to establish whether it offers any real advantage over monotherapy for mucormycosis.

In contrast to deferoxamine, the iron chelator deferasirox is fungicidal for clinical isolates of the Mucorales. In mice with DKA and disseminated mucormycosis, combination deferasirox-LAmB therapy resulted in synergistic improvement of survival rates. Enrollment in a double-blind, randomized, placebo-controlled, phase II safety/exploratory efficacy study of adjunctive deferasirox therapy (20 mg/kg per day for 14 days) [the Deferasirox-AmBisome Therapy for Mucormycosis (DEFEAT Mucor) Study, NCT00419770] has recently been completed; this study is likely to elucidate the potential risks and benefits of iron chelation therapy for mucormycosis.

Posaconazole is the only FDA-approved azole with in vitro activity against the Mucorales. However, pharmacokinetic/pharmacodynamic data raise concerns about the reliability of achieving adequate in vivo levels of orally administered posaconazole. Furthermore, posaconazole has been found to be inferior in efficacy to AmB for the treatment of murine mucormycosis and is not superior to placebo for treatment of murine infection with *R. oryzae*. Moreover, posaconazole-polyene combination therapy is not superior to polyene monotherapy for murine mucormycosis.

The roles of recombinant cytokines and neutrophil transfusions in the primary treatment of mucormycosis are not clear. Limited data indicate that hyperbaric oxygen may be useful in centers with the appropriate technical expertise and facilities.

In general, antifungal therapy for mucormycosis should be continued until all of the following objectives are attained: (1) resolution of clinical signs and symptoms of infection; (2) resolution or stabilization of residual radiographic signs of disease on serial imaging; and (3) resolution of underlying immunosuppression. For patients with mucormycosis who are receiving immunosuppressive medications, secondary antifungal prophylaxis is typically continued for as long as the immunosuppressive regimen is administered.

FURTHER READINGS

CHAMILOS G et al: Delaying amphotericin B–based frontline therapy significantly increases mortality among patients with hematologic malignancy who have zygomycosis. Clin Infect Dis 47:503, 2008

IBRAHIM AS et al: The iron chelator deferasirox protects mice from mucormycosis through iron starvation. J Clin Invest 117:2649, 2007

KONTOYIANNIS DP et al: Zygomycosis in a tertiary-care cancer center in the era of *Aspergillus*-active antifungal therapy: A case-control observational study of 27 recent cases. J Infect Dis 191:1350, 2005

MARR KA et al: Epidemiology and outcome of mould infections in hematopoietic stem cell transplant recipients. Clin Infect Dis 34:909, 2002

REED C et al: Combination polyene-caspofungin treatment of rhino-orbital-cerebral mucormycosis. Clin Infect Dis 47:364, 2008

RODEN MM et al: Epidemiology and outcome of zygomycosis: A review of 929 reported cases. Clin Infect Dis 41:634, 2005

SPELLBERG B et al: Recent advances in the management of mucormycosis: From bench to bedside. Clin Infect Dis 48:1743, 2009

SPELLBERG B, IBRAHIM AS: Recent advances in the treatment of mucormycosis. Curr Infect Dis Rep 12:423, 2010

CHAPTER 206

Superficial Mycoses and Less Common Systemic Mycoses

Carol A. Kauffman

ENDEMIC MYCOSES (DIMORPHIC FUNGI)

Dimorphic fungi exist in discrete environmental niches as molds that produce conidia, which are their infectious form. In tissues and at temperatures of >35°C, the mold converts to the yeast form. Other endemic mycoses—histoplasmosis, coccidioidomycosis, and blastomycosis—are discussed in Chaps. 199, 200, and 201, respectively.

■ SPOROTRICHOSIS

Etiologic agent

Sporothrix schenckii is a thermally dimorphic fungus that is found worldwide in sphagnum moss, decaying vegetation, and soil.

Epidemiology and pathogenesis

Sporotrichosis most commonly infects persons who participate in outdoor activities such as landscaping, gardening, and tree farming. Infected animals, especially cats, can transmit *S. schenckii* to humans. Sporotrichosis is primarily a localized infection of skin and subcutaneous tissues that follows traumatic inoculation of conidia. Osteoarticular sporotrichosis is uncommon, occurring most often in middle-aged men who abuse alcohol, and pulmonary sporotrichosis occurs almost exclusively in persons with chronic obstructive pulmonary disease who have inhaled the organism from the environment. Dissemination occurs rarely, almost always in markedly immunocompromised patients, especially those with AIDS.

Clinical manifestations

Days or weeks after inoculation, a papule develops at the site and then usually ulcerates but is not very painful. Similar lesions develop sequentially along the lymphatic channels proximal to the original lesion. Some patients develop a fixed cutaneous lesion that can be verrucous or ulcerative and that remains localized without lymphatic extension. The differential diagnosis of lymphocutaneous sporotrichosis includes nocardiosis, tularemia, nontuberculous mycobacterial infection (especially that due to *Mycobacterium marinum*), and leishmaniasis. Osteoarticular sporotrichosis can present as chronic synovitis or septic arthritis. Pulmonary sporotrichosis must be differentiated from tuberculosis or other fungal pneumonias. Numerous ulcerated skin lesions, with or without spread to visceral organs [including the central nervous system (CNS)], are characteristic of disseminated sporotrichosis.

Diagnosis

S. schenckii usually grows readily as a mold when material from a cutaneous lesion is incubated at room temperature. Histopathologic examination of biopsy material shows a mixed granulomatous and pyogenic reaction, and tiny oval or cigar-shaped yeasts are sometimes visualized with special stains. Serologic testing is not useful.

Treatment and prognosis

Guidelines for the management of the various forms of sporotrichosis have been published by the Infectious Diseases Society of America (Table 206-1). Itraconazole is the drug of choice for lymphocutaneous sporotrichosis. Fluconazole is less effective; voriconazole and posaconazole have not been used for sporotrichosis. Saturated solution of potassium iodide (SSKI) is also effective for lymphocutaneous infection and costs much less than itraconazole. However, SSKI is poorly tolerated because of adverse reactions, including metallic taste, salivary gland swelling, rash, and fever. Terbinafine appears to be effective but has been used in few patients. Treatment for lymphocutaneous sporotrichosis is continued for 2–4 weeks after all lesions have resolved, usually for a total of 3–6 months. Pulmonary and osteoarticular forms of sporotrichosis are treated with itraconazole for at least 1 year. Severe pulmonary infection and disseminated sporotrichosis, including that involving the CNS, are treated initially with amphotericin B (AmB), which is followed by itraconazole after improvement has been noted. Lifelong suppressive therapy with itraconazole is required for AIDS patients. The success rate for treatment of lymphocutaneous sporotrichosis is 90–100%, but other forms of the disease respond poorly to antifungal therapy.

■ PARACOCCIDIOIDOMYCOSIS

Etiologic agent

Paracoccidioides brasiliensis is a thermally dimorphic fungus that is endemic in humid areas of Central and South America, especially in Brazil.

Epidemiology and pathogenesis

A striking male-to-female ratio varies from 14:1 to as high as 70:1 (in rural Brazil). Most patients are middle-aged or elderly men from rural areas. Paracoccidioidomycosis develops after the inhalation of aerosolized conidia encountered in the environment. For most patients, disease rarely develops at the time of the initial infection but appears years later, presumably after reactivation of a latent infection.

Clinical manifestations

Two major syndromes are associated with paracoccidioidomycosis: the acute or juvenile form and the chronic or adult form. The acute form is uncommon, occurs mostly in persons <30 years old, and manifests as disseminated infection of the reticuloendothelial system. Immunocompromised individuals can also manifest this type of rapidly progressive disease. The chronic form of paracoccidioidomycosis accounts for ~90% of cases and predominantly affects older men. The primary manifestation is progressive pulmonary disease, primarily in the lower lobes, with fibrosis. Ulcerative and nodular mucocutaneous lesions in the nares and mouth—another common manifestation of chronic paracoccidioidomycosis—must be differentiated from leishmaniasis (Chap. 212) and squamous cell carcinoma (Chap. 87).

Diagnosis

The diagnosis is established by growth of the organism in culture. A presumptive diagnosis can be made by detection of the distinctive thick-walled yeast, with multiple narrow-necked buds attached circumferentially, in purulent material or tissue biopsies.

Treatment and prognosis

Itraconazole is the treatment of choice for paracoccidioidomycosis (Table 206-1). Ketoconazole is also effective but more toxic;

TABLE 206-1 Suggested Treatment for Endemic Mycoses

Disease	First-Line Therapy	Alternatives/Comments
Sporotrichosis		
Cutaneous, lymphocutaneous	Itraconazole, 200 mg/d until 2–4 weeks after lesions resolve	SSKI, increasing doses[a] Terbinafine, 500 mg bid
Pulmonary, osteoarticular	Itraconazole, 200 mg bid for 12 months	Lipid AmB[b] for severe pulmonary disease until stable; then itraconazole
Disseminated, central nervous system	Lipid AmB[b] for 4–6 weeks	Itraconazole, 200 mg bid after AmB for 12 months Itraconazole maintenance for AIDS patients: 200 mg/d until CD4+ T cell count is >200/µL for 12 months
Paracoccidioidomycosis		
Chronic (adult form)	Itraconazole, 100–200 mg/d for 6–12 months	TMP-SMX, 160/800 mg bid for 12–36 months
Acute (juvenile form)	AmB[c] until improvement	Itraconazole, 200 mg bid after AmB for 12 months
Penicilliosis		
Mild or moderate	Itraconazole, 200 mg bid for 12 weeks	Itraconazole maintenance for AIDS patients: 200 mg/d until CD4+ T cell count is >100/µL for 6 months
Severe	AmB[c] until improvement	Itraconazole, 200 mg bid after AmB for 12 weeks Itraconazole maintenance: as for mild or moderate disease

[a]The starting dosage is 5–10 drops tid in water or juice. The dosage is increased weekly by 10 drops per dose, as tolerated, up to 40–50 drops tid.
[b]The dosage of lipid AmB is 3–5 mg/kg daily; the higher dosage should be used when the central nervous system is involved.
[c]The dosage of AmB deoxycholate is 0.6–1.0 mg/kg daily.

Abbreviations: AmB, amphotericin B; SSKI, saturated solution of potassium iodide; TMP-SMX, trimethoprim-sulfamethoxazole.

voriconazole and posaconazole have been used with success in a few cases. Sulfonamides are also effective and are the least costly agents, but the response is slower and the relapse rate higher. Seriously ill patients should be treated with AmB initially. Patients with paracoccidioidomycosis have an excellent response to therapy, but pulmonary fibrosis is often progressive in those with chronic disease.

■ PENICILLIOSIS

Etiologic agent

Penicillium marneffei is a thermally dimorphic fungus that is endemic in the soil in certain areas of Vietnam, Thailand, and several other southeastern Asian countries.

Epidemiology and pathogenesis

The epidemiology of penicilliosis is linked to bamboo rats, which are infected with the fungus but rarely manifest disease. The disease occurs most often among persons living in rural areas in which the rats are found, but there is no evidence for transmission of the infection directly from rats to humans. Infection is rare in immunocompetent hosts, and most cases are reported in persons who have advanced AIDS. Infection results from the inhalation of conidia from the environment. The organism converts to the yeast phase in the lungs and then spreads hematogenously to the reticuloendothelial system.

Clinical manifestations

The clinical manifestations of penicilliosis mimic those of disseminated histoplasmosis and include fever, fatigue, weight loss, dyspnea, diarrhea (in some cases), lymphadenopathy, hepatosplenomegaly, and skin lesions, which appear as papules that often umbilicate and resemble molluscum contagiosum (Chap. 183).

Diagnosis

Penicilliosis is diagnosed by culture of *P. marneffei* from blood or from biopsy samples of skin, bone marrow, or lymph node. The organism usually grows within 1 week as a mold that produces a distinctive red pigment. Histopathologic examination of tissues and smears of blood or material from skin lesions shows oval or elliptical yeast-like organisms with central septation and can quickly establish a presumptive diagnosis.

Treatment and prognosis

Patients who have severe disease should be treated initially with AmB until their condition improves; therapy can then be changed to itraconazole (Table 206-1). Patients who have mild symptoms can be treated from the start with itraconazole. For patients with AIDS, suppressive therapy with itraconazole is recommended until immune reconstitution (related to successful therapy for HIV infection with antiretroviral drugs) is evident. Disseminated penicilliosis is usually fatal if not treated. With treatment, the mortality rate is ~10%.

PHAEOHYPHOMYCOSES

In these common soil organisms (also called *dematiaceous* fungi), melanin causes the hyphae and/or conidia to be darkly pigmented (brown/black). The term *phaeohyphomycosis* is used to describe any infection with a pigmented mold. This definition encompasses two specific syndromes—eumycetoma and chromoblastomycosis—as well as all other types of infections caused by these organisms. It is important to note that eumycetomas can be caused by hyaline molds as well as brown-black molds and that only about half of all mycetomas are due to fungi. Actinomycetes cause the remainder (Chap. 162). Most of these fungi cause localized subcutaneous infections after direct inoculation, but disseminated infection and serious visceral focal infections also occur, especially in immunocompromised patients.

Etiologic agents

A large number of pigmented molds can cause human infection. All are found in the soil or on plants, and some cause economically important plant diseases. The most common cause of eumycetoma is *Madurella* species, but hyaline molds such as *Scedosporium* species also cause this syndrome. *Fonsecaea* and *Cladophialophora* species are responsible for most cases of chromoblastomycosis. Disseminated infection and focal visceral infections are caused by a variety of dematiaceous fungi; *Alternaria*, *Exophiala*, *Curvularia*, and *Wangiella* species are among the more common molds reported to cause human infection.

Epidemiology and pathogenesis

Most infections, including all cases of eumycetoma and chromoblastomycosis, are acquired by inoculation through the skin. These two syndromes are seen almost entirely in tropical and subtropical areas and occur mostly in rural laborers who are frequently exposed to the organisms. Inhalation into the upper or lower respiratory tract leads to localized infection of sinuses and, in immunocompromised patients, to pneumonia and sometimes hematogenous dissemination. Several organisms, specifically *Cladophialophora bantiana* and *Rhinocladiella mackensiei*, are neurotropic and likely to cause CNS infection.

Clinical manifestations

Eumycetoma is a chronic subcutaneous and cutaneous infection that usually occurs on the lower extremities and that is characterized by swelling, development of sinus tracts, and the appearance of grains that are actually colonies of fungi discharged from the sinus tract. As the infection progresses, adjacent fascia and bony structures become involved. The disease is indolent and disfiguring, progressing slowly over years. Complications include fractures of infected bone and bacterial superinfections.

Chromoblastomycosis is an indolent subcutaneous infection characterized by nodular, verrucous, or plaque-like painless lesions that occur predominantly on the lower extremities and grow slowly over months or years. There is hardly ever extension to adjacent structures, as is seen with eumycetoma. Long-term consequences include bacterial superinfection, chronic lymphedema, and (rarely) the development of squamous cell carcinoma.

Dematiaceous molds are the most common cause of allergic fungal sinusitis and a less common cause of invasive fungal sinusitis. Keratitis occurs with corneal inoculation. Many patients, including some who are immunocompromised, develop only localized infection manifested by cyst-like subcutaneous lesions at the site of inoculation. Other immunocompromised patients have pneumonia and disseminated infection, including CNS involvement, and are quite ill.

Diagnosis

The specific diagnosis of infection with a pigmented mold is established by growth of the organism in culture. However, in eumycetoma, a tentative clinical diagnosis can be made when a patient presents with a lesion characterized by swelling, sinus tracts, and grains. Histopathologic examination and culture are necessary to ensure that the etiologic agent is a mold and not an actinomycete. In chromoblastomycosis, the diagnosis rests on the histologic demonstration of sclerotic bodies in the tissues; culture merely establishes which pigmented mold is causing the infection. Sclerotic bodies are dark brown, thick-walled, septate fungal forms that resemble large yeasts and define the syndrome. For disseminated infections and nonsubcutaneous focal infections, growth of the organism is essential to differentiate infection with a hyaline mold (e.g., *Aspergillus* or *Fusarium*) from that due to a pigmented mold. No serologic or non-culture-based methods are currently available to aid in the diagnosis of phaeohyphomycoses.

Treatment and prognosis

Treatment of eumycetoma and chromoblastomycosis involves both surgical extirpation of the lesion and use of antifungal agents. Surgical removal of the lesions of both eumycetoma and chromoblastomycosis is most effective if performed before extensive spread has occurred. In chromoblastomycosis, cryosurgery and laser therapy have been used with variable success. The antifungal agents of choice are itraconazole, voriconazole, and posaconazole. The most experience has accrued with itraconazole; there is less experience with the newer azoles, which are active in vitro and have been reported to be effective in a few patients. Flucytosine and terbinafine also have been used to treat chromoblastomycosis.

Disseminated and focal visceral infections are treated with the appropriate antifungal agent; the choice of agent is based on the location and extent of the infection, in vitro testing, and clinical experience with the specific infecting organism. AmB is not effective against many of these organisms but has been used successfully against others. Again, the most experience has been obtained with itraconazole, which is effective for localized infections. Voriconazole and posaconazole are likely to play an increasing role in therapy for both localized and disseminated infections. Chromoblastomycosis and eumycetoma are chronic indolent infections that are difficult to cure without surgical excision, but these are not life-threatening diseases. Disseminated or focal visceral infections with pigmented molds in immunocompromised patients are associated with high mortality rates unless immunosuppression can be diminished and effective antifungal agents prescribed promptly.

OPPORTUNISTIC FUNGAL INFECTIONS

Many environmental fungi can cause infection in markedly immunocompromised hosts, but two genera of hyaline (nonpigmented) molds, *Fusarium* and *Scedosporium*, and one yeast-like genus, *Trichosporon*, have become particularly prominent pathogens among such patients. *Fusarium* and *Scedosporium* species overlap with invasive aspergillosis in their clinical manifestations and, when seen in tissues, appear similar to *Aspergillus*. In the immunocompetent host, these fungi cause localized infections of skin, skin structures, and subcutaneous tissues, but their role in disseminated infection will be emphasized in this section.

■ FUSARIOSIS

Etiologic agent

Fusarium species, which are found worldwide in soil and on plants, have emerged as major opportunists in markedly immunocompromised patients.

Epidemiology and pathogenesis

Most human infections follow inhalation of conidia, but ingestion and direct inoculation can also lead to disease. An outbreak of severe *Fusarium* keratitis among soft contact lens wearers was traced back to a particular brand of contact lens solution and individual contact lens cases that had been contaminated. Disseminated infection is reported most often in patients who have a hematologic malignancy, are neutropenic, have received a stem cell or solid organ transplant, or have a severe burn.

Clinical manifestations

In immunocompetent persons, *Fusarium* species cause localized infections of various organs. These organisms commonly cause fungal keratitis, which can extend into the anterior chamber of the eye, cause loss of vision, and require corneal transplantation. Onychomycosis due to *Fusarium* species, while basically an annoyance in immunocompetent patients, is a source of subsequent hematogenous dissemination and should be aggressively sought and treated in neutropenic patients. In profoundly immunocompromised patients, fusariosis is angioinvasive, and clinical manifestations mimic those of aspergillosis. Pulmonary infection is characterized by multiple nodular lesions. Sinus infection is likely to lead to invasion of adjacent structures. Disseminated fusariosis occurs primarily in neutropenic patients with hematologic malignancies and in allogeneic stem cell transplant recipients, especially those with graft-versus-host disease. Disseminated fusariosis differs from disseminated aspergillosis in that skin lesions are extremely common with fusariosis; the lesions are nodular or necrotic, are usually painful, and appear over time in different locations.

Diagnosis

The diagnostic approach usually includes both documentation of the growth of *Fusarium* species from involved tissue and demonstration of invasion by histopathologic or microbiologic techniques that show septate hyphae in tissues or aspirates. The organism is difficult to differentiate from *Aspergillus* species in tissues; thus, identification with culture is imperative. An extremely helpful diagnostic clue is growth in blood cultures, which are positive in as many as 50% of patients with disseminated fusariosis. No serologic or non-culture-based techniques are currently available to aid in diagnosis.

Treatment and prognosis

Fusarium species are resistant to many antifungal agents. A lipid formulation of AmB (at least 5 mg/kg daily), voriconazole (200–400 mg twice daily), or posaconazole (400 mg twice daily) is recommended. Many physicians use both a lipid formulation of AmB and either voriconazole or posaconazole because susceptibility information is not available when therapy must be initiated. Serum drug levels should be monitored with either azole to ensure that absorption is adequate and with voriconazole to avoid toxicity. Mortality rates for disseminated fusariosis have been as high as 85%. With the antifungal therapy noted above, mortality rates have fallen to ~50%. However, if neutropenia persists, the mortality rate approaches 100%.

■ SCEDOSPORIOSIS

Etiologic agent

The genus *Scedosporium* includes several pathogens. The major causes of human infections are *Scedosporium apiospermum*, which in its sexual state is termed *Pseudallescheria boydii*, and *S. prolificans*. The *S. apiospermum* complex encompasses several species but will be referred to here simply as *S. apiospermum*.

Epidemiology and pathogenesis

S. apiospermum is found worldwide in temperate climates in tidal flats, swamps, ponds, manure, and soil. This organism is known as a cause of pneumonia, disseminated infection, and brain abscess in near-drowning victims. *S. prolificans* is also found in soil but is more geographically restricted; most cases are reported from Spain

and Australia. Infection occurs predominantly through inhalation of conidia, but direct inoculation through the skin or into the eye also can occur.

Clinical manifestations

Among immunocompetent persons, *Scedosporium* species are a prominent cause of eumycetoma. Keratitis as a result of accidental corneal inoculation is a sight-threatening infection. In patients who have hematologic malignancies (especially acute leukemia with neutropenia), recipients of solid organ or stem cell transplants, and patients receiving glucocorticoids, *Scedosporium* species are angioinvasive, causing pneumonia and widespread dissemination with abscesses. Pulmonary infection mimics that caused by aspergillosis; nodules, cavities, and lobar infiltrates are common. Disseminated infection involves the skin, heart, brain, and many other organs. Skin lesions are not as common or as painful as those of fusariosis.

Diagnosis

Diagnosis depends on the growth of *Scedosporium* species from involved tissue and the demonstration of invasion by histopathologic or microbiologic techniques that show septate hyphae in tissues or aspirates. Culture evidence is essential because *Scedosporium* species are difficult to differentiate from *Aspergillus* in tissues. Demonstration of tissue invasion is essential because these ubiquitous environmental molds can be mere contaminants or colonizers. *S. prolificans* can grow in blood cultures, but *S. apiospermum* usually does not. No serologic or non-culture-based diagnostic methods are available to aid in diagnosis.

Treatment and prognosis

Scedosporium species are resistant to AmB, echinocandins, and some azoles. Voriconazole is the agent of choice for *S. apiospermum*, and posaconazole has also been used for this infection. *S. prolificans* is resistant in vitro to almost every available antifungal agent; the addition of agents such as terbinafine to a voriconazole regimen has been attempted because in vitro data suggest possible synergy against some strains of *S. prolificans*. Mortality rates have been as high as 65–75% for *S. apiospermum* and 85–100% for *S. prolificans*. Mortality rates for *S. apiospermum* infection have decreased to 40–50% with the use of voriconazole, but those for disseminated *S. prolificans* infection remain extremely high.

■ TRICHOSPORONOSIS

Etiologic agent

The genus *Trichosporon* contains many species, some of which cause localized infection of hair and nails. The major pathogen responsible for invasive infection is *Trichosporon asahii*. *Trichosporon* species grow as yeast-like colonies in vitro; in vivo, however, hyphae, pseudohyphae, and arthroconidia can also be seen.

Epidemiology and pathogenesis

These yeasts are commonly found in soil, sewage, and water and in rare instances can colonize human skin and the human gastrointestinal tract. Most infections follow fungal inhalation or entry via central venous catheters. Systemic infection occurs almost exclusively in immunocompromised hosts, including those who have hematologic malignancies, are neutropenic, have received a solid organ transplant, or are receiving glucocorticoids.

Clinical manifestations

Disseminated trichosporonosis resembles invasive candidiasis, and fungemia is often the initial manifestation of infection. Pneumonia, skin lesions, and sepsis syndrome are common. The skin lesions begin as papules or nodules surrounded by erythema and progress to central necrosis. A chronic form of infection mimics hepatosplenic candidiasis (chronic disseminated candidiasis).

Diagnosis

The diagnosis of systemic *Trichosporon* infection is established by growth of the organism from involved tissues or from blood. Histopathologic examination of a skin lesion showing a mixture of yeast forms, arthroconidia, and hyphae can lead to an early presumptive diagnosis of trichosporonosis. The serum cryptococcal antigen latex agglutination test may be positive in patients with disseminated trichosporonosis because *T. asahii* and *Cryptococcus neoformans* share polysaccharide antigens.

Treatment and prognosis

Rates of response to AmB have been disappointing, and many *Trichosporon* isolates are resistant in vitro. Voriconazole appears to be the antifungal agent of choice and is used at a dosage of 200–400 mg twice daily. The mortality rates for disseminated *Trichosporon* infection have been as high as 70% but should decrease with the use of newer azoles, such as voriconazole; however, patients who remain neutropenic are likely to succumb to this infection.

SUPERFICIAL CUTANEOUS INFECTIONS

Fungal infections of the skin and skin structures are caused by molds and yeasts that do not invade deeper tissues but rather cause disease merely by inhabiting the superficial layers of skin, hair follicles, and nails. These agents are the most common cause of fungal diseases of humans but only rarely cause serious infections.

■ YEAST INFECTIONS

Etiologic agents

The lipophilic yeast *Malassezia* is actually dimorphic in that it lives on the skin in the yeast phase but transforms to the mold phase as it causes disease. Of the seven species, six are grouped together in some classification systems as the *M. furfur* complex; all six of these species require exogenous lipids for growth. The seventh species, *M. pachydermatis*, is also lipophilic but does not have an absolute requirement for lipids.

Epidemiology and pathogenesis

Malassezia species are part of the indigenous human flora found in the stratum corneum of the back, chest, scalp, and face—areas rich in sebaceous glands. Disease is more common in moist humid areas of the world. The organisms do not invade below the stratum corneum and generally elicit little if any inflammatory response.

Clinical manifestations

Malassezia species cause tinea versicolor (also called *pityriasis versicolor*), folliculitis, and seborrheic dermatitis. Tinea versicolor presents as flat round scaly patches of hypo- or hyperpigmented skin on the neck, chest, or upper arms. The lesions are usually asymptomatic but can be pruritic. They can be mistaken for vitiligo, but the latter is not scaly. Folliculitis occurs over the back and chest and mimics bacterial folliculitis. Seborrheic dermatitis manifests as erythematous pruritic scaly lesions in the eyebrows, moustache, nasolabial folds, and scalp. The scalp lesions are termed cradle cap in babies and dandruff in adults. Seborrheic dermatitis can be severe in patients with advanced AIDS. Fungemia and disseminated infection occur rarely with *Malassezia* species—almost always in premature neonates receiving parenteral lipid preparations through a central venous catheter.

Diagnosis

Malassezia infections are diagnosed clinically in most cases. If scrapings are collected on a microscope slide on which a drop of potassium hydroxide has been placed, a mixture of budding yeasts and short septate hyphae are seen. In order to culture *M. furfur* from those patients in whom disseminated infection is suspected, sterile olive oil must be added to the medium.

Treatment and prognosis

Topical creams and lotions, including selenium sulfide shampoo, ketoconazole shampoo or cream, terbinafine cream, and ciclopirox cream, are effective in treating *Malassezia* infections and are usually given for 2 weeks. Mild topical steroid creams are sometimes used to treat seborrheic dermatitis. For extensive disease, itraconazole (200 mg/d) or fluconazole (200 mg/d) can be used for 5–7 days. The rare cases of fungemia caused by *Malassezia* species are treated with AmB or fluconazole, prompt removal of the catheter, and discontinuance of parenteral lipid infusions. *Malassezia* skin infections are benign and self-limited, although recurrences are the rule. The outcome of systemic infection depends on the host's underlying conditions, but most infants do well.

■ DERMATOPHYTE (MOLD) INFECTIONS

Etiologic agents

The molds that cause skin infections in humans include the genera *Trichophyton*, *Microsporum*, and *Epidermophyton*. These organisms, which are not components of the normal skin flora, can live within the keratinized structures of the skin—hence the term *dermatophytes*.

Epidemiology and pathogenesis

Dermatophytes occur worldwide, and infections with these organisms are extremely common. Some organisms cause disease only in humans and can be transmitted by person-to-person contact and by fomites, such as hairbrushes or wet floors that have been contaminated by infected individuals. Several species cause infections in cats and dogs and can readily be transmitted from these animals to humans. Finally, some dermatophytes are spread from contact with soil. The characteristic ring shape of cutaneous lesions is the result of the organisms' outward growth in a centrifugal pattern in the stratum corneum. Fungal invasion of the nails usually occurs through the lateral or superficial nail plates and then spreads throughout the nails; when hair shafts are invaded, the organisms can be found either within the shaft or surrounding it. Symptoms are caused by the inflammatory reaction elicited by fungal antigens and not by tissue invasion. Dermatophyte infections occur more commonly in male than in female patients, and progesterone has been shown to inhibit dermatophyte growth.

Clinical manifestations

Dermatophyte infection of the skin is often called *ringworm*. This term is confusing because worms are not involved. *Tinea*, the Latin word for *worm*, describes the serpentine nature of the skin lesions and is a less confusing designation that is used in conjunction with the name of the body part affected—e.g., tinea capitis (head), tinea pedis (feet), tinea corporis (body), tinea cruris (crotch), and tinea unguium (nails, although infection at this site is more often termed *onychomycosis*).

Tinea capitis occurs most commonly in children 3–7 years old. Children with tinea capitis usually present with well-demarcated scaly patches in which hair shafts are broken off right above the skin; alopecia can result. Tinea corporis is manifested by well-demarcated, annular, pruritic, scaly lesions that undergo central clearing. Usually one or several small lesions are present. In some cases, tinea corporis can involve much of the trunk or manifest as

TABLE 206-2 Suggested Treatment for Extensive Tinea Infections and Onychomycosis

Antifungal Agent	Suggested Dosage	Comments
Extensive tinea skin infection		
Terbinafine	250 mg/d for 1–2 weeks	Adverse reactions minimal with short treatment period
Itraconazole[a]	200 mg/d for 1–2 weeks	Adverse reactions minimal with short treatment period except for drug interactions
Onychomycosis		
Terbinafine	250 mg/d for 3 months	Slightly superior to itraconazole; monitor for hepatotoxicity
Itraconazole[a]	200 mg/d for 3 months or 200 mg bid for 1 week each month for 3 months	Drug interactions frequent; monitor for hepatotoxicity; rarely causes hypokalemia, hypertension, edema; use with caution in patients with congestive heart failure

[a]Itraconazole capsules require food and gastric acid for absorption, whereas itraconazole solution is taken on an empty stomach.

folliculitis with pustule formation. The rash should be differentiated from contact dermatitis, eczema, and psoriasis. Tinea cruris is seen almost exclusively in men. The perineal rash is erythematous and pustular, has a discrete scaly border, is without satellite lesions, and is usually pruritic. The rash must be differentiated from intertriginous candidiasis, erythrasma, and psoriasis.

Tinea pedis also is more common among men than among women. It usually starts in the web spaces of the toes; peeling, maceration, and pruritus are followed by development of a scaly pruritic rash along the lateral and plantar surfaces of the feet. Hyperkeratosis of the soles of the feet often ensues. Tinea pedis has been implicated in lower-extremity cellulitis, as streptococci and staphylococci can gain entrance to the tissues through fissures between the toes. Onychomycosis affects toenails more often than fingernails and is most common among persons who have tinea pedis. The nail becomes thickened and discolored and may crumble; onycholysis almost always occurs. Onychomycosis is more common in older adults and in persons with vascular disease, diabetes mellitus, and trauma to the nails. Fungal infection must be differentiated from psoriasis, which can mimic onychomycosis but usually has associated skin lesions.

Diagnosis

Many dermatophyte infections are diagnosed by their clinical appearance. If the diagnosis is in doubt, as is often the case in children with tinea capitis, scrapings should be taken from the edge of a lesion with a scalpel blade, transferred to a slide to which a drop of potassium hydroxide is added, and examined under a microscope for the presence of hyphae. Cultures are indicated if an outbreak is suspected or the patient does not respond to therapy. Culture of the nail is especially useful as an aid to decisions about both diagnosis and treatment.

Treatment and prognosis

Dermatophyte infections usually respond to topical therapy. Lotions or sprays are easier than creams to apply to large or hairy areas. Particularly for tinea cruris, the affected area should be kept as dry as possible. When patients have extensive skin lesions, oral itraconazole or terbinafine can hasten resolution (Table 206-2). Terbinafine interacts with fewer drugs than itraconazole and is generally the first-line agent. Onychomycosis does not respond to topical therapy, although ciclopirox nail lacquer applied daily for a year is occasionally beneficial. Itraconazole and terbinafine both accumulate in the nail plate and can be used to treat onychomycosis (Table 206-2). These agents are more effective and better tolerated than griseofulvin and ketoconazole. The major decision to be made with regard to therapy is whether the extent of nail involvement justifies the use of systemic antifungal agents that have adverse effects, may interact with other drugs, and are costly. Treating for cosmetic reasons alone is discouraged. Relapses of tinea cruris and tinea pedis are common and should be treated early with topical creams to avoid development of more extensive disease. Relapses of onychomycosis follow treatment in 25–30% of cases.

FURTHER READINGS

BEN-AMI R et al: Phaeohyphomycosis in a tertiary care cancer center. Clin Infect Dis 48:1033, 2009

CHANG DC et al: Multistate outbreak of *Fusarium* keratitis associated with use of a contact lens solution. JAMA 296:953, 2006

CORTEZ KJ et al: Infections caused by *Scedosporium* species. Clin Microbiol Rev 21:157, 2008

DE BERKER D: Clinical practice. Fungal nail disease. N Engl J Med 360:2108, 2009

GARNICA M et al: Difficult mycoses of the skin: Advances in the epidemiology and management of eumycetoma, phaeohyphomycosis, and chromoblastomycosis. Curr Opin Infect Dis 22:559, 2009

KAUFFMAN CA et al: Clinical practice guidelines for the management of sporotrichosis: 2007 Update by the Infectious Diseases Society of America. Clin Infect Dis 45:1255, 2007

NUCCI M et al: *Fusarium* infections in hematopoietic stem cell transplant recipients. Clin Infect Dis 38:1237, 2004

RESTREPO A et al: Pulmonary paracoccidioidomycosis. Semin Respir Crit Care Med 29:182, 2008

RUAN SY et al: Invasive trichosporonosis caused by *Trichosporon asahii* and other unusual *Trichosporon* species at a medical center in Taiwan. Clin Infect Dis 49:1457, 2009

CHAPTER 207

Pneumocystis Infections

A. George Smulian

Peter D. Walzer

DEFINITION AND DESCRIPTION

Pneumocystis is an opportunistic fungal pulmonary pathogen that is an important cause of pneumonia in the immunocompromised host. Although organisms within the *Pneumocystis* genus are morphologically very similar, they are genetically diverse and host-specific. *P. jirovecii* infects humans, whereas *P. carinii*—the original species described in 1909—infects rats. For clarity, only the genus designation *Pneumocystis* will be used in this chapter.

Developmental stages of the organism include the trophic form, the cyst, and the precyst (an intermediate stage). The life cycle of *Pneumocystis* probably involves sexual and asexual reproduction, although definitive proof awaits the development of a reliable culture system. *Pneumocystis* contains several different antigen groups, the most prominent of which are the 95- to 140-kDa major surface glycoprotein (MSG) and kexin (KEX1).

EPIDEMIOLOGY

Serologic surveys have demonstrated that *Pneumocystis* has a worldwide distribution and that most healthy children have been exposed to the organism by 3–4 years of age. Airborne transmission of *Pneumocystis* has been documented in animal studies; person-to-person transmission has been suggested by hospital outbreaks of *Pneumocystis* pneumonia (PcP) and by molecular epidemiologic analysis of isolates. Data suggest that the cyst is the transmissible form.

PATHOGENESIS AND PATHOLOGY

Studies over the past several years have shown that *Pneumocystis* commonly colonizes patients who are immunosuppressed or who have chronic obstructive pulmonary disease. This colonization elicits an inflammatory response and is associated with a decline in lung function.

The host factors that predispose to the development of PcP include defects in cellular and humoral immunity. The risk of PcP among HIV-infected patients rises markedly when circulating CD4+ T cell counts fall below 200/μL. Other persons at risk for PcP are patients receiving immunosuppressive agents (particularly glucocorticoids) for cancer and organ transplantation; those receiving biologic agents such as infliximab and etanercept for rheumatoid arthritis and inflammatory bowel disease; children with primary immunodeficiency diseases; and premature malnourished infants.

The principal host effector cells against *Pneumocystis* are alveolar macrophages, which ingest and kill the organism, releasing a variety of inflammatory mediators. Proliferating organisms remain extracellular within the alveolus, attaching tightly to type I cells. Alveolar damage results in increased alveolar-capillary permeability and surfactant abnormalities, including a fall in phospholipids and an increase in surfactant proteins A and D. The host inflammatory response to lung injury leads to increases in levels of interleukin 8 and in neutrophil counts in bronchoalveolar lavage (BAL) fluid. These changes correlate with disease severity.

On lung sections stained with hematoxylin and eosin, the alveoli are filled with a typical foamy, vacuolated exudate. Severe disease may include interstitial edema, fibrosis, and hyaline membrane formation. The host inflammatory changes usually consist of hypertrophy of alveolar type II cells, a typical reparative response, and a mild mononuclear cell interstitial infiltrate. Malnourished infants display an intense plasma cell infiltrate that gave the disease its early name: interstitial plasma cell pneumonia.

CLINICAL FEATURES

Patients with PcP develop dyspnea, fever, and nonproductive cough. HIV-infected patients are usually ill for several weeks and may have relatively subtle manifestations. Symptoms in non-HIV-infected patients are of shorter duration and often begin after the glucocorticoid dose has been tapered. A high index of suspicion and a thorough history are key factors in early detection.

Physical findings include tachypnea, tachycardia, and cyanosis, but lung auscultation reveals few abnormalities. Reduced arterial oxygen pressure (Pa_{O_2}), increased alveolar-arterial oxygen gradient ($PA_{O_2} - Pa_{O_2}$), and respiratory alkalosis are evident. Diffusion capacity is reduced, and heightened uptake with nonspecific nuclear imaging techniques (gallium scan) may be noted. Elevated serum concentrations of lactate dehydrogenase, reflecting lung parenchymal damage, and β-D-glucan, a component of the fungal cell wall, have been reported; however, these elevations are not specific for PcP infection.

The classic findings on chest radiography consist of bilateral diffuse infiltrates beginning in the perihilar regions (Fig. 207-1*A*), but various atypical manifestations (nodular densities, cavitary lesions) have also been reported. Pneumothorax occurs, and its management is often difficult. Early in the course of PcP, the chest radiograph may be normal, although high-resolution CT of the lung may reveal ground-glass opacities at this stage (Fig. 207-1*B*).

While *Pneumocystis* usually remains confined to the lungs, cases of disseminated infection have occurred in both HIV-infected and non-HIV-infected patients. Common sites of involvement include the lymph nodes, spleen, liver, and bone marrow.

DIAGNOSIS

Because of the nonspecific nature of the clinical picture, the diagnosis must be based on specific identification of the organism. A definitive diagnosis is made by histopathologic staining. Traditional cell wall stains such as methenamine silver selectively stain the wall of *Pneumocystis* cysts, while reagents such as Wright-Giemsa stain the nuclei of all developmental stages. Immunofluorescence with monoclonal antibodies is more sensitive and specific than histologic staining. DNA amplification by PCR may become part of routine diagnostics but may not distinguish colonization from infection.

The successful diagnosis of PcP depends on the collection of proper specimens. In general, the yield from different diagnostic procedures is higher for HIV-infected patients than for non-HIV-infected patients because of the higher organism burden in the former group. Sputum induction and oral washes have gained popularity as simple, noninvasive techniques; however, these procedures require trained and dedicated personnel. Fiberoptic bronchoscopy with BAL, which provides information about the organism burden, the host inflammatory response, and the presence of other opportunistic infections, continues to be the mainstay of *Pneumocystis* diagnosis. Transbronchial biopsy and open lung biopsy, the most invasive procedures, are used only when a diagnosis cannot be made by BAL.

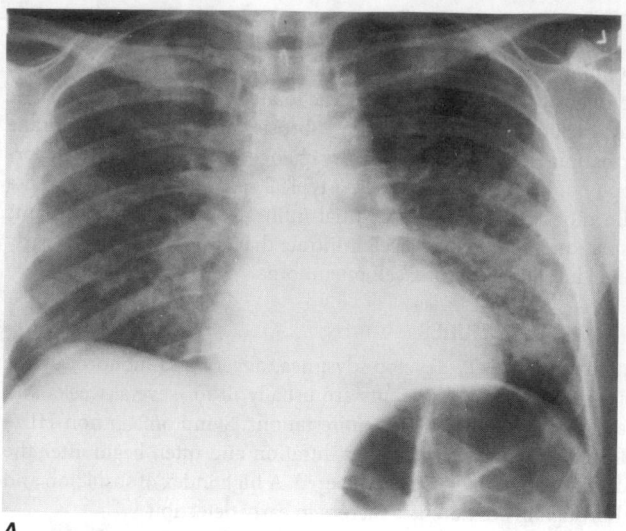

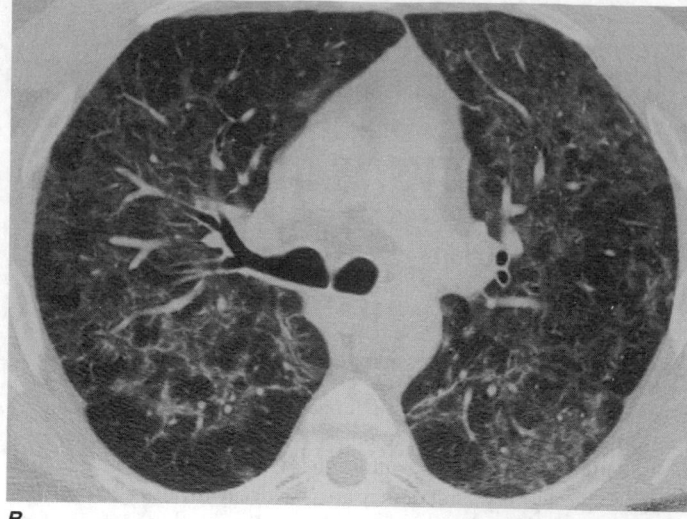

Figure 207-1 ***A.*** Chest radiograph depicting diffuse infiltrates in an HIV-infected patient with PcP. ***B.*** High-resolution CT of the lung showing ground-glass opacification in an HIV-infected patient with PcP. *(Courtesy of Dr. Cristopher Meyer, with permission.)*

■ COURSE AND PROGNOSIS

In the typical case of untreated PcP, progressive respiratory embarrassment leads to death. Therapy is most effective when instituted early, before there is extensive alveolar damage. If examination of induced sputum is nondiagnostic and BAL cannot be performed in a timely manner, empirical therapy for PcP is reasonable. However, this practice does not eliminate the need for a specific etiologic diagnosis. With improved management of HIV and its complications, mortality rates from PcP among HIV-infected patients are 0–15%. In contrast, rates of early death remain high among patients who require mechanical ventilation (60%) and among non-HIV-infected patients (40%).

TREATMENT ▶ *Pneumocystis* Infections

Trimethoprim-sulfamethoxazole (TMP-SMX), which acts by inhibiting folic acid synthesis, is considered the drug of choice for all forms of PcP (Table 207-1). Therapy is continued for 14 days in non-HIV-infected patients and for 21 days in persons infected with HIV. Since HIV-infected patients respond more slowly than non-HIV-infected patients, it is prudent to wait at least 7 days after the initiation of treatment before concluding that therapy has failed. TMP-SMX is well tolerated by non-HIV-infected patients, whereas more than half of HIV-infected patients experience serious adverse reactions.

Several alternative regimens are available for the treatment of mild to moderate cases of PcP (a Pa_{O_2} of >70 mmHg or a $PA_{O_2} - Pa_{O_2}$ of <35 mmHg while breathing room air). TMP plus dapsone and clindamycin plus primaquine are about as effective as TMP-SMX. Dapsone and primaquine should not be administered to patients with glucose-6-phosphate dehydrogenase (G6PD) deficiency. Atovaquone is less effective than TMP-SMX but is better tolerated. Since *Pneumocystis* lacks ergosterol, it is not susceptible to antifungal agents that inhibit ergosterol synthesis.

Alternative regimens that are recommended for the treatment of moderate to severe PcP (a Pa_{O_2} of ≤70 mmHg or a $PA_{O_2} - Pa_{O_2}$ of ≥35 mmHg) are parenteral pentamidine, parenteral clindamycin plus primaquine, or trimetrexate plus leucovorin. Parenteral clindamycin plus primaquine may be more efficacious than pentamidine.

Molecular evidence of resistance to sulfonamides and to atovaquone has emerged among clinical *Pneumocystis* isolates. Although prior sulfonamide exposure is a risk factor, this resistance has also occurred in HIV-infected patients who have never received sulfonamides. The outcome of therapy appears to be linked more strongly to traditional measures—e.g., high Acute Physiology, Age, and Chronic Health Evaluation III (APACHE III) scores, need for positive-pressure ventilation, delayed intubation, and development of pneumothorax—than to the presence of molecular markers of sulfonamide resistance.

Early institution of antiretroviral therapy when HIV patients present with PcP has been associated with improved survival rates, but careful attention should be devoted to the possible development of the immune reconstitution inflammatory syndrome. HIV-infected patients frequently experience deterioration of respiratory function shortly after receiving anti-*Pneumocystis* drugs. The adjunctive administration of tapering doses of glucocorticoids to HIV-infected patients with moderate to severe PcP can prevent this problem and improve the rate of survival (Table 207-1). For maximal benefit, this adjunctive therapy should be started early in the course of the illness. The use of steroids as adjunctive therapy in HIV-infected patients with mild PcP or in non-HIV-infected patients remains to be evaluated.

■ PREVENTION

Prophylaxis is indicated for HIV-infected patients with CD4+ T cell counts of <200/μL or a history of oropharyngeal candidiasis and for both HIV-infected and non-HIV-infected patients who have recovered from PcP. Prophylaxis may be discontinued in

TABLE 207-1 Treatment of Pneumocystosis

Drug(s), Dose, Route	Adverse Effects
First Choice[a]	
TMP-SMX (TMP: 5 mg/kg; SMX: 25 mg/kg[b]) q6–8 h PO or IV	Fever, rash, cytopenias, hepatitis, hyperkalemia, GI disturbances
Other Agents[a]	
TMP, 5 mg/kg q6–8h; plus dapsone, 100 mg qd PO	Hemolysis (G6PD deficiency), methemoglobinemia, fever, rash, GI disturbances
Atovaquone, 750 mg bid PO	Rash, fever, GI and hepatic disturbances
Clindamycin, 300–450 mg q6h PO or 600 mg q6–8h IV; plus primaquine, 15–30 mg qd PO	Hemolysis (G6PD deficiency), methemoglobinemia, rash, colitis, neutropenia
Pentamidine, 3–4 mg/kg qd IV	Hypotension, azotemia, cardiac arrhythmias, pancreatitis, dysglycemias, hypocalcemia, neutropenia, hepatitis
Trimetrexate, 45 mg/m^2 qd IV; plus leucovorin,[c] 20 mg/kg q6h PO or IV	Cytopenias, peripheral neuropathy, hepatic disturbances
Adjunctive Agent	
Prednisone, 40 mg bid × 5 d, 40 mg qd × 5 d, 20 mg qd × 11 d; PO or IV	Immunosuppression, peptic ulcer, hyperglycemia, mood changes, hypertension

[a]Therapy is administered for 14 days to non-HIV-infected patients and for 21 days to HIV-infected patients.
[b]Equivalent of 2 double-strength (DS) tablets. (One DS tablet contains 160 mg of TMP and 800 mg of SMX.)
[c]Leucovorin prevents bone marrow toxicity from trimetrexate.
Abbreviations: GI, gastrointestinal; G6PD, glucose-6-phosphate dehydrogenase; TMP-SMX, trimethoprim-sulfamethoxazole.

HIV-infected patients once CD4+ T cell counts have risen to >200/μL and remained at that level for ≥3 months. Primary prophylaxis guidelines for immunocompromised hosts not infected with HIV are less clear.

TMP-SMX is the drug of choice for primary and secondary prophylaxis (Table 207-2). This agent also provides protection against toxoplasmosis and some bacterial infections. Alternative regimens are available for individuals intolerant of TMP-SMX (Table 207-2). Although there are no specific recommendations for preventing the spread of *Pneumocystis* in health care facilities, it seems prudent to prevent direct contact between patients with PcP and other susceptible hosts.

TABLE 207-2 Prophylaxis of Pneumocystosis[a]

Drug(s), Dose, Route	Comments
First Choice	
TMP-SMX, 1 DS tablet or 1 SS tablet qd PO[b]	TMP-SMX can be safely reintroduced for treatment of some patients who have had mild to moderate side effects.
Other Agents	
Dapsone, 50 mg bid or 100 mg qd PO	—
Dapsone, 50 mg qd PO; plus pyrimethamine, 50 mg weekly PO; plus leucovorin, 25 mg weekly PO	Leucovorin prevents bone marrow toxicity from pyrimethamine.
Dapsone, 200 mg weekly PO; plus pyrimethamine, 75 mg weekly PO; plus leucovorin, 25 mg weekly PO	Leucovorin prevents bone marrow toxicity from pyrimethamine.
Pentamidine, 300 mg monthly via Respirgard II nebulizer	Adverse reactions include cough and bronchospasm.
Atovaquone, 1500 mg qd PO	—
TMP-SMX, 1 DS tablet three times weekly PO	TMP-SMX can be safely reintroduced for treatment of some patients who have had mild to moderate side effects.

[a]For a list of adverse effects, see Table 207-1.
[b]One DS tablet contains 160 mg of TMP and 800 mg of SMX.
Abbreviations: DS, double-strength; SS, single-strength; TMP-SMX, trimethoprim-sulfamethoxazole.

FURTHER READINGS

CUSHION MT et al: Echinocandin treatment of *Pneumocystis* pneumonia in rodent models depletes cysts leaving trophic burdens that cannot transmit the infection. PloS One 5:e8524, 2010

HELWEG-LARSEN J et al: Clinical efficacy of first- and second-line treatments for HIV-associated *Pneumocystis jirovecii* pneumonia: A tri-centre cohort study. J Antimicrob Chemother 64:1282, 2009

KAPLAN JE et al: Guidelines for prevention and treatment of opportunistic infections in HIV-infected adults and adolescents: Recommendations from CDC, the National Institutes of Health, and the HIV Medicine Association of the Infectious Diseases Society of America. MMWR Recomm Rep 58(RR-4):1–207; quiz CE1–4, 2009 [whole issue]

KRAJICEK BJ et al: *Pneumocystis* pneumonia: Current concepts in pathogenesis, diagnosis, and treatment. Clin Chest Med 30:265, vi, 2009

MILLER RF et al: Improved survival for HIV infected patients with severe *Pneumocystis jirovecii* pneumonias independent of highly active antiretroviral therapy. Thorax 61:716, 2006

MORRIS A et al: Epidemiology and clinical significance of *Pneumocystis* colonization. J Infect Dis 197:10, 2008

TIPIRNENI R et al: Healthcare worker occupation and immune response to *Pneumcystis jirovecii*. Emerg Infect Dis 15:1590, 2009

WALZER PD et al: Early predictors of mortality from *Pneumocystis jirovecii* pneumonia in HIV-infected patients: 1985–2006. Clin Infect Dis 46:634, 2008

YAZAKI H et al: Outbreak of *Pneumocystis jiroveci* pneumonia in renal transplant recipients: *P. jiroveci* is contagious to the susceptible host. Transplantation 88:380, 2009

ZOLOPA A et al: Early antiretroviral therapy reduces AIDS progression/death in individuals with acute opportunistic infections; a multicenter randomized strategy trial. PloS One 4:e5575, 2009

CHAPTER 208

Agents Used to Treat Parasitic Infections

Thomas A. Moore

Parasitic infections afflict more than half of the world's population and impose a substantial health burden, particularly in underdeveloped nations, where they are most prevalent. The reach of some parasitic diseases, including malaria, has expanded over the past few decades as a result of factors such as deforestation, population shifts, global warming, and other climatic events. Despite major efforts at vaccine development and vector control, chemotherapy remains the single most effective means of controlling parasitic infections. Efforts to combat the spread of some diseases are hindered by the development and spread of drug resistance, the limited introduction of new antiparasitic agents, and the proliferation of counterfeit medications. However, there are good reasons to be optimistic. The past 10 years have witnessed the launch of ambitious global initiatives aimed at controlling or eliminating threats such as AIDS, tuberculosis, and malaria. Recognition of the substantial burden imposed by the "neglected" tropical diseases has generated multinational partnerships to develop and deploy effective antiparasitic agents. Vaccines against several tropical diseases are being developed, and clinical trials have begun for vaccines against schistosomiasis, hookworm, and leishmaniasis.

This chapter deals exclusively with the agents used to treat infections due to parasites. Specific treatment recommendations for the parasitic diseases of humans are listed in subsequent chapters. The pharmacology of the antiparasitic agents is discussed in great detail in Chap. e26.

Table 208-1 presents a brief overview of each agent (including some drugs that are covered in other chapters), along with its major toxicities, spectrum of activity, and safety for use during pregnancy and lactation. Many of the agents are approved by the U.S. Food and Drug Administration but are considered investigational for the treatment of certain infections; these drugs are marked accordingly in the table. In addition, drugs available only through the Centers for Disease Control and Prevention (CDC) Drug Service (telephone: 404-639-3670 or 404-639-2888; *www.cdc.gov/laboratory/drugservice/*) or only through their manufacturers (whose contact information may be available from the CDC) are specified by footnotes in the table.

TABLE 208-1 Overview of Agents Used for the Treatment of Parasitic Infections

Drugs by Class	Parasitic Infection(s)	Adverse Effects	Major Drug-Drug Interactions	Pregnancy Class[a]	Breast Milk
4-Aminoquinolines					
Amodiaquine	Malaria[b]	Agranulocytosis, hepatotoxicity	No information	Not assigned	No information
Chloroquine	Malaria[b]	*Occasional:* pruritus, nausea, vomiting, headache, hair depigmentation, exfoliative dermatitis, reversible corneal opacity. *Rare:* irreversible retinal injury, nail discoloration, blood dyscrasias	Antacids and kaolin: reduced absorption of chloroquine / Ampicillin: bioavailability reduced by chloroquine / Cimetidine: increased serum levels of chloroquine / Cyclosporine: serum levels increased by chloroquine	Not assigned[c]	Yes
8-Aminoquinolines					
Primaquine	Malaria[b]	*Frequent:* hemolysis in patients with G6PD deficiency. *Occasional:* methemoglobinemia, GI disturbances. *Rare:* CNS symptoms	Quinacrine: potentiated toxicity of primaquine	Contraindicated	No information
Tafenoquine	Malaria[b]	*Frequent:* hemolysis in patients with G6PD deficiency, mild GI upset. *Occasional:* methemoglobinemia, headaches	No information	Not assigned	No information

(continued)

Drugs by Class	Parasitic Infection(s)	Adverse Effects	Major Drug-Drug Interactions	Pregnancy Class[a]	Breast Milk
Aminoalcohols					
Halofantrine	Malaria[b]	*Frequent:* abdominal pain, diarrhea. *Occasional:* ECG disturbances (dose-related prolongation of QTc and PR interval), nausea, pruritus. Contraindicated in persons who have cardiac disease or who have taken mefloquine in the preceding 3 weeks	Concomitant use of agents that prolong QTc interval contraindicated	C	No information
Lumefantrine	Malaria[b]	*Occasional:* nausea, vomiting, diarrhea, abdominal pain, anorexia, headache, dizziness	No major interactions	Not assigned	No information
Aminoglycosides					
Paromomycin	Amebiasis,[b] infection with *Dientamoeba fragilis*, giardiasis, cryptosporidiosis, leishmaniasis	*Frequent:* GI disturbances (oral dosing only). *Occasional:* nephrotoxicity, ototoxicity, vestibular toxicity (parenteral dosing only)	No major interactions	Not assigned[c]	No information
Amphotericin B	Leishmaniasis,[d] amebic meningoencephalitis	*Frequent:* fever, chills, hypokalemia, hypomagnesemia, nephrotoxicity. *Occasional:* vomiting, dyspnea, hypotension	Antineoplastic agents: renal toxicity, bronchospasm, hypotension	B	No information
Amphotericin B deoxycholate					
Amphotec (InterMune)			Glucocorticoids, ACTH, digitalis: hypokalemia		
Amphotericin B lipid complex, ABLC (Abelcet)			Zidovudine: increased myelo- and nephrotoxicity		
Amphotericin B, liposomal (AmBisome)					
Antimonials	Leishmaniasis				
Pentavalent antimony[e]		*Frequent:* arthralgias/myalgias, pancreatitis, ECG changes (QT prolongation, T wave flattening or inversion)	No major interactions	Not assigned	Yes
Meglumine antimoniate		*Frequent:* arthralgias/myalgias, pancreatitis, ECG changes (QT prolongation, T wave flattening or inversion)	Antiarrhythmics and tricyclic antidepressants: increased risk of cardiotoxicity	Not assigned	No information
Artemisinin and derivatives	Malaria[f]	*Occasional:* neurotoxicity (ataxia, convulsions), nausea, vomiting, anorexia, contact dermatitis			
Arteether			No information	Not assigned	Yes[g]
Artemether			No clinically significant interactions	C	Yes[g]
Artesunate[e]			Mefloquine: levels decreased and clearance accelerated by artesunate	C	Yes[g]
Dihydroartemisinin			Mefloquine: increased absorption	Not assigned	Yes[g]
Atovaquone	Malaria,[b] babesiosis	*Frequent:* nausea, vomiting. *Occasional:* abdominal pain, headache	Plasma levels decreased by rifampin, tetracycline; bioavailability decreased by metoclopramide	C	No information

(*continued*)

Drugs by Class	Parasitic Infection(s)	Adverse Effects	Major Drug-Drug Interactions	Pregnancy Class[a]	Breast Milk
Azoles Fluconazole Itraconazole Ketoconazole	Leishmaniasis	*Serious:* hepatotoxicity. *Rare:* exfoliative skin disorders, anaphylaxis	Warfarin, oral hypoglycemics, phenytoin, cyclosporine, theophylline, digoxin, dofetilide, quinidine, carbamazepine, rifabutin, busulfan, docetaxel, vinca alkaloids, pimozide, alprazolam, diazepam, midazolam, triazolam, verapamil, atorvastatin, cerivastatin, lovastatin, simvastatin, tacrolimus, sirolimus, indinavir, ritonavir, saquinavir, alfentanil, buspirone, methylprednisolone, trimetrexate: plasma levels increased by azoles Carbamazepine, phenobarbital, phenytoin, isoniazid, rifabutin, rifampin, antacids, H2-receptor antagonists, proton pump inhibitors, nevirapine: decreased plasma levels of azoles Clarithromycin, erythromycin, indinavir, ritonavir: increased plasma levels of azoles	C	Yes
Benzimidazoles Albendazole	Ascariasis, capillariasis, clonorchiasis, cutaneous larva migrans, cysticercosis,[b] echinococcosis,[b] enterobiasis, eosinophilic enterocolitis, gnathostomiasis, hookworm, lymphatic filariasis, microsporidiosis, strongyloidiasis, trichinellosis, trichostrongyliasis, trichuriasis, visceral larva migrans	*Occasional:* nausea, vomiting, abdominal pain, headache, reversible alopecia, elevated aminotransferases. *Rare:* leukopenia, rash	Dexamethasone, praziquantel: plasma level of albendazole sulfoxide increased by ~50%	C	Yes[g]
Mebendazole	Ascariasis,[b] capillariasis, eosinophilic enterocolitis, enterobiasis,[b] hookworm,[b] trichinellosis, trichostrongyliasis, trichuriasis,[b] visceral larva migrans	*Occasional:* diarrhea, abdominal pain, elevated aminotransferases. *Rare:* agranulocytosis, thrombocytopenia, alopecia	Cimetidine: inhibited mebendazole metabolism	C	No information
Thiabendazole	Strongyloidiasis,[b] cutaneous larva migrans,[b] visceral larva migrans[b]	*Frequent:* anorexia, nausea, vomiting, diarrhea, headache, dizziness, asparagus-like urine odor. *Occasional:* drowsiness, giddiness, crystalluria, elevated aminotransferases, psychosis. *Rare:* hepatitis, seizures, angioneurotic edema, Stevens-Johnson syndrome, tinnitus	Theophylline: serum levels increased by thiabendazole	C	No information

(*continued*)

Drugs by Class	Parasitic Infection(s)	Adverse Effects	Major Drug-Drug Interactions	Pregnancy Class[a]	Breast Milk
Triclabendazole	Fascioliasis, paragonimiasis	*Occasional:* abdominal cramps, diarrhea, biliary colic, transient headache	No information	Not assigned	Yes
Benznidazole	Chagas' disease	*Frequent:* rash, pruritus, nausea, leukopenia, paresthesias	No major interactions	Not assigned	No information
Bithionol[e]	Fascioliasis, paragonimiasis	Diarrhea, abdominal cramps (usually mild and transient)			
Clindamycin	Babesiosis, malaria, toxoplasmosis	*Occasional:* pseudomembranous colitis, abdominal pain, diarrhea, nausea/vomiting. *Rare:* pruritus, skin rashes	No major interactions	B	Yes[g]
Diloxanide furoate	Amebiasis	*Frequent:* flatulence. *Occasional:* nausea, vomiting, diarrhea. *Rare:* pruritus	None reported	Contraindicated	No information
Eflornithine[h] (difluoromethylornithine, DFMO)	Trypanosomiasis	*Frequent:* pancytopenia. *Occasional:* diarrhea, seizures. *Rare:* transient hearing loss	No major interactions	Contraindicated	No information
Emetine and dehydroemetine[e]	Amebiasis, fascioliasis	*Severe:* cardiotoxicity. *Frequent:* pain at injection site. *Occasional:* dizziness, headache, GI symptoms	None reported	X	No information
Folate antagonists					
Dihydrofolate reductase inhibitors					
Pyrimethamine	Malaria,[b] isosporiasis, toxoplasmosis[b]	*Occasional:* folate deficiency. *Rare:* rash, seizures, severe skin reactions (toxic epidermal necrolysis, erythema multiforme, Stevens-Johnson syndrome)	Sulfonamides, proguanil, zidovudine: increased risk of bone marrow suppression when used concomitantly	C	Yes
Proguanil and chlorproguanil	Malaria	*Occasional:* urticaria. *Rare:* hematuria, GI disturbances	No major interactions	C	Yes
Trimethoprim	Cyclosporiasis, isosporiasis	Hyperkalemia, GI upset, mild stomatitis	Methotrexate: reduced clearance Warfarin: effect prolonged Phenytoin: hepatic metabolism increased	C	Yes
Dihydropteroate synthetase inhibitors: sulfonamides Sulfadiazine Sulfamethoxazole Sulfadoxine	Malaria,[b] toxoplasmosis[b]	*Frequent:* GI disturbances, allergic skin reactions, crystalluria. *Rare:* severe skin reactions (toxic epidermal necrolysis, erythema multiforme, Stevens-Johnson syndrome), agranulocytosis, aplastic anemia, hypersensitivity of the respiratory tract, hepatitis, interstitial nephritis, hypoglycemia, aseptic meningitis	Thiazide diuretics: increased risk of thrombocytopenia in elderly patients Warfarin: effect prolonged by sulfonamides Methotrexate: levels increased by sulfonamides Phenytoin: metabolism impaired by sulfonamides Sulfonylureas: effect prolonged by sulfonamides	B	Yes
Dihydropteroate synthetase inhibitors: sulfones Dapsone	Leishmaniasis, malaria, toxoplasmosis	*Frequent:* rash, anorexia. *Occasional:* hemolysis, methemoglobinemia, neuropathy, allergic dermatitis, anorexia, nausea, vomiting, tachycardia, headache, insomnia, psychosis, hepatitis. *Rare:* agranulocytosis	Rifampin: lowered plasma levels of dapsone	C	Yes

(*continued*)

Drugs by Class	Parasitic Infection(s)	Adverse Effects	Major Drug-Drug Interactions	Pregnancy Class[a]	Breast Milk
Fumagillin	Microsporidiosis	*Rare:* neutropenia, thrombocytopenia	None reported	No information	No information
Furazolidone	Giardiasis	*Frequent:* nausea/vomiting, brown urine. *Occasional:* rectal itching, headache. *Rare:* hemolytic anemia, disulfiram-like reactions, MAO-inhibitor interactions	Risk of hypertensive crisis when administered for >5 days with MAO inhibitors	C	No information
Iodoquinol	Amebiasis,[b] balantidiasis, *D. fragilis* infection	*Occasional:* headache, rash, pruritus, thyrotoxicosis, nausea, vomiting, abdominal pain, diarrhea. *Rare:* optic neuritis, peripheral neuropathy, seizures, encephalopathy	No major interactions	C	No information
Ivermectin	Ascariasis, cutaneous larva migrans, gnathostomiasis, loiasis, lymphatic filariasis, onchocerciasis,[b] scabies, strongyloidiasis,[b] trichuriasis	*Occasional:* fever, pruritus, headache, myalgias. *Rare:* hypotension	No major interactions	C	Yes[g]
Levamisole	Ascariasis, hookworm	*Frequent:* GI disturbances, dizziness, headache. *Rare:* agranulocytosis, peripheral neuropathy	Alcohol: disulfiram-like effect Warfarin: prolonged prothrombin time	C	No information
Macrolides					
Azithromycin	Babesiosis	*Occasional:* nausea, vomiting, diarrhea, abdominal pain. *Rare:* angioedema, cholestatic jaundice	Cyclosporine and digoxin: levels increased by azithromycin Nelfinavir: increased levels of azithromycin	B	Yes
Spiramycin[h]	Toxoplasmosis	*Occasional:* GI disturbances, transient skin eruptions. *Rare:* thrombocytopenia, QT prolongation in an infant, cholestatic hepatitis	No major interactions	Not assigned[c]	Yes[g]
Mefloquine	Malaria[b]	*Frequent:* lightheadedness, nausea, headache. *Occasional:* confusion; nightmares; insomnia; visual disturbance; transient and clinically silent ECG abnormalities, including sinus bradycardia, sinus arrhythmia, first-degree AV block, prolongation of QTc interval, and abnormal T waves. *Rare:* psychosis, convulsions, hypotension	Administration of halofantrine <3 weeks after mefloquine use may produce fatal QTc prolongation. Mefloquine may lower plasma levels of anticonvulsants. Levels decreased and clearance accelerated by artesunate	C	Yes
Melarsoprol[e]	Trypanosomiasis	*Frequent:* myocardial injury, encephalopathy, peripheral neuropathy, hypertension. *Occasional:* G6PD-induced hemolysis, erythema nodosum leprosum. *Rare:* hypotension	No major interactions	Not assigned	No information
Metrifonate	Schistosomiasis	*Frequent:* abdominal pain, nausea, vomiting, diarrhea, headache, vertigo, bronchospasm. *Rare:* cholinergic symptoms	No major interactions	B	No

(continued)

Drugs by Class	Parasitic Infection(s)	Adverse Effects	Major Drug-Drug Interactions	Pregnancy Class[a]	Breast Milk
Miltefosine	Leishmaniasis	*Frequent:* mild and transient (1–2 days) GI disturbances within first 2 weeks of therapy (resolve after treatment completion); motion sickness. *Occasional:* reversible elevations of creatinine and aminotransferases	No major interactions	Not assigned	No information
Niclosamide	Intestinal cestodes[b]	*Occasional:* nausea, vomiting, dizziness, pruritus	No major interactions	B	No information
Nifurtimox[e]	Chagas' disease	*Frequent:* nausea, vomiting, abdominal pain, insomnia, paresthesias, weakness, tremors. *Rare:* seizures (all are reversible and dose-related)	No major interactions	Not assigned	No information
Nitazoxanide	Cryptosporidiosis,[b] giardiasis[b]	*Occasional:* abdominal pain, diarrhea. *Rare:* vomiting, headache	No major interactions	B	No information
Nitroimidazoles					
Metronidazole	Amebiasis,[b] balantidiasis, dracunculiasis, giardiasis, trichomoniasis,[b] *D. fragilis* infection	*Frequent:* nausea, headache, anorexia, metallic aftertaste. *Occasional:* vomiting, insomnia, vertigo, paresthesias, disulfiram-like effects. *Rare:* seizures, peripheral neuropathy	Warfarin: effect enhanced by metronidazole Disulfiram: psychotic reaction Phenobarbital, phenytoin: accelerate elimination of metronidazole Lithium: serum levels elevated by metronidazole Cimetidine: prolonged half-life of metronidazole	B	Yes
Tinidazole	Amebiasis,[b] giardiasis, trichomoniasis	*Occasional:* nausea, vomiting, metallic taste	See metronidazole	C	Yes
Oxamniquine	Schistosomiasis	*Occasional:* dizziness, drowsiness, headache, orange urine, elevated aminotransferases. *Rare:* seizures	No major interactions	C	No information
Paromomycin	Amebiasis,[b] *D. fragilis* infection, giardiasis, cryptosporidiosis, leishmaniasis	*Frequent:* GI disturbances (oral dosing only). *Occasional:* nephrotoxicity, ototoxicity, vestibular toxicity (parenteral dosing only)	No major interactions	Oral: B Parenteral: not assigned[c]	No information
Pentamidine isethionate	Leishmaniasis, trypanosomiasis	*Frequent:* hypotension, hypoglycemia, pancreatitis, sterile abscesses at IM injection sites, GI disturbances, reversible renal failure. *Occasional:* hepatotoxicity, cardiotoxicity, delirium. *Rare:* anaphylaxis	No major interactions	C	No information
Piperazine and derivatives					
Piperazine	Ascariasis, enterobiasis	*Occasional:* nausea, vomiting, diarrhea, abdominal pain, headache. *Rare:* neurotoxicity, seizures	None reported	C	No information
Diethylcarbamazine[e]	Lymphatic filariasis, loiasis, tropical pulmonary eosinophilia	*Frequent:* dose-related nausea, vomiting. *Rare:* fever, chills, arthralgias, headaches	None reported	Not assigned[c]	No information

(continued)

Drugs by Class	Parasitic Infection(s)	Adverse Effects	Major Drug-Drug Interactions	Pregnancy Class[a]	Breast Milk
Praziquantel	Clonorchiasis,[b] cysticercosis, diphyllobothriasis, hymenolepiasis, taeniasis, opisthorchiasis, intestinal trematodes, paragonimiasis, schistosomiasis[b]	*Frequent:* abdominal pain, diarrhea, dizziness, headache, malaise. *Occasional:* fever, nausea. *Rare:* pruritus, singultus	No major interactions	B	Yes
Pyrantel pamoate	Ascariasis, eosinophilic enterocolitis, enterobiasis,[b] hookworm, trichostrongyliasis	*Occasional:* GI disturbances, headache, dizziness, elevated aminotransferases	No major interactions	C	No information
Quinacrine[h]	Giardiasis[b]	*Frequent:* headache, nausea, vomiting, bitter taste. *Occasional:* yellow-orange discoloration of skin, sclerae, urine; begins after 1 week of treatment and lasts up to 4 months after drug discontinuation. *Rare:* psychosis, exfoliative dermatitis, retinopathy, G6PD-induced hemolysis, exacerbation of psoriasis, disulfiram-like effects	Primaquine: toxicity potentiated by quinacrine	C	No information
Quinine and quinidine	Malaria, babesiosis	*Frequent:* cinchonism (tinnitus, high-tone deafness, headache, dysphoria, nausea, vomiting, abdominal pain, visual disturbances, postural hypotension), hyperinsulinemia resulting in life-threatening hypoglycemia. *Occasional:* deafness, hemolytic anemia, arrhythmias, hypotension due to rapid IV infusion	Carbonic-anhydrase inhibitors, thiazide diuretics: reduced renal elimination of quinidine Amiodarone, cimetidine: increased quinidine levels Nifedipine: decreased quinidine levels; quinidine slows metabolism of nifedipine Phenobarbital, phenytoin, rifampin: accelerated hepatic elimination of quinidine Verapamil: reduced hepatic clearance of quinidine Diltiazem: decreased clearance of quinidine	X	Yes[g]
Quinolones					
Ciprofloxacin	Cyclosporiasis, isosporiasis	*Occasional:* nausea, diarrhea, vomiting, abdominal pain/discomfort, headache, restlessness, rash. *Rare:* myalgias/arthralgias, tendon rupture, CNS symptoms (nervousness, agitation, insomnia, anxiety, nightmares or paranoia); convulsions	Probenecid: increased serum levels of ciprofloxacin Theophylline, warfarin: serum levels increased by ciprofloxacin	C	Yes
Suramin[e]	Trypanosomiasis	*Frequent:* immediate: fever, urticaria, nausea, vomiting, hypotension; delayed (up to 24 h): exfoliative dermatitis, stomatitis, paresthesias, photophobia, renal dysfunction. *Occasional:* nephrotoxicity, adrenal toxicity, optic atrophy, anaphylaxis	No major interactions	Not assigned	No information

(*continued*)

TABLE 208-1 Overview of Agents Used for the Treatment of Parasitic Infections (*Continued*)

Drugs by Class	Parasitic Infection(s)	Adverse Effects	Major Drug-Drug Interactions	Pregnancy Class[a]	Breast Milk
Tetracyclines	Balantidiasis, *D. fragilis* infection, malaria; lymphatic filariasis (doxycycline)	*Frequent:* GI disturbances. *Occasional:* photosensitivity dermatitis. *Rare:* exfoliative dermatitis, esophagitis, hepatotoxicity	Warfarin: effect prolonged by tetracyclines	D	Yes

[a]Based on U.S. Food and Drug Administration pregnancy categories of A–D, X.

[b]Approved by the FDA for this indication.

[c]Use in pregnancy is recommended by international organizations outside the United States.

[d]Only AmBisome has been approved by the FDA for this indication.

[e]Available through the CDC.

[f]Only artemether (in combination with lumefantrine) and artesunate have been approved by the FDA for this indication.

[g]Not believed to be harmful.

[h]Available through the manufacturer.

Abbreviations: ACTH, adrenocorticotropic hormone; AV, atrioventricular; CNS, central nervous system; ECG, electrocardiogram; G6PD, glucose 6-phosphate dehydrogenase; MAO, monoamine oxidase.

FURTHER READINGS

ABRAMOWICZ M (ed): Drugs for parasitic infections. Med Lett Drugs Ther 5:e1, 2007

HOTEZ PJ et al: Control of neglected tropical diseases. N Engl J Med 357:1018, 2007

KEISER J, UTZINGER J: Efficacy of current drugs against soil-transmitted helminth infections. JAMA 299:1937, 2008

CHAPTER 209

Amebiasis and Infection With Free-Living Amebas

Samuel L. Stanley, Jr.

AMEBIASIS

■ DEFINITION

Amebiasis is infection with the parasitic intestinal protozoan *Entamoeba histolytica* (the "tissue-lysing ameba"). Most infections are probably asymptomatic, but *E. histolytica* can cause disease ranging from dysentery to extraintestinal infections, including liver abscesses.

■ LIFE CYCLE AND TRANSMISSION

E. histolytica exists in two stages: a hardy multinucleate cyst form (Fig. 209-1) and the motile trophozoite stage (Fig. 209-2). Infection (of which humans are the natural hosts) is acquired by ingestion of cysts contained in fecally contaminated food or water or, more rarely, through oral-anal sexual contact. Cysts survive stomach acidity and excyst within the small intestine to form the 20- to 50-μm trophozoite stage. Trophozoites can live within the large-bowel lumen without causing disease or can invade the intestinal mucosa, causing amebic colitis. In some cases, *E. histolytica* trophozoites invade through the mucosa and into the bloodstream, traveling through the portal circulation to reach the liver and causing amebic liver abscesses. Motile trophozoites may be excreted into the stool—a diagnostically important event—but are rapidly killed upon exposure to air or stomach acid and therefore are not infectious. Trophozoite cysts within the large bowel are excreted in the stool, continuing the life cycle.

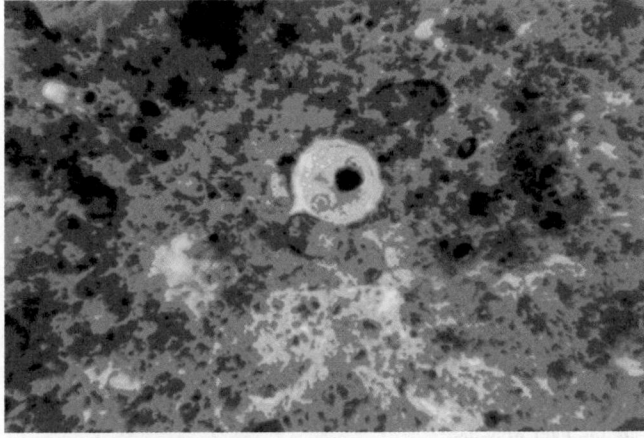

Figure 209-1   *Entamoeba* cyst. Three of the four nuclei are clearly visible. *(Courtesy of Dr. George Healy, Centers for Disease Control and Prevention.)*

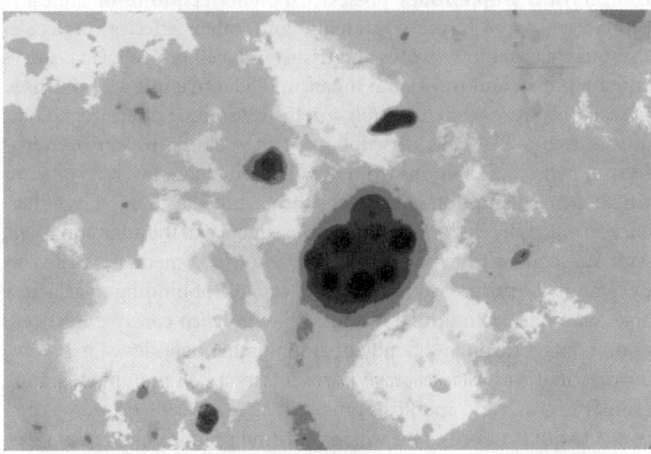

Figure 209-2   *E. histolytica* trophozoite with ingested red blood cells. Note the single nucleus with central nucleolus. *(Courtesy of the Centers for Disease Control and Prevention.)*

■ EPIDEMIOLOGY

Molecular diagnostics continue to clarify what was once a confusing picture of the true incidence and prevalence of *E. histolytica* infection and disease. It was a staple of most textbooks that 10% of the world's population was infected with *E. histolytica*. We now know that most asymptomatic individuals harboring amebic trophozoites or cysts in their stools are infected with a noninvasive species: *Entamoeba dispar* or *Entamoeba moshkovskii*. *E. dispar* appears not to cause disease, even in the most profoundly immunosuppressed individuals; furthermore, at this time, there is little evidence to suggest that *E. moshkovskii* causes disease, although epidemiologic studies of this species are in their infancy. In contrast, *E. histolytica* infection can cause disease, although not all patients develop symptoms. It remains unclear how frequently people infected with *E. histolytica* do develop symptoms; in one study in a highly endemic area, only 10% of infected patients developed symptoms over a 1-year observation period. A remarkable feature of amebiasis is its more common occurrence in men than in women, although the prevalence of infection with *E. histolytica* does not appear to differ between the sexes. This pattern is particularly pronounced for amebic liver abscess, whose prevalence is ~7 times higher among men than among women. The explanation for this difference remains unknown, but less efficient complement-mediated killing of amebic trophozoites by serum from men than by serum from women has been reported.

E. histolytica infections are most common in areas of the world where poor sanitation and crowding compromise the barriers to contamination of food and drinking water with human feces. Endemic areas include parts of Mexico, India, and nations in the tropical regions of Africa, South and Central America, and Asia. *E. histolytica* was present in ~2.1% of individuals presenting with diarrhea in a large series from Bangladesh and in 1.4% of the asymptomatic control group. In 2007, amebiasis was listed as the sixth most common cause of disease in Mexico, with an incidence of ~544 cases per 100,000 population. In the United States and other developed countries, disease is unusual and is found almost exclusively in travelers or immigrants from endemic areas.

Rarely, outbreaks take place in institutionalized populations, and infections have been documented with increased frequency among men who have sex with men; however, most of the latter cases have been asymptomatic and probably represent *E. dispar* infections.

■ PATHOGENESIS AND PATHOLOGY

E. histolytica trophozoites possess a potent repertoire of adhesins, proteinases, pore-forming proteins, and other effector molecules that enable them to lyse cells and tissue, induce both cellular necrosis and apoptosis, and resist both innate and adaptive immune defenses. Disease begins when *E. histolytica* trophozoites adhere to colonic mucosal epithelial cells. Disruption of the colonic mucin barrier is seen in pathologic sections from the diseased colon, but it is not clear whether this disruption is caused by the parasite, facilitating its adherence to mucosal cells, or occurs as a consequence of the adhesion event, with subsequent mucosal damage. Adherence is mediated primarily by a family of surface lectin molecules capable of binding to galactose and *N*-acetylgalactosamine residues. *E. histolytica* can lyse host cells upon contact through a family of amphipathic peptides called *amoebapores* that form barrel-stave pores in target cell membranes. Both cellular necrosis and apoptosis can occur after *E. histolytica* comes into contact with host cells, and which outcome predominates may relate to inherent characteristics of the target cell or the tissue environment. One consistent and unequivocal finding is the important role played by amebic cysteine proteinases in the disease process. *E. histolytica* possesses a large family of cysteine proteinases that are capable of lysing the extracellular matrix between host cells (thus detaching cells and facilitating invasion) and cleaving host defense molecules (including complement components and antibodies). Studies in animal models, including chimeric mice with human intestinal xenografts, have shown that inhibition of *E. histolytica* cysteine proteinase activity, via either direct gene targeting or chemical inhibitors, significantly reduces disease. The ultimate effect of all these amebic virulence factors on the human colon is the production of small ulcers that have heaped borders and contain focal areas of epithelial cell loss, a modest inflammatory response, and mucosal hemorrhage. The intervening mucosa is usually normal, but diffuse hyperemia is sometimes seen. *E. histolytica* trophozoites can then invade laterally through the submucosal layer, creating the classic flask-shaped ulcers that appear on pathologic examination as narrow-necked lesions, broadening in the submucosal region, with *E. histolytica* trophozoites at the margins between dead and live tissues (Fig. 209-3). Ulcers tend to stop at the muscularis layer, and full-thickness lesions and colonic perforation

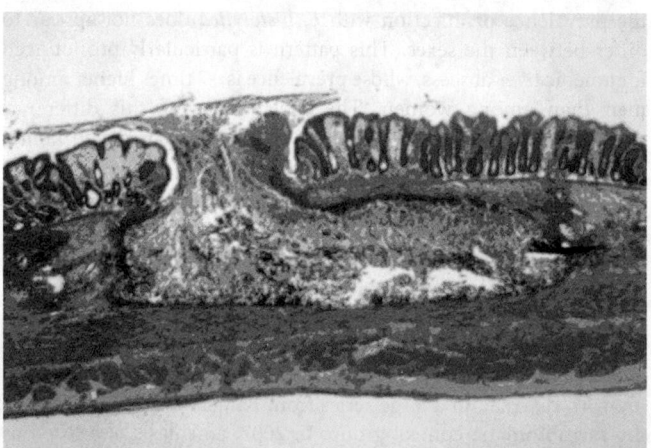

Figure 209-3 *E. histolytica* **flask-shaped intestinal ulceration** from a kitten. *(Courtesy of Dr. Mae Melvin, Centers for Disease Control and Prevention.)*

are unusual. Amebomas, a rare complication of intestinal disease, are granulomatous mass lesions protruding into the bowel lumen, with a thickened edematous and hemorrhagic bowel wall that can cause obstructive symptoms.

In some individuals with *E. histolytica* colonic infection, trophozoites invade the portal venous system and reach the liver, where they cause amebic liver abscesses. *E. histolytica* trophozoites must resist lysis by serum complement to survive in the bloodstream. Amebic liver abscesses have a characteristic appearance on pathologic examination: the roughly circular abscesses contain a large necrotic center resembling anchovy paste that is surrounded by a narrow ring of a few inflammatory cells, fibrosis, and occasionally a few amebic trophozoites. The adjacent liver parenchyma is usually completely normal. Results in experimental rodent models of amebic liver abscess suggest that initial lesions may have more inflammatory cells and that lysis of neutrophils by *E. histolytica* trophozoites may contribute to tissue damage. In murine models of disease, apoptosis is a prominent component of hepatocyte death and the blockade of caspase activity can significantly reduce liver abscess formation, but whether any of these factors is applicable to human disease is unclear.

The role of innate and adaptive immunity in preventing *E. histolytica* infection or controlling disease needs further clarification. Studies of children in a highly endemic area have suggested that prior *E. histolytica* intestinal infection may stimulate mucosal IgA antibodies to amebic antigens, thereby reducing the likelihood of subsequent infections; this protection is relatively short lived. In contrast, among individuals in an area of Vietnam with a high prevalence of amebic liver abscess, a prior episode of disease did not reduce the risk of a second case, despite the presence of serum antibodies. Studies of animal models suggest that cell-mediated immunity may play a role in host defense, and glucocorticoid use has been associated with worse outcomes in patients with amebic colitis. However, individuals with HIV/AIDS do not appear to be at increased risk for infection with *E. histolytica*, and there is no evidence that they develop more severe disease than do immunocompetent hosts.

■ CLINICAL SYNDROMES

Intestinal amebiasis

Most patients harboring *Entamoeba* species are asymptomatic, but individuals with *E. histolytica* infection can develop disease. Symptoms of amebic colitis generally appear 2–6 weeks after ingestion of the cyst form of the parasite. Diarrhea (classically heme-positive) and lower abdominal pain are the most common symptoms. Malaise and weight loss may be noted as disease progresses. Severe dysentery, with 10–12 small-volume, blood- and mucus-containing stools daily, may develop, but only ~40% of patients are febrile. Fulminant amebic colitis, with even more profuse diarrhea, severe abdominal pain (including peritoneal signs), fever, and pronounced leukocytosis are rare, disproportionately affecting young children, pregnant women, individuals being treated with glucocorticoids, and possibly individuals with diabetes or alcoholism. Paralytic ileus and colonic mucosal sloughing may be seen; intestinal perforation occurs in >75% of patients with this fulminant form of disease. Mortality rates from fulminant amebic colitis exceed 40% in some series. Recognized complications of amebic colitis also include toxic megacolon (documented in ~0.5% of patients with colitis), with severe bowel dilation and intramural air, and the aforementioned ameboma, which presents as an abdominal mass that may be confused with colon cancer.

Amebic liver abscess

Just a century ago, amebic liver abscess—the most common extraintestinal manifestation of amebiasis—was almost always fatal; however, with current rapid diagnostic methods and effective medical treatment, mortality rates are now 1–3%. Disease begins when *E. histolytica* trophozoites penetrate through the colonic mucosa, travel through the portal circulation, and reach the liver. Most individuals with amebic liver abscess do not have concurrent signs or symptoms of colitis, and most do not have *E. histolytica* trophozoites in their stools. The exceptions are individuals with fulminant amebic colitis, in which concurrent amebic liver abscess is not uncommon. Disease can arise from months to years after travel to or residence in an endemic area; therefore, a careful travel history is key in making the diagnosis. The classic presentations of amebic liver abscess are right-upper-quadrant pain, fever, and hepatic tenderness. The pace of disease is usually acute, with symptoms lasting <10 days. However, a more chronic presentation, with weight loss and anorexia as prominent accompanying features, does occur. Jaundice is unusual, but dullness and rales at the right lung base (secondary to pleural effusion) are common. The most common laboratory findings are leukocytosis (without eosinophilia), an elevated alkaline phosphatase level, mild anemia, and an elevated erythrocyte sedimentation rate.

Other extraintestinal complications of amebiasis

Right-sided pleural effusions and atelectasis are common in cases of amebic liver abscess and generally require no treatment. However, the abscess ruptures through the diaphragm in ~10% of patients, causing pleuropulmonary amebiasis. Suggestive symptoms are sudden-onset cough, pleuritic chest pain, and shortness of breath. In some patients, pleuropulmonary amebiasis is the presenting manifestation of amebic liver abscess and may be confused with bacterial pneumonia and empyema. A dramatic complication is the development of a hepatobronchial fistula, in which patients can cough up the contents of the liver abscess—copious amounts of brown sputum that may contain *E. histolytica* trophozoites. In ~1–3% of cases, the amebic liver abscess ruptures into the peritoneum, and peritoneal signs and shock develop. Even rarer is rupture of an amebic liver abscess into the pericardium; the signs and symptoms are those commonly seen with pericarditis (chest pain, pericardial rub, dyspnea, tachypnea, or cardiac tamponade), and nearly 30% of cases end in death. Cerebral abscesses complicate <0.1% of cases of amebic liver abscess and are associated with the sudden onset of headache, vomiting, seizures, and mental status changes and a high mortality rate. Cutaneous amebiasis (which usually involves the anal and perianal regions), genital disease (including rectovaginal fistulas), and urinary tract lesions are rare but reported complications of amebiasis.

■ DIAGNOSTIC TESTS

The diagnosis of amebic colitis has traditionally been based on the demonstration of *E. histolytica* trophozoites or cysts in the stool or colonic mucosa of patients with diarrhea. However, the inability of microscopy to differentiate between *E. histolytica* and other *Entamoeba* species, such as *E. dispar* and *E. moshkovskii*, limits its effectiveness as a sole diagnostic method. Examination of three stool samples improves sensitivity for the detection of *Entamoeba* species, and it has been argued that the presence of amebic trophozoites containing red blood cells in a diarrheal stool is highly suggestive of *E. histolytica* infection. However, because trophozoites containing red blood cells are not found in most patients with *E. histolytica* infection, the applicability of this finding is limited.

Despite these inherent limitations, microscopy, often combined with serologic testing, remains the standard diagnostic approach in many hospitals and clinics worldwide. Culture of stools for *E. histolytica* trophozoites serves as a research tool but is generally not available for clinical use. PCR assay for DNA in stool samples is currently the most sensitive and specific method for identifying *E. histolytica* infection and has become a valuable epidemiologic and research tool; probes can be configured to detect *E. dispar* and *E. moshkovskii* as well. While significant advances are being made in reducing the costs of PCR-based diagnostics, this method still is not feasible for clinical diagnosis in most endemic areas. Commercially available tests that use enzyme-linked immunosorbent assays (ELISAs) or immunochromatographic techniques to detect *Entamoeba* antigens are less expensive and more easily performed and are being used with increasing frequency. Greater sensitivity than microscopy and the ability to detect *E. histolytica* specifically are claimed by some of the leading kits, representing significant advantages over microscopy. Unfortunately, not all clinical studies have supported these claims, concerns have been raised about the specificity of the tests in nonendemic areas, and the ELISAs are less sensitive and specific than are PCR-based diagnostics. At this point, antigen detection–based ELISAs that can specifically identify *E. histolytica* in stool probably represent the best choice in endemic areas; however, the results of any of these diagnostic tests need to be interpreted in light of clinical presentation, and a second confirmatory test (e.g., microscopy and/or amebic serology) may be prudent. In instances in which amebiasis is suspected on clinical grounds in a patient with acute colitis but initial stool samples are negative, colonoscopy with examination of brushings or mucosal biopsies for *E. histolytica* trophozoites may be helpful in making the diagnosis or in identifying other diseases, such as inflammatory bowel disease or pseudomembranous colitis.

The diagnosis of amebic liver abscess is based on the detection (generally by ultrasound or CT; Fig. 209-4) of one or more space-occupying lesions in the liver and a positive serologic test for antibodies to *E. histolytica* antigens. As has been noted, amebiasis can present months or years after travel to or residence in an endemic area, and so a careful travel history is mandatory when anyone presents with a liver abscess. Amebic liver abscesses are classically described as single, large, and located in the right lobe of the liver, but sensitive imaging techniques have shown that multiple abscesses are more common than previously suspected. When a patient has a space-occupying lesion of the liver, a positive amebic serology is highly sensitive (>94%) and highly specific (>95%) for the diagnosis of amebic liver abscess. False-negative serologic tests have been reported when serum samples were obtained very early in the course of abscess (within 7–10 days of onset), but repeat tests are almost always positive.

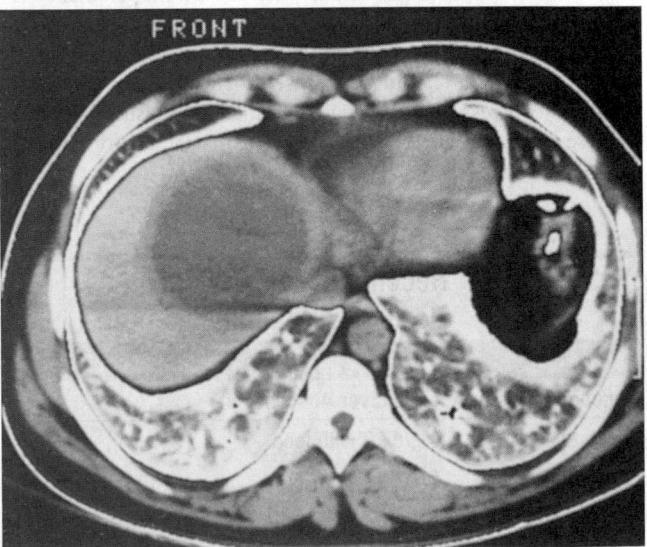

Figure 209-4 Large amebic abscess in the right lobe of the liver visualized by CT. *(Courtesy of Dr. M. M. Reeder, International Registry of Tropical Imaging.)*

■ DIFFERENTIAL DIAGNOSIS

The differential diagnosis of amebic colitis includes bacterial dysentery (e.g., *Shigella* and *Campylobacter* infections), schistosomiasis, *Balantidium coli* infection, pseudomembranous colitis, inflammatory bowel disease, and ischemic colitis. Stool cultures for bacterial pathogens, microscopic examination of stools, and amebic serology help differentiate amebic colitis from these other entities. Amebomas may be confused with colonic carcinoma; several case reports describe instances in which amebomas and associated liver abscesses were initially considered to be colon cancer with liver metastases. Amebic liver abscess must be distinguished from pyogenic liver abscess, echinococcal cysts, and primary or metastatic liver tumors. It is difficult to differentiate pyogenic from amebic liver abscesses on purely clinical grounds, but amebic serology is usually the key test in excluding or diagnosing amebic liver abscess. Abscesses that rupture into the pleural space may be accompanied by cough, sputum production, and dyspnea and may initially be diagnosed as bronchopneumonia.

TREATMENT   Amebiasis

The nitroimidazole compounds tinidazole and metronidazole are the drugs of choice for the treatment of amebic colitis and amebic liver abscess (Table 209-1). To date, *E. histolytica* has not demonstrated resistance to any of the commonly used agents—a situation that greatly simplifies treatment. Tinidazole appears to be better tolerated and slightly more effective than metronidazole for amebic colitis and amebic liver abscess. Metronidazole is available as a parenteral formulation for patients who cannot take oral medications. Whenever possible, fulminant amebic colitis is managed conservatively, even in the presence of perforation, with the addition of antibiotics to treat gut bacteria and percutaneous catheter drainage of fluid collections if needed.

Remarkably, given the large size of amebic liver abscesses, treatment with tinidazole or metronidazole in the same doses used for amebic colitis is almost always successful. More than 90% of patients respond with a decrease in abdominal pain and fever within 72 h of the initiation of therapy. Drainage of amebic liver abscesses is rarely needed; in one large series, neither time to becoming afebrile nor length of hospitalization was significantly different for patients who underwent percutaneous radiography-guided aspiration of the abscess accompanied by medical therapy than for those who received medical therapy alone. Aspiration should be reserved for individuals in whom pyogenic abscess or a bacterial superinfection is suspected but whose diagnosis is uncertain, for patients failing to respond to tinidazole or metronidazole (i.e., those who have persistent fever or abdominal pain after 4 days of treatment), for individuals with large liver abscesses in the left lobe (because of the risk of rupture into the pericardium), and for patients whose large abscesses and accelerated clinical course raise concerns about imminent rupture. In contrast, aspiration and/or percutaneous catheter drainage improves outcomes in patients with pleuropulmonary amebiasis and empyema (where amebic liver abscesses have ruptured into the pleural space), and percutaneous catheter or surgical drainage is absolutely indicated for cases of amebic pericarditis. Rupture of an amebic liver abscess into the peritoneum is generally managed conservatively, with medical therapy and percutaneous catheter drainage of fluid collections as needed.

Neither metronidazole nor tinidazole reaches high levels in the gut lumen; therefore, patients with amebic colitis or amebic liver abscess should also receive treatment with a luminal agent (paromomycin or iodoquinol) to ensure eradication of the infection (Table 209-1). Paromomycin is the preferred agent. Asymptomatic individuals with documented *E. histolytica* infection should be treated because of the risks of developing amebic colitis or amebic liver abscess in the future and of transmitting the infection to others. Paromomycin or iodoquinol in the doses listed in the table should be used in these cases.

Nitazoxanide, a broad-spectrum antiparasitic drug, is efficacious against *E. histolytica* trophozoites in both tissue and gut lumen and may become an important addition to the therapeutic repertoire. However, clinical experience with nitazoxanide for the treatment of *E. histolytica* infection remains limited at this point.

■ PREVENTION

Avoidance of the ingestion of food and water contaminated with human feces is the only way to prevent *E. histolytica* infection. Travelers to endemic areas should exercise the same measures used to reduce the risk of travelers' diarrhea (Chap. 117). Treatment of asymptomatic persons who pass *E. histolytica* cysts in the stool may help reduce opportunities for disease transmission. There is no evidence for any effective prophylaxis, and no vaccine is available.

INFECTION WITH FREE-LIVING AMEBAS

 In contrast to the trophozoites of the parasitic *E. histolytica*, which can survive only in humans and some other primate hosts, free-living amebas of the genera *Naegleria*, *Acanthamoeba*, and *Balamuthia* live in brackish or freshwater habitats around the world (including lakes, tap water, swimming pools, and air conditioning and heating ducts) and are accidental and opportunistic agents of disease.

■ *NAEGLERIA* INFECTIONS

Naegleria (the "brain-eating ameba") is the causative agent of primary amebic meningoencephalitis (PAM). Nearly always fatal but quite rare, cases of PAM have been reported from 15 countries and from all continents except Antarctica; 35 cases were reported in the United States between 1998 and 2009. *Naegleria* prefers warm freshwater, and most cases occur in otherwise healthy children, who usually have swum in lakes or swimming pools during the previous 2 weeks. *Naegleria* enters the central nervous system via water inhaled or splashed into the nose, with trophozoites disrupting the olfactory mucosa, invading through the cribriform plate, and ascending via the olfactory nerves into the brain. The earliest manifestations are anosmia (usually perceived as alterations in taste), headache, fever, photophobia, nausea, and

---

TABLE 209-1 Recommended Therapeutic Dosages of Antiamebic Drugs

Drug	Dosage	Duration, Days
Amebic Colitis or Amebic Liver Abscess		
Tinidazole	2 g/d PO with food	3
Metronidazole	750 mg tid PO or IV	5–10
***Entamoeba histolytica* Luminal Infection**		
Paromomycin	30 mg/kg qd PO in 3 divided doses	5–10
Iodoquinol	650 mg PO tid	20

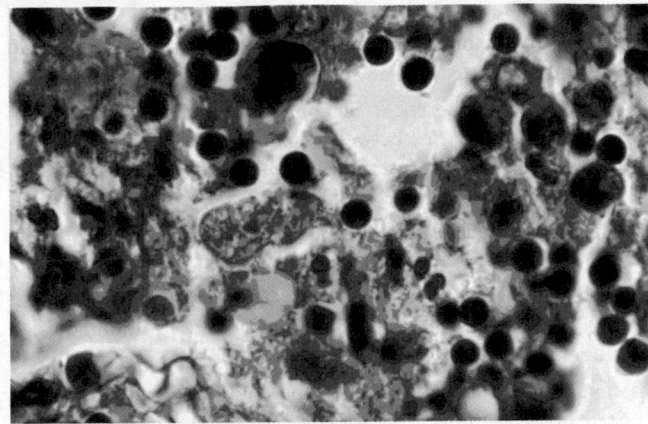

Figure 209-5 *Naegleria* **in a section of human brain tissue** from a patient with primary amebic meningoencephalitis. *(Courtesy of Dr. George Healy, Centers for Disease Control and Prevention.)*

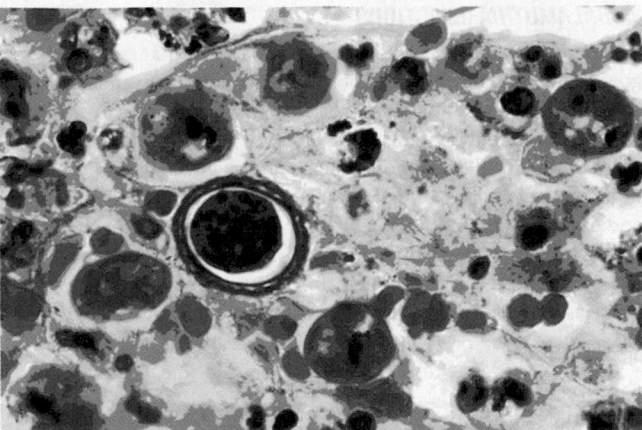

Figure 209-6 *Acanthamoeba* **cyst in brain tissue** from a patient with granulomatous amebic encephalitis. *(Courtesy of Dr. George Healy, Centers for Disease Control and Prevention.)*

vomiting. Cranial nerve palsies, especially of the third, fourth, and sixth nerves, are documented and rapid progression of disease, with seizures, coma, and death within 7–10 days of the onset of symptoms, are common. Pathologic examination reveals hemorrhagic necrosis of brain tissue (often most prominent in the olfactory bulbs), evidence of increased intracranial pressure, scant purulent material that may contain a few amebas, and marked leptomeningitis (Fig. 209-5).

The diagnosis of PAM is based on the finding of motile *Naegleria* trophozoites in wet mounts of freshly obtained cerebrospinal fluid (CSF). Laboratory findings in the CSF resemble those in bacterial meningitis, with high opening pressures, low glucose levels, high protein concentrations, and elevated polymorphonuclear cell–predominant white blood cell counts. PAM should be suspected in any patient who has an appropriate history and purulent meningoencephalitis with negative gram stains, negative antigen detection and PCR tests for other pathogens, and negative bacterial cultures. Unfortunately, the prognosis for PAM is dismal. The few survivors who have been reported were treated with high-dose amphotericin B and rifampin in combination.

◼ *ACANTHAMOEBA* INFECTIONS

Acanthamoeba species are free-living amebas that cause two major clinical syndromes: granulomatous amebic encephalitis and keratitis. Granulomatous amebic encephalitis occurs in debilitated, chronically ill, and immunosuppressed individuals who may be undergoing chemotherapy, receiving glucocorticoids, or suffering from lymphoproliferative diseases, systemic lupus erythematosus, or AIDS. It is believed that *Acanthamoeba* reaches the central nervous system through the bloodstream, traveling from a primary site of infection in the nares, skin, sinuses, or lungs. The pace of infection is indolent compared with that of PAM. Granulomatous amebic encephalitis tends to present as a space-occupying lesion in the brain. Common symptoms include altered mental status, stiff neck, and headache along with focal findings including hemiparesis, ataxia, and cranial nerve palsies. Seizures and coma often precede death. Pathologic findings in the brain include cerebral edema and multiple areas of necrosis and hemorrhage. Amebic trophozoites and cysts are scattered throughout the tissue and are often located near blood vessels (Fig. 209-6). Multinucleated giant cells forming granulomas give the syndrome its name but are seen less often in highly immunocompromised patients. The

diagnosis is usually made by detection of *Acanthamoeba* trophozoites or cysts in biopsy specimens; a fluorescein-labeled antiserum is available from the Centers for Disease Control and Prevention (CDC) to help identify *Acanthamoeba* in microscopic sections. *Acanthamoeba* trophozoites and cysts are occasionally seen in CSF, but samples from most patients with granulomatous amebic encephalitis show mild lymphocyte-predominant pleocytosis, slightly elevated protein levels, and normal or slightly depressed glucose concentrations without the presence of amebas. CT findings vary, with hypodense lesions that resemble infarcts in some patients and multiple enhancing lesions that resemble toxoplasmosis in others. Unfortunately, there are no therapies with proven efficacy against this disease, and almost all cases have ended in death. There have been case reports of survivors treated with multidrug combinations that included pentamidine, sulfadiazine, flucytosine, rifampin, and fluconazole.

Acanthamoeba keratitis is associated with corneal injuries complicated by exposure to water or soil and with the wearing of contact lenses. In contact lens–associated infection, extended wear, breaches in hygiene and disinfection procedures, swimming with contact lenses in place, and the use of homemade saline solutions contaminated with *Acanthamoeba* are important risk factors. The incidence of *Acanthamoeba* keratitis varies from 1.65–2.01 cases per million contact lens users in the United States to 17.53–19.5 cases per million users in the United Kingdom. Unilateral photophobia, excessive tearing, redness, and foreign-body sensation are the earliest signs and symptoms; disease is bilateral in some contact lens users. *Acanthamoeba* keratitis can progress rapidly; abscesses, hypopyon, scleritis, and corneal perforation with vision loss can develop within weeks. The disease may be diagnosed by identification of the polygonal cyst form in corneal scrapings or biopsy material, by culture of biopsy samples or contact lenses on *Escherichia coli*–seeded agar plates, by confocal microscopy, and by PCR. The differential diagnosis includes bacterial, fungal, mycobacterial, and viral (particularly herpetic) causes. Current therapy involves topical administration of a cationic antiseptic agent such as a biguanide or chlorhexidine, with or without a diamidine agent. The persistence of the cyst form of *Acanthamoeba* complicates treatment, and long durations of therapy (6 months to 1 year) are required. In severe cases, particularly when vision is threatened or already diminished, penetrating keratoplasty may be indicated.

Balamuthia mandrillaris is a free-living ameba that causes meningoencephalitis in both immunosuppressed and immunocompetent hosts, particularly children and the elderly. The disease presents similarly to granulomatous amebic encephalitis caused by *Acanthamoeba*, and essentially all of the points made above with regard to the latter organism—in terms of clinical presentation, pathologic findings, and lack of proven therapies—apply to *Balamuthia* infections as well. Most cases are identified post mortem; the few cases identified before death have been found during histologic examination of brain biopsy specimens. A specific antiserum is available from the CDC to aid in identifying *B. mandrillaris* in clinical specimens.

FURTHER READINGS

DART JKG et al: *Acanthamoeba* keratitis: Diagnosis and treatment update 2009. Am J Ophthalmol 148:487, 2009

FOTEDAR R et al: Laboratory diagnostic techniques for *Entamoeba* species. Clin Microbiol Rev 20:511, 2007

HAQUE R et al: Prospective case-control study of the association between common enteric protozoal parasites and diarrhea in Bangladesh. J Infect Dis 48:1191, 2009

SNOW M et al: Differences in complement-mediated killing of *Entamoeba histolytica* between men and women—an explanation for the increased susceptibility of men to invasive amebiasis? Am J Trop Med Hyg 78:922, 2008

STANLEY SL: Amoebiasis. Lancet 361:1025, 2003

VISVESVARA GS et al: Pathogenic and opportunistic free-living amoebae: *Acanthamoeba* spp., *Balamuthia mandrillaris*, *Naegleria fowleri*, and *Sappinia diploidea*. FEMS Immunol Med Microbiol 50:1, 2007

XIMÉNEZ C et al: Reassessment of the epidemiology of amebiasis: State of the art. Infect Genet Evol 9:1023, 2009

ZHANG Z et al: *Entamoeba histolytica* cysteine proteinases with interleukin-1 beta converting enzyme (ICE) activity cause intestinal inflammation and tissue damage in amoebiasis. Mol Microbiol 37:542, 2000

CHAPTER **210**

Malaria

Nicholas J. White
Joel G. Breman

Humanity has but three great enemies: Fever, famine and war; of these by far the greatest, by far the most terrible, is fever.

William Osler

Malaria is a protozoan disease transmitted by the bite of infected *Anopheles* mosquitoes. The most important of the parasitic diseases of humans, it is transmitted in 108 countries containing 3 billion people and causes nearly 1 million deaths each year. Malaria has been eliminated from the United States, Canada, Europe, and Russia; in the late twentieth and early twenty-first centuries, however, its prevalence rose in many parts of the tropics. Despite enormous control efforts, increases in the drug resistance of the parasite, the insecticide resistance of its vectors, and human travel and migration have contributed to this resurgence. Occasional local transmission after importation of malaria has occurred in several southern and eastern areas of the United States and in Europe, indicating the continual danger to nonmalarious countries. Although there are many promising new control and research initiatives, malaria remains today, as it has been for centuries, a heavy burden on tropical communities, a threat to nonendemic countries, and a danger to travelers.

ETIOLOGY AND PATHOGENESIS

Five species of the genus *Plasmodium* cause nearly all malarial infections in humans. These are *P. falciparum*, *P. vivax*, *P. ovale*, *P. malariae*, and—in Southeast Asia—the monkey malaria parasite *P. knowlesi*, which can be reliably identified only by molecular methods (Table 210-1). Almost all deaths are caused by falciparum malaria. Human infection begins when a female anopheline mosquito inoculates plasmodial *sporozoites* from its salivary gland during a blood meal (Fig. 210-1). These microscopic motile forms of the malarial parasite are carried rapidly via the bloodstream to the liver, where they invade hepatic parenchymal cells and begin a period of asexual reproduction. By this amplification process (known as *intrahepatic* or *preerythrocytic schizogony* or *merogony*), a single sporozoite eventually may produce from 10,000 to >30,000 daughter merozoites. The swollen infected liver cell eventually bursts, discharging motile *merozoites* into the bloodstream. These merozoites then invade the red blood cells (RBCs) and multiply six- to twentyfold every 48–72 h. When the parasites reach densities of ~50/μL of blood (~100 million parasites in the blood of an adult), the symptomatic stage of the infection begins. In *P. vivax* and *P. ovale* infections, a proportion of the intrahepatic forms do not divide immediately but remain dormant for a period ranging from 3 weeks to a year or longer before reproduction begins. These dormant forms, or *hypnozoites*, are the cause of the relapses that characterize infection with these two species.

After entry into the bloodstream, merozoites rapidly invade erythrocytes and become *trophozoites*. Attachment is mediated via a specific erythrocyte surface receptor. In the case of *P. vivax*, this receptor is related to the Duffy blood-group antigen Fy^a or Fy^b. Most West Africans and people with origins in that region carry the Duffy-negative FyFy phenotype and are therefore resistant to *P. vivax* malaria. During the early stage of intraerythrocytic development, the small "ring forms" of the different parasitic species appear similar under light microscopy. As the trophozoites enlarge, species-specific characteristics become evident, pigment becomes visible, and the parasite assumes an irregular or ameboid shape. By the end of the 48-h intraerythrocytic life cycle (24 h for *P. knowlesi*, 72 h for *P. malariae*), the parasite has consumed two-thirds of the RBC's hemoglobin and has grown to occupy most of the cell. It is now called a *schizont*. Multiple nuclear divisions have taken place (*schizogony* or *merogony*), and the RBC then ruptures to release 6–30 daughter merozoites, each potentially capable of invading a new RBC and repeating the cycle. The disease in human beings is caused by the direct effects of RBC invasion and destruction by the asexual parasite and the host's reaction. After a series of asexual cycles (*P. falciparum*) or immediately after release from the liver (*P. vivax*, *P. ovale*, *P. malariae*, *P. knowlesi*), some of the parasites develop into morphologically distinct, longer-lived sexual forms (*gametocytes*) that can transmit malaria.

TABLE 210-1 Characteristics of *Plasmodium* Species Infecting Humans

Characteristic	Finding for Indicated Species[a]			
	P. falciparum	*P. vivax*	*P. ovale*	*P. malariae*
Duration of intrahepatic phase (days)	5.5	8	9	15
Number of merozoites released per infected hepatocyte	30,000	10,000	15,000	15,000
Duration of erythrocytic cycle (hours)	48	48	50	72
Red cell preference	Younger cells (but can invade cells of all ages)	Reticulocytes and cells up to 2 weeks old	Reticulocytes	Older cells
Morphology	Usually only ring forms[b]; banana-shaped gametocytes	Irregularly shaped large rings and trophozoites; enlarged erythrocytes; Schüffner's dots	Infected erythrocytes, enlarged and oval with tufted ends; Schüffner's dots	Band or rectangular forms of trophozoites common
Pigment color	Black	Yellow-brown	Dark brown	Brown-black
Ability to cause relapses	No	Yes	Yes	No

[a]In Southeast Asia, the monkey malaria parasite *P. knowlesi* also causes disease in humans.
[b]Parasitemias of >2% are suggestive of *P. falciparum* infection.

After being ingested in the blood meal of a biting female anopheline mosquito, the male and female gametocytes form a zygote in the insect's midgut. This zygote matures into an ookinete, which penetrates and encysts in the mosquito's gut wall. The resulting oocyst expands by asexual division until it bursts to liberate myriad motile sporozoites, which then migrate in the hemolymph to the salivary gland of the mosquito to await inoculation into another human at the next feeding.

EPIDEMIOLOGY

Malaria occurs throughout most of the tropical regions of the world (Fig. 210-2). *P. falciparum* predominates in Africa, New Guinea, and Hispaniola (i.e., the Dominican Republic and Haiti); *P. vivax* is more common in Central America. The prevalence of these two species is approximately equal in South America, the Indian subcontinent, eastern Asia, and Oceania. *P. malariae* is found in most endemic areas, especially throughout sub-Saharan Africa, but is

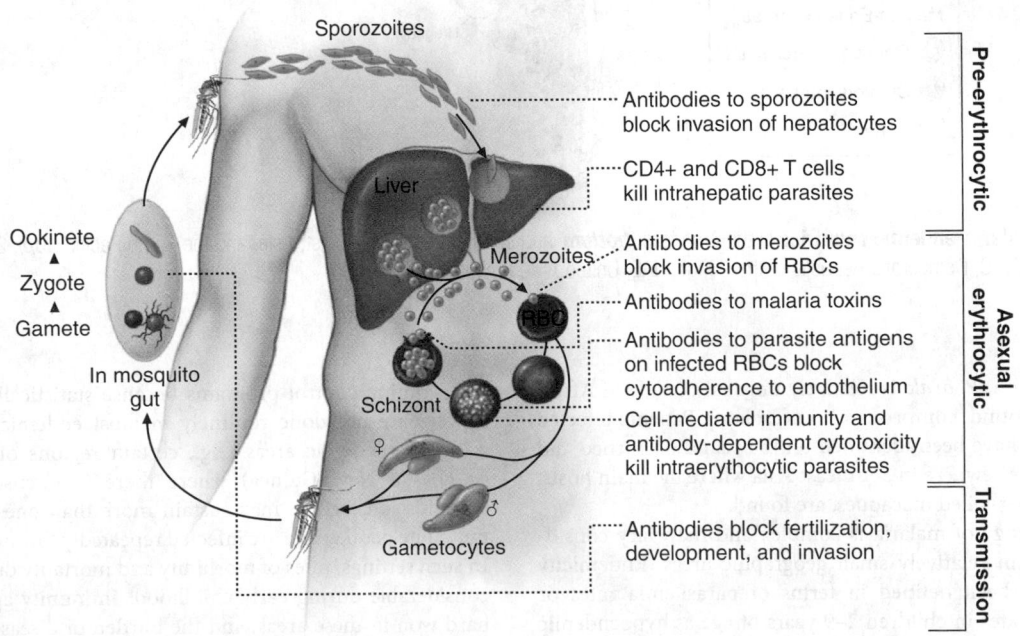

Sporozoites

Antibodies to sporozoites block invasion of hepatocytes

CD4+ and CD8+ T cells kill intrahepatic parasites

Liver

Ookinete
▲
Zygote
▲
Gamete

In mosquito gut

Merozoites

Antibodies to merozoites block invasion of RBCs

Antibodies to malaria toxins

RBC

Antibodies to parasite antigens on infected RBCs block cytoadherence to endothelium

Schizont

Cell-mediated immunity and antibody-dependent cytotoxicity kill intraerythrocytic parasites

Gametocytes

Antibodies block fertilization, development, and invasion

Pre-erythrocytic

Asexual erythrocytic

Transmission

Figure 210-1 The malaria transmission cycle from mosquito to human. RBC, red blood cell.

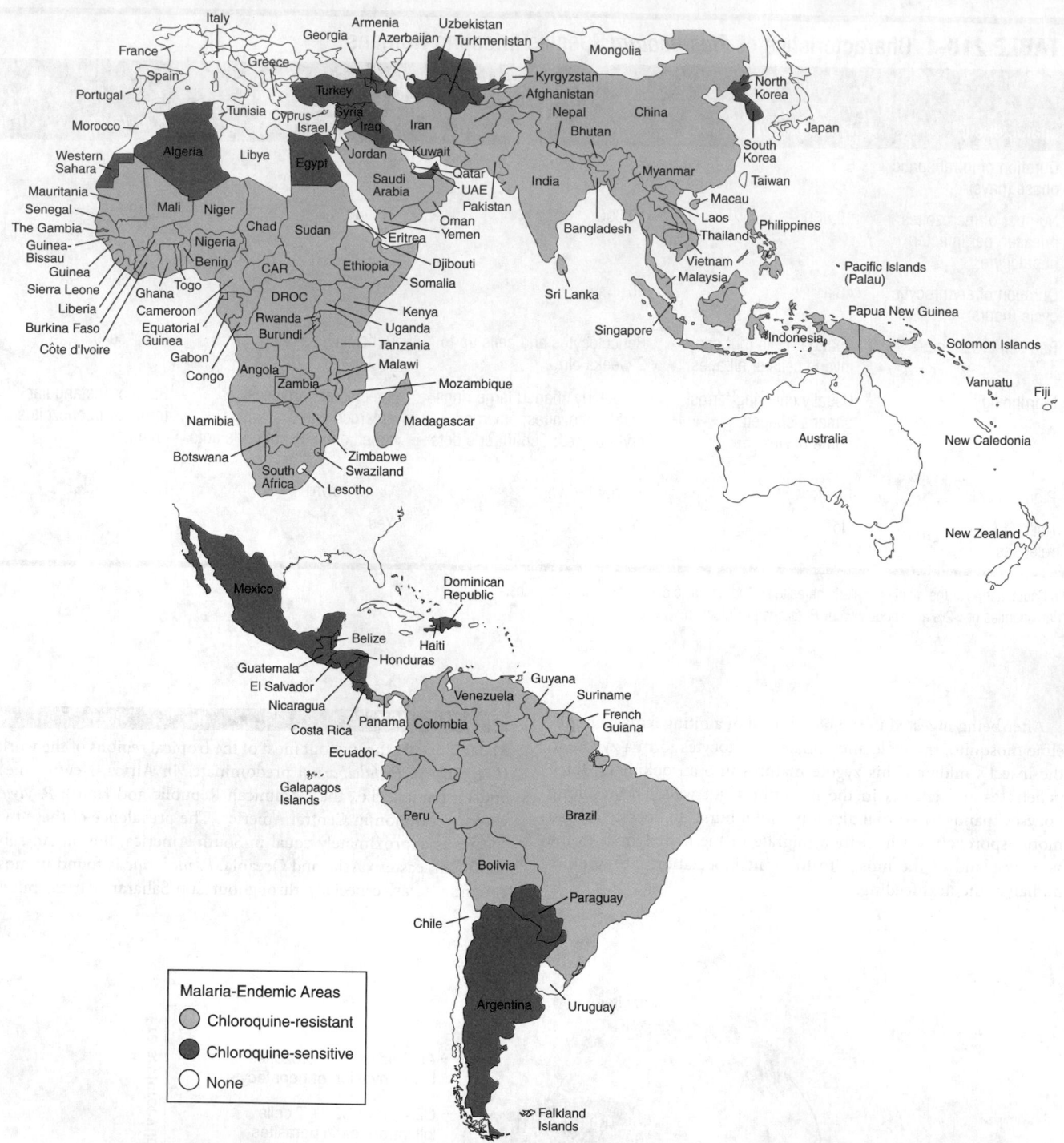

Figure 210-2   Malaria-endemic countries in the Americas (**bottom**) and in Africa, the Middle East, Asia, and the South Pacific (**top**), 2007. CAR, Central African Republic; DROC, Democratic Republic of the Congo; UAE, United Arab Emirates.

much less common. *P. ovale* is relatively unusual outside of Africa and, where it is found, comprises <1% of isolates. Patients infected with *P. knowlesi* have been identified on the island of Borneo and to a lesser extent elsewhere in Southeast Asia where the main hosts, long-tailed and pig-tailed macaques, are found.

The epidemiology of malaria is complex and may vary considerably even within relatively small geographic areas. Endemicity traditionally has been defined in terms of parasitemia rates or palpable-spleen rates in children 2–9 years of age as hypoendemic (<10%), mesoendemic (11–50%), hyperendemic (51–75%), and holoendemic (>75%); however, it is uncommon to use these indices

for planning control programs because statistically valid national surveys are not done routinely in most endemic areas. In holo- and hyperendemic areas (e.g., certain regions of tropical Africa or coastal New Guinea) where there is intense *P. falciparum* transmission, people may sustain more than one infectious mosquito bite per day and are infected repeatedly throughout their lives. In such settings, rates of morbidity and mortality due to malaria are considerable during early childhood. Immunity against disease is hard won in these areas, and the burden of disease in young children is high; by adulthood, however, most malarial infections are asymptomatic. Constant, frequent, year-round infection is termed *stable transmission*. In areas where transmission is low, erratic, or focal, full protective immunity is not acquired, and symptomatic disease may occur at all ages. This situation usually exists in hypoendemic areas and is termed *unstable transmission*. Even in stable transmission areas, there is often an increased incidence of symptomatic malaria coinciding with increased mosquito breeding and transmission during the rainy season. Malaria can behave like an epidemic disease in some areas, particularly those with unstable malaria, such as northern India (the state of Rajasthan), Sri Lanka, Iraq, Turkey, the horn of Africa, Rwanda, Burundi, southern Africa, Madagascar, and central Asia. An epidemic can develop when there are changes in environmental, economic, or social conditions, such as heavy rains following drought or migrations (usually of refugees or workers) from a nonmalarious region to an area of high transmission; a breakdown in malaria control and prevention services can intensify epidemic conditions. This situation usually results in considerable mortality among all age groups.

The principal determinants of the epidemiology of malaria are the number (density), the human-biting habits, and the longevity of the anopheline mosquito vectors. Not all of the >400 anophelines can transmit malaria, and the ~40 species that do so vary considerably in their efficiency as malaria vectors. More specifically, the transmission of malaria is directly proportional to the density of the vector, the square of the number of human bites per day per mosquito, and the tenth power of the probability of the mosquito's surviving for 1 day. Mosquito longevity is particularly important because the portion of the parasite's life cycle that takes place within the mosquito—from gametocyte ingestion to subsequent inoculation (*sporogony*)—lasts 8–30 days, depending on ambient temperature; thus, to transmit malaria, the mosquito must survive for >7 days. Sporogony is not completed at cooler temperatures—i.e., <16°C for *P. vivax* and <21°C for *P. falciparum*; thus transmission does not occur below these temperatures, although malaria outbreaks and transmission have occurred in the highlands (>1500 m) of east Africa, which were previously free of vectors. The most effective mosquito vectors of malaria are those, such as *Anopheles gambiae* in Africa, which are long-lived, occur in high densities in tropical climates, breed readily, and bite humans in preference to other animals. The entomologic inoculation rate (EIR; the number of sporozoite-positive mosquito bites per person per year) is the most common measure of malaria transmission and varies from <1 in some parts of Latin America and Southeast Asia to >300 in parts of tropical Africa.

ERYTHROCYTE CHANGES IN MALARIA

After invading an erythrocyte, the growing malarial parasite progressively consumes and degrades intracellular proteins, principally hemoglobin. The potentially toxic heme is detoxified by lipid-mediated crystallization to biologically inert hemozoin (malaria pigment). The parasite also alters the RBC membrane by changing its transport properties, exposing cryptic surface antigens, and inserting new parasite-derived proteins. The RBC becomes more irregular in shape, more antigenic, and less deformable.

In *P. falciparum* infections, membrane protuberances appear on the erythrocyte's surface 12–15 h after the cell's invasion. These "knobs" extrude a high-molecular-weight, antigenically variant, strain-specific erythrocyte membrane adhesive protein (PfEMP1) that mediates attachment to receptors on venular and capillary endothelium—an event termed *cytoadherence*. Several vascular receptors have been identified, of which intercellular adhesion molecule 1 (ICAM-1) is probably the most important in the brain, chondroitin sulfate B in the placenta, and CD36 in most other organs. Thus, the infected erythrocytes stick inside and eventually block capillaries and venules. At the same stage, these

P. falciparum–infected RBCs may also adhere to uninfected RBCs (to form rosettes) and to other parasitized erythrocytes (agglutination). The processes of cytoadherence, rosetting, and agglutination are central to the pathogenesis of falciparum malaria. They result in the sequestration of RBCs containing mature forms of the parasite in vital organs (particularly the brain), where they interfere with microcirculatory flow and metabolism. Sequestered parasites continue to develop out of reach of the principal host defense mechanism: splenic processing and filtration. As a consequence, only the younger ring forms of the asexual parasites are seen circulating in the peripheral blood in falciparum malaria, and the level of peripheral parasitemia underestimates the true number of parasites within the body. Severe malaria is also associated with reduced deformability of the uninfected erythrocytes, which compromises their passage through the partially obstructed capillaries and venules and shortens RBC survival.

In the other three ("benign") human malarias, sequestration does not occur, and all stages of the parasite's development are evident on peripheral-blood smears. Whereas *P. vivax*, *P. ovale*, and *P. malariae* show a marked predilection for either young RBCs (*P. vivax*, *P. ovale*) or old cells (*P. malariae*) and produce a level of parasitemia that is seldom >2%, *P. falciparum* can invade erythrocytes of all ages and may be associated with very high levels of parasitemia.

HOST RESPONSE

Initially, the host responds to plasmodial infection by activating nonspecific defense mechanisms. Splenic immunologic and filtrative clearance functions are augmented in malaria, and the removal of both parasitized and uninfected erythrocytes is accelerated. The parasitized cells escaping splenic removal are destroyed when the schizont ruptures. The material released induces the activation of macrophages and the release of proinflammatory mononuclear cell–derived cytokines, which cause fever and exert other pathologic effects. Temperatures of ≥40°C damage mature parasites; in untreated infections, the effect of such temperatures is to further synchronize the parasitic cycle, with eventual production of the regular fever spikes and rigors that originally served to characterize the different malarias. These regular fever patterns (tertian, every 2 days; quartan, every 3 days) are seldom seen today in patients who receive prompt and effective antimalarial treatment.

The geographic distributions of sickle cell disease, hemoglobins C and E, hereditary ovalocytosis, the thalassemias, and glucose-6-phosphate dehydrogenase (G6PD) deficiency closely resemble that of falciparum malaria before the introduction of control measures. This similarity suggests that these genetic disorders confer protection against death from falciparum malaria. For example, HbA/S heterozygotes (sickle cell trait) have a sixfold reduction in the risk of dying from severe falciparum malaria. This decrease in risk appears to be related to impaired parasite growth at low oxygen tensions and reduced parasitized red cell cytoadherence. Parasite multiplication in HbA/E heterozygotes is reduced at high parasite densities. In Melanesia, children with α-thalassemia appear to have more frequent malaria (both vivax and falciparum) in the early years of life, and this pattern of infection appears to protect them against severe disease. In Melanesian ovalocytosis, rigid erythrocytes resist merozoite invasion, and the intraerythrocytic milieu is hostile.

Nonspecific host defense mechanisms stop the infection's expansion, and the subsequent strain-specific immune response then controls the infection. Eventually, exposure to sufficient strains confers protection from high-level parasitemia and disease but not from infection. As a result of this state of infection without illness (*premunition*), asymptomatic parasitemia is common among adults and older children living in regions with stable and intense transmission (i.e., holo- or hyperendemic areas). Immunity is mainly specific for both the species and the strain of infecting malarial parasite. Both humoral immunity and cellular immunity are necessary for protection, but the mechanisms of each are incompletely understood (Fig. 210-1). Immune individuals have a polyclonal increase in serum levels of IgM, IgG, and IgA, although much of this antibody is unrelated to protection. Antibodies to a variety of parasitic antigens presumably act in concert to limit in vivo replication of the parasite. In the case of falciparum malaria, the most important of these antigens is the surface adhesin—the variant protein PfEMP1 mentioned above. Passively transferred IgG from immune adults has been shown to reduce levels of parasitemia in children; although parasitemia in very young infants can occur, passive transfer of maternal antibody contributes to the relative (but not complete) protection of infants from severe malaria in the first months of life. This complex immunity to disease declines when a person lives outside an endemic area for several months or longer.

Several factors retard the development of cellular immunity to malaria. These factors include the absence of major histocompatibility antigens on the surface of infected RBCs, which precludes direct T cell recognition; malaria antigen–specific immune unresponsiveness; and the enormous strain diversity of malarial parasites, along with the ability of the parasites to express variant immunodominant antigens on the erythrocyte surface that change during the period of infection. Parasites may persist in the blood for months (or, in the case of *P. malariae*, for many years) if treatment is not given. The complexity of the immune response in malaria, the sophistication of the parasites' evasion mechanisms, and the lack of a good in vitro correlate with clinical immunity have all slowed progress toward an effective vaccine.

CLINICAL FEATURES

Malaria is a very common cause of fever in tropical countries. The first symptoms of malaria are nonspecific; the lack of a sense of well-being, headache, fatigue, abdominal discomfort, and muscle aches followed by fever are all similar to the symptoms of a minor viral illness. In some instances, a prominence of headache, chest pain, abdominal pain, arthralgia, myalgia, or diarrhea may suggest another diagnosis. Although headache may be severe in malaria, there is not neck stiffness or photophobia as occurs in meningitis. While myalgia may be prominent, it is not usually as severe as in dengue fever, and the muscles are not tender as in leptospirosis or typhus. Nausea, vomiting, and orthostatic hypotension are common. The classic malarial paroxysms, in which fever spikes, chills, and rigors occur at regular intervals, are relatively unusual and suggest infection with *P. vivax* or *P. ovale*. The fever is irregular at first (that of falciparum malaria may never become regular); the temperature of nonimmune individuals and children often rises above 40°C in conjunction with tachycardia and sometimes delirium. Although childhood febrile convulsions may occur with any of the malarias, generalized seizures are specifically associated with falciparum malaria and may herald the development of encephalopathy (cerebral malaria). Many clinical abnormalities have been described in acute malaria, but most patients with uncomplicated infections have few abnormal physical findings other than fever, malaise, mild anemia, and (in some cases) a palpable spleen. Anemia is common among young children living in areas with stable transmission, particularly where resistance has compromised the efficacy of antimalarial drugs. In nonimmune individuals with acute malaria, the spleen takes several days to become palpable, but splenic enlargement is found in a high proportion of otherwise healthy individuals in malaria-endemic areas and reflects repeated infections. Slight enlargement of the liver is also common, particularly among young children. Mild jaundice is common among adults; it may develop in patients with otherwise uncomplicated malaria and usually resolves

over 1–3 weeks. Malaria is not associated with a rash like those seen in meningococcal septicemia, typhus, enteric fever, viral exanthems, and drug reactions. Petechial hemorrhages in the skin or mucous membranes—features of viral hemorrhagic fevers and leptospirosis—develop only rarely in severe falciparum malaria.

SEVERE FALCIPARUM MALARIA

Appropriately and promptly treated, uncomplicated falciparum malaria (i.e., the patient can swallow medicines and food) carries a mortality rate of ~0.1%. However, once vital-organ dysfunction occurs or the total proportion of erythrocytes infected increases to >2% (a level corresponding to >10^{12} parasites in an adult), mortality risk rises steeply. The major manifestations of severe falciparum malaria are shown in Table 210-2, and features indicating a poor prognosis are listed in Table 210-3.

Cerebral malaria

Coma is a characteristic and ominous feature of falciparum malaria and, despite treatment, is associated with death rates of ~20% among adults and 15% among children. Any obtundation, delirium, or abnormal behavior should be taken very seriously. The onset may be gradual or sudden following a convulsion.

Cerebral malaria manifests as diffuse symmetric encephalopathy; focal neurologic signs are unusual. Although some passive resistance to head flexion may be detected, signs of meningeal irritation are absent. The eyes may be divergent and a pout reflex is common, but other primitive reflexes are usually absent. The corneal reflexes are preserved, except in deep coma. Muscle tone may be either increased or decreased. The tendon reflexes are variable, and the plantar reflexes may be flexor or extensor; the abdominal and cremasteric reflexes are absent. Flexor or extensor posturing may be seen. On routine funduscopy, ~15% of patients have retinal hemorrhages; with pupillary dilatation and indirect ophthalmoscopy, this figure increases to 30–40%. Other funduscopic abnormalities (Fig. 210-3) include discrete spots of retinal opacification (30–60%), papilledema (8% among children, rare among adults), cotton wool spots (<5%), and decolorization of a retinal vessel or segment of vessel (occasional cases). Convulsions, usually generalized and often repeated, occur in ~10% of adults and up to 50% of children with cerebral malaria. More covert seizure activity is also common, particularly among children, and may manifest as repetitive tonic-clonic eye movements or even hypersalivation. Whereas adults rarely (i.e., in <3% of cases) suffer neurologic sequelae, ~5% of children surviving cerebral malaria—especially those with hypoglycemia, severe anemia, repeated seizures, and deep coma—have residual neurologic deficit when they regain consciousness; hemiplegia, cerebral palsy, cortical blindness, deafness, and impaired cognition and learning (all of varying duration) have been reported. The majority of these deficits improve markedly or resolve completely within 6 months. Approximately 10% of children surviving cerebral malaria have a persistent language deficit. The incidence of epilepsy is increased and the life expectancy decreased among these children.

Hypoglycemia

Hypoglycemia, an important and common complication of severe malaria, is associated with a poor prognosis and is particularly problematic in children and pregnant women. Hypoglycemia in malaria results from a failure of hepatic gluconeogenesis and an increase in the consumption of glucose by both host and, to a much lesser extent, the malaria parasites. To compound the situation, quinine (and quinidine), which is still widely used for the treatment of both severe and uncomplicated falciparum malaria, is a powerful stimulant of pancreatic insulin secretion. Hyperinsulinemic hypoglycemia is

TABLE 210-2 Manifestations of Severe Falciparum Malaria

Signs	Manifestations
Major	
Unarousable coma/cerebral malaria	Failure to localize or respond appropriately to noxious stimuli; coma persisting for >30 min after generalized convulsion
Acidemia/acidosis	Arterial pH of <7.25 or plasma bicarbonate level of <15 mmol/L; venous lactate level of >5 mmol/L; manifests as labored deep breathing, often termed "respiratory distress"
Severe normochromic, normocytic anemia	Hematocrit of <15% or hemoglobin level of <50 g/L (<5 g/dL) with parasitemia level of >100,000/μL
Renal failure	Urine output (24 h) of <400 mL in adults or <12 mL/kg in children; no improvement with rehydration; serum creatinine level of >265 μmol/L (>3 mg/dL)
Pulmonary edema/adult respiratory distress syndrome	Noncardiogenic pulmonary edema, often aggravated by overhydration
Hypoglycemia	Plasma glucose level of <2.2 mmol/L (<40 mg/dL)
Hypotension/shock	Systolic blood pressure of <50 mmHg in children 1–5 years or <80 mmHg in adults; core/skin temperature difference of >10°C; capillary refill >2 s
Bleeding/disseminated intravascular coagulation	Significant bleeding and hemorrhage from the gums, nose, and gastrointestinal tract and/or evidence of disseminated intravascular coagulation
Convulsions	More than two generalized seizures in 24 h; signs of continued seizure activity sometimes subtle (e.g., tonic-clonic eye movements without limb or face movement)
Hemoglobinuria[a]	Macroscopic black, brown, or red urine; not associated with effects of oxidant drugs and red blood cell enzyme defects (such as G6PD deficiency)
Other	
Impaired consciousness/arousable	Unable to sit or stand without support
Extreme weakness	Prostration; inability to sit unaided[b]
Hyperparasitemia	Parasitemia level of >5% in nonimmune patients (>20% in any patient)
Jaundice	Serum bilirubin level of >50 mmol/L (>3 mg/dL) if combined with other evidence of vital-organ dysfunction

[a]Hemoglobinuria may occur in uncomplicated malaria.

[b]In a child who is normally able to sit.

Abbreviation: G6PD, glucose-6-phosphate dehydrogenase.

especially troublesome in pregnant women receiving quinine treatment. In severe disease, the clinical diagnosis of hypoglycemia is difficult: the usual physical signs (sweating, gooseflesh, tachycardia) are absent, and the neurologic impairment caused by hypoglycemia cannot be distinguished from that caused by malaria.

Acidosis

Acidosis, an important cause of death from severe malaria, results from accumulation of organic acids. Hyperlactatemia commonly coexists with hypoglycemia. In adults, coexisting renal impairment often compounds the acidosis; in children, ketoacidosis may also contribute. Other still-unidentified organic acids are major contributors to acidosis. Acidotic breathing, sometimes called respiratory distress, is a sign of poor prognosis. It is often followed by circulatory failure refractory to volume expansion or inotropic drug treatment and ultimately by respiratory arrest. The plasma concentrations of bicarbonate or lactate are the best biochemical prognosticators in severe malaria. Lactic acidosis is caused by the combination of anaerobic glycolysis in tissues where sequestered parasites interfere with microcirculatory flow, hypovolemia, lactate production by the parasites, and a failure of hepatic and renal lactate clearance. The prognosis of severe acidosis is poor.

Noncardiogenic pulmonary edema

Adults with severe falciparum malaria may develop noncardiogenic pulmonary edema even after several days of antimalarial therapy. The pathogenesis of this variant of the adult respiratory distress syndrome is unclear. The mortality rate is >80%. This condition can be aggravated by overly vigorous administration of IV fluid. Noncardiogenic pulmonary edema can also develop in otherwise uncomplicated vivax malaria, where recovery is usual.

Renal impairment

Renal impairment is common among adults with severe falciparum malaria but rare among children. The pathogenesis of renal failure is unclear but may be related to erythrocyte sequestration and agglutination interfering with renal microcirculatory flow and metabolism. Clinically and pathologically, this syndrome manifests as acute tubular necrosis. Renal cortical necrosis never develops. Acute renal failure may occur simultaneously with other vital-organ dysfunction (in which case the mortality risk is high) or may progress as other disease manifestations resolve. In survivors, urine flow resumes in a median of 4 days, and serum creatinine levels return to normal in a mean of 17 days (Chap. 279). Early dialysis or hemofiltration considerably enhances the likelihood of a patient's survival, particularly in acute hypercatabolic renal failure.

Hematologic abnormalities

Anemia results from accelerated RBC removal by the spleen, obligatory RBC destruction at parasite schizogony, and ineffective erythropoiesis. In severe malaria, both infected and uninfected RBCs

TABLE 210-3 Features Indicating a Poor Prognosis in Severe Falciparum Malaria

Clinical

   Marked agitation

   Hyperventilation (respiratory distress)

   Hypothermia (<36.5°C)

   Bleeding

   Deep coma

   Repeated convulsions

   Anuria

   Shock

Laboratory

   Biochemistry

      Hypoglycemia (<2.2 mmol/L)

      Hyperlactatemia (>5 mmol/L)

      Acidosis (arterial pH <7.3, serum HCO_3 <15 mmol/L)

      Elevated serum creatinine (>265 μmol/L)

      Elevated total bilirubin (>50 μmol/L)

      Elevated liver enzymes (AST/ALT 3 times upper limit of normal)

      Elevated muscle enzymes (CPK ↑, myoglobin ↑)

      Elevated urate (>600 μmol/L)

   Hematology

      Leukocytosis (>12,000/μL)

      Severe anemia (PCV <15%)

      Coagulopathy

         Decreased platelet count (<50,000/μL)

         Prolonged prothrombin time (>3 s)

         Prolonged partial thromboplastin time

         Decreased fibrinogen (<200 mg/dL)

   Parasitology

      Hyperparasitemia

         Increased mortality at >100,000/μL

         High mortality at >500,000/μL

         >20% of parasites identified as pigment-containing trophozoites and schizonts

         >5% of neutrophils with visible pigment

Abbreviations: ALT, alanine aminotransferase; AST, aspartate aminotransferase; CPK, creatine phosphokinase; PCV, packed cell volume.

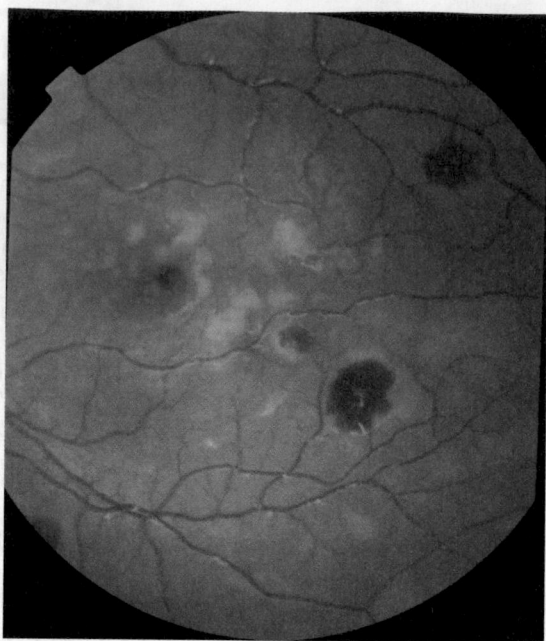

Figure 210-3 The eye in cerebral malaria: perimacular whitening and pale-centered retinal hemorrhages. *(Courtesy of N. Beare, T. Taylor, S. Harding, S. Lewallen, and M. Molyneux; with permission.)*

adults than among children; and results from hemolysis, hepatocyte injury, and cholestasis. When accompanied by other vital-organ dysfunction (often renal impairment), liver dysfunction carries a poor prognosis. Hepatic dysfunction contributes to hypoglycemia, lactic acidosis, and impaired drug metabolism. Occasional patients with falciparum malaria may develop deep jaundice (with hemolytic, hepatic, and cholestatic components) without evidence of other vital-organ dysfunction.

Other complications

HIV/AIDS predisposes to more severe malaria in nonimmune individuals. Malaria anemia is worsened by concurrent infections with intestinal helminths, hookworm in particular. Septicemia may complicate severe malaria, particularly in children. Differentiating severe malaria from sepsis with incidental parasitemia in childhood is very difficult. In endemic areas, *Salmonella* bacteremia has been associated specifically with *P. falciparum* infections. Chest infections and catheter-induced urinary tract infections are common among patients who are unconscious for >3 days. Aspiration pneumonia may follow generalized convulsions. The frequency of complications of severe falciparum malaria is summarized in Table 210-4.

show reduced deformability, which correlates with prognosis and development of anemia. Splenic clearance of all RBCs is increased. In nonimmune individuals and in areas with unstable transmission, anemia can develop rapidly and transfusion is often required. As a consequence of repeated malarial infections, children in many areas of Africa may develop severe anemia resulting from both shortened survival of uninfected RBCs and marked dyserythropoiesis. Anemia is a common consequence of antimalarial drug resistance, which results in repeated or continued infection.

Slight coagulation abnormalities are common in falciparum malaria, and mild thrombocytopenia is usual. Of patients with severe malaria, <5% have significant bleeding with evidence of disseminated intravascular coagulation. Hematemesis from stress ulceration or acute gastric erosions may also occur rarely.

Liver dysfunction

Mild hemolytic jaundice is common in malaria. Severe jaundice is associated with *P. falciparum* infections; is more common among

TABLE 210-4 Relative Incidence of Severe Complications of Falciparum Malaria

Complication	Nonpregnant Adults	Pregnant Women	Children
Anemia	+	++	+++
Convulsions	+	+	+++
Hypoglycemia	+	+++	+++
Jaundice	+++	+++	+
Renal failure	+++	+++	−
Pulmonary edema	++	+++	+

Note: −, rare; +, infrequent; ++, frequent; +++, very frequent.

MALARIA IN PREGNANCY

In areas of high malaria transmission, falciparum malaria in primi- and secundigravid women is associated with low birth weight (average reduction, ~170 g) and consequently increased infant and childhood mortality rates. In general, infected mothers in areas of stable transmission remain asymptomatic despite intense accumulation of parasitized erythrocytes in the placental microcirculation. Maternal HIV infection predisposes pregnant women to malaria, predisposes their newborns to congenital malarial infection, and exacerbates the reduction in birth weight associated with malaria.

In areas with unstable transmission of malaria, pregnant women are prone to severe infections and are particularly vulnerable to high-level parasitemia with anemia, hypoglycemia, and acute pulmonary edema. Fetal distress, premature labor, and stillbirth or low birth weight are common results. Fetal death is usual in severe malaria. Congenital malaria occurs in <5% of newborns whose mothers are infected; its frequency and the level of parasitemia are related directly to the parasite density in maternal blood and in the placenta. *P. vivax* malaria in pregnancy is also associated with a reduction in birth weight (average, 110 g), but, in contrast to the situation in falciparum malaria, this effect is more pronounced in multigravid than in primigravid women. About 150,000 women die in childbirth yearly, with most deaths occurring in low-income countries; maternal death from hemorrhage at childbirth is correlated with malaria-induced anemia.

MALARIA IN CHILDREN

Most of the nearly 1 million persons who die of falciparum malaria each year are young African children. Convulsions, coma, hypoglycemia, metabolic acidosis, and severe anemia are relatively common among children with severe malaria, whereas deep jaundice, acute renal failure, and acute pulmonary edema are unusual. Severely anemic children may present with labored deep breathing, which in the past has been attributed incorrectly to "anemic congestive cardiac failure" but in fact is usually caused by metabolic acidosis, often compounded by hypovolemia. In general, children tolerate antimalarial drugs well and respond rapidly to treatment.

TRANSFUSION MALARIA

Malaria can be transmitted by blood transfusion, needle-stick injury, sharing of needles by infected injection drug users, or organ transplantation. The incubation period in these settings is often short because there is no preerythrocytic stage of development. The clinical features and management of these cases are the same as for naturally acquired infections. Radical chemotherapy with primaquine is unnecessary for transfusion-transmitted *P. vivax* and *P. ovale* infections.

CHRONIC COMPLICATIONS OF MALARIA

TROPICAL SPLENOMEGALY (HYPERREACTIVE MALARIAL SPLENOMEGALY)

Chronic or repeated malarial infections produce hypergamma-globulinemia; normochromic, normocytic anemia; and, in certain situations, splenomegaly. Some residents of malaria-endemic areas in tropical Africa and Asia exhibit an abnormal immunologic response to repeated infections that is characterized by massive splenomegaly, hepatomegaly, marked elevations in serum titers of IgM and malarial antibody, hepatic sinusoidal lymphocytosis, and (in Africa) peripheral B cell lymphocytosis. This syndrome has been associated with the production of cytotoxic IgM antibodies to CD8+ T lymphocytes, antibodies to CD5+ T lymphocytes, and an increase in the ratio of CD4+ T cells to CD8+ T cells. These events may lead to uninhibited B cell production of IgM and the formation of cryoglobulins (IgM aggregates and

immune complexes). This immunologic process stimulates reticuloendothelial hyperplasia and clearance activity and eventually produces splenomegaly. Patients with hyperreactive malarial splenomegaly (HMS) present with an abdominal mass or a dragging sensation in the abdomen and occasional sharp abdominal pains suggesting perisplenitis. Anemia and some degree of pancytopenia are usually evident, and in some cases malarial parasites cannot be found in peripheral-blood smears. Vulnerability to respiratory and skin infections is increased; many patients die of overwhelming sepsis. Persons with HMS who are living in endemic areas should receive antimalarial chemoprophylaxis; the results are usually good. In nonendemic areas, antimalarial treatment is advised. In some cases refractory to therapy, clonal lymphoproliferation may develop and then evolve into a malignant lymphoproliferative disorder.

QUARTAN MALARIAL NEPHROPATHY

Chronic or repeated infections with *P. malariae* (and possibly with other malarial species) may cause soluble immune-complex injury to the renal glomeruli, resulting in the nephrotic syndrome. Other unidentified factors must contribute to this process since only a very small proportion of infected patients develop renal disease. The histologic appearance is that of focal or segmental glomerulonephritis with splitting of the capillary basement membrane. Subendothelial dense deposits are seen on electron microscopy, and immunofluorescence reveals deposits of complement and immunoglobulins; in samples of renal tissue from children, *P. malariae* antigens are often visible. A coarse-granular pattern of basement membrane immunofluorescent deposits (predominantly IgG3) with selective proteinuria carries a better prognosis than a fine-granular, predominantly IgG2 pattern with nonselective proteinuria. Quartan nephropathy usually responds poorly to treatment with either antimalarial agents or glucocorticoids and cytotoxic drugs.

BURKITT'S LYMPHOMA AND EPSTEIN-BARR VIRUS INFECTION

It is possible that malaria-related immune dysregulation provokes infection with lymphoma viruses. Burkitt's lymphoma is strongly associated with Epstein-Barr virus. The prevalence of this childhood tumor is high in malarious areas of Africa.

DIAGNOSIS

DEMONSTRATION OF THE PARASITE

The diagnosis of malaria rests on the demonstration of asexual forms of the parasite in stained peripheral-blood smears. After a negative blood smear, repeat smears should be made if there is a high degree of suspicion. Of the Romanowsky stains, Giemsa at pH 7.2 is preferred; Field's, Wright's, or Leishman's stain can also be used. Both thin (Figs. 210-4 and 210-5; see also Figs. e27-3 and e27-4) and thick (Figs. 210-6, 210-7, 210-8, and 210-9) blood smears should be examined. The thin blood smear should be rapidly air-dried, fixed in anhydrous methanol, and stained; the RBCs in the tail of the film should then be examined under oil immersion (×1000 magnification). The level of parasitemia is expressed as the number of parasitized erythrocytes per 1000 RBCs. The thick blood film should be of uneven thickness. The smear should be dried thoroughly and stained without fixing. As many layers of erythrocytes overlie one another and are lysed during the staining procedure, the thick film has the advantage of concentrating the parasites (by 40- to 100-fold compared with a thin blood film) and thus increasing diagnostic sensitivity. Both parasites and white blood cells (WBCs) are counted, and the number of parasites per unit volume is calculated from the total leukocyte count. Alternatively, a WBC count of 8000/μL is assumed. This figure is converted to the number of parasitized erythrocytes per microliter. A minimum of 200 WBCs should be counted under

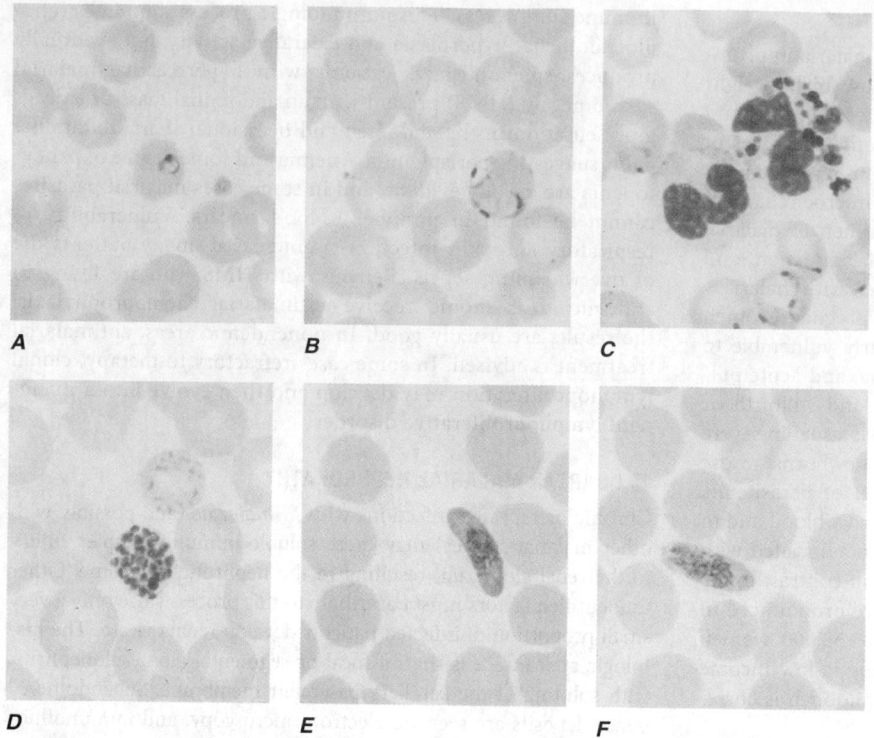

Figure 210-4 Thin blood films of *Plasmodium falciparum*. A. Young trophozoites. **B.** Old trophozoites. **C.** Pigment in polymorphonuclear cells and trophozoites. **D.** Mature schizonts. **E.** Female gametocytes. **F.** Male gametocytes. *(Reproduced from Bench Aids for the Diagnosis of Malaria Infections, 2nd ed, with the permission of the World Health Organization.)*

The relationship between parasitemia and prognosis is complex; in general, patients with >10^5 parasites/μL are at increased risk of dying, but nonimmune patients may die with much lower counts, and partially immune persons may tolerate parasitemia levels many times higher with only minor symptoms. In severe malaria, a poor prognosis is indicated by a predominance of more mature *P. falciparum* parasites (i.e., >20% of parasites with visible pigment) in the peripheral-blood film or by the presence of phagocytosed malarial pigment in >5% of neutrophils. In *P. falciparum* infections, gametocytemia peaks 1 week after the peak of asexual parasites. Because the mature gametocytes of *P. falciparum* are not affected by most antimalarial drugs, their persistence does not constitute evidence of drug resistance. Phagocytosed malarial pigment is sometimes seen inside peripheral-blood monocytes or polymorphonuclear leukocytes and may provide a clue to recent infection if malaria parasites are not detectable. After the clearance of the parasites, this intraphagocytic malarial pigment is often evident for several days in the peripheral blood or for longer in bone marrow aspirates or smears of fluid expressed after intradermal puncture. Staining of parasites with the fluorescent dye acridine orange allows more rapid diagnosis of malaria (but not speciation of the infection) in patients with low-level parasitemia.

oil immersion. Interpretation of blood smear films requires some experience because artifacts are common. Before a thick smear is judged to be negative, 100–200 fields should be examined under oil immersion. In high-transmission areas, the presence of up to 10,000 parasites/μL of blood may be tolerated without symptoms or signs in partially immune individuals. Thus in these areas the detection of malaria parasites is sensitive but has low specificity in identifying malaria as the cause of illness. Low-density parasitemia is common in other conditions causing fever.

Rapid, simple, sensitive, and specific antibody-based diagnostic stick or card tests that detect *P. falciparum*–specific, histidine-rich protein 2 (PfHRP2) or lactate dehydrogenase antigens in finger-prick blood samples are now being used widely in control programs (Table 210-5). Some of these rapid diagnostic tests (RDTs) carry a second antibody, which allows falciparum malaria to be distinguished from the less dangerous malarias. PfHRP2-based tests may remain positive for several weeks after acute infection. This feature is a disadvantage in high-transmission areas where infections are frequent but is of value in the diagnosis of severe malaria in patients who have taken antimalarial drugs and cleared peripheral parasitemia (but in whom the PfHRP2 test remains strongly positive). RDTs are replacing microscopy in many areas because of their simplicity and speed, but they are relatively expensive and do not quantify parasitemia.

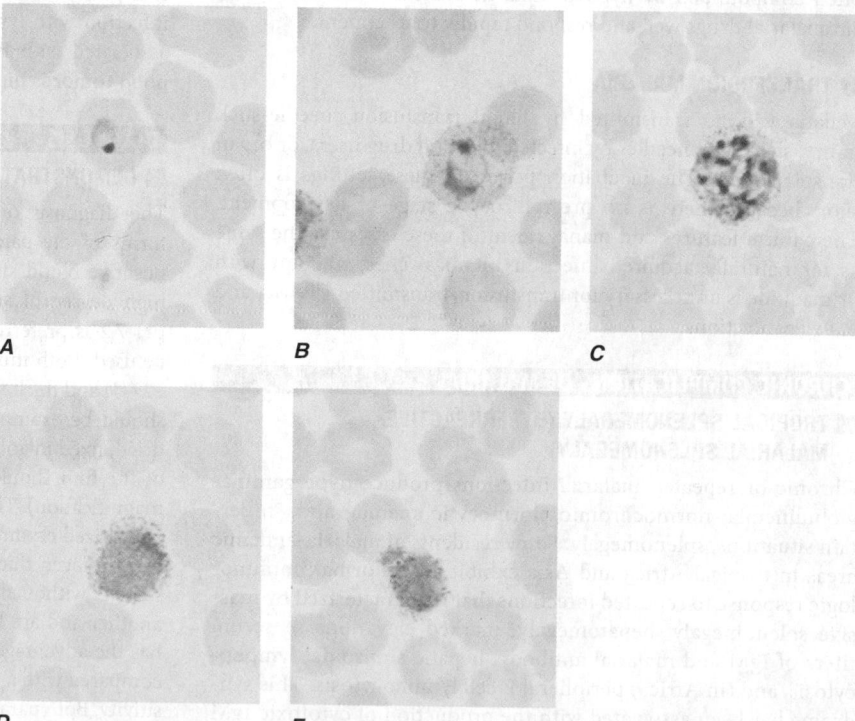

Figure 210-5 Thin blood films of *Plasmodium vivax*. A. Young trophozoites. **B.** Old trophozoites. **C.** Mature schizonts. **D.** Female gametocytes. **E.** Male gametocytes. *(Reproduced from Bench Aids for the Diagnosis of Malaria Infections, 2nd ed, with the permission of the World Health Organization.)*

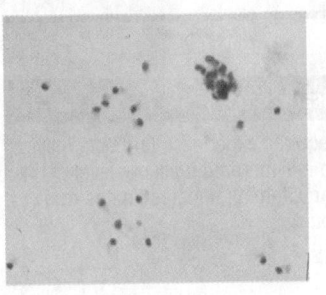 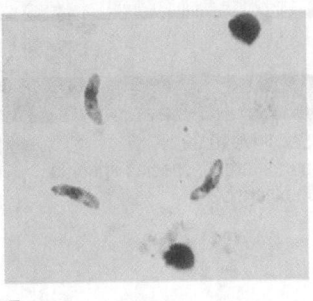

Figure 210-6 Thick blood films of *Plasmodium falciparum.* **A.** Trophozoites. **B.** Gametocytes. *(Reproduced from Bench Aids for the Diagnosis of Malaria Infections, 2nd ed, with the permission of the World Health Organization.)*

■ LABORATORY FINDINGS

Normochromic, normocytic anemia is usual. The leukocyte count is generally normal, although it may be raised in very severe infections. There is slight monocytosis, lymphopenia, and eosinopenia, with reactive lymphocytosis and eosinophilia in the weeks after the acute infection. The erythrocyte sedimentation rate, plasma viscosity, and levels of C-reactive protein and other acute-phase proteins are high. The platelet count is usually reduced to ~10^5/μL. Severe infections may be accompanied by prolonged prothrombin and partial thromboplastin times and by more severe thrombocytopenia. Levels of antithrombin III are reduced even in mild infection. In uncomplicated malaria, plasma concentrations of electrolytes, blood urea nitrogen (BUN), and creatinine are usually normal. Findings in severe malaria may include metabolic acidosis, with low plasma concentrations of glucose, sodium, bicarbonate, calcium, phosphate, and albumin together with elevations in lactate, BUN, creatinine, urate, muscle and liver enzymes, and conjugated and unconjugated bilirubin. Hypergammaglobulinemia is usual in immune and semi-immune subjects. Urinalysis generally gives normal results. In adults and children with cerebral malaria, the mean opening pressure at lumbar puncture is ~160 mm of cerebrospinal fluid (CSF); usually the CSF is normal or has a slightly elevated total protein level [<1.0 g/L (<100 mg/dL)] and cell count (<20/μL).

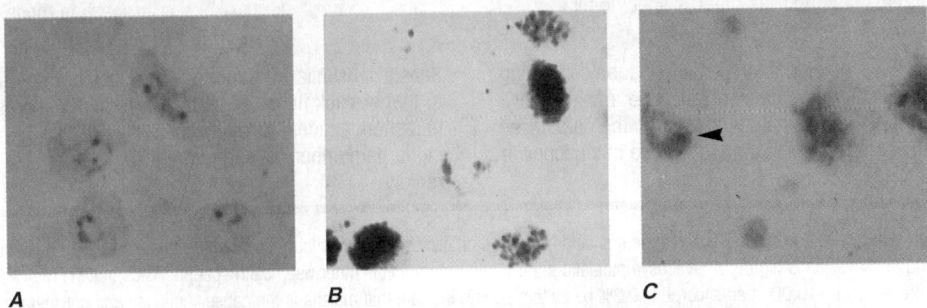

Figure 210-7   Thick blood films of *Plasmodium vivax*. A. Trophozoites. **B.** Schizonts. **C.** Gametocytes. *(Reproduced from Bench Aids for the Diagnosis of Malaria Infections, 2nd ed, with the permission of the World Health Organization.)*

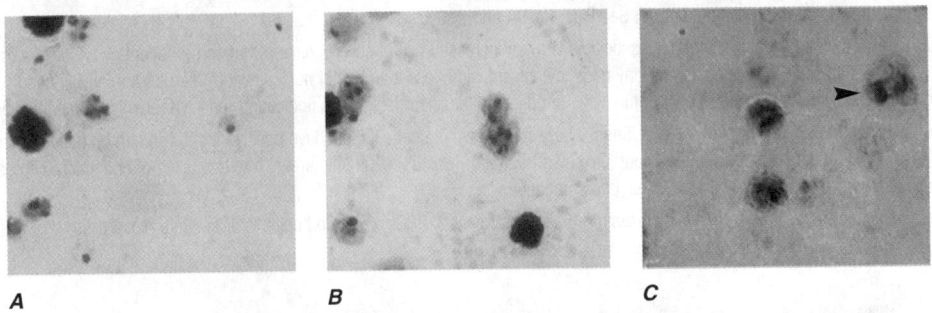

Figure 210-8   Thick blood films of *Plasmodium ovale*. A. Trophozoites. **B.** Schizonts. **C.** Gametocytes. *(Reproduced from Bench Aids for the Diagnosis of Malaria Infections, 2nd ed, with the permission of the World Health Organization.)*

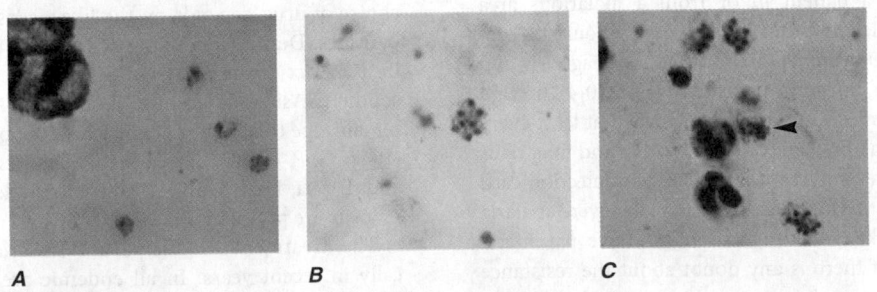

Figure 210-9   Thick blood films of *Plasmodium malariae*. A. Trophozoites. **B.** Schizonts. **C.** Gametocytes. *(Reproduced from Bench Aids for the Diagnosis of Malaria Infections, 2nd ed, with the permission of the World Health Organization.)*

TABLE 210-5 Methods for the Diagnosis of Malaria[a]

Method	Procedure	Advantages	Disadvantages
Thick blood film[b]	Blood should be uneven in thickness but sufficiently thin to read the hands of a watch through part of the spot. Stain dried, unfixed blood spot with Giemsa, Field's, or another Romanowsky stain. Count number of asexual parasites per 200 WBCs (or per 500 at low densities). Count gametocytes separately.[c]	Sensitive (0.001% parasitemia); species specific; inexpensive	Requires experience (artifacts may be misinterpreted as low-level parasitemia); underestimates true count
Thin blood film[d]	Stain fixed smear with Giemsa, Field's, or another Romanowsky stain. Count number of RBCs containing asexual parasites per 1000 RBCs. In severe malaria, assess stage of parasite development and count neutrophils containing malaria pigment.[e] Count gametocytes separately.[c]	Rapid; species specific; inexpensive; in severe malaria, provides prognostic information[e]	Insensitive (<0.05% parasitemia); uneven distribution of *P. vivax*, as enlarged infected red cells concentrate at leading edge
PfHRP2 dipstick or card test	A drop of blood is placed on the stick or card, which is then immersed in washing solutions. Monoclonal antibody captures the parasite antigen and reads out as a colored band.	Robust and relatively inexpensive; rapid; sensitivity similar to or slightly lower than that of thick films (~0.001% parasitemia)	Detects only *Plasmodium falciparum*; remains positive for weeks after infection[f]; does not quantitate *P. falciparum* parasitemia
Plasmodium LDH dipstick or card test	A drop of blood is placed on the stick or card, which is then immersed in washing solutions. Monoclonal antibodies capture the parasite antigens and read out as colored bands. One band is genus specific (all malarias), and the other is specific for *P. falciparum*.	Rapid; sensitivity similar to or slightly lower than that of thick films for *P. falciparum* (~0.001% parasitemia)	Slightly more difficult preparation than PfHRP2 tests; may miss low-level parasitemia with *P. vivax, P. ovale*, and *P. malariae* and does not speciate these organisms; does not quantitate *P. falciparum* parasitemia
Microtube concentration methods with acridine orange staining	Blood is collected in a specialized tube containing acridine orange, anticoagulant, and a float. After centrifugation, which concentrates the parasitized cells around the float, fluorescence microscopy is performed.	Sensitivity similar or superior to that of thick films (~0.001% parasitemia); ideal for processing large numbers of samples rapidly	Does not speciate or quantitate; requires fluorescence microscopy

[a]Malaria cannot be diagnosed clinically with accuracy, but treatment should be started on clinical grounds if laboratory confirmation is likely to be delayed. In areas of the world where malaria is endemic and transmission is high, low-level asymptomatic parasitemia is common in otherwise healthy people. Thus malaria may not be the cause of a fever, although in this context the presence of >10,000 parasites/μL (~0.2% parasitemia) *does* indicate that malaria is the cause. Antibody and polymerase chain reaction tests have no role in the diagnosis of malaria except that PCR is increasingly used for genotyping and speciation in mixed infections.

[b]Asexual parasites/200 WBCs × 40 = parasite count/μL (assumes a WBC count of 8000/μL). See Figs. 210-6 through 210-9.

[c]Gametocytemia may persist for days or weeks after clearance of asexual parasites. Gametocytemia without asexual parasitemia does not indicate active infection.

[d]Parasitized RBCs (%) × hematocrit × 1256 = parasite count/μL. See Figs. 210-4 and 210-5.

[e]The presence of >100,000 parasites/μL (~2% parasitemia) is associated with an increased risk of severe malaria, but some patients have severe malaria with lower counts. At any level of parasitemia, the finding that >50% of parasites are tiny rings (cytoplasm width less than half of nucleus width) carries a relatively good prognosis. The presence of visible pigment in >20% of parasites or of phagocytosed pigment in >5% of polymorphonuclear leukocytes (indicating massive recent schizogony) carries a worse prognosis.

[f]Persistence of PfHRP2 is a disadvantage in high-transmission settings, where many asymptomatic people have positive tests, but can be used to diagnostic advantage in low-transmission settings when a sick patient has received previous unknown treatment (which, in endemic areas, often consists of antimalarial drugs). A positive PfHRP2 test indicates that the illness is falciparum malaria, even if the blood smear is negative.

Abbreviations: LDH, lactate dehydrogenase; PfHRP2, *P. falciparum* histidine-rich protein 2; RBCs, red blood cells; WBCs, white blood cells.

TREATMENT   Malaria

(Table 210-6) When a patient in or from a malarious area presents with fever, thick and thin blood smears should be prepared and *examined immediately* to confirm the diagnosis and identify the species of infecting parasite (Figs. 210-4 through 210-9). Repeat blood smears should be performed at least every 12–24 h for 2 days if the first smears are negative and malaria is strongly suspected. Alternatively, a rapid antigen detection card or stick test should be performed. Patients with severe malaria or those unable to take oral drugs should receive parenteral antimalarial therapy. If there is any doubt about the resistance status of the infecting organism, it should be considered resistant. Antimalarial drug susceptibility testing can be performed but is rarely available, has poor predictive value in an individual case, and yields results too slowly to influence the choice of treatment. Several drugs are available for oral treatment. The choice of drug depends on the likely sensitivity of the infecting parasites. Despite increasing evidence of chloroquine resistance in *P. vivax* (from parts of Indonesia, Oceania, eastern and southern Asia, and Central and South America), chloroquine remains the treatment of choice for the non-falciparum malarias (*P. vivax, P. ovale, P. malariae, P. knowlesi*) except in Indonesia and Papua New Guinea, where high levels of resistance in *P. vivax* are prevalent.

The treatment of falciparum malaria has changed radically in recent years. In all endemic areas, the World Health Organization (WHO) now recommends artemisinin-based combinations as first-line treatment for uncomplicated

TABLE 210-6 Regimens for the Treatment of Malaria

Type of Disease or Treatment	Regimen(s)
Uncomplicated Malaria	
Known chloroquine-sensitive strains of *Plasmodium vivax, P. malariae, P. ovale, P. knowlesi, P. falciparum*[a]	Chloroquine (10 mg of base/kg stat followed by 5 mg/kg at 12, 24, and 36 h or by 10 mg/kg at 24 h and 5 mg/kg at 48 h) *or* Amodiaquine (10–12 mg of base/kg qd for 3 days)
Radical treatment for *P. vivax* or *P. ovale* infection	In addition to chloroquine or amodiaquine as detailed above, primaquine (0.5 mg of base/kg qd) should be given for 14 days to prevent relapse. In mild G6PD deficiency, 0.75 mg of base/kg should be given once weekly for 6–8 weeks. Primaquine should not be given in severe G6PD deficiency.
Sensitive *P. falciparum* malaria[b]	Artesunate[c] (4 mg/kg qd for 3 days) plus sulfadoxine (25 mg/kg)/pyrimethamine (1.25 mg/kg) as a single dose *or* Artesunate[c] (4 mg/kg qd for 3 days) plus amodiaquine (10 mg of base/kg qd for 3 days)[d]
Multidrug-resistant *P. falciparum* malaria	Either artemether-lumefantrine[c] (1.5/9 mg/kg bid for 3 days with food) *or* Artesunate[c] (4 mg/kg qd for 3 days) *plus* Mefloquine (25 mg of base/kg—either 8 mg/kg qd for 3 days or 15 mg/kg on day 2 and then 10 mg/kg on day 3)[d]
Second-line treatment/treatment of imported malaria	Either artesunate[c] (2 mg/kg qd for 7 days) or quinine (10 mg of salt/kg tid for 7 days) *plus 1 of the following 3:* 1. Tetracycline[e] (4 mg/kg qid for 7 days) 2. Doxycycline[e] (3 mg/kg qd for 7 days) 3. Clindamycin (10 mg/kg bid for 7 days) *or* Atovaquone-proguanil (20/8 mg/kg qd for 3 days with food)
Severe Falciparum Malaria[f]	
	Artesunate[c] (2.4 mg/kg stat IV followed by 2.4 mg/kg at 12 and 24 h and then daily if necessary)[g] *or, if unavailable, one of the following:* Artemether[c] (3.2 mg/kg stat IM followed by 1.6 mg/kg qd) *or* Quinine dihydrochloride (20 mg of salt/kg[h] infused over 4 h, followed by 10 mg of salt/kg infused over 2–8 h q8h[i]) *or* Quinidine (10 mg of base/kg[h] infused over 1–2 h, followed by 1.2 mg of base/kg per hour[i] with electrocardiographic monitoring)

[a]Very few areas now have chloroquine-sensitive *P. falciparum* malaria (Fig. 210-2).

[b]In areas where the partner drug to artesunate is known to be effective.

[c]Artemisinin derivatives are not readily available in some temperate countries.

[d]Fixed-dose coformulated combinations are available. The World Health Organization now recommends artemisinin combination regimens as first-line therapy for falciparum malaria in all tropical countries and advocates use of fixed-dose combinations.

[e]Tetracycline and doxycycline should not be given to pregnant women or to children <8 years of age.

[f]Oral treatment should be substituted as soon as the patient recovers sufficiently to take fluids by mouth.

[g]Artesunate is the drug of choice when available. The data from large studies in Southeast Asia showed a 35% lower mortality rate than with quinine, and very large studies in Africa showed a 22.5% reduction in mortality rate compared with quinine.

[h]A loading dose should not be given if therapeutic doses of quinine or quinidine have definitely been administered in the previous 24 h. Some authorities recommend a lower dose of quinidine.

[i]Infusions can be given in 0.9% saline and 5–10% dextrose in water. Infusion rates for quinine and quinidine should be carefully controlled.

Abbreviation: G6PD, glucose-6-phosphate dehydrogenase.

falciparum malaria. These rapidly and reliably effective drugs are sometimes unavailable in temperate countries, where treatment recommendations are limited by the registered available drugs. Fake or substandard antimalarials are commonly sold in many Asian and African countries. Thus, careful attention is required at the time of purchase and later, especially when the patient fails to respond as expected. Characteristics of antimalarial drugs are shown in Table 210-7.

TABLE 210-7 Properties of Antimalarial Drugs

Drug(s)	Pharmacokinetic Properties	Antimalarial Activity	Minor Toxicity	Major Toxicity
Quinine, quinidine	Good oral and IM absorption (quinine); Cl and V_d reduced, but plasma protein binding (principally to $\propto 1$ acid glycoprotein) increased (90%) in malaria; quinine $t_{1/2}$: 16 h in malaria, 11 h in healthy persons; quinidine $t_{1/2}$: 13 h in malaria, 8 h in healthy persons	Acts mainly on trophozoite blood stage; kills gametocytes of *P. vivax*, *P. ovale*, and *P. malariae* (but not *P. falciparum*); no action on liver stages	*Common:* "Cinchonism": tinnitus, high-tone hearing loss, nausea, vomiting, dysphoria, postural hypotension; ECG QT_c interval prolongation (quinine usually by <10% but quinidine by up to 25%) *Rare:* Diarrhea, visual disturbance, rashes *Note:* Very bitter taste	*Common:* Hypoglycemia *Rare:* Hypotension, blindness, deafness, cardiac arrhythmias, thrombocytopenia, hemolysis, hemolytic-uremic syndrome, vasculitis, cholestatic hepatitis, neuromuscular paralysis *Note:* Quinidine more cardiotoxic
Chloroquine	Good oral absorption, very rapid IM and SC absorption; complex pharmacokinetics; enormous Cl and V_d (unaffected by malaria); blood concentration profile determined by distribution processes in malaria; $t_{1/2}$: 1–2 months	As for quinine but acts slightly earlier in asexual cycle	*Common:* Nausea, dysphoria, pruritus in dark-skinned patients, postural hypotension *Rare:* Accommodation difficulties, keratopathy, rash *Note:* Bitter taste, well tolerated	*Acute:* Hypotensive shock (parenteral), cardiac arrhythmias, neuropsychiatric reactions *Chronic:* Retinopathy (cumulative dose, >100 g), skeletal and cardiac myopathy
Piperaquine	Adequate oral absorption, enhanced by fats; similar pharmacokinetics to chloroquine; $t_{1/2}$: 21–28 days	As for chloroquine, but retains activity against multidrug-resistant *P. falciparum*	Epigastric pain, diarrhea, slight ECG QT_c prolongation	None identified
Amodiaquine	Good oral absorption; largely converted to active metabolite desethylamodiaquine	As for chloroquine	Nausea (tastes better than chloroquine)	Agranulocytosis; hepatitis, mainly with prophylactic use; should not be used with efavirenz
Primaquine	Complete oral absorption; active metabolite not known; $t_{1/2}$: 7 h	Radical cure; eradicates hepatic forms of *P. vivax* and *P. ovale*; kills all stages of gametocyte development of *P. falciparum*	Nausea, vomiting, diarrhea, abdominal pain, hemolysis, methemoglobinemia	Massive hemolysis in subjects with severe G6PD deficiency
Mefloquine	Adequate oral absorption; no parenteral preparation; $t_{1/2}$: 14–20 days (shorter in malaria)	As for quinine	Nausea, giddiness, dysphoria, fuzzy thinking, sleeplessness, nightmares, sense of dissociation	Neuropsychiatric reactions, convulsions, encephalopathy
Halofantrine[b]	Highly variable absorption related to fat intake; $t_{1/2}$: 1–3 days (active desbutyl metabolite $t_{1/2}$: 3–7 days)	As for quinine	Diarrhea	Cardiac conduction disturbances; atrioventricular block; ECG QT_c interval prolongation; potentially lethal ventricular tachyarrhythmias
Lumefantrine	Highly variable absorption related to fat intake; $t_{1/2}$: 3–4 days	As for quinine	None identified	None identified
Artemisinin and derivatives (artemether, artesunate)	Good oral absorption, slow and variable absorption of IM artemether; artesunate and artemether biotransformed to active metabolite dihydroartemisinin; all drugs eliminated very rapidly; $t_{1/2}$: <1 h	Broader stage specificity and more rapid than other drugs; no action on liver stages; kills all but fully mature gametocytes of *P. falciparum*	Reduction in reticulocyte count (but not anemia); neutropenia at high doses	Anaphylaxis, urticaria, fever
Pyrimethamine	Good oral absorption, variable IM absorption; $t_{1/2}$: 4 days	For blood stages, acts mainly on mature forms; causal prophylactic	Well tolerated	Megaloblastic anemia, pancytopenia, pulmonary infiltration
Proguanil (chloroguanide)	Good oral absorption; biotransformed to active metabolite cycloguanil; $t_{1/2}$: 16 h; biotransformation reduced by oral contraceptive use and in pregnancy	Causal prophylactic; not used alone for treatment	Well tolerated; mouth ulcers and rare alopecia	Megaloblastic anemia in renal failure

(*continued*)

TABLE 210-7 Properties of Antimalarial Drugs (*Continued*)

Drug(s)	Pharmacokinetic Properties	Antimalarial Activity	Minor Toxicity	Major Toxicity
Atovaquone	Highly variable absorption related to fat intake; $t_{1/2}$: 30–70 h	Acts mainly on trophozoite blood stage	None identified	None identified
Tetracycline, doxycycline[a]	Excellent absorption; $t_{1/2}$: 8 h for tetracycline, 18 h for doxycycline	Weak antimalarial activity; should not be used alone for treatment	Gastrointestinal intolerance, deposition in growing bones and teeth, photosensitivity, moniliasis, benign intracranial hypertension	Renal failure in patients with impaired renal function (tetracycline)

[a]Tetracycline and doxycycline should not be given to pregnant women or to children <8 years of age.

[b]Halofantrine should not be used by patients with long ECG QT_c intervals or known conduction disturbances or by those taking drugs that may affect ventricular repolarization, e.g., quinidine, quinine, mefloquine, chloroquine, neuroleptics, antiarrhythmics, tricyclic antidepressants, terfenidine, or astemizole.

Abbreviations: *Cl*, systemic clearance; ECG, electrocardiogram; G6PD, glucose-6-phosphate dehydrogenase; V_d, total apparent volume of distribution.

SEVERE MALARIA In large studies conducted in Asia, parenteral artesunate, a water-soluble artemisinin derivative, has been shown to reduce mortality rates in severe falciparum malaria among adults by 35% from rates obtained with quinine. Recently, the largest trial ever in severe malaria showed that parenteral artesunate reduced the mortality rate among African children by 22.5% compared with that obtained with quinine. Artesunate has, therefore, become the drug of choice for all patients with severe malaria everywhere. Artesunate is given by IV injection but can also be given by IM injection. Artemether and the closely related drug artemotil (arteether) are oil-based formulations given by IM injection; they are erratically absorbed and do not confer the same survival benefit as artesunate. A rectal formulation of artesunate has been developed as a community-based pre-referral treatment for patients in the rural tropics who cannot take oral medications. Pre-referral administration of rectal artesunate has been shown to decrease mortality risk among severely ill children in communities without access to immediate parenteral treatment. Although the artemisinin compounds are safer than quinine and considerably safer than quinidine, only one formulation is available in the United States. IV artesunate has been approved by the U.S. Food and Drug Administration for emergency use against severe malaria through the Centers for Disease Control and Prevention (CDC) Drug Service (see end of chapter for contact information). The antiarrhythmic quinidine gluconate is as effective as quinine and, as it was more readily available, replaced quinine for the treatment of malaria in the United States. The administration of quinidine must be closely monitored if dysrhythmias and hypotension are to be avoided. A total plasma level >8 μg/mL, a QT_c interval >0.6 s, or QRS widening beyond 25% of baseline is an indication for slowing infusion rates. If arrhythmia or saline-unresponsive hypotension develops, treatment with this drug should be discontinued. Quinine is safer than quinidine; cardiovascular monitoring is not required except when the recipient has cardiac disease.

Severe falciparum malaria constitutes a medical emergency requiring intensive nursing care and careful management. The patient should be weighed and, if comatose, placed on his or her side or prone. Frequent evaluation of the patient's condition is essential. Ancillary drugs such as high-dose glucocorticoids, urea, heparin, dextran, desferrioxamine, antibody to tumor necrosis factor α, and high-dose phenobarbital (20 mg/kg) have proved either ineffective or harmful in clinical trials and should not be used. In acute renal failure or severe metabolic acidosis, hemofiltration or hemodialysis should be started as early as possible.

Parenteral antimalarial treatment should be started as soon as possible. Artesunate, given by either IV or IM injection, is the agent of choice; it is simple to administer, safe, and rapidly effective. If artesunate is unavailable and artemether, quinine, or quinidine is used, an initial loading dose must be given so that therapeutic concentrations are reached as soon as possible. Both quinine and quinidine will cause dangerous hypotension if injected rapidly; when given IV, they must be administered carefully by rate-controlled infusion only. If this approach is not possible, quinine may be given by deep IM injections into the anterior thigh. The optimal therapeutic range for quinine and quinidine in severe malaria is not known with certainty, but total plasma concentrations of 8–15 mg/L for quinine and 3.5–8.0 mg/L for quinidine are effective and do not cause serious toxicity. The systemic clearance and apparent volume of distribution of these alkaloids are markedly reduced and plasma protein binding is increased in severe malaria, so that the blood concentrations attained with a given dose are higher. If the patient remains seriously ill or in acute renal failure for >2 days, maintenance doses of quinine or quinidine should be reduced by 30–50% to prevent toxic accumulation of the drug. The initial doses should never be reduced. If one of the artemisinin derivatives is given, dose reductions are unnecessary, even in renal failure. Exchange transfusion may be considered for severely ill patients, although the precise indications for this procedure have not been agreed upon. It has been recommended that—if safe and feasible—exchange should be considered for patients with severe malaria, but there is no clear evidence that this measure is beneficial, particularly if artesunate is used. The role of prophylactic anticonvulsants in children is also uncertain. If respiratory support is not available, then a full loading dose of phenobarbital (20 mg/kg) to prevent convulsions should not be given as it may cause respiratory arrest.

When the patient is unconscious, the blood glucose level should be measured every 4–6 h. All patients should receive a continuous infusion of dextrose, and blood concentrations ideally should be maintained above 4 mmol/L. Hypoglycemia (<2.2 mmol/L or 40 mg/dL) should be treated immediately with bolus glucose. The parasite count and hematocrit level should be measured every 6–12 h. Anemia develops rapidly; if the hematocrit falls to <20%, then whole blood (preferably fresh) or packed cells should be transfused slowly, with careful attention to circulatory status. Renal function should be checked daily. Children presenting with severe anemia and acidotic breathing are often hypovolemic; in this situation, resuscitation with crystalloids or blood is indicated. Accurate assessment is vital. Management of fluid balance is difficult in severe malaria, particularly in adults, because of the thin dividing line between overhydration (leading to pulmonary edema) and underhydration (contributing to renal impairment). As soon as the patient can take fluids, oral therapy should be substituted for parenteral treatment.

UNCOMPLICATED MALARIA Infections due to *P. vivax*, *P. knowlesi*, *P. malariae*, and *P. ovale* should be treated with oral chloroquine (total dose, 25 mg of base/kg). In much of the tropics, drug-resistant *P. falciparum* has been increasing in distribution, frequency, and intensity. It is now accepted that, to prevent resistance, falciparum malaria should be treated with drug combinations and not with single drugs in endemic areas; the same rationale has been applied successfully to the treatment of tuberculosis, HIV/AIDS, and cancers. This combination strategy is based on simultaneous use of two or more drugs with different modes of action. Artemisinin combination treatment (ACT) regimens are now recommended as first-line treatment for falciparum malaria throughout the malaria-affected world. The artemisinin component is usually an artemisinin derivative (artesunate, artemether, or dihydroartemisinin) given for 3 days, and the partner drug is usually a slower-acting antimalarial to which *P. falciparum* is sensitive. Five ACT regimens are currently recommended by the WHO. In areas with multidrug-resistant falciparum malaria (parts of Asia and South America, including those with mefloquine-resistant parasites; Fig. 210-10), artemether-lumefantrine, artesunate-mefloquine, or dihydroartemisinin-piperaquine should be used; these regimens provide cure rates of >90%. In areas with sensitive parasites, the aforementioned combinations, artesunate-sulfadoxine-pyrimethamine, or artesunate-amodiaquine may also be used. Atovaquone-proguanil is also highly effective everywhere, although it is seldom used in endemic areas because of its high cost. Of great concern is the emergence of artemisinin-resistant *P. falciparum* in western Cambodia and adjacent Thailand. Infections with these parasites are cleared slowly from the blood, with clearance times typically exceeding 3 days.

The 3-day ACT regimens are all well tolerated, although mefloquine is associated with increased rates of vomiting and dizziness. As second-line treatments for recrudescence following first-line therapy, a different ACT regimen may be given; another alternative is a 7-day course of either artesunate or quinine plus tetracycline, doxycycline, or clindamycin. Tetracycline and doxycycline cannot be given to pregnant women or to children <8 years of age. Oral quinine is extremely bitter and regularly produces cinchonism comprising tinnitus, high-tone deafness, nausea, vomiting, and dysphoria. Adherence is poor with the required 7-day regimens of quinine.

Patients should be monitored for vomiting for 1 h after the administration of any oral antimalarial drug. If there is vomiting, the dose should be repeated. Symptom-based treatment, with tepid sponging and acetaminophen administration, lowers fever and thereby reduces the patient's propensity to vomit these drugs. Minor central nervous system reactions (nausea, dizziness, sleep disturbances) are common. The incidence of serious adverse neuropsychiatric reactions to mefloquine treatment is ~1 in 1000 in Asia but may be as high as 1 in 200 among Africans and Caucasians. All the antimalarial quinolines (chloroquine, mefloquine, and quinine) exacerbate the orthostatic hypotension associated with malaria, and all are tolerated better by children than by adults. Pregnant women, young children, patients unable to tolerate oral therapy, and nonimmune individuals (e.g., travelers) with suspected malaria should be evaluated carefully and hospitalization considered. If there is any doubt as to the identity of the infecting malarial species, treatment for falciparum malaria should be given. A negative blood smear makes malaria unlikely but does not rule it out completely; thick blood films should be checked again 1 and 2 days later to exclude the diagnosis. Nonimmune patients receiving treatment for malaria should have daily parasite counts performed until the thick films are negative. If the level of parasitemia does not fall below 25% of the admission value in 48 h or if parasitemia has not cleared by 7 days (and adherence is assured), drug resistance is likely and the regimen should be changed.

To eradicate persistent liver stages and prevent relapse (radical treatment), primaquine (0.5 mg of base/kg, adult dose) should be given daily for 14 days to patients with *P. vivax* or *P. ovale* infections after laboratory tests for G6PD deficiency have proved negative. If the patient has a mild variant of G6PD deficiency, primaquine can be given in a dose of 0.75 mg of base/kg (45 mg maximum) once weekly for 6 weeks. Pregnant women with vivax or ovale malaria should not be given primaquine but should receive suppressive prophylaxis with chloroquine (5 mg of base/kg per week) until delivery, after which radical treatment can be given.

COMPLICATIONS

Acute Renal Failure If the level of BUN or creatinine rises despite adequate rehydration, fluid administration should be restricted to prevent volume overload. As in other forms of hypercatabolic acute renal failure, renal replacement therapy is best performed early (Chap. 279). Hemofiltration and hemodialysis are more effective than peritoneal dialysis and are associated with lower mortality. Some patients with renal impairment pass small volumes of urine sufficient to allow control of fluid balance; these cases can be managed conservatively if other indications for dialysis do not arise. Renal function usually improves within days, but full recovery may take weeks.

Acute Pulmonary Edema (Acute Respiratory Distress Syndrome) Patients should be positioned with the head of the bed

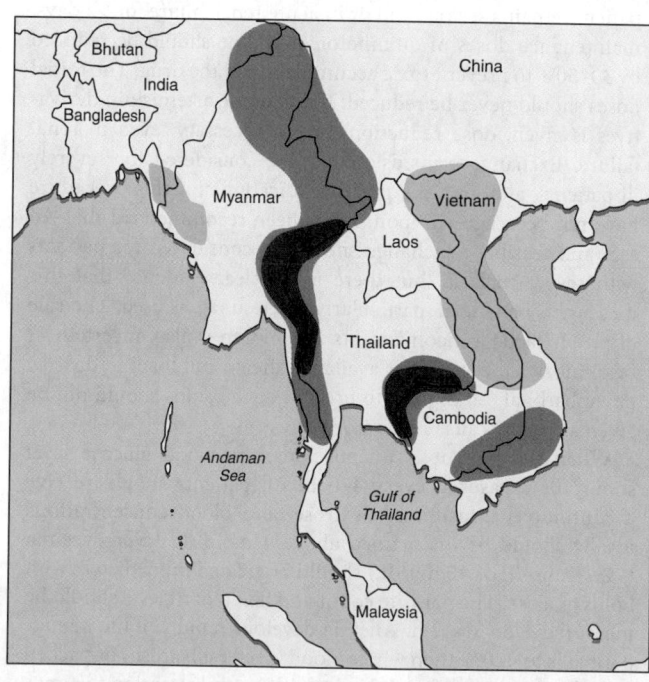

Figure 210-10 Mefloquine resistance in *Plasmodium falciparum* in Southeast Asia: high-level mefloquine resistance (*brown*), low-level mefloquine resistance (*red*), and mefloquine sensitivity (failure rate, <20%; *green*). There is insufficient information for other areas.

at a 45° elevation and given oxygen and IV diuretics. Pulmonary artery occlusion pressures may be normal, indicating increased pulmonary capillary permeability. Positive-pressure ventilation should be started early if the immediate measures fail (Chap. 235).

Hypoglycemia An initial slow injection of 50% dextrose (0.5 g/kg) should be followed by an infusion of 10% dextrose (0.10 g/kg per hour). The blood glucose level should be checked regularly thereafter as recurrent hypoglycemia is common, particularly among patients receiving quinine or quinidine. In severely ill patients, hypoglycemia commonly occurs together with metabolic (lactic) acidosis and carries a poor prognosis.

Other Complications Patients who develop spontaneous bleeding should be given fresh blood and IV vitamin K. Convulsions should be treated with IV or rectal benzodiazepines and, if necessary, respiratory support. Aspiration pneumonia should be suspected in any unconscious patient with convulsions, particularly with persistent hyperventilation; IV antimicrobial agents and oxygen should be administered, and pulmonary toilet should be undertaken. Hypoglycemia or gram-negative septicemia should be suspected when the condition of any patient suddenly deteriorates for no obvious reason during antimalarial treatment. In malaria-endemic areas where a high proportion of children are parasitemic, it is usually impossible to distinguish severe malaria from bacterial sepsis with confidence. It is increasingly accepted that these children should be treated with both antimalarials and broad-spectrum antibiotics from the outset. Because nontyphoidal *Salmonella* infections are particularly common, empirical antibiotics should be selected to cover these organisms. Antibiotics should be considered for severely ill patients of any age who are not responding to antimalarial treatment.

PREVENTION

In recent years, considerable progress has been made in malaria prevention, control, and research. New drugs have been discovered and developed, and one vaccine candidate has reached the stage of advanced field testing. Highly effective drugs, insecticide-treated nets, and insecticides for spraying dwellings are being purchased for endemic countries by the Global Fund to Fight AIDS, Tuberculosis, and Malaria; the President's Malaria Initiative; UNICEF; and other organizations. Malaria research and control are being strongly supported by the National Institute of Allergy and Infectious Diseases, the Wellcome Trust, the Bill & Melinda Gates Foundation, the WHO, the Multilateral Initiative on Malaria, the Roll Back Malaria Partnership, and the Global Health Council, among others. Still, the eradication of malaria is not feasible in the immediate future because of the widespread distribution of *Anopheles* breeding sites; the great number of infected persons; the continued use of ineffective antimalarial drugs; and inadequacies in human and material resources, infrastructure, and control programs. The call for and commitment to ultimate eradication of malaria by the Gates Foundation in 2007—seconded by Margaret Chan, Director General of the WHO—added great impetus to all malaria initiatives, especially those aimed at discovery and implementation of new interventions and other critical goals. Malaria may be contained by judicious use of insecticides to kill the mosquito vector, rapid diagnosis, appropriate patient management, and—where effective and feasible—administration of intermittent preventive treatment or chemoprophylaxis to high-risk groups such as pregnant women, young children, and travelers from nonendemic regions. Malaria researchers are intensifying their efforts to gain a better understanding of parasite-human-mosquito interactions and to develop more effective control and prevention interventions. Despite the enormous investment in efforts to develop a malaria vaccine and the 30–60% efficacy of

a recombinant protein sporozoite-targeted adjuvanted vaccine in limited field trials, no safe, effective, long-lasting vaccine is likely to be available for general use in the near future (Chap. 122). While there is great promise for one or more malaria vaccines on the more distant horizon, prevention and control measures continue to rely on antivector and drug-use strategies.

■ PERSONAL PROTECTION AGAINST MALARIA

Simple measures to reduce the frequency of infected-mosquito bites in malarious areas are very important. These measures include the avoidance of exposure to mosquitoes at their peak feeding times (usually dusk to dawn) as well as the use of insect repellents containing 10–35% DEET (or, if DEET is unacceptable, 7% picaridin), suitable clothing, and insecticide-impregnated bed nets or other materials. Widespread use of bed nets treated with residual pyrethroids reduces the incidence of malaria in areas where vectors bite indoors at night and has been shown to reduce mortality rates in western and eastern Africa.

■ CHEMOPROPHYLAXIS

(Table 210-8; *wwwnc.cdc.gov/travel/yellowbook/2010/chapter-2/malaria.aspx*) Recommendations for prophylaxis depend on knowledge of local patterns of *Plasmodium* species drug sensitivity and the likelihood of acquiring malarial infection. When there is uncertainty, drugs effective against resistant *P. falciparum* should be used [atovaquone-proguanil (Malarone), doxycycline, or mefloquine]. Chemoprophylaxis is never entirely reliable, and malaria should always be considered in the differential diagnosis of fever in patients who have traveled to endemic areas, even if they are taking prophylactic antimalarial drugs.

Pregnant women traveling to malarious areas should be warned about the potential risks. All pregnant women at risk in endemic areas should be encouraged to attend regular antenatal clinics. Mefloquine is the only drug advised for pregnant women traveling to areas with drug-resistant malaria; this drug is generally considered safe in the second and third trimesters of pregnancy, and the data on first-trimester exposure, although limited, are reassuring. Chloroquine and proguanil are regarded as safe. The safety of other prophylactic antimalarial agents in pregnancy has not been established. Antimalarial prophylaxis has been shown to reduce mortality rates among children between the ages of 3 months and 4 years in malaria-endemic areas; however, it is not a logistically or economically feasible option in many countries. The alternative—to give intermittent treatment doses [intermittent preventive treatment (IPT)]—shows promise for more widespread use in infants, young children, and pregnant women. Children born to nonimmune mothers in endemic areas (usually expatriates moving to malaria-endemic areas) should receive prophylaxis from birth.

Travelers should start taking antimalarial drugs 2 days to 2 weeks before departure so that any untoward reactions can be detected and so that therapeutic antimalarial blood concentrations will be present when needed (Table 210-8). Antimalarial prophylaxis should continue for 4 weeks after the traveler has left the endemic area, except if atovaquone-proguanil or primaquine has been taken; these drugs have significant activities against the liver stage of the infection (causal prophylaxis) and can be discontinued 1 week after departure from the endemic area. If suspected malaria develops while a traveler is abroad, obtaining a reliable diagnosis and antimalarial treatment locally is a top priority. Presumptive self-treatment for malaria with atovaquone-proguanil (for 3 consecutive days) or another drug can be considered under special circumstances; medical advice on self-treatment should be sought before departure for malarious areas and as soon as possible after illness begins. Every effort should be made to confirm the diagnosis by parasitologic studies.

TABLE 210-8 Drugs Used in the Prophylaxis of Malaria

Drug	Usage	Adult Dose	Pediatric Dose	Comments
Atovaquone/ proguanil (Malarone)	Prophylaxis in areas with chloroquine- or mefloquine-resistant *Plasmodium falciparum*	1 adult tablet PO[a]	5–8 kg: 1/2 pediatric tablet[b] daily ≥8–10 kg: 3/4 pediatric tablet daily ≥10–20 kg: 1 pediatric tablet daily ≥20–30 kg: 2 pediatric tablets daily ≥30–40 kg: 3 pediatric tablets daily ≥40 kg: 1 adult tablet daily	Begin 1–2 days before travel to malarious areas. Take daily at the same time each day while in the malarious areas and for 7 days after leaving such areas. Atovaquone-proguanil is contraindicated in persons with severe renal impairment (creatinine clearance rate <30 mL/min). In the absence of data, it is not recommended for children weighing <5 kg, pregnant women, or women breast-feeding infants weighing <5 kg. Atovaquone/ proguanil should be taken with food or a milky drink.
Chloroquine phosphate (Aralen and generic)	Prophylaxis only in areas with chloroquine-sensitive *P. falciparum*[c] or *P. vivax* only	300 mg of base (500 mg of salt) PO once weekly	5 mg/kg of base (8.3 mg of salt/kg) PO once weekly, up to maximum adult dose of 300 mg of base	Begin 1–2 weeks before travel to malarious areas. Take weekly on the same day of the week while in the malarious areas and for 4 weeks after leaving such areas. Chloroquine phosphate may exacerbate psoriasis.
Doxycycline (many brand names and generic)	Prophylaxis in areas with chloroquine- or mefloquine-resistant *P. falciparum*[c]	100 mg PO qd	≥8 years of age: 2 mg/kg, up to adult dose	Begin 1–2 days before travel to malarious areas. Take daily at the same time each day while in the malarious areas and for 4 weeks after leaving such areas. Doxycycline is contraindicated in children <8 years of age and in pregnant women.
Hydroxychloroquine sulfate (Plaquenil)	An alternative to chloroquine for primary prophylaxis only in areas with chloroquine-sensitive *P. falciparum*[c] or *P. vivax* only	310 mg of base (400 mg of salt) PO once weekly	5 mg of base/kg (6.5 mg of salt/kg) PO once weekly, up to maximum adult dose of 310 mg of base	Begin 1–2 weeks before travel to malarious areas. Take weekly on the same day of the week while in the malarious areas and for 4 weeks after leaving such areas. Hydroxychloroquine may exacerbate psoriasis.
Mefloquine (Lariam and generic)	Prophylaxis in areas with chloroquine-resistant *P. falciparum*	228 mg of base (250 mg of salt) PO once weekly	≤9 kg: 4.6 mg of base/kg (5 mg of salt/kg) PO once weekly 10–19 kg: 1/4 tablet once weekly 20–30 kg: 1/2 tablet once weekly 31–45 kg: 3/4 tablet once weekly ≥46 kg: 1 tablet once weekly	Begin 1–2 weeks before travel to malarious areas. Take weekly on the same day of the week while in the malarious areas and for 4 weeks after leaving such areas. Mefloquine is contraindicated in persons allergic to this drug or related compounds (e.g., quinine and quinidine) and in persons with active or recent depression, generalized anxiety disorder, psychosis, schizophrenia, other major psychiatric disorders, or seizures. Use with caution in persons with psychiatric disturbances or a history of depression. Mefloquine is not recommended for persons with cardiac conduction abnormalities.
Primaquine	For prevention of malaria in areas with mainly *P. vivax*	30 mg of base (52.6 mg of salt) PO qd	0.5 mg of base/kg (0.8 mg of salt/kg) PO qd, up to adult dose; should be taken with food	Begin 1–2 days before travel to malarious areas. Take daily at the same time each day while in the malarious areas and for 7 days after leaving such areas. Primaquine is contraindicated in persons with G6PD deficiency. It is also contraindicated during pregnancy and in lactation unless the infant being breast-fed has a documented normal G6PD level.
Primaquine	Used for presumptive antirelapse therapy (terminal prophylaxis) to decrease risk of relapses of *P. vivax* and *P. ovale*	30 mg of base (52.6 mg of salt) PO qd for 14 days after departure from the malarious area	0.5 mg of base/kg (0.8 mg of salt/kg), up to adult dose, PO qd for 14 days after departure from the malarious area	This therapy is indicated for persons who have had prolonged exposure to *P. vivax* and/or *P. ovale*. It is contraindicated in persons with G6PD deficiency as well as during pregnancy and in lactation unless the infant being breast-fed has a documented normal G6PD level.

[a]An adult tablet contains 250 mg of atovaquone and 100 mg of proguanil hydrochloride.

[b]A pediatric tablet contains 62.5 mg of atovaquone and 25 mg of proguanil hydrochloride.

[c]Very few areas now have chloroquine-sensitive malaria (Fig. 210-2).

Source: CDC: http://wwwn.cdc.gov/travel/contentMalariaDrugsHC.aspx.

Atovaquone-proguanil (Malarone; 3.75/1.5 mg/kg or 250/100 mg, daily adult dose) is a fixed-combination, once-daily prophylactic agent that is very well tolerated by adults and children, with fewer adverse gastrointestinal effects than chloroquine-proguanil and fewer adverse central nervous system effects than mefloquine. It is proguanil itself, rather than the antifolate metabolite cycloguanil, that acts synergistically with atovaquone. This combination is effective against all types of malaria, including multidrug-resistant falciparum malaria. Atovaquone-proguanil is best taken with food or a milky drink to optimize absorption. There are insufficient data on the safety of this regimen in pregnancy.

Mefloquine (250 mg of salt weekly, adult dose) has been widely used for malarial prophylaxis because it is usually effective against multidrug-resistant falciparum malaria and is reasonably well tolerated. The drug has been associated with rare episodes of psychosis and seizures at prophylactic doses; these reactions are more frequent at the higher doses used for treatment. More common side effects with prophylactic doses of mefloquine include mild nausea, dizziness, fuzzy thinking, disturbed sleep patterns, vivid dreams, and malaise. The drug is contraindicated for use by travelers with known hypersensitivity to mefloquine or related compounds (e.g., quinine, quinidine) and by persons with active or recent depression, anxiety disorder, psychosis, schizophrenia, another major psychiatric disorder, or seizures; mefloquine is not recommended for persons with cardiac conduction abnormalities. The role of mefloquine prophylaxis during pregnancy remains uncertain; in studies in Africa, mefloquine prophylaxis was found to be effective and safe during pregnancy. However, in one study from Thailand, treatment of malaria with mefloquine was associated with an increased risk of stillbirth.

Daily administration of doxycycline (100 mg daily, adult dose) is an effective alternative to atovaquone-proguanil or mefloquine. Doxycycline is generally well tolerated but may cause vulvovaginal thrush, diarrhea, and photosensitivity and cannot be used by children <8 years old or by pregnant women.

Chloroquine can no longer be relied upon to prevent *P. falciparum* infections in most areas but is used to prevent and treat malaria due to the other human *Plasmodium* species and for *P. falciparum* malaria in Central American countries west and north of the Panama Canal, Caribbean countries, and some countries in the Middle East. Chloroquine-resistant *P. vivax* has been reported from parts of eastern Asia, Oceania, and Central and South America. This drug is generally well tolerated, although some patients cannot take it because of malaise, headache, visual symptoms (due to reversible keratopathy), gastrointestinal intolerance, or pruritus. Chloroquine is considered safe in pregnancy. With chronic administration for >5 years, a characteristic dose-related retinopathy may develop, but this condition is rare at the doses used for antimalarial prophylaxis. Idiosyncratic or allergic reactions are also rare. Skeletal and/or cardiac myopathy is a potential problem with protracted prophylactic use; they are more likely to occur at the high doses used in the treatment of rheumatoid arthritis. Neuropsychiatric reactions and skin rashes are unusual. When used continuously, amodiaquine, a related aminoquinoline, is associated with a high risk of agranulocytosis (~1 person in 2000) and hepatotoxicity (~1 person in 16,000); thus this agent should not be used for prophylaxis.

Primaquine (daily adult dose, 0.5 mg of base/kg or 30 mg taken with food), an 8-aminoquinoline compound, has proved safe and effective in the prevention of drug-resistant falciparum and vivax malaria in adults. This drug can be considered for persons who are traveling to areas with or without drug-resistant *P. falciparum* and who are intolerant to other recommended drugs. Abdominal pain and oxidant hemolysis—the principal adverse effects—are not common as long as the drug is taken with food and is not given to G6PD-deficient persons, in whom it can cause hemolysis that is sometimes fatal. Travelers must be tested for G6PD deficiency

and be shown to have a level in the normal range before receiving primaquine. Primaquine should not be given to pregnant women or neonates. The 8-aminoquinolines (primaquine, tafenoquine) given in a single dose with ACT are being considered for widespread use in treatment regimens in malaria elimination programs because of their gametocytocidal effect on *P. falciparum.*

In the past, the dihydrofolate reductase inhibitors pyrimethamine and proguanil (chloroguanide) were administered widely, but the rapid selection of resistance in both *P. falciparum* and *P. vivax* has limited their use. Whereas antimalarial quinolines such as chloroquine (a 4-aminoquinoline) act on the erythrocyte stage of parasitic development, the dihydrofolate reductase inhibitors also inhibit preerythrocytic growth in the liver (causal prophylaxis) and development in the mosquito (sporontocidal activity). Proguanil is safe and well tolerated, although mouth ulceration occurs in ~8% of persons using this drug; it is considered safe for antimalarial prophylaxis in pregnancy. The prophylactic use of the combination of pyrimethamine and sulfadoxine is not recommended because of an unacceptable incidence of severe toxicity, principally exfoliative dermatitis and other skin rashes, agranulocytosis, hepatitis, and pulmonary eosinophilia (incidence, 1:7000; fatal reactions, 1:18,000). The combination of pyrimethamine with dapsone (0.2/1.5 mg/kg weekly; 12.5/100 mg, adult dose) has been used in some countries. Dapsone may cause methemoglobinemia and allergic reactions and (at higher doses) may pose a significant risk of agranulocytosis. Proguanil and the pyrimethamine-dapsone combination are not available in the United States.

Because of the increasing spread and intensity of antimalarial drug resistance (Figs. 210-2 and 210-10), the CDC recommends that travelers and their providers consider their destination, type of travel, and current medications and health risks when choosing antimalarial chemoprophylaxis. Consultation for the evaluation of prophylaxis failures or treatment of malaria can be obtained from state and local health departments and the CDC Malaria Hotline (770-488-7788) or the CDC Emergency Operations Center (770-488-7100).

FURTHER READINGS

BAIRD JK et al: Prevention and treatment of vivax malaria. Curr Infect Dis Rep 9:39, 2007

BREMAN JG: Eradicating malaria. Sci Prog 92:1, 2009

CENTERS FOR DISEASE CONTROL AND PREVENTION: Treatment of malaria (guidelines for clinicians). Atlanta, Department of Health and Human Services, 2010; available online at *wwwnc. cdc.gov/travel/yellowbook/2010/chapter-2/malaria.aspx*

DONDORP A et al: Artesunate versus quinine in the treatment of severe falciparum malaria in African children (AQUAMAT): An open-label randomized trial. Lancet 376:1647, 2010 (erratum Lancet 377:126, 2011)

GOMES MS et al: Pre-referral rectal artesunate to prevent death and disability in severe malaria: A placebo-controlled trial. Lancet 373:557, 2009

WHITE NJ: How antimalarial drug resistance affects post-treatment prophylaxis. Mal J 7:9, 2008

———: The assessment of antimalarial drug efficacy. Trends Parasitol 18:865, 2002

WORLD HEALTH ORGANIZATION: *Guidelines for the Treatment of Malaria*, 2nd ed. Geneva, World Health Organization, 2010 (*who.int/malaria/publications/atoz/9789241547925/en/*)

———: Assessment and monitoring of antimalarial drug efficacy for the treatment of uncomplicated falciparum malaria. WHO/HTM/RBM/2003.50; available online at *www.who.int/malaria/publications/atoz/whohtmrbm200350/en/*

CHAPTER 211

Babesiosis

Edouard Vannier
Jeffrey A. Gelfand

Babesiosis is a tick-borne infectious disease caused by parasites of the genus *Babesia*. These protozoans are obligate parasites of red blood cells (RBCs). Wild and domestic animals are the natural reservoirs of *Babesia*. Transmission to humans is incidental and was recognized only half a century ago. The vast majority of cases occur in the United States, where babesiosis has the status of an emerging infectious disease. Sporadic cases are reported in Europe and the rest of the world (see "Global Considerations," below).

■ EPIDEMIOLOGY

Geographic distribution

Babesia microti, a parasite of small rodents, is the etiologic agent of babesiosis in the northeastern United States. Highly endemic areas include Nantucket Island, Martha's Vineyard, Block Island, Shelter Island, eastern Long Island, and Fire Island. On the mainland, babesiosis is endemic in southeastern Massachusetts, coastal Rhode Island and Connecticut, central New Jersey, Wisconsin, and Minnesota. On the West Coast, the etiologic agent is *Babesia duncani*, a species closely related to those found in wildlife. The index case of infection with this species was reported from Washington State. Several cases were identified in northern California, and one case may have been contracted in central Oregon. Three cases of babesiosis caused by *Babesia divergens*–like organisms—from Washington State, Missouri, and Kentucky, respectively—have been reported.

Prevalence

The number of cases of *B. microti* illness has increased steadily over the last decade. In 2009, more than 700 cases were reported to the public health departments in endemic states. The prevalence of babesiosis caused by *B. microti* is underestimated because young healthy individuals typically experience a mild and self-limiting illness and may not seek medical attention. Accordingly, seroprevalence is much higher than the prevalence of clinical babesiosis.

Modes of transmission

The nymphal stage of the deer tick *Ixodes scapularis* is the primary vector for transmission of *B. microti*. Transmission occurs from May through September. The incubation period is 1–6 weeks long, with three-fourths of cases presenting in June and July. The vectors for transmission of *B. duncani* and *B. divergens*–like organisms remain unknown.

Babesiosis is occasionally acquired by transfusion of blood products, primarily packed RBCs; more than 70 such cases have been caused by *B. microti*, and two cases caused by *B. duncani* have been transmitted by this route. The incubation period lasts 1–9 weeks. Most cases occur in endemic areas during fall and winter. Some cases are diagnosed in nonendemic areas to which blood products have been imported from endemic areas. Of the 11 transfusion-related babesiosis deaths reported to the U.S. Food and Drug Administration since 1998, 10 have occurred since 2005.

Three cases of congenital babesiosis have been attributed to *B. microti*. Other cases of neonatal babesiosis have been acquired by transfusion or tick bite.

■ CLINICAL MANIFESTATIONS

Mild *B. microti* illness

Patients experience a gradual onset of malaise, fatigue, and weakness. Fever exceeds 38°C, can reach 40.6°C, and is accompanied by one or several of the following: chills, sweats, headache, myalgia, anorexia, dry cough, arthralgia, and nausea. Less common symptoms include neck stiffness, sore throat, shortness of breath, abdominal pain, and weight loss. On physical examination, fever is the salient feature. Development of *erythema chronicum migrans* is suggestive of intercurrent Lyme disease. Ecchymoses and petechiae have been reported. Mild splenomegaly and hepatomegaly are occasionally noted. Lymphadenopathy is absent. Jaundice, slight pharyngeal erythema, retinal infarcts, and retinopathy with splinter hemorrhages are rare.

Severe *B. microti* illness

Severe babesiosis is associated with parasitemia levels of >4% and requires hospitalization. Risk factors include an age of >50 years, male gender, asplenia, HIV/AIDS, malignancy, and immunosuppression. Compared with patients hospitalized for other febrile illnesses, patients with severe babesiosis are more likely to report malaise, myalgia or arthralgia, and shortness of breath. Complications develop in ~40% of hospitalized patients. Risk factors for complications are severe anemia (hemoglobin level ≤10 g/dL) and high-level parasitemia (>10%). Acute respiratory distress syndrome is the most common complication. Other complications include disseminated intravascular coagulation, congestive heart failure, and renal failure. Splenic infarcts and rupture have been reported. Strong predictors of poor outcome—defined as hospitalization for >2 weeks, stay in an intensive care unit for >2 days, or death—are male gender, alkaline phosphatase levels of >125 U/L, and white blood cell (WBC) counts of >5 × 10⁹/L. The fatality rate is 5% among all hospitalized patients but is much higher (20%) among immunocompromised patients.

Other babesial infections

Cases of *B. duncani* infection range in severity from asymptomatic to fatal. Clinical manifestations are those reported for *B. microti*. All three reported patients infected with *B. divergens*–like organisms required hospitalization; one died.

■ DIAGNOSIS

A diagnosis of babesiosis should be considered for any patient who (1) presents with flu-like symptoms and has recently resided in or traveled to an endemic area or received a blood transfusion or (2) presents with symptoms of or has been diagnosed with Lyme disease or human granulocytotropic anaplasmosis.

Babesiosis is diagnosed by microscopic examination of Giemsa-stained thin blood smears, on which *Babesia* species appear as round or pear-shaped organisms. The ring form is most common and lacks the central brownish deposit (hemozoin) typical of *Plasmodium falciparum* trophozoites (Chap. e27). Other distinguishing features are the absence of schizonts and gametocytes and the occasional presence of tetrads ("Maltese crosses"), which are pathognomonic of infection with *B. microti* or *B. duncani* but are also noted in human RBCs infected with *B. divergens*–like organisms. When parasitized RBCs are rare (particularly at the onset of symptoms), identification of the parasite may require multiple blood smears over several days. If babesiosis is suspected but the parasite cannot be identified by microscopy, amplification of babesial 18S rRNA by polymerase chain reaction (PCR) is recommended. Serology is useful to confirm the diagnosis. An indirect immunofluorescent antibody test for *B. microti* is available through the Centers for Disease Control and Prevention. IgM titers of ≥1:64 and IgG titers of ≥1:1024 signify active or recent infection. Titers typically decline over 6–12 months. Titers of <1:64 suggest complete clearance. Titers that remain positive (≥1:64) suggest persistent low-level parasitemia. Antibodies to *B. microti* do not react with *B. duncani* or *B. divergens*–like organisms.

Parasitemia levels typically range from 1% to 20% in immunocompetent hosts but can reach 85% in asplenic patients. Low hematocrit, low hemoglobin, low haptoglobin, and elevated lactate dehydrogenase levels are consistent with hemolytic anemia. Reticulocyte counts are elevated; thrombocytopenia is common. WBC counts are normal or slightly depressed. Liver function tests (alkaline phosphatase, aspartate and alanine aminotransferases, bilirubin) yield elevated values. Urinalysis may detect hemoglobinuria, excess urobilinogen, and proteinuria. Elevated concentrations of blood urea nitrogen and serum creatinine indicate renal compromise.

TREATMENT **Babesiosis**

(See Table 211-1) Whether *B. microti* infection should be treated depends on the clinical context. Asymptomatic infections need not be treated unless *Babesia* organisms are detected on blood smear or by PCR for >3 months. Symptomatic infections need not be treated if *Babesia* is not detected, despite positive serology. When *Babesia* is detected in symptomatic patients, treatment should be initiated.

MILD *B. MICROTI* ILLNESS The recommended regimen for treatment of mild illness due to *B. microti* is oral atovaquone plus azithromycin for 7–10 days. Clindamycin plus quinine is the second choice. The two regimens are equally effective, but atovaquone plus azithromycin is better tolerated. Symptoms should begin to abate within 48 h of the initiation of therapy and should resolve within 3 months. For immunocompromised patients, high-dose azithromycin (600–1000 mg/d) is recommended. Relevant antimicrobial therapy should be initiated when patients are also diagnosed with Lyme disease (Chap. 173) or human granulocytotropic anaplasmosis (Chap. 174)—conditions that should be sought whenever *B. microti* is diagnosed.

SEVERE *B. MICROTI* ILLNESS The recommended regimen for treatment of severe illness caused by *B. microti* is IV clindamycin plus oral quinine for 7–10 days. Oral quinine may be replaced with IV quinidine. Partial or complete RBC exchange transfusion is advised in cases of high-level parasitemia (>10%); severe anemia (hemoglobin, ≤10 g/dL); or pulmonary, hepatic, or renal compromise. Parasitemia and hematocrit should be monitored every day or every other day until symptoms recede and the parasitemia level is <5%.

A single course of standard antimicrobial therapy is often insufficient to eradicate symptoms and parasitemia in patients immunocompromised by splenectomy, HIV/AIDS, malignancy, or immunosuppressive therapy, including rituximab (anti-CD20) therapy for B cell lymphomas. In these patients, cure is more likely when therapy is administered for at least 6 weeks, including 2 weeks after parasites are no longer observed on blood smear. In immunocompromised patients with relapsing babesiosis, a second course of atovaquone plus azithromycin may fail to result in cure, despite >28 days of uninterrupted therapy. In the setting of severe disease, consideration should always be given to the possibility of intercurrent Lyme disease or human granulocytotropic anaplasmosis and empirical therapy for these infections considered until they are excluded.

TABLE 211-1 Treatment of Human Babesiosis

Organism	Severity	Adults	Children
B. microti	Mild[a]	Atovaquone (750 mg q12h PO)	Atovaquone (20 mg/kg q12h PO; maximum, 750 mg/dose)
		plus	*plus*
		Azithromycin (500–1000 mg/d PO on day 1, 250 mg/d PO thereafter)	Azithromycin [10 mg/kg qd PO on day 1 (maximum, 500 mg/dose), 5 mg/kg qd PO thereafter (maximum, 250 mg/dose)]
	Severe[a]	Clindamycin (300–600 mg q6h IV or 600 mg q8h PO)	Clindamycin (7–10 mg/kg q6–8h IV or 7–10 mg/kg q6–8h PO; maximum, 600 mg/dose)
		plus	*plus*
		Quinine (650 mg q6–8h PO)	Quinine (8 mg/kg q8h PO; maximum, 650 mg/dose)
		plus	*plus*
		Consider RBC exchange transfusion	Consider RBC exchange transfusion
B. divergens[b]		Immediate complete RBC exchange transfusion	Immediate complete RBC exchange transfusion
		plus	*plus*
		Clindamycin (600 mg q6–8h IV)	Clindamycin (7–10 mg/kg q6–8h IV; maximum, 600 mg/dose)
		plus	*plus*
		Quinine (650 mg q8h PO)	Quinine (8 mg/kg q8h PO; maximum, 650 mg/dose)

[a]Treatment for 7–10 days. In asplenic individuals and in immunocompromised patients, therapy should last for at least 6 weeks, including 2 weeks after parasites are no longer detected on blood smear.

[b]Treatment for 7–10 days, but duration may vary.

Abbreviation: RBC, red blood cell.

When clindamycin plus quinine fails to clear *B. microti* or when quinine must be discontinued, alternative regimens have been successful according to anecdotal reports. These empirical regimens have consisted of two- or three-drug combinations such as azithromycin plus quinine and clindamycin plus azithromycin added to doxycycline. In one immunocompromised patient, *B. microti* was cleared after administration of a five-drug regimen that consisted of clindamycin, quinine, azithromycin, atovaquone, and the combination of atovaquone-proguanil.

OTHER BABESIAL INFECTIONS The regimen for *B. duncani* infections typically consists of IV clindamycin (600 mg tid/qid or 1200 mg bid) plus oral quinine (600–650 mg tid) for 7–10 days. One relapse was cured with IV clindamycin (1200 mg tid) for 10 days. A pediatric case was successfully treated with IV clindamycin (40 mg/kg per day) plus oral quinine (25 mg/kg per day) for 15 days. The regimen for *B. divergens*–like infections typically consists of IV clindamycin (600 mg tid/qid, 900 mg tid, or 1200 mg bid) plus oral quinine or quinidine (650 mg tid).

■ PREVENTION

No vaccine is available for human use. There is no role for antibiotic prophylaxis. Individuals who reside in or travel to endemic areas, especially those at risk for severe babesiosis, should wear clothing that covers the lower part of the body, apply tick repellents (such as DEET) to clothing, and limit outdoor activities from May through September. A thorough skin examination should be conducted after outdoor activities and ticks removed using tweezers. Individuals with a history of symptomatic babesiosis or with positive antibody titers are indefinitely deferred from donating blood.

■ GLOBAL CONSIDERATIONS

Europe

About 30 cases of babesiosis have been attributed to *B. divergens*, a pathogen of cattle. Most cases have occurred in France, Ireland, and Great Britain. Sporadic cases have been reported from Croatia (index case), Spain, Portugal, and Sweden. Three cases—in Italy, Austria, and Germany, respectively—were caused by *Babesia* EU1, a parasite of roe deer. Both parasites are transmitted by the sheep tick *Ixodes ricinus*. The single reported case of *B. microti* infection was probably acquired by transfusion of a contaminated platelet concentrate.

Asplenia is a major risk factor for symptomatic *B. divergens* infection. The incubation period is 1–3 weeks long. The onset of hemoglobinuria and jaundice is sudden. Other symptoms include persistent fever (>41°C), shaking chills, drenching sweats, headache, myalgia, and lumbar and abdominal pain. Mild hepatomegaly may be noted. If the infection is not rapidly treated, the patient's condition deteriorates, with pulmonary edema and renal failure. In the past, most patients with severe cases died. Since exchange transfusion has been combined with chemotherapy, fatal cases have been rare. The overall fatality rate remains ~40%. All patients infected

with *Babesia* EU1 had been splenectomized, but their illness ranged from mild to severe; none died.

Because *B. divergens* infections are fulminant, the parasite is readily identified on blood smears. The parasitemia level may reach 80%. Serology is of no use because symptoms appear before antibody levels rise. In *Babesia* EU1 infection, the parasitemia level ranges from 1% to 30%. No serologic test specific for *Babesia* EU1 is available, but sera from patients infected with *Babesia* EU1 react with *B. divergens* antigen.

Babesiosis caused by *B. divergens* is a medical emergency. The recommended treatment is immediate complete blood exchange transfusion and therapy with IV clindamycin plus oral quinine or IV quinidine. In some cases, cure has been obtained with exchange transfusion and clindamycin monotherapy. Although uninfected RBCs are introduced by exchange transfusion, anemia may persist for >1 month. If so, additional transfusion is needed. One mild case was cured with IV pentamidine plus oral trimethoprim-sulfamethoxazole. *Babesia* EU1 infections have been treated with IV or oral clindamycin (600 mg tid) alone or in combination with oral quinine (650 mg tid). One patient who became intolerant to quinine was treated with oral atovaquone (750 mg bid) plus oral azithromycin (500 mg/d).

Rest of the world

A case of *B. divergens*–like infection has been identified on the Canary Islands, and isolated cases have been reported from South Africa, Mozambique, Egypt, and India. Two cases of *B. microti*–like infection have been reported in Taiwan and another in Japan. A patient in South Korea was infected with a *Babesia* species (KO1) related to species found in sheep. Asymptomatic infections have been identified in Mexico (*B. bigemina*, *B. canis*) and Colombia (*B. bigemina*, *B. bovis*). A case of *B. microti* infection diagnosed in Poland most likely was imported from Brazil.

FURTHER READINGS

Gubernot DM et al: Transfusion-transmitted babesiosis in the United States: Summary of a workshop. Transfusion 49:2759, 2009

Krause PJ et al: Persistent and relapsing babesiosis in immunocompromised patients. Clin Infect Dis 46:370, 2008

Tonnetti L et al: Transfusion-transmitted *Babesia microti* identified through hemovigilance. Transfusion 49:2557, 2009

Vannier E et al: Human babesiosis. Infect Dis Clin North Am 22:469, 2008

Wormser GP et al: Emergence of resistance to azithromycin–atovaquone in immunocompromised patients with *Babesia microti* infection. Clin Infect Dis 50:381, 2010

——— et al: The clinical assessment, treatment, and prevention of Lyme disease, human granulocytic anaplasmosis, and babesiosis: Clinical practice guidelines by the Infectious Diseases Society of America. Clin Infect Dis 43:1089, 2006

CHAPTER **212**

Leishmaniasis

Shyam Sundar

■ DEFINITION

Encompassing a complex group of disorders, leishmaniasis is caused by unicellular eukaryotic obligatory intracellular protozoa of the genus *Leishmania* and primarily affects the host's reticuloendothelial system. *Leishmania* species produce widely varying clinical syndromes ranging from self-healing cutaneous ulcers to fatal visceral disease. These syndromes fall into three broad categories: visceral leishmaniasis (VL), cutaneous leishmaniasis (CL), and mucosal leishmaniasis (ML).

■ ETIOLOGY AND LIFE CYCLE

Leishmaniasis is caused by ~20 species of the genus *Leishmania* in the order Kinetoplastida and the family Trypanosomatidae (Table 212-1). Several clinically important species are of the subspecies *Viannia*. The organisms are transmitted by phlebotomine sandflies of the genus *Phlebotomus* in the "Old World" (Asia, Africa, and Europe) and the genus *Lutzomyia* in the "New World" (the Americas). Transmission may be anthroponotic (i.e., the vector transmits the infection from infected humans to healthy humans) or zoonotic (i.e., the vector transmits the infection from an animal reservoir to humans). Human-to-human transmission via shared infected needles has been documented in IV drug users in the Mediterranean region. In utero transmission to the fetus occurs rarely.

Leishmania organisms occur in two forms: extracellular, flagellate promastigotes (length, 10–20 μm) in the sandfly vector and intracellular, nonflagellate amastigotes (length, 2–4 μm; Fig. 212-1) in vertebrate hosts, including humans. Promastigotes are introduced through the proboscis of the female sandfly into the skin of the vertebrate host. Neutrophils predominate among the host cells that first encounter and take up promastigotes at the site of parasite delivery. The infected neutrophils may undergo apoptosis and release viable parasites that are taken up by macrophages, or the apoptotic cells may themselves be taken up by macrophages and dendritic cells. The parasites multiply as amastigotes inside macrophages, causing cell rupture with subsequent invasion of other macrophages. While feeding on infected hosts, sandflies pick up amastigotes, which transform into the flagellate form in the flies' posterior midgut and multiply by binary fission; the promastigotes then migrate to the anterior midgut and can infect a new host when flies take another blood meal.

■ EPIDEMIOLOGY

Leishmaniasis occurs in 98 countries—most of them developing—in tropical and temperate regions (Fig. 212-2). Two million cases occur annually, of which 1–1.5 million are CL (and its variations) and 500,000 are VL. More than 350 million people are at risk, with an overall prevalence of 12 million. Although the distribution of *Leishmania* is limited by the distribution of sandfly vectors, human leishmaniasis is on the increase worldwide.

■ VISCERAL LEISHMANIASIS

VL (also known as *kala-azar*, a Hindi term meaning "black fever") is caused by the *L. donovani* complex, which includes *L. donovani* and *L. infantum* (the latter designated *L. chagasi* in the New World); these species are responsible for anthroponotic and zoonotic transmission, respectively. India and neighboring Nepal, Bangladesh, Sudan, and Brazil are the four largest foci of VL and account for 90% of the world's VL burden, with India the worst affected. Zoonotic VL is reported from all countries in the Middle East, Pakistan, and other countries from western Asia to China. Endemic foci also exist in the independent states of the former Soviet Union, mainly Georgia and Azerbaijan. In the Horn of Africa, Sudan, Ethiopia, Kenya, Uganda, and Somalia report VL. In Sudan, large outbreaks are thought to be anthroponotic, although zoonotic transmission also occurs. VL is rare in West and sub-Saharan Africa.

Mediterranean VL, long an established endemic disease due to *L. infantum*, has a large canine reservoir and was seen primarily in infants before the advent of HIV. In Mediterranean Europe, 70% of adult VL cases are associated with HIV co-infection. The combination is deadly because of the impact of the two infections together on the immune system. IV drug users are at particular risk. Other forms of immunosuppression (e.g., that associated with organ transplantation) also predispose to VL. In the Americas, disease caused by *L. infantum* is endemic from Mexico to Argentina, but 90% of cases in the New World are reported from northeastern Brazil.

Immunopathogenesis

The majority of individuals infected by *L. donovani* or *L. infantum* mount a successful immune response and control the infection, never developing symptomatic disease. Forty-eight hours after intradermal injection of killed promastigotes, these individuals exhibit delayed-type hypersensitivity (DTH) to leishmanial antigens in the leishmanin skin test (also called the Montenegro skin test). Results in mouse models indicate that the development of acquired resistance to leishmanial infection is controlled by the production of interleukin (IL) 12 by antigen-presenting cells and the subsequent secretion of interferon (IFN) γ, tumor necrosis factor (TNF) α, and other proinflammatory cytokines by the T helper 1 (T_H1) subset of T lymphocytes. The immune response in patients developing active VL is complex; in addition to increased production of multiple proinflammatory cytokines and chemokines, patients with active disease have markedly elevated levels of IL-10 in serum as well as enhanced IL-10 mRNA expression in lesional tissues. The main disease-promoting activity of IL-10 in VL may be to condition host macrophages for enhanced survival and growth of the parasite. IL-10 can render macrophages unresponsive to activation signals and inhibit killing of amastigotes by downregulating the production of TNF-α and nitric oxide. Multiple antigen-presentation functions of dendritic cells and macrophages are also suppressed by IL-10. Patients with such suppression do not have positive leishmanin skin tests, nor do their peripheral-blood mononuclear cells respond to leishmanial antigens in vitro. Organs of the reticuloendothelial system are predominantly affected, with remarkable enlargement of the spleen, the liver, and lymph nodes in some regions. The tonsils and intestinal submucosa are also heavily infiltrated with parasites. Bone marrow dysfunction results in pancytopenia.

Clinical features

On the Indian subcontinent and in the Horn of Africa, persons of all ages are affected by VL. In endemic areas of the Americas and the Mediterranean basin, immunocompetent infants and small children and immunodeficient adults are affected especially often. The most common presentation of VL is an abrupt onset of moderate- to high-grade fever associated with rigor and chills. Fever may continue for several weeks with decreasing intensity, and the patient may become afebrile for a short period before experiencing another bout of fever. The spleen may be palpable by the second

TABLE 212-1 Geographic Distribution and Characteristic Epidemiology of Leishmaniases

Organism, Endemic Region	Clinical Syndrome	Species	Vector	Reservoir	Transmission	Setting
L. donovani Complex						
South Asia	VL, PKDL	L. donovani	Phlebotomus argentipes	Humans	Anthroponotic	Rural, domestic
Sudan, Somalia, Ethiopia, Kenya, Uganda	VL, PKDL	L. donovani	P. orientalis, P. martini	Humans, rodents in Sudan, canines	Anthroponotic, occasionally zoonotic	Majority peridomestic, occasionally sylvatic
Mediterranean basin, Middle East, Central Asia, China	VL, CL	L. infantum	P. perniciosus, P. ariasi	Dogs, foxes, jackals	Zoonotic	Domestic, peridomestic
Middle East, Saudi Arabia, Yemen	VL	L. donovani	P. perniciosus, P. ariasi	Dogs, foxes, jackals	Zoonotic	Domestic, peridomestic
Central and South America	VL, CL	L. infantum	Lutzomyia longipalpis	Foxes, dogs, opossums	Zoonotic	Domestic, peridomestic, periurban
Azerbaijan, Armenia, Georgia, Kazakhstan, Kyrgyzstan, Tajikistan, Turkmenistan, Uzbekistan	VL	L. infantum	P. turanicus	Humans, dogs, foxes	Anthroponotic, zoonotic	Domestic
L. tropica						
Western India to Turkey, parts of North and East Africa	CL, leishmaniasis recidivans	L. tropica	P. sergenti	Humans	Anthroponotic	Urban domestic, peridomestic
L. major						
Western and Central Asia, North and sub-Saharan Africa	CL	L. major	P. papatasi, P. duboscqi	Nile rats, rodents	Zoonotic	Sylvatic, peridomestic
Kazakhstan, Turkmenistan, and Uzbekistan	CL	L. major	P. papatasi, P. duboscqi	Gerbils	Zoonotic	Rural
L. aethiopica						
Ethiopia, Uganda, Kenya	CL, DCL	L. aethiopica	P. longipes, P. pedifer	Hyraxes	Zoonotic	Sylvatic, peridomestic
Subspecies Viannia						
Peru, Ecuador	CL, ML	L. (V.) peruviana	Lutzomyia verrucarum, L. peruensis	Wild rodents	Zoonotic	Andean Valleys
Guyana, Surinam, French Guyana, Ecuador, Brazil, Colombia, Bolivia	CL, ML	L. (V.) guyanensis	L. umbratilis	Sloths, arboreal anteaters, opossums	Zoonotic	Tropical forests
Central America, Ecuador, Colombia	CL, ML	L. (V.) panamensis	L. trapidoi	Sloths	Zoonotic	Tropical forest and deforested areas
South and Central America	CL, ML	L. (V.) braziliensis	Lutzomyia spp., L. umbratilis, Psychodopygus wellcomei	Forest rodents, peridomestic animals	Zoonotic	Tropical forest and deforested areas
L. mexicana Complex						
Central America and northern parts of South America	CL, ML, DCL	L. amazonensis	L. flaviscutellata	Forest rodents	Zoonotic	Tropical forest and deforested areas
	CL, ML, DCL	L. mexicana	L. olmeca	Variety of forest rodents and marsupials	Zoonotic	
	CL, DCL	L. pifanoi	L. olmeca	Variety of forest rodents and marsupials	Zoonotic	Tropical forest and deforested areas

Abbreviations: CL, cutaneous leishmaniasis; DCL, diffuse cutaneous leishmaniasis; ML, mucosal leishmaniasis; PKDL, post–kala-azar dermal leishmaniasis; VL, visceral leishmaniasis.

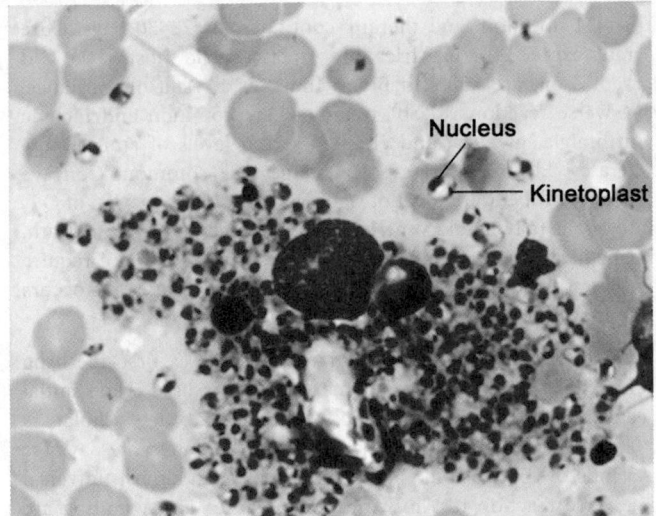

Figure 212-1 A macrophage with numerous intracellular amastigotes (2–4 μm) in a Giemsa-stained splenic smear from a patient with visceral leishmaniasis. Each amastigote contains a nucleus and a characteristic kinetoplast consisting of multiple copies of mitochondrial DNA. A few extracellular parasites are also visible.

week of illness and, depending on the duration of illness, may become hugely enlarged (Fig. 212-3). Hepatomegaly (usually moderate in degree) soon follows. Lymphadenopathy is common in most endemic regions of the world except the Indian subcontinent, where it is rare. Patients lose weight and feel weak, and the skin gradually develops dark discoloration due to hyperpigmentation that is most easily seen in brown-skinned individuals. In advanced illness, hypoalbuminemia may manifest as pedal edema and ascites. Anemia appears early and may become severe enough to cause congestive heart failure. Epistaxis, retinal hemorrhages, and gastrointestinal bleeding are associated with thrombocytopenia. Secondary infections such as measles, pneumonia, tuberculosis, bacillary or amebic dysentery, and gastroenteritis are common. Herpes zoster, chickenpox, boils in the skin, and scabies may also occur. Untreated, the disease is fatal in most patients, including 100% of those with HIV co-infection.

Leukopenia and anemia occur early and are followed by thrombocytopenia. There is a marked polyclonal increase in serum immunoglobulins. Serum levels of hepatic aminotransferases are raised in a significant proportion of patients, and serum bilirubin levels are elevated occasionally. Renal dysfunction is uncommon.

Laboratory diagnosis

Demonstration of amastigotes in smears of tissue aspirates is the gold standard for the diagnosis of VL (Fig. 212-1). The sensitivity of splenic smears is >95%, whereas smears of bone marrow (60–85%) and lymph node aspirates (50%) are less sensitive. Culture of tissue aspirates increases sensitivity. Splenic aspiration is invasive and may be dangerous in untrained hands. Several serologic techniques are currently used to detect antibodies to *Leishmania*. An enzyme-linked immunosorbent assay (ELISA) and the indirect immunofluorescent antibody test (IFAT) are used in sophisticated laboratories. In the field, however, a rapid immunochromatographic test based on the detection of antibodies to a recombinant antigen (rK39) consisting of 39 amino acids conserved in the kinesin region of *L. infantum* is used worldwide. The test requires only a drop of finger-prick blood or serum, and the result can be read within 15 minutes. Except in East Africa (where both its sensitivity and its specificity are lower), the sensitivity of the rK39 rapid diagnostic test in immunocompetent individuals is ~98% and its specificity is 90%. Qualitative detection of leishmanial nucleic acid by polymerase chain reaction (PCR) and quantitative detection by real-time PCR are confined to specialized laboratories and have yet to be used for routine diagnosis of VL in endemic areas. PCR can distinguish among the major species of *Leishmania* infecting humans.

Differential diagnosis

VL is easily mistaken for malaria. Other febrile illnesses that may mimic VL include typhoid fever, tuberculosis, brucellosis, schistosomiasis, and histoplasmosis. Splenomegaly due to portal hypertension, chronic myeloid leukemia, tropical splenomegaly syndrome, and (in Africa) schistosomiasis may also be confused with VL. Fever with neutropenia or pancytopenia in patients from an endemic region strongly suggests a diagnosis of VL; hypergammaglobulinemia in patients with long-standing illness strengthens the diagnosis. In nonendemic countries, a careful travel history is essential when any patient presents with fever.

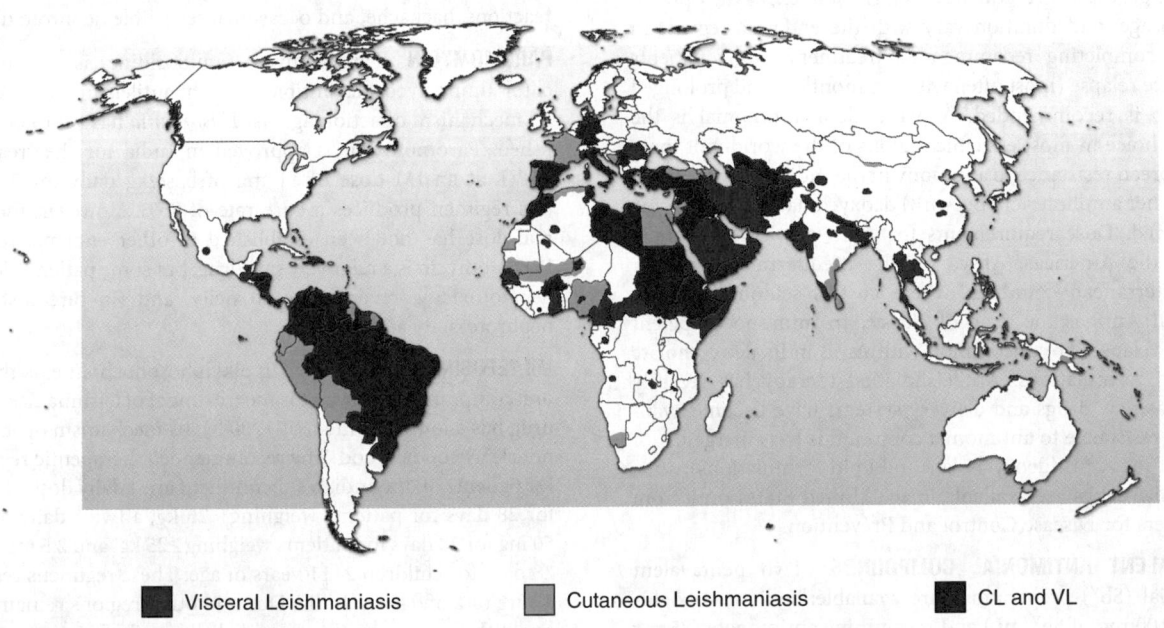

■ Visceral Leishmaniasis   ■ Cutaneous Leishmaniasis   ■ CL and VL

Figure 212-2 Worldwide distribution of human leishmaniasis.

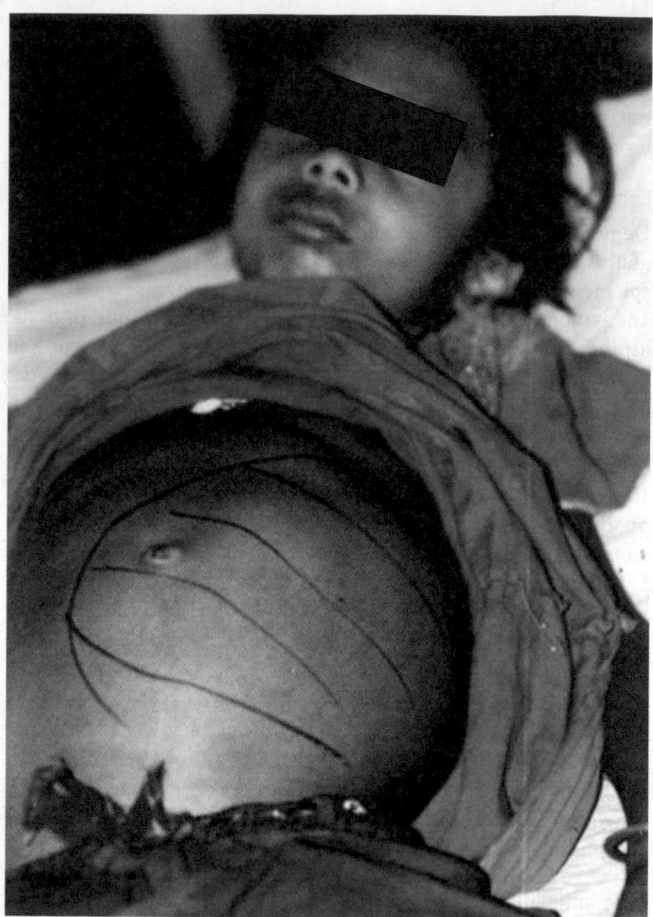

Figure 212-3 A patient with visceral leishmaniasis has a hugely enlarged spleen visible through the surface of the abdomen. Splenomegaly is the most important feature of visceral leishmaniasis.

TREATMENT   Visceral Leishmaniasis

GENERAL CONSIDERATIONS   Severe anemia should be corrected by blood transfusion, and other comorbid conditions should be managed promptly. Treatment of VL is complex, as the optimal drug, dosage, and duration vary with the endemic region. In spite of completing recommended treatment, some patients experience relapse (most often within 6 months), and prolonged follow-up is recommended. A pentavalent antimonial is the drug of choice in most endemic regions of the world, but there is widespread resistance to antimony in the Indian state of Bihar, where either amphotericin B (AmB) deoxycholate or miltefosine is preferred. Dose requirements for AmB are lower in India than in the Americas, Africa, or the Mediterranean region. In Mediterranean countries, where cost is seldom an issue, liposomal AmB is the drug of choice. In immunocompetent patients, relapses are uncommon with AmB in its deoxycholate and lipid formulations. Antileishmanial therapy has recently evolved as new drugs and delivery systems have become available and resistance to antimonial compounds has emerged.

Except for AmB (deoxycholate and lipid formulations), antileishmanial drugs are available in the United States only from the Centers for Disease Control and Prevention.

PENTAVALENT ANTIMONIAL COMPOUNDS   Two pentavalent antimonial (Sb^V) preparations are available: sodium stibogluconate (100 mg of Sb^V/mL) and meglumine antimonate (85 mg of Sb^V/mL). The daily dose is 20 mg/kg by rapid IV infusion

or IM injection, and therapy continues for 28–30 days. Cure rates exceed 90% in Africa, the Americas, and most of the Old World but are <50% in Bihar, India, as a result of resistance. Adverse reactions to Sb^V treatment are common and include arthralgia, myalgia, and elevated serum levels of aminotransferases. Electrocardiographic changes are common. Concave ST segment elevation is not significant, but prolongation of QT_c to >0.5 s may herald ventricular arrhythmia and sudden death. Chemical pancreatitis is common but usually does not require discontinuation of treatment; severe clinical pancreatitis occurs in immunosuppressed patients.

AMPHOTERICIN B   AmB is currently used as a first-line drug in Bihar. In others parts of the world, it is used when initial antimonial treatment fails. Conventional AmB deoxycholate is administered in doses of 0.75–1.0 mg/kg on alternate days for a total of 15 infusions. Fever with chills is an almost universal adverse reaction to AmB infusions. Nausea and vomiting are also common, as is thrombophlebitis in the infused veins. Acute toxicities can be minimized by administration of antihistamines like chlorpheniramine and antipyretic agents like acetaminophen before each infusion. AmB can cause renal dysfunction and hypokalemia and in rare instances elicits hypersensitivity reactions, bone marrow suppression, and myocarditis, all of which can be fatal.

The several lipid formulations of AmB developed to replace the deoxycholate formulation are preferentially taken up by reticuloendothelial tissues. Because very little free drug is available to cause toxicity, a large amount of drug can be delivered over a short period. Liposomal AmB has been used extensively to treat VL in all parts of the world. With a terminal half-life of ~150 h, liposomal AmB can be detected in the liver and spleen of animals for several weeks after a single dose. This is the only drug approved by the U.S. Food and Drug Administration (FDA) for the treatment of VL; the regimen is 3 mg/kg daily on days 1–5, 14, and 21 (total dose, 21 mg/kg). However, the total dose requirement for different regions of the world varies widely. In Asia, it is 10–15 mg/kg; in Africa, ~18 mg/kg; and in Mediterranean/American regions, not less than 20 mg/kg. The daily dose is flexible (1–10 mg/kg). In a study in India, a single dose of 10 mg/kg cured infection in 96% of patients. Adverse effects of liposomal AmB are usually mild and include infusion reactions, backache, and occasional reversible nephrotoxicity.

PAROMOMYCIN   Paromomycin (aminosidine) is an aminocyclitol-aminoglycoside antibiotic with antileishmanial activity. Its mechanism of action against *Leishmania* has yet to be established. Paromomycin is approved in India for the treatment of VL at an IM dose of 11 mg of base/kg daily for 21 days; this regimen produces a cure rate of 95%. However, the optimal dose has not been established in other endemic regions. Paromomycin is a relatively safe drug, but some patients develop hepatotoxicity, reversible ototoxicity, and (in rare instances) nephrotoxicity and tetany.

MILTEFOSINE   Miltefosine, an alkylphosphocholine, is the first oral compound approved for the treatment of leishmaniasis. This drug has a long half-life (150–200 h); its mechanism of action is not clearly understood. The recommended therapeutic regimens for patients on the Indian subcontinent are a daily dose of 50 mg for 28 days for patients weighing <25 kg, a twice-daily dose of 50 mg for 28 days for patients weighing ≥25 kg, and 2.5 mg/kg for 28 days for children 2–11 years of age. These regimens result in a cure rate of 94% in India. Doses in other regions remain to be established. Because of its long half-life, miltefosine is prone to induce resistance in *Leishmania*. Its adverse effects include mild to moderate vomiting and diarrhea in 40% and 20% of patients, respectively; these reactions usually clear spontaneously after a few days. Rare cases of severe allergic dermatitis, hepatotoxicity, and nephrotoxicity have been reported. Because miltefosine is expensive and is associated with significant adverse events, it is best administered as directly observed therapy to ensure completion of treatment and to minimize the risk of resistance induction. Because miltefosine is teratogenic in rats, its use is contraindicated during pregnancy and (unless contraceptive measures are strictly adhered to for at least 3 months after treatment) in women of childbearing age.

MULTIDRUG THERAPY Multidrug therapy for leishmaniasis is likely to be preferred in the future. Its potential advantages in VL include (1) better compliance and lower costs associated with shorter treatment courses and decreased hospitalization, (2) less toxicity due to lower drug doses and/or shorter duration of treatment, and (3) a reduced likelihood that resistance to either agent will develop. Trials of multidrug therapy are under way in Asia and Africa.

PROGNOSIS OF TREATED VL PATIENTS Recovery from VL is quick. Within a week of the start of treatment, defervescence, regression of splenomegaly, weight gain, and recovery of hematologic parameters are evident. With effective treatment, no parasites are recovered from tissue aspirates at the post-treatment evaluation. Continued clinical improvement over 6–12 months is suggestive of cure. A small percentage of patients (with the exact figure depending on the regimen used) relapse but respond well to treatment with AmB deoxycholate or lipid formulations.

VL IN THE IMMUNOCOMPROMISED HOST HIV/VL co-infection has been reported from 35 countries. VL behaves as an opportunistic infection in HIV-1-infected patients where both infections are endemic. HIV infection can increase the risk of developing VL severalfold in endemic areas. Co-infected patients usually show the classic signs of VL, but they may present with atypical features due to loss of immunity and involvement of unusual anatomic locations, with, for example, infiltration of the skin, oral mucosa, gastrointestinal tract, lungs, and other organs. Serodiagnostic tests are commonly negative. Parasites can be recovered from unusual sites such as bronchoalveolar lavage fluid and buffy coat. Liposomal AmB is the drug of choice for HIV/VL co-infection—both for primary treatment and for treatment of relapses. A total dose of 40 mg/kg, administered as 4 mg/kg on days 1–5, 10, 17, 24, 31, and 38, is considered optimal and is approved by the FDA, but most patients relapse within 1 year. Pentavalent antimonials and AmB deoxycholate can also be used where liposomal AmB is not accessible. Reconstitution of patients' immunity by antiretroviral therapy has led to a dramatic decline in the incidence of co-infection in the Mediterranean basin. In contrast, HIV/VL co-infection is on the rise in African and Asian countries. Ethiopia is worst affected: up to 30% of VL patients are also infected with HIV. Since restoration of the CD4+ T cell count to >200/µL does decrease the frequency of relapse, antiretroviral therapy (in addition to antileishmanial therapy) is a cornerstone for the management of HIV/VL co-infection. Secondary prophylaxis with liposomal AmB has been shown to delay relapses, but no regimen has been established as optimal.

■ **POST–KALA-AZAR DERMAL LEISHMANIASIS**

On the Indian subcontinent and in Sudan and other East African countries, 2–50% of patients develop skin lesions concurrent with

TABLE 212-2 Clinical, Epidemiologic, and Therapeutic Features of Post–Kala-Azar Dermal Leishmaniasis: East Africa and the Indian Subcontinent

Feature	East Africa	Indian Subcontinent
Most affected country	Sudan	Bangladesh
Incidence among patients with VL	~50%	~2%
Interval between VL and PKDL	During VL to 6 months	6 months to 3 years
Age distribution	Mainly children	Any age
History of prior VL	Yes	Not necessarily
Rashes of PKDL in presence of active VL	Yes	No
Treatment with sodium stibogluconate	2–3 months	2–4 months
Natural course	Spontaneous cure in majority of patients	Spontaneous cure not reported

Abbreviations: PKDL, post–kala-azar dermal leishmaniasis; VL, visceral leishmaniasis.

or after the cure of VL. Most common are hypopigmented macules, papules, and/or nodules or diffuse infiltration of the skin and sometimes of the oral mucosa. The African and Indian diseases differ in several respects; important features of post–kala-azar dermal leishmaniasis (PKDL) in these two regions are listed in Table 212-2, and disease in an Indian patient is depicted in Fig. 212-4.

In PKDL, parasites are scanty in hypopigmented macules but may be seen and cultured more easily from nodular lesions. Cellular infiltrates are heavier in nodules than in macules. Lymphocytes are the dominant cells; next most common are histiocytes and plasma cells. In about half of cases, epithelioid cells—scattered individually or forming compact granulomas—are seen. The diagnosis is based on history and clinical findings, but rK39 and other serologic tests are positive in most cases. Indian PKDL is treated with pentavalent antimonials for 60–120 days. This prolonged course frequently leads to noncompliance. The alternative—several courses of AmB spread over several months—is expensive and unacceptable for most patients. In East Africa, a majority of patients experience spontaneous healing. In those with persistent lesions, the response to 60 days of treatment with a pentavalent antimonial is good.

■ **CUTANEOUS LEISHMANIASIS**

CL can be broadly divided into Old World and New World forms. Old World CL caused by *L. tropica* is anthroponotic and is confined to urban or suburban areas throughout its range. Zoonotic CL is most commonly due to *L. major*, which naturally parasitizes several species of desert rodents that act as reservoirs over wide areas of the Middle East, Africa, and central and southern Asia. Local outbreaks of human disease are common. Major outbreaks currently affect Afghanistan and Pakistan in association with refugees and population movement. CL is increasingly seen in tourists and military personnel on mission in CL-endemic regions of countries like Afghanistan and Iraq and as a co-infection in HIV-infected patients. *L. aethiopica* is restricted to the highlands of Ethiopia, Kenya, and Uganda, where it is a natural parasite of hyraxes.

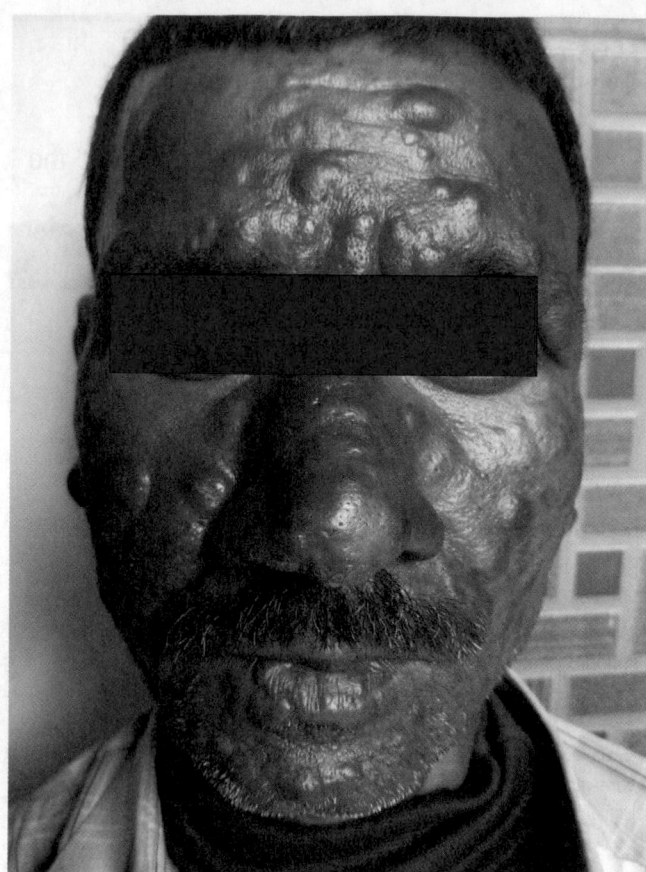

Figure 212-4 Post–kala-azar dermal leishmaniasis in an Indian patient. Note nodules of varying size involving the entire face. The face is erythematous, and the surface of some of the large nodules is discolored.

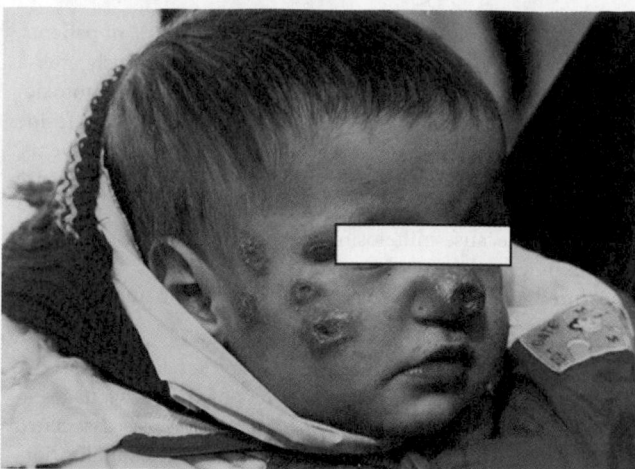

Figure 212-5 Cutaneous leishmaniasis in a Bolivian child. There are multiple ulcers resulting from several sandfly bites. The edges of the ulcers are raised. *(Courtesy of P. Desjeux.)*

New World CL is mainly zoonotic and is most often caused by *L. mexicana*, *L. (V.) panamensis*, and *L. amazonensis*. A wide range of forest animals act as reservoirs, and human infections with these species are predominantly rural. As a result of extensive urbanization and deforestation, *L. (V.) braziliensis* has adapted to peridomestic and urban animals, and CL due to this organism is increasingly becoming an urban disease. In the United States, a few cases of CL have been acquired indigenously in Texas.

Immunopathogenesis

As in VL, the proinflammatory (T$_H$1) response in CL may result in either asymptomatic or subclinical infection. However, in some individuals, the immune response causes ulcerative skin lesions, the majority of which will heal spontaneously, leaving a scar. Healing is usually followed by immunity to reinfection with that species of parasite.

Clinical features

A few days or weeks after the bite of a sandfly, a papule develops and grows into a nodule that ulcerates over some weeks or months. The base of the ulcer, which is usually painless, consists of necrotic tissue and crusted serum, but secondary bacterial infection sometimes occurs. The margins of the ulcer are raised and indurated. Lesions may be single or multiple and vary in size from 0.5 to >3 cm (Fig. 212-5). Lymphatic spread and lymph gland involvement may be palpable and may precede the appearance of the skin lesion. There may be satellite lesions, especially in *L. major* and *L. tropica* infections. The lesions usually heal spontaneously after 2–15 months. Lesions due to *L. major* and *L. mexicana* tend to heal rapidly, while those due to *L. tropica* and

parasites of subspecies *Viannia* heal more slowly. In CL caused by *L. tropica*, new lesions—usually scaly, erythematous papules and nodules—develop in the center or periphery of a healed sore, a condition known as *leishmaniasis recidivans*. Lesions of *L. mexicana* and *L. (V.) peruviana* closely resemble those seen in the Old World; however, lesions on the pinna of the ear are common, chronic, and destructive in the former infections. *L. mexicana* is responsible for chiclero's ulcer, the so-called self-healing sore of Mexico. CL lesions on exposed body parts (e.g., the face and hands), permanent scar formation, and social stigmatization may cause anxiety and depression and may affect the quality of life of CL patients.

Differential diagnosis

A typical history (an insect bite followed by the events leading to ulceration) in a resident of or a traveler to an endemic focus strongly suggests CL. Cutaneous tuberculosis, fungal infections, leprosy, sarcoidosis, and malignant ulcers are sometimes mistaken for CL.

Laboratory diagnosis

Demonstration of amastigotes in material obtained from a lesion remains the diagnostic gold standard. Microscopic examination of slit skin smears, aspirates, or biopsies of the lesion is used for detection of parasites. Culture of smear or biopsy material may yield *Leishmania*. PCR is more sensitive than microscopy and culture and allows identification of *Leishmania* to the species level. This information is important in decisions about therapy since responses to treatment can vary with the species. Isoenzyme profiling is used to determine species for research purposes.

TREATMENT Cutaneous Leishmaniasis

Although lesions heal spontaneously in the majority of cases, their spread or persistence indicates that treatment may be needed. One or a few small lesions due to "self-healing species" can be treated with topical agents. Systemic treatment is required for lesions over the face, hands, or joints; multiple lesions; large ulcers; lymphatic spread; New World CL with the potential for development of ML; and CL in HIV co-infected patients.

A pentavalent antimonial is the first-line drug for all forms of CL and is used in a dose of 20 mg/kg for 20 days, as for VL. The exceptions to this rule are CL caused by *L. (V.) guyanensis*, for which pentamidine isethionate is the drug of choice (two injections of 4 mg of salt/kg separated by a 48-h interval), and CL due to *L. aethiopica*, which responds to paromomycin (16 mg/kg daily) but not to antimonials. Relapses usually respond to a second course of treatment. In Peru, topical imiquimod (5–7.5%) plus parenteral antimonials have been shown to cure CL more rapidly than antimonials alone. Azoles and triazoles have been used with mixed responses in both Old and New World CL but have not been adequately assessed for this indication in clinical trials. In *L. major* infection, oral fluconazole (200 mg/d for 6 weeks) resulted in a higher rate of cure than placebo (79% vs. 34%) and also cured infection faster. Adverse effects include gastrointestinal symptoms and hepatotoxicity. Ketoconazole (600 mg/d for 28 days) is 76–90% effective in CL due to *L. (V.) panamensis* and *L. mexicana* in Panama and Guatemala. Miltefosine has been used in CL in doses of 2.5 mg/kg for 28 days. This agent is effective against *L. major* infections. In Colombia, where CL is due to *L. (V.) panamensis*, miltefosine was also effective, with a cure rate of 91%. For *L. (V.) braziliensis* infections, however, the results with miltefosine are less consistent. Other drugs, such as dapsone, allopurinol, rifampin, azithromycin, and pentoxifylline, have been used either alone or in combinations, but most of the relevant studies have had design limitations that preclude meaningful conclusions.

Small lesions (≤3 cm in diameter) may conveniently be treated weekly until cure with an intralesional injection of a pentavalent antimonial at a dose adequate to blanch the lesion (0.2–2.0 mL). An ointment containing 15% paromomycin sulfate plus 12% methylbenzonium chloride cures 70% of lesions due to *L. major* in 20 days and may be suitable for lesions caused by other species. Heat therapy with an FDA-approved radiofrequency generator and cryotherapy with liquid nitrogen have also been used successfully.

Diffuse cutaneous leishmaniasis (DCL)

DCL is a rare form of leishmaniasis caused by *L. amazonensis* and *L. mexicana* in South and Central America and by *L. aethiopica* in Ethiopia and Kenya. DCL is characterized by the lack of a cell-mediated immune response to the parasite, the uncontrolled multiplication of which thus continues unabated. The DTH response is negative, and lymphocytes do not respond to leishmanial antigens in vitro. DCL patients have a polarized immune response with high levels of immunosuppressive cytokines, including IL-10, transforming growth factor (TGF) β, and IL-4, and low concentrations of IFN-γ. Profound immunosuppression leads to widespread cutaneous disease. Lesions may initially be confined to the face or a limb but spread over months or years to other areas of the skin. They may be symmetrically or asymmetrically distributed and include papules, nodules, plaques, and areas of diffuse infiltration. These lesions do not ulcerate. The overlying skin is usually erythematous in pale-skinned patients. The lesions are teeming with parasites, which are therefore easy to recover. DCL does not heal spontaneously and is difficult to treat. If relapse and drug resistance are to be prevented, treatment should be continued for some time after lesions have healed and parasites can no longer be isolated. In the New World, repeated 20-day courses of pentavalent antimonials are given, with an intervening drug-free period of 10 days. Miltefosine has been used for several months with a good initial response. Combinations should be tried. In Ethiopia, a combination of paromomycin (14 mg/kg per day) and sodium stibogluconate (10 mg/kg per day) is effective.

■ MUCOSAL LEISHMANIASIS

The subgenus *Viannia* is widespread from the Amazon basin to Paraguay and Costa Rica and is responsible for deep sores and for ML (Table 212-1). In *L. (V.) braziliensis* infections, cutaneous lesions may be simultaneously accompanied by mucosal spread of the disease or followed by spread years later. ML is caused typically by *L. (V.) braziliensis* and rarely by *L. amazonensis*, *L. (V.) guyanensis*, and *L. (V.) panamensis*. Young men with chronic lesions of CL are at particular risk. Overall, ~3% of infected persons develop ML. Not every patient with ML has a history of prior CL. ML is almost entirely confined to the Americas. In rare cases, ML may also be caused by Old World species like *L. major*, *L. infantum*, or *L. donovani*.

Immunopathogenesis and clinical features

The immune response is polarized toward a T$_H$1 response, with marked increases of IFN-γ and TNF-α and varying levels of T$_H$2 cytokines (IL-10 and TGF-β). Patients have a stronger DTH response with ML than with CL, and their peripheral-blood mononuclear cells respond strongly to leishmanial antigens. The parasite spreads via the lymphatics or the bloodstream to mucosal tissues of the upper respiratory tract. Intense inflammation leads to destruction, and severe disability ensues. Lesions in or around the nose or mouth (espundia; Fig. 212-6) are the typical presentation of ML.

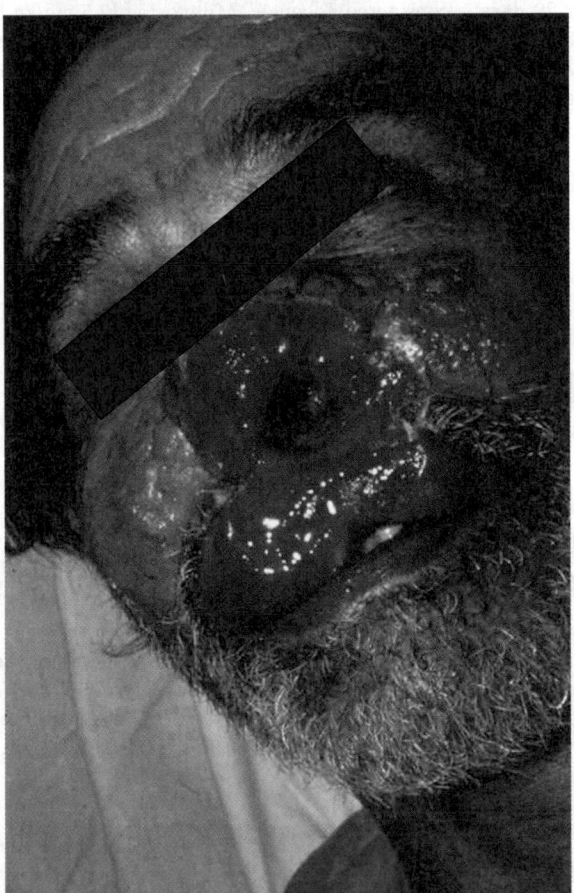

Figure 212-6 Mucosal leishmaniasis in a Brazilian patient. There is extensive inflammation around the nose and mouth, destruction of the nasal mucosa, ulceration of the upper lip and nose, and destruction of the nasal septum. *(Courtesy of R. Dietz.)*

Patients usually provide a history of self-healed CL preceding ML by 1–5 years. Typically, ML presents as nasal stuffiness and bleeding followed by destruction of nasal cartilage, perforation of the nasal septum, and collapse of the nasal bridge. Subsequent involvement of the pharynx and larynx leads to difficulty in swallowing and phonation. The lips, cheeks, and soft palate may also be affected. Secondary bacterial infection is common, and aspiration pneumonia may be fatal. Despite the high degree of T_H1 immunity and the strong DTH response, ML does not heal spontaneously.

Laboratory diagnosis

Tissue biopsy is essential for identification of parasites, but the rate of detection is poor unless PCR techniques are used. The strongly positive DTH response fails to distinguish between past and present infection.

TREATMENT	Mucosal Leishmaniasis

The regimen of choice is a pentavalent antimonial agent administered at a dose of 20 mg of Sb^V/kg for 30 days. Patients with ML require long-term follow-up with repeated oropharyngeal and nasal examination. With failure of therapy or relapse, patients may receive another course of an antimonial but then become unresponsive, presumably because of resistance in the parasite. In this situation, AmB should be used. An AmB deoxycholate dose totaling 25–45 mg/kg is appropriate. There are no controlled trials of liposomal AmB, but administration of 2–3 mg/kg for 20 days is considered adequate. Miltefosine (2.5 mg/kg for 28 days) cured 71% of ML patients in Bolivia. The more extensive the disease, the worse the prognosis; thus prompt, effective treatment and regular follow-up are essential.

■ PREVENTION OF LEISHMANIASIS

No vaccine is available for any form of leishmaniasis. Inoculation with live *L. major* ("leishmanization") is practiced in Iran. Anthroponotic leishmaniasis is controlled by case finding, treatment, and vector control with insecticide-impregnated bed nets and curtains and residual insecticide spraying. Control of zoonotic leishmaniasis is more difficult. Use of insecticide-impregnated collars for dogs, treatment of infected domestic dogs, and culling of street dogs are measures that have been used with uncertain efficacy to prevent transmission of *L. infantum*. Personal prophylaxis with bed nets and repellents may reduce the risk of CL infections in the New World.

FURTHER READINGS

ALVAR J et al: The relationship between leishmaniasis and AIDS: The second 10 years. Clin Microbiol Rev 21:334, 2008

AMATO VS et al: Mucosal leishmaniasis. Current scenario and prospects for treatment. Acta Trop 105:1, 2008

CHAPPUIS F et al: Visceral leishmaniasis: What are the needs for diagnosis, treatment and control? Nat Rev Microbiol 11:873, 2007

DEN BOER ML et al: Developments in the treatment of visceral leishmaniasis. Expert Opin Emerg Drugs 14:395, 2009

MAGILL AJ: *Leishmania* species: Visceral (kala-azar), cutaneous and mucosal leishmaniasis, in *Principles and Practice of Infectious Diseases*, 7th ed, GL Mandell et al (eds). Philadelphia, Churchill Livingstone Elsevier, 2010, pp 3463–3480

REITHINGER R et al: Cutaneous leishmaniasis. Lancet Infect Dis 7:581, 2007

SUNDAR S et al: Single-dose liposomal amphotericin B for visceral leishmaniasis in India. N Engl J Med 362:504, 2010

CHAPTER **213**

Chagas' Disease and Trypanosomiasis

Louis V. Kirchhoff

Anis Rassi, Jr.

Although the genus *Trypanosoma* contains many species of protozoans, only *T. cruzi*, *T. brucei gambiense*, and *T. brucei rhodesiense* cause disease in humans. *T. cruzi* is the etiologic agent of Chagas' disease in the Americas; *T. b. gambiense* and *T. b. rhodesiense* cause African trypanosomiasis.

CHAGAS' DISEASE

■ DEFINITION

Chagas' disease, or American trypanosomiasis, is a zoonosis caused by the protozoan parasite *T. cruzi*. Acute Chagas' disease is usually a mild febrile illness that results from initial infection with the organism. After spontaneous resolution of the acute illness, most infected persons remain for life in the indeterminate phase of chronic Chagas' disease, which is characterized by subpatent parasitemia, easily detectable antibodies to *T. cruzi*, and an absence of associated signs and symptoms. In 10–30% of chronically infected patients, cardiac and/or gastrointestinal lesions develop that can result in serious morbidity and even death.

■ LIFE CYCLE AND TRANSMISSION

T. cruzi is transmitted among its mammalian hosts by hematophagous triatomine insects, often called reduviid bugs. The insects become infected by sucking blood from animals or humans who have circulating parasites. Ingested organisms multiply in the gut of the triatomines, and infective forms are discharged with the feces at the time of subsequent blood meals. Transmission to a second vertebrate host occurs when breaks in the skin, mucous membranes, or conjunctivae become contaminated with bug feces that contain infective parasites. *T. cruzi* can also be transmitted by the transfusion of blood donated by infected persons, by organ transplantation, from mother to unborn child, by ingestion of contaminated food or drink, and in laboratory accidents.

■ PATHOLOGY

Initial infection at the site of parasite entry is characterized by local histologic changes that include the presence of parasites within leukocytes and cells of subcutaneous tissues and the development of interstitial edema, lymphocytic infiltration, and reactive hyperplasia of adjacent lymph nodes. After dissemination of the organisms

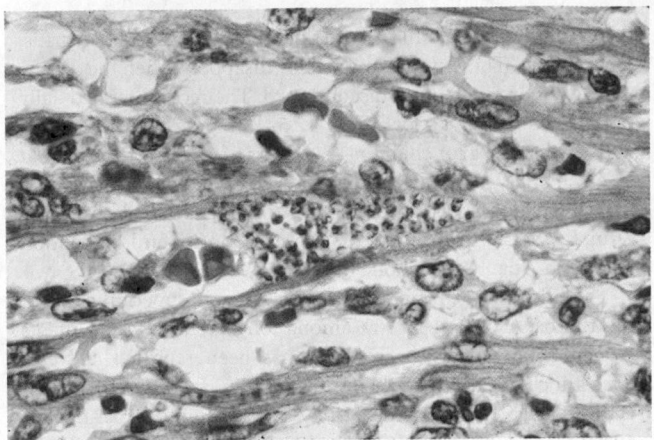

Figure 213-1 *Trypanosoma cruzi* in the heart muscle of a child who died of acute Chagas' myocarditis. An infected myocyte containing several dozen *T. cruzi* amastigotes is in the center of the field (hematoxylin and eosin, 900×).

through the lymphatics and the bloodstream, primarily muscles (including the myocardium) (Fig. 213-1) and ganglion cells may become heavily parasitized. The characteristic pseudocysts present in sections of infected tissues are intracellular aggregates of multiplying parasites.

In individuals with chronic *T. cruzi* infections who develop related clinical manifestations, the heart is the organ most commonly affected. Changes include thinning of the ventricular walls, biventricular enlargement, apical aneurysms, and mural thrombi. Widespread lymphocytic infiltration, diffuse interstitial fibrosis, and atrophy of myocardial cells are often apparent, but parasites are difficult to find in myocardial tissue by conventional histologic methods. Conduction-system abnormalities often affect the right branch and the left anterior branch of the bundle of His. In chronic Chagas' disease of the gastrointestinal tract (megadisease), the esophagus and colon may exhibit varying degrees of dilatation. On microscopic examination, focal inflammatory lesions with lymphocytic infiltration are seen, and the number of neurons in the myenteric plexus may be markedly reduced. Accumulating evidence implicates the persistence of parasites and the accompanying chronic inflammation—rather than autoimmune mechanisms—as the basis for the pathology in patients with chronic *T. cruzi* infection.

■ EPIDEMIOLOGY

T. cruzi is found only in the Americas. Wild and domestic mammals harboring *T. cruzi* and infected triatomines are found in spotty distributions from the southern United States to southern Argentina. Humans become involved in the cycle of transmission when infected vectors take up residence in the primitive wood, adobe, and stone houses common in much of Latin America. Thus human *T. cruzi* infection is a health problem primarily among the poor in rural areas of Mexico and Central and South America. Most new *T. cruzi* infections in rural settings occur in children, but the incidence is unknown because most cases go undiagnosed. Historically, transfusion-associated transmission of *T. cruzi* was a serious public health problem in many endemic countries. However, with some notable exceptions, transmission by this route has been essentially eliminated as effective programs for the screening of donated blood have been implemented. Several dozen patients with HIV and chronic *T. cruzi* infections who underwent acute recrudescence of the latter have been described. These

patients generally presented with *T. cruzi* brain abscesses, a manifestation of the illness that does not occur in immunocompetent persons. Currently, it is estimated that 8 million people are chronically infected with *T. cruzi* and that 14,000 deaths due to the illness occur each year. The resulting morbidity and mortality make Chagas' disease the most important parasitic disease burden in Latin America.

In recent years, the rate of *T. cruzi* transmission has decreased markedly in several endemic countries as a result of successful programs involving vector control, blood-bank screening, and education of at-risk populations. A major program, which began in 1991 in the "southern cone" nations of South America (Uruguay, Paraguay, Bolivia, Brazil, Chile, and Argentina), has provided the framework for much of this progress. Uruguay and Chile were certified free of transmission by the main domiciliary vector species (*Triatoma infestans*) in the late 1990s, and Brazil was declared transmission-free in 2006. Transmission has been reduced markedly in Argentina as well. Similar control programs have been initiated in the countries of northern South America and in the Central American nations.

Acute Chagas' disease is rare in the United States. Five cases of autochthonous transmission and five instances of transmission by blood transfusion have been reported. Moreover, *T. cruzi* was transmitted to five recipients of organs from three *T. cruzi*–infected donors. Two of these recipients became infected through cardiac transplants. Acute Chagas' disease has not been reported in tourists returning to the United States from Latin America, although three such instances have been reported in Europe. In contrast, the prevalence of chronic *T. cruzi* infections in the United States has increased considerably in recent years. An estimated 23 million immigrants from Chagas'-endemic countries currently live in the United States, ~17 million of whom are Mexicans. The total number of *T. cruzi*–infected persons living in the United States is estimated to be 300,000. Screening of the U.S. blood supply for *T. cruzi* infection began in January 2007. The overall prevalence of *T. cruzi* infection among donors is about 1 in 29,000, and to date more than 1200 infected donors have been identified and deferred permanently (see "Diagnosis," below).

■ CLINICAL COURSE

The first signs of acute Chagas' disease develop at least 1 week after invasion by the parasites. When the organisms enter through a break in the skin, an indurated area of erythema and swelling (the chagoma), accompanied by local lymphadenopathy, may appear. *Romaña's sign*—the classic finding in acute Chagas' disease, which consists of unilateral painless edema of the palpebrae and periocular tissues—can result when the conjunctiva is the portal of entry. These initial local signs may be followed by malaise, fever, anorexia, and edema of the face and lower extremities. Generalized lymphadenopathy and hepatosplenomegaly may develop. Severe myocarditis develops rarely; most deaths in acute Chagas' disease are due to heart failure. Neurologic signs are not common, but meningoencephalitis occurs occasionally, especially in children <2 years old. Usually within 4–8 weeks, acute signs and symptoms resolve spontaneously in virtually all patients, who then enter the asymptomatic or indeterminate phase of chronic *T. cruzi* infection.

Symptomatic chronic Chagas' disease becomes apparent years or even decades after the initial infection. The heart is commonly involved, and symptoms are caused by rhythm disturbances, segmental or dilated cardiomyopathy, and thromboembolism. Right bundle-branch block is a common electrocardiographic abnormality, but other types of intraventricular and atrioventricular blocks, premature ventricular contractions, and tachy- and bradyarrhythmias occur frequently. Cardiomyopathy often results in biventricular heart failure with a predominance of right-sided failure at advanced stages. Embolization of mural thrombi to the brain or other areas may take place. Sudden death is the main cause of death in Chagas' heart disease. Patients with megaesophagus suffer from dysphagia, odynophagia, chest pain, and regurgitation. Aspiration can occur (especially during sleep) in patients with severe esophageal dysfunction, and repeated episodes of aspiration pneumonitis are common. Weight loss, cachexia, and pulmonary infection can result in death. Patients with megacolon are plagued by abdominal pain and chronic constipation, which predisposes to fecaloma formation. Advanced megacolon can cause obstruction, volvulus, septicemia, and death.

■ DIAGNOSIS

The diagnosis of acute Chagas' disease requires the detection of parasites. Microscopic examination of fresh anticoagulated blood or the buffy coat is the simplest way to see the motile organisms. Parasites also can be seen in Giemsa-stained thin and thick blood smears. Microhematocrit tubes containing acridine orange as a stain can be used for the same purpose. When used by experienced personnel, all of these methods yield positive results in a high proportion of cases of acute Chagas' disease. Serologic testing plays no role in diagnosing acute Chagas' disease.

Chronic Chagas' disease is diagnosed by the detection of specific IgG antibodies that bind to *T. cruzi* antigens. Demonstration of the parasite is not of primary importance. In Latin America, ~30 assays are commercially available, including several based on recombinant antigens. Although these tests usually show good sensitivity and reasonable specificity, false-positive reactions may occur—typically with samples from patients who have other infectious and parasitic diseases or autoimmune disorders. In addition, confirmatory testing has presented a persistent challenge. For these reasons, the World Health Organization recommends that specimens be tested in at least two assays and that well-characterized positive and negative comparison samples be included in each run. The radioimmune precipitation assay (Chagas RIPA) is a highly sensitive and specific confirmatory method for detecting antibodies to *T. cruzi* (approved under the Clinical Laboratory Improvement Amendment and available in the authors' laboratory). In December 2006, the U.S. Food and Drug Administration (FDA) approved a test to screen blood and organ donors for *T. cruzi* infection (Ortho *T. cruzi* ELISA Test System, Ortho-Clinical Diagnostics, Raritan, NJ). Since January 2007, the vast majority of U.S. blood donors have been screened with the Ortho test, and positive units have undergone confirmatory testing in the Chagas RIPA. A second test for donor screening was approved by the FDA in April 2010 (Abbott PRISM® Chagas Assay, Abbott Laboratories, Abbott Park, IL). The use of PCR assays to detect *T. cruzi* DNA in chronically infected persons has been studied extensively. The sensitivity of this approach has not been shown to be reliably greater than that of serology, and no PCR assays are commercially available.

| TREATMENT | Chagas' Disease |

Therapy for Chagas' disease is still unsatisfactory. For many years now, only two drugs—nifurtimox and benznidazole—have been available for this purpose. Unfortunately, both drugs lack efficacy and may cause bothersome side effects.

In acute Chagas' disease, nifurtimox markedly reduces the duration of symptoms and parasitemia and decreases the mortality rate. Nevertheless, limited studies have shown that only ~70% of acute infections are cured parasitologically by a full course of treatment. Common adverse effects of nifurtimox include anorexia, nausea, vomiting, weight loss, and abdominal pain. Neurologic reactions to the drug may include restlessness,

disorientation, insomnia, twitching, paresthesia, polyneuritis, and seizures. These symptoms usually disappear when the dosage is reduced or treatment is discontinued. The recommended daily dosage is 8–10 mg/kg for adults, 12.5–15 mg/kg for adolescents, and 15–20 mg/kg for children 1–10 years of age. The drug should be given orally in four divided doses each day, and therapy should be continued for 90–120 days. Nifurtimox is available from the Drug Service of the Centers for Disease Control and Prevention (CDC) in Atlanta (telephone number, 404-639-3670).

The efficacy of benznidazole is similar or even superior to that of nifurtimox. A cure rate of 90% among congenitally infected infants treated before their first birthday has been reported. Adverse effects include rash, peripheral neuropathy, and rarely granulocytopenia. The recommended oral dosage is 5 mg/kg per day for 60 days for adults and 5–10 mg/kg per day for 60 days for children, with administration of two or three divided doses. Benznidazole is generally considered the drug of choice in Latin America.

The question of whether adults in the indeterminate or chronic symptomatic phase of Chagas' disease should be treated with nifurtimox or benznidazole has been debated for years. The fact that parasitologic cure rates in chronically infected persons are notably inferior to those in patients with acute or recent chronic infection is central to this controversy. No convincing evidence from randomized controlled trials indicates that nifurtimox or benznidazole treatment of adults in the indeterminate or chronic symptomatic phase reduces either the appearance and progression of symptoms or mortality rates. On the basis of results of some observational studies, a panel of experts convened by the CDC in 2006 recommended that adults <50 years old with presumably long-standing indeterminate *T. cruzi* infections—or even with mild to moderate disease—be offered treatment. A large randomized clinical trial (the BENEFIT multicenter trial) designed to assess the parasitologic and clinical efficacy of benznidazole in adults (18–75 years old) with chronic Chagas' heart disease (without advanced lesions) is being performed in Brazil, Argentina, Colombia, and Bolivia, but results will not be available until 2012 at the earliest. In contrast, randomized studies have shown that treatment of children is useful, and the current consensus of Latin American authorities is that all *T. cruzi*–infected persons up to 18 years old and all adults known to have become infected recently should be given benznidazole or nifurtimox.

The usefulness of antifungal azoles for the treatment of Chagas' disease has been studied in laboratory animals and to a lesser extent in humans. To date, none of these drugs has exhibited a level of anti–*T. cruzi* activity that would justify its use in humans. Several newer drugs in this class have shown promise in animal studies and are likely to undergo human trials in the near future.

Patients who develop cardiac and/or gastrointestinal disease in association with *T. cruzi* infection should be referred to appropriate subspecialists for further evaluation and treatment. Cardiac transplantation is an option for patients with end-stage chagasic cardiomyopathy; more than 150 such transplantations have been done in Brazil and the United States. The survival rate among Chagas' disease cardiac transplant recipients seems to be higher than that among persons receiving cardiac transplants for other reasons. This better outcome may be due to the fact that lesions are limited to the heart in most patients with symptomatic chronic Chagas' disease.

■ PREVENTION

Since drug therapy has limitations and vaccines are not available, the control of *T. cruzi* transmission in endemic countries depends on the reduction of domiciliary vector populations by spraying of insecticides, improvements in housing, and education of at-risk persons. As noted above, these measures, coupled with serologic screening of blood donors, have markedly reduced transmission of the parasite in many endemic countries. Tourists would be wise to avoid sleeping in dilapidated houses in rural areas of endemic countries. Mosquito nets and insect repellent can provide additional protection.

In view of the possibly serious consequences of chronic *T. cruzi* infection, it would be prudent for all immigrants from endemic regions who are living in the United States to be tested for evidence of infection. Identification of persons harboring the parasite would permit periodic electrocardiographic monitoring, which can be important because pacemakers benefit some patients who develop ominous rhythm disturbances. The possibility of congenital transmission is yet another justification for screening. *T. cruzi* is classified as a Risk Group 2 agent in the United States and a Risk Group 3 agent in some European countries. Laboratory staff should work with the parasite or infected vectors at containment levels consistent with the risk group designation in their areas.

SLEEPING SICKNESS

■ DEFINITION

Sleeping sickness, or human African trypanosomiasis (HAT), is caused by flagellated protozoan parasites that belong to the *T. brucei* complex and are transmitted to humans by tsetse flies. In untreated patients, the trypanosomes first cause a febrile illness that is followed months or years later by progressive neurologic impairment and death.

■ THE PARASITES AND THEIR TRANSMISSION

The East African (*rhodesiense*) and the West African (*gambiense*) forms of sleeping sickness are caused, respectively, by two trypanosome subspecies: *T. b. rhodesiense* and *T. b. gambiense*. These subspecies are morphologically indistinguishable but cause illnesses that are epidemiologically and clinically distinct (Table 213-1). The parasites are transmitted by blood-sucking

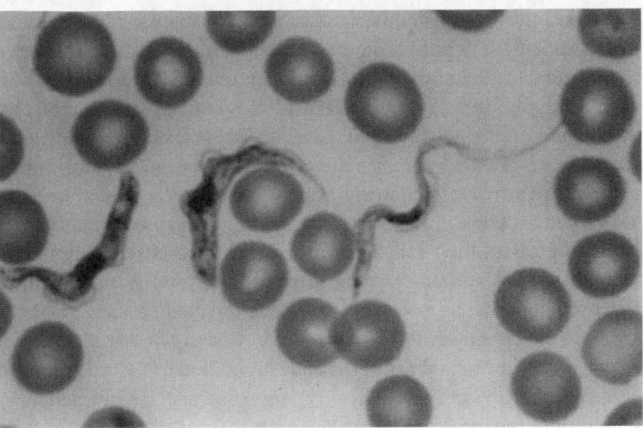

Figure 213-2 *Trypanosoma brucei rhodesiense* parasites in rat blood. The slender parasite is thought to be the form that multiplies in mammalian hosts, while the stumpy forms are nondividing and are capable of infecting insect vectors (Giemsa, 1200×). *(Courtesy of Dr. G. A. Cook, Madison, WI; with permission.)*

tsetse flies of the genus *Glossina*. The insects acquire the infection when they ingest blood from infected mammalian hosts. After many cycles of multiplication in the midgut of the vector, the parasites migrate to the salivary glands. Their transmission takes place when they are inoculated into a mammalian host during a subsequent blood meal. The injected trypanosomes multiply in the blood (Fig. 213-2) and other extracellular spaces and evade immune destruction for long periods by undergoing antigenic variation, a process driven by gene switching in which the antigenic structure of the organisms' surface coat of glycoproteins changes periodically.

■ PATHOGENESIS AND PATHOLOGY

A self-limited inflammatory lesion (trypanosomal chancre) may appear a week or so after the bite of an infected tsetse fly. A systemic febrile illness then evolves as the parasites are disseminated through the lymphatics and bloodstream. Systemic HAT without central nervous system (CNS) involvement is generally referred to as *stage I disease*. In this stage, widespread lymphadenopathy and splenomegaly reflect marked lymphocytic and histiocytic proliferation and invasion of morular cells, which are plasmacytes that may be involved in the production of IgM. Endarteritis, with perivascular infiltration of both parasites and lymphocytes, may develop in lymph nodes and the spleen. Myocarditis develops frequently in patients with stage I disease and is especially common in *T. b. rhodesiense* infections.

Hematologic manifestations that accompany stage I HAT include moderate leukocytosis, thrombocytopenia, and anemia. High levels of immunoglobulins, consisting primarily of polyclonal IgM, are a constant feature, and heterophile antibodies, antibodies to DNA, and rheumatoid factor are often detected. High levels of antigen-antibody complexes may play a role in the tissue damage and increased vascular permeability that facilitate dissemination of the parasites.

Stage II disease involves invasion of the CNS. The presence of trypanosomes in perivascular areas is accompanied by intense infiltration of mononuclear cells. Abnormalities in cerebrospinal fluid (CSF) include increased pressure, elevated total protein concentration, and pleocytosis. In addition, trypanosomes are frequently found in CSF.

■ EPIDEMIOLOGY

The trypanosomes that cause sleeping sickness are found only in sub-Saharan Africa. After its near-eradication in the mid-1960s, sleeping sickness underwent a resurgence in the

TABLE 213-1 Comparison of West African and East African Trypanosomiases

Point of Comparison	West African (Gambiense)	East African (Rhodesiense)
Organism	*T. b. gambiense*	*T. b. rhodesiense*
Vectors	Tsetse flies (palpalis group)	Tsetse flies (morsitans group)
Primary reservoir	Humans	Antelope and cattle
Human illness	Chronic (late CNS disease)	Acute (early CNS disease)
Duration of illness	Months to years	<9 months
Lymphadenopathy	Prominent	Minimal
Parasitemia	Low	High
Diagnosis by rodent inoculation	No	Yes
Epidemiology	Rural populations	Workers in wild areas, rural populations, tourists in game parks

Abbreviation: CNS, central nervous system.

Source: Reprinted with permission from LV Kirchhoff in GL Mandell et al (eds): *Principles and Practice of Infectious Diseases*, 7th ed. Philadelphia, Elsevier Churchill Livingstone, 2010.

1990s, primarily in Uganda, Sudan, the Central African Republic, the Democratic Republic of the Congo, and Angola. Although a subsequent increase in control activities reduced the incidence in many endemic areas, the World Health Organization estimated that there were 50,000–70,000 new cases in 2004, the vast majority of which were caused by *T. b. gambiense*. Approximately 50 million persons are at risk of acquiring HAT.

Humans are the only reservoir of *T. b. gambiense*, which occurs in widely distributed foci in tropical rain forests of Central and West Africa. *Gambiense* trypanosomiasis is primarily a problem in rural populations; tourists rarely become infected. Trypanotolerant antelope species in savanna and woodland areas of Central and East Africa are the principal reservoir of *T. b. rhodesiense*. Cattle can also be infected with this and other trypanosome species but generally succumb to the infection. Since risk results from contact with tsetse flies that feed on wild animals, humans acquire *T. b. rhodesiense* infection only incidentally, usually while visiting or working in areas where infected game and vectors are present. Roughly one or two imported cases of HAT acquired in East African parks are reported to the CDC each year.

■ CLINICAL COURSE

A painful trypanosomal chancre appears in some patients at the site of inoculation of the parasite. Hematogenous and lymphatic dissemination (stage I disease) is marked by the onset of fever. Typically, bouts of high temperatures lasting several days are separated by afebrile periods. Lymphadenopathy is prominent in *T. b. gambiense* trypanosomiasis. The nodes are discrete, movable, rubbery, and nontender. Cervical nodes are often visible, and enlargement of the nodes of the posterior cervical triangle, or *Winterbottom's sign*, is a classic finding. Pruritus and maculopapular rashes are common. Inconstant findings include malaise, headache, arthralgias, weight loss, edema, hepatosplenomegaly, and tachycardia. The differential diagnosis of stage I HAT includes many diseases that are common in the tropics and are associated with fevers. HIV infection, malaria, and typhoid fever are common in populations at risk for HAT and need to be considered.

CNS invasion (stage II disease) is characterized by the insidious development of protean neurologic manifestations that are accompanied by progressive abnormalities in the CSF. A picture of progressive indifference and daytime somnolence develops (hence the designation "sleeping sickness"), sometimes alternating with restlessness and insomnia at night. A listless gaze accompanies a loss of spontaneity, and speech may become halting and indistinct. Extrapyramidal signs may include choreiform movements, tremors, and fasciculations. Ataxia is frequent, and the patient may appear to have Parkinson's disease, with a shuffling gait, hypertonia, and tremors. In the final phase, progressive neurologic impairment ends in coma and death.

The most striking difference between the *gambiense* and *rhodesiense* forms of HAT is that the latter illness tends to follow a more acute course. Typically, in tourists with *T. b. rhodesiense* disease, systemic signs of infection, such as fever, malaise, and headache, appear before the end of the trip or shortly after the return home. Persistent tachycardia unrelated to fever is common early in the course of *T. b. rhodesiense* trypanosomiasis, and death may result from arrhythmias and congestive heart failure before CNS disease develops. In general, untreated *T. b. rhodesiense* trypanosomiasis leads to death in a matter of weeks to months, often without a clear distinction between the hemolymphatic and CNS stages. In contrast, *T. b. gambiense* disease can smolder for many months or even for years.

■ DIAGNOSIS

A definitive diagnosis of HAT requires detection of the parasite. If a chancre is present, fluid should be expressed and examined directly by light microscopy for the highly motile trypanosomes. The fluid also should be fixed and stained with Giemsa. Material obtained by needle aspiration of lymph nodes early in the illness should be examined similarly. Examination of wet preparations and Giemsa-stained thin and thick films of serial blood samples is also useful. If parasites are not seen initially in blood, efforts should be made to concentrate the organisms, which can be done in microhematocrit tubes containing acridine orange. Alternatively, the buffy coat from 10–15 mL of anticoagulated blood can be examined directly under a microscope. The likelihood of finding parasites in blood is higher in stage I than in stage II disease and in patients infected with *T. b. rhodesiense* rather than *T. b. gambiense*. Trypanosomes may also be seen in material aspirated from the bone marrow; the aspirate can be inoculated into liquid culture medium, as can blood, buffy coat, lymph node aspirates, and CSF. Finally, *T. b. rhodesiense* infection can be detected by inoculation of these specimens into mice or rats, which—when positive—results in patent parasitemias in a week or two. Although this method is highly sensitive for the detection of *T. b. rhodesiense*, it does not detect *T. b. gambiense* because of host specificity.

It is essential to examine CSF from all patients in whom HAT is suspected. Abnormalities in the CSF that may be associated with stage II disease include an increase in the CSF mononuclear cell count as well as increases in opening pressure and in levels of total protein and IgM. Trypanosomes may be seen in the sediment of centrifuged CSF. Any CSF abnormality in a patient in whom trypanosomes have been found at other sites must be viewed as pathognomonic for CNS involvement and thus must prompt specific treatment for CNS disease. In patients with CSF pleocytosis in whom parasites are not found, tuberculous meningitis and HIV-associated CNS infections such as cryptococcosis should be considered in the differential diagnosis.

A number of serologic assays, such as the card agglutination test for trypanosomes (CATT) for *T. b. gambiense*, are available to aid in the diagnosis of HAT, but their variable sensitivity and specificity mandate that decisions about treatment be based on demonstration of the parasite. These tests are of value for epidemiologic surveys. PCR assays for detecting African trypanosomes in humans have been developed, but none is commercially available.

TREATMENT   Sleeping Sickness

The drugs used for treatment of HAT are suramin, pentamidine, eflornithine, and the organic arsenical melarsoprol. In the United States, these drugs can be obtained from the CDC. Therapy for HAT must be individualized on the basis of the infecting subspecies, the presence or absence of CNS disease, adverse reactions, and occasionally drug resistance. The choices of drugs for the treatment of HAT are summarized in Table 213-2.

Suramin is highly effective against stage I *rhodesiense* HAT. However, it can cause serious adverse effects and must be administered under the close supervision of a physician. A 100- to 200-mg IV test dose should be given to detect hypersensitivity. The dosage for adults is 20 mg/kg on days 1, 5, 12, 18, and 26. The drug is given by slow IV infusion of a freshly prepared 10% aqueous solution. Approximately 1 patient in 20,000 has an immediate, severe, and potentially fatal reaction to the drug, developing nausea, vomiting, shock, and seizures. Less severe reactions include fever, photophobia, pruritus, arthralgias, and skin eruptions. Renal damage is the most common important adverse effect of suramin. Transient proteinuria often appears during treatment. A urinalysis should be done before each dose, and treatment should be discontinued if proteinuria increases or

TABLE 213-2 Treatment of Human African Trypanosomiases[a]

Causative Organism	Clinical Stage	
	I (Normal CSF)	II (Abnormal CSF)
T. brucei gambiense (West African)	Pentamidine Alternative: Suramin	Eflornithine Alternative: Melarsoprol
T. brucei rhodesiense (East African)	Suramin	Melarsoprol

[a]For doses and duration, see text.
Abbreviation: CSF, cerebrospinal fluid.

if casts and red cells appear in the sediment. Suramin should not be given to patients with renal insufficiency.

Pentamidine is the first-line drug for treatment of stage I *gambiense* HAT. The dose for both adults and children is 4 mg/kg per day, given IM or IV for 7–10 days. Frequent, immediate adverse reactions include nausea, vomiting, tachycardia, and hypotension. These reactions are usually transient and do not warrant cessation of therapy. Other adverse reactions include nephrotoxicity, abnormal liver function tests, neutropenia, rashes, hypoglycemia, and sterile abscesses. Suramin is an alternative agent for stage I *T. b. gambiense* disease.

Eflornithine is highly effective for treatment of both stages of *gambiense* sleeping sickness. In the trials on which the FDA based its approval, this agent cured >90% of 600 patients with stage II disease. The recommended treatment schedule is 400 mg/kg per day, given IV in four divided doses, for 2 weeks. Adverse reactions include diarrhea, anemia, thrombocytopenia, seizures, and hearing loss. The high dosage and duration of therapy required are disadvantages that make widespread use of eflornithine difficult. A randomized trial comparing the standard eflornithine regimen (400 mg/kg per day infused over 6 h for 14 days) with nifurtimox-eflornithine combination therapy (oral nifurtimox, 15 mg/kg per day for 10 days; plus eflornithine, 400 mg/kg per day infused over 12 h for 7 days) in adults with stage II *gambiense* HAT showed improved efficacy and reduced adverse effects with combination therapy, making it suitable for first-line use.

The arsenical melarsoprol is the drug of choice for the treatment of *rhodesiense* HAT with CNS involvement and is an alternative agent for stage II *gambiense* disease. For *rhodesiense* disease, the drug should be given to adults in three courses of 3 days each. The dosage is 2.0–3.6 mg/kg per day, given IV in three divided doses for 3 days and followed 1 week later by 3.6 mg/kg per day, also in three divided doses and for 3 days. The latter course is repeated 7 days later. In debilitated patients, suramin is administered for 2–4 days before therapy with melarsoprol is initiated; an 18-mg initial dose of the latter drug, followed by progressive increases to the standard dose, has been recommended. For children, a total of 18–25 mg/kg should be given over 1 month. An IV starting dose of 0.36 mg/kg should be increased gradually to a maximum of 3.6 mg/kg at 1- to 5-day intervals, for a total of 9 or 10 doses. The regimen for *gambiense* disease is 2.2 mg/kg per day, given IV for 10 days.

Melarsoprol is highly toxic and should be administered with great care. To reduce the likelihood of drug-induced encephalopathy, all patients receiving melarsoprol should be given prednisolone at a dose of 1 mg/kg (up to 40 mg) per day, beginning 1–2 days before the first dose of melarsoprol and continuing through the last dose. Without prednisolone prophylaxis, the incidence of reactive encephalopathy has been reported to be as high as 18% in some series. Clinical manifestations of reactive encephalopathy include high fever, headache, tremor, impaired speech, seizures, and even coma and death. Treatment with melarsoprol should be discontinued at the first sign of encephalopathy but may be restarted cautiously at lower doses a few days after signs have resolved. Extravasation of the drug results in intense local reactions. Vomiting, abdominal pain, nephrotoxicity, and myocardial damage can occur.

■ PREVENTION

HAT poses complex public-health and epizootic problems in Africa. Considerable progress has been made in some areas through control programs that focus on eradication of vectors and drug treatment of infected humans. People can reduce their risk of acquiring trypanosomiasis by avoiding areas known to harbor infected insects, by wearing protective clothing, and by using insect repellent. Chemoprophylaxis is not recommended, and no vaccine is available to prevent transmission of the parasites.

FURTHER READINGS

BACAL F et al: Transplantation for Chagas' disease: An overview of immunosuppression and reactivation in the last two decades. Clin Transplant 24:E29, 2010

BERN C et al: Evaluation and treatment of Chagas disease in the United States: A systematic review. JAMA 298:2171, 2007

———, MONTGOMERY SP: An estimate of the burden of Chagas disease in the United States. Clin Infect Dis 49:e52, 2009

BRUN R et al: Human African trypanosomiasis. Lancet 375:148, 2010

CHANG CD et al: Evaluation of a prototype *Trypanosoma cruzi* antibody assay with recombinant antigens on a fully automated chemiluminescence analyzer for blood donor screening. Transfusion 46:1737, 2006

KIRCHHOFF LV et al: Transfusion-associated Chagas' disease (American trypanosomiasis) in Mexico: Implications for transfusion medicine in the United States. Transfusion 46:298, 2006

PRIOTTO G et al: Nifurtimox-eflornithine combination therapy for second-stage African *Trypanosoma brucei gambiense* trypanosomiasis: A multicentre, randomised, phase III, non-inferiority trial. Lancet 374:56, 2009

RASSI A JR et al: Development and validation of a risk score for predicting death in Chagas' heart disease. N Engl J Med 355:799, 2006

——— et al: Chagas disease. Lancet 375:1388, 2010

SARTORI AM et al: Manifestations of Chagas disease (American trypanosomiasis) in patients with HIV/AIDS. Ann Trop Med Hyg 101:31, 2007

CHAPTER **214**

Toxoplasma Infections

Kami Kim

Lloyd H. Kasper

■ DEFINITION

Toxoplasmosis is caused by infection with the obligate intracellular parasite *Toxoplasma gondii*. Acute infection acquired after birth may be asymptomatic but is thought to result in the lifelong chronic persistence of cysts in the host's tissues. In both acute and chronic toxoplasmosis, the parasite is responsible for clinically evident disease, including lymphadenopathy, encephalitis, myocarditis, and pneumonitis. Congenital toxoplasmosis is an infection of newborns that results from the transplacental passage of parasites from an infected mother to the fetus. These infants may be asymptomatic at birth, but most later manifest a wide range of signs and symptoms, including chorioretinitis, strabismus, epilepsy, and psychomotor retardation. In immunocompetent individuals, toxoplasmosis can also present as acute disease (typically chorioretinitis) associated with food- or waterborne sources.

■ ETIOLOGY

T. gondii is an intracellular coccidian that infects both birds and mammals. There are two distinct stages in the life cycle of *T. gondii* (Fig. 214-1). In the *nonfeline* stage, tissue cysts that contain bradyzoites or sporulated oocysts are ingested by an intermediate host (e.g., a human, mouse, sheep, pig, or bird). The cyst is rapidly digested by the acidic-pH gastric secretions. Bradyzoites or sporozoites are released, enter the small-intestinal epithelium, and transform into rapidly dividing tachyzoites. The tachyzoites can infect and replicate in all mammalian cells except red blood cells. Once attached to the host cell, the parasite penetrates the cell and forms a parasitophorous vacuole within which it divides. Parasite replication continues until the number of parasites within the cell approaches a critical mass and the cell ruptures, releasing parasites that infect adjoining cells. As a result of this process, an infected organ soon shows evidence of cytopathology. Most tachyzoites are eliminated by the host's humoral and cell-mediated immune responses. Tissue cysts containing many bradyzoites develop 7–10 days after systemic tachyzoite infection. These tissue cysts occur in various host organs but persist principally within the central nervous system (CNS) and muscle. The development of this chronic stage completes the nonfeline portion of the life cycle. Active infection in the immunocompromised host is most likely to be due to the spontaneous release of encysted parasites that undergo rapid transformation into tachyzoites within the CNS.

The principal (*feline*) stage in the life cycle takes place in the cat (the definitive host) and its prey. The parasite's sexual phase is defined by the formation of oocysts within the feline host. This enteroepithelial cycle begins with the ingestion of the bradyzoite tissue cysts and culminates (after several intermediate stages) in the production of gametes. Gamete fusion produces a zygote, which envelops itself in a rigid wall and is secreted in the feces as an unsporulated oocyst. After 2–3 days of exposure to air at ambient temperature, the noninfectious oocyst sporulates to produce eight sporozoite progeny. The sporulated oocyst can be ingested by an intermediate host, such as a person emptying a cat's litter box or a pig rummaging in a barnyard. It is in the intermediate host that *T. gondii* completes its life cycle. Sporulated oocysts, which are environmentally hardy and very infectious, are thought to be sources of waterborne outbreaks such as those reported in Victoria (British Columbia, Canada) and in South America.

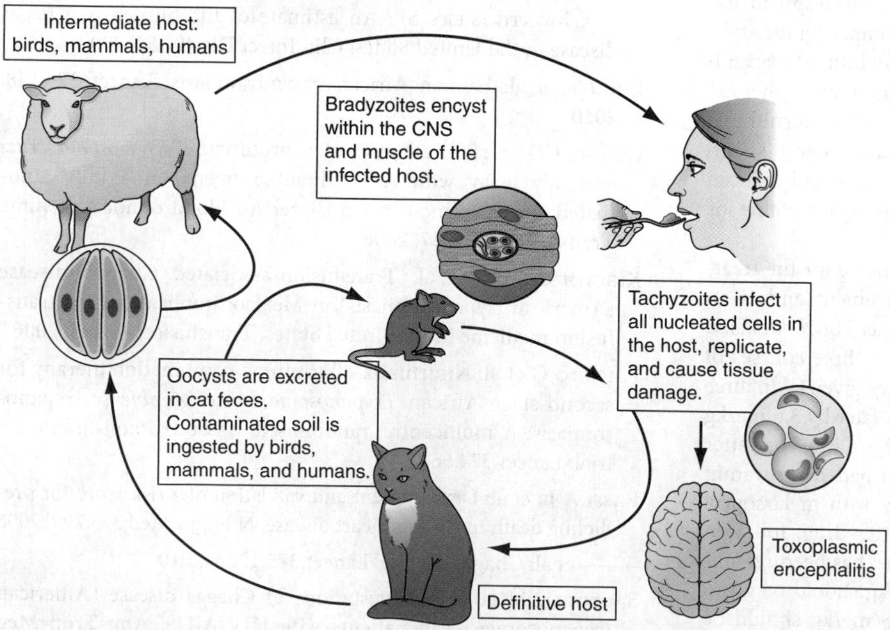

■ EPIDEMIOLOGY

T. gondii infects a wide range of mammals and birds. Its seroprevalence depends on the locale and the age of the population. Generally, hot arid climatic conditions are associated with a low prevalence of infection. In the United States and most European countries, the seroprevalence increases with age and exposure. For example, in the United States, 5–30% of individuals 10–19 years old and 10–67% of those >50 years old have serologic evidence of exposure. In Central America, France, Turkey, and Brazil, the seroprevalence is higher. Because of increased awareness of food-borne infections, the prevalence of seropositivity has decreased worldwide. There may be as many as 2100 cases of toxoplasmic encephalitis (TE) each year in the United States.

Figure 214-1 Life cycle of *Toxoplasma gondii*. The cat is the definitive host in which the sexual phase of the cycle is completed. Oocysts shed in cat feces can infect a wide range of animals, including birds, rodents, grazing domestic animals, and humans. The bradyzoites found in the muscle of food animals may infect humans who eat insufficiently cooked meat products, particularly lamb and pork. Although human disease can take many forms, congenital infection and encephalitis from reactivation of latent infection in the brains of immunosuppressed persons are the most important manifestations. CNS, central nervous system. *(Courtesy of Dominique Buzoni-Gatel, Institut Pasteur, Paris; with permission.)*

Labels in figure:
- Intermediate host: birds, mammals, humans
- Bradyzoites encyst within the CNS and muscle of the infected host.
- Tachyzoites infect all nucleated cells in the host, replicate, and cause tissue damage.
- Oocysts are excreted in cat feces. Contaminated soil is ingested by birds, mammals, and humans.
- Toxoplasmic encephalitis
- Definitive host

■ TRANSMISSION

Oral transmission

The principal source of human *Toxoplasma* infection remains uncertain, but infection is thought to occur by the oral route. Transmission can be attributable to ingestion of either sporulated oocysts from contaminated soil, food, or water or bradyzoites from undercooked meat. During acute feline infection, a cat may excrete as many as 100 million parasites per day. These very stable sporozoite-containing oocysts are highly infectious and may remain viable for many years in soil or water. Humans infected during a well-documented outbreak of oocyst-transmitted infection develop stage-specific antibodies to the oocyst/sporozoite.

Children and adults also can acquire infection from tissue cysts containing bradyzoites. The ingestion of a single cyst is all that is required for human infection. Undercooking or insufficient freezing of meat is an important source of infection in the developed world. In the United States, lamb products and pork products may show evidence of cysts that contain bradyzoites, but the overall prevalence of *T. gondii* has been gradually decreasing. The incidence in beef is much lower—perhaps as low as 1%. Direct ingestion of bradyzoite cysts in these various meat products leads to acute infection.

Transmission via blood or organs

In addition to being transmitted orally, *T. gondii* can be transmitted directly from a seropositive donor to a seronegative recipient in a transplanted heart, heart-lung, kidney, liver, or pancreas. Viable parasites can be cultured from refrigerated anticoagulated blood, which may be a source of infection in individuals receiving blood transfusions. *T. gondii* reactivation has been reported in bone marrow, hematopoietic stem cell, and liver transplant recipients as well as in individuals with AIDS. Although antibody titers generally are not useful in monitoring *T. gondii* infection, individuals with higher antibody titers reportedly may be at relatively high risk for reactivation after hematopoietic stem cell transplantation; thus routine polymerase chain reaction (PCR) screening of blood from these patients may be in order. Finally, laboratory personnel can be infected after contact with contaminated needles or glassware or with infected tissue.

Transplacental transmission

On average, about one-third of all women who acquire infection with *T. gondii* during pregnancy transmit the parasite to the fetus; the remainder give birth to normal, uninfected babies. Of the various factors that influence fetal outcome, gestational age at the time of infection is the most critical (see below). Few data support a role for recrudescent maternal infection as the source of congenital disease, although rare cases of transmission by immunocompromised women (e.g., those infected with HIV or those receiving high-dose glucocorticoids) have been reported. Thus, women who are seropositive before pregnancy usually are protected against acute infection and do not give birth to congenitally infected neonates.

The following general guidelines can be used to evaluate congenital infection. There is essentially no risk if the mother becomes infected ≥6 months before conception. If infection is acquired <6 months before conception, the likelihood of transplacental infection increases as the interval between infection and conception decreases. In pregnancy, if the mother becomes infected during the first trimester, the incidence of transplacental infection is lowest (~15%), but the disease in the neonate is most severe. If maternal infection occurs during the third trimester, the incidence of transplacental infection is greatest (65%), but the infant is usually asymptomatic at birth. Infected infants who are normal at birth may have a higher incidence of learning disabilities and chronic neurologic sequelae than uninfected children. Only a small proportion (20%) of women infected with *T. gondii* develop clinical signs of infection. Often the diagnosis is first appreciated when routine postconception serologic tests show evidence of specific antibody.

■ PATHOGENESIS

Upon the host's ingestion of either tissue cysts containing bradyzoites or oocysts containing sporozoites, the parasites are released from the cysts by a digestive process. Bradyzoites are resistant to the effect of pepsin and invade the host's gastrointestinal tract. Within enterocytes (or other gut-associated cells), the parasites undergo morphologic transformation, giving rise to invasive tachyzoites. These tachyzoites induce a parasite-specific secretory IgA response. From the gastrointestinal tract, parasites are disseminated to a variety of organs, particularly lymphatic tissue, skeletal muscle, myocardium, retina, placenta, and the CNS. At these sites, the parasite infects host cells, replicates, and invades the adjoining cells. In this fashion, the hallmarks of the infection develop: cell death and focal necrosis surrounded by an acute inflammatory response.

In the immunocompetent host, both the humoral and the cellular immune responses control infection; parasite virulence and tissue tropism may be strain specific. Tachyzoites are sequestered by a variety of immune mechanisms, including induction of parasiticidal antibody, activation of macrophages with radical intermediates, production of interferon γ (IFN-γ), and stimulation of CD8+ cytotoxic T lymphocytes. These antigen-specific lymphocytes are capable of killing both extracellular parasites and target cells infected with parasites. As tachyzoites are cleared from the acutely infected host, tissue cysts containing bradyzoites begin to appear, usually within the CNS and the retina. Studies indicate that *Toxoplasma* secretes signaling molecules into infected host cells and that these molecules modulate host gene expression, host metabolism, and host immune response.

In the immunocompromised or fetal host, the immune factors necessary to control the spread of tachyzoite infection are lacking. This altered immune state allows the persistence of tachyzoites and gives rise to progressive focal destruction that results in organ failure (i.e., necrotizing encephalitis, pneumonia, and myocarditis).

Persistence of infection with cysts containing bradyzoites is common in the immunocompetent host. This lifelong infection usually remains subclinical. Although bradyzoites are in a slow metabolic phase, cysts do degenerate and rupture within the CNS. This degenerative process, with the development of new bradyzoite-containing cysts, is the most probable source of recrudescent infection in immunocompromised individuals and the most likely stimulus for the persistence of antibody titers in the immunocompetent host. Although the concept is controversial, the persistence of toxoplasmosis has been hypothesized to be a contributing factor to a variety of neuropsychiatric conditions, including schizophrenia and bipolar disease. In rodents, infection clearly has significant effects on behavior, increasing predation.

■ PATHOLOGY

Cell death and focal necrosis due to replicating tachyzoites induce an intense mononuclear inflammatory response in any tissue or cell type infected. Tachyzoites rarely can be visualized by routine histopathologic staining of these inflammatory lesions. However, immunofluorescent staining with parasitic antigen–specific antibodies can reveal either the organism itself or evidence of antigen. In contrast to this inflammatory process caused by tachyzoites, bradyzoite-containing cysts cause inflammation only at the early stages of development, and even this inflammation may be a response to the presence of tachyzoite antigens. Once the cysts reach maturity, the inflammatory process can no longer be detected, and the cysts remain immunologically quiescent within the brain matrix until they rupture.

Lymph nodes

During acute infection, lymph node biopsy demonstrates characteristic findings, including follicular hyperplasia and irregular clusters of tissue macrophages with eosinophilic cytoplasm. Granulomas rarely are evident in these specimens. Although tachyzoites are not usually visible, they can be sought either by subinoculation of infected tissue into mice, with resultant disease, or by PCR. PCR amplification of DNA fragments of *Toxoplasma* genes is effective and sensitive in establishing lymph node infection by tachyzoites.

Eyes

In the eye, infiltrates of monocytes, lymphocytes, and plasma cells may produce uni- or multifocal lesions. Granulomatous lesions and chorioretinitis can be observed in the posterior chamber after acute necrotizing retinitis. Other ocular complications include iridocyclitis, cataracts, and glaucoma.

Central nervous system

During CNS involvement, both focal and diffuse meningoencephalitis can be documented, with evidence of necrosis and microglial nodules. Necrotizing encephalitis in patients without AIDS is characterized by small diffuse lesions with perivascular cuffing in contiguous areas. In the AIDS population, polymorphonuclear leukocytes may be present in addition to monocytes, lymphocytes, and plasma cells. Cysts containing bradyzoites frequently are found contiguous with the necrotic tissue border. As stated previously, it is estimated that there are as many as 2100 cases of TE in the United States each year.

Lungs and heart

Among patients with AIDS who die of toxoplasmosis, 40–70% have involvement of the lungs and heart. Interstitial pneumonitis can develop in neonates and immunocompromised patients. Thickened and edematous alveolar septa infiltrated with mononuclear and plasma cells are apparent. This inflammation may extend to the endothelial walls. Tachyzoites and bradyzoite-containing cysts have been observed within the alveolar membrane. Superimposed bronchopneumonia can be caused by other microbial agents. Cysts and aggregates of parasites in cardiac muscle tissue are evident in patients with AIDS who die of toxoplasmosis. Focal necrosis surrounded by inflammatory cells is associated with hyaline necrosis and disrupted myocardial cells. Pericarditis is associated with toxoplasmosis in some patients.

Gastrointestinal tract

Rare cases of human gastrointestinal tract infection with *T. gondii* have presented as ulcerations in the mucosa. Acute infection in certain strains of inbred mice (C57BL/6) results in lethal ileitis within 7–9 days. This inflammatory bowel disease has been recognized in several other mammalian species, including pigs and nonhuman primates. Although the association between human inflammatory bowel disease and either acute or recurrent *Toxoplasma* infection has not been established, studies have demonstrated recognition of the infection by human intestinal epithelial cells, as evidenced by mitogen-activated protein kinase phosphorylation, nuclear factor κB translocation, and interleukin 8 (IL-8) secretion.

Other sites

Pathologic changes during disseminated infection are similar to those described for the lymph nodes, eyes, and CNS. In patients

with AIDS, the skeletal muscle, pancreas, stomach, and kidneys can be involved, with necrosis, invasion by inflammatory cells, and (rarely) tachyzoites detectable by routine staining. Large necrotic lesions may cause direct tissue destruction. In addition, secondary effects from acute infection of these various organs, including pancreatitis, myositis, and glomerulonephritis, have been reported.

▣ HOST IMMUNE RESPONSE

Acute *Toxoplasma* infection evokes a cascade of protective immune responses in the immunocompetent host. *Toxoplasma* enters the host at the gut mucosal level and evokes a mucosal immune response that includes the production of antigen-specific secretory IgA. Titers of serum IgA antibody directed at p30 (SAG-1) are a useful marker for congenital and acute toxoplasmosis. Milk-whey IgA from acutely infected mothers contains a high titer of antibody to *T. gondii* and can block infection of enterocytes in vitro. In mice, IgA intestinal secretions directed at the parasite are abundant and are associated with the induction of mucosal T cells.

Within the host, *T. gondii* rapidly induces detectable levels of both IgM and IgG serum antibodies. Monoclonal gammopathy of the IgG class can occur in congenitally infected infants. IgM levels may be increased in newborns with congenital infection. The polyclonal IgG antibodies evoked by infection are parasiticidal in vitro in the presence of serum complement and are the basis for the Sabin-Feldman dye test. However, cell-mediated immunity is the major protective response evoked by the parasite during host infection. Macrophages are activated after phagocytosis of antibody-opsonized parasites. This activation can lead to death of the parasite by either an oxygen-dependent or an oxygen-independent process. If the parasite is not phagocytosed and enters the macrophage by active penetration, it continues to replicate, and this replication may represent the mechanism for transport and dissemination to distant organs. *Toxoplasma* stimulates a robust IL-12 response by human dendritic cells. The requirement for costimulation via CD40/154 has been established. The CD4+ and CD8+ T cell responses are antigen-specific and further stimulate the production of a variety of important lymphokines that expand the T cell and natural killer cell repertoire. *T. gondii* is a potent inducer of a T_H1 phenotype, with IL-12 and IFN-γ playing an essential role in the control of the parasites' growth in the host. Regulation of the inflammatory response is at least partially under the control of a T_H2 response that includes the production of IL-4 and IL-10 in seropositive individuals. Both asymptomatic patients and those with active infection may have a depressed CD4+-to-CD8+ ratio. This shift may be correlated with a disease syndrome but is not necessarily correlated with disease outcome. Human T cell clones of both the CD4+ and the CD8+ phenotypes are cytolytic against parasite-infected macrophages. These T cell clones produce cytokines that are "microbistatic." IL-18, IL-7, and IL-15 upregulate the production of IFN-γ and may be important during acute and chronic infection. The effect of IFN-γ may be paradoxical, with stimulation of a host downregulatory response as well.

Although in patients with AIDS *T. gondii* infection is believed to be recrudescent, determination of antibody titers generally is not helpful in establishing reactivation. Because of the severe depletion in CD4+ T cells, quite frequently there is no observed increase in antibody titer during exacerbation of infection. T cells from AIDS patients with reactivation of toxoplasmosis fail to secrete both IFN-γ and IL-2. This alteration in the production of these critical immune cytokines contributes to the persistence of infection. *Toxoplasma* infection frequently develops late in the course of AIDS, when the loss of T cell–dependent protective mechanisms, particularly CD8+ T cells, becomes most pronounced.

◼ CLINICAL MANIFESTATIONS

In persons whose immune systems are intact, acute toxoplasmosis is usually asymptomatic and self-limited. This condition can go unrecognized in 80–90% of adults and children with acquired infection. The asymptomatic nature of this infection makes diagnosis difficult in mothers infected during pregnancy. In contrast, the wide range of clinical manifestations in congenitally infected children includes severe neurologic complications such as hydrocephalus, microcephaly, mental retardation, and chorioretinitis. If prenatal infection is severe, multiorgan failure and subsequent intrauterine fetal death can occur. In children and adults, chronic infection can persist throughout life, with little consequence to the immunocompetent host.

Toxoplasmosis in immunocompetent patients

The most common manifestation of acute toxoplasmosis is cervical lymphadenopathy. The nodes may be single or multiple, are usually nontender, are discrete, and vary in firmness. Lymphadenopathy also may be found in suboccipital, supraclavicular, inguinal, and mediastinal areas. Generalized lymphadenopathy occurs in 20–30% of symptomatic patients. Between 20 and 40% of patients with lymphadenopathy also have headache, malaise, fatigue, and fever [usually with a temperature of <40°C (<104°F)]. A smaller proportion of symptomatic individuals have myalgia, sore throat, abdominal pain, maculopapular rash, meningoencephalitis, and confusion. Rare complications associated with infection in the normal immune host include pneumonia, myocarditis, encephalopathy, pericarditis, and polymyositis. Signs and symptoms associated with acute infection usually resolve within several weeks, although the lymphadenopathy may persist for some months. In one epidemic, toxoplasmosis was diagnosed correctly in only 3 of the 25 patients who consulted physicians. If toxoplasmosis is considered in the differential diagnosis, routine laboratory and serologic screening should precede node biopsy. It is now appreciated that genotypes of *T. gondii* prevalent in South America may be more virulent than those typically seen in North America or Europe. These genotypes may be associated with acute or recurrent ocular disease in immunocompetent individuals. Thus a detailed history is critical for establishing a diagnosis.

The results of routine laboratory studies are usually unremarkable except for minimal lymphocytosis, an elevated erythrocyte sedimentation rate, and a nominal increase in serum aminotransferase levels. Evaluation of cerebrospinal fluid (CSF) in cases with evidence of encephalopathy or meningoencephalitis shows an elevation of intracranial pressure, mononuclear pleocytosis (10–50 cells/mL), a slight increase in protein concentration, and (occasionally) an increase in the gamma globulin level. PCR amplification of the *Toxoplasma* DNA target sequence in CSF may be beneficial. The CSF of chronically infected individuals is normal.

Infection of immunocompromised patients

Patients with AIDS and those receiving immunosuppressive therapy for lymphoproliferative disorders are at greatest risk for developing acute toxoplasmosis. This predilection may be due either to reactivation of latent infection or to acquisition of parasites from exogenous sources such as blood or transplanted organs. In individuals with AIDS, >95% of cases of TE are believed to be due to recrudescent infection. In most of these cases, encephalitis develops when the CD4+ T cell count falls below 100/μL. In immunocompromised hosts, the disease may be rapidly fatal if untreated. Thus, accurate diagnosis and initiation of appropriate therapy are necessary to prevent fulminant infection.

Toxoplasmosis is a principal opportunistic infection of the CNS in persons with AIDS. Although geographic origin may be related to frequency of infection, it has no correlation with the severity of disease in immunocompromised hosts. Individuals with AIDS who are seropositive for *T. gondii* are at high risk for encephalitis. Before the advent of current combination antiretroviral treatment (ART), about one-third of the 15–40% of adult AIDS patients in the United States who were latently infected with *T. gondii* developed TE. TE may still be a presenting infection in individuals who are unaware of their positive HIV status.

The signs and symptoms of acute toxoplasmosis in immunocompromised patients principally involve the CNS (Fig. 214-2). More than 50% of patients with clinical manifestations have intracerebral involvement. Clinical findings at presentation range from nonfocal to focal dysfunction. CNS findings include encephalopathy, meningoencephalitis, and mass lesions. Patients may present with altered mental status (75%), fever (10–72%), seizures (33%), headaches (56%), and focal neurologic findings (60%), including motor deficits, cranial nerve palsies, movement disorders, dysmetria, visual-field loss, and aphasia. Patients who present with evidence of diffuse cortical dysfunction develop evidence of focal neurologic disease as infection progresses. This altered condition is due not only to the necrotizing encephalitis caused by direct invasion by the parasite but also to secondary effects, including vasculitis, edema, and hemorrhage. The onset of infection can range from an insidious process over several weeks to an acute confusional state with fulminant focal deficits, including hemiparesis, hemiplegia, visual-field defects, localized headache, and focal seizures.

Although lesions can occur anywhere in the CNS, the areas most often involved appear to be the brainstem, basal ganglia, pituitary gland, and corticomedullary junction. Brainstem involvement gives rise to a variety of neurologic dysfunctions, including cranial nerve palsy, dysmetria, and ataxia. With basal ganglionic infection, patients may develop hydrocephalus, choreiform movements, and choreoathetosis. Because *Toxoplasma* usually causes encephalitis, meningeal involvement is uncommon, and thus CSF findings may be unremarkable or may include a modest increase in cell count and in protein—but not glucose—concentration.

Cerebral toxoplasmosis must be differentiated from other opportunistic infections or tumors in the CNS of AIDS patients. The differential diagnosis includes herpes simplex encephalitis,

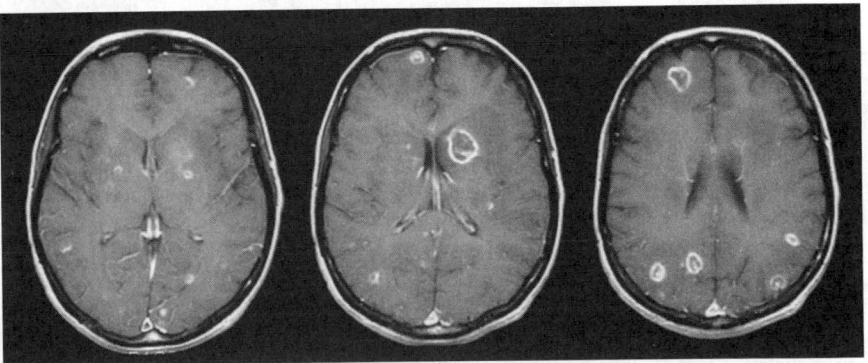

Figure 214-2 Toxoplasmic encephalitis in a 36-year-old patient with AIDS. The multiple lesions are demonstrated by magnetic resonance scanning (T1 weighted with gadolinium enhancement). *(Courtesy of Clifford Eskey, Dartmouth Hitchcock Medical Center, Hanover, NH; with permission.)*

cryptococcal meningitis, progressive multifocal leukoencephalopathy, and primary CNS lymphoma. Involvement of the pituitary gland can give rise to panhypopituitarism and hyponatremia from inappropriate secretion of vasopressin (antidiuretic hormone). HIV-associated neurocognitive disorder (HAND) may present as cognitive impairment, attention loss, and altered memory. Brain biopsy in patients who have been treated for TE but who continue to exhibit neurologic dysfunction often fails to identify organisms.

Autopsies of *Toxoplasma*-infected patients have demonstrated the involvement of multiple organs, including the lungs, gastrointestinal tract, pancreas, skin, eyes, heart, and liver. *Toxoplasma* pneumonia can be confused with *Pneumocystis* pneumonia (PcP). Respiratory involvement usually presents as dyspnea, fever, and a nonproductive cough and may rapidly progress to acute respiratory failure with hemoptysis, metabolic acidosis, hypotension, and (occasionally) disseminated intravascular coagulation. Histopathologic studies demonstrate necrosis and a mixed cellular infiltrate. The presence of organisms is a helpful diagnostic indicator, but organisms can also be found in healthy tissue. Infection of the heart is usually asymptomatic but can be associated with cardiac tamponade or biventricular failure. Infections of the gastrointestinal tract and the liver have been documented.

Congenital toxoplasmosis

Between 400 and 4000 infants born each year in the United States are affected by congenital toxoplasmosis. Acute infection in mothers acquiring *T. gondii* during pregnancy is usually asymptomatic; most such women are diagnosed via prenatal serologic screening. Infection of the placenta leads to hematogenous infection of the fetus. As gestation proceeds, the proportion of fetuses that become infected increases but the clinical severity of the infection declines. Although infected children may initially be asymptomatic, the persistence of *T. gondii* can result in reactivation and clinical disease—most frequently chorioretinitis—decades later. Factors associated with relatively severe disabilities include delays in diagnosis and in initiation of therapy, neonatal hypoxia and hypoglycemia, profound visual impairment (see "Ocular Infection," below), uncorrected hydrocephalus, and increased intracranial pressure. If treated appropriately, upwards of 70% of children have normal developmental, neurologic, and ophthalmologic findings at follow-up evaluations. Treatment for 1 year with pyrimethamine, a sulfonamide, and folinic acid is tolerated with minimal toxicity (see "Treatment," below).

Ocular infection

Infection with *T. gondii* is estimated to cause 35% of all cases of chorioretinitis in the United States and Europe. Most ocular involvement is believed to be due to congenital infection, but acquired infection can be associated with outbreaks of ocular disease even in immunocompetent individuals (as seen in Victoria, British Columbia, and in South America). A variety of ocular manifestations are documented, including blurred vision, scotoma, photophobia, and eye pain. Macular involvement occurs, with loss of central vision, and nystagmus is secondary to poor fixation. Involvement of the extraocular muscles may lead to disorders of convergence and to strabismus. Ophthalmologic examination should be undertaken in newborns with suspected congenital infection. As the inflammation resolves, vision improves, but episodic flare-ups of chorioretinitis, which progressively destroy retinal tissue and lead to glaucoma, are common. The ophthalmologic examination reveals yellow-white, cotton-like patches with indistinct margins of hyperemia. As the lesions age, white plaques with distinct borders and black spots within the retinal pigment become more apparent. Lesions usually are located near the posterior pole

of the retina; they may be single but are more commonly multiple. Congenital lesions may be unilateral or bilateral and show evidence of massive chorioretinal degeneration with extensive fibrosis. Surrounding these areas of involvement are a normal retina and vasculature. In patients with AIDS, retinal lesions are often large, with diffuse retinal necrosis, and include both free tachyzoites and cysts containing bradyzoites. Toxoplasmic chorioretinitis may be a prodrome to the development of encephalitis.

◼ DIAGNOSIS

Tissue and body fluids

The differential diagnosis of acute toxoplasmosis can be made by appropriate culture, serologic testing, and PCR (Table 214-1). Although difficult and available only at specialized laboratories, the isolation of *T. gondii* from blood or other body fluids can be accomplished after subinoculation of the sample into the peritoneal cavity of mice. If no parasites are found in the mouse's peritoneal fluid 6–10 days after inoculation, its anti-*Toxoplasma* serum titer can be evaluated 4–6 weeks after inoculation. Isolation of *T. gondii* from

TABLE 214-1 Differential Laboratory Diagnosis of Toxoplasmosis

Clinical Setting	Alternative Diagnosis	Distinguishing Characteristics
Mononucleosis syndrome	Epstein-Barr virus	Serology
	Cytomegalovirus	Serology/PCR or culture
	HIV	Serology/viral load
	Bartonella (cat-scratch disease)	Biopsy (PCR or culture)/serology
	Lymphoma	Biopsy
Congenital infection	Cytomegalovirus	Viral culture/PCR
	Herpes simplex virus	Viral culture/PCR
	Rubella virus	Viral culture/serology
	Syphilis	Serology
	Listeriosis	Bacterial culture
Chorioretinitis in immunocompetent individual	Tuberculosis	Bacterial culture
	Syphilis	Serology
	Histoplasmosis	Serology/culture
Chorioretinitis in AIDS patient	Cytomegalovirus	Viral culture/PCR
	Syphilis	Serology
	Herpes simplex virus	Viral culture/PCR
	Varicella-zoster virus	Viral culture/PCR
	Fungal infection	Culture
CNS lesions in AIDS patient	Lymphoma or metastatic tumor	Tissue biopsy
	Brain abscess	Bacterial culture
	Progressive multifocal leukoencephalopathy	PCR for JC Virus
	Fungal infection	Biopsy and culture
	Mycobacterial infection	Biopsy and culture

Source: Adapted from JD Schwartzman: Toxoplasmosis, *in Principles and Practice of Clinical Parasitology.* Hoboken, Wiley, 2001.

the patient's body fluids reflects acute infection, whereas isolation from biopsied tissue is an indication only of the presence of tissue cysts and should not be misinterpreted as evidence of acute toxoplasmosis. Persistent parasitemia in patients with latent, asymptomatic infection is rare. Histologic examination of lymph nodes may suggest the characteristic changes described above. Demonstration of tachyzoites in lymph nodes establishes the diagnosis of acute toxoplasmosis. Like subinoculation into mice, histologic demonstration of cysts containing bradyzoites confirms prior infection with *T. gondii* but is nondiagnostic for acute infection.

Serology

The procedures mentioned above have great diagnostic value but are limited by difficulties encountered either in the growth of parasites in vivo or in the identification of tachyzoites by histochemical methods. Serologic testing has become the routine method of diagnosis.

Diagnosis of acute infection with *T. gondii* can be established by detection of the simultaneous presence of IgG and IgM antibodies to *Toxoplasma* in serum. The presence of circulating IgA favors the diagnosis of an acute infection. The Sabin-Feldman dye test, the indirect fluorescent antibody test, and the enzyme-linked immunosorbent assay (ELISA) all satisfactorily measure circulating IgG antibody to *Toxoplasma*. Positive IgG titers (>1:10) can be detected as early as 2–3 weeks after infection. These titers usually peak at 6–8 weeks and decline slowly to a new baseline level that persists for life. Antibody avidity increases with time and can be useful in difficult cases during pregnancy for establishing when infection may have occurred. The serum IgM titer should be measured in concert with the IgG titer to better establish the time of infection; either the double-sandwich IgM-ELISA or the IgM-immunosorbent assay (IgM-ISAGA) should be used. Both assays are specific and sensitive, with fewer false-positive results than other commercial tests. The double-sandwich IgA-ELISA is more sensitive than the IgM-ELISA for detecting congenital infection in the fetus and newborn. Although a negative IgM result with a positive IgG titer indicates distant infection, IgM can persist for >1 year and should not necessarily be considered a reflection of acute disease. If acute toxoplasmosis is suspected, a more extensive panel of serologic tests can be performed at the *Toxoplasma* reference laboratory at the Palo Alto Medical Foundation (*http://www.pamf.org/serology/clinicianguide.html*).

Molecular diagnostics

Molecular approaches can directly detect *T. gondii* in biologic samples independent of the serologic response. Results obtained with PCR have suggested high sensitivity, specificity, and clinical utility in the diagnosis of TE in resource-poor settings. Real-time PCR is a promising technique that can provide quantitative results. Isolates can be genotyped and polymorphic sequences can be obtained, with consequent identification of the precise strain. Molecular epidemiologic studies with polymorphic markers have been useful in correlating clinical signs and symptoms of disease with different *T. gondii* genotypes.

The immunocompetent adult or child

For the patient who presents with lymphadenopathy only, a positive IgM titer is an indication of acute infection—and an indication for therapy, if clinically warranted (see "Treatment," below). The serum IgM titer should be determined again in 3 weeks. An elevation in the IgG titer without an increase in the IgM titer suggests that infection is present but is not acute. If there is a borderline increase in either IgG or IgM, the titers should be reassessed in 3–4 weeks.

The immunocompromised host

A presumptive clinical diagnosis of TE in patients with AIDS is based on clinical presentation, history of exposure (as evidenced by positive serology), and radiologic evaluation. To detect latent infection with *T. gondii*, HIV-infected persons should be tested for IgG antibody to *Toxoplasma* soon after HIV infection is diagnosed. When these criteria are used, the predictive value is as high as 80%. More than 97% of patients with AIDS and toxoplasmosis have IgG antibody to *T. gondii* in serum. IgM serum antibody usually is not detectable. Although IgG titers do not correlate with active infection, serologic evidence of infection virtually always precedes the development of TE. It is therefore important to determine the *Toxoplasma* antibody status of all patients infected with HIV. Antibody titers may range from negative to 1:1024 in patients with AIDS and TE. Fewer than 3% of patients have no demonstrable antibody to *Toxoplasma* at diagnosis of TE.

Patients with TE have focal or multifocal abnormalities demonstrable by CT or MRI. Neuroradiologic evaluation should include double-dose contrast CT of the head. By this test, single and frequently multiple contrast-enhancing lesions (<2 cm) may be identified. MRI usually demonstrates multiple lesions located in both hemispheres, with the basal ganglia and corticomedullary junction most commonly involved; MRI provides a more sensitive evaluation of the efficacy of therapy than does CT (Fig. 214-2). These findings are not pathognomonic of *Toxoplasma* infection, since 40% of CNS lymphomas are multifocal and 50% are ring-enhancing. For both MRI and CT scans, the rate of false-negative results is ~10%. The finding of a single lesion on an MRI scan increases the likelihood of primary CNS lymphoma (in which solitary lesions are four times more likely than in TE) and strengthens the argument for the performance of a brain biopsy. A therapeutic trial of anti-*Toxoplasma* medications is frequently used to assess the diagnosis. Treatment of presumptive TE with pyrimethamine plus sulfadiazine or clindamycin results in quantifiable clinical improvement in >50% of patients by day 3. By day 7, >90% of treated patients show evidence of improvement. In contrast, if patients fail to respond or have lymphoma, clinical signs and symptoms worsen by day 7. Patients in this category require brain biopsy with or without a change in therapy. This procedure can now be performed by a stereotactic CT-guided method that reduces the potential for complications. Brain biopsy for *T. gondii* identifies organisms in 50–75% of cases. PCR amplification of CSF may also confirm toxoplasmosis or suggest alternative diagnoses, such as progressive multifocal leukoencephalopathy (JC virus positive) or primary CNS lymphoma (Epstein-Barr virus positive).

Both positron emission tomography (PET) and single-photon emission CT (SPECT) have been touted as means of detecting or ruling out *Toxoplasma* infection when a CNS lesion is suspected. However, CT and MRI are currently the standard diagnostic imaging tests for TE. As in other conditions, the radiologic response may lag behind the clinical response. Resolution of lesions may take from 3 weeks to 6 months. Some patients show clinical improvement despite worsening radiographic findings.

Congenital infection

The issue of concern when a pregnant woman has evidence of recent *T. gondii* infection is whether the fetus is infected. PCR analysis of the amniotic fluid for the B1 gene of *T. gondii* has replaced fetal blood sampling. Serologic diagnosis is based on the persistence of IgG antibody or a positive IgM titer after the first week of life (a time frame that excludes placental leak). The IgG determination should be repeated every 2 months. An increase in IgM beyond the first week of life is indicative of acute infection. However, up to 25% of infected newborns may be seronegative and have normal routine physical examinations. Thus assessment of the eye and the brain, with ophthalmologic testing, CSF evaluation, and radiologic studies, is important in establishing the diagnosis.

Ocular toxoplasmosis

The serum antibody titer may not correlate with the presence of active lesions in the fundus, particularly in cases of congenital toxoplasmosis. In general, a positive IgG titer (measured in undiluted serum if necessary) in conjunction with typical lesions establishes the diagnosis. Antibody production in ocular fluids, expressed in terms of the Goldmann-Witmer coefficient, can also be used for diagnosis of ocular disease. Confirmation of local specific antibody production in the eye indicates that the site of inflammatory activity is localized to this organ. However, two-thirds of patients without evidence of specific antibody production at initial clinical presentation later develop a detectable titer. If lesions are atypical and the titer is in the low-positive range, the diagnosis is presumptive. The parasitic antigen–specific polyclonal IgG assay as well as parasitic antigen–specific PCR may facilitate the diagnosis. Accordingly, the clinical diagnosis of ocular toxoplasmosis can be supported in 60–90% of cases by laboratory tests, depending on the time of anterior chamber puncture and the panel of antibody analyses used. In the remaining cases, the possibility of a falsely negative laboratory diagnosis or of an incorrect clinical diagnosis cannot be clarified further.

| TREATMENT | Toxoplasmosis |

CONGENITAL INFECTION Congenitally infected neonates are treated with daily oral pyrimethamine (1 mg/kg) and sulfadiazine (100 mg/kg) with folinic acid for 1 year. Depending on the signs and symptoms, prednisone (1 mg/kg per day) may be used for congenital infection. Some U.S. states and some countries routinely screen pregnant women (France, Austria) and/or newborns (Denmark, Massachusetts). Management and treatment regimens vary with the country and the treatment center. Most experts use spiramycin to treat pregnant women who have acute toxoplasmosis early in pregnancy and use pyrimethamine/sulfadiazine/folinic acid to treat women who seroconvert after 18 weeks of pregnancy or in cases of documented fetal infection. This treatment is somewhat controversial: clinical studies, which have included few untreated women, have not proven the efficacy of such therapy in preventing congenital toxoplasmosis. However, studies do suggest that treatment during pregnancy decreases the severity of infection. Many women who are infected in the first trimester elect termination of pregnancy. Those who do not terminate pregnancy are offered prenatal antibiotic therapy to reduce the frequency and severity of *Toxoplasma* infection in the infant.

INFECTION IN IMMUNOCOMPETENT PATIENTS Immunologically competent adults and older children who have only lymphadenopathy do not require specific therapy unless they have persistent, severe symptoms. Patients with ocular toxoplasmosis are usually treated for 1 month with pyrimethamine plus either sulfadiazine or clindamycin and sometimes with prednisone. Treatment should be supervised by an ophthalmologist familiar with *Toxoplasma* disease. Ocular disease can be self-limited without treatment, but therapy is typically considered for lesions that are severe or close to the fovea or optic disc.

INFECTION IN IMMUNOCOMPROMISED PATIENTS

Primary Prophylaxis Patients with AIDS should be treated for acute toxoplasmosis; in immunocompromised patients,

toxoplasmosis is rapidly fatal if untreated. Before the introduction of ART, the median survival time was >1 year for patients who could tolerate treatment for TE. Despite their toxicity, the drugs used to treat TE were required for survival prior to ART. The incidence of TE has declined as the survival of patients with HIV infection has increased through the use of ART.

In Africa, many patients are diagnosed with HIV infection only after developing opportunistic infections such as TE. Hence, the optimal management of these opportunistic infections is important if the benefits of subsequent ART are to be realized. AIDS patients who are seropositive for T. gondii and who have a CD4+ T lymphocyte count of <100/μL should receive prophylaxis against TE.

Of the currently available agents, trimethoprim-sulfamethoxazole (TMP-SMX) appears to be an effective alternative for treatment of TE in resource-poor settings where the preferred combination of pyrimethamine plus sulfadiazine is not available. The daily dose of TMP-SMX recommended as the preferred regimen for PcP prophylaxis (one double-strength tablet) is effective against TE. If patients cannot tolerate TMP-SMX, the recommended alternative is dapsone-pyrimethamine, which is also effective against PcP. Atovaquone with or without pyrimethamine also can be considered. Prophylactic monotherapy with dapsone, pyrimethamine, azithromycin, clarithromycin, or aerosolized pentamidine is probably insufficient. AIDS patients who are seronegative for *Toxoplasma* and are not receiving prophylaxis for PcP should be retested for IgG antibody to *Toxoplasma* if their CD4+ T cell count drops to <100/μL. If seroconversion has taken place, then the patient should be given prophylaxis as described above.

Discontinuing Primary Prophylaxis Current studies indicate that prophylaxis against TE can be discontinued in patients who have responded to ART and whose CD4+ T lymphocyte count has been >200/μL for 3 months. Although patients with CD4+ T lymphocyte counts of <100/μL are at greatest risk for developing TE, the risk that this condition will develop when the count has increased to 100–200/μL has not been established. Thus, prophylaxis should be discontinued when the count has increased to >200/μL. Discontinuation of therapy reduces the pill burden; the potential for drug toxicity, drug interaction, or selection of drug-resistant pathogens; and cost. Prophylaxis should be recommenced if the CD4+ T lymphocyte count again decreases to <100–200/μL.

Individuals who have completed initial therapy for TE should receive treatment indefinitely unless immune reconstitution, with a CD4+ T cell count of >200/μL, occurs as a consequence of ART. Combination therapy with pyrimethamine plus sulfadiazine plus leucovorin is effective for this purpose. An alternative to sulfadiazine in this regimen is clindamycin.

Discontinuing Secondary Prophylaxis (Long-Term Maintenance Therapy) Patients receiving secondary prophylaxis for TE are at low risk for recurrence when they have completed initial therapy for TE, remain asymptomatic, and have a CD4+ T lymphocyte count of >200/μL for at least 6 months after ART. This recommendation is based on recent observations in a large cohort (381 patients) and is consistent with more extensive data indicating the safety of discontinuing secondary prophylaxis for other opportunistic infections during advanced HIV disease. Discontinuation of long-term maintenance therapy among these patients appears reasonable. A repeat MRI brain scan is recommended. Secondary prophylaxis should be reintroduced if the CD4+ T lymphocyte count decreases to <200/μL.

PREVENTION

All HIV-infected persons, including those who lack IgG antibody to *Toxoplasma*, should be counseled regarding sources of *Toxoplasma* infection. The chances of primary infection with *Toxoplasma* can be reduced by not eating undercooked meat and by avoiding oocyst-contaminated material (i.e., a cat's litter box). Specifically, lamb, beef, and pork should be cooked to an internal temperature of 165°–170°F; from a more practical perspective, meat cooked until it is no longer pink inside usually satisfies this requirement. Hands should be washed thoroughly after work in the garden, and all fruits and vegetables should be washed. Ingestion of raw shellfish is a risk factor for toxoplasmosis, given that the filter-feeding mechanism of clams and mussels concentrates oocysts.

If the patient owns a cat, the litter box should be cleaned or changed daily, preferably by an HIV-negative, nonpregnant person; alternatively, patients should wash their hands thoroughly after changing the litter box. Litter boxes should be changed daily if possible, as freshly excreted oocysts will not have sporulated and will not be infectious. Patients should be encouraged to keep their cats inside and not to adopt or handle stray cats. Cats should be fed only canned or dried commercial food or well-cooked table food, not raw or undercooked meats. Patients need not be advised to part with their cats or to have their cats tested for toxoplasmosis. Blood intended for transfusion into *Toxoplasma*-seronegative immunocompromised individuals should be screened for antibody to *T. gondii*. Although such serologic screening is not routinely performed, seronegative women should be screened for evidence of infection several times during pregnancy if they are exposed to environmental conditions that put them at risk for infection with *T. gondii*. HIV-positive individuals should adhere closely to these preventive measures.

FURTHER READINGS

DEDICOAT M: Management of toxoplasmic encephalitis in HIV-infected adults (with an emphasis on resource-poor settings). Cochrane Database Syst Rev 3:CD005420, 2006

JONES JL et al: *Toxoplasma gondii* infection in the United States, 1999–2004, decline from the prior decade. Am J Trop Med Hyg 77:405, 2007

—— et al: Risk factors for *Toxoplasma gondii* infection in the United States. Clin Infect Dis 49:878, 2009

KAPLAN JE et al: Guidelines for prevention and treatment of opportunistic infections in HIV-infected adults and adolescents. Recommendations from CDC, the National Institutes of Health, and the HIV Medicine Association of the Infectious Diseases Society of America. MMWR Recomm Rep 58:1–207, 2009

LEHMANN T et al: Globalization and the population structure of *Toxoplasma gondii*. Proc Natl Acad Sci USA 103:11423, 2006

MCLEOD R et al: Outcome of treatment for congenital toxoplasmosis, 1981–2004: The National Collaborative Chicago-Based, Congenital Toxoplasmosis Study. Clin Infect Dis 42:1383, 2006

MEERS S et al: Myeloablative conditioning predisposes patients for *Toxoplasma gondii* reactivation after allogeneic stem cell transplantation. Clin Infect Dis 50:1127, 2010

MONTOYA JG, REMINGTON JS: Management of *Toxoplasma gondii* infection during pregnancy. Clin Infect Dis 47:554, 2008

CHAPTER 215

Protozoal Intestinal Infections and Trichomoniasis

Peter F. Weller

PROTOZOAL INFECTIONS

GIARDIASIS

Giardia intestinalis (also known as *G. lamblia* or *G. duodenalis*) is a cosmopolitan protozoal parasite that inhabits the small intestines of humans and other mammals. Giardiasis is one of the most common parasitic diseases in both developed and developing countries worldwide, causing both endemic and epidemic intestinal disease and diarrhea.

Life cycle and epidemiology

(Fig. 215-1) Infection follows the ingestion of environmentally hardy cysts, which excyst in the small intestine, releasing flagellated trophozoites (Fig. 215-2) that multiply by binary fission. *Giardia* remains a pathogen of the proximal small bowel and does not disseminate hematogenously. Trophozoites remain free in the lumen or attach to the mucosal epithelium by means of a ventral sucking disk. As a trophozoite encounters altered conditions, it forms a morphologically distinct cyst, which is the stage of the parasite usually found in the feces. Trophozoites may be present and even predominate in loose or watery stools, but it is the resistant cyst that survives outside the body and is responsible for transmission. Cysts do not tolerate heating, desiccation, or continued exposure to feces but do remain viable for months in cold fresh water. The number of cysts excreted varies widely but can approach 10^7 per gram of stool.

Ingestion of as few as 10 cysts is sufficient to cause infection in humans. Because cysts are infectious when excreted, person-to-person transmission occurs where fecal hygiene is poor. Giardiasis (symptomatic or asymptomatic) is especially prevalent in day-care centers; person-to-person spread also takes place in other institutional settings with poor fecal hygiene and during anal-oral contact. If food is contaminated with *Giardia* cysts after cooking or preparation, food-borne transmission can occur. Waterborne transmission accounts for episodic infections (e.g., in campers and travelers) and for major epidemics in metropolitan areas. Surface water, ranging from mountain streams to large municipal reservoirs, can become contaminated with fecally derived *Giardia* cysts; outmoded water systems are subject to cross-contamination from leaking sewer lines. The efficacy of water as a means of transmission is enhanced by the small infectious inoculum of *Giardia*, the prolonged survival of cysts in cold water, and the resistance of cysts to killing by routine chlorination methods that are adequate for controlling bacteria. Viable cysts can be eradicated from water by either boiling or filtration. In the United States, *Giardia* (like *Cryptosporidium*; see below) is a common cause of waterborne epidemics of gastroenteritis.

Giardia is common in developing countries, and infections may be acquired by travelers.

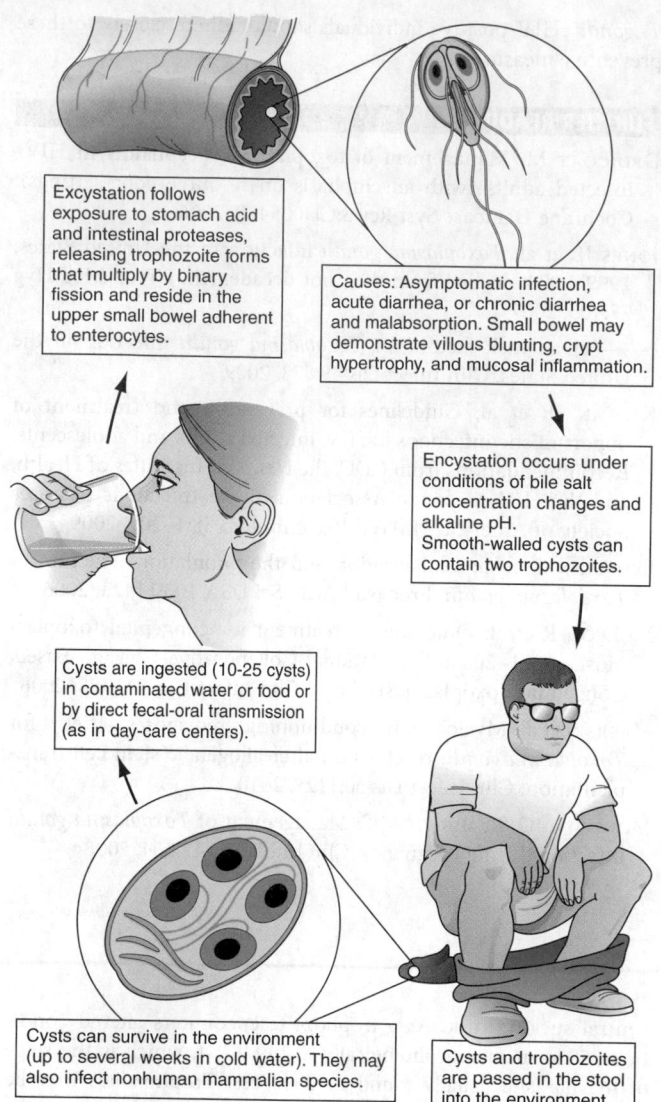

Excystation follows exposure to stomach acid and intestinal proteases, releasing trophozoite forms that multiply by binary fission and reside in the upper small bowel adherent to enterocytes.

Causes: Asymptomatic infection, acute diarrhea, or chronic diarrhea and malabsorption. Small bowel may demonstrate villous blunting, crypt hypertrophy, and mucosal inflammation.

Encystation occurs under conditions of bile salt concentration changes and alkaline pH. Smooth-walled cysts can contain two trophozoites.

Cysts are ingested (10-25 cysts) in contaminated water or food or by direct fecal-oral transmission (as in day-care centers).

Cysts can survive in the environment (up to several weeks in cold water). They may also infect nonhuman mammalian species.

Cysts and trophozoites are passed in the stool into the environment.

Figure 215-1 **Life cycle of** *Giardia.* *(Reprinted from RL Guerrant et al: Tropical Infectious Disease: Principles, Pathogens and Practice, 2nd ed, 2006, p 987, with permission from Elsevier Science.)*

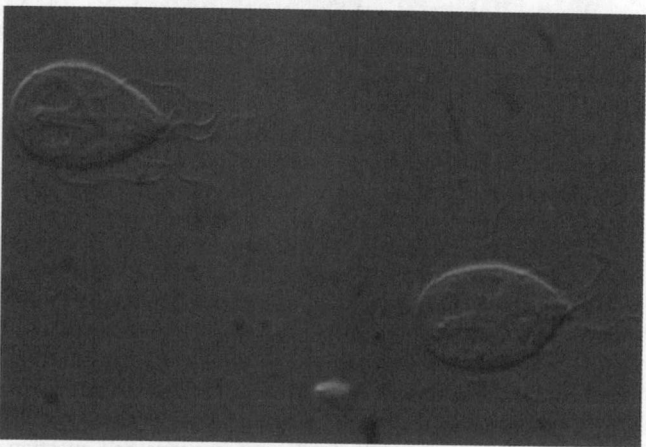

Figure 215-2 Flagellated, binucleate *Giardia* trophozoites.

Giardia parasites genotypically similar to those in humans are found in many mammals, including beavers from reservoirs implicated in epidemics. The importance of dogs and cats as sources of infection for humans is unclear.

Giardiasis, like cryptosporidiosis, creates a significant economic burden because of the costs incurred in the installation of water filtration systems required to prevent waterborne epidemics, in the management of epidemics that involve large communities, and in the evaluation and treatment of endemic infections.

Pathophysiology

The reasons that some, but not all, infected patients develop clinical manifestations and the mechanisms by which *Giardia* causes alterations in small-bowel function are largely unknown. Although trophozoites adhere to the epithelium, they do not cause invasive or locally destructive alterations. The lactose intolerance and, in a minority of infected adults and children, significant malabsorption that develop are clinical signs of the loss of brush-border enzyme activities. In most infections, the morphology of the bowel is unaltered; however, in a few cases (usually in chronically infected, symptomatic patients), the histopathologic findings (including flattened villi) and the clinical manifestations resemble those of tropical sprue and gluten-sensitive enteropathy. The pathogenesis of diarrhea in giardiasis is not known.

The natural history of *Giardia* infection varies markedly. Infections may be aborted, transient, recurrent, or chronic. Parasite as well as host factors may be important in determining the course of infection and disease. Both cellular and humoral responses develop in human infections, but their precise roles in the control of infection and/or disease are unknown. Because patients with hypogammaglobulinemia suffer from prolonged, severe infections that are poorly responsive to treatment, humoral immune responses appear to be important. The greater susceptibility of the young than of the old and of newly exposed persons than of chronically exposed populations suggests that at least partial protective immunity may develop. *Giardia* isolates vary genotypically, biochemically, and biologically, and variations among isolates may contribute to different courses of infection.

Clinical manifestations

Disease manifestations of giardiasis range from asymptomatic carriage to fulminant diarrhea and malabsorption. Most infected persons are asymptomatic, but in epidemics the proportion of symptomatic cases may be higher. Symptoms may develop suddenly or gradually. In persons with acute giardiasis, symptoms develop after an incubation period that lasts at least 5–6 days and usually 1–3 weeks. Prominent early symptoms include diarrhea, abdominal pain, bloating, belching, flatus, nausea, and vomiting. Although diarrhea is common, upper intestinal manifestations such as nausea, vomiting, bloating, and abdominal pain may predominate. The duration of acute giardiasis is usually >1 week, although diarrhea often subsides. Individuals with chronic giardiasis may present with or without having experienced an antecedent acute symptomatic episode. Diarrhea is not necessarily prominent, but increased flatus, loose stools, sulfurous belching, and (in some instances) weight loss occur. Symptoms may be continual or episodic and can persist for years. Some persons who have relatively mild symptoms for long periods recognize the extent of their discomfort only in retrospect. Fever, the presence of blood and/or mucus in the stools, and other signs and symptoms of colitis are uncommon and suggest a different diagnosis or a concomitant illness. Symptoms tend to be intermittent yet recurring and gradually debilitating, in contrast with the acute disabling symptoms associated with many enteric bacterial infections. Because of the less severe illness and the propensity for chronic infections, patients may seek medical advice late in the course of the illness; however, disease can be severe, resulting in

TABLE 215-1 Diagnosis of Intestinal Protozoal Infections

Parasite	Stool O+P[a]	Fecal Acid-Fast Stain	Stool Antigen Immunoassays	Other
Giardia	+		+	
Cryptosporidium	−	+	+	
Isospora	−	+		
Cyclospora	−	+		
Microsporidia	−			Special fecal stains, tissue biopsies

[a]O+P, ova and parasites.

malabsorption, weight loss, growth retardation, and dehydration. A number of extraintestinal manifestations have been described, such as urticaria, anterior uveitis, and arthritis; whether these are caused by giardiasis or concomitant processes is unclear.

Giardiasis can be severe in patients with hypogammaglobulinemia and can complicate other preexisting intestinal diseases, such as that occurring in cystic fibrosis. In patients with AIDS, *Giardia* can cause enteric illness that is refractory to treatment.

Diagnosis

(Table 215-1) Giardiasis is diagnosed by detection of parasite antigens in the feces or by identification of cysts in the feces or of trophozoites in the feces or small intestines. Cysts are oval, measure 8–12 μm × 7–10 μm, and characteristically contain four nuclei. Trophozoites are pear-shaped, dorsally convex, flattened parasites with two nuclei and four pairs of flagella (Fig. 215-2). The diagnosis is sometimes difficult to establish. Direct examination of fresh or properly preserved stools as well as concentration methods should be used. Because cyst excretion is variable and may be undetectable at times, repeated examination of stool, sampling of duodenal fluid, and biopsy of the small intestine may be required to detect the parasite. Tests for parasitic antigens in stool are at least as sensitive and specific as good microscopic examinations and are easier to perform. All of these methods occasionally yield false-negative results.

TREATMENT **Giardiasis**

Cure rates with metronidazole (250 mg thrice daily for 5 days) are usually >90%. Tinidazole (2 g once by mouth) is reportedly more effective than metronidazole. Nitazoxanide (500 mg twice daily for 3 days) is an alternative agent for treatment of giardiasis. Paromomycin, an oral aminoglycoside that is not well absorbed, can be given to symptomatic pregnant patients, although information is limited on how effectively this agent eradicates infection.

Almost all patients respond to therapy and are cured, although some with chronic giardiasis experience delayed resolution of symptoms after eradication of *Giardia*. For many of the latter patients, residual symptoms probably reflect delayed regeneration of intestinal brush-border enzymes. Continued infection should be documented by stool examinations before treatment is repeated. Patients who remain infected after repeated treatments should be evaluated for reinfection through family members, close personal contacts, and environmental sources as well as for hypogammaglobulinemia. In cases refractory to multiple treatment courses, prolonged therapy with metronidazole (750 mg thrice daily for 21 days) has been successful.

Prevention

Although giardiasis is extremely infectious, disease can be prevented by consumption of noncontaminated food and water and by personal hygiene when caring for infected children. Boiling or filtering potentially contaminated water prevents infection.

■ CRYPTOSPORIDIOSIS

The coccidian parasite *Cryptosporidium* causes diarrheal disease that is self-limited in immunocompetent human hosts but can be severe in persons with AIDS or other forms of immunodeficiency. Two species of *Cryptosporidium*, *C. hominis* and *C. parvum*, cause most human infections.

Life cycle and epidemiology

Cryptosporidium species are widely distributed in the world. Cryptosporidiosis is acquired by the consumption of oocysts (50% infectious dose: ~132 oocysts in nonimmune individuals), which excyst to liberate sporozoites that in turn enter and infect intestinal epithelial cells. The parasite's further development involves both asexual and sexual cycles, which produce forms capable of infecting other epithelial cells and of generating oocysts that are passed in the feces. *Cryptosporidium* species infect a number of animals, and *C. parvum* can spread from infected animals to humans. Since oocysts are immediately infectious when passed in feces, person-to-person transmission takes place in day-care centers and among household contacts and medical providers. Waterborne transmission (especially that of *C. hominis*) accounts for infections in travelers and for common-source epidemics. Oocysts are quite hardy and resist killing by routine chlorination. Both drinking water and recreational water (e.g., pools, waterslides) have been increasingly recognized as sources of infection.

Pathophysiology

Although intestinal epithelial cells harbor cryptosporidia in an intracellular vacuole, the means by which secretory diarrhea is elicited remain uncertain. No characteristic pathologic changes are found by biopsy. The distribution of infection can be spotty within the principal site of infection, the small bowel. Cryptosporidia are found in the pharynx, stomach, and large bowel of some patients and at times in the respiratory tract. Especially in patients with AIDS, involvement of the biliary tract can cause papillary stenosis, sclerosing cholangitis, or cholecystitis.

Clinical manifestations

Asymptomatic infections can occur in both immunocompetent and immunocompromised hosts. In immunocompetent persons, symptoms develop after an incubation period of ~1 week and consist principally of watery nonbloody diarrhea, sometimes in conjunction with abdominal pain, nausea, anorexia, fever, and/or weight loss. In these hosts, the illness usually subsides after 1–2 weeks. In contrast, in immunocompromised hosts (especially those with AIDS and CD4+ T cell counts <100/μL), diarrhea can be chronic, persistent, and remarkably profuse, causing clinically significant fluid and electrolyte depletion. Stool volumes may range from 1 to 25 L/d. Weight loss, wasting, and abdominal pain may be severe. Biliary tract involvement can manifest as midepigastric or right-upper-quadrant pain.

Diagnosis

(Table 215-1) Evaluation starts with fecal examination for small oocysts, which are smaller (4–5 μm in diameter) than the fecal stages of most other parasites. Because conventional stool examination for ova and parasites does not detect *Cryptosporidium*, specific testing must be requested. Detection is enhanced by evaluation of stools (obtained on multiple days) by several techniques, including modified acid-fast and direct immunofluorescent stains and enzyme immunoassays. Cryptosporidia can also be identified by light and electron microscopy at the apical surfaces of intestinal epithelium from biopsy specimens of the small bowel and, less frequently, the large bowel.

TREATMENT ▶ Cryptosporidiosis

Nitazoxanide is approved by the U.S. Food and Drug Administration for the treatment of cryptosporidiosis and is available in tablet form for adults (500 mg twice daily for 3 days) and as an elixir for children. To date, however, this agent has not been effective for the treatment of HIV-infected patients, in whom improved immune status due to antiretroviral therapy can lead to amelioration of cryptosporidiosis. Otherwise, treatment includes supportive care with replacement of fluids and electrolytes and administration of antidiarrheal agents. Biliary tract obstruction may require papillotomy or T-tube placement. Prevention requires minimizing exposure to infectious oocysts in human or animal feces. Use of submicron water filters may minimize acquisition of infection from drinking water.

▇ ISOSPORIASIS

The coccidian parasite *Isospora belli* causes human intestinal disease. Infection is acquired by the consumption of oocysts, after which the parasite invades intestinal epithelial cells and undergoes both sexual and asexual cycles of development. Oocysts excreted in stool are not immediately infectious but must undergo further maturation.

Although *I. belli* infects many animals, little is known about the epidemiology or prevalence of this parasite in humans. It appears to be most common in tropical and subtropical countries. Acute infections can begin abruptly with fever, abdominal pain, and watery nonbloody diarrhea and can last for weeks or months. In patients who have AIDS or are immunocompromised for other reasons, infections often are not self-limited but rather resemble cryptosporidiosis, with chronic, profuse watery diarrhea. Eosinophilia, which is not found in other enteric protozoan infections, may be detectable. The diagnosis (Table 215-1) is usually made by detection of the large (~25-μm) oocysts in stool by modified acid-fast staining. Oocyst excretion may be low-level and intermittent; if repeated stool examinations are unrevealing, sampling of duodenal contents by aspiration or small-bowel biopsy (often with electron-microscopic examination) may be necessary.

TREATMENT ▶ Isosporiasis

Trimethoprim-sulfamethoxazole (TMP-SMX, 160/800 mg four times daily for 10 days; and for HIV-infected patients, then three times daily for 3 weeks) is effective. For patients intolerant of sulfonamides, pyrimethamine (50–75 mg/d) can be used. Relapses can occur in persons with AIDS and necessitate maintenance therapy with TMP-SMX (160/800 mg three times per week).

▇ CYCLOSPORIASIS

Cyclospora cayetanensis, a cause of diarrheal illness, is globally distributed: illness due to *C. cayetanensis* has been reported in the United States, Asia, Africa, Latin America, and Europe. The epidemiology of this parasite has not yet been fully defined, but waterborne transmission and food-borne transmission by basil and imported raspberries have been recognized. The full spectrum of illness attributable to *Cyclospora* has not been delineated. Some patients may harbor the infection without symptoms, but many have diarrhea, flulike symptoms, and flatulence and belching. The illness can be self-limited, can wax and wane, or in many cases can involve prolonged diarrhea, anorexia, and upper gastrointestinal symptoms, with sustained fatigue and weight loss in some instances. Diarrheal illness may persist for >1 month. *Cyclospora* can cause enteric illness in patients infected with HIV.

The parasite is detectable in epithelial cells of small-bowel biopsy samples and elicits secretory diarrhea by unknown means. The absence of fecal blood and leukocytes indicates that disease due to *Cyclospora* is not caused by destruction of the small-bowel mucosa. The diagnosis (Table 215-1) can be made by detection of spherical 8- to 10-μm oocysts in the stool, although routine stool ova and parasite (O+P) examinations are not sufficient. Specific fecal examinations must be requested to detect the oocysts, which are variably acid-fast and are fluorescent when viewed with ultraviolet light microscopy. Cyclosporiasis should be considered in the differential diagnosis of prolonged diarrhea, with or without a history of travel by the patient to other countries.

TREATMENT ▶ Cyclosporiasis

Cyclosporiasis is treated with TMP-SMX (160/800 mg twice daily for 7 days). HIV-infected patients may experience relapses after such treatment and thus may require longer-term suppressive maintenance therapy.

▇ MICROSPORIDIOSIS

Microsporidia are obligate intracellular spore-forming protozoa that infect many animals and cause disease in humans, especially as opportunistic pathogens in AIDS. Microsporidia are members of a distinct phylum, Microspora, which contains dozens of genera and hundreds of species. The various microsporidia are differentiated by their developmental life cycles, ultrastructural features, and molecular taxonomy based on ribosomal RNA. The complex life cycles of the organisms result in the production of infectious spores (Fig. 215-3). Currently, eight genera of microsporidia—*Encephalitozoon, Pleistophora, Nosema, Vittaforma, Trachipleistophora, Brachiola, Microsporidium,* and *Enterocytozoon*—are recognized as causes of human disease. Although some microsporidia are probably prevalent causes of self-limited or asymptomatic infections in immunocompetent patients, little is known about how microsporidiosis is acquired.

Microsporidiosis is most common among patients with AIDS, less common among patients with other types of immunocompromise, and rare among immunocompetent hosts. In patients with AIDS, intestinal infections with *Enterocytozoon bieneusi* and *Encephalitozoon* (formerly *Septata*) *intestinalis* are recognized to contribute to chronic diarrhea and wasting; these infections are found in 10–40% of patients with chronic diarrhea. Both organisms have been found in the biliary tracts of patients with cholecystitis. *E. intestinalis* may also disseminate to cause fever, diarrhea, sinusitis, cholangitis, and bronchiolitis. In patients with AIDS, *Encephalitozoon hellem* has caused superficial keratoconjunctivitis as well as sinusitis, respiratory tract disease, and disseminated infection. Myositis due to *Pleistophora* has been documented. *Nosema, Vittaforma,* and *Microsporidium* have caused stromal keratitis associated with trauma in immunocompetent patients.

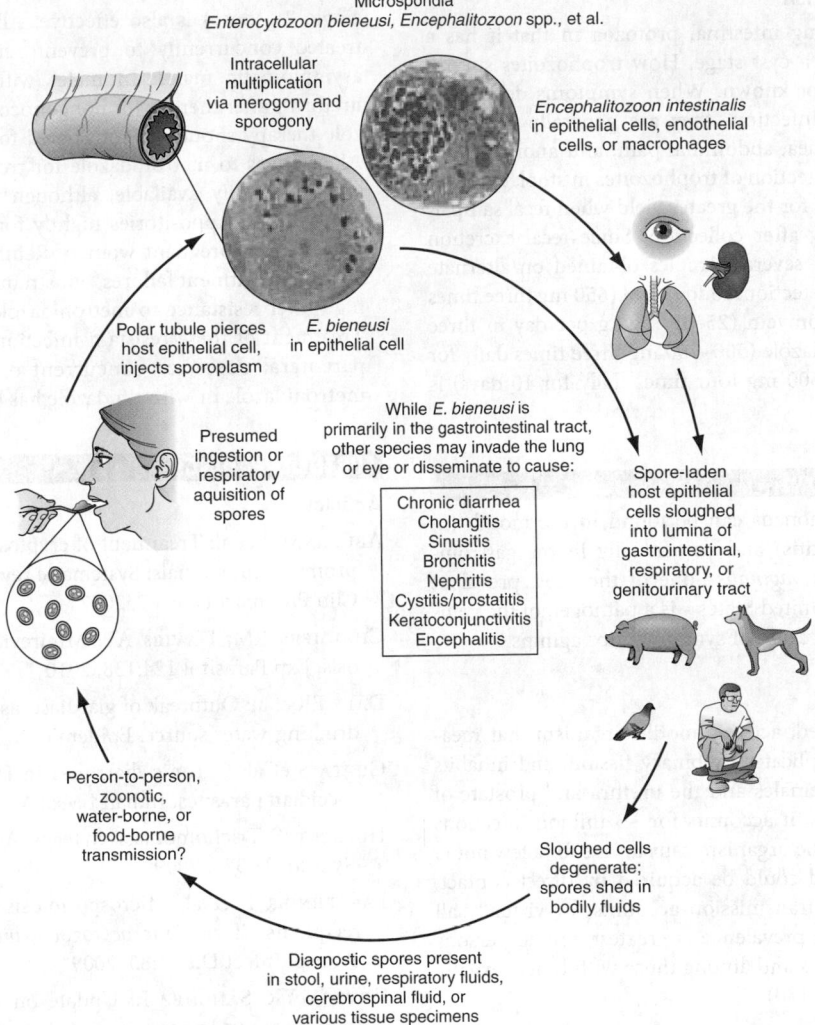

Microsporidia
Enterocytozoon bieneusi, Encephalitozoon spp., et al.

Intracellular multiplication via merogony and sporogony

Polar tubule pierces host epithelial cell, injects sporoplasm

E. bieneusi in epithelial cell

Encephalitozoon intestinalis in epithelial cells, endothelial cells, or macrophages

Presumed ingestion or respiratory aquisition of spores

While *E. bieneusi* is primarily in the gastrointestinal tract, other species may invade the lung or eye or disseminate to cause:

Chronic diarrhea
Cholangitis
Sinusitis
Bronchitis
Nephritis
Cystitis/prostatitis
Keratoconjunctivitis
Encephalitis

Spore-laden host epithelial cells sloughed into lumina of gastrointestinal, respiratory, or genitourinary tract

Person-to-person, zoonotic, water-borne, or food-borne transmission?

Sloughed cells degenerate; spores shed in bodily fluids

Diagnostic spores present in stool, urine, respiratory fluids, cerebrospinal fluid, or various tissue specimens

Figure 215-3   Life cycle of microsporidia. *(Reprinted from RL Guerrant et al: Tropical Infectious Disease: Principles, Pathogens and Practice, 2nd ed, 2006, p 1128, with permission from Elsevier Science.)*

Microsporidia are small gram-positive organisms with mature spores measuring 0.5–2 μm × 1–4 μm. Diagnosis of microsporidial infections in tissue often requires electron microscopy, although intracellular spores can be visualized by light microscopy with hematoxylin and eosin, Giemsa, or tissue Gram's stain. For the diagnosis of intestinal microsporidiosis, modified trichrome or chromotrope 2R-based staining and Uvitex 2B or calcofluor fluorescent staining reveal spores in smears of feces or duodenal aspirates. Definitive therapies for microsporidial infections remain to be established. For superficial keratoconjunctivitis due to *E. hellem*, topical therapy with fumagillin suspension has shown promise (Chap. 208). For enteric infections with *E. bieneusi* and *E. intestinalis* in HIV-infected patients, therapy with albendazole may be efficacious (Chap. 208).

OTHER INTESTINAL PROTOZOA

Balantidiasis

Balantidium coli is a large ciliated protozoal parasite that can produce a spectrum of large-intestinal disease analogous to amebiasis. The parasite is widely distributed in the world. Since it infects pigs, cases in humans are more common where pigs are raised. Infective cysts can be transmitted from person to person and through water, but many cases are due to the ingestion of cysts derived from porcine feces in association with slaughtering, with use of pig feces for fertilizer, or with contamination of water supplies by pig feces.

Ingested cysts liberate trophozoites, which reside and replicate in the large bowel. Many patients remain asymptomatic, but some have persisting intermittent diarrhea, and a few develop more fulminant dysentery. In symptomatic individuals, the pathology in the bowel—both gross and microscopic—is similar to that seen in amebiasis, with varying degrees of mucosal invasion, focal necrosis, and ulceration. Balantidiasis, unlike amebiasis, does not spread hematogenously to other organs. The diagnosis is made by detection of the trophozoite stage in stool or sampled colonic tissue. Tetracycline (500 mg four times daily for 10 days) is an effective therapeutic agent.

Blastocystis hominis infection

B. hominis, while believed by some to be a protozoan capable of causing intestinal disease, remains an organism of uncertain pathogenicity. Some patients who pass *B. hominis* in their stools are asymptomatic, whereas others have diarrhea and associated intestinal symptoms. Diligent evaluation reveals other potential bacterial, viral, or protozoal causes of diarrhea in some but not all patients with symptoms. Because the pathogenicity of *B. hominis* is uncertain and because therapy for *Blastocystis* infection is neither specific nor uniformly effective, patients with prominent intestinal symptoms should be fully evaluated for other infectious causes of diarrhea. If diarrheal symptoms associated with *Blastocystis* are prominent, either metronidazole (750 mg thrice daily for 10 days) or TMP-SMX (160 mg/800 mg twice daily for 7 days) can be used.

Dientamoeba fragilis infection

D. fragilis is unique among intestinal protozoa in that it has a trophozoite stage but not a cyst stage. How trophozoites survive to transmit infection is not known. When symptoms develop in patients with *D. fragilis* infection, they are generally mild and include intermittent diarrhea, abdominal pain, and anorexia. The diagnosis is made by the detection of trophozoites in stool; the lability of these forms accounts for the greater yield when fecal samples are preserved immediately after collection. Since fecal excretion rates vary, examination of several samples obtained on alternate days increases the rate of detection. Iodoquinol (650 mg three times daily for 20 days), paromomycin (25–35 mg/kg per day in three doses for 7 days), metronidazole (500–750 mg three times daily for 10 days), or tetracycline (500 mg four times daily for 10 days) is appropriate for treatment.

TRICHOMONIASIS

Various species of trichomonads can be found in the mouth (in association with periodontitis) and occasionally in the gastrointestinal tract. *Trichomonas vaginalis*—one of the most prevalent protozoal parasites in the United States—is a pathogen of the genitourinary tract and a major cause of symptomatic vaginitis.

Life cycle and epidemiology

T. vaginalis is a pear-shaped, actively motile organism that measures about 10×7 μm, replicates by binary fission, and inhabits the lower genital tract of females and the urethra and prostate of males. In the United States, it accounts for ~3 million infections per year in women. While the organism can survive for a few hours in moist environments and could be acquired by direct contact, person-to-person venereal transmission accounts for virtually all cases of trichomoniasis. Its prevalence is greatest among persons with multiple sexual partners and among those with other sexually transmitted diseases (Chap. 130).

Clinical manifestations

Many men infected with *T. vaginalis* are asymptomatic, although some develop urethritis and a few have epididymitis or prostatitis. In contrast, infection in women, which has an incubation period of 5–28 days, is usually symptomatic and manifests with malodorous vaginal discharge (often yellow), vulvar erythema and itching, dysuria or urinary frequency (in 30–50% of patients), and dyspareunia. These manifestations, however, do not clearly distinguish trichomoniasis from other types of infectious vaginitis.

Diagnosis

Detection of motile trichomonads by microscopic examination of wet mounts of vaginal or prostatic secretions has been the conventional means of diagnosis. Although this approach provides an immediate diagnosis, its sensitivity for the detection of *T. vaginalis* is only ~50–60% in routine evaluations of vaginal secretions. Direct immunofluorescent antibody staining is more sensitive (70–90%) than wet-mount examinations. *T. vaginalis* can be recovered from the urethra of both males and females and is detectable in males after prostatic massage. Culture of the parasite is the most sensitive means of detection; however, facilities for culture are not generally available, and detection of the organism takes 3–7 days.

TREATMENT   Trichomoniasis

Metronidazole, given either as a single 2-g dose or in 500-mg doses twice daily for 7 days, is usually effective. Tinidazole (a single 2-g dose) is also effective. All sexual partners must be treated concurrently to prevent reinfection, especially from asymptomatic males. In males with persistent symptomatic urethritis after therapy for nongonococcal urethritis, metronidazole therapy should be considered for possible trichomoniasis. Alternatives to metronidazole for treatment during pregnancy are not readily available, although use of 100-mg clotrimazole vaginal suppositories nightly for 2 weeks may cure some infections in pregnant women. Reinfection often accounts for apparent treatment failures, but strains of *T. vaginalis* exhibiting high-level resistance to metronidazole have been encountered. Treatment of these resistant infections with higher oral doses, parenteral doses, or concurrent oral and vaginal doses of metronidazole or with tinidazole has been successful.

FURTHER READINGS

Articles

ABUBAKAR I et al: Treatment of cryptosporidiosis in immunocompromised individuals: Systematic review and meta-analysis. Br J Clin Pharmacol 63:387, 2007

CHALMERS RM, DAVIES AP: Minireview: Clinical cryptosporidiosis. Exp Parasitol 124:138, 2010

DALY ER et al: Outbreak of giardiasis associated with a community drinking-water source. Epidemiol Infect 138:491, 2010

GUPTA S et al: Chronic diarrhoea in HIV patients: Prevalence of coccidian parasites. Indian J Med Microbiol 26:172, 2008

HUPPERT JS: Trichomoniasis in teens: An update. Curr Opin Obstet Gynecol 21:371, 2009

LANTERNIER F et al: Microsporidiosis in solid organ transplant recipients: Two *Enterocytozoon bieneusi* cases and review. Transpl Infect Dis 11:83, 2009

ORTEGA YR, SANCHEZ R: Update on *Cyclospora cayetanensis*, a food-borne and waterborne parasite. Clin Microbiol Rev 23:218, 2010

ROBERTSON LJ et al: Giardiasis—Why do the symptoms sometimes never stop? Trends Parasitol 26:75, 2010

SCHUSTER FL, RAMIREZ-AVILA L: Current world status of *Balantidium coli*. Clin Microbiol Rev 21:626, 2008

TAN KS: New insights on classification, identification, and clinical relevance of *Blastocystis* spp. Clin Microbiol Rev 21:639, 2008

VANDENBERG O et al: Clinical and microbiological features of dientamoebiasis in patients suspected of suffering from a parasitic gastrointestinal illness: A comparison of *Dientamoeba fragilis* and *Giardia lamblia* infections. Int J Infect Dis 10:255, 2006

WEITZEL T et al: Epidemiological and clinical features of travel-associated cryptosporidiosis. Clin Microbiol Infect 12:921, 2006

YODER JS, BEACH MJ: *Cryptosporidium* surveillance and risk factors in the United States. Exp Parasitol 124:31, 2010

———, ———: Giardiasis surveillance—United States, 2003–2005. MMWR Surveill Summ 56:11, 2007

Book

WEISS LM, SCHWARTZ DA: Microsporidiosis, in *Tropical Infectious Diseases: Principles, Pathogens and Practice*, 2nd ed, RL Guerrant et al (eds). Elsevier, Philadelphia, 2006, pp 1126–1140

Web Site

CDC DIVISION OF PARASITIC DISEASES. *http://www.cdc.gov/ncidod/dpd/default.htm*

CHAPTER **216**

Trichinellosis and Other Tissue Nematode Infections

Peter F. Weller

Nematodes are elongated, symmetric roundworms. Parasitic nematodes of medical significance may be broadly classified as either predominantly intestinal or tissue nematodes. This chapter covers the tissue nematodes that cause trichinellosis, visceral and ocular larva migrans, cutaneous larva migrans, cerebral angiostrongyliasis, and gnathostomiasis. All of these zoonotic infections result from incidental exposure to infectious nematodes. The clinical symptoms of these infections are due largely to invasive larval stages that (except in the case of *Trichinella*) do not reach maturity in humans.

TRICHINELLOSIS

Trichinellosis develops after the ingestion of meat containing cysts of *Trichinella* (e.g., pork or other meat from a carnivore). Although most infections are mild and asymptomatic, heavy infections can cause severe enteritis, periorbital edema, myositis, and (infrequently) death.

Life cycle and epidemiology

Eight species of *Trichinella* are recognized as causes of infection in humans. Two species are distributed worldwide: *T. spiralis*, which is found in a great variety of carnivorous and omnivorous animals, and *T. pseudospiralis*, which is found in mammals and birds. *T. nativa* is present in Arctic regions and infects bears; *T. nelsoni* is found in equatorial eastern Africa, where it is common among felid predators and scavengers such as hyenas and bush pigs; and *T. britovi* is found in Europe, western Africa, and western Asia among carnivores but not among domestic swine. *T. murrelli* is present in North American game animals.

After human consumption of trichinous meat, encysted larvae are liberated by digestive acid and proteases (Fig. 216-1). The larvae invade the small-bowel mucosa and mature into adult worms. After ~1 week, female worms release newborn larvae that migrate via the circulation to striated muscle. The larvae of all species except *T. pseudospiralis*, *T. papuae*, and

T. zimbabwensis then encyst by inducing a radical transformation in the muscle cell architecture. Although host immune responses may help to expel intestinal adult worms, they have little effect on muscle-dwelling larvae.

Human trichinellosis is often caused by the ingestion of infected pork products and thus can occur in almost any location where the meat of domestic or wild swine is eaten. Human trichinellosis also may be acquired from the meat of other animals, including dogs (in parts of Asia and Africa), horses (in Italy and France), and bears and walruses (in northern regions). Although cattle (being herbivores) are not natural hosts of *Trichinella*, beef has been implicated in outbreaks when contaminated or adulterated with trichinous pork. Laws that prohibit the feeding of uncooked garbage to pigs have greatly reduced the transmission of trichinellosis in the United States. About 12 cases of trichinellosis are reported annually in this country, but most mild cases probably remain undiagnosed. Recent U.S. and Canadian outbreaks have been attributable to consumption of wild game (especially bear meat) and, less frequently, of pork.

Pathogenesis and clinical features

Clinical symptoms of trichinellosis arise from the successive phases of parasite enteric invasion, larval migration, and muscle encystment (Fig. 216-1). Most light infections (those with <10 larvae per

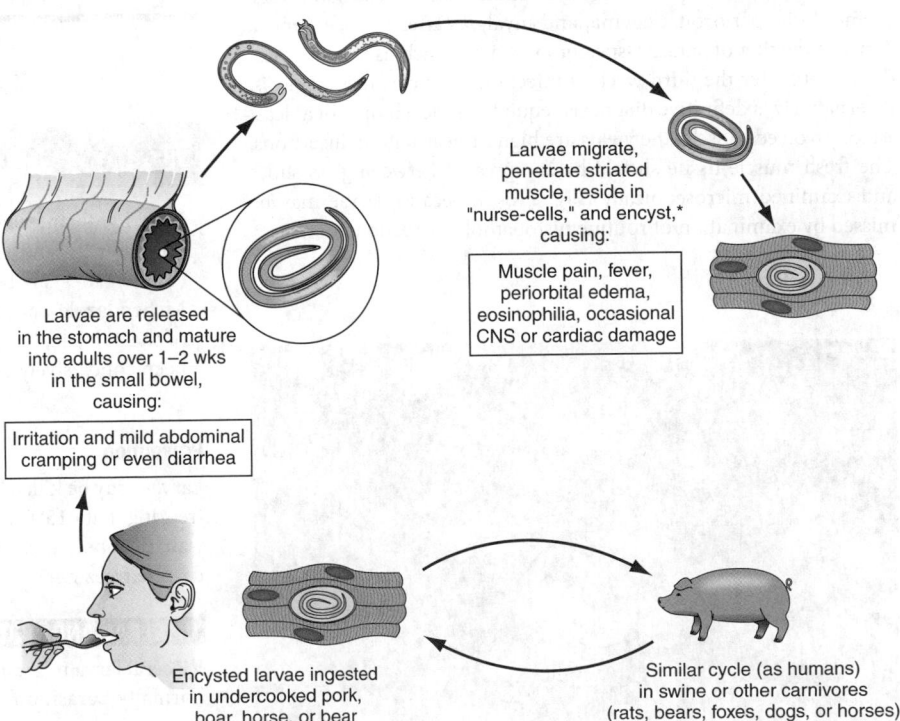

Figure 216-1 Life cycle of Trichinella spiralis (cosmopolitan); *nelsoni* (equatorial Africa); *britovi* (Europe, western Africa, western Asia); *nativa* (Arctic); *murrelli* (North America); *papuae* (Papua New Guinea); *zimbabwensis* (Tanzania); and *pseudospiralis* (cosmopolitan). CNS, central nervous system. [Reprinted from Guerrant RL et al (eds): Tropical Infectious Diseases: Principles, Pathogens and Practice, 2nd ed, p 1218. © 2006, with permission from Elsevier Science.]

gram of muscle) are asymptomatic, whereas heavy infections (which can involve >50 larvae per gram of muscle) can be life-threatening. Invasion of the gut by large numbers of parasites occasionally provokes diarrhea during the first week after infection. Abdominal pain, constipation, nausea, or vomiting also may be prominent.

Symptoms due to larval migration and muscle invasion begin to appear in the second week after infection. The migrating *Trichinella* larvae provoke a marked local and systemic hypersensitivity reaction, with fever and hypereosinophilia. Periorbital and facial edema is common, as are hemorrhages in the subconjunctivae, retina, and nail beds ("splinter" hemorrhages). A maculopapular rash, headache, cough, dyspnea, or dysphagia sometimes develops. Myocarditis with tachyarrhythmias or heart failure—and, less commonly, encephalitis or pneumonitis—may develop and accounts for most deaths of patients with trichinellosis.

Upon onset of larval encystment in muscle 2–3 weeks after infection, symptoms of myositis with myalgias, muscle edema, and weakness develop, usually overlapping with the inflammatory reactions to migrating larvae. The most commonly involved muscle groups include the extraocular muscles; the biceps; and the muscles of the jaw, neck, lower back, and diaphragm. Peaking ~3 weeks after infection, symptoms subside only gradually during a prolonged convalescence. Uncommon infections with *T. pseudospiralis*, whose larvae do not encapsulate in muscles, elicit prolonged polymyositis-like illness.

Laboratory findings and diagnosis

Blood eosinophilia develops in >90% of patients with symptomatic trichinellosis and may peak at a level of >50% 2–4 weeks after infection. Serum levels of muscle enzymes, including creatine phosphokinase, are elevated in most symptomatic patients. Patients should be questioned thoroughly about their consumption of pork or wild animal meat and about illness in other individuals who ate the same meat. A presumptive clinical diagnosis can be based on fevers, eosinophilia, periorbital edema, and myalgias after a suspect meal. A rise in the titer of parasite-specific antibody, which usually does not occur until after the third week of infection, confirms the diagnosis. Alternatively, a definitive diagnosis requires surgical biopsy of at least 1 g of involved muscle; the yields are highest near tendon insertions. The fresh muscle tissue should be compressed between glass slides and examined microscopically (Fig. 216-2), because larvae may be missed by examination of routine histopathologic sections alone.

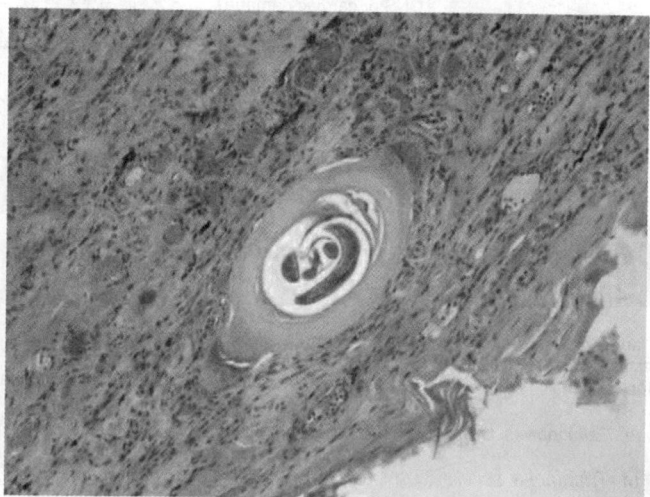

Figure 216-2 *Trichinella* **larva** encysted in a characteristic hyalinized capsule in striated muscle tissue. *(Photo/Wadsworth Center, New York State Department of Health. Reprinted from MMWR 53:606, 2004; public domain.)*

TABLE 216-1 Therapy for Tissue Nematode Infections

Infection	Severity	Treatment
Trichinellosis	Mild	Supportive
	Moderate	Albendazole (400 mg bid × 8–14 days) or
		Mebendazole (200–400 mg tid × 3 days, then 400 mg tid × 8–14 days)
	Severe	Add glucocorticoids (e.g., prednisone, 1 mg/kg qd × 5 days)
Visceral larva migrans	Mild to moderate	Supportive
	Severe	Glucocorticoids (as above)
	Ocular	Not fully defined; albendazole (800 mg bid for adults, 400 mg bid for children) with glucocorticoids × 5–20 days has been effective
Cutaneous larva migrans		Ivermectin (single dose, 200 µg/kg) or
		Albendazole (200 mg bid × 3 days)
Angiostrongyliasis	Mild to moderate	Supportive
	Severe	Glucocorticoids (as above)
Gnathostomiasis		Ivermectin (200 µg/kg per day × 2 days) or
		Albendazole (400 mg bid × 21 days)

TREATMENT   Trichinellosis

Most lightly infected patients recover uneventfully with bed rest, antipyretics, and analgesics. Glucocorticoids like prednisone (Table 216-1) are beneficial for severe myositis and myocarditis. Mebendazole and albendazole are active against enteric stages of the parasite, but their efficacy against encysted larvae has not been conclusively demonstrated.

Prevention

Larvae may be killed by cooking pork until it is no longer pink or by freezing it at –15°C for 3 weeks. However, Arctic *T. nativa* larvae in walrus or bear meat are relatively resistant and may remain viable despite freezing.

VISCERAL AND OCULAR LARVA MIGRANS

Visceral larva migrans is a syndrome caused by nematodes that are normally parasitic for nonhuman host species. In humans, these nematode larvae do not develop into adult worms but instead migrate through host tissues and elicit eosinophilic inflammation. The most common form of visceral larva migrans is toxocariasis due to larvae of the canine ascarid *Toxocara canis*; the syndrome is due less commonly to the feline ascarid *T. cati* and even less commonly to the pig ascarid *Ascaris suum*. Rare cases with eosinophilic meningoencephalitis have been caused by the raccoon ascarid *Baylisascaris procyonis*.

Life cycle and epidemiology

The canine roundworm *T. canis* is distributed among dogs worldwide. Ingestion of infective eggs by dogs is followed by liberation of *Toxocara* larvae, which penetrate the gut wall and migrate intravascularly into canine tissues, where most remain in a developmentally arrested state. During pregnancy, some larvae resume migration in bitches and infect puppies prenatally (through transplacental transmission) or after birth (through suckling). Thus, in lactating bitches and puppies, larvae return to the intestinal tract and develop into adult worms, which produce eggs that are released in the feces. Eggs must undergo embryonation over several weeks to become infectious. Humans acquire toxocariasis mainly by eating soil contaminated by puppy feces that contains infective *T. canis* eggs. Visceral larva migrans is most common among children who habitually eat dirt.

Pathogenesis and clinical features

Clinical disease most commonly afflicts preschool children. After humans ingest *Toxocara* eggs, the larvae hatch and penetrate the intestinal mucosa, from which they are carried by the circulation to a wide variety of organs and tissues. The larvae invade the liver, lungs, central nervous system (CNS), and other sites, provoking intense local eosinophilic granulomatous responses. The degree of clinical illness depends on larval number and tissue distribution, reinfection, and host immune responses. Most light infections are asymptomatic and may be manifest only by blood eosinophilia. Characteristic symptoms of visceral larva migrans include fever, malaise, anorexia and weight loss, cough, wheezing, and rashes. Hepatosplenomegaly is common. These features are often accompanied by extraordinary peripheral eosinophilia, which may approach 90%. Uncommonly, seizures or behavioral disorders develop. Rare deaths are due to severe neurologic, pneumonic, or myocardial involvement.

The ocular form of the larva migrans syndrome occurs when *Toxocara* larvae invade the eye. An eosinophilic granulomatous mass, most commonly in the posterior pole of the retina, develops around the entrapped larva. The retinal lesion can mimic retinoblastoma in appearance, and mistaken diagnosis of the latter condition can lead to unnecessary enucleation. The spectrum of eye involvement also includes endophthalmitis, uveitis, and chorioretinitis. Unilateral visual disturbances, strabismus, and eye pain are the most common presenting symptoms. In contrast to visceral larva migrans, ocular toxocariasis usually develops in older children or young adults with no history of pica; these patients seldom have eosinophilia or visceral manifestations.

Diagnosis

In addition to eosinophilia, leukocytosis and hypergammaglobulinemia may be evident. Transient pulmonary infiltrates are apparent on chest x-rays of about one-half of patients with symptoms of pneumonitis. The clinical diagnosis can be confirmed by an enzyme-linked immunosorbent assay for toxocaral antibodies. Stool examination for parasite eggs, while important in the evaluation of unexplained eosinophilia, is worthless for toxocariasis, since the larvae do not develop into egg-producing adults in humans.

| TREATMENT | Visceral and Ocular Larva Migrans |

The vast majority of *Toxocara* infections are self-limited and resolve without specific therapy. In patients with severe myocardial, CNS, or pulmonary involvement, glucocorticoids may be employed to reduce inflammatory complications. Available antihelminthic drugs, including mebendazole and albendazole,

have not been shown conclusively to alter the course of larva migrans. Control measures include prohibiting dog excreta in public parks and playgrounds, deworming dogs, and preventing pica in children. Treatment of ocular disease is not fully defined, but the administration of albendazole in conjunction with glucocorticoids has been effective (Table 216-1).

CUTANEOUS LARVA MIGRANS

Cutaneous larva migrans ("creeping eruption") is a serpiginous skin eruption caused by burrowing larvae of animal hookworms, usually the dog and cat hookworm *Ancylostoma braziliense*. The larvae hatch from eggs passed in dog and cat feces and mature in the soil. Humans become infected after skin contact with soil in areas frequented by dogs and cats, such as areas underneath house porches. Cutaneous larva migrans is prevalent among children and travelers in regions with warm humid climates, including the southeastern United States.

After larvae penetrate the skin, erythematous lesions form along the tortuous tracks of their migration through the dermal-epidermal junction; the larvae advance several centimeters in a day. The intensely pruritic lesions may occur anywhere on the body and can be numerous if the patient has lain on the ground. Vesicles and bullae may form later. The animal hookworm larvae do not mature in humans and, without treatment, will die after an interval ranging from weeks to a couple of months, with resolution of skin lesions. The diagnosis is made on clinical grounds. Skin biopsies only rarely detect diagnostic larvae. Symptoms can be alleviated by ivermectin or albendazole (Table 216-1).

ANGIOSTRONGYLIASIS

Angiostrongylus cantonensis, the rat lungworm, is the most common cause of human eosinophilic meningitis (Fig. 216-3).

Life cycle and epidemiology

This infection occurs principally in Southeast Asia and the Pacific Basin but has spread to other areas of the world. *A. cantonensis* larvae produced by adult worms in the rat lung migrate to the gastrointestinal tract and are expelled with the feces. They develop into infective larvae in land snails and slugs. Humans acquire the infection by ingesting raw infected mollusks; vegetables contaminated by mollusk slime; or crabs, freshwater shrimp, and certain marine fish that have themselves eaten infected mollusks. The larvae then migrate to the brain.

Pathogenesis and clinical features

The parasites eventually die in the CNS, but not before initiating pathologic consequences that, in heavy infections, can result in permanent neurologic sequelae or death. Migrating larvae cause marked local eosinophilic inflammation and hemorrhage, with subsequent necrosis and granuloma formation around dying worms. Clinical symptoms develop 2–35 days after the ingestion of larvae. Patients usually present with an insidious or abrupt excruciating frontal, occipital, or bitemporal headache. Neck stiffness, nausea and vomiting, and paresthesias are also common. Fever, cranial and extraocular nerve palsies, seizures, paralysis, and lethargy are uncommon.

Laboratory findings

Examination of cerebrospinal fluid (CSF) is mandatory in suspected cases and usually reveals an elevated opening pressure, a white blood cell count of 150–2000/μL, and an eosinophilic pleocytosis of >20%. The protein concentration is usually elevated and the glucose

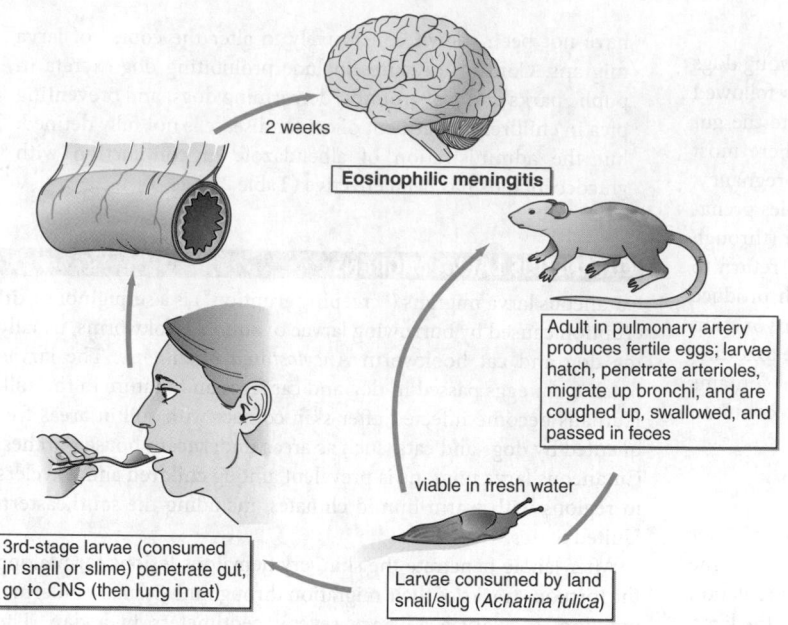

Figure 216-3 Life cycle of *Angiostrongylus cantonensis* (rat lung worm), found in Southeast Asia, Pacific Islands, Cuba, Australia, Japan, China, Mauritius, and U.S. ports. CNS, central nervous system. *[Reprinted from Guerrant RL et al (eds): Tropical Infectious Diseases: Principles, Pathogens and Practice, 2nd ed, p 1225. © 2006, with permission from Elsevier Science.]*

Figure labels

2 weeks

Eosinophilic meningitis

Adult in pulmonary artery produces fertile eggs; larvae hatch, penetrate arterioles, migrate up bronchi, and are coughed up, swallowed, and passed in feces

viable in fresh water

3rd-stage larvae (consumed in snail or slime) penetrate gut, go to CNS (then lung in rat)

Larvae consumed by land snail/slug (*Achatina fulica*)

level normal. The larvae of *A. cantonensis* are only rarely seen in CSF. Peripheral-blood eosinophilia may be mild. The diagnosis is generally based on the clinical presentation of eosinophilic meningitis together with a compatible epidemiologic history.

TREATMENT   Angiostrongyliasis

Specific chemotherapy is not of benefit in angiostrongyliasis; larvicidal agents may exacerbate inflammatory brain lesions. Management consists of supportive measures, including the administration of analgesics, sedatives, and—in severe cases—glucocorticoids (Table 216-1). Repeated lumbar punctures with removal of CSF can relieve symptoms. In most patients, cerebral angiostrongyliasis has a self-limited course, and recovery is complete. The infection may be prevented by adequately cooking snails, crabs, and prawns and inspecting vegetables for mollusk infestation. Other parasitic or fungal causes of eosinophilic meningitis in endemic areas may include gnathostomiasis (see below), paragonimiasis (Chap. 219), schistosomiasis (Chap. 219), neurocysticercosis (Chap. 220), and coccidioidomycosis (Chap. 200).

GNATHOSTOMIASIS

Infection of human tissues with larvae of *Gnathostoma spinigerum* can cause eosinophilic meningoencephalitis, migratory cutaneous swellings, or invasive masses of the eye and visceral organs.

Life cycle and epidemiology

Human gnathostomiasis occurs in many countries and is notably endemic in Southeast Asia and parts of China and Japan. In nature, the mature adult worms parasitize the gastrointestinal tract of dogs and cats. First-stage larvae hatch from eggs passed into water and are ingested by *Cyclops* species (water fleas). Infective third-stage larvae develop in the flesh of many animal species (including fish, frogs, eels, snakes, chickens, and ducks) that have eaten either infected *Cyclops* or another infected second intermediate host. Humans typically acquire the infection by eating raw or undercooked fish or poultry. Raw fish dishes, such as *som fak* in Thailand and *sashimi* in Japan, account for many cases of human gnathostomiasis. Some cases in Thailand result from the local practice of applying frog or snake flesh as a poultice.

Pathogenesis and clinical features

Clinical symptoms are due to the aberrant migration of a single larva into cutaneous, visceral, neural, or ocular tissues. After invasion, larval migration may cause local inflammation, with pain, cough, or hematuria accompanied by fever and eosinophilia. Painful, itchy, migratory swellings may develop in the skin, particularly in the distal extremities or periorbital area. Cutaneous swellings usually last ~1 week but often recur intermittently over many years. Larval invasion of the eye can provoke a sight-threatening inflammatory response. Invasion of the CNS results in eosinophilic meningitis with myeloencephalitis, a serious complication due to ascending larval migration along a large nerve track. Patients characteristically present with agonizing radicular pain and paresthesias in the trunk or a limb, which are followed shortly by paraplegia. Cerebral involvement, with focal hemorrhages and tissue destruction, is often fatal.

Diagnosis and treatment

Cutaneous migratory swellings with marked peripheral eosinophilia, supported by an appropriate geographic and dietary history, generally constitute an adequate basis for a clinical diagnosis of gnathostomiasis. However, patients may present with ocular or cerebrospinal involvement without antecedent cutaneous swellings. In the latter case, eosinophilic pleocytosis is demonstrable (usually along with hemorrhagic or xanthochromic CSF), but worms are almost never recovered from CSF. Surgical removal of the parasite from subcutaneous or ocular tissue, though rarely feasible, is both diagnostic and therapeutic. Albendazole or ivermectin may be helpful (Table 216-1). At present, cerebrospinal involvement is managed with supportive measures and generally with a course of glucocorticoids. Gnathostomiasis can be prevented by adequate cooking of fish and poultry in endemic areas.

FURTHER READINGS

Articles

Bouchard O et al: Cutaneous larva migrans in travelers: A prospective study, with assessment of therapy with ivermectin. Clin Infect Dis 31:493, 2000

Bowman DD et al: Hookworms of dogs and cats as agents of cutaneous larva migrans. Trends Parasitol 26:162, 2010

Herman JS, Chiodini PL: Gnathostomiasis, another emerging imported disease. Clin Microbiol Rev 22:484, 2009

Kennedy ED et al: Trichinellosis surveillance—United States, 2002–2007. MMWR Surveill Summ 58:1, 2009

Lederman ER et al: Dermatologic conditions of the ill returned traveler: An analysis from the GeoSentinel Surveillance Network. Int J Infect Dis 12:593, 2008

Ramirez-Avila L et al: Eosinophilic meningitis due to *Angiostrongylus* and *Gnathostoma* species. Clin Infect Dis 48:322, 2009

Rubinsky-Elefant G et al: Human toxocariasis: Diagnosis, worldwide seroprevalences and clinical expression of the systemic and ocular forms. Ann Trop Med Parasitol 104:3, 2010

Sakai S et al: Pulmonary lesions associated with visceral larva migrans due to *Ascaris suum* or *Toxocara canis*: Imaging of six cases. AJR Am J Roentgenol 186:1697, 2006

Shimoni Z et al: The use of prednisone in the treatment of trichinellosis. Isr Med Assoc J 9:537, 2007

Wang QP et al: Human angiostrongyliasis. Lancet Infect Dis 8:621, 2008

Won KY et al: National seroprevalence and risk factors for zoonotic *Toxocara* spp. infection. Am J Trop Med Hyg 79:552, 2008

Web Sites

CDC Division of Parasitic Diseases. *http://www.cdc.gov/ncidod/dpd/default.htm*

CHAPTER **217**

Intestinal Nematode Infections

Peter F. Weller
Thomas B. Nutman

More than a billion persons worldwide are infected with one or more species of intestinal nematodes. Table 217-1 summarizes biologic and clinical features of infections due to the major intestinal parasitic nematodes. These parasites are most common in regions with poor fecal sanitation, particularly in resource-poor countries in the tropics and subtropics, but they have also been seen with increasing frequency among immigrants and refugees to resource-rich countries. Although nematode infections are not usually fatal, they contribute to malnutrition and diminished work capacity. It is interesting that these helminth infections may protect some individuals from allergic disease. Humans may on occasion be infected with nematode parasites that ordinarily infect animals; these zoonotic infections produce diseases such as trichostrongyliasis, anisakiasis, capillariasis, and abdominal angiostrongyliasis.

Intestinal nematodes are roundworms; they range in length from 1 mm to many centimeters when mature (Table 217-1). Their life cycles are complex and highly varied; some species, including *Strongyloides stercoralis* and *Enterobius vermicularis*, can be transmitted directly from person to person, while others, such as *Ascaris lumbricoides*, *Necator americanus*, and *Ancylostoma duodenale*, require a soil phase for development. Because most helminth parasites do not self-replicate, the acquisition of a heavy burden of adult worms requires repeated exposure to the parasite in its infectious stage, whether larval or egg. Hence, clinical disease, as opposed to asymptomatic infection, generally develops only with prolonged residence in an endemic area and is typically related to infection intensity. In persons with marginal nutrition, intestinal helminth infections may impair growth and development. Eosinophilia and elevated serum IgE levels are features of many helminth infections and, when unexplained, should always prompt a search for intestinal helminths. Significant protective immunity to intestinal nematodes appears not to develop in humans, although mechanisms of parasite immune evasion and host immune responses to these infections have not been elucidated in detail.

ASCARIASIS

A. lumbricoides is the largest intestinal nematode parasite of humans, reaching up to 40 cm in length. Most infected individuals have low worm burdens and are asymptomatic. Clinical disease arises from larval migration in the lungs or effects of the adult worms in the intestines.

Life cycle

Adult worms live in the lumen of the small intestine. Mature female *Ascaris* worms are extraordinarily fecund, each producing up to 240,000 eggs a day, which pass with the feces. Ascarid eggs, which are remarkably resistant to environmental stresses, become infective after several weeks of maturation in the soil and can remain infective for years. After infective eggs are swallowed, larvae hatched in the intestine invade the mucosa, migrate through the circulation to the lungs, break into the alveoli, ascend the bronchial tree, and return—through swallowing—to the small intestine, where they develop into adult worms. Between 2 and 3 months elapse between initial infection and egg production. Adult worms live for 1–2 years.

Epidemiology

Ascaris is widely distributed in tropical and subtropical regions as well as in other humid areas, including the rural southeastern United States. Transmission typically occurs through fecally contaminated soil and is due either to a lack of sanitary facilities or to the use of human feces as fertilizer. With their propensity for hand-to-mouth fecal carriage, younger children are most affected. Infection outside endemic areas, though uncommon, can occur when eggs on transported vegetables are ingested.

Clinical features

During the lung phase of larval migration, ~9–12 days after egg ingestion, patients may develop an irritating nonproductive cough and burning substernal discomfort that is aggravated by coughing or deep inspiration. Dyspnea and blood-tinged sputum are less common. Fever is usually reported. Eosinophilia develops during this symptomatic phase and subsides slowly over weeks. Chest x-rays may reveal evidence of eosinophilic pneumonitis (Löffler's syndrome), with rounded infiltrates a few millimeters to several centimeters in size. These infiltrates may be transient and intermittent, clearing after several weeks. Where there is seasonal transmission of the parasite, seasonal pneumonitis with eosinophilia may develop in previously infected and sensitized hosts.

In established infections, adult worms in the small intestine usually cause no symptoms. In heavy infections, particularly in children, a large bolus of entangled worms can cause pain and small-bowel obstruction, sometimes complicated by perforation, intussusception, or volvulus. Single worms may cause disease when they migrate into aberrant sites. A large worm can enter and occlude the biliary tree, causing biliary colic, cholecystitis, cholangitis, pancreatitis, or (rarely) intrahepatic abscesses. Migration of

TABLE 217-1 Major Human Intestinal Parasitic Nematodes

Feature	Parasitic Nematode				
	Ascaris lumbricoides (Roundworm)	*Necator americanus, Ancylostoma duodenale* (Hookworm)	*Strongyloides stercoralis*	*Trichuris trichiura* (Whipworm)	*Enterobius vermicularis* (Pinworm)
Global prevalence in humans (millions)	807	576	100	604	209
Endemic areas	Worldwide	Hot, humid regions	Hot, humid regions	Worldwide	Worldwide
Infective stage	Egg	Filariform larva	Filariform larva	Egg	Egg
Route of infection	Oral	Percutaneous	Percutaneous or autoinfection	Oral	Oral
Gastrointestinal location of worms	Jejunal lumen	Jejunal mucosa	Small-bowel mucosa	Cecum, colonic mucosa	Cecum, appendix
Adult worm size	15–40 cm	7–12 mm	2 mm	30–50 mm	8–13 mm (female)
Pulmonary passage of larvae	Yes	Yes	Yes	No	No
Incubation period[a] (days)	60–75	40–100	17–28	70–90	35–45
Longevity	1 y	*N. americanus*: 2–5 y *A. duodenale*: 6–8 y	Decades (owing to autoinfection)	5 y	2 months
Fecundity (eggs/day/worm)	240,000	*N. americanus*: 4000–10,000 *A. duodenale*: 10,000–25,000	5000–10,000	3000–7000	2000
Principal symptoms	Rarely gastrointestinal or biliary obstruction	Iron-deficiency anemia in heavy infection	Gastrointestinal symptoms; malabsorption or sepsis in hyperinfection	Gastrointestinal symptoms, anemia	Perianal pruritus
Diagnostic stage	Eggs in stool	Eggs in fresh stool, larvae in old stool	Larvae in stool or duodenal aspirate; sputum in hyperinfection	Eggs in stool	Eggs from perianal skin on cellulose acetate tape
Treatment	Mebendazole Albendazole Pyrantel pamoate Ivermectin Nitazoxanide	Mebendazole Pyrantel pamoate Albendazole	1. Ivermectin 2. Albendazole	Mebendazole Albendazole Ivermectin	Mebendazole Pyrantel pamoate Albendazole

[a]Time from infection to egg production by mature female worm.

an adult worm up the esophagus can provoke coughing and oral expulsion of the worm. In highly endemic areas, intestinal and biliary ascariasis can rival acute appendicitis and gallstones as causes of surgical acute abdomen.

Laboratory findings

Most cases of ascariasis can be diagnosed by microscopic detection of characteristic *Ascaris* eggs (65 by 45 μm) in fecal samples. Occasionally, patients present after passing an adult worm—identifiable by its large size and smooth cream-colored surface—in the stool or through the mouth or nose. During the early transpulmonary migratory phase, when eosinophilic pneumonitis occurs, larvae can be found in sputum or gastric aspirates before diagnostic eggs appear in the stool. The eosinophilia that is prominent during this early stage usually decreases to minimal levels in established infection. Adult worms may be visualized, occasionally serendipitously, on contrast studies of the gastrointestinal tract. A plain abdominal film may reveal masses of worms in gas-filled loops of bowel in patients with intestinal obstruction. Pancreaticobiliary worms can be detected by ultrasound and endoscopic retrograde cholangiopancreatography; the latter method also has been used to extract biliary *Ascaris* worms.

TREATMENT   Ascariasis

Ascariasis should always be treated to prevent potentially serious complications. Albendazole (400 mg once), mebendazole (100 g twice daily for 3 days or 500 mg once), or ivermectin (150–200 μg/kg once) is effective. These medications are contraindicated in pregnancy, however. Pyrantel pamoate (11 mg/kg once; maximum, 1 g) is safe in pregnancy. Nitazoxanide (7.5 mg/kg once; maximum, 500 mg) has also been used in ascariasis. Mild diarrhea and abdominal pain are uncommon side effects of these agents. Partial intestinal obstruction should be managed with nasogastric suction, IV fluid administration, and instillation of piperazine through the nasogastric tube, but complete obstruction and its severe complications require immediate surgical intervention.

HOOKWORM

Two hookworm species (*A. duodenale* and *N. americanus*) are responsible for human infections. Most infected individuals are asymptomatic. Hookworm disease develops from a combination of factors—a heavy worm burden, a prolonged duration of infection, and an inadequate iron intake—and results in iron-deficiency anemia and, on occasion, hypoproteinemia.

Life cycle

Adult hookworms, which are ~1 cm long, use buccal teeth (*Ancylostoma*) or cutting plates (*Necator*) to attach to the small-bowel mucosa and suck blood (0.2 mL/d per *Ancylostoma* adult) and interstitial fluid. The adult hookworms produce thousands of eggs daily. The eggs are deposited with feces in soil, where rhabditiform larvae hatch and develop over a 1-week period into infectious filariform larvae. Infective larvae penetrate the skin and reach the lungs by way of the bloodstream. There they invade alveoli and ascend the airways before being swallowed and reaching the small intestine. The prepatent period from skin invasion to appearance of eggs in the feces is ~6–8 weeks, but it may be longer with *A. duodenale*. Larvae of *A. duodenale*, if swallowed, can survive and develop directly in the intestinal mucosa. Adult hookworms may survive over a decade but usually live ~6–8 years for *A. duodenale* and 2–5 years for *N. americanus*.

Epidemiology

 A. duodenale is prevalent in southern Europe, North Africa, and northern Asia, and *N. americanus* is the predominant species in the Western Hemisphere and equatorial Africa. The two species overlap in many tropical regions, particularly Southeast Asia. In most areas, older children have the highest incidence and greatest intensity of hookworm infection. In rural areas where fields are fertilized with human feces, older working adults also may be heavily infected.

Clinical features

Most hookworm infections are asymptomatic. Infective larvae may provoke pruritic maculopapular dermatitis ("ground itch") at the site of skin penetration as well as serpiginous tracks of subcutaneous migration (similar to those of cutaneous larva migrans; Chap. 216) in previously sensitized hosts. Larvae migrating through the lungs occasionally cause mild transient pneumonitis, but this condition develops less frequently in hookworm infection than in ascariasis. In the early intestinal phase, infected persons may develop epigastric pain (often with postprandial accentuation), inflammatory diarrhea, or other abdominal symptoms accompanied by eosinophilia. The major consequence of chronic hookworm infection is iron deficiency. Symptoms are minimal if iron intake is adequate, but marginally nourished individuals develop symptoms of progressive iron-deficiency anemia and hypoproteinemia, including weakness and shortness of breath.

Laboratory findings

The diagnosis is established by the finding of characteristic 40-by 60-μm oval hookworm eggs in the feces. Stool-concentration procedures may be required to detect light infections. Eggs of the two species are indistinguishable by light microscopy. In a stool sample that is not fresh, the eggs may have hatched to release rhabditiform larvae, which need to be differentiated from those of *S. stercoralis*. Hypochromic microcytic anemia, occasionally with eosinophilia or hypoalbuminemia, is characteristic of hookworm disease.

TREATMENT   Hookworm Infection

Hookworm infection can be eradicated with several safe and highly effective antihelminthic drugs, including albendazole (400 mg once), mebendazole (500 mg once), and pyrantel pamoate (11 mg/kg for 3 days). Mild iron-deficiency anemia can often be treated with oral iron alone. Severe hookworm disease with protein loss and malabsorption necessitates nutritional support and oral iron replacement along with deworming. There is some concern that the benzimidazoles (mebendazole and albendazole) are becoming less effective against human hookworms than in the past.

Ancylostoma caninum and *Ancylostoma braziliense*

A. caninum, the canine hookworm, has been identified as a cause of human eosinophilic enteritis, especially in northeastern Australia. In this zoonotic infection, adult hookworms attach to the small intestine (where they may be visualized by endoscopy) and elicit abdominal pain and intense local eosinophilia. Treatment with mebendazole (100 mg twice daily for 3 days) or albendazole (400 mg once) or endoscopic removal is effective. Both of these animal hookworm species can cause cutaneous larva migrans ("creeping eruption"; Chap. 216).

STRONGYLOIDIASIS

S. stercoralis is distinguished by its ability—unique among helminths (except for *Capillaria*; see below)—to replicate in the human host. This capacity permits ongoing cycles of autoinfection as infective larvae are internally produced. Strongyloidiasis can thus persist for decades without further exposure of the host to exogenous infective larvae. In immunocompromised hosts, large numbers of invasive *Strongyloides* larvae can disseminate widely and can be fatal.

Life cycle

In addition to a parasitic cycle of development, *Strongyloides* can undergo a free-living cycle of development in the soil (Fig. 217-1). This adaptability facilitates the parasite's survival in the absence of mammalian hosts. Rhabditiform larvae passed in feces can transform into infectious filariform larvae either directly or after a free-living phase of development. Humans acquire strongyloidiasis when filariform larvae in fecally contaminated soil penetrate the skin or mucous membranes. The larvae then travel through the bloodstream to the lungs, where they break into the alveolar spaces, ascend the bronchial tree, are swallowed, and thereby reach the small intestine. There the larvae mature into adult worms that penetrate the mucosa of the proximal small bowel. The minute (2-mm-long) parasitic adult female worms reproduce by parthenogenesis; adult males do not exist. Eggs hatch in the intestinal mucosa, releasing rhabditiform larvae that migrate to the lumen and pass with the feces into soil. Alternatively, rhabditiform larvae in the bowel can develop directly into filariform larvae that penetrate the colonic wall or perianal skin and enter the circulation to repeat the migration that establishes ongoing internal reinfection. This autoinfection cycle allows strongyloidiasis to persist for decades.

Epidemiology

 S. stercoralis is spottily distributed in tropical areas and other hot, humid regions and is particularly common in Southeast Asia, sub-Saharan Africa, and Brazil. In the United States, the parasite is endemic in parts of the Southeast and is found in immigrants, refugees, travelers, and military personnel who have lived in endemic areas.

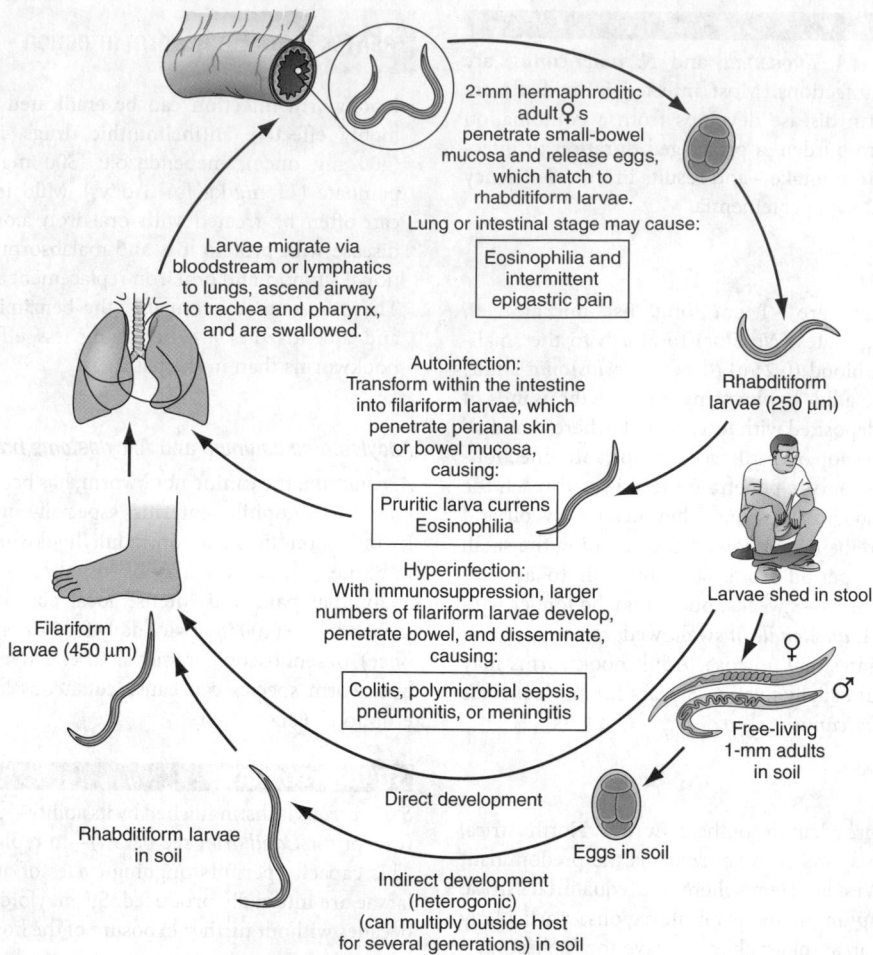

Figure 217-1 **Life cycle of** *Strongyloides stercoralis.* *(Adapted from Guerrant RL et al (eds): Tropical Infectious Diseases: Principles, Pathogens and Practice, 2nd ed, p 1276. © 2006, with permission from Elsevier Science.)*

Clinical features

In uncomplicated strongyloidiasis, many patients are asymptomatic or have mild cutaneous and/or abdominal symptoms. Recurrent urticaria, often involving the buttocks and wrists, is the most common cutaneous manifestation. Migrating larvae can elicit a pathognomonic serpiginous eruption, *larva currens* ("running larva"). This pruritic, raised, erythematous lesion advances as rapidly as 10 cm/h along the course of larval migration. Adult parasites burrow into the duodenojejunal mucosa and can cause abdominal (usually midepigastric) pain, which resembles peptic ulcer pain except that it is aggravated by food ingestion. Nausea, diarrhea, gastrointestinal bleeding, mild chronic colitis, and weight loss can occur. Small-bowel obstruction may develop with early, heavy infection. Pulmonary symptoms are rare in uncomplicated strongyloidiasis. Eosinophilia is common, with levels fluctuating over time.

The ongoing autoinfection cycle of strongyloidiasis is normally constrained by unknown factors of the host's immune system. Abrogation of host immunity, especially with glucocorticoid therapy and much less commonly with other immunosuppressive medications, leads to hyperinfection, with the generation of large numbers of filariform larvae. Colitis, enteritis, or malabsorption may develop. In disseminated strongyloidiasis, larvae may invade not only gastrointestinal tissues and the lungs but also the central nervous system, peritoneum, liver, and kidneys. Moreover, bacteremia may develop because of the passage of enteric flora through disrupted mucosal barriers. Gram-negative sepsis, pneumonia, or meningitis may complicate or dominate the clinical course. Eosinophilia is

often absent in severely infected patients. Disseminated strongyloidiasis, particularly in patients with unsuspected infection who are given glucocorticoids, can be fatal. Strongyloidiasis is a frequent complication of infection with human T cell lymphotropic virus type I, but disseminated strongyloidiasis is not common among patients infected with HIV-1.

Diagnosis

In uncomplicated strongyloidiasis, the finding of rhabditiform larvae in feces is diagnostic. Rhabditiform larvae are ~250 μm long, with a short buccal cavity that distinguishes them from hookworm larvae. In uncomplicated infections, few larvae are passed and single stool examinations detect only about one-third of cases. Serial examinations and the use of the agar plate detection method improve the sensitivity of stool diagnosis. In uncomplicated strongyloidiasis (but not in hyperinfection), stool examinations may be repeatedly negative. *Strongyloides* larvae may also be found by sampling of the duodenojejunal contents by aspiration or biopsy. An enzyme-linked immunosorbent assay for serum antibodies to antigens of *Strongyloides* is a sensitive method of diagnosing uncomplicated infections. Such serologic testing should be performed for patients whose geographic histories indicate potential exposure, especially those who exhibit eosinophilia and/or are candidates for glucocorticoid treatment of other conditions. In disseminated strongyloidiasis, filariform larvae should be sought in stool as well as in samples obtained from sites of potential larval migration, including sputum, bronchoalveolar lavage fluid, or surgical drainage fluid.

Strongyloidiasis

Even in the asymptomatic state, strongyloidiasis must be treated because of the potential for subsequent fatal hyperinfection. Ivermectin (200 μg/kg daily for 2 days) is more effective than albendazole (400 mg daily for 3 days). For disseminated strongyloidiasis, treatment with ivermectin should be extended for at least 5–7 days or until the parasites are eradicated.

TRICHURIASIS

Most infections with *Trichuris trichiura* are asymptomatic, but heavy infections may cause gastrointestinal symptoms. Like the other soil-transmitted helminths, whipworm is distributed globally in the tropics and subtropics and is most common among poor children from resource-poor regions of the world.

Life cycle

Adult *Trichuris* worms reside in the colon and cecum, the anterior portions threaded into the superficial mucosa. Thousands of eggs laid daily by adult female worms pass with the feces and mature in the soil. After ingestion, infective eggs hatch in the duodenum, releasing larvae that mature before migrating to the large bowel. The entire cycle takes ~3 months, and adult worms may live for several years.

Clinical features

Tissue reactions to *Trichuris* are mild. Most infected individuals have no symptoms or eosinophilia. Heavy infections may result in abdominal pain, anorexia, and bloody or mucoid diarrhea resembling inflammatory bowel disease. Rectal prolapse can result from massive infections in children, who often suffer from malnourishment and other diarrheal illnesses. Moderately heavy *Trichuris* burdens also contribute to growth retardation.

Diagnosis and treatment

The characteristic 50- by 20-μm lemon-shaped *Trichuris* eggs are readily detected on stool examination. Adult worms, which are 3–5 cm long, are occasionally seen on proctoscopy. Mebendazole (500 mg once) or albendazole (400 mg daily for 3 doses) is safe and moderately effective for treatment, with cure rates of 70–90%. Ivermectin (200 μg/kg daily for 3 doses) is also safe but is not quite as efficacious as the benzimidazoles.

ENTEROBIASIS (PINWORM)

E. vermicularis is more common in temperate countries than in the tropics. In the United States, ~40 million persons are infected with pinworms, with a disproportionate number of cases among children.

Life cycle and epidemiology

Enterobius adult worms are ~1 cm long and dwell in the cecum. Gravid female worms migrate nocturnally into the perianal region and release up to 10,000 immature eggs each. The eggs become infective within hours and are transmitted by hand-to-mouth passage. From ingested eggs, larvae hatch and mature into adults. This life cycle takes ~1 month, and adult worms survive for ~2 months. Self-infection results from perianal scratching and transport of infective eggs on the hands or under the nails to the mouth. Because of the ease of person-to-person spread, pinworm infections are common among family members.

Clinical features

Most pinworm infections are asymptomatic. Perianal pruritus is the cardinal symptom. The itching, which is often worse at night as a result of the nocturnal migration of the female worms, may lead to excoriation and bacterial superinfection. Heavy infections have been claimed to cause abdominal pain and weight loss. On rare occasions, pinworms invade the female genital tract, causing vulvovaginitis and pelvic or peritoneal granulomas. Eosinophilia is uncommon.

Diagnosis

Since pinworm eggs are not released in feces, the diagnosis cannot be made by conventional fecal ova and parasite tests. Instead, eggs are detected by the application of clear cellulose acetate tape to the perianal region in the morning. After the tape is transferred to a slide, microscopic examination will detect pinworm eggs, which are oval, measure 55 by 25 μm, and are flattened along one side.

Enterobiasis

Infected children and adults should be treated with mebendazole (100 mg once), albendazole (400 mg once), or pyrantel pamoate (11 mg/kg once; maximum, 1 g), with the same treatment repeated after 2 weeks. Treatment of household members is advocated to eliminate asymptomatic reservoirs of potential reinfection.

TRICHOSTRONGYLIASIS

Trichostrongylus species, which are normally parasites of herbivorous animals, occasionally infect humans, particularly in Asia and Africa. Humans acquire the infection by accidentally ingesting *Trichostrongylus* larvae on contaminated leafy vegetables. The larvae do not migrate in humans but mature directly into adult worms in the small bowel. These worms ingest far less blood than hookworms; most infected persons are asymptomatic, but heavy infections may give rise to mild anemia and eosinophilia. *Trichostrongylus* eggs in stool examinations resemble those of hookworms but are larger (85 by 115 μm). Treatment consists of mebendazole or albendazole (Chap. 208).

ANISAKIASIS

Anisakiasis is a gastrointestinal infection caused by the accidental ingestion in uncooked saltwater fish of nematode larvae belonging to the family Anisakidae. The incidence of anisakiasis in the United States has increased as a result of the growing popularity of raw fish dishes. Most cases occur in Japan, the Netherlands, and Chile, where raw fish—sashimi, pickled green herring, and ceviche, respectively—are national culinary staples. Anisakid nematodes parasitize large sea mammals such as whales, dolphins, and seals. As part of a complex parasitic life cycle involving marine food chains, infectious larvae migrate to the musculature of a variety of fish. Both *Anisakis simplex* and *Pseudoterranova decipiens* have been implicated in human anisakiasis, but an identical gastric syndrome may be caused by the red larvae of eustrongylid parasites of fish-eating birds.

When humans consume infected raw fish, live larvae may be coughed up within 48 h. Alternatively, larvae may immediately penetrate the mucosa of the stomach. Within hours, violent upper abdominal pain accompanied by nausea and occasionally vomiting ensues, mimicking an acute abdomen. The diagnosis can be established by direct visualization on upper endoscopy, outlining of the worm by contrast radiographic studies, or histopathologic examination of extracted tissue. Extraction of the burrowing larvae during endoscopy is curative. In addition, larvae may pass to the small bowel, where they penetrate the mucosa and provoke a vigorous eosinophilic granulomatous response. Symptoms may appear 1–2 weeks after the infective meal, with intermittent abdominal pain, diarrhea, nausea, and fever resembling the manifestations of Crohn's disease. The diagnosis may be suggested by barium studies and confirmed by curative surgical resection of a granuloma in which the worm is embedded. Anisakid eggs are not found in the stool, since the larvae do not mature in humans. Serologic tests have been developed but are not widely available.

Anisakid larvae in saltwater fish are killed by cooking to 60°C, freezing at −20°C for 3 days, or commercial blast freezing, but not usually by salting, marinating, or cold smoking. No medical treatment is available; surgical or endoscopic removal should be undertaken.

CAPILLARIASIS

Intestinal capillariasis is caused by ingestion of raw fish infected with *Capillaria philippinensis*. Subsequent autoinfection can lead to a severe wasting syndrome. The disease occurs in the Philippines and Thailand and, on occasion, elsewhere in Asia. The natural cycle of *C. philippinensis* involves fish from fresh and brackish water. When humans eat infected raw fish, the larvae mature in the intestine into adult worms, which produce invasive larvae that cause intestinal inflammation and villus loss. Capillariasis has an insidious onset with nonspecific abdominal pain and watery diarrhea. If untreated, progressive autoinfection can lead to protein-losing enteropathy, severe malabsorption, and ultimately death from cachexia, cardiac failure, or superinfection. The diagnosis is established by identification of the characteristic peanut-shaped (20- by 40-μm) eggs on stool examination. Severely ill patients require hospitalization and supportive therapy in addition to prolonged antihelminthic treatment with albendazole (200 mg twice daily for 10 days; Chap. 208).

ABDOMINAL ANGIOSTRONGYLIASIS

Abdominal angiostrongyliasis is found in Latin America and Africa. The zoonotic parasite *Angiostrongylus costaricensis* causes eosinophilic ileocolitis after the ingestion of contaminated vegetation. *A. costaricensis* normally parasitizes the cotton rat and other rodents, with slugs and snails serving as intermediate hosts. Humans become infected by accidentally ingesting infective larvae in mollusk slime deposited on fruits and vegetables; children are at highest risk. The larvae penetrate the gut wall and migrate to the mesenteric artery, where they develop into adult worms. Eggs deposited in the gut wall provoke an intense eosinophilic

granulomatous reaction, and adult worms may cause mesenteric arteritis, thrombosis, or frank bowel infarction. Symptoms may mimic those of appendicitis, including abdominal pain and tenderness, fever, vomiting, and a palpable mass in the right iliac fossa. Leukocytosis and eosinophilia are prominent. CT with contrast medium typically shows inflamed bowel, often with concomitant obstruction, but a definitive diagnosis is usually made surgically with partial bowel resection. Pathologic study reveals a thickened bowel wall with eosinophilic granulomas surrounding the *Angiostrongylus* eggs. In nonsurgical cases, the diagnosis rests solely on clinical grounds because larvae and eggs cannot be detected in the stool. Medical therapy for abdominal angiostrongyliasis is of uncertain efficacy. Careful observation and surgical resection for severe symptoms are the mainstays of treatment.

FURTHER READINGS

AUDICANA MT, KENNEDY MW: *Anisakis* simplex: From obscure infectious worm to inducer of immune hypersensitivity. Clin Microbiol Rev 21:360, 2008

BETHONY J et al: Soil-transmitted helminth infections: Ascariasis, trichuriasis, and hookworm. Lancet 367:1521, 2006

FOX LM, SARAVOLATZ LD: Nitazoxanide: A new thiazolide antiparasitic agent. Clin Infect Dis 40:1173, 2005

HARHAY MO et al: Epidemiology and control of human gastrointestinal parasites in children. Expert Rev Anti Infect Ther 8:219, 2010

HOTEZ PJ et al: Hookworm infection. N Engl J Med 351:799, 2004

KEISER J, UTZINGER J: Efficacy of current drugs against soil-transmitted helminth infections: Systematic review and meta-analysis. JAMA 299:1937, 2008

LU LH et al: Human intestinal capillariasis (*Capillaria philippinensis*) in Taiwan. Am J Trop Med Hyg 74:810, 2006

RAMANATHAN R, NUTMAN T: *Strongyloides stercoralis* infection in the immunocompromised host. Curr Infect Dis Rep 10:105, 2008

ROXBY AC et al: Strongyloidiasis in transplant patients. Clin Infect Dis 49:1411, 2009

SAICHUA P et al: Human intestinal capillariasis in Thailand. World J Gastroenterol 14:506, 2008

CHAPTER **218**

Filarial and Related Infections

Thomas B. Nutman

Peter F. Weller

Filarial worms are nematodes that dwell in the subcutaneous tissues and the lymphatics. Eight filarial species infect humans (Table 218-1); of these, four—*Wuchereria bancrofti*, *Brugia malayi*, *Onchocerca volvulus*, and *Loa loa*—are responsible for most serious filarial infections. Filarial parasites, which infect an estimated 170 million persons worldwide, are transmitted by specific species of mosquitoes or other arthropods and have a complex life cycle, including infective larval stages carried by insects and adult worms that reside in either lymphatic or subcutaneous tissues of humans. The offspring of adults are microfilariae, which, depending on their species, are 200–250 μm long and 5–7 μm wide, may or may not be enveloped in a loose sheath, and either circulate in the blood or migrate through the skin (Table 218-1). To complete the life cycle, microfilariae are ingested by the arthropod vector and develop over 1–2 weeks into new infective larvae. Adult worms live for many years, whereas microfilariae survive for 3–36 months. The *Rickettsia*-like endosymbiont *Wolbachia* has been found intracellularly in all stages of *Brugia*, *Wuchereria*, *Mansonella*, and *Onchocerca* and has become a target for antifilarial chemotherapy.

Usually, infection is established only with repeated, prolonged exposures to infective larvae. Since the clinical manifestations of filarial diseases develop relatively slowly, these infections should be considered to induce chronic diseases with possible long-term debilitating effects. In terms of the nature, severity, and timing of clinical manifestations, patients with filarial infections who are native to endemic areas and have lifelong exposure may differ significantly from those who are travelers or who have recently moved to these areas. Characteristically, filarial disease is more acute and intense in newly exposed individuals than in natives of endemic areas.

LYMPHATIC FILARIASIS

Lymphatic filariasis is caused by *W. bancrofti*, *B. malayi*, or *B. timori*. The threadlike adult parasites reside in lymphatic channels or lymph nodes, where they may remain viable for more than two decades.

■ EPIDEMIOLOGY

W. bancrofti, the most widely distributed filarial parasite of humans, affects an estimated 110 million people and is found throughout the tropics and subtropics, including Asia and the Pacific Islands, Africa, areas of South America, and the Caribbean basin. Humans are the only definitive host for the parasite. Generally, the subperiodic form is found only in the Pacific Islands; elsewhere, *W. bancrofti* is nocturnally periodic. (Nocturnally periodic forms of microfilariae are scarce in peripheral blood by day and increase at night, whereas subperiodic forms are present in peripheral blood at all times and reach maximal levels in the afternoon.) Natural vectors for *W. bancrofti* are *Culex fatigans* mosquitoes in urban settings and anopheline or aedean mosquitoes in rural areas.

TABLE 218-1 Characteristics of the Filariae

Organism	Periodicity	Distribution	Vector	Location of Adult	Microfilarial Location	Sheath
Wuchereria bancrofti	Nocturnal	Cosmopolitan areas worldwide, including South America, Africa, southern Asia, Papua New Guinea, China, Indonesia	*Culex, Anopheles* (mosquitoes)	Lymphatic tissue	Blood	+
	Subperiodic	Eastern Pacific	*Aedes* (mosquitoes)	Lymphatic tissue	Blood	+
Brugia malayi	Nocturnal	Southeast Asia, Indonesia, India	*Mansonia, Anopheles* (mosquitoes)	Lymphatic tissue	Blood	+
	Subperiodic	Indonesia, Southeast Asia	*Coquillettidia, Mansonia* (mosquitoes)	Lymphatic tissue	Blood	+
B. timori	Nocturnal	Indonesia	*Anopheles* (mosquitoes)	Lymphatic tissue	Blood	+
Loa loa	Diurnal	West and Central Africa	*Chrysops* (deerflies)	Subcutaneous tissue	Blood	+
Onchocerca volvulus	None	South and Central America, Africa	*Simulium* (blackflies)	Subcutaneous tissue	Skin, eye	−
Mansonella ozzardi	None	South and Central America	*Culicoides* (midges)	Undetermined site	Blood	−
		Caribbean	*Simulium* (blackflies)			
M. perstans	None	South and Central America, Africa	*Culicoides* (midges)	Body cavities, mesentery, perirenal tissue	Blood	−
M. streptocerca	None	West and Central Africa	*Culicoides* (midges)	Subcutaneous tissue	Skin	−

Brugian filariasis due to *B. malayi* occurs primarily in eastern India, Indonesia, Malaysia, and the Philippines. *B. malayi* also has two forms distinguished by the periodicity of microfilaremia. The more common nocturnal form is transmitted in areas of coastal rice fields, while the subperiodic form is found in forests. *B. malayi* naturally infects cats as well as humans. The distribution of *B. timori* is limited to the islands of southeastern Indonesia.

■ PATHOLOGY

The principal pathologic changes result from inflammatory damage to the lymphatics, which is typically caused by adult worms and not by microfilariae. Adult worms live in afferent lymphatics or sinuses of lymph nodes and cause lymphatic dilatation and thickening of the vessel walls. The infiltration of plasma cells, eosinophils, and macrophages in and around the infected vessels, along with endothelial and connective tissue proliferation, leads to tortuosity of the lymphatics and damaged or incompetent lymph valves. Lymphedema and chronic stasis changes with hard or brawny edema develop in the overlying skin. These consequences of filarial infection are due both to the direct effects of the worms and to the host's inflammatory response to the parasite. Inflammatory responses are believed to cause the granulomatous and proliferative processes that precede total lymphatic obstruction. It is thought that the lymphatic vessel remains patent as long as the worm remains viable and that the death of the worm leads to enhanced granulomatous reaction and fibrosis. Lymphatic obstruction results, and, despite collateralization of the lymphatics, lymphatic function is compromised.

■ CLINICAL FEATURES

The most common presentations of the lymphatic filariases are asymptomatic (or subclinical) microfilaremia, hydrocele (Fig. 218-1), acute adenolymphangitis (ADL), and chronic lymphatic disease. In areas where *W. bancrofti* or *B. malayi* is endemic, the overwhelming majority of infected individuals have few overt clinical manifestations of filarial infection despite large numbers of circulating microfilariae in the peripheral blood. Although they may be clinically asymptomatic, virtually all persons with *W. bancrofti* or *B. malayi* microfilaremia have some degree of subclinical disease that includes microscopic hematuria and/or proteinuria, dilated (and tortuous) lymphatics (visualized by imaging), and—in men with *W. bancrofti* infection—scrotal lymphangiectasia (detectable by ultrasound). In spite of these findings, the majority of individuals appear to remain clinically asymptomatic for years; in relatively few does the infection progress to either acute or chronic disease.

ADL is characterized by high fever, lymphatic inflammation (lymphangitis and lymphadenitis), and transient local edema. The lymphangitis is retrograde, extending peripherally from the lymph node draining the area where the adult parasites reside. Regional lymph nodes are often enlarged, and the entire lymphatic channel can become indurated and inflamed. Concomitant local thrombophlebitis can occur as well. In brugian filariasis, a single local abscess may form along the involved lymphatic tract and subsequently rupture to the surface. The lymphadenitis and lymphangitis can involve both the upper and lower extremities in both bancroftian and brugian filariasis, but involvement of the genital lymphatics occurs almost exclusively with *W. bancrofti* infection. This genital involvement can be manifested by funiculitis, epididymitis, and scrotal pain and tenderness. In endemic areas, another type of acute disease—dermatolymphangioadenitis (DLA)—is recognized as a syndrome that includes high fever, chills, myalgias, and headache. Edematous inflammatory plaques clearly demarcated from normal skin are seen. Vesicles, ulcers, and hyperpigmentation may also be noted. There is often a history of trauma, burns, radiation, insect bites, punctiform lesions, or chemical injury. Entry lesions, especially in the interdigital area, are common. DLA is often diagnosed as cellulitis.

If lymphatic damage progresses, transient lymphedema can develop into lymphatic obstruction and the permanent changes associated with elephantiasis (Fig. 218-2). Brawny edema follows

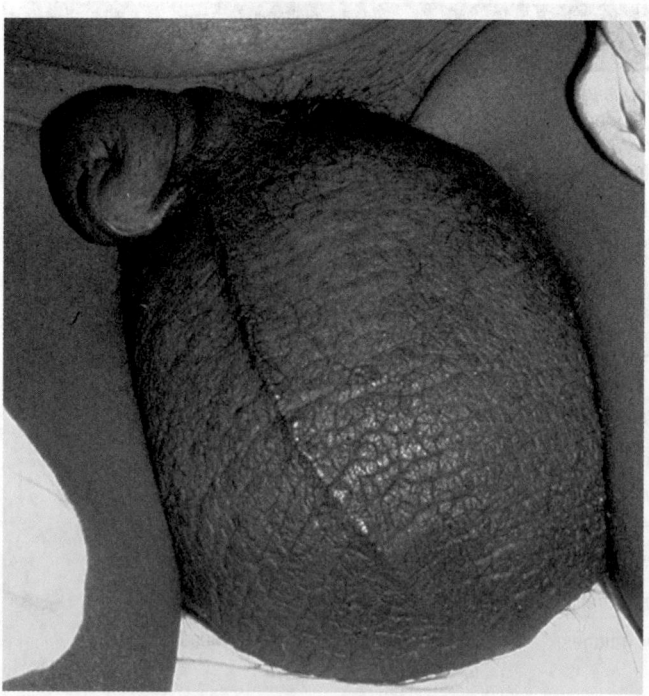

Figure 218-1   Hydrocele associated with *Wuchereria bancrofti* infection.

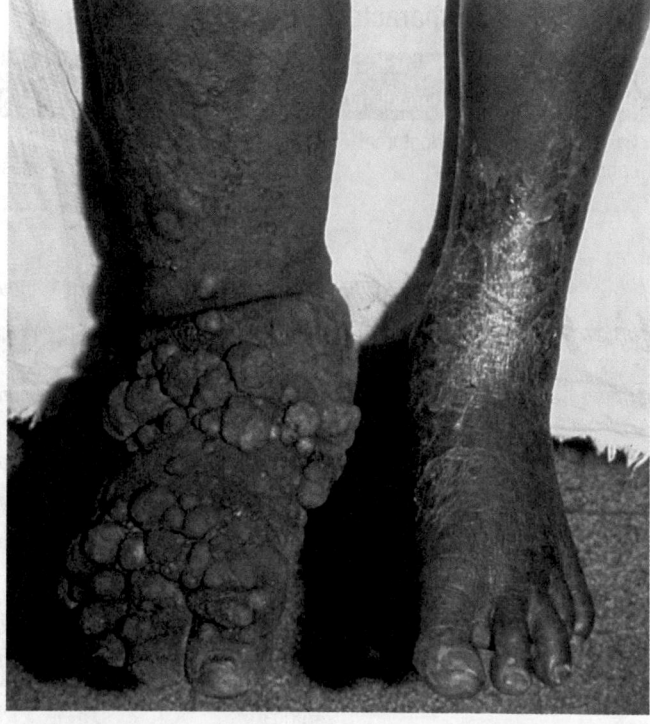

Figure 218-2   Elephantiasis of the lower extremity associated with *Wuchereria bancrofti* infection.

early pitting edema, and thickening of the subcutaneous tissues and hyperkeratosis occur. Fissuring of the skin develops, as do hyperplastic changes. Superinfection of these poorly vascularized tissues becomes a problem. In bancroftian filariasis, in which genital involvement is common, hydroceles may develop (Fig. 218-1); in advanced stages, this condition may evolve into scrotal lymphedema and scrotal elephantiasis. Furthermore, if there is obstruction of the retroperitoneal lymphatics, increased renal lymphatic pressure leads to rupture of the renal lymphatics and the development of chyluria, which is usually intermittent and most prominent in the morning.

The clinical manifestations of filarial infections in travelers or transmigrants who have recently entered an endemic region are distinctive. Given a sufficient number of bites by infected vectors, usually over a 3- to 6-month period, recently exposed patients can develop acute lymphatic or scrotal inflammation with or without urticaria and localized angioedema. Lymphadenitis of epitrochlear, axillary, femoral, or inguinal lymph nodes is often followed by retrogradely evolving lymphangitis. Acute attacks are short-lived and are not usually accompanied by fever. With prolonged exposure to infected mosquitoes, these attacks, if untreated, become more severe and lead to permanent lymphatic inflammation and obstruction.

■ DIAGNOSIS

A definitive diagnosis can be made only by detection of the parasites and hence can be difficult. Adult worms localized in lymphatic vessels or nodes are largely inaccessible. Microfilariae can be found in blood, in hydrocele fluid, or (occasionally) in other body fluids. Such fluids can be examined microscopically, either directly or—for greater sensitivity—after concentration of the parasites by the passage of fluid through a polycarbonate cylindrical-pore filter (pore size, 3 μm) or by the centrifugation of fluid fixed in 2% formalin (Knott's concentration technique). The timing of blood collection is critical and should be based on the periodicity of the microfilariae in the endemic region involved. Many infected individuals do not have microfilaremia, and definitive diagnosis in such cases can be difficult. Assays for circulating antigens of W. bancrofti permit the diagnosis of microfilaremic and cryptic (amicrofilaremic) infection. Two tests are commercially available: an enzyme-linked immunosorbent assay (ELISA) and a rapid-format immunochromatographic card test. Both assays have sensitivities of 93–100% and specificities approaching 100%. There are currently no tests for circulating antigens in brugian filariasis.

Polymerase chain reaction (PCR)-based assays for DNA of W. bancrofti and B. malayi in blood have been developed. A number of studies indicate that the sensitivity of this diagnostic method is equivalent to or greater than that of parasitologic methods.

In cases of suspected lymphatic filariasis, examination of the scrotum, the lymph nodes, or (in female patients) the breast by means of high-frequency ultrasound in conjunction with Doppler techniques may result in the identification of motile adult worms within dilated lymphatics. Worms may be visualized in the lymphatics of the spermatic cord in up to 80% of men infected with W. bancrofti. Live adult worms have a distinctive pattern of movement within the lymphatic vessels (termed the *filaria dance sign*). Radionuclide lymphoscintigraphic imaging of the limbs reliably demonstrates widespread lymphatic abnormalities in both subclinical microfilaremic persons and those with clinical manifestations of lymphatic pathology. While of potential utility in the delineation of anatomic changes associated with infection, lymphoscintigraphy is unlikely to assume primacy in the diagnostic evaluation of individuals with suspected infection; it is principally a research tool, although it has been used more widely for assessment of lymphedema of any cause. Eosinophilia and elevated serum concentrations of IgE and antifilarial antibody support the diagnosis of lymphatic

filariasis. There is, however, extensive cross-reactivity between filarial antigens and antigens of other helminths, including the common intestinal roundworms; thus, interpretations of serologic findings can be difficult. In addition, residents of endemic areas can become sensitized to filarial antigens (and thus be serologically positive) through exposure to infected mosquitoes without having patent filarial infections.

The ADL associated with lymphatic filariasis must be distinguished from thrombophlebitis, infection, and trauma. Retrograde evolution is a characteristic feature that helps distinguish filarial lymphangitis from ascending bacterial lymphangitis. Chronic filarial lymphedema must also be distinguished from the lymphedema of malignancy, postoperative scarring, trauma, chronic edematous states, and congenital lymphatic system abnormalities.

TREATMENT   Lymphatic Filariasis

With newer definitions of clinical syndromes in lymphatic filariasis and new tools to assess clinical status (e.g., ultrasound, lymphoscintigraphy, circulating filarial antigen assays, PCR), approaches to treatment based on infection status can be considered.

Diethylcarbamazine [(DEC), 6 mg/kg daily for 12 days], which has both macro- and microfilaricidal properties, remains the drug of choice for the treatment of active lymphatic filariasis (defined by microfilaremia, antigen positivity, or adult worms on ultrasound), although albendazole (400 mg twice daily for 21 days) has also demonstrated macrofilaricidal efficacy. A 4- to 6-week course of doxycycline (targeting the intracellular *Wolbachia*) also has significant macrofilaricidal activity, as has DEC/albendazole used daily for 7 days. The addition of DEC to a 3-week course of doxycycline has recently been shown to be efficacious in lymphatic filariasis.

Regimens that combine single doses of albendazole (400 mg) with either DEC (6 mg/kg) or ivermectin (200 μg/kg) all have a sustained microfilaricidal effect and are the mainstay of programs for the eradication of lymphatic filariasis in Africa (albendazole/ivermectin) and elsewhere (albendazole/DEC) (see "Prevention and Control," below).

As has already been mentioned, a growing body of evidence indicates that, although they may be asymptomatic, virtually all persons with W. bancrofti or B. malayi microfilaremia have some degree of subclinical disease (hematuria, proteinuria, abnormalities on lymphoscintigraphy). Thus, early treatment of asymptomatic persons is recommended to prevent further lymphatic damage. For ADL, supportive treatment (including the administration of antipyretics and analgesics) is recommended, as is antibiotic therapy if secondary bacterial infection is likely. Similarly, because lymphatic disease is associated with the presence of adult worms, treatment with DEC is recommended for microfilaria-negative carriers of adult worms.

In persons with chronic manifestations of lymphatic filariasis, treatment regimens that emphasize hygiene, prevention of secondary bacterial infections, and physiotherapy have gained wide acceptance for morbidity control. These regimens are similar to those recommended for lymphedema of most nonfilarial causes and known by a variety of names, including *complex decongestive physiotherapy* and *complex lymphedema therapy*. Hydroceles (Fig. 218-1) can be managed surgically. With chronic manifestations of lymphatic filariasis, drug treatment should be reserved for individuals with evidence of active infection.

Side effects of DEC treatment include fever, chills, arthralgias, headaches, nausea, and vomiting. Both the development and the severity of these reactions are directly related to the number of microfilariae circulating in the bloodstream. The adverse reactions may represent either an acute hypersensitivity reaction to the antigens being released by dead and dying parasites or an inflammatory reaction induced by the intracellular *Wolbachia* endosymbionts freed from their intracellular niche.

Ivermectin has a side effect profile similar to that of DEC when used in lymphatic filariasis. In patients infected with *L. loa*, who have high levels of *Loa* microfilaremia, DEC—like ivermectin (see "Loiasis," below)—can elicit severe encephalopathic complications. When used in single-dose regimens for the treatment of lymphatic filariasis, albendazole is associated with relatively few side effects.

■ PREVENTION AND CONTROL

To protect themselves against filarial infection, individuals must avoid contact with infected mosquitoes by using personal protective measures including bed nets, particularly those impregnated with insecticides such as permethrin. Community-based intervention is the current approach to elimination of lymphatic filariasis as a public health problem. The underlying tenet of this approach is that mass annual distribution of antimicrofilarial chemotherapy—albendazole with either DEC (for all areas except those where onchocerciasis is coendemic; see section on onchocerciasis treatment, below) or ivermectin—will profoundly suppress microfilaremia. If the suppression is sustained, then transmission can be interrupted.

Created by the World Health Organization in 1997, the Global Programme to Eliminate Lymphatic Filariasis is based on mass administration of single annual doses of DEC plus albendazole in non-African regions and of albendazole plus ivermectin in Africa. Available information at the end of 2008 indicated that >695 million persons in 51 countries had thus far participated. Not only has lymphatic filariasis been eliminated in some defined areas, but collateral benefits—avoidance of disability and treatment of intestinal helminths and other conditions (e.g., scabies and louse infestation)—have also been noted. The strategy of the global program is being refined, and attempts are being made to integrate this effort with other mass-treatment strategies (e.g., deworming programs, malaria control, and trachoma control).

TROPICAL PULMONARY EOSINOPHILIA

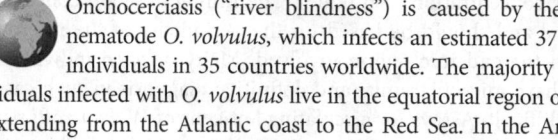

Tropical pulmonary eosinophilia (TPE) is a distinct syndrome that develops in some individuals infected with the lymphatic-dwelling filarial species. This syndrome affects males and females in a ratio of 4:1, often during the third decade of life. The majority of cases have been reported from India, Pakistan, Sri Lanka, Brazil, Guyana, and Southeast Asia.

■ CLINICAL FEATURES

The main features include a history of residence in filarial-endemic regions, paroxysmal cough and wheezing (usually nocturnal and probably related to the nocturnal periodicity of microfilariae), weight loss, low-grade fever, lymphadenopathy, and pronounced blood eosinophilia (>3000 eosinophils/µL). Chest x-rays or CT scans may be normal but generally show increased bronchovascular markings. Diffuse miliary lesions or mottled opacities may be present in the middle and lower lung fields. Tests of pulmonary function show restrictive abnormalities in most cases and obstructive defects in half. Characteristically, total serum IgE levels (10,000–100,000 ng/mL) and antifilarial antibody titers are markedly elevated.

■ PATHOLOGY

In TPE, microfilariae and parasite antigens are rapidly cleared from the bloodstream by the lungs. The clinical symptoms result from allergic and inflammatory reactions elicited by the cleared parasites. In some patients, trapping of microfilariae in other reticuloendothelial organs can cause hepatomegaly, splenomegaly, or lymphadenopathy. A prominent, eosinophil-enriched, intraalveolar infiltrate is often reported, and with it comes the release of cytotoxic proinflammatory eosinophil granule proteins that may mediate some of the pathology seen in TPE. In the absence of successful treatment, interstitial fibrosis can lead to progressive pulmonary damage.

■ DIFFERENTIAL DIAGNOSIS

TPE must be distinguished from asthma, Löffler's syndrome, allergic bronchopulmonary aspergillosis, allergic granulomatosis with angiitis (Churg-Strauss syndrome), the systemic vasculitides [most notably periarteritis nodosa and granulomatosis with polyangiitis (Wegener's)], chronic eosinophilic pneumonia, and the idiopathic hypereosinophilic syndrome.

TREATMENT   Tropical Pulmonary Eosinophilia

DEC is used at a daily dosage of 4–6 mg/kg for 14 days. Symptoms usually resolve within 3–7 days after the initiation of therapy. Relapse, which occurs in ~12–25% of cases (sometimes after an interval of years), requires re-treatment.

ONCHOCERCIASIS

■ EPIDEMIOLOGY

Onchocerciasis ("river blindness") is caused by the filarial nematode *O. volvulus*, which infects an estimated 37 million individuals in 35 countries worldwide. The majority of individuals infected with *O. volvulus* live in the equatorial region of Africa extending from the Atlantic coast to the Red Sea. In the Americas, isolated foci have been identified in Mexico, Guatemala, Colombia, Ecuador, Venezuela, and Brazil. The infection is also found in Yemen.

■ ETIOLOGY

Infection in humans begins with the deposition of infective larvae on the skin by the bite of an infected blackfly. The larvae develop into adults, which are typically found in subcutaneous nodules. About 7 months to 3 years after infection, the gravid female releases microfilariae that migrate out of the nodule and throughout the tissues, concentrating in the dermis. Infection is transmitted to other persons when a female fly ingests microfilariae from the host's skin and these microfilariae then develop into infective larvae. Adult *O. volvulus* females and males are ~40–60 cm and ~3–6 cm in length, respectively. The life span of adults can be as long as 18 years, with an average of ~9 years. Because the blackfly vector breeds along free-flowing rivers and streams (particularly in rapids) and generally restricts its flight to an area within several kilometers of these breeding sites, both biting and disease transmission are most intense in these locations.

■ PATHOLOGY

Onchocerciasis primarily affects the skin, eyes, and lymph nodes. In contrast to the pathology in lymphatic filariasis, the damage in onchocerciasis is elicited by microfilariae and not by adult parasites. In the skin, there are mild but chronic inflammatory changes that can result in loss of elastic fibers, atrophy, and fibrosis. The subcutaneous nodules, or onchocercomata, consist primarily of fibrous tissues surrounding the adult worm, often with a peripheral ring of inflammatory cells (characterized as lymphatic in origin) surrounded by an endothelial layer. In the eye, neovascularization and corneal scarring lead to corneal opacities and blindness. Inflammation in the anterior and posterior chambers frequently results in anterior uveitis, chorioretinitis, and optic atrophy. Although punctate opacities are due to an inflammatory reaction surrounding dead or dying microfilariae, the pathogenesis of most manifestations of onchocerciasis is still unclear.

◼ CLINICAL FEATURES

Skin

Pruritus and rash are the most common manifestations of onchocerciasis. The pruritus can be incapacitating; the rash is typically a papular eruption (Fig. 218-3) that is generalized rather than localized to a particular region of the body. Long-term infection results in exaggerated and premature wrinkling of the skin, loss of elastic fibers, and epidermal atrophy that can lead to loose, redundant skin and hypo- or hyperpigmentation. Localized eczematoid dermatitis can cause hyperkeratosis, scaling, and pigmentary changes. In an immunologically hyperreactive form of onchodermatitis (commonly termed *sowdah* or localized onchodermatitis), the affected skin darkens as a consequence of the profound inflammation that occurs as microfilariae in the skin are cleared.

Onchocercomata

These subcutaneous nodules, which can be palpable and/or visible, contain the adult worm. In African patients, they are common over the coccyx and sacrum, the trochanter of the femur, the lateral anterior crest, and other bony prominences; in patients from South and Central America, nodules tend to develop preferentially in the upper part of the body, particularly on the head, neck, and shoulders. Nodules vary in size and characteristically are firm and not tender. It has been estimated that, for every palpable nodule, there are four deeper nonpalpable ones.

Ocular tissue

Visual impairment is the most serious complication of onchocerciasis and usually affects only those persons with moderate or heavy

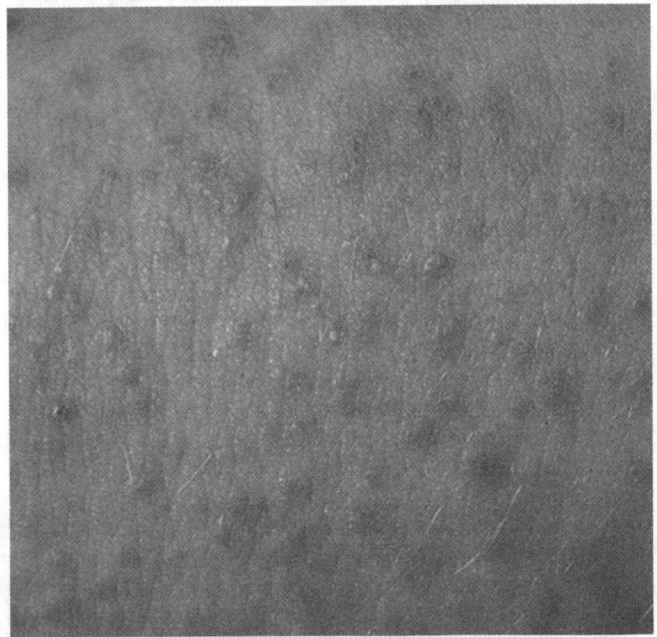

Figure 218-3 **Papular eruption** as a consequence of onchocerciasis.

infections. Lesions may develop in all parts of the eye. The most common early finding is conjunctivitis with photophobia. Punctate keratitis—acute inflammatory reactions surrounding dying microfilariae and manifested as "snowflake" opacities—is common among younger patients and resolves without apparent complications.

Sclerosing keratitis occurs in 1–5% of infected persons and is the leading cause of onchocercal blindness in Africa. Anterior uveitis and iridocyclitis develop in ~5% of infected persons in Africa. In Latin America, complications of the anterior uveal tract (pupillary deformity) may cause secondary glaucoma. Characteristic chorioretinal lesions develop as a result of atrophy and hyperpigmentation of the retinal pigment epithelium. Constriction of the visual fields and overt optic atrophy may occur.

Lymph nodes

Mild to moderate lymphadenopathy is common, particularly in the inguinal and femoral areas, where the enlarged nodes may hang down in response to gravity ("hanging groin"), sometimes predisposing to inguinal and femoral hernias.

Systemic manifestations

Some heavily infected individuals develop cachexia with loss of adipose tissue and muscle mass. Among adults who become blind, there is a three- to fourfold increase in the mortality rate.

◼ DIAGNOSIS

Definitive diagnosis depends on the detection of an adult worm in an excised nodule or, more commonly, of microfilariae in a skin snip. Skin snips are obtained with a corneal-scleral punch, which collects a blood-free skin biopsy sample extending to just below the epidermis, or by lifting of the skin with the tip of a needle and excision of a small (1- to 3-mm) piece with a sterile scalpel blade. The biopsy tissue is incubated in tissue culture medium or in saline on a glass slide or flat-bottomed microtiter plate. After incubation for 2–4 h (or occasionally overnight in light infections), microfilariae emergent from the skin can be seen by low-power microscopy.

Eosinophilia and elevated serum IgE levels are common but, because they occur in many parasitic infections, are not diagnostic in themselves. Assays to detect specific antibodies to *Onchocerca* and PCR to detect onchocercal DNA in skin snips are used in specialized laboratories and are highly sensitive and specific.

◼ TREATMENT

The main goals of therapy are to prevent the development of irreversible lesions and to alleviate symptoms. Surgical excision is recommended when nodules are located on the head (because of the proximity of microfilaria-producing adult worms to the eye), but chemotherapy is the mainstay of management. Ivermectin, a semisynthetic macrocyclic lactone active against microfilariae, is the first-line agent for the treatment of onchocerciasis. It is given orally in a single dose of 150 µg/kg, either yearly or semiannually. Recently, more frequent ivermectin administration (every 3 months) has been suggested to ameliorate pruritus and skin disease. Moreover, quadrennial administration of ivermectin has some macrofilaricidal activity.

After treatment, most individuals have few or no reactions. Pruritus, cutaneous edema, and/or maculopapular rash occurs in ~1–10% of treated individuals. In areas of Africa coendemic for *O. volvulus* and *L. loa*, however, ivermectin is contraindicated (as it is for pregnant or breast-feeding women) because of severe posttreatment encephalopathy seen in patients, especially children, who are heavily microfilaremic for *L. loa* (>2000–5000 microfilariae/mL). Although ivermectin treatment results in a marked drop in microfilarial density, its effect can be short-lived (<3 months in some cases). Thus, it is occasionally necessary to give ivermectin more frequently for persistent symptoms.

A 6-week course of doxycycline is macrofilaristatic, rendering female adult worms sterile for long periods. Because this agent targets the *Wolbachia* endosymbiont of the filarial parasite, new approaches for definitive treatment (i.e., cure) may become available.

■ PREVENTION

Vector control has been beneficial in highly endemic areas in which breeding sites are vulnerable to insecticide spraying, but most areas endemic for onchocerciasis are not suited to this type of control. Community-based administration of ivermectin every 6–12 months is being used to interrupt transmission in endemic areas. This measure, in conjunction with vector control, has already helped reduce the prevalence of disease in endemic foci in Africa and Latin America. No drug has proved useful for prophylaxis of *O. volvulus* infection.

LOIASIS

■ ETIOLOGY AND EPIDEMIOLOGY

Loiasis is caused by *L. loa* (the African eye worm), which is present in the rain forests of West and Central Africa. Adult parasites (females, 50–70 mm long and 0.5 mm wide; males, 25–35 mm long and 0.25 mm wide) live in subcutaneous tissues. Microfilariae circulate in the blood with a diurnal periodicity that peaks between 12:00 noon and 2:00 P.M.

■ CLINICAL FEATURES

Manifestations of loiasis in natives of endemic areas may differ from those in temporary residents or visitors. Among the indigenous population, loiasis is often an asymptomatic infection with microfilaremia. Infection may be recognized only after subconjunctival migration of an adult worm (Fig. 218-4) or may be manifested by episodic Calabar swellings—evanescent localized areas of angioedema and erythema developing on the extremities and less frequently at other sites. Nephropathy, encephalopathy, and cardiomyopathy can occur but are rare. In patients who are not residents of endemic areas, allergic symptoms predominate, episodes of Calabar swelling tend to be more frequent and debilitating, microfilaremia is less common, and eosinophilia and increased levels of antifilarial antibodies are characteristic.

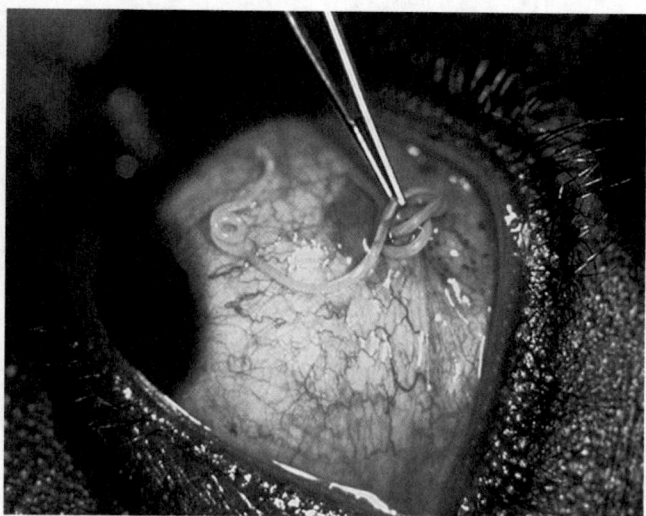

Figure 218-4   Adult *Loa loa* being surgically removed after its subconjunctival migration.

■ PATHOLOGY

The pathogenesis of the manifestations of loiasis is poorly understood. Calabar swellings are thought to result from a hypersensitivity reaction to adult worm antigens.

■ DIAGNOSIS

Definitive diagnosis of loiasis requires the detection of microfilariae in the peripheral blood or the isolation of the adult worm from the eye (Fig. 218-4) or from a subcutaneous biopsy specimen from a site of swelling developing after treatment. PCR-based assays for the detection of *L. loa* DNA in blood are available in specialized laboratories and are highly sensitive and specific, as are some newer recombinant antigen–based serologic techniques. In practice, the diagnosis must often be based on a characteristic history and clinical presentation, blood eosinophilia, and elevated levels of antifilarial antibodies, particularly in travelers to an endemic region, who are usually amicrofilaremic. Other clinical findings in the travelers include hypergammaglobulinemia, elevated levels of serum IgE, and elevated leukocyte and eosinophil counts.

TREATMENT	Loiasis

DEC (8–10 mg/kg per day for 21 days) is effective against both the adult and the microfilarial forms of *L. loa*, but multiple courses are frequently necessary before loiasis resolves completely. In cases of heavy microfilaremia, allergic or other inflammatory reactions can take place during treatment, including central nervous system involvement with coma and encephalitis. Heavy infections can be treated initially with apheresis to remove the microfilariae and with glucocorticoids (40–60 mg of prednisone per day) followed by doses of DEC (0.5 mg/kg per day). If antifilarial treatment has no adverse effects, the prednisone dose can be rapidly tapered and the dose of DEC gradually increased to 8–10 mg/kg per day.

Albendazole or ivermectin is effective in reducing microfilarial loads, although neither is approved for this purpose by the U.S. Food and Drug Administration. Moreover, ivermectin is contraindicated in patients with >5000 microfilariae/mL because this drug has been associated with >1200 deaths in heavily infected patients with loiasis in West and Central Africa. DEC (300 mg weekly) is an effective prophylactic regimen for loiasis.

STREPTOCERCIASIS

Mansonella streptocerca, found mainly in the tropical forest belt of Africa from Ghana to the Democratic Republic of the Congo, is transmitted by biting midges. The major clinical manifestations involve the skin and include pruritus, papular rashes, and pigmentation changes. Many infected individuals have inguinal adenopathy, although most are asymptomatic. The diagnosis is made by detection of the characteristic microfilariae in skin snips. Ivermectin at a single dose of 150 μg/kg leads to sustained suppression of microfilariae in the skin and is probably the treatment of choice for streptocerciasis.

MANSONELLA PERSTANS INFECTION

M. perstans, distributed across the center of Africa and in northeastern South America, is transmitted by midges. Adult worms reside in serous cavities—pericardial, pleural, and peritoneal—as well as in the mesentery and the perirenal and retroperitoneal tissues. Microfilariae circulate in the blood without periodicity. The clinical and pathologic features of the infection are poorly defined. Most patients appear to be asymptomatic, but manifestations may include transient angioedema and pruritus of the arms, face, or other parts of the body (analogous to the Calabar swellings of loiasis); fever; headache; arthralgias; and right-upper-quadrant pain. Occasionally, pericarditis and hepatitis occur. The diagnosis is based on the demonstration of microfilariae in blood or serosal effusions. Perstans filariasis is often associated with peripheral-blood eosinophilia and antifilarial antibody elevations.

With the identification of a *Wolbachia* endosymbiont in *M. perstans*, doxycycline (200 mg twice a day) for 6 weeks has been established as the first effective treatment for this infection.

MANSONELLA OZZARDI INFECTION

The distribution of *M. ozzardi* is restricted to Central and South America and certain Caribbean islands. Adult worms are rarely recovered from humans. Microfilariae circulate in the blood without periodicity. Although this organism has often been considered nonpathogenic, headache, articular pain, fever, pulmonary symptoms, adenopathy, hepatomegaly, pruritus, and eosinophilia have been ascribed to *M. ozzardi* infection. The diagnosis is made by detection of microfilariae in peripheral blood. Ivermectin (a single dose of 6 mg) is effective in treating this infection.

DRACUNCULIASIS (GUINEA WORM INFECTION)

ETIOLOGY AND EPIDEMIOLOGY

The incidence of dracunculiasis, caused by *Dracunculus medinensis*, has declined dramatically because of global eradication efforts. Current estimates suggest that there are slightly more than 3000 cases worldwide; the infection is endemic only in Ethiopia, Ghana, Mali, Niger, Nigeria, and Sudan. Asia has now been deemed dracunculiasis-free.

Humans acquire *D. medinensis* when they ingest water containing infective larvae derived from *Cyclops*, a crustacean that is the intermediate host. Larvae penetrate the stomach or intestinal wall, mate, and mature. The adult male probably dies; the female worm develops over a year and migrates to subcutaneous tissues, usually in the lower extremity. As the thin female worm, ranging in length from 30 cm to 1 m, approaches the skin, a blister forms that, over days, breaks down and forms an ulcer. When the blister opens, large numbers of motile, rhabditiform larvae can be released into stagnant water; ingestion by *Cyclops* completes the life cycle.

CLINICAL FEATURES

Few or no clinical manifestations of dracunculiasis are evident until just before the blister forms, when there is an onset of fever and generalized allergic symptoms, including periorbital edema, wheezing, and urticaria. The emergence of the worm is associated with local pain and swelling. When the blister ruptures (usually as a result of immersion in water) and the adult worm releases larva-rich fluid, symptoms are relieved. The shallow ulcer surrounding the emerging adult worm heals over weeks to months. Such ulcers, however, can become secondarily infected, the result being cellulitis, local inflammation, abscess formation, or (uncommonly) tetanus. Occasionally, the adult worm does not emerge but becomes encapsulated and calcified.

DIAGNOSIS

The diagnosis is based on the findings developing with the emergence of the adult worm, as described above.

TREATMENT

Gradual extraction of the worm by winding of a few centimeters on a stick each day remains the common and effective practice. Worms may be excised surgically. No drug is effective in treating dracunculiasis.

PREVENTION

Prevention, which remains the only real control measure, depends on the provision of safe drinking water.

ZOONOTIC FILARIAL INFECTIONS

Dirofilariae that affect primarily dogs, cats, and raccoons occasionally infect humans incidentally, as do *Brugia* and *Onchocerca* parasites that affect small mammals. Because humans are an abnormal host, the parasites never develop fully. Pulmonary dirofilarial infection caused by the canine heartworm *Dirofilaria immitis* generally presents in humans as a solitary pulmonary nodule. Chest pain, hemoptysis, and cough are uncommon. Infections with *D. repens* (from dogs) or *D. tenuis* (from raccoons) can cause local subcutaneous nodules in humans. Zoonotic *Brugia* infection can produce isolated lymph node enlargement, whereas zoonotic *Onchocerca* can cause subconjunctival masses. Eosinophilia levels and antifilarial antibody titers are not commonly elevated. Excisional biopsy is both diagnostic and curative. These infections usually do not respond to chemotherapy.

FURTHER READINGS

COULIBALY YI et al: A randomized trial of doxycycline for *Mansonella perstans* infection. N Engl J Med 361:1448, 2009

DREYER G et al: Pathogenesis of lymphatic disease in bancroftian filariasis: A clinical perspective. Parasitol Today 16:544, 2000

GARDON J et al: Serious reactions after mass treatment of onchocerciasis with ivermectin in an area endemic for *Loa loa* infection. Lancet 350:18, 1997

GONZALEZ RJ et al: Successful interruption of transmission of *Onchocerca volvulus* in the Escuintla-Guatemala focus, Guatemala. PLoS Negl Trop Dis 3:e404, 2009

HOERAUF A: Filariasis: New drugs and new opportunities for lymphatic filariasis and onchocerciasis. Curr Opin Infect Dis 21:673, 2008

—— et al: Depletion of *Wolbachia* endobacteria in *Onchocerca volvulus* by doxycycline and microfilaridermia after ivermectin treatment. Lancet 357:1415, 2001

HOOPER PJ et al: The Global Programme to Eliminate Lymphatic Filariasis: Health impact during its first 8 years (2000–2007). Ann Trop Med Parasitol 103(Suppl 1):S17, 2009

OTTESEN EA: Lymphatic filariasis: Treatment, control and elimination. Adv Parasitol 61:395, 2006

STINGL P: Onchocerciasis: Developments in diagnosis, treatment and control. Int J Dermatol 48:393, 2009

TAYLOR MJ et al: Lymphatic filariasis and onchocerciasis. Lancet 376:1175, 2010

—— et al: Macrofilaricidal activity after doxycycline treatment of *Wuchereria bancrofti*: A double-blind, randomised placebo-controlled trial. Lancet 365:2116, 2005

VIJAYAN VK: Tropical pulmonary eosinophilia: Pathogenesis, diagnosis and management. Curr Opin Pulm Med 13:428, 2007

WEIL GJ, RAMZY RM: Diagnostic tools for filariasis elimination programs. Trends Parasitol 23:78, 2007

CHAPTER **219**

Schistosomiasis and Other Trematode Infections

Adel A. F. Mahmoud

Trematodes, or flatworms, are a group of morphologically and biologically heterogeneous organisms that belong to the phylum Platyhelminthes. Human infection with trematodes occurs in many geographic areas and can cause considerable morbidity and mortality. The dependence on one drug—praziquantel—for treatment of most infections caused by helminths, including trematodes, raises the specter of developing resistance in these worms; several instances of reduced drug efficacy have already been reported.

ETIOLOGIC AGENTS AND THEIR LIFE CYCLES

For clinical purposes, significant trematode infections of humans may be divided according to tissues invaded by adult flukes: blood, biliary tree, intestines, and lungs (Table 219-1). Trematodes share some common morphologic features, including macroscopic size (from one to several centimeters); dorsoventral, flattened, bilaterally symmetric bodies (adult worms); and the prominence of two suckers. Except for schistosomes, all human parasitic trematodes

are hermaphroditic. Their life cycles involve a definitive host (mammalian/human), in which adult worms initiate sexual reproduction, and an intermediate host (snails), in which asexual multiplication of larvae occurs. More than one intermediate host may be necessary for some species of trematodes. Human infection is initiated either by direct penetration of intact skin or by ingestion. Upon maturation within humans, adult flukes initiate sexual reproduction and egg production. Helminth ova leave the definitive host in excreta or sputum and, upon reaching suitable environmental conditions, they hatch, releasing free-living miracidia that seek specific snail intermediate hosts. After asexual reproduction, cercariae are released from infected snails. In certain species, these organisms infect humans; in others, they find a second intermediate host to allow encystment into metacercariae—the infective stage.

The host-parasite relationship in trematode infections is a product of certain biologic features of these organisms: they are multicellular, undergo several developmental changes within the host, and usually result in chronic infections. In general, the distribution of worm infections in human populations is *overdispersed*; i.e., it follows a negative binomial mathematical relationship in which most infected individuals harbor low worm burdens while a small percentage are heavily infected. It is the heavily infected minority who are particularly prone to disease sequelae and who constitute an epidemiologically significant reservoir of infection in endemic areas. Equally important is an appreciation that worms do not multiply within the definitive host and that they have a relatively long life span, ranging from a few months to a few years. Morbidity and death due to trematode infections reflect a multifactorial process that results from the tipping of a delicate balance between intensity of infection and host reactions, which initiate and modulate immunologic and pathologic outcome. Furthermore, the genetics

TABLE 219-1 Major Human Trematode Infections

Trematode	Transmission	Endemic Area(s)
Blood Flukes		
Schistosoma mansoni	Skin penetration by cercariae released from snails	Africa, South America, Middle East
S. japonicum	Skin penetration by cercariae released from snails	China, Philippines, Indonesia
S. intercalatum	Skin penetration by cercariae released from snails	West Africa
S. mekongi	Skin penetration by cercariae released from snails	Southeast Asia
S. haematobium	Skin penetration by cercariae released from snails	Africa, Middle East
Biliary (Hepatic) Flukes		
Clonorchis sinensis	Ingestion of metacercariae in freshwater fish	Far East
Opisthorchis viverrini	Ingestion of metacercariae in freshwater fish	Far East, Thailand
O. felineus	Ingestion of metacercariae in freshwater fish	Far East, Europe
Fasciola hepatica	Ingestion of metacercariae on aquatic plants or in water	Worldwide
F. gigantica	Ingestion of metacercariae on aquatic plants or in water	Sporadic, Africa
Intestinal Flukes		
Fasciolopsis buski	Ingestion of metacercariae on aquatic plants	Southeast Asia
Heterophyes heterophyes	Ingestion of metacercariae in freshwater or brackish-water fish	Far East, North Africa
Lung Flukes		
Paragonimus westermani	Ingestion of metacercariae in crayfish or crabs	Global except North America and Europe

of the parasite and of the human host contribute to the outcome of infection and disease. Infections with trematodes that migrate through or reside in host tissues are associated with a moderate to high degree of peripheral-blood eosinophilia; this association is of significance in protective and immunopathologic sequelae and is a useful clinical indicator of infection.

Trematode Infection

The approach to individuals with suspected trematode infection begins with a question: Where have you been? Details of geographic history, exposure to freshwater bodies, and indulgence in local eating habits without ensuring safety of food and drink are all essential elements eliciting the history of present illness. The workup plan must include a detailed physical examination and tests appropriate for suspected infection. Diagnosis is based either on detection of the relevant stage of the parasite in excreta, sputum, or (rarely) tissue samples or on sensitive and specific serologic tests. Consultation with physicians familiar with these infections or with the U.S. Centers for Disease Control and Prevention (CDC) is helpful in guiding diagnosis and selecting therapy.

BLOOD FLUKES: SCHISTOSOMIASIS

Human schistosomiasis is caused by five species of the parasitic trematode genus *Schistosoma*: the intestinal species *S. mansoni*, *S. japonicum*, *S. mekongi*, and *S. intercalatum* and the urinary species *S. haematobium*. Infection may cause considerable morbidity in the intestines, liver, and urinary tract, and a proportion of affected individuals die. Other schistosomes (e.g., avian species) may invade human skin but then die in subcutaneous tissue, producing only self-limiting cutaneous manifestations.

■ ETIOLOGY

Human infection is initiated by penetration of intact skin with infective cercariae. These organisms, which are released from infected snails in freshwater bodies, measure ~2 mm in length and possess an anterior and a ventral sucker that attach to the skin and facilitate penetration.

Once in subcutaneous tissue, cercariae transform into schistosomula, with morphologic, membrane, and immunologic changes. The cercarial outer membrane changes from a trilaminar to a heptalaminar structure that is then maintained throughout the organism's life span in humans. This transformation is thought to be the schistosome's main adaptive mechanism for survival in humans. Schistosomula begin their migration within 2–4 days via venous or lymphatic vessels, reaching the lungs and finally the liver parenchyma. Sexually mature worms descend into the venous system at specific anatomic locations: intestinal veins (*S. mansoni*, *S. japonicum*, *S. mekongi*, and *S. intercalatum*) and vesical veins (*S. haematobium*). After mating, adult gravid females travel against venous blood flow to small tributaries, where they deposit their ova intravascularly. Schistosome ova (Fig. 219-1) have specific morphologic features that vary with the species. Aided by enzymatic secretions through minipores in eggshells, ova move through the venous wall, traversing host tissues to reach the lumen of the intestinal or urinary tract, and are voided with stools or urine. Approximately 50% of ova are retained in host tissues locally (intestines or urinary tract) or are carried by venous blood flow to the liver and other organs. Schistosome ova that reach freshwater bodies hatch, releasing free-living miracidia that seek the snail intermediate host and undergo several cycles of asexual multiplication. Finally, infective cercariae are shed from snails.

Adult schistosomes are ~1–2 cm long. Males are slightly shorter than females, with flattened bodies and anteriorly curved edges forming the gynecophoral canal, in which mature adult females are usually held. Females are longer, slender, and rounded in cross-section. The precise nature of biochemical and reproductive exchanges between the two sexes is unknown, as are the regulatory mechanisms for pairing. Adult schistosomes parasitize specific sites in the host venous system. What guides adult intestinal schistosomes to branches of the superior or inferior mesenteric veins or adult *S. haematobium* worms to the vesical plexus is unknown. In addition, adult worms inhibit the coagulation cascade and evade the effector arms of the host immune responses by still-undetermined mechanisms. The genome of schistosomes is relatively large (~270 Mb) and is arrayed on seven pairs of autosomes and one pair of sex chromosomes. Sequencing of the *S. japonicum* and *S. mansoni* genomes has provided the first insight into the worms' genomic and proteomic features, offering an opportunity to discover new drug targets and to understand the molecular basis of pathogenesis.

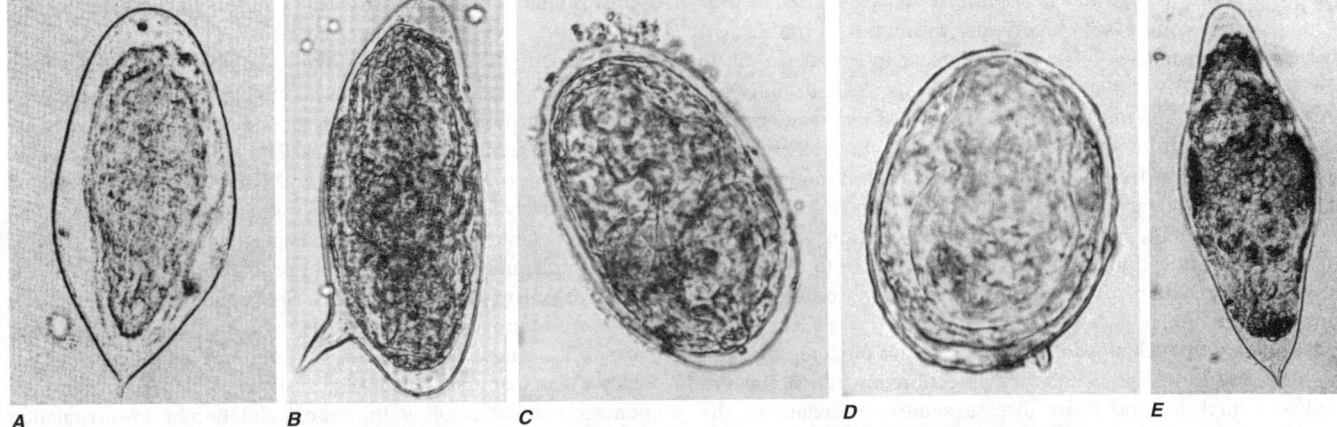

Figure 219-1 Morphology of schistosome eggs, the diagnostic stage of the parasite's life cycle. **A.** *S. haematobium* egg (in a urine sample) is large (~140 mm long), with a terminal spine. **B.** *S. mansoni* egg (in a fecal sample) is large (~150 mm long), with a thin shell and lateral spine. **C.** *S. japonicum* egg (fecal) is smaller than that of *S. mansoni* (~90 mm long), with a small spine or hooklike structure. **D.** *S. mekongi* egg (fecal) is similar to that of *S. japonicum* but smaller (~65 mm long). **E.** *S. intercalatum* egg (fecal) is larger than that of *S. haematobium* (~190 mm long), with a longer, sharply pointed spine. (*From LR Ash, TC Orihel: Atlas of Human Parasitology, 3rd ed. Chicago, ASCP Press, 1990; with permission.*)

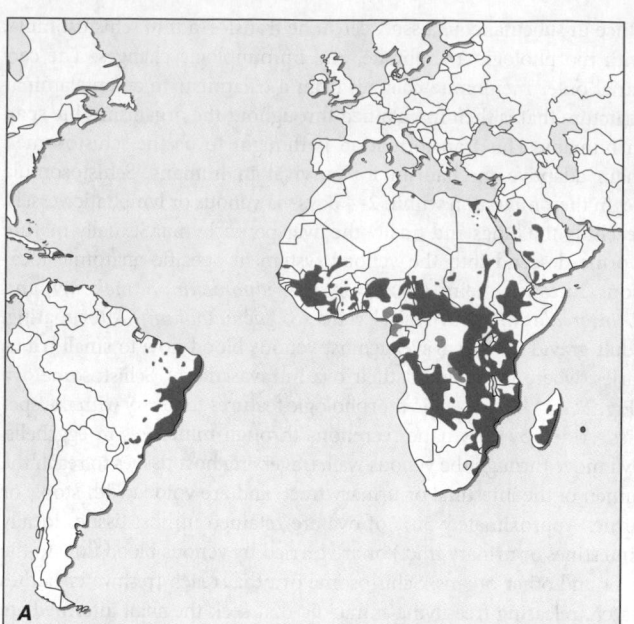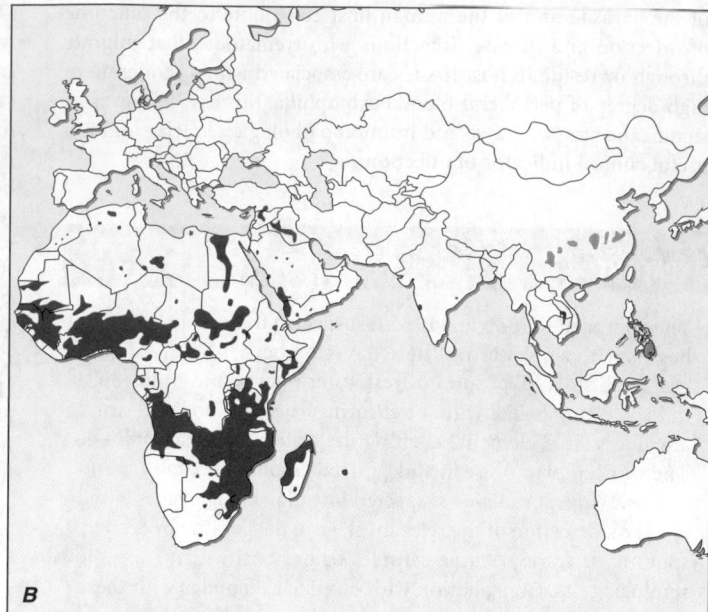

Figure 219-2 Global distribution of schistosomiasis. *A.* *S. mansoni* infection (*dark blue*) is endemic in Africa, the Middle East, South America, and a few Caribbean countries. *S. intercalatum* infection (*green*) is endemic in sporadic foci in West and Central Africa. ***B.*** *S. haematobium* infection (*purple*) is endemic in Africa and the Middle East. The major endemic countries for *S. japonicum* infection (*green*) are China, the Philippines, and Indonesia. *S. mekongi* infection (*red*) is endemic in sporadic foci in Southeast Asia.

EPIDEMIOLOGY

The global distribution of schistosome infection in human populations (Fig. 219-2) is dependent on both parasite and host factors. Information on prevalence and global distribution is inexact. The five *Schistosoma* species are estimated to infect 200–300 million individuals in South America, the Caribbean, Africa, the Middle East, and Southeast Asia. The total population living under conditions favoring transmission approximates double or triple that number—a fact reflecting the public health significance of schistosomiasis.

In endemic areas, the rate of yearly onset of new infection, or incidence, is generally low. Prevalence, on the other hand, starts to be appreciable by the age of 3–4 years and builds to a maximum that varies by endemic region (up to 100%) in the 15- to 20-year age group. Prevalence then stabilizes or decreases slightly in older age groups (>40 years). Intensity of infection (as measured by fecal or urinary egg counts, which correlate with adult worm burdens in most circumstances) follows the increase in prevalence up to the age of 15–20 years and then declines markedly in older age groups. This decline may reflect acquisition of resistance or may be due to changes in water contact patterns, since older people have less exposure. Infection with schistosomes in human populations has a peculiar pattern. Most infected individuals harbor low worm burdens, and only a small proportion suffer from high-intensity infection. This pattern may be due to differences in worm infectivity or to a spectrum of genetic susceptibilities in human populations.

Disease due to schistosome infection is the outcome of parasitologic, host, and associated viral infections or nutritional and environmental factors. Most disease syndromes relate to the presence of one or more of the parasite stages in humans. Disease manifestations in the populations of endemic areas correlate, in general, with intensity and duration of infection as well as with age and genetic susceptibility of the host. Overall, disease manifestations are clinically relevant in only a small proportion of persons infected with any of the intestinal schistosomes. In contrast, urinary schistosomiasis manifests clinically in most infected individuals. Estimates of total morbidity due to chronic schistosomiasis indicate a significantly greater burden than was previously appreciated.

Patients with both HIV infection and schistosomiasis excrete far fewer eggs in their stools than those infected with *S. mansoni* alone; the mechanism underlying this difference is unknown. Treatment with praziquantel may result in reduced HIV replication and increased CD4+ T lymphocyte counts.

PATHOGENESIS AND IMMUNITY

Cercarial invasion is associated with dermatitis arising from dermal and subdermal inflammatory responses, both humoral and cell-mediated. As the parasites approach sexual maturity in the liver of infected individuals and as oviposition commences, acute schistosomiasis or Katayama fever (a serum sickness–like illness; see "Clinical Features," below) may occur. The associated antigen excess results in formation of soluble immune complexes, which may be deposited in several tissues, initiating multiple pathologic events. In chronic schistosomiasis, most disease manifestations are due to eggs retained in host tissues. The granulomatous response around these ova is cell-mediated and is regulated both positively and negatively by a cascade of cytokine, cellular, and humoral responses. Granuloma formation begins with recruitment of a host of inflammatory cells in response to antigens secreted by the living organism within the ova. Cells recruited initially include phagocytes, antigen-specific T cells, and eosinophils. Fibroblasts, giant cells, and B lymphocytes predominate later. These lesions reach a size many times that of parasite eggs, thus inducing organomegaly and obstruction. Immunomodulation or downregulation of host responses to schistosome eggs plays a significant role in limiting the extent of the granulomatous lesions—and consequently disease—in chronically infected experimental animals or humans. The underlying mechanisms involve another cascade of regulatory cytokines and idiotypic antibodies. Subsequent to the granulomatous response, fibrosis sets in, resulting in more permanent disease sequelae. Because schistosomiasis is also a chronic infection, the accumulation of antigen-antibody complexes results in deposits in renal glomeruli and may cause significant kidney disease.

The better-studied pathologic sequelae in schistosomiasis are those observed in liver disease. Ova that are carried by portal blood embolize to the liver. Because of their size (~150 × 60 μm in the case of *S. mansoni*), they lodge at presinusoidal sites, where granulomas are formed. These granulomas contribute to the hepatomegaly observed in infected individuals (Fig. 219-3). Schistosomal liver enlargement is also associated with certain class I and class II human leukocyte antigen (HLA) haplotypes and markers; its genetic basis appears to be multigenic. Presinusoidal portal blockage causes several hemodynamic changes, including portal hypertension and associated development of portosystemic collaterals at the esophagogastric junction and other sites. Esophageal varices are most likely to break and cause repeated episodes of hematemesis. Because changes in hepatic portal blood flow occur slowly, compensatory arterialization of the blood flow through the liver is established. While this compensatory mechanism may be associated with certain metabolic side effects, retention of hepatocyte perfusion permits maintenance of normal liver function for several years.

The second most significant pathologic change in the liver relates to fibrosis. It is characteristically periportal (Symmers' clay pipe–stem fibrosis) but may be diffuse. Fibrosis, when diffuse, may be seen in areas of egg deposition and granuloma formation but is also seen in distant locations such as portal tracts. Schistosomiasis results in pure fibrotic lesions in the liver; cirrhosis occurs when other nutritional factors or infectious agents (e.g., hepatitis B or C virus) are involved. Deposition of fibrotic tissue in the extracellular matrix results from the interaction of T lymphocytes with cells of the fibroblast series; several cytokines, such as interleukin (IL) 2, IL-4, IL-1, and transforming growth factor β (TGF-β), are known to stimulate fibrogenesis. The process may be dependent on the genetic constitution of the host. Furthermore, regulatory cytokines that can suppress fibrogenesis, such as interferon γ (IFN-γ) or IL-12, may play a role in modulating the response.

While the above description focuses on granuloma formation and fibrosis of the liver, similar processes occur in urinary schistosomiasis. Granuloma formation at the lower end of the ureters obstructs urinary flow, with subsequent development of hydroureter and hydronephrosis. Similar lesions in the urinary bladder cause the protrusion of papillomatous structures into its cavity; these may ulcerate and/or bleed. The chronic stage of infection is associated with scarring and deposition of calcium in the bladder wall.

Studies on immunity to schistosomiasis, whether innate or adaptive, have expanded our knowledge of the components of these responses and target antigens. The critical question, however, is whether humans acquire immunity to schistosomes. Epidemiologic data suggest the onset of acquired immunity during the course of infection in young adults. Curative treatment of infected populations in endemic areas is followed by differentiation in the pattern of reinfection. Some (susceptible) individuals acquire reinfection rapidly, whereas other (resistant) individuals are reinfected slowly. This difference may be explained by differences in transmission, immunologic response, or genetic susceptibility. The mechanism of acquired immunity involves antibodies, complement, and several effector cells, particularly eosinophils. Furthermore, the intensity of schistosome infection has been correlated with a region in chromosome 5. In several studies, a few protective schistosome antigens have been identified as vaccine candidates, but none has been evaluated in human populations to date.

CLINICAL FEATURES

In general, disease manifestations of schistosomiasis occur in three stages, which vary not only by species but also by intensity of infection and other host factors, such as age and genetics. During the phase of cercarial invasion, a form of dermatitis may be observed. This so-called swimmers' itch occurs most often with *S. mansoni* and *S. japonicum* infections, manifesting 2 or 3 days after invasion as an itchy maculopapular rash on the affected areas of the skin. The condition is particularly severe when humans are exposed to avian schistosomes. This form of cercarial dermatitis is also seen around freshwater lakes in the northern United States, particularly in the spring. Cercarial dermatitis is a self-limiting clinical entity. During worm maturation and at the beginning of oviposition (i.e., 4–8 weeks after skin invasion), acute schistosomiasis or Katayama fever—a serum sickness–like syndrome with fever, generalized lymphadenopathy, and hepatosplenomegaly—may develop. Individuals with acute schistosomiasis show a high degree of peripheral-blood eosinophilia. Parasite-specific antibodies may be detected before schistosome eggs are identified in excreta.

Acute schistosomiasis has become an important clinical entity worldwide because of increased travel to endemic areas. Travelers are exposed to parasites while swimming or wading in freshwater bodies and upon their return present with acute manifestations. The course of acute schistosomiasis is generally benign, but deaths are occasionally reported in association with heavy exposure to schistosomes.

The main clinical manifestations of chronic schistosomiasis are species-dependent. Intestinal species (*S. mansoni*, *S. japonicum*, *S. mekongi*, and *S. intercalatum*) cause intestinal and hepatosplenic disease as well as several manifestations associated with portal hypertension. During the intestinal phase, which may begin a few months after infection and may last for years, symptomatic patients characteristically have colicky abdominal pain, bloody diarrhea, and anemia. Patients may also report fatigue and an inability to perform daily routine functions and may

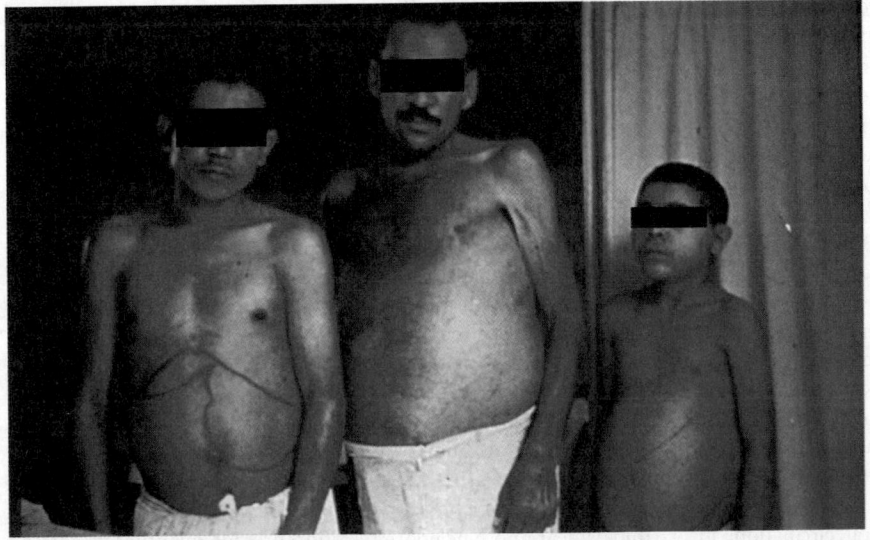

Figure 219-3   Chronic hepatosplenomegaly caused by schistosomiasis mansoni. Liver and spleen enlargement, ascites, and wasting are characteristically seen in patients with chronic *S. mansoni* infection.

show evidence of growth retardation. Schistosomiasis morbidity is generally underappreciated. The severity of intestinal schistosomiasis is often related to the intensity of the worm burden. The disease runs a chronic course and may result in colonic polyposis, which has been reported from some endemic areas, such as Egypt.

The hepatosplenic phase of disease manifests early (during the first year of infection, particularly in children) with liver enlargement due to parasite-induced granulomatous lesions. Hepatomegaly is seen in ~15–20% of infected individuals; it correlates roughly with intensity of infection, occurs more often in children, and may be related to specific HLA haplotypes. In subsequent phases of infection, presinusoidal blockage of blood flow leads to portal hypertension and splenomegaly (Fig. 219-3). Moreover, portal hypertension may lead to varices at the lower end of the esophagus and at other sites. Patients with schistosomal liver disease may have right-upper-quadrant "dragging" pain during the hepatomegaly phase, and this pain may move to the left upper quadrant as splenomegaly progresses. Bleeding from esophageal varices may, however, be the first clinical manifestation of this phase. Patients may experience repeated bleeding but seem to tolerate its impact, since an adequate total hepatic blood flow permits normal liver function for a considerable duration. In late-stage disease, typical fibrotic changes occur along with liver function deterioration and the onset of ascites, hypoalbuminemia, and defects in coagulation. Intercurrent viral infections of the liver (especially hepatitis B and C) or nutritional deficiencies may well accelerate or exacerbate the deterioration of hepatic function.

The extent and severity of intestinal and hepatic disease in schistosomiasis mansoni and japonica have been well described. While it was originally thought that S. japonicum might induce more severe disease manifestations because the adult worms can produce 10 times more eggs than S. mansoni, subsequent field studies have not supported this claim. Clinical observations of individuals infected with S. mekongi or S. intercalatum have been less detailed, partly because of the limited geographic distribution of these organisms.

The clinical manifestations of S. haematobium infection occur relatively early and involve a high percentage of infected individuals. Up to 80% of children infected with S. haematobium have dysuria, frequency, and hematuria, which may be terminal. Urine examination reveals blood and albumin as well as an unusually high frequency of bacterial urinary tract infection and urinary sediment cellular metaplasia. These manifestations correlate with intensity of infection, the presence of urinary bladder granulomas, and subsequent ulceration. Along with local effects of granuloma formation in the urinary bladder, obstruction of the lower end of the ureters results in hydroureter and hydronephrosis, which may be seen in 25–50% of infected children. As infection progresses, bladder granulomas undergo fibrosis, which results in typical sandy patches visible on cystoscopy. In many endemic areas, an association between squamous cell carcinoma of the bladder and S. haematobium infection has been observed. Such malignancy is detected in a younger age group than is transitional cell carcinoma. In fact, S. haematobium has now been classified as a human carcinogen.

Significant disease may occur in other organs during chronic schistosomiasis. Lung and central nervous system (CNS) disease have been documented; other sites, such as the skin and the genital organs, are far less frequently affected. In pulmonary schistosomiasis, embolized eggs lodge in small arterioles, producing acute necrotizing arteriolitis and granuloma formation. During S. mansoni and S. japonicum infection, schistosome eggs reach the lungs after the development of portosystemic collateral circulation; in S. haematobium infection, ova may reach the lungs directly via connections between the vesical and systemic circulation. Subsequent fibrous tissue deposition leads to endarteritis obliterans, pulmonary

hypertension, and cor pulmonale. The most common symptoms are cough, fever, and dyspnea. Cor pulmonale may be diagnosed radiologically on the basis of prominence of the right side of the heart and dilation of the pulmonary artery. Frank evidence of right-sided heart failure may be seen in late cases.

Although less common than pulmonary manifestations, CNS schistosomiasis is important, characteristically occurring in association with S. japonicum infection. Migratory worms deposit eggs in the brain and induce a granulomatous response. The frequency of this manifestation among infected individuals in some endemic areas (e.g., the Philippines) is calculated at 2–4%. Jacksonian epilepsy due to S. japonicum infection is the second most common cause of epilepsy in these areas. S. mansoni and S. haematobium infections have been associated with transverse myelitis. This syndrome is thought to be due to eggs traveling to the venous plexus around the spinal cord. In schistosomiasis mansoni, transverse myelitis is usually seen in the chronic stage after the development of portal hypertension and portosystemic shunts, which allow ova to travel to the spinal cord veins. This proposed sequence of events has been challenged because of a few reports of transverse myelitis occurring early in the course of S. mansoni infection. More information is needed to confirm these observations. During schistosomiasis haematobia, ova may travel through communication between vesical and systemic veins, resulting in spinal cord disease that may be detected at any stage of infection. Pathologic study of lesions in schistosomal transverse myelitis may reveal eggs along with necrotic or granulomatous lesions. Patients usually present with acute or rapidly progressing lower-leg weakness accompanied by sphincter dysfunction.

■ DIAGNOSIS

Physicians in areas not endemic for schistosomiasis face considerable diagnostic challenges. In the most common clinical presentation, a traveler returns with symptoms and signs of acute syndromes of schistosomiasis—namely, cercarial dermatitis or Katayama fever. Central to a correct diagnosis is a thorough inquiry into the patient's history of travel and exposure to freshwater bodies—whether slow- or fast-running—in a nonendemic area. Differential diagnosis of fever in returned travelers includes a spectrum of infections whose etiologies are viral (e.g., Dengue fever), bacterial (e.g., enteric fever, leptospirosis), rickettsial, or protozoal (e.g., malaria). In cases of Katayama fever, prompt diagnosis is essential and is based on clinical presentation, high-level peripheral-blood eosinophilia, and a positive serologic assay for schistosomal antibodies. Two tests are available at the CDC: the Falcon assay screening test/enzyme-linked immunosorbent assay (FAST-ELISA) and the confirmatory enzyme-linked immunoelectrotransfer blot (EITB). Both tests are highly sensitive and ~96% specific. In some instances, examination of stool or urine for ova may yield positive results.

Individuals with established infection are diagnosed by a combination of geographic history, characteristic clinical presentation, and presence of schistosome ova in excreta. The diagnosis may also be established with the serologic assays mentioned above or with those that detect circulating schistosome antigens. These assays can be applied either to blood or to other body fluids (e.g., cerebrospinal fluid). For suspected schistosome infection, stool examination by the Kato thick smear or any other concentration method generally identifies all but the most lightly infected individuals. For S. haematobium, urine may be examined by microscopy of sediment or by filtration of a known volume through Nuclepore filters. Kato thick smear and Nuclepore filtration provide quantitative data on the intensity of infection, which is of value in assessing the degree of tissue damage and in monitoring the effect of chemotherapy. Schistosome infection may also be diagnosed by examination of tissue samples, typically rectal biopsies; other biopsy procedures (e.g., liver biopsy) are not needed, except in rare circumstances.

The differential diagnosis of schistosomal hepatomegaly must include viral hepatitis of all etiologies, miliary tuberculosis, malaria, visceral leishmaniasis, ethanol abuse, and causes of hepatic and portal vein obstruction. The differential diagnosis of hematuria in *S. haematobium* infection includes bacterial cystitis, tuberculosis, urinary stones, and malignancy.

TREATMENT   Schistosomiasis

Treatment of schistosomiasis depends on the stage of infection and the clinical presentation. Other than topical dermatologic applications for relief of itching, no specific treatment is indicated for cercarial dermatitis caused by avian schistosomes. Therapy for acute schistosomiasis or Katayama fever needs to be adjusted appropriately for each case. While antischistosomal chemotherapy may be used, it does not have a significant impact on maturing worms. In severe acute schistosomiasis, management in an acute-care setting is necessary, with supportive measures and consideration of glucocorticoid treatment. Once the acute critical phase is over, specific chemotherapy is indicated for parasite elimination. For all individuals with established infection, treatment to eradicate the parasite should be administered. The drug of choice is praziquantel, which—depending on the infecting species (Table 219-2)—is administered PO as a total of 40 or 60 mg/kg in two or three doses over a single day. Praziquantel treatment results in parasitologic cure in ~85% of cases and reduces egg counts by >90%. Few side effects have been encountered, and those that do develop usually do not interfere with completion of treatment. Dependence on a single chemotherapeutic agent has raised the possibility of development of resistance in schistosomes; to date, such resistance does not seem to be clinically

significant. The effect of antischistosomal treatment on disease manifestations varies by stage. Early hepatomegaly and bladder lesions are known to resolve after chemotherapy, but the late established manifestations, such as fibrosis, do not recede. Additional management modalities are needed for individuals with other manifestations, such as hepatocellular failure or recurrent hematemesis. The use of these interventions is guided by general medical and surgical principles.

■ PREVENTION AND CONTROL

Transmission of schistosomiasis is dependent on human behavior. Since the geographic distribution of infections in endemic regions of the world is not clearly demarcated, it is prudent for travelers to endemic areas to avoid contact with all freshwater bodies, irrespective of the speed of water flow or unsubstantiated claims of safety. Some topical agents, when applied to skin, may inhibit cercarial penetration, but none is currently available. If exposure occurs, a follow-up visit with a health care provider is strongly recommended. Prevention of infection in inhabitants of endemic areas is a significant challenge. Residents of these regions use freshwater bodies for sanitary, domestic, recreational, and agricultural purposes. Several control measures have been used, including application of molluscicides, provision of sanitary water and sewage disposal, chemotherapy, and health education. Current recommendations to countries endemic for schistosomiasis emphasize the use of multiple approaches. With the advent of an oral, safe, and effective antischistosomal agent, chemotherapy has been most successful in reducing the intensity of infection and reversing disease. The duration of this positive impact depends on the transmission dynamics of the parasite in any specific endemic region. The ultimate goal of research on prevention and control is the development of a vaccine. Although there are a few promising leads, this goal is probably not within reach during the next decade or so.

LIVER (BILIARY) FLUKES

Several species of biliary fluke infecting humans are particularly common in Southeast Asia and Russia. Other species are transmitted in Europe, Africa, and the Americas. On the basis of their migratory pathway in humans, these infections may be divided into the *Clonorchis* and *Fasciola* groups (Table 219-1).

■ CLONORCHIASIS AND OPISTHORCHIASIS

Infection with *Clonorchis sinensis*, the Chinese or oriental fluke, is endemic among fish-eating mammals in Southeast Asia. Humans are an incidental host; the prevalence of human infection is highest in China, Vietnam, and Korea. Infection with *Opisthorchis viverrini* and *O. felineus* is zoonotic in cats and dogs. Transmission to humans occurs occasionally, particularly in Thailand (*O. viverrini*) and in Southeast Asia and eastern Europe (*O. felineus*). Data on the exact geographic distribution of these infectious agents in human populations are rudimentary.

Infection with any of these three species is established by ingestion of raw or inadequately cooked freshwater fish harboring metacercariae. These organisms excyst in the duodenum, releasing larvae that travel through the ampulla of Vater and mature into adult worms in bile canaliculi. Mature flukes are flat and elongated, measuring 1–2 cm in length. The hermaphroditic worms reproduce by releasing small operculated eggs, which pass with bile into the intestines and are voided with stools. The life cycle is completed in the environment in specific freshwater snails (the first intermediate host) and encystment of metacercariae in freshwater fish.

Except for late sequelae, the exact clinical syndromes caused by clonorchiasis and opisthorchiasis are not well defined. Since

TABLE 219-2   Drug Therapy for Human Trematode Infections

Infection	Drug of Choice	Adult Dose and Duration
Blood Flukes		
S. mansoni, S. intercalatum, S. haematobium	Praziquantel	20 mg/kg, 2 doses in 1 day
S. japonicum, S. mekongi	Praziquantel	20 mg/kg, 3 doses in 1 day
Biliary (Hepatic) Flukes		
C. sinensis, O. viverrini, O. felineus	Praziquantel	25 mg/kg, 3 doses in 1 day
F. hepatica, F. gigantica	Triclabendazole	10 mg/kg once
Intestinal Flukes		
F. buski, H. heterophyes	Praziquantel	25 mg/kg, 3 doses in 1 day
Lung Flukes		
P. westermani	Praziquantel	25 mg/kg, 3 doses per day for 2 days

most infected individuals harbor a low worm burden, many are asymptomatic. Moderate to heavy infection may be associated with vague right-upper-quadrant pain. In contrast, chronic or repeated infection is associated with manifestations such as cholangitis, cholangiohepatitis, and biliary obstruction. Cholangiocarcinoma is epidemiologically related to *C. sinensis* infection in China and to *O. viverrini* infection in northeastern Thailand. This association has resulted in classification of these infectious agents as human carcinogens.

■ FASCIOLIASIS

Infections with *Fasciola hepatica* and *F. gigantica* are worldwide zoonoses that are particularly endemic in sheep-raising countries. Human cases have been reported in South America, Europe, Africa, Australia, and the Far East. Recent estimates indicate a worldwide prevalence of 17 million cases. High endemicity has been reported in certain areas of Peru and Bolivia. In most endemic areas the predominant species is *F. hepatica*, but in Asia and Africa a varying degree of overlap with *F. gigantica* has been observed.

Humans acquire fascioliasis by ingestion of metacercariae attached to certain aquatic plants, such as watercress. Infection may also be acquired by consumption of contaminated water or ingestion of food items washed with such water. Acquisition of human infection through consumption of freshly prepared raw liver containing immature flukes has been reported. Infection is initiated when metacercariae excyst, penetrate the gut wall, and travel through the peritoneal cavity to invade the liver capsule. Adult worms finally reach bile ducts, where they produce large operculated eggs, which are voided in bile through the gastrointestinal tract to the outside environment. The flukes' life cycle is completed in specific snails (the first intermediate host) and encystment on aquatic plants.

Clinical features of fascioliasis relate to the stage and intensity of infection. Acute disease develops during parasite migration (1–2 weeks after infection) and includes fever, right-upper-quadrant pain, hepatomegaly, and eosinophilia. CT of the liver may show migratory tracks. Symptoms and signs usually subside as the parasites reach their final habitat. In individuals with chronic infection, bile duct obstruction and biliary cirrhosis are infrequently demonstrated. No relation to hepatic malignancy has been ascribed to fascioliasis.

■ DIAGNOSIS

Diagnosis of infection with any of the biliary flukes depends on a high degree of suspicion, elicitation of an appropriate geographic history, and stool examination for characteristically shaped parasite ova. Additional evidence may be obtained by documenting peripheral-blood eosinophilia or imaging the liver. Serologic testing is helpful, particularly in lightly infected individuals.

TREATMENT   Biliary Flukes

Drug therapy (praziquantel or triclabendazole) is summarized in Table 219-2. Patients with anatomic lesions in the biliary tract or malignancy are managed according to general medical guidelines.

INTESTINAL FLUKES

Two species of intestinal flukes cause human infection in defined geographic areas worldwide (Table 219-1). The large *Fasciolopsis buski* (adults measure 2 × 7 cm) is endemic in Southeast Asia, while the smaller *Heterophyes heterophyes* is found in the Nile Delta of Egypt and in the Far East.

Infection is initiated by ingestion of metacercariae attached to aquatic plants (*F. buski*) or encysted in freshwater or brackish-water fish (*H. heterophyes*). Flukes mature in human intestines, and eggs are passed with stools. Most individuals infected with intestinal flukes are asymptomatic. In heavy *F. buski* infection, diarrhea, abdominal pain, and malabsorption may be encountered. Heavy infection with *H. heterophyes* may be associated with abdominal pain and mucous diarrhea. The diagnosis is established by detection of characteristically shaped ova in stool samples. The drug of choice for treatment is praziquantel (Table 219-2).

LUNG FLUKES

Infection with the lung fluke *Paragonimus westermani* (Table 219-1) and related species (e.g., *P. africanus*) is endemic in many parts of the world, excluding North America and Europe. Endemicity is particularly noticeable in West Africa, Central and South America, and Asia. In nature, the reservoir hosts of *P. westermani* are wild and domestic felines. In Africa, *P. africanus* has been found in other species, such as dogs. Adult lung flukes, which are 7–12 mm in length, are found encapsulated in the lungs of infected persons. In rare circumstances, flukes are found encysted in the CNS (cerebral paragonimiasis) or the abdominal cavity. Humans acquire lung fluke infection by ingesting infective metacercariae encysted in the muscles and viscera of crayfish and freshwater crabs. In endemic areas, these crustaceans are consumed either raw or pickled. Once the organisms reach the duodenum, they excyst, penetrate the gut wall, and travel through the peritoneal cavity, diaphragm, and pleural space to reach the lungs. Mature flukes are found in the bronchioles surrounded by cystic lesions. Parasite eggs are either expectorated with sputum or swallowed and passed to the outside environment with feces. The life cycle is completed in snails and freshwater crustacea.

When maturing flukes lodge in lung tissues, they cause hemorrhage and necrosis, resulting in cyst formation. The adjacent lung parenchyma shows evidence of inflammatory infiltration, predominantly by eosinophils. Cysts usually measure 1–2 cm in diameter and may contain one or two worms each. With the onset of oviposition, cysts usually rupture in adjacent bronchioles—an event allowing ova to exit the human host. Older cysts develop thickened walls, which may undergo calcification. During the active phase of paragonimiasis, lung tissues surrounding parasite cysts may show evidence of pneumonia, bronchitis, bronchiectasis, and fibrosis.

Pulmonary paragonimiasis is particularly symptomatic in persons with moderate to heavy infection. Productive cough with brownish sputum or frank hemoptysis associated with peripheral-blood eosinophilia is usually the presenting feature. Chest examination may reveal signs of pleurisy. In chronic cases, bronchitis or bronchiectasis may predominate, but these conditions rarely proceed to lung abscess. Imaging of the lungs demonstrates characteristic features, including patchy densities, cavities, pleural effusion, and ring shadows. Cerebral paragonimiasis presents as either space-occupying lesions or epilepsy.

■ DIAGNOSIS

Pulmonary paragonimiasis is diagnosed by detection of parasite ova in sputum and/or stools. Serology is of considerable help in egg-negative cases and in cerebral paragonimiasis.

TREATMENT   Lung Flukes

The drug of choice for treatment is praziquantel (Table 219-2). Other medical or surgical management may be needed for pulmonary or cerebral lesions.

CONTROL AND PREVENTION OF TISSUE FLUKES

For residents of nonendemic areas who are visiting an endemic region, the only effective preventive measure is to avoid ingestion of local plants, fish, or crustaceans; if their ingestion is necessary, these items should be washed or cooked thoroughly. Instruction on water and food preparation and consumption should be included in physicians' advice to travelers (Chap. 123). Interruption of transmission among residents of endemic areas depends on avoiding ingestion of infective stages and disposing of feces and sputum appropriately to prevent hatching of eggs in the environment. These two approaches rely greatly on socioeconomic development and health education. In countries where economic progress has resulted in financial and social improvements, transmission has decreased. The third approach to control in endemic communities entails selective use of chemotherapy for individuals posing the highest risk of transmission (i.e., those with heavy infections). The availability of praziquantel—a broad-spectrum, safe, and effective anthelmintic agent—provides a means for reducing the reservoirs of infection in human populations. However, the existence of most of these helminthic infections as zoonoses in several animal species complicates control efforts.

FURTHER READINGS

Curtale F et al: Comprehensive primary health care, a viable strategy for the elimination of schistosomiasis. Trans R Soc Trop Med Hyg 104:70, 2010

King CH: Lifting the burden of schistosomiasis—defining elements of infection-associated disease and the benefits of antiparasite treatment. J Infect Dis 196:653, 2007

Lim JH et al: Parasitic diseases of the biliary tract. AJR Am J Roentgenol 188:1596, 2007

Lun ZR et al: Clonorchiasis: A key foodborne zoonosis in China. Lancet Infect Dis 5:31, 2005

Robinson MW, Dalton JP: Zoonotic helminth infections with particular emphasis on fasciolosis and other trematodiases. Philos Trans R Soc Lond B Biol Sci 364:2763, 2009

Schistosoma japonicum Genome Sequencing and Functional Analysis Consortium: The Schistosoma japonicum genome reveals features of host-parasite interplay. Nature 460:345, 2009

Stauffer WM et al: Biliary liver flukes (opisthorchiasis and clonorchiasis) in immigrants in the United States: Often subtle and diagnosed years after arrival. J Travel Med 11:157, 2004

Walson JL et al: Prevalence and correlates of helminth co-infection in Kenyan HIV-1 infected adults. PLoS Negl Trop Dis 4:e644, 2010

Wilson S et al: Health implications of chronic hepatosplenomegaly in Kenyan school-aged children chronically exposed to malarial infections and Schistosoma mansoni. Trans R Soc Trop Med Hyg 104:110, 2010

Web Sites

Centers for Disease Control and Prevention: http://www.cdc.gov/ncidod/dpd

CHAPTER **220**

Cestode Infections

A. Clinton White, Jr.
Peter F. Weller

Cestodes, or tapeworms, are segmented worms. The adults reside in the gastrointestinal tract, but the larvae can be found in almost any organ. Human tapeworm infections can be divided into two major clinical groups. In one group, humans are the definitive hosts, with the adult tapeworms living in the gastrointestinal tract (*Taenia saginata, Diphyllobothrium, Hymenolepis,* and *Dipylidium caninum*). In the other, humans are intermediate hosts, with larval-stage parasites present in the tissues; diseases in this category include echinococcosis, sparganosis, and coenurosis. Humans may be either the definitive or the intermediate hosts for *Taenia solium.* Both stages of *Hymenolepis nana* are found simultaneously in the human intestines.

The ribbon-shaped tapeworm attaches to the intestinal mucosa by means of sucking cups or hooks located on the scolex. Behind the scolex is a short, narrow neck from which proglottids (segments) form. As each proglottid matures, it is displaced further back from the neck by the formation of new, less mature segments. The progressively elongating chain of attached proglottids, called the *strobila,* constitutes the bulk of the tapeworm. The length varies among species. In some, the tapeworm may consist of more than 1000 proglottids and may be several meters long. The mature proglottids are hermaphroditic and produce eggs, which are subsequently released. Since eggs of the different *Taenia* species are morphologically identical, differences in the morphology of the scolex or proglottids provide the basis for diagnostic identification to the species level.

Most human tapeworms require at least one intermediate host for complete larval development. After ingestion of the eggs or proglottids by an intermediate host, the larval oncospheres are activated, escape the egg, and penetrate the intestinal mucosa. The oncosphere migrates to tissues and develops into an encysted form known as a *cysticercus* (single scolex), a *coenurus* (multiple scolices), or a *hydatid* (cyst with daughter cysts, each containing several protoscolices). Ingestion by the definitive host of tissues containing a cyst enables a scolex to develop into a tapeworm.

■ TAENIASIS SAGINATA AND TAENIASIS ASIATICA

The beef tapeworm *T. saginata* occurs in all countries where raw or undercooked beef is eaten. It is most prevalent in sub-Saharan African and Middle Eastern countries. *T. asiatica* is closely related to *T. saginata* and is found in Asia with pigs as intermediate hosts. The clinical manifestations and morphology of these two species are very similar and are therefore discussed together.

Etiology and pathogenesis

Humans are the only definitive host for the adult stage of *T. saginata* and *T. asiatica.* The tapeworms, which can reach 8 m in length with 1000–2000 proglottids, inhabit the upper jejunum. The scolex of *T. saginata* has four prominent suckers, whereas *T. asiatica* has an unarmed rostellum. Each gravid segment has 15–30 uterine branches (in contrast to 8–12 for *T. solium*). The eggs are indistinguishable from those of *T. solium*; they measure 30–40 μm, contain the oncosphere, and have a thick brown striated shell. Eggs deposited on vegetation can live for months or years until they are ingested by cattle or other herbivores (*T. saginata*) or pigs (*T. asiatica*). The embryo released after ingestion invades the intestinal wall and is carried to striated muscle or viscera, where it transforms into the cysticercus. When ingested in raw or undercooked meat, this form can infect humans. After the cysticercus is ingested, it takes ~2 months for the mature adult worm to develop.

Clinical manifestations

Patients become aware of the infection most commonly by noting passage of proglottids in their feces. The proglottids are often motile, and patients may experience perianal discomfort when proglottids are discharged. Mild abdominal pain or discomfort, nausea, change in appetite, weakness, and weight loss can occur.

Diagnosis

The diagnosis is made by the detection of eggs or proglottids in the stool. Eggs may also be present in the perianal area; thus, if proglottids or eggs are not found in the stool, the perianal region should be examined with use of a cellophane-tape swab (as in pinworm infection; Chap. 217). Distinguishing *T. saginata* or *T. asiatica* from *T. solium* requires examination of mature proglottids. All three species can be distinguished by examining the scolex. Available serologic tests are not helpful diagnostically. Eosinophilia and elevated levels of serum IgE may be detected.

TREATMENT   **Taeniasis Saginata and Taeniasis Asiatica**

A single dose of praziquantel (10 mg/kg) is highly effective.

Prevention

The major method of preventing infection is the adequate cooking of beef or pork viscera; exposure to temperatures as low as 56°C for 5 min will destroy cysticerci. Refrigeration or salting for long periods or freezing at –10°C for 9 days also kills cysticerci in beef. General preventive measures include inspection of beef and proper disposal of human feces.

■ TAENIASIS SOLIUM AND CYSTICERCOSIS

The pork tapeworm *T. solium* can cause two distinct forms of infection in humans: adult tapeworms in the intestine or larval forms in the tissues (cysticercosis). Humans are the only definitive hosts for *T. solium*; pigs are the usual intermediate hosts, although other animals may harbor the larval forms.

T. solium exists worldwide but is most prevalent in Latin America, sub-Saharan Africa, China, India, and Southeast Asia.

Cysticercosis occurs in industrialized nations largely as a result of the immigration of infected persons from endemic areas.

Etiology and pathogenesis

The adult tapeworm generally resides in the upper jejunum. The scolex attaches by both sucking disks and two rows of hooklets. Often only one adult worm is present, but that worm may live for years. The tapeworm, usually ~3 m in length, may have as many as 1000 proglottids, each of which produces up to 50,000 eggs. Groups of 3–5 proglottids are generally released and excreted into the feces, and the eggs in these proglottids are infective for both humans and animals. The eggs may survive in the environment for several months. After ingestion of eggs by the pig intermediate host, the larvae are activated, escape the egg, penetrate the intestinal wall, and are carried to many tissues; they are most frequently identified in striated muscle of the neck, tongue, and trunk. Within 60–90 days, the encysted larval stage develops. These cysticerci can survive for months to years. By ingesting undercooked pork containing cysticerci, humans acquire infections that lead to intestinal tapeworms. Infections that cause human cysticercosis follow the ingestion of *T. solium* eggs, usually from close contact with a tapeworm carrier. Autoinfection may occur if an individual with an egg-producing tapeworm ingests eggs derived from his or her own feces.

Clinical manifestations

Intestinal infections with *T. solium* may be asymptomatic. Fecal passage of proglottids may be noted by patients. Other symptoms are infrequent.

In cysticercosis, the clinical manifestations are variable. Cysticerci can be found anywhere in the body but are most commonly detected in the brain, cerebrospinal fluid (CSF), skeletal muscle, subcutaneous tissue, or eye. The clinical presentation of cysticercosis depends on the number and location of cysticerci as well as the extent of associated inflammatory responses or scarring. Neurologic manifestations are the most common (Fig. 220-1). Seizures are associated with inflammation surrounding cysticerci in the brain parenchyma. These seizures may be generalized, focal, or Jacksonian. Hydrocephalus results from CSF flow obstruction by cysticerci and accompanying inflammation or by CSF outflow obstruction from arachnoiditis. Signs of increased intracranial pressure, including headache, nausea,

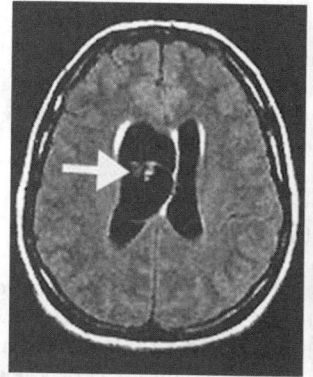 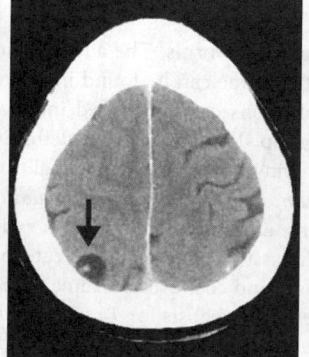 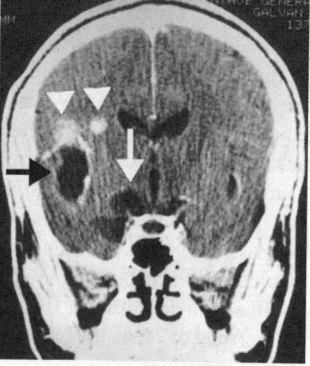

Figure 220-1   **Neurocysticercosis is caused by** *Taenia solium.* Neurologic infection can be classified on the basis of the location and viability of the parasites. When the parasites are in the ventricles, they often cause obstructive hydrocephalus. *Left:* MRI showing a cysticercus in the lateral ventricle, with resultant hydrocephalus. The arrow points to the scolex within the cystic parasite. *Center:* CT showing a parenchymal cysticercus, with enhancement of the cyst wall and an internal scolex (*arrow*). *Right:* Multiple cysticerci, including calcified lesions from prior infection (*arrowheads*), viable cysticerci in the basilar cisterns (*white arrow*), and a large degenerating cysticercus in the Sylvian fissure (*black arrow*). (*Modified with permission from JC Bandres et al: Clin Infect Dis 15:799, 1992. © The University of Chicago Press.*)

vomiting, changes in vision, dizziness, ataxia, or confusion, are often evident. Patients with hydrocephalus may develop papilledema or display altered mental status. When cysticerci develop at the base of the brain or in the subarachnoid space, they may cause chronic meningitis or arachnoiditis, communicating hydrocephalus, or strokes.

Diagnosis

The diagnosis of intestinal *T. solium* infection is made by the detection of eggs or proglottids, as described for *T. saginata*. More sensitive methods, including antigen-capture ELISA, PCR, and serology for tapeworm stage-specific antigens, are currently available only as research techniques. In cysticercosis, diagnosis can be difficult. A consensus conference has delineated absolute, major, minor, and epidemiologic criteria for diagnosis (Table 220-1). Diagnostic certainty is possible only with definite demonstration of the parasite (absolute criteria). This task can be accomplished by histologic observation of the parasite in excised tissue, by funduscopic visualization of the parasite in the eye (in the anterior chamber, vitreous, or subretinal spaces), or by neuroimaging studies demonstrating cystic lesions containing a characteristic scolex. With improving

TABLE 220-1 Diagnostic Criteria for Human Cysticercosis[a]

1. Absolute criteria

   a. Demonstration of cysticerci by histologic or microscopic examination of biopsy material

   b. Visualization of the parasite in the eye by funduscopy

   c. Neuroradiologic demonstration of cystic lesions containing a characteristic scolex

2. Major criteria

   a. Neuroradiologic lesions suggestive of neurocysticercosis

   b. Demonstration of antibodies to cysticerci in serum by enzyme-linked immunoelectrotransfer blot

   c. Resolution of intracranial cystic lesions spontaneously or after therapy with albendazole or praziquantel alone

3. Minor criteria

   a. Lesions compatible with neurocysticercosis detected by neuroimaging studies

   b. Clinical manifestations suggestive of neurocysticercosis

   c. Demonstration of antibodies to cysticerci or cysticercal antigen in cerebrospinal fluid by ELISA

   d. Evidence of cysticercosis outside the central nervous system (e.g., cigar-shaped soft-tissue calcifications)

4. Epidemiologic criteria

   a. Residence in a cysticercosis-endemic area

   b. Frequent travel to a cysticercosis-endemic area

   c. Household contact with an individual infected with *Taenia solium*

[a]Diagnosis is confirmed by either one absolute criterion or a combination of two major criteria, one minor criterion, and one epidemiologic criterion. A probable diagnosis is supported by the fulfillment of (1) one major criterion plus two minor criteria; (2) one major criterion plus one minor criterion and one epidemiologic criterion; or (3) three minor criteria plus one epidemiologic criterion.

Abbreviation: ELISA, enzyme-linked immunosorbent assay.
Source: Modified from Del Brutto et al., 2001.

resolution of neuroimaging studies, the scolex can now be identified in many cases. In other instances, a clinical diagnosis is made on the basis of a combination of clinical presentation, radiographic studies, serologic tests, and exposure history.

Neuroimaging findings suggestive of neurocysticercosis constitute the primary major diagnostic criterion. These findings include cystic lesions with or without enhancement (e.g., ring enhancement), one or more nodular calcifications (which may also have associated enhancement), or focal enhancing lesions. Cysticerci in the brain parenchyma are usually 5–20 mm in diameter and rounded. Cystic lesions in the subarachnoid space or fissures may enlarge up to 6 cm in diameter and may be lobulated. For cysticerci within the subarachnoid space or ventricles, the walls may be very thin and the cyst fluid is often isodense with CSF. Thus, obstructive hydrocephalus or enhancement of the basilar meninges may be the only finding on CT in extraparenchymal neurocysticercosis. Cysticerci in the ventricles or subarachnoid space are usually visible to an experienced neuroradiologist on MRI or on CT with intraventricular contrast injection. CT is more sensitive than MRI in identifying calcified lesions, whereas MRI is better for identifying cystic lesions, scolices, and enhancement.

The second major diagnostic criterion is detection of specific antibodies to cysticerci. While most tests employing unfractionated antigen have high rates of false-positive and false-negative results, this problem can be overcome by using the more specific immunoblot assay. An immunoblot assay using lentil-lectin purified glycoproteins has >99% specificity and is highly sensitive. However, patients with single intracranial lesions or with calcifications may be seronegative. With this assay, serum samples provide greater diagnostic sensitivity than CSF. All of the diagnostic antigens have been cloned, and assays using recombinant antigens are being developed. Antigen detection assays using monoclonal antibodies to detect parasite antigen in the blood or CSF may also facilitate diagnosis and patient follow-up. However, these assays are not widely available at present.

Studies have demonstrated that clinical criteria can aid in diagnosis in selected cases. In patients from endemic areas who had single enhancing lesions presenting with seizures, a normal physical examination, and no evidence of systemic disease (e.g., no fever, adenopathy, or chest radiographic abnormalities), the constellation of rounded CT lesions 5–20 mm in diameter with no midline shift was almost always caused by neurocysticercosis. Finally, spontaneous resolution or resolution after therapy with albendazole alone is consistent with neurocysticercosis.

Minor diagnostic criteria include neuroimaging findings consistent with but less characteristic of cysticercosis, clinical manifestations suggestive of neurocysticercosis (e.g., seizures, hydrocephalus, or altered mental status), evidence of cysticercosis outside the central nervous system (CNS) (e.g., cigar-shaped soft-tissue calcifications), or detection of antibody in CSF by ELISA. Epidemiologic criteria include exposure to a tapeworm carrier or household member infected with *T. solium*, current or prior residence in an endemic area, and frequent travel to an endemic area.

The diagnosis is confirmed in patients with either one absolute criterion or a combination of two major criteria, one minor criterion, and one epidemiologic criterion (Table 220-1). A probable diagnosis is supported by the fulfillment of (1) one major criterion plus two minor criteria; (2) one major criterion plus one minor criterion and one epidemiologic criterion; or (3) three minor criteria plus one epidemiologic criterion. While the CSF is usually abnormal in neurocysticercosis, CSF abnormalities are not pathognomonic. Patients may have CSF pleocytosis with a predominance of lymphocytes, neutrophils, or eosinophils. The protein level in CSF may be elevated; the glucose concentration is usually normal but may be depressed.

TREATMENT — Taeniasis Solium and Cysticercosis

Intestinal *T. solium* infection is treated with a single dose of praziquantel (10 mg/kg). However, praziquantel occasionally evokes an inflammatory response in the CNS if concomitant cryptic cysticercosis is present. Niclosamide (2 g) is also effective but is not widely available.

The initial management of neurocysticercosis should focus on symptom-based treatment of seizures or hydrocephalus. Seizures can usually be controlled with antiepileptic treatment. If parenchymal lesions resolve without development of calcifications and patients remain free of seizures, antiepileptic therapy can usually be discontinued after 1–2 years. Placebo-controlled trials are beginning to clarify the clinical advantage of antiparasitic drugs for parenchymal neurocysticercosis. Trends toward faster resolution of neuroradiologic abnormalities have been observed in most studies. The clinical benefits are less dramatic and consist mainly of shortening the period during which recurrent seizures occur and decreasing the number of patients who have many recurrent seizures. For the treatment of patients with brain parenchymal cysticerci, most authorities favor antiparasitic drugs, including albendazole (15 mg/kg per day for 8–28 days) or praziquantel (50–100 mg/kg daily in three divided doses for 15–30 days). Longer courses are often needed in patients with multiple subarachnoid cysticerci. Both agents may exacerbate the inflammatory response around the dying parasite, thereby exacerbating seizures or hydrocephalus as well. Thus, patients receiving these drugs should be carefully monitored, and high-dose glucocorticoids should be used during treatment. Since glucocorticoids induce first-pass metabolism of praziquantel and may decrease its antiparasitic effect, cimetidine should be co-administered to inhibit praziquantel metabolism. Pilot studies suggest that the two drugs in combination may be more effective than the individual agents.

For patients with hydrocephalus, the emergent reduction of intracranial pressure is the mainstay of therapy. In the case of obstructive hydrocephalus, the preferred approach is removal of the cysticercus via endoscopic surgery. However, this intervention is not always possible. An alternative approach is initially to perform a diverting procedure, such as ventriculoperitoneal shunting. Historically, shunts have usually failed, but low failure rates have been attained with administration of antiparasitic drugs and glucocorticoids. Open craniotomy to remove cysticerci is now required only infrequently. For patients with subarachnoid cysts or giant cysticerci, glucocorticoids are needed to reduce arachnoiditis and accompanying vasculitis. Most authorities recommend prolonged courses of antiparasitic drugs and shunting when hydrocephalus is present. Methotrexate can be used as a steroid-sparing agent in patients requiring prolonged therapy. In patients with diffuse cerebral edema and elevated intracranial pressure due to multiple inflamed lesions, glucocorticoids are the mainstay of therapy, and antiparasitic drugs should be avoided. For ocular and spinal medullary lesions, drug-induced inflammation may cause irreversible damage. Most patients should be managed surgically, although case reports have described cures with medical therapy.

Prevention

Measures for the prevention of intestinal *T. solium* infection consist of the application to pork of precautions similar to those described above for beef with regard to *T. saginata* infection. The prevention of cysticercosis involves minimizing the opportunities for ingestion of fecally derived eggs by means of good personal hygiene, effective fecal disposal, and treatment and prevention of human intestinal infections. Mass chemotherapy has been administered to human and porcine populations in efforts at disease eradication. Finally, vaccines to prevent porcine cysticercosis have shown promise in studies and are under development.

ECHINOCOCCOSIS

Echinococcosis is an infection caused in humans by the larval stage of the *Echinococcus granulosus* complex, *E. multilocularis*, or *E. vogeli*. *E. granulosus* complex parasites, which produce unilocular cystic lesions and are prevalent in areas where livestock is raised in association with dogs, cause cystic hydatid disease. Molecular evidence suggests that *E. granulosus* strains may actually belong to more than one species; specifically, strains from sheep, cattle, pigs, horses, and camels probably represent separate species. These parasites are found on all continents, with areas of high prevalence in China, central Asia, the Middle East, the Mediterranean region, eastern Africa, and parts of South America. *E. multilocularis*, which causes multilocular alveolar lesions that are locally invasive, is found in Alpine, sub-Arctic, or Arctic regions, including Canada, the United States, and central and northern Europe; China; and central Asia. *E. vogeli* causes polycystic hydatid disease and is found only in Central and South America.

Like other cestodes, echinococcal species have both intermediate and definitive hosts. The definitive hosts are canines that pass eggs in their feces. After the ingestion of eggs, cysts develop in the intermediate hosts—sheep, cattle, humans, goats, camels, and horses for the *E. granulosus* complex and mice and other rodents for *E. multilocularis*. When a dog (*E. granulosus*) or fox (*E. multilocularis*) ingests infected meat containing cysts, the life cycle is completed.

Etiology

The small (5-mm-long) adult *E. granulosus* complex worms, which live for 5–20 months in the jejunum of dogs, have only three proglottids: one immature, one mature, and one gravid. The gravid segment splits to release eggs that are morphologically similar to *Taenia* eggs and are extremely hardy. After humans ingest the eggs, embryos escape from the eggs, penetrate the intestinal mucosa, enter the portal circulation, and are carried to various organs, most commonly the liver and lungs. Larvae develop into fluid-filled unilocular hydatid cysts that consist of an external membrane and an inner germinal layer. Daughter cysts develop from the inner aspect of the germinal layer, as do germinating cystic structures called *brood capsules*. New larvae, called *protoscolices*, develop in large numbers within the brood capsule. The cysts expand slowly over a period of years.

The life cycle of *E. multilocularis* is similar except that wild canines, such as foxes, serve as the definitive hosts and small rodents serve as the intermediate hosts. The larval form of *E. multilocularis*, however, is quite different in that it remains in the proliferative phase, the parasite is always multilocular, and vesicles without brood capsule or protoscolices progressively invade the host tissue by peripheral extension of processes from the germinal layer.

Clinical manifestations

Slowly enlarging echinococcal cysts generally remain asymptomatic until their expanding size or their space-occupying effect in an involved organ elicits symptoms. The liver and the lungs are the most common sites of these cysts. The liver is involved in about two-thirds of *E. granulosus* infections and in nearly all *E. multilocularis* infections. Since a period of years elapses before cysts enlarge sufficiently to cause symptoms, they may be discovered incidentally on a routine x-ray or ultrasound study.

Patients with hepatic echinococcosis who are symptomatic most often present with abdominal pain or a palpable mass in the right upper quadrant. Compression of a bile duct or leakage of cyst fluid into the biliary tree may mimic recurrent cholelithiasis, and biliary obstruction can result in jaundice. Rupture of or episodic leakage from a hydatid cyst may produce fever, pruritus, urticaria, eosinophilia, or anaphylaxis. Pulmonary hydatid cysts may rupture into the bronchial tree or peritoneal cavity and produce cough, salty phlegm, dyspnea, chest pain, or hemoptysis. Rupture of hydatid cysts, which can occur spontaneously or at surgery, may lead to multifocal dissemination of protoscolices, which can form additional cysts. Other presentations are due to the involvement of bone (invasion of the medullary cavity with slow bone erosion producing pathologic fractures), the CNS (space-occupying lesions), the heart (conduction defects, pericarditis), and the pelvis (pelvic mass).

The larval forms of *E. multilocularis* characteristically present as a slowly growing hepatic tumor, with progressive destruction of the liver and extension into vital structures. Patients commonly report upper-quadrant and epigastric pain. Liver enlargement and obstructive jaundice may be apparent. The lesions may infiltrate adjoining organs (e.g., diaphragm, kidneys, or lungs) or may metastasize to the spleen, lungs, or brain.

Diagnosis

Radiographic and related imaging studies are important in detecting and evaluating echinococcal cysts. Plain x-rays will define pulmonary cysts of *E. granulosus*—usually as rounded masses of uniform density—but may miss cysts in other organs unless there is cyst wall calcification (as occurs in the liver). MRI, CT, and ultrasound reveal well-defined cysts with thick or thin walls. When older cysts contain a layer of hydatid sand that is rich in accumulated protoscolices, these imaging methods may detect this fluid layer of different density. However, the most pathognomonic finding, if demonstrable, is that of daughter cysts within the larger cyst. This finding, like eggshell or mural calcification on CT, is indicative of *E. granulosus* infection and helps to distinguish the cyst from carcinomas, bacterial or amebic liver abscesses, or hemangiomas. In contrast, ultrasound or CT of alveolar hydatid cysts reveals indistinct solid masses with central necrosis and plaquelike calcifications.

A specific diagnosis of *E. granulosus* infection can be made by the examination of aspirated fluids for protoscolices or hooklets, but diagnostic aspiration is not usually recommended because of the risk of fluid leakage resulting in either dissemination of infection or anaphylactic reactions. Serodiagnostic assays can be useful, although a negative test does not exclude the diagnosis of echinococcosis. Cysts in the liver elicit positive antibody responses in ~90% of cases, whereas up to 50% of individuals with cysts in the lungs are seronegative. Detection of antibody to specific echinococcal antigens by immunoblotting has the highest degree of specificity.

TREATMENT   Echinococcosis

Therapy for cystic echinococcosis is based on considerations of the size, location, and manifestations of cysts and the overall health of the patient. Surgery has traditionally been the principal definitive method of treatment. Currently, ultrasound staging is recommended for *E. granulosus* infections (Fig. 220-2). Small C1, CE1, and CE3 lesions may respond to chemotherapy with albendazole. For CE1 lesions and uncomplicated CE3 lesions, PAIR (*percutaneous aspiration, infusion of scolicidal agents, and reaspiration*) is now recommended instead of surgery. PAIR is contraindicated for superficially located cysts (because of the risk of rupture), for cysts with multiple thick internal septal divisions (honeycombing pattern), and for cysts communicating with the biliary tree. For prophylaxis of secondary peritoneal echinococcosis due to inadvertent spillage of fluid during PAIR, the administration of albendazole (15 mg/kg daily in two divided doses) should be initiated at least 4 days before the procedure and continued for at least 4 weeks afterward. Ultrasound- or CT-guided aspiration allows confirmation of the diagnosis by demonstration of protoscolices in the aspirate. After aspiration, contrast material should be injected to detect occult communications with the biliary tract. Alternatively, the fluid should be checked for bile

Echinococcosis cysts

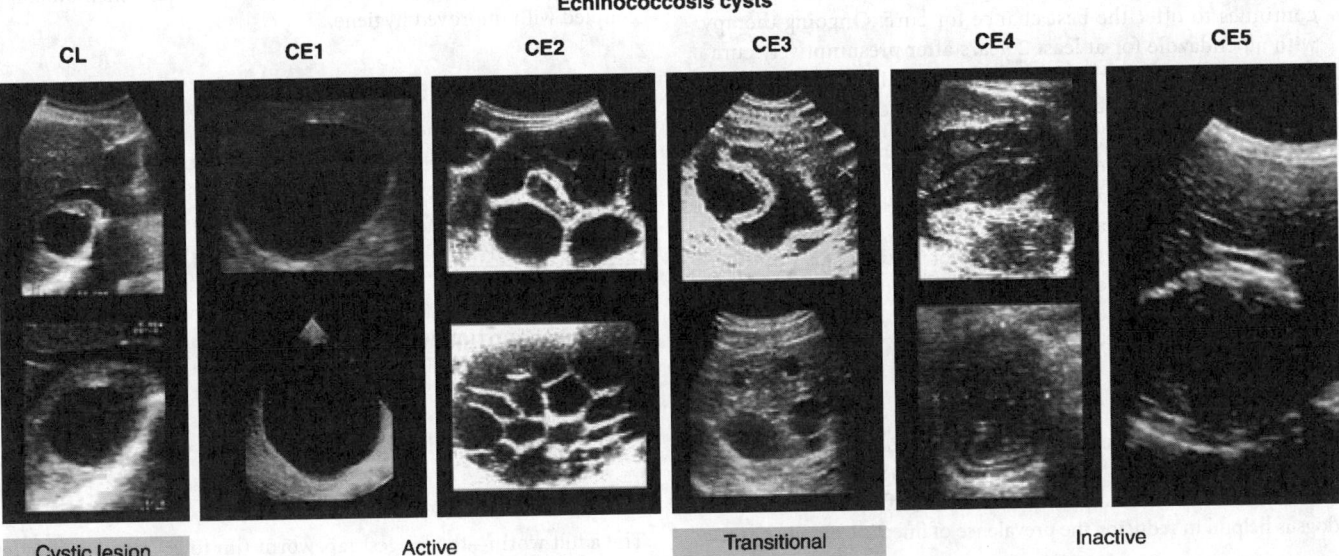

CL   CE1   CE2   CE3   CE4   CE5

Cystic lesion   Active   Transitional   Inactive

Figure 220-2 Management of cystic hydatid disease caused by *Echinococcus granulosus* should be based on viability of the parasite, which can be estimated from radiographic appearance. The ultrasound appearance includes lesions classified as active, transitional, and inactive. *Active* cysts include types CL (with a cystic lesion and no visible cyst wall), CE1 [with a visible cyst wall and internal echoes (snowflake sign)], and CE2 (with a visible cyst wall and internal septation). *Transitional cysts* (CE3) may have detached laminar membranes or may be partially collapsed. *Inactive cysts* include types CE4 (a nonhomogeneous mass) and CE5 (a cyst with a thick calcified wall). [*Adapted from RL Guerrant et al (eds): Tropical Infectious Diseases: Principles, Pathogens and Practice, 2nd ed, p 1312. © 2005, with permission from Elsevier Science.*]

staining by dipstick. If no bile is found and no communication visualized, the contrast material is reaspirated, with subsequent infusion of scolicidal agents (usually 95% ethanol; alternatively, hypertonic saline). This approach, when implemented by a skilled practitioner, yields rates of cure and relapse equivalent to those following surgery, with less perioperative morbidity and shorter hospitalization. In experienced hands, some CE2 lesions can be treated by aspiration with a trochar. Daughter cysts within the primary cyst may need to be punctured separately, and catheter drainage may be required.

Surgery remains the treatment of choice for complicated *E. granulosus* cysts (e.g., those communicating with the biliary tract) or for areas where PAIR is not possible. For *E. granulosus*, the preferred surgical approach is pericystectomy, in which the entire cyst and the surrounding fibrous tissue are removed. The risks posed by leakage of fluid during surgery or PAIR include anaphylaxis and dissemination of infectious protoscolices. The latter complication has been minimized by careful attention to the prevention of spillage of the cyst and by soaking of the drapes with hypertonic saline. Infusion of scolicidal agents is no longer recommended because of problems with hypernatremia, intoxication, or sclerosing cholangitis. Albendazole, which is active against *Echinococcus*, should be administered adjunctively, beginning several days before resection and continuing for several weeks for *E. granulosus*. Praziquantel (50 mg/kg daily for 2 weeks) may hasten the death of the protoscolices. Medical therapy with albendazole alone for 12 weeks to 6 months results in cure in ~30% of cases and in improvement in another 50%. In many instances of treatment failure, *E. granulosus* infections are subsequently treated successfully with PAIR or additional courses of medical therapy. Response to treatment is best assessed by serial imaging studies, with attention to cyst size and consistency. Some cysts may not demonstrate complete radiologic resolution even though no viable protoscolices are present. Some of these cysts with partial radiologic resolution (e.g., CE4 or CE5) can be managed with observation only.

Surgical resection remains the treatment of choice for *E. multilocularis* infection. Complete removal of the parasite continues to offer the best chance for cure. Ongoing therapy with albendazole for at least 2 years after presumptively curative surgery is recommended. Positron emission tomography (PET) scanning can be used to follow disease activity. Most cases are diagnosed at a stage at which complete resection is not possible; in these cases, albendazole treatment should be continued indefinitely, with careful monitoring. In some cases, liver transplantation has been used because of the size of the necessary liver resection. However, continuous immunosuppression favors the proliferation of *E. multilocularis* larvae and reinfection of the transplant. Thus, indefinite treatment with albendazole is required.

Prevention

In endemic areas, echinococcosis can be prevented by administering praziquantel to infected dogs, by denying dogs access to infected animals, or by vaccinating sheep. Limitation of the number of stray dogs is helpful in reducing the prevalence of infection among humans.

■ HYMENOLEPIASIS NANA

 Infection with *H. nana*, the dwarf tapeworm, is the most common of all the cestode infections. *H. nana* is endemic in both temperate and tropical regions of the world. Infection is spread by fecal/oral contamination and is common among institutionalized children.

Etiology and pathogenesis

H. nana is the only cestode of humans that does not require an intermediate host. Both the larval and adult phases of the life cycle take place in the human. The adult—the smallest tapeworm parasitizing humans—is ~2 cm long and dwells in the proximal ileum. Proglottids, which are quite small and are rarely seen in the stool, release spherical eggs 30–44 μm in diameter, each of which contains an oncosphere with six hooklets. The eggs are immediately infective and are unable to survive for >10 days in the external environment. When the egg is ingested by a new host, the oncosphere is freed and penetrates the intestinal villi, becoming a cysticercoid larva. Larvae migrate back into the intestinal lumen, attach to the mucosa, and mature into adult worms over 10–12 days. Eggs may also hatch before passing into the stool, causing internal autoinfection with increasing numbers of intestinal worms. Although the life span of adult *H. nana* worms is only ~4–10 weeks, the autoinfection cycle perpetuates the infection.

Clinical manifestations

H. nana infection, even with many intestinal worms, is usually asymptomatic. When infection is intense, anorexia, abdominal pain, and diarrhea develop.

Diagnosis

Infection is diagnosed by the finding of eggs in the stool.

TREATMENT	Hymenolepiasis Nana

Praziquantel (25 mg/kg once) is the treatment of choice, since it acts against both the adult worms and the cysticercoids in the intestinal villi. Nitazoxanide (500 mg bid for 3 days) may be used as an alternative.

Prevention

Good personal hygiene and improved sanitation can eradicate the disease. Epidemics have been controlled by mass chemotherapy coupled with improved hygiene.

■ HYMENOLEPIASIS DIMINUTA

Hymenolepis diminuta, a cestode of rodents, occasionally infects small children, who ingest the larvae in uncooked cereal foods contaminated by fleas and other insects in which larvae develop. Infection is usually asymptomatic and is diagnosed by the detection of eggs in the stool. Treatment with praziquantel results in cure in most cases.

■ DIPHYLLOBOTHRIASIS

Diphyllobothrium latum and other *Diphyllobothrium* species are found in the lakes, rivers, and deltas of the Northern Hemisphere, Central Africa, and South America.

Etiology and pathogenesis

The adult worm—the longest tapeworm (up to 25 m)—attaches to the ileal and occasionally to the jejunal mucosa by its suckers, which are located on its elongated scolex. The adult worm has 3000–4000 proglottids, which release ~1 million eggs daily into the feces. If an egg reaches water, it hatches and releases a free-swimming embryo that can be eaten by small freshwater crustaceans (*Cyclops* or *Diaptomus* species). After an infected crustacean containing a developed procercoid is swallowed by a fish, the larva migrates into the fish's flesh and grows into a plerocercoid, or sparganum larva. Humans acquire the infection by ingesting infected raw or smoked fish. Within 3–5 weeks, the tapeworm matures into an adult in the human intestine.

Clinical manifestations

Most *D. latum* infections are asymptomatic, although manifestations may include transient abdominal discomfort, diarrhea, vomiting, weakness, and weight loss. Occasionally, infection can cause acute abdominal pain and intestinal obstruction; in rare cases, cholangitis or cholecystitis may be produced by migrating proglottids. Because the tapeworm absorbs large quantities of vitamin B_{12} and interferes with ileal B_{12} absorption, vitamin B_{12} deficiency can develop, but this effect has been noted only in Scandinavia, where up to 2% of infected patients, especially the elderly, have megaloblastic anemia resembling pernicious anemia and may exhibit neurologic sequelae of B_{12} deficiency.

Diagnosis

The diagnosis is made readily by the detection of the characteristic eggs in the stool. The eggs possess a single shell with an operculum at one end and a knob at the other. Mild to moderate eosinophilia may be detected.

> **TREATMENT**   Diphyllobothriasis

Praziquantel (5–10 mg/kg once) is highly effective. Parenteral vitamin B_{12} should be given if B_{12} deficiency is manifest.

Prevention

Infection can be prevented by heating fish to 54°C for 5 min or by freezing it at –18°C for 24 h. Placing fish in brine with a high salt concentration for long periods kills the eggs.

■ DIPYLIDIASIS

Dipylidium caninum, a common tapeworm of dogs and cats, may accidentally infect humans. Dogs, cats, and occasionally humans become infected by ingesting fleas harboring cysticercoids. Children are more likely to become infected than adults. Most infections are asymptomatic, but abdominal pain, diarrhea, anal pruritus, urticaria, eosinophilia, or passage of segments in the stool may occur. The diagnosis is made by the detection of proglottids or ova in the stool. As in *D. latum* infection, therapy consists of praziquantel. Prevention requires anthelmintic treatment and flea control for pet dogs or cats.

■ SPARGANOSIS

Humans can be infected by the sparganum, or plerocercoid larva, of a diphyllobothrid tapeworm of the genus *Spirometra*. Infection can be acquired by the consumption of water containing infected *Cyclops*; by the ingestion of infected snakes, birds, or mammals; or by the application of infected flesh as poultices. The worm migrates slowly in tissues, and infection commonly presents as a subcutaneous swelling. Periorbital tissues can be involved, and ocular sparganosis may destroy the eye. Surgical excision is used to treat localized sparganosis.

■ COENUROSIS

This rare infection of humans by the larval stage (coenurus) of the dog tapeworm *Taenia multiceps* or *T. serialis* results in a space-occupying cystic lesion. As in cysticercosis, involvement of the CNS and subcutaneous tissue is most common. Both definitive diagnosis and treatment require surgical excision of the lesion. Chemotherapeutic agents generally are not effective.

FURTHER READINGS

Articles

BRUNETTI E et al: Expert consensus for the diagnosis and treatment of cystic and alveolar echinococcosis in humans. Acta Trop 114:1, 2010

CRAIG P, ITO A: Intestinal cestodes. Curr Opin Infect Dis 20:524, 2007

DEL BRUTTO OH et al: Proposed diagnostic criteria for neurocysticercosis. Neurology 57:177, 2001

—— et al: Meta-analysis: Cysticidal drugs for neurocysticercosis: Albendazole and praziquantel. Ann Intern Med 145:43, 2006

GARCIA HH et al: A trial of antiparasitic treatment to reduce the rate of seizures due to cerebral cysticercosis. N Engl J Med 350:249, 2004

NASH TE et al: Treatment of neurocysticercosis: Current status and future research needs. Neurology 67:1120, 2006

RANGEL-CASTILLA L et al: Contemporary neurosurgical approaches to neurocysticercosis. Am J Trop Med Hyg 80:373, 2009

SCHOLZ T et al: Update on the human broad tapeworm (genus *Diphyllobothrium*), including clinical relevance. Clin Microbiol Rev 22:146, 2009

SERPA JA et al: Neurocysticercosis in Houston, Texas: An update. Medicine (Baltimore) 90:81, 2011

WORLD HEALTH ORGANIZATION INFORMAL WORKING GROUP ON ECHINOCOCCOSIS: International classification of ultrasound images in cystic echinococcosis for application in clinical and field epidemiological settings. Acta Tropica 85:253, 2003

Web Sites

CDC Division of Parasitic Diseases. *www.cdc.gov/ncidod/dpd/default.htm*

PART 9
Terrorism and Clinical Medicine

CHAPTER **221**

Microbial Bioterrorism

H. Clifford Lane
Anthony S. Fauci

Descriptions of the use of microbial pathogens as potential weapons of war or terrorism date from ancient times. Among the most frequently cited of such episodes are the poisoning of water supplies in the sixth century B.C. with the fungus *Claviceps purpurea* (rye ergot) by the Assyrians, the hurling of the dead bodies of plague victims over the walls of the city of Kaffa by the Tartar army in 1346, and the efforts by the British to spread smallpox to the Native American population loyal to the French via contaminated blankets in 1767. Although the use of chemical weapons in wartime took place in the not-too-distant past (Chap. 222), the tragic events of September 11, 2001, followed closely by the mailing of letters containing anthrax spores to media and congressional offices through the U.S. Postal Service, dramatically changed the mindset of the American public regarding both our vulnerability to microbial bioterrorist attacks and the seriousness and intent of the federal government to protect its citizens against future attacks. Modern science has revealed methods of deliberately spreading or enhancing disease in ways not appreciated by our ancestors. The combination of basic research, good medical practice, and constant vigilance will be needed to defend against such attacks.

Although the potential impact of a bioterrorist attack could be enormous, leading to thousands of deaths and high morbidity rates, acts of bioterrorism would be expected to produce their greatest impact through the fear and terror they generate. In contrast to biowarfare, where the primary goal is destruction of the enemy through mass casualties, an important goal of bioterrorism is to destroy the morale of a society through fear and uncertainty. While the actual biologic impact of a single act may be small, the degree of disruption created by the realization that such an attack is possible may be enormous. This was readily apparent with the impact on the U.S. Postal Service and the functional interruption of the activities of the legislative branch of the United States government following the anthrax attacks noted above. Thus, the key to the defense against these attacks is a highly functioning system of public health surveillance and education so that attacks can be quickly recognized and effectively contained. This is complemented by the availability of appropriate countermeasures in the form of diagnostics, therapeutics, and vaccines, both in response to and in anticipation of bioterrorist attacks.

The Working Group for Civilian Biodefense has put together a list of key features that characterize the elements of biologic agents that make them particularly effective as weapons (Table 221-1). Included among these are the ease of spread and transmission of the agent as well as the presence of an adequate database to allow newcomers to the field to quickly apply the good science of others to bad intentions of their own. Agents of bioterrorism may be used in their naturally occurring forms or they can be deliberately modified to provide maximal impact. Among the approaches to maximizing the deleterious effects of biologic agents are the genetic modification of microbes for the purposes of antimicrobial resistance or evasion by the immune system, creation of fine-particle aerosols, chemical treatment to stabilize and prolong infectivity, and alteration of host range through changes in surface proteins.

TABLE 221-1 Key Features of Biologic Agents Used as Bioweapons

1. High morbidity and mortality rates
2. Potential for person-to-person spread
3. Low infective dose and highly infectious by aerosol
4. Lack of rapid diagnostic capability
5. Lack of universally available effective vaccine
6. Potential to cause anxiety
7. Availability of pathogen and feasibility of production
8. Environmental stability
9. Database of prior research and development
10. Potential to be "weaponized"

Source: From L Borio et al: JAMA 287:2391, 2002; with permission.

Certain of these approaches fall under the category of *weaponization*, which is a term generally used to describe the processing of microbes or toxins in a manner that would ensure a devastating effect of a release. For example, weaponization of anthrax by the Soviets comprised the production of vast amounts of spores in a form that maintained aerosolization for prolonged periods of time; the spores were of appropriate size to reach the lower respiratory tract easily and could be delivered in a massive release, such as via widely dispersed bomblets.

The U.S. Centers for Disease Control and Prevention (CDC) classifies potential biologic threats into three categories, A, B, and C (Table 221-2). Category A agents are the highest-priority pathogens. They pose the greatest risk to national security because they (1) can be easily disseminated or transmitted from person to person, (2) result in high mortality rates and have the potential for major public health impact, (3) might cause public panic and social disruption, and (4) require special action for public health preparedness. Category B agents are the second highest priority pathogens and include those that are moderately easy to disseminate, result in moderate morbidity rates and low mortality rates, and require specifically enhanced diagnostic capacity. Category C agents are the third highest priority. These include certain emerging pathogens to which the general population lacks immunity that could be engineered for mass dissemination in the future because of availability, ease of production, to ease of dissemination, and that have a major public health impact and the potential for high morbidity and mortality rates. It should be pointed out, however, that these A, B, and C designations are empirical, and, depending on evolving circumstances such as intelligence-based threat assessments, the priority rating of any given microbe or toxin could change. The CDC classification system also largely reflects the severity of illness produced by a given agent, rather than its accessibility to potential terrorists.

CATEGORY A AGENTS

■ ANTHRAX

See also Chap. 138.

Bacillus anthracis as a bioweapon

Anthrax may be the prototypic disease of bioterrorism. Although rarely, if ever, spread from person to person, the illness embodies the other major features of a disease introduced through terrorism, as outlined in Table 221-1. U.S. and British government scientists

TABLE 221-2 CDC Category A, B, and C Agents

Category A

Anthrax (*Bacillus anthracis*)

Botulism (*Clostridium botulinum* toxin)

Plague (*Yersinia pestis*)

Smallpox (*Variola major*)

Tularemia (*Francisella tularensis*)

Viral hemorrhagic fevers

  Arenaviruses: Lassa, New World (Machupo, Junin, Guanarito, and Sabia)

  Bunyaviridae: Crimean-Congo, Rift Valley

  Filoviridae: Ebola, Marburg

Category B

Brucellosis (*Brucella* spp.)

Epsilon toxin of *Clostridium perfringens*

Food safety threats (e.g., *Salmonella* spp., *Escherichia coli* 0157:H7, *Shigella*)

Glanders (*Burkholderia mallei*)

Melioidosis (*B. pseudomallei*)

Psittacosis (*Chlamydophila psittaci*)

Q fever (*Coxiella burnetii*)

Ricin toxin from *Ricinus communis* (castor beans)

Staphylococcal enterotoxin B

Typhus fever (*Rickettsia prowazekii*)

Viral encephalitis [alphaviruses (e.g., Venezuelan, eastern, and western equine encephalitis)]

Water safety threats (e.g., *Vibrio cholerae*, *Cryptosporidium parvum*)

Category C

Emerging infectious diseases threats such as Nipah, hantavirus, SARS coronavirus, and pandemic influenza.

Abbreviation: SARS, severe acute respiratory syndrome.

Source: Centers for Disease Control and Prevention and the National Institute of Allergy and Infectious Diseases.

studied anthrax as a potential biologic weapon beginning approximately at the time of World War II (WWII). Offensive bioweapons activity including bioweapons research on microbes and toxins in the United States ceased in 1969 as a result of two executive orders by President Richard M. Nixon. Although the 1972 Biological and Toxin Weapons Convention Treaty outlawed research of this type worldwide, the Soviet Union produced and stored tons of anthrax spores for potential use as a bioweapon until at least the late 1980s. At present, there is suspicion that research on anthrax as an agent of bioterrorism is ongoing by several nations and extremist groups. One example of this is the release of anthrax spores by the Aum Shinrikyo cult in Tokyo in 1993. Fortunately, there were no casualties associated with this episode because of the inadvertent use of a nonpathogenic strain of anthrax by the terrorists.

The potential impact of anthrax spores as a bioweapon was clearly demonstrated in 1979 following the accidental release of spores into the atmosphere from a Soviet Union bioweapons facility in Sverdlosk, Russia. While actual figures are not known, at least 77 cases of anthrax were diagnosed with certainty, of which 66 were

fatal. These victims were exposed in an area within 4 km downwind of the facility, and deaths due to anthrax were also noted in livestock up to 50 km further downwind. Based on recorded wind patterns, the interval between the time of exposure and development of clinical illness ranged from 2 to 43 days. The majority of cases were within the first 2 weeks. Death typically occurred within 1–4 days following the onset of symptoms. It is likely that the widespread use of postexposure penicillin prophylaxis limited the total number of cases. The extended period of time between exposure and disease in some individuals supports the data from nonhuman primate studies, suggesting that the anthrax spores can lie dormant in the respiratory tract for at least 4–6 weeks without evoking an immune response. This extended period of microbiologic latency following exposure poses a significant challenge for management of victims in the postexposure period.

In September 2001, the American public was exposed to anthrax spores as a bioweapon delivered through the U.S. Postal Service by an employee of the United States Army Research Institute for Infectious Diseases (USAMRIID) who had access to such materials and who committed suicide prior to being indicted for this crime. The CDC identified 22 confirmed or suspected cases of anthrax as a consequence of this attack. These included 11 patients with inhalational anthrax, of whom 5 died, and 11 patients with cutaneous anthrax (7 confirmed), all of whom survived (Fig. 221-1). Cases occurred in individuals who opened contaminated letters as well as in postal workers involved in the processing of mail. A minimum of five letters mailed from Trenton, NJ, served as the vehicles for these attacks. One of these letters was reported to contain 2 g of material, equivalent to 100 billion to 1 trillion weapon-grade spores. Since studies performed in the 1950s using monkeys exposed to aerosolized anthrax suggested that ~10,000 spores were required to produce lethal disease in 50% of animals exposed to this dose (the LD_{50}), the contents of one letter had the theoretical potential, under optimal conditions, of causing illness or death in up to 50 million individuals when one considers an LD_{50} of 10,000 spores. The strain used in this attack was the Ames strain. Although it was noted to have an inducible β-lactamase and to constitutively express a cephalosporinase, it was susceptible to all antibiotics standard for *B. anthracis*.

Microbiology and clinical features

Anthrax is caused by *B. anthracis*, a gram-positive, nonmotile, spore-forming rod that is found in soil and predominantly causes disease in herbivores such as cattle, goats, and sheep. Anthrax spores can remain viable for decades. The remarkable stability of these spores makes them an ideal bioweapon, and their destruction in decontamination activities can be a challenge. Naturally occurring human infection is generally the result of contact with anthrax-infected animals or animal products such as goat hair in textile mills or animal skins used in making drums. While an LD_{50} of 10,000 spores is a generally accepted number, it has also been suggested that as few as one to three spores may be adequate to cause disease in some settings. Advanced technology is likely to be necessary to generate spores of the optimal size (1–5 μm) to travel to the alveolar spaces as a bioweapon.

The three major clinical forms of anthrax are gastrointestinal, cutaneous, and inhalational. *Gastrointestinal anthrax* typically results from the ingestion of contaminated meat; the condition is rarely seen and is unlikely to be the result of a bioterrorism event. The lesion of *cutaneous anthrax* typically begins as a papule following the introduction of spores through an opening in the skin. This papule then evolves to a painless vesicle followed by the development of a coal-black, necrotic eschar (Fig. 221-2). It is the Greek word for coal (*anthrax*) that gives the organism and the disease its name. Cutaneous anthrax was ~20% fatal prior to the availability

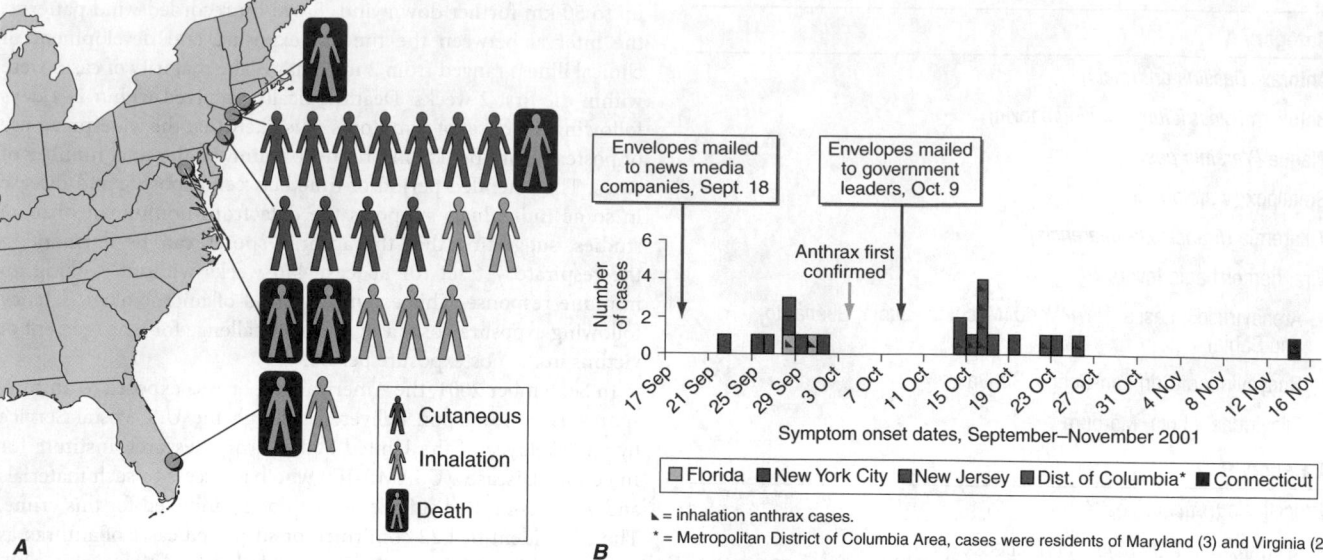

Figure 221-1 Confirmed anthrax cases associated with bioterrorism: United States, 2001. *A.* Geographic location, clinical manifestation, and outcome of the 11 cases of confirmed inhalational and 11 cases of confirmed cutaneous anthrax. *B.* Epidemic curve for 22 cases of anthrax. (*From DB Jernigan et al: Emerg Infect Dis 8:1019, 2002; with permission.*)

of antibiotics. *Inhalational anthrax* is the form most likely to be responsible for death in the setting of a bioterrorist attack. It occurs following the inhalation of spores that become deposited in the alveolar spaces. These spores are phagocytosed by macrophages and transported to the mediastinal and peribronchial lymph nodes where they germinate, leading to active bacterial growth and elaboration of the bacterial products edema toxin and lethal toxin. Subsequent hematogenous spread of bacteria is accompanied by cardiovascular collapse and death. The earliest symptoms are typically a viral-like prodrome with fever, malaise, and abdominal and/or chest symptoms that progress over the course of a few days to a moribund state. A characteristic finding is mediastinal widening and pleural effusions on chest x-ray (Fig. 221-3). While initially thought to be 100% fatal, the experiences at Sverdlosk in 1979 and in the United States in 2001 (see below) indicate that with prompt initiation of

antibiotic therapy, survival is possible. The characteristics of the 11 cases of inhalational anthrax diagnosed in the United States in 2001 following exposure to contaminated letters postmarked September 18 or October 9, 2001, followed the classic pattern established for this illness, with patients presenting with a rapidly progressive course characterized by fever, fatigue or malaise, nausea or vomiting, cough, and shortness of breath. At presentation, the total white blood cell counts were ~10,000 cells/μL; transaminases tended to be elevated, and all 11 had abnormal findings on chest x-ray and CT. Radiologic findings included infiltrates, mediastinal widening, and hemorrhagic pleural effusions. For cases in which the dates of exposure were known, symptoms appeared within 4–6 days. Death occurred within 7 days of diagnosis in the five fatal cases (overall mortality rate 55%). Rapid diagnosis and prompt initiation of antibiotic therapy were key to survival.

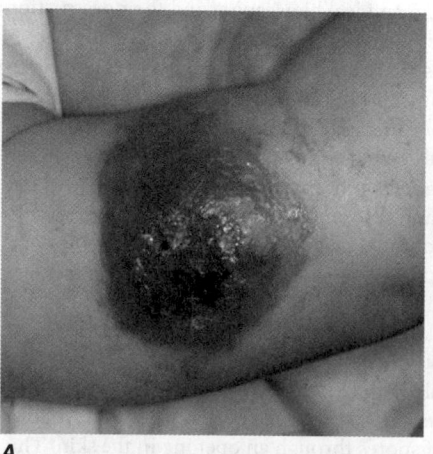
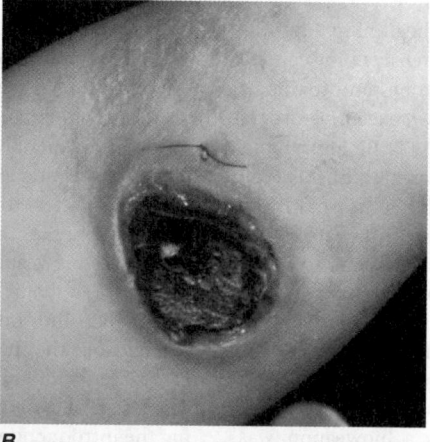
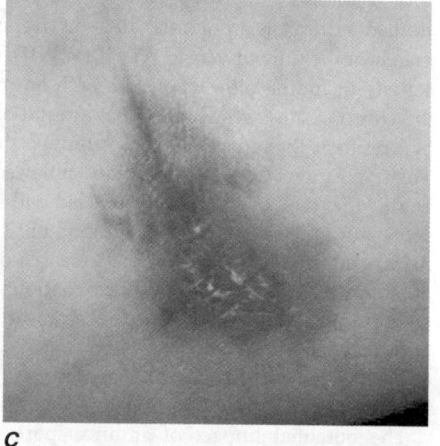

Figure 221-2 Clinical manifestations of a pediatric case of cutaneous anthrax associated with the bioterrorism attack of 2001. The lesion progresses from vesicular on day 5 (*A*) to necrotic with the classic black eschar on day 12 (*B*) to a healed scar 2 months later (*C*). (*Photographs provided by Dr. Mary Wu Chang and* (A) *reprinted with permission of the New England Journal of Medicine.*)

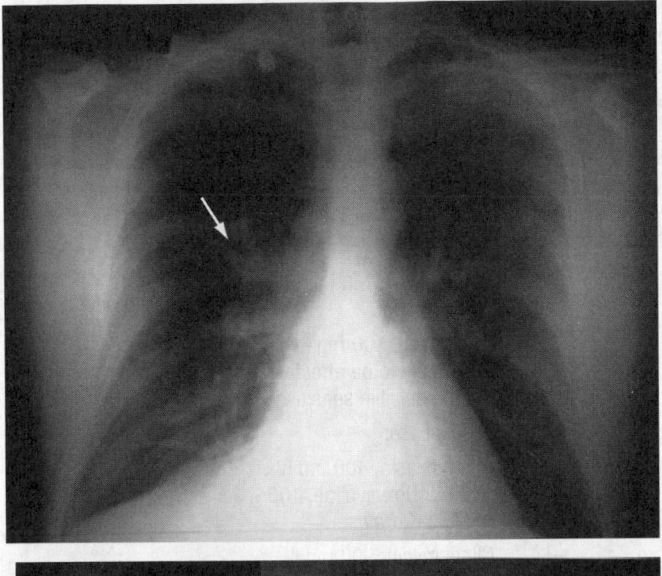
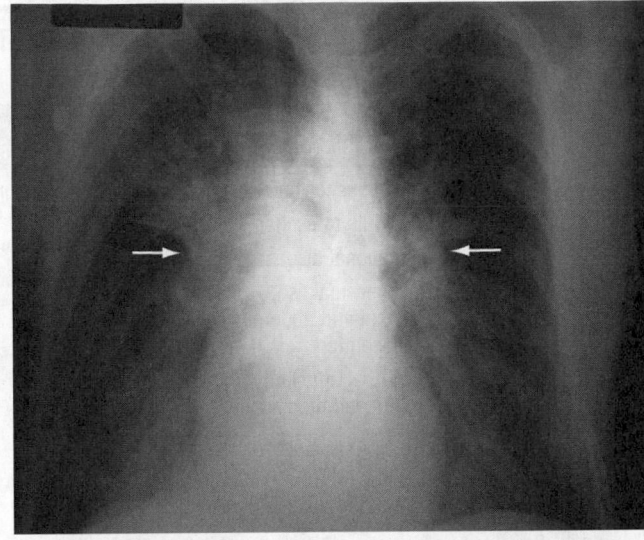
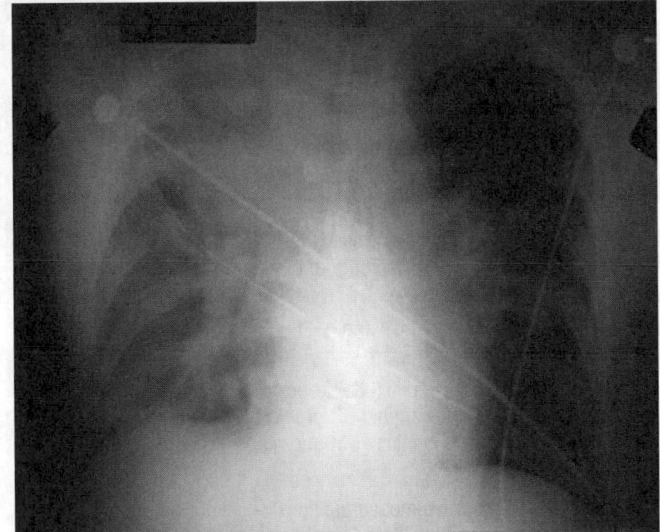
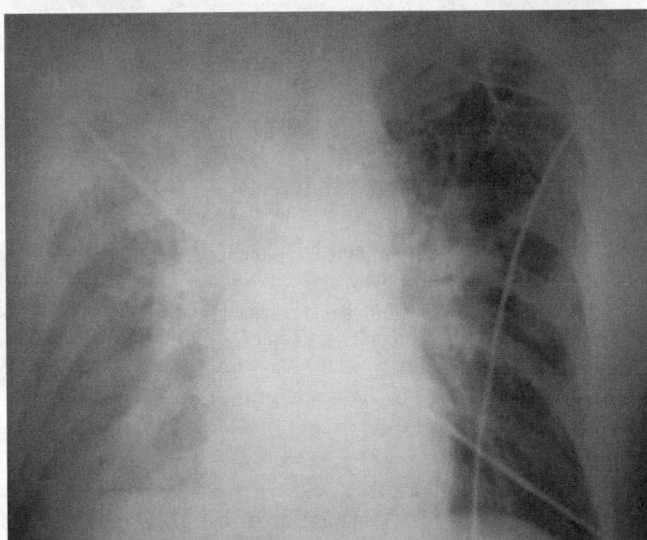

Figure 221-3 Progression of chest x-ray findings in a patient with inhalational anthrax. Findings evolved from subtle hilar prominence and right perihilar infiltrate to a progressively widened mediastinum, marked perihilar infiltrates, peribronchial cuffing, and air bronchograms. (*From L Borio et al: JAMA 286:2554, 2001; with permission.*)

TREATMENT ▸ Anthrax

Anthrax can be successfully treated if the disease is promptly recognized and appropriate therapy is initiated early. While penicillin, ciprofloxacin, and doxycycline are the currently licensed antibiotics for this indication, clindamycin and rifampin also have in vitro activity against the organism and have been used as part of treatment regimens. Until sensitivity results are known, suspected cases are best managed with a combination of broadly active agents (Table 221-3). Patients with inhalational anthrax are not contagious and do not require special isolation procedures.

Vaccination and prevention

The first successful vaccine for anthrax was developed for animals by Louis Pasteur in 1881. At present, the single vaccine licensed for human use is a product produced from the cell-free culture supernatant of an attenuated, nonencapsulated strain of *B. anthracis* (Stern strain), referred to as *anthrax vaccine adsorbed* (AVA).

Clinical trials for safety in humans and efficacy in animals are currently under way to evaluate the role of recombinant protective antigen (one of the major components, along with lethal factor and edema factor, of *B. anthracis* toxins) as an alternative to AVA. In a postexposure setting in non-human primates, a 2-week course of AVA + ciprofloxacin was found to be superior to ciprofloxacin alone in preventing the development of clinical disease and death. While the current recommendation for postexposure prophylaxis is 60 days of antibiotics, it would seem prudent to include immunization with anthrax vaccine if available. Given the potential for *B. anthracis* to be engineered to express penicillin resistance, the empirical regimen of choice in this setting is either ciprofloxacin or doxycycline.

■ PLAGUE

See also Chap. 159.

Yersinia pestis as a bioweapon

Although it lacks the environmental stability of anthrax, the highly contagious nature and high mortality rate of plague make it a close to

TABLE 221-3 Clinical Syndromes, Prevention, and Treatment Strategies for Diseases Caused by Category A Agents

Agent	Clinical Syndrome	Incubation Period	Diagnosis	Treatment	Prophylaxis

Bacillus anthracis (anthrax)	Cutaneous lesion:
	  Papule to eschar
	Inhalational disease:
	  Fever, malaise, chest and abdominal discomfort
	  Pleural effusion, widened mediastinum on chest x-ray
		1–12 days
		
		1–60 days
			Culture, Gram stain, PCR, Wright stain of peripheral smear	Postexposure:
				  Ciprofloxacin, 500 mg, PO bid × 60 d *or*
				  Doxycycline, 100 mg PO bid × 60 d or
				  Amoxicillin, 500 mg PO q8h, likely to be effective if strain penicillin sensitive
				Active disease:
				  Ciprofloxacin, 400 mg IV q12h *or* Doxycycline, 100 mg IV q12h *plus*
				  Clindamycin, 900 mg IV q8h and/or rifampin, 300 mg IV q12h; switch to PO when stable × 60 d total
				Antitoxin strategies:
				  Neutralizing monoclonal and polyclonal antibodies are under study
					Anthrax vaccine adsorbed
					Recombinant protective antigen vaccines are under study

Yersinia pestis (pneumonic plague)	Fever, cough, dyspnea, hemoptysis Infiltrates and consolidation on chest x-ray	1–6 days	Culture, Gram stain, direct fluorescent antibody, PCR	Gentamicin, 2.0 mg/kg IV loading then 1.7 mg/kg q8h IV *or* Streptomycin, 1.0 g q12h IM or IV Alternatives include doxycycline, 100 mg bid PO or IV; chloramphenicol, 500 mg qid PO or IV	Doxycycline, 100 mg PO bid (ciprofloxacin may also be active) Formalin-fixed vaccine (FDA licensed; not available)
Variola major (smallpox)	Fever, malaise, headache, backache, emesis Maculopapular to vesicular to pustular skin lesions	7–17 days	Culture, PCR, electron microscopy	Supportive measures; consideration for cidofovir, antivaccinia immunoglobulin	Vaccinia immunization
Francisella tularensis (tularemia)	Fever, chills, malaise, myalgia, chest discomfort, dyspnea, headache, skin rash, pharyngitis, conjunctivitis Hilar adenopathy on chest x-ray	1–14 days	Gram stain, culture, immunohistochemistry, PCR	Streptomycin, 1 g IM bid *or* Gentamicin, 5 mg/kg per day div q8h IV for 14 days *or* Doxycycline, 100 mg IV bid *or* Chloramphenicol, 15 mg/kg up to 1 gm IV qid *or* Ciprofloxacin, 400 mg IV bid	Doxycycline, 100 mg PO bid × 14 days *or* Ciprofloxacin, 500 mg PO bid × 14 days
Viral hemorrhagic fevers	Fever, myalgia, rash, encephalitis, prostration	2–21 days	RT-PCR, serologic testing for antigen or antibody Viral isolation by CDC or U.S. Army Medical Research Institute of Infectious Diseases (USAMRIID)	Supportive measures Ribavirin 30 mg/kg up to 2 g × 1, followed by 16 mg/kg IV up to 1 g q6h for 4 days, followed by 8 mg/kg IV up to 0.5 g q8h × 6 days	No known chemoprophylaxis Consideration for ribavirin in high-risk situations
Botulinum toxin (*Clostridium botulinum*)	Dry mouth, blurred vision, ptosis, weakness, dysarthria, dysphagia, dizziness, respiratory failure, progressive paralysis, dilated pupils	12–72 h	Mouse bioassay, toxin immunoassay	Supportive measures including ventilation, HBAT equine antitoxin from the CDC Emergency Operations Center, 770-488-7100	Administration of antitoxin

Abbreviations: CDC, U.S. Centers for Disease Control and Prevention; FDA, U.S. Food and Drug Administration; HBAT, heptavalent botulinum antitoxin; PCR, polymerase chain reaction; RT-PCR, reverse transcriptase PCR.

ideal agent of bioterrorism, particularly if delivered in a weaponized form. Occupying a unique place in history, plague has been alleged to have been used as a biologic weapon for centuries. The catapulting of plague-infected corpses into besieged fortresses is a practice that was first noted in 1346 during the assault of the city of Kaffa by the Tartars. Although unlikely to have resulted in disease transmission, some believe that this event may have played a role in the start of the Black Death pandemic of the fourteenth and fifteenth centuries in Europe. Given that plague was already moving across Asia toward Europe at this time, it is unclear whether such an allegation is accurate. During WWII, the infamous Unit 731 of the Japanese army was reported to have repeatedly dropped plague-infested fleas over parts of China, including Manchuria. These drops were associated with subsequent outbreaks of plague in the targeted areas. Following WWII, the United States and the Soviet Union conducted programs of research on how to create aerosolized *Y. pestis* that could be used as a bioweapon to cause primary pneumonic plague. As mentioned above, plague was thought to be an excellent bioweapon due to the fact that in addition to causing infection in those inhaling the aerosol, significant numbers of secondary cases of primary pneumonic plague would likely occur due to the contagious nature of the disease and person-to-person transmission via respiratory aerosol. Secondary reports of research conducted during that time suggest that organisms remain viable for up to 1 h and can be dispersed for distances up to 10 km. While the offensive bioweapons program in the United States was terminated prior to production of sufficient quantities of plague organisms for use as a weapon, it is believed that Soviet scientists did manufacture quantities sufficient for such a purpose. It has also been reported that more than 10 Soviet Institutes and >1000 scientists were working with plague as a biologic weapon. Of concern is the fact that in 1995 a microbiologist in Ohio was arrested for having obtained *Y. pestis* in the mail from the American Type Culture Collection, using a credit card and a false letterhead. In the wake of this incident, the U.S. Congress passed a law in 1997 requiring that anyone intending to send or receive any of 42 different agents that could potentially be used as bioweapons first register with the CDC.

Microbiology and clinical features

Plague is caused by *Y. pestis*, a nonmotile, gram-negative bacillus that exhibits bipolar, or "safety pin," staining with Wright, Giemsa, or Wayson stains. It has had a major impact on the course of history, thus adding to the element of fear evoked by its mention. The earliest reported plague epidemic was in 224 B.C. in China. The most infamous pandemic began in Europe in the fourteenth century, during which time one-third to one-half of the entire population of Europe was killed. During a plague outbreak in India in 1994, even though the number of confirmed cases was relatively small, it is estimated that 500,000 individuals fled their homes in fear of this disease.

The clinical syndromes of plague generally reflect the mode of infection. *Bubonic plague* is the consequence of an insect bite; primary *pneumonic plague* arises through the inhalation of bacteria. Most of the plague seen in the world today is bubonic plague and is the result of a bite by a plague-infected flea. In part as a consequence of past pandemics, plague infection of rodents exists widely in nature, including in the southwestern United States, and each year thousands of cases of plague occur worldwide through contact with infected animals or fleas. Following inoculation of regurgitated bacteria into the skin by a flea bite, organisms travel through the lymphatics to regional lymph nodes, where they are phagocytized but not destroyed. Inside the cell, they multiply rapidly leading to inflammation, painful

lymphadenopathy with necrosis, fever, bacteremia, septicemia, and death. The characteristic enlarged, inflamed lymph nodes, or *buboes*, give this form of plague its name. In some instances, patients may develop bacteremia without lymphadenopathy following infection, a condition referred to as *primary septicemic plague*. Extensive ecchymoses may develop due to disseminated intravascular coagulation, and gangrene of the digits and/or nose may develop in patients with advanced septicemic plague. It is thought that this appearance of some patients gave rise to the term *Black Death* in reference to the plague epidemic of the fourteenth and fifteenth centuries. Some patients may develop pneumonia (secondary pneumonic plague) as a complication of bubonic or septicemic plague. These patients may then transmit the agent to others via the respiratory route, causing cases of primary pneumonic plague. Primary pneumonic plague is the manifestation most likely to occur as the result of a bioterrorist attack, with an aerosol of bacteria spread over a wide area or a particular environment that is densely populated. In this setting, patients would be expected to develop fever, cough with hemoptysis, dyspnea, and gastrointestinal symptoms 1–6 days following exposure. Clinical features of pneumonia would be accompanied by pulmonary infiltrates and consolidation on chest x-ray. In the absence of antibiotics, the mortality rate of this disease is on the order of 85%, and death usually occurs within 2–6 days.

TREATMENT Plague

Streptomycin, tetracycline, and doxycycline are licensed by the U.S. Food and Drug Administration (FDA) for the treatment of plague. Multiple additional antibiotics licensed for other infections are commonly used and are likely effective. Among these are aminoglycosides such as gentamicin, cephalosporins, trimethoprim/sulfamethoxazole, chloramphenicol, and ciprofloxacin (Table 221-3). A multidrug-resistant strain of *Y. pestis* was identified in 1995 from a patient with bubonic plague in Madagascar. While this organism was resistant to streptomycin, ampicillin, chloramphenicol, sulfonamides, and tetracycline, it retained its susceptibility to other aminoglycosides and cephalosporins. Given the subsequent identification of a similar organism in 1997 coupled with the fact that this resistance is plasmid-mediated, it seems likely that genetically modifying *Y. pestis* to a multidrug-resistant form is possible. Unlike patients with inhalational anthrax (see above), patients with pulmonary plague should be cared for under conditions of strict respiratory isolation comparable to that used for multidrug-resistant tuberculosis.

Vaccination and prevention

A formalin-fixed, whole-organism vaccine was licensed by the FDA for the prevention of plague. That vaccine is no longer being manufactured, but its potential value as a current countermeasure against bioterrorism would likely have been modest at best as it was ineffective against animal models of primary pneumonic plague. Efforts are under way to develop a second generation of vaccines that will protect against aerosol challenge. Among the candidates being tested are recombinant forms of the F1 and V antigens of *Y. pestis*. It is likely that doxycycline or ciprofloxacin would provide coverage in a chemoprophylaxis setting. Unlike the case with anthrax, in which one has to be concerned about the persistence of ungerminated spores in the respiratory tract, the duration of prophylaxis against plague need only extend to 7 days following exposure.

■ SMALLPOX

See also Chap. 183.

Variola virus as a bioweapon

Given that most of the world's population was once vaccinated against smallpox, variola virus would not have been considered a good candidate as a bioweapon 30 years ago. However, with the cessation of immunization programs in the United States in 1972 and throughout the world in 1980 due to the successful global eradication of smallpox, close to 50% of the U.S. population is fully susceptible to smallpox today. Given its infectious nature and the 10–30% mortality rate in unimmunized individuals, the deliberate spread of this virus could have a devastating effect on our society and unleash a previously conquered deadly disease. It is estimated that an initial infection of 50–100 persons in a first generation of cases could expand by a factor of 10–20 with each succeeding generation in the absence of any effective containment measures. While the likely implementation of an effective public health response makes this scenario unlikely, it does illustrate the potential damage and disruption that can result from a smallpox outbreak.

In 1980, the World Health Organization (WHO) recommended that all immunization programs be terminated; that representative samples of variola virus be transferred to two locations, one at the CDC in Atlanta, GA, in the United States and the other at the Institute of Virus Preparations in the Soviet Union; and that all other stocks of smallpox be destroyed. Several years later, it was recommended that these two authorized collections be destroyed. However, these latter recommendations were placed on hold in the wake of increased concerns on the use of variola virus as a biologic weapon and thus the need to maintain an active program of defensive research. Many of these concerns were based upon allegations made by former Soviet officials that extensive programs had been in place in that country for the production and weaponization of large quantities of smallpox virus. The dismantling of these programs with the fall of the Soviet Union and the subsequent weakening of security measures led to fears that stocks of *V. major* may have made their way to other countries or terrorist organizations. In addition, accounts that efforts had been taken to produce recombinant strains of *Variola* that would be more virulent and more contagious than the wild-type virus have led to an increase in the need to be vigilant for the reemergence of this often fatal infectious disease.

Microbiology and clinical features

Smallpox is caused by one of two variants of variola virus, *V. major* and *V. minor*. Variola is a double-strand DNA virus and member of the *Orthopoxvirus* genus of the Poxviridae family. Infections with *V. minor* are generally less severe than those of *V. major*, with milder constitutional symptoms and lower mortality rates; thus *V. major* is the only one considered to be a viable bioweapon. Infection with *V. major* typically occurs following contact with an infected person. Patients are infectious from the time that a maculopapular rash appears on the skin and oropharynx through the resolution and scabbing of the pustular lesions. Infection occurs principally during close contact, through the inhalation of saliva droplets containing virus from the oropharyngeal exanthem. Aerosolized material from contaminated clothing or linen can also spread infection. Several days after exposure, a primary viremia is believed to occur that results in dissemination of virus to lymphoid tissues. A secondary viremia occurs ~4 days later that leads to localization of infection in the dermis. Approximately 12–14 days following the initial exposure, the patient develops high fever, malaise, vomiting, headache, backache, and a maculopapular rash that begins on the face and extremities and spreads to the trunk (centripetal) with lesions in the same developmental stage in any given location. This is in contrast to the rash of varicella (chickenpox) that begins on the trunk and face and spreads to the extremities (centrifugal) with lesions at all stages of development. The lesions are initially maculopapular and evolve to vesicles that eventually become pustules and then scabs. The oral mucosa also develops maculopapular lesions that evolve to ulcers. The lesions appear over a period of 1–2 days and evolve at the same rate. Although virus can be isolated from the scabs on the skin, the conventional thinking is that once the scabs have formed the patient is no longer contagious. Smallpox is associated with 10–30% mortality rates, with patients typically dying of severe systemic illness during the second week of symptoms. Historically, ~5–10% of naturally occurring smallpox cases take either of two highly virulent atypical forms, classified as *hemorrhagic* and *malignant*. These are difficult to diagnose because of their atypical presentations. The hemorrhagic form is uniformly fatal and begins with the relatively abrupt onset of a severely prostrating illness characterized by high fevers and severe headache and back and abdominal pain. This form of the illness resembles a severe systemic inflammatory syndrome, in which patients have a high viremia but die without developing the characteristic rash. Cutaneous erythema develops accompanied by petechiae and hemorrhages into the skin and mucous membranes. Death usually occurs within 5–6 days. The malignant, or "flat," form of smallpox is frequently fatal and has an onset similar to the hemorrhagic form, but with confluent skin lesions developing more slowly and never progressing to the pustular stage.

TREATMENT ▸ Smallpox

Given the infectious nature of smallpox and the extreme vulnerability of contemporary society, patients who are suspected cases should be handled with strict isolation procedures. While laboratory confirmation of a suspected case by culture, PCR and electron microscopy is essential, it is equally important that appropriate precautions be employed when obtaining samples for culture and laboratory testing. All health care and laboratory workers caring for patients should have been recently immunized with vaccinia, and all samples should be transported in doubly sealed containers. Patients should be cared for in negative-pressure rooms with strict isolation precautions.

There is no licensed specific therapy for smallpox, and historic treatments have focused solely on supportive care. While several antiviral agents, including cidofovir, that are licensed for other diseases have in vitro activity against *V. major*, they have never been tested in the setting of human disease. For this reason, it is difficult to predict whether or not they would be effective in cases of smallpox and, if effective, whether or not they would be of value in patients with advanced disease. Research programs studying the efficacy of new antiviral compounds (ST-246 and others) against *V. major* are currently under way.

Vaccination and prevention

In 1796, Edward Jenner demonstrated that deliberate infection with cowpox virus could prevent illness on subsequent exposure to smallpox. Today, smallpox is a preventable disease following immunization with vaccinia. The current dilemma facing our society regarding assessment of the risk and benefit of smallpox vaccination is that the degree of risk that someone will deliberately and effectively release smallpox into our society is unknown. As a prudent first step in preparedness for a smallpox attack, virtually all members of the U.S. armed services have received primary or booster immunizations with vaccinia. In addition, tens of thousands of civilian health care workers who comprise smallpox-response teams at the state and local public health level have been vaccinated.

Initial fears regarding the immunization of a segment of the American population with vaccinia when there are more individuals receiving immunosuppressive drugs and other immunocompromised patients than ever before were dispelled by the data generated from the military and civilian immunization campaigns of 2002–2004. Adverse event rates for the first 450,000 immunizations were similar to and, in certain categories of adverse events, even lower than those from prior historic data, in which most severe sequelae of vaccination occurred in young infants (Table 221-4). In addition, 11 patients with early-stage HIV infection were inadvertently immunized without problem. One significant concern during that immunization campaign, however, was the description of a syndrome of myopericarditis, which had not been appreciated during prior immunization campaigns with vaccinia. In an effort to provide a safer vaccine to protect against smallpox, ACAM 2000, a cloned virus propagated in tissue culture, was developed and became the first second-generation smallpox vaccine to be licensed. This vaccine is now used by the U.S. military and is part of the U.S. government stockpile. Research continues on attenuated forms of vaccinia such as modified vaccinia Ankara (MVA). Vaccinia immune globulin is available to treat those who experience a severe reaction to immunization with vaccinia.

TABLE 221-4 Complications From 438,134 Administrations of Vaccinia During the United States Department of Defense (DOD) Smallpox Immunization Campaign Initiated in December 2002

Complication	Number of Cases	DOD Rate per Million Vaccinees (95% Confidence Interval)	Historic Rate Per Million Vaccinees
Mild or temporary:			
Generalized vaccinia, mild	35	67 (52, 85)	45–212[a]
Inadvertent inoculation, self	62	119 (98, 142)	606[a]
Vaccinia transfer to contact	28	53 (40, 69)	8–27[a]
Moderate or serious:			
Encephalitis	1	2.2 (0.6, 7.2)	2.6–8.7[a]
Acute myopericarditis	69	131 (110, 155)	100[b]
Eczema vaccinatum	0	0 (0, 3.7)	2–35[a]
Progressive vaccinia	0	0 (0, 3.7)	1–7[a]
Death	1[c]	1.9 (0.2, 5.6)	1–2[a]

[a]Based on adolescent and adult smallpox vaccinations from 1968 studies, both primary and revaccinations.

[b]Based on case series in Finnish military recruits given the Finnish strain of smallpox vaccine.

[c]Potentially attributable to vaccination; after lupus-like illness.

Source: From JD Grabenstein and W Winkenwerder: http://www.smallpox.mil/event/SPSafetySum.asp.

TULAREMIA
See also Chap. 158.

Francisella tularensis as a bioweapon

Tularemia has been studied as an agent of bioterrorism since the mid-twentieth century. It has been speculated by some that the outbreak of tularemia among German and Soviet soldiers during fighting on the Eastern Front during WWII was the consequence of a deliberate release. Unit 731 of the Japanese Army studied the use of tularemia as a bioweapon during WWII. Large preparations were made for mass production of *F. tularensis* by the United States, but no stockpiling of any agent took place. Stocks of *F. tularensis* were reportedly generated by the Soviet Union in the mid-1950s. It has also been suggested that the Soviet program extended into the era of molecular biology and that some strains were engineered to be resistant to common antibiotics. *F. tularensis* is an extremely infectious organism, and human infections have occurred from merely examining an uncovered petri dish streaked with colonies. Given these facts, it is reasonable to conclude that this organism might be utilized as a bioweapon through either an aerosol or contamination of food or drinking water.

Microbiology and clinical features

While similar in many ways to anthrax and plague, tularemia, also referred to as rabbit fever or deer fly fever, is neither as lethal nor as fulminant as either of these other two category A bacterial infections. It is, however, extremely infectious, and as few as 10 organisms can lead to establishment of infection. Despite this fact, it is not spread from person to person. Tularemia is caused by *F. tularensis*, a small, nonmotile, gram-negative coccobacillus. Although it is not a spore-forming organism, it is a hardy bacterium that can survive for weeks in the environment. Infection typically comes from insect bites or contact with organisms in the environment. Infections have occurred in laboratory workers studying the agent. Large waterborne outbreaks have been recorded. It is most likely that the outbreak among German and Russian soldiers and Russian civilians noted above during WWII represented a large waterborne tularemia outbreak in a *Tularensis*-enzootic area devastated by warfare.

Humans can become infected through a variety of environmental sources. Infection is most common in rural areas where a variety of small mammals may serve as reservoirs. Human infections in the summer are often the result of insect bites from ticks, flies, or mosquitoes that have bitten infected animals. In colder months, infections are most likely the result of direct contact with infected mammals and are most common in hunters. In these settings, infection typically presents as a systemic illness with an area of inflammation and necrosis at the site of tissue entry. Drinking of contaminated water may lead to an oropharyngeal form of tularemia characterized by pharyngitis with cervical and/or retropharyngeal lymphadenopathy (Chap. 158). The most likely mode of dissemination of tularemia as a biologic weapon would be as an aerosol, as has occurred in a number of natural outbreaks in rural areas, including Martha's Vineyard in the United States. Approximately 1–14 days following exposure by this route, one would expect to see inflammation of the airways with pharyngitis, pleuritis, and bronchopneumonia. Typical symptoms would include the abrupt onset of fever, fatigue, chills, headache, and malaise (Table 221-3). Some patients might experience conjunctivitis with ulceration, pharyngitis, and/or cutaneous exanthems. A pulse-temperature dissociation might be present. Approximately 50% of patients would show a pulmonary infiltrate on chest x-ray. Hilar adenopathy might also be present, and a small percentage of patients could have adenopathy without infiltrates. The highly variable presentation makes acute recognition of aerosol-disseminated tularemia very difficult.

The diagnosis would likely be made by immunohistochemistry or culture of infected tissues or blood. Untreated, mortality rates range from 5 to 15% for cutaneous routes of infection and from 30 to 60% for infection by inhalation. Since the advent of antibiotic therapy, these rates have dropped to <2%.

TREATMENT   Tularemia

Both streptomycin and doxycycline are licensed for treatment of tularemia. Other agents likely to be effective include gentamicin, chloramphenicol, and ciprofloxacin (Table 221-3). Given the potential for genetic modification of this organism to yield antibiotic-resistant strains, broad-spectrum coverage should be the rule until sensitivities have been determined. As mentioned above, special isolation procedures are not required.

Vaccination and prevention

There are no vaccines currently licensed for the prevention of tularemia. While a live, attenuated strain of the organism has been used in the past with some reported success, there are inadequate data to support its widespread use at this time. Development of a vaccine for this agent is an important part of the current biodefense research agenda. In the absence of an effective vaccine, postexposure chemoprophylaxis with either doxycycline or ciprofloxacin appears to be a reasonable approach (Table 221-3).

■ VIRAL HEMORRHAGIC FEVERS
See also Chaps. 196 and 197.

Hemorrhagic fever viruses as bioweapons

Several of the hemorrhagic fever viruses have been reported to have been weaponized by the Soviet Union and the United States. Nonhuman primate studies indicate that infection can be established with very few virions and that infectious aerosol preparations can be produced. Under the guise of wanting to aid victims of an Ebola outbreak, members of the Aum Shinrikyo cult in Japan were reported to have traveled to central Africa in 1992 in an attempt to obtain Ebola virus for use in a bioterrorist attack. Thus, while there has been no evidence that these agents have ever been used in a biologic attack, there is clear interest in their potential for this purpose.

Microbiology and clinical features

The viral hemorrhagic fevers are a group of illnesses caused by any one of a number of similar viruses (Table 221-2). These viruses are all enveloped, single-strand RNA viruses that are thought to depend upon a host reservoir for long-term survival. While rodents or insects have been indentified as the hosts for some of these viruses, for others the hosts are unknown. These viruses tend to be geographically restricted according to the migration patterns of their hosts. Great apes are not a natural reservoir for Ebola virus, but large numbers of these animals in sub-Saharan Africa have died from Ebola infection over the past decade. Humans can become infected with hemorrhagic fever viruses if they come into contact with an infected host or other infected animals. Person-to-person transmission, largely through direct contact with virus-containing body fluids, has been documented for Ebola, Marburg, and Lassa viruses and rarely for the New World arenaviruses. While there is no clear evidence of respiratory spread among humans, these viruses have been shown in animal models to be highly infectious by the aerosol route. This, coupled with mortality rates as high as 90%, makes them excellent candidate agents of bioterrorism.

The clinical features of the viral hemorrhagic fevers vary depending upon the particular agent (Table 221-3). Initial signs and symptoms typically include fever, myalgia, prostration, and disseminated intravascular coagulation with thrombocytopenia and capillary hemorrhage. These findings are consistent with a cytokine-mediated systemic inflammatory syndrome. A variety of different maculopapular or erythematous rashes may be seen. Leukopenia, temperature-pulse dissociation, renal failure, and seizures may also be part of the clinical presentation.

Outbreaks of most of these diseases are sporadic and unpredictable. As a consequence, most studies of pathogenesis have been performed using laboratory animals. The diagnosis should be suspected in anyone with temperature >38.3°C for <3 weeks who also exhibits at least two of the following: hemorrhagic or purpuric rash, epistaxis, hematemesis, hemoptysis, or hematochezia in the absence of any other identifiable cause. In this setting, samples of blood should be sent after consultation to the CDC or the USAMRIID for serologic testing for antigen and antibody as well as reverse transcriptase polymerase chain reaction (RT-PCR) testing for hemorrhagic fever viruses. All samples should be handled with double-bagging. Given how little is known regarding the human-to-human transmission of these viruses, appropriate isolation measures would include full barrier precautions with negative-pressure rooms and use of powered air-purifying respirators (PAPRs). Unprotected skin contact with cadavers has been implicated in the transmission of certain hemorrhagic fever viruses such as Ebola, so it is recommended that autopsies of suspected cases be performed using the strictest measures for protection and that burial or cremation be performed promptly without embalming.

TREATMENT   Viral Hemorrhagic Fevers

There are no approved and effective antiviral therapies for this class of viruses (Table 221-3). While there are anecdotal reports of the efficacy of ribavirin, interferon-α, or hyperimmune immunoglobulin, definitive data are lacking. The best data for ribavirin are in arenavirus (Lassa and New World) infections. In some in vitro systems, specific immunoglobulin has been reported to enhance infectivity, and thus these potential treatments must be approached with caution.

Vaccination and prevention

There are no licensed and effective vaccines for these agents. Studies are currently under way examining the potential role of DNA, recombinant viruses, and attenuated viruses as vaccines for several of these infections. Among the most promising at present are vaccines for Argentine, Ebola, Rift Valley, and Kayasanur Forest viruses.

■ BOTULISM TOXIN (*Clostridium botulinum*)
See also Chap. 141.

Botulinum toxin as a bioweapon

In a bioterrorist attack, botulinum toxin would likely be dispersed as an aerosol or as contamination of a food supply. While contamination of a water supply is possible, it is likely that any toxin would be rapidly inactivated by the chlorine used to purify drinking water. Similarly, toxin can be inactivated by heating any food to >85°C for >5 min. Without external facilitation, the environmental decay rate is estimated at 1% per minute, and thus the time interval between weapon release and ingestion or inhalation needs to be rather short. The Japanese biologic warfare group, Unit 731, is reported to have conducted experiments on botulism poisoning in prisoners in the

1930s. The United States and the Soviet Union both acknowledged producing botulinum toxin, and there is some evidence that the Soviet Union attempted to create recombinant bacteria containing the gene for botulinum toxin. In records submitted to the United Nations, Iraq admitted to having produced 19,000 L of concentrated toxin—enough toxin to kill the entire population of the world three times over. By many accounts, botulinum toxin was the primary focus of the pre-1991 Iraqi bioweapons program. In addition to these examples of state-supported research into the use of botulinum toxin as a bioweapon, the Aum Shinrikyo cult unsuccessfully attempted on at least three occasions to disperse botulinum toxin into the civilian population of Tokyo.

Microbiology and clinical features

Unique among the category A agents for not being a live microorganism, botulinum toxin is one of the most potent toxins ever described and is thought by some to be the most poisonous substance in existence. It is estimated that 1 g of botulinum toxin would be sufficient to kill 1 million individuals if adequately dispersed. Botulinum toxin is produced by the gram-positive, spore-forming anaerobe *C. botulinum* (Chap. 141). Its natural habitat is soil. There are seven antigenically distinct forms of botulinum toxin, designated A–G. The majority of naturally occurring human cases are of types A, B, and E. Antitoxin directed toward one of these will have little to no activity against the others. The toxin is a 150-kDa zinc-containing protease that prevents the intracellular fusion of acetylcholine vesicles with the motor neuron membrane, thus preventing the release of acetylcholine. In the absence of acetylcholine-dependent triggering of muscle fibers, a flaccid paralysis develops. Although botulism does not spread from person to person, the ease of production of the toxin coupled with its high morbidity and 60–100% mortality make it a close to ideal bioweapon.

Botulism can result from the growth of *C. botulinum* infection in a wound or the intestine, the ingestion of contaminated food, or the inhalation of aerosolized toxin. The latter two forms are the most likely modes of transmission for bioterrorism. Once toxin is absorbed into the bloodstream, it binds to the neuronal cell membrane, enters the cell, and cleaves one of the proteins required for the intracellular binding of the synaptic vesicle to the cell membrane, thus preventing release of the neurotransmitter to the membrane of the adjacent muscle cell. Patients initially develop multiple cranial nerve palsies that are followed by a descending flaccid paralysis. The extent of the neuromuscular compromise is dependent upon the level of toxemia. The majority of patients experience diplopia, dysphagia, dysarthria, dry mouth, ptosis, dilated pupils, fatigue, and extremity weakness. There are minimal true central nervous system effects, and patients rarely show significant alterations in mental status. Severe cases can involve complete muscular collapse, loss of the gag reflex, and respiratory failure, requiring weeks or months of ventilator support. Recovery requires the regeneration of new motor neuron synapses with the muscle cell, a process that can take weeks to months. In the absence of secondary infections, which may be common during the protracted recovery phase of this illness, patients remain afebrile. The diagnosis is suspected on clinical grounds and confirmed by a mouse bioassay or toxin immunoassay.

TREATMENT ▶ Botulism

Treatment for botulism is mainly supportive and may require intubation, mechanical ventilation, and parenteral nutrition (Table 221-3). If diagnosed early enough, administration of equine antitoxin may reduce the extent of nerve injury and decrease the severity of disease. At present, a heptavalent botulinum antitoxin (HBAT) is available through the CDC as an investigational agent for treatment of naturally occurring noninfant botulism. HBAT contains horse serum–derived antibody fragments to all seven known botulinum toxins (A–G). It is composed of <2% intact immunoglobulin and ≥90% Fab and F(ab′)$_2$ immunoglobulin fragments. A single dose of antitoxin is usually adequate to neutralize any circulating toxin. Repeat dosing may be needed in a setting of continued toxin exposure. Given that this product is derived from horse serum, one needs to be vigilant for hypersensitivity reactions, including serum sickness and anaphylaxis following its administration. Once the damage to the nerve axon has been done, however, there is little possible in the way of specific therapy. At this point, vigilance for secondary complications such as infections during the protracted recovery phase is of the utmost importance. Due to their ability to worsen neuromuscular blockade, aminoglycosides and clindamycin should be avoided in the treatment of these infections.

Vaccination and prevention

A botulinum toxoid preparation has been used as a vaccine for laboratory workers at high risk of exposure and in certain military situations; however, it is not currently available in quantities that could be used for the general population. At present, early recognition of the clinical syndrome and use of appropriate equine antitoxin is the mainstay of prevention of full-blown disease in exposed individuals. The development of human monoclonal antibodies as a replacement for equine antitoxin antibodies is an area of active research interest.

CATEGORY B AND C AGENTS

The category B agents include those that are easy or moderately easy to disseminate and result in moderate morbidity and low mortality rates. A listing of the current category B agents is provided in Table 221-2. As can be seen, it includes a wide array of microorganisms and products of microorganisms. Several of these agents have been used in bioterrorist attacks, although never with the impact of the Category A agents described above. Among the more notorious of these was the contamination of salad bars in Oregon in 1984 with *Salmonella typhimurium* by the religious cult Rajneeshee. In this outbreak, which many consider to be the first bioterrorist attack against U.S. citizens, >750 individuals were poisoned and 40 were hospitalized in an effort to influence a local election. The intentional nature of this outbreak went unrecognized for more than a decade.

Category C agents are the third highest priority agents in the biodefense agenda. These agents include emerging pathogens to which little or no immunity exists in the general population, such as the severe acute respiratory syndrome (SARS) coronavirus or pandemic-potential strains of influenza that could be obtained from nature and deliberately disseminated. These agents are characterized as being relatively easy to produce and disseminate, having high morbidity and mortality rates and having a significant public health impact. There is no running list of category C agents at the present time.

PREVENTION AND PREPAREDNESS

As noted above, a large and diverse array of agents has the potential to be used in a bioterrorist attack. In contrast to the military situation with biowarfare, where the primary objective is to inflict mass casualties on a healthy and prepared militia, the objectives of bioterrorism are to harm civilians as well as to create fear and disruption among the civilian population. While the military needs only to prepare their troops to deal with the limited number of agents that pose a legitimate threat of biowarfare, the public health system needs to prepare the entire civilian population to deal with the multitude of agents and settings that could be utilized in a bioterrorism attack. This includes anticipating issues specific to the very young and the very old, the pregnant patient, and the immunocompromised individual. The challenges in this regard are enormous and immediate. While military preparedness emphasizes vaccines toward a limited number of agents, civilian preparedness needs to rely upon rapid diagnosis and treatment of a wide array of conditions.

The medical profession must maintain a high index of suspicion that unusual clinical presentations or the clustering of cases of a rare disease may not be a chance occurrence but rather the first sign of a bioterrorist event. This is particularly true when such diseases occur in traditionally healthy populations, when surprisingly large numbers of rare conditions occur, and when diseases commonly seen in rural settings appear in urban populations. Given the importance of rapid diagnosis and early treatment for many of these conditions, it is essential that the medical care team report any suspected cases of bioterrorism immediately to local and state health authorities and/or to the CDC (888-246-2675). Enhancements have been made to the public health surveillance network to facilitate the rapid sharing of information among public health agencies.

At present a series of efforts are in place to ensure the biomedical security of the civilian population of the United States. The Public Health Service is moving toward a more highly trained, fully deployable force. The Strategic National Stockpile (SNS) maintained by the CDC provides rapid access to quantities of pharmaceuticals, antidotes, vaccines, and other medical supplies that may be of value in the event of biologic or chemical terrorism. The SNS has two basic components. The first of these consists of "push packages" that can be deployed anywhere in the United States within 12 h. These push packages are a preassembled set of supplies, pharmaceuticals, and medical equipment ready for immediate delivery to the field. They provide treatment for a variety of conditions given the fact that an actual threat may not have been precisely identified at the time of stockpile deployment. The contents of the push packs are constantly updated to ensure that they reflect current needs as determined by national security threat assessments; they include antibiotics for treatment of anthrax, plague, and tularemia as well as a cache of vaccine to deal with a smallpox threat. The second component of the SNS comprises inventories managed by specific vendors and consists of the provision of additional pharmaceuticals, supplies, and/or products tailored to the specific attack.

The number of FDA-approved and -licensed drugs and vaccines for category A and B agents is currently limited and not reflective of the pharmacy of today. In an effort to speed the licensure of additional drugs and vaccines for these diseases, the FDA has a rule for the licensure of such countermeasures against agents of bioterrorism when adequate and well-controlled clinical efficacy studies cannot be ethically conducted in humans. This is commonly referred to as the "Animal Rule." Thus, for indications in which field trials of prophylaxis or therapy for a naturally occurring disease are not feasible, the FDA will rely on evidence solely from laboratory animal studies. For this rule to apply, it must be shown that (1) there are reasonably well-understood pathophysiologic

mechanisms for the condition and its treatment; (2) the effect of the intervention is independently substantiated in at least two animal species, including species expected to react with a response predictive for humans; (3) the animal study endpoint is clearly related to the desired benefit in humans; and (4) the data in animals allow selection of an effective dose in humans.

Finally, the Biomedical Advanced Research and Development Authority (BARDA) was established within the U.S. Department of Health and Human Services to provide an integrated, systematic approach to the development and purchase of the necessary vaccines, drugs, therapies, and diagnostic tools for public health medical emergencies. BARDA manages Project BioShield, an initiative established to facilitate biodefense research within the federal government, create a stable source of funding for the purchase of countermeasures against agents of bioterrorism, and create a category of "emergency use authorization" to allow the FDA to approve the use of unlicensed countermeasures during times of extraordinary unmet needs, as might be present in the context of a bioterrorist attack.

While the prospect of a deliberate attack on civilians with disease-producing agents may seem to be an act of incomprehensible evil, history shows us that it is something that has been done in the past and will likely be done again in the future. It is the responsibility of health care providers to be aware of this possibility, to be able to recognize early signs of a potential bioterrorist attack and alert the public health system, and to respond quickly to provide care to the individual patient. Among the web sites with current information on microbial bioterrorism are *www.bt.cdc.gov*, *www.niaid.nih.gov*, and *www.cidrap.umn.edu*.

FURTHER READINGS

ALIBEK K, HANDELMAN S: *Biohazard: The Chilling True Story of the Largest Covert Biological Weapons in the World, Told from the Inside by the Man Who Ran It.* New York, Random House, 1999

CRODDY E (WITH C PEREY-ARMENDARIZ AND J HART): *Chemical and Biological Warfare: A Comprehensive Survey for the Concerned Citizen.* New York, Copernicus Books, 2001

HENDERSON DA et al (eds): *Bioterrorism: Guidelines for Medical and Public Health Management.* JAMA and Archives Journals, AMA Press, 2002

JERNIGAN JA et al: Bioterrorism-related inhalational anthrax: The first 10 cases reported in the United States. Emerg Infect Dis 7:933, 2001

KENNEDY RB et al: Smallpox vaccines for biodefense. Vaccine 27: D73, 2009

NALCA A, ZUMBRUN EE: ACAM2000™: The new smallpox vaccine for United States Strategic National Stockpile. Drug Des Devel Ther 4:71, 2010

RUSNAK JM et al: Risk of occupationally acquired illnesses from biological threat agents in unvaccinated laboratory workers. Biosecur Bioterror 2:281, 2004

WILKENING DA: Sverdlovsk revisited: Modeling human inhalation anthrax. Proc Natl Acad Sci USA 103:20, 2006

CHAPTER 222

Chemical Terrorism

Charles G. Hurst
Jonathan Newmark
James A. Romano, Jr.

The use of chemical warfare agents (CWAs) in modern warfare dates back to World War I (WWI). Most recently, sulfur mustard and nerve agents were used by Iraq against the Iranian military and Kurdish civilians. Since the Japanese sarin attacks in 1994–1995 and the terrorist strikes of September 11, 2001, the all too real possibility of chemical or biological terrorism against civilian populations anywhere in the world has attracted increased attention.

Military planners consider the WWI blistering agent sulfur mustard and the organophosphorus nerve agents as the most likely agents to be used on the battlefield. In a civilian or terrorist scenario, the choice widens considerably. For example, many of the chemical warfare agents of WWI, including chlorine, phosgene, and cyanide, are used today in large amounts in industry. They are produced in chemical plants, are stockpiled in large tanks, and travel up and down highways and railways in large tanker cars. The rupture of any of these agents by accident or purposely could cause many injuries and deaths. Countless hazardous materials (HAZMATs) that are not used on the battlefield can be used as terrorist weapons. Some of them, including insecticides and ammonia, could wreak as much damage and injury as the weaponized chemical agents.

In a recent example, insurgents in Iraq used chlorine gas released from tankers after explosions as a crude form of chemical weaponry. Using this gas, they killed 12 people and intoxicated more than 140 others in three attacks in February 2007. Table 222-1 describes the physical appearance and initial physiologic effects, and Table 222-2 provides guidelines for immediate treatment of chlorine intoxication. Nonetheless, the focus of this chapter is on the blister and nerve chemical warfare agents, which have been employed in battle and against civilians and have demonstrated a significant public health impact.

Many mistakenly believe that chemical attacks will always be so severe that little can be done except to bury the dead. History proves the opposite. Even in WWI, when IV fluids, endotracheal tubes, and antibiotics were unavailable, the mortality rate among U.S. forces on the battlefield from chemical warfare agents, chiefly sulfur mustard and the pulmonary intoxicants, was only 1.9%. That was far lower than the 7% mortality rate from conventional wounds. In the 1995 Tokyo subway sarin incident, among the 5500 patients who sought medical attention at hospitals, 80% of whom were not actually symptomatic, only 12 died. Recent events should produce not a fatalistic attitude but a realistic wish to understand the pathophysiology of the syndromes these agents cause, with a view to treating expeditiously all patients who present for care and an expectation of saving the vast majority. As we prepare to defend our civilian population from the effects of chemical terrorism, we also must consider the fact that terrorism itself can produce sequelae such as physiologic or neurologic effects that may resemble the effects of nonlethal exposures to CWAs. These effects are due to a general fear of chemicals, fear of decontamination, fear of protective ensemble, or other phobic reactions.

Many writers have pointed out the increased difficulty in differentiating between stress reactions and nerve agent–induced organic brain syndromes. Knowledge of the behavioral effects of CWAs and their medical countermeasures is imperative to ensure that military and civilian medical and mental health organizations can deal with possible incidents involving weapons of mass destruction.

For the reader's benefit, the chemical warfare agents, their North Atlantic Treaty Organization (NATO) codes, and their initial effects are listed in Table 222-1.

◼ VESICANTS

Sulfur mustard

Sulfur mustard has been a military threat since it first appeared on the battlefield in Belgium during WWI. In modern times it remains a threat on the battlefield as well as a potential terrorist threat for bioterrorism because of simplicity of manufacture and extreme effectiveness. Sulfur mustard accounted for 70% of the 1.3 million chemical casualties in WWI. Occasional cases occur in the United States in people exposed to WWI and WWII-era munitions.

Mechanism Sulfur mustard constitutes both a vapor and a liquid threat to all exposed epithelial surfaces. The effects are delayed, appearing hours after exposure. The organs most commonly affected are the skin (with erythema and vesicles), eyes (ranging from mild conjunctivitis to severe eye damage), and airways (ranging from mild upper airway irritation to severe bronchiolar damage). After exposure to large quantities of mustard, precursor cells of the bone marrow are damaged, leading to pancytopenia and secondary infection. The gastrointestinal mucosa may be damaged, and there are sometimes central nervous system (CNS) signs of unknown mechanism. No specific antidotes exist; management is entirely supportive. Immediate decontamination of the liquid is the only way to reduce damage. Complete decontamination in 2 minutes stops clinical injury; decontamination at 5 minutes will reduce skin injury by ~50%. Table 222-2 lists approaches to decontamination of mustard and other CWAs.

Mustard dissolves slowly in aqueous media such as sweat, but once dissolved, it rapidly forms extremely reactive cyclic ethylene sulfonium ions, which react with cell proteins, cell membranes, and especially DNA in rapidly dividing cells. The ability of mustard to react with and alkylate DNA gives rise to the effects by which it has been characterized as "radiomimetic," similar to radiation injury. Mustard has many biologic actions, but its actual mechanism of action is largely unknown. Much of the biologic damage from mustard results from DNA alkylation and cross-linking in rapidly dividing cells: corneal epithelium, basal keratinocytes, bronchial mucosal epithelium, gastrointestinal mucosal epithelium, and bone marrow precursor cells. This may lead to cellular death and inflammatory reactions. In the skin, proteolytic digestion of anchoring filaments at the epidermal-dermal junction may be the major mechanism of action resulting in blister formation. Mustard also has mild cholinergic activity, which may be responsible for effects such as early gastrointestinal and CNS symptoms.

Mustard reacts with tissue within minutes of entering the body. Its circulating half-life in unaltered form is extremely brief.

Clinical features Topical effects of mustard occur in the skin, airways, and eyes, with the eyes being most sensitive, followed by the airways. Absorbed mustard may produce effects in the bone marrow, gastrointestinal tract, and CNS. Direct injury to the gastrointestinal tract also may occur after ingestion of the compound through contamination of water or food.

Erythema is the mildest and earliest form of mustard skin injury. It resembles sunburn and is associated with pruritus, burning, or

TABLE 222-1 Recognizing and Diagnosing Health Effects of Chemical Terrorism

Agent	Agent Name	Unique Characteristics	Initial Effects
Nerve	Cyclohexyl sarin (GF)[a] Sarin (GB) Soman (GD) Tabun (GA) VX VR	Miosis (pinpoint pupils) Copious secretions Muscle twitching/fasciculations	Miosis (pinpoint pupils) Blurred/dim vision Headache Nausea, vomiting, diarrhea Copious secretions/sweating Muscle twitching/fasciculations Breathing difficulty Seizures
Asphyxiant/blood	Arsine Cyanogen chloride Hydrogen cyanide	Possible cherry-red skin Possible cyanosis Possible frostbite[b]	Confusion Nausea Patients may gasp for air, similar to asphyxiation but more abrupt onset Seizures before death
Choking/pulmonary-damaging	Chlorine Hydrogen chloride Nitrogen oxides Phosgene	Chlorine is a greenish-yellow gas with pungent odor Phosgene gas smells like newly mown hay or grass Possible frostbite[a]	Eye and skin irritation Airway irritation Dyspnea, cough Sore throat Chest tightness
Blistering/vesicant	Mustard/sulfur mustard (HD, H) Mustard gas (H) Nitrogen mustard (HN-1, HN-2, HN-3) Lewisite (L) Phosgene oxime (CX)	Mustard (HD) has an odor like burning garlic or horseradish Lewisite (L) has an odor like penetrating geranium Phosgene oxime (CX) has a pepperish or pungent odor	Severe irritation Redness and blisters of the skin Tearing, conjunctivitis, corneal damage Mild respiratory distress to marked airway damage May cause death
Incapacitating/behavior-altering	Agent 15/BZ	May appear as mass drug intoxication with erratic behaviors, shared realistic and distinct hallucinations, disrobing, and confusion Hyperthermia Mydriasis (dilated pupils)	Dry mouth and skin Initial tachycardia Altered consciousness, delusions, denial of illness, belligerence Hyperthermia Ataxia (lack of coordination) Hallucinations Mydriasis (dilated pupils)

[a]Letters in parentheses indicate NATO codes for designated agents.

[b]Frostbite may occur from skin contact with liquid arsine, cyanogen chloride, or phosgene.

Source: State of New York, Department of Health, as modified by the Chemical Casualty Care Division, U.S. Army Medical Research Institute of Chemical Defense.

stinging pain. Erythema begins to appear within 2 hours to 2 days after vapor exposure. Time of onset depends on severity of exposure, ambient temperature and humidity, and type of skin. The most sensitive sites are the warm moist locations and thin delicate skin, such as the perineum, external genitalia, axillae, antecubital fossae, and neck.

Within the erythematous areas, small vesicles can develop, which may later coalesce to form bullae (Fig. 222-1). The typical bulla is large, dome-shaped, flaccid, thin-walled, translucent, and surrounded by erythema. The blister fluid, a transudate, is clear to straw colored and becomes yellow, tending to coagulate. The fluid does not contain mustard and is not itself a vesicant. Lesions from high-dose liquid exposure may develop a central zone of coagulation necrosis with blister formation at the periphery. These lesions take longer to heal and are more prone to secondary infection than

are the uncomplicated lesions seen at lower exposure levels. Severe lesions may require skin grafting.

The primary airway lesion is necrosis of the mucosa with possible damage to underlying smooth muscle. The damage begins in the upper airways and descends to the lower airways in a dose-dependent manner. Usually the terminal airways and alveoli are affected only as a terminal event. Pulmonary edema is not usually present unless the damage is very severe, and then it becomes hemorrhagic.

The earliest effects from mustard and perhaps the only effects from a low concentration involve the nose, sinuses, and pharynx. There may be irritation or burning of the nares, epistaxis, sinus pain, and pharyngeal pain. As the concentration increases, laryngitis, voice changes, and nonproductive cough develop. Damage to the trachea and upper bronchi leads to a productive cough. Lower

TABLE 222-2 Decontamination and Treatment of Chemical Terrorism

Agent	Decontamination	First Aid	Other Patient Considerations
Nerve	Remove clothing immediately Gently wash skin with soap and water Do not abrade skin For eyes, flush with plenty of water or normal saline	Atropine before other measures Pralidoxime (2-PAM) chloride	Onset of symptoms from dermal contact with liquid forms may be delayed Repeated antidote administration may be necessary
Asphyxiant/blood	Remove clothing immediately if no frostbite[a] Gently wash skin with soap and water Do not abrade skin For eyes, flush with plenty of water or normal saline	Rapid treatment with oxygen For cyanide, use antidotes (sodium nitrite and then sodium thiosulfate)	Arsine and cyanogen chloride may cause delayed pulmonary edema
Choking/pulmonary-damaging	Remove clothing immediately if no frostbite[a] Gently wash skin with soap and water Do not abrade skin For eyes, flush with plenty of water or normal saline	Fresh air, forced rest Semiupright position If signs of respiratory distress are present, oxygen with or without positive airway pressure may be needed Other supportive therapy, as needed	May cause delayed pulmonary edema, even after a symptom-free period that varies in duration with the amount inhaled
Blistering/vesicant	Immediate decontamination is essential to minimize damage Remove clothing immediately Gently wash skin with soap and water Do not abrade skin For eyes, flush with plenty of water or normal saline	Immediately decontaminate skin Flush eyes with water or normal saline for 10–15 min If breathing difficulty, give oxygen Supportive care	Mustard has an asymptomatic latent period There is no antidote or treatment for mustard Lewisite has immediate burning pain, blisters later Specific antidote British anti-lewisite (BAL) may decrease systemic effects of lewisite Phosgene oxime causes immediate pain Possible pulmonary edema
Incapacitating/behavior-altering	Remove clothing immediately Gently wash skin with water or soap and water Do not abrade skin	Remove heavy clothing Evaluate mental status Use restraints as needed Monitor core temperature carefully Supportive care	Hyperthermia and self-injury are largest risks Hard to detect because it is an odorless and nonirritating substance Possible serious arrhythmias Specific antidote (physostigmine) may be available

[a]For frostbite areas, DO NOT remove any adhering clothing. Wash area with plenty of warm water to release clothing.

Source: State of New York, Department of Health.

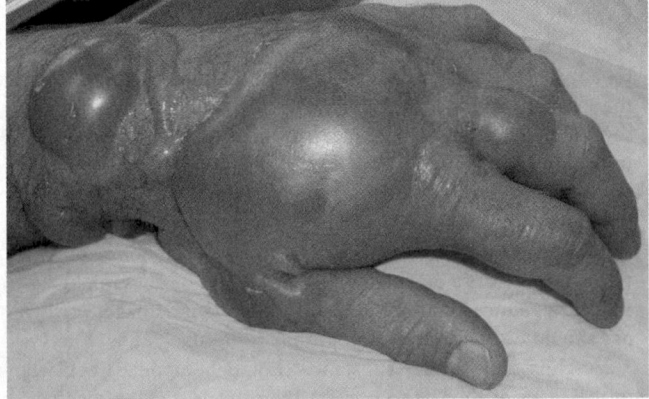

Figure 222-1   Large bulla formation from mustard burn in a patient. Although the blisters on this patient involved only 7% of the body surface area, this patient still required hospitalization in a burn intensive care unit.

airway involvement causes dyspnea, severe cough, and increasing quantities of sputum. Terminally, there may be necrosis of the smaller airways with hemorrhagic edema into surrounding alveoli. Hemorrhagic pulmonary edema is rare.

Necrosis of airway mucosa causes "pseudomembrane" formation. These membranes may cause obstruction of the bronchi. During WWI, high-dose mustard exposure caused acute death via this mechanism in a small minority of cases (Fig. 222-2).

The eyes are the organs most sensitive to mustard vapor injury. The latent period is shorter for eye injury than for skin injury and is also exposure concentration–dependent. After low-dose vapor exposure, irritation evidenced by reddening of the eyes may be the only effect. As the dose increases, the injury includes progressively more severe conjunctivitis, photophobia, blepharospasm, pain, and corneal damage (Fig. 222-3).

About 90% of eye injuries related to mustard heal in 2 weeks to 2 months without sequelae. Scarring between the iris and the lens may follow severe effects; this scarring may restrict pupillary movements

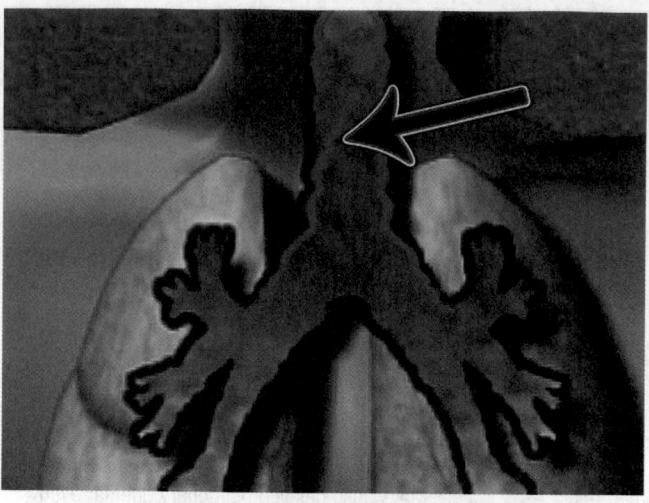

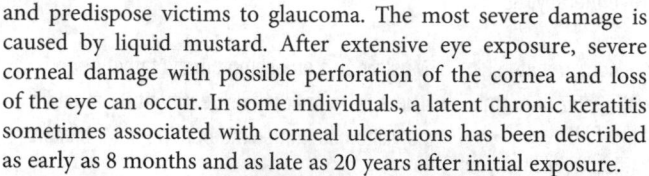

Figure 222-2 Schematic diagram of pseudomembrane formation as is seen in high-dose sulfur mustard vapor inhalation exposure. In World War I, severe inhalation exposure often caused death via obstruction of large airways.

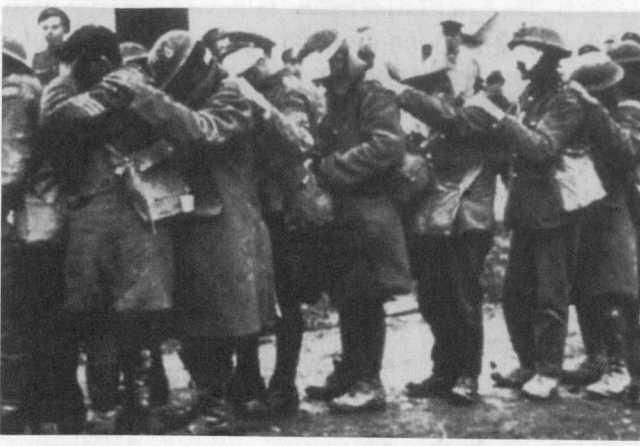

Figure 222-3 World War I photograph of troops exposed to sulfur mustard vapor. The vast majority of these troops survived with no long-term damage to the eyes; however, they were effectively rendered blind for days to weeks.

and predispose victims to glaucoma. The most severe damage is caused by liquid mustard. After extensive eye exposure, severe corneal damage with possible perforation of the cornea and loss of the eye can occur. In some individuals, a latent chronic keratitis sometimes associated with corneal ulcerations has been described as early as 8 months and as late as 20 years after initial exposure.

The mucosa of the gastrointestinal tract is susceptible to mustard damage from either systemic absorption or ingestion of the agent. Mustard exposure in small amounts will cause nausea and vomiting lasting up to 24 hours. The mechanism of the nausea and vomiting is not understood, but mustard does have a cholinergic-like effect. The CNS effects of mustard also remain poorly defined. Large exposures can cause seizures in animals. Reports from WWI and from the Iran-Iraq war described people exposed to small amounts of mustard acting sluggish, apathetic, and lethargic. These reports suggest that minor psychological problems could linger for a year or longer.

The cause of death in the majority of mustard poisoning cases is sepsis and respiratory failure. Mechanical obstruction via pseudomembrane formation and agent-induced laryngospasm is important in the first 24 hours, but only in cases of severe exposure. From the third through the fifth day after exposure, one can expect a secondary pneumonia due to bacterial invasion of denuded necrotic mucosa. The third wave of death is caused by agent-induced bone marrow suppression, which peaks 7–21 days after exposure and causes death via sepsis.

TREATMENT ▶ Sulfur Mustard

A patient severely ill from mustard poisoning requires the general supportive care provided for any severely ill patient as well as the specific care given to a burn patient. Liberal use of systemic analgesics, maintenance of fluid and electrolyte balance, nutrition, appropriate antibiotics, and other supportive measures are necessary (Table 222-2).

The management of a patient exposed to mustard may range from simple, as in the provision of symptomatic care for a sunburn-like erythema, to complex, as in providing total management for a severely ill patient with burns, immunosuppression, and multisystem involvement. Before raw denuded areas

of skin develop, especially with less severe exposures, topical cortisone creams or lotions may be of benefit. Some very basic research data point to the early use of anti-inflammatory preparations. Small blisters (<1–2 cm) should be left intact. Because larger bullae eventually will break, they should be unroofed carefully. Denuded areas should be irrigated three to four times daily with saline, other sterile solutions, or soapy water and then liberally covered with the topical antibiotic of choice, such as silver sulfadiazine or mafenide acetate, to a thickness of 1–2 mm. Some physicians advocate sterile needle drainage of large blisters, collapsing the blister roof to form a sterile dressing. Mustard blister fluid does not contain sulfur mustard, only sterile tissue fluid. Health care staff should not fear possible contamination. If an antibiotic cream is not available, sterile petrolatum will be useful. Modified Dakins solution (sodium hypochlorite 0.5%) was used both in WWI and in Iranian casualties (1984–1987) for field-expedient irrigation and antisepsis. Large areas of vesication require hospitalization, IV therapy, and whirlpool bath irrigation.

Systemic analgesics should be used liberally, particularly before manipulation of the patient. Monitoring of fluids and electrolytes is important in any sick patient, but it must be recognized that fluid loss is not of the magnitude seen with thermal burns. Overly rigorous hydration seems to have precipitated pulmonary edema in a few Iranian casualties sent to European hospitals.

Conjunctival irritation from a low vapor exposure will respond to any of a number of available ophthalmic solutions after the eyes are irrigated thoroughly. A topical antibiotic applied several times a day will reduce the incidence and severity of infection. Animal laboratory data have shown remarkable results with commercially available topical antibiotic/glucocorticoid ophthalmologic ointments applied early. An ophthalmologist should be consulted. Topical glucocorticoids are not of proven value, but their use during the first few hours or days might significantly reduce inflammation and subsequent damage. Further use should be relegated to an ophthalmologist.

Vaseline or a similar substance should be applied regularly to the edges of the lids to prevent them from sticking together. Topical analgesics may be useful initially if blepharospasm is too severe to permit an adequate examination; however, topical analgesics have limited value.

TABLE 222-3 Antidote Recommendations After Exposure to Cyanide

Patient	Mild (Conscious)	Severe (Unconscious)	Other Treatment
Child	If patient is conscious and has no other signs or symptoms, antidotes may not be necessary.	Sodium nitrite[a]: 0.12–0.33 mL/kg, not to exceed 10 mL of 3% solution[b] slow IV over no less than 5 min, or slower if hypotension develops *and* Sodium thiosulfate: 1.65 mL/kg of 25% solution IV over 10–20 min	Nasal oxygen supplementation For sodium nitrite–induced orthostatic hypotension, normal saline infusion and supine position are recommended. If still apneic after antidote administration, consider sodium bicarbonate for severe acidosis.
Adult	If patient is conscious and has no other signs or symptoms, antidotes may not be necessary.	Sodium nitrite[a]: 10–20 mL of 3% solution[b] slow IV over no less than 5 min, or slower if hypotension develops *and* Sodium thiosulfate: 50 mL of 25% solution IV over 10–20 min Alternate: hydroxocobalamin 5g in reconstituted solution IV over 15 minutes	For amyl nitrite, inhaled ampules titrated to need or until other forms of IV therapy are initiated

[a] If sodium nitrite is unavailable, administer amyl nitrite by inhalation from crushable ampoules.

[b] Available in Pasadena Cyanide Antidote Kit, formerly Lilly Cyanide Kit.

Note: Victims whose clothing or skin is contaminated with hydrogen cyanide liquid or solution can secondarily contaminate response personnel by direct contact or through off-gassing vapors. Avoid dermal contact with cyanide-contaminated victims or with gastric contents of victims who may have ingested cyanide-containing materials. Victims exposed only to hydrogen cyanide gas do not pose contamination risks to rescuers. *If the patient is a victim of recent smoke inhalation (may have high carboxyhemoglobin levels), administer only sodium thiosulfate.*

Source: State of New York, Department of Health.

A productive cough and dyspnea accompanied by fever and leukocytosis occurring within 12–24 hours are indicative of a chemical pneumonitis. The clinician must resist the urge to use prophylactic antibiotics for this process. Infection often occurs on the third to fifth day and is signaled by an increased fever, pulmonary infiltrate, and an increase in sputum production with a change in color. Appropriate antibiotic therapy should await confirmation by Gram stain and, later, positive culture and sensitivity.

Intubation may be necessary if laryngeal spasm or edema makes it difficult or becomes life threatening. Intubation permits better ventilation and facilitates suction of the necrotic and inflammatory debris. Early use of positive end-expiratory pressure (PEEP) or continuous positive airway pressure (CPAP) may be beneficial. Pseudomembrane formation may require fiberoptic bronchoscopy for suctioning of the necrotic debris.

Bronchodilators are of benefit for bronchospasm. If additional relief of bronchospasm is needed, glucocorticoids should be used. There is little evidence that the routine use of glucocorticoids is beneficial, except for additional relief of bronchospasm.

Leukopenia begins around day 3 with major systemic absorption. Marrow suppression peaks at 7–14 days. In the Iran-Iraq war, a white blood cell count of ≤200/μL usually resulted in death of the patient. Sterilization of the gut by nonabsorbable antibiotics should be considered to reduce the possibility of sepsis from enteric organisms. Cellular replacement (bone marrow transplants or transfusions) may be successful. Granulocyte colony-stimulating factor (G-CSF) produced a 50% reduction in the time for the bone marrow to recover in nonhuman primates exposed to sulfur mustard. Medication for nausea and vomiting may be necessary for gastrointestinal side effects. Lymphopenia precedes general leukopenia by a day or more, and may be a useful clinical tip-off to impending leukopenia.

Excellent assessments of the contributions of DNA alkylation, inflammation, activation of proteolytic enzymes, or lipid peroxidation to the mustard injury have been developed in the last 15–20 years. Some examples include (1) the demonstration of up to 75% reduction of inflammation and tissue damage in the mouse ear swelling test by vanilloid compounds and (2) the demonstration of 50–60% protection by *N*-acetylcysteine in the generation of free radicals within guinea pig lung exposed to mustard. In many cases, the demonstration of protection is dependent on the availability of sufficient amounts of drug with adequate half-lives. Strategies to enhance bioavailability include attachment of polyethylene glycol to the antioxidant drug/enzyme and delivery of the drug/enzyme in a liposome (or both).

■ NERVE AGENTS

The organophosphorus nerve agents are the deadliest of the CWAs. They work by inhibition of tissue synaptic acetylcholinesterase, creating an acute cholinergic crisis. Death ensues because of respiratory depression and can occur within seconds to minutes.

The nerve agents tabun and sarin were first used on the battlefield by Iraq against Iran during the first Persian Gulf War (1984–1987). Estimates of casualties from these agents range from 20,000–100,000. In 1994 and 1995, the Japanese cult Aum Shinrikyo used sarin in two terrorist attacks in Matsumoto and Tokyo. Two US soldiers were exposed to sarin while rendering safe an improvised explosive device in Iraq in 2004.

The "classic" nerve agents include tabun (GA), sarin (GB), soman (GD), cyclosarin (GF), and VX. VR, similar to VX, was manufactured in the former Soviet Union (Table 222-1). The two-letter codes were established by a NATO international convention and convey no clinical implications. All the nerve agents are organophosphorus compounds, which are liquid at standard temperature and pressure. The "G" agents evaporate at about the rate of water, except for GF, which is oily and thus probably will have evaporated within 24 hours after deposition on the ground. Their high volatility thus makes a spill of any amount a serious vapor hazard. In the Tokyo subway attack in which sarin was used, 100% of the symptomatic patients inhaled sarin vapor that spilled out on the floor of the subway cars. VX, an oily liquid, is the exception. Its low vapor pressure makes it much less of a vapor hazard but potentially a greater environmental hazard because it persists in the environment far longer.

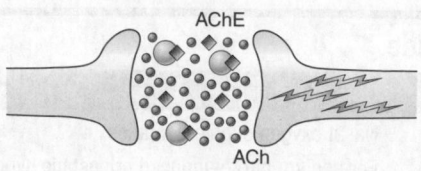

Figure 222-4   Schematic diagram of the pathophysiology of nerve agent exposure. Nerve agent (◆) binds to the active site of acetylcholinesterase (AChE), which is shown as floating free in space but is in reality a postsynaptic membrane-bound enzyme. As a result, acetylcholine (●), which normally is released from presynaptic membrane but normally is degraded, accumulates, and this leads (↯) to organ overstimulation and cholinergic crisis.

Mechanism   Acetylcholinesterase inhibition accounts for the major life-threatening effects of nerve agent poisoning. Reversal of this inhibition by antidotal therapy is effective, proving that this is the primary toxic action of these poisons. At cholinergic synapses, acetylcholinesterase, bound to the postsynaptic membrane, functions as a turn-off switch to regulate cholinergic transmission. Inhibition of acetylcholinesterases causes the released neurotransmitter, acetylcholine, to accumulate abnormally. End organ overstimulation, which is recognized by clinicians as a cholinergic crisis, ensues (Fig. 222-4).

Clinical features   Clinical effects of nerve agent exposure are identical for vapor and liquid exposure routes if the dose is sufficiently large. The speed and order of symptom onset will differ (Table 222-2).

Exposure of a patient to nerve agent vapor, overwhelmingly the more likely route of exposure in both battlefield and terrorist scenarios, will cause cholinergic symptoms in the order in which the toxin encounters cholinergic synapses. The most exposed synapses on the integument of the human are in the pupillary muscles. Nerve agent vapor easily crosses the cornea, interacts with these synapses, and produces miosis, described by Tokyo subway victims as "the world going black." Rarely, this also can cause eye pain and nausea. Exocrine glands in the nose, mouth, and pharynx next become exposed to the vapor, and cholinergic overload here causes increased secretions, rhinorrhea, excess salivation, and drooling. Next, toxin interacts with exocrine glands in the upper airway, causing bronchorrhea, and with bronchial smooth muscle, causing bronchospasm. This combination of events can cause hypoxia.

Once the victim has inhaled, vapor can passively cross the alveolar-capillary membrane, enter the bloodstream, and incidentally and asymptomatically inhibit circulating cholinesterases, particularly free butyrylcholinesterase and erythrocyte acetylcholinesterase, both of which can be assayed. Unfortunately, the assay may not be easily interpreted without a baseline, since cholinesterase levels vary enormously between subjects and over time in an individual, healthy patient.

Usually the first organ system to become symptomatic from bloodborne nerve agent exposure is the gastrointestinal tract, where cholinergic overload causes abdominal cramping and pain, nausea, vomiting, and diarrhea. After the gastrointestinal tract is involved, nerve agents will affect the heart, distant exocrine glands, muscles, and brain. Because there are cholinergic synapses on both the vagal (parasympathetic) and sympathetic sides of the autonomic input to the heart, one cannot predict how heart rate and blood pressure will change once intoxication has occurred. Remote exocrine activity will include oversecretion in the salivary, nasal, respiratory, and sweat glands—the patient will be "wet all over." Bloodborne nerve agents will overstimulate neuromuscular junctions in skeletal muscles, causing fasciculations followed by frank twitching. If the process goes on long enough, eventually ATP in muscles will be depleted and flaccid paralysis will ensue.

In the brain, since the cholinergic system is so widely distributed, bloodborne nerve agents will, in sufficient doses, cause rapid loss of consciousness, seizures, and central apnea leading to death within minutes. If respiration is supported, status epilepticus that does not respond to usual anticonvulsants may ensue (Chap. 369). If status epilepticus persists, neuronal death and permanent brain dysfunction may occur. Even in mild nerve agent intoxication, patients may recover but may experience weeks of irritability, sleep disturbance, and nonspecific neurobehavioral symptoms.

The time from exposure to development of the full-blown cholinergic crisis from nerve agent vapor inhalation can be minutes or even seconds, yet there is no depot effect. Since nerve agents have a short circulating half-life, if the patient is supported and, ideally, treated with antidotes, improvement should be rapid without subsequent deterioration.

Liquid exposure to nerve agents differs in speed and order of symptom onset. A nerve agent on intact skin will partially evaporate and partially begin to travel through the skin, causing localized sweating and then localized fasciculations when it encounters neuromuscular junctions. Once in muscle, it will cross into the circulation and cause gastrointestinal discomfort, respiratory distress, heart rate changes, generalized fasciculations and twitching, loss of consciousness, seizures, and central apnea. The time course will be much longer than with vapor inhalation; even a large, lethal droplet can take up to 30 minutes to have an effect, and a small, sublethal dose could continue to take effect over 18 hours. Clinical worsening that occurs hours after treatment has started is far more likely with liquid than with vapor exposure. Additionally, miosis, which is practically unavoidable with vapor exposure, is not always present with liquid exposure and may be the last symptom to present in this situation. This is due to the relative insulation of the pupillary muscle from the systemic circulation.

Unless removed by specific therapy (oximes), binding of a nerve agent to cholinesterase is essentially irreversible. Erythrocyte acetylcholinesterase activity recovers at about 1% per day. Plasma butyrylcholinesterase recovers more quickly and is a better guide to recovery of tissue enzyme activity.

TREATMENT   Nerve Agents

Acute nerve agent poisoning is treated by decontamination, respiratory support, and three antidotes: an anticholinergic, an oxime, and an anticonvulsant (Tables 222-3 and 222-4). In acute cases, all these forms of therapy may be given simultaneously.

DECONTAMINATION   Decontamination of a vapor is formally not necessary, but in the Tokyo subway attack, sarin vapor trapped in patients' clothing caused miosis in 10% of emergency personnel. Removal of clothing would have obviated most of this problem. Decontamination of liquid is accomplished in the military by using Reactive Skin Decontamination Lotion (RSDL), which absorbs liquid off skin. Civilian agencies now stockpile this product approved by the U.S. Food and Drug Administration (FDA). At hospitals, soap and copious amounts of water should suffice. RSDL is only approved for spot decontamination of small areas; whole-body decontamination requires water with or without soap. Physical removal of the agent is superior to all known decontamination solutions and lotions. In any event, decontamination must be accomplished before the patient enters the hospital facility to avoid contaminating the facility and its staff. In patients with contaminated wounds, one should extract potentially contaminated clothing and other foreign material that may serve as a depot for the liquid agent.

TABLE 222-4 Antidote Recommendations After Exposure to Nerve Agents

Patient Age	Antidotes Mild/Moderate Effects[a]	Severe Effects[b]	Other Treatment
Infants (0–2 years)	Atropine: 0.05 mg/kg IM, *or* 0.02 mg/kg IV; *and* 2-PAM chloride: 15 mg/kg IM *or* IV slowly	Atropine: 0.1 mg/kg IM, *or* 0.02 mg/kg IV; *and* 2-PAM chloride: 25 mg/kg IM, *or* 15 mg/kg IV slowly	Assisted ventilation after antidotes for severe exposure.
Child (2–10 years)	Atropine: 1 mg IM, *or* 0.02 mg/kg IV; *and* 2-PAM chloride[c]: 15 mg/kg IM *or* IV slowly	Atropine: 2 mg IM, *or* 0.02 mg/kg IV; *and* 2-PAM chloride[c]: 25 mg/kg IM, *or* 15 mg/kg IV slowly	Repeat atropine (2 mg IM, *or* 1 mg IM for infants) at 5- to 10-min intervals until secretions have diminished and breathing is comfortable *or* airway resistance has returned to near normal.
Adolescent (>10 years)	Atropine: 2 mg IM, *or* 0.02 mg/kg IV; *and* 2-PAM chloride[c]: 15 mg/kg IM *or* IV slowly	Atropine: 4 mg IM, *or* 0.02 mg/kg IV; *and* 2-PAM chloride[c]: 25 mg/kg IM, *or* 15 mg/kg IV slowly	
Adult	Atropine: 2 to 4 mg IM *or* IV; *and* 2-PAM chloride: 600 mg IM, *or* 15 mg/kg IV slowly	Atropine: 6 mg IM; *and* 2-PAM chloride: 1800 mg IM, *or* 15 mg/kg IV slowly	Phentolamine for 2-PAM-induced hypertension: (5 mg IV for adults; 1 mg IV for children). Diazepam for convulsions: (0.2 to 0.5 mg IV for infants <5 years: 1 mg IV for children >5 years; 5 mg IV for adults).
Elderly, frail	Atropine: 1 mg IM; *and* 2-PAM chloride: 10 mg/kg IM, *or* 5 to 10 mg/kg IV slowly	Atropine: 2 to 4 mg IM; *and* 2-PAM chloride: 25 mg/kg IM, *or* 5 to 10 mg/kg IV slowly	

[a]Mild/moderate effects include localized sweating, muscle fasciculations, nausea, vomiting, weakness, dyspnea.

[b]Severe effects include unconsciousness, convulsions, apnea, flaccid paralysis.

[c]If calculated dose exceeds the adult IM dose, adjust accordingly.

Note: 2-PAM chloride is pralidoxime chloride or protopam chloride.

Source: State of New York, Department of Health.

RESPIRATORY SUPPORT Death from nerve agent poisoning is almost always from respiratory causes. Ventilation will be complicated by increased resistance and secretions. Atropine should be given before ventilation or as ventilation begins, since it will make ventilation far easier.

ANTIDOTAL THERAPY

Atropine In theory, any anticholinergic could be used to treat nerve agent poisoning, but worldwide the choice is invariably atropine due to its wide temperature stability and rapid effectiveness either IM or IV and because inadvertent administration of this drug usually causes little CNS dysfunction (Table 222-4). Atropine rapidly reverses cholinergic overload at muscarinic synapses but has little effect at nicotinic synapses. Practically, this implies that atropine can quickly treat the life-threatening respiratory effects of nerve agents but probably will not help with neuromuscular and possibly sympathetic effects. In the field, military personnel are given MARK I kits (Fig. 222-5A) containing 2 mg atropine in autoinjector form for IM use. Civilian agencies are now stockpiling this FDA-approved product as well. The MARK 1 kit is being replaced for both civilian and military use by a combined autoinjector containing both 2.1 mg atropine and oxime (2-PAM Cl), licensed by the FDA under the trade name Duodote(TM). One can only give full autoinjector doses and not divide them. The field-loading dose is 2, 4, or 6 mg, with retreatment every 5–10 minutes until the patient's breathing and secretions improve. The Iranians used larger doses initially during the Iran-Iraq war, in which oximes were in short supply. When the patient reaches a level of medical care at which drugs can be given IV, this is the preferred route; in small children this may

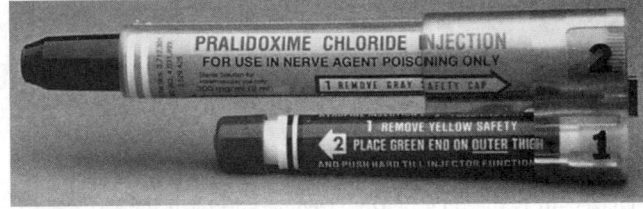

A

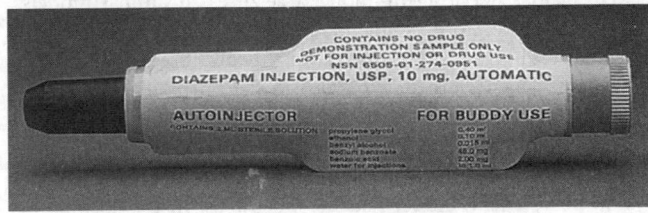

B

Figure 222-5 Antidotes to nerve agents. *A.* MARK I autoinjector set containing one 600-mg dose of 2-pralidoxime chloride and one 2-mg dose of atropine. Such sets are carried by all U.S. military forces in a potentially chemical battlefield and are being stockpiled by civilian first responders. *B.* Diazepam 10-mg autoinjector. These are carried by all U.S. military forces in a potential chemical battlefield and are being stockpiled by civilian first responders.

be the initial form of atropine therapy. However, pediatric auto-injectors of 0.5 mg and 1 mg are now manufactured. There is no upper limit to atropine therapy in a patient either IM or IV; however, a total average adult dose for a severely afflicted patient would usually be 20–30 mg.

In a mildly afflicted patient with miosis and no other systemic symptoms, atropine or homatropine eyedrops may suffice for therapy. This will produce ~24 hours of mydriasis. Frank miosis or imperfect accommodation may persist for weeks or even months after all other signs and symptoms have resolved.

Oxime Therapy Oximes are nucleophiles that reactivate the cholinesterase whose active site has been occupied and bound to nerve agent (Table 222-4). Therapy with oximes therefore restores normal enzyme function. Oxime therapy is limited by a second side reaction, called "aging," in which a side chain on nerve agents falls off the complex at a characteristic rate. "Aged" complexes are negatively charged, and oximes cannot reactivate negatively charged complexes. The practical effect of this differs from one nerve agent to another since each ages at a characteristic rate. VX, for practical purposes, never ages, sarin ages in 3–5 hours, and tabun ages over a longer period. All these are so much longer than the patient's expected life span after acute nerve agent toxicity that they may be ignored. Soman, in contrast, ages in 2 minutes. Thus, after only a few minutes after exposure, oximes are useless in treating soman poisoning. The oxime used varies by country; the United States has approved and fielded 2-pralidoxime chloride (2-PAM Cl). MARK 1 kits (Fig. 222-5A) and Duodotes(TM) both contain autoinjectors 600 mg 2-PAM Cl. Initial field loading doses are 600, 1200, and 1800 mg. Since blood pressure elevation may occur after administration of 45 mg/kg in adults, field use of 2-PAM Cl is restricted to 1800 mg, IM, per hour. During the time when more oxime cannot be given, atropine alone is recommended. In the hospital setting, 2.5–25 mg/kg IV 2-PAM Cl has been found to reactivate 50% of inhibited cholinesterase. The usual recommendation is 1000 mg through slow IV drip over 20–30 minutes, with ≤2500 mg over a period of 1–1.5 hours. Active research is ongoing to field a more effective and broader-spectrum oxime than 2-PAM Cl.

Anticonvulsants Nerve agent–induced seizures do not respond to the usual anticonvulsants used for status epilepticus, including phenytoin, phenobarbital, carbamazepine, valproic acid, and lamotrigine (Chap. 369). The only anticonvulsants that have been shown to stop this form of status are the benzodiazepines. Diazepam is the only benzodiazepine approved for seizures in humans, although other FDA-approved benzodiazepines work well against nerve agent–induced seizures in animal models. Diazepam therefore is manufactured in 10-mg injectors for IM use and given to U.S. forces for this purpose (Fig. 222-5B). Civilian agencies are stockpiling this field product (convulsive antidote for nerve agent, CANA), which generally is not used in hospital practice. Extrapolation from animal studies indicates that adults will probably require 30–40 mg diazepam, IM, to stop nerve agent–induced status epilepticus. In the hospital or in a small child unable to receive the autoinjector, IV diazepam may be used at similar doses. The clinician may confuse seizures with the neuromuscular signs of nerve agent poisoning. In the hospital, early electroencephalography is advised to distinguish among nonconvulsive status epilepticus, actual seizures, and postictal paralysis. Recent animal studies have shown that the most effective benzodiazepine in this situation is midazolam, which is not FDA-approved for seizures.

Peripheral neuropathy and the so-called intermediate syndrome, which are prominent long-term effects of insecticide poisoning, are not described in nerve agent survivors.

Recent research has explored approaches leading to a transient "immunity," or drugs that would provide protection against lethal nerve agents yet be devoid of side effects. A novel approach is to use enzymes to scavenge these highly toxic nerve agents before they attack their intended targets. The accumulated work has shown that if a scavenger is present at the time of nerve agent exposure, rapid reduction of toxicant levels is observed. This reduction is so rapid and profound that the need to administer a host of pharmacologically active drugs as antidotes is, according to laboratory studies, eliminated.

■ CYANIDE

Cyanide (CN^-) has become an agent of particular interest in terrorist scenarios because of its applicability to indoor targets. Attacks have occurred in recent years using this agent, for example, against the water supply of the U.S. Embassy in Italy. The 1993 World Trade Center bombing in New York may have been intended as a cyanide release as well.

Hydrogen cyanide and cyanogen chloride, the major forms of cyanide, are either true gases or liquids very close to their boiling points at standard room temperature. Hydrogen cyanide gas is lighter than air and does not remain concentrated outdoors for long; this makes it a poor military weapon but an effective weapon in an indoor space such as a train station or sports arena. Cyanide is also water-soluble and poses a threat to the food and water supply from either accidents or malign intent. It is well absorbed from the GI tract, through skin, or via inhalation, the preferred terrorist route. Cyanide smells like bitter almonds, but 50% of persons lack the ability to smell it.

Unique among chemical warfare agents, cyanide is a normal constituent of the environment and actually is a required cofactor in many compounds important in metabolism, including vitamin B_{12}. Cyanide is present in many plants; this explains why smokers, for instance, have three times the usual cyanide level chronically. In consequence, humans have evolved a detoxification mechanism for cyanide. Cyanide poisoning results if a large challenge of CN^- overwhelms this mechanism, while treatment of cyanide poisoning exploits it.

Mechanism

Cyanide directly poisons the last step in the mitochondrial electron transport chain, cytochrome a3, which results in a shutdown of cellular energy production. Tissues are poisoned in direct proportion to their metabolic rate, with the carotid baroreceptors and the brain, the most metabolically active tissues in the body, affected fastest and most severely. This results from cyanide's high affinity for certain metals, notably Co and Fe^{+++}. Cytochrome a3 contains Fe^{+++}, to which CN^- binds. Cyanide-poisoned tissues cannot extract oxygen from the blood; even though pulmonary oxygen exchange and cardiac function are preserved, cells die of hypoxia—of histotoxic rather than cardiopulmonary cause.

Clinical features

Approximately 15 seconds after inhalation of a high concentration of cyanide, there is a transient hyperpnea, followed within 15–30 s by the onset of convulsions and electrical status epilepticus. Respiratory activity stops 2–3 min later, and cardiac activity ceases several minutes after that. Exposure, especially via inhalation, to a large challenge of CN^- can cause death in as little as 8 min. Smaller challenges will cause symptoms spread over a longer period; very low doses may produce no effects at all because of the body's ability to detoxify small amounts. Cyanogen chloride additionally produces mucous membrane irritation. Many but not all patients will display a cherry red appearance because their venous blood remains oxygenated.

Differential diagnosis

In a mass casualty caused by a chemical agent, the primary differential diagnosis of cyanide poisoning will be nerve agent poisoning. Cyanide-poisoned patients lack the prominent cholinergic signs such as miosis and increased secretions seen in nerve agent poisoning. The cherry red appearance often seen in cyanide poisoning is never seen in nerve agent poisoning. Cyanosis, confusingly, is *not* a prominent early sign in cyanide poisoning.

TREATMENT   Cyanide

Treatment of cyanide poisoning may require simply evacuating the patient from the source of contamination. Decontamination of a true gas, other than clothing removal to avoid gas trapped in clothing air cells, is probably not a major concern.

Oxygen, via mask, nasal cannula, or endotracheal tube, has been shown to benefit patients, although the benefit is not explained by the known mechanism of action of CN^-.

ANTIDOTAL THERAPY Cyanide antidotes exploit the body's innate detoxification mechanism, the hepatic enzyme rhodanese. They also exploit cyanide's affinity for certain metal ions. The antidotes are summarized in Table 222-3.

The classic two-step cyanide antidote kit includes two IV solutions: sodium nitrite and sodium thiosulfate. It may also include amyl nitrite perles for inhalation.

Nitrites are methemoglobin formers. Giving a patient nitrite converts a fraction of the body's hemoglobin into methemoglobin by converting heme iron from Fe^{++} to Fe^{+++}. CN^- has a greater affinity for methemoglobin Fe^{+++} than for cytochrome a3. As a result, administration of nitrite creates a "sink" of cyanmethemoglobin; creation of methemoglobin pulls CN^- off mitochondrial cytochrome a3, allowing cellular respiration to resume. Recent work suggests that nitrites may also work via a second mechanism, involving the neurotransmitter nitrous oxide, which may explain why cyanide-poisoned patients improve after nitrite administration faster than is explained by the known rate of methemoglobin formation.

Nitrite administration may save the patient acutely but creates an unstable pool of cyanmethemoglobin, the elimination of which requires a sulfur donor: sodium thiosulfate. Sodium thiosulfate donates sulfur to the reaction catalyzed by rhodanese; this converts cyanide to thiocyanate, a compound the body eliminates harmlessly in urine. In fire victims—whose oxygen-carrying capacity is already reduced, and in whom the administration of nitrite may form so much methemoglobin as to make the blood unable to carry oxygen at all—sodium thiosulfate alone may be administered.

Hydroxocobalamin, or vitamin B_{12a}, has recently been approved for use as an alternate cyanide antidote. It must be reconstituted at the scene, unlike sodium nitrite or sodium thiosulfate. It lacks the propensity for hypotension of nitrites, but many of the cases in which it has been beneficial have also required the use of sodium thiosulfate. It causes an orange discoloration of the skin of no functional significance.

All of these antidotes require the placement of an IV line. Amyl nitrite is currently the only nonintravenous cyanide antidote available, although it has never been formally approved by the U.S. Food and Drug Administration. Cyanide antidote kits contain amyl nitrite perles that can be crushed and inhaled by a patient who is still breathing. Amyl nitrite can also be given through a respirator.

None of the cyanide antidotes is specifically approved for pediatric use.

Prognosis

Cyanide casualties tend to recover very quickly compared with casualties of other chemical agents. Many industrial cases have returned to work within the same shift. If a patient suffers a large challenge and expires, it is usually within minutes of exposure.

FURTHER READINGS

Hurst CG, Smith WJ: Health effects of exposure to vesicant agents, in *Chemical Warfare Agents: Chemistry, Pharmacology, Toxicology and Therapeutics*, JA Romano et al (eds). Boca Raton, FL, CRC Press, 2008

Karalliedde L et al: Possible immediate and long-term health effects following exposure to chemical warfare agents. Public Health 114:238–248, 2000

Lenz DE et al: Nerve agent bioscavengers: Progress in the development of a new mode of protection against organophosphorus poisoning, in *Chemical Warfare Agents: Chemistry, Pharmacology, Toxicology and Therapeutics*, JA Romano et al (eds). Boca Raton, FL, CRC Press, 2008

McDonough JH et al: Anticonvulsant treatment of nerve agent seizures: Anticholinergics versus diazepam in soman-intoxicated guinea pigs. Epilepsy Res 38:1–14, 2000

Newmark J: Nerve agents, in *Clinical Neurotoxicology: Syndromes, Substances, Environments*, MR Dobbs (ed). Philadelphia, Saunders-Elsevier, 2009, pp 646–659

Okumura T et al: Report on 640 victims of the Tokyo subway sarin attack. Ann Emerg Med 28:129–135, 1996

Russell D, Simpson J: Emergency planning and preparedness for the deliberate release of toxic industrial chemicals. Clin Toxicol 48:171–176, 2010

Sidell FR: Clinical considerations in nerve agent intoxication, in *Chemical Warfare Agents*, SM Somani (ed). San Diego, Academic Press, 1992, pp 156–194

Tuorinsky SD (ed.): *Medical Aspects of Chemical Warfare.* Walter Reed Army Medical Center, Washington, DC, Borden Institute, 2008. [Available on the website: http://ccc.apgea.army.mil]

U.S. Army Medical Research Institute of Chemical Defense, Chemical Casualty Care Division: *Medical Management of Chemical Casualties Handbook*, 4th ed. Aberdeen Proving Ground, MD, 2007 [Available on the website: http://ccc.apgea.army.mil]

Willems JL: Clinical management of mustard gas casualties. Ann Med Milit Belg 3(Suppl.):1–61, 1989

Wurzburg H. Treatment of cyanide poisoning in an industrial setting. Vet Human Toxicol 38:44–47, 1996

CHAPTER **223**

Radiation Terrorism

Zelig A. Tochner

Eli Glatstein

Terror attacks using nuclear or radiation-related devices are an unequivocal threat in the twenty-first century and are capable of having unique medical and psychological effects. This chapter will focus on the most probable scenarios of possible attacks and the medical principles of handling such threats.

There are two major categories of potential terrorist incidents with widespread radiologic consequences. The first is the use of radiologic dispersal devices. This could cause a purposeful dissemination of radioactive material without nuclear detonation by using conventional explosives with radionuclides, attacking fixed nuclear facilities, or attacking nuclear-powered surface vessels or submarines. Malfunctioning nuclear weapons that are detonated with no nuclear yield (nuclear "duds") and installation of radionuclides in food or water are also possible means of generating a terror attack. The second and less probable scenario is the actual use of nuclear weapons. Each scenario has its own medical aspects, including "conventional" blast or thermal injury, introduction to a radiation field, and exposure to either external or internal contamination from a radioactive explosion.

TYPES OF RADIOISOTOPIC RADIATION

Isotopes of atoms with uneven numbers of protons and/or neutrons are typically unstable; such isotopes discharge particles or energy to matter, a process that is defined as *radiation*. The main radiation types are alpha, beta, gamma, and neutrons.

Alpha (α) radiation consists of heavy, positively charged particles that contain two protons and two neutrons. Alpha particles usually are emitted from isotopes with an atomic number of ≥82, such as uranium and plutonium. Due to their large size, alpha particles have limited penetrating power. Fine obstacles such as cloth and human skin usually can stop them from penetrating into the body, and they represent a small risk with external exposure due to their limited penetration. If they somehow are internalized, alpha particles can cause significant cellular damage in their immediate proximity.

Beta (β) radiation consists of electrons, which are small, light, negatively charged particles (about 1/2000 the mass of a neutron or proton). They can travel only a short finite distance in tissue, depending on their energy. Exposure to beta particles is common in many radiation accidents. Radioactive iodine released in nuclear plant accidents is the best known member of this group. Plastic layers and clothing can stop most beta particles, and their penetration is measured to be a few millimeters. A large quantum of energy to the basal stratum of the skin can cause a burn that is similar to a thermal burn and is treated as such.

Gamma (γ) rays and *x-rays* (both photons) are similar. Gamma rays are uncharged electromagnetic radiation discharged from a nucleus as a wave or photons of energy. X-rays are the product of abrupt mechanical deceleration of electrons striking a heavy target such as tungsten. Gamma rays and x-rays have similar properties, (i.e., no charge and no mass, just energy). Both travel easily through matter, sometimes called *penetrating radiation*, and are the principal type of radiation that causes total-body exposure. If the energy of gamma rays and x-rays is the same, their biologic effects will be the same.

Neutron (η) particles are heavy and uncharged, often emitted during nuclear detonation. They possess a wide energy range; their ability to penetrate tissues is variable, depending on their energy. They are less likely to be present in most scenarios of radiation bioterrorism.

The ionization resulting from protons, electrons, and gamma rays is either a direct or an indirect (i.e., mediated through water) effect of particles or photons on DNA. Ionization of DNA resulting from neutrons is secondary to the neutrons knocking electrons out of their atomic orbit and the formation of free radicals, which can also damage DNA directly.

The commonly used units of radiation are the rad and the gray (Gy). The rad (radiation absorbed dose) is energy deposited within living matter and is equal to 100 ergs/g of tissue.

The traditional rad has been replaced by the Système Internationale (SI) unit of the gray; 100 rad = 1 Gy.

TYPES OF EXPOSURE

Whole-body exposure represents deposition of radiation energy over the entire body. Alpha and beta particles have limited penetration and do not cause significant noncutaneous injury unless emission results from an internalized source. Whole-body exposure from gamma rays, x-rays, or neutrons, which can penetrate through the body (depending on their energy), can result in damage to multiple tissues and organs. The tissue damage is proportional to the radiation exposure of the specific organ or tissue.

External contamination is a result of fallout of radioactive particles that land on the body surface, clothing, skin, and hair. This is the dominant element to consider in the mass casualty situation resulting from a radioactive terrorist strike. The common contaminants primarily emit alpha and beta radiation. Alpha particles do not penetrate beyond the skin and thus have minimal systemic effects. Beta emitters can cause significant cutaneous burns and scarring. Gamma emitters not only may cause local damage but also can cause whole-body radiation exposures and injury. The medical treatment is primarily decontamination of the body, including wounds and burns, to prevent the contamination from becoming internalized. Removing the contaminated clothing reduces the contamination significantly and is a first step in the decontamination process. Generally, patients will not constitute a significant radiation hazard to health care providers, and lifesaving treatment should not be delayed for fear of secondary contamination of the medical team. Any damage to health care personnel will depend directly on the duration of exposure and will be inversely proportional to the square of the distance from any radioactive source. Gowns that can be easily removed are essential to protect health care personnel.

Internal contamination will occur when radioactive material is inhaled or ingested or is able to enter the body through open wounds or burns or via skin absorption. In principle, any externally contaminated casualty should be evaluated for internal contamination. Some isotopes may have toxic effects on specific target organs due to their chemical properties, in addition to radiologic injury. The respiratory system is the main portal of entrance for internal contamination, and the lung is the organ at greatest risk. Aerosol particles <5 μm can reach the alveoli, whereas larger particles will remain in proximal airways. The tiny particles can be absorbed by the lymphatic system or the bloodstream. Bronchial lavage is often a helpful treatment in this situation. Radioactive material entering the gastrointestinal (GI) tract will be absorbed according to its chemical structure and solubility. The insoluble radionuclides may affect the lower GI tract. Intact skin is normally a good barrier to most radionuclides. Penetration through the skin usually takes place when wounds or burns have altered the skin barriers. Therefore, any skin erosion should be cleaned and decontaminated promptly.

Absorbed radioactive materials will travel throughout the body. Liver, kidney, adipose tissue, thyroid, and bone and bone marrow tend to bind and retain the radioactive material more than other tissues do. The medical treatment includes preventing absorption, reducing incorporation, and enhancing elimination (see below).

Localized exposure means close contact between a highly radioactive source and a part of the body, causing discrete damage to the skin and deeper tissues, similar to a thermal burn. Later signs include epilation, erythema, moist desquamation, ulceration, blistering, and necrosis in proportion to exposure. Alopecia, transient or permanent, is dose related and starts at cutaneous doses >3 Gy. Overt tissue damage can take weeks and even months to develop; the healing process can also be very slow, lasting for months. Long-term cutaneous changes, including keratosis, fibrosis, and telangiectasias, may appear years after the exposure. Treatment is based on analgesia and infection prophylaxis. Nevertheless, severe burns often require grafting or even amputation. Long-term radiation effects are characterized by cell loss and cell death.

■ RADIOLOGIC DISPERSAL EVENTS

Radiologic dispersal incidents are generally of two types, resulting from (1) small, usually localized sources or (2) wide dispersals over large areas. The radioactive materials can take the form of solid state, aerosol, gas, or liquid. They can be put into food or water, released from vehicles, or be spread by explosion. The principal route of exposure is usually direct contact between the victim's skin and the radioactive particles, although internal contamination could occur if the material were inhaled or ingested. The radiation field is also a potential source of whole-body exposure. The psychosocial effects that accompany such an event are significant and are beyond the scope of this chapter. A list of radioactive materials, including information on their major properties and medical treatment, is given in Table 223-1.

In a localized event, the amount and spread of the radioactive materials are usually limited and can be treated like a spill of hazardous material. Protective clothing prevents or minimizes the contamination of emergency responders.

The use of explosives coupled with a large amount of radioactive materials can result in wide dispersion of radiation, which is of far greater concern. Other potential sources of radiation are nuclear reactors, spent nuclear fuel, and transport vehicles. Less probable but still possible is the use of a large source of penetrating radiation without explosion. It is expected that most exposures would be low, and the principal health and psychosocial effects would be similar to those in the former scenario but on a larger scale.

Whenever an explosion is involved, conventional lifesaving treatment should be given first priority. Only then should decontamination and specific treatment be given for the radiation exposure.

Silent exposure represents a scenario in which a powerful radiologic source, often also called a radiologic exposure device, could be hidden in a crowded place and spread radioactive materials without any awareness or announcement. It might take a long time to recognize the event and the source of exposure. One of the major clues to this situation is the appearance of unusual clinical manifestations in many individuals; such manifestations are often nonspecific and include symptoms of acute radiation sickness (see below) such as headache, fatigue, malaise, and opportunistic infections. GI phenomena such as diarrhea, nausea, vomiting, and anorexia may occur. Dermatologic symptoms (burns, ulceration, and epilation) and hematopoietic manifestations such as bleeding tendency, thrombocytopenia, purpura, lymphopenia, and neutropenia are also possible and are dose related. Careful epidemiologic studies may be necessary to identify the source of such exposure.

■ NUCLEAR WEAPONS

The most likely scenario of nuclear terror would be the detonation of a single low-yield device. The estimated yield of such a device is anywhere between 0.01 and 10 kilotons of TNT, although the probability more likely would be toward the lower yield. Coping with such an event is certainly possible. The effects of such an explosion are a combination of several components: ground shock, air blast, thermal radiation, initial nuclear radiation, crater formation, and radioactive fallout.

The nuclear detonation, like a conventional explosion, will produce a shock wave that can further damage structures and cause many casualties. In addition, the detonation can produce an extremely hot fireball that can ignite materials and cause severe burns. The detonation also releases an intense pulse of ionizing radiation, mainly gamma rays and neutrons. The radiation produced in the first minute is termed *initial radiation*, whereas the ongoing radiation due to fallout is termed *residual radiation*. Both types of radiation can cause acute radiation sickness. The $LD_{50/30}$ (i.e., a dose that causes a 50% mortality rate at 30 days) is ~4 Gy for whole-body exposure without medical support; with medical support, the $LD_{50/30}$ ranges between 8 and 10 Gy. Winds can carry fallout and contaminate large areas.

On top of its effects, a massive blast forms a crater in the soil and usually produces a ground shock that compounds the damage and the number of casualties. Inhalation of large amounts of radioactive dust causes pneumonitis that can lead to pulmonary fibrosis. Use of a mask covering the mouth and nose can be very helpful. The intense flash of infrared and visible light can cause either temporary or permanent blindness. Cataracts can develop months to years later among those who survive.

■ ACUTE RADIATION SYNDROME

Radiation interactions with atoms can result in ionization and the formation of free radicals that damage tissue by disrupting chemical bonds and molecular structures in the cell, including DNA. Radiation damage can lead to cell death; the cells that recover may be mutated and at higher risk for subsequent cancer. Cell sensitivity increases as the replication rate increases and cell differentiation decreases. Bone marrow and mucosal surfaces of the GI tract, which have vast mitotic activity, are significantly more sensitive to radiation than are slowly dividing tissues such as bones and muscles. After exposure of either all or most of the human body to ionizing radiation, acute radiation syndrome (ARS) can develop. The clinical manifestations of ARS reflect the dose and type of radiation as well as the part of the body exposed.

ARS manifests as three major groups of signs and symptoms: hematopoietic, GI, and neurovascular. There are four major stages in ARS: prodrome, latent phase, illness, and recovery or death. The higher the radiation doses, the shorter and more severe each stage. The prodrome appears within minutes to 4 days after exposure, lasts from a few hours to a few days, and can include nausea, vomiting, anorexia, and diarrhea. At the end of the prodrome, ARS progresses to the latent phase. Minimal or no symptoms are present during the latent phase, which commonly lasts up to 2.5 weeks but can last up to 6 weeks. The duration depends on the radiation dose, the health of the patient, and the coexisting illness or injury. After the latent phase, the exposed person manifests illness that may eventuate in recovery or lead to death.

TABLE 223-1 Internal Contaminant Radionuclides: Properties and Treatment

Isotope Name	Symbol	Common Usage	Radiation Type $t_{1/2}$ Radiologic $t_{1/2}$ Biologic, days	Exposure Type	Mode of Contamination	Focal Accumulation in Body	Treatment
Manganese	Mn-56	Reactors, research laboratories	β, γ 2.6 h 5.7	External, internal	N/A	Liver	N/A
Cobalt	Co-60	Medical radiotherapy devices, commercial food irradiators	β, γ 5.26 y 9.5	External, internal	Lungs	Liver	Gastric lavage, purgatives; penicillamine in severe cases
Strontium	Sr-90	Fission product of uranium	β 28 y 18,000	Internal	Moderate GI tract	Bones—similar to calcium	Strontium, calcium, ammonium chloride
Molybdenum	Mo-99	Hospitals—scans	β, γ 66.7 h 3	External, internal	N/A	Kidneys	N/A
Technetium	Tc-99m	Hospitals—scans	β, γ 6.049 h 1	External, internal	IV administration	Kidneys, total body	Potassium perchlorate to reduce thyroid dose
Cesium	Cs-137	Medical radiotherapy devices	β, γ 30 y 70	External, internal	Lungs, GI tract, wounds, follows potassium	Renal excretion	Ion-exchange resins, Prussian blue
Gadolinium	Gd-153	Hospitals	β, γ 242 d 1000	External, internal	N/A	N/A	N/A
Iridium	Ir-192	Commercial radiography	β, γ 74 d 50	External, internal	N/A	Spleen	N/A
Radium	Ra-226	Instrument illumination, industrial applications, old medical equipment, former Soviet Union military equipment	α, β, γ 1602 y 16,400	External, internal	GI tract	Bones	$MgSO_4$ lavage, ammonium chloride, calcium alginates
Tritium	H-3	Luminescent gun sights, muzzle-velocity detectors, nuclear weapons	β 12.5 y 12	Internal	Inhalation, GI tract, wounds	Total body	Dilution with controlled water intake, diuretics
Iodine-131	131I	Reactor accidents, thyroid ablators	β, γ 8.1 d 138	Internal	Inhalation, GI tract, wounds	Thyroid	Potassium/sodium iodide, propylthiouracil, methimazole
Uranium	U-235	Depleted uranium, natural uranium, fuel rods, weapons-grade material	α, (α, β, γ) 7.1×10^8 y 15	Internal	GI tract	Kidneys, bones	$NaHCO_3$, chelation with EDTA
Plutonium	Pu-239	Produced from uranium in reactors, nuclear weapons	α 2.2×10^4 y 73,000	Internal	Limited lung absorption, high retention	Lungs, bones, bone marrow, liver, gonads	Chelating with DTPA or EDTA
Americium	Am-241	Smoke detectors, nuclear weapon detonation fallout	α 458 y 73,000	Internal	Inhalation, skin wounds	Lungs, liver, bones, bone marrow	Chelating with DTPA or EDTA
Polonium	Po-210	Calibration source	α 138.4 d 60	Internal	Inhalation, wounds	Spleen, kidneys	Lavage, dimercaprol
Thorium	Th-232	Calibration source	α 1.41×10^{10} y 73,000	Internal	N/A	N/A	N/A
Phosphorus	P-32	Research laboratories, medical facilities	β 14.3 d 1155	Internal	Inhalation, GI tract, wounds	Bones, bone marrow, rapidly replicating cells	Lavage, aluminum hydroxide, phosphate

Abbreviations: DTPA, diethylenetriamine pentaacetic acid; EDTA, ethylenediamine tetraacetic acid; GI, gastrointestinal; h, hours; N/A, not available; y, years.

With exposure to doses <1 Gy, ARS is generally mild. At this dose symptoms can be minimal or nonexistent even if the entire body is exposed to penetrating radiation. The clinical picture will mainly be transient depression of bone marrow (lymphopenia) that lasts up to 2 to 3 weeks and then improves.

ARS is significantly more acute and severe with exposure to very high doses: >30 Gy. At this dose the prodrome appears in minutes and is followed by 5 to 6 hours of latency before a cardiovascular collapse occurs secondary to irreversible damage to the microcirculation.

The type and dose of radiation and the part of the body exposed will determine not only the timing of the different stages of ARS but also the dominant clinical picture. At low radiation doses of 0.7–4 Gy, hematopoietic depression due to bone marrow suppression takes place and constitutes the main illness. The patient may develop infections and bleeding secondary to low leukocyte and platelet counts, respectively. The bone marrow eventually will recover in almost all patients if they are supported with transfusions and fluids; antibiotics are often needed in addition. With exposure to 6–8 Gy, the clinical picture is significantly more complicated. At these doses, the bone marrow will not always recover and death may ensue. A GI syndrome may accompany the hematopoietic manifestations and further worsen the patient's condition. Compromise of the absorptive layer of the gut alters absorption of fluids, electrolytes, and nutrients. GI injury can lead to vomiting, diarrhea, GI bleeding, sepsis, and electrolyte and fluid imbalance in a patient whose blood counts are compromised for a period of weeks, often leading to death. Whole-body exposure to doses >9–10 Gy is almost always fatal. Crucial elements of the bone marrow simply will not recover. In addition to the GI syndrome associated with very large exposures, patients may develop a neurovascular syndrome; the latter dominates with whole-body doses >20 Gy. Vascular collapse, seizures, confusion, and death usually occur within days. In this variant the prodrome and latent phase both shorten to a few hours.

| TREATMENT | Acute Radiation Sickness |

The treatment of ARS is focused on maintaining homeostasis, giving damaged organs a chance to recover. Aggressive support is given to every damaged system. Treatment for the hematopoietic system includes mainly therapy for neutropenia and infection, transfusion and blood products such as leukoreduced irradiated blood as needed, and hematopoietic growth factors. The value of bone marrow transplantation in this situation is questionable. None of the transplants that were performed among the victims of the nuclear reactor accident in Chernobyl proved successful. Bone marrow transplantation could be considered for casualties with whole-body exposure to 6–10 Gy when the hematopoietic syndrome is dominant and the bone marrow is less likely to recover with time. Another major component of the treatment of ARS is partial or total parenteral nutrition to bypass the damaged GI system. For blast and thermal injuries, standard therapy for trauma is given. Psychological support is essential in many cases.

■ MEDICAL MANAGEMENT OF RADIATION BIOTERRORISM

Victims of radiation bioterrorism can suffer from conventional thermal or blast injuries, exposure to radiation, and contamination by radioactive materials. Many will have combinations of the above, which can be synergistic and cause higher morbidity and mortality rates than is the case when they occur alone. The number of casualties will be a major factor in determining the response of the medical system to an act of radiation bioterrorism. If only a few persons are affected, no significant changes and adaptation of the system are needed to treat the victims. However, if a terror attack results in a large number (dozens or more) of casualties, an organized disaster plan at the local and state levels must be invoked to deal with the crisis properly. Useful U.S. planning documents that include many universal planning concepts can be found at *http://www.remm.nlm.gov/remm_Preplanning.htm*. Medical personnel should have a prior assignment and training and be prepared to function in a scenario with which they are familiar. Stockpiles of specific equipment and medications have to be preplanned (see the Centers for Disease Control and Prevention Web site at *http://www.bt.cdc.gov/stockpile/*). One of the goals of terrorists is to overwhelm medical facilities and minimize the salvage of casualties.

Initial management consists of *primary triage and transportation* of the wounded to medical facilities for treatment. The rationale behind the triage is to sort patients into classes according to the severity of injury for the purpose of expediting clinical care and maximizing the use of the available clinical services and facilities. Triage requires determination of the level of emergency care needed. The higher the number and range of casualties are, the more complex and difficult triage becomes. The mildly wounded and victims of contamination only can be sent to evacuation, registration with disaster response teams, and decontamination and treatment centers. Figure 223-1 illustrates evacuation in a multicasualties radiologic event. In this way, the hospitals can avoid being directly overwhelmed, and those who are severely wounded can receive better treatment. Emergency treatment will be administered initially according to the presence of conventional injuries such as wounds, trauma, and thermal or chemical burns. Individuals with such injuries should be stabilized, if possible, and immediately transported to a medical facility. Removing the victim's clothes and wrapping him or her in clean blankets or nylon sheets reduces both the exposure of the patient and the contamination risk to the staff. However, the possibility of contamination needs to be determined. Less severely injured victims should receive a preliminary decontamination before or during evacuation to a hospital.

One must remember that radionuclide contamination of the skin is commonly not an acute life-threatening situation for the patient or the personnel who care for the patient. Only powerful gamma emitters are likely to cause real damage from contamination. It is important to emphasize that exposure to a radiation field alone does not necessarily create any contamination. The exposed person, if not contaminated, is not radioactive and does not directly emit any radiation.

To protect the staff, protective gear (gowns, gloves, masks, and caps) should be used. Protective masks with filters and chemically protective overgarments provide excellent protection from contamination. Waterproof shoe covers are also important. Remaining in the contaminated area and dealing with lifesaving procedures should take place according to the "ALARA" principle: as low as reasonably achievable. It is better to send many people for short exposure times than to send a few people for longer periods of time to do the same job.

Decontamination of victims should take place in the field before their arrival at medical facilities, but radiologic decontamination should never interfere with medical care. Removal of outer clothing and shoes usually will reduce a patient's contamination by 80–90%. Contaminated clothes should be carefully removed by rolling them over themselves, placing them in marked plastic bags, and removing them to a predefined area for contaminated clothes and equipment. A radiation detector should then be used to check for the presence

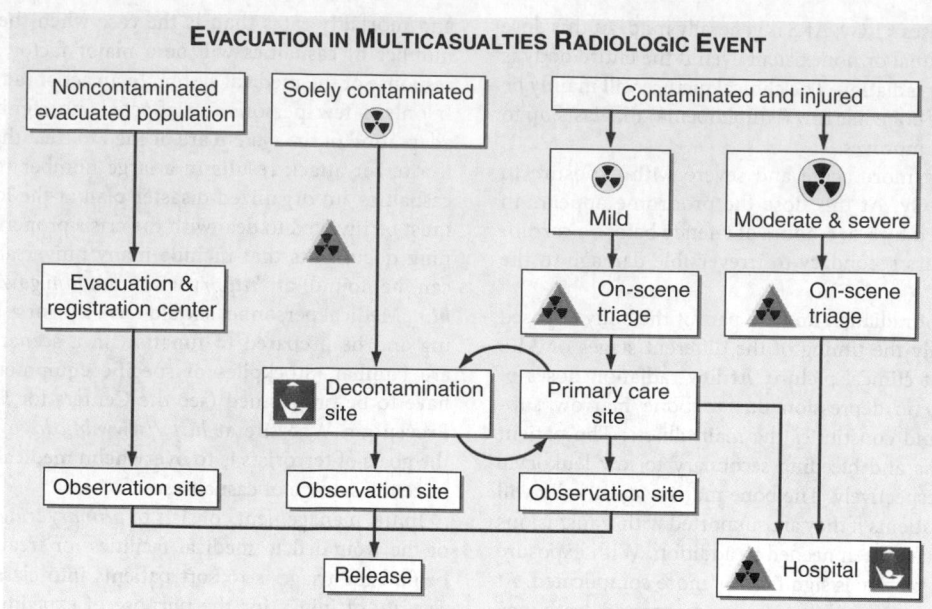

EVACUATION IN MULTICASUALTIES RADIOLOGIC EVENT

Figure 223-1 Algorithm for evacuation in a multicasualties radiologic event.

of any residual radiologic contamination on the patient's body. To prevent internalization of the radioactive materials, one should cover open wounds before decontamination. Showering or washing of the entire skin and hair is very important. The skin is dried and reassessed for residual contamination until no radiation is found. Contamination-removing chemical agents are more than sufficient to remove radiologic contamination.

Wound decontamination should be as conservative as possible. The main goal is to prevent both extensive local damage and internal contamination through lacerated skin. The bandages should be removed, and the wounds flushed. The wound should then be dried and assessed for radiation. This procedure can be repeated again and again until contamination is undetectable. Excision of contaminated wounds should be attempted only when surgically necessary. Radioactive shrapnel that can penetrate through the skin should be removed.

In the hospital, staff can wear normal hospital barrier clothing, including two pairs of gloves, a gown, shoe covers, a head cover, and a face mask. Eye protection is recommended. Decontamination of medical personnel is obligatory after emergency treatment and decontamination of the patient. All protective clothing should be placed after use in a designated container for contaminated clothing.

Radiation intensity decays rapidly with the square of the distance from the source, and increasing the distance from the source and decreasing the time spent near it are basic principles of radiation safety. Shielding with lead can be used as protection from small radioactive gamma sources. Geiger counters can detect gamma and beta radiation. Pocket chamber (pencil) dosimeters, film badges, and thermoluminescent dosimeters can measure accumulated exposure to gamma radiation. All these detectors are in common use in medical facilities and should be used to help define the level of contamination. Alpha radiation is harder to detect due to its poor penetration. An alpha scintillation counter, which is capable of detecting alpha radiation, is not commonly used in medical facilities.

■ GUIDELINES FOR HOSPITAL MANAGEMENT

Figure 223-2 shows a model for hospital arrangement for triage. Persons contaminated either externally or internally should

be identified, externally decontaminated, and, if needed, treated immediately and specifically for internal contamination. In all other cases, the need for treatment of radiation injuries does not constitute a medical emergency. Early actions, such as blood sampling both for assessing the degree of severity of the exposure and for blood type and cross-matching for possible transfusion, need to be taken promptly if ARS is evident or if exposure is suspected.

In the hospital entrance, a distinct decontamination area should be set up promptly. Separation between clean and contaminated areas is essential. Medical personnel in this area should wear protective gear as noted above. They also should be rotated in their assignments every 1 to 2 hours to ensure minimal exposure to radiation. If patients are critically wounded and require either surgery or resuscitation, they need to pass directly to "contaminated" operating rooms or resuscitation sites for lifesaving procedures. Once such patients are stable, they should be decontaminated. It is important to obtain details concerning the exposure, look for prodromal signs of radiation sickness, and do a physical examination. One of the best ways to estimate exposure clinically is to measure the time of prodromal appearance. The earlier the prodromal signs and symptoms appear, the higher the dose is of radiation exposure. A few laboratory tests need to be taken routinely, such as complete blood count and urinalysis. If internal contamination is suspected, specific treatment should be given, as outlined below.

TREATMENT ▶ Radionuclide Contamination

Treatment for internal radionuclide contamination, decorporation, should be started as soon as possible after suspected or known exposure. The approximate upper limit of radionuclide contamination that can reasonably be ignored from a radiation safety point of view is not well defined. These are judgments that will depend on the circumstances of the event and the resources available. One method to determine a level of internal contamination that will trigger decorporation would be the upper

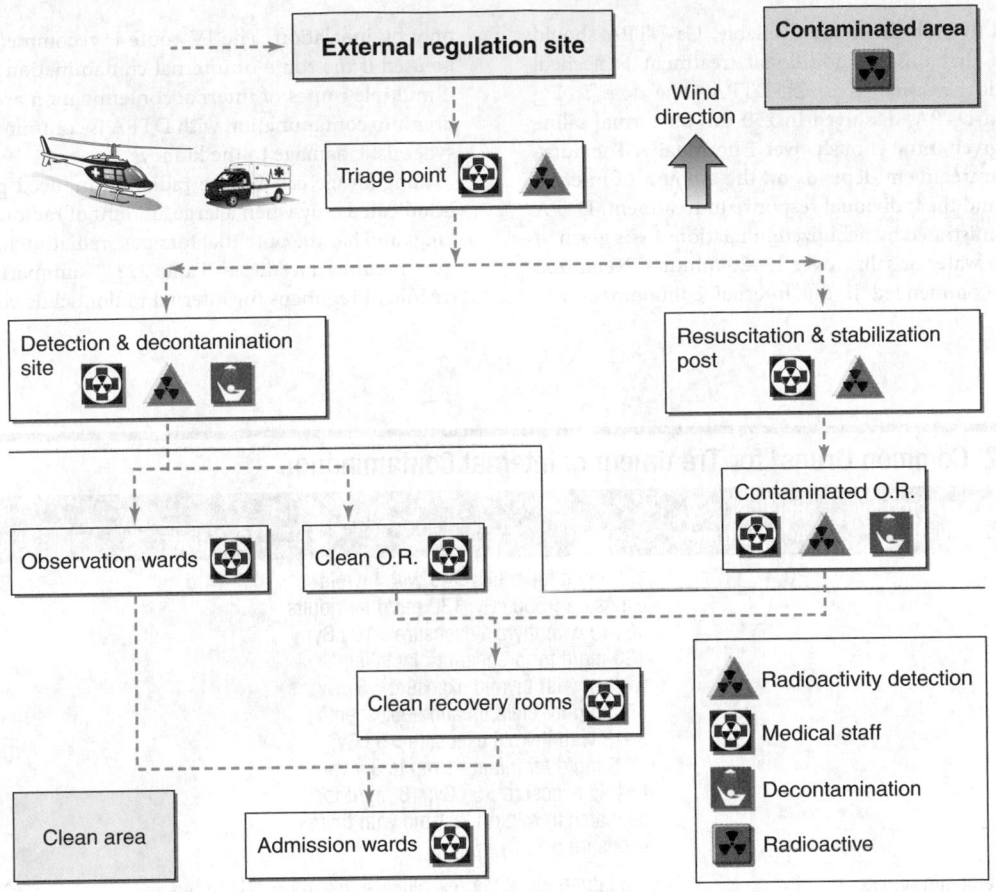

Figure 223-2 Flow chart of hospital triage. O.R., operating room.

limit of the yearly radionuclide contamination permitted for radiation workers [allowable levels of intake (ALIs)]. Radiation workers are permitted 50 times more radiation dose each year than are members of the general public. A new concept called the Clinical Decision Guide is contained in the National Council on Radiation Protection and Measurements (NCRP) Report 161 and is expected to replace the use of ALI.

The goal is to leave the smallest amount of radionuclides possible in the body. Treatment is given to reduce absorption and enhance elimination and excretion. Some of the decorporation agents are not U.S. Food and Drug Administration (FDA)-approved for these indications, and there is very little clinical data to support the efficacy of their use.

Clearance of the GI tract may be achieved by stomach lavage, with emetics (such as apomorphine, 5 to 10 mg, or ipecac, 1- to 2-g capsules or 15 mL in syrup), or by using purgatives, laxatives, ion exchangers, and aluminum antacids. Prussian blue, 1 g tid for a minimum of 3 weeks, is an ion exchanger used to treat cesium 137 internal contamination. Aluminum antacids (such as aluminum phosphate gel) may reduce strontium uptake in the gut if given immediately after exposure. Aluminum hydroxide is less effective.

Prevention or reversal of radionuclide interaction with tissues can be done by blocking, diluting, mobilizing, and chelating agents. *Blocking agents* prevent the entrance of radioactive materials. A good example is potassium iodide (KI), which blocks the uptake of radioactive iodine (^{131}I) by the thyroid. KI is most effective if taken within the first hour after exposure and is still effective 6 hours after exposure. The effectiveness subsequently

declines until 24 hours after exposure; however, it is recommended that KI be taken up to 48 hours after exposure. The KI dose is based on age, predicted thyroid exposure, and pregnancy and lactation status. Adults between the ages of 18–40 should receive 130 mg/d for 7–14 days if exposed to ≥10 cGy of radioactive iodine. Other thyroid-blocking agents include prophylthiouracil, 100 mg tid for 8 days, and methimazole, 10 mg tid for 2 days followed by 5 mg tid for 6 days, but they are somewhat less effective.

Diluting agents decrease the absorption of the radionuclide; for example, water may be used as a diluting agent in the treatment for tritium (^{3}H) contamination. The recommended amount is 3–4 L/d for at least 3 weeks.

Mobilizing agents are most effective when given immediately; however, they may be effective for up to 2 weeks after exposure. These agents include antithyroid drugs, parathyroid extract, glucocorticoids, ammonium chloride, diuretics, expectorants, and inhalants. All of them should induce the release of radionuclides from tissues.

Chelating agents can bind many radioactive materials, after which the complexes are excreted from the human body. In this regard, diethylenetriaminepentaacetic acid (DTPA) as either Ca-DTPA or Zn-DTPA is superior to ethylenediamine tetraacetic acid (EDTA); DTPA was approved by the FDA to treat internal contamination with plutonium, americium, and curium, but it also chelates berkelium, californium, and any material with an atomic number >92. Ca-DTPA is more effective than Zn-DTPA during the first 24 hours after internal contamination, and both drugs are equally effective after the initial 24 hours. If both drugs are available, Ca-DTPA should be given as the first dose. If additional treatment is needed, treatment should be switched to Zn-DTPA. The dose is 1 g Ca-DTPA or Zn-DTPA, dissolved in 250 mL of normal saline or 5% glucose, given intravenously over 1 hour daily. The duration of chelation treatment depends on the amount of internal contamination and the individual response to treatment. DTPA also can be administered by nebulized inhalation; 1 g is given in 1:1 dilution with water or saline over 15–20 minutes. Nebulized Zn-DTPA is recommended if the internal contamination is only by inhalation. The IV route is recommended and should be used if the route of internal contamination is not known or if multiple routes of internal contamination are likely. Treating uranium contamination with DTPA is contraindicated due to its synergistic damage to the kidneys.

Lung lavage can reduce radiation-induced pneumonitis and is indicated only when a large amount of radionuclide enters the lungs and has the potential for acute radiation injury. The procedure requires anesthesia. Table 223-2 summarizes the common treatment regimens for internal radionuclide contamination.

TABLE 223-2 Common Drugs^a for Treatment of Internal Contamination

Medication	Administered for Radionuclides	Route of Administration	Dosage	Duration	Mechanism of Action
KI	^{131}I	PO	130 mg/d for adults >40 with thyroid exposure >500 cGy; 130 mg/d for adults 18–40 with thyroid exposure >10 cGy; 130 mg/d for pregnant or lactating women with thyroid exposure >5 cGy; 65 mg/d for children and adolescents 3–18 with thyroid exposure >5 cGy; 32.5 mg/d for infants 1 mo to 3 y with thyroid exposure >5 cGy; 16 mg/d for neonates from birth to 1 mo with thyroid exposure >5 cGy	7–14 d	Blocking agent
Zn-DTPA	Plutonium, trans-plutonium, yttrium, americium, curium	IV	1 g in 250 mL NS or 5% glucose, given in 1–2 h, or bolus over 3–4 min	Up to 5 d	Chelating agent
		Inhalation	1 g in 1:1 dilution with water or NS over 15–20 min		
		IM	1 g; not recommended because of pain		
Ca-DTPA	Plutonium, trans-plutonium, yttrium, americium, curium	IV	1 g in 250 mL NS or 5% glucose, given in 1–2 h, or bolus over 3–4 min	Up to 5 d	Chelating agent
		Inhalation	1 g in 1:1 dilution with water or NS over 15–20 min		
		IM	1 g; not recommended because of pain		
Bicarbonate	Uranium	IV	2 ampoules sodium bicarbonate (44.3 meq each, 7.5%) in 1000 mL NS, 125 mL/L, or 1 ampoule of sodium bicarbonate (44.3 meq, 7.5%) in 500 mL NS, 500 mL/h	Usually IV for the first 24 h, PO for additional 2 d; continuation of treatment for >3 d is rare and can be done according to titration of uranium amounts in the body	Increased excretion via the kidneys
		PO	2 tablets every 4 h until urine pH = 7–8, or 4 g (8 tablets) 3 tid		
Prussian blue	Cesium-137	PO	1 g tid with 100–200 mL water, up to 10 g/d	=3 wk titrated by urine and fecal bioassay and whole-body counting	Ion exchanger
Water	Tritium (H-3)	PO	>3–4 L per d	3 wk	Excretion of water
Aluminum phosphate gel	Strontium	PO	100 mL immediately after exposure	Once	Decreased gut absorption
Aluminum hydroxide		PO	60–100 mL	Once	Decreased gut absorption

^{a}Excluding KI, these drugs have not been approved for this purpose by the U.S. Food and Drug Administration at the time of publication.

Abbreviations: NS, normal saline.

■ MEDICAL ASSAY OF THE RADIATION-EXPOSED PATIENT

One of the major difficulties in treating victims exposed to radiation is determination of the amount of exposure. Clinical assessment of the patient is the best approach. Biodosimetry, when available, can lead to better assessment of the level of exposure. The clinical assessment is based primarily on the timing and severity of the prodrome of ARS. Appearance of an early prodrome indicates high exposure to radiation. Victims who arrive at the hospital complaining of severe weakness, nausea, vomiting, diarrhea, or seizures probably will not survive despite supportive measures. Decontamination and the use of radiation-detection equipment are both very important. Few tests can be performed to estimate the radiation exposure and the contamination. Biodosimetry Assessment Tool (BAT) is a tool to aid treatment decisions during radiation exposure incidents; it was developed by the U.S. Armed Forces Radiobiology Research Institute (*http://www.afrri.usuhs.mil*). Baseline laboratory tests should include a complete blood count with differential and platelet count, renal evaluation, and determination of electrolytes. Urine and stool samples should be obtained if internal contamination is suspected. Nasal swabs should be taken from each nostril for determination of inhalation of radionuclides. The nasal swabs are useful if taken within the first 1–2 hours after the exposure. After exhalation, each swab is labeled and sealed in a plastic bag and sent for analysis to appropriate laboratories. Patients exposed to 0.7–4 Gy will develop pancytopenia from as early as 10 days to as long as 8 weeks after exposure. Lymphocytes show the most rapid decline, whereas other leukocytes and platelets decline less rapidly. Erythrocytes are the least vulnerable blood elements.

Absolute lymphocyte counts should be taken every 4–6 hours for 5–6 days; they are the most valuable early indicator because they are recognized to be a sensitive marker for radiation damage and correlate with both the exposure and the prognosis. A 50% drop in absolute lymphocyte count within the first 24 hours indicates a significant injury. HLA typing is necessary whenever there is suspicion of irreversible bone marrow damage. Lymphocyte chromosomal analysis can detect radiation exposure as low as 0.03–0.06 Gy, and 15 mL of blood should be drawn as early as possible in a heparinized collection tube and kept cool. Radiation-induced chromosomal aberrations in peripheral blood lymphocytes include dicentric chromosomes and ring forms that last for a few weeks. Calibration of a dose-response curve makes it possible to assess the radiation dose. Dicentric quantification requires multiple days to perform and is available only in select centers.

Another method for estimating exposure is the in vitro cytokinesis-block micronucleus assay. Micronuclei can be the result of small acentric chromosome fragments that arise during exposure to radiation. The technique to score the micronuclei in peripheral blood lymphocytes has been standardized in the last few years. It can be a useful tool in small-scale exposure but is not feasible in a mass casualty setting. An algorithm for the treatment of radiation casualties is shown in Fig. 223-3.

■ FOLLOW-UP

It is desirable to continue follow-up in some circumstances. In general, only persons who are exposed to <8–10 Gy whole-body irradiation have a chance to survive in the long term, and they are at risk of developing cataracts, sterility, and lung, kidney, and bone marrow problems. Based on their age, their gender, and

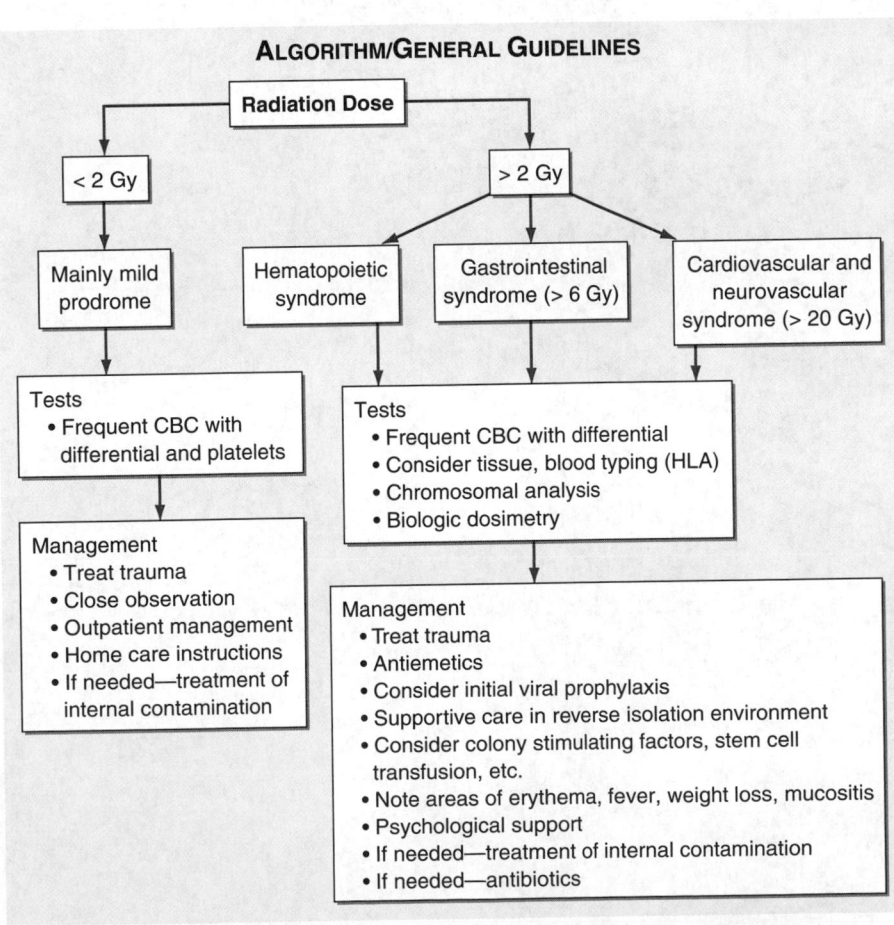

Figure 223-3 General guidelines for treatment of radiation casualties. CBC, complete blood count.

the amount and type of exposure, they should be followed for many years. A major public health issue is the risk of secondary malignancy in individuals and populations that were exposed to low doses of radiation. Leukemia and breast, brain, thyroid, and lung cancer are the most common, but the exposed population is at increased risk for many other cancers as well. Appropriate follow-up protocols should be developed, based on the type of exposure and the exposed population. In cases of internal contamination, the long-term follow-up should be focused on the organ at risk. Such is the case with uranium contamination, with its nephrotoxic properties.

FURTHER READINGS

DAINIAK N: Hematologic consequences of exposure to ionizing radiation. Exp Hematol 30:513, 2002

HARPER FT et al: Realistic radiological dispersal device hazard boundaries and ramifications for early consequence management decisions. Health Phys 93:1, 2007

HOMELAND SECURITY COUNCIL: Planning Guidance for Response to a Nuclear Detonation. *http://www.remm.nlm.gov/planning-guidance.pdf 1/2009*

LAWRENCE LIVERMORE NATIONAL LABORATORY: Key Response Planning Factors for the Aftermath of Nuclear Terrorism. *http://www.remm.nlm.gov/IND_ResponsePlanning_LLNL-TR-410067.pdf*

METTLER FA JR, VOELZ GL: Major radiation exposure—what to expect and how to respond. N Engl J Med 346:1554, 2002

MOULDER JE: Report on an interagency workshop on the radiobiology of nuclear terrorism: Molecular and Cellular Biology of Moderate Dose (1–10 Sv) Radiation and Potential Mechanisms of Radiation Protection (Bethesda, MD, December 17–18, 2001). Radiat Res 158:118, 2002

U.S. DEPARTMENT OF HEALTH AND HUMAN SERVICES: Radiation event medical management: Guidance on diagnosis & treatment for health care providers. *http://www.remm.nlm.gov/remm_Preplanning.htm*

INDEX

Bold numbers indicate the start of the main discussion of a topic; numbers followed by "f" or "t" refer to figures and tables; numbers preceded by "e" refer to the e-chapter pages on the DVD; "V" refers to the videos on the DVD.

A

AA amyloidosis, 945, 945t, 946f, **949**. *See also* Amyloidosis
AAP (alanine aminopeptidase), in acute kidney injury, 2304t
Abacavir
  adverse effects of
    cutaneous, 435, 436
    genetic factors in, 433, 2693t
  in HIV infection, 1555, 1571t, 1578
  genetic variations in response to, 42t, 44
  for HIV infection, 1571t, 1578
  molecular structure of, 1574f
  resistance to, 1576f, 1578
A band, of sarcomere, 1802
Abatacept, for rheumatoid arthritis, 2748t, 2749–2750
ABCA1 deficiency. *See* Tangier disease (ABCA1 deficiency)
ABCD rule, e16-6
ABCG5/G8 hemitransporter, 2616
Abciximab
  action of, 989f, 991–992
  adverse effects of, 967, 967t, 992
  dosage of, 992
  genetic variations in response to, 985t
  indications for, 992
  in PCI, 2036
  pharmacology of, 992t
  for UA/NSTEMI, 2019t
Abdomen
  auscultation of, 330
  inspection of, 330, 1822
  palpation of, 331, 1822
Abdominal pain, **108**
  in appendicitis, 2516, 2517t
  approach to the patient, 110–112
  differential diagnosis of , by location, 111t
  in gastrointestinal disease, 2404, 2404t
  history in, 110–111
  imaging in, 112
  in intestinal ischemia, 2511–2513
  in intestinal obstruction, 2514
  in irritable bowel syndrome, 2496
  in malabsorption syndromes, 2476t
  mechanisms of
    abdominal wall disorders, 109, 109t
    inflammation of parietal peritoneum, 108, 109t
    metabolic, 109t, 110
    neurogenic, 109t, 110
    obstruction of hollow viscera, 108, 109t
    toxic, 109t
    vascular disturbances, 108–109, 109t
  in pancreatitis, 2636
  in pelvic inflammatory disease, 1104
  in peptic ulcer disease, 2444–2445
  in peritonitis, 1076
  in pregnancy, 60
  referred, 109–110, 109t
Abdominal radiography
  in aortic aneurysm, 2062
  in gallbladder disease, 2619, 2619t, 2620f
  in pancreatic disease evaluation, 2630t, 2632
Abdominal swelling/distention, **330**. *See also* Ascites
  in appendicitis, 2517
  causes of, 330
  history in, 330
  imaging in, 331, 331f
  in intestinal obstruction, 2514
  physical examination in, 330–331
Abdominal wall disorders, 109, 305
Abducens nerve, examination of, 3236
Abducens nerve palsy, 239
Abducens nerve paresis, 238
Abduction and external rotation test, 2071
A-beta (Aβ) fibers, 93

Abetalipoproteinemia, **3153**
  clinical features of, 3153, e41-4f
  diarrhea in, 314
  genetic factors in, 3153
  pathophysiology of, 2464, 3153
  peripheral blood smear in, e17-5f
  small-intestinal mucosal biopsies in, 2468, 2468t
  treatment of, 603, 3153
  vitamin E deficiency in, 603
Aβ̣M amyloidosis, 950. *See also* Amyloidosis
Abiotrophia spp., 789, 1057, 1179–1180
Abiraterone acetate, for prostate cancer, 803
ABO blood group system, 951
Abortion
  septic, 1287, 1335
  spontaneous, 513, 514t, 3188
ABPA. *See* Allergic bronchopulmonary aspergillosis (ABPA)
Abruptio placenta, 56, 59
Abscess
  anorectal, 2508, 2509f
  antibiotic penetration into, 1141
  brain. *See* Brain abscess
  cerebral, 3244f
  dental, 159
  epidural. *See* Epidural abscess
  formation of, 1023
  hematogenous, 3429
  intraabdominal. *See* Intraabdominal abscess
  intraperitoneal. *See* Intraperitoneal abscess
  liver. *See* Liver abscess
  periapical, 268
  perinephric, 1081–1082
  peritonsillar, 264, 265, 1334
  perivalvular, 1054
  psoas, 1082
  renal, 1081–1082
  retropharyngeal, 267
  splenic. *See* Splenic abscess
  subperiosteal, 262
  tuboovarian, 1328, 1329f, 1335
Abscopal effect, 471
Absence seizures, 3251t, 3252
Absent (vanishing) testis syndrome, 3051
Absolute lymphocyte count, in radiation-exposed patient, 1795
Absolute risk reduction, 28, 3281, 3283
Absorption
  of carbohydrates, 2465–2466, 2465t
  disorders of, **2460**. *See also* Malabsorption syndromes
  of drugs, 34–35
  impaired, 2403
  of lipids, 2463–2465, 2463t, 2464f
  nutrient, **2461**
  of proteins, 2466
Absorption spectrum, 440
Abstract thought, assessment of, 3236
Abulia, 2247
Acalculia, 206
Acalculia, 206
Acamprosate, in alcoholism management, 3552
Acanthamoeba, 1687, 1687f, e25-4t, e25-6t, e25-7t
Acanthocytes, e17-1
Acanthocytosis, 2464, e17-5f
Acantholysis, 424
Acanthosis, 442
Acanthosis nigricans
  in diabetes mellitus, 2988
  disorders associated with, 412, e16-15
  in gastric cancer, 766
  hyperpigmentation in, 412, e16-15f
  in metabolic syndrome, 1995
  in obesity, 629
Acarbose
  adverse effects of, 2998
  for diabetes mellitus, 2996t, 2997–2998

Accelerated idioventricular rhythm, **1891,** 2032, e30-12f
Accelerated junctional rhythm, 1888, 2033
Accessory gene regulator *(agr),* 1161
Accessory genome, 1181
Accessory pathway-mediated tachycardia, 1889–1890, 1889f
Accidents
  deaths from, 50t, 51t, 67t
  in health care industry, **85,** 85f
ACE. *See* Angiotensin-converting enzyme (ACE)
Acebutolol
  dosage of, 1883t
  indications for, 1883t
  for ischemic heart disease, 2009t
  overdosage/poisoning with, e50-10t
  pharmacology of, 1883t
ACE inhibitors. *See* Angiotensin-converting enzyme (ACE) inhibitors
Aceruloplasminemia, 604
Acetabulum, Paget's disease of, e41-3f
Acetaminophen
  adverse effects of
    hepatotoxicity, 48, 328, 2560t, 2561–2563, 2563f
    lactic acidosis, 366
    nephrotoxicity, 97
    thrombocytopenia, 967t
  for back pain, 136, 137
  drug interactions of, 2835t
  for fever, 146, 147
  for influenza, 1498
  metabolism of, 532, 2561
  for migraine, 118t, 119
  for osteoarthritis, 2835, 2835t
  overdosage/poisoning with, 2563, 2563f
  for pain, 72, 97, 98t
  for spinal stenosis, 134
Acetaminophen-aspirin-caffeine, for migraine, 118t, 119
Acetate, in specialized nutritional support formulas, 617t
Acetazolamide
  action of, 2283
  for acute angle-closure glaucoma, 230
  adverse effects of, 343, 434
  for altitude illness, 217, e51-2
  for high-altitude pulmonary edema, e51-4
  for hyperkalemia, e15-3
  for hypokalemic periodic paralysis, 3505
  for metabolic alkalosis, 371
  for pseudotumor cerebri, 233
  for raised CSF pressure headache, 126
  for salicylate-induced acidosis, 367
Acetoacetate, 366
Acetohydroxamic acid, 2387
N-Acetyl-β-glucosaminidase (NAG), 2304t
Acetylcholine
  anatomic and clinical aspects of, 3227t
  deficiency of, in delirium, 197
  in neural control of gastrointestinal system, 308
  structure of, 3227t
  in swallowing, 298
Acetylcholine receptor, in myasthenia gravis, 3481
Acetylcholinesterase
  in nerve agent exposure, 1783–1784, 1784f
  test, in myasthenia gravis, 3481
Acetylcholinesterase inhibitors
  overdosage/poisoning with, e50-11t
  for snakebite, 3570, 3570t
N-Acetylcysteine, 48
  for acetaminophen overdose, 2563
  for prevention of contrast-induced nephropathy, 1854
  for sulfur mustard exposure, 1783
N-Acetylglutamate synthase deficiency, 3216t
N-Acetyl-benzoquinone-imine (NAPQI), 2561

INDEX

INDEX

INDEX

INDEX

INDEX

INDEX

INDEX

INDEX

INDEX

INDEX

INDEX

Ibutilide
action of, 1865t
adverse effects of, 1884t
for atrial fibrillation, 1882
dosage of, 1883t
indications for, 1883t
for pharmacologic cardioversion, 1886
ICAM-1 (intercellular adhesion molecule 1), 1011, 1534
ICD. *See* Implantable cardioverter-defibrillator (ICD)
Ice bath, 147
"Iceberg" disease, 2470
ICF (immunodeficiency, centromere instability, and facial anomalies) syndrome, 2701, e39-2
Ichthyosis, in HIV infection, 1557
Icodextrin, 2325
ICP. *See* Intracranial pressure (ICP)
ICS (immunochromatographic strip) test, treponemal, 1385
Icterus, in liver disease, 2523
Ictotest, 325
ICU patient. *See* Critically ill patient
ICU psychosis. *See* Delirium
Idarubicin, 698t, 702, 910
IDDM (insulin-dependent diabetes mellitus). *See* Diabetes mellitus, type 1
Idiopathic CD4+ T lymphocytopenia, 1567–1568
Idiopathic cutaneous vasculitis, **2798**
Idiopathic growth hormone deficiency (IGHD), 2892
Idiopathic hypercalcemia of infancy, 3108
Idiopathic pulmonary fibrosis
clinical features of, 2165
histologic findings in, 2165–2166
imaging of, e34-7f
lung transplantation for, 2191t
pathogenesis of, 2162f
treatment of, 2166
Idiopathic rapid eye movement behavioral sleep disorder. *See* REM sleep behavior disorder
Idiopathic thrombocytopenic purpura
H. pylori infection and, 1263
infections in patient with, 712t
in women, 53
Idiopathic thrombocytosis. *See* Essential thrombocytosis (ET)
Idiopathic torsion dystonia, 3328
IDLs (intermediate-density lipoproteins), 3145, 3145f, 3146t
IFN-α. *See* Interferon-α (IFN-α)
IFN-α2a. *See* Interferon-α2a (IFN-α2a)
IFN-α2b. *See* Interferon-α2b (IFN-α2b)
Ifosfamide
action of, 696
adverse effects of, 696, 697t, 708
cardiotoxicity, 838, 1962
cystitis, 840, 2277
hypokalemia, 352
nephrogenic diabetes insipidus, 350
nephrotoxicity, 2298
neurologic, 2272, 3394t
pulmonary, 839, 2276
dosage of, 697t
for Ewing's sarcoma, 820
for osteosarcoma, 819
for soft tissue sarcoma, 818
for testicular cancer, 809
Ig. *See* Immunoglobulin(s)
IGF. *See* Insulin-like growth factor (IGF)
IGHD (idiopathic growth hormone deficiency), 2892
IGRAs (interferon-γ release assays), 162–163, 1352, 1370
iKNRs (inhibitory NK cell receptors), in HIV infection, 1532
ILDs. *See* Interstitial lung diseases (ILDs)
Ileal resection, cobalamin deficiency after, 868
Ileocecal syndrome. *See* Neutropenic enterocolitis
Ileocolitis, in Crohn's disease, 2483
Ileorectostomy, 319
Ileus
abdominal swelling in, 330
adynamic, 2513–2516
gallstone, cholecystitis and, 2622
hypokalemia and, 353
postoperative, 99
Iliopsoas bursitis, 2860
Iliotibial band syndrome, 2861
Iloperidone, 3544t
Iloprost, for pulmonary hypertension, 2079
IMAGe syndrome, 2955t

Imatinib
action of
against *BCR-ABL*, 666
in CML, 915
kinase inhibition, 675
targets of, 677t, 705, 705f, 706
adverse effects of
cardiac, 705, 838
hepatic, 705
most common, 916
myelosuppression, 700t, 916
pulmonary, 705
for CML, 666, 675, 677t, 705, 915–917, 916t
dosage of, 700t
drug interactions of, 2272
for gastrointestinal stromal tumors, 675, 677t, 768
genetic variations in response to, 42t, 44
for hypereosinophilic syndrome, 481
resistance to, 675, 916–917
for small intestinal leiomyosarcoma, 776
for soft tissue sarcoma, 818
Imerslund-Gräsbeck syndrome, 868
IMF (International Monetary Fund), 9
Iminoglycinuria, 3221t
Imipenem
for anaerobic infections, 1339t
for bite-wound infections, e24-3
for *Campylobacter* infections, 1288
for glanders, 1269t
for health care–associated pneumonia, 2139t
indications for, 1144t
for melioidosis, 1269t
for *Nocardia* infections, 1326
for *P. aeruginosa* infections, 1269t, 2135t
for peritonitis, 1078
resistance to, 1144t
Imipenem-cilastin
for actinomycosis, 1330t
adverse effects of, 967t
in pregnancy, 1142t
for sepsis/septic shock, 2229t
Imipramine
adverse effects of, 329, 3531t
for depression, 3531t, 3538
for detrusor spasticity, 376
dosage of, 3531t, 3538
overdosage/poisoning with, e50-9t to e50-10t, e50-11t
for pain, 98t
for sleep enuresis, 221
Imiquimod
for basal cell carcinoma, 732
for genital warts, 403
Immersion (trench) foot, 169
Immortality, of stem cells, 536
Immune-complex formation, 2681, 2683t
Immune-mediated brachial plexus neuropathy (IBPN), 3470
Immune memory, 2651
Immune myelopathies, 3371–3372
Immune neuropathies, 3474, 3475f
Immune reconstitution inflammatory syndrome (IRIS)
in HIV infection, 1349–1350, 1372, 1548, 1556, 1556t
pathogenesis of, 1527, 1556
Immune response/immune system, **1008**. *See also* Cell-mediated immunity
adaptive, 2651, **2668**
cells triggering, 2656t
definition of, 2650
humor mediators of, 2673–2674, 2674t
vs. innate immune system, 2653, 2654t, 2655f, 2655t
intercellular interactions of, 2658f
primary immunodeficiencies of, 2696t, **2699**
B lymphocyte deficiencies. *See* B cell(s), deficiencies of
T lymphocyte deficiencies. *See* T cell(s), deficiencies of
PRRs in modulation of, 2655t
response to microbes, 1009t, 2678
T cells in, 2668–2672, 2669f
antitumor effects, 710
in celiac disease, 2470
cellular interactions in regulation of, 2674–2675
clinical evaluation of, 2683
components of, 2695
endogenous derangements of, 2719t, 2720
endothelium in, 1799
exogenous derangements of, 2719–2720, 2719t
gut-related dysfunction of, 2403

Immune response/immune system (*Cont.*):
in IBD, 2478–2479
innate, **2651**
vs. adaptive immune system, 2653, 2654t, 2655f, 2655t
cells triggering adaptive immunity, 2656t
components of, 2651, 2654t
definition of, 2650
effector cells of, **2654**
primary immunodeficiencies of. *See* Primary immunodeficiencies, of innate immune system
PRRs of, 2653–2654, 2654t
response to infection, 1008, 1009–1010t, 1010
introduction to, **2650**
in irritable bowel syndrome, 2498
macrophages in, 480
molecular defects of, 2680t
at mucosal surfaces, 2675, 2677–2678, 2678f
pattern recognition in, 2651, 2653–2654, 2654t–2657t, 2655f. *See also* Pattern recognition receptors (PRRs), of innate immune system
reference values for laboratory tests, 3588–3596t
in rheumatic fever, 2753, 2753f
terminology related to, **2650**
in women, 53
Immune thrombocytopenic purpura, 469, 968–969
Immune tolerance, 976, 2675
Immunization. *See also* Vaccine(s)
for adults, 30t, 1032
administration of, 1038–1039, 1039f
contraindications to, 1035–1037, 1036–1037t
determining need for, 1035
provider recommendation for, 1040
schedules for, 30t, 1032, 1033–1035f
system support for, 1040
timing of, 1035
for cancer patient, 713t, 722
for children, 2555–2556, 2555t
consumer access to and demand for, 1037f, 1039–1040
documentation of, 1040
for health care workers, 1040–1041, 1119
in HIV infection, 1033f, 1034f, 1046–1047
in nonmedical settings, 1041
performance monitoring, 1041
in pregnancy, 1033f, 1034f, 1035, 1037
for transplant recipient, 1131–1132, 1132t
for travelers, 1042–1044, 1043f
Immunoblastic lymphomas, in HIV infection, 1566. *See also* Diffuse large B cell lymphoma
Immunochromatographic strip (ICS) test, treponemal, 1385
Immunocompromised patient. *See also* Transplant recipient
actinomycosis in, 1329
adenovirus in, 1491–1492
antibiotic use in, 1141
bite-wound infection in, e24-1
Candida infections in, 402
diarrhea in, 310, 314, 1087
HRSV infection in, 1488
immunization in, 1037–1038
primary CNS lymphoma in, 3387–3388
rhinovirus infection in, 1486
sexual practices of, 722
sinusitis in, 257
skin cancer in, 443
Immunodeficiency, centromere instability, and facial anomalies (ICF) syndrome, 2701, e39-2
Immunodeficiency diseases, primary. *See* Primary immunodeficiencies
Immunodeficiency viruses, 1506, 1508f, 1509. *See also* HIV
Immunodysregulation polyendocrinopathy enteropathy X-linked syndrome (IPEX), 2705
Immunofluorescent antibody technique, e22-2
Immunoglobulin(s), 1010. *See also* Antibody(ies)
in adaptive immunity, 2673–2674
allotypes of, 936
hyperimmune, for viral hemorrhagic fever, 1772t
idiotypes of, 936
isotypes of, 936
properties of, 2674t
reference values, 3593t
replacement of, 2704
structure of, 936, 2673
Immunoglobulin A (IgA), 1010, 2673–2674, 2674t
Immunoglobulin A (IgA) deficiency, 310, 2704
Immunoglobulin A (IgA) nephropathy, 339, 2342–2343, 2343f, e14-3f

INDEX

INDEX

INDEX

INDEX

Ranolazine, for ischemic heart disease, 2011
RANTES, 2662t
Rapamycin
  action of, 676f
  for Kaposi's sarcoma, 1128
  lifespan enhancement and, 569, 585
  after liver transplantation, 2611
  mTOR signaling and, 569
  for prevention of EBV-B cell lymphoproliferative
    disease, 1125
Rapid acetylators, 44
Rapid plasma reagin (RPR) test, for syphilis, 1385, 1385f
RARA gene, 906–907
Rarefaction, 527t
RAS (reticular activating system), 2247
Rasburicase
  adverse effects of, 2274
  genetic variations in response to, 42t
  for tumor lysis syndrome treatment/prophylaxis,
    2274
  for uric acid nephropathy, 909
RAS gene, 664–665
Rash. *See also* Skin lesions; *specific diseases*
  arrangement of lesions, 148
  centrally distributed maculopapular eruptions,
    148, 149–151t, 157
  configuration of, 148
  confluent desquamative erythemas, 152–153t, 157
  distribution of, 148
  drug-induced, 434–435, 435f, e7-2f. *See also* Drug-
    induced illness, cutaneous
  fever and, **148,** e7-1
    approach to the patient, 148
    diseases associated with, 149–156t, 423, 1619–1621
  nodular eruptions, 155t
  peripheral eruptions, 151–152t, 157
  purpuric eruptions, 155–156t, 158, 1215t
  pustular eruptions, 153–154t, 157
  ulcers and eschars, 156t, 158
  urticarial-like eruptions, 154–155t, 158
  vesiculobullous eruptions, 153–154t, 157
Rasmussen's aneurysm, 1345
Rat-bite fever (sodoku, Haverhill fever), 150t, 152t,
  e24-2
Rat bite-wound, e24-2
Rat flea, 3582
Rathke's cyst, 2883
Rationing, 88
Rat lungworm. *See Angiostrongylus* spp. infections
Rattlesnake bite, 3566, 3566f, 3569t, 3571. *See also*
  Snakebites
R_{aw}. *See* Airway resistance (R_{aw})
Raynaud's disease, 279, 2071–2072
Raynaud's phenomenon, **2071**
  chemotherapy-related, 808, 841
  chilblain in, 169
  clinical features of, 2071
  cyanosis in, 289
  localized hypoxia in, 287
  pathophysiology of, 2071
  secondary causes of, 2072, 2072t
  in Sjögren's syndrome, 2771, 2771t
  in systemic sclerosis, 431, 2759, 2762–2763, 2763f
  treatment of, 2072
RB gene. *See* Retinoblastoma (RB) gene
RB tumor suppressor protein. *See* Retinoblastoma
  (RB) tumor suppressor protein
RCC. *See* Renal cell carcinoma (RCC)
RDW (red blood cell distribution width), 450, e17-1
Reactive arthritis (Reiter's syndrome), **2778, 2847**
  aortic aneurysm in, 2061
  aortitis in, 2065, e31-3 to e31-4
  C. trachomatis, 1423–1424, 1427t
  clinical features of, 2779
  diagnosis of, 2779–2780
  diarrhea in, 310
  epidemiology of, 2778
  etiology of, 2778–2779
  vs. gonococcal arthritis, 1224, 1224f
  historic background of, 2778
  in HIV infection, 1555
  HLA gene association with, 2693t
  laboratory findings in, 2779
  vs. Lyme arthritis, 1404
  ocular involvement in, 229
  oral manifestations of, 269
  pathogenesis of, 2778–2779
  pathology of, 2778
  radiographic findings in, 2779
  vs. relapsing polychondritis, 2805
  after *Salmonella* infections, 1279
  after *Shigella* infections, 1283

Reactive arthritis (Reiter's syndrome) (*Cont.*):
  skin manifestations of, 405, 405t
  after streptococcal infections, 2754
  treatment of, 2780
  after *Yersinia* infections, 1312, 1313
Reactive hyperemia, 2071
Reactive lymphocytes, e17-2
Reactive oxygen species (ROS)
  in aging, e18-10
  damage to mitochondrial DNA by, e18-9f, e18-9
    to e18-10
  in endothelium, 1799
  generation of, 441
  in hyperbaric oxygen therapy, e52-1 to e52-2, e52-2f
  skin damage caused by, 441
"Readback," 86
Reading, assessment of, 203
Rebound tenderness, 111
Rebuck skin window test, 482
Receiver operative characteristic curve, 23, 23f
Receptor tyrosine kinase, 675, 676f
Receptor tyrosine kinase receptors, 680f
Recessive disorders
  autosomal, 500–501, 500f
  X-linked, 501
RECIST criteria, 651
Recluse spider bite, 3579
Recombinant tissue plasminogen activator (rtPA).
    See Alteplase
Recombination, genetic, 489, 489f, 504
Recommended dietary allowance, **589**
Recoverin, 833t
Rectal bleeding
  colorectal cancer. *See* Colorectal cancer
  in hemorrhoidal disease. *See* Hemorrhoidal disease
  in rectal prolapse, 2505
  in ulcerative colitis, 2481–2482, 2482t
Rectal cancer. *See* Colorectal cancer
Rectal carcinoids, 3058t, 3061
Rectal prolapse, **2505**
  anatomy of, 2505
  clinical features of, 2505–2506, 2505f
  degree of, 2505f
  epidemiology of, 2505
  evaluation of, 2505–2506, 2505f
  incidence of, 2505
  pathophysiology of, 2505
  treatment of, 2506, 2506f
Rectal temperatures, 143
Rectoanal angle, 309, 309f, 318
Rectocele, 318
Rectopexy, for rectal prolapse, 2506, 2506f
Rectus sheath, hematoma of, 109
Red blood cell(s)
  agglutination of, e17-2, e17-4f
  in anemia, **448**
  antigens and antibodies, 951–952, 952t
  for chemotherapy-related anemia, 708
  complement activation and, 885f
  folate in, 870
  fragmented, e17-4f
  glycolysis in, 873, 873f
  hematopoietic differentiation of, 541f
  iron content in, 845
  life cycle of, 845
  life span of, 873–874
  mechanical destruction of, 881, 882f
  nucleated, e17-5f
  osmotic fragility of, 875
  in peripheral blood smear, e17-1 to e17-2, e17-2f
    to e17-7f
  polycythemia, **457**
  protoporphyrin levels in, 846f, 847
  redox metabolism in, 878f
  transfusions. *See* Transfusion(s)
  urinary casts, e14-10f
Red blood cell distribution width (RDW),
    450, e17-1
Red blood cell indices, 450, 450t
Red blood cell membrane/cytoskeleton complex
  abnormalities causing hemolytic anemia, 874–875,
    876f
  structure of, 874, 874f
Red blood cell scintigraphy, in gastrointestinal
  bleeding, 323
Red blood cell survival study, 874
Red clover, 461t
Red light, for basal cell carcinoma, 441
Red man syndrome, 437
Red pulp, of spleen, 467, 468f
Red tide, 3575
5α-Reductase, 381

5α-Reductase inhibitors
  adverse effects of, 376t
  for benign prostatic hypertrophy, 804–805
5α-Reductase type 2 deficiency, 3051
Reductionism, e19-1, e19-3
Reduviid bugs, 1958, 3582
Reed-Sternberg cells, 933f, e17-11f
Reentry, 1863, 1863f, 1879
  excitable gap, 1863f, 1864
  functional, 1864
  leading circle, 1864
Refeeding edema, 294
Refeeding syndrome, 606, 639
Referred pain, 95
  in abdominal diseases, 109–110
  to back, 130, 136
  convergence-projection hypothesis of, 95f
Reflex(es), testing of, 3237–3238, e45-7. *See also*
    specific reflexes
Reflexology, e2-2t
Reflex sympathetic dystrophy, 97, 2858, 3358–3359
Reflex syncope, 171. *See also* Syncope
Reflux nephropathy, 2371–2372, 2371f
Refractive state, 224
Refractory anemia, 895t
  with excess blasts, 894, 895t
  with ring sideroblasts, 894, 895t
Refractory cytopenia with multilineage dysplasia, 895t
Refractory neutropenia, 895t
Refractory thrombocytopenia, 895t
Refsum disease, 236, 3456, 3456t
Refusal of care, 79, e5-2
Refusal to swallow, 297
Regenerative medicine, **535**
Regional enteritis. *See* Crohn's disease
Regional wall motion abnormality
  in ischemic heart disease, 2005
  in myocardial infarction, 2034
Registries, 27
Regulatory failure, e3-1
Regurgitation, 301
  in achalasia, 2431
  in esophageal disease, 2427
  in GERD, 2433–2435
  nasal, 298
Rehabilitation
  of alcoholics, 3551–3552
  in ischemic stroke management, 3274
  pulmonary, 280, 2158
  of spinal cord disorders, **3375,** 3375t
Reifenstein syndrome, 3053
Reiter's syndrome. *See* Reactive arthritis (Reiter's
    syndrome)
Rejection
  inflammatory mediators in, 2682t
  in kidney transplantation, 2329
  in liver transplantation, 2612–2613, e38-3f
Relapsing fever
  approach to the patient, 1398
  clinical features of, 146, 150t, 1398–1399, 1398t
  complications of, 1399
  diagnosis of, 1399
  epidemiology of, 1398
  global features of, 1397, 1398
  pathogenesis of, 1397, 1397f
  prevention of, 1399–1400
  prognosis of, 1399
  treatment of, 1399, 1400f
Relapsing polychondritis, **2802**
  ANCA in, 2804
  aortic aneurysm in, 2061
  aortitis in, 2065
  auricular chondritis in, 1822, 2803, 2803t, 2804f
  cardiac valvular regurgitation in, 2804
  clinical features of, 2803–2804, 2803t, 2804f
  course of, 2805
  diagnosis of, 2804
  differential diagnosis of, 2804–2805
  disorders associated with, 2802t
  HLA-DR4 in, 2802
  incidence of, 2802
  joint involvement in, 2803–2804
  kidney disease in, 2804
  laboratory findings in, 2804
  laryngotracheobronchial involvement in, 2803t,
    2804
  nasal involvement in, 2803, 2803t, 2804f
  ocular involvement in, 229, 2803t, 2804
  pathogenesis of, 2802–2803
  pathology of, 2802–2803
  prognosis of, 2805
  saddlenose in, 2803, 2803t, 2804f

INDEX

INDEX

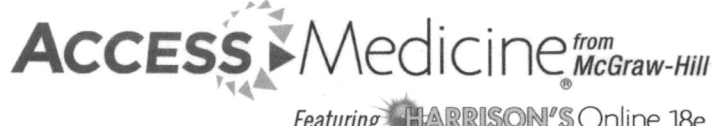
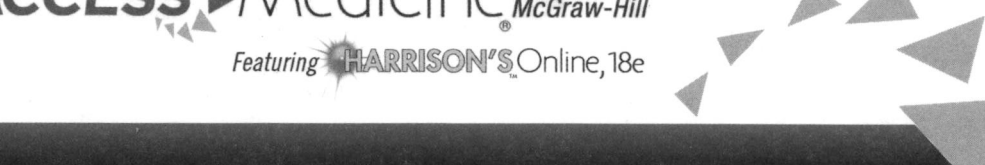
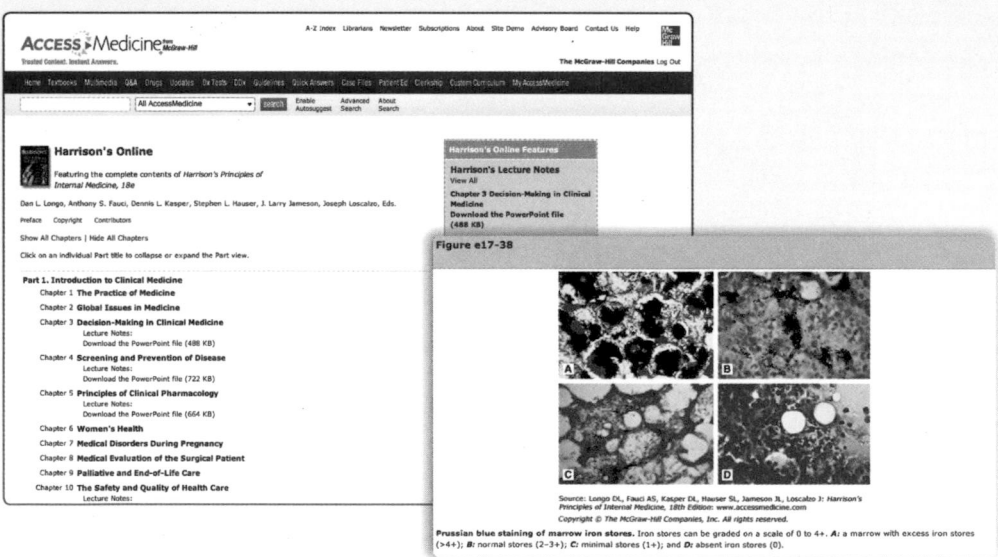
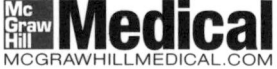